PRINCIPLES AND PRACTICE OF

INFECTIOUS DISEASES

THIRD EDITION

PRINCIPLES AND PRACTICE OF INFECTIOUS DISEASES

THIRD EDITION

Edited by

GERALD L. MANDELL, M.D.
Professor, Department of Internal Medicine
Owen R. Cheatham Professor of the Sciences
Head, Division of Infectious Diseases
University of Virginia School of Medicine
Charlottesville, Virginia

R. GORDON DOUGLAS, JR., M.D.
E. Hugh Luckey Distinguished Professor in Medicine
Chairman, Department of Medicine
Cornell University Medical College
Physician-in-Chief
The New York Hospital
New York, New York

JOHN E. BENNETT, M.D.
Head, Clinical Mycology Section
Laboratory of Clinical Investigation
National Institute of Allergy and Infectious Diseases
National Institutes of Health
Bethesda, Maryland

CHURCHILL LIVINGSTONE
New York, Edinburgh, London, Melbourne

Library of Congress Cataloging-in-Publication Data

Principles and practice of infectious diseases / edited by Gerald L.
Mandell, R. Gordon Douglas, Jr., John E. Bennett. — 3rd ed.
p. cm.
Includes bibliographies and index.
ISBN 0-443-08686-9 (single volume)
ISBN 0-443-08710-5 (two-volume set)
1. Communicable diseases. I. Mandell, Gerald L. II. Douglas, R.
Gordon (Robert Gordon), date. III. Bennett, John E. (John
Eugene), date.
[DNLM: 1. Communicable Diseases. WC 100 P957]
RC111.P78 1990
616.9—dc20
DNLM/DLC
for Library of Congress 89-15734
CIP

Distributed in the United Kingdom by Churchill Livingstone, Robert Stevenson House, 1–3 Baxter's Place, Leith Walk, Edinburgh EH1 3AF, and by associated companies, branches, and representatives throughout the world.

Accurate indications, adverse reactions, and dosage schedules for drugs are provided in this book, but it is possible that they may change. The reader is urged to review the package information data of the manufacturers of the medications mentioned.

The Publishers have made every effort to trace the copyright holders for borrowed material. If they have inadvertently overlooked any, they will be pleased to make the necessary arrangements at the first opportunity.

Acquisitions Editor: *Beth Kaufman Barry*
Assistant Editor: *Leslie Burgess*
Copy Editor: *David Terry*
Production Designer: *Charlie Lebeda*
Production Supervisor: *Jocelyn Eckstein*

Printed in the United States of America

First published in 1990

Fourth printing in 1990

CONTENTS

PART II. MAJOR CLINICAL SYNDROMES

SECTION A. FEVER

SECTION B. UPPER RESPIRATORY INFECTIONS

SECTION C. PLEUROPULMONARY AND BRONCHIAL INFECTIONS

SECTION D

SECTION E

SECTION F

SECTION G. CARDIOVASCULAR INFECTIONS

SECTION H. CENTRAL NERVOUS SYSTEM INFECTIONS

SECTION I. SKIN AND SOFT TISSUE INFECTIONS

SECTION G. PROTOZOAL DISEASES

SECTION H. DISEASES DUE TO HELMINTHS

SECTION I. ECTOPARASITES

SECTION J. DISEASES OF UNKNOWN ETIOLOGY

PART IV. SPECIAL PROBLEMS

SECTION A. NOSOCOMIAL INFECTIONS

CONTRIBUTORS

N. FRANKLIN ADKINSON, M.D.
Professor, Department of Medicine, Johns Hopkins University School of Medicine; Physician-in-Charge, Asthma and Allergy Clinics, Baltimore, Maryland

ROBERT H. ALFORD, M.D.
Clinical Professor, Department of Medicine, Vanderbilt University School of Medicine; Medical Director, Park View Medical Center, Nashville, Tennessee

DAVID M. ALLEN, M.D.
Senior Fellow in Infectious Diseases, Department of Medicine, Cornell University Medical College; Assistant Attending Physician and Chief Medical Resident, Department of Medicine, The New York Hospital, New York, New York

VINCENT T. ANDRIOLE, M.D.
Professor, Department of Medicine, Yale University School of Medicine; Attending Physician, Yale-New Haven Hospital, New Haven, Connecticut

MICHAEL A. APICELLA, M.D.
Professor of Medicine and Microbiology, Department of Medicine, State University of New York at Buffalo School of Medicine, Buffalo, New York

GORDON L. ARCHER, M.D.
Professor, Departments of Medicine and Microbiology/Immunology, Virginia Commonwealth University Medical College of Virginia School of Medicine, Richmond, Virginia

DONALD ARMSTRONG, M.D.
Professor, Department of Medicine, Cornell University Medical College; Chief, Infectious Disease Service, and Director, Microbiology Laboratory, Memorial Sloan-Kettering Cancer Center, New York, New York

LARRY M. BADDOUR, M.D.
Associate Professor, Department of Medicine, University of Missouri—Columbia School of Medicine, Columbia, Missouri

CAROL J. BAKER, M.D.
Professor, Departments of Pediatrics and Microbiology and Immunology, and Head, Section of Pediatric Infectious Diseases, Baylor College of Medicine, Houston, Texas

J. RICHARD BARINGER, M.D.
Professor and Chairman, Department of Neurology, University of Utah School of Medicine, Salt Lake City, Utah

KENNETH J. BART, M.D.
Agency Director for Health, Agency for International Development, Office of Health, Bureau for Science and Technology, Washington, D.C.

JOHN G. BARTLETT, M.D.
Professor, Department of Medicine, and Chief, Division of Infectious Diseases, Johns Hopkins University School of Medicine, Baltimore, Maryland

STEPHEN G. BAUM, M.D.
Professor, Department of Medicine, Mount Sinai School of Medicine of the City University of New York; Director, Department of Medicine, Beth Israel Medical Center, New York, New York

EDWIN H. BEACHEY, M.D.
Professor, Departments of Medicine and Microbiology and Immunology, and Chief, Division of Infectious Diseases, University of Tennessee College of Medicine; Associate Chief of Staff, Department of Research and Development, Veterans Administration Medical Center, Memphis, Tennessee

JOHN E. BENNETT, M.D.
Head, Clinical Mycology Section, Laboratory of Clinical Investigation, National Institute of Allergy and Infectious Diseases, National Institutes of Health, Bethesda, Maryland

KENNETH W. BERNARD, M.D., D.T.M. & H.
Medical Epidemiologist, International Health Program Office, Centers for Disease Control, Atlanta, Georgia; Consultant, Departments of Public Health Policy and Tropical Medicine, Peace Corps, Washington, D.C.

ROBERT F. BETTS, M.D.
Professor, Department of Medicine, University of Rochester School of Medicine and Dentistry; Attending Physician, Department of Medicine, Strong Memorial Hospital, Rochester, New York

ALAN L. BISNO, M.D.
Professor, Department of Medicine, University of Miami School of Medicine; Chief, Department of Medical Service, Miami Veterans Administration Medical Center, Miami, Florida

NEIL R. BLACKLOW, M.D.
Professor, Department of Medicine, and Director, Division of Infectious Diseases, University of Massachusetts Medical School, Worcester, Massachusetts

MARTIN J. BLASER, M.D.
Addison B. Scoville Professor of Medicine and Director, Division of Infectious Diseases, Department of Medicine; Professor, Department of Microbiology, Vanderbilt University School of Medicine, Nashville, Tennessee

WILLIAM BONNEZ, M.D.
Assistant Professor, Department of Medicine, University of Rochester School of Medicine and Dentistry; Attending Physician, Department of Medicine, Strong Memorial Hospital, Rochester, New York

RICHARD C. BOUCHER, M.D.
Professor, Department of Medicine, University of North Carolina at Chapel Hill School of Medicine, Chapel Hill, North Carolina

WILLIAM R. BOWIE, M.D.
Professor, Department of Medicine, University of British Columbia Faculty of Medicine, Vancouver, British Columbia, Canada

JOHN M. BOYCE, M.D.
Associate Professor, Department of Medicine, Brown University Program in Medicine; Associate Director, Infectious Diseases Section, Miriam Hospital, Providence, Rhode Island

PHILIP S. BRACHMAN, M.D.
Director, Epidemiology Program Office, Department of Health and Human Services, Centers for Disease Control, Atlanta, Georgia

BARRY D. BRAUSE, M.D.
Clinical Associate Professor, Department of Medicine, Cornell University Medical College; Associate Attending Physician, Department of Medicine, The New York Hospital for Special Surgery, New York, New York

ROBERT B. BREITENBUCHER, M.D.
Associate Professor, Department of Medicine, and Former Director, Division of Geriatric Medicine, University of Minnesota Medical School, Minneapolis, Minnesota

ARTHUR E. BROWN, M.D.
Associate Professor of Clinical Medicine and Clinical Pediatrics, Department of Medicine and Pediatrics, Cornell University Medical College; Attending Physician, Infectious Disease Service, Memorial Sloan-Kettering Cancer Center; Associate Attending Pediatrician, Department of Pediatrics, The New York Hospital, New York, New York

RALPH T. BRYAN, M.D.
Medical Epidemiologist, Parasitic Diseases Branch, Division of Parasitic Diseases, Centers for Disease Control, Atlanta, Georgia

RICHARD E. BRYANT, M.D.
Professor, Department of Medicine, and Director, Division of Infectious Disease, Oregon Health Sciences University School of Medicine, Portland, Oregon

WARD E. BULLOCK, M.D.
Professor, Department of Internal Medicine, and Director, Division of Infectious Disease, University of Cincinnati College of Medicine; Attending Physician, University of Cincinnati Medical Center, Cincinnati, Ohio

JAMES E. BURNS, M.D.
Department of Pediatrics, Division of Infectious Diseases, University of Virginia School of Medicine, Charlottesville, Virginia

LARRY M. BUSH, M.D.
Clinical Assistant Professor, Department of Medicine, Medical College of Pennsylvania, Philadelphia, Pennsylvania

THOMAS BUTLER, M.D.
Professor and Chief, Division of Infectious Diseases, Department of Internal Medicine, Texas Tech University Health Sciences Center School of Medicine, Lubbock, Texas

CHARLES C. J. CARPENTER, M.D.
Professor, Department of Medicine, Brown University Program in Medicine; Physician-in-Chief, Miriam Hospital, Providence, Rhode Island

THOMAS R. CATE, M.D.
Professor, Department of Medicine, Baylor College of Medicine, Houston, Texas

RICHARD E. CHAISSON, M.D.
Assistant Professor, Departments of Medicine and Epidemiology, Johns Hopkins University School of Medicine; Director, AIDS Service, Johns Hopkins Hospital, Baltimore, Maryland

MARY E. CHAMBERLAND, M.D., M.P.H.
Medical Epidemiologist, Surveillance and Evaluation Branch, AIDS Program, Centers for Disease Control, Atlanta, Georgia

STANLEY W. CHAPMAN, M.D.
Associate Professor, Department of Medicine, University of Mississippi School of Medicine; Chief, Medical Service and Infectious Diseases Section, Veterans Administration Medical Center, Jackson, Mississippi

ANTHONY W. CHOW, M.D., F.R.C.P.(C.)
Professor, Department of Medicine, and Head, Division of Infectious Diseases, University of British Columbia Faculty of Medicine; Head, Department of Medicine, Vancouver General Hospital, Vancouver, British Columbia, Canada

GORDON D. CHRISTENSEN, M.D.
Associate Professor, Departments of Medicine, Microbiology, and Immunology, University of Missouri-Columbia School of Medicine, Columbia, Missouri; Clinical Investigator, Research Service, Harry S. Truman Hospital, Columbia, Missouri

JEFFREY D. CHULAY, M.D., D.T.M. & H.
Associate Professor, Department of Medicine, Uniformed Services University of the Health Sciences F. Edward Hébert School of Medicine, Bethesda, Maryland; Chief, Department of Immunology, Walter Reed Army Institute of Research, Washington, D.C.

MARY LOU CLEMENTS, M.D., M.P.H.
Associate Professor, Department of International Health, Johns Hopkins University School of Hygiene and Public Health; Associate Professor, Department of Medicine, Johns Hopkins University School of Medicine; Director, Johns Hopkins University Center for Immunization Research, Baltimore, Maryland

C. GLENN COBBS, M.D.
Professor, Department of Medicine, and Director, Division of Infectious Diseases, University of Alabama School of Medicine, Birmingham, Alabama

MYRON S. COHEN, M.D.
Associate Professor, Departments of Medicine and Microbiology and Immunology, University of North Carolina at Chapel Hill School of Medicine, Chapel Hill, North Carolina

ROBERT B. COUCH, M.D.
Professor, Department of Medicine, and Chairman, Department of Microbiology and Immunology, Baylor College of Medicine, Houston, Texas

JAMES W. CURRAN, M.D., M.P.H.
Director, AIDS Program, and Associate Director for AIDS, Center for Infectious Diseases, Centers for Disease Control, Atlanta, Georgia

CARLOS DEL RIO, M.D.
Senior Associate, Department of Medicine, Emory University School of Medicine; Chief Resident, Department of Medicine, Crawford W. Long Memorial Hospital, Atlanta, Georgia

PETER DENSEN, M.D.
Associate Professor, Department of Internal Medicine, University of Iowa College of Medicine, Iowa City, Iowa

ROGER M. DES PREZ, M.D.
Professor, Department of Medicine, Vanderbilt University School of Medicine; Chief, Medical Service, Veterans Administration Medical Center, Nashville, Tennessee

RICHARD D. DIAMOND, M.D.
Professor, Departments of Medicine and Biochemistry, Boston University School of Medicine; Head, Section of Infectious Disease, Evans Memorial Department of Clinical Research, University Hospital, Boston, Massachusetts

CHARLES A. DINARELLO, M.D.
Professor, Departments of Medicine and Pediatrics, Tufts University School of Medicine; Staff Physician, Department of Medicine, New England Medical Center Hospital, Boston, Massachusetts

WILLIAM E. DISMUKES, M.D.
Professor and Vice-Chairman, Department of Medicine, University of Alabama School of Medicine; Director, Medical House Staff, University of Alabama Medical Center, Birmingham, Alabama

WILLIAM O. DOBBINS III, M.D.
Professor, Department of Internal Medicine, University of Michigan Medical School; Associate Chief of Staff for Research, Veterans Administration Medical Center, Ann Arbor, Michigan

JAY F. DOBKIN, M.D.
Associate Professor of Clinical Medicine, Department of Medicine, Columbia University College of Physicians and Surgeons; Medical Director, AIDS Center, Presbyterian Hospital, New York, New York

BRADLEY N. DOEBBELING, M.D.
Fellow Associate, University of Iowa Hospitals and Clinics, Iowa City, Iowa

RAPHAEL DOLIN, M.D.
Professor, Department of Medicine, and Director, Division of Infectious Diseases, University of Rochester School of Medicine and Dentistry; Head, Infectious Disease Unit, and Attending Physician, Department of Medicine, Strong Memorial Hospital, Rochester, New York

GERALD R. DONOWITZ, M.D.
Associate Professor, Department of Internal Medicine, and Associate Director, Hematology-Oncology Unit, University of Virginia School of Medicine, Charlottesville, Virginia

R. GORDON DOUGLAS, JR., M.D.
E. Hugh Luckey Distinguished Professor in Medicine and Chairman, Department of Medicine, Cornell University Medical College; Physician-in-Chief, The New York Hospital, New York, New York

J. STEPHEN DUMMER, M.D.
Associate Professor, Departments of Medicine and Surgery, University of Pittsburgh School of Medicine, Pittsburgh, Pennsylvania

HERBERT L. DuPONT, M.D.
Mary W. Kelsey Professor of the Medical Sciences, The University of Texas Medical School at Houston; Interim Chairman, Department of Internal Medicine, Director, Program in Infectious Diseases, and Interim Clinical Chief of the Internal Service, The Hermann Hospital, Houston, Texas

DAVID T. DURACK, M.B., D. PHIL.
Professor, Departments of Medicine and Microbiology and Immunology, and Chief, Division of Infectious Diseases, Duke University School of Medicine, Durham, North Carolina

JOHN E. EDWARDS, JR., M.D.
Professor, Department of Medicine, University of California, Los Angeles, UCLA School of Medicine, Los Angeles, California; Chief, Division of Infectious Diseases, Harbor-UCLA Medical Center, Torrance, California

MORVEN S. EDWARDS, M.D.
Associate Professor, Department of Pediatrics, Baylor College of Medicine, Houston, Texas

BARRY I. EISENSTEIN, M.D.
Professor and Chairman, Department of Microbiology and Immunology, and Professor, Department of Internal Medicine, University of Michigan Medical School, Ann Arbor, Michigan

JERROLD J. ELLNER, M.D.
Professor, Department of Medicine, Case Western Reserve University School of Medicine; Director, Division of Infectious Diseases, University Hospitals, Cleveland, Ohio

STANLEY FALKOW, PH.D.
Professor, Departments of Medicine and Microbiology and Immunology, Stanford University School of Medicine, Stanford, California

GUO-DONG FANG, M.D.
Associate Professor, Department of Medicine, Beijing Union Medical College, Beijing, China

BARRY M. FARR, M.D.
Associate Professor, Department of Medicine, University of Virginia School of Medicine, Charlottesville, Virginia

W. EDMUND FARRAR, M.D.
Professor, Department of Medicine, Medical University of South Carolina College of Medicine, Charleston, South Carolina

ANTHONY S. FAUCI, M.D.
Director, National Institute of Allergy and Infectious Diseases, National Institutes of Health, Bethesda, Maryland

STEPHEN M. FEINSTONE, M.D.
Medical Officer, Hepatitis Viruses Section, Laboratory of Infectious Diseases, National Institute of Allergy and Infectious Diseases, National Institutes of Health, Bethesda, Maryland

ROBERT FEKETY, M.D.
Professor, Department of Internal Medicine, and Head, Division of Infectious Diseases, University of Michigan Medical School; Chief, Adult Infectious Diseases Service, University Hospital, Ann Arbor, Michigan

BERNARD N. FIELDS, M.D.
Adele Lehman Professor and Chairman, Department of Microbiology and Molecular Genetics, and Professor, Department of Medicine, Harvard Medical School, Boston, Massachusetts

SYDNEY M. FINEGOLD, M.D.
Professor, Departments of Medicine and Microbiology, and Immunology, University of California, Los Angeles, UCLA School of Medicine; Associate Chief of Staff, Research and Development Service, Wadsworth Veterans Administration Medical Center, Los Angeles, California

GERALD W. FISCHER, M.D.
Professor, Department of Pediatrics, Uniformed Services University of the Health Sciences F. Edward Hébert School of Medicine, Bethesda, Maryland

DANIEL B. FISHBEIN, M.D.
Medical Epidemiologist, Viral and Rickettsial Zoonoses Branch, Division of Viral and Rickettsial Diseases, Center for Infectious Diseases, Centers for Disease Control, Atlanta, Georgia

L. NEAL FREEMAN, M.D.
Fellow in Ophthalmic Plastic and Reconstructive Surgery, Department of Ophthalmology, University of California, San Francisco, School of Medicine, San Francisco, California

JOHN I. GALLIN, M.D.
Director, Intramural Research Program, National Institute of Allergy and Infectious Diseases, and Senior Investigator, Bacterial Diseases Section, Laboratory of Clinical Investigation, National Institutes of Health, Bethesda, Maryland

HARRY A. GALLIS, M.D.
Associate Professor, Department of Internal Medicine, Duke University School of Medicine, Durham, North Carolina

ROBERT C. GALLO, M.D.
Chief, Laboratory of Tumor Cell Biology, National Cancer Institute, National Institutes of Health, Bethesda, Maryland

WALTER R. GAMMON, M.D.
Professor, Department of Dermatology, University of North Carolina at Chapel Hill School of Medicine, Chapel Hill, North Carolina

JEFFREY A. GELFAND, M.D.
Associate Professor, Department of Medicine, Tufts University School of Medicine; Physician, Department of Medicine, New England Medical Center, Boston, Massachusetts

ANNE A. GERSHON, M.D.
Professor, Department of Pediatrics, and Director, Division of Pediatric Infectious Diseases, Columbia University College of Physicians and Surgeons, New York, New York

PETER GILLIGAN, M.D.
Associate Professor, Departments of Microbiology and Immunology and Pathology, University of North Carolina at Chapel Hill School of Medicine, Chapel Hill, North Carolina

ALAN PAUL GLOMBICKI, M.D.
Assistant Professor, Department of Medicine, Baylor College of Medicine; Medical Director, Liver Transplant Unit, Texas Medical Center, Houston, Texas

ELLIE J. C. GOLDSTEIN, M.D.
Associate Clinical Professor, Department of Medicine, University of California, Los Angeles, UCLA School of Medicine, Los Angeles, California; Director, R. M. Alden Research Laboratory, Santa Monica Hospital Medical Center, Santa Monica, California

ROBERT A. GOODWIN, JR., M.D.
Professor Emeritus, Department of Medicine, Vanderbilt University School of Medicine, Nashville, Tennessee

W. RICHARD GREEN, M.D.
Professor, Department of Ophthalmology, and Associate Professor, Department of Pathology, Johns Hopkins University School of Medicine; Chief, Eye Pathology Laboratory, Johns Hopkins Hospital, Baltimore, Maryland

JOHN E. GREENLEE, M.D.
Professor, Department of Neurology, University of Utah School of Medicine; Chief, Neurology Service, Veterans Administration Medical Center, Salt Lake City, Utah

WILLIAM B. GREENOUGH III, M.D.
Professor, Department of Medicine, Johns Hopkins University School of Medicine, and Professor, Department of International Health, Johns Hopkins University School of Hygiene and Public Health, Baltimore, Maryland

DIANE E. GRIFFIN, M.D.
Professor, Departments of Medicine and Neurology, Johns Hopkins University School of Medicine, Baltimore, Maryland

DIETER H. M. GRÖSCHEL, M.D.
Professor, Departments of Pathology and Internal Medicine, and Director, Division of Clinical Microbiology, University of Virginia School of Medicine, Charlottesville, Virginia

DAVID I. GROVE, M.D.
Director of Postgraduate Medical Education, Sir Charles Gairdner Hospital, Nedlands, Western Australia

RICHARD L. GUERRANT, M.D.
Professor, Department of Internal Medicine, and Head, Division of Geographic Medicine, University of Virginia School of Medicine, Charlottesville, Virginia

JACK M. GWALTNEY, JR., M.D.
Professor, Department of Internal Medicine, and Head, Division of Epidemiology and Virology, University of Virginia School of Medicine, Charlottesville, Virginia

ASHLEY T. HAASE, M.D.
Professor and Head, Department of Microbiology, University of Minnesota Medical School, Minneapolis, Minnesota

CAROLINE BREESE HALL, M.D.
Professor, Departments of Pediatrics and Medicine, University of Rochester School of Medicine and Dentistry, Rochester, New York

WILLIAM J. HALL, M.D.
Professor of Medicine and Pulmonology, Department of Medicine, University of Rochester School of Medicine and Dentistry; Chairman, Department of Medicine, Rochester General Hospital, Rochester, New York

MARGARET A. HAMBURG, M.D.
Special Assistant to the Director, National Institute of Allergy and Infectious Diseases, National Institutes of Health, Bethesda, Maryland

W. LEE HAND, M.D.
Professor, Department of Medicine, and Director, Division of Infectious Diseases, Emory University School of Medicine; Chief, Infectious Diseases Section, Veterans Administration Medical Center, Atlanta, Georgia

H. HUNTER HANDSFIELD, M.D.
Professor, Department of Medicine, University of Washington School of Medicine; Director, Sexually Transmitted Disease Control Program, Seattle-King County Department of Public Health, Seattle, Washington

GAVIN HART, M.D., M.P.H.
Clinical Associate Professor, Department of Medicine, Flinders University School of Medicine; Director, STD Control Branch, South Australian Health Commission, Adelaide, South Australia

BARRY J. HARTMAN, M.D.
Associate Professor of Clinical Medicine, Department of Medicine, Cornell University Medical College; Associate Attending Physician, Department of Medicine, The New York Hospital, New York, New York

R. J. HAY, D.M., F.R.C.P.
Reader in Clinical Mycology, Department of Clinical Sciences, London School of Hygiene and Tropical Medicine; Consultant Dermatologist, Department of Microbial Diseases, St. Johns Hospital for Diseases of the Skin, London, England

FREDERICK G. HAYDEN, M.D.
Associate Professor, Departments of Internal Medicine and Pathology; Stuart S. Richardson Professor, Department of Internal Medicine; and Associate Director, Clinical Microbiology Laboratory (Virology), University of Virginia School of Medicine, Charlottesville, Virginia

CRAIG R. HEIM, M.D.
Associate Professor, Department of Medicine, Vanderbilt University School of Medicine; Attending Physician, Department of Medicine, Vanderbilt University Hospital, Nashville, Tennessee

FREDERICK P. HEINZEL, M.D.
Assistant Professor, Department of Medicine, University of California, San Francisco, School of Medicine, San Francisco, California

DAVID K. HENDERSON, M.D.
Associate Director for Quality Assurance and Hospital Epidemiology, Office of the Director, Clinical Center; Hospital Epidemiologist, Clinical Center; Investigator, Laboratory of Clinical Investigation, National Institute of Allergy and Infectious Diseases, National Institutes of Health, Bethesda, Maryland

J. OWEN HENDLEY, M.D.
Professor, Department of Pediatrics, and Head, Division of Pediatric Infectious Diseases, University of Virginia School of Medicine, Charlottesville, Virginia

JOHN E. HERRMANN, PH.D.
Associate Professor, Departments of Medicine and Molecular Genetics and Microbiology, University of Massachusetts Medical School, Worcester, Massachusetts

ERIK L. HEWLETT, M.D.
Professor, Departments of Internal Medicine and Pharmacology, and Head, Division of Clinical Pharmacology, University of Virginia School of Medicine, Charlottesville, Virginia

DAVID R. HILL, M.D.
Assistant Professor, Department of Medicine, University of Connecticut School of Medicine, Farmington, Connecticut

ALAN R. HINMAN, M.D., M.P.H.
Director, Center for Prevention Services, Centers for Disease Control, Atlanta, Georgia

MARTIN S. HIRSCH, M.D.
Professor, Department of Medicine, Harvard Medical School; Physician, Department of Medicine, Infectious Diseases Unit, Massachusetts General Hospital, Boston, Massachusetts

SHALOM Z. HIRSCHMAN, M.D.
Professor, Department of Medicine, and Director, Division of Infectious Diseases, Mount Sinai School of Medicine of the City University of New York, New York, New York

MONTO HO, M.D.
Professor and Chairman, Department of Microbiology; Professor, Department of Medicine; and Chief, Division of Infectious Diseases, University of Pittsburgh School of Medicine, Pittsburgh, Pennsylvania

GARY S. HOFFMAN, M.D.
Expert, Laboratory of Immunoregulation, National Institute of Allergy and Infectious Diseases, National Institutes of Health, Bethesda, Maryland

F. BLAINE HOLLINGER, M.D.
Professor, Departments of Medicine, Virology, and Epidemiology, and Head, Hepatitis and AIDS Research Units, Baylor College of Medicine, Houston, Texas

KING K. HOLMES, M.D., PH.D.
Professor and Vice Chairman, Department of Medicine, University of Washington School of Medicine, Physician-in-Chief, Harborview Medical Center, Seattle, Washington

JAY H. HOOFNAGLE, M.D.
Director, Division of Digestive Diseases and Nutrition, and Senior Investigator, Liver Diseases Section, National Institutes of Diabetes and Digestive and Kidney Diseases, National Institutes of Health, Bethesda, Maryland

EDWARD W. HOOK, M.D.
Professor and Chairman, Department of Internal Medicine, University of Virginia School of Medicine; Physician-in-Chief, University of Virginia Hospitals, Charlottesville, Virginia

EDWARD A. HOROWITZ, M.D.
Assistant Professor, Departments of Medicine and Medical Microbiology, Creighton University School of Medicine, Omaha, Nebraska

JAMES M. HUGHES, M.D.
Clinical Assistant Professor, Department of Medicine, Emory University School of Medicine; Deputy Director, Center for Infectious Diseases, Centers for Disease Control, Atlanta, Georgia

KARL M. JOHNSON, M.D.
Visiting Professor, Department of Tropical Medicine, Tulane University School of Public Health and Tropical Medicine, New Orleans, Louisiana; Consultant, Pharmaceutical Research and Development, Big Sky, Montana

RICHARD T. JOHNSON, M.D.
Dwight D. Eisenhower Professor, Department of Neurology, and Professor, Departments of Microbiology and Neuroscience, Johns Hopkins University School of Medicine, Baltimore, Maryland

WARREN D. JOHNSON, JR., M.D.
Professor, Department of Medicine, and Chief, Division of International Medicine, Cornell University Medical College; Attending Physician, Department of Medicine, The New York Hospital, New York, New York

THOMAS C. JONES, M.D.
Adjunct Professor, Department of Medicine, Cornell University Medical College, New York, New York; Head, Department of Allergy and Infectious Diseases, Sandoz, Ltd., Basle, Switzerland

ALLEN B. KAISER, M.D.
Associate Professor and Vice Chairman for Clinical Affairs, Department of Medicine, Vanderbilt University School of Medicine, Nashville, Tennessee

DENNIS L. KASPER, M.D.
Edward H. Kass Professor, Department of Medicine, Harvard Medical School; Co-Director, Channing Laboratory, Brigham and Women's Hospital, and Chief, Division of Infectious Diseases, Beth Israel Hospital, Boston, Massachusetts

MICHAEL KATZMAN, M.D.
Assistant Professor, Department of Medicine, Pennsylvania State University College of Medicine, Hershey, Pennsylvania

DONALD KAYE, M.D.
Professor and Chairman, Department of Medicine, Medical College of Pennsylvania; Chief, Department of Medicine, Hospital of the Medical College of Pennsylvania, Philadelphia, Pennsylvania

LOUIS V. KIRCHHOFF, M.D., M.P.H.
Associate Professor, Department of Internal Medicine, University of Iowa College of Medicine; Staff Physician, Department of Veterans, Affairs Medical Center, Iowa City, Iowa

JEROME O. KLEIN, M.D.
Professor, Department of Pediatrics, Boston University School of Medicine; Director, Division of Pediatric Infectious Diseases, Maxwell Finland Laboratory for Infectious Diseases, Boston City Hospital, Boston, Massachusetts

FREDERICK A. KLIPSTEIN, M.D.
Professor, Departments of Medicine and Microbiology, University of Rochester School of Medicine and Dentistry; Attending Physician, Department of Medicine, Strong Memorial Hospital, Rochester, New York

MICHAEL R. KNOWLES, M.D.
Associate Professor, Department of Medicine, University of North Carolina at Chapel Hill School of Medicine, Chapel Hill, North Carolina

SCOTT KOENIG, M.D., PH.D.
Senior Investigator, National Institute of Allergy and Infectious Diseases, National Institutes of Health, Bethesda, Maryland

JOHN N. KRIEGER, M.D.
Associate Professor, Department of Urology, University of Washington School of Medicine; Attending Surgeon, Department of Urology, University Hospital and Harborview Medical Center; Consultant, Division of Urology, Seattle Veterans Administration Medical Center, Seattle, Washington

CALVIN M. KUNIN, M.D.
Professor, Department of Internal Medicine, Ohio State University College of Medicine; Attending Physician, Department of Internal Medicine, Ohio State University Hospital, Columbus, Ohio

F. MARC LaFORCE, M.D.
Professor, Department of Medicine, University of Rochester School of Medicine and Dentistry; Physician-in-Chief, Genesee Hospital, Rochester, New York

WILLIAM J. LEDGER, M.D.
Professor, Department of Obstetrics and Gynecology, Cornell University Medical College; Obstetrician and Gynecologist-in-Chief, The New York Hospital, New York, New York

JAMES R. LEHRICH, M.D.
Associate Professor, Department of Neurology, Harvard Medical School; Director, Neurology Ambulatory Unit, Department of Neurology, Massachusetts General Hospital, Boston, Massachusetts

PHILLIP I. LERNER, M.D.
Professor, Department of Medicine, Case Western Reserve University School of Medicine; Chief, Division of Infectious Diseases, Mt. Sinai Hospital, Cleveland, Ohio

MATTHEW E. LEVISON, M.D.
Professor, Department of Medicine, and Chief, Division of Infectious Diseases, Medical College of Pennsylvania, Philadelphia, Pennsylvania

PAUL S. LIETMAN, M.D.
Professor, of Medicine, and Director, Division of Clinical Pharmacology, Johns Hopkins University School of Medicine, Baltimore, Maryland

NATHAN LITMAN, M.D.
Associate Professor, Department of Pediatrics, Albert Einstein College of Medicine of Yeshiva University; Assistant Chief of Service and Associate Director, Department of Pediatrics, Montefiore Medical Center, Bronx, New York

JACOB A. LOHR, M.D.
Professor, Vice Chairman, and Chief, Department of Pediatrics, University of Virginia School of Medicine, Charlottesville, Virginia

JAMES E. LOYD, M.D.
Assistant Professor, Department of Medicine, Vanderbilt University School of Medicine, Nashville, Tennessee

ROB ROY MacGREGOR, M.D.
Professor, Department of Medicine, and Chief, Division of Infectious Diseases, University of Pennsylvania School of Medicine, Philadelphia, Pennsylvania

EL SHEIKH MAHGOUB, M.D.
Professor, Department of Medical Microbiology and Parasitology, University of Khartoum School of Medicine, Khartoum, Sudan

ADEL A. F. MAHMOUD, M.D., PH.D.
John H. Hord Professor and Chairman, Department of Medicine, Case Western Reserve University School of Medicine; Physician-in-Chief, University Hospitals of Cleveland, Cleveland, Ohio

GERALD L. MANDELL, M.D.
Professor, Department of Internal Medicine; Owen R. Cheatham Professor of the Sciences; and Head, Division of Infectious Diseases, University of Virginia School of Medicine, Charlottesville, Virginia

THOMAS J. MARRIE, M.D.
Professor, Department of Medicine, Dalhousie University Faculty of Medicine; Head, Division of Infectious Diseases, Victoria General Hospital, Halifax, Nova Scotia, Canada

MICHAEL A. MARTIN, M.D.
Assistant Professor, Department of Medicine, University of Maryland School of Medicine; Hospital Epidemiologist, University of Maryland Hospital, Baltimore, Maryland

HENRY MASUR, M.D.
Professor, Department of Medicine, George Washington University School of Medicine, Washington, D.C.; Chief, Department of Critical Care Medicine, Clinical Center, National Institutes of Health, Bethesda, Maryland

GLENN E. MATHIESEN, M.D.
Assistant Professor, Department of Medicine, University of California, Los Angeles, UCLA School of Medicine, Los Angeles, California; Physician Specialist, Department of Medicine, Olive View Hospital, Sylmar, California

KENNETH H. MAYER, M.D.
Associate Professor, Department of Medicine, and Director, AIDS Program, Brown University Program in Medicine, Providence, Rhode Island; Chief, Division of Infectious Disease, Memorial Hospital, Pawtucket, Rhode Island

ROBERT E. McCABE, M.D.
Assistant Professor, Department of Medicine, University of California, Davis, School of Medicine, Davis, California; Chief, Infectious Diseases Section, Veterans Administration Medical Center, Martinez, California

J. BRUCE McCLAIN, M.D.
Associate Professor, Department of Clinical Medicine, Uniformed Services University of Health Sciences F. Edward Hébert School of Medicine, Bethesda, Maryland; Infectious Disease Officer, Walter Reed Army Institute of Research, Washington, D.C.

PETER J. McDONNELL, M.D.
Assistant Professor, Department of Ophthalmology, University of Southern California School of Medicine, Los Angeles, California

ZELL A. McGEE, M.D.
Professor, Departments of Medicine and Pathology, and Director, Center for Infectious Diseases, Division of Diagnostic Microbiology and Immunology, University of Utah School of Medicine, Salt Lake City, Utah

JOHN E. McGOWAN, JR., M.D.
Professor, Departments of Medicine and Pathology and Laboratory Medicine, Emory University School of Medicine; Director, Clinical Microbiology Section, Grady Memorial Hospital, Atlanta, Georgia

KENNETH McINTOSH, M.D.
Professor, Department of Pediatrics, Harvard Medical School; Chief, Division of Infectious Diseases, The Children's Hospital, Boston, Massachusetts

ANTONE A. MEDEIROS, M.D.
Professor, Department of Medicine, Brown University Program in Medicine; Chief, Division of Infectious Disease, Miriam Hospital, Providence, Rhode Island

MARILYN A. MENEGUS, M.D.
Associate Professor, Departments of Microbiology and Immunology; Pathology; and Pediatrics; Director, Clinical Microbiology Laboratories, University of Rochester School of Medicine and Dentistry, Rochester, New York

FRANÇOISE MEUNIER, M.D.
Chief, Division of Infectious Diseases and Microbiology Laboratory; Research Associate, Fund for Medical Scientific Research, Institute Jules Bordet, Brussels, Belgium

JOEL D. MEYERS, M.D.
Professor, Division of Infectious Diseases, Department of Medicine, University of Washington School of Medicine; Member and Head, Program in Infectious Diseases, Fred Hutchinson Cancer Research Center, Seattle, Washington

DENNIS J. MIKOLICH, M.D.
Clinical Assistant Professor, Department of Medicine, Brown University Program in Medicine, Providence, Rhode Island

JOHN F. MODLIN, M.D.
Associate Professor, Department of Pediatrics, Johns Hopkins University School of Medicine, Baltimore, Maryland

ROBERT C. MOELLERING, JR., M.D.
Shields Warren-Mallinckrodt Professor of Clinical Research, and Professor, Department of Medicine, Harvard Medical School; Physician-in-Chief, New England Deaconess Hospital, Boston, Massachusetts

THOMAS P. MONATH, M.D.
Chief, Division of Virology, U.S. Army Medical Research Institute of Infectious Diseases, Fort Detrick, Frederick, Maryland

E. RICHARD MOXON, M.D.
Professor, Department of Paediatrics, Oxford University Faculty of Medicine; Head, Department of Paediatrics, John Radcliffe Hospital, Headington, Oxford, England

MAURICE A. MUFSON, M.D.
Professor and Chairman, Department of Medicine, Marshall University School of Medicine; Associate Chief of Staff, Research and Development Section, Veterans Administration Medical Center, Huntington, West Virginia

DANIEL M. MUSHER, M.D.
Professor, Department of Medicine, Baylor College of Medicine; Chief, Infectious Diseases Section, Veterans Administration Hospital, Houston, Texas

THEODORE E. NASH, M.D.
Medical Officer and Senior Scientist, Laboratory of Parasitic Diseases, National Institute of Allergy and Infectious Diseases, National Institutes of Health, Bethesda, Maryland

JOHN M. NEFF, M.D.
Professor, Department of Pediatrics, and Associate Dean, University of Washington School of Medicine; Medical Director, The Children's Hospital and Medical Center; Seattle, Washington

HAROLD C. NEU, M.D.
Professor, Departments of Medicine and Pharmacology, Columbia University College of Physicians and Surgeons; Hospital Epidemiologist, Department of Epidemiology, Presbyterian Hospital, New York, New York

CHARLES H. NIGHTINGALE, PH.D.
Research Professor, University of Connecticut School of Pharmacy, Farmington, Connecticut; Vice President, Hartford Hospital, Hartford, Connecticut

CARL W. NORDEN, M.D.
Professor, Department of Medicine, University of Pittsburgh School of Medicine; Head, Division of Infectious Disease, Montefiore Hospital, Pittsburgh, Pennsylvania

SANDRA NORRIS, Pharm. D.
President, DataMed Scientific Communications, Inc., New York, New York

STEVEN M. OPAL, M.D.
Assistant Professor, Department of Medicine, Brown University Program in Medicine, Providence, Rhode Island; Hospital Epidemiologist and Infectious Disease Consultant, Memorial Hospital, Pawtucket, Rhode Island

WALTER A. ORENSTEIN, M.D.
Director, Division of Immunization, Center for Prevention Services, Centers for Disease Control, Atlanta, Georgia

MICHAEL N. OXMAN, M.D.
Professor, Departments of Medicine and Pathology, University of California, San Diego, School of Medicine; Chief, Infectious Diseases Section, Veterans Administration Medical Center, San Diego, California

RICHARD D. PEARSON, M.D.
Associate Professor, Departments of Internal Medicine and Pathology, University of Virginia School of Medicine, Charlottesville, Virginia

JAMES E. PENNINGTON, M.D.
Clinical Professor, Department of Medicine, University of California, San Francisco, School of Medicine, San Francisco, California; Director, Department of Medical Research, Cutter Biological, Berkeley, Calfornia

PHILLIP K. PETERSON, M.D.
Professor, Department of Medicine, University of Minnesota Medical School—Minneapolis; Director, Section of Infectious Diseases, Hennepin County Medical Center, Minneapolis, Minnesota

WILLIAM A. PETRI, JR., M.D.
Lucille P. Markey Scholar and Assistant Professor, Departments of Internal Medicine and Microbiology, University of Virginia School of Medicine, Charlottesville, Virginia

PHILIP A. PIZZO, M.D.
Head, Infectious Disease Section, and Chief, Pediatric Branch, National Cancer Institute, National Institutes of Health, Bethesda, Maryland

MATTHEW POLLACK, M.D.
Professor, Department of Medicine, Uniformed Services University of the Health Sciences F. Edward Hébert School of Medicine, Bethesda, Maryland

STEPHEN R. PREBLUD, M.D.
Surveillence, Investigation, and Research Branch, Division of Immunization, Center for Prevention Services, Centers for Disease Control, Atlanta, Georgia

D. RAOULT, M.D.
Unité des Rickettsies, Laboratoire de Bacteriologie-Sérologie-Virologie, Groupe Hospitalier de la Timone; Directeur, Centre National de Référence des Rickettsioses, Marseille, France

JONATHAN I. RAVDIN, M.D.
Associate Professor, Departments of Internal Medicine and Pharmacology, University of Virginia School of Medicine, Charlottesville, Virginia

RICHARD C. REICHMAN, M.D.
Associate Professor, Departments of Medicine and Microbiology and Immunology, University of Rochester School of Medicine and Dentistry; Attending Physician, Department of Medicine, Strong Memorial Hospital, Rochester, New York

MICHAEL F. REIN, M.D.
Professor, Department of Internal Medicine, University of Virginia School of Medicine, Charlottesville, Virginia

MARVIN S. REITZ, JR., PH.D.
Investigator, Laboratory of Tumor Cell Biology, Division of Cancer Etiology, National Cancer Institute, National Institutes of Health, Bethesda, Maryland

DAVID A. RELMAN, M.D.
Postdoctoral Fellow, Departments of Microbiology, Immunology, and Medicine, Standford University School of Medicine, Stanford, California

JACK S. REMINGTON, M.D.
Professor, Department of Medicine, Stanford University School of Medicine, Stanford, California; Chairman, Department of Immunology and Infectious Diseases, and Marcus A. Krupp Research Chair, Palo Alto Medical Foundation, Palo Alto, California

ANGELA RESTREPO M., PH.D.
Head, Mycology Laboratory, and Investigator, Corporacion para Investigaciones Biológicas, Medellín, Colombia

HERBERT Y. REYNOLDS, M.D.
Professor and Chairman, Department of Medicine, Pennsylvania State University College of Medicine, Hershey, Pennsylvania

NORBERT J. ROBERTS, JR., M.D.
Associate Professor, Department of Medicine, University of Rochester School of Medicine and Dentistry; Attending Physician, Strong Memorial Hospital, Rochester, New York

WILLIAM S. ROBINSON, M.D.
Professor, Department of Medicine, Stanford University School of Medicine, Stanford, California

RICHARD K. ROOT, M.D.
Professor and Chairman, Department of Medicine, University of California, San Francisco, School of Medicine, San Francisco, California

DANIEL ROTROSEN, M.D.
Senior Staff Fellow, Bacterial Diseases Section, Laboratory of Clinical Investigation, National Institute of Allergy and Infectious Diseases, National Institutes of Health, Bethesda, Maryland

ALFRED J. SAAH, M.D., M.P.H.
Associate Professor, Department of Epidemiology, Johns Hopkins University School of Hygiene and Public Health, and Associate Professor, Department of Medicine, Johns Hopkins University School of Medicine, Baltimore, Maryland

MERLE A. SANDE, M.D.
Professor and Vice Chairman, Department of Medicine, University of California, San Francisco, School of Medicine; Chief, Medical Service, San Francisco General Hospital, San Francisco, California

W. EUGENE SANDERS, JR., M.D.
Professor and Chairman, Department of Medical Microbiology, and Professor, Department of Medicine, Creighton University School of Medicine; Attending Physician, Department of Medicine, Veterans Administration Medical Center and St. Joseph Hospital, Omaha, Nebraska

JAY P. SANFORD, M.D.
Professor, Department of Medicine; President and Dean, Uniformed Services University of the Health Sciences F. Edward Hébert School of Medicine, Bethesda, Maryland

MARIA C. SAVOIA, M.D.
Assistant Adjunct Professor, Department of Medicine, University of California, San Diego, School of Medicine; Acting Chief, Department of Medicine, San Diego Veterans Administration Medical Center, San Diego, California

WILLIAM SCHAFFNER, M.D.
Professor and Chairman, Department of Preventive Medicine, and Professor, Department of Medicine, Vanderbilt University School of Medicine, Nashville, Tennessee

W. MICHAEL SCHELD, M.D.
Professor, Departments of Internal Medicine and Neurosurgery, University of Virginia School of Medicine, Charlottesville, Virginia

STEPHEN C. SCHIMPFF, M.D.
Professor, Departments of Medicine and Oncology, University of Maryland School of Medicine; Executive Vice President, University of Maryland Medical System, Baltimore, Maryland

CHARLES J. SCHLEUPNER, M.D.
Associate Professor, Department of Internal Medicine, University of Virginia School of Medicine, Charlottesville, Virginia; Chief, Infectious Diseases Section, Veterans Administration Medical Center, Salem, Virginia

ROBERT T. SCHOOLEY, M.D.
Associate Professor, Department of Medicine, Harvard Medical School; Assistant Physician, Infectious Disease Unit, Massachusetts General Hospital, Boston, Massachusetts

G. TOM SHIRES, M.D.
Lewis Atterbury Stimson Professor and Chairman, Department of Surgery, Cornell University Medical College; Surgeon-in-Chief, The New York Hospital, New York, New York

RICHARD L. SIMMONS, M.D.
George Vance Foster Professor and Chair, Department of Surgery, University of Pittsburgh School of Medicine; Chief of Surgery, Presbyterian-University Hospital, Pittsburgh, Pennsylvania

W. ANDREW SIMPSON, M.D.
Associate Professor, Departments of Medicine and Microbiology and Immunology, University of Missouri—Columbia School of Medicine, Columbia, Missouri

JAMES W. SMITH, M.D.
Professor, Department of Internal Medicine, University of Texas Health Science Center at Dallas Southwestern Medical School; Chief, Infectious Diseases Section, Veterans Administration Medical Center, Dallas, Texas

ROSEMARY SOAVE, M.D.
Assistant Professor, Departments of Medicine and Public Health, Cornell University Medical College; Assistant Attending Physician, Department of Medicine, The New York Hospital, New York, New York

JACK D. SOBEL, M.D.
Professor, Department of Medicine, and Chief, Division of Infectious Diseases, Wayne State University School of Medicine, Detroit, Michigan

ANASTACIO DE QUEIROZ SOUSA, M.D.
Assistant Professor, Department of Medicine, Federal University of Ceara, Fortaleza, Brazil

CAROL A. SPIEGEL, Ph.D., A.B.M.M.
Director, Clinical Microbiology Laboratory, University of Wisconsin Hospital and Clinics, Madison, Wisconsin

HAROLD C. STANDIFORD, M.D.
Professor, Department of Medicine, University of Maryland School of Medicine; Chief, Infectious Diseases Section, Veterans Administration Medical Center, Baltimore, Maryland

ALLEN C. STEERE, M.D.
Professor, Department of Medicine, and Chief, Department of Rheumatology and Immunology, Tufts University School of Medicine, Boston, Massachusetts

NEAL H. STEIGBIGEL, M.D.
Professor, Department of Medicine, Albert Einstein College of Medicine of Yeshiva University; Head, Division of Infectious Diseases, Montefiore Medical Center, Bronx, New York

DAVID A. STEVENS, M.D.
Professor, Department of Medicine, Stanford University School of Medicine, Stanford, California; Chief, Division of Infectious Diseases, Department of Medicine, Santa Clara Valley Medical Center; Principal Investigator, Infectious Diseases Research Laboratory, Institute for Medical Research, San Jose, California

MARK STOECKLE, M.D.
Assistant Professor, Department of Medicine, Cornell University Medical College; Attending Physician, Department of Medicine, The New York Hospital; Adjunct Faculty Member, Laboratory of Molecular Oncology, Rockefeller University, New York, New York

STEPHEN E. STRAUS, M.D.
Head, Medical Virology Section, Laboratory of Clinical Investigation, National Institute of Allergy and Infectious Diseases, National Institutes of Health, Bethesda, Maryland

STEPHEN A. STREED, M.S., C.I.C.
Manager, Epidemiology Systems, University of Iowa Hospital and Clinics, Iowa City, Iowa

ALAN M. SUGAR, M.D.
Associate Professor, Department of Medicine, Boston University School of Medicine, Boston, Massachusetts

BARRETT SUGARMAN, M.D.
Professor, Departments of Medicine, Microbiology, and Public Health, and Chief, Division of Infectious Diseases, Michigan State University College of Human Medicine, East Lansing, Michigan

MORTON N. SWARTZ, M.D.
Professor, Department of Medicine, Harvard Medical School; Chief, Department of Infectious Diseases, Massachusetts General Hospital, Boston, Massachusetts

ROBERT V. TAUXE, M.D.
Chief, Epidemiology Section, Enteric Diseases Branch, Division of Bacterial Diseases, Center for Infectious Diseases, Centers for Disease Control, Atlanta, Georgia

DAVID TAYLOR-ROBINSON, M.D.
Head, Division of Sexually Transmitted Diseases, MRC Clinical Research Centre, Harrow, Middlesex; Research Director, Jefferies Research Wing of the Praed Street Clinic, St. Mary's Hospital, London, England

MICHAEL G. THRELKELD, M.D.
Fellow, Department of Medicine, University of Alabama School of Medicine, Birmingham, Alabama

EDMUND C. TRAMONT, M.D.
Colonel, United States Army Medical Department; Professor, Department of Medicine, and Chief, Division of Infectious Diseases, Uniformed Services University of the Health Sciences F. Edward Hébert School of Medicine, Bethesda, Maryland; Associate Director, Walter Reed Army Institute of Research, Washington, D.C.

CARMELITA U. TUAZON, M.D.
Professor, Department of Medicine, and Director, Division of Infectious Disease, George Washington University School of Medicine and Health Sciences, Washington, D.C.

KENNETH L. TYLER, M.D.
Associate Professor, Department of Neurology-Neuroscience, Harvard Medical School; Assistant Neurologist, Department of Neurology, Massachusetts General Hospital, Boston, Massachusetts

DAVID E. VAN REKEN, M.D.
Clinical Associate Professor, Department of Pediatrics, Indiana University School of Medicine, Indianapolis, Indiana

PAUL A. VOLBERDING, M.D.
Associate Professor, Department of Medicine, and Chief, AIDS Activities Division, University of California, San Francisco, School of Medicine, San Francisco, California

KENNETH F. WAGNER, D.O.
Associate Professor, Department of Internal Medicine, Uniformed Services University of the Health Sciences F. Edward Hébert School of Medicine, Bethesda, Maryland; Senior Research Physician, HIV Research Program, Henry M. Jackson Foundation for the Advancement of Military Medicine, Bethesda, Maryland; Attending Physician, Department of Internal Medicine, Naval Hospital, Bethesda, Maryland, and Walter Reed Army Medical Center, Washington, D.C.

FRANCIS A. WALDVOGEL, M.D.
Professor, Department of Medicine, Faculty of Medicine, University of Geneva Medical School; Physician-in-Chief, Department of Medicine, Clinique Médicale Thérapeutique, University Hospital, Geneva, Switzerland

D. H. WALKER, M.D.
Professor and Chairman, Department of Pathology, University of Texas Medical School at Galveston, Galveston, Texas

PETER D. WALZER, M.D.
Professor, Department of Internal Medicine, University of Cincinnati College of Medicine; Chief, Division of Infectious Diseases, Department of Medical Services, Veterans Administration Medical Center, Cincinnati, Ohio

JOHN W. WARREN, M.D.
Associate Professor, Department of Medicine, and Head, Division of Infectious Diseases, University of Maryland School of Medicine, Baltimore, Maryland

KENNETH S. WARREN, M.D.
Professor, Department of Medicine, New York University School of Medicine; Adjunct Professor, Rockefeller University; Director for Science, Maxwell Communication Corporation, The Maxwell Foundation, New York, New York

RONALD G. WASHBURN, M.D.
Assistant Professor, Department of Medicine, Bowman Gray School of Medicine of Wake Forest University, Winston-Salem, North Carolina

JOHN A. WASHINGTON II, M.D.
Chairman, Department of Microbiology, The Cleveland Clinic Foundation, Cleveland, Ohio

PEYTON E. WEARY, M.D.
Professor and Chairman, Department of Dermatology, University of Virginia School of Medicine, Charlottesville, Virginia

DAVID J. WEBER, M.D., M.P.H.
Assistant Professor, Department of Medicine, University of North Carolina at Chapel Hill School of Medicine, Chapel Hill, North Carolina

CYNTHIA S. WEIKEL, M.D.
Assistant Professor, Department of Medicine, Johns Hopkins University School of Medicine, Baltimore, Maryland

MICHAEL E. WEISS, M.D.
Postdoctoral Fellow, Department of Medicine, Johns Hopkins University School of Medicine, Baltimore, Maryland

RICHARD P. WENZEL, M.D.
Professor, Department of Internal Medicine, and Director, Division of Clinical Epidemiology, University of Iowa College of Medicine; Hospital Epidemiologist, University of Iowa Hospitals and Clinics, Iowa City, Iowa

RICHARD J. WHITLEY, M.D.
Professor, Departments of Pediatrics and Microbiology, University of Alabama School of Medicine, Birmingham, Alabama

BARBARA BRAUNSTEIN WILSON, M.D.
Assistant Professor, Department of Dermatology, University of Virginia School of Medicine, Charlottesville, Virginia

CHRISTOPHER B. WILSON, M.D.
Professor, Department of Pediatrics, and Head, Division of Immunology and Rheumatology, University of Washington School of Medicine; Associate, Division of Infectious Disease, Children's Hospital and Medical Center, Seattle, Washington

BRIAN WISPELWEY, M.D.
Assistant Professor, Department of Internal Medicine, University of Virginia School of Medicine, Charlottesville, Virginia

MARTIN S. WOLFE, M.D.
Clinical Professor, Department of Medicine, George Washington University School of Medicine and Health Science, and Clinical Associate Professor, Department of Medicine, Georgetown University School of Medicine; Director, Traveler's Medical Service of Washington, Washington, D.C.

SHELDON M. WOLFF, M.D.
Endicott Professor and Chairman, Department of Medicine, Tufts University School of Medicine; Physician-in-Chief, New England Medical Center Hospital, Boston, Massachusetts

DAVID J. WYLER, M.D.
Professor, Department of Medicine, Tufts University School of Medicine; Physician and Director, Travelers' Health Service, New England Medical Center Hospitals, Boston, Massachusetts

LOWELL S. YOUNG, M.D.
Clinical Professor, Department of Medicine, University of California, San Francisco, School of Medicine; Chief, Division of Infectious Diseases, Pacific Presbyterian Medical Center, and Director, Kuzell Institute for Arthritis and Infectious Diseases, Medical Research Institute of San Francisco, San Francisco, California

VICTOR L. YU, M.D.
Professor, Department of Medicine, University of Pittsburgh School of Medicine; Chief, Infectious Disease Section, Veterans Administration Medical Center, Pittsburgh, Pennsylvania

ROGER W. YURT, M.D.
Associate Professor and Vice Chairman, Department of Surgery, Cornell University Medical College; Director, Trauma Center, The New York Hospital, New York, New York

DORI F. ZALEZNIK, M.D.
Assistant Professor, Department of Medicine, Harvard Medical School; Hospital Epidemiologist, Division of Infectious Diseases, Beth Israel Hospital, Boston, Massachusetts

STEPHEN H. ZINNER, M.D.
Professor, Department of Medicine, Brown University Program in Medicine; Director, Infectious Diseases Section, Department of Medicine, Roger Williams General Hospital; Consultant in Infectious Disease, Rhode Island Hospital, Veterans Administration Medical Center, Miriam Hospital, and Women and Infants Hospital, Providence, Rhode Island

PREFACE TO THE THIRD EDITION

This expanded and extensively rewritten third edition reflects the immense changes that have occurred in the field of infectious diseases in the five years since the second edition of *Principles and Practice of Infectious Diseases* was published. The authors have met the challenge of providing accurate, up-to-date information relative to the science and practice of infectious diseases. All of the chapters have been revised, rewritten, and updated. Many new authors have been added to the roster of outstanding clinician-scientists, and chapters have been added to thoroughly cover important new aspects of our specialty.

Part I of the book considers basic principles important for the diagnosis and management of infectious diseases. New chapters in this section include A Molecular Perspective of Microbial Pathogenicity; Evaluation of the Patient with Suspected Immunodeficiency; Mechanisms of Antibiotic Resistance; β-Lactam Allergy; and Quinolones. New additions to Part II, which covers Major Clinical Syndromes, include The Acutely Ill Patient with Fever and Rash; Cystic Fibrosis; Infections with Prostheses in Bones and Joints; Slow Infections of the Central Nervous System; and an extensive coverage of the acquired immunodeficiency syndrome that includes epidemiology and prevention, immunology, clinical manifestations, diagnostic tests for HIV infection, therapy, and vaccines.

Newly recognized pathogens discussed in Part III, Infectious Diseases and Their Etiologic Agents, include papillomaviruses; reovirus and orbivirus; parvoviruses; retroviruses including the lentiviruses, human immunodeficiency viruses types 1 and 2, the oncoviruses, and human T-cell leukemia virus types I and II; prions; TWAR; *Borellia burgdorferi*; cat scratch disease agent; microsporidia; and *Ehrlichia* species. Finally, new considerations under Part IV, Special Problems, include HIV nosocomial infections; infections in bone marrow recipients; infections in solid organ transplant recipients; infections in patients with spinal cord injuries; and infections in the elderly.

We are immensely pleased with the superb job our publisher, Churchill Livingstone Inc., has done in producing the third edition. Special thanks go to Leslie Burgess, David Terry, and Beth Barry for their tireless devotion to excellence.

Gerald L. Mandell, M.D.
R. Gordon Douglas, Jr., M.D.
John E. Bennett, M.D.

PREFACE TO THE FIRST EDITION

Infectious diseases traverse the usual boundaries established by medical specialists. All organ systems may be involved, and all physicians caring for patients may have to deal with infected patients. The format of this book was chosen with the intent that it would contain the necessary information to aid the practitioner in the understanding, diagnosis, and treatment of infectious diseases. Thus, internists, family or general practitioners, pediatricians, surgeons, obstetrician-gynecologists, urologists, residents and fellows in training, medical students, hospital infection control personnel, and clinical microbiologists should find the book a valuable reference.

In planning this book the editors considered several different patterns of organization. The system adopted allows the reader to approach an infected patient three different ways: (a) by major clinical syndrome, (b) by specific etiologic organism, and (c) by host characteristics for patients who are compromised.

Principles and Practice of Infectious Diseases consists of four major parts. The book may be perused as a whole, or individual chapters may be examined when the reader is concerned with a specific problem. Part I covers the basic principles necessary for a clear understanding of the concepts of diagnosis and management of infectious disease. Chapters dealing with microbial virulence factors, host defense mechanisms, the epidemiology of infectious diseases, and the clinician and the microbiology laboratory are included. In addition, there is a comprehensive discussion of anti-infective chemotherapy.

Part II considers major clinical syndromes. The syndromes are described, followed by a discussion of the potential etiologic agents, evaluation of differential diagnostic possibilities, and an outline of presumptive therapy. All major infectious diseases are discussed in this part of the book.

Part III describes all important pathogenic microbes for man and the diseases they cause. The pathogen is classified and described, the epidemiology is discussed, clinical manifestations are listed, and specific information on therapy and prevention is presented. The most comprehensive discussion of a disease entity can be found by reading about both the etiologic agent and the clinical syndrome. Thus, a comprehensive treatment of pneumococcal pneumonia could be found in reading the appropriate sections of the chapters on acute pneumonia and *Streptococcus pneumoniae*. We attempted to make the chapters dealing with etiologic agents and those dealing with syndromes complete. Therefore some repetition was unavoidable.

The final section, Part IV, covers special problems in infectious diseases including nosocomial infections, infections in impaired hosts, immunizations, and protection of travelers.

The editors are grateful to our expert contributors. These physicians are the world's leaders in their fields, and they diligently prepared carefully written, well-referenced "state of the art" chapters. Our secretaries were skillful and meticulous in their attention to the complexities of assembling *Principles and Practices of Infectious Diseases*. John de Carville, executive editor of John Wiley & Sons, encouraged, cajoled, and advised us from the formative steps all the way through to completion. Lastly, and perhaps most important, we are grateful to our wives and children for putting up with interminable editorial work and meetings.

Gerald L. Mandell, M.D.
R. Gordon Douglas, Jr., M.D.
John E. Bennett, M.D.

PRINCIPLES AND PRACTICE OF

INFECTIOUS DISEASES

THIRD EDITION

BASIC PRINCIPLES IN THE DIAGNOSIS AND MANAGEMENT OF INFECTIOUS DISEASES

PART I

SECTION A. MICROBIAL VIRULENCE FACTORS

1. TOXINS AND OTHER VIRULENCE FACTORS

ERIK L. HEWLETT

Although humans are continually exposed to a vast array of microorganisms in the environment, only a small proportion of those microbes are capable of interacting with the host in such a way that infection and disease result. The capacity to cause disease is determined by the production of a variety of virulence factors by the infecting organism. Although it was once thought that all microorganisms elicit their adverse effects on hosts by elaboration of toxins, it is now clear that the pathogenetic process is complex and represents a well-orchestrated sequence of events in which many microbial components are required.

The first step in this process is the initial interaction of host and parasite. The adherence of microorganisms to host surfaces or tissues is now recognized to be highly specific and essential for subsequent events in the pathogenetic process to occur.[1] The specificity, mechanisms, and pathogenetic significance of bacterial attachment will be addressed in Chapter 2.

For some bacteria, the attachment to a mucosal surface represents the final destination. These bacteria, such as *Vibrio cholerae, Bordetella pertussis,* and some *Escherichia coli,* remain attached to the mucosa and exert their ill effects by cell contact and/or elaboration of toxins that interact with adjacent or distant cells. For many other organisms, however, the attachment process represents only the establishment of a beachhead from which tissue penetration and/or cell invasion can be launched. Organisms such as *Salmonella, Shigella,* and *Yersinia* penetrate the anatomic barriers of the host and either enter cells or disseminate within the body. In order to survive under these conditions all of these organisms have special virulence factors that enable them to avoid or disarm host defenses. Some are true toxins, in the classic sense, that kill, damage, or alter the function of host cells, but others such as staphylococcal protein A and the polysaccharide capsule of a variety of bacteria provide protection without being directly harmful to individual cells.

Survival and continued proliferation of the infecting organisms are often accompanied by the production of toxins, that is, protein molecules capable of adversely affecting cells or tissues of the host. In some cases, these toxins only enhance the development of the disease process, whereas in others they are the sine qua non in that they appear to be totally responsible for the manifestations of disease. Examples in this latter group include diphtheria, cholera, tetanus, and botulinum toxins.

Finally, one of the following three outcomes results: (*1*) The proliferation of organisms and production of toxic products impair the host to such an extent that the host dies. (*2*) A state of relative equilibrium is reached with the establishment of a chronic infection. (*3*) Host defense mechanisms, with or without the aid of exogenous factors such as antibiotics, supervene, and the infecting organism is cleared. It is of note that in some cases elimination of the causative organism may not be sufficient to terminate the disease process because toxin effects or immunologic reactions may persist in the absence of microbes.

The remainder of this chapter is devoted to the role of bacterial toxins and other components such as virulence factors. Additional information on each example cited herein can be obtained from the chapters on specific causative organisms.

TOXINS

Classification and Structure of Toxins

The word *toxin* is derived from the Greek *toxikon,* bow poison, referring to poisonous material placed on arrows by Greek warriors. The implication of this choice of terms is that the bacterium produces a molecule that it "releases" to affect host cells at a distance. The term was first used by Roux and Yersin to describe the factor released into the culture medium by *Corynebacterium diphtheriae* that caused the death of recipient animals.[2] Subsequently, many toxins have been identified, and confusion has arisen concerning the terminology used to describe and classify different toxins. Exotoxin was previously used to refer to toxins produced by and released from gram-positive bacteria during growth, whereas endotoxin was used for the intracellular and cell-associated toxic components of gram-negative organisms, including the lipopolysaccharide component that now bears the name endotoxin. Because gram-negative bacteria are now recognized to elaborate classic protein toxins, it seems prudent that the term *exotoxin* be used for bacterial products that are protein in nature, are released from the bacterium during exponential growth, and are toxic for target cells or experimental animals. As noted earlier, this definition excludes protein toxins that are intracellular and released only with lysis of the bacterial cells (intracellular or cell-associated toxins), gram-negative bacterial lipopolysaccharide, and bacterial virulence factors that may be involved in attachment, local or systemic dissemination, and acquisition of nutrients but that possess no capacity for direct toxicity to the host.

Although exotoxins occur in many forms, there is a general structural model to which a number of the important exotoxins conform (Table 1). According to the A-B model described by Gill, each of these toxins is composed of a binding (B) domain, component, or subunit portion and an enzymatic (A) portion, which is responsible for the toxic effect once inside the cell.[12] Isolated A subunits are enzymatically active but lack binding and cell entry capability and thus have no biologic activity (the ability to intoxicate intact cells). Isolated B subunits, on the other hand, may bind to target cells and even block the action of holotoxin, but they are, in most instances, nontoxic and biologically inactive.

Other criteria by which toxins may be classified are their cellular or tissue target of action (i.e., enterotoxins, neurotoxins, leukotoxins), their mechanisms of action (ADP-ribosylating toxins, adenylate cyclase toxins, etc., Table 1), their major biologic effects (dermonecrotic toxin, edema-producing toxin, hemolytic toxin, lymphocytosis-promoting toxin), and the establishment of their contribution to the pathogenicity of the disease process (Table 2). Quite clearly the difficulties associated with describing and classifying these bacterial products reflect limitations in our knowledge of their production, target cell interaction, mechanism of action, and clinical significance. The available information on these aspects of bacterial toxins is discussed below.

Control of Synthesis and Release of Toxins

There are many variations in the genetic regulation of toxin production.[12] For example, both regulatory and structural genes

TABLE 1. Properties of A-B Type Bacterial Toxins

Toxin	Organism	Genetic Control	Subunit Structure	Target Cell Receptor	Enzymatic Activity	Biologic Effects
Anthrax toxins	*B. anthracis*	Plasmid	Three separate proteins (EF, LF, PA)[a]	Unknown, probably glycoprotein	EF is a calmodulin-dependent adenylate cyclase; LF enzyme activity is unknown	EF + PA: increase in target cell cAMP level, localized edema; LF + PA: death of target cells and experimental animals
Bordetella adenylate cyclase toxin	*Bordetella* species	Chromosomal	A-B[b]	Unknown, probably glycolipid	Calmodulin-activated cyclase	Increase in target cell cAMP level; modified cell function or cell death
Botulinum toxin	*C. botulinum*	Phage	A-B[c]	Possibly ganglioside (GD_{1b})	None known	Decrease in peripheral, presynaptic acetylcholine release; flaccid paralysis
Cholera toxin	*V. cholera*	Chromosomal	A-5B[d]	Ganglioside (GM_1)	ADP ribosylation of adenylate cyclase regulatory protein, G_s	Activation of adenylate cyclase, increase in cAMP level; secretory diarrhea
Diphtheria toxin	*C. diphtheriae*	Phage	A-B[e]	Probably glycoprotein	ADP ribosylation of elongation factor II	Inhibition of protein synthesis; cell death
Heat-labile enterotoxins[f]	*E. coli*	Plasmid	Similar or identical to cholera toxin			
Pertussis toxin	*B. pertussis*	Chromosomal	A-5B[g]	Unknown, probably glycoprotein	ADP ribosylation of signal-transducing G proteins	Block of signal transduction mediated by target G proteins
Pseudomonas exotoxin A	*P. aeruginosa*	Chromosomal	A-B	Unknown, but different from diphtheria toxin	Similar or identical to diphtheria toxin	
Shiga toxin	*S. dysenteriae*	Chromosomal	A-5B[h]	Glycoprotein or glycolipid	RNA *N*-glycosidase	Inhibition of protein synthesis, cell death
Shiga-like toxins	*Shigella* species, *E. coli*	Phage	Similar or identical to shiga toxin			
Tetanus toxin	*C. tetani*	Plasmid	A-B[c]	Ganglioside (GT_1 and/or GD_{1b})	None known	Decrease in neurotransmitter release from inhibitory neurons; spastic paralysis

[a] The binding component (known as protective antigen [PA]) catalyzes/facilitates the entry of either edema factor (EF) or lethal factor (LF).[3]
[b] Apparently synthesized as a single polypeptide with binding and catalytic (adenylate cyclase) domains.[4]
[c] Holotoxin is apparently synthesized as a single polypeptide and cleaved proteolytically as diphtheria toxin; subunits are referred to as L: light chain, A equivalent; H: heavy chain, B equivalent.[5,6]
[d] The A subunit is proteolytically cleaved into A_1 and A_2, with A_1 possessing the ADP-ribosyl transferase activity; the binding component is made up of five identical B units.
[e] Holotoxin is synthesized as a single polypeptide and cleaved proteolytically into A and B components held together by disulfide bonds.[7]
[f] The heat-labile enterotoxins of *E. coli* are now recognized to be a family of related molecules with identical mechanisms of action.[8]
[g] The binding portion is made up of two dissimilar heterodimers labeled S2-S3 and S2-S4 that are held together by a bridging peptide, S5.[9]
[h] Similar subunit composition and structure to cholera toxin.[10]

TABLE 2. Categorization of Bacterial Toxins according to Their Relative Contribution to Disease Pathogenesis

- Well-studied toxin with a clear role as a major effector
  - Diphtheria toxin
  - Botulinum toxin
  - Tetanus toxin
  - Enterotoxins
    - Cholera toxin
    - *E. coli* heat-labile toxin (LT)
    - *E. coli* heat-stable tosin (ST_a)
    - Staphylococcal enterotoxin (neurotoxin)
    - Clostridial enterotoxin
- Well-studied toxin with a contributory role
  - Anthrax toxins (edema factor, lethal factor, protective antigen)
  - *Pseudomonas* exotoxin A
- Well-studied toxin with a probable, but unproven role
  - Pertussis toxin and *Bordetella* extracytoplasmic adenylate cyclase
  - *Shigella* (shiga) toxin
  - Streptolysin O and other streptococcal toxins
  - Other clostridial toxins (including *C. difficile* cytotoxin)
  - Cholera-like enterotoxins produced by *Salmonella, Klebsiella, Aeromonas,* and *Citrobacter*
  - Yersinia toxins
  - Other staphylococcal toxins (toxic shock syndrome toxin, TSST-1)

for toxin synthesis and release may be chromosomal in location, as is the case for cholera toxin.[13] Production of the family of immunologically and functionally homologous heat-labile toxins of *E. coli,* on the other hand, is plasmid mediated.[13] The structural gene for diphtheria toxin is located on a β-phage, but toxin synthesis is inhibited by excess iron, apparently through interaction with a factor of bacterial origin.[7] The structural gene for tetanus toxin is located on a large (75 kilobase [kb]) plasmid.[14] The pertussis toxin gene is present in three *Bordetella* species but is expressed only in *B. pertussis* due to mutations in the promoter region of the gene in *B. parapertussis* and *B. bronchiseptica*.[15,16] Finally, the gene for staphylococcal enterotoxin may be either chromosomal or plasmid in location, but its production is regulated by genes on a plasmid.[17]

The question of how large proteins such as toxins are exported from the bacterial cell has been clarified by analysis of DNA sequences. There are two major hypotheses to explain the mechanism, the signal hypothesis and the membrane trigger hypothesis.[18] Many of the classic exotoxins are synthesized with an NH-terminal signal or leader sequence consisting of a few (1–3) charged amino acids and a stretch (14–20) of hydrophobic amino acids.[19] The signal sequence may bind and be inserted into the cytoplasmic membrane during translation such that the polypeptide is secreted while being synthesized. The signal peptide is then cleaved, which leaves the intact toxin molecule free in the periplasm. Alternatively (membrane trigger hypothesis), the protein may be synthesized intracytoplasmically. Subsequent binding via the leader sequence to the cytoplasmic membrane may cause a conformational change allowing the protein to traverse the membrane with or without the help of pores or transport molecules. The synthesis and release of some toxins such as *E. coli* hemolysin clearly entail a process requiring the products of multiple genes involved in processing and/or transport.[20] Some multicomponent toxins such as cholera toxin have their subunits secreted separately; they are then assembled in the periplasmic space. In gram-negative organisms, however, the outer membrane provides an additional barrier for escape of periplasmic protein molecules.

Middledorp and Witholt have proposed that some toxins such as *E. coli* heat-labile toxin may not be released but rather delivered to target cells while contained in vesicles of the outer membrane.[21] These vesicles would possess outer membrane-associated attachment factors enabling them to act as "bombs" capable of interacting with and possibly entering target cells to release their contents of toxin.

Attachment and Entry of Toxins

Some toxins such as the hemolytic phospholipases are bacterial exoenzymes that appear to interact with the external surface of host cell membranes by catalyzing their specific reactions and thereby eliciting their toxic effects without cell entry.[22] A number of toxins, however, act on intracellular substrates and thus require cell entry to be effective. Most of these conform to the A-B model described earlier[11] and have binding components that interact with specific receptors on the target cells such as the sialogangliosides GM_1 for cholera toxin, GT_1 for tetanus toxin, and probably GD_{1b} for botulinum toxin.[23] The relatively wide distribution of FM_1 ganglioside among cell types accounts for the apparent lack of specificity of cholera toxin in vitro. The specificity of the effect of cholera toxin during infection (secretory diarrhea), however, is due to the localization of the organisms and the toxin to the intestinal tract. Pertussis toxin has been shown to interact with sialic acid-containing glycoproteins,[23,24] which also must be widespread since most cells are sensitive to intoxication by pertussis toxin. Diphtheria toxin and *Pseudomonas* exotoxin A, on the other hand, catalyze the identical reaction intracellularly[7,25] and are both distributed systemically, yet the resultant disease processes are quite distinct. The differences between the two appear to reside, at least in part, at the level of target cell specificities.[26]

There are several different mechanisms by which the A subunits of A-B toxins enter the target cell. In each case, however, a large protein molecule must insert into or cross the lipid bilayer.[27] In some cases such as diphtheria toxin, there appears to be binding to a surface receptor, uptake into an endocytotic vesicle, and acidification of that vesicle so as to result in a conformational change that enables a part of the toxin molecule to traverse the membrane.[7] The final step in diphtheria toxin translocation is energy requiring and dependent upon membrane potential and a proton gradient.[28] A part of this process can be mimicked in vitro with diphtheria toxin B subunit, which makes artificial membranes permeable to small ions.[29] *Pseudomonas* exotoxin A appears to be internalized somewhat differently, by endocytosis into coated pits and vesicles.[27]

Often toxins with identical enzymatic mechanisms also enter cells by separate and distinct pathways. Adenylate cyclase toxins from *Bordetella pertussis* and *Bacillus anthracis* both catalyze the production of cAMP from host intracellular ATP stores.[4] Anthrax toxin (edema factor plus protective antigen [EF + PA]) enters by receptor-mediated endocytosis, whereas pertussis adenylate cyclase toxin has a different entry mechanism to traverse the cell membrane directly.[30] For many toxins such as pertussis toxin, tetanus toxin, and others, putative receptors have been identified, but the entry mechanisms remain a mystery.

Mechanism of Toxin Action and Role in Clinical Disease

As noted earlier, bacterial toxins can be categorized according to our concept of their relative contribution to the disease process with which they are associated (Table 2). In this section, individual toxins and families of toxins will be discussed by that classification scheme. The criteria indicating a major pathogenic role for a particular toxin include (*1*) production of the toxin by pathogenic organisms and not by avirulent ones, (*2*) avirulence of organisms specifically lacking the toxin, (*3*) protection against disease by antibody against the toxin, and (*4*) the ability of purified toxin to mimic the disease.[31]

Diphtheria Toxin. One of the most extensively studied of all toxins is that produced by β-phage–infected *C. diphtheriae*.[7] It is the prototype ADP-ribosylating toxin that inhibits cellular protein synthesis by catalyzing the transfer of ADP-ribose from nicotinamide adenine dinucleotide (NAD) to elongation factor II.[7] This single enzymatic reaction, which is responsible for the systemic toxicity in clinical diphtheria, does not occur in individuals infected with nontoxigenic strains. The widespread control of diphtheria with the use of diphtheria toxoid attests to the dominant role of this toxin both in the establishment of infection and in the systemic manifestations of disease. As noted in Table 1, exotoxin A of *Pseudomonas aeruginosa* catalyzes the identical reaction but is associated with a disease process quite different from diphtheria. These differences are felt to be due to different tissue (Target cell) specificities of the toxins[26] and to the fact that exotoxin A is only one of a number of virulence factors involved in *Pseudomonas*-induced disease.[32]

Tetanus Toxin. In contrast to diphtheria, immunization with tetanus toxin has no effect on the establishment of infection with *Clostridium tetani*. The resultant antibody response does, however, totally prevent the disease process of clinical tetanus, the major effector role of tetanus toxin. The toxin exhibits selectivity for neural tissue, being taken up at myoneural junctions and transported by retrograde axonal flow to alpha motoneuron synapses. It crosses the synapse where it acts presynaptically to impair inhibitory neurotransmitter release.[5] The toxin specificity is attributed to its binding domain, which interacts with cell surface ganglioside (GT_1 or GD_{1b}). Tetanus toxin can, however, at high enough concentrations cause the inhibition of acetylcholine release at the myoneural junction and flaccid paralysis equivalent to that elicited by botulinum toxin.[33] There are also structural homologies between the two toxins, which suggests that they may act by a similar, as yet unknown intracellular mechanism and may be derived from a common ancestral gene.[34] While tetanus toxin is not known to affect non-neuronal cells clinically, it can inhibit exocytosis when injected into adrenal chromaffin cells.[35] Furthermore, tetanus toxin causes the inhibition of lysozyme secretion from human macrophages and is associated with reduced protein kinase C activity.[36,37] Such studies provide a new approach for study of the mechanism of tetanus toxin action in vitro.

Botulinum Toxin. Botulinum toxin is among the most potent toxins known, with a human lethal dose (toxin type A) of approximately 1 ng/kg.[38] "Botulinum toxin" consists of a family of seven immunologically distinct molecules, most of which cause flaccid paralysis by inhibiting myoneural junction acetylcholine release.[6] The mechanism of this neurotoxic activity is unknown, but a related toxin from *C. botulinum,* botulinum C2 toxin, possesses ADP-ribosyl transferase activity, with G-actin as the target substrate.[39]

The classic presentation of clinical botulism results from the ingestion of preformed toxin in improperly prepared foods. A subacute intoxication can occur in infants (infant botulism) harboring *C. botulinum* in their gastrointestinal tracts.[40] In most cases the low-level toxin absorption results in listlessness and hypotonia, but the course can be fulminant, and infant botulism has been proposed as a cause of sudden infant death syndrome.[40]

Cholera Toxin and Escherichia coli Heat-Labile Toxin. Cholera and *E. coli* heat-labile enterotoxin (LT) are discussed together because their structures are similar and their mechanisms of action appear to be identical.[41] It has been recognized recently, however, that the heat-labile enterotoxins of *E. coli* represent a more heterogeneous group, with some (type II) being nonimmunologically cross-reactive and interacting with a different receptor despite operating by an apparently identical mechanism of action.[8] Cholera toxin and the LTs promote isotonic intestinal secretion by catalyzing the ADP ribosylation of the B-subunit of the stimulatory guanine nucleotide protein G_s.[41] This covalent modification causes semipermanent activation of the cellular adenylate cyclase and increased cAMP accumulation. While these enterotoxins reproduce the secretory diarrhea when administered experimentally, it is clear that multiple other bacterial components such as attachment factors, mucinase, etc., are required for establishment of infection and perhaps toxin delivery in order for the disease process to occur.

Enterotoxin effects can be prevented by the addition of specific antibody to toxin in animal assay systems,[42] but the use of parenteral toxoid immunization has been largely unsuccessful. The combination of killed whole *Vibrio cholerae* organisms and purified nontoxic B-subunit administered orally has shown limited efficacy in vaccine trials.[43] Genetically engineered vaccines consisting of organisms that produce inactive toxin are being evaluated for oral use at present.[44] Related enterotoxins are produced by a variety of other gram-negative organisms such as *Klebsiella, Salmonella, Aeromonas,* and *Plesiomonas,* but the incidence of diarrhea caused by these organisms and the roles of such toxins in that disease are unknown.

Escherichia coli Heat-Stable Toxin. A separate enterotoxin produced by *E. coli* causes diarrhea in humans. This heat-stable toxin, referred to as ST_a or ST-I, is a peptide of 18 or 19 amino acids.[45] It causes secretory diarrhea by promoting the activation of intestinal particulate guanylate cyclase and increasing cyclic guanosine monophosphate (GMP) levels in the jejunum and ileum.[46] Unlike cholera toxin and LT, ST_a exhibits striking target cell specificity with little activity in extraintestinal tissues.[47] The molecule is poorly immunogenic alone, but antitoxin antibody may develop against hybrid toxins in which St_a is covalently linked to LT B-subunits.[48] As with LT, other bacterial species such as *Yersinia enterocolitica,* non-01 *Vibrio cholerae,* and *Citrobacter freundii* can produce homologous molecules that are of unknown significance.[49]

There is a second heat-stable enterotoxin of *E. coli*, ST_b or ST-II, that is not a human pathogen but produces diarrhea in piglets by a noncyclic nucleotide mechanism.[50]

Toxins of Bordetella pertussis. *Bordetella pertussis,* the causative agent of whooping cough, produces several toxins that have striking effects in experimental systems and are hypothesized to be major contributors to the pathophysiology of the disease process. Pertussis toxin, also known as lymphocytosis-promoting factor, histamine-sensitizing factor, or islet-activating protein, is expressed only by *B. pertussis,* although a silent gene is present in *B. parapertussis*.[16] Pertussis toxin acts by ADP ribosylating several members of the family of guanine nucleotide-binding G proteins involved in cellular signal transduction.[9] The result of this covalent modification is inhibition of G protein function and consequently interruption of the signal from the receptor to inhibition of adenylate cyclase, activation of phospholipase, or modulation of ion channels.[9,51] Although pertussis toxin is clearly a virulence factor for *B. pertussis* and a protective antigen,[52,53] its role in clinical pertussis remains unclear. In contrast to tetanus and botulinum toxins, pertussis toxin can be given to human volunteers (1 μg/kg iv) without adverse effects.[54]

Bordetella species also produce an adenylate cylcase toxin that can enter target cells to catalyze the production of cAMP from endogenous ATP.[4] This toxin is also a virulence factor for *B. pertussis*[52] and is believed to contribute to both the evasion of host defenses by the organism and damage to the respiratory mucosa.[55]

Anthrax Toxins. *Bacillus anthracis* produces three toxin components that are novel in their interaction with cells.[3] None of the three components, edema factor (EF), lethal factor (LF), or protective antigen (PA) has toxin activity alone. Edema factor is a calmodulin-dependent adenylate cyclase analogous to *Bordetella* adenylate cyclase toxin and when combined with PA is able to enter target cells to increase cAMP levels.[3] Lethal factor when combined with PA is lethal for macrophages and experimental animals by unknown mechanisms.[56] Protective antigen serves as the binding subunit to facilitate the entry of either EF or LF into target cells. Protective antigen is so named because it is an important PA in anthrax vaccine. The genes for all three toxin components are located on plasmids.[57]

Shiga and Shiga-like Toxins. *Shigella dysenteriae* 1 produces a toxin, shiga toxin, that is responsible for a variety of biologic activities in experimental animals including neurotoxicity, enterotoxicity, and cytotoxicity.[58] The toxin conforms to the A-B model, with a subunit structure similar to cholera toxin (i.e., A-5B).[10] The A subunit causes inhibition of protein synthesis by enzymatic inactivation of 60S ribosomes within the target cell by a process (RNA *N*-glycosidase) analogous to that employed by ricin.[59,60] Despite the striking effects of shiga toxin in vitro, definition of its role in clinical shigellosis remains circumstantial.[61]

A family of related molecules designated shiga-like toxins (previously vero toxins) have been demonstrated in other *Shigella* species and *E. coli.*[10] These toxins have been implicated in enteropathogenic (EPEC)- and enterohemorrhagic (EHEC)-mediated disease as well as hemolytic–uremic syndrome.[10] Those shiga-like toxins that are neutralized by antishiga toxin serum are designated SLT-I, while those which are not immunologically cross-reactive are SLT-II.[10] As with other toxins, the genetic regulation is different in the different organisms; the shiga toxin gene in *S. dysenteriae* is chromosomal, while production of shiga-like toxin in *E. coli* is phage mediated.[62]

Other toxins. The list of toxins discussed in the preceding sections is, by no means, all inclusive. It is, however, representative of those toxins that are most extensively characterized with regard to their roles in pathogenesis. Additional toxins include toxins A and B of *Clostridium difficile*, which appear to be involved in psuedomembranes colitis but by unknown mechanisms.[63] There are other toxins, such as the heterogeneous group of molecules known as hemolysins, which are also important virulence factors. One group (i.e., *C. perfringens* α toxin) possesses phospholipase C activity and produces hemolysis by cleavage of membrane phospholipids on target cells.[63a] Another group (some of which are activated by sulfhydryl reagents) appear to act by inserting into host cell membranes. Examples include streptolysins S and O, staphylococcal α-toxin, and *E. coli* hemolysin.[64–65a] The hemolysins from intracellular pathogens such as *Shigella flexneri* and *Listeria monocytogenes* are virulence factors that are postulated to aid the organism in its disruption of phagosome membranes during entry into the cytoplasm.[65b,65c] Most hemolysins are also cytolytic for other host cells such as leukocytes. While there are many other toxins that have been identified, their contributions to the diseases caused by the respective organisms is, in many cases, uncertain.

OTHER VIRULENCE FACTORS

In contrast to toxins, ''other virulence factors'' are, by definition, not toxic to target cells. Although bacterial virulence is often quantitated by the number of organisms required to kill 50 percent of challenged experimental animals (LD_{50}), any single nontoxin virulence factor alone is likely to have little or no effect on a host animal. In most cases, the pathophysiologic process requires the concerted action of a variety of microbial products, including those involved in attachment (see Chapter 2), entry into the host and dissemination, acquisition of nutrients, proliferation, avoidance of host defenses, and production of tissue damage.[66] A loss of virulence in association with elimination of a specific bacterial component is strongly supportive of a major role for that factor in the pathogenic process. Production of one or more putative virulence factors by avirulent strains, however, does not mean that they are not, in fact, virulence factors. Because infection and disease result from a carefully orchestrated sequence of events, single factors are often inadequate to promote the development of disease without their supporting cast.

Many virulence factors do possess specific biologic activities that interfere with normal host function to the advantage of the microbe.[67,68] The discussion of these other virulence factors will focus on those responsible for circumventing major host defenses such as anatomic barriers, serum (humoral) factors, and phagocytic cells (Table 3). The examples are primarily those of pathogenic bacteria, and the reader is referred to specific reviews for information on viral and parasitic virulence mechanisms.[66,69,70] It is important to note that the current understanding of virulence mechanisms is frequently incomplete and there are many factors that have been demonstrated to be major virulence determinants yet have no biologic or biochemical activity yet identified.[67] Examples include the V protein and W lipoprotein of *Yersinia* species[68] and the Vi antigen of *Salmonella* species,[71] which have been postulated to contribute to cell invasion and avoidance of host clearance mechanisms. This deficiency in the knowledge of pathogenesis is being overcome by molecular biologic approaches to define the structure of these antigens and their role in the disease process.[72]

Virulence Factors for Overcoming Anatomic Barriers

The first line of host defense against microorganisms is the anatomic barrier of skin and mucous membranes. These "external" surfaces are colonized by normal flora, which in itself provides a barrier against the uncontrolled proliferation of potentially pathogenic bacteria. Thus, in order for pathogens to survive and proliferate to sufficient to numbers to cause disease, they must compete successfully with the other microorganisms present. Many bacteria produce bacteriocins, which are toxins directed at other microbes.[73] These products provide an adaptive advantage, and some even exhibit activity against host cells such as mononuclear phagocytes, which further explains their contribution to microbial virulence.[74]

Although many organisms are able to enter the body through skin disrupted by laceration, abrasion, a puncture wound, or an insect bite, there are no bacteria known to be capable of penetrating intact skin. In contrast, some parasites such as cercariae of *Schistosoma mansoni* and larvae of *Strongyloides stercoralis, Ancylostoma duodenale,* and *Necator americanus* do have this capability (direct penetration of intact skin), which represents a major mechanism for entry into the host.

Many bacteria gain access to the body through breaks in the mucosa of the respiratory, gastrointestinal, or genitourinary tracts and thus are not truly "invasive." In contrast, invasive organisms such as *Salmonella typhimurium, Shigella flexneri, Yersinia enterocolitica,* and some *Escherichia coli* strains have a special capacity for the penetration of intact cells.[72,75–78] When administered by the oral route, wild-type *S. flexneri* organisms are lethal for guinea pigs, whereas noninvasive mutants are without effect.[75] The importance of other virulence factors, however, is illustrated by the full virulence (lethality) of the noninvasive mutants when administered intraperitoneally to mice.[75] This process, which may be the sine qua non of virulence for these organisms, occurs by a poorly understood process.

Invasive strains of *E. coli* are restricted to a few serotypes and have been shown to share surface determinants with invasive shigellae, which suggests that these components may be involved in the invasion process.[75,76] In vitro models of invasiveness have been developed with the use of tissue culture cells, which allows for the screening of many strains for the invasiveness trait.[77,78] With this approach, large (>100 megadalton) plasmids have been demonstrated to be associated with invasiveness in several organisms.[72,79–81]

Bacterial proteins with a variety of enzymatic activities such as protease, hyaluronidase, neuraminidase, elastase, collagenase, and mucinase have been postulated to contribute to cell invasion. While these products are certainly contributory to virulence factors for many bacteria, their role appears to be in facilitating local tissue spread of the organisms rather than the primary invasion event.

Virulence Factors for Avoiding or Disrupting Humoral Defenses

One secondary line of defense against microbial infections is provided by humoral factors such as antibody, complement, complement-activated mediators, and an assortment of other soluble host proteins such as clotting factors, B-lysin, and transferrin. Several organisms have mechanisms that impair antibody production at different sites in the multistep process. These include induction of suppressor cells,[82] blockade of antigen processing,[83] and inhibition of lymphocyte mitogenesis.[84] Other bacteria possess antiphagocytic capsules that either prevent the binding of opsonic antibodies or allow them to penetrate the capsule and bind but prevent subsequent interaction with phagocytic cell receptors.[85]

While there is little complement present on mucosal surfaces, antibody such as secretory IgA may be active against microorganisms even before invasion. In response to this protective measure of the host, several organisms including *Neisseria gonorrhoeae, Streptococcus pneumonia,* and *Haemophilus influenzae* produce IgA-specific proteases that cleave and inactivate the secretory antibody.[86,87] Similarly, the ability of organisms to elaborate factors that modify or degrade serum components such as fibrin, heparin, and clotting factors is recognized to be associated with increased virulence. The binding of the F_c domains of host immunoglobulin by staphylococcal protein A is postulated to represent a protective mechanism. The production of protein A by a variety of virulent and avirulent staphylococcal strains, however, has prevented adequate assessment of this possibility.

One of the bacterial traits most clearly associated with virulence or systemic infections is resistance to the lytic effect of serum. It has long been recognized that most blood stream isolates are serum resistant.[88] This observation explains why the *N. gonorrhoeae* isolates from patients with disseminated disease are serum resistant while those isolated only from the genital tract are predomiantly serum sensitive.[89] The serum lytic

TABLE 3. Other Virulence Factors[a] and Their Activities

Penetration of anatomic barriers
Bacteriocins
Direct skin penetration activity
Mucosal invasiveness traits
Connective tissue-disrupting enzymes
Disruption or avoidance of humoral factors
Antibody-degrading enzymes
Enzymes that disrupt other humoral factors (fibrinolysin)
Serum resistance
Avoidance or inactivation of phagocytic cells
Components resulting in impaired phagocytosis
Factors preventing oxidative burst
Molecules preventing phagosome–lysosome fusion
Surfaces that are resistant to lysosomal enzymes

[a] Adherence factors are excluded here but are discussed in Chapter 2.

effect in gram-negative organisms is complement-mediated but can be activated by either of two pathways. Many organisms entering the blood stream activate complement by the classic pathway in an antibody-dependent manner and are lysed by the membrane attach complex (C_{5b}-C_9).[88–90] In contrast, some organisms are direct activators of the alternative pathway, but their killing may be enhanced by an antibody-mediated amplification.[91] Antibodies involved in both of these processes arise from prior exposure to the organisms or reflect cross-reactivity with antigens from common organisms in the environment.[92] Several mechanisms appear to be involved in serum resistance including (*1*) a failure to activate complement, (*2*) shedding of molecules that activate the system, (*3*) blockade of activation before the formation of C_{5b}-C_9, and (*4*) formation of a nonlytic complex.[93] In addition, some bacteria and parasites have been shown to invade host cells by using complement deposited on their surfaces to facilitate interaction with target cell complement receptors.[93a,93b] The structure and quantity of lipopolysaccharide (LPS) on the surface of gram-negative organisms, including that absorbed from the medium, may contribute to resistance.[94] Plasmids encoding some outer membrane proteins may enhance virulence by virtue of the binding of LPS to the induced surface components.[95] In other cases, serum resistance is mediated by masking of sensitive surface antigens by K antigens,[90,96] nonbactericidal blocking antibodies,[97] or sialic acid residues.[91] The latter modification creates a surface that is poor in its ability to activate the alternative pathway of complement.[91,93]

Nontoxin Virulence Factors Directed at Phagocytic Cells

Microbes that have penetrated the protection of anatomic barriers meet another main line of the host defenses, phagocytic cells including polymorphonuclear leukocytes, monocytes, and macrophages. The phagocytosis and killing of microorganisms are part of a specific sequence of events consisting of (*1*) attraction of the phagocyte in a chemotactic gradient of bacterial products, (*2*) movement of the phagocyte to the site, (*3*) contact between the organism and the phagocyte, (*4*) phagocytosis (ingestion), (*5*) development of an oxidative burst, (*6*) fusion of the phagosome and lysosome with degranulation of lysosomal contents, and (*7*) death and degradation of the ingested organism (see Chapter 7).[66,98] In the evolution of virulence mechanisms, microbes have developed methods to elude, inactivate, or ignore each of these steps.[98,99]

Parasites are particularly adept at disguising their surfaces to avoid recognition by immune effector cells.[100] Similarly, an array of microorganisms resists phagocytosis by protective surface components such as capsular polysaccharide or other antigens.[101–103] The capsule of *Bacteroides fragilis* is not only antiphagocytic but also plays a major role in the induction of abscess formation by this organism.[101] Other pathogenic parasites and bacteria such as *Toxoplasma gondii, Leishmania* sp., *Legionella pneumophila,* and *Listeria monocytogenes* either do not elicit or actively suppress the oxidative response associated with surface contact and phagocytosis.[102–104] In addition, many organisms produce enzymes such as catalase, glutathione peroxidase, and superoxide dismutase that destroy the reactive oxygen species generated in the oxidative burst, or they are individually resistant to those reactive lethal molecules.[103,104] Still other organisms survive intracellularly by inhibiting phagosome–lysosome fusions.[105] Several mycobacteria appear to do so by increasing phagocyte cAMP concentrations to inhibitory levels.[106] Finally, microbes such as *Mycobacterium leprae, Salmonella enteritidis* serotype *typhimurium,* and *Leishmania* sp. survive despite phagosome–lysosome fusion and degranulation, apparently by virtue of innate resistance to the lysosomal enzymes.[105,107] Although the mechanisms of these microbial defensive actions are largely unknown, it is clear that they play a major role in the establishment of intracellular infections.

Finally, as mentioned earlier, there are a number of recognized characteristics of microorganisms that are associated with virulence but are of unknown pathophysiologic significance such as the presence of large plasmids,[108] The complete understanding of the pathogenetic process and the role of these additional factors awaits future research efforts.

REFERENCES

1. Beachey EH, ed. Bacterial Adherence. London: Chapman & Hall; 1980:1.
2. Roux E, Yersin A. Contribution a l'étude de la diphtherie. Ann Inst Pasteur. 1988;2:629.
3. Leppla SH. *Bacillus anthracis* calmodulin-dependent adenylate cyclase: Chemical and enzymatic properties and interactions with eucaryotic cells. Adv Cyclic Nucleotide Prot Phos Res 1984;17:189.
4. Hewlett EL, Gordon VM. Adenylate cyclase toxin of *Bordetella pertussis.* In: Wardlaw AC, Parton R, eds. Pathogenesis and Immunity in Pertussis. Chichester, England: John Wiley & Sons; 1988:193.
5. van Heyningen S. Tetanus toxin. In: Dorner F, Drews J, eds. Pharmacology of Bacterial Toxins. IEPT Section 119. Oxford: Pergamon Press; 1986:549.
6. Sakaguchi G. *Clostridium botulinum* toxins. In: Dorner F, Drews J, eds. Pharmacology of Bacterial Toxins. IEPT Section 119. Oxford: Pergamon Press; 1986:519.
7. Uchida T. Diphtheria toxin. In: Dorner F, Drews J, eds. Pharmacology of Bacterial Toxins. IEPT Section 119. Oxford: Pergamon Press; 1986:693.
8. Holmes RK, Twiddy EM, Neill RJ. Recent advances in the study of heat-labile enterotoxins of *Escherichia coli.* In: Takeda Y, Minatoni, eds. Bacterial Diarrheal Diseases. Boston: Martinus Nijhoff Publishing; 1985:125.
9. Ui M. The multiple biological activities of pertussis toxin. In: Wardlaw AC, Parton R, eds. Pathogenesis and Immunity in Pertussis. Chichester, England: John Wilcy & Sons; 1988:121–145.
10. O'Brien AD, Holmes RK. Shiga and shiga-like toxins. Microbiol Rev. 1987;51:206.
11. Gill DM. Seven toxic peptides that cross cell membranes. In: Jeljaszewicz J, Wadstrom T, eds. Bacterial Toxins and Cell Membranes. New York: Academic Press; 1978:291.
12. Maas WK. Genetic aspects of toxigenesis in bacteria. In: Dorner F, Drews J, eds. Pharmacology of Bacterial Toxins. IEPT Section 119. Oxford, Pergamon Press; 1986:17.
13. Betley MJ, Miller VL, Mekalanos JJ. Genetics of bacterial enterotoxins. Annu Rev Microbiol. 1986;40:577.
14. Finn CW, Silver RP, Habig WH, et al. The structural gene for tetanus neurotoxin is on a plasmid. Science. 1984;224:881.
15. Locht C, Keith JM. Pertussis toxin gene: Nucleotide sequence and genetic organisation. Science. 1986;232:1258.
16. Arico B, Rappuoli R. *Bordetella parapertussis* and *Bordetella bronchiseptica* contain transcriptionally silent pertussis toxin genes. J Bacteriol. 1987; 169:2847.
17. Dyer DW, Iandolo JJ. Plasmid-chromosomal transition of genes important in staphylococcal enterotoxin B expression. Infect Immun. 1981;33:450.
18. Randall LL, Hardy SJS. Export of protein in bacteria. Microbiol Rev. 1984;48:290.
19. Oliver D. Protein secretion in *Escherichia coli.* Annu Rev Microbiol. 1985;39:615.
20. Cavalieri SJ, Bohach GA, Snyder IS. *Escherichia coli* α-hemolysin: Characteristics and probable role in pathogenicity. Microbiol Rev. 1984;48:326.
21. Middeldorp JM, Witholt B. K88-mediated binding of *Escherichia coli* outer membrane fragments to porcine intestinal epithelial cell brush borders. Infect Immun. 1981;31:42.
22. Mollby R. Bacterial phospholipases. In: Jeljaszewicz J, Wadstrom T, eds. Bacterial Toxins and Cell Membranes. New York: Academic Press; 1978:367.
23. Eidels L, Proia RL, Hart DA. Membrane receptors for bacterial toxins. Microbiol Rev. 1983;47:596.
24. Sekura RD, Zhang Y-L, Quentin-Millet M-JJ. Pertussis toxin: Structural elements involved in the interaction with cells. In: Sekura RD, Moss J, Vaughan M, eds. Pertussis Toxin. Orlando, FL: Academic Press; 1985:45.
25. Iglewski BH, Kabat D. NAD-dependent inhibition of protein synthesis by *Pseudomonas aeruginosa* toxin. Proc Natl Acad Sci USA. 1975;72:2284.
26. Middlebrook JL, Dorland RB. Response of cultured mammalian cells to the exotoxins of *Pseudomonas aeruginosa* and *Corynebacterium diphtheriae:* Differential cytotoxicity. Can J Microbiol. 1977;23:183.
27. Middlebrook JL, Dorland RB. Bacterial toxins: Cellular mechanisms of action. Microbiol Rev. 1984;48:199.
28. Hudson TH, Scharff J, Kimak MAG, et al. Energy requirements for diphtheria toxin translocation are coupled to the maintenance of a plasma membrane potential and a proton gradient. J Biol Chem. 1988;263:4773.
29. Kagan BL, Finkelstein A, Colombini M. Diphtheria toxin fragment forms large pores in phospholipid bilayer membranes. Proc Natl Acad Sci USA. 1981;78:4950.
30. Gordon VM, Leppla SH, Hewlett EH. Inhibitors of receptor-mediated endocytosis block the entry of *Bacillus anthracis* adenylate cyclase toxin but

not that of *Bordetella pertussis* adenylate cyclase toxin. Infect Immun. 1988;56:1066.
31. McDonel JL, Dorner F, Drews J. The role of toxins in bacterial pathogenesis. In: Dorner F, Drews J, eds. Pharmacology of Bacterial Toxins. IEPT Section 119. Oxford: Pergamon Press; 1986:1.
32. Pollack M, Young LS. Protective activity of antibodies to exotoxin A and lipopolysaccharide at the onset of Pseudomonas aeruginosa septicemia in man. J Clin Invest. 1979;863:276.
33. Habermann E, Dreyer F, Bigalke H. Tetanus toxin blocks the neuromuscular transmission in vitro like botulinum A toxin. Naunyn Schmiedebergs Arch Pharmacol. 1980;311:33.
34. Eisel U, Jaransch W, Goretzki K, et al. Tetanus toxin: Primary structure, expression in *E. coli* and homology with botulinum toxins. EMBO J. 1986;5:2495.
35. Penner R, Neher E, Dreyer F. Intracellularly injected tetanus toxin inhibits exocytosis in bovine adrenal chromaffin cells. Nature. 1986;324:76.
36. Ho JL, Klempner MS. Tetanus toxin inhibits secretion of lysosomal contents from human macrophages. J Infect Dis. 1985;152:922.
37. Ho JL, Klempner MS. Diminished activity of protein kinase C in tetanus toxin-treated macrophages and in spinal cord of mice manifesting generalized tetanus intoxication. J Infect Dis. 1988;157:925.
38. Gill DM. Bacterial toxins: A table of lethal amounts. Microbiol Rev. 1982;46:86.
39. Aktories K, Barmann M, Ohishi I, et al. Botulinum C2 toxin ADP-ribosylates actin. Nature. 1986;322:390.
40. Arnon SS. Infant botulism. Annu Rev Med. 1980;31:541.
41. Moss J, Vaughan M. Mechanism of action of choleragen and *E. coli* heat-labile enterotoxin: Activation of adenylate cyclase by ADP-ribosylation. Mol Cell Biochem. 1981;37:75.
42. Pierce NF, Cray WC Jr, Sacci JB Jr. Oral immunization of dogs with purified cholera toxin, its B-subunit or a crude culture filtrate of *Vibrio cholerae:* Evidence for synergistic protection by antitoxic and anti-bacterial mechanisms. Infect Immun. 1982;37:687.
43. Clemens JD, Harris JR, Sack DA, et al. Field trial of oral cholera vaccines in Bangladesh: results of one year of follow-up. J Infect Dis. 1988;158:60.
44. Levine MM, Kaper JB, Herrington D, et al. Volunteer studies of deletion mutants of *Vibrio cholerae* prepared by recombinant techniques. Infect Immun. 1988;56:161.
45. Greenberg RN, Guerrant RL. *E. coli* heat-stable enterotoxin. In: Dorner F, Drews J, eds. Pharmacology of Bacterial Toxins. IEPT Section 119. Oxford: Pergamon Press; 1986:115.
46. Hughes JM, Murad F, Cherry B, et al. Role of cyclic GMP in the action of heat-stable enterotoxin of *Escherichia coli.* Nature. 1978;271:755.
47. Guerrant RL, Hughes JM, Chang B, et al. Activation of rat and rabbit intestinal guanylate cyclase by the heat-stable enterotoxin of *Escherichia coli:* Studies of tissue specificity, potential receptors and intermediates. J Infect Dis. 1980;142:220.
48. Klipstein FA, Engert RF, Clemens JD, et al. Vaccine for enterotoxigenic *Escherichia coli* based on synthetic heat-stable toxin cross-linked to the B subunit of heat-labile toxin. J Infect Dis. 1983;147:318.
49. Guarino A, Caparo G, Malamisura B, et al. Production of *Escherichia coli* ST_a-like heat-stable enterotoxin by *Citrobacter freundii* isolated from humans. J Clin Microbiol. 1987;25:110.
50. Kennedy DJ, Greenberg RN, Dunn JA, et al. Effects of *Escherichia coli* heat stable enterotoxin ST_b on intestines of mice, rats, rabbits and piglets. Infect Immun. 1984;46:639.
51. Fain JN, Wallace MS, Wojcikiewics RJH. Evidence for involvement of guanine nucleotide-binding regulatory proteins in the activation of phospholipases by hormones. FASEB J 1988;2:2569.
52. Weiss AA, Hewlett EL, Myers GA, et al. Pertussis toxin and extracytoplasmic adenylate cyclase as virlence factors of *Bordetella pertussis.* J Infect Dis. 1984;150:219.
53. Sato Y, Izumiya K, Dato H, et al. Role of antibody to leukocytosis-promoting factor hemagglutinin and to filamentous hemagglutinin in immunity to pertussis. Infect Immun. 1981;31:1223.
54. Toyota T, Kai Y, Kakizaki M, et al. Effect of islet-activating protein (IAP) on blood blucose and plasma insulin in healthy volunteers (phase 1 studies). Tohoku J Exp Med. 1980;130:105.
55. Weiss AA, Hewlett EL. Virulence factors of *Bordetella pertussis.* Annu Rev Microbiol. 1986;40:661.
56. Friedlander AM. Macrophages are sensitive to anthrax lethal toxin through an acid-dependent process. J Biol Chem. 1986;201:7123.
57. Robertson DL, Leppla SH. Molecular cloning and expression in *Escherichia coli* of the lethal factor gene of *Bacillus anthracis.* Gene. 1986;44:71.
58. Keusch GT, Donohue-Rolfe A, Jacewicz M. *Shigella* toxin and the pathogenesis of shigellosis. In: Microbial Toxins and Diarrheal Disease. Ciba Foundation Symposium 112. London: Pitman; 1985:193.
59. Reisbig R, Olsnes S, Eiklid K. The cytotoxin activity of *Shigella* toxin. Evidence for catalytic inactivation of the 60S ribosomal subunit. J Biol Chem. 1981;256:8739.
60. Obrig TG, Morgan TP, Colinas RJ. Ribonuclease activity associated with the 60S ribosome-inactivating proteins ricin A, phytolaccin and Shiga toxin. Biochem Biophys Res Commun. 1985;130:879.
61. Cantey RJ. Shiga toxin—an expanding role in the pathogenesis of infectious diseases. J Infect Dis. 1985;151:766.
62. O'Brien AD, Newland JW, Miller SF, et al. Shiga-like toxin–converting phages from *Escherichia coli* strains that cause hemorrhagic colitis or infantile diarrhea. Science. 1984;226:694.
63. Chang WT, Bartlett JH, Sullivan NM, et al. *Clostridium difficile* toxin. In: Dorner F, Drews J, eds. Pharmacology of Bacterial Toxins. IEPT Section 119. Oxford: Pergamon Press; 1986:571–580.
63a. Mollby R: Bacterial phospholipases. In: Jeljaszewicz J, Wadstrom T, eds. *Bacterial Toxins and Cell Membranes.* New York: Academic Press; 1978:367.
64. Alouf JE. Streptococcal toxins (streptolysin O, streptolysin S, erythrogenic toxin). In: Dorner F, Drews J, eds. Pharmacology of Bacterial Toxins. IEPT Section 119. Oxford: Pergamon Press; 1986:635–692.
65. Freer JH, Arbuthnott JP. Toxins of *Staphylococcus aureus.* In: Dorner F, Drews J, eds. *Pharmacology of Bacterial Toxins.* IEPT Section 119. Oxford: Pergamon Press; 1986:581–634.
65a. Cavalieri SJ, Bohach GA, Synder IS. *Escherichia coli* α-hemolysin: Characteristics and probable role in pathogenicity. Microbiol Rev. 1984;48:326.
65b. Clerc PL, Ryter A, Mounier J, et al. Plasmid-mediated early killing of eucaryotic cells by *Shigella flexneri* as studied by infection of J774 macrophages. Infect Immun. 1987;55:521.
65c. Portnoy DA, Jacks PS, Hinrichs DJ. Role of hemolysin for the intracellular growth of *Listeria monocytogenes.* J Exp Med. 1988;167:1459.
66. Mims CA. The Pathogenesis of Infectious Disease. London: Academic Press; 1987.
67. Smith H. Biochemical challenge of microbial pathogenicity. Bacteriol Rev. 1968;32:164.
68. Brubaker RR. Mechanisms of bacterial virulence. Annu Rev Microbiol. 1985;39:21.
69. Sweet C, Smith H. Pathogenicity of influenza virus. Microbiol Rev. 1980;44:303.
70. Fields BN, Greene MI. Genetic and molecular mechanisms of viral pathogenesis: Implications for prevention and treatment. Nature. 1982;300:19.
71. Hornick RS, Greisman SE, Woodward TE, et al. Typhoid fever: Pathogenesis and immunologic control. N Engl J Med. 1970;283:686.
72. Falkow S, Small P, Isberg R, et al. A molecular strategy for the study of bacterial invasion. Rev Infect Dis. 1987;9(Suppl 5):5450.
73. Smith HW, Huggins MB. Further observations on the association of the colicine V plasmid of *Escherichia coli* with pathogenicity and with survival in the alimentary tract. J Gen Microbiol. 1976;92:335.
74. Aguerro ME, Cabello FC. Relative contribution of Col V plasmid and K1 antigen to the pathogenicity of *Escherichia coli.* Infect Immun. 1983;40:359.
75. Labre EH, Schneider H, Magnani TJ, et al. Epithelial cell penetration as an essential step in the pathogenesis of bacillary dysentery. J Bacteriol. 1964; 88:1503.
76. DuPont HL, Formal SB, Hornick RB, et al. Pathogenesis of *Escherichia coli* diarrhea. N Engl J Med. 1971;285:1.
77. Maki M, Gronroos P, Vesikari T. In vitro invasiveness of *Yersinia enterocolitica* isolated from children with diarrhea. J Infect Dis. 1978;138:677.
78. Giannella RA, Washington O, Gemski P, et al. Invasion of HeLa cells by *Salmonella typhimurium:* A model for study of invasiveness of *Salmonella.* J Infect Dis. 1973;128:69.
79. Zink DL, Feeley JC, Wells JG, et al. Plasmid-mediated tissue invasiveness in *Yersinia enterocolitica.* Nature. 1980;283:224.
80. Hale TL, Sansonett PJ, Schad PA, et al. Characterization of virulence plasmids and plasmid-associated outer membrane proteins in *Shigella flexneri, Shigella sonnei,* and *Escherichia coli.* Infect Immun. 1983;40:340.
81. Harris JR, Wachsmuth IK, Davis BR, et al. High-molecular weight plasmid correlates with *Escherichia coli* enteroinvasiveness. Infect Immun. 1982; 37:1295.
82. Garzelli C, Colizzi V, Campa M, et al. Depression of contact sensitivity by *Pseudomonas aeruginosa*–induced suppressor cells which affect the induction phase of immune response. Infect Immun. 1979;26:4.
83. Baugh RE, Musher DM. Aberrant secondary antibody response to sheep erythrocytes in rabbits with experimental syphilis. Infect Immun. 1979; 25:133.
84. Higerd TB, Vesole DH, Goust J-M. Inhibitory effects of extracellular products from oral bacteria on human fibroblasts and stimulated lymphocytes. Infect Immun. 1978;21:567.
85. Wilkinson BJ, Sisson SP, Kim Y, et al. Localization of the third component of complement on the cell wall of encapsulated *Staphylococcus aureus* M: Implications for the mechanism of resistance to phagocytosis. Infect Immun. 1979;26:1159.
86. Kilian M. Bacterial enzymes degrading human IgA. In: Robbins JR, Hill JC, Sadoff JC, eds. Seminars in Infectious Disease. v. 4. Bacterial Vaccines. New York: Thieme-Stratton; 1982:213–8.
87. Male C. *Streptococcus pneumoniae* and *Haemophilus influenzae* IgA_1, proteases and their possible role in pathogenesis. In: Robbins JB, Hill JC, Sadoff JC, eds. Seminars in Infectious Disease. v. 4. Bacterial Vaccines. New York: Thieme-Stratton; 1982:219–24.
88. Roantree RJ, Rantz LA. A study of the relationship of the normal bactericidal activity of human serum to bacterial infection. J Clin Invest. 1960;39:72.
89. Schoolnik GK, Buchanan TM, Holmes KK. Gonococci causing disseminated gonococcal infection are resistant to the bactericidal action of normal human sera. J Clin Invest. 1976;58:1163.
90. Frank M, Joiner K, Hammer C. The function of antibody and complement in the lysis of bacteria. Rev Infect Dis. 1987;9(Suppl 5):5537.
91. Fearon DT, Austen KF. The alternative pathway of complement: A system for host resistance to microbial infection. N Engl J Med. 1980;303:259.

92. Glode MP, Robbins JB, Liu TY, et al. Cross antigenicity between capsular polysaccharides of group C *Neisseria meningitidis* and *Escherichia coli* K92. J Infect Dis. 1977;135:94.
93. Joiner KA. Complement evasion by bacteria and parasites. Annu Rev Microbiol. 1988;42:201.
93a. Wozencraft AO, Sayers G, Blackwell JM: Macrophage type 3 complement receptors mediate serum-independent binding of *Leishmania donovani*. J Exp Med. 1986;164:1332.
93b. Payne NR, Bellinger-Kawahara C, Horwitz MA: Phagocytosis of *Legionella pneumophilia* is mediated by human monocyte complement receptors: J Exp Med. 1987;166:1377.
94. Allen RJ, Scott GK. Comparison of the effects of different lipopolysaccharides on the serum bactericidal reactions of two strains of *Escherichia coli*. Infect Immun. 1981;31:831.
95. Nilins AM, Savage DC. Serum resistance encoded by colicin V plasmids in *Escherichia coli* and its relationship to the plasmid transfer system. Infect Immun. 1984;43:547.
96. Howard CJ, Glynn AA. The virulence for mice of strains of *Escherichia coli* related to the effects of K antigens on their resistance ot phagocytosis and killing by complement. Immunology. 1971;20:767.
97. McCutchan JS, Katzenstein D, Norquist D, et al. Role of blocking antibody in disseminated gonococcal infection. J Immunol. 1978;121:1884.
98. Densen P, Mandell GL. Phagocyte strategy vs microbial tactics. Rev Infect Dis. 1980;2:817.
99. Quie PG. Perturbation of the normal mechanisms of intraleukocytic killing of bacteria. J Infect Dis. 1983;148:189.
100. Sher A, Hall BF, Vadas MA. Acquisition of murine major histocompatibility complex gene products by schistosomula of *Schistosoma mansoni*. J Exp Med. 1978;148:46.
101. Zalezwik DF, Kasper DL. The role of anaerobic bacteria in abscess formation. Annu Rev Med. 1982;33:217.
102. Wilson CW, Tsai V, Remington JS. Failure to trigger the oxidative metabolic burst by normal macrophages. J Exp Med. 1980;151:328.
103. Murray HW. How protozoa evade intracellular killing. Ann Intern Med. 1983;98:1016.
104. Murray HW, Nathan CF, Cohn ZA. Macrophage oxygen-dependent antimicrobial activity IV. Role of endogenous scavengers of oxygen intermediates. J Exp Med. 1980;152:1601.
105. Goren MB. Phagocyte lysosomes: Interactions with infectious agents, phagosomes, and experimental perturbations in function. Annu Rev Microbiol. 1977;31:507.
106. Lowrie DB, Aber VR, Jackett PS. Phagosome lysosome fusion and cyclic adenosine 3′:5′ monophosphate in macrophages infected with *Mycobacterium lepraemurium*. J Gen Microbiol. 1979;110:431.
107. Lewis DH, Peters W. The resistance of intracellular *Leishmania* parasites to digestion by lysosomal enzymes. Ann Trop Med Parasitol. 1977;71:295.
108. Elwell LP, Shipley PL. Plasmid-mediated factors associated with virulence of bacteria to animals. Annu Rev Microbiol. 1980;34:465.
109. Welch RA, Dellinger EP, Minshew B, et al. Haemolysin contributes to virulence of extraintestinal *E. coli* infections. Nature. 1981;294:665.
110. Macrina FL. Molecular cloning of bacterial antigens and virulence determinants. Annu Rev Microbiol. 1984;38:193.

2. MICROBIAL ADHERENCE

LARRY M. BADDOUR
GORDON D. CHRISTENSEN
W. ANDREW SIMPSON
EDWIN H. BEACHEY

The process by which microbes bind to surfaces is known as *adherence*. In 1908 Guyot first recognized that certain bacteria bind to erythrocytes, a process resulting in hemaglutination.[1] In 1935, ZoBell and Allen examined bacterial adherence in marine environments.[2] Medical interest in bacterial adherence dates to 1955 when Duguid and coworkers began a series of publications relating filamentous bacterial surface structures to intestinal cell adherence by certain gram-negative bacilli.[3–9] In the 1970s, Gibbons and van Houte reported that the selective attachment of bacteria to various oral surfaces resulted in dental disease.[10,11] Microbial adherence has been recently reviewed in several books,[12,16] monographs,[17–19] and articles.[20–22] Understanding this literature requires familiarity with the terms defined below:

1. *Adhesins*. Adhesins are microbial surface molecules or organelles that function to bind the organism to a surface.[6]
2. *Capsules*. Capsules are a subclass of extracellular polymeric substances that are generally polysaccharide in nature. Capsules cling closely to the surface and have a distinct outer margin. In general, capsules inhibit phagocytosis and adherence, although there are many exceptions.[23,24]
3. *Extracellular polymeric substances*. Extracellular polymeric substances are usually polysaccharides, may include slime or capsules, and are roughly synonymous with the extracellular glycocalyx.
4. *Fibrillae*. Fibrillae are the fine ''hairy'' structures on bacterial cells that are irregular in size and structure.[22]
5. *Fimbriae*. Fimbriae (or pili) are nonflagellar filamentous structures on bacterial cells that have a regular structure and diameter. Generally but not exclusively, they function as adhesins.[3]
6. *Glycocalyx*. The glycocalyx is the superficial polysaccharide-containing structure on the external surface of cells.[25] It includes the cuticle of invertebrates, cell walls of plants, epithelial cell basement membrane, intercellular cement, the carbohydrate-rich surface of mammalian cells,[26] and the carbohydrate-rich surface of prokaryotic cells.[21] It may be subdivided into the intrinsic glycocalyx, which is required for cell viability, and the extracellular or extraneous glycocalyx, which is not required for cell viability.[26] An overlap in definitions should be noted, see for example, definitions 2, 3, 9, and 12.
7. *Lectin*. Lectins are carbohydrate-binding proteins of nonimmune origin that agglutinate cells or precipitate polysaccharides or glycoproteins.[27]
8. *Ligand*. A ligand is a molecule that exhibits specific binding to a complementary substrate molecule.
9. *Mucous gel*. The mucous gel is the viscous layer composed of mucins, a class of glycoproteins, produced by specialized cells that cover animal mucosal surfaces.[28] It is equivalent to the extracellular glycocalyx.
10. *Sex pili*. Traditionally, sex pili are a subclass of fimbriae that bind prokaryotic cells to each other for the conjugative transfer of genetic information.[9,22]
11. *Receptors*. Receptors are the complementary substrate molecules that bind specific ligands or adhesins.
12. *Slime*. Slime is a subclass of extracellular polymeric substances that is generally polysaccharide in composition. Slime loosely associates with the bacterial surface and has an indistinct margin. Generally, slime mediates the nonspecific attachment of a bacterium to a surface in a slimy layer.[23,24]
13. *Substratum*. The substratum is the surface to which a cell binds.

THE ADHERENCE PROCESS

All immersed objects attract suspended particles, including microbes, to their surfaces. The colloidal theories of Derjaguin and Landau and of Verwey and Overbeek (DLVO theory) describe this attraction by postulating that two positions of thermodynamic stability exist near a submerged surface. (For a more complete discussion of the DLVO theory and the following material, see refs. 22, 29–34.) A variety of long-range nonspecific weak interactions that include gravitation, chemotaxis, London–van der Waals forces, electrostatic forces, and surface tension, for example, attract particles to surfaces (Fig. 1). At closer range, however, London–van der Waals repulsion and steric hindrance repel particles from the surface. In addition, if the particles share the same charge as the surface, which is the rule when negatively charged prokaryotic cells bind to negatively charged eukaryotic cells, charge repulsion between like charges strongly repels the particles from the surface. As a re-

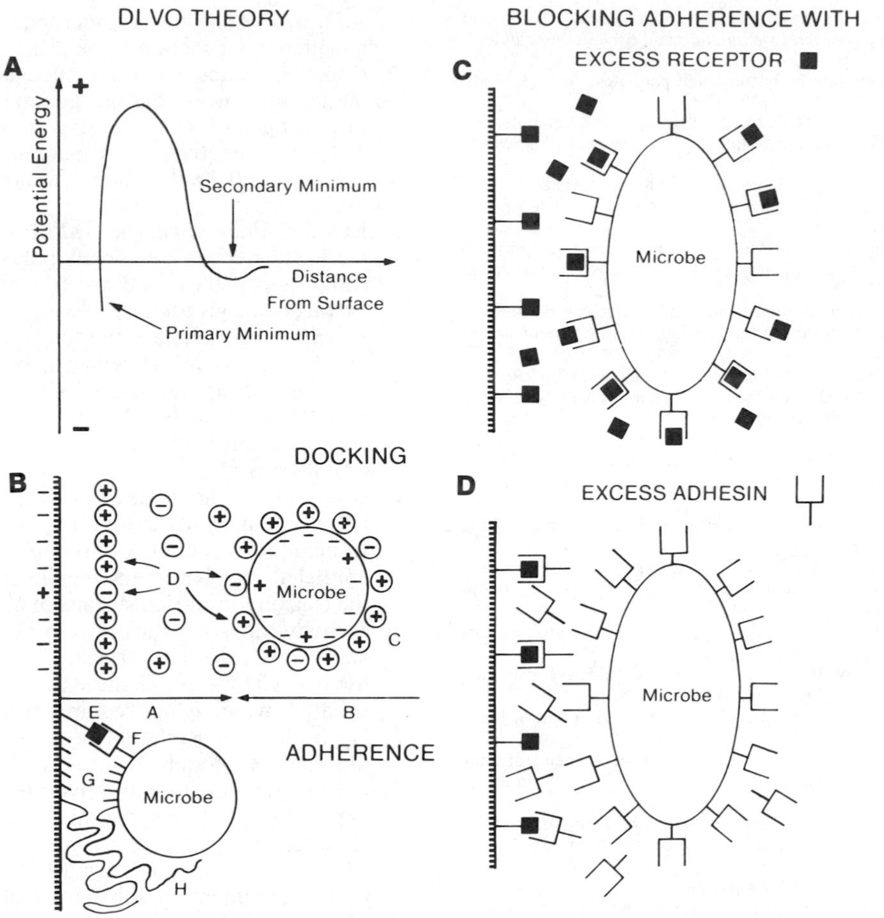

FIG. 1. (**A**) Illustration of the DLVO theory. Shown are the two points of low potential energy that lead to the association and attachment of soluble particles to surfaces. The low-energy point closest to the surface is the primary energy minimum; it is separated by a high-energy barrier from an additional point further away from the surface known as the secondary energy minimum. The precise shape and amplitude of this energy curve varies with local conditions, but the energy level of the secondary minimum is always higher than the energy level of the primary minimum. (**B**) The top portion of Fig. B shows a microbe surrounded by a charge field near a surface. This is the first stage in the attachment of a microbe to a surface in which the microbe "docks" at the surface by entering the secondary energy minimum. The particle is propelled into the secondary energy minimum by physical and chemical forces of repulsion and attraction, thereby resulting in the nonspecific and reversible adsorption of the particle to the surface. In this case, the adsorbed microbe also has an adhesin that extends beyond the surrounding charge field. The close proximity of the adsorbed microbe to the surface allows the adhesin to come into contact with surface structures. If a complementary surface structure is present, the adhesin binds to the surface receptor in a lock-and-key manner, drawing the microbe across the high-energy barrier and into the primary energy minimum. This process of microbial adherence is illustrated in the bottom portion of Fig. B. The microbe is now permanently attached to the surface. Adherence can be blocked by flooding the microbe with soluble receptors (**C**) or by flooding the surface with soluble adhesins (**D**).

sult, the forces of attraction and repulsion counterbalance each other, loosely holding the particle at the "secondary minimum" position just off the surface (Fig. 1). We refer to the concentration of particles at the secondary minimum as *adsorption* or *docking*. Characteristically, adsorption is a reversible process; particles may desorb as well as adsorb. If the particle overcomes the forces of repulsion, stronger but short-range forces of attraction bind the particle closely to the surface. These stronger, short-range forces include covalent, hydrogen, ionic, and hydrophobic binding. The DLVO theory describes this binding as the *primary minimum* (Fig. 1); particles held in this position are essentially irreversibly bound to the surface.

We refer to the process whereby particles leave the secondary minimum and enter the primary minimum as *adherence*. The energy barrier separating the secondary minimum from the primary minimum can be broached by several means. In a water environment such as on a mucosal surface, microbial surface hydrophobicity promotes the close association of microbes with lypophilic regions of eukaryotic cell membranes (see also below). In addition, many microbes excrete or extracellularly synthesize polymeric compounds such as "slime." The substrate adsorbs these compounds, which in turn embed the organism and "glue" it onto the surface. Perhaps the area of greatest interest is in the adhesive surface structures (adhesins) of microbes. Because of their smaller size, these adhesins are not subject to the forces of repulsion on the same scale as the microbe and can bridge the gap between microbe and substrate. These "bridging" adhesins include adhesive organelles and adhesive molecules or "ligands."

Generally, adhesins recognize only particular molecular conformations (receptors), and binding to these receptors is considered to be specific. The situation is analogous to the specific binding of an antigen by an antibody or a carbohydrate by a lectin. Indeed, in a very general sense, these two examples represent specific adherence systems. The former mediates the binding of a particle to a phagocyte; the latter mediates the binding of a commensal bacterium to a plant. The latter also mediates the binding of bacteria to epithelial cells as well as to phagocytes.[35] We can conclude that the binding is specific in any given circumstance if adherence is blocked by the following

1. A large excess of isolated receptor (or receptor analogue) or isolated adhesin (or adhesin analogue) (Fig. 1)
2. Specific chemical or enzymatic treatment of the microbe or substrate
3. Specific antireceptor or antiadhesin antibody

If the adhesin binds the organism to a wide variety of substrata, the binding is considered *nonspecific*. This term, however, is misleading. Many systems that appear superficially to be nonspecific are, in fact, quite specific. The reason is that all solid surfaces when exposed to fluids instantaneously adsorb macromolecules onto their surfaces, a process referred to as *conditioning*. These adsorbed molecules may, in turn, serve as receptors for microorganisms to bind to the surface.

Some authors describe a third stage in microbial surface colonization called *coaggregation*. In this stage, the microbe uses the same general processes involved in surface adherence, but rather than binding to a solid surface, the organism binds to other adherent organisms. Coaggregation allows for the accumulation of thick colonies of microorganisms on a surface.

Bacterial adherence is the first stage of bacterial invasion. To the microorganism's disadvantage, the same mechanisms that promote tissue adherence also may promote adherence to and ingestion by phagocytes. To overcome this potential liability, pathogenic microbes alter their surface characteristics by three general means. First, an organism may stop producing its adhesins and leave future generations with a surface free of adhesive structures. This can take place in response to environmental conditions (environmental regulation) or by switching on and off the adhesin gene (phase variation). Second, an organism may cover the adhesins with a capsule. Capsules, which for bacteria tend to be polysaccharides, also have some nonspecific functions. They increase the negative-charge density on the particle's surface and thereby increase the like-charge repulsion force. Capsules tend to be hydrophilic and cover surfaces that tend to be hydrophobic; capsules may mask surface structures that are antigenic or complement activating. Finally, pathogenic microbes can alter their surface by adsorbing host proteins. By covering adhesive, antigenic, or complement-activating sites, these proteins further "encapsulate" the organism's surface and immunologically confuse host defenses.

Examples of Microbial Adherence Mechanisms

Table 1 lists microorganisms that appear to rely upon adherence mechanisms to colonize and infect mammalian tissues. The specifics of the adherence process vary considerably from organism to organism, but the overall principles remain the same. Rather than discuss all the entries on Table 1, we will concentrate upon a few systems that exhibit certain basic principles, beginning with *Streptococcus pyogenes* as a paradigm of the adherence process.

Adherence Paradigm: Lipoteichoic Acid, a Streptococcal Adhesin. A fine irregular fuzz, or *fibrillae*, covers the streptococcal surface. Fibrillae bind streptococci to human epithelial cells[123,124] (Fig. 2) and are composed of M protein, lipoteichoic acid (LTA),[123] and other unidentified substances.

Because LTA is an amphipathic surface molecule that binds to virtually all eukaryotic cells, it makes an excellent candidate for a streptococcal adhesin.[125–127] An ester bond links LTA's hydrophilic polyglycerolphosphate "backbone" to its hydrophobic glycolipid "tail." The molecule is found with its tail buried in the bacterial cytoplasmic membrane of most gram-positive bacteria. LTA has a variety of biologic activities, mostly inflammatory in nature, all of which depend upon the integrity of the hydrophobic tail.

We might expect that in the native state the biologically active tail would be unavailable for binding, but apparently this is not so. The streptococcus constantly leaks LTA into the surrounding media,[128] and LTA can complex with M protein.[129] This suggests that as the LTA crosses the cell wall it might complex with surface proteins and make an about-face, thereby exposing the hydrophobic moiety.[8,129] Observations in support of this include the following: (*1*) the streptococcal cell wall is fatty acid rich,[130] (*2*) the unencapsulated streptococcal surface is very hydrophobic,[131,132] (*3*) the surface hydrophobicity is sensitive to proteolysis,[131,133] (*4*) the surface hydrophobicity correlates with surface LTA,[133] and (*5*) the selective inactivation of the hydrophobic tail converts the hydrophobic streptococcal surface into a hydrophilic one.[131]

As noted previously, hydrophobic surfaces promote prokaryotic–eukaryotic cell contact. In this regard, LTA's contribution to surface hydrophobicity and ultimately to bacterial adherence is important. Nevertheless, hydrophobic interactions are general processes and cannot by themselves explain the specificities of streptococcal adherence. For example, streptococcal cutaneous strains preferentially bind to cutaneous epithelial cells.[134] Furthermore, rheumatogenic strains bind preferentially to pharyngeal cells of rheumatic heart disease patients,[135] and streptococci bind to adult buccal epithelial cells but not to neonatal epithelial cells.[136] Finally, bound streptococci exhibit a highly nonuniform topographic distribution on epithelial cells, thus indicating the existence of privileged binding sites.[137] The specificity of this cellular attachment indicates that specific bacterial adhesins interact with specific cellular receptors. There is evidence that LTA also functions as one of these adhesins: LTA blocks streptococcal adherence to epithelial cells,[123,125,126,134] as does antibody to LTA.[123] Lipopolysaccharide from *Escherichia coli* and *Serratia marcescens*, streptococcal somatic antigens (M protein, C carbohydrate, and peptidoglycan sonicate), and M-type-specific and group A-specific antisera do not block adherence.[123] The inhibitory activity of LTA resides in its hydrophobic tail because the hydrophobic backbone alone (deacylated LTA) cannot block streptococcal adherence.[125]

Cellular binding of LTA is highly specific. For example, buccal epithelial cells from newborn infants bind only half as much LTA as do cells from 3-day-old infants and from adults.[126] Furthermore, LTA binds 10 times greater to right-side-out red blood cell (RBC) ghosts than to inside-out RBC ghosts,[138] thus indicating that LTA binds to a receptor on the exterior of the RBC rather than simply intercalating its tail into the lipid cell membrane. Finally, LTA binds to a single population of binding sites (receptors) on neutrophilic leukocytes,[139] RBCs,[140] platelets,[141] lymphocytes,[142] and oral epithelial cells.[126]

Fibronectin is a ubiquitous adhesive glycoprotein that also binds LTA, but not deacylated LTA,[143] via fatty acid receptors in a manner entirely analogous to albumin's binding of LTA.[144] Streptococci will bind soluble and surface-fixed fibronectin,[88] and fibronectin inhibits the adherence of streptococci to epithelial cells.[88] As we might expect, LTA but not deacylated LTA blocks the binding of fibronectin to streptococci.[88]

Previous work demonstrated that group A streptococci incubated in the presence of sublethal concentrations of penicillin released their surface LTA.[128] At the same time, the streptococci lost their ability to bind to oral epithelial cells.[145] More recent studies have examined the formation and release of LTA–fibronectin complexes from streptococcal surfaces in the presence of sublethal concentrations of penicillin.[146,147] The binding of fibronectin to penicillin-exposed streptococci decreased, and this decrease corresponded to a loss of LTA. Radiolabeling experiments using [^{3}H] fibronectin and antisera to LTA showed that cells of *S. pyogenes* that had been incubated in penicillin released the radiolabeled fibronectin and antiserum to LTA precipitated most of the released fibronectin. Examination of the fibronectin molecule has shown that *S. pyogenes* and *S. aureus* bind to the NH_2-terminal region of the fibronectin

TABLE 1. Partial List of Pathogenic and Commensal Microorganisms with Adherence Mechanisms

Microbe	*Adhesin*	*Receptor (Carrier)*	*Reference*
Viruses			
Orthomyxovirus (influenza)	Hemagglutinin	Sialic acid	36, 37
Picornavirus (poliovirus, rhinovirus, coxsackievirus)	Capsid protein	Four receptor "families"	36, 37
Adenovirus	Fiber protein	?	36, 37
Togavirus (Sindbis, Semliki Forest)	Glycoprotein spike	Phospholipid or cholesterol?	36, 37
Rhabdovirus (vesicular stomatitis virus)	Sialic acid residue on glycoprotein spike	Phospho- or glycolipid	36, 37
Intracellular bacteria and mycoplasma			
Chlamydia	Cell surface lectin	*N*-acetyl-D-glucosamine	38, 39
Mycoplasma			
M. gallisepticum	Tip structure	Sialic acid (glycophorin)	40
M. pneumoniae	Protein P-1 on tip structure	Sialic acid	40–42
Aerobic gram-negative bacilli			
Escherichia coli	Type I fimbriae	D-Mannose (Tamm-Horsfall glycoprotein)	43, 44
	K88 fimbriae	GM_1 ganglioside	18, 45
	K99 fimbriae	Galp-β(1–4)-GLcp-β(1–1)-ceramide	18, 46
	CFA/1 fimbriae	GM ganglioside	18, 47
	CFA/2 fimbriae	?	18
	987P fimbriae	Glycoprotein	48–51
	F41 fimbriae	?	52, 53
	PCF8775 fimbriae	?	54–56
	P fimbriae	P blood group glycolipid	57, 58
Enterobacteriaceae (*Salmonella, Shigella, Klebsiella, Citrobacter, Morganella, Aeromonas*)	Type I fimbriae	D-Mannose	59–63
Klebsiella aerogenes	Type III fimbriae	?	62
Serratia marcescens	Type III fimbriae	?	62
Proteus			
P. mirabilis	Fimbriae, type IV fimbriae	?	62, 64
P. vulgaris	Fimbriae	?	64
Providencia	Fimbriae	?	64, 65
Yersinia enterocolitica	Two types of fimbriae	?	66, 67
Pseudomonas aeruginosa	Fimbriae	?	68, 69
Pasteurella multocida	Fimbriae	*N*-acetyl-D-glucosamine	70
Bordetella pertussis	Fimbriae	?Sterol	71–73
Hemophilus influenzae	Fimbriae	?	74, 75
Vibrio cholera	Fimbriae	?	76
	Cholera lectin	?Protein	77, 78
Legionella pneumophila	Fimbriae	?	79
Aerobic gram-negative cocci			
Neisseria			
N. meningitidis	Fimbriae	?	80, 81
N. gonorrhoeae	Fimbriae	GD_1 ganglioside	62, 82
	Type II outer membrane	?	82, 83
	Protein	?	83
Moraxella	Fimbriae	?	62

(Continued)

structure.[148–150] Unlike *S. pyogenes, S. aureus* cells bind to an additional site close to the cell attachment region. It should be noted that the streptococci may not always be recognized by cell surface receptors such as fibronectin because their adhesin may be masked either by hyaluronate capsules[151] or by adsorbed host proteins once the organisms invade deeper tissue.[152]

Adhesive Organelles. As opposed to *S. pyogenes*, many organisms use a specific adhesive organelle, fimbriae (or pili), to mediate adherence. The archetypical fimbria is type I, or common fimbriae, and is expressed by most Enterobacteriaceae (Table 2). Originally recognized for their hemagglutinin properties, these adhesins enable the bacterium to attach to most of the protozoal, fungal, and animal cells and cell products so far tested. Characteristically, D-mannose, methyl-α-D-mannoside, yeast mannan, and other D-mannose derivatives inhibit this attachment.[174,175] As such, type I fimbriae from different genera exhibit close structural but limited antigenic similarities.[176] The precise oligosaccharide receptor also varies between genera.[177] Typically, bacteria have 50–400 of these filaments projecting from their surface. The filaments radiate outward from where their hydrophobic tips initiate contact with other cells and substrata. The phenotypic expression of type I fimbriae switches on and off from bacterial generation to bacterial generation (phase variation) so that under any given cultural condition a proportion of the bacterial population will always be fimbriated and nonfimbriated.[9,178] Although these organelles aid saprophytic and commensal bacterial colonization, their importance in pathogenicity remains controversial because many pathogenic Enterobacteriaceae do not express type I fimbriae.[9] However, almost all possess the ability to produce fimbriae.

Fimbria-mediated attachment is exemplified by *E. coli.* The organisms are richly endowed with fimbriae and may simultaneously exhibit several different kinds.[176,179–181] The structure and function of many of these fimbriae have only been partially characterized. The best described fimbriae fall into three groups: the common fimbriae, the enteric colonization fimbriae of enterotoxigenic E. coli (ETEC), and the P fimbriae of uropathogenic *E. coli* (Table 2).

Similar to other Enterobacteriaceae, most but not all strains of *E. coli* express type I fimbriae under appropriate cultural conditions.[9] They enable the organism to attach to almost all human tissues including white blood cells, buccal epithelial cells, enterocytes, uroepithelial cells, and uromucoid (Tamm-Horsfall glycoprotein). Although we would expect type I fimbriae to promote the colonization of epithelial surfaces by pathogenic *E. coli,*[18] investigators have not found type I fimbriae to be associated with ETEC diarrhae.[182] On the other hand, animal studies suggest that there is a role for type I fimbriae in the pathogenesis of urinary tract infections.[108,183,184] Rene and Silverblatt[185] reported an association between pyelonephritis in

TABLE 1. (Continued)

Microbe	*Adhesin*	*Receptor (Carrier)*	*Reference*
Aerobic gram-positive bacilli			
Corynebacterium renale	Fimbriae	?	84, 85
Aerobic gram-positive cocci			
Staphylococcus aureus	Lipotechoic acid (LTA)	?	86
Staphylococcus epidermidis	Slime	?	87
Streptococcus			
S. pyogenes	LTA-M protein complex		
	Fibrillae		88, 89
S. mitior			
S. salivarius			
S. mutans, groups C and G	?	?	90, 91
S. mutans	Glucosyltransferase and glucan-binding protein	Glucan	92–96
	Cell surface lectin	Galactose	97
S. sanguis	LTA, fibrillae	Salivary agglutinin	98, 99
	Cell surface lectin	Galactose, on *Actinomyces viscosus*	100
	Binding protein	*A. viscosus*	100
	Binding protein	Dental pellicle	101
S. salivarius	Cell surface lectin	Galactose, on *Veillonella alcalescens*	102, 103
	Binding protein	?	102
	Glucosyltransferase	Glucan	104
S. agalactiae	Protein	*N*-acetyl-D-glucosamine	105, 106
Enterococcus			
E. faecalis	Fimbriae	?	107
Anaerobic bacteria			
Bacteroides fragilis	Capsular polysaccharide	?	108
Eikenella corrodens	?	Galactose	109
Actinomyces			
A. viscosus	Fimbriae	Galactose on *S. sanguis*	100, 110
	Fimbriae	*S. sanguis*	100, 110
	Fimbriae	Dental pellicle	111
	Glucan-binding protein	Glucan	112
A. naeslundii	Fimbriae	Galactose on *S. sanguis*	100
	Fimbriae	*S. sanguis*	100
	Fimbriae	Dental pellicle	111
	Fimbriae	Epithelial cells	113
Spirochetes			
Treponema pallidum	P_1, P_2, P_3	Fibronectin	114, 115
Fungi			
Candida albicans	Mannan	?	116, 117
Protozoa			
Plasmodium			
P. falciparum	Apical complex	*N*-acetyl-D-glucosamine (glycophorin)	118, 119
P. vivax	Apical complex	Duffy blood group antigen	118
Entamoeba histolytica	Cell surface lectin	*N*-acetyl-glucosamine	120, 121
Giardia lamblia	Gripping disk	Mechanical	122

humans and type I fimbriated *E. coli*. They also noted a specific immune response to type I fimbriae in their infected patients.[185] Swedish investigators, however, have not found an association between urinary tract infection and type I fimbriae.[57,186] These organelles may be more important in the initiation of a urinary tract infection than in its persistence.[187] Type I fimbriated organisms have a particularly high affinity for the uromucoid that bathes the urinary tract.[43] This could encourage bacterial colonization, or alternatively, by entrapment and excretion uromucoid may actually be a nonspecific host defense against type I fimbriated bacteria.[188]

Enterotoxigenic *E. coli* cause traveler's diarrhea and infant diarrhea in humans and neonatal enteric colibacillosis of piglets, calves, and lambs. ETEC bacteria possess plasmids that code for the production of either or both heat-stable (ST) or heat-labile (LT) enterotoxin. The enterotoxin, in turn, causes a secretory diarrhea. Genetic manipulations demonstrate that the production of an enterotoxin alone is not sufficient for pathogenicity. The organism must also have an adhesin that binds the organism to the enterocyte so that the toxin can be expeditiously delivered to the target tissue.[189–192] These adhesins, or colonization factors, are fimbriae that exhibit host specificity. For example, the K88 fimbriae determine organ specificity (anterior portion of the small intestine) and host specificity (neonatal pigs).[193,194] Furthermore, the different antigenic types of K88, namely K88ab, K88ac, and K88ad, bind to different piglet phenotypes.[195] A number of colonization factors for human and animal ETEC strains have been described in addition to those listed in Table 2.[18,182] Unlike type I fimbriae, the agglutination is not inhibited by mannose; thus arises the term *mannose-resistant* adherence. Other common properties of this group include plasmid location of the fimbrial gene (generally not on the same plasmid as the enterotoxin gene), phenotypic expression of fimbriation at body temperature (37°C) but not at room temperature (18°C), and confinement of fimbriation to certain serogroups.[9,18] Despite these common functional properties, this is actually a heterogenous group. The fimbriae have different hemagglutinin patterns, mucosal receptors, antigens, and primary and quaternary structures (Table 2).[18,196] Human and animal studies indicate that the enteric colonization fimbriae mediate specific enterocyte adherence that is saturable, inhibited by homologous but not heterologous purified fimbriae, and inhibited by homologous but not heterologous antifimbrial antibodies.[53,197–200] Veterinary studies demonstrate an 80–100 percent protection of neonatal animals passively immunized by the ingestion of colostrum from mothers vaccinated with purified fimbriae of the homologous type.[200,201]

P fimbriae refers to a class of antigenically distinct (designated F-7 through F-12) uropathogenic *E. coli* adhesins that share the common property of agglutinating human RBCs carrying the ubiquitous P blood group antigen, which consists of globoseries glycolipids.[169] Characteristically, this agglutination is mannose resistant, but it is inhibited by the isolated and purified P blood group substance or by a synthetic Galα(1–4)Galβ-

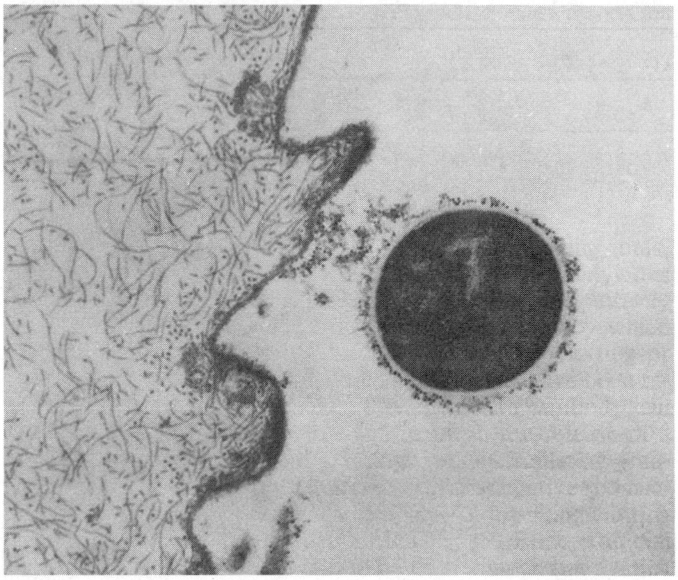

FIG. 2. Transmission electron micrograph of an ultrathin section of human buccal epithelial cells incubated with a suspension of *Streptococcus pyogenes* and treated first with rabbit antibody to fibronectin and then with ferritin-conjugated goat antibody to rabbit IgG. An *S. pyogenes* cell (center) is seen associated with an epithelial cell coated with ferritin particles, which indicates the presence of fibronectin. The rim of ferritin-labeled antibody around the bacterium appears to be due to the acquisition of fibronectin from epithelial cell surfaces during incubation.

ceramide derivative.[57,58,166,176,202] Coating a substrate with the natural or synthetic glycolipid promotes attachment of P fimbriated bacteria. The P antigen, the minimum structural determinant being a digalactose Galα(1–4)Galβ residue, is not only present on human RBCs but is also present on the kidney tissues of humans and mice (but not rats).[203] P. fimbriae are at least a marker for pyelonephritogenic *E. coli* that bind to human and mouse uroepithelial cells in a mannose-resistant but globoside-sensitive manner.[167,176] P-specific adherence is most commonly seen in collections of pyelonephritogenic *E. coli* strains[57,164,186] and is also frequently present in collections of cystitis and asymptomatic bacteruria strains.[57,164,186] In comparison, it is a rare finding in collections of fecal *E. coli* isolates. In an elegant study performed in mice, Swedish and U.S. investigators used genetically manipulated *E. coli* strains as tools to determine the importance of fimbriae in murine urinary tract infections. The P fimbriae served to localize the organism to the upper urinary tract, whereas both P fimbriae and common fimbriae localized the organism to the mouse bladder.[183]

The P fimbriae specificity determines the host specificity of these organisms. CBA mice have a higher concentration of P antigen than do BALB/c mice. CBA mice are also more predisposed to P-fimbriated *E. coli* experimental pyelonephritis than are BALB/c mice.[183] There is similar evidence that humans with high concentrations of P antigen are also particularly predisposed to pyelonephritis.[183,204] Thus, P fimbriae join the enteric colonization fimbriae as host-specific adhesins. P fimbriae also share with enteric colonization fimbriae the properties of serogroup restriction[179] and temperature-dependent expression of fimbriae.[205] P fimbriae, on the other hand, appear to be closely related to type I fimbriae. Both have chromosomal genetic codes,[165] and they share considerable primary structure homology[206] and similar quaternary structure.[168]

Another fimbrial type on *E. coli*, termed S fimbriae, is characterized by its specific binding to sialyl galactosides on human erythrocytes and is associated with *E. coli* serotype 018:K1:H7, which is commonly isolated from infants with meningitis and septicemia.[170–173,207–212] The major erythrocyte receptor for S-fimbriated *E. coli* is the NeuAcα(2–3)Galβ(1–3)GlcNac sequence of the *O*-linked oligosaccharide chains of glycophorin A.[173] S fimbriae, serum resistance, and hemolysin production are operative virulence factors of *E. coli* strains in the rat pyelonephritis model.[207] Binding sites for S fimbriae of *E. coli* to frozen sections of human kidney include epithelial and vascular endothelial cells.[208] The genetic determinant coding for the S-fimbrial adhesin has been cloned, and analysis of the DNA sequences are highly conserved in their coding and flanking regions and are identical, except for small alterations, in uropathogenic (06:K+) and meningitis (018:K1, 083:K1) strains.[209,210]

Recent data from the infant rat model examining the pathogenesis of *E. coli* bacteremia and meningitis are particularly intriguing and support a virulence role of S fimbriae.[211] Inocula subpopulations of strain IH3080, 018:K1:H7 organisms that contain S fimbriae, were the most virulent in this animal model as compared with subpopulations with type I fimbriae or nonfimbriated isolates. Fimbrial phase variation to the type S fimbriated forms was observed in all body fluids 6 hours after injection, while nonfimbriated forms were seen 1 hour after challenge, which led the investigators to speculate on the role of phase variation in establishing serious infections in this animal model. Moreover, three different cell types of the neonatal rat brain demonstrated specific binding sites for S fimbriae of *E. coli*.[212]

Tip Location of Fimbrial Adhesin Proteins. Until recently it was thought that the sugar binding sites of bacterial fimbriae were located within the major structural subunits. While this may be true for some fimbriae, new evidence suggests that the sugar binding sites of several fimbrial types (e.g., type I, P and S) reside in minor proteins that represent only 1/100–1000 of the total structural protein. That a protein other than the major subunit was involved was first shown by insertion and deletion mutation analyses of fimbrial clones. Mutants producing morphologically normal fimbriae that were nonadhesive lacked certain minor proteins. By using a combination of specific antibodies and gold-conjugated protein A as probes, the adhesin proteins of type I, P and S fimbriae were shown to be located at the tips of the respective organelles.[213–216a] Further studies of type I fimbriae have revealed that the antigenic structure of the adhesin protein of type I fimbriae is more highly conserved than is that of the major structural protein among different strains of *E. coli*. The vaccine implications of these findings are obvious; vaccines prepared from the shared adhesin proteins should be broadly protective against many strains of *E. coli* and perhaps other gram-negative bacillary infections.

Adherence as a Means of Toxin Delivery. The pathogenesis of cholera parallels the pathogenesis of diarrhea by ETEC; however, the adherence mechanisms are entirely different. Certain *Vibrio cholerae* biotypes, namely, classic and El Tor, colonize the human small intestine where they release an enterotoxin (choleragen). When the choleragen comes into contact with the host intestinal mucosa, it stimulates host adenyl cyclase and results in a secretory diarrhea. As with diarrhea caused by ETEC, the key to this chain of events is the successful delivery of toxin to the target cell.[217] Although we cannot be sure of the precise means by which the vibrios associate with the human intestinal mucosa in vivo, in vitro and animal model studies conducted primarily by Freter and Jones indicate a multistep process.[218] An overlying blanket of mucus (mucous gel) blocks contact between luminal bacteria and intestinal mucosa.[76,219,220] Vibrios possess flagella that can propel them through the mucous gel, providing that the organism can also follow a chemotactic gradient to the intestinal surface.[219] Nonmotile[219,221,222] or nonchemotactic[219,223] mutant vibrios are avirulent unless they spontaneously revert and recover their locomotive powers.[219,222] Having arrived at the mucosal surface, the organism

TABLE 2. Characteristics of Some *Escherichia coli* Fimbrial Adhesins

	Fimbrial Classes												
	Common	*Host Specific*											
		Enteropathogenic				*Uropathogenic*							
										PCF8775			
Characteristic	*Type 1*	*K88*	*K99*	*987P*	*F-41*	*CFA/I*	*CFA/II: CS1, CS2, CS3*	*CFA/III*	*AF/R1*	*CS4/CS6*	*CS5/CS6*	P. fimbriae *(F-7 to F-12 and Others)*	*S*
Host	Animals Plants Bacteria Fungi	Pigs	Calves Lambs Pigs	Pigs	Calves Lambs Pigs	Humans	Humans	Humans Mice Rabbits	Rabbits	Humans		Humans	Humans Rats
Target cells	Procarytoic cells, eucarytoic cells	Enterocytes, brush border membranes			Enterocytes	Uroepithelial cells							Uroepithelial cells, vascular endothelial cells
Serogroup restricted?	No	Yes	Yes	Yes	Yes	Yes	Yes	Yes	Yes	Yes		Yes	Yes
Phenotypic expression	Phase variation	Temperature dependent	Temperature dependent	Phase variation	Temperature dependent	Temperature dependent	Temperature dependent	Temperature dependent	Temperature dependent	Temperature dependent		Temperature dependent	Phase variation
Genetic control	Chromosomal	Plasmid		Chromosomal			Plasmid					Chromosomal	Chromosomal
Agglutination													
Yeast cells	MS	0	0	0	0	0	0	—	—	—	—	0	0
Human RBC	MS	0	0	0	MR	MR	0	0	0	MR	MR	MR	MR
Guinea pig RBC	MS	MR	0	0	MR	0	0	—	0	0	MR	0	—
Horse RBC	MS	0	MR	0	MR	0	0	—	—	—	—	0	—
Sheep RBC	MS	0	MR	0	MR	0	0	—	—	—	—	0	—
Chicken RBC	—	MR	0	0	0	MR	MR	—	0	—	—	0	—
Bovine RBC	—	0	0	0	0	MR	MR	0	0	MR	MR	0	—
Structure													
Shape	Tubular	Filament	Helical filament	Tubular	Filament	Filament	Filament	—	Filament	—		Tubular	Tubular
Diameter	7.0 nm	2.1 nm	4.8 nm	7.0 nm	3.2 nm	3.2 nm	3.2 nm	—	5 nm	7 nm		5–7 nm (variable with type)	5–7 nm
Subunit molecular weight	17,100	27,540	18,500	20,000	29,500	15,058	13,000	18,000	19,000	—		17,000–22,000	17,000
References	44, 153	18, 154	18, 155	18, 48	18, 52, 53	18, 156	18	157, 158	159–163	54–56		57, 165–169	170–173

Abbreviations: MS: mannose-sensitive agglutination; MR: mannose-resistant agglutination; 0: no agglutination; (—): no data available.

firmly adheres to the brush border membranes of the intestinal epithelium, first by the nonflagellar end and then sideways.[76] The adhesin that mediates this attachment appears to be fimbriae (see below). The adherence is specific,[224] temperature dependent,[225] and time dependent;[76,226] requires divalent cations;[225] and is saturable.[76,226,227] In animal models characterized by bowel stasis, the organisms disengage from the mucosa after 7–16 hours;[76,228] if bowel flow is unimpeded, however, adherence remains constant.[227] Adherence to intestinal epithelial tissue is closely but not absolutely linked to vibrio motility.[222,224,226,228] Generally, nonmotile organisms do not adhere, even if compacted upon the intestinal mucosa.[222] *Vibrio cholerae* produces one or more hemagglutinins, and hemagglutination correlates with intestinal epithelial adherence.[222,225] Mannose[222] and fucose[222] inhibit hemagglutination and intestinal epithelial cell adherence (although some investigators question the latter[229]). Recently, Finkelstein and Hanne[77] and Finkelstein et al.[78] found a multifunctional cholera surface protein (cholera lectin) with the properties of hemagglutination, hydrophobicity, and protease activity. Antibodies to this material block *V. cholerae* adherence to intestinal epithelial cells, which suggests it may be the long-sought cholera adhesin.[77,78] Booth and colleagues, using cultured human intestinal epithelial cells, demonstrated correlations between adhesion of *V. cholerae* and expression of hemagglutinin activity.[230] This in vitro system had been used previously to examine adherence mechanisms of enterotoxigenic *E. coli*.[231,232] Key studies recently demonstrated that the same gene product (*tox R*) is (*1*) required for production of a pilus colonization factor that is encoded by the *tcp A* gene and is important in intestinal colonization; (*2*) controls the production of cholera toxin by regulating the activity of the *ctx* operon, the transcriptional unit that encodes for cholera toxin; (*3*) and is necessary for the expression of an outer-membrane protein encoded by the *ompll* gene.[233,234] This "coupling" of enterotoxicity and colonization where the same regulatory gene controls the transcription of multiple virulence factors of *V. cholerae* is fascinating pathogenetically.[233] In a similar vein, linkage of the genes for toxin and adhesive antigen production on a plasmid has been shown in enterotoxigenic *E. coli* strains of human[56,236–239] and animal[240] origin.

Multiple Adhesins. In the preceding sections, we have taken the simplistic approach—that each microbe has its own variety of adhesin and that the display of the adhesin directly determines the adherence of the microbe. A microorganism, however, is not necessarily limited to one adhesin system, particularly since having two or more systems could be advantageous to the organism. A fastidious organism could increase both the specificity and range of its adherence by simultaneously and differentially using more than one adhesin. In the following discussion of *N. gonorrhoeae*, two surface structures determine the adherence of gonococci to tissues and also influence the antigenicity of the bacterial surface and its resistance to host defenses. The first structure is a fimbrial adhesin referred to as gonococcal pili (P); the second structure is a protein component of the outer membrane known as protein II (P.II). The expression or nonexpression of both of these structures is independently subject to spontaneous change through a process of phase variation. Both structures are also susceptible to spontaneous antigenic and functional changes.[241]

Gonococcal infections begin with bacterial adherence to mucous-secreting cells of the urogenital tract.[82,242,243] The attachment is species[244] and host[242,245] specific. Organisms freshly isolated from the male urethral mucosa generally produce small, high-domed, opaque colonies; after several transfers on fresh media, however, a variety of other colonial forms develop. Swanson demonstrated that this polymorphism reflects a change in piliation and P.II under in vitro conditions[246] (Fig. 3). Gonococci with pili (P+ and P.II+) produce small, high-domed colonies, whereas cells without pili (P−) produce low,

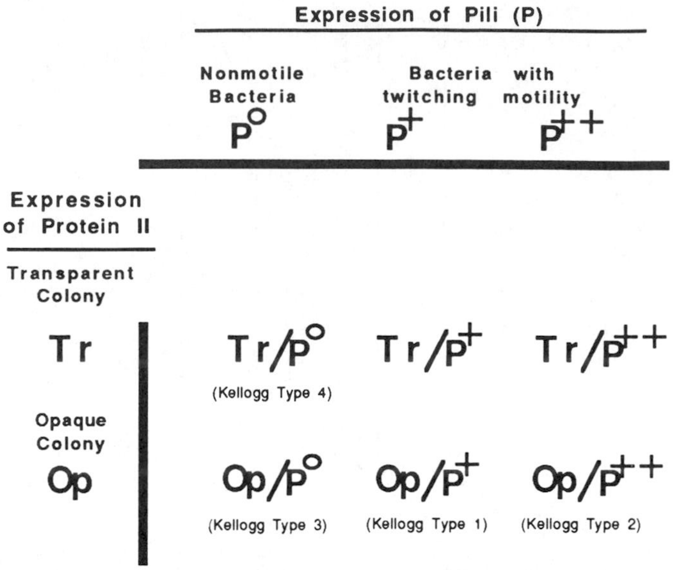

FIG. 3. The variety of colonial forms exhibited by *Neisseria gonorrhoeae* are organized on this chart according to the expression of two adhesins: pili and protein II. Gonococci without pili are nonmotile (P°), while gonococci with varying amounts of pili demonstrate twitching motility (P^+ and P^{++}). Most forms of protein II cause gonococci to aggregate and result in opaque (Op) colonies. If the gonococci do not produce protein II (or produce certain varieties of protein II), the cells do not aggregate, and the colony appears translucent (Tr). The independent expression of these two adhesins results in four to six colonial forms with different virulence properties.

broad colonies.[246] Particular types of P.II, on the other hand, cause the gonococci to adhere to one another, thereby resulting in highly aggregated opaque (Op) colonies.[246] Other types of P.II or the complete absence of P.II cause the organisms to grow separately and result in translucent (Tr) colonies.[246,247] Since both pili and opaque forms of P.II are conserved, the course of a natural gonococcal urethritis must select for these proteins.

We know that pili function as adhesins since cells with pili adhere better than do cells without pili.[248,249] Furthermore, purified pili preferentially adhere to human cells of buccal and genital (sperm, vaginal epithelium, fallopian tube mucosa) origin over a variety of other human cells (e.g., RBCs polymorphonuclear [PMN] leukocytes, and tissue culture cells.[250,251] This adherence has pH and temperature optimums and is saturable and promoted by multivalent ions (particularly ferric).[250,251] Anti-pilus antibodies are naturally present in the vaginal fluid of infected patients, and these antibodies inhibit gonococcal adherence.[252] This inhibition, however, is much greater for homologous than for heterologous strains, thus indicating that pili exhibit antigenic variation.[253] Spontaneous antigenic variation has also been observed in the course of natural infections.[247,254] This antigenic variation arises spontaneously from rearrangements of the pili gene,[255,256] which results in structural[257] and functional variation[258] along with antigenic variation. Despite this variability, different gonococcal pili have identical amino acid sequences that are shared at the aminotermini with the fimbriae of *Neisseria meningitidis, Moraxella nonliquifaciens,* and *Pseudomonas aeruginosa*.[259]

P.II actually includes a family of outer-membrane proteins that are structurally related[260] but antigenically[261] and functionally distinct.[83] For example, one particular P.II promotes gonococcal adherence to PMN leukocytes, whereas another P.II discourages it.[83] Individual P.II also influence antimicrobial resistance.[83] In general, P.II protects the gonococci from the lytic effect of serum[83] and promotes gonococcal adherence to buccal[83] and vaginal[262] epithelial cells. This adherence is selective. Opaque strains do not adhere as well to RBCs[83] and fallopian tube mucosa[82] as do transparent strains. Clones with different amounts and types of P.II arise spontaneously through the course of an infection[247,263] or its transmission.[264] Certain anatomic sites (male urethra) and metabolic conditions (cervical isolates from women at the midmenstrual cycle) seem to select for the expression of P.II, whereas other sites (fallopian tube) and metabolic conditions (cervical isolates from women during menses or from women using oral contraceptives) appear to exclude strains of P.II.[82,263] Even though pili are conserved under each of these conditions, they also undergo spontaneous antigenic and functional variation. Taken together, this evidence indicates that the quantitative and qualitative differential expression of P.II and pili enable the gonococci to infect and exploit a wide variety of human microenvironments by determining to which tissues the organism will adhere and its ability to repel host defenses.

Polymicrobial Adherence. So far, we have examined the topic of bacterial adherence by emphasizing the deployment and use of adhesins by individual pathogens as they launch their assault on the host. A much more common and wider application of bacterial adherence is in the coordination and construction of polymicrobial communities on surfaces. The best-studied example of this is in the microbiology of the human oropharynx.[10,11]

Infections of the gums and the teeth afflict more humans than do any other infectious disease. The causative agents are indigenous to our mouths and persist in that environment despite the constant scrubbing of our oral tissues by salivation and mastication. In the past, we ascribed this persistence to the organism's growth rate, that is, rapidly growing organisms replenish their losses and remain in place, whereas slowly growing organisms simply wash away.[10] Gibbons and Van Houte changed this concept by introducing evidence that the selective adherence of bacteria to the oral tissues determines the pattern of their oral colonization.[10] Abnormal conditions that accentuate or change this pattern, such as a sucrose-rich diet, result in dental disease.

Dental plaque, the provoking agent of dental disease, includes the bacterial accumulations in the crevices between tooth and gum (subgingival or supragingival plaque) and over the tooth's enamel surfaces (coronal plaque). By fixing bacteria onto oral surfaces, plaque allows microbial digestive and toxic products to cause dental dimineralization (caries) and mucosal inflammation (periodontitis and gingivitis). These bacterial accumulations should not be construed as amorphous conglomerates of random components. Rather, they represent microbial climax communities whose precise composition and organization varies in a predictable manner with certain factors such as oral location, host diet, and salivary secretions. For example, subgingival plaque is organized along three zones: the organisms next to the tooth are gram-positive, the organisms next to the gum are spirochetes and other motile bacteria, and the organisms in between are gram-negative.[10]

Specific molecular interactions dictate the plaque architecture. The interactions include bacterial cell to dental surface, bacterial cell to homologous cell, bacterial cell to heterologous cell, and bacterial cell to extracellular substance.[11] Extracellular substances are either host derived, such as secretory IgA, or bacterial derived, such as extracellular polymeric substances. Referred to as the plaque matrix, these substances give the bacterial biomass structural integrity in addition to influencing its overall design. Extracellular substances also play a role in anchoring the microbial plaque to the dental surface. As we mentioned earlier, all immersed solids adsorb dissolved materials to their surfaces. The teeth are no exception. A variety of salivary products of host and bacterial origin such as high-molecular-weight glycoproteins (salivary mucins), lysozyme, salivary agglutinins, IgA, fibronectin, and bacterial extracellular polymeric substances coat the dental surface and form a biofilm, or *pellicle*.[10,11,90] Consequently, these adsorbed substances function as either specific bacterial receptors or adherence blockers, thereby dictating the microbial composition of the adherent plaque. Two factors determine pellicle composition: first, hydroxyapatite, the major constituent of dental enamel, selectively adsorbs certain compounds such as acidic glycoproteins and acidic proteins. Second, the quality and quantity of various salivary constituents such as agglutinins and immunoglobulins vary greatly from person to person.[265–267]

The primary microbial constituents of dental plaque are streptococci (*S. mutans, S. mitis, S. mitior, S. sanguis,* and *S. salivarius*), actinomyces (*A. viscosus, A. naeslundii*), and veillonellae, but the microbial membership also includes *Lactobacillus, Neisseria, Bacteroides, Fusobacterium, Capnocytophaga, Actinobacillus, Selenomonas,* and *Campylobacter*, to name only a few.[10,11] The ecologic interactions among the oral bacteria, tissues, and secretions are far too complex and controversial to be discussed here. Instead, we will concentrate upon the proposed adherence mechanisms of three microorganisms—*S. mutans, S. sanguis,* and *A. viscosus*—as an illustration of the intricacies of plaque construction.

Streptococcus mutans produces dental caries in experimental animals only if the animals are fed a sucrose-rich diet. Curiously, when grown in vitro, the addition of sucrose—but not other carbohydrates—to laboratory media enables *S. mutans* to coat the media container with an adhesive layer of bacteria. This artificial plaque has attracted considerable attention because its form resembles dental plaque and because a similar processs in vivo could explain the association of dental caries with *S. mutans* and sucrose.[10,96] In sucrose media, *S. mutans* extracellular enzymes synthesize a number of polysaccharides, including glucans and fructans, that form part of the dental pellicle and the plaque matrix. The glucans may function as adhesins and bind *S. mutans* cells to each other through surface glucosyltransferases (GT)[95] and glucan-binding proteins (GBP),[92,94] which essentially act as cell surface lectins (or adhesins). *Streptococcus mutans* constantly release GT into the surrounding media where the GT remains active, creates more glucan, and perhaps further enmeshes the *S. mutans* and other bacteria.[10] As a component of the dental pellicle, glucan also functions as a receptor binding the *S. mutans* to the dental enamel[93] via GT and GBP. It appears, however, that a variety of other mechanisms may play a greater role in the adherence of *S. mutans* to teeth.[95] For example, hydroxyapatite adsorbs streptococci via cell surface teichoic acid in vitro and could thus bind the cells in vivo.[268] Furthermore, *S. mutans* adheres to pellicle proteins such as fibronectin[90] and to salivary agglutinins,[10] and antibodies to serotype antigens are known to interfere with adherence.[269] In a similar manner, a cell surface galactose-specific lectin binds *S. mutans* to pellicle carbohydrates, further tying the organisms to the dental surface.[97]

Streptococcus mutans dental adherence does not take place independently of other bacteria. Organisms such as *A. viscosus* can also bind to *S. mutans*-generated glucan via their own cell surface GBP.[112] If the microbe lacks GBP such as in the case of most *S. sanguis* strains, the organism may still bind to the glucan by adsorbing to its surface GT released from *S. mutans*.[270] *S. sanguis* and *A. viscosus* coaggregate, which further illustrates the complexity of dental plaque architecture. *Actinomyces viscosus* binds to *S. sanguis* surface carbohydrate by a fimbrial lactose-sensitive lectin[110,271,272] and by lactose-resistant fimbriae.[100] Isolation of phage-resistant mutants has allowed investigators to observe a functional relationship between phage receptors of *A. viscosus* and coaggregation.[273,274] Continuation of these studies should allow delineation of the molecular mechanisms involved in these interactions. The lactose-resistant fimbriae also appear to bind *A. viscosus* to the dental pellicle.[111] Recent work by Gibbons and Hay[275] suggests that both proline-rich proteins and statherin may act as pellicle receptors for *A. viscosus*. An interesting finding in these studies was that the proline-rich proteins apparently undergo a confirmational change upon binding to hydroxyapatite that allows the *A. viscosus* to recognize "hidden molecular segments" on these receptors.[275] *Streptococcus sanguis* seems to bind to the dental surface by mechanisms similar to *S. mutans*[90,93,276] and to possess fibrillae that bind salivary agglutinins, further fixing the organism to the dental plaque.[98,99] The sum of these adherence mechanisms, along with others that we have not described, is a tightly knit and highly organized microbial community. The host's secretions, diet, and tissues determine the array of exposed bacterial receptors, which in turn, guide the dental plaque architecture and composition by promoting the adherence of particular bacteria.

Receptor Specificity. The presence of microbial receptors on host tissue is just as much a determinant of microbial infectivity as is the microbe's display of adhesins. If the host does not express the correct receptor, binding and subsequent colonization and infection cannot take place. The host's display of microbial receptors may be genetically determined or subject to later modification or induction. These host receptors fall into two categories—cell surface sugar residues of the glycocalyx and cell surface proteins.

Table 1 demonstrates that, so far, sugar moieties are the primary residues identified as microbial receptors. Whereas many simple sugars are listed as receptors, more precisely, these receptors represent the simplest molecular structures exhibiting receptor activity. In actuality, these sugars are submolecular components of larger structures that function as the true receptor; the saccharide is simply the active site. The precise orientation of the sugar moiety on the molecule and the presence of neighboring submolecular structures primarily determines the specificity of the adhesin–receptor interaction. For example, Firon et al.[44] recently demonstrated that the combining site for *E. coli* contains a hydrophobic region and is in a form to best receive a D-mannose-containing trisaccharide, Manα(1–3)Manβ(1–4)GlcNac. The best receptor–fimbriae fits that they obtained were with short oligomannoside chains linked to a carrier molecule by *N*-glycoside.[44] Carrier molecules for sugar-specific receptors are either glycoproteins (e.g., glycophorin for *Mycoplasma gallisepticum*,[40] and *Plasmodium falciparum*[119], and Tam-Horsfall protein[43] and erythrocyte glycoprotein[227] for *E. coli* type I fimbriae) or glycolipids (e.g., the gangliosides: GM_1 for K88 fimbriae,[18] GM_2 for K99 and CFA/1 fimbriae,[18,47] GD_1 for *N. gonorrhoeae*,[62] and the glycolipid P blood group antigens for P fimbriae.[58])

As opposed to the variety of sugar-specific receptors, only one protein, fibronectin, has been promoted as a microbial receptor. Fibronectin has attracted considerable interest since it binds a variety of gram-positive cocci (*S. aureus*,[278–281] S. pyogenes,[89] *S. mutans*,[90] S. salivarius,[90] *S. mitior*,[90] and groups C and G streptococci[91]) rather than one or two selected microbial species. This binding is truly multivalent because different fragments of the fibronectin molecule bind different bacteria.[88,89] Fibronectin does not bind as well to gram-negative bacteria,[89,280] which suggests that one of fibronectin's functions is to fix gram-positive bacteria rather than gram-negative bacteria to the cell surface. Woods et al. first suggested that fibronectin functions as a modulator of the human oral microecology by selectively promoting gram-positive coccal adherence over gram-negative bacillary adherence.[282,283] They noted that by using trypsin they could digest cell-bound fibronectin and thereby increase the adherence of *P. aeruginosa* to oral epithelial cells. Fibronectin on the oral mucosa is confined to the exposed epithelial surface.[284] By scraping the buccal epithelium, Abraham et al.[285] found two populations of cells. One population was coated with fibronectin and probably represented superficial cells; a second population was not coated with fibronectin and may have been deeper, unexposed cells. The fibronectin-coated cells bound *S. pyogenes* but not *E. coli* and *P. aeruginosa*, whereas the uncoated cells could not bind *S. pyogenes* but did bind *E. coli* and *P. aeruginosa*.[285] These observations tie in with the well-known clinical observation that certain patients (hospitalized, ill, aged) have predominantly gram-negative bacilli colonizing their oropharynx rather than the usual gram-positive cocci seen in healthy people.[286] Whether this change is due to salivary proteases[282,283] or diminished fibronectin levels in oral secretions[90,287] remains to be determined.[288] Since the aged and infirm are also subject to gram-negative bacillary pneumonias, it does suggest that fibronectin protects the host from certain infections by selectively influencing the oral microecology toward less invasive organisms.

Nonspecific Adherence. Even though the stereospecific interlocking of complementary microbial and host surface molecules characterizes the infection process, we should bear in mind that, in microbiology, host–pathogen interactions are special cases. Microbes can and do adhere to a wide range of animate and inanimate surfaces in a very nonspecific manner. For example, the human parasite *S. pyogenes* not only adheres to human epithelial cells but also to the surface of hydrocarbon droplets.[289,290] The hydrocarbon-degrading saprophyte *Acinetobacter calcoaceticus* RAG-1, on the other hand, binds to human epithelial cells in addition to its normal habitat of hydrocarbon droplets.[289,290] Furthermore, if a RAG-1 variant loses the ability to adhere to hydrocarbon droplets, it also loses the ability to adhere to epithelial cells.[289] This demonstrates that certain common adherence mechanisms mediate the binding of many different kinds of microbes to many different substrata. Less attention has been paid in the medical literature to these nonspecific processes since they do not directly select for the host. Nevertheless, nonspecific processes such as hydrophobicity are important for their ability to potentiate more specific adherence processes and promote the colonization and infection of inanimate foreign bodies such as indwelling medical devices.

Hydrophobicity. Since the human host is an aqueous environment, suspended particles with hydrophobic surfaces, such as microbes, will tend to leave the water phase and associate with host tissues. The earlier cited example of bacterial adherence to hydrocarbon droplets is, itself, an indirect measurement of microbial surface hydrophobicity,[289–291] as are hydrophobic interaction chromatography[182,229,292–295] and phase partition studies.[296–298] Microorganisms determined to be hydrophobic by these means have a greater tendency to adhere to animal tissues than do hydrophilic particles. The microbial expression of hydrophobicity, like other adherence mechanisms, changes with the stage of growth,[229,289] in response to environmental[229] or genetic influences, and by display of adhesive structures.[299] For example, the streptococcal adhesin LTA[131,300] and the *E. coli* adhesins type I fimbriae,[182] CFA fimbriae,[301] and K88 fimbriae[294] have hydrophobic properties that increase the organisms's hydrophobicity and its tissue adherence. At the same time, the surface hydrophobicity and in vitro adherence vary greatly among *E. coli* strains with type I fimbriae.[302] Several authors have suggested that hydrophobicity promotes more specific binding by bringing the two surfaces together and stabilizing their juxtaposition so that specific interactions between complementary molecules can take place.[229,294,303] In this regard, Falkowski and colleagues[304] have provided evidence that there may be a hydrophobic binding domain for *E. coli* adherence to epithelial cells.

Adherence of Bacteria to Medical Devices. Microbial colonization and infection of medical devices probably do not depend upon specific substrate receptors but likely proceed through more nonspecific means. We know that the engineering and composition of the surfaces of various devices encourage or discourage microbial colonization. Studies of the in vitro adhesion of various microorganisms to urinary catheters,[305] prosthetic vascular grafts,[306] suture material,[307] myringotomy tubes,[308] and intravascular catheters[309,310] indicate that the device's roughness,[307–309] chemical composition,[305,310–313] and hydrophobicity[311,314,315] increase microbial colonization. More recent studies[316] of coagulase-negative staphylococci treated with antimicrobial agents measured hydrophobicity and showed an excellent correlation with adherence of these organisms to plastic tissue culture plates in vitro. This suggests that this adherence depends heavily on hydrophobic surface moieties. The precise method of microbe-to-device binding is unknown for most of these situations. In the case of coagulase-negative staphylococcal adherence to plastic catheters, however, the situation appears analogous to Fletcher's investigations into the formation of microbial slime layers on marine solid surfaces. Fletcher's study organism, a marine pseudomonad, bound to surfaces such as polystyrene and glass by producing extracellular adhesive polymeric substances.[317] In a similar manner, some but not all strains of coagulase-negative staphylococci bind in vitro to plastic, glass, and intravascular catheters in a slime layer consisting of polysaccharides.[87,318–321] Epidemiologic and animal studies suggest that this slime plays a role in the pathogenesis of coagulase-negative staphylococccal foreign-body infections.[87,318,322–324] Consistent with these findings are the observations of Bayston and Penny[325] and others[326–328] that, upon removal from the patient, cerebrospinal fluid shunts and intravascular catheters are covered with coagulase-negative staphylococci enmeshed in a slimy or mucoid deposit. Moreover, recent clinical evidence[329,330] demonstrates that medical treatment failures and shunt complications are more likely to occur in cerebrospinal fluid shunt infections due to slime-producing coagulase-negative staphylococci as compared with strains that fail to produce slime.

ANTIADHESIVE THERAPY

Now that a number of adhesin–receptor systems have been identified, workers are using this knowledge to design antiadhesive prophylactic strategies that interdict the infectious process before it begins.[331] Three areas of investigation to develop effective prophylactic strategies have included *(1)* immunization, including both passive and active vaccines, *(2)* antimicrobial therapy, and *(3)* novel antiadhesive therapies.

The identification and purification of bacterial adhesins have enabled the production of adhesin vaccines that could provide the host with long-lasting protection. In order to be effective, however, vaccine-generated antibodies must be released near the susceptible tissue and be able to block bacterial attachment. If the adhesin is characterized by antigenic variation (such as in *N. gonorrhoeae* fimbriae) or has multiple forms (as in *E. coli* fimbriae), then the successful vaccine will have to evoke an immune response to common epitopes of antigenic variants or be manufactured as a multivalent vaccine that includes all adhesin forms. These last two points have been the major stumbling blocks in the current efforts to produce effective antiadhesive vaccines. The recent discovery that some of the fimbrial types contain structurally conserved adhesion proteins[216] may overcome some of these obstacles; a vaccine prepared from a single adhesin protein may be protective against a broader variety of bacteria bearing fimbriae exhibiting the same sugar binding specificity.

Immunization experiments in humans demonstrated excellent vaccine efficacy against diarrhea caused by enterotoxigenic *E. coli*.[332] None of the 10 volunteers who previously received the lyophilized milk immunoglobulins that had been prepared from the colostrum of cows immunized with several *E. coli* virulence antigens developed diarrhea after an oral challenge with *E. coli* H10407. In contrast, 9 of 10 control volunteers who received an immunoglobulin concentrate with no anti-*E. coli* activity had diarrhea.

Bacterial adherence to tissues can be blocked by antibiotics. Subinhibitory concentrations of antibiotics poison a variety of biologic functions and result in profound effects upon the bacterial surface and adherence capabilities. These effects may be used to prevent bacterial adherence and infection, particularly if the host is only transiently and predictably at risk such as in the prophylaxis against bacterial endocarditis.

The effect of antibiotics on adherence is neither predictable nor readily explained. Some strains of *S. pyogenes*,[331] *S. mutans*,[333] *A. naeslundii*,[333] and *E. coli*[334] exhibit decreased adherence when grown in subinhibitory concentrations of penicillin. This antibiotic causes resting-phase *S. pyogenes* organisms to leak their adhesin, LTA, into the surrounding medium and become less adherent.[128] *Escherichia coli*, on the other hand, loses its fimbriae and mannose-sensitive adherence when grown in sublethal concentrations of various antibiotics including streptomycin.[123,331,335] Eisenstein et al.[336] noted that one streptomycin-resistant isolate of *E. coli* retained its fimbriation despite a concurrent loss in its adherence ability when the organisms were grown in streptomycin. Examination by electron microscopy indicated that the functionless fimbriae were twice the length of normal fimbriae.[336] Taken together, these reports indicate that sublethal antibiotics may induce the leakage of preformed adhesins from resting cells, suppress the formation or expression of adhesins in growing cells, or induce the formation of functionally aberrant forms. Alternatively, antibiotics may cause the organism to reveal hidden adhesins or induce adhesin formation.

In addition to the traditional therapeutic modalities of antibiotics and vaccination, novel approaches to the prophylaxis of infectious diseases may become possible through knowledge of the specific adherence mechanisms involved. Aronson et al. reasoned that mannose and its derivatives would act as receptor analogues and block the attachment of type I fimbriated *E. coli* to mouse bladder epithelial cells.[184] To test this hypothesis, they instilled *E. coli* with either the receptor analogue, α-methylmannoside or the control α-methylglucoside into mouse bladders. Animals receiving the receptor analogue had far fewer episodes of cystitis than did animals receiving the control carbohydrate. Receptor analogue therapy may become complicated if the receptor analogue binds to the cell and functions as a cell surface receptor or if the receptor analogue also blocks attachment of the bacterium to professional phagocytes. Bar-Shavit et al.[337] demonstrated that when type I fimbriated organisms were instilled into the peritoneal cavity of mice along with mannose the virulence of the organisms was accentuated. The alternative approach, using chemical modification of the surface, was elegantly demonstrated by Parsons et al.[338–340] They noted that the natural glycosaminoglycan layer covering the urinary bladder mucosa prevented the adherence of bacteria. Stripping the bladder of the cover increased bacterial adherence, but covering the denuded surface with natural (heparin) or synthetic glycoaminoglycans once again protected it from bacterial adherence.

ACKNOWLEDGMENTS

The authors would like to thank the following individuals who provided key suggestions in the revision of this chapter: Drs. Joel B. Baseman, James P. Duguid, Richard A. Finkelstein, Madilyn Fletcher, Anthony G. Gristina, Richard E. Isaacson, Kevin Marshall, Itzak Ofek, Barrett Sugarman, and John Swanson. We are also indebted to Susan Selig for reference review and Pamela Swann for her untiring efforts in the preparation of the chapter revision.

REFERENCES

1. Guyot G. Uber die bakterielle hemagglutination. Zbt Bakt Abt I Orig. 1908;47:640–53.
2. Zobell CE, Allen EC. The significance of marine bacteria in the fouling of submerged surfaces. J Bacteriol. 1935;29:239–51.
3. Duguid JP, Smith IW, Dempster G, et al. Non-flagellar filamentous appendages ("fimbriae") and haemagglutinating activity in *Bacterium coli*. J Pathol Bacteriol. 1955;70:335–48.
4. Duguid JP, Gillies RR. Fimbriae and adhesive properties in dysentery bacilli. J Pathol Bacteriol. 1957;74:397–411.
5. Duguid JP, Gillies RR. Fimbriae and haemagglutinating activity in *Salmonella, Klebsiella, Proteus* and *Chromobacterium*. J Pathol Bacteriol. 1958;75:519–20.
6. Duguid JP. Fimbriae and adhesive properties in klebsiella strains. J Gen Microbiol. 1959;21:271–86.
7. Duguid JP, Anderson ES. Fimbriae and adhesive properties in salmonellae. J Pathol Bacteriol. 1966;92:107–38.
8. Duguid JP, Anderson ES. Terminology of bacterial fimbriae, or pili, and their types. Nature. 1967;215:89–90.
9. Duguid JP, Old DC. Adhesive properties of Enterobacteriaceae. In: Beachey EH, ed. Bacterial Adherence (Receptors and Recognition). v. 6. ser. B. New York: Chapman & Hall; 1980:184–218.
10. Gibbons RJ, van Houte J. Bacterial adherence and the formation of dental plaques. In: Beachey EH, ed. Bacterial Adherence (Receptors and Recognition). v. 6. ser. B. New York: Chapman & Hall; 1980:60–104.
11. van Houte J. Bacterial adherence and dental plaque formation. Infection. 1982;10:252–60.
12. Beachey EH, ed. Bacterial Adherence (Receptors and Recognition). v. 6. ser. B. New York: Chapman & Hall; 1980.
13. Berkeley RCW, Lynch JM, Melling J, et al. Microbial Adhesion to Surfaces. Chichester, England: Ellis Horwood; 1980.
14. Bitton G, Marshall KC. Adsorption of Microorganisms to Surfaces. New York: John Wiley & Sons; 1980.
15. Marshall KC. Interfaces in Microbial Ecology. Cambridge, MA: Harvard University Press; 1976.
16. Elliot K, O'Connor M, Whelan J. Adhesion and Microorganisms Pathogenicity, Ciba Foundation Symposium 80. London: Pitman Medical; 1981.
17. Beachey EH, Eisenstein BI, Ofek I. Bacterial Adherence in Infectious Diseases, Current Concepts. Kalamazoo, MI: Upjohn; 1982.
18. Gaastra W, de Graaf FK. Host-specific fimbrial adhesins of noninvasive enterotoxigenic *Escherichia coli* strains. Microbiol Rev. 1982;46:129–61.
19. Smith H. Microbial surfaces in relation to pathogenicity. Bacteriol Rev. 1977;41:475–500.
20. Beachey EH. Bacterial adherence: Adhesin–receptor interactions mediating the attachment of bacteria to mucosal surfaces. J Infect Dis. 1981;143:325–45.
21. Costerton JW, Geesey GG, Cheng K-J. How bacteria stick. Sci Am. 1978;238:86–95.
22. Jones GW. The attachment of bacteria to the surface of animal cells. In: Reissig JL, ed. Microbial Intereactions (Receptors and Recognition). v. 3. ser. B. London: Chapman & Hall; 1977:139–76.
23. Geesey GG. Microbial exopolymers: Ecological and economic considerations. Am Soc Microbiol News. 1982;48:9–14.
24. Ward JB, Berkeley RCW. The microbial cell surface and adhesion. In: Berkeley RCW, Lynch JM, Melling J, et al, eds. Microbial Adhesion to Surfaces. Chichester, England: Ellis Horwood; 1980:48–60.
25. Bennet HS. Morphological aspects of extracellular polysaccharides. J Histochem Cytochem. 1963;11:14–23.
26. Ito S. Structure and function of the glycocalyx. Fed Proc. 1969;28:12–25.
27. Goldstein IJ, Hughes RC, Monsigny M, et al. What should be called a lectin? Nature. 1980;285:66.
28. Freter R. Mechanisms of association of bacteria with mucosal surfaces. In: Elliot K, O'Connor M, Whelan J, eds. Adhesion and Microorganism Pathogenicity, Ciba Foundation Symposium 80. London: Pitman Medical; 1981:36–55.
29. Marshall KC, Stout R, Mitchell R. Mechanism of the initial events in the sorption of marine bacteria to surfaces. J Gen Microbiol. 1971;68:337–48.
30. Fletcher M, Latham MJ, Lynch JM, et al. The characteristics of interfaces and their role in microbial attachment. In: Berkeley RCW, Lynch JM, Melling J, et al, eds. Microbial Adhesion to Surfaces. Chichester, England: Ellis Horwood; 1980:67–78.
31. Grieg RG, Jones MN. The possible role of steric forces in cellular cohesion. J Theor Biol. 1976;63:405–9.
32. Grieg RG, Jones MN. Mechanisms of intercellular adhesion. Biosystems. 1977;9:43–55.
33. Rutter PR, Vincent B. The adhesion of micro-organisms to surfaces: Physico-chemical aspects. In Berkeley RCW, Lynch JM, Melling J, et al, eds. Microbial Adhesion to Surfaces. Chichester, England: Ellis Horwood; 1980:79–92.
34. Tadros RF. Particle surface adhesion. In Berkeley RCW, Lynch JM, Melling J, et al, eds. Microbial Adhesion to Surfaces. Chichester, England: Ellis Horwood; 1980:93–116.
35. Ofek I, Sharon N. Lectinophagocytosis: A molecular mechanism of recognition between cell surface sugars and lectins in the phagocytosis of bacteria. Infect Immun. 1988;56:539–47.
36. Meager A, Hughes RC. Virus receptors. In: Cuatrecasas P, Greaves MF, eds. Receptors and Recognition, v. 4, ser. A. London: Chapman & Hall; 1977:143–59.
37. Crowell RL, Lonberg-Holm K. Viral Attachment and Entry Into Cells. Washington DC: American Society for Microbiology; 1986.
38. Levy NJ. Wheat germ agglutinin blockage of chlamydial attachment sites: antagonism by *N*-acetyl-D-glucosamine. Infect Immun. 1979;25:946–53.
39. Levy NJ, Moulder JW. Attachment of cell walls of *Chlamydia psittaci* to mouse fibroblasts (L cells). Infect Immun. 1982;37:1059–65.
40. Razin S, Kahane I, Banai M, et al. Adhesion of mycoplasms to eukaryotic cells. In: Elliot K, O'Connor M, Whelan J, eds. Adhesion and Microorganism Pathogenicity, Ciba Foundation symposium 80. London: Pitman Medical; 1981:98–106.
41. Krause DC, Baseman JB. Inhibition of *Mycoplasma pneumoniae* hemadsorption and adherence to respiratory epithelium by antibodies to a membrane protein. Infect Immun. 1983;39:1180–6.
42. Krause DC, Leith DK, Baseman JB. Reacquisition of specific proteins confers virulence in *Mycoplasma pneumoniae*. Infect Immun. 1983;39:830–6.
43. Chick S, Harber MJ, Mackenzie R, et al. Modified method for studying bacterial adhesion to isolated uroepithelial cells and uromucoid. Infect Immun. 1981;34:256–61.
44. Firon N, Ofek I, Sharon N. Interaction of mannose-containing oligosaccharides with the fimbrial lectin of *Escherichia coli*. Biochem Biophys Res Commun. 1982;105:1426–32.
45. Laux DC, McSweegan EF, Williams TJ, et al. Identification and characterization of mouse small intestine mucosal receptors for *Escherichia coli* K-12 (K88ab). Infect Immun. 1986;52:18–25.
46. Smit H, Gaastra W, Kamerling JP, et al. Isolation and structural characterization of the equine erythrocyte receptor for enterotoxigenic *Escherichia coli* K99 fimbrial adhesion. Infect Immun. 1984;46:578–84.
47. Faris A, Lindahl M, Wadstrom T. GM_2-like glycoconjugate as possible erythrocyte receptor for the CFA/I and K99 hemagglutinins of enterotoxigenic *Escherichia coli*. FEMS Microbiol Lett. 1980;7:265–9.
48. Isaacson RE, Richter P. *Escherichia coli* 987P pilus: Purification and partial characterization. J Bacteriol. 1981;146:784–9.
49. Dean EA, Isaacson RE. In vitro adhesion of piliated *Escherichia coli* to small intestinal villous epithelial cells from rabbits and the identification of a soluble 987P pilus receptor-containing fraction. Infect Immun. 1982;36:1192–8.
50. Dean EA, Isaacson RE. Purification and characterization of a receptor for the 987P pilus of *Escherichia coli*. Infect Immun. 1985;47:98–105.
51. Dean EA, Isaacson RE. Location and distribution of a receptor for the 987P pilus of *Escherichia coli* in small intestines. Infect Immun. 1985;47:345–8.
52. de Graaf F, Frits K, Roorda I. Production, purification, and characterization of the fimbrial adhesive antigen F41 isolated from calf enteropathogenic *Escherichia coli* strain B41M. Infect Immun. 1982;36:751–8.
53. Morris JA, Thorns C, Scott AC, et al. Adhesion *in vitro* and *in vivo* associated with an adhesive antigen (F41) produced by a K99 mutant of the reference strain *Escherichia coli* B41. Infect Immun. 1982;36:1146–53.
54. Thomas LV, Cravioto A, Scotland SM, et al. New fimbrial antigenic type (E8775) that may represent a colonization factor in enterotoxigenic *Escherichia coli* in humans. Infect Immun. 1982;35:1119–24.
55. Thomas LV, McConnell MM, Rowe B, Field AM. The possession of three novel coli surface antigens by enterotoxigenic *Escherichia coli* strains positive for the putative colonization factor PCF8775. J Gen Microbiol. 1985;131:2319–26.
56. Thomas LV, Rowe B, McConnell MM. In strains of *Escherichia coli* 0167 a single plasmid encodes for the coli surface antigens CS5 and CS6 of putative colonization factor PCF8775, heat-stable enterotoxin, and colicin IA. Infect Immun. 1987;55:1929–31.
57. Leffler H, Svanborg-Eden C. Glycolipid receptors for uropathogenic *Escherichia coli* on human erythrocytes and uroepithelial cells. Infect Immun. 1981;34:920–9.
58. Svenson SB, Hultberg H, Kallenius G, et al. P-fimbriae of pyelonephritogenic *Escherichia coli*: Identification and chemical characterization of receptors. Infection. 1983;11:61–7.
59. Fader RC, Duffy LK, Davis CP, et al. Purification and chemical characterization of type 1 pili isolated from *Klebsiella pneumoniae*. J Biol Chem. 1982;257:3301–5.
60. Korhonen TK, Lounatmaa K, Ranta H, et al. Characterization of type 1 pili of *Salmonella typhimurium* LT2. J. Bacteriol. 1980;144:800–5.
61. Mirelman D, Altmann G, Eshdat Y. Screening of bacterial isolates for mannose-specific lectin activity by agglutination of yeast. J Clin Microbiol. 1980;11:328–31.
62. Pearce WA, Buchanan TM. Structure and cell membrane-binding properties of bacterial fimbriae. In: Beachey EH, ed. Bacterial Adherence (Receptors and Recognition). v. 6. ser. B. New York: Chapman & Hall, 1980:289–344.
63. Pruzzo C, Debbia EA, Satta G. Identification of the major adherence ligand of *Klebsiella pneumoniae* in the receptor for coliphage T7 and alteration of *Klebsiella* adherence properties by lysogenic conversion. Infect Immun. 1980;30:562–71.
64. Old DC, Adegbola RA. Haemagglutinins and fimbriae of *Morganella, Proteus,* and *Providencia*. J Med Microbiol. 1982;15:551–64.
65. Old DC, Scott SS. Hemagglutinins and fimbriae of *Providencia* spp. J Bacteriol. 1981;146:404–8.
66. Maclagan RM, Old DC. Hemagglutinins and fimbriae in different serotypes and biotypes of *Yersinia enterocolitica*. J Appl Bacteriol. 1980;49:353–60.
67. Old DC, Robertson J. Adherence of fimbriate and non-fimbriate strains of

Yersinia enterocolitica to human epithelial cells. Microbiol Immunol. 1981;25:993–8.
68. Sastry PA, Pearlstone JR, Smillie LB, et al. Amino acid sequence of pilin isolated from *Pseudomonas aeruginosa* PAK. FEBS Lett. 1983;151:253–6.
69. Woods DE, Straus DC, Johanson WG Jr, et al. Role of pili in adherence of *Pseudomonas aeruginosa* to mammalian buccal epithelial cells. Infect Immun. 1980;29:1146–51.
70. Glorioso JC, Jones GW, Rush HG, et al. Adhesion of type A *Pasteurella multocida* to rabbit pharyngeal cells and its possible role in rabbit respiratory tract infections. Infect Immun. 1982;35:1103–9.
71. Muse KE, Collier AM, Baseman JB. Scanning electron microscopic study of hamster tracheal organ cultures infected with *Bordetella pertussis*. J Infect Dis. 1977;136:768–77.
72. Morse JH, Morse SI. Studies on the ultrastructure of *Bordetella pertussis*. I. Morphology, origin, and biological activity of structures present in the extracellular fluid of liquid cultures of *Bordetella pertussis*. J Exp Med. 1970;131:1342–57.
73. Sato Y, Sato H, Izumiya K, et al. Role of antibody of filamentous hemagglutinin in immunity to pertussis. In: Robbins JB, Hill JC, Sadoff JC, eds. Bacterial Vaccines (Symposium on Infectious Diseases). New York: Thieme; 1981:380–5.
74. Lampe RM, Mason EO Jr, Kaplan SL, et al. Adherence of *Haemophilus influenzae* to buccal epithelial cells. Infect Immun. 1982;35:166–72.
75. Pichichero ME, Loeb M, Anderson P, et al. Do pili play a role in pathogenicity of *Haemophilus influenzae* type B? Lancet. 1982;2:960–2.
76. Nelson ET, Clements JD, Finkelstein RA. *Vibrio cholerae* adherence and colonization in experimental cholera: Electron microscopic studies. Infect Immun. 1976;14:527–47.
77. Finkelstein RA, Hanne LF. Purification and characterization of the soluble hemagglutinin (cholera lectin) produced by *Vibrio cholerae*. Infect Immun. 1982;36:1199–208.
78. Finkelstein RA, Boesman-Finkelstein M, Holt P. *Vibrio cholera* hemagglutinin/lectin/protease hydrolyzes fibronectin and ovomucin: F. M. Burnet revisited. Proc Natl Acad Sci USA. 1983;80:1092–5.
79. Rodgers FG, Greaves PW, Macrae AD, Lewis MJ. Electron microscopic evidence of flagella and pili on *Legionella pneumophila*. J Clin Pathol. 1980;33:1184–8.
80. Stephens DS, McGee ZA. Attachment of *Neisseria meningitidis* to human mucosal surfaces: Influence of pili and type of receptor cell. J Infect Dis. 1981;143:525–32.
81. Salit IE, Morton G. Adherence of *Neisseria meningitidis* to human epithelial cells. Infect Immun. 1981;31:430–5.
82. Swanson J. Adhesion and entry of bacteria into cells: A model of the pathogenesis of gonorrhea. In: Smith H, Skehel JJ, Turner MJ, eds. The Molecular Basis of Microbial Pathogenicity, Dahlem Konferenzen. Weinheim: Verlag Chemie GmbH; 1980:17–40.
83. Lambden PR, Heckels JE, James LT, et al. Variations in surface protein composition associated with virulence properties in opacity types of *Neisseria gonorrhoeae*. J Gen Microbiol. 1979;114:305–12.
84. Sato H, Yanagawa R, Fukuyama H. Adhesion of *Corynebacterium renale, Corynebacterium pilosum,* and *Corynebacterium cystitidis* to bovine urinary bladder epithelial cells of various ages and levels of differentiation. Infect Immun. 1982;36:1241–5.
85. Honda E, Yanagawa R. Pili-mediated attachment of *Corynebacterium renale* to mucous membrane of urinary bladder of mice. Am J Vet Res. 1978;39:155–8.
86. Carruthers MM, Kabat WJ. Mediation of staphylococcal adherence to mucosal cells by lipoteichoic acid. Infect Immun. 1983;40:444–6.
87. Christensen GD, Simpson WA, Bisno AL, et al. Adherence to slime-producing strains of *Streptococcus epidermidis* to smooth surfaces. Infect Immun. 1982;37:318–26.
88. Simpson WA, Beachey EH. Adherence of group A streptococci to fibronectin on oral epithelial cells. Infect Immun. 1983;39:275–9.
89. Simpson WA, Hasty DL, Mason JM, et al. Fibronectin-mediated binding of group A streptococci to human polymorphonuclear leukocytes. Infect Immun. 1982;37:805–10.
90. Babu J, Simpson WA, Courtney HS, et al. Interaction of human plasma fibronectin with cariogenic and non-cariogenic oral streptococci. Infect Immun. 1983;41:162–8.
91. Switalski LM, Ljungh A, Ryden C, et al. Binding of fibronectin to the surface of group A, C, and G streptococci isolated from human infections. Eur J Clin Microbiol. 1982;1:381–7.
92. Germaine GR, Schachtele CF. *Streptococcus mutans* dextransucrase: Mode of interaction with high-molecular-weight dextran and role in cellular aggregation. Infect Immun. 1976;13:365–72.
93. Liljemark WF, Schauer SV. Competitive binding among oral streptococci to hydroxyapatite. J Dent Res. 1977;56:157–65.
94. McCabe MM, Hamelik RM, Smith EE. Purification of dextran-binding protein from cariogenic *Streptococcus mutans*. Biochem Biophys Res. Commun. 1977;78:273–8.
95. Staat RH, Langley SD, Doyle RJ. *Streptococcus mutans* adherence: Presumptive evidence for protein-mediated attachment followed by glucan-dependent cellular accumulation. Infect Immun. 1980;27:675–81.
96. Wenham DG, Davies RM, Cole JA. Insoluble glucan synthesis by mutansucrase as a determinant of the cariogenicity of *Streptococcus mutans*. J Gen Microbiol. 1981;127:407–15.
97. Gibbons RJ, Qureshi JV. Inhibition of adsorption of *Streptococcus mutans* strains to saliva-treated hydroxyapatite by galactose and certain amines. Infect Immun. 1979;26:1214–7.
98. Hogg SD, Embery G. Blood-group reactive glycoprotein from human saliva interacts with lipoteichoic acid on the surface of *Streptococcus sanguis* cells. Arch Oral Biol. 1982;27:261–8.
99. Hogg SD, Handley PS, Embery G. Surface fibrils may be responsible for the salivary glycoprotein-mediated aggregation of the oral bacterium *Streptococcus sanguis*. Arch Oral Biol. 1981;26:945–9.
100. Kolenbrander PE. Isolation and characterization of coaggregation detective mutants of *Actinomyces viscosus, Actinomyces naeslundii,* and *Streptococcus sanguis*. Infect Immun. 1982;37:1200–8.
101. Liljemark WF, Bloomquist CG. Isolation of a protein-containing cell surface component from *Streptococcus sanguis* which affects its adherence to saliva-coated hydroxyapatite. Infect Immun. 1981;34:428–34.
102. Weerkamp AH, Jacobs T. Cell wall-associated protein antigens of *Streptococcus salivarius*: Purification, properties, and function in adherence. Infect Immun. 1982; 38:233–42.
103. Weerkamp AH, McBride BC. Identification of a *Streptococcus salivarius* cell wall component mediating coaggregation with *Veillonella alcalescens* V-1. Infect Immun. 1981;32:723–30.
104. McCabe RM, Donkersloot JA. Adherence of *Veillonella* species mediated by extracellular glucosyltransferase from *Streptococcus salivarius*. Infect Immun. 1977;18:726–34.
105. Bagg J, Poxton IR, Weir DM, et al. Binding of type 111 group B streptococci to buccal epithelial cells. J Med Microbiol. 1982;15:363–72.
106. Broughton RA, Baker CJ. Role of adherence in the pathogenesis of neonatal group B streptococcal infection. Infect Immun. 1983;39:837–43.
107. Handley PS, Jacob AE. Some structural and physiological properties of fimbriae of *Streptococcus faecalis*. J Gen Microbiol. 1981;127(Pt 2):289–93.
108. Onderdonk AB, Moon NE, Kasper DL, et al. Adherence of *Bacteroides fragilis* in vivo. Infect Immun. 1978;19:1083–7.
109. Yamazaki Y, Ebisu S, Okada H. *Eikonella corrodens* adherence to human buccal epithelial cells. Infect Immun. 1981;31:21–7.
110. Revis GJ, Vatter AE, Crowle AJ, et al. Antibodies against the Ag2 fimbriae of *Actinomyces viscosus* T14V inhibit lactose-sensitive bacterial adherence. Infect Immun. 1982;36:1217–22.
111. Clark WB, Webb EL, Wheeler TT, et al. Role of surface fimbriae (fibrils) in the adsorption of *Actinomyces* species to saliva-treated hydroxyapatite surfaces. Infect Immun. 1981;33:908–17.
112. Bourgeau G, McBride BC. Dextran mediates interbacterial aggregation between dextran-synthesizing streptococci and *Actinomyces viscosus*. Infect Immun. 1976;13:1228–34.
113. Ellen RP, Walker DL, Chau KH. Association of long surface appendages with adherence related functions of the gram-positive species *Actinomyces naeslundii*. J Bacteriol. 1978;134:1171–5.
114. Thomas DD, Baseman JB, Alderette JF. Fibronectin mediates *Treponema pallidum* cytadherence through recognition of fibronectin cell-binding domain. J Exp Med. 1985;161:514–25.
115. Thomas DD, Baseman JB, Alderette JF. Putative *Treponema pallidum* cytadhesins share a common functional domain. Infect Immun. 1985;49:833–5.
116. Maisch PA, Calderone RA. Role of surface mannan in the adherence of *Candida albicans* to fibrin-platelet clots formed in vitro. Infect Immun. 1981;32:92–7.
117. Sandin RL, Rogers AL, Patterson RJ, et al. Evidence for mannose-mediated adherence of *Candida albicans* to human buccal cells in vitro. Infect Immun. 1982;35:79–85.
118. Howard RJ, Miller LH. Invasion of erythrocytes by malaria merozoites: Evidence for specific receptors involved in attachment and entry. In: Elliott K, O'Connor M, Whelan J, eds. Adhesion and Microbial Pathogenicity, Ciba Foundation Symposium 80. Tunbridge Well, England: Pitman Medical; 1981:202–14.
119. Jungery M, Pasvol G, Newbold CI, et al. A lectin-like receptor is involved in invasion of erythrocytes by *Plasmodium falciparum*. Proc Natl Acad Sci USA. 1983;80:1018–22.
120. Kobiler D, Mirelman D. Lectin activity in *Entamoeba histolytica* trophozoites. Infect Immun. 1980;29:221–5.
121. Kobiler D, Mirelman D. Adhesion of *Entamoeba histolytica* trophozoites to monolayers of human cells. J Infect Dis. 1981;144:539–46.
122. Erlandsen SL, Chase DG. Morphological alterations in the microvillous border of villous epithelial cells produced by intestinal microorganisms. Am J Clin Nutr. 1974;27:1277–86.
123. Beachey EH, Ofek I. Epithelial cell binding of group A streptococci by lipoteichoic acid on fimbriae denuded of M protein. J Exp Med. 1976;143:759–71.
124. Ellen RP, Gibbons RJ. Parameters affecting the adherence and tissue tropisms of *Streptococcus pyogenes*. Infect Immun. 1974;9:85–91.
125. Ofek I, Beachey EH, Jefferson W, et al. Cell membrane-binding properties of group A streptococcal lipoteichoic acid. J Exp Med. 1975;141:990–1003.
126. Simpson WA, Ofek I, Sarasohn C. Characteristics of the binding of streptococcal lipoteichoic acid to human oral epithelial cells. J Infect Dis. 1980;141:457–62.
127. Wicken AJ, Knox KW. Biological properties of lipoteichoic acids. In: Schlessinger D, ed. Microbiology. Washington, DC: American Society for Microbiology; 1977:360–365.
128. Alkan ML, Beachey EH. Excretion of lipoteichoic acid by group A strep-

tococci: Influence of penicillin on excretion and loss of ability to adhere to human oral epithelial cells. J Clin Invest. 1978;61:671–7.
129. Ofek I, Simpson WA, Beachey EH. Formation of molecular complexes between a structurally defined M protein and acylated or deacylated lipoteichoic acid of *Streptococcus pyogenes*. J Bacteriol. 1982;149:426–33.
130. Hill MJ, James AM, Maxted WR. Some physical investigations of the behaviour of bacterial surfaces. X. The occurrence of lipid in the streptococcal cell wall. Biochim Biophys Acta. 1963;75:414–24.
131. Ofek I, Whitnack E, Beachey EH. Hydrophobic interactions of group A streptococci with hexadecane droplets. J Bacteriol. 1983;154:139–45.
132. Tylewska S, Hjerten S, Wadstrom T. Contribution of M protein to the hydrophobic surface properties of *Streptococcus pyogenes*. FEMS Microbiol Lett. 1979;6:249–53.
133. Miorner H, Johansson G, Kronvall G. Lipoteichoic acid is the major cell wall component responsible for surface hydrophobicity of group A streptococci. Infect Immun. 1983;39:336–43.
134. Alkan M, Ofek I, Beachey EH. Adherence of pharyngeal and skin strains of group A streptococci to human skin and oral epithelial cells. Infect Immun. 1977;18:555–7.
135. Selinger DS, Julie N, Reed WP, et al. Adherence of group A streptococci to pharyngeal cells: A role in the pathogenesis of rheumatic fever. Science. 1978;201:455–7.
136. Ofek I, Beachey EH, Eyal F, et al. Postnatal development of binding of streptococci and lipoteichoic acid by oral mucosal cells of humans. J Infect Dis. 1977;135:267–74.
137. Beachey EH, Simpson WA, Ofek I. Interaction of surface polymers of *Streptococcus pyogenes* with animal cells. In: Berkeley RCW, Lynch JM, Melling J, et al, eds. Microbial Adhesion to Surfaces. London: Ellis Horwood; 1980:389–405.
138. Chiang TM, Alkan ML, Beachey EH. Binding of lipoteichoic acid of group A streptococci to isolated human erythrocyte membranes. Infect Immun. 1979;26:316–21.
139. Courtney H, Ofek I, Simpson WA, et al. Characterization of lipoteichoic acid binding to polymorphonuclear leukocytes of human blood. Infect Immun. 1981;32:625–31.
140. Beachey EH, Dale JB, Simpson WA, et al. Erythrocyte binding properties of streptococcal lipoteichoic acids. Infect Immun. 1979;23:618–25.
141. Beachey EH, Chiang TM, Ofek I, et al. Interaction of lipoteichoic acid of group A streptococci with human platelets. Infect Immun. 1977;16:649–54.
142. Beachey EH, Dale JB, Grebe S, et al. Lymphocyte binding and T-cell mitogenic properties of group A streptococcal lipoteichoic acid. J Immunol. 1979;122:189–95.
143. Simpson WA, Beachey EH. Adherence of group A streptococci to fibronectin on oral epithelial cells. Infect Immun. 1983;39:275–9.
144. Courtney HS, Simpson WA, Beachey EH. Binding of streptococcal lipoteichoic acid to fatty-binding sites on human plasma fibronectin. J Bacteriol. 1983;153:763–70.
145. Phillips GN Jr, Flicker PF, Cohen C, et al. Streptococcal M protein: alpha-helical coiled-coil structure and arrangement on the cell surface. Proc Natl Acad Sci USA. 1981;78:4689–93.
146. Nealon TJ, Beachey EH, Courtney HS, et al. Release of fibronectin-lipoteichoic acid complexes from group A streptococci with penicillin. Infect Immun. 1986;51:529–35.
147. Stanislawski L, Courtney HS, Simpson WA, et al. Hybridoma antibodies to the lipid-binding site(s) in the amino-terminal region of fibronectin inhibits binding of streptococcal lipoteichoic acid. J Infect Dis. 1987;156:344–9.
148. Mosher DF, Proctor RA. Binding and factor XIIIa-mediated cross-linking of a 27-kilodalton fragment of fibronectin to *Staphylococcus aureus*. Science. 1980;209:927–9.
149. Kuusela P, Vartio T, Vuento M, et al. Binding sites for streptococci and staphylococci in fibronectin. Infect Immun. 1984;45:433–6.
150. Hasty DL, Courtney HS, Simpson WA, et al. Immunochemical and ultrastructural mapping of the gelatin-binding and cell-attachment regions of human plasma fibronectin with monoclonal antibodies. J Cell Sci. 1986;81:125–41.
151. Whitnack E, Bisno AL, Beachey EH. Hyaluronate capsule prevents attachment of group A streptococci to mouse peritoneal macrophages. Infect Immun. 1981;31:985–91.
152. Whitnack E, Beachey EH. Antiopsonic activity of fibrinogen bound to M protein on the surface of group A streptococci. J Clin Invest. 1982;69:1042–5.
153. Davis CP, Avots-Avotins AE, Fader RC. Evidence for a bladder cell glycolipid receptor for *Escherichia coli* and the effect of neuraminic acid and colominic acid on adherence. Infect Immun. 1981;34:944–8.
154. Klemm P. The complete amino-acid sequence of the K88 antigen, a fimbrial protein from *Escherichia coli*. Eur J Biochem. 1981;117:617–27.
155. de Graaf FK, Klemm P, Gaastra W. Purification, characterization, and partial covalent structure of *Escherichia coli* adhesive antigen K99. Infect Immun. 1980;33:877–83.
156. Klemm P. Primary structure of the CFA-1 fimbrial protein from human enterotoxigenic *Escherichia coli* strains. Eur J Biochem. 1982;124:339–48.
157. Honda T, Khan MM, Takeda Y, et al. Grouping of enterotoxigenic *Escherichia coli* by hydrophobicity and its relation to hemagglutination and enterotoxin productions. FEMS Microbiol Lett. 1983;17:273–6.
158. Honda T, Arita M, Miwatani T. Characterization of new hydrophobic pili of human enterotoxigenic *Escherichia coli*: A possible new colonization factor. Infect Immun. 1984;43:959–65.
159. Cheney CP, Formal SB, Schad PA, et al. Genetic transfer of a mucosal adherence factor (R1) from an enteropathogenic *Escherichia coli* strain into a *Shigella flexneri* strain and the phenotypic suppression of this adherence factor. J Infect Dis. 1983;147:711–23.
160. Berendson R, Cheney CP, Schad PA, et al. Species-specific binding of purified pili (AF/R1) from the *Escherichia coli* RDEC-1 to rabbit intestinal mucosa. Gastroenterology 1983;85:837–45.
161. Sherman PM, Houston WL, Boedeker EC. Functional heterogeneity of intestinal *Escherichia coli* strains expressing type 1 somatic pili (fimbriae): Assessment of bacterial adherence to intestinal membranes and surface hydrophobicity. Infect Immun. 1985;49:797–804.
162. Inman LR, Cantey JR, Formal SB. Colonization, virulence, and mucosal interaction of an enteropathogenic *Escherichia coli* (strain RDEC-1) expressing shigella somatic antigen in the rabbit intestine. J Infect Dis. 1986;154:742–51.
163. Sherman PM, Boedeker EC. Pilus-mediated interactions of the *Escherichia coli* strain RDEC-1 with mucosal glycoproteins in the small intestine of rabbits. Gastroenterology 1987;93:734–43.
164. Kallenius G, Mollby R, Svenson SB, et al. Occurrence of P-fimbriated *Escherichia coli* in urinary tract infections. Lancet. 1981;2:1369–72.
165. Hull RA, Gill RE, Hsu P, et al. Construction and expression of recombinant plasmids encoding type 1 or D-mannose-resistant pili from a urinary tract infection *Escherichia coli* isolate. Infect Immun. 1981;33:933–8.
166. Klemm P, Orskov I, Orskov F. Isolation and characterization of F-12 adhesive fimbrial antigen from uropathogenic *Escherichia coli* strains. Infect Immun. 1983;40:91–6.
167. Korhonen TK, Vaisanen V, Kallio P, et al. The role of pili in the adhesion of *Escherichia coli* to human urinary tract epithelial cells. Scand J Infect Dis. 1982;33(Suppl):26–31.
168. Korhonen TK, Vaisanen V, Saxen H, et al. P-antigen–recognizing fimbriae from human uropathogenic *Escherichia coli* strains. Infect Immun. 1982;37:286–91.
169. Orskov I, Orskov F, Birch-Andersen A, et al. O, K, H and fimbrial antigens in *Escherichia coli* serotypes associated with pyelonephritis and cystitis. Scand J Infect Dis. 1982;33(Suppl):18–25.
170. Korhonen TK, Valtonen MV, Parkkinen J, et al. Serotypes, hemolysin production, and receptor recognition of *Escherichia coli* strains associated with neonatal sepsis and meningitis. Infect Immun. 1985;48:486–91.
171. Parkkinen J, Finne J, Achtman M, et al. *Escherichia coli* strains binding to neuraminyl 2-3 galactosides. Biochem Biophys Res Commun. 1983;111:456–61.
172. Korhonen TK, Vaisanen-Rhen V, Rhen M, et al. *Escherichia coli* fimbriae recognizing sialyl galactosides. J Bacteriol. 1984;159:762–6.
173. Parkkinen J, Rogers GN, Korhonen T, et al. Identification of the O-linked sialyloligosaccharides of glycophorin A as the erythrocyte receptors for S-fimbriated *Escherichia coli*. Infect Immun. 1986;54:37–42.
174. Sharon N, Ofek I. Mannose specific bacterial surface lectins. In Mirelman D, ed. Microbial Lectins. New York: John Wiley & Sons; 1986:55–81.
175. Sharon N. Bacterial lectins, cell-cell recognition and infectious diseases. FEBS Lett. 1987;217:145–57.
176. Korhonen TK, Leffler H, Svanborg-Eden C. Binding specificity of piliated strains of *Escherichia coli* and *Salmonella typhimurium* to epithelial cells, *Saccharomyces cerevisiae* cells and erythrocytes. Infect Immun. 1981;32:796–804.
177. Firon N, Ofek I, Sharon N. Carbohydrate-binding sites of the mannose-specific fimbrial lectins of enterobacteria. Infect Immun. 1984;43:1088–90.
178. Brinton CC Jr, Buzzell A, Lauffer MA. Electrophoresis and phage susceptibility studies on a filament-producing variant of the *E. coli* B bacterium. Biochim Biophys Acta. 1954;15:533–42.
179. Czirok E, Orskov I, Orskov F. O:K:H:F serotypes of fimbriated *Escherichia coli* strain isolated from infants with diarrhea. Infect Immun. 1982;37:519–25.
180. Jann K, Schmidt G, Blumenstock E, et al. *Escherichia coli* adhesion to *Saccharomyces cerevisiae* and mammalian cells: Role of piliation and surface hydrophobicity. Infect Immun. 1981;32:484–8.
181. Klemm P. Fimbrial colonization factor CFA/1 protein from human enteropathogenic *Escherichia coli* strains. FEBS Lett. 1979;108:107–10.
182. Bergman MJ, Updike WS, Wood SJ, et al. Attachment factors among enterotoxigenic *Escherichia coli* from patients with acute diarrhea from diverse geographic areas. Infect Immun. 1981;32:881–8.
183. Hagberg L, Hull R, Hull S, et al. Contribution of adhesion to bacterial persistence in the mouse urinary tract. Infect Immun. 1983;40:265–72.
184. Aronson M, Medalia O, Schori L, et al. Prevention of *E. coli* colonization of the urinary tract by blocking bacterial adherence with methyl alpha-D-mannopyranoside. J Infect Dis. 1979;139:329–32.
185. Rene P, Silverblatt FJ: Serological response to *Escherichia coli* pili in pyelonephritis. Infect Immun. 1982;37:749–54.
186. Hagberg L, Jodal U, Korhonen TK, et al. Adhesion, hemagglutination, and virulence of *Escherichia coli* causing urinary tract infections. Infect Immun. 1981;31:564–70.
187. Ofek I, Mosek A, Sharon N, Mannose-specific adherence to *Escherichia coli* freshly excreted in the urine of patients with urinary tract infections, and of isolates subcultured from the infected urine. Infect Immun. 1981;34:708–11.
188. Orskov I, Orskov F, Birch-Andersen A. Comparison of *Escherichia coli* fimbrial antigen F7 with type 1 fimbriae. Infect Immun. 1980;27:657–66.
189. Jones GW, Rutter JM. Role of the K88 antigen in the pathogenesis of neo-

natal diarrhea caused by *Escherichia coli* in piglets. Infect Immun. 1972;6:918–27.
190. Sellwood R. *Escherichia coli*-associated porcine neonatal diarrhea: Antibacterial activities of colostrum from generally susceptible and resistant sows. Infect Immun. 1982;35:396–401.
191. Smith HW, Huggins MB. The influence of plasmid-determined and other characteristics of enteropathogenic *Escherichia coli* on their ability to proliferate in the alimentary tracts of piglets, calves and lambs. J Med Microbiol. 1978;11:471–92.
192. Smith HW, Linggood MA. Observations on the pathogenic properties of the K88, Hly and Ent plasmids of *Escherichia coli* with particular reference to porcine diarrhoea. J Med Microbiol. 1971;4:467–85.
193. Sellwood R, Gibbons RA, Jones GW, et al. Adhesion of enteropathogenic *Escherichia coli* to pig intestinal brush borders: The existence of two pig phenotypes. J Med Microbiol. 1975;8:405–11.
194. Smith HW, Halls S. Observations by the ligated intestinal segment and oral inoculation methods in *Escherichia coli* infections in pigs, calves, lambs and rabbits. J Pathol Bacteriol. 1967;93:499–529.
195. Bijlsma IG, de Nijs A, Frik JF. Adhesion of *Escherichia coli* to porcine intestinal brush borders by means of serological variants of the K88 antigen. Antonie van Leeuwenhoek. 1981;47:467–8.
196. de Graaf FK, Roorda I. Production, purification and characterization of the fimbrial adhesive antigen F41 isolated from calf enteropathogenic *Escherichia coli* strain B41M. Infect Immun. 1982;36:751–8.
197. Cheney CP, Boedeker EC. Adherence of an enterotoxigenic *Escherichia coli* strain, serotype 078:H11, to purified human intestinal brush borders. Infect Immun. 1983;39:1280–4.
198. Isaacson RE, Fusco PC, Brinton CC, et al. In vitro adhesion of *Escherichia coli* to porcine small intestinal epithelial cells: Pili as adhesive factors. Infect Immun. 1978;21:392–7.
199. McNeish AS, Turner P, Fleming J, et al. Mucosal adherence of human enteropathogenic *Escherichia coli*. Lancet. 1975;2:946–8.
200. Wilson MR, Hohmann AW. Immunity to *Escherichia coli* in pigs. Adhesion of enteropathogenic *Escherichia coli* to isolated intestinal epithelial cells. Infect Immun. 1974;10:776–82.
201. Nagy B, Moon HW, Isaacson RE, et al. Immunization of suckling pigs against enterotoxigenic *Escherichia coli*-induced diarrheal disease by vaccinating dams with purified pili. Infect Immun. 1978;21:269–74.
202. Kallenius G, Mollby R, Svenson SB. Identification of a carbohydrate receptor recognized by uropathogenic *Escherichia coli*. Infection. 1980;8(Suppl 3):288–93.
203. Hagberg L, Engberg I, Freter R, et al. Ascending, unobstructed urinary tract infection in mice caused by pyelonephritogenic *Escherichia coli* of human origin. Infect Immun. 1983;40:273–83.
204. Lomberg H, Jodal U, Eden CS, et al. P_1 blood group and urinary tract infection. Lancet. 1981;1:551–2.
205. Kallenius G, Mollby R. Adhesion of *Escherichia coli* to human periurethral cells correlated to mannose-resistant agglutination of human erythrocytes. FEMS Microbiol Lett. 1979;5:295–9.
206. Klemm P, Orskov I, Orskov F. F-7 and type 1-like fimbriade from three *Escherichia coli* strains isolated from urinary tract infections: Protein chemical and immunological aspects. Infect Immun. 1982;36:462–8.
207. Marre R, Hacker J, Henkel W, et al. Contribution of cloned virulence factors from uropathogenic *Escherichia coli* strains to nephropathogenicity in an experimental rat pyelonephritis model. Infect Immun. 1986;54:761–7.
208. Korhonen TK, Parkkinen J, Hacker J, et al. Binding of *Escherichia coli* S fimbriae to human kidney epithelium. Infect Immun. 1986;54:322–7.
209. Hacker J, Schmidt G, Hughes C, et al: Cloning and characterization of genes involved in production of mannose-resistant, neuraminidase-susceptible (X) fimbriae from a uropathogenic 06:K15:H31 *Escherichia coli* strain. Infect Immun. 1985;47:434–40.
210. Ott M, Hacker J, Schmoll T, et al. Analysis of the genetic determinants coding for the S-fimbrial adhesin (*sfa*) in different *Escherichia coli* strains causing meningitis or urinary tract infections. Infect Immun. 1986;54:646–53.
211. Saukkonen KMJ, Nowicki B, Leinonen M. Role of type 1 and S fimbriae in the pathogenesis of *Escherichia coli* 018:K1 bacteremia and meningitis in the infant rat. Infect Immun. 1988;56:892–7.
212. Parkkinen J, Korhonen TK, Pere A, et al. Binding sites in the rat brain for *Escherichia coli* S fimbriae associated with neonatal meningitis. J Clin Invest. 1988;81:860–5.
213. Moch T, Hoschutzky H, Hacker J, et al. Isolation and characterization of the alpha-sialyl-beta-2,3-galactosyl-specific adhesin from fimbriated *Escherichia coli*. Proc Natl Acad Sci USA. 1987;84:3462–6.
214. Lindberg F, Lund B, Johansson B, et al. Localization of the receptor-binding protein adhesin at the tip of the bacterial pilus. Nature. 1987;328:84–7.
215. Abraham SN, Goguen JD, Sun D, et al. Identification of two ancillary subunits of *Escherichia coli* type 1 fimbriae by using antibodies against synthetic oligopeptides of *fim* gene products. J Bacteriol. 1987;169:5530–6.
216. Hanson MS, Brinton CC Jr. Identification and characterization of *E. coli* type 1 pilus tip adhesion protein. Nature. 1988;332:265–8.
216a. Abraham SN, Sun D, Dale JB, et al. Conservation of the D-mannose-adhesion protein among type I fimbriated members of the family *Enterobacteriaceae*. Nature. 1988;336:682–4.
217. Chitnis DS, Sharma KD, Kamat RS. Role of bacterial adhesion in the pathogenesis of cholera. J Med Microbiol. 1982;15:43–51.
218. Jones GW. The adhesive properties of *Vibrio cholerae* and other *Vibrio* species. In Beachey EH, ed. Bacterial Adherence. New York: Chapman & Hall; 1980:219–49.
219. Freter R, Allweiss B, O'Brien PCM, et al. Role of chemotaxis in the association of motile bacteria with intestinal mucosa: In vitro studies. Infect Immun. 1981;34:241–9.
220. Schrank GD, Verwey WF. Distribution of cholera organisms in experimental *Vibrio cholera* infections: Proposed mechanisms of pathogenesis and antibacterial immunity. Infect Immun. 1976;13:195–203.
221. Guentzel MN, Berry LJ. Motility as a virulence factor for *Vibrio cholerae*. Infect Immun. 1975;11:890–7.
227. Jones GW, Freter R: Adhesive properties of *Vibrio cholerae*: Nature of the interaction with isolated rabbit brush border membranes and human erythrocytes. Infect Immun. 1976;14:240–5.
223. Freter R, O'Brien PCM, Macsai MS. Role of chemotaxis in the association of motile bacteria with intestinal mucosa: In vivo studies. Infect Immun. 1981;34:234–40.
224. Freter R, Jones GW. Adhesive properties of *Vibrio cholerae*: Nature of the interaction with intact mucosal surfaces. Infect Immun. 1976;14:246–56.
225. Jones GW, Abrams GD, Freter R. Adhesive properties of *Vibrio cholerae*: Adhesion to isolated rabbit brush border membranes and hemagglutinating activity. Infect Immun. 1976;14:232–9.
226. Bhattacharjee JW, Srivastava BS. Adherence of wild-type and mutant strains of *Vibrio cholerae* to normal and immune intestinal tissue. Bull WHO. 1979;57:123–8.
227. Spira WM, Sack RB. Kinetics of early cholera infection in the removable intestinal tie–adult rabbit diarrhea model. Infect Immun. 1982;35:952–7.
228. Srivastava R, Sinha VB, Srivastava BS. Events in the pathogenesis of experimental cholera: Role of bacterial adherence and multiplication. J Med Microbiol. 1980;13:1–9.
229. Kabir S, Ali S. Characterization of surface properties of *Vibrio cholera*. Infect Immun. 1983;39:1048–58.
230. Booth BA, Dyer TJ, Finkelstein RA. Adhesion of *Vibrio cholerae* to cultured human cells. In: Advances in Research on Cholera and Related Diarrheas. Tokyo: KTK Scientific Publishers. In press.
231. Bergman MJ, Updike WS, Wood SJ, et al. Attachment factors among enterotoxigenic *Escherichia coli* from patients with acute diarrhea from diverse geographic areas. Infect Immun. 1981;32:381–8.
232. Bergman MJ, Evans DG, Mandell GL, et al. Attachment of *E. coli* to human intestinal epithelial cells: A functional in vitro test for intestinal colonization factor. Trans Assoc Am Physicians 1978;91:80–9.
233. Miller VL, Taylor RK, Mekalanos JJ. Cholera toxin transcriptional activator ToxR is a transmembrane DNA binding protein. Cell. 1987;48:271–9.
234. Taylor RK, Miller VL, Furlong DB, et al. Use of *phoA* gene fusions to identify a pilus colonization factor coordinately regulated with cholera toxin. Proc Natl Acad Sci USA. 1987;84:2833–7.
235. Betley MJ, Miller VL, Mekalanos JJ. Genetics of bacterial enterotoxins. Annu Rev Microbiol. 1986;40:577–605.
236. Smith HR, Cravioto A, Willshaw GA, et al. A plasmid coding for the production of colonization factor antigen I and heat-stable enterotoxin in strains of *Escherichia coli* of serogroup 078. FEMS Microbiol Lett. 1979;6:255–60.
237. McConnell MM, Smith HR, Field AM, et al: Plasmids coding for colonization factor antigen I and heat-stable enterotoxin production isolated from enterotoxigenic *Escherichia coli*: Comparison of their properties. Infect Immun. 1981;32:927–36.
238. Penaranda ME, Mann MB, Evans DG, Evans DJ. Transfer of an ST:LT:CFA/II plasmid into *Escherichia coli* K12 strain RRI by co-transformation with PSC301 plasmid DNA. FEMS Microbiol Lett. 1980;8:251–4.
239. Smith HR, Scotland SM, Rowe B. Plasmids that code for production of colonization factor antigen II and enterotoxin production in strains of *Escherichia coli*. Infect Immun. 1983;40:1236–9.
240. Harnett NM, Gyles GL. Linkage of genes coding for heat-stable enterotoxin, drug resistance, K99 antigen, and colicin in bovine and porcine strains of enterotoxigenic *Escherichia coli*. Am J Vet Res. 1985;46:428–33.
241. Sparling PF, Cannon JG, So M. Phase and antigenic variation of pili and outer membrane protein II of *Neisseria gonorrhoeae*. J Infect Dis. 1986;153:196–201.
242. Johnson AP, Taylor-Robinson D, McGee ZA. Species specificity of attachment and damage to oviduct mucosa by *Neisseria gonorrhoeae*. Infect Immun. 1977;18:833–9.
243. Watt PJ, Ward ME. Adherence to *Neisseria gonorrhoeae* and other *Neisseria* species to mammalian cells. In: Beachey EH, ed. Bacterial Adherence (Receptors and Recognition). v. 6. ser B. New York: Chapman & Hall; 1980:251–88.
244. McGee ZA, Melly A, Gregg CR, et al. Virulence factors of gonococci: Studies using human fallopian tube organ cultures. In: Brooks GF, Gotschlich EC, Holmes KK, et al, eds. Immunobiology of *Neisseria gonorrhoeae*. Washington, DC: American Society for Microbiology; 1978:258–62.
245. Johnson AP, Clark JB, Osborn MF, et al. A comparison of the association of *Neisseria gonorrhoeae* with human and guinea pig genital mucosa maintained in organ cultures. Br J Exp Pathol. 1980;61:521–7.
246. Swanson J. Studies on gonococcus infection. XII. Colony color and opacity variants of gonococci. Infect Immun. 1978;19:320–31.
247. Zak K, Diay J-L, Jackson D, et al. Antigenic variation during infection with *Neisseria gonorrhoeae*: Detection of antibodies to surface proteins in sera of patients with gonorrhea. J Infect Dis. 1984;149:166–74.
248. McGee ZA, Johnson AP, Taylor-Robinson D. Pathogenic mechanisms of

Neisseria gonorrhoeae: Observations on damage to human fallopian tubes in organ culture by gonococci of colony type 1 or type 4. J Infect Dis. 1981;143:413–22.
249. Trust TJ, Lambden PR, Watt PJ. The cohesive properties of variants of *Neisseria gonorrhoeae* strain P9: Specific pilus-mediated and non-specific interactions. J Gen Microbiol. 1980;119:179–87.
250. Buchanan TM, Pearce WA, Chen KC. Attachment of *Neisseria gonorrhoeae* pili to human cells and investigations of the chemical nature of the receptor for gonococcal pili. In: Brooks GF, Gotschlich EC, Holmes KK, et al, eds. Immunobiology of *Neisseria gonorrhoeae*. Washington DC: American Society for Microbiology; 1978:242–9.
251. Pearce WA, Buchanan TM. Attachment role of gonococci pili. J Clin Invest. 1978;61:931–43.
252. Tramont EC, Ciak J, Boslego J, et al. Antigenic specificity of antibodies in vaginal secretions during infection with *Neisseria gonorrhoeae*. J Infect Dis. 1980;143:23–31.
253. Tramont EC. Specificity of inhibition of epithelial cell adhesion of *Neisseria gonorrhoeae*. Infect Immun. 1976;14:593–5.
254. Swanson J, Robbins K, Barrera O, et al. Gonococcal pili variants in experimental gonorrhea. J Exp Med. 1987;165:1344–57.
255. Bergstrom S, Robbins K, Koomey JM, et al. Piliation control mechanisms in *Neisseria gonorrhoeae*. Proc Natl Acad Sci USA. 1986;83:3890–4.
256. Segal E, Hagblom P, Seifert HS, et al. Antigenic variation of gonococcal pilus involves assembly of separated silent gene segments. Proc Natl Acad Sci USA. 1986;83:2177–81.
257. Lambden PR. Biochemical comparison pili from variants of *Neisseria gonorrhoeae* P9. J Gen Microbiol. 1982;128:2105–11.
258. Lambden PR, Robertson JN, Watt PJ. Biological properties of two distinct pilus types produced by isogenic variants of *Neisseria gonorrhoeae* P9. J Bacteriol. 1980;141:393–6.
259. Hermodson MA, Chen KCS, Buchanan TM. *Neisseria* pili proteins: Amino-terminal amino acid sequences and identification of an unusual amino acid. Biochemistry. 1978;17:442–5.
260. Heckels JE. Structural comparison of *Neisseria gonorrhoeae* outer membrane proteins. J Bacteriol. 1981;145:736–42.
261. Diaz JL, Heckels JE. Antigenic variation of outer membrane protein II in colonial variants of *Neisseria gonorrhoeae* PA. J Gen Microbiol. 1982;128:585–91.
262. Forslin L, Danielsson D. In vitro studies of the adherence of *Neisseria gonorrhoeae* and other urogenital bacteria to vaginal and uroepithelial cells, with special regard to the menstrual cycle. Gynecol Obstet Invest. 1980;11:327–40.
263. James JF, Swanson J. Studies on gonococcus infection. XIII. Occurrence of color/opacity colonial variants in clinical cultures. Infect Immun. 1978;19:332–40.
264. Duckworth M, Jackson D, Zak K, et al. Structural variations in pili expressed during gonococcal infection. J Gen Microbiol. 1983;129:1593–6.
265. Gahnberg L, Olsson J, Krasse B, et al. Interference of salivary immunoglobulin A antibodies and other salivary fractions with adherence of *Streptococcus mutans* to hydroxyapatite. Infect Immun. 1982;37:401–6.
266. Malamud D, Appelbaum B, Kline R, et al. Bacterial aggregating activity in human saliva: Comparisons of bacterial species and strains. Infect Immun. 1981;31:1003–6.
267. Rosan B, Malamud D, Appelbaum B, et al. Characteristic differences between saliva-dependent aggregation and adhesion of streptococci. Infect Immun. 1982;35:86–90.
268. Ciardi JE, Rolla G, Bowen WH, et al. Adsorption of *Streptococcus mutans* lipoteichoic acid to hydroxyapatite. Scand J Dent Res. 1977;85:387–91.
269. Hamada S, Slade DH. Adherence of serotype e *Streptococcus mutans* and the inhibitory effect of Lancefield group E and *S. mutans* type e antiserum. J Dent Res. 1976;55:65.
270. Hamada S, Torii M, Kotani S, et al. Adherence of *Streptococcus sanguis* clinical isolates to smooth surfaces and interaction of the isolates with *Streptococcus mutans* glucosyltransferase. Infect Immun. 1981;32:364–72.
271. Heeb MJ, Costello AH, Gabriel O. Characterization of a galactose-specific lectin from *Actinomyces viscosus* by a model aggregation system. Infect Immun. 1982;38:993–1002.
272. McIntire FC, Crosby LK, Vatter AE. Inhibitors of coaggregation between *Actinomyces viscosus* T14V and *Streptococcus sanguis* 34: Beta-galactosides, related sugars, and anionic amphipathic compounds. Infect Immun. 1982;36:371–8.
273. Tylenda CA, Enriquez E, Kolenbrander PE, et al. Simultaneous loss of bacteriophage receptor and coaggregation mediator activities in *Actinomyces viscosus* MG-I. Infect Immun. 1985;48:228–33.
274. Delisle AL, Donkersloot JA, Kolenbrander PE, et al. Use of lytic bacteriophage for *Actinomyces viscosus* T140 as a probe for cell surface components mediating intergeneic coaggregation. Infect Immun. 1988;56:54–9.
275. Gibbons RJ, Hay DI. Human salivary acidic proline-rich proteins and statherin promote the attachment of *Actinomyces viscosus* L47 to apatite surfaces. Infect Immun. 1988;56:439–45.
276. Rolla G, Robrish SA, Bowen WH. Interaction of hydroxyapatite and protein-coated hydroxyapatite with *Streptococcus mutans* and *Streptococcus sanguis*. Acta Pathol Microbiol Scand [B]. 1977;85:341–6.
277. Giampapa CS, Abraham SN, Chiang TM, et al. Isolation and characterization of a receptor for type 1 fimbriae of *Escherichia coli* from guinea pig erythrocytes. J Biol Chem. 1988;263:5362–7.
278. Doran JE, Raynor RH. Fibronectin binding to protein A-containing staphylococci. Infect Immun. 1981;33:683–9.
279. Espersen F, Clemmensen I. Isolation of a fibronectin-binding protein from *Streptococcus aureus*. Infect Immun. 1982;37:526–31.
280. Kuusela P. Fibronectin binds to *Streptococcus aureus*. Nature. 1978;276:718–20.
281. Proctor RA, Mosher DF, Olbrantz PJ. Fibronectin binding to *Staphylococcus aureus*. J Biol Chem. 1982;257:14788–94.
282. Woods DE, Straus DC, Johanson WG Jr, et al. Role of salivary protease activity in adherence of gram-negative bacilli to mammalian buccal epithelial cells in vivo. J Clin Invest. 1981;68:1435–40.
283. Woods DE, Straus DC, Johanson WG Jr, et al. Role of fibronectin in the prevention of adherence of *Pseudomonas aeruginosa* to buccal cells. J Infect Dis. 1981;143:784–90.
284. Zetter BR, Daniels TE, Quadra-White C, et al. LETS protein in normal and pathological human oral epithelium. J Dent Res. 1979;58:484–8.
285. Abraham SN, Beachey EH, Simpson WA. Adherence of *Streptococcus pyogenes, Escherichia coli* and *Pseudomonas aeruginosa* to fibronectin-coated and uncoated epithelial cells. Infect Immun. 1983;41:1261–8.
286. Valenti WM, Trudell RG, Bentley DW. Factors predisposing to oropharyngeal colonization with gram negative bacilli in the aged. N Engl J Med. 1978;298:1108–11.
287. Simpson WA, Courtney H, Beachey EH. Fibronectin—a modulator of the oropharyngeal bacterial flora. In: Microbiology 1982. Washington, DC: American Society for Microbiology; 1982:346–7.
288. Woods DE. Role of fibronectin in the pathogenesis of gram-negative bacillary pneumonia. Rev Infect Dis. 1987;9(Suppl 4):386–90.
289. Rosenburg M, Perry A, Bayer EA, et al. Adherence of *Acinetobacter calcoaceticus* RAG-1 to human epithelial cells and to hexadecane. Infect Immun. 1981;33:29–33.
290. Rosenberg M, Gutnick D, Rosenberg E. Adherence of bacteria to hydrocarbons: A simple method for measuring cell surface hydrophobicity. FEMS Microbiol Lett. 1980;9:29–33.
291. Olsson J, Westergren G. Hydrophobic surface properties of oral streptococci. FEMS Microbiol Lett. 1982;15:319–23.
292. Kihlstrom E, Edebo L. Association of viable and inactivated *Salmonella typhimurium* 395 MS and MR 10 with HeLa cells. Infect Immun. 1976;14:851–7.
293. Perers L, Andaker L, Edebo O, et al. Association of some enterobacteria with the intestinal mucosa of mouse in relation to their partition in aqueous polymer two-phase systems. Acta Pathol Microbiol Scand [B]. 1977;85:308–16.
294. Smyth CJ, Jonsson P, Olsson E, et al. Differences in hydrophobic surface characteristics of porcine enteropathogenic *Escherichia coli* with or without K88 antigen as revealed by hydrophobic interaction chromatography. Infect Immun. 1978;22:462–72.
295. Tylewska SK, Wadstrom T, Hjerten S. The effect of subinhibitory concentrations of penicillin and rifampicin on bacterial cell surface hydrophobicity and on binding to pharyngeal epithelial cells. J Antimicrob Chemother. 1980;16:292–4.
296. Colleen S, Hovelius B, Wieslander A, et al. Surface properties of *Staphylococcus saprophyticus* and *Staphylococcus epidermidis* as studied by adherence tests and two-polymer, aqueous phase systems. Acta Pathol Microbiol Scand [B]. 1979;87:321–8.
297. Gerson DF, Akit J. Cell surface energy, contact angles and phase partition. II. Bacterial cells in biphasic aqueous mixtures. Biochim Biophys Acta. 1980;602:281–4.
298. Stendahl O, Tagesson C, Edebo M. Partition of *Salmonella typhimurium* in a two-polymer aqueous phase system in relation to liability to phagocytosis. Infect Immun. 1973;8:36–41.
299. Ohman L, Normann B, Stendahl O. Physicochemical surface properties of *Escherichia coli* strains isolated from different types of urinary tract infections. Infect Immun. 1981;32:951–5.
300. Miorner H, Myhre E, Bjorck L, et al. Effect of specific binding of human albumin, fibrinogen, and immunoglobulin G on surface characteristics of bacterial strains as revealed by partition experiments in polymer phase systems. Infect Immun. 1980;39:879–85.
301. Faris A, Wadstrom T, Freer JH. Hydrophobic adsorptive and hemagglutinating properties of *Escherichia coli* possessing colonization factors, antigen (CFA/I or CFA/II), type 1 pili or other pili. Curr Microbiol. 1981;5:67–72.
302. Sherman PM, Houston WL, Boedeker EC. Functional heterogeneity of intestinal *Escherichia coli* strains expressing type I somatic pili (fimbriae): Assessment of bacterial adherence to intestinal membranes and surface hydrophobicity. Infect Immun. 1985;49:797–804.
303. Nesbitt WE, Doyle RJ, Taylor KG. Hydrophobic interactions and the adherence of *Streptococcus sanguis* to hydroxyapatite. Infect Immun. 1982;38:637–44.
304. Falkowski W, Edwards M, Schaeffer AJ. Inhibitory effect of substituted aromatic hydrocarbons on adherence of *Escherichia coli* to human epithelial cells. Infect Immun. 1986;52:863–6.
305. Sugarman B. Adherence of bacteria to urinary catheters. Urol Res. 1982;10:37–40.
306. Sugarman B. In vitro adherence of bacteria to prosthetic vascular grafts. Infection. 1982;10:9–14.
307. Sugarman B, Musher D. Adherence of bacteria to suture materials (41141). Proc Soc Exp Biol Sci. 1981;167:156–60.

308. Karlan MS, Skobel A, Grizzard M, et al. Myringotomy tube materials: Bacterial adhesion and infection. Otolaryngol Head Neck Surg. 1980;88:783–94.
309. Locci R, Peters G, Pulverer G. Microbial colonization of prosthetic devices. III. Adhesion of staphylococci to lumina of intravenous catheters perfused with bacterial suspensions. Zentralbl Bakteriol Mikrobiol Hyg. 1981;172:300–7.
310. Sheth NK, Rose HD, Franson TF, et al. In vitro quantitative adherence of bacteria to intravascular catheters. J Surg Res. 1983;34:213–8.
311. Hogt AH, Feijen J, Dankert J, et al. Adhesion of *Staphylococcus epidermidis* and *Staphylococcus saprophyticus* onto FEP-Teflon and cellulose acetate. In: Proceedings of International Conference on Biomedical Polymers. London: Biological Engineers Society; 1982:39–47.
312. Rotrosen D, Gibson TR, Edwards JE Jr. Adherence of *Candida* species to intravenous catheters. J Infect Dis. 1983;147:594.
313. Gristina AG. Biomaterial-centered infection: Microbvial adhesion versus tissue integration. Science. 1987;237:1588–95.
314. van Loosdrecht MCM, Lyklema J, Norde W, et al. Electrophoretic mobility and hydrophobicity as a measure to predict the initial steps of bacterial adhesion. Appl Environ Microbiol. 1987;53:1898–1901.
315. van Loosdrecht MCM, Lyklema J, Norde W, et al. The role of bacterial cell wall hydrophobicity in adhesion. Appl Environ Microbiol. 1987;53:1893–7.
316. Schadow KH, Simpson WA, Christensen GD. Characteristics of adherence to plastic tissue culture plates of coagulase-negative staphylococci exposed to subinhibitory concentrations of antimicrobial agents. J Infect Dis. 1988;157:71–7.
317. Fletcher M. Adherence of marine micro-organisms to smooth surfaces. In: Beachey EH, ed. Bacterial Adherence (Receptors and Recognition). New York: Chapman & Hall; 1980:345–74.
318. Christensen GD, Simpson WA, Beachey EH, et al. Adherence to pathogenic *Streptococcus epidermidis* to smooth surfaces and to catheters implanted in mice (abstract). In: Proceedings of the 22nd Interscience Conference on Antimicrobial Agents and Chemotherapy. Washington, DC: American Society for Microbiology; 1982:649.
319. Peters G, Locci R, Pulverer G. Adherence and growth of coagulase-negative staphylococci on surfaces of intravenous catheters. J Infect Dis. 1982;146:479–82.
320. Peters G, Schumacher-Perdreau F, Jansen B, et al. Biology of *S. epidermidis* extracellular slime. In: Pulverer G, Quie PG, Peters G, eds. Pathogenicity and clinical significance of coagulase-negative staphylococci. Stuttgart: Gustav Fischer Verlag; 1987:15–32.
321. Tojo M, Yamashita N, Goldmann DA, et al. Isolation and characterization of a capsular polysaccharide adhesin from *Staphylococcus epidermidis*. J Infect Dis. 1988;157:713–22.
322. Christensen GD, Simpson WA, Bisno AL, et al. Experimental foreign body infections in mice challenged with slime-producing *Staphylococcus epidermidis*. Infect Immun. 1983;40:407–10.
323. Baddour LM, Smalley DL, Kraus AP Jr, et al. Comparison of microbiologic characteristics of pathogenic and saprophytic coagulase-negative staphylococci from patients on continuous ambulatory peritoneal dialysis. Diagn Microbiol Infect Dis. 1986;5:197–205.
324. Christensen GD, Baddour LM, Simpson WA. Phenotypic variation of *Staphylococcus epidermidis* slime production in vitro and in vivo. Infect Immun. 1987;55:2870–7.
325. Bayston R, Penny SR: Excessive production of mucoid substance in staphylococcus SIIA: A possible factor in colonisation of Holter shunts. Dev Med Child Neurol. 1972;14(Suppl 27):25–8.
326. Peters G, Locci R, Pulverer G. Microbial colonization of prosthetic devices. II. Scanning electron microscopy of naturally infected intravenous catheters. Zentralbl Bakteriol Mikrobiol Hyg. 1981;173:293–9.
327. Franson TR, Sheth NK, Rose HD, et al. Scanning electron microscopy of bacteria adherent to intravascular catheters. J Clin Microbiol. 1984;20:500–5.
328. Marrie TJ, Costerton JW. Scanning and transmission electron microscopy of in situ bacterial colonization of intravenous and intra-arterial catheters. J Clin Microbiol 1984;19:687–93.
329. Younger JJ, Christensen GD, Bartley DL, et al. Coagulase-negative staphylococci isolated from cerebrospinal fluid shunts: Importance of slime production, species identification, and shunt removal to clinical outcome. J Infect Dis. 1987;156:548–54.
330. Diaz-Mitoma F, Harding GKM, Hoban DJ, et al. Clinical significance of a test for slime production in ventriculoperitoneal shunt infections caused by coagulase-negative staphylococci. J Infect Dis. 1987;156:555–60.
331. Beachey EH, Eisenstein BI, Ofek I. I. Adherence of bacteria: Prevention of the adhesion of bacteria to mucosal surfaces: Influence of antimicrobial agents. In: Eickenberg HU, Hahn H, Opferkuch W, eds. The Influence of Antibiotics on the Host Parasite Relationship. Munich: Springer-Verlag; 1982:171–82.
332. Tacket CO, Losonsky G, Link H, et al. Protection by milk immunoglobulin concentrate against oral challenge with enterotoxigenic *Escherichia coli*. New Engl J Med. 1988;318:1240–3.
333. Peros WJ, Gibbons RJ. Influence of sublethal antibiotic concentrations on bacterial adherence to saliva treated hydroxyapatite. Infect Immun. 1982;35:326–34.
334. Vosbeck K, Handschin H, Menge EB, et al. Effects of subminimal inhibitory concentrations of antibiotics on adhesiveness of *Escherichia coli in vitro*. Rev Infect Dis. 1979;1:845–51.
335. Ofek I, Beachey EH, Eisenstein BI, et al. Suppression of bacterial adherence by subminimal inhibitory concentrations of beta-lactam and aminoglycoside antibiotics. Rev Infect Dis. 1979;1:832–7.
336. Eisenstein BI, Ofek I, Beachey EH. Loss of lectin-like activity in aberrant type 1 fimbriae of *Escherichia coli*. Infect Immun. 1981;31:792–7.
337. Bar-Shavit Z, Ofek I, Goldman R, et al. Mannose residues on phagocytes as receptors for the attachment of *Escherichia coli* and *Salmonella typhi*. Biochem Biophys Res Commun. 1977;78:455–60.
338. Parsons CL, Mulholland SG, Anwar H. Antibacterial activity of bladder surface mucin duplicated by exogenous glycosaminoglycan (heparin). Infect Immun. 1979;24:552–7.
339. Parsons CL, Pollen SS, Anwar H, et al. Antibacterial activity of bladder surface mucin duplicated in the rabbit bladder by exogenous glycosaminoglycan (sodium pentosanpolysulfate). Infect Immun. 1980;27:876–81.
340. Parsons CL, Stauffer C, Schmidt JD. Bladder-surface glycosaminoglycans: An efficient mechanism of environmental adaptation. Science. 1980;208:605–7.

3. A MOLECULAR PERSPECTIVE OF MICROBIAL PATHOGENICITY

DAVID A. RELMAN
STANLEY FALKOW

The study of microbial pathogenicity at the molecular level has altered the way we view the host–parasite relationship and forced the redefinition of some commonly used terms. Infection, infectious disease, and virulence have been defined and used in numerous and sometimes misleading ways. The essential feature of most infections, however, is the successful multiplication of a microbe on or within a host. This process is often of benefit to both participants. Thus, following birth, human exposure to a myriad of microorganisms leads to the establishment of a protective microbial flora, stimulates the immune system, and in addition, provides small amounts of human accessory growth factors. The human participants in these infections are most often asymptomatic or exhibit subclinical signs but are generally better off for their encounter with the infecting organism(s). It is probably fair to say that this is the usual outcome of most infections.

The term *infectious disease* applies when signs and symptoms result from infection and its associated damage or altered physiology. A *pathogen* is usually defined as any microorganism that has the capacity to cause disease. Yet not all pathogens have an equal probability of causing disease in the same host population. *Virulence* provides a quantitative measure of pathogenicity, or the likelihood of causing disease. For example, encapsulated pneumococci are more virulent than are nonencapsulated pneumococci, and type b encapsulated *Haemophilus influenzae* organisms are more virulent than are other *H. influenzae* capsular types. Virulence factors refer to the properties, i.e., gene products, that enable a microorganism to establish itself on or within a host of a particular species and enhance its potential to cause disease.

If one is to examine microbial pathogenicity in detail, it is useful to distinguish "principal" pathogens, which *regularly* cause disease in some proportion of susceptible individuals with apparently *intact* specific and nonspecific defense systems, from other potentially pathogenic microorganisms. Certain microorganisms do not meet this definition of a principal pathogen because they do not regularly cause disease in individuals with intact host defenses. *Pseudomonas aeruginosa* is a good example. This microorganism does not usually cause disease in people with intact host defense systems; yet it can clearly cause devastating disease in many hospitalized and immunocompromised patients. It is probable that virtually any microorganism with a capacity for sustained multiplication in humans can cause disease more readily in individuals with underlying chronic disease or who are otherwise compromised. The common term *opportunist* suits this category of pathogen well. One could extend this argument to say that, for most organisms classified as principal pathogens, for example, *Staphylococcus aureus* and the pneumococcus, there must be some impairment or local breakdown of the normal host defense mechanisms in order for these bacteria to cause disease. On the other hand, it seems clear that the capacity of certain microorganisms to cause disease in seemingly uncompromised human hosts on a regular basis reflects some fundamental difference in their virulence capabilities as compared with opportunists or nonpathogens.

THE ATTRIBUTES OF MICROBIAL PATHOGENS

To be successful a pathogen must find an appropriate host niche and multiply there. Disease is arguably only an inadvertent outcome of microbial multiplication. To cause infection, a microorganism must possess an interactive group of complementary genetic properties, sometimes coregulated, that promote its interaction with a particular host. For a given microorganism these genetic traits define unique attributes[1] that enable it to follow a common sequence of steps used by organisms that are successful in establishing infection or subsequent disease. These traits are reflected as phenotypes for which one or more genes and their gene products may be responsible. Elegant molecular techniques, many devised only since 1980, have permitted the identification, isolation, and characterization of many of these genes and their products. Precise manipulation of the pathogen's genome has led to the determination of the roles for some of these putative virulence factors.

An initial step required of a pathogen is for it to gain access to the host in sufficient numbers. Gaining access to a potential host requires that the microorganism not only make contact with an appropriate surface but also then reach its unique niche or microenvironment on or within the host. This requirement is not trivial. Some pathogens must survive for varying lengths of time in the external environment. Others have evolved an effective and suitable means of transmission. To accomplish this goal the infecting microbe may make use of chemotactic properties and adhesive structures, or adhesins, that mediate binding to specific eukaryotic cell receptors.[2] Pre-existing microorganisms, the normal flora, provide competition against establishment of the newcomer; in addition, the latter must adapt, at least temporarily, to the particular nutrient environment in which it now finds itself.

Normal host defense mechanisms pose the next and most difficult set of obstacles to the arriving pathogen. For any set of specific host defenses an individual pathogen may have devised a unique and distinctive counterstrategy. Some of the best known mechanisms for countering host defenses include the use of an antiphagocytic capsule and the elaboration of toxins and microbial enzymes that act on host immune cells and destroy anatomic barriers. In addition, microorganisms may employ subtle mechanisms to avoid or even subvert host defenses, including immunoglobulin-specific protease, iron sequestration mechanisms, or coating themselves with host proteins so as to confuse the immune surveillance system. Examples of these mechanisms include the production of IgA1 protease by *H. influenzae,* the use of receptors for iron-saturated human transferrin and lactoferrin by *Neisseria gonorrhoeae,* and the coating of *Treponema pallidum* with human soluble fibronectin. Antigenic variation and intracellular invasion are other common strategies used by successful pathogens to avoid immune detection.

The ability to multiply is a characteristic of all living organisms. Whether the pathogen's niche in the relevant host be intracellular or extracellular, mucosal or submucosal, within the blood stream or within a privileged anatomic site, the pathogen will have evolved a distinct set of biochemical tactics to achieve this goal. The success of a pathogen, indeed of any microorganism, is measured by the degree with which it can survive, usually with multiplication, upon reaching its specific niche.

Thus, the outcome of the events just described is determined by the degree to which the pathogen has perpetuated itself and by the nature of the relationship it has established with its host. The result may be altered host physiology, tissue damage, and even clinical manifestations of disease. Death of the host is a rare event and one that must be viewed as most often detrimental to both parties involved! The more usual outcome is sufficient multiplication of the pathogen to ensure its establishment within the host (transient or long-term colonization) or its successful transmission to a new susceptible host.

Why do some pathogens cause disease more readily than others do? The strategy used for multiplication on or within the host often defines fundamental differences between pathogens that commonly cause disease and those that do not. If a microorganism succeeds by multiplying within deep fascial planes, it is far more likely to cause disease than is a nontoxinogenic microorganism that is content to grow on a mucosal surface. If a microorganism has evolved a means to nullify or destroy phagocytic cells in order to multiply successfully, it is more likely a disease-causing pathogen. Furthermore, an organism that can reach and multiply in privileged anatomic sites away from the competitive environment of skin and some mucosal surfaces is likely to disrupt homeostasis in the host and cause disease. Commensal organisms are content to multiply just enough, in the midst of competing microflora, to persist but not damage the host's self-preserving homeostatic mechanisms. It is important to emphasize that a microorganism exceptionally equipped to cause infection may be an unexceptional pathogen and only infrequently, if ever, cause clinically manifested disease.

Why are some organisms like *Pseudomonas aeruginosa* only opportunists despite their impressive array of virulence factors? An organism has no presupposition about the state of the host defenses when it encounters a human host. For opportunistic pathogens that state is the main determinant of whether disease will be the outcome of their interaction with the host. This reflects the fact that these organisms may lack an effective means to overcome normal host defense mechanisms. Opportunists may be very adept at establishing an infection, but because of their preferred growth locale, e.g., the mucosal surface, and preferred growth conditions, e.g., a microaerophilic environment, they may have limited growth opportunities outside of their restricted niche in an unimpaired individual. As a result, disease may be only a rare consequence of the host–microbe encounter.

Pathogens were once viewed as organisms, largely unadapted to their hosts, that elaborated potent toxins or other powerful aggressive factors that caused the signs and symptoms of disease. The current view is that a microbial pathogen is a highly adapted organism that follows a strategy for survival requiring multiplication on or within another living organism. Occasionally this survival strategy produces overt damage to the host. Of course, some infectious diseases occur predominantly in dramatic epidemic form, arguing against the evolution of a balanced host-parasite relationship; however, in many such epidemics there are mitigating circumstances that involve herd immunity and other underlying social, economic, and political issues that impinge upon this relationship. Furthermore, some of the most serious infectious diseases occur when humans are infected by microorganisms that prefer and are better adapted to another mammalian host.

THE CLONAL NATURE OF BACTERIAL PATHOGENS

Pathogenicity is not a microbial trait that has appeared by chance. Instead, particular microbial strains and species have evolved to carry very specific arrays of virulence-associated genes. By examining the genetic organization of pathogens, opportunists, and nonpathogenic bacteria one can now begin to understand the origins of pathogenicity.

Techniques used in the study of genetic relatedness include primary protein or nucleic acid sequence comparisons and DNA hybridization methods. A technique gaining widespread use is multilocus enzyme electrophoresis by which chromosomal structure or genotype is deduced from the electrophoretic mobility variations in a number of common metabolic enzymes.[3] The grouping of strains according to electrophoretic type assumes the absence of selective pressure favoring any particular electrophoretic enzyme variant. On the other hand, it avoids comparisons of phenotype, i.e., gross observable characteristics of a microbe, which can be unreliable. When these techniques are employed, a consistent finding emerges concerning the population structure of microorganisms.

Most natural populations of microorganisms consist of a number of discrete clonal lineages with preserved genotypes.[4] This finding implies that the rates of recombination of chromosomal genes between different strains of the same species and between different bacterial species are very low. At first view, this may seem somewhat unexpected since there exist well-established naturally occurring mechanisms for horizontal genetic exchange between and within species, including transformation, transduction, and conjugation. But bacteria are haploid creatures. If horizontal transfer of genetic material and subsequent recombination were frequent occurrences, one would expect to see homogenization of bacterial species and little specialization. In fact, the opposite is true. Bacterial species have remained discrete and distinct taxonomic entities.[5] This is because the bacterial chromosome is a highly integrated and coadapted entity that has resisted rearrangement.

Analysis of natural populations of *Escherichia coli*[4,6] as well as other species with pathogenic potential including *Salmonella* sp.,[7] *Neisseria meningitidis, Bordetella pertussis, H. influenzae, Legionella* sp., and *Streptococcus* sp.[8] has revealed the prominent representation of a relatively few clones. In fact, most cases of serious disease may be caused by a small proportion of the total number of extant clones that constitute a pathogenic bacterial species (Table 1). For example, from 104 distinct *H. influenzae* type b clones identified in natural populations, only 6 are commonly recovered from patients with invasive disease. The differences between pathogenic and nonpathogenic clones of the same species should provide considerable insight into the virulence mechanisms of these microorganisms. It has been noted that, in many instances, the proper unit of study in bacterial pathogenicity is not a phenotypic trait such as biotype or serotype but rather the clone. Phenotypic traits do not correlate directly with genotype and do not distinguish one clonal lineage from another. Indeed, in some extreme cases all members of a species such as *Shigella sonnei* or *Bordetella pertussis* belong to the same electrophoretic type or small group of closely related types. Although it is true of most that have been studied, not all pathogenic bacterial species reveal this pattern of clonal organization. Two notable exceptions are *Neisseria gonorrhoeae* and *Pseudomonas aeruginosa,* which appear to use chromosomal recombination to increase their genetic diversity. In addition, while the members of the genus *Salmonella* are largely clonal, there is evidence indicating that some diversity seen among members of the same serogroup can be best explained by horizontal genetic transmission rather than by the presence of numerous discrete clonal subpopulations.

Clonal analysis using multilocus enzyme electrophoresis has generated other important conclusions concerning the evolution of bacterial species and pathogenic strains in particular. The study of *E. coli* populations in the human intestinal tract indicates that only a small number of clonal lineages persist while numerous unrelated cell lines appear and disappear.[4] The nonrandom association of particular versions of different genes within a distinct clone has led to speculation that this species has evolved, not by means of accumulated random recombinational events, but by "random sampling" of clonal populations from the environment with periodic selection and extinction. *Escherichia coli* urinary tract pathogens causing symptomatic disease in humans are even less genetically diverse than are *E. coli* strains found in the intestinal flora or those that cause asymptomatic urinary tract colonization.[4]

PLASMIDS, PHAGES, INSERTION ELEMENTS AND PATHOGENICITY

The study of natural populations of bacteria suggests that the genetic potential for pathogenicity within a bacterial species has arisen among a small number of unrelated clones. It has arisen through means that do not compromise the genetic individuality of the organism or its unique place in nature but nonetheless in a fashion that provides the microbe with genetic and biochemical flexibility for a competitive environment. How might this have happened? Although periodic selection of mutant clones may play some role in the evolution of pathogenesis, it does not explain many of the differences seen between pathogenic and nonpathogenic clones of the same species.

A number of separate observations indicate that microbes frequently carry virulence-associated genes on mobile genetic elements.[1] Bacteriophages and extrachromosomal elements such as bacterial plasmids are supplements to the bacterial genome that allow a microbe to maintain the integrity of its chromosome and still increase its genetic diversity. Some of these mobile elements are able to enter a wide variety of host organisms and may facilitate the transfer of genes that have been selected for their ability to function in diverse genetic backgrounds.[10] Clinicians are painfully aware that genes encoding

TABLE 1. Proportion of Certain Infectious Diseases Caused by Common Bacterial Clonal Types

Species	Total number of Clonal Types Identified	Number of Clonal Types Commonly Isolated from Cases of Disease	Percentage of Disease Due to Common Clonal Types
B. bronchiseptica	21	3	87
B. parapertussis	1	1	100
B. pertussis	2	2	100
H. influenzae type b			
North America	104	6	81
Europe	60	3	78
L. pneumophila			
Global	50	5	52
Wadsworth VA Hospital	10	1	86
N. meningitidis			
serogroups B and C (clone families)	192	7	85
S. sonnei	1	1	100

(Modified from Selander et al.,[9] with permission.)

TABLE 2. Examples of Plasmid and Phage-Encoded Virulence Determinants

Organism	*Virulence Factor*	*Biologic Function*
Plasmid-encoded		
Enterotoxigenic *E. coli*	Heat labile, heat-stable enterotoxins (LT, ST)	Activation of adenyl/guanylcyclase in the small bowel, which leads to diarrhea
	CFA/I and CFA/II	Adherence/colonization factors
Extraintestinal *E. coli*	Hemolysin	Cytotoxin
Shigella sp. and enteroinvasive *E. coli*	Gene products involved in invasion	Induces internalization by intestinal epithelial cells
Yersinia sp.	Adherence factors and gene products involved in invasion	Attachment/invasion
B. anthracis	Edema factor, lethal factor, and protective antigen	Edema factor has adenylcyclase activity
S. aureus	Exfoliative toxin	Causes toxic epidermal necrolysis
C. tetani	Tetanus neurotoxin	Blocks the release of inhibitory neurotransmitter, which leads to muscle spasms
Phage-encoded		
C. diphtheriae	Diphtheria toxin	Inhibition of eukaryotic protein synthesis
S. pyogenes	Erythrogenic toxin	Rash of scarlet fever
C. botulinum	Neurotoxin	Blocks synaptic acetylcholine release which leads to flaccid paralysis
Enterohemorrhagic *E. coli*	Shigalike toxin	Inhibition of eukaryotic protein synthesis

(Data from Elwell et al.,[11] Kopecko et al.,[12] and Falkow et al.[13])

antibiotic resistance are efficiently disseminated among different microbial species in nature by such means. The presence of virulence factors in pathogenic bacteria is also associated with the presence of plasmids,[11,12] transposons, and bacteriophages to a striking degree, both in gram-positive and gram-negative species (Table 2).

Comparisons of pathogenic and nonpathogenic representatives of a single genus or species usually demonstrate the nonpathogens to be totally devoid of genetic sequences encoding the pathogenic trait(s). Inactive mutational variants or portions of virulence-associated genes infrequently occur in nonpathogenic strains of the same species. Not uncommonly, virulence-specific sequences are bounded by repeated DNA segments, some of which represent known insertion elements. This suggests that these virulence genes were once associated with a mobile genetic element or that these genes formerly occupied another chromosomal locale in either the same species or another microorganism all together. Thus, it often seems that microbes gain pathogenic potential through the inheritance of unique genetic information. Acquisition of an adhesin, toxin, or serum-resistance factor might dictate that a previously nonpathogenic organism will cause disease in a host that had previously been insusceptible.

Plasmids, transposons, and phages provide bacteria with the potential for relatively rapid adaptation to an unfavorable, changing, or new environment. Although these mobile genetic elements are often dispensable to the host bacterium, they are typically conserved over substantial periods of time within diverse cell lineages.[14] This is hardly surprising if the mobile element enables the organism to multiply successfully in a host. Often the mobile element carries multiple virulence-associated genes as a coadapted block. When such gene blocks are accompanied by a separate self-regulatory system that is responsive to a changing microbial environment, they influence the pathogenic potential even more.

THE REGULATION OF BACTERIAL PATHOGENICITY

All bacteria respond to environmental changes with metabolic alterations. A successful host–parasite relationship demands that a pathogen be capable of sensing its local host environment; it must distinguish between conditions favorable to rapid growth and those that are threatening and require a protective response. Consequently, regulating the expression of virulence factors is an additional, yet essential complication of a pathogenic microbe's life. When it first encounters a host, a pathogen must adapt dramatically to its changed environment. A study of the environmental regulation of microbes should recognize biases that arise from the peculiarities of laboratory culture conditions. These conditions may be inappropriate or irrelevant to the natural environments encountered by a microorganism. Given these limitations, some studies indicate that bacteria may be found in a "viable but nonculturable state" in their natural external environment.[15] *Vibrio cholerae,* for example, is thought to persist in this state in brackish estuaries and other saline aquatic environments, sometimes associated with the chitinous exoskeleton of various marine organisms.[16–18] Transition from this milieu to the contrasting environment of the human small intestinal lumen must be accompanied by substantial genetic regulatory events.

Less dramatic changes in the surrounding environment affect the expression of the determinants of virulence. Some pathogens, e.g., *B. pertussis, V. cholerae, E. coli, Shigella* sp., and *Yersinia* sp., regulate their virulence determinants in response to changes in temperature, ionic conditions, pH, and iron and other metal concentrations. Other microbial pathogens periodically vary prominent antigenic components of their surface and, by so doing, may avoid the host immune response, e.g., *N. gonorrhoeae, Borrelia recurrentis,* and *Trypanosoma brucei.*

The number of well-characterized virulence regulatory systems is rapidly increasing. At the same time relatively little is known about both the specific environmental signals to which these systems respond and the rationale for these responses in the human host. The examples of regulation of bacterial virulence factors that are provided below illustrate two common themes for the response of prokaryotes to their environmental stimuli. First, the mechanism for transducing environmental signals typically involves a two-component regulatory system that acts on gene expression, usually at the transcriptional level. Such systems make use of similar pairs of proteins; one protein of the pair has a transmitter domain and may act as a sensor of environmental stimuli, whereas the other has a receiver domain and acts as the regulator. The first of these proteins transmits a signal to the second, usually by means of phosphorylation. The second protein, upon receiving this signal, may regulate the expression of a variety of genes. Systems of this type control, for example, the permeability properties of the *E. coli* cell envelope in response to osmotic stimuli (*envZ*/*ompR*), motor control involved in *E. coli* chemotaxis (*cheA*/*cheY*), the switch from vegetative growth to sporulation by *Bacillus subtilis* (an unidentified sensor/*spoOA*), and even the ability of the soil bacterium *Agrobacterium tumefaciens* to induce tumors in susceptible plant cells in response to plant wound exudates (*virA*/*virG*). The *toxR* gene of *V. cholerae* and the *vir* region of

B. pertussis share several features common to these systems, but they also retain significant differences.

The coordinated control of pathogenicity illustrates a second common feature of bacterial regulation, i.e., the *regulon.* A regulon is a group of operons controlled by a common regulator, usually a protein activator or repressor. This regulator may, in some cases, also be a receiver protein in a two-component system as described above. A regulon provides a means by which many genes can respond in concert to a particular stimulus. At other times the same genes may respond independently to other signals. The concept of a regulon is integral to the study of bacterial physiology. However, only recently has it been appreciated that microbial virulence determinants can be under the control of such a global regulatory network (Table 3).

Bordetella pertussis synthesizes a group of surface-associated or extracellular products that are responsible for the pathologic and clinical findings of pertussis. These products include pertussis toxin, filamentous hemagglutinin, adenylate cyclase, and fimbrial protein. A *trans*-acting regulatory locus, *vir,*[20] positively controls the coordinate expression of these virulence factors. In the few situations that have been studied *vir* activates expression at the level of transcription. The deduced amino acid sequence of genes within the *vir* locus demonstrates homologies to known transmitter and receiver domains in proteins of the two-component regulatory system; however, the exact mechanisms by which the *vir* proteins act are as yet unknown. Twenty or more unlinked chromosomal genes of *B. pertussis* and their gene products are involved in this global regulatory scheme.

The *vir* region mediates spontaneous phase variation and phenotypic modulation, both of which represent oscillation between full expression of all factors and a complete lack thereof. Phenotypic modulation occurs in response to environmental stimuli including temperature. At 37°C the full array of *vir*-regulated genes is expressed, while at 30°C these genes are silent. This regulatory response probably allows *B. pertussis* to cope with the diverse local conditions of the human upper respiratory mucosal surface, its natural site of infection.

Reversible regulation by temperature of the expression of virulence genes is a feature common to several bacterial pathogens, including enteropathogenic and uropathogenic *E. coli* (K-88 and K-99 fimbriae, pyelonephritis associated pilus (Pap) fimbriae, and K-1 capsular antigen), *Shigella* sp. (invasiveness and shiga toxin), and *Yersinia* sp. (virulence-associated determinants including a low calcium response and outer membrane proteins). Temperature-responsive regulation in *Shigella* sp. depends upon another *trans*-acting genetic locus, *vir*R, which exerts a negative regulatory effect upon a number of both chromosomal and plasmid virulence-associated genes.[21]

The regulation of the expression of virulence determinants by *Vibrio cholerae* also illustrates the use of a global regulatory protein that, in this case, serves a dual function. The *tox*R gene product is a transmembrane, DNA-binding protein that can activate transcription of the genes encoding cholera toxin, pilus colonization factor, and specific outer membrane proteins.[22] The *tox*R protein is also thought to sense a variety of other environmental regulatory signals including osmolarity, amino acid concentration, temperature, and pH.[23] At the level of amino acid sequence as well, the *tox*R protein contains features of both sensor and regulator proteins from the two-component sensory transduction system. The combination of these features into one protein may lead to an increased specificity of action.

Antigenic variation in *Salmonella typhimurium* and *Neisseria gonorrhoeae* provide examples of alternative molecular mechanisms, i.e., DNA rearrangements, that mediate the regulation of the expression of virulence factors. *Salmonella typhimurium* varies an immunodominant antigen by alternating between the expression of two different flagellin genes, H1 and H2. The mechanism for this form of variation has been well characterized: inversion of a 995 basepair (bp) chromosomal DNA sequence orients a promoter such that transcription of the H2 flagellin gene occurs together with that of a gene encoding a *trans*-acting repressor of the H1 gene.[24] The opposite orientation allows relief of H1 gene repression and prevents transcription of H2. Inversion is catalyzed by the *hin* gene product. It promotes site-specific recombination between the 14 bp inverted repeats that flank the invertible segment. In this manner, *S. typhimurium* avoids the host antibody response directed against it.

Pili are essential for virulence of the gonococcus in the human host, probably as a result of their role in adherence to the mucosal target surface.[25] They also elicit a specific local and systemic host antibody response.[26] Intermittent production of pili as well as variation in the antigenic type of pilus may be strategies used by the gonococcus to avoid the host immune response. The molecular mechanisms behind these strategies are complex. In general terms, phase and antigenic variation results from DNA rearrangements that move pilin-related sequences scattered around the gonococcal chromosome (in silent *pil*S loci) to the expression site (*pil*E locus).[27] Numerous different pilus types may be expressed by derivatives of a single *N. gonorrhoeae* strain. Gene conversion and other recombination mechanisms may be involved. Among other microbial pathogens DNA rearrangements account for the antigenic variation of variant surface glycoproteins of *Trypanosoma brucei*[28] and the antigenic variation of variable major proteins in *Borrelia* sp.[29] A DNA rearrangement is also associated with the expression of type I pili in *E. coli.*

THE IDENTIFICATION AND CHARACTERIZATION OF VIRULENCE GENES

The characterization of microbial pathogenicity at the molecular level begins with the identification of a virulence-associated phenotype. This may come from clinical observation, epidemiologic investigation, or the use of a model system that reliably reproduces the microbial phenotype in a manner similar to that seen in the natural infection. Traditionally, a virulent strain was compared with a naturally occurring avirulent variant. Such variants, however, may have complex genotypic alterations in-

TABLE 3. Examples of Bacterial Virulence Regulatory Systems

Organism	*Regulatory Gene(s)*	*Environmental Stimuli*	*Regulated Functions*
E. coli	ND	Temperature	Pyelonephritis-associated pili
	fur	Iron concentration	Shigalike toxin, siderophores
B. pertussis	*vir*	Temperature, ionic conditions, nicotinic acid	Pertussis toxin, filamentous hemagglutinin, adenylate cyclase, others
V. cholerae	*tox*R	Temperature, osmolarity, pH, amino acids	Cholera toxin, pili, outer membrane proteins
Yersinia sp.	*lcr* loci	Temperature, calcium	Outer membrane proteins
	ND	Temperature	Adherence, invasiveness
Shigella sp.	*vir*R	Temperature	Invasiveness
S. aureus	*agr*	ND	Alpha toxin, toxic shock syndrome toxin 1, protein A

Abbreviation: ND: not determined.
(Data from Miller et al.[19])

volving multiple genetic loci. The comparison of strains of naturally occurring virulent and nonvirulent organisms may be even more confounding since we now understand that they may represent entirely different clones.

Analysis using mutant strains of identical genetic background is a more desirable approach to the definition of virulence phenotypes. The goal is to define a single, well-defined genetic lesion that alters a recognizable phenotype and then test the effect of this alteration on the pathogenicity or virulence of the organism in an appropriate model system. The use of insertional elements, e.g., antibiotic-resistant transposons, as mutational agents is an attractive means of accomplishing this aim. Transposons are pieces of DNA that are able to translocate from one genomic site to another. Insertion into a gene usually disrupts its function. Transposons have the advantage of marking the mutagenized genetic locus with a new selectable phenotype, typically antibiotic resistance. The development of broad host range plasmid vectors carrying well-defined transposons has extended this method of analysis to a number of pathogenic species for which a method of genetic manipulation was not previously available.[30] Consequently, the comparison of organisms with identical genetic backgrounds, differing only in a single, defined mutation, is employed widely to identify putative virulence genes. Once identified, more precise characterization of such genes and the identification of the gene products usually follow.

Molecular cloning has been the method preferred by many investigators in recent years to isolate specific virulence genes and to modify them in a precise way.[31] A description of the methodologies available for the isolation and characterization of virulence genes is outside the scope of this discussion; however, it may be useful to point out several basic approaches.

Single genes are usually isolated by screening a "library" of overlapping pieces of a fragmented microbial genome that have been inserted into an appropriate plasmid or bacteriophage vector, which is then introduced into a carrier microorganism, typically *E. coli* K-12. In some instances only a few hundred carrier organisms bearing such recombinant molecules need to be examined to screen effectively an entire, average-sized bacterial genome.[32] Typical strategies for screening a genomic library may or may not depend upon expression of the cloned gene of interest by the carrier organisms.

Genes encoding putative virulence determinants may not express their gene products in the *E. coli* carrier strain, either because the product is lethal to the cell or because the appropriate mechanisms for transcription or translation are not available. Screening techniques based upon hybridization with DNA probes avoid the need for expression of the cloned gene, although not the possible lethal effects of expression. These probes may derive from previously isolated genes known to be homologous to the gene of interest,[33] from an oligonucleotide corresponding to the N-terminal amino acid sequence of the gene product,[34] or from DNA flanking an insertion element that has been used to mutagenize the gene in the original host.[30] In the case of the last method, DNA flanking a transposon-marked gene can be easily isolated by screening an initial genomic library for a clone with the appropriate antibiotic resistance phenotype.[35]

Screening recombinant clones for the presence of a cloned gene whose product is stable and expressed at adequate levels is often accomplished by using labeled antibodies directed against the gene product. Although transcription and translation of the cloned gene and stability of the gene product may be enhanced by special expression vectors,[36] appropriate antibodies are not always available. In some cases a recombinant host expressing the cloned gene will display a corresponding phenotype that can be exploited for screening purposes: expression of the cloned *inv* locus from *Yersinia pseudotuberculosis* confers on the *E. coli* host an ability to invade certain types of cultured eukaryotic cells in vitro.[37] The carrier organisms bearing the recombinant clones, once intracellular, are uniquely resistant to the killing effect of gentamicin, which acts only on extracellular bacteria.

To isolate the cloned gene on a DNA fragment of minimal size the boundaries of the gene must be mapped on the initial recombinant vector insert. Transposon mutagenesis may be used for this purpose. The smallest restriction endonuclease fragment that carries the virulence-associated gene is then subcloned. Further characterization at this point includes introducing specific mutations in the gene and defining their effect on a function of its protein product. Site-directed mutagenesis,[38] rapid DNA sequencing,[39] and in vitro coupled transcription–translation of plasmid-encoded proteins[40,41] are techniques that facilitate such analyses. Final proof, however, that the cloned and characterized gene is associated with pathogenicity requires its return to the strain of origin and that certain criteria be met.

ASSOCIATION OF GENES WITH VIRULENCE: PROOF BY A MOLECULAR FORM OF KOCH'S POSTULATES

Technical advances have brought about a proliferation of reports describing the cloning and sequencing of genes thought to be involved in microbial pathogenicity. At the same time these advances have dramatized the need for defined criteria by which genes may be assigned a role in pathogenesis. In a manner analogous to Koch's original postulates these criteria must include the return of the putative causal agent (the cloned virulence-associated gene, mutated or intact) to the host of origin. Unless one can demonstrate an effect on pathogenicity by this kind of controlled genetic manipulation, causality with respect to virulence has not been proved. Just as the original Henle-Koch postulates have provided a reference point for later revised criteria of microbial causality,[42] the criteria outlined below best serve as guidelines, in this case, for an experimental approach to the molecular genetic basis of pathogenicity.

A molecular form of Koch's postulates[43] can be stated as follows: (*1*) The phenotype or property under investigation should be associated significantly more often with pathogenic members of a genus or pathogenic strains of a species than with nonpathogenic members or strains. (*2*) Specific inactivation of the gene or genes associated with the suspected virulence trait should lead to a measurable decrease in virulence. If inactivation of the gene has taken place in a cloned copy carried by a recombinant host, then this mutated gene must be exchanged for the wild-type copy of the gene in the host of origin; the latter must suffer a loss of virulence following the exchange. (*3*) Restoration of full pathogenicity should accompany replacement of the mutated version of the gene with the wild-type version in the strain of origin.

Technical limitations often face the investigator who wishes to apply these postulates to an organism poorly characterized from a genetic standpoint. The ability to exchange alleles in the organism under investigation is crucial because it allows a virulence-associated gene to be studied in an isogenic background. Until recently this was an impossible task with the respiratory tract pathogen *Bordetella pertussis*. Although the complementation of chromosomal mutations was possible by using recombinant multiple-copy plasmids, there was no easy means of replacing a chromosomal gene with a cloned copy, thereby avoiding a multiple gene dose effect. The construction of a suicide vector, pRTP1,[44] provided a solution to this problem and illustrates some of the principles by which this kind of problem can be approached in other organisms.

Homologous recombination is the process by which a segment of DNA replaces an equivalent segment elsewhere that has identical or nearly identical nucleotide sequences. Enzymes that catalyze DNA repair and synthesis mediate this process. Cloned genes, carried into the strain of origin on plasmid vectors, are exchanged for the analogous chromosomal version of the same genes by means of homologous recombination. A suicide plasmid cloning vector can be used for this purpose. Such vectors carry DNA sequences responsible for transfer of the plasmid to a broad range of hosts so that the plasmid can be mated, by conjugation, into a variety of gram-negative organisms. A suicide plasmid also carries *E. coli* DNA sequences that allow it to replicate in this gram-negative organism but not many others. pRTP1 is such a plasmid vector that can be transferred to *B. pertussis* but cannot replicate there. When conjugation is performed in the presence of an antibiotic that selects for the presence of the suicide plasmid, the plasmid becomes recombined into the recipient organism's chromosome because of the homology with the cloned gene copy in the plasmid. Subsequent antibiotic selection against the presence of the suicide plasmid causes a second recombinational event to occur that results in excision of the plasmid and replacement of the original *B. pertussis* chromosomal gene copy with that carried by the plasmid. In this way, chromosomal virulence genes can be modified in a directed fashion.

Another difficulty in the application of a molecular form of Koch's postulates is similar to a problem that faced Koch in his own day: finding an appropriate animal model system. This is a problem that limits the study of microbial pathogenesis as much as any other. It does little good to return a carefully constructed virulence gene mutation to the original strain if there is no way to evaluate its effect on a particular virulence phenotype. A model must duplicate relevant pathology commonly observed in the normal host. The animal host must become consistently infected by using a natural route. Clearly, a model of this sort does not exist for many pathogens. At the same time, it should be remembered that exposure to a known human pathogen does not uniformly lead to disease in all humans.

The postulates just outlined are meant to provide principles by which one may study the genes and gene products associated with microbial pathogenesis. This kind of approach can also be used to analyze the internal structure of these genes and the corresponding functional domains of the encoded proteins.

UNDERSTANDING VIRULENCE: CLINICAL CORRELATIONS AND APPLICATIONS

Do these concepts of microbial pathogenicity have a practical impact on the practice of clinical infectious diseases? It is already apparent that studies of microbial pathogenicity at the molecular level have made substantial contributions to our understanding of the epidemiology, clinical manifestations, diagnosis, and immunoprophylaxis of infectious diseases.

Infectious disease epidemiology hinges upon clear definition of the clinical problem under study and, moreover, precise identification of the etiologic agent. Molecular techniques, including multilocus enzyme electrophoresis and diagnostic DNA probe hybridization, provide for both sensitive and specific detection of putative pathogens and a means for establishing relationships among multiple isolates of the same species. As a result, seemingly unrelated cases occurring during an outbreak have been connected; similarly, geographically or temporally distinct outbreaks have been linked to the same pathogenic clone. Molecular techniques have been employed in other epidemiologic investigations to study transmission mechanisms and the role of avirulent microbial variants in the spread of disease.

Multilocus enzyme electrophoresis has been used in epidemiologic investigation to define clonal relationships among pathogens in numerous outbreaks. These include *E. coli* 0157:H7 strains associated with hemorrhagic colitis and hemolytic uremic syndrome,[45] *N. meningitidis* strains causing epidemic disease,[46] and *Bordetella* sp. isolated from diverse hosts at different times and locations[47]; all demonstrate the prevalence of a relatively few distinct clonal lineages.

Specific DNA probes are available for an increasing number of microbial pathogens.[48] Probes linked to nonradioactive detection systems are readily applied to field investigations and are widely used in laboratory diagnosis. By creating DNA probes that detect sequences encoding virulence factors, investigations of outbreaks and field surveillance work can precisely target the presumed pathogen. One of the first examples of this approach was the detection of enterotoxinogenic *E. coli* by colony hybridization with a probe for the LT gene.[49] DNA probes offer the ability to detect sexually transmitted disease agents, for example, directly in clinical specimens.[50] The recent development of a *Y. pestis*-specific DNA probe allows rapid in situ detection of this pathogen in its normal host vector, the rat flea.[51] In addition, DNA probes have been used for strain identification in epidemiologic investigations: analysis of Swedish *C. diphtheriae* isolates from recent years by using a probe against a specific multicopy transposable DNA insertion element has linked most epidemic diphtheria cases to a single clonal strain and provided important information about the epidemiology of this disease.[52]

One of the most exciting technical advances in recent years is the development of the polymerase chain reaction (PCR) for amplification of a DNA sequence.[53] When using this technique it is possible to detect the presence of a single target DNA sequence in a sample of 10^5 cells. This should greatly benefit epidemiologic investigations that depend upon the screening of environmental material for a presumed pathogen. Other molecular techniques that are commonly used in infectious disease epidemiology include plasmid analysis[54] and restriction endonuclease analysis.[55] Recent investigations into the spread of chloramphenicol-resistant *Salmonella newport* in the food chain[54] and an outbreak of *Legionella* sp. prosthetic valve endocarditis[55] illustrate the usefulness of these methods.

The clinical manifestations of numerous infectious diseases are more readily understood as a result of the molecular analysis of microbial virulence factors. Methods by which genes encoding virulence determinants can be isolated, modified, and returned to the original strain have been described earlier. Further techniques are available to create specific internal mutations within these genes, e.g., site-directed mutagenesis.[38] In this manner, not only can virulence factors be correlated with specific manifestations of disease, but particular protein domains can be correlated with specific biologic activities. This kind of analysis is currently underway for the ADP-ribosylating protein pertussis toxin.[56]

Improvements in the diagnosis of infectious diseases have followed in step with many of the advances in epidemiologic investigation. In particular, DNA probe technology and PCR amplification techniques seem destined to have major impacts on diagnosis. The list of pathogens for which there are diagnostic DNA probes is already quite substantial.[48] Polymerase chain reaction amplification is quickly finding numerous applications, including the detection of human immunodeficiency virus sequences in clinical specimens.[57] As these two techniques become simplified and more widely used, it will be increasingly important to distinguish target sequences that are virulence associated from those that are not.

The application of molecular techniques and theory to infectious disease therapeutics and prophylaxis is in its infancy.[58] As virulence factors for essential steps in pathogenesis are identified in individual pathogens, it should be possible to interfere with their function. For example, one might design competitive inhibitors of microbial adherence factors or invasion-promoting proteins.[59] As they become better characterized, manipulation of global virulence regulatory systems may have therapeutic value. New acellular or recombinant live attenuated vaccines will likely result from the identification of immunoprotective antigens with molecular approaches. A growing understanding of microbial pathogenesis at the molecular level is expected to foster these kinds of practical developments. The result should be a more informed and effective approach to the detection and treatment of infectious diseases.

REFERENCES

1. Falkow S, Small P, Isberg R, et al. A molecular strategy for the study of bacterial invasion. Rev Infect Dis. 1987;9:450–5.
2. Jones GW, Isaacson RE. Proteinaceous bacterial adhesins and their receptors. CRC Crit Rev Microbiol. 1983;10:229–60.
3. Selander RK, Caugant DA, Ochman H, et al. Methods of multilocus enzyme electrophoresis for bacterial population genetics and systematics. Appl Environ Microbiol. 1986;51:873–84.
4. Selander RK, Caugant DA, Whittam TS. Genetic structure and variation in natural populations of *Escherichia coli*. In: Neidhardt FC, ed. *Escherichia coli* and *Salmonella typhimurium*. Washington, DC: American Society for Microbiology; 1987:1625–48.
5. Ochman H, Wilson AC. Evolutionary history of enteric bacteria. In: Neidhardt FC, ed. *Escherichia coli* and *Salmonella typhimurium*. Washington, DC: American Society for Microbiology; 1987:1649–54.
6. Ochman H, Selander RK. Evidence for clonal population structure in *Escherichia coli*. Proc Natl Acad Sci USA. 1984;81:198–201.
7. Beltran P, Musser JM, Helmuth R, et al. Toward a population genetic analysis of *Salmonella:* Genetic diversity and relationships among strains of serotypes *S. choleraesuis, S. derby, S. dublin, S. enteriditis, S. heidelberg, S. infantis, S. newport*, and *S. typhimurium*. Proc Natl Acad Sci USA. 1988;85:7753–7.
8. Selander RK, Musser JM, Caugant DA, et al. Population genetics of pathogenic bacteria. Microbial Pathogenesis. 1987;3:1–7.
9. Selander RK, Musser JM. The population genetics of bacterial pathogenesis. In: Iglewski BH, Clark VL, eds. Molecular Basis of Bacterial Pathogenesis. Orlando, FL: Academic Press. In press.
10. Campbell A. Evolutionary significance of accessory DNA, elements in bacteria. Annu Rev Microbiol. 1981;35:55–83.
11. Elwell LP, Shipley PL. Plasmid-mediated factors associated with virulence of bacteria to animals. Annu Rev Microbiol. 1980;34:465–96.
12. Kopecko DJ, Formal SB. Plasmids and the virulence of enteric and other bacterial pathogens (Editorial). Ann Intern Med. 1984;101:260–2.
13. Falkow S, Portnoy DA. Bacterial plasmids—an overview. Clin Invest Medicine. 1983;6:207–12.
14. Mercer AA, Morelli G, Heuzenroeder M, et al. Conservation of plasmids among *Escherichia coli* K1 isolates of diverse origins. Infect Immun. 1984;46:649–57.
15. Roszak DB, Colwell RR. Survival strategies of bacteria in the natural environment. Microbiol Rev. 1987;51:365–79.
16. Huq A, Small EB, West PA, et al. Ecological relationships between *Vibrio cholerae* and planktonic crustacean copepods. Appl Environ Microbiol. 1983;45:275–83.
17. Tamplin ML, Colwell RR. Effects of microcosm salinity and organic substrate concentration on production of *Vibrio cholerae* enterotoxin. Appl Environ Microbiol. 1986;52:297–301.
18. Perez-Rosas N, Hazen TC. In situ survival of *Vibrio cholerae* and *Escherichia coli* in tropical coral reefs. Appl Environ Microbiol. 1988;54:1–9.
19. Miller JF, Mekalanos JJ, Falkow S. Coordinate regulation and sensory transduction in the control of bacterial virulence. Science. 1989;243:916–22.
20. Weiss AA, Falkow S. Genetic analysis of phase change in *Bordetella pertussis*. Infect Immun. 1984;43:263–9.
21. Maurelli AT, Sansonetti PJ. Identification of a chromosomal gene controlling temperature-regulated expression of *Shigella* virulence. Proc Natl Acad Sci USA. 1988;85:2820–4.
22. Miller VL, Taylor RK, Mekalanos JJ. Cholera toxin transcriptional activator *tox*R is a transmembrane DNA binding protein. Cell 1987;48:271–9.
23. Miller VL, Mekalanos JJ. A novel suicide vector and its use in construction of insertion mutations: Osmoregulation of outer membrane proteins and virulence determinants in *Vibrio cholerae* requires *tox*R. J Bacteriol. 1988; 170:2575–83.
24. Simon M, Zieg J, Silverman M, et al. Phase variation: Evolution of a controlling element. Science. 1980;209:1370–4.
25. McGee ZA, Johnson AP, Taylor-Robinson D. Pathogenic mechanisms of *Neisseria gonorrhoeae:* Observations on damage to human fallopian tubes in organ culture by gonococci of colony type 1 or type 4. J Infect Dis. 1981;143:413–22.
26. McChesney D, Tramont EC, Boslego JW, et al. Genital antibody response to a parenteral gonococcal pilus vaccine. Infect Immun. 1982;36:1006–12.
27. Seifert HS, So M. Genetic mechanisms of bacterial antigenic variation. Microbiol Rev. 1988;52:327–36.
28. Borst P. Discontinuous transcription and antigenic variation in trypanosomes. Annu Rev Biochem. 1986;55:701–32.
29. Meier JT, Simon MI, Barbour AG. Antigenic variation is associated with DNA rearrangements in a relapsing fever borrelia. Cell. 1985;41:403–9.
30. Weiss AA, Hewlett EL, Myers GA, et al. *Tn*5-induced mutations affecting virulence factors of *Bordetella pertussis*. Infect Immun. 1983;42:33–41.
31. Macrina FL. Molecular cloning of bacterial antigens and virulence determinants. Annu Rev Microbiol. 1984;38:193–219.
32. Collins J. *Escherichia coli* plasmids packageable in vitro in lambda bacteriophage particles. Methods Enzymol. 1979;68:309–26.
33. Pearson GDN, Mekalanos JJ. Molecular cloning of *Vibrio cholerae* enterotoxin genes in *Escherichia coli* K-12. Proc Natl Acad Sci USA. 1982;79:2976–80.
34. Livey I, Duggleby CJ, Robinson A. Cloning and nucleotide sequence analysis of the serotype 2 fimbrial subunit gene of *Bordetella pertussis*. Mol Microbiol. 1987;1:203–9.
35. Stibitz S, Weiss AA, Falkow S. Genetic analysis of a region of the *Bordetella pertussis* chromosome encoding filamentous hemagglutinin and the pleiotropic regulatory locus *vir*. J Bacteriol. 1988;170:2904–13.
36. Shatzman AR, Rosenberg M. Expression, identification, and characterization of recombinant gene products in *Escherichia coli*. Methods Enzymol. 1987;152:661–73.
37. Isberg RR, Falkow S. A single genetic locus encoded by *Yersinia pseudotuberculosis* permits invasion of cultured animal cells by *Escherichia coli* K-12. Nature. 1985;317:262–4.
38. Botstein D, Shortle D. Strategies and applications of in vitro mutagenesis. Science. 1985;229:1193–201.
39. Sanger F, Nicklen S, Coulson AR. DNA sequencing with chain-terminating inhibitors. Proc Natl Acad Sci USA. 1977;74:5463–7.
40. Frazer AC, Curtiss R. Production, properties and utility of bacterial minicells. Curr Top Microbiol Immunol. 1975;69:1–84.
41. Sancar A, Hack AM, Rupp WD. Simple method for identification of plasmid-coded proteins. J Bacteriol. 1979;137:692–3.
42. Evans AS. Causation and disease: The Henle-Koch postulates revisited. Yale J Biol Med. 1976;49:175–95.
43. Falkow S. Molecular Koch's postulates applied to microbial pathogenicity. Rev Infect Dis. 1988;10(Suppl):274–6.
44. Stibitz S, Black W, Falkow S. The construction of a cloning vector designed for gene replacement in *Bordetella pertussis*. Gene. 1986;50:133–40.
45. Whittam TS, Wachsmuth IK, Wilson RA. Genetic evidence of clonal descent of *Escherichia coli* 0157:H7 associated with hemorrhagic colitis and hemolytic uremic syndrome. J Infect Dis. 1988;157:1124–33.
46. Caugant DA, Froholm LO, Bovre K, et al. Intercontinental spread of a genetically distinctive complex of clones of *Neisseria meningitidis* causing epidemic disease. Proc Natl Acad Sci USA. 1986;4927–31.
47. Musser JM, Hewlett EL, Peppler MS, et al. Genetic diversity and relationships in populations of *Bordetella* spp. J Bacteriol. 1986;166:230–7.
48. Tenover FC. Diagnostic deoxyribonucleic acid probes for infectious diseases. Clin Microbiol Rev. 1988;1:82–101.
49. Moseley SL, Huq I, Alim AR, et al. Detection of enterotoxigenic *Escherichia coli* by DNA colony hybridization. J Infect Dis. 1980;142:892–8.
50. Horn JE, Quinn T, Hammer M, et al. Use of nucleic acid probes for the detection of sexually transmitted infectious agents. Diagn Microbiol Infect Dis. 1986;4(Suppl):101–9.
51. McDonough KA, Schwan TG, Thomas RE, et al. Identification of a *Yersinia pestis*-specific DNA probe with potential for use in plague surveillance. J Clin Microbiol. 1988;26:2515–9.
52. Rappuoli R, Perugini M, Falsen E. Molecular epidemiology of the 1984–1986 outbreak of diphtheria in Sweden. N Engl J Med. 1988;318:12–4.
53. Saiki RK, Gelfand DH, Stoffel S, et al. Primer-directed enzymatic amplification of DNA with a thermostable DNA polymerase. Science. 1988;239:487–91.
54. Spika JS, Waterman SH, Hoo GW, et al. Chloramphenicol resistant *Salmonella newport* traced through hamburger to dairy farms. N Engl J Med. 1987; 316:565–70.
55. Tompkins LS, Roessler BJ, Redd SC, et al. *Legionella* prosthetic-valve endocarditis. N Engl J Med. 1988;318:530–5.
56. Black WJ, Munoz JJ, Peacock MG, et al. ADP-ribosyltransferase activity of pertussis toxin and immunomodulation by *Bordetella pertussis*. Science 1988;240:656–9.
57. Ou CY, Kwok S, Mitchell SW, et al. DNA amplification for direct detection of HIV-1 in DNA of peripheral blood mononuclear cells. Science. 1988;239:295–7.
58. Engleberg NC, Eisenstein BI. The impact of new cloning techniques on the diagnosis and treatment of infectious diseases. N Engl J Med. 1984;311:892–901.
59. Isberg RR, Voorhis DL, Falkow S. Identification of invasin: A protein that allows enteric bacteria to penetrate cultured mammalian cells. Cell. 1987;50:769–78.

SECTION B. HOST DEFENSE MECHANISMS

4. GENERAL OR NONSPECIFIC HOST DEFENSE MECHANISMS

EDMUND C. TRAMONT

General or nonspecific host defense mechanisms refer to a formidable array of host resistance factors that interfere with a microorganism's ability to invade and/or harm its host. The protective effects are due to innate resistance (i.e., intact skin) or are stimulated by the invading organism. In contrast to antibodies, they are not specifically directed against the invading organism (i.e., cytokines). These mechanisms are an important first encounter for a microorganism with its host and often represent the initial response elicited by the host. Because of their general nature, these nonspecific host defense mechanisms are difficult to quantitate, and because they are so efficient, they are often taken for granted (Table 1). Taken as a whole, the effect of this first line of defense is impressive; taken individually, each mechanism or factor is of a much smaller magnitude and much less dramatic than are responses that confer resistance to a specific infectious agent (i.e., antibodies).

NORMAL INDIGENOUS MICROBIAL FLORA

A microorganism in most cases must gain access into or onto the host in order to develop a particular relationship with that host (a preformed toxin such as that produced by *Clostridium botulinum* would be an exception). This host–parasite relationship may be *symbiotic*, *commensal*, or *parasitic*, depending upon the particular situation that is being described. For example, *Escherichia coli* is a commensal organism in the gastrointestinal tract, but it is a parasite in the lung. Certain organisms always behave in a predictable fashion. In humans, the rabies virus is always considered a pathogen, whereas the lactobacillus seldom is. From the point of view of the microorganism, the better adapted it becomes to exist in a symbiotic or commensal relationship with its host, the better its chances for survival.

The normal commensal flora plays an important role in protecting the host from microbial invasion by "pathogenic" organisms.[1] Mechanisms of this protection include the following: (*1*) competition for the same nutrients (interference), (*2*) competition for the same receptors on host cells (tropism), (*3*) production of bacteriocins, that is, bacterial products that are toxic to other organisms, usually of the same species, (*4*) continual stimulation of the immune system to maintain low but constant levels of class II histocompatibility (DR) molecule expression on macrophages and other accessory cells,[2] and (*5*) stimulation of cross-protective immune factors such as the so-called natural antibodies.

The ultimate effect of the first three protective mechanisms is to limit the quantity or dominance of any one species of organism. For example, broad-spectrum antibiotic therapy decreases the concentration of all sensitive bacteria in the gut. When the antibiotic therapy is stopped, a rebound results and the gut is repopulated, but to the advantage of the faster-growing aerobic Enterobacteriaceae over the slower-metabolizing anaerobes. A disproportion therefore is created that may be reflected in "rebound bacteremia," especially in immunocompromised hosts.[2] We might favorably influence the development of commensal flora in this case by stopping all antibiotics that have an anaerobic spectrum 24–36 hours before stopping aminoglycoside antibiotics that lack an anaerobic spectrum to allow anaerobic organisms to reestablish a competitive foothold.[3] Other examples include the purposeful recolonization of *Staphylococcus aureus* carriers with the relatively avirulent S. aureus strain 502A and the repopulation of gut flora with lactobacilli or normal fecal flora.

The microbial flora harbored by the host can be divided into two groups: (*1*) normal resident flora that is regularly found and, if disturbed, prompty reestablishes itself and (*2*) a transient flora that may colonize the host for periods ranging from hours to weeks but does not permanently establish itself.

The normal microbial flora that can be isolated from sites of the body are listed in Table 2. Certain organisms characteristically colonize certain sites (tropism). This is obviously taken into consideration when deciding whether a particular organism is behaving in a pathogenic fashion. Bacteria and fungi make up the great majority of commensal and symbiotic organisms. Mycoplasmas and viruses are much less prevalent. The presence of a member of the herpesvirus family usually reflects activation of latency rather than true colonization of mucosal surfaces. Protozoa are also less ubiquitous than bacteria and fungi, almost always reside in the gastrointestinal tract, and are more prevalent in underdeveloped countries.

The species that make up the normal flora are obviously influenced by environmental factors such as diet, sanitary conditions, air pollution, and hygienic habits. For example, lactobacilli are common intestinal commensals whenever dairy products make up a significant proportion of the dietary intake; protozoa are common intestinal inhabitants of those living where sanitation is poor; and a patient with underlying chronic bronchitis is more likely to harbor *Haemophilus influenzae* in the tracheobronchial tree.

The normal flora is also influenced by hormones. Premenarchal and postmenopausal vaginal flora differ significantly from that present during the childbearing period.

However, perhaps the ultimate effect of the normal flora on the immune system is to keep it "primed" and thus more rapid and efficient in its response to invading microorganisms. Antigens must be presented to the immune system in an ordered and specified way. T cells recognize antigens only after they

TABLE 1. Factors Contributing to Host Nonspecific Resistance to Infection

Normal indigenous microflora
Genetic factors
Natural antibodies
Morphologic integrity
Normal excretory secretions and flow
Phagocytosis
Natural killer (NK) cells
Nutrition
Non-antigen-specific immune response
Fibronectin
Hormonal factors

The views of the author do not purport to reflect the position of the Department of the Army or the Department of Defense (para 4–3. AR 360–5).

TABLE 2. Microorganisms That Commonly Colonize Healthy Human Body Surfaces (Normal Flora)

Skin	
Bacteria	
Staphylococcus epidermidis	+ + + +[a]
Diphtheroids	
Corynebacterium spp.	+ + + +
Propionibacterium acnes	+ + + +
Staphylococcus aureus	+ +
Streptococcus spp. including *S. pyogenes*	+
Peptococcus	+
Mycobacterium spp.	+
Bacillus spp.—soil or free-living bacteria	+
Acinetobacter	±
Enterobacteriaceae	±
Pseudomonas spp.	±
Fungi	
Malassezia furfur	+ + + +
Candida spp.	+
Mouth and oropharynx[b]	
Bacteria	
Streptococcus spp.	
St. mitus	+ + + +
Non-group A *Streptococcus*	+ +
St. pneumoniae	+ +
St. pyogenes	+
St. salivarius	+ + + +
Anaerobic gram-negative spp.	
Veillonella spp.	+ + + +
Bacteroidaceae spp.	+ +
Fusobacterium spp.	+ + + +
S. epidermidis	+ + +
Treponema spp.	+ + +
Lactobacillus spp.	+ +
Neisseria spp.	+ +
N. meningitidis	+
Nonpathogenic (*N. sicca*, etc.)	+ +
Haemophilus spp.	+
H. influenzae, non-group B	+
H. influenzae, group B	+
H. parainfluenzae	+
Anaerobic streptococci and micrococci	+
Peptococcus	+
Peptostreptococcus	+
Mycoplasma	±
Actinomycetes	+
S. aureus	+
Enterobaciaceae	±
Fungi	
Yeasts	
Candida spp. (*C. albicans*)	+ +
Virus	
Herpes simplex	±
Nose	
Bacteria	
Staphylococcus spp.	
S. epidermidis	+ + + +
S. aureus	+ +
Neisseria spp.	+
Streptococcus spp.	+ +
St. pneumoniae	+
St. pyogenes	+
Haemophilus spp.	+
Outer ear	
Bacteria	
S. epidermidis	+ + + +
Pseudomonas spp.	+
St. pneumoniae	±
Enterobacteriaceae	+
Conjunctivae	
Bacteria	
S. epidermidis	+ + +
Haemophilus spp.	+
S. aureus	+
Streptococcus spp.	±
St. pneumoniae	±
Group A streptococci	±
Neisseria spp.	±
Moraxella spp.	±
Enterobacteriaceae	±

(*Continued*)

TABLE 2. (Continued)

Esophagus and stomach	
Bacteria	
Low numbers of (10^4/ml)	
Surviving bacteria from upper respiratory tract and food	+
Mycobacterium spp.	+
Small intestine	
Bacteria	
Lactobacillus spp.	+ + +
Mycobacterium spp.	+ +
Enterobacteriaceae	+ +
S. aureus	±
Enterococcus	+ +
Gram-negative anaerobic spp.	+ + +
Bacteroides spp.	+ +
Clostridium spp.	+ +
Large intestine (95% or more of species are obligate anaerobes)	
Bacteria	
Gram-negative anaerobes	
Bacteroidaceae spp.	+ + + +
Fusobacterium spp.	+ + + +
Gram-positive anaerobes	
Peptococcus spp.	+ + + +
Peptostreptococcus spp.	+ + + +
Enterobacteriaceae	+ + + +
E. coli	+ + + +
Klebsiella spp.	+ + +
Proteus spp.	+ + +
Enterococcus	+ +
Lactobacillus	+ + +
Clostridium spp.	+ + + +
C. perfringens	+ + +
C. welchii	+ + +
Streptococcus spp.	+ +
Group B streptococci	±
Pseudomonas spp.	+
Aeromonas spp.	±
P. aeruginosa	
Alcaligenes spp.	+
Acinetobacter spp.	+
S. epidermidis	+
S. aureus	+
Campylobacter spp.	±
Arizona spp.	±
Mycobacterium spp.	+
Actinomycetes	+
Treponema spp.	+
Virus	
Adenovirus (in children)	±
Fungi	
Yeasts, especially *Candida* spp.	±
Protozoa[c]	
Giardia lamblia	±
Liver, gallbladder, pancreas (normally sterile or low numbers of anaerobic organisms)	
Vagina	
Bacteria	
Mycoplasma spp.	±
Ureaplasma urealyticum	±
Döderlein's bacillus	+ + + +
Lactobacillus spp.	+ + + +
Gram-positive anaerobic spp.	+ + +
Peptococcus	+ +
Peptostreptococcus	+
Bifidobacterium	+
Propionibacterium	+
Clostridium spp.	+ +
Streptococcus spp.	+
Enterococcus	+
S. epidermidis	+
Mobiluncus spp.	+
Diphtheroids	+ +
Gram-positive anaerobic spp.	+ +
Veillonella spp.	+
Bacteroidaceae	+
Gardnerella vaginale	+
Acinetobacter	+
Enterobacteriaceae	±
Neisseria spp.	±

(Continued)

TABLE 2. (Continued)

Fungi	
Candida spp.	+ +
Torulopsis spp.	+
Actinomycetes	+
Protozoa	
Trichomonas vaginalis	±
External genitalia and anterior urethra	
Bacteria	
Mycoplasma spp.	±
Ureaplasma urealyticum	±
"Skin flora"	+ + + +
Fusobacterium spp.	+
Gram-negative anaerobe spp.	+
Mycobacterium spp.[d]	+ +
Peptostreptococcus	+
Enterococcus	+
Enterobacteriaceae	±
Acinetobacter	±
Protozoa	
Trichomonas vaginalis	±

[a] Relative frequency of isolation: + + + +, almost always present; + + +, usually present; + +, frequently present; +, occasionally present; ±, rarely present.
[b] The presence of teeth affects the normal flora and anerobic organisms, *Fusobacterium* and *Treponema* being less prevalent in edentulous people.
[c] Protozoa are more prevalent in the intestines of people living in underdeveloped countries.
[d] Mycobacteria are particularly common in the smegma of uncircumcised boys and men.

are displayed on the surface of a macrophage (or other antigen-presenting cell) in physical association with a class II histocompatibility (DR) molecule. Normally, 75–85 percent of circulating monocytes in adults maintain relatively high levels of DR molecule expression. DR expression is much lower on monocytes in human newborns,[2] neonatal mice, and germ-free animals.[4] Thus, the constant stimulation by the host's indigenous microbial flora maintains the high level of DR molecule expression on macrophages and perhaps other antigen-presenting cells, and this serves to keep the immune system primed. This modulation is due, at least in part, to low-level production of γ-interferon, interleukin-4, and other cytokines by activated T cells (see below).

TISSUE TROPISMS AND HEREDITARY FACTORS

Receptors exist on tissues that permit the attachment of microorganisms. The attachment of a microorganism to a receptor is dependent upon the presence of a complementary ligand or adhesin on that microorganism.[5] (see Chapter 2). The ligand and the receptor vary independently as to their specificity—a receptor binding to one or many different organisms (ligands), a ligand binding one or many different receptors. Thus, most organisms preferentially colonize certain tissues and spare others. This phenomenon is referred to as *tissue tropism*. For example, influenza virus and mycoplasmas preferentially adhere to respiratory epithelial cells, *E. coli* and *Vibrio cholerae* to intestinal cells, and *Streptococcus mutans* to tooth enamel; also, gram-positive organisms more readily attach to heart valves than do gram-negative organisms.[6] *Treponema pallidum*, on the other hand, binds to many different tissue receptors, and untreated late syphilis may involve any organ.

Receptors on host cells may change. For example, there is evidence to suggest that viral illness may affect tissue tropisms of the oropharynx to allow easier colonization by gram-negative organisms.[7] Also, urinary epithelial cells from people prone to develop urinary tract infections support the attachment of urinary pathogens over urinary epithelial cells from healthy people.[8] The genetics of tissue tropisms are unknown. The role of these factors in determining susceptibilities of a host to a particular infection is obviously important.

The relationship of genetic factors to susceptibilities to infectious agents has been appreciated for many years.[9,10] Infections have been one of the strongest selective pressures in human evolution. The devastating effects of tuberculosis, measles, and smallpox on the native American populations was tantamount to genocide. Conversely, the protective effects of sickle cell trait on the outcome of falciparum malaria are well known.

Histocompatible antigens have been linked to a predisposition to some infectious complications. The HLA-B27 and reactive arthropathy or Reiter syndrome was one of the earliest associations that was recognized. There is evidence of HLA-linked determinants in tuberculoid leprosy,[11] acute glomerulonephritis,[12] paralytic poliomyelitis,[13,14] and responsiveness to antigenic stimulus.[15] The list is destined to grow. Genetic influences on other infectious processes are not as well understood.

Natural Antibodies

Natural antibodies are specific antibodies found in healthy people without a previous history of a compatible infection. These antibodies are of great importance in the immunity to many bacteria, especially encapsulated bacteria such as *Neisseria meningiditis* and *H. influenzae*, type b.

These antibodies are stimulated by colonization in the oropharynx, gut, or elsewhere of organisms sharing cross-reactive (cross-protective) antigens.[15] However, these antibodies are not always beneficial. There are data to suggest that specific serum IgA antibodies to *N. meningitidis* may predispose an otherwise immune person to become susceptible by preferentially attaching to the organism, thus blocking the beneficial bactericidal effect of the protective IgG and IgM antibodies.[16] The blood group antibodies are a consequence of colonization in the gut of microorganisms bearing cross-reactive antigens.

NATURAL BARRIERS TO THE ENTRY OF MICROORGANISMS INTO THE BODY

The morphologic integrity of the body surface is an important and effective first line of defense.

Skin and Mucous Membranes

The intact skin forms a very effective mechanical barrier to invasion by microorganisms. Since very few organisms have the innate ability to penetrate the skin, they must gain access by some physical means such as by an arthropod vector, a primary skin lesion such as eczema, trauma, a surgeon's incision, or an intravenous catheter. The papovavirus (warts) is an exception.

The specific antimicrobial properties of skin have not been exhaustively studied. However, the relative dryness or desiccating effect of skin, the mild acidity (acid mantle, pH 5–6), and the normal skin flora act in concert to form an effective prohibitive environment. Inflamed skin is more permeable to water and therefore leads to greater colonization. It has been speculated that oily skin may retard evaporation of water, resulting in increased numbers of organisms. The acidity of the skin results from the breakdown of lipids into fatty acids. Sebum contains few esterified fatty acids, but the normal skin flora partially hydrolyzes the triglycerides, thereby liberating fatty acids. Desquamation of skin scales also aids in the elimination of microorganisms.

The mucous membranes support a larger number of microorganisms but also offer mechanical resistance. Also, the mucosal surfaces are bathed in secretions with antimicrobial properties. For example, cervical mucus, prostatic fluid, and tears have been shown to be toxic to a large variety of microorganisms. One of the more potent antimicrobial substances is lysozyme, which is found in every local secretion. It is an enzyme that lyses bacteria by splitting the muramic acid B-(1–4)-*N*-acetylglucosamine linkage in the bacterial cell wall and is especially effective against gram-positive organisms. Local secretions also contain specific immunoglobulins, principally IgG and secretory IgA (which act primarily to block the attachment of organisms to host cells [ligands]) and significant amounts of iron-binding proteins. The importance of iron for microorganisms is well recognized, and all fluids that are potentially exposed to microbes are enriched with iron-binding proteins.[17]

Respiratory Tract

The respiratory tract has formidable antimicrobial defense mechanisms.[18] First, the inhaled particles must survive and penetrate the aerodynamic filtration system of the upper airway and tracheobronchial tree. The airflow in these areas is quite turbulent, causing large particles to impact on the mucosal surfaces. Humidification of the incoming air causes hydroscopic organisms to increase in size, thus aiding phagocytosis.

Once deposited, the mucociliary blanket transports the invading offender away from the lung. Coughing obviously aids this expulsion. This system is amazingly efficient: 90 percent of deposited material is cleared in less than 1 hour. In addition, the bronchial secretions contain various antimicrobial substances (e.g., lysozyme).

Once a particle reaches the alveoli, physical expulsion becomes much less effective, and the alveolar macrophage and tissue histiocytes play a more prominent role in protecting the host. When the lungs become inflamed, they are aided by the influx of polymorphonuclear leukocytes and monocytes, which become even more efficient when specific immune mechanisms such as opsonins are present.

Like all defense mechanisms, these nonspecific mechanisms can be overcome by the introduction of large numbers of invading organisms (e.g., contaminated respirator), particularly when exposed over an extended period of time. Furthermore, their effectiveness is decreased by air pollutants (e.g., cigarette smoke), mechanical respirators, tracheostomy, concomitant infection, and allergenic agents.

Intestinal Tract

The acid pH of the stomach, the antibacterial effect of the various pancreatic enzymes, and bile and intestinal secretions are effective antimicrobial factors. Peristalsis and the normal loss of epithelial cells also act to purge the intestinal tract of harmful microorganisms. Alteration of these parameters can lead to increased susceptibility of the host to infection. For example, *Salmonella* and tuberculosis infections are more common in achlorhydric patients, and slowing peristalsis with belladonna or opium alkaloids prolongs symptomatic shigellosis.[19] Intubated patients treated with inhibitors of gastric acid secretion have a higher incidence of aspiration pneumonia.

Normal bowel flora competition (10^{12} organisms per gram of feces) plays an extremely important protective role. Altering this flora with broad-spectrum antibiotics can lead to overgrowth with inherently pathogenic organisms (e.g., *Salmonella typhimurium*) or suprainfection with ordinarily commensal organisms (e.g., *Candida albicans*). The interfering competitive capacity of the normal flora can be overcome by large numbers of virulent organisms. For example, the rate of development of salmonellosis has been directly related to the number of *Salmonella* organisms ingested.[20]

Genitourinary Tract

Urine is normally sterile. The factors that contribute to the ability of the urinary tract to resist infection are quite complex. Urine may be bactericidal for some strains of bacteria. This is mostly due to the pH of the urine, but factors such as urea and other solutes may play a role.

The lower urinary tract is flushed with urine four to eight times each day, eliminating potential pathogenic organisms unless they are capable of firmly attaching to epithelial cells of the urinary tract, such as *N. gonorrhoeae* and certain strains of *E. coli*. The length of the male urethra (20 cm in the adult) also provides protection, and bacteria seldom gain access to the bladder in men unless introduced by instrumentation. The female urethra is much shorter (5 cm in the adult and more readily traversed by microorganisms, which may be one reason why urinary tract infections are 14 times more common in women than in men. The hypertonic state of the kidney medulla presents an unfavorable milieu for most microorganisms. Tamm-Horsfall protein is a glycoprotein produced by the kidneys and excreted in large amounts in urine (approximately 50 mg/liter). Certain bacteria avidly bind to it, suggesting that it prevents them from gaining a foothold in the urinary tract, thereby acting as a natural host defense mechanism against colonization and subsequent infection.[21]

The vagina has a unique mechanism of protection. Under hormonal influence, especially estrogens, the vaginal epithelium contains increased amounts of glycogen that Döderlein's bacilli and other commensals metabolize into lactic acid. *Döderlein's bacilli* is an all-encompassing term used to describe acidogenic gram-positive rods residing in the vagina. Normal vaginal secretions contain up to 10^8 of such bacteria per milliliter. Thus an acid environment that is unfavorable to most pathogenic bacteria is established. The vaginal secretions of women with nonspecific vaginitis are usually characterized by an elevated pH.

The Eye

Constant bathing of the eyes by tears is an effective means of protection. Foreign substances are continually diluted and washed away via the tear ducts into the nasal cavity. Tears also contain large amounts of lysozyme and other antimicrobial substances.[22]

NONSPECIFIC ASPECTS OF THE IMMUNE SYSTEM

The immune system is modulated by a large number of regulatory mediators known as *cytokines* (see Chapter 8), which act through a complicated bidirectional feedback network similar to the endocrine system to influence other cells, especially lymphoid cells and cells of the neuroendocrine system.

Cytokines

Cytokines are hormone-like polypeptides that are produced during the initial response to an invading foreign agent (microorganism) and participate in a variety of cellular responses, including modulation of the immune system (Fig. 1). They are produced by a growing list of different cells, but principally by macrophages and activated lymphocytes (Table 3). Many of the generalized symptoms (morbidity) associated with infections are attributable to this cytokine cascade (e.g., fever, sleepiness, muscle aches and pain) (Fig. 1). Unlike antibodies, whose chemical composition is specifically determined by the stimulating antigen, the chemical composition of cytokines is constant and independent of the stimulating antigen.[23]

Cytokines are usually named for the cell that produces them (e.g., lymphokines, monokines). Most cytokines have more than one biologic property and share a number of overlapping functions (Table 4). This is probably why no single disease state has ever been traced to a deficiency or overproduction of any single cytokine and why their individual functions could not be discerned until the recent advances in molecular biologic techniques were made. As foreign agents (e.g., toxins, microbial products) trigger the immune system, a non-antigen-specific cascading release of cytokines ensues, acting in concert to increase resistance to invading microorganisms (and neoplastic cells). Cytokines thus form the first line of defense of the immune system and their impact is a prelude to specific immune responses.

There is a constant low-level background sentinel-like activity that helps to maintain the host's steady state of good immunologic health. This steady-state background activity may be either diminished or augmented (i.e., dysregulated). For example, persons who are immunocompromised for any reason have their immune "thermostat" set much lower and/or their level of maximal response dampened; therefore, the efficiency of their response is clearly hampered. This can be measured clinically by examining their *cellular immune status*, although all components of the immune system are adversely affected.[24] The most convenient means to measure the state of one's cellular immune system is with skin tests.[25]

In the United States, end-stage cancer, renal disease, human immunodeficiency virus (HIV) infection (acquired immune deficiency syndrome, AIDS), liver disease, and alcoholism are the most common underlying illnesses resulting in diminished cellular immune responsiveness. Worldwide, malnutrition is the leading cause.[26,27] This is especially evident in malnourished children, who have increased susceptibility to and severity of several infections. These include life-threatening bacterial in-

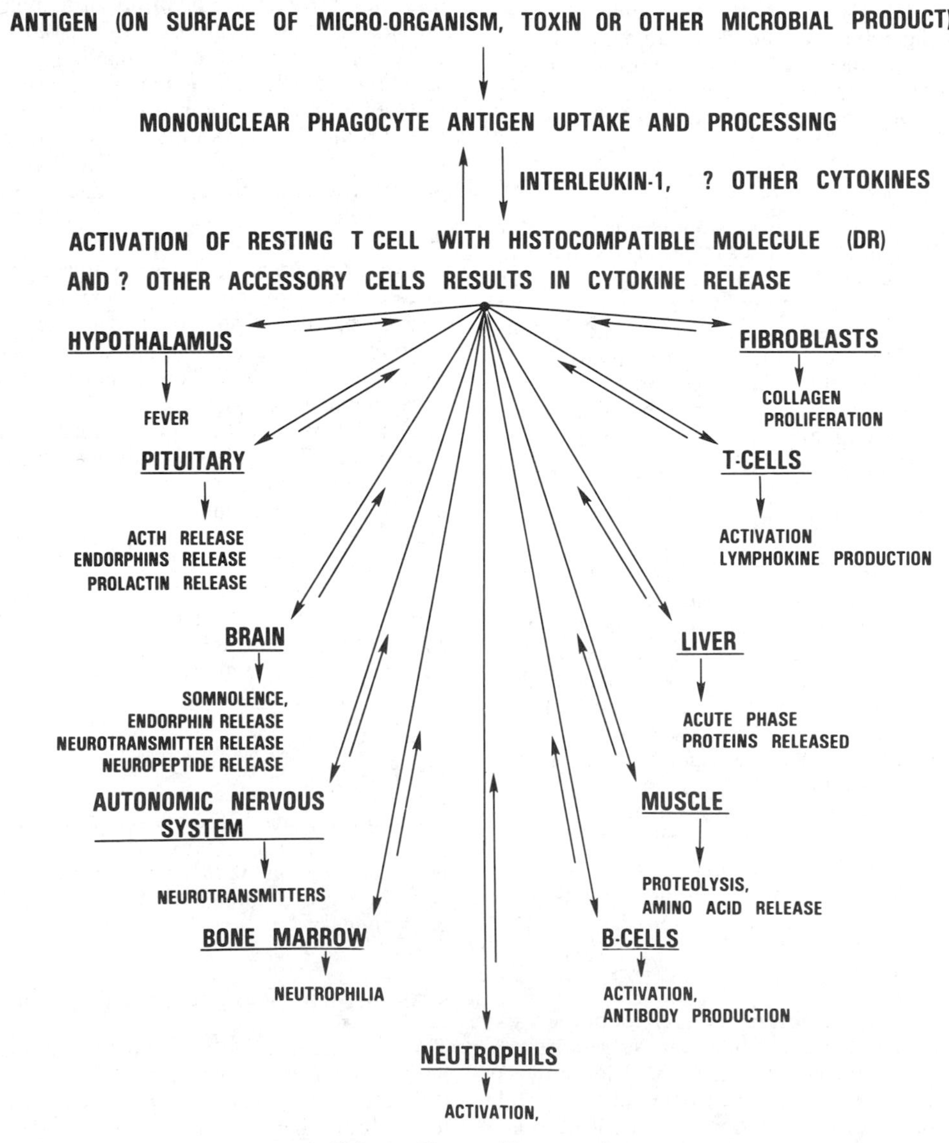

FIG. 1. The cytokine cascade.

TABLE 3. Cell Sources of Cytokines

Monocytes/macrophages
Lymphocytes
Langerhan cells
Histiocytes
Keratinocytes/epithelial cells
Corneal cells
Gingival epithelium
Melanocytes
Astrocytes
Microglial cells
Gliomal cells
Hypothalamus
Fibroblasts
Synovial cells
Neutrophils
Endothelial cells

fections of the middle ear, pervasive dental carries, and common childhood diseases, especially measles.[28]

Acute Phase Response

An easily recognized augmented non-antigen-specific response referred to as the *acute phase response* is a generalized but remarkably consistent host reaction that develops irrespective of the local or systemic nature of the inciting microorganism. It is mediated through an increased release of various cytokines, particularly interleukin-1 and tumor necrosis factor α (cachectin).[29,30]

Fever is the most obvious sign of the acute phase response and is the result of the action of cytokines, particularly interleukin-1, tumor necrosis factor, and α-interferon on the thermoregulatory center (hypothalamus) of the brain. The beneficial vs. detrimental effects of fever on the host have long been debated.[31] However, its role in upregulating the initial phase of an immune response appears to be critical (see Chapter 39).

An increase in the number and immaturity of circulating neutrophils is another readily demonstrated response (see Chapter 7) and is a direct consequence of the effect of cytokines, especially interleukin-1 and colony-stimulating factors, on the bone marrow. Other cytokines are involved in the activation of the neutrophils[31a] and promote and stimulate the colony formation of the various cell lines.

A decrease in serum iron and zinc and an increase in ceruloplasmin have long been recognized as components of the acute phase response. The virulence of many microorganisms is enhanced by increased availability of iron, and this has led to speculation that the host redistributes iron by an increased release of transferrin in an attempt to withhold this critical metal from the invader.[17] Furthermore, all normal mucosal secretions contain iron-binding proteins, suggesting a host defense mechanism to starve colonizing organisms. For example, gonococci disseminate most often in women during menstruation, a time when these organisms are exposed to increased amounts of free iron.

Zinc appears to be involved in wound healing, improves lymphocyte responsiveness, is required for hepatic RNA polymerase activity (increased during infection), and is implicated in the synthesis of protein, including acute phase globulins by the liver. Zinc also has been shown to affect phagocytosis. Thus, a deficiency of zinc, which is not stored in the body, influences the effectiveness of the immune response and aids with tissue repair.[25a]

The effects of the increased level of ceruloplasmin are not well understood, but it possibly increases the oxidation of catecholamines and therefore indirectly affects the redistribution of bood to vital organs.

During the acute phase response, the liver decreases albumin synthesis but dramatically increases the synthesis of other proteins, such as haptoglobin, complement components, amyloid A protein, C-reactive protein,[32] and certain protease inhibitors like α1-antitrypsin, α2-macroglobulins, and glycoproteins. Some of these derangements become quite prominent as the chronicity of the infection develops, (e.g., the decreased serum albumin levels noted in certain chronic infections).

A number of other systemic derangements are also evident during the acute phase response. These include increased production of thyroid-stimulating hormone, vasopressin, insulin, and glucagon, as well as a profound catabolism of muscle protein as a result of oxidation of amino acids from skeletal muscles. Prolonged infection results in muscle wasting, which can be clearly evident within days. Increased oxygen and caloric demands because of fever also contribute to this negative nitrogen balance. The increased circulating amino acids may be utilized by cells of the immune system.

Cytokines, especially interleukin-1 and tumor necrosis factor, also induce sleepiness through their effects on the central nervous system, a common host response leading to reduced energy demands.

The exact effects of cytokines on the brain and hypothalamus have not yet been fully elucidated. The release of ACTH, endorphins, prolactin, neurotransmitters, and growth hormone are induced by cytokines.[33] As the infectious process progresses, this nonspecific cytokine-driven response is augmented by the development of specific immunologic responses.[34]

Taken as a whole, this initial nonspecific response appears to be quite efficient and effective. The overlapping functions of the cytokines and their far-flung effects appear to be an evo-

TABLE 4. Biologic Properties of Cytokines Involved in the Non-Antigen-Specific Immune Response

Cytokine	*Biologic Properties*
Interleukin-1	Activates resting T cells; induces the acute phase response and sleep; stimulates the pituitary gland, ACTH, endorphin, prolactin release; stimulates the synthesis of other cytokines, collagen, and collagenases; activates macrophages; mediates inflammation; primes neutrophils.
Tumor necrosis factor α (cachectin)	Induces the acute phase response, sleep; is cytotoxic for some tumor cells; stimulates the synthesis of other cytokines, collagen, and collagenase; activates macrophages; mediates inflammation; primes neutrophils.
Interleukin-2	Induces cytokine synthesis; activates cytotoxic lymphocytes; is growth factor for activated T cells.
Interleukin-3	Growth factor for multilineage (pluripotent) cells and mast cells.
Interleukin-4	Growth factor for activated B cells, resting T cells, and mast cells; induces DR expression on B cells; enhances cytotoxic T cells; activates macrophages.
Interleukin-5	B-cell differentiating and growth factor; eosinophil differentiation.
Interleukin-6	B-cell maturation factor (stimulates antibody formation).
γ-Interferon	Induces class I and class II molecule (DR) on cells. Induces other antigens on cells; activates macrophages; enhances natural killer cell activity; enhances and inhibits other cytokines; exerts antiviral activity.
α- and β-Interferon	Exerts antiviral activity; augments natural killer cell activity; induces fever; induces class I antigen expression; inhibits protein synthesis.
Granulocyte–macrophage colony-stimulating factor (CSF)	Promotes growth of neutrophil, eosinophil, and monocyte bone marrow colonies; activates PMNs and macrophages. Primes neutrophil.
Granulocyte colony-stimulating factor (GSF)	Promotes growth of neutrophil colonies.
Macrophage colony-stimulating factor (MSF)	Promotes growth of macrophage colonies.

lutionary development resulting in effective backup systems that improve the host's chances of surviving in a potentially hostile environment. However, dysregulation can and does occur. For example, it may be the critical underlying defect leading to septic shock.[35,36]

Stress. There are studies that suggest that there is a link between mental state and susceptibility to infections,[37] and a growing body of evidence demonstrating a relationship between stress and immune function.[33,38,39]

Fibronectin. Fibronectin is a large molecular weight glycoprotein found in plasma and on cell surfaces. It mediates nonspecific clearance of bacterial and nonbacterial particulates such as fibrinogen–fibrin complexes, fragments of damaged cells, collagen debris, and altered platelets. It also covers the receptors of surface cells, blocking the attachment of many organisms, such as *Pseudomonas aeruginosa*, but it also enhances the binding of other organisms, such as *S. aureus*, to host cells.[40]

Hormones. Increased ACTH production occurs during the acute phase response and appears to augment the host's survival potential. The depressive effects of excess corticosteroids on inflammation and cellular immunity are well known. Estrogen affects the lining of the vagina, resulting in increased nonspecific resistance. Pregnant women develop weaker cell-mediated immune responses,[41] which may account for the severity of certain viral infections such as poliomyelitis and influenza. There is also speculation that the increased severity of influenza pneumonia in pregnant women may be due to increased pulmonary venous pressure. Certain other acute bacterial infections appear to be more serious during pregnancy. For example, group A β-hemolytic streptococci and *N. gonorrhoeae*, organisms that ordinarily colonize mucosal surfaces, are more prone to disseminate in the last trimester of pregnancy.

Phagocytosis. Microorganisms that enter the lymphatics, lung, or blood stream are engulfed by a variety of phagocytic cells, among them polymorphonuclear cells, wandering macrophages, and fixed macrophages (histiocytes). Phagocytosis that occurs independently of the action of opsonins is related to the contact angle between the microorganism and the surface upon which it rests, and therefore is most efficient when organisms are trapped in small tissue spaces (e.g., alveoli) as compared to smooth open surfaces (e.g., synovium).[42]

The reticuloendothelial system refers to a functional concept whereby mononuclear phagocytic cells in the blood, lymphoid tissue, liver, spleen, lung, bone marrow, and other tissues remove particulate matter from the lymph and blood stream. An example of a dramatic deleterious consequence of failure of this system occurs in asplenics (surgical or nonfunctional), whose blood stream is invaded by encapsulated bacteria such as pneumococci.

Natural Killer (NK) cells are interferon-induced leucocytes capable of recognizing cell surface changes, especially on virally infected cells. The NK cells bind to and lyse these target cells.[42a]

Age

The very young and the elderly are more susceptible to infection than persons in other age groups. The underlying defects, however, are usually different. Young children are at particular risk after their maternal antibody disappears and before they have had time to stimulate their own antibody production. This is particularly evident in acute infections with encapsulated organisms, especially *N. meningitidis* and *H. influenzae*.[44]

In the elderly, there is a functional decline in cell-mediated immunity. There is also a diminution in the physiologic functions of certain organ systems such as the lung.[45] Taken together, their reserve is severely taxed.

Complement. Complement refers to a group of upwards of 20 serum components that interact with each other in an orderly fashion and are referred to as the complement cascade. Although most often activated in conjunction with specific immunity through the classical pathway, complement can be spontaneously activated by the surface of some microorganisms and lyse them through the alternative complement pathway. Complement lyses microbial cells by destroying the cell wall.[46]

Inflammation. Inflammation is a complex reaction that directs elements of the immune system into sites of injury or infection. It is manifest by an increase in the local blood supply and capillary permeability that allows chemotactic peptides, especially the complement fragment C5a, to reach the site of irritation. Migration of polymorphonuclear leukocytes and later mononuclear cells (macrophages) to the site follows. Other consequences include local edema and fibrin deposition, which acts to limit the spread of infection. Other mediators of inflammation include cytokines and derivatives of arachidonic acids, including prostaglandins, thromboxanes, and leukotrienes.

REFERENCES

1. Mackowiak PA. The normal microbial flora. N Engl J Med. 1982;307:83–6.
2. Stiehm ER, Sztein MB, Steeg PS, et al. Deficient antigen expression on human cord blood monocytes. Reversal with lymphokines. Clin Immunol Immunopathol. 1984;30:430–6.
3. Quiot HR, van der Meer JW, Van Furth R. Selective antimicrobial modulation of human microbial flora: Infection prevention in patients with decreased host defense mechanisms by selective elimination of potentially pathogenic bacteria. J Infect Dis. 1981;143:644–54.
4. Steinman RM, Nogueira N, Witmer MD, et al. Lymphokine enhances the expression and synthesis of 1a antigens on cultured mouse peritoneal macrophages. J Exp Med. 1980;152:1248–61.
5. Beachley EH. Bacterial adherence: Adhesion–receptor interactions mediating the attachment of bacteria to mucosal surfaces. J Infect Dis. 1981;143:325.
6. Gould RC, Rameriez-Randa H, Holmes RK, et al. Adherence of bacteria to heart valves. J Clin Invest. 1978;56:1364.
7. Ramirez-Ronda CH, Fuxench-Lopez Z, Nevarez M. Increased pharyngeal bacterial colonization during viral illness. Arch Intern Med. 1981;141:1599.
8. Svanburg-Eden C, Jodal V. Attachment of E. coli to urinary sediment epithelial cells from urinary tract infection prone to healthy children. Infect Immun. 1979;26:837.
9. Kaslow RA, Shaw S. The role of histocompatibility antigens (HLA) in infection. Epidemiol Rev. 1981;3:90.
10. Whisnant JK, Rogentine N, Gradmick MA, et al. Host factors and antibody response to Haemophilus influenzae type B meningitidis and epiglottitis. J Infect Dis. 1976;133:488.
11. Van Eden W, de Vries RRP, Mehra NK, et al. HLA segregation of tuberculoid leprosy: Confirmation of the DR2 marker. J Infect Dis. 1980;141:693.
12. Sasazuki I, Hayose R, Wanto I, et al. HLA and acute poststreptococcal glomerulonephritis. N Engl J Med. 1979;301:1184.
13. Zander H, Gross-Wilde H, Kuntz B, et al. HLA-A -B, and -D antigens in paralytic poliomyelitis. Tissue Antigens. 1979;13:310.
14. de Vries RRP, Kreeftenberg HG, Loggen HG, et al. In vitro responsiveness to vaccinia virus and HLA. N Engl J Med. 1979;297:692.
15. Schneerson R, Robbins JB. Induction of serum haemophilus influenzae type b capsular antibodies in adult volunteers fed cross reacting Escherichia coli 075:K100:H5. N Engl J Med. 1975;292:1093.
16. Griffiss JM. Bactericidal activity by IgA of lytic antibody in human convalescent sera. J Immunol. 1975;114:1779.
17. Weinberg ED. Iron Witholdings: A defense against infection and neoplasia. Physiol Rev. 1984;64:65–102.
18. Green GM. In: Defense of the lung. Am Rev Respir Dis. 102:691, 1970.
19. Dupont HL, Hornick RB. Adverse effect of Lomotil therapy in shigellosis. JAMA. 1973;226:1525.
20. Hornick RB, Greisman SE, Woodward TE, et al. Typhoid fever: Pathogenesis and immunologic control. N Engl J Med. 1970;283:686.
21. Israde V, Darabi A, McCracken GH. The role of bacterial virulence factors and Tamm-Horsfall protein in the pathogenesis of *E. coli* urinary tract infections in infants. Am J Dis Child. 1987;147:1230–4.
22. Golden B, ed. Ocular Inflammatory Diseases. Springfield, Ill.: Charles C. Thomas, 1974.
23. Dinarello CA, Mier JW. Lymphokines. N Engl J Med. 1987;317:940–5.
24. Blackburn GL. Nutritional assessment and support during infection. Am J Clin Nutr. 1977;30:1943.

25. MacLean LD. Delayed type hypersensitivity testing in surgical patients. Surg Gyn Obs. 1988;166:285–293.
25a. Powanda MC. Changes in body balances of nitrogen and other key nutrients. Am J Clin Nutr. 1977;30:1254.
26. Corman LC. The relationship between nutrition, infection and immunity. Med Clin North Am. 1985;69:519–31.
27. Keenan RA, Moldawer H, Yang RD, et al. An altered response by peripheral leukocytes to synthesize or release leukocyte endogenesis mediator in critically ill, protein-malnourished patients. J Clin Lab Med. 1982;100:844–56.
28. Gordon JE, Scrimshan NS: Infectious disease in the malnourished. Med Clin North Am 1970;54:1495.
29. Dinarello CA. Interleukin-1 and the pathogenesis of the acute-phase response. N Engl J Med. 1984;311:1413–7.
30. Beutler B, Cerami A. Cachectin: More than a tumor necrosis factor. N Engl J Med. 1987;316:379–85.
31. Dinarello CA, Wolff SM. Molecular basis of fever in humans. Am J Med. 1981;72:799–819.
31a. Sullivan GW, Carper HT, Sullivan JA, et al. Both recombinant interleukin-1 (Beta) and purified human monocytc interleukin-1 prime human neutrophils for increased oxidative activity and promote neutrophil spreading. J Leukocyte Biol. 1989; Press.
32. Pepys MB, Baltz ML. Acute phase proteins with special reference to C-reactive protein and related proteins (pentaxins) and serum amyloid A protein. Adv Immunol. 1983;34:141–211.
33. Breder CD, Dinerello CA, Saper CB. Interleukin-1: Immuno-reactive innervation of the human hypothalamus. Science. 1988;240:321–3.
34. Rouse BT, Nordey S, Martin S. Antiviral cytotoxic T lymphocyte induction and vaccination. Rev Infect Dis. 1988;10:16–33.
35. Michie HR, Manogue KR, Spriggs DR, et al. Detection of circulating tumor necrosis factor after endotoxin administration. N Engl J Med. 1988;318:1481–6.
36. Tracey KJ, Lowry SF, Cerami A. Cachectin: A hormone that triggers acute shock and chronic cachexia. J Infect Dis. 1988;157:413–20.
37. Goetzl EJ, ed. Neuromodulation of immunity and hypersensitivity. J Immunol. 1985;135(Suppl):739–863.
38. Stein M, Keller SE, Schleifer SJ: Stress and immunomodulation: The role of depressive and neuroendocrine function. J Immunol. 1985;135(Suppl):827–33.
39. Pert CB, Ruff MR, Weber RJ, et al. Neuropeptides and their receptors: A psychosomatic network. J Immunol. 1985;135(Suppl):820–6.
40. Proctor RA. Fibronectin: A brief overview of its structure, function and physiology. Rev Infect Dis. 1984;9:S317–21.
41. Weingerg ED. Pregnancy—associated depression of cell-mediated immunity. Rev Infect Dis. 1984;6:814–31.
42. Van Oss CJ, Gillman CF. Phagocytosis as a surface phenomenon. I. Contact angles and phagocytosis of nonopsonized bacteria. J Reticuloendothel Soc. 1972;12:283.
43. Herberman RB. Immunoregulation and natural killer cells. Mol Immunol. 1982;19:1313–1321.
44. Goldschneider I, Gotschlich EC, Artenstein MS. Human immunity to the meningococcus. J Exp Med. 1969;129:1307.
45. Saltzman RL, Peterson PK. Immunodeficiency of the elderly. Rev Infect Dis. 1987;1127–39.
46. Frank MM. Complement. In: Samter M, Immunological Diseases. 4th ed. Boston: Little Brown; 1987:247–61.

5. ANTIBODIES

FREDERICK P. HEINZEL
RICHARD K. ROOT

Defense against infections involves nonspecific mechanisms mediated by mucocutaneous barriers, the phagocytic and complement systems, and responses that are specifically determined by the antigenic structures on invading microorganisms. The humoral immune response refers to that mediated by antibodies, i.e., immunoglobulins with binding specificity for microbial or other antigens. Such antibodies may be instrumental in aiding the host to eradicate the organism, directly or indirectly, as protection against subsequent challenge with the same organisms (immunity); in the diagnosis of infection by acting as a highly specific marker for the presence of a given organism; or in the pathogenesis of certain features of some infections (e.g., immune complex-mediated tissue injury). The mechanisms of antibody development and the essential features of the specific humoral immune response will be reviewed as they relate to these events. In addition, disorders of the antibody-forming capacity will be discussed.

IMMUNOGLOBULIN STRUCTURE

All antibodies are complex glycoproteins known as immunoglobulins. Although all normal immunoglobulins can be presumed to be capable of binding antigens, the term antibody is reserved for those immunoglobulins for which a target antigen has been identified. To date five major classes of immunoglobulins have been recognized and characterized: immunoglobulins G (IgG), M (IgM), A (IgA), D (IgD), and E (IgE). IgG immunoglobulins are made up of four subclasses and comprise 75 percent of the total in serum; IgA, 15 percent, with two subclasses; IgM, 10 percent, IgD, 0.2 percent; and IgE, only 0.004 percent. Of the four IgG subclasses, IgG_1 comprises the majority (approximately 80 percent of total IgG). These concentrations may be indicative of their relative importance to host defenses against infection, as will be discussed below. The chemical properties that permit this classification are summarized in Table 1, their metabolic properties in Table 2, and their biologic activities in Table 3 (for reviews see Refs. 1–4).

Regardless of class, every immunoglobulin molecule has the same basic unit structure, consisting of two longer peptide chains known as "heavy" or H-chains bound by disulfide bridges to two shorter peptide chains known as "light" or L-chains (Fig. 1). Depending on immunoglobulin class and subclass, a variable number of disulfide bridges bind the H-chains to each other, with the one closest to the amino terminus located in a region of the molecule known as the "hinge." Insertion of the disulfide bonds from the L-chains into this region theoretically permits, on antigen binding, their free rotation together with the corresponding amino-terminal segment of the H-chain.

On the basis of amino acid sequence, L-chains can be placed into one of two groups, known as "kappa" and "lambda." A single monomeric immunoglobulin molecule has two κ- or two λ-chains, never one of each. Each light chain has a chemically "constant" and "variable" region. The variable region is located at the amino terminus and is so named because it has an amino acid sequence that varies with different antibody molecules. This variability provides the basis of antibody specificity for different antigenic targets and comprises an intimate portion

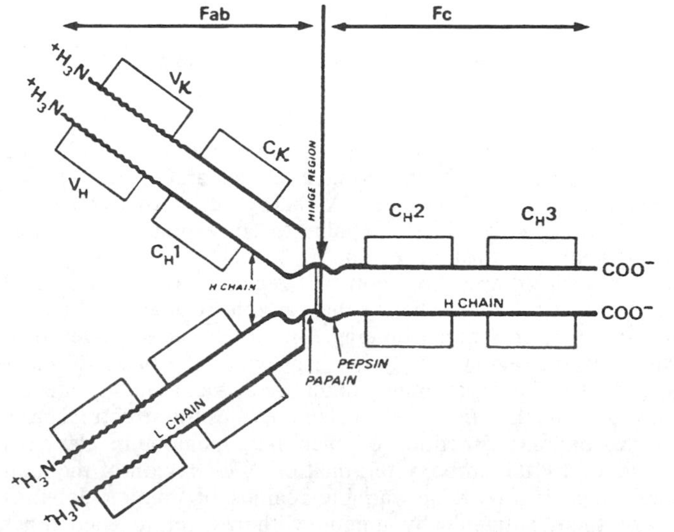

FIG. 1. A simplified model for an IgG_1 (κ) human antibody showing the four-chain basic structure and domains. V, variable region; C, constant region; vertical arrow, the hinge region; thick lines, H- and L-chains; thin lines, disulfide bonds. (From Stites et al.,[323] with permission.)

TABLE 1. Chemical Properties of Human Immunoglobulins

	IgG	*IgA*	*IgM*	*IgD*	*IgE*
Basic structure	Monomer	Monomer[a] Dimer[b]	Pentamer	Monomer	Monomer
Molecular weight	150,000	160,000[a] or 400,000[b]	900,000	180,000	190,000
Sedimentation coefficient(s)	6–7	7[a]	19	7–8	8
H-chain class	γ	α	μ	δ	ϵ
Subclass	$\gamma_1, \gamma_2, \gamma_3, \gamma_4$	α_1, α_2	μ_1, μ_2		
L-chain type	κ and λ	κ and λ	κ and λ	κ and λ	κ and λ
Molecular formula	γ_2L_2	α_2L_2[a] or $(\alpha_2L_2)_2$ SC J[c]	$(\mu_2L_2)_5J$	δ_2L_2	ϵ_2L_2
Electrophoretic mobility	γ	Fast γ and β	Fast γ to β	Fast γ	Fast γ

[a] Properties that belong to the monomeric form of IgA.
[b] Properties that belong to the dimeric form of IgA.
[c] Properties of secretory IgA. SC, secretory component; K, J-piece; a J-piece is also found in pentameric serum IgA.

TABLE 2. Metabolic Properties of Immunoglobulins

	IgG	*IgA*	*IgM*	*IgD*	*IgE*
Serum level mean (range) (mg/dl)	989 (600–1600)	200 (60–330)	100 (45–150)	3	0.008
Total body pool mean (range) (mg/kg)	1030 (570–2050)	210	36	1.1	0.01
Synthesis rate mean (range) (mg/kg/day)	36 (20–60)	28	2.2	0.4	0.004
Plasma half-life mean (range) (days)	21 (14–28)	5.9	5.1	2.8	2.4
Fractional turnover rate mean (range) (%/day)	6.9 (4.3–9.8)	24.0	10.6	37.0	72.0
Fraction in plasma[a] mean (range)	0.52 (0.32–0.64)	0.55	0.74	0.75	0.51

[a] This fraction represents the portion of the total immunoglobulins of each class that is found in the plasma.
(Adapted from Wells,[322] with permission.)

TABLE 3. Biologic Properties of Antibodies by Immunoglobulin Class

	IgG	*IgA*	*IgM*	*IgD*	*IgE*
Complement activation					
Classical pathway	++	0	++++	0	0
Alternative pathway	+	+	+	+	+
Opsonic activity	++++	0	+[a]	0	0
Lytic activity[a]	++	0	++++	0	0
Inhibition of bacterial adherence	+	+++	+	?	?
Viral neutralization	+++	+++	++	?	?
Reaginic activity	0	0	0	0	++++
Placental transfer	++++	0	0	0	0

[a] Through activation of complement after combining with cellular antigens.

of the antigen-binding site of the immunoglobulin molecule. The constant regions of L-chains have similar and specific amino acid sequences for all κ- and λ-chains, respectively. The disulfide bridges that bind L-chains to corresponding H-chains insert near the constant region.

One variable and three constant regions have been defined in H-chains.[2] Like L-chains, the variable regions of H-chains are involved in antigen binding. The amino acid sequence of the constant regions of H-chains provides the basis for class specificity of each immunoglobulin and is consistent within a class and subclass (isotype). It also provides the structural basis of the biologic functions of each immunoglobulin class, as mediated by the carboxy terminal or "Fc" region of the molecule (see below). The variable regions of immunoglobulins make them antigenically unique with respect to each other (idiotypes).

Soluble IgG, IgE, and IgD exist in serum and tissues as monomers. However, other immunoglobulins may polymerize or associate with nonimmunoglobulin accessory proteins. IgM is found in its monomeric form on the surface of B lymphocytes[5] but exists in serum as a pentamer. Whereas serum IgA is monomeric, IgA found on mucosal surfaces ("secretory") is largely dimeric. Polymeric IgM and IgA are linked, via disulfide bonds, with a 15 kD protein called J-chain[6] (Fig. 2). The J-chain is produced by B lymphocytes and is probably required to initiate polymerization and cellular secretion of IgM and dimeric IgA. No other function for the J-chain is currently known. Secretory component is another protein uniquely associated with mucosal IgA or IgM. It is synthesized by epithelial cells and serves as a membrane receptor for serum polymeric IgA or IgM, facilitating endocytosis, transport, and secretion of the immunoglobulin onto the mucosal surface.[7]

IMMUNOGLOBULIN METABOLISM AND DISTRIBUTION

The distribution and metabolism of the different immunoglobulin classes have been studied by a number of investigators (see

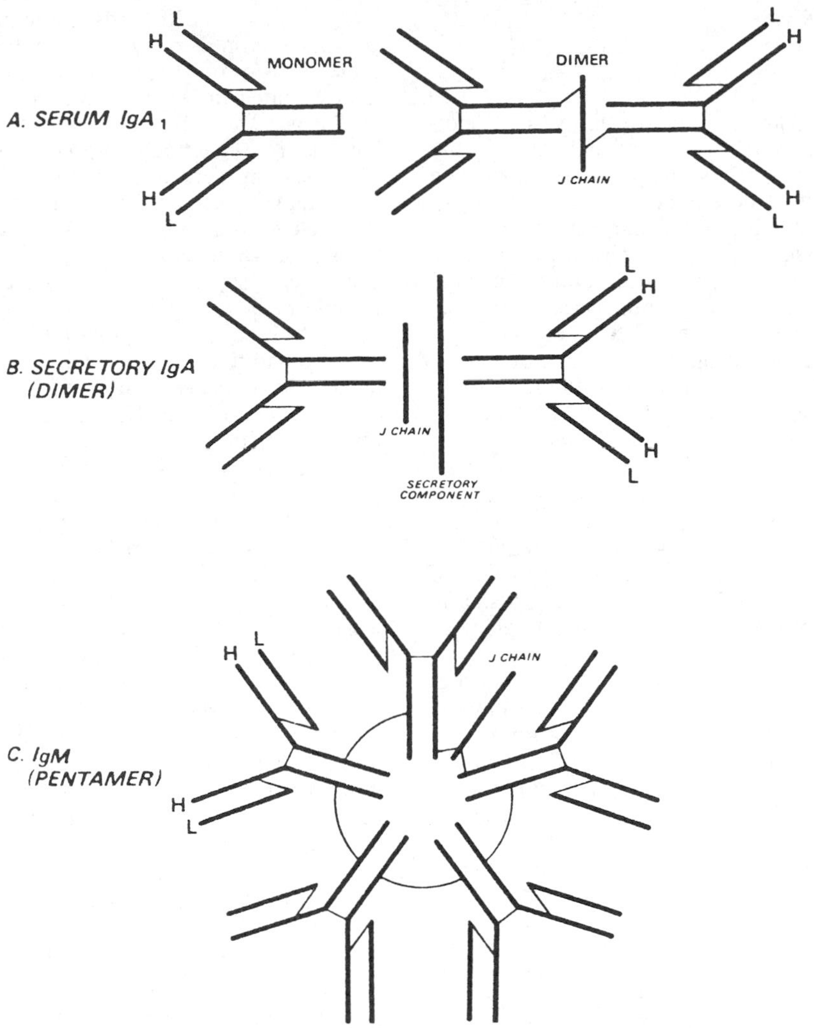

FIG. 2. Highly schematic illustration of polymeric immunoglobulins. Polypeptide chains are represented by lines; disulfide bonds linking different polypeptide chains are represented by thin lines. (From Stites et al.,[323] with permission.)

Refs. 8–10 for reviews). As noted in Table 2, under normal conditions both serum concentrations and the total body pool of IgG (in particular IgG) average 5 to 20 times higher than those of IgA and IgM and 1000 to 100,000 times higher than IgD and IgE, respectively. The differences in amounts of the separate immunoglobulin classes reflect differing rates of both synthesis and catabolism. These have been measured by infusing small amounts of radiolabeled immunoglobulin into normal subjects and measuring their clearance from the circulation. For example, the rates of synthesis of plasma IgA and IgG are almost identical (approximately 30 mg/kg/day); however, catabolic rates for IgA are almost fivefold higher. IgM is synthesized at one-tenth the rate of either IgA or IgG (approximately 2 mg/kg/day) and is catabolized four times as fast. Similarly, synthesis rates for IgE and IgD are low, and catabolic rates are high. A limitation of all of these studies is that they provide information only on those immunoglobulins that readily gain access to the circulation after production. At present there are no corresponding data for secretory immunoglobulins.

Using the same techniques of infusion of radiolabeled immunoglobulins, the intravascular vs. extravascular distribution of the immunoglobulins has been calculated. Approximately 50 percent of IgG, IgA (serum), and IgE is intravascular, compared with 75 percent of IgM and IgD. Thus the body pool of IgG is not only large, but it is well distributed in extravascular locations, particularly in lymphatic fluid.[11] IgG is the only immunoglobulin class to be actively transported across the placenta.[12] In contrast to the prevailing situation in the circulation, more IgA than IgG is isolated from saliva, tears, human colostrum or milk, and gastrointestinal secretions. In addition, secretory IgA is largely dimeric subclass IgA_2, whereas serum IgA is monomeric and mostly of the IgA_1 subclass.[13] These observations reflect the local production of secretory IgA_2 by plasma cells located beneath the lamina propria of the gut and serum IgA_1 by plasma cells in the bone marrow. During inflammation the secretions contain significantly higher amounts of IgG, as well as complement components, due to increased exudation from serum.[14]

These findings indicate that the major operational site of IgA in host defense against infection is on mucosal surfaces. IgM would appear to be involved primarily in intravascular defenses, particularly during the early phases of infection before the IgG antibody response develops. IgG, by virtue of its large amount, wide distribution, and penetration into inflamed tissues, is capable of operating in both the intravascular location and at tissue sites of active infection. The presence of long-lived IgG antibodies against many organisms can be correlated most closely with active "immunity" against these species or their toxins (see below). How these molecules can participate in host defense against infection will be discussed below.

FUNCTIONAL PROPERTIES OF IMMUNOGLOBULINS

Structure–Function Correlations

Immunoglobulins with antibody activity are bifunctional molecules: one function is to bind to specific antigenic targets; the other is to elicit a biologic response on the part of the host. The nature of this response will be determined by the type of immunoglobulin bound to the antigen and its interaction with specific host cells as well as with the serum complement system.

Through enzymatic cleavage of immunoglobulin molecules, the underlying structures that govern the bifunctional properties have been identified and characterized.[2,3] Treatment of immunoglobulins with the enzyme papain cleaves the molecule at the amino-terminal side of the inter-H-chain disulfide bond in the hinge region, thereby yielding two identical "Fab" (antigen-binding) fragments and a third "Fc" (crystallizable) fragment (Fig. 1). Each Fab fragment consists of a single complete L-chain and the variable and one constant ($C_H l$) domain of the amino-terminal portions of a single H-chain. The two peptide H-chains are bound to each other by a single interchain disulfide bridge. The Fc fragment consists of the remaining portion of the two H-chains, also bound together by interchain disulfide bridges and the carboxy-terminal region of the immunoglobulin molecule.

By virtue of specific amino acid sequences and tertiary structure contained within the "variable" domains, antigen binding occurs at the amino-terminal region of the Fab portion of immunoglobulin molecules. Each Fab fragment can bind a single antigenic determinant. The affinity of binding presumably depends upon the degree of "fit" of antigen structure into the binding site.[15] Cleavage of immunoglobulins by treatment with the enzyme pepsin results in a break of the molecule posterior to the inter-H-chain disulfide bridge or the hinge region. This results in a single large $F(ab)_2'$ fragment (i.e., the two single Fab fragments joined together by the disulfide bridge linking the H-chains (pFc fragments). As do single Fab fragments, $F(ab)_2'$ molecules also bind antigens and display affinities similar to the parent molecule. Both Fab and $F(ab)_2'$ fragments lack the capacity to generate certain critical biologic activites of intact immunoglobulins; such activities are contained within the Fc region.

The structure of the hinge region varies considerably between immunoglobulin classes and may determine some of the functions of the molecule. For instance, the short, inflexible hinge region of IgG_4 is predicted to hinder Fc portion accessibility to C1q (complement) and may account for the poor complement-fixing characteristics of IgG_4.[16] Similarly, the great length and flexibility of the hinge region in IgD may be important for effective cross-linking of membrane-bound IgD with antigen.[17]

The Fc fragment cannot bind antigens; however, it is because of the molecular characteristics of this region that certain subclasses of immunoglobulins possess the ability to bind C1q and to initiate activation of C1 of the complement system or to bind to and affect critical cells in the host immune or inflammatory system.[3,18]

Effects of Antibody Binding to Fc Receptors on Cells

Cells involved in the immune or inflammatory response possess surface molecules that can bind Fc portions of immunoglobulins (Fc receptors). These have been operationally demonstrated usually using aggregates of immunoglobulins or Ig-coated erythrocytes; monoclonal antibodies are also available that inhibit function or identify the presence of specific classes of Fc receptors.[19]

Considerable heterogeneity in isotope affinity, cellular distribution, and function of these receptors exists (Table 4). Three classes of Fc receptors for IgG (FcRI, -II, and -III) are recognized; all bind IgG_1 and IgG_3 with much higher affinity than IgG_2 or IgG_4.[20] FcRI binds monomeric IgG with high affinity, is expressed on monocytes and some neutrophils, and provides a mechanism for attachment to, and lysis of, appropriate antibody-coated target cells (antibody-dependent cell cytotoxicity—ADCC).[21] FcRII has low affinity for monomeric IgG but binds antigen–antibody complexes effectively. This receptor is expressed on monocytes, neutrophils, eosinophils, B lymphocytes, and platelets; receptor function differs on phagocytes and B cells. Cross-linking of FcRII on the surface of phagocytic cells by antigen–antibody complexes induces phagocytosis, discharge or lysosomal contents, and superoxide anion generation.[22] The binding of aggregated IgG or antigen–antibody complexes to B-cell Fc receptors inhibits the subsequent activation and proliferation of these cells and may serve as a feedback mechanism to prevent antibody-excess states.[23] The third class of IgG receptor is FcRIII (or FcRlo), which is present on macrophages, neutrophils, and cytotoxic lymphocytes. On phagocytes, this receptor binds and removes circulating immune complexes and is implicated in the clearance of Ig-coated blood cells during immune cytopenias.[24] FcRIII is also expressed on large granular lymphocytes (LGL) and CD3+ T cells with ADCC activity. FcR on these cells is required for antibody-directed cytotoxocity.[25] Certain of these IgG Fc receptors stimulate release of potent vasoactive and chemoattractant substances (PGE_2, LTC_4, and LTB_4) when bound to aggregated IgG.[26] This response may contribute to inflammation induced by immune complexes deposited in tissue.

Two classes of IgE receptor have been characterized. High-affinity FcR is present on mast cells and basophils and is important in mediating anaphylactic responses to allergenic antigen.[27] When receptor-bound IgE is cross-linked with antigen, an intracytoplasmic signal is generated that results in release of vasoactive amines and arachidonic acid derivatives. Low-affinity FcR_ϵ (CD23) is expressed on macrophages, eosinophils, platelets, and T and B lymphocytes.[28] FcR_ϵ on macrophages and eosinophils is involved in IgE-directed cytotoxicity against parasites.[29–31] In the presence of specific IgE, platelets possess cytotoxic activity against *Schistosoma mansoni*; this requires that antigen-specific IgE link the parasite to platelet FcR_ϵ.[32,33] The mechanisms of platelet cytotoxic behavior are not yet understood. T cells bearing FcR_ϵ are implicated in the regulation of IgE production, presumably via the secretion of IgE-binding proteins that promote or suppress IgE synthesis.[34]

In a similar fashion, T cells that express Fc receptors for IgA, IgD, IgM, and IgG may have analogous isotype-specific regulatory functions.[35,36] The release of heavy-chain binding factors for isotypes other than IgE has been described.[37] T lymphocytes bearing receptors for IgM possess "helper cell" activity and promote the production of IgG synthesis.[38] However, the expression of these surface antigens on T cells is inconstant; the presence of CD4 and CD8 membrane proteins has proven more reliable as a phenotypic marker.[38,39] Recently, IgA Fc receptors capable of mediating phagocytosis have been described on mucosal neutrophils and on circulating monocytes.[40–42]

Complement Fixation

The Fc regions of the immunoglobulin molecules have differing capabilities for binding to C1q and thus activating the classical complement pathway through assembly of the C1qrs molecular complex. On a molecular basis, IgM is the most effective in this regard, perhaps in part due to its pentameric structure.[4] IgG_1 and IgG_3 are more active than the other IgG subclasses in C1q binding and activation.[3,18] None of the other immunoglobulin subclasses are capable of classical pathway activation; however, aggregates of IgA, IgE, and IgD may activate the alternative pathway, perhaps because of their high substitution with sugar residues.[4] IgG bound to sialic acid moieties on nonac-

TABLE 4. Immunoglobulin Fc Receptors: Distribution and Function

Type	Synonyms	Cellular Distribution	Function
IgG Fc receptors ($IgG_1/IgG_3 \gg IgG_2/IgG_4$)			
Fcγ RI	High affinity[a] MoAb: 32	Monocytes[b]	Antibody-mediated cytotoxicity
Fcγ RII (CD_w 32)	Low affinity MoAb: IV.3, KuFc 79	Monocytes, neutrophils, eosinophils, B lymphocytes, platelets	Antibody-mediated cytotoxicity, phagocytosis, lysosomal discharge, superoxide anion generation, regulation of immunoglobulin production
Fcγ RIII (CD 16)	Low affinity MoAb: 3G8, 4F7, Leu11, B73, VEP13	Macrophages, neutrophils, large granular lymphocytes (LGL), T lymphocytes	Phagocytosis, removal of immune complexes, ADCC
IgE Fc receptors			
Fcε R (high affinity)		Mast cells, basophils	Degranulation, leukotriene production if cross-linked by IgE bound to antigen
Fcε R (low affinity) (CD 23)		T lymphocytes, B lymphocytes, macrophages, eosinophils, platelets	Regulation of IgE production, ADCC, phagocytosis
IgA Fc receptors			
Fcα R		T lymphocytes, monocytes, neutrophils[b]	Mediates phagocytosis and regulation of IgA production

[a] High affinity for monomeric IgG; low-affinity receptors bind immune complexes. MoAb, monoclonal antibodies specific for receptor.
[b] Inducible on neutrophils with cytokine treatment.

tivating bacteria may also trigger alternative pathway activation.[43,44]

ROLE OF ANTIBODIES IN PROTECTION AGAINST INFECTION

After binding to specific microbial antigens and depending on the immunoglobulin class, antibodies can either enlist the effector cells of the host or can activate the complement system or both to assist in the eradication of infecting organisms. The success of this defense system depends greatly on the efficacy with which these coordinated systems complete this task. There is no evidence to indicate that viable organisms that are in an intracellular location can be selectively reached or modified by extracellular antibody or complement without destroying the host cell as well. Thus if tissue damage is to be limited, the primary protective role of these factors must be directed against pathogens when they are in an extracellular location. Specific antibodies can be involved in this process by promoting the following:

1. Opsonization of organisms for ingestion and destruction by phagocytic cells
2. Cell-free lysis of susceptible organisms by the complement system
3. Neutralization of toxins
4. Inhibition of attachment of organisms to host cells
5. Inhibition of the infectivity of extracellular viruses (virus neutralization)

Once pathogens are in an intracellular location, they are, in most circumstances, in a sanctuary where they are protected against the action of antibodies and complement. They may then serve as a source of chronic antigenic stimulation for more antibody production, as well as for activation of the cellular immune system (see Chapter 8). In addition, organisms may modify the surface properties of cells that they invade so that an antibody response occurs against these infected cells. Antibodies directed against cells harboring organisms may be destroyed by an ADCC reaction. A potential role for IgE antibodies in protection of hosts from parasitic infections that uses none of these mechanisms has recently been postulated. In this section the various mechanisms outlined will be discussed as they apply to different species of infecting microorganisms.

Opsonization

To describe the role that serum factors play in promoting the ingestion of staphylococci by polymorphonuclear leukocytes, Wright and Douglas in 1903 coined the term "opsonin" from the Greek opsono meaning "I prepare victuals for."[45] Opsonization thus refers to the process by which organisms or other particles are coated by antibodies and/or complement or other factors and thereby are prepared for "recognition" and ingestion by phagocytic cells. The efficacy of this process as a mechanism of defense against infection depends on (*1*) the ability of specific antibodies, complement, and other proteins to promote these events, (*2*) the presence and phagocytic capacity of host polymorphonuclear leukocytes, monocytes, and macrophages, and (*3*) the susceptibility of organisms to intracellular killing, once ingested. These latter two areas will be subjects for discussion in Chapters 7 and 8. In their classic investigations with staphyloccoci, Wright and Douglas observed that some, but not all of the opsonic activity or normal serum was lost with heating.[45] Heat-labile and heat-stable components of the serum opsonic system were defined and for most organisms are now known to involve a role largely for antibody or complement, respectively. In addition, recent evidence indicates that for some organisms fibronectin[46] or C-reactive protein[47,48] may be opsonic.

Complement serves as an opsonin when the cleavage products of C3 convertase activity, C3b or C3bi, are deposited on the particle or cellular surface and engage the complementary CR1 or CR3 receptors on polymorphonuclear (PMN) and macrophage cell membranes.[49] The mechanisms by which these events occur are discussed in detail in Chapter 6. Antibodies bound to organism surfaces may be opsonic either indirectly through their ability to activate the complement system, directly through binding to Fc receptors on phagocytes for IgG, IgA, or IgE, or by a combination of both mechanisms.

Experiments utilizing C3b or IgG coated erythrocytes indicated that phagocytosis was triggered when the IgG FcR was engaged, with the C3b receptor serving as an adherence ligand only.[50,51] While antibody and complement often function synergistically in promoting opsonization in phagocytes, a requirement for dual receptor involvement is not essential for microbial ingestion. A number of organisms can be readily opsonized in serum that contains no measurable immunoglobulins.[52–56] For example, protein A-positive strains of staphylococci are often more effectively opsonized in agammaglobulinemic than in normal serum.[54] Protein A serves as an antiopsonic factor in normal serum by binding the Fc portion of IgG[54,57]; conversely, in agammaglobulinemic serum it can activate C1 directly.[54] Similarly, opsonization and ingestion of some strains of group B streptococci[58] and *Escherichia coli*[59] may proceed by direct activation of the classical complement pathway without a role for antibodies. Thus the requirements for both antibody and complement to serve as components in the opsonization process vary considerably from species to species and even from strain to strain of microorganisms.

Physicochemical factors between particles and phagocytes other than engagement of specific complement and Fc receptors may affect opsonization and phagocytosis. Encapsulated as opposed to "rough" bacteria have differences in surface charge. Rough organisms have a hydrophobic surface charge and can often be ingested without opsonization. A hydrophobic surface charge on encapsulated organisms develops upon opsonization with antibody and complement.[60–63] Binding of IgG and C3 to the surface of salmonellae allows these organisms to fuse with artificial liposomes that contain no specific receptors for IgG and C3.[64] Finally, some organisms also contain surface lectins that bind to glycoproteins on phagocytes, thereby promoting adherence and ingestion.[65]

Opsonic antibodies are almost invariably of the IgG_1, IgG_3, or IgM classes, corresponding to the specificity of FcR on phagocytes for IgG_1 and IgG_3 and the ability of these antibodies to activate the complement system.[66,67] With the exception of mucosal phagocytes, which display functional Fc receptors for IgA, IgA antibodies are not opsonic.[40] In fact, IgA antibodies bound to the surface of microorganisms may block the binding of complement-fixing IgM or IgG.[68] IgE antibodies may bind metazoan parasites to macrophages or platelets, as discussed above,[20–33] and in this sense are "opsonic"; however, most such organisms are too large to be ingested by phagocytes.

Identified microbial targets for opsonizing antibodies include capsular polysaccharides,[49,56,58,67,69–72] M protein of group A streptococci,[73] and peptidoglycans.[74] Purified polysaccharides of pneumococci,[75] meningococci, group B streptococci,[76] and *Haemophilus influenzae*[77] are normally effective immunogens in all but young infants and have been used as subunit antigens in vaccines that generate opsonizing (pneumococci, streptococci) or opsonizing plus lytic activity (meningococci, *H. influenzae*). Administration of IgG obtained from normal or specifically immunized subjects prevents recurrent bacterial infections in patients with hypogammaglobulinemia through provision of specific opsonins.[78–80] Antipseudomonal hyperimmune globulin works through a similar mechanism.[81] While opsonic antibodies can be demonstrated against viruses[82,83] and fungi,[84–86] their role in defense against infection with these organisms is uncertain. Opsonic antibodies are thus most effective against organisms that are rapidly destroyed by phagocytes upon ingestion, i.e., "obligate extracellular parasites."

Lysins

Antibodies that can initiate the activation of the complement system through the terminal component membrane attack mechanism can cause lysis of susceptible organisms or cells. Microbial susceptibility is usually unique to gram-negative bacterial species[87,88] and to some viruses[83]; the initiating antibodies are of the IgM or IgG classes. Gram-negative enteric organisms causing bacteremia are often resistant to lysis by complement in contrast to the commensal gut flora.[88] Bactericidal antibodies that operate through the complement system play a major role in protection against infections with *Neisseria* sp. and *H. influenzae* type B. It should be emphasized that it is not entirely clear in all cases whether antibodies that initiate the membrane attack system of complement are also opsonic or whether separate immunoglobulin molecules are involved in the respective responses. With respect to gram-positive species, coating of organisms with complement does not cause lysis but may render them more susceptible to intracellular killing[89] or to the lytic action of lysozyme.[90]

Finally, infections of target cells with some viruses may lead to an antibody response that destroys infected cells by lysis in the presence of complement.[83] The importance of this mechanism in vivo in the control of viral infections remains to be confirmed.

Toxin-Neutralizing Antibodies

The demonstration by Roux and Yersin in 1888 that the virulence of *Corynebacterium diphtheriae* was due to the production of a protein exotoxin led to development of the first successful treatment and prevention of a bacterial infection by the use of passive and active immunization. The function of antibodies contained in an equine antiserum or developed actively in the human host by immunization with formalinized diphtheria toxoid is to bind to circulating or locally produced toxin and to prevent either its attachment to receptor sites or host target cells or its entry into the cells. Since the mechanism of action of the toxin in inhibiting cellular protein synthesis depends on passage of the active "A" fragment into the cytosol of the target cell, inhibition of binding (by the "B" fragments) or entry of the A fragment blocks the toxic effect.[91] The presence of neutralizing antibodies in the immunized host may be detected in vivo by a negative reaction in the Schick test, which measures the local reaction to an intracutaneous injection of toxin.[92] These antibodies are predominantly of the IgG class. Similar principles apply to passive and active antitoxic therapy of tetanus, botulism, and histotoxic clostridial infections and will be discussed in more detail in the chapters dealing with these organisms.

It is difficult to identify a specific toxigenic mechanism in the pathogenesis of disease caused by most other organisms; however, the role of endotoxin in the production of the shock syndrome seen with gram-negative infections has been extensively studied.[93] Immunization of animals[94,95] and perhaps humans[96] with mutant bacteria that are deficient in all or most polysaccharides in the terminal and core portions of their endotoxins ("Re" mutants) provides broad protection against lethal infection with a variety of gram-negative bacteria. Furthermore, in nonimmunized human hosts, survival from bacteremic gram-negative infection can be correlated with the presence of antibodies that react with Re lipopolysaccharides.[97] Passive immunization with serum obtained from normal individuals vaccinated with a "rough" mutant *E. coli* J5 decreased the morbidity and mortality of gram-negative sepsis in a hospitalized patient population.[96,98] Passively administered monoclonal antibodies directed against surface epitopes of J5 *E. coli* are protective against lethal gram-negative sepsis in animals[99] and are currently undergoing trial in man. The precise mechanism of this protective effect is currently under active investigation; the data suggest that it operates not through an opsonic effect of the antibodies[100] but rather through "detoxification" of the LPS.

Adherence-Inhibiting Antibodies

The capacity of bacteria to colonize the mucosal surfaces of human and other mammalian hosts is dependent in part on their ability to adhere to the epithelial and endothelial cells that form their lining. The role of adherence in the pathogenicity of various bacterial species has been recently reviewed.[101] For example, M proteins and lipoteichoic acids in group A streptococci project from the cell walls in fimbria that adhere to the oral mucosa.[102] Pili of pathogenic gonococcal strains promote adherence to mucosal cells and leukocytes while inhibiting phagocytosis.[103] Nonpathogenic strains of gonococci lack pili and do not adhere to cells; they are promptly phagocytized and killed. Enteric bacteria that cause diarrhea have an adherence-promoting "intestinal colonization factor."[104] Organisms that lack this factor cannot cause diarrhea even if they contain pathogenic enterotoxins. The pathogenicity of gram-negative enteric organisms in urinary tract infections can be correlated with pili that adhere to mucosal carbohydrates such as mannose or galactose dimers.[105,106]

Secretory IgA may contain antibodies that bind to these adherence-promoting factors and block their ability to attach to cellular receptors.[106–108] This constitutes a major protective mechanism for IgA against infection by pathogenic bacteria and perhaps other species on mucosal surfaces.[101,109] Proteases that cleave the hinge region of IgA or IgA_2 and that block adherence-inhibiting activity may be important virulence factors in some bacteria.[109] IgG antibodies may also block adherence by similar mechanisms, but the relatively low concentration of IgG in secretions and on mucosal surfaces does not support a major role for IgG in this phenomenon.

Viral Neutralization

Antibodies of the IgG, IgM, or IgA (including secretory IgA) classes have been described that inhibit (i.e., neutralize) the ability of extracellular viruses to infect their target cells (see Refs. 83 and 110 for reviews). Fixation of classical pathway complement components, in particular C4b, to the virus may aid in the neutralization process.[83,111–113] Infection of cells may be inhibited by antibodies because the virus does not fix to key cell membrane targets, or because of interference with entry or uncoating.[110,114] The development of neutralizing antibodies is instrumental in limiting the capacity of viruses to spread from an extracellular focus to an intracellular location, whether it be from a mucosal surface or by a hematogenous route.

The production of neutralizing antibody is synonymous with immunity against infection with viruses causing the common childhood exanthems or polio.[110] It should be emphasized that neutralizing antibodies can only aid against viruses that have a cell-free location in their spread ("type II" transfer). Those that are spread directly from one cell to another ("type I" transfer) are not likely to be directly neutralized in the presence of antibody (e.g., human immunodeficiency virus [HIV], herpesvirus). Cellular immune mechanisms become much more important in controlling infection caused by these viruses as well as in inhibiting viruses in an intracellular location. These mechanisms may involve a cooperative role for antibody, as noted below.[83,115]

Antibody-Dependent Cell-Mediated Cytotoxicity

Certain viruses may cause changes in the surface properties of infected target cells that lead to the development of an antibody response directed against the infected cell. Lysis of the infected cell may be achieved by the combined action of antibody and complement[83] or by the antibody-directed binding of effector "killer" lymphocytes, neutrophils, or macrophages via their Fc regions to the altered target cell (ADCC).[116–118] Cytotoxic lymphocytes possess cytoplasmic granules that contain serine proteinases similar to the complement proteins. These are discharged onto the target cell surface and assemble into membrane-bound complexes that induce osmotic lysis in a fashion akin to complement.[119,120]

IgE and Parasitic Infections

Immune mechanisms against parasites are only partially understood. Cellular immunity appears to play a major role in the containment of infections caused by protozoa. A role for humoral immunity in some protozoan infections is suggested by the high frequency of chronic intestinal giardiasis in patients with primary hypogammaglobulinemia.[121] In addition, *Pneumocystis carinii* infections may occur spontaneously in patients with isolated hypogammaglobulinemia.[122] The exact mechanisms of protection by antibodies in these infections remains to be ascertained.

Helminthic infections, particularly those that have a tissue invasive phase, are often associated with both eosinophilia and elevated levels of IgE.[123] Eosinophils are capable of destroying schistosomules in the presence of immune serum by binding to the surface of the organism and discharging their lysosomal granules.[30,31,124,125] The nature of the antibody promoting binding appears to be IgG, which can act in concert with complement to mediate the cytotoxic effect.[22,126,127] Similarly, cytophilic IgE may play a role in macrophage-dependent and platelet-dependent killing of schistosomes by serving as a ligand between the organism and the cells.[33,128]

The binding of antigen to IgE on mast cells and basophils triggers their degranulation with the release of a variety of amines that act on smooth muscle or affect vascular permeability.[27] It has been suggested that local amine release may be a protective mechanism in the gut to aid in expelling worms.[129] Increased vascular permeability may enhance the delivery of cells and serum components to local sites of infestation to participate in an attack on the parasite. In support of these suggestions, basophils and mast cells can be observed in gut mucosa at the site of invasion by nematodes in experimental infections.[130] Furthermore, treatment with drugs that inhibit histamine activity may impair elimination of the worms.[129,130] Definition of antiparasitic host defense mechanisms remains an important area for future investigation.

IMMUNOGLOBULIN GENETICS

Antibody diversity is created by a process of random genetic recombination that takes place in immunoglobulin genes during the early development of B lymphocytes. An estimated 10^8 possible antigen-binding specificities (idiotypes) result from the variable joining of 1100 component genes contained in the germ line DNA of all B-cell precursors.[131–133] Similar mechanisms have proved central to the generation of diversity in another immunologically important class of molecules, the T-cell receptor.[134] Certain constant portions of the immunoglobulin gene have also been incorporated into a large variety of surface receptor and identity proteins, such as the mixed major histocompatibility complexes (MHC). This aggregate of related genes thus constitutes an "immunoglobulin supergene family."[135] Beyond explaining the mechanism underlying antibody diversity, these observations have also provided understanding of antibody isotypic switching and affinity maturation during the course of repeated immune responses.

The gene complexes encoding the two light chains of immunoglobulin reside on separate chromosomes, with the genes for κ constant (C_κ) and variable regions (V_κ) on chromosome 22 and the genes for λ constant (C_λ) and variable (V_λ) regions on chromosome 2. There are several hundred V DNA segments and 5–10 short joining (J) segments contained in each light chain gene complex. The κ complex has one C_κ gene and the λ complex has six or more C_λ genes. During B-cell maturation, one of the light chain complexes undergoes recombination, a process whereby a single V and J segment will joint with a C_λ gene. Together, these form a single linear array, which constitutes the mature light chain gene. Both V and J DNA contribute to the final variable region of the light chain; therefore the number of possible V regions is the product of the numbers of V and J segments. Additional diversity is created through the inaccuracy of the joining process and the resultant random choice of amino acids at the splice site. Only one of the four light chain complexes present in each B cell (one κ and λ complex for each set of parental chromosomes) will undergo rearrangement at a time. The other gene complexes are activated only if a functional recombination does not occur, but are "turned off" for the life of the cell otherwise.

The genes of the heavy chain complex rearrange in a fashion that is similar in principle to light chain recombination. The heavy chain complex consists of about 1000 V_H genes and 4 J_H segments located on chromosome 14 (Fig. 3). In addition, there are 10 or more short, diversity-generating (D_H) segments. One of each is joined together in the order V-D-J during rearrange-

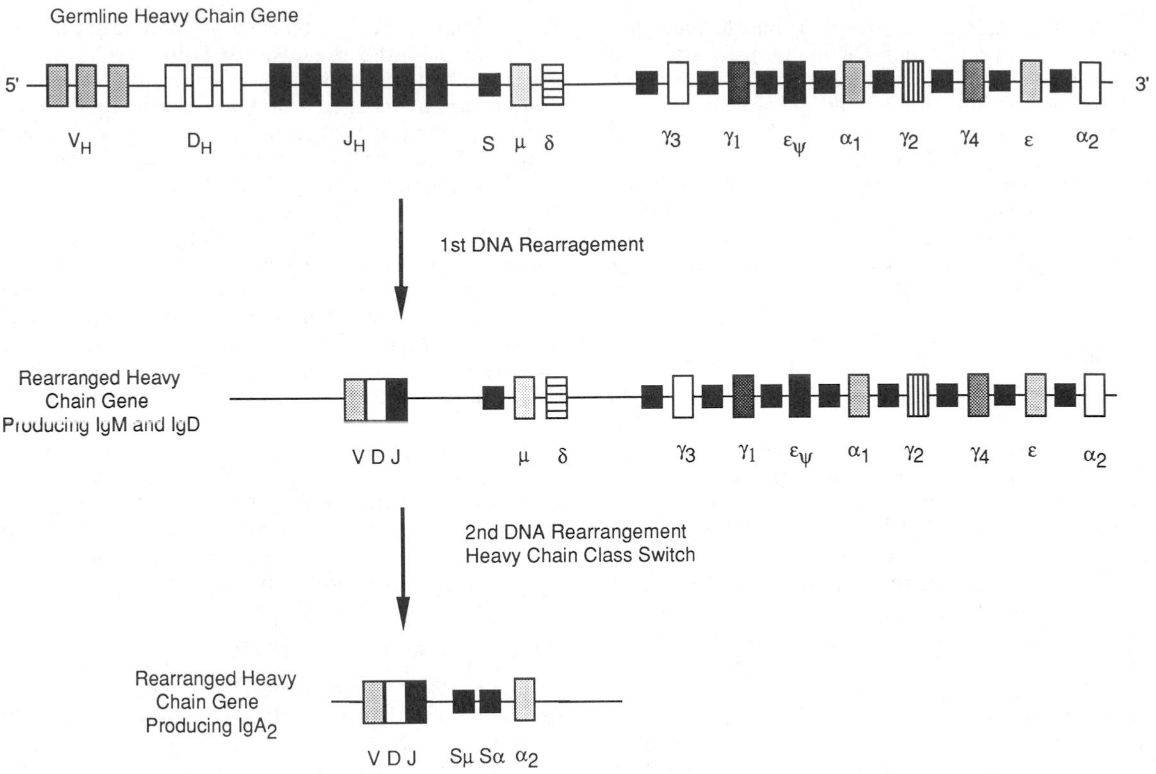

FIG. 3. Schematic illustration showing how immunoglobulin heavy chain genes recombine to create antibody diversity. During the first DNA rearrangement, single units from each set of variable (V_H), diversity (D_H), and joining (J_H) segments are joined together (VDJ) to form an active variable region gene. RNA transcribed from the variable region through the proximal heavy chain constant regions (μ and δ) generates either IgM or IgD heavy chains, depending on RNA processing. A second DNA rearrangement is illustrated to show the juxtaposition of the same variable region gene to a switch site (S) immediately before the α_2 constant region. Intervening genes are deleted. Transcription of the recombined gene results in production of IgA_2 heavy chain with unaltered antigen specificity. (Adapted from Waldmann et al.,[324] with permission.)

ment, and this combination encodes the mature heavy chain variable gene. The addition of D segments increases the potential number of combinations. The rearranged variable gene is linked with an available C_H gene to form the complete heavy chain gene. The C_H genes are arranged in linear fashion, in the following order: C_μ, C_δ, $C_{\gamma 3}$, $C_{\gamma 1}$, $C_{\epsilon\psi}$, $C_{\alpha 1}$, $C_{\gamma 2}$, $C_{\gamma 4}$, C_ϵ, and $C_{\alpha 2}$ (the $C_{\epsilon\psi}$ gene is a nonfunctional duplication of the C_ϵ gene). The rearranged variable region gene is initially joined with the C_μ and C_δ genes. The length of DNA encompassing the variable gene and both heavy chain genes is transcribed into messenger RNA. Splicing of the RNA transcript then determines whether IgM or IgD, or both, are produced.[136] Later, during B-cell differentiation, the variable gene can be spliced into proximity with distal heavy chain genes at defined "switch" regions; the intervening DNA is excised. The completed heavy chain gene, whatever the isotype, is capable of producing both membrane-bound and soluble immunoglobulin. This is regulated by the inclusion or deletion of a short segment of RNA encoding a 40-residue hydrophobic "tail" that promotes anchorage in the plasma membrane of the B cell.[137]

The structure of the heavy chain complex explains how isotypic switches occur during B-cell differentiation. The order of C_H genes approximates the order of appearance of isotypes during maturation of B cells. IgM and IgD are the first classes to be produced and are replaced by IgG, IgE, or IgA during subsequent differentiation. B cells producing the latter immunoglobulin classes have not been observed to revert to earlier isotypes. This is understandable given the order of heavy chain genes and the fact that they are deleted during recombination. The antigen-binding specificity is preserved during isotypic switches, as there is no alteration of the variable genes for heavy and light chains. It is unclear if a switch to distal genes occur in one step or via multiple, transient recombinations with intervening genes. The mechanisms that control isotypes switches are also not well understood, although T-cell products may play key roles in augmenting IgE or IgA production from stimulated B cells.[34,37] Thus B cell production of IgA in the intestinal lymphoid tissue may reflect the presence of IgA-promoting T cells ("switch cells").

In summary, antigen-binding diversity is generated through the recombination of diverse V, D, and J sequences, the inexact junction of these segments, and the combination of V_H and V_L regions that occurs during final assembly of the immunoglobulin molecule. However, a fourth mechanism can create further diversity after recombination has taken place; this occurs via somatic mutation of the variable regions. Comparisons of immunoglobulin gene sequences before and after secondary antigen challenges demonstrate single base pair mutations in previously rearranged variable regions of light and heavy chains. These mutations occur at frequencies considerably greater than those observed for constant region genes.[138,139] Mutations resulting in greater immunoglobulin affinity for a specific antigen may therefore generate a B cell more easily activated to proliferate and to produce that antibody. This will result in selection of higher-affinity antibodies during repeated cycles of immune stimulation with a single antigen, so-called "affinity maturation."

CELLULAR MECHANISMS IN ANTIBODY PRODUCTION

Antibodies must be produced promptly in response to the introduction of foreign protein and polysaccharide antigens on microbial invaders. There is need for economy and specificity in this response. The humoral immune response to infection must therefore direct antibodies to the relevant antigens, prevent self-directed responses, and control the classes of antibodies produced. When the need is past, the antibody response must be attenuated and a pool of memory cells reserved to allow brisk and specific recall of immunoglobulin production for future needs. Not surprisingly, intricate control mechanisms have evolved to serve this immunologic mandate. These mechanisms depend on the participation of three major cellular components: B cells, T cells, and accessory cells.

B cells are bone marrow-derived lymphocytes responsible for manufacturing antibody. The cardinal feature of mature B cells is the expression of surface-bound immunoglobulin with single antigen specificity and the ability of the cells to secrete soluble immunoglobulin of the same specificity when the cells are stimulated by antigen.[140,141] The antigen binds to surface immunoglobulin and triggers a series of chemical reactions and ionic events that stimulate the B cell into proliferative and antibody secretory activity; this initial signaling event is termed "activation." A subsequent proliferative phase precedes terminal differentiation of the B cell into the antibody-secreting plasma cells (for reviews see Refs. 142–144).

Thymus-derived or T lymphocytes are mononuclear cells, also derived from hematopoietic stem cells, that undergo precursor growth and maturation in the thymus.[144,145] T cells do not display surface Ig but instead express an antigen-binding protein, the T-cell receptor (TcR), which belongs to the immunoglobulin gene "family" and which derives clonal specificity through the same diversity-generating rearrangements as occur in B cells.[134] T-cell receptors are not secreted but remain associated on the T-cell membrane. Binding of specific antigen to the TcR also initiates a cascade of activation events, inducing T cells to proliferate and differentiate along a variety of functional lines. Unlike B cells, which bind to soluble, intact antigen, T-cell receptors recognize antigen that is displayed on accessory cell surfaces in close proximity with (perhaps even bound to) the class II histocompatibility antigen (HLA-DR). T cells additionally displaying the CD4 surface marker (OKT4, Leu3), participate or "help" in the activation or differentiation of B cells and are broadly referred to as T-helper cells.[39,146] This participation occurs in the form of either direct cell-to-cell contact or in the production of soluble immunoregulatory proteins called lymphokines, which are received via specific receptors on the target B cell. Another subset of T cells, which displays the surface CD8 marker (OKT8, Leu2), includes some cells that can inhibit B-cell antibody production.[147] The suppression may be specific for a single antigen response or may serve to limit production of selected or all subclasses of immunoglobulin. The mechanisms of suppression are heterogenous and poorly understood in humans but may function via elaborated antigen-specific inhibitory proteins.[148]

Accessory cells constitute the third group of cells important to activation of B cells; the best known and studied accessory cells are blood monocytes and tissue macrophages, but this group also includes dendritic cells, endothelial cells, and Langerhans cells.[149,150] These cells continually monitor the internal milieu through endocytosis and display of available proteins, in partially digested form, on their cell surface for T-cell scrutiny. An important feature of the accessory cell is the presence on its membrane of MHC class II antigen.[151] These surface proteins constitute the HLA-D (DR, DP, DQ) antigens in humans. When T-cell receptors recognize foreign antigen in close association with MHC, a TcR–antigen–MHC trimolecular complex is formed, and the lymphocyte receives the first of several signals necessary for activation to occur. Mature T cells only express TcR that recognizes the unique host MHC antigen—"MHC restriction." Accessory cells assist in B-cell activation by both direct and indirect means. B-cell activation is assisted by the presence of interleukin-1 (IL-1), which is produced by many types of accessory cells.[152] Accessory cells may indirectly participate in B-cell function by activating T cells, which produce many of the activation, growth, and differentiation factors required for B-cell development.[153,154] B cells are also capable of functioning as accessory cells to T lymphocytes. Soluble antigen can be specifically bound to surface Ig of B cells, internalized by endocytosis, and presented on the surface in conjunction with MHC antigen in a form recognizable by T cells.[155]

Ontogeny of B Cells

B cells, as well as T cells and the cells of hematopoiesis, are derived from pluripotent stem cells. Precursor, or pre-B cells develop in the fetal liver until the time of birth, when B-cell production shifts to the bone marrow. In this location, stem cells continuously produce new B cells throughout life; the daily yield is estimated to be more than one billion cells.[142] Proliferation and maturation of pre-B cells are supported by growth factors produced by stromal cells in the marrow microenvironment.[154,156] Pre-B cells are defined as B cells prior to the expression of surface Ig.[142] It is at this stage that immunoglobulin gene rearrangement takes place. The first gene to undergo recombination is the heavy chain complex; therefore IgM heavy chains are the first Ig products detectable in the cytoplasm of the pre-B cell. Light chains appear next when successful recombination takes place. When both light and heavy chains are present in the cytoplasm, Ig is assembled and displayed on the cell membrane, cell proliferation ceases, and the B-cell phenotype, as defined by the presence of surface Ig, is apparent. With further maturation, B cells express first IgM and then both IgM and IgD surface antibodies. Expression of other Ig isotypes occurs after activation and differentiation of the B cell.

Other important surface molecules on mature B cells include complement receptors and Fc receptors. The complement receptor CR1, which binds the proteins C3b and C4b, is expressed on the cell membrane of B cells.[157] CR2, which binds C3d, occurs only on B cells and is the receptor for Epstein-Barr virus.[158] Cross-linked C3d ligand binds to its receptor and promotes B-cell growth; soluble C3d inhibits B-cell growth.[159] A variety of Fc receptors have been described on B cells; many of these receptors are specific for a single isotype and are implicated in regulation of antibody production. In general, binding of the Fc portion of immunoglobulin to the B-cell FcR inhibits cellular functioning and may function to prevent antibody overproduction. Class II MHC is displayed on mature B cells and is enhanced when B cells are activated by antigen or IL-4. Possession of this surface complex allows B cells to function as accessory cells to T cells. A subpopulation of human B lymphocytes express the T-cell marker CD5 (Leu1), which may identify B cells committed to produce rheumatoid factor antibody.[160]

B-Cell Activation

There are many different activating signals, and B cells may require a specific combination and sequence of stimulations or signals before cell division can occur (for reviews, see Refs. 142 and 161). In general, activation may be antigen-specific or -nonspecific (polyclonal activation). The activation pathway can be additionally categorized according to the need for the presence of T cells (T-dependent) or activation in the absence of T cells (T-independent activation).

The central event in antigen-specific B-cell activation is the binding of antigen to surface Ig at a time when the B cell has matured sufficiently.[17] Antigen binding early in B-cell development generates an inhibitory signal and results in B-cell unresponsiveness to further stimulation.[162] This mechanism may function to ensure tolerance to host antigens that are present during early B-cell development. If no early inhibitory signal is received, the B cell activates when antigen cross-links surface

Ig and initiates a series of intracellular molecular events. Phospholipids of the cellular membrane are cleaved by phospholipase C to form inositol polyphosphates and diacylglycerol, which are potent intracellular second messengers. These molecules induce increases in intracellular calcium and mediate activation of functionally important proteins that prompt the cell to synthesize RNA and enter G_1 of the cell cycle. Activation of the cell also results in the expression of receptors for various growth factors, including IL-2, IL-4, transferrin, and B-cell stimulatory factor (BSF)-2.[163–165] Binding of these receptors with the appropriate growth factor initiates the proliferative phase of the B-cell response.

Antigen-specific B-cell activation (Fig. 4) can occur in the absence of T cells upon stimulation with certain antigens, usually polysaccharides that consist of repeating subunits; these are referred to as T-independent antigens.[166] These include polysaccharide molecules derived from the capsules of pathogenic bacteria such as *H. influenzae* and *Streptococcus pneumoniae*. The dependence of B-cell activation on the polymeric nature of these antigens suggests that extensive cross-linking of surface Ig is an important feature for T-independent B-cell responses. Such cellular responses are only T-independent in that T-cell contact is not required for activation. T-cell products are probably necessary for proliferation and maturation of B cells into plasma cells after activation occurs; the T cells involved need not be antigen-specific or matched for DR antigen. Activation of this pathway results in the appearance of B cells producing only certain isotypes of immunoglobulin.[167] Normal humans challenged with pneumococcal capsular polysaccharide vaccine, for instance, develop an antibody response consisting largely of IgG_2 molecules,[168] whereas T-dependent protein vaccines, such as tetanus toxoid, elicit IgG_1 subclass production.[167] In addition, secondary antibody responses to protein antigen tend to be greater than those following polysaccharide antigen immunization.[169] Polysaccharide vaccines therefore have been conjugated with protein antigens to increase the variety and magnitude of the antibodies produced during immunization.[169] In hosts devoid of T cells, B-cell activation occurs but results in a diminished antibody response, wholly of the IgM isotype.[166]

T-dependent B-cell activation (Fig. 4) largely requires contact of B and T cells—"cognate" activation.[170] B cells ingest and process antigen bound to surface immunoglobulin and present the immunogen in conjunction with B cell MHC protein.[171] Antigen-specific T-cell receptors on CD4+ cells recognize this molecular combination and prompt binding of T and B cells. The bicellular complex is stabilized by nonspecific interactions between CD4 on the T cell with nonpolymorphic portions of the B cell MHC molecules. The cellular adhesion molecule LFA-1 is also a necessary factor for cellular binding.[172,173] The T-cell receptor does not necessarily identify the same portion or epitope of the antigen recognized by B-cell surface antibody. This interaction is the probable molecular equivalent of the classic description of hapten-carrier cooperation.[174] The intimate binding of T and B cells provides greater opportunity for delivery of activation signals in either direction, and it is likely that each member of the pair simultaneously activates the other. The production of lymphokines by the T cell would then assist in subsequent proliferation and maturation of the B cell, even when contact is severed.

Cognate B-cell activation seems to be the major pathway responsible for formation of antibodies directed toward protein antigens, as patients who lack LFA-1 (and therefore do not form T:B cell complexes) produce only small quantities of specific antibody following vaccination with protein antigens, such as

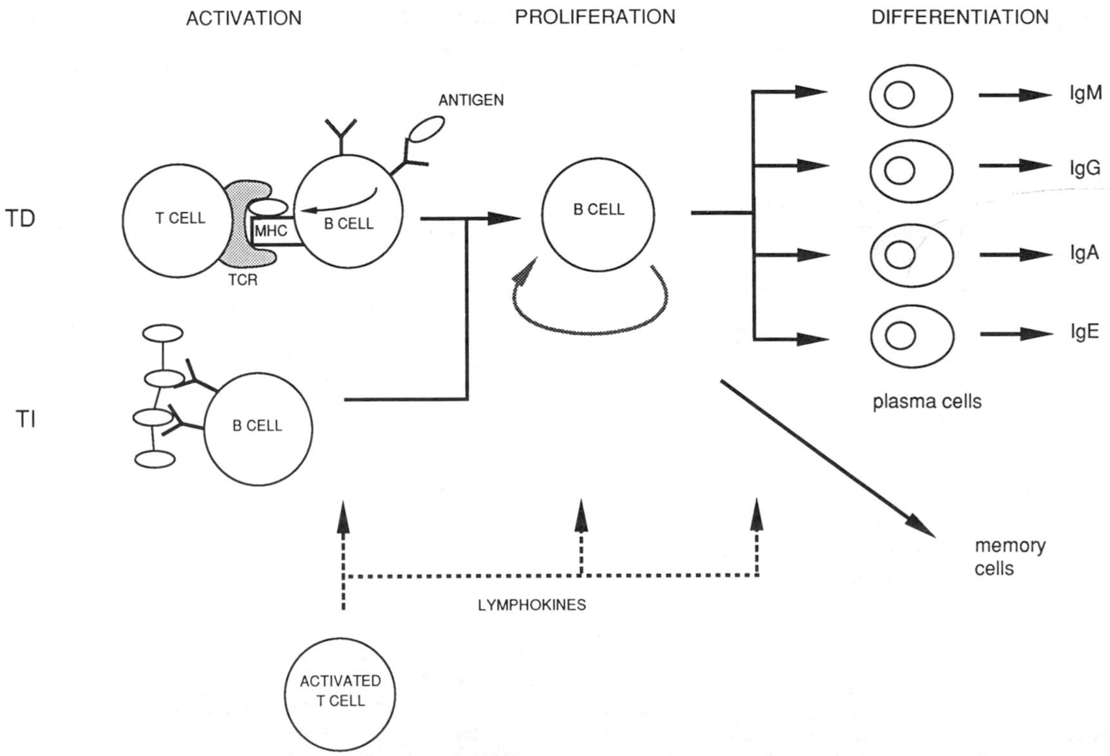

FIG. 4. Cooperation of B and T cells during immunoglobulin production. During T-dependent B-cell activation (TD), antigen binds to antibody receptors on antigen-specific B cells and is internalized, processed, and displayed on the B-cell surface in conjunction with the major histocompatibility complex antigen (MHC). T-helper cells bearing antigen-specific T-cell receptor (TCR) recognize the antigen–MHC complex and stimulate B-cell activation. During T-independent B-cell activation (TI), surface Ig is cross-linked by polymeric antigen, resulting in B-cell activation without T-cell contact. Either pathway of activation results in repeated cycles of B-cell proliferation, followed by differentiation of B cells into Ig-secreting plasma cells or long-lived memory cells. All stages of B-cell function are influenced by lymphokines secreted by activated T cells (dashed line).

tetanus toxoid, pertussis toxin, diphtheria toxin, purified protein derivative of tuberculin (PPD), and influenza vaccine.[173] However, these patients generate antibody to T-independent antigens, such as mannan and isohemagglutinin polysaccharides.

Other types of activation occur upon exposure to nonspecific mitogens of B cells, such as phorbol esters and lipopolysaccharide (LPS), which bypass the need for binding with surface antibody and directly activate regulatory proteins in the cell.[161] B cells can also be nonspecifically activated with anti-IgM/IgD immunoglobulin or with staphylococcal protein A, which are capable of multivalent binding of human Ig. These reagents activate B cells in a polyclonal fashion that may not be physiologic but that provides useful models for in vitro experimentation.[175]

The activated B cell next enters a proliferative phase that amplifies, by clonal expansion of antigen-specific cells, the quantity of antibody produced. Whatever the mode of activation, the subsequent proliferative phase is dependent on the presence of B-cell growth factors.[153,154] Several of these factors have been isolated and cloned, allowing for careful functional studies (Table 5). Many of these factors are not functionally restricted to B-cell stimulation, as IL-2 and IL-4 also induce T-cell proliferation, nor is their action on B cells specific for a single stage: IL-4 is capable of supporting activation, proliferation, and differentiation. The expression of regulatory surface molecules, such as membrane IgD, CR2, and MHC, diminishes during proliferation and subsequent differentiation of the activated cells.

One outcome of growth and differentiation of B cells is that they become nondividing plasma cells within 3–4 days after initial activation of the cell. The plasma cell is evolved for the single purpose of producing large quantities of immunoglobulin. The cytoplasm is crowded with ribosomes and a massive golgi apparatus, displacing the nucleus into its characteristic eccentric location. Certain other activated B cells are differentiated into long-lived memory cells that are capable of rapidly producing mature antibody isotypes upon restimulation with antigen.[142,143] Because IgM is the isotype first expressed by activated B cells, it constitutes the first class of antibody to be observed in the serum following primary antigenic challenge. IgM levels peak at 5–7 days after exposure and decline thereafter. IgG antibodies first appear at 7–14 days following antigenic exposure, consistent with the longer time necessary for B cells to differentiate into IgG-synthesizing cells. Secondary antigenic exposures, by virtue of pre-existing memory B cells, produce prompt IgG responses. The association of IgM with acute exposure has importance in the serodiagnosis of certain infections.

Control mechanisms have evolved to direct the type of antibodies produced by the fully differentiated B cell. Certain T-cell lymphokines function as B-cell differentiation factors and influence isotype commitment during maturation (Table 5). For example, the lymphokine IL-4 induces experimentally activated murine B-cell populations to preferentially produce IgG_1 and IgE.[176] This interaction may be central to the elevated levels of IgE in mammals infected with helminths, as has been shown in experimental *Nippostrongylus nipponensis* infection.[177] Interferon-γ, in contrast, is antagonistic to IL-4 isotype selection and separately induces the production of other Ig classes.[178] Similarly, IL-5 augments IgA secretion from activated B cells.[179]

In addition to producing these characterized lymphokines, T cells secrete heavy chain binding factors that can either augment or inhibit the production of certain immunoglobulin isotypes. The best characterized of these bind IgE or IgA. IgE binding factors are produced by CD4+ T lymphocytes that possess surface receptors for the Fc portion of IgE ($Fc_\epsilon R$).[39] The binding factor has stimulatory or inhibitory activity, depending on the state of glycosylation. A similar network regulating IgA synthesis has been proposed. T cells bearing IgA Fc receptors ($Fc_\alpha R$) have been indentified that also secrete factors that bind and regulate IgA production. The increased numbers of $Fc_\alpha R$+ T cells in the intestinal lymphoid tissue may therefore account for the increased production of IgA in that location.[37] Peyer's patch T cells also produce increased amounts of IL-5, which may additionally stimulate IgA production.[180,181]

B cells are also subject to various inhibitory mechanisms that prevent self-directed immune responses or excessive immunoglobulin synthesis. Inhibitory networks that act on B cells at different stages of development have been described. Tolerance to self-antigen may occur during early B-cell development and result from the selective deletion of self-reactive B-cell clones. An excess of foreign antigen may accomplish the same result—"immune paralysis."[182] At a second level, mature B-cell function can be actively inhibited by suppressor T cells. These cells suppress antibody production in either an antigen-specific or -nonspecific fashion and may act either directly on B cells or on other, antibody-promoting T cells. The exact suppressor mechanism is poorly characterized, partly because of its complexity. Although the effector cell in the suppressor circuit is typically CD8+, interactions with CD4+ cells may be required, and the final inhibitory signal may be mediated by soluble suppressor factors.[147,148,183]

Antibody production may also be regulated by other immunoglobulins that specifically recognize the variable region of the first, or idiotypic antibody. These anti-idiotypic antibodies have been observed during native immune responses and are speculated to modulate antibody production.[182,184] Because the variable region of anti-idiotype antibodies may mimic the original antigen epitope, these immunoglobulins have been used as experimental vaccines.[185,186] Finally, circulating antibodies or immune complexes may provide an inhibitory signal to B cells by binding to surface Fc receptors, an interaction that suppresses B-cell activation and development.[17,23]

TABLE 5. Cytokine Involvement in B-Cell Activation, Proliferation and Antibody Secretion

Cytokine	*Synonyms*	*Cell of Origin*	*Effect on B Cell*
Interleukin-1 (α and β)	Lymphocyte activating factor	Macrophages, B cells	Activation and proliferation
Interleukin-2	T-cell growth factor	T cells	Proliferation
Interleukin-4	(BSF-1, BCGF I)	T cells, mast cells	Activation (increases HLA-DR, CD 23), proliferation, differentiation (stimulates IgE production)
Interleukin-5	(BCGF II, TRF)	T cells	Differentiation (stimulates IgA production)
Interleukin-6	BSF-2, hybridoma growth factor, IFN-β_2	Fibroblasts, T cells, macrophages	Proliferation, differentiation
$BCGF_{low}$		T cells	Proliferation
γ-Interferon	Macrophage activating factor	T cells	Proliferation, differentiation (inhibits IL-4 action)

Abbreviations: BSF: B-cell stimulatory factor; BCGF: B-cell growth factor; TRF: T-cell replacing factor; HLA: human leukocyte antigen; CD: common determinant.

Diagnosis of Disease

With organisms that may be difficult to identify by standard culture methods, the identification of a specific humoral immune response may be instrumental in the diagnosis of infection. This technique is particularly useful in the diagnosis of viral infections, since most laboratories are not equipped to grow the organisms in tissue culture. A high IgM response is characteristic of most acute or recrudescent viral infections, whereas the presence of IgG antibodies can only be correlated with established, chronic, quiescent, or resolved infection.[187]

Tissue Injury

Chronic antigenic stimulation of B lymphocytes results in the production of large amounts of polyclonal antibodies (polyclonal gammopathy), as well as the related production of immune complexes and rheumatoid factor. Polyclonal gammopathy is the most commonly recognized disorder of serum immunoglobulin levels and is associated with a large number of infectious, neoplastic, and inflammatory states.[188] Prolonged activation of antigen-specific B and T cells is hypothesized to result in the nonspecific recruitment of "bystander" B-cell clones, many of which produce autoantibodies or antibody to unrelated antigens. Several chronic infectious diseases induce a polyclonal gammopathy, as exemplified by infective endocarditis.[189,190] Although IgG responses predominate, helminthic infections additionally induce elevated levels of polyclonal IgE.[191] Certain viruses, such as Epstein-Barr virus,[192] interact directly with B cells to stimulate polyspecific antibody generation during acute infection. Polyclonal gammopathy can be a prominent feature of symptomatic infection with HIV (see Chapter 108).

Antibody and antigen bind together to form immune complexes. Circulating immune complexes are apparent during many infectious processes, but are clinically significant in only a minority of patients.[193,194] The pathologic potential of immune complexes depends on size, valency, charge characteristics, and site of formation of the complex.[193] Immune complexes can initiate a cascade of proinflammatory events through interaction with Fc receptors on phagocytic cells or by activating complement. Binding of immune complexes to Fc receptor induces granulocytes to discharge lysosomal contents and generate reactive oxidative products. Macrophages are similarly stimulated by immune complexes to produce proinflammatory agents such as IL-1 and arachidonic acid derivatives.[195] Immune complexes containing IgM or IgG can also activate the classical pathway of complement and generate C3a and C5a, which contribute to inflammatory responses through their chemotaxic and anaphylatoxic properties.

Immune complex-mediated damage is most evident in the wide spectrum of glomerular disease that complicates the course of various acute and chronic infections. The prototypic lesion is that of poststreptococcal glomerulonephritis, which is caused when bacterial antigen–antibody complexes are deposited in the glomerular capillary wall. Local damage is presumably mediated by complement and mesangial cell products triggered by the immobilized complexes.[196] Immune complex glomerulonephritis is also associated with infections that cause prolonged antigenemia, such as infective endocarditis,[189] ventriculoatrial shunt infections ("shunt nephritis"),[193] and hepatitis B.[197]

Rheumatoid factors are IgM or IgG antibodies distinguished by their specificity for the Fc portion of autologous IgG.[198] A population of Leu1+ B cells may be uniquely evolved for rheumatoid factor synthesis.[160] IgM rheumatoid factors are normal products of secondary humoral immune reactions. Production only becomes pathologic when prolonged and elevated levels result.[198,199] Molecular analysis has shown that the genes encoding the variable (antigen-binding) portions of rheumatoid factor light chains are highly conserved during B-cell ontogeny, so that remarkable homology is evident in rheumatoid factors elicited from different individuals or from different B-cell hybridomas.[200] This degree of conservation suggests that important immune functions may be served by rheumatoid factor, a teleologic argument supported in part by animal studies.[201] For example, the opsonizing and cytolytic capacity of complement-nonreactive IgG may be increased when bound to an IgM molecule that efficiently activates the classical pathway of complement.[200] Rheumatoid factor may also improve the antigen-binding performance of low-affinity IgG by increasing valency. Finally, rheumatoid factor may facilitate the removal of soluble immune complexes by accelerating complement activation on the complex and thus promoting uptake by complement receptor-bearing phagocytes. Rheumatoid factor production accompanies polyclonal B-cell activation and immune complex formation and is frequently present during prolonged infection. No direct pathologic role is usually evident. When rheumatoid factor associates with circulating antigen–antibody complexes, cryoglobulins may result.[193] The mixed cryoglobulinemia that accompanies chronic infection is usually benign, but has been associated with hypersensitivity vasculitis and severe glomerulonephritis during hepatitis B infection.[202]

Certain infectious agents are hypothesized to induce autoimmunity because they share antigenic determinants with host tissue—"molecular mimicry."[203] For instance, streptococcal M proteins share determinants with myocardial sarcolemma proteins,[204] *Klebsiella pneumoniae* epitopes cross react with HLA-B27,[205] and monoclonal antibodies against any of several viruses bind to several different normal human tissues.[206] Although circulating antibodies that are cross-reactive with these antigens have been recognized in some patients, these instances of molecular mimicry have not yet proven to be causal in the pathogenesis of autoimmune disease.

IMMUNOGLOBULIN AND ANTIBODY DEFICIENCY STATES

Interference with any of the stages of antigen processing, cellular proliferation, or regulation of the formation of immunoglobulins or specific antibodies may lead to a deficiency of the humoral immune responses. The consequences to the host may range from a loss of function of a specific antibody or immunoglobulin class to all classes depending on the nature of the defect. The loss of the IgG class has the most serious effects when compared with the other classes. A variety of disorders that involve the humoral immune system as it relates to antibody formation or action have been described and are indicated in Table 6 (for reviews see Refs. 207–209).

When the capacity to develop IgM or, in particular, IgG antibodies is lacking, then the host is unable to generate specific antibody-mediated serum opsonic, lytic, or neutralizing activities as they relate to these molecules. The serum of agammaglobulinemic patients is not capable of fixing complement by the classical pathway unless C1 is activated by an non-immunoglobulin-dependent mechanism; the ability to activate the complement system through the alternative pathway is retained, however. The end result of such deletions in the host defense system is the development of recurrent infections involving encapsulated bacteria and, to a lesser extent, gram-negative organisms in which opsonic and lytic defenses are important. These infections often involve the sinopulmonary tract, and the causative organisms may enter the blood stream with subsequent wide dissemination to other sites.[210] Thus patients who have unusually severe or recurrent infections with pneumococci, streptococci, *H. influenzae*, or meningococci should be examined carefully for possible defects in humoral immunity.

Even though the development of neutralizing antibodies of the IgG class is the hallmark of measurable long-standing protection against reinfection by specific viruses,[187] with some important exceptions[211–213] unusually severe disseminated or re-

TABLE 6. Disorders Involving the Humoral Immune System

	Consequences to Host Defense
Primary	
Pure antibody-mediated B-cell disorders	
X-linked hypogammaglobulinemia	Major[a]
Transient hypogammaglobulinemia of infancy	Variable[b]
Common variable hypogammaglobulinemia	Major
X-linked immunodeficiency with hyper-IgM	Major
Selective IgA deficiency	Minor[c]
Selective IgM deficiency	Minor
Selective deficiency of IgG subclasses	Variable
Mixed antibody-mediated (B-cell) and cell-mediated (T-cell) immunodeficiency disorders	
Severe combined immunodeficiency disease	Major
Nezelof syndrome	Major
Ataxia–telangectasia	Variable
Wiskott-Aldrich syndrome	Major
Short-limbed dwarfism	Major
Episodic lymphocytopenia with lymphotoxin	Major
Secondary to another disease or therapy	
Pure (B-cell) disorders	
Multiple myeloma	Major
Waldenström's macroglobulinemia	Variable
Heavy chain disease	Major
Chronic lymphocytic leukemia	Major
Some lymphomas	Major
Nephrotic syndrome	Variable
Splenectomy	Variable
Mixed disorders	
Cytotoxic therapy	Variable
Corticosteroid therapy	Variable
Severe burns	Major
Graft-vs.-host disease	Variable
Intestinal lymphangiectasia	Major
Acquired immunodeficiency syndrome	Major

[a] Antibody and/or cellular immune deficiency is routinely so severe that major infections result.
[b] Deficiency of antibodies or cellular immunity varies from patient to patient.
[c] Most patients have no significant increase in susceptibility to infection.

current viral infections are not characteristic of most patients with immunoglobulin deficiency. This finding suggests that cellular immune mechanisms may play a more important role in limiting the extent and severity of viral infection than do humoral mechanisms, a point substantiated by the observation that patients who are deficient in cellular immunity are at great risk for serious viral infections.

Likewise, the humoral immune deficiencies are not particularly associated with recurrent or severe fungal or parasitic infections, with two exceptions: patients who are hypogammaglobulinemic may develop pneumonia due to *P. carinii* or may be plagued with recurrent severe intestinal giardiasis.[121,122] Gastrointestinal giardiasis in patients with dysgammaglobulinemia or hypogammaglobulinemia may lead to prolonged malabsorption. In patients with acquired hypogammaglobulinemia, a peculiar nodular hyperplasia of lymphoid tissues in the submucosa of the small intestine may be seen with giardiasis.[121,210] Malabsorption may occur in humorally deficient patients in the absence of giardiasis, however, and has been associated with a sprue-like histologic pattern on intestinal biopsy specimens.[210,214] Treatment of such patients with replacement immunoglobulin theory may not only reduce the susceptibility to infection but may also reverse the malabsorption syndromes. This suggests that the intestinal mucosal changes may be related to chronic low-grade bacterial infection. When antibodies such as serum IgA function to clear or block environmental antigens, their loss may result in undesirable allergic responses. IgA deficiency is accompanied by a high rate of atopic disorders.

Clinical Features

Table 6 lists the major immunodeficiency disorders affecting the synthesis or function of antibody. They have been classified into primary diseases or secondary disorders, which represent complications of other disease states or therapy.

Primary Disorders: Pure Antibody Deficiency. X-LINKED HYPOGAMMAGLOBULINEMIA. Originally described by Bruton in 1952,[215] this represents the first immunodeficiency disorder to be characterized. The genetic origin of this disorder has been mapped to a locus on the long arm of the X chromosome.[216] Possession of this genotype in males results in defective maturation of B cells as a result of abortive heavy chain assembly.[217] As a consequence, B cells and plasma cells are absent from lymphoid tissue and bone marrow. Due to passive transfer of maternal IgG, affected infants are usually asymptomatic until 5–6 months of age, at which time maternal antibodies are almost completely cleared from the system.[218] The hypogammaglobulinemia will then usually manifest as recurrent middle ear, sinopulmonary, and gastrointestinal tract infections with or without complicating bacteremia, meningitis, and cellulitis.[219] Less commonly, such patients may not develop these recurrent infections until later in childhood, when they have other disorders such as chronic conjunctivitis, dental caries, or malabsorption. Because of severe pulmonary infection some patients may have bronchiectasis by the time hypogammaglobulinemia in diagnosed. Severe enteroviral infections are characteristic of this group of patients. Echovirus, in particular, is associated with a prolonged meningoencephalitis or a disseminated infection producing a dermatomyositis-like syndrome.[212,220,221] Other patients may have a chronic recurring type of arthritis syndrome that can resemble rheumatoid arthritis; *Mycoplasma* and *Ureaplasma* have been isolated from the joint fluid of some of these patients.[222,223] The futility of serodiagnosis makes it likely that additional viral complications are underrecognized. Mortality commonly occurs in the second or third decade and results from chronic pulmonary disease or from disseminated viral infections.

A diagnosis of this disease is made by demonstrating that there is a marked absence or deficiency of all five immunoglobulin classes. IgG levels in particular are usually less than 200 mg/dl, a level below which antibody-dependent serum opsonization is severely affected. These patients are incapable of antibody formation after specific antigenic stimulation. Biopsy specimens from appropriate tissues will demonstrate a complete absence of plasma cells in the germinal centers of lymph nodes and the lamina propria of the gut. An absence of circulating B cells, with normal or elevated levels of circulating T cells, is also characteristic.[224] Cellular immunity is completely intact.[218] Related syndromes include X-linked hypogammaglobulinemia with isolated growth hormone deficiency[225] and autosomal recessive hypogammaglobulinemia.[208]

Historically, replacement IgG was provided by intramuscular gammaglobulin. However, the limited volume tolerable by this route of delivery made normalization of serum IgG levels unrealistic. Immunoglobulin preparations for intravenous injection are now available that can be administered in quantities that result in normal serum IgG levels.[226,227] These preparations are 95–99 percent IgG, with trace quantities of IgA, IgM, IgD, and IgE; the half-life of the delivered IgG is variable but averages about 20 days. Maintenance doses start at 200 mg/kg in monthly infusions, but may need to be increased up to 500 mg/kg/month to achieve protection. A comparative study has shown that a higher-dose regimen resulted in improved pulmonary function. The incidence of acute infection diminished when serum levels were 500 mg/dl or higher.[228]

Intravenous immunoglobulin is typically well tolerated and can be self-administered at home after appropriate training of the patient or family. About 3–12 percent of patients experience fever, chills, headache, myalgia, and nausea with infusion.[226] When symptoms are severe enough, pretreatment with acetaminophen, antihistamines, or hydrocortisone is justified in order to reduce these side effects.[229] A few cases of non-A, non-B hepatitis have been transmitted by intravenous immunoglobulin, apparently due to contamination of isolated lots of infusate.[227] Otherwise the infectious risk of intravenous immunoglobulin is very small; no known instances of HIV transmission from IgG have occurred. In addition to immunoglobulin replacement therapy, specific infections must be treated with appropriate antimicrobials. The efficacy of maintenance prophylactic antimicrobials in the long-term management of these patients is questionable, and this practice may lead to superinfections with resistant bacteria.

TRANSIENT HYPOGAMMAGLOBULINEMIA OF INFANCY. This is an exaggerated form of the normal reduction in serum IgG levels that occurs at approximately 5–6 months of age.[208,230] In normal infants, serum IgG levels may fall to as low as 350 mg/dl before such patients begin to generate substantial amounts of IgG antibody from their own plasma cells. Occasionally the onset of IgG synthesis is delayed, resulting in a pathologically significant decrease in its level for a period of time. As a result, the patients may be subjected to the same type of infections as children with X-linked hypogammaglobulinemia. Suggested mechanisms for a delay in IgG production include immaturities in macrophage function,[231,232] reduced T-helper cells,[233] or exaggerated suppressor function.[234] Because of a risk of active infection, these children should not receive immunizations with live virus vaccine until a normal immunocompetency has been established.[235] Treatment with immune serum globulin is required when these patients are symptomatic with infection, but concern exists that such treatment may suppress subsequent production of endogenous immunoglobulin.[236]

COMMON VARIABLE UNCLASSIFIABLE IMMUNODEFICIENCY. This disorder is also called "acquired" hypogammaglobulinemia and appears to have a familial pattern, although the mechanism of inheritance has not been clearly established.[208,237] This disease is usually not apparent until the age of 15–35 years. Affected persons appear to have an unusually high frequency of autoimmune disorders in addition to an increased susceptibility to pyogenic infections.[210] While IgG levels are invariably below 250 mg/dl in symptomatic patients, and the levels of other immunoglobulins are also very low, this pattern is less pronounced or consistent when compared with that of patients with X-linked hypogammaglobulinemia. They also differ from these subjects in having detectable B cells in the peripheral circulation. However, the numbers of mature plasma cells in lymphoid tissues are decreased, consistent with a defect in B-cell maturation and differentiation. This disorder is probably heterogenous with respect to pathogenesis. Increased T-suppressor numbers and function[225,238] or reduced T-helper cell activity[239] have been described; other patients have intrinsic B-cell defects. A very few patients have anti-B-cell antibodies.

The disease affects men and women with approximately equal frequency. Its manifestation is often more subtle than that of X-linked hypogammaglobulinemia, with many patients merely experiencing an increased number or severity of sinopulmonary infections. Other patients may have chronic bacterial conjunctivitis, severe malabsorption, or a rheumatoid arthritis-like disorder. Systemic lupus erythematosus, idiopathic thrombocytopenia purpura, dermatomyositis, hemolytic anemia, or pernicious anemia have been described in some. In contrast to patients with X-linked hypogammaglobulinemia, many patients with acquired hypogammaglobulinemia have significant lymphadenopathy, splenomegaly, and intestinal lymphoid nodular hyperplasia rather than absence of lymphatic tissue.[210,221,235] Histologic examination of the lymph nodes reveals a marked accumulation of macrophages, immature B cells, and both CD4+ and CD8+ T cells.[206,208] The treatment of patients with the acquired form is similar to that of those with X-linked hypogammaglobulinemia. Successful treatment results in amelioration of infections as well as lymphadenopathy and splenomegaly.[206] In addition, affected patients may require therapy for associated autoimmune disorders. Some patients who have been appropriately treated have survived for a long time. Besides acute infection, a major complication appears to be chronic lung disease. An increased incidence of malignant disease has also been noted.[235,237] For patients with increased suppressor cell activity, cimetidine treatment has resulted in increased production of immunoglobulin.[240]

HYPER-IgM WITH IgG DEFICIENCY. A syndrome characterized by high IgM levels and very low IgG and IgA levels has been described. In most patients the inheritance appears to be sex-linked, and the manifestation is characterized by recurrent pyogenic infections.[241] There is an apparent inability of B cells and their successor plasma cells to form IgG and IgA after initial IgM and IgD synthesis. A deficiency in the heavy chain gene switch mechanism is thus suggested and may be caused by the absence of switch T cells in these patients.[242] This syndrome can be separated diagnostically from the other disorders by the characteristic increase in serum IgM concentrations, with low-to-absent levels of IgA and IgG. Treatment is similar to that of the other hypogammaglobulinemic disorders outlined above.

SELECTIVE IgA DEFICIENCY. This is the most common immunodeficiency disorder, with an incidence of about 1:600 in the normal population.[243] Whereas the majority of people with IgA deficiency are clinically normal, it is clear that this defect predisposes to a variety of diseases including (*1*) recurrent sinopulmonary infections, (*2*) atopy, (*3*) gastrointestinal tract disease, (*4*) autoimmune disorders (e.g., systemic lupus erythematosus, rheumatoid arthritis, pernicious anemia), and (*5*) malignancy (diffuse histiocytic lymphona or gastrointestinal carcinoma).[243–245] These clinical manifestations are probably due to the absence of protective IgA on mucosal surfaces and the loss of serum IgA blocking antibody directed against environmental antigens.[246] Affected patients have markedly reduced levels of IgA in both serum (< 5 mg/dl) and secretions, with normal or increased values of the other immunoglobulin classes. Most patients have decreases in both IgA_1 and IgA_2. Cellular immune functions and B- and T-cell numbers are usually normal. Some patients with IgA deficiency also have decreased levels of IgG_2, IgG_4, and/or IgE, indicative of a more generalized disorder affecting isotypic switching of immunoglobulins and further contributing to the heterogeneity of clinical manifestations.[247,248] A few of these cases may be caused by deletions of heavy chain genes.[249,250] These patients should not receive immune serum globulin therapy, since IgG levels are normal-to-elevated, and dangerous anaphylactic responses to transfused IgA may ensue. Similarly, treatment with plasma or blood may lead to anaphylactic transfusion reactions because of IgE antibodies to IgA in the recipient's circulation.[251] No effective replacement therapy is yet available; therefore treatment is directed primarily at complications.

SELECTIVE IgM DEFICIENCY. This is a rare disorder. Affected patients exhibit a susceptibility to autoimmune diseases or to severe infection with organisms that have polysaccharide capsules.[252] Cellular immunity is intact, and other classes of immunoglobulins are synthesized normally. The pathogenesis is unknown, but antibody production to T-independent antigens is impaired. Treatment is preventive and directed toward the complicating infections. No replacement therapy is available, except possibly with plasma.

SELECTIVE DEFICIENCY OF IgG SUBCLASSES. Isolated deficiency of IgG_1 is very rare and results in total IgG levels that are reduced, since this subtype accounts for approximately 70 percent of the IgG class. Patients with this disorder experience an increased incidence of infections with encapsulated bacteria, like hypogammaglobulinemic patients.[253] The pathogenesis is not known. Replacement gammaglobulin therapy is usually effective in reducing the incidence of infections.

The use of sensitive and specific IgG subclass immunoassays has uncovered selective deficiencies of IgG_2 and IgG_4, often coexisting with IgA and IgE deficiencies, in patients suffering from recurrent bacterial infections.[247,254] In most cases, the total levels of IgG were in the normal range. IgG_2 deficiency has been linked to impaired antibody responses to polysaccharide vaccines.[255]

MIXED DISORDERS WITH ANTIBODY DEFICIENCY. A number of primary immunodeficiency disorders have been described in which both antibody production and cellular immunity are impaired. Affected patients are susceptible to severe, recurrent, and often fatal infections with all classes of organisms, including obligate extracellular parasites as well as organisms that are capable of intracellular survival. They have both impaired antibody formation as well as defects in cellular immunity.

COMBINED IMMUNODEFICIENCY OF INFANCY. This is the most severe of the mixed immunodeficiency disorders and is discussed in Chapter 8 as well. Described inheritance patterns are either sex-linked or autosomal recessive. Typical patients are markedly lymphopenic and lack both B and T cells in their lymph nodes, thymus, or blood[208,209]; other patients exhibit only immature T-cell precursors in their circulation.[224,256] Normal immunologic competence has been restored in some patients by bone marrow transplantation, consistent with a stem cell defect.[257] About one-half of the patients with the autosomal recessive form of severe combined immunodeficiency lack enzymatic activities involved in adenosine nucleoside metabolism.[258] Adenosine deaminase deficiency causes lymphocyte depletion by allowing toxic levels of deoxyadenosine triphosphate to accumulate in the cells of these patients. Transfusion of normal erythrocytes to patients with adenosine deaminase deficiency has resulted in immunologic and clinical improvement,[259] based on the fact that the nucleosides pass freely through cell membranes, enter the erythrocytes, and are there metabolized by donor enzyme. Bone marrow transplantation is curative and the treatment of choice if a suitable donor is available.[260] A related metabolic cause of severe immunodeficiency in childhood is purine–nucleoside phosphorylase deficiency.[258,261] This rare syndrome similarly results in accumulations of nucleotides, which are selectively toxic for T cells. In contrast to the other forms of severe combined immunodeficiency, B-cell numbers and serum immunoglobulin levels may be normal in this disorder.

CELLULAR IMMUNODEFICIENCY WITH ABNORMAL IMMUNOGLOBULIN SYNTHESIS: NEZELOF SYNDROME. A variety of patients have been described who have marked impairments in cellular immunity with variable depression of antibody-forming capacity. They are grouped loosely under the eponym of "Nezelof syndrome," unless other characteristic features permit a different classification.[262] No specific genetic pattern can be demonstrated, and both affected males and females have been described. On a pathogenetic basis, it has been suggested that the defect in immunoglobulin synthesis is a consequence of the loss of function of the helper T-cell population, although this notion requires further definition. In contrast to the patients described above with severe combined immunodeficiency, most affected patients have lymphoid hypertrophy and hepatosplenomegaly, with macrophage infiltration and granuloma formation. Circulating B and T cells are usually normal in number, and immunoglobulin levels may be normal or reduced. Markedly depressed cellular immunity is characteristic, and most patients are incapable of mounting a humoral immune response to new antigens, although evidence of prior antibody formation may be found (e.g., isohemagglutinins).

WISKOTT-ALDRICH SYNDROME. This is an X-linked recessive disorder in which both cellular immunity and antibody synthesis are impaired. In contrast to Nezelof syndrome, affected patients also have thrombocytopenia and chronic eczematoid dermatitis. The precise mechanism involved in the defect in this syndrome is unknown, although a specific glycoprotein is missing from the surface of platelets and lymphocytes in these patients.[263] Affected patients have normal numbers of B and T cells. Immunoglobulin levels are in the low-normal range; however, patients have a characteristic difficulty in the synthesis of antibodies to T-independent antigens (e.g., polysaccharides).[264,265] They have major problems due to severe infection with encapsulated bacteria such as the pneumococcus and *H. influenzae*, since they cannot generate opsonic antibody against these organisms. Patients have had both the hematologic and immunologic abnormalities corrected by bone marrow transplantation.[266]

ATAXIA-TELANGIECTASIA. Patients with this neurologic disorder have variable deficiencies of IgG, IgA, and/or IgE levels, decreased humoral immune responses to new antigens, and diminished cellular immunity.[267,268] These findings suggest the existence of abnormal T-lymphocyte function affecting both IgA and IgE synthesis and immunity to cellular antigens. This disease may be caused by deficient DNA repair mechanisms, and chromosomal damage near the T-cell receptor and immunoglobulin genes may contribute to the immune defects.[269,270] Selective deficiencies of IgG_2 in this syndrome may be associated with chronic infections.[271] No effective treatment has been devised for the immune disorders in this disease.

OTHER COMBINED IMMUNODEFICIENCIES. There are a variety of other disorders of combined immunodeficiency, as outlined in Table 6. As far as the infectious complications are concerned, their manifestations are similar to those already described. For a more detailed description the interested reader is referred to several reviews.[147,208,209] The syndrome of hyper-IgE with eosinophilia, deficient chemotaxis, and recurrent staphylococcal infections is described in more detail in Chapter 7. Evidence supports the concept that this is due to a T-cell immunoregulatory defect involving impaired control of IgE synthesis as well as the production of a neutrophil chemotactic inhibitor.[272]

Humoral Deficiency Secondary to Other Diseases or Treatment. PURE B-CELL DISORDERS. Certain disorders may characteristically impair the humoral immune response as one of their central features. Accordingly, affected patients may develop severe or recurrent infections with organisms that are similar to those seen in hypogammaglobulinemic states. Two major types of disorders are seen: (*1*) those that affect immunoglobulin or antibody synthesis, and (*2*) those that increase the rate of immunoglobulin catabolism. Prime examples of the former are seen in a variety of malignant conditions affecting the lymphoreticular or hematopoietic systems.[273] Some patients with certain types of lymphoma, lymphosarcoma, thymoma, or chronic lymphocytic leukemia will be incapable of production of one or more classes of immunoglobulins and will become hypogammaglobulinemic.[274,275] Such abnormalities could be due to a primary involvement of the B-cell system in unregulated proliferation without maturation or increased suppressor activity. Besides treatment of the primary disease, such patients may benefit from regular administration of intravenous immunoglobulin.[275a] Conversely, patients with primary immunodeficiencies, in particular those involving the T-lymphocyte system, have a higher incidence of hematopoietic and lymphatic malignancies.[276]

In multiple myeloma, Waldenstrom's macroglobulinemia, and the various "heavy chain diseases," overproduction of a given class or subcomponent of an immunoglobulin occurs because of unregulated expansion and production of these proteins by a malignant clone of plasma cells or their precursors. When intact, the immunoglobulins produced in these diseases characteristically bear only a single L-chain type and have no effective antibody activity.[277] The expansion of the malignant plasma cell pool occurs at the expense of normal cells and diminishes the activity of the latter. In addition, disordered immunoregulation has been reported in myeloma.[278] Infections with encapsulated and gram-negative bacteria are prominent in these patients.[274,279,280] Immune serum globulin therapy is of little help, since catabolic rates of immunoglobulins are increased (particularly in the case of IgG myeloma),[8] and little additive effect of exogenous IgG can be defined.[281]

Immunoglobulin catabolism is also increased in some patients with severe burns,[282] protein-losing enteropathies,[8] or the nephrotic syndrome.[8,283] In burned patients, immunoglobulins are lost excessively into the burn site, whereas gastrointestinal or urinary tract losses of IgG are responsible for hypogammaglobulinemia in the other disorders. Treatment of the primary disease process will bring about a reversal of these conditions. Therapy with immune serum globulin may be desirable but is of no proven benefit.

SPLENECTOMY. The spleen performs several important host defense functions. As a phagocytic filter it can nonspecifically survey and present intravascular antigen to the large numbers of T and B cells that reside in or transit through this lymphoid organ.[284] It removes senescent or defective red blood cells, including those infected with intraerythrocytic parasites during malaria or babesiosis.[285,286] Although the liver may contain a greater total mass of phagocytic cells, the spleen is more efficient at removing poorly or unopsonized pathogens.[287] The spleen is also an important site of IgM production and memory B-cell differentiation during primary humoral responses. In particular, it is responsible for generating antibody responses to polysaccharide antigens.[288]

Some splenectomized patients are susceptible to severe infections with pneumococci, other streptococci, *H. influenzae*, meningococci, and the capnophilic gram-negative bacterium DF-2.[289] They are also susceptible to severe infection with *Babesia microttii*.[286] These infections are particularly prominent when splenectomy is performed in children for congenital hemolytic anemia[290] or Hodgkin's disease[291] and in some adults within the first 3 years after an incidental or post-traumatic splenectomy.[292] Sickle cell patients, who are functionally asplenic following infarction of that organ, also suffer from an increased incidence and severity of pneumococcal, *Haemophilus*, and meningococcal infections.[293] The increased susceptibility to infection in these patients have been attributed to the removal or dysfunction of an organ important for the clearance of intravascular organisms, to poor antibody responses to capsular polysaccharides, and to deficient serum opsonizing activity. Impaired antibody formation may be the central factor responsible for the observed serum opsonizing defects.[294] Tuftsin is an immunoglobulin-derived tetrapeptide produced in the spleen that stimulates phagocyte cell functions. Tuftsin levels are decreased following splenectomy and may also contribute to immunoincompetence.[295]

The improvement in intravascular clearance of organisms or foreign cells with specific immunization of splenectomized subjects[296,297] indicates that they should be considered as candidates for immunization with bacterial capsular polysaccharides. Satisfactory antibody levels, as measured by immunoassay, were reported in splenectomized subjects who received pneumococcal or meningococcal vaccine, provided they were not receiving cytotoxic or lymph node irradiation therapy.[298–300] However, even following vaccination, serum opsonic activity of asplenic hosts can still be deficient.[294,301] Although pneumococcal vaccine is protective in sickle cell patients, it has not yet been proved of benefit in splenectomized subjects.[299] Thus vaccination with capsular antigens does not remove the need for continued surveillance of splenectomized or asplenic subjects for possible sepsis with organisms included in the vaccine preparations. A decrease in infection incidence has been noted in sickle cell patients treated prophylactically with daily oral penicillin.[302]

Mixed Cellular and Humoral Deficiency Secondary to Disease or Therapy

Patients with generalized lymphomas may have both impaired cellular as well as humoral immunity.[273,275] Lymphopenia may occur in severely burned patients, leading to similar impairments.[303] Other disorders that can affect both limbs of the immune response in the absence of disease treatment are quite rare. One such disease is the disorder known as intestinal lymphangiectasia. Small lymphocytes, the majority of which are T cells, are lost in the gastrointestinal tract through dilated lymphatic channels. Patients with these disorders become markedly lymphopenic and can suffer from the same infections as patients with primary combined immunodeficiency.[304]

The majority of patients with secondary impairments in both humoral and cellular immunity are receiving cytotoxic, irradiation, or corticosteroid therapy.[274,275,305–307] By reducing the lymphocyte mass and by providing particular effectiveness against rapidly proliferating cells, cytotoxic agents can markedly impair the immune response. This is especially true when the host is faced with newer antigens for which a rapid proliferative response is called. Secondary responses are less affected by cytotoxic treatment both with respect to cellular and humoral immune components. Whereas patients receiving cytotoxic therapy may experience a reduction in the levels of circulating immunoglobulins, frank hypogammaglobulinemia is rarely seen, and established antibodies remain.[305,307]

Corticosteroid therapy exerts its major immunosuppressive effects against the T-lymphocyte population and against macrophages.[308,309] T-cell "traffic" is markedly disrupted by glucocorticoids.[310] Monocyte traffic, including egress from the circulation, is similarly disrupted, potentially creating a second level of impairment in tissue macrophage–lymphocyte interactions. Macrophage and lymphocyte production of immunoregulatory cytokines may be markedly diminished.[311,312] Glucocorticoid therapy can also reduce polymorphonuclear inflammatory responses; however, because this population is rapidly repleted, the effects are of short duration.[309] The consequences are most evident if glucocorticoid doses exceed 0.3 mg/kg/day/dose of prednisone or its equivalent.[313] A marked increase in susceptibility to a wide variety of infections is experienced within several weeks of steroid therapy if the dosages are in excess of 1 mg/kg/day and is the major cause of infection in patients undergoing renal transplantation[314] or treatment for lupus.[315]

Infection with HIV, the causative agent of AIDS, is associated with aberrant immunoglobulin production.[316] Patients most notably demonstrate polyclonal gammopathy, but specific antibody responses to new antigens are impaired.[317,318] In some patients, this results in an increased frequency of pneumonias caused by encapsulated bacteria.[319] For a more detailed discussion of these phenomena see Chapter 108.

Evaluation and Treatment of Disorders of Humoral Immunity

A summary of common practices used to evaluate and treat disorders of humoral immunity is given in Table 6, and a brief description follows. Chronic, unusually severe, or recurrent infections with bacteria and viruses can be caused by deficiencies in immunoglobulin, complement, or phagocyte-mediated immunity. Abnormal T-cell function is more commonly associated with fungal, protozoan, or viral illnesses. Certain nonimmunologic abnormalities, such as ciliary dyskinesis syndrome and cystic fibrosis, can additionally result in infectious complications. Therefore the measurement of serum immunoglobulin levels should not occur in isolation but must be part of a coordinated diagnostic strategy in the evaluation of suspected immunodeficiencies.[205]

Diagnosis

Information on immunoglobulin synthesis and antibody formation can be derived from a number of readily available studies. Serum protein electrophoresis can be used to screen for grossly hypogammaglobulinemic conditions and for the presence of paraproteins[188]; however, important selective immunoglobulin deficiencies can be missed. Instead, the separate amounts of IgM, IgG, and IgA can be quantitated directly by radial diffusion assay, immunoelectrophoresis, or automated laser nephelometry,[188] and these tests should be used to diagnose Ig class deficiencies. IgG subclasses (IgG_1, IgG_2, IgG_3, and IgG_4) and IgE must be measured using very sensitive enzyme-linked immunosorbent assays (ELISA) or radioimmunoassays that utilize isotype-specific monoclonal antibody reagents.[255] Because normal values for immunoglobulin concentrations vary with age, adjusted reference values must be used. Specific antibody formation against previously experienced antigens can be evaluated by measurements of A and B isohemagglutinins (IgM) or by application of a Schick test in an immunized patient (IgG). Primary responses to new antigens such as keyhole limpet hemocyanin can be evaluated, but this is an investigative procedure. Lymphocyte numbers can be estimated or quantitated by total lymphocyte counts and by enumeration of the circulating B and T cells using fluorescent monoclonal antibodies or other markers as described.[320] Measurement of in vitro responses of B cells to mitogens by immunoglobulin production is a research tool available in a number of centers, as is the quantitation of helper and suppressor T lymphocytes and their functions.[320] In some cases, a rectal or intestinal biopsy will allow further classification of immunodeficiency by providing lymphatic tissue for histologic study. When these tests are coupled with assays of complement, phagocyte, and T-lymphocyte function, a complete picture of the host defense system can be assembled.

REFERENCES

1. Natvig JB, Kunkel HG. Immunoglobulins: classes, subclasses, genetic variants and idiotypes. Adv Immunol. 1973;16:1–59.
2. Porter, RR. Structural studies of immunoglobulins. Science. 1973;180: 713–6.
3. Spiegelberg HL. Biological activities of immunoglobulins of different classes and subclasses. Adv Immunol. 1974;19:259–94.
4. Goodman JW. Immunoglobulins I: Structure and function. In Stites DP, Stobo JD, Wells JV, eds. Basic and Clinical Immunology. ed. 6th Los Altos, CA: Appleton & Lange; 1987:27–36.
5. Fu SM. Occurrence of IgM and IgD on human lymphocytes. J Exp Med. 1974;139:451–6.
6. Koshland ME. The coming of age of the immunoglobulin J chain. Annu Rev Immunol. 1985;3:425–53.
7. Underdown BJ, Schiff MJ. Immunoglobulin A: strategic defense initiative at the mucosal surface. Annu Rev Immunol. 1986;4:389–417.
8. Waldmann TA, Strober W. Metabolism of immunoglobulins. Prog Allergy. 1969;13:1–27.
9. Waldmann TE. The metabolism of IgE: studies in normal individuals and in a patient with IgE myeloma. J Immunol. 1976;117:1139–44.
10. Moller G, ed. Immunoglobulin D: structure, synthesis, membrane representation and function. Immunol Rev. 1977;37:1–62.
11. Yoffey YM, Courtice FC, eds. Lymphatics, Lymph and the Lymphomyeloid Complex. New York: Academic Press; 1970.
12. Virella G, Nunes MAS, Tamagini G. Placental transfer of IgG subclasses. Clin Exp Immunol. 1972;10:475–9.
13. Conley ME, Delacroix DL. Intravascular and mucosal immunoglobulin A: two separate but related systems of immune defense? Ann Intern Med. 1987;106:892–9.
14. Reynolds HY. Immunoglobulin G and its function in the human respiratory tract. Mayo Clin Proc. 1988;63:161–74.
15. Goodman JW. Antigenic determinants and antibody combining sites. In Sela M, ed. The Antigens. vol. 3. New York: Academic Press; 1975;127.
16. Isenman DE, Dorrington KJ, Painter RH. The structure and function of immunoglobulin domains: II. The importance of interchain disulfide bonds and the possible role of molecular flexibility in the interaction between immunoglobulin G and complement. J Immunol. 1975;114:1726–31.
17. Finkelman, FD, Vitetta ES. Role of surface immunoglobulin in B lymphocyte activation. Fed Proc. 1984;43:2624–32.
18. Bruggemann M, Williams GT, Bindon CI, et al. Comparison of the effector functions of human immunoglobulins using a matched set of chimeric antibodies. J Exp Med. 1987;166:1351–61.
19. Morgan EL, Weigle WO. Biological activities residing in the Fc region of immunoglobulin. Adv Immunol. 1987;40:61–134.
20. Anderson CL, Loon JR. Human leukocyte IgG Fc receptors. Immunol Today. 1986;7:264–6.
21. Shen L, Guyre PM, Fanger MW. Polymorphonuclear leukocyte function triggered through the high affinity Fc receptor for monomeric IgG. J Immunol. 1987;139:534–8.
22. Willis HE, Browder B, Feister AJ, et al. Monoclonal antibody to human IgG Fc receptors: cross-linking of receptors induces lysosomal enzyme release and superoxide generation by neutrophils. J Immunol. 1988;140:234–9.
23. Ryan JL, Henkart PA. Fc receptor mediated inhibition of murine B lymphocyte activation. J Exp Med. 1976;144:768–75.
24. Clarkson SB, Ory PA. Developmentally regulated IgG Fc receptors on cultured human monocytes. J Exp Med. 1988;167:408–17.
25. Lanier LL, Phillips JH. Evidence for three types of human cytotoxic lymphocytes. Immunol Today. 1986;7:132–4.
26. Ferreri NR, Howland WC, Spiegelberg HL. Release of leukotrienes C_4 and B_4 and prostaglandin E_2 from human monocytes stimulated with aggregated IgG, IgA, and IgE. J Immunol. 1986;136:4188–92.
27. Metzger H, Alcaraz G, Hohman R, et al. The receptor with high affinity for immunoglobulin E. Annu Rev Immunol. 1986;4:419–70.
28. Bonnefoy JY, Aubry JP, Peronne C, et al. Production and characterization of a monoclonal antibody specific for the human lymphocyte low affinity receptor for IgE: CD 23 is a low affinity receptor for IgE. J Immunol 1987;138:2970–8.
29. Spiegelberg HL, Boltz-Nitulescu G, Plummer JM, et al. Characterization of the IgE Fc receptors on monocytes and macrophages. Fed Proc. 1983;42:124–8.
30. Butterworth AE, David JR, Franks D, et al. Antibody-dependent eosinophil mediated damage to 51 Cr labeled schistosomula by *Schistosoma mansoni*: damage by purified eosinophils. J Exp Med. 1977;145:136–50.
31. Densen P, Mahmoud AAF, Sullivan J, et al. Demonstration of eosinophil degranulation on the surface of opsonized schistosomules by phase-contrast cinemicrography. Infect Immun. 1978;22:282–5.
32. Joseph M, Capron A, Ameisen JC, et al. The receptor for IgE on blood platelets. Eur J Immunol. 1986;16:306–12.
33. Joseph M, Auriault C, Capron A, et al. A new function for platelets: IgE-dependent killing of schistosomes. Nature. 1983;303:810–12.
34. Ishizaka K. Twenty years with IgE: from the identification of IgE to regulatory factors for the IgE response. J Immunol. 1985;135:i–x.
35. Lum LG, Muchmore AV, Keren D, et al. A receptor for IgA on human T lymphocytes. J Immunol. 1979;122:65–71.
36. Daeron M, Yodoi J, Neauport-Sautes C, et al. Receptors for immunoglobulin isotypes (FcR) on murine T cells. Eur J Immunol. 1985;15:662–7.
37. Kiyono H, Mosteller-Barnum IM, Pitts AM, et al. Isotype-specific immunoregulation: IgA-binding factors produced by Fc receptor-positive T cell hybridomas regulate IgA responses. J Exp Med. 1985;161:731–47.
38. Moretta L, Webb SR, Grossi CE, et al. Functional analysis of two human T cell subpopulations: help and suppression of B cell responses by T cells bearing receptors for IgM or IgG. J Exp Med. 1977;146:184–200.
39. Moretta L, Mingari MC, Moretta A, et al. Human lymphocyte surface markers. Semin Hematol. 1982;19:273–84.
40. Fanger MW, Goldstone SN, Shen L. Cytofluorographic analysis of receptors for IgA on human polymorphonuclear cells and monocytes and the correlation of receptor expression with phagocytosis. Mol Immunol. 1983;20:1019–27.
41. Maliszewski CR, Shen L, Fanger MW. The expression of receptors for IgA on human monocytes and calcitrol-treated HL-60 cells. J Immunol. 1985;135:3878–81.
42. Weisbart RH, Kacena A, Schuh A, et al. GM-CSF induces human neutrophil IgA-mediated phagocytosis by an IgA Fc receptor activation mechanism. Nature. 1988;332:647–8.
43. Edwards MS, Nicholson-Weller A, Baker CJ, et al. The role of specific antibody in alternative complement pathway-mediated opsonophagocytosis of type III, group B streptococcus. J Exp Med. 1980;151:1275–87.
44. Winkelstein JA, Shin HS. The role of immunoglobulin in the interaction of pneumococci and the properdin pathway: evidence for its specificity and lack of requirement for the Fc portion of the molecule. J Immunol. 1974;112:1635–42.
45. Wright AE, Douglas SR. An experimental investigation of the role of the body fluids in connection with phagocytosis. Proc R Soc Lond. 1903;72:357.
46. Proctor RA. Fibronectin: an enhancer of phagocyte function. Rev Infect Dis. 1987;9:S412–9.
47. Kilpatrick JM, Volanakis JE. Opsonic properties of C-reactive protein. Simulation by phorbol myristate acetate enables human neutrophils to phagocytize C-reactive protein-coated cells. J Immunol. 1985;134:3364–70.
48. Horowitz J, Volanakis JE, Brites DE. Blood clearance of *Streptococcus pneumoniae* by C-reactive protein. J Immunol. 1987;138:2598–603.
49. Horowitz MA. Phagocytosis of microrganisms. Rev Infect Dis. 1982;4:104–18.
50. Griffin FM, Blanco C, Silverstein SC. Characterization of the macrophage receptor for complement and demonstration of its functional independence from the receptor for the Fc portion of immunoglobulin G. J Exp Med. 1975;141:1269–77.
51. Mantovani B. Different roles of IgG and complement receptors in phagocytosis by polymorphonuclear leukocytes. J Immunol. 1975;115:15–7.
52. Guckian JC, Christensen WD, Fine DP. Evidence for quantitative variability of bacterial opsonic requirements. Infect Immun. 1978;19:822.
53. Jasin HE. Human heat labile opsonins: evidence for their mediation via the alternate pathway of complement activation. J Immunol. 1972;109:26.
54. Peterson PK, Verhoef J, Sabath LD, et al. Effect of protein A on staphylococcal opsonization. Infect Immun. 1977;15:760–4.
55. Williams RC, Quie PG. Opsonic activity of agammaglobulinemic human sera. J Immunol. 1971;106:51–5.
56. Giebink GS, Verhoef J, Peterson PK, et al. Opsonic requirements for phagocytosis of *Streptococcus pneumoniae* types VI, XVIII, XXIII, and XXV. Infect Immun. 1977;18:291–7.

57. Verhoef J, Peterson PK, Kim Y, et al. Opsonic requirements for staphylococcal phagocytosis: heterogeneity among strains. Immunology. 1977;33:191–7.
58. Baker CJ, Edwards MS, Webb BJ, et al. Antibody-independent classical pathway-mediated opsonophagocytosis of type 1a, group B streptococcus. J Clin Invest. 1982;69:394–404.
59. Leist-Welsh P, Bjornson AB. Immunoglobulin-independent utilization of the classical complement pathway in opsonophagocytosis of *Escherichia coli* by human peripheral leukocytes. J Immunol. 1982;128:2643–51.
60. Stjernstrom I, Magnusson KE, Stendahl O, et al. Liability to hydrophobic and charge interaction of smooth *Salmonella typhimurium* 395 MS sensitized with anti-MS immunoglobulin G and complement. Infect Immun. 1977; 18:261–72.
61. Van Oss CJ, Gillman CF. Phagocytosis as a surface phenomenon. II. Contact angles and phagocytosis of encapsulated bacteria before and after opsonization by specific antiserum and complement. J Reticuloendothel Soc. 1972;12:497–502.
62. Stendahl O, Tagesson C, Edebo L. Influence of hyperimmune immunoglobulin G on the physicochemical properties of the surface of *Salmonella typhimurium* 395 MS in relation to interaction with phagocytic cells. Infect Immun. 1974;10:316–9.
63. Absolom CJ, Van Oss CJ, Zingg W, et al. Phagocytosis as a surface phenomenon: opsonization by a specific absorption of IgG as a function of bacterial hydrophobicity. J Reticuloendothel Soc. 1982;31:59–64.
64. Tagesson C, Magnusson KE, Stendahl O. Physicochemical consequences of opsonization. Perturbation of liposomal membranes by *Salmonella ty phimurium* 395 MS opsonized with IgG antibodies. J Immunol. 1977; 119:609–13.
65. Ofeck I, Sharon N. Lectinophagocytosis: a molecular mechanism of recognition between cell surface sugars and lectins in the phagocytosis of bacteria. Infect Immun. 1988;56:539–47.
66. Quie PG, Messner RP, Williams RK. Phagocytosis in subacute bacterial endocarditis: localization of the primary opsonic site to Fc fragment. J Exp Med. 1968;128:553–70.
67. Shigeoka AO, Hall RT, Hemming VG, et al. Role of antibody and complement in opsonization of group B streptococci. Infect Immun. 1978;21:34.
68. Griffis JM. Epidemic meningococcal disease: synthesis of a hypothetical immunoepidemiologic model. Rev Infect Dis. 1982;4:159–79.
69. Johnston RB Jr, Klemperer MR, Alper CA, et al. The enhancement of bacterial phagocytosis by serum: the role of complement components and two cofactors. J Exp Med. 1969;129:1275–90.
70. Young LS. Human immunity to *Pseudomonas aeruginosa*. II. Relationship between heat stable opsonins and type-specific lipopolysaccharides. J Infect Dis. 1972;126:277–87.
71. Anderson P, Johnston RB Jr. Human serum activities against *Hemophilus influenzae*, type B. J Clin Invest. 1972;51:31–8.
72. Hemming VG, Hall RT, Rhodes PG. Assessment of group B streptococcal opsonins in human and rabbit serum by neutrophil chemiluminescence. J Clin Invest. 1976;58:1379–87.
73. Fischetti VA, Gottschlich EC, Siviglia G, et al. Streptococcal M protein: an antiphagocytic molecule assembled on the cell wall. J Infect Dis. 1977; 136:S222–33.
74. Peterson PK, Wilkinson BJ, Kim Y, et al. The key role of peptidoglycan in the opsonization of *Staphylococcus aureus*. J Clin Invest. 1978;61:597–609.
75. Schwartz JS. Pneumococcal vaccine: clinical efficacy and effectiveness. Ann Intern Med. 1982;96:208–20.
76. Baker CJ, Kasper DL. Group B streptococcal vaccines. Rev Infect Dis. 1985;7:458–67.
77. Hill JC. Summary of a workshop on *Haemophilius influenzae* type B vaccines. J Infect Dis. 1983;148:167–75.
78. van Furth R, Leijh PCJ, Klein F. Correlation between opsonic activity for various microorganisms and composition of gammaglobulin preparations for intravenous use. J Infect Dis. 1984;149:511–7.
79. Hill HR, Bathras JM. Protective and opsonic activities of a native, pH 4.25 intravenous immunoglobulin G preparation against common bacterial pathogens. Rev Infect Dis. 1986;8:S396–400.
80. Cunningham-Rundles C, Siegal FP, Smithwick EM, et al. Efficacy of intravenous immunoglobulin in primary immunodeficiency disease. Ann Intern Med. 1984;101:435–9.
81. Pennington JE, Pier GB, Sadoff JC, et al. Active and passive immunization strategies for *Pseudomonas aeruginosa* pneumonia. Rev Infect Dis. 1986;8:S426–33.
82. Allison AC. On the role of mononuclear phagocytes in immunity against viruses. Prog Med Virol. 1974;18:15–7.
83. Sissons JGP, Oldstone MBA. Killing of virus infected cells. The role of antiviral and complement in limiting virus infection. J Infect Dis. 1980;142:442–8.
84. Lehrer RI, Cline MJ. Interaction of *Candida albicans* with human leukocytes and serum. J Bacteriol. 1969;98:996.
85. Diamond RD, Root RK, Bennett JE. Factors influencing killing of *Cryptococcus neoformans* by human leukocytes in vitro. J Infect Dis. 1972;125:367–76.
86. Davies SF, Clifford DP, Hoidal JR, et al. Opsonic requirements for the uptake of *Cryptococcus neoformans* by human polymorphonuclear leukocytes and monocytes. J Infect Dis. 1982;145:870–4.
87. Roantree RJ, Rantz LA. A study of the relationship of the normal bactericidal activity of human serum to bacterial infection. J Clin Invest. 1960;39:72–81.
88. Frank MM, Joiner K, Hammer C. The function of antibody and complement in the lysis of bacteria. Rev Infect Dis. 1987;9:S537–45.
89. Li IW, Mudd S. The heat labile serum factor associated with intracellular killing of *Staphylococcus aureus*. J Immunol. 1965;94:852–62.
90. Wilson LA, Spitznagel JK. Molecular and structural damage to *Escherichia coli* produced by antibody, complement and lysozyme systems. J Bacteriol. 1969;96:1339–42.
91. Pappenheimer AM, Gill DM. Diphtheria. Science. 1973;182:353–8.
92. Pappenheimer AM Jr. The Schick test 1913–1958. Int Arch Allergy Appl Immunol. 1958;12:35–7.
93. Morrison DC. Endotoxins and disease mechanisms. Annu Rev Med. 1987;38:417–32.
94. McCabe WR, Bruins SC, Cralven DE, et al. Cross reactive antigens: their potential for immunization induced immunity to gram negative bacteria. J Infect Dis. 1977;136:S161–76.
95. Braude AI, Ziegler EJ, Douglas H, et al. Antibody to cell wall glycolipid of gram negative bacteria: induction of immunity to bacteremia and endotoxemia. J Infect Dis. 1977;136:S167–73.
96. Ziegler EJ, McCutchan JA, Fierer J, et al. Treatment of gram-negative bacteremia and shock with human antiserum to a mutant *Escherichia coli*. N Engl J Med. 1982;307:1225–30.
97. McCabe WR, Kreger BE, Johns M. Type specific and cross-reactive antibodies in gram negative bacteremia. N Engl J Med. 1972;287:261–7.
98. Baumgartner JD, Glauser MP, McCutchan JA, et al. Prevention of gram-negative shock and death in surgical patients by antibody to endotoxin core glycolipid. Lancet. 1985;2:59–63.
99. Teng NNH, Kaplan HS, Hebert JM, et al. Protection against gram-negative bacteremia and endotoxemia with human monoclonal IgM antibodies. Proc Natl Acad Sci USA. 1985;82:1790–4.
100. Proctor RA. Role of antibody in the prevention and pathogenesis of endotoxin and gram-negative septic shock. In: RA Proctor, ed. Handbook of Endotoxin. Vol 4. New York: Elsevier Science Publishers; 1986:161–84.
101. Beachey EH. Bacterial adherence: adhesion-receptor interactions mediating the attachment of bacteria to mucosal surfaces. J Infect Dis. 1981;143:325–45.
102. Beachey EH, Ofek I: Epithelial cell binding of group A streptococci by lipoteichoic acid on fimbriae denuded of M protein. J Exp Med. 1976;143:759–71.
103. Densen P, Mandell GL. Gonococcal interactions with polymorphonuclear neutrophils. Importance of the phagosome for bactericidal activity. J Clin Invest. 1978;62:1161–71.
104. Levine, MM. Escherichia coli that cause diarrhea: Enterotoxigenic, enteropathogenic, enteroinvasive, enterohemorrhagic and enteroadherent. J Infect Dis. 1987;155:377–88.
105. O'Hanley P, Low D, Romero I, et al. Gal-Gal binding and hemolysin phenotypes and genotypes associated with uropathogenic escherichia coli. N Engl J Med. 1985;313:414–20.
106. Abraham SN, Beachey EH. Host defenses against adhesion of bacteria to mucosal surfaces. In: Gallin JI, Fauci AS, eds. Advances in Host Defense Mechanisms. Vol. 4, New York: Raven Press; 1985:63–88.
107. Williams RC, Gibbons RJ. Inhibition of bacterial adherence by secretory immunoglobulin A: Mechanism of antigen disposal. Science. 1972;177: 697–9.
108. Tramont EC. Inhibition of adherence of *Neisseria gonorrhoeae* by human genital secretions. J Clin Invest. 1977;59:117–24.
109. Kilian M, Mesteoky J, Russell MW. Defense mechanisms involving Fc-dependent functions of immunoglobulin A and their subversion by bacterial immunoglobulin A proteases. Microbiol Rev. 1988;52:296–303.
110. Dimmock NJ. Mechanisms of neutralization of animal viruses. J Gen Virol. 1984;65:1015–22.
111. Daniels CA. Neutralization of sensitized virus by purified components of complement. Proc Natl Acad Sci USA. 1970;65:528–35.
112. Nemerow GR, Jensen FC, Cooper NR. Neutralization of Epstein-Barr virus by nonimmune human serum. J Clin Invest. 1982;70:1081–91.
113. Beebe DP, Schrieber RD, Cooper NR. Neutralization of influenza virus by normal human sera: mechanisms involving antibody and complement. J Immunol. 1983;130:1317–27.
114. Svehag S. Formation and dissociation of virus-antibody complexes with special reference to the neutralization process. Prog Med Virol. 1968;10:1–11.
115. Sissons JGP, Oldstone MBA. Killing of virus infected cells by cytotoxic lymphocytes. J Infect Dis. 1980;142:114–9.
116. Shore SL, Melewicz FM, Gordon DS. The mononculear cell in human blood which mediates antibody-dependent cellular cytotoxicity to virus-infected target cells. I. Identification of the population of effector cells. J Immunol. 1977;118:558–66.
117. Kohl SS, Starr SE, Oleske JM, et al. Human monocyte-macrophage-mediated antibody-dependent cytotoxicity to herpes simplex virus-infected cells. J Immunol. 1977;118:729–35.
118. Clark RA, Klebanoff SJ. Studies on the mechanism of antibody-dependent polymorphonuclear leukocyte-mediated cytotoxicity. J Immunol. 1977; 119:1413–8.
119. Tschopp J, Masson D, Stanley KK. Structural/functional similarity between proteins involved in complement- and cytotoxic T-lymphocyte-mediated cytolysis. Nature. 1986;322:831–4.
120. Podack ER. Molecular mechanisms of cytolysis by complement and by cytolytic lymphocytes. J Cell Biochem. 1986;30:133–70.

121. Ochs HD, Ament ME, Davis ID. Giardiasis with malabsorption in X-linked agammaglobulinemia. N Engl J Med. 1972;287:341–2.
122. Burke BA, Good RA. *Pneumocystis carinii* infection. Medicine. 1973;52:23.
123. Olgilvie BM. Immunity to parasites (helminths and arthropods). Prog Immunol. 1974;2:127–37.
124. Hsu SYL, Hsu HF, Isacson P, et al. In vitro schistomulicidal effect of immune serum and eosinophils, neutrophils and lymphocytes. J Reticuloendothel Soc. 1977;21:153–9.
125. Sher A, Butterworth AE, Colley DG, et al. Immune responses during human schistosomiasis mansoni. II. Occurrence of eosinophil-dependent cytotoxic antibodies in relation to intensity and duration of infection. Am J Trop Med Hyg. 1977;26:909–15.
126. Ottesen EA, Stanley AM, Gelfand JA, et al. Immunoglobulin and complement receptors on human eosinophils and their role in cellular adherence to schistosomules. Am J Trop Med Hyg. 1977;26:135–41.
127. Vadas MA, Butterworth AE, Sherry B, et al. Interactions between human eosinophils and schistosomula of *Schistosoma mansoni*. I. Stable and irreversible antibody-dependent adherence. J Immunol. 1980;124:1441–8.
128. Capron A, Dessaint JP, Capron M. Specific IgE antibodies in immune adherence of normal macrophages to *Schistosoma mansoni* schistosomules. Nature. 1975;253:474–5.
129. Rothwell TLW, Dineen JK, Love RJ. The role of pharmacologically active amines in resistance to *Trichostrongulus colubriformis* in the guinea pig. Immunology. 1971;21:925–32.
130. Murray M, Jarrett WFH, Jennings FW. Mast cells and macromolecular leak in intestinal immunological reactions. Immunology. 1971;21:17–21.
131. Tonegawa S. Somatic generation of antibody diversity. Nature. 1983; 302:575–81.
132. Milstein C. From antibody structure to immunological diversification of immune response. Science. 1986;231:1261–8.
133. Korsmeyer SJ, Waldmann TA. Immunoglobulins II: Gene organization and assembly. In: Stites DP, Stobo JD, Wells JV, eds. Los Altos, CA: Appleton & Lange; 1987.
134. Marrack P, Kappler J. The T cell receptor. Science. 1987;238:1073–9.
135. Williams AF. A year in the life of the immunoglobulin superfamily. Immunol Today. 1987;8:298–302.
136. Yuan D, Gilliam AC, Tucker PW. Regulation of expression of immunoglobulins M and D in murine B cells. Fed Proc. 1985;44:2652–9.
137. McCune M, Fu SM, Kunkel HG, et al. Biogenesis of membrane-bound and secreted immunoglobulins: two primary translation products of the human chain, differentially N-glycosylated to four discrete forms *in vivo* and *in vitro*. Proc Natl Acad Sci USA. 1981;78:5127–31.
138. Griffith GM, Berek C, Kaartinen M, et al. Somatic mutation and the maturation of immune response to 2-phenyl oxazolone. Nature. 1984;312: 271–5.
139. Siekevitz M, Kocks C, Rajewsky K, et al. Analysis of somatic mutation and class switching in naive and memory B cells generating adaptive primary and secondary responses. Cell. 1987;48:757–70.
140. Fu SM, Kunkel HG. Membrane immunoglobulin of B lymphocytes. J Exp Med. 1974;140:895–903.
141. Raff MC, Feldmann M, DePetris S. Monospecificity of B lymphocytes. J Exp Med. 1973;137:1024–30.
142. Cooper MD. B lymphocytes: normal development and function. N Engl J Med. 1987;317:1452–6.
143. Cooper MD, Kearney J, Scher I. B lymphocytes. In: Paul WE, ed. Fundamental Immunology. New York: Raven Press; 1984:43–55.
144. Stobo JD. Lymphocytes. In: Stites DP, Stobo JD, Wells JV, eds. Basic and Clinical Immunology. 6th ed. Los Altos, CA: Appleton & Lane; 1987.
145. Royer HD, Reinherz EL. T lymphocytes: ontogeny, function, and relevance to clinical disorders. N Engl J Med. 1987;317:1136–42.
146. Haynes BF. Human T lymphocyte antigens as defined by monoclonal antibodies. Immunol Rev. 1981;57:127–58.
147. Reinherz EL, Schlossman SF. Regulation of the immune response: inducer and suppressor T-lymphocyte subsets in human beings. N Engl J Med. 1980;303:370–4.
148. Lynch RG. Immunoglobulin-specific suppressor T cells. Adv Immunol. 1987;40:135–51.
149. Shevach EM. Macrophages and other accessory cells. In: Paul WE, eds. Fundamental Immunology. New York: Raven Press; 1984.
150. Unanue ER, Allen PM. The basis for the immunoregulatory role of macrophages and other accessory cells. Science. 236:551–7.
151. Shackleford AA, Kaufman JF, Korman AJ, et al. HLA-DR antigens: structure, separation of subpopulations, gene cloning and function. Immunol Rev. 1982;66:133–52.
152. Dinarello CA. Interleukin-1 and the pathogenesis of the acute-phase response. N Engl J Med. 311:1413–8.
153. O'Garra A, Umland S, DeFrance T, et al. B-cell factors are pleiotropic. Immunol Today. 1988;9:45–54.
154. Kishimoto T. B-cell stimulatory factors (BSFs): molecular structure, biological function, and regulation of expression. J Clin Immunol. 1987;7:343–55.
155. Chestnut RW, Grey HM. Antigen presentation by B cells and its significance in T-B interactions. Adv Immunol. 1986;39:51–95.
156. Hunt P, Robertson D, Weiss D, et al. A single bone marrow-derived stromal cell type supports the in vitro growth of early lymphoid and myeloid cells. Cell. 1987;48:997–1007.
157. Ross GP, Polley MJ, Rabellino EM, et al. Two different complement receptors on human lymphocytes. J Exp Med. 1973;138:798–818.
158. Fingeroth JD, Weiss JJ, Tedder TF, et al. Epstein-Barr virus receptor of human B lymphocytes is the C3d receptor CR2. Proc Natl Acad Sci USA. 1984;81:4510–4.
159. Melchers F, Erdei A, Schulz T. Growth control of activated, synchronized murine B cells by the C3d fragment of human complement. Nature. 1985;317:264–7.
160. Casali P, Burastero E, Nakamura M, et al. Human lymphocytes making rheumatoid factor and antibody to ssDNA belong to Leu-1 + B-cell subset. Science. 1987;236:77–80.
161. DeFranco AL. Molecular aspects of B-lymphocyte activation. Annu Rev Cell Biol. 1987;3:143–78.
162. Maruyama S, Kubagawa H, Cooper MD. Activation of human B cells and inhibition of their terminal differentiation by monoclonal anti-antibodies. J Immunol. 1985;135:192–6.
163. Mingari MC, Gerosa F, Carra G, et al. Human interleukin-2 promotes proliferation of activated B cells via surface receptors similar to those of activated T cells. Nature. 1984;312:641–3.
164. Park LS, Friend D, Sassenfeld HM. Characterization of the human B cell stimulatory factor 1 receptor. J Exp Med. 1987;166:476–88.
165. Taga T, Kawanishi Y, Hardy RR, et al. Receptors for B cell stimulatory factor 2: quantification, specificity, distribution, and regulation of their expression. J Exp Med. 1987;166:967–81.
166. Feldmann M, Basten A, Phil D. The relationship between antigenic structure and the requirement for thymus-derived cells in the immune response. J Exp Med. 1971;134:103–19.
167. Yount WJ, Dorner MM, Kunkel HG, et al. Studies on human antibodies: selective variations in subgroup composition and genetic markers. J Exp Med. 1968;127:633–46.
168. Riesen WF, Skvaril F, Braun DG. Natural infection of man with group A streptococci. Levels; Restriction in class, subclass, and type; and clonal appearance of polysaccharide group-specific antibodies. Scand J Immunol. 1976;5:383–90.
169. Makela O, Mattila P, Rautonen N, et al. Isotype concentrations of human antibodies to *Haemophilus influenzae* type b polysaccharide (Hib) in young adults immunized with the polysaccharide as such or conjugated to a protein (diphtheria) toxoid. J Immunol. 1987;139:1999–2004.
170. Abbas AK. A reassessment of the mechanisms of antigen-specific T-cell dependent B-cell activation. Immunol Today. 1988;9:89–91.
171. Jones B. Cooperation between T and B cells. A minimal model. Immunol Rev. 1987;99:5–18.
172. Sanders VM, Snyder JM, Uhr JW, et al. Characterization of the physical interaction between antigen-specific B and T cells. J Immunol. 1986; 137:2395–404.
173. Fischer A, Durandy A, Sterkers G. Role of the LFA-1 molecule in cellular interactions required for antibody production in humans. J Immunol. 1986;136:3198–203.
174. Mitchison NA. The carrier effect in the secondary response to hapten-carrier conjugates. II. Cellular cooperation. Eur J Immunol. 1971;1:18–26.
175. DeFranco AL, Gold MR, Jakway JP. B-lymphocyte signal transduction in response to anti-immunoglobulin and bacterial lipopolysaccharide. Immunol Rev. 1987;95:161–76.
176. Coffman RL, Ohara J, Bond MW, et al. B cell stimulatory factor-1 enhances the IgE response of lipopolysaccharide-activated B cells. J Immunol. 1986;136:4538–41.
177. Finkelman FD, Katona IM, Urban JF, et al. Suppression of *in vivo* polyclonal IgE responses by monoclonal antibody to the lymphokine B-cell stimulatory factor 1. Proc Natl Acad Sci USA. 1986;83:9675–8.
178. Snapper CM, Paul WE. Interferon-γ and B cell stimulatory factor-1 reciprocally regulate Ig isotype production. Science. 1987;236:944–7.
179. Coffman RL, Shrader B, Carty J, et al. A mouse T cell product that preferentially enhances IgA production. I. Biologic characterization. J Immunol. 1987;139:3685–90.
180. Harriman GR, Strober W. Commentary: Interleukin 5, a mucosal lymphokine? J Immunol. 1987;139:3553–5.
181. Murray PD, McKenzie DT, Swain SL, et al. Interleukin 5 and interleukin 4 produced by Peyer's patch T cells selectively enhance immunoglobulin A expression. J Immunol. 1987;139:2669–74.
182. Siskind GW. Immunologic tolerance. In: Paul WE, ed. Fundamental Immunology. New York: Raven Press; 1984:537–58.
183. Schaper HW, Pierre CW, Aune TM. Identification and initial characterization of concanavalin A- and interferon-induced human suppressor factors: evidence for a human equivalent of murine soluble immune response suppressor (SIRS). J Immunol. 1984;132:2429–34.
184. Burdette S, Schwartz RS. Current concepts: immunology. Idiotypes and idiotypic networks. N Engl J Med. 1987;317:219–24.
185. McNamara MK, Ward RE, Kohler H. Monoclonal idiotype vaccine against *Streptococcus pneumoniae* infection. Science. 1984;226:1325–6.
186. Kennedy RC, Melnick SL, Preesman GR. Antibody to hepatitis B virus induced by injecting antibodies to the idiotype. Science. 1984;223:930–1.
187. McIntosh K. Diagnostic virology. In: Fields BN, et al., eds. Virology 1985. New York: Raven Press; 1985:309–22.
188. Ritzmann SE. Pathology of Immunoglobulins: Diagnostic and Clinical Aspects. New York: Alan R. Liss; 1982:1–10.
189. Bach A. Immunologic manifestations. In: Sande MA, Kaye D, Root RK, eds. Endocarditis. New York: Churchill Livingstone; 1984:33–58.

190. Phair JP, Clarke J. Immunology of infective endocarditis. Prog Cardiovasc Dis. 1979;22:137–44.
191. Turner KS, Feddema L, Quinn EH. Nonspecific potentiation of IgE by parasitic infections in man. Int Arch Allergy Appl Immunol. 1979;58:232–6.
192. Rosen A, Gergely P, Jondal M, et al. Polyclonal Ig production after Epstein-Barr virus infection of human lymphocytes *in vitro*. Nature. 1977;267:52–5.
193. Theofilopoulos AN, Dixon FJ. The biology and detection of immune complexes. Adv Immunol. 1979;28:89–220.
194. Hoiby N, Doring G, Schiotz. The role of immune complexes in the pathogenesis of bacterial infections. Annu Rev Microbiol. 1986;40:29–53.
195. Arnend WP, Joslin FG, Massoni RJ. Effects of immune complexes on production by human monocytes of interleukin 1 or an interleukin 1 inhibitor. J Immunol. 1985;134:3868–75.
196. Couser WG. Mechanisms of glomerular injury in immune-complex disease. Kidney Int. 1985;28:569–83.
197. Gocke DJ. Extrahepatic manifestations of viral hepatitis. Am J Med Sci. 1975;270:49–60.
198. Carson DA, Chen PP, Fox RI, et al. Rheumatoid factor and immune networks. Annu Rev Immunol. 1987;5:109–26.
199. Coulie PG, Van Snick J. Rheumatoid factor (RF) production during anamnestic immune responses in the mouse. III. Activation of RF precursor cells is induced by their interaction with immune complexes and carrier-specific helper T cells. J Exp Med. 1985;161:88–97.
200. Radoux V, Chen PP, Sorge JA, et al. A conserved human germline V gene directly encodes rheumatoid factor light chains. J Exp Med. 1986;164:2119–24.
201. Clarkson AB, Mellow GH. Rheumatoid factor-like immunoglobulin M protects previously uninfected rat pups and dams from *Trypanosoma lewisi*. Science. 1981;214:186–8.
202. Levo Y, Gorevic PD, Kassal HJ, et al. Association between hepatitis B virus and essential mixed cryoglobulinemia. N Engl J Med. 1977;296:1501–3.
203. Oldstone MBA, Molecular mimicry and autoimmune disease. Cell. 1987;50:819–20.
204. Dale JB, Beachey EH. Multiple, heart-cross-reactive epitopes of streptococcal M proteins. J Exp Med. 1985;161:113–23.
205. Schwimmbeck PL, Yu DTY, Oldstone MBA. Autoantibodies to HLA B27 in the sera of HLA B27 patients with ankylosing spondylitis and Reiter's syndrome: Molecular mimicry with *Klebsiella pneumoniae* as potential mechanism of autoimmune disease. J Exp Med. 1987;166:173–81.
206. Srinvasappa J, Saegusa J, Prabhakar BS, et al. Molecular mimicry: frequency of reactivity of monoclonal antiviral antibodies with normal tissues. J Virol. 1986;57:397–401.
207. WHO Scientific Group on Immunodeficiency. Primary immunodeficiency diseases: report of a world health organization scientific group. Clin Immunol Immunopathol. 1986;40:166–96.
208. Rosen FS, Cooper MD, Wedgwood RJP. Medical progress: the primary immunodeficiencies. N Engl J Med. 1984;311:235–42, 300–10.
209. Ammann AJ. Immunodeficiency Diseases. In: Stites DP, Stobo JD, Wells JV, eds. Basic and Clinical Immunology. 6th ed. 1987:317–55.
210. Hermans PE, Diaz-Buxo JA, Stobo JD. Idiopathic late onset immunoglobulin deficiency. Clinical observations in 50 patients. Am J Med. 1976;61:221–32.
211. Davis LE, Bodian D, Price D, et al. Chronic progressive poliomyelitis secondary to vaccination of an immunodeficient child. N Engl J. Med. 1977; 297:241–5.
212. Wilfert CM, Buckley RH, Mohanakumar T, et al. Persistent and fatal central nervous system echo virus infections in patients with agammaglobulinemia. N Engl J Med. 1977;296:1485–9.
213. Saulsbury FT, Winkelstein JA, Yolken RH. Chronic rotavirus infection in immunodeficiency. Pediatrics. 1980;97:61–5.
214. Ament ME, Ochs HD, Davis SD. Structure and function of the gastrointestinal tract in primary immunodeficiency syndromes. Medicine. 1973; 52:227–48.
215. Bruton OC. Agammaglobulinemia. Pediatrics. 1952;9:722–30.
216. Fearon ER, Winkelstein JA, Civin CI, et al. Carrier detection in X-linked agammaglobulinemia by analysis of X-chromosome inactivation. N Engl J Med. 1987;316:427–31.
217. Schwaber J, Molgaard H, Orkin SH, et al. Early pre-B cells from normal and X-linked agammaglobulinaemia produce C without an attached V region. Nature. 1983;304:355–7.
218. Gail-Pezcalskak Lim JD, Good RA. B lymphocytes in primary and secondary deficiencies of humoral immunity. Birth Defects. 1975;11:33.
219. Lederman HM, Winkelstein JA. X-linked agammaglobulinemia: an analysis of 96 patients. Medicine. 1985;64:145–56.
220. Crennan JM, Van Scoy RE, McKenna CH, et al. Echovirus polymyositis in patients with hypogammaglobulinemia: failure of high-dose intravenous gammaglobulin therapy and review of the literature. Am J Med. 1986;81:35–42.
221. McKinney RE, Katz SL, Wilfert CM. Chronic enteroviral meningoencephalitis in agammaglobulinemic patients. Rev Infect Dis. 1987;9:334–56.
222. Roifman CM, Rao CP, Lederman HM, et al. Increased susceptibility to mycoplasma infection in patients with hypogammaglobulinemia. Am J Med. 1986;80:590–4.
223. Taylor-Robinson D, Furr PM, Webster AD. *Ureaplasma urealyticum* in the immunocompromised host. Pediatr Infect Dis 1986;5:236–8.
224. Reinherz EL, Cooper MD, Schlossman SF, et al. Abnormalities of T cell maturation and regulation in human beings with immunodeficiency disorders. J Clin Invest. 1981;68:699–705.
225. Fleisher TA, White RM, Broder S, et al. X-linked hypogammaglobulinemia and isolated growth hormone deficiency. N Engl J Med. 1980;302:1492–34.
226. Stiehm RE, Ashida E, Kim KS, et al. Intravenous immunoglobulins as therapeutic agents. Ann Intern Med. 1987;107:367–82.
227. Wedgwood RJ. Intravenous immunoglobulin. Clin Immunol Immunopathol. 1986;40:147–50.
228. Roifman CM, Levison H, Gelfand EW. High-dose versus low-dose intravenous immunoglobulin in hypogammaglobulinaemia and chronic lung disease. Lancet. 1987;I:1075–7.
229. Lederman HM, Roifman CH, Lari S, et al. Corticosteroids for prevention of adverse reactions to intravenous immune serum globulin infusions in hypogammaglobulinemic patients. Am J Med. 1986;81:443–7.
230. Tiller TL, Buckley RH. Transient hypogammaglobulinemia of infancy: review of the literature, clinical and immunologic features of 11 new cases, and long-term follow-up. J Pedatr. 1978;92:347–53.
231. Wilson CB, Remington JS. Effects of monocytes from human neonates on lymphocyte transformation. Clin Exp Immunol. 1979;36:511–6.
232. Ferguson AC, Cheung SSC. Modulation of immunoglobulin M and G synthesis by monocytes and T lymphocytes in the newborn infant. J Pediatr. 1981;98:385–95.
233. Siegel RL, Issekutz T, Schwaber J, et al. Deficiency of T helper cells in transient hypogammaglobulinemia of infancy. N Engl J Med. 1981;305:1307–13.
234. Rodriquez MA, Bankhurst AD, Cueppens JL, et al. Characterization of the suppressor activity in human cord blood lymphocytes. J Clin Invest. 1981;68:1577–85.
235. Good RA, Zak SJ, Condie RM, et al. Clinical investigation of patients with agammaglobulinemia and hypogammaglobulinemia. Pediatr Clin North Am. 1960;7:397–416.
236. Buckley RH. Humoral immunodeficiency. Clin Immunol Immunopathol. 1986;40:13–24.
237. Geha RS, Schneeberger E, Merter E, et al. Heterogeneity of "acquired" or common variable agammaglobulinemia. N Engl J Med. 1974;291:1–6.
238. Waldmann TA, Durm M, Broder S, et al. Role of suppressor T cells in pathogenesis of common variable hypogammaglobulinaemia. Lancet. 1974;2:609.
239. Reinharz EL, Geha R, Wohl ME, et al. Immunodeficiency associated with loss of T4+ inducer-T cell function. N Engl J Med. 1981;304:811–6.
240. White WB, Ballow M. Modulation of suppressor-cell activity by cimetidine in patients with common variable hypogammaglobulinemia. N Engl J Med. 1985;312:198–202.
241. Stiehm ER, Fudenberg HH. Clinical and immunologic features of dysgammaglobulinemia type I. Am J Med. 1966;40:805–17.
242. Mayer L, Kwan SP, Thompson C, et al. Evidence for a defect in "switch" T cells in patients with immunodeficiency and hyperimmunoglobulinemia M. N Engl J Med. 1986;314:409–13.
243. Burks AW, Steele RW. Selective IgA deficiency. Ann Allergy. 1986;57: 3–8.
244. Vanthiel DH, Smith WI Jr., Rabin BS, et al. A syndrome of immunoglobulin A deficiency, diabetes mellitus, malabsorption, a common HLA haplotype. Immunologic and genetic studies of forty-three family members. Ann Intern Med. 1977;86:10–4.
245. Ammann AJ, Hong R. Selective IgA deficiency: presentation of 30 cases and a review of the literature. Medicine. 1971;50:223–36.
246. Walker WA, Isselbacher KJ, Block KJ. Intestinal uptake of macromolecules: effect of oral immunization. Science. 1972;177:608–10.
247. Oxelius VA, Laurell AB, Lindquist B, et al. IgG subclasses in selective IgA deficiency. Importance of IgG_2-IgA deficiency. N Engl J Med. 1981; 304:1476–7.
248. Bjorkander J, Bake B, Oxelius VA, et al. Impaired lung function in patients with IgA deficiency and low levels of IgG2 or IgG3. N Engl J Med. 1985;313:720–4.
249. Migane N, Oliviero S, DeLange G, et al. Multiple-gene deletions within the human immunoglobulin heavy chain cluster. Proc Natl Acad Sci USA. 1984;81:5811–5.
250. Carbonara AO, Demarchi M. Genetics and techniques: Ig isotypes deficiency caused by gene deletions. Monogr Allergy. 1986;20:13–7.
251. Burks AW, Sampson HA, Buckley RH. Anaphylactic reactions after gammaglobulin administration in patients with hypogammaglobulinemia: detection of IgE antibodies to IgA. N Engl J Med. 1986;314:560–3.
252. Hobbs JR, Milner RDG, Watt PJ. Gamma-M deficiency predisposing to meningococcal septicemia. Br Med J. 1967;2:583–5.
253. Schur PH, Borel H, Gelfand EW, et al. Selective gamma-G globulin deficiencies in patients with recurrent pyogenic infections. N Engl J Med. 1970;283:631–4.
254. Ochs HD, Wedgwood RJ. IgG subclass deficiencies. Annu Rev Med. 1987; 38:325–40.
255. Umetsu DT, Ambrosino DM, Quinti I, et al. Recurrent sinopulmonary infection and impaired antibody response to bacterial capsular polysaccharide antigen in children with selective IgG-subclass deficiency. N Engl J Med. 1985;313:1247–51.
256. Pahwa RN, Pahwa SG, Good RA. T-lymphocyte differentiation in severe combined immunodeficiency: defects of stem cells. J Clin Invest. 1979; 64:1632–41.

257. Good RA, Bach FH. Bone marrow and thymus transplants: cellular engineering to correct primary immunodeficiency. Clin Immunobiol. 1974;2:63.
258. Hirschhorn R. Inherited enzyme deficiencies and immunodeficiency: adenosine deaminase (ADA) and purine nucleoside phosphorylase (PNP) deficiencies. Clin Immunol Immunopathol. 1986;40:157–65.
259. Polmar SH, Stem RC, Schwartz AL, et al. Enzyme replacement therapy for adenosine deaminase deficiency and severe combined immunodeficiency. N Engl J Med. 1976;295:1337–43.
260. Gatti RA, Allen HD, Meuwissen HJ, et al. Immunological reconstitution of sex-linked lymphopenic immunological deficiency. Lancet. 1968;2:1366–9.
261. Stoop JW, Zegers BJ, Hendrix GF, et al. Purine nucleoside phosphorylase deficiency associated with selective cellular immune deficiency. N Engl J Med. 1977;296:651–5.
262. Lawlor GJ Jr, Amman AJ, Wright WC Jr. The syndrome of cellular immunodeficiency with immunoglobulins. J Pediatr. 1974;84:183–7.
263. Remold-O'Donnell E, Davis AE, Kenney D, et al. Purification and chemical composition of gpL115, the human lymphocyte surface sialoglycoprotein that is defective in Wiskott-Aldrich syndrome. J Biol Chem. 1986;261:7526–30.
264. Cooper MD, Chase HP, Lowman JT, et al. Wiskott-Aldrich syndrome: an immunologic disease involving the afferent limb of immunity. Am J Med. 1968;44:499–506.
265. Blaese RM, Strober W, Brown RS, et al. Wiskott-Aldrich syndrome. Lancet. 1968;1:1056–7.
266. Parkman R, Rappeport J, Geha R, et al. Correction of the Wiskott-Aldrich syndrome by bone-marrow transplantation. N Engl J Med. 1978;298:291–8.
267. Biggar WD, Good RA. Immunodeficiency in ataxia-telangiectasia. Birth Defects. 1975;11:271–7.
268. Berkel AI. Studies of IgG subclasses in ataxia-telangiectasia patients. Monogr Allergy. 1986;20:100–5.
269. Davis MM, Gatti RA, Sparkes RS. Neoplasia and chromosomal breakage in ataxia-telangiectasia: a 2-14 translocation. In: Gatti RA, Swift M, eds. Ataxia-Telangiectasia: Genetics, Neuropathology, and Immunology of a Degenerative Disease of Childhood. New York: Alan R Liss; 1985:197–203.
270. McKinnon PJ. Ataxia-telangiectasia: an inherited disorder of ionizing-radiation sensitivity in man. Hum Genet. 1987;75:197–207.
271. Oxelius VA, Berkel AI, Hanson LA. IgG2 deficiency in ataxia-telangiectasia. N Engl J Med. 1982;306:515–7.
272. Donabedian H, Gallin JI. The hyperimmunoglobulin E recurrent infection (Job's) syndrome. A review of the NIH experience and the literature. Medicine. 1983;62:195–212.
273. Levine AS, Graw RG Jr, Young RC. Management of infections in patients with leukemia and lymphoma: current concepts and experimental approaches. Semin Hematol. 1972;9:141–26.
274. Miller DG. Patterns of immunologic deficiency in lymphomas and leukemias. Ann Intern Med. 1972;57:703–6.
275. Weitzman SA, Aisenberg AC, Siber GR, et al. Impaired humoral immunity in treated Hodgkin's disease. N Engl J Med. 1977;297:245–8.
275a. Cooperative group for the study of immunoglobulin in chronic lymphocytic leukemia. Intravenous immunoglobulin for the prevention of infection in chronic lymphocytic leukemia. N Engl J Med. 1988;319:902–7.
276. Louie S, Schwartz RS. Immunodeficiency and the pathogenesis of lymphoma and leukemia. Semin Hematol. 1978;15:117–28.
277. Bergsagel DE. Lymphoreticular disorders—malignant proliferative response and/or abnormal immunoglobulin synthesis—plasma cell dyscrasias. In Williams WJ, et al, eds. Hematology. 2nd ed. New York: McGraw-Hill; 1977 :1087.
278. Paglieroni T, MacKenzie MR. Studies on the pathogenesis of an immune defect in multiple myeloma. J Clin Invest. 1977;59:1120–33.
279. Glenchur H, Zinneman HH, Hall WH. A review of fifty-one cases of multiple myeloma: emphasis on pneumonia and other infections as complications. Arch Intern Med. 1959;103:173–9.
280. Myers BR, Hirshman SZ, Azelrod JA. Current patterns of infection in multiple myeloma. Am J Med. 1972;52:87–97.
281. Salmon SE, Samal BA, Hayes D, et al. Role of gammaglobulin for immunoprophylaxis in multiple myelona. N Engl J Med. 1968;277:1336–40.
282. Bjornson AB, Altemeier WA, Bjornson HS. Changes in humoral components of host defense following burn trauma. Ann Surg. 1977;186:88–96.
283. Wilfert CM, Katz SL. Etiology of bacterial sepsis in nephrotic children, 1963–1967. Pediatrics. 1968;42:840–59.
284. Lockwood CM. Immunological functions of the spleen. Clin Haematol. 1983;12:449–65.
285. Bohnsack JF, Brown EJ. The role of the spleen in resistance to infection. Annu Rev Med. 1986;37:49–59.
286. Rosner F, Zarrabi MH, Benach JL, et al. Babesiosis in splenectomized adults: review of 22 reported cases. Am J Med. 1984;76:696–702.
287. Brown EJ, Hosea SW, Frank MM. The role of complement in the localization of pneumococci in the splanchnic reticuloendothelial system during experimental bacteremia. J Immunol. 1981;126:2230–6.
288. Likhite VV. Immunological impairment and susceptibility to infection after splenectomy. JAMA. 1976;236:1376.
289. Martone WJ, Zuehl RW, Minson GE. Postsplenectomy sepsis with DF-2: report of a case with isolation of the organism from the patient's dog. Ann Intern Med. 1980;93:457–8.
290. Eraklis AJ, Kevy SV, Diamond LK, et al. Hazard of overwhelming infection after splenectomy in childhood. N Engl J Med. 1967;276:1225–9.
291. Chilcote RR, Baehner RL, Hammond D, et al. Septicemia and meningitis in children splenectomized for Hodgkin's disease. N Engl J Med. 1976; 295:802.
292. Bisno AL, Gopol V. Fulminant pneumococcal infection in "normal" asplenic hosts. Arch Intern Med. 1977;137:1526–32.
293. Pearson HA, Spencer RP, Cornelius EA. Functional asplenia in sickle-cell anemia. N Engl J Med. 1969;281:923–7.
294. Bjornson AB, Lobel JS. Direct evidence that decreased serum opsonization of *Streptococcus pneumoniae* via the alternative complement pathway in sickle cell disease is related to antibody deficiency. J Clin Invest. 1987;79:388–98.
295. Spirer Z, Zakuth V, Diamant S, et al. Decreased tuftsin concentrations in patients who have undergone splenectomy. Br Med J. 1977;2:1574–6.
296. Brown EJ, Hosea SW, Frank MM. The role of the spleen in experimental pneumococcal bacteremia. J Clin Invest. 1981;67:975–82.
297. Hosea SE, Brown EJ, Hamburger MI, et al. Opsonic requirements for intravascular clearance after splenectomy. N Engl J Med. 1981;304–245.
298. Siber GR, Weitzman SA, Aisenberg CA, et al. Impaired antibody response to pneumococcal vaccine after treatment for Hodgkin's disease. N Engl J Med. 1978;299:442–8.
299. Amman AJ, Addiego J, Wara DW, et al. Polyvalent pneumococcal-polysaccharide immunization of patients with sickle-cell anemia and patients with splenectomy. N Engl J Med. 1977;297:897–900.
300. Ruben FL, Hankins WA, Zeigler Z, et al. Antibody responses to meningococcal polysaccharide vaccine in adults without a spleen. Am J Med. 1984;76:115–21.
301. Giebink GS, Foker JE, Kim Y, et al. Serum antibody and opsonic responses to vaccination with pneumococcal polysaccharide in normal and splenectomized children. J Infect Dis. 1980;141:404–12.
302. Gaston MH, Verter JI, Woods G, et al. Prophylaxis with oral penicillin in children with sickle cell anemia: a randomized trial. N Engl J Med. 1986;314:1593–9.
303. Alexander JW. Immunologic considerations and the role of vaccination in burn injury. In Polk HC, Stone HH, eds. Contemporary Burn Management. Boston: Little, Brown; 1971:265.
304. Strober W, Wochner RD, Carbone PP, et al. Intestinal lymphangiectasia: a protein-losing enteropathy with hypogammaglobulinemia, lymphocytopenia, and impaired homograft rejection. J Clin Invest. 1967;46:1643–56.
305. Heppner GH, Calabresi P. Selective suppression of humoral immunity by antineoplastic drugs. Annu Rev Pharmacol Toxicol. 1976;16:367.
306. Stewart CC, Perez CA. Effect of irradiation on immune responses. Radiology. 1976;118:201–11.
307. Order SE. The effects of therapeutic irradiation on lymphocytes and immunity. Cancer. 1977;39:737–45.
308. Webb DR, Winkelstein A. Immunosuppression, immunopotentiation, and antiinflammatory drugs. In Stites DP, Stobo JD, Wells JV, eds. Basic and Clinical Immunology. 4th ed. Los Altos, CA: Appleton & Lange, 1982:277.
309. Fauci AS, Dale DC, Balow JE. Glucocorticosteroid therapy: mechanisms of action and clinical considerations. Ann Intern Med. 1976;84:304–15.
310. Haynes BF, Fauci AS. The differential effect of in vivo hydrocortisone on the kinetics of subpopulations of human peripheral blood thymus-derived lymphocytes. J Clin Invest. 1978;61:703–10.
311. Arya SK, Wong-Staal F, Gallo RC. Dexamethasone-mediated inhibition of human T cell growth factor and interferon messenger RNA. J Immunol. 1984;133:273–6.
312. Snyder DS, Unanue ER. Corticosteroids inhibit murine macrophage Ia expression and interleukin 1 production. J Immunol. 1982;129:1803–5.
313. Dale DC, Fauci AS, Wolff SM. Alternate day prednisone: leukocyte kinetics and susceptibility to infections. N Engl J Med. 1974;291:1154–8.
314. Anderson RJ, Schafer LA, Olin DB, et al. Infectious risk factors in the immunosuppressed host. Am J Med. 1973;54:453–62.
315. Staples PJ, Gerding DN, Decker JL, et al. Incidence of infection in systemic lupus erythematosus. Arthritis Rheum. 1974;17:1–11.
316. Lane HC, Masur H, Edgar LC, et al. Abnormalities of B-cell activation and immunoregulation in patients with the acquired immunodeficiency syndrome. N Engl J Med. 1983;309:453–8.
317. Ammann AJ, Schiffman G, Abrams D, et al. B-cell immunodeficiency in acquired immune deficiency syndrome. JAMA. 1984;251:1447–9.
318. Pahwa SG, Quilop MTJ, Lange M. Defective B-lymphocyte function in homosexual men in relation to the acquired immunodeficiency syndrome. Ann Intern Med. 1984;101:757–63.
319. Polsky B, Gold JWM, Whimbey E, et al. Bacterial pneumonia in patients with acquired immunodeficiency syndrome. Ann Intern Med. 1986;104:38–41.
320. Buckley RH. Advances in the diagnosis and treatment of primary immunodeficiency diseases. Arch Intern Med. 1986;146:377–84.
321. Waldmann TA, Korsmeyer SJ, Bakhshi A, et al. Molecular genetic analysis of human lymphoid neoplasms. Immunoglobulin genes and the c-myc oncogene. Ann Intern Med. 1985;102:497–510.
322. Wells JV. Metabolism of immunoglobulins. In: Fudenberg HH, et al., eds. Basic and Clinical Immunology. 2nd ed. Los Altos, CA: Lange; 1978:237.
323. Stites DP, Stobo JD, Wells JV, eds. Basic and Clinical Immunology. 6th ed. Los Altos, CA: Appleton & Lange; 1987.
324. Waldmann TA, Korsmeyer SJ, Bakhshi A, et al. Molecular genetic analysis of human lymphoid neoplasms. Ann Intern Med. 1985;102:497–510.

6. COMPLEMENT

PETER DENSEN

Functional activity attributable to the complement system was first described in the period between 1888 and 1894.[1] These experiments demonstrated that fresh serum contained a heat-labile bactericidal factor termed *alexin*. Subsequently it was shown that a heat-stable factor present in convalescent serum also contributed to bactericidal activity. At the turn of the century Paul Erlich employed the term *complement* to describe the heat-labile factor and *amboceptor* (antibody) to describe the heat-stable factor. The early part of the nineteenth century saw the demonstration that complement consisted of more than one component. However, it was not until 1941 that Louis Pillemer was able to separate functionally distinct components of the classical pathway from various serum fractions. In the early 1950s Pillemer and coworkers also described and characterized an antibody-independent mechanism for activating complement that they termed the *properdin pathway*.[1–3] However, the protein purification techniques then available were unable to provide complement components of sufficient purity to convince others of the existence of this pathway. The 1960s and 1970s saw the development of a mathematical model capable of describing the sequential activation of complement as well as new techniques for the purification of the individual complement components. The latter development led to the rediscovery of Pillemer's work, and the characterization of these proteins and the mechanisms controlling the activity of this pathway. With the 1980's has come the recognition that the complement system consists not only of plasma proteins capable of being deposited upon the surface of invading microbes but also of membrane proteins that protect host cells from the detrimental effects of complement activation.

At the present time the complement system is known to consist of 19 plasma and at least 9 membrane proteins (Table 1). Activation of the system results in the sequential triggering of the various proteins and in this regard exhibits many similarities to the clotting cascade. The beneficial effects of complement activation for the host include the development of an inflammatory response and the elimination of microbial pathogens and immune complexes.

The antibody and complement systems are grouped together because of their historical and functional association as well as because they both occur as soluble proteins in serum.[4] However, a number of important differences distinguish the two systems. Antibody-mediated events are characterized by a high degree of specificity dictated by a given antibody for a given antigenic epitope. Consequently, after initial exposure to antigen there is a significant delay while protective antibody is synthesized to influence the course of the disease. In contrast, the complement system is activated by a wide variety of chemically diverse substances even in the absence of antibody. Consequently, the multiplicity of its physiologic effects is felt early in the course of infection. In many instances antibody and complement are synergistic in providing effective host defense. The presence of specific antibody leads to more rapid and efficient complement activation and serves to direct complement deposition to appropriate sites on the surface of invading pathogens. Opsonization of infectious agents with both antibody and complement leads to more efficient ingestion and killing of these microbes than does opsonization with either substance alone. Similarly, the presence of receptors on lymphocytes for immunoglobulin and complement suggest a cooperative role for these substances in both the affector and effector pathways of the immune response. "In such a way a highly specific response mediated by the tertiary structure of an antibody molecule can be coupled with the more general cellular or humoral responses of the phagocytic and complement system to eradicate attacking organisms."[4]

COMPLEMENT SYNTHESIS, CATABOLISM, AND DISTRIBUTION

Studies employing human hepatic cells in culture have demonstrated that most of the complement components can be synthesized by the liver.[5,6] Moreover, examination of complement component polymorphisms in patients before and after orthotopic liver transplantation has shown that hepatic synthesis accounts for at least 90 percent of the quantity of these components in plasma.[7] The normal concentration of many individual complement components may fluctuate widely in a given individual over time. In part this fluctuation reflects the fact that many components are acute-phase reactants, and their synthesis can be modulated by a variety of immune modulators. These substances, including interleukin-1β (IL-1β), tumor necrosis and dexamethasone, can increase hepatic synthesis of these components two- to fivefold.[8,9]

Complement synthesis has also been demonstrated in a variety of other cells, most notably monocytes and macrophages.[10] These cells synthesize C1q, C4, C2, factors D and B, C3, and C5.[6] Synthesis varies with the site of isolation of the cell. For example, bronchoalveolar fluid, breast milk, and monocyte-derived macrophages differ with respect to the proportion of the cells secreting C2, average rate of C2 production per cell, and the amount of C2-specific RNA.[11] Complement synthesis by monocytes can be modulated by γ-interferon and the lipid A component of endotoxin.[12,13] The exact mechanism by which complement synthesis is enhanced has not been delineated in most cases but appears to occur at a pretranslational level.[13] Other sites of complement component synthesis that have been demonstrated on an experimental basis include intestinal and uroepithelial cells and fibroblasts.[6]

Synthesis of the early components of both activating pathways of complement by mononuclear phagocyte cells is believed to be an important aspect of complement-mediated host defense in tissues. In vitro studies have demonstrated that these cells can synthesize sufficient amounts of these components to promote opsonization, ingestion, and killing of bacteria or other target cells with which they have been coincubated.[14]

A detailed examination of the metabolic fate of all complement components has not been carried out. However, studies have demonstrated fractional catabolic rates for C3, C4, C5, and factor B that range from 1 to 2 percent per hour, thus indicating that they are among the most rapidly metabolized of all plasma proteins. Catabolic rates of C3 and C4 are independent of serum levels, whereas their synthetic rates correlate with serum levels, which indicates that in healthy people the rate of synthesis is the major determinant of plasma concentration.[15]

In healthy individuals the vast majority of complement is found in blood. Concentrations of complement proteins in normal mucosal secretions are approximately 5–10 percent of serum levels and in normal spinal fluid even lower, perhaps 1 percent or less of serum levels. In the presence of local infection or inflammation complement levels in mucosal secretions and in cerebrospinal fluid increase, most likely as a result of alterations in vascular permeability barriers as well as by enhanced synthesis and secretion of these components by local mononuclear cells.

Serum complement activity is reduced in preterm infants in proportion to the magnitude of their immaturity.[16] In contrast, complement levels in healthy term infants range from 60 to 100 percent of those in healthy adults. Despite these nearly normal levels, defective complement activation via either the classical or alternative pathway has been noted in as many as 40 percent of such infants.[17–19]

TABLE 1. Complement Components Present in Serum

Component	Approximate Serum Concentration (μg/ml)	Molecular Weight	Chain Structure[a]	Number of Genetic Loci	Chromosomal Assignment[b]
Classical Pathway					
C1q	70	410,000	(A, B, C) × 6	3 (A, B, C)	1p
C1r	34	170,000	Dimer of 2 identical chains	1	12p
C1s	31	85,000	2 identical chains	1	12p
C4	600	206,000	β-α-γ	2 (C4A, C4B)	6p
C2	25	117,000	1 chain	1	6p
Alternative pathway					
D	1	24,000	1 chain	1	ND
C3	1300	195,000	β-α	1	19q
B	200	95,000	1 chain	1	6p
Membrane attack complex					
C5	80	180,000	β-α	1	9q
C6	60	128,000	1 chain	1	ND
C7	55	120,000	1 chain	1	ND
C8	65	150,000	3 nonidentical chains α---γ, β	3 (α, β, γ)	1p (γ-ND)
C9	60	79,000	1 chain	1	ND
Control proteins					
Positive regulation					
Properdin	25	220,000	Cyclic polymers of a single 57 kD chain	1	Xp
Negative regulation					
C1 INH	200	105,000	1 chain	1	11q
C4 BP	250	550,000	7 identical chains	1	1q
Factor H	500	150,000	1 chain	1	1q
Factor I	34	90,000	β-γ	1	4
Anaphylatoxin inactivator (carboxypeptidase B)	35	280,000	Dimer of 2 nonidentical chains (H, L) × 2	ND	ND
S protein (vitronectin)	500	80,000	1 chain	1	ND

[a] For multichain components parentheses are used to indicate subunit structure; commas indicate noncovalent linkage of chains arising from separate genes; solid lines indicate covalent linkage of chains arising from post-translational cleavage of a proenzyme molecule, chains being listed in order beginning at the amino terminus of the proenzyme molecular; dashed lines indicate covalent linkage of chains arising from separate genes.
[b] p indicates the short arm and q the long arm of the chromosome.
Abbreviations: ND: not determined; C1-INH: C1 inhibitor.

COMPLEMENT ACTIVATION

Generation of the Classical Pathway C3 Convertase

Activation of the classical pathway occurs most commonly as the result of an immunologic reaction between antibody and antigen (Fig. 1). Of the various isotypes only IgM and certain subclasses of IgG (3 > 1 > 2) bind C1 and initiate complement activation.[20,21] C1 in serum is a trimolecular complex containing one molecule of C1q and two molecules each of the C1r and C1s subunits. C1q is the subunit responsible for binding to antibody. The C1q molecule consists of a central core with six radiating pods that terminate in globular heads. The globular heads contain the antibody binding site.[21,22]

The mechanism by which the interaction of antibody with antigen facilitates C1q binding and complement activation differs between the two antibody isotypes. In solution or under conditions of antigen excess IgM exists as a planar pentameric structure and displays a weak C1q binding site in the CH3 or CH4 region of each monomeric IgM subunit. Binding of IgM to several antigen molecules on the same particle causes IgM to assume a "staple" configuration. This change results in the appearance of at least two additional C1q binding sites and the firm association of C1q with IgM. In contrast IgG possesses two C1q binding sites in the CH2 domain of its Fc fragment, but functionally effective C1q binding requires that two IgG molecules be cross linked via the globular heads on C1q. This requirement dictates that thousands of IgG molecules be bound to a target particle to ensure sufficient proximity for doublet formation. At a functional level this requirement means that complement activation by IgG is less efficient than that by IgM since the latter requires only that a single molecule be bound in the correct configuration.[21,22]

C1 binding by antibody results in a change in the structural configuration of the C1q molecule such that the C1r and C1s tetramer contained within the cagelike structure formed by the radiating pods of C1q becomes autocatalytically active. This structural alteration may involve the release of C1 inhibitor which binds reversibly to proenzyme C1. C1r and C1s are structurally related molecules consisting of a head bearing the serine esterase enzymatic site and a tail bearing the binding site. The subunits are aligned linearly such that the central portion of the tetramer is formed by two C1r subunits linked through their catalytic domains. Each C1r molecule is joined to a C1s molecule via the binding site in the tail region of the respective subunits. This linear arrangement allows the tetramer to assume a figure eight configuration such that all four catalytic domains are in close proximity. In this configuration each C1r molecule is believed to activate the other C1r molecule, which in turn then activates C1s.[21,23,24]

Expression of enzymatic activity by C1r and C1s represents the initial activation and amplification step in the classical pathway. Thus many molecules of substrate are cleaved by a given enzyme complex, which results in the fixation of subsequent components in the complement cascade to the surface of the target particle in close proximity to the antibody binding site. Hence antibody serves not only to activate complement in a kinetically efficient manner but also to direct complement deposition to specific sites on the target surface.

Activated C1s cleaves a 9 kD fragment, C4a, from the amino terminus of the α-chain of C4. This results in the exposure of an internal thiolester bond linking the SH group of a cysteine residue with the terminal COOH group of glutamic acid. This bond is subject to nucleophilic attack by hydroxyl or amino groups, which leads to the formation of covalent ester or amide linkages.[20,21,25] Through this reaction and the analogous one involving C3 (Fig. 2), the complement system acquires a chemically stable association with the target surface. Of interest with regard to the formation of these covalent bonds is that due to

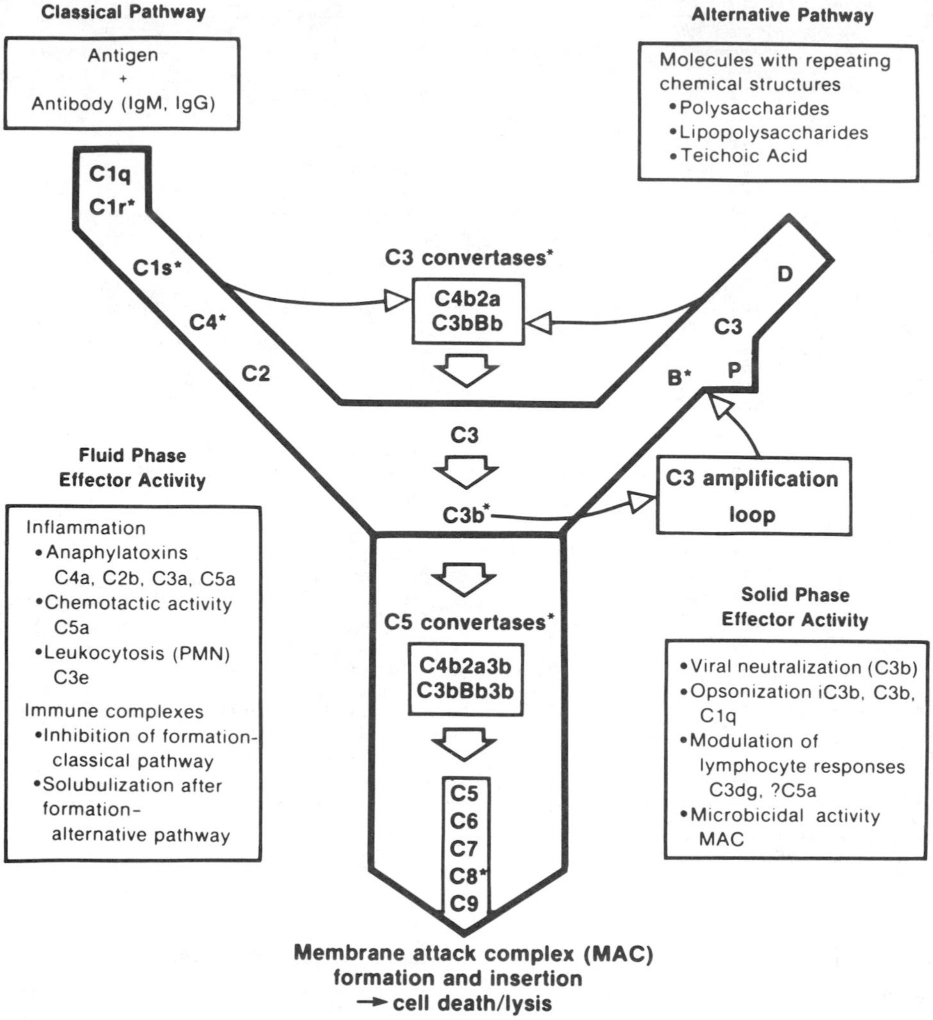

FIG. 1. The complement cascade. Within each pathway the components are arranged in order of their activation and aligned opposite their functional and structural analogue in the opposite pathway. Asterisks (*) indicate sites of downregulation of complement activity (see Table 2).

gene duplication there are two slightly different C4 genes, C4A and C4B. The product of the C4A gene preferentially forms amide bonds with target surfaces and is hemolytically less active than is the product of the C4B gene, which preferentially forms ester bonds.[27–29] Consequently, C4A binds more effectively to proteins, for example, antigen–antibody complexes, than does C4B.[28,30,31] The molecular basis for this difference in binding efficiency appears to be the presence of an aspartic acid residue in the C4A molecule and a histidine residue in the C4B molecule at a site distant from the thiolester. Although distant from the thiolester in the primary structure of C4, the tertiary configuration of the molecule probably brings these charged amino acids into close proximity with the thiolester such that they influence the nucleophilic attack of the thiolester bond by amino or hydroxyl groups on the target surface. The difference in reactivity of the C4A and C4B molecules may play a role in determining the clinical picture observed in patients with inherited deficiencies of these respective genes.[32]

Activated C1s also cleaves C2 to produce a small fragment, C2b, which is released into the environment, and a larger fragment, C2a, which binds to C4b on the surface of the target particle. This complex, C4b2a, is the classical pathway C3 convertase (Fig. 1). It is inherently labile, but after its dissociation C4b can bind fresh C2a derived from further cleavage of C2 by C1s.[20,21]

Generation of the Alternative-Pathway C3 Convertase

Activation of complement by the alternative pathway displays several unique features. First, antibody is not required, although it can facilitate the activation process. Second, activation proceeds both in the fluid phase as well as on cell surfaces. Fluid-phase activation occurs continuously at a low rate that is controlled by regulator proteins in plasma. Spillover from the fluid phase results in complement deposition on cells of the host as well as intruding microorganisms. Thus host cells must possess a mechanism to limit the effects of complement fixation (i.e., they are "nonactivators"), whereas intruding cells must provide a surface that allows complement activation to proceed further (i.e., they are "activators").[20,33,34] Third, a component of the activation process, C3b, is also a product of the reaction, thereby generating a positive-feedback system that amplifies the activation process. Consequently, C3b deposition resulting from C3 cleavage by either the alternative- or the classical-pathway C3 convertase can initiate the alternative-pathway amplification loop (Fig. 1).[20,33,34] The time required until amplification occurs makes complement activation via the alternative pathway three to five times kinetically less efficient than via the classical pathway on the same target.[35] This delay in activation is characteristic for a given target and differs among different target particles.[33,34] Fourth, in contrast to the classical pathway in which antibody directs covalent C4b binding in clus-

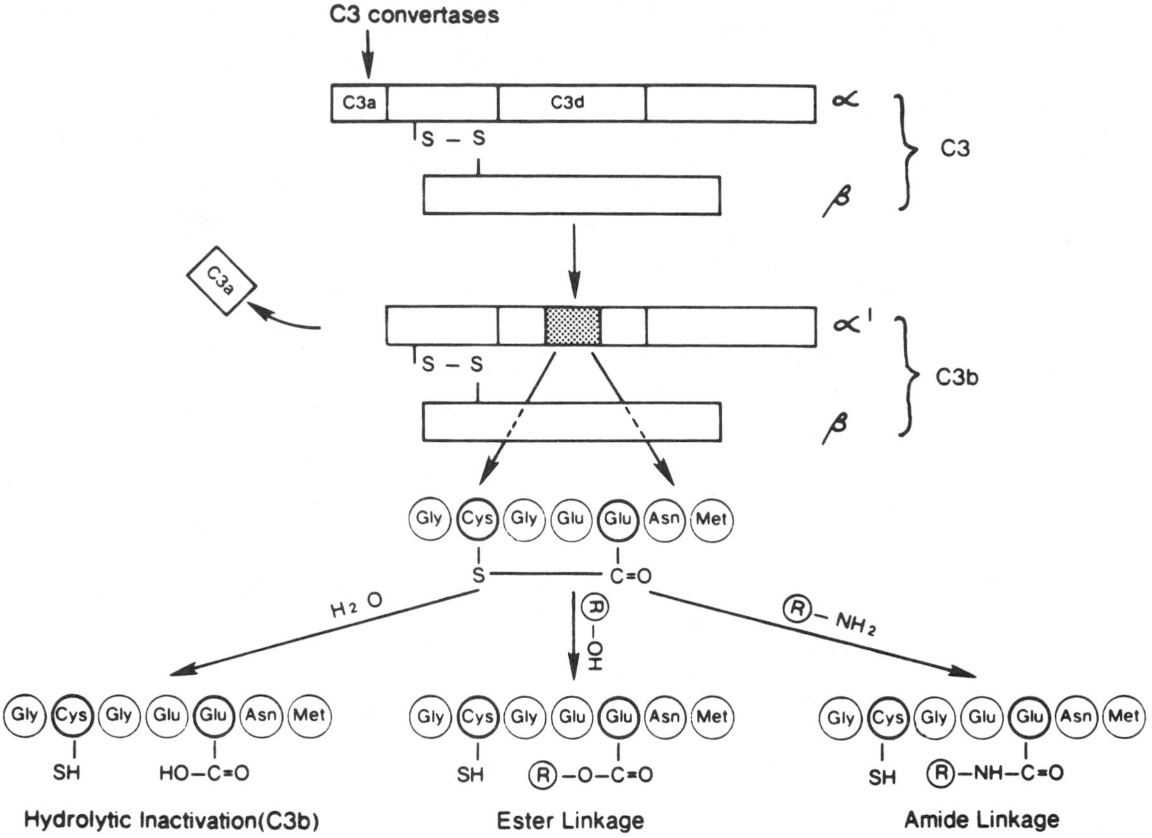

FIG. 2. C3 activation and fate of the internal thiolester bond. During activation C3a is released from the amino terminus of the α-chain of C3. The exposed internal thiolester bond becomes accessible to nucleophilic attack and can react with water or available hydroxyl or amine groups on cell surfaces. Analogous reactions occur with C4. Together these reactions involving C3 and C4 are responsible for covalently linking complement deposition to the cell surface. (From Gordon et al.,[26] with permission.)

ters about the antibody binding site, covalent C3b binding mediated by the alternative pathway occurs randomly over the surface of the target particle.[33,34] The random nature of this process contributes in part to the delay in complement activation via this pathway.

C3 is the critical reactant of the alternative pathway. It is structurally and functionally analogous to C4 (Fig. 1) and contains the same internal thiolester bond within its α-chain. This internal thiolester bond undergoes spontaneous low-rate hydrolysis to form C3(H_2O) as shown in Figure 2. For a brief moment before its inactivation by the control proteins factors H and I, C3(H_2O) can form a complex with factor B. Once bound to C3, factor B can be cleaved by factor D to yield C3 (H_2O) Bb—the fluid-phase C3 convertase. C3(H_2O)Bb reacts with intact C3 to cleave a 9 kD peptide fragment, C3a, from the amino terminus of the α-chain.[33,34] Analogous to the situation with C4, this process results in the exposure of the internal thiolester in the α-chain. The resulting metastable C3b can form covalent ester or amide linkages with appropriate chemical constituents on the surface of nearby cells. Surface-bound C3b can bind additional factor B, which in turn can be cleaved by factor D to produce C3bBb. This complex is the alternative-pathway C3 convertase, which is capable of cleaving additional C3, thereby initiating the amplification phase of the alternative pathway. Like its classical-pathway analogue, this convertase is inherently labile and has a half-life of approximately 90 seconds. Properdin binding to C3bBb stabilizes the complex and prolongs its half-life by 5- to 10-fold,[36,37] thereby providing reaction conditions sufficient for further C3 cleavage and signaling the initiation of the amplification phase of alternative-pathway activation.

From these considerations it is apparent that any substance that stabilizes the alternative-pathway convertase will also promote C3 consumption. This situation arises in patients who develop autoantibodies to C3bBb that stabilize the convertase.[38] In addition, cobra venom contains a C3b-like factor that forms an extremely stable complex with factor B that functions as a C3 convertase except that it is resistant to the action of the control proteins. Thus, the addition of cobra venom factor to serum leads to the dramatic consumption of C3.[33,39–41] Consequently, infusion of this factor can be used in experimental animals to delineate the role of the complement cascade in host defense or other disease processes.

Although antibody is not required for activation of the alternative pathway, it acts synergistically with properdin to facilitate the activation process.[42,43] Facilitation is dependent upon the Fab portion of the antibody molecule rather than the Fc fragment responsible for classical-pathway activation.[43–47] Not all antibodies can enhance activation, for example, guinea pig IgG1 but not IgG2 can augment alternative-pathway activation.[48] The molecular basis for facilitation is uncertain but probably requires carbohydrate moieties present on IgG.[49] Antibody deposited on target surfaces can itself become a potential binding site for the covalent linkage of C3.[44] Moreover, the alternative-pathway C3 convertase, C3bBb that is formed on IgG is relatively resistant to the action of the regulatory proteins.[50,51] This property may contribute to the ability of antibody to facilitate alternative-pathway activation.

C3—The Linchpin of the Complement System

The critical importance of C3 in the complement cascade is evident from its position at the convergence of the classical and alternative pathways, its role in activating and amplifying alternative-pathway activation, the multitude of functional activities associated with its various cleavage products, the fact that it is a major point of regulation of complement activity (Fig. 1), and the fact that its concentration in plasma (1.6 mg/ml) exceeds by 2 to 10-fold the concentration of all other complement components (Table 1).[52] The α-chain of C3b is subject to proteolytic cleavage by factor I to yield iC3b and by less well defined proteases to C3dg and C3d. Each of these progressively smaller C3 fragments remains linked to the cell surface via the original covalent bond. Each of these C3 cleavage products (C3b, iC3b, C3dg, and C3d) can react with specific receptors on phagocytic and lymphocytic cells, but only C3b perpetuates complement activation. C3b binding to the C3 convertases generates new complexes, C4bC2aC3b and C3bBbC3b, the C5 convertases, which are responsible for cleaving C5 and initiating assembly of the membrane attack complex (MAC). Enzymes present in neutrophil granules can proteolytically inactivate C3. Cleavage products have been detected in areas of pus formation such as empyema and may contribute to the impaired ingestion of bacteria in abscesses.[53,54]

Assembly of the Membrane Attack Complex

C5 is the structural hemologue of C4 and C3 except that its α-chain does not contain an internal thiolester bond. Instead, the amino acids cysteine and glutamine, which form the internal thiolester in C4 and C3, have been replaced by serine and alanine.[55,56] Analogous to C4 and C3, activation of C5 proceeds via cleavage of an 11.2 kD fragment, C5a, from the amino terminus of its α-chain. The resulting C5b binds noncovalently to the surface of the target particle.[57] The remaining terminal complement components C6, C7, C8β, C8α-γ, and C9 share a high level of structural organization at both the DNA and protein levels.[58–60] Unlike the early components of the classical and alternative pathways these proteins lack enzymatic activity but as a group are characterized by their amphipathic properties. They circulate in plasma in a hydrophilic form but undergo hydrophobic transformation upon binding to the nascent MAC.[57] Assembly of the MAC begins when C5b binds to hydrophobic sites on the cell surface and expresses a metastable binding site for C6. After C6 binding, C7 also binds to C5b, which results in the formation of a stable trimolecular complex, C5b67.[57] Subsequently, C8 binds to C5b via a site on its β-chain.[61,62] In the final step, C8 initiates polymerization of C9 through a binding site on C8α-γ.[63] A current model of this process suggests that the function of C5b-8 is to create a discontinuity in the membrane lipid bilayer, thereby establishing an environment for the stepwise unfolding, insertion, and polymerization of monomeric C9.[64] In its completely assembled state the MAC consists of a single molecule each of C5b-C8 and multiple (1–18) molecules of C9.[57]

Fully inserted and polymerized C9 has a tubular shape and the properties of an integral membrane protein.[57,64] It is responsible for the characteristic electron microscopic appearance of the membrane holes that appear during effective complement activation. The inner aspect of this tubular structural is hydrophilic and allows the passage of water and ions, whereas the outer surface of the structure is hydrophobic and causes varying degrees of membrane disorganization during insertion.[57,64] Both of these effects are thought to contribute to the microbicidal and cytolytic properties of the MAC. A functionally and structurally related protein called perforin has been isolated from the granules of natural killer (NK) cells. Translocation of this protein from NK cells to the membrane of target cells occurs during the cytolytic process.[58,65–67]

REGULATION OF COMPLEMENT ACTIVATION

Regulation of C1 Activation

As described earlier, C1 esterase inhibitor (C1-INH) binds reversibly to pro-C1, thereby preventing its spontaneous activation.[22] Binding of C1q to antibody subverts this control by causing dissociation of C1-INH from pro-C1 and allowing autocatalytic cleavage to proceed. At some point after C1 activation C1-INH binds to the serine esterase sites on C1r and C1s and inactivates their catalytic function. Complete inactivation requires the binding of four molecules of C1-INH per C1rC1s tetramer (one per catalytic site). In contrast to its reversible binding to pro-C1, C1-INH binding to C1r and C1s is irreversible, thereby preventing cleavage of C4 and controlling the initial amplification step of classical-pathway activation.[22,68]

Regulation of the C3 Convertases

As indicated in Figure 1 the classical- and alternative-pathway C3 convertases are functionally analogous molecules. Control of their activity occurs by three basic mechanisms and uses functionally identical or shared regulator proteins (Table 2).[20,33,34,38] First, both of the convertases are inherently labile and undergo spontaneous decay with the loss of C2a or Bb from the complex. Second, the rate of spontaneous decay can be accelerated by the binding of C4 binding protein (C4bp) or factor H to C4b or C3b, respectively. These regulatory proteins compete with C2a and Bb for binding sites on C4b and C3b, respectively, thereby inhibiting new convertase formation and enhancing the rate of dissociation of the already formed convertases. Third, functionally active C3b and C4b remaining on the cell surface after dissociation of the convertases are proteolytically cleaved by factor I. C4bp, factor H, complement receptor type 1 (CR1), and membrane cofactor protein (MCP) function as cofactors in mediating this reaction.[20,33,34,38,69] Proteolysis results in the display of an array of covalently bound C4b and C3b cleavage fragments that can promote additional complement-mediated functions when present on the appropriate target particle.

C4bp and factor H are soluble molecules that exert their regulatory influence over both fluid-phase and surface-bound C3 convertases.[20,33,69,70] Functionally analogous molecules are present in the membrane of host cells. These proteins include the C3b receptor (CR1), MCP (or GP45-70), and decay accelerating factor (DAF).[71] CR1 is present primarily on peripheral blood cells and facilitates the clearance of immune complexes. MCP and DAF enjoy a wider tissue distribution and play a major role in the inactivation of C3b deposited on host cells during complement activation.[69,70] Thus they serve to distinguish self from nonself with respect to the deleterious effects of complement activation.[70] Like C4bp and factor H all three proteins function to inhibit the assembly and accelerate the decay of the C3 convertases, but unlike the soluble regulator proteins, the membrane-bound proteins do not exhibit pathway specificity.[69,70] Of the membrane-bound proteins, DAF exhibits specificity for C3b and C4b only when these molecules are bound to the same cell on which the DAF is located (intrinsic activity), whereas CR1 and MCP exhibit extrinsic activity. Although the soluble regulator proteins C4bp and factor H contribute to the regulation of cell-bound C3 convertases, their principal role is to control the formation and activity of these convertases in the fluid phase, whereas the membrane-bound regulatory proteins primarily regulate cell-bound C3b and C4b.[69,70] The multiplicity of proteins involved and the existence of both fluid-phase and membrane-bound regulatory proteins all with activity specific for the C3 convertases serve to emphasize the critical importance of the convertases in amplifying complement activation.

Recently the assembly and insertion of the MAC has been shown to inhibit C3 convertase formation and to accelerate the decay of the alternative-pathway convertase. Feedback inhibition of this sort may serve to protect the host from the detrimental affects of continued complement activation.[72,73]

The Basis for Discriminating between Host and Microbial Cell Surfaces

The capacity of C4 and C3 to form covalent bonds with reactive groups on cell surfaces, thereby establishing the nidus for C3

TABLE 2. Plasma and Membrane Proteins That Regulate or Mediate Complement Activity

Location *Protein*	*Specificity*	*Function*
Plasma		
C1-INH	C1r, C1s	Binds to and removes C1r and C1s from C1 complex
C4bp	C4b	Inhibits assembly and accelerates decay of C4b2a Cofactor for C4b cleavage by factor I
Factor H	C3b	Inhibits assembly and accelerates decay of C3bBb Cofactor for C3b cleavage by factor I
Factor I	C4b, C3b	Proteolytic inactivation of C4b and C3b
S protein	C5b-7	Binds fluid-phase C5b-7; prevents attachment of SC5b-7, C5b-9 to membranes
Carboxypeptidase N	C4a, C3a, C5a	Inactivates these anaphylatoxins by removal of C terminal arginine
Cell Membranes		
CR1	C3b, C4b, iC3b	Inhibit assembly and accelerate decay of C3 convertases
MCP	C3b, C4b	Cofactor for cleavage of C4b/C3b by factor I
DAF	C4b2a, C3bBb	
CR1	C3b, C4b, iC3b	Binds immune complexes to erythrocytes; phagocytosis
CR2	C3d, C3dg, iC3b, C3b	Phagocytosis Modulates B-cell responses Epstein-Barr virus receptor
CR3	iC3b	Phagocytosis
CR4 (p150, 95)	C3dg, C3d	Unknown
HRF	C8 in C5b-8	? Binds to C8 Inhibits polymerization of C9
C3a/C4a receptor	C3a, C4a	Vasodilation
C5a receptor	C5a, C5a des-arg	Chemotaxis
C1qR	C1q	Phagocytosis

convertase formation, is inherently incapable of distinguishing between host and microbial cells. Consequently, in order for the beneficial effects of complement activation to be expressed as an effective host defense mechanism additional factors must allow the discrimination between self and nonself[76]: inhibiting activation of complement amplification on host cells ("nonactivators") yet permitting amplification on the surface of microbial organisms ("activators"). One element of this discriminatory process is the presence of the complement regulatory proteins in the membranes of host cells but not on the cells of microbial organisms.[70] The other important determinant of complement activation is the chemical composition of the cell surface. Moreover, since covalent bond formation is nondiscriminatory, the basis for discrimination must lie in the capacity for chemical differences to affect the outcome of the competition between factor B and factor H for the binding site on C3b, which in turn determines C3 convertase formation or decay and whether or not a particular cell surface will activate the alternative pathway. For example, C3b bound to the surface of a nonactivating particle binds factor H with about a 100-fold greater affinity than C3b bound to an activator particle. Consequently, factor B binding and subsequent amplification of complement activation is favored on the latter particle.[20,33,34,38]

Chemical constituents that influence the competition between factor B and factor H for C3b include sialic acid and sulfated acid mucopolysaccharides (e.g., heparin sulfate). These chemical molecules are present on most human cells and enhance the affinity of factor H for C3b, thereby contributing to the nonactivator status of host cells.[74–76] From the standpoint of infectious diseases it is interesting that sialic acid is a prominent chemical constituent of the capsular polysaccharides present on type 3 group B streptococci, K1 *Escherichia coli*, and group B and C meningococci.[38] Consequently, the capsules of these organisms are nonactivators of the alternative pathway and, being a constituent of host cells, constitute a poor stimulus for antibody production. In this context it is noteworthy that K1 *E. coli*, group B streptococci, and group B meningococci are prominent causes of neonatal and infant sepsis and meningitis. Moreover, the frequent absence in these individuals of specific antibody to activate the classic pathway coupled with bacterial sialic acid–mediated inhibition of alternative-pathway activity may provide the ideal clinical setting for infection with these organisms.

Chemical constituents other than sialic acid must also affect the outcome of the competition between factors B and H for C3b. For example, sheep and human erythrocytes contain an extensive amount of sialic acid on their surface and are normally nonactivators of the alternative pathway.[74,77] Enzymatic removal of sialic acid from these cells converts sheep but not human erythrocytes into activating particles. Moreover, the chemical introduction of lipopolysaccharide molecules capable of activating the alternative pathway into the membrane of sheep erythrocytes converts them from a nonactivating to an activating particle despite the presence of sialic acid.[77]

In summary, the C3 convertases represent the major site of both complement amplification and regulation. The membranes of host cells contain both unique proteins that act specifically to downregulate the C3 convertases and other chemical constituents that enhance the affinity of fluid-phase factor H for surface-bound C3b and promote its regulatory activity. In contrast, most microbial surfaces lack specific factors capable of downregulating complement activation and possess a chemical composition that decreases the affinity of factor H for cell-bound C3b. Thus, factor B binding to C3b and alternative-pathway activation and amplification are favored on microbial surfaces. The composition of the cell surface also influences the efficiency of complement activation by the classic pathway. The mechanism of this modulation is less clearly understood but appears to occur at the level of cellbound C4b.[78]

Regulation of the Membrane Attack Complex

Control of the assembly of the MAC is exerted at two levels. First, S protein in plasma binds to lipophilic sites on the fluid-phase trimolecular C5b-7 complex. This interaction inhibits the binding of C5b-7 to membranes and prevents the assembly of the MAC on innocent bystander cells of the host.[57] Second, homologous restriction protein (HRP) present on many types of peripheral blood cells binds C8 and prevents C9 polymerization.[79–81] This protein was discovered as a result of the observation that appropriately sensitized erythrocytes from a given species were lysed less well when the complement source, in particular the C8 and C9, was derived from the same species rather than from another species.[82]

Nucleated eukaryotic cells are quite resistant to complement-mediated cytolysis even in the face of a nonhomologous complement source. Resistance is associated with the capacity of the cell to maintain high synthetic rates of membrane lipids and the ability to shed MAC from the cell surface.[83–85] Insertion of the MAC in eukaryotic cell membranes is accompanied by a rapid influx of calcium and stimulation of arachidonic acid metabolism.[86–90] These events may contribute to host cell injury in certain disease states.[86]

COMPLEMENT RECEPTORS

During the 1980's, an increasing number of membrane receptors have been recognized for the products of complement activation.[91–93] These receptors have been described primarily on peripheral blood cells including erythrocytes, neutrophils, monocytes, B and T lymphocytes, and platelets. They fall into two broad categories: those that bind complement components deposited on cell surfaces such that the component serves as a bifunctional ligand linking the target cell to the receptor and those that bind diffusable complement fragments released during activation of the complement cascade. The latter are responsible for many of the manifestations of the inflammatory response.

The former category of receptor includes C1qR, CR1, CR2, CR3, and CR4. Little is known about C1qR other than that it is present on phagocytic cells and that binding results from the interaction of the receptor with the central collagenlike core of the molecule. Recent evidence suggests that interaction of C1q with its receptor on granulocytes may mediate particle ingestion and stimulate a respiratory burst in these cells (see Chapter 7).[91,92]

Receptors for the cleavage products of C3 and C4 (CR1, CR2, CR3, and CR4) have been studied more extensively. Despite recognizing closely related ligands each of these receptors is structurally distinct and exhibits a unique pattern of distribution on peripheral blood cells.[93,94] A portion of these receptors is linked to the cellular cytoskeleton, an association that is probably important in the transduction of the binding signal into a cellular response.[95]

CR1, the C3b receptor, is present on erythrocytes, neutrophils, monocytes, B lymphocytes, subpopulations of T lymphocytes, follicular dendritic cells, and glomerular podocytes. It also recognizes C4b and iC3b but with less affinity than for C3b. This receptor mediates immune complex binding and clearance and ingestion of particles bearing C3b and presumably modulates certain immune lymphocyte responses.[91,93,94]

CR3, the iC3b receptor, is the major complement receptor mediating phagocytosis by phagocytic cells.[91,93,94] It is a heterodimer and has recently been shown to be a member of the integrin family[96] It recognizes a three–amino acid sequence, arg-gly-asp, present on C3[97] and other ligands important in adhesion.[98] In addition to recognizing iC3b it plays an important role in the adherence-related functions of neutrophils and is covered more extensively in Chapter 7.

CR4 is the C3dg receptor. It is present on phagocytic cells and appears to be synonomous with p150,95.[99] More CR4 is present on culture-derived macrophages than on freshly isolated monocytes. CR2, the C3d receptor, is present on B lymphocytes and follicular dendritic cells. Its stimulation appears to modulate antibody production by these lymphocytes. It also serves as the Epstein-Barr virus receptor, and its stimulation during viral entry may contribute to the polyclonal gammopathy observed early in the course of infectious mononucleosis.[100,101]

Receptors for complement-derived mediators of the inflammatory response including C4a, C3a, and C5a have also been described. Of these the C5a receptor has been best studied. It is present on neutrophils and monocytes, and its pertubation causes directed migration (chemotaxis) of these cells in the direction of increasing C5a concentration. Experimental evidence suggests the presence of receptors for C3a on guinea pig ileum, vascular endothelium, and mast cells.[102]

FAMILIES OF COMPLEMENT PROTEINS

The preceding material and the representation of the complement cascade presented in Figure 1 emphasize features shared by both pathways with respect to their activation and regulation. It is apparent from these similarities that a number of complement components belong to several different protein families. These include the serine protease family (C1r, C1s, C2, factor D, factor B, and factor I); multichained disulfide-linked molecules with homology to an ancestral protein that contain an internal thiolester bond (C4, C3, and C5); proteins that are the products of class 3 major histocompatibility complex (MHC) genes located on chromosome 6 (C2, factor B, C4A, and C4B); proteins that bind C3 and C4 fragments that belong to a closely clustered supergene family located on the long arm of chromosome 1 (C4bp, factor H, DAF, MCP, CR1, and CR2); and proteins sharing homology with the low-density lipoprotein (LDL) receptor (C9, C8α, C8β, C7, and probably C6). These families also include a number of noncomplement homologues.[103]

Of these families current interest has focused on those components that are the products of the class 3 MHC genes, the regulatory protein supergene family on chromosome 1, and the proteins with homology to the LDL receptor. Class 3 MHC genes are located between the class 1 and class 2 loci on the short arm of chromosome 6 (Fig. 3).[104] The genetic material in this region is of particular interest because it appears to have undergone two duplication events resulting on the one hand in the structurally and functionally related proteins C2 and factor B and on the other hand the C4 and 21-hydroxylase A and B variants.[103–105] The gene for tumor necrosis factor/cachectin has also been localized to this region of chromosome 6.[106] Recombinant events in this region of the chromosome tend to be suppressed, thereby leading to the usual inheritance of the entire region intact from each parent.[107] The polymorphic variants of the complement components encoded by these genes in a given individual are referred to as complotypes.[108] The association of specific complotypes with specific products of the class 1 and 2 MHC genes probably contributes to the association of specific complotypes with certain disease states (e.g., systemic lupus erythematosus [SLE])[109]

Proteins encoded by the complement regulatory protein loci on the long arm of chromosome 1 share a common organization with each other, with other proteins capable of binding to C3 and C4 (e.g., C2 and factor B), and with some complement and noncomplement proteins that do not bind these two components.[110,111] All of these proteins contain tandem repeats of approximately 60 amino acids that share a consensus sequence. Each of these 60 amino acid repeats are encoded within separate exons, and the number of repeats varies from as few as 2 and 3 in C1r and C2/factor B, respectively, to as many as 20 in factor H, although CR1 may contain up to 36 repeats. The functional significance of these repeating structures, particularly with respect to their C3 and C4 binding properties, remains to be delineated.[111]

The LDL receptor-related complement proteins are cysteine-rich molecules. Each molecule contains an even number of cysteine residues that are clustered at the amino and carboxy terminal portions of the protein and participate in disulfide bond formation. Those clustered at the amino terminus of the molecule share homology with epidermal growth factor, while those at the carboxy terminus share homology with the LDL receptor. The large number of disulfide bonds in these molecules is thought to convey a tertiary structure that facilitates the hydrophilic–hydrophobic transition that occurs upon their inter-

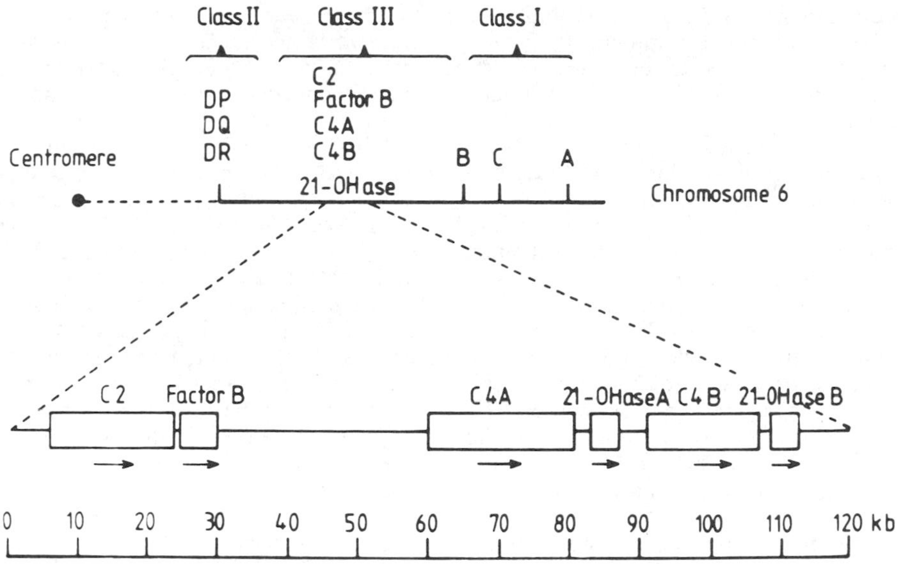

FIG. 3. Organization of the human MHC genes on chromosome 6. The proximity of the class 3 genes to one another and to the class 2 and 1 genes is apparent. C2 and factor B are tightly linked and probably represent duplication of the phylogenetically older factor B gene. Genetic duplication is also apparent in the paired arrangement of the C4 and 21-hydroxylase genes. (From Campbell,[104] with permission.)

action with lipid membranes during the assembly of the MAC.[58,59,102]

COMPLEMENT-MEDIATED FUNCTIONS

Complement plays a major role in initiating the inflammatory response, clearing immune complexes, modulating immunoglobulin production, opsonizing microbial pathogens, and killing certain gram-negative bacteria (Fig. 1). Small, diffusable peptide fragments released from C4, C3, C5, and probably C2 during their activation help mediate the inflammatory response.[102] Collectively C4a, C3a, and C5a are referred to as anaphylatoxins, and together they stimulate histamine release from mast cells (C3a), promote vascular dilation (C3a, C4a), increase endothelial permeability (C3a), and stimulate neutrophil responses (C5a, e.g., adhesiveness, chemotaxis, degranulation, and oxidative burst; see Chapter 7). Each of these structurally related anaphylatoxins contains an arginine residue at its carboxy terminus. Removal of this terminal amino acid by carboxypeptidase B in serum abrogates their functional activity by preventing their interaction with specific receptors.[102] However, in the case of C5a des-arg (the inactivated form of C5a), chemotactic activity is restored by association with a cochemotaxin present in serum[112] that has recently been identified as a vitamin D binding protein.[113,114] The chemotactic activity of this complex can be inhibited by free Bb, a situation that occurs in the sera of some patients with SLE.[115]

The incorporation of complement in immune complexes enhances their clearance and helps to minimize their potential for causing tissue damage.[116,117] This process includes the inhibition of immune complex precipitation from solution, the solubilization of immune complexes, and the clearance of C3b-bearing immune complexes via the CR1 receptor. Under conditions of antibody excess or antibody–antigen equivalence the attachment of both antigen binding sites on a single antibody to epitopes on a single antigen and the binding of multiple antibody molecules to a given molecule of antigen provide an opportunity for antibody–antibody interactions via their Fc fragments, a condition that leads to immune complex precipitation.[117] C1q binding inhibits these Fc–Fc interactions and leads to complement activation with covalent binding of C3b to the immune complex. Subsequent recruitment of the alternative pathway via the C3b amplification loop promotes further C3b deposition within the immune complex lattice, thereby reducing the forces holding the lattice together and causing separation (solubilization) of smaller complexes from the lattice network. Thus the classic pathway functions to inhibit immune complex precipitation, whereas the alternative pathway promotes solubilization of the immune complex.[116,117]

Small immune complexes bearing C3b are bound to cells bearing C3b receptors (CR1). The number of these receptors per cell varies from a low of 950 for erythrocytes to a high of 57,000 for neutrophils.[118] However, since red cells outnumber white cells by a thousandfold, 95 percent of the total CR1 receptors in the peripheral circulation are located on red cells. Consequently, immune complexes bearing C3b are 500–1000 times more likely of being removed from the circulation via red cells than white cells.[118] These complexes are removed from the red cell during passage through the liver by an as yet undefined mechanism.[119]

Most evidence implicates C3 as the major complement-derived stimulus involved in modulating immune responses. These studies suggest that C3 or its fragments may enhance or inhibit both T- and B-cell-mediated immune responses, the observed effect perhaps depending upon the concentration of the relevant C3 fragment.[120,121] This evidence includes the observation that the trapping of aggregated human IgG within splenic germinal centers is dependent upon the presence of C3[122] and the demonstration that lymphocytes, particularly B cells, possess receptors (CR2) with ligand specificity for C3dg and C3d.[100] In addition, impaired antibody responses have been demonstrated after primary immunization with a T-cell-dependent antigen, bacteriophage ϕX174, in C2-, C4-, and C3-deficient guinea pigs[123,124] as well as in a limited number of patients with analogous deficiencies.[125] Moreover, dogs with inherited C3 deficiency or animals rendered C3 deficient by the infusion of cobra venom factor were also unable to respond normally to ϕX174.[124,124a] Immune responsiveness in deficient animals could be restored by repletion of the complement system with the missing component or by increasing the dose of antigen during primary immunization.[123] In addition to the impaired response to primary antigenic exposure, complement-deficient animals exhibit an abnormal anamestic response and fail to demonstrate isotype switching after secondary antigenic presentation.[124] Impaired antibody responses in C3-deficient dogs were also observed after primary and secondary immunization with a T-cell independent antigen. In contrast to the results with T-cell dependent antigens, the impaired response to T-cell independent antigens could not be overcome by increasing the dose of antigen or changing the route of administration.[124a] These results clearly demonstrate a critical role for C3 in the generation of a normal humoral immune response.

Finally, a small fragment, C3e, derived from the α-chain of C3 promotes the development of leukocytosis. This observation may account for the failure of some C3-deficient patients to develop leukocytosis in response to infection.[20]

Cell-bound fragments of C3, particularly C3b and iC3b, serve as bifunctional ligands linking target particles with cells bearing receptors for these fragments. In the case of bacteria, opsonization with C3b or iC3b, especially in conjunction with IgG, promotes ingestion of the organism and triggers the microbicidal mechanisms of phagocytic cells (see Chapter 7). Ingestion is more efficient when the organism is opsonized with iC3b than with C3b.[26,126]

The complete activation of the complement cascade with the assembly of the MAC and its effective insertion into cell membranes results in the death and eventual lysis of the cell. Death and lysis are independent events, and in the case of prokaryotes some evidence suggests that a metabolic response of the organism is required before the lethal effects of the MAC can be expressed.[127] For some organisms the assembly of the MAC through C8 is sufficient to kill the organism[128]; however, in all cases the incorporation of C9 accelerates this process. Complement-mediated virucidal activity has also been well described and frequently requires deposition of only the early components of the classic pathway.[129]

MICROBIAL INTERACTIONS WITH THE COMPLEMENT SYSTEM

A common theme encountered in the pathogenesis of many infectious agents is the evolution of strategies to neutralize or elude normal host defense mechanisms. An example of this principle and one of the first to suggest an important role of the bactericidal capacity of complement in host defense was the demonstration by Roantree and Rance that gram-negative bacteria isolated from the blood of infected patients were almost always resistant to serum (complement)-mediated killing.[130] In contrast, two-thirds of the gram-negative bacteria isolated from mucosal surfaces could be killed by normal serum. This finding has been confirmed many times in relationship to other invasive bacterial infections, although different organisms employ a variety of molecular strategies to achieve this end.

Resistance to the bactericidal effect of complement is influenced by the structural organization and chemical composition of the outer membrane, the capacity of the organism to activate the alternative pathway, and the presence of bactericidal antibody. Virtually all gram-positive organisms and fungi are resistant to complement-mediated killing, not because they fail to activate complement, but because a thick outer membrane prevents access of the MAC to their inner membrane.[131]

Gram-negative bacilli, for example, *Salmonella*, owe their serum resistance to the long 0-antigen side chains on their lipopolysaccharides. These chains lead to complement activation at sites distant from the outer membrane and hinder access of C5b-9 complexes to it.[132] The failure of these complexes to localize to hydrophobic domains in the bacterial outer membrane results in their shedding and the survival of the organism.[133]

Gram-negative bacteria possessing truncated lipopolysaccharide molecules, for example, *Haemophilus influenzae*, meningococci, and gonococci, are not innately resistant to the bactericidal effects of the complement system but require antibody for effective sensitization and complement deposition. Thus, the absence of bactericidal antibody renders these organisms serum resistant and contributes to the greater frequency of *H. influenzae* and meningococcal disease during the first several years of life. Gonococci isolated from individuals with disseminated gonococcal infection are resistant to the bactericidal activity of normal human serum, whereas those isolated from individuals with symptomatic local genital disease are serum sensitive.[134] The MAC is assembled on the surface of both types of gonococci but fails to insert properly in the outer membrane of the resistant isolates.[135,136] However, insertion and killing occur normally in the presence of IgG antilipooligosaccharide antibody found in the convalescent serum of some individuals with this infection.[137,138] These findings emphasize the importance of both the composition of the outer membrane of gram-negative bacteria in determining sensitivity to complement-mediated killing and the importance to the host of specific antibody in overcoming the resistance of these organisms to killing.[139]

Other strains of serum-resistant gonococci appear to owe their serum resistance to the presence in some sera of an IgG specific for protein 3 in the gonococcal outer membrane.[140,141] This antibody competes with bactericidal antibody for binding sites on the surface of the organism, thereby blocking its bactericidal effect. Although the blocking antibody promotes complement deposition on the organism, it apparently does so at sites that do not lead to the killing of the organism.[142] Blocking antibody also appears to account for the resistance of meningococci to killing by the serum of many adults who acquire this infection.[143,144] In contrast to the situation with gonococci, this antibody is a non-complement-fixing IgA that competes with killing antibody for bactericidal sites on the capsular polysaccharide.[144–146]

The importance of the interaction of antibody with different antigenic structures in determining the effectiveness of complement in promoting host defense mechanisms is further emphasized by the observation that both antipneumococcal cell wall antibody and antipneumococcal capsular antibody promote the efficient deposition of C3b on the pneumococcal surface. However, only C3b deposited on the surface of the pneumococcal capsule is opsonically effective. These results imply that the pneumococcal capsule interferes with the interaction of cell wall–bound C3b with receptors on phagocytic cells.[147]

Protozoan parasites, which undergo dramatic metamorphosis from insect to human infective forms, provide a striking testimony to the importance of serum resistance. For example epimastigotes, the insect infective form of *Trypanosoma cruzi*, are efficiently killed in nonimmune normal human serum as a consequence of complement activation via the alternative pathway. In contrast, trypomastigotes, the human infective form of *T. cruzi*, are not killed under identical circumstances.[148] The basis for this difference is the capacity of trypomastigotes but not epimastigotes to *N*- glycosylate a 72 kD surface protein[149] that serves as the C3b acceptor site on both forms of *T. cruzi*.[148] Although C3b is deposited on both organisms, the presence of the glycosylated 72 kD protein on the invasive trypomastigotes reduces the affinity of C3b for factor B, thereby promoting its cleavage to iC3b.[150] Consequently, amplification of the alternative pathway, MAC formation, and killing occurs only on the serum-sensitive epimastigotes containing the unglycosylated 72 kD protein.

Although serum resistance is an important virulence factor for many organisms, this property by itself cannot account for the difference in virulence among various smooth gram-negative bacilli, all of which have outer membranes containing long-chain lipopolysaccharide molecules. This issue has been addressed in experiments correlating virulence with lipopolysaccharide composition and complement activation by three *Salmonella typhimurium* transductants and recombinants.[151] These organisms share identical outer membrane protein patterns but possess lipopolysaccharide side chains that differ in their chemical structure. The relative in vivo virulence of these three isolates was inversely proportional to their ability to activate complement via the alternative pathway. The rates and extent of C3 consumption and C3b deposition on the surface of these bacteria paralleled one another, the greatest consumption and deposition occurring on the least virulent strain.[152–154] Subsequent studies demonstrated that the magnitude of C3b binding was a function of the fine structure of the lipopolysaccharide O antigen and that while this structure affected C3 binding it had no effect on the subsequent cleavage and breakdown of the bound C3b. The effect of O antigen structure was expressed at the level of alternative-pathway amplification rather than degradation as shown by a greater affinity of factor B for C3b on the surface of the least virulent as compared with the most virulent strains, whereas the affinity of factor H for C3b was the same on all strains.[155,156]

The chemical composition of other structures on the bacterial surface also affects complement activation. Thus, K-1 *E. coli*, type 3 group B streptococci, and group B meningococci that possess sialylated capsular polysaccharides are poor activators of the alternative pathway[157,158] due to the higher affinity of C3b for factor H than for factor B in this setting.[38,74–76] Studies of alternative-pathway activation by pneumococci have demonstrated an effect of the chemical composition of the capsule on both the extent and the degradation of C3b. An interesting observation of these studies is an apparent inverse relationship between the degree of C3b degradation on a given capsular polysaccharide and the ability of that capsular polysaccharide to elicit an immune response when administered as part of the polyvalent pneumococcal vaccine.[159]

In addition to the capacity of the microbial surface to modulate the activity of bound C3, some organisms possess glycoproteins that bind C3 noncovalently. These proteins are antigenically similar to C3 receptors on human cells as shown by their ability to bind monoclonal, receptor-specific antibodies.[160–162] In the case of herpes simplex viruses expression of a complement binding protein (glycoprotein C) is associated with resistance to neutralization by complement.[163] In the case of *Candida albicans* the presence of these surface proteins is associated with resistance to phagocytosis.[164]

COMPLEMENT DEFICIENCY STATES

Frequency

Complement deficiency states may be either acquired or inherited. Acquired deficiency states can occur acutely, as part of an abrupt insult such as infection, or in conjunction with more chronic diseases such as rheumatologic or autoimmune processes. The frequency of inherited complement deficiencies in the general population is about 0.03 percent. Since these states are rare, the utility of screening tests is greatest in populations that contain the clinical correlates of abnormal complement inheritance, that is, persons with rheumatologic diseases and/or recurrent bacterial infections.[165] In one such study, a single individual with a homozygous complement deficiency was detected among 545 patients with rheumatologic diseases.[166] This frequency (0.2 percent) is approximately 10-fold greater than that in the general population. In addition, 19 individuals with a definite, probable, or possible heterozygous C2 deficiency state were detected among the 545 rheumatologic patients as compared with only 6 possible heterozygotes among 509 individuals without these diseases. Thus, this study provides clear support for the association of complement deficiency states with certain rheumatologic disorders, in particular, SLE.[166]

Reports of an association between systemic meningococcal and gonococcal infections and an inherited deficiency of C5, C6, C7, or C8[165,167] have led to several studies of the frequency of these deficiencies among patients with these infections. Such studies have uncovered as few as 0 of 47 (<2 percent) to as many as 3 of 20 (15 percent) individuals presenting with a first episode of documented meningococcal disease.[168–171] The wide range in frequency is probably related to the age of the patients in the studies, the relatively small number of patients studied, and a disproportionate genetic influence in relatively insular populations.[165] The best estimate of the frequency of inherited complement deficiency states among patients with endemic neisserial disease is about 5–10 percent, although the likelihood of a complement deficiency increases dramatically (31 percent) among patients who have had more than one episode of meningococcal infection.[172]

Classical-Pathway Deficiencies

The association of immune disorders, in particular SLE, with complement deficiency states is most evident in individuals lacking C1, C4, C2, or C3 (Table 3). The clinical presentation of SLE in individuals with a deficiency of one of these components differs from that in the general population in that males are commonly affected, renal disease is less severe, antinuclear antibody titers are low or absent, and there is an increased prevalence of Ro antibodies.[173–175]

In contrast to the relationship with infection in which an association is apparent only in homozygous deficient individuals, an increased frequency of collagen vascular diseases is apparent in individuals with either homozygous or heterozygous deficiency. The basis for this phenomenon has not been precisely delineated, although impaired immune complex handling and the tight genetic linkage of the C2 and C4 loci with the class I and II MHC genes appear to contribute to the association.[176] Of these variables, impaired immune complex clearance probably exerts a greater impact since the association is apparent for all four of these complement proteins whereas only C4 and C2 are MHC linked (see Fig. 3). The role of the early components of the classical pathway in inhibiting immune complex precipitation has been confirmed in the sera from patients with these deficiencies.[177,178] Moreover, abnormal humoral immune system regulation and the presence of autoantibodies, including rheumatoid factors, have been demonstrated in C2- and C4-deficient guinea pigs.[179]

Consequent to the linkage disequilibrium with other MHC loci, the C2 and C4 null genes occur predominantly as part of distinct extended haplotypes. For C2 deficiency, this haplotype is DR2;C2Q0;BfS;C4A-4;C4B-2;B18;A25,[180] and for C4 deficiency it is DR3;C2C;BfS;C4AQ0;C4B-1;B8.[181] Multivariate analysis of DR and C4 gene types has confirmed an independent contribution of the C4AQ0 and the DR2 antigens to the development of SLE. The C4B null gene (C4Q0) was not associated with SLE.[182] The chemical preference of the internal thiolester in C4A to form amide bonds during complement activation and to react with immune complexes may account for the contribution of the C4A null gene to the development of SLE.[28,30,31]

A preliminary report suggests that C4B deficiency may occur with increased frequency among children with bacterial meningitis. This report is particularly intriguing given the preference of C4B to form covalent ester bonds during complement activation and the abundance of available hydroxyl groups on the surface of the bacterial pathogens usually responsible for meningitis.[183]

The low frequency of infection (20 percent) in individuals with a deficiency of C1, C4, or C2 as compared with other component deficiencies (Table 3) is attributed to the presence of an intact alternative pathway in these patients. When present, bacterial infection is usually caused by encapsulated bacteria, especially *Streptococcus pneumoniae*, and may be recurrent. The most common sites of infection are the sinopulmonary tree, meninges, and blood.[165]

The molecular basis fo C4A deficiency involves gene deletion.[181] In contrast, the C2 gene appears intact in individuals with C2 deficiency and data suggest that this deficiency may be due to a defect in transcription.[184] The existence of two separate C4 genes dictates that complete C4 deficiency, that is, the

TABLE 3. Complement Deficiency States

Component	*Number of Reported Patients*	*Mode of Inheritance*	*Functional Defect*	*Disease Associations*
Classical pathway				
C1qrs	29	ACD	Impaired IC handling	CVD, 48%
C4	20	ACD	Delayed C′ activation	Infection (encaps bact), 22%
C2	90	ACD	Impaired immune response	Both, 18% Healthy, 12%
Alternative pathway				
D	2	ACD	Impaired C′ activation	Infection (meningococcal), 74%
P	41	XL	In absence of specific antibody	Healthy, 26%
Junction of classical and alternative pathways				
C3	14	ACD	Impaired IC handling opson/phag; granulocytosis, CTX, immune response, and absent SBA	CVD, 79% Recurrent infection (encaps bact), 71%
Terminal components				
C5	17	ACD	Impaired CTX; absent SBA	Infection (*Neisseria*—primarily meningococcal), 69% CVD, 4%
C6	64	ACD	Absent SBA	Both, 1%
C7	47	ACD	Absent SBA	Healthy, 25%
C8	55	ACD	Absent SBA	
C9	12	ACD	Impaired SBA	Healthy, 92% Infection, 8%
Plasma proteins regulating C′ activation				
C1-INH	Many	AD acq	Uncontrolled generation of an inflammatory mediator upon C′ act	Hereditary angioedema
H	5	ACD	Uncontrolled AP act → low C3[a]	CVD, 40% CVD + infection (encaps bact), 40% Healthy, 20%
I	9	ACD	Uncontrolled AP act → low C3[a]	Infection (encaps bact), 100%
Membrane proteins regulating C′ activation				
DAF HRF	Many	acq	Impaired regulation of C3b and C8 deposited on host RBC, PMN platelets → cell lysis	Paroxysmal nocturnal hemoglobinuria
CR3	>20	ACD	Impaired PMN adhesive functions i.e., margination, CTX, iC3b-mediated opson/phag	Infection (*S. aureus, Pseudomonas* sp.), 100%
Autoantibodies				
C3 nephritic factors	>59	acq	Stabilizes AP C3 convertase → low C3[a]	MPGN, 41%; PLD, 25%; infection (encaps bact), 16% MPGN + PLD, 10%; PLD + infection, 5%; MPGN + PLD + infection, 3%; MPGN + infection, 2%
C4 nephritic factor	4	acq	Stabilizes CP C3 convertase → low C3[a]	Glomerulonephritis, 50% CVD, 50%

Abbreviations: ACD: autosomal codominant; XL: X-linked; AD: autosomal dominant; acq: acquired; IC: immune complex; C′: complement; act: activation; opson/phag: opsonophagocytosis; CTX: chemotaxis; SBA: serum bactericidal activity; AP: alternative pathway; RBC: red blood cells; PMN: polymorphonuclear neutrophils; CVD: collagen vascular disease; encaps bact: encapsulated bacteria; MPGN: membrane proliferative glomerulonephritis; PLD: partial lymphodystrophy.
[a] See Table 3, Section III.
(Data updated to June 1988 from Ross et al.[165])

absence of the products of all four C4 genetic loci, is extremely rare. Conversely, the heterozygous C4 deficiency state is very common and occurs in approximately 25 percent of the general population.[185]

ALTERNATIVE-PATHWAY DEFICIENCIES

Inherited deficiencies of the components of the alternative pathway appear to be less common than those of other complement proteins, and to date, no individuals with homozygous factor B deficiency have been identified (Table 3). In the presence of specific antibody, individuals with alternative-pathway defects can activate the classic pathway normally, but the absence of antibody, coupled with the defect in alternative-pathway activation, leads to a profound defect in complement activation and serum bactericidal activity. Consequently, infection in such individuals might be expected to have dire consequences, a prediction borne out in properdin-deficient individuals (Table 4).

Properdin deficiency is unique because it is an X-linked trait. Three-quarters of properdin-deficient individuals experience infections, most of which are caused by *Neisseria meningitidis*. These infections are frequently characterized by a fulminant course and high mortality rate. Consequently, recurrent infections are uncommon.[186,187] Three properdin-deficient variants have been described: type 1 is characterized by extremely low properdin levels (<0.1 μg/ml) and absent properdin function.[186,187] The serum from individuals with type 2 deficiency contains low levels (~2 μg/ml) of antigenically detectable and functionally altered properdin. Properdin from these individuals has a normal monomeric molecular weight, but oligomer formation and size are altered. Functionally these molecules do not support alternative-pathway activation in the fluid phase but do on target particles, albeit at a slow rate.[188] Type 3 de-

TABLE 4. Comparison of Meningococcal Disease In Normal, Late Complement Component, and Properdin-Deficient Individuals

Characteristic	*Normal*	*LCCD*[a]	*Properdin Deficient*[b]
Number of homozygotes	—	195	41
Number with meningococcal disease	—	124	14–26
Frequency of infection (%)	.0072	64	34–63
Male:female ratio	1.3:1	2.8:1	14:0–25:1
Median age (yr)—first episode	3	17	14–11.5
Recurrence rate (%)	0.34	46.2	0(<2.4)
Relapse rate (%)	0.6	4.7–5.8	0(<2.4)
Mortality/100 episodes (%)	19	1.6–2.7[c]	43–65
Infecting serogroup			
# of isolates	3184	48	11
% B	50.2	20.8	27.3
% Y	4.4	41.7	27.3

[a] Late complement component deficient.
[b] Where a range is given, the first number (e.g., 14) refers to documented cases of meningococcal infection, and the second number (e.g., 26) refers to documented plus probable and possible cases of meningococcal disease.
[c] Larger estimate includes two deaths in individuals with unconfirmed LCCD. The corresponding mortality rate per 100 patients is 2.4–4.0 percent.

ficiency is characterized by normal amounts of antigenically detectable properdin (~25 μg/ml) but absent function.[189]

C3 Deficiency

C3 deficiency is uncommon (see Table 3). As expected from its position and function as the linchpin of the complement cascade, almost all individuals with this defect are seriously ill.[165] Approximately three-quarters develop SLE or a related rheumatologic syndrome. Moreover, the inability to use either the classic or alternative pathway results in a multitude of severe defects in host defense, including impairments in opsonization, immune response, neutrophil chemotaxis, and the ability to generate serum bactericidal activity. Consequently, severe and recurrent pneumococcal, *H. influenzae*, and meningococcal infections involving the sinopulmonary tree, meninges, and blood stream are common, occurring in about 70 percent of such patients.[165]

A comparable clinical picture is observed in individuals with an inherited deficiency of either factor H or factor I and in individuals who develop autoantibody to C3 (C3 nephritic factor).[165] The similar clinical picture results from uncontrolled alternative-pathway activation and the resultant low levels of C3 (less than 10 percent) in serum. Recurrent infection and collagen vascular disorders occur less commonly in individuals with C3 nephritic factor, presumably due to the somewhat higher levels of C3 in these patients. Patients with autoantibody to C3 have an increased incidence of membranoproliferative glomerulonephritis and/or partial lipodystrophy (see Table 3), although the basis for these associations has not been elucidated.[190,191]

Late Complement Component Deficiencies

With the exception of C9, individuals with a deficiency of one of the terminal complement components exhibit a striking susceptibility to systemic neisserial infection, especially meningococcal disease.[33,165] The basis for this association is the inability to express complement-dependent serum bactericidal activity. Support for this conclusion stems from the observation that the serum from C9-deficient individuals can kill meningococci, albeit at a slower rate than is normal, a finding that is consistent with the fact that C9 is not absolutely required for complement-mediated lysis of red cells and presumably accounts for the relative lack of meningococcal infection in these individuals.[128]

Complement-dependent opsonization is unimpaired in late complement component–deficient sera.[192] Nevertheless, phagocytic cells in the tissues and reticuloendothelial system do not seem to prevent neisserial infection in these patients. The reason for this apparent failure seems to be that the serum from unvaccinated and previously uninfected late component–deficient patients as well as healthy individuals contains inadequate amounts of specific IgG anticapsular antibodies. As a result C3 is not deposited on the capsule of these organisms, thereby leading to impaired opsonization as discussed earlier.[147] Bactericidal activity in healthy individuals is mediated primarily by antibodies directed at subcapsular antigens on meningococci. The level of these antibodies in healthy individuals and late complement component–deficient patients who have not experienced previous meningococcal infection are comparable.[193] Thus, the complement deficiency and resulting absence of serum bactericidal activity account for the susceptibility of these patients to meningococcal disease, but the associated lack of anticapsular antibody contributes to this susceptibility by impairing effective elimination of this organism by phagocytes. Conversely, stimulation of an anticapsular antibody response via vaccination may help to protect these individuals by recruiting the phagocytic arm of host defense.[194]

Meningococcal Infection in Complement Deficiency States

Meningococcal disease is the most common infection experienced by complement-deficient individuals (see Table 3).[165] The clinical pattern of the disease is different in complement-deficient and healthy individuals (Table 4). In particular, meningococcal disease in properdin-deficient individuals occurs in males and the first episode of infection usually occurs during the teenage years.[187] The clinical course is frequently fulminant, and there is an associated high mortality,[186,187] presumably as a consequence of low levels of specific outer membrane and anticapsular antibodies, which leads to an impaired capacity to use the classical pathway to opsonize bacteria and develop serum bactericidal activity. The severity of the disease in these individuals contrasts with that in individuals with late complement component deficiencies, presumably because the former are unable to effectively recruit any C3-dependent host defense mechanisms whereas the latter can express some of these activities.

A striking finding in individuals with late complement component deficiencies is the low mortality of meningococcal disease in these individuals as compared with healthy people.[165,171,195] This observation suggests that exuberant complement activation, which occurs frequently in meningococcal disease,[169] may contribute to mortality in healthy individuals and that this contribution is dependent in part upon assembly of an intact MAC. The first occurrence of meningococcal disease at an older age in complement-deficient individuals as compared with healthy people has not been fully explained. Group Y meningococcal disease is relatively more common among complement-deficient than among healthy individuals. The basis for the altered distribution of meningococcal serogroups appears to stem in part from the fact that group Y organisms are more serum sensitive but exhibit a more stringent requirement for elimination by phagocytic cells than do group B strains.[193] However, the absence of complement-dependent bactericidal activity in individuals with late complement component deficiencies does not automatically provide access to the blood stream by the multitude of serum-sensitive organisms present on mucosal membranes.[196] This observation suggests that the serum-sensitive organisms normally present on mucosal surfaces lack factors in addition to serum resistance determinants (e.g., tissue invasion determinants) that contribute to the pathogenesis of infection.

Other Complement Deficiency States

Hereditary Angioedema–C1 Inhibitor Deficiency. Individuals lacking C1-INH present with a distinctive noninfectious, nonrheumatologic clinical picture historically referred to as hereditary angioneurotic edema (HANE or HAE).[197] The hereditary form of this disease was recognized over 100 years ago, whereas an acquired variant has been identified as a distinct entity only within the last 25 years. The genetic form of the disease is inherited as an autosomal dominant trait and exhibits two variants. Type 1 HAE is more common and accounts for 75–85 percent of cases and is characterized by the presence of low (5–30 percent) or normal plasma levels of normally functioning C1-INH protein. In contrast, type 2 HAE is characterized by the presence of normal to elevated levels of antigenic C1-INH that is functionally abnormal.[68,197–199] The acquired forms of this disorder occur considerably less commonly, and two variants are recognized. One, occurring in association with B-lymphocyte disorders, is due to a reaction of circulating anti-idiotype antibodies, with the monoclonal immunoglobulin expressed on the surface of the abnormal B cells.[200] The resulting immune complex leads to C1-INH consumption and secondarily to the clinical picture of angioedema. The second type derives from the presence of autoantibody to the C1-INH. In this situation, angioedema develops as a consequence of inhibition of C1-INH activity.[201]

Since the hereditary form of this disorder is inherited as an autosomal dominant trait, the serum from all of these individuals contains some normally functioning C1-INH.[68] In contrast, individuals with the acquired variants have markedly reduced or absent functional C1-INH activity in their serum. As a consequence of this basic difference, the serum from individuals with the hereditary form of this disorder contains normal amounts of C1 and C1q but reduced levels of C4 and C2, whereas the serum from individuals with the acquired variants contains strikingly reduced amounts of C1, C1q, C4, and C2.[68,197–199]

The health of individuals with this disorder is punctuated by attacks of nonpitting, nonpruritic, and nonpainful edema of the extremities, face, or larynx. Angioedema of the larynx is the most severe complication of the disorder and is a common cause of death in these individuals. The gastrointestional tract may also be affected, and such attacks present as episodes of acute, crampy abdominal pain frequently associated with nausea, vomiting, and occasionally diarrhea. In the inherited form of the disorder, attacks generally begin in childhood, increase in frequency and worsen in severity during adolescence, increase during menstruation, are markedly reduced during pregnancy, and diminish gradually in the fifth and sixth decades of life. A typical attack lasts 2–3 days. Impeded androgens increase the biosynthesis of c1-INH in vitro and have been employed successfully to treat individuals with the hereditary form of the disease.[68,197]

Although C1-INH is the only recognized inhibitor of C1 esterase activity, it also participates in regulating the plasma kinin system and some of the enzymes in the coagulation and fibrinolytic cascades.[68,197] Plasma from these patients exhibits an impaired ability to inactivate kallikrein, and it has been suggested that this impairment is responsible for the manifestations of HAE. However, subcutaneous injection of bradykinin produces pain and swelling, and intravenous infusion induces hypotension, none of which are characteristic of HAE.[68] In contrast, intradermal injection of activated C1s leads to nonpainful, nonpruritic swelling in both humans and guinea pigs. This response does not occur if activated C1 is injected into C2-deficient individuals or guinea pigs, but it was observed upon injection into a C3-deficient patient.[202] Consequently, these data favor the hypothesis that the clinical manifestations of this disorder are due to the release of an anaphylatoxic-like peptide from the C2b fragment of the C2 molecule. It is also possible that symptoms result from the interaction of several factors from these cascade systems.[68]

Studies employing a cDNA probe to examine Southern digests of DNA from families with type 1 HAE[203] and studies of mutant C1-INH molecules from unrelated families with type 2 HAE[204] have shown that the genetic basis for both types of this disorder is an alteration in the structural gene for C1-INH. These studies also make it clear that the molecular basis for this alteration frequently differs among unrelated families.[204]

Paroxysmal Nocturnal Hemoglobinuria. Another syndrome in which the function of complement regulatory proteins is deranged is paroxysmal nocturnal hemoglobinuria (PNH).[205,206] The basic problem in such individuals is an increased susceptibility of their red blood cells to hemolysis. The disease is uncommon but usually presents in young adults during the third to fifth decades. Occasionally it may be observed in association with drug-induced aplastic anemia, but in most instances there is no apparent inciting event. Classically, individuals present with bouts of hemolysis that are worse at night and last for several days to weeks. The precipitating events responsible for these bouts of hemolysis are usually inapparent, although they are occasionally associated with infection. The basis for the increased hemolysis at nighttime is not clear but may relate to a lower pH in the small vessels of the peripheral venous circulation. Although this is the classic picture of the disease, the more common presentation, occurring in about half of the patients, is one of chronic hemolysis. Patients may have back pain, crampy abdominal pain, and headaches. Some of these individuals are prone to venous thrombosis, especially after surgery, while others may have slightly more frequent infections. Thrombocytopenia and/or leukopenia develop in most individuals at some point during their illness.[205,206]

The peripheral blood of individuals with PNH contains varying proportions of three populations of red blood cells. PNH type 1 cells are normal, whereas type 2 and type 3 PNH cells exhibit a 3- to 6- and 15- to 25-fold increase in sensitivity to complement-mediated lysis, respectively. The severity of the clinical picture correlates best with the proportion of type 3 cells present in the peripheral circulation.[207]

Identification of surface proteins that downregulate the effect of C3b deposited on host cells led to the discovery that types 2 and 3 PNH cells lack one of these proteins, decay-accelerating factor (DAF).[208–210] Moreover, if normal erythrocytes are treated with antibody to DAF, they behave like PNH type 2 cells, and if DAF is inserted in the membrane of type 2 cells, they behave like normal (type 1) cells. However, insertion of DAF into the membrane of PNH type 3 cells, while circumventing increased C3b uptake, has no effect on their increased susceptibility to complement-mediated lysis.[211] Thus although both PNH type 2 and 3 cells lack DAF, the greatly increased sensitivity to complement-mediated lysis, which is the physiologic basis[207,211] for the clinical manifestations of the disorder, is determined by another factor. This factor appears to be the absence of a second complement-regulatory protein, homologous restriction protein (HRP or C8 binding protein), from PNH type 3 cells.[212] Thus, the latter cells are missing two important membrane proteins that protect host cells from complement-mediated damage. Other studies have demonstrated that these cells are missing or have reduced amounts of additional surface proteins including acetycholinesterase, alkaline phosphatase, and lymphocyte function-associated antigen 3 (LFA-3).[207,211,213] Some of these molecules are missing from the surface of platelets and neutrophils isolated from patients with PNH,[209,214] a finding that may help to explain the increased susceptibility of these individuals to episodes of venous thrombosis and infection.

The fact that these molecules are present in normal amounts on human cells, for example, endothelial cells, that are not bone marrow derived supports the origin of this disorder as a clonal abnormality within bone marrow precursor cells. Recently it has been established that the surface molecules that are absent or present in reduced amounts on PNH cells are unique in that they are bound to the membrane through a carboxy terminal glycolipid linkage.[215] Thus, although the physiologic basis for the clinical symptomatology observed in this disorder is the absence of the complement-regulatory proteins from PNH cells, the molecular basis for the absence of these proteins is probably an abnormality in the metabolic pathway by which these surface proteins become anchored to the cell membrane through glycolipid linkages[216] or to a basic defect in the membrane lipids themselves, which secondarily affects this process.

Miscellaneous Deficiency States. Additional deficiency states related to the complement system include the neutrophil iC3b (CR3) receptor deficiency[217] (see Chapter 7), the deficiency of a C5a inhibitor molecule in familial Mediterranean fever,[218,219] and a deficiency of anaphylatoxin inactivator (carboxypeptidase B).[220]

COMPLEMENT IN DISEASE STATES

Complement activation has been demonstrated in a wide variety of diseases, which suggests that products of this activation may play a role in the development of symptoms or in the outcome of these disorders. Evidence supporting this suggestion includes the fact that the extent of complement activation parallels disease activity, that complement deposition can be demonstrated at the site of tissue injury, the finding of altered complement metabolism in various disease states, and the demonstration that complement activation modulates the course of disease in animal models of these disorders. In this context, the role of complement has been most extensively studied in infectious diseases, rheumatologic conditions, renal diseases, and hemolytic states. The recent demonstration of the MAC in ischemic myocardium,[221–225] renal tissue in various immune and nonimmunologic renal diseases,[226–233] the skin of individuals with immunologically mediated dermatitis,[234] the cerebrospinal fluid of individuals with central nervous system lupus erythematosus,[235] and the serum and peripheral nerves of individuals with Guillain-Barré syndrome as well as other demyelinating diseases[236–238] implicates this complex in tissue damage in these disorders.

Infectious Diseases

Complement activation probably occurs during most infections but can be particularly impressive in diseases like dengue fever, bacterial endocarditis, and bacteremia in which the organisms or their products react with antibodies to form circulating immune complexes and initiate complement consumption. Complement consumption is particularly striking in meningococcal disease and other forms of gram-negative bacteremia. Complement activation via the alternative pathway has been well documented in gram-negative sepsis, with the greatest degree of activation occurring in patients with shock.[239] Whether complement activation contributes to shock or is a consequence of the development of shock itself has been a matter of debate. Circulating C5a has been associated with the development of the acute respiratory distress syndrome in humans[240,241] and in a monkey model of gram-negative shock.[242] In the latter, mortality could be prevented and morbidity attenuated by the administration of antibody to C5a.[243] The observation that individuals with inherited C5, C6, C7, or C8 deficiency have a 6000-fold greater frequency of meningococcal disease, but 10-fold less mortality than do persons with a normal complement system (see Table 4) suggests that the ability to assemble the MAC may increase mortality.[165] The increase in mortality may relate to the release of endotoxin, which occurs upon insertion of the MAC in the outer membrane of gram-negative bacteria. Endotoxin release under such circumstances may contribute to the development of shock via its role as a potent stimulus for tumor necrosis factor synthesis[243,244] and by the continued activation of both complement pathways.

Complement, in conjunction with the organs of the reticuloendothelial system, plays a critical role in the removal of encapsulated bacteria from the blood stream.[245] Delineation of the contribution of these variables to the clearance process has been accomplished in an animal model of pneumococcal bacteremia and has demonstrated that the more virulent the organism, the greater the role of the spleen in performing this clearance function.[246,247] Complement depletion of the animals led to a significant decrease in the number of pneumococci needed to kill 50 percent of the animals, thus demonstrating an important role for complement in the clearance function. In addition, clearance of pneumococci was similar in healthy and C4-deficient animals, thus indicating that complement activation and fixation to the bacteria via the alternative pathway was particularly relevant in this process. Last, the presence of immune antibody shifted the burden of clearance from the spleen to the liver, but this effect was absolutely dependent upon a functional alternative complement pathway.[248]

An increased susceptibility to infection is observed both in individuals undergoing splenectomy as well as in individuals with intact but nonfunctioning spleens, for example, patients with sickle cell anemia.[249,250] The incidence of infection varies from a low of approximately 1 percent in individuals undergoing incidental splenectomy to a high of approximately 25 percent in individuals undergoing splenectomy as treatment for thalassemia.[250] The mortality rate in these individuals varies between 40 and 80 percent depending on the underlying condition prompting splenectomy. A wide variety of organisms have been reported to cause overwhelming sepsis in splenectomized individuals, but the pneumococcus accounts for 50–70 percent of such infections, with the bulk of the remainder being accounted for by the meningococcus, *H. influenzae*, and to a lesser extent *E. coli*.[250] The typical presentation of such individuals is that of septic shock, disseminated intravascular coagulopathy, and the adult respiratory distress syndrome occurring in the absence of a primary site of infection.[251]

Rheumatologic Disorders

Substantial clinical and experimental evidence links complement deficiency syndromes and complement activation to a variety of rheumatologic diseases, most notably SLE.[252] Additional support for this relationship is the finding that pharmacologic agents, for example, hydralazine and isoniazid, associated with the drug-induced form of SLE inactivate C4 by nucleophilic attack on its internal thiolester and formation of amide bonds.[253] Evidence that complement activation may be associated with the manifestations of the disease and tissue injury includes the demonstration of C3 and immune complex deposition at the dermal–epidermal junction in the cutaneous lesions from patients with both SLE and discoid lupus erthyematosus. Similar immunohistochemical alterations have been demonstrated in biopsy specimens of healthy skin from the same individuals. However, the recent finding of MACs in areas of affected but not unaffected skin from these individuals strengthens the hypothesis that complement activation may partly mediate tissue injury in these disorders.[235]

In addition to these effects in the tissues, the sera from about 40 percent of patients with SLE contain an inhibitor of C5a-derived chemotactic activity.[254–256] Its presence correlates with disease activity and the resultant chemotactic defect with the enhanced susceptibility of these patients to infection. The inhibitor has been identified as the Bb fragment of factor B, and it exerts its effect by blocking the interaction of C5a des-arg with its cochemotaxin in serum.[115] The presence of free Bb in the serum of these individuals reflects alternative-pathway activation and substantiates the utility of complement component quantitation in assessing disease activity.

Incorporation of C3 into immune complexes promotes their binding to C3b receptors (CR1) on erythrocytes, and the number of these receptors is reduced in individuals with disorders like SLE that are characterized by circulating immune complexes.[253,257] The degree of CR1 reduction correlates well with disease activity and the extent of complement activation. These and other data indicate that erythrocyte CR1 is removed along with immune complexes during passage through the liver and spleen. The decrease in CR1 coupled with the inability of circulating red cells to resynthesize them further exacerbates the defect in immune complex clearance, thereby promoting their deposition in the tissues, with resultant damage to the host.

Renal Disorders

Complement deposition in renal disease associated with immune disorders is related to the deposition of immune complexes within the kidney,[226–229,231–233] whereas complement deposition in the absence of immune complexes is postulated to occur by activation of the alternative pathway.[230] Recently, a rat model of chronic tubulointerstitial disease has been used to investigate the mode of complement deposition and its role in producing injury.[230] In the diseased rats, the loss of renal mass and function was correlated with increased ammonia production and systemic acidosis. Under these conditions, peritubular deposition of C3 and the MAC was readily demonstrated. However, deposition of these components and evidence of tubulointerstitial inflammation were markedly decreased in diseased animals treated with sodium bicarbonate. These and other results suggest that ammonia attacks the C3 internal thiolester to form amidated C3. Amidated C3 serves to activate the alternative complement pathway in the fluid phase, leads to C3 and C5b-9 deposition in the tissue, and elicits an inflammatory response and tissue injury.[230,258] The resulting intrarenal complement depletion may also contribute to the development of chronic bacterial pyelonephritis.[259]

Local ammonia production may also play a role in complement deposition in ischemic tissue. The mechanism of ammonia formation in such tissues involves the release of adenosine from affected cells and its deamination to ammonia by the adenosine deamidase present in circulating erthyrocytes.[260,261]

The use of C6-sufficient and -deficient rabbits and the infusion of C8-deficient serum into rats has clearly demonstrated that the development of proteinuria in membranous glomerulonephritis is dependent upon the assembly and deposition of a complete MAC on the glomerular epithelial cells.[228,232] A substantial portion of this injury results from MAC-mediated stimulation of prostaglandin and thromboxane synthesis since the proteinuria could be inhibited by treatment with indomethacin, an inhibitor of cyclo-oxygenase.[262]

Many patients with chronic renal disease ultimately require hemodialysis. Exposure of plasma to first-use filter membranes during dialysis results in complement activation.[263] Anaphylatoxins released during this process, for example, C5a, have been associated in a concentration-dependent and temporal fashion with the onset of respiratory distress in some dialysis patients.[241,263,264] This association is believed to relate in part to C5a-dependent neutrophil aggregation and stimulation and the formation of microemboli and their deposition in the lung[241] (see Chapter 7).

EVALUATION AND TREATMENT OF COMPLEMENT DISORDERS

Evaluation

Evaluation of the complement system is indicated when the diagnosis of a complement deficiency state is being considered or when specific measures of complement proteins are being used to assess disease activity or response to therapy. As pointed out earlier, several clinical clues should lead the clinician to suspect a complement deficiency state.[165] Foremost among these is a medical or family history of recurrent systemic infection caused by encapsulated bacteria, especially meningococci. A family history of fulminant meningococcal disease occurring in males in skipped generations should suggest the possibility of X-linked properdin deficiency. Meningococcal disease occurring in individuals over 10 years of age, especially when caused by non-group B meningococci, warrants evaluation of the complement system since 5–10 percent of these individuals will have a complement deficiency state, even in the absence of recurrent disease. Likewise, a history of SLE in family members or the occurrence of atypical features of SLE should also suggest the need to evaluate the complement system. Specific syndromes including partial lipodystrophy, angioedema, and PNH are other indications for the specific measurement of complement function or related activities.

Since any of a number of specific complement deficiencies can produce one of the typical clinical syndromes associated with these disorders, it is important to use a test that measures the function of the entire complement cascade during the initial evaluation of such patients. The most common of these tests is the CH_{50}, which measures the function of the classical and terminal complement pathways. When defects in the alternative pathway are being considered, an analogous test evaluating alternative-pathway function should be requested. Many hospital laboratories do not perform the latter test, so it may be necessary to contact a research or commercial laboratory with specific expertise in this area. A negative or extremely low result in either of these two assays warrants further diagnostic evaluation. The combined results of the tests of classical- and alternative-pathway function should suggest which additional tests need to be performed. If both the classical- and alternative-pathway CH_{50} values are extremely low, the defect must lie in one of the components shared by both pathways, i.e., C3 through C9 (see Fig. 1). If the alternative pathway is normal but the classical pathway is not, the deficient component must be either C1, C2, or C4. Conversely, a normal classical but defective alternative pathway suggests a defect in factors D or B, or properdin. The diagnosis of these specific defects can frequently be accomplished by using immunochemical methods to demonstrate an absence of the relevant antigen. However, several complement deficiency states involve absent function in the presence of normal amounts of antigenic protein; thus confirmation of the diagnosis of a specific component deficiency should be documented by using functional assays for the protein under consideration. Such assays usually require the expertise of a complement laboratory.

Treatment

There are two aspects of the treatment of complement deficiency states: replacement of the missing protein and prevention of infection. Although advances in our knowledge of the molecular basis for the various complement deficiency states may provide an alternative means of therapy in the future, replacement of a deficient component at the present time generally requires the infusion of fresh frozen plasma. This approach has been successfully employed in therapy for acute attacks of angioedema[68,197] and in restoring C3 levels toward normal in individuals with C3 deficiency. This approach suffers from several drawbacks. First, the half-life of most complement proteins in vivo is short,[15] although a notable exception occurs in patients with low C3 levels secondary to factor I deficiency. In these patients, replacement therapy restores factor I activity, thereby markedly reducing the accelerated breakdown of C3 that is observed in this disorder.[265] Second, replacement of a genetically absent protein may stimulate the production of antibody to the missing component, thereby limiting the value of subsequent therapy. This consideration is of limited concern in individuals with autosomally inherited disorders such as hereditary angioedema whose serum contains some normal protein or in individuals with other complement deficiency disorders characterized by the presence of antigenically normal amounts of a dysfunctional protein. Third, the relative infrequency of infection in most of these individuals must be balanced against the potential risk of acquiring non-A, non-B hepatitis or human immunodeficiency virus (HIV) infection during plasma infusion, especially since alternative modes of therapy are available. Whether the acute infusion of fresh frozen plasma might be beneficial in the treatment of life-threatening infections,[266] especially in properdin-deficient patients, remains an untested possibility. The use of impeded androgens to enhance the in vivo biosynthesis of C1-INH provides a long-term alternative approach to the replacement of this protein.[68,197,267]

Prevention of infection in complement-deficient patients is best achieved through vaccination. Deficient individuals should be vaccinated with the tetravalent meningococcal, polyvalent pneumococcal, and *Haemophilus influenzae* capsular polysaccharide vaccines. Successful vaccination leads to the production of anticapsular antibodies that promote utilization of the classical pathway in individuals with an alternative-pathway defect and facilitate alternative-pathway utilization in individuals lacking one of the classical-pathway components.[42,187] In such individuals, these antibodies may promote bactericidal activity as well as microbial elimination by enhancing opsonophagocytosis. Although anticapsular antibody cannot enhance serum bactericidal activity in individuals with a deficiency of one of the terminal complement proteins, it should promote opsonization and killing of these organisms by phagocytic cells.[193] In view of experimental evidence indicating a suboptimal response to protein and polysaccharide antigens in C1-, C2-, C4-, and C3-deficient humans and animals, documentation of the patient's response to vaccination with these antigens seems prudent.

Anecdotal evidence suggests that prophylactic antibiotics may have use in the rare complement-deficient patient who experiences several episodes of systemic infection over a short period of time.[268] However, the use of this approach is unlikely to be successful in preventing infections for prolonged periods. A potentially more important use of appropriate antibiotics is to eliminate the carrier state in complement-deficient individuals receiving treatment for systemic infections caused by meningococci or *Haemophilus influenzae*.

REFERENCES

1. Ross GD. Introduction and history of complement research. In: Ross GD, ed. Immunobiology of the Complement System. Orlando, FL: Academic Press; 1986:1–20.
2. Ratnoff WD. A war with the molecules: Louis Pillemer and the history of properdin. Perspect Biol Med. 1980;23:638–57.
3. Lepow IH. Louis Pillemer, properdin, and scientific controversy. J Immunol. 1980;125:471–8.
4. Root RK, Ryan JL. Humoral immunity and complement. In: Mandell GL, Douglas RG Jr, Bennett JE, eds. Principles and Practice of Infectious Diseases. 2nd ed. New York: Churchill Livingstone; 1985:31–56.
5. Morris KM, Aden DP, Knowles BB, et al. Complement biosynthesis by the human hepatoma-derived cell line HepG2. J Clin Invest. 1982;70:906–13.
6. Perlmutter DH, Colten HR. Molecular immunobiology of complement biosynthesis: A model of single-cell control of effector–inhibitor balance. Annu Rev Immunol. 1986;4:231–51.
7. Alper CA, Raum D, Awdeh ZL, et al. Studies of hepatic synthesis in vivo of plasma proteins, including orosomucoid, transferrin, α_1-antitrypsin, C8, and factor B. Clin Immunol Immunopathol. 1980;16:84–9.
8. Mier JW, Dinarello CA, Atkins MB, et al. Regulation of hepatic acute phase protein synthesis by products of interleukin 2 (IL 2)-stimulated human peripheral blood mononuclear cells. J Immunol. 1987;139:1268–72.
9. Baumann H, Richards C, Gauldie J. Interaction among hepatocyte-stimulating factors, interleukin 1, and glucocorticoids for regulation of acute phase plasma proteins in human hepatoma (HepG2) cells. J Immunol. 1987;139:4122–8.
10. Beatty DW, Davis AE III, Cole FS, et al. Biosynthesis of complement by human monocytes. Clin Immunol Immunopathol. 1981;18:334–43.
11. Cole FS, Auerbach HS, Goldberger G, et al. Tissue-specific pretranslational regulation of complement production in human mononuclear phagocytes. J Immunol. 1985;134:2610–6.
12. Strunk RC, Cole FS, Perlmutter DH, et al. γ-Interferon increases expression of class III complement genes C2 and factor B in human monocytes and in murine fibroblasts transfected with human C2 and factor B genes. J Biol. Chem. 1985;260:15280–5.
13. Strunk RC, Whitehead AS, Cole FS. Pretranslational regulation of the synthesis of the third component of complement in human mononuclear phagocytes by the lipid A portion of lipopolysaccharide. J Clin Invest. 1985;76:985–90.
14. Hetland G, Eskeland T. Formation of the functional alternative pathway of complement by human monocytes in vitro as demonstrated by phagocytosis of agarose beads. Scand J Immunol. 1986;23:301–8.
15. Ruddy S, Carpenter CB, Chin KW, et al. Human complement metabolism: An analysis of 144 studies. Medicine (Baltimore). 1975;54:165–78.
16. Notarangelo LD, Chirico G, Chaira A, et al. Activity of classical and alternative pathways of complement in preterm and small for gestational age infants. Pediatr Res. 1984;18:281–5.
17. Johnston RB Jr, Altenburger KM, Atkinson AW Jr, et al. Complement in the newborn infant. Pediatrics. 1979;64(Pt 2, Suppl):781–6.
18. Mills EL, Björksten B, Quie PG. Deficient alternative complement pathway activity in newborn sera. Pediatr Res. 1979;13:1341–4.
19. Edwards MS, Buffone GJ, Fuselier PA, et al. Deficient classical complement pathway activity in newborn sera. Pediatr Res. 1983;17:685–8.
20. Fearon DT. Complement. J Allergy Clin Immunol. 1983;71:520–9.
21. Lachmann PJ, Hughes-Jones NC. Initiation of complement activation. Springer Semin Immunopathol. 1984;7:143–62.
22. Cooper NR. The classical complement pathway: Activation and regulation of the first complement component. Adv Immunol. 1985;37:151–216.
23. Arlaud GJ, Colomb MG, Gagnon J. A functional model of the human C1 complex. Immunol Today. 1987;8:106–11.
24. Schumaker VN, Zavodszky, P, Poon RH. Activation of the first component of complement. Annu Rev Immunol. 1987;5:21–42.
25. Müller-Eberhard HJ. Molecular organization and function of the complement system. Annu Rev Biochem. 1988;57:321–47.
26. Gordon DL, Hostetter MK. Complement and host defense against microorganisms. *Pathology*. 1986,18:365–75.
27. Isenman DE, Young JR. The molecular basis for the difference in immune hemolysis activity of the Chido and Rodgers isotypes of human complement component C4. J Immunol. 1984;132:3019–27.
28. Law SKA, Dodds AW, Porter RR. A comparison of the properties of two classes, C4A and C4B, of the human complement component C4. EMBO J. 1984;3:1819–23.
29. Dodds AW, Law SK, Porter RR. The origin of the very variable haemolytic activities of the common human complement component C4 allotypes including C4-A6. EMBO J. 1985;4:2239–44.
30. Schifferli JA, Steiger G, Paccaud J-P, et al. Difference in the biological properties of the two forms of the fourth component of human complement (C4). Clin Exp Immunol. 1986;63:473–7.
31. Schifferli JA, Hauptmann G, Paccaud J-P. Complement-mediated adherence of immune complexes to human erythrocytes. FEBS Lett. 1987;213:415–8.
32. Naama JK, Niven IP, Zoma A, et al. Complement, antigen–antibody complexes and immune complex disease. J Clin Lab Immunol. 1985;17:59–67.
33. Pangburn MK, Müller-Eberhard HJ. The alternative pathway of complement. Springer Semin Immunopathol. 1984;7:163–92.
34. Pangburn MK. The alternative pathway. In: Ross GD, ed. Immunobiology of the Complement System. Orlando, FL: Academic Press; 1986:45–62.
35. Densen P, McRill C, Ross SC. The contribution of the alternative and classical complement pathways to gonococcal killing and C3 fixation. In: Poolman JT, Zanen HC, Meyer TF, et al, eds. Gonococci and Meningococci. Dordrecht: Kluwer Academic Publishers; 1988:693–7.
36. Fearon DT, Austen KF. Properdin: Initiation of alternative complement pathway. Immunology. 1975;72:3220–4.
37. Fearon DT, Austen KF. Properdin: Binding to C3b and stabilization of the C3b-dependent C3 convertase. J Exp Med. 1975;142:856–63.
38. Fearon DT, Austen KF. The alternative pathway of complement—a system for host resistance to microbial infection. N Engl J Med. 1980;303:259–63.
39. Hunsicker LG, Ruddy S, Austen KF. Alternate complement pathway: Factors involved in cobra venom factor (CoVF) activation of the third component of complement (C3). J Immunol. 1973;110:128–38.
40. Müller-Eberhard HJ, Schreiber. Molecular biology and chemistry of the alternative pathway of complement. Adv Immunol. 1980;29:1–53.
41. Vogel C-W, Smith CA, Müller-Eberhard HJ. Cobra venom factor: Structural homology with the third component of human complement. J Immunol. 1984;133:3235–41.
42. Söderström C, Braconier JH, Danielsson D, et al. Bactericidal activity for *Neisseria meningitidis* in properdin-deficient sera. J Infect Dis. 1987;156:107–12.
43. Schenkein HA, Ruddy S. The role of immunoglobulins in alternative complement pathway activation by zymosan. II. The effect of IgG on the kinetics of the alternative pathway. J Immunol. 1981;126:11–5.
44. Ratnoff WD, Fearon DT, Austen KF. The role of antibody in the activation of the alternative complement pathway. Springer Semin Immunopathol. 1983;6:361–71.

45. Winkelstein JA, Shin HS. The role of immunoglobulin in the interaction of pneumococci and the properdin pathway: Evidence for its specificity and lack of requirement for the Fc portion of the molecule. J Immunol. 1974;112:1635–42.
46. Nelson B, Ruddy S. Enhancing role of IgG in lysis of rabbit erythrocytes by the alternative pathway of human complement. J Immunol. 1979;122:1994–9.
47. Schenkein HA, Ruddy S. The role of immunoglobulins in alternative complement pathway activation by zymosan. I. Human IgG with specificity for zymosan enhances alternative pathway activation by zymosan. J Immunol. 1981;126:7–10.
48. Nicholson-Weller A, Daha MR, Austen KF. Different functions for specific guinea pig IgG1 and IgG2 in the lysis of sheep erythrocytes by C4-deficient guinea pig serum. J Immunol. 1981;126:1800–4.
49. Capel PJA, Groeneboer O, Grosveld G, et al. The binding of activated C3 to polysaccharides and immunoglobulins. J Immunol. 1978;121:2566–72.
50. Fries LF, Gaither TA, Hammer CH, et al. C3b covalently bound to IgG demonstrates a reduced rate of inactivation by factors H and I. J Exp Med. 1984;160:1640–55.
51. Joiner KA, Fries LF, Schmetz MA, et al. IgG bearing covalently bound C3b has enhanced bactericidal activity for *Escherichia coli* 0111. J Exp Med. 1985;162:877–89.
52. Lambris JD, Müller-Eberhard HJ. The multifunctional role of C3: Structural analysis of its interactions with physiological ligands. Mol Immunol. 1986;23:1237–42.
53. Suter S, Nydegger UE, Roux L, et al. Cleavage of C3 by neutral proteases from granulocytes in pleural empyema. J Infect Dis. 1981;144:499–508.
54. Manthei U, Strunk RC, Giclas PC. Acute local inflammation alters synthesis, distribution, and catabolism of the third component of complement in rabbits. J Clin Invest. 1984;74:424–3.
55. Wetsel RA, Lemons RS, Le Beau MM, et al. Molecular analysis of human complement component C5: Localization of the structural gene to chromosome 9. Biochemistry. 1988;27:1474–82.
56. Lundwall AB, Wetsel RA, Kristensen T, et al. Isolation and sequence analysis of a cDNA clone encoding the fifth complement component. J Biol Chem. 1985;260:2108–12.
57. Müller-Eberhard HJ. The membrane attack complex of complement. Annu Rev Immunol. 1986;4:503–28.
58. Stanley K, Luzio P. A family of killer proteins. Nature. 1988;334:475–6.
59. Tschopp J, Mollnes T-E. Antigenic crossreactivity of the α subunit of complement component C8 with the cysteine-rich domain shared by complement component C9 and low density lipoprotein receptor. Proc Natl Acad Sci USA. 1986;83:4223–7.
60. Haefliger J-A, Tschopp J, Nardelli D, et al. Complementary DNA cloning of complement C8β and its sequence homology to C9. Biochemistry. 1987;26:3551–6.
61. Monahan JB, Sodetz JM. Binding of the eighth component of human complement to the soluble cytolytic complex is mediated by its β subunit. J Biol Chem. 1980;255:10579–82.
62. Stewart JL, Kolb WP, Sodetz JM. Evidence that C5b recognizes and mediates C8 incorporation into the cytolytic complex of complement. J Immunol. 1987;139:1960–4.
63. Stewart JL, Sodetz JM. Analysis of the specific association of the eighth and ninth components of human complement: Identification of a direct role for the α subunit of C8. Biochemistry 1985;24:4598–602.
64. Stanley KK, Page M, Campbell AK, et al. A mechanism for the insertion of complement component C9 into target membranes. Mol Immunol. 1986;23:451–8.
65. Podack ER. The molecular mechanism of lymphocyte-mediated tumor cell lysis. Immunol Today. 1985;6:21–7.
66. Tschopp J, Masson D, Stanley KK. Structural/functional similarity between proteins involved in complement- and cytotoxic T-lymphocyte-mediated cytolysis. Nature 1986;322:831–4.
67. Shinkai Y, Takio K, Okumura K. Homology of perforin to the ninth component of complement (C9). Nature. 1988;334:525–7.
68. Davis AE III. C1 inhibitor and hereditary angioneurotic edema. Annu Rev Immunol 1988;6:595–628.
69. Holers VM, Cole JL, Lublin DM, et al. Human C3b- and C4b-regulatory proteins: A new multi-gene family. Immunol Today. 1985;6:188–92.
70. Atkinson JP, Farries T. Separation of self from non-self in the complement system. Immunol Today. 1987;8:212–5.
71. Nicholson-Weller A, Burge J, Fearon DT, et al. Isolation of a human erythrocyte membrane glycoprotein with decay-accelerating activity for C3 convertases of the complement system. J Immunol. 1982;129:184–9.
72. Bhakdi S, Maillet F, Muhly M, et al. The cytolytic C5b-9 complement complex: Feedback inhibition of complement activation. Proc Natl Acad Sci USA. 1988;85:1912–6.
73. Densen P, McRill CM, Ross SC. Assembly of the membrane attack complex promotes decay of the alternative pathway C3 convertase on *Neisseria gonorrhoeae*. J Immunol. 1988;141:3902–9.
74. Fearon DT, Austen KF. Activation of the alternative complement pathway with rabbit erythrocytes by circumvention of the regulatory action of endogenous control proteins. J Exp Med 1977;146:22–33.
75. Fearon DT. Regulation by membrane sialic acid of β1H-dependent decay-dissociation of amplification C3 convertase of the alternative complement pathway. Proc Natl Acad Sci USA. 1978;75:1971–5.
76. Kazatchkine MD, Fearon DT, Austen KF. Human alternative complement pathway: membrane-associated sialic acid regulates the competition between B and β1H for cell-bound C3b. J Immunol 1979;122:75–81.
77. Pangburn MK, Morrison DC, Schreiber RD, et al. Activation of the alternative complement pathway: Recognition of surface structures on activators by bound C3b. J Immunol. 1980;124:977–82.
78. Brown EJ, Ramsey J, Hammer CH, et al. Surface modulation of classical pathway activation: C2 and C3 convertase formation and regulation on sheep, guinea pig, and human erythrocytes. J Immunol. 1983;131:403–8.
79. Schönermark S, Rauterberg EW, Shin ML, et al. Homologous species restriction in lysis of human erythrocytes: A membrane-derived protein with C8-binding capacity functions as an inhibitor. J Immunol. 1986;136:1772–6.
80. Shin ML, Hänsch G, Hu VW, et al. Membrane factors responsible for homologous species restriction of complement-mediated lysis: Evidence for a factor other than DAF operating at the stage of C8 and C9. J Immunol. 1986;136:1777–82.
81. Zalman LS, Wood LM, Müller-Eberhard HJ. Isolation of a human erythrocyte membrane protein capable of inhibiting expression of homologous complement transmembrane channels. Proc. Natl Acad Sci USA. 1986;83:6975–9.
82. Hänsch GM, Hammer CH, Vanguri P, et al. Homologous species restriction in lysis of erythrocytes by terminal complement proteins. Proc Natl Acad Sci USA. 1981;78:5118–21.
83. Carney DF, Koski CL, Shin ML. Elimination of terminal complement intermediates from the plasma membrane of nucleated cells: The rate of disappearance differs for cells carrying C5b-7 or C5b-8 or a mixture of C5b-8 with a limited number of C5b-9. J Immunol 1985;134:1804–9.
84. Ramm LE, Whitlow MB, Koski CL, et al. Elimination of complement channels from the plasma membranes of U937, a nucleated mammalian cell line: Temperature dependence of the elimination rate. J Immunol. 1983;131:1411–5.
85. Schlager SI, Ohanian SH, Borsos T. Correlations between the ability of tumor cells to resist humoral immune attack and their ability to synthesize lipid. J Immunol. 1978;120:463–71.
86. Campbell AK, Luzio JP. Intracellular free calcium as a pathogen in cell damage initiated by the immune system. Experientia. 1981;37:1110–2.
87. Imagawa DK, Osifchin NE, Paznekas WA, et al. Consequences of cell membrane attack by complement: Release of arachidonate and formation of inflammatory derivatives. Proc Natl Acad Sci USA. 1983;80:6647–51.
88. Betz M, Hansch GM. Release of arachidonic acid: A new function of the late complement components. Immunobiology. 1984;166:473–83.
89. Hänsch GM, Seitz M, Martinotti G, et al. Macrophages release arachidonic acid, prostaglandin E_2, and thromboxane in response to late complement components. J Immunol. 1984;133:2145–50.
90. Suttorp N, Seeger W, Zinsky S, et al. Complement complex C5b-8 induces PGI_2 formation in cultured endothelial cells. Am J Physiol. 1987;253:13–32.
91. Fearon DT, Wong WW. Complement ligand-receptor interactions that mediate biological responses. Annu Rev Immunol. 1983;1:243–71.
92. Gresham HD, Volanakis JE. Structure and function of human complement receptors: 1985. Year Immunol. 1986;2:177–86.
93. Ross GD, Medof ME. Membrane complement receptors specific for bound fragments of C3. Adv Immunol. 1985;37:217–67.
94. Wilson JG, Andriopoulos NA, Fearon DT. CR1 and the cell membrane proteins that bind C3 and C4. A basic and clinical review. Immunol Res. 1987;6:192–209.
95. Jack RM, Ezzell RM, Hartwig J, et al. Differential interaction of the C3b/C4b receptor and MHC class I with the cytoskeleton of human neutrophils. J Immunol. 1986;137:3996–4003.
96. Hynes RO. Integrins: A family of cell surface receptors. Cell 1987;48:549–54.
97. Wright SD, Reddy A, Jong MTC, et al. C3bi receptor (complement receptor type 3) recognizes a region of complement protein C3 containing the sequence Arg-Gly-Asp. Proc Natl Acad Sci USA. 1987;84:1965–68.
98. Ruoslahti E, Pierschbacher MD. Arg-Gly-Asp: A versatile cell recognition signal. Cell. 1986;44:517–8.
99. Myones BL, Dalzell JG, Hogg N, et al. Neutrophil and monocyte cell surface p150,95 has iC3b-receptor (CR4) activity resembling CR3. J Clin Invest. 1988;81:640–51.
100. Cooper NR, Moore MD, Nemerow GR. Immunobiology of CR2, the B lymphocyte receptor for Epstein-Barr virus and the C3d complement fragment. Annu Rev Immunol. 1988;6:85–113.
101. Fingeroth JD, Weis JJ, Tedder TF, et al. Epstein-Barr virus receptor of human B lymphocytes is the C3d receptor CR2. Proc Natl Acad Sci USA. 1984;81:4510–4.
102. Hugli TE. Biological activities of fragments derived from human complement components. Prog Immunol. 1983:419–26.
103. Perlmutter DH, Colten HR. Complement molecular genetics. In: Gallin JI, Goldstein IM, Snyderman R, eds. Inflammation: Basic Principles and Clinical Correlates. New York: Raven Press; 1988:75–88.
104. Campbell RD. The molecular genetics and polymorphism of C2 and Factor B. Br Med Bull. 1987;43:37–49.
105. Campbell RD, Law SKA, Reid KBM et al. Structure, organization, and regulation of the complement genes. Annu Rev Immunol. 1988;6:161–95.
106. Spies T, Morton CC, Nedospasov SA, et al. Genes for the tumor necrosis factors α and β are linked to the human major histocompatibility complex. Proc Natl Acad Sci USA. 1986;83:8699–702.
107. Awdeh ZL, Raum D, Yunis EJ, et al. Extended HLA/complement allele

haplotypes: Evidence for T/t-like complex in man. Proc Natl Acad Sci USA. 1983;80:259–63.
108. Alper CA, Raum D, Karp S, et al. Serum complement 'supergenes' of the major histocompatibility complex in man (complotypes). Vox Sang. 1983;45:62–7.
109. Porter RR. Complement polymorphism, the major histocompatibility complex and associated diseases: A speculation. Mol Biol Med. 1983;1:161–68.
110. Kristensen T, D'Eustachio P, Ogata RT, et al. The superfamily of C3b/C4b-binding proteins. Fed Proc. 1987;46:2463–9
111. Reid KBM, Bentley DR, Campbell RD, et al. Complement system proteins which interact with C3b or C4b. A superfamily of structurally related proteins. Immunol Today. 1986;7:230–4.
112. Perez HD, Chenoweth DE, Goldstein IM. Attachment of human C5a des Arg to its cochemotaxin is required for maximum expression of chemotactic activity. J Clin Invest. 1986;78:1589–95.
113. Perez HD, Kelly E, Chenoweth D, et al. Identification of the C5a des Arg cochemotaxin. Homology with vitamin D-binding protein (group-specific component globulin). J Clin Invest. 1988;82:360–3.
114. Kew RR, Webster RO. Ge-globulin (vitamin D-binding protein) enhances the neutrophil chemotactic activity of C5a and C5a des Arg. J Clin Invest. 1988;82:364–9.
115. Perez HD, Hooper C, Volanakis J, et al. Specific inhibitor of complement (C5)-derived chemotactic activity in systemic lupus erythematosus related antigenically to the Bb fragment of human factor B. J Immunol. 1987;139:484–9.
116. Miller GW, Nusenzweig V. A new complement function: Solubilization of antigen–antibody aggregates. Proc Natl Acad Sci USA. 1975;72:418–22.
117. Schifferli JA, Ng YC, Peters DK. The role of complement and its receptor in the elimination of immune complexes. N Engl J Med. 1986;315:488–95.
118. Siegel I, Liu TL, Gleicher N. The red-cell immune system. Lancet. 1981;2:556–9.
119. Cornacoff JB, Hebert LA, Smead WL, et al. Primate erythrocyte-immune complex-clearing mechanism. J Clin Invest. 1983;71:236–47.
120. Weiler JM, Ballas ZK, Needleman BW, et al. Complement fragments suppress lymphocyte immune responses. Immunol Today. 1982;3:238–43.
121. Laham MN, Caldwell JR, Panush RS. Modulation of lymphocyte proliferative responses to mitogens and antigens by complement components C1, C4 and C2. J Clin Lab Immunol. 1982;9:39–47.
122. Papamichail M, Gutierrez C, Embling P, et al. Complement dependence of localisation of aggregated IgG in germinal centres. Scand J Immunol. 1975;4:343–7.
123. Ochs HD, Wedgwood RJ, Frank MM, et al. The role of complement in the induction of antibody responses. Clin Exp Immunol. 1983;53:208–16.
124. Böttger EC, Bitter-Suermann D. Complement and the regulation of humoral immune responses. Immunol Today. 1987;8:261–4.
124a. O'Neil KM, Ochs HD, Heller SR, et al. Role of C3 in humoral immunity defective antibody production in C3–deficient dogs. J Immunol. 1988;140:1939–45.
125. Ochs HD, Wedgwood RJ, Heller SR, et al. Complement, membrane glycoproteins, and complement receptors: Their role in regulation of the immune response. Clin Immunol Immunopathol. 1986;40:94–104.
126. Hostetter MK, Krueger RA, Schmeling DJ. The biochemistry of opsonization: Central role of the reactive thiolester of the third component of complement. J Infect Dis. 1984;150:653–61.
127. Taylor PW. Bactericidal and bacteriolytic activity of serum against gram-negative bacteria. Microbiol Rev. 1983;47:46–83.
128. Harriman GR, Esser AF, Podack ER, et al. The role of C9 in complement-mediated killing of *Neisseria*. J Immunol. 1981;127:2386–90.
129. Cooper NR, Nemerow GR. Complement-dependent mechanisms of virus neutralization. In: Ross GD, ed. Immunobiology of the Complement System. Orlando, FL: Academic Press; 1986:139–62.
130. Roantree RJ, Rantz LA. A study of the relationship of the normal bactericidal activity of human serum to bacterial infection. J Clin Invest. 1960;39:72–81.
131. Brown EJ. Interaction of gram-positive microorganisms with complement. Curr Top Microbiol Immunol. 1985;121:159–87.
132. Joiner KA, Grossman N, Schmetz M, et al. C3 binds preferentially to long-chain lipopolysaccharide during alternative pathway activation by *Salmonella montevideo*. J Immunol. 1986;136:710–5.
133. Brown EJ, Joiner KA, Frank MM. The role of complement in host resistance to bacteria. Springer Semin Immunopathol. 1983;6:349–60.
134. Schoolnik GK, Buchanan TM, Holmes KK. Gonococci causing disseminated gonococcal infection are resistant to the bactericidal action of normal human sera. J Clin Invest. 1976;58:1163–73.
135. Joiner KA, Warren KA, Brown EJ, et al. Studies on the mechanism of bacterial resistance to complement-mediated killing. IV. C5b-9 forms high molecular weight complexes with bacterial outer membrane constituents on serum-resistant but not on serum-sensitive *Neisseria gonorrhoeae*. J Immunol. 1983;131:1443–51.
136. Harriman GR, Podack ER, Braude AI, et al. Activation of complement by serum-resistant *Neisseria gonorrhoeae*. J Exp Med. 1982;156:1235–49.
137. Rice PA, Kasper DL. Characterization of gonococcal antigens responsible for induction of bactericidal antibody in disseminated infection. J Clin Invest. 1977;60:1149–58.
138. Densen P, Gulati S, Rice PA. Specificity of antibodies against *Neisseria gonorrhoeae* that stimulate neutrophil chemotaxis. Role of antibodies directed against lipooligosaccharides. J Clin Invest. 1987;80:78–87.
139. Frank MM, Joiner K, Hammer C. The function of antibody and complement in the lysis of bacteria. Rev Infect Dis. 1987;9(Suppl5):537–45.
140. Rice PA, Kasper KL. Characterization of serum resistance of *Neisseria gonorrhoeae* that disseminate. Roles of blocking antibody and gonococcal outer membrane proteins. J Clin Invest. 1982;70:157–67.
141. Rice PA, Vayo HE, Tam MR, et al. Immunoglobulin G antibodies directed against protein III block killing of serum-resistant *Neisseria gonorrhoeae* by immune serum. J Exp Med. 1986;164:1735–48.
142. Joiner KA, Scales R, Warren KA, et al. Mechanism of action of blocking immunoglobulin G for *Neisseria gonorrhoeae*. J Clin Invest. 1985;76:1765–72.
143. Griffiss MJ, Bertram MA. Immunoepidemiology of meningococcal disease in military recruits. II. Blocking of serum bactericidal activity by circulating IgA early in the course of invasive disease. J Infect Dis. 1977;136:733–9.
144. Griffiss JM. Epidemic meningococcal disease: Synthesis of a hypothetical immunoepidemiologic model. Rev Infect Dis. 1982;4:159–72.
145. Griffiss JM, Goroff DK. IgA blocks IgM and IgG-initiated immune lysis by separate molecular mechanisms. J Immunol. 1983;130:2882–5.
146. Griffiss JM. Bactericidal activity of meningococcal antisera. Blocking by IgA of lytic antibody in human convalescent sera. J Immunol. 1975;114:1779–84.
147. Brown EJ, Joiner KA, Cole RM, et al. Localization of complement component 3 on *Streptococcus pneumoniae*: Anti-capsular antibody causes complement deposition on the pneumococcal capsule. Infect Immun. 1983;39:403–9.
148. Joiner K, Hieny S, Kirchhoff LV, et al. gp72, the 72 kilodalton glycoprotein, is the membrane acceptor site for C3 on *Trypanosoma cruzi* epimastigotes. J Exp Med. 1985;161:1196–212.
149. Sher A, Hieny S, Joiner K. Evasion of the alternative complement pathway by metacyclic trypomastigotes of *Trypanosoma cruzi*: Dependence on the developmentally regulated synthesis of surface protein and N-linked carbohydrate. J Immunol. 1986;137:2961–7.
150. Joiner K, Sher A, Gaither T, et al. Evasion of alternative complement pathway by *Trypanosoma cruzi* results from inefficient binding of Factor B. Proc Natl Acad Sci USA. 1986;83:6593–7.
151. Leive LL, Jimenez-Lucho VE. Lipopolysaccharide O-antigen structure controls alternative pathway activation of complement: Effects on phagocytosis and virulence of *Salmonella*. In: Leive L, ed. Microbiology. Washington, DC: American Society for Microbiology; 1986:14–7.
152. Liang-Takasaki C-J, Mäkelä PH, Leive L. Phagocytosis of bacteria by macrophages: Changing the carbohydrate of lipopolysaccharide alters interaction with complement and macrophages. J Immunol. 1982;128:1229–35.
153. Liang-Takasaki C-J, Saxén H, Mäkelä PH, et al. Complement activation by polysaccharide of lipopolysaccharide: An important virulence determinant of *Salmonella*. Infect Immun. 1983;41:563–9.
154. Grossman N, Leive L. Complement activation via the alternative pathway by purified *Salmonella* lipopolysaccharide is affected by its structure but not its O-antigen length. J Immunol. 1984;132:376–85.
155. Grossman N, Joiner KA, Frank MM, et al. C3b binding, but not its breakdown, is affected by the structure of the O-antigen polysaccharide in lipopolysaccharide from *Salmonella*. J Immunol. 1986;136:2208–15.
156. Jimenez-Lucho VE, Joiner KA, Foulds J, et al. C3b generation is affected by the structure of the O-antigen polysaccharide in lipopolysaccharide from *Samonella*. J Immunol. 1987;139:1253–9.
157. Jarvis GA, Vedros NA. Sialic acid of group B *Neisseria meningitidis* regulates alternative complement pathway activation. Infect Immun. 1987;55:174–80.
158. Edwards MS, Kasper DL, Jennings HJ, et al. Capsular sialic acid prevents activation of the alternative complement pathway by type III, group B streptococci. J Immunol. 1982;128:1278–83.
159. Hostetter MK. Serotypic variations among virulent pneumococci in deposition and degradation of covalently bound C3b: Implications for phagocytosis and antibody production. J Infect Dis. 1986;153:682–93.
160. Friedman HM, Cohen GH, Eisenberg RJ, et al. Glycoprotein C of herpes simplex virus 1 acts as a receptor for the C3b complement component on infected cells. Nature. 1984;309:633–5.
161. Friedman HM, Glorioso JC, Cohen GH, et al. Binding of complement component C3b to glycoprotein gC of herpes simplex virus type 1: Mapping of gC-binding sites and demonstration of conserved C3b binding in low-passage clinical isolates. J Virol. 1986;60:470–5.
162. Edwards JE Jr, Gaither TA, O'Shea JJ, et al. Expression of specific binding sites on candida with functional and antigenic characteristics of human complement receptors. J Immunol. 1986;137:3577–83.
163. McNearney TA, Odell C, Holers VM, et al. Herpes simplex virus glycoproteins gC-1 and gC-2 bind to the third component of complement and provide protection against complement-mediated neutralization of viral infectivity. J Exp Med. 1987;166:1525–35.
164. Gilmore BJ, Retsinas EM, Lorenz JS, et al. An iC3b receptor on *Candida albicans*: Structure, function, and correlates for pathogenicity. J Infect Dis. 1988;157:38–46.
165. Ross SC, Densen P. Complement deficiency states and infection: Epidemiology, pathogenesis and consequences of neisserial and other infections in an immune deficiency. Medicine (Baltimore). 1984;63:243–73.
166. Glass D, Raum D, Gibson D, et al. Inherited deficiency of the second component of complement. J Clin Invest. 1976;58:853–61.
167. Cornacoff JB, Hebert LA, Smead WL, et al. Primate erythrocyte-immune complex-clearing mechanism. J Clin Invest 1983;71:236–47.

168. Ellison RT III, Kohler PF, Curd JG, et al. Prevalence of congenital or acquired complement deficiency in patients with sporadic meningococcal disease. N Engl J Med. 1983;308:913–6.
169. Beatty DW, Rynder CR, Hesse HDV. Complement abnormalities during an epidemic of group B meningococcal infection in children. Clin Exp Immunol. 1985;64:465–70.
170. Møller M, Rasmussen J, Brandslund I, et al. Screening for complement deficiencies in unselected patients with meningitis. Clin Exp Immunol. 1987;68:437–45.
171. Zimran A, Rudensky B, Kramer MR, et al. Hereditary complement deficiency in survivors of meningococcal disease: High prevalence of C7/C8 deficiency in sephardic (Moroccan) Jews. Q J Med. 1987;63:349–58.
172. Merino J, Rodriguez-Valverde V, Lamelas JA, et al. Prevalence of deficits of complement components in patients with recurrent meningococcal infections. J Infect Dis. 1983;148:331.
173. Agnello v. Complement deficiency states. Medicine (Baltimore). 1978;57:1–23.
174. Agnello V. Lupus diseases associated with hereditary and acquired deficiencies of complement. Springer Semin Immunopathol. 1986;9:161–78.
175. Provost TT, Arnett FC, Reichlin M. Homozygous C2 deficiency, lupus erythematosus, and anti-Ro (SSA) antibodies. Arthritis Rheum. 1983;26:1279–82.
176. Davis AE III. The efficiency of complement activation in MHC-linked diseases. Immunol Today. 1983;4:250–2.
177. Schifferli JA, Peters DK. Complement, the immune-complex lattice, and the pathophysiology of complement-deficiency syndromes. Lancet. 1983;2:957–9.
178. Schifferli JA, Steiger G, Hauptmann G, et al. Formation of soluble immune complexes by complement in sera of patients with various hypocomplementemic states. J Clin Invest. 1985;76:2127–33.
179. Böttger EC, Hoffmann T, Hadding U, et al. Guinea pigs with inherited deficiencies of complement components C2 or C4 have characteristics of immune complex disease. J Clin Invest. 1986;78:689–95.
180. Awdeh ZL, Raum DD, Glass D, et al. Complement-human histocompatibility antigen haplotypes in C2 deficiency. J Clin Invest. 1981;67:581–3.
181. Kemp ME, Atkinson JP, Skanes VM, et al. Deletion of C4A genes in patients with systemic lupus erythematosus. Arthritis Rheum. 1987;30:1015–22.
182. Howard PF, Hochberg MC, Bias WB, et al. Relationship between C4 null genes, HLA-D region antigens, and genetic susceptibility to systemic lupus erythematosus in Caucasian and Black Americans. Am J Med. 1986;81:187–93.
183. Rowe PC, McLean RH, Wood RA, et al. Association of C4B deficiency with bacterial meningitis (Abstract). Pediatr Res. 1988;23:360.
184. Cole FS, Whitehead AS, Auerbach HS, et al. The molecular basis for genetic deficiency of the second component of human complement. N Engl J Med. 1985;313:11–6.
185. Hauptmann G, Goetz J, Uring-Lambert B, et al. Component deficiencies. 2. The fourth component. Progr Allergy. 1986;39:232–49.
186. Sjöholm, AG, Braconier J-H, Söderström C. Properdin deficiency in a family with fulminant meningococcal infections. Clin Exp Immunol. 1982;50:291–7.
187. Densen P, Weiler JM, Griffiss JM, et al. Familial properdin deficiency and fatal meningococcemia. Correction of the bactericidal defect by vaccination. N Engl J Med. 1987;316:922–6.
188. Sjöholm, AG, Söderström, C. Nilsson L-A. A second variant of properdin deficiency: The detection of properdin at low concentration in affected males. Complement. 1988;5:130–40.
189. Sjöholm AG, Kuijper EJ, Tijssen CC, et al. Dysfunctional properdin in a Dutch family with meningococcal disease. N Engl J Med. 1988;319:33–7.
190. Sissons JGP, West RJ, Fallow J, et al. The complement abnormalities of lipodystrophy. N Engl J Med. 1976;294:461–5.
191. Ipp MM, Minta JO, Gelfand EW. Disorders of the complement system in lipodystrophy. Clin Immunol Immunopathol. 1977;7:281–7.
192. Nicholson A, Lepow IH. Host defense against *Neisseria meningitidis* requires a complement-dependent bactericidal activity. Science. 1979;205:298–9.
193. Densen P. Interaction of complement with *Neisseria meningitidis* and *Neisseria gonorrhoeae*. Clin Microbiol Rev. 1989;2:(April, in press).
194. Ross SC, Rosenthal PJ, Berberich HM, et al. Killing of *Neisseria meningitidis* by human neutrophils: Implications for normal and complement-deficient individuals. J Infect Dis. 1987;155:1266–75.
195. Orren A, Potter PC, Cooper RC, et al. Deficiency of the sixth component of complement and susceptibility to *Neisseria meningitidis* infections: Studies in 10 families and five isolated cases. Immunology. 1987;62:249–53.
196. Ross SC, Berberich HM, Densen P. Natural serum bactericidal activity against *Neisseria meningitidis* isolates from disseminated infections in normal and complement-deficient hosts. J Infect Dis. 1985;152:1332–5.
197. Frank MM, Gelfand JA, Atkinson JP. Hereditary angioedema: The clinical syndrome and its management. Ann Intern Med. 1976;84:580–93.
198. Frank MM. C1 esterase inhibitor: Clinical clues to the pathophysiology of angioedema. J Allergy Clin Immunol. 1986;78:848–50.
199. Frank MM. The C1 esterase inhibitor and hereditary angioedema. J Clin Immunol. 1982;2:65–8.
200. Geha RS, Quinti I, Austen KF, et al. Acquired C1-inhibitor deficiency associated with antiidiotypic antibody to monoclonal immunoglobulins. N Engl J Med. 1985;312:534–40.
201. Alsenz J, Bork K, Loos M. Autoantibody-mediated acquired deficiency of C1 inhibitor. N Engl J Med. 1987;316:1360–6.
202. Strang CJ, Auerbach HS, Rosen FS. C1s-induced vascular permeability in C2-deficient guinea pigs. J Immunol. 1986;137:631–5.
203. Stoppa-Lyonnet D, Tosi M, Laurent J, et al. Altered C1 inhibitor genes in type I hereditary angioedema. N Engl J Med. 1987;317:1–6.
204. Donaldson VH, Harrison RA, Rosen FS. Variability in purified dysfunctional C1-inhibitor proteins from patients with hereditary angioneurotic edema. Functional and analytical gel studies. J Clin Invest. 1985;75:124–32.
205. Rosse WF. Paroxysmal nocturnal hemoglobinuria. In: Williams WJ, Beutler E, Erslev AJ, Rundles RW, eds. Hematology. New York: McGraw-Hill; 1972;460–74.
206. Rosse WF, Parker CJ. Paroxysmal nocturnal haemoglobinuria. Clin Haematol. 1985;14:105–25.
207. Rosse WF. The control of complement activation by the blood cells in paroxysmal nocturnal hemoglobinuria. Blood. 1986;67:268–9.
208. Nicholson-Weller A, March JP, Rosenfeld SI, et al. Affected erythrocytes of patients with paroxysmal nocturnal hemoglobinuria are deficient in the complement regulatory protein, decay accelerating factor. Proc Natl Acad Sci USA. 1983;80:5066–70.
209. Nicholson-Weller A, Spicer DB, Austen KF. Deficiency of the complement regulatory protein, "decay-accelerating factor," on membranes of granulocytes, monocytes, and platelets in paroxysmal nocturnal hemoglobinuria. N Engl J Med. 312:1091–7.
210. Pangburn MK, Schreiber RD, Müller-Eberhard HJ. Deficiency of an erythrocyte membrane protein with complement regulatory activity in paroxysmal nocturnal hemoglobinuria. Proc Natl Acad Sci USA. 1983;80:5430–4.
211. Medof ME, Gottlieb A, Kinoshita T, et al. Relationship between decay accelerating factor deficiency, diminished acetylcholinesterase activity, and defective terminal complement pathway restriction in paroxysmal nocturnal hemoglobinuria erythrocytes. J Clin Invest. 1987;80:165–74.
212. Hänsch GM, Schönermark S, Roelcke D. Paroxysmal nocturnal hemoglobinuria type III. Lack of an erythrocyte membrane protein restricting the lysis of C5b-9. J Clin Invest. 1987;80:7–12.
213. Selvaraj P, Dustin ML, Silber R, et al. Deficiency of lymphocyte function-associated antigen 3 (LFA-3) in paroxysmal nocturnal hemoglobinuria. Functional correlates and evidence for a phosphatidylinositol membrane anchor. J Exp Med. 1987;166:1011–25.
214. Kinoshita T, Medof ME, Silber R, et al. Distribution of decay-accelerating factor in the peripheral blood of normal individuals and patients with paroxysmal nocturnal hemoglobinuria. J Exp Med. 1985;162:75–92.
215. Medof ME, Walter EI, Roberts WL, et al. Decay accelerating factor of complement is anchored to cells by a C-terminal glycolipid. Biochemistry. 1986;25:6740–7.
216. Low MG. Biochemistry of the glycosyl-phosphatidylinositol membrane protein anchors. Biochem J. 1987;244:1–13.
217. Anderson DC, Schmalsteig FC, Finegold MJ. The severe and moderate phenotypes of heritable Mac-1, LFA-1 deficiency: Their quantitative definition and relation to leukocyte dysfunction and clinical features. J Infect Dis. 1985;152:668–89.
218. Matzner Y, Brzezinski A. C5a-inhibitor deficiency in peritoneal fluids from patients with familial Mediterranean fever. N Engl J Med. 1984;311:287–90.
219. Schwabe AD, Lehman TJA. C5a-inhibitor deficiency—a role in familial Mediterranean fever? N Engl J Med. 1984;311:325–6.
220. Mathews KP. Anaphylatoxin inactivator. In: Rother K, Rother U, eds. Hereditary and Acquired Complement Deficiencies in Animals and Man. Basel: S Karger AG; 1986:344–51.
221. Schafer H, Mathey D, Bhakdi HF. Deposition of the terminal C5b-9 complement complex in infarcted areas of human myocardium. J Immunol. 1986;137:1945–9.
222. Rus HG, Niculescu F, Vlaicu R. Presence of C5b-9 complement complex and S-protein in human myocardial areas with necrosis and sclerosis. Immunol Lett. 1987;16:15–20.
223. Rus HG, Niculescu F, Constantinescu E, et al. Immunoelectron-microscopic localization of the terminal C5b-9 complement complex in human atherosclerotic fibrous plaque. Atherosclerosis. 1986;61:35–42.
224. Maroko PR, Carpenter CB, Chiariello M, et al. Reduction by cobra venom factor of myocardial necrosis after coronary artery occlusion. J Clin Invest. 1978;61:661–70.
225. Pinckard RN, O'Rourke RA, Crawford MH, et al. Complement localization and mediation of ischemic injury in baboon myocardium. J Clin Invest. 1980;66:1050–6.
226. Biesecker G, Katz S, Koffler D. Renal localization of the membrane attack complex in systemic lupus erythematosus nephritis. J Exp Med. 1981;151:1790–1.
227. Falk RJ, Dalmasso AP, Kim Y, et al. Neoantigen of the polymerized ninth component of complement. Characterization of a monoclonal antibody and immunohistochemical localization in renal disease. J Clin Invest. 1983;72:560–73.
228. Groggel GC, Adler S, Rennke HG, et al. Role of the terminal complement pathway in experimental membranous nephropathy in the rabbit. J Clin Invest. 1983;72:1948–57.
229. Adler S, Baker PJ, Pritzl P, et al. Detection of terminal complement components in experimental immune glomerular injury. Kidney Int. 1984;26:830–7.
230. Nath KA, Hostetter MK, Hostetter TH. Pathophysiology of chronic tubulo-

interstitial disease in rats. Interactions of dietary acid load, ammonia, and complement component C3. J Clin Invest. 1985;76:667–75.
231. Cybulsky AV, Rennke HG, Feintzeig ID, et al. Complement-induced glomerular epithelial cell injury. Role of the membrane attack complex in rat membranous nephropathy. J Clin Invest. 1986;77:1096–1107.
232. Cybulsky AV, Quigg RJ, Salant DJ. The membrane attack complex in complement-mediated glomerular epithelial cell injury: Formation and stability of C5b-9 and C5b-7 in rat membranous nephropathy. J Immunol. 1986;137:1511–6.
233. Rus HG, Niculescu F, Nanulescu M, et al. Immunohistochemical detection of the terminal C5b-9 complement complex in children with glomerular diseases. Clin Exp Immunol. 1986;65:66–72.
234. Biesecker G, Lavin L, Ziskind M, et al. Cutaneous localization of the membrane attack complex in discoid and systemic lupus erythematosus. N Engl J Med. 1982;306:264–70.
235. Sanders ME, Alexander EL, Koski CL, et al. Detection of activated terminal complement (C5b-9) in cerebrospinal fluid from patients with central nervous system involvement of primary Sjögren's syndrome or systemic lupus erythematosus. J Immunol. 1987;138:2095–9.
236. Koski CL, Sanders ME, Swoveland PT, et al. Activation of terminal components of complement in patients with Guillain-Barré syndrome and other demyelinating neuropathies. J Clin Invest. 1987;80:1492–7.
237. Cammer W, Brosnan CF, Basile C, et al. Complement potentiates the degradation of myelin proteins by plasmin: Implications for a mechanism of inflammatory demyelination. Brain Res. 1986;364:91–101.
238. Mollnes TE, Vandvik B, Lea T, et al. Intrathecal complement activation in neurological diseases evaluated by analysis of the terminal complement complex. J Neurol Sci. 1987;78:17–28.
239. Fearon DT, Ruddy S, Schur PH, et al. Activation of the properdin pathway of complement in patients with gram-negative bacteremia. N Engl J Med. 1975;292:937–40.
240. Weaver LJ, Craddock PR, Jacob HS. Association of complement activation and elevated plasma-C5a with adult respiratory distress syndrome. Pathophysiological relevance and possible prognostic value. Lancet. 1980;1:947–9.
241. Jacob HS, Craddock PR, Hammerschmidt DE, et al. Complement-induced granulocyte aggregation. An unsuspected mechanism of disease. N Engl J Med. 1980;302:789–94.
242. Stevens JH, O'Hanley P, Shapiro JM, et al. Effects of anti-C5a antibodies on the adult respiratory distress syndrome in septic primates. J Clin Invest 1986;77:1812–6.
243. Beutler B, Cerami A. The endogenous mediator of endotoxic shock. Clin Res. 1987;35:192–7.
244. Beutler B, Milsark IW, Cerami AC. Passive immunization against cachectin/tumor necrosis factor protects mice from lethal effect of endotoxin. Science. 1985;229:869–71.
245. Hosea SW, Brown EJ, Frank MM. The critical role of complement in experimental pneumococcal sepsis. J Infect Dis. 1980;142:903–9.
246. Brown EJ, Hosea SW, Frank MM. The role of the spleen in experimental pneumococcal bacteremia. J Clin Invest. 1981;67:975–82.
247. Bohnsack JF, Brown EJ. The role of the spleen in resistance to infection. Annu Rev Med. 1986;37:49–59.
248. Brown EJ, Hosea SW, Frank MM. The role of antibody and complement in the reticuloendothelial clearance of pneumococci from the bloodstream. Rev Infect Dis. 1983;5(Suppl):797–805.
249. Singer DB. Postsplenectomy sepsis. Perspect Pediatr Pathol. 1973;1:285–311.
250. Winkelstein JA, Drachman RH. Deficiency of pneumococcal serum opsonizing activity in sickle-cell disease. N Engl J Med. 1968;279:459–66.
251. Bisno AL, Freeman JC. The syndrome of asplenia, pneumococcal sepsis, and disseminated intravascular coagulation. Ann Intern Med. 1970;72:389–93.
252. Atkinson JP. Complement activation and complement receptors in systemic lupus erythematosus. Springer Semin Immunopathol. 1986;9:179–94.
253. Sim E, Gill EW, Sim RB. Drugs that induce systemic lupus erythematosus inhibit complement component C4. Lancet 1984;2:422–4.
254. Clark RA, Kimball HR, Decker JL. Neutrophil chemotaxis in systemic lupus erythematosus. Ann Rheum Dis. 1974;33:167–172.
255. Perez HD, Lipton M, Goldstein IM. A specific inhibitor of complement (C5)-derived chemotactic activity in serum from patients with systemic lupus erythematosus. J Clin Invest. 1978;62:29–38.
256. Perez HD, Goldstein IM. Polymorphonuclear leukocyte chemotaxis in systemic lupus erythematosus. J Rheumatol. 1987;14:53–8.
257. Ross GD, Yount WJ, Walport MJ, et al. Disease-associated loss of erythrocyte complement receptors (CR1, C3b receptors) in patients with systemic lupus erythematosus and other diseases involving autoantibodies and/or complement activation. J Immunol. 1985;135:2005–14.
258. Gordon DL, Krueger RA, Quie PG, et al. Amidation of C3 at the thiolester site: Stimulation of chemiluminescence and phagocytosis by a new inflammatory mediator. J Immunol. 1985;134:3339–45.
259. Beeson PB, Rowley D. The anticomplementary effect of kidney tissue. Its association with ammonia production. J Exp Med. 1959;110:685–98.
260. Hostetter MK, Gordon DL. Biochemistry of C3 and related thiolester proteins in infection and inflammation. Rev Infect Dis. 1987;9:97–109.
261. Rubio R, Berne RM, Katori M. Release of adenosine in reactive hyperemia of the dog. Am J Physiol. 1969;216:56–62.
262. Cybulsky AV, Lieberthal W, Quigg RJ, et al. A role for thromboxane in complement-mediated glomerular injury. Am J Pathol. 1987;128:45–51.
263. Hakim RM, Breillatt J, Lazarus MJ, et al. Complement activation and hypersensitivity reactions to dialysis membranes. N Engl J Med. 1984;311:878–82.
264. Craddock PR. Complement and granulocyte activation and deactivation during hemodialysis. In: Lysaght MJ, Gurland JG, eds. Plasma Separation and Plasma Fractionation. Basel: S Karger AG; 1983;14–21.
265. Barrett DJ, Boyle MDP. Restoration of complement function in vivo by plasma infusion in factor I (C3b inactivator) deficiency. J Pediatr. 1984;104:76–81.
266. Rao CP, Minta JO, Laski B, et al. Inherited C8β subunit deficiency in a patient with recurrent meningococcal infections: In vivo functional kinetic analysis of C8. Clin Exp Immunol. 1985;60:183–90.
267. Pitts JS, Donaldson VH, Forristal J, et al. Remissions induced in hereditary angioneurotic edema with an attenuated androgen (danazol): Correlation between concentrations of C1-inhibitor and the fourth and second components of complement. J Lab Clin Med. 1978;92:501–7.
268. Densen P, Brown EJ, O'Neill GJ. Inherited deficiency of C8 in a patient with recurrent meningococcal infections: Further evidence for a dysfunctional C8 molecule and nonlinkage to the HLA system. J Clin Immunol. 1983;3:90–9.

7. GRANULOCYTIC PHAGOCYTES

PETER DENSEN
GERALD L. MANDELL

Granulocytes are the most numerous leukocytes in the peripheral circulation. The granulocytic cell series consists of basophils, eosinophils, and neutrophils. These cells share in common a multilobed nucleus, the presence of numerous membrane-bound, characteristically staining cytoplasmic granules, as well as a primary site of action in the tissues. Functionally, however, their differences are greater than are their similarities.

White cells were first recognized in blood in the 1760s by William Hewson in England. A century later, Elya Metchnikoff reported his observations on phagocytosis and formulated his theory of cellular immunity. In 1903–1904, Wright and Douglas demonstrated the importance of serum factors in phagocytosis and coined the term *opsonins* for these factors. Their work provided the impetus for the experimental resolution of the conflict between the theories of cellular and humoral immunity.[1,2] The past 20 years have seen the progressive understanding of neutrophil function in biochemical terms. Central to this understanding has been the clinical recognition of qualitative defects in neutrophil function and the experimental elucidation of the basis for these defects.

NEUTROPHILS

Development

Neutrophils are derived from pluripotential stem cells located in the bone marrow. Granulocyte development and maturation in the bone marrow occurs in two phases, a mitotic phase and a nonmitotic phase. Each phase lasts approximately 1 week. During the mitotic phase, cells mature sequentially from myeloblasts into promyelocytes and myelocytes.[3] Maturation is associated with the appearance of the characteristic granules in the cytoplasm of neutrophils, basophils, and eosinophils. The nonmitotic phase of development includes metamyelocytes, band (or immature) neutrophils, and mature neutrophils.

Morphologic development is accompanied by changes in the physical properties of the cell, the appearance of specific cell surface antigens[4–6] and maturation of cell function.[7] Thus, IgG Fc receptors appear as the cells develop into promyelocytes;

phagocytic ingestion in the early myelocyte stage; complement receptors in the late myelocyte and metamyelocyte stage; oxygen-independent microbicidal activity in the early metamyelocyte stage; oxidative activity and oxygen-dependent microbicidal activity at the metamyelocyte stage; and increased adhesiveness, cell motility, and chemotactic responses in the late metamyelocyte–band stage.[7,8] Morphologically mature neutrophils in the bone marrow exhibit lower stimulated oxidative responses than do mature neutrophils in the peripheral circulation.[8] A reduction in net surface charge, due primarily to the loss of sialic acid, occurs during maturation and has been implicated in the release of cells from the bone marrow.[9,10]

Morphologic and Structural Characteristics

Neutrophils contain two major granule populations, primary or azurophil granules and specific or secondary granules.[11] Careful studies using differential centrifugation, electron microscopy, and biochemical markers have suggested the existence of additional types or subtypes of granules.[12–16] In particular, a gelatinase-containing tertiary granule has been described that is morphologically similar to specific granules but degranulates upon very mild stimulation.[15] The possible role that the tertiary granules play in neutrophil priming requires further delineation.

The characteristics of the two major granule types are summarized in Table 1. Primary granules appear first, stain blue, and are subject to reduction in number during mitosis. Specific granules arise during the nonmitotic stage of cell development and thus do not undergo numerical reduction. Consequently in the mature neutrophil, specific granules outnumber primary granules 2–3 : 1.[3,11] Primary granules are true lysosomes since they contain acid hydrolases in addition to neutral proteases, myeloperoxidase, cationic proteins, lysozyme and acid mucopolysaccharide. Specific granules contain lactoferrin, lysozyme, vitamin B_{12} binding protein, and cytochrome b, and their membranes serve as a source of receptors. In general, the contents of the primary granule have a lower pH optimum than do those of the specific granule.

During maturation, the nucleus becomes segmented and cytoskeletal elements—microfilaments and microtubules—appear in the cytoplasm. A meshwork of microfilaments makes up the clear cortical veil that surrounds the cell and forms the lamellipodium of an advancing cell (Fig. 1). These structures are polymers of actin, a protein representing 5–10 percent of the total cellular protein. Actin, together with a number of other interacting proteins, constitutes the contractile machinery of the cell that generates locomotion.[17–19] Actin monomers (G-actin), in the presence of actin binding protein, polymerize to form cross-linked actin filaments (F-actin). Regulation of the length of the filaments and the degree of cross-linking provide for the physicochemical fluctuation of actin between the gel and sol states. Filament length is controlled by several different proteins. Profilin serves to sequester G-actin and may provide a mechanism for rapid transport of actin to sites of polymerization. Acumentin, by initiating multiple sites of filament formation (nucleation) and preferentially inhibiting actin monomer exchange from the "slow growing" end of elongating filaments, maintains actin in short filaments. Gelsolin, a calcium-modulated protein that initiates filament nucleation, binds to the "fast growing" end of the filaments and can split preformed actin filaments. In the presence of ATP, myosin repetitively dissociates and binds to cross-linked actin. Myosin binding changes the cross-linking angle between actin filaments from 90 to 45 degrees, which results in movement of the filaments. Thus myosin serves to harness the changes in the physicochemical state of actin to give directionality to cell movement. Changes in calcium concentration that occur with membrane perturbation, directly and in concert with calmodulin, exert control over the contractile process by regulating myosin kinase and gelsolin. As a result, intracellular calcium gradients provide for an increase in polymerized actin in regions of high calcium concentrations.[17–19]

Actin filaments are associated with the cytoskeleton or with the plasma membrane via membrane skeletal proteins.[20] Stimulation of the cell with chemotactic factors causes an abrupt increase in the amount of actin associated with the cytoskeleton[21] and a shift in microfilament organization from a parallel strand to a crosshatched meshwork most evident at the leading edge of the directionally polarized cell.[22]

Microtubules are large, hollow structures composed of dimers of tubulin. In contrast to the role of microfilaments in directed locomotion and changes in cell shape, microtubules appear necessary for the initial orientation of the cell in a chemotactic gradient as well as the spatial organization of structures within the cell during locomotion. They also may be involved in degranulation and in the regulation of cell surface microviscosity during phagocytosis.[23–26]

Mature neutrophils (Figs. 1 and 2) are characterized by a paucity of ribosomal material and mitochondria, which reflects the relative lack of synthetic processes in these cells. Glycogen granules fill the cytoplasm and serve as a source of energy for neutrophil function.

Receptors with specificity for a number of humoral sub-

TABLE 1. Characteristics of Neutrophil Granules

Characteristics	*Primary (Azurophil)*	*Specific (Secondary)*
Contents	Acid hydrolases	Lactoferrin
	β-glucuronidase	Lysozyme
		Vitamin B_{12} binding protein
	α-Mannosidase	
	Arylsulfatase	
	5′-Nucleotidase	Collagenase (?)
		Monocyte chemotactic factor
	Acid protease (cathepsin)	
		C3 and C5 cleaving proteases
	Neutral proteases	
		Membrane bound receptors
	Cathepsin G	
	Elastase	CR-3
	Collagenase (?)	C5a
	Myeloperoxidase	FMLP
	Cationic proteins	Laminin
		Membrane-bound components of NADPH oxidase system
	Lysozyme	
	Acid mucopolysaccharide	Cytochrome b_{558}
pH optimum	5.5–6.5	7.0–7.5
Degranulation	Degranulation delayed >50% Into Phagosome	Degranulates first >90% Exocytosis
Function	Microbial killing Digestion	Inflammatory process

Abbreviation: FMLF: formylmethyl-leucyl-phenylalanine.

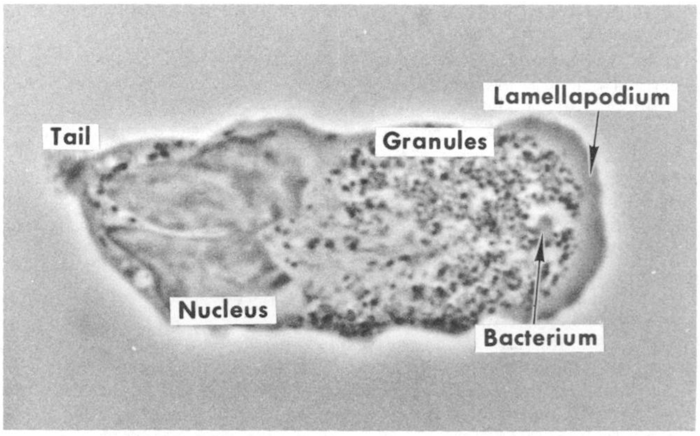

FIG. 1. Phase-contrast photomicrograph of a human neutrophil.

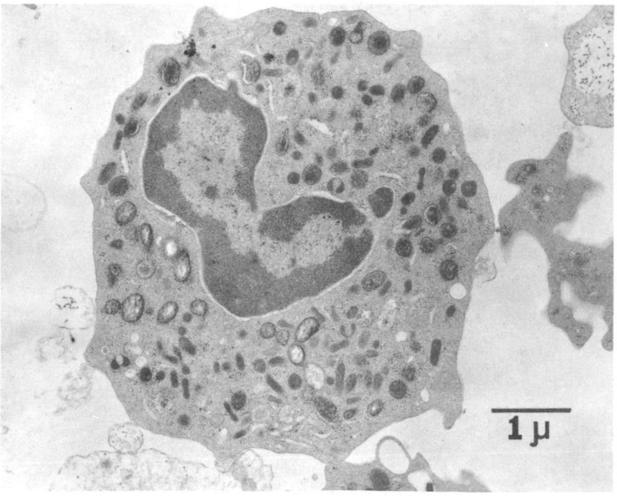

FIG. 2. Electron micrograph of a human neutrophil. Note the granules (large oval structures), glycogen particles (small dark particles), but few other visible organelles.

stances, including IgG, IgA, C3b, iC3b, and several chemotactic factors,[27–31] have been identified and characterized both functionally and structurally. These receptors are homogeneously distributed over the surface of the resting cell. Upon polarization of the cell in response to a chemotactic stimulus, receptors for IgG and concanavalin A undergo an asymmetric clustering at the front of the cell. It is now clear that the distribution of receptors with different ligand specificity can be independently regulated even though stimulation via these receptors may result in similar functional effects.[32–34] Moreover, the various neutrophil functional responses exhibit differential requirements for receptor occupancy. Thus, maximal degranulation requires brief receptor occupancy whereas sustained oxidative responses are dependent upon continuous ligand binding to the receptor.[35]

Neutrophil Kinetics

The daily production of mature neutrophils (PMNs) is on the order of 10^{11} cells. This granulocyte reserve contains up to 10 times the normal daily neutrophil requirement. During acute infection or other inflammatory stresses, neutrophils are mobilized from the marrow reservoir. In the face of a continuing stimulus this reserve may be depleted, thus necessitating additional means for increasing delivery to meet demands. Increased stem cell input, increased mitoses during the mitotic stage of development, use of a store of cells whose maturation had been inhibited (so-called hiatal cells), and shortening of the maturation time within the marrow may all occur.[36] Multiplication and differentiation of stem cells is stimulated by a family of proteins called colony-stimulating factors. These factors are produced by peripheral blood monocytes, tissue macrophages, and stimulated lymphocytes and exhibit a hierarchy with respect to the type(s) of myeloid cells that they stimulate.[36,37] Different proteins induce growth and differentiation, and the interaction of these factors determines the balance between immature and mature cells.[37] Lithium carbonate, a drug used primarily for the treatment of manic-depressive disorders, accelerates neutrophil production by stimulating clonal proliferation. This effect leads to an increase in the total circulating neutrophil mass without a reduction in the delivery of cells to sites of inflammation.[38,39]

Intravascular neutrophils are present in a circulating pool and a marginating pool. The circulating pool contains about 22×10^7 cells/kg and the marginating pool (which can be released with exercise or epinephrine) about 17×10^7 cells/kg. In contrast, more than 1000×10^7 PMNs and PMN percursors/kg are found in the marrow. The half-life of intravascular neutrophils is 6–8 hours. Mature neutrophils leave the body via the gut, respiratory secretions, and urine, and senescent cells may be engulfed by other phagocytic cells in the tissues. Estimates of extravascular survival range from 7 hours to 4 days.

In addition to infection, granulocytosis can be produced by a number of pharmacologic and physiologic stimuli. Most of these situations do not involve an increase in cell production but rather cause granulocytosis by altering the distribution of cells in the various granulocyte pools. Thus, the acute administration of corticosteroids and endotoxin induces the release of cells from a marrow granulocyte reserve, which is analogous to the redistribution observed during acute inflammatory processes. Chronic steroid administration, however, inhibits granulocyte egress from the circulation. Exercise, stress, epinephrine, alcohol, and hypoxia all produce granulocytosis by mobilizing marginating granulocytes. Steroids, aspirin, and alcohol also decrease granulocyte adherence.

Delivery to the Inflammatory Site

The circulating and marginating pools are heterogeneous, being composed of a large subpopulation (80 percent) of neutrophils with IgG rosetting properties and a smaller population lacking this characteristic.[40] It is not clear whether this heterogeneity represents different cellular subsets or is due to maturational differences within a single cell line. The functional significance of neutrophil heterogeneity is uncertain, but differences in the distribution of these cells may contribute to the development of "impaired" neutrophil function in certain disease states.[41] In contrast to circulating granulocytes, tissue neutrophils are homogeneous, greater than 96 percent being capable of IgG rosette formation.[40] Tissue neutrophils contain fewer lysosomal granules but up to 10-fold greater amounts of glycogen than their circulating counterparts have.[42] Anaerobic glycolysis of these glycogen stores provides the energy for neutrophil locomotion.

Although neutrophils within the marginating pool stick to vascular endothelium, they are not truly adherent; rather, they tumble slowly along the vessel wall. After, a local insult these neutrophils become firmly adherent to the side of the vessel wall closest to the injury. Plasma factors,[43] neutrophil and endothelial cell products, and surface glycoproteins on neutrophils and endothelial cells all combine to modulate neutrophil adherence to the endothelium.[44] Inflammatory mediators and chemotactic factors stimulate the limited release of specific granules and probably tertiary granules from neutrophils in the local circulation. The consequences of this degranulation include decreased surface charge, increased neutrophil adhesiveness, and an increase in a number of membrane receptors. The functional result of these changes is a cell that has been primed to a state of enhanced responsiveness.[45–48] Increased expression of the laminin receptor coupled with the release of granule enzymes may facilitate limited digestion of laminin, an endothelial matrix protein, thereby facilitating diapedesis and entry of the neutrophil into the tissues.[44] Several neutrophil surface glycoproteins promote neutrophil-dependent adherence to endothelial cells. These include an 80–100 kD protein, also found on monocytes, eosinophils, and lymphocytes,[49] and the CDw18 glycoproteins (Mo1, MAC-1/LFA-1, GP150,95) that are variably present on granulocytes, monocytes, macrophages, T lymphocytes, and large granular lymphocytes.[50] Mo1 is synonymous with the complement receptor for iC3b, CR3. The CDw18 proteins are heterodimers composed of a common 95 kD β-chain and unique 150–180 kD α-chains. The β-chain exhibits a high degree of structural homology with other cellular adhesion proteins belonging to the integrin family of cell surface receptors.[51,52] Many of these receptors recognize the tripeptide amino acid sequence arg-gly-asp.[53] A 90–110 kD glycoprotein having a broad tissue distribution and termed intercellular adhesion molecule (ICAM-1) facilitates neutrophil adherence to endothelial cells. Surface expression of this molecule is up regulated by interleukin-1 (IL-1)), tumor necrosis factor (TNF), and interferon-γ (IFN-γ).[54] Thus neutrophil adherence to endothelial cells is promoted by glycoproteins present on the surface of both cells.[55]

Neutrophils can arrive at an inflammatory site either by increasing their overall random movement (chemokinesis) or by following a concentration gradient of inflammatory substances in a directional manner (chemotaxis). Most substances that stimulate directed movement on the part of the neutrophil also stimulate an increase in overall motility.[56]

Directed movement of neutrophils requires cell polarization and the orderly making and breaking of cell–substrate contact. There is no evidence that neutrophils can swim, and progress appears to be made either by gliding along a surface with caudad displacement of dorsal folds or cycles of partial release of the lamellipodium from the substrate with anterior advance followed by lamellipodial reassociation with the substrate.[57]

Chemotactic factors fall into two categories: (1) chemotaxins, which act directly to stimulate chemotaxis, and (2) chemotaxigens, which induce the formation of chemotaxins. Bacterial factors may fall into either category. The tripeptide formylmethionyl-leucyl-phenylalanine (FMLP) is directly chemotactic for neutrophils at concentrations as low as 10^{-11} M. Since bacteria and mitochondria initiate protein synthesis with formylmethionine at the N-terminus, it has been suggested that bacterial or mitochondrial proteins released during cell death are responsible for stimulating neutrophil chemotaxis.[58]

The interaction of bacteria or their products with complement generates the chemotactic factor C5a. This fragment is converted rapidly to C5a des arg, which has little inherent chemotactic activity but combines with an anionic polypeptide cochemotaxin via sialic acid residues to form the bulk of chemotactic activity present in activated normal serum.[59,60] Biologically active lipids generated from arachidonic acid are potent mediators of a variety of inflammatory reactions. Products of arachidonic acid metabolism, particularly the hydroxyeicosatetranoic acids (HETEs) and leukotriene B_4 (LTB_4) are potent mediators of the inflammatory response. These substances influence a number of neutrophil functions including chemokinesis, chemotaxis, granule release, and iC3b receptor expression.[61] Substances released during neutrophil degranulation can, either by direct action or via cleavage of C5a from C5, attract other cells to the site of bacterial invasion.[62]

Chemotactic factor concentration differences as little as 0.1–1.0 percent across the neutrophil are sufficient to produce cellular orientation and directed movement (Figs. 3 and 4). The mechanism by which transduction of chemotactic factor binding to specific receptors produces a chemotactic response is unclear, but calcium fluxes and transmethylation of phospholipids appear essential.[24] Fusion of granule and cell membranes during limited degranulation increases the number of chemotactic receptors.[46] As the cell moves in an increasing chemotactic gradient, these receptors become occupied and are rapidly internalized. The resultant decrease in receptor number and perhaps a decrease in affinity of the remaining receptors may control chemotactic responsiveness.[63] Occupied receptors are internalized, stripped of ligand, and recycled to the cell surface.[64,65] Recycling is facilitated by sialic acid on membrane glycoproteins.[65] The oxidative and degranulation responses induced in the neutrophil by increasing concentrations of mediators (Fig. 4) promote the inactivation of unbound chemotactic mediators.[61,66,67] In addition, lysozyme release dampens both the chemotactic and oxidative responsiveness of the cell.[68] In concert, this multitude of effects serves to attract and keep the neutrophil at the site of bacterial invasion.

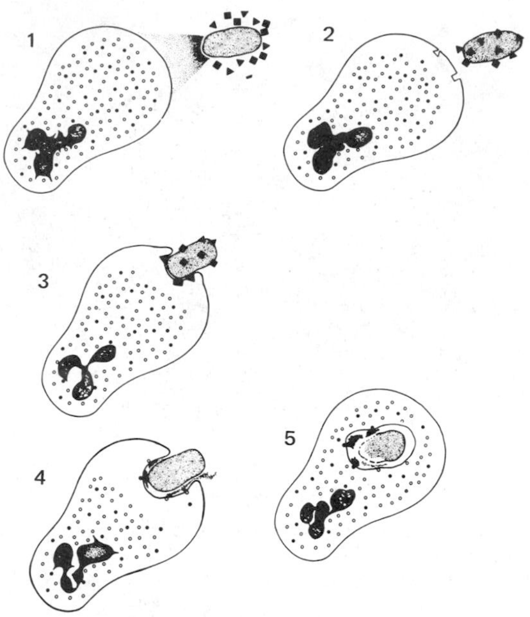

FIG. 4. **(1)** A neutrophil approaching a bacterium is guided by a concentration gradient of chemotactic factors emanating from the microbe. **(2)** Antibody and complement attaching to the surface of the bacterium to opsonize the organism. **(3)** Ingestion taking place by sequential binding of receptors on the neutrophil to opsonins on the bacterium. **(4)** Early degranulation. Specific granules (open circles) are discharging before the phagocytic vacuole is closed, and thus much of the granule contents are found outside of the cell—"regurgitation during feeding." **(5)** Later degranulation and destruction of ingested bacteria. Primary granules fire into the closed phagosome. This, in conjunction with an oxidative burst of activity, results in bactericidal activity.

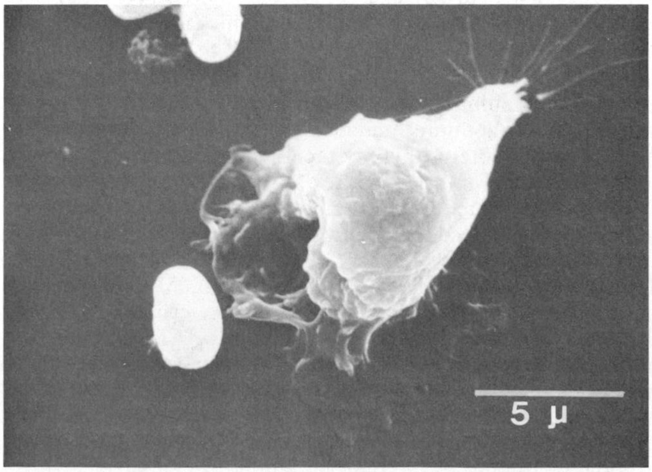

FIG. 3. Scanning electron micrograph of a neutrophil extending a pseudopod toward *Candida albicans.*

Phagocytosis

Phagocytosis is a two-step process involving attachment and engulfment of the phagocytic particle. Ingestion but not attachment is an active process requiring energy from anaerobic glycolysis. Optimal ingestion requires the presence of calcium and magnesium ions. Some microorganisms and inert particles may be ingested by neutrophils in the absence of serum factors, but most bacteria must be coated with opsonins (humoral substances that enhance microbial ingestion) for attachment to and ingestion by neutrophils to occur.

Specific IgG and complement are the major opsonic factors promoting recognition and ingestion of microorganisms by neutrophils. Antibody promotes phagocytic uptake by neutralization of antiphagocytic molecules on the bacterial surface, e.g., capsular polysaccharide; physically linking the organism to the neutrophils; efficiently activating the classical pathway of complement and promoting deposition of opsonic fragments of C3 on the bacterial surface; and by activating the neutrophil ingestion mechanism through interaction of IgG with its receptor in the neutrophil membrane (Fig. 4). Activation of complement via either the alternative or classical pathways leads to C3b and iC3b deposition on the microbial surface (Chapter 6). In addition C1q deposition enhances Fc receptor-dependent ingestion.[69]

Receptors for IgG (FcγRI-III), but not other immunoglobulins, and for C3b (CR-1) and iC3b (CR-3) are present in the neutrophil membrane.[27,28,70] These receptors are biochemically, topographically, and functionally distinct. Recent evidence suggests that FcγRs mediate phagocytosis via calcium-dependent pathways whereas CR-1 and 3 use calcium-independent pathways.[71] FcγRII and -III are low to moderate affinity receptors normally present on the cell surface, whereas the high-affinity FcγRI is found on the surface of IFN-γ-stimulated neutrophils.[70] Intracellular pools of Fc receptors have not been identified. In contrast, such pools have been described for both CR-1 and CR-3, the latter clearly being associated with the specific granules.[72,73] These receptor pools are rapidly mobilized to the surface after stimulation of the cell by a variety of inflammatory mediators.[73] It is likely that C3 receptors enjoy only low-level expression on circulating neutrophils and that differences in resting expression levels are attributable to the presence of miniscule amounts of mediators (e.g., endotoxin) in the isolation procedures used during neutrophil purification.

In contrast to upregulation, which occurs primarily through an increase in receptor numbers, downregulation of receptor-mediated processes occurs principally via diminished receptor function. Receptor oxidation as a consequence of the normal stimulation of the neutrophil oxidative burst contributes to decreased receptor function. Consequently, neutrophil receptor half-life and function are enhanced in individuals with either impaired oxidase activity (e.g., chronic granulomatous disease) or in whom the generation of certain oxidative reactants is depressed (e.g., myeloperoxidase deficiency).[74,75] The balance between these regulating events is probably an important modulating factor in the inflammatory response and in limiting tissue damage.

Both IgG and C3 binding increase the rate of phagocytosis of appropriately sensitized erythrocytes, but in the unprimed cell only interactions via the Fc receptor initiate microfilament polymerization and ingestion of this target.[76–78] However, complement deposition alone is sufficient to promote ingestion of a number of bacteria, a finding that emphasizes the heterogeneity among opsonic requirements for different particles. In most cases phagocytosis is most efficient when organisms are coated with both IgG and C3, thereby allowing cooperative interaction of the two types of receptors. In fact, recent data suggest that a subpopulation of CR3 and Fc receptors are physically associated within the membrane.[79]

Ingestion is the result of the sequential interaction between opsonic ligands distributed homogeneously over the particle surface and their receptors on the phagocyte membrane. The sequential interaction of these opsonic ligands with their receptors in the phagocytic membrane initiates polymerization of actin microfilaments in the cytoplasm underlying the site of a particle attachment and results in the circumferential flow of the cell membrane about the opsonized particle and its enclosure within a phagosome (Figs. 4 and 5).[18,80,81]

In addition to acting as ligands between the phagocytic particle and the phagocyte, complement and specific immunoglobulin alter the surface characteristics of the phagocytic particle. The surface of bacteria, which has antiphagocytic properties, is hydrophilic relative to the surface of the neutrophil. Upon opsonization the surface of these bacteria becomes relatively more hydrophobic than that of the neutrophil, and they are readily engulfed. Alterations in surface properties may also promote ingestion by reducing charge repulsion between the particle and the phagocyte.[82] Different bacterial species, as well as mutants within the same species, may vary in their opsonic requirements for optimal phagocytosis.

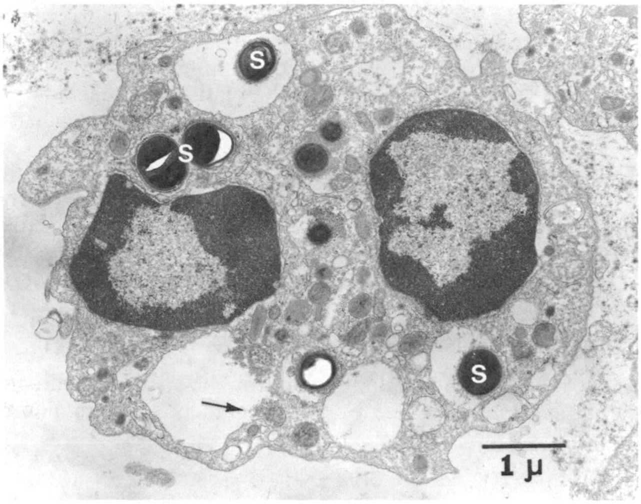

FIG. 5. Electron micrograph of a neutrophil that has ingested *Staphylococcus aureus* (S). Bacteria are in phagocytic vacuoles formed by invagination of external cell membrane. Degranulation into a phagocytic vacuole can be seen at the lower left (arrow).

Increased attention has been paid to the important role that nonspecific factors play in the phagocytic process, especially in soft tissues where the functional impact of the neutrophil is most critical. Chief among these factors are fibronectin and laminin, proteins that constitute part of the extracellular matrix secreted by endothelial cells. These proteins contain the arg-gly-asp amino acid recognition sequence through which they bind to specific but separate membrane receptors.[53] Since the different receptors recognize the same binding sequence, specificity must be conferred by other aspects of the structure of these matrix proteins.[53] In the fluid phase or by themselves these proteins fail to promote ingestion of target particles. However, when neutrophils adherent to surfaces coated with these proteins are stimulated with a variety of chemotactic factors, their capacity to ingest either IgG- or C3-coated particles, in particular, the latter, is substantially enhanced. This effect requires neutrophil adherence to the matrix protein but not the interaction of the matrix protein with the target particles or an increase in FcγR or C3 receptor number. Hence these proteins are not opsonins. Rather, they enhance phagocytosis primarily by promoting the conversion of C3 receptors from a binding to an ingesting function. Thus chemotactic mediators and extracellular matrix proteins cooperate to prepare neutrophils for their primary phagocytic function as they migrate from the circulation to sites of infection.[83,84]

Postphagocytic Events

The term *postphagocytic events* refers to the burst of metabolic activity and the discharge of granule contents that occurs during and after phagocytosis. These events are initiated by the attachment of opsonized microbes to the cell membrane as well as by an array of soluble mediators such as C5a, LTB_4, and platelet activating factor.

The metabolic or respiratory burst is a series of enzymatic

reactions used by stimulated phagocytes to convert oxygen to various active metabolites critical for bactericidal activity. A number of other events including chemiluminescence, iodination of protein, lipid turnover, and the binding and degradation of some hormones are increased during phagocytosis but are secondary to the reduction of oxygen.

The basic series of reactions of the respiratory burst results in (1) oxygen consumption, (2) superoxide production, (3) hydrogen peroxide production, and (4) stimulation of the hexose monophosphate shunt. Oxygen is consumed and reduced to the superoxide anion radical $O_2^{\overline{\cdot}}$ by the one electron transfer to oxygen from the reduced pyridine nucleotide NADPH:

$$2O_2 + NADPH \rightarrow 2O_2^{\overline{\cdot}} + H^+ + NADP^+$$

At the acidic pH present in the phagocytic vacuole, hydrogen peroxide is rapidly formed by the spontaneous dismutation of superoxide.

$$2O_2^{\overline{\cdot}} + 2H^+ \rightarrow H_2O_2 + O_2$$

Detoxification of superoxide and hydrogen peroxide as they diffuse into the surrounding cytoplasm is accomplished by cellular antioxidant systems. At neutral pH, superoxide dismutase catalyzes the above reaction to eliminate superoxide, whereas hydrogen peroxide is destroyed by the glutathione peroxide system.

$$H_2O_2 + 2GSH \rightarrow 2H_2O + GSSG$$

Reduced glutathione (GSH) is regenerated by glutathione (GSSG) reductase.

$$GSSG + 2NADPH \rightarrow 2GSH + 2NADP^+$$

Thus, NADPH serves a critical role both in the primary reduction of oxygen as well as in the protection of the cell from toxic metabolites of oxygen.[85]

The hexose monophosphate shunt, a series of reactions oxidizing glucose to a five-carbon sugar and carbon dioxide, serves to regenerate NADPH. In resting neutrophils only 1–2 percent of glucose metabolism occurs via the hexose monophosphate shunt, but during phagocytosis glucose use via this pathway increases 15- to 30-fold.[86]

The NADPH oxidase lies dormant in resting neutrophils. Stimulation of the cell is followed by a 30–60 second lag during which the dormant enzyme is activated, thereby resulting in the characteristic burst of respiratory activity. In its active state the oxidase is associated with the plasma membrane. Current evidence supports the view that the oxidase is a multicomponent electron transport system. A component on the cytoplasmic face of the cell membrane[87] catalyzes the oxidation of NADPH generated by the hexose monophosphate shunt and initiates the flow of electrons through the membrane via other components to environmental oxygen as the terminal electron acceptor.[88–90] Superoxide is the product of this terminal reduction of oxygen. Evidence supporting a role for a flavoprotein, quinones, cytosolic factors, and cytochrome b_{-558} (previously termed cytochrome b_{-245}) has been generated from several laboratories.[91–95] However, the identity of the individual components in the putative transport chain is a matter of a debate.[89,90] Evidence supporting the participation of a flavoprotein, cytosolic factors, and cytochrome b_{-558} in a multicomponent oxidase system derives from studies of the chronic granulomatous diseases (CGD). Neutrophils from patients with these disorders lack oxidase activity, and this phenotype has been associated with the absence of each of the three aforementioned components.[96–99]

The organization of the components of the oxidase within the membrane requires further delineation. However, it is clear that the NADPH binding site lies on the inner face of the cytoplasmic membrane.[87] Studies using an NADPH analog in chemical cross-linking experiments have identified a 65-kD NADPH membrane binding protein in guinea pig neutrophils.[100] The relationship of this protein to the reported components of the oxidase system is uncertain. The outer face of the plasma membrane must contain the component responsible for the direct transfer of electrons to oxygen. The low midpoint potential of cytochrome b_{-558} argues for its role in this function and thus as the terminal constituent of the transport chain.[89,90] Recent work indicates that the human cytochrome is a 120–135 kD protein composed of two tightly associated polypeptide chains, α (22 kD) and β (91 kD).[101] The α-chain is encoded on chromosome 16 and probably bears the cytochrome heme binding site, whereas the heavily glycosylated β-chain is encoded by an X-linked gene.[102–105]

A major question concerns the mechanism of oxidase activation after stimulation of the cell. Activation appears to involve multiple steps and several pathways since multiple substances, each with a characteristic lag time, can initiate the burst and patients have been identified whose granulocytes respond with a burst to some but not all stimuli.[85,106] Transient depolarization of the cell membrane occurs within 5 to 10 seconds of stimulation, precedes the earliest detectable changes in oxygen metabolism, and seems to be a necessary although insufficient condition for activation.[107,108] The demonstration that 70–90 percent of the cytochrome b_{-558} activity is located in the specific granules[88,109,110] implies that degranulation with translocation of the cytochrome from the granule to the cell membrane may be involved in the assembly and activation of the oxidase system.[109] However, the oxidative burst can occur in the apparent absence of degranulation,[111,112] and certain substances can reversibly activate the oxidase system.[113,114] Hence degranulation alone is not the sole determinant of oxidase activation. In addition not all investigators have found cytochrome b_{-558} associated with specific granules.[115,116]

Evidence is accumulating that suggests that there is more than one pathway for activating the oxidase system.[89,117,118] This conclusion is based on the observations that different stimuli exhibit markedly disparate kinetics for activation[118] and that a comparison of a number of parameters (e.g., phosphoinositide turnover, calcium fluctuations, inhibition by pertussis toxin and protein kinase C dependency) for each of the different stimuli yields a pattern that cannot be accounted for by a simple, stepwise activation pathway.[89] A protein kinase C dependent pathway clearly involves receptors, phosphoinositide metabolism, G proteins and calcium.[117,119] A second pathway used by arachidonic acid and sodium dodecyl sulfate (SDS) is protein kinase C independent.[117] It has been suggested that these latter two stimuli may activate the oxidase by virtue of their detergent properties or by producing changes in membrane fluidity in the vicinity of the oxidase.[120,121] Inactivation of the oxidase may occur by a poorly characterized desensitization mechanism[122] or by myeloperoxidase-dependent oxidation of critical determinants of oxidase activity.[123]

Degranulation, the other major postphagocytic event, is also initiated before completion of ingestion. Ninety percent of the contents released from specific granules during phagocytosis can be found outside the cell. These substances function optimally at the pH encountered extracellularly. Thus specific granules appear to function principally as secretory granules. In contrast, greater than 50 percent of the contents released from primary granules during phagocytosis can be recovered from the phagosome.[124] These enzymes function best at the low pH (6.0–6.5) found in phagosomes. Consequently, the contents of the primary granule appear to function principally in microbial killing and digestion.

Recent evidence links degranulation to calcium fluxes and depolarization of the neutrophil membrane.[125,126] Changes in the intracellular levels of cyclic nucleotides also influence degranulation, perhaps by modulating microtubule assembly, but these changes are unlikely to account directly for granule release induced by stimulation of the cell.[127,128] Inhibition of microtubule assembly by colchicine interferes with degranulation;

however, microtubule assembly does not induce granule release in the absence of surface adherence.[129] Hence, microtubule assembly is necessary but not sufficient for degranulation. Microtubules are believed to promote granule movement toward the phagosome, but microfilaments probably are also involved in the degranulation process.[130] Fusion of the cytoplasmic granules with the phagosome results in the melding of the two membranes, an increase in the size of the phagocytic vacuole, activation of membrane-bound enzymes, and discharge of granule contents into the phagosome.

The extracellular release of the constituents of neutrophil granules occurs by two different routes.[131] The first, known as "regurgitation during feeding," occurs by virtue of granule discharge into the nascent phagosome before closure of the phagosome around the phagocytic particle. Exocytosis may also involve the direct fusion of lysosomes with the external cell membrane and subsequent extracellular extrusion of granule contents. This process is called "reverse endocytosis" or "frustrated phagocytosis." Granule extrusion occurs over a large area of membrane surface and may involve greater quantities of enzyme release than with the regurgitation route.

Signal Transduction

The major neutrophil functions depicted in Figure 4 (chemotaxis, phagocytosis, degranulation, and the oxidative burst) are initiated by the interaction of mediators with specific receptors in the cell membrane. The transduction of a given signal into a specific response has elements unique to the stimulus as well as aspects shared with other stimuli.[132] For example, chemotactic stimuli promote directed cell movement but may also stimulate degranulation or the oxidative burst.

As with other cells a major transduction pathway involves the phosphoinositide–protein kinase C (PKC) system,[133–135] but as discussed above, PKC-independent, calcium-dependent pathways also exist. The basic components of the phosphoinositide pathway include a receptor that communicates via G protein(s) with membrane-bound phospholipase C. Agonist binding to the receptor promotes phosphatidyl-4,5-biphosphate (IP_2) cleavage by phospholipase C, which results in the release of diacylglycerol (DAG) and inositol triphosphate (IP_3), the latter of which can be further converted to IP_4. IP_3 and IP_4 mediate increases in free intracellular calcium by respectively stimulating its release from unique intracellular compartments called calcisomes and by promoting its influx from the cell exterior.[136,137] The increase in intracellular calcium is greatest at the region of stimulation, for example, at the leading edge of the cell during chemotaxis or periphagosomally during phagocytosis, as might be anticipated from the role of calcium in actin polymerization and the importance of microfilaments in cell movement and ingestion.[138]

Free intracellular calcium also acts in conjunction with DAG to promote translocation of PKC from the cytosol to the cell membrane where it functions to phosphorylate critical proteins, thereby regulating the activity of these molecules. Current research is directed at establishing the identity of the phosphorylated molecules in order to delineate their function. That this approach is likely to yield important insights is attested to by the recent demonstration of an association between one form of CGD and failure to phosphorylate a 44–48 kD membrane protein.[139–141] Phorbol myristate acetate, an agent commonly used to activate a variety of neutrophil responses, substitutes for DAG in the phosphoinositide pathway, thereby bypassing the steps between the receptor and PKC activation.[133,134] Pertussis toxin, another commonly used reagent, binds to certain G proteins, thereby inhibiting neutrophil responses.[142]

Priming of Neutrophil Responses

Recently obtained data have emphasized that concentrations of mediators sufficiently low enough not to stimulate neutrophils directly nevertheless prepare the cell for an enhanced response to a second unrelated stimulus.[143,144] This phenomenon is referred to as priming and is likely to be important in vivo since it appears to be cell specific. That is, bacterial infection primes neutrophils, whereas parasitic infection or allergic responses prime eosinophils.[145] A broad array of inflammatory mediators including chemotactic factors, endotoxin, cytokines, and certain lipids can prime the neutrophil, and the primed state exists with respect to each of the major aspects of neutrophil function (Fig. 4). This state of enhanced responsiveness persists for an extended period of time (>20 minutes) relative to the response elicited by direct stimulation of the cell.[122,143] Presentation of the same agonist in both the priming and stimulating steps results in decreased cellular responses indicating the existence of chemical pathways for desensitization in addition to those for priming.[122] The chemical basis for these different pathways is uncertain. Current evidence suggests that, in contrast to directly stimulated responses, primed responses are independent of PKC activation and translocation.[145] Changes in the physicochemical properties of the lipid bilayer have been invoked as the physiologic basis for this phenomenon.[145]

Microbicidal Mechanisms

The postphagocytic events described above are designed to deliver the products of degranulation and the respiratory burst to the phagocytic vacuole. The phagosome plays an important role in this process because it provides a closed space in which an ingested microbe is exposed to high concentrations of toxic substances and the exposure of the phagocyte and other cells to these metabolites is minimized (Fig. 5).[146]

Oxygen-dependent bactericidal mechanisms can be divided into myeloperoxidase-dependent and -independent reactions.[147] The essential requirements for the myeloperoxidase-mediated bactericidal mechanisms as first described by Klebanoff are myeloperoxidase, released from the primary granule; hydrogen peroxide, generated by the respiratory burst; and a halide ion. In addition, the low pH present in the phagocytic vacuole enhances myeloperoxidase activity. Hydrogen peroxide by itself has bactericidal properties, but in the presence of myeloperoxidase the potency of this system for bacteria is enhanced 50-fold. The halide used in the myeloperoxidase–hydrogen peroxide reaction also has an effect on the bactericidal potency in decreasing order of efficacy—ioide, bromide, and chloride. However, on the basis of concentration, chloride appears to be the physiologic cofactor for this reaction in the cell.[147]

Hypochlorous acid, formed by the neutrophil when chloride is the relevant halide, is a potent oxidizing and microbicidal agent.[147] The microbicidal activity of this system probably results from halogenation or oxidation of critical iron-rich catalytic components of the electron transport chain within the microbial membrane. Oxidation of these molecules leads to the release of free iron, which can then participate in the formation of the highly reactive hydroxyl radical.[148–151] In addition to these well-defined effects, the myeloperoxidase-hydrogen peroxide-halide system promotes the formation of singlet oxygen, decarboxylation of amino acids to form toxic aldehydes, and the generation of chloramines.[152,153] These effects probably contribute to neutrophil microbicidal activity.[147,154,155]

Metabolites of oxygen for which a role in neutrophil bactericidal activity has been suggested include hydrogen peroxide, superoxide, singlet oxygen, and hydroxyl radical. The fact that catalase, which destroys hydrogen peroxide, protects bacteria from the bactericidal effects of neutrophils[156] and that the bactericidal activity of myeloperoxidase-deficient neutrophils remains high are strong pieces of evidence supporting a direct germicidal effect of hydrogen peroxide. Superoxide, by itself, is thought to play little role in the killing of microorganisms. This conclusion is based on the demonstration that bacteria incubated in a cell-free, superoxide-generating system survive normally. However, under appropriate conditions superoxide can react with other products of oxygen to generate hydroxyl radical and singlet oxygen. The bactericidal effect of these oxygen-derived free radicals may be due to the initiation of a chain of oxidizing events in the bacterial cell wall.[147,154,155] Hydroxyl radical is a potent bactericidal agent that can be formed by the direct reaction of superoxide with hydrogen peroxide. This reaction occurs too slowly to be of biologic importance, but it can be catalyzed by ferric salts.[157,158] Recent studies support this scenario since hydroxyl radical formation by stimulated neutrophils occurred only in the presence of free iron.[159] Thus the formation of this highly reactive species in vivo is probably determined by the availability of free iron in the environment or its release from oxidatively injured organisms.[158] The demonstration that neutrophils emit light during the metabolic burst and the fact that the relaxation of oxygen from an excited singlet state to the ground state produces light led to the suggestion that neutrophil chemiluminescence was due to singlet oxygen. Both superoxide- and myeloperoxidase-dependent reactions have been implicated in the formation of singlet oxygen. Myeloperoxidase-dependent reactions are clearly an important source of chemiluminsecence, but available evidence at present suggests that chemiluminescence is not directly related to singlet oxygen.[154]

The presence of oxygen-independent microbicidal mechanisms in neutrophils is clearly demonstrated by the ability of these cells to kill some organisms under anaerobic conditions.[160] Substances contributing to oxygen-independent microbicidal activity include acid, lactoferrin, lysozyme, and cationic proteins. In human neutrophils, the pH in the phagosome decreases to about 6.0.[161] Although pneumococci are readily killed by the effect of acid alone, most bacteria are little affected by the acid environment. The main effect of the low pH in the phagocytic vacuole appears to be enhancement of the activity of the granule enzymes important in the killing and digestion of ingested microorganisms.

Lactoferrin is an iron-binding protein found in secretions bathing mucosal membranes as well as in neutrophils.[162] Its presence in the specific granules of neutrophils suggests that the primary site of its action lies extracellularly. Lactoferrin's bacteriostatic effect is related to its ability to deprive bacteria of the iron required for growth, and this effect is eliminated by saturation of both iron binding sites.[162] Lactoferrin plays a role in the alteration of the physicochemical properties of the neutrophil membrane that occurs during degranulation,[163] the modulation of hydroxyl radical production,[158] the regulation of granulopoiesis,[164] and the modulation of complement function.[165]

Lysozyme is found mainly in the specific granules but is also present in the primary granules. This enzyme hydrolyzes the glycoside bond between *N*-acetylmuramic acid and *N*-acetylglucosamine, a component of the peptidoglycan in bacterial cell walls. The bactericidal properties of lysozyme are due to this reaction. However, in most bacteria, peptide substitutions on the *N*-acetylmuramic acid residue make this bond inaccessible to lysozyme. The bacteriolytic properties of lysozyme are correspondingly limited. The action of lysozyme is enhanced by the presence of other substances, for example, complement, which damages the bacterial cell wall, thereby allowing access of lysozyme to its site of action.[147]

A number of highly cationic proteins have been isolated from neutrophil primary granules.[166–168] The reaction of these proteins with acidic groups on the bacterial surface is associated with inhibition of bacterial growth. Some of these proteins preferentially inhibit specific bacterial species.[169] These proteins include a 37 kD cation antimicrobial protein, the activity of which is favored by the intraphagosomal acid pH[166,170,172]; a 59 kD "bactericidal permeability increasing" protein, the activity of which resides in a 25 kD amino terminal fragment[167,172]; and a family of small (3–4 kD) cysteine- and arginine-rich peptides dubbed "defensins".[168,173] The former two proteins are active only against gram-negative bacteria and are more active against strains with a rough (incomplete) rather than a smooth (complete) lipopolysaccharide. Their exact mode of action is incompletely understood but involves temperature-independent binding to the organism via ionic interactions followed by temperature-dependent insertion into the outer membrane via hydrophobic interactions.[166,167,174] These events result in increased permeability of the bacterial outer membrane which in turn is associated with death of the organism. In contrast, the defensins exhibit antimicrobial activity against both gram-negative and gram-positive organisms as well as fungi and viruses.[168,173] The structure of these peptides is highly conserved among different and within the same animal species.[168,175] The mode of action of these peptides may relate more to their detergent-like properties than their cationic nature.[168] Intracellular killing of bacteria may also be enhanced by antibody and complement independently of the role of these ligands in opsonization and triggering the respiratory burst.[176,177]

Microbial Defenses against Phagocytes

In general, microbes involved in the pathogenesis of acute infections must remain extracellular if they are to produce an infection, whereas chronic infections are typically produced by organisms whose pathogenic potential necessitates an intracellular environment, usually in monocytes or macrophages. Both types of microbes possess virulence factors that enable them to persist in their respective locations. Bacteria may elude neutrophils by failing to stimulate chemotaxis or by circumventing attachment or ingestion. Organisms that inhibit degranulation or the oxidative burst may survive inside neutrophils or monocytes and generally cause chronic infections (Table 2).[178]

Tissue Injury—The Dark Side of Neutrophil Function

Ordinarily, degranulation and the oxidative burst are restricted to the points of contact between an opsonized organism and the developing phagolyosome.[179,180] Downregulation of receptor-mediated events during continuous exposure to homologous stimuli (desensitization)[122] and during exposure to products of the oxidative burst,[75] oxidative inactivation of inflammatory mediators[66,181] and the oxidase itself,[74,123] and the release of lactoferrin to bind environmental iron in a form in which it is not available to catalyze hydroxyl radical formation[158,182,183] further limit neutrophil activation and confine the toxic effects of oxygen-dependent and -independent microbicidal systems to the vicinity of the organism. However, the toxic potential of these microbicidal systems can be unleashed and cause damage to host tissues in diseases associated with autoantibody formation, immune complex deposition, the intravascular release of excessive quantities of inflammatory mediators, or chronic low-grade inflammation. Thus various granule proteins and products of the neutrophil oxidative burst have been implicated in the pathogenesis of immune- and non-immune-mediated arthropathies and nephropathies as well as pulmonary and cardiac injury.[184,185]

Inflammatory cytokines such as tumor necrosis factor and interleukin-1 activate neutrophils and may contribute to tissue damage.

The intravascular activation of complement and generation of circulating C5a that can occur during the initiation of hemodialysis, cardiopulmonary bypass, or septic shock has been shown to stimulate neutrophil aggregation, oxidative activity, and degranulation. Aggregation of neutrophils leads to the formation of microemboli that lodge in the lung and accounts for the neutropenia observed in these situations. The release of toxic products of oxygen metabolism, coupled with the discharge of granule contents from aggregated neutrophils in the pulmonary circulation, leads to endothelial damage and has been implicated in the development of the adult respiratory dis-

TABLE 2. Tactics of Microorganisms against Strategies of Phagocytic Cells and the Microbes That Use Them

Function of Phagocyte Inhibited									
						Microbial Activity by Resistance to		*Tactic of Microbe*	
Recognition	*Chemotaxis*	*Attachment and Ingestion*	*Ingestion (Despite Attachment)*	*Oxidative Burst*	*Degranulation*	*Oxidative Attack*	*Granule Substance*	*Escape from Phagosome*	*Leukotoxicity*
Schistosome	*Salmonella typhi* *Neisseria meningitidis* *Neisseria gonorrhoeae* *Pseudomonas aeruginosa* *Serratia* species *Mycobacterium tuberculosis* *Staphylococcus aureus* *Capnocytophaga*[a] *Escherichia coli* *Vibrio cholera* *Bordetella pertussis*	*Streptococcus pneumoniae* *Streptococcus pyogenes* *N. gonorrhoeae* *N. meningitidis* *Klebsiella pneumoniae* *S. aureus* *Haemophilus influenzae* *E. coli* *Yersinia pectis* *Bacillus anthracis* *Campylobacter fetus* *Cryptococcus neoformans* *P. aeruginosa* *Pasteurella multocida* *Bacteroides fragilis* *B. pertussis*	*N. gonorrhoeae* *Mycoplasma* Influenza virus	*S. typhi* *Brucella abortus* Newcastle disease virus Vaccinia virus Herpes simplex virus Reovirus *B. pertussis* *Legionella micdadei*	*M. tuberculosis* *Mycobacterium microti* *Mycobacterium bovis* *Toxoplasma gondii* *L. pneumophila*	*S. aureus* *Listeria monocytogenes* *E. coli* *Sarcina lutea* *B. abortus*	*Salmonella typhimurium* *Salmonella minnesota* *Mycobacterium leprae* *Mycobacterium lepraemurium* *M. tuberculosis*	*M. bovis* *Rickettsia tsutsugamushi* Vaccinia virus Reovirus	*S. pneumoniae* *S. pyogenes* *S. aureus* *P. aeruginosa* *Entamoeba histolytica*

[a] Known also as *Bacteroides ochraceus*.

tress syndrome both in vitro and in vivo.[186–189] However, the occurrence of the adult respiratory distress syndrome in neutropenic patients indicates that factors other than intravascular neutrophil aggregates also contribute to the development of this syndrome.[190] Substantial evidence implicates neutrophil products in the development of pulmonary emphysema. In this scenario neutrophils infiltrate the lung and are activated consequent to inflammation-provoking substances in cigarette smoke. Cigarette smoke and products of activated neutrophils inactivate α_1-antitrypsin, the major inhibitor of neutrophil elastase. Neutrophil elastase released during cellular stimulation then promotes proteolytic destruction of the lung architecture.[191–194]

Defects in Neutrophil Function

Defects in neutrophil function can result from decreased numbers of mature neutrophils or abnormalities in chemotaxis, ingestion, or bactericidal mechanisms.[195,196] Table 3 summarizes these defects. Infections resulting from quantitative or qualitative defects in neutrophil function share in common a tendency to be prolonged, to respond slowly to antibiotics, and to be recurrent. Staphylococci, gram-negative organisms, and fungi are the usual organisms responsible for these infections. Patients with defective opsonic activity suffer from infections due to encapsulated bacteria.

Qualitative defects may be intrinsic or extrinsic to the neutrophil. In general, the intrinsic defects of qualitative neutrophil function are more severe than are the extrinsic defects. Chemotactic defects are frequently expressed as cutaneous infections with associated adenitis. Unlike quantitative defects or defects in phagocytosis or intracellular killing, they rarely result in bacteremia or metastatic spread of infection. This is probably due to the fact that, although neutrophil accumulation is delayed, phagocytosis and bactericidal activity frequently proceed normally once neutrophils encounter the microorganism.

TABLE 3. Defects in Neutrophil Function

- Neutropenia
  - Acquired
    - Drug induced
    - Autoimmune
    - Cancer related
  - Hereditary
    - Infantile genetic agranulocytosis
    - Familial neutropenia
    - Cyclic neutropenia
- Qualitative defects
  - Adhesion defects
    - Leukocyte adhesion deficiency
  - Chemotactic defects
    - Humoral
      - Complement deficiency
      - Inhibitors
      - Immune complexes
      - Hyperimmunoglobulinemia E (Job's) syndrome
    - Cellular
      - Chédiak-Higashi syndrome
      - Hypophosphatemia
      - Lazy leukocyte syndrome
  - Opsonic defects
    - Complement deficiency
    - Antibody deficiency
  - Defects in intracellular killing
    - Abnormal respiratory burst
      - Chronic granulomatous disease
      - G6PD deficiency
    - Granule abnormalities
      - Myeloperoxidase deficiency
      - Specific granule deficiency
      - Chédiak-Higashi syndrome

Abbreviation: G6PD: glucose-6-phosphate dehydrogenase.

NEUTROPENIA

The most common granulocyte defect encountered is the absolute reduction of circulating neutrophils. The lower limit of normal for circulating neutrophils is 1500–2000/mm^3. The risk of acquiring an infection increases progressively with both the duration and the magnitude of the granulocytopenia below 1500 cells/mm^3. Below 500 neutrophils/mm^3, there is a dramatic increase in the incidence of infection.[197]

The acquired neutropenias are most often related to drug therapy and may be a predictable result of therapy or an idiosyncratic reaction. The former are frequently encountered during chemotherapy for various neoplastic and immunologic disorders. Neutropenia as a result of an idiosyncratic drug reaction is observed with phenothiazines, sulfonamides, penicillins, cephalosporins, and vancomycin. Chloramphenicol can cause both a predictable and an idiosyncratic neutropenia. The latter is uncommon but is frequently fatal. Increased granulocyte destruction may occur as a result of splenic sequestration. Splenic sequestration of neutrophils may be immunologically mediated by antibody[198,199] or secondary to any of the causes of hypersplenism. Splenectomy may be beneficial in restoring neutrophil counts toward normal.

Hereditary neutropenias are observed either as solitary defects or in association with other defects, for example, orotic aciduria. The neutropenia may be severe as in infantile genetic agranulocytosis, moderate as in familial (benign) neutropenia, or cyclic. Infantile genetic agranulocytosis is an autosomal recessive disorder characterized by granulocyte maturation arrest and severe infection with death in infancy. Some hereditary neutropenias are accompanied by an apparent compensatory monocytosis. Cyclic neutropenia is a rare autosomal dominant defect of myelopoiesis that is characterized by the periodic disappearance of neutrophils and other blood elements from the circulation. Early granulocyte precursors are present in the marrow during the neutropenia, which suggests a transient maturation arrest. The duration of neutropenia ranges from 5 to 8 days, followed by a 2- to 5-week period with normal numbers of circulating neutrophils. In a given patient, the periodic oscillations are constant. During the neutropenic state, the patients suffer from aphthous stomatitis, fever, malaise, and cutaneous infections. The disease is usually recognized during childhood, and there is no amelioration with age. Alternate-day predinosolone (25 mg qod) therapy attenuates the oscillation in neutrophil maturation.[200]

LEUKOCYTE ADHESION (Mo-1,Mac-1,LFA-1) DEFICIENCY SYNDROME

The development of monoclonal antibodies to neutrophil antigens and the use of these reagents to probe the cell surface in patients with neutrophil defects has led to the recognition of a new category of neutrophil dysfunction.[50] Previously the defect in these patients had been variously ascribed to actin, chemotactic, or phagocytic dysfunction.[201–205] It is now appreciated that the basic abnormality involves surface glycoproteins that mediate the adherence-related functions of the cell. Thus neutrophil adhesion, chemotaxis, and phagocytosis are all impaired in these patients.

The disorder is inherited in an autosomal recessive manner, and there is frequently a history of consanguinity. Severe and moderate phenotypes are recognized. Patients with this syndrome typically present with prolonged and/or recurrent staphylococcal and *Pseudomonas* infections beginning in infancy, often in the perinatal period. Patients with the severe phenotype often have delayed separation of the umbilical cord and may develop omphalitis. Infections involving the soft tissues, mucosal surfaces, and the intestinal tract are common. Cutaneous infections frequently become necrotic. Initially they may resemble ecthyma gangrenosum, whereas later they may assume a pyoderma gangrenosum appearance. Individuals surviving infancy universally develop acute gingivitis with eruption of primary dentition. The ginivitis persists and results in progressive gingival hypertrophy and alveolar bone loss. Individuals expressing the severe phenotype may also exhibit poor wound healing. Although survival into adulthood is well described, particularly in patients with the moderate phenotype, 41 percent of affected individuals die before the age of 2 years.[50,206]

A hallmark of the disease is a markedly and persistently elevated peripheral white blood cell count. Cell counts typically range from 2 to 20 times normal and remain elevated even in the absence of infection, probably due to impaired cellular margination and egress from the vascular tree. Evaluation of neutrophil function demonstrates impaired adherence to artificial substrates, impaired chemotaxis in vivo and in vitro, and an impaired respiratory burst in response to the ingestion of particles coated with iC3b but not IgG.[50,195,196] Affected neutrophils exhibit an above- or below-normal burst in oxidative metabolism after stimulation with soluble stimuli, depending on which stimulus is used and the nature of the association between its receptor and the cytoskeleton.[207]

The basis for this syndrome is the absence of a family of surface glycoproteins on the neutrophils from affected individuals. These proteins are important molecular determinants of adhesion-related functions and include the iC3b receptor (CR3, Mo-1, or Mac-1), lymphocyte function-associated antigen 1 (LFA-1), and p150,95. The proteins are α,β-heterodimers sharing identical β-chains but possessing distinct α-chains. The β-chain and each α-chain are the products of separate genes located on chromosomes 21 and 16, respectively. All three proteins are normally present on granulocytes and monocytes, whereas only LFA-1 is present on lymphocytes.

Leukocytes from individuals with the severe phenotypic expression of this disorder have less than 0.3 percent of the normal quantity of all three proteins on their surface, whereas moderately affected individuals express levels 2.5–6 percent of that in healthy people.[206] In affected individuals the surface expression of both the α- and β-chains is abnormal. However the α- but not the β-chain can be found in normal amounts within the cell. This finding indicates that the basis for the syndrome lies in the synthesis of the β-chain and that assembly of the α,β-heterodimer is required for transport of the α-chain to the cell surface.[208] Molecular analysis of the abnormal β-gene from a number of patients with this disorder has demonstrated a spectrum of mutations in the β-gene that range from the failure to produce mRNA in some individuals with the severe disease phenotype, to the production of an abnormally sized precursor β-protein, and to no readily apparent defect in some patients with either disease phenotype.[209]

CHEMOTACTIC DEFECTS

Extrinsic Abnormalities

Neutrophil chemotactic defects due to factors extrinsic to the cell may be secondary to abnormalities involving the complement cascade. These include genetic deficiencies (C3, C5), as well as decreased synthesis (cirrhosis, kwashiorkor, premature infants), hypercatabolism, and increased loss (severe burns) of serum proteins. Some investigators have noted a depression in neutrophil chemotactic responses in patients with diabetes mellitus that is independent of serum osmolality. The defect is mild and is most readily demonstrated in juvenile-onset diabetics. Chemotactic responsiveness of diabetic neutrophils can be restored in vitro by incubation with insulin.[210–212]

Chemotactic inhibitors may express their effect directly or indirectly by neutralizing the chemotactic effect of complement. Polymeric IgA is cytophilic for neutrophils and can markedly depress chemotaxis.[213] Defective chemotaxis has been described in a number of diseases characterized by circulating immune complexes. These include rheumatoid arthritis, systemic lupus erythematosus, and subacute bacterial endocarditis. Neutrophils exposed to immune complexes have high rates of oxidative metabolism and granule release in the resting state as well as an abnormal response to chemotactic stimuli. The sera from about 40 percent of patients with systemic lupus erythematosus contain an inhibitor that is specific for C5-derived chemotactic activity. This inhibitory factor does not interfere with the expression of other C5-mediated functions. Its presence correlates with disease activity and the resultant chemotactic defect with the enhanced susceptibility of these patients to infection.[214,215] The inhibitor has been identified as the Bb fragment of complement factor B, and it exerts its effect by inhibiting the interaction of C5a des arg with cochemotaxin in serum.[216,217]

A chemotactic defect has been described in patients with juvenile periodontitis, a familial disorder characterized by periodontitis occurring in the absence of severe dental disease. Serum from some of these patients contains an inhibitor of chemotaxis, and the resultant defect in chemotaxis has been postulated to play a role in the pathogenesis of this disease.[218,219] In addition, neutrophils from some of these patients bear fewer chemotactic receptors as compared with cells from unaffected individuals.[220] Of particular note in this regard is the report of an acquired neutrophil chemotactic defect in two adults with gingival infection due to *Capnocytophaga* (Bacteroides ochraceus). Eradication of infection resulted in a return to normal of neutrophil function. Sonicates of *Capnocytophaga* and filtrates of broth in which the organism had been grown inhibited the chemotactic response of normal neutrophils. These findings suggest that the chemotactic defect associated with some forms of periodontal disease may be due to the presence of bacterial products in the circulation.[221]

Chemotactic inhibitors whose mode of action appears to be the inactivation of chemotactic substances have been described in Hodgkin's disease, sarcoidosis, leprosy, and cirrhosis. These inhibitors are usually present in low concentration in normal serum and affect chemotaxis only when present in high concentrations.[212] Recurrent skin infections and abnormal neutrophil chemotaxis have also been associated with an IgG antineutrophil antibody.[222]

A number of pharmacologic agents including alcohol, steroids, tetracyclines, and amphotericin B inhibit chemotaxis in vitro. Alcohol may exert its effect by elevating cyclic AMP levels. The inhibitory effect of tetracyclines may be related to their ability to chelate calcium.

Intrinsic Abnormalities

Chédiak-Higashi Syndrome. The Chédiak-Higashi syndrome is a rare autosomal recessive trait involving a generalized dysfunction of granule-containing cells. Giant granules have been found in melanocytes, Schwann cells, renal tubular cells, thyroid cells, and all types of leukocytes (Fig. 6). These abnormal granules account for many of the physical findings including partial oculocutaneous albinism, rotatory nystagmus, peripheral neuropathy (both sensory and motor), and recurrent infection. In neutrophils, they are formed during cell maturation by fusion of the two granule types.[223] Laboratory abnormalities include anemia, leukopenia, thrombocytopenia, and evidence of intramedullary destruction of all blood elements with an associated elevation in serum lysozyme levels and deficiencies in iron and folate concentrations. Abnormal natural killer (NK) cell function has also been reported.[224] In a number of patients with the Chédiak-Higashi syndrome, the disease undergoes a transformation to an accelerated phase. This phase is characterized by hepatosplenomegaly, lymphadenopathy, and lymphocytic organ infiltration. Unexplained febrile episodes occur, and patients frequently die of infection or less commonly of hemorrhage at an early age.[225]

Neutrophils from patients with the Chédiak-Higashi syndrome exhibit a defective chemotactic response, but ingestion occurs normally.[226] Many bacteria, including both catalase-positive and catalase-negative species, exhibit prolonged survival within these neutrophils. Bacterial killing rates are most abnormal during the first 20 minutes of contact in vitro but approach normal levels at 2 hours. The faulty release of the large neutrophil granules is associated with the delayed appearance of myeloperoxidase within phagocytic vacuoles. The metabolic burst is normal.[227] The intracellular killing defect thus appears primarily due to delayed delivery of granule enzymes to the phagosome.

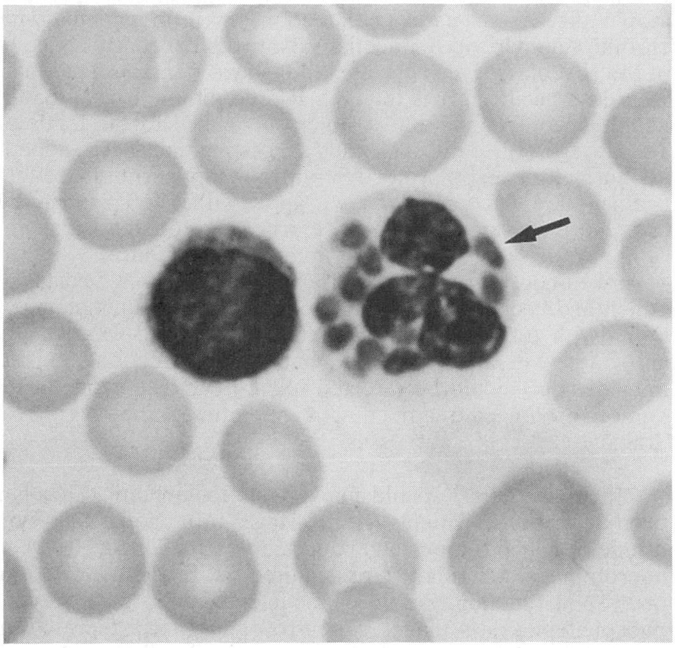

FIG. 6. Neutrophil and lymphocyte from a patient with Chédiak-Higashi syndrome. Note the large abnormal granules (arrow).

The biochemical abnormality underlying the neutrophil dysfunction in the Chédiak-Higashi syndrome is unknown. Abnormal function of a diverse number of cell types suggests that the defect involves some basic aspect of cell function. The bulk of current evidence suggests that the defect involves the microtubule apparatus: cell ultrastructure studies confirm a decreased number of centriole-associated microtubules in some patients; membrane fluidity is enhanced and has been suggested as a possible explanation for the abnormal fusion of the azurophil and specific granules; the level of tyrosylated tubulin is abnormally high; and pharmacologic agents, such as ascorbic acid, that affect microtubule assembly may improve cell function in occasional patients. In addition, agents that decrease the cyclic AMP/GMP ratio have been reported to improve neutrophil function. Many of these agents also affect microtubule assembly, and changes in cyclic nucleotide metabolism now appear to be a consequence of these alterations.[210,228–230]

Hyperimmunoglobulinemia E with Impaired Chemotaxis (Job's Syndrome). Job's syndrome, as originally described, is an affliction of fair-skinned, red-haired females that is characterized by eczema, recurrent "cold" staphylococcal skin abscesses, sinusitis, and otitis media.[231,232] However, the disorder occurs in blacks and males as well. Many of the patients have coarse facial features and a broad nasal bridge. In addition to cutaneous staphylococcal infection, recurrent pneumonia and mucocutaneous candidiasis are common. Patients may have mild eosinophilia, and although variable, the neutrophils of most patients exhibit a chemotactic abnormality. The chemotactic defect appears to correlate best with the severity of the eczema, and patients have been reported in whom a chemotactic defect could be demonstrated only during relapses of their dermatitis.[211] Mononuclear cells from these patients but not from individuals either with or without atopy spontaneously produce a factor that inhibits the chemotactic responses of normal neutrophils and monocytes.[233] All patients have markedly elevated (>10 times normal) serum levels of IgE due to a decreased fractional catabolic rate of this immunoglobulin.[234] Antistaphylococcal and anti-*Candida* IgE antibodies have been demonstrated in the serum from patients with Job's syndrome but not from healthy people, from patients with hyperimmunoglobulinemia E due to atopic disease or parasitic infection, or from patients with chronic staphylococcal infections. Antistaphylococcal antibody of the IgM class is also elevated in the sera from these patients, whereas specific IgA is low and IgG no different from that in healthy people. Infection is inversely related to the levels of specific IgE, IgA, and IgM, thus suggesting that these antibodies normally exert a protective rather than a permissive effect against staphylococci.[235] Thus it appears that Job's syndrome does not represent an intrinsic defect of neutrophil function but rather is the result of aberrant immune regulation.

A well-controlled clinical trial established that levamisol, which had been reported to improve neutrophil function in patients with Job's syndrome, failed to reduce and was actually associated with an increase in the number of infections.[236] Thus management should be directed toward early detection of infection, prolonged treatment with antibiotics, and early surgical drainage of "cold" abscesses.[232]

Other Disorders. A mild and variable chemotactic defect has been described in patients with Kartagener (immotile cilia) syndrome in which there is an abnormality in the linkage between microtubules and cilia.[210] An acquired but reversible defect in neutrophil function has been documented with severe hypophosphatemia (less than 1 mg/dl) secondary to phosphate-free hyperalimentation. The defect in these cells is thought to be due to an inability to generate ATP from anaerobic glycolysis.[237]

Abnormal Phagocytosis

Defective opsonization occurs with inherited or acquired deficiencies of the early complement components (especially C3) or immunoglobulin. Similar derangements accompany the paraproteinemias as well as a number of other neoplastic and nonneoplastic disorders characterized by hypoglobulinemia and/or hypocomplementemia. Anatomic or functional asplenia results in a deficiency of opsonic factors for a number of encapsulated bacteria. Splenectomy also results in a deficiency in tuftsin, a tetrapeptide synthesized in the spleen and reported to facilitate ingestion of staphylococci.[238] Patients with opsonic disorders frequently have recurrent infections with encapsulated bacteria, particularly pneumococci and *Haemophilus influenzae*. Infection with these organisms in the splenectomized person can present as a fulminant bacteremia or meningitis accompanied by disseminated intravascular coagulation.[239]

Defects in Intracellular Killing

Abnormal Respiratory Burst. CHRONIC GRANULOMATOUS DISEASES OF CHILDHOOD. The chronic granulomatous diseases of childhood (CGDs) are a group of disorders characterized by recurrent infections attributable to defects in neutrophil oxygen-dependent microbicidal activity. The classic form of this disease is an X-linked recessive disorder, but a clinically indistinguishable variant affecting females as well as males exhibits an autosomal mode of inheritance. The relative frequency of these two forms of the disease is uncertain. The disease usually presents early in childhood, 78 percent of affected individuals manifesting recurrent and often prolonged infection during the first year of life. Although an infectious agent is not isolated during the majority of most febrile episodes,[240] the microbiology of this disorder is distinctive for the paucity of infections caused by the encapsulated or catalase-negative organisms (e.g., *S. pneumoniae*) that ordinarily predominate in this age group. Rather, *Staphylococcus aureus* is the causative agent in 52 percent of the infections with an identifiable etiology. Other primary infecting agents include *Salmonella, Pseudomonas aeruginosa, Serratia marcescens, Nocardia asteroides,* and *Aspergillus*. Although *S. aureus* is the pathogen most commonly isolated from infected sites, gram-negative bacteria account for 73 percent of all bacteremic episodes and for 80 percent of fatal septicemias.[241] Pyogenic dermatitis, suppurative adenitis, recurrent pneumonia with abscess formation, stomatitis, enteritis, and colitis are common. Intestinal obstruction secondary to inflammatory masses, especially in the perirectal area, has been reported. A third of the patients have deep-seated abscesses in the liver or perihepatic region. Obstructive uropathy and xanthogranulomatous pyelonephritis also occur. Osteomyelitis is common and is noteworthy for its relatively frequent causation by *Serratia marcescens* and involvement of the metacarpal and metatarsal bones.[242] Physical findings commonly include dermatitis, adenopathy, hepatosplenomegaly, and "failure to thrive." Routine laboratory studies show leukocytosis, anemia of chronic disease, and hyperglobulinemia. Pathologic examination of affected tissues reveals noncaseating granulomas. Although recurrent infection with death by an average age of 3.7 years was the rule in 1955–1965, the average life expectancy in the period 1975–1982 was 9.5 years. The disorder has been diagnosed in adults presenting with "idiopathic" pulmonary fibrosis. These patients frequently have a history of recurrent infections in childhood, but infections seem to occur less frequently during adulthood. Thus, the increased life expectancy in this disease probably reflects both an improvement in medical management and the recognition of milder forms of the disease.[85,106,243]

Female carriers of X-linked CGD have both normal and abnormally functioning neutrophils. Most of these women display no undue susceptibility to infection, although an association with discoid lupus erythematosus has been noted in several reports.[97,244,245] The greater frequency of infection that occurs in some carriers correlates with an increase in the population of defective neutrophils. This increase appears due to the chance inactivation of a disproportionate number of normal X chromosomes as predicted by the Lyon hypothesis.[246]

The defect in CGD is an inability of neutrophils, other granulocytes, and monocytes to display the respiratory burst during phagocytosis. All oxidative events associated with the burst (oxygen consumption, chemiluminescence, production of toxic oxygen species, hexose monophosphate shunt activity, and microbial halogenation) are absent in CGD neutrophils. These cells also fail to undergo membrane depolarization during phagocytosis. Chemotaxis, phagocytosis, and degranulation are normal. Infections caused by catalase-negative organisms are uncommon because hydrogen peroxide produced by these bacteria effectively circumvents the biochemical lesion and reacts with myeloperoxidase and a halide in the phagosome to regenerate microbicidal activity.

Recognition of the complexity of the oxidase system coupled with the identification of patients with CGD due to different biochemical defects has led to the classification of these disorders on the basis of whether they involve oxidase activation pathways or the oxidase system itself (Table 4).[85,89,106] Disorders involving the activation pathways may be due to a defect in signal recognition or transduction. The defect is usually inapparent upon stimulation of the cell with soluble agents but becomes evident when a phagocytic particle is used as the stimulus. This contrasts with disorders involving the oxidase system itself in which neither particulate nor soluble stimuli activate the respiratory burst. Neutrophils from patients with the leukocyte adhesion deficiency syndrome lack CR3 and do not respond to iC3b-coated particles but exhibit a normal oxidative burst upon stimulation with phorbol myristate acetate (PMA). Thus they are representative of the former category of CGD.[201–205] This type of defect emphasizes the importance of using more than one type of stimulus when considering the diagnosis of CGD.

Defects involving the oxidase itself are subclassified as to whether oxidase activity is impaired or totally absent (Table 4). The former category is represented by a clinically mild variant of X-linked CGD described in two unrelated males whose neutrophils exhibited normal membrane depolarization and a nor-

TABLE 4. Classification of the Chronic Granulomatous Diseases

Type of Defect in the Oxidase System	*Relative Frequency[a] (%)*	*Inheritance*	*Oxidase Response to Stimuli*		*Cytochrome b_{-558}*		*Flavo-protein*	*Cytosolic Factor*	*Phosphorylation of 48 kD Membrane Protein*
			Particulate	*Soluble*					
Impaired activation									
LAD syndrome	<3.3	AR	abs/imp	nl/super nl	nl		nl	nl	depends on stimulus
Abnormal oxidase activity									
Impaired activity	<3.3–18	XL	imp	imp	"abs"–low		nl	nl	imp
Absent activity									
Cytochrome b_{-558} absent					Chain α	β			
a	23–64	XL	abs	abs	abs	abs[b]	nl	nl	imp
b	<3.3–3.3	AR	abs	abs	ND[c]	ND	nl	nl	ND
c	13–18	XL	abs	abs	abs	abs	low	nl	ND
Cytochrome b_{-558} present	18–60								abs
a		AR	abs	abs	nl	nl	nl	47 kD prot—abs 65 kD prot—nl	ND
b		AR	abs	abs	nl	nl	nl	47 kD prot—nl 65 kD prot—abs	ND

[a] Among individuals with the CGD syndrome.[98,247]
[b] The primary defect involes the β-chain encoded by a gene on the X chromosome.
[c] The primary defect probably involves the α-chain encoded by a gene on chromosome 16.
Abbreviations: LAD: leukocyte adhesion deficiency; AR: autosomal recessive; XL: X-linked; abs: absent; imp: impaired; nl: normal; ND: not determined.

mal lag time between stimulation and onset of the respiratory burst. However, the magnitude of the burst was substantially reduced. A reduced affinity of the oxidase system for NADPH was felt to account for this defect.[248,249] An unexplained finding in these two patients has been the associated absence of the b cytochrome.[249]

CGD due to the total absence of neutrophil oxidase activity is inherited in either an X-linked or autosomal manner. That different biochemical lesions underlie these two genetic variants of CGD was originally most clearly demonstrated in a cooperative European study of 27 CGD patients and their families. The b cytochrome was absent from the neutrophils of patients with X-linked CGD and present in half-normal amounts in female carriers of this form of the disease. In contrast, neutrophils from patients with the autosomal recessive form of the disease contained normal quantities of an apparently normal b cytochrome.[97] Subsequently it was shown that oxidase activity could be restored by cross-hybridization of monocytes from patients with different inherited forms of CGD.[250] These studies demonstrated that at least three separate biochemical defects could result in absent oxidase activity.[251] As detailed above, substantial evidence supports a role for cytochrome b_{-558}, a flavoprotein, and cytosolic factors as constituents of the oxidase system. Cytochrome b_{-558} is an α,β-heterodimer consisting of a 22 kD α-chain that contains the heme group responsible for the cytochrome spectral signal and a 91 kD β-chain. These chains appear to be tightly but noncovalently associated in the intact cytochrome.[101,103,104] The α-chain is encoded by a gene on chromosome 16 and the β-chain by an X-linked gene.[102] Neutrophils from patients with X-linked CGD are missing both the α- and the β-chains of the cytochrome as determined by both immunoprecipitation studies and detection of the cytochrome spectral signal.[101,252] The absence of the 22 kD product of a gene on chromosome 16 in X-linked CGD suggests that the 91 kD β-chain, which is the product of the X-linked gene, may be required for cellular processing of the α-chain.[101] Recently four patients with autosomal CGD due to cytochrome b_{-558} deficiency have been identified on the basis of an absent spectral signal for the cytochrome.[247,251] Neither of these reports examined neutrophil membranes for the presence of the α- or the β-chain of the cytochrome. On the basis of the chromosomal location of the genes for the respective polypeptide chains one might speculate that this form of CGD may be due to an abnormality involving the α-gene on chromosome 16 and that the β-chain might be present in these neutrophils. Finally, some patients with X-linked cytochrome b deficiency have an associated flavoprotein deficiency (Table 4).[91,98,247]

Cytochrome b_{-558} and flavoprotein levels are normal in most patients with autosomal recessive CGD.[247] These patients may have a clinically milder form of the disease,[99,106,253] although this is not supported by all studies.[98] Neutrophils from these patients are missing either a 47 kD or 65 kD cytosolic factor that must be translocated to the cell membrane in order to activate the oxidase system.[99,254–256] This type of CGD is associated with the failure of these neutrophils or their cytosol to phosphorylate an uncharacterized 48 kD membrane protein(s)[139,254]; however, the factor does not appear to be protein kinase C since the activity of this enzyme is normal in neutrophils from some of these patients.[254] Although further characterization is obviously required, it is of interest that the molecular size of the 65 kD protein is consistent with that described for the NADPH membrane binding protein in guinea pigs.[100] There is evidence supporting a defect in the phosphorylation of a 48 kD membrane protein in X-linked CGD as well.[257] On the other hand, some investigators have failed to detect such an abnormality in any form of CGD.[258] Thus the role of phosphorylation in the activation of the oxidase system requires further delineation.

The diagnosis of CGD is readily made by using the nitroblue tetrazolium dye (NBT) test.[259] This test depends on the ability of normal neutrophils to reduce the yellow dye, nitroblue tetrazolium, to blue formazan. NBT reduction by neutrophils is primarily dependent on the production of superoxide; therefore, the NBT test is negative in CGD. A properly performed, negative NBT test with appropriate controls is very strong evidence for the diagnosis of CGD. It should be confirmed by the demonstration of normal phagocytosis and a marked reduction in the parameters of the metabolic burst. In order to detect abnormalities in the activation mechanism, both soluble and particulate stimuli should be used in tests of oxidative function.

GLUCOSE-6-PHOSPHATE DEHYDROGENASE DEFICIENCY. Although erythrocyte and leukocyte glucose-6-phosphate dehydrogenase (G6PD) are products of the same gene, the common form of G6PD deficiency that presents as a hemolytic anemia in blacks is not associated with neutrophil dysfunction. This discrepancy is explained by the fact that this deficiency is due to an unstable enzyme, the activity of which diminishes over a period of time that exceeds the life expectancy of the neutrophil. Neutrophil dysfunction does occur in rare cases of G6PD deficiency in whites missing or having less than 5 percent of the normal levels of G6PD. The basis for neutrophil dysfunction in this disorder is that in the absence of G6PD glucose cannot be metabolized via the hexose monophosphate shunt. As a consequence, NADPH, used by the oxidase, cannot be regenerated from NADP. Aside from the presence of a hemolytic anemia, the clinical, laboratory, and genetic (X-linked) presentation is very similar to CGD. The NBT test is negative or low, as are other parameters of the respiratory burst. The failure of methylene blue to stimulate hexose monophosphate shunt activity and low levels of G6PD distinguish this defect from CGD.[85,260]

Granule Abnormalities. MYELOPEROXIDASE DEFICIENCY. Once thought to be a rare disorder, neutrophil myeloperoxidase (MPO) deficiency is now recognized as the most common of all neutrophil functional disorders, with a frequency of 1 per 2000–4000 people for whom leukocyte counts are performed. This discrepancy is accounted for by the fact that the overwhelming majority of such individuals are healthy and that detection of this condition has been greatly facilitated by the widespread use of flow cytometry techniques that use peroxidase staining for leukocyte differential counts.[261] Eosinophil peroxidase is not affected in this disorder. An autosomal recessive manner of inheritance has been reported, but the heterogeneous expression of the defect has led to the suggestion that inheritance may be under polygenic control. Of all the patients recognized with this disorder, only six have had serious infections. Systemic candidiasis occurred in four of these patients, three of whom had diabetes mellitus. This association suggests that diabetics with serious fungal infection should be screened for MPO deficiency and, conversely, that MPO-deficient individuals receiving broad-spectrum antibiotics may be at increased risk for fungal superinfection.[262]

Since the cell is devoid of MPO-dependent but not other oxidative killing mechanisms, there is delayed but not absent intracellular killing in MPO-deficient neutrophils. Delayed killing is more pronounced for fungi than for bacteria,[263] which suggests an explanation for the clinical findings in this disorder. Chemotaxis, phagocytosis, and degranulation are normal, but the respiratory burst is enhanced. The supranormal oxidative metabolism may be due to absent MPO-dependent inactivation of the oxidase system[123] and may help explain the lack of clinical expression of this defect in most patients.

Normal MPO is the product of a single gene on chromosome 17.[264] Post-translational cleavage of a glycosylated (89 kD) primary gene product results in a mature molecule containing heavy α (59 kD) and light β (13.5 kD) chains.[262,265,266] The current structural model suggests that the chain content of mature MPO is $\alpha_2\beta_2$, but this is a matter of some debate.[262,267] Granule extracts from normal neutrophils contain an 80–90 kD MPO-related peptide in addition to the mature α- and β-chains, whereas similar extracts from completely deficient MPO neutrophils contain only the 80–90 kD peptide.[265] This finding strongly suggests that MPO deficiency is due to a defect in the post-translational modification of the 89 kD precursor protein. Restriction endonuclease DNA mapping and analysis of MPO-specific mRNA obtained from the bone marrow of deficient individuals indicates that a number of heterogeneous molecular defects are responsible for the phenotypic deficit in processing.[262] MPO deficiency has also been recognized as an acquired defect accompanying some myeloproliferative disorders, particularly acute myelogenous leukemia (AML). In the leukemic but not the preleukemic state this deficiency is associated with an increased risk of infection.[262] This finding coupled with analogous observations in the inherited form of the disorder indicates that the occurrence of MPO deficiency by itself does not alter the host's susceptibility to infection but in conjunction with an additional insult (e.g., diabetes mellitus, AML) may tip the balance in favor of infection.

SPECIFIC GRANULE DEFICIENCY. The absence of specific granules has been recognized in five patients with recurrent infection.[268] The peripheral white blood cell count in such individuals is normal when they are uninfected, and the diagnosis is established by the apparent absence of intracellular granules on routine Wright stain (primary granules do not take up Wright stain). Close examination reveals a bilobed nuclear morphology with nuclear blocks and clefts. Specific granule contents (e.g., lactoferrin, vitamin B_{12}-binding protein) are absent, as is membrane alkaline phosphatase.[164,268,269] This finding coupled with the presence of apparently empty granule vesicles in one of these patients and the abnormal nuclear morphology suggests that the defect may be a more general disorder involving membrane assembly rather than a defect unique to specific granules.[268]

Specific granules are a rich source of substances that modulate the inflammatory response, and their membranes contain receptors for a number of opsonic ligands and inflammatory mediators. Hence it is not surprising that in vitro upregulation of these receptors is impaired and that there are associated impairments in chemotaxis, phagocytosis, and oxidase activity with certain stimuli. Of particular note, however, is the demonstration of an in vivo chemotactic defect for both neutrophils and monocytes from patients with this disorder, whereas only neutrophils exhibit a chemotactic defect in vitro. This finding supports a role for defective chemotaxis in the genesis of infection in these patients and further suggests that a constitutent of specific granules may normally modulate monocyte infiltration to sites of inflammation.[268] Neutrophils from severely burned patients and from neonates share some of the characteristics of specific granule-deficient cells.[268]

Therapy for Neutrophil Defects

Antimicrobial Therapy. The recurrent and severe infections that occur in many patients with abnormal neutrophil function has made the administration of prophylactic antibiotics common despite concerns about colonization and infection with resistant microorganisms. The low prevalence of these disorders has made controlled trials of prophylactic antibiotics nearly impossible, although one study evaluating cloxacillin prophylaxis in the Chédiak-Higashi syndrome did not show any benefit.[270] The administration of lipid-soluble antibiotics such as rifampin and trimethoprim-sulfamethoxazole that penetrate phagocytic cells[271,272] has been advocated for patients with impaired neutrophil bactericidal activity. In this regard, the broad antimicrobial spectrum of trimethoprim-sulfamethoxazole against both gram-positive and gram-negative bacteria, coupled with its penetration and concentration within neutrophils probably explains its apparent effectiveness in reducing infections in patients with CGD.[273,274] Prophylactic antibiotic therapy in patients with CGD has been associated with an increase in the infection-free interval from 9.6 to 40 months.[240] The effect of antibiotics on the intracellular killing mechanisms has received attention with the demonstration that staphylococci exposed to sublethal concentrations of cell wall-active antibiotics for a short time were more readily killed by neutrophils than were staphylococci grown in the absence of antibiotics. Improved killing was due to an enhancement in nonoxidative bactericidal mechanisms and was both organism and antibiotic specific.[275,276] The significance of these findings for patient management is unknown.

Cytokine Therapy. Incubation of IFN-γ with granulocytic cells from patients with CGD enhances superoxide production, restores killing of *S. aureus* and increases cytochrome b_{-558} content. In total, cells from 15 of 18 patients with cytochrome b positive (primarily autosomal) CGD but only 7 of 21 individuals with cytochrome b negative (primarily X-linked) CGD responded to IFN-γ. In vitro testing appeared predictive of a response in vivo in five patients who received subcutaneous injections of recombinant human IFN-γ. Moreover in vivo responses persisted for 3 to 5 weeks following cessation of therapy.[277,277a,277b] Clinical trials evaluating drug toxicity and efficacy in ameliorating the infectious consequences of this disease are currently in progress.

Granulocyte Transfusion. Granylocyte transfusions have been used therapeutically in febrile granulocytopenic patients. To achieve a theoretic blood neutrophil count of 1000 cells/mm^3 after transfusion, approximately 1×10^{10} neutrophils (all the neutrophils in 2–3 liters of blood) are required for the average adult per day. However, many patients will show no significant rise in the peripheral white cell count after transfusion of this number of cells.[278] Two basic methods of procurement have been devised—centrifugation and filtration leukopheresis. The former method uses differences in density among blood cells to achieve separation. Filtration uses the ability of neutrophils to adhere to nylon wool to achieve separation from other cells. Cells obtained by both procedures are functional both in vitro and in vivo, but those obtained by filtration leukopheresis exhibit cytoplasmic vacuolization and surface distortion as well as a loss of granule contents and reduced bactericidal capacity.[278,279] In addition, up to 75 percent of the recipients of cells obtained by leukopheresis will have transfusion reactions, predominantly fever and chills, as compared with 15 percent of the recipients of cells obtained by centrifugation.[280] Despite these differences, administration of cells obtained by either method to granulocytopenic patients with infection has been beneficial in some but not all controlled trials.[281,282] Granulocytopenic patients with proven bacterial infection who received daily granulocyte transfusions for the duration of their infection survived longer than did infected nontransfused control patients. Both groups received therapy appropriate for their infection.[280,283] Leukocyte transfusions have also been therapeutically successful when administered to a limited number of patients with neutrophil bactericidal defects and progressive infection. By using a positive NBT test as a marker, delivery to and persistence of transfused normal leukocytes at the site of infection has been documented in a patient with CGD.[284]

Although leukocyte transfusions may be lifesaving in certain infected granulocytopenic patients, associated complications have limited their routine use in these febrile patients. These complications include (1) transfusion-associated cytomegalovirus infection; (2) allosensitization to HLA antigens; (3) difficulties in locating adequate numbers of suitable donors; (4) risks to the donor; (5) extreme cost of the procedure; and (6) an increased incidence of acute pulmonary reactions when transfusions are given in conjunction with amphotericin B.[285–287] This latter complication is a major concern since one accepted indication for the use of leukocyte transfusions is the treatment of unrelenting fungal infection in the neutropenic host. This reaction most commonly occurs when amphotericin B treatment is initiated simultaneously with or after transfusion. It is characterized by the acute onset of respiratory decompensation, pulmonary infiltrates, and intra-alveolar hemorrhage.[287] A potentially serious complication of red cell or white cell transfusions in patients with CGD is related to the Kell-related antigen, K_X. This antigen is present on the surface of red and white cells from healthy people and patients with autosomally transmitted CGD. K_X is absent from the neutrophils of most patients with the X-linked form of the disease due to the close linkage of the CGD and X_k genes on the X chromosone.[288–290] Failure to recognize this antigenic abnormality can result in severe transfusion reactions.[291] As a consequence of these complicating aspects, leukocyte transfusion seems best reserved for the patient with severe granulocytopenia or functionally defective neutrophils who has a serious bacterial or fungal infection that has not responded to appropriate antimicrobial therapy.

TABLE 5. Evaluation of Neutrophil Function

White blood cell count and differential count
Migration to site[295]
Chemotaxis[296]
Phagocytosis and bactericidal activity[297]
Postphagocytic activity
Oxygen consumption[298]
Hexose monophosphate shunt[299]
Iodination[300]
NBT reduction[259,301]
Degranulation[302]
Chemiluminescence[303]

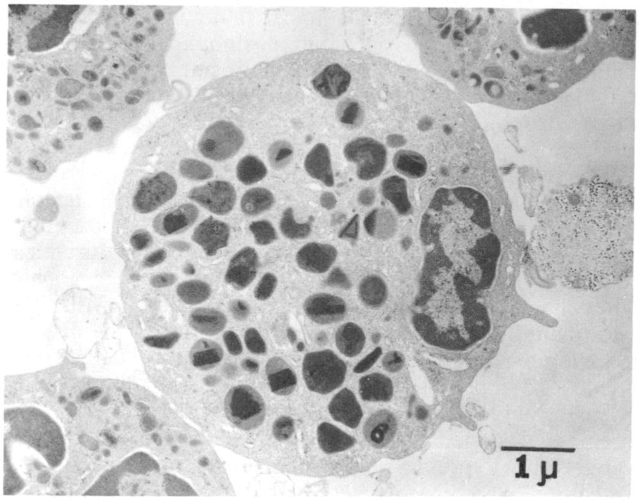

FIG. 7. Electron micrograph of a human eosinophil. Note the prominent granules with crystalloid cores.

Bone Marrow Transplantation. Several patients, one with leukocyte adhesion deficiency[201] and three with CGD,[292–294] have undergone successful bone marrow engraftment and clinical improvement. Two of the latter patients ultimately rejected their transplant but continued to enjoy clinical improvement.[292,294] This result illustrates the difficulty in the meaningful evaluation of this procedure in these types of patients. Moreover, given the increased infection-free interval and survival observed with the use of prophylactic antibiotics in CGD,[240] it seems reasonable to reserve such aggressive therapy for unusual situations.

Evaluating Phagocyte Function

The single most important test in the evaluation of possible abnormalities of neutrophil function is a white blood cell count with a differential count. Serum immunoglobulin and complement levels should be determined. An NBT test, requiring only a drop or two of blood, is simple and can be performed quickly. Further evaluation depends on the results of these simple screening tests (Table 5).[294]

EOSINOPHILS

Eosinophils are primarily tissue-based granulocytes, the ratio of tissue to blood eosinophils being 100 to 1 in humans.[304] Eosinophils differentiate from stem cells in the bone marrow over the course of 5 to 6 days.[305] Maturation is accompanied by the development of cytoplasmic granules and surface receptors for complement and IgG.[304] The number of these receptors is upregulated during specific stimulation of the eosinophil. There are at least two types of granules present in the cytoplasm of eosinophils. The larger, more numerous eosinophil granules contain an electron-dense crystalloid core (Fig. 7) composed of major basic protein. The crystalloid core is surrounded by a less dense, regularly arranged matrix that contains a number of highly cationic proteins including eosinophil cationic protein, eosinophil-derived neurotoxin, and eosinophil myeloperoxidase. This peroxidase is antigenically and genetically distinct from neutrophil myeloperoxidase. A second, smaller and more homogenous granule containing arylsulfatase B and acid phosphatase is also present in the cytoplasm.[306] Other enzymes and nonenzymatic proteins isolated in relatively greater quantities from eosinophils than from neutrophils include phospholipase D, lysophospholipase, histaminase, and cationic proteins.[304] Oxidative metabolism in resting and stimulated eosinophils is higher than that of neutrophils; the significance of this observation is unknown but may relate to the underlying disease in the patients with hypersinophilia from whom the cells were obtained.[307] Two populations of eosinophils, normodense and hypodense, have been recognized on the basis of their different densities. Hypodense cells are eosinophils that have been activated. They express a greater number of complement and immunoglobulin receptors, have a higher resting level of oxidative metabolism, and predominate in the blood and tissues of individuals with eosinophilia.[306] The half-life of eosinophils in blood is 2 hours.[304] After leaving the circulation, eosinophils are found along with IgE-bearing mast cells and basophils subjacent to the skin and mucosal lining of the respiratory and gastrointestinal tracts.[304,308] The development of eosinophilia[309,310] is dependent in part on a specific cytokine released from sensitized T lymphocytes. An eosinophilopoietin has also been isolated and characterized.[311] These factors produce eosinophilia by increasing eosinophil release from the bone marrow and spleen, shortening the marrow maturation time, and increasing eosinophil production. Eosinophil colony-stimulating factor both stimulates the differentiation of eosinophil precursors and promotes activation of mature eosinophils in the circulation.[306] Certain products of complement activation are chemotactic for eosinophils as they are for neutrophils. Substances specifically chemotactic for eosinophils are released in substantial quantities during immediate hypersensitivity reactions. These substances include eosinophil chemotactic factor of anaphylaxis (ECF-A), histamine, lymphokines, and lipoxygenase metabolites of arachidonic acid, particularly the hydroxyeicosatetranoic acids.[61,304]

Substantial evidence supports a role for eosinophils in immunity to helminthic parasites,[312–314] for modulation of type I hypersensitivity reactions, [304,315] and for the production of tissue damage in certain disease states.[304,306,308,315–317] Although eosinophils can phagocytose bacteria in vitro, they are less efficient in this regard than are neutrophils[307] and probably do not play a role in host defense against bacteria.[316] In contrast, they are a major effector of immunity to helminthic infections as demonstrated by the greater worm burden and tissue damage in animals whose eosinophils have been eliminated by treatment with antieosinophil serum.[314] This conclusion is buttressed by the presence of eosinophils on and around degenerating parasites in vivo and by the ability of eosinophils to kill these organisms in vitro. Killing is also antibody and complement dependent,[312,313] but the transfer of passive immunity requires the presence of eosinophils in the recipient.[314]

Killing of parasites is related to exocytosis of eosinophil granule contents onto the parasite surface while it is in close opposition to the eosinophils.[318,319] The eosinophil peroxidase, hydrogen peroxide, halide oxidation, system plays a minor role in anthelminthic activity.[304,306,308,316] Rather, the cationic granule proteins are responsible for the bulk of this activity. These proteins appear to have different sites of action as inferred from different morphologic alterations in the parasite surface and internal tissues that are observed upon incubation of the organism with purified preparations of the various proteins. Synergistic activity among proteins with different loci of action may occur. On a molar basis eosinophil cationic protein exerts a more potent anthelminthic effect than does major basic protein, but the greater quantity of the latter in the eosinophil makes its contribution more significant.[306] The effect of these proteins is also specific for different stages in the life cycle of the parasite.[306,320]

Recognition that eosinophil granules contain a number of substances capable of inactivating the chemical mediators of anaphylaxis has led to the suggestion that the eosinophil may modulate the severity of type I hypersensitivity reactions.[304,306,317] In this scenario, stimulation of basophils and mast cells by the interaction of surface IgE with specific antigen results in the release of substances important in type I hypersensitivity reactions. These include vasoactive amines, slow-reacting substance of anaphylaxis (leukotrienes C, D, and E), platelet activating factor (PAF), and ECF-A. Histamine and ECF-A attract eosinophils to the site of antigen reaction with basophils and mast cells. ECF-A can also stimulate eosinophil degranulation, as can immune complexes that the eosinophil phagocytizes. Histaminase secreted by the eosinophil may inactivate local histamine, and further histamine secretion by basophils may be inhibited by a substance present in eosinophils. Arylsulfatase and phospholipase present in the smaller eosinophil granules are capable of inactivating leukotrienes C, D, and E and PAF. Thus, eosinophils may modulate immediate hypersensitivity reactions by inhibiting the release of mediators of the type I reaction as well as by destroying mediators that have already been released.[304,315]

The association of eosinophilia of several weeks' duration with the development of endocardial lesions and the isolation of an eosinophil-derived neurotoxin capable of reproducing the neurologic picture observed in patients with cerebrospinal fluid eosinophilia strongly supports a role for the eosinophil in the pathogenesis of tissue injury in certain disorders.[306] Most prominent among these disorders is bronchial asthma. Here substantial evidence indicates that eosinophil major basic protein (MBP) is an important mediator of tissue injury. This evidence can be summarized as follows. (1) Nanomolar concentrations of MBP but not other cationic proteins cause exfoliation of epithelial cells and impaired ciliary function in tracheal ring explants. (2) Immunofluorescent staining of bronchial epithelium in autopsy specimens from patients dying of asthma reveals extensive deposition of MBP in the peribronchial areas and overlying regions of bronchial epithelial denuclation. These findings were not observed in autopsy material obtained from patients whose death was related to other pulmonary diseases. The importance of epithelial denudation lies in the resultant enhanced responsiveness of the underlying bronchial smooth muscle to contractile agonists including leukotriene C_4 produced by eosinophils. (3) Increased quantities of MBP are detectable in the bronchial washings from patients with asthma but not other pulmonary disorders.[306]

BASOPHILS

Basophils are tissue-based granulocytes related to mast cells. Although capable of phagocytosis, they perform this function poorly. Basophil granules are rich in heparin and vasoactive amines, particularly histamine. Basophils circulate with IgE bound to their membrane; recognition of antigen by this cytophilic immunoglobulin results in the external secretion of the contents of the granules. While the pharmacologic actions and importance of these vasoactive amines are well recognized, their physiologic role and the role of the basophils in secreting them is less well understood.[321] Although basophils do not appear to have a primary role in dealing with infection, recent evidence suggests that they may play a role in immunity to ticks.[322]

REFERENCES

1. Silverstein AM. Cellular versus humoral immunity: Determinants and consequences of an epic 19th century battle. Cell Immunol. 1979;48:208.

2. Hirsch JG. Host resistance to infectious diseases—a centennial. Adv Host Defense Mech. 1982;1:1.
3. Bainton DF. Differentiation of human neutrophilic granulocytes: Normal and abnormal. Prog Clin Biol Res. 1977;13:1.
4. Cotter TG, Spears P, Henson PJ. A monoclonal antibody inhibiting human neutrophil chemotaxis and degranulation. J Immunol. 1981;127:1355.
5. Cotter TG, Keeling PG, Henson PM. A monoclonal antibody–inhibiting FMLP-induced chemotaxis of human neutrophils. J Immunol. 1981;127:2241.
6. Nauseef WM, Root RK, Newman SL, et al. Inhibition of zymosan activation of human neutrophil oxidative metabolism by a mouse monoclonal antibody. Blood. 1983;62:635.
7. Glasser L, Fiederlein RL. Functional differentiation of normal human neutrophils. Blood. 1987;69:937–44.
8. Zakhireh B, Root RK. Development of oxidase activity by human bone marrow granulocytes. Blood. 1979;54:429.
9. Lichtman MA, Weed RI. Alteration of the cell periphery during granulocyte maturation: Relationship to cell function. Blood. 1972;39:301.
10. Lichtman MA, Chamberlain JK, Weed RI, et al. The regulation of the release of granulocytes from normal marrow. Prog Clin Biol Res. 1977;13:53.
11. Bainton DF, Farquhar MG. Origin of granules in polymorphonuclear leukocytes. J Cell Biol. 1966;28:277.
12. Bretz U, Baggiolini M. Biochemical and morphological characterization of azurophil and specific granules of human neutrophilic polymorphonuclear leukocytes. J Cell Biol. 1974;63:251.
13. Spitznagel JK, Dalldorf FG, Leffell MS, et al. Character of azurophil and specific granules purified from human polymorphonuclear leukocytes. Lab Invest. 1974;30:774.
14. West BC, Rosenthal AS, Gelb NA, et al. Separation and characterization of human neutrophil granules. Am J Pathol. 1974;77:41.
15. Dewald B, Bretz U, Baggiolini M. Release of gelatinase from a novel secretory compartment of human neutrophils. J Clin Invest. 1982;70:518–25.
16. Brederoo P, van der Meulen J, Mommaas-Kienhuis AM. Development of the granule population in neutrophil granulocytes from human bone marrow. Cell Tissue Res. 1983;234:469–96.
17. Weeds A. Actin-binding proteins—regulators of cell architecture and motility. Nature. 1982;296:811.
18. Southwick FS, Stossel TP. Contractile proteins in leukocyte function. Semin Hematol. 1983;20:305.
19. Stossel TP, Hartwig JH, Yin HL, et al. The motor of leukocytes. Fed Proc. 1984;43:2760–3.
20. Stevenson KB, Nauseef WM, Clark RA. Fodrin and band 4.1 in a plasma membrane–associated fraction of human neutrophils. Submitted for publication.
21. White JR, Naccache PH, Sha'afi RI. Stimulation by chemotactic factor of actin association with the cytoskeleton in rabbit neutrophils. J Biol Chem. 1983;258:14041–7.
22. Ryder MI, Weinreb RN, Niederman R. The organization of actin filaments in human polymorphonuclear leukocytes. Anat Rec. 1984;209:7–20.
23. Berlin RD, Fera JP. Changes in membrane microviscosity associated with phagocytosis: Effects of colchicine. Proc Natl Acad Sci USA. 1977;74:1072.
24. Snyderman R, Goetzl EJ. Molecular and cellular mechanisms of leukocyte chemotaxis. Science. 1981;213:830.
25. Bucher NLR. Microtubules. N Engl J Med. 1972;287:195.
26. Malfunctioning microtubules (Editorial). Lancet. 1978;1:697.
27. Messner RP, Jelinek J. Receptors for human gamma-globulin on human neutrophils. J Clin Invest. 1970;49:2165.
28. Spiegelberg NL, Lawrence DA, Henson P. Cytophilic properties of IgA to human neutrophils. Adv Exp Biol Med. 1974;45:67.
29. Lay WH, Nussenzweig V. Receptors for complement on leukocytes. J Exp Med. 1968;129:991.
30. Williams LT, Snyderman R, Pike MC, et al. Specific receptor sites for chemotactic peptides on human polymorphonuclear leukocytes. Proc Natl Acad Sci USA. 1977;74:1204.
31. Chenoweth DE, Hugli TE. Demonstration of specific C5a receptor on intact human polymorphonuclear leukocytes. Proc Natl Acad Sci USA. 1978;75:3943.
32. Walter RJ, Berlin RD, Oliver JM. Asymmetric Fc receptor distribution on human PMN oriented in a chemotactic gradient. Nature. 1980;286:724.
33. Weinbaum DL, Sullivan JA, Mandell GL. Receptors for concanavalin A cluster at the front of polarized neutrophils. Nature. 1980;286:725.
34. Bender JG, Van Epps DE, Chenoweth DE. Independent regulation of human neutrophil chemotactic receptors after activation. J Immunol. 1987;139:3028–33.
35. Korchak HM, Wildenfeld C, Rich AM, et al. Stimulus response coupling in the human neutrophil. J Biol Chem. 1984;259:7439–45.
36. Walker RI, Willemze R. Neutrophil kinetics and the regulation of granulopoiesis. Rev Infect Dis. 1980;2:282–92.
37. Sachs L. The molecular control of blood cell development. Science. 1987;238:1374–9.
38. Rothstein G, Clarkson DR, Larsen W, et al. Effect of lithium on neutrophil mass and production. N Engl J Med 1978;298:178.
39. Barr RD, Koekebakker M, Brown EA, et al. Putative role for lithium in human hematopoiesis. J Lab Clin Med. 1987;109:159–63.
40. Klempner MS, Gallin JI. Separation and functional characterization of human neutrophil subpopulations. Blood. 1978;51:659.
41. Gallin JI. Human neutrophil heterogeneity exists, but is it meaningful? Blood. 1984;63:977–83.
42. Robinson JM, Karnovsky ML, Karnovsky MJ. Glycogen accumulation in polymorphonuclear leukocytes, and other intracellular alterations that occur during inflammation. J Cell Biol. 1982;95:933.
43. Lentnek AL, Schreiber AD, MacGregor RR: Induction of augmented granulocyte adherence by inflammation. J Clin Invest. 1976;47:1098.
44. Harlan JM. Leukocyte-endothelial interactions. Blood. 1985;65:513–25.
45. Gallin JI. Degranulating stimuli decrease the negative surface charge and increase the adhesiveness of human neutrophils. J Clin Invest. 1980;65:298.
46. Fletcher MP, Gallin JI. Degranulating stimuli increase the availability of human neutrophils for the chemoattractant f-met-leu-phe. J Immunol. 1980;124:1585.
47. Bockenstedt KL, Goetzl EJ. Constituents of human neutrophils that mediate enhanced adherence to surfaces. J Clin Invest. 1980;65:1372.
48. Zimmerli W, Seligmann B, Gallin JI. Exudation primes human and guinea pig neutrophils for subsequent responsiveness to the chemotactic peptide *N*-formylmethionylleucylphenylalanine and increases complement component C3bi receptor expression. J Clin Invest 1986;77:925–33.
49. Lewinsohn DM, Bargatze RF, Butcher EC. Leukocyte–endothelial cell recognition: Evidence of a common molecular mechanism shared by neutrophils, lymphocytes, and other leukocytes. J Immunol. 1987;138:4313–21.
50. Anderson DC, Springer TA. Leukocyte adhesion deficiency: An inherited defect in the Mac-1, LFA-1, and p169,95 glycoproteins. Annu Rev Med. 1987;38:1975–94.
51. Kishimoto TK, O'Connor K, Lee A, et al. Cloning of β subunit of the leukocyte adhesion proteins: Homology to an extracellular matrix receptor defines a novel supergene family. Cell. 1987;48:681–90.
52. Hynes RO. Integrins. A family of cell surface receptors. Cell. 1987;48:549–54.
53. Ruoslahti E, Pierschbacher MD. Arg-Gly-Asp: A versatile cell recognition signal. Cell. 1986;44:517–8.
54. Dustin ML, Rothlein R, Bhan AK, et al. Induction of IL 1 and interferon-γ: Tissue distribution, biochemistry, and function of a natural adherence molecule (ICAM-1). J Immunol. 1986;137:245–54.
55. Zimmerman GA, McIntyre TM. Neutrophil adherence to human endothelium in vitro occurs by CDw18 (Mol, MAC-1/LFA-1/GP 150,95) glycoprotein-dependent and -independent mechanisms. J Clin Invest. 1988;81:531–7.
56. Zigmond SH. Chemotaxis by polymorphonuclear leukocytes. J Cell Biol. 1978;77:269.
57. Sullivan JA, Mandell GL. Motility of human polymorphonuclear neutrophils. J Reticuloendothel Soc. 1983;3:31.
58. Schiffmann E, Corcoran BA, Wahl SM. Formylmethionyl peptides as chemoattractants for leukocytes. Proc Natl Acad Sci USA. 1975;72:1059.
59. Perez HD, Goldstein IM, Webster RO, et al. Enhancement of the chemotactic activity of human C5a des arg by an anionic polypeptide ("cochemotaxin") in normal serum and plasma. J Immunol. 1981;126:800.
60. Perez HD, Chenoweth DE, Goldstein IM. Attachment of human C5a des Arg to its cochemotaxin is required for maximum expression of chemotactic activity. J Clin Invest. 1986;78:1589–95.
61. Goetzl EJ. Mediators of immediate hypersensitivity derived from arachidonic acid. N Engl J Med. 1980;303:822.
62. Wright DG, Gallin JI. A functional differentiation of human neutrophil granules: Generation of C5a by a specific (secondary) granule product and inactivation of C5a by azurophil (primary) granule products. J Immunol. 1977;119:1068.
63. Donabedian H, Gallin JI. Deactivation of human neutrophil chemotaxis by chemoattractants: Effect on receptors for the chemotactic factor f-met-leu-phe. J Immunol. 1981;127:839.
64. Jesaitis AJ, Naemura JR, Painter RG, et al. The fate of an *N*-formylated chemotactic peptide in stimulated human granulocytes. J Biol Chem. 1983;258:1968–77.
65. Perez HD, Elfman F, Lobo E. Removal of human polymorphonuclear leukocyte surface sialic acid inhibits reexpression (or recycling) of formyl peptide receptors. J Immunol. 1987;139:1978–84.
66. Clark RA. Chemotactic factors trigger their own oxidative inactivation by human neutrophils. J Immunol. 1982;129:2725.
67. Lee CW, Lewis RA, Corey EJ, et al. Oxidative inactivation of leukotriene C4 by stimulated human polymorphonuclear leukocytes. Proc Natl Acad Sci USA. 1982;79:4166.
68. Gordon LI, Douglas SD, Kay NE, et al. Modulation of neutrophil function by lysozyme. J Clin Invest. 1979;64:226.
69. Bobak DA, Gaither TA, Frank MM, et al. Modulation of FcR function by complement: Subcomponent C1q enhances the phagocytosis of IgG-opsonized targets by human monocytes and culture-derived macrophages. J Immunol. 1987;138:1150–56.
70. Petroni KC, Shen L, Guyre PM. Modulation of human polymorphonuclear leukocyte IgG Fc receptors and Fc receptor-mediated functions by IFN-γ and glucocorticoids. J Immunol. 1988;140:3467–72.
71. Lew DP, Andersson T, Hed J, et al. Ca^{2+}-dependent and Ca^{2+}-independent phagocytosis in human neutrophils. Nature. 1985;315:509–11.
72. Berger M, O'Shea J, Cross AS, et al. Human neutrophils increase expression of C3bi as well as C3b receptors upon activation. J Clin Invest. 1984;74:1566–71.
73. O'Shea JJ, Brown EJ, Seligmann BE, et al. Evidence for distinct intracellular

pools of receptors for C3b and C3bi in human neutrophils. J Immunol. 1985;134:2580–7.
74. Stendahl O, Coble B-I, Dahlgren C, et al. Myeloperoxidase modulates the phagocytic activity of polymorphonuclear neutrophil leukocytes. Studies with cells from a myeloperoxidase-deficient patient. J Clin Invest. 1984;73:366–73.
75. Gaither TA, Medley SR, Gallin JI, et al. Studies of phagocytosis in chronic granulomatous disease. Inflammation. 1987;11:211–27.
76. Lawrence WD, Packman CH, Rowe JM, et al. Attachment of particle bound IgG and complement to human neutrophils. Blood. 1981;58:772.
77. Stossel TP. Phagocytosis recognition and ingestion. Semin Hematol. 1975;12:83.
78. Newman S, Johnston RB Jr. Role of binding through C3b and IgG in polymorphonuclear neutrophil function: Studies with trypsin generated C3b. J Immunol. 1979;123:1839.
79. Brown EJ, Bohnsack JF, Gresham HD. Mechanism of inhibition of immunoglobulin G-mediated phagocytosis by monoclonal antibodies that recognize the Mac-1 antigen. J Clin Invest. 1988;81:365–75.
80. Griffin FM, Griffin JH, Leider JE, et al. Studies on the mechanism of phagocytosis. I. Requirements for circumferential attachment of particle bound ligands to specific receptors on the macrophage plasma membrane. J Exp Med. 1975;142:1263.
81. Griffin FM, Griffin JA, Silverstein SC. Studies on the mechanism of phagocytosis. II. The interaction of macrophages with anti-immunoglobulin IgG-coated bone marrow derived lymphocytes. J Exp Med. 1976;144:788.
82. van Oss CJ. Phagocytosis as a surface phenomenon. Annu Rev Microbiol. 1978;32:19.
83. Wright SD, Griffin FM. Activation of phagocytic cells' C3 receptors for phagocytosis. J Leukocyte Biol. 1985;38:327–39.
84. Brown EJ. The role of extracellular matrix proteins in the control of phagocytosis. J Leukocyte Biol. 1986;39:579–91.
85. Babior GL, Crowley CA. Chronic granulomatous disease and other disorders of killing by phagocytes. In: Steinbury JB, Wyngaarden JB, Frederickson DS, et al, eds. The Metabolic Basis of Inherited Disease. 5th ed. New York: McGraw-Hill; 1983:1969.
86. Eggleston LV, Krebs AA. Regulation of the pentose phosphate cycle. Biochem J. 1974;138:424.
87. Babior BM, Rosin RE, McMurrich BJ, et al. Arrangement of the respiratory burst oxidase in the plasma membrane of the neutrophil. J Clin Invest. 1981;67:1724.
88. Borregaard N, Tauber AI. Subcellular localization of the human neutrophil NADPH oxidase. J Biol Chem. 1984;259:47–52.
89. Rossi F. The $O_2^{\cdot-}$-forming NADPH oxidase of the pahgocytes: Nature, mechanisms of activation and function. Biochim Biophys Acta. 1986;853:65–89.
90. Bellavite P. The superoxide-forming enzymatic system of phagocytes. Free Radic Biol Med. 1988;4:225–261.
91. Cross AR, Jones OTG, Garcia R, et al. The association of the FAD with the cytochrome b_{-245} of human neutrophils. Biochem J. 1982;208:759.
92. Gabig TG, Schervish EW, Santinga JT. Functional relationship of the cytochrome b to the superoxide-generating oxidase of human neutrophils. J Biol Chem. 1982;257:4114–9.
93. McPhail LC, Shirley PS, Clayton CC, et al. Activation of the respiratory burst enzyme from human neutrophils in a cell-free system. J Clin Invest. 1985;75:1735–9.
94. Curnutte JT. Activation of human neutrophil nicotinamide adenine dinucleotide phosphate, reduced (triphosphopyridine nucleotide, reduced) oxidase by arachidonic acid in a cell-free system. J Clin Invest. 1985;75:1740–43.
95. Clark RA, Leidal KG, Pearson DW, et al. NADPH oxidase of human neutrophils. J Biol Chem. 1987;262:4065–74.
96. Segal AW, Jones OTG, Webster D, et al. Absence of a newly described cytochrome b from neutrophils of patients with chronic granulomatous disease. Lancet. 1978;2:446–9.
97. Segal AW, Cross AR, Garcia RD, et al. Absence of cytochrome b_{-245} in chronic granulomatous disease: A multicenter European evaluation of its incidence and relevance. N Engl J Med. 1983;308:245.
98. Ohno Y, Buescher ES, Roberts R, et al. Reevaluation of cytochrome b and flavin adenine dinucleotide in neutrophils from patients with chronic granulomatous disease and description of a family with probable autosomal recessive inheritance of cytochrome b deficiency. Blood. 1986;67:1132–8.
99. Curnutte JT, Berkow RL, Roberts RL, et al. Chronic granulomatous disease due to a defect in the cytosolic factor required for nicotinamide adenine dinucleotide phosphate oxidase activation. J Clin Invest. 1988;81:606–10.
100. Umei T, Takeshige K, Minakami S. NADPH binding component of neutrophil superoxide-generating oxidase. J Biol Chem. 1984;261:5229–32.
101. Parkos CA, Allen RA, Cochrane CG, et al. Purified cytochrome b from human granulocyte plasma membrane is comprised of two polypeptides with relative molecular weights of 91,000 and 22,000. J Clin Invest. 1987;80:732–42.
102. Royer-Pokora B, Kunkel LM, Monaco AP, et al. Cloning the gene for an inherited human disorder–chronic granulomatous disease—on the basis of its chromosomal location. Nature. 1986;322:32–8.
103. Dinauer MC, Orkin SH, Brown R, et al. The glycoprotein encoded by the X-linked chronic granulomatous disease locus is a component of the neutrophil cytochrome b complex. Nature. 1987;327:717–20.
104. Teahan C, Rowe P, Parker P, et al. The X-linked chronic granulomatous disease gene codes for the β-chain of cytochrome b_{-245}. Nature. 1987;327:720–1.
105. Harper AM, Chaplin MF, Segal AW. Cytochrome b_{-245} from human neutrophils is a glycoprotein. Biochem J. 1985;227:783–8.
106. Tauber AI, Borregaard N, Simons ER, et al. Phagocyte oxidase deficiency syndrome (PODS): A revised nosology of chronic granulomatous disease and related acquired disorders. Medicine (Baltimore). 1983;62:286–309.
107. Whitin JC, Chapman CE, Simons ER, et al. Correlation between membrane potential changes and superoxide production in human granulocytes stimulated by phorbol myristate acetate. J Biol Chem. 1980;255:1874.
108. Seligmann BE, Gallin JI. Use of lipophilic probes of membrane potential to assess human neutrophil activation. J Clin Invest. 1980;66:493.
109. Borregaard N, Heiple JM, Simons ER, et al. Subcellular localization of the b-cytochrome component of the human neutrophil microbicidal oxidase: Translocation during activation. J Cell Biol. 1983;97:52.
110. Ohno Y, Seligmann BE, Gallin JI. Cytochrome b translocation to human neutrophil plasma membranes and superoxide release. J Biol Chem. 1985;260:2409–14.
111. Goldstein IM, Kaplan HB, Radin A, et al. Independent effects of IgG and complement upon human PMN leukocyte function. J Immunol. 1976;177:1282.
112. Henson PM, Oades ZG. Stimulation of human neutrophils by soluble and insoluble immunoglobulin aggregates. J Clin Invest. 1975;56:1053.
113. Curnutte JT, Babior BM, Karnovsky ML. Fluoride-mediated activation of the respiratory burst in human neutrophils. A reversible process. J Clin Invest. 1979;63:637.
114. Badwey J, Curnutte JT, Karnovsky ML. *Cis*-polyunsaturated fatty acids induce high levels of superoxide production by human neutrophils. J Biol Chem. 1981;256:12640.
115. Mollinedo F, Schneider DL. Subcellular localization of cytochrome b and ubiquinone in a tertiary granule of resting human neutrophils and evidence for a proton pump ATPase. J Biol Chem. 1984;259:7143–50.
116. Yamaguchi T, Kaneda M, Kakinuma K. Is cytochrome b_{-558} translocated into the plasma membrane from granules during the activation of neutrophils? J Biochem. 1986;99:953–9.
117. Tauber AI. Protein kinase C and the activation of the human neutrophil NADPH-oxidase. Blood. 1987;69:711–20.
118. McPhail LC, Snyderman R. Activation of the respiratory burst enzyme in human polymorphonuclear leukocytes by chemoattractants and other soluble stimuli. J Clin Invest. 1983;72:192–200.
119. Clark RA, Volpp BD, Leidal KG, et al. NADPH oxidase in subcellular fractions of human neutrophils: Evidence for a guanine and adenine nucleotide-dependent activation event (Abstract). Clin Res. 1987;35:655.
120. Badwey JA, Curnutte JT, Robinson JM, et al. Effect of free fatty acids on release of superoxide and on change of shape by human neutrophils. Reversibility by albumin. J Biol Chem. 1984;259:7870.
121. Bromberg Y, Pick E. Activation of NADPH-dependent superoxide production in a cell-free system by sodium dodecyl sulfate. J Biol Chem. 1985;260:13539.
122. McPhail LC, Clayton CC, Snyderman R. The NADPH oxidase of human polymorphonuclear leukocytes. J Biol Chem. 1984;259:5768–75.
123. Jandl RC, Andre-Schwartz J, Borges-Dubois L, et al. Termination of the respiratory burst in human neutrophils. J Clin Invest. 1978;61:1176.
124. Leffell MS, Spitznagel JK. Fate of human lactoferrin and myeloperoxidase in phagocytizing human neutrophils: Effects of immunoglobulin G subclasses and immune complexes coated on latex beads. Infect Immun. 1975;12:813.
125. Naccache PH, Showell HJ, Becker EL, et al. Changes in ionic movements across rabbit polymorphonuclear leukocyte membranes during lysosomal enzyme release. J Cell Biol. 1977;75:665.
126. Korchak HM, Weissmann G. Changes in membrane potential of human granulocytes antecede the metabolic responses to surface stimulation. Proc Natl Acad Sci USA. 1978;75:3818.
127. Weissmann G, Smolen JE, Korchak HM. Release of inflammatory mediators from stimulated neutrophils. N Engl J Med. 1980;303:27.
128. Wright DG. The neutrophil as a secretory organ of host defense. Adv Host Defense Mech. 1982;1:75.
129. Goldstein IM, Hoffstein ST, Weissmann G. Influence of divalent cations upon complement-mediated enzyme release from human PMN leukocytes. J Immunol. 1975;115:665.
130. Moore PL, Bank HL, Brissie NT, et al. Association of microfilament bundles with lysosomes in PMN leukocytes. J Cell Biol. 1976;71:659.
131. Goldstein IM. Polymorphonuclear leukocyte lysosomes and immune tissue injury. Prog Allergy. 1976;20:301.
132. Becker EL. Leukocyte stimulation: Receptor, membrane, and metabolic events. Fed Proc. 1986;7:2148–50.
133. Bell RM. Protein kinase C activation by diacylglycerol second messengers. Cell. 1986;45:631–2.
134. Marx JL. Polyphospoinositide research updated. Science. 1987;235:974–6.
135. Casey PJ, Gilman AG. G protein involvement in receptor-effector coupling. J Biol Chem. 1988;263:2577–80.
136. Krause K-H, Lew PD. Subcellular distribution of Ca^{2+} pumping sites in human neutrophils. J Clin Invest. 1987;80:107–16.
137. Volpe P, Krause K-H, Hashimoto S, et al. "Calciosome," a cytoplasmic organelle: The inositol 1,4,5-trisphosphate–sensitive Ca^{2+} store of nonmuscle cells? Proc Natl Acad Sci USA. 1988;85:1091–5.
138. Sawyer DW, Sullivan JA, Mandell GL. Intracellular free calcium localization in neutrophils during phagocytosis. Science. 1985;230:663–6.

139. Segal AW, Heyworth PG, Cockcroft S, et al. Stimulated neutrophils from patients with autosomal recessive chronic granulomatous disease fail to phosphorylate a M_r-44,000 protein. Nature 1985;316:547–9.
140. Hayakawa T, Suzuki K, Suzuki S, et al. A possible role for protein phosphorylation in the activation of the respiratory burst in human neutrophils. J Biol Chem. 1986;261:9109–15.
141. Caldwell SE, McCall CE, Hendricks CL, et al. Coregulation of NADPH oxidase activation and phosphorylation of a 48-kD protein(s) by a cytosolic factor defective in autosomal recessive chronic granulomatous disease. J Clin Invest. 1988;81:1485–96.
142. Becker EL, Kermode JC, Naccache PH, et al. Pertussis toxin as a probe of neutrophil activation. Fed Proc. 1986;45:2151–5.
143. Van Epps DE, Garcia ML. Enhancement of neutrophil function as a result of prior exposure to chemotactic factor. J Clin Invest. 1980;66:167–75.
144. Bender JG, McPhail LC, Van Epps DE. Exposure of human neutrophils to chemotactic factors potentiates activation of the respiratory burst enzyme. J Immunol. 1983;130:2316–23.
145. Bass DA, Gerard C, Olbrantz P, et al. Priming of the respiratory burst of neutrophils by diacylglycerol. J Biol Chem. 1987;262:6643–9.
146. Densen P, Mandell GL. Gonococcal interactions with polymorphonuclear neutrophils. Importance of the phagosome for bactericidal activity. J Clin Invest. 1978;62:1161.
147. Klebanoff SJ. Antimicrobial mechanisms in neutrophilic PMN leukocytes. Semin Hematol. 1975;12:117.
148. Rosen H, Klebanoff SJ. Oxidation of *Escherichia coli* iron centers by the myeloperoxidase-mediated microbicidal system. J Biol Chem. 1982;257:13731–5.
149. Rosen H, Klebanoff SJ. Oxidation of microbial iron-sulfur centers by the myeloperoxidase-H_2O_2-halide antimicrobial system. Infect Immun. 1985;47:613–8.
150. Rosen H, Rakita RM, Waltersdorph AM, et al. Myeloperoxidase-mediated damage to the succinate oxidase system of *Escherichia coli.* J Biol Chem. 1987;262:15004–10.
151. Repine JE, Fox RB, Berger EM. Hydrogen peroxide kills *Staphylococcus aureus* by reacting with staphylococcal iron to form hydroxyl radical. J Biol Chem. 1981;256:7094–6.
152. Thomas EL, Jefferson MM, Grisham MB. Myeloperoxidase-catalyzed incorporation of amines into proteins: Role of hypochlorous acid and dichloramines. Biochemistry. 1982;24:6299–6308.
153. Grisham MB, Jefferson MM, Melton DF, et al. Chlorination of endogenous amines by isolated neutrophils. J Biol Chem. 1984;259:10404–13.
154. Klebanoff SJ. Oxygen-dependent cytotoxic mechanisms of phagocytes. Adv Host Defense Mech. 1982;1:111.
155. Babior BM. Oxygen-dependent microbial killing by phagocytes. N Engl J Med. 1978;298:659, 721.
156. Mandell GL. Catalase, superoxide dismutase, and virulence of *S. aureus*. J Clin Invest. 1975;55:561.
157. Klebanoff SJ. The iron-H_2O_2-iodide cytotoxic system. J Exp Med. 1982;156:1262–7.
158. Cohen MS, Britigan BE, Hassett DJ, et al. Phagocytes, O_2 reduction, and hydroxyl radical. Rev Infect Dis. 1988;10:1088.
159. Britigan BE, Rosen GM, Chai Y, et al. Do human neutrophils make hydroxyl radical? J Biol Chem. 1986;261:4426–31.
160. Mandell GL. Bactericidal activity of aerobic and anaerobic polymorphonuclear neutrophils. Infect Immun. 1974;9:337.
161. Mandell GL. Intraphagosomal pH of human polymorphonuclear neutrophils. Proc Soc Exp Biol Med. 1970;134:447.
162. Oram JD, Reiter B. Inhibition of bacteria by lactoferrin and other iron-chelating agents. Biochim Biophys Acta. 1968;170:351.
163. Boxer LA, Coates TD, Haak RA, et al. Lactoferrin deficiency associated with altered granulocyte function. N Engl J Med. 1982;387:404.
164. Broxmeyer HE, Smithyman A, Eger RR, et al. Identification of lactoferrin as the granulocyte-derived inhibitor of colony-stimulating activity production. J Exp Med. 1978;148:1052.
165. Kijlstra A, Jeurissen HM. Modulation of classical C3 convertase of complement by tear lactoferrin. Immunology. 1982;47:263.
166. Sptiznagel JK, Shafer WM. Neutrophil killing of bacteria by oxygen-independent mechanisms: A historical summary. Rev Infect Dis 1985;7:398.
167. Elsbach P, Weiss J. Oxygen-independent bactericidal systems of polymorphonuclear leukocytes. In: Weissmann G, ed. Advances in Inflammation Research. v. 2. New York: Raven Press; 1981:95.
168. Ganz T, Selsted ME, Lehrer RI. Antimicrobial activity of phagocyte granule proteins. Semin Respir Infect 1986;1:107.
169. Zeya AT, Spitznagel JK. Arginine-rich proteins of PMN leukocyte lysosomes. J Exp Med. 1968;127:927.
170. Shafer WM, Martin LE, Spitznagel JK. Cationic antimicrobial proteins isolated from human neutrophil granulocytes in the presence of diisopropyl flurophosphate. Infect Immun. 1984;45:29.
171. Shafer WM, Martin LE, Spitznagel JK. Late intraphagosomal hydrogen ion concentration favors the in vitro antimicrobial capacity of a 37-kilodalton cationic granule protein of human neutrophil granulocytes. Infect Immun. 1986;53:651.
172. Ooi CE, Weiss J, Elsbach P, et al. A 25-kD NH_2-terminal fragment carries all the antibacterial activities of the human neutrophil 60-kD bactericidal/permeability-increasing protein. J Biol Chem. 1987;262:14891.
173. Ganz T, Selsted ME, Szklarek D, et al. Defensins. Natural peptide antibiotics of human neutrophils. J Clin Invest. 1985;76:1427.
174. Weiss J, Victor M, Elsbach P. Role of charge and hydrophobic interactions in the action of the bactericidal/permeability-increasing protein of neutrophils on gram-negative bacteria. J Clin Invest. 1983;71:540.
175. Selsted ME, Harwig SSL, Ganz T, et al. Primary structures of three human neutrophil defensins. J Clin Invest. 1985;76:1436.
176. Leijh PCJ, van den Barselaar MTh, van Zwet TL, et al. Requirement of extracellular complement and immunoglobulin for intracellular killing of microorganisms by human monocytes. J Clin Invest. 1979;63:772.
177. Tedesco F, Rottini G, Patriarca P. Modulating effect of the late acting components of the complement system on the bactericidal activity of human polymorphonuclear leukocytes on *E. coli* 0111:34. J Immunol. 1981;127:1910.
178. Densen P, Mandell GL. Phagocyte strategy vs. microbial tactics. Rev Infect Dis. 1980;2:817.
179. Bellavite P, Serra MC, Davoli A, et al. Selective enrichment of NADPH oxidase activity in phagosomes from guinea pig polymorphonuclear leukocytes. Inflammation. 1982;6:21.
180. Ohno YI, Hirai KI, Kanoh T, et al. Subcellular localization of H_2O_2 production in human neutrophils stimulated with particles and an effect of cytochalasin-B on the cells. Blood. 1982;60:253.
181. Clark RA. Extracellular effects of the myeloperoxidase-hydrogen peroxide-halide system. In: Weissmann G, ed. v. 5. Advances in Inflammation Research. New York: Raven Press; 1983;107.
182. Britigan BE, Rosen GM, Thompson BY, et al. Stimulated human neutrophils limit iron-catalyzed hydroxyl radical formation as detected by spin-trapping techniques. J Biol Chem. 1986;261:17026.
183. Britigan BE, Hassett DJ, Rosen GM, et al. Neutrophil degranulation inhibits potential hydroxyl radical formation: Differential impact of myeloperoxidase and lactoferrin release on hydroxyl radical production by iron supplemented neutrophils assessed by spin trapping techniques. Submitted for publication.
184. Henson PM, Johnston RB Jr. Tissue injury in inflammation. J Clin Invest. 1987;79:669.
185. Cross CE, Halliwell B, Borish ET, et al. Oxygen radicals and human disease. Ann Intern Med. 1987;107:526.
186. Jacob HS, Craddock PR, Hammerschmidt DE, et al. Complement induced granulocyte aggregation. An unsuspected mechanism of disease. N Engl J Med. 1980;302:789.
187. Zimmerman G, Renzetti AD, Hill HR. Functional and metabolic activity of granulocytes from patients with adult respiratory distress syndrome. Evidence for activated neutrophils in the pulmonary circulation. Am Rev Respir Dis. 1983;127:290.
188. Hammerschmidt DE. Activation of the complement system and of granulocytes in lung injury: The adult respiratory distress syndrome. In: Weissmann G, ed. Advances in Inflammation Research v. 5. New York: Raven Press; 1983:147.
189. Smedley LA, Tonnesen MG, Sandhaus RA, et al. Neutrophil-mediated injury to endothelial cells: Enhancement by endotoxin and essential role of neutrophil elastase. J Clin Invest. 1968;77:1233.
190. Ognibene FP, Martin SE, Parker MM, et al. Adult respiratory distress syndrome in patients with severe neutropenia. N Engl J Med. 1986;315:547.
191. Janoff A. Elastase in tissue injury. Annu Rev Med. 1985;36:207.
192. Wewers MD, Gadek JE. The protease theory of emphysema. Ann Intern Med. 1987;107:761.
193. Carrell RW. α_1-Antitrypsin: Molecular pathology, leukocytes and tissue damage. J Clin Invest. 1986;78:1427.
194. Desrochers PE, Weiss SJ. Proteolytic inactivation of alpha-1-proteinase inhibitor by a neutrophil metalloproteinase. J Clin Invest. 1988;81:1646.
195. Rotrosen D, Gallin JI. Disorders of phagocyte function. Annu Rev Immunol. 1987;5:127.
196. Malech HL, Gallin JI. Neutrophils in human diseases. N Engl J Med. 1987;317:687.
197. Bodey GP, Buckley M, Sathe YS, et al. Quantitative relationships between circulating leukocytes and infection in patients with acute leukemia. Ann Intern Med. 1966;64:328.
198. Cines DB, Passero F, DuPont GM, et al. Granulocyte-associated IgG in neutropenic disorders. Blood. 1982;59:124.
199. Wright DG. Autoimmune leukopenia. In Lichtenstein LM, Fauci AS, eds: Current Therapy in Allergy and Immunology. Toronto: BC Decker; 1983:277.
200. Wright DG, Fauci AS, Dale DC, et al. Correction of human cyclic neutropenia with prednisolone. N Engl J Med. 1978;298:295.
201. Boxer LA, Hedley-Whyte T, Stossel TP: Neutrophil actin dysfunction and abnormal neutrophil behavior. N Engl J Med. 1974;291:1093.
202. Crowley CA, Curnutte JT, Rosin RE, et al. An inherited abnormality of neutrophil adhesion. N Engl J Med. 1980;302:1163.
203. Arnaout MA, Pitt J, Cohen HJ, et al. Deficiency of a granulocyte-membranc glycoprotein (gp-150) in a boy with recurrent bacterial infections. N Engl J Med. 1982;306:693.
204. Weening RS, Roos D, Weemoes CMR, et al. Defective imitation of the metabolic stimulation in phagocytizing granulocytes: A new congenital defect. J Lab Clin Med. 1976;88:757.
205. Harvath L, Andersen BR. Defective initiation of oxidative metabolism in polymorphonuclear leukocytes. N Engl J Med. 1979;300:1130.
206. Anderson DC, Schmalsteig FC, Finegold MJ, et al. The severe and moderate phenotypes of heritable Mac-1, LFA-1 deficiency: Their quantitative definition and relation to leukocyte dysfunction and clinical features. J Infect Dis. 1985;152:668.

207. Nauseef WM, de Alarcon P, Bale JF, et al. Aberrant activation and regulation of the oxidative burst in neutrophils with Mo1 glycoprotein deficiency. J Immunol. 1986;137:636.
208. Springer TA, Thompson WS, Miller LJ, et al. Inherited deficiency of the Mac-1, LFA-1, p150,95 glycoprotein family and its molecular basis. J Exp Med. 1984;160:1901.
209. Kishimoto TK, Hollander N, Roberts TM, et al. Heterogeneous mutations in the β subunit common to the LFA-1, Mac-1, and p150,95 glycoproteins cause leukocyte adhesion deficiency. Cell. 1987;50:193.
210. Gallin JI. Abnormal phagocyte chemotaxis: Pathophysiology, clinical manifestations, and management of patients. Rev Infect Dis. 1981;3:1196.
211. Quie PG, Cates KL. Clinical conditions associated with defective PMN leukocyte chemotaxis. Am J Pathol. 1977;88:711.
212. Ward PA. Leukotaxis and leukotactic disorders. Am J Pathol. 1974;77:520.
213. Van Epps DE, Williams RC. Suppression of leukocyte chemotaxis by human IgA myeloma components. J Exp Med. 1976;144:1227.
214. Clark RA, Kimball HR, Decker JL. Neutrophil chemotaxis in systemic lupus erythematosus. Ann Rheum Dis. 1974;33:167.
215. Perez HD, Lipton M, Goldstein IM. A specific inhibitor of complemennt (C5)-derived chemotactic activity in serum from patients with systemic lupus erythematosus. J Clin Invest. 1978;62:29.
216. Perez HD, Hooper C, Volanakis J, et al. Specific inhibitor of complement derived chemotactic activity in systemic lupus erythematosus related antigenically to the Bb fragment of human factor B. J Immunol. 1987;139:484.
217. Perez HD, Goldstein IM. Polymorphonuclear leukocyte chemotaxis in systemic lupus erythematosus. J Rheumatol. 1987;14:53.
218. Cianciola LJ, Genco RJ, Patters MR, et al. Defective polymorphonuclear leukocyte function in a human periodontal disease. Nature. 1977;265:445.
219. Clark RA, Page RC, Wilde G. Defective neutrophil chemotaxis in juvenile periodontis. Infect Immun. 1977;18:694.
220. Van Dyke TE. Role of the neutrophil in oral disease: Receptor deficiency in leukocytes from patients with juvenile periodontitis. Rev Infect Dis. 1985;7:419.
221. Shurin SB, Socransky SS, Sweeney E, et al. A neutrophil disorder induced by capnocytophaga; a dental micro-organism. N Engl J Med. 1979;301:849.
222. Kramer N, Perez HD, Goldstein IM. An immunoglobulin (IgG) inhibitor of polymorphonuclear leukocyte motility in a patient with recurrent infection. N Engl J Med. 1980;303:1253.
223. Rausch PG, Pryzwansky KB, Spitznagel JK. Immunochemical characterization of Chédiak-Higashi neutrophils. N Engl J Med. 1978;298:693.
224. Haliotis T, Roder J, Klein M, et al. Chédiak-Higashi gene in humans. I. Impairment of natural killer function. J Exp Med. 1980;151:1039.
225. Blume RS, Wolff SM. The Chédiak-Higashi syndrome: Studies in four patients and a review of the literature. Medicine (Baltimore). 1972;51:247.
226. Clark RA, Kimball HR. Defective granulocyte chemotaxis in the Chédiak-Higashi syndrome. J Clin Invest. 1971;50:2645.
227. Root RK, Rosenthal AS, Balestra DJ. Abnormal bactericidal, metabolic, and lysosomal functions of Chédiak-Higashi syndrome leukocytes. J Clin Invest. 1972;51:649.
228. Oliver JM. Cell biology of leukocyte abnormalities—membrane and cytoskeletal functions in normal and defective cells. Am J Pathol. 1978;93:219.
229. Baehner RL, Boxer LA. Disorders of polymorphonuclear leukocyte function related to alterations in the integrated reactions of cytoplasmic constituents with the plasma membrane. Semin Hematol. 1979;16:148.
230. Pryzwansky KB, Schliwa M, Boxer LA. Microtubule organization of unstimulated and stimulated adherent human neutrophils in Chédiak-Higashi syndrome. Blood. 1985;66:1398.
231. Davis SD, Schaller J, Wedgwood RJ. Job's syndrome. Recurrent "cold" staphylococcal abscesses. Lancet. 1966;1:1013.
232. Donabedian H, Gallin JI. The hyperimmunoglobulin E recurrent-infection (Job's) syndrome. Medicine (Baltimore). 1983;62:195.
233. Donabedian H, Gallin JI. Mononuclear cells from patients with the hyperimmunoglobulinemia E recurrent infection syndrome produce an inhibitor of leukocyte chemotaxis. J Clin Invest. 1982;69:1155.
234. Dreskin SC, Goldsmith PK, Strober W, et al. Metabolism of immunoglobulin E in patients with markedly elevated serum immunoglobulin E levels. J Clin Invest. 1987;79:1764.
235. Dreskin SC, Goldsmith PK, Gallin JI. Immunoglobulins in the hyperimmunoglobulin E and recurrent infection (Job's) syndrome. J Clin Invest. 1985;75:26.
236. Donabedian H, Alling DW, Gallin JI. Levamisole is inferior to placebo in the hyperimmunoglobulin E recurrent-infection (Job's) syndrome. N Engl J Med. 1982;307:290.
237. Craddock PR, Yawata P, Van Santen L, et al. Acquired phagocyte dysfunction. A complication of the hypophosphatemia of parenteral hyperalimentation. N Engl J Med. 1974;290:1403.
238. Najjar VA, Constantopoulos A. A new phagocytosis stimulating tetrapeptide hormone, tuftsin and its role in disease. J Reticuloendothel Soc. 1972;12:197.
239. Bisno AL, Freeman JC. The syndrome of asplenia, pneumococcal sepsis, and disseminated intravascular coagulation. Ann Intern Med. 1970;72:389.
240. Gallin JI, Buescher ES, Seligmann BE, et al. Recent advances in chronic granulomatous disease. Ann Intern Med. 1983;99:657–74.
241. Lazarus GM, Neu HM. Agents responsible for infection in chronic granulomatous disease of childhood. J Pediatr. 1975;86:415.
242. Johnston RB Jr, Newman SL. Chronic granulomatous disease. Pediatr Clin North Am 1977;24:365.
243. Dilworth JA, Mandell GL. Adults with chronic granulomatous disease of childhood. Am J Med. 1977;63:233.
244. Schaller J. Illness resembling lupus erythematosus in mothers of boys with chronic granulomatous disease. Ann Intern Med. 1972;76:747.
245. Kragballe K, Borregaard N, Brandrup F, et al. Relation of monocyte and neutrophil oxidative metabolism to skin and oral lesions in carriers of chronic granulomatous disease. Clin Exp Immunol. 1981;43:390.
246. Johnston RB Jr. Unusual forms of an uncommon disease (chronic granulomatous disease). J Pediatr. 1976;88:172.
247. Bohler M-C, Seger RA, Mouy R, et al. A study of 25 patients with chronic granulomatous disease: A new classification by correlating respiratory burst, cytochrome b, and flavoprotein. J Clin Immunol. 1986;6:136.
248. Lew PD, Southwick FS, Stossel TP, et al. A variant of chronic granulomatous disease: Deficient oxidative metabolism due to a low-affinity NADPH oxidase. N Engl J Med. 1981;305:1329.
249. Seger RA, Tiefenauer L, Matsunaga T, et al. Chronic granulomatous disease due to granulocytes with abnormal NADPH oxidase activity and deficient cytochrome b. Blood. 1983;61:423.
250. Hamers MN, de Boer M, Meerhof LJ, et al. Complementation in monocyte hybrids revealing genetic heterogeneity in chronic granulomatous disease. Nature. 1984;307:553–5.
251. Weening RS, Corbeel L, De Boer M, et al. Cytochrome b deficiency in an autosomal form of chronic granulomatous disease. J Clin Invest. 1985;75:915–20.
252. Segal AW. Absence of both cytochrome b_{-245} subunits from neutrophils in X-linked chronic granulomatous disease. Nature. 1987;326:88.
253. Weenings RS, Adriaansz LH, Weemaes CMR, et al. Clinical differences in chronic granulomatous disease in patients with cytochrome b-negative or cytochrome b-positive neutrophils. J Pediatr. 1985;107:102.
254. Caldwell SE, McCall CE, Hendricks CL. Coregulation of NADPH oxidase activation and phosphorylation of a 48-kD protein(s) by a cytosolic factor defective in autosomal recessive chronic granulomatous disease. J Clin Invest. 1988;81:1485.
255. Curnutte JT, Kuver R, Scott PJ. Activation of neutrophil NADPH oxidase in a cell-free system. Partial purification of components and characterization of the activation process. J Biol Chem. 1987;262:5563.
256. Gabig TG, English D, Akard LP, et al. Regulation of neutrophil NADPH oxidase activation in a cell free system by guanine nucleotides and fluoride: Evidence for participation of a pertussis and cholera toxin–insensitive G protein. J Biol Chem. 1987;262:1685.
257. Hayakawa T, Suzuki K, Suzuki S, et al. A possible role for protein phosphorylation in the activation of the respiratory burst in human neutrophils. Evidence from studies with cell from patients with chronic granulomatous disease. J Biol Chem. 1986;261:9109.
258. Ishii E, Juta K, Fujita I, et al. Protein phosphorylation of neutrophils from normal children and patients with chronic granulomatous disease. Eur J Pediatr. 1986;145:22.
259. Ochs HD, Igo RP. The NBT slide test: A simple screening method for detecting chronic granulomatous disease and female carriers. J Pediatr. 1973;83:77.
260. Cooper MR, DeChatelet LR, McCall CE, et al. Complete deficiency of leukocyte glucose-6-phosphate dehydrogenase with defective bactericidal activity. J Clin Invest. 1972;51:769.
261. Parry MF, Root RK, Metcalf JA, et al. Myeloperoxidase deficiency. Prevalance and clinical significance. Ann Intern Med. 1981;95:293.
262. Nauseef WM. Myeloperoxidase deficiency. Hematol Oncol Clinics North Am. 1988;2:135.
263. Lehrer RJ, Cline MJ. Leukocyte myeloperoxidase deficiency and disseminated candidiasis: The role of myeloperoxidase in resistance to candida infection. J Clin Invest. 1969;48:1478.
264. van Tuinen P, Johnson KR, Ledbetter S, et al. Localization of myeloperoxidase to the long arm of human chromosome 17: Relationship to the 15:17 translocation of acute promyelocytic leukemia. Oncogene. 1987;1:319.
265. Nauseef WM, Root RK, Malech HL. Biochemical and immunologic analysis of hereditary myeloperoxidase deficiency. J Clin Invest. 1983;71:1297.
266. Koeffler HP, Ranyard J, Pertcheck M. Myeloperoxidase: Its structure and expression during myeloid differentiation. Blood. 1985;65:484.
267. Nauseef WM, Malech HL. Analysis of the peptide subunits of human neutrophil myeloperoxidase. Blood. 1986;67:1504.
268. Gallin JI. Neutrophil specific granule deficiency. Annu Rev Med. 1985; 36:263.
269. Gallin JI, Fletcher MP, Seligmann BE, et al. Human neutrophil-specific granule deficiency: A model to assess the role of neutrophil-specific granules in the evolution of the inflammatory response. Blood. 1982;59.1317.
270. Wolff SM, Dale DC, Clark RA, et al. The Chédiak-Higashi syndrome: Studies of host defenses. Ann Intern Med. 1972;76:293.
271. Ezer G, Soothill JF. Intracellular bactericidal effects of rifampicin in both normal and chronic granulomatous disease polymorphs. Arch Dis Child. 1974;49:463.
272. Mandell GL: Interaction of intraleukocytic bacteria and antibiotics. J Clin Invest. 1973;52:1673.
273. Johnston R, Wilfert CM, Buckley RH, et al. Enhanced bactericidal activity of phagocytes from patients with chronic granulomatous disease in the presence of sulphisoxazole. Lancet. 1975;1:824.
274. Gmümder RK, Seger RA. Chronic granulomatous disease: Mode of action of sulfamethoxazole/trimethoprim. Pediatr Res. 1981;15:1533.

275. Root RK, Isturiz R, Molavi A, et al. Interactions between antibiotics and human neutrophils in the killing of staphylococci. J Clin Invest. 1981;67:247.
276. Yourtee EL, Root RK. Antibiotic-neutrophil interactions in microbial killing. Adv Host Defense Mech. 1982;1:187.
277. Ezekowitz RAB, Orkin SH, Newburger PE. Recombinant interferon gamma augments phagocyte superoxide production and X-chronic granulomatous disease gene expression in X-linked variant chronic granulomatous disease. J Clin Invest. 1987;80:1009.
277a. Sechler JMG, Malech HL, White CJ, et al. Recombinant human interferon-gamma reconstitutes defective phagocyte function in patients with chronic granulomatous disease of childhood. Proc Natl Acad Sci USA. 1988; 85:4874–8.
277b. Ezekowitz RAB, Dinauer MC, Jaffe HS, et al. Partial correction of the phagocyte defect in patients with X-linked chronic granulomatous disease by subcutaneous interferon gamma. N Engl J Med. 1988;319:146.
278. Herzig GP, Graw RG. Granulocyte transfusion for bacterial infections. Prog Hematol. 1975;9:207.
279. Klock JC, Bainton DF. Degranulation and abnormal bactericidal function of granulocytes procured by reversible adhesion to nylon wool. Blood. 1976;48:149.
280. Herzig RH, Herzig GP, Grano RG, et al. Successful granulocyte transfusion therapy for gram-negative septicemia. N Engl J Med. 1977;296:701.
281. Strauss RG, Connett JE, Gale RP, et al: A controlled trial of prophylactic granulocyte transfusions during initial induction chemotherapy for acute myelogenous leukemia. N Engl J Med. 1981;305:597.
282. Winston DJ, Winston GH, Gale RP: Therapeutic granulocyte transfusions for documented infections. Ann Intern Med. 1982;97:509.
283. Alavi JB, Root RK, Djerassi I, et al. A randomized clinical trial of granulocyte transfusions for infections in acute leukemia. N Engl J Med. 1977;296:706.
284. Buescher ES, Gallin JI. Leukocyte transfusion in chronic granulomatous disease. N Engl J Med. 1982;307:800.
285. Young LS. Prophylactic granulocytes in the neutropenic host. Ann Intern Med. 1982;96:240.
286. Rosenshein MS, Farewell VT, Price TH, et al. The cost effectiveness of therapeutic and prophylactic leukocyte transfusion. N Engl J Med. 1980;302:1058.
287. Wright DG, Robichaud KJ, Pizzo PA, et al. Lethal pulmonary reactions associated with the combined use of amphotericin B and leukocyte transfusions. N Engl J Med. 1981;304:1185.
288. Marsh WL, Oyen R, Nichols ME. K_X antigen, the McLeod phenotype, and chronic granulomatous disease: Further studies. Vox Sang. 1976;31:356.
289. Densen P, Wilkinson-Kroovand S, Mandell GL, et al. K_X: Its relationship to chronic granulomatous disease and genetic linkage with Xg. Blood. 1981;58:34.
290. Frey D, Machler M, Seger R, et al. Gene deletion in a patient with chronic granulomatous disease and McLeod syndrome: Fine mapping of the Xk gene locus. Blood. 1988;71:252.
291. Giblett ER, Klebanoff SJ, Pincus SH, et al. Kell phenotypes in chronic granulomatous disease: A potential transfusion hazard. Lancet. 1971;1:1235.
292. Westminster Hospitals Bone Marrow Transplant Team. Bone marrow transplant from an unrelated donor for chronic granulomatous disease. Lancet, 1977;1:210.
293. Kamani N, August CS, Douglas SD, et al. Bone marrow transplantation in chronic granulomatous disease. J Pediatr. 1984;105:42.
294. van der Meer JWM, van den Broek PJ. Present status of the management of patients with defective phagocyte function. Rev Infect Dis. 1984;6:107.
295. Rebuck JW, Crowley JH. A method of studying leukocyte functions in vivo. Ann NY Acad Sci. 1955;59:757.
296. Nelson RB, Quie PG, Simmons RL. Chemotaxis under agarose: A new and simple method for measuring chemotaxis and spontaneous migration of human polymorphonuclear leukocytes and monocytes. J Immunol. 1975;155:1650.
297. Mandell GL, Hook EW. Leukocyte function in chronic granulomatous disease of childhood. Studies on a 17 year old boy. Am J Med. 1969;47:473.
298. Holmes B, Page A, Good R. Studies of the metabolic activity of leukocytes from patients with genetic abnormality of phagocytic function. J Clin Invest. 1967;46:1422.
299. Root RK, Rosenthal AS, Balestra DJ. Abnormal bactericidal metabolic and lysosomal functions of Chédiak-Higashi syndrome leukocyte. J Clin Invest. 1972;51:649.
300. Klebanoff SJ, Clark RA. Iodination of human polymorphonuclear leukocytes: A re-evaluation. J Lab Clin Med. 1977;89:675.
301. Baehner RL, Nathan DG. Quantitative nitroblue tetrazolium dye test in chronic granulomatous disease. N Engl J Med. 1968;278:971.
302. Stossel TP, Root RK, Vaughan M. Phagocytosis in chronic granulomatous disease and the Chédiak-Higashi syndrome. N Engl J Med. 1972;286:120.
303. Allen RC, Loose LD. Phagocytic activation of a luminol-dependent chemiluminescence in rabbit alveolar and peritoneal macrophages. Biochem Biophys Res Commun. 1976;69:245.
304. Weller PF, Goetzl EJ. The human eosinophil. Roles in host defense and tissue injury. Am J Pathol. 1980;100:790.
305. Spry CJE. Mechanisms of eosinophilia. V. Kinetics of normal and accelerated eosinopoiesis. Cell Tissue Kinet. 1971;4:351.
306. Gleich GJ, Adolphson CR. The eosinophilic leukocyte: Structure and function. Adv Immunol. 1986;39:177.
307. Mickenberg ID, Root RK, Wolff SM. Bactericidal and metabolic properties of human eosinophils. Blood. 1972;39:67.
308. Ackerman SJ, Durack DT, Gleich GJ. Eosinophil effector mechanisms in health and disease. Adv Host Defense Mech. 1982;1:269.
309. Basten A, Boyer MH, Beeson PB. Mechanisms of eosinophilia. I. Factors affecting the eosinophil response of rats to *Trichinella spiralis*. J Exp Med. 1970;131:1271.
310. Basten A, Beeson PB. Mechanisms of eosinophilia. II. Role of the lymphocyte. J Exp Med. 1970;131:1288.
311. Mahmoud AAF, Stone MK, Kellermeyer RW. Eosinophilopoietin. A circulating low molecular weight peptide-like substance which stimulates the production of eosinophils in mice. J Clin Invest. 1977;60:675.
312. Butterworth AE, Sturrock RV, Houba V, et al. Eosinophils as mediators of antibody dependent damage to schistosomula. Nature. 1975;257:727.
313. David JR, Vadas MA, Butterworth AE, et al. Enhanced helminthotoxic capacity of eosinophils from patient with eosinophilia. N Engl J Med. 1980;303:1147.
314. Mahmoud AAF, Warren KS, Peters PA. A role for the eosinophil in acquired resistance to *Schistosoma mansoni* infection as determined by antieosinophil serum. J Exp Med. 1975;142:805.
315. Goetzl EJ, Wasserman SI, Austen KF. Eosinophil polymorphonuclear leukocyte function in immediate hypersensitivity. Arch Pathol. 1975;99:1.
316. Bass DA. Eosinophil behavior during host defense reactions. Adv Host Defense Mech. 1982;1:211.
317. Butterworth AE, David JR. Eosinophil function. N Engl J Med. 1981; 304:154.
318. McLaren DJ, MacKenzie CD, Ramalho-Pinto FJ. Ultrastructural observations on the in vitro interaction between rat eosinophils and some parasitic helminths (*Schistosoma mansoni, Trichinella spiralis* and *Nippostrongylus brasiliensis*). Clin Exp Immunol. 1977;30:105.
319. Densen P, Mahmoud AAF, Sullivan J, et al. Demonstration of eosinophil degranulation on the surface of opsonized schistosomules by phase-contrast cinemicrography. Infect Immun. 1978;22:282.
320. Grove DI, Mahmoud AAF, Warren KS. Eosinophils and resistance to *Trichinella spiralis*. J Exp Med. 1977;145:755.
321. Dvorak HF, Dvorak AM. Basophilic leucocytes: Structure, function and role in disease. Clin Haematol. 1975;4:651.
322. Brown SJ, Galli SJ, Gleich GJ, et al. Ablation of immunity to *Ambylomna americanum* by antibasophil serum. Cooperation between basophils and eosinophils in expression of immunity to ectoparasites (tubo) in guinea pigs. J Immunol. 1982;129:790–796.

BIBLIOGRAPHY

Klebanoff SJ, Clark RA: The Neutrophil. Function and Clinical Disorders. Amsterdam: North Holland; 1978.

8. THE CELLULAR IMMUNE SYSTEM AND ITS ROLE IN HOST DEFENSE*

CHRISTOPHER B. WILSON

TERMS

Cell Types

Dendritic cell. Bone-marrow-derived, adherent cell that is nonphagocytic, expresses class II HLA (Ia) molecules, and lacks Fc receptors for IgG and receptors for the third component of complement. It is antigenically and morphologically distinct from macrophages, occupies different areas of the spleen from macrophages, and is a potent accessory cell in antigen-specific T-cell proliferation. It stimulates syngeneic and allogeneic mixed lymphocyte reactions and induces specific cytotoxic T cells and cells that mediate delayed-type hypersensitivity (DTH).

Macrophage. Bone-marrow-derived tissue phagocyte that begins as a monocyte progenitor cell in bone marrow. Has class II HLA (Ia) molecules and receptors for IgG (Fc receptors) and for the third component of complement on its

* Parts of this chapter are based on the chapter by McLeod, Wing, and Remington in the second edition.

surface. Presents antigens to lymphocytes and inhibits or kills microorganisms.

Monocyte. Circulating bone-marrow-derived phagocyte that begins as a monocyte progenitor cell in bone marrow and differentiates into macrophage in tissue.

Mononuclear phagocytes. Monocytes, tissue macrophages, and macrophage-like cells (e.g., microglia).

Natural killer (NK) cell. Large granular lymphocyte with distinct surface antigens. It is cytotoxic to tumor cells, certain virus-infected cells, and certain protozoa.

Null cell. Lymphocyte that lacks surface markers of B or T lymphocytes.

T cell. Thymus-derived lymphocyte that bears a receptor (T-cell antigen receptor, TCR) that recognizes and triggers a response to a specific antigen in the context of host HLA molecules.

T4 cell. T cell that expresses the surface CD4 molecule and recognizes antigen in the context of class II HLA molecules; these cells are commonly called helper T cells but are functionally heterogeneous (see text).

T8 cell. T cell that expresses the surface CD8 molecule and recognizes antigen in the context of class I HLA molecules; these cells are commonly called cytotoxic cells and include cells that inhibit (suppress) B- and T-cell responses.

Genetic Restriction of Cell-Mediated Immunity

Cell-mediated immunity (CMI). Immunity conferred by T lymphocytes and effected by lymphocytes and macrophages.

Major histocompatibility complex (MHC). Cluster of gene loci that encodes class I and class II determinants that provide context for antigen recognition by T lymphocytes.

Class I HLA determinants. Glycoprotein antigens that are encoded by the A, B, and C regions of the MHC of humans, are integral membrane proteins, and restrict interactions of T8 cells.

Class II HLA determinants. Glycoprotein antigens that are encoded by the D region of the MHC of humans, are integral membrane proteins, and restrict interactions of T4 cells.

Haplotype. Constellation of alleles in a particular MHC (i.e., groups of genes that are adjacent and therefore inherited together).

HLA-A, HLA-B, HLA-C. MHC loci encoding class I histocompatibility determinants in humans.

HLA-D. MHC loci encoding class II histocompatibility determinants in humans.

Human leukocyte antigen (HLA) region. MHC region of humans.

I region associated (a) molecule. Product of the Ir gene (D region in humans), which is the I region in mice.

Miscellaneous Terms

Cytokine/lymphokines. Hormone-like or neurotransmitter-like proteins or glycoproteins, secreted by lymphocytes or macrophages, that act as molecular signals for communication between cells of the immune system and as mediators of the systemic response to infection/inflammation.

Epitope. Unique antigenic structure.

T-cell antigen receptor (TCR). Dimeric molecule that contains a unique receptor for antigen and a variable portion of the MHC.

CELL-MEDIATED IMMUNITY

CMI collectively refers to those aspects of the immune response in which T lymphocytes and mononuclear phagocytes induce, regulate, or mediate host response(s), either directly or indirectly, by their effects on other aspects of the immune system. Although CMI is generally thought to play a primary role in protecting against microbes that replicate within host cells (intracellular pathogens),[1–4] including those outlined in Table 1, it has become increasingly apparent that CMI plays a pivotal role in regulating all aspects of the immune system. Central to this role is the critical importance of helper T cells (CD4 antigen-positive cells, hereafter referred to as *T4 cells* or *T4 lymphocytes*) in the induction of specific immune responses[5]; this is clearly illustrated by the devastating effect that selective ablation of functional T4 cells has on all aspects of immunity in acquired immunodeficiency syndrome (AIDS).[6] Thus, although not part of the classic cellular immune system, the optimal function of B lymphocytes, which are the source of specific humoral immunity, and to a lesser degree of granulocytes, which function to ingest and kill antibody-coated microbes, is dependent on intact T4 lymphocyte function.

Historically, CMI was recognized by the delayed-type hypersensitivity (DTH) response, in which, approximately 2 days after intradermal injection of antigen, erythema and induration are detected. This correlates with an influx of lymphocytes and macrophages into the site and can be passively transferred with T lymphocytes but not with serum. Resistance to certain intracellular pathogens can be transferred in a similar fashion.[1–3] Recently, with the rapid increase in knowledge made possible by advances in cell culture, cell cloning, monoclonal antibody techniques, and molecular and structural biologic techniques, our understanding of the cellular immune system and its effects on all aspects of the host response has increased markedly. These discoveries have served to illustrate the complexity of this system. Accordingly, current knowledge, as summarized in this chapter, is necessarily an incomplete and simplistic overview of an elegant system that functions in concert with other aspects of immunity to protect us from the complex microbial environment in which we live. Both T lymphocytes and mononuclear phagocytes function in the inductive and effector phases of the immune response. This chapter discusses these functions separately after describing the origin and differentiation of these cell types and the molecular basis for specific antigen recognition.

T LYMPHOCYTES

T lymphocytes both mediate specific immune functions and modulate those of other cells in the immune system, thereby regulating most aspects of specific immune recognition. These cells recognize antigen via a cell surface receptor for specific antigen, which is structurally similar to immunoglobulin.[7] When activated by antigen in an appropriate context, T cells are stimulated to replicate and/or to mediate one of three principal functions: helping, by stimulating the immune responses of other cells; suppression, by inhibiting the immune response of other cells; and cytotoxicity, by direct killing of target cells. The helper functions are mediated primarily by a subset of T-cell helpers that express the CD4 (T4) surface antigen, whereas the suppressor and cytotoxic functions are mediated primarily by cells expressing the CD8 (T8) surface antigen.[5] However, recent data indicate that the functions of these subsets in part overlap.[8,9] The CD4 molecule is expressed on cells that recognize antigen associated with human leukocyte antigen (HLA) class II molecules; T4 cells can act as helper cells for B-cell responses, as cells that induce other T cells to suppress immune responses and, less commonly, as cytotoxic cells. The CD8 molecule is expressed on cells that respond to antigens (such as viruses) in association with HLA class I antigens and can act as cytotoxic or suppressor cells.

T-Cell Receptors

Structure. Unlike immunoglobulin, the antigen receptor for B cells, the T-cell antigen receptor (TCR) requires simultaneous recognition of antigen with self-major histocompatibility com-

TABLE 1. Pathogens Against Which Cell-Mediated Immunity Contributes to Host Defense in Humans or Experimental Animals

Intracellular					*Extracellular*			
Bacteria	*Viruses*	*Fungi*	*Protozoa*	*Other*	*Bacteria*	*Fungi*	*Protozoa*	*Helminths*
Brucella spp.	Cytomegalovirus	*Blastomyces dermatidis*[a]	*Leishmania*[a]	*Chlamydia*[a]	*Pseudomonas aeruginosa*	*Aspergillus*	*Plasmodia*[a]	*Schistosoma* spp.[a]
Erysipelothrix rhusiopathiae	Herpes simplex	*Candida* spp.	*Toxoplasma gondii*[a]	*Rickettsia*[a]	*Bacteroides fragilis*	*Zygomycetes*	*Giardia*	*Strongyloides stercorales*
Francisella tularenis	Varicella-zoster	*Coccidioides immitis*[a]	*Trypanosoma cruzi*[a]	*Treponema pallidum*			*Entamoeba histolytica*[a]	*Trichinella spiralis*
Listeria monocytogenes[a]	Epstein-Barr	*Cryptococcus neoformans*[a]						
Legionella pneumophila[a]	Rubeola (measles)	*Histoplasma capsulatum*[a]						
Mycobacteria, including	Vaccinia	*Paracoccidioides brasiliensis*[a]						
M. tuberculosis[a]								
M. leprae[a]								
M. avium intracellulare								
Nocardia asteroides								
Pseudomonas pseudomallei								
Pseudomonas mallei								
Salmonella spp.[a]								
Yersinia spp.								

[a] Organisms susceptible to the IFN-γ-activated monocyte/macrophage in vitro.
(Adapted from Murray,[4] with permission.)

plex (self-MHC).[10] Like immunoglobulin, the TCR is a heterodimer (reviewed in Refs. 7 and 11). Most T cells (more than 95 percent in healthy people) express a heterodimer composed of an α- and a β-chain[7,11,12]; the remainder express a receptor composed of a γ- and a δ-chain.[11,13] TCR chains are synthesized independently from separate genes and then associate to form the TCR molecule (Fig. 1). Both chains have a variable and a constant region. The β- and δ-chain variable regions are derived, like immunoglobulin heavy chains, by sequential rearrangement of diversity (D), joining (J), and variable (V) gene segments to form a contiguous VDJ gene segment; this rearrangement of germ line genomic DNA occurs during thymic development only in cells of the T-cell lineage. The derived variable region and the adjacent constant (C) region, which includes the transmembrane (TM) and cytoplasmic (CY) domains, is then transcribed to form the β- or the δ-chain messenger RNA. The α- and δ-chains are formed by a similar mechanism, although to date no α- or δ-chain D regions have been found, suggesting that these chains, like immunoglobulin light chains, are derived from VJC segments only. Rearrangement of TCR genes appears to be mediated by an enzyme(s) similar or identical to that mediating immunoglubulin gene rearrangement.[14] The mechanisms determining whether a cell will rearrange its immunoglobulin genes and become a B cell, or its TCR genes and become a T cell, is not known. It is also not known with certainty what determines which TCR gene will be rearranged to form a functional receptor.

Gene transfer studies using the α, β TCR indicate that these two chains are sufficient to dictate specific recognition of antigen and HLA[15,16]; this recognition process is discussed more fully below. Specific recognition is thought to be mediated by three hypervariable regions that, because they determine complementary interaction with antigen-HLA, are known as *complementarity-determining regions* (CDR 1, 2, and 3), as shown in Figure 1 for the TCR α-chain. The CDR regions appear to be closely approximated spatially to form the recognition site.[11]

TCR genes are expressed on the surface of T cells in an obligatory fashion with a complex of molecules, the CD3 (T3) complex, that appears to consist of five chains: δ, γ, ε, and either two ζ-chains or a ζ plus an η-chain.[17] The CD3 complex appears to act as the signal transduction mechanism whereby antigen binding to the TCR activates T cells.

TCR Diversity. A variety of mechanisms are used to generate the diversity in the nucleotide and the resultant polypeptide sequence of TCR genes sufficient to allow recognition of the variety of antigens to which we are exposed. These include the use of different V, D, and J segments and imprecise joining together of these segments to form the variable region of the TCR. A great deal more information is known about the mouse compared to humans regarding the organization of the genes and the diversity in the V gene segments (Table 2). In the mouse there are estimated to be about 100 Vα and about 25 Vβ gene segments. There are about 50 Jα gene segments and a single Cα. There are two Cβ gene segments, each preceded by one Dβ and six Jβ gene segments. All potential recombinations appear to be possible. The number of γ-chain variable segments appears to be more limited, with three Jγ and Cγ pairs. The TCR δ-locus is located within the TCR α-locus, and certain V segments may be shared. As in the γ-chain, the number of δ-chain V genes appears to be limited. Estimates of potential diversity in humans, although not identical, are similar.[18] As in immunoglobulin, the phenomenon of allelic exclusion appears to be operative, so that a given cell expresses only one αβ or γδ heterodimer.

Additional diversity in the TCR is provided by imprecise joining together of V, D, and J segments so that addition or deletion of nucleotides occurs, producing N-region diversity; this is probably mediated by terminal transferase.[7] However, in contrast to B cells, somatic hypermutation appears either not to occur or to be infrequent in TCR V regions. Nevertheless, the estimated diversity of TCR genes is greater than that of immunoglobulin genes[11] because of greater N-region diversity. This is particularly true for the γδ TCR, which compensates for its more limited V-region repertoire by increased junctional diversity.

Both T4 (helper) cells and T8 (suppressor/cytotoxic) cells can use the same V-region gene segments.[19–21] This suggests that specificity and HLA class I or class II restriction are not determined by the V-region segment alone. Specificity appears to be determined by both the α- and β-chains; specificity is affected both by the germ line gene segments used and by junctional diversity and nucleotide addition or deletion during rearrangement.[15,22,23] A working hypothesis for the mechanism of TCR recognition has recently been published.[11]

Role of Accessory Molecules, Including CD4 and CD8, in T-Cell Recognition

Mature T cells express on their surface accessory molecules that function to enhance T-cell recognition of other cells. The

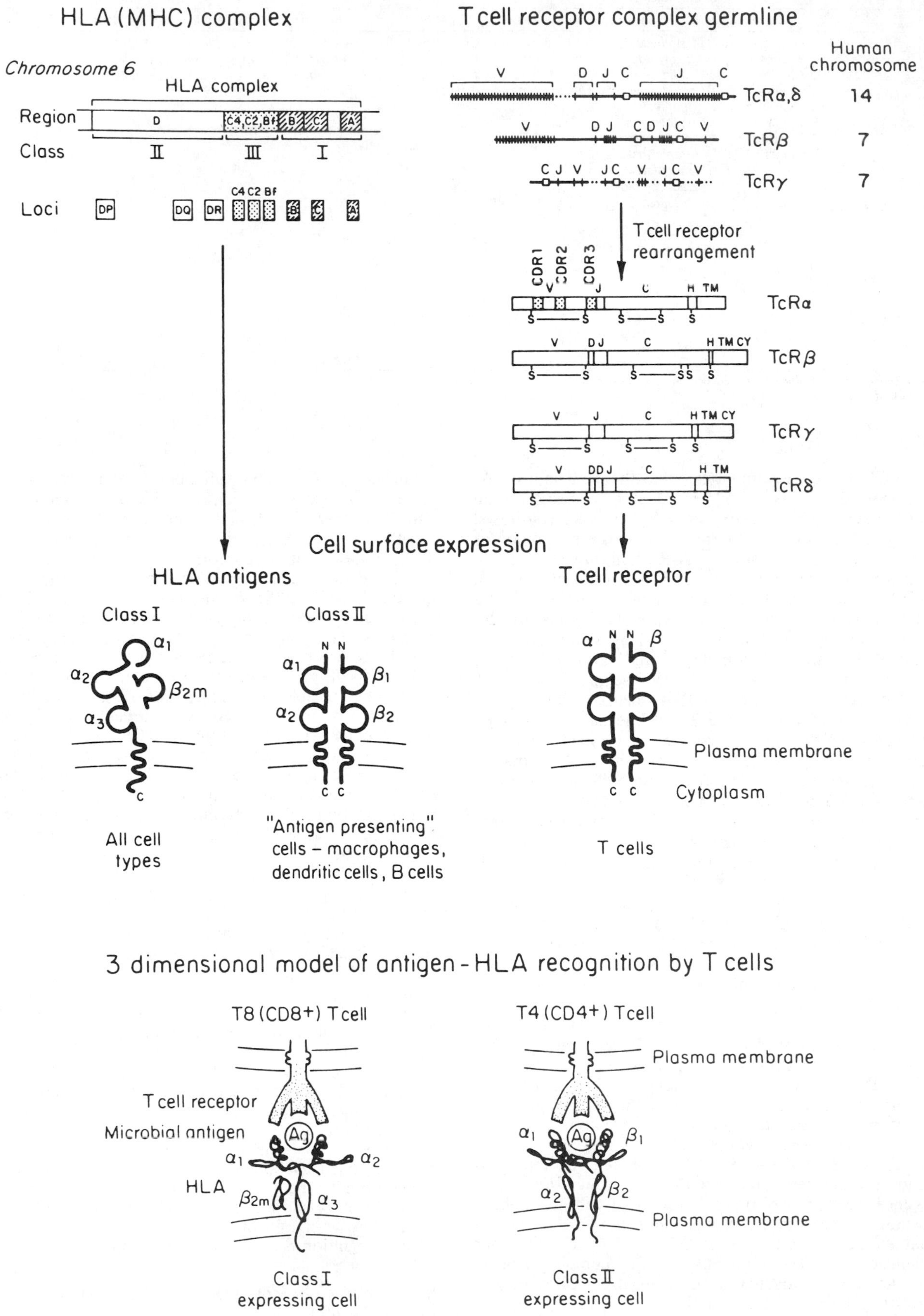
HLA (MHC) complex
Chromosome 6
HLA complex
Region
D
C4, C2, Bf
B
C
A
Class
II
III
I
Loci
DP
DQ
DR
C4 C2 Bf
T cell receptor complex germline
Human chromosome
V
D J C
J
C
TcRα,δ
14
V
D J
C D J C
V
TcRβ
7
C J V
J C
V
J C
V
TcRγ
7
T cell receptor rearrangement
CDR1
CDR2
CDR3
V
J
C
H TM
TcRα
V
D J
C
H TM CY
TcRβ
V
J
C
H TM CY
TcRγ
V
DD J
C
H TM
TcRδ
S
Cell surface expression
HLA antigens
T cell receptor
Class I
α1
α2
β2m
α3
c
Class II
N N
α1
β1
α2
β2
c c
α
N N
β
Plasma membrane
c c
Cytoplasm
All cell types
"Antigen presenting" cells – macrophages, dendritic cells, B cells
T cells
3 dimensional model of antigen-HLA recognition by T cells
T8 (CD8+) T cell
T4 (CD4+) T cell
Plasma membrane
T cell receptor
Microbial antigen
Ag
α1
α2
HLA
β2m
α3
α1
Ag
β1
α2
β2
Plasma membrane
Class I expressing cell
Class II expressing cell

TABLE 2. Sequence Diversity in T-Cell Receptor and Immunoglobulin Genes in the Mouse

	IG[a]		*TCR I*		*TCR II*	
	H	κ	α	β	γ	δ
Variable segments	250–1000[b]	250	100	25	7	10
Diversity segments	10	0	0	2	0	2
D's read in all frames	Rarely	—	—	Often	—	Often
N-region addition	V–D, D–J	None	V–J	V–D, D–J	V–J	V–D1, D1–2, D1–J
Joining segments	4	4	50	12	3	2
Variable region combinations	62,500–250,000		2500		70	
Junctional combinations	~10^{11}		~10^{15}		~10^{18}	

[a] Immunoglobulin heavy chain.
[b] Number of gene segments.
(From Davis and Bjorkman,[11] with permission.)

CD4 and CD8 molecules are expressed in a mutually exclusive manner on T4 and T8 T cells, respectively. The CD4 and CD8 molecules have structural homology to the immunoglobulin gene superfamily[24–26] but are not variable, as are TCR and HLA molecules. They are believed to act, in part, as a stabilizing ligand for T-cell binding to HLA class II (CD4) or class I (CD8) molecules.[8] This is believed to be mediated by binding of these molecules to nonpolymorphic (nonvariable) regions of the HLA molecule.[16,27] Such interactions may be particularly important in stabilizing binding of T cells to antigen–HLA when the TCR does not have a high affinity for the particular antigen–HLA complex. The importance of these accessory molecules was illustrated in gene transfer experiments in which it was necessary to transfer both the TCR α- and β-chains and the CD8 molecule in order to achieve functional interaction of T cells with an antigen–MHC class I expressing target cell.[16,27] These and other studies have illustrated that the CD4 and CD8 molecules are most closely associated with recognition of antigen in the context of class II and class I MHC molecules, respectively, rather than as determinants of specific types of helper (CD4) or cytotoxic/suppressor (CD8) T-cell function.

The CD2 (sheep erythrocyte receptor) may also facilitate T-cell activation. Recent studies have identified the LFA-3 molecule as its natural ligand.[28] Both have recently been cloned.[29–31] CD2–LFA-3 interaction also may play a role in thymocyte differentiation and selection, an accessory role in T-cell activation, and a primary role in activation of NK cells as discussed below.[31–33] Other T-cell surface molecules,[34–36] particularly the LFA-1 molecule,[37–39] may play ancillary roles in T-cell function by their effects on interaction with other cells, on activation, and on migration.

Derivation of T Cells from Thymocytes

T cells are originally derived from bone marrow precursors (prothymocytes) that migrate to and mature in the thymus. The mass of the thymus relative to body mass is greatest in late fetal life and infancy. The relatively large size of this organ appears to reflect the need for rapid expansion of the T-cell pool at this age. The stages of thymocyte differentiation and the mechanisms leading to differentiation remain to be clearly defined. Much of the work has been performed in the mouse,[39,40] but more recent studies in humans reveal a similar pattern of differentiation.[5,41,42]

Putative pathways of differentiation in the postnatal thymus are schematically depicted in Figure 2. This scheme is a modification of stages originally proposed for humans based on cell surface marker data[5] that has been modified to incorporate recent information from murine studies[39,40] and studies of T-cell receptor gene expression. This represents a working hypothesis rather than established fact.

Prothymocyte precursors are derived from the bone marrow.[41,42] Such cells, as well as all thymocytes and T cells, can be detected by expression of the CD7 surface antigen.[42] In the thymus, cells initially acquire T10 (type 1). Thereafter, CD2 and subsequently a series of different antigens are acquired. The precise precursor–product relationship of cells from type 2 to mature T cell has not been defined. Models in humans[5] and mice[40] in which cells mature sequentially from type 1 to mature T cells seem not to explain fully the heterogeneity recently described in thymocytes. Similarly, the view that immature cells first enter the thymic cortex, mature, and migrate to the medulla, from which they exit, may be overly simplistic.[39,40,43] This complexity is best exemplified by recent findings regarding two aspects of thymocyte development: the TCR and homing receptors. Conventionally, type 1 and type 2 thymocytes, which do not express either CD4 or CD8 (double-negative cells), were thought to be the most immature thymocytes. Support for this belief comes from observations in the mouse. In irradiated mice, transplanted double-negative cells give rise to all other thymocyte populations.[39] If thymus from day 13 or day 14 fetal mice (gestation = 20 days) is cultured in vitro for 7 days, the phenotype of the cells changes from 100 percent double-negative cells to include all types of thymocytes in a proportion similar to that of the mature thymus.[44,45] That mature T cells (CD3+ and either CD4 or CD8+) may also derive from double-positive cells (CD4+, CD8+) under certain conditions is sug-

FIG. 1. Representation of the genetic organization of the HLA and TCR complex, TCR rearrangement, HLA and TCR expression, and TCR recognition of the antigen–HLA complex. In humans, the HLA complex is on chromosome 6; the class I (A, B, and C) antigen locus is separated from the class II (DR, DQ, DP) locus by genes for certain complement components (also called *class III genes*) and for the cytokines, TNF, and lymphotoxin (not shown). Surface expression of class I HLA antigens is ubiquitous (with rare exceptions; see text), whereas class II HLA antigens are restricted in their expression to antigen-presenting cells, primarily macrophages, dendritic cells, and B cells (see text).

The TCR genes are on chromosome 14 (α, δ) or 7 β, γ). The Vα and Vδ gene segments are adjacent to each other on chromosome 14. The Dδ, Jδ, and Cδ gene segments lie between the Vα and Vδ segments and the Jα and Cα segments; the β and γ regions on chromosome 7 do not overlap. In the upper portion of the figure, the germ line configuration of the TCR genes is shown; this is the configuration found in non-T cells. The specific chromosomal relationships are shown for the mouse but are similar in humans. The TCR genes are rearranged in T cells during thymic development in a way that juxtaposes the VDJC (β, δ) or VJC (α, γ) gene segments, usually by deletion of the intervening germ line segments. Following productive rearrangement, a TCR, shown here as an αβ heterodimer, is expressed on the T-cell surface. A model of T-cell recognition of antigen in the context of HLA molecules is shown schematically, based on that proposed by Davis and Bjorkman.[11] It is proposed that the CDR3 region of the TCR is that portion that contacts antigen, and the CDR1 and CDR2 regions contact HLA. Not shown are the T cell accessory molecules CD8 and CD4, which are believed to stabilize the bicellular complex by binding to nonvariable regions of class I and class II HLA molecules, respectively.

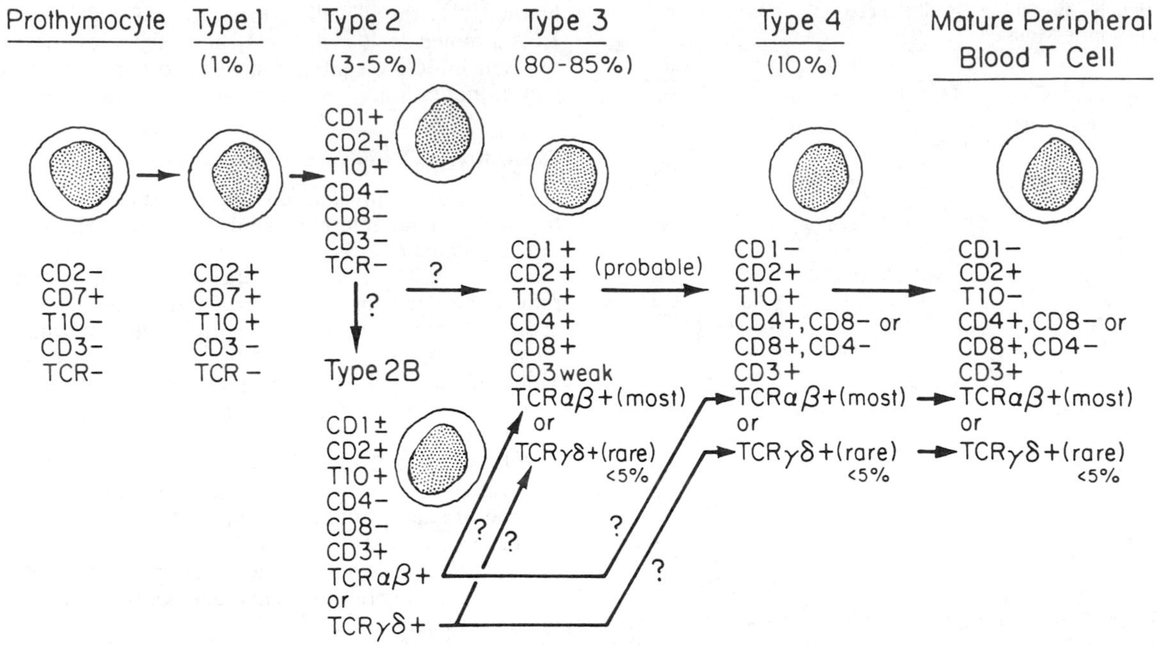

FIG. 2. Putative stages of thymocyte differentiation in postnatal humans. Types of thymocytes are defined by their expression of certain surface antigens. The T cell receptor (TCR), usually composed of an αβ heterodimer or, less commonly, of a γδ heterodimer, is expressed in association with the CD3 surface antigens. Pathways of maturation are indicated by arrows. (?)-uncertain.

gested by in vitro studies.[46] However, in the murine thymus, most double-positive thymocytes die[39,40] and do not differentiate into more mature cells. Thus, it is unclear whether type 4 cells are derived from type 3 or type 2 cells or both. The mechanism determining which thymocytes differentiate into T cells and which die is unknown. Failure to productively rearrange TCR genes and to express cell surface TCR or expression may lead to thymocyte death, but other selection mechanisms also appear to determine which cells survive and mature. One such mechanism is the "education" of cells by self-MHC molecules. Mice that are treated as neonates with antibodies to class I or class II MHC do not develop normal numbers of T8 or T4 cells, respectively; they are accordingly deficient in helper or cytotoxic T-cell function, respectively.[47] Thus, MHC molecules appear to be important in the development of type 4 thymocytes and mature T cells. In addition to this "positive" selection, thymocytes strongly reactive with self-MHC molecules are deleted during thymic maturation.

Recent studies also indicate that type 2 cells are not a single population. Rather, they include a CD3-negative subset, which is the most immature, and two CD3-positive subsets; each of the CD3-positive subsets appears to represent a separate pathway of T-cell development. One of the CD3-positive, CD4- and CD8-negative thymocytes express the uncommon type of TCR composed of the Tγ chain in association with the newly described protein Tδ.[48–52] Even as mature cells, most of these δT lymphocytes with the γδ TCR do not express either the CD4 or the CD8 accessory molecule; a few express the CD8 molecule.[52] The other CD3-positive, CD4- and CD8-negative thymocyte subset expresses the common α-β TCR; these are precursors of most (about 97 percent) mature T cells—those that express the α-β TCR and either the CD4 or the CD8 accessory molecule. The cells expressing the γδ TCR constitute about 3 percent of the circulating T cells.[52,53] The function of the γδ TCR-bearing T cells compared to the α-β TCR-bearing T cells is not clear. Such cells are markedly increased in number in nude mice and in certain patients with primary immunodeficiency.[48]

During fetal development, prothymocytes are first detected in the thymus at 8 weeks in the human[42] and at 14 days in the mouse.[39,40] At this stage, the phenotype of most thymocytes is immature.[42] Data on the sequential appearance of thymocyte types is more complete in the mouse than in the human. There is sequential rearrangement of γ and then β TCR genes, and subsequent expression of their mRNA followed by that of α. At this stage the α-β TCR can first be detected on the surface of thymocytes,[54] and surface expression of CD4 and CD8 is first revealed. The percentage of cells gradually changes to reach values similar to those of adults by about 7 days of postnatal age in the mouse[55] and probably by 12–16 weeks of gestation in humans.[42]

During thymic development in the fetus, T cells that recognize self-antigens appear to be deleted. This has been convincingly shown in mice. Two groups demonstrated the selective loss during thymic maturation of thymocytes bearing a specific TCR variable region gene in inbred mice of one genetic type of histocompatibility antigen but not in those with a different genetic type.[56–59] Although other mechanisms of tolerance to self-antigens are possible, these results suggest that deletion of T cells expressing strongly self-reactive receptors is likely to be the major mechanism.

MONONUCLEAR PHAGOCYTES AND DENDRITIC CELLS

Origin and Differentiation

The mononuclear phagocyte system includes bone marrow precursors, circulating monocytes, and macrophages. In the adult, the promonocyte is the first recognizable marrow precursor cell, although it presumably is derived from a myeloid stem cell precursor. Promonocytes are actively dividing cells that mature into nonreplicating monocytes. Under steady-state conditions, monocytes are released from the marrow within 24 hours and circulate in the blood for 1–3 days before moving to the tissues.[60] Their growth and maturation in the marrow are regulated by specific colony-stimulating factors, as discussed in the section on cytokines.

Once they have left the blood, monocytes do not recirculate but differentiate into macrophages, which are present in all tissues. The estimated life span of macrophages in the tissues is 4–12 weeks. Under steady-state conditions, more than 95 percent of mononuclear phagocytes are mature tissue macrophages and less than 2 percent are monocytes.[60,61] Data from bone marrow transplants indicate that tissue macrophages are ultimately derived from blood monocyte precursors[62]; however, tissue macrophages appear capable of limited replication and self-renewal.[62,63]

Differentiation of monocytes into macrophages is associated with some common maturational changes and others that are unique to the tissue in which they are located. For example, all monocytes lose granule myeloperoxidase as they differentiate into tissue macrophages.[64] Monocytes and peritoneal macrophages rely primarily on anaerobic glycolysis, whereas alveolar (lung) macrophages use aerobic cytochrome oxidation as well.[62] The function of macrophages is readily modulated by lymphokines and they are capable of fusing to form multinucleated giant cells.[60] Thus, unlike granulocytes, mononuclear phagocytes are relatively long-lived cells capable of limited self-renewal and of morphologic and functional modulation, depending on local conditions.

Dendritic cells are also derived from bone marrow precursors.[64] They represent a very small fraction of blood mononuclear cells (less than 1 percent). Like monocytes and macrophages, they express class II MHC molecules and are highly efficient antigen-presenting cells. However, they are phenotypically distinct since they have a dendritic morphology and do not have surface receptors for IgG (Fc receptors) or for the third component of complement. They are found in lymphoid tissue in association with T-lymphocyte-rich areas. Compared to mononuclear phagocytes, less is known regarding their progenitor cells in the bone marrow and their life span in the tissues.

Langerhans cells are related to but phenotypically distinct from macrophages and dendritic cells. They express class II MHC antigens and are efficient antigen-presenting cells.[65] Like macrophages, they express Fc receptors for IgG and receptors for the third component of complement, but they also express the CD1 and S100 antigens not found on other antigen-presenting cells.[66,67] Langerhans cells are abundant in skin, and similar cells are found in the thymus and lymph nodes. They are the normal counterpart of the malignant cells found in histiocytosis X.[66–68]

THE MAJOR HISTOCOMPATIBILITY COMPLEX MOLECULES RESTRICT AND DETERMINE THE CAPACITY FOR THE IMMUNE RESPONSE TO ANTIGENS

Nature of Major Histocompatibility Complex Genes and Molecules

The major histocompatibility complex (MHC) is a cluster of genetic loci, located in humans on the short arm of chromosome 6, that encode genetically polymorphic cell membrane molecules involved in antigen binding and T-cell recognition; these molecules are known in humans as *human leukocyte antigens* (HLAs). These molecules were discovered when investigators studying the rejection of organ transplants in inbred strains of mice found that the capacity to discriminate self from non-self mapped to the MHC. Subsequently, studies by McDevitt and Benacerraf revealed that the capacity to develop an immune response to simple exogenous antigens mapped to a region within the MHC locus, which they named the immune response (Ir) gene locus.[69] Subsequent studies revealed that the Ir locus was identical to the MHC region containing class II MHC molecules.

The MHC locus encodes two structurally distinct types of polymorphic molecules, referred to as *class I* and *class II molecules*.[70–72] As shown in Figure 1, each class contains several individual antigens. The class I molecules in humans are denoted HLA-A, -B, and -C, and the class II molecules are denoted HLA-DR, -DQ, and -DP. The genes for class I and class II molecules are in separate clusters on chromosome 6 and are separated by genes for complement factor C2, C4, and B, and by genes for the lymphokines, tumor necrosis factor α and β. Additional HLA genetic elements are also present, but those studied to date appear not to be functional genes. Each chromosome contains a complete set of these molecules. Accordingly, two alleles each of HLA-A, -B, and -C, and HLA-DR, -DP, and -DQ, are simultaneously present on the cells of each individual. The number of alleles for each HLA molecule varies: at least 50 B but only about 10 C and intermediate numbers of A alleles are known; the number of D region alleles is less well known, but DR appears to be the most diverse. The diversity provided by two alleles of each HLA antigen is sufficient to permit immune recognition by most individuals of the entire array of microbes and antigens that they encounter.

Structure. Structurally, each HLA molecule is a heterodimer, that is, is composed of two different molecules (Fig. 1). Class I molecules are composed of a polymorphic α-chain 45 kD in size that is an integral membrane protein; it is associated on the cell surface with a smaller (12 kD) invariant molecule, β_2-microglobulin by a noncovalent interaction that appears to stabilize the α-chain structure. Class II molecules are composed of an α- (about 30 kD) and a β- (about 26 kD) chain, both of which are polymorphic and are integral membrane proteins. The genes for the α- and β-chains of class II molecules are adjacent to each other on chromosome 6 and are inherited as a paired set.

Both class I and class II molecules contain paired regions that resemble immunoglobulin.[26] Such regions are about 100 amino acids in length and are folded into regions with sheet-like (β-pleated sheets) domains by intramolecular disulfide bonds. The importance of this structure has recently been demonstrated by x-ray crystallographic analysis of the HLA-A2 molecule, the first MHC molecule for which precise structural data are known. These studies showed that the β-pleated sheets of the α_1 and α_2 domains of the molecule, which are exposed on its surface, form an antigen-binding platform within a groove formed by other parts of the molecule.[73] Molecular modeling predicts a similar structure for class II molecules in which the platform is formed by the α_1 and β_1 domains[74] (Fig. 1).

Distribution and Regulation of Expression. In general, class I molecules are expressed by most nucleated cells. However, certain tissues express few or no class I antigens; these include the villous trophoblast, central nervous system neurons, corneal endothelium, and most endocrine cells, including pancreatic β-cells. Expression of class II molecules is much more restricted. B cells express these molecules in a relatively invariant manner; antigen-presenting macrophages, dendritic cells, and Langerhans cells also ordinarily express class II molecules, but expression on cells from different tissues varies in intensity and in which of the three classes (DR, DP, and DQ) are expressed.[75–77] Class II antigen expression is commonly less intense on tissue macrophages than on blood monocytes.[75]

The intensity of HLA antigen expression is an important determinant of the intensity of T-cell recognition and response; this is particularly important for class II antigen expression. Accordingly, the intensity of class II expression can be modulated reciprocally. Interferon-γ (IFN-γ) increases expression on macrophages and dendritic antigen-presenting cells[75,77,78] and can induce expression on cells that ordinarily are class II negative, such as endothelial, epithelial, and endocrine cells. This allows such cells to function as antigen-presenting cells at times of need but to be class II negative normally. Aberrant expression of class II molecules by such cells may be undesirable by leading to autoimmune injury, as seen in models of insulin-dependent diabetes.[79] Class II expression on B cells is not increased by IFN-γ but by another lymphokine, interleukin-4 (see section on lymphokines). Class I expression is increased by IFN-γ, but unlike class II molecules, class I expression is also increased by IFN-α, IFN-β, and tumor necrosis factor (see section on lymphokines). Class II expression is under reciprocal negative control by bacterial lipopolysaccharides, prostaglandins, and glucocorticoids. This system of regulatory controls, particularly for class II molecules, underscores their importance in immune response control.

Interaction of MHC Molecules with T-Cell Subsets

The cell and tissue distribution of class I compared to class II HLA molecules appears to be functionally related to their interaction with T-cell subsets. As noted above, class I and class II molecules restrict antigen recognition by T8 and T4 cells, respectively. T8 cells function primarily as cytotoxic T cells that recognize and destroy virus-infected cells, allogeneic grafts, or tumor cells. Since these target cells may include nucleated cells of all types, it is important that all or most nucleated cells express class I molecules, which they do.

In contrast, T4 cells are critical regulators of the function of other cell types, such as B cells and cytotoxic T cells—both enhancing the response (helper function) or inhibiting the response (suppressor inducer function).[80–83] By limiting class II HLA expression to a few cell types that are present at sites of potential microbial entry or entrapment (skin, lymphoid tissue, and spleen),[64,84–86] the amplitude and location of T4 compared to T8 cell stimulation may be more finely controlled; the ability of the lymphokines IFN-γ and interleukin-4 to induce or increase expression provides a mechanism for increasing the capacity of class II-dependent antigen- presentation at times of need.

Once induced to express class II MHC molecules, cells such as endothelial cells and fibroblasts can also present antigen to helper T cells.[84] Data derived from experiments in which class II MHC genes were expressed in fibroblasts by recombinant DNA techniques or peptide antigens were presented on artificial membranes containing class II suggest that MHC class II expression may be the only absolute requirement for a cell to function in antigen presentation to T4 cells.[10,84,87]

ROLE OF MACROPHAGES AND OTHER ANTIGEN-PRESENTING CELLS IN THE INDUCTIVE PHASE OF THE SPECIFIC IMMUNE RESPONSE

Antigen

Recognition of antigen by T cells differs fundamentally from recognition of antigen by B cells.[10,86,88–90] In most cases, B cells recognize intact antigens, frequently the confirmational determinants provided by the secondary and tertiary structures of the molecule. In contrast, T-cell recognition appears to depend on the primary amino acid sequence, and a relatively small number (about 10–20) of sequential amino acids are recognized in association with a specific MHC molecule.

Antigen Presentation to T4 (Helper) Cells. T4 cells that regulate all immune responses and are necessary for the induction of a primary response to antigen recognize the primary amino acid sequence only in association with class II HLA molecules.[10,86,87,91,92] Therefore, necessary requirements for induction of a primary T-cell response are that antigen-presenting cells both alter complex antigens so that the specific primary sequence is accessible and express class II MHC molecules on their surface. Optimal presentation of most antigens appears to require three important functional components: antigen processing, class II antigen expression, and cytokine (e.g., interleukins-1 and -6) production.[86]

Antigen processing appears most often to involve partial proteolysis or denaturation of an antigen.[88] This appears to take place in acidic endosomes within antigen-presenting cells[90] following endocytosis of microbes or other complex antigens. Such processing appears to be required for most globular proteins. Nonglobular hydrophilic proteins may not require such processing in all cases, as the recognized amino acids may be exposed and not cryptic, as in globular proteins. The efficiency of antigen uptake and subsequent processing by macrophages, Langerhans cells, and B cells may be facilitated by surface receptors for IgG (Fc receptors) and for derivatives of the third component of complement. These opsonic receptors facilitate phagocytosis of microbes or other particulate antigens. Such receptors are absent from other antigen-presenting cells.

The function of processing is to create peptides that will bind to MHC molecules and in so doing display a conformation that is recognized (i.e., that will bind to a specific T-cell antigen receptor).[86,89] Experiments with synthetic peptides derived from the sequences of known antigens, such as viral proteins of influenza and human immunodeficiency virus (HIV), suggest that 10–20 sequential amino acids are sufficient for both binding to MHC and recognition by T cells.[89,92,93]

Binding of processed antigen to class II MHC molecules is thought to occur in most cases intracellularly; then the antigen bound to the class II molecule is transported to the cell surface.[86,89] Such intracellular binding may be required because processed antigen binds to MHC with relatively low affinity (about 10^{-3} to 10^{-6} M), and both binding and release of antigen from MHC occur slowly over hours.[84,94] Thus, on the cell surface, MHC molecules probably have antigen bound at all times, limiting the access of newly processed antigens to newly synthesized or recycled MHC molecules within the cell.

Antigen Presentation to T8 Cytotoxic Cells. Antigens recognized in the context of class I MHC molecules are commonly derived from proteins synthesized within the cell on which they are presented. This is true for viral proteins[94–96] and for proteins of the MHC that are recognized as foreign in an allogeneic host.[97] However, recent studies indicate that the viral antigens recognized by cytotoxic T cells, including those of influenza[96,98] and HIV-1,[99] are often internal viral proteins rather than or in addition to those on the viral envelope or host cell plasma membrane.[95,98] These results suggest that viral or MHC antigens, newly synthesized within the cell but most likely in an incomplete or proteolytically processed form, may associate within the cell with host cell MHC class I molecules. MHC class I antigen complex would then be transported to the cell surface. In this manner, both internal and external viral antigens may be targets for recognition and destruction by cytotoxic T cells. This fact has obvious implications for viral vaccine strategies, since internal viral antigens may be suitable candidates in diseases such as influenza and HIV, in which surface antigens vary considerably among strains.[96,98,99]

MHC Molecular Polymorphism Regulates Responsiveness to Different Antigens

Early studies showed that helper T cells sensitized by immunization in vivo responded to a specific antigen only in the presence of autologous macrophages or macrophages bearing class II MHC molecules of the same allele (haplotypes). The T-cell response was said to be restricted by a specific MHC molecule. Molecular analyses indicate that a single amino acid substitution either in the MHC molecule or in the recognized portion of the antigen molecule is sufficient to alter recognition by T cells.[10,77,86,89,93] Structural analysis of the MHC molecules[73,74,100] and molecular manipulation of antigens[88,91] suggest that this restriction is mediated by variation in the binding affinity of MHC alleles for specific antigenic peptides. This variability is such that a given region of a processed complex antigen may bind strongly, weakly, or not at all; antigens that do not bind cannot be presented by that MHC molecule.

Antigen is predicted to bind in an antigen-binding groove at the exterior surface of the MHC molecule.[73,74] Further, many of the antigenic peptide sequences recognized by T cells are predicted to exist in an amphipathic α-helical conformation[89,92] such that one side of the antigen molecule binds to the MHC molecule and the opposite side binds to the T cell receptor. This is shown schematically in Figure 1. This model illustrates the basic nature of MHC restriction: the structure of the MHC molecule dictates which portions of an antigen will bind in the antigen-binding groove and, once bound, which portion and side of the antigen will be available for recognition by the T-cell receptor.

The Basis for T-Cell Recognition of the Antigen–MHC Complex

As noted, the potential diversity of T-cell receptors (about 10^{15}–10^{18} different possible receptors) is similar to the potential diversity of immunoglobulin.[11] However, unlike immunoglobulin, the diversity within the T-cell receptor genes is more heavily concentrated in the junctional regions, which are the location of the third complementarity determining region (CDR3) and is much more limited in the variable regions, the location of CDR1 and CDR2. Specific recognition of the MHC–antigen complex is mediated entirely by the two-chain T-cell receptor molecule. The recent evidence that antigen binds in a groove in the MHC molecule and other molecular modeling data suggested to Davis and Bjorkman[11] that the highly variable CDR3 region might bind to antigen as it lies within the groove and that the less variable CDR1 and CDR2 regions might contact the MHC molecule on the sides of the groove (Fig. 1). This model is appealing since it would explain the concentration of variability in the CDR3 region of the receptor. Compatible with this model are recent data indicating that for a series of T-cell clones recognizing a specific antigen, the CDR3 regions have been highly conserved.[23] Further experimental data are needed to determine the general applicability of this model.

There is a high degree of specificity present in this system: a specific antigenic peptide–MHC molecule complex is recognized by a given T cell. Although each T cell recognizes only a short peptide region of a larger molecule, each molecule may have many regions capable of binding to one or another of the host's MHC alleles. The T-cell receptor repertoire contains sufficient diversity that in most cases any complex microbial antigen will contain several peptide regions that bind to one or both MHC molecules of an individual and are recognized by T cells with the appropriate receptor. However, as noted above, inbred rodents with certain MHC class II alleles will not respond to a specific antigen; they lack an immune response gene (MHC class II allele) necessary for that response. Such occurrences are likely to be uncommon in highly outbred human populations. However, the association of specific diseases, most commonly autoimmune diseases, with specific HLA alleles in humans suggests that such differences may also account in part for increased susceptibility to certain infectious pathogens in humans.

T-Cell Activation and Proliferation

Binding of the TCR to antigen–MHC triggers a series of intracellular events that ultimately lead to lymphokine production and replication or, in the case of cytolytic T cells, trigger the cytolytic mechanism. Collectively, this process is referred to as *T-cell activation.*[101,102] Transduction of the signal from the T-cell receptor appears to be mediated by the CD3 (T3) complex.[17,101] There follows a series of associated biochemical events, critical among which appear to be an increase in intracellular free calcium concentration[103] and translocation of protein kinase C from cytosol to plasma membrane, whereby the T cell is activated.[104] Together these two events act, through as yet poorly characterized intracellular pathways, to induce transcription of a series of genes, among which are those for interleukin-2, the interleukin-2 receptor, and other lymphokines.[101,102] As described below ("The Role of Cytokines in T-Cell Proliferation"), binding of interleukin-2 to its receptor appears to be the critical event driving T cells to proliferate.

Both the increase in intracellular calcium and the activation of protein kinase C follow the activation of a cell membrane-associated phospholipase C, which releases inositol phosphates and diacylglycerol from membrane phospholipids. Inositol phosphates trigger the intracellular increase in calcium; diacylglycerol and calcium act together to activate membrane-associated protein kinase C.[101,102] This pathway is a common mechanism of intracellular signaling in many cell types. Although these pathways were deduced initially from studies in which stimuli other than the antigen–MHC complex were used to activate T cells, studies in which antigen was used have yielded similar results.[105,106]

The CD4 and CD8 molecules appear to play an accessory role in T-cell activation. Their major role may be to enhance adhesion between the T cell and the antigen-presenting cell or target cell by binding to nonpolymorphic regions of class II or class I MHC molecules, respectively. However, recent data suggest that they may modulate signaling through the T-cell receptor, enhancing the signal in the presence of antigen–MHC, inhibiting the signal in the absence of MHC molecules.[9,37,107–109] The CD2 surface molecule (the sheep erythrocyte receptor) also appears to function as an accessory signal for T-cell activation[32,33,37] and may be important in activation of NK cells.[110]

LYMPHOKINES AND CYTOKINES

Definitions and Overview

Lymphokines are proteins (or glycoproteins) secreted by lymphocytes that act as molecular signals for communication between cells of the immune system and as systemic mediators of the host's response to infection; as such, their function is analogous to that of neurotransmitters and hormones, respectively. It is now clear that other cell types, particularly mononuclear phagocytes, release and/or respond to such substances. In recognition of this, *cytokines*, a more general term that includes lymphokines, monokines (cytokines produced by mononuclear phagocytes), and other such mediators, is now in common use. The two terms are often used interchangeably.

Cytokines were originally detected in experimental systems that defined them by a specific biologic effect. An example is T-cell growth factor, now called *interleukin-2*. Biologic assays were used to monitor purification procedures for this molecule, which was found to be a glycoprotein of about 15 kD.[111] Modern molecular biologic techniques have resulted in the molecular cloning of this lymphokine and subsequently of many others. Once recombinant materials were made available, it became apparent that in most cases more than one lymphokine can mediate a biologic effect previously ascribed to a specific molecule. An example is the ability of interleukin-4 to act as a T-cell growth factor.[112,113] Conversely, many biologic effects originally thought to be mediated by different molecules were subsequently found to be the properties of one. For example, a molecule causing hemorrhagic necrosis of tumors, tumor necrosis factor (TNF), was found to be identical to a molecule causing wasting in rabbits with trypanosomiasis, cachectin.[114,115] Thus, definitions based solely on biologic effects can be misleading. Until it is cloned and molecularly characterized, a cytokine is generally referred to as a *factor* and is named according to its biologic effect(s), recognizing that this may or may not represent a single molecule. Once the amino acid sequence of the human form has been determined, it may be assigned an interleukin (IL) number.[116] However, some lymphokines, including the interferons, TNF, and msot of the colony-stimulating factors, have retained their original names even though cloned and molecularly characterized. For purposes of clarity and because many of the important lymphokines originally described as factors have been cloned in the past few years, this chapter focuses on those that have been molecularly defined. The reader should recognize that this necessarily oversimplifies the true complexity of the system; many factors that are not molecularly characterized and not fully discussed are likely to play a role in the processes that will be discussed.

Cytokines Act to Amplify or Attenuate Immune Responses

Cytokines bind to specific receptors on the surface of cells. In most cases, each cytokine has a unique receptor to which only it will bind with high affinity. However, there are at present two examples of related cytokines that exhibit minimal molecular homology but bind to a common receptor and appear to mediate similar biologic effects. IL-1 biologic activity is mediated by two molecules, IL-1α and IL-1β,[117,118] which are 26 percent homologous at the amino acid level but bind to a common receptor with similar affinities.[119,120] Similarly, TNF/cachectin biologic activity is mediated by two molecules, TNF-α and TNF-β (also called *lymphotoxin*), which are 30 percent homologous at the amino acid level.[121,122] TNF-α and -β bind to a common receptor. Although many of the biologic activities of TNF are also common to IL-1, the receptors for TNF are distinct from those for IL-1 and are not shared with other cytokines. Many cytokine receptors are present in low numbers (less than 500) and increase minimally on stimulated cells, suggesting that few molecules are required to mediate the biologic effect. An exception to this is the high-affinity receptor for IL-2, which is absent on resting T cells but present in moderately high numbers (more than 1000/cell) on activated T cells.[111] Up- and down-regulation of receptor numbers are two mechanisms by which the response to cytokines may be modulated. The molecular mechanism by which the cytokines alter cell function after binding is not well characterized, although receptor internalization after binding is a common feature often required for action.

The actions of cytokines are not antigen specific. However, their effects in many cases serve to transduce antigen-specific signals. Such is the case for the T-cell-derived lymphokines, since their production is stimulated by specific antigen in the context of HLA antigens. Also, in certain cases, their actions are restricted to cells that have first been primed to respond by specific antigen stimulation. Examples are IL-2, which stimulates proliferation of T cells primed to express high-affinity IL-2 receptors by antigen stimulation,[111] and B cells, which respond to IL-5 and IL-6 after antigen-triggered activation.[123] However, in many cases, cytokines act not only on antigen-triggered T and B cells but also on a wide variety of other cell types to amplify specific or nonspecific immune responses or to mediate more general host responses. In addition, many cytokines are produced by NK cells, mononuclear phagocytes, and certain nonimmune system cells in response to infections or inflammatory stimuli of a nonspecific nature. Thus, cytokines serve as transducing or modulating signals in the immune system, mediating both antigen-specific and non-antigen-specific effects.

Table 3 lists the principal cytokines that have been molecularly characterized and describes their basic characteristics, the major cell sources and stimuli triggering their secretion, and their major biologic effects. It should be emphasized that the effects listed are representative of those currently described that appear to be of biologic importance. In many cases, specific receptors for these molecules are much more widely distributed on cells than are the known biologic effects. Thus, it is to be anticipated that additional effects of importance will be discovered with time. The biochemistry, sources, production, and actions of TNF-α,[114,115,123] IL-1,[116,125] IL-2,[111] IL-4, IL-5, IL-6,[123,126,127] the interferons,[4,128–130] and the colony-stimulating factors (CSF), including IL-3,[131–133] have recently been reviewed. Progress in this field has been rapid. I will focus on a general overview of cytokines, including regulation of their production and their role in specific immune pathways relevant to host defense. New findings not available when the cited reviews were prepared have been included where informative.

General Biochemical Properties of Cytokines

Cytokines are not stored preformed within cells. Their production requires new protein and in most cases new mRNA synthesis. As expected from their role as humoral mediators of cellular immunity, they are encoded as propeptides, and with the exception of IL-1 (discussed below) and perhaps TNF-α,[134] they have an NH_2-terminal sequence dictating their transport to the Golgi apparatus, where they are glycosylated (for those that are glycoproteins) and promptly secreted. At this time the signal peptide sequence is removed to yield the mature protein of a lower molecular mass. Each cytokine is encoded by a unique mRNA and those described to date are encoded by a single gene. Monocyte CSF (M-CSF) is actually two different proteins, which are encoded by a single gene and derived by alternate mRNA processing.

Specific Cytokines Produced by Mononuclear Phagocytes and Mechanisms Regulating Their Production

Monocytes and macrophages are important sources of IL-1, IL-6, IFN-α, TNF-α, GM-CSF, G-CSF and M-CSF. Studies performed primarily in vitro indicate that each of these cytokines is also produced by other human cells types; human endothelial and fibroblasts are probably important sources of CSFs,[132,133,135] IL-1,[117,125] and IL-6[127]; B lymphocytes of IL-1,[117,125,136] T lymphocytes of TNF-α[137–139] and probably of IL-6[127,139]; and NK cells of TNF-α.[138] IFN-β, which is a molecule related to IFN-α with similar biologic activity, is produced by fibroblasts and epithelial cells. Other cell types may produce one or more of these cytokines; this may be of physiologic importance in specific anatomic sites. Most cytokines produced by mononuclear phagocytes have potent and diverse systemic effects in addition to their effects on immune function.

In general, appropriate stimulation of mononuclear phagocytes induces synthesis of specific cytokine mRNAs and proteins, followed rapidly by cytokine secretion. In addition, as illustrated by TNF-α, unstimulated monocytes and macrophages isolated from humans[140] and mice[141] appear to contain small amounts of mRNA for TNF-α but produce little or no detectable TNF-α protein until stimulated; stimulation induces increased TNF-α mRNA synthesis and enhances translation of preexisting and newly synthesized TNF-α mRNA. Low-level expression of mRNA in the absence of stimulation has been seen with other macrophage cytokines, including IL-1α and IL-1β,[117] IL-6,[127] M-CSF, and G-CSF in vitro (135, unpubl. obs.); it is not known if this actually occurs in vivo or is an artifact of the procedures used to isolate or culture the cells. Preexisting mRNA may allow more rapid production of cytokine protein by mononuclear phagocytes in response to infectious or inflammatory stimuli in vivo than would be possible if all protein was derived from newly synthesized mRNA.

A common set of stimuli lead to the production of cytokines by mononuclear phagocytes. Bacteria and their products, such as lipopolysaccharide and toxic shock syndrome toxin,[142] are potent inducers of TNF-α,[140,141] IL-1,[117,125,143] IL-6,[144,145] IFN-α/β,[128,146] and M-CSF, G-CSF, and GM-CSF[132,133,135] production by mononuclear phagocytes. Viruses and polynucleotides also induce IFN-α/β[146–148] and perhaps IL-1.[117] An interesting and important property of these cytokines is the capacity to induce or enhance their own or each other's production. Thus, TNF-α and IL-1 directly induce production of IL-1,[143,149–152] TNF-α,[143] IL-6,[144,145] GM-CSF, G-CSF, and M-CSF[132,133,135,153] by human mononuclear phagocytes, endothelial cells, and fibroblasts. Similar results have been observed in many cases with experimental animals in vivo.[149,154] In addition to directly stimulating cytokine production, cytokines can enhance production induced by other stimuli. GM-CSF and INF-γ enhance production of TNF-α and IL-1[140,155] and of M-CSF and G-CSF.[156,157] Activated complement components and immune complexes also stimulate cytokine production by human mononuclear phagocytes.[158]

Under most conditions, stimulation of macrophages induces the coordinate release of each of these cytokines. Although teleologically appealing, examples of selective cytokine production by macrophages are limited. IFN-α/β are in part differentially regulated from other cytokines, since their production is efficiently induced by certain stimuli (viruses) that do not induce or only weakly induce the other macrophage-derived cytokines. Differentially diminished IL-1 relative to TNF production and secretion has also been described. Human monocytes infected with *Leishmania donovani* or cultured under resting conditions have impaired IL-1 but not TNF-α production.[140,159,160] IFN-γ enhances TNF-α production under all conditions[140] and reverses the block in IL-1 production induced by *Leishmania*.[160] There is no clear evidence for subsets of blood monocytes that produce only one or a few cytokines and not others. Differential regulation of cytokine production in tissue macrophages resulting from differences in local conditions is suggested by the studies with cultured monocytes but has not been directly determined.

Stimulation of macrophage cytokine production by microbial products with amplification by other cytokines may be important for a rapid response to minimal microbial invasion but also has the potential for overproduction in response to maximal microbial challenge; this may contribute to some of the deleterious host responses to infection discussed below. However, the host also has pathways for down-regulating production, and for limiting systemic release of these mediators, while focusing their production at the site(s) of infection.

One mechanism for focusing the effects of the cytokines would be to limit their production to the local site. This is accomplished in part by the positive feedback system described above. Resting tissue macrophages appear to have a more limited capacity to release TNF-α, and particularly IL-1, than do inflammatory macrophages and monocytes.[140] The higher capacity of inflammatory macrophages may relate in part to their more recent derivation from monocytes and to their exposure to high local concentrations of microbial products, chemotactic complement components, and cytokines. The end result is that the greatest production will be by macrophages at inflammatory sites. In addition, only part of the IL-1 produced is secreted; the remainder is cell-associated, at least in part, as an integral plasma membrane protein.[161] This is possible because both IL-1α and IL-1β lack a signal peptide sequence directing secretion.[118,125] The pathways by which IL-1α and IL-1β are processed from precursor forms of about 31 kD to their secreted low molecular weight forms (about 17.5 kD) and how they reach the cell membrane or are secreted is unclear.[125,162] However this occurs, the effects of IL-1 are thereby focused, allowing it to act locally to enhance T-cell activation in response to antigen while minimizing systemic effects. We have found that cultured human monocytes as a model of resting macrophages secrete a much smaller fraction of total IL-1 produced than do circulating blood monocytes[140]; results with tissue macrophages were intermediate between those of fresh and cultured monocytes. Thus, in the absence of an influx of large numbers of inflammatory macrophages, IL-1 may be highly focused at local sites of infection. Consistent with this is the finding that alveolar macrophages from people with inflammatory processes secrete greater amounts of IL-1 in response to stimulation than do macrophages from healthy people.[163] Similar to IL-1, a small fraction of TNF-α may be initially expressed as an integral membrane protein.[134]

Cytokines also induce the production of compounds that down-regulate their own production. Both TNF-α and IL-1 induce production of prostaglandins, particularly PGE_2, which down-regulates their production.[114,124,125] PGE_2 also inhibits certain effects of IL-1, such as T-cell activation.[164] IL-1 appears to be unique in its ability to enhance production of certain pituitary hormones, including ACTH and α-melanocyte stimulating hormone.[117,125,165–167] ACTH, by enhancing glucocorticoid production, can negatively regulate production of itself, TNF, and other cytokines, including the CSFs, interferons, and IL-2 to IL-6. In addition to inhibiting cytokine production, glucocorticoids and α-melanocyte stimulating hormone inhibit the effects of IL-1 on many cell types. Other substances may act as endogenous negative regulators of cytokine production and effects, but their precise role in vivo remains to be determined.[168–170] The effects of excessive TNF and IL-1 production are also attenuated by their ability to down-regulate their own receptors.

The relative role that each of these processes plays in vivo in attenuating the potential adverse systemic effects of overproduction of TNF, IL-1, and other macrophage-derived cytokines remains to be determined.

Lymphokines Produced by T Cells and Mechanisms Regulating Their Production

With the exception of certain tumors, T lymphocytes are the sole source of IL-2, -3, and -5 and lymphotoxin (TNF-β), and are the major source of IFN-γ; along with macrophages and NK cells, they produce TNF-α; they are the major source of IL-4, which is also produced by mast cells.[126] Unlike macrophages, which produce and secrete cytokines in response to a number of stimuli, T cells secrete lymphokines in response to activation by antigen in the context of HLA. The molecular events that transduce these signals and mediate the initial events in T-cell activation have been discussed above. Following activation, the genes encoding these lymphokines are transcribed within a few hours, followed rapidly by their production and prompt secretion. Production continues to increase over the first 24–72 hours after stimulation, depending on the conditions, and then declines.

Activation of a mixed population of T lymphocytes and antigen-presenting cells, such as blood, tonsillar, or splenic mononuclear cells, usually leads to coordinate production of each of these lymphokines, although the rate and time to maximal production of each vary slightly. This reflects the aggregate production of lymphokines by all cells in the population. However, evidence suggests that the production of individual lymphokines may be regulated, in part, differentially.

T4 cells of humans and mice produce each of these lymphokines[171–175]; However, the capacity to secrete specific lymphokines may be restricted to subsets of T4 cells. Initially, data derived from murine T-cell clones in vitro indicated that certain ones (known as *TH1 clones*) produced IL-2, IFN-γ, TNF-α, TNF-β (lymphotoxin), and GM-CSF, whereas others (known as *TH2 clones*) produced IL-4 and IL-5; both produced IL-3.[173–175] Interestingly, evidence (discussed below) suggests that this selective lymphokine production may have functional significance in that the lymphokines produced by TH2 cells enhance production of antibody isotypes that sensitize mast cells and eosinophils (IgG1 and IgE in the mouse) and stimulate mar-

TABLE 3. Properties of Lymphokines and Cytokines

Name	*Physicochemical Characteristics (Human)*	*Principal Cell Sources*	*Stimuli Inducing Release*	*Major Biologic Effects*
Interleukin-1 (Lymphocyte-activating factor, endogenous pyrogen hemopo etin 1)	Two proteins: α and β, both Mr ~17.5 kD; α more acidic than β	Many cell types; mononuclear phagocytes are a major source	Bacteria and their products (e.g., endotoxin), antigens, other cytokines (e.g., TNF)	Induces catabolic state, fever, acute phase protein synthesis, and ACTH release; is a cofactor for T-cell activation, B-cell proliferation, and bone marrow stem cell proliferation; induces PMN release from bone marrow; enhances or induces TNF, IL-1, IFN and CSF production; increases endothelial adherence and procoagulant properties
Interleukin-2 (T-cell growth factor)	Glycoprotein Mr ~15 kD	T cells	Antigen–MHC	Major mediator of T-cell proliferation; promotes production of other T-cell lymphokines; enhances cytotoxic T-cell production and differentiation; enhances NK function; cofactor for B-cell proliferation and immunoglobulin secretion
Interleukin-4 (B-cell stimulating factor, B-cell growth factor I)	Glycoprotein ~20 kD	T cells	Antigen–MHC	Promotes proliferation of B cells; induces IgE isotype synthesis; enhances cytotoxic T-cell production and differentiation; enhances B-cell surface HLA class II and IgE receptors; enhances mast cell production; cofactor with other colony stimulating factors in the mouse
Interleukin-5 (B-cell growth factor II, T-cell replacing factor)	Glycoprotein ~18 kD (circulates as a homodimer)	T cells	Antigen–MHC	Induces IgA and IgM isotype synthesis; enhances eosinophil production and function; unclear whether it promotes proliferation of B cells and immunoglobulin secretion in humans
Interleukin-6 (B-cell stimulating factor 2, interferon-β-2, B-cell differentiation factor)	Glycoprotein 21–29 kD	Mononuclear phagocytes; fibroblasts; T cells; certain tumors	Low-level constitutive, increased by viruses, bacteria and their products, IL-1, TNF, IFN, PDGF	Induces immunoglobulin production in activated B cells; little or no interferon activity; induces fever, acute phase protein synthesis, and ACTH release
Interferon-α	Family of peptides 8–20 kD	Mononuclear phagocytes; lymphocytes	Bacteria and their products, viruses, double stranded RNA, other	Interferes with viral replication; decreases cell replication; increases class I MHC expression;

Interferon-β	Glycoprotein 23 kD	Fibroblasts; epithelial cells	cytokines	increases NK cell function; induces fever
Interferon-γ	Glycoprotein 20–25 kD	T cells; NK cells	Antigen–MHC; NK targets	Same as α and β; also increases class II MHC expression, enhances macrophage functions, enhances IgG subtype production
Tumor necrosis factors (TNF) α (cachectin)	Peptide 17 kD	Mononuclear phagocytes; T cells; NK cells	Bacteria and their products, other cytokines, (e.g., IL-1, CSFs, IFN-γ) Antigen–MHC; NK targets	Induces catabolic state, fever, acute phase protein synthesis; major mediator of septic shock; has direct antiviral and antitumor activity; increases endothelial cell adherence and procoagulant properties; enhances B-cell proliferation and immunoglobulin production; enhances PMN adherence and cidal activity (α > β); increases class I MHC expression; enhances or induces TNF, IL-1, IFN and colony stimulating factor production (α > β); inhibits bone marrow cell proliferation
β (lymphotoxin)	Glycoprotein 25 kD	T cells	Antigen–MHC	
Interleukin-3 (multi-CSF)	Glycoprotein 14–28 kD	T cells	Antigen–MHC	Promotes proliferation of pluripotent marrow stem cells
GM-CSF (granulocyte-macrophage-CSF)	Glycoprotein 14–35 kD	T cells; endothelial cells; mononuclear phagocytes; fibroblasts	Antigen–MHC; bacterial products, other cytokines (e.g., TNF, IL-1, IFN-γ)	Promotes proliferation of neutrophil, macrophage, and eosinophil precursors; enhances neutrophil, eosinophil, and macrophage function
M-CSF (macrophage CSF, CSF-1)	Glycoprotein, two forms: 35–45 kD and 20–25 kD (one gene); both circulate as homodimers	Mononuclear phagocytes; fibroblasts; endothelial cells	Constitutive production, increased in response to bacterial products, other cytokines	Promotes proliferation of monocytes; enhances macrophage function
G-CSF (granulocyte CSF)	Glycoprotein 19 kD	Mononuclear phagocytes; epithelial cells; fibroblasts	Low-level constitutive production increased in response to bacterial products, other cytokines	Promotes proliferation of granulocytes; enhances granulocyte function

row production of eosinophils and mast cells.[126,171–176] In contrast, TH1 cells produce INF-γ, which preferentially enhances production of a complement-fixing antibody isotype (IgG2a in the mouse), thought to be important in antiviral and antibacterial defense.[126,177] There is no direct evidence to date that selective lymphokine production is a property of T cells that have not been passaged and cloned in vitro. However, in the rat, a subset of T4 cells that expresses the surface marker OX22 produces IL-2 but does not support immunoglobulin production by B cells, whereas the subset lacking OX22 does not produce IL-2 but does support immunoglobulin synthesis.[178] The situation in the human may be somewhat different. An antigen analogous to OX22, CD45R (detected by the monoclonal antibody 2H4), is absent on T4 cells that support immunoglobulin production and is present on those that do not.[83] We have recently found that IL-4 production is restricted to a small subpopulation (about 5 percent) of human T4 cells; although IL-4-producing cells are almost all CD45R negative, only 6–8 percent of CD45R-negative T4 cells produce IL-4.[172] In contrast, about 30–50 percent CD45R-positive or -negative T4 cells produce IL-2 and IFN-γ. Initial data with cloned human T4 cells also suggest that there is more overlap in production of lymphokines than in the mouse clones. A single T4 cell clone produced IL-4, IL-5 and GM-CSF, but not IL-2, IL-3, and IFN-γ, whereas all other clones produced IL-2, IL-4, and IFN-γ.[171] Nevertheless, these data indicate that production of specific lymphokines by T cells may be regulated, in part, by differences in the capacity of an individual T cell to produce specific lymphokines.

There is a more clear distinction in the capacity for lymphokine production between T4 and T8 cells than within subsets of T4 cells. Although both T4 and T8 cells produce IL-2 and IFN-γ when stimulated with nonspecific mitogens or in response to allogeneic cells,[179,180] production of IL-2 in response to antigens appears to be restricted primarily to T4 cells. Production of other lymphokines by T8 cells in response to antigens but not nonspecific mitogens appears to be almost completely dependent on IL-2 production by T4 cells.[181–183] These findings highlight the critical importance of T4 (helper) cells in lymphokine production, as in T-cell proliferation (see below), and provide an explanation for the devastating effects that result from ablation of this T-cell subset in AIDS. In addition, to the requirement for IL-2, other cytokines may enhance lymphokine production. IL-1 acts to increase production of IL-2, particularly when antigen or antigen-presenting cells are limiting,[116,184,185] and thereby indirectly augments production of other lymphokines. In addition, IFN-γ and TNF-α and -β augment the production of each other.[116,137,186]

Differential regulation of lymphokine production may also be determined, in part, by differences in the way antigen is presented. For example, antigen-presenting cells that have had surface molecules altered by chemical agents have altered antigen-presenting properties such that they induce little or no IL-2 production, whereas IFN-γ, IL-3, and IL2-R are normally induced.[187] Other evidence suggests that the state of T-cell activation or T-cell surface molecules, which could bind to and be affected differently by altered antigen-presenting cells, may act to regulate in part which lymphokines, are produced.[188] How these changes lead to selective induction of certain lymphokines is unclear, although altered production of putative second mediators, such as arachidonic acid metabolites for IFN-γ production,[189] has been proposed.

Since T cells produce IL-2, which augments production of other T-cell-derived lymphokines, there is a potential for overproduction. Important regulatory mechanisms act to attenuate the response. First, IL-2 does not stimulate its own production.[111] In addition, with mouse T-cell clones, the capacity of IL-2 to enhance lymphokine production is maximum within the first 24–48 hours after T cells have been activated by antigen stimulation and is virtually absent 7 days later.[188,190] Reciprocally, exposure of T cells to high concentrations of IL-2 impairs their activation through the antigen receptor.[191] In addition, activated T cells (192, 193) produce transforming growth factor-β early after activation.[192,193] This factor inhibits IL-2-induced T-cell proliferation and inhibits preferentially IFN-γ production, with less inhibition of TNF-α and TNF-β (lymphotoxin) production. In addition, monocytes that are exposed to IFN-γ produce PGE_2 and 1,25 dihydroxy vitamin D_3 (calcitriol), which inhibit IL-2 and IFN-γ production and the T-cell response to IL-2.[164,194,195] Thus, like the production of cytokines by macrophages, both positive and negative regulatory signals act to modulate the strength and duration of T-cell lymphokine production.

Cytokine Production by NK Cells and B Cells

The repertoire of lymphokines that NK and B cells produce is more limited. Binding to target cells induces NK cells to secret TNF-α but apparently not TNF-β.[138,196] However, unlike T cells, most mitogens are poor inducers of TNF-α production by NK cells.[138] IL-2 and inflammatory stimuli induce NK cells to produce IFNγ.[130,197] B cells and NK cells may release low levels of IL-1 constitutively.[136] It is likely that these cells also release additional cytokines, since tumor cell lines of these lineages have been reported to secrete such lymphokines as IL-6,[123] lymphotoxin,[121] and GM-CSF.[198]

IMPORTANT IMMUNOLOGIC RESPONSE PATHWAYS ARE REGULATED BY CYTOKINES

To provide a conceptual framework for understanding the function of cytokines in the immune response, several examples of cytokine-regulated responses are discussed below. These discussions are necessarily oversimplified. Additional complexity due to the interaction of cell types and cytokines that are not shown, or are still not cloned or molecularly characterized, is likely. The role of cytokines in modifying effector cell function is discussed in the section on these cells.

Fever, the Systemic Acute Phase Response to Infection and Septic Shock

The role of cytokines in the pathogenesis of fever has recently been reviewed (see Chapter 39).[154] Fever is associated with an elevation of the normal temperature set point for an individual; although the mean body temperature is increased, the normal diurnal fluctuation of temperature is not altered. Fever may play a beneficial role in host resistance to infection both by inhibiting the growth of certain microorganisms directly and by enhancing certain aspects of host immune responses.[199,200] The elevation of temperature is mediated primarily by endogenous pyrogens. Studies to define the pyrogenic molecules have, by necessity, been done largely in experimental animals. TNF-α and TNF-β and IL-1α and IL-1β are directly pyrogenic in rabbits. They appear to act directly on vascular endothelial cells in the hypothalamic area to cause local production of PGE_2, which then acts on cells within the anterior hypothalamus to cause fever. The antipyretics, such as aspirin and acetaminophen, act by blocking the production of PGE_2 in the brain. In addition to inducing fever directly, TNF stimulates IL-1 production, accounting for the biphasic fever observed in animals administered TNF. The major mediators of bacterial lipopolysaccharide-induced fever appear to be TNF and IL-1; lipopolysaccharide also acts directly on the hypothalamus to induce fever, accounting for the biphasic fever in response to this substance. Other cytokines, including interferons and IL-6, cause fever in experimental animals,[154,201] although they are less potent, and in the case of IFN-γ perhaps act indirectly by inducing TNF or IL-1 release. The pyrogenic effects of TNF and the interferons have been demonstrated in humans.[154]

The *acute phase reaction* is a term describing collectively a range of metabolic changes occurring in response to infection and inflammation (see Chapter 4). Striking effects include those on hepatic protein synthesis, lipid metabolism, and tissue catabolism. TNF, IL-1, and IL-6 all play a role in altering hepatic protein synthesis. Albumin synthesis is decreased and, concomitantly, synthesis of complement components C3 and factor B, metallothionein, serum amyloid A, α_1-antitrypsin, haptoglobin, fibrinogen, C-reactive protein, and others is increased in human hepatoma cell lines in vitro or in experimental animals in vivo.[117,125,201–205] Both TNF and IL-1 also inhibit lipoprotein lipase production, thereby causing lipemia, which is characteristic of certain chronic infections, including experimental trypanosomiasis.[114,115,117,205] The role of TNF-α in cachexia related to infection or malignancy has been postulated based on its effects on food intake and catabolism; this has been directly demonstrated in experimental transgenic mice bearing tumors continually secreting TNF-α in which progressive anorexia and wasting occurred.[206] It is likely that IL-1 also contributes to the wasting seen in chronic inflammatory conditions.[117]

A striking effect of TNF, which is augmented by IL-1, is its ability to produce profound vascular effects. Both increase the adhesive properties of endothelial cells, due in part to increased synthesis of cell adhesion molecules.[207] TNF increases the adhesiveness of circulating granulocytes, due in part to increased surface expression of the leukocyte cell adhesion molecules (LCAM) of the Mac-1, LFA-1 family.[208,209] Endothelial cell procoagulant activity and platelet activating factor production are also increased by TNF and IL-1.[210,211] These and additional effects likely act to induce granulocyte adhesion, capillary leakage, vessel thrombosis, and hemorrhagic necrosis at local sites of administration in experimental animals.[114,115,125] Systemic administration of TNF to rodents produces a syndrome resembling septic shock and disseminated intravascular coagulation; this is characterized by hemorrhagic necrosis, particularly in the gastrointestinal tract, hypotension, hypoglycemia, and lactic acidosis terminating in death.[212–214] IL-1,[117] IFN-γ,[215] and lipopolysaccharide enhance these toxic effects of TNF. The most convincing evidence for a role for TNF in the pathogenesis of septic shock comes from studies in baboons with experimentally induced *Echerichia coli* bacteremia. In such animals treated with antibody to TNF-α 2 hours before infection, death associated with hypotension, and cardiopulmonary and renal failure were completely prevented, whereas they were observed in 100 percent of controls.[213] Circulating TNF-α concentrations were markedly elevated in controls and were not detectable in the treated animals. It is likely that the effects of TNF-α are mediated, at least in part, indirectly. Data support an important role for cyclooxygenase products in TNF-α-induced septic shock in rats; in this model, PGE_2 concentrations in plasma are markedly increased; this increase and the rapidly fatal course are largely blocked in animals that are pretreated with the cyclooxygenase inhibitors indomethacin or ibuprofen.[216] Other mediators, such as lipoxygenase products of arachidonic acid, platelet activating factor, and kinins, are likely to be involved.

Hematopoiesis

Hematopoietic cells are derived from pluripotent stem cells in the bone marrow. The growth and differentiation of hematopoietic cells are under the control of specific cytokines[132,133,135] (Fig. 3). IL-1α,[217,218] IL-6,[219] and IL-3[220] stimulate proliferation of early pluripotent stem cells; IL-3 and GM-CSF stimulate proliferation of cells capable of forming granulocytes, erythrocytes, macrophages, and megakaryocytes[132,133]; GM-CSF stimulates granulocyte and macrophage precursors to proliferate[221]; M-CSF and G-CSF stimulate proliferation of their respective committed precursors[222–224]; IL-5 stimulates eosinophil production.[176] TNF and interferons may act as negative feedback signals to impede marrow cell growth. Note that the factors acting on the most mature precursors of phagocytes (M-CSF and G-CSF) are rapidly produced by macrophages and other nonhematopoietic cells in response to microbial or inflammatory stimuli. This may be important in allowing rapid mobilization of marrow reserves in response to infection. In contrast, the T-cell-derived products act either to augment production of cells at earlier stages of differentiation (IL-3 and GM-CSF) or to stimulate production of eosinophils (IL-5).

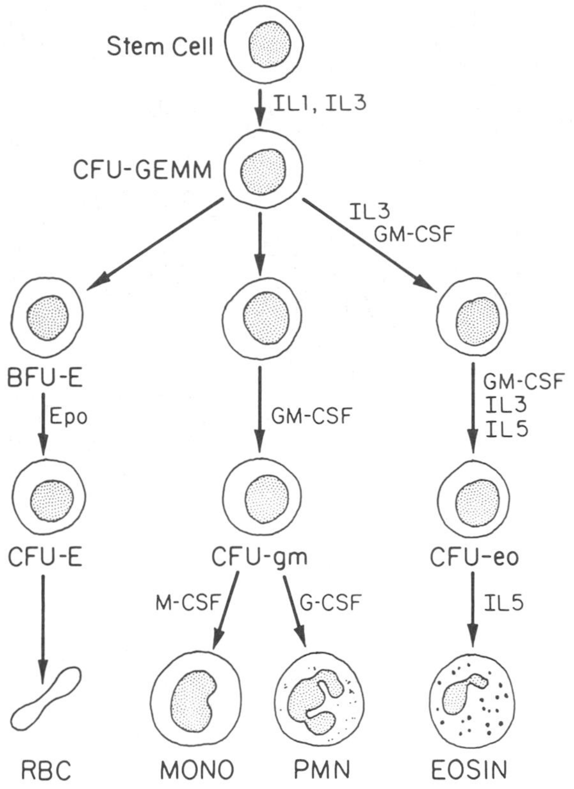

FIG. 3. The role of lymphokines in marrow growth and differentiation. IL, interleukin; CSF, colony-stimulating factor; G, granulocyte; M, monocyte/macrophage.

The Role of Cytokines in T-Cell Proliferation

As discussed above, T cells are activated by antigen in the context of HLA antigens on macrophages or other antigen-presenting cells to produce cytokines, most importantly IL-2, and to express IL-2 receptors on their plasma membrane (Fig. 4). Cognate interaction of T cells with antigen associated with MHC on the antigen-presenting macrophages induces IL-1 production by the macrophages[162,225]; this may be mediated by a direct cell contact mechanism and perhaps also by an as yet undefined soluble factor(s) that T cells release in response to this interaction. IL-1 appears to be most important in enhancing T-cell activation when antigen is limiting.[162] It acts both to increase IL-2 and high-affinity IL-2 receptor expression by T cells. However, IL-1 cannot completely replace antigen-presenting cells in most experimental systems even if a direct signal to the T cell is delivered by a monoclonal antibody that activates the T-cell receptor complex; this indicates that antigen-presenting cells facilitate T-cell activation at multiple levels.

T-cell proliferation appears to be closely regulated by the amount of free IL-2 and by the number and affinity of IL-2 receptors.[112] Since T4 (helper) cells appear to be the primary source of IL-2 produced in response to antigen stimulation, it follows that they are critical to one component of this process—the amount of free IL-2. High-affinity IL-2 receptors are expressed in response to stimulation both by T4 and by T8 (cytotoxic) T cells. High-affinity receptors are composed of two

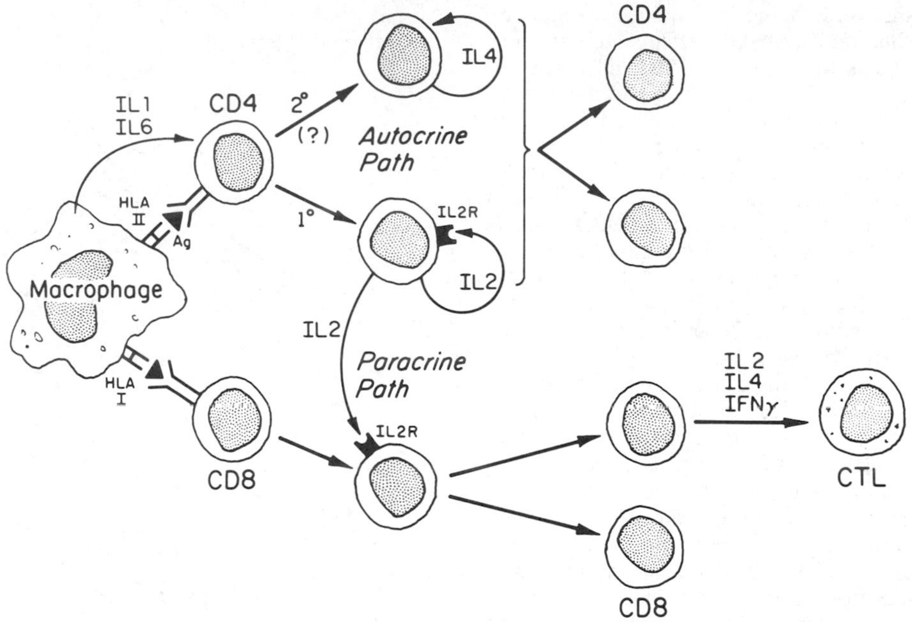

FIG. 4. The role of lymphokines in T-cell proliferation and differentiation. IL: interleukin; IFN-γ: interferon-γ: IL-2R, interleukin-2 receptor; CD4 and CD8: T4 (helper) and T8 (cytotoxic) T cells, respectively; CTL: cytotoxic T lymphocyte.

chains: one of about 55 kD and another of about 70–75 kD.[236–238] Little if any of either chain is present on resting T cells.[229] In the absence of the other, either chain can bind IL-2—the 55 kD chain rapidly but with low affinity and the 70 kD chain slowly and with medium affinity.[230,231] Together they form a receptor with high affinity, which binds IL-2 rapidly but releases it slowly. Current data suggest that the 70 kD chain is critical for induction of IL-2 driven proliferation.[231] Such a receptor permits maximal expression of high-affinity receptors when desirable, shortly after antigen-triggered T-cell activation, that are down-regulated within a few days unless T cells are restimulated by antigen. Thus, when recently triggered by antigen, all T cells express high-affinity receptors and can be driven to proliferate by IL-2. Conversely, the response to IL-2 is limited to cells recently activated by antigen, thereby preventing nonspecific proliferation of T cells not activated by antigen and excessive, sustained proliferation of antigen-activated T cells. This process of negative control is likely to be even more complex, since for a period late after antigen activation, T cells may become refractory to IL-2-driven proliferation even though they still express high-affinity IL-2 receptors; likewise, T cells recently stimulated by high concentrations of IL-2 may be temporarily refractory to antigen-induced activation.[191] The mechanism by which this refractoriness is mediated is not yet clear, but it may be due to a block in signal transduction.

Recent data indicate that there may be alternative pathways by which T-cell proliferation may be driven. IL-4 may augment or replace the need for IL-2 in T-cell proliferation.[112,113] A role for IL-6 has also been suggested.[232] However, it is likely that IL-2 is the major lymphokine required for T-cell proliferation under most conditions. The role of cytokines in differentiation of cytotoxic T cells is discussed in the section on "Cytotoxic T Cells."

Role of Cytokines in B-Cell Activation and Differentiation into Antibody-Secreting Cells

B cells are activated by specific antigens through surface immunoglobulin that acts as an antigen receptor. Once activated, they replicate and then differentiate into immunoglobulin-secreting B cells, and subsequently into memory B cells or plasma cells. This process is controlled by T cells, macrophages, and cytokines from these cells, as shown in Figure 5 (reviewed in Ref. 233). This appears to be a sequential process involving first antigen-induced activation and then DNA synthesis and proliferation, followed by differentiation into immunoglobulin-secreting cells. The requirements for activation vary with the nature of the antigen. Many of the steps were first deduced in the murine system; the relative requirement for T-cell help has been less well studied in humans. It is clear that the actions of specific lymphokines in this process may differ somewhat between the two species; this may reflect species differences or differences in the source of cells and culture conditions used in the in vitro studies. The data shown for the lymphokines are those derived from studies with human cells. The studies on T-cell-independent vs. T-cell-dependent responses are largely extrapolated from those in the mouse; available human data are consistent with these distinctions but require confirmation.

The activation step may be fully T cell independent or dependent on T cells to provide lymphokines (partially T cell independent, type II), or dependent on direct cognate T cell–B cell interaction[234]; cognate T cell–B cell interaction requires that processed antigen be presented in association with class II MHC antigens on B cells to T cells that bind antigen through their antigen receptor. It is unclear if naturally occurring, fully T-cell-independent (type I) antigens exist in humans, although lipopolysaccharide may be an example; in the mouse such antigens are usually large, multivalent, synthetic molecules. Partially T-cell-independent (type II) antigens are oligovalent antigens with repetitive sites, such as the polysaccharide antigens of encapsulated bacteria. Other antigens, including most proteins, are T cell dependent. The activation step triggered by antigen is often mimicked in studies in vitro by antibody to B cell surface IgM or by staphylococcal protein A. These stimuli, like soluble antigen, provide the first signals in B-cell activation, and full activation is facilitated by IL-4. In T-cell-dependent activation, murine studies suggest that cognate T cell–B cell interaction appears to provide one signal independent of IL-4[235,236]; however, IL-4 appears to provide an additional signal and may regulate this process both positively and negatively.[237,238]

Once activated, B cells become responsive to the prolifera-

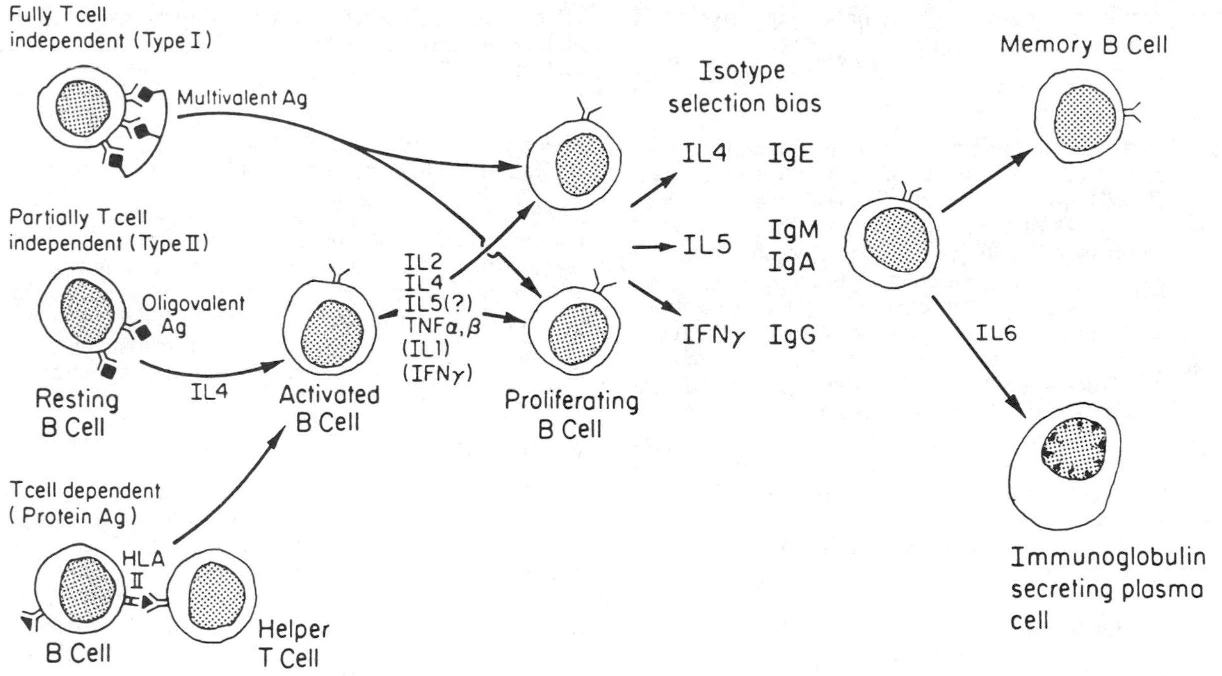

FIG. 5. The role of lymphokines in B-cell growth and differentiation. IL: interleukin; TNF: tumor necrosis factor; IFN-γ: interferon-γ; Ig: immunoglobulin.

tive effects of several lymphokines. In humans, IL-2,[239–242] IL-4,[243,244] and TNF-α[245] and -β[246] appear able to serve as independent signals for proliferation of activated B cells. The effects of one are frequently augmented by those of the others or by the effects of IL-1[233,247] and IFN-γ,[248] which act as cofactors for B-cell proliferation. IL-5, which is a major mediator of B-cell proliferation in the mouse, has not yet been shown to have such activity in the human[233]; conversely, TNF-α and -β have not been shown to drive murine B-cell proliferation, and IFN-γ inhibits this proliferation. After proliferation, B cells either become quiescent memory B cells or differentiate into antibody-secreting plasma cells. IL-6 appears to enhance differentiation into plasma cells and supports the growth of antibody-secreting cells.[249,250] Other lymphokines, such as IFN-γ and IL-2, may also act together to increase the secretion of immunoglobulin.[239]

Lymphokines also influence and may in part determine the class of immunoglobulin secreted. This has most clearly been shown for IL-4, which appears to stimulate a switch from IgM to IgE production in the mouse and in the human.[171,233] In contrast, this switch is antagonized by IFN-γ, which preferentially increases production of IgG in the human[171,233]; in the mouse, IFN-γ increases production of IgG2a, a complement-fixing IgG subclass implicated in antiviral and perhaps antibacterial defenses.[126] IL-5 enhances IgM and IgA production in both species.[176,233,251] There is clearly greater complexity in the system. For example, IL-4 also appears to be important in the B-cell response to polysaccharide antigens such as those of encapsulated bacteria[252]; antibodies to such organisms are commonly of the IgG2 and IgG4 subclasses in humans. Further, with T-cell-dependent antigens, IL-4 may enhance IgM secretion while inhibiting production of all IgG subclasses. These latter effects of IL-4 have been described in the mouse but have not yet been studied in the human.

THE IMMUNOREGULATORY FUNCTION OF T CELLS AND MACROPHAGES

T-cell functions have commonly been divided into three categories: helper, suppressor, or cytotoxic function. The first two roles are immunoregulatory and the final is a direct effector role. These functions correlate in part with surface expression of the CD4 (T4 helper) and CD8 (T8 suppressor/cytotoxic) surface molecules.

T-Cell Help

Traditionally, help is defined as the ability of certain T cells to enhance immunoglobulin synthesis by B cells.[253–256] This capacity appears to be restricted to T4 cells, hence their designation as helper T cells. As discussed above, T4 cells are heterogeneous in that B-cell help is mediated by some but not all T4 cells.[83,173] This heterogeneity has been discerned by assays in which B-cell help is provided only by those cells defined as helper-inducer T cells, which express surface antigens detected by the monoclonal antibodies 4B4 and UCHL1[83]; similarly, heterogeneity has been found in the production by T4 cell clones of specific lymphokines known to regulate B-cell growth and differentiation.[171–175] B-cell help may be both antigen specific and antigen nonspecific. Both types of help appear to be provided by helper-inducer T cells: the antigen-specific help appears to require direct "cognate" interaction through concomitant binding of T cells and B cells to different components of the same complex antigen; the nonspecific help is mediated by release of certain lymphokines. Lymphokines also appear to play a role in antigen-specific help, as discussed more fully in the section on role of lymphokines in B-cell help.

A broader definition of T-cell help includes the role of T4 cells in differentiation of T8 cells[257–259] or macrophages into more competent antigen-presenting or effector cells. It is likely that these effects are mediated primarily by lymphokines. Thus, heterogeneity in the production of certain lymphokines may be one reason why T-cell help for B cells, cytotoxic T cells, and macrophages is not directly correlated. A characteristic of cells in the helper-inducer subset of T4 cells (as defined by the surface antigens detected by monoclonal antibodies 4B4 and UCHL1) is their capacity to respond to soluble antigen. In the absence of these cells, other T4 and T8 cells do not respond to specific antigens, leading to the suggestion that "memory," recognition of antigens to which the individual has previously been exposed, is restricted to these cells.[83] This observation may explain the pivotal role these cells play in helping other T and B cells to respond.

T-Cell Suppression

The proper function of the immune system is efficient destruction of microbial pathogens with minimal injury to host tissues. Accordingly, T cells also attenuate the immune response to balance the potential risks of excessive tissue injury.

Although suppressor T cells are well described from in vivo and in vitro studies, there is no area of immunology more controversial than that regarding the existence, characterization, and specificity of these cells.[260] Suppressor T cells are thought to regulate the immune response by inhibiting the promoting effects of helper T cells on growth and differentiation of T and B cells. These effects were initially defined in bulk cell culture studies in vitro[260] or in adoptive transfer studies of experimental infections, including those due to mycobacteria, fungi, and protozoa.[261] However, it was not possible to produce clones or lines of antigen-induced suppressor T cells by the techniques used to develop helper and cytotoxic T-cell clones,[260] calling the existence of a distinct suppressor T-cell lineage into question.

Initial studies suggested that suppression is mediated by T8 cells, which are known to recognize antigen in the context of class I MHC antigens and to include most functionally cytotoxic T cells. Recent studies propose a complex network whereby a subset of soluble, antigen-responsive T4 cells induce a subset of T8 cells to inhibit the response of the CD4 helper T cells in an antigen-specific fashion; it is suggested that the specificity derives from recognition of the TCR on the helper T cell as antigen by the TCR of the T8 suppressor cells.[260,262] Further complexity may be provided by a network of contrasuppressor cells that block the suppressive effect of the T8 cells on the antigen-specific helper T cells.[263] The requirement for both T4 and T8 cells for suppression induction/mediation may explain the differences in requirements for these subsets to inhibit responses in different animal models of infection (e.g., suppression of resistance to *Leishmania* by T4 cells in BALB-c mice).[264] There is some evidence that antigen-induced enhancement of response occurs with optimum doses of antigen and that attenuation (suppression) occurs with much lower or higher doses of antigen.[260]

The molecular mechanism responsible for antigen-specific suppression is as yet uncharacterized. Direct cell-to-cell interaction is thought to be one mechanism of suppression.[260] Soluble antigen-specific suppressor factors have also been described,[265] but as yet none have been molecularly characterized or cloned convincingly. It is also unclear whether the mechanisms mediating antigen-specific suppression of helper T-cell function and of B-cell growth and differentiation are the same; certain evidence suggests that they are not.[257–260]

Non-antigen-specific suppression of T-cell and B-cell responses by soluble T-cell-derived products has also been described. One well-characterized factor is transforming growth factor-β.[266,267] Other factors that are not yet molecularly characterized are likely to function as attenuators of the immune response. One such factor is a product of T cells that is inactive until modified by oxygen metabolites apparently derived from macrophages.[268] This factor may play a role in attenuating responses in human infection and may be overproduced in AIDS[269]; it is suggested that its effects can be overcome by lymphokine growth factors.[270]

Suppressive Macrophage–Lymphocyte Interactions. The effect of macrophages on lymphocyte responses is dependent on the macrophage-to-lymphocyte ratio in vitro. Low ratios appear to enhance lymphocyte responses, whereas high ratios suppress them. Activated macrophages have an increased capacity to both enhance and suppress lymphocyte responses.[12] Inhibitory effects may be mediated in part by production of PGE_2[164,271] and by oxidative modification of the T-cell-derived suppressor factor.

Effector Cells and Cytokines Mediate the Antimicrobial Activity of the Cellular Immune System

The preceding discussion has focused on the role of CMI in the induction and regulation of host defenses. In addition, CMI plays a direct and often a primary role in controlling infection with pathogens, many of which survive and replicate within host cells. Immunity to these intracellular pathogens is mediated by effector cells, including antigen-specific cytotoxic T cells, NK cells and activated macrophages, and cytokines.

Cytotoxic T Cells

Most cytotoxic T cells express CD8 and recognize antigen in the context of class I MHC antigens found on nearly all cells of the body. As isolated from the blood or tissues, T8 cells are not capable of cytolysis. However, after antigen injection into experimental animals, T8 cells with cytolytic capacity can be isolated. Restimulation with antigen in vitro further enhances cytotoxicity; primary induction of cytotoxic T cells can also be affected in vitro by antigen stimulation. Under most conditions, T4 cells are required for differentiation of T8 cells into cytotoxic cells; this reflects the need for IL-2 for this process in vitro and in vivo[272–274] (Fig. 4). However, IL-2 alone is not sufficient.[272,273] Other factors that appear to play a role as indicated by studies in the human and the mouse, include IL-4,[275–277] produced by a subset of helper T cells,[171,172] IFN-γ,[130,272] and perhaps IL-6.[278] As noted for T-cell proliferation, the ability of these lymphokines to trigger differentiation of T8 cells into cytotoxic cells may be regulated in part by their expression of receptors for the respective lymphokines. As noted, expression of IL-2 receptors is tightly regulated by antigen-induced activation in a time-dependent fashion. However, receptors for IL-4, IFN-γ, and probably IL-6 appear to be constitutively expressed,[279] although they increase in number with activation. Thus, the effects of these cytokines may not be as tightly regulated, indicating the critical role of IL-2 and its receptor in the regulation of this differentiative process as well.

The biochemical processes accounting for the differentiated state of cytotoxic T cells and the mechanisms by which lymphokines mediate this process are only partly understood. Cytotoxic T cells differentiated in vitro have cytoplasmic granules that contain a protein termed *perforin*, which polymerizes to form pores in the membranes of target cells and organisms; these pores resemble those produced by terminal complement components.[280,281] These molecules have been best defined in murine cells but also appear to be present in human cytotoxic T cells.[281,282] Differentiated cytotoxic T cells also contain a family of serine esterases in their granules.[283] Development of cytotoxic function in mouse T cells in vitro correlates with the acquisition of granules containing pore-forming activity but not with serine esterase activity,[284] suggesting that the esterases may not have a direct cytotoxic role. Differentiated cytotoxic T cells may also secrete TNF-α, lymphotoxin (TNF-β), and molecules with activity related to but apparently distinct from those of TNF-α and TNF-β.[285] The precise role that each plays in the cytotoxic function of these cells is not clear. In addition, cytotoxic T cells raised entirely in vivo appear to lack the pore-forming protein but are cytotoxic nevertheless, indicating that other mechanisms are sufficient, if not solely responsible, for cytotoxic activity.[286] Data are not available to determine which properties of differentiated cytotoxic T cells are induced by specific lymphokines. Both IL-2 and IL-4 act, at least in part, by increasing the number of cytotoxic T cells generated in response to antigen stimulation.[285–287]

NK Cells

Natural killer (NK) cells constitute 10–15 percent of blood lymphocytes in adult humans. They are nonadherent, nonphagocytic cells and morphologically are large, granular lymphocytes. They express some surface antigens common to T cells, monocytes, and granulocytes; specifically, most express surface CD2 (the sheep erythrocyte receptor found on all T cells), OKM1, a marker found on monocytes, and CD16 (Leull), a receptor for IgG-Fc found only on NK cells and granulocytes.[287–289] CD16 can be used to define the NK cells in a mixed mononuclear cell population, as can a second antigen, NKH1.[287,288] Only a small portion of NK cells express CD3 and TCR[289–291]; some of these are CD3 cells expressing the unique γδ receptor.[48,52] Other evidence indicating that most NK cells are not T cells includes their lack of T-cell receptor gene rearrangement and messenger RNA expression,[289–291] the presence of normal or increased numbers of NK cells and NK cell precursors in mice that lack mature T and B cells,[290] and differential modulation of T cell and NK cell cytotoxicity.[292]

NK cells were originally defined by their ability to lyse target cells in a manner not restricted by HLA antigens and not requiring presensitization.[293] Recent data suggest that absent or abnormal cell surface HLA antigens, as occur on certain tumor cells and virus-infected cells, are associated with susceptibility to lysis by NK cells; cells expressing abundant, normal HLA antigens are not lysed.[294,295] The molecules that mediate binding of NK cells to targets have not been fully defined, although the leukocyte cell adhesion molecule (LCAM) family plays a role.[296] The CD2 molecule may also be important in NK cell binding and activation.[110]

Studies in experimental animals support a role for these cells in controlling resistance to tumors and viruses,[293] including cytomegalovirus[297] and herpes simplex virus,[298] in vivo. They may also play a role in resistance to other infectious agents, including *Toxoplasma*.[299] The cytolytic mechanisms of NK cells appear to be similar if not identical to those of cytotoxic T cells. IFN-α, -β, or -γ and IL-2 augment NK activity.[130,300–302]

In addition to their cytolytic function, NK cells produce certain lymphokines, as noted above; replicate in response to IL-2, augment cytolytic T-cell responses, inhibit T- and B-cell growth and differentiation, and inhibit hematopoietic cell growth and maturation.[292,303,304] However, their precise functions in vivo have not been fully defined.

NK cells also mediate, in part, antibody-dependent cell-mediated cytotoxicity (ADCC).[293] Cells to which IgG antibodies are bound are lysed. This process is more efficient than antibody-independent NK lysis, presumably because of the increased binding of effector cells to the target. Other cell types, including granulocytes and monocytes, may mediate antibody-dependent cytolysis. Human NK cytotoxicity is most commonly measured against a K562 erythroleukemia cell target. NK and ADCC have also been assessed using cells infected with herpes simplex virus or cytomegaloviruses. In these studies, the cells mediating the cytolytic activity against virus-infected targets appear to be NK cells.[298,305–307]

Monocytes and Activated Macrophages

Properties and Functions of Resting Macrophages as Effector Cells. Resting macrophages play an important role in clearing small numbers of microbes that gain access to tissues and in removing damaged or affected cells and extracellular tissue matrix. Accordingly, these cells contain surface receptors for IgG-Fc, for the derivatives of the third component of complement (C3), and for cell surface carbohydrates (e.g., mannose and frucose) and glycoproteins.[308] These receptors allow marcophages to internalize macromolecules and larger particles that exist in the extracellular environment by pinocytosis and phagocytosis. Pinocytosis consists of the incorporation of small amounts of extracellular material by invagination of a portion of cell membrane and the formation of a cytoplasmic vesicle 1–2 μm in size. Phagocytosis involves larger particles and is greatly enhanced when the particle to be phagocytosed is coated with antibody and/or complement, thereby allowing binding by Fc or C3b receptors on the macrophage surface. The process of phagocytosis involves binding of a particle to macrophage membrane receptors, circumferential enclosure of a particle by a portion of the cell membrane, internalization with formation of a phagosome, fusion of the phagosome with a lysosome, and subsequent digestion. Mechanisms by which macrophages inhibit or kill and degrade phagocytosed organisms include the actions of toxic oxygen metabolites and lysosomal enzymes (e.g., lysozyme). There is some evidence that deprivation of nutrients needed for growth of the organisms, but without which the host cell can survive, might also be involved in some cases.[4,309] Whether killing and/or degradation of phagocytosed organisms is effective depends at least in part on the characteristics of the organisms, the mononuclear phagocytes' innate functional capabilities, the receptor involved in attachment and uptake of the organism, whether the phagocytosing macrophage is activated, and the susceptibility of the particle to the host's microbicidal or digestive mechanisms. Because the macrophage's microbicidal mechanisms may also injure host tissues, it is important that tissue macrophages be limited in the potency of these toxic microbicidal mechanisms. Conversely, resting tissue macrophages are rich in components needed for tissue remodeling, including a wide variety of proteases.

Macrophage Activation and the Role of IFN-γ. At times of infectious challenge, the macrophage adapts. This process, whereby antimicrobial activity is increased at times of need, is known as *macrophage activation*. It was first described by Mackaness and colleagues in the 1960s[310] and has recently been reviewed by others[4,124,308,311]; it is a lymphokine-dependent process central to cellular immunity. The lymphokine dependence of this process was initially suggested by in vivo studies with experimental animals, which indicated that resistance to infection with intracellular pathogens, such as *Mycobacteria, Listeria*, and *Toxoplasma*, could be adoptively transferred by T lymphocytes and did not develop in T-cell-deficient nude mice. Macrophages were also required for resistance. Dissection of this process in vitro indicated that antigen-stimulated T cells secrete lymphokines that alter the macrophage so that it is primed to a state of enhanced microbicidal activity.[4,311,312] Subsequent exposure to microbes or to microbial products, particularly lipopolysaccharide, may either trigger microbial killing directly or provide a second stimulus that fully activates macrophages to lyse tumors or other targets such as virus-infected cells.

It is now apparent that the principal lymphokine that activates macrophages is IFN-γ[313–316] (reviewed in Ref. 4). Macrophages activated by IFN-γ have increased activity against a wide variety of microbes, as indicated in Table 1. The extent to which activated macrophages can kill or inhibit the growth of these organisms varies; for example, activated human macrophages are microbicidal for *Toxoplasma gondii* and *Leshmania donovani*, inhibit but do not kill *Chlamydia psittaci*, and have minimal activity against *Mycobacteria* in vitro. Two types of studies in experimental animals support a role for IFN-γ in resistance to intracellular pathogens. In the first type of study, IFN-γ, when given before or immediately after experimental infection, produced varying degrees of protection against *Listeria*,[317] *T. gondii*,[318] *Mycobacterium intracellulare* or *M. tuberculosis*,[319,320] *L. donovani*,[321] *Salmonella typhimurium*,[322] and *Franciscella tularesis*.[323] In the second type of study, animals treated with antibodies that neutralize IFN-γ had more severe infection with *Listeria*,[324] *L. donovani*,[325] *T. gondii*,[326] and *Rickettsia conarii*.[327] It should be noted that treatment with IFN-γ did not usually protect completely, nor did anti-IFN-γ antibody completely ablate resistance, suggesting IFN-γ-independent mechanisms of resistance. It is also likely that effects of IFN-γ other than macrophage activation, including enhancement of antigen presentation, T-cell help, and cytotoxic T-cell activity, and effects on the survival of pathogens in cells other than macrophages, play an important role.

Although IFN-γ appears to be the lymphokine that induces the broadest range of macrophage antimicrobial activity, other lymphokines activate macrophage activity against a more restricted range of pathogens. TNF enhances macrophage activity against *Trypanosoma cruzi*[328] and *M. avium-intracellulare*,[329] and GM-CSF enhances macrophage activity against *T. cruzi*[330] and *Leshmania tropica* or *L. donovani*[331,332] In contrast, to date only IFN-γ has been shown to activate macrophage anti-*Toxoplasma* activity.[316]

Characteristics of Activated Macrophages. The properties and functions of mononuclear phagocytes and the effects of macrophage activation on them are shown in Table 4.[308] It is evident that activation is associated with a wide variety of changes that enhance the capacity of these cells to migrate to sites of infection, phagocytose particles coated with IgG or C3 more efficiently, and release increased amounts of potentially microbicidal oxygen metabolites, proteases, and cytokines. The role of enhanced release of oxygen metabolites in the microbicidal activity of activated macrophages has been well characterized (reviewed in Ref. 4). Oxygen-independent mechanisms have been less well characterized but include the degradation of tryptophan, which contributes to activity against *T. gondii* and *C. psittaci* in human cells,[309,333,334] limiting iron availability, which contributes to activity against *Legionella*[335] and arginine catabolism,[336] which contributes to anticryptococcal activity. It is likely that the tissue source, state of activation, and varying susceptibility of given pathogens to different antimicrobial mechanisms determine the relative importance of individual mechanisms in a particular circumstance.

ROLE OF CMI IN DEFENSE AGAINST SPECIFIC TYPES OF INFECTIOUS PATHOGENS

In general, cellular immunity is important in resistance to those infectious pathogens that replicate intracellularly, either in an obligate or a facultative manner. Mechanisms of resistance to intracellular viral pathogens differ somewhat from those to nonviral intracellular pathogens. Accordingly, these will be discussed separately, as will the role of cellular immunity in resistance to certain extracellular pathogens. This section uses representative examples of pathogens in each class to illustrate general concepts. Important differences will be noted, but it should be recognized that this overview is by nature simplistic, and more details are provided in the chapters discussing specific pathogens. Potential approaches for future trials of immunologic intervention are discussed.

TABLE 4. Major Functions of Mononuclear Phagocytes and Their Modification by the Process of Activation[a]

Microbicidal activity (↑)
Tumoricidal activity (↑)
Chemotaxis (↑)
Phagocytosis (varies with particle)
Pinocytosis (↑)
Glucose transport and metabolism (↑)
Microbicidal oxygen-metabolite production (↑)
Antigen presentation (↑)
Secretion
Lysozyme (NC)
Prostaglandins, leukotrienes (↓)
Apolipoprotein E and lipoprotein lipase (↓)
Elastase (↓)
Complement components (↑ or NC)
Acid hydrolases (↑)
Collagenase (↑)
Plasminogen activator (↑)
Cytolytic proteinase (↑)
Arginase (↑)
Fibronectin (↑)
Interleukin-1 (↑ when stimulated)
Tumor necrosis factor-cachectin (↑ when stimulated)
Interferon-α and -β (↑)
Angiogenesis factor (↑)
Colony stimulating factors (↑ when stimulated)

[a] ↑ Indicates that the activity or constituent is increased in activated macrophages, ↓ indicates that it is decreased, and NC indicates no change. This list is based primarily on studies with macrophages from animals and humans infected with intracellular parasites; in some cases, the findings have been confirmed by the addition of IFN-γ in vitro.
(Adapted from Johnston,[308] with permission.)

Nonviral Pathogens—Intracellular

In addition to viruses, certain organisms, facultative and obligate intracellular pathogens, respectively, are capable of or are restricted to replication within cells. Of those noted in Table 1, the intracellular protozoa, *Chlamydia* and *Rickettsia*, are obligate intracellular pathogens, and the remaining organisms are facultative intracellular pathogens. Unlike pyogenic bacteria, for which phagocytosis usually represents death, phagocytosis may represent entry into a comfortable home for these organisms.

Overview of Defense Mechanisms. Animal studies indicate that control of infection with these nonviral organisms is mediated primarily by T lymphocytes, monocytes, and macrophages. The critical role of macrophages has been established in animal studies in which depletion of macrophages increased susceptibility to *Listeria*.[1] The critical role of T lymphocytes is indicated by the marked susceptibility of athymic animals[1] and by passive transfer of resistance with T lymphocytes.[337] Similarly, the important role of T lymphocytes in protecting humans from *Toxoplasma* is suggested by the marked increase in the incidence of severe infection in patients with AIDS,[338] who have a deficiency in helper T4 cells.

In the first days of infection, the rate at which monocytes are recruited to the site of infection and the microbicidal activity of these cells appear to be important in controlling *Listeria* and *Toxoplasma* infection in animals. These findings correlate with the greater microbicidal activity of human monocytes compared with macrophages against *Toxoplasma* and *Listeria*.

Subsequently, resolution of active infection and development of protective immunity in animals depend on appropriate interaction between macrophages and T lymphocytes. On the basis of studies initially performed in animal cells but since reproduced with human cells in vitro, it is thought that this interaction, which is both antigen and host specific, leads to the production of macrophage- and T-cell-derived cytokines. After ingestion and killing by local macrophages, organisms are degraded by these cells. Microbial antigens are then displayed on the macrophage surface in association with class II (HLA-DR) major histocompatibility epitopes. Macrophages stimulated by phagocytosis or by microbial products release IL-1. In the presence of IL-1 and microbial antigen displayed on class II MHC-bearing macrophages, antigen-specific T4 cells are recruited to the site of infection, where they secrete IL-2. Interleukin-2 binds to IL-2 receptors on these and other antigen-activated T lymphocytes, both of the T4 and T8 phenotypes, and stimulates these cells to divide, to release more IL-2, and to release factors that recruit and focus monocytes and macrophages to the site of infection, and enhance monocyte and macrophage microbicidal activity. Interferon-γ appears to be the most important factor mediating these effects on macrophages. In mice, resistance correlates directly with the amount of IFN-γ produced during infection, IFN-γ is protective, and antibody to IFN-γ markedly impairs resistance to *Listeria, Leishmania*, and *Toxoplasma*.[324–326] In addition, depletion of T4 cells in mice causes reactivation of central nervous system toxoplasmosis, illustrating the central role of these cells, as suggested by the frequency and severity of this infection in patients with AIDS.[339]

In contrast to the production by T cells of chemotactic factors and IFN-γ, which are host cell and pathogen specific, monocyte recruitment and macrophage activation are nonspecific.[1] Once recruited to the site of infection and activated, macrophages have increased activity against a wide range of microbes. The basis for the enhanced activity of activated macrophages appears to be multifactorial; both increased generation of microbicidal oxygen metabolites and oxygen-independent mechanisms appear to contribute (reviewed in Ref. 308).

Roles of Cytokines and Mononuclear Phagocytes. Recent studies in patients with leprosy appear to illustrate the importance of these processes. Leprosy is a disease in which the clinical features vary between two polar forms. Patients with the tuberculoid form have a strong cellular immune response, few lesions, and very small numbers of *Mycobacterium leprae*, whereas patients with the lepromatous form have a selective absence of cellular immunity and a high body burden of *M. leprae*.[340] Antibody offers no apparent protection, since patients with lepromatous disease have higher titers than those with tuberculoid disease. Because the disease has major cutaneous manifestations, it has been possible to assess the cellular immune response in vivo as well as in vitro.[341–343] In vitro T cells from tuberculoid but not lepromatous patients fail to produce IL-2 or IFN-γ in response to *M. leprae* antigen, whereas T cells from patients with both types produce these lymphokines in response to other antigens and mitogens.[344,345] In contrast to lesions from tuberculoid patients, biopsied lesions from lepromatous patients have many *M. leprae*. In addition, compared to tuberculoid lesions, in lepromatous lesions the expression of class II MHC antigen on overlying keratinocytes and the number of class II MHC-bearing macrophages and T cells is low. Fewer of the T cells are of the T4 phenotype, and of these, most do not express the 4B4+ phenotype, characteristic of memory T cells with the helper-inducer phenotype, but rather express the CD45R+ phenotype, characteristic of suppressor-inducer cells. Accordingly, fewer T cells in lepromatous lesions are producing IL-2. Addition of IL-2 to T cells from lepromatous patients in vitro allows these cells to proliferate and secrete IFN-γ in response to *M. leprae* antigen.[345] Injection of IFN-γ but not placebo into lepromatous lesions leads to an enhanced mononuclear infiltrate, increased expression of class II MHC on keratinocytes, and a variable decrease in the number of *M. leprae*.

In addition to IFN-γ and IL-2, other cytokines and blood monocytes are likely to be important in the control of nonviral intracellular pathogens. This is suggested by the inability of IFN-γ alone to induce macrophages from mice to be fully activated to kill *Listeria monocytogenes* or *S. typhimurium*, even though these cells are active against *T. gondii*.[346,347] These results are compatible with other data indicating the importance of macrophages derived from newly recruited monocytes rather than from resident macrophages in resistance to *Listeria*.[1] Monocytes have greater antimicrobial activity than resting tissue macrophages against many intracellular pathogens, including *Toxoplasma*[348] and *Leishmania*.[349] Recent data suggest that the CSFs, produced early in the response of mice that resist *Listeria* but later in more susceptible mice, may be important in stimulating the production of monocytes and enhancing their activity[350,351]; production of these CSFs was dependent on T4 cells. As noted in the section on activated macrophages, GM-CSF and TNF-α may contribute to resistance against certain organisms by enhancing macrophage function; in contrast, M-CSF does not appear to enhance activity against *L. tropica* or *T. gondii*.[352]

It is unclear in most cases why certain lymphokines enhance macrophage activity against one pathogen but not another. This may relate in part to differences in the still incompletely characterized effects of specific lymphokines on molecular events associated with macrophage activity. In addition, the nonviral obligate and facultative intracellular pathogens appear to use a wide variety of strategies to survive within the cell.[353,354] For example, *T. gondii* evades killing by several mechanisms: it is relatively resistant to reactive oxygen metabolites,[355] and it does not effectively trigger production of reactive oxygen metabolites (respiratory burst) or phagolysosome fusion in resting macrophages.[348,356] *Leishmania donovani* promastigotes, but not the intracellular amastigotes, are easily killed by oxygen metabolites[4]; promastigotes, but not amastigotes, trigger a respiratory burst in resting macrophages. Both forms are resistant to killing by lysosomes that fuse with phagosomes in which they reside. *Trypanosoma cruzi* evades oxygen metabolites and lysosomal enzymes by escaping from the phagocytic vacuole to reside within the cytoplasm. Other intracellular pathogens, including *Listeria, Legionella, Mycobacteria*, fungi, *Rickettsia*, and *Chlamydia*, use one or more of these strategies to survive within macrophages and other cells. In addition, each pathogen appears to have particular metabolic requirements that are supplied by the host cell and that, in most cases, are still uncharacterized. These differences among pathogens in the mechanisms for establishing intracellular parasitism are likely to provide different targets for attack and thereby dictate which mechanisms must be affected by a lymphokine(s) for it to activate macrophages to kill that organism.

The broad range of pathogens susceptible to IFN-γ-activated macrophages are indicated by an asterisk in Table 1. This broad activity of IFN-γ may relate in part to its much greater capacity, compared to that of other lymphokines, to increase the macrophage production of reactive oxygen metabolites and to uniquely enhance an apparent variety of oxygen-independent mechanisms.[4] Interferon-γ induces expression of a multitude of new proteins in murine and human macrophages[357] and other cell types, some of which are unique and some of which are induced by other lymphokines, including TNF. Further study of these proteins should help elucidate the molecular basis of IFN-γ-induced macrophage activation.

Role of Other Cell Types in Resistance. Activated macrophages may not be sufficient to control infection completely. This may occur either because the pathogen is capable of invading host cells other than macrophages and granulocytes or because activated macrophages are not sufficiently microbicidal. Infection of cells other than macrophages and granulocytes is the rule for infection with *Toxoplasma, Chlamydia*, and *Rickettsia* but may also occur to a limited extent in infections with other nonviral intracellular pathogens. An example is infection of Schwann cells in tuberculoid leprosy.

One mechanism by which infection is controlled in nonmacrophage cells may be the induction of microbistatic or microbicidal activity in fibroblasts and in endothelial, epithelial, and parenchymal cells by IFN-γ (reviewed in Ref. 4). This has been demonstrated for *Toxoplasma, Chlamydia*, and *Rickettsia*.

An alternative control mechanism may be the lysis of infected cells or extracellular organisms by T cells and NK cells. Kaufmann has demonstrated that murine macrophages infected with *L. monocytogenes, M. tuberculosis*, and *M. leprae* are recognized by specific T-cell clones both of the T4 and T8 phenotypes and that both can lyse infected macrophages in an antigen- and MHC-restricted manner.[353] *Nocardia asteroides* also appears to be sensitive to killing by cytotoxic T cells.[358] NK cells may play a role in resistance to *Cryptococcus neoformans, Leishmania, Plasmodium berghei*, and *T. cruzi* in experimental animals (reviewed in Ref. 359). They may act to lyse extracellular organisms directly, such as *T. cruzi* and *T. gondii*[299,359] or to lyse infected cells, particularly in the presence of antibody. This process may be beneficial to the host if liberated organisms are then killed by another mechanism; however, cytotoxic T-cell activity could lead to pathologic tissue damage. The potential role of NK cells is not well established.

The Role of Antibody. Lymphokine-dependent cellular immunity appears to be the sole mechanism for resistance of animals to *Listeria* and *M. tuberculosis*. Antibody appears to play no role.[310] Based on studies with animals and with human cells in vitro, antibody may play a limited role in protection against other intracellular bacterial pathogens, including *Salmonella* and *Legionella*,[360–362] although this is an area of controversy.

Antibody does contribute to protection against protozoa, including *Toxoplasma*, in experimental animals. Mice that cannot mount an antibody response are slightly more susceptible to late death from *Toxoplasma* than are normal mice. Antibody and complement lyse extracellular *Toxoplasma*, and antibody-coated *Toxoplasma* organisms are killed by resting mouse and human macrophages.[363] Antibody alone provides minimal protection in adult and newborn mice, but antibody enhances protection by activated macrophages.[364] T-lymphocyte-deficient mice are much more susceptible than are antibody-deficient animals and are not protected by antibody.

Leishmania donovani promastigotes are lysed by naturally occurring antibody and complement, but the intracellular amastigote forms are resistant.[349] However, antibody may contribute to protection against amastigotes by inhibiting uptake of amastigotes into resting macrophages in which they replicate.[365] Antibodies also inhibit motility and nucleic acid synthesis by *T. cruzi*.

Nonviral Pathogens—Extracellular Helminths and Bacteria

CMI appears to play an important role in resistance to certain extracellular protozoa and helminths (Table 1).

Of the protozoa, the mechanisms of immunity to *Plasmodia* are the best characterized. Sterile immunity to the sporozoite form (the form passed from the mosquito to the host) of the rodent parasites *P. berghei* and *P. yoelii* requires antibody and T8 but not T4 cells[366–368]; antibody alone or T cells alone may be sufficient to prevent infection with a very small inoculum. T8 cells may act in part by cytotoxic mechanisms and in part by lymphokine production. Interferon-γ appears to play an important role in this process, since antibody to IFN-γ blocks protection in immunized mice and in mice passively protected by antibody and immune T cells.[368] Interferon-γ acts in part by causing destruction of exo-erythrocytic forms within hepatic parenchymal cells. Interferon-γ also activates human and murine macrophages to kill erythrocytic forms of *Plasmodia*.[369] TNF-α has antiplasmodial activity and is detectable in the serum of infected humans.[370] However, data in mice infected with *P. berghei* suggest that overproduction of TNF-α may be an important cause of fatal cerebral malaria by causing cerebrovascular accumulation of macrophages containing phagocytosed, parasitized erythrocytes.[371] Anti-TNF-α antibody protects against cerebral malaria without increasing parasitemia. This illustrates the delicate balance needed in the CMI response to provide protection without excessive tissue injury.

CMI appears to be important in conferring protection but may also contribute to tissue damage in response to helminths. In patients with more intense infections with *Schistosoma mansoni*, killing of schistosomula by monocytes and lymphocytes and the response to schistosome antigens are depressed compared to those with less intense infection[372]; however, it is not known whether this is a cause or an effect of more severe infection. Interferon-γ-activated macrophages have antischistosomal activity,[4] and TNF, released in greater amounts by activated macrophages, enhances eosinophil killing of *S. mansoni* larvae in vitro.[373] In addition to CMI, eosinophils, neutrophils, and IgE antibodies contribute to resistance to schistosomes.[372] Since IgE and eosinophil production is controlled by the T4-cell-derived lymphokines IL-4 and -5, respectively (see above), it is likely that these cells play an important role in resistance to schistosomiasis, as they do in mice infected with *Nippostrongylus brasiliensis* and *Trichinella spiralis*[374]; in these infections, IgE, eosinophils, and immune lymphocytes cause worm expulsion from the intestine of infected rodents.[374–378] An important component of the immune response to schistosomiasis is downmodulation of hepatic CMI. This attenuates the granulomatous response to schistosome larvae that develops in the liver, which may lead to cirrhosis. In mice, attenuation of the granulomatous response appears to correlate with decreased IFN-γ and IL-2 production by T cells. This is mediated by antigen- and MHC-specific T8 (suppressor) cells in *S. mansoni* infection, and by this mechanism and antibody-induced suppression in *S. japonicum* infection.[375]

Recent studies indicate that T cells may also participate directly in defenses against certain pyogenic bacteria. For example, T cells regulate the development of abscesses induced by *Bacteroides fragilis* in mice[379,380]; similar to the studies with schistosome-induced hepatic granulomas, T cells act both to induce abscess formation in naive mice and to inhibit abscess formation in immune mice. In addition, in a murine model, specific immune T8 cells protect against intraperitoneal infection with *Pseudomonas aeruginosa*.[381] Immune T cells alone are protective in the absence of antibody and in granulocytopenic mice.[381–383] The T cells appear to act by secreting a still uncharacterized lymphokine with bactericidal activity. Induction of the lymphokine is antigen specific, but it is protective against a variety of bacteria. In other murine models, lymphokines, including IL-1[384] and IL-2,[385] increase resistance to pyogenic bacterial infections. However, the mechanism by which resistance is increased is unknown.

Viruses

The immune response to certain viral infections, particularly those in which viral transmission occurs by cell-to-cell contact rather than by release of virus into the extracellular environment, appears to be cell mediated. For a particular virus, an individual function or combination of functions of sensitized T lymphocytes may be important; these functions may include (*1*) mobilization and activation of macrophages, (*2*) direct cytotoxicity against virus-infected cells, and (*3*) release of interferon (Table 5). Because they are the most common severe viral infections in patients with cellular immune dysfunction, including neonates and the aged, transplant recipients and individuals with AIDS, infections with the herpes viruses provide

TABLE 5. Mechanisms of Host Defense Against Viruses

	Mechanism	Target: Extracellular Virus	Target: Infected Cells
Humoral			
Antibody	Neutralize	+	−
	ADCC	−	+
Interferon	Inhibit viral replication	−	+
Cellular			
Monocytes/macrophages	Ingest and clear virus	+	−
	Inhibit viral replication	−	+
	Lyse infected cells ADCC NK cytotoxicity	−	+
Lymphocytes			
NK cells	Lyse infected cells ADCC NKC	−	+
T lymphocytes	Specific cell-mediated cytotoxicity	−	+

Abbreviations: ADCC: antibody-dependent cell-mediated cytotoxicity; NK: natural killer cell.

models for the role of CMI in viral defenses and have recently been reviewed.[386]

Antibody can neutralize extracellular virus or sensitize virus-infected cells to lysis by complement (IgG and IgM) or by effector cels (IgG only).[387] In animal models, T cells appear to be important in herpes simplex virus (HSV) and cytomegalovirus (CMV) infection because depletion of complement does not alter the protective effect of antibody,[388] whereas depletion of T cells by irradiation or by antithymocyte serum does.[389]

Intracellular viral replication may be prevented by noncytotoxic mechanisms and by mechanisms that lyse infected cells. The best-characterized noncytotoxic mechanism is interferon-mediated inhibition of viral replication. Interferon is produced by macrophages, fibroblasts, and nonimmune lymphocytes in response to viral challenge (IFN-α and -β) and by specifically sensitized lymphocytes in response to antigen (IFN-γ)[390]. IFN-β and -γ are highly species specific, whereas IFN-α has some activity in cells from other species.

Ingestion of HSV by human monocytes (and perhaps polymorphonuclear leukocytes, PMNs) is associated with abortive infection, thus effectively clearing extracellular virus.[391] Unlike the monocytes from which they are derived, macrophages may support viral replication. Mouse macrophages can inhibit viral replication within other cells by a noninterferon, noncytotoxic mechanism[392]; human cells have not been studied. Mouse and human lymphocytes and monocytes (and perhaps PMNs) can lyse HSV- and CMV-infected cells in the presence of specific antibody by ADCC.[387] Although less efficient, cell-mediated lysis of virus-infected cells also occurs in the absence of specific antibody by NK cytotoxicity,[393,394] thought to be important in controlling early infection in mice before specific immunity develops.[387] NK cells are the major effector cell of ADCC and NK cytotoxicity in mice and humans; macrophages may also mediate cytotoxicity. Cells from nonimmune humans are as effective[394] or almost as effective in ADCC and NK cytotoxicity as cells from immune individuals.[393] Both ADCC and NK cytotoxicity are augmented by interferon.

Nude mice, which lack T lymphocytes, are more resistant than controls to early overwhelming infection; this is thought to result from high NK cytotoxicity. However, nude mice commonly die late in the infectious process, when specific T-cell-mediated cellular cytotoxicity, which they lack, normally develops.[387]

The relative roles of these processes in protection are not established in humans. Neither humans with isolated T lymphocyte deficiency (DiGeorge syndrome) nor those with isolated immunoglobulin or complement deficiency develop disseminated primary HSV infection.[387] In contrast, primary infection is severe in patients with combined immunodeficiency.[387,395]

In adults, Merigan and coworkers[396] have shown that increased HSV-specific induction of IFN-γ in vivo and in vitro correlates with a longer interval to recurrence of HSV infection; the IFN-γ appeared to be produced primarily by T4 cells. In contrast, IFN-α production did not correlate with time to next recurrence. Human neonates develop severe and often fatal HSV infection, whereas in adults primary HSV infection is much less severe. We have recently found that neonates with HSV infection compared to adults with primary HSV infection have markedly delayed and diminished production of IFN-γ in response to HSV.[397] They also produce less TNF in response to HSV. TNF and IFN-γ-synergistically inhibit HSV replication and lyse HSV-infected cells in vitro.[398] At the time of primary infection nearly all neonates have detectable HSV antibody, whereas antibody is absent in the adults with primary infection.[397] These data suggest a more important role for T-cell-dependent lymphokine production than for antibody in resistance to primary and recurrent HSV infection. The importance of cellular and humoral immunity is also suggested by studies in mice.[399,400]

Overall, based on animal and human data, the following may be hypothesized for HSV infection. High-titer antibody may prevent infection with a low inoculum. With a higher inoculum or in the absence of antibody, infection develops. NK cytotoxicity (and if passively derived antibody is present, as in some neonates, ADCC) may limit the initial spread of infection. Eradication of acute infection and establishment and maintenance of latency may depend on or at least be markedly facilitated by specific cytotoxic T lymphocytes and T-cell-dependent lymphokine production. Further basic and clinical studies are needed to determine the validity of these hypotheses.

Similar mechanisms appear operative in CMV infection.[401,402] Specific HLA-restricted, cytotoxic T lymphocytes have been more strongly implicated in the control of severe CMV[401] than HSV infection, and antibody appears to have a limited role in resistance to CMV infection.[401] Resistance to Epstein-Barr virus (EBV) also appears to be mediated principally by CMI. T8 cells act to restrict EBV-induced polyclonal B cell proliferation.[386] Attenuation of T-cell defenses by cyclosporine in transplant patients is associated with EBV-induced polyclonal B-cell proliferation, which is reversible on discontinuation of the drug. An X-linked defect, apparently in the CMI response to EBV infection, is seen in the X-linked lymphoproliferative syndrome.[403] The precise mechanisms that are aberrant in this syndrome are not known; it appears that some patients have an excessive CMI response associated with fatal infectious mononucleosis or hypogammaglobulinemia and that others have an inadequate CMI response associated with B-cell lymphoma. Impaired production of immune interferon has been proposed as a mechanism in one patient with this syndrome and B-cell lymphoma.[404] Impaired T-cell control of EBV replication may also contribute to EBV-associated complications in AIDS.[405]

In addition to the herpes group viruses, CMI has been shown to play an important role in influenza virus infection. Development of virus-specific, HLA-restricted, cytotoxic T cells appears to be important for resistance.[406,407] Specific antigenic epitopes of influenza recognized by cytotoxic T cells have been extensively studied as models,[408] and results indicate that both internal viral antigens, such as nucleoproteins, as well as surface antigens are recognized.[95,96]

Defense mechanisms acting against HIV infection are reviewed in Chapter 107. They include T8 cells that suppress HIV replication in T4 cells[409] or lyse infected T4 cells[99,410] and perhaps contribute to helper T-cell depletion. Recent studies indicate that IFN-γ, production of which is impaired in those with progressive AIDS, inhibits HIV replication.[411] With IFN-γ, TNF synergistically inhibits HIV replication in T cells.[411] GM-CSF synergistically inhibits HIV infection in the monocytic cell line U937 but increases HIV infection in U1, which is derived from U937.[412]

Cell-mediated cytotoxicity may contribute to tissue damage when directed against critical host cells, as in AIDS. This is an established mechanism for tissue injury in lymphocytic choriomeningitis infection[413] and may play a role in rabies.[414]

PROSPECTS FOR IMMUNOLOGIC INTERVENTION

Cytokines, including purified IL-2 and IFN-γ, TNF, and CSFs, are now available in large quantities through recombinant DNA methods, and clinical trials have been initiated.

Interferon-γ

Interferon-γ has been used in treatment trials of patients with cancer, leprosy, chronic granulomatous disease, and AIDS (reviewed in Ref. 4). In patients with cancer or leprosy who received doses ranging from 10 to 1000 units/M^2, circulating monocytes produced increased amounts of potentially microbicidal oxygen metabolites when stimulated[415–417] and had increased activity against allogeneic tumor cells in vitro.[418] Variable decreases in the number of *M. leprae* organisms were seen in patients receiving intralesional IFN-γ.[340] Blood monocytes from patients with AIDS receiving intermittent IFN-γ intravenously had increased activity against *T. gondii* and *L. donovani*[419] and enhanced NK-cell[420] and T-cell function.[421,422]

However, patients with AIDS have not been fully protected from opportunistic infections by IFN-γ, since cryptococcal meningitis and *Pneumocystis* pneumonia have developed in the first week of therapy[419,421] or during low-dose therapy,[421] and IFN-γ did not affect established CMV infection.[419] The failure of IFN-γ to protect may be due in part to the short interval between initiation of treatment and infection, failure to focus delivery at the site of infection, or lack of activity of IFN-γ or IFN-γ-activated effector cells against *Pneumocystis* and CMV.[4]

The effects of IFN-γ on immune functions does not correlate clearly with the dosage or the dosage interval.[4] This is particularly true in patients with chronic granulomatous disease (CGD). Although these patients suffer from frequent pyogenic infections, infections with intracellular pathogens, such as *Mycobacteria* and *Nocardia*, may also be problematic. Administration of IFN-γ often results in increased microbicidal activity of phagocytes from CGD patients that lasts for 2 or more weeks suggesting actions in addition to direct effects on mature macrophages.[423,423a,423b]

Toxicity of IFN-γ includes fever, fatigue, myalgias, and headaches at dosages greater than 10 $\mu g/m^2$ and appears to be dose limiting at dosages of 500 $\mu g/m^2$ or greater. Granulocytopenia also develops, as do other transient laboratory abnormalities.

Interleukin-2

Because it enhances T-cell growth and cytotoxic T-cell function, IL-2 is an attractive candidate for immune intervention. Administration of IL-2 to experimental animals has increased resistance to viral, bacterial, and protozoan pathogens. However, therapeutic trials in humans, including AIDS patients, have not yet shown convincing evidence of efficacy. Some increase in the number of lymphocytes in lymph nodes proximal to the site of administration was seen in a child with immunodeficiency, possibly due to Nezeloff syndrome or to AIDS, who had received a bone marrow transplant that did not engraft; the child died of overwhelming infections 5 days after IL-2 therapy was initiated.[424] In the same series, another patient with AIDS had improvement in CMV retinitis while receiving IL-2 but *Salmonella* sepsis subsequently developed. Although no toxicity was seen in this study, which used relatively low dosages of purified IL-2, toxicity has been a significant problem in cancer patients receiving high dosages in conjunction with LAK cells (up to 100,000 units/kg every 8 hours). Severe fluid retention associated with capillary leakage appears to be dose limiting; fever and neuropsychiatric effects have also been problems.[425,426] However, if LAK cells are omitted, toxicity of IL-2 appears to be greatly reduced (C. Henney, personal communication.

More promising is the potential use of the IL-2 gene in recombinant vaccines.[427,428] This strategy involves the incorporation of the IL-2 gene in a vaccinia virus recombinant. Such vaccines result in the localized production of IL-2 only at sites of viral replication; local control of viral replication then stops IL-2 production, thereby focusing its effects both locally and temporally. In T-cell-deficient nude mice given vaccinia virus progressive disease resulted. However, in these mice the infection completely resolved with vaccinia virus recombinants containing the IL-2 gene. In one study, influenza virus hemagglutinin or nucleoprotein genes were included in the recombinant vaccinia virus vectors[427]; in studies also containing the IL-2 gene, antibody production was increased under conditions in which the response to vaccines without the IL-2 gene was often suboptimal. The precise mechanisms by which IL-2 acted are not yet known. However, these results suggest potential sechanisms by which lymphokine therapy can be directed to enhance a specific desired response and limit its undesirable systemic effects.

Colony-Stimulating Factors

The CSFs have been used in clinical trials in patients with AIDS, cancer, and bone marrow transplants. Experience with GM-CSF suggests that it is well tolerated at dosages that increase circulating monocyte and neutrophil counts.[429,430] Whether delivery of monocytes to sites of infection increases resistance to infection with intracellular pathogens remains to be determined. Interleukin-1-α acts early in the hematopoietic pathway to increase production. This may account for its radioprotective effect in experimental animals[217] and may suggest a potential role in limiting the duration and severity of myelosuppression in individuals receiving radiotherapy. However, there is concern about the potential for causing recrudescence of hematologic malignancies by the use of exogenous CSFs to limit therapy-induced cytopenias. Accordingly, trials in patients treated for solid tumors are receiving greater initial attention.

Other Cytokines

TNF-α has been used initially in trials for the treatment of cancer. Toxicity has been problematic and the response minimal. Because of its synergistic activity with IFN-γ, an initial trial of these agents is being undertaken in AIDS patients. Low doses of TNF-α have reduced infection in mice with experimental malaria.[431]

Future studies will need to determine the optimal means for giving cytokines. It may be possible to partially target delivery to sites of infection by administering them in an appropriate vehicle, as in vaccinia virus—IL-2 recombinants. Another example may be the use of lymphokines targeted to the reticuloendothelial system or to the lung. Further, antimicrobial chemotherapy is currently used for many intracellular infections with varying degrees of success. Synergistic effects have been observed in vitro with IFN-γ and antimicrobials.[4] It will be important to determine the potential for synergistic or antagonistic interaction between immunologic and antimicrobial therapy in vivo. It is also likely that combined use of IFN-γ and other cytokines, such as IL-2 or CSFs, may be advantageous.

Noncytokine Immunopotentiators

Use of other nonspecific immunoenhancers has been attempted, but to date success has been limited and has often been overshadowed by toxicity. *Corynebacterium parvum* (killed) and Calmette-Guerin bacillus (BCG) (live or various extracts) are immunologic adjuvants and appear to stimulate both the afferent and efferent limbs of CMI. Although *C. parvum* has been used extensively for immunotherapy in cancer patients, its use for infections in humans has been limited. In one study it had no effect on the chronic carriage of hepatitis B surface antigen. Similarly, transfer factor, an uncharacterized crude extract of peripheral blood leukocytes, was suggested to be useful in certain patients with congenital immunodeficiency,[432] in the treatment of varicella zoster in children with cancer,[433] and in certain other infections with intracellular infections. However, its use has never been properly studied in multicenter controlled trials and in the absence of molecular characterization it is primarily of historical interest. Similarly, studies to date with levamisole and other chemical immune potentiators and with thymic hormones have been limited and have not provided clear evidence of benefit.

Immunoattenuation

In certain disease states, an excessive immune response results in tissue damage and attenuation rather than enhancement is desirable. An example is septic shock (see Chapter 59). Cytokines, particularly TNF-α, appear to be major mediators. In experimental animals, either early administration of corticosteroids, which blocks production of TNF, IL-1, and other cytokines, or specific antibody to TNF-α prevents the development of fatal septic shock. Unfortunately, delay in administration of these treatments until after the disease is established is less successful and may account for the failure of corticosteroids to clearly benefit humans. Whether agents with specific activities, like antibodies to cytokines, or a combination of agents would be more effective must be determined in clinical trials. The use of reagents more specific than corticosteroids offers the potential for relatively selective inhibition of undesirable responses with retention of those critical to resistance. Examples include immunotoxins in which lymphokines or specific monoclonal antibodies may be fused to a toxin. By so doing, the toxin can be targeted to cells expressing specific lymphokine receptors or surface molecules recognized by the antibodies.

Immunoattenuating therapy may be more beneficial in patients with less rapidly progressive diseases. For example, corticosteroids appear to be beneficial in decreasing the severity of lung dysfunction in AIDS patients with *Pneumocystis* pneumonia[434] or lymphoid interstitial pneumonitis.[435]

DEFECTS IN THE FUNCTION OF CMI

The thorough review of this topic by McLeod et al.[311] in the previous edition of this book has been updated and material on the physiologic "immunodeficiency" of infancy and the aged has been added.

Physiologically Diminished CMI in Infants and the Aged

The human fetus and the neonate are unduly susceptible to severe infection with multiple pathogens, including those against which CMI is the major mechanism of host defense. These include *Toxoplasma, Listeria, Treponema pallidum*, and the herpes group viruses. The rate of disease progression in neonates with HIV infection is also more rapid than in older individuals, with a median survival time for infants with AIDS of 6.5 months.[436]

Deficiencies in the cytokine-dependent interaction between T lymphocytes and macrophages have been demonstrated with human neonatal cells in vitro (reviewed in Ref. 437). Interleukin-1 production by monocytes from most newborn infants is normal,[140] and although the density of HLA-DR on neonatal monocytes is somewhat less than on adult monocytes, they support a normal proliferative response of T lymphocytes to microbial antigens. The proliferative response of neonatal T cells to nonspecific mitogens and of T cells from most infants with congenital *Toxoplasma* infections to *Toxoplasma* antigen is normal. However, the response to *Toxoplasma* antigen is less consistent in infants younger than 2 months, and in infants with other congenital or neonatal infections, the proliferative response to specific antigens is often absent or diminished. In contrast, production of the major macrophage activation factor, IFN-γ, by T cells from neonates at birth and in the first weeks of life is markedly decreased.[438] This immaturity of lymphokine production is relatively selective, since production of other T-cell- and macrophage-derived cytokines is similar or only slightly less than by adult cells, with the exception of IL-4.[439]

Human neonatal monocytes migrate somewhat less well than adult monocytes; both efficiently ingest and kill *Toxoplasma*.[356] Macrophages derived from neonatal monocytes and fetal macrophages from the placenta can be activated in vitro by macrophage activiation factor produced by adult lymphocytes or by recombinant or purified IFN-γ.[356] Once activated, these cells are as effective at killing or inhibiting the replication of *Toxoplasma* as are adult cells.[356] These studies suggest that defects in delivery and activation of macrophages at sites of infection may contribute to the susceptibility of the fetus and neonate to infection with nonviral intracellular pathogens.

Antiviral cellular defenses are also immature in the neonate. Although production of IFN-α and -β by human neonatal cells is normal,[440] production of IFN-γ is markedly decreased. Further, IFN-α less consistently inhibits viral replication[441] and enhances cytotoxic activity in human neonatal cells compared with adult cells.[394] In mice, development of interferon soon after challenge is important in conferring protection from large inocula[442] and is delayed in neonates[443]; such data are not available in humans.

Some studies suggest that monocytes[444] and alveolar macrophages from human newborn infants[445] may not clear extracellular virus, as adult cells do. The validity of these results is uncertain, either because the cell preparations contained both monocytes and lymphocytes[444] or because alveolar macrophages from only three patients were studied at the time of death.[445] We have found no consistent difference in this function between adult and neonatal monocytes and macrophages.[446]

More consistent defects have been found in the ability of neonatal human lymphocytes and monocytes to lyse HSV-infected cells. In the extensive studies by Ching and Lopez[447] and by Kohl et al.,[394] neonatal cells had clearly less NK cytotoxicity than did adult cells; ADCC was less severely decreased. However, the total number and percentage of NK cells in neonatal blood are similar to those in adult blood.[448] The relevance of these observations is suggested by studies in newborn mice, which have deficient NK and ADCC cytotoxicity. Newborn mice are protected against lethal HSV infection by either antibody, acyclovir, or interferon in combination with lymphocytes or monocytes from human adults but not from human neonates.[298] The development of specific cytotoxic T cells has not been documented in human neonates; however, lymphocyte proliferation and production of IFN-γ and TNF in response to HSV is delayed in neonates compaed to adults with primary HSV infection.[397]

In summary, the failure of neonates to control HSV may be related in part to decreased production of or reduced response to interferon or to decreased activity of nonimmune and immune cellular cytotoxic mechanisms. In addition, infection with HSV occurs more often in infants born to mothers with primary rather than secondary infection; the lack of passively acquired antibody in such infants is a possible but unproved susceptibility factor. Similarly, infection with *Toxoplasma* and intracellular bacterial pathogens, such as *Listeria*, may be more severe because of the decreased generation of lymphokines and interleukins, which attract macrophages to the site of infection and enable them to kill these organisms. Much of the data on neonatal immunity are based on in vitro and animal studies and summarize current information in a rapidly changing field rather than stating established fact. The data suggest that immature CMI may contribute to the neonate's susceptibility. The precise age at which most of the immune functions discussed reach maturity is unknown. However, the risk of severe infection with these pathogens appears to wane by 2–3 months of age. Although this may partly reflect decreased exposure, it is possible that immune functions that are mature by this age are those most critical for protection.

Aged individuals also have diminished CMI responses in vitro and delayed hypersensitivity skin test responses in vivo.[449] The major consistent change appears to be a decline in proliferative responses to antigens and certain mitogens; this appears to reflect diminished production of and response to IL-2.[450] There is an associated decrease in cytotoxic T-cell generation.[451] Altered T-cell-mediated immunoregulation may contribute to the increased incidence of autoantibodies and to the enhanced susceptibility to viral and nonviral intracellular pathogens seen in the aged.[451]

CMI is also decreased physiologically during pregnancy in response to antigens and less consistently to mitogens. This is associated with an apparent increase in susceptibility to infections, including those due to varicella-zoster virus, *C. immitis*, and *M. leprae*.[452]

Congenital Disorders

A number of congenital disorders of CMI and their associated laboratory abnormalities are listed in Table 6. DiGeorge syndrome, a classic example of a congenital disease with defective CMI, results when the third and part of the fourth pharyngeal pouch fail to develop during embryogenesis. This results in the absence of the thymus and parathyroid glands. Severe hypocalcemia and tetany secondary to hypoparathyroidism occur in the neonatal period and are early clues to the diagnosis. Absence of the thymus gland prevents differentiation of T-lymphocyte precursors into T lymphocytes; lack of T lymphocytes prevents expression of a normal cellular immune response. Children with this disorder are lymphopenic, and thymic-dependent areas of their lymph nodes show depletion of lymphocytes. Their lymphocytes do not undergo transformation when exposed to either mitogen or antigen or when placed in mixed lymphocyte culture. A common feature of this and other disorders affecting T-cell function is defective production of lymphokines, including IFN-γ.[4] DTH skin reactivity to antigens, including streptokinase-streptodornase and candidin, is absent, and they cannot be sensitized with dinitrochlorobenzene. The CMI defects in these patients are associated with increased susceptibility to life-threatening infections by pathogens against which CMI is important, including herpes simplex virus, varicella-zoster virus, *Candida albicans*, and *Pneumocystis carinii*. Other congenital diseases that affect CMI are associated with variable defects in resistance to intracellular pathogens (Table 7). One important clinical corollary in the management of patients suspected or known to have disorders of CMI is the danger associated with their receiving live vaccines such as BCG, vaccinia, measles, rubella, and mumps. The attenuated organisms in these vaccines may disseminate, with fatal consequences in patients with defects in CMI.

Abnormalities of regulatory T cells and T-cell maturation have recently been identified as the possible mechanisms of the immunodeficiency in the common-variable forms of combined immunodeficiency syndrome, DiGeorge syndrome, and acquired agammaglobulinemia.[453] In one study,[453] several disorders of T-cell differentiation occurred in patients with combined immunodeficiency. One subtype of combined immunodeficiency was associated with failure to develop lymphocytes that expressed any thymus-specific antigens; another subtype was associated with failure to differentiate beyond the early prothymocyte–thymocyte stage; a third subtype was associated with failure to differentiate beyond a late thymocyte stage. In contrast, patients with thymic aplasia (DiGeorge syndrome) had a diminished but detectable population of mature T cells. Imbalances in immunoregulatory T cells with a relative excess of suppressor cells were found in approximately half of a group of patients with spontaneously occurring acquired agammaglobulinemia. In one of the latter group, there was an activated suppressor T-cell population that expressed Ia antigens. Another had no inducer (T4) cells. Patients with X-linked agammaglobulinema frequently had an abnormal ratio of inducer to suppressor cells, as well as an absence of circulating surface immunoglobulin-bearing cells. Common variable immunodeficiency is heterogeneous with defects in both cellular and humoral immunity; humoral immune defects may result from B-cell abnormalities or abnormalities in the production of regulatory T-cell lymphokines. Low lytic efficiency of mature NK cells[454] has recently been identified as another facet of immune dysfunction in Chédiak-Higashi syndrome, and defects of secretion of IFN-γ and NK cell activities have been identified in patients with recurrent and unusually severe viral and bacterial infections.[403]

Certain immune deficiency diseases have been associated with a deficiency of particular cellular enzymes. For example, severe combined immunodeficiency disease has been associated with a lack of the enzyme adenosine deaminase. In a patient with severe combined immunodeficiency disease and lack of adenosine deaminase, replacement therapy for the enzyme, using frozen irradiated human red blood cells as a source of adenosine deaminase, restored humoral immunity and CMI.[455] Other examples of defective T-lymphocyte function associated with enzyme deficiencies occurred in patients who lacked purine nucleoside phosphorylase and had abnormal CMI[456] and occurred in two siblings with an autosomally recessive error of pyrimidine metabolism, hereditary orotic aciduria, who had cellular immunodeficiency.[457] A less severe defect in CMI is seen in Down syndrome.[458]

Patients with Chédiak-Higashi syndrome,[454] LCAM deficiency,[459] and chronic granulomatous disease[460] suffer most from severe infection with extracellular bacterial pathogens. However, cytotoxic lymphocyte function is also abnormal in the former two disorders and may explain their greater susceptibility to viral pathogens. Intracellular bacterial pathogens including *Nocardia*, Mycobacteria and *Legionella* also cause serious infections in these patients.[461,469]

Acquired Disorders

Infections. Among the causes of defective CMI that are acquired after birth is infection itself.[462] These infections known to depress DTH skin tests and in vitro lymphocyte transformation to either mitogens or antigens are listed in Table 7; these include infectious mononucleosis and influenza; bacterial infections including tuberculosis, leprosy, bacterial pneumonia, and syphilis; and fungal infections including coccidioidomycosis. Although most studies of the suppression of CMI that occurs during infection have demonstrated defects in response to DTH skin tests and in lymphocyte transformation, data have accumulated that also reveal the presence of acquired defects in monocyte and macrophage function. Suppression of in vitro chemotaxis has been described in monocytes from patients acutely infected with influenza virus. This defect persists for approximately 3 weeks.[463] Suppression of phagocytosis by macrophages from animals infected with viruses is well described.[464] Thus, both lymphocyte and macrophage function may be abnormal during and after acute infections. It is unclear in most cases whether suppression of these in vivo and in vitro correlates of CMI by a given infection results in an increased susceptibility to other organisms or even to the original infecting organism.

Viral infection can inhibit CMI either directly, by infecting lymphocytes and macrophages and thereby altering their function, or indirectly, by altering immune regulatory mechanisms (reviewed in Ref. 465). AIDS is an example of the first mechanism and is discussed fully in Chapter 107. Another example in which viral infection of lymphocytes may be important is measles. Measles virus does this in part by reducing DTH and the response of lymphocytes to mitogens and antigens, as well as by suppression of the number of circulating T lymphocytes by noncytolytic infection, transforming lymphocytes and thereby suppressing lymphocyte transformation and proliferation.[465] Ratios of circulating T-lymphocyte subsets remain normal in measles.[466] The possible clinical relevance of abnormalities in tests of CMI during measles infection is controversial.

Viruses, including influenza, respiratory syncytial virus, and CMV, may inhibit the accessory functions of macrophages for T-cell responses in vitro[465,467–469]; however, results in vivo do

TABLE 6. Congenital Disorders of Cell-Mediated Immunity

	Di George Syndrome[a]	*Nezelof Syndrome*[b]	*Cartilage Hair Hypoplasia*	*Chronic Mucocutaneous Candidiasis*	*Wiskott-Aldrich Syndrome*[c]	*Ataxia Telangiectasia*[d]	*Severe Combined Immunodeficiency Disease (SCID)*	*Adenosine Deaminase Deficiency*[e]	*Purine Nucleoside Phosphorylase Deficiency*[f]	*Chédiak-Higashi Syndrome*[g]	*LCAM Deficiency*[h]	*Chronic Granulomatous Disease of Childhood*[i]
Increased incidence or severity of infections due to												
intracellular bacteria		Yes					Yes	Yes	Yes	Yes	Yes	Yes
Viruses	Yes	Yes	Yes		Yes	Yes	Yes	Yes	Yes	Yes	Yes	
Fungi	Yes	Yes		Yes			Yes	Yes				Yes
Protozoa	Yes	Yes			Yes		Yes	Yes				
Lymphopenia	Yes	Yes	Yes	Variable	Variable	Variable	Yes	Yes	Yes	Yes		
Absent delayed-type hypersensitivity	Yes	Yes	Variable	Variable	Variable	Variable	Yes	Yes	Yes			
Absent lymphocyte transformation to:												
Phytohemagglutinin	Yes	Yes	Variable	Variable	Variable	Variable	Yes	Yes	Yes			
Antigen	Yes	Yes	Yes (Varicella)	Variable	Variable	Variable	Yes	Yes	Yes			

[a] Thymic hypoplasia. Other features include congenital cardiac defects and hypocalcemia.
[b] Autosomal recessive lymphopenia.
[c] Immunodeficiency with thrombocytopenia. Other features include X-linked thrombocytopenia and death in childhood.
[d] Other features include cerebellar ataxia (infancy), cutaneous telangiectasia, sinopulmonary infections, lymphomas, carcinomas, maldevelopment of thymus, ovarian agenesis, increased α-fetoprotein, susceptibility to radiation-induced chromosomal damage.
[e] Other features include symptoms in the first 6 months of life, death in the first year of life, bony abnormalities (cupping of the ribs at the costochondral junctions, abnormal metaphyses, short extremities). Causes one-third of autosoma recessive severe combined immunodeficiency disease. Prenatal diagnosis with amniotic fluid cells. Treatment is bone marrow transplantation or transfusion of normal erythrocytes
[f] Appears normal at birth, but progressive depletion of T lymphocytes occurs between first and second years of life with recurrent infections. Autoimmune hemolytic anemia. It is a rare autosomal recessive trait.
[g] Autosomal inheritance; giant lysosomal granules in leukocytes, melanocytes, Schwann cells, and possibly other tissues; partial oculocutaneous albinism and a lymphoma-like phase with widespread mononuclear cell infiltration. Ascorbic acid, which increases cGMP, is reported to improve a chemotactic defect. There is also defective NK cell function.
[h] Leukocyte cell adhesion molecule deficiency; LCAM are three different molecules composed of a variable α and a common β subunit; the most common defect is autosomal recessive β-chain deficiency, causing deficiency of all three molecules.
[i] More commonly X-linked recessive but also autosomal recessive inheritance, generalized lymphadenopathy, frequent hepatosplenomegaly with granulomas. Inability of monocytes and PMNs to generate superoxide and hydrogen peroxide. Common X-linked form is due to absence of b cytochrome heavy chain.

TABLE 7. Some Infections and Vaccines That May Be Associated with Depressed Delayed-Type Hypersensitivity or CMI

Viral	Bacterial
Human immunodeficiency viruses	Tuberculosis
Measles (and vaccine)	Leprosy
Mumps	Syphilis
Chickenpox	Streptococcal infection
Influenza	Brucellosis
Infectious mononucleosis	Bacterial pneumonia
Yellow fever	Typhoid fever
Rubella vaccine	Other
Measles-mumps-rubella vaccine	Schistosomiasis
Chronic hepatitis B	Toxoplasmosis
Cytomegalovirus infection	Malaria
Fungal	Filiariasis
Coccidioidomycosis	Leishmaniasis
Histoplasmosis	
Blastomycosis	

not always parallel those in vitro, as indicated by the failure of influenza infection to impair induction of the DTH skin test response.[470] Viruses, including influenza virus, may also impair human monocyte migration, phagocytosis, and microbicidal activity[471]; however, the microbicidal activity of human alveolar macrophages is not impaired.[472] Thus, caution is advisable in extrapolation of these variable results to human disease.

Diminished CMI also occurs in patients with infectious mononucleosis due to EBV.[386,403] This virus infects B lymphocytes, which have a specific receptor for the virus, the type 2 complement receptor. Infected B lymphocytes are polyclonally activated to secrete immunoglobulin and are immortalized in vitro; this may account for the development of heterophilic antibodies and autoantibodies in this infection. In vivo cytotoxic/suppressor T8 cells increase in number and act to inhibit infected B cells but may also inhibit other T-cell responses.

In two forms of the X-linked lymphoproliferative syndrome,[403] an accentuation of the T8 response appears to result in fatal infectious mononucleosis or hypogammaglobulinemia. In patients with acute CMV mononucleosis, there are decreased numbers of helper T4 lymphocytes and increased numbers of cytotoxic/suppressor T8 lymphocytes in conjunction with depressed concanavalin A responsiveness, all of which return to normal in convalescence.[473] Parasitic disease as a cause of immunosuppression has recently been reviewed.[474] Immunodepression and alteration of T-cell subsets occur during some *Toxoplasma* infections in humans[475] and in some animal models. A novel mechanism of immunosuppression in malaria is the appearance of cold reactive lymphocytotoxic antibodies.[476]

Malignancies. Malignancies may adversely affect both humoral and cellular immunity (e.g., Hodgkin's disease[477–479]). In patients with Hodgkin's disease, there is lymphopenia, low NK cell activity, depressed DTH, decreased ability to be sensitized to dinitrochlorobenzene, and diminished in vitro lymphocyte transformation to antigens and mitogens and in mixed lymphocyte culture. Depressed lymphocyte function due to Hodgkin's disease has been attributed variously to serum factors,[477] to an adherent mononuclear cell population,[478] to a prostaglandin-producing adherent suppressor cell, and to suppressor T lymphocytes.[479] Lymphocyte responsiveness has been restored by incubating T lymphocytes in fetal calf serum and levamisole, demonstrating that the alteration of T lymphocytes is reversible. Another in vitro correlate of CMI, production of chemotactic factor, is normal in Hodgkin's disease even when responsiveness to mitogens is abnormal. High levels of a naturally occurring chemotactic factor inactivator have been detected in the sera of patients with Hodgkin's disease, which may result in a generalized defect in the ability to mobilize inflammatory cells in these patients. The abnormalities in CMI described above are associated with an increased susceptibility of patients with Hodgkin's disease to a variety of intracellular pathogens.

Although defects in cellular immunity have been clearly established in patients with Hodgkin's disease and certain other lymphomas, they are less well described in other malignancies, and results of testing CMI in many such patients have been reported to be normal. Some patients with advanced neoplasms (e.g., those with squamous cell carcinoma of the head and neck, intracranial tumors, and melanoma) have depressed DTH and/or mitogen-stimulated lymphocyte transformation. In some reports that describe cancer patients, washing lymphocytes has improved lymphocyte responsiveness, suggesting the presence of an elutable inhibitor factor. In addition, monocyte function has been reported to be suppressed in patients with malignancy. In animal models and/or in vitro, tumor cells and/or their products have been reported to block accumulation of macrophages in vivo, inhibit development of macrophage activation, reduce release of lytic substances from macrophages or inhibit injurious effects of these mediators once they have been released, and suppress macrophage anti-microbial activity against *Leishmania* and *Toxoplasma* in conjunction with suppression of oxidative mechanisms.[480]

Pharmacologic Agents and Radiation. CYTOTOXIC AGENTS, CORTICOSTEROIDS, AND RADIATION. Cytotoxic drugs and corticosteroids may have profound effects on CMI.[481–483] Two chemotherapeutic drugs that are highly immunosuppressive, cyclophosphamide and methotrexate, differ both qualitatively and quantitatively in their effects on the immune system and will be used here as examples. Cyclophosphamide is a cycle-specific agent that is toxic to cells in either proliferating or resting stages but has a preferential effect on proliferating cells. Cyclophosphamide inhibits T-lymphocyte proliferation and production of many lymphokines and depletes the intermitotic circulating T-lymphocyte pool, thereby decreasing the number of previously committed lymphocytes as well as those available for sensitization.

Methotrexate is a phase-specific drug that acts primarily on dividing cells. If the drug is administered for 7 days after an animal is exposed to a new antigen, suppression of DTH and antigen-specific lymphocyte transformation occurs; if it is administered before or after the 7-day induction period, no effect on CMI function is seen. Therefore, methotrexate usually will not affect the CMI response to an antigen when sensitization has already been established.

Administration of corticosteroids results in lymphopenia and the shrinkage of organs of the reticuloendothelial system in certain animals. However, there are large differences among different species of animals with regard to susceptibility of the immune system to corticosteroids; the principal effect of administration of the drug in humans is to cause transient lymphopenia by redistribution of lymphocytes.[481] Corticosteroids decrease expression of DTH. The production of most cytokines by lymphocytes and mononuclear phagocytes is inhibited.[484] The effects of cytokines on target cells also may be blocked[485]; however, this varies since corticosteroids do not block IFN-γ-induced activity of human macrophages against *Listeria* but do block IFN-γ-induced activity against *Nocardia* and *Salmonella*. Target cells may be protected from direct cytotoxicity by T lymphocytes without directly affecting the T lymphocytes themselves. Corticosteroids cause monocytopenia, decreased clearance of particulate material, and decreased bactericidal and fungicidal activity of monocytes in vitro.

In animals, increased susceptibility to infection, as well as increased risk of reactivation of latent infections, can result from administration of corticosteroids.[482] Although this is also true in humans, the incidence of infection depends largely on the underlying disease for which the corticosteroids are being administered.

Cytotoxic agents and corticosteroids are frequently administered in combination, and it is the total effect of all the drugs in this combination that dictates the degree and nature of immunosuppression. Studies with combinations of these drugs in the treatment of malignancy in humans show that immunosuppression occurs during therapy but that immunologic competence may return after therapy. In some cases (e.g., patients who have received combined-modality therapy for Hodgkin's disease and who have depressed responses to vaccines many years after completion of therapy), either the underlying diseases or the therapy continues to cause depressed immune function. Continuous therapy has longer, more profound effects than intermittent therapy.[483]

As would be expected from the above, when immunosuppressive agents are given before or simultaneously with experimental infections, CMI fails to develop and mortality frequently increases. Numerous experimental infections produced by intracellular pathogens are exacerbated by immunosuppressive agents. In humans, there is evidence of increased susceptibility to infection with the use of cytotoxic drugs. Transplant recipients who receive immunosuppressive drugs to prevent tissue rejection have a striking susceptibility to opportunistic infections, although the incidence of such infections has decreased with the change to a less immunosuppressive regimen that includes cyclosporin A (see below under "Other Pharmacologic Agents"[486]). In children with acute lymphocytic leukemia, the incidence of *P. carinii* pneumonia increases when the number of cytotoxic agents used to combat the leukemia is increased. In addition, in patients with herpes zoster and stage 3 or 4 lymphoma, a randomized trial revealed that treatment with cytosine arabinoside increased the time for resolution of zoster lesions. The antiviral effects of the drug were apparently less important than its immunosuppressive effect.

Radiation therapy also predisposes the patient to infections by affecting proliferating and nonproliferating lymphoid cell populations and consequently depressing CMI. In animals, suppression of established DTH and interference with initial sensitization of lymphocytes occur as a result of irradiation. The combination of radiation and drugs such as cortisone and nitrogen mustard more frequently resulted in relapse of latent infection with *Toxoplasma* in hamsters than radiation or drugs alone.[482] Extrapolation of these findings to humans is difficult because of the differences in the doses of radiation given to humans and to experimental animals and because of the deficiencies in CMI secondary to the underlying disease process in humans for which the radiation is being administered.

ANTIMICROBIAL AGENTS. Certain antimicrobial agents are associated with abnormalities of CMI.[487,488] The meaning, clinical relevance, and significance of the changes observed are not yet clear. Results have been conflicting, and few controlled clinical studies have been carried out to determine the effect of antibiotics on the immune response in humans. There is a need for better understanding of the influence of antibiotics on the immune response. This is especially important for patients who receive antibiotic therapy for prolonged periods and for immunosuppressed patients.

OTHER PHARMACOLOGIC AGENTS. Cyclosporin A is used to suppress allograft rejection and alters helper T cells, effector T cells, and NK cells.[489] It is a fungal metabolite of *Trichoderma polysporum* and is a cyclic polypeptide containing 11 amino acids. It is an effective immunosuppressant with low myelotoxicity and has been used successfully as the primary drug to suppress the rejection of transplants of nonmatched cadaver kidneys, as well as heart, lung, bone marrow, and liver transplants. It prevents the response of T lymphocytes to alloantigens and certain mitogens. The synthesis of IL-2, the expression of receptors for IL-2 on the cell membrane, and the response to IL-2 are inhibited by cyclosporin A. These effects appear to reflect inhibition of calcium-dependent T-cell activation pathways.[490] Interferon -γ and IL-3 but not GM-CSF production is also inhibited.[491] Allograft recipients treated with cyclosporin A rather than with the more cytotoxic regimens used formerly have less pronounced immunodepression and a reduced incidence of opportunistic infections.[486] It is of interest that cyclosporin A also has antimicrobial effects against malaria, schistosomes, and *Toxoplasma*. Whether this has any effect on the patterns of opportunistic infections that allograft recipients acquire remains to be determined.

Other Disorders. In addition to those factors discussed above, leukocytosis, anemia, and fever depress DTH skin responses. Autoantibodies may alter CMI (e.g., a patient with acquired agammaglobulinemia had an autoantibody to T4 cells and subsequently to T8 cells). Uremia,[492] diabetes mellitus,[493] surgery and anesthesia,[494] sarcoidosis,[495] cystic fibrosis,[496] and prolonged but not brief zinc deficiency[497] have also been reported to be associated with depressed CMI. Anergy, zinc deficiency, and decreased nucleoside phosphorylase activity have been found in patients with sickle cell anemia.[498]

Nutritional status has a profound effect on immune function.[499–501] Chronic protein-calorie malnutrition exerts a suppressive effect on functions of T lymphocytes (e.g., DTH reactions, lymphocyte proliferative responses to mitogens and antigens, and T-cell-dependent antibody responses are all decreased by protein-calorie malnutrition) and to a lesser extent on macrophage function. Depressed T-lymphocyte function has also been documented in deficiencies of trace elements such as copper (as well as zinc; see above) and certain vitamins, such as thiamine and folate. Replacement of deficient nutritional components results in restoration of immune function.

An increasing body of data indicates that the nervous and immune systems interact. As described above, immune cytokines act on the central nervous system to induce fever, sleep, and changes in alertness. Reciprocally, neural transmitters released in response to stress may alter CMI. Norepinephrine and epinephrine block induction by IFN-γ of mouse macrophage activity against herpes simplex virus-infected cells, an effect apparently mediated by increased intracellular cyclic AMP.[502] Cyclic AMP negatively regulates many aspects of CMI, including IL-2 production[503]; thus, adrenergic agents may have more general down-modulating effects on CMI. Deficiency of prolactin, secretion of which is induced by stress and other neuroactive compounds, appears to impair CMI and resistance to the intracellular pathogen *L. monocytogenes* in mice[504]; a major mechanism appears to be impaired IFN-γ production and as a consequence, impaired macrophage activation. Certain opioid peptides enhance IFN-γ production by human mononuclear cells.[505] Another example of neuroregulation of the immune response is the stimulation by IL-1 of adrenocorticotrophic hormone (ACTH) and glucocorticoid release,[166,167] which act to inhibit IL-1 production.[506]

Patients with autoimmune disorders have variable deficiencies of CMI. Interferon-γ production by the cells of patients with systemic lupus erythematosus, rheumatoid arthritis and connective tissue disease, and psoriasis is diminished.[4] CMI in these patients may be further impaired by treatment.

Certain types of infections (e.g., with cytomegalovirus or fungi) appear to occur most frequently at identifiable intervals following bone marrow transplantation, which in part reflects immunosuppressive therapy and in part the development of a graft vs. host (GvH) reaction. In the first phase of GvH disease, recognition of allogeneic MHC antigens activates a potent suppressive signal that rapidly abrogates immunity. The number of helper T4 cells decreases, and the number of regulatory macrophages increases.[507] Acutely, there is a lack of suppressor T-cell activity that leads to increased levels of serum IgE. In the second phase, macrophage production of PGE_2 increases, and later this terminates. In the third phase there is destruction of thymic medullary epithelium, disruption of T-cell maturation, functional defects in B-cell maturation, neutrophil development, chemotaxis, formation of autoantibodies, and more frequently, development of neoplasia (e.g., B-cell lymphomas and mammary carcinomas[507]).

TABLE 8. Evaluation of the Capacity for Immune Response[a]

History
- Increased frequency and severity of infections
- Abnormal responses to live vaccines (e.g., vaccinia)
- Frequent infections with less common pathogens (e.g., fungi)
- Recurrent diarrhea
- Family history of increased susceptibility to infection
- Sexual preference
- Intravenous drug abuse
- Blood product transfusions

Physical examination
- Signs of chronic infection
- Absence of lymphoid tissue
- Signs associated with specific immunodeficiency disorders (see Chapter 9)

Laboratory

I. Preliminary screen[a]
  - A. Complete blood cell count with differential smear
  - B. Quantitative immunoglobulin levels

II. Readily available studies
  - A. B-cell function
    1. Natural or commonly acquired antibodies: isohemagglutinins, "febrile" agglutinins, antibodies to common viruses (rubella, rubeola, influenza), and toxins (diphtheria, tetanus)
    2. Response to immunization (typhoid, polio, diphtheria-tetanus vaccines)
    3. Determination of total B cells by immunofluorescence
  - B. T-cell function
    1. Skin tests (PPD, *Candidin, Trichophyton*, streptokinase-streptodornase), tetanus toxoid (1:100 dilution)
    2. Chest x-ray film (thymus shadow in infants, thymoma in adults)
    3. T-cell subsets CD4, CD8 by immunofluorescence
  - C. Complement
    1. C3
    2. CH_{50} (total hemolytic complement)
  - D. Phagocyte function
    1. Reduction of nitroblue tetrazolium
    2. Inflammatory skin window (Rebuck)
    3. LCAM expression by immunofluorescence
    4. Class II HLA expression on monocytes
  - E. Infectious agents causing immunodeficiency
    1. Antibodies to HIV-1, HIV-2, Epstein-Barr virus (isolation of virus also at reference laboratories)

III. In-depth investigation
  - A. B cell
    1. Pre-B-cell examination in bone marrow samples
    2. B-lymphocyte membrane markers: IgM, IgD, IgG, IgA; receptors for aggregated IgG (Fc receptor), C3; antigens detected by anti-B antibodies
    3. Induction of B-lymphocyte differentiation in vitro stimulated by pokeweed mitogen, Epstein-Barr virus, or other polyclonal B-cell activators
    4. Kinetics and immunoglobulin class of antibody produced in response to specific primary and secondary immunization
    5. Measurement of IgG subclasses and κ:λ ratio
    6. Histologic and immunofluorescent examination of biopsy specimens (intestinal mucosa, lymph node, bone marrow)
  - B. T cell
    1. Surface markers for T-helper subsets: 4B4, 2H4
    2. In vitro correlates of delayed hypersensitivity
       - a. Proliferative response to mitogens; phytohemagglutinin, ConA, specific antigens (purified protein derivative, *Candida*, tetanus); allogeneic cells (one-way mixed lymphocyte response)
       - b. Quantification of lymphokines (interferon, IL-2, etc.) or lymphokine mRNA
       - c. Induction of killer cells by stimulation with allogeneic lymphocytes
    3. Measurement of thymus hormones
    4. Assays for T-cell helper function using supernatants of antigen-activated T cells or T cells plus pokeweed mitogen or antigens to trigger B-lymphocyte differentiation
    5. Skin graft rejection
  - C. Phagocytes and complement
    1. Chemotactic response in vitro
    2. Bactericidal function
    3. Classic and alternative pathway complement components
  - D. Natural killer cells
    1. Enumeration with monoclonal antibodies
    2. Functional assay using appropriate target cells
  - E. Miscellaneous
    1. Lymphocytotoxic antibodies
    2. Measurement of adenosine deaminase and purine nucleoside phosphorylase enzyme activities

[a] Analyses of complement, B, T, and phagocytic cells are included because of interrelated syndromes.
(Adapted from Cooper and Lawton,[508] with permission.)

Evaluation of the Patient with Suspected Deficiency of CMI

Immunodeficiency syndromes—congenital, spontaneously acquired, or iatrogenic—are characterized by unusual susceptibility to infection. Autoimmune disease and lymphoreticular malignancies sometimes occur. The types of infection often provide an early clue to the immunologic defect. T-cell deficiency is almost always accompanied by some abnormality of antibody responses. Since many antibody responses require T-cell help, this may explain in part why patients with primary T-cell defects also develop overwhelming infection with bacterial species against which antibody plays a major role in resistance. An outline of important considerations in the evaluation of patients with suspected defects in CMI is presented in Table 8.[508] It is important to obtain a careful history and to perform a thorough physical examination, as these may indicate whether the antibody–complement–phagocyte system or CMI is defective. A normal response to smallpox vaccination or contact dermatitis due to poison ivy suggests intact cellular immunity. Lymphopenia, absence of palpable lymph nodes or diffuse lymphoid hyperplasia, and signs of specific infections are relevant.

Since at least 80 percent of the population have been sensitized to one of the following—*Candida, Trichophyton*, streptokinase-streptodornase, or purified protein derivative (PPD)—using these antigens for skin tests to elicit DTH is useful in evaluation of CMI. A positive skin test indicates prior sensitization of helper T cells to antigens of the organism. Absence of skin reactivity to these antigen indicates either a defect in CMI, failure to properly inject the antigen intradermally, or a defect in the ability of the patient to develop a nonspecific inflammatory skin response. (The last defect can be tested by placing irritating substances such as benzalkonium chloride on the skin.) For skin testing, an initial evaluation should be made at 2–6 hours after injection of the antigen for immediate hypersensitivity reactions that are not due to CMI and may result in false-positive readings 24–48 hours later.

Basic in vitro tests of CMI are becoming more widely available since the onset of the AIDS epidemic. These include determination of T-cell subsets (T4 and T8), B-cell and NK-cell number, expression of class II HLA antigens, and proliferative responses to mitogens. Tests commonly performed by research or reference laboratories for in-depth investigation are also indicated in Table 8. In certain conditions associated with defects in CMI, there may be a negative correlation between the DTH response in vivo and results of in vitro correlates of DTH (e.g., in mucocutaneous candidiasis, the candidin skin test may be negative in a patient whose lymphocytes transform to candidin antigen in vitro).

ACKNOWLEDGMENT

This chapter was supported in part by grants from the National Institutes of Health.

REFERENCES

1. Hahn H, Kaufmann SHE. The role of cell-mediated immunity in bacterial infections. Rev Infect Dis. 1981;3:1221–50.
2. Blanden RV. Mechanisms of recovery from a generalized viral infection: Mouse-pox-I. The effects of anti-thymocyte serum. J Exp Med. 1970; 132:1035–50.
3. Ruskin J, McIntosh J, Remington JS. Studies on the mechanisms of resistance to phylogenetically diverse intracellular organisms. J Immunol. 1969;103:252–9.
4. Murray HW. Interferon-gamma, the activated macrophage, and the host defense against microbial challenge. Ann Intern Med. 1988;108:595–608.
5. Royer HD, Reinherz EL. T lymphocytes: Ontogeny, function, and relevance to clinical disorders. N Engl J Med. 1987;317:1136–42.
6. Fauci AS. The human immunodeficiency virus: Infectivity and mechanisms of pathogenesis. Science. 1988;239:617.
7. Kronenberg M, Siu G, Hood LE, et al. The molecular genetics of the T-cell

antigen receptor and T-cell antigen recognition. Ann Rev Immunol. 1986;4:529–91.
8. Swain SL. T-cell subsets and the recognition of MHC class. Immunol Rev. 1983;74:129.
9. Fleischer B, Schrezenmeier H, Wagner H. Function of the CD4 and CD8 molecules on human cytotoxic T lymphocytes: Regulation of T cell triggering. J Immunol. 1986;136:1625–8.
10. Schwartz RH. T-lymphocyte recognition of antigen in association with gene products of the major histocompatibility complex. Ann Rev Immunol. 1985;3:237–61.
11. Davis MM, Bjorkman PJ. T cell antigen receptor genes and T cell recognition. Nature. 1988;334:395–402.
12. Fitch FW. T-cell clones and T-cell receptors. Microbiol Rev. 1986;50:50–69.
13. Elliott JF, Rock EP, Patten PA, et al. The adult T-cell receptor δ-chain is diverse and distinct from that of fetal thymocytes. Nature. 1988;331:627–31.
14. Yancopoulous GD, Blackwell TK, Heikyung S, et al. Introduced T cell receptor variable region gene segments recombine in pre-B cells: Evidence that T and B cells use a common recombinase. Cell. 1986;44:251–9.
15. Dembic Z, Haas W, Weiss S, et al. Transfer of specificity by murine alpha and beta T-cell receptor genes. Nature. 1986;320:232–8.
16. Gabert J, Langlet C, Zamoyska R, et al. Reconstitution of MHC Class I specificity by transfer of the T cell receptor and Lyt-2 genes. Cell. 1987;50:545–54.
17. Clevers H, Alarcon B, Wileman T, et al. The T cell receptor/CD3 complex: A dynamic protein ensemble. Ann Rev. Immunol. 1988;6:629–62.
18. Wilson RK, Lai E, Concannon P, et al. Structure, organization and polymorphism of murine and human T-cell receptor alpha and beta chain gene families. Immunol Rev. 1988;101:149–72.
19. Gefter M, Marrack P. Development and modification of the lymphocyte repertoire. Nature. 1986;321:116–8.
20. Garman RD, Ko JL, Vulpe CD, et al. T-cell receptor variable region gene usage in T-cell populations. Proc Natl Acad Sci USA. 1986;83:3987–91.
21. Rupp F, Acha-Obeo H, Hengartner H, et al. Identical Vβ T-cell receptor genes used in alloreactive cytotoxic and antigen plus I-A specific helper T cells. Nature. 1985;315:425–7.
22. Epplen JT, Bartels F, Becker A, et al. Change in antigen specificity of cytotoxic T lymphocytes is associated with the rearrangement and expression of a T-cell receptor beta-chain gene. Proc Natl Acad Sci USA. 1986;83:4441–5.
23. Hedrick SM, Engel I, McElligott DL, et al. Selection of amino acid sequences in the beta chain of the T cell antigen receptor. Science. 1988;239:1541–4.
24. Maddon MJ, Littman DR, Godfrey M, et al. The isolation and nucleotide sequence of a cDNA encoding the T cell surface protein T4: A new member of the immunoglobulin gene family. Cell. 1985;42:93–104.
25. Littman DR, Thomas Y, Maddon PJ, et al. The isolation and sequence of the gene encoding T8: A molecule defining functional classes of T lymphocytes. Cell. 1985;40:237–46.
26. William AF, Barclay AN. The immunoglbulin superfamily—domains for cell surface recognition. Ann Rev Immunol. 1988;6:381–405.
27. Gay D, Maddon P, Sekaly R, et al. Functional interaction between human T-cell protein CD4 and the major histocompatibility complex HLA-DR antigen. Nature. 1987;328:626–9.
28. Shaw S, Ginther GE. The lymphocyte function-associated antigen (LFA)-1 and CD2/LFA-3 pathways of antigen-independent human T cell adhesion. J Immunol. 1987;139:1037–45.
29. Peterson A, Seed B. Monoclonal antibody and ligand binding sites of the T cell erythrocyte receptor (CD2). Nature. 1987;329:842–6.
30. Sewell WA, Brown MH, Dunne J. Molecular cloning of the human T-lymphocyte surface CD2 (T11) antigen. Proc Natl Acad Sci USA. 1986;83:8718–22.
31. Wallner BP, Frey AZ, Tizard R, et al. Primary structure of lymphocyte function-associated antigen 3 (LFA-3). The ligand of the T lymphocyte CD2 glycoprotein. J Exp Med. 1987;166:923–32.
32. Yang SY, Chouaib S, Dupont B. A common pathway for T lymphocyte activation involving both the CD3-Ti complex and CD2 sheep erythrocyte receptor determinants. J Immunol. 1986;137:1097–1100.
33. Fox DA, Scholossman SF, Reinherz EL. Regulation of the alternative pathway of T cell activation by anti-T3 monoclonal antibody. J Immunol. 1986;136:1945–50.
34. June CH, Rabinovitch PS, Ledbetter JA. CD5 antibodies increase intracellular ionized calcium concentration in T cells. J Immunol. 1987;138:2782–92.
35. Martin PJ, Ledbetter JA, Morishita Y, et al. A 44 kilodalton cell surface homodimer regulates interleukin 2 production by activated human T lymphocytes. J Immunol. 1986;136:3282–7.
36. Springer TA, Teplow DB, Dreyer WJ. Sequence homology of the LFA-1 and Mac-1 leukocyte adhesion glycoproteins and unexpected relation to leukocyte interferon. Nature. 1985;314:540–2.
37. Bierer BE, Mentzer SJ, Greenstein JL, et al. Year Immunol. 1986:39–59.
38. Blanchard D, van Els C, Borst J, et al. The role of the T cell receptor, CD8, and LFA-1 in different stages of the cytolytic reaction mediated by alloreactive T lymphocyte clones. J Immunol. 1987;138:2417–21.
39. Fowlkes BJ, Mathieson BJ. Intrathymic differentiation: Thymocyte heterogeneity and the characterization of early T-cell precursors. Surv Immunol Res. 1985;4:96–109.
40. Rothenberg E, Lugo JP. Differentiation and cell division in the mammalian thymus. Dev Biol. 1985;112:1–17.
41. Haynes BF. The human thymic microenvironment. Adv Immunol. 1984; 36:87–142.
42. Lobach DF, Hensley LL, Ho W, et al. Human T cell antigen expression during the early stages of fetal thymic maturation. J Immunol. 1985;135:1752–9.
43. Gallatin M, St. John TP, Siegelman M. Lymphocyte homing receptors. Cell. 1986;44:673–80.
44. Kisielow P, Leiserson W, von Boehmer H. Differentiation of thymocytes in fetal organ culture: Analysis of phenotypic changes accompanying the appearance of cytolytic and interleukin 2-producing cells. J Immunol. 1984;133:1117–23.
45. Kingston R, Jenkinson EJ, Owen JJT. A single stem cell can recolonize an embryonic thymus, producing phenotypically distinct T-cell populations. Nature. 1985;317:811–3.
46. Blue ML, Daley JF, Levinc H, et al. Class II major histocompatibility complex molecules regulate the development of the $T4^+T8^-$ inducer phenotype of cultured human thymocytes. Proc Natl Acad Sci USA. 1985;82:8178–82.
47. Marusic-Galesic S, Stephany DA, Longo DL, et al. Development of $CD4^-CD8^+$ cytotoxic T cells requires interactions with class I MHC determinants. Nature. 1988;333:180–3.
48. Brenner MB, McLean J, Scheft H, et al. Two forms of the T-cell receptor gamma protein found on peripheral blood cytotoxic T lymphocytes. Nature. 1987;325:6898.
49. Brenner MB, McLean J, Dialynas DP, et al. Identification of a putative second T-cell receptor. Nature. 1986;322:145–9.
50. Bank I, DePinho RA, Brenner MB, et al. A functional T3 molecule associated with a novel heterodimer on the surface of immature human thymocytes. Nature. 1986;322:179–81.
51. Weiss A, Newton M, Crommie D. Expression of T3 in association with a molecule distinct from the T-cell antigen receptor heterodimer. Proc Natl Acad Sci USA. 1986;83:6998–7002.
52. Borst J, van Dongen JJM, Bolhuis RLH, et al. Distinct molecular forms of human T cell receptor γ/δ detected on viable T cells by a monoclonal antibody. J Exp Med. 1988;167:1625–44.
53. Lanier LL, Ruitenberg JJ, Phillips JH. Human $CD3^+$ T lymphocytes that express neither CD4 nor CD8 antigens. J Exp Med. 1986;164:339–44.
54. Roehm N, Herron L, Cambier J. The major histocompatibility complex-restricted antigen receptor on T cells: Distribution on thymus and peripheral T cells. Cell. 1984;38:577–84.
55. Lugo JP, Krishnan SN, Sailor RD, et al. Early precursor thymocytes can produce interleukin 2 upon stimulation with calcium ionophore and phorbol ester. Proc Natl Acad Sci USA. 1986;83:1862–6.
56. Kappler JW, Roehm N, Marrack P. T cell tolerance by clonal elimination in the thymus. Cell. 1987;49:273–80.
57. MacDonald HR, Schneider R, Lees RK, et al. T-cell receptor Vβ use predicts reactivity and tolerance to Mls^{α}-encoded antigens. Nature. 1988;332:40–45.
58. Kappler JW, Staerz U, White J, et al. Self-tolerance eliminates T cells specific for Mls-modified products of the major histocompatibility complex. Nature. 1988;332:35–40.
59. Robertson M. Tolerance, restriction and the Mls enigma. Nature. 1988;332:18–9.
60. Hocking WG, Golde DW. The pulmonary–alveolar macrophage. N Engl J Med. 1979;301:580–646.
61. Bitterman PB, Saltzman LE, Adelberg S, et al. Alveolar macrophage replication. One mechanism for the expansion of the mononuclear phagocyte population in the chronically inflamed lung. J Clin Invest. 1984;74:460–9.
62. Nichols BA, Bainton DF, Farquhar MG. Differentiation of monocytes. J Cell Biol. 1984;50:498–515.
63. Keleman E, Janossa M. Macrophages are the first differentiated blood cells formed in human embryonic liver. Exp Hematol. 1980;8:996–1000.
64. Brooks CF, Moore M. Differential MHC class II expression on human peripheral blood monocytes and dendritic cells. Immunology. 1988;63:303–11.
65. Wolff K, Stingl G. The Langerhans cell. J Invest Dermatol. 1983;80:17s–21s.
66. Braathen LR, Bjercke S, Thorsby E. The antigen-presenting function of human Langerhans cells. Immunobiology. 1984;168:301–12.
67. Jaffe R. Pathology of histiocytosis X. Perspect Pediatr Pathol. 1987;9:4–47.
68. Favara BE, McCarthy RC, Mierau GW. Histiocytosis X. Hum Pathol. 1983;14:663–76.
69. McDevitt HO. Regulation of the immune response by the major histocompatibility system. N Engl J Med. 1980;303:1514.
70. Srivastava R, Duceman BW, Biro PA, et al. Molecular organization of the class I genes of human major histocompatibility complex. Immunol Rev. 1985;84:93–120.
71. Bell JI, Denny DW, McDevitt HO. Structure and polymorphism of murine and human class II major histocompatibility antigens. Immunol Rev. 1985;84:52–70.
72. Lee JS, Cohen EB, Hume CR, et al. Organization, polymorphism, and regulation of class II genes of the major histocompatibility complex. Year Immunol. 1986;2:205–21.
73. Bjorkman PJ, Saper MA, Samraoui B, et al. The foreign antigen binding site and T cell recognition regions of class I histocompatibility antigens. Nature. 1987;329:512.

74. Brown JH, Jardetzky T, Saper MA, et al. A hypothetical model of the foreign antigen binding site of class II histocompatibility molecules. Nature. 1988;332:845–50.
75. Glover DM, Brownstein D, Burchett SK, et al. Expression of HLA class II antigens and secretion of interleukin 1 by monocytes and macrophages from adults and neonates. Immunology. 1987;61:195–201.
76. Eckels DD, Lake P, Lamb JR, et al. SB-restricted presentation of influenza and herpes simplex virus antigens to human T-lymphocyte clones. Nature. 1983;301:716–8.
77. Brown MA, Glimcher LA, Nielsen EA, et al. T-cell recognition of Ia molecules selectively altered by a single amino acid substitution. Science 1986;231:255–8.
78. Lyons CR, Ball EJ, Toews GB, et al. Inability of human alveolar macrophages to stimulate resting T cells correlates with decreased antigen-specific T cell macrophage binding. J Immunol. 1986;137:1173–80.
79. Sarvetnick N, Liggitt D, Pitts SL, et al. Insulin-dependent diabetes mellitus induced in transgenic mice by ectopic expression of class II MHC and interferon-gamma. Cell. 1988;52:773–82.
80. Morimoto C, Letvin NL, Distaso JA, et al. The isolation and characterization of the human suppressor inducer T cell subset. J Immunol. 1985;134:1508–15.
81. Morimoto C, Letvin NL, Rudd CE, et al. The role of the 2H4 molecule in the generation of suppressor function in Con A-activated T cells. J Immunol. 1986;137:3247–53.
82. Morimoto C, Letvin NL, Boyd AW, et al. The isolation and characterization of the human helper inducer T cell subset. J Immunol. 1985;134:3762–9.
83. Rudd CE, Morimoto C, Wong LL, et al. The subdivision of the T4 (CD4) subset on the basis of the differential expression of L-C/T200 antigens. J Exp Med. 1987;166:1758–73.
84. Grey HM, Chesnut R. Antigen processing and presentation to T cells. Immunol Today. 1985;6:101–6.
85. Chesnut RW, Grey HM. Antigen presentation by B cells and its significance in T–B interactions. Adv Immunol. 1986;236:3951–94.
86. Unanue ER, Allen PM. The basis for the immunoregulatory role of macrophages and other accessory cells. Science. 1987;236:551–7.
87. Fox BS, Quill H, Carlson L, et al. Quantitative analysis of the T cell response to antigen and planar membranes containing purified Ia molecules. J Immunol. 1987;138:3367–74.
88. Allen PM. Antigen processing at the molecular level. Immunol Today. 1987;8:270–3.
89. Rothbard JB, Taylor WR. A sequence pattern common to T cell epitopes. EMBO J. 1988;7:93–100.
90. Cresswell P. Antigen recognition by T lymphocytes. Immunol Today. 1987;8:67–9.
91. Buus S, Sette A, Colon SM, et al. The relation between major histocompatibility complex (MHC) restriction and the capacity of Ia to bind immunogenic peptides. Science. 1987;235:1353–8.
92. Berzofsky JA. Structural features of protein antigenic sites recognized by helper T cells: What makes a site immunodominant? Year Immunol. 1986;2:28–38.
93. Rothbard JB, Lechler RI, Hoiwland, K, et al. Structural model of HLA-DR1 restricted T cell antigen recognition. Cell. 1988;52:515–23.
94. Buus S, Sette A, Colon SM, et al. Isolation and characterization of antigen–Ia complexes involved in T cell recognition. Cell. 1986;47:1071–7.
95. Rouse BT, Norley S, Martin S. Antiviral cytotoxic T lymphocyte induction and vaccination. Rev Infect Dis. 1988;10:16–33.
96. Yewdell JW, Bennink JR, Hosaka Y. Cells process exogenous proteins for recognition by cytotoxic T lymphocytes. Science. 1988;239:637–40.
97. Maryanski JL, Pala P, Corradin G, et al. H-2-restricted cytolytic T cells specific for HLA can recognize a synthetic HLA peptide. Nature. 1986;324:578–9.
98. Wraith DC. The recognition of influenza A virus-infected cells by cytotoxic T lymphocytes. Immunol Today. 1987;8:239–45
99. Walker BD, Flexner C, Paradis TJ. HIV-1 reverse transcriptase is a target for cytotoxic T lymphocytes in infected individuals. Science. 1988;240:64–6.
100. Bjorkamn PJ, Sasper MA, Samraoui B, et al. Structure of the human class I histocompatibility antigen, HLA-A2. Nature. 1987;329:506–16.
101. Weiss A, Imboden J, Hardy K, et al. The role of the T3/antigen receptor complex in T-cell activation. Ann Rev Immunol. 1986;4:593–619.
102. MacDonald HR. T-cell activation. Ann Rev Cell Biol. 1986;2:231–53.
103. Imboden JB, Weiss A, Stobo JD. The antigen receptor on a human T cell line initiates activation by increasing cytoplasmic free calcium. J Immunol. 1985;134:663–5.
104. Manger B, Weiss A, Imboden J, et al. The role of protein kinase C in transmembrane signaling by the T cell antigen–receptor complex. J Immunol. 1987;139:2755–60.
105. Utsunomiya N, Tsuboi M, Nakanishi M. Early transmembrane events in alloimmune cytotoxic T-lymphocyte activation as revealed by stopped-flow fluorometry. Proc Natl Acad Sci USA. 1986;83:1877–80.
106. Nisbet-Brown E, Cheung RK, Lee JWW, et al. Antigen-dependent increase in cytosolic free calcium in specific human T-lymphocyte clones. Nature. 1985;316:545–7.
107. Rosoff PM, Burakoff SJ, Greenstein JL. The role of the L3T4 molecule in mitogen- and antigen-activated signal transduction. Cell. 1987;49:845–53.
108. Takada S, Engleman EG. Evidence for an association between CD8 molecules and the T cell receptor complex on cytotoxic T cells. J Immunol. 1987;139:3231–5.
109. Leo O, Foo M, Henkart PA, et al. Role of accessory molecules in signal transduction of cytolytic T lymphocyte by anti-T cell receptor and anti-Ly-6.2C monoclonal antibodies. J Immunol. 1987;139:3556–63.
110. Siliciano RF, Pratt JC, Schmidt RE, et al. Activation of cytolytic T lymphocyte and natural killer cell function through the T11 sheep erythrocyte binding protein. Nature 1985;317:428–30.
111. Smith KA. Interleukin 2. Ann Rev Immunol. 1984;2:319–33.
112. Hu-Li J, Shevach EM, Mizuguchi J, et al. B cell stimulatory factor I (interleukin 4) is a potent costimulant for normal resting T lymphocytes. J Exp Med. 1987;165:157–72.
113. Spits H, Yssel H, Takebe Y, et al. Recombinant interleukin 4 promotes the growth of human T cells. J Immunol. 1987;139:1142–7.
114. Beutler B, Cerami A. Cachectin and tumour necrosis factor as two sides of the same biological coin. Nature. 1986;320:584–8.
115. Beutler B, Cerami A. Cachectin: More than a tumor necrosis factor. N Engl J Med. 1987;316:379–85.
116. Dinarello CA, Mier JW. Lymphokines. N Engl J Med. 1987;317:940–5.
117. Dinarello CA. Biology of interleukin 1. FASEB J. 1988;2:108–15.
118. March CJ, Mosley B, Larsen A, et al. Cloning, sequence and expression of two distinct human interleukin-1 complementary DNAs. Nature. 1985; 315:641–7.
119. Bird TA, Saklatvala J. Identification of a common class of high affinity receptors for both types of porcine interleukin-1 on connective tissue cells. Nature. 1986;324:263–6.
120. Dower SK, Kronheim SR, Hopp TP, et al. The cell surface receptors for interleukin-1α and interleukin-β are identical. Nature. 1986;324:266–8.
121. Gray PW, Aggarwal BB, Benton CV, et al. Cloning and expression of cDNA for human lymphotoxin, a lymphokine and tumour necrosis activity. Nature. 1984;312:721–4.
122. Pennica D, Nedwin GE, Hayflick JS, et al. Human tumour necrosis factor: Precursor structure, expression and homology to lymphotoxin. Nature. 1984;312:724–9.
123. Kishimoto T. B-cell stimulatory factors (BSFs): Molecular structure, biological function, and regulation of expression. J Clin Immunol. 1987;7:343–55.
124. Nathan CF. Secretory products of macrophages. J Clin Invest. 1987;79:319–26.
125. Dinarello CA. Interleukin-1: Amino acid sequences, multiple biological activities and comparison with tumor necrosis factor (cachectin). Year Immunol. 1986;2:68–89.
126. Paul WE. Interleukin 4 B cell stimulatory factor 1: One lymphokine, many functions. FASEB J. 1987;1:456–61.
127. Sehgal PB, May LT, Tamm I, et al. Human β^2 interferon and B-cell differentiation factor BSF-2 are identical. Science. 1987;235:731–2.
128. Epstein LB. The comparative biology of immune and classical interferons, in: Cohen S, Pich E, Oppenheim JJ, eds. Biology of the Lymphokines. New York: Academic Press, 1979:443–514.
129. Gray PW, Leung DW, Pennica D, et al. Expression of human immune interferon cDNA in *E. coli* and monkey cells. Nature. 1982;295:503–8.
130. Trinchieri G, Perussia B. Immune interferon: A pleiotropic lymphokine with multiple effects. Immunol Today. 1985;6:131–35
131. Metcalf D. The granulocyte–macrophage colony-stimulating factors. Science. 1985;229:16–22.
132. Sieff CA. Hematopoietic growth factors. J Clin Invest. 1987;79:1549–57.
133. Clark SC, Kamen R. The human hematopoietic colony-stimulating factors. Science. 1987;236:1229–37.
134. Kriegler M, Perez C, DeFay K, et al. A novel form of TNF/cachectin is a cell surface cytotoxic transmembrane protein: Ramifications for the complex physiology of TNF. Cell. 1988;53:45–53.
135. Kaushansky K, Lin N, Adamson JW. Interleukin 1 stimulates fibroblasts to synthesize granulocyte–macrophage and granulocyte colony-stimulating factors. J Clin Invest. 1988;81:92–7.
136. Pistoia V, Cozzolino F, Rubartelli A, et al. In vitro production of interleukin 1 by normal and malignant human B lymphocytes. J Immunol. 1986; 136:1688–92.
137. Nedwin GE, Svedersky LP, Bringman TS, et al. Effect of interleukin 2, interferon-γ and mitogens on the production of tumor necrosis factors α and β. J Immunol. 1985;135:2492–7.
138. Cuturi MC, Murphy M, Costa-Giomi MP, et al. Independent regulation of tumor necrosis factor and lymphotoxin production by human peripheral blood lymphocytes. J Exp Med. 1987;165:1581–94.
139. Hirano T, Yasukawa K, Harada YH, et al. Complementary DNA for a novel human interleukin (BSF-2) that induces B lymphocytes to produce immunoglobulin. Nature. 1986;324:73–6.
140. Burchett SK, Weaver WM, Westall JA, et al. Regulation of tumor necrosis factor/cachectin and interleukin 1 secretion in human mononuclear phagocytes. J Immunol. 1988;140:3473–7.
141. Beutler B, Krochin N, Milsark IW, et al. Control of cachectin (tumor necrosis factor) synthesis: Mechanisms of endotoxin resistance. Science. 1986;232:977–80.
142. Ikejima T, Dinarello CA, Gill DM, et al. Induction of human interleukin-1 by a product of *Staphylococcus aureua* associated with toxic shock syndrome. J Clin Invest. 1984;73:1312–20.
143. Philip RM, Epstein LB. Tumour necrosis factor as immunomodulator and

mediator of monocyte cytotoxicity induced by itself, γ-interferon and interleukin-1. Nature. 1986;323:86–9.
144. Van Damme J, Opdenakker G, Simpson RJ, et al. Identification of the human 26-kD protein, interferon β^2 (IFN-β^2), as a B cell hybridoma/plasmacytoma growth factor induced by interleukin 1 and tumor necrosis factor. J Exp Med. 1987;165:914–9.
145. Tosato G, Seamon KB, Goldman ND, et al. Monocyte-derived human B-cell growth factor identified as interferon-β^2 (BSF-2, IL-6). Science. 1987; 239:502–4.
146. Abb J, Abb H, Deinhardt F. Phenotype of human α-interferon producing leucocytes identified by monoclonal antibodies. Clin Exp Immunol. 1983;52:179–84.
147. Bell DM, Roberts NJ Jr, Hall CB. Different antiviral spectra of human macrophage interferon activities. Nature. 1983;305:319–21.
148. Stevenson HC, Dekaban GA, Miller PJ, et al. Analysis of human blood monocyte activation at the level of gene expression. J Exp Med. 1985;161:503–13.
149. Dinarello CA, Cannon JG, Wolff SM, et al. Tumor necrosis factor (cachectin) is an endogenous pyrogen and induces production of interleukin 1. J Exp Med. 1986;163:1433–50.
150. Broudy VC, Harlan JM, Adamson JW. Disparate effects of tumor necrosis factor-α cachectin and tumor necrosis factor-β lymphotoxin on hematopoietic growth factor production and neutrophil adhesion molecule expression by cultured human endothelial cells. J Immunol. 1987;136:4298–4302.
151. Locksley RM, Heinzel FP, Shepard HM, et al. Tumor necrosis factors α and β differ in their capacities to generate interleukin 1 release from human endothelial cells. J Immunol. 1987;139:1891–5.
152. Kurt-Jones EA, Fiers W, Pober JS. Membrane interleukin 1 induction on human endothelial cells and dermal fibroblasts. J Immunol. 1987;139:2317–24.
153. Munker R, Gasson J, Ogawa M, et al. Recombinant human TNF induces production of granulocyte–monocyte colony-stimulating factor. Nature. 1986;323:79–82.
154. Dinarello CA, Cannon JG, Wolff SM. New concepts on the pathogenesis of fever. Rev Infect Dis. 1988;10:168–89.
155. Cannistra SA, Rambaldi A, Spriggs DR, et al. Human granulocyte–macrophage colony-stimulating factor induces expression of the tumor necrosis factor gene by the U937 cell line and by normal human monocytes. J Clin Invest. 1987;79:1720–8.
156. Herrmann F, Cannistra SA, Griffin JD. T cell–monocyte interactions in the production of humoral factors regulating human granulopoiesis in vitro. J Immunol. 1986;136:2856–61.
157. Horiguchi J, Warren MK, Kufe D. Expression of the macrophage-specific colony-stimulating factor in human monocytes treated with granulocyte–macrophage colony-stimulating factor. Blood. 1987;69:1259–62.
158. Okusawa S, Dinarello CA, Yancey KB, et al. C5a induction of human interleukin 1. J Immunol. 1987;139:2635–40.
159. Crawford GD, Wyler DJ, Dinarello CA. Parasite–monocyte interactions in human leishmaniasis: Production of interleukin-1 in vitro. J Infect Dis 1985;152:315–22.
160. Reiner NE, Behm EA, Ng W, et al. Human monocytes treated with recombinant interferon gamma become responsive to *Leishmania donovani* for the production of interleukin 1 and tumor necrosis factor alpha. Clin Res. 1988;36:468A.
161. Kurt-Jones EA, Virgin HW IV, Unanua ER. In vivo and in vitro expression of macrophage membrane interleukin 1 in response to soluble and particulate stimuli. J Immunol. 1986;137:10–14.
162. Mizel SB. Interleukin 1 and T-cell activation. Immunol Today. 1987;8:330–1.
163. Eden E, Turino GM, Interleukin 1 secretion from huma alveolar macrophages in lung disease. J Clin Immunol. 1986;6:326–33.
164. Goodwin JS, Ceuppens JL, Gualde N. Control of the immune response in humans by prostaglandins. Adv Inflamm Res. 1984;7:79–92.
165. Bernton EW, Beach JE, Holaday JW, et al. Release of multiple hormones by a direct action of interleukin-1 on pituitary cells. Science. 1987;238:519–21.
166. Besedovsky H, del Rey A, Sorkin E, et al. Immunoregulatory feedback between interleukin-1 and glucocorticoid hormones. Science. 1986;233:652–3.
167. Woloski BMRNJ, Smith EM, Meyer WJ III, et al. Corticotropin-releasing activity of monokines. Science. 1985;230:1035–7.
168. Roberts NJ Jr, Prill AH, Mann TN. Interleukin 1 and interleukin 1 inhibitor production by human macrophages exposed to influenza virus or respiratory syncytial virus. J Exp Med. 1986;163:511–9.
169. Fujiwara H, Ellner JJ. Spontaneous production of a suppressor factor by the human macrophage-like cell line U937: I. Suppression of interleukin 1, interleukin 2, and mitogen-induced blastogenesis in mouse thymocytes. J Immunol. 1986;136:181–5.
170. Pennica D, Kohr WJ, Kuang W-J, et al. Identification of human uromodulin as the Tamm-Horsfall urinary glycoprotein. Science. 1987;236:83–8.
171. Jabara HH, Ackerman SJ, Vercelli D, et al. Induction of IgE synthesis and eosinophil differentiation by supernatants of an IL-4, IL-5 producing human helper T cell clone. J Immunol. 1988;140:4211–16.
172. Lewis DB, Prickett K, Larsen A, et al. Restricted production of interleukin-4 by activated T cells. Proc Natl Acad Sci USA. 1988;85:9743–47.
173. Mosmann TR, Cherwinski H, Bond MW, et al. Two types of murine helper T cell clone. I. Definition according to profiles of lymphokine activities and secreted proteins. J Immunol. 1986;136:2348.
174. Cherwinski HM, Schumacher JH, Brown KD, et al. Two types of mouse helper T cell clone. III. Further differences in lymphokine synthesis between Th1 and Th2 clones revealed by RNA hybridization, functionally monospecific bioassays, and monoclonal antibodies. J Exp Med. 1987;166:1229–44.
175. Kurt-Jones EA, Hamberg S, Ohara J, et al. Heterogeneity of helper/inducer T lymphcoytes. I. Lymphokine production and lymphokine responsiveness. J Exp Med. 1987;166:1774–87.
176. Yokota T, Coffman TL, Hagiwara H, et al. Isolation and characterization of lymphokine cDNA clones encoding mouse and human IgA-enhancing factor and eosinophil colony-stimulating factor activities: Relationship to interleukin 5. Proc Natl Acad Sci USA. 1987;84:7388–92.
177. Snapper CM, Paul WE. Interferon-γ and B cell stimulatory factor-1 reciprocally regulate Ig isotype production. Science. 1987;236:944–7.
178. Arthur RP, Mason D. T cells that help B cell responses to soluble antigen are distinguishable from those producing interleukin 2 on mitogenic or allogeneic stimulation. J Exp Med. 1986;163:774–6.
179. Luger TA, Smolen JS, Chused TM, et al. Human lymphocytes with either the OKT4 and OKT8 phenotype produce interleukin 2 in culture. J Clin Invest. 1982;70:470–3.
180. Mizuochi T, Ono S, Malek TR, et al. Characterization of two distinct primary T cell populations that secrete interleukin 2 upon recognition of class I or class II major histocompatibility antigens. J Exp Med. 1986;163:603–19.
181. Kasahara T, Hooks JJ, Dougherty SF, et al. Interleukin-2-mediated immune interferon (IFN-γ) production by human T cells and T cell subsets. J Immunol. 1983;130:1784–9.
182. Vilcek J, Henriksen-Destefano D, Siegal D, et al. Regulation of IFN-γ induction in human peripheral blood cells by exogenous and endogenously produced interleukin 2. J Immunol. 1985;135:1851–6.
183. Kelly CD, Welte K, Murray HW. Antigen-induced human interferon-γ production. Differential dependence on interleukin 2 and its receptor. J Immunol. 1987;139:2325–8.
184. Smith KA, Lachman LB, Oppenheim JJ, et al. The functional relationship of the interleukins. J Exp Med. 1980;151:1551–6.
185. Hagiwara H, Huang H-JS, Arai N, et al. Interleukin 1 modulates messenger RNA levels of lymphokines and of other molecules associated with T cells activation in the T cell lymphoma LBRM33-1A5. J Immunol. 1987;138:2514–9.
186. Scheurich P, Thoma B, Ucer U, et al. Immunoregulatory activity of recombinant human tumor necrosis factor (TNF)-α: Induction of TNF receptors on human T cells and TNF-α-mediated enhancement of T cell responses. J Immunol. 1987;138:1786–90.
187. Jenkins MK, Pardoll DM, Mizuguchi J, et al. Molecular events in the induction of a nonresponsive state in interleukin 2-producing helper T-lymphocyte clones. Proc Natl Acad Sci USA. 1987;84:5409–13.
188. Heckford SE, Gelmann EP, Agnor CL, et al. Distinct signals are required for proliferation and lymphokine gene expression in murine T cell clones. J Immunol. 1986;137:3652–63.
189. Rola-Pleszczynski M. Immunoregulation by leukotrienes and other lipoxygenase metabolites. Immunol Today. 1985;6:302–7.
190. Harris DT, Kozumbo WJ, Cerutti P, et al. Molecular mechanisms involved in T cell activation. I. Evidence for independent signal-transducing pathways in lymphokine production vs proliferation in cloned cytotoxic T lymphocytes. J Immunol. 1987;138:600–5.
191. Otten G, Herold KC, Fitch FW. Interleukin 2 inhibits antigen-stimulated lymphokine synthesis in helper T cells by inhibiting calcium-dependent signalling. J Immunol. 1987;139:1348–53.
192. Derynck R, Harrett JA, Chen EY, et al. Human transforming growth factor-β-complementary DNA sequence and expression in normal and transformed cells. Nature. 1985;316:701–5.
193. Kehrl JH, Wakefield LM, Roberts AB, et al. Production of transforming growth factor β by human T lymphocytes and its potential role in the regulation of T cell growth. J Exp Med. 1986;163:1037–50.
194. Wolf M, Falk W, Mannel D, et al. Inhibition of interleukin 2 production by prostaglandin E_2^- is not absolute but depends on the strength of the stimulating signal. Cell Immunol. 1985;90:190–5.
195. Rigby WFC. The immunobiology of vitamin D. Immunol Today. 1988;9:54–6.
196. Peters PM, Ortaldo JR, Shalaby R, et al. Natural killer-sensitive targets stimulate production of TNF-α but not TNF-β (lymphotoxin) by highly purified human peripheral blood large granular lymphocytes. J Immunol. 1986;137:2592–8.
197. Munakata T, Semba U, Shibuya Y, et al. Induction of interferon-γ production by human natural killer cells stimulated by hydrogen peroxide. J Immunol. 1985;134:2449–51.
198. Bickel M, Amstad P, Tsuda H, et al. Induction of granulocyte–macrophage colony-stimulating factor by lipopolysaccharide and anti-immunoglobulin M-stimulated murine B cell lines. J Immunol. 1987;139:2984–8.
199. Mackowiak PA. Direct effects of hyperthermia on pathogenic microorganisms: Teleologic implications with regard to fever. Rev Infect Dis. 1981;3:508–20.
200. Roberts NJ Jr. Temperature and host defense. Microbiol Rev. 1979;43:241–59.
201. Marx JL. Orphan interferon finds a new home. Science. 1988;239:25–6.
202. Perlmutter DH, Goldberger G, Dinarello CA, et al. Regulation of class III

major histocompatibility complex gene products by interleukin-1. Science. 1986;232:850–2.
203. Perlmutter DH, Dinarello CA, Punsal PI, et al. Cachectin/tumor necrosis regulates hepatic acute-phase gene expression. J Clin Invest. 1986;78:1349–54.
204. Baumann H, Richards C, Gauldie J. Interaction among hepatocyte-stimulating factors, interleukin 1, and glucocorticoids for regulation of acute phase plasma proteins in human hepatoma (HepG2) cells. J Immunol. 1987;139:4122–8.
205. Beutler BA, Cerami A. Recombinant interleukin 1 suppresses lipoprotein lipase activity in 3T3-L1 cells. J Immunol. 1985;135:3969–71.
206. Oliff A, Defeo-Jones D, Boyer M, et al. Tumors secreting human TNF/cachectin induce cachexia in mice. Cell. 1987;50:555–63.
207. Dustin ML, Rothlein R, Bhan AK, et al. Induction by IL 1 and interferon-γ: Tissue distribution, biochemistry, and function of a natural adherence molecule (ICAM-1). J Immunol. 1986;137:245–54.
208. Gamble JR, Harlan JM, Klebanoff SJ, et al. Stimulation of the adherence of neutrophils to umbilical vein endothelium by human recombinant tumor necrosis factor. Proc Natl Acad Sci USA. 1985;82:8667–71.
209. Pohlman TH, Stanness KA, Beatty PG, et al. An endothelial cell surface factor(s) induced in vitro by lipopolysaccharide, interleukin 1 and tumor necrosis factor-α increases neutrophil adherence by a CDw18-dependent mechanism. J Immunol. 1986;136:4548–53.
210. Nawroth PP, Stern DM. Modulation of endothelial cell hemostatic properties by tumor necrosis factor. J Exp Med. 1986;163:740–5.
211. Bevilacqua MP, Pober JS, Majeau GR, et al. Recombinant tumor necrosis factor induces procoagulant activity in cultured human vascular endothelium: Characterization and comparison with the actions of interleukin 1. Proc Natl Acad Sci USA. 1986;83:4533–7.
212. Tracey KJ, Beutler B, Lowry SF, et al. Shock and tissue injury induced by recombinant human cachectin. Science. 1986;234:470–4.
213. Tracey KJ, Fong Y, Hesse DG, et al. Anti-cachectin/TNF monoclonal antibodies prevent septic shock during lethal bacteraemia. Nature. 1987;330:662–4.
214. Rothstein JL, Schreiber H. Synergy between tumor necrosis factor and bacterial products causes hemorrhagic necrosis and lethal shock in normal mice. Proc Natl Acad Sci USA. 1988;85:607–11.
215. Billiau A. Not just cachectin involved in toxic shock. Nature. 1988;331:665.
216. Kettelhut IC, Fiers W, Goldberg AL. The toxic effects of tumor necrosis factor in vivo and their prevention by cyclooxygenase inhibitors. Proc Natl Acad Sci USA. 1987;84:4273–7.
217. Neta R, Oppenheim JJ, Douches SD. Interdependence of the radioprotective effects of human recombinant interleukin 1α, tumor necrosis factor α, granulocyte colony-stimulating factor, and murine recombinant granulocyte–macrophage colony-stimulating factor. J Immunol. 1988;140:108–11.
218. Mochizuki DY, Eisenman JR, Conlon PJ, et al. Interleukin 1 regulates hematopoietic activity, a role previously ascribed to hemopoietin 1. Proc Natl Acad Sci USA. 1987;84:5267–71.
219. Ikebuchi K, Wong GG, Clark SC, et al. Interleukin 6 enhancement of interleukin 3-dependent proliferation of multipotential hemopoietic progenitors. Proc Natl Acad Sci USA. 1987;84:9035–9.
220. Yang Y-C, Ciarletta AB, Temple PA, et al. Human IL-3 (Multi-CSF): Identification by expression cloning of a novel hematopoietic growth factor related to murine IL-3, Cell. 1986;47:3–10.
221. Vadhan-Raj S, Keating M, LeMaistre A, et al. Effects of recombinant human granulocyte–macrophage colony-stimulating factor in patients with myelodysplastic syndromes. N Engl J Med. 1987;317:1545–52.
222. Caracciolo D, Shirsat N, Wong GG, et al. Recombinant human macrophage colony-stimulating factor (M-CSF) requires subliminal concentrations of granulocyte–macrophage (GM) CSF for optimal subliminal concentrations of granulocyte–macrophage (GM) CSF for optimal stimulation of human macrophage colony formation in vitro. J Exp Med. 1987;166:1851–60.
223. Welte K, Bonilla MA, Gillio AP, et al. Recombinant human granulocyte colony-stimulating factor. J Exp Med. 1987;165:941–8.
224. Souza LM, Boone TC, Gabrilove J, et al. Recombinant human granulocyte colony-stimulating factor: Effects on normal and leukemic myeloid cells. Science. 1986;232:61–5.
225. Weaver CT, Unanue ER. T cell induction of membrane IL 1 on macrophages. J Immunol. 1986;137:3868–73.
226. Leonard WJ, Depper JM, Crabtree GR, et al. Molecular cloning and expression of cDNAs for the human interleukin-2 receptor. Nature. 1984;311:626–31.
227. Sharon M, Klausner RD, Cullen BR, et al. Novel interleukin-2 receptor subunit detected by cross-linking under high-affinity conditions. Science. 1986;234:859–63.
228. Teshigawara K, Wang H-M, Kato K, et al. Interleukin 2 high-affinity receptor expression requires two distinct binding proteins. J Exp Med. 1987;165:223–38.
229. Tsudo M, Kozak RW, Goldman CK, et al. Demonstration of a non-Tac peptide that binds interleukin 2: A potential participant in a multichain interleukin 2 receptor complex. Proc Natl Acad Sci USA. 1986;83:9693–8.
230. Lowenthal JW, Greene WC. Contrasting interleukin 2 binding properties of the α (p55) and β (p70) protein subunits of the human high-affinity interleukin 2 receptor. J Exp Med. 1987;166:1156–61.
231. Wang H-M, Smith KA. The interleukin 2 receptor. J Exp Med. 1987;166:1055–69.
232. Lotz M, Jirik F, Kabouridis P, et al. B cell stimulating factor 2/interleukin 6 is a costimulant for human thymocytes and T lymphocytes. J Exp Med. 1988;167:1253–8.
233. O'Garra A, Umland Sh, De France T, et al. "B-cell factors" are pleiotropic. Immunol Today. 1988;9:45–54.
234. Stein P, Dubois P, Greenblatt D, et al. Induction of antigen-specific proliferation in affinity-purified small B lymphocytes: Requirement for BSF-1 by type 2 but not type 1 thymus-independent antigens. J Immunol. 1986;136:2080–9.
235. Krusemeier M, Snow EC. Induction of lymphokine responsiveness of hapten-specific B lymphocytes promoted through an antigen-mediated T helper lymphocyte interaction. J Immunol. 1988;140:367–75.
236. Brian AA. Stimulation of B-cell proliferation by membrane-associated molecules from activated T cells. Proc Natl Acad Sci USA. 1988;85:564–8.
237. Asano Y, Nakayam T, Kubo M, et al. Analysis of two distinct B cell activation pathways mediated by a monoclonal T helper cell. II. T helper cell secretion of interleukin 4 selectively inhibits antigen-specific B cell activation by cognate, but not noncognate, interactions with T cells. J Immunol. 1988;140:419–26.
238. Sanders VM, Fernandez-Botran R, Uhr JW, et al. Interleukin 4 enhances the ability of antigen-specific B cells to form conjugates with T cells. J Immunol. 1987;139:2349–54.
239. Bich-Thuy L, Fauci AS. Recombinant interleukin 2 and gamma-interferon act synergistically on distinct steps of in vitro terminal human B cell maturation. J Clin Invest. 1986;77:1173–9.
240. Jelinek DF, Lipsky PE. Comparative activation requirements of human peripheral blood, spleen, and lymph node B cells. J Immunol. 1987;139:1005–13.
241. Pike BL, Raubitschek A, Nossal GJV. Human interleukin 2 can promote the growth and differentiation of single hapten-specific B cells in the presence of specific antigen. Proc Natl Acad Sci USA. 1984;81:7917–21.
242. Mingari MC, Gerosa F, Carra G, et al. Human interleukin-2 promotes proliferation of activated B cells via surface receptors similar to those of activated T cells. Nature. 1984;312:641–3.
243. Defrance T, Vanbervliet B, Aubry J-P, et al. B cell growth-promoting activity of recombinant human interleukin 4. J Immunol. 1987;139:1135–41.
244. Yokota T, Otsuka T, Mosmann T, et al. Isolation and characterization of a human interleukin cDNA clone, homologous to mouse B-cell stimulatory factor 1, that expresses B-cell- and T-cell-stimulating activities. Proc Natl Acad Sci USA. 1986;83:5894–8.
245. Kehrl JH, Miller A, Fauci AS. Effect of tumor necrosis factor α on mitogen-activated human B cells. J Exp Med. 1987;166:786–91.
246. Kehrl JH, Alvarez-Mon M, Delsing GA, et al. Lymphotoxin is an important T cell-derived growth factor for human B cells. Science. 1987;238:1144–6.
247. Pike BL, Nossal GJB. Interleukin 1 can act as a B-cell growth and differentiation factor. Proc Natl Acad Sci USA. 1985;82:8153–7.
248. Defrance T, Aubry J-P, Vanbervliet B, et al. Human interferon-γ acts as a B cell growth factor in the anti-IgM antibody co-stimulatory assay but has no direct B cell differentiation activity. J Immunol. 1986;137:3861–7.
249. Kawano M, Hirano T, Matsuda T, et al. Autocrine generation and requirement of BSF-2/IL-6 for human multiple myelomas. Nature. 1988;332:83–5.
250. Poupart P, Vandenabeele P, Cayphas S, et al. B cell growth modulating and differentiating activity of recombinant human 26-kd protein (BSF-2, HuIFN-β^2, HPGF). EMBO J. 1987;6:1219–24.
251. Azuma C, Tanabe T, Konishi M, et al. Cloning of cDNA for human T-cell replacing factor (interleukin-5) and comparison with the murine homologue. Nucleic Acid Res. 1986;14:9149–58.
252. Stein P, Dubois P, Greenblatt D, et al. Induction of antigen-specific proliferation in affinity-purified small B lymphocytes: Requirement for BSF-1 by type 2 but not type 1 thymus-independent antigens. J Immunol. 1986;136:2080–9.
253. Reinherz EL, Schlossmann SF. Regulation of the immune response: Inducer and suppressor T lymphocyte subsets in man. N Engl J Med. 1980;303:370.
254. Reinherz EL, Kung PC, Goldstein G, et al. A monoclonal antibody reactive with the human cytotoxic/suppressor T cell subset previously defined by heteroantiserum termed TH^2. J Immunol. 1980;124:1301.
255. Thomas Y, Sosman J, Irigoyen O, et al. Functional analysis of human T cell subsets defined by monoclonal antibodies. I. Collaborative T–T interactions in the immunoregulation of B cell differentiation. J Immunol. 1980;125:2402.
256. Ledbetter J, Evans RL, Lipinski M, et al. Evolutionary conservation of surface molecules that distinguish T lymphocyte inducer and cytotoxic/suppressor subpopulations in mouse and man. J Exp Med. 1981;153:310.
257. Damle NK, Childs AL, Doyle LV. Immunoregulatory T lymphocytes in man: Soluble antigen-specific suppressor inducer T lymphocytes are derived from the CD4 CD45R p80 subpopulation. J Immunol. 1987;139:1501–8.
258. Takeuchi T, Rudd CE, Schlossman SF, et al. Induction of suppression following autologous mixed lymphocyte reaction; role of a novel 2H4 antigen. Eur J Immunol. 1987;17:97–103.
259. Morimoto C, Letvin NL, Distaso JA, et al. The cellular basis for the induction of antigen-specific T8 suppressor cells. Eur J Immunol. 1986;16:198–204.
260. Damle NK. Suppressor T lymphocytes in man. Year Immunol. 1986;2:60–7.
261. Ellner JJ. Suppressor cells of man. Clin Immunol Dev. 1981;1:119–41.
262. Damle NK, Childs AL, Doyle LV. Immunoregulatory T lymphocytes in man. Soluble antigen-specific suppressor-inducer T lymphocytes are derived from the CD4 CD45R p80 subpopulation. J Immunol. 1987;139:1501–8.

263. Green DR, Flood PM, Gershon RK. Immunoregulatory T-cell pathways. Ann Rev Immunol. 1983;1:439–64.
264. Sathish M, Bhutani LK, Sharma AK, et al. Monocyte-derived soluble suppressor factor(s) in patients with lepromatous leprosy. Infect Immun. 1983;42:890–9.
265. Kapp JA, Pierce CW, Sorensen CM. Antigen-specific suppressor T-cell factors. Hosp Pract. 1984;19-8:85–98.
266. Espevik T, Figari IS, Shalaby MR, et al. Inhibition of cytokine production by cyclosporin A and transforming growth factor β. J Exp Med. 1987; 166:571–6.
267. Lee G, Ellingsworth LR, Gillis S, et al. β Transforming growth factors are potential regulators of B lymphopoiesis. J Exp Med. 1987;166:1290–9.
268. Schnaper HW, Pierce CW, Aune TM. Identification and initial characterization of concanavalin A- and interferon-induced human suppressor factors: Evidence for a human equivalent of murine soluble immune response suppressor (SIRS). J Immunol. 1984;132:2429–35.
269. Laurence J, Mayer L. Immunoregulatory lymphokines of T hybridomas from AIDS patients: Constitutive and inducible suppressor factors. Science. 1984;225:66–9.
270. Aune TM. Inhibition of soluble immune response suppressor activity by growth factors. Proc Natl Acad Sci USA. 1985;82:6260–4.
271. Chouaib S, Chatenoud L, Klatzmann D, et al. The mechanisms of inhibition of human IL2 production. II. PGE_2 induction of suppressor T lymphocytes. J Immunol. 1984;132:1851–7.
272. Gromo G, Geller RL, Inverardi L, et al. Signal requirements in the stepwise functional maturation of cytotoxic T lymphocytes. Nature. 1987;327:424–6.
273. Gately MK, Wilson DE, Wong HL. Synergy between recombinant interleukin 2 (rIL 2) and IL 2-depleted lymphokine-containing supernatants in facilitating allogeneic human cytolytic T lymphocyte responses in vitro. J Immunol. 1986;136:1274–82.
274. Hefeneider SH, Conlon PJ, Henney CS, et al. In vivo interleukin 2 administration augments the generation of alloreactive cytolytic T lymphocytes and resident natural killer cells. J Immunol. 1983;130:222–7.
275. Widmer MB, Grabstein KH. Regulation of cytolytic T-lymphocyte generation by B-cell stimulatory factor. Nature. 1987;326:795–8.
276. Widmer MB, Acres RB, Sassenfeld HM, et al. Regulation of cytolytic cell populations from human peripheral blood by B cell stimulatory factor 1 (interleukin 4). J Exp Med. 1987;166:1447–55.
277. Pfeifer JD, McKenzie DT, Swain SL, et al. B cell stimulatory factor 1 (interleukin 4) is sufficient for the proliferation and differentiation of lectin-stimulated cytolytic T lymphocyte precursors. J Exp Med. 1987;166:1464–70.
278. Takai Y, Wong GG, Clark SC, et al. B cell stimulatory factor-2 is involved in the differentiation of cytotoxic T lymphocytes. J Immunol. 1988;140:508–12.
279. Park LS, Friend D, Sassenfeld HM, et al. Characterization of the human B cell stimulatory factor 1 receptor. J Exp Med. 1987;166:476–88.
280. Podack ER. Molecular mechanisms of cytolysis by complement and by cytolytic lymphocytes. J Cell Biochem. 1986;30:133–70.
281. Young JDE, Hengartner H, Podack ER, et al. Purification and characterization of a cytolytic pore-forming protein from granules of cloned lymphocytes with natural killer activity. Cell. 1986;44:849–59.
282. Martin DE, Zalman LS, Jung G, et al. Induction of synthesis of the cytolytic C9 (ninth component of complement)-related protein in human peripheral mononuclear cells by monoclonal antibody OKT3 or interleukin 2: Correlation with cytotoxicity and lymphocyte phenotype. Proc Natl Acad Sci USA. 1987;84:2946–50.
283. Masson D, Tschopp J. A family of serine esterases in lytic granules of cytolytic T lymphocytes. Cell. 1987;49:679–85.
284. Garcia-Sanz JA, Plaetinck G, Velotti F, et al. Perforin is present only in normal activated Lyt2 T lymphocytes and not in L3T4 cells, but the serine protease granzyme A is made by both subsets. EMBO J. 1987;6:933–8.
285. Young JD-E, Liu C-C. How do cytotoxic T lymphocytes avoid self-lysis? Immunol Today. 1988;9:14–15.
286. Dennert G, Anderson CG, Prochazka G. High activity of *N*-benzyloxycarbonyl-L-lysine thiobenzyl ester serine esterase and cytolytic perforin in cloned cell lines is not demonstrable in in vivo-induced cytotoxic effector cells. Proc Natl Acad Sci USA. 1987;84:5004–8.
287. Lanier LL, Le AM, Civin CI, et al. The relationship of CD16 (LEU-11) and LEU-19 (NKH-1) antigen expression on human peripheral blood NK cells and cytotoxic T lymphocytes. J Immunol. 1986;136:4480–6.
288. Lanier LL, Kipps TJ, Phillips JH. Functional properties of a unique subset of cytotoxic CD3 lymphocytes that express Fc receptors for IgG (CD16/LEU-11 antigen). J Exp Med. 1985;162:2089–2106.
289. Lanier LL, Cwirla S, Federspiel N, et al. Human natural killer cells isolated from peripheral blood do not rearrange T cell antigen receptor β chain genes. J Exp Med. 1986;163:209–14.
290. Hackett J, Bosma GC, Bosma MJ, et al. Transplantable progenitors of natural killer cells are distinct from those of T and B lymphocytes. Proc Natl Acad Sci USA. 1986;83:3427–31.
291. Ritz J, Campen TJ, Schmidt RE. Analysis of T-cell receptor gene rearrangement and expression in human natural killer clones. Science. 1985;228:1540–3.
292. Bensussen A, Tourveille B, Chen LI, et al. Phorbol ester induces a differential effect on the effector function of human allospecific cytotoxic T lymphcyte and natural killer clones. Immunology 1985;66:42–6.
293. Herberman RB, Ortaldo JR. Natural killer cells: Their role in defenses against disease. Science. 1981;214:24–30.
294. Bellan AH, Quilct A, Marchiol C, et al. Natural killer susceptibility of human cells may be regulated by genes in the HLA region on chromosome 6. Proc Natl Acad Sci USA. 1986;83:5688–92.
295. Stern P, Gidlund M, Orn A, et al. Natural killer cells mediate lysis of embryonal carcinoma cells lacking MHC. Nature. 1980;285:341–2.
296. Springer TA, Anderson DC. The importance of the Mac-1, LFA-1, glycoprotein family in monocyte and granulocyte adherence, chemotaxis, and migration into inflammatory sites: Insights from an experiment of nature. Ciba Found Symp. 1986;118:102–26.
297. Bukowski JF, Warner JR, Dennert G, et al. Adoptive transfer studies demonstrating the antiviral effect of natural killer cells in vivo. J Exp Med. 1985;161:40–52.
298. Kohl S. Herpes simplex virus immunology: Problems, progress and promises. J Infect Dis. 1985;152:435–40.
299. Hauser WE, Tsai V. Acute toxoplasma infection of mice induces spleen NK cells that are cytotoxic for *T. gondii* in vitro. J Immunol. 1986;136:313–9.
300. Seki H, Ueno Y, Taga K, et al. Mode of in vitro augmentation of natural killer cell activity by recombinant human interleukin 2: A comparative study of LEU-11$^+$ and LEU-11$^-$ cell populations in cord blood and adult peripheral blood. J Immunol. 1985;135:2351–6.
301. Herberman RB, Ortaldo JR, Mantovani A, et al. Effect of human recombinant interferon on cytotoxic activity of natural killer (NK) cells and monocytes. Cell Immunol. 1982;67:160–7.
302. Targan S, Stebbing N. In vitro interactions of purified cloned human interferons on NK cells: Enhanced activation. J Immunol. 1982;129:934–5.
303. Shah PD, Gilbertson SM, Rowley DA. Dendritic cells that have interacted with antigen are targets for natural killer cells. J Exp Med. 1985;162:625–36.
304. Callewaert DM. Purification and characterization of NK cells. In: Herberman R, ed. Mechanisms of Cytotoxicity by NK Cells. New York: Academic Press, 1985:17–28.
305. Starr SE, Garrabrant T. Natural killing of cytomegalovirus-infected fibroblasts by human mononuclear leucocytes. Clin Exp Immunol. 1981;46:484–92.
306. Lopez CC. Natural killing of herpes simplex virus type 1-infected target cells: normal human responses and influence of antiviral antibody. Infect Immun. 1979;26:49.
307. Kohl S, Shaban SS, Starr SE, et al. Human neonatal and maternal monocyte–macrophage and lymphocyte-mediated antibody-dependent cytotoxicity to cells infected with herpes simplex. J Pediatr. 1978;93:206–10.
308. Johnston RB Jr. Monocytes and macrophages. N Engl J Med. 1988;318:747–52.
309. Pfefferkorn ER. Interferon-γ blocks the growth of *Toxoplasma gondii* in human fibroblasts by inducing the host cells to degrade tryptophan. Proc Natl Acad Sci USA. 1984;81:908–12.
310. Mackaness GB. The immunological basis of acquired cellular immunity. J Exp Med. 1964;120:105–20.
311. McLeod RE, Wing J, Remington JS. Lymphocytes and macrophages in cell-mediated immunity. In: Mandell GL, Douglas RG Jr, Bennett JE, eds. Principles and Practice of Infectious Diseases. 2nd ed. New York: Churchill Livingstone; 1985:72–93.
312. Hamilton TA, Adams DO. Molecular mechanisms of signal transduction in macrophages. Immunol Today. 1987;8:151–8.
313. Murray HW, Rubin BY, Rothermel CD. Killing of intracellular *Leishmania donovani* by lymphokine-stimulated human mononuclear phagocytes. J Clin Invest. 1983;72:1506–10.
314. Wilson CB, Haas JE. Cellular defenses against *Toxoplasma gondii* in newborns. J Clin Invest. 1984;73:1606–16.
315. Wilson CB, Westall J. Activation of neonatal and adult human macrophages by alpha, beta, and gamma interferons. Infect Immun. 1985;49:351–6.
316. Nathan CF, Prendergast TJ, Wiebe ME, et al. Activation of human macrophages. Comparison of other cytokines with interferon-γ. J Exp Med. 1984;160:600–5.
317. Roberts WK, Vasil A. Evidence for the identity of murine gamma interferon and macrophage activating factor. J Interferon Res. 1982;2:519–32.
318. Edwards CK III, Hedegaard HB, Zlotnik A, et al. Chronic infection due to *Mycobacterium intracellulare* in mice: Association with macrophage release of prostaglandin E_2 and reversal by injection of indomethacin, muramyl dipeptide, or interferon-gamma. J Immunol. 1986;136:1820–7.
319. McCabe RE, Luft BJ, Remington JS. Effect of murine interferon-γ on murine toxoplasmosis. J Infect Dis. 1984;150:961–2.
320. Khor M, Lowrie DB, Coates AR, et al. Recombinant interferon-gamma and chemotherapy with isoniazid and rifampicin in experimental murine tuberculosis. Br J Exp Pathol. 1986;67:587–96.
321. Murray HW, Stern JJ, Welte K, et al. Experimental visceral leishmaniasis: Production of interleukin 2 and interferon-γ, tissue immune reaction, and response to treatment with interleukin 2 and interferon-γ. J Immunol. 1987;138:2290–7.
322. Gould CL, Sonnenfeld G. Effect of treatment with interferon-gamma and concanavalin A on the course of infection of mice with *Salmonella typhimurium* strain LT-2. J Interferon Res. 1987;7:255–60.
323. Anthony LSD, Ghadirian E, Kongshavn PAL. Effect of gamma-interferon treatment on the resistance of mice to experimental tularemia (Abstract). J Leukocyte Biol. 1987;42:415.
324. Buchmeier NA, Schreiber RD. Requirement of endogenous interferon-

gamma production for resolution of *Listeria monocytogenes* infection. Proc Natl Acad Sci USA. 1985;82:7404–8.
325. Squires KE, Schreiber RD, McElrath MJ, et al. Role of endogenous interferon-γ in murine visceral leishmaniasis (Abstract). Clin Res. 1987;35:492.
326. Suzuki Y, Orellana MA, Schreiber RD, et al. Interferon-γ: The major mediator of resistance against *Toxoplasma gondii*. Science. 1988;240:516–8.
327. Li H, Jerrells TR, Spitalny GL, et al. Gamma interferon as a crucial host defense against *Rickettsia conorii* in vivo. Infect Immun. 1987;55:1252–5.
328. De Titto E, Catterall JR, Remington JS. Activity of recombinant tumor necrosis factor on *Toxoplasma gondii* and *Trypanosoma cruzi*. J Immunol. 1986;1342–5.
329. Bermudez LEM, Young LS. Tumor necrosis factor, alone or in combination with IL-2, but not IFN-γ, is associated with macrophage killing of *Mycobacterium avium* complex. J Immunol. 1988;140:3006–13.
330. Reed SG, Nathan CF, Pihl DL, et al. Recombinant granulocyte/macrophage colony-stimulating factor activates macrophages to inhibit *Trypanosoma cruzi* and release hydrogen peroxide. J Exp Med. 1987;166:1734–46.
331. Handman E, Burgess AW. Stimulation by granulocyte–macrophage colony-stimulating factor of *Leishmania tropica* killing by macrophages. J Immunol. 1979;22:1134–7.
332. Weiser WY, Van Niel A, Clark SC, et al. Recombinant human granulocyte/macrophage colony-stimulating factor activates intracellular killing of *Leishmania donovani* by human monocyte-derived macrophages. J Exp Med. 1987;166:1436–46.
333. Byrne GI, Lehmann LK, Landry GJ. Induction of tryptophan catabolism is the mechanism for gamma-interferon-mediated inhibition of intracellular *Chlamydia psittaci* replication in T24 cells. Infect Immun. 1986;53:347–51.
334. Niesel DW, Hess CB, Cho YJ, et al. Natural and recombinant interferons inhibit epithelial cell invasion by *Shigella* spp. Infect Immun. 1986;52:828–33.
335. Byrd TF, Horwitz MA. Intracellular multiplication of *Legionella pneumophila* in human monocytes is iron-dependent and the capacity of activated monocytes to inhibit intracellular multiplication is reversed by iron-transferrin (Abstract). Clin Res. 1987;35:613.
336. Granger DL, Hibbs JB Jr, Perfect JR, et al. Specific amino acid requirement for the microbistatic activity of murine macrophages. J Clin Invest. 1988;81:1129–36.
337. Frenkel JK. Adoptive immunity of intracellular infection. J Immunol. 1966;98:1309–19.
338. Luft BJ, Brooks RG, Conley FK, et al. Toxoplasmic encephalitis in patients with acquired immune deficiency syndrome. JAMA. 1984;252:913–7.
339. Vollmer TL, Waldor MK, Steinman L, et al. Depletion of T-4 lymphocytes with monoclonal antibody reactivates toxoplasmosis in the central nervous system: A model of superinfection in AIDS. J Immunol. 1987;138:3737–41.
340. Sansonetti P, Lagrange PH. The immunology of leprosy: Speculations on the leprosy spectrum. Rev Infect Dis. 1981;3:422–69.
341. Nathan CF, Kaplan G, Levis W, et al. Local and systemic effects of intradermal recombinant interferon-γ in patients with lepromatous leprosy. N Engl J Med. 1986;315:6–15.
342. Modlin RL, Hofman RM, Horwitz DA, et al. In situ identification of cells in human leprosy granulomas with monoclonal antibodies to interleukin 2 and its receptor. J Immunol. 1984;132:3085–90.
343. Modlin RL, Melancon-Kaplan J, Young SMM, et al. Learning from lesions: Patterns of tissue inflammation in leprosy. Proc Natl Acad Sci USA. 1988;85:1213–7.
344. Haregewoin A, Godal T, Mustafa AS, et al. T-cell conditioned media reverse T-cell unresponsiveness in lepromatous leprosy. Nature. 1983;303:342–4.
345. Nogueira N, Kaplan G, Levy E, et al. Defective γ interferon production in leprosy. J Exp Med. 1983;158:2165–70.
346. van Dissel JT, Stikkelbroeck JM, van den Barselaar MT, et al. Divergent changes in antimicrobial activity after immunologic activation of mouse peritoneal macrophages. J Immunol. 1987;139:1665–72.
347. van Dissel JT, Stikkelbroeck JM, Michel BC, et al. Inability of recombinant interferon-γ to activate the antibacterial activity of mouse peritoneal macrophages against *Listeria monocytogenes* and *Salmonella typhimurium*. J Immunol. 1987;139:1673–8.
348. Wilson CB, Tsai V, Remington JS. Failure to trigger the oxidative metabolic burst by normal macrophages. J Exp Med. 1980;151:328–46.
349. Pearson RD, Wheeler DA, Harrison LH, et al. The immunobiology of *Leishmania*. Rev Infect Dis. 1983;5:907–27.
350. Cheers C, Haigh AM, Kelso A, et al. Production of colony-stimulating factors (CSFs) during infection: Separate determinations of macrophage-, granulocyte-, granulocyte macrophage-, and multi-CSFs. Infect Immun. 1988;56:247–51.
351. Magee DM, Wing EJ. Antigen-specific production of colony-stimulating factors by *Listeria monocytogenes*-immune, L3T4-positive cells. J Infect Dis. 1988;157:941–9.
352. Wing EJ, Ampel NM, Waheed A, et al. Macrophage colony-stimulating factor (M-CSF) enhances the capacity of murine macrophages to secrete oxygen reduction products. J Immunol. 1985;135:2052–6.
353. Kaufmann SHE. Possible role of helper and cytolytic T lymphocytes in antibacterial defense: Conclusions based on a murine model of listeriosis. Rev Infect Dis. 1987;9(S5):S650–9.
354. Moulder JW. Comparative biology of intracellular parasitism. Microbiol Rev. 1985;49:298–337.
355. Murray HW. How protozoa evade intracellular killing. Ann Intern Med. 1983;98:1016–8.
356. Wilson CB, Haas JE. Cellular defenses against *Toxoplasma gondii* in newborns. J Clin Invest. 1984;73:1606 16.
357. MacKay RJ, Russell SW. Protein changes associated with stages of activation of mouse macrophages for tumor cell killing. J Immunol. 1986;137:1392–8.
358. Deem RL, Doughty FA, Beaman BL. Immunologically specific direct T lymphocyte-mediated killing of *Nocardia asteroides*. J Immunol. 1983;130:2401–6.
359. Albright JW, Munger WE, Henkart PA, et al. The toxicity of rat large granular lymphocyte tumor cells and their cytoplasmic for rodent and African trypanosomes. J Immunol. 1988;140:2774–8.
360. Eisenstein TK, Tamada R, Meissler J, et al. Vaccination against *Legionella pneumophila*: Serum antibody correlates with protection induced by heat-killed or acetone-killed cells against intraperitoneal but not aerosol infection in guinea pigs. Infect Immun. 1984;45:685–91.
361. Eisenstein TK, Killar LM, Sultzer BM. Immunity to infection with *Salmonella typhimurium*: Mouse-strain differences in vaccine- and serum-mediated protection. J Infect Dis. 1984;150:425–35.
362. Horwitz MA, Silverstein SC. Interaction of the Legionnaires' disease bacterium (*Legionella pneumophila*) with human phagocytes. II. Antibody promotes binding of *L. pneumophila* to monocytes but does not inhibit intracellular multiplication. J Exp Med. 1981;153:398–406.
363. Frenkel JK, Taylor DW. Toxoplasmosis in immunoglobulin M-suppressed mice. Infect Immun. 1982;38:360.
364. Eisenhauer P, Mack DG, McLeod R. Prevention of peroral and congenital acquisition of *Toxoplasma gondii* by antibody and activated macrophages. Infect Immun. 1988;56:83–7.
365. Change K-P. Antibody-mediated inhibition of phagocytosis in *Leishmania donovani*–human phagocyte interactions *in vitro*. Am J Trop Med Hyg. 1981;30(2):334–9.
366. Weiss WR, Sedegah M, Beaudoin RL, et al. CD8 T cells (cytotoxic/suppressors) are required for protection in mice immunized with malaria sporozoites. Proc Natl Acad Sci USA. 1988;85:573–6.
367. Cox FEG. Which way for malaria? Nature. 1988;331:486–7.
368. Schofield L, Villaquiran J, Ferreira A, et al. γ-Interferon, CD8 T cells and antibodies required for immunity to malaria sporozoites. Nature. 1987;330:664.
369. Ockenhouse CF, Schulman S, Shea HL. Induction of crisis forms in the human malaria parasite *Plasmodium falciparum* by γ-interferon-activated, monocyte-derived macrophages. J Immunol. 1984;133:1601–8.
370. Scuderi P, Lam KS, Ryan KJ, et al. Raised serum levels of tumour necrosis factor in parasitic infections. Lancet. 1986;1:1364–5.
371. Grau GE, Fajardo LF, Piguet P-F, et al. Tumor necrosis factor (cachectin) as an essential mediator in murine cerebral malaria. Science. 1987;237:1210–2.
372. Ellner JJ. Immunology of human schistosomiasis. Clin Immunol Newsletter. 1983;4:108–17.
373. Silberstein DS, David JR. Tumor necrosis factor enhances eosinophil toxicity to *Schistosoma mansoni* larvae. Proc Natl Acad Sci USA. 1986; 83:1055–9.
374. Katona IM, Urban JF Jr, Finkelman FD. The role of L3T4 and Lyt-2 cells in the IgE response and immunity to *Nippostrongylus brasiliensis*. J Immunol. 1988;140:3206–11.
375. Stavitsky AB. Immune regulation in *Schistosoma japonica*. Immunol Today. 1987;8:228–32.
376. Ogilvie BM, Love RJ. Cooperation between antibodies and cells in immunity to a nematode parasite. Transplant Rev. 1974;19:147.
377. Wakelin D, Wilson MM. Transfer of immunity to *Trichinella spiralis* in the mouse with mesenteric lymph node cells. Time of appearance of effective cells in donors and expression of immunity in recipients. Parasitology. 1977;74:215.
378. Wing EJ, Remington JS. A role for activated macrophages in resistance against *Trichinella spiralis*. Infect Immun. 1978;21:398.
379. Shapiro ME, Kasper DL, Zaleznik DF, et al. Cellular control of abscess formation: Role of T cells in the regulation of abscesses formed in response to *Bacteroides fragilis*. J Immunol. 1986;137:341–6.
380. Onderdonk AB, Markham RB, Zeleznik DF, et al. Evidence for T cell-dependent immunity to *Bacteroides fragilis* in an intraabdominal abscess model. J Clin Invest. 1982;69:9–16.
381. Powderly WG, Schreiber JR, Pier GB, et al. T cells recognizing polysaccharide-specific B cells function as contrasuppressor cells in the generation of T cell immunity to *Pseudomonas aeruginosa*. J Immunol. 1988;140:2746–52.
382. Markham RB, Powderly WG. Exposure of mice to live *Pseudomonas aeruginosa* generates protective cell-mediated immunity in the absence of an antibody response. J Immunol. 1988;140:2039–45.
383. Powderly WG, Pier GB, Markham RB. T lymphocyte-mediated protection against *Pseudomonas aeruginosa* infection in granulocytopenic mice. J Clin Invest. 1986;78:375–80.
384. Ozaki Y, Ohashi T, Minami A, et al. Enhanced resistance of mice to bacterial infection induced by recombinant human interleukin-α. Infect Immun. 1987;55:1436–1450.
385. Iizawa Y, Nishi T, Kondo M, et al. Effect of recombinant human interleukin-2 on the course of experimental chronic respiratory tract infection caused by *Klebsiella pneumoniae* in mice. Infect Immun. 1988;56:45–50.
386. Finberg R, Hom R. The role of T cell immunity in infection with the herpes group viruses. Year Immunol. 1986;2:267–78.

387. Shore SL, Feorino PM. Immunology of primary herpes virus infections in human. In: Nahmias AJ, Dowdle WR, Schinazi RF, eds. The Human Herpes Viruses. New York: Elsevier, 1981;267–8.
388. Oakes JE, Lausch RN. Role of Fc fragments in antibody-mediated recovery from ocular and subcutaneous herpes simplex virus infection. Infect Immun. 1981;33:109.
389. Oakes JE, Davis WB, Taylor JA, et al. Lymphocyte reactivity contributes to protection conferred by specific antibody passively transferred to herpes simplex virus-infected mice. Infect Immun. 1980;29:642.
390. Epstein LB. The comparative biology of immune and classical interferons. In: Cohen S, Pich E, Oppenheim JJ, eds. Biology of the Lymphokines. New York: Academic Press, 1979;443–514.
391. Daniels CA: Kleinerman ES, Snyderman R: Abortive and productive infections of human mononuclear phagocytes by type I herpes simplex virus. Am J Pathol. 1978;91:119.
392. Morahan PS, Morse SS, McGeorge MB. Macrophage extrinsic activity during herpes simplex virus infection. J Gen Virol. 1980;46:291.
393. Ching C, Lopez C. Natural killing of herpes simplex virus type 1-infected target cells: normal human responses and influence of antiviral antibody. Infect Immun. 1979;26:49.
394. Kohl S, Frazier JJ, Greenberg SB, et al. Interferon induction of natural killer cytotoxicity in human neonates. J Pediatr. 1981;98:379–84.
395. St. Geme JW, Prince JT, Burke BA, et al. Impaired cellular resistance to herpes-simplex virus in Wiskott-Aldrich syndrome. N Engl J Med. 1965; 273:229.
396. Torseth JW, Merigan TC. Significance of local γ interferon in recurrent herpes simplex infection. J Infect Dis. 1986;153:979–84.
397. Burchett SK, Mohan K, Corey L, et al. Delayed production of interferon-gamma (IFNγ) and tumor necrosis factor (TNFα) by mononuclear cells (MC) of herpes simplex virus (HSV) infected neonates (NB). Pediatr Res. 1987;21:309A.
398. Wong GHW, Goeddel DV. Tumour necrosis factors α and β inhibit virus replication and synergize with interferons. Nature. 1986;323:819–22.
399. Hayashi Y, Wada T, Mori R. Protection of newborn mice against herpes simplex virus infection by prenatal and postnatal transmission of antibody. J Gen Virol. 1983;64:1007.
400. Kohl S, Loo LS. The relative role of transplacental and mild immune transfer in protection against lethal neonatal herpes simplex virus infection in mice. J Infect Dis. 1984;149:38.
401. Quinnan GV, Kirmani N, Rook AH, et al. Cytotoxic T cells in cytomegalovirus infection. N Engl J Med. 1982;307:7–12.
402. Winston DJ, Ho WG, Lin CH, et al. Intravenous immune globulin for prevention of cytomegalovirus infection and interstitial pneumonia after bone marrow transplantation. Ann Intern Med. 1987;106:12–18.
403. Grierson H, Purtilo DT. Epstein-Barr virus infections in males with the X-linked lymphoproliferative syndrome. Ann Intern Med. 1987;106:538–45.
404. Virelizier J-L, Lenoir G, Griscelli C. Persistent Epstein-Barr virus infection in a child with hypergammaglobulinemia and immunoblastic proliferation associated with a selective defect in immune interferon secretion. Lancet. 1978;2:231–4.
405. Birx DL, Redfield RR, Tosato G. Defective regulation of Epstein-Barr virus infection in patients with acquired immunodeficiency syndrome (AIDS) or AIDS-related disorders. N Engl J Med. 1986;314:874–9.
406. Ennis FA, Yi-Hua Q, Riley D, et al. HLA-restricted virus-specific cytotoxic T-lymphocyte responses to live and inactivated influenza vaccines. Lancet. 1981;2:88–91.
407. McMichael AJ, Gotch FM, Noble GR, et al. Cytotoxic T-cell immunity to influenza. N Engl J Med. 1983;309:13–7.
408. Ennis FA, Martin J, Verbonitz MW, et al. Specificity studies on cytotoxic thymus-derived lymphocytes reactive with influenza virus-infected cells: Evidence for dual recognition of H-2 and viral hemagglutinin antigens. Proc Natl Acad Sci USA. 1977;74:3006–10.
409. Walker CM, Moody DJ, Stites, DP, et al. CD8 lymphocytes can control HIV infection in vitro by suppressing virus replication. Science. 1986;234:1563–6.
410. Walker BD, Chakrabarti S, Moss B, et al. HIV-specific cytotoxic T lymphocytes in seropositive individuals. Nature. 1987;328:345–8.
411. Wong GHW, Krowka FJ, Stites DP, et al. In vitro anti-human immunodeficiency virus activities of tumor necrosis factor-α and interferon-γ. J Immunol. 1988;140:120–4.
412. Folks TM, Justement J, Kinter A, et al. Cytokine-induced expression of HIV-1 in a chronically infected promonocyte cell line. Science. 1987; 238:800–2.
413. Oldstone MBA, Tishon A, Buchmeier MJ. Virus-induced alterations in homeostasis and differentiated functions of infected cells in vivo. Science. 1982;218:1125–9.
414. Hemachudha T, Phanuphak P, Sriwanthana B, et al. Immunologic study of human encephalitic and paralytic rabies. Am J Med. 1988;84:563–77.
415. Nathan CF, Kaplan G, Levis WR, et al. Local and systemic effects of intradermal recombinant interferon-γ in patients with lepromtous leprosy. N Engl J Med. 1986;315:6–15.
416. Nathan CF, Horowitz CR, de la Harpe, et al. Administration of recombinant interferon-γ to cancer patients enhances monocyte secretion of hydrogen peroxide. Proc Natl Acad Sci USA. 1985;82:8686–90.
417. Maluish AE, Urba WJ, Gordon K, et al. Determination of an optimal biological response modifying dose of interferon gamma in melanoma patients (Abstract). In: Abstracts of the Proceedings of the American Society of Chemotherapy and Oncology. V. 6. Chicago: American Society of Chemotherapy and Oncology, 1987:251.
418. Kleinerman ES, Kurzrock R, Wyatt D, et al. Activation or suppression of the tumoricidal properties of monocytes from cancer patients following treatment with human recombinant γ-interferon. Cancer Res. 1986;46:5401–5.
419. Murray HW, Scavuzzo D, Jacobs JL, et al. In vitro and in vivo activation of human mononuclear phagocytes by gamma interferon: Studies with normal and AIDS monocytes. J Immunol. 1987;138:2457–62.
420. Lane HC, Sherwin SA, Masur H, et al. A phase I trial of recombinant immune (γ) interferon in patients with the acquired immunodeficiency syndrome (Abstract). Clin Res. 1985;33:408.
421. Parkin JM, Eales LJ, Moshtael O, et al. A preliminary report of the use of interferon-gamma in patients with the acquired immune deficiency syndrome. In: Staquet MJ, Hemmer R, Baert AE, eds. Clinical Aspects of AIDS and AIDS-Related Complex. Oxford: Oxford University Press, 1986:167–74.
422. Murray HW, Roberts RB. Interferon-γ and interleukin 2 treatment in AIDS: Clinical toxicity and T lymphocyte effects (Abstract). Clin Res. 1987;35:610.
423. Ezekowitz RAB, Orkin SH, Newburger PE. Recombinant interferon gamma augments phagocyte superoxide production and XO chronic granulomatous disease gene expression in X-linked variant chronic granulomatous disease. J Clin Invest. 1987;80:1009–16.
423a Ezekowitz RAB, Newburger PE. New perspectives in chronic granulomatous disease. J Clin Immunol. 1988;8:419–425
423b Sechler JMG, Malech HL, White CJ, Gallin JI. Recombinant human interferon-γ reconstitutes defective phagocyte function in patients with chronic granulomatous disease of childhood. Proc Natl Acad Sci USA. 1988;85:4874–78.
424. Welte K, Mertelsmann T. Human interleukin 2: Biochemistry, physiology, and possible pathogenetic role in immunodeficiency syndromes. Cancer Invest. 1985;3:35–49.
425. Rosenberg SA, Lotze MT, Muul LM, et al. Observations on the systemic administration of autologous lymphokine activated killer cells and recombinant interleukin-2 to patients with metastatic cancer. N Engl J Med. 1985;313:1485–92.
426. Denicoff KD, Rubinow DR, Papa MZ, et al. The neuropsychiatric effects of treatment with interleukin-2 and lymphokine-activated killer cells. Ann Intern Med. 1987;107:293–300.
427. Flexner C, Hugin A, Moss B. Prevention of vaccinia virus infection in immunodeficient mice by vector-directed IL-2 expression. Nature. 1987; 330:259–62.
428. Ramshaw IA, Andrew ME, Phillips SM, et al. Recovery of immunodeficient mice from a vaccinia virus/IL-2 recombinant infection. Nature. 1987; 329:545–6.
429. Groopman JE, Mitsuyasu RT, DeLeo MJ, et al. Effect of recombinant human granulocyte–macrophage colony-stimulating factor on myelopoiesis in the acquired immunodeficiency syndrome. N Engl J Med. 1987;317:593–8.
430. Brandt SJ, Peters WP, Atwater SK, et al. Effect of recombinant human granulocyte–macrophage colony-stimulating factor on hematopoietic reconstitution after high-dose chemotherapy and autologous bone marrow transplantation. N Engl J Med. 1988;318:869–76.
431. Cerami A, Beutler B. The role of cachectin/TNF in endotoxic shock and cachexia. Immunol Today. 1988;9:28–31.
432. Balow M, Hyman LR. Combination immunotherapy in chronic mucocutaneous candidiasis; synergism between transfer factor and fetal thymus tissue. Clin Immunol Immunopathol. 1977;8:504.
433. Steele RW, Myers MG, Vincent MM. Transfer factor for the prevention of varicella-zoster infection in childhood leukemia. N Engl J Med. 1980;1303–355.
434. MacFadden DK, Hyland RH, Inouye T, et al. Corticosteroids as adjunctive therapy in treatment of *Pneumocystis carinii* pneumonia in patients with acquired immunodeficiency syndrome. Lancet. 1987;1:1477–9.
435. Scott GB. Management of HIV infection in children. In: Schimazi RF, Nahmias AJ, eds. AIDS in Children Adolescents, and Heterosexual Adults. Amsterdam: Elsevier; 1988:264–70.
436. Rogers MF, Thomas PA, Starcher ET, et al. Acquired immunodeficiency syndrome in children: Report of the Centers for Disease Control national surveillance, 1982 to 1985. Pediatrics. 1987;79:1008–14.
437. Wilson CB. Developmental Immunology and Role of Host Defenses in Neonatal Susceptibility. Philadelphia: WB Saunders Co; in press.
438. Wilson CB, Westall J, Johnston L, et al. Decreased production of interferon-gamma by human neonatal cells. J Clin Invest. 1986;77:860–7.
439. Lewis DB, Wilson CB. Molecular basis for decreased interleukin-4 (IL4) and interferon-gamma (IFNγ) production by neonatal T cells. Pediatr Res. 1988;23:356A.
440. Handzel ZT, Levin S, Dolphin Z, et al. Immune competence of newborn lymphocytes. Pediatrics. 1980;65:491.
441. Thorley-Lawson DA. The transformation of adult but not newborn human lymphocytes by Epstein-Barr virus and phytohemagglutinin is inhibited by interferon: The early suppression by T cells of Epstein-Barr infection is mediated by interferon. J Immunol. 1981;1126:829–33.
442. Zawatzky R, DeMaeyer E, Kirchner H. The role of interferon in the resistance of C57BL/6 mice to various doses of herpes simplex virus type 1. J Infect Dis. 1982;146:405–10.
443. Pedersen EB, Haahr S, Mogensen SC. X-linked resistance of mice to high doses of herpes simplex virus type 2 correlates with early interferon production. Infect Immun. 1983;142:740–6.

444. Trofatter KF, Daniels CA, Williams RJ, et al. Growth of type 2 herpes simplex virus in newborn and adult mononuclear leukocytes. Intervirology. 1979;11:117–25.
445. Mintz L, Drew WL, Hoo R, et al. Age-dependent resistance of human alveolar macrophages to herpes simplex virus. Infect Immun. 1980;28:417.
446. Cottman GW, Westall J, Corey L, et al. Replication of HSV2 in mononuclear phagocytes from newborns and adults. Clin Res. 1984;32:108A.
447. Ching C, Lopez C. Natural killing of herpes simplex virus type 1-infected target cells: normal human responses and influence of antiviral antibody. Infect Immun. 1979;26:49–56.
448. Perussia B, Starr S, Abraham S, et al. Human natural killer cells analyzed by B73.1, a monoclonal antibody blocking Fc receptor functions. J Immunol. 1983;130:2133–41.
449. Joris F, Girard JP. Immune response in aged and young subjects following administration of large doses of tuberculin. Int Arch Allergy Appl Immunol. 1975;48:584.
450. Gillis S, Kozak R, Durante M, et al. Decreased production of and response to T cell growth factor by lymphocytes from aged humans. J Clin Invest. 1981;67:937–42.
451. Gardner ID. The effect of aging on susceptibility to infection. Rev Infect Dis. 1980;2:801–10.
452. Brunham RC, Martin DH, Hubbard TW, et al. Depression of the lymphocyte transformation response to microbial antigens and to phytohemagglutinin during pregnancy. J Clin Invest. 1983;72:1629–38.
453. Reinherz EL, Cooper MD, Schlossman SF, et al. Abnormalities of T cell maturation and regulation in human beings with immunodeficiency disorders. J Clin Invest. 1981;68:699.
454. Brahmi Z. Nature of natural killer cell hyporesponsiveness in the Chediak-Higashi syndrome. In: Human Immunology. V. 6. New York: Elsevier; 1983:45.
455. Polmar SH, Stern RC, Schwartz AL, et al. Enzyme replacement therapy for adenosine deaminase deficiency and severe combined immunodeficiency. N Engl J Med. 1976;295:1337.
456. Stoop JW, Zegers BJM, Hendricks GFM, et al. Purine nucleoside deficiency associated with selective cellular immunodeficiency. N Engl J Med. 1977;296:651.
457. Girot R, Hamet M, Perignon JL, et al. Cellular immune deficiency in two siblings with hereditary orotic aciduria. N Engl J Med. 1983;308:700.
458. Lockitch G, Singh VK, Putterman ML, et al. Age-related changes in humoral and cell-mediated immunity in Down syndrome children living at home. Pediatr Res. 1987;22:536–40.
459. Anderson DC, Schmalsteig FC, Finegold MJ, et al. The severe and moderate phenotypes of heritable Mac-1, LFA-1 deficiency: Their quantitative definition and relation to leukocyte dysfunction and clinical features. J Infect Dis. 1985;152:668–89.
460. Gallin JI, Buescher S, Seligmann BE, et al. Recent advances in chronic granulomatous disease. Ann Intern Med. 1983;99:657–74.
461. Peerless AG, Liebhaber M, Anderson S, et al. Legionella pneumonia in chronic granulomatous disease. J Pediatr. 1985;106:783–5.
462. Mackowiak PA. Microbial synergism in human infections. N Engl J Med. 1978;298:21.
463. Pike MC, Daniels CA, Sydnerman R. Influenza-induced depression of monocyte chemotaxis: Reversal by levamisole. Cell Immunol. 1977;32:234–40.
464. Warshauer D, Goldstein E, Akers T, et al. Effect of influenza viral infection on the ingestion and killing of bacteria by alveolar macrophages. Am Rev Respir Dis. 1977;115:269–77.
465. Rouse BT, Horohov DW. Immunosuppression in viral infections. Rev Infect Dis. 1986;8:850–73.
466. Arneborn P, Biberfeld G. T-lymphocyte subpopulations in relation to immunosuppression in measles and varicella. Infect Immun. 1983;39:29–37.
467. Roberts NJ. Different effects of influenza virus, respiratory syncytial virus, and Sendai virus on huuman lymphocytes and macrophages. Infect Immun. 1982;35:1142–6.
468. Roberts NJ, Diamond ME, Douglas RG, et al. Mitogen responses and interferon production after exposure of human macrophages to infections and inactivated influenza viruses. J Med Virol. 1980;5:17–23.
469. Roberts NJ, Prill AH, Mann TN. Interleukin 1 and interleukin 1 inhibitor production by human macrophages exposed to influenza virus or respiratory syncytial virus. J Exp Med. 1986;163:511–9.
470. Cate TR, Couch RB. Lack of effect of influenza virus infection on induction and expression of delayed hypersensitivity. J Infect Dis. 1981;144:280.
471. Gardner ID, Lawton JWM. Depressed human monocyte function after influenza infection in vitro. J Reticuloendothel Soc 1982;32:443–48.
472. Nugent KM, Pesanti EL. Effect of influenza infection on the phagocytic and bactericidal activities of pulmonary macrophages. Infect Immun. 1979; 26:651–7.
473. Carney WP, Rubin RH, Hoffman RA, et al. Analysis of T lymphocyte subsets in cytomegalovirus mononucleosis. J Immunol. 1981;126:2114.
474. Nussenzweig RS. Parasitic disease as a cause of immunosuppression. N Engl J Med. 1982;306:423–4.
475. Luft BJ, Kansas G, Engleman EG, et al. Functional and quantitative alterations in T lymphocyte subpopulations in acute toxoplasmosis. J Infect Dis. 1984;150:761–7.
476. Gibreath MJ, Pavanand K, Macdermott RP, et al. Characterization of cold reactive lymphocytotoxic antibodies in malaria. Clin Exp Immunol. 1983; 51:232.
477. Gaines JD, Gilmer MA, Remington JS. Deficiency of lymphocyte antigen recognition in Hodgkin's disease. In: International Symposium on Hodgkin's Disease. National Cancer Institute Monograph 36. 1973:117.
478. Twomey JJ, Laughter AH, Farrow S, et al. Hodgkin's disease: An immunodepleting and immunosuppressive disorders. J Clin Invest. 1975;56:467.
479. Engleman EJ, Benike CJ, Hoppe RT, et al. Autologous mixed lymphocyte reaction in patients with Hodgkin's disease. J Clin Invest. 1980;66:149.
480. Szuro-Sudol A, Murray HW, Nathan CF. Suppression of macrophage antimicrobial activity by a tumor cell product. J Immunol. 1983;131:384.
481. Fauci AS, Dale DC, Balow JE. Glucocorticosteroid therapy: Mechanisms of action and clinical considerations (NIH conference). Ann Intern Med. 1976;84:304.
482. Frenkel JK, Nelson BM, Arias-Stella J. Immunosuppression and toxoplasmic encephalitis, clinical experimental aspects. Hum Pathol. 1975;6:97.
483. Bodey GP, Hersh EM, Valdivieso M, et al. Effects of cytotoxic and immunosupressive agents on the immune system. Postgrad Med. 1975;58:67.
484. Lew W, Oppenheim JJ, Matsushima K. Analysis of the suppression of IL-1α and Il-1β production in human peripheral blood mononuclear adherent cells by a glucocorticoid hormone. J Immunol. 1988;140:1895–1902.
485. Schaffner A, Schaffner T. Glucocorticoid-induced impairment of macrophage antimicrobial activity: Mechanisms and dependence on the stage of activation. Rev Infect Dis. 1987;9:S620–9.
486. Preiksaitis JK, Rosno G, Grumet C, et al. Infections due to herpesviruses in cardiac transplant recipients: Role of the donor heart and immunosuppressive therapy. J Infect Dis. 1983;147:974.
487. Wilson CB, Jacobs RF, Smith AL. Cellular antibiotic pharmacology. Semin Perinatol. 1982;6:205–13.
488. Hauser WE, Remington JS. Effects of antibiotics on the immune response. Am J Med. 1982;72:711–6.
489. Britton S, Palacios R. Cyclosporin A: Usefulness, risks and mechanism of action. Immunol Rev. 1982;65:5.
490. Manger B, Hardy KJ, Weiss A, et al. Differential effect of cyclosporin A on activation signaling in human T cell lines. J Clin Invest. 1986;77:1501–6.
491. Bickel M, Tsuda H, Amstad P, et al. Differential regulation of colony-stimulating factors and interleukin 2 production by cyclosporin A. Proc Natl Acad Sci USA. 1987;84:3274–7.
492. Alevy YG, Hutcheson P, Mueller KR, et al. Suppressor alveolar macrophages in experimentally induced uremia. J Reticuloendothel Soc. 1983; 33:11.
493. MacCuish AC, Urbaniak SJ, Campbell CJ, et al. Phytohemagglutinin transformation and a circulating lymphocyte subpopulation in insulin-dependent diabetic patients. Diabetes. 1974;23:708.
494. Vose BM, Mondgil GC. Postoperative depression of antibody dependent lymphocyte cytotoxicity following minor surgery and anesthesia. Immunology. 1976;30:123.
495. Kataria YP, Sagne AL, LoBuglio AR, et al. In vitro observations on sarcoid lymphocytes and their correlation with cutaneous anergy and clinical severity of disease. Am Rev Respir Dis. 1973;108:767.
496. Lieberman J, Kaneshiro W. Abnormal response of cultured lymphocytes to phytohemagglutinin and autologous serum in cystic fibrosis. Am Rev Respir Dis. 1977;116:1047.
497. Sugarman B. Zinc and infection. Rev Infect Dis. 1983;5:137.
498. Ballester OF, Prasad AS. Anergy, zinc deficiency, and decreased nucleoside phosphorylase activity in patients with sickle cell anemia. Ann Intern Med. 1983;98:180.
499. Chandra RK. Nutrition, immunity and infection: Present knowledge and future directions. Lancet. 1983;1:688–91.
500. Keusch GT, Scrimshaw NS. Selective primary health care strategies for control for disease in the developing world. XXIII. Control of infection to reduce the prevalence of infantile and childhood malnutrition. Rev Infect Dis. 1986;8:273–87.
501. Beisei WR, Edelman R, Nauss K, et al. Single-nutrient effects on immunologic functions. JAMA. 1981;1:53–8.
502. Koff WC, Dunegan MA. Neuroendocrine hormones suppress macrophage-mediated lysis of herpes simplex virus-infected cells. J Immunol. 1986;136:705–9.
503. Mary D, Aussel C, Ferrua B, et al. Regulation of interleukin 2 synthesis by cAMP in human T cells. J Immunol. 1987;4:1179–84.
504. Bernton EW, Meltzer MS, Holaday JW. Suppression of macrophage activation and T-lymphocyte function in hypoprolactinemic mice. Science. 1988;239:401–4.
505. Brown SL, VanEpps DE. Opioid peptides modulate production of interferon-γ by human mononuclear cells. Cell Immunol. 1986;103:1926.
506. Kern JA, Lamb RJ, Reed JC, et al. Dexamethasone inhibition of interleukin-1 beta production by human monocytes. J Clin Invest. 1988;81:237–44.
507. Seemayer TA, Gartner JG, Lapp WA. The graft versus host reaction. Hum Pathol. 1983;14:3.
508. Cooper MD, Lawton AR. Immune deficiency diseases. In: Braunwald E, Isselbacher KJ, Petersdorf RG, et al, eds. Harrison's Principles of Internal Medicine. 11th ed. New York: McGraw-Hill; 1987:1385–92.

9. EVALUATION OF THE PATIENT WITH SUSPECTED IMMUNODEFICIENCY

DANIEL ROTROSEN
JOHN I. GALLIN

Pediatricians, internists, and infectious disease specialists are occasionally involved in the diagnostic evaluation of the patient with suspected immunodeficiency. With the exception of the acquired immunodeficiency syndrome (AIDS), the well-characterized immunodeficiency syndromes are, for the most part, exceedingly uncommon. As a result, physicians generally lack the clinical experience to readily recognize these disorders or proceed toward a diagnosis in an orderly, stepwise fashion. Our experience at a referral center specializing in phagocytic cell disorders suggests that simple, inexpensive, and widely available tests are underused in the initial evaluation of patients with suspected defects in host defense mechanisms. Furthermore, many texts describe a bewildering array of specialized procedures to assess immune function, but their diagnostic utility is limited, and specific guidelines for their application are neither available nor uniformly accepted. As a result, the correct diagnosis may be unduly delayed and patients subjected to repetitive, costly, and inappropriate testing.

With the exception of transplantation of immunocompetent tissue in severe combined immunodeficiency, curative therapy is not available for any of the primary immunodeficiency disorders, and adequate replacement or immunomodulatory treatments remain remote possibilities in all but a few. Nonetheless, a diligent attempt at specific diagnosis still seems warranted in all cases of suspected immunodeficiency. Early diagnosis is critical in treatable forms of severe immunodeficiency to prevent life-threatening infections and morbid complications. In several instances the underlying defects are now understood at a biochemical level, and genes encoding missing or defective proteins have been cloned. Recognition of heterozygote carriers is important for early (in some cases, antenatal) diagnosis and essential for sound genetic counseling. The rare immunodeficiency diseases are rightly viewed as "experiments in nature," and further advances will certainly depend on continued identification of individuals with these disorders. Finally, as in other areas of medicine, earlier diagnosis of affected individuals is likely to result in lesser morbidity and mortality, even without the advent of specific therapies.

GOALS IN THE INITIAL EVALUATION OF PATIENTS WITH SUSPECTED IMMUNODEFICIENCY

Clinical evaluation of patients with recurrent or unusual infections should be grounded on the realization that nearly all of the primary immunodeficiencies are uncommon. Appropriate goals in the initial screening of such patients include the following: (*1*) recognition of clinical features truly indicative of an abnormal frequency or severity of infection and differentiation of these from the range of normal, (*2*) early identification of features suggestive of defects in nonspecific host defense mechanisms (integrity of normal mucocutaneous barriers or clearance mechanisms, for example) that may direct the immediate evaluation away from the immune system, and (*3*) recognition of clinical features suggestive of defects within a particular limb of immune defenses. In addition, a realistic goal in the initial laboratory evaluation of such patients is to expeditiously gather data sufficient to profile immune function despite the fact that neither a precise classification nor specific therapy may be an immediate possibility. These aims should take into account the likelihood that thorough evaluation, accurate diagnosis, and management of patients with unusual, poorly characterized, or clinically severe primary immunodeficiencies are often possible only in specialized research facilities.

INITIAL CLINICAL SCREENING

Despite thorough evaluation the vast majority of patients in whom an immunodeficiency is suspected on the basis of a history of chronic or recurrent infection will not have a clearly defined disorder. A detailed history is always indicated to determine the frequency and severity of infections, sites and organ systems involved, etiologic agents, and age at onset. As a rule, severe congenital immunodeficiencies present with life-threatening infection within the first year of life. In most congenital immunodeficiencies, a convincing history of recurrent or unusual infection dates to early childhood, although in some disorders patients with clinically less severe "variants" may not be recognized until adolescence. Primary immunodeficiency with clinical onset in adulthood occurs (e.g., common variable hypogammaglobulinemia and hypogammaglobulinemia with thymoma) but is the exception.

It is important to appreciate that normal school-age children may have 6–12 respiratory infections per year.[1] Attack rates decline with age and reach adult rates of two to four infections per year by adolescence.[1,2] Furthermore, common colds, nonnecrotizing pharyngitis, and tonsillitis are rarely if ever serious problems in individuals with well-characterized immunodeficiencies. Recurrent skin infections due to gram-positive cocci, without a history of extracutaneous infection, are rarely indicative of immunodeficiency. Likewise, recurrent urinary tract and biliary tree infections suggest obstructive lesions and are unlikely to be due to defects in immune defense mechanisms. Factitious illness may warrant consideration in adults with recurrent infection.

A thorough family history is essential to document consanguinity, to identify risk factors for vertical transmission of AIDS, and to identify relatives with recurrent infections, connective tissue disorders, malignancies, and early demise. Laboratory evaluation of family members may be necessary to assess modes of inheritance and to provide a data base for appropriate genetic counseling.

The clinical presentation may be indicative of deficiencies within a particular limb of host defense. The guidelines in Table 1 and the following discussion are generally useful in directing the emphasis to a given system and in suggesting common disorders of nonimmune defenses that should be excluded. However, due to the complex interdependencies embodied in the immune response there may be considerable overlap in the clinical features of disorders arising from pathophysiologically discrete but functionally interrelated defects in host defenses. For this reason, a complete and encompassing algorithm for the evaluation of patients with suspected immunodeficiency is probably neither possible nor advisable.

Recurrent sinopulmonary infections, meningitis, and bacteremia due to encapsulated organisms suggest deficiencies of complement or antibody and certain types of phagocytic cell dysfunction. In the absence of pneumonia, chronic otitis media, or systemic infection, recurrent sinusitis alone is rarely indicative of immunodeficiency because it occurs so frequently in normal individuals. In such patients anatomic abnormalities of the sinuses and allergic disorders should be considered potential contributing factors. Bronchial obstruction, underlying cystic and cavitary diseases, and disorders of bronchopulmonary clearance such as cystic fibrosis and immotile cilia syndrome should be considered in patients with recurrent pneumonia. Recurrent pneumonia in the same pulmonary lobe suggests an anatomic abnormality as opposed to immunodeficiency.

Recurrent staphylococcal skin infection associated with subcutaneous extension or deep-organ infection suggests phago-

TABLE 1. Common Clinical Syndromes Associated with Immune Deficiency

	Common Clinical Syndromes
B lymphocytes	Sinopulmonary infection due to encapsulated bacteria, chronic otitis media Giardiasis Repeated episodes of common viral illnesses[3] Chronic enteroviral encephalitis[4–7]
Complement	Sinopulmonary infection due to encapsulated bacteria, chronic otitis Neisserial bacteremia and meningitis Autoimmune syndromes, glomerulonephritis
Phagocytic cells	
CR3 deficiency	Delayed separation of the umbilical stump, patent urachus Leukocytosis, necrotizing infections without pus, periodontitis, pneumonitis, perianal abscesses
Chronic granulomatous disease	Infection due to catalase-positive bacteria (e.g., staphylococci, (Enterobacteriaceae), *Nocardia, Candida, Aspergillus* Cellulitis, suppurative lymphadenitis, draining sinuses, osteomyelitis, visceral and brain abscesses, periodontitis Recurrent granulomas
Chédiak-Higashi syndrome Neutrophil-specific granule deficieny	Moderate neutropenia Skin and deep-organ bacterial infection (no particular class of organisms) Periodontitis Oculocutaneous albinism and neuropathy (CHS only)
Myeloperoxidase deficiency	No significant increased susceptibility to infection (perhaps fungal infection in association with immunocompromising systemic illness, e.g., diabetes mellitus)
T lymphocytes	Disseminated infection due to intracellular pathogens, protozoans, opportunistic fungi, normally benign DNA viruses Protracted diarrhea, eczema, endocrinopathy Graft-vs.-host disease after transfusions Malignancies

cytic cell dysfunction. Children with clinically significant phagocytic cell defects generally have moderate to severe periodontal disease, a finding usually lacking in individuals with recurrent skin infections but without phagocyte dysfunction.[8] Most patients with recurrent infection limited to the skin do not have a significant or well-characterized immunodeficiency. In such patients other predisposing factors should be sought. These include chronic nasal carriage of staphylococci phage identical to those in the lesions, needle use, draining sinuses, apocrine gland obstruction, foreign bodies, and chronic excoriating or bullous skin disorders.

Disseminated infection with intracellular pathogens, protozoans, opportunistic fungi, or ordinarily benign viruses strongly suggests defective cell-mediated immunity. Hypocalcemia in the newborn (in DiGeorge syndrome) or intrauterine graft-vs.-host disease (scaling erythroderma and total alopecia) are useful early signs of severe T-cell deficiency. Children with primary disorders of cell-mediated immunity may have failure to thrive, wasting, diarrhea, severe eczema, chronic mucocutaneous candidiasis, a high incidence of malignancies, and early demise.[5–7] This clinical presentation is so striking that confusion with infectious illnesses in immunocompetent individuals is usually not an issue.

CLINICAL AND LABORATORY ASSESSMENT OF B-CELL FUNCTION

Specific humoral immunodeficiency syndromes are considered in detail in Chapters 5 and 6. Antibody deficiencies are the most common and constitute approximately one-half of patients with primary immunodeficiencies.

With rare exceptions, deficiency of humoral immunity is accompanied by decreased levels of one or more classes of serum immunoglobulin. The widely available techniques to measure immunoglobulins use commercially available and well-standardized, immunoglobulin class-specific antisera. Most clinical laboratories quantitate immunoglobulins by radial diffusion or nephelometrically by determination of changes in light scattering that occur in dilute solutions of immunoglobulin on mixing with class-specific antisera. Nephelometry may yield spurious results in the presence of circulating immune complexes, but for most clinical purposes the techniques are essentially equivalent.[9,10] IgE is measured by radioimmunoassay. While immunoelectrophoresis allows detection of three immunoglobulin classes, it is not quantitative and is not a satisfactory technique for the measurement of immunoglobulins. Because serum immunoglobulin concentrations vary among normal individuals and with age, difficulties arise in defining the lower limits of normal. Reasonable estimates for low normal values in adults are 40 mg/dl for IgM, 500 mg/dl for IgG, and 50 mg/dl for IgA; serum immunoglobulins are detectable in the primary hypogammaglobulinemic and agammaglobulinemic disorders but are below the 95 percent confidence limits for age- and race-matched controls. Corresponding normal values in prepubertal children are ≈30–80 percent of adult levels and increase with age.[3,10–12] In protein-losing states with depression of immunoglobulins, IgM levels usually remain normal or are only slightly diminished. Simultaneous determination of serum albumin and transferrin levels may be helpful in identifying these conditions.

A major goal of screening for antibody deficiency is the identification of the subset of patients in whom replacement therapy will be helpful. In all such situations the benefits of therapy (i.e., provision of protective antibody) need to be weighed against the potential risks (suppression of endogenous antibody formation and induction of anti-IgG allotype antibodies). As a general rule, patients with B-cell disorders in which replacement therapy is indicated do not have IgG or IgM antibodies. Knowledge of the IgA concentration is also of pivotal help in guiding initial evaluation because a normal serum IgA content excludes not only isolated IgA deficiency but all of the permanent types of agammaglobulinemia since IgA is low or absent in those conditions as well.[4,6]

Humoral immunodeficiency may exist in the presence of normal or near-normal concentrations of most or all five immunoglobulin classes, as demonstrated by patients with the Wiskott-Aldrich syndrome.[5,6,13] In the presence of borderline immunoglobulin concentrations or if the suspicion of antibody deficiency is strong, humoral immunity should be assessed by responses to ''natural'' antigens to which the population is commonly exposed or after active immunization. Active immunization should be considered as a diagnostic maneuver only with the following caveats: (*1*) live vaccines (Calmette-Guérin bacillus [BCG], poliomyelitis, measles, rubella, mumps, and smallpox) should never be given when primary or severe secondary immunodeficiency is suspected, (*2*) polysaccharide antigens are ineffective in infants less than 1 year old, (*3*) the capacity to make antibody to T-cell-independent polysaccharide antigens is acquired late in infancy and results in predominantly IgM responses associated with little immunologic memory, and (*4*) immunization of infants (as opposed to adults) with protein antigens results primarily in the production of IgM antibodies with a relatively slow progression to an IgG response.[5,14–16]

Nearly all hospital blood banks can measure isohemagglutinins. These are predominantly IgM antibodies (normally detectable in infants by 6 months of age) against bacterial polysaccharides cross-reactive with type A and B red blood cells. Most hospital laboratories can also measure anti-streptolysin O and febrile agglutinins. Antibody against typhoid H and O antigens can be measured before and after immunization with typhoid vaccine. Production of diphtheria toxin-specific IgG can be demonstrated by the Schick test, and most state and local health department laboratories can titer antibodies to common viral agents, diphtheria/tetanus toxoid, *Escherichia coli*, and pneumococcal polysaccharides. Except in previously unimmunized children, antigen challenge assesses the capacity for secondary (recall) responses. If results are normal, the patient is unlikely to have a clinically significant deficit in antibody production. The primary response can be assessed on an investigational basis by using keyhole limpet hemocyanin, or bacteriophage ϕX174.[7,17] The use of bacteriophage ϕX174 demonstrates the capacity for isotype switch (T cell dependent) and allows quantitation of antigen clearance and an assessment of primary and secondary responses. Based on these responses, identification of those who will benefit from IgG replacement is possible. A presumptive diagnosis of B-cell deficiency can be made in the neonate since healthy subjects clear bacteriophage ϕX174 immediately whereas abnormal subjects show phage persistence for more than 1 week.[17]

IgA deficiency may occur in association with isolated deficits in specific IgG subclasses. In these cases, specific subclass determinations may be necessary to demonstrate the deficiency. Unfortunately, antisera suitable for subclass determinations are neither widely available nor well standardized. An effort by the World Health Organization is likely to improve this situation in the near future.[7] It is important to assess the severity of the deficiency in such individuals by measuring the recall response to a panel of antigens. Because safe replacement therapy (i.e., subclass-specific IgG) is not available, failure to identify patients with deficits in specific IgG subclasses but without severe antibody deficiency is of limited clinical impact.

Measuring levels of antigen-specific antibody may be useful in particular settings. For example, high titers of *Staphylococcus aureus*- and *Candida*-specific IgE or low titers of *S. aureus*-specific IgA may be useful in distinguishing patients with hyperimmunoglobulin E (Job) syndrome from those with atopy, chronic eczema, and elevated IgE levels.[18]

Circulating B cells can be quantitated by immunofluorescence; the information obtained may be useful in classification but is usually not critical to an initial assessment of the level of immunodeficiency. In an investigational setting, mitogen-driven B-cell proliferation has been useful in characterizing B-cell defects and T-"helper" and -"suppressor" function in humoral immunodeficiency, but is not generally useful in initial screening.

TABLE 2. Delayed Cutaneous Hypersensitivity Testing (DCH)

Agent	*Dilution*[a]	*Comments*
Tuberculin	2 IU Tween-stabilized PPD	If negative, repeat with 50 IU
Candida[b]	1:100	If no reaction, repeat with 1:10 dilution
Trichophyton[b]	1:30	
Mumps[c]	Undiluted	Read at 6–8 hr for early Arthus reaction (antibody mediated) Read at 48 hr for DCH
Tetanus/diphtheria toxoids[d]	1:100	Ascertain immunization status, repeat DCH testing after active immunization if initially negative
Keyhole limpet hemocyanin[a]	100 ug	DCH testing 2 wk after subcutaneous immuniztion with 2.5 mg KLH

[a] All skin tests intradermal injection of 0.1 ml of antigen diluted in Hollister-Stier–buffered saline.
[b] Hollister-Stier Laboratories.
[c] Mumps skin test, Eli Lilly & Company. Immunization with live viral vaccines is contraindicated in all patients with severe combined or cell-mediated immunodeficiency.
[d] Pediatric diphtheria and tetanus toxoid, Wyeth Laboratories.
[e] Sigma Chemical Company or Calbiochem-Behring, not currently licensed by FDA for use in humans.
(Data from Rosen et al.[7] and deShazo et al.[9])

TABLE 3. In Vitro Lymphocyte Proliferation

Stimulus	*Interpretation*
Mitogens	
Phytohemagglutinin Concanavalin A Anti-thymocyte globulin	Nonspecific stimulation of both helper and suppressor subsets, predominantly T-cell mitogens in humans; response indicates that some of the normal populations are present.
Pokeweed	Stimulates T cells for B-cell help required for immunoglobulin synthesis and secretion.
Staphylococcus aureus (Cowan I strain)	Direct stimulation of B-cell proliferation and polyclonal activation.
Allogenic lymphocytes	Proliferative stimulus to T-helper cells resulting in generation of specific cytotoxic cells against the stimulating histocompatibility antigens. Response may be normal even in the presence of severe T-cell immunodeficiency.
Antigens	Response requires genetically restricted antigen-presenting cell. Most stringent test of immunologic competence and correlates better with state of health than do other tests.

CLINICAL AND LABORATORY EVALUATION OF CELL-MEDIATED IMMUNITY

Cell-mediated and combined immunodeficiency syndromes are considered in detail in Chapter 8. Cellular deficiencies constitute ≈40 percent of patients with primary immunodeficiencies. Of these, approximately three-quarters have associated antibody deficiencies.

Delayed cutaneous hypersensitivity (DCH) testing represents the most informative and cost-effective approach in the initial evaluation of cell-mediated immunity. All skin tests are by intradermal injection of 0.1 ml of antigen and should be read at 48–72 hours for maximum induration. A positive skin test response, defined as induration greater than 5 mm at 48–72 hours, indicates intact cell-mediated immunity. Erythema is not an indication of DCH. To demonstrate defective cell-mediated immunity several antigens must be used; widely available and commonly used preparations are shown in Table 2. Response to sensitization with dinitrochlorobenzene is no longer recommended because it is mutagenic and causes necrosis.[7] An assessment of response after primary sensitization can be made after immunization with keyhole limpet hemocyanin (KLH), but this is an investigational procedure, and KLH preparations are not currently licensed by the Food and Drug Administration (FDA) for use in humans.

Tuberculin reactivity should be ascertained early in all patients with suspected immunodeficiency to identify those who would benefit from chemoprophylaxis.

For practical purposes, normal DCH responses to a panel of test antigens excludes significant cellular immunodeficiency. With rare exceptions in vitro evaluation of T-cell or macrophage function in such patients is not indicated. Selective anergy to specific pathogens appears to play a role (albeit poorly defined) in the impaired immune response in chronic mucocutaneous candidiasis and lepromatous leprosy,[6,7,19] but with rare exceptions defective cell-mediated immunity is not likely to be a significant factor underlying infection in individuals with otherwise normal DCH responses.

DCH testing is of limited value in infants because of inadequate natural sensitization and because they are uniformly anergic during the first few weeks of life regardless of antigen exposure. However, the total lymphocyte count of peripheral blood is normally $\geq 1200/mm^3$, regardless of age. In infants and patients with absent or borderline DCH, further assessment of cell-mediated immunity generally requires T-cell profiling and in vitro functional testing (Table 3). These tests have been useful in elucidating the basic mechanisms of disease and in classification but are not usually essential for the diagnosis of primary immunodeficiency. In vitro functional responses are influenced by steroid administration; viral, bacterial, and fungal infection; or recent vaccination.[3,6,9] In vitro functional studies should be obtained only after consultation with specialists who have reviewed the clinical aspects of the case and who are familiar with the techniques, limitations, and interpretation of such studies. Recent experience in AIDS suggests that changes in the number of CD4+ ("helper") T cells may be a clinically useful predictor of the relative risk of opportunistic infection, but guidelines for periodic T-lymphocyte profiling, based on controlled studies, are not available in AIDS or in other immunodeficiencies. Limited data suggest that determination of the CD4+/CD8+ cell ratio may be helpful in distinguishing certain primary immunodeficiencies from AIDS, particularly in pediatric patients.[20]

The chest radiograph or tomography may be useful in identifying adults with thymoma. In children the thymic shadow (retrosternal lucency) is more easily appreciated on the lateral chest projection than on the frontal view. However, the absence of a thymic shadow on the chest radiograph is of limited predictive value due to rapid involution in normal infants during a stressful illness.[21] Thymic biopsy and lymph node biopsy may be highly informative in infants with signs of severe immunodeficiency but should be performed by experienced surgeons only after careful consideration of diagnostic alternatives. Biopsy should be performed on rapidly enlarging lymph nodes in any patient with immunodeficiency to exclude infection, malignancy, or lymphoreticular hyperplasia. For standardization, lymph node biopsy should be performed 5–7 days after local antigenic challenge with diphtheria/tetanus toxoids and morphologic assessment based on the published criteria of the World Health Organization.[21]

In particular situations additional studies may be diagnostic of specific immunodeficiency disorders. Erythrocyte adenosine deaminase (ADA) levels should be determined in all infants with the clinical features of severe combined immunodeficiency to exclude ADA deficiency as the underlying biochemical lesion. Early diagnosis and treatment are essential in this instance to prevent significant morbidity. Likewise, purine nucleoside phosphorylase (PNP) levels should be determined in all infants with T-cell deficiency or features of Diamond-Blackfan aplastic anemia.[7,22] Other immunodeficiency disorders that are both treatable and associated with specific and easily demonstrated biochemical lesions include transcobalamine II deficiency and acrodermatitis enteropathica (associated with a deficiency of serum zinc). Serum α-fetoprotein (AFP) levels are helpful in distinguishing ataxia teleangiectasia (AFP levels elevated in ≥95 percent) from other neurologic disorders.[7]

Endocrinopathy associated with disorders of impaired cell-mediated immunity (e.g., chronic mucocutaneous candidiasis) may precede or follow clinically apparent immunodeficiency. In addition, endocrine dysfunction in this setting is progressive, thus necessitating careful observation for treatable endocrine dysfunction in patients with immunodeficiency and vice versa.[23]

The role of a number of cytokines and inflammatory mediators in normal immune function is being increasingly recognized.[24–31] Some of these factors have been characterized at the molecular level and their specific receptors on immunocompetent cells identified. Very likely, immunodeficiency disorders due to a lack (or overproduction) of these factors or their corresponding receptors will eventually be recognized. However, outside of specific investigational settings there are presently no indications for measurement of such factors in serum or tissues.

CLINICAL AND LABORATORY EVALUATION OF PATIENTS WITH SUSPECTED COMPLEMENT DEFICIENCY

The synthesis and function of the components of the complement system are described in detail in Chapter 6 and in recent reviews.[32,33] Complement components do not cross the placenta. Total hemolytic complement (CH_{50}) determinations and the levels of most components in term infants correspond to ≈60–80 percent of normal adult levels; levels of C8 and C9 are lower and correspond to ≈10 percent of normal adult levels.[34]

With the exception of properdin, which is X-linked, complement proteins are encoded by genes inherited in an autosomal codominant fashion.[33,35] Congenital deficiency is the consequence of inheritance of a null allele, which codes for nonsynthesis of the protein.[33] In part due to the prevalence of null alleles, the normal range of complement proteins is broad, usually ±50 percent of the normal mean.[34] Since diminished levels but not the absence of complement proteins are adequate for normal host defense mechanisms, complement deficiency syndromes (with the exception of properdin deficiency) are characterized phenotypically by an apparent autosomal recessive pattern of inheritance. In general, absence of the early components is primarily but not strictly associated with autoimmune disease, thus reflecting the overlapping role of the alternative pathway in protection against bacterial infection. In contrast, deficiencies of late components or alternative-pathway factors generally present with a strikingly increased suseptibility to infection accompanied by less prominent autoimmune manifestations.[33,36] Due to the pivotal role C3 plays in both complement activation pathways and the opsonic and pro-inflammatory properties of C3 fragments, C3 deficiency has among the most severe consequences of all the complement deficiency disorders. All homozygous C3-deficient individuals described to date have experienced serious complications including recurrent infection or autoimmune disorders.[33] Individual complement component deficiencies associated with an increased risk of infection are discussed in detail in Chapter 6.

A CH_{50} determination should be the initial step in the laboratory evaluation of all patients with a suspected complement deficiency. Appropriate sample handling is important. Blood should be allowed to clot at room temperature (cold activation of complement may occur at 0°C), centrifuged at 4°C, and serum frozen in aliquots at −70°C. Deficiencies of classical pathway components profound enough to account for infectious complications are easily detected by the CH_{50} assay, but the test is relatively insensitive to even moderate depression of individual components. The CH_{50} value will be 0 or extremely low in the absence of classical pathway or terminal components.[33] If the CH_{50} value is low, levels of individual components should be measured. In homozygous complement component deficiencies, the deficient component will be essentially absent on either antigenic or functional testing. Heterozygotes usually exhibit below-normal levels on careful antigenic or functional testing for the component in question.[33,34] Ideally, the initial investigation of individual components should be based on the clinical presentation and known gene frequencies. Individual components can be assayed by radial immunodiffusion or nephelometry using commercially available antibodies. Assays for C3 and C4 are widely available; antigenic assays for other components and functional titration of individual components are reliable and sensitive tests but are largely confined to reference laboratories. In contrast to the role of structural variants in C1 inhibitor deficiency (hereditary angioedema), reports of immune impairment due to dysfunctional structural variants are exceedingly rare.[33,35]

Routine CH_{50} determinations do not assess alternative-pathway components. Commercial kits for the assay of factor B and properdin are available, but determinations of these and other alternative pathway components are usually done by specialized facilities.

Simultaneous depression of more than a single complement component argues strongly against a hereditary deficiency and is more consistent with consumptive disorders or diminished complement synthesis.

PHAGOCYTIC CELL DYSFUNCTION

Nearly all of the clinically significant and well-characterized defects in phagocytic cell defenses can be identified by widely available and easily performed screening tests. Specific syndromes and appropriate screening procedures are discussed in the following sections.

Neutrophil Kinetics and Neutropenia

Neutropenia is the most commonly encountered defect in phagocytic cell host defenses. The normal range of peripheral blood neutrophil counts is from 1500 to 8000/mm^3 but can be as low as 1000/mm^3 in healthy black individuals.[37–40] The increased risk of bacterial and fungal infection in patients with profound neutropenia secondary to cytotoxic chemotherapy dramatically underscores the central role that phagocytes play in host defense. A moderate neutropenia commonly accompanies clinically significant T-cell deficiency; the underlying mechanisms are poorly understood. Detailed approaches for the evaluation of causes of neutropenia are provided elsewhere.[38]

A severe neutropenia of the newborn occurs as a result of maternal antibody response to neutrophil-specific antigens. This is a self-limited process resolving over several weeks as maternal antibodies are cleared. However, the risk of infection is significant during the neutropenic period. Similar neutrophil-specific antibodies may occur in autoimmune neutropenia as a primary disorder or in association with other immune disorders such as systemic lupus erythematosus.

A complete blood count and white blood cell differential will identify all patients with neutropenia; sequential testing (3 days per week over an 8- to 12-week period) may be necessary to demonstrate cycling and to document the periodicity and duration of neutropenia. Normal neutrophil counts vary among individuals but remain relatively constant in a particular individual followed over a period of several years. Idiopathic acute neutropenia (particularly in the elderly or debilitated) should prompt a work-up for sepsis, even when other signs of infection are lacking. Bone marrow aspiration and biopsy for histology and culture are essential parts of the work-up of neutropenia but may be delayed in some cases of acute neutropenia where a presumptive cause is obvious and recovery likely.

Screening for autoimmune disease is indicated in all neonates and in patients with chronic neutropenia; the evaluation should include lymphocyte profiling with assessment of natural killer cell number. Anti-neutrophil antibodies should be sought by fluorescence-activated cell sorting using patient serum directed against autologous and normal donor cells and by induction of leukoagglutination in normal neutrophils.[41,42]

Bone marrow biopsy is the most direct and informative procedure to assess myeloid maturation and marrow reserves. Kinetic studies (challenge with endotoxin, steroids, or epinephrine) have been used to evaluate marrow reserves and the size of the marginated pool but require close monitoring by experienced physicians.[37–40] Clinical experience with kinetic studies is limited (relative to bone marrow biopsy), and interpretation of abnormal results can be problematic. Nonetheless, used in an investigational setting these tests have been critical to a current understanding of neutrophil kinetics and will likely be important in evaluating the physiologic response to newly described inflammatory mediators and cytokines.

Chronic Granulomatous Disease

Since the initial descriptions of chronic granulomatous disease (CGD) (see Chapter 7) more than 30 years ago well over 300 cases have been reported.[43–45] This is a rare disorder with a frequency of 1:500,000 to 1:1,000,000. Nonetheless, the disease has engendered tremendous interest as a prototype for abnormalities of phagocyte oxidative metabolism, and elucidation of the underlying defects has been critical to an understanding of the activation, structure, and function of the respiratory burst oxidase. Recent studies indicate that CGD represents a genetically heterogenous group of disorders potentially affecting the entire cascade of events leading to the production of toxic oxygen metabolites.[46,47]

Patients with the "classic" form of CGD develop serious infections due to catalase-positive microorganisms. The onset of serious infections is usually within the first year of life. Common infectious syndromes include pneumonia and lung abscesses, skin and soft tissue infections, lymphadenopathy and suppurative lymphadenitis, visceral abscesses, and osteomyelitis, usually involving the small bones of the hands and feet. Septicemia, meningitis, and brain abscesses are less common. Although severe, infection in CGD may follow a rather indolent course characterized only by malaise, low-grade fever, and a mild leukocytosis, but the erythrocyte sedimentation rate is nearly always elevated during infection. There may be incomplete resolution of the inflammatory process (even after infection has been eliminated) that leads to granuloma formation. The resulting granulomatous lesions occasionally cause esophageal, antral, or genitourinary tract obstruction. "Variant" clinical forms of the disease have been recognized including presentation in adolescence or young adulthood; such patients usually have a history of infection since childhood, although typically less severe than in the "classic" form of the disease.[43–45]

Staphylococcus aureus and gram-negative bacilli account for most infections in CGD, but infection due to *Aspergillus, Candida*, and *Nocardia* is not uncommon. Organisms that produce H_2O_2 but are catalase-negative (e.g., streptococci, pneumococci, and lactobacilli) are not major pathogens in CGD; the persistence of H_2O_2 within the phagosome in concert with host cell myeloperoxidase may result in bactericidal activity against these organisms. Alternatively, oxygen-independent microbicidal mechanisms may be sufficient in CGD to kill certain pathogens. In preliminary studies subcutaneous interferon-γ treatment partially corrected the defects in superoxide production and bactericidal activity in neutrophils obtained from some CGD patients and, in vitro, improved function of their cultured monocytes.[48,49] A multicenter cooperative trial of interferon-γ in CGD has been started.

CGD is X chromosome linked in ≈65 percent of cases and autosomal recessively inherited in ≈35 percent of cases. A kindred with probable autosomal dominant inheritance has been described.[44] As a group, patients with autosomal recessive inheritance may have a less severe clinical course than those with X-linked inheritance, but in the individual patient severity of infectious episodes does not reliably predict the mode of inheritance.

Essentially all patients with CGD can be identified on screening by the nitroblue tetrazolium (NBT) dye reduction test.[43–45] Positive tests (no reduction of NBT by neutrophils) should be confirmed by quantitative determination of superoxide production and an assessment of respiratory burst kinetics. Female carriers can be identified by the NBT slide test with the caveat that certain affected individuals (because of chance inactivation of the normal or defective X chromosome) may display an apparently normal or CGD phenotype. A severe deficiency of glucose-6-phosphate dehydrogenase (G6PD) has been reported to result in the phenotypic expression of CGD. These reports predated current concepts of the molecular and genetic heterogeneity of CGD, and in retrospect, it is thought that such patients probably had autosomal recessive CGD. The clinical features in such cases were attributed to impaired activity of the hexose-monophosphate shunt, which normally furnishes reducing equivalents (NADPH) required for oxidase activity. However, NADPH oxidase activity is normal in G6PD deficiency, and such patients would be readily distinguished from those with classic CGD by the history of severe hemolytic anemia, by quantitation of G6PD, and by a failure to stimulate hexose-monophosphate shunt activity with methylene blue. As recent advances have demonstrated, a more complete understanding of the respiratory burst oxidase and elucidation of the underlying genetic and biochemical defects in CGD will depend on continued identification and investigation of patients with unique lesions.

iC3b Receptor (CR3) Deficiency

The adherence of neutrophils to opsonized particles, endothelial cells, and plastic and glass surfaces is mediated in part by a family of cell surface glycoproteins that includes complement receptor type 3 (CR3), lymphocyte function-associated antigen 1 (LFA-1), and p150,95 (see Chapter 7). Neutrophil CR3 deficiency is associated with abnormalities of adherence-related functions including aggregation, margination, chemotaxis, spreading, and phagocytosis of opsonized particles.[50–52] The clinical features include a history of delayed separation of the umbilical stump and patent urachus (sometimes requiring surgical excision and closure), poor wound healing, and the absence of pus formation in a setting of recurrent bacterial and fungal infections. Focal or spreading skin and subcutaneous infections, otitis, mucositis, gingivitis, and periodontitis are common; systemic and deep-seated infections including meningitis, pneumonitis, and perianal abscess formation occur less frequently. The intravascular marginated pool of neutrophils is absent or markedly diminished in CR3 deficiency, and patients have a persistent neutrophilia even in the absence of infection and a striking leukocytosis (up to ≈150,000/mm^3) in its presence. Impaired T-cell cytotoxicity and abnormal B-cell function are also seen.[50,51]

A patient from one kindred who was initially shown to have a disorder of neutrophil actin polymerization was later found to be deficient in CR3 as well.[53,54] Neutrophils deficient in CR3 demonstrate a prolonged respiratory burst[55] and fail to adapt normally to repetitive stimulation with formylpeptide chemoattractants.[56] These observations suggest that the CR3 family of adherence-related glycoproteins may additionally be involved in the modulation of cytoskeletal assembly and receptor processing.

Patients with CR3 deficiency are easily recognized by immunofluorescence microscopy or fluorescence-activated cell sorter analysis using commercially available antibodies to CR3 epitopes.[50,51] Since patients may have moderate or profound deficits in CR3 expression, these tests should be performed by laboratories familiar with their interpretation. In the absence of immediate access to such facilities, presumptive evidence supporting the diagnosis can be obtained by the failure of neutrophils to stick and spread normally on glass or a failure to aggregate, despite shape change, upon stimulation with formylpeptide chemoattractants.[57]

Neutrophil-Specific Granule Deficiency

The first granules to appear during neutrophil maturation are the primary or azurophil granules, which account for about one-third of all granules in the mature cell. Azurophil granules are lysosome-like and contain acid hydrolases and a diverse group of degradative enzymes as well as distinct antimicrobial cationic proteins, the defensins, and bactericidal/permeability increasing factor.[58,59] Azurophil granules function primarily in the intracellular milieu (in the phagolysosomal vacuole) where they are involved in the killing and degradation of microorganisms and ultimately in the inactivation of the inflammatory response.

Neutrophil secondary granules appear at approximately the metamyelocyte stage of maturation and have been designated "specific" by virtue of their unique contents, lactoferrin and vitamin B_{12} binding protein.[60] Lactoferrin facilitates the production of hydroxyl radicals and chelates the iron necessary for microbial growth. In addition, specific granules contain lysozyme and collagenase, components of azurophil granules.[61] Recent evidence supports the existence of a population of gelatinase-containing tertiary granules that undergoes exocytosis in response to mild stimuli.[62,63] Neutrophils also contain an intracellular reservoir of various proteins (including receptors for iC3b, laminin, formylpeptide chemoattractants, signal-transducing G-proteins, cytochrome b_{558}, plasminogen activator, and alkaline phosphatase) whose translocation to the cell surface may be important in chemotaxis, activation of microbicidal pathways, and regulation of the inflammatory response.[64–69] Specific granules have been considered the intracellular reservoir for some of these proteins, but other, as yet poorly characterized intracellular membrane vescicles may also be involved.

The importance of neutrophil-specific granules in host defenses is dramatized by the congenital syndrome of specific granule deficiency.[60] This is an exceedingly rare disorder characterized by diminished inflammatory responses and severe bacterial infections of skin and deep tissues without predisposition to a particular class of organisms. Cell motility to all stimuli is strikingly diminished in congenital specific granule deficiency. Decreasing bactericidal activity and a failure to generate chemoattractants and inflammatory mediators from plasma probably also contribute to the increased susceptibility to infection.[60,61]

There is evidence for heterogeneity in the genesis of this disorder since neutrophils from one patient described appear to contain "empty" secondary granules, whereas neutrophils from other patients lack the granule-limiting membrane in addition to granule contents.[70] Azurophil granules from patients with specific granule deficiency are of lighter than normal density, and neutrophils from the few patients studied lack gelatinase and defensins, normally components of tertiary and azurophil granules, respectively.[71] The defect appears to be limited to cells of myeloid lineage since lactoferrin is found in normal amounts in parotid and nasolacrimal secretions in patients with neutrophil-specific granule deficiency.[71] Lactoferrin mRNA is totally absent or greatly diminished in bone marrow cultures of patients with specific granule deficiency, which suggests that the disorder involves regulatory defects in the transcription of specific mRNAs normally produced at a particular stage of myelogenesis.[71]

Neutrophil secondary granules but not primary granules are visualized by Wright staining of peripheral blood. Hence, patients with specific granule deficiency can be recognized because their neutrophils appear devoid of granules on Wright stain but stain normally with peroxidase. Nuclei are bilobed, and the nuclear membrane may be distorted by blebs, clefts, and pockets.[60] The absence of neutrophil-specific granules should be confirmed by a quantitative determination of vitamin B_{12} binding protein (by radioisotope binding) and lactoferrin (by enzyme-linked immunoassay or immunoblot analysis using commercially available antibodies).

Chédiak-Higashi Syndrome

The Chédiak-Higashi syndrome (CHS) is a rare disorder characterized by autosomal recessive inheritance, recurrent infections, moderate neutropenia, characteristic giant lysosomes in many tissues, partial occulocutaneous albinism, and central and peripheral neuropathy. In most patients the disease eventually enters an accelerated phase characterized by extensive non-neoplastic lymphoid infiltration, pancytopenia, serious infection, and progressive peripheral neuropathy.[72,73] In CHS, neutrophils are deficient in elastase (a normal component of azurophil granules that may be important in the degradation of endothelial basement membrane and neutrophil diapedesis[74]) and the giant neutrophil lysosomes contain other constituents normally segregated between azurophil and specific granules.[73] In addition, in vitro abnormalities of cell deformability and microtubule assembly, impaired chemotaxis, and phagolysosomal fusion probably contribute to the increased susceptibility to infection in vivo.

In the appropriate clinical setting examination of the peripheral blood smear is sufficient to identify all patients with CHS. The giant blue-gray lysosomes in granulocytes can be confused with Döhle or May-Hegglin bodies, but in the absence of the characteristic clinical features of CHS the latter abnormalities will be easily distinguished. Moreover, in CHS, giant lysosomes are found within lymphocytes and erythrocytes, whereas Döhle bodies are limited to neutrophils and May-Hegglin bodies to cells of granulocytic lineage.[75]

Myeloperoxidase Deficiency

In the presence of halide, myeloperoxidase (MPO) catalyzes the conversion of H_2O_2 to hypochlorous acid.[46,47] The MPO-halide-H_2O_2 system can damage microorganisms by incorporation of halide into the cell wall, but other mechanisms probably account for the microbicidal potency of the system. In addition to hypochlorous acid, other toxic moieties are ultimately produced including chlorine and potent long-lived *N*-chloro oxidants.[76] MPO is an iron-containing heme protein that is responsible for the peroxidase activity of azurophil granules and for the greenish color of these granules and of pus. Hereditary MPO deficiency is a relatively common disorder occurring as a total (≈1:4000) or a partial (≈1:2000) absence of MPO in neutrophils and monocytes.[77] The MPO gene is on chromosome 17.[78] A full-length cDNA probe has been cloned and used to show that the endonuclease cleavage pattern of genomic DNA from individuals deficient in MPO differs from that of normal individuals in the region of the MPO gene.[78] Native MPO consists of large and small peptide subunits. The relationship between subunits and the location of the heme binding regions have not been fully established. Since myeloid cells from individuals with a complete deficiency of MPO produce normal-sized mRNA for MPO but do not contain mature MPO peptides, hereditary MPO deficiency may represent a genetic defect that affects post-translational processing of an abnormal precursor protein.[79]

In complete MPO deficiency the respiratory burst is prolonged, which supports the concept that MPO plays a role in inactivation of the inflammatory response.[80–82] Otherwise healthy individuals with a complete deficiency of MPO are not at an increased risk of infection, but deep fungal infections have been noted infrequently in poorly controlled diabetics with MPO deficiency. Better identification of MPO-deficient individuals would have little impact on clinical practice since optimal management depends only on careful control of any underlying immunosuppressive diseases. MPO deficiency is easily recognized by peroxidase stains.

Localized Juvenile Periodontitis

Moderate to severe gingivitis, periodontitis, and mucositis are frequent findings in patients with significant neutropenia or phagocytic cell dysfunction. In most cases intraoral infection is associated with recurrent infection at other sites. In contrast, localized juvenile periodontitis (LJP) is a disease of adolescents that is characterized by severe alveolar bone loss limited primarily to the first molars and incisors.[8] Patients are not predisposed to extraoral infection. Patients with LJP have a moderate but reproducible impairment of chemotaxis stimulated by formylpeptides and C5a; neutrophil adherence in LJP is normal. Defective chemotaxis in LJP persists after aggressive local therapy (in distinction to the chemotactic defect described in patients with intraoral *Capnocytophaga* infection[83]) and has been demonstrated in siblings of index patients before the development of clinical disease.[8] Limited data suggest that chemoattractant receptor numbers and affinities are normal in LJP but that receptor processing may be impaired.[84,85] It is unclear whether the latter abnormalities are causally related to the chemotactic defect in LJP or reflect a more fundamental abnormality in membrane processing.

TABLE 4. Secondary Immunodeficiency

Clinical Setting	*Observed Functional Deficiencies*
Infection	
Acute viral infection	Lymphopenia, decreased circulating T cells, depressed CD4/CD8 ratio in some, abnormal monocyte function with influenza and herpes simplex
HIV infection	Lymphopenia, decreased circulating T cells, depressed CD4/CD8 ratio
Tuberculosis, leprosy	Decreased DCH
Malignancy	
Hodgkin's disease	Decreased DCH, impaired antibody response to certain antigens, treatment and splenectomy may contribute to deficits
Leukemia	Variable immunoglobulin levels
Myeloma	Impaired antibody response, decreased immunoglobulins and/or complement
Solid tumors	Impaired monocyte chemotaxis
Autoimmune disorders	
SLE	Decreased DCH, decreased T cells, immunoglobulins usually increased, may be associated with complement deficiency
Rheumatoid arthritis	Decreased DCH, immunoglobulins usually increased, normal response to antigens, abnormal neutrophil chemotaxis
Protein-losing states	Decreased immunoglobulins, complement, and DCH
Immunosuppressive therapy	
Corticosteroids	Transient T-cell sequestration, decreased immunoglobulin synthesis, decreased neutrophil adherence and degranulation
Cytotoxic agents Radiation	Variable decrease in T-cell, B-cell, and granulocyte numbers and function
Anti-thymocyte globulin	Decreased T-cell numbers and function, B-cell function variably impaired
Cyclosporine	Decreased T-cell function and T-cell-dependent B-cell function
Dilantin, penicillamine	IgA deficiency, hypogammaglobulinemia
Miscellaneous	
Sickle cell disease Splenectomy	Decreased antibody response, opsonization
Thermal injury Neonates	Decreased neutrophil chemotaxis and degranulation
Diabetes	Decreased neutrophil chemotaxis and phagocytosis
Aging	Decreased antibody response to certain antigens, decreased DCH

Abbreviations: HIV: human immunodeficiency virus; DCH: delayed cutaneous hypersensitivity; SLE, systemic lupus erythematosus.

ADDITIONAL STUDIES OF PHAGOCYTE FUNCTION

Assays of neutrophil or monocyte chemotaxis, phagocytosis, and microbicidal activity, although frequently recommended in evaluation of patients with suspected immunodeficiency, are of limited value in screening. In an investigational setting such studies have been critical to the current understanding of leukocyte physiology. However, these assays are poorly standardized for clinical testing, are technically demanding, and are subject to considerable biologic variability, even in experienced hands. Unless in vitro function is profoundly impaired, the extent to which the demonstrated abnormalities contribute to impaired host defenses in vivo is usually unclear. Moreover, in and of themselves, the demonstrated abnormalities are not diagnostic of any of the well-characterized disorders of phagocyte function. Migration of leukocytes into Rebuck skin windows or skin blisters is occasionally informative but not essential for diagnosis. These procedures establish a potential portal of entry for microbes and may be hazardous in immunodeficient patients. The foregoing notwithstanding, several poorly understood syndromes of phagocyte dysfunction (e.g., lazy leukocyte syndrome, Papillon-Lefevre syndrome, icthyosis, mannosidosis, Down syndrome) lack specific biochemical markers and were initially characterized on the basis of clinical features accompanied by in vitro deficits in chemotaxis, phagocytosis, or killing.[86,87] These appear to be exceedingly rare conditions and, for practical purposes, may be largely of historic interest. Were such patients studied within a contemporary technical and conceptual framework, other diagnoses would, in some instances, probably be apparent.

CLINICAL ASSESSMENT OF IMMUNOCOMPETENCE IN PATIENTS WITH SYSTEMIC ILLNESS

Aging, systemic illness, and the use of immunosuppressive agents may be accompanied by a decline in immunocompetence (Table 4). In some instances the particular limb or component of the immune system that is involved has been identified. Beyond simple screening (complete blood count and differential, DCH testing, and possibly an assessment of immunoglobulins) there is no advantage to routine immunologic testing. Recognition of the increased risk of infection and attention to immunization status are important. Assays of immune function may provide critical insights into the natural history and basic mechanisms of disease but do not aid in the care of the individual patient.

REFERENCES

1. Dingle JH, Badger GF, Jordan WS Jr. Illness in the Home: Study of 25,000 Illnesses in a Group of Cleveland Families. Cleveland: Western Reserve University Press; 1964:1.
2. Gwaltney JM Jr, Hendley JO, Simon G, et al. Rhinovirus infections in an industrial population. I. The occurrence of illness. N Engl J Med. 1966;275:1261.
3. Cooper MD, Lawton AR III. Immune deficiency diseases. In: Braunwald E, Isselbacher KJ, Petersdorf RG, et al., eds. Harrison's Principles of Internal Medicine. 11th ed. New York: McGraw-Hill; 1987:1385.
4. Buckley RH. Humoral immunodeficiency. Clin Immunol Immunopathol. 1986;40:13.
5. Rosen FS, Cooper MD, Wedgwood, RJP. The primary immunodeficiencies. N Engl J Med. 1984;311:235, 300.
6. Buckley RH: Immunodeficiency diseases. JAMA. 1987;258:2841.
7. Rosen FS, Wedgwood RJ, Eibl M, et al. Primary immunodeficiency diseases: Report of a World Health Organization Scientific Group. Clin Immunol Immunopathol. 1986;40:166.
8. Van Dyke TE, Levine MJ, Genco RJ. Neutrophil function and oral disease. J Oral Pathol. 1985;14:95.
9. deShazo RD, Lopez M, Salvaggio JE. Use and interpretation of diagnostic immunologic laboratory tests. JAMA. 1987;258:3011.
10. Check IJ, Piper M. Quantitation of immunoglobulins. In: Rose NR, Friedman H, Fahey JL, eds. Manual of Clinical Laboratory Immunology. 3rd ed. Washington DC: American Society for Microbiology 1986:138.
11. Stiehm ER, Fudenberg HH. Serum levels of immune globulins in health and disease: A survey. Pediatrics. 1966;37:715.
12. Stiehm ER. Immunodeficiency—general considerations. In: Stiehm ER, Fulginetti VA, eds. Immunologic Disorders in Infants and Children. Philadelphia: WB Saunders; 1980.
13. Nahn MH, Blaese RM, Crain MJ, et al. Patients with Wiskott-Aldrich syndrome have normal IgG2 levels. J Immunol. 1986;137:3484.
14. Claman HN. The biology of the immune response. JAMA. 1987;258:2835.
15. Wall R, Kuehl M. Biosynthesis and regulation of immunoglobulins. Annu Rev Immunol. 1983;1:393.
16. Gathings WE, Kubagawa H, Cooper MD. A distinctive pattern of B-cell immaturity in perinatal humans. Immunol Rev. 1981;57:107.
17. Wedgwood RJ, Ochs HD, Davis SD. The recognition and classification of immunodeficiency diseases with bacteriophage ϕX174. I: Bergsma D, Good RA, Finstad J, eds. Immunodeficiency in Man and Animals. Sunderland, MA: Sinauer Associates; 1975:331.
18. Dreskin SC, Goldsmith PK, Gallin JI. Immunoglobulins in the hyperimmunoglobulin E and recurrent infection (Job's) syndrome. J Clin Invest. 1985;75:26.
19. Nathan CF, Kaplan G, Levis WR, et al. Local and systemic effects of intradermal recombinant interferon-γ in patients with lepromatous leprosy. N Engl J Med. 1986;315:6.
20. Buckley RH. Advances in the diagnosis and treatment of immunodeficiency diseases. Arch Intern Med. 1986;146:377.
21. Hong R. Immunodeficiency. In: Rose NR, Friedman H, Fahey JL, eds. Manual of Clinical Laboratory Immunology. 3rd ed. Washington DC: American Society for Microbiology. 1986:702.
22. Hirschorn R. Inherited enzyme deficiencies and immunodeficiency: Adenosine deaminase (ADA) and purine nucleoside phosphorylase (PNP) deficiencies. Clin Immunol Immunopathol. 1986;40:157.
23. Ammann AJ. Immunodeficiency diseases. In: Stites DP, Stobo JD, Wells JV, eds. Basic & Clinical Immunology. 6th ed. Norwalk, CT: Appleton & Lange; 1987:317.
24. Dinarello CA, Mier JW. Current concepts: Lymphokines. N Engl J Med. 1987;317:940.
25. Johnston RB Jr. Current concepts—immunology: Monocytes and macrophages. N Engl J Med. 1988;318:747.
26. Beutler B, Cerami A. Cachectin and tumor necrosis as two sides of the same biological coin. Nature. 1986;320:584.
27. Adams DO, Hamilton TA. The cell biology of macrophage activation. Annu Rev Immunol. 1984;2:283.
28. Metcalf D. The granulocyte-macrophage colony stimulating factors. Science. 1985;229:16.
29. Walz A, Peveri P, Aschauer W, et al. Purification and amino acid sequencing of NAF, a novel neutrophil-activating factor produced by monocytes. Biochem Biophys Res Commun. 1987;149:755.
30. Yoshimura T, Matsushima K, Oppenheim JJ, et al. Neutrophil chemotactic factor produced by lipopolysaccharide (LPS)-stimulated human blood mononuclear leukocytes: Partial characterization and separation from interleukin 1 (IL 1). J Immunol. 1987;139:788.
31. Murray HW. Interferon-gamma, the activated macrophage, and host defense against microbial challenge. Ann Intern Med. 1988;108:595.
32. Joiner KA, Brown EJ, Frank MM. Complement and bacteria: Chemistry and biology in host defense. Annu Rev Immunol. 1984;2:461.
33. Fries LF, Frank MM. Complement and related proteins: Inherited deficiencies. In: Gallin JI, Goldstein IM, Snyderman R, eds. Inflammation: Basic Principles and Clinical Correlates. New York: Raven Press; 1988:89.
34. Ruddy S. Complement. In: Rose NR, Friedman H, Fahey JL, eds. Manual of Clinical Laboratory Immunology. 3rd ed. Washington DC: American Society for Microbiology. 1986:175.
35. Sjiholm AG, Kuijper EJ, Tijssen CC, et al. Dysfunctional properdin in a Dutch Family with meningococcal disease. N Engl J Med. 1988;319:33.
36. Ross SC, Densen P. Complement deficiency states and infection: Epidemiology, pathogenesis and consequences of neisserial and other infections in an immune deficiency. Medicine (Baltimore). 1984;63:243.
37. Cartwright GE, Athens JW, Wintrobe MM. The kinetics of neutrophilic cells. Blood. 1964;24:780.
38. Finch SC. Granulocytopenia. In: Williams WJ, Beutler E, Erslev AJ, et al., eds. Hematology. 2nd ed. New York: McGraw-Hill; 1977:717.
39. Dancey JT, Deubelbeiss KA, Harker LA, et al. Neutrophil kinetics in man. J Clin Invest. 1976;58:705.
40. Joyce RA, Boggs DR, Hasiba U, et al. Marginal neutrophil pool size in normal subjects and neutropenic patients as measured by epinephrine infusion. J Lab Clin Med. 1976;88:614.
41. Minchinton RM, McGrath KM. Alloimmune neonatal neutropenia—a neglected diagnosis? Med J Aust. 1987;147:139.
42. Ducos R, Madyastha PR, Warrier RP, et al. Neutrophil agglutinins in idiopathic chronic neutropenia of early childhood. Am J Dis Child. 1986;140:65.
43. Gallin JI, Fauci AS, eds. Advances in Host Defense Mechanisms. v. 3. In: Chronic Granulomatous Disease. New York: Raven Press; 1982:262.
44. Gallin JI, Buescher ES, Seligmann BE, et al. Recent advances in chronic granulomatous disease. Ann Intern Med. 1983;99:657.
45. Tauber AI, Borregaard N, Simons E, et al. Chronic granulomatous disease; a syndrome of phagocyte oxidase deficiencies. Medicine (Baltimore). 1983;62:286.
46. Klebanoff SJ. Oxygen metabolism and the toxic properties of phagocytes. Ann Intern Med. 1980;93:480.
47. Babior BM. The respiratory burst of phagocytes. J Clin Invest. 1984;73:599.
48. Ezekowitz RAB, Orkin SH, Newburger PE. Recombinant interferon gamma augments phagocyte superoxide production and X-chronic granulomatous disease gene expression in X-linked variant chronic granulomatous disease. J Clin Invest. 1987;80:1009.
49. Sechler JMG, Malech HL, White CJ, et al. Recombinant interferon-γ reconstitutes defective phagocyte function in patients with chronic granulomatous disease of childhood. Proc Natl Acad Sci USA. 1988;85:4874.

50. Anderson DC, Schmalstieg FC, Finegold MJ, et al. The severe and moderate phenotypes of heritable Mac-1, LFA-1, p150,95 deficiency: Their qualitative definition and relation to leukocyte dysfunction and clinical features. J Infect Dis. 1985;152:668.
51. Anderson DC, Springer TA. Leukocyte adhesion deficiency: An inherited defect in the Mac-1, LFA-1, and p150,95 glycoproteins. Annu Rev Med. 1987;38:175.
52. Harlan JM, Killen PD, Senecal FM, et al. The role of neutrophil membrane glycoprotein GP-150 in neutrophil adherence to endothelium in vitro. Blood. 1985;66:167.
53. Boxer LA, Hedley-Whyte ET, Stossel TP. Neutrophil actin dysfunction and abnormal neutrophil behavior. N Engl J Med. 1974;291:1093.
54. Southwick FS, Holbrook T, Howard T, et al. Neutrophil actin dysfunction is associated with a deficiency of Mol (Abstract). Clin Res. 1986;34:533.
55. Nauseef WM, DeAlarcon P, Bale JF, et al. Aberrant activation and regulation of the oxidative burst in neutrophils with Mol glycoprotein deficiency. J Immunol. 1986;137:636–42.
56. Seligmann B, Gallin JI. Neutrophils from a CR3 (C3bi) receptor deficient patient exhibit low ED-50 values for fmet-leu-phe stimulated responses and do not exhibit affinity adaption (Abstract). Clin Res. 1986;34:679.
57. Rotrosen D, Gallin JI. Disorders of phagocyte function. Annu Rev Immunol. 1987;5:127.
58. Weiss J, Victor M, Elsbach P. Role of charge and hydrophobic interactions in the action of the bactericidal/permeability increasing protein of neutrophils on gram-negative bacteria. J Clin Invest. 1981;71:540.
59. Ganz T, Selsted ME, Szklarek D, et al. Defensins: Natural peptide antibiotics of human neutrophils. J Clin Invest. 1985;76:1427.
60. Gallin JI. Neutrophil specific granule deficiency. Annu Rev Med. 1985;36:263.
61. Wright DG, Gallin JI. A functional differentiation of human neutrophil granules: Generation of C5a by a specific (secondary) granule product and inactivation of C5a by azurophil (primary) granule products. J Immunol. 1977;119:1068.
62. DeWald B, Bretz U, Baggiolini M. Release of gelatinase from a novel secretory compartment of human neutrophils. J Clin Invest. 1982;70:518.
63. Yoon PS, Boxer LA, Mayo LA, et al. Human neutrophil laminin receptors: Activation-dependent receptor expression. J Immunol. 1987;138:259.
64. Borregaard N, Heiple JM, Simons ER, et al. Subcellular localization of the b-cytochrome component of the human neutrophil microbicidal oxidase: Translocation during activation. J Cell Biol. 1983;97:52.
65. Borregaard N, Miller LJ, Springer TA. Chemoattractant-regulated mobilization of a novel intracellular compartment in human neutrophils. Science. 1987;237:1204.
66. Fletcher MP, Gallin JI. Human neutrophils contain an intracellular pool of putative receptors for the chemoattractant N-formyl-methionyl-leucyl-phenylalanine. Blood. 1983;62:792.
67. Heiple JM, Ossowski L. Human neutrophil plasminogen activator is localized in specific granules and is translocated to the cell surface by exocytosis. J Exp Med. 1986;164:826.
68. Ohno Y, Seligmann BE, Gallin JI. Cytochrome b translocation to human neutrophil plasma membranes and superoxide release. J Biol Chem. 1985;260:2409.
69. Rotrosen D, Gallin JI, Spiegel AM, et al. Subcellular localization of Giα in human neutrophils. J Biol Chem. 1988;263:10958.
70. Parmley RT, Tzeng DY, Baehner RL, et al. Abnormal distribution of complex carbohydrates in neutrophils of a patient with lactoferrin deficiency. Blood. 1983;62:538.
71. Lomax KJ, Gallin JI, Rotrosen D, et al. A selective defect in myeloid cell lactoferrin gene expression in neutrophil specific granule deficiency. J Clin Invest. 1989;83:514–519.
72. Blume RS, Wolff SM. The Chédiak-Higashi syndrome: Studies in four patients and a review of the literature. Medicine (Baltimore). 1972;51:247.
73. Klebanoff SJ, Clark RA. Chédiak-Higashi syndrome. In: The Neutrophil: Function and Clinical Disorders. Amsterdam: Elsevier Biomedical; 1978.
74. Smedly LA, Tonnesen MG, Sandhaus RA, et al. Neutrophil mediated injury to endothelial cells: Enhancement by endotoxin and essential role of neutrophil elastase. J Clin Invest. 1986;77:1233.
75. Wintrobe MM, Lee RG, Bithell TC, et al. eds. Clinical Hematology. 7th ed. Philadelphia: Lee & Febriger; 1975:221.
76. Test ST, Lampert MB, Ossanna PJ, et al. Generation of nitrogen-chlorine oxidants by human phagocytes. J Clin Invest. 1984;74:1341.
77. Parry MF, Root RK, Metcalf JA. Myeloperoxidase deficiency. Prevalence and clinical significance. Ann Intern Med. 1981;95:293.
78. Weil SC, Rosner GL, Reid MS, et al. cDNA cloning of human myeloperoxidase: Decrease in myeloperoxidase in RNA upon induction of HL-60 cells. Proc Natl Acad Sci USA. 1987;84:2057.
79. Nauseef WM. Myeloperoxidase biosynthesis by a human promyelocytic leukemia cell line: Insight into myeloperoxidase deficiency. Blood. 1986;67:865.
80. Clark RA, Klebanoff SJ. Chemotactic factor inactivation by the myeloperoxidase-hydrogen peroxide-halide system. J Clin Invest. 1979;64:913.
81. Henderson WR, Klebanoff SJ. Leukotriene production and inactivation by normal, chronic granulomatous disease and myeloperoxidase-deficient neutrophils. J Biol Chem. 1983;258:13522.
82. Clark RA, Borregaard N. Neutrophils autoinactivate secretory products by myeloperoxidase-catalyzed oxidation. Blood. 1985;65:375.
83. Shurin SB, Socransky SS, Sweeney E, et al. A neutrophil disorder induced by capnocytophaga, a dental micro-organism. N Engl J Med. 1979;301:849.
84. Van Dyke TE, Levine MJ, Tabak LA, et al. Reduced chemotactic peptide binding in juvenile periodontitis: A model for neutrophil function. Biochem Biophys Res Commun. 1981;100:1278.
85. Van Dyke TE. Role of the neutrophil in oral disease: Receptor deficiency in leukocytes from patients with juvenile periodontitis. Rev Infect Dis. 1985;7:419.
86. Gallin JI. Abnormalities of phagocyte chemotaxis: Pathophysiology, clinical manifestations, and management of patients. Rev Infect Dis. 1981;3:1196.
87. Elmostehy MR. Papillon-Lefevre syndrome. Precocious periodontosis with epidermal lesions: Review of literature and presentation of five cases. Egypt Dent J. 1976;22:49.

SECTION C. EPIDEMIOLOGY OF INFECTIOUS DISEASE

10. PRINCIPLES AND METHODS

PHILIP S. BRACHMAN

Epidemiology is the evaluation of the determinants, occurrence, distribution, and control of health and disease in a defined population. The word *epidemiology* is derived from the Greek (*epi*, upon; *demos*, people; *logy*, study); it is the study of anything that happens to people.

The science of epidemiology can be applied to the study of any disease or condition, acute or chronic, infectious or noninfectious, communicable or noncommunicable, and to the study of health as well. It is a science of rates, in which, for example, the numerator is the number of cases of a disease that occur in a given period of time and the denominator is the total population at risk, that is, exposed to the etiologic agent.

Epidemiologists should be working colleagues of clinicians. A clinician who sees an individual patient may not relate that patient's condition to the community in which he or she lives. The insularity of the clinician may inhibit definition of a common disease problem occurring among a group of people and thus delay or inhibit the institution of appropriate control and prevention measures. Multiple cases of a single disease entity may appear simultaneously in a population who have had a common exposure to the etiologic agent. If the individual cases diagnosed by different physicians are not reported, no association among the cases can be made. If, however, the individual cases are reported and can be investigated as a group in an *epidemiologic investigation*, the epidemic has a better chance of being characterized, the cases related, and control measures instituted.

Once the outbreak has been identified and the diagnosis confirmed, other cases that are not diagnosable with certainty by themselves may become diagnosable by their similarities with the cases initially identified as epidemic cases. This development of *consensus diagnosis* has obvious benefits for the individual patient as well as allowing a better characterization of the epidemic.

Evaluation of a single case of an infectious disease may not identify the method of transmission since diseases can be transmitted by various routes; however, if multiple cases have occurred and each is investigated, analysis of the combined data may identify the route of transmission.

Additionally, evaluation of multiple cases of the same disease may identify predisposing host factors; with this information, cases may be prevented by removing or protecting people at risk against the predisposing factor.

The epidemiologic investigation provides the opportunity of collating information from cases temporally related into a coherent narrative, examination of which should describe the cause, transmission, and host factors that may suggest an intervention point leading to control and prevention. Without an epidemiologic investigation, cases may continue to occur until the disease has run its natural course and/or there are no susceptibles left in the population.

A parallel may be drawn between the professional activities of the private practitioner or clinician and the practitioner of epidemiology. The private practitioner's initial contact with the situation is through an individual patient, whereas the epidemiologist usually becomes involved because of a collection of cases. The clinician obtains the patient's history, conducts a physical examination, and orders laboratory tests, all of which are necessary in investigating the illness of an individual patient. The epidemiologist is also interested in the history, physical examination, and results of laboratory tests, but he or she collects these data for all the patients involved in the outbreak. The private practitioner considers the results of the examination of one patient, makes a diagnosis, and prescribes appropriate therapy for that person. The epidemiologist analyzes available data from the community of patients and others at risk, makes a prediction as to additional cases, and then prescribes intervention measures for the involved population. The private practitioner is concerned with the prognosis for the patient, whereas the epidemiologist is concerned with the trend of the disease in the community.

It should be apparent that the clinician and the epidemiologist are dependent on each other. The epidemiologist is dependent on the clinician to make the diagnosis and to report the case; the accumulation of individual reports of cases allows the epidemiologist to practice his or her profession. The clinician is dependent on the epidemiologist to investigate a collection of cases of a similar nature and to prescribe the proper control and prevention measures. However, these two professionals should not be isolated within their own specialties. The clinician should know something about epidemiology, just as the epidemiologist should be knowledgeable about clinical medicine. At the same time they need to recognize their own limitations and to consult freely with one another. In this way they both may practice their professions to the advantage of the community in controlling and preventing disease.

The epidemiologist can serve as a connection between the clinicians and their patients, the community, and all the patients ultimately involved in the specific disease problem. It should be apparent that epidemiologic investigations should be beneficial to the patient and to the physician, as well as to the community. In addition to reducing the incidence of disease, there should be financial savings to all involved in the health care system and, ultimately, better use of health resources.

DEFINITIONS

Infection means the presence and replication of microorganisms in the tissues of a host. The host response to infection is highly variable, depending on the interrelationship of many host and agent factors, and ranges from subclinical or inapparent infection to disease. *Disease* is the clinical expression of infection and indicates that not only are microorganisms present and replicating but they also are disrupting the host to the extent that signs and symptoms are being produced. Disease may vary from mild to severe with the most severe form leading to death.

A *subclinical infection* indicates a reaction between the agent and the host limited to an immune response that can only be diagnosed by serologic means with demonstration of either a single high titer or a fourfold rise in titer to the infecting agent.

Colonization indicates the presence of an organism without clinical or subclinical disease. However, the organism is replicating in or on the tissues of the host and can be identified by culture in the laboratory. *Contamination* refers to the presence of microorganisms on a body surface without tissue invasion or reaction or to their presence on the surface of inanimate objects.

A *carrier* is a person who is colonized with an organism but shows no evidence of disease, although disease may have been present earlier. The organisms can be recovered by culture. Carriage may be transient, that is, the organism is carried for a short period of time, intermittent (sporadic), or long term (chronic). The factors that influence the length of carriage are not well defined but may represent partial immunity or be a result of partial therapy directed against the organism. Recovery from clinical disease may result in short-term carriage (*Shigella*) or occasionally in chronic carriage (*Salmonella typhi*).

Dissemination of microorganisms can occur from either a person who is infected or has disease.[1] Usually dissemination is greatest during the latter part of the incubation period, just before the infection becomes clinically apparent. Once disease is evident, dissemination usually decreases, sometimes rather dramatically. However, with some diseases, dissemination may be a serious problem during the clinical phase and until treatment is initiated. A person with disease will arouse suspicion of dissemination, and appropriate precautions can be taken. However, the silent disseminator, that is, the infected person without overt evidence of disease, causes the greatest concern because dissemination can be demonstrated only by special shedding studies or if secondary cases of infection can be proved to have resulted from contact with this person.[2] Dissemination from a carrier may be enhanced by infection or disease with a second microorganism, by development of another (noninfectious) disease, or as a result of unknown causes.[3]

A carrier not disseminating is not necessarily dangerous, and special precautions may be unwarranted. A judgment as to therapy, isolation, or other special actions directed against a carrier should reflect proven dissemination and not just carriage. Special culture surveys to define carriage may lead to an inappropriate decision if there is no evidence of dissemination from the carrier.

Multiple cases of a disease can occur infrequently, at irregular or regular intervals, or at an increased frequency. *Sporadic occurrence* refers to the occasional cases of disease at irregular intervals. *Endemic frequency* refers to a low-level frequency of disease at moderately regular intervals. *Hyperendemic* refers to a gradual increase in the occurrence of a disease beyond the endemic level but not currently at epidemic proportions. The *epidemic occurrence* of disease refers to the sudden increase in incidence of the disease above the expected incidence. *Pandemic disease* is epidemic disease that has spread among continents. For example, the current occurrence of cholera in Africa, Asia, and southern Europe reflects the seventh pandemic of cholera that began in the Celebes Islands in the Pacific.

Disease prevalence refers to the number of cases of the disease that are active at a particular point in time (point prevalence) or that occur over a defined period of time (period prevalence). *Disease incidence* is a rate that reflects the number of new cases of the disease in a defined time period within a specific population.

TECHNIQUES OF EPIDEMIOLOGIC PRACTICE

Three basic epidemiologic techniques—descriptive, analytic, and experimental—are used individually or collectively to investigate an epidemic.

Descriptive Epidemiology

The descriptive technique is most frequently applied initially. If the problem is not solved or if additional questions arise as a result of the initial analysis of the data, then the analytic or the experimental method or both may be applied to the problem.

In descriptive epidemiology, all pertinent data are collected and described according to time, place, and person. In describing time, there are four trends that need to be considered—secular, periodic, seasonal, and acute. The secular trend refers to the long-term variation in the occurrence of the disease; the time interval is years. For example, the secular trend of tetanus shows a gradual but steady decrease in incidence from 1954 to 1987 (Fig. 1).[4] In general, the secular trend is influenced by the overall immunity level of the population and by nonspecific factors, such as socioeconomic, nutritional, and hygienic status.

Periodic trends are the temporary variations in the occurrence of the disease that disrupt the secular trend of the disease. Periodic trends will occur over a time frame of several months to several years. An example is the periodic increase in the incidence of influenza A every 2–3 years, which reflects antigenic drifts in the predominant strain as well as changes in the immunity level of the population.[5] Another example is periodic change in death rates associated with influenza that reflect changes in circulating influenza viruses as well as changes in immunity in the population (Fig. 2).

Seasonal trends are the variations based on climatic factors that directly or indirectly influence disease transmission. Thus, food-borne diseases are more likely to occur in warm months because of the favorable temperature conditions for microorganisms to multiply to disease-producing levels in unrefrigerated foods (Fig. 3).

The acute trend describes the sudden rise in the incidence (rate) of a disease. This trend is referred to as an *epidemic*. The graphic portrayal of these data is called an epidemic curve, which commonly is an analysis of the time of onset (abscissa or horizontal axis) plotted against the number of cases (ordinate or vertical axis).

The time scale for analyzing epidemiologic data varies from minutes for diseases with short incubation periods, such as chemical gastroenteritis, to years for diseases with extremely long incubation periods, such as leprosy. Analysis of these data may allow a judgment to be made as to the mode of transmission.

Frequently the epidemiologist becomes involved in the investigation after the peak of the epidemic has occurred, and the epidemiologic analysis is mainly retrospective; however, if cases are continuing to occur, knowing something about the epidemiology of the disease, including the method of transmission and the shape of its epidemic curve, may allow predictions to be made about the occurrence of additional cases and institution of appropriate controls.

Description of epidemiologic data by place refers to the geographic area in which the contact between the susceptible host and the etiologic agent occurred. This may be a home, public building, or restaurant; a water distribution district; a sanitary district; a political subdivision such as a city, county, region, and so on. The place in which the actual contact between the organism and the person took place may be different from the place in which the vehicle of infection became contaminated. This differentiation may be important with regard to instituting control and prevention measures. For example, a food item contaminated in a delicatessen may have been taken home and then eaten, which would result in the home being the site in which the vehicle of infection came into contact with the susceptible host(s). However, the primary effort toward prevention of additional cases would involve identifying the delicatessen as the site in which the food became contaminated and in which control efforts need to be directed. Place in which exposure to the organism occurred becomes of even greater importance when long-distance travel is considered. Exposure to an infectious agent can occur in one country with the onset of symptoms days

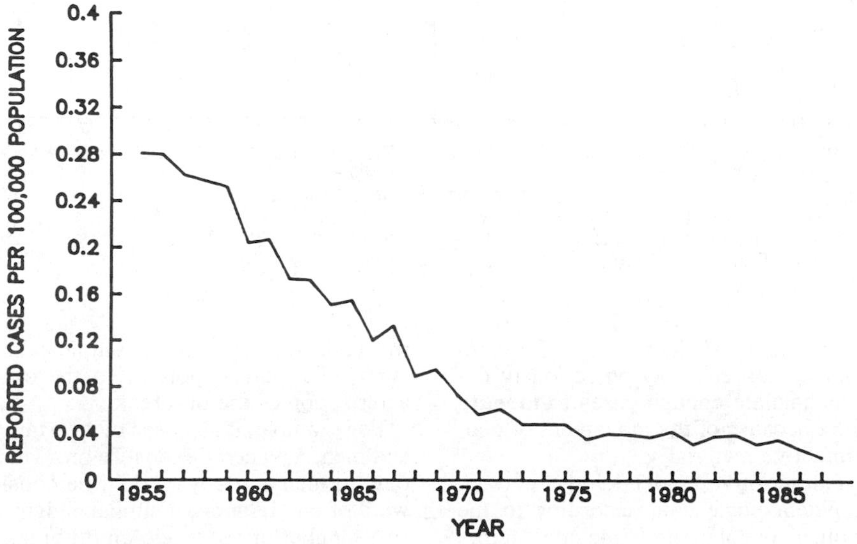

FIG. 1. Reported tetanus cases by year: United States, 1954–1987. (Courtesy of Centers for Disease Control, Epidemiology Program Office, Division of Surveillance and Epidemiologic Studies, Atlanta, GA.)

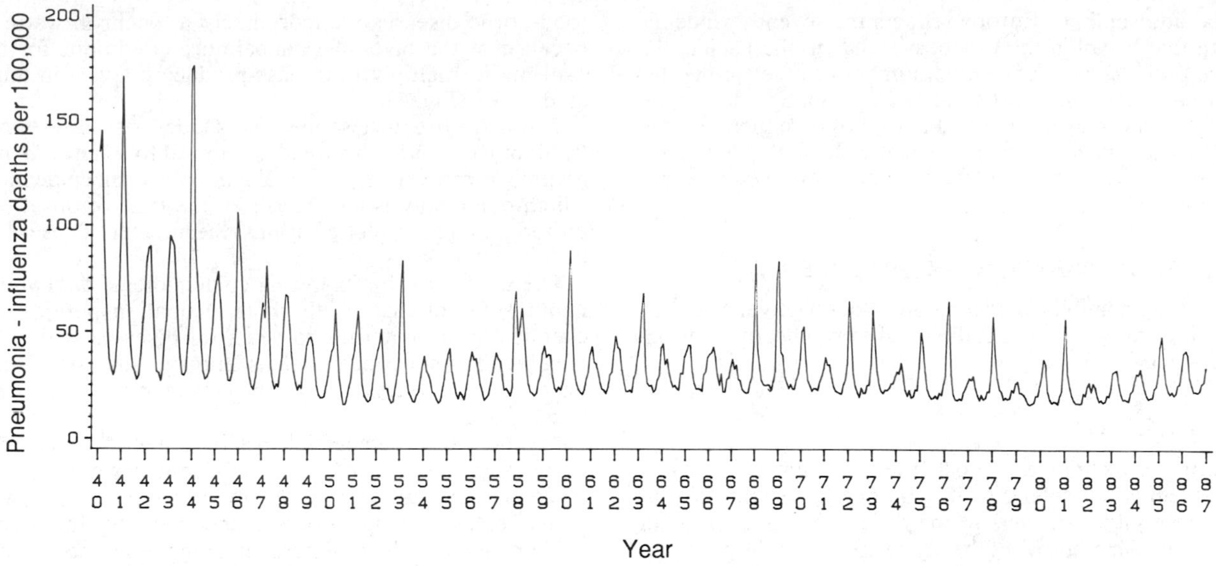

FIG. 2. Pneumonia-influenza death rates by month in the United States, 1940–1987. Monthly rates; annual base. (Courtesy of Centers for Disease Control, Biometrics Activity and Epidemiology Office, Division of Viral Diseases, Atlanta, GA.)

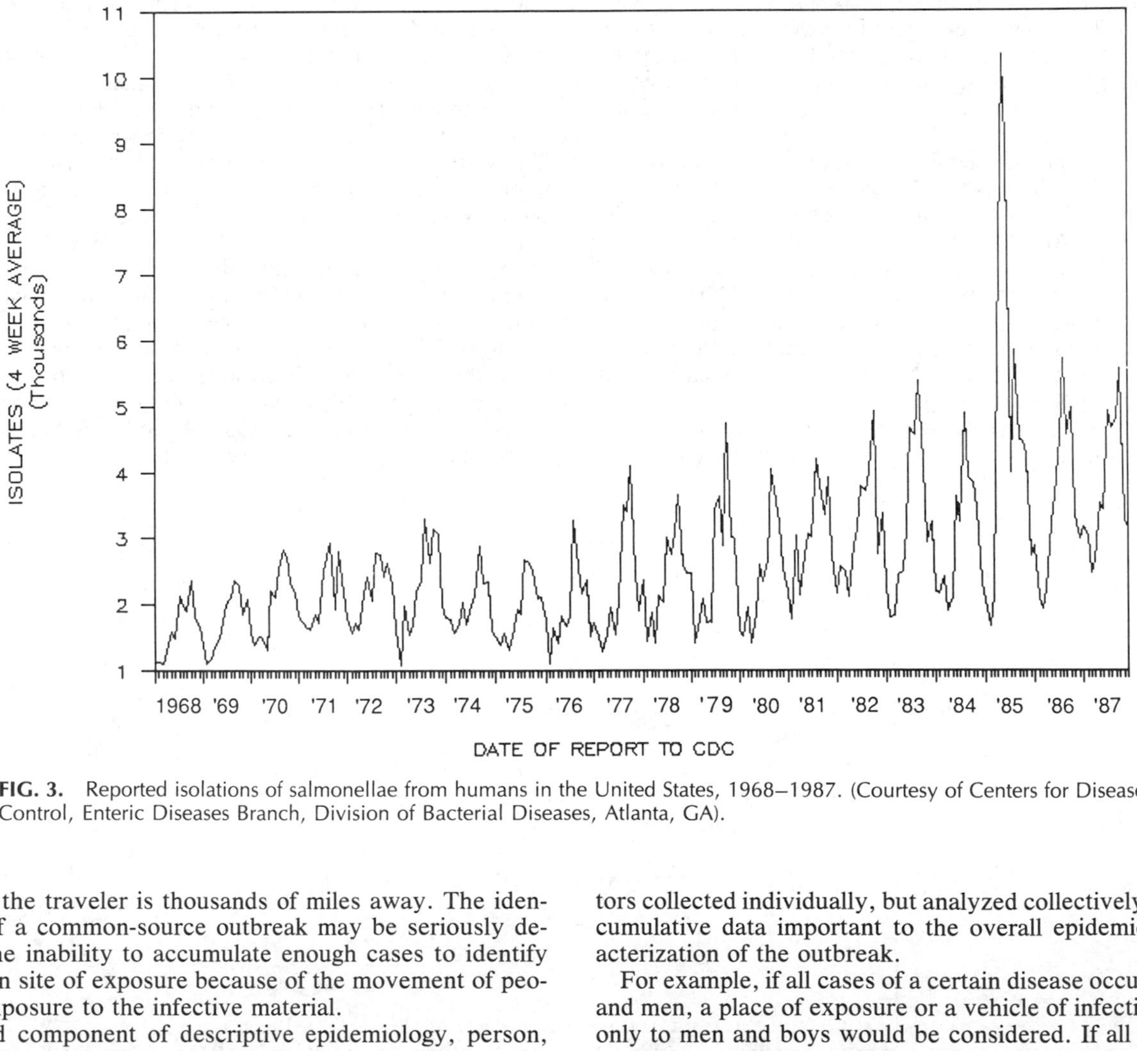

FIG. 3. Reported isolations of salmonellae from humans in the United States, 1968–1987. (Courtesy of Centers for Disease Control, Enteric Diseases Branch, Division of Bacterial Diseases, Atlanta, GA).

later when the traveler is thousands of miles away. The identification of a common-source outbreak may be seriously delayed by the inability to accumulate enough cases to identify the common site of exposure because of the movement of people after exposure to the infective material.

The third component of descriptive epidemiology, person, refers to organizing the epidemiologic data according to the characteristics of the involved people; these include factors such as age, sex, individual susceptibility, race, religion, socioeconomic status, occupation, and social history. These factors collected individually, but analyzed collectively, may show cumulative data important to the overall epidemiologic characterization of the outbreak.

For example, if all cases of a certain disease occurred in boys and men, a place of exposure or a vehicle of infection common only to men and boys would be considered. If all the patients were of one religion, a similar judgment would be made.

A number of years ago an outbreak of gastroenteritis due to *Salmonella new brunswick*, a rare serotype, involving people in eight states occurred.[6] Age-specific attack rates clearly indicated that the cases had primarily occurred in infants; there were three times as many cases in this age group as would be expected. This suggested that the vehicle of infection was something common to infants, commercially distributed over a wide area. These clues led to the identification of the vehicle as a particular batch of powdered skim milk distributed under a variety of brand names but that originated from one processing factory. The source of infection was identified, intervention measures were introduced, and the epidemic was terminated.

The accurate description of the epidemiologic data by personal characteristics may reveal important clues that help to answer the questions of why the epidemic occurred and how to control it and to prevent further spread.

Analytic Epidemiology

The second epidemiologic technique is analytic epidemiology, which is used to investigate the relationships between cause and effect and to evaluate risk factors and disease.[7,8] There are two basic analytic epidemiologic methods—the case-control study and the cohort study. In the case-control method, the investigation starts with an effect and attempts to identify the cause that resulted in that effect. This is conceptually referred to as a *retrospective study*, going back in time to determine what events occurred that resulted in the specific effect. In this type of study, new records are not created; the investigation involves a review of existing records. A critical part of this investigation is the selection of the control group (or comparison group, which is a more accurate term); it is absolutely necessary to avoid having overt or covert bias enter into the selection process. The purpose of a comparison group is to allow comparison with the group to whom the effect occurred to identify quantifiable difference(s) between the two groups that should explain why the effect developed. The comparison group is selected so that it resembles the case group as closely as possible, except that the former group does not have the effect. Thus, if the comparison group is carefully matched to the case group except for the presence of the effect, the reason the case group developed the disease, but the comparison group did not, should become apparent. Case-control studies are used in acute- as well as chronic-disease investigations.

An example of a case-control study is the investigation of an outbreak of gastroenteritis among people at a picnic. It may be difficult or impossible by obtaining food histories only from those ill to identify the common vehicle that transmitted the infection; no one food item may stand out as the contaminated item. Selecting a comparison group of picnickers who selected their meals from the same menu, ate at the same time, were generally of the same age, lived in the same area of town, but were not ill, and obtaining their food histories for the same period of time, should reveal data that incriminate a certain food as the vehicle of infection. That is, those who are ill should have a statistically higher consumption rate of the suspected food than the comparison group.

The second analytic method is the cohort study, which is conceptually referred to as a prospective study. In this method, a population exposed to a specific presumed cause is followed to identify resulting effects. In this type of investigation new records are created. Again, we select a comparison group of people who are similar to the exposed cohort except that they do not have contact with the cause being investigated. Both groups are followed to note the effect of the supposed cause. The comparison group should remain free of the effect. For example, a hospital is experiencing an increase in septicemia and suspects that the cause may be related to use of a certain lot of intravenous fluids. The study cohort is made up of those who receive the suspect fluids; the comparison group should be patients who match them in age, sex, underlying diagnosis, location within the hospital, and other therapeutic procedures but who do not receive the suspect intravenous fluid. If the suspect intravenous fluid is actually contaminated, then some of the group who receive it should develop septicemia, whereas people in the comparison group should not, though some could develop septicemia due to other causes; however, the rates should be statistically significantly different. The difference in attack rates for septicemia between the two groups should be attributable to having received the contaminated fluids.

The case-control study has the advantages over the prospective cohort study of being easier and quicker to conduct and less expensive. One potential difficulty is in selecting an appropriate comparison group without allowing bias to develop in the selection process. Another problem is asking people questions about previous activities, which is fraught with the dangers of poor memory. Another potential problem is inadvertently including subclinical cases among the controls.

The prospective cohort study does not depend on the memory of people and makes it possible to obtain the necessary epidemiologic data as it occurs—not retrospectively. We do have to be careful that there is no bias in selecting the comparison group and in determining the diagnosis. Another problem is the possible need to follow the two groups for a long time. If the incubation period is long, there is the need to follow the participants for an equal or longer period of time. Some of the participants may leave the study, reducing the number of people in the study. Additionally, because of the time involved and the chance of negative findings, the cohort study is usually more expensive to conduct.

Another type of cohort study is a retrospective cohort study in which the effect (disease) occurs and a study is conducted to show whether there is a relationship between the effect and a specific cause. A population exposed to the suspected cause is identified; a comparison group is selected, matching for various factors except that the comparison group lacks exposure to the suspected cause; and the incidence of the effect is calculated. This method of study uses existing records to establish the history of exposure to the cause and then measures the effect of that exposure. Conceptually, this is a cohort study, but temporally, it is a retrospective study.

An additional study method is the cross-sectional study which examines the relationships between cause and effect in a defined population at a specific point in time. This study describes prevalence relationships and allows a direct measurement of the variables.

Experimental Epidemiology

The third epidemiologic technique, the experimental method, involves stating a hypothesis, developing an experimental model that allows for manipulation of one or several factors, and then noting the resultant effect. In this method, the hypothesis is tested. An example is the evaluation of a drug in the treatment of a certain disease. Patients with the disease are selected randomly and divided into two groups; one group is treated with the drug, and the other group is given a placebo. The resultant difference(s) between the two groups is attributed to the drug itself. Animals may be used in experimental epidemiology; if this technique is used on humans, careful consideration must be given to the ethics of the experiment as concerns real or potential danger to the human subjects.

EPIDEMIC INVESTIGATIONS

The objectives of investigating an outbreak of disease are to identify the problem, to ascertain its cause and the method of transmission, and to define the extent of involvement in terms of time, place, and person. The ultimate purpose of the investigation is to determine the appropriate measures necessary to control the outbreak and to prevent similar outbreaks from occurring.

The following paragraphs describe various elements of an epidemic investigation that form the skeleton for investigating the outbreak. There is no rigid rule that an investigation must be investigated in a particular order; it may be appropriate to change the sequence of the elements to meet certain exigencies of the investigation or of the ongoing occurrence of the disease itself. The actual elements may be telescoped or expanded. Additionally, it is important to consider whether control measures can be instituted before completion of the epidemic investigation to prevent the occurrence of additional cases.

An epidemic is an increase in the incidence of a disease above the expected incidence in a specific geographic area within a defined time period. The background occurrence (endemicity) of the disease in the population must be known in order for a judgment to be made as to whether the increased incidence is an epidemic or only normal variation. For example, an increase in the number of *Salmonella* isolates in August in a community may represent the normal increase for that time of year and not an unusual event.

An investigation may be carried out by the physician whose patients are involved, or the local or state health department may be notified and may provide support. Initially, an epidemiologist may be the only resource necessary; however, depending on the complexities of the outbreak, additional personnel may be needed, including nurses, veterinarians, sanitarians, environmental engineers, industrial hygienists, interviewers, statisticians, and laboratorians.

The first element in the investigation is to establish the existence of an epidemic. The initial and possibly other reporting sources should be consulted. This may involve contacting a physician, a health officer, patients, and relatives of patients; examining laboratory reports; reviewing hospital records; and checking absenteeism in industries or schools. This initial effort may be carried out very quickly.

The second element is to verify the diagnosis by obtaining clinical histories, examining patients, and obtaining appropriate specimens for laboratory study. A case definition needs to be developed; it should be broad enough to include all cases that may be important to the overall investigation. In setting a case definition it is important to remember the variability of host responses and that some cases may have been modified by reason of treatment or partial immunity. It is important for the epidemiologist to see "cases" and to discuss the diagnosis with the attending physician(s). It may be that some "noncases" should also be seen to refine the case definition. It might be appropriate to establish a classification system for cases under the headings of definite, probable, and suspected. In reviewing the laboratory data, it must be remembered that the laboratory results may not always be correct because of inadequacies in collection of the laboratory specimens, improper labeling, or improper handling or processing in the laboratory.

The next element is to do a rough case count to get an idea of the magnitude of the problem. Much time should not be spent on individual case data. These data should then be oriented according to time, place, and person (descriptive epidemiology). Time refers to determining the incubation period and graphing the epidemic curve. The shape of the curve may suggest the method of transmission and allow a prediction to be made about the course of the epidemic. As for place, plotting a spot map of the location of cases (where infection occurred) may provide important clues about the reservoir, the source, and the method of transmission. The data should also be oriented according to personal characteristics, that is, age, sex, occupation, socioeconomic status, and so on. It may be possible to make some preliminary judgments not only about the disease but also about intervention points for the institution of control measures that should perhaps be implemented at this time. In spite of implementation of any control measures, it is important to complete the epidemic investigation, not only to develop further information on the outbreak but also to evaluate the effectiveness of the implemented control measures.

The next element is to identify the population at risk, that is, the population exposed to the infectious agent, so attack rates can be calculated. The population may be determined by geographic area, such as those exposed to a specific water distribution area or those who work in a certain building. However, the exposed population may be more diffuse and difficult to identify, such as people who ate in a certain restaurant or who had contact with a certain commercially distributed food. It may be necessary to conduct a survey to determine the population at risk.

At this stage, a tentative hypothesis should be proposed by considering the data developed on the source and the reservoir of the agent, the mode of transmission, and the relevant host factors. Preferably the tentative hypothesis should be one that involves a single explanation for the outbreak. The hypothesis should allow for the best fit of all the data developed up to this point.

The next element is to plan and to conduct more systematic or specific investigations, including surveys, laboratory analyses, environmental examinations, and analytic epidemiologic studies. It may be necessary to reexamine patients or to seek out additional patients who may have been missed. The case definition may need to be narrowed, or cases that were previously listed as probable or suspected may now need to be included. The development of a comparison group may be important. New data should be combined with the previously analyzed data and reanalyzed. The analysis may involve hand tabulation of the data, use of McBee cards, or use of a computer. It may be appropriate to subject the analyzed data to statistical testing. The specific tests used will depend on various factors including the interrelationships between these factors and the quantity and complexity of the data.

The results of this analysis should confirm or challenge the tentative hypothesis. The hypothesis may be further tested by instituting specific control measures, which if successful, would result in a reduction of the number of cases. Knowledge of the past history of the disease in the population is necessary to know whether the change in the occurrence of cases was due to chance or was related to the control measures. If the hypothesis is correct, then it should be possible to predict the duration of the outbreak.

In testing the hypothesis it is important that the hypothesis be compatible with all the known facts. If this is not the case, the areas of incompatibility should be carefully reanalyzed to see whether an error was made in the analyses, whether some facts were missing, or whether some facts were wrong.

The local public health officials should be kept informed as to the progress of the investigation. A report of the investigation and recommended control measures should be prepared and distributed. At the appropriate time, the state and federal public health officials should be made aware of the epidemic and be provided with a copy of the report. Releasing publicity for general consumption may be a positive factor and should be considered.

Preventive measures should be considered, and an appropriate program should be planned and instituted. There may be need for a special surveillance program to evaluate the effectiveness of the recommended control measures. Education and training programs may be considered for selected groups of people.

SURVEILLANCE

General Aspects

Surveillance is a dynamic activity that includes gathering information on the occurrence of disease in a defined population, collating and analyzing these data, and summarizing the publishable findings.[9] If no action resulted from surveillance activities, it would be purely an archival function. Surveillance should be closely tied to control and prevention actions. Surveillance should either stimulate appropriate action or be used to evaluate actions already instituted.

The person responsible for reporting the occurrence of a reportable disease is the health care provider, usually a physician, who sees the patient and makes the diagnosis. The actual reporter, however, may be a representative of the physician, such as an assistant or secretary, a nurse, or hospital personnel. The list of reportable diseases varies from state to state and is modified at intervals. All physicians are required to report the occurrence of the three quarantinable diseases (cholera, plague, and yellow fever), and state health officials have agreed to collect and to report to federal officials cases of certain other communicable diseases. Additionally, depending on the need for additional data in some states, other communicable diseases may be reportable by individual state law.

A question often asked is why the private practitioner should report the occurrence of diseases, since filing a report takes time, and the physician frequently does not reap any noticeable benefits from participating in a surveillance program. An active surveillance program should provide physicians the opportunity to see the relationships of their cases to the occurrence of that disease in the community and should allow them to be more effective providers of health care. They should be interested in knowing whether their patient represents a single case of that disease or whether there are other cases that have occurred or are occurring.

Active surveillance may provide important information about therapy. For example, several years ago there was an epidemic of bacillary dysentery due to *Shigella dysenteriae* 1 in Mexico.[10] Some U.S. travelers became infected in Mexico and then returned to the United States, where clinical disease developed. This particular strain of *Shigella* had an unusual antibiotic resistance pattern (resistant to penicillin, tetracycline, chloramphenicol, and sulfonamide). Since the disease was under surveillance, cases had been reported, and since the organism had been studied in a laboratory, it was possible to recommend specific chemotherapy (ampicillin) when the diagnosis was first suspect. Thus it was not necessary to withhold specific therapy until the patient's organism had been isolated and its antibiogram had been determined.

Surveillance may provide information suggesting the need for institution of specific control and prevention measures, such as vaccination and prophylactic antibiotics. If surveillance reveals an increase in the occurrence of meningococcal meningitis, vaccination of highly susceptible groups of people with type-specific vaccine may clearly be indicated to prevent the occurrence of additional cases. Surveillance of hepatitis B may reveal an increasing incidence, which when investigated may identify a common source. Accordingly, those that have had contact with the common source within a prescribed period of time may be offered prophylactic immune serum or hepatitis B vaccine.

Current surveillance information may show the ineffectiveness of past or present disease control measures against the occurrence of a disease. Analysis of measles surveillance data, for example, has indicated that vaccination at less than 1 year of age did not, because of the presence of maternal antibody, provide all recipients with long-lasting immunity. Thus surveillance had identified a group of children who had been considered to be immune and who needed to be revaccinated.

Reporting may also make it possible to recognize epidemiologically related cases of a disease that without being reported to a central office would be considered sporadic cases. If this association is not recognized, the epidemic could continue smoldering and spreading. A number of years ago, an outbreak of staphylococcal skin infections developed in a newborn nursery, but the infants were being discharged before the infections became clinically apparent. Different pediatricians were seeing the infants, and it was not until two cases were reported by two pediatricians that the extensive outbreak was uncovered.

Surveillance data can be useful to health departments in their use of resources, including personnel, equipment, and money that should lead not only to increased efficiency but also to better control of the diseases under surveillance.

Collection of Data

There are 10 basic sources of surveillance information, some or all of which will be useful in describing a specific disease.[11]

The first element and the one most commonly used is morbidity data. Morbidity data are generated from case reports from health practitioners who report the occurrence of disease by various methods. These data, the backbone of any surveillance program, are dependent on the diagnosis being made by the health practitioner. Reporting methods vary. The traditional method has been the use of a simple card or form that a physician fills out and sends to the local or state health department. Other methods include reporting by telephone using a toll-free number. To encourage reporting, if the telephone report is being made at other than normal working hours, a recording device can be used to transcribe the data; if more information is desired, the physician can be called back.

Another method of obtaining morbidity data is the use of sentinel-physician reporting; a random selection of physicians from among those who are more likely to see infectious diseases (pediatricians, internists, family practice physicians, infectious disease specialists) are contacted and asked to report regularly the occurrence of reportable diseases.

These methods are passive methods: the reporter is asked to report cases when they occur. Active surveillance can be instituted by regularly contacting the reporters, usually by telephone, and asking if they have seen cases of specific diseases. This method may be very useful when attempting to develop information concerning the occurrence of a new disease or during an epidemic of a disease.

The second source of surveillance information is mortality data. Validity is dependent on the accuracy and completeness of the listing of the cause of death on death certificates. An example of the usefulness of this method is the collection of mortality data by the Centers for Disease Control (CDC) from 121 cities throughout the United States as part of the influenza surveillance program.[12] Knowing that excess mortality in the winter is usually due to influenza has made these data very useful in portraying the occurrence of epidemic influenza.

The third method of collecting surveillance data is case investigation. The occurrence of certain diseases, such as poliomyelitis, botulism, and plague, will always be investigated. The specific case investigation may uncover other cases of the same disease that would not have been diagnosed without the case investigation.

The fourth method of developing surveillance data is reporting of epidemics. Not all epidemics will be investigated, possibly because it is felt that nothing new will be gained from a particular investigation or because the health department does not have enough personnel available. During the influenza season, after the initial cases have been confirmed and laboratory specimens collected, it is quite possible that epidemics will be recorded but will not be investigated further unless some unusual feature occurs. Even without a specific investigation, the report of the epidemic will add important data to the surveillance program.

Another method of obtaining surveillance data is from an epidemic investigation. The initial report will indicate the occurrence of a certain number of cases; however, field investigation may result in a significant increase in the case count. In 1965, an outbreak of gastroenteritis due to *Salmonella typhimurium* occurred in Riverside, California.[13] Less than 1000 cases were or would have been reported had there been no further investigation. Because of the need to identify the source of infection, a field investigation was conducted, which included a community survey. As a result of the survey, more than 16,000 cases of gastroenteritis due to *S. typhimurium* were projected to have occurred. Since the majority of acute disease epidemics are not investigated, this method of obtaining surveillance data is undoubtedly underused.

The sixth method of gathering surveillance information is that of reviewing laboratory reports. For some diseases the laboratory identification of the etiologic agent is necessary if the disease is to be diagnosed at all or with any degree of accuracy. For example, it is difficult if not impossible to be specific as to the cause of gastroenteritis without laboratory assistance. An example of a successful surveillance program based on laboratory identification of the etiologic agent is that of salmonellosis. Not only is identification of the genus important but serotype identification of salmonella may show a cluster of cases due to the same serotype; identification of a rare serotype may trigger a specific field investigation. Laboratory identification of the antigenic makeup of influenza viruses is the only way that specific information concerning the occurrence and/or spread of specific types can be documented. These data are of significant value in deciding the formulation and subsequent use of influenza vaccines. The laboratory may also play a valuable part by characterizing the antibiotic sensitivity of organisms.

The seventh method of obtaining surveillance information is that of conducting population surveys to determine who has had a certain illness and to delineate characteristics that are key to the development of an illness.[14] Not all people in the community need actually be questioned; a statistically valid sample can be identified and questioned. If the survey group was properly selected, analysis of the data should produce data that are applicable to the entire population.

The eighth method for consideration is animal and vector disease occurrence data, which may be obtained from surveys of the appropriate populations, from observation of the occurrence of the disease in these populations, or from knowledge of carriage of the infectious agent among animals or vectors. In general, the surveillance of zoonotic diseases is enhanced by maintaining knowledge of the status of the disease in its host animals or insect vectors. For example, reports of tularemia would be investigated if cases of animal tularemia were not being reported from the area.

The ninth method of surveillance is that of noting the usage of certain biologics. For example, by noting requests for specific antitoxin, botulism surveillance is maintained.

The tenth method of surveillance is the use of demographic data that portrays the characteristics of a population. Demographic data may be useful in evaluating surveillance data and in projecting the anticipated occurrence of a disease in the population.

Another source of information that may provide surveillance data is local publicity. As reporters are frequently interested in the occurrence of disease, information from newspapers, radio, or television stations may provide the initial clue to the occurrence of a disease that may not have been reported.

Not all these methods of surveillance will be used to maintain surveillance for any one disease. Most frequently morbidity reporting is the main method used, supported by laboratory reports. The methods used will vary according to the type of surveillance data desired, the use to which it will be put, the sensitivity and specificity desired, and the available resources. Additional methods may be incorporated depending on the occurrence or on the anticipated occurrence of the disease.

The sensitivity and specificity of the surveillance system varies according to the disease, the method of reporting—including the reporting official, the circumstances of disease occurrence, and other nonpredictable factors. In disease of low frequency, such as poliomyelitis, plague, and anthrax, sensitivity is probably quite high, with close to 100 percent of the actual cases being reported. Diseases that occur with a high frequency, such as hepatitis, rubella, and salmonellosis, have a low reporting sensitivity. For example, only approximately 1 percent of the cases of salmonellosis are cultured and subsequently reported, and approximately 10 percent of cases of viral hepatitis are reported. The development of surveillance information is basically to show the linear trends of occurrence of disease. If the surveillance techniques remain fairly consistent, then the data will be adequate for comparison with previously collected data, for defining health problems, and for developing and evaluating control and prevention techniques. However, if there is a significant change in the surveillance technique, then there is need to be concerned about comparing data that may have been developed after the change occurred. For example, when *Shigella* surveillance was initiated in the United States, one-third of the states entered the program. Over the next several years, the other states joined, and there was a significant increase in the number of *Shigella* organisms identified in laboratories and reported to the surveillance system. Without knowing something about the expanding surveillance program throughout the country, we would have interpreted the surveillance data as showing a significant increase in shigellosis in the United States.

ANALYSIS OF DATA

The data, having been collected, must be collated and analyzed for those characteristics of the disease for which the surveillance program was initiated. The data should not be analyzed to any greater extent than they will be used. Depending on the complexities of the data and of the analyses, the statistical treatment of the data may be by hand or by computer. The data should be analyzed at intervals that allow development of relevant and timely information. If surveillance data are collected at weekly intervals, these data must be analyzed weekly. Frequency of analysis should be dictated by the use of the data.

Once the data have been analyzed, a report discussing those data and their analyses should be prepared. Additionally, the reports can provide comparisons with similarly collected data from previous years, discuss control and prevention measures, recount interesting aspects of the disease, and summarize outbreak investigations. The reports should be distributed to people who assisted in obtaining the data, as well as to those who need to see the results of surveillance activities in reference to their roles in control and prevention. Reports may be distributed at weekly or less frequent intervals. The CDC prepares a weekly surveillance report (*Morbidity and Mortality Weekly Report*) that summarizes the data reported weekly by the states and contains surveillance summaries, reports of current field investigations, international summaries, and quarantine-regulation information. Additionallly, the annual summary of these data compares the current year with others. The CDC also prepares quarterly and special surveillance reports at varying intervals for approximately 25 diseases.

Special surveillance programs may be established to meet the need for specific information over a limited period of time. For example, during the fall and winter, when influenza is prevalent, school and factory absenteeism is reported in selected areas. Routine reporting of excess mortality and review of laboratory isolates continues, but the additional data are useful in portraying the epidemic occurrence of influenza. Special surveillance programs may be developed for diseases that become of specific importance to public health such as legionnaires' disease, toxic shock syndrome, Reye syndrome, and acquired immunodeficiency syndrome (AIDS).

International surveillance through the World Health Organization is maintained on the three quarantinable diseases (cholera, plague, and yellow fever) and other diseases such as influenza and salmonellosis.

REFERENCES

1. Williams REO. Airborne staphylococci in the surgical ward. J Hyg (Camb). 1967;65:207.
2. Noble WZ. Dispersal and acquisition of microorganisms. In: Brachman PS, Eickhoff TC, eds. Proceedings of the International Conference on Nosocomial Infections. Chicago: American Hospital Association; 1971:193.
3. Eichenwald HF, Kotsevalov O, Fasso LA. The "cloud baby": an example of bacterial-viral interaction. Am J Dis Child. 1960;100:161.
4. Centers for Disease Control. Epidemiology Program Office, Division of Surveillance & Epidemiologic Studies.
5. Dowdle WR, Coleman MT, Gregg MB. Natural history of influenza type A in the United States, 1957–1972. Prog Med Virol. 1974;17:91.
6. Collins RN, Treger MD, Goldsby JB, et al. Interstate outbreak of *Salmonella new brunswick* infection traced to powdered milk. JAMA. 1968;203:838.
7. Fox JP, Hall CE, Elveback LR. Epidemiology: Man and Disease. New York: Macmillan; 1970:6.
8. MacMahon B, Pugh TF. Epidemiology Principles and Methods. Boston: Little Brown; 1970:41.
9. Thacker SB, Choi K, Brachman PS. The surveillance of infectious diseases. JAMA. 1983;249:1181.
10. Weissman JB, Marton KI, Lewis JN, et al. Impact in the United States of the Shiga dysentery pandemic of Central America and Mexico: a review of surveillance data through 1972. J Infect Dis. 1974;129:218.
11. World Health Organization. The surveillance of communicable diseases. WHO Chron. 1968;22:439.
12. Serfling RE. Methods for current statistical analysis of excess pneumonia-influenza deaths. Public Health Rep. 1963;78:494.
13. A waterborne epidemic of salmonellosis in Riverside, California, 1965, epidemiologic aspects, a collaborative report. Am J Epidemiol. 1971;93:33.
14. Serfling RE, Sherman IL. Attribute Sampling Methods, Publication No. 1230, US Department of Health, Education and Welfare, Public Health Service, 1965.

11. TRANSMISSION AND PRINCIPLES OF CONTROL

PHILIP S. BRACHMAN

Infectious disease results from the interaction between an infectious agent and a susceptible host. If the agent already resides in the host (endogenous infection), disease may develop due to changes in the relationship between the agent and the host. If the agent is transported from an external source to the host (exogenous infection) and if the balance between agent and host favors the agent, disease develops. The relationships among the agent, transmission, and the host may be considered the chain of infection.

There are four exogenous routes by which microorganisms are transmitted from the source to the host: contact, common vehicle, air, and vector. The environment plays an all-encompassing role, impacting on the agent, the route of transmission, and the host. Control and prevention of infections depend on defining the interaction of these factors. The most effective, practical, and appropriate means of interrupting the development of infection can then be identified and implemented. The relationships of these interrelating factors (chain of infection) will be discussed in this chapter.

AGENT

The agent, the first link in the chain of infection, is any microorganism—bacterium, virus, fungus, parasite, rickettsia or *Chlamydia*. The pathogenicity of an agent describes its ability to cause disease. An organism with high pathogenicity is the smallpox virus. There is no known human carrier state for this agent; once infected with the virus, the host will develop disease. Thus its presence in a human is always associated with disease. An organism of low pathogenicity is *Staphylococcus epidermidis,* an organism associated with a high colonization rate but not frequently associated with significant disease. Pathogenicity may be further described by noting the organism's virulence and invasiveness. Virulence may be described according to epidemiologic factors of morbidity, mortality, and communicability and by clinical factors, noting the severity of the disease.

In considering all organisms, there is a spectrum of virulence from low to high. Some organisms are described as avirulent; however, avirulence is a relative term, dependent on agent, host, and possibly other factors. An organism considered to be avirulent when in contact with a normally healthy person may cause disease in a highly susceptible person. For example, years ago *Serratia marcescens* organisms were used for air tracer studies because they were thought to be avirulent and their cultural characteristics made them distinctively identifiable. However, disease has been found to result from infection with *S. marcescens,* primarily in people with increased susceptibility to infectious agents.

Invasiveness is the ability of the agent to enter and to move through tissue. Some organisms move with relative ease, whereas others are likely to remain at the point of first tissue contact. For example, *Vibrio cholerae* organisms are not invasive but remain localized on the intestinal mucosa and produce toxin that on reacting with tissues results in the production of signs and symptoms. On the other hand, *Shigella* organisms are highly invasive and, when they locate on the mucosal surface of the intestine, will invade the submucosal tissue, become established, and cause disease.

Other agent factors to be considered in evaluating the role of the agent in causing infection are the infective dose, physical characteristics, organism specificity, antigenic variations of the organism, elaboration of enzymes and toxins, and genetic factors such as resistance transfer plasmids.

The infective dose, that is, the number of organisms necessary to cause an infection, vary according to the route and conditions of transmission and according to host susceptibility. The influence of transmission on the infective dose is exemplified by the susceptibility of enteric organisms to gastric acidity. For example, if the organisms are freely exposed to the gastric contents, a higher oral infective dose will be necessary than if they are transported through the stomach in milk, which will protect them from the acidity of the gastric contents.[1]

Physical characteristics of agents may influence the occurrence of disease. Some agents such as *Bacillus anthracis* can survive in soil for years, whereas most viruses generally do not survive for long within the inanimate environment.

Agent specificity refers to host preference as shown by some agents. For example, *Salmonella typhi* is host-specific for humans, whereas *Salmonella dublin* has a predilection for cattle. The smallpox virus was found only in humans. *Clostridium botulinum* types A, B, E, and F are associated with human disease, whereas types C and D are associated with disease in birds and mammals.

Within one species there may be antigenic variations that reflect differences in the pathogenicity of that organism. For example, among pneumococci there are 83 different serotypes (U.S. typing system); however, 80 percent of the cases of pneumococcal pneumonia are associated with only 14 types.

Other organisms may show antigenic variations over time. Influenza A virus shows minor antigenic drifts every 2–3 years and major changes or shifts every 7–10 years (A/Japan/305/57 H2N2, 1958–1959, A/Hong Kong/68 H3N2, 1968–1969, and so on).[2] These variations are reflected in changes in the occurrence of influenza A, which are further influenced by the immunity level of the population, which will vary according to the past experiences with that particular virus strain and with the use of influenza vaccines.

Some organisms elaborate enzymes that challenge the defense mechanisms of the host; other organisms produce toxins that damage the host's tissues. Resistance transfer plasmids may have a direct influence on antibiotic resistance and thus have an influence on the pathogenicity of bacterial organisms.

It is important to differentiate between the *reservoir* and the *source* of an organism if control measures are to be effectively directed against the organism. The reservoir is the location in which the organism is normally found, that is, where it becomes established, metabolizes, and multiplies. The source is the location from which the organism is immediately transmitted to the host either directly or indirectly through a vehicle (see below). The reservoir of *C. botulinum* is in the environment, specifically, in soil; the source of *C. botulinum* organisms for human infection is usually improperly processed food contaminated by soil. The reservoir and source may have the same location, such as a nasal carrier of *Staphylococcus aureus* who is disseminating organisms. However, if they have different locations, eradication of the organism at its source may not prevent further spread of infection, since the reservoir may remain and be capable of reinfecting the previous source or establishing new sources.

The presence of an organism depicts a potential for transmission, but the important event is the actual dissemination of the agent. Dissemination is influenced by various factors, including the number of organisms present, physical activity, stress, environmental factors, and the presence of another infection.

The period of infectivity refers to the time during which the source (usually refers to a human source) is infectious or is disseminating organisms. This is usually during the incubation period and the first days of the clinical period of disease as seen in hepatitis A and measles. A patient with influenza is usually only infectious during the clinical period. Some patients may remain infectious during the convalescent period, such as in shigellosis.

The portals of exit of organisms are most likely the respiratory, gastrointestinal, and genitourinary tracts. Additionally, the skin and wounds and blood can be the portals of exit.

TRANSMISSION

Transmission is the second link in the chain of infection, and there are four main routes of infection: contact, common vehicle, airborne, and vector-borne. Identification of the route by which microorganisms are transmitted from the source to the host may allow for specific control measures that are designed to interrupt transmission.

The contact route implies contact between the source and the host; that contact is by direct contact, indirect contact, or droplets. Direct contact means that the source and the host come in physical contact, allowing for direct transfer of microorganisms; this route is frequently called person-to-person. For example, a physician with a staphylococcal furuncle on a finger may directly infect a patient while performing a physical examination.

Indirect contact refers to the transmission of microorganisms from the source to the host via passive transfer—usually on an inanimate object. An example would be a common shaving brush that has become contaminated with *Pseudomonas* organisms and serves to transfer the organisms from an initial human source to the host.[3]

Droplet-spread organisms are those particles usually larger than 5 μm whose route of transmission is through the air, but only for very short distances. Because of their relatively large size, they rapidly settle out because they cannot travel in the air further than approximately 1 m. Transfer of microorganisms by droplets occurs because of the close proximity of the source and the host; droplets are usually produced by talking or sneezing. Measles and streptococcal infection are examples of droplet-spread diseases. When many people are exposed to a single source of droplets, attack rates will show a gradation from high for those closest to the source to low for those furthest away. For example, in a study of streptococcal transmission in an army barracks, where transmission was by the droplet route, susceptible soldiers whose beds were located nearest the source had the highest rates of acquiring streptococci.[4]

In common-vehicle spread, a single inanimate vehicle serves to transmit the infectious agent to multiple hosts. The vehicle may be actively involved in transmission by means of multiplication of the agent in the vehicle (direct), such as *Clostridium perfringens* in gravy, or may be passively involved (indirect) and only serve as a means by which the agent is transmitted to hosts, such as hepatitis A virus in food. The most frequently involved common vehicles are food and water; however, lots or batches of blood, blood products, intravenous fluids, and drugs may be prepared from a single contaminated source and serve as a "common vehicle," resulting in multiple infections.

In airborne transmission, the etiologic agent is truly airborne in its transmission from the source to the host. The airborne infected particles are either contained in droplet nuclei or dust and travel over 1 m in the air from the disseminating source to the host. Droplet nuclei are small particles—less than 5 μm in diameter—that represent the residua resulting from evaporation of larger particles (droplets). Dust represents material that settles out from the air and becomes resuspended by physical forces. Skin squames may also serve as airborne vehicles of infectious agents. The distance airborne particles are carried in the air depends on the force with which the particles are propelled into the air. In some outbreaks of airborne disease, the infective particles were carried several miles from the source to the susceptible hosts.

Humans, animals, and inanimate objects can be sources of airborne agents. When humans and animals are the source, the agent can be propelled by coughing and sneezing into the air from the respiratory tract. Tuberculosis is an example of an airborne spread disease from a human source. Usually the organisms become airborne by coughing. In one case, tubercule bacilli became airborne from a singer whose lesion was on a vocal chord, and he only disseminated when he sang. An example of human disease resulting from the airborne spread of the agent from an animal is psittacosis among bird owners, the source of the agent being psittacine birds.

An example of an inanimate source of airborne particles is an outbreak of Q fever, in which equipment in a rendering plant in which contaminated animal products were being processed produced aerosols containing *Coxsiella burnetii* that were being carried up to 10 miles downwind by the prevailing winds and resulted in 75 cases of disease.[5]

Insects are the source of vector-borne agents, and vector-borne transmission includes external and internal transmission. In external or mechanical transmission, the agent is carried on the body of the insect vector. Carriage is passive, with no change in the organism during transmission. Flies carrying *Salmonella* or *Shigella* organisms on their appendages from a fecal source to food would be an example of external carriage. In internal transmission, the etiologic agent is carried within the insect vector, and there is either harborage or a biologic transmission phase. In harborage transmission, the organism is ingested by the insect but undergoes no changes within the vector while being carried. An example of harborage transmission is carriage of *Yersinia pestis* within a flea during the transmission of plague. The organisms are picked up by the flea while it is feeding on a "source" and carried in the flea gut until deposited on the skin of a host, but they undergo no changes while in the flea.

Biologic transmission indicates that the etiologic agent goes through physiologic changes in the vector, such as in malaria, in which there is maturation of the agent within the mosquito. In investigating vector-borne disease in which there is a true biologic transmission phase, it is important to consider the incubation period of the etiologic agent within the vector, which is known as the extrinsic incubation period, as distinct from the intrinsic incubation period, which is the incubation period within the susceptible host after transmission has occurred.

Usually the route of transmission is predictable; however, some microorganisms may be transmitted by one of several different routes. For example, staphylococci are usually transmitted by direct (person-to-person) contact; however, they can also be transported by the airborne route. Salmonellae are usually transported by means of a common vehicle, but they can also be transported by direct contact and by the airborne route; they also have been reported to be transmitted by vectors (external). Malaria parasites are most frequently transmitted by vectors, but they have also been transmitted in transfused contaminated blood. Knowledge of the most likely route of transmission can be important in rapidly controlling the occurrence of additional cases if it is not possible to conduct definitive studies to define all the circumstances of the epidemic.

HOST

The host is the last link in the chain of infection. The site of entrance of the agent may be the skin, mucous membranes, respiratory tract, urinary tract, or gastrointestinal tract. Some organisms, such as *Leptospira,* are able to penetrate the intact skin, whereas other organisms can only enter the skin through breaks in the integrity of the skin. Microorganisms may also be introduced through the skin by the parenteral route such as by means of contaminated blood (hepatitis B virus) or intravenous fluids (gram-negative organisms or yeasts). Insect vectors may inject organisms through the skin (malaria).

Organisms may be deposited on the mucous membranes by movement through the air (adenovirus 8) or by contact with inanimate objects, such as instruments or medications. Organisms inhaled into the lungs will be deposited at various levels of the pulmonary tree in relation to their size. The larger particles may not reach the bronchi but impinge on the nasal cilia and travel no further; the majority of the smaller particles (less than 5 μm in diameter) will reach the terminal alveoli where they may be deposited and cause disease or be carried across the aveolar membranes in macrophages and may either be deposited in local lymph nodes or spread systemically throughout the body.

Organisms may also enter the host via the urinary tract during the process of catheterization or instrumentation or may travel retrogressively through a urinary catheter. Organisms may be ingested with contaminated food or water or through contamination of an instrument introduced into the gastrointestinal tract.

Infection may also be transmitted via the transplacental route such as rubella viruses and *Toxoplasma* parasites.[6] Transplantation may also result in the introduction of organisms into the body, such as a kidney contaminated with cytomegalovirus or a heart valve contaminated with *S. epidermidis* organisms.

Microorganisms may colonize one site without any evidence of disease, but the same organism located in another site may cause symptomatic disease. For example, *S. aureus* may colonize the external nares without any evidence of disease, but the same organism located beneath the skin may result in a skin infection.

The host defense mechanisms may be categorized as either nonspecific or specific (see Section B for a more complete discussion of host defense mechanisms). Nonspecific mechanisms include the skin, body secretions such as tears, mucus, and saliva, and nasal cilia. Inflammation is another nonspecific action the body uses to mobilize defense mechanisms against microorganisms. Nonspecific defense mechanisms are also influenced by age, sex, genetic factors, nutrition, and behavioral patterns.

Specific defense mechanisms include natural and artificial im munity. Natural immunity follows the natural occurrence of disease, such as measles, rubella, and poliomyelitis. Natural immunity usually has a long duration, at times for the life of the host, and can be demonstrated by specific serologic studies. It may also be demonstrated by noting the lack of the occurrence of disease in a population previously naturally exposed to the agent. For example, people exposed to the HlNl influenza viruses that circulated throughout the world from late 1946 to early 1957 now show relative immunity to the new prevalent strain A/USSR/7/77(HlNl), which is antigenetically related to the prior HlNl virus.[7]

Artificial immunity is either active or passive. Active artificial immunity results from vaccination using killed vaccines (typhoid fever or pertussis), attenuated vaccines (Calmette-Guérin/bacillus—BCG or poliomyelitis), or toxoids (diphtheria, tetanus). Passive immunity is associated with the use of immunoglobulins, antitoxins, or material antibody in newborn infants.

A more complete discussion of immunization will be found in Chapter 296.

The spectrum of host response to infection depends on agent and host factors and varies from subclinical, or inapparent infection, to severe disease with the most severe involvement being death. Subclinical infection can be determined by serologic means. Also, a carrier state may develop. If a host has partial immunity that may develop following imperfect immunization or incomplete therapy and if infection develops, it may result in modified or atypical disease. Also, prophylactic or therapeutic treatment after exposure to an infectious agent may result in an atypical clinical expression of the disease.

ROLE OF THE ENVIRONMENT

Infection develops within the milieu of the environment, and thus any of the determinants involved in the occurrence of an infection may be influenced by environmental factors such as heat, cold, moisture, radiation, air pressure, movement and velocity of the air, and presence of chemicals, gases, and toxins. The influence may promote the development of infection or it may inhibit, limit, or prevent the development of infection.

Environmental factors in effect at the agent's reservoir, such as temperature, humidity, and nutrients, may be beneficial or inhibitory to the growth and multiplication of the agent. The movement of the agent from the source to the susceptible host may be influenced by air velocity, humidity, radiation, and temperature. The host may also be influenced by environmental factors, such as low humidity, which may increase the permeability of mucous membranes to infectious agents.

Environmental studies should be conducted to define the precise role of the environment so control efforts can be directed specifically if indicated and not randomly at the appropriate environmental factor. In hospitals, for example, it is not unusual to find an extremely complex—but random—environmental control program in operation; such programs are more expensive and less effective than programs directed at preventing specific infections. Not only do catchall programs cost more but they may also lead to a false sense of security.

Some hospitals have relied heavily on routine environmental culturing in their efforts to prevent nosocomial infections. They have set unsubstantiated standards for recovery of microorganisms from these environmental specimens and have predicted that when recovery does exceed the standard, disease will result unless special decontamination efforts are instituted. Generally, however, setting such standards is not based on factual data. Another example of the overemphasis on the environment was the promotion of full-room ultraviolet irradiation in operating theaters as a technique to prevent the development of postoperative infections.[8] Full-room irradiation does reduce the number of airborne bacteria, but a double-blind study conducted by the National Research Council indicated that there was no difference in the overall rate of postoperative wound infections. There was a difference in the postoperative wound infection rate for operations with the highest risk of developing postoperative wound infections (''dirty wounds''—such as those where the bowel was transected), but it did not show any statistically valid effect for the rest of the operations, and thus there was no justification for using full-room irradiation for all operative procedures.

There are some appropriate standards, such as the number of coliform organisms in water, which are acceptable as standards for human use. Some routine environmental cultures can be meaningful, such as regular bacteriologic checks of autoclaves and/or hospital-prepared infant formula. Some environmental cultures may be useful in training programs to demonstrate the potential role of the inanimate environment in causing disease.

The environment can play an important role in the development of infections, but before strenuous nonspecific control efforts aimed at influencing environmental factors are instituted, appropriate studies must be conducted to demonstrate the specific role that the environmental factors play in the development of infections. Only after these studies have been completed should measures be adopted aimed at influencing the environmental factors. The environmental emphasis should be in concert with knowledge of the specific role of the environment in particular disease outbreak situations.

CONTROL

Since the development of infections is multifactorial, designing control measures is complex. We have to consider available resources, cost effectiveness, time constraints, adverse effects or complications of the proposed control measures, and effect on prevention of future cases (or epidemics). Control activities may reflect compromises among competing measures. For the most appropriate, effective, and acceptable decision, all the interrelated parameters related to the occurrence of the particular infection (or epidemic) need to be identified. Only then can an intelligent decision be made. Basically, control measures should be directed against the part of the infection cycle most susceptible to such actions. However, other considerations, such as cost and availability of personnel may indicate otherwise.

Control efforts may best be directed toward controlling or eradicating the agent at its reservoir or source. If the reservoir or source is human, then therapy or isolation techniques may be the best method of preventing the spread of infection.[9] If the reservoir or source is an inanimate object, then it may be controlled by either decontamination procedures or by using disposable materials.

If the route of transmission seems to be the best area for approaching control, then the specific type of transmission needs to be identified, for methods of control will vary depending on the route. If the disease is spread by the contact route, then control measures need to be directed toward people or inanimate objects associated with transmission. Personal factors may reflect the need for education or antibiotic therapy. If an inanimate object is involved, improved disinfection or sterilization methods may be necessary. If there is a common-vehicle-spread disease, then the vehicle must be decontaminated by better processing, sterilization, and improved training of humans to prevent contamination from occurring. If airborne infection is involved, effective filtering of the contaminated air or other treatment of the air needs to be instituted. If the disease is spread by vector, the vector must be controlled by spraying or other techniques.

If the best way to control infection is to increase the resistance of the host, then the primary defense mechanisms may need to be strengthened. It may be necessary to improve secondary host defenses by vaccination, either actively or passively.

Thus control must be directed toward the part of the pathway of infection that is most susceptible to the development of infection.

One of the most important areas of control is education, not only for new employees but ongoing, continuing education for all employees. All need to be reminded of old techniques and taught new techniques. Changing human behavioral patterns by education can be a very effective way to reduce the risk of infection.

REFERENCES

1. Hornick RB, Greisman SE, Woodward TE, et al. Typhoid fever: pathogenesis and immunologic control. N Engl J Med. 1970;283:686.
2. Dowdle WR, Coleman MT, Gregg MB. Natural history of influenza type A in the United States, 1957–1972. Prog Med Virol. 1974;17:91.
3. Ayliffe CAJ, Lowbury EJL, Hamilton JG, et al. Hospital infection with *Pseudonomas aeruginosa* in neurosurgery. Lancet. 1965;1:365.
4. Rammelkamp CH Jr, Mortimer EA Jr, Wolinsky E. Transmission of streptococcal and staphylococcal infections. Ann Intern Med. 1964;60:753.
5. Wellock CE. Epidemiology of Q-fever in the urban East Bay area. California Health. 1960;18:73.
6. Benenson AS, ed. Control of Communicable Diseases in Man. 13th ed. Washington, DC: APHA; 1980:296, 356.
7. Gregg MB, Hinman AR, Craven RB. The Russian flu: its history and implications for this year's influenza season. JAMA. 1978;240:2260.
8. Postoperative Wound Infections. The influence of ultraviolet irradiation of the operating room and of various other factors. Report of an ad hoc committee. Ann Surg. 1964;Suppl, August.
9. CDC Guidelines for Isolation Precautions in Hospitals. US Department of Health and Human Services, Public Health Service, Centers for Disease Control; 1983:81.

12. PRINCIPLES OF CHEMOPROPHYLAXIS AND IMMUNOPROPHYLAXIS

PHILIP S. BRACHMAN

CHEMOPROPHYLAXIS

Chemoprophylaxis is the treatment with a drug before, during, or shortly after exposure to an infectious agent or agents in an attempt to prevent the development of infection due to that agent. Chemoprophylaxis may be specific, that is, directed against a specific microorganism—usually an exogenous organism such as *Neisseria meningitidis*—or it may be nonspecific—when more than one organism, any one of which may cause an infection, may be present. These organisms are usually endogenous (or autogenous). An example of nonspecific prophylaxis is the preoperative use of antibiotics to prevent postoperative wound infections.

The greatest possibility for success occurs when chemoprophylaxis is directed against a specific organism with known antibiotic sensitivities. When nonspecific chemoprophylaxis is directed against various organisms, usually the host's nonspecific defense mechanisms have been compromised. If the antibiotic sensitivities of the organisms vary, then the choice of the prophylactic drug is a difficult one. If prophylaxis directed against two or more organisms is not effective against all of them, one or several of the surviving species may multiply to fill the niche vacated by the eradicated organism. This may lead to the development of disease due to the replacement organism.

Other potential problems related to specific or nonspecific prophylaxis are that the prolonged use of a chemoprophylactic agent may lead to the development of hypersensitivity to that agent or to the development of resistant strains for which the specific prophylaxis is no longer effective. Other considerations include the expense of prophylaxis and the development of adverse reactions, such as hepatitis following exposure to isonicotinic acid hydrazide (INH).

When to start, how much to give, which to give, and how long to continue prophylactic therapy depend on the microorganism or microorganisms involved, the period during which it or they may be infectious to the patient, the mode of transmission, and the period during which the patient is susceptible to infection. The patient's susceptibility will reflect the defense mechanisms. These may be normal, but due to a high degree of pathogenicity of the organism, the development of disease is a definite possibility. However, the host's defenses may be compromised as a result of hereditary factors, disease, malnutrition, or therapy, making possible an infection with an organism of low pathogenicity, such as *Staphylococcus epidermidis*. Prophylaxis is often started before potential exposure to the infectious agent, such as preoperatively, but it may be given during exposure, such as chloroquine during travel in a malarious area, or after exposure, such as after contact with a person with gonorrhea.

A potential problem in making a decision about prophylaxis may be in determining the degree of contact the person actually had with the microorganism. The decision to initiate prophylactic therapy is at times made on the basis of an emotional response to the potential pathogenicity of the organism and not on the basis of the actual degree of contact with the organism. When considering chemoprophylaxis, a judgment should be made as to whether the benefits outweigh the possible adverse effects.

Specific Chemoprophylaxis

Specific chemoprophylaxis has been shown to be effective in cholera,[1] gonorrhea (Chapter 190)[2] *Haemophilus influenza* (Chapter 201),[3] influenza (Chapter 142),[4] leprosy (Chapter 230),[5] malaria (Chapter 251),[6] meningococcal infections (Chapter 189),[7] rheumatic fever (Chapter 177), syphilis (Chapter 213),[8,9] and tuberculosis (Chapter 229).[10]

Chemoprophylaxis has also been shown to be effective in preventing certain nosocomial infections. For example, it may be very effective in preventing wound infections after clean-contaminated surgical procedures and has shown effectiveness following some clean surgical procedures. This subject is reviewed in detail by Eickhoff.[11] Prophylactic doxycycline has been reported to be effective in preventing travelers' diarrhea in some areas.[12] However, there is concern over the extrapolation of these results to other areas; the prophylactic use of antibiotics for travelers' diarrhea should be approached with caution.

There are also some infections for which chemoprophylaxis is used, but its effectiveness in preventing infections has not been proven. One example is in contacts of pneumonic plague among whom the use of tetracycline has been recommended.

IMMUNOPROPHYLAXIS

Immunoprophylaxis is the use of vaccines, toxoids, and immune serum to protect otherwise susceptible people against specific diseases. (A more detailed discussion of specific immunoprophylaxis will be found in Chapter 296.) Occurrence of the natural disease usually results in the production of protective antibody against that disease; this usually persists for years and possibly for the life of the person. If one lacks natural antibody against a disease, then active or passive immunoprophylaxis may help provide immunologic protection. In active immunoprophylaxis the body's immune system is stimulated to develop antibody against the antigen. The antigen can be live, or inactivated (killed), or a toxoid. An antibody so produced varies in the duration of effectiveness from months, as in the case of some cholera vaccines, to years, as in the case of diphtheria or tetanus toxoid. With certain vaccines, especially the killed vaccines and toxoids, booster inoculations are necessary to maintain protection. In passive immunoprophylaxis, antibody formed in another host, animal or human, is given to a susceptible person and provides protection for the life (relatively short) of the passively infused antibodies. An example of this is immunoglobulin used against hepatitis A.

Control of current and prevention of future epidemics of some infectious diseases may result from increasing the immunity level (herd immunity) of groups of susceptible people by means of community vaccination programs. These are especially important today in populations in which there may be significant numbers of people susceptible to diseases of relatively high prevalence, such as measles and rubella. In diseases of low prevalence, such as diphtheria and poliomyelitis, there may be small pockets of susceptible people who should be vaccinated to prevent focal epidemics from occurring. Vaccination campaigns supported by public health authorities, medical societies, and other groups have been successful in raising immunity levels and in preventing serious large epidemics of these diseases. However, many of these diseases occur at a frequency that clearly indicates a need to continue to stimulate health care providers to promote routine vaccination actively for their patients as a part of good preventive care. Some of the newer vaccines have been used to control outbreaks of disease in selected populations, such as the outbreak of meningococcal disease in Brazil[13] and in other populations[14] and outbreaks of pneumococcal disease in military recruits.[15]

Active or passive immunization may afford only partial protection, which means that subsequent exposure to the specific etiologic agent may result in the disease or in a modified clinical form of the disease. In some cases the modified or atypical clinical manifestations may be as severe or more severe than the natural disease. For example, this has been seen in some people initially vaccinated with live measles vaccine in combination with measles immune serum globulin who subsequently were exposed to naturally occurring measles virus.

Active Immunoprophylaxis

Recommendations for the use of an active immunizing agent depend on the potential for exposure to that pathogen. The vaccine should be administered far enough in advance of exposure for protective antibody to develop; antibody responses usually take 7–21 days. There are some diseases for which the vaccine should be given as part of a regular ''childhood vaccination'' program (diphtheria, pertussis, tetanus, poliomyelitis, measles, rubella, mumps; in some countries Calmette-Guérin bacillus [BCG] is considered part of the regular vaccination program).[16] Other vaccines such as cholera, plague, typhoid fever, and yellow fever, should be given as necessary, depending on exposure potential related to travel. At times residence may necessitate recommendations for certain vaccines because of the prevalence of certain diseases in the area such as plague and yellow fever. Professional activity may dictate the need for vaccination programs. In a laboratory in which pathogenic organisms are handled, vaccines against them, if they exist, should be routinely used for the personnel or for those people who may have contact with this laboratory or with the specific agents. These diseases include anthrax, cholera, hepatitis B, plague, rabies, Rocky Mountain spotted fever, typhoid fever, typhus, and yellow fever. Additionally, anthrax vaccination is indicated for people who are exposed to certain imported raw animal materials, and rabies vaccine should be given to people whose occupations may bring them into contact with possibly rabid animals, either domestic or wild.

Some vaccines should be used in selected populations, depending on the disease occurrence and on the population characteristics. Influenza vaccine should be considered for use on an annual basis for those people with chronic debilitating conditions such as pulmonary disease, cardiovascular disease, and metabolic diseases.[17] Additionally, elderly people should be routinely given the current vaccine. Consideration should be given to vaccinating people, such as policemen, firemen, hospital personnel, and utility repair personnel, who provide essential community services. Meningococcal vaccine should be considered in areas of population groups in which the disease is of moderate prevalence, such as in some military recruit populations[18] or in some families with a risk of secondary cases.[19] In some elderly populations, pneumococcal vaccines are recommended as a regular immunization program.[20] In some hospitals, some vaccines are recommended or mandated for employees who work in specific high-risk areas. These include hepatitis B, measles, and rubella vaccines.[21] In some countries, BCG vaccine is recommended for children due to the prevalence of active disease among the population.[16] In addition to some professional groups in hospitals, there are other high-risk groups for which hepatitis B vaccine is recommended.[22]

Passive Immunoprophylaxis

Passive immunoprophylaxis is recommended in circumstances in which a susceptible person is exposed to an infectious agent and there is inadequate time to allow for immunization and antibody formation or there is no appropriate vaccine with which to immunize that person actively. In these instances there should be documentation of the actual exposure before use of the passive immunizing agent. It may be necessary to use epidemiologic evidence to decide whether the passive immunizing agent should be used. For example, when rabies exposure stems from animal contact and the animal is not available for diagnostic studies, a judgment has to be made as to the likelihood of that animal being rabid. In circumstances in which a definite judgment cannot be made, it is usually best to err on the side of providing therapy.

The diseases for which passive immunoprophylaxis should be considered are botulism, diphtheria, viral hepatitis, measles, rabies, tetanus, and varicella-zoster.

It is recommended that a serum sample be taken before the patient is given the passive immunizing agent so diagnostic or therapeutic studies can be conducted if appropriate.

Maternal antibodies are forms of passive immunization that are important in certain situations. For example, in some countries the passive transfer of maternal tetanus antibody is of prophylactic importance in preventing neonatal tetanus. The presence and relative persistence of maternal antibody will influence the effectiveness of active vaccination, which has to be considered in planning the regular vaccination schedule for newborns. This has been of particular importance in scheduling use of measles vaccine.

REFERENCES

1. McCormick WM, Chowdhury AM, Hahangir N, et al. Tetracycline prophylaxis in families of cholera patients. Bull WHO. 1968;38:787.
2. Centers for Disease Control. Sexually Transmitted Diseases Treatment Guidelines—1982. MMWR. 1982;31(Suppl):375.
3. Centers for Disease Control. Prevention of secondary cases of *Haemophilus influenzae* type b disease. MWWR. 1982;31:672.
4. Jackson GG, Stanley ED. Prevention and control of influenza by chemoprophylaxis and chemotherapy. JAMA. 1976;235:2739.
5. Noorden SK. Chemoprophylaxis in leprosy. Lepr India. 1969;41:247.
6. Centers for Disease Control. Prevention of malaria in travelers. MMWR. 1982;31(Suppl):3s.
7. Meningococcal Disease Surveillance Group. Analysis of endemic meningococcal disease by serogroup and evaluation of chemoprophylaxis. J Infect Dis. 1976;134:201.
8. Centers for Disease Control. Sexually Transmitted Diseases Treatment Guidelines—1982. MMWR. 1982;31(Suppl):50s.
9. Elliott WC. Treatment of primary syphilis. J Am Venereal Dis. 1976;3:128.
10. American Thoracic Society/Centers for Disease Control. Treatment of tuberculosis and other mycobacterial diseases. Am Rev Respir Dis. 1983;127:793.
11. Eickhoff TC. Antibiotics and nosocomial infections. In: Bennett JV, Brachman PS, eds. Hospital Infections. Boston: Little, Brown; 1979:195–221.
12. Sack DA, Kaminsky DC, Sack RB, et al. Prophylactic doxycycline for travelers' diarrhea. N Engl J Med. 1978;298:758.
13. Meningococcal meningitis vaccine: Brazil. Bull Pan Am Health Organ. 1976;10:20.
14. Makela PH, Kayhty H, Weckstrom P, et al. Effect of group-A meningococcal vaccine in army recruits in Finland. Lancet. 1975;1:883.
15. MacLeod CM, Hodges RG, Heidelberger M, et al. Prevention of pneumococcal pneumonia by immunization with specific capsular polysaccharides. J Exp Med. 1945;82:445.
16. American Thoracic Society/Centers for Disease Control. Treatment of tuberculosis and other mycobacterial diseases. Am Rev Respir Dis. 1983;127:795.
17. Centers for Disease Control. Influenza vaccines. MMWR. 1983;32:333.
18. Centers for Disease Control. Meningococcal polysaccharides vaccines. Recommendations of the Public Health Service Advisory Committee on Immunization Practices. MMWR. 1978;27:327.
19. Greenwood BM, Hassan-King M, Whittle HC. Prevention of secondary cases of meningococcal disease in household contacts by vaccination. Br Med J. 1978;1:1317.
20. Centers for Disease Control. Pneumococcal polysaccharide vaccine. Recommendation of the Public Health Service Advisory Committee on Immunization Practices. MMWR. 1981;30:410.
21. CDC Guideline for Infection Control in Hospital Personnel. US Dept Health and Human Services, Public Health Service, Centers for Disease Control; 1983:17–8.
22. Centers for Disease Control. Inactivated hepatitis B viral vaccine. Recommendations of the Immunizations Practice Advisory Committee (APIC). MMWR. 1982;31:317–27.

SECTION D. THE CLINICIAN AND THE MICROBIOLOGY LABORATORY

13. BACTERIA, FUNGI, AND PARASITES

JOHN A. WASHINGTON II

The purpose of the microbiology laboratory is to isolate and identify microorganisms that cause disease and to determine their susceptibility to antimicrobial agents that assist in their eradication. There is, however, no other area of the clinical laboratory in which specimen sources and types are so diverse, in which specimen selection and collection are so important, and in which close communication with the clinician is so vital.

SPECIMEN COLLECTION AND PROCESSING

There are several general guidelines on selection and collection of the specimen that bear emphasis. First of all, the specimen selected should be representative of the disease process. Material swabbed from the orifice of a sinus tract is, for example, more apt to yield harmless saprophytic microorganisms present on the skin than would material obtained by curettage or biopsy of the base of the tract. Second, an adequate quantity of material should be obtained for complete examination. All too frequently, a small or even invisible amount of material is obtained with a swab, which makes it nearly impossible for the laboratory to make appropriate smears and adequate cultures. Characteristically, chronic lesions contain few organisms. These may be missed readily in smears, cultures, and histopathologic sections. Third, scrupulous attention must be given to avoiding contamination of the specimen by the many varieties of organisms indigenous to the skin and mucous membranes (Table 1), culture of which may often be more confusing and misleading than helpful. Sterile equipment and aseptic technique should be used for collecting specimens, particularly those from normally sterile sites. Fourth, material should be forwarded promptly to the laboratory. Fastidious organisms may not survive prolonged storage or may be overgrown by less fastidious organisms before cultures can be made. Last, specimens should be obtained before antimicrobial agents have been administered.

Other factors may impair the laboratory's ability to establish the cause of an infectious disease. First, sampling difficulties may preclude obtaining a specimen representative of the disease process. Second, it may be impossible to obtain a specimen that is not contaminated with flora indigenous to the site of infection. Third, patients with serious underlying diseases often become colonized with gram-negative bacilli, so their indigenous flora contains potentially pathogenic bacteria not ordinarily encountered on healthy human body surfaces. A somewhat different problem in the compromised host is that infections may be caused by organisms ordinarily considered to be indigenous on healthy human body surfaces; therefore, the more attention given to collecting the specimen, the greater the level of confidence we can place on the results of its culture. Fourth, technical errors of various types can interfere with the recovery of organisms causing disease. Examples include patients to whom antimicrobials were being administered at the time of specimen collection, the application of topical anesthetics to infected sites before specimen collection, the use of saline or another irrigating solution containing a preservative to collect the specimen, improper transport or storage of specimens, and the inappropriate selection of culture media.

A final limitation on the laboratory's ability to determine the cause of an infectious disease relates to the laboratory's capability of recovering a rare, unusual, or fastidious organism. It is unreasonable to expect equal capabilities from all microbiology laboratories, and varying extents or levels of capability have been recognized in bacteriology, mycobacteriology, mycology, virology, and parasitology by national laboratory accreditation agencies. Thus, a laboratory offering level I service in mycobacteriology, for example, develops a proficiency in the collection of adequate clinical specimens and in their prompt transport to a more specialized laboratory. With existing and anticipated regulations requiring inspection, proficiency testing, and accreditation, we may anticipate that an increased number of clinical laboratories will establish extents and levels of performance and refer materials or cultures to be examined for rare, fastidious, or otherwise unusual organisms to specialized laboratories. Although it is essential for laboratories to recognize their own limitations, it also behooves the clinician to be aware of these limitations and to recommend referral of material or cultures to specialized laboratories when a diagnosis is suspected that cannot be established by the laboratory facilities at hand. It is essential that diagnostic specimens sent to reference laboratories be shipped according to minimum packaging requirements specified by federal regulation.[1]

Hospital procedure guides should contain reasonably precise guidelines for the collection and transport of specimens from various sites (Table 2). There are numerous kinds of devices and containers available for this purpose. Swabs of every description and composition are available. Many commercially manufactured swab tubes contain a transport medium that is designed to preserve a variety of organisms and to prevent the multiplication of rapidly growing organisms. The swab, however, should be limited in its use to collecting material from the skin and mucous membranes, principally because the amount of material that can be collected with it is limited and is often negligible in practice. It should never be submitted in lieu of curettings, biopsy material, pus, or fluid or tissue removed surgically. All too frequently, biopsy specimens or excised materials are placed in their entirety into formalin for histopatho-

TABLE 1. Microorganisms Encountered on Healthy Human Body Surfaces

Organism	*Skin*	*Conjunctiva*	*Upper Respiratory Tract*	*Mouth*	*Intestine*	*External Genitalia*	*Anterior Urethra*	*Vagina*
Bacteria								
Actinomyces			+	+	±			
Bacteroides			+	++	++	+	+	+
Bifidobacteria				+	++			
Clostridia	±			±	++		±	±
Corynebacteria	++	+	+	+	+	+	+	+
Enterobacteriaceae	±		±	±	++	+	+	±
Fusobacteria			+	++	+	+	+	±
Haemophilus		±	++	+				
Lactobacilli				+	+		±	++
Mycoplasmas			+	+			+	+
Neisseriae		±	++	+			+	±
Propionibacteria	++		+	±	±		±	
Staphylococci	++	+	+	+	±	++	+	+
Streptococci								
Enterococcal			±	+	+	+	+	+
Pyogenic			±	±				±
Viridans group	±	±	+	++	+	+	+	+
Spirochetes				+	+			
Cocci, anaerobic								
Gram-positive	+		+	++	++	+	±	+
Gram-negative			+	++	+		±	+
Fungi								
Aspergillus	±	+		+				
Candida	±	+	+	++	+			+
Cryptococcus	±			±				
Penicillium	+	+		+				
Rhodotorula	±	+		+				
Torulopsis	±			+	±			±

Symbols: ±: irregular; +: common; ++: prominent.

TABLE 2. Guidelines for Microbiologic Specimen Collection and Transport

Specimen	*Container or Transport Device*	*Volume (ml)*	*Other Considerations*
Respiratory tract			
Nasopharynx	Flexible wire calcium alginate tipped swab or no. 8 French 16" suction catheter in sterile jar	NA	Used to detect carrier states of *Streptococcus pyogenes, Neisseria meningitidis, Corynebacterium diphtheriae,* and *Bordetella pertussis*. Aspirates are useful in the diagnosis of pertussis.
Sinus aspirate	Anaerobic transport vial	NA	
Tympanocentesis	Anaerobic transport vial	NA	
Oral cavity	Swab	NA	
Throat	Swab	NA	Swab tonsils, tonsillar areas, posterior pharynx, and areas of inflammation, exudation, ulceration, or capsule formation. Notify laboratory when diphtheria, pertussis, or gonococcal pharyngitis is suspected clinically.
Tracheal aspirate	Sterile, screw-capped tube or jar	NA	Specimen unsuitable for anaerobic culture.
Bronchial washings	Sterile, screw-capped tube or jar	NA	Specimen unsuitable for anaerobic culture unless obtained with double-lumen, distally occluded catheter.
Transtracheal apirate	Anaerobic transport vial	3–5	
Sputum			
Bacteria	Sterile, screw-capped jar	NA	Collect fresh specimen resulting from deep cough. Instruct patient not to expectorate saliva or postnasal discharge into container. Specimen unsuitable for anaerobic culture.
Mycobacteria	Sterile, screw-capped jar	5–10	Collect three early morning, fresh specimens resulting from deep cough or induced by heated aerosol of 10% glycerin and 15% NaCl. Send to laboratory promptly or store under refrigeration. DO NOT COLLECT 24-HOUR SPECIMENS.
Fungi	Sterile, screw-capped jar	3–5	
Lung abscess, empyema fluid	Anaerobic transport vial	NA	
Urinary tract			
Clean-voided midstream urine or urine obtained by catheterization or cystoscopy for	Sterile, screw-capped tube or jar		Send to laboratory promptly or store under refrigeration. DO NOT COLLECT 24-HOUR SPECIMENS. Specimen unsuitable for anaerobic cultures.
Bacteria		1–10	
Mycobacteria		>20	
Fungi		>20	
Suprapubic aspirate	Anaerobic transport vial	(As above)	Only valid means of establishing diagnosis of anaerobic bacteriuria.
Voided urine for parasites	Clean, screw-capped container	24-hour collection	Primarily collected to detect eggs of *Schistosoma haematobium,* trophozoites of *Trichomonas vaginalis* in the male, and microfilariae of *Onchocerca volvulus*.
Blood			
Cultures for			
Bacteria	Blood culture bottles containing broth or lysis–centrifugation tube	20–30 from adults, 1–3 from infants and children	Collect three separate blood samples during a 24-hour period; intervals between cultures are determined by urgency of clinical situation. More than three cultures per 24 hours are rarely necessary.
Brucellae and fungi	Lysis–centrifugation tube or biphasic blood culture bottle	(As for bacteria)	(As for bacteria)
Leptospires	Sterile, heparinized tube	1	(As for bacteria)
Examination for			
Borreliae	Peripheral smear	NA	Examine wet mount by darkfield microscopy or smear stained with aniline dyes
Malaria	Thick and thin films on clean glass slide	NA	
Filaria, Trypanosomes	Sterile tube containing anticoagulant (citrate, oxalate, heparin)	5	Wet mount of drop of blood or concentrated hemolyzed blood preferable to stained thick and thin films.
Fluids			
Exudates, transudates, drainage, pus	Anaerobic transport vial	1–5	
Abdomen, chest	Anaerobic transport vial	1–5 for bacteria, >10 for mycobacteria or fungi	
Synovial	Anaerobic transport vial	1–5 for bacteria, >10 for mycobacteria or fungi	Inoculate modifed Thayer-Martin medium in cases of suspected gonococcal arthritis.
Cerebrospinal	Sterile, screw-capped tube	1–2 for bacteria, >2 for mycobacteria or fungi	Send to laboratory immediately.

(Continued)

logic examination, and the microbiology laboratory receives one swab for a variety of smears and cultures.

Because of the frequency with which anaerobic bacteria play a role in causing infectious diseases, fluids or pus from the brain, thoracic and abdominal cavities, transtracheal and suprapubic aspirations, the pelvis, and the musculoskeletal system should be placed into a transport vial or tube in which anaerobes can survive for several hours. Alternatively, the syringe used to aspirate such materials may be used for their transport to the laboratory, provided the transport time is short. Anaerobe transport vials or tubes are available commercially, or they may be prepared in the laboratory. These contain gaseous mixtures of hydrogen, nitrogen, and carbon dioxide or deoxygenated carbon dioxide alone. Vials should contain a transport medium

TABLE 2. *(Continued)*

Specimen	*Container or Transport Device*	*Volume (ml)*	*Other Considerations*
Catheters			
Intravascular	Sterile, screw-capped tube; Culterette (with swab removed)	NA	Disinfect skin entry site, remove catheter, clip off end into tube.
Suction, drainage	Sterile, screw-capped tube	NA	
Skin and soft tissues			
Cultures	Swab	NA	
	Anaerobic transport vial	NA	
Scrapings for dermatophytes	Sterile Petri dish	NA	
Gastrointestinal tract			
Stool culture or examination for			
Bacteria	Sterile, screw-capped jar Transport medium swab	NA	Freshly collected specimen mandatory; transport medium less desirable. Request cultures for vibrios when suspected clinically.
Fungi	Sterile, screw-capped tube		Refrigerate if storage time exceeds 1 hour.
Ova and parasites	Stool carton sealed in plastic bag PVA preservative	NA	Collect saline purged stools on 3 consecutive days.
Anal swab for pinworm	Sterile plastic swab in tube (SWUBE)	NA	Swab perianal area, preferably on arising in morning and before bathing or defecation.
Sexually transmitted diseases			
Neisseria gonorrhoeae	Swab; modified Thayer-Martin medium (Transgrow, JEMBEC)	NA	Women Cervix—moisten speculum with water; insert swab into cervical canal. Anal canal—insert swab approximately 1 in. to sample anal crypts. Urethral or vaginal—culture if cervix not accessible. Men Urethral—obtain material for smear and culture with swab or a sterile bacteriologic loop, which is used to inoculate medium directly and for preparing smears of exudates from men.
Gardnerella vaginalis	Swab	NA	
Haemophilus ducreyi	Swab	NA	
Treponema pallidum	Serous exudate on clean glass slide or in capillary pipet	NA	Abrade lesion with clean dry sponge. Examine preparation by darkfield microscopy *immediately*.
Chlamydia trachomatis	Sucrose-phosphate solution (2 SP)	NA	Extract urethral or cervical material on swab in solution and refrigerate during storage.
Ureaplasma urealyticum	(As for *Chlamydia*)	(As for *Chlamydia*)	(As for *Chlamydia*)
Candida albicans	Swab	NA	
Trichmonas vaginalis	Swab	NA	
Genitourinary tract excluding sexually transmitted diseases			
Cervical, vaginal discharge	Swab	NA	Specimen unsuitable for anaerobic culture.
Culdocentesis fluid	Anaerobic transport vial	NA	
Abscess			
Pelvic, tubal, ovarian	Anaerobic transport vial	NA	
Prostatic secretion	Sterile, screw-capped bottle	NA	
Eye			
Corneal lesion or scraping	Material should be inoculated directly onto appropriate media and applied directly to clean microscope slides for staining and microscopic examination.		
Conjunctiva examination for			
Bacteria, fungi	Swab		
Neisseria gonorrhoeae	Modified Thayer-Martin medium (Transgrow, JEMBEC)	NA	Inoculate swab directly onto medium.
Chlamydia trachomatis	Sucrose-phosphate solution (2 SP)	NA	Extract material on swab in solution and refrigerate during storage.
Tissue	Sterile, screw-capped bottle	Representative samples	Specimen must be of sufficient size to ensure recovery of small numbers of organisms.

Abbreviations: NA: not applicable; PVA: polyvinyl alcohol.

with an indicator, for example, resazurin, which in its colorless state shows that the interior of the vial is anaerobic at the time a specimen is introduced. Anaerobic swab devices are also commercially available; however, their use is inadvisable because of the limited amount of material generally collected on swabs. Specimen containers should be sterile; they should not contain nonviable but stainable organisms that may provide misleading results.

Protection of Laboratory Workers from Infectious Diseases

Although microbiology laboratory workers are trained to practice aseptic technique and to handle specimens and cultures as being potentially infectious, the advent of infections due to human immune deficiency virus (HIV) and of the practice of universal precautions for preventing infection due to HIV, hepatitis B virus (HBV), and other blood-borne pathogens has led to changes in safety practices in clinical laboratories.

Under universal precautions, blood and body fluids are considered potentially infectious for HIV, HBV, and other blood-borne pathogens. Treating all such specimens as potentially infectious eliminates the need for warning labels on specimen containers. Specimens to which universal precautions should apply are blood and the following fluids: cerebrospinal, synovial, pleural, bronchial (including bronchoalveolar lavage), pericardial, peritoneal, and amniotic as well as vaginal secretions and semen. Universal precautions do not apply to upper respiratory secretions, sputum, urine, and feces unless they contain visible blood.

Specimens should be placed into sturdy, leak-proof containers, and care should be taken not to contaminate the external surface of containers during collection and handling of specimens. Specimen containers should routinely be checked to ensure they are leak-proof before any bulk purchase agreement with manufacturers. When contamination of the external surface of a specimen container is likely, the primary container should be placed into a secondary container such as a plastic sealable bag. In such cases, the specimen requisition should be affixed to the outside of the secondary container.

Laboratory workers should use appropriate barrier protection when handling specimens. In most instances, wearing gloves and a laboratory gown or coat is sufficient; however, the use of masks and protective eyewear or face shields and wearing aprons may be necessary if there is a high degree of likelihood that splashing may occur. Gloves should be removed if they become visibly contaminated with blood or if punctured or torn and the hands washed immediately.

Laboratory-specific precautions also include the use of mechanical pipetting devices (no mouth pipetting); restricted use of needles and syringes; prohibition of eating, drinking, or smoking in the laboratory; and biosafety level 2 practices, including the use of a class I or II biologic safety cabinet when there is a high probability of producing infectious droplets (e.g., homogenization of tissue, vigorous mixing, blending, sonicating), decontamination of work surfaces on a daily basis or after a spill of blood or a body fluid, the use of biohazard disposal techniques, handwashing after completing work and before leaving the laboratory, and the use of laboratory coats and gowns, which should be removed before leaving the laboratory.

More specific guidelines for the protection of laboratory workers are available from the National Committee for Clinical Laboratory Standards (NCCLS, Villanova, PA), the Centers for Disease Control (Atlanta, GA), and for laboratories performing HIV testing, the Division of Safety at the National Institutes of health (Bethesda, MD).

SPECIFIC GUIDELINES FOR SPECIMEN COLLECTION AND PROCESSING

Respiratory Tract

Many types of specimens originate from the respiratory tract. The means of their collection and transport are outlined in Table 2, whereas the procedures recommended for their microscopic examination and culture are listed in Table 3.

Nasopharynx. Cultures of the nose are occasionally made to detect carriers of *Staphylococcus aureus;* however, the results of such cultures are seldom of any epidemiologic value and are not indicated except when serious focal outbreaks of nosocomially acquired staphylococcal infections occur. The results of cultures of the nose have been shown by Evans et al.[2]

TABLE 3. Recommended Procedures for the Isolation and Identification of Respiratory Tract Pathogens

		Microscopic Examination					
Source	*Organism Sought or Disease Suspected*	*Gram Stain*	*FA*[a]	*Acid-Fast*	*KOH*	*Toluidine Blue*	*Methenamine Silver*
Nasopharynx	*Streptococcus pyogenes*		+				
	Neisseria meningitidis						
	Corynebacterium diphtheriae						
	Bordetella pertussis		+				
Paranasal sinus (aspirate)	Sinusitis	+					
Ear (aspirate)	Otitis media	+					
Mouth	Acute necrotizing ulcerative gingivitis (Vincent's)	+					
	Thrush				+		
Throat	*S. pyogenes*		+				
	N. gonorrhoeae						
	C. diphtheriae						
	Mycoplasma pneumoniae						
Sputum	Bacteria	+					
	Legionella		+				
	Mycobacteria			+			
	Nocardia			+[c]			
	Fungi				+		
	Mycoplasma						
Tracheal aspirate	Pneumonitis	+					
Transtracheal aspirate	Pneumonitis, abscess	+				±	
Bronchial washings, lavage, aspirate	Bacteria	+					
	Legionella						
	Mycobacteria			+			
	Nocardia			+[c]			
	Fungi				+		+
	Pneumocystis carinii					+	+
Pleural fluid	Empyema						
	Nonsurgical	+		+			
	Surgical	+					
Lung tissue		+	+	+	+	+	+

Abbreviations: BA: Blood agar; CBA: chocolate blood agar; EMB: eosin–methylene blue (MacConkey's is an acceptable alternative); CNA: colistin–nalidixic acid BA; BCYE: buffered yeast extract medium; BMPA: BCYE with antibiotics; L-J: Lowenstein-Jensen agar; 7H11: Middlebrook 7H11 agar; BHI: brain–heart infusion agar with and without antibiotics; Sab: Sabouraud agar.

[a] Immunofluorescence with specific labeled conjugates can be performed directly with smears prepared from specimens indicated, although *S. pyogenes* is best detected in smears prepared from centrifuged sediment of a 2–4 hour broth culture of the swab.

[b] Anaerobic media: thioglycolate supplemented with vitamin K and hemin; BA with vitamin K and hemin; BA with gentamicin and vancomycin; phenylethyl alcohol agar (PEA).

[c] Modified acid-fast stain.

to correlate poorly with those of sinus aspirates and are, therefore, of little value in establishing the microbial etiology of sinusitis. Since aerobic, anaerobic, and facultatively anaerobic bacteria as well as fungi and viruses have been shown to cause sinusitis,[2] it is necessary to take appropriate precautions with sinus aspirates to ensure the recovery of such a variety of organisms. There is similarly little value in making cultures of the nose to establish the microbial cause of otitis media.[3] Although seldom necessary in acute cases because of the rather predictable findings of *Haemophilus influenzae, Streptococcus pneumoniae,* and *Streptococcus pyogenes,* tympanocentesis is probably warranted in cases with chronic otitis media due to this condition's variable bacteriologic etiology.

Cultures of the nasopharynx may be used to detect carriers of *S. pyogenes* (i.e., group A streptococci), *Neisseria meningitidis, Corynebacterium diphtheriae,* and *Bordetella pertussis.* Some have advocated their use in determining the cause of pneumonia in infants and children; however, nasotracheal aspiration is likely to provide material that is more representative of the disease process. Nasopharyngeal suction, as described by Auger,[4] is preferred for establishing the bacteriologic diagnosis of pertussis. A no. 8 French 16 in. suction catheter with a safety valve is satisfactory in most cases. It is important to remember that cultures for *N. meningitidis, C. diphtheriae,* and *B. pertussis* must be requested specifically since these organisms either will not grow or will fail to be recognized on conventional bacteriologic media. Pertussis may be accurately and rapidly diagnosed by staining a smear of nasopharyngeal aspirate with anti-*B. pertussis* fluorescein-labeled conjugate.

Oral Cavity. Cultures of the oral cavity are seldom helpful because of the millions of microorganisms normally resident in it (Table 1). Direct examination of potassium hydroxide (KOH) preparations may, however, be helpful in confirming the diagnosis of oral thrush, and a Gram or methylene blue-stained smear may be helpful in the diagnosis of acute necrotizing ulcerative gingivitis (Vincent's angina or fusospirochetal disease).

Throat. Most cultures of the throat are made to diagnose streptococcal pharyngitis since its clinical presentation is highly variable and is often indistinguishable from that of viral pharyngitis. Moreover, it is not at all uncommon for there to be concurrent viral and group A streptococcal infections of the throat. Sampling errors in swabbing the throat are frequent, and the patient's interests are best served by vigorous rather than gentle application of the swab to the posterior portion of the pharynx, tonsillar areas, and areas of ulceration, exudation, and membrane formation. Gram-stained smears are of little use or reliability since streptococci of all kinds occur normally and in

Media												
BA	*CBA*	*EMB*	*CNA*	*BCYE, BMPA*	*Anaerobic[b]*	*Loeffler, Tellurite*	*Thayer-Martin*	*Charcoal or Bordet-Gengou*	*L-J, 7H11*	*BHI or Sab*	*Mycoplasma*	*Comments and Other Procedures*
+												
							+					
						+						
								+				
+	+				+							
+	+				+							
										+		
+												Antigen test
							+					
						+						
											+	Serology
+	+	+										
				+								Serology
+									+			PPD
									+	+		
										+		
											+	Serology
+	+	+	+									
+	+	+	+		+							
+	+		+									
									+			PPD
									+	+		
										+		
+	+		+		+				+	+		
+	+	+	+									
+	+	+	+	+					+	+	+	Selection of tests based on clinical and histopathologic findings

large numbers in the mouth and there is little that is distinctive about the microscopic appearance of group A streptococci.

A large number of rapid group A streptococcal antigen detection kits are commercially available for direct testing of throat swabs. Although these tests are highly specific, their sensitivity ranges from 45 to 100 percent, depending on the population studied, culture method used for comparison purposes, and the criteria (i.e., number of colonies) used to define a positive culture. Since the sensitivity of antigen detection kits is directly correlated with the number of group A streptococci present in the specimen, kit sensitivity is lowest with specimens yielding few colonies of group A streptococci in cultures. Manufacturers have tended to discount false-negative kit test results under these circumstances as clinically unimportant; however, since the seroconversion (antistreptolysin O [ASO] and/or anti-DNase B) rate in children with both positive antigen test and culture results is virtually identical to that in children with negative antigen test results and positive cultures,[5] the number of group A streptococci in the specimen often reflect sampling variation and are seldom helpful in distinguishing between infection and colonization or the carrier state. Thus, although antigen tests have a high positive predictive value (100 percent), their negative predictive value may be substantially lower. Antigen tests may, therefore, not be acceptable as a culture substitute, particularly in areas in which there has been a resurgence of acute rheumatic fever. Although it has been shown that the treatment rate is markedly higher for cases detected by antigen tests than for those detected by culture,[6] it is likely that inappropriate treatment rates are also markedly higher when a screening test is known to have a sensitivity of only 45 percent.

In expert hands, a Loeffler's alkaline methylene blue smear of material collected from the margin of a membrane may suggest the diagnosis of diphtheria; however, such expertise is rare in the United States today, and culture remains the principal means of establishing this diagnosis.

It must also be remembered that acute pharyngitis may be caused by *Neisseria gonorrhoeae,* which will not grow on media usually used for throat cultures. If gonococcal pharyngitis is suspected on clinical or epidemiologic grounds, the laboratory should be notified accordingly; however, it is preferable to inoculate modified Thayer-Martin medium directly at the time the swab is taken.

Sputum. The microbiologic examination of sputum is fraught with numerous problems. The patient is usually poorly instructed as to the type of specimen required; supervision is generally lacking during specimen collection; and the specimen often remains on the patient's night table for hours before being delivered to the laboratory, during which time it becomes overgrown with bacteria normally present in saliva. Ideally, patients should be instructed to rinse out their mouths with water and to provide only material resulting from a deep cough. Several attempts may be necessary before a suitable specimen of sputum is obtained. The specimen should then be transported to the laboratory promptly. If bacterial infection is suspected clinically, examination under low power (×100) of a Gram-stained smear of a carefully selected aliquot of the specimen, as described by Chodosh,[7] is a rapid means of determining its suitability for culture (Fig. 1). The presence of many squamous epithelial cells (>25 per low-power field[lpf]) indicates that the specimen consists substantially of saliva and contains an abundance of oropharyngeal microflora.[8,9] It is advisable not to culture this specimen but to try to collect another one. If few squamous epithelial cells (<25/lpf) are present, the smear should be examined carefully under oil immersion (×1000) to determine whether bacteria morphologically typical of certain species (e.g., pneumococci, staphylococci) are present and the specimen should be cultured. In cases of suspected pneumococcal pneumonia it may be helpful to examine a wet mount of sputum that has been mixed with pneumococcal antiserum for evidence of the quellung reaction. In cases of suspected legionellosis, a smear of sputum should be examined by immunofluorescence or genetic probe, and cultures should be made on buffered charcoal yeast extract medium containing antibiotics (BMPA medium). The most important consideration, however, in the laboratory diagnosis of pneumococcal and other bacterial pneumonias is the attention given to proper specimen collection.[10]

Although the degree of oropharyngeal contamination is not as critical in sputum specimens submitted for mycobacterial or fungal examination, every effort should still be made to collect material resulting from a deep cough and to minimize the specimen's contamination since the overgrowth by aerobic and facultatively anaerobic bacteria of mycobacterial and fungal cultures may severely limit the laboratory's ability to recover these pathogens. Twenty-four-hour specimens should not be collected for mycobacterial or fungal cultures. In some cases collection of sputum induced by a heated aqueous aerosol of 10% glycerin and 15% sodium chloride is useful for recovering mycobacteria and fungi. Specimens that cannot be processed within 1 or 2 hours after collection should be refrigerated during their storage and transport; failure to do so may result in a decreased yield of mycobacteria or fungi.

In suspected mycobacterial or fungal disease, appropriately prepared smears should be examined. A fluorochrome stain provides the most rapid means of examining a smear for mycobacteria, while phase-contrast microscopy of a KOH preparation represents the best means of looking for fungi (Fig. 2). It is important to remember that *Nocardia,* which may be seen in Gram-stained smears or KOH preparations (Fig. 3) of respiratory tract specimens, may not be seen in carbol fuchsin (Ziehl-Neelsen or Kinyoun) acid-fast stained smears unless decolorized with 0.5–1% sulfuric acid.

Mycoplasma pneumoniae may be isolated on special media from sputum or from throat swabs from patients with pneumonia due to this organism. Because the growth and isolation of *M. pneumoniae* can be quite slow, it is suggested that serodiagnosis also be attempted by testing acute and convalescent sera for a fourfold or greater increase in complement fixing or immunofluorescent antibody activity.

Transtracheal Aspirate. A transtracheal aspirate (TTA) provides a means of bypassing the upper respiratory tract and obtaining lower respiratory secretions that are suitable for culture of aerobic and anaerobic bacteria as well as mycobacteria and some fungi other than *Candida.*[11] The procedure does require technical expertise and should be reserved for situations in which other less invasive procedures have provided inconclusive results.

Bronchoscopy. Bronchoscopy is a relatively safe technique that provides secretions directly from bronchial drainage sites of infection. Examination of bronchoscopy specimens should be considered in two categories: (*1*) studies to detect microorganisms (e.g., *Legionella, Mycobacterium, Pneumocystis carinii*) that pose no problem in interpretation even in the presence of upper respiratory contamination and (*2*) studies for bacteria that may comprise upper respiratory flora but in which differentiation between upper and lower respiratory origin is necessary.[12] Bronchoscopy, including washings, biopsy, or lavage procedures, is suitable for the first category of examination, whereas bronchoscopy with a double-lumen catheter and a distal occluding plug is useful in the second category, particularly when accompanied by quantitative cultures for aerobic and anaerobic bacteria.[12]

Pleural Fluid. Pleural or empyema fluid is of particular value in the diagnosis of anaerobic pleuropulmonary infections and legionnaires' disease. In such cases, a Gram-stained smear can be very helpful, although it is necessary to prolong the period

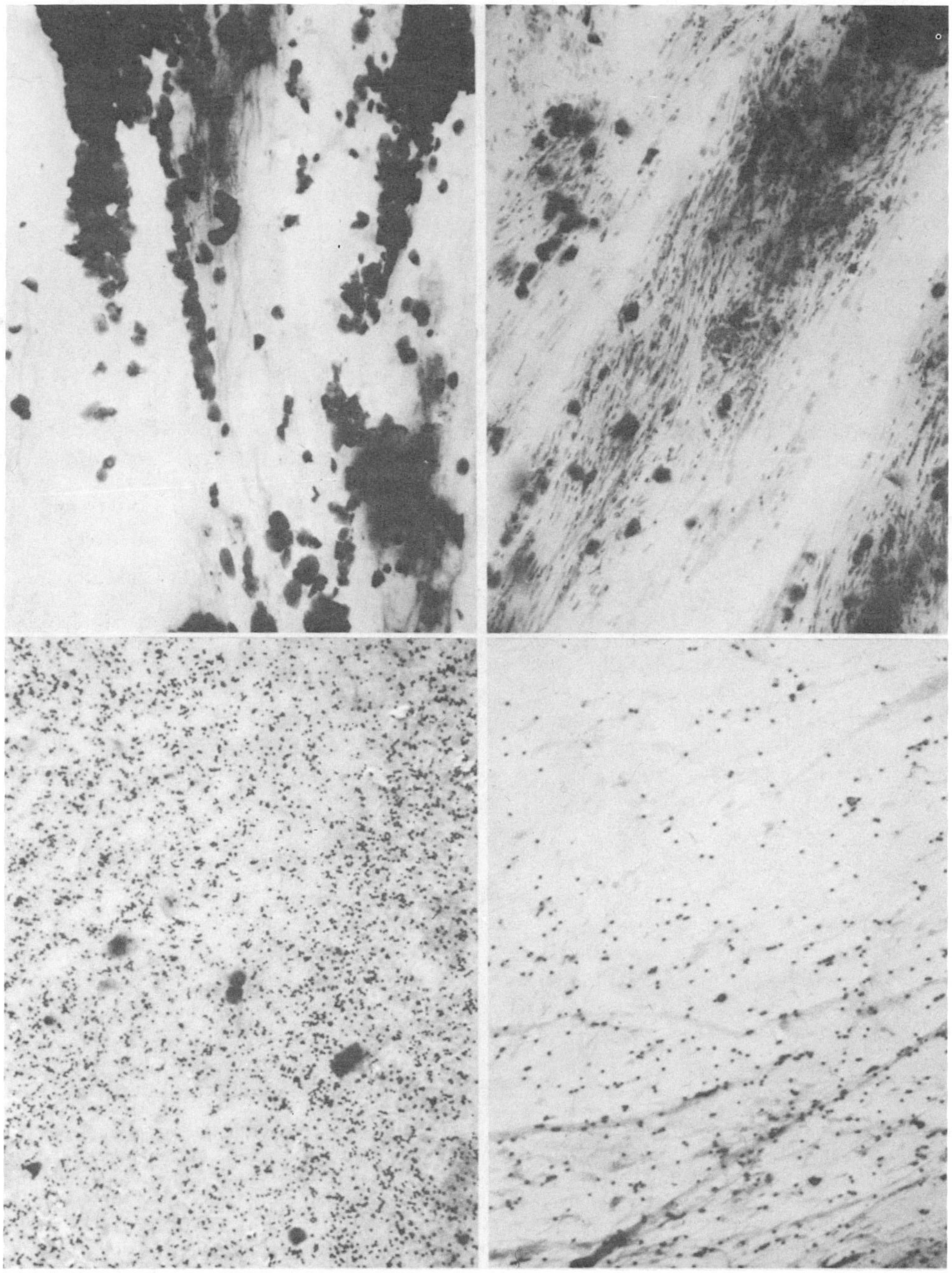

A B C D

FIG. 1. Smears of representative sputum specimens. (Gram stain, ×100) **(A)** Group 1: leukocytes, <10; epithelial cells, >25. **(B)** Group 3: leukocytes, >25; epithelial cells, >25. **(C)** Group 4: leukocytes, >25; epithelial cells, 10–25. **(D)** Group 5: leukocytes, >25; epithelial cells, <10. (From Murray et al.,[8] with permission.)

of counterstaining with safranin for several minutes to detect *Legionella*. A more specific approach to the diagnosis of this disease is by direct immunofluorescent staining of a smear of pleural fluid. Obviously, pleural or empyema fluid can be examined and cultured for other etiologic agents of pulmonary disease.

Lung Tissue. Obtained at substantial cost and some risk to the patient, lung tissue specimens warrant special attention by all concerned.[12] The microbiologist needs to know the suspected clinical diagnosis and what the histopathologic studies show. It should be stressed that few organisms may be present in a chronic inflammatory lesion and that an adequate quantity of the lesion should be submitted for examination and cultures. Impression smears of tissue are especially useful in the diagnosis of *Pneumocystis carinii* infections and legionnaires' disease. Although *P. carinii* is readily seen in Gomori methenamine silver-stained smears, smears stained with toluidine blue 0 can be easily and rapidly prepared and examined in the microbiology laboratory.[13] Impression smears for *Legionella* are fixed with 10% formalin for 10 minutes and are stained with specific fluorescein-labeled conjugate.

Gram stain, an acid-fast stain, and Gomori methenamine silver stain are satisfactory for screening tissue sections for microorganisms.[12] Dieterle silver-impregnation stain will demonstrate *Legionella* in paraffinized tissue sections.[12]

Tissue for culture is finely minced with sterile scissors and is then ground in a tissue grinder or with a small amount of sterile abrasive (alundum) in a sterile mortar with a pestle. A 10–20 percent suspension is prepared with nutrient broth and is used to inoculate cultures. Alternatively, tissue may be ma-

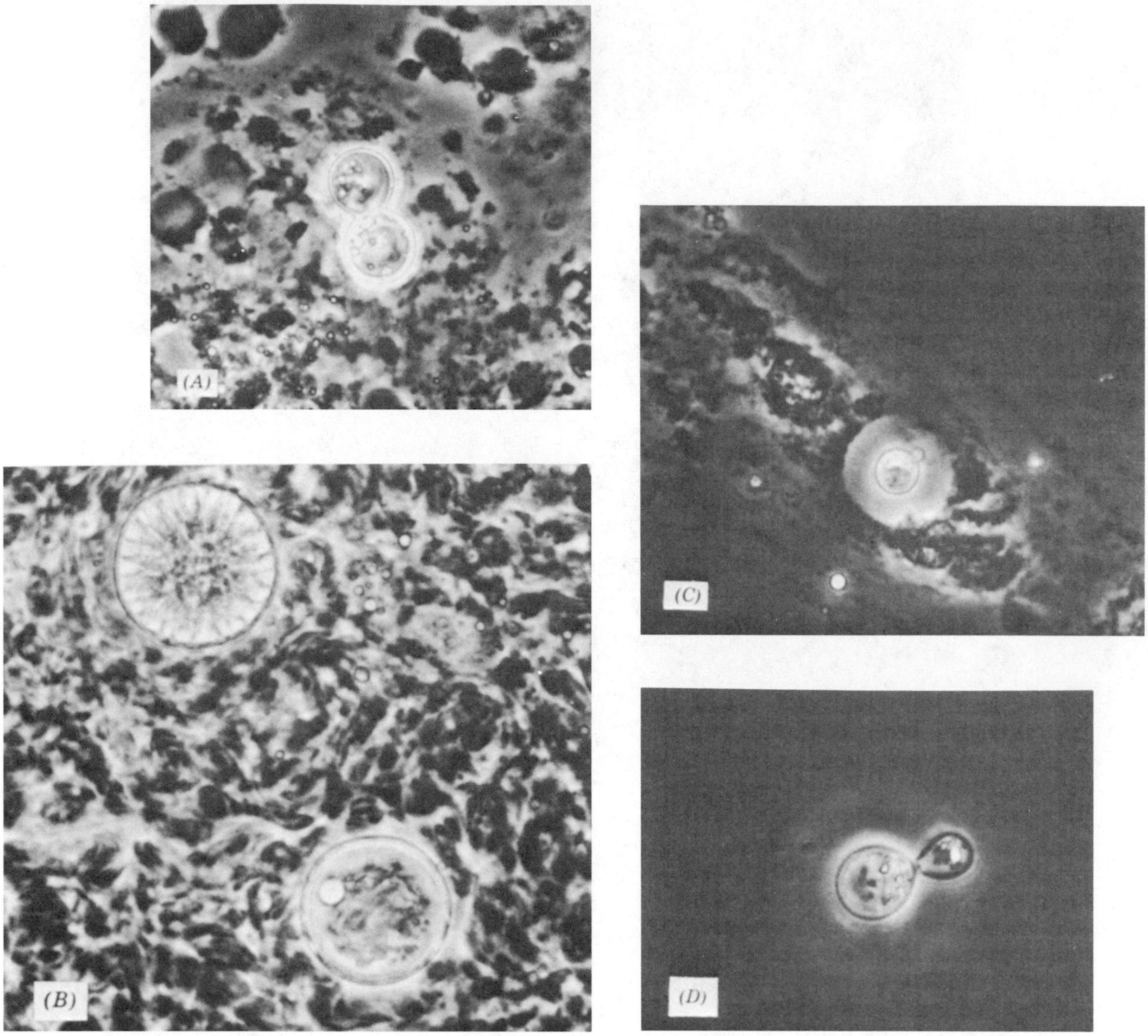

FIG. 2. Phase-contrast microscopy of clinical specimens. (×2000) **(A)** *Blastomyces dermatitidis* in sputum. The characteristic yeast form has a budding cell attached by a broad base. Also note the "double contoured" appearance of the cell wall. **(B)** *Coccidioides immitis* in sputum. Large thick-walled spherules with few endospores are scattered within the interior of the spherule (lower) or cleavage furrows developing along the periphery to form endospores (upper). **(C)** *Cryptococcus neoformans* in sputum. Spherical yeast is surrounded by a large capsule with a small bud arising from the parent cell. **(D)** *C. neoformans* in sputum. An encapsulated yeast form has a budding cell attached by a narrow base. (*Figure continues*)

cerated in a stomaching device and the extract used for microbiologic examination. Such suspensions are saved, most conveniently in a sterile 60 ml dropper bottle, until after the tissue sections and special stains have been reviewed in case additional cultures are indicated.

Urinary Tract

Clean-voided midstream urine is preferred for bacterial, mycobacterial, and fungal cultures. Twenty-four-hour collections are suitable only for parasitologic study (Table 2). Catheterization is not recommended for obtaining urine unless the procedure fulfills a diagnostic or therapeutic purpose. Suprapubic aspiration is recommended for establishing the diagnosis of bacteriuria in infants and small children, for determining the significance of borderline counts of bacteria in repeated clean-voided midstream specimens, and for determining the presence of anaerobic bacteriuria.

Because the distal urethra of both men and women is normally colonized with large numbers of aerobic, facultatively anaerobic, and anaerobic bacteria, the diagnosis of clinically significant bacteriuria in a clean-voided, midstream specimen requires quantitative smears and cultures. A Gram stain of a drop (allow to dry without spreading) of well-mixed urine will not only provide a means of determining the adequacy of its collection but also will provide the diagnosis of significant bacteriuria (≥100,000 cfu/ml) when at least two bacteria per oil immersion (×1000) field are found. The correlation of the results of this test in expert hands with those of quantitative cultures should be at least 90 percent. Essential to the validity of these results is proper specimen collection and transport to the laboratory. Unless refrigerated during storage and transport, no urine arriving in the laboratory more than 2 hours after its collection should be cultured. The presence of many squamous epithelial cells on microscopic examination of the urine is indicative of poor technique in its collection, and another specimen should be requested.

Quantitation of bacteriuria in cultures can be most conveniently accomplished by streaking a measured volume (e.g., 0.01

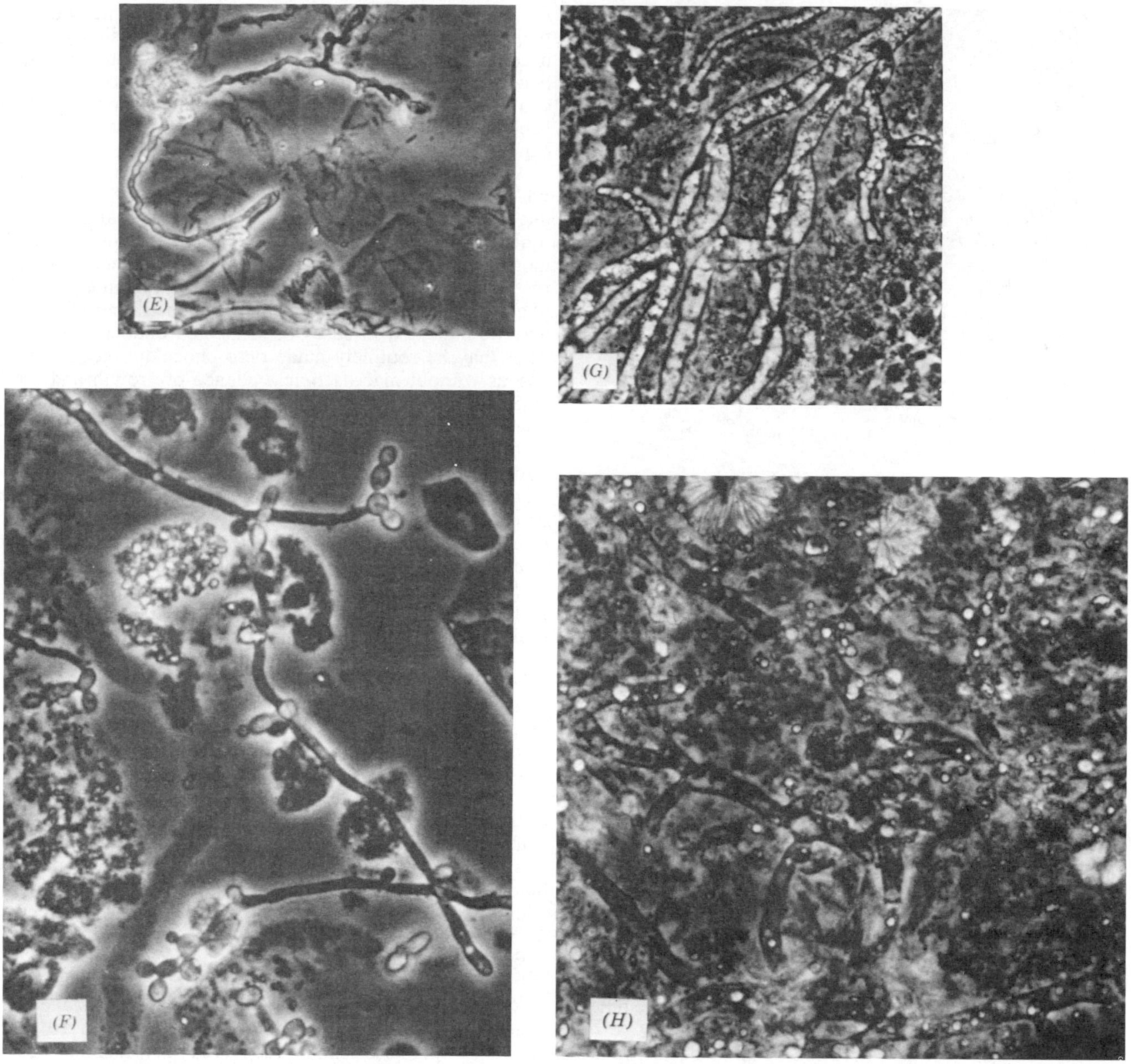

FIG. 2 (*Continued*). **(E)** Dermatophyte in a skin scraping. Septate hyphae intertwine among squamous cells. **(F)** *Candida albicans* in urine. Hyphae and budding yeasts appear among epithelial cells. **(G)** *Mucor* sp. in pus from a skin lesion. The large, branching, ribbonlike aseptate hyphae are indicative of a zygomycete. **(H)** *Aspergillus fumigatus* in sputum. The septate hyphae show dichotomous branching. (Courtesy of Dr. Glenn D. Roberts, Rochester, MN.)

or 0.001 ml) of well-mixed urine onto the surface of culture media with a calibrated milk dilution platinum loop. A general-purpose medium (e.g., blood agar) and a gram-negative differential medium (e.g., eosin–methylene blue [EMB] or MacConkey) should be used. Broth cultures of clean-voided urine are meaningless and should not be made since the growth of even a few bacteria of urethral origin will render the broth turbid and will provide misleading results. Precision in reporting the number of colonies isolated on solid media is unnecessary, and the results can be reported as approximate colony counts (e.g., $<10^3$, 10^4–10^5, $>10^5$ cfu/ml). Provided the specimen has been properly collected, colony counts of $\geq 10^4$/ml are usually significant; however, as few as 100 cfu/ml may be significant in women with the acute dysuric syndrome.

Commercially available screening tests for significant bacteriuria include bioluminescence, miniaturized culture systems, dipstick method for nitrite and leukocyte esterase (Chemstrip L-N) and staining of bacteria and leukocytes on filter paper (Bac-T-Screen, Filtra Check-UTI). Regardless of the principle involved in the test, sensitivity is maximal with at least 10^5 cfu/ml, although it may vary with the populations of patients studied. The sensitivity of the L-N test may be enhanced by using the additional tests for blood and protein that are available on the Chemstrip 9.[14]

Despite the fact that cultures of the urine for other microorganisms (e.g., brucellae, leptospires, mycobacteria, fungi, mycoplasmas, and viruses) entail selective processes for their isolation, the same requirements for careful specimen collection and transport apply because selective procedures are not uniformly successful in eliminating any bacterial contamination that may be present and that may overgrow cultures or otherwise interfere with the isolation of these other microorganisms. Decontamination and selective isolation procedures for these other organisms are described in detail elsewhere.[15]

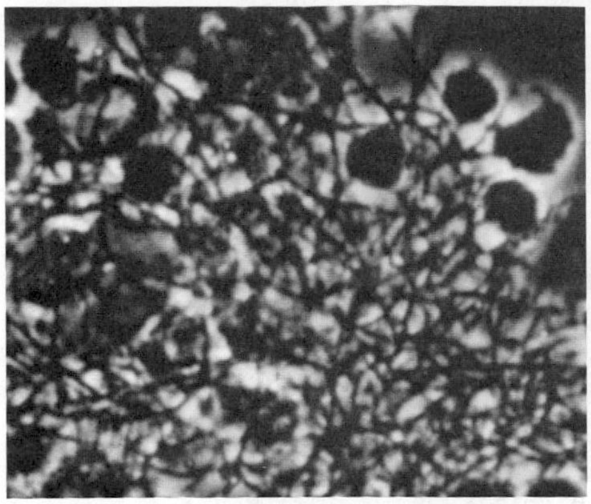

FIG. 3. Phase-contrast microscopy of sputum containing *Nocardia asteroides* shows slender, branching filaments. (×2000) (Courtesy of Dr. Glenn D. Roberts, Rochester, MN.)

Septicemia

The successful isolation of microorganisms from blood requires an understanding of the intermittency and low order of magnitude of most bacteremias, the great variety of organisms capable of causing septicemia, and a broad range of microbiologic considerations involved in the isolation of microorganisms from blood. Each of these factors is reviewed in detail elsewhere.[16,17] There are two major variables that warrant emphasis here: timing of blood collections and the volume of blood collected for culture. Most bacteremias are intermittent, so blood collections for culture should be made intermittently during a 24-hour period. Studies have shown that the sensitivity of two to three separately collected blood cultures within a 24-hour period in establishing the cause of clinically significant bacteremias is nearly 100 percent and that the sensitivity of a single blood culture within this same time period is approximately 80 to 90 percent. The bacteremia associated with subacute bacterial endocarditis is usually continuous, so only two cultures will yield the etiologic agent in nearly all cases. It is apparent, therefore, that two and preferably three separate blood cultures should be collected within a 24-hour period and that it is seldom necessary to perform more than three blood cultures within this same time period.

Most bacteremias, with the exception of those occurring in infants, are of a very low order of magnitude; therefore, an adequate volume of blood should be collected for each set of cultures. It is suggested that 20 ml be obtained from adults and that 1–3 ml be obtained from infants and small children. It is important to consider the volume of blood cultured and the number of blood cultures obtained as independent variables; therefore, we should avoid the obvious temptation to use one venipuncture to obtain an unusually large volume of blood that is then inoculated into several sets of cultures. Although the rate of recovery of bacteria from blood is directly related to the volume of blood cultured, the yield from several separate sets of blood cultures is related, in turn, to the usual intermittency of bacteremia. Both factors, therefore, must be kept in mind when making blood cultures.

The proposed venipuncture site requires careful disinfection since bacteria normally resident in the skin include species that frequently are associated with infections of implanted prosthetic material. Their isolation from blood cultures can cause considerable confusion unless the skin has been carefully prepared for venipuncture with a suitable antiseptic agent and multiple sets of blood cultures have been inoculated with blood obtained from separate venipunctures.

Proper selection of blood culture bottles, although important, is difficult because of differences among manufacturers in their formulations of media, use of additives, and methods of bottling. Published evaluations of media are impossible to interpret if comparisons were made sequentially or if cultures were inoculated with different volumes of blood. Other variables, for example, atmosphere of incubation, timing, and frequency of subcultures, require careful scrutiny before broad conclusions can be drawn.

As a general rule, blood should be inoculated on a 10 percent vol/vol basis into two vacuum bottles, one of which remains unvented (relatively anaerobic) during incubation while the other is vented transiently to permit the growth of pseudomonads and yeasts. Cultures should be examined daily for macroscopic, infrared spectrophotometric, or radiometric evidence of growth for a minimum of 1 week; longer periods of incubation may be indicated in cases of suspected endocarditis. Subcultures may be routinely made onto chocolate blood agar from bottles without macroscopic evidence of growth and are best made between 6 and 24 hours after the initial inoculation. Routine subcultures of anaerobic bottles are not useful. With the early subculture, routine Gram-stained smears are unnecessary. Subcultures of bottles yielding growth should be made onto media suitable for the growth of aerobic, facultatively anaerobic, and anaerobic bacteria and for the differentiation of mixtures of different species of bacteria since polymicrobial bacteremia occurs in nearly 10 percent of the cases. Turbid broth or colonies from bottles yielding growth may be used for direct antimicrobial susceptibility testing after a short incubation period and adjustment of the inoculum size to that used in standardized methodology.

In cases of suspected meningococcemia or gonococcemia, media without sodium polyanetholesulfonate (SPS) should be inoculated because of this polyanion's inhibitory effects on some strains of pathogenic neisseriae. Otherwise, SPS, which has antiphagocytic, anticomplement, and anticoagulant activity, should be incorporated at concentrations of 0.025–0.05 percent into all blood culture media. The use of sodium amylosulfate (SAS) in lieu of SPS appears to be contraindicated at this time. The value of penicillinase in media inoculated with blood from patients receiving penicillins is uncertain, but its addition is probably advisable provided it is tested concurrently for its sterility.

Brucellae are most likely to be recovered from blood that is cultured early in the course of the disease and that has been inoculated into a bottle containing biphasic (Castaneda principle) soybean-casein digest medium and 10 percent carbon dioxide. Leptospires can be recovered only in some cases during the first week of illness and from essentially none thereafter. Cultures should be made by inoculating a few drops of fresh or anticoagulated blood into each of several tubes containing a leptospiral semisolid culture medium such as Fletcher's. Cultures should be incubated at 30°C for 2 or 3 weeks and should be examined with darkfield or immunofluorescent microscopy twice weekly. Direct darkfield microscopic examination of blood or blood cultures should be interpreted very cautiously because of the formation of motile "pseudospirochetes" from blood components.

In cases in which fungal sepsis is suspected, blood should be inoculated into bottles that contain biphasic brain–heart infusion (BHI) medium and that are vented and incubated at 30°C for 1 month. Most yeasts will grow in media in conventional blood culture bottles provided these bottles are vented if under vacuum; however, the growth of yeasts in vented vacuum bottles is significantly slower than in bottles containing biphasic media.

Techniques that lyse blood cells and concentrate the residue by filtration or centrifugation for culture have generally proved more sensitive methods than those of conventional broth culture in detecting bacteria and fungi present in blood. A lysis–centrifugation device is available commercially (Isolator, DuPont) and has generally been found to increase and accelerate the detection of bacteria and, particularly, fungi in blood.[17] Disadvantages of this system include the need for processing specimens within several hours of blood collection, increased yield of presumed contaminants (primarily *Staphylococcus epidermidis*), and decreased yield of *S. pneumoniae,* nutritionally deficient streptococci, *Listeria monocytogenes,* and anaerobic bacteria. For these reasons, it is advisable for the system to be used in conjunction with a suitable vacuum blood culture bottle.

Intra-abdominal Infections

According to Finegold,[18] the incidence of infections involving anaerobic bacteria in this site generally is 86 percent. Anaerobes are involved in pyogenic abscesses of the liver in 50–100 percent of the cases and in at least 90 percent of tuboovarian and pelvic abscesses. Appropriate measures must, therefore, be taken to ensure the survival of anaerobes during the specimen's transport to the laboratory. Fluid or pus should be aspirated into a syringe, and air bubbles expelled, and the syringe transported directly to the laboratory, or its contents should be injected into an anaerobic vial or tube for transport to the laboratory. Swabs are generally not suitable for this purpose.

Granulomatous lesions of the liver, spleen, or lymph nodes should be cultured for mycobacteria, brucellae, and fungi as well as for aerobic and facultatively anaerobic bacteria. Complete microbiologic examination of material removed surgically is essential in patients undergoing abdominal exploration for fever of unexplained origin (Table 4). Because the distribution of organisms in tissue may not be uniform, generous portions of tissue should be removed for histologic and microbiologic examination.

Amebic abscesses of the liver are rarely confused histologically with pyogenic abscesses and are mainly composed of necrotic granular and eosinophilic material with considerable nuclear debris and few or no cells. The amebae are usually found near the capsule and not in the central necrotic material. Microscopic examination of the pus may be facilitated by its enzymatic digestion with streptodornase and the preparation of wet mounts from centrifuged sediment. Indirect hemagglutination titers are usually elevated in sera from patients with extraintestinal amebiasis.

Central Nervous System Infections

The cerebrospinal fluid (CSF) from a patient suspected of having meningitis demands immediate attention from the microbiologist. This urgency is dictated by the lethality of acute bacterial meningitis if untreated, its morbidity if inadequately treated, and its curability if treated early with appropriate antimicrobial agents. The prompt detection, isolation, and identification of the etiologic agent and determination of its antimicrobial susceptibility play a crucial role in the management of meningitis.

Cerebrospinal fluid must be collected aseptically, both to prevent the inadvertent introduction of organisms into the central nervous system and to avoid contamination with organisms indigenous to the skin or other body surfaces, culture of which may delay or confuse the diagnosis. Aspirations of cerebrospinal fluid shunts must be made very carefully since bacteria associated with infections of such shunts frequently belong to species that are ordinarily indigenous to the skin. Careful preparation of the skin must be carried out with a suitable antiseptic such as tincture of iodine or an iodophor; aqueous benzalkonium chloride should be avoided for skin antisepsis.

Specimen containers in lumbar puncture trays, whether prepared in-house or commercially, should be randomly tested by the microbiology laboratory for sterility, absence of stainable but nonviable bacteria, and effectiveness of closure to prevent leakage during transport. Many hospitals now use pneumatic tube systems to transport medically urgent specimens to the laboratory, and it is not uncommon for leakage from certain kinds of tubes to occur under these conditions. Cerebrospinal fluid should not be stored or refrigerated, and it should be transported to the laboratory for examination as rapidly as possible.

Although the number of bacteria per milliliter of cerebrospinal fluid in cases with meningitis usually exceeds 10^5 cfu, numbers significantly below this level do occur.[19] Moreover, if present, the numbers of mycobacteria and fungi in cerebrospinal fluid are often few. It is, therefore, important for a sufficient volume (Table 2) of fluid to be sent to the laboratory to ensure its proper examination. Additional fluid is, of course, required for cell counts and biochemical analyses. Ideally, fluid for microbiologic studies should be placed in separate containers from that needed for other studies to expedite processing and to minimize contamination.

Fluid should be examined microscopically in the laboratory (Table 5). Procedures to be followed for the laboratory diagnosis of viral meningitis and encephalitis are described elsewhere (Chapter 14). Centrifuged sediment is generally examined microscopically; however, it is important to realize that some bacteria usually require a force of at least 10,000 $\times g$ for 10 minutes to sediment and that 60 minutes may be required to accomplish the same purpose with the conventional bench-top laboratory centrifuge, which develops a maximum force of only 1000 $\times g$. In most cases, the presence of inflammatory cells will hasten the sedimentation process; however, there may only be a few polymorphonuclear leukocytes in the cerebrospinal fluid early in the course of acute bacterial meningitis. Published reports of the sensitivity of the Gram-stained smear of cerebrospinal fluid sediment from patients with acute bacterial meningitis vary but approximate 70 percent. For this reason as well as because of possible misinterpretation of findings in the smear, other methods of bacterial detection in cerebrospinal fluid have been developed, the most rapid and specific of which are immunologic.

Counterimmunoelectrophoresis (CIE), latex particle agglutination (LPA), and coagglutination (CoA) tests have been positive upon initial evaluation of cerebrospinal fluid in 82 (range, 68–94), 95 (range, 78–100), and 94 (range, 83–100) percent, respectively, of patients with *Haemophilus influenzae* meningitis.[20] The corresponding figures for CIE, LPA, and CoA in meningococcal meningitis are 60 (range, 17–100), 78 (range, 20–100), and 39 (range, 33–50) percent, respectively, and for pneu-

TABLE 4. Recommended Procedures for Examination and Culture of Intra-abdominal Fluids and Tissue

Type of Lesion	Microscopic Examination	Culture Media[a] BA	CBA	EMB	CNA	Thayer-Martin	Anaerobic	L-J, 7H11	BHI or Sab	Brucella[b]
Pyogenic										
Abdominal	Gram stain	X	X	X	X		X			
Pelvic	Gram stain	X	X	X	X	X	X			
Granulomatous	Acid-fast and methenamine silver							X	X	X

[a] Abbreviations as in Table 3.
[b] Brucella media: blood–heart infusion agar, W medium.[15]

TABLE 5. Microbiologic Examination of Cerebrospinal Fluid

Suspected Cause	Detection Procedures: Essential	Detection Procedures: Supplemental	Media
Bacterial	Gram-stained smear	Quellung reaction, immunofluorescence, counterimmunoelectrophoresis, coagglutination, latex agglutination, and limulus lysate assay	BA, CBA, Thiogly/S, MHB/S
Leptospiral	Darkfield microscopy	Macroscopic agglutination for antibody in serum	Fletcher's semisolid medium or albumin fatty acid broth (Ellinghausen)
Mycobacterial	Acid-fast stained smear		L-J, 7H11
Fungal	India ink wet mount	Latex agglutination for cryptococcal antigen in CSF, complement fixation for coccidioidal antibody in CSF	BHI,[a] Sab
Amebae	Phase-contrast microscopy	Cocultivation on plain agar with *E. coli*	1.5% agar in distilled water

Abbreviations: Thiogly/S: thioglycollate medium supplemented with rabbit serum; MHB/S: Mueller-Hinton broth with supplement C; others as in Table 3.
[a] BHI without cycloheximide should be included.

mococcal meningitis are 67 (range, 20–100), 67 (range, 50–100), and 82 (range, 60–100) percent, respectively.[20] The sensitivity of CIE, LPA, and CoA is much less in cases in which the Gram-stained smear of cerebrospinal fluid was negative than in those in which the smear was positive.[20] False-positive immunologic test results (i.e., positive for antigen and a negative culture) on cerebrospinal fluid are uncommon. Whether such false-positive results actually represent false-negative cultures, technical errors, cross-reactions, or in the case of tests of urine in which false-positives occur more frequently, antigenuria in asymptomatic carriers or recently immunized children remains uncertain.[20,21]

The major question regarding rapid antigen tests of cerebrospinal fluid is how the information they provide is used clinically. In one study of this question, appropriate therapy for *H. influenzae* type b meningitis was initiated before the results of latex particle agglutination were known, and in no case did the results of the test alter therapy.[21] Granoff et al. concluded that physicians believed that the risks of error in the test were not acceptable in the management of an infection that is potentially fatal without appropriate antimicrobial therapy and that culture results rather than antigen test results were being used for management decisions.[21] Antigen tests of cerebrospinal fluid may be helpful in partially treated patients and when cerebrospinal fluid indices do not distinguish between bacterial and nonbacterial meningitis.

A high level of sensitivity in the diagnosis of meningitis due to *N. meningitidis*, *H. influenzae*, and other gram-negative bacteria can be obtained with the limulus lysate test, in which a lysate prepared from amebocytes of the horseshoe crab, *Limulus polyphemus*, undergoes gelation when exposed to endotoxin. A positive response to a limulus lysate test is obviously nonspecific and, therefore, provides less information than do the more specific immunologic tests.

In suspected fungal meningitis, an India ink wet mount preparation of cerebrospinal fluid sediment should be examined carefully for the presence of encapsulated, budding yeasts resembling cryptococci (Chapter 241). Care must be taken not to confuse red blood cells, white blood cells, or starch granules with the characteristically encapsulated cryptococci. The sensitivity of this procedure, however, is only approximately 50 percent; therefore, it is important to supplement it with a latex agglutination test for cryptococcal antigen. Properly controlled, the sensitivity of this test approximates that of culture. Wet mount preparations are not usually useful in establishing the diagnosis of coccidioidal meningitis. Cultures should be made, and most patients develop complement-fixing antibodies to *Coccidioides* in their spinal fluid.

Darkfield microscopy of cerebrospinal fluid may be helpful in establishing the diagnosis of leptospirosis; however, the presence of leptospires in cerebrospinal fluid closely parallels that in blood. Darkfield examinations and cultures should therefore be made during the first week of illness.

The motile amebae (*Naegleria, Hartmannella-Acanthamoeba* group) may be seen with phase microscopy. They may be cultured on plain agar by placing a drop of cerebrospinal fluid onto a loopful of *E. coli* spread in a 1 cm^2 area in the center of the plate.

Brain abscesses contain anaerobic bacteria in nearly 90 percent of cases.[18] Often their presence is suggested in Gram-stained smears made directly with pus from the abscess. Appropriate precautions must be taken to ensure the survival of anaerobes during the specimen's transport to the laboratory, and anaerobic cultures should be prepared.

Media to be inoculated with cerebrospinal fluid are listed in Table 5 according to the etiologic agent suspected. It is important to concentrate the specimen before its inoculation either by centrifugation or by membrane filtration. In the latter case, fluid is forced through a 0.45 μm disposable membrane filter device (e.g., Swinnex, Millipore Corporation), and the filter is cultured by placing it "upstream" side down on the agar surface. After 24–48 hours of incubation, the filter is moved to determine whether colonies may have arisen at its site of application.

Musculoskeletal Infections

Most musculoskeletal infections are due to bacteria (aerobic, facultatively anaerobic, anaerobic, and mycobacterial) and less frequently to fungi. Microorganisms are usually recovered from previously unopened and undrained abscesses, provided the pus has been properly collected and transported to the laboratory. "Sterile" pus is usually due to carelessness on the part of the person collecting the specimen or to the ineptness of the laboratory personnel examining it. In chronic lesions the number of organisms is often small, so an adequate quantity of specimen should be obtained. Swabs are usually unsatisfactory for this purpose, and material should be collected with a sterile syringe and needle. If necessary, irrigation of the lesion with bacteriostat-free saline or Ringer lactate solution is satisfactory. Sinus tracts often originate in bone or lymph nodes, and their microbial cause is seldom elucidated by swabbing the tract's orifice.[22] The orifice should be cleansed with an antiseptic, and curettings should be taken of the tract as close to its base as possible. A biopsy specimen is preferable. Cultures of swabs of ulcers may also be misleading, and it is suggested that curetting or biopsy specimens be taken from the base or undermined edge of such lesions. Cultures of previously opened abscesses usually yield a great variety of microorganisms, identification of which taxes the technologist and defies rational antimicrobial therapy. Again, a carefully collected specimen does much to minimize confusion.

Wounds, both traumatic and nosocomial in origin, are increasingly found to be infected with gram-negative bacilli and anaerobic bacteria. Media appropriate for the isolation and identification of these bacteria should be used for cultures of wound material (see Table 4 for suitable bacteriologic media). Quantitative bacteriology of biopsy specimens from acute and chronic wounds has been shown to provide valuable prognostic information on the risk of sepsis at the time of closure.[23] In addition, quantitative bacteriology of biopsy specimens of burn wounds has been found to reflect infection more accurately than have surface culture techniques.[24] As a general rule, the risk of wound sepsis increases significantly if there are more than 10^5 cfu/g of tissue, whereas wounds with fewer than 10^5 cfu/g have little risk of developing sepsis when closed primarily.[23] Gram-stained smears of biopsy material may be made to provide quantitative results within 30 minutes after receipt of the specimen in the laboratory.[23]

Post-traumatic mycobacterial infections are often due to the *Mycobacterium fortuitum-chelonae* complex and to *Mycobacterium marinum*.[25] Sources of the former group of mycobacteria have included soil, lower animals, dirty skin, foreign bodies, contaminated needles or syringes, and contaminated injectable material, whereas those of *M. marinum* have included tropical fish aquariums, swimming pools, and tributaries. When granulomas are suspected of being due to *M. marinum,* the laboratory should be notified so cultures are incubated at 25°–30°C; *M. marinum* grows slowly if at all at 37°C. Colonies of *M. marinum* require 2 weeks or longer to develop, whereas those of the *M. fortuitum-chelonae* complex will usually appear within 7 days of incubation. Mycobacterial infections of the bones and joints may also be due to several species including *M. tuberculosis, M. bovis,* and *M. kansasii*.[25] Their growth requires at least 2 weeks.

The significance of mycobacteria other than tubercle bacilli that are isolated from the musculoskeletal system and wounds must be interpreted cautiously because of their occurrence in nature as well as in clinically asymptomatic humans, especially in superficial lesions. Their significance is increased if isolated from an abscess or closed lesion, when present in large numbers, and if isolated in repeated cultures. Acid-fast bacteria may not be seen in as many as half of the tissues from which tubercle bacilli are isolated, so acid-fast stains are helpful only when positive.

Osseous lesions may occur in disseminated forms of brucellosis, cryptococcosis, coccidioidomycosis, blastomycosis, and sporotrichosis. The presence of granulomas in frozen sections of bone should therefore prompt a request for cultures for mycobacteria, brucellae, and fungi (see Table 4 for suitable media).

Acute-Onset Diarrhea

Acute-onset diarrhea may be caused by a variety of bacterial, parasitic, and viral agents. Included among bacterial etiologic agents are *Bacillus cereus, Campylobacter jejuni, Clostridium difficile, Clostridium perfringens,* enterotoxigenic and enteroinvasive *E. coli,* salmonellae, shigellae, *Vibrio cholerae* and halophilic vibrios, and *Yersinia enterocolitica*. Among parasitic agents, those most frequently encountered in the United States are *Giardia lamblia* and *Entamoeba histolytica;* however, cryptosporidiosis has become a serious problem in patients with the acquired immunodeficiency syndrome (AIDS). Viral causes of acute-onset diarrhea are rotavirus, Norwalk and similar agents, calicivirus, and adenovirus. With certain exceptions, serotypes of *E. coli,* which were formerly described as "enteropathogenic," have been shown not to be pathogenic and should therefore no longer be routinely identified in stool cultures. Identification of enterotoxigenicity in *B. cereus* or *E. coli* and of cytotoxicity in *C. difficile* requires inoculation of tissue culture cell lines, whereas identification of enteroinvasive *E. coli* requires animal inoculation. Alternative methods for detecting *C. difficile* toxin have included counterimmunoelectrophoresis, which generally lacks sensitivity (41–100 percent) and specificity (78–95 percent), enzyme immunoassay, which has variable sensitivity (56–100 percent) but appears to be highly specific (98–100 percent), and a commercially available latex agglutination that is relatively specific (92–98 percent) and moderately sensitive (80–91 percent) but appears to react with a protein that is not associated with either toxin A or toxin B.[26,27] Although the latex agglutination test is simple and rapid to perform, its use should probably be limited to laboratories that are unable to perform a cytotoxin assay. Although culture for *C. difficile* is the most sensitive test for antibiotic-associated gastroenteritis, isolation of the organism is a nonspecific finding; therefore, testing is usually limited to toxin detection.

DNA hybridization appears to be a highly sensitive and specific approach to the detection of enterotoxigenic *E. coli;* however, reagents for this purpose are as yet not commercially available.

To examine stool for the more conventional pathogenic bacteria, the laboratory should receive a freshly passed stool or freshly collected rectal swab. It may be helpful in distinguishing between diarrhea due to invasive and toxigenic bacteria to examine a fleck of mucus or stool mixed with Loeffler methylene blue stain for the presence of leukocytes.[28] The specimen should then be inoculated onto blood agar, a gram-negative differential medium (EMB or MacConkey agar), a selective medium for *Salmonella* and *Shigella* (xylose-lysine-deoxycholate [XLD] or Hektoen enteric [HE] agar), and enrichment broth (gram-negative [GN] or selenite), and selective media for *C. jejuni* and, when specifically requested, *Y. enterocolitica*. Should infection with vibrios be suspected on the basis of recent travel in an endemic area (*V. cholerae*) or recent ingestion of raw seafood or shellfish (*Vibrio parahaemolyticus*), the laboratory should be so notified so that thiosulfate-citrate-bile salts (TCBS) agar can also be inoculated. *Bacillus cereus* food poisoning has been only infrequently recognized in the United States but becomes manifested either by upper gastrointestinal tract symptoms, similar to those seen in staphylococcal food poisoning, or by lower intestinal tract symptoms, similar to those seen in clostridial food poisoning. Diagnosis of the former syndrome can only be established by the isolation of large numbers of *B. cereus* in incriminated food; however, diagnosis of the latter syndrome is limited to isolation of the organism from stool and determining whether it is enterotoxigenic.

In suspected parasitic infections, loose watery stools should be promptly submitted to the laboratory since protozoan trophozoites may degenerate rapidly, especially at room or incubation temperatures. If the stools are formed, it is preferable to obtain a saline-purged stool on each of 3 consecutive days after having the patient ingest 15 ml of magnesium sulfate (Epsom salt) early in the day. Specimens that are mailed or in which delivery is delayed should be placed in 10% formalin or polyvinyl alcohol (PVA) fixative in a small, plastic, screw-capped container. For brief periods of storage ($\leq$2 hours), refrigeration is advisable. A negative report based on examination of a single specimen is unreliable. Specimens are examined grossly for the presence of proglottids or adult worms and for areas of blood or mucus that should be examined microscopically in direct and concentrated wet mounts and in permanently stained smears. Concentration procedures by formalin-ether sedimentation or zinc sulfate flotation techniques increase the likelihood of detection of protozoan cysts and helminthic eggs and larvae. Trichrome and iron hematoxylin are commonly used for preparing permanent stains.

Norwalk-like agents are important causes of epidemic gastroenteritis but require special immune electron microscopy or radioimmunoassay techniques for their detection (see Chapter 14). Rotavirus causes a syndrome characterized by diarrhea, fever, and vomiting but may also be shed asymptomatically; thus, detection of rotavirus in feces may have little utility in distinguishing between those who are infected (as evidenced by antibody titer rise) and those who are carriers.[29,30] Nonetheless, detection of rotavirus has epidemiologic utility since viral shedding is the major means of transmission of the virus. The major diagnostic tests available commercially for detection of rotavirus in feces are enzyme immunoassay and latex agglutination. Latex agglutination is comparable to enzyme immunoassay in the acute phase of rotaviral infection since large amounts of antigen are excreted during the first days of illness; however, latex agglutination has less sensitivity than does enzyme immunoassay later in the course of disease or in the detection of asymptomatic carriers.[31]

Despite the many advances that have been made in determining the etiology of diarrheal disease, the diagnostic capabilities of the clinical laboratory remain limited to cultures for *Salmonella, Shigella, Campylobacter, Yersinia,* and *Vibrio;* examination for ova and parasites; and detection of *C. difficile* toxin and rotavirus antigen. Detection of enterotoxigenic, enteroinvasive, enterohemorrhagic, and enteropathogenic strains of *E. coli,* Norwalk-like agents, caliciviruses, astroviruses, and adenoviruses await further technologic developments.

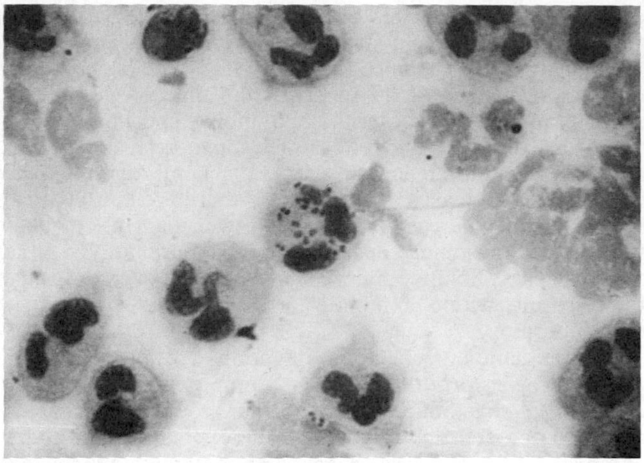

FIG. 4. Intracellular diplococci in a smear of urethral exudate from a male with gonorrhea. (Gram stain, ×1000) (From Washington,[33] with permission.)

Genital Infections

Changing social mores, AIDS, and other poorly definable factors have resulted in significant increases in the incidence of sexually transmitted diseases. At the same time, technical developments in the isolation of anaerobic bacteria and *Chlamydia* have increased our understanding of the cause of these diseases. The laboratory must therefore be prepared to handle a variety of specimens and process them appropriately according to the disease suspected clinically.

Syphilis. Although usually diagnosed serologically, syphilis can in its primary and secondary stages be diagnosed by darkfield or direct fluorescent antibody microscopic examination of serous exudate from infectious lesions. Lesions should be abraded with a dry sponge to provoke exudation; however, it is important to minimize bleeding since the presence of red cells will make the examination more difficult. The exudate is applied directly to a clean coverslip that is inverted on a glass slide. The edges of the coverslip can be sealed to minimize evaporation since *Treponema pallidum* is very sensitive to desiccation. The slide should, at any rate, be examined as soon as possible. Spirochetes of *T. pallidum* are motile, 6–15 μm in length, and have 5–20 rigid and regular spirals. Because of the normal presence of nonpathogenic treponemes in the mouth, darkfield microscopic examinations of material from this source should not be performed.

Serologic tests for syphilis are divided into nontreponemal tests, including the Venereal Disease Research Laboratory (VDRL) test, and treponemal tests, including the fluorescent treponemal antibody absorption (FTA-ABS) test and microhemagglutination tests such as MHA-TP. The sensitivity of the VDRL test is high in secondary syphilis and early latent syphilis and less sensitive in primary syphilis. Its specificity is high (99.5–100 percent) in healthy persons but reduced (75–85 percent) in sick persons.[32] The VDRL test is the preferred test for screening asymptomatic persons and, when positive, should be confirmed by a hemagglutination test. The VDRL should then be followed at 3, 6, and 12 months to determine the adequacy of treatment.[32] Although the CSF-VDRL test is a highly specific indicator of neurosyphilis, it is positive in only 22–69 percent of patients with active neurosyphilis.[32] Because of its lack of specificity, the CSF-FTA-ABS is not recommended for use in this country.[32]

Gonorrhea. The diagnosis of gonorrhea in men can be established presumptively by the findings of gram-negative intracellular diplococci in stained smears of urethral discharge (Fig. 4). Gram-stained smears of cervical drainage lack sensitivity and specificity,[34] and it is probably advisable for laboratories other than those in sexually transmitted disease clinics not to make them at all. Nonpathogenic neisseriae, anaerobic cocci, overdecolorized gram-positive cocci, and short forms of gram-negative bacilli that may normally be found in the vagina and may appear to be within or adherent to leukocytes render interpretation of Gram-stained smears of this area especially difficult and are subject to potentially serious error. To confirm the diagnosis in men and to establish it in women, it is necessary to make cultures for *N. gonorrhoeae*. The sites and types of examination recommended for various gonococcal syndromes are shown in Table 6. In the absence of a urethral discharge, which may sometimes be obtained by "milking" the urethra, material should be obtained either by inserting a thin calcium alginate swab or small-diameter, smooth bacteriologic loop into the urethra. Cervical material should be obtained by direct visualization with the aid of a speculum. In all women and in homosexual men suspected of having gonorrhea it is also recommended that the anal crypts be swabbed for culture since this may be the only site from which gonococci may be recovered. In cases of suspected gonococcal pharyngitis, the posterior portion of the pharynx and tonsillar areas should be vigorously swabbed as for any throat culture. In cases of suspected gonococcemia, blood should be inoculated into media without SPS, as has already been described (see "Septicemia").

Specimens from sites normally inhabited by fungi or other bacteria should be inoculated promptly onto selective media such as modified Thayer-Martin medium (MTM) containing vancomycin (3 μg/ml), colistin (7.5 μg/ml), and nystatin (12.5 units/ml) or, preferably, anisomycin (10 μg/ml). The addition of trimethoprim (5 μg/ml) to MTM is desirable to prevent swarming by *Proteus*. Concurrent inoculation of chocolate blood agar without antibiotics is also recommended to allow growth of vancomycin-susceptible gonococci, another cause of false-positive smears. Incubation in an atmosphere of at least 70 percent humidity and 3–7 percent carbon dioxide should be done as quickly as possible. Gonococci are sensitive to drying and wide fluctuations in temperature.

Several devices are available commercially that permit the physician to inoculate MTM directly with clinical material. The necessary carbon dioxide is either already provided in the device by its manufacturer (e.g., Transgrow) or by placing a carbon dioxide–generating effervescent tablet in a chamber at the time the MTM is inoculated (e.g., JEMBEC). Such devices may then be transported to a laboratory for examination; however, it is important that they be incubated at 35°C overnight before mailing, and failure to do so will significantly decrease recovery of *N. gonorrhoeae*.

An enzyme immunoassay (EIA) for the detection of gonococcal antigen is commercially available and has been found to

TABLE 6. Recommended Specimens for Laboratory Evaluation of Specific Sexually Transmitted Disease Syndromes

	Urethral		*Cervical*		*First-Voided Urine*		*Rectal*	*Pharyngeal*	*Orogastric Aspirate*		*Serous or Synovial Exudate*		*Abscess Pus*		*Conjunctival*		*Biopsy*		*Blood Culture*
Syndrome	*S*	*C*	*S*	*C*	*S*	*C*	*C*	*C*	*S*	*C*	*S*	*C*	*S*	*C*	*S*	*C*	*S*	*C*	*C*
Men																			
Acute urethritis	R	±			±	±													
Chronic urethritis	R	R			±	±													
Suspected gonorrhea in homosexuals without urethritis	±	R					R	R											
Women																			
Acute symptomatic GU gonorrhea	±	R	R	R	±	±	R	±											
Asymptomatic suspected GU gonorrhea (e.g., contact)	—	±	—	R	±	±	R	±											
Bartholin's abscess	±	R	±	R			±						R[a]	R[a]					
Pelvic inflammatory disease	R	R	R	R			R				R[a]	R[a]					R[a]	R[a]	
Both sexes																			
Pharyngitis	R	R	R	R				R											
Suspected neonatal sepsis							±		R	R									R
Neonatal conjunctivitis															R	R			
Disseminated gonococcal infection	R	R	R	R							R[a]	R[a]	R[a]	R[a]			R[a]	R[a]	R
Men																			
Heterosexual	—	R																	
Homosexual	—	R					R												
Women	—	±	—	R															

Abbreviations: S: Gram-stained smear; R: routine examinations; C: culture; ±: optional examinations; GU: genitourinary.
[a] If sites are believed to be infected
(From Kellogg et al.,[34] with permission.)

be as sensitive as Gram-stained smears of male urethral specimens and more sensitive than are Gram-stained smears of cervical specimens for the detection of *N. gonorrhoeae*. Compared with culture of endocervical specimens, the sensitivity of EIA has varied between 75 and 100 percent, whereas specificity has varied between 95 and 99 percent. False-positives in endocervical specimens have been troublesome and appear to be due to cross-reactive gram-negative bacteria. Whether EIA can serve as a culture substitute depends upon multiple factors, including the prevalence of gonorrhea in the population being examined, the incidence of antibiotic resistance of isolates from cultures, laboratory resources, turnaround time, and cost. A small false-positive rate may be acceptable in a high-prevalence population seen in a sexually transmitted disease clinic but may be unacceptable in a low-prevalence private practice setting. The turnaround time of the EIA is 4 hours but may be considerably longer if tests are batched to reduce the per-test cost. Even on a batched basis, however, cost of the EIA exceeds that of Gram-stained smear and culture. Finally, if screening for *N. gonorrhoeae* is by EIA only, this obviously precludes determining β-lactamase activity or the susceptibility of gonococci to other antimicrobial agents.

Chlamydia. Infection due to *Chlamydia trachomatis* is most accurately detected by culture (see Chapter 14). Specimens should be collected by rubbing a swab vigorously over the suspected site of infection. In collecting specimens from the cervix it is especially important to remove excess discharge and to rub the swab vigorously along the walls of the endocervical canal. Failure to do so will substantially reduce the detection of *C. trachomatis,* especially when sought in smears stained with the fluorescent antibody technique. Specimens that cannot be cultured immediately should be stored in sucrose-phosphate (2 SP) transport medium at 5°C for up to 72 hours or at −70°C if for longer than 72 hours.[35] Cultures are made by inoculating with centrifugation aliquots of 2 SP onto cycloheximide-treated McCoy cells, incubating for 48 to 72 hours, and then staining the cells with the fluorescent antibody technique or iodine to detect inclusions.[35]

Tests for detecting chlamydial antigen in specimens include enzyme immunoassay (EIA) and direct fluorescent antibody staining (DFA). Although their specificities are generally ≥95 percent, their sensitivities vary from nearly 70 to 100 percent,[36,37] depending upon the quality of the specimen and the skill of the person performing the DFA. EIA is easier to perform than DFA is, but the DFA provides the faster turnaround time and is less expensive to perform than is EIA, regardless of batching. Although culture is less expensive than either antigen detection test, many laboratories do not have tissue culture capabilities. Since the specificity of antigen tests is not 100 percent, only a culture performed in a competent laboratory should be used in evaluating chlamydial infection in sexually abused children.[38]

Mycoplasma. The role of the genital mycoplasmas in producting urethritis and pelvic inflammatory disease remains unclear, although there are circumstantial data implicating *Ureaplasma urealyticum* (T-strain mycoplasmas) in nongonococcal urethritis. Swabs transported in 2 SP are suitable for culture of genital mycoplasmas; however, the results of cultures should be interpreted cautiously because of the frequency of isolation of mycoplasmas from genital sources.

Gardnerella vaginalis. The role of *Gardnerella vaginalis* in causing bacterial vaginosis remains uncertain since it is found in the vaginal flora of many asymptomatic women and since the entity of bacterial vaginosis appears to be associated with the isolation of *G. vaginalis,* anaerobic curved rods, and anaerobic gram-negative bacilli. Amsel et al.[39] have proposed three of the four following criteria adequate for a diagnosis of bacterial vaginosis: (*1*) vaginal pH greater than 4.5; (*2*) thin, homogeneous, milklike discharge; (*3*) release of fishy amine odor on addition of a drop of KOH (10% solution) to a drop of vaginal discharge; and/or (*4*) the presence microscopically of clue cells in a saline wet mount of the vaginal discharge. Culture is not currently recommended for diagnostic purposes.

Pelvic Inflammatory Disease. The cause of pelvic inflammatory disease is difficult to determine and varies according to the population of patients studied, the types of specimens examined, and the investigator bias as to the types of microorganisms being studied. Pelvic inflammatory disease may be classified as gonococcal and nongonococcal or as sexually transmitted and nonsexually transmitted.[40] The major causes of the sexually transmitted disease are *Neisseria gonorrhoeae* and *Chlamydia trachomatis*. The possible roles of *Mycoplasma hominis* and *Ureaplasma urealyticum* remain controversial.[40] The major causes of nonsexually transmitted pelvic inflammatory disease are aerobic and anaerobic bacteria, often in mixed culture.[40] Diagnosis of gonococcal disease is facilitated by the isolation of *N. gonorrhoeae* from the endocervix, while the preferred method of diagnosis of disease due to aerobic and anaerobic bacteria is by aspiration with a needle and syringe or surgical incision and drainage or excision.[18] Anaerobic cultures should be routinely performed with such specimens as well as with material obtained by culdocentesis. Cultures of material aspirated from the uterine cavity should be limited to those obtained with a double-lumen, distally occluded catheter, which will minimize contamination of the specimen by normal vaginal and cervical flora.

Both *Chlamydia trachomatis* and genital tract mycoplasmas have been implicated as causes of acute salpingitis after their recovery from material obtained by laparoscopy.[41] Cultures of endocervical or tubal material for *C. trachomatis* are therefore of value in elucidating the cause of salpingitis. The interpretation of endocervical cultures yielding mycoplasmas, however, remains problematic because of the frequency of isolation of this group of organisms from asymptomatic women.

Ocular Infections

The difficulties of determining the cause of conjunctivitis on the basis of Gram-stained smears and bacteriologic cultures have been emphasized by Leibowitz et al.[42] who found a poor correlation between the initial clinical impression and the results of microbiologic studies and between the findings in Gram-stained smears and in cultures. Although bacteriologic studies of conjunctivitis are useful primarily in gonococcal conjunctivitis, microbiologic studies for chlamydiae and viruses (e.g., adenovirus, herpesvirus) are often warranted. Although Giemsa stains demonstrate chlamydiae in a very high percentage of neonates with inclusion blennorrhea, they are considerably less sensitive than are tissue culture in detecting chlamydiae in adults with follicular conjunctivitis due to *C. trachomatis*. Direct fluorescent antibody-stained smears are highly sensitive in either case.

Corneal ulcers require careful laboratory studies as described elsewhere by Jones et al.[43] and by François and Rysselaere.[44] The microbiologist should ensure that the following materials are available to the ophthalmologist for these studies: sterile swabs, spatula, clean glass microscopic slides and coverslips, proparacaine hydrochloride (Ophthaine, 0.5%), alcohol lamp, and media suitable for cultivation of bacteria, mycobacteria, and fungi. The swabs are used for obtaining conjunctival and lid cultures. Corneal scrapings are taken with the aid of a slit lamp and are spread gently over a small area of each slide and medium to be examined. Multiple areas of the ulcer should be sampled. One slide each should be stained by the Gram and Giemsa methods. Scrapings on a third slide are examined under a coverslip in a potassium hydroxide preparation. If indicated, the remaining slides may be stained with a fluorochrome or carbol fuchsin technique for mycobacteria and by a silver impregnation method for fungi.

Intraocular infections, including those related to surgery, may be due to a variety of microorganisms. Material obtained by ocular paracentesis requires scrupulous attention with appropriate smears and cultures for bacteria (including anaerobic), mycobacteria, fungi, and viruses.

IDENTIFICATION OF ORGANISMS

The laboratory can provide preliminary or definitive identification of etiologic agents based on: (*1*) microscopic examination of specimens, of growth occurring in cultures of those specimens, or of indirect evidence of growth in tissue culture (e.g., cytopathic effects); (*2*) immunologic techniques that detect microbial antigens or antibodies in body fluids or in cultures of those fluids; (*3*) DNA probes to detect microorganisms or genetically encoded characteristics of microorganisms in specimens or cultures; and (*4*) growth or biochemical characteristics of organisms isolated in cultures.

Microscopy

Unstained. Wet mount preparations of specimens can be examined with an ordinary light microscope for evidence of fungi or parasites. The substage condenser should be raised and lowered during examination to achieve optimal illumination and contrast. Practical applications include direct examination for fungi or sputum and other body fluids, transtracheal and bronchial aspirates, skin and hair scrapings, and urinary sediments mixed with 10% potassium hydroxide on a clean glass microscopic slide. A coverslip is placed over the mixture, and the slide is gently heated by passing it through a flame. Wet mounts are also used for examining fecal material for the presence of protozoan trophozoites and helminth larvae. Contrast can be increased in examining cerebrospinal fluid for cryptococci by mixing centrifuged sediment with India ink. Contrast can also be enhanced with phase microscopy (Figs. 2 and 3) or with darkfield microscopy, the latter being the procedure of choice for the detection of spirochetes in skin lesions in early cases of syphilis or in the cerebrospinal fluid or urine in early cases of leptospirosis.

Wet mounts of urinary sediment, with or without methylene blue, will provide reliable evidence of the presence of significant bacteriuria when at least 20 bacteria per high dry objective field (×430) are seen. Capsular swelling (quellung reaction) of pneumococci occurs in wet mounts of cerebrospinal fluid or sputum when polyvalent or type-specific antibody is added to the specimen.

In each of these cases microscopy can provide rapid and definitive identification of an etiologic agent in a specimen, assuming, of course, that organisms display typical morphologic characteristics. All these procedures are limited by the occurrence of small or rare numbers of organisms in the specimen, by the findings of artifacts that may resemble organisms, and by the presence of atypical forms of organisms that are not readily identifiable. Training and experience are required to prevent over- or underinterpretation of findings.

Stained. Innumerable stains have been described for the examination of specimens or organisms. Only those in frequent use will be described here, and the interested reader is referred to standard references for details about reagents and procedures for other stains.

ACID-FAST STAINS

A. Kinyoun carbol fuchsin

Reagents

1. Carbol fuchsin

Basic fuchsin	4 g
Phenol, melted	8 ml
Ethyl alcohol, 95%	20 ml
Distilled water	68 ml

Mix the phenol and alcohol in 50 ml of water in a flask or bottle; add the dye, shake, and allow to stand overnight at room temperature. Add the rest of the water, and filter through coarse paper. Store in the bottle.

2. Decolorizer*

HCl, concentrated	12 ml
Ethyl alcohol, 95%	388 ml

3. Counterstain

Methylene blue	4 g
Water	400 ml

Procedure

1. Air-dry the smears on new, clean glass microscope slides, and heat fix by passing through a flame.
2. Cover the slides with strips of coarse filter paper and flood with carbol fuchsin for 5 minutes.
3. Remove the filter paper and rinse the slide with tap water.
4. Decolorize until thick portions of the smear are clear.
5. Rinse the slide with tap water.
6. Flood the slide with counterstain for 1 minute.
7. Rinse the slide with tap water, drain, and blot dry.

B. Auramine-rhodamine (fluorochrome)

Reagents

1. Auramine-rhodamine

Auramine O (C.I. 41000)	1.5 g
Rhodamine B (C.I. 45170)	0.75 g
Glycerol	75 ml
Phenol, melted	10 ml
Distilled water	50 ml

Dissolve the phenol in water, add dyes, and mix. Add glycerol in 25 ml water and mix with a magnetic stirrer or shake periodically for several hours. Filter through glass wool. Store in the bottle.

2. Decolorizer*

HCl, concentrated	2.5 ml
Ethyl alcohol, 70%	500 ml

3. Counterstain

Potassium permanganate	5 g
Distilled water	1000 ml

* One percent sulfuric acid is used as a decolorizer for acid-fast stains of *Nocardia*.

Procedure

1. Air-dry the smears on new, clean glass microscope slide and heat-fix by passing through a flame.
2. Flood the slide with auramine-rhodamine for 15 minutes.
3. Rinse the slide with distilled water.
4. Flood the slide with decolorizer for 2 minutes.
5. Rinse the slide with distilled water.
6. Flood the slide with counterstain for 2 minutes.
7. Rinse the slide with tap water, drain, and blot dry.

The sensitivity and specificity of the carbol fuchsin and fluorochrome stains are approximately equal. However, because carbol fuchsin stains must be examined with the ×100 oil immersion objective and fluorochrome stains are examined with a ×25 objective, the latter is a far more rapid and efficient method of screening smears. Moreover, the fluorochrome stain may be more sensitive in some observer's hands because of the greater contrast it provides.

GIEMSA STAIN FOR MALARIA AND OTHER ORGANISMS

Reagents

1. Stock Giemsa stain solution (commercially available)
2. Methyl alcohol, absolute
3. Phosphate buffer, M/15, pH 7.0

Working solution is prepared by mixing 15 ml of stock solution in 35 ml phosphate buffer. Filter if necessary.

Procedure

1. Puncture the skin with a sterile, disposable lancet.
2. Apply a drop of blood to surface of a clean (with alcohol or acetone) glass microscope slide.
3. Stir the drop of blood vigorously in a circular motion with the corner of another glass slide so as to cover a surface approximately 1.5 cm in diameter. A proper thick film should be thin enough for newsprint to be read through it.
4. Prepare a thin film as for a conventional hematologic smear.
5. Allow the films to dry gently.
6. Fix the thin film with methyl alcohol (3 minutes). Do not fix the thick film, and if both films are on the same slide, protect the thick film from the alcohol or its fumes.
7. Place the slides into a Coplin jar containing working Giemsa solution for a minimum of 30 minutes.
8. Remove the slides, and rinse in phosphate buffer.
9. Drain the slides, and allow to air-dry.
10. Examine with low power (×100) for microfilariae and with high power (×430) and oil immersion (×1000) for blood and tissue protozoa.

Smears should be prepared whenever malaria is suspected; however, the optimal time is midway between attacks, and the least favorable time is during or immediately after an episode of fever. Care must be taken to differentiate malaria forms from normal blood components (e.g., platelets).

GRAM STAIN

Reagents

1. Crystal violet solution

Crystal violet, 90% dye content	10 g
Methyl alcohol, absolute	500 ml

2. Iodine solution

Iodine crystals	6 g
Potassium iodide	12 g
Distilled water	1800 ml

3. Decolorizer†

Acetone	400 ml
Ethyl alcohol, 95%	1200 ml

4. Counterstain

Safranin, 99% dye content	10 g
Distilled water	1000 ml

Procedure

1. Air-dry smears of clean glass microscope slides and heat-fix by passing through a flame.
2. Flood the slide with crystal violet solution for at least 10 seconds.
3. Rinse the slide with tap water.
4. Flood the slide with iodine solution for at least 10 seconds.
5. Rinse the slide with tap water.
6. Decolorize until no more blue color comes off thin portions of the smear, and rinse immediately with tap water.
7. Flood the slide with counterstain for 10 seconds.
8. Rinse the slide with tap water, drain, and blot dry.

This stain should be used routinely by the bacteriology laboratory in examining material from normally sterile body fluids, abscesses, wounds, sputum, and tissue. The finding of at least two bacteria per oil immersion field (×1000) in well-mixed properly collected and stored urine represents significant bacteriuria (≥70,000 cfu/ml). Although the finding of gram-positive or gram-negative bacteria is not specific, it is often possible to surmise on the basis of the patient's clinical presentation and source of the material examined what the organisms seen in the smear are likely to be. Those inexperienced with the Gram stain technique are most apt to have difficulty with the decolorization step and to over- or underdecolorize. Artifacts such as deposited crystal violet may be misinterpreted as being cocci or bacilli.

PNEUMOCYSTIS CARINII STAIN

A. Toluidine blue[13,45]

Reagents

1. Sulfation reagent

Glacial acetic acid	45 ml
Sulfuric acid, concentrated	15 ml

Pour glacial acetic acid into a Coplin jar that has been placed in a plastic tub containing cool tap water (≥10°C). Add 15 ml concentrated sulfuric acid slowly and mix with a glass rod. Seal the jar with petroleum jelly, and store at room temperature. The reagent should be replaced after 1 week's use.

2. Toluidine blue

Toluidine blue 0	0.3 g
Hydrochloric acid	2 ml
Ethyl alcohol	140 ml
Distilled water	60 ml

Mix the dye in water, and then add acid and finally alcohol. Store at room temperature. The reagent should be replaced after 1 year's use.

Procedure

1. Air-dry the smear and touch preparations on clean glass microscope slides for 30 minutes.
2. Place the slides in sulfation reagent for 10 minutes.
3. Rinse the slides gently with tap water for 5 minutes.
4. Stain the slides in toluidine blue for 3 minutes.
5. Decolorize by dipping once into 95% ethyl alcohol and once into absolute alcohol, each for approximately 10 seconds.
6. Dip in and out of Xyless (Columbia Diagnostics, Inc., Springfield, VA) twice each for approximately 10 seconds, and allow to evaporate.
7. Mount in a suitable mounting medium (e.g., Permount) with a coverslip.

Pneumocystis carinii cysts stain lavender. In contrast with yeasts, which also are stained by toluidine blue, cysts of *P. carinii* do not bud. Nevertheless, a diagnosis of *P. carinii* infection should not be made when specimens contain yeast cells unless at least one cluster of *P. carinii* cysts in seen.[12]

Other stains for *P. carinii* include Giemsa, which demonstrates the internal contents of the cyst and the trophozoite forms but which requires considerable experience on the part of the microscopist for accurate interpretation, and the Gomori methenamine silver (GMS), which provides the most reliable detection of cysts in touch preparations and tissue section. Although GMS staining is usually performed in histopathology laboratories, a simple and reliable rapid method is available that can be readily performed in the clinical laboratory.[46]

TISSUE SECTION STAINS. Hematoxylin and eosin (H&E) is a useful stain for screening tissue to determine whether a lesion is malignant or inflammatory and, if so, whether it is granulomatous or suppurative. Bacteria may be stained by various modifications of the Brown and Brenn Gram stain as well as by the Dieterle stain. The fluorochrome procedure can be used to examine tissue homogenate for mycobacteria; however, the sensitivity of this procedure is less than 50 percent as compared with culture of tissue from non-AIDS patients. Gomori methenamine silver stain is used to detect and characterize actinomycetes, fungi, and *Pneumocystis carinii*. Direct fluorescent antibody stain is the most specific method for detecting *Legionella pneumophila* in tissue sections.

INTESTINAL PARASITE STAINS. Wet preparations can be made by mixing a small quantity of feces on a glass microscope slide with a drop or two of freshly mixed 0.1% eosin in saline. A coverslip is placed over the mixture, which is then examined under low power (×100). The eosin is nontoxic for protozoa and worms and provides a contrasting reddish background for the normally pale green parasites. Concentration procedures are recommended to enhance the detection of cysts, eggs, and larvae. The zinc sulfate centrifugal flotation and the acid–ether centrifugal sedimentation methods are those most widely used in the United States. There are also a variety of permanent staining techniques, of which Heidenhain's iron hematoxylin and the Wheatley trichrome stains are widely used. Concentration methods and stains are described in detail in a number of standard references in parasitology. Care must be exercised in the examination of smears to avoid over- and underinterpretation. Unless skilled examiners are available, it is strongly recommended that the specimen be mixed in 10% formalin or polyvinyl alcohol (PVA) fixative for shipment to a reference laboratory. Laboratories engaging in parasitologic work should have photographs and other illustrated material available. (An excellent three-volume *Atlas of Diagnostic Medical Parasitology* may be obtained from the American Society of Clinical Pathologists.)

Care should be taken not to examine specimens from patients who have had recent cleansing or barium enemas, antidiarrheal compounds, antiparasitic medications, laxatives, or antibiotics. These compounds or procedures will either interfere with the visualization of parasites in stool or cause their disappearance at the time stool is collected for examination.

† Ninety-five percent alcohol may be used instead of acetone-alcohol to reduce the risk of overdecolorization.

LOEFFLER'S METHYLENE BLUE STAIN

Reagents

Methylene blue, certified	0.3 g
Potassium hydroxide, 10% solution	0.1 ml
Ethyl alcohol, 95%	30 ml
Distilled water	100 ml

Dissolve methylene blue with alcohol with a mortar and pestle and transfer to a flask. Add potassium hydroxide to water, wash the mortar, and pour the washings with the remainder of the water into the flask. Filter the mixture through paper 24 hours later.

Procedure

A small fleck of mucus or liquid stool is placed on a clean glass microscope slide and mixed thoroughly with the stain. A coverslip is applied, and after 2 or 3 minutes, the slide is examined under high power (×430) for leukocytes.[28]

Immunoassays and DNA Probe Hybridization Techniques

New technologies that provide rapid detection or identification of specified microorganisms or specific characteristics of microorganisms (e.g., *E. coli* enterotoxins) are exciting developments that are likely to substantially alter the practice of medical microbiology. As new immunoassays and DNA probes are developed, however, certain critical issues need to be addressed before these technologies can be implemented in the clinical laboratory. These issues include the sensitivity, specificity, predictive values, and confidence intervals of the new test in relation to an accepted reference method. The confidence interval allows one to assess the relative precision of the different point estimates provided by an investigator evaluating the test or the manufacturer selling the product.[47] With the appropriate statistical data, it is then possible to assess the clinical value of the test and to decide whether to implement the test in the laboratory. It is important to determine whether the test will be used for screening purposes or for confirming or ruling out a diagnosis. In the former instance a sensitive test is desirable, while in the latter instance a specific test is desirable. A highly sensitive test should be used when knowledge of the disease present is highly important in the management of the patient, while a highly specific test should be used if no confirmatory test is available or there would be serious adverse consequences from a false-positive result. These issues must be addressed whether the test is used to detect a particular microorganism that is either difficult or easy to culture and when there is any question about whether an immunoassay or DNA probe might serve as a culture substitute. For example, DNA probes for *E. coli* enterotoxins appear to be highly specific and to be as, if not more, sensitive than are traditional methods involving culture isolation of colonies of *E. coli* that are then tested for toxinogenicity in either tissue culture or animals. DNA hybridization allows the processing of a large number of specimens on a batch basis in a much shorter period of time than do traditional methods; therefore, a DNA probe for *E. coli* enterotoxin has the attributes of high sensitivity, high specificity, and cost-effectiveness required for its implementation in laboratories investigating diarrheal disease. In contrast, the commercially available *Legionella* probe, although highly specific, has a sensitivity of 60–80 percent and can therefore only be used as a screening test, with culture and/or serology serving as confirmatory tests. Thus, the *Legionella* probe must be compared with the *Legionella* direct immunofluorescent antibody (DFA) test for screening purposes. The sensitivity of both tests is 60–80 percent, while the specificities of the probe and the monoclonal DFA for *L. pneumophila* are >99 percent (specificity of the polyclonal DFA may be ≥97 percent).[48] Since the procedure for the probe requires less technical expertise than that for DFA, the probe may be the preferred screening test, provided the batch size allows for complete utilization of the test kit and the frequency of testing allows for complete utilization of the radiolabeled reagents within the product's short shelf life. If neither of these conditions is met, the per-test cost of the probe is substantially higher than for DFA. In other words, DFA is the most cost-effective procedure for the laboratory processing an average of two to four specimens a day, provided the technical expertise in immunofluorescence microscopy is available in the laboratory. The same considerations arise when comparing DFA and enzyme immunoassay to screen for *Chlamydia trachomatis*.

Replacement of isotopically labeled probes with nonisotopically labeled probes should eventually reduce equipment and reagent expense. Ultimately, however, the use of probes and immunoassays as culture substitutes will depend on improved sensitivity and specificity, simplification of specimen processing, and automation of procedures. As long as these techniques remain culture supplements (vs. substitutes), they represent added costs that may be difficult to implement unless a clear-cut clinical benefit can be demonstrated from their use.

Other Immunologic Techniques

Direct Immunofluorescence. Direct immunofluorescence technique involves the attachment of antigen or antibody labeled with fluorescein isothiocyanate (FITC) to its antibody or antigen, respectively, and detection of the labeled product with fluorescence microscopy. Practical applications of direct staining include the identification of *S. pyogenes* (group A) in throat swabs or cultures; *B. pertussis* in nasopharyngeal swabs, aspirates, or cultures; *H. influenzae, L. monocytogenes, N. meningitidis, S. agalactiae* (group B), and *S. pneumoniae* in cerebrospinal fluid; *T. pallidum* in lesions of early syphilis; *Brucella, Francisella tularensis,* and *Yersinia pestis* in clinical specimens; *Legionella* in lung tissue; colonies of *N. gonorrhoeae* in cultures of genital sources; and *C. trachomatis* in ocular, nasopharyngeal, and genital specimens.

Direct immunofluorescence is a rapid and sensitive method of staining organisms in specimens or cultures. Fluorescent antibody procedures for screening clinical material and cultures for fungi have been described by Kaufman and Reiss at the Centers for Disease Control[49]; however, labeled reagents are not yet available from commercial sources. The accuracy of immunofluorescence depends on many factors, including technical expertise, properly functioning equipment, the sensitivity of the reagents and their specificity, and the source of the specimen being examined. Immunofluorescence is not necessarily a substitute for culture since it does not yield a viable organism for antimicrobial susceptibility testing or other specific studies. Nonetheless, it can provide rapid detection and often at least presumptive identification of many microorganisms, and it has become an indispensable tool for many laboratories.

Reagents for some specific antigen–antibody reactions are only available in larger nongovernmental reference laboratories and in state or federal public health facilities. Specimens or cultures that are mailed to such laboratories must be shipped in accordance with federal packaging requirements.[1]

Agglutination. Agglutination tests to identify etiologic agents in specimens are limited in number. The most important one in use today is the latex agglutination test for *Cryptococcus neoformans* antigen in cerebrospinal fluid and serum. The sensitivity of this test exceeds that of the India ink preparation for examination of cerebrospinal fluid. Specificity of the cryptococcal latex agglutination test may be reduced by the presence of rheumatoid factor or other interfering proteins; however, treatment of the specimen with a protease (pronase) will eliminate false-positive results due to interfering proteins.[49a]

As discussed earlier, latex and coagglutination may be useful in the diagnosis of bacterial meningitis of partially treated children or in those children in whom the inflammatory response and various biochemical indices in the cerebrospinal fluid do not clearly distinguish between bacterial and viral meningitis.

Latex agglutination, coagglutination, the quellung reaction and counterimmunoelectrophoresis have been used to detect pneumococcal antigen in sputum from patients with suspected pneumococcal pneumonia. The sensitivity of each of these tests relative to documented pneumococcal pneumonia is approximately 80 percent and is therefore higher than that of a Gram-stained smear (approximately 50 percent) in which a positive result is defined by a predominance of lancet-shaped diplococci in each of several oil immersion fields (× 1000). Specificities of the antigen tests may, however, be only about 70 percent since false-positive results occur, particularly in patients with chronic bronchitis and pneumococci in their sputum. Latex agglutination tests for group A streptococci are widely available commercially. Although highly specific, these tests are only relatively sensitive, so antigen-negative tests should be backed up by cultures, particularly in areas in which there is a high prevalence of acute rheumatic fever or in which there has been a resurgence of acute rheumatic fever.

Latex agglutination has also been used to detect *Candida* antigenemia; however, differences in study populations and criteria for defining invasive candidiasis have made interpretation of published evaluations difficult. Although fairly specific, antigen tests, including a commercially available product, appear to be relatively insensitive, even if patients with candidemias unrelated to intravascular devices are included in the invasive category of disease. The transient nature of antigenemia and its detection relatively late in the course of disease appear to limit the test's utility in the differentiation between invasive and noninvasive candidiasis.[50,51]

Growth or Biochemical Characteristics

The presence of growth can usually be readily recognized by the development of colonies on solid media and colonies or turbidity in liquid media; however, the rate of growth is a function of the original inoculum size and the group of organisms involved. Most pathogenic bacteria, for example, require only a few hours to produce visible growth, whereas it may take many weeks for colonies of mycobacteria to become evident. It is important for the clinician to know what are reasonable reporting times for various kinds of cultures (Table 7). It is equally important for the laboratory to establish a system for reporting important preliminary results by telephone and in writing.

TABLE 7. Reporting Times for Various Microbiologic Procedures

Procedure	*Time*
Microscopic	
Acid-fast	4–6 hr
Gram stain	½ hr
India ink	1 hr
Toluidine blue (*Pneumocystis*)	1 hr
Direct fluorescent antibody (*Legionella, Chlamydia trachomatis*)	1 hr
Culture	
Actinomyces	10 days
Anaerobic bacteria	2–14 days
Brucella	21 days
Other bacteria	2–7 days
Leptospires	30 days
Mycobacteria	8 wk
Chlamydia	2–3 days
Mycoplasma	30 days
Fungi	4–6 wk
Viruses	2–14 days

The initial identity of an organism may be suggested by the source of the material cultured, its pattern of growth on nutrient and selective media, its colonial morphology on the various media inoculated, its hemolytic or fermentative properties, and its microscopic appearance. This process requires careful training and experience and provides information that is essential for all further procedures required to identify the organism. The experienced microbiologist can often provide a reasonably accurate preliminary identification of an organism at this point.

Bacteria. Most clinically important bacteria grow under both aerobic and anaerobic conditions and are called facultatively anaerobic. Some, such as *Pseudomonas aeruginosa,* are strict aerobes. For practical purposes, anaerobic bacteria are those that grow only in an atmosphere of reduced oxygen tension and do not grow on solid media in an atmosphere with 10% CO_2 in air.[18] The term *microaerophilic* has no standard meaning but is commonly applied to bacteria preferring an incubation atmosphere of 10% CO_2 in air to aerobic or anaerobic atmospheres of incubation. General schemes for differentiating the major groups of gram-positive and gram-negative bacteria are shown in Figures 5 and 6.

AEROBIC AND FACULTATIVELY ANAEROBIC BACTERIA. *Gram-Positive Cocci.* The gram-positive cocci usually grow satisfactorily on blood agar and are inhibited in their growth on gram-negative differential media such as EMB and MacConkey agar. Staphylococci possess catalase that produces oxygen bubbles when a drop of hydrogen peroxide (H_2O_2) is placed on a colony on a glass microscope slide or on a medium without red blood cells; streptococci are catalase-negative. Staphylococci may or may not exhibit hemolytic properties. Streptococci may display β-hemolytic (complete), α-hemolytic (partial), or nonhemolytic (called γ) properties on blood agar. This method of classifying streptococci is complicated by other schema that place them into pyogenes, viridans, and enterococcal groups based on their biologic properties and into serologic (Lancefield) groups based on group-specific carbohydrate precipitin patterns. Although many β-hemolytic strains are pyogenic and belong to a specific Lancefield group, Lancefield's group D includes β- and nonhemolytic strains. Both α- and nonhemolytic strains (other than those belonging to group D) are frequently classified as viridans streptococci.

More recent changes in streptococcal taxonomy include the reclassification of what were formerly salt-tolerant group D streptococci into the genus *Enterococcus,* including the species *E. faecalis, E. faecium,* and *E. durans,* and the reclassification, by some workers, of "*S. milleri,*" *S. intermedius, S. constellatus,* and minute or small colony-forming β-hemolytic streptococci that are nongroupable or possess the group A, C, F, or G antigens into the species *S. anginosus.* (see Chapter 182).

Most clinical laboratories perform the coagulase test directly with catalase-positive cocci resembling staphylococci and report *Staphylococcus aureus* or coagulase-negative *Staphylococcus* accordingly. Although *S. epidermidis* constitutes the predominant coagulase-negative staphylococcal species of clinical importance, *S. saprophyticus* is an important cause of the acute dysuric syndrome. Other coagulase-negative species of *Staphylococcus* are infrequently pathogenic. The novobiocin test for presumptive identification of *S. saprophyticus* can be limited to urinary isolates of coagulase-negative staphylococci from young female outpatients in the sexually active age group. Otherwise, speciation of coagulase-negative staphylococci is seldom indicated.

Bile solubility may be performed by observing lysis of colonies of streptococci when a solution of 10% deoxycholate is applied to the agar surface. Pneumococci are also inhibited by low concentrations of ethyl hydrocuprein hydrochloride or optochin. Presumptive identification of group A streptococci can be made on the basis of their inhibition by low concentrations

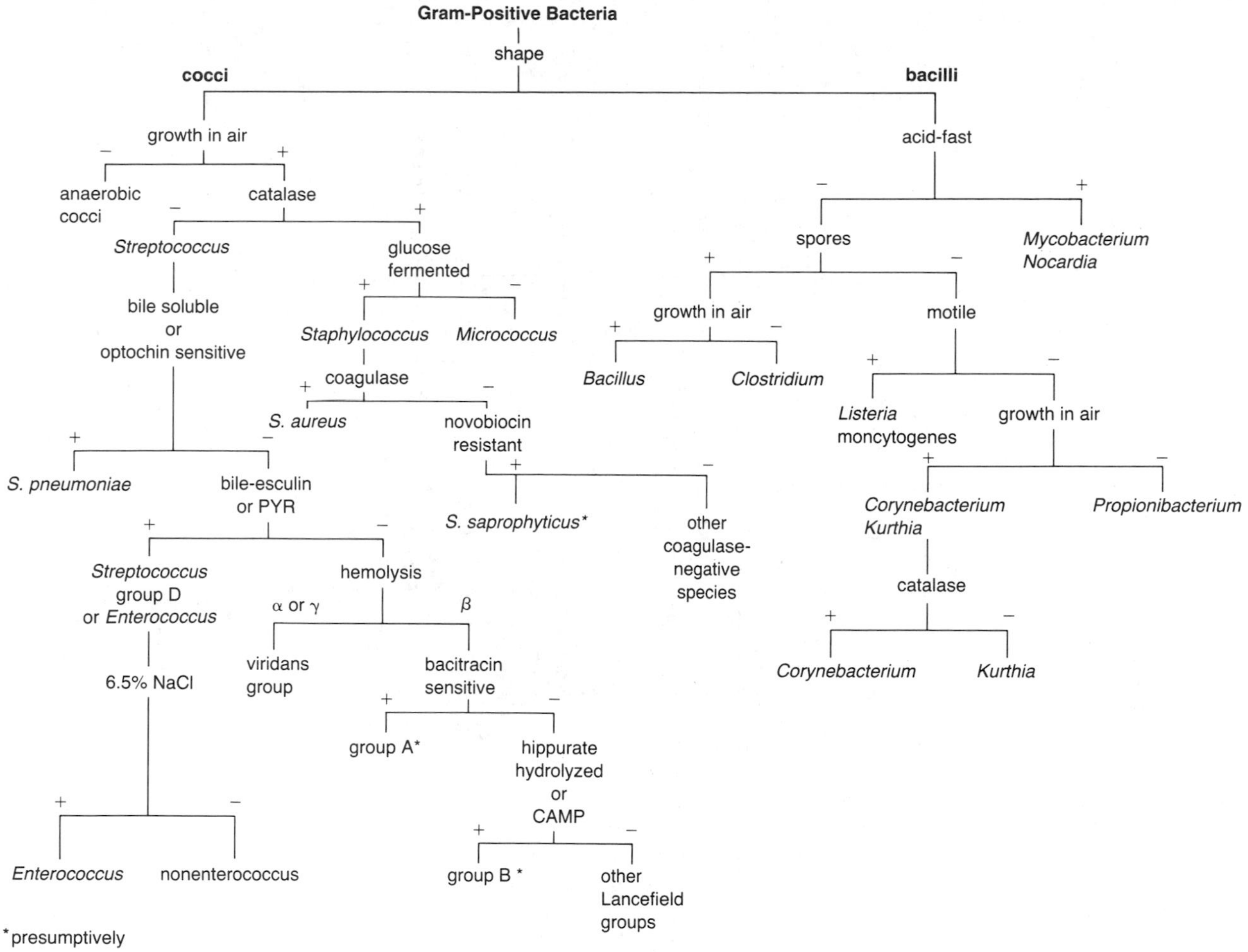

FIG. 5. Schematic outline for the identification of gram-positive bacteria. (From Washington,[15] with permission.)

of bacitracin contained in a paper disk that is applied to the surface of agar to which the organism has been subcultured. Although it is rare for a group A *Streptococcus* to be resistant to bacitracin, between 5 and 10 percent of nongroup A β-hemolytic streptococci (generally belonging to groups B, C, and G) are inhibited. Group B β-hemolytic streptococci can be identified on the basis of their ability to hydrolyze hippurate. Group D streptococci tolerate 40% bile and hydrolyze esculin; those growing in the presence of 6.5% sodium chloride or hydrolyzing L-pyrrolidonyl-β-naphthalamide (PYR) represent enterococcal species. Viridans streptococci represent a group of at least nine species, including *S. pneumoniae*. Most so-called microaerophilic strains belong to these species. In practice, however, it is sufficient to call them viridans streptococci.

Immunofluorescence, latex agglutination, or coagglutination can be used for the rapid identification of group A and group B β-hemolytic streptococci. Lancefield grouping is otherwise performed by capillary precipitin techniques. Typing of group A streptococci, based on their M proteins, may be useful for epidemiologic purposes.

Gram-Negative Cocci. Presumptive identification of the pathogenic neisseriae is based on the growth of gram-negative cocci on modified Thayer-Martin medium and a positive oxidase reaction. Definitive identification and differentiation of *N. gonorrhoeae* and *N. meningitidis* require carbohydrate utilization tests. Immunofluorescence can be used to identify colonies of *N. gonorrhoeae;* however, anti-*N. meningitidis* fluorescein-labeled conjugates tend to cross-react with *N. gonorrhoeae*. Another species, *Neisseria lactamica,* also grows on Thayer-Martin agar and closely resembles *N. meningitidis* in its carbohydrate utilization properties; however, it utilizes lactose, which *N. meningitidis* does not. *Neisseria lactamica* is rarely pathogenic. *Branhamella* (or *Moraxella*) *catarrhalis* has assumed increasing importance in otitis media and as an opportunistic lower respiratory pathogen; it frequently produces β-lactamase.

Gram-Negative Bacilli. The identification of gram-negative bacilli is complex and is based on the interpretation of numerous biochemical tests. The number of tests required for speciation of the various groups in Figure 6 depends on technical expertise, interest, economics, epidemiologic necessity, and clinical relevance. Commercially prepared devices containing multiple tests for identifying the Enterobacteriaceae have become widely used and have generally proved to be convenient and accurate. In most kits individual test results are reduced to profile or code numbers. It should be emphasized that the reproducibility of these numbers reflects the reproducibility of individual test reactions and that some of these reactions are sufficiently variable to render unreliable the use of the numbers ("biotypes") for epidemiologic purposes. Devices are also available for the identification of nonfermenters; however, the identification of these organisms remains rather complex, and the tests provided in the devices often need to be supplemented with other tests to obtain a definitive identification.

There are, in addition, gram-negative bacilli that require enriched media and, in many cases, added carbon dioxide during incubation for their growth. Included in this group are *Campylobacter, Haemophilus, Cardiobacterium, Actinobacillus, Bordetella, Brucella,* and *Francisella*.

Species of *Haemophilus* of clinical importance are *H. influ-*

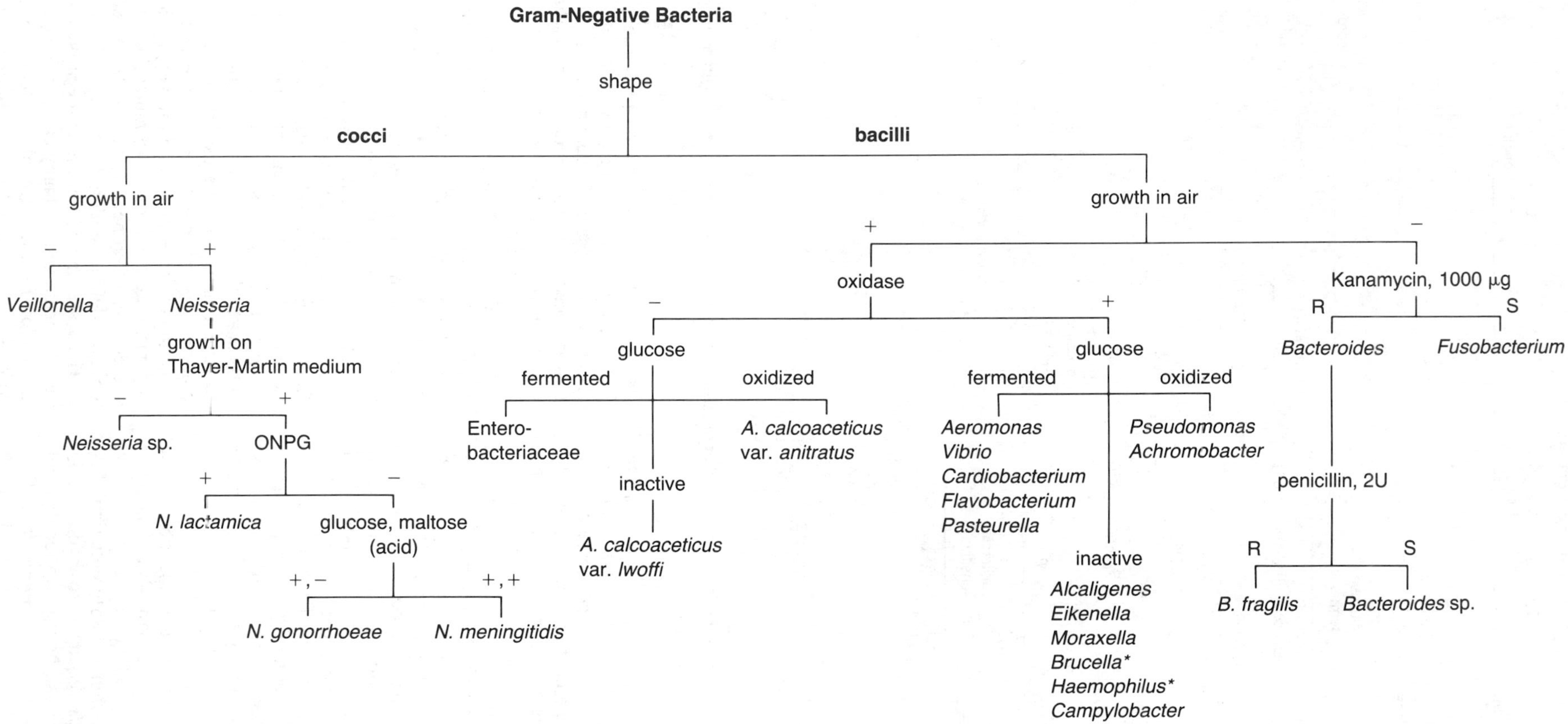

*Carbohydrate utilization not important for differentiation or speciation and can only be demonstrated in special media.

FIG. 6. Schematic outline for the identification of gram-negative bacteria. (From Washington,[17] with permission.)

enzae, H. parainfluenzae, H. aphrophilus, H. paraphrophilus, and *H. ducreyi.* Although *H. influenzae* is readily identifiable on the basis of its colonial morphology, characteristic odor, oxidase activity, requirements for hemin (X factor) and nicotinamide adenine dinucleotide (V factor), and antigenic characteristics, the other species are not and require a more complex series of tests for their differentiation. These species are being recognized increasingly, along with *Actinobacillus, Cardiobacterium,* and *Eikenella,* for their role in causing endocarditis. The identification of *Brucella* and *Francisella* can be expedited with direct immunofluorescent staining.

Gram-Positive Bacilli. Gram-positive bacilli are either sporulating or nonsporulating. The most commonly isolated nonsporulating bacilli are the corynebacteria ("diphtheroids") that normally inhabit the skin but may cause infections of implanted prosthetic material, a possibility that is strongly suggested by their repeated isolation from normally sterile fluids or sites. When isolated from blood or cerebrospinal fluid, it is important to distinguish corynebacteria, which produce catalase and are usually not motile, from another nonsporulating gram-positive bacillus, *L. monocytogenes,* which is motile at room temperature and may cause meningitis in newborn infants and in immunosuppressed hosts.

The isolation of *C. diphtheriae,* a nonsporulating rod, or *Bacillus anthracis,* a large sporulating rod, requires that the laboratory be notified so appropriate media are inoculated and toxigenicity tests performed. Otherwise, these organisms, if isolated, are apt to be discarded as contaminants.

ANAEROBIC BACTERIA. Most infections occurring in proximity to a mucosal surface, particularly those in the abdomen and the pelvis, are due to a combination of facultatively anaerobic (e.g., *E. coli* and *Enterococcus*) and anaerobic bacteria, including *Bacteroides* species, fusobacteria, anaerobic cocci, clostridia, and nonsporulating gram-positive bacilli. The presence of anaerobic bacteria is often suspected on the basis of their pleomorphism in Gram-stained smears of appropriately collected specimens and is subsequently confirmed in cultures on selective and nonselective media. Since cultures are often mixed and since definitive identification of anaerobic bacteria is time-consuming and expensive, the extent of identification provided must first reflect clinical need and then laboratory resources. When several different groups of anaerobic bacteria are present in a culture, it may be sufficient to characterize them superficially according to their Gram-stained morphology and to determine whether any anaerobic gram-negative bacilli that may be present produce β-lactamase. Although not necessarily predictive of β-lactam activity, a positive β-lactamase test (nitrocefin) finding is generally indicative of the presence of the *Bacteroides fragilis* group in the culture. In the case of perirectal lesions and sacral decubiti, it may be sufficient to report the presence of mixed fecal flora. Definitive identification may be reserved for isolates in pure culture and those from blood, brain abscesses, and other critical areas and may be carried out with one of several commercially available rapid identification kits.

Because of continuing debate about the relevance of in vitro susceptibility test results to clinical response, the variability of results provided by the different methods that are available for susceptibility testing of anaerobic bacteria, disagreement over break points for defining susceptibility, and the relatively slow turnaround time for isolating and performing susceptibility test of individual isolates of anaerobic bacteria, testing should be limited to those isolates from brain abscesses, bone and joint infections, infections of implanted prosthetic materials or devices, endocarditis, and persistent or recurrent bacteremia. Otherwise, susceptibility testing should be done to monitor susceptibility patterns on a regional or local basis and to evaluate the activity of new antimicrobial agents.

Mycobacteria. The extent to which laboratories should engage in mycobacterial isolation and identification should reflect the number of specimens received, the frequency of isolation of mycobacteria, technical expertise, availability of suitable facilities to process cultures and identify mycobacteria safely, and accessibility to suitable reference laboratories. Limits of mycobacteriologic services have been suggested by the College of American Pathologists and the American Thoracic Society. These suggested limits range from no services or services limited to acid-fast smears on site with transmittal of specimens to a reference laboratory, the isolation and identification of *M. tuberculosis,* and preliminary grouping of other species on site to isolation, identification, and drug susceptibility testing of isolates on site.

Identification of mycobacteria is based on microscopy, optimal temperature for growth, colonial morphology and pigmentation, growth in liquid medium, cord formation, niacin production, and other tests described elsewhere.[52]

The isolation after 2 or more weeks of incubation of slowly growing, nonpigmented, and rough colonies is strongly suggestive of *M. tuberculosis,* confirmation of which is obtained with a positive niacin test result. Calmette-Guérin bacillus (BCG) mutants of *M. bovis* have been isolated from patients receiving immunotherapy for cancer and are distinguishable from *M. tuberculosis* in that they are inhibited by thiophene-2-carboxylic acid hydrazide (TCH). *Mycobacterium kansasii,* which causes lesions resembling tuberculosis, grows slowly (2–3 weeks) and produces raised, rough, colorless, or buff-colored colonies that become yellow when exposed to light (photochromogenic). Similar characteristics are displayed by *M. marinum,* which, however, grows best at 30°C and is usually isolated from superficial lesions. Also photochromogenic at 25°C is *Mycobacterium szulgai,* which produces lesions resembling tuberculosis; this organism grows slowly and produces pale yellow colonies (scotochromogenic) whether exposed to light or not when incubated at 37°C. *Mycobacterium scrofulaceum* is a slowly growing (1–3 weeks) scotochromogen that is widely distributed in nature and may cause cervical adenitis in children.

Mycobacterium xenopi is a slowly growing (3–4 weeks) organism that grows best at 42°–45°C, is found in water, and has been associated with pulmonary lesions. It resembles *Mycobacterium intracellulare,* which is closely related to *M. avium,* hence the term *M. avium-intracellulare* complex ("Battey bacillus"). Although members of the *M. avium-intracellular* complex are highly resistant to most antimicrobial agents, *M. xenopi* is not.

Mycobacterium fortuitum is a rapidly growing (1–3 days) soil mycobacterium that is closely related to *Mycobacterium chelonae* and for which the term *M. fortuitum-chelonae* has been proposed. Rarely the cause of pulmonary disease, this group of organisms has caused wound infections, postinjection abscesses, and contamination of porcine valves used for heart valve replacement in humans.

Mycobacterium ulcerans grows slowly (3–4 weeks) at 30°C but not at 37°C, is nonphotochromogenic, and produces chronic skin ulcers ("Buruli ulcer") on the extremities of patients living in the tropics. *Mycobacterium leprae* causes leprosy in humans but cannot be cultured on artificial media. It is identified in tissue sections and smears by the arrangement of acid-fast bacilli in intracellular bundles called "globi." Bacilli may be abundant in lepromatous leprosy but are rare in tuberculoid lesions.

Fungi. The diagnosis of fungal infection can often be made by mixing a portion of the specimen with a drop of 10% potassium hydroxide on a clean glass microscope slide, applying a coverslip, gently flaming the slide, and examining the material microscopically (Fig. 2). Fungal cultures most often yield yeasts, the most frequently isolated species of which is *Candida albicans,* followed by *Torulopsis glabrata, C. tropicalis, C. parapsilosis, C. krusei,* and *Saccharomyces.* The interpretation of these results is complicated by the normal occurrence of these yeasts in the oropharynx, gastrointestinal tract, and vagina.

However we decide to identify isolates from these sources, a minimal requirement is that all clinical laboratories should be able to isolate and identify *Cryptococcus neoformans* and *C. albicans* from normally sterile body fluids and tissues. Yeasts isolated from these sources should be screened for urease production. The production of urease should strongly suggest *C. neoformans,* the identification of which should be confirmed with carbohydrate and nitrate assimilation tests or Niger seed agar.[15] *Candida albicans* is identified by inoculating a colony into 0.5 ml of normal human serum, incubating the test at 37°C for 3 hours, and examining the suspension microscopically for germ tube formation. Carbohydrate assimilation and fermentation tests may be used to identify other species of *Candida.*[15]

The identification of the filamentous fungi is more complex and time-consuming. Their colonial morphology is seldom characteristic and is highly medium dependent. Rates of growth vary widely. *Coccidioides immitis* colonies may appear after only a day's incubation, whereas colonies of *Blastomyces dermatitidis* and *Histoplasma capsulatum* may take as long as a month to appear. Definitive identification is based therefore on microscopic examination of the hyphae and the arrangement and appearance of the spores. Demonstration of the saprobic and parasitic forms of the dimorphic fungi is usually required. In some cases animals, most often mice, must be inoculated to convert the dimorphic fungi to the parasitic or yeast form. Recognition of the morphology characteristic of the various species requires experience, and it is suggested that photographs and other illustrative material be used as reference material with which to compare the morphology of isolates. An excellent six-volume *Atlas of Clinical Mycology* may be obtained for this purpose from the American Society of Clinical Pathologists.

DETECTION OF ANTIBODIES

Cultures of certain bacteria, fungi, parasites, and viruses may be unavailable because the methodology remains undeveloped (e.g., *T. pallidum,* hepatitis and Epstein-Barr viruses), is unsafe (e.g., rickettsiae), or is impractical for all but a few research and reference laboratories. Moreover, cultures may be negative because of prior antimicrobial therapy or because of the chronic state of the disease. Under these circumstances, the detection of nonspecific (Table 8) or specific antibodies may be of considerable diagnostic and epidemiologic use. Antibody response to infection is, however, quite variable, so serologic tests may vary considerably in sensitivity and specificity. An elevated single antibody titer usually does not permit a distinction to be made between active and past infection, and the absence of a measurable antibody titer may reflect a lack of immunogenicity of the etiologic agent, the use of an inappropriate test for detecting the antibody, or insufficient time from the onset of infection for an antibody response to have occurred. For these reasons, test selection and timing of the collection of specimens are essential to the proper use and interpretation of serologic tests. As a general rule, therefore, tests should be performed concurrently with a specimen taken during the acute phase of the disease and a specimen (convalescent) taken 1 or more weeks thereafter. A fourfold or greater rise in antibody titer usually provides unequivocal evidence of recent infection. Serologic testing is for this reason often of confirmatory or epidemiologic value.

Antibodies may be detected by agglutination, immunodiffusion, immunofluorescence, immunoassay, and many other techniques. No single technique is universally applicable for measuring antibody responses to all microorganisms. Techniques are selected on the basis of their sensitivity, specificity, ease and speed of performance, and cost-effectiveness.

The commonly available bacterial antibody tests are described in Table 9. Antibodies to the 0 antigens of *Proteus vulgaris* (Table 8), *Brucella, Francisella,* and *Salmonella* have commonly been included in a "febrile agglutinin" test battery, which, either because of the infrequency of the diseases involved or the lack of specificity of the tests involved, has very limited use and the individual components of which should be selectively ordered when clinically indicated. Moreover, certain tests within the battery should be replaced by more specific tests (e.g., rickettsial group-specific complement fixation or immunofluorescent antibody for *P. vulgaris* agglutinins [Weil-Felix test]) or eliminated (*Salmonella* agglutinins [Widal test]).

The commonly available fungal serologic tests are described in Table 10. Those pertinent to virology are discussed elsewhere (Chapter 14).

DETERMINATIONS OF ANTIMICROBIAL ACTIVITY

Susceptibility Tests

General indications for performing susceptibility tests are (*1*) the isolation of organisms with unpredictable susceptibility to antimicrobial agents (e.g., staphylococci, Enterobacteriaceae, and pseudomonads) and (*2*) the isolation of organisms of clinical significance (e.g., isolates from normally sterile sources, wounds and abscesses, and urine if present in significant numbers). Susceptibility tests are usually performed with organisms that grow rapidly and well on artificial media, so variables such as inoculum size, medium, atmosphere and duration of incubation, and interpretative criteria can be standardized. Standards, therefore, have been established for testing the rapidly growing aerobic and facultatively anaerobic bacteria.[54,55] Standards are under development for testing anaerobic bacteria, mycobacteria and fungi, although procedures have been described in the literature for testing these organisms.

Susceptibility testing of anaerobic bacteria should be limited to isolates from more serious or persistent infections (e.g., bacteremia); brain abscess; and bone, joint, or intraocular infections. Periodic testing of large numbers of anaerobes should be carried out by large reference laboratories to determine whether any alterations in susceptibility have occurred.

TABLE 8. Nonspecific Antibody Tests

Disease	*Test*	*Antigen or Hapten*	*Comments*
Infectious mononucleosis	Heterophile agglutination	Sheep erythrocytes	Test is negative in about 10% of cases
Inflammation disorder, acute infection	C-reactive protein	C-reactive protein	Nonspecific indicator of active tissue-damaging process
Mycoplasma pneumoniae	Cold agglutinins	Human O erythrocytes	Titers rise in only about 50% of cases and may rise in cases with hemolytic anemias and liver disease
Rickettsial diseases	Weil-Felix	O antigen of *Proteus vulgaris* OX 2, OX 19, and OX K	Nonspecific; questionable reliability unless more than fourfold rise in titer occurs
Syphilis	Nontreponemal (VDRL, RPR, ART)	Cardiolipin	If reactive, test should be confirmed with specific treponemal antigen test

Abbreviations: RPR: rapid plasma reagin; ART: automated reagin test.

TABLE 9. Commonly Available Bacterial Serologic Tests

Disease	*Antigen(s)*	*Test(s)*	*Interpretation*
Brucellosis	*Brucella abortus*	Agglutination	Titers of more than 1:80 are suggestive of past infection, whereas titers of more than 1:160 are highly suggestive of active infection. Titers of less than 1:80 occur occasionally in cases of active infection. Cross-reactions occur in patients with *Francisella, Yersinia,* or *Vibrio* infections or immunizations.
Tularemia	*Francisella tularensis*	Agglutination	Titers of 1:40 or more are indicative of past infection; titers usually rise to more than 1:160 during active infection. Minor cross-reactions occur in patients with *Brucella* infection or immunization.
Legionellosis	*Legionella pneumophila* and other species	Immunofluorescence	Fourfold titer rise to 1:128 is indicative of recent infection. Titers of 1:256 or more may occur in asymptomatic population.
Leptospirosis	Multiple *Leptospira* serovars	Agglutination	Titers of 1:100 or more are indicative of recent or past infection.
Rickettsioses	Group specific	Immunofluorescence	Fourfold titer rise, single titer of 1:128 or more, or any IgM titer is indicative of infection.
		Complement fixation	Fourfold titer rise is significant; however, CF test is less sensitive and specific than is the immunofluorescent antibody test.
Salmonellosis	O and H antigens of *Salmonella typhi* and *S. enteritidis,* bioser *paratyphi* A–C	Agglutination (Widal)	Elevated titers may represent a cross-reaction from past infection with group A, C, or nontyphoidal D *Salmonella* or result from past immunization with typhoid–paratyphoid vaccine. Early antibiotic therapy may prevent a titer rise. *Salmonella* agglutinins are the least accurate of any diagnostic test for typhoid–paratyphoid fever.
Streptococcal infection (group A)	Streptolysin O DNase B	Neutralization (ASO) Neutralization (anti-DNase B)	Approximately 45% of children with pharyngitis and positive throat cultures for group A streptococci have a fourfold rise in ASO and/or anti-DNase B titers. Approximately 10% of such children will have a fourfold rise in ASO but not in anti-DNase B titer or vice versa. ASO titers usually do not rise in cases of streptococcal pyoderma.
	"Extracellular products"	Agglutination (streptozyme)	Sensitivity is equivalent to but the specificity is less than either ASO or anti-DNase B. False-positives may be due to non-group A β-hemolytic streptococci.
Syphilis	*Treponema pallidum*	Immunofluorescence (FTA-ABS) Hemagglutination (MHA-TP)	These tests are used to confirm positive nontreponemal or reagin test.
Psittacosis	*Chlamydia trachomatis* (LGV-1)	Immunofluorescence (Micro-IF)	Fourfold titer rise (IgG) or presence of IgM antibody is indicative of recent chlamydial infection. LGV-1 antigen cannot distinguish between infection by *C. trachomatis* and *C. psittaci.*
Other chlamydial	*Chlamydia trachomatis* (LGV-1)	Immunofluorescence (Micro-IF)	There is a high incidence of seroreactors among venereal disease populations. IgM antibody (>1:32) and IgG antibody (≥1:2000) titers occur in patients with active lymphogranuloma venereum. IgM antibody titers of 1:128 or more occur in infants with *C. trachomatis* pneumonitis.
Mycoplasmal	*Mycoplasma pneumoniae*	Complement fixation	Fourfold titer rise is indicative of recent infection. High titers may persist for more than 1 year.

Mycobacteria usually do not require susceptibility testing when isolated from previously untreated patients; however, susceptibility testing is probably indicated for mycobacteria isolated from previously treated patients who have relapsed after a course of chemotherapy, from patients whose sputum smears continue to show acid-fast bacilli after 2–3 months of treatment or whose cultures are persistently positive after 5 or 6 months of treatment, and from patients who acquired their disease outside the United States or from possible contacts with drug-resistant tuberculosis. Because they are often resistant to the commonly recommended antimycobacterial agents, clinically significant mycobacteria other than *M. tuberculosis* probably should be tested. Susceptibility testing of mycobacteria is based on the principle that when more than 1 percent of tubercle bacilli are drug resistant in vitro therapy with that agent is not likely to be effective. Inocula of mycobacteria are therefore adjusted so that colony-forming units can be enumerated, and the percentage or proportion surviving in the presence of various agents is calculated.[52] Direct drug susceptibility studies of specimens may be performed if the initial smear demonstrates that sufficient numbers of acid-fast bacilli are present. Radiometric procedures are suitable alternatives for testing *M. tuberculosis.*[52] Agents to be tested against mycobacteria include the primary antituberculous drugs, isoniazid, streptomycin, rifampin, and ethambutol. The secondary drugs include ethionamide, kanamycin, capreomycin, cycloserine, pyrazinamide, and para-aminosalicylic acid and are usually only given in cases with infections due to mycobacteria that are resistant to the primary drugs. As has already been discussed, susceptibility testing of mycobacteria should be limited to laboratories expert in this area.

The indications for performing susceptibility tests of fungi are quite limited, probably reflecting the small number of antifungal agents available, the limited number of people expert in their administration, and the technical difficulties involved in testing yeasts and, especially, filamentous fungi reproducibly. Amphotericin B has a broad range of activity in vitro against fungi, including the yeasts, dimorphic fungi, and strictly filamentous

TABLE 10. Commonly Available Fungal Serologic Tests

Infection	*Antigen(s)*	*Test(s)*	*Interpretation*
Aspergillosis	*Aspergillus fumigatus* *Aspergillus niger* *Aspergillus flavus*	Immunodiffusion	One or more precipitin bands is suggestive of active infection. Precipitin bands have been shown to correlate with complement fixation titers—the greater the number of bands, the higher the titer. Preciptins can be found in 95% of the fungus ball cases and 50% of the allergic bronchopulmonary cases. They are sometimes positive in invasive infection, depending on the immunologic status of the patient.
Blastomycosis	*Blastomyces dermatitidis* Yeast form	Complement fixation	Titers of 1:8 to 1:16 are highly suggestive of active infection; titers of 1:32 or greater are indicative. Cross-reactions occur in patients having coccidioidomycosis or histoplasmosis; however, titers are usually lower. A decreasing titer is indicative of regression. Most patients (75%) having blastomycosis have negative test findings.
	Yeast culture filtrate	Immunodiffusion	An A precipitin band may occur in as many as 80% of proven cases of blastomycosis.
Candidiasis	*Candida albicans*	Immunodiffusion, CIE	The test is difficult to interpret because precipitins are found in 20–30% of the normal population, and reports in the literature are conflicting. Clinical correlation must exist for the test to be useful.
Coccidioidomycosis	Coccidioidin	Complement fixation	Titers of 1:2 to 1:4 have been seen in active infection. Low titers should be followed by repeat testing at 2–3 wk intervals. Titers of greater than 1:16 are usually indicative of active infection. Cross-reactions occur in patients having histoplasmosis, and false-negative results occur in patients with solitary pulmonary lesions. Titer parallels the severity of infection.
	Coccidioidin	Immunodiffusion	Results correlate with complement fixation test and can be used as a screening test—should be confirmed by performing complement fixation test. A concentration (8- to 10-fold) of specimen enhances antibody detection.
	Coccidioidin	Latex agglutination	Precipitins occur during first 3 wk of infection and are diagnostic but not prognostic—useful as a screening test for precipitins in early infection. False-positive tests are frequent when diluted serum or cerebrospinal fluid specimens are used.
Cryptococcosis	No antigen—latex particles coated with hyperimmune anticryptococcal globulin	Latex agglutination for cryptococcal antigen	The presence of cryptococcal polysaccharide in body fluids is indicative of cryptococcosis. Rheumatoid factor presents false-positive reactions, and an RA test must be performed as a control. A decrease in antigen titer indicates regression. Positive tests (in CSF) have been seen in 95% of cryptococcal meningitis cases and 30% of nonmeningitis cases. Serum is less frequently positive than CSF. Disseminated infections usually present positive results in serum. The test may be performed by using serum and CSF, and is more sensitive than the India ink preparation.
Histoplasmosis	Histoplasmin and yeast form of *Histoplasma capsulatum*	Complement fixation	Titers of 1:8 to 1:16 are highly suspicious of infection; however, titers of 1:32 or greater are usually indicative of active infection. Cross-reactions occur in patients having aspergillosis, blastomycosis, and coccidioidomycosis, but titers are usually lower. Several follow-up serum samples should be tested—drawn at 2–3 week intervals. Rising titers indicate progressive infection, and decreasing titers indicate regression. Some disseminated infections are nonreactive to the complement fixation test. Recent skin tests in persons who have had prior exposure to *H. capsulatum* will cause an elevation in the complement fixation titer. This occurs in 17–20% of persons tested. The yeast antigen gives positive reactions in 75–80% of cases, and the histoplasmin gives positive reactions in 10–15% of cases. In 10% of cases both are positive simultaneously.
	Histoplasmin	Immunodiffusion	H and M bands appearing simultaneously are indicative of active infection. M band may appear alone and can indicate early infection or chronic infection. Also the M band may appear after a recent skin test. The H band appears later than the M band does and disappears earlier, and its disappearance may indicate regression of the infection.
	Histoplasmin	Latex agglutination	The test is unreliable. Many false-positive and negative test results may be observed. Any positive test result should be confirmed by the complement fixation test.
Sporotrichosis	Yeast of *Sporothrix schenckii*	Agglutination	Titers of 1:80 or greater are usually indicative of active infection. Some cutaneous infections present negative test findings; however, extracutaneous infections present positive test results.

(From Koneman et al.,[53] with permission.)

fungi; therefore, determination of its antifungal activity is rarely indicated in clinical practice. Although most clinically significant yeasts are initially susceptible to flucytosine, resistance is acquired during therapy in a substantial number of cases. For this reason, the drug is seldom administered alone, and it is usually used in conjunction with amphotericin B, with which it acts synergistically unless the organism is resistant to it. It is therefore probably important to determine the susceptibility to flucytosine of yeasts isolated from serious infections so that its use with amphotericin B can be considered. A standard method has not been agreed on; however, the choice of medium is important since some media are inhibitory to flucytosine. Most authors seem to agree on the use of yeast nitrogen base (YNB) for this purpose. The activity of ketoconazole is also highly medium dependent. Be that as it may, it seems reasonable to suggest that susceptibility testing of fungi be limited to those centers with expertise in antifungal chemotherapy.

Because of the specialized nature of antimycobacterial and antifungal susceptibility testing, the remainder of this discussion will be limited to antibacterial susceptibility tests.

Selection of Antimicrobial Agents

Agents selected for susceptibility testing should be confined to those that are clinically useful and relevant to the kind of bacterium isolated as well as to its source. Closely related analogues with activity in vitro that do not differ significantly from that of the parent or an established compound should not be tested routinely. Suggested guidelines for selecting agents to be tested are listed in Table 11. Additions to and perhaps deletions from this list can be anticipated as new agents are introduced and older ones become infrequently used. Close coordination between the laboratory and the hospital formulary committee is of utmost importance for the final selection of antimicrobial agents to be tested. Sulfonamides, except in combination with trimethoprim, are not included in this list because their principal use is in the treatment of uncomplicated lower urinary tract infections that are usually due to susceptible strains of *E. coli,* the most accurate susceptibility test of which is their eradication within the first 48–72 hours of therapy. Oxacillin or nafcillin is preferable to methicillin because of its greater stability in disks or solution. Resistance of staphylococci to the penicillinase-resistant penicillins often requires the addition of NaCl (2% in broth, 4% in agar) to Mueller-Hinton medium and incubation at temperatures not exceeding 35°C. Cephalosporins, imipenem, and some β-lactam/β-lactamase inhibitor combinations may appear to be active against methicillin-resistant staphylococci in vitro; however, there is clinical evidence that these compounds are not effective in treating serious infections due to methicillin-resistant staphylococci. Thus, staphylococci that are resistant in vitro to oxacillin, nafcillin, or methicillin should be considered resistant to other β-lactams and reported as such. Because of this characteristic, cephalosporins are not tested in some laboratories against staphylococci, and all oxacillin-, nafcillin-, or methicillin-susceptible staphylococci are considered to be susceptible to cephalosporins.

Of the currently available aminoglycosides, only three—gentamicin, tobramycin, and amikacin—generally appear in hospital formularies. Testing of any one or all of these should depend on which one or ones are in the formulary, which might, in turn, reflect the local prevalence of resistance to gentamicin or tobramycin and local bias regarding the relative toxicity of each aminoglycoside. Since resistance of enterococci to the synergistic activity of penicillin or ampicillin plus streptomycin or gentamicin can be predicted from their resistance to 2000 μg streptomycin/ml or 500 μg gentamicin/ml, it is suggested that susceptibility testing of enterococci from blood, tissue, and normally sterile body fluid cultures be tested at these high concentrations of streptomycin and gentamicin. Netilmicin may be tested if local resistance patterns to other aminoglycosides indicate that netilmicin may be useful.

The most complex issue facing formulary committees and microbiologists is the proliferation of expanded-spectrum β-lactams. Selection of a few from among the many for the hospital formulary and for laboratory testing requires familiarity with their similarities and dissimilarities in vitro and in vivo and a substantial amount of commitment and fortitude. Aztreonam and all third-generation cephalosporins available to date are equally active in vitro against the Enterobacteriaceae; therefore, aztreonam, cefotaxime, ceftazidime, ceftizoxime, ceftriaxone, or moxalactam could be selected for testing. Although cefotaxime, ceftriaxone, or moxalactam could be selected for testing against *Pseudomonas,* aztreonam has somewhat greater activity, and cefoperazone and ceftazidime have substantially greater activity than do other third-generation cephalosporins, and it would be advisable to test either cefoperazone or ceftazidime against *Pseudomonas*. Whether to test aztreonam against *Pseudomonas* in this instance might reflect its position in the formulary, and it might simply not be relevant to test cefotaxime, ceftriaxone, or moxalactam against *Pseudomonas*. Although neither aztreonam nor all third-generation cephalosporins are listed as primary antibiotics in Table 11, there are probably few settings in which one or more of these compounds are not included in the formulary and are not being tested. The situation with the *Pseudomonas*-active penicillins is complicated by some similarities and dissimilarities in their activity in vitro, their usual administration with an aminoglycoside, and the general lack of much clinical data, even among febrile granulocytopenic patients, that demonstrate statistically significant differences among them. Thus, selection of the one for the formulary and for testing should probably not be based solely on in vitro activity and could be based on competitive bidding.

Resistance among microorganisms such as *Haemophilus influenzae, Neisseria gonorrhoeae,* and *Streptococcus pneumoniae* that were previously considered to be uniformly susceptible to penicillins and some other commonly recommended alternatives has created a need for determining their susceptibility on a more routine basis. Initially, it was sufficient to test isolates of *H. influenzae* and *N. gonorrhoeae* to detect plasmid-mediated β-lactamases; however, chromosomally mediated resistance to penicillins, which is not related to β-lactamase production and is, therefore, not detectable by β-lactamase testing, has occurred in both species so that susceptibility testing of β-lactamase–negative isolates to penicillins is becoming necessary. Moreover, resistance of *H. influenzae* to cefuroxime and chloramphenicol and of *N. gonorrhoeae* to tetracycline and spectinomycin has been reported, so additional testing may be indicated in certain instances. Although susceptibility testing of *H. influenzae* by diffusion or dilution methods is reasonably well standardized and readily accomplished in most clinical laboratories, the same is not true of susceptibility testing of *N. gonorrhoeae* in which lot-to-lot differences in GC medium base produce highly variable results. Although isolates of pneumococci with penicillin minimal inhibitory concentrations (MICs) between 0.12 and 1.0 have been recognized for many years, strains with penicillin MICs of ≥2 μg/ml have only been recognized in recent years, initially in South Africa but subsequently in other parts of the world including the United States. Since pneumococci with MICs of 0.12–1.0 μg/ml may not respond to penicillin therapy in cases of meningitis and since infections due to penicillin-resistant pneumococci fail to repond to therapy with penicillin and antibiotics other than vanco-

TABLE 11. Guidelines for Selection of Antibacterial Agents for Susceptibility Testing

Agent	*Staphylococci*	*Enterococci*	*Nonenterococcal Streptococci*	*Pseudomonads*	Enterobacteriaceae
Amikacin				P	P
Ampicillin	S	P			P
Ampicillin/sulbactam (or amoxicillin/clavulanate)	S				S
Azlocillin (or mezlocillin, carbenicillin, piperacillin or ticarcillin)				P	
Aztreonam				S	S
Cefamandole (or cefonicid or cefuroxime)					S
Cefotaxime (or cefoperazone, ceftazidime, ceftizoxime, ceftriaxone, or moxalactam)					P
Cefoxitin (or cefotetan)					S
Ceftazidime (or cefoperazone)				P	
Cephalothin	P[a]		P		P[b]
Chloramphenicol	S			S	S
Ciprofloxacin	S			S	S
Clindamycin	P		P		
Erythromycin	P	U	P		
Gentamicin (or tobramycin)	S	S[c]		P	P
Imipenem				S	S
Mezlocillin (or piperacillin or ticarcillin)					P
Netilmicin				S	S
Oxacillin (or methicillin or nafcillin)	P[b]				
Penicillin G	P		P		
Tetracycline	S				S, U
Ticarcillin/clavulanate					S
Trimethoprim/sulfamethoxazole	S			S[d]	P
Vancomycin	P	S			
Cinoxacin (or nalidixic acid)					U
Nitrofurantoin	U	U	U		U
Norfloxacin	U	U	U	U	U
Trimethoprim	U				U

Abbreviations: P: primary agents to be tested routinely; S: secondary agents to be tested under special circumstances such as in institutions harboring endemic or epidemic resistance to one or more of the primary agents, for therapy for patients allergic to a primary agent, or as an epidemiologic aid; U: urinary tract–specific agent to be tested against urinary isolates only.

[a] Oxacillin (or methicillin- or nafcillin)-resistant staphylococci should be considered resistant to cephalosporins, penicillins (including combinations with β-lactamase inhibitors), and imipenem.

[b] Although cephalothin can be used to predict the in vitro activity of other first-generation cephalosporins, cefazolin should not be used for the same purpose because cefazolin is more active than are other first-generation cephalosporins vs. *E. coli*.

[c] Gentamicin should be tested at concentration of 500 or 2000 μg/ml to detect high-level resistant strains that are not synergistically affected by the combination of a penicillin and gentamicin.

[d] Applies only to species other than *P. aeruginosa*.

(Data from National Committee for Clinical Laboratory Standards.[54,55])

mycin, it is imperative for the laboratory to test clinically significant isolates of pneumococci against penicillin.

Methods

Dilution. The principle of dilution tests is to determine the lowest or minimal concentration of antimicrobial agent that is required to inhibit the growth of a microorganism. The MIC is usually expressed in micrograms per milliliter, although SI units may be used in the future. Approved standards describing the methods to be used for dilution testing have been published by the National Committee for Clinical Laboratory Standards.[55] Dilution tests may be performed in agar or in broth, the latter of which can be readily adapted to microdilution, which is currently in widespread use in clinical and research laboratories. Dilution tests are often preferred because they are incorrectly perceived as being more accurate than disk diffusion tests are and because laboratory personnel incorrectly assume that MICs are preferred by clinicians. In fact, dilution and diffusion tests are directly correlated, and most clinicians other than those with subspecialty interest in infectious diseases require interpretation of MICs. Thus, the indications for dilution testing are (*1*) investigations of new antimicrobial agents, (*2*) testing of microorganisms that grow slowly or have special growth requirements, (*3*) determination of precise susceptibility when the preferred therapy is with a relatively nontoxic but not highly active β-lactam, and (*4*) as an alternative to disk diffusion testing when inocula replica plating is deemed cost-effective. Replicate inoculation of a single microorganism into microwells containing biochemical substrates for microbial identification and antimicrobial agents for susceptibility testing is a common feature of many commercially available devices today.

Discrepancies between dilution methods in broth and in agar are largely limited to tests of aminoglycosides against *Pseudomonas aeruginosa*. Tests in Mueller-Hinton broth that has been supplemented with Ca^{2+} and Mg^{2+} at concentrations of 50 and 25 mg/liter, respectively, appear to provide an unacceptably high false-resistance rate relative to results obtained with a reference lot of Mueller-Hinton agar when aminoglycosides are tested against *P. aeruginosa*. As a consequence, the recommended concentrations of Ca^{2+} and Mg^{2+} will be reduced so as to bring the results of testing with agar and broth into agreement.[55]

Interpretative guidelines for translating MIC results into susceptible, moderately susceptible, intermediate, or resistant categories have been published by the National Committee for Clinical Laboratory Standards.[55] As a rule, these interpretative criteria should be made available in laboratory reports of MICs.

With appropriate modifications of media and the duration and atmosphere of incubation, dilution procedures may be adapted for use with slow-growing or fastidious microorganisms.

The greatest day-to-day variability in MICs is due to variations in inoculum size. The recommended inoculum is approximately 5×10^5 cfu/ml,[55] and it is not sufficient to rely on a manufacturer's directions for attaining this inoculum size, particularly when performing microdilution methods. It is incumbent on each user of a susceptibility testing device to establish procedures through quantitative studies that ensure a final inoculum of approximately 5×10^5 cfu/ml. Attainment of this inoculum is critical to the accurate detection of penicillin- and methicillin-resistant staphylococci as well as of mutants of Enterobacteriaceae and *P. aeruginosa* that are selectively derepressed for the chromosomal class I β-lactamase and that are resistant to expanded-spectrum β-lactam antibiotics. Conversely, preparation of the inoculum of *Haemophilus influenzae* by visual comparison with the recommended McFarland standard is likely to yield an inoculum exceeding 1×10^6 cfu/ml and result in false resistance to expanded-spectrum cephalosporins.

Disk Diffusion. The principle of the disk diffusion technique is that the diameter of a zone of inhibition about an antimicrobial-impreganated paper disk relates approximately linearly to the antimicrobial's $\log_2$ MIC. Zone diameters are interpreted as signifying susceptibility, intermediate susceptibility, or resistance to each antimicrobial agent tested according to published criteria. Obviously, these criteria retain their validity only as long as standard procedures are followed.[54] It should be equally obvious that the interpretative criteria apply only to organisms that grow rapidly on Mueller-Hinton agar, with or without whole or chocolatized blood, when incubated at 35°C for 16–18 hours in room air, that is, staphylococci, Enterobacteriaceae, and pseudomonads. The disk diffusion test may also be used reliably to determine whether *H. influenzae* is susceptible to ampicillin. No disk diffusion method is uniformly reliable for determining the susceptibility of anaerobic bacteria.

Disk Elution. Elution of antimicrobial agents into liquid or solid media occurs rapidly and completely. The concept has been applied to automated rapid susceptibility testing using procedures including the Organon Teknika Autobac and the Abbott MS-2 as well as to the testing of anaerobic bacteria.

Quality Control. All susceptibility tests must undergo frequent performance controls to ensure accurate and reproducible results. Methods for quality control of disk diffusion methods are described elsewhere[54] and involve the testing on weekly basis of *S. aureus* (ATCC 25923), *E. coli* (ATCC 25922), and *P. aeruginosa* (ATCC 27853), for which acceptable zone diameter control limits have been established. Control of dilution tests is performed with *S. aureus* (ATCC 29213), *S. faecalis* (ATCC 29212), *E. coli* (ATCC 25922), and *P. aeruginosa* (ATCC 27853).[55] *E. coli* (ATCC 35218) should be included when testing β-lactam/β-lactamase inhibitor combinations.

Bactericidal Tests

Broth. The principle of this test is to determine the lowest or minimal concentration of antimicrobial agent that kills ≥99.9 percent of the inoculum used for the test. The minimal bactericidal concentration (MBC) or minimal lethal concentration (MLC) is obtained by subculturing measured aliquots from broth in tubes containing no visible growth (inhibitory phase) to antimicrobial-free media. Although the inhibitory phase of this test has been standardized, the volume of the aliquot subcultured, the subculture medium, the subculture method (pour vs. streak plates), and the duration of incubation have not. There are consequently numerous technical variations of this test in the literature. Most investigators agree on the need to quantify the original inoculum to determine the lowest concentration of antimicrobial agent that destroys at least 99.9 percent of it. Recommended procedures for performing bactericidal tests have been described by Pearson et al.[56] and in a proposed guideline published by the National Committee for Clinical Laboratory Standards.[57] Critical components of the methodology include an inoculum of at least 5×10^5 cfu/ml and a subculture volume of 0.01 ml to allow accurate estimation of ≥99.9 percent killing.[56,57]

There are very few indications for bactericidal testing. Although the MBC is an accepted parameter in the evaluation of a new antimicrobial agent, its clinical value is debatable, especially since the test is so method dependent and interpretation of the results is not well defined. A related issue is that of tolerance, about which much has been written but about which there are substantial definitional problems.[58,59] Among the technical problems involved are (*1*) the fact that stationary-phase cultures result in diminished killing rates, (*2*) bacteria may escape exposure to the antibiotic by adhering to the side of the tube above the meniscus, (*3*) sufficient antibiotic may be transferred in subcultures to inhibit surviving organisms, and (*4*) the rate of bactericidal activity may vary according to duration of incubation, medium content, and pH.[58,59] For all of these reasons it appears that the most reliable method for determining tolerance, defined as a reduced rate of killing, is by timed killing curve studies in which an exponential phase of growth of the organism is adjusted to provide an inoculum of approximately 5×10^5 cfu/ml that is exposed to a concentration of the antibiotic that is eight times its MIC and the number of survivors after 4 to 6 hours of incubation is compared with those at 2-hour or 0 time.[59] Determination of the number of persisters can be made by quantitative subculture after 24 hours of incubation.[59]

Combination Studies. Studies of combinations of antimicrobial agents are performed when there is multiple resistance to antimicrobials singly, when there are contraindications to the use of preferred antimicrobials, when therapeutic failure has occurred with a current antimicrobial regimen, and when the potential for toxicity exists during a prolonged therapeutic regimen.

There are two major approaches to performing combination studies.[60]

METHODS WITH SOLID MEDIUM. Antimicrobials can be combined in a single disk to determine whether their activity is greater (or less) than that of either agent singly. A frequently used example of this approach is the cotrimoxazole (trimethoprim-sulfamethoxazole) disk. The synergistic interaction of this combination can be seen if its components are tested separately by placing disks containing each proximately on the seeded agar surface. A modification of this technique is to place two filter paper strips, each containing a different antimicrobial, at right angles to one another on the seeded agar surface. Bacteriostatic synergism is indicated by inhibition of growth within the angle formed by the two strips. Bactericidal interactions between two antimicrobial agents may be determined by the cellophane transfer technique wherein a cellophane tambour inoculated on the inside with the test organism is applied to an agar surface into which antimicrobials have prediffused from filter paper

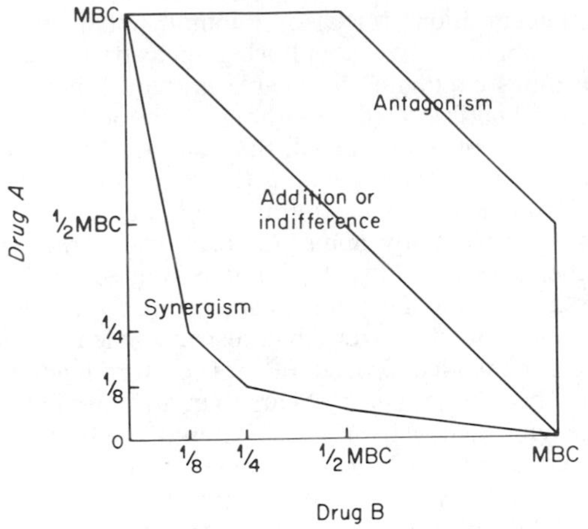

FIG. 7. Isobologram depicting three possible interactions between two antimicrobial agents when tested in combination by the two-dimensional ("checkerboard") technique. (From Washington,[15] with permission.)

strips placed at right angles.[60] The antimicrobials and nutrients from the agar diffuse through the cellophane. After overnight incubation, the tambour is removed from the agar surface, transferred to an antimicrobial-free medium, and incubated for an additional 24 hours. Synergism is indicated when growth is absent within the area formerly encompassed by the angle formed by the two antimicrobial-containing strips.

METHODS WITH LIQUID MEDIUM. There are two techniques for combination studies in liquid medium.[60] In the two-dimensional ("checkerboard") method serial, twofold dilutions of two agents, alone and in combination, are inoculated with the test organism. After incubation for 16–18 hours, those tubes containing broth without visible growth are subcultured, as for the MBC, to antimicrobial-free media. The results are then depicted according to isobologram criteria as demonstrating synergy, antagonism, or indifference (Fig. 7). In the timed killing curve two or more fixed concentrations of two or more antimicrobials, singly and in combination, are inoculated with the test organism and subcultured quantitatively over time to compare the rate of killing by the combinations with that of either antimicrobial by itself[61] (Fig. 8).

Synergism is usually defined by the significantly greater activity of the combination than would be expected from the sum of the separate effects of the antimicrobials being tested.[60] In the checkerboard method, synergism is defined when the fractional inhibitory concentration (FIC) or fractional bactericidal concentration (FBC) index is ≤ 0.5, whereas in killing curve studies synergy is defined as a $\geq 2 \log_{10}$ cfu/ml decrease between the combination and its most active component after 24 hours of incubation, assuming that at least one of the antimicrobials in the combination does not produce inhibitory or killing activity by itself. Antagonism is defined in the checkerboard method by an FIC or FBC index of >4.0 and in the killing curve method by $\leq 2 \log_{10}$ decrease in killing by the combination at 24 hours as compared with the most active antimicrobial by itself. Between synergy and antagonism are additive and indifferent effects.[60]

In either test it is important to standardize the inoculum. In the case of the checkerboard method, all of the variables discussed previously in determining MBCs apply. In killing curve studies, it is important to define the lower threshold of sensitivity of the detectable number of colony-forming units per milliliter and to limit the effects of antimicrobial carryover either by inactivating one or both antimicrobials in the subculture or serially diluting subcultures to the point at which each antimicrobial is present only in subinhibitory concentrations.

Although the interpretative results of both the checkerboard and timed killing curve methods often agree, differences do occur, often reflecting differences between methods in inoculum size and growth phase as well as in sampling times.[62] Because of the extremely laborious nature of these methods and because of difficulties in applying the results in clinical practice, their use should probably be restricted to investigational studies.

Serum Bactericidal Test. The dilution of serum that is inhibitory or bactericidal to an organism isolated from a patient receiving antimicrobial therapy has been used for years as an indirect method of monitoring the antimicrobial dosage. First described by Schlichter et al.[63] as a test of the serum's bacteriostatic activity at the anticipated trough level of antibiotics, the test has undergone innumerable modifications as regards the timing of blood collection, inoculum size, serum diluent, subculture volume and medium, and end points. Proposed guidelines for performing the test have been published by the National Committee for Clinical Laboratory Standards[64]; however, the interpretative guidelines provided are limited by sev-

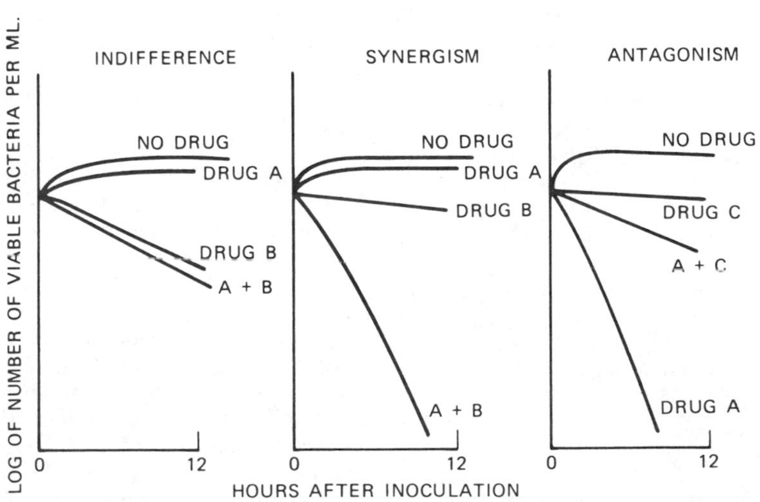

FIG. 8. Schematic representation of bactericidal action in vitro shows the possible types of results seen when one drug or two drugs act on a homogeneous population of bacteria under conditions permitting growth. (From Jawetz,[61] with permission.)

eral factors. First, exclusive of infections associated with implanted prosthetic materials, most cases of endocarditis and osteomyelitis are successfully treated with currently recommended antibiotic regimens, so the correlation between treatment failure and any range of titers is based on a very small sample. Accordingly although the predictive value of a titer, for example, ≥1:16, for cure may be high, that for failure with a lesser titer is not, particularly when confidence limits are applied to any published predictive values for failure related to titers below 1:16. Second, although the serum bactericidal test is considered an indirect assay of antimicrobial activity in vitro, the test is subject to all of the methodological variables that have been described for the MBC. Third, there is an inherent risk in promoting a particular minimal acceptable titer in that efforts to increase a low titer might result in an inappropriate increase in the dosage of a potentially toxic antibiotic. In conclusion, although the determination of serum bactericidal titers may provide another piece of information about the antimicrobial properties in vivo of a new investigational antimicrobial agent, there are few clinical indications for their use.

Assays

Assays of antimicrobial concentrations in serum should be made when there is dysfunction of excretory or metabolic organs or systems, when there is an in vivo response that is inconsistent with in vitro susceptibility test results, when there is variability in the pharmacokinetics of an antimicrobial agent, and when potentially toxic antimicrobial agents are being administered. Assays are particularly useful when therapeutic concentrations of an agent approximate its potentially toxic concentrations. For example, therapeutic concentrations of gentamicin are in the range of 4–6 μg/ml, whereas potentially toxic concentrations are 12 μg/ml or greater. Assays in this case assist in adjusting the antibiotic dosage to achieve therapeutic concentrations in serum and, at the same time, provide a means of monitoring the dosage to ensure that potentially toxic levels are not being attained. Although many formulas have been published to assist in adjusting antibiotic dosage, changing renal status often renders these calculations invalid, and assays should be made to monitor antimicrobial therapy.

There are many methods for performing antimicrobial assays, the details of which are described in several excellent books devoted to the subject.[15,65–69] The methods most frequently used in clinical laboratories are microbiologic assay or bioassay, radioenzymatic assay (REA), radioimmunoassay (RIA), chromatography, and nonisotopic immunoassays (e.g., fluorescence polarization).

Bioassay. Bioassays compare the response of a highly susceptible test organism to known concentrations of an antimicrobial with the response of the same organism under identical test conditions to an unknown concentration of the same antimicrobial. Bioassays may be made by serial dilution methods (Table 12); however, since the reproducibility of such methods is ±1 $\log_2$ dilutions, their accuracy is generally not suitable for

TABLE 12. Sample Protocol for Broth Dilution Assay Method

	Tube Number							
Series	*1*	*2*	*3*	*4*	*5*	*6*	*7*	*8*
First								
Antimicrobial (μg/ml)	4	2	1	0.5	0.25	0.12	0.06	0.03
Second								
Serum (reciprocal titer)	4	8	16	32	64	128	256	512

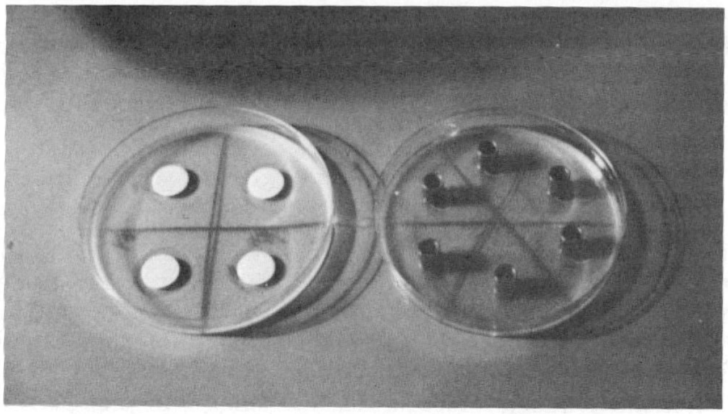

FIG. 9. Agar diffusion assays using stainless steel cylinders (right) and paper disks (left) to contain the standards and samples to be tested.

assays of agents with narrow toxic:therapeutic ratios. In the example shown (Table 12), the antimicrobial to be assayed is serially diluted, as is the patient's serum containing an unknown concentration of the antimicrobial. Both series of tubes are inoculated with a standardized suspension of the test organism. Should the organism be inhibited after overnight incubation by 0.12 μg/ml of the antibiotic and by a 1:16 dilution of the patient's serum, the concentration of the antibiotic in the patient's serum would be 1.9 μg/ml (16 × 0.12).

Many bioassays are performed by the diffusion method, which is more accurate and reproducible than is the dilution method because response is measured as a zone of inhibition and therefore as a progression of antimicrobial activity in agar. In the diffusion assay a standard curve is constructed from the inhibitory zone diameters produced by standards with varying concentrations of antimicrobial. The zone diameter of inhibition produced by an unknown sample is extrapolated from the standard curve to a concentration (μg/ml). Standards and unknown materials to be assayed are placed into a cylinder or onto a paper disk applied to the seeded agar surface (Fig. 9). Alternatively, samples can be placed into wells punched out of the seeded agar. By increasing the inoculum size, it is often possible to shorten the incubation time of the bioassay. Most aminoglycosides, for example, can be assayed within a 4-hour period.

Fluids to be assayed often contain more than one antimicrobial agent. In the bioassay this problem is circumvented by selecting a test organism that is very susceptible to the agent to be assayed and resistant to other agents, by inactivating interfering antimicrobials, or by diluting the fluid to eliminate detectable activity of any agents present in low concentrations to assay one that is present in high concentrations. In practice, the first two approaches are commonly used. Organisms with the desired susceptibility patterns can be obtained from reference laboratories or can be selected from isolates encountered in the laboratory. These organisms should be tested at regular intervals to ensure that they have retained their original susceptibility patterns. Penicillins and cephalosporins can be inactivated with β-lactamases, whereas aminoglycosides can be inactivated with calcium hydroxide or sodium polyanetholsulfonate.

It is essential for physicians ordering assays to provide the laboratory with information on the dosage and time interval since the last dose of the antimicrobial to be assayed as well as what other antimicrobials are being administered concurrently. Failure to do so may not only delay completion of the assay but can also lead to spurious results.

Radioenzymatic Assay. In the REA a radiolabeled functional group, for example, ^{14}C-adenosine triphosphate (ATP), that serves as the source of an adenyl or acetyl group is transferred enzymatically to an aminoglycoside. The adenylylated or acetylated aminoglycoside is strongly cationic and binds to phosphocellulose paper; therefore, phosphocellulose-bound radioactivity measures the amount of aminoglycoside present. The procedure is rapid, accurate, and reproducible but requires access to a liquid scintillation spectrometer.

Radioimmunoassay. The RIA depends on the noncovalent binding of an antigen, the antimicrobial agent, by a specific antibody. If the amount of antibody is limited and kept constant, the percentage of antigen bound will be inversely related to the total amount of antigen present in the standard or sample. This distribution is determined by adding a small amount of radiolabeled antigen as a tracer so that the amount of radioactivity in the bound fraction can be counted and expressed as a percentage of total counts.

The RIA is rapid, accurate, and reproducible. As with the REA, access to a liquid scintillation spectrometer is required. The RIA is expensive to perform unless large numbers of specimens can be tested in batches. Neither the REA nor the RIA are particularly well suited for handling single specimens on demand, as often occurs in hospital practice. Alternatives to assays requiring radioisotopes and scintillation spectrometry are highly desirable.

Chromatography. Chromatographic assays are very sensitive, rapid, and specific and lend themselves readily to handling single specimens on demand. In contrast to REA and RIA, chromatography usually requires only a single internal standard that is run with each specimen. The two types of chromatography that have been developed to the point of practicality for antimicrobial assays are gas–liquid (GLC) and high-pressure liquid (HPLC) chromatography, the latter of which does not require volatility of the antimicrobial or derivatization and is, therefore, simpler and more rapid. Antimicrobial agents that may be assayed by GLC include clindamycin, chloramphenicol, thiamphenicol, sulfonamides, flucytosine, miconazole, griseofulvin, and metronidazole. HPLC methodology exists for assay of most antibacterial, antimycobacterial, antifungal, and antiparasitic agents.

Nonisotopic Immunoassays. Nonisotopic immunoassays differ from radioimmunoassays in that the drug is labeled with a fluorophore or enzyme instead of a radionuclide. Because of the greater stability of nonisotopic labels, the lack of potential exposure to radioactive materials, and the more moderate equipment costs, nonisotopic immunoassays have replaced radioimmunoassays for measuring aminoglycoside and vancomycin levels.[69]

Chemical Tests for β-Lactamase

The determination of production of β-lactamase by staphylococci, *H. influenzae,* and *N. gonorrhoeae* is of considerable clinical value in the treatment of diseases caused by these organisms. There are both rapid acidimetric and iodometric methods, as well as a rapid chromogenic cephalosporin test, available for this purpose. These can be used with isolated colonies of bacteria and provide results within a few minutes.

REFERENCES

1. Huffaker RH, ed. Collection, Handling and Shipment of Microbiological Specimens. Atlanta: US Department of Health, Education, and Welfare. Public Health Service. Centers for Disease Control. DHEW Publication No. CDC 75-8263; 1974.
2. Evans FO, Sydnor JB, Moore WEC, et al. Sinusitis of the maxillary antrum. N Engl J Med. 1975;293:735–9.
3. Schwartz R, Rodriguez WJ, Mann R, et al. The nasopharyngeal culture in acute otitis media: A reappraisal of its usefulness. JAMA. 1979;241:2170–3.
4. Auger WJ. An original method of obtaining sputum from infants and children with reference to the incidence of pneumococci in the nasopharynx. J Pediatr. 1939;15:640–5.
5. Gerber MA. Rapid diagnosis of group A beta-hemolytic streptococcal pharyngitis. Use of antigen detection tests. Diagn Microbiol Infect Dis. 1986;4(Suppl):5–15.
6. Lieu TA, Fleisher GR, Schwartz JS. Clinical performance and effect on treatment rates of latex agglutination testing for streptococcal pharyngitis in an emergency department. Pediatr Infect Dis. 1986;5:655–9.
7. Chodosh S. Examination of sputum cells. N Engl J Med. 1970;282:854–7.
8. Murray PR, Washington JA II. Microscopic and bacteriologic analysis of sputum. Mayo Clin Proc. 1975;50:339–44.
9. Geckler RW, Gremillion DH, McAllister CK, et al. Microscopic and bacteriological comparison of paired sputa and transtracheal aspirates. J Clin Microbiol. 1977;6:396–9.
10. Thorsteinsson SB, Musher DM, Fagan T. The diagnostic value of sputum culture in acute pneumonia. JAMA. 1975;233:894–5.
11. Bartlett JG, Rosenblatt JE, Finegold SM. Percutaneous transtracheal aspiration in the diagnosis of anaerobic pulmonary infection. Ann Intern Med. 1973;79:535–40.
12. Bartlett JG, Ryan KJ, Smith TF, et al. Cumitech 7A. In: Washington JA II, ed. Laboratory Diagnosis of Lower Respiratory Tract Infections. Washington: American Society for Microbiology; 1987.
13. Chalvardjian AM, Grawe LA: A new procedure for the identification of *Pneumocystis carinii* cysts in tissue sections and smears. J Clin Pathol. 1963;16:383–4.
14. Jones RN. Contemporary perspectives on clinical laboratory diagnosis of urinary tract infections: Two protocols that function in a cost-containment outpatient medical practice. In: Smith JW, ed. The Role of Clinical Microbiology in Cost-Effective Health Care. Skokie, IL: College of American Pathologists; 1985:427–36.
15. Washington JA II (ed): Laboratory Procedures in Clinical Microbiology, 2nd ed. New York: Springer-Verlag; 1985.
16. Reller LB, Murray PR, MacLowry JD. Cumitech 1A. In: Washington JA II, ed. Blood Cultures II. Washington: American Society for Microbiology; 1982.
17. Washington JA II. Blood cultures: Issues and controversies. Rev Infect Dis. 1986;8:792–802.
18. Finegold SM: Anaerobic bacteria in Human Disease. New York: Academic Press; 1977.
19. Feldman WE. Concentrations of bacteria in cerebrospinal fluid of patients with bacterial meningitis. J Pediatr. 1976;88:549–52.
20. Wilson CB, Smith AL. Rapid tests for the diagnosis of bacterial meningitis. In: Remington JS, Swartz MN, eds. Current clinical topics in infectious diseases 7. New York: McGraw Hill; 1986:134–56.
21. Granoff DM, Murphy TV, Ingram DL, et al. Use of rapidly generated results in patient management. Diagn Microbiol Infect Dis. 1986;4(Suppl):157–66.
22. Mackowiak PA, Jones SR, Smith JW. Diagnostic value of sinus-tract cultures in chronic osteomyelitis. JAMA. 1978;239:2772–5.
23. Krizek TJ, Robson MC: Evolution of quantitative bacteriology in wound management. Am J Surg. 1975;130:579–84.
24. Loebel EC, Marvin JA, Heck EL, et al. The method of quantitative burn-wound biopsy cultures and its routine use in the care of the burned patient. Am J Clin Pathol. 1974;61:20–4.
25. Woods GL, Washington JA II. Mycobacteria other than *Mycobacterium tuberculosis:* Review of microbiologic and clinical aspects. Rev Infect Dis 1987;9:275–94.
26. Ryan RW. Considerations in the laboratory diagnosis of antibiotic-associated gastroenteritis. Diagn Microbiol Infect Dis. 1986;4(Suppl):79–86.
27. Lyerly DM, Ball DW, Toth J, et al. Characterization of cross-reactive proteins detected by Culturette brand rapid latex test for *Clostridium difficile.* J Clin Microbiol. 1988;26:397–400.
28. Harris JC, DuPont HL, Hornick RB: Fecal leukocytes in diarrheal illness. Ann Intern Med. 1972;76:697–703.
29. Champsaur H, Questiaux E, Prevot J, et al. Rotavirus carriage, asymptomatic infection, and disease in the first two years of life. I. Virus shedding. J Infect Dis. 1984;149:667–74.
30. Champsaur H, Henry-Amar M, Goldszmidt D, et al. Rotavirus carriage, asymptomatic infection, and disease in the first two years of life. II. Serological response. J Infect Dis. 1984;149:675–82.
31. Yolken RH, Miotti P, Viscidi R. Immunoassays for the diagnosis and study of viral gastroenteritis. Pediatr Infect Dis. 1986;5(Suppl):46–52.
32. Hart G. Syphilis tests in diagnostic and therapeutic decision making. Ann Intern Med. 1986;104:368–76.
33. Washington JA II. What can you reasonably ask and expect of the microbiology laboratory? Med Times. 1977;105:20–7.
34. Kellogg DS, Holmes KK, Hill GA: Cumitech 4. In: Marcus S, Sherris JC, eds. Laboratory Diagnosis of Gonorrhea. Washington: American Society for Microbiology; 1976.
35. Clyde WA Jr, Kenny GE, Schachter J. Cumitech 19. In: Drew L, ed. Laboratory Diagnosis of Chlamydial and Mycoplasmal Infection. Washington: American Society for Microbiology; 1984.
36. Chernesky MA, Mahony JB, Castriciano S, et al. Detection of *Chlamydia trachomatis* antigens by enzyme immunoassay and immunofluorescence in

genital specimens from symptomatic and asymptomatic men and women. J Infect Dis. 1986;154:141–8.
37. Tilton RC, Judson FN, Barnes RC, et al. Multicenter comparative evaluation of two microscopic methods and culture for detection of *Chlamydia trachomatis* in patient specimens. J Clin Microbiol. 1988;26:167–70.
38. Hammerschlag MR, Rettig PJ, Shields ME. False positive results with the use of chlamydial antigen detection tests in the evaluation of suspected sexual absue in children. Pediatr Infect Dis. 1988;7:11–14.
39. Amsel R, Totten PA, Spiegel CA, et al. Nonspecific vaginitis: Diagnostic criteria and microbial and epidemiologic associations. Am J Med. 1983;74:14–22.
40. Burnakis TG, Hildebrandt NB. Pelvic inflammatory disease: A review with emphasis on antimicrobial therapy. Rev Infect Dis. 1986;8:86–116.
41. Mardh P-A. An overview of infectious agents of salpingitis, their biology, and recent advances in methods of detection. Am J Obstet Gynecol. 1980;138:933–51.
42. Leibowitz HM, Pratt MV, Flagstad IJ, et al. Human conjunctivitis. I. Diagnostic evaluation. Arch Ophthalmol. 1976;94:1747–9.
43. Jones DB, Liesegang TJ, Robinson NM. Cumitech 13. In: Washington JA II, ed. Laboratory Diagnosis of Ocular Infections. Washington: American Society for Microbiology; 1981.
44. François J, Rysselaere M: Oculomycoses. Springfield, IL, Charles C Thomas; 1972.
45. Gosey LL, Howard RM, Witebsky FG, et al. Advantages of a modified toluidine blue O stain and bronchoalveolar lavage for the diagnosis of *Pneumocystis carinii* pneumonia. J Clin Microbiol. 1985;22:803–7.
46. Shimono LH, Hartman B. A simple and reliable rapid methenamine silver stain for *Pneumocystis carinii* and fungi. Arch Pathol Lab Med. 1986;110:855–6.
47. Braitman LE. Confidence intervals extract clinically useful information from data. Ann Intern Med. 1988;108:296–8.
48. Edelstein PH. The laboratory diagnosis of legionnaires' disease. Semin Respir Infect 1987;2:235–41.
49. Kaufman L, Reiss E. Serodiagnosis of fungal diseases. In: Rose NR, Friedman H, Fahey JL, eds. Manual of Clinical Immunology. 3rd ed. Washington: American Society for Microbiology; 1986;446–66.
49a. Stockman L, Roberts GD. Specificity of latex test for cryptococcal antigen: A rapid, simple method for eliminating interference factors. J Clin Microbiol. 1982;16:965–7.
50. Bailey JW, Sada E, Brass C, et al. Diagnosis of systemic candidiasis by latex agglutination for serum antigen. J Clin Microbiol. 1985;21:749–52.
51. Kahn FW, Jones JM. Latex agglutination for detection of *Candida* antigens in sera of patients with invasive candidiasis. J Infect Dis. 1986;153:579–85.
52. Sommers HM, Good RC. *Mycobacterium*. In Lennette EH, Balows A, Hausler WJ Jr, et al., eds. Manual of Clinical Microbiology. 4th ed. Washington: American Society for Microbiology; 1985;216–48.
53. Koneman EW, Roberts GD. Clinical and laboratory diagnosis of mycotic disease. In: Henry JB, ed. Clinical Diagnosis and Management by Laboratory Methods. 16th ed. Philadelphia: WB Saunders; 1979:1276–7.
54. National Committee for Clinical Laboratory Standards. Performance Standards for Antimicrobial Disk Susceptibility Tests. Tentative Standard NCCLS Publication M2T4. Villanova, PA: NCCLS; 1988.
55. National Committee for Clinical Laboratory Standards. Methods for Dilution Antimicrobial Susceptibility Tests for Bacteria That Grow Aerobically. Tentative Standard NCCLS Publication M7-T2. Villanova, PA: NCCLS; 1988.
56. Pearson RD, Steigbigel RT, Davis HT, et al. Method for reliable determination of minimal lethal concentrations. Antimicrob Agents Chemother. 1980;18:699–708.
57. National Committee for Clinical Laboratory Standards. Methods for Determining Bactericidal Activity of Antimicrobial Agents. Proposed Guideline. NCCLS Document M26-P. Villanova, PA: NCCLS; 1987.
58. Handwerger S, Tomasz A. Antibiotic tolerance among clinical isolates of bacteria. Rev Infect Dis. 1985;7:368–86.
59. Sherris JC. Problems in in vitro determination of antibiotic tolerance in clinical isolates. Antimicrob Agents Chemother. 1986;30:633–7.
60. Krogstad DJ, Moellering RC Jr. Antimicrobial combinations. In Lorian V, ed. Antibiotics in Laboratory Medicine. 2nd ed. Baltimore: Williams & Wilkins; 1986;537–95.
61. Jawetz E. Combined antibiotic action. Some definitions and correlations between laboratory and clinical results. Antimicrob Agents Chemother. 1967:203–9.
62. Bayer AS, Morrison JO. Disparity between timed-kill and checkerboard methods for determination of in vitro bactericidal interactions of vancomycin plus rifampin versus methicillin-susceptible and -resistant *Staphylococcus aureus*. Antimicrob Agents Chemother. 1984;26:220–3.
63. Schlichter JG, Maclean H, Milzer A. Effective penicillin therapy in subacute bacterial endocarditis and other chronic infections. Am J Med Sci. 1949;217:600–8.
64. National Committee for Clinical Laboratory Standards. Methodology on the Serum Bactericidal Test. Proposed Guideline. NCCLS Document M21-P. Villanova, PA: NCCLS; 1987.
65. Grove DC, Randall WA: Assay Methods of Antibiotics: A Laboratory Manual (Anitibiotics Monograph 2). New York: Medical Encyclopedia; 1955.
66. Kavanagh F, ed. Analytical Microbiology. New York: Academic Press; 1963.
67. Kavanagh F, ed. Analytical Microbiology. v. 2. New York: Academic Press; 1972.
68. Hash JH, ed. Antibiotics. Methods in Enzymology. V. 43. New York: Academic Press; 1975.
69. Edberg SC. The measurement of antibiotics in human body fluids: Techniques and significance. In Lorian V, ed. Antibiotics in Laboratory Medicine. 2nd ed. Baltimore: Williams & Wilkins; 1986;381–476.

14. VIRUSES, RICKETTSIAE, CHLAMYDIAE, AND MYCOPLASMAS

MARILYN A. MENEGUS
R. GORDON DOUGLAS, JR.

VIRUSES

As a result of discovery of the viral etiology of a number of diseases and of the increasing interest in antiviral chemotherapy, a number of hospitals and health care facilities now have active viral diagnostic laboratories. Currently, the major emphasis is placed on isolation of viruses and on serologic tests.[1–6] Serologic tests suffer from the requirement for convalescent serum, usually obtained 10 or more days after the acute serum specimen, thus providing diagnoses in retrospect. Viral isolation techniques, on the other hand, are expensive and relatively slow because of the dependence on the rate of replication of virus in cell cultures. Today, techniques such as electron microscopy (EM), immunofluorescence (IFA), radioimmunoassay (RIA), enzyme-linked immunosorbent assay (ELISA), and nucleic acid hybridization (NAH) are being adapted to detect viruses in clinical specimens.[7–11] Using these techniques, results can be obtained rapidly, often on the day the specimen is submitted. The isolation of viruses in cell culture systems, however, remains the most widely available system; it is sensitive and highly specific and is the "gold standard" against which all new techniques must be measured. The relative efficiency with which the common human viruses can be isolated in cell culture systems is shown in Table 1. Appropriate choice of specimen and proper collection and transportation of such specimens to the laboratory are essential to viral diagnosis. Communication between laboratory personnel and clinicians is critical to ensuring that these processes are carried out properly.

General Principles

The first step in making a viral diagnosis is to decide the following: (*1*) Are viral studies warranted for this patient at this time? (*2*) If so, what specimens should be collected? (*3*) How should specimens be cared for until they reach the laboratory?

Since virus shedding may be of short duration, it is important to collect specimens early in illness. Virus is excreted or shed at its highest titer at this time, and quantities generally diminish as illness progresses. Thus, sampling late in the course of an illness may result in false-negative reports. Because nosocomial viral infections are reasonably common,[12] special care should be taken to collect specimens from the hospitalized patient as close to the time of admission as possible. The dilemma of whether a positive virus isolation should be attributed to the illness that required admission or to a nosocomially acquired infection is thus avoided.

Choosing the type of specimen to be collected is also important in viral diagnosis. In contrast to bacteriologic diagnosis, fluid specimens rather than swabs are inoculated onto cell mon-

TABLE 1. Relative Efficacy of the Viral Diagnostic Laboratory in the Isolation of Human Viral Pathogens

Viruses commonly and easily isolated by routine cell culture technique
Adenoviruses
Coxsackieviruses
type A (few types)
type B
Echoviruses
Herpes simplex virus types 1 and 2
Influenza viruses types A and B
Polioviruses
Vaccinia virus
Reovirus
Viruses more difficult to isolate by virtue of viral instability or requirement of specialized culture conditions
Cytomegalovirus
Measles virus
Mumps virus
Parainfluenzaviruses
Respiratory syncytial virus
Rhinovirus
Rubella virus
Varicella-zoster virus
Viruses best isolated in animal systems
Bunyaviruses
Coxsackievirus type A (most types)
Lymphocytic choriomeningitis virus
Orbivirus
Rabies virus
Togaviruses
Viruses that are only isolated by specialized laboratories
Coronavirus (some types)
Epstein-Barr virus
Coronavirus (most)
Virus of progressive multifocal leukoencephalopathy
Virus of subacute sclerosing panancephalitis
Hepatitis A
Rotavirus
Human immunodeficiency viruses
Viruses that cannot be isolated
Hepatitis B
Molluscum contagiosum
Human papillomavirus
Paravaccinia
Parvovirus
Norwalk-like viruses

olayers. Thus, if swab specimens are collected, the secretions and cells that adhere to the cotton or Dacron swab are eluted by vigorously agitating the swab in a fluid-transport medium, usually contained in a tube or a vial. On the other hand, specimens that are fluid by nature, such as urine or cerebrospinal fluid, are satisfactory as obtained from the patient. Solid specimens or those containing mucus such as sputum are processed by homogenizing in a glass tissue grinder in the presence of transport medium followed by centrifugation to obtain a fluid specimen.

Gross contamination of specimens with bacteria or fungi may result in the growth of the contaminating microorganisms in cell culture with destruction of the cell monolayers. To help minimize contamination, grossly contaminated specimens are usually centrifuged to remove bacteria, fungi, and cell debris before inoculation of cell cultures. In addition, both transport media and cell culture media usually contain broad-spectrum antibiotics for this purpose. A frequently used combination is penicillin, gentamicin, and amphotericin B.

Many viral transport media have been devised. Although they may differ from laboratory to laboratory, the basic elements are similar. One of the most widely used is veal infusion broth, although Hanks' or Earle's balanced salt solutions are satisfactory.[13] In either case, the medium is supplemented with antibiotics as indicated above, and a protein such as gelatin or albumin is added to stabilize virus and to preserve viral infectivity. Transport media should be stored in a refrigerator or freezer to maintain the antibiotic potency. Phenol red is often used as a pH indicator, giving viral transport media its characteristic pink color. Since viral transport media contain several potential allergens, instruments or swabs should not be immersed in transport media before obtaining specimens from patients. It should also be noted that the antibiotics generally contained in viral transport media make specimens placed in it unsuitable for the isolation of most other infectious agents, such as fungi, bacteria, mycoplasmas, and chlamydiae. Thus, it is often necessary to obtain more than one specimen from a single site if multiorganism etiology is suspected.

Many viruses are thermolabile, and a large decrease in the amount of virus in a specimen may occur even after storage for only a few minutes at room temperature. Optimally, specimens for virus isolation should be taken to the laboratory immediately after collection, because the delays in transportation often encountered in busy hospitals explain some of the inability to make a viral diagnosis. Either a special system that provides rapid transportation for specimens for viral diagnosis must be devised or, as is more often practical, specimens should be placed in wet ice (0°C) as soon as they are collected and until they arrive in the laboratory. If delay in delivery is unavoidable and will not exceed 24 hours, the specimens should be refrigerated (4°C); if delay will exceed 24 hours, the specimens should be frozen, preferably at −70°C. It should be remembered, however, that freezing and thawing reduces the infectivity of many viruses; thus, the yield is less frequent from specimens exposed to a freeze–thaw cycle. Repeated freezing and thawing should definitely be avoided.

Specimens

Respiratory Tract. Specimens from the respiratory tract are commonly collected for virus isolation procedures and include throat swabs and washings, nasopharyngeal swabs and washings, and sputum. Throat and nasal swabs must be placed in transport medium after collection. Such swabs when well collected are saturated with approximately 0.1–0.15 ml of secretions. In contrast, washings contain larger quantities of secretions, up to 1.0 ml and are superior for that reason for isolation of many viruses. Swab specimens may be preferred by patients because of familiarity with the technique; however, it should be noted that a vigorously applied swab may be more uncomfortable than a washing technique.

Some viruses, for example, rhinoviruses and respiratory syncytial virus, are best isolated from nasopharyngeal washings. On the other hand, a throat swab is the specimen of choice for the isolation of others, for example, adenoviruses and enteroviruses, probably because these viruses replicate to a greater extent in the pharynx than in the nose.[14,15] Unfortunately, the optimal specimen is not always easily obtained. An uncooperative patient or the lack of equipment often makes nasal washings or sputum difficult to obtain. Also, due to the multiple etiology of respiratory tract syndromes, the optimum specimen is not always easy to establish.[16] Probably the best compromise is a vigorously obtained nasopharyngeal swab specimen and a throat swab specimen that are then combined in a single container of transport medium. Fortunately, unlike the parallel situation in bacteriology and mycology, specimens from the upper respiratory tract can be quite useful in the diagnosis of lower respiratory infections. Isolation of a virus from the upper respiratory tract generally indicates recent infection, since shedding of most viruses from this site usually ceases 10–14 days after onset of illness. Subclinical infections occur, but shedding ceases after several days in these cases as well.[15,17–20] The only virus that can properly be called "normal flora" of the upper respiratory tract is herpes simplex virus in that it may be recovered from 5 percent of normal adults.[21]

Nasal swab specimens are collected by inserting a dry swab into the nares until resistance is met at the level of the turbinates, then swabbing the entire surface of the cavity at that level, and repeating the process on the other side. Throat swab specimens are best obtained with direct visualization and, without a tongue blade if possible, swabbing first one, then the other tonsil or tonsillar crypt, and finally the posterior pharyngeal wall with a dry swab. Gagging or coughing frequently ensues. Nasal washings are performed by instilling 5 ml of sterile saline (not containing antibiotics) into each nostril with the head hyperextended and the subject told not to swallow, then tilting the head forward, allowing the fluid to run out of the nares into a sterile container. Saline washes are then placed in an equal volume of viral transport media.[22,23]

Tissue. Virtually any type of tissue can be tested for the presence of viruses. The standard method of processing tissue consists of making a 10 percent suspension of tissue in cell culture medium, homogenizing it in a glass tissue grinder, sedimenting larger debris by centrifugation, and then testing the supernatant fluid for presence of viruses.[1,3,5,6] Whenever possible, at least 1 g of tissue should be sent to the laboratory, either hand-carried by the physician immediately or transported in a sterile container on wet ice. If tissues from several organs are sent for examination, each should be taken with a separate set of instruments and should be put into individual sterile containers. Large specimens can be transported intact, but if only a small amount of tissue can be obtained, care should be taken to keep it from drying out before it reaches the laboratory. This can be done by placing the specimen in a sterile Petri dish on a gauze wetted with saline or directly into a vial of transport medium. In some instances viruses are more easily isolated by outgrowth of the tissue itself (see "Cocultivation" and "Organ Culture" below). This special procedure is available in few institutions, and the laboratory should be contacted in advance.

Cerebrospinal Fluid (CSF). The diagnosis of viral meningitis or encephalitis is presumptive until virus is isolated from a central nervous system (CNS) source. Because of its diagnostic value, therefore, CSF should always be sent for viral culture in suspected cases of CNS infection. Controversy exists among virologists over the frequency of recovery of virus from the CSF. Some have reported poor rates of isolation,[17] while others detected virus in CSF more frequently.[24–26] The rate of isolation varies with the etiologic agent. Mumps virus, for example, is relatively easy to recover from CSF, and in one series was isolated in up to 77 percent of the cases examined.[27] On the other hand, herpes simplex virus, poliovirus, and many togaviruses are isolated only rarely from the CSF.[28–30] A major impediment to successful isolation frequently encountered by the laboratory is the small amount of CSF submitted. At least 1 ml is required for adequate testing. Since CSF is usually a bacteriologically sterile fluid, the specimen is generally tested unprocessed.

Feces. Fecal specimens for virus isolation have been recommended in a number of clinical situations, but, in fact, they are useful in very few. The viruses most commonly associated with viral gastroenteritis (rotavirus and Norwalk-like agents) cannot be isolated by conventional cultural methods.[31,32] Because virus is shed in stools for a long time after the onset of illness and after oropharyngeal excretion has ceased, fecal specimens have been said to be useful for the diagnosis of enteroviral aseptic meningitis, encephalitis, and pericarditis, and adenoviral pneumonia.[1,4,6] It is just this prolonged shedding, however, that minimizes the diagnostic value of the stool specimen isolate. For example, as many as 15–20 percent of well children sampled in the summertime, when enteroviruses are prevalent, may be found to be shedding these viruses in their stools.[29,33] Although generally not useful for diagnosis in the individual patient, stools and sewage have been used for surveillance of enteroviral activity in the community.[34] Either bulk stool or an anal swab specimen in viral transport medium can be sent for culture. In the former case, stool is homogenized in transport medium and centrifuged by the laboratory before inoculation of cell culture. Anal swabs are obtained by inserting a dry cotton or Dacron swab several centimeters in the anal canal, twirling it, and then eluting the absorbed material in transport medium. Like stool specimens, anal swab specimens are centrifuged before inoculation of cell cultures.

Vesicular Fluid and Lesion Swabs. The virus most commonly isolated from vesicular fluids and swabs of skin lesions is herpes simplex. It is easily isolated from such specimens taken in the early stages of the illness. Even later, when scabs have already formed, removal of the scab and vigorous rubbing of the vesicle base with a swab will occasionally lead to recovery of virus. Although not a common diagnostic problem, vaccinia virus is also readily isolated from swab specimens. On the other hand, coxsackieviruses, echoviruses, and varicella-zoster virus are generally more difficult to recover from such lesions, but recovery can be accomplished if proper technique is used. If infection with one of these agents is suspected, obtaining vesicular fluid rather than a swab specimen is recommended. Fluid should be obtained by puncturing the intact vesicle with a sterile needle, expressing the fluid through the puncture hole, and then drawing it up with a syringe or capillary pipette. The advantage of using a capillary pipette is that the amount of fluid obtained can be easily visualized. Even if the amount obtained may be too little to see when collected with a syringe, washing of the needle and syringe several times, by moving the plunger back and forth with the needle immersed in transport medium, will remove the fluid trapped in the needle. Although collection of vesicular fluid in transport medium is adequate for those viruses that are more difficult to isolate, direct inoculation into cell cultures is ideal and should be arranged with the laboratory if at all possible.

Eye. The most common causes of viral conjunctivitis are adenovirus and herpes simplex virus infections. Varicella-zoster, vaccinia, cytomegalovirus, and enterovirus 70 have also been isolated from ocular specimens. Conjunctival swabs or corneal scrapings may be used for isolation of viruses from the eye. Studies suggest that corneal scraping is superior for the isolation of herpes simplex virus, but these studies have not been extended to include other viruses.

Conjunctival swab specimens should be collected by placing a dry sterile swab in the lower medial conjunctival sac so as to occlude the nasolacrimal duct and waiting until the swab is saturated or nearly saturated with fluid. The swab is then placed in viral transport medium. Corneal scrapings should be obtained by an ophthalmologist or other experienced person with a sterile spatula, which is then washed off in viral transport medium. It should be remembered that viral transport media generally contain antibiotics and foreign protein and should not be introduced into the eye during the process of specimen collection.

Urine. Urine is commonly used only for the isolation of cytomegalovirus. It can be useful, as well, for isolation of mumps virus because urinary excretion often continues for weeks after oral excretion has ceased. Enteroviruses, adenoviruses, and herpes simplex have also been isolated from urine specimens, but generally these isolates represent contamination from fecal or genital sources. Adenovirus, however, has been cultured from the urine of patients with acute hemorrhagic cystitis and is thought to be etiologically related to this syndrome.

Clean-voided urine samples, collected in conventional containers, are satisfactory for virus isolation. Like other specimens, urine should be kept at 4°C until it can be delivered to the laboratory, but unlike other specimens, it should not be frozen, even if delivery is delayed.

Blood. Blood cultures are not commonly used in the diagnosis of virus infections, but recent studies suggest they may be quite useful, particularly in young children with enterovirus infection and in the immunocompromised host.[35–37] Buffy coat preparations, separated subpopulations of leukocytes, and serum have all been successfully used to demonstrate viremia in patients with a number of different virus infections. Depending on the virus sought, either serum or anticoagulated whole blood should be submitted to the laboratory for culture.

Other Specimens. Occasionally other specimens such as pleural fluid, semen, cervical secretions, and urethral secretions are submitted for viral culture. If sufficient fluid can be obtained, that fluid is a satisfactory specimen; if not, a swab can be used to absorb secretions and then can be immersed in transport medium.

Isolation and Identification. Viruses require living cells to support their replication. Several methods of using living cells for viral isolation are available: cell cultures, embryonated hen's eggs, and experimental animals. Cell culture is by far the most widely used technique.

Cell Cultures. Cell cultures, often inappropriately called tissue cultures, are initiated by dissociating tissue with proteolytic enzymes and chelating agents, generally trypsin and ethylenediamine-tetraacetic acid (EDTA), into a suspension of single cells. The dissociating agents are removed by centrifugation, and the cells are resuspended in cell culture medium that is basically a balanced salt solution containing glucose, vitamins, amino acids, antibacterial and antifungal agents, sodium bicarbonate as a buffer, and phenol red as a pH indicator. The suspended cells are placed in culture vessels, which for most diagnostic laboratories, consist of 130 × 15 mm screw cap tubes. The cells settle on and attach to the surface of the vessel and replicate, eventually forming a single layer (monolayer) of firmly adherent cells.

Cell cultures are divided into three general classes:

1. *Primary cultures*. These consist of cells derived directly from tissue (e.g., kidney, lung). They generally contain a mixed cell population of epithelial cells, fibroblasts, and trapped leukocytes.
2. *Semicontinuous cell cultures*. These are obtained by "splitting" (dissociating and dividing) or subculturing of primary cultures; epithelial cells and trapped leukocytes do not survive, so generally these cell populations consist of fibroblasts that are diploid and undergo a finite number of subpassages.
3. *Continuous cell cultures*. These are derived from malignant tissue that is generally epithelial in origin. They grow rapidly, are heteroploid, and can be subpassaged indefinitely.

Cell cultures can be prepared in the diagnostic laboratory or can be purchased from commercial sources. Most virus laboratories have available a primary monkey (rhesus, African green, or cynomolgus) kidney cell culture, a semicontinuous cell line such as WI-38 human embryonic lung fibroblast or human foreskin fibroblast, and one or more continuous cell lines such as KB human nasopharyngeal carcinoma, HeLa human cervical carcinoma. Hep-2 human epidermoid laryngeal carcinoma, or Madin–Darby canine kidney (MDCK). In addition, many also use primary human embryonic kidney cells. Each type of cell culture has its own spectrum of viral sensitivity, just as different bacteriologic media have differing selective and restrictive properties for growth of bacteria (Table 2).

Specimen Inoculation and Viral Effects. Based on clinical history, the clinician, in consultation with the virologist, decides which viruses may be responsible for the patient's illness (Table 3) and then selects and collects the appropriate specimen(s), as indicated in Table 4. The virologist selects for inoculation a combination of cell cultures with the appropriate sensitivity range (Table 2), and the cell cultures are inoculated with the fluid specimen. Viruses contained in the specimen are then free to attach to and to penetrate the cells and begin their replicative cycle. Depending on the viruses sought, the cultures are incubated for 7–21 days at either 33°C or 36°C. The cells are examined daily or every other day at a total magnification of 40×–100× using a conventional light microscope.

The presence of viral replication in cell cultures is tradition-

TABLE 2. Optimal System for Primary Isolation of Human Viral Pathogens

Virus Family	*Virus Type*	*Suckling Mouse*	*Embryonated Egg*	*Primary Monkey Kidney*	*Primary Human Embryonic Kidney*	*Semicontinuous Human Diploid*	*Continuous Human Heteroploid*
Picornaviridae	Rhinovirus		0	+	±	+ +	0 to + +
	Polioviruses 1–3	0	0	+ +	+ +	+ +	+ +
	Coxsackievirus A1–24	+ +	0	0 to + +[a]	0 to + +[a]	0 to + +[a]	0 to + +[a]
	Coxsackievirus B1–6	+ +	0	+ +	+ +	±	+ +
	Echovirus 1–32	0 to + +	0	+ +	+	+ +	0
						±	
Orthomyxoviridae	Influenza A, B, C	0	+ +	0 to + +	±	±	0
Paramyxoviridae	Parainfluenza 1,2,3,4	0	0	+ +	+	+	±
	Respirtory syncytial	0	0	+	+	+ +	+ +
	Measles	0	0	+	+ +	0	±
	Mumps	0	+ +	+ +	+ +	+	0
Adenoviridae	Adenovirus types 1–34	0	0	± to +	+ +	+	+
Herpesviridae	Herpes simplex	0	+ +	0 to + +	+ +	+ +	0 to + +
	Varicella-zoster	0	0	0	+	+ +	0
	Cytomegalovirus	0	0	0	0	+ +	0
Togaviridae	Rubella virus	0	0	+	+	0	0
	Eastern equine encephalitis	+ +	0	±		0	±
	Western equine encephalitis	+ +	0	+		0	+
	St. Louis encephalitis	+ +	0	0		0	+
Bunyaviridae	California encephalitis virus	+ +	0	0		0	+
Reoviridae	Rotavirus	0	0	0	0	0	0
	Colorado tick fever	+	0	0	0	0	0
Poxviridae	Vaccinia	+	+ +	+ +	+ +	+ +	+ +
Arenaviridae	Lymphocytic choriomeningitis	+ +	+ +	+ +	+ +	+ +	+ +

Key: 0: not suitable for isolation; ±: some strains may be recovered; +: many strains may be recovered; + +: most strains will be recovered.

[a] Coxsackievirus A-7, A-9, and A-16 strains grow well in cell culture.

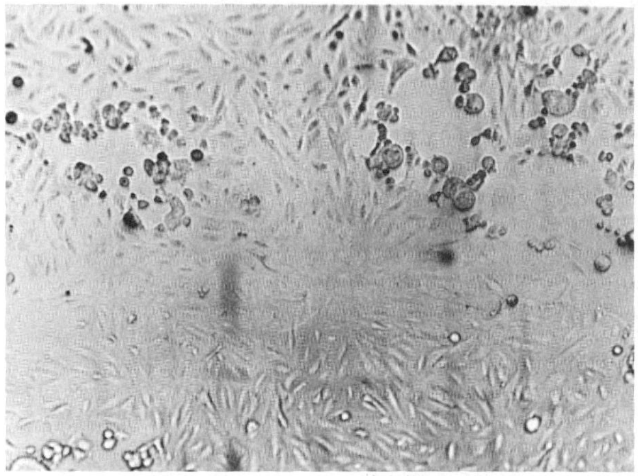

FIG. 1. Human embryonic kidney cell culture infected with herpes simplex. The focal rounding seen is the typical CPE of this virus. This photograph was taken 24 hours after inoculation of the cell culture with a specimen obtained from an ulcerative penile lesion.

ally detected in three ways: (*1*) by the observation of cytopathic effect (CPE), (*2*) by hemadsorption, and (*3*) by the use of interference. In addition, more recently, EM, immunoassays, and NAH (described in detail later in this chapter) have been applied to cell cultures to detect the presence of virus.

Cytopathic Effect. Cytopathic effect, generally a prelude to cell death, is an observable change that occurs in cells as a result of viral replication. Among the changes that occur are rounding, ballooning, syncytial formation, and clustering. The CPE of herpes simplex virus is illustrated in Figure 1. Because cells are examined live and unstained, if a suspected area of CPE is observed, the culture can be further incubated and reexamined for progression of the effect. The nature of the CPE, is rapidity of development, and the cell types in which it occurs all aid the virologist in identifying the putative virus. Some viruses exhibit such characteristic patterns of CPE that definitive identification can be based on CPE alone. For example, herpes simplex virus can often be identified on this basis.[38] Others, however, such as adenoviruses and picornaviruses, produce a CPE characteristic of the virus family, and serologic methods, which can take several weeks to complete, must be used for specific identification of virus type.[1–3,5,6] The tendency, especially among hospital-based laboratories, is to issue a preliminary report when definite CPE is observed, followed by a final report when serotyping is completed.

Hemadsorption. As well as examining cell cultures for the development of CPE at staggered intervals during the incubation period, a suspension of red blood cells (usually guinea pig) is added to selected cultures. Several viruses during their replicative cycle alter the cell membrane in such a way that red blood cells adhere firmly to it. When this phenomenon, called *hemadsorption*, is observed, the virologist issues a preliminary report stating that a hemadsorbing virus has been isolated. Specific serologic typing is then carried out, and a final report is issued. The commonly encountered hemadsorbing viruses include influenza virus types A and B, parainfluenza virus types 1, 2, and 3, and mumps virus.

Interference. Some viruses produce no CPE and cause no hemadorption in cell culture. Cells infected with these viruses, although they appear normal, are resistant to superinfection with certain other cytopathic viruses. This phenomenon, known as *interference,* is used by the diagnostic laboratory primarily for the detection of rubella virus. When interference is found, a preliminary report that an interfering virus has been isolated is issued; following serologic typing, a final report is sent.

Isolation of viruses in cell cultures can be achieved far more rapidly than is commonly appreciated. Table 5 summarizes some of our recent experience with the more frequently isolated virus types. As can be seen, a positive report can often be issued within several days of receipt of specimen.

Embryonated Hen's Eggs. Before the advent of cell cultures, embryonated hen's eggs were widely used for virus isolation. Because cell cultures provide a broader range of sensitivity (Table 2) and are easier to maintain, most laboratories have abandoned eggs in lieu of cell cultures. Even in the case of influenza virus, where embryonated hen's eggs were thought to be the optimal system for isolation, equivalent or superior rates of virus isolation from clinical specimens with A/H1N1 and A/H3N2 and B strains have been achieved using rhesus monkey kidney, cynomolgus monkey kidney, or MDCK cells.[39] There are three main routes of egg inoculation for virus isolation: (*1*) the allantoic cavity, (*2*) the amniotic cavity, and (*3*) the chorioallantoic membrane. Virus replication is recognized by the development of pocks on the chorioallantoic membrane,

TABLE 3. Viruses Associated with Different Categories of Disease

	Associated Virus	
Disease Category	*Common*	*Less Common*
Respiratory tract		
Upper respiratory infection (including common cold and pharyngitis)	Rhinoviruses Parainfluenza 1–3 Influenza A, B Herpes simplex Adenoviruses[a] Echoviruses[a] Coxsackieviruses[a] Epstein-Barr virus Respiratory syncytial	Coronaviruses Influenza C Parainfluenza 4 Echoviruses[b] Coxsackieviruses[b] Adenoviruses[b]
Croup	Influenza A, B Respiratory syncytial Parainfluenza 1–3	Measles Adenovirus[a]
Bronchiolitis	Respiratory syncytial Parainfluenza 1–3	Influenza A
Pneumonia (adults)	Influenza A	Adenovirus Herpes simplex[c] Varicella-zoster[c] Cytomegalovirus[c]
Pneumonia (children)	Respiratory syncytial Parainfluenza 1–3 Influenza A	Measles Varicella-zoster Adenovirus

(*Continued*)

TABLE 3. (Continued)

Disease Category	Associated Virus: Common	Associated Virus: Less Common
Central nervous system		
Aseptic meningitis	Mumps Coxsackievirus B1–5 Coxsackievirus A9 Echovirus 4, 6, 9, 11, 14, 18, 30, 31	Human immunodeficiency virus Other enteroviruses Herpes simplex 2 (adults) Lymphocytic choriomeningitis Varicella-zoster Many other viruses
Paralysis	Polio 1–3	Enterovirus 71 Coxsackievirus A7 Many other enteroviruses (rarely)
Encephalitis and encephalopathy	Human immunodeficiency virus Alphaviruses, Flaviviruses, Bunyaviruses (formerly arboviruses) Herpes simplex 1 Enterovirus 71 Mumps	Rabies Herpes virus B Enteroviruses (rarely) Polyomaviruses (BK and JC)[c]
Genitourinary tract		
Vulvovaginitis, cervicitis	Herpes simplex 2	Herpes simplex 1 Cytomegalovirus (?)[d]
Penile and vulvar lesions	Herpes simplex 2 Molluscum contagiosum Warts	Herpes simplex 1
Acute hemorrhagic cystitis	Adenovirus 11	Adenovirus 2, 21
Glomerulonephritis		Hepatitis B
Ocular		
Conjunctivitis	Adenovirus 3, 4, 7, 8, 19 Herpes simplex Varicella-zoster Enterovirus 70 Measles	Vaccinia Dengue Newcastle disease virus
Subacute opticoneuropathy	New herpetovirus (?)[d]	
Gastrointestinal tract		
Gastroenteritis	Rotavirus Norwalk-like viruses Adenoviruses	Enteroviruses (?)[d]
Hepatitis	Hepatitis A Hepatitis B Delta hepatitis virus Epstein-Barr virus Cytomegalovirus[c]	Herpes simplex[c] Arenaviruses Togaviruses (e.g., yellow fever)
Skin		
Maculopapular rash	Measles Rubella Parvovirus Echoviruses[a] Coxsackievirus[a]	Adenovirus Epstein-Barr virus Cytomegalovirus
Vesicular rash	Varicella-zoster Herpes simplex Coxsackievirus A16 Enterovirus 71	Vaccinia Coxsackieviruses A and B[a] Echovirus[a]
Hemorrhagic rash	Alphavirus, Bunyavirus, Flaviviruses[a] (formerly arboviruses)	
Localized lesions	Herpes simplex Warts Molluscum contagiosum Varicella-zoster virus	Cowpox Milker's nodule ORF
Neonatal		
Teratogenic effects	Rubella Cytomegalovirus	Others (?)[d]
Disseminated disease	Coxsackievirus B1–5 Echoviruses[a] Hepatitis B Parvovirus Cytomegalovirus	Varicella Herpes simplex Adenovirus
Lower respiratory disease	Respiratory syncytial Influenza	Adenovirus Measles Parainfluenza 1–3
Enteritis	Rotavirus	
Other		
Arthritis	Rubella Parvovirus Hepatitis B	
Myositis	Togaviruses Influenza B	Coxsackieviruses
Carditis	Coxsackievirus B	Other enteroviruses
Parotitis, pancreatitis, and orchitis	Mumps	Coxsackieviruses

[a] Several serotypes.
[b] Many serotypes.
[c] Particularly in the "compromised host."
[d] (?) Association questioned.

TABLE 4. Clinical Specimen(s) to Be Obtained for Viral Diagnosis

Disease Category	*Specimens that Should Be Taken Routinely*	*Specimens Also of Value*[a]	*Comment*
Respiratory tract	Nasal wash *or* throat wash *or* nasal/throat swab *or* sputum	Bronchial brush *or* wash, bronchoalveolar lavage transtracheal aspirate, lung biopsy	Urine if cytomegalovirus is suspected
Central nervous system			
Aseptic meningitis	Cerebrospinal fluid, throat swab, rectal swab	Urine (for mumps virus)	Adults should be examined for genital lesions (see genitourinary tract); whole blood should be obtained in cases of suspected toga and bunya viral meningitis
Encephalitis	Cerebrospinal fluid, throat swab, rectal swab	Brain biopsy, whole blood	
Genitourinary tract			
Vaginitis and cervicitis	Cervicovaginal swab		
Penile and vulvar lesions	Lesion swab		
Acute hemorrhagic cystitis	Urine	Throat swab, rectal swab *or* stool	
Ocular			
Conjunctivitis	Conjunctival swab *or* corneal scraping	Throat swab	
Gastrointestinal			
Gastroenteritis	Stool[b]		Most viruses associated with these syndromes not diagnosed by conventional isolation techniques; antigen detection and serologic techniques currently most useful for diagnosis
Hepatitis	Serum	Urine (for cytomegalovirus)	
Skin			
Maculopapular rash	Throat swab	Rectal swab *or* stool, urine	
Vesicular rash	Vesicular fluid	Throat swab, rectal swab *or* stool	
Hemorrhagic rash	Whole blood		
Localized lesions	Vesicular fluid *or* lesion swab		
Neonatal disease			
Teratogenic effects	Nasal/throat swab and urine		Virus isolation techniques generally more useful than serodiagnostic procedures for the diagnosis of neonatal disease
Disseminated disease	Cerebrospinal fluid, nasal/throat swab, urine, blood		
Lower respiratory disease	Stool *or* rectal swab, nasal/throat swab, urine		
Other			
Arthritis	Nasal/throat swab		
Myositis	Nasal/throat swab, rectal swab *or* stool		
Carditis	Throat swab, rectal swab *or* stool		
Parotitis, pancreatitis and orchitis	Throat swab, urine	Stool *or* rectal swab	

[a] Autopsy tissues may often be useful in cases of death thought to be associated with viral infection. The value of serodiagnostic procedures varies widely based on the agent sought. Always consider serodiagnositc procedures.
[b] If electronmicroscopy or other rapid diagnostic techniques are available.

by the development of hemagglutinins in the allantoic and amniotic fluid, and by death of the embryo.

Laboratory Animals. Laboratory animals, especially infant mice, were also widely used for virus isolation before the advent of cell cultures. Although they, too, have been largely supplanted by cell cultures, there are a number of viruses that are best isolated in laboratory animals, among them, many members of the Togaviridae and Bunyaviridae families, most of the 24 types of coxsackievirus A, and several members of the Arenaviridae family. Inoculated animals are observed for specific signs of disease or death. For some viruses, hemagglutinins can be extracted from infected tissues for serotyping. Others, once isolated in laboratory animals, can be adapted to growth in cell cultures and then serotyped. A few viruses remain, however, that can be serotyped only by using laboratory animals as the indicator system, an expensive and laborious procedure.

Cocultivation. Cocultivation consists of the incorporation of cells from a diagnostic tissue specimen into an already established cell culture. The established culture serves to support and maintain the viability of the cells under investigation and sometimes as an indicator for viral replication. This technique gained prominence after its successful use for the detection of SV40 virus in experimental tumors in animals and of measles virus in brain tissue of patients with subacute sclerosing panencephalitis.[40] It is now widely used by research laboratories attempting to demonstrate latent virus infection. Although most viral diagnostic laboratories do not routinely perform cocultivation techniques, some have the capabilities and attempt cocultivation on special request.

Organ Culture. Certain viruses (e.g., coronaviruses and rotaviruses), although they do not replicate in conventional cell monolayers, do replicate in tissue whose normal architecture has been preserved; such cultures are called *organ cultures*. Organ culture is accomplished by placing small fragments of organs (e.g., tracheal rings, intestinal rings) intact into cell culture medium. Specimens are then inoculated into the cell culture medium. Loss of ciliary function, histopathologic changes, electron microscopy, and serologic tests have all been used as measures of viral replication in organ culture. This technique is generally available only in specialized research laboratories.

Organ culture has also been used to reveal latent virus. The best known example of this is the demonstration of herpes simplex virus in sensory ganglia.[41] The ganglia are removed and placed intact in cell culture medium. Virus replication is assessed by removing aliquots of the medium in which the ganglion is being maintained and inoculating the aliquots onto indicator cultures.

TABLE 5. Rate of Development of Reportable Cytopathic Effect for Different Viruses[a]

Virus or Virus Group	*No. of Isolates Examined*	*Earliest Day of Positivity*	*Day ≥50% Cultures Positive*	*Day ≥90% Cultures Positive*
Adenoviruses	30	1	5	13
Cytomegalovirus	60	2	7	13
Enteroviruses (echovirus, coxsackievirus, poliovirus)	80	1	3	6
Herpes simplex virus	100	1	2	4
Influenza virus	80	1	3	5
Parainfluenza virus	30	3	7	14
Respiratory syncytial virus	40	3	7	14
Rhinovirus	20	2	6	14
Varicella-zoster virus	40	3	5	10

[a] Based on readings made daily for the first 7 days and every fourth day thereafter.

Practical Application of Virus Culture

Although more widely available than in the past, viral diagnostic laboratories are still not often present in hospitals. When they are, the frequency with which they are used generally increases rather rapidly, indicating that they can produce important diagnostic information. For example, at the Strong Memorial Hospital and Monroe County Department of Health Viral Diagnostic Laboratory in Rochester, New York, the number of specimens submitted for virus isolation has increased from 354 specimens in 1970 to approximately 6800 specimens in 1983. This laboratory serves as the only viral diagnostic facility serving a community of 750,000 people with 2500 hospital beds.

The frequency of isolation and spectrum of viruses isolated from clinical specimens in a current hospital diagnostic facility are illustrated in Table 6. In this laboratory, primary cynomolgus monkey kidney, primary human embryonic kidney, and human embryonic fibroblast cell cultures are used routinely. Hep-2 cells are added in the winter months, primarily for the detection of respiratory syncytial virus. The isolation rate achieved is affected by both the season and the type of specimen submitted. A broad spectrum of viruses can be obtained especially from specimens from the respiratory tract. Diagnostic laboratories differ significantly in their ability to isolate certain viruses, depending on experience and on the spectrum of cell cultures used. If a particular agent that is more difficult to isolate (Table 1) is being sought, the laboratory should be consulted about its experience with the agent.

Other Methods for Detection of Virus and Viral Components

Electron Microscopy. Many investigators recommend EM as a tool for rapid diagnosis. One advantage is that EM is more frequently found in hospitals than in the viral diagnostic laboratory. Using EM, viruses have been demonstrated by the direct negative-staining technique in a wide variety of specimens including spinal fluid, urine, tissue, stools, nasal secretions, and throat swabs.[42–47] A diagnosis can often be made within hours of receiving the specimen. Direct EM, however, has its limitations. It requires expensive equipment, highly trained technicians, and is only applicable to specimens in which a high density of intact virus (10^6 virions/ml of specimen or greater) are present. The sensitivity of direct EM can be increased by application of several techniques including ultracentrifugation, agar gel diffusion, and immune electron microscopy.[43,44,46] Immune EM can also be used for virus identification. Unfortunately, each of these methods is time-consuming and therefore cannot be used routinely.

Specimens for EM examination may also be embedded and sectioned, but because this technique is also quite time-consuming, only carefully selected specimens should be submitted. Cold gluteraldehyde is the most widely recommended fixative, but the herpesviruses, the viruses of progressive multifocal leucoencephalopathy (PML) and subacute sclerosing panencephalitis (SSPE), and adenoviruses, among others, have been successfuly demonstrated in formalin-fixed and even paraffin-embedded tissue. Figure 2 illustrates adenovirus particles in a lung specimen that had been formalin-fixed before EM study. Although tissue architecture is sometimes lost in suboptimally fixed specimens, viral morphologic characteristics are generally well preserved.

A valuable contribution of the EM to viral diagnosis has been the detection of viruses that are difficult or even impossible to culture by conventional methods. Examples include hepatitis A virus, a number of viruses associated with gastroenteritis including rotaviruses and Norwalk-like agents, the viruses of PML and SSPE, and wart virus.

Immunofluorescence. Detection of viral antigen in clinical specimens by immunofluorescence (FA) can be used to demonstrate infection with a number of viruses including respiratory syncytial virus, influenza viruses, parainfluenza virus, mumps virus, measles virus, rabies virus, herpesviruses, variola virus,, adenoviruses, rubella virus, and some togaviruses.[11,48] Both direct and indirect methods are used. In the direct test, specific antiserum is tagged with the fluorescein label. In the indirect test, an unlabeled, virus-specific antiserum is allowed to react with antigen, and fluorescein-labeled antibody to the specific antiviral antiserum is then added.

The great advantage of FA is speed; often results are available within a few hours of specimen collection. In practice, FA is

TABLE 6. Types of Virus Isolated from Clinical Specimens over a 1-Year Period (1980) by the Strong Memorial Hospital—Monroe County Health Department Virus Laboratory

Type of Specimen Submitted	*Number Submitted*	*Percentage Yielding Virus*	*Number and Type of Viruses Isolated*
Genital culture	1,149	27.8	304 Herpes simplex 15 Cytomegalovirus
Eye culture	76	9.2	5 Herpes simplex 2 Adenovirus
Urine and saliva	365	9.0	26 Cytomegalovirus 4 Enterovirus 2 Herpes simplex 1 Adenovirus
Fecal	630	12.9	55 Enterovirus 19 Adenovirus 4 Herpes simplex 2 Reovirus 1 Cytomegalovirus (22 Poliovirus)[a]
CSF	362	7.2	25 Enterovirus 1 Herpes simplex
Lesion culture and vesicular fluid (extragenital)	338	42.3	126 Herpes simplex 15 Varicella-zoster 2 Enterovirus
Respiratory tract culture	1,324	24.3	71 Influenza B 61 Enterovirus 44 Herpes simplex 39 Rhinovirus 28 Parainfluenza virus 27 Respiratory syncytial virus 24 Adenovirus 17 Cytomegalovirus 11 Influenza A (6 Poliovirus)[a]
Tissues and effusions	172	6.4	8 Herpes simplex 2 Cytomegalovirus 1 Enterovirus

[a] Presumed to be vaccine strain, not included in calculating percentage of specimens yielding virus.

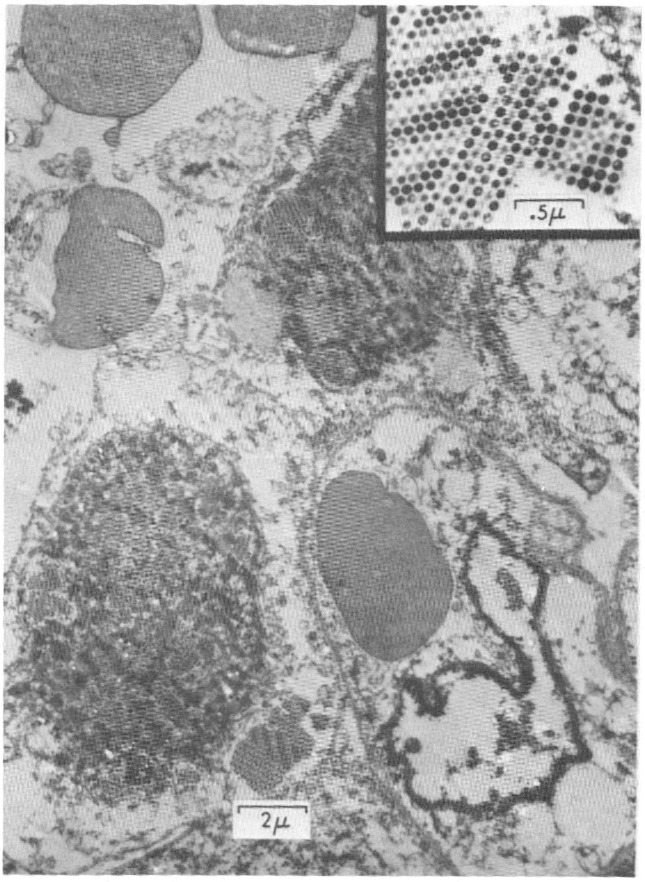

FIG. 2. Crystaline arrays of adenovirus particles seen in the lung of an infant with fatal adenovirus pneumonia. Although the tissue was fixed in formalin before preparation for electron microscopy, viral structure is well preserved.

very successful in the hands of experienced personnel, however, it does have some serious drawbacks. FA requires highly trained and experienced personnel to interpret the results. Although specific and sensitive when tested against virus grown in cell culture, there are problems of nonspecific absorption to leukocytes, mucus, and other materials in clinical specimens that make interpretation of results an "art." Finally, FA is dependent on collection of adequate numbers of intact infected cells rather than extracellular fluids containing viruses. This necessitates specialized specimen collecting and processing techniques, time-consuming for both the laboratory and those obtaining the specimens.

Immunohistochemical Assay. A modification of immunofluorescent staining using indicator antibody conjugated with an enzyme rather than a fluorescent tag has been developed.[49] After addition of the enzyme-labeled antibody, the appropriate substrate is added, and, if positive, a fixed color reaction develops that can be read with an ordinary light microscope. The advantages of this technique are that it does not require a fluorescent microscope and that fixed slides can be permanently mounted and kept indefinitely.

Radioimmunoassay. The first widespread application of RIA for the diagnosis of viral infections was for the detection of HBsAg. A number of RIA formats have been described, but the one most frequently used for antigen detection is the indirect solid-phase RIA.[50] The indirect solid-phase RIA uses the "sandwich" principle, in which test samples are added to plastic tubes or beads coated with a "capture" antibody directed against the antigen being sought. After a suitable incubation period, the sample is removed, and the tubes or beads are washed. Antibody to the antigen in question labeled with radioisotope (generally ^{125}I) is then added. Following a second incubation and washing step, the tubes or beads are counted in a gamma counter. The counts are compared with counts given by known negative specimens to establish a cut-off point for distinguishing negative from positive specimens.

The major advantage of RIA is its high degree of sensitivity. RIA never gained widespread acceptance by routine diagnostic laboratories for other than HBsAg detection. Lack of standardized commercially available reagents, high equipment costs, and instability of reagents are major contributing factors to the limited use of RIA in routine diagnosis. RIA has for the most part been replaced by ELISA for routine diagnostic purposes.

Enzyme-Linked Immunosorbent Assay. A relatively new technique, ELISA is similar in principle to the solid-phase RIA and is now widely used for the detection of both antibody and antigen in clinical specimens.[51,52] It makes use of enzyme-labeled rather than radioactively labeled reagents. Commonly used enzymes include peroxidase and alkaline phosphatase. Enzyme activity is easily assayed by color change, obviating the need for expensive radioactive counting equipment. Reagents are stable and relatively easy to standardize. Commercial ELISA kits are already available for the detection of several viruses including hepatitis B, rotavirus, and respiratory syncytial virus. The use of monoclonal antibodies has improved the sensitivity and specificity of current methods and led to the more widespread use of ELISA as a diagnostic tool.[53]

Nucleic Acid Technology

In recent years, nucleic acid techniques have been used to address a variety of problems in clinical microbiology. Although many methods remain research tools, a number are already in use in clinical laboratories. The general principles of such tests and their applications are summarized below.

Restriction Endonuclease Analysis. Restriction endonucleases are enzymes that recognize defined DNA nucleotide sequences and cleave viral nucleic acid at specific sites. Once cleaved, the fragmented viral genome can be separated on gels based on the fragment size. When identical patterns result, regardless of the number of enzymes used, the viruses under analysis are considered identical. Identity is more certain if it is established with a number of enzymes with different specificities.[54] Restriction enzyme analysis has been used to establish epidemiologic links among cases of viral infection[55] and to resolve questions surrounding the reactivation of latent infection and reinfection.[56]

Nucleic Acid Hybridization. Through the advances that have been made in recent years in the field of molecular biology, it is now possible to demonstrate viral nucleic acid as well as viral antigen in clinical specimens. The technique used, NAH, makes use of labeled, single-stranded DNA or RNA probes (specific viral nucleic acid sequences) for virus detection. The probe is applied to the clinical specimen, and hybridization takes place if a complementary strand of viral nucleic acid is present. A variety of hybridization techniques, including filter, Southern blot, Northern blot, and in situ hybridization are now in common use, and each exploits the technology in a slightly different way.[9]

Many viruses, including herpes simplex virus,[57] cytomegalovirus,[58] rotavirus,[59] papillomavirus,[60] and human immunodeficiency virus (HIV)[61] have been detected in clinical specimens by NAH techniques and at least one commercial NAH assay has already been approved for diagnostic use by the Food and Drug Administration. Like antigen detection methods, NAH is particularly useful for the diagnosis of viruses that cannot be readily grown in cell culture. Unfortunately, while NAH appears to be slightly more specific than antigen detection for the demonstration of viruses in clinical specimens, its sensitivity in most cases is comparable to antigen detection methods and significantly less than that of cell culture. The recent development of biotinylated (nonradioactive) probes has made NAH much more practical for use in the routine diagnostic laboratory.[62,63]

Polymerase Chain Reaction. PCR, first described in 1985, is a novel method for the *in vitro* amplification of specific DNA sequences.[64–66] In 1986 a modification of the technique (the thermolabile DNA polymerase initially used was replaced by the thermostable DNA polymerase *Taq*) greatly simplified the procedure and permitted automation of the reaction.[67] Now, within a few hours, a single viral DNA sequence in a clinical specimen can be amplified to over a million copies. The procedure involves repeated cycles of heat denaturation of the targeted DNA, annealing of the primers to their complementary sequences, and extension of the annealed primers with a DNA polymerase. The specificity of PCR is based on the selection of the viral oligonucleotide sequences used to prime the reaction. Once amplified, the product DNA can be detected and characterized by a variety of methods, including NAH and endonuclease restriction analysis.

The extraordinary sensitivity of PCR is also the basis for one of its limitations. Since even a single DNA sequence is amplified a million times during one reaction, contamination of the sample being examined even with minute amounts of DNA will create false-positive reactions. For this reason scrupulous care must be taken to avoid the introduction of extraneous DNA into the sample being examined.

Despite its very recent discovery, PCR has already been used to detect HIV-1,[68] HTLV-1,[69] and cytomegalovirus[70] in fresh clinical specimens. Concurrent infection with HIV-1 and HIV-2 has also been demonstrated.[71] In addition, PCR has also been used to detect human papillomavirus (HPV) DNA in thin sections of formalin-fixed, paraffin-embedded material, underscoring the power and flexibility of the technique.[72] Within the next few years, PCR will undoubtedly assume a prominent place in the clinical virology laboratory.

Virus Serology

In years past, serology was the primary laboratory means used to diagnose viral infections.[2] However, with the shift from remote diagnostic facilities to hospital-based laboratories, greater emphasis is now being placed on testing methods such as culture, EM, and antigen detection, which can provide results in time to influence patient management. Although serologic results are for the most part retrospective, there are still clinical situations in which they can be quite helpful.

General Considerations. A large number of tests and test formats are available.[1,3,5,6] The criteria used for interpreting results depend not only on the test used but also on the virus substrate. The best approach for detecting antibody to specific viruses should be sought in the chapters in Part III.

Clotted blood is the preferred specimens for all serologic tests. Whole blood can be refrigerated for several days; however, if a longer delay in sending the specimen to the laboratory is anticipated, the blood should be centrifuged and the serum should be frozen at −20°C. Anticoagulants should be avoided because they are incompatible with many serologic tests. CSF specimens can also be tested for virus-specific antibody, but, with the exception of measles titers in patients with subacute sclerosing panencephalitis, there is very little basis for interpreting the results. Any efforts to draw conclusions based on CSF antibody titers should take into account the integrity of the blood-brain barrier.[73]

Virus serology is often the preferred diagnostic method for viruses that are difficult to isolate in cell culture (Table 1). In addition, it may be a useful alternative to culture if optimal conditions of storage and transport of isolation specimens are not available.

Even in instances in which virus isolation in cell culture is more desirable, serology can contribute to a more accurate diagnosis by establishing the significance of an isolate. Some viruses such as cytomegalovirus and enterovirus can be shed for prolonged periods, and a rise in antibody titer strengthens the etiologic association with disease.

Virus serology can be used to diagnose acute infection and to determine immune status.

Diagnosis of Acute Infection. The serodiagnosis of viral infections is best accomplished by demonstrating a significant rise in antibody titer between sera collected during the acute phase of the patient's illness and convalescence. The acute serum should be collected as early as possible, and the convalescent specimen should be obtained 2–3 weeks later. The examiner risks missing a titer rise if sera are more closely spaced and may have difficulty determining when the infection occurred if the sera are taken too far apart. Test-to-test variation is common. Therefore, paired sera must be tested in parallel in the same test run. Results cannot be interpreted reliably unless this is done.

Traditional serologic tests (e.g., complement fixation) employ serial twofold dilutions of serum, and titers are expressed as the reciprocal of the highest serum dilution that produces a positive reaction. For such tests, a fourfold rise in titer is considered diagnostic. However, many of the newer serologic tests (e.g., ELISA) measure antibody concentration using a linear scale. The criteria for interpreting such tests are not yet standardized; therefore most laboratories provide an interpretation with the numerical test results.

In some cases, serodiagnosis can be accomplished by testing a single acute-phase serum. Virus-specific IgM appears early during primary infection, persists for a short time, and then declines to undetectable levels. Therefore, demonstration of specific IgM correlates well with primary infection. Many assay systems have been decribed for this purpose.[74–77] However, a number of factors limits the reliable interpretation of results.[75,77,78] Caution in the interpretation of results should always be exercised when using specific IgM tests as a diagnostic tool.

Immune Status Testing. In a number of clinical situations, knowing the immune status of a patient for a particular virus is important. Immunization with rubella vaccine is advised for all women of childbearing age with negative antibody titers unless, of course, they are pregnant. The cytomegalovirus antibody status of both donor and recipient is an important consideration in transplantation and blood transfusion in neonates.[79,80] Varicella-zoster immune status results are used to establish if exposed immunocompromised patients require passive immunization and to guide institution of infection control precautions.[81] Finally, the enormous consequences associated with a positive test for HIV have made the examination of sera for antibody to this virus the single most important test of immune status performed in the clinical laboratory. Sophisticated and extremely accurate protocols for determining the immune status of individuals to HIV are now in routine use throughout the world.[82]

The ideal antibody status test should be highly sensitive and highly specific; however, selecting for sensitivity sometimes compromises specificity and vice versa. The selection of the test that provides the appropriate balance between the two should be based on which is more undesirable from a clinical standpoint—a false-negative or a false-positive result.

RICKETTSIAE

Rickettsial diseases can be diagnosed serologically and by isolation of the organism. Because isolation is both hazardous to laboratory personnel and expensive, serodiagnostic methods are preferred. Isolation of rickettsiae is generally confined to reference laboratories and specialized research laboratories.

Although rickettsiae can be propaged in embryonated hen's eggs and some cell cultures, inoculation of adult male guinea pigs or adult white mice is the method of choice for the isolation of all known species of rickettsiae, save for *R. quintana,* which can be cultivated on artificial medium. Several animals per specimen are inoculated and observed daily for 14 days for signs of illness. On the second or third day of illness, one animal is sacrificed, a postmortem examination is performed, and smears are made for microscopic examination. *Rickettsia mooseri* and the members of the spotted fever group evoke scrotal edema and erythema in the guinea pig that may be useful in preliminary identification. Generally, however, postmortem examination reveals only mild peritonitis. Smears are made by touching the serosal surface of the spleen, the parietal peritoneum, and in the guinea pig, the tunica vaginalis to glass slides. The slides are stained either with analine dyes (Macchiavello or Giemsa stains) or with fluorescent antibody reagents. The organisms are found intracytoplasmically in serosal cells. Several passages in animals are often required before organisms can be detected with certainty. Inoculated animals are examined for evidence of seroresponse as well as for the presence of organisms.

Definitive identification of isolates can be established by complement-fixation and agglutination tests with specific antigens, in some cases by type-specific fluorescent antibody tests, and by toxin neutralization and cross-protection tests in mice.

A rickettsemia is associated with the early febrile period of all rickettsial infections in humans. For isolation attempts, 20–30 ml of clotted blood should be taken at this time. It is important that the blood be drawn before treatment with antibiotics. The serum and clot should be separated as soon as possible. The clot should be "snap" frozen in either a dry ice–alcohol bath or liquid nitrogen. Since loss of viability occurs at higher temperatures, storage at −70°C is recommended. The serum can be stored at 4–20°C for serodiagnosis. Tissue specimens should be taken aseptically and also "snap" frozen and stored at −70°C. Because of the unique epidemiology of rickettsial disease, information on the patient's travel history and possible exposure to vectors can aid the laboratory significantly.[83]

Immunofluorescence of skin specimens in cases of Rocky Mountain spotted fever may be positive as early as the third or fourth day of illness, and if the reagents are available, the diagnosis may be established in a few hours.[84]

CHLAMYDIAE

The increased emphasis on chlamydiae as etiologic agents of nongonococcal urethritis, cervicitis, and pelvic inflammatory disease in adults and of conjunctivitis and pneumonia in children as well as their well-recognized association with psittacosis and lymphogranuloma venereum has resulted in the widespread availability of diagnostic services for this class of organisms.[85] Although culture is still accepted as the most sensitive and specific technique for the laboratory diagnosis of chlamydia infections, immunodetection methods (direct fluorescent antibody [DFA] and ELISA) have supplanted the use of culture in many laboratories because such tests are in general more rapid, easier to perform, and less costly than culture.

A variety of cell cultures and methods can be used for the cultivation of chlamydiae.[85,86] The most commonly employed protocol includes inoculation of the clinical specimen into cyclohexamide-treated McCoy cells, centrifugation of the inoculum into the cell monolayer, and incubation of the culture for 2–3 days. Following the incubation period, chlamydiae are detected by examining the cell monolayer for cytoplasmic inclusions stained with either iodine, Giemsa, or immunofluorescent stains. The sensitivity of cell culture varies somewhat from laboratory to laboratory depending on the methods used, but, as with most other culture methods, the specificity is usually equal or close to 100 percent. Although cell culture is the most sensitive diagnostic test available, there is ample evidence that its sensitivity is not 100 percent. Therefore, a negative culture result does not reliably exclude infection.[85]

Many immunodiagnostic kits and reagents are now commercially available for the direct detection of clinical specimens of chlamydia antigens. Most use either a DFA or an ELISA format. For the DFA tests fluorescein-conjugated antibodies specific for *C. trachomatis* are used to stain smears prepared from the clinical specimen. The smears are then examined for elementary bodies (rather than inclusions) by a microscopist. The quality of the results obtained with DFA tests depends a great deal on the interpretative skills of the microscopist. ELISA tests for the direct detection of chlamydiae in clinical specimens are available in a variety of configurations for use in the clinical laboratory. In addition, very simple ELISA tests (similar in format to those described to detect rotavirus), which take only minutes to perform, have recently been approved by the Food and Drug Administration and are now being actively marketed for use in the office setting.[87] ELISA methods have the advantage of being far less subject to interpreter variation than DFA tests. Many studies of DFA and ELISA for the detection of *C. trachomatis* have been published, and most conclude that the sensitivity and specificity of the two methods are essentially equal and range from 70 to 95 percent and from 90 to 100 percent, respectively, relative to cell culture.[88–93]

MYCOPLASMAS

Mycoplasma and *Ureaplasma* species comprise the two genera of the family Mycoplasmataceae. Although many mycoplasma species have been isolated from humans, only three—*Mycoplasma pneumoniae, Ureaplasma urealyticum,* and *Mycoplasma hominis*—have been associated with disease.

Mycoplasma pneumoniae is well established as a cause of upper and lower respiratory tract disease, but the role played by *U. urealyticum* and *M. hominis* as human pathogens remains poorly defined. *Ureaplasma urealyticum* and *M. hominis* are frequently found in specimens obtained from the respiratory and genital tract both in the presence and absence of disease. In addition, *U. urealyticum* and *M. hominis* have been recovered from the blood of women with postpartum fever, from the lower respiratory tract, blood, and CSF of newborn infants, and from postoperative wound infections.[94–99]

Unlike most other organisms discussed in this chapter, mycoplasmas can be grown on artificial media. However, they are significantly more fastitidious than most bacteria, and the media used for their isolation must be supplemented with horse serum and yeast extract to assure growth. In addition, antibiotics and inhibitors must be added to the medium to prevent overgrowth by bacteria and fungi.

Unfortunately, no single medium can be used for the recovery of all mycoplasmas because of their heterogeneous growth requirements. The medium most frequently used for the recovery of *M. pneumoniae* is the diphasic medium (an agar layer covered by broth), SP-4.[100] Specimens are inoculated into the broth phase, and growth is indicated by a change in the pH of the fluid phase. The presence of *M. pneumoniae* is then confirmed by subculture of the broth phase to an agar plate and the observation of colonies with a typical morphology. Recovery of the organism usually takes 8–15 days. *Ureaplasma urealyticum* and *M. hominis* are less fastidious than *M. pneumoniae*. Consequently, they can be recovered on a variety of different media.[101,102] One, A-7, has been found useful for the recovery of both organisms and is presently the medium most widely used by clinical laboratories.[102] However, some investigators still prefer the use of two media to prevent overgrowth of *U. urealyticum* by *M. hominis*. *Ureaplasma urealyticum* and *M. hominis* are easily distinguished by their unique colonial morphology; they usually take 2–3 days to grow.

Mycoplasmas produce small characteristic colonies on agar, which are barely visible to the naked eye and are best seen using 40× –100× magnification. The organisms do not stain well with ordinary bacterial stains but can be stained with specialized mycoplasma stains (Dienes and Romanovksy).

Although definitive identification of *Mycoplasma* species is established by serologic methods, *M. pneumoniae* can be tentatively identified by its ability (*1*) to grow in the presence of methylene blue under aerobic conditions, (*2*) to rapidly hemolyze guinea pig erythrocytes, and (*3*) to adsorb guinea pig erythrocytes. The serologic methods used for definitive identification of mycoplasmal isolates include growth inhibition (the most widely used), immunofluorescence, and metabolic inhibition.

Recently, NAH technology has been applied to the detection of *M. pneumoniae* in clinical specimens with some success.[103] The major advantage offered by this technique is the speed with which the diagnosis can be made.

Specimens for *Mycoplasma* isolation are best collected in veal infusion broth containing no antibiotics, in contrast to the transport medium used for viral isolation procedures. If the broth is kept cold during transport to the laboratory, growth of bacteria is minimized, and the specimen may be used for the isolation of viruses and other organisms. If, however, there is a risk that specimens will remain at room temperature for prolonged periods, thallium acetate and/or penicillin should be added to the medium to prevent bacterial overgrowth. For best results specimens should be tested soon after they are obtained; if this cannot be done, they should be frozen and stored at −70°C until such tests can be performed.

REFERENCES

1. Grist NR, Ross CA, Bell EJ, et al. Diagnostic Methods in Clinical Virology. 2nd ed. Oxford: Blackwell; 1974.
2. Herrmann EC Jr. The tragedy of viral diagnosis. Postgrad Med. 1970;46:545.
3. Hsuing GD. Diagnostic Virology: An Illustrated Handbook. 3rd ed. New Haven: Yale University Press; 1982.
4. Timbury M. Notes on Medical Virology. 7th ed. Edinburgh: Churchill Livingstone; 1983.
5. Lennette EH. Manual of Clinical Microbiology. 4th ed. Washington, DC: American Society for Microbiology; 1985.
6. Lennette EH, Schmidt NJ. Diagnostic Procedures for Viral and Rickettsial Infections. 5th ed. New York: American Public Health Association; 1979.
7. World Health Organization. Rapid laboratory techniques for the diagnosis of virus infections. WHO Tech Rep Ser. 1981;661.
8. Atanasiu P, Avrameas S, Beale J, et al. Progress in the rapid diagnosis of viral infections: A memorandum. Bull WHO. 1978;56:241–4.
9. Zwadyk P Jr, Cooksey RC. Nucleic acid probes in clinical microbiology. Clin Lab Sci. 1987;25:71.
10. McIntosh K, Wilfert C, Chernesky M, et al. Summary of a workshop on new and useful methods in viral diagnosis. J Infect Dis. 1980;142:793–802.
11. Gardner PS. Rapid viral diagnosis. J Gen Virol. 1977;36:1–28.
12. Douglas RG Jr, Betts RF, Hruska JF, et al. Epidemiology of nosocomial viral infections. In: Weinstein L, ed. Seminars in Infectious Disease. New York: Stratton Intercontinental; 1979.
13. Baxter BD, Couch RB, Greenberg SB, et al. Maintenance of viability and comparison of identification methods for influenza and other respiratory viruses of humans. J Clin Microbiol. 1977;6:19–22.
14. Jackson GG, Muldoon RL. Viruses Causing Common Respiratory Infections in Man. New York: University of Chicago Press; 1975.
15. Wenner HA, Behbehani AM. Echoviruses. In: Gard S, Hallaner C, Meyer KF, eds. Virology Monographs 1. New York: Springer-Verlag; 1968.
16. Report of a WHO Scientific Group. Respiratory viruses. WHO Tech Rep Ser. 1969;408.
17. Herrmann EC Jr, Herrmann JA. Laboratory diagnosis of viral disease. In: Drew WL, ed. Viral Infections. Philadelphia: FA Davis; 1976:23–45.
18. Douglas RG Jr, Cate TR, Gerone PJ, et al. Quantitative rhinovirus shedding patterns in volunteers. Am Rev Respir Dis. 1966;94:159–67.
19. Knight V, Kasel JA. Influenza. In: Knight V, ed. Viral and Mycoplasmal Infections of the Respiratory Tract. Philadelphia: Lea & Febiger; 1973:87–123.
20. Hall CB, Douglas RG Jr, Geiman JM. Quantitative shedding patterns of respiratory syncytial virus in infants. J Infect Dis. 1975;132:151–6.
21. Douglas RG Jr, Couch RB. A prospective study of chronic herpes simplex virus infection and recurrent herpes labialis in humans. J Immunol. 1970;104:289–95.
22. Cate TR, Couch RB, Johnson KM. Studies with rhinoviruses in volunteers: production of illness, effect of naturally acquired antibody and determination of a protective effect not associated with serum antibody. J Clin Invest. 1964;43:56–67.
23. Hall CB, Douglas RG Jr. Clinically useful method for the isolation of respiratory syncytialvirus. J Infect Dis. 1975;131:1–5.
24. Haynes RE, Cramblett HG, Kronfol HJ. Echovirus 9 meningoencephalitis in infants and children. JAMA. 1969;208:1657–60.
25. Chonmaitree T, Menegus MA, Powell KR. The clinical relevance of "CSF viral culture." JAMA. 1982;247:1843–47.
26. Lake AM, Lauer BA, Clark JC, et al. Enterovirus infections in neonates. J Pediatr. 1976;89:787–91.
27. Wolontis S, Bjorvatn B. Mumps meningoencephalitis in Stockholm, November 1964–July 1971. Scand J Infect Dis. 1973;5:261–71.
28. Johnson RT, Olson LC, Buescher EL. Herpes simplex infections of the nervous system: problems in laboratory diagnosis. Arch Neurol. 1968;18:260–4.
29. Melnick JL. Enteroviruses. In: Evans AS, ed. Viral Infections of Humans. New York: Plenum; 1982;187–251.
30. Downs WB. Arboviruses. In: Evans AS, ed. Viral Infections of Humans. New York: Plenum; 1982;95–126.
31. Cukor G, Blacklow NR. Human viral gastroenteritis. Microbiol Rev. 1984;48:157–79.
32. Madeley CR. Viruses and diarrhoea: problems of proving causation. In: de la Maza LM, Peterson EM, eds. Medical Virology II. New York: Elsevier Biomedical; 1983;81–109.
33. Kepfer PD, Hable KA, Smith TF. Viral isolation rates during summer from children with acute upper respiratory tract disease and healthy children. Am J Clin Pathol. 1974;61:1–5.
34. Lund E, Hedström C-E, Strannegord O. A comparison between virus isolations from sewage and from fecal specimens from patients. Am J Epidemiol. 1966;84:282–66.
35. Prather SL, Jenista JA, Menegus MA. The isolation of nonpolio enteroviruses from serum. Diagn Microbiol Infect Dis. 1984;2:353–7.
36. Murray DL, Zonana J, Seidel JS, et al. Relative importance of bacteremia and viremia in the course of acute fevers of unknown origin in outpatient children. Pediatrics. 1981;68:157–60.
37. Howell CL, Miller MJ, Martin WJ. Comparison of rates of virus isolation from leukocyte subpopulations separated from blood by conventional and Ficoll-Paque/macrodex methods. J Clin Microbiol. 1979;10:533–7.
38. Herrmann EC Jr. Experiences in the laboratory diagnosis of herpes simplex, varicella-zoster, and vaccinia virus infections in routine medical practice. Mayo Clin Proc. 1967;42:744–53.
39. Frank AL, Couch RB, Griffis CA, et al. Comparison of different tissue cultures for isolation and quantitation of influenza and parainfluenza viruses. J Clin Microbiol. 1979;10:32–6.
40. Horta-Barbosa L, Fuccilo DA, Sever JL, et al. Subacute sclerosing panencephalitis: isolation of measles virus from a brain biopsy. Nature. 1969;221:974.
41. Stevens JG, Cook ML. Latent herpes simplex virus in the spinal ganglia of mice. Science. 1971;173:843–5.
42. Chernesky MA. The role of electronmicroscopy in diagnostic virology. In: Lennette D, Specter S, Thompson K, eds. Diagnosis of Viral Infections: The Role of the Clinical Laboratory. Baltimore: University Park Press; 1979;125–42.
43. Doane FW, Anderson N. Electron and immune electron microscopic procedures for diagnosis of viral infections. In: Kurstak E, Kurstak C, eds. Comparative Diagnosis of Viral Diseases. New York: Academic Press; 1977:2:505–39.
44. Hsuing GD, Fong CKY, August MJ. The use of electronmicroscopy for the diagnosis of virus infections: an overview. In: Melnick JL, ed. Progress in Medical Virology. Basal: S Karger; 1979:25:133–59.
45. Almeida JD. Practical aspects of diagnostic electron microscopy. Yale J Biol Med. 1980;53:5–25.
46. Field AM. Diagnostic virology using electron microscopic technique. In: Lauffer MA, Maramorosch K, Bang FB, et al., eds. Advances in Virus Research. New York: Academic Press; 1982:7:1–69.
47. Yunis EJ, Hashida Y, Haas J. The role of electronmicroscopy in the identification of viruses in human disease. In: Sommers SC, Rosen PP, eds. Pathology Annual. New York: Appleton-Century-Crofts; 1977:311–30.
48. Gardner PS, McQuillin J. Rapid Virus Diagnosis. London: Butterworths; 1974.
49. Nakane PK. Recent progress in the perioxidase-labeled antibody method. In: Hijmans W, Schaeffer M, eds. Fifth International Conference on Immunofluorescence and Related Staining Techniques. Ann NY Acad Sci. 1975;254:203–11.
50. Halonen P, Meurman O. Radioimmunoassay in diagnostic virology. In: Howard CR, ed. New Developments in Practical Virology. New York: Alan R Liss, Inc; 1982;83–124.

51. Voller A, Bidwell DE, Bartlett A. ELISA techniques in virology. In: Howard CR, ed. New Developments in Practical Virology. New York: Alan R Liss; 1982;59–81.
52. Avrameas S. Enzyme immunoassays and related techniques: Development and limitations. In: Bachman PA, ed. Current Topics in Microbiology and Immunology: New Developments in Diagnostic Virology. Berlin: Springer-Verlag; 1983;93–9.
53. Yolken RH. Use of monoclonal antibodies for viral diagnosis. In: Bachman PA, ed. Current Topics in Microbiology and Immunology: New Developments in Diagnostic Virology. Berlin: Springer-Verlag; 1983;177–95.
54. Wilhelm JM. Introduction to methods or characterization of viruses and viral macromolecules. In: Belshe RB, ed. Textbook of Human Virology. Littleton, MA: PSG Publishing Co; 1984;29–48.
55. Buchman TG, Roizman B, Adams G, et al. Restriction endonuclease fingerprinting of herpes simplex virus DNA: a novel epidemiological tool applied to a nosocomial outbreak. J Infect Dis. 1978;138:488–98.
56. Yow MD, Lakeman AD, Stagno S, et al. Use of restriction enzymes to investigate the source of a primary cytomegalovirus infection in a pediatric nurse. Pediatrics. 1982;70:713–6.
57. Redfield DC, Richman DD, Albinil S, et al. Detection of herpes simplex virus in clinical specimens by DNA hybridization. Diagn Microbiol Infect Dis. 1983;1:117–28.
58. Chou S, Merrigan TC. Rapid detection and quantitation of human cytomegalovirus in urine through DNA hybridization. N Engl J Med. 1983;308:921–5.
59. Flores J, Goeggeman E, Purcell RH, et al. A dot hybridization assay for detection of rotavirus. Lancet. 1983;1:55–7.
60. Lörincz AT. Detection of human papillomavirus infection by nucleic acid hybridization. In: Reid R, ed. Obstetrics and Gynecology Clinics of North America. Philadelphia: WB Saunders; 1987;14:451–69.
61. Pezzella M, Pezzella F, Galli C, et al. In situ hybridization of human immunodeficiency virus (HTLV-III) in cryostat sections of lymph nodes of lymphadenopathy syndrome patients. J Med Virol. 1987;22:135–42.
62. Langer PR, Waldrop AA, Ward DC. Enzymatic synthesis of biotin-labeled polynucleotides. Novel nucleic acid affinity probes. Proc Natl Acad Sci USA. 1981;78:6633–7.
63. Leary JJ, Brigati DJ, Ward DC. Rapid and sensitive colorimetric method for visualizing biotin-labeled DNA probes hybridized to DNA or RNA immobilized on nitrocellulose: bioblots. Proc Natl Acad Sci USA. 1983;80:4045–9.
64. Marx JL. Multiplying genes by leaps and bounds. Science. 1988;240:1408.
65. Erlich HA, Gelfand DH, Saiki RK. Specific DNA amplification. Nature. 1988;331:461–2.
66. Schochetman G, Ou CY, Jones W. Polymerase chain reaction. J Infect Dis. 1988;158:1154–7.
67. Saiki RK, Gelfand DH, Stoffel S, et al. Primer-directed enzymatic amplification of DNA with a thermostable DNA polymerase. Science. 1988;239:487–91.
68. Ou CY, Kwok S, Mitchell SW, et al. DNA amplification for direct detection of HIV-1 in DNA of peripheral blood mononuclear cells. Science. 1988;239:295–7.
69. Kwok S, Ehrlich G, Poiesz B, et al. Enzymatic amplification of HTLV-1 viral sequences from peripheral blood mononuclear cells and infected tissues. Blood. 1988;72:1117–23.
70. Demmler GJ, Buffone GJ, Schimbor CM, et al. Detection of cytomegalovirus in the urine of newborns by using polymerase chain reaction amplification. J Infect Dis. 1988;1177–84.
71. Rayfield M, DeCock K, Heyward W, et al. Mixed human immunodeficiency virus (HIV) infection of an individual: demonstration of both HIV type 1 and type 2 proviral sequences by using polymerase chain reaction. J Infect Dis. 1988;158:1170–6.
72. Shibata DK, Arnheim N, Martin WJ. Detection of human papilloma virus in paraffin-embedded tissue using the polymerase chain reaction. J Exp Med. 1988;167:225–30.
73. Eickhoff K, Heipertz R. Discrimination of elevated immunoglobulin concentrations in CSF due to inflammatory reaction of the central nervous system and blood-brain-barrier dysfunction. ACTA Neurol Scand. 1977;56:475–82.
74. Ziegler DW. Determination of IgM antibodies in diagnostic virology. In: Lennette D, Specter S, Thompson D, eds. Diagnosis of Viral Infections: The Role of the Clinical Laboratory. Baltimore: University Park Press; 1979:63–73.
75. Schmidt NJ. Application of class-specific antibody assays to viral serodiagnosis. Clin Immunol Newsl. 1980;1:1–3.
76. Handsher R, Fogel A. Modified staphylococcal absorption method used for detecting rubella-specific immunoglobulin M antibodies during a rubella epidemic. J Clin Microbiol. 1977;5:588–92.
77. Herrmann, KL. Problems associated with immunoglobulin M detection in the diagnosis of acute viral infections. In: Schlessinger D, ed. Microbiology. Washington, DC: American Society for Microbiology; 1981;280–9.
78. Salonen EM, Vaheri A, Suni J, et al. Rheumatoid factor in acute viral infections: interference with determination of IgM, IgG, and IgA antibodies in an enzyme immunoassay. J Infect Dis. 1980;142:250–5.
79. Stagno S, Pass RF, Reynolds DW, et al. Comparative study of diagnostic procedures for congenital cytomegalovirus infection. Pediatrics. 1980;65:251–7.
80. Yeager AS, Grumet FC, Hafleigh EB, et al. Prevention of transfusion acquired cytomegalovirus infection in new born infants. J Pediatr. 1981;98:281–7.
81. Grandien M, Appelgren P, Espmark A, et al. Determination of varicella immunity by the indirect immunofluorescence test in urgent clinical situations. Scand J Infect Dis. 1976;8:65–9.
82. Hausler WJ Jr. Report of the third consensus conference on HIV testing sponsored by the association of state and terratorial public health laboratory directors. Infect Control Hosp Epidemiol. 1988;9:345–9.
83. Elisberg BL, Bozeman FM. Rickettsiae. In: Lennette EH, Schmidt NJ, eds. Diagnostic Procedures for Viral and Rickettsial Infections. 5th ed. New York: American Public Health Association; 1979;1061–108.
84. Woodward TE, Pederson CE Jr, Oster CN, et al. Prompt confirmation of Rocky Mountain spotted fever: identification of rickettsiae in skin tissues. J Infect Dis. 1976;134:297–305.
85. Batteiger BE, Jones RB. Chlamydial infections. Infect Dis Clin North Am. 1987;1:55–81.
86. Clyde WA Jr, Kenny GE, Schacter J. Laboratory diagnosis of chlamydial and mycoplasmal infections. In: Drew WL, ed. Cumitech 19. Washington, DC: American Society for Microbiology; 1984;1–5.
87. Chernesky M, Castriciano S, Mahony J, et al. Ability of Testpack Rotavirus enzyme immunoassay to diagnose rotavirus gastroenteritis. J Clin Microbiol. 1988;26:2459–61.
88. Chernesky MA, Mahony JB, Castrciano S, et al. Detection of *Chlamydia trachomatis* antigens by enzyme immunoassay and immunofluoresence in genital specimens from symptomatic and asymptomatic men and women. J Infect Dis. 1986;154:141–8.
89. Lipkin ES, Moncada JV, Shafer MA et al. Comparison of monoclonal antibody staining and culture in diagnosing cervical chlamydial infection. J Clin Microbiol. 1986;23:114–7.
90. Tilton RC, Judson FN, Barnes BC, et al. Multicenter comparative of two rapid microscopic methods and culture for detection of *Chlamydia trachomatis* in patient specimens. J Clin Microbiol. 1988;26:167–9.
91. Forbes BA, Bartholomoa N, McMillan J, et al. Evaluation of a monoclonal antibody test to detect chlamydia in cervical and urethral specimens. J Clin Microbiol. 1986;23:1136–7.
92. Quinn TC, Warfield P, Kappus E, et al. Screening for *Chlamydia trachomatis* infection in an inner city population: a comparison of diagnostic methods. J Infect Dis. 1984;152:419–23.
93. Stamm WE, Tam M, Koester M, et al. Diagnosis of *Chlamydia trachomatis* infections by direct immunofluoresence staining of genital secretions: a multi-center trial. Ann Intern Med. 1984;101:638–41.
94. Moller BR. The role of mycoplasmas in the upper genital tract of women. Sex Transm Dis. 1983;10:281–4.
95. Mufson MA. *Mycoplasma hominis*: a review of its role as a respiratory tract pathogen of humans. Sex Transm Dis. 1983;10:335–40.
96. Taylor-Robinson D, McCormack WM. Medical progress: the genital mycoplasmas. N Engl J Med. 1980;302:1003–10,1063–7.
97. Cassell GH, Cole BC. Mycoplasmas as agents of human disease. N Engl J Med. 1981;304:80–9.
98. Murray HW, Masur H, Senterfit LB, et al. The protean manifestations of *Mycoplasma pneumoniae* infection in adults. Am J Med. 1975;58:229–42.
99. Kenny GE. Mycoplasmas: In: Lennette EH, Balows A, Hausler WJ Jr, Shadomy HJ, eds. Manual of Clinical Microbiology. Washington, DC: American Society for Microbiology; 1985;407–11.
100. Tulley JG, Rose DL, Witcomb RF, et al. Enhanced isolation of *Mycoplasma pneumoniae* from throat washings with a newly modified culture medium. J Infect Dis. 1979;139:478–82.
101. Phillips LE, Goodrich KH, Turner RM, et al. The isolation of *Mycoplasma* species and *Ureaplasma urealyticum* from obstetrical and gynecological patients by using commercially available medium formulations. J Clin Microbiol. 1986;24:377–9.
102. Yajko DM, Balston E, Wood D, et al. Evaluation of PPLO, A7B, E, and NYC agar media for the isolation of *Ureaplasma urealyticum* and *Mycoplasma* species from the genital tract. J Clin Microbiol. 1984;19:73–6.
103. Dular R, Kajioka R, and Kasatiya S. Comparison of Gen-Probe commercial kit and culture technique for the diagnosis of *Mycoplasma pneumoniae* infection. J Clin Microbiol. 1988;26:1068–9.

SECTION E. ANTI-INFECTIVE THERAPY

15. PRINCIPLES OF ANTI-INFECTIVE THERAPY

ROBERT C. MOELLERING, JR.

Although the discovery of effective agents to prevent and treat infection caused by bacteria and other pathogenic microorganisms is one of the most important developments of modern medicine, the use of such agents has not been limited to the present era. Substances with anti-infective potential have been applied medically for thousands of years. Indeed, more than 2500 years ago the Chinese were aware of the therapeutic properties of moldy soybean curd applied to carbuncles, boils, and other infections,[1] and the ancient Greek physicians, including Hypocrates, routinely used substances with antimicrobial activity including wine, myrrh, and inorganic salts in their treatment of wounds.[2] Until the discovery of the microbiologic basis of infections in the nineteenth century, however, the therapy for infections remained strictly empirical. Heavy metals such as arsenic and bismuth were found to be useful against a number of infections including syphilis in the early 1900s; but the modern era of chemotherapy did not really begin until the discovery and initial clinical use of the sulfonamides in 1936.[1] This was followed in the 1940s by the discovery of the therapeutic value of penicillin and streptomycin, and by 1950 the "golden age" of antimicrobial chemotherapy was well underway.

It is the result of the relatively recent work in this area since 1936 that forms the basis for this and each of the succeeding chapters on anti-infective therapy. The major emphasis in this chapter is on antibacterial agents because there are more data available on these drugs. However, many of the principles to be discussed can also be applied to the use of antifungal, antiviral, and to some extent, antiparasitic drugs.

CHOICE OF THE PROPER ANTIMICROBIAL AGENT

In choosing the appropriate antimicrobial agent for therapy for a given infection, a number of important factors must be considered. First, the identity of the infecting organism must be known, or at the very least, it must be possible to arrive at a reasonable statistical guess as to its identity on the basis of clinical information. Second, we must have as accurate information as possible about the antimicrobial susceptibility (or potential susceptibility) of the infecting organism. Finally, a series of so-called host factors must be taken into consideration to arrive at the optimal choice of antimicrobial agent. Each of these items will be considered in this section.

Identification of the Infecting Organism

Several methods for the rapid identification of pathogenic bacteria in clinical specimens are available. A Gram stain preparation is perhaps the simplest, least expensive, and most useful of all the "rapid methods" of identification of bacterial (and some fungal) pathogens. This technique can be used to identify the presence and morphologic features of microorganisms in body fluids that are normally sterile (cerebrospinal fluid, pleural fluid, synovial fluid, peritoneal fluid, urine). On occasion, Gram staining of a buffy coat preparation of blood will reveal phagocytosed organisms in the polymorphonuclear leukocytes of patients with bacteremia or fungemia. Similar preparations of sputum will also be helpful in revealing the nature of the infecting organism in patients with bacterial bronchitis or pneumonia. Gram stain of a stool specimen may also produce useful information. In patients with staphylococcal enterocolitis, the Gram stain reveals sheets of gram-positive cocci replacing the normal stool flora. The presence of polymorphonuclear leukocytes in the stool also provides a helpful clue to the cause of certain cases of diarrhea. Polymorphonuclear leukocytes are not found in normal stools. When present, they suggest the possibility of a bacterial gastroenteritis such as shigellosis, salmonellosis, or campylobacteriosis, or invasive *Escherichia coli* gastroenteritis. Polymorphonuclear leukocytes are not found in the stools of patients with viral gastroenteritis, food poisoning, cholera, and diarrhea due to noninvasive toxigenic *E. coli*.[3] *Campylobacter* may be identified in the stools of patients by its characteristic gull-wing appearance on smears of stool.[4]

Immunologic methods for antigen detection (such as enzyme-linked immunoabsorbent assay [ELISA] or latex agglutination) may also provide clues for the rapid identification of the infecting pathogens. Final and definitive identification of pathogenic organisms usually requires cultural techniques. It is thus imperative that appropriate specimens be obtained for culture before beginning antimicrobial therapy. Once anti-infective therapy has been started, cultures often are rendered sterile, even though viable organisms remain in the host.

In most cases, it may be impossible to determine the exact nature of the infecting organisms before the institution of antimicrobial therapy. In these cases the use of bacteriologic statistics may be particularly helpful.[5,6] The term *bacteriologic statistics* refers to the application of knowledge of the organisms most likely to cause infection in a given clinical setting. For example, a person with normal host defense mechanisms who develops cellulitis of the arm after a minor abrasion most likely has an infection due to *Staphylococcus aureus* or group A streptococci, and antimicrobial therapy should be tailored accordingly, even though there is no material available for examination with Gram stain. Similarly, a young child with acute otitis media almost certainly has an infection due to either a virus or to one of four major bacterial pathogens: *Haemophilus influenzae, Streptococcus pneumoniae, Branhamella catarrhalis,* or a group A streptococcus.

Determination of Antimicrobial Susceptibility of Infecting Organisms

Since different organisms vary in their susceptibility to antimicrobial agents, it is imperative that we have some means for determining the antimicrobial susceptibility of the actual (or presumed) infecting organism(s). If the pathogen is isolated from a culture, it can be subjected to direct susceptibility testing as described in Chapter 13. A number of methods for determining antimicrobial susceptibility are available. The commonly used disk-diffusion method is simple to perform and is relatively inexpensive, but it provides at best only semiquantitative or qualitative data about the susceptibility of a given organism to a given agent. It is not useful for slow-growing or fastidious organisms and has not been standardized for anaerobes. Nonetheless, if the test is carefully done, it provides data that are clinically useful. Quantitative data are provided by methods that incorporate serial dilutions of antimicrobials in agar-containing or broth culture media. The lowest concentration of the antimicrobial agent that prevents visible growth after an 18- to 24-hour incubation period is known as the minimal inhibitory concentration (MIC). The minimal bacterial concentration (MBC) or minimal lethal concentration (MLC) may be determined in broth dilution tests by subculturing the containers that show no growth onto antibiotic-free agar-containing media. The lowest concentration of antimicrobial that totally suppresses growth on antibiotic-free media (or results in a 99.9 percent or greater decline in colony count) after overnight incubation is known as the MBC (or MLC). The aforementioned techniques are based on an 18- to 24-hour incubation period. A variety of "rapid methods" are now available as well.[7] These are based on a determination of changes in bacterial growth rates caused by antimicrobial agents and can provide susceptibility in 4 to 8 hours.

Susceptibility testing is particularly important for certain organisms such as *S. aureus* and the various facultative and aerobic gram-negative bacilli. The widespread clinical and agricultural use of antibiotics since the 1930s and 1940s has resulted in the emergence of many strains of bacteria resistant to one or more antimicrobial agents.[8] In most cases in which adequate studies have been done, it appears that the role of antimicrobial agents is to exert selective pressure that results in the emergence of resistant organisms. In some cases the organisms are naturally resistant to the antibiotic used. Examples of this include gram-positive organisms such as staphylococci and streptococci, which are naturally resistant to the polymyxins. Many gram-negative bacilli are naturally resistant to penicillin G, erythromycin, and clindamycin. In other cases the resistant bacterial strains have acquired R factors or plasmids that enable them to resist antimicrobial inhibition. These plasmids may provide the organisms with the ability to synthesize enzymes that modify or inactivate the antimicrobial agent; they may result in changes in the bacterial cell's ability to accumulate the antimicrobial agent or may permit the cell to produce metabolic enzymes resistant to inhibition by the antimicrobial agent.[8] Examples of each of these mechanisms of resistance are well known. Most strains of *S. aureus* that are resistant to penicillin contain plasmids that enable them to produce an extracellular β-lactamase that hydrolyzes and inactivates penicillin G.[8] Many gram-negative bacilli that are resistant to aminoglycosidic aminocyclitol antibiotics such as streptomycin, kanamycin, tobramycin, gentamicin, and amikacin contain plasmids that code for the production of periplasmic enzymes that catalyze a modification of the aminoglycosidic aminocyclitols by phosphorylation, acetylation, or adenylylation.[8] R-factor–mediated tetracycline resistance in both gram-negative bacilli and *S. aureus* involves an inducible decrease in the uptake of tetracycline, although the actual mechanism for this decreased uptake is not yet understood.[8] *Escherichia coli* organisms resistant to trimethoprim have been found to contain R factors that enable them to synthesize a new dihydrofolate reductase (the enzyme specifically inhibited by trimethoprim) that is 10,000 times less susceptible to the in vitro effects of trimethoprim than is the host bacteria's own chromosomal enzyme.[8]

The aforementioned developments provide the rationale for performing tests of antimicrobial susceptibility whenever there is reasonable doubt about the susceptibility of a given organism. There are certain cases in which routine susceptibility testing need not be done, but they make up an ever-diminishing list. All group A streptococci remain susceptible to the penicillins and cephalosporins; meningococci likewise are universally susceptible to chloramphenicol; virtually all anaerobes except *Bacteroides* species are susceptible to penicillin G. Thus, testing these organisms against the agents listed need not be routinely carried out at the present time. Even a statement such as this is fraught with a certain amount of danger. The discoveries of penicillin-resistant meningococci and pneumococci in South Africa, the emergence of penicillin-resistant gonococci in Asia and Africa, the rapid spread of ampicillin-resistant (and even chloramphenicol-resistant) strains of *H. influenzae* in the United States and Europe and the proliferation of vancomycin-resistant enterococci and staphylococci make us realize that, in time, strains of virtually any organism may be found that are resistant to antimicrobial agents that previously had been effective against them.[9]

It is important to consider geographic differences in patterns of susceptibility of organisms when choosing antimicrobial agents. In many cases, there may be variations in susceptibility patterns between hospitals and the community or among hospitals themselves. The emergence of gram-negative bacilli that are resistant to gentamicin is a good example of this. Most of the aminoglycoside-resistant organisms are found in hospitals, whereas most isolates from nonhospitalized patients remain susceptible to gentamicin.[8,10] The possibility of significant geographic variations in antimicrobial susceptibility must be remembered as we examine Table 1, which is a compendium of antimicrobial agents of choice for various commonly encountered infectious agents. The data in this table are based on material accumulated primarily in the United States and are similar in many aspects to data published periodically in the *Medical Letter on Drugs and Therapeutics*.[11]

Host Factors

It is obviously important to determine the identity and antimicrobial susceptibility of the organism(s) causing a given infection. However, optimal therapy is impossible unless we also consider a number of host factors that may influence the efficacy and toxicity of antimicrobial agents.[12]

History of Previous Adverse Reactions to Antimicrobial Agents. Simply obtaining an adequate history of previous adverse reactions to drugs may prevent the inadvertent administration of an antimicrobial agent to which the patient is allergic. A failure to do so can have serious (and sometimes fatal) consequences.

Age. The age of the patient is a major factor to consider in the choice of antimicrobial agents. Gastric acidity varies with age. The pH of gastric secretions is higher in young children and does not reach adult levels of acidity until approximately the age of 3 years. At the other end of the age spectrum, there is also a decline in gastric acidity such that gastric achlorhydria is found in 5.3 percent of people 20–29 years of age, in 16 percent of those 40–49, and in 35.4 percent of those over 60.[12] The absorption of a number of antimicrobials via the oral route depends on their acid stability and the pH of gastric secretions. Penicillin G is an excellent example of this phenomenon. The oral absorption of penicillin G is markedly reduced by gastric acid. However, in young children and in older achlorhydric patients, the absorption of the drug is markedly enhanced. As a result, various orally administered penicillins will produce high serum levels in young children and in elderly patients who have achlorhydria. It makes no sense to give such a patient the more expensive acid-resistant forms of penicillin such as phenoxymethyl penicillin (penicillin V) since these drugs will not be absorbed any better than the less expensive penicillin G. The absorption of other orally administered β-lactam antibiotics is probably also enhanced in achlorhydric patients; however, evidence is convincing only in the case of the penicillins.[13] Gastric acidity does not always have a negative influence on the absorption of antimicrobials. Drugs that are weak acids such as ketoconazole may be better absorbed at a low pH. Thus, absorption of ketoconazole is impaired by the administration of antacids, cimetidine, or even food.[14]

Renal function, likewise, varies with age. It is relatively diminished in premature and newborn children and reaches "adult levels" between 2 and 12 months of age.[12] Thus the serum half-lives of drugs that are primarily excreted by the kidneys may be considerably increased in neonates. As a result, doses of antimicrobial agents such as penicillin G and its various

TABLE 1. Antimicrobial Agents of Choice

Organism	*Antimicrobial of Choice*	*Alternative Agents*
Gram-positive cocci		
Staphylococcus aureus		
Non-penicillinase producing	Penicillin	A cephalosporin,[a] vancomycin, clindamycin, imipenem, erythromycin
Penicillinase producing	A penicillinase-resistant penicillin[b]	A cephalosporin,[a] vancomycin, clindamycin, imipenem, erythromycin
β-Streptococci (groups A, B, C, and G)	Penicillin	A cephalosporin,[a] erythromycin, vancomycin
α-Streptococci (*Streptococcus viridans*)	Penicillin	A cephalosporin,[a] vancomycin, erythromycin
Streptococcus bovis	Penicillin	A cephalosporin,[a] vancomycin, erythromycin
Enterococci		
Endocarditis or other serious infection	Penicillin (or ampicillin) plus gentamicin or streptomycin	Vancomycin plus gentamicin or streptomycin
Uncomplicated urinary tract infection	Ampicillin or amoxicillin	Nitrofurantoin, erythromycin
Streptococcus pneumoniae	Penicillin	A cephalosporin,[a] erythromycin, chloramphenicol, vancomycin
Gram-negative cocci		
Neisseria meningitidis	Penicillin	Chloramphenicol, cefuroxime, ceftriaxone, cefotaxime, moxalactam, a sulfonamide
Neisseria gonorrhoeae		
Non-β-lactamase producing	Penicillin	Spectinomycin, ampicillin, amoxicillin, cefoxitin, ceftriaxone, cefuroxime, cefotaxime, trimethoprim-sulfamethoxazole, ciprofloxacin
β-Lactamase producing	Ceftriaxone	Cefoxitin, cefuroxime, amoxicillin clavulanate, spectinomycin, chloramphenicol, cefotaxime, trimethoprim-sulfamethoxazole, ciprofloxacin
Gram-negative bacilli		
Acinetobacter sp. (*Mima, Herellea*)	Imipenem	Tobramycin or kanamycin (± carbenicillin), sulfisoxazole, trimethoprim-sulfamethoxazole, ticarcillin, mezlocillin, piperacillin, doxycycline
Brucella sp.	Tetracycline (± streptomycin)	Chloramphenicol (± streptomycin)
Campylobacter jejuni	Erythromyycin	Ciprofloxacin[c,f], tetracycline, chloramphenicol, gentamicin
Enterobacter sp.	Gentamicin or tobramycin	Carbenicillin, ticarcillin, mezlocillin, piperacillin, netilmicin, amikacin, third-generation cephalosporin,[d] cefoperazone, tetracycline, chloramphenicol, imipenem, trimethoprim-sulfamethoxazole, ciprofloxacin
Escherichia coli		
Uncomplicated urinary tract infection	Ampicillin, amoxicillin, or trimethoprim-sulfamethoxazole	A cephalosporin,[a] a tetracycline, trimethoprim, sulfisoxazole
Systemic infection	Ampicillin or amoxicillin (for serious infections, third-generation cephalosporin[d], cefoperazone)	A cephalosporin,[a] carbenicillin, mezlocillin, piperacillin, gentamicin, tobramycin, kanamycin, amikacin, netilmicin, ciprofloxacin, imipenem, aztreonam
Francisella tularensis	Streptomycin	Tetracycline, chloramphenicol
Haemophilus influenzae		
Meningitis	Chloramphenicol, third-generation cephalosporin[d]	Ampicillin (if β-lactamase–negative), cefuroxime
Other infections	Ampicillin or amoxicillin[e]	Trimethoprim-sulfmethoxazole, cefuroxime cefaclor, cefamandole, sulfisoxazole, amoxicillin clavulanate, ciprofloxacin
Klebsiella pneumonia	A cephalosporin[a] (for serious infections, third-generation cepholosporin[d])	Imipenem, aztreonam, trimetheprim-sulfamethoxazole, cefuroxime, cefamandole, amikacin, netilmicin, gentamicin, tobramycin, ciprofloxacin, chloramphenicol, tetracycline
Legionella sp.	Erythromycin	Rifampin plus erythromycin, trimethoprim-sulfamethoxazole
Proteus mirabilis	Ampicillin	Gentamicin or tobramycin, a cephalosporin,[a] imipenem, aztreonam, ticarcillin, mezlocillin, piperacillin
Other *Proteus* sp. (*P. rettgeri, M. morganii, P. vulgaris*	Gentamicin or tobramycin	Third-generation cephalosporin,[d] carbenicillin, ticarcillin, mezlocillin, piperacillin, amikacin, kanancycin, netilmicin, imipenem, aztreonam, trimethoprim-sulfamethoxazole, chloramphenicol, ciprofloxacin
Providencia sp.	Gentamicin or tobramycin	Third-generation cephalosporin,[d] amikacin, kanamcycin, netilmicin, carbenicillin, ticarcillin, mezlocillin, piperacillin, imipenem, aztreonam, trimethoprim-sulfamethoxazole, chloramphenicol, ciprofloxacin
Pseudomonas aeruginosa	Tobramycin or gentamicin plus ticarcillin, carbenicillin, azlocillin, mezlocillin, or piperacillin	Amikacin, netilmicin, imipenem, aztreonam, ceftazidime, ciprofloxacin
Salmonella sp.	Chloramphenicol	Ampicillin or amoxicillin, trimethoprim-sulfamethoxazole,[f] ciprofloxacin

(*Continued*)

TABLE 1. (Continued)

Organism	*Antimicrobial of Choice*	*Alternative Agents*
Serratia marcescens	Gentamicin or amikacin	Third-generation cephalosporin,[d] carbenicillin, ticarcillin, mezlocillin, piperacillin, imipenem, aztreonam, tobramycin, netilmicin, chloramphenicol
Shigella sp.	Trimethoprim-sulfamethoxazole	Ciprofloxacin, ampicillin, chloramphenicol, nalidixic acid
Yersinia pestis	Streptomycin	Tetracycline, chloramphenicol, gentamicin
Anaerobes		
Anaerobic streptococci	Penicillin	Clindamycin, erythromycin, chloramphenicol, a cephalosporin,[a] tetracycline
Bacteroides sp.		
Oropharyngeal stains	Penicillin	Clindamycin, tetracycline, chloramphenicol metronidazole, cefoxitin, cefotetan
Gastrointestinal strains	Clindamycin or metronidazole	Chloramphenicol, cefoxitin, cefotetan, moxalactam, carbenicillin, ticarcillin, piperacillin, mezlocillin, imipenam, ticarcillin clavulanate, ampicillin-sulbactam
Clostridium sp.	Penicillin	Chloramphenicol, clindamycin, metronidazole

[a] The term *cephalosporin* refers to the first-generation cephalosporins cephalothin, cefazolin, cephapirin, cephradine, cephalexin, cefaclor, and cefadroxil.
[b] Methicillin, nafcillin, oxacillin, or dicloxacillin.
[c] For adults.
[d] The term *third-generation cephalosporin* refers to ceftriaxone, cefotaxime, ceftizoxime, ceftazidime, and moxalactam.
[e] For strains that do not produce β-lactamase.
[f] Not approved for this indication by the U.S. Food and Drug Administration.

semisynthetic derivatives as well as the aminoglycosides must be altered in neonates.

Aging results in the decline of a number of physiologic processes, including renal function.[13] It is especially important to realize that creatinine clearance may be significantly reduced in elderly patients even though they have normal blood urea nitrogen (BUN) or serum creatinine concentrations. In view of this, high doses of the penicillins or cephalosporins must be given with caution to elderly patients to prevent the development of excessively high serum levels that may produce severe neurotoxic reactions such as myoclonus, seizures, and coma.[12,13] It is likewise possible that other adverse reactions to the penicillins such as reversible neutropenia may be dose related and may occur with increased frequency when high doses of such drugs are given to elderly patients with physiologic renal impairment.[13] This, however, has not been proved. Impaired renal excretion of the aminoglycoside antibiotics may result in elevated serum concentrations, which in turn may be associated with an increasing incidence of ototoxicity in elderly patients.[15]

In addition to the toxicity that may result from impaired renal excretion in neonates and elderly patients, other adverse effects of antimicrobial agents may also be age related.[14,16] Hepatic function in the neonate is underdeveloped by adult standards. This can result in difficulties if such patients are administered drugs that are normally excreted or inactivated by the liver. Chloramphenicol is inactivated by conjugation to the glucuronide form in the liver. However, in the neonate, hepatic levels of glucuronyl transferase are relatively insufficient. Thus when neonates are given large doses of chloramphenicol, high serum levels of unconjugated chloramphenicol result. Such high concentrations of unconjugated chloramphenicol are toxic and can result in shock, cardiovascular collapse, and death (the so-called gray syndrome).[12,17] For this reason, chloramphenicol should be avoided if possible in the neonate. If it is necessary to use the drug, however, it may be safely administered if given in a dosage that has been reduced appropriately for the patient's age.[17,18]

The sulfonamides compete with bilirubin for binding sites on serum albumin. When given to neonates, they produce increased serum levels of unbound bilirubin that predispose the child to kernicterus.[17,18] For this reason, these agents should not be administered to neonates. Hyperbilirubinemia per se may be associated with the administration of novobiocin to neonates.[17] This is due to the ability of this drug to inhibit hepatic glucuronyl transferase, which in turn diminishes the ability of the liver to conjugate and excrete bilirubin. Hence, novobiocin should be avoided in newborn infants.

The tetracyclines are avidly bound to developing bone and tooth structures. As they bind to developing teeth, tetracyclines may cause a number of adverse effects ranging from purplish to brownish discoloration of the teeth to actual enamel hypoplasia.[12,17] The tetracyclines readily cross the placenta.[19] Thus, when administered during the latter half of pregnancy or from birth to the age of 6 months, they may cause these effects on the deciduous teeth of the infant. From the age of 6 months to 6–8 years, similar damage to the permanent teeth may occur. In view of this, tetracycline should be avoided, if possible, in young children.

The quinolone antimicrobials including the newer agents such as ciprofloxacin, norfloxacin, ofloxacin, pefloxacin, and others have been shown to cause cartilage damage and arthropathy in young animals. As a result, they are not recommended for use in prepubertal children.[20]

Adverse effects due to a number of antimicrobial agents have been noted to occur with increased incidence in the elderly.[13] In some cases (and perhaps in all if adequately studied), this relationship may be shown to be due to specific disease states or to impairment of physiologic processes associated with aging as noted earlier. However, in certain cases no specific factors other than age can be identified. The hepatotoxicity associated with isoniazid administration is a good example of this. A small percentage of patients receiving isoniazid develop toxic hepatitis that may be fatal if not recognized in time.[21] Liver damage from isoniazid almost never occurs in patients under 20 years of age. In patients 20–34 years of age, the incidence of isoniazid hepatotoxicity is 0.3 percent and rises steadily with age to reach 2.3 percent in patients 50 years of age or more. Because of this, it is currently recommended that routine prophylactic use of isoniazid for patients discovered to have positive tuberculin test reactions be limited to people under the age of 35.[22]

Nephrotoxic reactions to certain antimicrobial agents likewise appear to be more frequent or to occur with lower doses of drugs among the elderly. This has been demonstrated to occur with cephaloridine[23] and colistin[12,24] and may be true for other nephrotoxic antimicrobials as well.

Finally, hypersensitivity reactions to antimicrobial agents also appear to be more common in elderly than in younger patients.[12] This appears to be due to the fact that older patients are more likely to have been previously exposed and, thus, sensitized to these agents. In addition, prior exposure to drugs such as the aminoglycosidic aminocyclitols, which produce irreversible cochlear damage, can result in cumulative toxicity on repeat exposure.[13]

Genetic or Metabolic Abnormalities. The presence of genetic or metabolic abnormalities may also have a significant effect on the use or toxicity of a given antimicrobial agent. The rate at which isoniazid is conjugated and biologically inactivated by acetylation in the liver is genetically determined.[12] Rapid acetylators are more commonly found among Oriental populations, whereas 45–65 percent of U.S. and North European populations are slow acetylators. Several studies have suggested that polyneuritis is seen more frequently as a complication of isoniazid therapy in slow than in rapid acetylators.[12] It was once thought that hepatotoxicity due to isoniazid is related to the conversion of isoniazid to acetylhydrazine and other related hepatoxic derivatives and is more common among rapid acetylators,[25] but this does not appear to be true.

A number of antimicrobial agents have been shown to be capable of provoking hemolysis in patients with glucose-6-phosphate dehydrogenase (G6PD) deficiency, including the sulfonamides, nitrofurantoin, furazolidone, diaminodiphenylsulfone, and chloramphenicol.[12] Sulfonamides may likewise cause hemolytic reactions in the presence of certain hemoglobinopathies, including hemoglobin Zurich and hemoglobin H.[12]

The presence of metabolic disorders such as diabetes mellitus may also pose problems in antimicrobial therapy. Certain agents such as the sulfonamides (especially the long-acting types) and chloramphenicol can potentiate the hypoglycemic activity of sulfonylurea hypoglycemic agents such as tolbutamide and chlorpropamide.[13] In the case of the sulfonamides, this action may be related to their structural similarity to the sulfonylurea drugs. Chloramphenicol inhibits microsomal enzyme activity in the liver, and this impairs the metabolism of the sulfonylurea hypoglycemic agents. The dextrose load infused with intravenous antibiotics dissolved in dextrose-containing vehicles may be sufficient to produce hyperglycemia and glucosuria in diabetic patients. Another kind of "glucosuria" can occur in patients receiving antimicrobial agents. The cephalosporins, chloramphenicol, isoniazid, nalidixic acid, nitrofurantoin, penicillin, streptomycin, sulfanilimide, and the tetracyclines can all cause false-positive test results when urine sugar levels are determined by a method (such as the Benedict test or Clinitest) that measures reducing substances in the urine.[23] Tests that are specific for glucose (i.e., that use glucose oxidase) such as Dextrostix or Labstix are not affected by antimicrobial agents.

The absorption of intramuscularly administered antibiotics may be impaired in diabetic patients. Diabetics with bacterial endocarditis who failed to respond to intramuscular penicillin have been described.[12] Administration of the same dose of penicillin by the intravenous route, however, resulted in bacterial eradication.[12] Because of the potential impaired absorption of intramuscularly administered antimicrobial agents, it is probably prudent to initiate therapy by the intravenous route when using drugs such as the aminoglycosides to treat diabetic patients with gram-negative bacteremia (especially if accompanied by hypotension) or other serious infections.

The concomitant administration of chloramphenicol has been noted to delay the reticulocyte response to vitamin B_{12} or iron therapy in patients with pernicious anemia or iron deficiency anemia.[12] As noted previously, patients with pernicious anemia and gastric achlorhydria may exhibit enhanced serum levels of antimicrobials such as penicillin G when given by the oral route.

Rifampin may increase the hepatic metabolism and therefore decrease the effect of oral anticoagulants, oral contraceptives, and barbiturates. See Rizack and Hilman[27] for a comprehensive list of drug interactions.

Pregnancy. Patients who are pregnant and nursing mothers also pose certain problems in the selection of appropriate antimicrobial agents. All antimicrobial agents cross the placenta in varying degrees.[28,29] Thus, the use of such agents in pregnant women provides direct exposure of the fetus to the adverse effects of the drug. Although there are few solid data on the teratogenic potential of most antimicrobial agents in humans, experience suggests that certain drugs such as the penicillins (with the possible exception of ticarcillin[30]), the cephalosporins, and erythromycin are unlikely to be teratogenic and are safe for pregnant women to use.[17,28,29] Metronidazole and ticarcillin have been shown to be teratogenic in rodents and thus should be avoided in pregnancy.[30,31] The teratogenic potential of many other drugs in humans, including rifampin and trimethoprim, is simply unknown.

A number of antimicrobials have been shown to be deleterious in pregnancy. Tetracycline heads the list. The possible adverse effects of this drug on fetal dentition have already been noted. In addition, pregnant women receiving tetracycline are particularly vulnerable to certain toxic effects including acute fatty necrosis of the liver, pancreatitis, and probably renal damage,[12] The liver damage may be severe and can result in death. When administered to patients with impaired renal function, these effects may be magnified, particularly if the agent is one of the tetracyclines that is primarily excreted by the kidneys. These adverse effects are dose related and may be more frequent after intravenous administration. Although it has been suggested that tetracyclines may be given to pregnant women by the oral route in doses of 1 g or less per 24 hours, it is probably safer to avoid these agents entirely in pregnancy.[12,17]

The aminoglycosidic aminocyclitol antibiotics cross the placenta. So far fetal toxicity has been reported only for streptomycin when used to treat tuberculosis in pregnant women. Even in that setting, the toxicity has been mild, detectable only by formal vestibular testing or by an audiogram.[32] Psychomotor retardation, myoclonus, and convulsions have been reported in a small uncontrolled series of children whose mothers received isoniazid for tuberculosis during pregnancy.[33] This observation has not been confirmed to date.

Another aspect of drug therapy in pregnancy has recently been examined. It has been found that serum levels after a given dose of ampicillin are lower in pregnant than in nonpregnant women.[34] This is related to more rapid clearance of the drug and to a greater volume of distribution (probably due to increased plasma volume) in pregnancy. Thus, higher doses of ampicillin are required to achieve therapeutic blood levels in pregnancy. It is likely that these observations will also apply to other antimicrobial agents, but data on this are not presently available.

Virtually all antimicrobial agents appear in measurable concentrations in breast milk when administered in therapeutic doses to nursing women.[35] The amount of drug excreted into breast milk depends on its degree of ionization, its molecular weight, and its solubility in fat and water. Under usual circumstances, the concentrations of antibiotics found in breast milk are quite low. However, even these small amounts may cause significant adverse reactions in the nursing infant. Nalidixic acid and the sulfonamides in breast milk have been shown to cause hemolysis in infants with G6PD deficiency. Sulfonamides in breast milk may be dangerous to premature babies because even small doses of ingested sulfonamides may produce increased levels of unbound bilirubin by displacing bilirubin from its albumin binding sites. As noted previously, this predisposes the child to kernicterus.[35] The possibility that antimicrobial agents in breast milk can sensitize newborn children is a theoretic one, but it has not been convincingly demonstrated. Although tetracycline is excreted in breast milk, it is unlikely to produce damage to the nursing child's bones or teeth because the calcium in the milk forms an insoluble chelate with tetracyclines, which is not absorbable by the oral route.[35]

Renal and Hepatic Function. The ability of the patient to metabolize or excrete antimicrobial agents is one of the most important host factors to consider, especially when high serum or tissue concentrations of the administered drugs are potentially toxic. From a practical point of view, this means that one must carefully assess the patient's renal and hepatic function since these organs serve as the major (and in most cases the *only*) routes of excretion and/or inactivation of antimicrobials. Renal excretion is the most important route of elimination for most antimicrobial agents.[36–41] Table 2 lists those drugs that must be used with particular care in patients with decreased renal function. Doses for these drugs may be found in the chapters dealing with the individual agents and in Chapter 38. In general those agents that require no dosage change in impaired renal function are excreted effectively by extrarenal routes (usually the hepatobiliary system) in patients with renal failure. Their use in normal doses does not result in the appearance of toxic serum levels in this situation, although the urine levels of a number of these agents such as doxycycline and chloramphenicol may be significantly diminished.

Toxic serum levels of the remaining agents may develop if they are used without dosage modification in patients with impaired renal function. Excessive serum levels of penicillin G, carbenicillin, or imipenem may be associated with neuromuscular hyperexcitability, myoclonus, seizures, or coma.[12] Excessive serum levels of semisynthetic penicillins such as carbenicillin and ticarcillin or of cephalothin or moxalactam may cause hemostatic defects in patients with impaired renal failure because of interference with platelet function.[42,43] Elevated serum levels of aminoglycosidic aminocyclitol antibiotics or vancomycin may result in eighth nerve damage.[15,41] Neurotoxic reactions including respiratory arrest and death may occur in patients with excessive serum levels of certain aminoglycosidic aminocyclitols or the polymyxins.[12,24] Bone marrow suppression may occur in patients with renal failure who receive inappropriately high doses of 5-fluorocytosin.[44] In all the above situations, the possibility of toxic reactions can be significantly lessened or eliminated if the doses of the antimicrobial agents are appropriately reduced in the presence of renal insufficiency.

The tetracyclines (except doxycycline and possibly minocycline) are contraindicated in patients with impaired renal function because the elevated serum levels that result may produce a significant worsening of the uremic state due to their antianabolic effect. Moreover, they may cause enhanced hepatotoxicity in this situation.[12] Cephaloridine and the long-acting sulfonamides should be avoided in this situation because they are potentially nephrotoxic.

Certain antimicrobial agents, including erythromycin, chloramphenicol, lincomycin, and clindamycin, should be used with caution in patients with impaired hepatic function.[45] These drugs are primarily excreted or detoxified in the liver. Bone marrow suppression due to chloramphenicol is much more likely to occur in patients with impaired hepatic function; because of this, it has been suggested that the dose of chloramphenicol be cut at least in half in patients with cirrhosis and other severe liver disease.[46] The serum half-life of clindamycin is increased in patients with severe liver disease; because of this, the dose should be decreased in this situation. The tetracyclines may produce elevations in serum transaminase levels in patients recovering from viral hepatitis.[12] They should be avoided or used with extreme caution in patients with underlying liver disease. The serum half-lives of both rifampin and isoniazid are prolonged in patients with cirrhosis.[47] Other drugs that should be used with caution or for which serum levels should be monitored in patients with severe liver disease include metronidazole, ketoconazole, miconazole, nitrofurantoin, fusidic acid, and pyrazinamide.[45] Hepatobiliary disease influences antimicrobic therapy in still another way. The biliary concentrations of many antimicrobial agents, including ampicillin and nafcillin, that are normally excreted in high concentration in the bile may be significantly reduced in patients with liver disease or biliary obstruction.[12]

TABLE 2. Antimicrobial Use in Patients with Varying Degrees of Impaired Renal Function

Antimicrobial agents requiring no dosage change regardless of renal function
Erythromycin, clindamycin, chloramphenicol, doxycycline, cefoperazone, oxacillin, cloxacillin, dicloxacillin, nafcillin, rifampin, amphotericin B,[a] cefaclor, ceftriaxone, metronidazole
Antimicrobial agents requiring dosage change only with severe renal failure
Penicillin G, amoxicillin, ampicillin, methicillin, cephalothin, cephalexin, cefamandole, cefoxitin, cefotaxime, ceftizoxime, piperacillin, isoniazid, ethambutol, trimethoprim-sulfamethoxazole, cefotetan, ceftazidime, cefuroxime, cefonicid, mezlocillin, nalidixic acid, ciprofloxacin, norfloxacin
Antimicrobial agents requiring dosage change with impaired renal function
Carbenicillin, ticarcillin, cefazolin, moxalactan, streptomycin, kanamycin, gentamicin, tobramycin, amikacin, netilmicin, polymxyin B, colistin, vancomycin, flucytosine, imipenem
Antimicrobial agents contraindicated in renal failure
Tetracyclines (except doxycycline and possibly minocycline), nitrofurantoin, cephaloridine, long-acting sulfonamides, methenamine, para-aminosalicyclic acid

[a] Even though amphotericin B is excreted primarily by nonrenal means, this drug must be used with caution in patients with impaired renal function because of its nephrotoxicity.

Site of Infection. Of all the host factors to be considered in the choice of an antimicrobial agent, none is more important than the site of infection. The locus of the infectious process determines not only the choice of the agent but also its dose and the route by which it should be administered. For antimicrobial therapy to be effective, an adequate concentration of the drug must be delivered to the site of infection. In most cases, this means that the local concentration of the antimicrobial agent should at least equal the MIC of the infecting organism. Concentrations representing multiples of the MIC are generally felt more likely to be efficacious, but in many cases such local concentrations may be difficult or impossible to achieve. A failure to achieve local concentrations of antibiotics higher than the MIC of the infecting organism may not always be disastrous, however, because there is evidence that subinhibitory concentrations of drugs may produce antimicrobial effects that aid the host defenses against infections. It has been clearly demonstrated that subinhibitory concentrations of antibiotics can alter bacterial morphology,[48] adherence properties,[49] and opsonic requirements[50]; can enhance phagocytosis[51]; and can even aid intracellular killing of bacteria by polymorphonuclear leukocytes.[52] This may explain the clinical observation that, on occasion, doses of antimicrobials that produce seemingly inadequate serum levels may still result in clinical cure. In spite of such observations, most infectious disease clinicians feel that optimal therapy requires concentrations of antimicrobials that are above the MIC.

Serum concentrations of antimicrobial agents are relatively easy to determine and therefore are often used as a guide in the therapy. However, except in cases of bacteremia, antimicrobial efficacy is more likely determined by the tissue concentration than by blood level, as noted earlier. Moreover, there are some agents such as spiromycin and certain macrolides that are effective in vivo despite an inability to achieve serum levels above the MICs of certain organisms. This may be explained by the ability to achieve intracellular and tissue concentrations that far exceed those obtained in serum.[53] Binding to serum proteins may affect both the tissue distribution and the activity of antimicrobial agents in the blood. Although much careful investigation has been done on protein binding, the precise clinical significance of this phenomenon remains to be determined. For example, it has been shown that only the unbound form of a given antimicrobial agent is active in vitro (and presumably also in vivo) against infecting organisms.[54] However, since protein binding is rapidly reversible,[55] the activity of even highly protein-bound agents may not be absolutely limited by protein binding. The penetration of antimicrobial agents into interstitial fluid and lymph is related to protein binding since only the free form of the agent is able to pass through the capillary wall.[54] Penetration of antibiotics into fibrin clots (which may be analogous to the penetration of the drugs to reach the site of infection in patients with bacterial endocarditis) is likewise related to the amount of unbound antibiotic in the surrounding fluid.[56] Nevertheless, it is often difficult to correlate therapeutic outcome with in vitro susceptibility and protein binding unless several variables are carefully controlled.[51,58] The reason for this is simply that it is the concentration of antibiotic at the site of infection that is the major determinant in the successful therapy. Such concentrations are often difficult to assess because they are the result of a complex interaction between local factors that may bind, inactivate, or enhance the activity of a given antimicrobial agent. The ability of an antibiotic to pass through membranes by nonionic diffusion is related to its lipid solubility. Thus, lipid-soluble agents such as chloramphenicol, rifampin, trimethoprim, and isoniazid are all more adept at penetrating membranes than are the more highly ionized compounds.[54] These agents rapidly cross the blood-brain barrier and produce better cerebrospinal fluid levels than do more highly ionized compounds such as the aminoglycosidic aminocyclitols. Except in neonates, none of the aminoglycosides produces effective cerebrospinal fluid levels when given parenterally. To be effective for the treatment of meningitis, they must be given via the intrathecal or intraventricular route in adults.[59] This is an excellent example of the importance of the site of infection in determining the most efficacious antimicrobial therapy. For the treatment of bacterial meningitis in adults, we either must choose agents such as chloramphenicol or the third-generation cephalosporins (e.g., cefotaxime, ceftriaxone, or ceftazidime) that cross the blood-brain barrier reasonably well, or we must use high concentrations of parenteral doses of drugs such as penicillin G, ampicillin, or nafcillin that penetrate into the cerebrospinal fluid only with difficulty. Agents such as the aminoglycosidic aminocyclitols and first-generation cephalosporins that produce inadequate cerebrospinal fluid levels even after high-dose parenteral therapy must be administered directly into the cerebrospinal fluid or must be avoided entirely.

The vegetations of bacterial endocarditis, bones, and devitalized tissue represent examples of other areas in which the penetration of antimicrobial agents to the site of infection may be borderline or inadequate. Because of this, high-dose and prolonged parenteral therapy is usually required for the effective treatment of bacterial endocarditis and osteomyelitis. In some cases, we may take advantage of the physiologic handling of antimicrobials to achieve therapeutic success. Agents that are excreted by the liver and are concentrated in the bile such as ampicillin or doxycycline may be more effective in treating cholangitis than are agents such as the first-generation cephalosporins or aminoglycosidic aminocyclitols that are not greatly concentrated in bile. The new fluoroquinolones may owe some of their effectiveness in the treatment of osteomyelitis to their ability to achieve superior concentrations in bone.[60]

Even the achievement of "therapeutic concentrations" of antimicrobial agents at the site of infection may not be sufficient for cure. The reason for this is that a number of local factors may influence the activity of antimicrobial agents. These, too, must be considered in designing an appropriate therapeutic regimen. Aminoglycosidic aminocyclitols and the polymyxins are bound to and inactivated by purulent material.[61] This is one of many reasons why surgical drainage is imperative when treating abscesses with agents such as these. Interestingly, carbenicillin does not lose activity in pus.[61] Although carbenicillin (and other penicillins) may be more active in purulent material, clinical experience strongly suggests that appropriate drainage procedures greatly enhance the efficacy of these agents as well. Although penicillin G, like carbenicillin, is not inactivated by purulent material per se,[54] recent studies suggest that the presence of β-lactamase–producing organisms such as *Bacteroides fragilis* in abscesses may result in local inactivation of penicillin G and other β-lactam antibiotics.[62]

Pencillins and tetracyclines are also bound by hemoglobin and thus may be less effective in the presence of significant hematoma formation.[54] In vitro *Pseudomonas aeruginosa* is protected from the action of the aminoglycosidic aminocyclitols and polymyxins by high concentrations of calcium or magnesium in the culture medium.[63] The clinical significance of this observation, if any, remains to be determined. Local decreases in oxygen tension such as occur in abscesses and intraperitoneal infections may also have an effect on the activity of certain antimicrobial agents. The aminoglycosidic aminocyclitols, for example, are inactive against anaerobes and may also be less effective against facultative organisms under anaerobic conditions because oxygen is required for the transport of these agents into the bacterial cell.[64]

Local alterations in pH such as occur in abscesses and especially in the urine may have an important effect on the activity of a number of antimicrobial agents. Methenamine, nitrofurantoin, novobiocin, and chlortetracycline are more active at an acid pH, whereas alkalinization enhances the activity of erythromycin, lincomycin, clindamycin, and the aminoglycosidic aminocyclitol antibiotics. Indeed, the aminoglycosidic aminocyclitols show a marked loss of activity at a low pH. These observations have been used in treating patients with urinary tract infections, a situation in which the local pH can be altered by the addition of acidifying or alkalinizing agents.[65,66]

The presence of foreign bodies also has a profound effect on the activity of antimicrobial agents. Thus, it is often necessary to remove the foreign material to cure an infection in the vicinity of a prosthetic heart valve or joint implant.[67] The mechanism by which foreign bodies potentiate infection is not clear, but they probably cause localized impairment of host defense mechanisms.[68] In addition, the foreign body often serves as a nidus on which organisms can adhere and produce extracellular substances such as glycocalyx or slime that may interfere with phagocytosis and impair the penetration of antibiotics to the underlying organisms.[69] It has also been demonstrated that antimicrobial agents themselves may cause alterations in host defenses. Clinically achievable concentrations of many different agents have been shown to have adverse effects on leukocyte chemotaxis, lymphocyte transformation, monocyte transformation, delayed hypersensitivity, antibody production, phagocytosis, and the microbicidal action of polymorphonuclear leukocytes.[70–76] It is not clear, however, whether any of these effects (largely demonstrated by in vitro studies) are of clinical significance.[76] Nonetheless, the possibility that antimicrobial agents can cause immunosuppression exists, and this fact should discourage the indiscriminate use of antibiotics, especially in patients who are already immunosuppressed because of their underlying disease or because of their concomitant drug therapy.[74]

ANTIMICROBIAL COMBINATIONS

Most infections in humans can be treated with a single antimicrobial agent, but there are clear-cut (as well as borderline) indications for the use of combinations (usually two) of antimicrobials. Because combinations may provide more broad-spectrum coverage than single agents can, the physician is often tempted to use combinations for the sense of security they provide, even in situations in which they are not indicated. Such inappropriate use of antimicrobial combinations may have significantly deleterious effects. In this section we will examine indications for the use of combinations and the potential disadvantages of this approach to therapy.

In Vitro Results of Combination Therapy

When two antimicrobial agents are combined, they may have one of three types of activity against a given organism in vitro: (*1*) an additive effect (sometimes called an indifferent effect), (*2*) synergism, and (*3*) antagonism.[77] Two drugs are said to be additive when the activity of the drugs in combination is equal to the sum (or a partial sum) of their independent activities when studied separately. The combined effect of a synergistic pair of antimicrobials is greater than the sum of their independent activities when measured separately. If two drugs are antagonistic, the activity of the combination is less than the sum of their independent effects when measured alone. These concepts are illustrated by "time-kill curves" in Figure 1. The various methods used to determine the in vitro effects of antibiotic combinations are beyond the scope of this chapter but have been reviewed in detail.[78]

Indications for the Clinical Use of Antimicrobial Combinations

Five reasons have been advanced to justify the use of antimicrobial combinations. The first three of these are discussed in detail in other chapters and, therefore, will be given only brief mention here.

Prevention of the Emergence of Resistant Organisms. Although the use of antimicrobial agents to prevent the emergence of resistant organisms would seem to be a major indication for the use of such therapy, combination therapy has been clearly documented as effective in preventing resistance only during the treatment of tuberculosis (see Chapters 32 and 229). There is somewhat less epidemiologic evidence in support of this concept as it applies to the use of rifampin for the treatment of nonmycobacterial infections, but it nonetheless appears that one of the major benefits of using rifampin in combination with a second agent for treating staphylococcal infections, for example, is that the combination prevents the rapid emergence of resistance to rifampin, which is evident when this drug is used alone.[80,81]

Polymicrobial Infections. In most infections, even those due to more than one organism, a single effective agent can be found. For example, cellulitis due to *S. aureus* and group A streptococci can be treated with a penicillinase-resistant penicillin alone. However, there are certain types of infections due to such a broad variety of organisms that more than one antimicrobial agent may be required to provide adequate coverage. Examples of such infections include intraperitoneal and pelvic infections due to mixed bowel flora and certain brain abscesses (see Chapters 60, 70, and 96).

Initial Therapy. In neutropenic patients or other patients with presumed infection in whom the nature of the infection is not clear, it may be reasonable to begin broad-spectrum coverage, usually with two agents such as ticarcillin plus gentamicin or tobramycin while awaiting the results of cultures. In this setting, it is often possible to discontinue treatment with one of the agents or to switch to an alternate single drug after the results of cultures are available (see Chapter 29). The development of new drugs with broad spectra of activity makes it possible to use a single agent for most cases of initial therapy, but it would be premature to advocate a general application of this concept at present.

Decreased Toxicity. Many of the drugs used in therapy for infections are potentially toxic (e.g., aminoglycosidic aminocyclitols). Therefore, a major goal of combination therapy has been to reduce the amount of drug required for treatment and, thus, to reduce dose-related toxicity. Unfortunately, at present there are no data from clinical trials that establish beyond doubt that combination therapy with different agents permits a reduction of the drug dose sufficient to reduce dose-related toxicity. There is evidence that the use of a mixture of similar agents (e.g., triple sulfonamides) can reduce the incidence of a dose-related complication: crystalluria with stone formation.[82] The explanation for this effect is that the solubility of each component (sulfadiazine, sulfamerazine, sulfamethazine) in urine is independent of the others, although their antibacterial activity is cumulative.

Synergism. The use of synergistic combinations of antimicrobial agents to treat infections due to resistant or relatively resistant organisms represents one of the most appealing ways to use these agents. There are numerous examples of in vitro synergism, but thus far synergistic antimicrobial combinations have proved more effective than are single agents in only a limited number of clinical settings.[79,83]

Perhaps the best known application of synergistic combinations of antimicrobial agents is for the treatment of enterococcal endocarditis. Treatment of this disease with penicillin alone results in an unacceptable relapse rate because enterococci are relatively resistant to penicillin.[84] Indeed, penicillin alone seems to act as a bacteriostatic and not a bactericidal agent.[85] The addition of an aminoglycoside such as streptomycin or gentamicin results in both in vitro and in vivo synergism and yields clinical cure rates comparable to those achieved for endocarditis caused by less resistant streptococci.[84,85] Penicillin enhances the uptake of aminoglycosides by enterococci; the result of this interaction is the synergistic killing of the organisms.[86] In recent years some enterococci have been found to be resistant to penicillin-streptomycin, penicillin-kanamycin, and penicillin-amikacin synergism due to high-level resistance (MIC > 2000 μg/ml) to streptomycin and/or to kanamycin.[87] Strains may resist synergism if they are ribosomally resistant to streptomycin[88] or if they contain plasmid-mediated enzymes

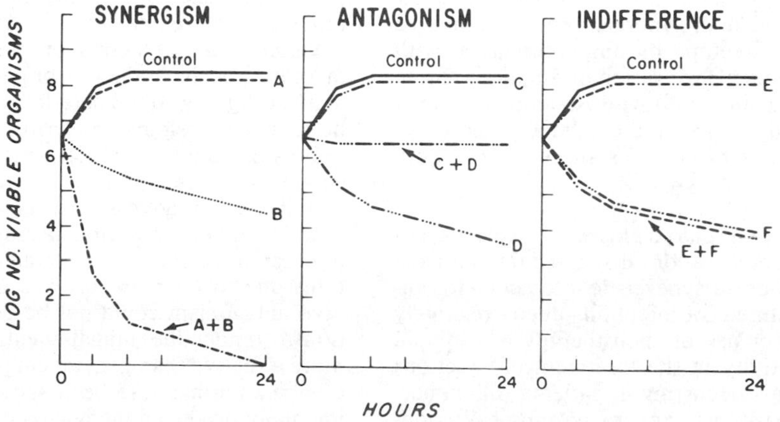

FIG. 1. Antibacterial effects of antibiotic combinations. *Left* (A and B): synergism; *center* (C and D): antagonism; *right* (E and F): indifference (additive). (From Moellering,[79] with permission.)

that inactivate streptomycin, kanamycin, or amikacin.[89] The prevalence of enterococci with high-level resistance to gentamicin appears to be increasing rapidly.[91] Moreover, the use of penicillin-gentamicin therapy in such patients may result in a failure to eradicate the infecting organisms.[92] Therefore it is important to test for high-level resistance to streptomycin and gentamicin before embarking on a therapeutic regimen for enterococcal endocarditis or meningitis.

Penicillin-streptomycin combinations are also synergistic against viridans streptococci and have been used for the treatment of endocarditis due to these organisms.[83] However, viridans streptococci are usually very susceptible to penicillin, and penicillin alone has been used successfully for treatment of this kind of endocarditis.[93,94]

A similar type of synergism occurs when semisynthetic penicillinase-resistant penicillins such as nafcillin or oxacillin are combined with gentamicin against *S. aureus*.[95] So far there are no data to document that the use of combination therapy for *S. aureus* infections in humans has any advantage over therapy with a penicillin or cephalosporin alone.[96]

Combinations of carbenicillin, ticarcillin, mezlocillin, azlocillin, or piperacillin with gentamicin, tobramycin, or amikacin exhibit synergism against many strains of *P. aeruginosa*.[97,98] The mechanism of synergism in this setting is similar to that described for enterococci (i.e., enhanced uptake of the aminoglycoside in the presence of the antipseudomonal penicillin). Studies with experimental animals convincingly demonstrate the superiority of such combinations for the treatment of serious *Pseudomonas* infections.[99] Although the information available from limited human trials to date is also consistent with enhanced activity of these combinations for *Pseudomonas* infections, this form of therapy has not been subjected to definitive controlled study.[78]

Synergism occurs by a different mechanism when sulfonamides are combined with trimethoprim. In this case, the two agents are synergistic because they act to inhibit sequential steps in the microbial pathway of folic acid metabolism.[100] As a result, combinations of sulfonamides with trimethoprim are often useful for the treatment of infections due to organisms that may be resistant to sulfonamides alone. A fixed combination of sulfamethoxazole and trimethoprim is available for clinical use and has been shown effective for the treatment and prevention of chronic urinary tract infections, even when due to sulfonamide-resistant organisms.[101] The combination has also been shown to be useful for the treatment of typhoid fever and shigellosis caused by organisms resistant to ampicillin and/or chloramphenicol, for the treatment of infections due to ampicillin-resistant *H. influenzae* and for therapy for a wide variety of other infections as well.[78,102–104]

Combinations of amphotericin B with a number of other agents including 5-fluorocytosine, rifampin, and tetracycline have been shown to result in enhanced antimicrobial activity against fungi.[105] The mechanism of synergism seems to involve damage to the fungal cell envelope by amphotericin B, with resultant enhanced intracellular penetration of 5-fluorocytosine and other agents.[105] Flucytosine and low-dose amphotericin B have been used successfully in treating candidiasis and cryptococcosis when the patient's isolate was susceptible to both drugs.[106,107]

Synergism and Infections in Impaired Hosts. The clinical applications of antimicrobial combinations discussed thus far have all represented attempts to use a synergistic interaction for enhanced efficacy in the treatment of infections due to relatively resistant organisms. Another use of such therapy is to obtain enhanced antimicrobial activity in the treatment of infections due to susceptible organisms occurring in patients with abnormalities of host defense systems. Several groups have conducted randomized trials of various combinations of two agents chosen from among carbenicillin, ticarcillin, piperacillin, the cephalosporins, gentamicin, tobramycin, and amikacin for the treatment of severe infections in patients with impaired host defense mechanisms. Both Lau et al.[108] and Klastersky et al.[109] have demonstrated improved survival rates in such patients treated with combinations that were synergistic against the infecting organisms as compared with patients receiving nonsynergistic combinations. These studies add strong support to the concept that synergistic combinations of antimicrobials may be an important determinant of success in the treatment of serious infections, especially when due to gram-negative organisms in patients with impaired host defenses. However, there is no absolute proof that synergistic combinations are more effective in this setting than are single agents that have a sufficiently broad spectrum and that produce sufficiently high serum bactericidal titers against the infecting organisms.[110]

Disadvantages of the Inappropriate Use of Antimicrobial Combinations

Whereas the clinical use of synergistic combinations of antimicrobial agents may have beneficial results as noted above, the inappropriate use of antimicrobial combinations may have important adverse effects, three of which will be discussed below.

Antagonism. The medical literature contains a large number of reports of in vitro antagonism between antimicrobial agents.[79,83] In view of this, it is surprising that there are only a few well-documented clinical examples of antagonism. Perhaps the most impressive is the study of Lepper and Dowling, who demonstrated conclusively in 1951 that penicillin is more effective than is the combination of penicillin with chlortetracycline for the treatment of pneumococcal meningitis.[111] The fatality among patients treated with penicillin alone was 21 percent, whereas that among patients treated with penicillin plus chlortetracycline was 79 percent. A study of childhood meningitis has also demonstrated the superiority of single-drug therapy. Mathies et al. treated a group of children suffering from bacterial meningitis with either ampicillin alone or a combination of ampicillin, chloramphenicol, and streptomycin.[112] The mortality among 140 children treated with ampicillin alone was 4.3 percent, whereas the mortality among 124 children receiving the antibiotic combination was 10.5 percent, a difference that reached statistical significance. There are several other reports of the influence of antagonism on the treatment of urinary tract infections and streptococcal pharyngitis, but none are particularly impressive.[79] Considering the extensive clinical use of antimicrobial combinations and especially in view of the large number of reports of in vitro antagonism, it is surprising that there are so few reports of in vivo antagonism. This may be due in part to the paucity of well-controlled studies in this area or to the reluctance of investigators to report adverse results. Another possible explanation is simply that clinically significant antagonism is not a common event. In most cases, in vitro antagonism results in the loss or partial loss of activity of the most active drug (e.g., the bactericidal activity of such an agent may be reduced to simple bacteriostasis), but the combination still retains some antimicrobial activity. As long as the patient receiving such therapy has normal host defense mechanisms, it is unlikely that adverse effects will be seen. This has been the case in studies using an antagonistic combination of antibiotics (chloramphenicol plus gentamicin) to treat experimental infections due to *Proteus mirabilis* in mice.[113] In healthy mice, in vivo antagonism could not be demonstrated, but after irradiation to render the animals neutropenic, gentamicin alone was more effective than gentamicin plus chloramphenicol was. This combination has also been shown to be antagonistic in experimentally produced meningitis due to *P. mirabilis* in rabbits.[114] Thus, it seems that clinically important antagonism is most likely to be manifested in patients with generalized impairment of host defense mechanisms (such as seen in leukemia, cancer patients who are neutropenic, etc.) or in patients with infections such as meningitis or endocarditis where localized host defenses may be inadequate.

The observation of in vivo antagonism in the treatment of bacterial meningitis raises some questions about the recommendations of the use of ampicillin plus chloramphenicol in the initial treatment of childhood meningitis (see Chapter 66) because of the emergence of ampicillin-resistant strains of *H. influenzae*.[8] Combinations of penicillin plus chloramphenicol have been shown to exhibit in vitro antagonism against pneumococci and other organisms.[83] However, this antagonism takes the form of lessened bactericidal activity of penicillin in the presence of chloramphenicol. Since chloramphenicol alone is quite active against the organisms likely to cause childhood meningitis. (*H. influenzae, S. pneumoniae, Neisseria meningitidis*) and since there is no evidence that penicillin or ampicillin antagonizes the activity of chloramphenicol, it seems unlikely that the current recommendations for pediatric meningitis will result in in vivo antagonism when used to treat meningitis due to the organisms listed above.[83]

Studies documenting the effectiveness of some of the newer cephalosporins such as cefuroxime and ceftriazone[115,116] for childhood meningitis may ultimately make it unnecessary to continue to use combination therapy in this setting.

There has been a recent upsurge of interest in the use of the newer broad-spectrum β-lactams in combination with each other to obtain broad-spectrum coverage without exposing the patient to the possible toxicity of an agent such as chloramphenicol or an aminoglycosidic aminocyclitol.[117] For the most part, this seems reasonable. However, there is in vitro and in vivo evidence that some β-lactam–β-lactam combinations may be antagonistic against certain organisms such as *Enterobacter, Serratia,* or *Pseudomonas*. This antagonism seems to be the result of the induction or derepression inactivation of the second.[118] The exact clinical significance of this phenomenon is not presently clear, but it must be kept in mind when one considers the clinical use of such combinations.

Most of the examples of in vitro antagonism are the result of interactions of the antimicrobial agents as they react at a subcellular level on a given microorganism. However, another type of antagonism should also be included in this discussion. This may result from the direct interaction of drugs before they reach the microorganism. If chloramphenicol and erythromycin are inadvertently mixed together in the same parenteral infusion solution, they form insoluble precipitates and hence lose activity. In recent years, it has become clear that the mixing of penicillins (especially carbenicillin or ticarcillin) with aminoglycosides results in the inactivation of the aminoglycoside.[119] Because the reaction occurs slowly, this is usually not a problem in vivo, provided the drugs are given by separate routes of administration. However, in uremic patients in whom the serum half-life of aminoglycosides is greatly prolonged, in vivo inactivation can occur.[120] The clinical significance of this observation, however, has not yet been elucidated.

Cost. With the possible exception of penicillin G and certain of the tetracyclines and sulfonamides, antimicrobials are expensive drugs. Thus the inappropriate use of antimicrobial combinations (when a single agent would be adequate) can add greatly to the cost of the patient's illness. This important consideration is discussed in greater detail in Chapter 37.

Adverse Effects. It has been estimated that approximately 5 percent of the patients receiving a given antibiotic in the hospital will experience some sort of adverse reaction.[14,121] Obviously the possibility of such adverse reactions (including hypersensitivity reactions and direct toxic effects) is increased without any enhanced therapeutic benefit when one inappropriately uses combinations of antimicrobial agents. Moreover, when an adverse reaction occurs in a patient receiving more than one drug, it is often difficult to be certain of the agent that caused the reaction. This may mean that treatment with several or all drugs must be stopped. If combination drug therapy is to be used in such a patient, each drug must be tested carefully before use to make certain that it was not the cause of the original adverse reaction. This is time-consuming and expensive and may needlessly deprive the patient of the benefits of a useful agent.

CHOICE OF APPROPRIATE ROUTE OF ADMINISTRATION OF ANTIMICROBIAL AGENTS AND EVALUATION OF EFFICACY

Route of Administration

Once the physician has determined the most appropriate drug or drugs with which to treat a given infection, he must decide which route of administration to use to obtain maximum benefits from the therapy. In most cases this is a choice between oral and parenteral routes. In general, the oral route of administration is chosen for those infections that are mild and can be treated on an outpatient basis. Not all antibiotics can be administered in this way. Drugs such as vancomycin, the polymyxins, the aminoglycosidic aminocyclitols, and amphotericin B are absorbed so poorly from the gastrointestinal tract that they cannot be administered orally to treat systemic infections. When drugs are administered by the oral route, the physician must ascertain that the patient will reliably take them as ordered. The absorption of certain agents such as penicillin G is markedly impaired if taken with meals, whereas the absorption of acid-stable penicillins such as penicillin V is not affected by food or gastric acidity. The concomitant administration of antacids or iron-containing preparations may severely impair the absorption of tetracycline since this drug forms insoluble chelates in the presence of Mg^{2+}, Ca^{2+}, or Fe^{2+} ions. Antacids and histamine antagonists may also interfere with the absorption of the fluoroquinolones such as ciprofloxacin and norfloxacin.[122] More detailed information on the oral absorption of antimicrobial agents may be found in the chapters on the individual drugs.

The parenteral route of administration is used for agents that are inefficiently absorbed from the gastrointestinal tract and for the treatment of patients with serious infections in whom high serum concentrations of antimicrobial agents are required. The aminoglycosidic aminocyclitols and polymyxins may be given by intramuscular injection and are well tolerated when given this way. For most infections, adequate serum concentrations are achieved after the intramuscular administration of these drugs. However, in life-threatening infections, especially in the presence of shock (or in diabetic patients as discussed earlier), intravenous administration is preferred. Intravenous administration allows large doses of drugs to be given with a minimum of discomfort to the patient when high serum concentrations are required for the effective treatment of disease processes such as meningitis, endocarditis, and osteomyelitis. Whether intravenously administered drugs should be given by continuous infusion or by intermittent bolus infusion remains a matter of controversy. The former method has the advantage of simplicity; because pulses containing very high concentrations of drugs are avoided, it may result in less venous irritation and phlebitis. Studies in animal models suggest that the concentration of drugs such as penicillins and cephalosporins in fibrin clots is related to the peak serum levels achieved. Thus, greater concentrations of drugs are achieved in the clots in the face of intermittent bolus therapy.[123] It has been suggested that this data may be applicable to therapy for infective endocarditis and other infections in which high tissue concentrations of antibiotics are required. Convincing clinical proof of this concept, however, does not exist.

As discussed earlier, the intrathecal or intraventricular route of administration may be necessary for the treatment of meningeal infections with drugs such as the aminoglycosidic aminocyclitols, polymyxins, bacitracin, and possibly vancomycin, all of which cross the blood-brain barrier with considerable difficulty. The parenteral administration of antimicrobial agents results in adequate concentrations in pleural, peritoneal, pericardial, and synovial fluids. Thus, direct instillation of antibiotics into these areas is not necessary.

Monitoring the Response of the Patient to Antimicrobial Therapy

Although several laboratory tests are available to assist in the monitoring of antimicrobial therapy, clinical assessment remains the most important method for determining the efficacy of treatment. It is not uncommon to see patients fail to respond in the face of laboratory studies that suggest adequate therapy and vice versa. The reasons for this may usually be found among the many host factors that affect therapy as described earlier.

Nonetheless, the measurement of serum concentrations of antimicrobial agents and a determination of serum bactericidal titers are often of considerable use. The details concerning these tests are given in Chapter 13 and will not be repeated here. The major value of the direct determination of serum concentrations of antimicrobial agents is to avoid toxicity from excessive levels of agents such as the aminoglycosidic aminocyclitols and vancomycin, especially in patients with impaired renal or hepatic function. These tests are also useful for determining inadequate serum levels due to insufficient dosing or unusually rapid clearance.

Another method used to monitor the effectiveness of antimicrobial therapy is the serum bactericidal titer (sometimes called the serum antimicrobial dilution titer). This test was originally described by Schlichter and MacLean as a guide for effective therapy for subacute bacterial endocarditis.[126] Subsequently this test has been used to monitor therapy in patients with infective endocarditis, osteomyelitis, septic arthritis, empyema, and bacteremia.[109,127] In this test, serial dilutions of the patient's serum are incubated with an inoculum of the infecting organism; after incubation, the highest dilution that inhibits and/or kills the organism is determined. Most investigators feel that a serum bactericidal titer of at least 1:8 can be correlated with a successful therapeutic outcome.[109,126,128,130] A more recent multicenter study has suggested that peak and trough titers of at least 1:64 and 1:32, respectively, are good predictors of a successful therapeutic outcome in patients with infective endocarditis.[129] However, a lack of standardization and a lack of consistency in specifying the point (peak, trough, or midpoint serum levels) at which the test should be done have hindered attempts at more widespread application and evaluation of this test.[131–134]

CONCLUSION

Optimal use of antimicrobial agents demands consideration of a large number of important factors that may influence the choice of an appropriate agent and that determine the most effective dose and route of administration of a drug. A number of these factors have been outlined in this chapter. In the final analysis, sound clinical judgment remains the most important determinant of a successful outcome.

REFERENCES

1. Weinstein L. General considerations. In: Goodman LS, Gilman A, eds. The Pharmacological Basis of Therapeutics. New York. Macmillan; 1970:1154.
2. Majno G. The Healing Hand: Man and Wound in the Ancient World. Cambridge, MA: Harvard University Press; 1975:154,215.
3. Harris JC, Dupont HL, Hornick RB. Fecal leukocytes in diarrheal illness. Ann Intern Med. 1972;76:697.
4. Ho D, Ault MJ, Ault MA, et al. *Campylobacter* enteritis. Early diagnosis with Gram's stain. Arch Intern Med. 1982;142:1858.
5. Weinstein L. Common sense (clinical judgment) in the diagnosis and antibiotic therapy of etiologically undefined infections. Pediatr Clin North Am. 1968;15:141.
6. Moellering RC Jr. A rational approach to the choice of antimicrobial agents in bacterial infections. In: Seminar on Gram-Negative Infections. St Louis: 1974:5.
7. Thornsberry C. Automated procedures for antimicrobial susceptibility tests. In: Lennette EH, Balows A, Hausler WJ Jr, et al., eds. Manual of Clinical Microbiology. Washington DC: American Society for Microbiology; 1985:1015.
8. Murray BE, Moellering RC Jr. Patterns and mechanisms of antibiotic resistance. Med Clin North Am. 1978;62:899.
9. Puoff KL. Gram-positive vancomycin-resistant clinical isolates. Clin Microbiol Newsletter. 1989;11:1.
10. Moellering RC Jr, Kunz LJ, Poitras JW, et al. Microbiologic basis for the rational use of antibiotics. South Med J. 1977;70(Suppl):8.
11. Abramowicz M, ed. The choice of antimicrobial drugs. Med Lett. 1988;30:33.
12. Weinstein L, Dalton AC. Host determinants of response to antimicrobial agents. N Engl J Med. 1968;279:467.
13. Moellering RC Jr. Factors influencing the clinical use of antimicrobial agents in elderly patients. Geriatrics. 1978;33:83.
14. Mannisto PT, Mantyla R, Nykanen S, et al. Impairing effect of food on ketoconazole absorption. Antimicrob Agents Chemother. 1982;21:730.
15. Jackson GG, Arcieri G. Ototoxicity of gentamicin in man: A survey and controlled analysis of clinical experience in the United States. J Infect Dis. 1969;119:432.
16. Calderwood S, Moellering RC Jr. Common adverse effects of antibacterial agents on major organ systems. Surg Clin North Am. 1980;60:65.
17. Moellering RC Jr. Antimicrobial agents in pregnancy and the postpartum period. Clin Obstet Gynecol. 1989;22:277.
18. McCracken GH Jr. Pharmacologic basis for antimicrobial therapy in newborn infants. Am J Dis Child. 1974;128:407.
19. Kline AH, Blattner RJ, Lunin M. Transplacental effect of tetracyclines on teeth. JAMA. 1964;118:178.
20. Hoyer D, Walfson J. Adverse effects of quinolone antibiotics. In: Hooper D, Wolfson J, eds. Quinolone Antimicrobial Agents. Washington DC: American Society for Microbiology; 1989:249–271.
21. Garibaldi RA, Drusin RE, Ferebee SH, et al. Isoniazid-associated hepatitis. Am Rev Respir Dis. 1972;106:357.
22. Anonymous. Preventive therapy of tuberculous infection. MMWR. 1975;24:71.
23. Foord RD. Cephaloridine, cephalothin and the kidney. J Antimicrob Chemother. 1975;1(Suppl):119.
24. Koch-Weser J, Sidel VW, Federman EB, et al. Adverse effects of sodium colistimethate. Ann Intern Med. 1970;72:857.
25. Van Scoy RE. Antituberculous agents. Mayo Clin Proc. 1977;52:694.
26. Young DS, Thomas DW, Friedman RB, et al. Effects of drugs on clinical laboratory tests. Clin Chem. 1972;18:1041.
27. Rizack MA, Hilman CDM. The Medical Letter Handbook of Drug Interactions. New Rochelle, NY: The Medical Letter; 1983.
28. Sabath LD. Antibiotics in obstetric practice. In: Charles D, Finland M, eds. Obstetric and Perinatal Infections. Philadelphia: Lea & Febiger; 1973:563.
29. Monif GRG. Infectious Diseases in Obstetrics and Gynecology. Hagerstown, MD: Harper & Row; 1974:18.
30. Anonymous. Ticarcillin. Med Lett. 1977;19:17.
31. Anonymous. Is Flagyl dangerous? Med Lett. 1975;17:53.
32. Conway N, Birt BD. Streptomycin in pregnancy: Effect in foetal ear. Br Med J. 1965:2:260.
33. Monnet P, Kalb JC, Pujol M. Toxic influence of isoniazid on fetus. Lyon Med. 1967;218:431.
34. Philipson A. Pharmakokinetics of ampicillin during pregnancy. J Infect Dis. 1977;136:370.
35. Vorherr H. Drug excretion in breast milk. Postgrad Med. 1974;56:97.
36. Reeves DS. The effect of renal failure on the pharmacokinetics of antibiotics. J Antimicrob Chemother. 1988;21:5.
37. Jackson EA, McLeod DC. Pharmacokinetics and dosing of antimicrobial agents in renal impairment, part i. Am J Hosp Pharm. 1974;31:36.
38. Jackson EA, McLeod DC. Pharmacokinetics and dosing of antimicrobial agents in renal impairment, part ii. Am J Hosp Pharm. 1974;31:137.
39. Cheigh J. Drug administration in renal failure. Am J Med. 1977;62:555.
40. Bennett WM, Singer I, Coggins CJ. A guide to drug therapy in renal failure. JAMA. 1974;230:1544.
41. Appel GB, Neu HC. The nephrotoxicity of antimicrobial agents. N Engl J Med. 1977;296:663,722.
42. Natelson EA, Brown CH III, Bradshaw MW, et al. Influence of cephalosporin antibiotics on blood coagulation and platelet function. Antimicrob Agents Chemother. 1976;9:91.
43. Neu HC. Adverse effects of new cephalosporins. Ann Intern Med. 1983;98:415.
44. Kaufman CA, Frame PT. Bone marrow toxicity associated with 5-fluorocytosine therapy. Antimicrob Agents Chemother. 1977;11:244.
45. Davey PG. Pharmacokinetics in liver disease. J Antimicrob Chemother. 1988;21:1.
46. Suhrland LG, Weisberger AS. Choramphenicol toxicity in liver and renal disease. Arch Intern Med. 1963;112:747.

47. Pessayre D, Allemand H, Benhamou J-P. Effets des maladies du foie et des voies biliaires sur le métabolisme des médicaments. Nouv Presse Med. 1977;35:3209.
48. Lorian V, Atkinson B. Killing of oxacillin-exposed staphylococci in human polymorphonuclear leukocytes. Antimicrob Agents Chemother. 1980;18:807.
49. Ofek IE, Beachey H, Eisenstein BI, et al. Suppression of bacterial adherence by subminimal inhibitory concentration of β-lactam and aminoglycoside antibiotics. Rev Infect Dis. 1979;1:832.
50. Gemmell CG, Peterson PK, Schmeling DJ, et al. Potentiation of opsonization and phagocytosis of *Streptococcus pyogenes* following growth in the presence of clindamycin. J Clin Invest. 1981;67:1249.
51. Friedman HH, Warren GH. Enhanced susceptibility of penicillin-resistant staphylococci to phagocytosis after in vitro incubation with low dose of nafcillin. Proc Soc Exp Biol Med. 1974;146:707.
52. Elliott GR, Peterson PK, Verbrugh HA, et al. Influence of subinhibitory concentrations of penicillin, cephalothin, and clindamycin on *Staphyloccus aureus* growth in human phagocytic cells. Antimicrob Agents Chemother. 1982;22:781.
53. Smith CR. The spiramycin paradox. J Antimicrob Chemother. 1988;22(Suppl B):141.
54. Craig WA, Kunin CM. Significance of serum protein and tissue binding of antimicrobial agents. Annu Rev Med. 1976;27:287.
55. Peterson LR, Gerding DN. Interaction of cephalosporins with human and canine serum proteins. J Infect Dis. 1978;137:452.
56. Barza M, Samuelson T, Weinstein L. Penetration of antibiotics into fibrin loci in vivo. II. Comparison of nine antibiotics: Effect of dose and degree of protein binding. J Infect Dis. 1974;129:66.
57. Kunst MW, Mattie H. Cefazolin and cephradine. Relationship between antibacterial activity in vitro and in mice experimentally infected with *Escherichia coli*. J Infect Dis. 1978;137:391.
58. Merrikin DJ, Briant J, Rolinson GN. Effect of protein binding on antibiotic activity in vivo. J Antimicrob Chemother. 1983;11:233.
59. Kaiser AB, McGee ZA. Aminoglycoside therapy of gram-negative bacillary meningitis. N Engl J Med. 1975;293:1215.
60. Waldvogel FW. Treatment of osteomyelitis and septic arthritis with quinolone antimicrobial agents. In: Hooper D, Wolfson J, eds. Quinolone antimicrobial Agents. Washington DC: American Society for Microbiology; 1989:177–86.
61. Bryant RE, Howard D. Interaction of purulent material with antibiotics used to treat *Pseudomonas* infections. Antimicrob Agents Chemother. 1974;6:702.
62. O'Keefe JP, Tally FP, Barza M, et al. Inactivation of penicillin G during experimental infection with *Bacteroides fragilis*. J Infect Dis. 1978;137:437.
63. Zimelis VM, Jackson GG. Activity of aminoglycoside antibiotics against *Pseudomonas aeruginosa*. Specificity and site of calcium and magnesium antagonism. J Infect Dis. 1973;127:663.
64. Bryan LE, Van Den Elzen HM. Streptomycin accumulation in susceptible and resistant strains of *Escherichia coli* and *Pseudomonas aeruginosa*. Antimicrob Agents Chemother. 1976;9:928.
65. Zinner SH, Sabath LD, Casey JI, et al. Erythromycin and alkalinization of the urine in the treatment of urinary tract infections due to gram-negative bacilli. Lancet. 1971;1:1267.
66. Sabath LD, Gerstein DA, Leaf CD, et al. Increasing the usefulness of antibiotics: Treatment of infections caused by gram-negative bacilli. Clin Pharmacol Ther. 1970;11:161.
67. Karchmer AW, Dismukes WE, Buckley MJ, et al. Late prosthetic valve endocarditis. Am J Med. 1978;64:99.
68. Zimmerli W, Waldvogel FA, Vaudaux P, et al. Pathogenesis of foreign body infection: Description and characteristics of an animal model. J Infect Dis. 1982;146:487.
69. Dickinson GM, Bisno AL. Infections associated with indwelling medical devices. Antimicrob Agents Chemother. In press.
70. Forsgren A, Schmeling D, Quie PG. Effect of tetracycline on the phagocytic function of human leukocytes. J Infect Dis. 1974;130:412.
71. Seklecki MM, Quintiliani R, Maderazo EG. Aminoglycoside antibiotics moderately impair granulocyte function. Antimicrob Agents Chemother. 1978;13:552.
72. Chaperon EA, Sanders WE Jr. Suppression of lymphoctye responses by cephalosporins. Infect Immun. 1978;19:378.
73. Mandell LA. Effects of antimicrobial and antineoplastic drugs on the phagocytic and microbicidal function of the polymorphonuclear leukocyte. Rev Infect Dis. 1982;4:683.
74. Hauser WE, Remington JS. Effect of antibiotics on the immune response. Am J Med. 1982;72:711.
75. Manzella JP, Clark JK. Effects of moxalactam and cefuroxime on mitogen-stimulated human mononuclear leukocytes. Antimicrob Agents Chemother. 1983;23:360.
76. Daschner FD. Antibiotics and host defense with special reference to phagocytosis by human polymorphonuclear leukocyte function in vivo. Antimicrob Agents Chemother. 1985;27:712.
77. Jawetz E. Combined antibiotic action: Some definitions and correlations between laboratory and clinical results. Antimicrob Agents Chemother. 1967,1968;203.
78. Krogstad DJ, Moellering RC Jr. Antimicrobial combinations. In: Lorian V, ed. Antibiotics in Laboratory Medicine. 2nd ed. Baltimore: Williams & Wilkins; 1986:537–95.
79. Moellering RC Jr. Use and abuse of antibiotic combinations. RI Med J. 1972;55:341.
80. VanderAuwera P, Meunier-Carpentier F, Klastersky J. Clinical study of combination therapy with oxacillin and rifampin for staphylococcal infections. Rev Infect Dis. 1983;5(Suppl 3):515.
81. Karchmer AW, Archer GL, Dimukes WE. Rifampin treatment of prosthetic valve endocarditis due to *Staphylococcus epidermidis*. Rev Infect Dis. 1983;5(Suppl 3):543.
82. Lehr D. Inhibition of drug precipitation in the urinary tract by the use of sulfonamide mixtures. I. Sulfathiazole-sulfadiazine mixture. Proc Soc Exp Biol Med. 1945;58:11.
83. Rahal JJ Jr. Antibiotic combinations: The clinical relevance of synergy and antagonism. Medicine (Baltimore). 1978;57:179.
84. Mandell GL, Kaye D, Levison ME, et al. Enterococcal endocarditis. An analysis of 38 patients observed at the New York Hospital–Cornell Medical Center. Arch Intern Med. 1970;125:258.
85. Moellering RC Jr, Wennersten C, Weinberg AN. Studies on antibiotic synergism against enterococci: I. Bacteriologic studies. J Lab Clin Med. 1971;77:821.
86. Moellering RC Jr, Weinberg AN. Studies on antibiotic synergism against enterococci: II. Effect of various antibiotics on the uptake of ^{14}C-labelled streptomycin by enterococci. J Clin Invest. 1971;50:2580.
87. Moellering RC Jr, Wennersten CBG, Medrek T, et al. Prevalence of high-level resistance ot aminoglycosides in clinical isolates of enterococci. Antimicrob Agents Chemother. 1970, 1971;335.
88. Zimmermann RA, Moellering RC Jr, Weinberg AN. Mechanism of resistance to antibiotic synergism in enterococci. J Bacteriol. 1971;105:873.
89. Krogstad DJ, Korfhagen TR, Moellering RC Jr, et al. Aminoglycoside-inactivating enzymes: An explanation for resistance to penicillin-aminoglycoside synergism in enterococci. J Clin Invest. 1978;62:480.
90. Mederski-Samoraj BD, Murray BE. High-level resistance to gentamicin in clinical isolates of enterococci. J Infect Dis. 1983;147:751.
91. Moellering RC Jr. The enterococcus: High-level resistance to gentamicin and production of beta-lactamase. Clin Microbiol Newsletter. 1988;10:129.
92. Fernandez-Guerrero ML, Barros C, Tudela JLR, et al. Aortic endocarditis caused by gentamicin-resistant *Enterococcus*. Eur J Clin Microbiol. 1988;7:525.
93. Wolfe JC, Johnson WD Jr. Penicillin-sensitive streptococcal endocarditis. Ann Intern Med. 1974;81:178.
94. Karchmer AW, Moellering RC Jr, Maki D, et al. Single antibiotic therapy of streptococcal endocarditis. JAMA. 1979;241:1801.
95. Watanakunakorn C, Glotzbecker C. Enhancement of the effects of antistaphylococcal antibiotics by aminoglycosides. Antimicrob Agents Chemother. 1974;6:802.
96. Korzeniowski O, Sande MA. The National Collaborative Endocarditis Study Group: Combination antimicrobial therapy for *Staphylococcus aureus* endocarditis in patients addicted to parenteral drugs and in nonaddicts. Ann Intern Med. 1982;97:496.
97. Smith CB, Dans PE, Wilfert JN, et al. Use of gentamicin in combination with other antibiotics. J Infect Dis. 1969;119:370.
98. Eliopoulos GM, Moellering RC Jr. Azlocillin, mezlocillin and piperacillin: New broad-spectrum penicillins. Ann Intern Med. 1982;97:755.
99. Adriole VT. Antibiotic synergy in experimental infection with *Pseudomonas:* II. The effect of carbenicillin, cephalothin or cephanone combined with tobramycin or gentamicin. J Infect Dis. 1974;129:124.
100. Then R. Synergism between trimethoprim and sulfonamides. Science. 1977;197:1301.
101. Harding GKM, Ronald AR. A controlled study of antimicrobial prophylaxis of recurrent urinary tract infections in women. N Engl J Med. 1974;291:597.
102. Gilman RN, Terminel M, Levine MM, et al. Comparison of trimethoprim-sulfamethoxazole and amoxicillin in therapy of chloramphenicol-resistant and chloramphenicol-sensitive typhoid fever. J Infect Dis. 1975;132:630.
103. Chang MJ, Dunkle LM, Van Reken D, et al. Trimethoprim-sulfamethoxazole compared to ampicillin in the treatment of shigellosis. Pediatrics. 1977;59:726.
104. Quintiliani R, Levite RE, Nightingale CH. Potential role of trimethoprim-sulfamethoxazole in the treatment of serious hospital-acquired infections. Rev Infect Dis. 9(Suppl 2):S160, 1987;9(Suppl 2):160.
105. Kwan CN, Medoff G, Kobayashi G, et al. Potentiation of the anti-fungal effects of antibiotics by amphotericin B. Antimicrob Agents Chemother. 1972;2:61.
106. Titsworth E, Grunberg E. Chemotherapeutic activity of 5-fluorocytosine and amphotericin B against *Candida albicans* in mice. Antimicrob Agents Chemother. 1973;4:306.
107. Bennett J, Dismukes W, Duma R, et al. A comparison of amphotericin B alone with amphotericin B plus flucytosine in the treatment of cryptoccal meningitis. N Engl J Med. 1979;301:126.
108. Lau WK, Young LS, Block RE, et al. Comparative efficacy and toxicity of amikacin/carbenicillin versus gentamicin/carbenicillin in leukopenic patients. Am J Med. 1977;62:959.
109. Klastersky J, Hensgens C, Meunier-Carpentier F. Comparative effectiveness of combinations of amikacin with penicillin G and amikacin with carbenicillin in gram-negative septicemia: Double-blind clinical trial. J Infect Dis. 1976;134(Suppl):433.
110. Moellering RC Jr. Monotherapy with expanded-spectrum cephalosporins for empiric treatment of serious infections diseases. In Hoepelman IM, Moell-

ering RC Jr, eds. New Directions in Cephalosporin Therapy: The Expanded Spectrum Cephalosporins. Winchester, UK: Theracom; 1988:49.
111. Lepper MH, Dowling HF. Treatment of pneumococcic meningitis with penicillin compared with penicillin plus aureomycin. Arch Intern Med. 1951;88:489.
112. Mathies AW Jr, Leedom JM, Ivier D, et al. Antibiotic antagonism in bacterial meningitis. Antimicrob Agents Chemother. 1967;7:218.
113. Sande MA, Overton JW. In vivo antagonism between gentamicin and chloramphenicol in neutropenic mice. J Infect Dis. 1973;128:247.
114. Strausbaugh LJ, Sande MA. Factors influencing the therapy of experimental *Proteus mirabilis* meningitis in rabbits. J Infect Dis. 1978;137:251.
115. Swedish Study Group: Cefuroxime versus ampicillin and chloramphenicol for the treatment of bacterial meningitis. Lancet. 1982;1:295.
116. Del Rio MDL, Chrane D, Shelton S, et al. Ceftriaxone versus ampicillin and chloramphenicol for treatment of bacterial meningitis in children. Lancet. 1983;1:1241.
117. Moellering RC Jr. Rationale for the use of antibiotic combinations. Am J Med. 1983;75(2A):4.
118. Sanders CC. Novel resistance selected by the new expanded spectrum cephalosporins: A concern. J Infect Dis. 1983;147:585.
119. McLaughlin JE, Reeves DS. Clinical and laboratory evidence for inactivation of gentamicin by carbenicillin. Lancet. 1971;1:261.
120. Riff LJ, Jackson GG. Laboratory and clinical conditions for gentamicin inactivation by carbenicillin. Arch Intern Med. 1972;130:887.
121. Seidl LG, Thornton GF, Smith SW, et al. Studies on epidemiology of adverse drug reactions. III. Reactions in patients on general medical service. Bull Johns Hopkins Hosp. 1966;119:299.
122. Drusano GL. Pharmacokinetics of quinolone antimicrobial agents. In: Hooper D, Wolfson J, eds. Quinolone Antimicrobial Agents. Washington DC: American Society for Microbiology; 1989:71–105.
123. Barza M, Brusch J, Bergeron M, et al. Penetration of antibiotics into fibrin loci in vivo. III. Intermittent versus continuous infusion and the effect of probenicid. J Infect Dis. 1974;129:73.
124. Nelson JD. Antibiotic concentrations in septic joint effusions. N Engl J Med. 1971;284:349.
125. Gerding DN, Hall WH. The penetration of antibiotics into peritoneal fluid. Bull NY Acad Med. 1975;51:1016.
126. Schlichter JG, MacLean H. A method of determining the effective therapeutic level in the treatment of subacute bacterial endocarditis with penicillin. Am Heart J. 1947;34:209.
127. Reller LB, Stratton CW. Serum dilution test for bactericidal activity. II. Standardization and correlation with antimicrobial assays and susceptibility tests. J Infect Dis. 1977;136:196.
128. Carrizosa J, Kaye D. Antibiotic concentrations in serum, serum bactericidal activity, and results of therapy of streptococcal endocarditis in rabbits. Antimicrob Agents Chemother. 1977;12:479.
129. Weinstein MP, Stratton CW, Ackley A, et al. Multicenter collaborative evaluation of a standardized serum bactericidal test as a prognostic indicator in infective endocarditis. Am J Med 1985;78:262.
130. Levy J, Klastersky J. Serum bactericidal test: A review with emphasis on its role in the evaluation of antibiotic combination. In: Klastersky J, Staquet MJ, eds. Combination Antibiotic Therapy in the Compromised Host. New York: Raven Press; 1982:43.
131. Pien FD, Vosti KL. Variation in performance of the serum bactericidal test. Antimicrob Agents Chemother. 1974;6:330.
132. Stratton CW, Reller LB. Serum dilution test for bactericidal activity. I. Selection of a physiologic diluent. J Infect Dis. 1977;136:187.
133. Mellors JW, Colman DL, Andriole VT. Value of the serum bactericidal test in management of patients with bacterial endocarditis. Eur J Clin Microbiol. 1986;5:67.
134. Reller LB. The serum bactericidal test. Rev Infect Dis. 1986;8:803.

16. MECHANISMS OF ANTIBIOTIC RESISTANCE

KENNETH H. MAYER
STEVEN M. OPAL
ANTONE A. MEDEIROS

MOLECULAR GENETICS OF ANTIBIOTIC RESISTANCE

Genetic variability is essential in order for microbial evolution to occur. Antimicrobial agents exert strong selective pressures upon bacterial populations and favor those organisms that are capable of resisting them.[1,2] Genetic variability may occur by a variety of mechanisms. Point mutation may occur at a nucleotide base pair, a process referred to as microevolutionary change. Point mutations may alter the target site of an antimicrobial agent, thereby interfering with its activity.

A second level of genomic variability in bacteria is referred to as a macroevolutionary change and results in whole-scale rearrangements of large segments of DNA as a single event. Such rearrangements may include inversions, duplications, insertions, deletions, or transpositions of large sequences of DNA from one location of the bacterial chromosome to another. These whole-scale rearrangements of large segments of the bacterial chromosome are frequently created by specialized genetic elements known as transposons, or insertion sequences that have the capacity to move independently of the rest of the bacterial chromosome.[2]

A third level of genetic variability in bacteria is created by the acquisition of foreign DNA carried by plasmids, bacteriophages, or transposable genetic elements. Inheritance of these extrachromosomal elements further contributes to the organism's ability to cope with selection pressures imposed by antimicrobial agents.[3] These mechanisms endow bacteria with the seemingly unlimited capacity to develop resistance to any antimicrobial agent. Once an antibiotic resistance gene evolves, this resistance determinant may spread to other bacteria by transformation, transduction, conjugation, or transposition. Favored clones of bacteria may then proliferate in the flora of patients exposed to antibiotics.

Plasmids

Extrachromosomal elements were present in bacteria before the advent of antibiotics.[4] However, the introduction of antibiotics into clinical medicine over the past five decades has created selection pressures that favored the dissemination of antibiotic resistance genes via mobile genetic elements, i.e., plasmids and transposons. Rapid increases in the spread of antibiotic resistance within species and between species is often correlated with the dissemination of resistance (R). Plasmids are particularly well adapted to serve as agents of genetic evolution and resistance gene dissemination.[5] Plasmids are extrachromosomal genetic elements that are made of circular double-stranded DNA molecules that range in size from less than 10 to greater than 400 kilobase pairs and are extremely common in bacteria.[6] While multiple copies of a specific plasmid and/or multiple different plasmids may be found in a single bacterial cell, closely related plasmids often cannot coexist in the same cell. This observation has led to a classification scheme of plasmids that is based upon incompatibility groups.[7]

Plasmids may determine a wide range of functions besides antibiotic resistance, including virulence and metabolic capacities. Plasmids are autonomous, self-reproducing genetic elements that require an origin of replication and a region of the plasmid that is essential for its stable maintenance in host bacteria.[7] Conjugative plasmids require additional genes that can initiate self-transfer.[8]

The transfer of plasmid DNA between bacterial species is a complex process, and thus conjugative plasmids tend to be larger than nonconjugative plasmids. Some small plasmids may be able to use the conjugation apparatus of a coresident conjugative plasmid. Many plasmid-encoded functions enable bacterial strains to persist in the environment by resisting noxious agents. Compounds such as hexachlorophene are used as topical bacteriostatic agents, and plasmid-mediated resistance to these agents has increased significantly in recent years.[9]

Plasmids may be involved in the dissemination of antibiotic resistance in several ways (Fig. 1). A single clone of a specific organism may become resistant by mutation or by the inheritance of a resistance plasmid. The resultant resistant organism may have genes that are particularly well adapted to a specific niche and thus be able to disseminate widely. The single clone

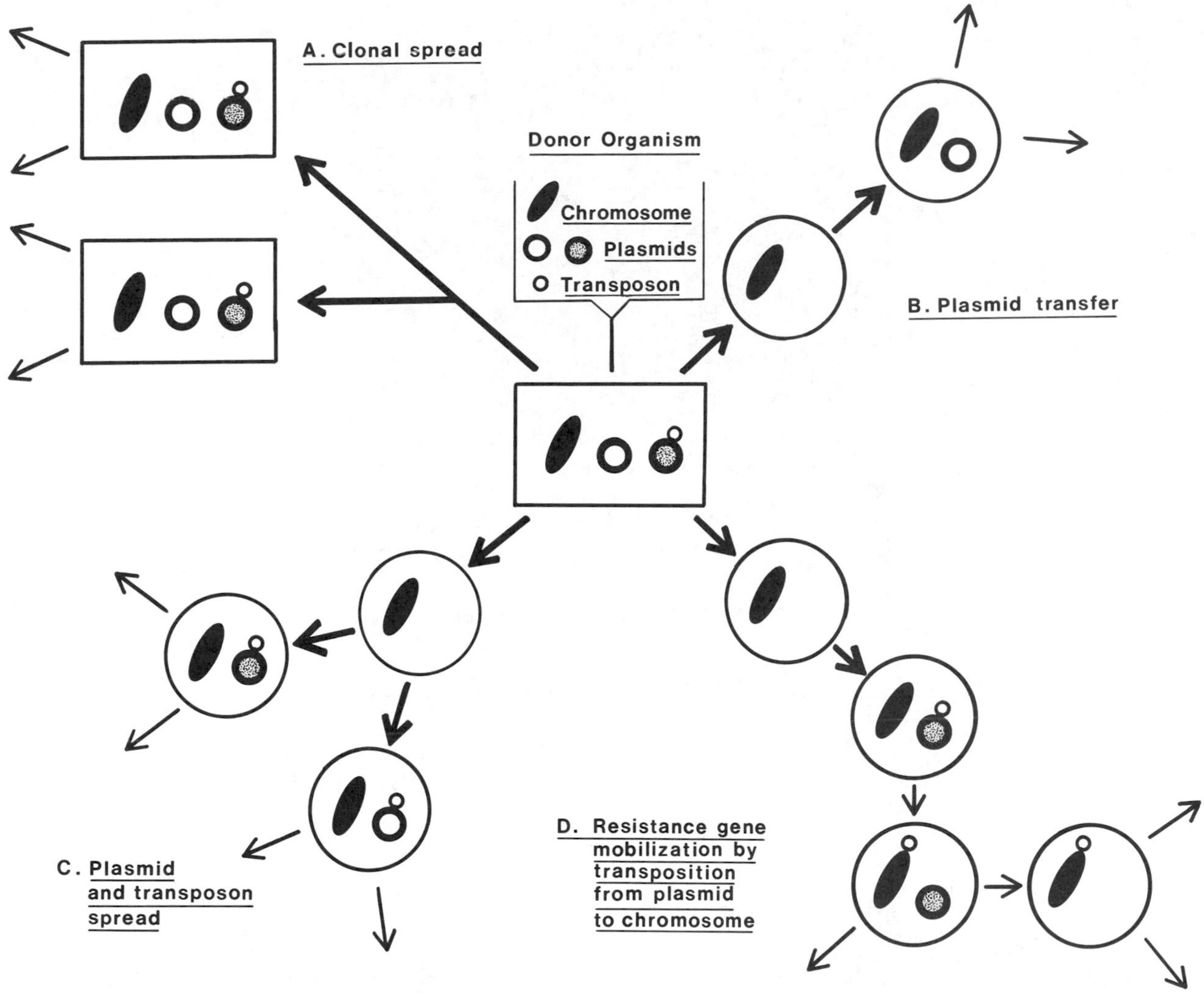

FIG. 1. Examples of the molecular spread of antibiotic resistance. The donor organism has a chromosome, two plasmids, and a transposon. If it is well adapted to a particular niche, it may remain stable in the environment and continue to replicate itself and thus disseminate through clonal spread **(A)**. If the organism comes into close physical contact with another bacterium that may not possess extrachromosomal DNA, attachment between the two cells from different bacterial species may allow for the introduction of one of the plasmids by conjugation **(B)**. The donor organism may be able to spread resistance genes through several mechanisms including the spread of transposons as well as plasmids **(C)**. Transposons may be able to hop between plasmids **(C)**, or they may be able to allow for the mobilization of resistance genes by being transferred on a conjugative plasmid into new bacterial species and then hop from the plasmid to the chromosome **(D)**. Some transposons may subsequently become integrated into the host chromosome and be spread as a stable genetic element in the chromosome without any subsequent transfer via plasmid DNA.

may be responsible for multiple outbreaks of antibiotic resistance. Conjugative plasmids may be transferred from one species to another and result in new outbreaks of antibiotic-resistant organisms.[10] Transposons create the potential for even wider dissemination of antibiotic resistance genes.[11]

Transposable Genetic Elements

Transposons can translocate from one area of the bacterial chromosome to another or between the chromosome and plasmid or bacteriophage DNA. Transposable genetic elements possess a specialized system of recombination that is independent of the generalized recombination system that classically permits recombination of largely homologous sequences of DNA by crossover events (the recA system of bacteria). The recA-independent recombination system of transposable elements usually occurs in a random fashion between nonhomologous sequences of DNA and results in whole-scale modifications of large sequences of DNA as a single event (Fig. 2).[1,3]

There are two types of transposable genetic elements, referred to as transposons and insertion sequences, that have similar characteristics. Transposons (Tn) differ from insertion sequences in that they mediate a recognizable phenotypic characteristic such as an antibiotic resistance marker. Either element can translocate as an independent unit. Transposons and insertion sequences are incapable of autonomous self-replication and therefore must exist on a replicon such as the chromosome, bacteriophage, or plasmid in order to be replicated and maintained in a bacterial population. Recently, a new class of transposable elements has been described that have the capability to move from the chromosome of one bacterium to another without being part of a plasmid or bacteriophage. These elements are referred to as "conjugative" transposons and have been found in aerobic and anaerobic gram-positive organisms.[12,13]

Transposition usually results in localized replication of the transposable element from the original donor sequence of DNA as well as the insertion of a copy of the transposable element

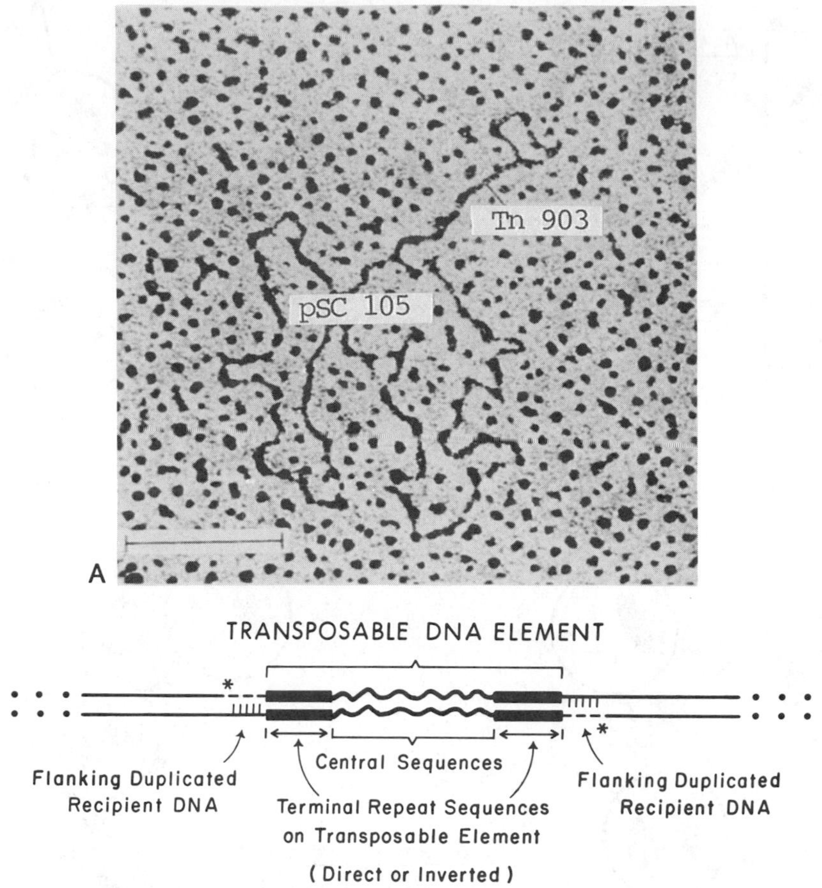

FIG. 2. **(A)** Characteristic appearance of a transposon by electron microscopy showing the stem-loop configuration. The kanamycin resistance transposon Tn903 is inserted into a small plasmid (pSC105). After denaturation, intrastrand annealing of the complementary, 1000 base pair, inverted repeat terminal sequences of the transposon form the stem structure. The kanamycin resistance gene and the genes necessary for transposition are located in the central loop structure. **(B)** The structure of a transposable element inserted into a recipient DNA sequence. The transposon (depicted by the rectangles and wavy lines) consists of a central sequence containing the phenotypic marker gene(s) (antibiotic resistance gene) and the "transposase" genes. The terminal repeat sequences of the transposon flank the central sequences on both sides. Insertion of the transposon results in single-strand, staggered cuts in the recipient DNA (marked by asterisks). Subsequent gap-filling DNA synthesis and ligation results in duplication of a short sequence of recipient DNA at either end of the transposon. (From Kopecko,[1] with permission.)

into the recipient sequence of DNA (replicative transposition).[1–3] Transposition is a continuous and ongoing process in bacterial populations. A recent example of this phenomenon is the spread of a tetracycline resistance transposon among *Neisseria gonorrhoeae, Mycoplasma hominis,* and *Ureaplasma urealyticum*.[14,15] Transposons are also essential in the evolution of R plasmids that contain multiple antibiotic resistance determinants.[11] Single transposons may encode multiple antibiotic resistance determinants within their inverted repeat termini as well.[3]

MECHANISMS OF ANTIBIOTIC RESISTANCE

At least seven distinctive mechanisms of antibiotic resistance have been described in bacteria (Table 1).

Enzymatic Inhibition

β-Lactamases. Resistance to β-lactam antibiotics is due mainly to the production of β-lactamases, enzymes that inactivate these antibiotics by splitting the amide bond of the β-lactam ring. Numerous β-lactamases exist, encoded either by chromosomal genes or by transferable genes located on plasmids or transposons.[17]

Three evolutionarily distinct classes of β-lactamases have been defined on the basis of amino acid and nucleotide sequence studies. Class A β-lactamases have molecular weights around 29,000, possess a serine residue at their active site, and preferentially hydrolyze penicillins. An example is the TEM-1 β-lactamase widely prevalent in gram-negative bacilli. Class B β-lactamase is a metalloenzyme with a molecular weight of 23,000 that attacks cephalosporins preferentially. Class C includes the chromosomally determined β-lactamase of *Escherichia coli,* which shares extensive sequence homology with chromosomally mediated β-lactamases of *Shigella* and *Klebsiella* species. These enzymes are large proteins with molecular weights about 39,000 and also have serine at their active site but share no homology with the class A β-lactamases.[18]

GRAM-POSITIVE BACTERIA. Among the gram-positive bacteria staphylococci are the major pathogens that produce β-lactamase. Staphylococcal β-lactamases preferentially hydrolyze penicillins. Most are inducible and are excreted extracellularly.[17] The genes that determine staphylococcal β-lactamases are usually carried on small plasmids that can be transferred from cell to cell by transduction. Larger plasmids encoding β-lactamase and other resistances also exist and can transfer by conjugation, not only between strains of *Staphylococcus aureus* but also between *S. aureus* and *Staphylococcus epidermidis*.[19]

TABLE 1. Major Mechanisms of Antibiotic Resistance

	Type of Antibiotic											
Resistance Mechanism	*β-Lactams*	*Amino-glycosides*	*Chloram-phenicol*	*Macrolides*	*Lincos-amides*	*Sulfon-amides*	*Trimetho-prim*	*Tetra-cyclines*	*Quino-lones*	*Vanco-mycin*[a]	*Rifampin*	*Polymyxin*
1. Enzymatic inhibition	B	B	P	P	—	—	—	—	—	—	—	—
2. Membrane impermeability	C	C	P	—	—	C	C	B	—	C	—	C
3. Alteration in intracellular target site	—	C	C	B	B	—	—	B	—	—	—	C
4. Alteration in target enzyme	B	—	—	—	—	B	B	—	C	—	C	—
5. Overproduction of target enzyme	—	—	—	—	—	C	C	—	—	—	—	—
6. Auxotrophs that bypass inhibited steps	—	—	—	—	—	B	B	—	—	—	—	—
7. Active pumping out of substrate	—	—	—	—	—	—	—	B	—	—	—	—

[a] Plasmid-mediated vancomycin resistance has been described, but its mechanism has not yet been characterized.[16]
Abbreviations: P: plasmid mediated; C: chromosomally mediated; B: both; —: not yet described.

The streptococci also produce β-lactamase; an *Enterococcus faecalis* strain produces a plasmid-determined β-lactamase that appears to be of staphylococcal origin.[20]

GRAM-NEGATIVE BACTERIA. Gram-negative bacteria produce a much greater variety of β-lactamases than do gram-positive bacteria. This diversity has led to several classification schemes. Over 30 different plasmid-determined β-lactamases have been discovered.[21] All are produced constitutively and can be grouped into three broad classes: (*1*) those that hydrolyze benzylpenicillin and cephaloridine at similar rates (broad-spectrum enzymes), (*2*) those that hydrolyze oxacillin and related penicillins rapidly (oxacillinases), and (*3*) those that break down carbenicillin readily (carbenicillinases). The properties of the plasmid-determined β-lactamases are summarized in Table 2.

ANAEROBIC BACTERIA. The resistance of anaerobic bacteria to β-lactam antibiotics also involves the production of β-lactamases. The β-lactamases of fusobacteria and clostridia are principally penicillinases. Those produced by *Bacteroides fragilis* are predominantly cephalosporinases, some of which have been found to hydrolyze cefoxitin and imipenem and may be transferable.[22,23]

DISTRIBUTION IN CLINICAL ISOLATES. The existence of β-lactamase genes on plasmids and transposons ensures that a β-lactamase originally confined to one group of bacteria sooner or later may appear in other groups. The widespread use of antibiotics fosters selection of the resistant organisms, which rise in prevalence locally and then spread worldwide. A prime example of this process occurred with the TEM-1 β-lactamase, which has spread from the Enterobacteriaceae to *Haemophilus influenzae*[24] and *N. gonorrhoeae*.[25] Clinical isolates may produce two and even three plasmid-determined β-lactamases. In nearly all cases TEM-1 is one of the β-lactamases produced. A large number of strains from South America and the Far East have had novel and/or multiple plasmid β-lactamases.[19]

The success of the pharmaceutical industry in developing new β-lactams resistant to hydrolysis by β-lactamases led to the introduction into clinical use of the third-generation cephalosporins around 1978 in Europe and 1981 in the United States. These antibiotics were very resistant to hydrolysis by the known plasmid-determined β-lactamases. Then in 1983 in Germany, isolates of *Klebsiella pneumoniae* and then other Enterobacteriaceae were discovered that produced a plasmid-determined β-lactamase that hydrolyzed cefotaxime as well as other newer cephalosporins. This new β-lactamase, called SHV-2, derived from a mutation in the well-known SHV-1 β-lactamase commonly found in *Klebsiella*. The mutation resulted in an enhanced affinity of the SHV-1 β-lactamase for cefotaxime.[26] More recently, cefotaxime-resistant strains of *K. pneumoniae* producing a novel plasmid-encoded, TEM-like, cefotaxime-hydrolyzing β-lactamase, designated CTX-1, have been recovered from several French hospitals.[27] Also, three novel plasmid-encoded β-lactamases that hydrolyze ceftazidime and aztreonam have appeared in clinical isolates from France and Germany.[28,29] On the basis of DNA hybridization studies these new β-lactamases appear to be derivatives of the TEM-2 β-lactamase.[30] Thus, in response to new selection pressures engendered by the frequent use of third-generation cephalosporins, mutations have occurred among the well-established plasmid-determined β-lactamases, which has resulted in the dissemination of novel transferable β-lactamases with an expanded spectrum of activity.

β-LACTAMASES DETERMINED BY CHROMOSOMAL GENES. Virtually all gram-negative bacteria produce some chromosomally determined β-lactamase. Furthermore, the types of β-lactamase produced are often specific for species and sometimes for subspecies. β-Lactamase activity is frequently very low, particularly in ampicillin-susceptible isolates, but may increase due to induction or to alterations in the number of β-lactamase genes on the chromosome; also, mutation of genes that regulate induction may lead to constitutive hyperproduction of inducible β-lactamases.[31] Most of the chromosomally determined β-lactamases preferentially hydrolyze cephalosporins, including many of the third-generation agents that are resistant to hydrolysis by the plasmid-determined β-lactamases (Table 3).[31a]

Chromosomally determined β-lactamases nearly always differ in their biochemical properties from the plasmid-determined enzymes. The exception is a chromosomal β-lactamase found in many isolates of *K. pneumoniae* that is indistinguishable from the SHV-1 β-lactamase. It may be that the SHV-1 β-lactamase gene evolved as a chromosomal gene in *Klebsiella* and was later incorporated into a plasmid.[32] As yet no such ancestral chromosomal gene has been found for the much more common TEM-1 β-lactamase or for any of the other plasmid-determined β-lactamases.

CONTRIBUTION OF β-LACTAMASES TO β-LACTAM ANTIBIOTIC RESISTANCE. The level of antibiotic resistance mediated by a particular β-lactamase in a population of bacteria is determined by several variables. The efficiency of the β-lactamase in hydrolyzing an antibiotic depends on both its rate of hydrolysis (V_{max}) and its affinity for the antibiotic (K_m). Other variables are the amount of β-lactamase produced by the bacterial cell, the susceptibility of the target protein (penicillin binding protein [PBP]) to the antibiotic, and the rate of diffusion of the antibiotic into the periplasm of the cell.

Within the bacterial cell, β-lactamases contribute to antibiotic resistance in several ways. The simplest model is that of penicillinase-producing staphylococci in which the bacteria, upon exposure to penicillin, begin to produce β-lactamase, which they excrete extracellularly. Two events then take place concurrently: (*1*) penicillin lyses bacteria, and (*2*) β-lactamase hydrolyzes penicillin. If viable bacterial cells remain after the level

TABLE 2. Properties of Plasmid-Determined β-Lactamases

β-Lactamase	*pI*	*Prevalence*	*Host Bacteria*	*Specific Features*
Broad Spectrum				
HMS-1	5.2	Rare	Enterobacteriaceae	
TEM-1	5.4	Very common	Enterobacteriaceae *P. aeruginosa* *H. influenzae* *N. gonorrhoeae* *Vibrio cholerae*	Most common type in nearly all bacterial species
TLE-1	5.55	Rare	*E. coli*	Closely related to TEM-1
TEM-2	5.6	Common	Enterobacteriaceae	Differs from TEM-1 by 1 amino acid
LCR-1	5.85	Rare	*P. aeruginosa*	
NPS-1	6.5	Rare	*P. aeruginosa*	Cefsulodin induces conformational change
TLE-2	6.5	Rare	*K. pneumoniae*	High affinity for cefsulodin and cefotetan
LXA-1	6.7	Uncommon	Enterobacteriaceae	Very low affinity for benzylpenicillin confers low-level β-lactam resistance
OHIO-1	7.0	Uncommon	Enterobacteriaceae	Only found in isolates from Ohio
SHV-1	7.6	Common	Enterobacteriaceae	Often encoded by chromosomal genes in *K. pneumoniae*
ROB-1	8.1	Uncommon	*H. influenzae* *H. pleuropneumoniae* *P. multocida*	Found in both human and animal isolates
Oxacillinase				
Unnamed (Gn11499)	6.9	Rare	*B. fragilis*	
OXA-3	7.1	Uncommon	Enterobacteriaceae *P. aeruginosa*	
OXA-1	7.4	Common	Enterobacteriaceae *P. aeruginosa*	Second most common type in *E. coli*
OXA-4	7.45	Rare	Enterobacteriaceae	Closely related to OXA-1
OXA-5	7.62	Rare	*P. aeruginosa*	
OXA-7	7.65	Rare	*E. coli*	
OXA-6	7.68	Rare	*P. aeruginosa*	
OXA-2	7.7	Common	Enterobacteriaceae *P. aeruginosa*	Second most common type in salmonellae
Carbenicillinase				
CARB-4	4.3	Rare	*P. aeruginosa*	Confers resistance to cefsulodin
SAR-1	4.9	Rare	*V. cholerae*	
PSE-4 (CARB-1)	5.3	Uncommon	*P. aeruginosa* Enterobacteriaceae	
BRO-1	5.6	Common	*Branhamella* *Moraxella*	Confers resistance to ampicillin and cefaclor
PSE-1 (CARB-2)	5.7	Common	*P. aeruginosa* Enterobacteriaceae	Most common type in *P. aeruginosa*
CARB-3	5.75	Rare	*P. aeruginosa*	
AER-1	5.9	Rare	*A. hydrophila*	
Unnamed (N-3)	6.0 (5.73)	Rare	*P. mirabilis*	Similar to PSE-1
PSE-2	6.1	Uncommon	*P. aeruginosa* Enterobacteriaceae	Hydrolyzes oxacillin rapidly
PSE-3	6.9	Uncommon	*P. aeruginosa* Enterobacteriaceae	
Unnamed (N-29)	6.9 (6.93)	Rare	*P. mirabilis*	
Cephalosporinase				
CEP-1	8.0	Rare	*P. mirabilis*	
CEP-2	8.1	Rare	*Achromobacter*	
Cefotaximase				
RHH-1	5.5	Rare	Enterobacteriaceae	
CAZ-1	5.55	Common (France)	Enterobacteriaceae	Derivative of TEM-2
CAZ	5.85	Uncommon (Germany)	Enterobacteriaceae	Derivative of TEM-2
CTX-1	6.3	Common (France)	Enterobacteriaceae	Derivative of TEM-2
SHV-2	7.6	Uncommon but widespread (Germany, France, Greece, Chile, China)	Enterobacteriaceae	Derivative of SHV-1

TABLE 3. Classification of Chromosomal β-Lactamases

Broad-spectrum cephalosporinases—hydrolyze benzylpenicillin, ampicillin, and carbenicillin as well as cephalosporins
- *P. vulgaris*
- *K. pneumoniae*
- *K. oxytoca*
- *K. aerogenes* K-1

Typical cephalosporinases—little or no activity against penicillins
- Constitutive
  - *E. coli*
  - *B. fragilis*
- Inducible
  - *E. aerogenes*
  - *E. cloacae*
  - *P. rettgeri*
  - *P. aeruginosa*
  - *A. anitratus*
  - *S. marcescens*

(Data from Sawai.[31a])

of penicillin has fallen below the minimal inhibitory concentration, regrowth of bacteria occurs.[18]

Another model is exemplified by gram-negative bacilli, which (*1*) produce a β-lactamase that remains trapped in the periplasmic space and (*2*) have no barrier to antibiotic penetration. An example is *H. influenzae* strains that produce the TEM-1 β-lactamase.[33] In both this model and the first one discussed, a marked inoculum effect occurs in that the minimal inhibitory concentration (MIC) for a large inoculum (10^6 organisms/ml) may be 1000-fold greater than with a small inoculum (10^2 organisms/ml). The low level of resistance of single cells has made it possible for ampicillin to cure some infections caused by β-lactamase-producing strains of *H. influenzae* when the inoculum of infecting bacteria was low.

Another model is exemplified by ampicillin resistance of *E. coli* strains that produce the TEM-1 β-lactamase. These bacteria have a barrier to the entry of β-lactam molecules (the outer membrane), and they produce a β-lactamase that remains localized to the periplasmic space. In this model, the kinetics are more complicated. The enzyme is strategically situated between the barrier to antibiotic penetration (outer membrane) and the antibiotic targets (penicillin binding proteins on the cytoplasmic membrane). In this position the enzyme can sequentially destroy antibiotic molecules as they make their way through the barrier in a manner analogous to a sharpshooter with abundant ammunition who aims at targets passing through a single entry point. As a consequence, high levels of resistance occur with single bacterial cells, unlike the previous example.[18]

Variations on this model may occur when the amount of β-lactamase produced increases with exposure to a β-lactam (induction) as occurs in *Enterobacter* and *Pseudomonas* species. High levels of β-lactamase are produced only after a period of exposure to the inducing antibiotic, and hence resistance may be expressed late. When *Enterobacter* strains are exposed to two β-lactam antibiotics, one of which is a potent inducer (e.g., cefamandole), antagonism between the two antibiotics may result.[34]

Aminoglycoside Resistance-Modifying Enzymes. Among aerobic bacteria, aminoglycoside resistance is most commonly due to modifying enzymes that are coded by genes on plasmids or the chromosome.[35] Several of the aminoglycoside-modifying enzymes have been shown to be carried on transposons.[11]

More than two dozen aminoglycoside-modifying enzymes that have been identified are capable of three general reactions: *N*-acetylation, *O*-nucleotidylation, and *O*-phosphorylation. For each of these general reactions there are several different enzymes that attack a specific amino or hydroxyl group. The nomenclature for these enzymes lists the molecular site where the modification occurs after the type of enzymatic activity. For example an aminoglycoside acetyltransferase (AAC) that acts at the 3′ site is designated AAC(3′)[36] (Table 4). However, there may be more than one enzyme that will catalyze the same reaction, and thus roman numerals may be necessary (e.g., AAC(3′)-IV).

Enzymatic aminoglycoside resistance is achieved by modification of the antibiotic in the process of transport across the cytoplasmic membrane.[35] Resistance to a particular aminoglycoside is a function of two different rates, that of drug uptake vs. that of drug inactivation. An important factor in determining the level of resistance is the affinity of the modifying enzyme for the antibiotic. If an enzyme has a high affinity for the specific aminoglycoside, then drug inactivation can occur at very low concentrations.

The differences in the worldwide distribution of aminoglycoside-modifying enzymes may partially be a function of antibiotic selection pressures and have had profound implications on the choice of antibiotics used at specific centers.[37] APH(3′) and APH(3″) are widely distributed among gram-positive and gram-negative species worldwide and thus have led to decreased utilization of kanamycin and streptomycin. The ANT(2″) gene has been associated with multiple nosocomial outbreaks over the past decade across the United States.AAC(6′)-I gene has been found to be more prevalent in East Asia.[38] The AAC(3) group of enzymes have been responsible for outbreaks of antibiotic resistance in South America, Western Europe, and the United States. Although each outbreak of aminoglycoside-resistant Enterobacteriaceae in the United States has its own pattern, the most typical manner of spread has been the appearance of a plasmid-carrying aminoglycoside-resistant strain of *K. pneumoniae,* usually carrying the ANT(2″) gene, with subsequent dissemination to other strains of the species and further spread later to other species and genera of Enterobacteriaceae.[39] A recent global survey detected an increased prevalence of amikacin-resistant isolates from hospitals in the United States and Western Europe,[39a] reflecting ongoing changes in the deployment of different aminoglycoside-modifying enzymes among gram-negative bacilli.

Chloramphenicol Acetyltransferase. Resistance to chloramphenicol in gram-positive and gram-negative organisms is primarily mediated by an inactivating enzyme known as chloramphenicol acetyltransferase. This is an intracellular enzyme that inactivates the drug by 3-*O*-acetylation[40] and is encoded by plasmid-borne or chromosomal genes. Despite homology at the active site of this enzyme, there is considerable diversity between chloramphenicol acetyltransferase enzymes isolated from gram-positive and gram-negative organisms.[41]

Erythromycin Esterase. While resistance to erythromycin and other macrolides is generally the result of an alteration in the ribosomal target site, an additional mechanism of resistance

TABLE 4. Examples of Where Common Aminoglycoside-Modifying Enzymes Are Found

Enzymes	*Usual Antibiotics Modified*	*Common Genera*
Phosphorylation		
APH(2″)	K, T, G	SA, SR
APH(3′)-I	K	E, PS, SA, SR
APH(3′)-III	K, + A	E, PS, SA, SR
Acetylation		
AAC(2′)	G	PR
AAC(3)-I	± T, G	E, PS
AAC(3)-III, IV, or -V	K, T, G	E, PS
AAC(6′)	K, T, ± A	E, PS, SA
Adenylation		
ANT(2″)	K, T, G	E, PS
ANT(4′)	K, T, A	SA

Abbreviations: K: kanamycin; T: tobramycin; G: gentamicin; A: amikacin; E: Enterobacteriaceae; SA: staphylococci; SR: streptococci; PS: pseudomonads; PR: providencia/proteus.

that is based upon enzymatic destruction has recently been characterized. An enzyme known as erythromycin esterase has been isolated from *E. coli* that hydrolyzes the lactone ring of the antibiotic, thereby resulting in its inactivation.[42] This is a plasmid-mediated resistance determinant that is constitutively produced and results in high-level resistance to erythromycin (MIC > 2000 μg/ml).[43] This resistance determinant may limit the utility of oral erythromycin in reducing the aerobic gram-negative flora of the intestinal tract before gastrointestinal surgical procedures.

Alterations in Bacterial Membranes

Outer Membrane Permeability. It was recognized early in the history of antibiotic development that penicillin was effective against gram-positive bacteria but not against gram-negative bacteria.[44] This difference in susceptibility to penicillin is due in large part to the outer membrane, a lipid bilayer that acts as a barrier to the penetration of antibiotics into the cell.[45] Situated outside the peptidoglycan cell wall of gram-negative bacteria, this outer membrane is absent in gram-positive bacteria. The outer portion of this lipid bilayer is composed principally of lipopolysaccharide made up of tightly bound hydrocarbon molecules that impede the entry of hydrophobic antibiotics such as nafcillin or erythromycin.[46,47] Agents that disrupt the integrity of the lipopolysaccharide layer such as polymyxin or mutations that lead to the production of defective lipopolysaccharide result in increased permeability of hydrophobic antibiotics.[48]

The passage of hydrophilic antibiotics through this outer membrane is facilitated by the presence of porins, proteins that are arranged so as to form water-filled diffusion channels through which antibiotics may traverse.[49] Bacteria usually produce a large number of porins; approximately 10^5 porin molecules are present in a single cell of *E. coli*. Bacteria are able to regulate the relative number of different porins in response to the osmolarity of the surrounding media. Thus, in hyperosmolar media *E. coli* may repress production of the larger porins (OmpF) while continuing to express smaller ones (OmpC).[50]

The rate of diffusion of antibiotics through this outer membrane is a function not only of the number and properties of the porin channels but also of the physicochemical characteristics of the antibiotic. Generally, the larger the antibiotic molecule, the more negative the charges, and the greater the degree of hydrophobicity, the less likely it is to penetrate through the outer membrane.[45,51] Small, hydrophilic molecules with a zwitterionic charge such as imipenem are highly permeable. Conversely, larger highly charged molecules such as carbenicillin are much less permeable.

Mutations resulting in the loss of specific porins can occur in clinical isolates and determine increased resistance to β-lactam antibiotics. For example, a strain of *Salmonella typhimurium* obtained from a perirenal abscess became resistant to various cephalosporins during therapy with cephalexin.[52] The parent strain produced both OmpF and OmpC proteins, but the mutant produced only OmpF. The mutant was resistant to β-lactam antibiotics only when tested in media of high osmolarity, comparable to that in the patient's tissues. Under these conditions the production of the OmpF protein was repressed completely, leaving the microorganism devoid of either species of porin and impermeable to the cephalosporins. Resistance to aminoglycosides and carbapenems that emerges during therapy has also been associated with a lack of production of outer membrane proteins, probably by mechanisms other than diffusion through porins.[53,54]

Resistance to nalidixic acid and other quinolones may also be associated with alterations of outer membrane proteins.[55] Plasmid-mediated chloramphenicol resistance due to decreased permeability has been demonstrated in *E. coli*.[56] The mechanism by which plasmid-mediated vancomycin and teicoplanin resistance in *Enterococcus faecium* occurs has not yet been elucidated but may be related to outer membrane impermeability.[16]

Inner Membrane Permeability. The rate of entry of aminoglycoside molecules into bacterial cells is a function of their binding to a usually nonsaturable anionic transporter whereupon they retain their positive charge and are subsequently "pulled" across the cytoplasmic membrane by the internal negative charge of the cell.[57] This process requires energy and a threshold minimal level of internal negative charge of the cell that has to be present before significant transport occurs ("proton motive force").[58] The level of the internal charge that is required may depend on the actual aminoglycoside concentration at a given time. The energy generation or the proton motive force that is required for substrate transport into the cell may be altered in mutants resistant to aminoglycosides.

These aminoglycoside-resistant isolates with altered proton motive force occur rarely but develop in the course of long-term aminoglycoside therapy.[59] These isolates usually have a "small-colony" phenotype due to their reduced rate of growth. They may be unstable and revert back to a sensitive phenotype in the absence of selective amingolycoside pressure. The clinical significance of these isolates is not clear. They may retain some virulence[60] and may cause fatal bacteremia rarely.[61] Because oxidative metabolism is essential for aminoglycoside uptake, *Pseudomonas* mutants deficient in specific cytochrome action as well as cell growth and development have been found.[57] Resistant mutants with defective electron transport systems have been described in *E. coli, S. aureus,* and *Salmonella* species. Facultative organisms grown anaerobically are resistant to aminoglycosides because of a marked reduction of the uptake of the antibiotic.[35]

Promotion of Antibiotic Efflux

The major mechanism of resistance to tetracycline found in enteric gram-negative organisms results from the decreased accumulation of tetracycline. This reduced uptake is an energy-dependent process that is related to the generation of an inner membrane protein produced by the tetracycline resistance determinant. The primary mechanism for decreased accumulation of tetracycline is due mainly to active efflux of the antibiotic across the cell membrane.[62,63] Decreased uptake of tetracycline from the extracellular environment also accounts for decreased accumulation of tetracycline inside resistant cells. These resistance determinants may be found on the chromosome or plasmids and are frequently found on transposable genetic elements. Tetracycline resistance genes are generally inducible by subinhibitory concentrations of tetracycline. An active efflux system for the removal of fluoroquinolones has recently been demonstrated in *E. coli*.[64] This system may represent a potential mechanism for resistance to the newer quinolone antimicrobial agents.

Alteration in Ribosomal Target Sites

Resistance to a wide variety of antimicrobial agents including tetracyclines, macrolides, lincosamides, and the aminoglycosides may result from an alteration in ribosomal binding sites. Failure of the antibiotic to bind to its target site(s) on the ribosome disrupts its ability to inhibit protein synthesis and cell growth. For the macrolides (such as erythromycin) and lincosamides (such as clindamycin), this is the principal mechanism of resistance among gram-positive organisms.[65] Resistance occurs as the result of a methylase enzyme that dimethylates adenine residues on the 23S ribosomal RNA of the 50S subunit of the prokaryotic ribosome, thereby disrupting the binding of macrolides and lincosamides to the ribosome. There are four classes of this resistance determinant that may be located on plasmids or the bacterial chromosome.[66] Tetracycline resistance may also occur by a mechanism that interferes with the ability of tetracycline to bind to the ribosome. The ubiquitous *tetM* resistance gene protects the ribosome from tetracycline action. The precise mechanism of action of this resistance gene is unclear at present.[67] The *tetM* determinant is widely dispersed in gram-positive organisms[67] in addition to *Mycoplasma,*[68] *Ureaplasma,*[15] *Campylobacter,*[69] and *Neisseria* spp.[14]

Resistance to aminoglycosides may also be mediated at the ribosomal level. Mutations of the S12 protein of the 30S subunit has been shown to interfere with binding streptomycin to the ribosome. Ribosomal resistance to streptomycin may be a significant cause of streptomycin resistance among enterococcal isolates.[70] Ribosomal resistance to the 2-deoxystreptamine aminoglycosides (gentamicin, tobramycin, amikacin) appears to be uncommon and may require multiple mutations in that these aminoglycosides appear to bind to several sites on the 30S and 50S subunits of the prokaryotic ribosome. Ribosomal resistance is often associated with decreased intracellular accumulation of the drug.[71]

Alteration in Target Enzymes

β-Lactams. β-Lactam antibiotics inhibit bacteria by binding covalently to penicillin binding proteins (PBPs) in the cytoplasmic membrane. These target proteins catalyze the synthesis of the peptidoglycan that forms the cell wall of bacteria.[72] Alterations in PBPs can lead to β-lactam antibiotic resistance.[73]

In gram-positive bacteria, resistance to β-lactam antibiotics may be associated either with a decrease in the affinity of the PBP for the antibiotic[74] or with a change in the amount of PBP produced by the bacterium.[75] Multiple mechanisms appear to be present in some clinical isolates. For example, penicillin-resistant strains of *Streptococcus pneumoniae* isolated in South Africa have shown several changes in their PBPs, i.e., decreased affinity of some PBPs, loss of others, and appearance of PBPs not present in the more susceptible cells.[76] In *S. aureus*[77–79] and *Enterococcus faecium*[79,80] additional PBPs may be inducible, i.e., their production is stimulated by exposure of the microorganism to the β-lactam antibiotic. These inducible PBPs have a lower affinity for β-lactam antibiotics, which makes them less susceptible to inhibition by low concentrations of drug. Changes in the types of PBPs observed in susceptible and resistant strains have also been seen with a viridans streptococcal species, *S. mitis*.[81]

Factors that regulate the induction of PBPs are poorly understood. The induction of a low-affinity PBP in methicillin-resistant *S. aureus* (MRSA) occurs to a larger extent when the microorganisms are grown at 32°C rather than at 37°C, conditions known to favor the expression of methicillin resistance.[82] There is evidence that the production of this inducible PBP is under the control of plasmid-borne genes that regulate staphylococcal penicillinase production. The structural gene that determines the low-affinity PBP of MRSA shares extensive sequence homology with a PBP of *E. coli,* and the genes that regulate the production of the low-affinity PBP have considerable sequence homology with the genes that regulate the production of staphylococcal penicillinase.[83] Thus, the production of this low-affinity penicillin-binding protein in MRSA may be mediated by a fusion of genes scavenged from *E. coli* and *S. aureus*.

The PBPs of chromosomally mediated, penicillin-resistant strains of *N. gonorrhoeae* have shown reduced penicillin binding of some of their PBPs.[84] Mutations leading to a loss of outer membrane proteins may also be associated with acquisition of penicillin resistance in non-penicillinase-producing strains of *N. gonorrhoeae,* thus suggesting that altered permeability may also contribute to the resistance.[85] Permeability changes and a decreased affinity of PBPs are mechanisms jointly found in clinical isolates of *P. aeruginosa*[86] and non beta-lactamase producing strains of *H. influenzae* as well.[87] Thus, multiple mutations may be necessary in order to effect this type of resistance.

Sulfonamides and Trimethoprim. Sulfonamides compete with para-aminobenzoic acid to bind the enzyme dihydropteroate synthetase, thereby halting the generation of pteridines and nucleic acids. Sulfonamide resistance may be mediated by the production of a dihydropteroate synthetase that is resistant to binding by sulfonamides.[88] The high prevalence of resistance to sulfonamides among gram-negative bacteria may be attributed to the spread of R plasmids that contain genes that elaborate resistant enzymes. The most common mechanism of transferable trimethoprim resistance occurs in a similar fashion, by making a drug-resistant dihydrofolate reductase (DHFR).[89] Trimethoprim-resistant DHFRs have been found on the chromosome, and multiple forms have been found to be plasmid mediated.[90]

Quinolones. DNA gyrase is necessary for the supercoiling of chromosomal DNA in bacteria in order to have efficient cell division.[91] This enzyme consists of two A subunits encoded by the *gyr* A gene and two B subunits encoded by the *gyr* B gene. Although spontaneous mutations in the *gyr* A locus have resulted in resistance to multiple fluoroquinolones, B-subunit alterations may also affect resistance to these drugs. Mutations in a variety of chromosomal loci have been described that result in altered DNA gyrases that are resistant to nalidixic acid and the newer fluoroquinolones in Enterobacteriaceae and *P. aeruginosa*.[92,93]

Bypass of Antibiotic Inhibition

Another mechanism for acquiring resistance to specific antibiotics is by the development of auxotrophs, which have growth factor requirements different from those of the wild strain. These mutants require substrates that normally are synthesized by the target enzymes, and thus if the substrates are present in the environment, the organisms are able to grow despite inhibition of the synthetic enzyme. For example, bacteria that lose the enzyme thymidilate synthetase are "thymine dependent" and cannot synthesize thymidilate in the usual way. They therefore require exogenous supplies of thymidine to synthesize thymidilate via salvage pathways and are thus highly resistant to trimethoprim.[94]

CONTROL OF ANTIBIOTIC RESISTANCE

Although the emergence of antibiotic-resistant bacteria has generally been correlated with the rise and fall of specific antibiotic use in clinical practice, the chain of causality is not always clear-cut.[95] Bacterial strains contain complex aggregations of genes that may be linked together. Thus the use of one antibiotic may select for the emergence of resistance to another. Although the development of antibiotic resistance may be inevitable, the rate at which it develops may be diminished by the rational use of antibiotics.[96]

The wider accessibility of minicomputers as well as the ability to track antibiotic resistance genes with molecular techniques has enhanced the ability to track the spread of antibiotic resistance. With the appropriate computerized surveillance, a hospital laboratory may be able to rapidly detect the emergence of a new type of resistance or the presence of a new microbial strain within a specific unit or patient population. Techniques such as restriction endonuclease digestion analyses of bacterial plasmids and chromosomes and genetic probes of resistance genes make it possible to confirm the presence of new genes in the environment. This information may then be correlated with the phenotypic measures determined by the clinical microbiology surveillance system.[97] Utilization of molecular techniques greatly augments routine surveillance (Fig. 3) since large data

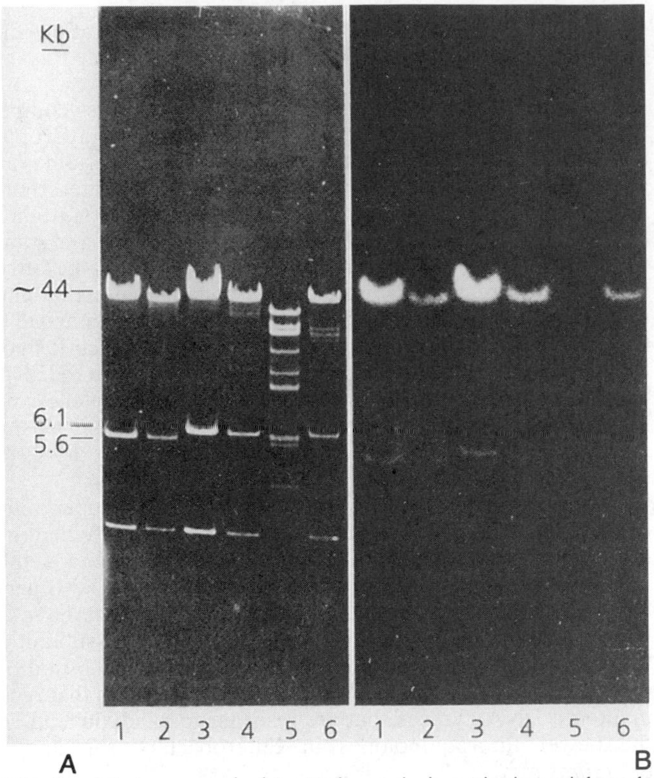

FIG. 3. **(A)** Agarose gel of *Eco*RI-digested plasmids derived from four isolates that contain a nosocomial trimethoprim resistance plasmid (known as pBWH10) from a Boston hospital (lanes 1–4). Another nosocomial plasmid from the same hospital that does not contain trimethoprim resistance genes (lane 5), and one in which both the trimethoprim-resistant and -sensitive plasmids are present in the same isolate (lane 6). **(B)** In order to show that the "fingerprints" from the trimethoprim-resistant plasmids in lanes 1–4 and 6 contain the same gene, DNA–DNA hybridization of the same six plasmids was performed by using a type II DHFR probe. The probe and the restriction endonuclease analyses helped to pinpoint the location and genetic homology of this trimethoprim resistance gene. (From Mayer et al.,[98] with permission.)

sets may obscure subtle changes ("miniepidemics") that may be more amenable to the institution of stringent infection control measures.

Study of the genetics of antibiotic resistance, particularly the awareness of the great mobility of plasmids and transposons, leads one to the conclusion that ultimately each antibiotic used may inexorably alter its microenvironment and create selective advantages for resistant organisms. Since prokaryotic organisms all contribute to a common "gene pool," favorable genes mediating antibiotic resistance may disseminate among bacterial populations. In less than a decade, newly used inexpensive drugs such as trimethoprim have gone from being highly effective in the treatment of dysentery in developing countries to becoming unusable in several of these areas.[99] Rational antibiotic usage policies would suggest the curtailment of the unnecessary use of antibiotics in situations such as animal husbandry, although the causal link between the use of antibiotics for animal growth promotion and their augmentation of the resistance in human pathogens has been disputed.[100] New drug discoveries have allowed us to be one step ahead of the bacterial pathogens. Nonetheless, the rapid evolution of resistance has limited the duration of the effectiveness of specific agents against certain pathogens. The best hope for the future is the development of greater understanding of how antimicrobial resistance spreads and the implementation of effective infection control strategies. Newer antimicrobial agents have had a substantial impact in decreasing human morbidity and mortality over the past half century. It behooves us to expand our surveillance of antibiotic resistance determinants and to exercise caution in dispensing antibiotics in order to maximize their continued efficacy.

REFERENCES

1. Kopecko D. Specialized genetic recombination systems in bacteria: Their involvement in gene expression and evolution. Prog Mol Subcell Biol. 1980;7:135–243.
2. Kopecko DJ. Involvement of specialized recombination in the evolution and expression of bacterial genes. In: Stuttgart C, Rozel KR, eds. Plasmids and Transposons. New York: Academic Press; 1980:165–206.
3. Lupski JR. Molecular mechanisms for transposition of drug-resistance genes and other movable genetic elements. Rev Infect Dis. 1987;9:357–68.
4. Datta N. Plasmids as organisms. In: Helinski DR, Cohen SN, Clevwell DB, et al., eds. *Plasmids in Bacteria.* New York: Plenum Press; 1985:383–95.
5. O'Brien T, del Pilar Pla M, Mayer KH, et al. Intercontinental spread of a new antibiotic resistance gene on an epidemic plasmid. Science. 1985; 230:87–8.
6. Timmis KN, Gonzalez-Carrero MI, Sekizaki T, et al. Biological activities specified by antibiotic resistance plasmids. J Antimicrob Chemother. 1986;18:1–12.
7. Nordstrom K. Replication, incompatibility and partition. In: Helinski DR, Cohen SN, Clewell DB, et al., eds. Plasmids in Bacteria. New York: Plenum Press; 1985:119–23.
8. Thompson R. R plasmid transfer. J Antimicrob Chemother. 1986;18:13–23.
9. Foster TJ. Plasmid-determined resistance to antimicrobial drugs and toxic metal ions in bacteria. Microbiol Rev. 1983;43:361–409.
10. Mayer KH, Hopkins JD, Gilleece ES, et al. Molecular evolution, species distribution and clinical consequences of an endemic aminoglycoside resistance plasmid. Antimicrob Agents Chemother. 1986;29:628–33.
11. Rubens CE, McNeill WF, Farrar WE Jr. Evolution of multiple-antibiotic-resistance plasmids mediated by transposable plasmid deoxyribonucleic acid sequences. J Bacteriol. 1979;140:713–9.
12. Franke AE, Clewell DB. Evidence for a chromosome-borne resistance transposon (Tn916) in *Streptococcus faecalis* that is capable of "conjugal" transfer in the absence of a conjugative plasmid. J Bacteriol. 1981;145:494–502.
13. Solh NE, Allignet J, Bismuth R, et al. Conjugative transfer of staphylococcal antibiotic resistance markers in the absence of detectable plasmid DNA. Antimicrob Agents Chemother. 1986;30:161–69.
14. Morse SA, Johnson SR, Biddle JW, et al. High-level tetracycline resistance in *Neisseria gonorrhoeae* is the result of acquisition of streptococcal *tetM* determinant. Antimicrob Agents Chemother. 1986;30:664–70.
15. Roberts MC, Kenny GE. Dissemination of the *tetM* tetracycline resistance determinant to *Ureaplasma urealyticum*. Antimicrob Agents Chemother. 1986;29:350–52.
16. Lecleq R, Derlot E, Duval J, et al. Plasmid-mediated resistance to vancomycin and teicoplanin in *Enterococcus faecium*. N Engl J Med. 1988;319:157–61.
17. Medeiros AA. Beta-lactamases. Br Med Bull. 1984;40:18–27.
18. Sykes RB, Matthew M. The beta-lactamases of gram-negative bacteria and their role in resistance to beta-lactam antibiotics. J Antimicrob Chemother. 1976;2:115–57.
19. McDonnell RW, Sweendy HM, Cohen S. Conjugational transfer of gentamicin resistance plasmids intra- and interspecifically in *Staphylococcus aureus* and *Staphylococcus epidermidis*. Antimicrob Agents Chemother. 1983;23:151–60.
20. Murray BE, Mederski-Samoraj B, Foster SK, et al. In-vitro studies of plasmid-mediated penicillinase from *Streptococcus faecalis* suggest a staphylococcal origin. J Clin Invest. 1986;77:289–93.
21. Medeiros AA. Plasmid-determined beta-lactamases. Microbial resistance to drugs. In: Bryan LE, ed. Handbook of Experimental Pharmacology. Berlin: Springer-Verlag. 1989:102–27.
22. Cuchural GJ Jr, Tally FP, Storey JR, et al. Transfer of beta-lactamase-associated cefoxitin resistance in *Bacteroides fragilis*. Antimicrob Agents Chemother. 1986;29:918–20.
23. Cuchural GJ Jr, Mulamy MH, Tally FP. Beta-lactamase-mediated imipenem resistance in *Bacteroides fragilis*. Antimicrob Agents Chemother. 1986; 30:645–48.
24. Medeiros AA, O'Brien TF. Ampicillin-resistant *Haemophilus influenzae* type B possessing a TEM-type beta-lactamase but little permeability barrier to ampicillin, Lancet. 1975;1:716.
25. Elwell LP, Roberts M, Mayer LW, et al. Plasmid-mediated beta-lactamase production in *Neisseria gonorrhoeae*. Antimicrob Agents Chemother. 1977;11:528–33.
26. Kliebe C, Nies BA, Meyer JF, et al. Evolution of plasmid-coded resistance to broad-spectrum cephalosporins. Antimicrob Agents Chemother. 1985; 28:302–7.
27. Brun-Buisson C, Legrand P, Philippon A, et al. Transferable enzymatic resistance to third-generation cephalosporins during nosocomial outbreak of multiresistant *Klebsiella pneumoniae*. Lancet. 1987;302–6.
28. Bauernfeind A, Horl G. Novel R-factor borne beta-lactamase of *Escherichia coli* conferring resistance to cephalosporins. Infection. 1987;15:257–9.
29. Sirot J, Labia R, Thabaut A. *Klebsiella pneumoniae* strains more resistant to ceftazidime than to other third-generation cephalosporins (Abstract). J Antimicrob Chemother. 1987;20:611–2.

30. Goussard S, Sougakoff W, Gerbaud G, et al. CTX-1, a wide-substrate-range enzyme, is a derivative of a TEM beta-lactamase (Abstract). Proceedings of the 27th Interscience Conference on Antimicrobial Agents and Chemotherapy. New York: American Society for Microbiology; 1987.
31. Jaurin B, Grundstrom T, Edlund T, et al. The *E. coli* beta-lactamase attenuator mediates growth rate–dependent regulation. Nature. 1981;290:221–5.
31a. Sawai T, Kanno M, Tsukamoto K. Characterization of eight beta-lactamases of gram-negative bacteria J. Bacteriol. 1982;152:567–71.
32. Nugent ME, Hedges RW. The nature of the genetic determinant for the SHV-1 beta-lactamase. Mol Gen Genet. 1979;175:239–43.
33. Moxon ER, Medeiros AA, O'Brien TF. Beta-lactamase effect on ampicillin treatment of *Haemophilus influenzae* B bacteremia and meningitis in infant rats. Antimicrob Agents Chemother. 1977;12:461–4.
34. Sanders CC, Sanders WE, Goering RV. In vitro antagonism of beta-lactam antibiotics by cefoxitin. Antimicrob Agents Chemother. 1982;21:968–75.
35. Bryan LE. Aminoglycoside resistance. In: Bryan LE, ed. Antimicrobial Drug Resistance. Orlando, FL: Academic Press; 1984:241–77.
36. Davies J, Smith DI. Plasmid-determined resistance to antimicrobial agents. Annu Rev Biochem. 1978;32:469.
37. Mayer KH. Review of epidemic aminoglycoside resistance worldwide. Am J Med. 1986;80(Suppl 6B):56–64.
38. Shimizu K, Kumada T, Hsieh W, et al. Comparison of aminoglycoside resistance patterns in Japan, Formosa, and Korea, Chile, and the United States. Antimicrob Agents Chemother. 1985;28:282–8.
39. John JF Jr, Twitty JA. Plasmids as epidemiologic markers in nosocomial gram-negative bacilli: Experience at a university and review of the literature. Rev Infect Dis. 1986;8:693–704.
39a. Hare RS, Shaw KJ, Miller GH, et al. The activity of isepamicin (ISM) against amikacin resistant gram-negative bacteria from the USA, Europe, Argentina, and Japan (Abstract). Proceedings of the 28th Interscience Conference on Antimicrobial Agents and Chemotherapy. Los Angeles: American Society for Microbiology. 1988:Abstract 1495;376.
40. Gaffney DF, Foster TJ, Shaw WV. Chloramphenicol acetyl transferases determined by R-plasmids from gram (−) bacteria. J Gen Microbiol. 1978;109:351–8.
41. Davies J. General mechanisms of antimicrobial resistance. Rev Infect Dis. 1979;1:23–7.
42. Barthelemy P, Autissier D, Gerbaud G, et al. Enzymatic hydrolysis of erythromycin by a strain of *Escherichia coli*: A new mechanism of resistance. J Antibiot. 1984;37:1692–6.
43. Andremont A, Gerbaud G, Courvalin P. Plasmid-mediated high-level resistance to erythromycin in *Escherichia coli*. Antimicrob Agents Chemother. 1986;29:515–8.
44. Fleming A. On the antibacterial action of cultures of a *Penicillium*, with special reference to their use in the isolation of *B. influenzae*. Br J Exp Pathol. 1929;10:226–36.
45. Nikaido H. Role of permeability barriers in resistance to beta-lactam antibiotics. Pharmacol Ther. 1985;27:197–231.
46. Labischinski H, Barnickel G, Bradaczek H, et al. High state of order of isolated bacterial lipopolysaccharide and its possible contribution to the permeation barrier property of the outermembrane. J Bacteriol. 1985;162:9–20.
47. Takeuchi Y, Nikaido H. Physical interaction between lipid A and phospholipids: A study with spin-labeled phospholipids. Rev Infect Dis. 1984;6:488–92.
48. Vaara M. Polymyxin B nonapeptide complexes with lipopolysaccharide (Letter). FEMS Microbiol. 1983;18:117–21.
49. Nikaido H, Vaara M. Molecular basis of the permeability of outer membrane permeability. Microbiol Rev. 1985;49:1–32.
50. Hasegawa Y, Yamada H, Mizushima S. Interactions of outer membrane proteins 0-8 and 0-9 with peptidoglycan sacculus of *Escherichia coli* K-12. J Biochem. 1976;80:1401–9.
51. Yoshimura F, Nikaido H. Diffusion of beta-lactam antibiotics through the porin channels of *Escherichia coli* K-12. Antimicrob Agents Chemother. 1985;27:84–92.
52. Medeiros AA, O'Brien TF, Rosenberg EY, et al. Loss of OmpC porin in a strain of *Salmonella typhimurium* causes increased resistance to cephalosporins during therapy. J Infect Dis. 1987;156:751–7.
53. Goldstein FW, Gutmann L, Williamson R, et al. In vivo and in vitro emergence of simultaneous resistance to both beta-lactam and aminoglycoside antibiotics in a strain of *Serratia marcescens* (Abstract). Ann Microbiol (Paris). 1983;134:329–37.
54. Quinn JP, Dudek EJ, DiVincenzo CA, et al. Emergence of resistance to imipenem during therapy for *Pseudomonas aeruginosa* infections. J Infect Dis. 1986;154:289–94.
55. Sanders CC, Sanders WE Jr, Goering RV, et al. Selection of multiple antibiotic resistance by quinolones, beta-lactams, and aminoglycosides with special reference to cross-resistance between unrelated drug classes. Antimicrobial Agents Chemother. 1984;26:797–801.
56. Gaffney DF, Cundiffe E, Foster TJ. Chloramphenicol resistance that does not involve chloramphenicol acetyltransferase encoded by plasmids from gram (−) bacteria. J Gen Microbiol. 1981;125:113–121.
57. Bryan LE, Kwan S. Roles of ribosomal binding membrane potential and electron transport in bacterial uptake of streptomycin and gentamicin. Antimicrob Agents Chemother. 1983;23:835–45.
58. Mates SM, Esenberg ES, Mandel LF, et al. Membrane potential and gentamicin uptake in *Staphylococcus aureus*. Proc Natl Acad Sci USA. 1982;79:6693–7.
59. Rusthoven JJ, Davies A, Lerner SA. Clinical isolation and characterization of aminoglycoside-resistant small colony variants of *Enterobacter aerogenes*. Am J Med. 1979;67:702–6.
60. Musher DN, Baughan RE, Merrell GL. Selection of small-colony variants of Enterobacteriaceae by *in vitro* exposure to aminoglycosides: Pathogenicity for experimental animals. J Infect Dis. 1979;140:209–14.
61. Funada H, Hattori K, Kosaki N. Catalase-negative *Escherichia coli* isolated from the blood. J Clin Microbiol. 1978;7:474–8.
62. McMurry L, Petrucci RE, Levy SB. Active efflux of tetracycline encoded by four genetically different tetracycline resistance determinants in *Escherichia coli*. Proc Natl Acad Sci USA. 1980;71:3974–7.
63. McMurry LM, Park BH, Burdette V, et al. Energy-dependent efflux mediated by Class L (*tetL*) tetracycline resistance determinant from streptococci. Antimicrob Agents Chemother. 1987;31:1648–50.
64. Cohen SP, Hooper DC, Wolfson JS, et al. Endogenous active efflux of norfloxacin in susceptible *Escherichia coli*. Antimicrob Agents Chemother. 1988;32:1187–90.
65. Engel HWB, Soedirman N, Rost JA, et al. Transferability of macrolide, lincomycin, and streptogramin resistances between group A, B, and D streptococci, *Streptococcus pneumoniae*, and *Staphylococcus aureus*. J Bacteriol. 1980;142:407–13.
66. Weisblum B. Inducible resistance to macrolides, lincosamides and streptogramin type B antibiotics: The resistance phenotype, its biological diversity, and structural elements that regulate expression—a review. J Antimicrob Chemother. 1985;16(Suppl A):63–90.
67. Burdette V. Streptoccal tetracycline resistance mediated at the level of protein synthesis. J Bacteriol. 1986;165:564–9.
68. Roberts MC, Koutsy LA, Holmes KK, et al. Tetracycline-resistant *Mycoplasma hominis* strains contain streptococcal *tetM* sequences. Antimicrob Agents Chemother. 1985;28:141–3.
69. Taylor DE, Kiratsuka K, Ray H, et al. Characterization and expression of a cloned tetracycline resistance determinant from *Campylobacter jejuni* plasmid pUA466. J Bacteriol. 1987;169:2984–9.
70. Eliopoulos GM, Farber BF, Murray BE, et al. Ribosomal resistance of clinical enterococcal isolates to streptomycin. Antimicrob Agents Chemother. 1984;25:398–9.
71. Ahmad MH, Rechenmacher A, Boch A. Interaction between aminoglycoside uptake and ribosomal resistance mutations. Antimicrob Agents Chemother. 1980;18:798–806.
72. Waxman DJ, Strominger JL. Penicillin-binding proteins and the mechanism of action of beta-lactam antibiotics. Annu Rev Biochem 1983;52:825–69.
73. Malouin F, Bryan LE. Modification of penicillin-binding proteins as mechanisms of beta-lactam resistance. Antimicrob Agents Chemother. 1986;30: 1–5.
74. Williamson R. Resistance of *Clostridium perfringens* to beta-lactam antibiotics mediated by a decreased affinity of a single essential penicillin-binding protein. J Gen Microbiol. 1983;129:2339–42.
75. Giles AF, Reynolds PE. *Bacillus megaterium* resistance to cloxacillin accompanied by a compensatory change in penicillin binding proteins. Nature. 1979;280:167–8.
76. Hakenbeck R, Tarpay M, Tomasz A. Multiple changes of penicillin-binding proteins in penicillin-resistant clinical isolates of *Streptococcus pneumoniae*. Antimicrob Agents Chemother. 1980;17:364–71.
77. Hartman BJ, Tomasz A. Low-affinity penicillin-binding protein associated with beta-lactam resistance in *Staphylococcus aureus*. J Bacteriol. 1984;158:513–6.
78. Ubukata K, Yamashita N, Konno M. Occurrence of a beta-lactam-inducible penicillin-binding protein in methicillin-resistant staphylococci. Antimicrob Agents Chemother. 1985;27:851–7.
79. Fontana R. Penicillin-binding proteins and the intrinsic resistance to beta-lactams in gram positive cocci. J Antimicrob Chemother. 1985;16:412–6.
80. Fontana R, Grossato A, Rossi L, et al. Transition from resistance to hypersusceptibility to beta-lactam antibiotics associated with loss of low-affinity penicillin-binding protein in a *Streptococcus faecium* mutant highly resistant to penicillin. Antimicrob Agents Chemother. 1985;28:678–83.
81. Farber BF, GM Eliopoulos, Ward JI, et al. Multiply resistant viridans streptococci: Susceptibility to beta-lactam antibiotics and comparison of penicillin-binding protein patterns. Antimicrob Agents Chemother. 1983;24:702–5.
82. Sabath LD. Chemical and physical factors influencing methicillin resistance of *Staphylococcus aureus* and *Staphylococcus epidermidis*. J Antimicrob Chemother. 1977;3(Suppl C):47–51.
83. Song MD, Wachi M, Doi M, et al. Evolution of an inducible penicillin target protein in methicillin-resistant *Staphylococcus aureus* by gene fusion. FEBS Lett. 1987;226:167–71.
84. Dougherty TJ, Koller AE, Tomasz A. Penicillin binding proteins of penicillin-susceptible and intrinsically resistant *Neisseria gonorrhoeae*. Antimicrob Agents Chemother. 1980;18:730–7.
85. Faruki H, Kohmescher RN, McKinney WP, et al. A community based outbreak of infection with penicillin-resistant *Neisseria gonorrhoeae* not producing penicillinase (chromosomally mediated resistance). N Engl J Med. 1985;313:607–11.
86. Mirelman D, Nuchamowitz Y, Rubinstein E. Insensitivity of peptidoglycan biosynthetic reactions to beta-lactam antibiotics in a clinical isolate of *Pseudomonas aeruginosa*. Antimicrob Agents Chemother. 1981;19:687–95.
87. Parr TR, Bryan LE. Mechanism of resistance of an ampicillin-resistant beta-

lactamase-negative clinical isolate of *Haemophilus influenzae* type b to beta-lactam antibiotics. Antimicrob Agents Chemother. 1984;25:747–53.
88. Hamilton-Miller JMT. Resistance to antibacterial agents acting on antifolate metabolism. In: Bryan LE, ed. Antimicrobial Drug Resistance. Orlando, FL: Academic Press; 1984:173–88.
89. Huovinen P. Trimethoprim resistance. Antimicrob Agents Chemother. 1987;31:1451–6.
90. Steen R, Skold O. Plasmid-borne or chromosomally mediated resistance by Tn7 is the most common response to ubiquitous use of trimethoprim. Antimicrob Agents Chemother. 1985;27:933–7.
91. Wolfson JS, Hooper DC. The fluoroquinolones: Structures, mechanisms of action and resistance, and spectra of activity in vitro. Antimicrob Agents Chemother. 1985;28:581–6.
92. Hane MW, Wood TH. *Escherichia coli* K-12 mutants resistant to nalidixic acid: Genetic mapping and dominance studies. J Bacteriol. 1969;99:238–41.
93. Robillard NJ, Scarpa AL. Genetic and physiological characterization of ciprofloxacin resistance in *Pseudomonas aeruginosa* PAO. Antimicrob Agents Chemother. 1988;32:535–9.
94. Maskell R, Okubagejo OA, Payne RH. Human infections with thymine-requiring bacteria. J Med Microbiol. 1978;11:33–42.
95. McGowan JE. Antimicrobial resistance in hospital organisms and its relation to antimicrobial use. Rev Infect Dis. 1983;5:1033–48.
96. Levy SB. Resistance to the tetracyclines. In: Bryan LE, ed. Antimicrobial Drug Resistance. Orlando, FL: Academic Press; 1984:192–234.
97. Mayer KH, Hopkins JD, Gilleece ES, et al. Computer-assisted correlations between antibiotypes of clinical isolates and the endonuclease restriction fragment of types of their plasmids. In: Mitsuhasi S, Rosival L, Krcmery V, eds. Transferrable Antibiotic Resistance: Plasmids and Gene Manipulation. Prague and Heidelberg: Czechoslovak Press and Springer-Verlag; 1984:163–9.
98. Mayer KH, Fling ME, Hopkins JD, et al: Trimethoprim resistance in multiple genera of Enterobacteriaceae at a U.S. hospital: Spread of type II dihydrofolate reductase gene by a single plasmid. J Infect Dis. 1985;151:783–89.
99. Murray BE, Alvarado T, Kim K-H. Increasing resistance to trimethoprim-sulfamethoxazole among isolates of *Escherichia coli* in developing countries. J Infect Dis. 1985;152:1107–13.
100. Holmberg SD, Solomon SL, Blake PA. Health and economic impacts of antimicrobial resistance. Rev Infect Dis. 1987;6:1065–78.

17. PHARMACOKINETICS OF ANTIMICROBIAL AGENTS

PAUL S. LIETMAN

The pharmacokinetics of antimicrobial agents should be considered in terms of the time-dependent interactions with both microorganisms and humans.

The time-dependent interactions of antimicrobial agents with microorganisms are important to the effectiveness of the drug.[1] This effectiveness is influenced by both the kinetics of microbial growth and the drug concentration in the environment of the microbe. Usually, the drug concentration in the environment of the microbe changes over time, with peaks and troughs that roughly parallel the plasma levels when intermittent doses are administered. Although much is unknown about the interplay between microbial growth kinetics and constantly changing drug concentrations in the microbial environment, some generalizations can be made. Penicillin G (and probably other penicillins, β-lactams, and inhibitors of cell wall synthesis) can inhibit bacterial cell growth and can produce cell lysis even though the concentration of antibiotic drops quite low during some of each dosing interval if the target organism is *Staphylococcus* sp., *Streptococcus pyogenes,* or *Streptococcus pneumoniae*.[2] With these organisms and drugs, the physician does not need to keep the level of these antibiotics above the minimum bacteriostatic concentration (MIC) throughout all of each dosing interval. Although there is insufficient evidence about any other drugs and these organisms, it can be assumed that the level of drug in the environment of these bacteria should be maintained above the MIC throughout each dosing interval. The MIC should be considered as the lowest concentration, which, if constantly maintained adjacent to the bacterium, will prevent bacterial growth. β-Lactam antibiotics behave quite differently with gram-negative bacilli, and there is mounting evidence that bacterial regrowth begins as soon as the concentration of drug falls below the MIC.[2,3] In these situations, the β-lactam level should be maintained above the MIC throughout each dosing interval. Aminoglycoside antibiotics also appear to be dependent on the bacterial species being treated. When aminoglycosides interact with *Pseudomonas aeruginosa,* there is a significant lag between the time the bacteria begin to regrow and the time the antibiotic concentration falls below the MIC.[2] With *Escherichia coli,* however, and probably other Enterobacteriaceae as well, bacterial regrowth commences very quickly after the adjacent antibiotic concentration falls below the MIC.[2] Since data exist for only a very few combinations of antimicrobial agents and microbes, the physician is often forced to act without the benefit of adequate information. Thus, a dosing regimen that would maintain the drug level above the MIC throughout each entire dosing interval would be the conservative approach.

The time-dependent interactions of antimicrobial agents with humans are important to both effectiveness and toxicity. The interactions of drugs and microorganisms depend on attaining antibiotic concentrations immediately adjacent to bacteria, and consequently these levels depend on human drug interactions including absorption, distribution, metabolism, and excretion. In addition, the plasma and tissue concentrations of drugs may correlate with dose-related toxicities. The time-dependent interactions with humans can also be used to construct dosing regimens.

Although the precise description of the pharmacokinetics of any drug can be exceedingly complex, the clinician can benefit considerably from approximations that are reasonably accurate and yet comprehensible. The goal of this chapter is to provide a foundation of pharmacokinetics of chemotherapeutic agents that is useful in the construction of therapeutic regimens and in the modification of these regimens for individualization of antimicrobial therapy. More extensive discussions of pharmacokinetics can be found in several excellent books.[4–6]

VOLUME OF DISTRIBUTION (V_D)

The volume of distribution (V_D) of a drug is defined as that volume in which the total amount of drug in the body (A) would have to be uniformly distributed in order to give the observed plasma concentration (C_P).

$$V_D = \frac{A}{C_p} \tag{1}$$

Thus if 140 mg of gentamicin were given to a 70 kg patient and the plasma concentration was found to be 8 μg/ml (= 8 mg/liter), then the volume of distribution would be (140 mg) ÷ (8 mg/liter) = 17.5 liters.

The volume of distribution is often expressed in terms of the body weight, liters/kg. If expressed as liters/kg, then the actual V_D is obtained simply by multiplying the volume of distribution per kg by the body weight.

By rearranging Equation 1, the dose (or amount) necessary to produce any desired plasma concentration can be calculated with a drug whose volume of distribution is known or the plasma concentration that can be expected with any chosen dose. Thus, if the goal is to produce a plasma gentamicin concentration of 10 μg/ml (= 10 mg/liter) in a 70 kg man and the V_D is known to be 0.25 liter/kg, then the dose must = (V_D)(C_P) = (0.25 liter/kg)(70 kg)(10 mg/liter) = 175 mg.

The volume of distribution need not and usually does not correspond to any actual anatomic or physiologic space. It is simply a mathematical tool.

Most antimicrobial agents have volumes of distribution of

between 0.15 liter/kg and 0.40 liter/kg. However, a few have larger volumes of distribution. For example, flucytosine, isoniazid, and erythromycin have volumes of distribution of 0.6 liter/kg to 0.7 liter/kg while chloramphenicol, doxycycline, nafcillin, and tetracycline have volumes of distribution of about 1 liter/kg. A few antimicrobial agents have volumes of distribution that exceed the body weight. Trimethoprim, ethambutol, and rifampin have volumes of distribution of 1.6 liters/kg to 1.8 liters/kg, and amphotericin B has a V_D of 4 liters/kg.

The important clinical use of the V_D is that it provides an initial or loading dose that promptly provides a therapeutic plasma concentration. The V_D is also useful, as is described below, in calculating subsequent or maintenance doses to achieve therapeutic and yet safe plasma concentrations.

HALF-LIFE ($T_{\frac{1}{2}}$)

The half-life of a drug is defined as the time required for the plasma concentration to fall to one-half its former value as it is being eliminated from the body.

It is usually assumed that the half-life associated with a drug is the half-life of the predominant phase of drug elimination, that absorption of the drug is completed, and that the distribution of the drug throughout the entire volume of distribution has been completed. It is also assumed that the fall in the plasma concentration parallels the fall in the total amount of drug in the body.

The half-life of a drug remains constant over time if there has been no change in the processes of drug elimination. During each half-life, 50 percent of the total amount of drug in the body is eliminated, and the plasma concentration falls by 50 percent. Generally, a constant percentage (or fraction) of drug is eliminated from the body in any constant period of time.

The half-lives of antimicrobial agents vary considerably. All of the currently marketed β-lactam antibiotics except ceftriaxone have very short half-lives (usually <1.5 hours). The aminoglycosides have somewhat longer half-lives (2–3 hours). Ceftriaxone, chloramphenicol, flucytosine, sulfisoxazole, and vancomycin have half-lives of 3–6 hours. Sulfamethoxazole, tetracycline, and trimethoprim have half-lives of 6–12 hours. Doxycycline has a relatively long half-life of 20 hours.

The usually quoted half-life of a drug is applicable as a generalization to young adults without renal or hepatic dysfunction. Clinically significant prolongation of a drug's half-life often accompanies renal dysfunction and occasionally occurs with hepatic dysfunction. The half-life may also be influenced by age with prolongations of the half-life in the newborn and the elderly and with shortened half-lives in young children when compared with young adult values. Other drugs administered concomitantly can also alter a drug's half-life as, for example, probenecid prolongs the half-life of many β-lactam antibiotics.

The half-life data are used to calculate continuing (or maintenance) doses of a drug and provide important information about oscillations of plasma concentrations of a drug given intermittently and repetitively.

REPETITIVE DOSING: THE PLATEAU PRINCIPLE

With repetitive dosing of a drug at regular intervals, the maximal or peak plasma concentrations and the minimal or trough plasma concentrations rise to a steady state or plateau, and after such a plateau is reached, the peak and trough plasma concentrations remain constant if the dose remains constant and if there is no change in the rate of drug elimination. The attainment of a plateau is also applicable to continuous dosing at a constant rate where the plasma concentrations climb until a plateau is reached and then remain constant.

The rate at which the plateau is attained is a function exclusively of the half-life of drug elimination and is independent of the rate of drug administration. Thus, giving twice as much drug per dose or per unit of time ultimately provides a higher plasma concentration at the plateau but the plateau is still reached at the same time. A useful concept is that the plateau is reached after four half-lives. Actually, after one half-life the peak and trough or mean plasma concentrations are about 50 percent, after three half-lives 88 percent, and after four half-lives 94 percent of the ultimate plateau levels. Similarly, when a dosage change is made or when a drug is discontinued, the new plateau is reached after about four half-lives.

The plateau principle is especially important in antimicrobial chemotherapy where the physician often wishes to provide therapeutic levels of the antimicrobial agent very promptly and where waiting four half-lives to achieve a desired level may be disastrous. In such situations an initial, or loading dose, of the drug should be given in order to achieve quickly the desired therapeutic level of the antimicrobial agent. As mentioned above, the loading dose is determined exclusively by the volume of distribution and not by the half-life.

Clearly, the plateau principle has greater clinical significance when a half-life is several hours or longer than when the half-life is an hour or less. As a generalization in antimicrobial chemotherapy, a loading dose should be considered whenever the half-life of the chosen drug in the patient is estimated to be longer than 3 hours and whenever a delay of 12 hours or longer to achieve a therapeutic level is unacceptable. A loading dose should also be considered whenever the half-life of the chosen drug is estimated to be prolonged beyond 3 hours by renal or hepatic dysfunction.

It is often useful to estimate the peak and trough plasma concentrations that can be expected with a chosen dose and dosing interval. This can be easily calculated if the volume of distribution and half-life are known. At steady state the minimal plasma concentrations (C_{min}) or trough levels are related to the V_D, $T_{\frac{1}{2}}$ and dose (D) by the following equation where n equals the dosing interval expressed in half-lives.

$$C_{min} = \frac{D}{(V_D)(2^n - 1)} \qquad (2)$$

Thus, if a 6 g dose of carbenicillin (V_D = 0.18 liter/kg; $T_{\frac{1}{2}}$ = 1.0 hour) is given every 6 hours (i.e., every six half-lives; n = 6) to an 80 kg man, the minimal of trough plasma concentration can be anticipated to be (6000 mg) ÷ (0.18 liter/kg)(80 kg)(2^6 − 1) = 6.6 mg/liter = 6.6 μg/ml.

The relationship between the maximal plasma concentrations (C_{max}) or peak levels and the minimal plasma concentrations (C_{min}) or trough levels is given by Equation 3 where n is again the dosing interval expressed in half-lives.

$$\frac{C_{max}}{C_{min}} = 2^n \qquad (3)$$

Thus, to continue with the example of carbenicillin given above, the drug was to be given every six half-lives and the ratio of C_{max} to C_{min} = 2^6 or 64. Thus, the peak plasma levels at steady state will be 64 times the trough levels of (64)(6.6 μg/ml) = 422 μg/ml. The oscillations during every dosing interval of 6 hours at steady state will be from a peak of 422 μg/ml to a trough of 6.6 μg/ml.

It may be desirable to give an antimicrobial agent by continuous intravenous infusion rather than intermittently. In such a case a plateau can be reached in about four half-lives as with intermittent dosing but there will be no peaks and troughs but only a plasma concentration at steady state (C_{ss}). The plasma concentration can also be easily estimated from a fourth simple equation.

$$C_{ss} = \frac{\text{Dose per half-life}}{(0.693)(V_D)} \qquad (4)$$

Thus, to extend the example of carbenicillin cited above, assume that the same total daily dose (i.e., 24 g) is given by continuous intravenous infusion without a loading dose. The dose per half-life is then 1 g/hr, and the plasma concentration at steady state will be 1000 mg ÷ (0.693)(V_D) = 1000 mg ÷ (0.693)(0.18 liter/kg)(80 kg) = 100 mg/liter = 100 μg/ml.

By rearranging Equations 3 or 4, it is easy to solve for the dose that needs to be given to achieve any desired plasma concentration or alternatively the dosing interval that can provide any desired oscillation from peak to trough level.

DOSE-RELATED KINETICS

Most antimicrobial agents behave pharmacokinetically in a manner that can be described with reasonable accuracy by the above four equations. However, Equations 2, 3, and 4 all used the half-life, and we have stated that the half-life in constant over time. This constancy of the half-life is dependent on there being no process of elimination (renal, hepatic, or other) that is saturable at the concentrations of drug realized. If, however, the concentration of drug begins to exceed that which can be removed from the body, then the drug is said to exhibit dose-related kinetics. With dose-related kinetics, it is as if the half-life of the drug were not constant. Although it is theoretically possible to exceed the renal secretory mechanism or the renal reabsorption mechanism, this is rarely, if ever, seen in clinical practice. The hepatic drug metabolizing capacity is, however, occasionally exceeded, in which case the drug may exhibit dose-related kinetics. A specific example is chloramphenicol where at high plasma concentrations the half-life is prolonged. This is especially pertinent to the newborn or the patient with hepatic disease.

ALTERATIONS OF DOSE WITH RENAL OR LIVER DISEASE

In general, antibiotics are eliminated from the body either into the gut after secretion into the bile or into the urine. In either case, the drug may be eliminated unchanged or may be metabolized, usually by the liver, before excretion. Thus, liver disease can impair drug elimination either as a result of impaired drug metabolism or impaired drug secretion into the bile. Kidney disease can impair drug elimination as a result of impaired glomerular filtration or, occasionally, impaired tubular secretion. The extent to which renal or hepatic processes are rate-limiting is quite variable for different drugs and is pivotal in the construction of a dosing regimen in the presence of reduced renal or hepatic function. In the presence of liver disease, the elimination of a few antimicrobial agents is slowed, that is, the half-life is prolonged. There are, however, no clear and useful correlations between any test of liver structure or function and the rate of drug elimination from the body. Thus, in a patient with known liver disease, the examiner cannot predict how the half-life of any drug will be affected, and the patient must be monitored, either clinically or with plasma drug levels, in order to be provided with safe and effective dosing.

In the presence of renal disease the elimination of many antimicrobial agents is slowed and the half-life prolonged. The prolongation of the half-life can often be estimated, however, and rational dosing adjustments can be calculated.

REFERENCES

1. Drusano GL. Role of pharmacokinetics in the outcome of infections. Antimicrob Agents Chemother. 1988;32:289.
2. Bundtzen RW, Gerber AU, Cohn DL, et al. Postantibiotic suppression of bacterial growth. Rev Infect Dis. 1981;3:28.
3. Rolinson GN. Plasma concentrations of penicillin in relation to the antibacterial effect. In Davies DS, Pritchard BNC, eds. Biological Effects of Drugs in Relation to Their Plasma Concentrations. Baltimore: University Park Press; 1973:183.
4. Gladtke E, von Hattingberg HM. Pharmacokinetics: An Introduction. New York: Springer-Verlag; 1979.
5. Rowland M, Tozer TN. Clinical Pharmacokinetics: Concepts and Applications. Philadelphia: Lea & Febiger; 1980.
6. Tedrell T, Dedrick RL, Condliffe PG. Pharmacology and Pharmacokinetics. New York: Plenum Press; 1974.

18. PENICILLINS

HAROLD C. NEU

Penicillin was isolated from *Penicillium notatum* by Fleming in 1929. The fortuitous isolation of this compound did not bear fruit until the work of Florey, Chain, and associates in 1941 made possible the commercial production of penicillin G. In 1928 Fleming found that the mold *Penicillium* produced a substance, which he named penicillin, that inhibited the growth of *Staphylococcus aureus*.[1] Fleming was not successful in attempts to obtain significant amounts of the agent and let the matter rest while he continued his work on lysozyme. In 1939 Florey at the Sir William Dunn School of Pathology began to work out the isolation, structure, and properties of the compound. In 1940 his group showed that penicillin protected mice experimentally infected with streptococci, and by 1941 they had produced enough penicillin to treat a few patients, the first of whom was a British policeman infected with both staphylococci and streptococci. As a result of the war, production of penicillin was undertaken in the United States. Initial clinical trials at Yale and the Mayo Clinic were so successful that the U.S. Army began to use the material to treat streptococcal, gonococcal, and treponemal infections. As fermentation techniques improved, production of large amounts of pure drug became possible, and by the end of the 1940s penicillin G was available for general use in the United States.

Initial production of penicillin was from *P. notatum*, but it was discovered that greater yields could be achieved from *Penicillium chrysogenum* and from growing the organism in different media. It was soon apparent that the growth medium affected the type of natural penicillin produced. Although a number of penicillins were found, for example, F, X, N, K, none of these were superior to the benzylpenicillin that was designated as penicillin G.

CHEMISTRY

The basic structure of the majority of commercially available penicillins is a nucleus that consists of three components—a thiazolidine ring, the β-lactam ring, and a side chain (Fig. 1). The side chain determines in large part the antibacterial spectrum and pharmacologic properties of a particular penicillin. The penicillin nucleus is a condensation of alanine and β-dimethylcysteine. Penicillins currently in use are dextrorotatory and usually exist as salts combined with alkaline earth metals such as sodium or potassium. The β-lactam nucleus is essential for antibacterial activity. Although biosynthesis of penicillin has been achieved, it has not proved to be a useful technique, and fermentation remains the method of production of penicillin G.

The appearance of β-lactamase-producing organisms, particularly of *S. aureus*, prompted studies to develop compounds with resistance to hydrolysis by β-lactamases and also to find agents that had increased activity over that of penicillin G against gram-negative species. In 1959 Batchelor et al.[2] isolated the penicillin nucleus 6-amino-penicillanic acid from a precursor-depleted fermentation of *P. chrysogenum*. This made possible the production and testing of numerous semisynthetic penicillins, the first of which was methicillin, active against β-lactamase-producing *S. aureus*; followed by ampicillin, active

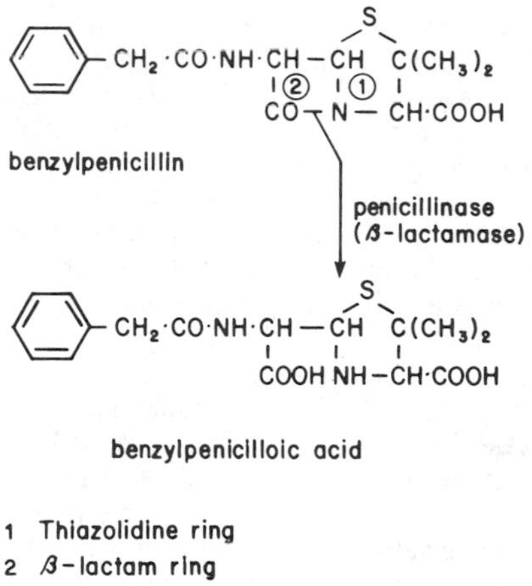

FIG. 1. Structure of penicillin and site of β-lactamase attack.

against selected gram-negative bacilli; and in 1957 by carbenicillin, which had activity against *Pseudomonas aeruginosa*. The past few years have seen the development of a score of agents with different pharmacologic and antimicrobial properties, which will be discussed subsequently in this chapter.

MECHANISM OF ACTION

We do not know precisely how penicillins kill bacterial cells. Study of the action of penicillins has elucidated many aspects of bacterial physiology, but recent advances suggest that the concept that penicillin inhibited the last step in cell wall synthesis is a simplistic one. The cell wall of bacteria is assembled in a series of enzymatic steps that involve at least 30 enzymes.

Bacterial Cell Walls

The cell walls of both gram-positive and gram-negative bacteria are held in a rigid manner protecting against osmotic rupture by the peptidoglycan, also called murein sacculus.[3,4] The cell wall of gram-positive bacteria is a large, 50–100 molecular layer, whereas the peptidoglycan component of gram-negative bacteria is only 1 or 2 molecules thick.

There is an outer lipopolysaccharide layer on top of the peptidoglycan in gram-negative species such as Enterobacteriaceae and the pseudomonads, which is absent in gram-positive species.

All peptidoglycans are long polysaccharide chains in which *N*-acetylglucosamine (NAG) and *N*-acetylmuramic (NAM) acid alternate in a linear form. These long chains are cross-linked by short peptides linked in amide linkage to the D-alanyl group of the *N*-acetylmuramic acid. In gram-negative species the 6-amino group of diaminopimelic acid is linked to the carboxyalanine terminus of another chain.[4] Interestingly, cross-linking is less common in *Escherichia coli* (25 percent), compared with the 90 percent cross-linking in *S. aureus*.[5]

Peptidoglycan synthesis has been divided into three stages. The first is the synthesis of the nucleotide precursors with uridine diphosphate (UDP) by cytoplasmic enzymes to make UDP-*N*-acetylmuramyl-LAra-Disglu-LX-DAla-Dala and UDP-*N*-acetylglucosamine. The "X" in gram-negative species is diaminopimelic acid. The next step is the translocation of the NAM-pentapeptide and NAG across the cytoplasmic membrane by a lipid-soluble carrier, which is a C_{55} isoprenyl alcohol phosphate. Transglycosylation into peptidoglycan polymer occurs at this stage. The final reaction is the incorporation of new peptidoglycan into the existing peptidoglycan. In this final reaction a free amino group on the third amino acid of the NAM-pentapeptide of one strand displaces the terminal D-alanine from a pentapeptide of a second strand in a transpeptidation reaction. This final step was the step thought to be the sole penicillin-sensitive reaction, but we now realize that the other earlier steps also can be inhibited.

It has been shown that penicillin can inhibit transpeptidation without altering transglycosylation of the disaccharide units. There appear to be distinct transpeptidases that provide for anchoring of new peptidoglycan to old, that cross-link special structures, and that make the cell wall septum. Although there are other penicillin-susceptible reactions, such as the effects on carboxypeptidase, these reactions do not seem to be critical in gram-negative species. The most telling argument that penicillin inactivates transpeptidases was the stereo chemistry modeling of Strominger's group,[6] which supports an acylenzyme intermediate because of the structural similarity of penicillin and the acyl-D-alanyl-D-alanine.

Penicillin-Binding Proteins

In 1972 Suginaka and Blumberg and Strominger detected penicillin-binding proteins (PBPs). Subsequently Spratt's studies[7,8] of the PBPs in *E. coli* provided the biggest advance in our understanding of the effect of β-lactams on cell walls. Since then the PBPs of almost all species have been studied.

The PBPs of a given organism are numbered in order of decreasing molecular weight, for example, PBP-1 weighs about 120,000 and PBP-6 weighs 40,000. The particular number of a PBP will not readily relate from one species to another, and the PBP numbering system of gram-positive bacteria bears no relation to the PBP numbering of gram-negative bacteria. The PBPs probably account for only 1 percent of the membrane protein.

The PBPs vary greatly in the amount present. In *E. coli* and *P. aeruginosa*, high molecular weight PBPs, that is, 1, 2, 3, are in low amounts compared with PBPs 5 and 6, which account for 78 percent of the PBPs in *E. coli*. The PBPs also vary greatly in their affinity for certain β-lactams. In general, the affinity of a β-lactam to a particular PBP has been expressed as the concentration of antibiotic needed to reduce the ^{14}C-penicillin G binding to that PBP. The PBPs bind β-lactams covalently. It is believed that penicillins bind to PBPs through the carbonyl as a penicilloyl moiety and the binding of penicilloyl moiety is to a serine residue in the PBP via a bimolecular reaction.

Since the 1940s it has been known that low concentrations of penicillins cause filamentation of *E. coli*, whereas at high concentrations lysis occurs. It seems most likely that binding of a β-lactam to PBP-1Bs, or its substitute enzyme PBP-1A, results in rapid cell lysis and that this PBP is the most important protein for cell elongation.[8]

The role of PBP-2 in cell shape of bacteria was delineated by the availability of amdinocillin (mecillinam). *Escherichia coli* in the presence of amdinocillin form osmotically stable large round forms.[9] After several hours in the presence of amdinocillin, these bacteria lyse. It is probable that PBP-2 catalyzes a specific topologically restricted transpeptidase or carboxypeptidase reaction during a particular part of the cell cycle of division.

The third major PBP is PBP-3, which is important in cell division of *E. coli* and other enterobacteriaceae and pseudomonads. The PBP-3 is activated upon completion of DNA replication and subsequently catalyzes a carboxypeptidase reaction needed for the special peptidoglycan synthesis that ensues when cells divide.[10] The other low molecular weight PBPs have been thought to lack importance in the killing events associated with β-lactam binding to the proteins since mutants lacking PBP-4, -5, -6 have been isolated and grow well.[11]

The PBPs that are important in gram-positive organisms are PBPs-1, -2, and -4, since their antibiotic susceptibility closely resembles the effect of the agents on whole organisms.[12] In general, low molecular PBP-5, the carboxypeptidases, are not killing targets. Analysis of the lack of activity of β-lactams such as amdinocillin or aztreonam against gram-positive species and anaerobes shows that these agents fail to bind to PBPs of gram-positive species and anaerobes.[13]

The high activity of penicillins such as penicillin G against staphylococci can be correlated with binding to essential PBPs in these agents. Alteration of PBPs in gram-positive species has been correlated with resistance of *Streptococcus pneumoniae*, *S. aureus*, coagulase-negative staphylococci, and *Enterococcus faecium* to penicillin.

"Unleashing" of bacterial autolysins by β-lactam antibiotics may be responsible for cell death in certain species.

BACTERIAL RESISTANCE

Since there are many components involved in cell wall synthesis, variation in the composition of the wall components among bacteria accounts for some of the differences in susceptibility of individual bacterial strains to a particular penicillin. The differential binding of specific penicillins to target sites also accounts for differences in activity of different penicillins against a single organism or species. Mutation in a gene that specifies a binding site may lead to resistance to a penicillin, but this has been uncommon since most penicillins attack more than one of the peptidoglycan targets, and a coordinated mutation in a number of genes is an unlikely event. Resistant organisms with altered penicillin-binding proteins have been shown to produce an altered peptidoglycan structure.[14]

Some organisms are resistant to penicillins because the penicillin fails to reach its receptor site. Failure of a penicillin to reach its target is unlikely to be a mechanism of resistance in gram-positive species since the peptidoglycan layer lies outside the bacterial membrane,[15] but in gram-negative bacteria, two membranes compose the cell envelope, and the peptidoglycan lies inside the outer membrane. Thus in gram-negative bacteria a penicillin must pass through the outer membrane to reach its target site. Formerly it was supposed that lipophilicity of a molecule determined its activity. We now know that the protein layers on the outer surface of the bacterial membrane are held together by protein molecules that pass through the structure from one surface to the other. It is probable that penicillins that conform to the structural and charge properties of these stability proteins pass through to their receptor sites, whereas those β-lactam antibiotics that are structurally "different" do not enter the envelope and hence fail to reach a receptor site. Changes in structural protein components of the outer membrane due to mutations yield organisms more or less susceptible to penicillins. It is uncommon for naturally occurring resistant bacterial strains to owe their resistance to an alteration in membrane properties that prevents the particular penicillin from reaching its target.

The most important mechanism of bacterial resistance to penicillins is enzymatic hydrolysis of the β-lactam bond by β-lactamases with loss of antibiotic activity of the molecule.[16] A classification of β-lactamases is shown in Figure 2. The enzymes are classified on the basis of affinity for specific β-lactam compounds and amino acid composition. In gram-positive bacteria such as staphylococci, β-lactamase production is plasmid-mediated. The enzyme is both inducible and is an exoenzyme, that is, it is liberated into the surrounding medium in which it carries out its protective role by destroying the penicillins in the environment before they reach the cell surface. This mechanism of production of an exoenzyme is a protective one for bacteria such as staphylococci since they produce a large amount of enzyme with a very high affinity for penicillins.

On the other hand, β-lactamases of gram-negative bacteria are located in the periplasmic space that lies between the inner and outer membranes of gram-negative bacteria. Thus the enzymes are strategically located to protect the β-lactam target. Gram-negative β-lactamases may be either chromosomally or plasmid-mediated, constitutive or inducible enzymes, with an affinity for penicillins or for cephalosporins or both types of compounds. It is probable that all gram-negative species contain small amounts of a β-lactamase. The activity of the β-lactamase stable compounds, methicillin, and the isoxazolyl penicillins against staphylococci, is due to their β-lactamase stability. Differences in β-lactamase stability also account for some of the differences in activity of different penicillins against gram-negative bacteria. For example, carbenicillin is destroyed at a much slower rate than is ampicillin by *Enterobacter cloacae* or *Morganella morganii*.

Increased β-lactamase stability may decrease overall antibacterial activity since addition of bulky side chains that prevent β-lactamase hydrolysis also interfere with passage of the molecule across the outer membrane of gram-negative bacteria.[17] In general, increased activity of penicillins against β-lactamase-producing gram-negative bacteria is not associated with stability against β-lactamase hydrolysis but with affinity to penicillin receptor proteins and with increased entry into the bacterial cell. The one exception is temocillin, which contains a methoxy group on the β-lactam ring. Plasmid β-lactamases have markedly increased in number in the past decade, and some of the recent enzymes will destroy many cephalosporins as well as penicillins.

One final mechanism of resistance to penicillins seen in some gram-positive species is that of tolerance. This has been reported primarily for *S. aureus* and *S. pneumoniae*. Bacterial loss of viability, that is, cell death, is the result of secondary responses to inhibition of cell wall assembly. In some organisms the lytic effect of β-lactam antibiotics can be eliminated by inactivation of peptidoglycan hydrolyases (autolysins). For example, in pneumococci, lipoteichoic acids inhibit amidases. These acids are secreted into the surrounding milieu when penicillins are present. Suppression of autolytic activity protects the bacterium from the lytic effect of cell wall inhibition by penicillin. Thus an isolate that lacks autolysins will be inhibited but not killed by penicillin, that is, it is tolerant. At certain pHs the cellular autolysins are inactive and the bacteria although inhibited are not killed. The relevance of these observations to clinical situations is unclear.

CLASSIFICATION

Penicillins can be conveniently divided into classes on the basis of antibacterial activity (Table 1). Great overlaps do exist among the groups, but differences within a group usually are of a pharmacologic nature, although one compound in a group may be more active than another.

The susceptibility patterns of various species of microorganisms are given in Tables 2, 3, and 4. Gram-positive bacteria inhibited by natural penicillins in general are more susceptible to these penicillins than to semisynthetic penicillins.[18–23] Penicillin V (used orally) can be substituted for penicillin G, except against gram-negative species since it is less active than penicillin G against *Neisseria* and *Haemophilus*. Semisynthetic penicillinase-resistant penicillins are the drugs of choice only for penicillin-resistant *S. aureus* and *Staphylococcus epidermidis*, even though they will inhibit streptococci at concentrations below that needed to inhibit staphylococci.[19,20] Carboxypenicillins such as carbenicillin and ticarcillin are less active than the ureidopenicillins against streptococcal and *Haemophilus* species. The susceptible gram-negative organisms that are members of the Enterobacteriaceae or *Pseudomonas* vary from hospital to hospital and from community to community. Most of the anaerobic gram-positive bacteria are susceptible to all the penicillins. Gram-negative anaerobic bacteria are susceptible to most penicillins with the exception of isolates of *Bacteroides fragilis*, which are inhibited by high levels of penicillin G or the semisynthetic anti-*Pseudomonas* agents—azlocillin, carbenicillin, mezlocillin, piperacillin, and ticarcillin.[22] *Fusobacterium varium* often are resistant to all penicillins.

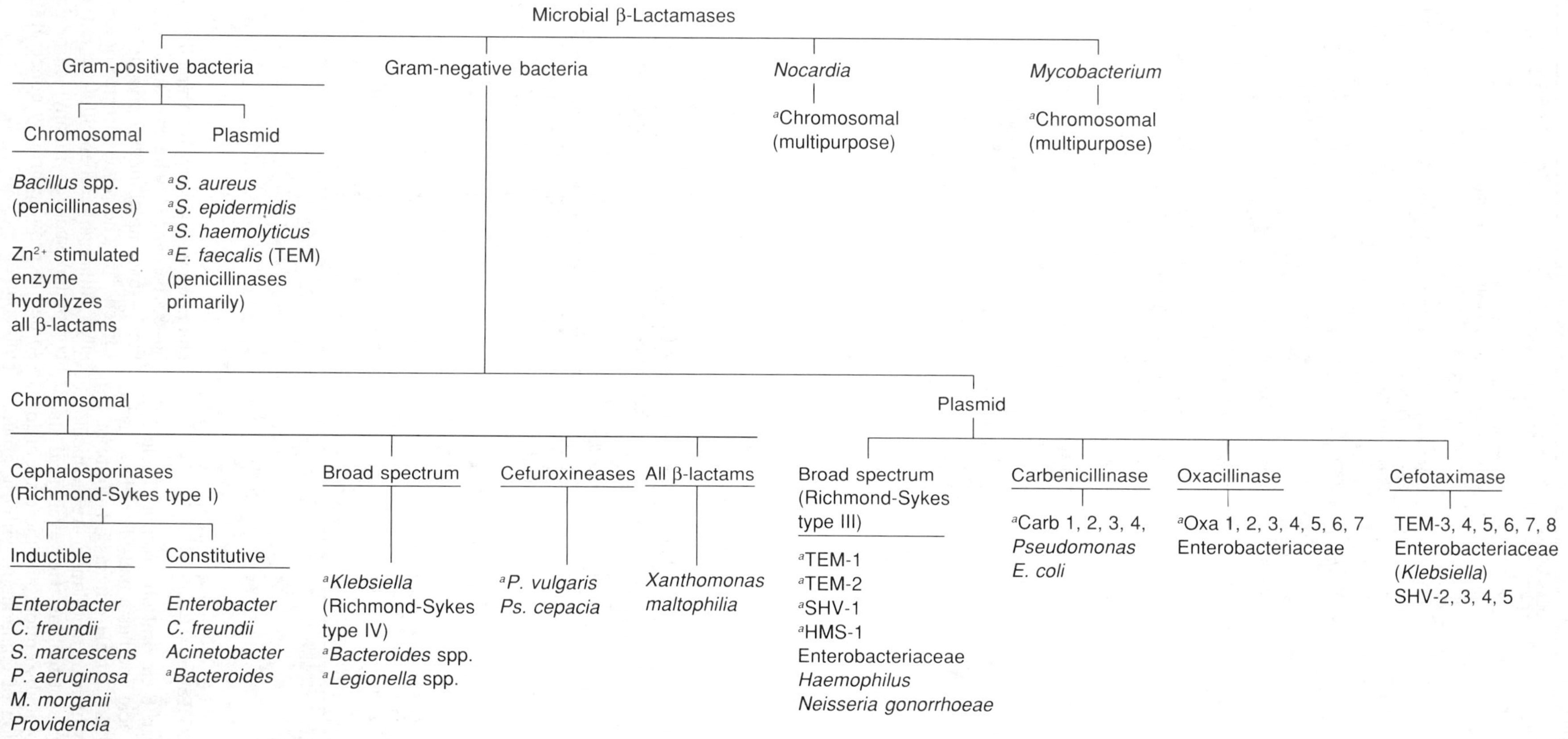

FIG. 2. Diagrammatic representation of β-lactamases.

[a] Inhibited by clavulanate, sulbactam, and tazobactam

TABLE 1. Classification of Penicillins

	Routes of Use	*Trade Names*
Natural penicillins		
Penicillin G	PO	Pfizerpen, Pentids, Kesso-Pen
	IM	Procaine—Wycillin, Duracillin, Crysticillin
	IM	Benzathine—Permapen, Bicillin
Penicillin G potassium or sodium	IV	
Penicillin V	PO	Ledercillin, Compocillin, Betapen, V-cillin, Veetids, Uticillin, S-K penicillin, Robicillin, Pen-Vee, Penapar
Phenethicillin	PO	Broxil, Syncillin, Maxipen, Pensig
Penicillinase-resistant penicillins		
Methicillin	IM, IV	Staphcillin, Celbenin
Nafcillin	IM, IV	Unipen
Isoxazolyl penicillins		
Cloxacillin	PO	Tegopen
Dicloxacillin	PO	Veracillin, Pathocil, Dynapen
Flucloxacillin	PO	
Oxacillin	PO, IM, IV	Prostaphlin, Bactocill
Aminopenicillins		
Ampicillin	IM, IV	Alpen, Amcil, Pen A/N, Omipen, Totacillin, Supen, S-K ampicillin, Principen, Probampcin, Polycillin, Pensyn, Penbritin
Amoxicillin	PO	Amoxil, Larotid, Polymox
Bacampicillin	PO	Spectrobid
Cyclacillin	PO	Cyclapen
Epicillin	PO	
Hetacillin	PO	Versapen
Pivampicillin	PO	
Anti-Pseudomonas penicillins		
Azlocillin	IM, IV	Azlin
Carbenicillin	IM, IV	Pyopen, Geopen
Indanylcarbenicillin	PO	Geocillin
Ticarcillin	IM, IV	Ticar
Extended-spectrum penicillins		
Mezlocillin	IM, IV	Mezlin
Piperacillin	IM, IV	Pipral, Pipracil
Amidino penicillins		
Amdinocillin	IM, IV	
Pivamdinocillin	PO	
Stable against gram-negative β-lactamases		
Temocillin	IM IV	

TABLE 2. Usual Minimal Inhibitory Concentrations (MIC) of Penicillins Against Cocci

	Mean Minimum Inhibitory Concentration (μg/ml)							
	Penicillin G	*Penicillin V*	*Ampicillin, Amoxicillin*	*Methicillin*	*Oxacillin, Cloxacillin Dicloxacillin*	*Nafcillin*	*Carbenicillin, Ticarcillin*	*Azlocillin Mezlocillin, Piperacillin*
Streptococcus pneumoniae	0.01[a]	0.02[a]	0.02[a]	0.1[a]	0.04	0.02	0.4	0.02
Streptococcus pyogenes	0.005	0.01	0.02	0.2	0.04	0.02	0.2	0.02
Streptococcus agalactiae	0.005	0.01	0.02	0.2	0.06	0.02	0.2	0.15
Viridans streptococci	0.01	0.01	0.05	0.1	0.1	0.06	0.2	0.12
Enterococcus faecalis	3.0	6.0	1.5[c]	>25	>25	>25	50	1.5
Peptostreptococcus	0.2	0.5	0.2	2.0	0.6	0.5	0.4	0.8
Staphylococcus aureus								
Penase-negative	0.02	0.02	0.05	1.0	0.3	0.25	1.2	0.8
Penase-positive	>25	>25	>25	2.0	0.4	0.25	25	25
Staphylococcus epidermidis	0.02[b]	0.02[b]	0.05[b]	0.8[b]	0.2[b]	0.2[b]	0.8[b]	1.6[b]
Neisseria gonorrhoeae[d]	0.01[b]	0.1	0.03[b]	12.0	12.0	12.0	0.3[b]	0.05[b]
Neisseria meningitidis	0.05	0.25	0.05	6.0	6.0	6.0	0.1	0.05

[a] Rare isolates resistant to penicillins have been found MIC >5 μg/ml.
[b] Many isolates resistant.
[c] Amoxicillin has a mean MIC of 0.4.
[d] Can range from 0.005 to 100.

PHARMACOLOGIC PROPERTIES

Penicillins differ markedly in their oral absorption (Table 5). Penicillin G is not stable to acid and has a half-life of less than 20 minutes at pH 2. In contrast, at pH 4 it has a half-life of 1 hour. The other penicillins, which are acid-labile, are methicillin and all the anti-*Pseudomonas* penicillins. However, acid stability is not a guarantee of oral absorption, and there are major differences in oral absorption of compounds within a group. Penicillin V is well absorbed even when ingested with food, and the greatest absorption of penicillin V is with the potassium salt.[24] The semisynthetic penicillins, with the exception of nafcillin, are well absorbed. Ampicillin is only partially absorbed, 30–60 percent,[19] whereas amoxicillin and the "proampicillins"—bacampicillin and pivampicillin—are almost totally absorbed.[23,25] The pivaloyl ester of amdinocillin is absorbed orally. Although carbenicillin is not absorbed, esters of the compound such as indanyl carbenicillin are adequately absorbed to provide urinary concentration to treat urinary tract infections.[26]

The majority of penicillins are absorbed so they yield peak levels 1–2 hours after ingestion. When ingested with food, absorption is delayed to yield peak serum levels 2–3 hours after

TABLE 3. Activity of Penicillins Against Selected Bacilli and Anaerobic Organisms

	Mean Minimum Inhibitory Level (μg/ml)				
Organism	*Penicillin G*	*Ampicillin, Amoxicillin*[a]	*Oxacillin*[b]	*Carbenicillin, Ticarcillin*[a]	*Azlocillin, Mezlocillin, Piperacillin*[a]
Clostridium perfringens	0.5	0.05	0.5	0.5	0.05
Corynebacterium diphtheriae	0.1	0.02	0.1	0.1	1.0
Listeria monocytogenes	0.5	0.5	4.0	4	0.5
Haemophilus influenzae[c]	0.8	0.5	25	0.5	0.1
Bacteroides melaninogenicus	0.5	0.5	25	0.5	0.2
Fusobacterium nucleatum	0.5	0.1	>100	0.5	0.5
Bacteroides fragilis	32	32	>500	64	32

[a] Minor differences do occur.
[b] Oxacillin is used as representative of isoxazoyl penicillins.
[c] β-lactamase-producing strains occur and are resistant to the penicillins.

TABLE 4. Activity of Penicillins Against Enterobacteriaceae and *Pseudomonas*

	Mean Minimum Inhibitory Levels (μg/ml)						
	Penicillin G	*Ampicillin, Amoxicillin*	*Oxacillin*[a]	*Carbenicillin, Ticarcillin*	*Azlocillin,*[d] *Mezlocillin, Piperacillin*	*Amdinocillin*	*Temocillin*
Escherichia coli[b]	100	3	>1000	6	8	0.5	10
Proteus mirabilis	50	3	>1000	1.5	1	25	5
Klebsiella spp.	>400	200	>1000	>400	16	1.5	10
Enterobacter spp.	>500	>500	>1000	50	16	1.5	10
Citrobacter diversus	>500	>100	>1000	12	8	1.5	2.5
Citrobacter freundii	>500	50	>1000	12	32	1.5	2.5
Serratia	>500	>500	>1000	100	32	100	25
Salmonella[b]	10	1.5	>1000	3	4	1	5
Shigella[b]	20	1.5	>1000	3	8	1	5
Proteus vulgaris	>500	>500	>1000	12	16	100	2.5
Providencia	>500	>500	>1000	12	8	100	2.5
Morganella	>500	200	>1000	25	8	8	2.5
Pseudomonas, other	>500	>500	>500	100	>100	>100	<100
Acinetobacter	>500	250	>1000	25	32	400	>100
Pseudomonas aeruginosa	>500	>500	>1000	50[c]	16[a]	100	>100

[a] Used as representative antistaphylococcal penicillin.
[b] Amoxicillin is twofold more active against *Salmonella* and twofold less active against *Shigella*. Strains containing the TEM plasmid β-lactamase are resistant except to temocillin.
[c] Ticarcillin two- to fourfold more active.
[d] Some isolates, particularly *Klebsiella*, are resistant to azlocillin but susceptible to mezlocillin and piperacillin.
[e] Mezlocillin is less active than azlocillin or piperacillin.

ingestion, and peak levels are lower, except for the pivaloyl esters and amoxicillin.

Repository forms of penicillin G are available. These are procaine penicillin G and benzathine penicillin G. These are absorbed more slowly from intramuscular sites than are the crystalline salts. Procaine or lidocaine can also be used as a diluent for intramuscular injection of anti-*Pseudomonas* penicillins, but the half-life of these drugs is not prolonged by this maneuver.

Penicillins are bound to protein in varying degrees from 17 percent for the aminopenicillins to 97 percent for dicloxacillin (Table 5). The major protein to which they bind is albumin.[19] Only an unbound (free) drug exerts antibacterial activity, since the bound drug cannot reach a receptor site within the bacteria. However, protein binding is a reversible process, and it is possible for bound penicillin to be released and to kill bacteria in tissue or in the blood stream. Penicillins are metabolized to a minor degree.[27] However, differences in metabolism explain the differences in half-lives in the presence of renal failure. The major mechanism by which they are removed from the body is by excretion as intact molecules via the kidney.[28] Biliary excretion of penicillins does occur, but it probably is important only for nafcillin and the anti-*Pseudomonas* penicillins.[29]

The mechanism of excretion of penicillins is via renal tubular cells. Penicillins are rapidly excreted into urine, and hence they have a short half-life, ranging from less than 30 minutes for penicillin to 72 minutes for carbenicillin. The one exception is temocillin, which has a half-life of 4 hours in healthy people.[30] The ability of the renal tubular cells to excrete penicillin varies with the agents, but up to 4 g/hr of penicillin G can be excreted. This excretion can be blocked by probenecid, which prolongs the serum half-life of all the penicillins.[31] Probenecid also competes for binding sites on albumin; hence, there is more free drug in the presence of probenecid. Renal excretion of all penicillins by the newborn is markedly less than in older children since tubular function is not fully developed. Hence, the dosage programs for penicillins must be modified when given to newborns or low birth weight infants.

Reduction in renal function is an important consideration in the administration of certain penicillins, namely, carbenicillin, ticarcillin, and temocillin. If the creatinine clearance is greater than 10 ml/min, it is necessary to make only minor adjustments in the dosage of other penicillins. In the presence of anuria, reduction in total daily dose of the natural penicillins, of many of the penicillinase-resistant penicillins, and of the aminopenicillins is necessary[32] (Table 6).

Peritoneal dialysis removes variable amounts of the penicillins. In general, after peritoneal dialysis only the dosage programs of carbenicillin and ticarcillin need to be adjusted. After hemodialysis it is necessary to replace the dialyzed penicillin G, ampicillin, amoxicillin, carbenicillin, ticarcillin, azlocillin, mezlocillin, piperacillin, and temocillin, but not nafcillin or the isoxazolyl penicillins.[32]

Penicillins are well distributed to most areas of the body such as lung, liver, kidney, muscle, bone, and placenta. The levels

TABLE 5. Pharmacokinetic Properties of Penicillins

					Serum Level[a]		Serum $T_{1/2}$ (hr)[b]			
Antibiotic	*Oral Adsorption (%)*	*Food Decreases Adsorption*	*Protein Binding (%)*	*Percentage of Dose Metabolized (%)*	*Total Drug (μg/ml)*	*Free Drug (μg/ml)*	*Normal ($C_{cr} > 90$ ml/min)*	*Renal Failure ($C_{cr} < 10$ ml/min)*	*Liver Impairment Increases ($T_{1/2}$)*	*Na^+ Content[d] (mEq/g)*
Penicillin G	20	Yes	55	20	2	0.9	0.5	10	+	2.7
Penicillin V	60	No	80	55	4	0.8	1	4		
Methicillin	Nil		35	10			0.5	4		3.1
Oxacillin	30	Yes	93	45	6	0.4	0.5	1		
Cloxacillin	50	Yes	94	20	10	0.6	0.5	1	+ +	
Dicloxacillin	50	Yes	97	10	15	0.45	0.5	1.5	+ +	
Nafcillin	Erratic	Yes	87				0.5	1.5	+ + +	
Ampicillin[c]	40	Yes	17	10	3.5	2.9	1	8	+ +	3.4
Amoxicillin	75	No	17	10	7.5	6.2	1	8	+	
Carbenicillin	Nil		50	2			1.1	15	+ +, 18–20 hr	4.7
Indanyl carbenicillin	30	No	50		15	7.5	1.1	15	+ +	
Ticarcillin	Nil		50	15			1.2	15	+ +, 18–20 hr	4.7
Amdinocillin	Nil		20				0.8	4	+	
Pivamdinocillin	50	No	20		3		1	4	+	
Mezlocillin	Nil		50				1.1	4	+ +	1.8
Piperacillin	Nil		50				1.3	4	+ +	1.8
Azlocillin	Nil		20				0.8	4	+ +	2.2
Temocillin	Nil		85	10			4	17	+ +	

[a] After 500 mg dose taken fasting.
[b] Values have been rounded of to approximate values.
[c] Proampicillins (bacampicillin, pivampicillin) are absorbed twice as well as ampicillin and food does not decrease absorption, but other properties are those of the parent ampicillin. Bacampicillin would give a serum level of 9 μg/ml after 500 mg.
[d] Na^+ content based on IV preparations.

TABLE 6. Antibiotic Dosage Change in Renal Disease and after Dialysis

	Dosage Change in Renal Failure[a]		
Agent	*Creatinine Clearance (30–50 ml/min)*	*Creatinine Clearance (<10 ml/min)*	*Dosage after Hemodialysis*
Penicillin G	NC	1.6×10^6 units/6 hr	Yes (1.6×10^6 units)
Penicillin V	NC	250 mg/6 hr	Yes (250 mg)
Methicillin	NC	2 g/8 hr	Slight (2 g)
Oxacillin	NC	NC	Slight (as in uremia)
Cloxacillin	NC	NC	Slight (as in uremia)
Dicloxacillin	NC	NC	Slight (as in uremia)
Nafcillin	NC	NC	Slight (as in uremia)
Ampicillin[c]	NC	0.5–1 g/8 hr	Yes (500 mg)
Amoxicillin	NC	500 mg/12 hr	Yes (250 mg)
Carbenicillin[b]	3 g/4 hr	2 g/8 hr	Yes (2 g)
Ticarcillin[b]	2 g/4 hr	2 g/12 hr	Yes (2 g)
Indanyl carbenicillin	NC	Avoid	
Azlocillin	NC	3 g/8–12 hr	Yes (2 g)
Mezlocillin	NC	3 g/8–12 hr	Yes (2 g)
Piperacillin	NC	3 g/8–12 hr	Yes (2 g)
Temocillin	1 g/24 hr	1 g/48 hr	Yes (1 g)
Amdinocillin	NC	1 g/8 hr	Yes (1 g)

[a] Refers to maximum dose used.
[b] Only carbenicillin and ticarcillin need adjustment of dosage after peritoneal dialysis.
[c] Dosage adjustments of "pivampicillins" should be the same as those of amoxicillin.
Abbreviations: NC: no change.

of penicillins in abscesses, middle ear, and pleural, peritoneal, and synovial fluids are sufficient in the presence of inflammation to inhibit most susceptible bacteria.[33–37] Most penicillins are relatively insoluble in lipid and so do not penetrate cells, including polymorphonuclear cells. Distribution of all the penicillins to eye, brain, cerebrospinal fluid, or prostate is nil in the absence of inflammation.[38] Inflammation alters normal barriers, permitting entry of penicillins, but more importantly it interferes with the anion pump that removes penicillins from areas such as cerebrospinal fluid. Low protein-bound penicillins reach levels in fetal serum equivalent to levels in maternal serum 30–60 minutes after injection. In contrast, the highly protein-bound semisynthetic penicillins achieve low concentrations in both amniotic fluid and fetal serum.[39]

Urinary concentrations of all penicillins are high, even in the presence of moderately reduced renal function, but in people with creatinine clearances below 10 ml/min the urinary levels may not exceed those in the blood. Cortical and medullary concentrations of penicillins during normal hydration and in hydropenia exceed serum levels.[40]

Most penicillins are actively secreted into the bile, yielding biliary concentrations well in excess of those in serum. The levels of penicillin G, ampicillin, and amoxicillin are at least 10 times those in the serum, and the levels of nafcillin and mezlocillin are as high as 100 times the simultaneous serum level. In the presence of common duct obstruction, the levels of all penicillins in bile are markedly reduced. Since the biliary transport system is a saturable one, at very high serum levels the biliary levels are not significantly increased over those obtained at lower serum levels.

UNTOWARD REACTIONS

The major adverse effects of the penicillins are hypersensitivity reactions, which range in severity from rash to immediate anaphylaxis (Table 7)[41,42] (see Chapter 21). Penicillins are capable of acting as haptens to combine with proteins contaminating the solution or with human protein after the penicillin has been administered to humans. The most important antigenic component of penicillins is the penicolloyl determinant, which is produced through opening of the β-lactam ring, thereby allowing amide linkage to body proteins (Fig. 3). Penicillanic acid and derivatives of penicillanic acid are produced when reconstituted penicillins break down in solution due to acidity or temperature elevation. The penicillolyl and penicillanic derivatives are the major determinants of penicillin allergy. Minor determinants of allergy are benzyl penicillin itself or sodium benzyl penicilloate, which can act either as sensitizing agents or on their own elicit an allergic reaction.[41,42] Both major and minor determinants may be involved in anaphylactic reactions, as well as in urticarial reactions. These reactions are mediated by IgE antibody. Minor determinants are the major cause of anaphylactic reactions. When a person has been sensitized by the hapten–carrier complex, he or she can have a reaction to penicillin alone or to penicillin that has formed dimers or polymers in

TABLE 7. Adverse Reactions to Penicillins

Type of Reaction	*Frequency (%)*	*Occurs Most Frequently with*[a]
Allergic		
IgE antibody	0.004–0.4	Penicillin G
Anaphylaxis		
Early urticaria (<72 hr)		
Cytotoxic antibody	Rare	Penicillin G
Hemolytic anemia		
Ag-Ab complex disease	Rare	Penicillin G
Serum sickness		
Delayed hypersensitivity	4–8	Ampicillin
Contact dermatitis		
Idiopathic	4–8	Ampicillin
Skin rash		
Fever		
Late onset urticaria		
Gastrointestinal	2–5	
Diarrhea	2–5	Ampicillin
Enterocolitis	<1	Ampicillin
Hematologic		
Hemolytic anemia	Rare	Penicillin G
Neutropenia	1–4	Penicillin G
		Oxacillin
		Piperacillin
Platelet dysfunction	3	Carbenicillin
Hepatic		
Elevated SGOT level	1–4	Oxacillin
		Nafcillin
		Carbenicillin
Electrolyte disturbance		
Sodium overload	Variable	Carbenicillin
Hypokalemia	Variable	Carbenicillin
Hyperkalemia—acute	Rare	Penicillin G
Neurologic		
Seizures	Rare	Penicillin G
Bizarre sensations		Procaine Penicillin
Renal		
Interstitial nephritis	1–2	Methicillin
Hemorrhagic cystitis	Rare	Methicillin

[a] All the reactions can occur with any of the penicillins.

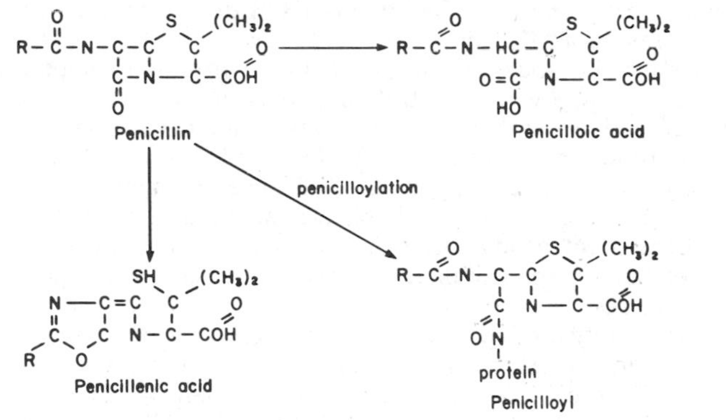

FIG. 3. Mechanisms for formation of antigens from penicillins.

solution. Anaphylactic reactions to penicillins are uncommon, occurring in only 0.2 percent of 10,000 courses of treatment, with 0.001 percent out of 100,000 cases resulting in fatality.[43] People with atopic dermatitis or allergic rhinitis appear not to be at increased risk of a penicillin reaction.[44]

Serum sickness does occur with penicillins, but it is very uncommon today. It probably is due to IgG antibodies to the benzyl penicilloyl hapten. The illness is characterized by fever, urticaria, joint pains, and angioneurotic edema. Exfoliative dermatitis and Stevens-Johnson syndrome are rare forms of allergic reactions to penicillins. The morbilliform eruptions that develop after penicillin therapy probably are due to IgM antibody to the benzyl penicilloyl hapten and to the minor determinants. In many patients these rashes will disappear, even if the penicillin is continued, due to the production of IgG blocking antibody. There is a risk, however, that the rash could progress to generalized desquamation. If an allergic reaction does occur, epinephrine given intramuscularly or intravenously will usually abort the reaction. Antihistamines and corticosteroids have not been shown to be of benefit.

Another allergic reaction to penicillins is that of allergic vasculitis with development of cutaneous and visceral lesions similar to that found with periarteritis nodosa. This reaction is extremely rare.

Hematologic toxicity is rare, although neutropenia has been encountered with the use of all types of penicillins, particularly when large doses are used.[45] The mechanism of the neutropenia is unknown, and white blood cell counts return to normal rapidly if the offending agent is discontinued. Sometimes a lower dose of drug can be used without production of neutropenia. Coombs-positive hemolytic anemia occurs rarely.[46] All penicillins at high concentrations, but particularly carbenicillin and ticarcillin, bind to the adenosine diphosphate receptor site in platelets, preventing normal platelet aggregation. A clinically significant bleeding disorder occurs relatively infrequently.[47]

Renal toxicity from penicillins has varied from allergic angiitis to interstitial nephritis.[48,49] Interstitial nephritis has occurred most commonly with the use of methicillin, but it has been seen with all penicillins. The clinical syndrome is one of fever, macular rash, eosinophilia, proteinuria, eosinophiluria, and hematuria. Initially the reaction is one of nonoliguric renal failure with a decrease in creatinine clearance and a rise in serum urea nitrogen and serum creatinine concentrations. This reaction can progress to anuria and renal failure. Biopsy specimens of the kidney show an interstitial infiltrate of mononuclear and eosinophilic cells with tubular damage but no glomerular lesions. Discontinuation of the penicillin will result in the return of renal function to normal in the majority of situations.[50]

Administration of massive doses of any penicillin, but most often carbenicillin and ticarcillin, may result in hypokalemia due to the large dose of nonreabsorbable anion presented to the distal renal tubules, which alters [H^+] excretion and secondarily results in K^+ loss.[48]

Central nervous system toxicity in the form of myoclonic seizures can follow administration of massive doses of penicillin G, ampicillin, carbenicillin, or methicillin. If there is reduced renal function, the drugs accumulate, and this toxicity is more likely.[51] Direct instillation of small doses of methicillin, oxacillin, or nafcillin into the ventricles at the time of surgery for placement of atrioventricular shunts has not resulted in seizures. Direct application of penicillin to the cortex will provoke seizure activity.

Gastrointestinal disturbances have followed the use of any of the oral forms but have been most pronounced with ampicillin. Enterocolitis due to *Clostridium difficile* has followed the use of all of the penicillins (see Chapter 83). All the penicillins used at high doses for prolonged periods will abolish normal bacterial flora with resulting colonization with resistant gram-negative bacilli and/or with fungi such as *Candida*. Abnormalities in hepatic function tests such as elevation of the alkaline phosphatase and serum glutamic oxaloacetic (SGOT) levels have been reported most often after the use of oxacillin and carbenicillin.[45,52] The pathogenesis of the hepatic reaction is unknown. Major hepatic injury is very uncommon, and liver enzymes return to normal values within a few days of stopping therapy.

CLINICAL USE

Table 8 lists some uses of penicillins. Penicillin G remains the primary agent for treatment of *Streptococcus pyogenes* and *S. pneumoniae* infections (regardless of the site). None of the newer penicillins or agents in other classes has been shown to be more effective. *Streptococcus pneumoniae* resistant to penicillin have been isolated in South Africa and the United States, but these are rarely encountered. In the United States *S. pneumoniae* of relative resistance to penicillin, minimum inhibitory concentration (MIC) values of 0.1–1 μg/ml, have been seen. Much higher doses of penicillin are required to kill these organisms. Nearly all *Neisseria meningitidis* strains are susceptible to penicillin G. *Neisseria gonorrhoeae* vary in susceptibility to penicillin G. Strains can be resistant due to β-lactamase production, to altered PBPs, or to membrane changes (see Chapter 16). Penicillin G is the drug of choice for treponemal infection in all its forms. Puerperal infections due to anaerobic streptococci or group B streptococci (*Streptococcus agalactiae*), as well as genital clostridial infections, are treated with penicillin G. Infections produced by anaerobic mouth flora including gram-positive and gram-negative cocci and the *Actinomyces* can be treated with penicillin G, although *Bacteroides melaninogenicus* producing a β-lactamase and resistant to penicillin are being encountered.

PROPHYLACTIC USE

Penicillins have been used in a number of situations for prevention of infection. Oral administration of 200,000 units of penicillin G or penicillin V every 12 hours has resulted in a significant reduction in recurrences of rheumatic fever. Because of the problems with compliance with oral therapy, intramuscular injections of 1.2 or 2.4 million units of benzathine penicillin given once each month have also been used with excellent results.

Outbreaks of streptococcal infection due to *S. pyogenes* have been aborted by the use of oral penicillin G or V given twice a day for 5 days, by single injections of procaine penicillin daily, or by administration of benzathine penicillin.

One of the most important prophylactic uses of penicillin is for prevention of bacterial endocarditis (see Chapter 63).

Antistaphylococcal penicillins may be used prophylactically at the time of implantation of an artificial joint or heart valve. These agents should be given just before the surgery, during the procedure, and in the immediate postoperative period. There are no studies that delineate the best penicillin agent for such procedures, and many physicians prefer to use a cephalosporin (see Chapter 285).

Ampicillin or amoxicillin has been administered orally to asplenic children or to children with agammaglobulinemia to prevent infections caused by *H. influenzae* and *S. pneumoniae*.

Penicillin prophylaxis has not been of benefit in prevention of meningococcal infection, bacterial infection after viral respiratory infection, or pneumonia after coma, shock, or congestive heart failure.

PROPERTIES OF INDIVIDUAL PENICILLINS

Dosages of penicillins are given in Tables 9 and 10.

Natural Penicillins

Penicillin G. Penicillin G or benzylpenicillin G (Fig. 4) is available in oral, parenteral, and respository salts. Oral salts are either the sodium or potassium forms, which are available as suspensions for pediatric use or as tablets in doses of 50,000 to 1 million units (200,00 units equals 125 mg). Penicillin G should be used orally only if it is taken 1 hour before or 2 hours after a meal to prevent its destruction by gastric acid. There is little reason to use oral penicillin G for acute infection at the present time, and penicillin V should be the oral preparation used.

Crystalline penicillin G in aqueous solution has been used intramuscularly, subcutaneously, intravenously, and intrathecally. It is available either as the potassium or sodium salt. The sodium salt is much more expensive than the potassium salt, and it rarely needs to be used since the amount of potassium present in 6 million units, an amount a patient with reduced renal function would receive, is less than 10 mEq. Given intramuscularly as an aqueous solution, penicillin G is very rapidly cleared from the body, and it is preferable to use a repository form. It is available as sterile dry powder in ampules or vials containing 200,000–20 million units per vial. Each million units of penicillin G contains 1.7 mEq of sodium or potassium.

Repository penicillins provide tissue depots from which the drug is absorbed over hours in the case of procaine penicillin or over days in the case of benzathine penicillin. Repository penicillins are only for intramuscular use and cannot be used intravenously or subcutaneously or to irrigate wounds. Procaine penicillin is a mixture of equal molar parts of procaine and penicillin. Thus 300,000 units contains 120 mg of procaine. Use of this suspension delays the peak of activity but provides serum and tissues levels for at least 12 hours. Doubling the dose of procaine penicillin given at a single injection site does not double the serum level. To increase the peak level it is necessary to use two body sites as was done in the treatment of gonorrhea, for example, with 2.4 million units of procaine penicillin given in each buttock. Marketed procaine penicillin preparations are of two types: One is an aqueous solution of the crystalline salt, and the other contains 2% aluminum monosterate as a dispensing agent. The preparations are marketed in cartridges and vials in doses of 300,000, 500,000, and 600,000 units in 1–4 ml and as 2.4 million units/4 ml.

Benzathine penicillin is a repository form of penicillin, which is a combination of 1 mole of penicillin and 2 moles of an ammonium base. It is available for intramuscular injection in 10 ml vials containing 300,000 units/ml and as prefilled syringes containing 600,000 units/ml in 1-, 2-, and 4 ml sizes. It provides detectable serum levels for 15–30 days depending on the size of the dose. Concentrations of penicillin G in the spinal fluid after use of benzathine penicillin probably are inadequate to treat treponemal infections of the nervous system.

TABLE 8. Antimicrobial Spectrum of Penicillins[a]

Organisms	*Penicillin of Choice*	*Alternate Acceptable Penicillin*	*Frequency of Resistance to Penicillins (%)*
Gram-positive cocci			
Streptpcoccus pneumoniae	G	V	Uncommon
Streptococcus pyogenes (A)	G	V	None
Streptococcus agalactiae (B)	G	Ampicillin	None
Viridans streptococci	G		None
Streptococcus bovis (D)	G		None
Enterococcus faecalis	Ampicillin	Mezlocillin	Rare, <1
Staphylococcus aureus (nonpenicillinase)	G	Penase-resistant	80
Staphylococcus aureus (penicillinase)	Penase-resistant		100
Staphylococcus aureus (methicillin-resistant)	None	None	100
Staphylococcus epidermidis	Penase-resistant		80
Staphylococcus epidermidis (methicillin-resistant)	None	None	100
Gram-negative cocci			
Neisseria meningitidis	G	Ampicillin	Very rare
Neisseria gonorrhoeae	G	Ampicillin	1–40
Gram-positive bacilli			
Bacillus anthracis	G		None
Corynebacterium diphtheriae	G		None
Listeria monocytogenes	Ampicillin	G	None
Anaerobic species			
Peptostreptoccoccus	G	Ampicillin	None
Actinomyces israeli	G	V	None
Bacteroides melaninogenicus	G	C, T	10
Fusobacterium	G	Ampicillin	1–10
Bacteroides fragilis	M, PA		75
Clostridium	G	Ampicillin	<1
Gram-negative bacilli			
Haemophilus	Ampicillin	G	5–30
Escherichia coli	Ampicillin		30
Proteus mirabilis	Ampicillin	G	<5
Salmonella typhi	Ampicillin		20
Salmonella, other sp.	Ampicillin		20
Klebsiella	None		95
Enterobacter spp.	M, P, T, C		70
Citrobacter freundii	M, P, T		80
Proteus, indole-positive	M, P, T, C		20
Serratia	M, P, T, C		90
Pseudomonas aeruginosa	A, P, T		20–30
Pseudomonas, other	None		95
Acinetobacter	T	A, G, P	50
Providencia	M, P, TC		20–30
Xanothomonas	None		95
Other organisms infrequently encountered			
Erysipelothrix	G	Ampicillin	None
Pasturella multocida	G		Rare, <1
Streptobacillus moniliformis	G		None
Spirillum minus	G		None
Fucospirochetes	G	Ampicillin	None
Treponema pallidum	G		None

[a] In each case it is assumed that a route of administration would be used that would achieve levels in serum and tissue to eradicate the organism. If there is no entry in the alternate column, it means that an antibiotic in another class would be a more appropriate choice. Amoxicillin can be used in place of ampicillin in all situations except with *Shigella*.
Abbreviations: A: azlocillin; C: carbenicillan; M: mezlocillin, P: piperacillin; T: ticarcillin.

Penicillin V. Phenoxymethyl penicillin (Fig. 4) is available only for oral use as sodium or potassium salts in suspension or tablets in doses of 125, 250, and 500 mg. The potassium salt produces higher blood levels than the other salts. Serum levels are from two to five times those obtained with penicillin G. Absorbed penicillin V is handled in the body similarly to penicillin G. Penicillin V can be substituted for penicillin G in most situations in which it is reasonable to treat an infection by the oral route. However, penicillin V is less active than penicillin G against *Haemophilus*, *Neisseria*, and enteric organisms. Blood levels after 500 mg given to an adult are equivalent to the levels achieved with 600,000 units of procaine penicillin given intramuscularly. The usual dosage for children is 25–50 mg/kg/day and for adults, 1–4 g/day. The interval between dosages is 6–8 hours.

Phenethicillin. This phenoxyethyl analogue of penicillin G (Fig. 4) has microbiologic properties similar to penicillin G. It is acid-stable and better absorbed from the gastrointestinal tract. Blood levels are high, but food delays its absorption. It is available only as the potassium salt in the form of 125 and 250 mg tablets and an oral suspension of 125 mg in 5 ml. Once absorbed it is handled in the body the same way as is penicillin G.

Penicillanse-Resistant Penicillins (Fig. 5)

Methicillin. Methicillin (2,6-dimethoxyphenylpenicillin) is a penicillin resistant to staphylococcal β-lactamase.[36] Its activity against staphylococci is low, with most strains inhibited by 2–3 μg/ml. Methicillin-resistant *S. aureus* are resistant not because of β-lactamase activity but by virtue of altered penicillin-binding proteins. These organisms have become a serious problem in some parts of the United States. Methicillin inhibits *S. pyogenes* and *S. pneumoniae* at levels of 0.2 μg/ml, but it has no activity against *Enterococcus fecalis* and gram-negative bacilli. Methicillin is acid-unstable and must be given parenterally. Absorption after an intramuscular injection is rapid, as is excretion, with peak levels after 1 g of 17 μg/ml but subinhibitory levels by 4 hours. Methicillin is less protein bound than the

TABLE 9. Dosage of Penicillins

Compound	*Oral*	*Intramuscular*	*Intravenous*
Penicillin G			25,000–500,000 units/kg/day, 6 doses
Procaine		300,000–600,000 units every 12 hr	
Benzathine		1.2–2.4 mega units every 15–20 days	
Pencillin V	Infant: 50 mg/kg/day, 3 doses 125–500, 4 doses		
Ampicillin[a]	25–200 mg/kg/day, 4 doses	100–200 mg/kg/day, 4 doses	100–400 mg/kg/day, 6 doses
Amoxicillin	25–50 mg/kg/day, 3 doses		
Methicillin Oxacillin Nafcillin		100 mg/kg/day, 4 doses	100–300 mg/kg/day, 6 doses
Cloxacillin	25–100 mg/kg/day, 4 doses		
Dicloxacillin	12–25 mg/kg/day, 4 doses		
Carbenicillin		50–100 mg/kg/day, 4 doses	50–500 mg/kg/day, 6 doses
Ticarcillin		50–100 mg/kg/day, 4 doses	50–300 mg/kg/day, 6 doses
Indanylcarbenicillin	50–65 mg/kg/day, 4 doses		
Azlocillin		50–100 mg/kg/day, 4 doses	200–300 mg/kg/day, 4 doses
Mezlocillin		50–100 mg/kg/day, 4 doses	200–300 mg/kg/day, 4 doses
Piperacillin		50–100 mg/kg/day, 4 doses	200–300 mg/kg/day, 4 doses

[a] Proampicillins are given at the same dose as amoxicillin.

TABLE 10. Dosage of Antibiotics in Newborn Infants

	Infants Less than 1 Week Old		*Infants 1 Week–1 Month Old*	
Compound	*Dose (per kg/day)*	*Interval between Doses (in hours)*	*Dose (per kg day)*	*Interval between Doses (in hours)*
Penicillin G	50,000–100,000 units	12	100,000 units	8
Ampicillin	100 mg	12	200 mg	6
Oxacillin	100 mg	12	200 mg	6
Methicillin	100 mg	12	300 mg	6
Nafcillin	100 mg	12	200 mg	6
Carbenicillin	250 mg	8	400 mg	6
Ticarcillin	150 mg	8	300 mg	6
Mezlocillin	75 mg	12	300 mg	6
Azlocillin	75–100 mg	12	300 mg	6

other antistaphylococcal penicillins, and although its intrinsic activity is less than the other antistaphylococcal penicillins, it is as active in the presence of serum as are the more intrinsically active oxacillin and nafcillin. Methicillin is available as a sodium salt, but since it is unstable in acidic media, it is used as a buffered solution. It is packaged as 1, 4, and 6 g vials and can be diluted with sodium chloride or dextrose in water. When diluted, buffered solutions are stable at room temperature for 8 hours. It is preferable to administer the drug every 4 hours if

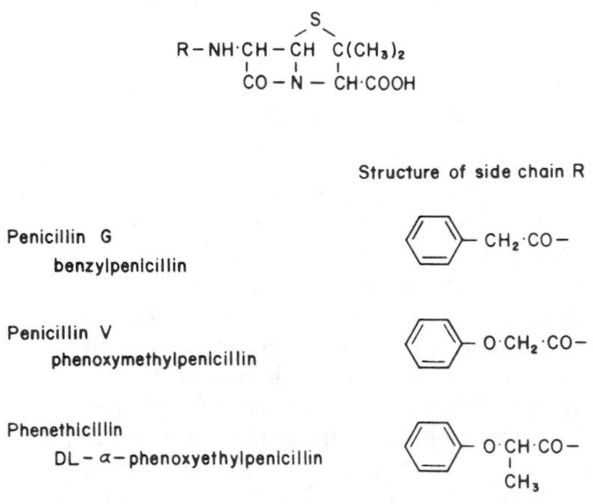

FIG. 4. Structure of penicillin G, penicillin V, and phenethicillin.

used intravenously. Methicillin should be used only for the treatment of penicillin G-resistant staphylococcal infections. Toxicity is that seen with any penicillin, although interstitial nephritis may be more common. The usual dosage is 4–12 g/day for adults and 200–300 mg/kg/day for children given in 4 or 6 doses.

Nafcillin. Nafcillin (2-ethoxy-1-naphthylpenicillin) has more intrinsic activity than methicillin against both staphylococci and streptococci but is not active against gram-negative bacteria. Nafcillin is highly protein bound, and in the presence of serum its activity is similar to methicillin. Although nafcillin is absorbed when taken by mouth, absorption is erratic whether the drug is taken fasting or with food, and hence serum levels are low.[36] Levels after intramuscular injection are low, and the preferred route of administration is intravenously. The antibiotic is primarily excreted by the liver and to a lesser extent by the kidney. Serum levels are elevated and the half-life is prolonged by probenecid. Although available as capsules (250 mg) and a suspension, one of the other agents in this class would be preferred for oral use. Sterile vials of 500 mg/1, 2, or 4 g of the sodium salt can be reconstituted in most solutions and are stable for up to 4 hours at room temperature. The usual dosage of nafcillin is 4–9 g/day, depending on the severity of the infection, and 100–200 mg/kg/day for children.

Isoxazolyl Penicillins. All these agents are stable to staphylococcal β-lactamase and inhibit both penicillin-sensitive and penicillin-resistant staphylococci at mean concentrations of 0.2–0.4 μg/ml. Methicillin-resistant *S. aureus* is resistant to

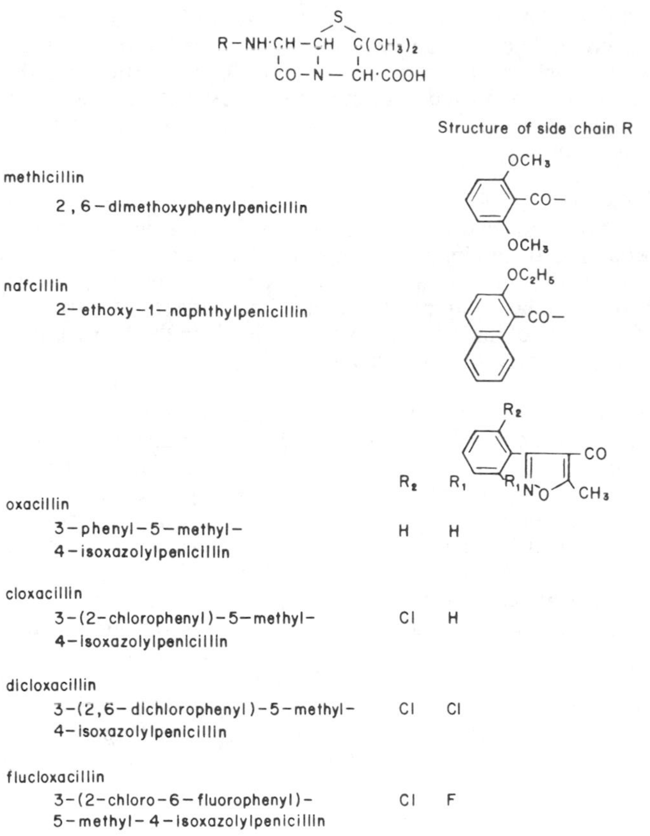

FIG. 5. Antistaphylococcal penicillins.

these penicillins. Recently an increasing number of *S. epidermidis* isolates resistant to these penicillins has been found as the cause of serious infections. The mechanism of resistance is altered PBPs. Isoxazolyl penicillins inhibit streptococci and pneumococci but are virtually inactive against gram-negative bacilli. All are absorbed after oral administration, but absorption is adversely affected by food. There are differences in serum levels among the drugs after oral ingestion, with the serum level of cloxacillin twice that of oxacillin and the levels of dicloxacillin and flucloxacillin twice that of cloxacillin; all the drugs are highly bound to serum proteins; oxacillin, cloxacillin, and flucloxacillin are equally bound, but dicloxacillin is bound to a greater extent. Thus, actual free serum concentrations of the drugs are greatest for flucloxacillin followed by cloxacillin and dicloxacillin as equals and oxacillin the least (Table 5). After intravenous infusion of 1 g over 15 minutes, peak serum levels are 70–100 μg/ml, with levels of 25 μg/ml at 1 hour and less than 1 μg/ml at 6 hours. The isoxazolyl penicillins undergo some metabolism but are excreted primarily by the kidney with slight biliary excretion. Oxacillin undergoes more rapid degradation in the body than does cloxacillin or dicloxacillin.

OXACILLIN. Oxacillin is available as a sodium salt for oral use in 250 and 500 mg capsules and as a powder for suspension at 250 mg/5 ml. It should be taken 1–2 hours before meals. The daily dosage for adults is 1–4 g taken in four parts. The dosage for children is 50–100 mg/kg/day taken in four parts. Oxacillin sodium for injection may be given intramuscularly or intravenously. It is available in 500 mg and 1, 2, or 4 g vials and is stable in most saline and dextrose solutions for 6 hours at room temperature. Adult dosage is 2–12 g/day and for children, 100–300 mg/kg/day given every 4–6 hours.

CLOXACILLIN. Cloxacillin sodium is available in the United States only as an oral solution (125 mg/5 ml), or capsules of 250 and 500 mg. Dosage for children is 50–100 mg/kg/day given as four equal doses. Dosage for adults is 1–4 g/day given as four equal doses. In Europe cloxacillin is available as a parenteral for intramuscular or intravenous administration in 250 mg vials. It yields serum levels similar to those achieved with oxacillin.

DICLOXACILLIN. Dicloxacillin sodium is available as a suspension (62.5 mg/5 ml) and as capsules of 125 and 250 mg. The dosage for children less than 40 kg is 25 mg/kg/day given as four doses. Some authorities recommend doses as above for cloxacillin. For adults, a dosage of 250 mg–1 g every 6 hours can be given, depending on the severity of the infection.

FLUCLOXACILLIN. Flucloxacillin sodium is not available in the United States. It is available in Europe in the form of suspension and capsules similar to the forms of cloxacillin, 250 mg capsules, and for parenteral use in 250 mg vials.

Aminopenicillins (Fig. 6)

The antibacterial activity of all these penicillins is similar.[53] They are not stable to β-lactamases of either gram-positive or gram-negative bacteria. The aminopenicillins are only slightly less active than penicillin G against *S. pyogenes*, *S. pneumoniae*, and *S. agalactiae*. They are more active against *E. fecalis*. Activity of the compounds against clostridial species, *Actinomyces*, corynebacteria, and *N. meningitidis* is equal to that of penicillin G. They are more active than penicillin G against *Listeria monocytogenes*. Sensitivity of *N. gonorrhoeae* (see Chapter 190) varies from highly sensitive to completely resistant strains that bear a plasmid-mediating production of a β-lactamase. *Haemophilus influenzae* (both typeable and nontypeable strains) and *Haemophilus parainfluenzae* are usually susceptible, except for the isolates that produce β-lactamases (see Chapter 201). Although many domiciliary *E. coli* are sensitive to aminopenicillins, plasmid resistance is common in hospital isolates. *Shigella sonnei*, many salmonellae, including many *Salmonella typhi*, are resistant because of β-lactamases. Most *Klebsiella, Serratia, Acinetobacter*, indole-positive *Proteus, Pseudomonas*, and *B. fragilis* are resistant to the penicillins of this class.

Ampicillin. Ampicillin is moderately well absorbed after oral administration, but peak levels are delayed and lowered if it is ingested with food. Peak blood levels of 3 μg/ml occur 1–2 hours after ingestion of 0.5 g. Peak blood levels occur later in diabetic patients with neurologic disease and in patients with renal failure. Drug can be detected in the serum for 4–6 hours. After intramuscular injection of 0.5 g peak levels of 10 μg are achieved in 1 hour and persist for 4 hours. Probenecid increases the height of peak levels and prolongs the period in which the drug can be detected in serum. Ampicillin is well distributed to body compartments and achieves therapeutic concentrations in cerebrospinal fluid (CSF) and in pleural, joint, and peritoneal fluids

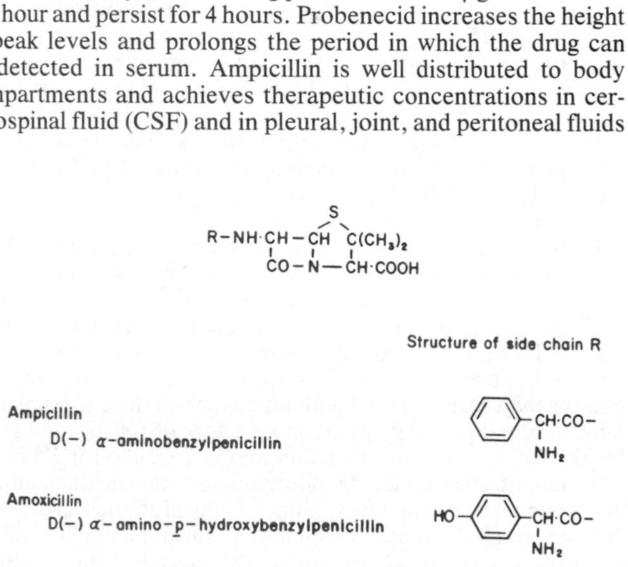

FIG. 6. Aminopenicillins.

in the presence of inflammation after parenteral administration. Urinary levels are high even in the presence of markedly reduced renal function. Peritoneal dialysis is ineffective in removing the drug, but hemodialysis removes approximately 40 percent in a 6 hour period.

Ampicillin is available for oral use as the sodium salt or as the trihydrate in capsules of 125, 250, and 500 mg, as a suspension of 125 and 250 mg/5 ml, as drops of 100 mg/ml, and as 125 mg chewable tablets. It is also prepared as a suspension, which contains 3.5 g of ampicillin trihydrate and 1 g of probenecid. It is available as ampicillin trihydrate in 2.5 g vials only for intramuscular use. As a sodium salt in vials of 0.125, 0.5, 2, and 4 g it can be used either intramuscularly or intravenously. It is stable in sodium chloride for 8 hours at concentrations up to 30 mg/ml, but for intravenous use at concentrations greater than 2 mg/ml it is stable at room temperature for less than 4 hours and hence would preferably be administered by "piggy back" within 0.5–1 hour. Dosage varies with the age of the patients, the status of renal function, and the severity of the disease. For children above 1 month of age the oral dosage is 50–100 mg/kg/day in four doses; the intramuscular or intravenous dosage is 100–400 mg/kg/day in four or six doses. For adults the oral dosage is 2–4 g/day given in a dose every 6 hours. For severe infection the parenteral dosage is 6–12 g/day given in divided doses every 4 hours. See Chapter 20 for a discussion of ampicillin–sulbactam.

Hetacillin. This is a condensation product of ampicillin and acetone that is rapidly hydrolyzed to ampicillin either as it crosses the gastrointestinal mucosa or in the serum.[54] It offers no advantage over ampicillin.

Pivampicillin. The pivaloyloxymethyl ester of ampicillin—pivampicillin—is stable in aqueous acid but undergoes rapid hydrolysis in serum and tissue.[55] Pivampicillin is absorbed intact and is rapidly hydrolyzed by nonspecific esterases in cells and blood to yield pivalic acid and the hydroxyl methyl ester of ampicillin, which are rapidly hydrolyzed to ampicillin and formaldehyde. At no time does the concentration of ester in the blood exceed 2 percent of the ampicillin, and within 15 minutes more than 99 percent of the compound has been converted to ampicillin. Pivampicillin is more rapidly absorbed than ampicillin, with peak levels at 1 hour, and serum levels are approximately twice those achieved with a comparable oral dose of ampicillin and are equal to those achieved with a comparable intramuscular dose of ampicillin. Urinary recovery and levels are twice those achieved with the same dose of ampicillin. In terms of distribution in the body, the compound is identical to ampicillin. Side effects due to the drug are those encountered with ampicillin, although there may be more gastric intolerance than with ampicillin, especially if not taken with food, but diarrhea is less. The drug is not available in the United States. In Europe it is available in capsules of 178 and 358 mg, which contain 125 and 250 mg of ampicillin. An advantage for the drug has not been established.

Bacampicillin. Bacampicillin is the hydrochloride of the 1-ethoxycarboxyloxyethyl ester of ampicillin. It has no antibacterial activity, but when it is adminsitered orally it is totally hydrolyzed to free ampicillin. It is better absorbed in the presence of food, with peak serum levels occurring earlier than with ampicillin and approximately from one and a half to two times greater than that achieved with an equimolar dose of ampicillin. Peak serum levels of 9 μg/ml follow a dose of 500 mg, and serum levels exceed those of ampicillin and amoxicillin for 2.5 hours, but thereafter serum levels of ampicillin from bacampicillin are equivalent to those of amoxicillin.[25] Clinical studies have shown efficacy similar to that of ampicillin.[56] Bacampicillin is available as an oral suspension containing 125 mg per 5 ml as 400 mg tablets, which is the equivalent of 280 mg of ampicillin.

Talampicillin. This is the phthalidyl ester of ampicillin. It has no antibacterial activity but is hydrolyzed to free ampicillin as it is absorbed. It produces serum levels earlier and three times those achieved with equimolar doses of ampicillin. It is not available in the United States. It has no merit over ampicillin.

Epicillin. Epicillin is a compound in which the benzene ring has been replaced by a 1,4-cyclohexadienyl ring. It has a bacterial spectrum similar to ampicillin. It is acid-stable and has oral absorption, serum binding, excretion, and tissue distribution similar to ampicillin. It has been effective in treatment of a variety of infections. It is not available in the United States. It has no value over ampicillin.

Cyclacillin. Cyclacillin, 6-(1-aminocyclohexande carboxyamido) penicillanic acid, is an acid-stable aminopenicillin with antibacterial activity similar to ampicillin. It is the most rapidly absorbed aminopenicillin, with levels of 10–18 μg/ml 30 minutes after ingestion of 500 mg—levels four times that of ampicillin. However, it is extremely rapidly cleared, and levels at 2 hours are less than those achieved with a comparable dose of ampicillin. Probenecid causes appreciably less delay in excretion than with other penicillins. It has no merit over ampicillin.

Amoxicillin. Amoxicillin differs from ampicillin only in the presence of a hydroxyl group in the para position of the benzene side chain. It has in vitro activity similar to ampicillin. It is significantly better absorbed when given by mouth than is ampicillin.[23] Peak blood levels are from two to two and a half times those achieved with a similar dose of ampicillin, and food does not decrease absorption. Oral amoxicillin produces blood levels similar to those produced by intramuscularly administered sodium ampicillin or ampicillin trihydrate. Urinary excretion of amoxicillin is greater than that of ampicillin. Tissue distribution is similar to that of ampicillin. Clinical studies with amoxicillin have been extensive, and it has been used in the treatment of otitis media, bronchitis, pneumonia, typhoid, gonorrhea, and urinary tract infections.[57] It has been used as a single 3 g dose for therapy for bacterial cystitis in women.[59] It is not useful as treatment of shigellosis. Side effects of amoxicillin are similar to those seen with ampicillin, although diarrhea may be less common than with ampicillin. It is available as the trihydrate in suspensions of 125 and 250 mg/5 ml, as drops of 50 mg/ml, and as capsules of 250 and 500 mg. Usual dosage for children is 20–40 mg/kg/day given in three doses every 8 hours, and for adults the dosage is 250 mg every 8 hours, although it has been used in doses up to 1 g every 4 hours. It has been useful in pediatric infections, except for shigellosis, and may be preferred to ampicillin. In adult infections its use would depend on cost factors and tolerance. See Chapter 20 for a discussion of amoxicillin–clavulanate.

Carboxy Penicillins (Fig. 7)

Carbenicillin. Carbenicillin was the first penicillin with activity against *P. aeruginosa* and certain indole-positive *Proteus* species that were not susceptible to other penicillins or to the cephalosporins.[37] It is destroyed by β-lactamases of both gram-positive and gram-negative organisms, but it is more stable against hydrolysis by the β-lactamases of species such as *Pseudomonas, Enterobacter, Morganella*, and *Proteus-Providencia*, which function primarily as cephalosprorinases. Carbenicillin is less active than ampicillin against *S. pyogenes, S. pneumoniae*, and *E. fecalis*. It is less active than the ureidopenicillins against streptococcal species and *Listeria*. Its activity against *Haemophilus, N. gonorrhoeae*, and *N. meningitidis* is similar to ampicillin. It has gram-negative activity similar to ampicillin against *E. coli, Proteus mirabilis, Salmonella* species, and *Shigella* species, but it is inactive against *Klebsiella*.

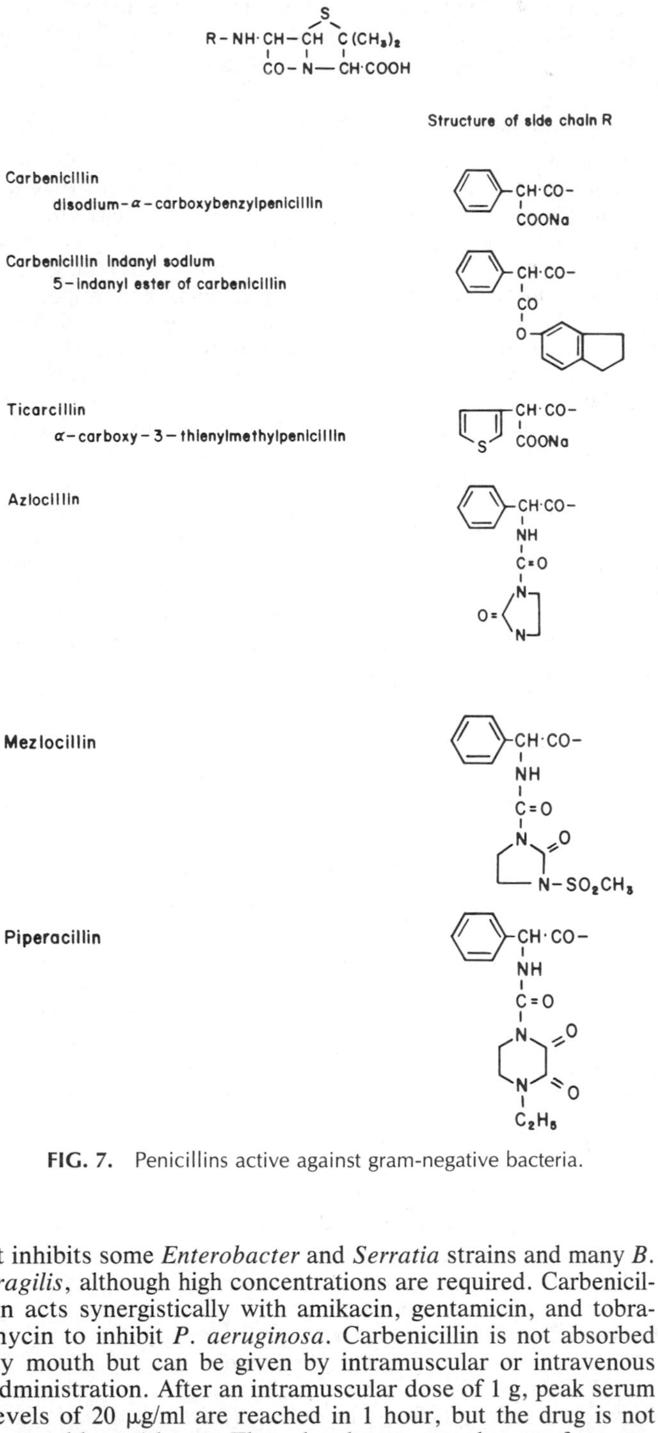

FIG. 7. Penicillins active against gram-negative bacteria.

It inhibits some *Enterobacter* and *Serratia* strains and many *B. fragilis*, although high concentrations are required. Carbenicillin acts synergistically with amikacin, gentamicin, and tobramycin to inhibit *P. aeruginosa*. Carbenicillin is not absorbed by mouth but can be given by intramuscular or intravenous administration. After an intramuscular dose of 1 g, peak serum levels of 20 μg/ml are reached in 1 hour, but the drug is not detectable at 4 hours. These levels are not adequate for treatment of tissue *Pseudomonas* infections, but levels of 2000–4000 μg/ml are achieved in the urine, and, therefore, it could be used by this route for urinary infections. Serum levels of 150–200 μg/ml will be maintained when it is given at dosages of 70–100 mg/kg over 1–2 hours. Carbenicillin is excreted by renal tubules, but since less is converted to penicilloic acid, its half-life (72 minutes) is longer than that of penicillin G, and it accumulates in the presence of renal failure.[37,60] Greater accumulation occurs if there is combined hepatic and renal dysfunction. Hemodialysis reduces plasma concentrations. Probenecid delays renal excretion and increases serum concentrations. Tissue distribution is simlar to ampicillin, but concentrations in the cerebrospinal fluid are not adequate for *Pseudomonas*. Side effects due to carbenicillin are similar to those seen with penicillins, but since it is a disodium salt and each gram contains 4.7 mEq of sodium, when administered at doses of 30–40 g/day congestive failure may occur. Carbenicillin causes more hypokalemia than other penicillins due to the load of nonreabsorbable anion in the distal tubule. Carbenicillin binds to the adenosine 5′-diphosphate (ADP) receptor site on platelets and prevents normal contraction; hence, bleeding occurs on occasion in the presence of high serum levels such as may occur in renal failure.

Carbenicillin is available as the disodium salt in vials of 1, 2, 5, and 10 g. It should never be mixed or administered in the same solution with aminoglycosides, since it complexes with these drugs and the activity of both compounds is inhibited. Intravenous dosages of 400–600 mg/kg/day given over 1–2 hours every 4 hours are used for treatment of systemic *Pseudomonas* infections. In the presence of markedly decreased renal function (creatinine clearance less than 10 ml/min) 2 g every 8 hours will provide adequate levels without toxicity. It should be replaced by one of the following agents.

Ticarcillin. The antibacterial spectrum of ticarcillin is identical to that of carbenicillin, except that it is from two to four times more active against *P. aeruginosa*.[61] The pharmacokinetics of ticarcillin and carbenicillin are virtually identical, as are side effects.[62] Ticarcillin can be used at dosages of 200–300 mg/kg/day. It is available in 1, 3, and 6 g vials. The advantage of ticarcillin over carbenicillin is that it inhibits some *Pseudomonas* that could be achieved with safety.[63] Another advantage is a reduced dose of ticarcillin (with the same therapeutic efficacy) resulting in less platelet dysfunction and less hypokalemia. See Chapter 20 for a discussion of ticarcillin-clavulanate.

Oral Antipseudomonas Penicillins

Indanyl Carbenicillin. Indanyl carbenicillin (carindacillin) is an α-carboxy ester of carbenicillin. It has no intrinsic activity of its own, but as a sodium ester it is highly acid-stable and relatively well absorbed from the gastrointestinal tract. Ingestion with food may actually enhance absorption. The ester is immediately hydrolyzed to free carbenicillin, and only trace amounts of ester are found in serum or urine. Peak serum levels after 1 g taken orally are 10 μg at 1–2 hours. Urine levels are 300–1000 μg/ml with 30 percent of a dose recovered in the first 6 hours. The compound does not provide adequate serum or tissue levels for systemic infections, and it is useful only for the treatment of urinary tract infections. In the presence of decreased renal function, urine levels are lower and may be inadequate to treat *Pseudomonas* infections. Side effects are those of all the penicillins, but gastrointestinal irritation has been a problem in some people. It is available as 500 mg capsules (containing 382 mg of carbenicillin). The usual dosage is 1 g every 6 hours for adults. Quinolones should replace this agent for treatment of urinary tract infections and prostatitis.

Carfecillin. Carfecillin is the phenyl ester of carbenicillin. It is also well absorbed and rapidly hydrolyzed to yield carbenicillin. Serum levels are similar to those of the indanyl ester. It is useful only to treat urinary infections due to *Pseudomonas*. It has been better tolerated due to a less bitter taste. It is not available in the United States.

Ureidopenicillins

Azlocillin. Azlocillin is an acylureido penicillin that is 8–16 times more active than carbenicillin against *P. aeruginosa* and is less active against indole-positive *Proteus* species. It has the same activity as ampicillin against streptococcal species.[64] It is destroyed by β-lactamases of both gram-positive and gram-negative bacteria. It is not orally absorbed and must be given by the intravenous route to provide adequate serum levels to treat

Pseudomonas infection. The half-life is approximately 50 minutes, and administration of 4 g yields peak levels of 285 μg/ml.

Azlocillin shows nonlinear pharmacokinetics. The peak serum concentrations and the area under the drug curve are not proportional; that is, a 4 or 5 g dose produces serum levels that are greater than four or five times the 1 g dose.[65] The drug thus could be administered in larger doses at intervals of 6 hours rather than the 4 hour intervals used for carbenicillin. Azlocillin also does not accumulate in renal failure to the same degree as do carbenicillin and ticarcillin since its half-life rises only to 4 hours with creatinine clearances below 7 ml/min.[66–68] Azlocillin enters the cerebrospinal fluid in the presence of meningeal inflammation, but levels are only 10 percent of the serum level. Azlocillin also causes less increase in bleeding time than does carbenicillin since it apparently has less affinity for the ADP receptor site. Azlocillin is used primarily to treat *Pseudomonas* infections. It has proved to be a useful drug in a variety of clinical situations.[67] It is available as 1, 2, 3, and 4 g vials, which contain 2.17 mEq sodium per gram of drug.

Mezlocillin. Mezlocillin is an acylureido penicillin similar in antibacterial spectrum to carbenicillin and ticarcillin but with some significant differences.[64] It is more active in vitro against *E. faecalis* than either of the above-mentioned agents. It inhibits about 75 percent of *Klebsiella* species at a concentration of 25 μg/ml, whereas less than 5 percent would be inhibited by 100 μg/ml of carbenicillin.[69] It is also more active than carbenicillin or ticarcillin against *H. influenzae* and is more active than carbenicillin against *B. fragilis*. It is, however, not more stable to β-lactamase hydrolysis than is carbenicillin; hence its greater intrinsic activity is due to other factors such as greater affinity for penicillin-binding proteins and better entry into the bacterial periplasmic space. It acts synergistically against gram-negative bacteria when combined with aminoglycosides. The drug must be given parenterally. Its pharmacokinetics are different from carbenicillin since, like azlocillin and piperacillin, it shows dose-related nonlinear kinetics. Peak serum levels, half-life, and area under the time curve are greater with larger doses. Administration of 4 g produces peak levels of 300 μg/ml.[70] Its half-life increases only to 4 hours in patients in renal failure. Mezlocillin is the least likely of the broad-spectrum penicillins to alter bleeding times. Clinical studies in the United States and Europe have shown that it is effective therapy for respiratory, urinary, gynecologic, and surgical infections.[67,71–76] It causes less increase in bleeding time than does carbenicillin. Usual doses have been 12–18 g/day for adults. It is available as 1, 2, 3, and 5 g vials, which contain 1.85 mEq of sodium per gram.

Piperacillin. Piperacillin is an acylureido penicillin derivative that is similar in activity to ampicillin against gram-positive species.[77] It has excellent activity against streptococcal species and against *Neisseria* and *Haemophilus* and many Enterobacteriaceae. It also has excellent activity against both cocci and bacilli anaerobic species. It inhibits 60 percent of *Pseudomonas* species at 3 μg/ml and 90 percent at 12 μg/ml.[77,78] It is hydrolyzed by plasmid-mediated β-lactamases of gram-positive and gram-negative bacteria. Its acts synergistically against *Pseudomonas* and against some of the Enterobacteriaceae when combined with aminoglycosides.[77] The human pharmacology of piperacillin is similar to that of azlocillin and mezlocillin.[79–82] Administration of 4 g by the intravenous route produces peak serum levels of 300 μg/ml. It shows kinetics that are dose-dependent. It accumulates in renal failure to a lesser degree than does carbenicillin, and its half-life is only 4 hours in renal failure.[83] It is removed by hemodialysis. Piperacillin has shown adverse reactions similar to those of the other penicillins noted earlier. After prolonged administration at high doses neutropenia has been reported. Alteration of bleeding time and hypokalemia occur but less frequently than with carbenicillin. Clinical studies have shown that it is a useful agent in treatment of a variety of infections.[67,84–90] It is administered in daily doses to adults of 12–18 g. It is available in vials of 2, 3, and 4 g, which contain 1.85 mEq of sodium per gram of drug.

Amdinopenicillanic Acid Derivatives

Amdinocillin, formerly called mecillinam, is a 6-β-acylaminopenicillanic acid. It has unusual antibacterial properties for a penicillin.[91,92] It has poor antigram-positive activity. In situations in which 0.01 μg/ml of penicillin G inhibits *S. pyogenes*, 6 μg/ml of amdinocillin are needed to inhibit streptococci. It does not bind to the penicillin-binding proteins of gram-positive species. It has poor activity against *Haemophilus* and *Neisseria*. However, it is extremely active against *E. coli*, inhibiting many β-lactamase-containing strains even though it is hydrolyzed by the plasmid-mediated β-lactamases. The reason for its activity is that it binds only to PBP-2 in Enterobacteriaceae, and this protein is critical in cell wall production in these species. Amdinocillin is active against many ampicillin-resistant *Shigella* and *Salmonella* species. In contrast to ampicillin, it is active against many *Klebsiella, Enterobacter*, and *Citrobacter* species. It has variable activity against *Proteus*, both *P. mirabilis* and the indole-positive *Proteus*, and it fails to inhibit *Pseudomonas* and anaerobic species such as *B. fragilis* and *Clostridium*. Amdinocillin acts synergistically with other penicillins such as ampicillin or carbenicillin and also with cephalosporins.[92] It does not act synergistically with aminoglycosides nor is its activity inhibited by chloramphenicol.

Amdinocillin is not acid-stable and cannot be used orally except in the form of a pivaloyl ester. This ester is well absorbed and immediately hydrolyzed, yielding free compound in the serum. Serum levels of pivamdinocillin after ingestion are equivalent to those obtained with pivampicillin (see above), and absorption is improved in the presence of food. Amdinocillin administered parenterally as a sodium salt yields serum levels comparable to those achieved with equimolar doses of ampicillin.[93,94] The compound is renally excreted similarly to ampicillin and is distributed within the body in the same manner as ampicillin. Clinical studies have shown the compound to be effective in the treatment of infections caused by susceptible microorganisms.[95,96] It is available in Europe as the pivaloyl ester for oral use and as the sodium salt for parenteral administration.

6-Methoxy Penicillin Derivatives

Temocillin is a 6-α-methoxy derivative of ticarcillin. The presence of the methoxy group on the β-lactam ring renders the compound extremely resistant to hydrolysis by both plasmid and chromosomally mediated β-lactamases. However, there has been a marked loss in activity against gram-positive species and *Pseudomonas*.[97,98] Temocillin inhibits the majority of *E. coli, Klebsiella, Enterobacter* species, *Proteus, Serratia*, and *Citrobacter* species at 10 μg/ml or less. *Haemophilus* and *Branhamella* are inhibited by less than 1 μg/ml. *Bacteroides* species are resistant. Temocillin is not hydrolyzed by the common chromosomal and plasmid β-lactamases. It is not destroyed by the cefotaxine–ceftazidime-destroying β-lactamases. Although it does not inhibit *Pseudomonas*, this is due to failure to cross the outer cell wall.

Peak serum concentrations of temocillin after 500 mg and 1 g are administered by the intramuscular route average 50 and 70 μg/ml, respectively.[30,99] Serum half-life of temocillin after intramuscular administration ranges from 4 to 6 hours. After bolus intravenous administration of temocillin peak serum concentrations have been 75 μg/ml for 500 mg and 170 μg/ml for 1 g. Serum half-life after intravenous administration averages 4½ hours. Urinary recovery of temocillin is 70–80 percent, with urine concentrations of 100–500 μg/ml for 12 hours after a 500 mg intramuscular injection. Temocillin accumulates in the presence of renal failure with serum half-life reaching 15–20 hours.[30] It is partially removed by hemodialysis but not by peritoneal dialysis. Temocillin has been used in Europe to treat urinary infections and tissue infections due to gram-negative bacilli.[100–102] It is not available in the United States.

REFERENCES

1. Fleming A. On the antibacterial action of cultures of a penicillium, with special reference to their use in the isolation of *B. influenzae*. Br J Exp Pathol. 1929;10:226.
2. Batchelor FR, Doyle FP, Naylor JHC, et al. Synthesis of penicillin: 6-aminopenicillanic acid in penicillin fermentations. Nature. 1959;183:257.
3. Tipper DJ, Wright A. The structure and biosynthesis of bacterial cell walls. In: Sokatch JR, Ornstein LA, eds. The Bacteria. v. 7. New York: Academic Press; 1979:291.
4. Strominger JL. Penicillin-sensitive enzymatic reactions in bacterial cell wall synthesis. Harvey Lect. 1970;64:179.
5. Mirelman D. Biosynthesis and assembly of cell wall peptidoglycan. In: Inouye M, ed. Bacterial Outer Membranes. New York: John Wiley & Sons; 1980:166.
6. Waxman DL, Yocum RR, Stominger JL. Penicillins and cephalosporins are active site-directed acylating agents: evidence in support of the substrate analogue hypothesis. Philos Trans R Soc Lond [Biol]. 1980;289:257.
7. Spratt BG. Distinct penicillin binding proteins involved in the division, elongation and shape of *Escherichia coli*, K 12. Proc Natl Acad Sci USA. 1975;72:2999.
8. Spratt BG. Biochemical and genetical approaches to the mechanism of action of penicillin. Philos Trans R Soc Lond (Biol). 1980;289:273.
9. Tamaki S, Nakajima S, Matsuhashi M. Thermosensitive mutation in *Escherichia coli* simultaneously causing defects in penicillin-binding protein 1 Bs and in enzyme activity for peptidoglycan synthesis in vivo. Proc Natl Acad Sci USA. 1977;74:5472.
10. Spratt BG, Bowler LB, Edelman A, et al. Membrane topology of PBPs 7B and 3 of *E. coli* and the production of water-soluble forms of high molecular weight PBPs. In: Shockman GD, ed. Antibiotic Inhibition of Bacterial Cell Surface Assembly and Function. Washington, DC: American Society for Microbiology; 1988:292–300.
11. Suzuki H, Nishimuka Y, Hirota Y. On the process of cellular division in *Escherichia coli*: a series of mutants of *E. coli* altered in penicillin-binding proteins. Proc Natl Acad Sci USA. 1978;75:664.
12. Yocum RR, Waxman DW, Strominger JL. The mechanism of action of penicillin. J Biol Chem. 1980;255:3977.
13. Georgopapadakou NH, Liu FY. Binding of β-lactam antibiotics to penicillin-binding proteins of *Staphylococcus aureus* and *Streptococcus faecalis* in relation to antibacterial activity. Antimicrob Agents Chemother. 1980;18:834.
14. Garcia-Bustos JF, Chait BT, Tomasz A. Altered peptidoglycan structure in a pneumococcal transformant resistant to penicillin. J Bacteriol. 1989; 170:2143–7.
15. Tomaz A. Penicillin tolerance and the control of the murein hydrolases. In: Salton M, Shockman GD, eds. Beta-lactam Antibiotics. New York: Academic Press; 1980:227–47.
16. Sykes RB, Matthew M. The β-lactamases of gram-negative bacteria and their role in resistance to β-lactam antibiotics. J Antimicrob Agents Chemother. 1976;2:115.
17. Neu HC. β-Lactam antibiotics: structural relationships affecting in vitro activity and pharmacologic properties. Rev Infect Dis. 1986;8(Suppl 3):237–59.
18. Barber M, Waterworth PM. Antibacterial activity of the penicillins. Br Med J. 1962;1:1159.
19. Rolinson GN, Sutherland R. Semisynthetic penicillins. Adv Pharmacol Chemother. 1973;11:152.
20. Marcy SM, Klein JO. The isoxazolyl penicillins: oxacillin, cloxacillin and dicloxacillin. Med Clin North Am. 1970;54:1127.
21. Finland M, Garner C, Wolcox C, et al. Susceptibility of pneumococci and *Haemophilus influenzae* to antibacterial agents. Antimicrob Agents Chemother. 1976;9:274.
22. Sutter VL, Finegold SM. Susceptibility of anaerobic bacteria to 23 antimicrobial agents. Antimicrob Agents Chemother. 1976;10:736.
23. Neu HC. Antimicrobial activity and human pharmacology of amoxicillin. J Infect Dis. 1974;129 (Suppl):123.
24. McCarthy CG, Finland M. Absorption and excretion of four penicillins: penicillin G, penicillin V, phenethicillin and phenylmercaptomethyl penicillin. N Engl J Med. 1960;263:315.
25. Neu HC. The pharmacokinetics of bacampicillin. Rev Infect Dis. 1981;3:110.
26. Butler K, English AR, Briggs B, et al. Indanyl carbenicillin: chemistry and laboratory studies with a new semisynthetic penicillin. J Infect Dis. 1973;127(Suppl):97.
27. Cole M, Kening MD, Hewitt VA. Metabolism of penicillins to penicilloic acidosis and 6-aminopenicillanic acid in man and its significance in assessing penicillin absorption. Antimicrob Agents Chemother. 1973;3:463.
28. Eagle H, Newman E. Renal clearance of penicillin F, G, K, and X in rabbits and man. J Clin Invest. 1947;26:903.
29. Acocella G, Mattiussi R, Nichols FB, et al. Biliary excretion of antibiotics in man. Gut. 1968;9:536.
30. Bodaert J, Daneels R, Schurgers M, et al. The pharmacokinetics of temocillin in patients with normal and impaired renal function. J Antimicrob Chemother. 1983;11:349.
31. Gilbaldi M, Swartz MA. Apparent effect of probenecid on the distribution of penicillins in man. Clin Pharmacol Ther. 1968;9:345.
32. Appel GB, Neu HC. Infections and antibiotic usage in patients with renal diseases. In: Martinez-Maldonado M, ed. Handbook of Renal Therpeutics. New York: Plenum; 1983:227.
33. Parker RH, Schmid FR. Antibacterial activity of synovial fluid during therapy of septic arthritis. Arthritis Rheum. 1971;14:96.
34. Barza M, Weinstein L. Penetration of antibiotics into fibrin loci in vivo. I. Comparison of penetration of ampicillin into fibrin clots, abscesses and interstitial fluid. J Infect Dis. 1974;129:59.
35. Pancoast SJ, Neu HC. Antibiotic levels in human bone and synovial fluid. Orthopedics Rev. 1980;9:49.
36. Neu HC. Antistaphylococcal penicillins. Med Clin North Am. 1982; 66:51.
37. Neu HC. Carbenicillin and ticarcillin. Med Clin North Am. 1982;66:61.
38. Fishman RA. Blood-brain and CSF barriers to penicillin and related organic acids. Arch Neurol. 1966;15:13.
39. Depp R, Kind AC, Kirby WMM, et al. Transplacental passage of methicillin and dicloxacillin into the fetus and amniotic fluid. Am J Obstet Gynecol. 1970;197:1054.
40. Whelton A, Carter GG, Bryant HH, et al. Carbenicillin concentrations in normal and diseased kidneys. A therapeutic consideration. Ann Intern Med. 1973;78:659.
41. Levine BB, Redmond AP, Feller MF, et al. Penicillin allergy and the heterogeneous immune response of man to benzylpenicillin. J Clin Invest. 1966;45:1895.
42. Saxon A. Immediate hypersensitivity reactions to β-lactam antibiotics. Rev Infect Dis. 1983;5(Suppl 2):368.
43. Idsoe O, Gothe T, Wilcox RR, et al. Nature and extent of penicillin side reactions with particular reference to fatalities from anaphylactic shock. Bull WHO. 1968;38:159.
44. Green GR, Rosenblum A. Report of the penicillin study group, American Academy of Allergy. J Allergy Clin Immunol. 1971;48:331.
45. Parry MF, Neu HC. The safety and tolerance of mezlocillin. J Antimicrob Chemother. 1982;9(Suppl A):273.
46. Kerr RO, Cardamone J, Dalmasso AP, et al. Two mechanisms of erthrocyte destruction in penicillin-induced hemolytic anemia. N Engl J Med. 1972;287:1322.
47. Brown CH, Natelson EA, Bradshaw W, et al. The hemostatic defect produced by carbenicillin. N Engl J Med. 1974;291:265.
48. Appel GB, Neu HC. The nephrotoxicity of antimicrobial agents. N Engl J Med. 1977;296:63.
49. Appel GB, Neu HC. Acute interstitial nephritis induced by β-lactam antibiotics. In: Fillastre JP, ed. Nephrotoxicity-ototoxicity of Drugs. Rouen: Inserum Publ de l'Université de Rouen; 1981:195.
50. Baldwin DS, Levine BB, McCluskey RT, et al. Renal failure and interstitial nephritis due to penicillin and methicillin. N Engl J Med. 1968;279:1245.
51. Bloomer HA, Barton LJ, Maddock RJ Jr. Penicillin-induced encephalopathy in uremic patients. JAMA. 1967;200:121.
52. Wilson FM, Belamavic J, Lauter CB, et al. Anicteric carbenicillin hepatitis. Eight episodes in four patients. JAMA. 1967;232:818.
53. New HC. Aminopenicillins: clinical pharmacology and use in disease states. Int J Clin Pharmacol Biopharm. 1975;11:132.
54. Tuano SD, Johnson LD, Brodie JL, et al. Comparative blood levels of hetacillin, ampicillin and penicillin G. N Engl J Med. 1966;275:635.
55. Daehne W von, Godfredsen WO, Rotrott K, et al. Pivampicillin, a new orally active ampicillin ester. Antimicrob Agents Chemother. 1971;10:431.
56. Scheife RT, Neu HC. Bacampicillin hydrochloride: chemistry, pharmacology and clinical use. Pharmacotherapy. 1982;2:313.
57. Prince AS, Neu HC. New penicillins and their use in pediatrics. Pediatr Clin North Am. 1983;30:3.
58. McCracken GH Jr. Selection of antimicrobial agents for treatment of acute otitis media with effusion. Pediatr Infect Dis J. 1987;6:985–8.
59. Fang LST, Tolokoff-Rubin NE, Rubin RH. Efficacy of single-dose and conventional amoxicillin therapy in urinary tract infection localized by antibody-coated bacteria technique. N Engl J Med. 1978;298:413.
60. Hoffman TA, Cestero R, Bullock WE. Pharmacodynamics of carbenicillin in patients with hepatic and renal failure. Ann Intern Med. 1970;73:173.
61. Fuchs PC, Thornsberry C, Barry AL, et al. Ticarcillin: a collaborative in vitro comparison with carbenicillin against 9,000 clinical bacterial isolates. Am J Med Sci. 1977;274:255.
62. Neu HC, Garvey GG. Comparative in vitro activity and clinical pharmacology of ticarcillin and carbenicillin. Antimicrob Agents Chemother. 1975;8:457.
63. Parry MF, Neu HC. Ticarcillin for treatment of serious infections with gram-negative bacteria. J Infect Dis. 1976;134:476.
64. Fu KP, Neu HC. Azlocillin and mezlocillin: new ureido penicillins. Antimicrob Agents Chemother. 1978;13:930.
65. Bergen T. Review of the pharmacokinetics and dose dependency of azlocillin in normal subjects and patients with renal insufficiency. J Antimicrob Agents. 1983;11(Suppl B):101.
66. Whelton A, Stout RL, Delgado FA. Azlocillin kinetics during extracorporeal haemodialysis and peritoneal dialysis. J Antimicrob Chemother. 1983;11(Suppl B):89.

67. Drusano GL, Schimpff SC, Hewitt WL. The acylampicillins: mezlocillin, piperacillin, and azlocillin. Rev Infect Dis. 1984;6:13–32.
68. Lowenbraun S, Fox N, Cunitz D. Azlocillin, cephalothin and tobramycin therapy in solid tumor patients with chemotherapy-induced leukopenia. Cancer. 1987;60:14–7.
69. Parry MF, Folta D. The in vitro activity of mezlocillin against community hospital isolates in comparison to other penicillins and cephalosporins. J Antimicrob Chemother. 1983;11(Suppl C):97.
70. Meyers BR, Mendelson MH, Srulevitch-Chin E, et al. Pharmacokinetic properties of mezlocillin in ambulatory elderly subjects. J Clin Pharmacol. 1987;27:678–81.
71. Pancoast SJ, Jahre JA, Neu HC. Mezlocillin in the therapy of serious infections. Am J Med. 1979;67:747.
72. Issell BF, Bodey GP. Mezlocillin for treatment of infections in cancer patients. Antimicrob Agents Chemother. 1980;17:1008.
73. Melikian V, Wise R, Allum WH, et al. Mezlocillin and gentamicin in the treatment of infections in seriously ill and immunosuppressed patients. J Antimicrob Chemother. 1981;7:657.
74. Ramirez-Ronda CH, Gotierrez J, Bermudez RH. Comparative effectiveness, safety and tolerance of mezlocillin and ticarcillin: a prospective randomized trial. J Antimicrob Chemother. 1982;9 (Suppl A):125.
75. Faro S, Phillips LE, Baker JL, et al. Comparative efficacy and safety of mezlocillin, cefoxitin, and clindamycin plus gentamicin in post-partum endometritis. Obstet Gynecol. 1987;69:760–6.
76. Alvarez RD, Kilgore LC, Huddlestone JF. A comparison of mezlocillin versus clindamycin/gentamicin for the treatment of post-caesarean endomyometritis. Am J Obst Gynecol. 1988;158:425–9.
77. Fu KP, Neu HC. Piperacillin, a new penicillin active against many bacteria resistant to other penicillins. Antimicrob Agents Chemother. 1978;13:358.
78. Verbist L. Comparison of the activities of the new ureido-penicillins—piperacillin, mezlocillin, azlocillin and Bay K4999—against gram-negative organisms. Antimicrob Agents Chemother. 1979;16:115.
79. Bergen T. Overview of acylureidopenicillin pharmacokinetics. Scand J Infect Dis. 1981;29:33.
80. Tjandramaga TB, Mollie A, Verbesselt R, et al. Piperacillin pharmacokinetics after intravenous and intramuscular administration. Antimicrob Agents Chemother. 1978;14:829.
81. Martens MG, Faro S, Feldman S, et al. Pharmacokinetics of the acylureidopenicillins piperacillin and mezlocillin in the post-partum patient. Antimicrob Agents Chemother. 1987;31:2015–7.
82. Brattstrom C, Malmborg AS, Tyden G. Penetration of clindamycin, cefoxitin, and piperacillin into pancreatic juice in man. Surgery. 1988;103:563–7.
83. Francke EL, Appel GB, Neu HC. Pharmacokinetics of intravenous piperacillin in patients undergoing chronic hemodialysis. Antimicrob Agents Chemother. 1979;16:788.
84. Winston DJ, Murphy W, Young LS, et al. Piperacillin therapy for serious bacterial infections. Am J Med. 1980;69:255.
85. Wade JC, Schimpff SC, Newman KA, et al. Piperacillin or ticarcillin plus amikacin: a double blind prospective comparison of empiric antibiotic therapy for febrile granulocytopenic cancer patients. Am J Med. 1981;71:983.
86. Pancoast SJ, Prince AS, Francke EL, et al. Clinical evaluation of piperacillin for therapy of infection. Arch Intern Med. 1981;141:1447.
87. Prince AS, Neu HC. Use of piperacillin, a semisynthetic penicillin, in the therapy of acute exacerbations of pulmonary disease in patients with cystic fibrosis. J Pediatr. 1980;97:148.
88. Hemsell DL, Hemsell PG, Heard MC. Piperacillin and a combination of clindamycin and gentamicin for the treatment of hospital and community-acquired acute pelvic infections including pelvic abscess. Surg Gynecol Obstet. 1987;165:223–9.
89. Menichetti F, Del Favero A, Guerciolini R, et al. Empiric antimicrobial therapy in febrile granulocytopenic patients. Randomized prospective comparison of amikacin plus piperacillin with or without parenteral trimethoprim/sulfamethoxazole. Infection. 1986;14:61–267.
90. Holmes B, Richard DM, Brodgen RN, et al. Piperacillin: a review of its antibacterial activity, pharmacokinetic properties, and their therapeutic use. Drugs. 1984;28:375–425.
91. Neu HC. Mecillinam, a novel penicillanic acid derivative with unusual activity against gram-negative bacteria. Antimicrob Agents Chemother. 1976;9:793.
92. Neu HC. Mecillinam: an amdinocillin which acts synergistically with other β-lactam compounds. J Antimicrob Cheother. 1977;3(Suppl B):43.
93. Neu HC, Srinivasan S, Francke EL, et al. Pharmacokinetics of amdinocillin and pivamdinocillin in normal volunteers. Am J Med. 1983;75(Suppl 2A):60.
94. Moukhtar I, Nawishy S, Sabbour M. Pharmacokinetics of mecillinam after a single intravenous dose in patients with impaired renal function. Int J Clin Pharmacol Res. 1987;7:59–62.
95. Demos CH, Green E. Review of clinical experience with amdinocillin monotherapy and comparative studies. Am J Med. 1983;75(Suppl 2A):72.
96. King JW, Beam TR Jr, Neu HC, et al. Systemic infections treated with amdinocillin in combination with other beta-lactam antibiotics. Am J Med. 1983;75(Suppl 2A):90.
97. Jules K, Neu HC. Antibacterial activity and β-lactamase stability of temocillin. Antimicrob Agents Chemother. 1982;22:453.
98. Gobernado M, Conton E. Comparative in vitro activity of temocillin. Drugs. 1985;29(Suppl 5):24–31.
99. Hampel B, Feike M, Koeppe P, et al. Pharmacokinetics of temocillin in volunteers. Drugs. 1985;29(Suppl 5):99–102.
100. Kosmidis J. The treatment of complicated and uncomplicated urinary tract infections with temocillin. Drugs. 1985;29(Suppl 5):172–4.
101. VanLanduyt HW, Lambert A, vanCouter A, et al. Temocillin in the treatment of gram-negative septicemia. Drugs. 1985;29(Suppl 5):182–5.
102. Lindsay G, Beattie AD, Taylor EW. Temocillin in the treatment of serious gram-negative infections. Drugs. 1985;29(Suppl 5):191–3.

19. CEPHALOSPORINS

GERALD R. DONOWITZ
GERALD L. MANDELL

Most of the new antibiotics introduced for clinical use in recent years are cephalosporins. These agents are now the most prescribed of all antimicrobials and account for a large segment of the health care budget. It all started in 1945 when Professor Giuseppe Brotzu began searching for antibiotic-producing microorganisms. He hypothesized that the process of self-purification of water might be due in part to substances produced by certain organisms inhibiting other microbes. He isolated a fungus, *Cephalosporium acremonium*, from seawater near a sewage outlet in Kaglara, Sardinia, and found that this organism inhibited the growth of a variety of gram-positive and gram-negative bacteria. Broth cultures produced a filtrate that showed some antibacterial effect on infections in animals and later in patients.

Professor Brotzu sent a culture of his organism to Oxford in 1948, and attempts were made by several workers, led by Professor Edward P. Abraham, to isolate the active antibacterial factors. Several different antibiotic fractions were isolated from these broth cultures. These included cephalosporin C, which is the parent substance from which the first cephalosporins for clinical use were derived. In addition to its fairly broad range of antimicrobial activity, it had the interesting features of being relatively acid stable and resistant to penicillinase.[1]

CLASSIFICATION

Cephalosporins may be classified by their chemical structure, major differences in clinical pharmacology, β-lactamase resis-

TABLE 1. Selected Cephalosporins Listed by Generation

Generic Name	*Proprietary Name*
First generation	
Cefazolin	Ancef, Kefzol
Cephalothin	Keflin, Seffin
Cephapirin	Cefadyl
Cefadroxil	Duricef
Cephalexin	Keflex
Cephradine	Anspor, Velasef
Second generation	
Cefamandole	Mandol
Cefoxitin	Mefoxin
Cefuroxime	Zinacef, Kefurox
Cefotetan	Cefotan
Cefonicid	Monocid
Cefaclor	Ceclor
Cefuroxime axetil	Ceftin
Third generation	
Cefotaxime	Claforan
Ceftizoxime	Cefizox
Ceftriaxone	Rocephin
Moxalactam	Moxam
Ceftazidime	Fortaz, Taxidime, Tazicef
Cefoperazone	Cefobid
Cefpirome	—
Cefpiramide	—
Cefixime	Suprax

tance, or antibacterial spectrum. The well-accepted "generations scheme" is a somewhat arbitrary but useful way to classify these agents (Table 1). *Generations* are based on antimicrobial activity and not on the time of introduction of the agents.

CHEMISTRY

The three active fermentation products of *Cephalosporium* were identified as cephalosporin C, cephalosporin N, and cephalosporin P. Cephalosporin N is actually a penicillin, with an aminocarboxybutyl side chain. Cephalosporin P is a steroid with a very narrow range of antibacterial activity. Cephalosporin C is the major product, and it is the basis for the new cephalosporins. Cephalosporin C resembles a penicillin since it has a β-lactam structure, but the five-member thiazolidine ring characteristic of the penicillins is replaced by a six-member dihydrothiazine ring (Fig. 1). Previous experience has shown that the potency of penicillins was improved by substitution of different groups at the 6-acylamino function adjacent to the β-lactam ring. Attempts were made to cleave the side chain off enzymatically, but these failed. Acid treatment, however, did hydrolyze cephalosporin C to 7-aminocephalosporanic acid (7-ACA) (Fig. 2). This compound has been subsequently modified with different side chains to create a whole family of cephalosporin antibiotics. In general, modifications at position 7 of the 7-aminocephalosporanic acid nucleus are associated with alteration in antibacterial activity, and substitutions at position 3 of the dihydrothiazine ring are associated with changes in the pharmacokinetics and the metabolic parameters of the drug (Fig. 3).[2,3] Hepatic metabolism occurs at the 3-acetoxymethyl position. There has been an association made with certain adverse side effects such as disulfuram-like (Antabuse) reactions, and the potential for bleeding associated with the methylthiotetrazole group at position 3 of the dihydrothiazoladine ring.[4] Molecules with a methoxy group in position 7 of the 7-aminocephalosporanic acid nucleus are called cephamycins.

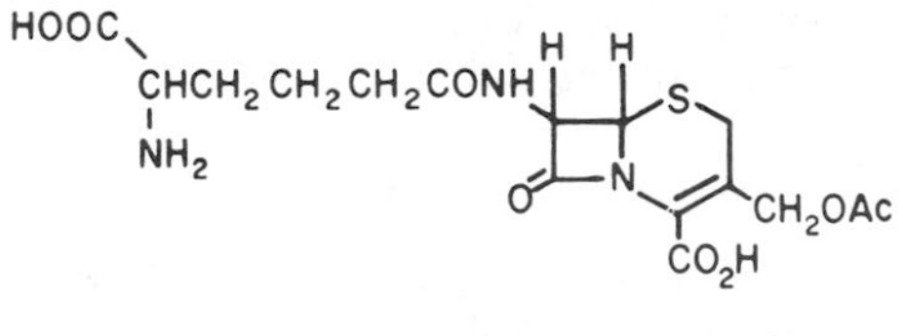

FIG. 1. Structure of cephalosporin C.

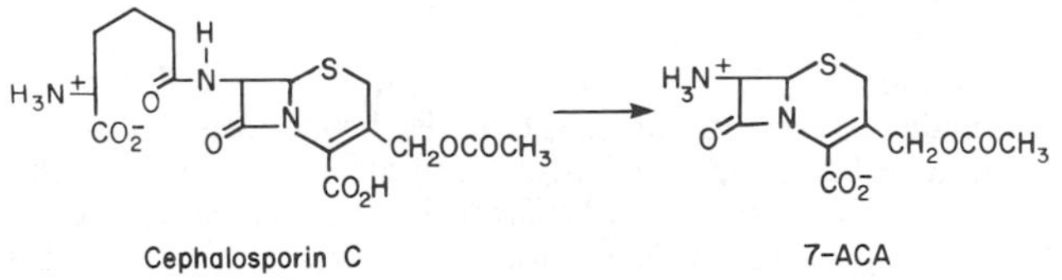

FIG. 2. Preparation of 7-aminocephalosporanic acid (7-ACA) from cephalosporin C.

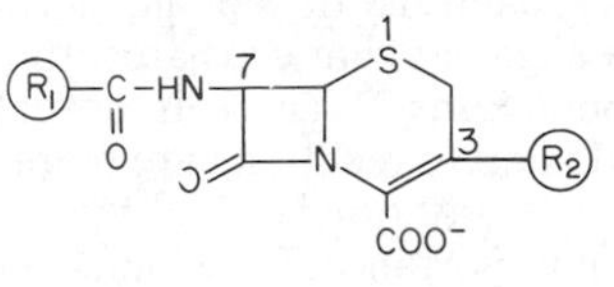

FIG. 3. Basic structure of a cephalosporin.

MECHANISM OF ACTION

The mechanism of action of the β-lactam antibiotics could be explained with confidence and precision a decade ago. It was thought that all β-lactam antibiotics had the same mechanism of action and that this was related to interference with cell wall structure. A brilliant series of experiments by a number of investigators identified the particular step in the cross-linking of the peptidoglycan polymer that was interfered with by the β-lactam antibiotics.[5] It was thought that these weak or defective cell walls then allowed for growth of bizarre bacterial forms with subsequent lysis and death of bacterial cells.

It became clear that this explanation of the mechanism of action of the β-lactam antibiotics was oversimplified and failed to explain various observations of drug–bacteria interactions. First, antibiotic-induced lysis of bacteria appeared to be an enzymatic process rather than a process resulting from a weakened bacterial cell wall.[6] It also became clear that multiple targets for β-lactam molecules existed within bacteria and differed from each other biochemically and functionally.[7,8] Furthermore, different agents produced greatly different effects on bacteria. Some β-lactam antibiotics produced lytic effects such as those seen with cephalothin acting on *Staphylococcus aureus*. Other agents, such as cephalexin, produced long filamentous forms when they interacted with *Escherichia coli*, while yet other agents such as amdinocillin produced round, osmotically fragile forms.

At present, our understanding of the specific mechanisms involved in the antibacterial activity of β-lactam antibiotics, including the cephalosporins, remains incomplete. However, several basic elements have been established. These agents act by binding to and inactivating specific targets located on the inner aspect of the bacterial cell membrane.[7,8] These targets, or penicillin-binding proteins (PBPs), are enzymes, including transpeptidases, carboxypeptidases, and endopeptidases, that are important for the biosynthesis of the peptidoglycan component of the bacterial cell wall. β-Lactam antibiotics have different binding affinities to the various PBPs. The effect of an antibiotic on a bacterium is, in part, dependent on which PBP or combination of PBPs are bound and inactivated.[9–11] Some PBPs (PBP1A, -1BS, -2, and -3) are of critical importance, and their inactivation leads to cell death. Other PBPs (PBP4, -5, and -6) are not essential for bacterial survival, and their inhibition causes nonlethal changes.[12,13] Actual lysis of a bacterium by a β-lactam appears to involve inhibition of protein synthesis and the loss from the cell of an inhibitor of an enzyme that functions as an autolysin. Bacterial cells containing the autolysins are often lysed by the activity of the β-lactam antibiotics. Bacterial cells not containing the autolysin may develop bizarre forms, and their growth may be only inhibited.[14,15] Thus the β-lactam exhibits a bacteriostatic effect rather than a bactericidal effect. This phenomenon has been called tolerance.

Some of the newer concepts of the mechanism of action of the β-lactam antibiotics may be of clinical importance. In the past it was thought that there would be no reason to combine β-lactam antibiotics, since it was thought that they all worked in an identical fashion and thus true synergism would not be seen. However, since these agents may bind to different proteins in the bacterial cell, it may be feasible to use two β-lactam antibiotics together to achieve a synergistic effect.[16]

MECHANISM OF BACTERIAL RESISTANCE TO THE CEPHALOSPORINS

The antibacterial activity of cephalosporins is dependent on their ability to penetrate the bacterial cell wall, resist inactivation by bacterial enzymes known as β-lactamases, and bind to and inactivate penicillin-binding proteins. Bacterial resistance may develop at each of these steps. The peptidoglycan structure of the cell wall of gram-positive organisms offers little resistance to the entry of antibiotic molecules. In contrast, the outer cell wall of gram-negative organisms, consisting of lipids, proteins, and polysaccharides, represents a formidable barrier to entry of many molecules, including cephalosporins.[17] Passage of these agents through the cell wall occurs through channels lined by proteins called porins. Porin channels allow selective movement of molecules through the bacterial cell wall based on size, change, and hydrophilic properties.[18] This selective permeability of the cell wall may be an inherent property of a bacterium but may also result from changes caused by exposure to antibiotics. Difficulty in penetration may by itself offer a means of resistance for bacteria like *Pseudomonas aeruginosa* and *Enterobacter cloacae*. This mechanism may also interact synergistically with other bacterial mechanisms of resistance.[19]

Decreased binding affinity of penicillin-binding proteins for antibiotics is another mechanism of bacterial resistance and is the reason that cephalosporins are ineffective against methicillin-resistant *S. aureus*. Exposure of these organisms to β-lactam antibiotics stimulates the production of a novel PBP termed PBP2′ or PBP2a, which has a markedly lowered binding affinity for cephalosporins as well as penicillinase-resistant penicillins.[20,21] The most important bacterial mechanism of resistance to the cephalosporins is the production of β-lactamases.[22–25] These enzymes are present in virtually all gram-negative and gram-positive bacteria and hydrolyze the cyclic amide bond of the β-lactam ring, rendering it inactive. Among gram-positive organisms, the staphylococcal β-lactamses are the most significant and are released into the surrounding media. While the penicillins are highly susceptible to these enzymes, most cephalosporins, with the exception of cephaloridine, are poorly hydrolyzed. Gram-negative bacilli produce a variety of β-lactamses that may be encoded chromosomally or extrachromosomally via plasmids or transposons. Although gram-negative organisms seem to produce less β-lactamase, the location of their β-lactamases in the periplasmic space makes the enzymes more effective in destroying cephalosporins as they attempt to reach their target on the inner membrane.[22]

The cephalosporins have variable susceptibility to β-lactamase. Cephaloridine is the most sensitive to both gram-positive and gram-negative β-lactamases, and thus more antibiotic is hydrolyzed by the enzyme. Cefazolin is more susceptible to hydrolysis by β-lactamases from *S. aureus* than is cephalothin.[26] Cefoxitin, cefuroxime, and the third-generation cephalosporins are the most resistant to hydrolysis by the β-lactamases produced by gram-negative organisms.[27] However, the correlation between antimicrobial activity and β-lactamase resistance is not linear. Some bacterial strains that fail to hydrolyze the antibiotics are nevertheless resistant. Conversely, some bacteria with β-lactamases that can destroy cephalosporins are susceptible to the cephalosporins.[28]

Although most of the third-generation cephalosporins are relatively resistant to hydrolysis by bacterial β-lactamases, there are increasing reports of development of resistance to the third-generation cephalosporins by *Enterobacter, Serratia, Citrobacter*, and *Pseudomonas* species.[27] Sanders and Sanders[29] have suggested that the derepression of chromosomally mediated β-lactamases in these organisms has resulted in the production of large amounts of enzyme that have a high affinity for the antibiotics although they slowly hydrolyze them. They propose that the complex of a β-lactamase and a cephalosporin prevents binding to penicillin-binding proteins, thereby leading to antibiotic resistance.[30,31] That the binding of a drug rather than its hydrolysis can be a major factor in the development of resistance is still debated.[32]

It is important to remember that cephalosporins do not have reliable activity or effectiveness against penicillin-resistant *Streptococcus pneumoniae*, methicillin-resistant *S. aureus*, methicillin-resistant *Staphylococcus epidermidis, Enterococcus faecalis, Listeria monocytogenes, Legionella pneumophila, Legionella micdadei, Clostridium difficile, Xanthomonas maltophila, Pseudomonas putida, Campylobacter jejuni*, and, of course, *Candida albicans*.

PHARMACOLOGY

The pharmacologic features of selected cephalosporins are shown in Table 2.[33–48] Six of the agents may be absorbed orally and include the first-generation agents cephradine, cephalexin, and cefadroxil, the second-generation agents cefaclor and cefuroxime axetil, and the third-generation agent cefixime. The remaining drugs must be given parenterally. Cephalothin and cephapirin are painful when given intramuscularly and are therefore restricted to intravenous use. The rest of the agents may be administered intramuscularly and intravenously.

Peak serum levels for most of these agents are similar for a given dose and route of administration. Serum levels about 100 μg/ml can be expected for parenteral doses of 2 g.

Several cephalosporins penetrate into cerebrospinal fluid in sufficient amounts to be useful for treating meningitis. These include cefuroxime, moxalactam, cefotaxime, ceftriaxone, and ceftazidime.

Cephalosporins are found in high concentrations across the placenta and in synovial[49] and pericardial fluid. Penetration into the aqueous humor of the eye after systemic administration is relatively good for third-generation cephalosporins, but vitreous penetration is poor. There is some evidence that therapeutic levels for eye infections due to gram-positive and certain gram-negative organisms can be achieved after systemic administration. Bile levels are usually high, with those after cefoperazone administration being the highest.

Most cephalosporins are excreted primarily via the kidneys. Probenecid slows their renal excretion and may be used to increase serum levels. These agents require dosage adjustments in patients with renal failure. Two cephalosporins with different means of elimination are cefoperazone and ceftriaxone, which are eliminated primarily in the liver. Neither of these agents requires dosage adjustments in renal failure.

Agents with the acetyl group at the R2 position, including cephalothin, cephapirin, and cefotaxime (Figs. 4 and 5) undergo in vivo metabolism to the desacetyl forms, which have less biologic activity than the parent compounds.

ADVERSE REACTIONS

The cephalosporins are relatively safe drugs. Thrombophlebitis occurs with intravenous administration of all the cephalosporins. There are no conclusive data indicating significant differences.[50,51]

Hypersensitivity reactions related to the cephalosporins are the most common systemic side effects.[52] Unlike the penicillins, where metabolites of the bicyclic core structure are the major allergenic determinents, the acyl side chains of the cephalosporins appear to be important determinants as well.[53–56]

Immediate reactions of anaphylaxis, bronchospasm, and urticaria have been reported. More commonly, patients develop maculopapular rash, usually after several days of therapy. These patients may or may not have fever and eosinophilia. Fever and lymphadenopathy have been associated with cephalosporin administration without other manifestations of allergic phenomena.[57]

The specific haptens involved in producing allergic responses to cephalosporins are unknown. It is therefore difficult to assess the degree of cross-reactivity of cephalosporins with each other. Limited evidence suggests that cross-reactivity is less than that noted with the penicillins.[58] There is no data to suggest that immune-mediated allergic reactions are more common with one cephalosporin versus any other.

Of major clinical importance is the incidence of cross-reacting allergic responses occurring in penicillin-allergic patients who

TABLE 2. Pharmacologic Properties of the Cephalosporins

Generic Name	*Adult Dose for Serious Infection*[a]	*Peak Serum Concentration*[b] *(μg/ml)*	*Half-Life (hr)*	*Cerebrospinal Fluid Concentration (μg/ml)*	*Route of Excretion*
First generation					
Cefazolin	1g q8h	80 (1)	1.5	NA	Renal
Cephalothin	1g q4h	30 (1)	0.6	NA	Renal
Cefadroxil	0.5g q12h PO	16 (1)	1.2	NA	Renal
Cephalexin	0.5–1g q6h PO	18 (1)	0.75	NA	Renal
Cephradine	0.5g q6h PO	(18) (1)	0.7	NA	Renal
Second generation					
Cefamandole	1g 4q–6h	150 (2)	0.8	NA	Renal
Cefonicid	1–2g q24h	260 (2)	4.5	NA	Renal
Cefotetan	2–3g q12h	230 (2)	3.5	NA	Renal
Cefoxitin	2g q6–8h	150 (2)	0.8	NA	Renal
Cefuroxime	1.5g q8h	100 (1.5)	1.3	7	Renal
Cefaclor	0.25–0.5g q8h PO	13 (0.5)	0.8	NA	Renal
Cefuroxime axetil	0.25–0.5g q12h PO	8–9 (0.5)	1.3	NA	Renal
Third generation					
Cefixime	0.4g q24h PO	3.9 (0.4)	3.0	Data not available	Renal (15–20%); other?
Cefotaxime	2g q6–8h	130 (2)	1.0	44	Renal
Ceftizoxime	2g q8–12h	130 (2)	1.7	29	Renal
Ceftriaxone	1–2g q12h	250 (2)	8.0	10	Renal (50%); hepatic (40%)
Moxalactam	1–2g q8h	200 (2)	2.2	65	Renal
Third-generation cephlasporins with anti-Pseudomonas activity					
Cefoperazone	2g q8–12	250 (2)	2.0	8	Hepatic (70%); renal (25%)
Cefpiramide[c]	1–4g q12–24h	166 (1)	4.4	Data not available	Biliary (80%); renal (20%)
Cefpirome[c]	1–2g q12h	100 (1)	2.0	Data not available	Renal
Ceftazidime	2g q8h	160 (2)	1.8	40	Renal

[a] All doses are parenteral unless otherwise stated.
[b] Level after noted gram amount (in parentheses) of drug is given intravenously or, where noted in column 2, orally. Peak serum concentrations reported in the literature vary, depending on the time over which drug is given and time of serum sampling. Represented values are noted.
[c] Not yet available.
Abbreviations: NA: not clinically applicable.

receive a cephalosporin. Unfortunately, definitive data on this point is lacking. Early series indicated that the incidence of allergic reactions to cephalosporins was higher in patients with a history of penicillin allergy (5–16 percent) than in patients with no history of penicillin allergy (1–2.5 percent).[59,60] Flaws in these studies make evaluation difficult. Since only 15–40 percent of patients with a history of penicillin allergy will have positive skin tests,[61,62] many patients listed as penicillin-allergic were probably not. In addition, not all reactions described as allergic were shown to be immune-mediated. Adverse drug reactions in general are three times more common in patients with a penicillin allergy even when the drugs used are immunologically dissimilar to penicillin.[63] The increased incidence of reactions to cephalosporins in these studies may therefore have been due in part to this predisposition, rather than true allergic cross-reactivity.[64]

Cephalosporins have been given to patients in whom penicillin allergy was documented with skin testing including penicilloyl polylysine.[64–66] While the numbers of patients have been small, only one of ninety-nine (1 percent) developed a clinically significant reaction. Since IgE antibodies diminish over time, fewer allergic reactions to cephalosporins may occur in patients whose allergic reactions to penicillin were in the distant past.[67] Until the specific haptens involved in cephalosporin allergy have been identified and until testing for cephalosporin allergy is standardized, all that can be said definitively is that allergic reactions to cephalosporins do occur in penicillin-allergic patients, the incidence appears to be low, and mechanisms for the accurate prediction of allergic cross-reactions are not available.

Use of cephalosporins in penicillin-allergic patients should be guided by the severity of the allergy to penicillin, the availability of effective noncephalosporin treatment regimens, and clinical judgment. In most instances, a non-β-lactam agent should be used in patients with a definite history of severe penicillin or cephalosporin allergy. If possible, a history of penicillin allergy should be documented by skin testing with penicilloyl polylysine and a minor determinant mixture (See Chapter 21). Patients having no immediate reaction to either test probably can be given a cephalosporin safely. Practices differ when one of the tests is positive. There are insufficient data to make a reliable decision. Some experts do not recommend use of a cephalosporin under these circumstances (see Chapter 21). We feel that if a patient is skin test-positive to penicillin but has no history of anaphalaxis or other significant IgE-mediated reaction to penicillin, cephalosporins may be used with caution *if* no other suitable regimen is available. Where skin test positivity to penicillin is associated with a recent history of a severe IgE-mediated response, alternative, noncephalosporin regimens should be sought.

A positive Coombs reaction appears frequently in patients receiving large doses of cephalosporin drugs. Hemolysis is not usually associated with this phenomenon, although it has been reported. Rare cases of bone marrow depression characterized by granulocytopenia have been reported.

The cephalosporins have been implicated as potentially nephrotoxic agents, although they are not nearly as toxic to the kidney as are the aminoglycosides or the polymyxins.[68] Renal tubular necrosis has been described with cephaloridine in doses greater than 4 g/day. Other cephalosporins are much less toxic and, in recommended doses, rarely produce significant renal toxicity when used by themselves. High doses of cephalothin have produced acute tubular necrosis in certain cases, and usual doses (8–12 g/day) have been nephrotoxic in patients with preexisting renal disease[69] There is fairly good evidence that the combination of cephalothin plus gentamicin or tobramycin is synergistically nephrotoxic.[70] Interstitial nephritis, identical to that occurring during therapy with semisynthetic penicillins, may result from cephalosporin therapy. This is especially marked in patients over 60 years of age. Diarrhea has been reported with cephalosporin administration and may be more frequent with cefoperazone, perhaps because of its greater biliary excretion. Alcohol intolerance (a disulfuram-like reaction) has been noted with cefamandole, moxalactam, and cefotetan.

Ceftriaxone has recently been associated with the formation of biliary sludge in the gallbladder, which may lead to signs and symptoms of cholecystitis. This phenomenon appears to be unusual and is reversible once the drug is discontinued.[71–73] Ceftriaxone competes with bilirubin for albumin binding sites,

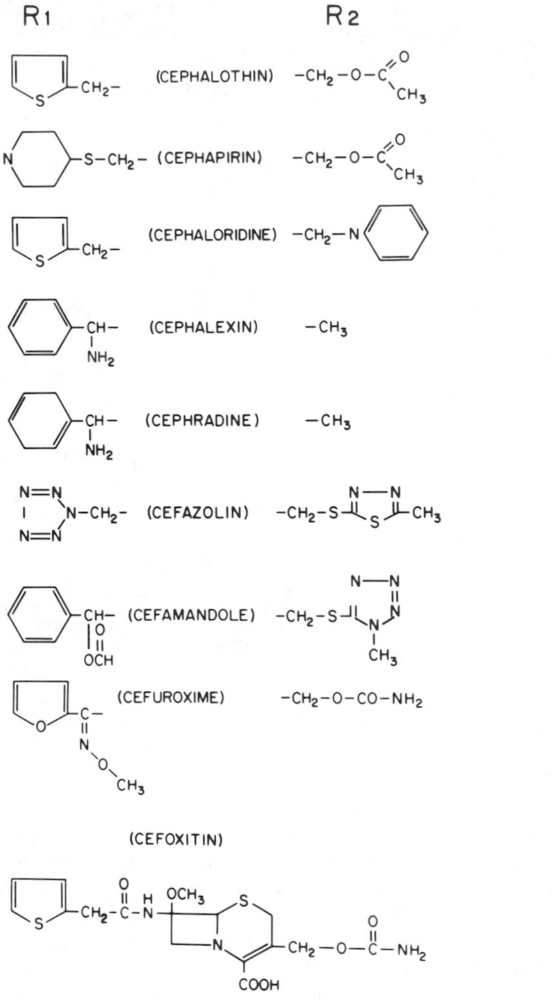

FIG. 4. Structures of selected first- and second-generation cephalosporins (see Fig. 3).

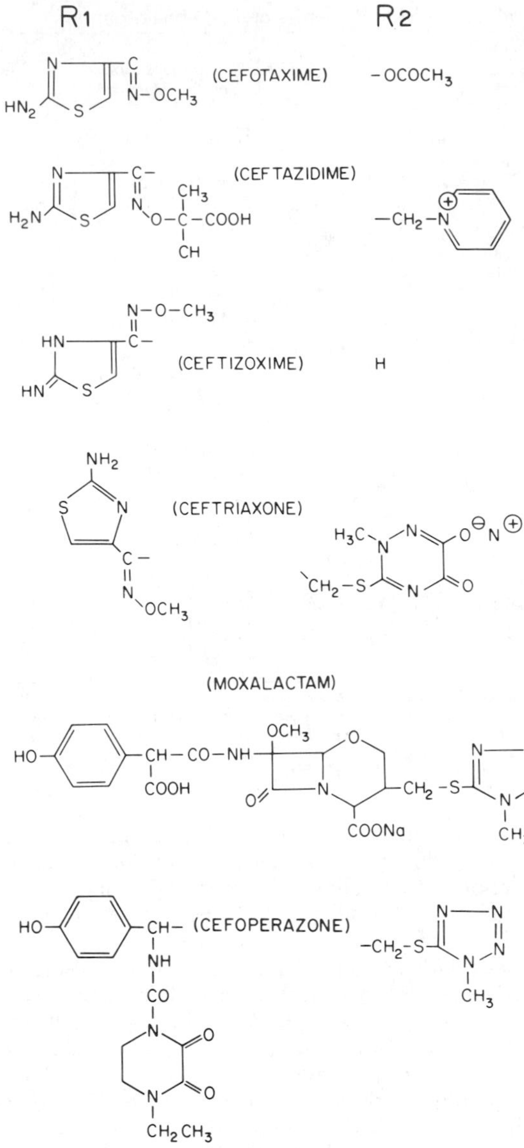

FIG. 5. Structures of selected third-generation cephalosporins (see Fig. 3).

which in neonates could theoretically be a factor in the development of bilirubin encephalopathy.[74,75] Its use in the neonate has therefore been discouraged.

Bleeding due to hypoprothrombinemia, platelet aggregation abnormalities, and thrombocytopenia have been associated with cephalosporin use.[76–78] The cause of hypoprothrombinemia is due to several factors. Inhibition of vitamin K synthesis by suppression of gut flora may occur with any of these agents.[79] The methylthiotetrazole side chain in cefamandole, cefotetan, moxalactam, and cefoperazone may inhibit the conversion of clotting factors II, VII, IX, and X to their active form and may also inhibit the formation of active vitamin K from its inactive precursor.[80–83] Use of these agents has been associated with abnormal coagulation parameters in 20–60 percent of patients.[84,85] Consequently vitamin K prophylaxis has been recommended when these agents are used in nutritionally deprived or otherwise seriously ill patients. Platelet aggregation abnormalities have been seen only with moxalactam among the cephalosporins.[86,87] This agent, more than any other of the cephalosporins, has been associated with significant bleeding[76] and for this reason has been removed from many formularies.

MODIFICATION OF DOSE WITH RENAL INSUFFICIENCY

The cephalosporins, although largely excreted by the kidney, require only moderate dose reduction in patients with renal insufficiency (see Chapter 38).

FIRST-GENERATION CEPHALOSPORINS

First-generation cephalosporins are the most active cephalosporins against gram-positive cocci, including *S. aureus* and streptococci[88] (Table 3). Two important exceptions to this are methicillin-resistant staphylococci and penicillin-resistant *S. pneumoniae*, which are not usually sensitive.[89] First-generation agents have moderate activity against a limited number of aerobic gram-negative bacilli, including *E. coli, Klebsiella pneumoniae*, and indole-negative *Proteus*.[90,91] Both parenteral and oral preparations of first-generation agents are available.

Cephalothin (Keflin) is not well absorbed orally and is available only in parenteral form. Because of pain on intramuscular injection, it is rarely administered via that route. After intravenous use, cephalothin has a large volume of distribution, indicating wide dispersal throughout body tissues and fluids. Cephalothin has a short half-life (30–40 minutes) and is actively metabolized in addition to being excreted. From 20 to 30 percent of cephalothin is excreted as the desacetyl metabolite. Unmetabolized active cephalothin does not appreciably enter the cerebrospinal fluid, and thus this drug and other first-generation

TABLE 3. In Vitro Activities of Selected Cephalosporins[a]

	S. aureus	*S. epidermidis*	*S. pyogenes*	*H. influenzae*	*E. coli*	*K. pneumoniae*	*S. marcesens*	*P. aeruginosa*	*B. fragilis*
First generation									
Cefazolin	1.0	0.8	0.1	10	5.0	6.0	>100	>100	>100
Cephalothin	1.0	0.5	0.1	10	5.0	32	>100	>100	>100
Second generation									
Cefamandole	1.0	2.0	0.06	1.0	4.0	8.0	>100	>100	>100
Cefoxitin	3.0	12.5	0.7	6.0	8.0	5.0	>100	>100	16
Cefuroxime	2.0	1.0	0.06	2.0	4.0	4.0	>100	>100	>100
Cefotetan	8.0	32	2.0	1.6	0.5	0.5	16	>100	16
Third generation									
Cefotaxime	2.0	8.0	0.03	0.03	0.25	0.25	2.0	>32	64
Ceftizoxime	3.0	2.5	0.03	0.01	0.13	0.25	2.0	>32	32
Moxalactam	8.0	32	2.0	0.1	0.25	0.25	4.0	64	16
Ceftriaxone	4.0	16	0.03	0.1	0.1	0.1	4.0	>32	>64
Third generation with good anti-*Pseudomonas* activity									
Cefoperazone	4.0	8.0	0.12	0.06	2.0	4.0	16	32	>64
Ceftazidime	16.0	32	0.25	0.1	0.5	0.5	1	4	>64
Cefpirome	1.0	2.0	0.1	0.03	0.06	0.03	0.12	16	32
Cefpiramide	8.0	8.0	0.25	0.25	32	32	>128	16	>256

[a] Minimum inhibitory concentration (μg/ml) for 90 percent of strains (MIC_{90}).
Values are approximations and are derived from Refs. 46, 88, 90–92, 94, 95, 105, 113, 117, 143, 147, 149, 150, 153, 154, 164, 165, 167.

cephalosporins should not be used for the treatment of meningitis. Since cephalothin is the cephalosporin most impervious to attack by staphylococcal β-lactamase, some authorities consider it to be the cephalosporin of choice in severe staphylococcal infections such as endocarditis.

Cefazolin (Ancef and Kefzol) has a spectrum of activity similar to that of cephalothin. However, cefazolin is more active against *E. coli* and *Klebsiella* species.[92] Cefazolin is somewhat more sensitive to staphylococcal penicillinase than is cephalothin.[93,94] Serum levels of cefazolin are higher after intramuscular and intravenous injections than are levels of cephalothin due in part to a smaller volume of distribution. The half-life is also appreciably longer, being 1.8 hours as compared with 0.5 hour for cephalothin.[95] The renal clearance of cefazolin is lower than that of cephalothin. This is probably related to the fact that cefazolin is excreted by glomerular filtration, whereas cephalothin is also excreted by the kidney tubule. Cefazolin is highly (about 80 percent) protein-bound. Cefazolin is relatively well tolerated after intramuscular or intravenous injections. It is the usually preferred first-generation cephalosporin since it can be administered less frequently.[96]

Cephradine (Anspor—oral,Velosef—oral and parenteral) is similar in structure to cephalexin, and its in vitro activity is almost identical. Cephradine is unmetabolized and after rapid oral absorption is excreted unchanged in the urine. Cephradine can be administered intramuscularly or intravenously. When administered by mouth the clinical pharmacology of cephradine is very much like that of cephalexin. Because cephradine is so well absorbed, the serum levels after an oral or intramuscular dose are nearly equivalent (about 10–18 μg/ml after 0.5 g orally or intramuscularly). The peak serum level for the oral dose is actually higher, but the area under the curve for both routes of administration is equivalent.[97]

Cephapirin (Cefadyl) is very similar to cephalothin. Like cephalothin, it is painful after intramuscular injection. Also like cephalothin, it is metabolized as the desacetyl derivative, which is about half as active as the parent compound. The half-life and excretion pattern of cephapirin are like that of cephalothin.[98]

Cefadroxil monohydrate (Duricef, Ultracef) is the parahydroxy analogue of cephalexin. Serum and urine concentrations of cefadroxil are somewhat more sustained than those noted with cephalexin. The drug may be used once or twice a day for treatment of urinary tract infections. In vitro activity is similar to that of cephalexin.[99]

Cephalexin (Keflex) is a cephalosporin for oral use that has the same antibacterial spectrum as other first-generation cephalosporins. It is less active, however, against penicillinase-producing staphylococci. Oral cephalexin therapy (0.5 g) results in peak serum levels of 16 μg/ml, which are adequate for the inhibition of many cephalosporin-sensitive gram-positive and gram-negative pathogens. The drug is unmetabolized, and more than 90 percent is excreted in the urine.[100]

Clinical Uses

The first-generation cephalosporins most commonly in use are the parenteral agents cefazolin and cephalothin and the oral agent cephalexin. Because of their activity against gram-positive cocci, they are useful alternatives to penicillin for therapy of a variety of infections due to staphylococci and nonenterococcal streptococci. The first-generation cephalosporins are the agents of choice for prophylaxis of most surgical procedures including orthopaedic and cardiovascular operations.[101–104] Because cefazolin has a longer half-life than cephalothin, it is the preferred agent in this regard. For procedures in which anaerobic infections are likely (colorectal surgery, appendectomies), agents with better anaerobic coverage such as cefoxitin or cefotetan are suggested. The first-generation agents can be used to treat a variety of infections caused by susceptible aerobic gram-negative bacilli, but the activity of these drugs against gram-negative rods is inconsistent and their empiric use is not suggested.

SECOND-GENERATION CEPHALOSPORINS

As a group, the second-generation cephalosporins are more potent than first-generation cephalosporins against *E. coli, Klebsiella* sp., and indole-negative *Proteus* (Table 3). Individual members of the second generation extend the spectrum of activity of first-generation agents to include strains of *Haemophilus influenzae, Enterobacter* sp., *Serratia* sp., indole-positive *Proteus*, anaerobes, *Neisseria meningitidis*, and *Neisseria gonorrhoeae*. None of the agents has activity against *Pseudomonas* sp.[44,105,106]

Specific Agents

Cefamandole (Mandol) is more active than the first-generation cephalosporins against certain species of gram-negative organisms. This is especially evident for *H. influenzae*,[107] *Enterobacter* sp., indole-positive *Proteus* sp., *E. coli*, and *Klebsiella* sp.[108] Its activity against β-lactamase-producing, ampicillin-resistant *H. influenzae* is inconsistent, and heavy bacterial inocula show decreased susceptibility. Most gram-positive cocci are susceptible to cefamandole.

Cefoxitin (Mefoxin) is a cefamycin produced by *Streptomyces lactamdurans*. It is highly resistant to β-lactamases produced by gram-negative rods.[109] This antibiotic is more active than cephalothin against certain gram-negative organisms, including *E. coli, Klebsiella*, indole-positive and -negative *Proteus*, and *Serratia* sp. It is less active than cefamandole against *Enterobacter* sp. and many strains of *H. influenzae*. It is also less active than both cefamandole and the older cephalosporins against gram-positive bacteria. Cefoxitin is more active than other first-, second-, and most third-generation agents against anaerobes, especially *Bacteroides fragilis*. Cefoxitin's special role seems to be for treatment of certain mixed anaerobic–aerobic infections.[110–112]

Cefuroxime (Zinacef, Kefurox) is similar to cefamandole in structure and antibacterial activity.[113] It is relatively more resistant to β-lactamases than is cefamandole, including those produced by ampicillin-resistant *H. influenzae*. Its serum half-life is longer (1.5 vs. 0.5 hours), and the drug may be given every 8 hours. Cefuroxime is the only second-generation cephalosporin with consistent penetration into cerebrospinal fluid.

Cefuroxime axetil (Ceftin) is the 1-acetoxyethyl ester of cefuroxime. Taken orally, cefuroxime axetil is hydrolyzed to cefuroxime after absorption.[114–116] Bioavailability varies between 30 and 50 percent and is increased after food ingestion. Mean peak serum levels occur 1.5–2.5 hours after a 500 mg dose. The half-life is 1.2 hours, but adequate serum levels persist long enough to allow for twice a day dosing.

Cefotetan (Cefotan) is a cephamycin that has characteristics of both second- and third-generation agents.[117,118] Its activity against gram-positive cocci and *B. fragilis* is similar to that of cefoxitin. It is less active than cefoxitin against other *Bacteroides* species.[119] Its activity against aerobic gram-negative bacilli is superior to that of cefoxitin and most other second-generation agents. Its half-life is 3.3 hours, and it may be used with twice daily dosing.

Cefaclor (Ceclor) is a cephalosporin for oral administration. The serum levels after an oral dose are about 50 percent of those achieved after equivalent oral doses of cephalexin. However, cefaclor is more active against gram-negative bacilli. This may be especially important for *H. influenzae, E. coli*, and *Proteus mirabilis*, although some β-lactamase-producing strains of *H. influenzae* may be resistant.[120]

Ceforanide (Precef) is similar in structure and antimicrobial activity to cefamandole. However, it is less active against strains of *H. influenzae*. Peak plasma concentrations after 1 g given intramuscularly are approximately 65 μg/ml. Ninety percent of a dose is excreted unchanged in the urine, and the half-life is approximately 3 hours. The drug has been effective when administered every 12 hours.[121]

Cefonicid (Monicid) has similar in vitro activity to cefamandole. The plasma half-life of the drug is about 4½ hours, and one dose a day has been effective for certain infections caused by susceptible organisms.[122]

Clinical Uses

Cefuroxime, because of its activity against *S. pneumoniae, S. aureus*, and *H. influenzae*, including ampicillin-resistant strains, has been used widely as therapy for community-acquired pneumonia when a specific pathogen is not suggested by sputum examination.[123,124] Cefamandole's relative lack of efficacy against some strains of ampicillin-resistant *H. influenzae* makes it a less attractive alternative in this situation.[125] Cefuroxime has been used to treat meningitis caused by *H. influenzae, S. pneumoniae*, and *N. meningitidis*, but since third-generation agents have greater activity and better penetration into the cerebrospinal fluid, these agents are usually preferred.[126–128]

Cefuroxime axetil has been used to treat a variety of mild-to-moderate infections including skin and soft tissue infections, urinary tract infections, pneumonia, bronchitis, otitis media, and uncomplicated gonococcal urethritis.[129,130] In most but not all of these cases, cefuroxime has proved at least as effective as other oral agents including cefaclor and amoxicillin with and without clavulanic acid. Failure to cure cases of purulent bronchitis and recurrent urinary tract infections has been reported, and its utility in more serious infections remains to be proved.[131,132]

Cefoxitin has been used successfully to treat mixed aerobic–anaerobic infections. It has often been used with an aminoglycoside to maximize coverage of aerobic gram-negative bacilli. Intra-abdominal infections, pelvic infections, nosocomial aspiration pneumonia, and foot infections in the diabetic have all been successfully treated.[133,134] Because of its anaerobic activity cefoxitin has been suggested as the agent of choice for prophylaxis of colorectal surgery, appendectomies, and procedures in which anaerobic infections are likely.[135] Cefoxitin has been used as effective therapy for gonorrhea including disease caused by penicillin-resistant strains.[136,137] Cefotetan has been suggested as a replacement for cefoxitin because of its similar spectrum of activity against anaerobes and its longer half-life. It has proven to be as effective as cefoxitin for prophylaxis in pelvic and abdominal surgery and is as effective as either cefoxitin or moxalactam for therapy of obstetric and gynecologic infections and intra-abdominal infections.[138–141]

THIRD-GENERATION CEPHALOSPORINS

The third-generation cephalosporins have the broadest spectrum and most potent activity of all cephalosporins against gram-negative bacilli[44,46] (Table 3). They are resistant to many of the β-lactamases produced by gram-negative bacteria and retain their activity against organisms resistant to first- and second-generation agents, aminoglycosides, and extended spectrum penicillins. Their activity against gram-positive cocci adds nothing to that of first- and second-generation agents. Activity against anaerobes is agent-dependent but is usually no better than that provided by cefoxitin. The third-generation agents may be divided into two groups, based on their activity against *P. aeruginosa*. Cefotaxime, ceftizoxime, ceftriaxone, moxalactam, and the oral agent cefixime have poor anti-*Pseudomonas* activity. (Moxalactam is an oxa-β-lactam and not a true cephalosporin since it has an oxygen molecule instead of a sulphur molecule at the C_1 position of the dihydrothiazine ring [see Fig. 5]. It is usually placed in this group due to similar antimicrobial activity and pharmacologic properties.) Ceftazidime, cefoperazone, and the investigational agents cefpirome and cefpiramide are third-generation agents with activity against *P. aeruginosa*.

Specific Agents

Cefotaxime (Claforan) was the first of the third-generation cephalosporins to become available in the United States and is the agent with which there has been the greatest experience. Cefotaxime is highly resistant to bacterial β-lactamases and has good activity against gram-positive organisms, with the exception of enterococci and *Listeria monocytogenes*, and to gram-negative aerobic organisms, with the exception of all strains of *Pseudomonas*.[142,143] Ninety to one hundred percent of strains of *E. coli, Klebsiella*, indole-positive and -negative *Proteus, H. influenzae, N. meningitidis*, and *N. gonorrhoeae* are inhibited. *Enterobacter cloacae* and strains of *Acinetobacter* show moderate susceptibility to the drug. The majority of strains of *P. aeruginosa* are resistant. While peptococci and peptostreptococci are usually susceptible to cefotaxime, many strains of anaerobes are resistant. Cefotaxime penetrates reliably into cerebrospinal fluid.[144]

Moxalactam (Moxam) has a unique structure (designated

oxa-β-lactam), which is created by the substitution of an oxygen for the sulfur atom in the six-membered ring of the cephem nucleus (see Fig. 5). Moxalactam has the broad antimicrobial activity characteristic of the third-generation cephalosporins.[145] In comparison with cefotaxime, it is less active against gram-positive organisms including streptococci and staphylococci. It is somewhat less active against *H. influenzae* and has very similar activity against most of the Enterobacteraceae. It is slightly more active against *Pseudomonas* and appreciably more active against *B. fragilis* than is cefotaxime. Clinically significant bleeding has been reported with moxalactam administration and for this reason we no longer recommend it for clinical use.[146]

Ceftizoxime (Cefizox) has in vitro activity similar to that of cefotaxime, with more activity against strains of *Serratia marcescens* and *Bacteroides*.[147] Like cefotaxime, ceftizoxime penetrates well into the cerebrospinal fluid.[148] Its half-life is slightly longer than that of cefotaxime, allowing it to be dosed at 8 hour intervals.

Ceftriaxone (Rocephin) has a spectrum of activity that mirrors that of cefotaxime and ceftizoxime.[149,150] It is the most potent agent against both *N. meningitidis* and *N. gonorrhoeae*, with an MIC_{90} of 0.025 μg/liter. Like cefotaxime and ceftizoxime, reliable cerebrospinal fluid levels can be attained. The truly outstanding feature of ceftriaxone is its half-life of 8 hours, significantly longer than any other cephalosporin. This has allowed serious infections to be treated with once a day, or twice a day dosing.

Cefixime (Suprax) is the first oral third-generation cephalosporin. Its spectrum of activity against aerobic gram-negative rods is similar to that of ceftizoxime and superior to those of cephalexin, cefaclor, and cefuraxime axetil—the other oral cephalosporins.[151,152] Its activity against nonenterococcal streptococci is similar to that of other oral cephalosporins, but its activity against *S. aureus* is inferior. Clinical experience is limited.

Specific Agents with Anti-Pseudomonas Activity

Cefoperazone (Cefobid) is less active than cefotaxime against gram-positive cocci and the majority of aerobic gram-negative rods.[46,153–156] Cefoperazone does, however, have activity against *P. aeruginosa*, with greater than 50 percent of strains susceptible to ≤16 μg/ml. Activity against anaerobes is not different from that of cefotaxime and is inferior to that of cefoxitin. Cefoperazone's half-life of 2 hours allows for twice a day dosing for selected situations, although severe infections should be treated with shorter dosing intervals. Serum levels are among the highest for all cephalosporins, and its biliary levels are greater than any other currently available third-generation agent.[157] Penetration into the cerebrospinal fluid is poor and mitigates against its use in meningitis. As with other agents containing a methylthiotetrazole side chain at the C_3 position, cefoperazone causes a disulfiram-like reaction in patients ingesting alcohol. Bleeding abnormalities due to hypoprothrombinemia have been reported,[158–161] and prophylactic vitamin K has been recommended when the drug is used in seriously ill or malnourished patients.

Ceftazidime (Fortaz, Taxidime, Tazicef) is the most active third-generation cephalosporin against *P. aeruginosa*.[46,162] Approximately 90 percent of strains will be inhibited by 4 μg/ml. Ceftazidime's activity against other gram-negative bacilli is comparable to that of cefotaxime. Ceftazidime is the least active third-generation agent against *S. aureus* and has little activity against anaerobes. Peak serum levels are comparable to that of other third-generation agents. Penetration into cerebrospinal fluid is adequate to treat meningitis.[163]

Cefpiramide is a new third-generation agent with activity against *P. aeruginosa* that is comparable to that of cefoperazone.[164,165] In general, it is less active than many of the other third-generation agents against other gram-negative organisms. This agent has consistent activity against gram-positive cocci and is unique in that it has activity against *Enterococcus* sp.

Cefpirome is a new cephalosporin with an extremely wide spectrum of activity.[166–168] Its activity against gram-positive cocci is similar to that of first- and second-generation agents but includes *Enterococcus* sp. The activity of cefpirome against most anaerobes and aerobic gram-negative bacteria is comparable to that of cefotaxime and is better than cefotaxime for strains of *Enterobacter, Acinetobacter*, and *Serratia*. It possesses activity against *Pseudomonas* comparable to that of cefoperazone but is inferior to that of ceftazidime.

Clinical Uses

The major use of the third-generation cephalosporins is in the therapy of serious aerobic gram-negative infections. The third-generation agents should not be used for most community-acquired infections. Multiply-resistant organisms are unusual in this circumstance, and agents with a narrower spectrum of activity and equal efficacy are available.

Cefotaxime, ceftriaxone, and ceftazidime have been successfully used to treat meningitis caused by *H. influenzae, S. pneumoniae*, and *N. meningitidis*. In children, these drugs appear to be as effective as the standard combination regimens of ampicillin and chloramphenicol or ampicillin and gentamicin.[144,169–176] Delayed sterilization of cerebrospinal fluid has been noted in small numbers of patients treated with ceftriaxone and, at the very least, suggests that close scrutiny of patients treated for meningitis is needed.[177] Ceftizoxime has also proved effective for meningitis, although experience with this drug remains limited.[148]

Third-generation cephalosporins, especially cefotaxime and ceftazidime, are the drugs of choice for the therapy of meningitis in adults caused by aerobic gram-negative bacilli.[144,169,170,172] Success rates of 80–90 percent have been reported with disease caused by *E. coli, Klebsiella pneumoniae*, and *Serratia* sp. Lower response rates have been noted with *Enterobacter* and *Salmonella*. This is in marked contrast to the 60–80 percent mortality noted in cases treated before the development of these agents.[178] Because of its excellent penetration into the cerebrospinal fluid and excellent activity against *Pseudomonas*, ceftazidime has been used to treat *P. aeruginosa* meningitis with responses rates of approximately 80 percent.[172,179]

The third-generation agents are extremely useful for therapy of nocosomial infections, especially those caused by multiply-resistant gram-negative organisms, where aminoglycosides and extended spectrum penicillins may be of limited use. Pneumonias, bacteremias, urinary tract infections, intra-abdominal infections, and skin and soft tissues have all been treated with success rates of over 80–90 percent.[180–192] It remains unclear whether these agents should be used in conjunction with other β-lactam antibiotics or aminoglycosides for maximum efficacy. There is no convincing data to indicate clinical superiority of any specific third-generation agent in the therapy of a given disease.

Because of its extended half-life ceftriaxone may be used to treat a variety of severe infections with once daily or twice daily dosing; it has been used successfully and with demonstrated cost savings for outpatient therapy of skin and soft-tissue infections and urinary tract infections.[193–195] Because of its potent activity against penicillin-sensitive and -resistant strains of *N. gonorrhoeae*, ceftriaxone has become the agent of choice for treating uncomplicated urethral, anorectal, and pharyngeal gonorrhoeae.[196,197] Limited data suggest that ceftriaxone may be effective in eradicating oropharyngeal carriage of *N. meningitidis*.[198] Ceftriaxone is effective therapy for Lyme disease.

Cefoperazone and ceftazadime have been used in patients when *P. aeruginosa* infections are suspected. When used as monotherapy in neutropenic patients, cefoperazone has led to resonse rates lower than those usually seen with antibiotic combinations.[199,200] Combination regimens of cefoperazone plus mezlocillin and cefoperazone plus aminoglycoside have proved as efficacious as other combination regimens.[201,202] Ceftazadime has been used as monotherapy or as modified monotherapy (used with an aminoglycoside for 3 days and then continued as monotherapy thereafter) in patients with fever and neutropenia.[203,204] The findings suggest that ceftazidime alone is adequate for the majority of infections, but its use with an aminoglycoside may be more effective in documented gram-negative rod bacteremia.

REFERENCES

1. Abraham EP, Loder PB. Cephalosporin C. In: Flynn EH, ed. Cephalosporins and Penicillins. New York: Academic Press; 1972:2.
2. Huber FM, Chauvette RR, Jackson BG. Preparative methods for 7-aminocephalosporanic acid and 6-aminopenicillanic acid. In: Flynn EH, ed. Cephalosporins and Penicillins. New York: Academic Press; 1972:27.
3. Neu HC. Structure-activity relations of new beta-lactam compounds and in vitro activity against common bacteria. Rev Infect Dis. 1983;5(Suppl):S319–37.
4. Neu HC. The new beta-lactamase-stable cephalosporins. Ann Intern Med. 1982;97:408–17.
5. Strominger JL. How penicillin kills bacteria: a short history. In: Schlessinger D, ed. Microbiology—1977. Washington, DC: ASM Publications; 1977:177.
6. Tomasz A, Albino A, Zanatle E. Multiple antibiotic resistance in a bacterium with suppressed autolytic system. Nature. 1970;227:138–40.
7. Tomasz A. The mechanism of the irreversible antimicrobial effects of penicillins: how the beta-lactam antibiotics kill and lyse bacteria. Annu Rev Microbiol. 1979;33:113–37.
8. Blumberg PM, Strominger JL. Interaction of penicillin with the bacterial cell: penicillin-binding proteins and penicillin-sensitive enzymes. Bacteriol Rev. 1974;38:291–335.
9. Spratt BG. Proerties of the penicillin-binding proteins of *Escherichia coli* K 12. Eur J Biochem. 1977;72:341–52.
10. Neu HC. Penicillin-binding proteins and role of amdinocillin in causing bacterial cell death. Am J Med. 1983;75:(Suppl 2A):9–20.
11. Matsuhashi S, Kamiryo T, Blumberg PM, et al. Mechanism of action and development of resistance to a new amidino penicillin. J Bacteriol. 1974;117:578–87.
12. Waxman DJ, Strominger JL. Penicillin-binding proteins and the mechanism of action of β-lactam antibiotics. Annu Rev Biochem. 1983;52:825–69.
13. Tomasz A. Penicillin-binding proteins and the antibacterial effectiveness of β-lactam antibiotics. Rev Infect Dis. 1986;8(Suppl 3):S260–78.
14. Tomasz A, Waks S. Enzyme replacement in a bacterium: phenotypic correction by the experimental introduction of the wild type enzyme into a live enzyme defective mutant pneumococcus. Biochem Biophys Res Commun. 1975;65:1311–9.
15. Tomasz A, Holtje SV. Murein hydrolases and the lytic and killing action of penicillin. In: Schlessinger D, ed. Microbiology—1977. Washington, DC: American Society for Microbiology; 1977:209–15.
16. Tomasz A. Penicillin-binding proteins in bacteria. Ann Intern Med. 1982;96:502–4.
17. Nikaido H, Nakae T. The outer membrane of gram-negative bacteria. Adv Microb Physiol. 1979;20:163–250.
18. Nikaido H, Rosenberg EY, Foulds J. Porin channels in *Escherichia coli*: studies with β-lactams in intact cells. J Bacteriol. 1983;153:232–40.
19. Sawai T, Yamaguchi A, Hiruma R. Effect of interaction between outer membrane permeability and β-lactamase production on resistance to β-lactam agents in gram-negative bacteria. Rev Infect Dis. 1988;10:761–4.
20. Hartman BJ, Tomasz A. Low affinity penicillin binding protein associated with β-lactam resistance in *Staphylococcus aureus*. J Bacteriol. 1984;158:513–6.
21. Utsui Y, Yokota T. Role of an altered penicillin-binding protein in methicillin and cephem-resistant *Staphylococcus aureus*. Antimicrob Agents Chemother. 1985;28:397–403.
22. Richmond MH, Sykes RB. The beta-lactamases of gram-negative bacteria and their possible physiological role. Adv Microb Physiol. 1973;9:31–88.
23. Sykes RM, Matthew M. The β-lactamases of gram-negative bacteria and their role in resistance to β-lactam antibiotics. J Antimicrob Chemother. 1976;2:115–57.
24. Novick RP, Richmond MH. Nature and interactions of the genetic elements governing penicillinase synthesis in *Staphylococcus aureus*. J Bacteriol. 1965;90:467–80.
25. Dyke KGH. β-lactamases of *Staphylococcus aureus*. In: Hamilton-Miller JMT, Smith JT, eds. Beta-Lactamases. New York: Academic Press; 1979:291–310.
26. Farrar WE Jr, O'Dell NM. Comparative beta-lactamase resistance and antistaphylococcal activities of parenterally and orally administered cephalosporins. J Infect Dis. 1978;137:490–3.
27. Sykes RB, Bush K. Interaction of new cephalosporins with beta-lactamases and beta lactamase-producing gram-negative bacilli. Rev Infect Dis. 1983;5(Suppl 5):S356–67.
28. Farrar WE, Krause JM. Relationship between beta-lactamase activity and resistance of *Enterobacter* to cephalothin. Infect Immun. 1970;2;610–6.
29. Sanders CC, Sanders WE. Emergence of resistance during therapy with the newer beta-lactam antibiotics: role inducible beta-lactamases and implications for the future. Rev Infect Dis. 1983;5:639–48.
30. Sanders CC. Inducible β-lactamases and non-hydrolytic resistance mechanisms. J Antimicrob Chemother. 1984;13:1–3.
31. Sanders CC, Sanders WE Jr. Trapping and hydrolysis are not mutually exclusive mechanisms for β-lactamase-mediated resistance (Letter). J Antimicrob Chemother. 1986;17:121–2.
32. Charnas RL, Then RL. Mechanism of inhibition of chromosomal β-lactamases by third-generation cephalosporins. Rev Infect Dis. 1988;10:752–60.
33. Brumfitt W, Kosmidis J, Hamilton-Miller JMT, et al. Cefoxitin and cephalothin: antimicrobial activity, human pharmacokinetics, and toxicology. Antimicrob Agents Chemother. 1974;6:290–9.
34. Tauber MG, Hackbarth CJ, Scott KG, et al. New cephalosporins cefotaxime, cefpirizole, BMY 289142, and HR 810 in experimental pneumococcal meningitis in rabbits. Antimicrob Agents Chemother. 1985;27:340–2.
35. Bodian M, Molerczyk V, Collins JD, et al. Safety, tolerance and pharmacokinetics of 2.0 g of cefpirome (HR810) after single and multiple dosing. Chemotheray 1988;34:367–73.
36. Nakagawa K, Koyama M, Matsui H, et al. Pharmacokinetics of cefpiramide (SM-1652) in humans. Antimicrob Agents Chemother. 1984;25:221–5.
37. Barza M, Srikumaran M, Berger S, et al. Comparative pharmacokinetics of cefamandole, cephapirin and cephalothin in healthy subjects and effect of repeated dosing. Antimicrob Agents Chemother. 1976;10:421–5.
38. Pitkin D, Dubb J, Altor P, et al. Kinetics and renal handling of cefonicid. Clin Pharmacol Ther. 1981;30:587–93.
39. Malerczyk V, Maab L, Verho M, et al. Single and multiple dose pharmacokinetics of intravenous cefpirome (HR810), a novel cephalosporin derivative. Infection 1987;15:211–4.
40. Maab L, Malerczyk V, Verho M. Pharmacokinetics of cefpirome (HR810), a new cephalosporin deriative administered intramuscularly and intravenously to healthy volunteers. Infection. 1987;15:207–10.
41. Yates RA, Adam HK, Donnelly RJ, et al. Pharmacokinetics and tolerance of single intravenous doses of cefotetan disodium in male Caucasian volunteers. J Antimicrob Chemother. 1983;11(Suppl A):185–91.
42. Sommers DK, Van Wyk M, Williams PEO et al. Pharmacokinetics and tolerance of cefuroxime axetil in volunteers during repeated dosing. Antimicrob Agents Chemother. 1987;25:374–7.
43. Jones RN, Antimicrobial activity, spectrum and pharmacokinetics of old and new orally administered cephems. Antimicrob Newsletter. 1988;5:1–7.
44. Thompson RL, Wright AJ. Cephalosporin antibiotics. Mayo Clin Proc. 1983;58:79–87.
45. Fried JS, Hinthrom DR. The cephalosporins. DM. 1985;31:1–60.
46. Donowitz GR, Mandell GL. Beta-lactam antibiotics. N Engl J Med. 1988;318(2 Pt 2):490–500.
47. Fong IW, Ralph ED, Engelking FR, et al. Clinical pharmacology of cefamandole as compared with cephalothin. Antimicrob Agents Chemother. 1976;9:65–9.
48. Neu HC. Comparison of the pharmacokinetics of cefamandole and other cephalosporin compounds. J Infect Dis. 1978;137(Suppl):S80–7.
49. Nelson JD. Antibiotic concentration in spectic joint effusion. N Engl J Med. 1971;284:349.
50. Berger S, Ernest E, Barza M. Comparative incidence of phlebitis due to buffered cephalothin, cephapirin and cefamandole. Antimicrob Agents Chemother. 1976;9:575–9.
51. Carrizosa J, Levison ME, Kaye D. Double-blind controlled comparison of phlebitis produced by cephapirin and cephalothin. Antimicrob Agents Chemother. 1973;3:306–7.
52. Petz LD. Immunologic cross-reactivity between penicillins and cephalosporins: a review. J Infect Dis. 1978;137(Suppl):S74–9.
53. Petersen BH, Graham J. Immunologic cross-reactivity of cephalosporin and penicillin. J Lab Clin Med. 1974;833:860–70.
54. Iwata M, Tokiwa H, Matuhasi T. Detection and characterization of polymers in cephalothin by passive cutaneous anaphylaxis in mice. Int Arch Allergy Appl Immunol. 1983;70:132–7.
55. Batchelor FR, Dewdney JM, Weston RD, et al. The immunogenicity of cephalosporin derivatives and their cross-reaction with penicillin. Immunology 1966;10:21–33.
56. Hamilton-Miller JMT, Abraham EP. Specificities of haemagglutinating antibodies evolved by members of the cephalosporin C family and benzyl penicillin. Biochem J. 1971;123:183–90.
57. Sanders WE, Johnson JE, Taggart JG. Adverse reactions to cephalothin and cephapirin. N Engl J Med. 1974;290:424.
58. Scholond JF, Tennenbaum JL, Cerilliu GJ. Anaphylaxis to cephalothin in a patient allergic to penicillin. JAMA. 1968;206:130–2.
59. Thoburn R, Johnson JE, Cliff LE. Studies on the epidemiology of adverse drug reactions. JAMA. 1966;198:345–8.
60. Petz LD. Immunologic reactions of humans to cephalosporins. Postgrad Med J. 1971; Feb[Suppl]64–9.
61. Sullivan TJ, Wedner HJ, Shatz GS, et al. Skin testing to detect penicillin allergy. J Allergy Clin Immunol. 1981;68:171–80.
62. Sogn DD. Prevention of allergic reactions to penicillin. J Allergy Clin Immunol. 1986;78:1051–2.
63. Smith JW, Johnson JE, Cliff LE. Studies on the epidemiology of adverse

drug reactions. II. An evaluation of penicillin allergy. N Engl J Med. 1966;274:998–1002.
64. Saxon A, Beall GN, Rohn AS, et al. Immediate hypersensitivity reaction to beta-lactam antibiotics. Ann Intern Med. 1987;107:204–15.
65. Solley GO, Cleich GJ, Van Dellen RG. Penicillin allergy-clinical experience with a battery of skin-test reagents. J Allergy Clin Immunol. 1982;69:238–44.
66. Saxon A. Immediate hypersensitivity reactions to beta-lactam antibiotics. Rev Infect Dis. 1983;5:S368–78.
67. Finke SR, Grieco MH, Connel JT, et al. Results of comparative skin tests with penicilloyl-polylysine and penicillin in patients with penicillin allergy. Am J Med. 1965;38:71–82.
68. Barza M. The nephrotoxicity of cephalosporins: an overview. J Infect Dis. 1978;137(Suppl):S60–S73.
69. Pasternack DP, Stephen BG. Reversible nephrotoxicity associated with cephalothin therapy. Arch Intern Med. 1975;135:599–602.
70. Wade JC, Petty BG, Conrad G, et al. Cephalothin plus an aminoglycside is more nephrotoxic than methicillin plus an aminoglycoside. Lancet. 1978;2:604–6.
71. Jacobs RF. Ceftriaxone-associated cholecystitis. Pediatr Infect Dis J. 1988;7:434–6.
72. Schaad UB, Tschappeler H, Lentze MJ. Transient formation of precipitations in the gallbladder associated with ceftriaxone therapy. Pediatr Infect Dis J. 1986;5:708–10.
73. Schaad UB, Gianella-Borradori A, Sutter S. Ceftriaxone versus cefuroxime for bacterial meningitis in infants and children. 27th Interscience Conference on Antimicrobial Agents and Chemotherapy. 1987;#789:234.
74. Finke S, Karp W, Robertson A. Ceftriaxone effect in bilirubin-albumin binding. Pediatrics 1987;80:873–5.
75. Gulian JM, Dalmasso C, Pontier F, et al. Displacement effect of ceftriaxone on bilirubin bound to human serum albumin. Chemotherapy 1986;32:399–403.
76. Sattler FR, Weitekamp MR, Ballard JO. Potential for bleeding with the new beta-lactam antibiotics. Ann Intern Med. 1986;105:924–31.
77. Nichols RL, Wikler MA, McDevitt JT, et al. Coagulopathy associated with extended-spectrum cephalosporins in patients with serious infections. Antimicrob Agents Chemother. 1987;31:231–5.
78. Bank NU, Kammer RB. Hematologic complications associated with betalactam antibiotics. Rev Infect Dis. 1983;5(Suppl 2):S380–93.
79. Conly JM, Ramotar K, Chubb H, et al. Hypoprothrombinemia in febrile, neutropenic patients with cancer: association with antimicrobial suppression of intestinal microflora. J Infect Dis. 1984;150:202–12.
80. Lipsky JJ, Lewis JC, Novick WJ Jr. Production of hypoprothrombinemia by moxalactam and 1-methyl-5-thiotetrazole in rats. Antimicrob Agents Chemother. 1984;25:380–1.
81. Bechtold H, Andrassy K, Jahnchen E, et al. Evidence for impaired hepatic vitamin K_1 metabolism in patients treated with N-methyl-thiotetrazole cephalosporins. Thromb Haemost. 1984;51:358–61.
82. Barza M, Furie B, Brown AE, et al. Defects in vitamin K-dependent carboxylation associated with moxalactam treatment. J Infect Dis. 1986;153:1166–9.
83. Agnelli G, Del Favero A, Parise P, et al. Cephalosporin-induced hypoprothrombinemia: is the N-methylthiotetrazole side chain the culprit? Antimicrob Agents Chemother. 1986;29:1108–9.
84. Sattler FR, Colao DJ, Caputo GM, et al. Cefoperazone for empiric therapy in patients with impaired renal function. Am J Med. 1986;81:229–36.
85. Baxter JG, Marble DA, Whitfield LR, et al. Clinical risk factors for prolonged PT/PTT in abdominal sepsis patients treated with moxalactam or tobramycin plus clindamycin. Ann Surg. 1985;201:96–102.
86. Meyers BR. Comparative toxicities of third-generation cephalosporins. Am J Med. 1985;79(Suppl 2A):96–103.
87. Weitekamp MR, Caputo GM, Al-Mondhiry HA, et al. The effect of latamoxef, cefotaxime, and cefoperazone on platelet function and coagulation in normal volunteers. J Antimicrob Chemother. 1985;16:95–101.
88. Moellering RC Jr, Swartz MN. The newer cephalosporins. N Engl J Med. 1976;294:24–8.
89. Hartman B, Tomasz A. Altered penicillin-binding proteins in methicillin-resistant strains of *Staphylococcus aureus*. Antimicrob Agents Chemother. 1981;19:726–35.
90. Chang TW, Weinstein L. In vitro biological activity of cephalothin. J Bacteriol. 1963;85:1022.
91. Klein JO, Eickhoff TC, Tilles JG, et al. Cephalothin: activity in vitro, absorption and excretion in normal subjects and clinical observations in 40 patients. Am J Med Sci. 1964;248:640.
92. Sabath LD, Wilcox C, Garner C, et al. In vitro activity of cefazolin against recent clinical bacterial isolates. J Infect Dis. 1973;128(Suppl):S320–6.
93. Regamey C, Libke RD, Engelking ER, et al. Inactivation of cefazolin, cephaloridine, and cephalothin by methicillin-sensitive and methicillin-resistant strains of *Staphylococcus aureus*. J Infect Dis. 1975;131:291–4.
94. Fong IW, Engelking ER, Kirby WMM. Relative inactivation by *Staphylococcus aureus* of eight cephalosporin antibiotics. Antimicrob Agents Chemother. 1976;9:939–44.
95. Bergeron MG, Brusch JL, Barza M, et al. Bactericidal activity and pharmacology of cefazolin. Antimicrob Agents Chemother. 1973;4:396–401.
96. Quintiliani R, Nightingale CH. Cefazolin: diagnosis and treatment. Ann Intern Med. 1978;89:650–6.
97. Neiss E. Cephradine: summary of preclinical studies and clinical pharmacology. J Irish Med Assoc. 1973;66(Suppl):1–12.
98. Renzini G, Ravagnan G, Oliva B. In vitro and in vivo microbiological evaluation of cephapirin, a new antibiotic. Chemotherapy. 1975;21:289.
99. Hartstein AI, Patrick KE, Jones SR, et al. Comparison of pharmacological and antimicrobial properties of cefadroxil and cephalexin. Antimicrob Agents Chemother. 1977;12:93–7.
100. Meyers BR, Kaplan K, Weinstein L. Cephalexin microbiological effects and pharmacologic parameters in man. Clin Pharmacol Ther. 1969;10:810.
101. Cartwright PS, Pittaway DE, Jones HW III, et al. The use of prophylactic antibiotics in obstetrics and gynecology: a review. Obstet Gynecol Surv. 1984;39:537–4.
102. DiPiro JT, Bowden TA Jr, Hooks VH III. Prophylactic parenteral cephalosporins in surgery: are the newer agents better? JAMA. 1984;252:3277–9.
103. Gilbert DN. Current status of antibiotic prophylaxis in surgical patients. Bull NY Acad Med. 1984;60:340–57.
104. Norden CW. A critical review of antibiotic prophylaxis in orthopedic surgery. Rev Infect Dis. 1983;5:928–32.
105. Sanders CV, Greenberg RN, Marier RL. Cefamandole and cefoxitin. Ann Intern Med. 1985;103:70–8.
106. Fraser DG. Drug therapy reviews: antimicrobial spectrum, pharmacology and therapeutic use of cefamandole and cefoxitin. Am J Hosp Pharm. 1979;36:1503–8.
107. Delgado DG, Crau CJ, Cobbs CG, et al. Clinical and laboratory evaluation of cefamandole in the therapy of *Haemophilus* sp. Bronchopulmonary infections. Antimicrob Agents Chemother. 1979;15:807–12.
108. Meyers BR, Hirschman SZ. Antibacterial activity of cefamandole in vitro. J Infect Dis. 1978;137(Suppl):S25–31.
109. Kass EH, Evans DA. Future prospects and past problems in antimicrobial therapy: the role of cefoxitin. Rev Infect Dis. 1979;1:1.
110. Chow AW, Bednorz D. Comparative in vitro activity of newer cephalosporins against anaerobic bacteria. Anttimicrob Agents Chemother. 1978;14:668–71.
111. Sutter VL, Finegold SM. Susceptibility of anaerobic bacteria to carbenicillin, cefoxitin, and related drugs. J Infect Dis. 1975;131:417–22.
112. Bach VT, Roy I, Thadepalli H. Susceptibility of anaerobic bacteria to cefoxitin and related compounds. Antimicrob Agents Chemother. 1977;11:912–3.
113. Smith BR, LeFrock JL. Cefuroxime: antimicrobial activity, pharmacology, and clinical efficacy. Ther Drug Monit. 1983;5:149–60.
114. Williams PEO, Harding SM. The absolute bioavailability of oral cefuroxime axetil in male and female volunteers after fasting and after food. J Antimicrob Chemother. 1984;13:191–6.
115. Harding SM, Williams PEO, Ayrton J. Pharmacology of cefuroxime as the 1-acetoxyethyl ester in volunteers. Antimicrob Agents Chemother. 1984;25:78–82.
116. Sommers D, Van Wyk M, Williams PEO, Harding SM. Pharmacokinetics and tolerance of cefuroxime axetil in volunteers during repeated dosing. Antimicrob Agents Chemother. 1984;25:344–7.
117. Morel C, Vergnaud M, Langeard MM, et al. Cefotetan: comparative study in vitro against 266 gram-negative clinical isolates. J Antimicrob Chemother. 1983;11(Suppl A):31–6.
118. Ruckdeschel G. Activity in vitro of cefotetan against nonsporing anaerobes: a comparative study. J Antimicrob Chemother. 1983;11(Suppl A):117–24.
119. Wexler HM, Finegold SM. In vitro activity of cefotetan compared with that of other antimicrobial agents against anaerobic bacteria. Antimicrob Agents Chemother. 1988;32:601–4.
120. Silver MS, Counts GW, Zeleznik D, et al. Comparison of in vitro antibacterial activity of three oral cephalosporins: cefaclor, cephalexin, and cephradine. Antimicrob Agents Chemother. 1977;12:591–6.
121. Barriere SL, Mills J. Ceforanide: antibacterial activity, pharmacology, and clinical efficacy. Pharmacotherapy. 1982;2:322–7.
122. Gremillion DH, Winn RE, Vandenbout E. Clinical trial of cefonicid for treatment of skin infections. Antimicrob Agents Chemother. 1983;23:944–6.
123. Pines A, Raafat HH, Khorasani M, et al. Cefuroxime and ampicillin compared in a double-blind study in the treatment of lower respiratory tract infections. Chemotherapy. 1981;27:459–65.
124. Mehtar S, Parr JH, Morgan DJR. A comparison of cefuroxime and cotrimoxazole in severe respiratory tract infections. J Antimicrob Chemother. 1982;9:479–84.
125. Bergeron MG, Claveau S, Simard P. Limited in vitro activity of cefamandole against 100 beta-lactamase and non-beta-lactamase producing *H. influenzae* strains: Comparison of moxalactam, chloramphonical and ampicillin. Antimicrob Agents Chemother. 1981;19:101–5.
126. Swedish Study Group, Cefuroxime versus ampicillin and chloramphonical for the treatment of bacterial meningitis. Lancet. 1982;1:295–9.
127. Pfenninger J, Schaad UB, Lutschg J, et al. Cefuroxime in bacterial meningitis. Arch Dis Child. 1982;57:539–45.
128. Sirinavin S, Chiemchanya S, Visudhipan P, et al. Cefuroxime treatment of bacterial meningitis in infants and children. Antimicrob Agents Chemother. 1984;25:273–5.
129. Schleupner CJ, Anthony WC, Tan J, et al. Blinded comparison of cefuroxime to cefaclor for lower respiration tract infections. Arch Intern Med. 1988;148:343–8.
130. Reichman RC, Nolte FS, Wolinsky SM, et al. Single dose cefuroxime axetil for treatment of uncomplicated gonorrhea: a controlled trial. Sex Transm Dis. 1985;12:184–7.

131. Davies BL, Maesen FDV, Teengs JP. Cefuroxime axetil in acute purulent exacerbations of chronic bronchitis infections. 1987;15:253–6.
132. Brumfitt W, Hamilton-Miller JMT, Smith GW. Comparative trial of cefuroxime axetil in recurrent urinary tract infections, illustrating the importance of 6-week follow-up. Antimicrob Agents Chemother. 1987;31:1442–3.
133. Lefrock JL, Blais F, Schell RD, et al. Cefoxitin in the treatment of diabetic patients with lower extremity infections. Infect Surg. 1983;2:361–74.
134. Drusano GL, Warren W, Saah AJ, et al. A prospective randomized controlled trial of cefoxitin versus clindamycin-aminoglycoside in mixed anaerobic-aerobic infections. Surg Gynecol Obstet. 1982;154:715–20.
135. Antimicrobial prophylaxis in surgery. Med Lett. 1987;29(Issue 750):91.
136. Rice RJ, Thompson SE. Treatment of uncomplicated infections due to *Neisseria gonorrhoeae*: a review of clinical efficacy and in vitro susceptibility studies from 1982 through 1985. JAMA. 1986;255:1739–46.
137. Sanchez PL, Wingall FS, Zajdowicz TR, et al. One gram of cefoxitin cures uncomplicated gonococcal urethritis caused by penicillinase-producing *Neisseria gonorrhoeae* (PPNG). Sex Transm Dis. 1973;10:135–7.
138. Orr JW, Varner RE, Kilgore LC, et al. Cefotetan versus cefoxitin as prophylaxis in hysterectomy. Am J Obstet Gynecol. 1986;154:960–3.
139. McGregor JA, French JI, Makowski F. Single dose cefotetan versus multidose cefoxitin for prophylaxis in cesarean section in high risk patients. Am J Obstet Gynecol. 1986;154:955–60.
140. Wilson SE, Boswick JA, Duma RJ, et al. Cephalosporin therapy in intraabdominal infections: a multicenter randomized, comparative study of cefotetan, moxalactam and cefoxitin. Am J Surg. 1988;155(Suppl 5A):61–6.
141. Sweet R, Gall SA, Gobbs RS, et al. Multicenter clinical trial comparing cefotetan with moxalactam or cefoxitin as therapy for obstetric and gynecologic infections. Am J Surg. 1988;155(Suppl 5A):56–60.
142. Richmond MH. β-Lactamase stability of cefotaxime. J Antimicrob Chemother. 1980;6(Suppl A):13–7.
143. Schrinner E, Limbert M, Penasse L, et al. Antibacterial activity of cefotaxime and other newer cephalosporins (in vitro and in vivo). J Antimicrob Chemother. 1980;6(Suppl A):25–30.
144. Mullaney DT, John JF. Cefotaxime therapy: evaluation of its effects on bacterial meningitis, CSF drug levels, and bactericidal activity. Arch Intern Med. 1983;143:1705–8.
145. Moellering RC, Young LS. Moxalactam international symposium. Rev Infect Dis. 1982;4:S489–90.
146. Weitekamp MR, Aber RC. Prolonged bleeding times and bleeding diathesis associated with moxalactam administration. JAMA. 1983;249:69
147. Fu KP, Neu HC. Antibacterial activity of ceftizoxime, a β-lactamase stable cephalosporin. Antimicrob Agents Chemother. 1980;17:583–90.
148. Overturf GD, Cable DC, Forthal DN, et al. Treatment of bacterial meningitis with ceftizoxime. Antimicrob Agents Chemother. 1984;25:158–61.
149. Cleeland R, Squires E. Antimicrobial activity of ceftriaxone, a review. Am J Med. 1984;77:3–11.
150. Neu HC, Meropol NJ, Fu KP. Antibacterial activity of ceftriaxone (Ro 13-9904) a β-lactamase stable cephalosporin. Antimicrob Agents Chemother. 1981;19:414–23.
151. Neu HC, Chin NX, Labthavikul P. Comparative in vitro activity and β-lactamase stability of FR 17027, a new orally active cephalosporin. Antimicrob Agents Chemother. 1984;26:174–80.
152. Jones RN. Antimicrobial activity spectrum and pharmacokinetics of old and new orally administered cephens. Antimicrob Newslett. 1988;5:1–8.
153. Neu HC. The new beta-lactamase stable cephalosporins. Ann Intern Med. 1982;97:408–19.
154. Fass RJ. Comparative in vitro activities of third generation cephalosporins. Arch Intern Med. 1983;143:1743–5.
155. Trabulsi LR, Almada NP, Marqus LRM. Inhibitory concentrations of cefoperazone, cefazolin, cefamandole, cephaloridine and cefoxitin for 300 gram-negative clinical isolates. Clin Ther. 1980;3:145–8.
156. Brogden RN, Carmine A, Heel RC, et al. Cefoperazone, a review of its in vitro antimicrobial activity, pharmacological properties and therapeutic efficacy. Drugs. 1981;22:423–60.
157. Kemmerich B, Lode H, Borner K, et al. Biliary excretion and pharmacokinetics of cefoperazone in humans. J Antimicrob Chemother. 1983;12:27–37.
158. Sattler FN, Weitekamp MR, Ballard JO. Potential for bleeding with the new beta-lactam antibiotics. Ann Intern Med. 1986;105:924–30.
159. Shenkenberg TD, Mackowiak PA, Smith JW. Coagulopathy and hemorrhage associated with cefoperazone therapy in a patient with renal failure. South Med J. 1985;78:488–9.
160. Osborne JC. Hypoprothrombinemia and bleeding due to cefoperazone. Ann Intern Med. 1985;102:721–2.
161. Sattler FR, Colao DJ, Caputo GM, et al. Cefoperazone for empiric therapy in patients with impaired renal function. Am J Med. 1986;81:229–36.
162. Neu HC, Labthavikul P. Antibacterial activity and beta-lactamase stability of ceftazidime, an aminothiazolyl cephalosporin potentially active against *Pseudomonas aeruginosa*. Antimicrob Agents Chemother. 1982;21:11–8.
163. Modai J, Vittecoq D, DeCazes JM, et al. Penetration of ceftazidime into cerebral spinal fluid of patients with bacterial meningitis. Antimicrob Agents Chemother. 1983;24:126–8.
164. Pfaller MA, Niles AC, Murray PR. In vitro antibacterial activity of cefpiramide. Antimicrob Agents Chemother. 1984;25:368–72.
165. Fukasawa M, Noguchi H, Okuda T, et al. In vitro antibacterial activity of SM-1652 a new broad-spectrum cephalosporin with anti-pseudomonal activity. Antimicrob Agents Chemother. 1983;3:195–200.
166. Jones RN, Thornsberry C, Barry AL. In vitro evaluation of HR810, a new wide-spectrum aminothiazolyl—methoxyimino cephalosporin. Antimicrob Agents Chemother. 1984;25:710–8.
167. Jones RN, Gerlach EH. Antimicrobial activity of HR810 against 419 strict anaerobic bacteria. Antimicrob Agents Chemother. 1985;27:413–5.
168. Bauernfeind A. Susceptibility of gram positive aerobic cocci to the new cephalosporin HR810. Eur J Clin Microbiol. 1988;2:354–5.
169. Lecour H, Seara A, Miranda AM, et al. Treatment of 160 cases of acute bacterial meningitis with cefotaxime. J Antimicrob Chemother. 1984;14(Suppl B):195–202.
170. Belohradsky BH, Geiss D, Marget W, et al. Intravenous cefotaxime in children with bacterial meningitis. Lancet. 1980;i:61–3.
171. Rodriquez WJ, Khan WN, Gold B, et al. Ceftazidime in the treatment of meningitis in infants and children over one month of age. Am J Med. 1985;79(Suppl 2A):52–5.
172. Norrby SR. Role of cephalosporins in the treatment of bacterial meningitis in adults: overview with special emphasis on ceftazidime. Am J Med. 1985;(Suppl 2A):56–61.
173. Jacobs RF, Wells TG, Steele RW, et al. A prospective randomized comparison of cefotaxime vs ampicillin and chloramphenicol for bacterial meningitis in children. J Pediatr. 1985;107:129–33.
174. Barson WJ, Miller MA, Brady MT, et al. Prospective comparative trial of ceftriaxone vs conventional therapy for treatment of bacterial meningitis in children. Pediatr Infect Dis. 1986;4:362–8.
175. Congeni BL. Comparison of ceftriaxone and traditional therapy of bacterial meningitis. Antimicrob Agents Chemother. 1984;25:40–4.
176. Bryan JP, Rocha H, da Silva HR, et al. Comarison of ceftriaxone and ampicillin plus chloramphenicol for therapy of acute bacterial meningitis. Antimicrob Agents Chemother. 1985;28:361–8.
177. Jacobs RF, Wright MW, Deskin RL, et al. Delayed sterilization of *Haemophilus influenzae* type B meningitis with twice-daily ceftriaxone. JAMA. 1988;259:392–4.
178. Cherubin CE, Marr JS, Sierra MF, et al. *Listeria* and gram-negative bacillary meningitis in New York City 1972–1979: frequent causes of meningitis in adults. Am J Med. 1981;71:199–209.
179. Fong IW, Tompkins KB. Review of *Pseudomonas aeruginosa* meningitis with special emphasis on treatment with ceftazidime. Rev Infect Dis. 1985;7:604–12.
180. Francke EL, Neu HC. Use of cefotaxime, a β-lactamase stable cephalosporin in the therapy of serious infections, including those due to multiresistant organisms. Am J Med. 1981;71:435–42.
181. Young JPW, Husson JM, Bruch K, et al. The evaluation of efficacy and safety of cefotaxime: a review of 2500 cases. J Antimicrob Chemother. 1980;6(Suppl A):293–300.
182. Daikos GK, Kosmidis J, Giamarellou H, et al. Evaluation of cefotaxime in a hospital with high antibiotic resistance rates. J Antimicrob Chemother. 1980;6(Suppl A):255–61.
183. Scully BE, Neu HC. The use of ceftizoxime in the treatment of critically ill patients infected with multiply antibiotic resistant bacteria. J Antimicrob Chemother. 1982;10(Suppl C):141–50.
184. Johnson ES, Smith LG. Ceftrizoxime in moderate-to-severe infections. J Antimicrob Chemother. 1982;10(Suppl C):151–7.
185. Baumgartner J-D, Glauser MP. Single daily dose treatment of severe refractory infections with ceftriaxone: cost savings and possible parenteral outpatient treatment. Arch Intern Med 1983;143:1868–73.
186. Eron LJ, Park CH, Goldenberg RI, et al. Ceftriaxone therapy of serious bacterial infections. J Antimicrob Chemother. 1983;12:65–78.
187. Cohen MS, Washton HE, Barranco SF. Multicenter clinical trial of cefoperazone sodium in the United States. Am J Med. 1984;77(Suppl 1B):35–41.
188. Warren JW, Miller EH Jr, Fitzpatrick B, et al. A randomized, controlled in trial of cefoperazone vs cefamandole-tobramycin in the treatment of putative, severe infections with gram-negative bacilli. Rev Infect Dis. 1983;5(Suppl 1):S173–80.
189. Mangi RJ, Greco T, Ryan J, et al. Cefoperazone versus combination antibiotic therapy of hospital acquired pneumonia. Am J Med. 1988;84:68–74.
190. Bergeron MG, Mendelson J, Harding GK, et al. Cefoperazone compared with ampicillin plus tobromycin for severe biliary tract infections. Antimicrob Agents Chemother. 1988;32:1231–6.
191. Scully BE, Neu HC. Clinical efficacy of ceftazidime: treatment of serious infection due to multiresistant pseudomonas and other gram negative bacteria. Arch Intern Med. 1984;144:57–62.
192. Young LS. Ceftazidime in the treatment of nosocomial sepsis. Am J Med. 1985;79(Suppl 2A):89–95.
193. Bradsher RW JR, Snow RM. Ceftriaxone treatment of skin and soft tissue infections in a once daily regimen. Am J Med. 1984;77(Suppl 4C):63–7.
194. Eron LJ, Park CH, Hixon DL, et al. Ceftriaxone therapy of bone and soft tissue infections in hospital and outpatient settings. Antimicrob Agents Chemother. 1983;23:731–7.
195. Poretz DM, Woolard D, Eron LJ, et al. Outpatient use of ceftriaxone: a cost-benefit analysis. Am J Med. 1984;77(Suppl 4C):77–83.
196. Judson FN, Ehret JM, Handsfield HH. Comparative study of ceftriaxone and spectinomycin for treatment of uncomplicated gonorrhoea in men. Lancet. 1983;2:67–70.
197. Collier AC, Judson FN, Murphy VL, et al. Comparative study of ceftriaxone and spectinomycin in the treatment of uncomplicated gonorrhea in women. Am J Med. 1984;77(Suppl 4C):68–72.
198. Schwartz B, Al-Ruwais A, A'ashi J, et al. Comparative efficacy of ceftriax-

one and rifampian in eradicating pharyngeal carriage of group A *Neisseria meningitidis*. Lancet. 1988;1:1239–45.
199. Bolivar R, Fainstein V, Elting L, et al. Cefoperazone for the treatment of nfections in patients with cancer. Rev Infect Dis. 1983;5(Suppl 1):S181–7.
200. Piccart M, Klastersky J, Meunier F, et al. Single-drug versus combination empirical therapy for gram-negative bacillary infections in febrile cancer patients with and without granulocytopenia. Antimicrob Agents Chemother. 1984;26:870–5.
201. Gucalp R, Lia S, McKitrick JC, et al. Cefoperaxone plus tobramycin versus ticarcillin plus tobramycin in febrile granulocytopenic cancer patients. Am J Med. 1988;85(Suppl 1A):31–3.
202. Winston DJ, Ho WG, Bruckner DA, et al. Controlled trials of double beta-lactam therapy with cefoperazone plus piperacillin in febrile granulocytopenic patients. Am J Med. 1988;85(Suppl 1A):21–30.
203. Pizzo PA, Hathorn JW, Hiemenz J, et al. A randomized trial comparing ceftazidime alone with combination antibiotic therapy in cancer patients with fever and neutropenia. N Engl J Med. 1986;315:552–8.
204. EORTC International Antimicrobial Therapy Cooperative Group. Ceftazidime combined with a short or long course of amikacin for empirical therapy of gram-negative bacteremia in cancer patients with granulocytopenia. N Engl J Med. 1987;317:1692–8.

20. OTHER β-LACTAM ANTIBIOTICS

HAROLD C. NEU

Several antimicrobial agents belonging to the β-lactam class of antibiotics have been developed in recent years. Since these agents differ widely in their antibacterial and pharmacologic properties, they will be discussed as separate entities.

CARBAPENEMS

Imipenem is the prototype drug of this class of compounds. In the early 1970s scientists in Spain discovered a new *Streptomyces* species called *Streptomyces cattleya*, which produced a carbapenem compound that was subsequently named thienamycin.[1]

Chemistry

Figure 1 shows the chemical structure of the stable *N*-formimidoyl derivative of thienamycin. The presence of an azetidiome group caused thienamycin to undergo aminolysis of the β-lactam ring through reaction of the amino group of one molecule with another. *N*-formimidoyl thienamycin is called imipenem.

Carbapenems possess novel stereochemical features that differentiate them from penicillins and cephalosporins. They are in an S transconfiguration, and the endocyclic sulfur is replaced by a methylene group, with the sulfur adjacent to the bicyclic ring system.

Antibacterial Activity

Imipenem has excellent in vitro activity against aerobic grampositve species such as the hemolytic streptococci of the Lancefield classifications A, B, C, and G, with minimal inhibitory values (MICs) of 0.2 μg/ml or less (Table 1).[2,3] *Streptococcus*

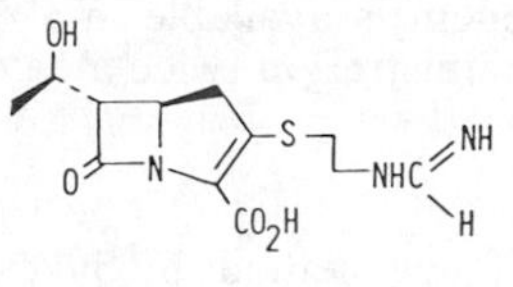

FIG. 1. Imipenem (*N*-formimidoyl thienamycin).

TABLE 1. Activity of Imipenem against Aerobic and Anaerobic Bacteria

Organism	*MIC$_{90}$ (μg/ml)*
Staphylococcus aureus[a]	0.1
S. epidermidis[a]	0.2
Streptococcus pyogenes	0.1
S. agalactiae	0.1
Viridans streptococci	0.1
S. pneumoniae	0.01
S. bovis	0.1
Enterococcus faecalis	0.8
Haemophilus influenzae	0.1
Neisseria gonorrhoeae	0.1
N. meningitidis	0.02
Listeria monocytogenes	0.02
Klebsiella pneumoniae[a]	0.4
Enterobacter cloacae[a]	1.6
E. aerogenes[a]	0.2
E. agglomerans[a]	0.4
E. hafnia[a]	0.4
Escherichia coli[a]	0.4
Klebsiella oxytoca[a]	0.2
Arizona hinshawii[a]	0.1
Aeromonas hydrophila[a]	0.1
Citrobacter freundii	1.6
C. diversus[a]	0.2
Serratia marcescens[a]	6.3
Proteus mirabilis	1.6
Morganella morganii[a]	1.6
Proteus rettgeri[a]	1.6
P. vulgaris[a]	0.6
Providencia stuart[a]	1.6
Salmonella	0.1
Shigella	0.2
Acinetobacter	0.8
Pseudomonas aeruginosa[a]	12.5
P. maltophilia	>50
P. cepacia	>50
Bacteroides fragilis	1
Bacteroides bivius	0.03
Bacteroides melaninogenicus	0.12
Bacteroides disiens	0.03
Bacteroides thetaiotamicron	1
Bacteroides vulgatus, B. ovatus	1
Fusobacterium nucleatum	0.25
Fusobacterium species	0.5
Veillonella species	1
Clostridium difficile	16
Clostridium perfringens	1
Clostridium species	2
Peptostreptococci	0.12
Peptococci	0.12
Propionibacterium species	0.01
Eikenella corrodens	0.25
Campylobacter fetus	0.12

[a] Both β-lactamase- and non-β-lactamase-containing strains.

pneumoniae organisms are inhibited by less than 0.1 μg/ml, and *S. pneumoniae* strains resistant to by penicillin (MIC values >4 μg/ml) are inhibited by 1 μg/ml or less. *Enterococcus faecalis* organisms are inhibited by less than 1.5 μg/ml, but there is a discrepancy between inhibitory and bactericidal levels just as exists for ampicillin and vancomycin, and *Enterococcus faecium* strains resistant to ampicillin are resistant to imipenem. *Staphylococcus aureus* and *Staphylococcus epidermidis* are inhibited by less than 0.2 and 1.5 μg/ml, respectively. Methicillin-resistant staphylococci are resistant and have MICs of ≥16 μg/ml. *Listeria* and *Bacillus* sp. are also inhibited by less than 1 μg/ml.[4]

Most of the Enterobacteriaceae are inhibited by concentrations of imipenem less than or equal to 1 μg/ml. Some *Proteus* strains have MIC values of 2–4 μg/ml. *Haemophilus infuenzae* and *Neisseria gonorrhoeae*, including their β-lactamase–producing isolates, are inhibited by less than 0.5 μg/ml.

Pseudomonas aeruginosa, including strains resistant to penicillins such as piperacillin and to cephalosporins such as ceftazidime and cefsulodin, are inhibited by 1–6 μg/ml.[5] Some *Pseudomonas cepacia* strains are inhibited by imipenem, but

Pseudomonas maltophilia is resistant. Most *Acinetobacter* organisms are inhibited by less than 1 μg/ml.

Imipenem inhibits most anaerobic species, including *Bacteroides fragilis* and some isolates resistant to moxalactam and cefoxitin, at concentrations of less than 0.5 μg/ml.[6,7] Most *Clostridium* sp. are inhibited by 1 μg/ml or less, with the exception of *Clostridium difficile*, which requires 6–8 μg/ml. *Fusobacterium, Actinomyces, Campylobacter*, and *Yersinia* are inhibited by imipenem, and many *Nocardia asteroides* strains are inhibited by 1 μg/ml. It also inhibits *Mycobacterium-avium* and some *Legionella* spp.

Mechanism of Action

Imipenem binds to penicillin-binding protein 2 (PBP-2) of gram-negative aerobic bacteria and to critical PBPs in *S. aureus* and streptococci. Unlike the situation with amdinocillin, imipenem causes rapid death of bacteria, and there is no major discrepancy between inhibitory and bactericidal activity. Imipenem shows a marked postantibiotic effect on both gram-positive and gram-negative bacteria.

Imipenem is not hydrolyzed by most β-lactamases, penicillinases, cephalosporinases, plasmid or chromosomally mediated, of *S. aureus, Escherichia coli, Enterobacter cloacae, Citrobacter freundii, Proteus rettgeri, Serratia marcescens, Proteus vulgaris, Klebsiella oxytoca, P. aeruginosa, P. cepacia* and *B. fragilis*. It is hydrolyzed by a *P. maltophilia* β-lactamase, some *Bacillus*, and *Bacteroides* enzymes.

Pharmacology

Imipenem cannot be absorbed after oral ingestion due to its instability in gastric acid. Although initial studies of imipenem after iv infusion showed high serum levels, urinary recovery was only 6–38 percent of an administered dose. Extrarenal metabolism is minimal but renal peptidase, dehydropeptidase-1, which hydrolyzes L-L and L-D dipeptides, is located on the brush border of the proximal renal tubules. After imipenem is removed from the circulation by glomerular filtration and secretion, it is hydrolyzed. Metabolites of imipenem in the absence of cilastatin are nephrotoxic.

Imipenem in the circulation is not destroyed and is widely distributed to various body compartments.[8,9] There is minimal biliary secretion of imipenem, and there is minimal change in bowel flora. In the absence of meningeal inflammation only minor amounts of imipenem enter the cerebrospinal fluid (CSF). In the presence of meningeal inflammation CSF levels of 1–5 μg/ml have been recorded. Imipenem has a high affinity for brain cells.

To overcome the problem of the destruction of imipenem in urine, a dehydropeptidase inhibitor was synthesized. This molecule, called cilastatin, is administered in equal amounts to imipenem. Cilastatin has no antibacterial activity, nor does it alter the antibacterial activity of imipenem. Cilastatin does not affect zinc metalloenzyme peptidases or angiotensin-converting enzymes.

After 20–30 minutes of infusion of 250 mg imipenem plus 250 mg cilastatin, mean peak serum levels of imipenem are 13 μg/ml. After 500 mg, mean peak serum levels are 33 μg/ml; 1000 mg produces a peak concentration of 52 μg/ml[10,11]; the half-life of imipenem is 1 hour in healthy people. The serum half-life increases to 4 hours with a fall in creatinine clearance in patients whose creatinine clearance is less than 10 ml/min. The half-life of cilastatin increases to a much greater extent than does that of imipenem and reaches 16 hours in anuria.[12] Imipenem is removed from the body by hemodialysis. Cilastatin is also removed by dialysis less completely. With dialysis the half-life of imipenem is 2.5 hours, and for cilastatin it is 3.8 hours.

In the presence of cilastatin, urinary recovery of imipenem is 70 percent, with a 25–29 percent recovery of the metabolites. Fecal elimination of imipenem is less than 1 percent.[13]

Adverse Reactions. Imipenem has generally been well tolerated.[14] It causes minimal phlebitis when used iv. It can cause immediate hypersensitivity,[15] and cross-reactions with penicillins have occurred. No major adverse effects such as diarrhea, pseudomembranous colitis, coagulation abnormalities, nephrotoxicity, or hepatotoxicity have been reported. Rapid infusion of imipenem has produced nausea and emesis in about 1 percent of patients. About 2–4 percent of imipenem-treated patients will have from a one- to two-fold elevation of serum glutamic-oxaloacetic transaminase and/or serum glutamic-pyruvic transaminase (SGOT, SGPT) values. Leukopenia has occurred, but infrequently. No drug interactions have been reported. The most serious toxicity is seizure, which occurs infrequently but most often in patients with underlying central nervous system pathology and in individuals with decreased renal function in whom dose adjustment has not been made.

Clinical Use. Animal infection studies have demonstrated the utility of imipenem in therapy for staphylococcal endocarditis (but not enterococcal endocarditis where high relapse rates were noted),[16,17] bacteremia due to *P. aeruginosa* in neutropenic rats,[18] and pyelonephritis in rats.

These observations have been extended to humans where imipenem has been found to be useful in the treatment of bone and soft tissue infections,[19,20] obstetric and gynecologic infections,[21] complicated urinary tract infections,[22] intra-abdominal sepsis,[23] pneumonia,[24] and endocarditis due to *S. aureus*.[25] In addition, imipenem has been found to be effective as a single agent in the treatment of febrile neutropenic patients, although the number of patients treated to date has been small.[26]

Since imipenem is not active against *Chlamydia trachomatis* a tetracycline would also have to be administered for the treatment of pelvic inflammatory disease. Imipenem has activity against *Nocardia asteroides* in vitro and in a murine model of cerebral infection.[27] Clinical experience is limited.[28]

In cystic fibrosis patients receiving imipenem as a single agent for the treatment of pulmonary exacerbations, a significant number of *P. aeruginosa* isolates resistant to imipenem have been encountered.[29] In addition, the treatment of pneumonia due to *P. aeruginosa* in non-cystic fibosis patients with imipenem as a single agent has had a disappointingly low success rate.[30] These observations suggest that imipenem not be used alone in therapy for serious pseudomonal infections, particularly those involving the respiratory tract.

The use of imipenem is most appropriate in the treatment of infections due to cephalosporin-resistant *Enterobacteriaceae*, particularly those due to *Citrobacter freundii* and *Enterobacter* spp.; as empirical therapy in the treatment of serious infections in patients previously treated with multiple antibiotics because the likelihood of encountering organisms resistant to more conventional β-lactams is high; possibly as a single agent in the treatment of febrile, neutropenic patient, although this is not clearly established at present; and in the treatment of polymicrobial infections where otherwise multiple-drug regimens of higher cost and potentially more adverse side effects would be necessary.

Based on their pharmacokinetic profiles, imipenem/cilastatin can be administered safely on an q6h or q8h basis to patients with normal renal function. Based on the available MIC data and the knowledge that a 500 mg infusion of imipenem results in a peak serum concentration of about 35 μg/ml, most infections can be treated with a regimen of 500 mg every 6 hours.

In Europe imipenem is available in a different formulation that permits im administration twice a day.

MONOBACTAMS

The development of new methods by Sykes and his colleagues[31] to screen large numbers of organisms for the production of β-lactam antibiotics showed that a number of bacteria, particularly *Gluconobacter* and *Acinetobacter*, produced monocyclic β-lactam antibiotics with antibacterial activity. From *Chromobacterium violaceum* a monocyclic compound was isolated and the structure confirmed. This compound was subsequently modified to yield a highly active therapeutic agent, aztreonam.

AZTREONAM

Chemistry

Aztreonam is a monocyclic β-lactam (Fig. 2) in which there is a sulfate group affixed to the nitrogen at position 1, an acyl side chain at position 3 that consists of an aminothiazolyl nucleus and an iminocarboxypropyl group, and a methyl group at position 4 of the ring.

Mechanism of Action

Aztreonam has no appreciable antibacterial activity against gram-positive or anaerobic bacteria. This is because it does not bind to penicillin-binding proteins in these species. Aztreonam binds primarily to PBP-3 in Enterobacteriaceae, *Pseudomonas*, and other gram-negative aerobic organisms. It produces long filamentous structures that are not viable. Aztreonam readily passes through the outer wall of gram-negative species, and it is not hydrolyzed by most plasmid and chromosomal β-lactamases but is hydrolyzed by some *K. oxytoca* and *P. cepacia* and the cefotaxime-hydrolyzing plasmid enzymes.

TABLE 2. In Vitro Activity of Aztreonam

Organism	*MIC₉₀ (μg/ml)*
Escherichia coli	0.25
Klebsiella pneumoniae	1
K. oxytoca	1
Enterobacter cloacae	16
E. aerogenes	8
E. agglomerans	1
Citrobacter freundii	8
C. diversus	0.25
Serratia marcescens	4
Proteus mirabilis	0.01
P. vulgaris	0.12
P. rettgeri	0.12
Morganella morganii	0.25
Providencia	0.025
Salmonella enteritidis	0.25
Shigella	0.12
Arizona hinshawii	0.12
Aeromonas hydrophila	0.12
A. shigelloides	0.12
Yersinia enterocolitica	2
Pasteurella multocida	0.12
Salmonella typhi	0.12
Haemophilus influenzae	0.12
Neisseria gonorrhoeae	0.25
N. meningitidis	0.025
Pseudomonas aeruginosa	16
P. maltophilia	>128
Pseudomonas, other (*P. cepacia, P. diminuta, P. stutzeri, P. fluorescens*)	>128
S. pyogenes	16
S. pneumoniae	16
Enterococci	>128
Clostridium	>128
Bacteroides sp.	>128

Antibacterial Activity

Aztreonam inhibits most Enterobacteriaceae at concentrations below 0.5 μg/ml (Table 2); some *P. aeruginosa. E. cloacae*, and *C. freundii* strains are resistant. Most *P. aeruginosa* organisms are inhibited by less than 16 μg/ml. Most *C. cepacia* and *P. maltophilia* are resistant, as are many *Aceintobacter* sp.; *Haemophilus* and *Neisseria*, including β-lactamase–producing isolates, are inhibited by less than 0.2 μg/ml. *Yersinia* and *Aeromonas* are inhibited by less than 0.5 μg/ml. In general, the antibacterial activity is minimally affected by inoculum size except for *P. aeruginosa*, and there is no major difference between MIC and minimum bactericidal concentration (MBC) values.[32,34] Aztreonam acts synergistically with aminoglycosides against *P. aeruginosa* and some *Enterobacteriaceae*. It also acts synergistically with amdinocillin against *Enterobacteriaceae*.

Bacterial Resistance. *Enterobacteriaceae* and *P. aeruginosa* can be resistant due to a failure to cross the outer cell wall, destruction by β-lactamases i.e., *P. maltophilia*, CTX-1, and related enzymes, and a failure to bind to PBPs.

Adverse Reactions

No new major adverse reactions to aztreonam have been reported.[35] Skin rashes have occurred. Neither anaphylaxis nor rashes have followed its use in patients with positive skin test reactions to penicillins (see Chapter 21). About 2–4 percent of patients will have increases in serum transaminase values two times above normal when receiving aztreonam. No hematologic, gastrointestinal, nephrotoxic, or neurotoxic reactions have been noted with this agent.

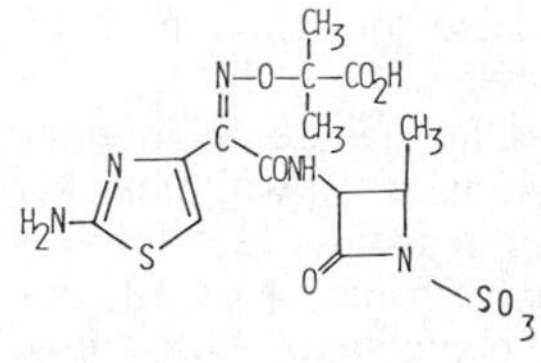

FIG. 2. Aztreonam.

Pharmacokinetics

Aztreonam is not absorbed from the gastrointestinal tract. It is rapidly and completely absorbed after im administration, with peak serum concentrations attained within 1 hour.[37–40] A 500 mg im aztreonam dose produces serum concentrations of 21–27 μg/ml at 1 hour, 3.8–5.9 μg/ml at 6 hours, 1.5–3.3 μg/ml at 8 hours, and 0.1–1.7 μg/ml at 12 hours. A 1 g im dose yields peaks of 3.5 μg/ml at 8 hours and 0.7 μg/ml at 12 hours.[40] Aztreonam serum concentrations 1 hour after an im dose are the same as after an iv dose.

After iv infusion of a single 0.5, 1, or 2 g dose of aztreonam in healthy adults over a period of 30 minutes, peak serum concentrations of the drug immediately after completion of the infusion average 55–65, 90–160, or 200–255 μg/ml, respectively.[40] After repeated dosing the drug does not accumulate. In healthy adults receiving 1 or 2 g doses of aztreonam im or iv every 8 hours, steady-state trough serum concentrations of the drug average 1–1.8 and 2.5–3.8 μg/ml, respectively.[37]

Aztreonam is widely distributed into body tissues and fluids.[37] Therapeutic levels are present in adipose tissue, bone, gallbladder, liver, lungs, kidney, heart, intestinal tissue, and prostatic tissue. It is also present in saliva, sputum, bronchial secretions, bile, and pericardial, pleural, peritoneal, and synovial fluids.

Azteonam enters the CSF after iv administration, with CSF concentrations at 1 and 4 hours after a 2 g dose of 2 and 3.2 μg/ml, respectively.[41] In neonates and children 3 months to 2 years of age with bacterial meningitis who received a 30 mg/kg dose of aztreonam by iv injection over a period of 3 minutes, CSF aztreonam concentrations ranged from 2.1 to 20.8 μg/ml at 0.8 to 4.3 hours after the dose.[42]

Aztreonam concentrations in peritoneal fluid are approximately equal to concurrent serum concentrations of the drug,[37] and concentrations 1 hour after a 2 g dose average 300 μg/ml in common duct bile and 100 μg/ml in gallbladder bile. At serum concentrations of 1–100 μg/ml aztreonam is 45–60 percent bound to serum proteins in patients with normal serum albumin levels, but in patients with impaired renal function and decreased serum albumin concentrations, aztreonam is 22–40 percent bound.[37] Aztreonam is primarily removed from the body by renal mechanisms of both glomerular filtration and tubular secretion. No active metabolites have been found in serum or urine. In adults with normal renal and hepatic function, the distribution half-life of aztreonam averages 0.2–0.7 hours, and the elimination half-life averages 1.3–2.2 hours.

The half-life of aztreonam averages 1.7 hours in children 2 months to 12 years of age.[42] In neonates 7 days old, the half-life of aztreonam averages 5.5–9.9 hours in neonates weighing less than 2.5 kg.[42]

Serum concentrations of aztreonam are higher and the serum half-life prolonged in patients with renal impairment.[43,44] In adults with renal impairment, the half-life of aztreonam averages 3.5, 5.6, 7.8, and 8.5 hours in adults with creatinine clearances of 30–80, 10–30, ≤10, and 2 ml/min, respectively. The half-life of aztreonam is only slightly prolonged in patients with hepatic impairment.

Aztreonam is excreted as unchanged drug by both glomeruler filtration and tubular secretion, with approximately 58–74 percent of the dose excreted unchanged and 1–7 percent as open ring metabolites.[37] In adults with normal renal function, urinary concentrations of aztreonam after a single 0.5 or 1 g iv dose average 250–330 and 710–720 μg/ml, respectively 4–6 hours after the dose.[40]

Aztreonam and its renal metabolite are removed by hemodialysis.[43,44] The amount of the drug removed depends on the type of coil used and the dialysis flow rate. The serum half-life of aztreonam averages 2.7 hours during hemodialysis and 6–8 hours between dialysis sessions. A 4-hour period of hemodialysis removes 25–50 percent of a dose. Aztreonam is removed to a lesser extent by peritoneal dialysis. With a 6-hour dwell time, about 10 percent of a single 1 g iv dose of aztreonam is removed.[45]

Clinical Use

Aztreonam has been used for the treatment of a variety of infections such as urinary tract infections (including pyelonephritis and cystitis), lower respiratory tract infections including pneumonia and bronchitis, septicemia, skin and skin structure infections including those associated with postoperative wounds or ulcers and burns, intra-abdominal infection including peritonitis, and gynecologic infections including endometritis and pelvic cellulitis due to gram-negative aerobic bacteria.[35,46–55]

Because aztreonam has a spectrum of activity limited to aerobic gram-negative bacteria, the drug should not be used singly for empirical therapy in seriously ill patients if there is any possibility that the infection may be caused by gram-positive aerobic bacteria or if a mixed aerobic–anaerobic bacterial infection is suspected, an anti-infective agent effective against the suspected organism(s) should be used concomitantly. Aztreonam has been used safely and effectively in conjunction with clindamycin, erythromycin, metronidazole, penicillins, and vancomycin.

β-LACTAMASE INHIBITORS

Clavulanate

Clavulanate (Fig. 3) is a β-lactamase inhibitor. This compound was found in cultures of *Streptomyces clavuligerus*. It showed only a low level of antibacterial action, but when the compound was combined with penicillin G, inhibition of a *Klebsiella* isolate normally resistant to penicillin was noted. Clavulanate has subsequently been shown to inhibit β-lactamases from a number of clinically important gram-positive and gram-negative organisms.[56,57]

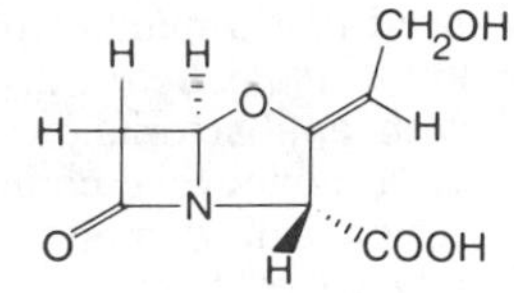

FIG. 3. Clavulanate.

Mechanism of Action. β-Lactamases account for the major form of resistance to penicillins and cephalosporins. These enzymes hydrolyze the cyclic amide bond in β-lactam–containing molecules. When the β-lactam ring is hydrolyzed, an inactive penicilloate is produced, or in the case of cephalosporins because of the unsaturated bond between carbons 3 and 4, both rings decompose to smaller fragments.

β-Lactamases of gram-positive species are exoenzymes, and in *S. aureus* the enzyme is plasmid mediated and inducible. Generally endemic hospital *S. aureus* produces large amounts of β-lactamase. The β-lactamases of gram-negative bacteria, aerobic and anaerobic, are situated in the periplasmic space and are either of chromosomal or plasmid origin. Richmond and Sykes developed a classification for gram-negative β-lactamases that lists them as I–V.[58] The most important chromosomal β-lactamases, most of which fall into class I, are present in *Acinetobacter, Citrobacter, Enterobacter, Proteus, Pseudomonas*, and *Serratia*. These are inducible enzymes and are not inhibited by clavulanate except at very high concentrations, which are only possible in test tube conditions. β-Lactamases are produced constitutively by some *Enterobacter, E. coli*, and *Shigella*. These are not inhibited by clavulanate. Conversely, β-lactamases of *Legionella* and *Bacteroides* are inhibited by clavulanate. Other important chromosomally mediated β-lactamases are the class IV enzymes produced by *Klebsiella*. These are also inhibited by clavulanate.[59–62]

Plasmid-mediated β-lactamases are of a number of types. The most common is TEM-1, so-called for the initials of the original patient from whom the *E. coli* β-lactamase–containing isolate was derived. There are also TEM-2; oxacillin-hydrolyzing enzymes; OXA-1, -2, and -3; sulfhydro-inhibited enzymes SHV-1 and HMS; and finally PSE-1, PSE-2, PSE-3, and PSE-4, originally felt to be enzymes found only in *Pseudomonas* but now found occasionally in *E. coli*. All of these plasmid enzymes are inhibited by clavulanate (Table 3), as are the new cefotaxime-ceftazidime hydrolyzing enzymes TEM-3, -4, -5, -6, -7, and -8 and SHV-2, -3, -4, and -5. Concentrations needed to inhibit bacteria are shown in Table 4.

Since clavulanate inhibits β-lactamases, it has been shown to act synergistically with amoxicillin, ampicillin, piperacillin, mezlocillin, and cefoperazone, all of which can be destroyed by *Staphylococcus, Klebsiella*, or plasmid-mediated β-lactamases.

The mode of inhibition of a β-lactamase by clavulanate is characteristic of the particular enzyme studied.[60] Although competitive inhibition is seen, clavulanate primarily acts as a suicide inhibitor that, after forming an acyl enzyme intermediate with the enzyme, causes destruction of the enzyme.

Pharmacology. Clavulanate is moderately well absorbed from the gastrointestinal tract, with peak serum levels occurring 40–120 minutes after ingestion. Mean peak serum levels for 62.5 mg are 1 μg/ml; for 125 mg, 4 μg/ml; and for 250 mg, 6 μg/ml.[63,64] Combining clavulanate with amoxicillin does not significantly alter the pharmacologic parameters of either drug.

TABLE 3. Inhibition of β-Lactamases by β-Lactam inhibitors

β-Lactamases	Name	Organisms	Inhibited by Clavulanate-Sulbactam
Plasmid		*S. aureus*	Yes
Plasmid	TEM-1	*E. coli*	Yes
		Haemophilus	
		N. gonorrhoeae	
		Salmonella	
		Shigella	
Plasmid	TEM-2	*E. coli*	Yes
Plasmid	TEM-3 to -8	*Klebsiella*	Yes
Plasmid	SHV-1	*Klebsiella*	Yes
Plasmid	SHV-2 to -5	Enterobacteriaceae	Yes
Plasmid	OXA-1, 2, 3	*E. coli*	Variable
Plasmid	PSE-1, 2, 3	*Pseudomonas*	Variable
Chromosomal	Type 1a[a]	*Enterobacter*	No
		Morganella	
		Citrobacter	
		Serratia	
Chromosomal	Type Id[a]	*Pseudomonas*	No
Chromosomal	Type IV, K1[a]	*Klebsiella*	Yes
Chromosomal		*Bacteroides*	Yes
Chromosomal		*Legionella*	Yes
Chromosomal		*Branhamella*	Yes

[a] Richmond-Sykes classification.[58]

The pharmacokinetics of orally administered clavulanate in children in terms of peak serum levels and plasma half-lives of the drug are similar to those in adults.[65,66]

The absorption of clavulanate in the adult is unaffected by the simultaneous administration of food, milk, or aluminum hydroxide–containing antacids. After iv infusion of calvulanate combined either with amoxicillin or ticarcillin, the drug is rapidly distributed. Peak serum concentration are approximately 11 μg/ml after a 200 mg iv dose, with drug detectable to levels of 0.2 μg/ml at 6 hours.[67,68] Peak serum concentrations of clavulanate in children receiving 5 mg/kg have been 19 μg/ml with less than 1 μg/ml present at 3 hours.[66]

The serum half-life of clavulanate is slightly less than that of amoxicillin, 0.76–1.4 hours. No accumulation of clavulanate occurs until creatinine clearances fall below 10 ml/min.[69] Dose adjustment usually is made by adjustment for amoxicillin or ticarcillin. Clavulanate has been shown to be degraded in vivo in animals, with metabolites being excreted via lung, feces, and urine and only 20–60 percent appearing unchanged in urine 6 hours after an oral dose. After a dose of 125 mg of clavulanate urine levels are 115–508 μg/ml for 0–2 hours and 45–74 μg/ml for 4–6 hours.[69]

Concentrations less than 1 μg/ml of clavulanate are achieved in sputum after the oral administration of amoxicillin-clavulanate, but pleural fluid levels are 46–91 percent of peak serum levels. There is rapid penetration of clavulanate into peritoneal fluid, with mean peritoneal fluid levels of clavulanate 66 percent of serum levels.[67,70] After 200 mg of clavulanate, peritoneal fluid levels fall below 5 μg/ml after about 0.5 hours and below 1 μg/ml after about 3 hours. Clavulanate does not penetrate noninflamed meninges, but after large iv doses in patients with meningitis, CSF levels of clavulanate have been in the range of 1 μg/ml. Clavulanate produces therapeutic levels in bile, middle ear fluid, and tonsil tissue.[70]

Clavulanate crosses the placenta and may be found in the cord blood of newborns and in the amniotic fluid, but no clavulanate can be detected in breast milk.

Adverse Reactions. No new or major adverse reactions to the use of clavulanate combined with amoxicillin or of clavulanate combined with ticarcillin have been reported. The incidence of skin reactions has been similar to that of penicillin used alone. Diarrhea has followed the use of 250 mg clavulanate given three times daily, and some nausea has occurred with this dose program. Parenteral amoxicillin-clavulanate and ticarcillin-clavulanate have not caused undue diarrhea.

Amoxicillin-Clavulanate

Amoxicillin-clavulanate (Augmentin) has been used in a number of different clinical settings. The combination has proved useful as therapy for acute otitis media in children that is caused by β-lactamase–producing *Haemophilus influenzae* and *Branhamella catarrhalis*.[71] It has also been used to treat sinusitis and, rarely, pharyngitis in individuals where large tonsillar tissue contains β-lactamase–producing *Bacteroides melaninogenicus*.[71] Amoxicillin-clavulanate has proved useful in lower respiratory tract infections such as exacerbations of bacterial bronchitis or pneumonitis due to β-lactamase–producing bacteria. It has proved particularly useful to treat bite wounds of human or animal origin. Skin structure infections due to streptococci and staphylococci have responded to amoxicillin-clavulanate with results comparable to oral antistaphylococcal agents and oral cephalosporins.[72] Amoxicillin-clavulanate has been used to treat diabetic foot infections since it has activity against staphylococci, anaerobes, and aerobic gram-negative bacteria.

Amoxicillin-clavulanate is available as a parenteral agent in many countries and has been used to treat gynecologic infections and intra-abdominal infections.

Ticarcillin-Clavulanate

Ticarcillin-clavulanate has been used as treatment of community- and hospital-acquired pneumonia, particularly where there has been aspiration of oral secretions and aerobic gram-negative bacilli.[73] Intra-abdominal infections and gynecologic infections have been treated successfully, as have skin structure infections and osteomyelitis.[74,75] When ticarcillin-clavulanate has been used to treat febrile neutropenic patients, it has been necessary to combine it with an aminoglycoside. The usual doses are either 3.1 or 3.2 g administered every 4 or 6 hours.

TABLE 4. Activity of Augmentin against Amoxicillin-Resistant Organisms

Organism	Amoxicillin	Augmentin[a]
Staphylococcus aureus	256	1.0
Staphylococcus epidermidis	256	2.0
Staphylococcus aureus (MRSA)	256	16.0
Haemophilus influenzae	64	0.5
Branhamella catarrhalis	16	0.25
Neisseria gonorrhoeae	128	1.0
Escherichia coli	>256	8.0
Klebsiella pneumoniae	128	4.0
Proteus mirabilis	>256	4.0
Proteus vulgaris	>256	2.0
Bacteroides fragilis	32	0.5
Enterobacter, Citrobacter, Serratia sp. and *Pseudomonas aeruginosa*	>128	>128

[a] Contains amoxicillin and clavulanate in a 2:1 ratio.

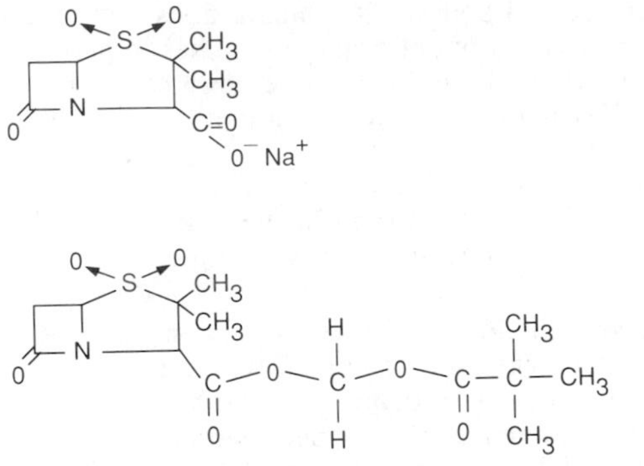

FIG. 4. Sulbactam and sulbactam oral ester (lower).

Adverse Reactions. The clinical studies of the combination of sulbactam plus ampicillin have reported no major hematologic, renal, hepatic, or central nervous system reactions.[81–83] Diarrhea has not been a major problem after iv use. Skin reactions are similar to those found for ampicillin, and there is occasional elevation of transaminase levels.

Clinical Use. Sulbactam-ampicillin in the United States is available only as a parenteral agent where it is used primarily intravenously. It has been used in treatment of mixed bacterial infections such as intra-abdominal infections, obstetric and gynecologic infections, and soft tissue and bone infections.[84,85] It has been used to treat meningitis in infants and children and to treat epiglottitis and selected other pediatric infections.[86,87] However, the pediatric experience is limited, and it would seem that third-generation cephalosporins would be preferred in such infections.

Sulbactam

Sulbactam (Fig. 4) is a 6-desaminopenicillin sulfone that resembles clavulanate structurally by a lack of substitution at carbon 6 of the β-lactam ring and by the presence of an activated center at carbon 5. Sulbactam has weak antibacterial activity against most gram-positive cocci, Enterobacteriaceae, and *Pseudomonas* but has reasonable activity against *Neisseria* sp., *Bacteroides* sp., and some *Acinetobacter* sp.[76–78]

Sulbactam acts similarly to clavulanate as a suicide inhibitor of certain plasmid- and chromosomally mediated β-lactamases. It does not inhibit β-lactamases of the Richmond-Sykes type Ia classification. These are chromosomally mediated β-lactamases of *Enterobacter, Citrobacter freundii*, and the indole-positive *Proteus-Providencia* organisms. Like clavulanate, it inhibits the β-lactamases of *Staphylococcus aureus*, Enterobacteriaceae with TEM-1 to -8 and SHV-1 to -5, *Klebsiella, Bacteroides, Branhmaella, Legionella*, and *Mycobacterium*. It does not inhibit the *Pseudomonas maltophilia* β-lactamase.

Sulbactam does not induce β-lactamases, nor does it select for derepressed β-lactamase–producing bacteria.

Sulbactam penetrates some bacteria less well than does clavulanate, particularly some *Klebsiella* species, but like clavulanate, it is a suicide inhibitor.

Sulbactam acts synergistically with penicillins and cephalosporins that are degraded by β-lactamases. In the presence of 8 μg/ml of sulbactam and 16 μg/ml of ampicillin, most staphylococci, *Klebsiella, Haemophilus, E. coli*, and *Bacteroides* sp. that would normally be resistant to ampicillin are inhibited.[77,78]

Pharmacology. Sulbactam has pharmacokinetics in humans similar to ampicillin.[79,80] Peak serum levels after 250 mg are 6.4 μg/ml, with 1.1 μg/ml at 4 hours.[79] Peak serum levels after im injections of 0.250 and 0.5 g are 7 and 13 μg/ml, respectively, with a serum half-life of 1.1–1.3 hours. After the iv infusion of 0.5 g, peak serum levels of 30 μg/ml are achieved, and after 1 g, 68 μg/ml are achieved. The serum half-life is 1 hours. Sulbactam is excreted by the kidney and has a urinary recovery of 70–80 percent of a dose. Biliary excretion is minimal, and metabolism is $<$25 percent. Concentrations of sulbactam in interstitial fluid and peritoneal secretions are comparable to levels in serum. Penetration of sulbactam into inflamed meninges is low, with levels of 0.1–10 μg/ml found in the CSF after a 1 g infusion. Excretion is blocked by probenecid. The half-life does not increase down to creatinine clearances of 30 ml/min. With clearances between 15 and 30, the half-life is 5.1 hours; with clearances of 5–15, the half-life is 9.2 hours, and the half-life of anuric patients is 20 hours. It can be removed by hemodialysis.

REFERENCES

1. Kahan JS, Kahan FM, Goegleman R, et al. Thienamycin, a new beta-lactam antibiotic. 1. Discovery, isolation and physical properties. J Antibiot. 1979;32:1–12.
2. Neu HC, Labthavikul P. Comparative in vitro activity of *N*-formimidoyl thienamycin against gram-positive and gram-negative aerobic and anaerobic species and its beta-lactamase stability. Antimicrob Agents Chemother. 1982;21:180–7.
3. Wise R, Andrews JM, Patel N. *N*-formimidoyl thienamycin a novel beta-lactam: An in vitro comparison with other beta-lactam antibiotics. J Antmicrob Chemother. 1981;7:521–9.
4. Jones RN. Review of the in vitro spectrum of activity of imipenem. Am J Med. 1985;78:22–32.
5. Prince AS, Neu HC. Activities of new beta-lactam antibiotics against isolates of *Pseudomonas aeruginosa* from patients with cystic fibrosis. Antimicrob Agents Chemother. 1981;20:545–6.
6. Brown JE, Del Benes VE, Collins CD. In vitro activity of *N*-formimidoyl thienamycin, moxalactam and other new beta-lactam agents against *Bacteroides fragilis*: Contribution of beta-lactamase to resistance. Antimicrob Agents Chemother. 1981;19:248–52.
7. Kesado T, Hashizume T, Ashi Y, et al. Susceptibilities of anaerobic bacteria to *N*-formimidoyl thienamycin (MK0787) and to other antibiotics. Antimicrob Agents Chemother. 1982;21:1016–22.
8. Norrby SR, Alestig K, Björngard B, et al. Urinary recovery of *N*-formimidoyl thienamycin (MK0787) as affected by coadminstration of *N*-formimidoyl thienamycin dehydropeptidase inhibitors. Antimicrob Agents Chemother. 1983;23:300–7.
9. Norrby SR, Alestig K, Ferber F, et al. Pharmacokinetics and tolerance of *N*-formimidoyl thienamycin (MK0787) in humans. Antimicrob Agents Chemother. 1983;23:293–9.
10. Drusano GL, Standiford HC, Ruslamante C, et al. Multiple dose kinetics of imipenem/cilastatin. Antimicrob Agents Chemother. 1984;26:715–21.
11. Drusano GL, Standiford HC. Pharmacokinetic profile of imipenem/cilastatin in normal volunteers. Am J Med. 1985;78:47–53.
12. Berman SJ, Sugihara JG, Nakumara JM, et al. Multiple dose study of imipenem/cilastatin in patients with end-stage renal disease undergoing long-term hemodialysis. Am J Med. 1985;78:105–8.
13. Norrby SR, Rogers JD, Ferber F, et al. Disposition of radio labeled imipenem and cilastatin in normal human volunteers. Antimicrob Agents Chemother. 1985;26:707–14.
14. Calandra GB, Ricci FM, Wang C, et al. Safety and tolerance comparison of imipenem-cilastatin to cephalothin and cefazolin. J Antimicrob Chemother. 1983;12(Suppl D):125–31.
15. Sadon A, Gilden BN, Rohr AS, et al. Immediate hypersensitivity reactions to beta-lactam antibiotics. Ann Intern Med. 1987;127:204–15.
16. Baumgardner JD, Galuser MP. Comparative imipenem treatment of *Staphylococcus aureus* endocarditis in the rat. J Antimicrob Chemother. 1983;12(Suppl D):79–87.
17. Scheld WM, Keely J. Imipenem therapy of experimental *Staphylococcus aureus* and *Streptococcus faecalis* endocarditis. J Antimicrob Chemother. 1983;12(Suppl D):69–78.
18. Johnson DE, Calia IM, Snyder MJ, et al. Imipenem therapy of *Pseudomonas aeruginosa* bacteremia in neutropenic rats. J Antimicrob Chemother. 1983;12(Suppl D):89–96.
19. MacGregor RR, Gentry LO. Imipenem/cilastatin in the treatment of osteomyelitis. Am J Med. 1985;78:92–5.
20. Marier RL. Role of impenem in the treatment of soft tissue infections. Am J Med. 1985;78:132–6.
21. Berkeley AS, Freedman K, Hirsch J, et al. Imipenem/cilastatin in the treatment of obstetric and gynecologic infections. Am J Med. 1985;78:71–6.

22. Cox CE, Corrado ML. Safety and efficacy of imipenem/cilastatin in treatment of complicated urinary tract infections. Am J Med. 1985;78:84–91.
23. Kager L, Nord CE. Imipenem/cilastatin in the treatment of intraabdominal infections: A review of worldwide experience. Rev Infect Dis. 1985;7(Suppl 3):518–21.
24. Salata RA, Gebhart RC, Palmer DL, et al. Pneumonia treated with imipenem/cilastatin. Am J Med. 1985;78:96–101.
25. Dickson G, Rodriguez K, Arcey S, et al. Efficacy of imipenem/cilastatin in endocarditis. Am J Med. 1985;78:109–18.
26. Bodey GP, Alvarez ME, Jones PG, et al. Imipenem/cilastatin as initial therapy for febrile cancer patients. Antimicrob Agents Chemother. 1986;30:211–4.
27. Gombert ME, Aulicino TM, duBouchet L, et al. Therapy of experimental cerebral nocardiosis with imipenum, amikacin, trimethoprim-sulfamethoxazole, and minocycline. Antimicrob Agents Chemother. 1986;30:270–3.
28. Ertl G, Schall K, Kochsiek K. Nocardial endocarditis of an aortic valve prosthesis. Br Heart J. 1987;57:384–6.
29. Krilov LR, Blumer JL, Stern RC, et al. Imipenem/cilastatin in acute pulmonary exacerbations of cystic fibrosis. Rev Infect Dis. 1985;7(Suppl 3):482–9.
30. Acar JF. Therapy for lower respiratory tract infections with imipenem/cilastatin: A review of worldwide experience. Rev Infect Dis. 1985;7:S513–7.
31. Sykes RB, Cimarausti CM, Bonner DP, et al. Monocyclic beta-lactam antibiotics produced by bacteria. Nature. 1981;291:489–91.
32. Neu HC, Labthavikul P. Antibacterial activity of a monocyclic beta-lactam SQ 26,776. J Antimicrob Chemother. 1981;9(Suppl E):111–2.
33. Barry AL, Thornsberry C, Jones RN, et al. Aztreonam: Antibacterial activity, beta-lactamase stability, and interpretive standards and quality control guidelines for disk-diffusion susceptibility tests. Rev Infect Dis. 1985;7(Suppl 4):594–604.
34. Sykes RB, Bonner DP, Bush K, et al. Aztreonam (SQ 26,776), a synthetic monobactam specifically active against aerobic gram-negative bacteria. Antimicrob Agents Chemother. 1982;21:85–92.
35. Henry SA, Bendush CB. Aztreonam: Worldwide overview of the treatment of patients with gram-negative infections. Am J Med. 1985;78(Suppl 2A):57–64.
36. Swabb EA, Sugerman AA, Stern M. Oral bioavailability of the monobactam aztreonam (SQ 26,776) in healthy subjects. Antimicrob Agents Chemother. 1983;23:548–550.
37. Swabb EA. Review of the clinical pharmacology of the monobactam antibiotic aztreonam. Am J Med. 1985;78(Suppl 2A):11–8.
38. Jones PG, Bodey GP, Swabb EA, et al. Clinical pharmacokinetics of aztreonam in cancer patients. Antimicrob Agents Chemother. 1984;26:455–61.
39. Janicke DM, Cafarell RF, Parker SW, et al. Pharmacokinetics of aztreonam in patients with gram-negative infections. Antimicrob Agents Chemother. 1985;27:16–20.
40. Scully BE, Swabb EA, Neu HC. Pharmacology of aztreonam after intravenous infusion. Antimicrob Agents Chemother. 1983;24:18–22.
41. Duma RJ, Berry AJ, Smith SM, et al. Penetration of aztreonam into cerebrospinal fluid of patients with and without inflammed meninges. Antimicrob Agents Chemother. 1984;26:730–3.
42. Stutman HR, Marks MI, Swabb EA. Single-dose pharmacokinetics of aztreonam in pediatric patients. Antimicrob Agents Chemother. 1984;26:196–9.
43. Fillastre JP, Leroy A, Baudoin C, et al. Pharmacokinetics of aztreonam in patients with chronic renal failure. Clin Pharmacokinet. 1985;10:91–100.
44. Mihindu JC, Scheld WM, Bolton ND, et al. Pharmacokinetics of aztreonam in patients with various degrees of renal dysfunction. Antimicrob Agents Chemother. 1983;24:252–61.
45. Gerig JS, Bolton ND, Swabb EA, et al. Effect of hemodialysis and peritoneal dialysis on aztreonam pharmacokinetics. Kidney Int. 1984;26:308–18.
46. Daikos GK. Clinical experience with aztreonam in four Mediterranean countries. Rev Infect Dis. 1985;7(Suppl 4):831–9.
47. Giamarellou H, Galanakis N, Douzinas E, et al. Evaluation of aztreonam in difficult-to-treat infections with prolonged post-treatment follow-up. Antimicrob Agents Chemother. 1984;26:245–9.
48. Gibbs RS, Blanco JD, Bernstein S. Role of aerobic gram-negative bacilli in endometritis after cesarean section. Rev Infect Dis. 1985;7(Suppl E):690–5.
49. Rodriguez JR, Ramirez-Ronda CH. Efficacy and safety of aztreonam versus tobramycin for aerobic gram-negative bacilli lower respiratory tract infections. Am J Med. 1985;78(Suppl 2A):42–3.
50. Romero-Vivas J, Rodriguez-Creixems M, Bouza E, et al. Evaluation of aztreonam in the treatment of severe bacterial infections. Antimicrob Agents Chemother. 1985;28:222–6.
51. Scully BE, Henry SA. Clinical experience with aztreonam in the treatment of gram-negative bacteremia. Rev Infect Dis. 1985;7(Suppl 4):789–93.
52. Scully BE, Neu HC. Use of aztreonam in the treatment of serious infections due to multiresistant gram-negative organisms, including *Pseudomonas aeruginosa*. Am J Med. 1985;78:251–61.
53. Scully BE, Ores CN, Prince AS, et al. Treatment of lower respiratory tract infections due to *Pseudomonas aeruginosa* in patients with cystic fibrosis. Rev Infect Dis. 1985;7(Suppl):669–74.
54. Simons WJ, Lee TJ. Aztreonam in the treatment of bone and joint infections caused by gram-negative bacilli. Rev Infect Dis. 1985;7(Suppl 4):783–8.
55. Gudiol F, Pallares R, Ariza X, et al. Comparative clinical evaluation of aztreonam versus aminoglycosides in gram-negative septicaemia. J Antimicrob Chemother. 1986;17:661–71.
56. Reading C, Cole M. Clavulanic acid: A beta-lactamase inhibiting beta-lactam from *Streptomyces clavuligerus*. Antimicrob Agents Chemother. 1977;11:852–7.
57. Neu HC, Fu KP. Clavulanic acid: A beta-lactamase–inhibiting beta-lactamase. Antimicrob Agents Chemother. 1978;14:650–5.
58. Richmond MM, Sykes RB. The beta-lactamases of gram-negative bacteria and their possible physiological role. Adv Microb Physiol. 1973;9:31–88.
59. Neu HC. The contribution of beta-lactamases to bacterial resistance and mechanisms to inhibit beta-lactamases. Am J Med. 1986;79(Suppl 5B):2–12.
60. Neu HC. The role of beta-lactamase inhibitors in chemotherapy. In: Tipper PJ, ed. Antibiotic Inhibitors of Bacterial Cell Wall Biosynthesis. Oxford: Pergamon Press; 1987:241–58.
61. Neu HC. Penicillin-binding proteins and beta-lactamases: Their effects on the use of cephalosporins and other new beta-lactams. In: Remington JS, Swartz MN, eds. Current Clinical Topics in Infectious Diseases. New York: McGraw-Hill; 1987:37–83.
62. Bush K: Recent developments in beta-lactamase research and their implications for the future. Rev Infect Dis. 1988;10:681–90.
63. Munch P, Luthy R, Blaser J, et al. Human pharmacokinetics and CSF penetration of clavulanic acid. J Antimicrob Chemother. 1981;8:29–37.
64. Adam D, Visser I, Koeppe P. Pharmacokinetics of amoxicillin and clavulanic acid administered alone and in combination. Antimicrob Agents Chemother. 1982;22:353–7.
65. Nelson JD, Kusmiesz H, Shelton S. Pharmacokinetics of potassium clavulanate in combination with amoxicillin in pediatric patients. Antimicrob Agents Chemother. 1982;21:681–2.
66. Schaad UB, Casey PA, Copper DL. Single-dose pharmacokinetics of intravenous clavulanic acid with amoxicillin in pediatric patients. Antimicrob Agents Chemother. 1983;23:252–5.
67. Bennett S, Wise R, Weston D, et al. Pharmacokinetics and tissue penetration of ticarcillin combined with clavulanic acid. Antimicrob Agents Chemother. 1983;23:831–4.
68. Scully BE, Chin NX, Neu HC. Pharmacology of ticarcillin combined with clavulanic acid in humans. Am J Med. 1985;79(Suppl 5B):39–43.
69. Jackson D, Cockburn A, Cooper DL, et al. Clinical pharmacology and safety evaluation of Timentin. Am J Med. 1985;79(Suppl 5B):44–55.
70. Walsted RA, Hellum KB, Thurmann-Nielson E, et al. Pharmacokinetics and tissue penetration of Timentin: A simultaneous study of serum, urine, lymph, suction blister, and subcutaneous treatment fluid. J Antimicrob Chemother. 1986;17(Suppl C):71–80.
71. Kaleida PH, Bluestone DC, Rockette HE, et al. Amoxicillin-clavulanate potassium compared with cefaclor for acute otitis media in infants and children. Pediatr Infect Dis. 1987;6:265–71.
72. Neu HC, ed. Progress and perspectives on beta-lactamase inhibition: a review of Augmentin. Postgrad Med. 1984;3–295.
73. Neu HC, ed. Beta-lactamase inhibition: Therapeutic advances. Am J Med. 1985;79(Suppl 5B):1–196.
74. Gentry LO, Macko V, Lind R, et al. Ticarcillin plus clavulanic acid (Timentin) therapy for osteomyelitis. Am J Med. 1985;79(Suppl 5B):116–21.
75. Leigh DA, Phillips I, Wise R, eds. Timentin-ticarcillin plus clavulanic acid, a laboratory and clinical perspective. J Antimicrob Chemother. 1986;17(Suppl C):1–244.
76. Aswapokee N, Neu HC. A sulfone, beta-lactam compound which acts as a beta-lactamase inhibitor. J Antibiot. 1978;31:1238–43.
77. Retsema VA, English AR, Girard AR. CP-45,899 in combination with penicillin or ampicillin against penicillin-resistant staphylococci. Antimicrob Agents Chemother. 1980;17:615–22.
78. Jones RN. In vitro evaluation of aminopenicillin–beta-lactamase inhibitor combinations. Drugs. 1988;36(Suppl 7):17–26.
79. Foulds G, Stankewich JP, Marshall DC, et al. Pharmacokinetics of sulbactam in humans. Antimicrob Agents Chemother. 1983;23:692–9.
80. Hampel B, Lode H, Bruchnor G, et al. Comparative pharmacokinetics of sulbactam/ampicillin and clavulanic acid/amoxicillin in human volunteers. Drugs. 1988;35(Suppl 7):29–33.
81. Guneren MF. Clinical experience with intramuscular sulbactam/ampicillin in the out-patient treatment of various infections: A multicenter trial. Drugs. 1988;35(Suppl 7):57–68.
82. Dajani AS. Sulbactam/ampicillin in pediatric infections. Drugs. 1988;35(Suppl 7):35–8.
83. Kass EH, Lode H, eds. Enzyme-mediated resistance to beta-lactam antibiotics: A symposium on sulbactam/ampicillin. Rev Infect Dis. 1986;8(Suppl 5):465–650.
84. Reinhardt JF, Johnston L, Ruane P, et al. A randomized, double-blind comparison of sulbactam/ampicillin and clindamycin for the treatment of aerobic and aerobic-anaerobic infections. Rev Infect Dis. 1986;8(Suppl 5):569–75.
85. Hemsell DL, Heard MC, Hemsell PG, et al. Sulbactam/ampicillin versus cefoxitin for uncomplicated and complicated acute pelvic inflammatory disease. Drugs. 1988;35(Suppl 7):39–42.
86. Rodriguez WJ, Kahn WN, Puig N, et al. Sulbactam/ampicillin vs. chloramphenicol/ampicillin for the treatment of meningitis in infants and children. Rev Infect Dis. 1986;8(Suppl 5):620–9.
87. Wald E, Reilly JS, Bluestone CD, et al. Sulbactam/ampicillin in the treatment of acute epiglottis in children. Rev Infect Dis. 1986;8(Suppl 5):617–9.

21. β-LACTAM ALLERGY

MICHAEL E. WEISS
N. FRANKLIN ADKINSON

After the clinical introduction of penicillin in the mid-1940s, it soon became clear that its principal toxicity was allergic in origin. The first reported case of anaphylaxis due to penicillin was in 1946,[1] and the first reported death was in 1949.[2] Subsequently, a broad spectrum of allergic reactions to β-lactam antibiotics have been recognized. Allergic reactions occur in 0.7–4 percent of penicillin treatment courses.[3]

REACTIONS

Gell and Coombs have classified four types of immunopathologic reactions,[4] all of which have been seen with penicillin (Table 1).

Type I—Immediate Hypersensitivity

These reactions result from the interaction of penicillin haptenic determinants with preformed penicillin-specific IgE antibodies that are bound to tissue mast cells and/or circulating basophils via high-affinity IgE receptors. Cross-linking of two or more IgE receptors by penicillin antigens leads to the release of both preformed (histamine, proteases, and chemotactic factors) and newly generated (prostaglandins, leukotrienes, and platelet activating factor) mediators from cell membrane phospholipids.[5] Release of these mediators can lead to urticaria, laryngeal edema, and bronchospasm with or without cardiovascular collapse. Anaphylactic reactions occur in 0.004–0.015 percent of penicillin treatment courses.[6] Fatality from penicillin anaphylaxis occurs about once in every 50,000–100,000 treatment courses.[6] β-Adrenergic antagonists apparently increase the risk of a fatal outcome from anaphylaxis by rendering treatment more difficult.[7] IgE-mediated reactions may be the most important allergic reaction to β-lactam drugs clinically, because of the risk of life-threatening anaphylaxis.

Type II—Cytotoxic Antibodies (Usually IgG and/or IgM)

Penicillin determinants can become chemically bound to circulating blood cells (or renal interstitial cells), leading to their accelerated destruction via IgG or IgM antibodies and complement. Long-term, high-dose penicillin treatment is usually required for this form of immunopathology. Interstitial nephritis, seen most frequently with methicillin, may also be caused by a type II mechanism.

Type III—Immune Complexes

Penicillin-specific IgG or IgM antibodies form circulating complexes with penicillin haptenized to serum proteins, largely albumin. These circulating complexes can fix complement and then lodge in tissue sites, causing serum sickness and possibly drug fever. Immune complex reactions typically appear 7–14 days after the initiation of high-dose β-lactam therapy; the syndrome sometimes appears after termination of therapy.

Type IV—Cell-mediated Hypersensitivity

Contact dermatitis from penicillin involves drug-sensitized, thymus-derived lymphocytes. The high rate of penicillin contact dermatitis (5–10 percent) in the 1940s led to the discontinuation of its use as a topical antibiotic. Contact dermatitis is still occasionally seen in individuals who are occupationally exposed to penicillins, particularly those involved in antibiotic manufacturing and packaging.[6,8]

Idiopathic Reactions

Some reactions to β-lactam antibiotics have an obscure pathogenesis. Among these are the very common maculopapular rash that appears late in the treatment course in 2–3 percent of penicillin treatments. Ampicillin-induced rashes occur with much greater frequency (5.2–9.5 percent of treatment courses in uncomplicated cases).[9–11] When ampicillin is given during infections with Epstein-Barr virus or cytomegalovirus, or to patients with acute lymphocytic leukemia, a much higher incidence of rash (69–100 percent) occurs.[12] The participation of immune mechanisms in the origin of the measles-like (non-urticarial) rash is unclear. Exfoliative dermatitis and the Stevens-Johnson syndrome also have obscure immunologic origins. Pseudoanaphylactic reactions have been observed after im or inadvertent iv injection of procaine penicillin. These reactions are probably due to a combination of toxic and embolic phenomena from procaine.[13]

Levine proposed a classification of adverse reactions to penicillin according to their time of onset[14] (Table 2). Immediate reactions occur within the first hour after penicillin administration, and they are almost always IgE-mediated (anaphylaxis and urticaria). Accelerated reactions occur 1–72 hours after initial treatment with penicillin; they most commonly involve urticaria. Late reactions begin more than 72 hours after the onset of penicillin therapy. Anaphylaxis does not occur later in the course of continuous β-lactam therapy; maculopapular erup-

TABLE 1. Classification of Immunopathologic Reactions to Penicillin

Type[a] of reaction	Description	Primary Effector Mechanism(s): Antibody	Cells	Other	Clinical Reactions
I	Anaphylactic (reaginic) hypersensitivity	IgE	Basophils, mast cells		Anaphylaxis, urticaria
II	Cytotoxic or cytolytic damage	IgG IgM	Any cell with isoantigen	C′, RES	Coombs + hemolytic anemia; drug-induced nephritis
III	Immune complex disease	Soluble immune complexes (Ag-Ab)	None directly	C′	Serum sickness; drug fever
IV	"Delayed" or cell-mediated hypersensitivity	None known	Sensitized T lymphocytes		Contact dermatitis
V	Idiopathic	IgM(?) ? ? ?	? ? ? ?	? ? ? ?	Maculopapular eruptions Eosinophilia Stevens-Johnson syndrome Exfoliative dermatitis

[a] According to the scheme of Gell and Coombs.[4]
Abbreviations: C′: complement; RES: reticuloendothelial system; Ag-Ab: antigen-antibody; (?): immunopathologic mechanism in doubt.

TABLE 2. Classification of Allergic Reactions to Penicillin

Reaction Type	*Onset*	*Spectrum of Clinical Reactions*
Immediate	0–1 hr	Anaphylaxis Hypotension Laryngeal edema Urticarial/angioedema Wheezing
Accelerated	1–72 hr	Urticaria/angioedema Laryngeal edema Wheezing
Late	>72 hr	Morbilliform rash Interstitial nephritis Hemolytic anemia Neutropenia Thrombocytopenia Serum Sickness Drug fever Stevens-Johnson syndrome Exfoliative dermatitis

(Adapted from Levine,[14] with permission.)

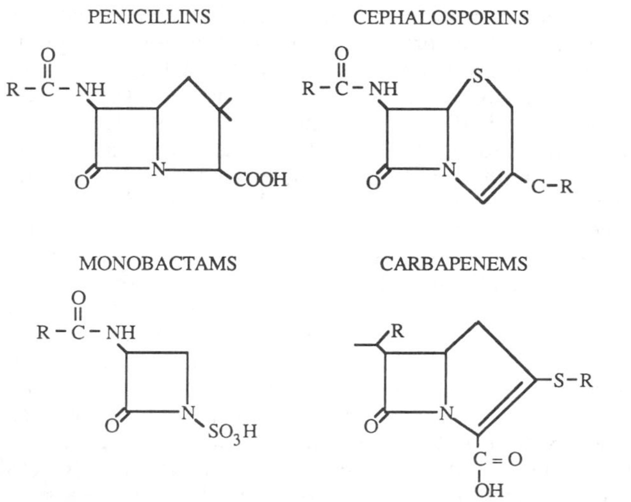

FIG. 1. Structure of the four classes of β-lactam antibiotics in use today. All contain the four-membered β-lactam ring.

tions are most common, but types II–IV reactions also occur in this time frame.

IMMUNOCHEMISTRY

Penicillins consist of a β-lactam ring, on which antimicrobial activity depends, and a five-membered thiazolidine ring (Fig. 1). Penicillin (MW 356) is a low molecular weight chemical and as such must first covalently combine with tissue macromolecules (presumably proteins) to produce multivalent hapten-protein complexes, which are required both for the induction of an immune response and the elicitation of an allergic reaction.[15]

Levine and Parker showed that the β-lactam ring spontaneously opens under physiologic conditions forming the penicilloyl group.[16] This penicilloyl group has been designated the *major determinant* because about 95 percent of the penicillin molecules that irreversibly combine with protein form penicilloyl groups (Fig. 2).[14] Recent evidence suggests that penicillin haptenization is facilitated by dializable serum molecules.[16a] This reaction occurs with the prototype benzylpenicillin and virtually all semisynthetic penicillins. Multiple penicilloyl determinants have been synthetically coupled to a weakly immunogenic polylysine carrier molecule to form penicilloyl-polylysine (PPL), which has been successfully used as a skin test reagent for the detection of penicilloyl IgE antibody.[17]

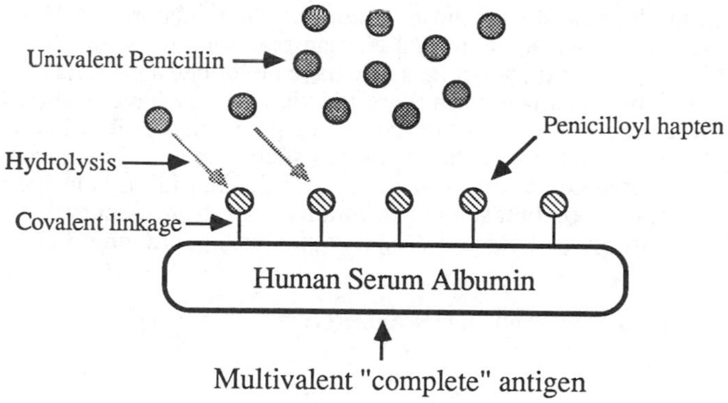

FIG. 2. Formation of penicilloyl-protein conjugates.

Benzylpenicillin can also be degraded by other metabolic pathways to form additional antigenic determinants.[18] These derivatives are formed in small quantities and stimulate a variable immune response; hence they have been termed the *minor determinants*. Because some of the determinants are labile and cannot be readily synthesized in multivalent form, skin testing for minor determinant specificities is usually accomplished using a mixture of benzylpenicillin, its alkaline hydrolysis product (benzylpenicilloate), and its acid hydrolysis product (benzylpenilloate), collectively called the *minor determinant mixture* (MDM). Therefore, for penicillin and other β-lactams, IgE antibodies can be produced against a number of haptenic derivatives labeled the major and minor determinants.

Anaphylactic reactions to penicillin are usually mediated by IgE antibodies directed against minor determinants, although some anaphylactic reactions have occurred in patients with only penicilloyl-specific IgE antibodies.[14,18,19] Accelerated and late urticarial reactions are generally mediated by penicilloyl-specific IgE antibody (major determinant).[14]

RISK FACTORS FOR IgE-DEPENDENT PENICILLIN REACTIONS

It is generally agreed, despite sparse evidence, that penicillin reactions occur less frequently in both children and the elderly than in nonelderly adults.[20,21] Although the frequency of anaphylactic reactions may be less in the elderly, fatal outcomes are more common due to compromised cardiopulmonary reserve.

Serial measurements in patients who mounted an immune response to penicillin showed that the half-life of penicilloyl-specific IgE antibody ranged from as short as 10 days to an indeterminantly long interval (more than 1,000 days).[22] An individual whose penicillin-specific IgE antibody response persists is at greater cumulative risk for allergic reactions to penicillin than one whose IgE antibody quickly disappears. Recent evidence suggests that as a group, patients allergic to penicillin dehaptenate penicillin determinants from albumin more slowly than non-penicillin-allergic subjects.[23]

A history of atopy does not seem to be an independent risk factor for the development of penicillin allergy,[20,22] although atopic individuals may be predisposed to fatal reactions to penicillin should anaphylaxis occur.[6]

Parenteral administration of penicillin produces more allergic reactions than orally administered penicillin.[24] Recent evidence suggests that this may be more related to dose than route of administration. When higher oral doses are given, as in the treatment of gonorrhea, the incidence of allergic reactions is no different from that of im procaine penicillin at a comparable dose.[25]

Individuals with a history of a prior penicillin reaction have a four- to sixfold increased risk of subsequent reactions to penicillin compared with those without previous histories.[20] However, most serious and fatal allergic reactions to β-lactam antibiotics occur in individuals who have never had a prior allergic reaction. Sensitization in these individuals may have occurred from their last therapeutic course of penicillin or (less likely) via occult environmental exposures such as milk or meat from cows treated with penicillin,[26] penicillin in other food sources,[2,27] or breast milk in infants,[21] or from occupational exposure in medical and drug manufacturing personnel.[8]

TESTING FOR PENICILLIN ALLERGY

Skin Tests

The most useful single piece of information in assessing an individual's potential for an immediate IgE-mediated reaction is his skin test response to major (PPL) and minor (MDM) penicillin determinants. When therapeutic doses of penicillin are given to patients with histories of penicillin allergy but with negative skin tests to PPL and MDM, IgE-mediated reactions occur very rarely and are almost always mild and self-limited. About 1 percent of skin test-negative patients will develop accelerated urticarial reactions, and approximately 3 percent will develop other mild reactions.[28] Penicillin anaphylaxis has not been reported in skin test-negative patients. Therefore negative skin tests indicate that β-lactam antibiotics may be safely given.

A limited number of skin test-positive patients have been treated with therapeutic doses of penicillin. The risk of an acute immediate or accelerated allergic reaction ranges from about 10 percent in history-negative subjects to 50–70 percent in history-positive subjects (Fig. 3).[28] The risk appears, with limited experience, to be somewhat higher when patients have positive skin tests to minor determinant reagents.[29] Therefore, if skin tests are positive, an equally effective, non-cross reacting antibiotic should be substituted when available. Since semisynthetic penicillins contain the same nucleus as penicillin G, and since the nuclear conformation determines the major antigenic specificity, skin testing with reagents derived from semisynthetic penicillins is generally not necessary.[30]

Skin testing to penicillin preferably should be done immediately before its intended use and repeated before each course of β-lactam therapy in patients with a history of an IgE-dependent reaction. Patients with a history of exfoliative dermatitis or Stevens-Johnson or Lyell syndromes, reactions that constitute nearly absolute contraindications for penicillin administration, should not be evaluated by skin testing. Skin tests have no predictive value in non-IgE-mediated reactions, such as serum sickness, hemolytic anemia, drug fever, interstitial nephritis, contact dermatitis, exfoliative dermatitis, or maculopapular exanthems.

In numerous studies in which both PPL and minor determinant skin tests were performed, only 7–35 percent of patients who gave histories of penicillin allergy were skin test-positive to either reagent,[28] although one study found a positive rate of 63 percent.[31] In general, with increasing time from the allergic reaction to penicillin, the prevalence of positive skin tests to penicillin determinants decreases, although some patients have penicillin-specific IgE antibody indefinitely.[31,32] Therefore skin tests in patients who gave a history of penicillin allergy confirm that 65–93 percent can safely be given a β-lactam antibiotic. With negative histories of penicillin allergy, the rate of positive skin tests is about 2 percent (Fig. 3).[33]

Ideally, all patients should be skin tested before receiving β-lactam drugs, but a systematic study of routine skin testing in history-negative patients from a sexually transmitted disease clinic indicated that such testing is probably not cost-effective.[33] Therefore we believe skin testing should be restricted to patients with a history of prior penicillin allergy for whom a β-lactam antibiotic is presently the indicated drug of choice.

A scratch or puncture (epicutaneous) test should be performed first. If there is no induration (or systemic symptoms) after 15 minutes, duplicate intradermal injections are placed, raising 3–4-mm blebs. Testing should be done with PPL, MDM, a positive control (histamine phosphate, 100 μg/ml), and a negative diluent control. The diameter of induration at 15–20 minutes is read; if it is greater than 5 mm, the test is considered positive.[34] Antihistamines, tricyclic antidepressants, and adrenergic drugs, all of which may inhibit skin test results, should be discontinued at least 24 hours prior to skin testing. Antihistamines with long half-lives (hydroxyzine, terfenadine, astemazole, etc.) may attenuate skin test results up to a week, or longer after discontinuation. Unfortunately, a minor determinant mixture is not commercially available in the United States at present. A minor determinant mixture can be prepared as described previously,[34] or benzylpenicillin can be used as the sole minor determinant reagent.

Presently only PPL (PRE-PEN; Kremers-Urban) at a concentration of 6×10^{-5} M (re: penicilloyl) is commercially available in the United States for use as a skin test reagent. Use of PPL alone would miss between 10 and 25 percent of all positive

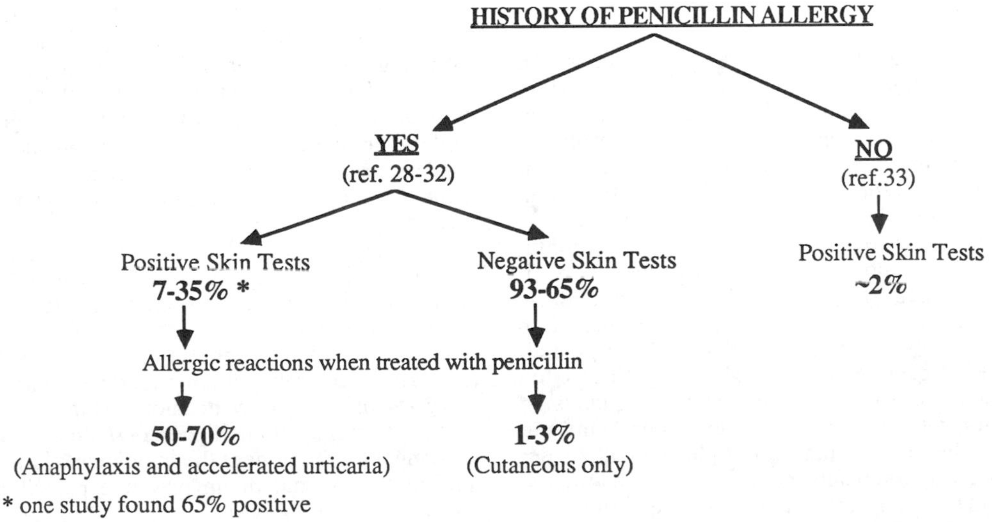

FIG. 3. Prevalence of positive and negative skin tests, and subsequent allergic reactions in patients treated with penicillin (based on studies using both penicilloyl-polylysine and minor determinant mixture as skin test reagents).

skin test reactions.[3,31] If one uses benzylpenicillin diluted to a concentration of 10,000 units/ml (10^{-2} M) as the sole minor determinant reagent, about 5–10 percent of skin test-reactive patients will be missed.[3,31] However, some of those missed may be at risk for serious, anaphylactic reactions.[35] Nevertheless, this is a reasonable alternative to MDM for use in patients *without* impressive histories of IgE-mediated reactions. Unfortunately, the lack of general access to a licensed minor determinant reagent has hindered the general application of penicillin skin testing for risk assessment.

When properly performed with due consideration for preliminary scratch tests and appropriate dilutions, skin testing with penicillin reagents can almost always be safely accomplished. Systemic reactions accompany about 1 percent of positive skin tests[36]; these are usually mild but can be serious. Therefore skin tests should be done in the presence of a physician and with immediate access to medications and equipment needed to treat anaphylaxis.

Other Tests

Solid-phase immunoassays such as the radioallergosorbent test (RAST) have been developed to detect serum IgE antibodies directed against the penicilloyl determinant. At present there is no in vitro RAST for minor determinant antibodies.[34] The penicilloyl-specific RAST is positive in 60–95 percent of patients with a positive skin test to PPL. Because it is more time-consuming, more expensive, less sensitive for detection of the major determinant IgE than skin testing, and unavailable for minor determinant detection, the RAST and other in vitro analogs have limited clinical utility.

MONITORING PATIENTS TREATED WITH β-LACTAM ANTIBIOTICS

Traditionally, outpatients treated with parenteral β-lactam antibiotics have been observed for 30 minutes following treatment. As most anaphylactic reactions to β-lactam antibiotics occur within 30 minutes of dosing,[6] this is a reasonable observation period. We have shown that a high-dose oral treatment (e.g., ampicillin 3.5 g with probenecid) is as likely to cause allergic reactions as comparable doses of parenteral procaine penicillin.[25] Therefore it is suggested that patients treated with high-dose oral β-lactam antibiotics be observed for 30 minutes also. More worrisome patients, such as those with histories of acute allergic reactions to penicillin in whom skin testing has not been done, should be observed for longer periods if they must receive β-lactams without skin testing. For such patients treated orally or parenterally as outpatients, 2 hours is a reasonable period for observation. For hospitalized patients considered at risk, the first intravenous dose may be infused slowly over a 1–2-hour period, sacrificing the initial peak antibiotic level, to observe for signs of an allergic reaction.

TABLE 3. Oral Desensitization Protocol

Step[a]	Phenoxymethyl Penicillin (units/ml)	Amount (ml)	Dose (units)	Cumulative Dosage (units)
1	1,000	0.1	100	100
2	1,000	0.2	200	300
3	1,000	0.4	400	700
4	1,000	0.8	800	1,500
5	1,000	1.6	1,600	3,100
6	1,000	3.2	3,200	6,300
7	1,000	6.4	6,400	12,700
8	10,000	1.2	12,000	24,700
9	10,000	2.4	24,000	48,700
10	10,000	4.8	48,000	96,700
11	80,000	1.0	80,000	176,700
12	80,000	2.0	160,000	336,700
13	80,000	4.0	320,000	656,700
14	80,000	8.0	640,000	1,296,700
Observe patient for 30 minutes				
Change to benzylpenicillin G iv				
15	500,000	0.25	125,000	
16	500,000	0.50	250,000	
17	500,000	1.00	500,000	
18	500,000	2.25	1,125,000	

[a] Interval between steps, 15 min.
(Adapted from Sullivan,[36] with permission.)

TABLE 4. Parenteral Desensitization Protocol: Typical Schedule

Injection No.	Benzylpenicillin Concentration (units/ml)	Vol. and Route (cc)[a]
1[b]	100	0.1 id
2	↓	0.2 sc
3	↓	0.4 sc
4	↓	0.8 sc
5[b]	1,000	0.1 id
6	↓	0.3 sc
7	↓	0.6 sc
8[b]	10,000	0.1 id
9	↓	0.2 sc
10	↓	0.4 sc
11	↓	0.8 sc
12[b]	100,000	0.1 id
13	↓	0.3 sc
14	↓	0.6 sc
15[b]	1,000,000	0.1 id
16	↓	0.2 sc
17	↓	0.2 im
18	↓	0.4 im
19	Continuous iv infusion (1,,000,000 units/hr)	

[a] Administer progressive doses at intervals of not less than 20 minutes
[b] Observe and record skin wheal and flare response to intradermal dose.
Abbreviations: id: intradermal; sc: subcutaneous; im: intramuscular; iv: intravenous.

PENICILLIN DESENSITIZATION

Effective, non-cross reacting alternative antibiotics to penicillin are usually available for patients with positive penicillin skin tests. If alternative drugs fail, induce unacceptable side effects, or are clearly less effective, then the administration of a penicillin using a desensitization protocol may be justified. Infections in which this may be considered include subacute bacterial endocarditis due to enterococci, brain abscess, bacterial meningitis, overwhelming infections with staphylococci or *Pseudomonas* organisms such as osteomyelitis or sepsis, *Listeria* infections, neurosyphilis, or syphilis during pregnancy. Use of a desensitization protocol for penicillin skin test-positive patients markedly reduces the risk of anaphylaxis.

Acute penicillin desensitization should only be performed in an intensive care setting. Any remedial risk factor should be corrected. All β-adrenergic antagonists such as propranolol or even timolol ophthalmic drops should be discontinued. Asthmatic patients should be under optimal control. An intravenous line should be established, baseline electrocardiogram (ECG) and spirometry should be performed, and continuous ECG monitoring should be instituted. Premedication with antihistamines or steroids is not recommended, as these drugs have not proven effective in suppressing severe reactions but may mask early signs of reactivity that would otherwise result in a modification of the protocol.[37,38]

Protocols have been developed for penicillin desensitization using both the oral and parenteral route[24,39] (Tables 3 and 4). As of 1987 there were 93 reported cases of oral desensitization, 74 of which were done by Sullivan and his collaborators.[40] Of these 74 patients, 32 percent experienced a transient allergic reaction either during desensitization (one-third) or during penicillin treatment after desensitization (two-thirds). These reactions were usually mild and self-limited in nature. Only one

IgE-mediated reaction (wheezing and bronchospasm) required discontinuation of the procedure before desensitization could be completed.[41] It has been argued that oral desensitization may be safer than parenteral desensitization,[39] but most patients can also be safely desensitized by the parenteral route.[42]

During desensitization any dose that causes mild systemic reactions such as pruritus, fleeting urticaria, rhinitis, or mild wheezing should be repeated until the patient tolerates the dose without systemic symptoms or signs. More serious reactions such as hypotension, laryngeal edema, or asthma require appropriate treatment, and if desensitization is continued, the dose should be decreased by at least 10-fold and withheld until the patient is stable.[39]

Once desensitized, the patient's treatment with penicillin must not lapse or the risk of an allergic reaction increases. If the patient requires a β-lactam antibiotic in the future and still remains skin test-positive to penicillin reagents, desensitization would be required again.

Several patients have been maintained on long-term, low-dose penicillin therapy (usually bid-tid) to sustain a chronic state of desensitization. Such individuals usually require chronic desensitization because of continuous occupationally related exposures to β-lactam drugs.[43,44]

ALLERGY TO OTHER β-LACTAM ANTIBIOTICS

Cephalosporins

Like penicillin, cephalosporins possess a β-lactam ring, but the five-member thiazolidine ring is replaced by the six-member dihydrothiazine ring (Fig. 1). Shortly after the cephalosporins came into clinical use, allergic reactions including anaphylaxis were reported, and the question of cross-reactivity between cephalosporins and penicillins was raised.[45] Complicating matters, the early cephalosporin antibiotics were contaminated with trace amounts of penicillin,[46] potentially leading to overestimates of the degree of cross-reactivity. Nevertheless, studies in both animals and man have clearly demonstrated cross-reactivity between penicillins and the cephalosporins using immuno- and bioassays to evaluate IgG, IgM, and IgE antibodies.[47–49]

When patients with positive skin tests to any penicillin reagents are skin tested with native cephalosporins (relevant degradation products are unknown), approximately 50 percent are positive,[31,50] but some of these studies used concentrations of cephalosporins above 1 mg/ml, which tends to give irritative, false-positive reactions in the skin. Very few cephalosporin skin test-positive individuals have been challenged with cephalosporins to allow estimation of the predictive value of a positive skin test. Small numbers of penicillin skin test-positive patients have been treated with cephalosporin antibiotics without allergic reactions.[51,52] Primary cephalosporin allergy in non-penicillin-allergic patients has been reported, but the exact incidence is not clear.[53,54]

The incidence of clinically relevant cross-reactivity between the penicillins and the cephalosporins is probably small, but rare cases of life-threatening anaphylactic cross-reactivity have occurred. There is no proven test to predict cephalosporin hypersensitivity. Patients with positive skin tests to any penicillin reagents probably should not receive cephalosporin antibiotics unless alternative drugs are clearly less desirable. If cephalosporin drugs are to be used, they should be administered with caution using a modified desensitization protocol.

Monobactams

The monobactams are a new group of β-lactam antibiotics that contain a monocyclic ring structure rather than the bicyclic structure of the penicillins and cephalosporins (Fig. 2). In animal studies, aztreonam, a monobactam prototype, showed negligible cross-reactivity with either benzylpenicillin or cephalothin.[55] Skin tests with azetreonam determinants analogous to the major and minor penicillin determinants were undertaken in patients with positive skin tests to penicillin; these tests also failed to demonstrate appreciable cross-reactivity between penicillin and aztreonam.[56] Out of 72 penicillin-allergic patients, 4 showed weak skin test responses to one or more aztreonam reagents.[56,57] In a subsequent trial, 20 patients with positive penicillin skin tests were treated with therapeutic doses of aztreonam, and none had IgE-mediated reactions.[57] Taken together, these data suggest weak cross-reactivity between aztreonam and other β-lactam antibiotics and indicate that aztreonam may be safely administered to most if not all penicillin-allergic subjects. Preliminary studies also suggest that the immunogenicity of aztreonam appears to be lower than penicillins and cephalosporins.[55]

Carbapenems

Another new class of β-lactam antibiotics are the carbapenems, of which imipenem is the prototype. Like penicillin, this class of β-lactams has a bicyclic nucleus containing a β-lactam ring and an adjacent five-membered ring (Fig. 1). Recent studies showed that 9 of 20 penicillin skin test-positive patients had positive skin reactions to analogous imipenem determinants, suggesting appreciable cross-reactivity and indicating the prudence of withholding carbapenems from penicillin skin test-positive patients.[58]

REFERENCES

1. Gorevic PD. Drug-induced autoimmune disease. In: Kaplan A, ed. Allergy. New York: Churchill Livingston; 1985:480.
2. Schwartz HJ, Sher TH. Anaphylaxis to penicillin in a frozen dinner. Ann Allergy. 1984;52:342–3.
3. Parker CW. Drug therapy (first of three parts). N Engl J Med. 1975;292:511.
4. Gell PGH, Coombs RRA. Classification of allergic reactions responsible for clinical hypersensitivity and disease. In: Gell PGH, Coombs RRA, Hachmann PJ, eds. Clinical Aspects of Immunology. Oxford: Blackwell Scientific Publications; 1975:761–82.
5. Plaut M, Lichtenstein LM. Cellular and chemical basis of the allergic inflammatory response. In: Middleton E Jr, Reed CE, Ellis EF, eds. Allergy: Principles and Practice. St. Louis: CV Mosby; 1983:119–46.
6. Idsoe O, Guthe T, Willcox RR, et al. Nature and extent of penicillin side-reactions, with particular reference to fatalities from anaphylactic shock. Bull World Health Org. 1968;38:159–88.
7. Jacobs RL, Geoffrey WR Jr, Fournier DC, et al. Potentiated anaphylaxis in patients with drug-induced beta-adrenergic blockade. J Allergy Clin Immunol. 1981;68:125–7.
8. Shmunes E, Taylor JS, Petz LD, et al. Immunologic reactions in penicillin factory workers. Ann Allergy. 1976;36:313.
9. Levine B. Skin rashes with penicillin therapy: current management. N Engl J Med. 1972;286:42.
10. Shapiro S, Siskin V, Slone D, et al. Drug rash with ampicillin and other penicillins. Lancet. 1969; 2:7628.
11. Arndt KA, Jick H. Rates of cutaneous reactions to drugs. A report from the Boston Collaborative Drug Surveillance Program. JAMA. 1976;235:918–22.
12. Kerns DL, Shira JE, Go S, et al. Ampicillin rash in children. Relationship to penicillin allergy and infectious mononucleosis. Am J Dis Child. 1973;125:187.
13. Galpin JE, Chow AW, Yoshikawa TT, et al. "Pseudoanaphylactic" reactions from inadvertent infusion of procaine penicillin G. Ann Intern Med. 1974;81:358.
14. Levine BB. Immunologic mechanisms of penicillin allergy. A haptenic model system for the study of allergic diseases of man. N Engl J Med. 1987;275:1115.
15. Eisen HN. Hypersensitivity to simple chemicals. In: Lawrence HS, ed. Cellular and Humoral Aspects of the Hypersensitive States. New York: PB Hoeber, 1959.
16. Levine BB. Immunochemical mechanisms involved in penicillin hypersensitivity in experimental animals and in human beings. Fed Proc. 1965;24:45.

16a. Lee M, Sullivan T. Facilitated haptenation of human proteins by penicillin (Abstract). J Allergy Clin Immunol. 1989;83:255.

17. Parker CW. The immunochemical basis for penicillin allergy. Postgrad Med J. 1964;40:141–55.
18. Levine BB, Redmond AP. Minor haptenic determinant-specific reagins of penicillin hypersensitivity in man. Int Arch Allergy. 1969;35:445–55.
19. Levine BB, Redmond AP, Fellner MJ, et al. Penicillin allergy and the heterogeneous immune responses of man to benzylpenicillin. J Clin Invest. 1966;45:1895.

20. Sogn DD. Prevention of allergic reactions to penicillin. J Allergy Clin Immunol. 1987;78:1051.
21. Sogn DD. Penicillin allergy. J Allergy Clin Immunol. 1984;74:589.
22. Adkinson NF Jr. Risk factors for drug allergy. J Allergy Clin Immunol. 1984;74:567–72.
23. Sullivan TJ. Dehaptenation of albumin substituted with benzylpenicillin G determinants (Abstract). J Allergy Clin Immunol. 1988;81:222.
24. Sullivan TJ, Yecies LD, Shatz GS, et al. Desensitization of patients allergic to penicillin using orally administered beta-lactam antibiotics. J Allergy Clin Immunol. 1982;69:275–82.
25. Adkinson NF Jr, Wheeler B. Risk factors for IgE-dependent reactions to penicillin. In: Kerr JW, Ganderton MA, eds. XI International Congress of Allergology and Clinical Immunology. London: Macmillan; 1983;55–9.
26. Wicher K, Reisman RE, Arbesman CE. Allergic reaction to penicillin present in milk. JAMA. 1969;208:143–5.
27. Wicher K, Reisman RE. Anaphylactic reaction to penicillin (or penicillin-like substance) in a soft drink. J Allergy Clin Immunol. 1980;66:155–7.
28. Weiss ME, Adkinson NF Jr. Immediate hypersensitivity reactions to penicillin and related antibiotics. Clin Allergy. 1988;18:515–40.
29. Levine BB, Zolov DM. Prediction of penicillin allergy by immunological tests. J Allergy. 1969;43:231.
30. Warrington RJ, Simons FER, Ho HW, et al. Diagnosis of penicillin allergy by skin testing: the Manitoba experience. CMA J. 1978;11:787.
31. Sullivan TJ, Wedner HJ, Shatz GS, et al. Skin testing to detect penicillin allergy. J Allergy Clin Immunol. 1981;68:171–80.
32. Chandra RK, Joglekar SA, Tomas E. Penicillin allergy: antipenicillin IgE antibodies and immediate hypersensitivity skin reactions employing major and minor determinants of penicillin. Arch Dis Child. 1980;55:857–60.
33. Adkinson NF Jr, Spence M, Wheeler B. Randomized clinical trial of routine penicillin skin testing (Abstract). J Allergy Clin Immunol. 1984;73:163.
34. Adkinson NF Jr. Tests for immunological drug reactions. In: Rose NF, Friedman H, eds. Manual of Clinical Immunology. Washington, DC: American Society for Microbiology; 1986:692–7.
35. Gorevic PD, Levine BB. Desensitization of anaphylactic hypersensitivity specific for the penicilloate minor determinant of penicillin and carbenicillin. J Allergy Clin Immunol. 1981;68:267–72.
36. Sullivan TJ. Penicillin allergy. In: Lichtenstein LM, Fauci A, eds. Current Therapy in Allergy. Philadelphia: BC Decker, 1985:57.
37. Mathews KP, Hemphill FM, Lovell RG, et al. A controlled study on the use of parenteral and oral antihistamines in preventing penicillin reactions. J Allergy. 1956;27:1.
38. Sciple GW, Knox JM, Montgomery CH. Incidence of penicillin reactions after an antihistaminic simultaneously administered parenterally. N Engl J Med. 1959;261:1123.
39. Adkinson NF Jr. Penicillin allergy. In: Lichtenstein LM, Fauci A, eds. Current Therapy in Allergy, Immunology and Rheumatology. Ontario, Canada: BS Decker; 1983:57–62.
40. Stark BJ, Earl HS, Gross GN, et al. Acute and chronic desensitization of penicillin-allergic patients using oral penicillin. J Allergy Clin Immunol. 1987;79:523–32.
41. Earl HS, Sullivan TJ. Acute desensitization of a patient with cystic fibrosis allergic to both beta-lactam and aminoglycoside antibiotics. J Allergy Clin Immunol. 1987;79:477–83.
42. Graybill JR, Sande MA, Reinarz JA, et al. Controlled penicillin anaphylaxis leading to desensitization. South Med J. 1974;67:62–4.
43. Naclerio R, Mizrahi EA, Adkinson NF Jr. Immunologic observations during desensitization and maintenance of clinical tolerance to penicillin. J Allergy Clin Immunol. 1983;71:294–301.
44. O'Driscoll BJ. Desensitization of nurses allergic to penicillin. Br Med J. 1955;2:473.
45. Grieco MH. Cross-allergenicity of the penicillins and the cephalosporins. Arch Intern Med. 1967;119:141.
46. Pedersen-Bjergaard J. Cephalothin in the treatment of penicillin sensitive patients. Acta Allergol. 1967;XXII:299–306.
47. Petz L. Immunologic cross-reactivity between penicillins and cephalosporins: A review. J Infect Dis. 1978;137:S74.
48. Shibata K, Atsumi T, Itorivchi Y, et al. Immunological cross-reactivities of cephalothin and its related compounds with benzylpenicillin (penicillin G). Nature. 1966;212:491.
49. Abraham GN, Petz LD, Fudenberg HH. Immunohaematological cross-allergenicity between penicillin and cephalothin in humans. Clin Exp Immunol. 1968;3:343–57.
50. Assem ESK, Vickers MR. Tests for penicillin allergy in man. II. The immunological cross-reaction between penicillins and cephalosporins. Immunology 1964;27:255.
51. Saxon A. Immediate hypersensitivity reactions to beta-lactam antibiotics. Rev Infect Dis. 1983;5:S368.
52. Solley GO, Gleich GJ, Van Dellen RG. Penicillin allergy: clinical experience with a battery of skin-test reagents. J Allergy Clin Immunol. 1982;69:238–44.
53. Abraham GN, Petz LD, Fudenberg HH. Cephalothin hypersensitivity associated with anti-cephalothin antibodies. Int Arch Allergy. 1968;34:65–74.
54. Ong R, Sullivan T. Detection and characterization of human IgE to cephalosporin determinants (Abstract). J Allergy Clin Immunol 1988;81:222.
55. Adkinson NF Jr, Swabb EA, Sugerman AA. Immunology of the monobactam aztreonam. Antimicrob Agents Chemother. 1984;25:93–7.
56. Saxon A, Hassner A, Swabb EA, et al. Lack of cross-reactivity between aztreonam, a monobactam antibiotic, and penicillin in penicillin-allergic subjects. J Infect Dis. 1984;149:16–22.
57. Adkinson NF Jr, Wheeler B, Swabb EA. Clinical tolerance of themonobactam aztreonam in penicillin allergic subjects (Abstract WS-26-4). Presented at the 14th International Congress of Chemotherapy, June 23–28, 1985, Kyoto, Japan.
58. Saxon A, Beall GN, Rohr AS, et al. Immediate hypersensitivity reactions to beta-lactam antibiotics. Ann Intern Med. 1987;107:204–215.

22. AMINOGLYCOSIDES AND SPECTINOMYCIN: AMINOCYCLITOLS

PAUL S. LIETMAN

Since the introduction of streptomycin in the mid-1940s, one or another of the aminoglycosides has been a mainstay in our therapeutic armamentarium. Their bactericidal activity against aerobic gram-negative bacilli, their coverage of *Pseudomonas* species, and their antitubercular activity are their three most acclaimed attributes. However, their dose-related toxicity is a major consideration, limiting their dosage and making them prime targets for competition by other, and presumably safer, classes of antibiotics. Nevertheless, they continue to be widely used in serious infections.

HISTORY

Waksman and colleagues derived streptomycin from *Streptomyces griseus* in 1943. This drug was used for tuberculosis but resistance rapidly emerged when used alone. In 1949 neomycin was isolated from *Streptomyces fradiae*. The agent proved to be too toxic for systemic administration. Kanamycin was isolated by Japanese investigators in 1957 and became the dominant aminoglycoside until its replacement by newer agents, including gentamicin, tobramycin, netilmicin, and amikacin. [Fig. 1]

STRUCTURES

The family of aminoglycoside antibiotics is defined by the presence of two or more aminosugars linked by glycosidic bonds to an aminocyclitol ring.[1–3] The six-member aminocyclitol ring is either streptidine (as in streptomycin) or 2-deoxystreptamine (as in neomycin, kanamycin, gentamicin, tobramycin, amikacin, and netilmicin). Spectinomycin is often included as a member of the family, although it contains no aminosugar and no glycosidic bond. Since spectinomycin does contain an aminocyclitol ring, as do the aminoglycosides, a general term that includes both aminoglycosides and spectinomycin is *aminocyclitol antibiotics*. However, the term *aminoglycoside* is sanctioned by common usage.

Streptomycin, neomycin, kanamycin, and tobramycin have each been isolated from a different species of *Streptomyces*, whereas the gentamicins and netilmicin have been isolated from *Micromonospora* species. The spelling of gentamicin and netilmicin with -micin rather than -mycin denotes this difference in origin. The two newest aminoglycosides, amikacin and netilmicin, are semisynthetic aminoglycosides since they are both artificial derivatives of naturally occurring aminoglycosides. Amikacin is the 1-*N*-hydroxyaminobutyric acid derivative of kanamycin A, and netilmicin is the 1-*N*-ethyl derivative of si-

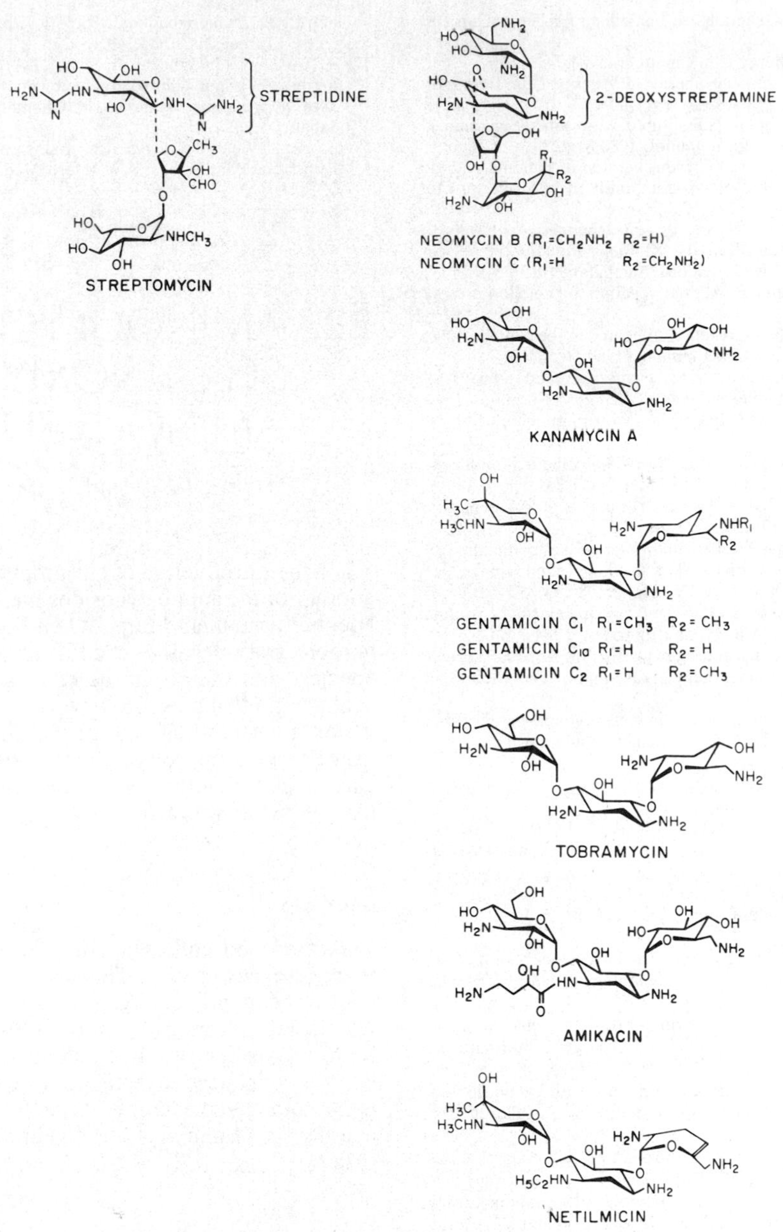

FIG. 1. Structures of aminoglycosides.

somicin, a naturally occurring aminoglycoside derived from a *Micromonospora* species.[4]

The structure–activity relationships of the aminoglycosides are incompletely understood, but the importance of the several hydroxyl and amino groups attached to the various rings is established by the loss of antibacterial activity when these groups are modified, either by synthetic chemists or by numerous bacterial enzymes.[4,5] Numerous intriguing similarities between aminoglycosides and polyamines such as spermine and spermidine suggest that aminoglycosides might be viewed as unusual polyamines with respect to their interactions with both bacteria and humans.

The groups of aminoglycosides differ from one another in the nature of the aminosugars that are linked to the central aminocyclitol ring. Structures of the aminoglycosides currently marketed in the United States are shown in Figure 1.

Although most of the aminoglycosides are unique chemical entities, gentamicin consists of a mixture of roughly equal amounts of three individual components, gentamicin C_1, C_{1a}, and C_2, and neomycin consists of roughly equal amounts of neomycin B and neomycin C. The inherent difficulties in separating the closely related gentamicins and neomycins have accounted for the inclusion of two or three components in the commercial formulations of each.

INTERACTIONS WITH MICROBES

Mechanism of Action

The precise biochemical mechanism of action of the aminoglycosides remains enigmatic in spite of an enormous amount of sophisticated attention. The difficulty lies in an inability to correlate the known biochemical effects of aminoglycosides with their lethal action. Aminoglycosides clearly inhibit bacterial protein synthesis, and this effect appears to be a necessary component of the lethal event. However, inhibition of bacterial protein synthesis is not a sufficient explanation for aminoglycoside lethality, and a second target for aminoglycoside effect appears to be necessary. The second target has remained elusive.[6–10]

Aminoglycosides inhibit protein synthesis after interacting

with one or more ribosomal binding sites. The interactions appear to be specifically localized to the interface between the smaller ribosomal subunit and the larger ribosomal subunit, an area that includes individual proteins of the smaller ribosomal unit (S3, S4, S5, and S12), as well as at least one protein of the larger ribosomal subunit (L6).[10–14] Streptomycin binds specifically, rapidly, tightly, and reversibly in a 1:1 stoichiometric ratio with the smaller 30s ribosomal subunit.[15,16] The binding of streptomycin is dependent on the S12 protein, although the actual binding is not to this protein but to an adjacent area in the vicinity of S3 and S5.[17,18] The other aminoglycosides that have been studied (including neomycin, kanamycin, gentamicin, and tobramycin) appear to bind to multiple ribosomal binding sites on both the larger and smaller ribosomal subunits and fail to compete with streptomycin binding to the smaller subunit.[15] Thus the exact site of aminoglycoside binding may differ among the aminoglycosides, and there appear to be at least two different types of ribosomal binding, one unique to streptomycin and one shared by other aminoglycosides.

The consequences of the interactions of aminoglycosides with ribosomes are numerous.[7,8] The two best documented consequences are the inhibition of protein synthesis and an infidelity in correctly reading the genetic code.

Streptomycin prevents the maintenance of polysomal function by stimulating polysome breakdown to monosomes, thereby precluding effective peptide bond formation and chain elongation.[19] These "streptomycin monosomes" dissociate into ribosomal subunits more slowly than do normally released monosomes.[20] Furthermore, "streptomycin monosomes" may be considered as abortive initiation complexes, since effective initiation cannot occur.[20–22] The effects of the deoxystreptamine-containing aminoglycosides on protein synthesis are less well understood. In general, there is less of an effect of these aminoglycosides on protein synthesis and more of an effect on the fidelity of reading the genetic code.[10]

The effects of aminoglycosides on the correct reading of the genetic code have also received considerable attention. The localization of interactions to the area of the interface between the smaller ribosomal subunit and the larger ribosomal subunit appears quite relevant to the fidelity with which the genetic code is read. This area is believed to consist of messenger RNA (mRNA) binding sites and aminoacyl transfer RNA (tRNA) acceptor sites. The faithful translation of the RNA depends on the error-free interaction between ribosomes, RNA, and the anticodon associated with each incoming aminoacyl tRNA.[10–13] The identification of ribosomal protein L6 as a protein involved with the fidelity of codon–anticodon recognition and its function in terms of determining aminoglycoside sensitivity or resistance suggests an important role for this protein in the process of aminoglycoside-induced misreading of the genetic code.[12] As a result of faulty codon–anticodon recognition, "fraudulent" proteins and proteins of abnormal length are synthesized in the presence of aminoglycosides. These effects of aminoglycosides are less prominent with streptomycin and more prominent with deoxystreptamine-containing members of the family.

Unfortunately, the relationship between either of the two prominent ribosomal effects of aminoglycosides and aminoglycoside lethality remains inconclusive.[7,8,10] Other antibacterial agents inhibit protein synthesis at least as effectively as do the aminoglycosides and yet fail to cause a lethal event, that is, produce only bacteriostasis. Thus the inhibition of protein synthesis appears insufficient to explain the bactericidal effect of aminoglycosides. Similarly, the production of "fraudulent" proteins correlates imperfectly with lethality. Based on the inadequacy of either of these two ribosomal effects to explain lethality, other targets for aminoglycoside action must be considered. Hancock has recently provided a thoughtful review of the issues involved in identifying the second target for aminoglycoside lethality.[7] Its nature, however, remains speculative.[8,10]

Although the precise biochemical events leading to aminoglycoside lethality remain to be divined, it is clear that an essential element in the process leading to lethality is the transport of aminoglycosides from the external milieu across the cell membrane and into the interior of the bacterium.[6,7,11,23,24] Aminoglycoside transport by bacteria results in the accumulation of aminoglycosides inside bacterial cells to concentrations far in excess of the external concentration. Ineffective transport precludes aminoglycoside lethality.

The transport process is energy-dependent, and the energetics of transport depend on an electrochemical gradient of protons (designated Δu_{H+}) that is generated by proton extrusion during respiration or adenosine 5′-triphosphate (ATP) hydrolysis.[9,23,25,26] The electrochemical gradient of protons is composed of both an electrical potential (designated $\Delta\Psi$) and a chemical component (designated ΔpH), which represents the difference in proton concentrations across a membrane. The transport of aminoglycosides is well correlated with the electrical potential ($\Delta\Psi$), and the effects of several situations in which aminoglycoside transport is impaired can be rationalized by considering this component of the electrochemical gradient of protons.[25,26] For example, anaerobiasis is associated with a low magnitude of $\Delta\Psi$ and impaired aminoglycoside transport, a low external pH is associated with a diminution of $\Delta\Psi$ and impaired aminoglycoside transport, an increase in the osmolarity of the environment is associated with a lower $\Delta\Psi$ and less aminoglycoside transport, and bacterial mutants that are unable to maintain a proton gradient are unable to generate a $\Delta\Psi$ or transport aminoglycosides. In each of these situations in which the electrical potential ($\Delta\Psi$) is diminished, aminoglycoside transport is impaired, and relative aminoglycoside resistance is seen.

The transport of aminoglycosides also appears to involve a transporter molecule to which the aminoglycosides bind during their internalization. Although the nature of this putative carrier molecule has not been defined, it seems likely that both divalent calcium or magnesium and polyvalent polyamines bind to the same carrier.[6,7,24,27] This competition could explain the fact that high external concentrations of calcium, magnesium, or polyamines prevent aminoglycoside transport. The interactions with calcium and magnesium are particularly relevant to the creation of appropriate and consistent media for the in vitro assessment of minimum inhibitory or minimum bacteriocidal concentrations (MIC or MBC) of aminoglycosides.

Aminoglycoside transport is also blocked by low and clinically relevant concentrations of chloramphenicol.[24,28] Thus, in the presence of chloramphenicol, the aminoglycosides will be ineffective, at least in those organisms sensitive to chloramphenicol. Whether or not the same phenomenon exists in bacteria resistant to chloramphenicol is unknown.

Mechanisms of Resistance

The usefulness of aminoglycosides depends on their selective toxicity to bacteria as opposed to eucaryotic (including human) cells. This selective toxicity to bacterial cells or, conversely, this selective resistance of eucaryotic cells is due to the inability of the cells of most human organs to transport aminoglycosides and to the failure of aminoglycosides to interact with eucaryotic cytosoline ribosomes.[10] Although mitochondrial ribosomes are sensitive to aminoglycosides, mitochondria cannot transport aminoglycosides, and mitochondrial protein synthesis is probably unaffected in vivo, even in the few tissues (such as the proximal renal tubule and cochlea) that can internalize aminoglycosides.

Bacterial resistance to aminoglycosides can occur by at least three different mechanisms: ribosomal resistance, ineffective transport, or enzymologic modification of the aminoglycoside.[29–31]

Ribosomal resistance to streptomycin is dependent on one specific aberrant protein (S12) in the smaller ribosomal subunit. A mutation in S12 leads to loss of ribosomal binding of streptomycin and to very high levels of resistance in a single mutational event.[17] At a clinical level, this type of streptomycin resistance is very uncommon in gram-negative bacilli. Ribosomal resistance can also exist for the deoxystreptamine group of aminoglycosides. In contrast to the ribosomal resistance to streptomycin, however, this resistance requires multiple mutational events before high-level resistance is seen, suggesting that more than one site must be altered.[12–14] This type of ribosomal resistance is also exceedingly uncommon clinically.

Resistance due to ineffective transport appears to be uncommon in most geographic areas, although a few centers have reported that this is the most common mechanism for aminoglycoside resistance. Genetic defects associated with ineffective transport can be localized to any of numerous proteins that have in common an involvement in bacterial electron transport or adenosine triphosphatase (ATPase) activity.[6,7,9] An inability to maintain the requisite electrical potential appears to be pivotal to each of the known mutants. It is fortunate that this mechanism for aminoglycoside resistance is uncommon, since these transport mutants are defective in the transport of all aminoglycosides.

The most common mechanism for aminoglycoside resistance involves the conjugation of the aminoglycoside with one of three groups, an acetyl group, an adenyl group, or a phosphoryl group, thereby rendering the aminoglycoside inactive.[29–32] The conjugation, in each case, is catalyzed by an enzyme produced in the bacterial cell from information contained in an extrachromasomal plasmid. Plasmid-mediated resistance is particularly worrisome because the responsible plasmids can infect other gram-negative bacteria, even of different species, and because information for multiple-resistance mechanisms involving other antibacterial classes can be simultaneously introduced into bacterial cells. A very large number of individual enzymes has been identified, each of which catalyzes the addition of one of the above groups onto a specific site on one or more than one aminoglycoside. The overlapping substrate specificities of the individual inactivating enzymes leads to a bewildering array of possibilities for cross-resistance to several aminoglycosides.[29–32] For example, an enzyme capable of acetylating an aminoglycoside at the 6′ position (i.e., the 6 position of one of the aminosugar rings adjacent to the deoxystreptamine ring) can inactivate neomycin, kanamycin, tobramycin, amikacin, and netilmicin but not streptomycin or gentamicin. An enzyme capable of phosphorylating the 3′ position, however, can inactivate only neomycin and kanamycin. To complicate the picture even further, isoenzymes have been identified for many of the specific enzymatic functions. Thus there may be several unique isoenzymes, each capable of catalyzing the addition of an acetyl group to the 6 prime position of an aminoglycoside but each possessing different substrate specificity so that one might inactivate kanamycin where as another might inactivate tobramycin. Thus an incredible multiplicity of possibilities exists for cross-resistance to multiple aminoglycosides.

The prevalence of individual aminoglycoside-inactivating enzymes varies widely with respect to both place and time. Thus, whereas 2″-adenyltransferase, 3-acetyltransferase, and 6′-acetyltransferase are predominant in that order in the United States, 6′-acetyltransferase is most common in Japan, and 3-acetyltransferase is most common in Chile.[31] Further geographic variability exists between hospitals in any one country, state, or city and even between wards in one hospital. The reasons for this variability have remained an enigma. A simple relationship to patterns of aminoglycoside usage does not exist. This may be explicable in part by the overlapping of aminoglycoside resistance generated by each of the inactivating enzymes. Thus the prevalence of resistance to amikacin might be expected to be lessened by the infrequent use of amikacin and the consequent diminished genetic pressure for the emergence of amikacin-inactivating enzymes. This may well be partially negated by the continued use of other aminoglycosides that can also be inactivated by the same enzymes that are capable of inactivating amikacin. For example, the continued use of kanamycin, tobramycin, or netilmicin should provide genetic pressure for the emergence of 6′-acetylating enzyme; the continued use of kanamycin or tobramycin should provide pressure for the emergence of a 4′-adenylating enzyme; and the continued use of any of the available deoxystreptamine-containing aminoglycosides should provide pressure for the emergence of a 2″-phosphorylating enzyme.

At a clinical level, several conclusions are justified by the current information on aminoglycoside resistance.

First, we cannot predict the precise enzymologic mechanism responsible for aminoglycoside resistance in an individual patient. Although resistance patterns may be known for a particular time and place, these patterns can be helpful only in the selection of an initial aminoglycoside to be used before the determination of the specific sensitivity of the individual patient's pathogen.

Second, it is seldom feasible to determine the precise enzymologic mechanism responsible for aminoglycoside resistance, and we must rely on more general tests of sensitivity and resistance such as the MIC or MBC.

Third, it may be futile to reserve an individual aminoglycoside for future use in hopes of delaying the emergence of resistance, since the continued use of other aminoglycosides that are inactivated by the same enzyme may provide sufficient genetic pressure for the emergence of the enzyme that can inactivate the reserved drug.

Sepectrum of In Vitro Activity

The spectrum of in vitro activity of the aminoglycosides includes primarily aerobic and facultative gram-negative bacilli and *Staphylococcus aureus*. A representative summary of MICs at which 75 or 100 percent of the strains of various bacteria are sensitive in one laboratory is shown in Table 1.[33] Some hospitals have more aminoglycoside resistance than that shown in the table. In general, aminoglycosides are not often used for known staphylococcal infections since a number of alternative antibiotics has considerably more data backing clinical efficacy. Aminoglycosides are considered excellent choices for serious infections caused by aerobic or facultative gram-negative bacilli and especially those caused by *Pseudomonas aeruginosa*. For these latter infections, in spite of some in vitro differences in MICs, there is no clinical evidence to substantiate an advantage for anyone of the aminoglycosides in treating an infection due to a susceptible organism. Thus, although the percentage of resistant strains in a given locale may dictate the most rational initial aminoglycoside to be used, equivalent effectiveness should be expected from any of this group in treating a patient with a sensitive organism. Nevertheless, differences in in vitro activity do exist with respect to some bacteria. Streptomycin has the greatest in vitro activity against *Mycobacterium tuberculosis*, is considered the drug of choice for *Francisella tularensis* and *Yersinia pestis*, and is often used in brucellosis.[34] Streptomycin is seldom used for aerobic or facultative gram-negative bacillary infections due to the frequency of resistance.[34] Kanamycin is limited in its spectrum, compared with the other 2-deoxystreptamine-containing aminoglycosides, because of the common resistance of *P. aeruginosa*.[34] Kanamycin is also inactivated by a large number of the plasmid-mediated enzymes, and consequently kanamycin resistance among other gram-negative bacilli is prevalent in many locales. Gentamicin and tobramycin share very similar in vitro profiles, although gentamicin is somewhat more potent in vitro against *Serratia* species and tobramycin somewhat more potent against *P. aeruginosa*.[33] However, these minor differences in in vitro potencies

TABLE 1. In Vitro Susceptibility of Various Bacteria to Five Aminoglycosides[a]

	Kanamycin		*Gentamicin*		*Tobramycin*		*Amikacin*		*Netilmicin*	
Organism (No.)	*75%*	*100%*	*75%*	*100%*	*75%*	*100%*	*75%*	*100%*	*75%*	*100%*
Staphylococcus aureus (25)	1.6	3.1	≤0.2	0.8	≤0.2	6.2	1.6	3.1	0.4	0.8
Enterococci (20)	12.5	>50	3.1	6.2	6.2	12.5	25	50	3.1	6.2
Neisseria gonorrhoeae (20)	12.5	25	6.2	12.5	6.2	12.5	25	50	6.2	12.5
Escherichia coli (40)	12.5	>50	1.6	6.2	3.1	12.5	6.2	12.5	1.6	6.2
Klebsiella sp. (20)	3.1	>50	0.4	1.6	0.4	1.6	1.6	6.2	0.4	0.8
Enterobacter sp. (40)	3.1	>50	0.8	1.6	1.6	6.2	1.6	6.2	0.4	6.2
Citrobacter sp. (15)	12.5	25	1.6	6.2	1.6	1.6	3.1	6.2	0.8	3.1
Serratia sp. (15)	3.1	6.2	1.6	1.6	3.1	6.2	3.1	6.2	1.6	3.2
Proteus mirabilis (20)	3.1	25	1.6	3.1	1.6	3.1	6.2	12.5	1.6	3.1
Morganella morganii (29)	3.1	6.2	0.8	0.8	0.8	1.6	3.1	6.2	0.8	1.6
Proteus vulgaris (6)	6.2	6.2	1.6	1.6	1.6	3.1	3.1	6.2	0.8	0.8
Providencia rettgeri (6)	3.1	3.1	3.1	6.2	3.1	6.2	1.6	1.6	12.5	12.5
Providencia stuartii (8)	1.6	3.1	3.1	6.2	3.1	12.5	3.1	3.1	3.1	12.5
Pseudomonas aeruginosa (40)	ND	ND	0.8	3.1	≤0.2	1.6	0.8	12.5	0.8	6.2

[a] MIC (μg/ml) for percent of strains indicated.
(Data from Sanders et al.[33])

have not been demonstrated to correlate with greater in vivo effectiveness. Since gentamicin and tobramycin are both susceptible to the same enzymologic modifications (save for a few uncommon enzymes that can inactivate gentamicin and not tobramycin), the percentage of resistant strains to these two aminoglycosides is also quite similar.[33] Amikacin has a clear advantage over gentamicin or tobramycin as a result of its resistance to many of the common plasmid-mediated enzymes. Consequently, the percentage of strains susceptible to amikacin is significantly greater for amikacin compared with gentamicin or tobramycin.[33] The in vitro potency of amikacin with respect to many of the gram-negative bacilli is less than that of gentamicin or tobramycin, but the dose that is allowed by its lesser toxicity (i.e., three to four times the dose of gentamicin or tobramycin) compensates for this lesser potency. Again, there is no clinical evidence to suggest lesser or greater effectiveness against sensitive bacteria. Netilmicin shares the spectrum of gentamicin and tobramycin in general. However, netilmicin is resistant to aminoglycoside-adenylating enzymes and as a result some *Escherichia coli*, *Klebsiella*, *Enterobacter*, and *Citrobacter* isolates that are resistant to gentamicin remain sensitive to netilmicin.[32] Gentamicin-resistant *Serratia*, *Proteus*, *Providencia*, and *Pseudomonas* strains are, however, usually also netilmicin-resistant.[35]

In vitro sensitivity and resistance to aminoglycosides is usually determined as a minimum inhibitory concentration. Since the minimum bacteriocidal concentration is nearly always close to the MIC, there is no advantage associated with this more cumbersome technique. The MIC is most frequently assessed by a disk diffusion method but may be more accurately quantified by either agar dilution or broth dilution methods.[34] For the disk diffusion method, standards have been set for the aminoglycoside content of the individual disks, zone diameters, and agar composition.[36] Standardization of agar diffusion and broth dilution methods is also important, since several variables in the media can significantly influence the MIC, especially pH and cation concentration.[37] These variables affect the MIC determinations primarily by affecting transport of the aminoglycosides into the bacteria. An acid pH of the media will provide erroneously high MICs, whereas an alkaline pH will give an erroneously low MIC. The pH of the agar or broth should be kept at pH 7.3–7.5. High concentrations of cations, especially calcium, magnesium, and sodium, yield erroneously high MICs, especially with *P. aeruginosa*.[37] Standardization of the calcium salt concentration at about 50 μg/ml and the magnesium salt concentration at about 25 μg/ml has been proposed.[37] The number of bacteria used should also be standardized, although the "inoculum effect" is far less important with aminoglycosides than with β-lactams.[34] The relative lack of inoculum effect is attributable to the failure of aminoglycoside-inactivating enzymes to be released into the medium. Thus the concentration of aminoglycoside in the medium will remain nearly constant, even with large inocula of resistant bacteria.

Time Course of Antibacterial Effects

Each of the routine methods of determining an MIC provides a constant concentration of antibiotic adjacent to the bacterium for the entire period of incubation. Thus the MIC should be interpreted as the lowest concentration that inhibits bacterial growth *if constantly adjacent to the bacterium*.

Recent interest has focused on more sophisticated systems to assess both the in vitro effects and the in vivo effects in laboratory animals of changing concentrations of antibiotics over time.[38–55] Although these systems are not feasible for the routine definition of sensitivity and resistance to antibiotics, they contribute significantly to an understanding of the complex interrelationships between the pharmacokinetics of the antibiotic and the kinetics of bacterial growth. In these systems, with continuously changing aminoglycoside concentrations adjacent to continuously growing bacteria, there is evidence of a significant "postantibiotic effect" by aminoglycosides on *P. aeruginosa*. There is also a suggestion that a lesser, but potentially significant, "postantibiotic effect" is exerted by aminoglycosides on *E. coli* and *Klebsiella pneumoniae*.[50–52] The presence of such a "postantibiotic effect" would support the possible feasibility of longer dosing intervals (12 or even 24 hours) for aminoglycosides in man. While preliminary human studies have been compatible with both the safety and the effectiveness of a 24-hourly dosing regimen, larger clinical trials are needed to ascertain the true comparative value of such regimens compared with the existing standard regimen using an 8-hourly dosing regimen.[49]

Synergism

Aminoglycosides frequently exhibit synergism with other antibiotics. Especially noteworthy is the synergism usually found in enterococcal species between penicillin or vancomycin and the aminoglycosides.[56] The mechanism of this synergism involves the enhancement of aminoglycoside uptake into cells whose wall has been damaged by the cell wall inhibitor.[57] Numerous other synergistic combinations involving an aminoglycoside also exist.

INTERACTIONS WITH HUMANS

Pharmacokinetics

The pharmacokinetics of all of the aminoglycosides are quite similar. Subtle differences among individual members of the family may have importance with respect to the pathophysiology of their toxicities, but these minor differences are unimportant with respect to rational dosing.

Absorption. The extent of absorption of oral aminoglycosides is unpredictable but always low.[58–62] Consequently, aminoglycosides are generally considered nonabsorbable antibiotics and are occasionally used to alter the gut flora. In the presence of impaired elimination, however, even a small amount of absorbed aminoglycoside may accumulate to toxic levels.[63–66]

Absorption after intramuscular aminoglycoside administration is both complete and rapid, with maximal plasma levels achieved between 30 and 90 minutes.[67–68] Impaired tissue perfusion, as in shock, delays the absorption of intramuscular aminoglycosides.

Intravenous aminoglycoside administration is frequently used in patients with serious infections, and the dose is completely delivered to the vascular space. When the intravenous infusion lasts for 20–30 minutes, the plasma levels are similar to those achieved by intramuscular administration.

Topical aminoglycosides generally either are not absorbed or only minimally absorbed. Exceptions include patients with extensive epidermal loss due to burns or epidermolysis and patients with open wounds in which significant absorption can occur.[69,70]

Intraperitoneal or intrapleural aminoglycosides are rapidly absorbed, quickly providing plasma levels that are dependent on the concentration of drug instilled into the peritoneal or pleural fluid.[71,72] Administration of large amounts of aminoglycosides can result in very high plasma levels and toxicity.

Bladder irrigation is not associated with significant aminoglycoside absorption,[73] intratracheal or aerosolized aminoglycosides are poorly absorbed,[74,75] and intrathecal or intraventricular aminoglycosides produce negligible plasma levels.[76]

Distribution. Aminoglycosides are freely distributed in the vascular space and are relatively freely distributed in the interstitial spaces of most tissues. Although the mean aminoglycoside concentration in interstitial fluids approximates the mean plasma concentration at steady state with repetitive dosing, the peak concentrations are lower, the oscillations between peak and trough concentrations are less, and the rate of elimination is lower from interstitial fluids.[77]

Because of their size and polycationic charge, aminoglycosides cross biologic membranes that lack transport mechanisms very poorly. This accounts for their low intracellular concentrations in nearly all human tissues. An exception is the proximal renal tubular cell, which appears to have a unique transport mechanism and can concentrate aminoglycosides to levels far in excess of plasma or interstitial fluid levels.[78]

Aminoglycosides enter bronchial secretions poorly, attaining mean levels approximately 20 percent of mean plasma levels.[79] Intermittent administration produces higher peak levels in bronchial secretions than does continuous infusion, but areas under the concentration versus time curves as similar.[79,80] Neither mode of delivery produces high aminoglycoside levels in bronchial secretions, however, and the direct intratracheal administration of aminoglycosides to patients with serious gram-negative pneumonitis has been advocated on the basis of higher levels in bronchial secretions and greater clinical effectiveness.[80]

Intravenous or intramuscular administration of aminoglycosides to adults produces very low aminoglycoside levels in the cerebrospinal fluid.[76,81,82] In newborns cerebrospinal fluid levels are higher relative to plasma levels.[83] Intrathecal administration in the lumbar area produces high lumbar cerebrospinal fluid levels but poor intraventricular levels, whereas intraventricular administration produces high levels in both ventricular fluid and lumbar cerebrospinal fluid.[81] Based on these findings, intraventricular aminoglycoside administration has been proposed for gram-negative bacillary meningitis in adults.[81,82] In the newborn, intraventricular aminoglycoside administration has been shown to be no more effective and possibly more toxic than intravenous administration alone.[83]

Aminoglycoside distribution in the eye has been studied after repetitive intramuscular or continuous intravenous dosing in the rabbit. The cornea and aqueous fluids attain levels approximating serum levels, whereas entry into vitreous fluid is slow, and mean vitreous levels are only about 40 percent of serum levels over a 12-hour period.[84] Subconjunctival injection produces high aqueous fluid levels of aminoglycosides in humans.[85] However, neither systemic nor subconjunctival aminoglycoside administration in single doses produces reliable levels in the vitreous humor of humans, and intravitreal injection has been advocated in the treatment of endophthalmitis.[86]

Aminoglycosides enter the synovial fluid rather easily and achieve levels only modestly less than simultaneously measured plasma levels.[87–91]

Aminoglycosides penetrate into prostatic fluid poorly, and levels are low compared with plasma levels.[92]

Aminoglycosides do not enter saliva.[93]

The biliary concentrations of aminoglycosides are significantly less than the plasma levels.[94,95]

Urinary concentrations of aminoglycosides reach levels about 25–100 times peak plasma aminoglycoside concentrations within an hour after dosing and remain well above therapeutic levels for several days after even a single dose.[96–99] After termination of a multiple dosing regimen, urinary aminoglycoside concentrations remain above therapeutic levels for many days, with a terminal half-life of about 48–200 hours.[97–100]

Metabolism. Aminoglycosides are not metabolized by humans.

Excretion. Aminoglycosides are eliminated entirely as unchanged drugs and almost entirely from the kidneys. Less than 1 percent of a parenterally administered dose appears in the feces and none in saliva.[101,102]

Aminoglycosides are filtered by the glomerulus. Although they are negligibly protein bound, their filtration is not completely free, since their polycationic nature appears to impede filtration through the glomerular capillary wall.[103] After entering the luminal fluid of the proximal renal tubule, a small but toxicologically important portion of the total filtered aminoglycoside is reabsorbed exclusively into the proximal renal tubular cells.[78,104,105] This reabsorption appears to involve binding of the aminoglycosides to negatively charged phospholipids in the renal tubular brush border membranes, with subsequent internalization by pinocytosis.[106–110] There is no conclusive evidence for secretion of aminoglycosides into the urine. Quantitatively, most of the filtered aminoglycoside is excreted into the urine.

Overall Pharmacokinetics

The overall pharmacokinetics of aminoglycosides can be quite accurately described as a composite of contributions from absorption and three phases of elimination.[111,112] Since absorption is predictably complete and rapid after either intramuscular or intermittent intravenous administration, it is the three phases of elimination that deserve emphasis.

The three phases of aminoglycoside elimination can be considered to be related to three connected compartments in the commonly used model of the pharmacokinetic behavior of drugs or simply as mathematical components of a triexponential equation that has been found to fit the experimentally derived decay curve of plasma aminoglycoside levels versus time. Although neither of the above approaches allows the designation of anatomic or physiologic spaces for the compartments or for the components of the equation, it is clearly of practical value to consider the disposition of aminoglycosides in physiologic terms. The first (or alpha or distributive) phase of aminoglycoside elimination is made up predominantly of the process of drug distribution from the vascular space to some extravascular space. Since aminoglycosides enter most cells poorly, the extravascular space may be considered to be similar to the extracellular fluid volume. The time course of this phase can be described as having a half-life of about 15–30 minutes.[111–113] Measurement of plasma aminoglycoside levels after the end of this phase provides levels that approach the levels in interstitial fluid and avoids the rapidly changing plasma levels that occur earlier. For this reason it has been suggested that "peak" aminoglycoside levels should be drawn 30 minutes to 1 hour after the end of an intravenous infusion.[114]

The second (or beta) phase of aminoglycoside elimination involves the excretion of the drug from the plasma and simultaneously from most of the extravascular space. The time course of this beta phase is determined nearly exclusively by the glomular filtration rate, and it is this phase that is most important in terms of clinical dosing. It is also this phase that is altered by a number of clinically important factors, as discussed below. In the young healthy adult with normal renal function, this phase can be reasonably described by a small number of pharmacokinetic parameters. The volume of distribution is about 25–30 percent of body weight,[115–117] the half-life is 1.5–3.5 hours,[115–118] and the plasma clearance is about 1 ml/min/kg.[119] Each of these pharmacokinetic parameters can be altered, however, by a number of clinically important conditions, and rational dosing of the aminoglycosides must take cognizance of these alterations, which are described below.

The third (or gamma) phase of aminoglycoside elimination involves the prolonged and slow excretion of the drug from the plasma and simultaneously from a relatively small portion of an extravascular space either through the plasma space or directly into the urine. This portion of the extravascular space has been termed a *deep compartment* to distinguish it from the portion of the extravascular space that readily equilibrates with the vascular space. It has also been considered to represent primarily the kidneys, since aminoglycosides accumulate in kidney parenchymal tissue and leave very slowly. The importance of this third phase of aminoglycoside elimination has been clearly demonstrated in terms of rigorously describing the overall pharmacokinetics of aminoglycoside elimination.[111,120–122] However, the importance of this phase in terms of rational aminoglycoside dosing remains unclear. The third phase can be described in pharmacokinetic terms as having a large volume of distribution (the volume of distribution at steady state) of 45–100 percent of the body weight, a very long half-life of 35–200 hours, and a clearance of about 1 ml/min/kg.[100,101,109–111] The influence of various clinical conditions on the pharmacokinetics of the third phase has not been defined, although individual aminoglycosides appear to vary with respect to their volumes of distribution at steady state.[111,112,120–122]

Alterations with Age. The pharmacokinetics of aminoglycosides in both children and the elderly differ significantly from those in young healthy adults. The differences are attributable to known differences in glomerular function in newborns, children, and the elderly and are seen primarily as deviations during the second phase of elimination.

In the newborn the volume of distribution is considerably larger as a percentage of body weight (34–78 percent), and the half-life of the second phase is significantly prolonged (3–14 hours). Both the volume of distribution and the half-life of the second phase are inversely correlated with either gestational age or postnatal age.[123–131]

After the newborn period, infants and children have volumes of distribution that are close to those of young adults and half-lives that are shorter (.4–3 hours) than those of young adults.[123,131–141]

In the elderly the volumes of distribution are similar to those of young adults, but the half-lives are considerably longer due to decreased glomerular function with age.[142] Since the diminution in glomerular function in the elderly is not necessarily reflected in a higher serum creatinine (Cr) (due to a decrease in creatinine production in the elderly), it is important to use a calculated creatinine clearance (C_{cr}) in order to estimate the half-life or clearance of an aminoglycoside in the elderly.[143] The equation of Cockcroft and Gault is as follows:

$$C_{cr}(\text{ml/min}) = \frac{(140 - \text{age}) \times \text{weight}}{\text{Cr} \times 72}$$

The modification by Spyker and Guerrant is

$$C_{cr}(\text{ml/min}) = \frac{(140 - \text{age}) \times (1.03 - 0.053 \times \text{Cr})}{\text{Cr}}$$

The nomogram of Siersbaek-Nielson et al. is useful in calculating the creatinine clearance.[143–145] In the above equations weight is in kilograms, creatinine in milligrams per deciliter, and age in years.

Alterations with Disease States. Kidney disease with glomerular dysfunction is the most common disease state associated with altered aminoglycoside pharmacokinetics. The clearance of an aminoglycoside is linearly related to the clearance of creatinine since aminoglycosides are nearly entirely eliminated renally and their elimination rate is highly dependent on the glomerular filtration rate. A useful estimation of aminoglycoside clearance[146] is given by the following equation:

$$\text{Aminoglycoside clearance} = (C_{cr})\,(0.6) + 10$$

Since the creatinine clearance, as a measure of glomerular filtration rate, can also be calculated reasonably accurately using the equation of Cockcroft and Gault (given above), we can easily estimate the clearance of an aminoglycoside in a patient with renal disease. The volume of distribution as a percent of body weight of an aminoglycoside may be increased in patients with marked renal dysfunction.[146–148] The half-life, which is a function of the ratio of the volume of distribution to clearance, is prolonged in patients with renal disease and may in fact be somewhat longer than would be predicted on the basis of the creatinine clearance alone due to the somewhat larger volume of distribution.

In obese patients, the volume of distribution of aminoglycosides as a fraction of the total body weight is about 75 percent of that seen in nonobese patients, or about 20 percent of total body weight. The rates of elimination and half-lives, however, are similar in obese and nonobese patients.[149,150]

Conversely, in protein–calorie malnutrition (marasmus), the volume of distribution of aminoglycosides as a fraction of the total body weight is about 120 percent of that seen in well-nourished patients.[151]

Fever appears to alter aminoglycoside pharmacokinetics. Lower plasma aminoglycoside levels are found in febrile patients.[152]

In severe burns the glomerular filtration rate and consequently the rate of elimination of aminoglycosides may be markedly enhanced.[153,154]

Alterations with Other Drugs. The aminoglycosides can be inactivated by many of the β-lactam antibiotics in vitro and to a lesser extent in vivo. The inactivation occurs because a covalent bond is formed between the carboxyl group of a broken β-lactam ring and an amino group on the aminoglycoside. The reaction occurs at high molar ratios of β-lactam to aminoglycoside and is thus especially important when carbenicillin or ticarcillin is used with an aminoglycoside, since large doses of these β-lactams provide the requisite high molar ratios. Since 1 mol of β-lactam is inactivated at the same time that 1 mol of aminoglycoside is being inactivated, theoretically there should be a loss of both activities. The disproportionate number of β-lactam molecules, however, is not significantly diminished by having lost a few molecules through these interactions. The reaction occurs more readily in a protein-free setting, and therefore the reaction is more relevant to the situation in an intravenous bottle containing both drugs than to the patient containing both drugs. The rapid elimination of most β-lactams also tends to minimize the ability of the β-lactam to inactivate the aminoglycoside, since the required molar ratios of the two antibiotics exist for only a brief period in patients with normal renal function. The shortening of the half-life of the aminoglycoside in patients with renal failure may be clinically significant.

DOSING

Extensive pharmacokinetic data on aminoglycosides permit the construction of dosage regimens that will achieve and maintain plasma aminoglycoside levels within practically any desired range. Numerous dosage regimens have been proposed, and extensive and rigorous clinical trials have been conducted with a few of the proposed regimens. However, studies comparing one regimen with another with respect to both effectiveness and safety are virtually nonexistent. A dosage regimen that has been used extensively and rigorously and that has been carefully assessed with respect to both effectiveness and toxicity is presented as one approach.[114,155] Although other regimens may be equally or even more effective and equally or even less toxic, there is currently no comparative information to verify such differences.

Initiation of therapy should involve the administration of a loading dose of aminoglycoside in order to achieve therapeutic aminoglycoside plasma levels quickly. This principle is especially relevant when elimination of the aminoglycoside is delayed, since in such situations it will take many hours to achieve a plateau level unless a loading dose is given. The loading dose will be determined exclusively by the volume of distribution of the aminoglycoside and the desired maximum plasma aminoglycoside level. Considerable evidence suggests that a reasonable goal in terms of the maximum plasma aminoglycoside level is between 5 and 10 μg/ml for gentamicin, tobramycin, and netilmicin and between 20 and 40 μg/ml for kanamycin and amikacin.[156–162] Based on an average volume of distribution of 25 percent of the body weight, a loading dose of 1.5–2 mg/kg for gentamicin, tobramycin, or netilmicin or 7.5–8 mg/kg for kanamycin or amikacin will provide plasma levels of 6–8 and 30–32 μg/ml, respectively.

Several aspects of the loading dose deserve emphasis. First, the loading dose should be the same whether or not there is reason to believe that elimination will be impaired. Thus, no matter what the degree of renal dysfunction, the same loading dose should be given. Second, in calculating a loading dose, we should aim at the maximal plasma level desired, since some drug will be eliminated before the first maintenance dose and we would not choose to provide suboptimal levels during the critical initiation of aminoglycoside therapy. Third, the loading dose should be given intravenously over 20–30 minutes or intramuscularly rather than as a rapid intravenous bolus in order to minimize the risk of transient neuromuscular paralysis.

The next step is to calculate a maintenance dosage regimen, including the size of individual doses and the dosing intervals. In adult patients with normal renal function, a dose of 1.5–2 mg/kg of gentamicin, tobramycin, or netilmicin given every 8 hours or 7.5–8 mg/kg of kanamycin or amikacin given every 12 hours will provide levels that oscillate between peaks of about 8 or 32 μg/ml, respectively, and troughs of about 1 or 4 μg/ml, respectively.

In patients with diminished renal glomerular function, the total daily dose of aminoglycosides must be reduced. A convenient method of calculating the appropriate daily dose of an aminoglycoside in the presence of renal glomerular dysfunction is to multiply the usual daily dose for a patient with normal renal function by the ratio of the clearance of the drug in renal insufficiency to the clearance of the drug with normal renal function. Since the clearance of aminoglycosides is linearly related to the endogenous creatinine clearance, the ratio of the patient's creatinine clearance to normal creatinine clearance will closely approximate the ratio of aminoglycoside clearances. Thus, if the calculated creatinine clearance, taking into account the patient's age, sex, weight, and serum creatinine, is 40 ml/min/1.73 m^2, the appropriate ratio is (40 ml/min/1.73 m^2)/(100 ml/min/1.73 m^2) = 0.4, and the total daily aminoglycoside dose should be 0.4 times or 40 percent of the usual daily aminoglycoside dose. Instead of 4.5–6 mg/kg/day, the reduced dose should be 1.8–2.4 mg/kg/day.

Having derived a reduced daily maintenance dose, there are two commonly advocated methods of giving the reduced dose. One can either reduce the individual dose given at the usual dosage interval or give the usual individual dose at less frequent intervals. There is currently no evidence to support one method over the other.

It must be emphasized that any calculation of dosage reduction will be approximate and should only be used to provide an estimate of the appropriate maintenance dose. As soon as convenient (usually within 24–48 hours), plasma aminoglycoside levels should be measured and the maintenance doses adjusted to provide selected plasma levels. Plasma levels of 5–10 μg/ml 30 minutes to 1 hour after the end of an intravenous infusion over 20–30 minutes or after an intramuscular injection of gentamicin, tobramycin, or netilmicin have been associated with effectiveness and acceptibly low toxicity as have plasma levels of 20–40 μg/ml for amikacin (and presumably kanamycin).[114,155]

TOXICITY

All aminoglycosides share three principal toxicities, although there are quantitative differences among individual aminoglycosides for each of the three. The principal toxicities are neuromuscular paralysis, ototoxicity, and nephrotoxicity. Although the detailed mechanisms involved in these toxicities remain to be defined, an intriguing thread that appears to run through each involves the interactions of the polycationic aminoglycosides, polyamines, calcium, and magnesium with the polyanionic phosphatidylinositol, phosphatidylinositol diphosphate, and phosphatidylinositol triphosphate.

Neuromuscular Paralysis

The aminoglycosides are all capable of producing clinically significant neuromuscular paralysis. Although this phenomenon is rare, it is potentially quite serious.

The mechanism responsible for aminoglycoside-induced neuromuscular paralysis appears to involve both an inhibition of the presynaptic release of acetylcholine and a blockade of the postsynaptic receptor sites for acetylcholine. The presynaptic site of inhibition is dependent on the ability of an aminoglycoside to inhibit the internalization of calcium into the presynaptic region of the neuronal axon, thus preventing an event that necessarily precedes the release of acetylcholine.[163] This presynaptic effect is manifest more by neomycin or tobramycin than by streptomycin and is prevented or reversed by the provision of additional local calcium.[150–152] The postsynaptic site of blockade involves an effect on the postsynaptic receptor for acetylcholine such that the response to acetylcholine is blunted. The postsynaptic effect is produced more potently by streptomycin or netilmicin than by neomycin.[164,165]

The neuromuscular paralysis associated with aminoglycosides is enhanced by the presence of curare-like drugs, succinylcholine, and magnesium, by the simultaneous presence of botulin toxin in patients with botulism, and in patients with myasthenia gravis.[166–171]

The neuromuscular paralysis of aminoglycosides is clearly associated with the presence of very high concentrations of drug at the neuromuscular junctions. Sufficiently high concentrations are achieved only by the very rapid intravenous administration of a bolus of aminoglycoside or as a result of absorption of the drug from the pleural or peritoneal space after instillation of a highly concentrated solution.

The neuromuscular paralysis of aminoglycosides can be prevented by administering intravenous doses over 20–30 minutes, by the intramuscular administration of the drugs, and by the instillation of less concentrated solutions into the pleural or peritoneal spaces.

Once manifest, the neuromuscular paralysis of aminoglycosides can be treated by the prompt administration of calcium. Neostigmine has also been advocated, but neostigmine may be less rational if it is the presynaptic release of acetylcholine that is inhibited by aminoglycosides.

Aminoglycosides are capable of inhibiting both myocardial and vascular smooth muscle contractility in experimental situations, but the clinical relevance is uncertain.[172–174]

Ototoxicity

All aminoglycosides are capable of causing ototoxicity. Although individual aminoglycosides preferentially reduce either auditory toxicity or vestibular toxicity in experimental animals, all aminoglycosides are capable of producing both in humans. Although relatively uncommon, ototoxicity is especially worrisome because of its frequent irreversibility, its occurrence even after discontinuation of the drug, and its cumulative nature with repeated courses of the drug.[175]

The mechanism of auditory toxicity of aminoglycosides involves the selective destruction of the outer hair cells of the organ of Corti, especially those located in the basal turn.[175–178] Subsequently, retrograde degeneration of the auditory nerve occurs.[179] Inner hair cells and cells of the stria vascularis are affected with more extensive damage. The vestibular system is affected primarily by damage to type I hair cells of the summit of the ampullar cristae.[180] Neither cochlear nor ampullar cells can regenerate once they have been destroyed, thus accounting for irreversibility.

The cellular damage may be related to the concentrations of aminoglycosides in the perilymph and endolymph that bathe the relevant cells. Aminoglycosides enter and leave the perilymph slowly, compared with their pharmacokinetics in plasma.[181] Endolymph levels rise and disappear even more slowly.[181] Thus cells bathed by these fluids may be exposed to aminoglycosides for prolonged periods of time even after discontinuation of the drug.

The biochemical events associated with aminoglycoside ototoxicity appear to be biphasic, with an immediate effect that is reversible by calcium and a subsequent irreversible event that may involve binding of the aminoglycoside by phosphatidylinositol biphosphate.[182,183] An inhibition of a sodium–potassium ATPase has also been found.[184] This inhibition might lead to alterations in endolymph or perilymph ion gradients with subsequent effects on the integrity of cochlear cells.

The incidence of aminoglycoside-induced auditory and vestibular toxicity in humans is quite low if clinically detectable hearing loss or vestibular dysfunction is required, but it is clearly higher if more sensitive measures of auditory or vestibular function, such as audiometry or electronystagmography, are used. Large prospective comparative clinical trials of aminoglycosides, usually using rigorous dosing regimens, have delineated relative incidents of aminoglycoside ototoxicity and have also contributed significantly to an understanding of the clinical course of the ototoxicity and risk factors involved with the development of ototoxicity.

Clinically detectable toxicity has been reported to occur in 3–5 percent of patients receiving gentamicin, tobramycin, or amikacin in whom audiometric testing could be performed.[185,186] In other extensive clinical trials of gentamicin, tobramycin, and amikacin, only 3 patients with clinically detectable hearing loss were seen out of a total of 674 patients receiving an aminoglycoside. Thus another estimate of the incidence of clinically detectable hearing loss is less than 0.5 percent of those receiving an aminoglycoside.[114,155]

Using audiometric testing, the incidence of auditory toxicity in patients receiving gentamicin, tobramycin, or amikacin has not been shown to differ significantly when individual aminoglycosides are directly compared.[114,155,185,186] Netilmicin, however, has been shown to produce auditory toxicity less frequently than tobramycin in one multicenter study.[187]

Vestibular dysfunction has been reported as clinically significant in 0.4 percent of patients receiving gentamicin, tobramycin, or amikacin[185,186] and present by electronystagmography in 4 percent of patients receiving gentamicin and 6 percent of patients receiving amikacin.[172] In a prospective but unblinded study tobramycin produced vestibular dysfunction significantly less frequently than did gentamicin.[186]

Auditory toxicity associated with aminoglycosides is seen clinically as hearing loss. Although tinnitus and a feeling of fullness in the ears have been said to precede hearing loss, these are clearly unreliable premonitors of auditory toxicity since they often occur without subsequent hearing loss and hearing loss often occurs without these symptoms. The hearing loss is usually bilateral, although unilateral hearing loss has been reported and usually involves the loss of high-tone hearing before the loss of low-tone hearing. The occurrence and severity of the hearing loss are related to the dose and duration of aminoglycoside therapy.[187,188] There is, however, a somewhat less clear relationship between plasma aminoglycoside levels and auditory toxicity. In prospective clinical trials in which aminoglycoside levels have been carefully monitored and adjusted, there has been no correlation of auditory toxicity and plasma aminoglycoside levels within the narrow range of levels seen. However, if plasma aminoglycoside levels are not carefully adjusted, high plasma levels would surely be associated with greater auditory toxicity. Transient aminoglycoside levels above the usual limits of 10 μg/ml for gentamicin, tobramycin, and netilmicin or 40 μg/ml for amikacin (and presumably kanamycin) are unlikely to be ototoxic.

Even when plasma aminoglycoside levels are carefully monitored, some patients will suffer hearing loss by audiometry and even clinical hearing loss. Risk factors for the development of auditory toxicity include the duration of aminoglycoside use, the presence of bacteremia, fever, liver dysfunction, and the ratio of serum urea nitrogen to serum creatinine as a measure of hypovolemia.[189]

Another important risk factor for auditory aminoglycoside toxicity is the concurrent use of ethacyrnic acid.[190–192] Fortunately, furosemide at clinically used doses and with proper attention to hydration does not appear to be associated with enhanced aminoglycoside auditory toxicity.[192]

Several other potential risk factors that have been identified in experimental animals but that have not yet been proven in humans include noise and age, with increased susceptibility in the very young and the elderly.[193–196]

It should be emphasized that auditory toxicity is cumulative. Thus, with repeated aminoglycoside courses, hearing loss may become detectable as a result of cumulative damage even during a carefully monitored course of therapy.[186–189] This is surely related to the inability of damaged or destroyed cochlear hair cells to regenerate.

Vestibular dysfunction is manifest clinically by nausea, vomiting, vertigo, dizziness, and an unsteady gait with nystagmus. These symptoms and signs are difficult to evaluate in ill patients. More sophisticated laboratory tests are too cumbersome for use in most ill patients.[188]

As with auditory toxicity, vestibular toxicity is dose-related, duration-related, and probably related to plasma levels outside the therapeutic range. However, because of the difficulties of evaluating vestibular function, it has been less well defined than has been auditory toxicity.

Nephrotoxicity

All aminoglycosides are capable of causing nephrotoxicity, although individual differences exist among members of the family with respect to nephrotoxic potential.

The mechanisms involved in aminoglycoside nephrotoxicity include the rapid transport, extensive accumulation, and avid retention of aminoglycosides for prolonged periods of time. In addition, the aminoglycosides are assumed to produce biochemical effects on proximal tubular metabolism that lead to pathophysiologic effects linking proximal tubular damage to diminished glomerular function.

The transport of aminoglycosides is primarily across the luminal brush border of the proximal renal tubular cells and involves an initial binding of the positively charged aminoglycoside to the negatively charged phosphatidylinositol within the membrane.[104,106,107,110] Internalization is believed to occur by pinocytosis into vesicles that eventually coalesce with lysosomes whose highly negative interior effectively traps the aminoglycoside.[105,197] The extensive accumulation of aminoglycosides is confined to the renal cortex, where concentrations 5–50-fold higher than plasma concentrations are found.[198] Within the renal cortex the aminoglycosides are further localized exclusively to the proximal renal tubular cells.[78,105]

It remains unclear whether the proximal tubular cell damage that is characteristic of the aminoglycosides is attributable to lysosomal or extralysosomal effects. Lysosomes may be a primary site of aminoglycoside toxicity or may be salvage organelles responsible for keeping the intracellular aminoglycoside in a nontoxic site. Morphologically, aminoglycosides cause an accumulation of multilamellar structures within lysosomes called myeloid bodies.[197,199,200] Biochemically, aminoglycosides inhibit lysosomal phospholipases A_1, A_2, and C_1 and are also associated with a loss of sphingomyelinase activity.[201,202] Extralysosomal effects of aminoglycosides include both structural and functional effects on mitochondria,[203–205] the inhibition of a sodium–potassium adenosine triphosphatase localized on the basolateral portion of the plasma membrane,[206] and the inhibition of a cytosolic phosphatidylinositol specific phospholipase C.[207] The inhibition of this cytosolic phospholipase may be particularly important since this enzyme may be responsible for an early and pivotal step in the biosynthesis of prostaglandins and prostacyclin. Such an effect might be quite relevant to the reduction of glomerular filtration that is produced by the aminoglycosides subsequent to proximal tubular damage, since an inhibition of the production of vasodilatory prostaglandins would allow the unopposed vasoconstrictor action of angiotensin II, leading to arteriolar vasoconstriction and a decrease in glomerular filtration.[208] Structural and functional alterations of glomeruli have also been identified and may be directly related to aminoglycosides or secondary to effects on prostaglandin or angiotensin systems.[209–212]

Clinical nephrotoxicity, as defined by a reduced glomerular filtration rate (GFR), occurs in between 5 and 25 percent of aminoglycoside recipients.[114,155] The earliest manifestation of an effect of aminoglycosides on the kidney is an increase in the urinary excretion of several renal tubular enzymes, including alanine aminopeptidase, B-D-glucosaminidase, and alkaline phosphatase.[213] In addition, the reabsorption of β_2-microglobulin is competitively inhibited, and its excretion is enhanced.[214] These early indicators of renal effects are too sensitive and too nonspecific to be of clinical value, since every patient receiving an aminoglycoside will exhibit these effects.[213] It appears to be more useful to define aminoglycoside nephrotoxicity in terms of a reduction in GFR as reflected by a rise in serum creatinine, and the serum creatinine is an adequate and convenient parameter to follow when monitoring for aminoglycoside nephrotoxicity.

The onset of glomerular dysfunction usually occurs several days after the initiation of therapy, although a more rapid onset is possible. The glomerular dysfunction in humans increases in severity over a few days, although in experimental animals a cyclic phenomenon of damage and repair occurs even with continuing administration of the aminoglycoside.[215] Whether the same phenomenon occurs in humans remains unknown.

The extent of human kidney damage associated with aminoglycosides is most often mild, occasionally moderate, and rarely severe.[216] It appears that severe nephrotoxicity does not occur if the aminoglycoside dosage is carefully adjusted for changing glomerular function.

The degree of reversibility of renal dysfunction associated with aminoglycosides is remarkable, since the potential of the proximal renal tubule for regeneration is extensive and no or very little irreversible damage is associated with aminoglycosides. The type of renal dysfunction is nonoliguric.

Although individual functions served by the proximal renal tubule such as glucose reabsorption or amino acid reabsorption have been abnormal in experimental animals, these individual proximal tubular functions are usually remarkably well preserved in humans. A syndrome of hypokalemia, hypocalcemia, and hypomagnesemia has been reported in a very few patients.[217–221]

Considerable attention has centered on risk factors in an effort to identify patients who are likely to develop renal dysfunction while receiving an aminoglycoside. Risk factors include older age, female sex, concomitant liver disease, and concomitant hypotension at the onset of aminoglycoside therapy.[222–224] Concomitant cephalothin administration has been reported to be associated with an increased incidence of renal dysfunction.[225] Other nephrotoxic drugs including *cis*-platinum, amphotericin B, and cyclosporin also contribute to the renal dysfunction associated with aminoglycosides.

In addition, different aminoglycosides possess differing degrees of inherent nephrotoxic potential. Of the currently available aminoglycosides, gentamicin is more nephrotoxic than tobramycin.[155] Amikacin is also less nephrotoxic than gentamicin on a weight basis in animals. At a clinical level, however, higher doses of amikacin are allowed because of this lesser nephrotoxicity, and at least some of the difference may be abolished. Netilmicin is also less nephrotoxic than gentamicin in animal studies, but the evidence in humans is currently unconvincing.

Since aminoglycoside nephrotoxicity is usually mild and reversible, we should not err on the side of undertreatment as a result of excessive fear of this adverse effect.

INDIVIDUAL DRUGS

Streptomycin

Streptomycin is available as streptomycin sulfate for intramuscular administration in vials either premixed or to be reconstituted to concentrations of 400 or 500 mg/ml.

Streptomycin is primarily considered as an antituberculous drug with good activity against both *M. tuberculosis* and *Mycobacterium bovis* and less activity against atypical mycobacteria. Streptomycin is also considered the drug of choice for *F. tubarensis* (tularemia) and *Y. pestis* (plague) and is often used for infections caused by *Brucella*. In addition, streptomycin is frequently used, in combination with penicillin or vancomycin, for infections caused by *Enterococcus* (*Streptococcus*) *faecalis* or *Streptococcus viridans*, especially endocarditis, and in prophylactic regimens designed to prevent endocarditis. Enterococcal resistance to streptomycin in some areas, however, may preclude the use of streptomycin and favor gentamicin.[46]

The dosage of streptomycin for tuberculosis is generally 1

g/day followed in a few weeks by 1 g three times a week. For tularemia an accepted dosage is 2 g/day in divided doses (12 hourly), for plague 2 g/day in divided doses (12 hourly), and for brucellosis 1 g/day in divided doses (12 hourly) along with tetracycline. For the treatment of enterococcal endocarditis a recommended dosage regimen is 1 g/day in divided doses (12 hourly) for 4–6 weeks. Enterococci may be highly resistant to streptomycin, and gentamicin is usually recommended for treatment of endocarditis caused by streptomycin-resistant organisms. For the prevention of endocarditis, a recommended dosage regimen of streptomycin is 1 g given ½–1 hour before dental or surgical intervention and for genitourinary or gastrointestinal surgery an additional 1 g at 12 hours and again at 24 hours postoperatively.

As with other aminoglycosides, the dosage should be reduced in the elderly, in newborns, and in patients with diminished glomerular function.

Neomycin

Neomycin is available as neomycin sulfate for oral administration in tablets containing 500 mg each. In addition, neomycin sulfate is available either alone or in combination with other agents in numerous ophthalmologic, otic, and dermatologic formulations for topical application.

For preoperative suppression of intestinal bacteria a dosage regimen of 6 g/day (divided four hourly) for 2–3 days has been recommended. In hepatic coma a dosage regimen of 4–12 g/day (divided four or six hourly) has been recommended. It is imperative to recognize that a small percentage of the oral dose of neomycin will be absorbed and that this may provide toxic systemic levels in a patient with renal dysfunction.

Kanamycin

Kanamycin is available as kanamycin sulfate in both parenteral and oral formulations. For parenteral use kanamycin sulfate is available at concentrations of 250, 333, or 37.5 mg/ml. All parenteral formulations contain sodium bisulfite as a preservative. For oral use kanamycin sulfate is available in capsules of 500 mg each.

The place of kanamycin for treatment of systemic infections is debatable. Its widespread usage during the 1960s was sharply curtailed in the 1970s as a result of the relatively common emergence of resistance in common gram-negative bacillary organisms in conjunction with the usual resistance of *Pseudomonas* species. With its disuse, however, the level of resistance has decreased in many areas, and it has again enjoyed some increase in use in infections unlikely to be associated with *Pseudomonas* species. In general, however, its place has been taken by gentamicin, tobramycin, and amikacin.

The dosage of kanamycin (either intramuscularly or intravenously) for systemic infections has been 15 mg/kg/day in divided doses (usually 12 hourly) with a maximal dose of 1.5 g/day. If given intravenously, the dose should be administered over at least 30 minutes.

The parenteral formulation of kanamycin sulfate may be diluted with sterile distilled water to provide solutions for intraperitoneal instillation or for the irrigation of abscess cavities, pleural or peritoneal spaces, the bladder, or wounds. Although concentrations of 25 mg/ml for intraperitoneal instillation and 2.5 mg/ml for irrigating solutions have been recommended, it is important to recognize that absorption can occur, especially from the peritoneum, pleura, or open wounds, and that very large daily systemic doses can be achieved inadvertently with these concentrated solutions. It would seem more prudent to use solutions of 25 μg/ml since this is the peak level achieved in plasma with systemic dosing and since this level is unlikely to produce toxicity in the absence of renal dysfunction.

The oral dose of kanamycin for the suppression of intestinal bacteria preoperatively or in hepatic coma is 8–12 g/day in divided doses (four or six hourly). As with neomycin, some kanamycin will be absorbed, and toxic systemic levels may result in patients with renal dysfunction.

As with all aminoglycosides, the systemic dosing of kanamycin must be adjusted for renal glomerular dysfunction, including that seen in the elderly and the newborn.

Gentamicin

Gentamicin is available as gentamicin sulfate for parenteral and topical use. For parenteral use gentamicin sulfate is available in concentrations of 2 mg/ml (without methyl and propylparabens, ethylenediaminetetraacetic acid (EDTA), and sodium bisulfite as preservatives) for intrathecal or intraventricular use, 10 mg/ml (pediatric), 40 mg/ml (intravenous or intramuscular), or 1 mg/ml (intravenous piggyback without preservative) in various sized vials, prefilled syringes, or piggyback units.

Gentamicin sulfate is also available in several topical formulations for ophthalmologic or dermatologic use.

Gentamicin remains a mainstay in the treatment of gram-negative bacillary infections, in part because of its relatively low cost after the expiration of its patent.

Gentamicin dosing is discussed above.

Tobramycin

Tobramycin is available as tobramycin sulfate for parenteral or topical use. For parenteral use tobramycin sulfate is available in concentrations of 10 mg/ml (pediatric) and 40 mg/ml (intravenous or intramuscular) in vials or prefilled syringes. Each of these formulations contains phenol, EDTA, and sodium bisulfite as preservatives. In addition, a powder for injection is available, which can be reconstituted with sterile water to a concentration of 40 mg/ml. This formulation contains no preservatives and may be a more reasonable choice for intrathecal or intraventricular injections.

Tobramycin sulfate is also available as ophthalmic drops containing 3 mg/mg.

Tobramycin is widely used in the treatment of gram-negative bacillary infections. At a clinical level there is no evidence for its superiority or inferiority when compared with gentamicin, amikacin, or netilmicin with respect to effectiveness in infections caused by susceptible organisms. Its in vitro activity is somewhat greater than gentamicin for *P. aeruginosa* and somewhat less for *Serratia*, but this has not led to demonstrable differences in clinical effectiveness. A few organisms are resistant to gentamicin and yet sensitive to tobramycin, but the resistance profiles of the two are highly similar. Tobramycin is somewhat less nephrotoxic than gentamicin and may be somewhat less ototoxic as well, but the lesser ototoxicity that exists in animals has been supported only with respect to vestibular dysfunction in humans.

Tobramycin dosing is discussed above and is identical to gentamicin dosing.

Amikacin

Amikacin is available as amikacin sulfate for parenteral use in solutions containing 50 or 250 mg/ml. Only one formulation of amikacin sulfate contains no preservatives (sodium bisulfite and sulfuric acid), and this is probably the preferred formulation for intrathecal or intraventricular use.

Amikacin is widely used in the treatment of gram-negative bacillary infections. At a clinical level there is no evidence for its superiority or inferiority when compared with gentamicin, tobramycin, or netilmicin with respect to effectiveness in infections caused by susceptible organisms. Although its in vitro potency is somewhat less, or a weight basis, than that of gentamicin, tobramycin, or netilmicin, the larger dosages used compensate for this lesser potency. A clear advantage of amikacin lies in its resistance profile. Many of the aminoglycoside-inactivating enzymes that inactivate other aminoglycosides cannot inactivate amikacin, and consequently many organisms that are resistant to gentamicin, tobramycin, or netilmicin remain sensitive to amikacin. Thus amikacin has clear-cut advantages in treating infections caused by organisms known to be resistant to other aminoglycosides and in nosocomial infections in which the likelihood of resistant organisms is increased. The use of amikacin in other and more general settings currently presents a dilemma for the clinician. On the one hand, the restriction of amikacin usage is often believed to be wise in order to delay the emergence of resistance to this valuable drug. On the other hand, there is no evidence that the restriction of amikacin usage will delay the emergence of resistance, and there is a theoretical reason that resistance may not be delayed. This is based on the fact that each of the relatively few aminoglycoside-inactivating enzymes that can inactivate amikacin can also inactivate other aminoglycosides. Thus the continued use of other aminoglycosides may provide ecologic pressure for the development of those enzymes capable of inactivating amikacin even though amikacin use is restricted.

With respect to toxicity, amikacin is probably less nephrotoxic and less ototoxic than gentamicin on a weight basis. However, since larger doses of amikacin are used, the differences on a weight basis may be at least partially lost. On a clinical level there have been no direct prospective and blinded comparisons between amikacin and either tobramycin or netilmicin with respect to toxicity. Therefore, the precise placement of amikacin with respect to its relative toxicity remains unclear.

Netilmicin

Netilmicin is available as netilmicin sulfate for parenteral use, in formulations containing 10 mg/ml (neonatal; with sodium metabisulfite and sodium sulfite as preservatives), 25 mg/ml (pediatric; with methyl and propyl parabens, EDTA, sodium metabisulfite, and sodium sulfite as preservatives) and 100 mg/ml (with benzyl alcohol, EDTA, sodium metabisulfite, and sodium sulfite as preservatives) in vials or prefilled syringes.

Netilmicin has only recently been marketed, and its place in therapy is yet to be established. Its clinical effectiveness is probably similar to gentamicin, tobramycin, and amikacin. In vitro its resistance profile resembles gentamicin and tobramycin, with only a few strains of bacteria being resistant to gentamicin or tobramycin and sensitive to netilmicin. From a toxicologic point of view, netilmicin is less nephrotoxic than gentamicin in experimental animals, but this has not been confirmed in humans. Subclinical auditory toxicity, as detected by audiometry, is less with netilmicin than with tobramycin.[187] Clinically detectable auditory toxicity is very rare with any of the commonly used aminoglycosides if dosing is appropriately controlled.

Spectinomycin

Spectinomycin is isolated from *Streptomyces spectabilis* and is classified as an aminocyclitol antibiotic but is not an aminoglycoside since it contains neither an aminosugar nor a glycosidic bond (Fig. 2).[226,227]

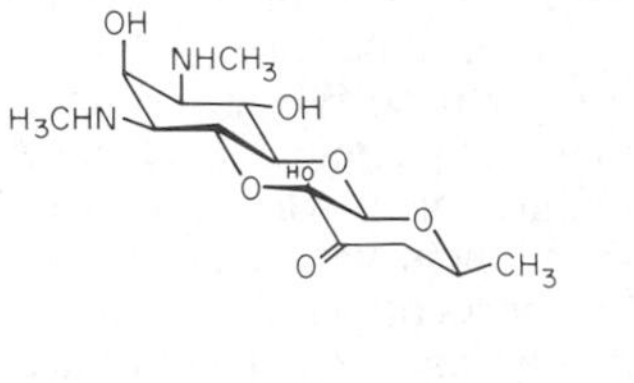

FIG. 2. Structure of spectinomycin—an aminocyclitol.

The site of action of spectinomycin may be similar to the aminoglycosides since spectinomycin binds to the smaller (30s) ribosomal subunits, and protein synthesis is inhibited.[228] However, misreading of the genetic code does not occur, and a membrane effect does appear to exist by electron microscopy.[229]

Resistance to spectinomycin is rarely seen in *Neisseria gonorrhoea*, and there is no cross-resistance with penicillins.[226]

Although the spectrum of activity of spectinomycin is broader, spectinomycin is used only as an agent for infections caused by *N. gonorrhoea*. Significantly, it is not effective against *Treponema pallidum* or *Chlamydia trachomatis*, but it may be somewhat effective against *Ureaplasma urealyticum* and *Gardnerella vaginalis*.[226,227,230]

Spectinomycin is rapidly and completely absorbed after intramuscular administration.[231] Its volume of distribution is about 0.33 liter/kg and its half-life about 1 hour.[216] It is not metabolized and is excreted completely into the urine as unchanged drug. Spectinomycin does not enter saliva and is not predictably effective in eliminating pharyngeal *Neisseria*.[212]

Toxicologically, spectinomycin differs considerably from the aminoglycosides in that it is neither ototoxic nor nephrotoxic, and, in fact, few side effects exist with the usual dosing of the drug. Urticaria, chills, fever, dizziness, nausea, and insomnia have been reported.

Therapeutically, spectinomycin is clearly highly effective in the treatment of uncomplicated gonorrhea and disseminated gonococcal infection. It is unpredictable in the treatment of pharyngeal gonorrhea. Spectinomycin is the drug of choice in the treatment of penicillinase-producing gonococcal infections and in the treatment of patients who fail to respond to treatment.

Spectinomycin is available as spectinomycin hydrochloride in a powder form that is reconstituted with 0.9% benzyl alcohol as a diluent to a concentration of 400 mg/ml. It can be given only intramuscularly.

For uncomplicated gonorrheal infections 2 g as a single intramuscular dose is recommended. For disseminated gonococcal infections the recommended dose is 4 g/day in divided doses (12 hourly) for 3 days.

REFERENCES

1. Rinehart KL. Comparative chemistry of the aminoglycoside and aminocyclitol antibiotics. J Infect Dis. 1969;119:345.
2. Daniels PJL: Antibiotics (aminoglycosides). In: Grayson M, ed. Kirk-Othmer: Encyclopedia of Chemical Technology. v. 5. 3rd ed. New York: John Wiley Sons; 1978:819.
3. Hooper IR. The naturally occurring aminoglycoside antibiotics. In: Umezawa H, Hooper IR, eds. Aminoglycoside Antibiotics. New York: Springer-Verlag; 1982:1.
4. Umezawa S, Tsuchiya T. Total synthesis and chemical modification of the aminoglycoside antibiotics. In: Umezawa H, Hooper IR, eds. Aminoglycoside Antibiotics. New York: Springer-Verlag; 1982:37.
5. Price KE, Godfrey JC, Kawaguchi H. Effect of structural modifications on the biological properties of aminoglycoside antibiotics containing 2-deoxystreptamine. Adv Appl Microbiol. 1974;18:191.
6. Hancock REW. Aminoglycoside uptake and mode of action: with special reference to streptomycin and gentamicin. I. Antagonists and mutants. J Antimicrob Chemother. 1981;8:249.
7. Hancock REW. Aminoglycoside uptake and mode of action: with special reference to streptomycin and gentamicin. II. Effects of aminoglycosides on cells. J Antimicrob Chemother. 1981;8:429.
8. Davis BD. The lethal action of aminoglycosides. J Antimicrob Chemother. 1988;22:1.
9. Nichols WW. On the mechanism of translocation of dihydrostreptomycin across the bacterial cytoplasmic membrane. Biochim Biophys Acta. 1987;895:11.
10. Pestka S. Inhibitors of protein synthesis. In: Weissback H, Pestka S, eds. Molecular Mechanisms of Protein Synthesis. New York: Academic Press; 1977:467.
11. Stoffler G, Wittmann HG. Primary structure and three-dimensional arrangement of proteins within the *Escherichia coli* ribosome. In: Weissbach H, Pestka S, eds. Molecular Mechanisms of Protein Synthesis. New York: Academic Press; 1977:117.
12. Hummel H, Piepersberg W, Bock A. 30s subunit mutations relieving restriction of ribosomal misreading caused by L6 mutations. Mol Gen Genet. 1980;179:147.
13. Kuhberger R, Piepersberg W, Petzet A, et al. Alteration of ribosomal protein

L6 in gentamicin-resistant strains of *Escherichia coli*. Effects on fidelity of protein synthesis. Biochemistry. 1979;18:187.
14. Tai P-C, Davis BD. Triphasic concentration effects of gentamicin on activity and misreading in protein synthesis. Biochemistry. 1979;18:193.
15. Chang FN, Flaks JG. Binding of dihydrostreptomycin to *Escherichia coli* ribosomes: characteristics and equilibrium of the reaction. Antimicrob Agents Chemother. 1972;2:294.
16. Chang FN, Flaks JG. Binding of dihydrostreptomycin to *Escherichia coli* ribosomes: kinetics of the reaction. Antimicrob Agents Chemother. 1972;2:308.
17. Ozaki M, Mizushima S, Nomura M. Identification and functional characterization of the protein controlled by the streptomycin-resistant locus in *E. coli*. Nature. 1969;222:333.
18. Schreiner G, Nierhaus KH. Protein involved in the binding of dihydrostreptomycin to ribosomes of *Escherichia coli*. J Mol Biol. 1973;81:71.
19. Wallace BJ, David BD. Cyclic blockade of initiation sites by streptomycin-damaged ribosomes in *Escherichia coli*: an explanation for dominance of sensitivity. J Mol Biol. 1973;75:377.
20. Wallace BJ, Tai P-C, Davis BD. Effect of streptomycin on the response of *Escherichia coli* ribosomes to the dissociation factor. J Mol Biol. 1973;75:391.
21. Luzzatto L, Apirion D, Schlessinger D. Mechanism of action of streptomycin in *E. coli*: Interruption of the ribosome cycle of the initiation of protein synthesis. Proc Natl Acad Sci USA. 1968;60:873.
22. Luzzatto L, Apirion D, Schlessinger D. Polyribosome depletion and blockage of the ribosome cycle by streptomycin in *Escherichia coli*. J Mol Biol. 1969;42:315.
23. Bryan LE, van den Elzen HM. Effects of membrane-energy mutations and cations on streptomycin and gentamicin accumulation by bacteria: a model for entry of streptomycin and gentamicin in susceptible and resistant bacteria. Antimicrob Agents Chemother. 1977;12:163.
24. Mak L, Lietman PS. Aminoglycoside transport by bacteria. In: Fillastre J-P, ed. Nephrotoxicité et Ototoxicité Medicamenteuses. Rouen: Editions INSERM; 1981:55.
25. Damper PD, Epstein W. Role of the membrane potential in bacterial resistance to aminglycoside antibiotics. Antimicrob Agents Chemother. 1981;20:803.
26. Mates SM, Patel L, Kaback HR, et al. Membrane potential in anaerobically growing *Staphylococcus aureus* and its relationship to gentamicin uptake. Antimicrob Agents Chemother. 1983;23:526.
27. Holtje J-V. Regulation of polamine and streptomycin transport during stringent and relaxed control in *Escherichia coli*. J Bacteriol. 1979;137:661.
28. Hurwitz C, Rosano CL. Chloramphenicol-sensitive and -insensitive phases of the lethal action of streptomycin. J Bacteriol. 1962;83:1202.
29. Bryan LE. General mechanisms of resistance to antibiotics. J Antimicrob Chemother. 1988;22(Suppl A):1.
30. Mitsuhashi S, Kawabe H. Aminoglycoside antibiotic resistance in bacteria. In: Whelton A, New HC, eds. The Aminoglycosides. New York: Marcel Dekker; 1983:97.
31. Davies JE. Resistance to aminoglycosides: mechanism and frequency. Rev Infect Dis. 1983;5(Suppl):3261.
32. Kabins SA, Nathan C, Cohen S. *In vitro* comparison of netilmicin, a semisynthetic derivative of sisomicin, and four other aminoglycoside antibiotics. Antimicrob Agents Chemother. 1976;10:139.
33. Sanders CC, Sanders WE, Jr, Goering RV. *In vitro* studies with Sch 21420 and Sch 22591: activity in comparison with six other aminoglycosides and synergy with penicillin against enterococci. Antimicrob Agents Chemother. 1978;14:178.
34. Moellering RC Jr. Clinical microbiology and the *in vitro* activity of aminoglycosides. In: Whelton A, Neu HC, eds. The Aminoglycosides: Microbiology, Clinical Use, and Toxicology. New York: Marcel Dekker; 1982:65.
35. Fu K, Neu HC. *In vitro* study of netilmicin compared with other aminoglycosides. Antimicrob Agents Chemother. 1976;10:526.
36. National Committee for Clinical Laboratory Standards. Performance standards for antimicrobial disc susceptibility tests. Approved Standard: ASM-2, Villanova, PA, 1979.
37. Thornsberry C, Gavan TL, Gerlach EH, et al. New developments in antimicrobial agent susceptibility testing. In: Sherris JC, ed. Cumitech 6. Washington, DC: American Society of Microbiology; 1977:1.
38. McDonald PJ, Craig WA, Konin CM. Persistent effect of antibiotics on *Staphylococcus aureus* after exposure for limited periods of time. J Infect Dis. 1977;135:217.
39. Grasso S, Meinardi G, DeCarneri J, et al. New *in vitro* model to study the effect of antibiotic concentration and rate of elimination on antibacterial activity. Antimicrob Agents Chemother. 1978;13:570.
40. Al-Asadi MJS, Greenwood D, O'Grady F. *In vitro* model simulating the form of exposure of bacteria to antimicrobial drugs encountered in infection. Antimicrob Agents Chemother. 1979;16:77.
41. Murakawa T, Sakamoto H, Hinrose T, et al. New *in vitro* model for evaluating bactericidal efficacy of antibiotics. Antimicrob Agents Chemother. 1980;18:77.
42. Bergan T, Carlsen IB, Fuglesang JE. An *in vitro* model for monitoring bacterial responses to antibiotic agents under simulated *in vivo* conditions. Infection. 1980;8(Suppl 1):S96.
43. Longstreth JA. Interaction of aminoglycoside pharmacokinetics and bacterial population kinetics in a chemostat. PhD dissertation. Johns Hopkins University, 1982.
44. Hammond BJ, Kogot M, Lightbown JW. Analogue computer studies of the growth characteristics of *Escherichia coli* following dihydrostreptomycin treatment. J Gen Microbiol. 1967;48:189.
45. Kogot M, Lightbown JW, Isaacson P. Effects of dihydrostreptomycin treatment on the growth of *Escherichia coli* after removal of extracellular antibiotic. J Gen Microbiol. 1965;39:165.
46. Bundtzen RW, Gerber AU, Cohn DL, et al. Postantibiotic suppression of bacterial growth. Rev Infect Dis. 1981;3:28.
47. Gerber AU, Wippraechtiger P, Stettler U, et al. Constant infusions versus intermittent doses of gentamicin against Pseudomonas *in vitro*. J Infect Dis. 1982;145:554.
48. Gerber AU, Craig WA, Brugger H-P, et al. Impact of dosing intervals on activity of gentamicin and ticarcillin against *Pseudomonas aeruginosa* in granulocytopenic mice. J Infect Dis. 1983;147:910.
49. Powell SH, Thompson WL, Luthe MA, et al. Once-daily versus continuous aminoglycoside dosing: efficacy and toxicity in animal and clinical studies of gentamicin, netilmicin and tobramycin. J Infect Dis. 1983;147:918.
50. Vogelman BS, Craig WA. Postantibiotic effects. J Antimicrob Chemother. 1985;15(Suppl A):37.
51. Blaser J, Stone BB, Zinner SH. Efficacy of intermittent versus continuous administration of netilmicin in a two-compartment *in vitro* model. Antimicrob Agents Chemother. 1985;27:343.
52. Craig WA, Vogelman B. The postantibiotic effect. Ann Intern Med. 1987;106:900.
53. Vogelman B, Gudmundsson S, Turnidge J, et al. *In vivo* postantibiotic effect in a thigh infection in neutropenic mice. J Infect Dis. 1988;157:287.
54. Isaksson B, Nilsson L, Maller R, et al. Postantibiotic effect of aminoglycosides on Gram-negative bacteria evaluated by a new method. J Antimicrob Chemother. 1988;22:23.
55. Wood CA, Norton DR, Kohlhepp SJ, et al. The influence of tobramycin dosage regimens on nephrotoxicity, ototoxicity and antibacterial efficacy in a rat model of subcutaneous abscess. J Infect Dis. 1988;158:13.
56. Klastersky J, Cappel R, Danpau D. Clinical significance of *in vitro* synergism between antibiotics in gram-negative infections. Antimicrob Agents Chemother. 1972;2:470.
57. Moellering RC Jr, Wennerstein C, Weinberg AN. Studies on antibiotic synergism against enterococci: I. Bacteriologic studies. J Lab Clin Med. 1971;77:821.
58. Kunin CM, Chalmers TC, Leevy CM. Absorption of orally administered neomycin and kanamycin. N Engl J Med. 1960;262:380.
59. Last PM, Sherlock S. Systemic absorption of orally administered neomycin in liver disease. N Engl J Med. 1960;262:385.
60. Kunin CM. Absorption, distribution, excretion and fate of kanamycin. Ann NY Acad Sci. 1966;132:811.
61. Breen KF, Bryant RE, Levinson JD, et al. Neomycin absorption in man. Ann Intern Med. 1972;76:211.
62. Mitch WE, Lietman PS, Walser M. Effects of oral neomycin and kanamycin in chronic uremic patients. I. Urea metabolism. Kidney Int. 1977;11:116.
63. King JT. Severe deafness in an infant following oral administration of neomycin. J Med Assoc Ga. 1962;51:530.
64. Ruben RJ, Daly JF. Neomycin ototoxicity and nephrotoxicity. Laryngoscope. 1968;78:1734.
65. Kalbian VV. Deafness following oral use of neomycin. South Med J. 1972;65:499.
66. Ward KM, Rounthwaite FJ. Neomycin ototoxicity. Ann Otol. 1978;87:211.
67. Doluisio JT, Dittert LW, LaPiana JC. Pharmacokinetics of kanamycin following intramuscular administration. J Pharmacokinet Biopharm. 1973;1:253.
68. Barza M, Lauermann M. Why monitor serum levels of gentamicin. Clin Pharmacokinet. 1978;3:202.
69. Little PJ, Lynn KL. Neomycin toxicity. NZ Med J. 1975;81:445.
70. Bamford MFM, Jones LF. Deafness and biochemical imbalance after burns treatment with topical antibiotics in young children. Arch Dis Child. 1978;53:326.
71. Somani P, Shapiro RS, Stockard H, et al. Unidirectional absorption of gentamicin from the peritoneum during continuous ambulatory peritoneal dialysis. Clin Pharmacol Ther. 1982;32:113.
72. DePaepe M, Lameire N, Belpaire F, et al. Peritoneal pharmacokinetics of gentamicin in man. Clin Nephrol. 1983;19:107.
73. Chamberlain G, Needham P. The absorption of antibiotics from the bladder. J Urol. 1976;116:172.
74. Lifschitz MI, Denning CR. Safety of kanamycin aerosol. Clin Pharmacol Ther. 1971;12:91.
75. Odio W, VanLeier E, Klastersky J. Concentrations of gentamicin in bronchial secretions after intramuscular and endotracheal administration. J Clin Pharmacol. 1975;15:518.
76. Rahal JJ Jr, Hyams PJ, Simberkoff MS, et al. Combined intrathecal and intramuscular gentamicin for gram-negative meningitis. N Engl J Med. 1974;290:1394.
77. Van Etta LL, Kravitz GR, Russ TE, et al. Effect of method of administration on extravascular penetration of four antibiotics. Antimicrob Agents Chemother. 1982;21:873.
78. Kuhar MJ, Mak LL, Lietman PS. Localization of ^{3}H-gentamicin in the proximal renal tubule of the mouse. Antimicrob Agents Chemother. 1979;15:131.
79. Thys JP, Klastersky J, Mombelli G. Peak or sustained antibiotic levels for optimal tissue penetration. J Antimicrob Chemother. 1981;8(Suppl C):29.
80. Klastersky J, Meunier-Carpentier F, Kahan-Coppens L, et al. Endotra-

cheally administered antibiotics for gram negative bronchopneumonia. Chest. 1979;75:586.
81. Kaiser AB, McGee ZA. Aminoglycoside therapy of gram-negative bacillary meningitis. N Engl J Med. 1975;293:1215.
82. Wirt TC, McGee ZA, Oldfield EH, et al. Intraventricular administration of amikacin for complicated gram-negative meningitis and ventriculitis. J Neurosurg. 1979;50:95.
83. McCracken GH Jr, Mize S, Threlkeld N. Intraventricular gentamicin therapy in gram-negative bacillary meningitis of infancy. Lancet. 1980;i:787.
84. Barza M, Kane A, Baum J. Comparison of the effects of continuous and intermittent systemic administration on the penetration of gentamicin into infected rabbit eyes. J Infect Dis. 1983;147:144.
85. Gorden TB, Cunningham RD. Tobramycin levels in aqueous humor after subconjunctival injection in humans. Am J Ophthalmol. 1982;93:107.
86. Rubenstein E, Goldfarb J, Keren G, et al. The penetration of gentamicin into the vitreous humor in man. Invest Ophthalmol Vis Sci. 1983;24:637.
87. Marsh DC Jr, Matthew EB, Perselin RA. Transport of gentamicin into synovial fluid. JAMA. 1974;228:607.
88. Dee TH, Koein F. Gentamicin and tobramycin penetration into synovial fluid. Antimicrob Agents Chemother. 1977;12:548.
89. Chow A, Hecht R, Witners R. Gentamicin and carbenicillin penetration into the septic joint. N Engl J Med. 1971;285:178.
90. Baciocco EA, Iles RI. Ampicillin and kanamycin concentration in joint fluid. Clin Pharmacol Ther. 1971;12:858.
91. Schurman DJ, Wheeler R. Bone and joint gram-negative infection and amikacin treatment. Am J Med. 1977;62(Suppl):160.
92. Alftan O, Renkonen OV, Sironen A. Concentration of gentamicin in serum, urine and urogenital tissue in man. Acta Pathol Microbiol Scand [B]. 1973;81(Suppl 241):92.
93. Mahmod S, Al-Hakiem MHH, Landon J, et al. Aminoglycoside antibiotics do not appear in saliva. Clin Chem. 1983;29:988.
94. Pitt HA, Roberts RB, Johnson WD Jr. Gentamicin levels in the human biliary tract. J Infect Dis. 1973;127:299.
95. Mendelson J, Portnoy J, Sigman H. Pharmacology of gentamicin in the biliary tract of humans. Antimicrob Agents Chemother. 1973;4:538.
96. Wood MJ, Farrell W. Comparison of urinary excretion of tobramycin and gentamicin in adults. J Infect Dis. 1976;134(Suppl):S133.
97. Kahlmeter G, Kamme C. Prolonged excretion of gentamicin in a patient with unimpaired renal function. Lancet. 1975;i:286.
98. Kahlmeter G, Jonsson S, Kamme C. Multiple-compartment pharmacokinetics of tobramycin. J Antimicrob Chemother. 1978;4(Suppl A):5.
99. Kahlmeter G. Netilmicin: clinical pharmacokinetics and aspects on dosage schedules. An overview. Scand J Infect Dis. 1980;23:74.
100. Laskin OL, Longstreth JA, Smith CR, et al. Netilmicin and gentamicin multidose kinetics in normal subjects. Clin Pharmacol Ther. 1983;34:644.
101. Wilson TW, Mahon WA, Inaba T, et al. Elimination of tritiated gentamicin in normal human subjects and in patients with severely impaired renal function. Clin Pharmacol Ther. 1973;14:815.
102. Kahlmeter G. Gentamicin and tobramycin: clinical pharmacokinetics and nephrotoxicity: aspects on assay techniques. Thesis, Department of Medical Microbiology, University of Lund, Sweden, 1979.
103. Pastoriza-Munoz E, Timmerman D, Feldman S, et al. Ultrafiltration of gentamicin and netilmicin *in vivo*. J Pharmacol Exp Ther. 1982;220:604.
104. Collier VU, Lietman PS, Mitch WE. Evidence for luminal uptake of gentamicin in perfused rat kidney. J Pharmacol Exp Ther. 1979;210:247.
105. Silverblatt FJ, Kuehn C. Autoradiography of gentamicin uptake by the rat proximal tubular cell. Kidney Int. 1979;15:335.
106. Lipsky JJ, Cheng L, Saktor B, et al. Gentamicin uptake by renal tubule brush border membrane vesicles. J Pharmacol Exp Ther. 1980;215:390.
107. Sastrasinh M, Knauss TC, Weinberg JM, et al. Identification of the aminoglycoside binding site in rat renal brush border membranes. J Pharmacol Exp Ther. 1982;222:350.
108. Senekjian HO, Knight TF, Weinman EJ. Micropuncture study of the handling of gentamicin by the rat kidney. Kidney Int. 1981;19:416.
109. Pastoriza-Munoz E, Bowman RL, Kaloyanides GJ. Renal tubular transport of gentamicin in the rat. Kidney Int. 1979;16:440.
110. Frommer JP, Senekjian HO, Babino H, et al. Intratubular microinjection study of gentamicin transport in the rat. Mineral Electrolyte Metab. 1983;9:108.
111. Wenk M, Spring P, Vozeh S, et al. Multicompartment pharmacokinetics of netilmicin. Eur J Clin Pharmacol. 1979;16:331.
112. Laskin OL, Longstreth JA, Smith CR, et al. Netilmicin and gentamicin multidose kinetics in normal subjects. Clin Pharmacol Ther. 1983;34:644.
113. Lanao JM, Dominguez-Gil A, Tobernero JM, et al. Pharmacokinetics of amikacin (BB-K8) in patients with normal or impaired renal function. Int J Clin Pharmacol Biopharm. 1979;17:171.
114. Smith CR, Baughman KL, Edwards CQ, et al. Controlled comparison of amikacin and gentamicin. N Engl J Med. 1977;296:349.
115. Gyselynck A-M, Forrey A, Cutler R. Pharmacokinetics of gentamicin: distribution and plasma and renal clearance. J Infect Dis. 1971;124(Suppl):S70.
116. Plantier J, Forrey AW, O'Neill MA, et al: Pharmacokinetics of amikacin in patients with normal or impaired renal function: radioenzymatic acetylation assay. J Infect Dis. 1976;134(Suppl):S323.
117. Barza M, Brown RB, Shen D, et al. Predictability of blood levels of gentamicin in man. J Infect Dis. 1975;132:165.
118. Clarke JT, Libke RD, Regamey C, et al. Comparative pharmacokinetics of amikacin and kanamycin. Clin Pharmacol Ther. 1974;15:610.
119. Walker JM, Wise R, Mitchard M. The pharmacokinetics of amikacin and gentamicin in volunteers: a comparison of individual differences. J Antimicrob Chemother. 1979;5:95.
120. Kahlmeter G, Jonsson S, Kamme C. Multiple-compartment pharmacokinetics of tobramycin. J Antimicrob Chemother. 1978;4(Suppl A):5.
121. Kahlmeter G. Gentamicin and Tobramycin: Clinical Pharmacokinetics and Nephrotoxicity: Aspects on Assay Techniques. Lund; Berlings; 1979.
122. Adelman M, Evans E, Schentag JJ. Two-compartment comparison of gentamicin and tobramycin in normal volunteers. Antimicrob Agents Chemother. 1982;22:800.
123. Assael BM, Cavanna G, Jusko WJ, et al. Multiexponential elimination of gentamicin. A kinetic study during development. Dev Pharmacol Ther. 1980;1:171.
124. Driessen OMJ, Sorgedrager N, Michel MF, et al. Pharmacokinetic aspects of therapy with ampicillin and kanamycin in new-born infants. Eur J Clin Pharmacol. 1978;13:449.
125. Haughey DB, Hilligoss DM, Grassi A, et al. Two compartment gentamicin pharmacokinetics in premature neonates. A comparison to adults with decreased glomerular filtration rate. J Pediatr. 1980;96:325.
126. Herngren L, Boreaus LO, Jalling B, et al. Pharmacokinetic aspects of streptomycin treatment of neonatal septicemia. Scand J Infect Dis. 1977;9:301.
127. Howard JB, McCracken GH. Reappraisal of kanamycin usage in neonates. J Pediatr. 1975;86:949.
128. Howard JB, McCracken GH, Trujillo H, et al. Amikacin in newborn infants: comparative pharmacology with kanamycin and clinical efficacy in 45 neonates with bacterial diseases. Antimicrob Agents Chemother. 1976;10:205.
129. McCracken GH Jr, Gay Jones L. Gentamicin in the neonatal period. Am J Dis Child. 1970;120:524.
130. McCracken GH Jr, Nelson JD. Antimicrobial Therapy for Newborns: Practical Application of Pharmacology to Clinical Use. New York: Grune & Stratton; 1977.
131. Yoshioka H, Takimoto M, Matsudi I, et al. Dosage schedule of gentamicin for chronic renal insufficiency in children. Arch Dis Child. 1978;53:334.
132. Echeverria P, Siber GR, Paisley J, et al. Age dependent dose response to gentamicin. J Pediatr. 1975;87:805.
133. Evans WE, Feldman S, Barker LF, et al. Use of gentamicin serum levels to individualize therapy in children. J Pediatr. 1978;93:133.
134. Evans WE, Huntley Taylor R, Feldman S, et al. A model for dosing gentamicin in children and adolescents that adjusts for tissue accumulation with continuous dosing. Clin Pharmacokinet. 1980;5:295.
135. Hoecker JL, Pickering LK, Swaney J, et al. Clinical pharmacology of tobramycin in children. J Infect Dis. 1978;137:592.
136. Karetzis DA, Sinaniotis CA, Papadatos CJ, et al. Pharmacokinetics of amikacin in infants and preschool children. Acta Paediatr Scand. 1979;68:419.
137. Kramer WG, Cleary T, Frankel LS, et al. Multiple-dose amikacin kinetics in pediatric oncology patients. Clin Pharmacol Ther. 1979;26:635.
138. Marks MI, Vose A, Hammerberg S, et al. Clinico-pharmacological studies of sisomicin in ill children. Antimicrob Agents Chemother. 1978;13:753.
139. McCracken GH Jr. Clinical pharmacology of gentamicin in infants 2 to 24 months of age. Am J Dis Child. 1972;124:884.
140. Siber GR, Echeverria P, Smith AL, et al. Pharmacokinetics of gentamicin in children and adults. J Infect Dis. 1975;132:637.
141. Vogelstein B, Kowarski AA, Lietman PS. The pharmacokinetics of amikacin in children. J Pediatr. 1977;91:333.
142. Wellilng PG, Baumueller A, Lau CC, et al. Netilmicin pharmacokinetics after single intravenous doses to elderly male patients. Antimicrob Agents Chemother. 1977;12:328.
143. Spyker DA, Guerrant RL. Dosage nomograms for aminoglycoside antibiotics. Hosp Formulary. 1981;16:132.
144. Cockcroft DW, Gault MH. Prediction of creatinine clearance from serum creatinine. Nephron. 1976;16:31.
145. Siersbaek-Nielsen K, Molholm-Hansen J, Kampmann J. Rapid evaluation of creatinine clearance. Lancet. 1971;i:1133.
146. Plantier J, Forrey AW, O'Neill MA, et al. Pharmacokinetics of amikacin in patients with normal or impaired renal function: radioenzymatic acetylation assay. J Infect Dis. 1976;134(Suppl):5323.
147. Gyscelynck A-M, Forrey A, Cutler R. Pharmacokinetics of gentamicin: distribution and plasma and renal clearance. J Infect Dis. 1971;124(Suppl):570.
148. Lanao JM, Dominguez-Gil A, Tabernero JM, et al. Pharmacokinetics of amikacin (BB-K8) in patients with normal or impaired renal function. Int J Clin Pharmacol Biopharm. 1979;17:171.
149. Schwartz SN, Pazin GJ, Lyon JA, et al. A controlled investigation of the pharmacokinetics of gentamicin and tobramycin in obese subjects. J Infect Dis. 1978;138:499.
150. Blouin RA, Mann HJ, Griffen WO Jr, et al. Tobramycin pharmacokinetics in morbidly obese patients. Clin Pharmacol Ther. 1979;26:508.
151. Bravo ME, Arancibia A, Jarpa S, et al. Pharmacokinetics of gentamicin in malnourished infants. Eur J Clin Pharmacol. 1982;21:499.
152. Pennington JE, Dale DC, Reynolds HY, et al. Gentamicin sulfate pharmacokinetics: lower levels of gentamicin in blood during fever. J Infect Dis. 1975;132:270.
153. Sawchuk RJ, Zaske DE. Pharmacokinetics of dosing regimens which utilize multiple intravenous infusions: gentamicin in burn patients. J Pharmacokinet Biopharm. 1976;4:183.
154. Loirat P, Rohan J, Baillet A, et al. Increased glomerular filtration rate in patients with major burns and its effect on the pharmacokinetics of tobramycin. N Engl J Med. 1978;299:915.

155. Smith CR, Lipsky JJ, Laskin OL, et al. Double-blind comparison of the nephrotoxicity and auditory toxicity of gentamicin and tobramycin. N Engl J Med. 1980;302:106.
156. Noone P, Parsons TMC, Pattison JR, et al. Experience in monitoring gentamicin therapy during treatment of series gram-negative sepsis. Br Med J. 1974;1:477.
157. Tally FP, Louie TJ, Weinstein WM, et al. Amikacin therapy for severe gram-negative sepsis. Ann Intern Med. 1975;83:484.
158. Anderson ET, Young LS, Hewitt WL. Simultaneous antibiotic levels in "breakthrough" gram-negative and bacteremia. Am J Med. 1976;61:493.
159. Klastersky J, Meunier-Carpentier F, Prevase J. Significance of antimicrobial synergism for the outcome of gram-negative sepsis. Am J Med Sci. 1977;273:157.
160. Moore RD, Smith CR, Lietman PS. The association of aminoglycoside plasma levels with mortality in patients with gram-negative bacteremia. J Infect Dis. 1984;149:443.
161. Moore RD, Smith CR, Lietman PS. Association of aminoglycoside plasma levels with therapeutic outcome in gram-negative pneumonia. Am J Med. 1984;77:657.
162. Moore RD, Lietman PS, Smith CR. Clinical response to aminoglycoside therapy: importance of the ratio of peak concentration to minimal inhibitory concentration. J Infect Dis. 1987;155:93.
163. Wright JM, Collier B. The effects of neomycin upon transmitter release and action. J Pharmacol Exp Ther. 1977;200:576.
164. Lee C, DeSilva JC. Acute and subchronic neuromuscular blocking characteristics of streptomycin: a comparison with neomycin. Br J Anaesth. 1979;51:431.
165. Caputy AJ, Kim YI, Sanders DB. The neuromuscular blocking effects of therapeutic concentrations of various antibiotics on normal rat skeletal muscle: a quantitative comparison. J Pharmacol Exp Ther. 1981;217:369.
166. Chinyanga HM, Stoyka WW. The effect of colymycin M, gentamycin and kanamycin on depression of neuromuscular transmission induced by pancuronium bromide. Can Anaesth Soc J. 1974;21:569.
167. L'Hommedieu CS, Huber PA, Rasch DK. Potentiation of magnesium-induced neuromuscular weakness by gentamicin. Crit Care Med. 1983;11:55.
168. L'Hommedieu C, Stough R, Brown L, et al. Potentiation of neuromuscular weakness in infant botulism by aminoglycosides. J Pediatr. 1979;95:1065.
169. Hokkanen E. The aggravating effect of some antibiotics on the neuromuscular blockade in myasthenia gravis. Acta Neurol Scand. 1964;40:346.
170. Sanders DB, Kim YI, Howard JF, et al. Intercostal muscle biopsy studies in myasthenia gravis: clinical correlations and the direct effects of drugs and myasthenic serum. Ann NY Acad Sci. 1981;377:544.
171. Pittinger CB, Adamson R. Antibiotic blockade of neuromuscular function. Annu Rev Pharmacol. 1972;12:169.
172. Adams HR. Direct myocardial depressant effects of gentamicin. Eur J Pharmacol. 1975;30:272.
173. Descotes J, Evreux JC. Cardiac depressant effects of some recent aminoglycoside antibiotics. J Antimicrob Chemother. 1981;7:197.
174. Adams HR, Goodman FR, Wass GB. Alteration of contractile function and calcium ion movements in vascular smooth muscle by gentamicin and other aminoglycoside antibiotics. Antimicrob Agents Chemother. 1974;5:640.
175. Lerner SA, Matz GJ, Hawkins JE, eds. Aminoglycoside Ototoxicity. Boston: Little, Brown and Company; 1981.
176. Brummett RE, Meikle MM, Vernon JA. Ototoxicity of tobramycin in guinea pigs. Arch Otolaryngol. 1971;94:59.
177. Theopold HM. Comparative surface studies of ototoxic effects of various aminoglycoside antibiotics on the organ of Corti in the guinea pig. Acta Otolaryngol. 1977;84:57.
178. Johnson L-G, Hawkins JE Jr, Kinesley TC, et al. Aminoglycoside-induced cochlear pathology in man. Acta Otolaryngol [Suppl] (Stockh). 1981;383:1.
179. Koitchev K, Guilhaume A, Cazals Y, et al. Spiral ganglion changes after massive aminoglycoside treatment in the guinea pig. Acta Otolaryngol (Stockh). 1982;94:431.
180. Igarashi M. Vestibular ototoxicity in primates. Audiology. 1973;12:337.
181. Tran Ba Hay P, Muelemans A, Wassef M, et al. Gentamicin persistence in rat endolymph and perilymph after a two-day constant infusion. Antimicrob Agents Chemother. 1983;23:344.
182. Takada A, Sachacht J. Calcium antagonism and reversibility of gentamicin-induced loss of cochlear microphonics in the guinea pig. Hear Res. 1982;8:179.
183. Schacht J. Biochemistry of neomycin ototoxicity. J Acoust Soc Am. 1978;59:940.
184. Iinuma T, Mizukoshi O, Daly JF. Possible effects of various ototoxic drugs upon the ATP-hydrolyzing system in the stria vascularis and spiral ligament of the guinea pig. Laryngoscope. 1967;77:159.
185. Matz GJ, Lerner SA. Prospective studies of aminoglycoside ototoxicity in adults. In: Lerner SA, Matz GJ, Hawkins JE, eds. Aminoglycoside Ototoxicity. Boston: Little Brown and Company; 1981:327.
186. Fee WE Jr. Aminoglycoside ototoxicity in the human. Laryngoscope. 1980;90(Suppl 24):1.
187. Lerner AM, Reyes MP, Cone LA, et al. Randomized, controlled trial of the comparative efficacy, auditory toxicity, and nephrotoxicity of tobramycin and netilmicin. Lancet. 1983;i:1123.
188. Bendush CL. Ototoxicity: clinical considerations and comparative information. In: Whelton A, Neu HC, eds. The Aminoglycosides. New York: Marcel Dekker; 1982:453.
189. Moore RD, Smith CR, Lietman PS. Risk factors for the development of auditory toxicity in patients receiving aminoglycosides. J Infect Dis. 1984;149:23.
190. Mathog RH, Klein WJ, Jr. Ototoxicity of ethacrynic acid and aminoglycoside antibiotics in uremia. N Engl J Med. 1969;280:1223.
191. Brummett RE, Brown RT, Himes DL. Quantitative relationships of the ototoxic interaction of kanamycin and ethacrynic acid. Arch Otolaryngol. 1979;105:240.
192. Smith CR, Lietman PS. Effect of furosemide on aminoglycoside-induced nephrotoxicity and auditory toxicity in humans. Antimicrob Agents Chemother. 1983;23:133.
193. Dodson HC, Bannister LH, Dovek EE. The effects of combined gentamicin and white noise on the spiral organ of young guinea pigs. Acta Otolaryngol (Stockh). 1982;94:193.
194. Ryan AF, Bone RC. Non-simultaneous interaction of exposure to noise and kanamycin intoxication in the chinchilla. Am J Otolaryngol. 1982;3:264.
195. Henry KR, Chole RA, McGinn MD, et al. Increased ototoxicity in both young and old mice. Arch Otolaryngol. 1981;107:92.
196. Dumas G, Charachon R. Ototoxicity of kanamycin in developing guinea pigs: an electrophysiological study. Acta Otolaryngol (Stockh). 1982;94:203.
197. Silverblatt F. Pathogenesis of nephrotoxicity of cephalosporins and aminoglycosides. A review of current concepts. Rev Infect Dis. 1982;4(Suppl):S360.
198. Edwards CQ, Smith CR, Baughman KL, et al. Concentrations of gentamicin and amikacin in human kidneys. Antimicrob Agents Chemother. 1976;9:925.
199. Luft FC, Yun MN, Walker PD, et al. Gentamicin gradient patterns and morphological changes in human kidneys. Nephron. 1977;18:167.
200. Houghton DC, Campbell-Boswell MV, Bennett WM, et al. Myeloid bodies in the renal tubules of humans: relationship to gentamicin therapy. Clin Nephrol. 1978;10:140.
201. Aubert-Tulkens G, Van Hoof F, Tulkens P. Gentamicin-induced lysosomal phospholipidosis in cultured rat fibroblasts. Quantitative ultrastructural and biochemical study. Lab Invest. 1979;40:481.
202. Carlier MB, Laurent G, Claes PJ, et al. Inhibition of lysosomal phospholipases by aminoglycoside antibiotics: *in vitro* comparative studies. Antimicrob Agents Chemother. 1983;23:440.
203. Bennett WM, Gilbert DN, Houghton D, et al. Gentamicin nephrotoxicity: morphologic and pharmacologic features. West J Med. 1977;126:65.
204. Wellwood JM, Simpson PM, Tighe JR, et al. Evidence of gentamicin nephrotoxicity in patients with renal allographs. Br Med J. 1975;3:278.
205. Simmons CF, Bogusky RT, Humes HD. Inhibitory effects of gentamicin on renal mitochondrial oxidative phosphorylation. J Pharmacol Exp Ther. 1980;214:709.
206. Lipsky JJ, Lietman PS. Neomycin inhibition of adenosine triphosphatase: evidence for a neomycin-phospholipid interaction. Antimicrob Agents Chemother. 1980;18:532.
207. Lipsky JJ, Lietman PS. Aminoglycoside inhibition of a renal phophatidylinositol phospholipase C. J Pharmacol Exp Ther. 1981;220:287.
208. McNeil JS, Jackson B, Nelson L, et al. The role of prostaglandins in gentamicin-induced nephrotoxicity in the dog. Nephron. 1983;33:202.
209. Baylis C, Rennke HR, Brenner BM. Mechanism of the defect in glomerular ultrafiltration associated with aminoglycoside administration. Kidney Int. 1977;12:344.
210. Cojocel C, Hook JB. Differential effect of aminoglycoside treatment on glomerular filtration and renal reabsorption of lysozyme in rats. Toxicity. 1981;22:261.
211. Luft FC, Aronoff GR, Evan AP, et al. The effect of aminoglycosides on glomerular endothelium: a comparative study. Res Commun Chem Pathol Pharmacol. 1981;34:89.
212. Cojocel C, Dociu N, Maita K, et al. Effects of aminoglycosides on glomerular permeability, tubular reabsorption, and intracellular catabolism of the cation low-molecular-weight protein lysozyme. Toxicol Appl Pharmacol. 1983;68:96.
213. Carlier B, Ninane G. Effects of aminoglycosides on enzymuria and beta 2 microglobulinuria. Acta Clin Belg. 1982;37:23.
214. Walenkamp GHIM, Vree TB, Guelen PJM, et al. Interaction between the renal excretion rates of beta-2-microglobulin and gentamicin in man. Clin Chim Acta. 1983;127:229.
215. Elliott WC, Houghton DC, Gilbert DN, et al. Gentamicin nephrotoxicity: 1. Degree and permanence of acquired insensitivity. J Lab Clin Med. 1982;100:501.
216. Lietman PS, Smith CR. Aminoglycoside nephrotoxicity in humans. J Infect Dis. 1983;5(Suppl 2):S284.
217. Holmes AM, Hesling CM, Wilson TM. Drug-induced secondary hyperaldosteronism in patients with pulmonary tuberculosis. Q J Med. 1970;39:299.
218. Bar RS, Wilson HE, Mazzaferri EL. Hypomagnesemic hypocalcemia secondary to renal magnesium wasting: a possible consequence of high-dose gentamicin therapy. Ann Intern Med. 1975;82:646.
219. Roediger WEW, Ludwin D, Hinder RA. Hypocalcaemic response to streptomycin in malignant hypercalcaemia. Postgrad Med J. 1975;51:399.
220. Keating MJ, Seth MR, Bodey GP, et al. Hypocalcemia with hypoparathyroidism and renal tubular dysfunction associated with aminoglycoside therapy. Cancer. 1977;39:1410.
221. Patel R, Savage A. Symptomatic hypomagnesemia associated with gentamicin therapy. Nephron. 1979;23:50.
222. Moore RD, Smith CR, Lipsky JJ, et al. Risk factors for renal dysfunction in patients treated with aminoglycosides. Ann Intern Med. 1984;100:352.

223. Moore RD, Smith CR, Lietman PS. Increased risk of renal dysfunction due to interaction of liver disease and aminoglycosides. Am J Med. 1986;80:1093.
224. Lietman PS. Liver disease, aminoglycoside antibiotics, and renal dysfunction. Hepatology. 1988;8:966.
225. Wade JC, Petty BG, Conrad G, et al. Cephalothin plus an aminoglycoside is more nephrotoxic than methicillin plus an aminoglycoside. Lancet. 1978;ii:604.
226. Davies J, Anderson P, Davis BD. Inhibition of protein synthesis by spectinomycin. Science. 1965;149:1096.
227. Ward ME. The bactericidal action of spectinomycin on *Neisseria gonorrhoeae*. J Antimicrob Chemother. 1977;3:323.
228. Holloway WJ. Spectinomycin. Med Clin North Am. 1982;66:169.
229. McCormack WM, Finland M. Spectinomycin. Ann Intern Med. 1976;84:712.
230. Virtanen S. Sensitivity of *Haemophilus vaginalis* (*Corynebacterium vaginale*) to oleandomycin and spectinomycin. Pathol Microbiol. 1975;42:36.
231. Wagner JG, Novak E, Leslie LG. Absorption, distribution and elimination of spectinomycin dihydrochloride in man. Int J Clin Pharmacol Biopharm. 1967;14:261.

23. TETRACYCLINES AND CHLORAMPHENICOL

HAROLD C. STANDIFORD

THE TETRACYCLINES

All the tetracyclines are primarily bacteriostatic at therapeutic concentrations and have a broad spectrum that includes gram-positive, gram-negative, aerobic, and anaerobic bacteria, spirochetes, mycoplasmas, rickettsia, chlamydiae, and some protozoa. The analogues can be divided into three groups based on differences in their pharmacology: (*1*) the short-acting compounds chlortetracycline, oxytetracycline, and tetracycline; (*2*) an intermediate group consisting of demeclocycline and methacycline; and (*3*) the more recently discovered, longer-acting compounds doxycycline and minocycline.

Structure, Derivation, Nomenclature, and Brand Names

Unlike the fortuitous discovery of penicillin by Flemming, the first tetracycline, chlortetracycline, was discovered by screening organisms obtained from the soil for their antimicrobial properties. Benjamin M. Duggar, a meticulous mycologist in his 70s, noted unusual antimicrobial activity from organisms that formed a golden yellow colony.[1] He designated the organism *Streptomyces aureofaciens* (L. *aurum*, golden) and named the product aureomycin. Oxytetracycline was derived from *Streptomyces rimosus* in 1950, and tetracycline was produced by the catalytic dehalogenation of chlortetracyline in 1953. The two long-acting compounds were derived semisynthetically: doxycycline in 1966 and minocycline in 1967. The generic names of the analogues are determined by the substitutions on the basic structure of tetracycline, which consists of a hydronaphthacene nucleus containing four fused rings (Fig. 1). The compounds currently available in the United States and their major brand names, doses, and costs are listed in Table 1. Of these, tetracycline HCl and doxycycline have emerged as the most useful clinically. Chlortetracycline (aureomycin), the first member of the family, is no longer available except for topical use.

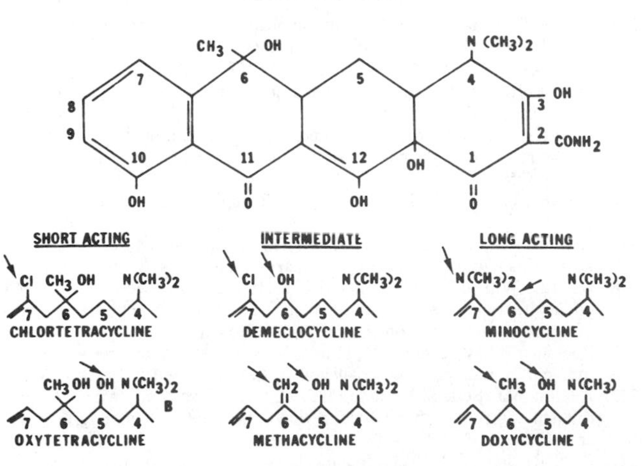

FIG. 1. The chemical structure of the tetracyclines. The analogues differ from tetracycline at the fifth, sixth, or seventh position, as indicated by the arrows.

TABLE 1. The Names, Preparations, Usual Adult Oral Dose, and Costs for the Tetracyclines Currently Available in the United States

Generic Name (Major Brand Name[a])	*Oral Preparations*	*Usual Adult Oral Dose*	*Cost for 10 Days[f]*
Short acting[b]			
Oxytetracycline (Terramycin, Pfizer)	Capsules: 125, 250 mg	500 mg q6h	45.00
Tetracyclone HCl[c] (Achromycin V, Lederle)	Capsules: 100, 250, 500 mg	500 mg q6h	7.50[g]
	Syrup: 125 mg/5 ml		5.75
Intermediate			
Methacycline (Rondomycin, Wallace)	Capsules: 150, 300 mg	300 mg q12h	31.50
Demeclocycline HCl (Declomycine, Lederle)	Capsules: 150 mg Tablets: 150, 300 mg	300 mg q12h	71.90
Long Acting[d]			
Doxycycline (Vibramycin, Pfizer)	Capsules (hyclate): 50, 100 mg	200 mg (or 100 q12h for first day), then 100 mg q24h[e]	25.60
	Syrup (calcium): 50 mg/5 ml Suspension (monohydrate): 25 mg/5 ml		5.65[g]
Minocycline (Minocin, Lederle)	Capsules and tablets: 50, 100 mg Suspension: 50 mg/5 ml	200 mg, then 100 mg q12h	35.65

[a] Many other brands are available for some of the analogues.
[b] The short-acting tetracyclines are also available for intravenous administration at usual doses of 500 mg every 6–12 hours not to exceed 2 g daily. However, most prefer doxycycline for this route of administration. Preparations combined with a local anesthetic agent can be given intramuscularly, but these are not recommended.
[c] Tetracycline is also available as a tetracycline phosphate complex (Tetrex, Bristol) intended to enhance absorption, but its superiority has not been established.
[d] The longer-acting agents can be given intravenously in the same doses that are recommended for oral therapy. Doxycycline is available at 100 or 200 mg per vial and minocycline at 100 mg per vial.
[e] The treatment schedules for sexually transmitted diseases use 100 mg twice daily.
[f] The costs (in dollars) are those for a 10-day adult treatment regimen when the antibiotics are purchased by the patient at a community pharmacy. (Courtesy of Robert Plummer, Dell's Pharmacy, Aberdeen, MD.)
[g] Cost for the generic form.

Mechanism of Action

The tetracyclines enter bacteria by an initial rapid phase driven by the proton-motive force followed by a slower accumulation over a period of hours that is energy dependent.[2] Once within the cell, they reversibly bind primarily to the 30S ribosomal subunit at a position that blocks the binding of the aminoacyl-tRNA to the accepter site on the mRNA–ribosome complex.[3] This prevents the addition of new amino acids into the growing peptide chain. The tetracyclines also inhibit protein synthesis in mammalian cells but do not accumulate within these cells by an active process.[4] This may partially explain the difference in the degree of protein inhibition produced in the host and in the microorganism.

In Vitro Activity

The antimicrobial spectra of all the tetracyclines are almost identical. Some differences, however, in the degree of activity against these organisms do exist among the analogues. In general, the lipophilic congeners are more active than are those that are more hydrophilic. It follows, therefore, that minocycline is the most active of the analogues, closely followed by doxycycline. The minimum inhibitory concentration (MIC) of the more hydrophilic congeners oxytetracycline and tetracycline are two- to fourfold higher against many bacteria and are the least-active analogues. Despite these differences, for cost reasons, it is recommended that tetracycline be used in the clinical microbiology laboratory to evaluate susceptibility for all the analogues.[5] Minimum inhibitory concentrations of tetracycline and doxycycline for many aerobic bacteria are given in Table 2. For the activity of the other analogues, the reader is referred to the extensive work from the laboratory of Finland et al.[7–9]

Although many of the aerobic and facultative anaerobic organisms are within the spectrum of the tetracyclines, more effective agents are available for the treatment of infections caused by most of these bacteria. The pneumonococci and many *Haemophilus influenzae* can be inhibited by concentrations of tetracyclines achieved in the serum, and this provides a rationale for their use in sinusitis and acute exacerbations of chronic bronchitis.[13] Gonococci and meningococci are extremely susceptible; unfortunately, gonococci resistant to penicillin G also tend to be resistant to tetracycline and are becoming more common.[6,14] Most *Escherichia coli* acquired outside the hospital setting can be inhibited by concentrations achieved in the serum or urine. Tetracyclines, therefore, are useful agents for the treatment of acute, uncomplicated, urinary tract infections. *Pseudomonas pseudomallei* organisms are generally sensitive, and this has therapeutic importance, as does the high degree of susceptibility of *Brucella* sp.[10,15] *Vibrio cholerae, vulnificus*, and other vibrios are generally susceptible, and the tetracyclines are important for therapy for diseases caused by this group of organisms.[16] Although *Campylobacter* sp. are generally susceptible, a high percentage of resistant isolates has been noted in some countries.[11,17,18] Therefore, it is not the drug of choice for infections caused by these bacteria. *Shigella* organisms have become increasingly resistant to these agents.[12] *Mycobacterium marinum* is susceptible and appears to respond clinically.[19]

The tetracyclines have activity against many anaerobic organisms[20] (Table 3). Their activity against *Actinomyces* is particularly relevant clinically. Doxycycline is more active against *Bacteroides fragilis* than tetracycline is, but clindamycin or metronidazole are the preferred agents for infections caused by this organism. The activity of the tetracyclines against anaerobic bacteria, however, may be partially responsible for the effectiveness of the neomycin–tetracycline combination and doxycycline alone as oral presurgical bowel preparations.[21,22] Many pathogenic spirochetes are susceptible including *Borrelia burgdorferi*, the agent of Lyme disease.[23] Other organisms generally inhibited by this group of antibiotics include rickettsia, chlamydiae, mycoplasmas, and to a limited degree protzoa (malariae and *Entamoeba histotytica)*.[24]

Bacteria develop resistance to the tetracyclines predominantly by preventing the accumulation of tetracycline within the cell. This is accomplished by decreasing the influx transport system and/or increasing the ability of the cell to export the antibiotic. Rarely if ever are the tetracyclines inactivated bio-

TABLE 2. Minimum Inhibitory Concentration of Tetracycline and Doxycycline for Common Aerobic and Facultative Anaerobic Bacteria[a]

Organism	Number of Strains	Antibiotic	Cumulative Percentage Inhibited by Indicated Concentrations (μg/ml)						
			0.4	0.8	1.6	3.1	6.3	12.5	25
Gram-positive									
S. aureus	56	Tetracycline	0	2	20	65	67	67	67
		Doxycycline	2	25	63	65	68	80	87
S. pyogenes[b]	63	Tetracycline	10	50	80	87	90	92	98
		Doxycycline	56	90	90	95	95	98	100
S. pneumoniae[c]	35	Tetracycline	70	96	96	100			
		Doxycycline	100						
Streptococcus (group B)	12	Tetracycline	0	0	50	50	50	50	75
		Doxycycline	0	50	50	50	50	58	100
Streptococcus (group D)	36	Tetracycline	0	0	0	0	10	15	15
		Doxycycline	0	0	0	0	10	18	22
Gram-negative[d]									
N. gonorrhoeae[e]	25	Tetracycline	5	60	85	88	100		
		Doxycycline	60	75	80	92	100		
N. meningitidis[f]	10	Tetracycline	0	50		100			
		Doxycycline	0		50		100		
H. influenzae	15	Tetracycline	0	0	0	33	87	100	
		Doxycycline	0	0	60	93	100		
E. coli	48	Tetracycline	0	0	0	5	35	60	65
		Doxycycline	0	0	0	5	35	60	70
K. pneumoniae	17	Tetracycline	0	0	0	0	5	30	40
		Doxycycline	0	0	0	0	12	35	40
Enterobacter sp.	10	Tetracycline	0	10	30	50	70	80	90
		Doxycycline	0	0	0	0	10	30	60
Pseudomonas pseudomallei	10	Tetracycline	0	0	60	100			
Campylobacter jejuni	172	Tetracycline	44	62	74	81	84	85	88
	107	Doxycycline	68	74	79	80	86	98	100
Shigella sp.	213	Tetracycline	0	10	12	50	50	55	62

[a] Organisms should be considered susceptible if the MICs are 4 μg/ml or less. A moderate susceptibility range of up to 8 μg/ml may be useful for the treatment of urinary tract infections.[5]
[b] More recent series indicate that 20–40 percent of *S. pyogenes* have become resistant to the tetracyclines.
[c] Tetracycline-resistant *S. pneumoniae* strains are more common in some areas.
[d] *Proteus mirabilis*, indole-positive *Proteus* sp., and *P. aeruginosa* are generally resistant to 25 μg/ml.
[e] Many individual cases and clusters of tetracycline-resistant *Neisseria gonorrhoeae* have been reported.[6]
[f] The medium inhibitory concentration of minocycline for meningococci is 1.6 μg/ml (range, 0.8–1.6 μg/ml).
(Data from refs. 7–12.)

TABLE 3. Minimum Inhibitory Concentrations of Tetracycline and Doxycycline for Common Anaerobic Bacteria[a]

Organism	*Number of Strains*	*Antibiotic*	*Cumulative Percentage Susceptible to Indicated Concentration (μg/ml)* 0.5	1.0	2.0	4.0	8.0	16.0	32.0
Gram-positive									
Peptococcus and *Gaffkya*	59	Tetracycline	25	29	36	36	37	61	92
		Doxycycline	28	35	40	70	93	98	100
Peptostreptococcus	29	Tetracycline	38	41	48	52	72	86	97
		Doxycycline	45	45	66	79	97	100	
Streptococci, anaerobic and microaerophilic	10	Tetracycline	50	60	70	90	90	90	100
		Doxycycline	70	90	90	90	100		
Eubacterium	17	Tetracycline	24	59	65	65	77	82	94
		Doxycycline	59	65	77	82	88	100	
Propioni bacterium	12	Tetracycline	58	75	83	83	83	83	100
		Doxycycline	75	83	83	92	92	92	100
Clostridium perfringens	9	Tetracycline	22	22	56	67	67	78	78
		Doxycycline	67	67	67	78	89	100	
Other clostridia	33	Tetracycline	36	46	49	52	61	67	76
		Doxycycline	49	52	61	68	82	97	97
Actinomyces	16	Tetracycline	56	69	94	94	94	100	
		Doxycycline	63	69	94	100			
Gram-negative									
Gram-negative cocci	26	Tetracycline	54	69	73	73	73	85	92
		Doxycycline	58	69	73	81	96	100	
Fusobacterium	34	Tetracycline	94	97	97	97	97	100	
		Doxycycline	94	94	94	94	100		
Bacteroides fragilis	76	Tetracycline	25	40	40	42	46	68	63
		Doxycycline	41	42	50	75	88	97	100
Bacteroides melaninogenicus	67	Tetracycline	75	76	79	87	94	96	99
		Doxycycline	75	78	90	96	97	99	99
Other *Bacteroides*, *Selenomonas*	72	Tetracycline	33	35	43	50	60	75	93
		Doxycycline	40	43	53	68	79	85	96

[a] An organism with a MIC of 4 μg/ml or less should be considered susceptible.
(Modified from Sutter et al.,[20] with permission.)

logically or altered chemically by resistant bacteria.[25–28] Resistance to one tetracycline usually implies resistance to all, although there are marked differences in the degree of resistance among species. The resistance among bacteria can be mediated by transferable resistance plasmids, a mechanism particularly important for *Shigella*. The tetracyclines have been widely used in feeds to promote growth in animals. This may be a major factor in providing selective antibiotic pressure for the spread of plasmid-mediated resistance to these and other antibiotics.[29–31]

Pharmacology

Serum levels achieved by usual oral doses in adults are seen in Figure 2. Absorption occurs primarily in the proximal small bowel and produces peak serum concentrations 1–3 hours after administration. The commonly used 500 mg therapeutic dose of tetracycline gives a serum level of 4 μg/ml, highest of all the short-acting analogues.[32] Doxycycline and minocycline (200 mg) achieve serum levels of about 2.5 μg/ml, slightly higher than levels attained by the larger therapeutic doses of the intermediate agents.[33–37]

After the intravenous administration of 500 mg, serum levels of the short-acting agents (not shown) are approximately 8 μg/ml at 30 minutes and decrease to 2–3 μg/ml by 5 hours.[38] Intravenous injection of the usual 200 mg loading dose of the long-acting agents doxycycline and minocycline produces serum levels of approximately 4 μg/ml at 30 minutes. Once tissue distribution occurs for the long-acting analogues, levels are almost identical to concentrations achieved orally.[33,39] Thrombophlebitis is a frequent complication of the intravenous preparations. Intramuscular preparations are available for the short-acting compounds but are not recommended because of the severe pain produced on injection, even when they are mixed with local anesthetics.

Some of the pharmacokinetic properties of the tetracyclines are compared in Table 4. The high levels obtained orally with tetracycline as compared with other short-acting agents are due primarily to better absorption from the gastrointestinal tract. The long-acting analogues doxycycline and minocycline are absorbed almost completely; thus, high serum levels are achieved with relatively small doses.[33,34] The tetracyclines can be differentiated into three groups on the basis of their different half-lives. Doxycycline has the longest of all and allows therapeutic levels to be maintained with a single daily dose.[33] The 8-hour half-life of tetracycline[38] suggests that the dosage interval could

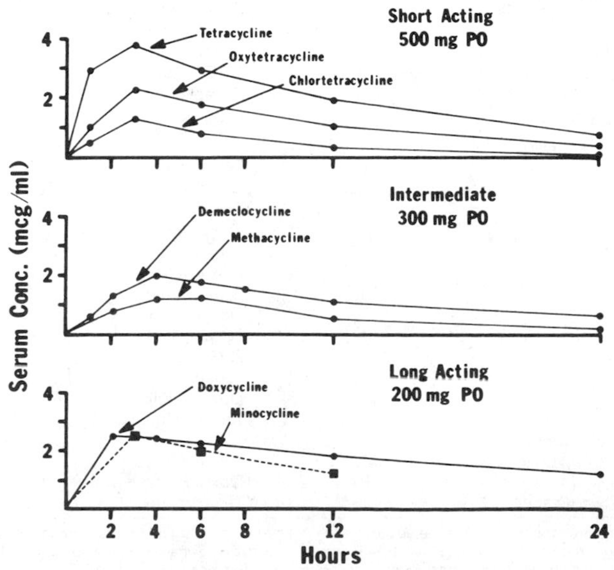

FIG. 2. Serum levels achieved with the usually recommended oral doses of the tetracyclines. Chlortetracycline is no longer available for oral or parenteral administration. (Data from refs. 32–36.)

TABLE 4. Pharmacokinetic Features of the Tetracyclines[a]

Antibiotic	*GI Absorption (%)*	*Half-Life (hr)*	*Renal Clearance[b] (ml/min/1.73 m²)*	*Urinary Recovery (%)*	*Apparent Volume of Distribution[b] (Liters)*	*Protein Binding[c] (%)*
Short acting						
Chlortetracycline	30	6	32	18	100	47
Oxytetracycline	58	9	99	70	128	35
Tetracycline	77	8	74	60	108	65
Intermediate						
Demeclocycline	66	12	35	39	121	91
Methacycline	58	14	31	60	79	90
Long acting						
Doxycycline	93	18	20	42	50	93
Minocycline	95	16	9	6	60	76

[a] The pharmacokinetic values vary considerably from laboratory to laboratory. These values were selected in most instances because comparative data were available from reliable investigators.
[b] After single-dose intravenous administration.
[c] Ultrafiltration technique.
(Data from refs. 33–35 and 38–41.)

be 8 hours for this antibiotic when it is used to treat minor infections. The half-lives of the compounds are determined mainly by the rate of excretion by the kidneys. Chlortetracycline is an exception: it has a short half-life despite a slow rate of clearance as a result of the marked instability of the compound in vitro as well as in vivo.[38] With the possible exception of chlortetracycline and minocycline, adequate therapeutic concentrations of all the tetracyclines are achieved in the urine for treatment of urinary tract infections caused by sensitive organisms. The degree of protein binding of the analogues is variable, depending on the methods used for the determination, but it tends to be greater for the intermediate and long-acting compounds.[39–41] This may be one of the factors that determines their slow rate of renal excretion. The apparent volume of distribution for most of the tetracyclines is greater than that of extracellular body water, thus indicating sequestration in tissues, presumably the liver.[38] Minocycline and doxycycline have the smallest volume of distribution, another factor that tends to enhance their serum levels.[39]

Tissue Distribution. The tetracyclines can be found in small amounts in many tissues and fluids, including the lung, liver, kidney, brain, sputum, and mucosal fluid. For tetracycline, the levels in the cerebral spinal fluid are approximately 10–26 percent of the serum levels,[42,43] whereas concentrations in synovial fluid and the maxillary sinus mucosa approach serum levels.[44,45] All the tetracyclines are concentrated in unobstructed bile and produce levels in this fluid 5–20 times those obtained in the serum. It has been suggested that lipid solubility is a primary determinant for the diffusion in many tissues. Minocycline, followed by doxycycline, is more lipophilic at a physiologic pH than are the other drugs. This may explain why minocycline reaches sufficient concentrations in saliva and tears to eradicate the meningococcal carrier state whereas the other tetracyclines do not.[46,47] The tetracyclines cross the placenta, accumulate in fetal bone and teeth, and therefore, should not be given during pregnancy.[48] Because they are excreted in breast milk, caution is advised in the postpartum period.

Renal and Hepatic Insufficiency. The tetracyclines should not be used in patients with renal failure. Doxycycline, the only exception, is excreted in the gastrointestinal tract under these circumstances. Neither the half-life nor the therapeutic dose of this antibiotic varies with alterations in renal function.[49] The tetracyclines are slowly removed by hemodialysis but not effectively by peritoneal dialysis. Hepatic disease is not known to cause elevated serum levels of the tetracyclines. However, they should be used very cautiously in such situations because they have been noted to cause hepatic toxicity.

Assay

The tetracyclines generally are measured by bioassay using *Bacillis cereus* as the test organism.[50] A spectrofluorometric assay is available for some of the analogues,[51] but monitoring of serum levels during therapy is rarely indicated.

Toxicity

Skin and Allergy. Hypersensitivity reactions including anaphylaxis, urticuria, periorbital edema, fixed drug eruptions, and morbilliform rashes occur with tetracyclines but are not common.[52–54] When a patient is allergic to one analogue, he should be considered to be allergic to all. Photosensitivity reactions consisting of a red rash on areas exposed to sunlight that is frequently associated with onycholysis are most common in patients receiving demeclocycline but occur with all analogues.[55,56] They appear to be a toxic rather than an allergic reaction. Prolonged administration of minocycline has been noted rarely to cause nail, skin, and scleral pigmentation, which is usually reversible, as well as an asymptomatic black pigmentation of the thyroid.[57,58]

Teeth and Bones. A gray-brown to yellow discoloration of the teeth has been noted in 80 percent of the children taking tetracyclines in some communities.[59] This side effect is permanent and may be associated with hypoplasia of the enamel[55,60] and depression of skeletal growth in premature infants.[61] The darkening effect of tetracyclines on permanent teeth appears to be related to the total dose of the antibiotic administered. In a retrospective study, cosmetically noticeable, but mild darkening of the permanent teeth occurred in 3 of 14 children receiving five courses of tetracycline, whereas 4 of 6 children receiving eight courses had moderate darkening of the enamel.[62] Primary teeth generally show more darkening than do the larger, thicker, and more opaque permanent teeth. Since there is some variability in staining with similar tetracycline exposure, it is prudent not to administer these agents to pregnant women and to children up to the age of 8 years, the period when tooth enamel is being formed. For this reason, the Food and Drug Administration (FDA) has withdrawn from the market the concentrated liquid dosage forms (drops) specifically intended for pediatric use.[63] It is not unreasonable, however, to administer a single course of tetracycline therapy to young children for specifically defined indications where the alternative regime may produce more severe toxicity. Thus, the tetracyclines are indicated for children suspected of having Rocky Mountain spotted fever who can tolerate oral medications. Doxycycline binds less with calcium than do other tetracyclines and may cause dental changes less frequently in children.[64]

Gastrointestinal. The tetracyclines are irritative substances and frequently produce gastrointestinal symptoms after oral administration. Esophageal ulcerations that are manifested as retrosternal pain exacerbated by swallowing have been clearly documented after tetracycline and doxycycline administration. In most cases, the patients were taking the capsules with little or no fluid just before going to bed. A word of caution to the patient is indicated in order to prevent this toxicity. The complication may also occur in patients with esophageal obstruction or motility disorders.[65,66] Nausea, vomiting, and epigastric distress are dose related and limit the dose of most the analogues. The administration of food with doxycycline, minocycline, or oxytetracycline may ameliorate some of these symptoms, but food seriously decreases the absorption of the other tetracyclines. Diarrhea is most often associated with analogues that are poorly absorbed and appears to be related to alterations in the enteric flora. Doxycycline produces less of an effect on bowel flora than does tetracycline.[67] The diarrhea usually subsides when treatment with the antibiotic is stopped, but prolonged symptoms due to pseudomembranous colitis have been reported.[68] Tetracycline also has been noted, rarely, to cause pancreatitis with or without overt liver disease.[69]

Liver. The hepatoxicity of the tetracyclines, first described in patients receiving intravenous chlortetracycline but now described with other analogues, appears pathologically as a fine droplet fatty metamorphosis and results in a high mortality.[70,71] The administration of less than 2 g/day intravenously is not associated with liver dysfunction or injury except in pregnant women, who are particularly at risk,[72] and in patients with an excessive serum level due to renal failure.[73]

Renal Function. The tetracyclines aggravate pre-exisitng renal failure by inhibiting protein synthesis, which increases the azotemia from amino acid metabolism.[74] Nephrogenic diabetes insipidus is produced by demeclocycline, a side effect that has been used therapeutically to reverse chronic inappropriate antidiuretic hormone secretion[75]; renal failure has complicated its use for this purpose in patients with cirrhosis.[76] Outdated tetracycline has produced a reversible Fanconi-like syndrome with renal tubular acidosis, but tetracycline formulations producing this syndrome have been modified. It is unlikely that this complication will recur.[49]

Nervous and Sensory Systems. Vertigo is a side effect unique to minocycline. Symptoms of light-headedness, loss of balance, dizziness, and tinnitus usually begin on the second and third days of therapy and have been noted more frequently in women (70 percent) than in men (28 percent). The symptoms are reversible within several days after discontinuation of therapy with the antibiotic, but this side effect has seriously limited the use of minocycline.[77] Benign intracranial hypertension (pseudotumor cerebri) has been described in infants and adults with many of the analogues.[78,79]

Superinfection. Colonization by tetracycline-resistant organisms is a frequent occurrence during tetracycline therapy and is generally of little clinical significance. Rarely, a fulminating diarrhea resulting from staphylococcal enteritis may occur after oral or parenteral therapy.[80,81] More often and less serious, oral or vaginal monaliasis complicates treatment, a complication that may require specific therapy.

Significant Drug Interactions

Food adversely affects the absorption of tetracycline, chlortetracycline, methacycline, and demeclocycline. All the tetracyclines form complexes with divalent or tivalent cations. Therefore, absorption is markedly decreased when these drugs are administered simultaneously with calcium, magnesium, and aluminum in antacids, milk, or iron and iron-containing tonics.[82] Sodium bicarbonate also has an adverse effect on absorption and should not be administered simultaneously.[83] Cimetidine has been shown to decrease the absorption of tetracycline, but this is unlikely to be significant in the clinical situation.[84] Carbamazepine (Tegretol), diphenylhydantoin, and barbiturates decrease the normal half-life of doxycycline to almost one-half by increasing the hepatic metabolism of the antibiotic.[85,86] Chronic ethanol ingestion has also resulted in a shorter half-life of doxycycline but not tetracycline, presumably also through induction of hepatic microsomal enzymes.[87] Methyoxyflurane anesthesia may cause nephrotoxicity when administered with tetracyclines.[88] It has been suggested that this adverse interaction occurs with the newer, less nephrotoxic fluorinated anesthetic agents as well.[89] The use of these antibiotics concurrently with diuretics produces an elevated blood urea nitrogen (BUN) level, although th exact mechanism has not been determined.[90] It has been reported that women receiving oral contraceptives have become pregnant while receiving tetracycline. This may be caused by the reduction in bacterial hydrolysis of conjugated estrogen in the intestine.[91,92]

Indications

The tetracyclines are the drugs of choice or effective alternative therapy for a wide variety of infections (Table 5). Their role in the therapy for many of the sexually transmitted diseases, including infections caused by the gonococci and chlamydiae, and for the treatment of the syndromes of acute pelvic inflammatory disease, nonspecific urethritis, and sexually transmitted epididymo-orchitis in young adults is particularly noteworthy.[93] The reader is referred to the specific chapter for details. They have no role in the treatment of viral or fungal diseases. Tetracycline, the least expensive of the analogues, is sometimes preferred for oral administration. Doxycycline, however, ap-

TABLE 5. Major Therapeutic Indications for the Tetracyclines[a]

Therapy of Choice	*Effective Therapy*
Brucellosis (with streptomycin in seriously ill patients	Acne, severe
Chlamydial infections	Actinomycosis
Ornithosis	Anthrax
Trachoma	*Campylobacter fetus, jejuni*
Urethral, endocervical, or rectal infections in adults	Chronic bronchitis (acute exacerbations)
Cholera	Glanders (*Pseudomonas mallei*)
Lymphogranuloma venereum	Gonococcal infections (resistance is a problem)
Epididymitis, acute (sexually transmitted form)	*Pasteurella multocida*
Granuloma inguinale	Prostatitis
Leptospirosis	Rat-bite fever (*Spirillum minus, Streptococcus moniliformis*)
Lyme disease (early stages)	Syphilis
Melioidosis (with chloramphenicol in seriously ill patients)	Tularemia
Mycobacterium marinum (minocycline)	Vincent's infection
Mycoplasma pneumoniae (some prefer erythromycin)	Whipple's disease
Pelvic inflammatory disease (acute, in combination with other antibiotics)	Yaws, nasopalatal
Relapsing fever (*Borrelia recurrentis*)	*Yersinia enterocolitica*
Rickettsial infections (some prefer chloramphenicol for severe infections)	*Effective Alternative Prophylaxis*
Rocky Mountain spotted fever	Oral bowel preparation for intestinal surgery (tetracycline in combination with neomycin or doxycycline alone)
Typhus fever	Meningococcal disease (only minocycline)
Q fever	Traveler's diarrhea (doxycycline)
Rickettsial pox	
Ehrlichiosis	
Urethritis, nonspecific	
Urethral syndrome (dysuria-frequency syndrome)	
Vibrio vulnificus	

[a] Unless otherwise specified, tetracycline hydrochloride is the preferred analogue for oral administration.

pears equally effective and is preferred by most when intravenous administration is required.

CHLORAMPHENICOL

Soon after chloramphenicol was released in the United States in 1949, reports linked this highly effective agent with aplastic anemia, and it quickly fell into disfavor. The increased awareness of the pathogenicity of anaerobic organisms and the development of ampicillin-resistant *H. influenzae* accounted for an increase in the use of the compound. However, the availability of other agents for anaerobic infections has reduced the need for chloramphenicol for this indication, and its use for ampicillin-resistant *H. influenzae* is currently being challenged by the newer cephalosporins. Chloramphenicol remains a useful antibiotic, but only for well-defined indications in seriously ill patients.

Structure, Derivation, Brand Names, and Preparations

Like the early tetracyclines, chloramphenicol was discovered by screening organisms for their antimicrobial activity. Isolated independently by Burkholder from a mulched field near Caracas, Venezuela,[94] and by workers at the University of Illinois from compost,[95] the organism producing the active compound was named *Streptomyces venezuelae*.[96] The structure of chloramphenicol is shown in Figure 3. It was the first antibiotic whose chemical synthesis was economically and technically practical for large-scale production.[97] Preparations currently available and the usual doses are given in Table 6.

Thiamphenical, not available in the United States, is an analogue in which the *p*-nitro group on the benzene ring is replaced by a methylsulfonyl group. Its spectrum of activity is similar to chloramphenicol, but it has not been reported to cause aplastic anemia.

Mechanism of Action

Chloramphenicol appears to enter the cell by an energy-dependent process.[98] Once within the cell it inhibits protein synthesis. This is accomplished by reversibly binding to the larger 50S subunit of the 70S ribosome at a locus that prevents the attachment of the amino acid-containing end of the aminoacyl-tRNA to its binding region. Without this attachment, the association of the amino acid substrate with peptidyl transferase does not occur, and peptide bond formation is prevented.[2] This block in protein synthesis produces a static effect against most sensitive microorganisms. However, in vitro evidence indicates that chloramphenicol is bactericidal against some meningeal pathogens such as *H. influenzae, Streptococcus pneumoniae*, and *Neisseria meningitidis* but not group B streptococci or enteric gram-negative bacilli at concentrations that can be achieved therapeutically.[99–101] Although mammalian cells contain primarily 80S ribosomes that are unaffected by chloramphenicol, the mitochondria do contain 70S particles. The effect of chloramphenicol on these has been suggested as a cause for the dose-related bone marrow suppression of the compound but not the idiosyncratic aplastic anemia.[102]

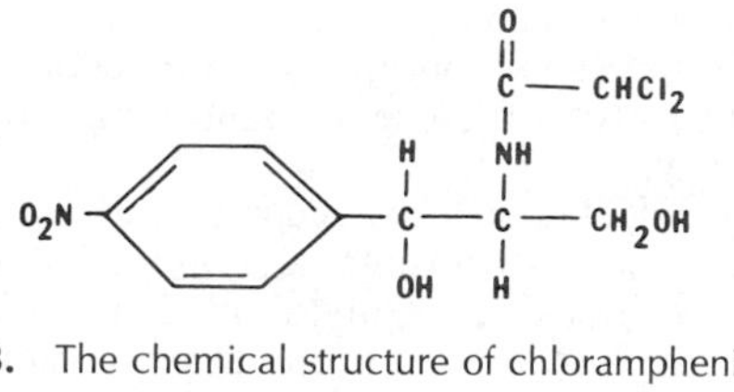

FIG. 3. The chemical structure of chloramphenicol.

TABLE 6. Systemic Chloramphenicol Preparations Currently Available in the United States[a]

Preparation	How Supplied	Usual Dose
Oral		
Capsules		
Chloromycetin (Parke-Davis)	250 mg	25 mg/kg/day for neonates less than 1 wk old; 25 mg/kg q12h for infants 1–4 wk; 50 mg/kg/day in 6-hr intervals for older children and adults; 100 mg/kg/day for older children and adults with meningitis
Mychel (Rachelle)	250 mg	
Suspension		
Chloromycetin Palmitate (Parke-Davis)	150 mg/5 ml	Same as above
Parenteral (intravenous)		
Chloromycetin Sodium Succinate (Parke-Davis)	1 g (powder)	Same as above

[a] Other pharmaceutical companies also make chloramphenicol.

In Vitro Activity

Chloramphenicol is extremely active against a variety of organisms, including bacteria, spirochetes, richettsia, chlamydiae, and mycoplasmas. The MICs required for bacteria are listed in Table 7. Most of the gram-positive and gram-negative aerobic bacteria are inhibited by concentrations easily achieved in the serum of patients, but more active or less toxic therapeutic agents are available for most of these pathogens.[8–10,20,97,103–107] Salmonellae icluding *Salmonella typhi* are generally susceptible.[105] In the United States, resistant strains occasionally occur,[109] but imported strains may be highly resistant. The three most common organisms causing meningitis in childhood (*H. influenzae, S. pneumoniae*, and *N. meningitidis*) are highly susceptible,[9,110,111] although rare resistant strains of each species have been reported. The overall rate of *H. influenzae* resistance among clinical strains in the United States is approximately 0.6 percent.[112] Indeed, strains of *H. influenzae* that cause clinical infections and are resistant to both chloramphenicol and ampicillin have been isolated in several parts of the world.[113–115] These resistant isolates are rare in the United States but rather frequent in Spain.[116–118] Chloramphenicol is one of the most active antibiotics against anaerobic bacteria including *B. fragilis*, but clindamycin, metronidazole, and imipenem have become more important clinically to treat infections caused by these bacteria.[20,108,119,120]

Bacteria develop resistance to chloramphenicol by becoming impermeable to the drug or by producing an enzyme, acetyltransferase, that acetylates the antibiotic to an inactive diacetyl derivative.[121,122] This latter mechanism has been R factor–mediated and has been responsible for widespread epidemics of chloramphenicol-resistant typhoid fever and *Shigella* dysentery in Central and South America, Vietnam, and other countries.[123–126] It has been suggested that the unrestricted over-the-counter sale of chloramphenicol in the countries involved may be an important factor that provides antibiotic pressure for the development of these resistant strains.[125,126] In the United States, chloramphenicol resistance in *Salmonella* has been traced to the use of chloramphenicol on dairy farms.[31]

Pharmacology

Chloramphenicol serum levels achieved by different routes of administration and with different product forms are listed in Figure 4. Chloramphenicol in the encapsulated form is well absorbed from the gastrointestinal tract and results in peak serum levels of 12 μg/ml of active antibiotic after a 1 g dose.[127,128] Since

TABLE 7. Activity of Chloramphenicol against Bacteria[a]

Bacteria	Number of Strains	*Cumulative Percentage Inhibited at Indicated Concentration (μg/ml)*						
		0.4	*0.8*	*1.6*	*3.1*	*6.3*	*12.5*	*25*
Aerobic bacteria								
Gram-positive								
S. aureus	291	0	0	0	5	55	95	96
S. aureus (methicillin-resistant)	22	0	0	0	0	20	20	20
S. pyogenes	303	0	0	20	92	99	100	
Streptococci, group B	146	0	0	0	85	99	100	
S. viridans	193	0	0	0	60	90	100	
Streptococci, group D	382	0	0	0	0	0	12	48
S. pneumoniae	78				50	100		
Gram-negative								
H. influenzae	17			50	100			
N. meningitidis	7		50		100			
N. gonorrhoeae	106	5	52	97	100			
E. coli	71	0	0	5	30	75	95	95
K. pneumoniae	35	0	0	6	70	75	75	75
Enterobacter	10	0	0	0	10	20	50	80
Serratia marcescens	111	0	0	0	0	5	33	60
P. mirabilis	209	0	0	0	20	60	90	95
Proteus (indole-positive)	32	0	0	0	10	40	50	65
Salmonella typhosa	81	0	0	0	50	95	100	
S. paratyphi A	31				28	97	97	97
Shigella sp.	44		20	30	75	90	90	95
Vibrio cholera	64					84		89
Brucella sp.	25	0	0	28	92	100		
P. aeruginosa	11	0	0	0	0	0	0	0
P. pseudomallei	10	0	0	0	0	50	100	
Bordetella pertussia	31	20	45	85	97	99		
Anaerobic bacteria								
Gram-positive								
Peptococcus sp.	145	8	25	67	97	98	98	99
Peptostreptococcus sp.	72	11	37	63	96	100		
Propionibacterium acnes	16	12	31	94	100			
Eubacterium lentum	14	14	14	28	71	100		
Clostridium perfringens	34	0	0	15	100			
Clostridium sp.	17	12	12	53	88	100		
Gram-negative								
Veillonella sp.	13	23	46	85	100			
B. fragilis	195	0	1	2	23	98	100	
B. melaninogenicus	29	14	31	93	96	100		
Fusobacterium fusiforme	18	39	44	56	89	100		

[a] The National Committee for Clinical Laboratory Standards suggests that 4 μg/ml or less be considered susceptible when testing *H. influenzae* and 12 μg/ml or less be considered susceptible when testing other organisms.[5]
(Data from refs. 8–10, 12, 20, 97, and 103–108.)

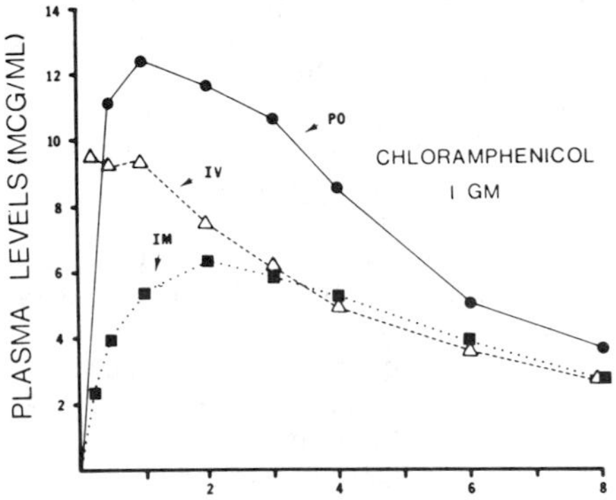

FIG. 4. Plasma levels of active chloramphenicol achieved with 1 g of chloramphenicol administered orally (Chloromycetin Kapseals) and with chloramphenicol sodium succcinate intravenously (iv) and intramuscularly (im). (Modified from Glazko,[127] with permission.)

it is a very bitter substance, aqueous solutions may not be accepted by children. A tasteless suspension in the form of chloramphenicol palmitate is available. This preparation must be hydrolized in the intestine to produce active chloramphenicol. Although earlier formulations sometimes produced erratic serum levels, the bioavailability of chloramphenicol palmitate in the current formulation is the same as in the capsules and is effective for children with *H. influenzae* meningitis (A. J. Glazko, Warner-Lambert/Parke-Davis Pharmaceutical Research Division, Ann Arbor, Michigan, personal communication).[129,130]

The intravenous preparation of the drug is the soluble but inactive chloramphenicol succinate ester that is rapidly hydrolized within the body to biologically active chloramphenicol.[131] This preparation produces active chloramphenicol levels in the serum that are 70 percent of those obtained after oral administration due to incomplete hydrolysis.[127] Intramuscular injection is well tolerated and in most studies produces peak serum levels and areas under the serum level curve similar to intravenous administration.[132–136] One study in adults, however, showed peak concentrations of only one-half to two-thirds of those obtained by the intravenous route, and this was associated with a delayed therapeutic response and increased relapse rate of typhoid fever.[137] Since 30 percent of the unhydrolyzed inactive succinate ester is found in the urine regardless of which parenteral route is used, the lower serum levels produced by intramuscular injection appear to be due to delayed absorption of the ester from the site of injection rather than to decreased hydrolysis.[127] The intramuscular route should be used cautiously.

Chloramphenicol is metabolized primarily by the liver where it is conjugated with glucuronic acid and is excreted in this inactive form by the kidney. Only about 5–10 percent of the administered dose is recovered in the urine as biologically active chloramphenicol. Nevertheless, in the absence of renal disease, concentrations of 150–200 μg/ml of active drug are achieved, which is sufficient to treat urinary tract infections if necessary. Urinary concentrations are markedly diminished, however, in patients with renal failure.[138]

The increased use of chloramphenicol in children has led to a better understanding of the pharmacokinetics. It is clear that there is a wide variation in the metabolism and excretion in that age group. Dosage requirements may vary threefold in children of the same age, with even greater variation noted in newborn and young infants. Because they metabolize the antibiotic at a slow rate, the initial dose for newborns less than 1 week old should be 25 mg/kg every 24 hours and for infants from 1–4 weeks old, 25 mg/kg every 12 hours instead of the usual 50 mg/kg/day divided into 6-hour dosing intervals for older children and adults. However, the wide variation makes monitoring serum levels imperative.[136,139,140]

Chloramphenicol has a half-life in adults of 4.1 hours after single intravenous injections, is not highly bound to protein (25–50 percent), and has an apparent volume of distribution of 100 liters.[97,127,141] The antibiotic diffuses well into many tissues and body fluids. Kramer et al.[142] have shown levels in the brain to be 36 μg/ml, whereas corresponding serum levels were 4 μg/ml. These high levels may reflect the antibiotic's high degree of lipid solubility in conjunction with low protein binding and small molecular size.[143] Levels in the cerebral spinal fluid even without inflamed meninges are generally 30–50 percent of serum concentrations, much higher than those of most other antibiotics.[97] Therapeutic levels are obtained in pleural, ascitic, and synovial fluids.[97,144] In the aqueous humor levels are approximately 50 percent of those in the serum,[145] but studies in rabbits and humans suggest that topical administration may be more efficient in providing high aqueous concentrations.[146,147] Subconjuctival injections are not satisfactory.[148] The antibiotic crosses the placenta to the fetal circulation but produces negligible amounts in the amniotic fluid.Only small amounts of active chloramphenicol are recovered in the bile (0.14 percent of a 1 g dose).[97]

Renal and Hepatic Insufficiency. The half-life of biologically active chloramphenicol in patients with renal disease differs only slightly from healthy subjects, whereas its metabolites increase markedly. The dose, however, should not be modified if therapeutic levels of the active drug are to be maintained. Fortunately, the metabolites do not appear to be as toxic as the active compound. Neither peritoneal nor hemodialysis alters serum levels sufficiently to require dose alterations.[141,149]

Patients with hepatic failure, as evidenced by jaundice or ascites, conjugate chloramphenicol at a slower rate. Serum levels of active chloramphenicol increase to levels capable of bone marrow suppression.[150] The regimen suggested for adults with hepatic insufficiency is an initial 1 g loading dose followed by 500 mg every 6 hours. The course of therapy should be limited where possible to 10–14 days.

Assay

Because of the narrow therapeutic-to-toxic ratio, it is important to monitor serum levels of this antibiotic, particularly in newborn and premature infants, in patients with hepatic disease, and in those patients taking interacting drugs. There are a number of very effective assays that can be used, including bioassays, radioenzymatic assays, competitive enzyme-linked immunoassays, and high-performance chromotography.[151–158] Serum levels in most cases should be maintained between 10 and 30 μg/ml.

Toxicity

Hematologic. The most important toxic effects of chloramphenicol occur in the bone marrow. The effects can be divided into two types. The first is a reversible bone marrow depression due to a direct pharmacologic effect of the antibiotic as a result of inhibition of mitochondrial protein synthesis. It is manifested by reticulocytopenia, anemia, leukopenia, thrombocytopenia, or any combination thereof. There is an increase in serum iron in association with a reduced uptake of radioactive iron by the red blood cells, thus indicating diminished hemoglobin synthesis. The bone marrow reveals vacuolization of the erythyroid and myeloid precursors, but these changes are not specific for chloramphenicol. This type of toxicity is extremely common, occurs during the course of therapy, and is dose related.[159] It is more likely to occur in patients receiving 4 g or more per day or in patients in whom serum levels are above 25 μg/ml, a level that may occur in patients with severe liver disease who are receiving usual doses. It is reversible when treatment with the antibiotic is discontinued.[160]

The second type of toxicity is a rare but generally fatal "idiosyncratic" response that is most frequently manifested as aplastic anemia.[161] Indeed, chloramphenicol is the most common cause of this syndrome. According to the best epidemiologic studies in the United States, aplastic anemia occurs once in 24,500–40,800 patients who receive the antibiotic, a risk about 13 times greater than that for aplastic anemia in the general population.[162] The aplastic anemia most commonly occurs weeks to months after completion of therapy and is not necessarily dose related. It appears that this toxic effect is caused by a mechanism different from the direct bone marrow suppression previously described. Although the pathogenesis of this idiosyncratic response is not known, there have been several observations and theories that deserve comment. This type of toxicity has occurred in identical twins, which suggests a genetic predisposition.[163] Morley et al.[164] have observed that mice given chloramphenicol after treatment with busulfan had a progressive decrease in the number of pluripotential stem cells whereas control mice did not. Since most of the animals had entirely normal hemograms before receiving chloramphenicol, they suggest that the aplastic anemia might result in patients with unrecognized pre-existing residual marrow damage either genetic or acquired. In 1967 Holt observed that the aplastic anemia occurred only after oral administration of the antibiotic.[165] He postulates that the fatal reaction may be caused by the absorption of toxic products produced by enzymatic degradation of chloramphenicol, perhaps as a result of specific types of bacteria colonizing the gut of affected people. Supporting this hypothesis, Jimenez and colleagues have shown that one of chloramphenicol's metabolites, dehydrochloramphenicol, is 10- to 20-fold more cytotoxic than chloramphenicol is yet only one-third as effective in inhibiting protein synthesis, thus suggesting that this metabolite and perhaps others may play a significant role in this toxicity.[166] However, a number of cases of aplastic anemia from parenteral chloramphenicol and after the administration of eye drops have also been reported. Although the number of cases reported is greater after oral therapy, the parenteral form of the antibiotic should also be considered to be potentially toxic.[167–169] It has been speculated that the nitrobenzene moiety of chloramphenicol may be the culprit responsible for the aplastic anemia. Thiamphenicol, an analogue of chloramphenicol that is currently used in Europe and Japan, has the nitro group on the benzene ring replaced by methysulfone. This analogue produces the reversible bone marrow suppression as readily as chloramphenicol does but has not been associated with the aplastic anemia.[170] Although most cases of aplastic anemia from chloramphenicol become apparent after the completion of therapy, it should be emphasized that 22 percent of the cases occur concurrently with antibiotic administration.[161,169] Whether some of these episodes can be prevented by checking the blood counts of patients is not known. Until the pathogenesis of the toxicity is clearly understood, it is recommended that a complete blood count be obtained on a twice-a-week basis on all patients receiving chloramphenicol. If the white blood cell count decreases below 2500/mm^3, it is desirable to discontinue treatment with the antibiotic if the clinical condition allows. It should be recognized, however, that low numbers of white blood cells may occur in illnesses for which chloramphenicol is used such as typhoid fever.

Also of concern are the reports of childhood leukemia after the use of chloramphenicol. Although these cases generally follow the aplastic anemia, a recent population-based case control interview study of 309 childhood leukemia cases and 618 age- and sex-matched controls showed a significant dose-response relation between chloramphenicol and the risk of both acute lymphocytic and nonlymphocytic leukemia, particularly after treatment for greater than 10 days in children without prior aplastic anemia. Until this is more clearly defined, it seems prudent to change therapy as quickly as possible to alternate agents when organisms prove susceptible to other equally effective and less toxic antibiotics.[171]

Chloramphenicol may also produce a hemolytic anemia in patients with the Mediterranean form of glucose-6-phosphate dehydrogenase (G6PD) deficiency. This apparently does not occur with the milder A type G6PD deficiency, which is the most common form in blacks.[172]

Gray Baby Syndrome. The gray baby syndrome of neonates is characterized by abdominal distension, vomiting, flaccidity, cynosis, circulatory collapse, and death. The side effect results from a diminished ability of neonates to conjugate chloramphenicol and to excrete the active form in the urine.[173] If chloramphenicol is necessary in premature infants and neonates, the dose should be reduced to 25 mg/kg/day, and the antibiotic levels should be monitored. This syndrome has also been recognized in toddlers and after accidental overdoses in adults.[174,175] It is generally associated with serum concentrations of chloramphenicol of greater than 50 μg/ml and may present with unexplained metabolic acidosis.[176] Large-volume exchange transfusions or charcoal hemoperfusion has been used to accelerate drug removal.[177,178]

Optic Neuritis. Optic neuritis resulting in decreased visual acuity has been described in patients receiving prolonged chloramphenicol therapy.[179] The symptoms are generally reversible, but a loss of vision has occurred. Other neurologic sequelae such as peripheral neuritis, headache, depression, opthalmoplegia, and mental confusion have also been described.

Other Types. Hypersensitivity reactions including rashes and drug fevers and anaphylaxis are rare. Herxheimer-like responses during therapy for syphilis, brucellosis, and typhoid fever have been observed. Symptoms involving the gastrointestinal tract, including nausea, vomiting and diarrhea, glossitis, and stomatitis, occur but have not been a major problem. Bleeding due to decreased vitamin K synthesis has resulted from prolonged administration.

Significant Drug Interactions

Chloramphenicol prolongs the half-life of tolbutamide, chlorpropamide, phenytoin, cyclophosphamide, and warfarin (Coumadin), apparently by inhibiting hepatic microsomal enzymes.[180–183] Severe toxicity and death have occurred. Phenytoin, rifampin, and phenobarbital have been observed to decrease the serum concentration and increase the total body clearance of chloramphenicol, perhaps by inducing hepatic microsomal enzymes. Serum concentrations should be monitored when these drugs are administered concurrently.[184,185] The physician should be on the alert for toxicity from other agents that are metabolized by the liver when administering this agent and should monitor serum levels when these drugs are administered concurrently. Chloramphenicol may delay the response of anemias to iron, folic acid, and vitamin B_{12}.[186]

TABLE 8. Indications for Chloramphenicol

Indication	*Usual Adult Dose*	*Comment*
Therapy of choice		
Brain abscess	100 mg/kg/day	Used with a penicillin; some prefer penicillin plus metronidazole for this indication
Typhoid fever and invasive salmonellosis	50 mg/kg/day	Strains in some areas may be chloramphenicol resistant; not used for gastroenteritis or carrier state
Effective alternative therapy		
Bacterial meningitis *H. influenzae* *S. pneumoniae* *N. meningitidis*	100 mg/kg/day	For penicillin-allergic patients; can be used for empirical therapy when these pathogens are suspected; also used for *S. pneumoniae* relatively resistant to penicillin
Rickettsial infections Rocky Mountain spotted fever Typhus (murine) Scrub typhus Tick bite fever Q fever	50 mg/kg/day	Preferred drug when patients require parenteral therapy, in pregnancy, and in young children
Melioidosis, acute	50 mg/kg/day	Used with tetracycline

Chloramphenicol is primarily a bacteriostatic agent and will antagonize in vitro the bactericidal activity of the penicillins, cephalosporins, and aminoglycoside antibiotics. This has doubtful clinical significance in most instances. However, care should be exercised in the use of such combinations for infections that require bactericidal activity for efficacy such as for infections in the granulocytopenic host or in the treatment of endocarditis.[187] In the treatment of meningitis, the bacteriostatic activity of chloramphenicol against group B streptococci and its in vitro antagonism with ampicillin against this organism are of concern and should be considered in selecting therapy when this organism is likely to be a pathogen.[101]

Indications

The clinical indications for the use of chloramphenicol are listed in Table 8. In most cases, these indications are clearly defined. Many experts feel that the third-generation cephalosporins have superseded chloramphenicol for the treatment of bacterial meningitis in infants and children. The antibiotic is still used for the treatment of meningitis in the penicillin-allergic patients, for meningitis cases by relatively penicillin-resistant pneumococci, and as an oral alternative where the use of parenteral therapy is impossible.[188–190] Occasionally, the antibiotic is useful when the differential diagnosis includes both meningococcemia and Rocky Mountain spotted fever, diseases that may be difficult to distinguish on clinical characteristics. It also may be useful in the place of a nephrotoxic agent for the treatment of severe infections due to sensitive organisms in patients with decreased renal function.

Chloramphenicol is a valuable antimicrobial agent. Like many other agents, it is toxic and can cause death. When the rare clinical indications are present, however, the antibiotic should not be avoided because of its possible toxicity.

REFERENCES

1. Finland M. Twenty-fifth anniversary of the discovery of Aureomycin: The place of the tetracyclines in antimicrobial therapy. Clin Pharmacol Ther. 1974;15:3.
2. Pratt WB, Fekety R. The Antimicrobial Drugs. New York: Oxford University Press; 1986:205–8.
3. Craven GR, Gavin R, Fanning T. The transfer RNA binding site of the 30

s ribosome and the site of tetracycline inhibition. Symp Quant Biol. 1969;34:129.
4. Beard HS, Armentrout SA, Weisberger. Inhibition of mammalian protein synthesis by antibiotics. Pharmacol Rev. 1969;21:213.
5. National Committee for Clinical Laboratory Standards. Methods for dilution antimicrobial susceptibility tests for bacteria that grow aerobically: Approved standard. NCCLS Publication M7-A. Villanova, PA: NCCLS; 1985.
6. Centers for Disease Control. Antibiotic-resistant strains of *Neisseria gonorrhoeae*. MMWR. 1987;36(Suppl 55)1–18.
7. Steigbigel NH, Reed CR, Finland M. Susceptibility of common pathogenic bacteria to seven tetracycline antibiotics in vitro. Am J Med Sci. 1968;255:179.
8. Finland M. Changing patterns of susceptibility of common bacterial pathogens to antimicrobial agents. Ann Intern Med. 1972;76:1009.
9. Sabath LD, Stumpf LL, Wallace SJ, et al. Susceptibility of *Diplococcus pneumoniae, Haemophilus influenzae*, and *Neisseria meningitidis* to 23 antibiotics. Antimicrob Agents Chemother. 1970, 1971;53.
10. Eickhoff TC, Bennett JV, Hayes PS, et al. *Pseudomonas pseudomallei* susceptibility to chemotherapeutic agents. J Infect Dis. 1970;121:95.
11. Karmali MA, DeGrandis S, Fleming PC. Antimicrobial susceptibility of *Campylobacter jejuni* with special reference to resistance patterns of Canadian isolates. Antimicrob Agents Chemother. 1981;19:593.
12. Gordon RC, Thompson TR, Carlson W, et al. Antimicrobial resistance of shigellae isolated in Michigan. JAMA. 1975;231:1159.
13. Neu HC. A symposium on the tetracyclines: A major appraisal. Introduction. Bull NY Acad Med. 1978;54:141.
14. Sparling PF. Antibiotic resistance in *Neisseria gonorrhoeae*. Med Clin North Am. 1972;56:1133.
15. Farrell ID, Hinchliffe PM, Robertson L. Susceptibility of *Brucella* spp. to tetracycline and its analogues. J Clin Pathol. 1976;29:1097.
16. Morris J Glenn Jr, Black RE. Chloera and other vibrioses in the United States, N Engl J Med. 1985;312:343–50.
17. Chow AW, Patten V, Dominick B. Susceptibility of *Campylobacter fetus* to twenty-two antimicrobial agents. Antimicrob Agents Chemother. 1978;13:416.
18. Michel J, Rogol M, Dickman D. Susceptibility of clinical isolates of *Campylobacter jejuni* to sixteen antimicrobial agents. Antimicrob Agents Chemother. 1983;23:796.
19. Wallace RJ, Wiss K. Susceptibility of *Mycobacterium marinum* to tetracyclines and aminoglycosides. Antimicrob Agents Chemother. 1981;20:610.
20. Sutter VL, Finegold SM. Susceptibility of anaerobic bacteria to 23 antimicrobial agents. Antimicrob Agents Chemother. 1976;10:736.
21. Washington JA, Dearing WH, Judd ES, et al. Effect of preoperative antibiotic regimen on development of infection after intestinal surgery: Prospective, randomized, double-blind study. Ann Surg. 1974;180:567.
22. Hojer H, Wetterfors J. Systemic prophylaxis with doxycycline in surgery of the colon and rectum. Ann Surg. 1978;187:362.
23. Johnson SE, Klein GP, Schmid GP, et al. Susceptibility of the Lyme disease spirochete to seven antimicrobial agents. Yale J Biol Med. 1984;57:549–53.
24. Pang LW, Limsomwong N, Boudreau EF, et al. Doxycycline prophylaxis for *falciparum malaria*: Lancet. 1987;1:1161–4.
25. Benveniste R, Davies J. Mechanisms of antibiotic resistance in bacteria. Annu Rev Biochem. 1973;42:471.
26. Sompolinsky D, Zemira S. Plasmid-determined resistance to tetracycline. Microbios. 1981;30:109.
27. Park BH, Hendricks M, Malamy MH, et al. Cryptic tetracycline resistance determinant (class F) isolated from *Bacteroides fragilis* mediates resistance in *Escherichia coli* by actively reducing tetracycline accumulation. Antimicrob Agents Chemother. 1987;31:1739–43.
28. Roberts MC, Kenny GE, Tet M. Tetracycline resistance determinants in *Ureaplasma urealyticum*. Antimicrob Agents Chemother. 1986:29:350–2.
29. Rapoport MI, Calia FM. The use of antibiotics in animal feeds. JAMA. 1974;229:1212.
30. VanLeeuwen WJ, VanEmbden J, Guinee PAM, et al. Decrease in drug resistance in *Salmonella* in the Netherlands. Antimicrob Agents Chemother. 1979;16:237.
31. Spika JS, Waterman SH, Soo Hoo GW, et al. Chloramphenicol-resistant *Salmonella newport* traced through hamburger to dairy farms. N Engl J Med. 1987;316:565–70.
32. Finland M, Garrod LP. Demethylchlortetracycline. Br Med J. 1960;2:959.
33. Fabre J, Milek E, Kalfopoulos P, et al. The kinetics of tetracyclines in man: Digestive absorption and serum concentrations. In: Doxycycline (Vibramycin): A Compendium of Clinical Evaluation. New York: Pfizer Laboratories; 1973:13.
34. Lederle Laboratories. Minocin: Minocycline. Pearl River, NY: Lederle Laboratories; 1975.
35. Rosenblatt JE, Barrett JE, Brodie JL, et al. Comparison of in vitro activity and clinical pharmacology of doxycycline with other tetracyclines. Antimicrob Agents Chemother. 1966, 1967;134.
36. Kirby WMM, Roberts CE, Burdick RE. Comparison of two new tetracyclines with tetracycline and demethylchlortetracycline. Antimicrob Agents Chemother. 1961,1962;286.
37. Fabre J, Pitton JS, Junz JP, et al. Distribution and excretion of doxycycline in man. Chemotherapia. 1966;11:73.
38. Kunin CM, Dornbush AC, Finland M. Distribution and excretion of four tetracycline analogues in normal young men. J Clin Invest. 1959;38:1950.
39. MacDonald H, Kelley RG, Allen ES, et al. Pharmacokinetic studies on minocycline in man. Clin Pharmacol Ther. 1973;14:852.
40. Kunin CM. Comparative serum binding distribution and excretion of tetracycline and a new analogue methacycline. Proc Soc Exp Biol Med. 1962;110:311.
41. Bennett JV, Mickewait JS, Barrett JE, et al. Comparative serum binding of four tetracyclines under simulated in vivo conditions. Antimicrob Agents Chemother. 1965, 1966;180.
42. Wood WS, Kipnis GR. The concentrations of tetracycline, chlortetracycline and oxytetracycline in the cerebrospinal fluid after intravenous administration. In: Antibiotics Annual, 1953–1954. New York: Medical Encyclopedia; 1953:98.
43. Yim CW, Flynn NM, Fitzgerald FT. Penetration of oral doxycycline into the cerebrospinal fluid of patients with latent or neurosyphilis. Antimicrob Agents Chemother. 1985;28:347.
44. Parker RH, Schmid F. Antimicrobial activity of synovial fluid during therapy of septic arthritis. Arthritis Rheum. 1971;14:96.
45. Lundberg C, Malmburg A, Ivemark BI. Antibiotic concentrations in relation to structural changes in maxillary sinus mucosa folowing intramuscular or peroral treatment. Scand J Infect Dis. 1974;6:187.
46. Fabre J, Milek E, Kalopoulos P, et al. The kinetics of tetracyclines in man II. Excretion, penetration in normal and inflammatory tissues, behavior in renal insufficiency and hemodialysis. In: Doxycycline (Vibramycin): A Compendium of Clinical Evaluations. New York: Pfizer Laboratories; 1973:19.
47. Hoeprich PD, Warshauer DM. Entry of four tetracyclines into saliva and tears. Antimicrob Agents Chemother. 1974;5:330.
48. LeBlanc AL, Perry JE. Transfer of tetracycline across the human placenta. Tex Rep Biol Med. 1967;25:541.
49. Whelton A. Tetracyclines in renal insufficiency: Resolution of a therapeutic dilemma. Bull NY Acad Med. 1978;54:223.
50. Bennett JV, Brodie JL, Benner EJ, et al. Simplified accurate method for antibiotic assay of clinical specimens. Appl Microbiol. 1966;14:170.
51. Kohn KW. Determination of tetracyclines by extraction of fluorescent complexes: Application to biological materials. Anal Chem. 1961;33:862.
52. Csonka GW, Rosedale N, Walkden L. Balanitis due to fixed drug eruption associated with tetracycline therapy. Br J Vener Dis. 1970;47:42.
53. Fellner MJ, Baer RL. Anaphylactic reaction to tetracycline in a penicillin-allergic patient: Immunologic studies. JAMA. 1965;192:997.
54. Furey WW, Tan C. Anaphylactic shock due to oral demethylchlortetracycline. Ann Intern Med. 1969;70:357.
55. Carey BW. Photodynamic response of a new tetracycline. JAMA. 1960;172:1196.
56. Frost P, Weinstein GD, Gomez EC. Phototoxic potential of minocycline and doxycycline. Arch Dermatol. 1972;105:681.
57. Angeloni VL, Salasche SJ, Ortiz R. Nail, skin and scleral pigmentation induced by minocycline. Cutis. 1987;40:229–33.
58. Atwood HD, Dennet X. A black thyroid and minocycline treatment. Br Med J. 1976;2:1109.
59. Brearley LJ, Storey E. Tetracycline-induced tooth changes: Part 2. Prevalence, localization and nature of staining in extracted deciduous teeth. Med J Aust. 1968;2:714.
60. Witkop CJ, Wolf RO. Hypoplasia and intrinsic staining of enamel following tetracycline therapy. JAMA. 1963;185:1008.
61. Cohan S, Bevelander G, Tiamsic T. Growth inhibition of prematures receiving tetracycline. Am J Dis Child. 1963;105:453.
62. Grossman ER, Walcheck A, Freedman H. Tetracycline and permanent teeth: The relationship between doses and tooth color. Pediatrics. 1971;47:567.
63. Department of Health Education and Welfare. Tetracycline pediatric drops to be withdrawn from the market. FDA Drug Bull. 1978;8:23.
64. Forti G, Benincori C. Doxycycline and the teeth. Lancet. 1969;1:782.
65. Schneider R. Doxycycline esophageal ulcers. Am J Dig Dis. 1977;22:805.
66. Winckler K. Tetracycline ulcers of the oesophagus: Endoscopy, histology, and reoentgenology in two cases, and review of the literature. Endoscopy. 1981;13:225.
67. Hinton NA. The effect of oral tetracycline HCl and doxycycline on the intestinal flora. Curr Ther Res. 1970;12:341.
68. Gorbach SL, Bartlett JG. Anaerobic infections. N Engl J Med. 1974;290:1289.
69. Elmore MF, Rogge JD. Tetracycline induced pancreatitis. Gastroenterology. 1981;81:1134.
70. Lepper MH, Wolfe CK, Zimmerman HJ, et al. Effect of large doses of Aureomycin on human liver. Arch Intern Med. 1951;88:271.
71. Schultz JC, Adamson JS Jr, Workman WW, et al. Fatal liver disease after intravenous administration of tetracycline in high doses. N Engl J Med. 1963;269:999.
72. Whalley PJ, Adams RH, Combes B. Tetracycline toxicity in pregnancy: Liver and pancreatic dysfunction. JAMA. 1964;189:357.
73. Damjanov I, Arnold R, Faour M. Tetracycline toxicity in a non-pregnant woman. JAMA. 1968;204:934.
74. Shils ME. Renal disease and the metabolic effects of tetracycline. Ann Intern Med. 1963;58:389.
75. Forrest JN, Cox M, Hong C, et al. Superiority of demeclocycline over lithium in the treatment of chronic syndrome of inappropriate secretion of antidiuretic hormone. N Engl J Med. 1978;298:173.
76. Carrilho F, Bosch J, Arroyo V, et al. Renal failure associated with demeclocycline in cirrhosis. Ann Intern Med. 1977;87:195.

77. Fanning WL, Gump DW, Sofferman RA. Side effects of minocycline: A double blind study. Antimicrob Agents Chemother. 1977;11:712.
78. Koch-Weser J, Gilmore EB. Benign intracranial hypertension in an adult after tetracycline therapy. JAMA. 1967;200:345.
79. Walters BNJ, Gubbay SS. Tetracycline and benign intracranial hypertension: Report of five cases. Br Med J. 1981;282:19.
80. Jackson GG, Haight TH, Kass EH, et al. Tetramycin therapy of pneumonia: Clinical and bacteriologic studies in 91 cases. Ann Intern Med. 1951;35:1175.
81. Lundsgaard-Hansen P, Senn A, Roos B, et al. Staphylococcal enteritis: Report of six cases with two fatalities after intravenous administration of *N*-(pyrrolidinomethyl) tetracycline. JAMA. 1960;173:1008.
82. Neuvonen PJ, Gothoni G, Hackman R, et al. Interference of iron with the absorption of tetracyclines in man. Br Med J. 1970;4:532.
83. Bar WH, Adir J, Garrettson L. Decrease of tetracycline in man by sodium bicarbonate. Clin Pharmacol Ther. 1971;12:779.
84. Fisher P, House F, Inns P, et al. Effect of cimetidine on the absorption of orally administered tetracycline. Br J Clin Pharmacol. 1980;9:153.
85. Neuvonen PJ, Pentitila O. Interaction between doxycycline and barbiturates. Br Med J. 1974;1:535.
86. Pentitla O, Neuvonen PJ, Lehtovaara R. Interaction between doxcycline and some antiepileptic drugs. Br Med J. 1974;2:470.
87. Neuvonen PJ, Penttila O, Roos M. Effect of long-term alcohol consumption on the half-life of tetracycline and doxycycline in man. Int J Clin Pharmacol. 1976;14:303.
88. Kuzucu EY. Methoxyflurane, tetracycline and renal failure. JAMA. 1970;211:1162.
89. Semel JD. Renal failure and multiple organ toxicity associated with tetracycline operative prophylaxis. Infect Surg. 1988;June:405–8.
90. Boston collaborative drug surveillance program. Tetracycline and drug-attributed rises in blood urea nitrogen. JAMA. 1972;220:377.
91. Bacon JF, Chenfield GM. Pregnancy attributable to interaction between tetracycline and oral contraceptives. Br Med J. 1980;280:293.
92. Hansen PD. Drug Interactions. 5th ed. Philadelphia: Lea & Febiger; 1985:239.
93. U.S. Department of Health and Human Services. 1985 STD treatment guidelines. MMWR. 1985;34(Suppl 4):81–6.
94. Ehrlich J, Bartz QR, Smith RM, et al. Chloromycetin, a new antibiotic from a soil actinomycete. Science. 1947;106:417.
95. Carter HE, Gottliebb D, Anderson HW. Comments and communications. Science. 107;113:947.
96. Ehrlich J, Gottlieb D, Burkholder PR, et al. *Streptomyces venezuelae*, N. sp., the source of Chloromycetin. J Bacteriol. 1948;56:467.
97. Woodward TE, Wisseman CL. Chloromycetin (Chloramphenicol). New York: Medical Encyclopedia; 1958.
98. Abdel-Sayed S. Transport of chloramphenicol into sensitive strains of *Escherichia coli* and *Pseudomonas aeruginosa*. J Antimicrob Chemother. 1987;19:7–20.
99. Turk DC. A comparison of chloramphenicol and ampicillin as bactericidal agents for *Haemophilus influenzae* type B. J Med Microbiol. 1977;10:127.
100. Rahal JJ, Simberkoff MS. Bactericidal and bacteriostatic action of chloramphenicol against meningeal pathogens. Antimicrob Agents Chemother. 1979;16:13.
101. Weeks JL, Mason EO Jr, Baker CJ. Antagonism of ampicillin and chloramphenicol for meningeal isolates of group B streptococci. Antimicrob Agents Chemother. 1981;20:281.
102. Roodyn DB, Wilkie D. The Biogenesis of Mitochondria. London: Methuen; 1968.
103. McGowan JE, Garner C, Wilcox C, et al. Antibiotic susceptibility of gram negative bacilli isolated from blood cultures: Results of tests with 35 agents and strains from 169 patients at Boston City Hospital during 1972. Am J Med. 1974;57:225.
104. Yow EM, Spink WW. Experimental studies on the action of streptomycin, Aureomycin and Chloromycetin on *Brucella*. J Clin Invest. 1949;28:871.
105. Robertson RP, Wahab MFA, Raasch FO. Evaluation of chloramphenicol and ampicillin in *Salmonella* enteric fever. N Engl J Med. 1968;278:171.
106. Rubinstein E, Shainberg B. In vitro activity of cinoxacin, ampicillin, and chloramphenicol against *Shigella* and non-typhoid *Salmonella*. Antimicrob Agents Chemother. 1977;11:577.
107. Wells EB, Chang SM, Jackson GG, et al. Antibiotic spectrum of *Hemophilus pertussis*. J Pediatr. 1950;36:752.
108. Martin WJ, Gardner M, Washington JA II. In vitro antimicrobial susceptibility of anaerobic bacteria isolated from clinical specimens. Antimicrob Agents Chemother. 1972;1:148.
109. Cherubin CE, Neu HC, Rahal JJ, et al. Emergence of resistance to chloramphenicol in *Salmonella*. J Infect Dis. 1977;135:807.
110. Long SS, Phillips SE. Chloramphenicol-resistant *Hemophilus influenzae*. J Pediatr. 1976;90:1030.
111. Mathies AW Jr. Penicillins in the treatment of bacterial meningitis. *J R Coll Physicians Lond.* 1972;6:139.
112. Doern GV, Jorgensen JH, Thornsberry C, et al. Prevalance of antimicrobial resistance among clinical isolates of *Haemophilus influenzae*: A collaborative study. Diagn Microbiol Infect Dis. 1986;4:95–107.
113. MacMahon P, Sills J, Hall E, et al. *Haemophilus influenzae* type b resistant to both chloramphenicol and ampicillin in Britain. Br Med J. 1982;24:1229.
114. Bergeron MC, Claveau S, Simard P. Limited in vitro activity of cefamandole against 100 beta-lactamase and non–beta-lactamase-producing *Haemophilus influenzae* strains: Comparison of moxalactam, chloramphenicol and ampicillin. Antimicrob Agents Chemother. 1981;19:101.
115. Kenny JF, Isburg CD, Michaels RH. Meningitis due to *Haemophilus influenzae* type b resistant to both ampicillin and chloramphenicol. Pediatrics. 1980;66:14.
116. Campos J, Garcia-Tornel S, San Feliu I. Susceptibility studies of multiply resistant *Haemophilus influenzae* isolated from pediatric patients and contacts. Antimicrob Agents Chemother. 1984;25:706.
117. Centers for Disease Control. Ampicillin and chloramphenicol resistance in systemic *Haemophilus influenzae* disease. MMWR. 1984;33:35.
118. Williams JD, Mossdeen F. Antibiotic resistance in *Haemophilus influenzae*; epidemiology, mechanisms, and therapeutic possibilities. Rev Infect Dis. 1986;8(Suppl 5):555–61.
119. Cuchural GJ Jr, Talley FP, Jacobus NV, et al. Susceptibility of the *Bacteroides fragilis* group in the United States: Analysis by site of isolation. Antimicrob Agents Chemother. 1988;32:717–22.
120. Finegold SM, Wexler HM. Therapeutic implications of bacteriologic findings in mixed aerobic-anaerobic infections. Antimicrob Agents Chemother. 1988;32:611–6.
121. Okamoto S, Mizuno D. Mechanism of chloramphenicol and tetracycline resistance in *Escherichia coli*. J Gen Microbiol. 1964;35:125.
122. Okamoto S, Suzuki Y. Chloramphenicol-, dihydrostreptomycin-, and kanamycin-inactivating enzymes from multiple drug-resistant *Escherichia coli* carrying episome "R." Nature. 1965;208:1301.
123. Gangarosa EJ, Bennett JV, Wyatt C, et al. An epidemic-associated episome? J Infect Dis. 1972;126:215.
124. Butler T, Linh NN, Arnold K, et al. Chloramphenicol-resistant typhoid fever in Vietnam associated with R-factor. Lancet. 1973;2:983.
125. Editorial: Drug resistance in salmonellas. Lancet. 1982;1:1391.
126. Anderson ES, Smith HR. Chloramphenicol resistance in the typhoid bacillus. Br Med J. 1972;3:329.
127. Glazko AJ, Dill WA, Kinkel AW, et al. Absorption and excretion of parenteral doses of chloramphenicol sodium succinate in comparison with peroral doses of chloramphenicol (Abstract). Clin Pharmacol Ther. 1977;21:104.
128. Bartelloni PJ, Calia FM, Minchew BH, et al. Absorption and excretion of two chloramphenicol products in humans after oral administration. Am J Med Sci. 1969;258:203.
129. Pickering LK, Hoecker JL, Kramer WG, et al. Clinical pharmacology of two chloramphenicol preparations in children: Sodium succinate (IV) and palmitate (oral) esters. J Pediatr. 1980;96:757.
130. Tuomen EI, Powell KR, Marks MI, et al. Oral chloramphenicol in the treatment of *Haemophilus influzenae* meningitis. J Pediatr. 1981;99:968.
131. McCrumb FR, Snyder MJ, Hicken WJ. The use of chloramphenicol acid succinate in the treatment of acute infections. In: Antibiotics Annual, 1957–1958. New York: Medical Encyclopedia; 1958:837.
132. Ross S, Puig JR, Zarembra EA. Chloramphenicol acid succinate (sodium salt); some preliminary clinical and laboratory observations in infants and children. In Antibiotics Annual, 1957–1958. New York: Medical Encyclopedia; 1958:803–19.
133. McCrumb FR Jr, Snyder MJ, Hicken WJ. The use of chloramphenicol acid succinate in the treatment of acute infections. In Antibiotics Annual, 1957–1958. New York: Medical Encyclopedia; 1958:837.
134. Ciocatto E, Marchiaro G. Chloramphenicol in resuscitation and cardiac surgery. Postgrad Med J. 1967;43(Suppl):90–3.
135. Shann F, Linnenmann V, MacKenzie A, et al. Absorption of chloramphenicol sodium succinate after intramuscular administration in children. N Engl J Med. 1985;313:410–4.
136. Smith AL, Weber A. Pharmacology of chloramphenicol. Pediatr Clin North Am. 1983;30:209–36.
137. DuPont HL, Hornick RB, Weiss CF, et al. Evaluation of chloramphenicol acid succinate therapy of induced typhoid fever and Rocky Mountain spotted fever. N Engl J Med. 1970;282:53.
138. Lindberg AA, Nilsson LH, Bucht H, et al. Concentration of chloramphenicol in the urine and blood in relation to renal function. Br Med J. 1966;2:724.
139. Kauffman RE, Miceti JN, Strebel L, et al. Pharmacokinetics of chloramphenicol and chloramphenicol succinate in infants and children. J Pediatr. 1981;98:315.
140. Kauffman RE, Thirumoorthi MC, Buckley JA, et al. Relative bioavailability of intravenous chloramphenicol succinate and oral chloramphenicol palmitate in infants and children. J Pediatr. 1981;99:363.
141. Kunin CM. A guide to use of antibiotics in patients with renal disease. Ann Intern Med. 1967;67:151.
142. Kramer PW, Griffith RS, Campbell RL, et al. Antibiotic penetration of the brain: A comparative study. J Neurosurg. 1969;31:295.
143. Braude AI: Antimicrobial Drug Therapy. Philadelphia: WB Saunders; 1976:82.
144. Rapp GF, Griffith RS, Hebble WM. The permeability of traumatically inflamed synovial membrane to commonly used antibiotics. J Bone Joint Surg [Am]. 1966;48:1534.
145. Abraham RK, Burnett HH. Tetracycline and chloramphenicol studies on rabbit and human eyes. Arch Ophthalmol. 1955;54:641.
146. Beasley H, Boltralik JJ, Baldwin HA. Chloramphenicol in aqueous humor after topical application. Arch Ophthalmol. 1975;93:184.
147. George FJ, Hanna C. Ocular penetration of chloramphenicol. Arch Ophthalmol. 1977;95:879.
148. McPherson SD Jr, Presley GD, Crawford JR. Aqueous humor assays of subconjunctival antibiotics. Am J Ophthalmol. 1968;66:430.

149. Kunin CM, Glazko AJ, Finland M. Persistence of antibiotics in blood of patients with acute renal failure. II. Chloramphenicol and its metabolic products in the blood of patients with severe renal disease or hepatic cirrhosis. J Clin Invest. 1959;38:1498.
150. Suhrland LG, Weisberger AS. Chloramphenicol toxicity in liver and renal disease. Arch Intern Med. 1963;112:161.
151. Louie TJ, Tally FP, Bartlett JG, et al. Rapid microbiological assay for chloramphenicol and tetracyclines. Antimicrob Agents Chemother. 1976;9:874.
152. Jorgensen JH, Alexander GA. Rapid bioassay for chloramphenicol in the presence of other antibiotics. Am J Clin Pathol. 1981;76:474.
153. Lietman PS, White TJ, Shaw WV. Chloramphenicol: An enzymological microassay. Antimicrob Agents Chemother. 1976;10:347.
154. Smith AL, Smith DH. Improved enzymatic analysis of chloramphenicol. Clin Chem. 1978;24:1452.
155. Aravind MK, Miceli JN, Kauffman RE, et al. Simultaneous measurements of chloramphenicol and chloramphenicol succinate in body fluids utilizing HPLC. J Chromatogr. 1980;221:176.
156. Nahata MC, Powell DA. Simultaneous determination of chloramphenicol and its succinate ester by high-performance liquid chromatography. J Chromatogr. 1981;223:247.
157. Cambell GS, Mageau RP, Schwab B, et al. Detection and quantitation of chloramphenicol by competitive enzyme-linked immunoassay. Antimicrob Agents Chemother. 1984;25:205–11.
158. Abou-Khalil S, Abou-Khalil WH, Masoud AM, et al. High-performance liquid chromatographic determination of chloramphenicol and four analogues usingg reductive and oxidative electrochemical and ultraviolet detection. J Chromatogr. 1987;417:111–9.
159. Yunis AA. Chloramphenicol-induced bone marrow suppression. Semin Hematol. 1973;10:225.
160. Scott JL, Finegold SM, Belkin GA, et al. A controlled double-blind study of the hematologic toxicity of chloramphenicol. N Engl J Med. 1965;272:1137.
161. Best WR. Chloramphenicol-associated blood dyscrasias. A review of cases submitted to the American Medical Association Registry. JAMA. 1967;201:181.
162. Wallerstein RO, Condit PK, Kasper CK, et al. Statewide study of chloramphenicol therapy and fatal aplastic anemia. JAMA. 1969;208:2045.
163. Nagao T, Mauer AM. Concordance for drug-induced aplastic anemia in identical twins. N Engl J Med. 1969;281:7.
164. Morley A, Trainor K, Remes J. Residual marrow damage: Possible explanation for idiosyncrasy to chloramphenicol. Br J Haematol. 1976;32:525.
165. Holt R. The bacterial degradation of chloramphenicol. Lancet. 1967;1:1259.
166. Jimenez JJ, Arimura GK, Abou-Khalil WH, et al. Chloramphenicol-induced bone marrow injury: Possible role of bacterial metabolites of chloramphenicol. Blood. 1987;70:1180–5.
167. Polin HB, Plaut ME. Chloramphenicol. NY State J Med. 1977;77:378.
168. Plaut ME, Best WR. Aplastic anemia after parenteral chloramphenicol: Warning renewal (Letter). N Engl J Med. 1982;306:1486.
169. Daum RS, Cohen DL, Smith AL. Fatal aplastic anemia following apparent "dose-related" chloramphenicol toxicity. J Pediatr. 1979;94:403.
170. Keiser G. Introduction: Symposium on thiamphenicol. Postgrad Med J. 1974;50(Suppl 5):13.
171. Shu XO, Linet MS, Gao RN, et al. Chloramphenicol use and childhood leukaemia in Shanghai. Lancet. 1987;2:934–7.
172. Beutler E. Glucose 6-phosphate dehydrogenase deficiency. In: Williams WJ, Beutler E, Erslev AJ, et al., eds. Hematology. New York: McGraw-Hill; 1977:466.
173. Burns LE, Hodgman JE, Cass AB. Fatal circulatory collapse in premature infants receiving chloramphenicol. N Engl J Med. 1959;261:1318.
174. Craft AW, Brocklebank JT, Hey EN, et al. The "grey toddler": Chloramphenicol toxicity. Arch Dis Child. 1974;49:235.
175. Thompson WL, Anderson SE, Lipsky JJ, et al. Overdoses of chloramphenicol. JAMA. 1975;234:149.
176. Evans LS, Kleiman MB. Acidosis as a presenting feature of chloramphenicol toxicity. J Pediatr. 1986;108:475–7.
177. Stevens DC, Kleinman MB, Lietman PS, ett al. Exchange transfusion in acute chloramphenicol toxicity. J Pediatr. 1981;99:651.
178. Freundlick M, Cynamon H, Tamer A, et al. Management of chloramphenicol intoxication in infancy by charcoal hemoperfusion. J Pediatr. 1983;103:485.
179. Chloramphenicol blindness (Editorial). Br Med J. 1965;1:1511.
180. Christensen LK, Skovsted L. Inhibition of drug metabolism by chloramphenicol. Lancet. 1969;2:1397.
181. Petitpierre B, Fabre J. Chlorpropamide and chloramphenicol. Lancet. 1970;1:789.
182. Rose JQ, Choi HK, Schentag JJ. Intoxication caused by interaction of chloramphenicol and phenytoin. JAMA. 1977;237:2630.
183. Faber OK, Mouridsen HT, Skovsted L, et al. The effect of chloramphenicol and sulphaphenazole on the biotransformation of cyclophosphamide in man. Br J Clin Pharmacol. 1975;2:281.
184. Powell DA, Nahata MC, Durrell DC, et al. Interactions among chloramphenicol, phenytoin and phenobarbital in a pediatric patient. J Pediatr. 1981;98:1001.
185. Prober CG. Effect of rifampin on chloramphenicol levels. N Engl J Med. 1985;312:788–9.
186. JiJi RM, Gangarosa EJ, de la Macorra F. Chloramphenicol and its sulfamoyl analogue. Report of reversible erythropoietic toxicity in healthy volunteers. Arch Intern Med. 1963;11:70.
187. Sande MA, Overton JW. In vivo antagonism between gentamicin and chloramphenicol in neutropenic mice. J Infect Dis. 1973;128:247.
188. del Rio M, Chrane D, Shelton S, et al. Ceftriaxone versus ampicillin and chloramphenicol for treatment of bacterial meningitis in children. Lancet. 1983;1:1241–4.
189. Odio CM, Faingezicht I, Salas JL, et al. Cefotaxime versus conventional therapy for the treatment of bacterial meningitis of infants and children. Pediatr Infect Dis. 1986;5:402.
190. McCracken GH, Nelson JD, Kaplan SL, et al. Consensus report: Antimicrobial therapy for bacterial meningitis in infants and children. Pediatr Infect Dis J. 1987;6:501–5.

24. RIFAMYCINS

BARRY M. FARR
GERALD L. MANDELL

Rifampin is a semisynthetic derivative of rifamycin B, a macrocyclic antibiotic compound produced by the mold *Streptomyces mediterranei*. First isolated from fermentation culture of a soil isolate in 1957, rifamycins were named for a then current French movie, *Le Riffi*.[1] Rifampin, which is the 3-4-methyl-piperazinyl-iminomethyl derivative of rifamycin SV, is more soluble and active in vitro than is its parent compound[2] (Fig. 1). Rifampin is a zwitterion (inner salt) that is soluble in acidic aqueous solution, is even more soluble in organic solvents, and displays remarkable diffusion through lipids.[3]

MECHANISM OF ACTION

The rifamycins exert a bactericidal effect by inhibition of DNA-dependent RNA polymerase at the β-subunit, which prevents chain initiation but not elongation.[4] Mammalian mitochondrial RNA synthesis is not impaired at clinically achievable concentrations.

PHARMACOLOGY

Rifampin is available in the United States as a capsule of orange-red powder that is almost completely absorbed from the gastrointestinal tract to yield peak plasma concentrations of approximately 7–10 μg/ml (range, 4–32) within 1–4 hours after ingestion of 600 mg in adults or 10 mg/kg of body weight in children. Higher doses such as 1200 mg in adults result in a similar, more-than-proportional increase in the peak (≥30 μg/ml) serum concentration because such doses exceed the biliary Tm for excretion of rifampin.[5] The area under the curve (AUC) shows a similar, more-than-proportional increase after saturation of the biliary Tm. For this reason, a single daily dose of 1200 mg results in higher AUC values for rifampin than does divided doses totaling 1200 mg.

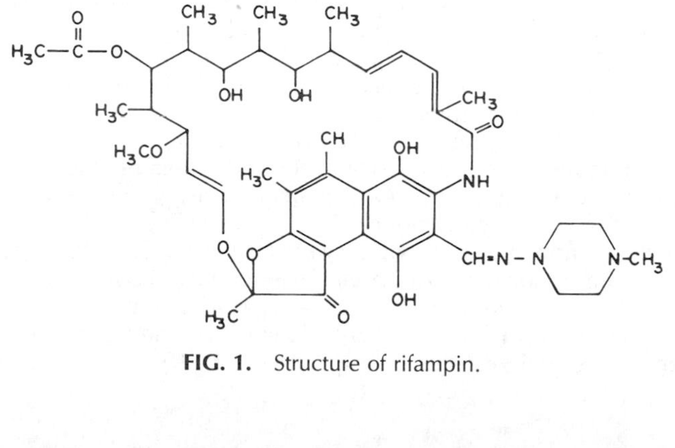

FIG. 1. Structure of rifampin.

The recommended dosage is usually 10 to 20 mg/kg (600 mg maximum) in a single daily administration. A 1% weight/volume oral suspension containing 10 mg/ml may be prepared by mixing the contents of four 300 mg capsules with 120 ml of any of several commercially available syrups according to the directions in the package insert or the *Physician's Desk Reference*.[6] Dosage adjustment is unnecessary in renal failure, but rifampin should be avoided or used with caution (perhaps at a lower dosage) in patients with hepatic dysfunction. Food with a high fat concentration interferes with absorption by lowering and delaying peak blood levels.[7] Para-aminosalicylic acid also interferes with absorption.

The drug is 80 percent protein bound in serum and distributes into a volume calculated to be 160 percent of body weight. Plasma clearance is through hepatic uptake, deacetylation to an active metabolite, and biliary excretion. Deacetylation diminishes reabsorption and increases fecal excretion, but there is significant enterohepatic circulation. The half-life is initially 2–5 hours, but it decreases by 40 percent during the first 2 weeks of therapy due to enhanced biliary excretion. Slow acetylators of isoniazid have an accelerated clearance of rifampin. From 6 to 30 percent of a dose is excreted in the urine. Probenecid does not consistently affect rifampin serum levels. Renal excretion is reduced in the elderly, but serum levels remain similar to those in young adults because of hepatic clearance.[8] Pharmacokinetics in pediatric patients are similar to those in adults.[9] An intravenous preparation commercially available in several countries but not yet licensed in the United States yields higher peak concentrations of about 27 μg/ml but otherwise similar pharmocokinetics.[10] An investigational parenteral formulation is available from Merrell Dow Laboratories in the United States.

Rifampin penetrates well into almost all body tissues. It achieves concentrations in lung, liver, bile, cholecystic wall, and urine that exceed peak blood levels.[11] Peak concentrations average 300–350 μg/ml in urine.[5] The concentration in tears is similar to that in serum, and salivary concentrations are about 20 percent of those in serum. It achieves therapeutic levels in pleural exudate, sputum,[5] ascites, cavity fluid, milk, urinary bladder wall, skin blister fluid,[12] and soft tissues. It penetrates bone, with higher levels being reached in the presence of osteomyelitis.[11] Levels in cerebrospinal fluid (CSF) of 0–0.5 μg/ml have been achieved in healthy people, and higher levels (up to 1.3 μg/ml) have been observed during meningitis after a standard oral dosage of 600 mg/day. Rifampin has also been shown to penetrate and sterilize abscess fluid more readily than do most other antibiotics with similar antibacterial activity.[13,14] This may relate both to the drug's high lipid solubility and to its relatively unusual ability to enter living phagocytes and kill intracellular bacteria.[3,12,15]

TABLE 1. Susceptibility of Various Bacteria to Rifampin

Species (n)	MICs (μg/ml) Range (Mode)	MIC_{50}	MIC_{90}
Gram-positive bacteria			
Staphylococcus aureus (26)	0.008–0.015 (0.015)	0.015	0.015
Staphylococcus epidermidis (25)	0.004–0.015 (0.015)	0.015	0.015
Group A streptococci (25)	0.03–0.12 (0.12)	0.12	0.12
Group B streptococci (25)	0.25–1 (1)	1.0	1.0
Streptococcus pneumoniae (28)	0.06–32 (0.06)	0.12	4.0
Viridans group Streptococci (34)	0.03–8 (0.06)	0.06	0.12
Enterococcus faecalis (16)	1.0–8 (2)	2.0	8.0
Haemophilus influenzae (26)	0.5–64 (1)	1.0	1.0
Neisseria gonorrhoeae (29)	0.06–2 (0.25)	0.25	0.5
Neisseria meningitidis (26)	0.015–1 (0.03)	0.03	0.5
Listeria monocytogenes (40)	≤0.12–0.25 (≤0.12)	≤0.12	0.25
Mycobacterium fortuitum (18)	16.0–>64 (>64)	>64	>64
Mycobacterium chelonae (15)	>64 (>64)	>64	>64
Gram-negative bacteria			
Escherichia coli (15)	8–16 (8)	8	16
Klebsiella pneumoniae (14)	16–32 (32)	32	32
Enterobacter agglomerans (14)	8–64 (32)	32	64
Enterobacter cloacae (13)	16–64 (32)	64	64
Enterobacter aerogenes (15)	16–64 (32)	32	64
Citrobacter freundii (4)	32 (32)	32	32
Citrobacter diversus (4)	32 (32)	32	32
Proteus mirabilis (15)	4–8 (4)	4	8
Proteus vulgaris (17)	8–32 (32)	16	32
Morganella morganii (15)	8–32 (32)	16	32
Providencia rettgeri (15)	8–64 (8, 16)	16	32
Providencia stuartii (15)	4–16 (8)	8	16
Serratia marcescens (15)	32–64 (64)	64	64
Acinetobacter species (15)	4–16 (8)	8	8
Pseudomonas aeruginosa (17)	32–>64 (32)	32	64
Pseudomonas species (12)	4–>64 (8)	8	32

Abbreviation: MIC: minimal inhibitory concentration.
(From Thornsberry et al.,[17] with permission.)

ANTIMICROBIAL ACTIVITY

Rifampin exhibits bactericidal activity against a wide range of organisms (Table 1).[16,17] It is extremely active against staphylococci (both coagulase-positive and coagulase-negative strains) and is also effective against other gram-positive cocci, although somewhat less so than penicillin. *Neisseria meningitidis, Neisseria gonorrhoeae*, and *Haemophilus influenzae* are the most sensitive gram-negative species. Rifampin has less activity than tetracycline, chloramphenicol, or aminoglycosides do against most gram-negative aerobic bacilli.

Rifampin is the most active agent known against the various species and strains of *Legionella*, being clearly more active than erythromycin, the drug of choice for legionellosis.[17] It is as active as vancomycin in vitro against *Clostridium difficile*, the organism associated with pseudomembranous colitis.

Mycobacterium tuberculosis has remained quite sensitive to rifampin, with most epidemiologic surveys finding less than 1 percent initial resistance to the drug.[18,19] *Mycobacterium ulcerans* is equally sensitive. A spiropiperidyl rifamycin called rifabutin (ansamycin) has remarkable in vitro activity against many mycobacteria including the *Mycobacterium avium-intracellulare* complex and *Mycobacterium fortuitum*.[20]

The rifamycins possess antiviral and possible antitumor activity, which have not proved clinically useful at usual therapeutic levels. Rifampin is among the most active agents against *Chlamydia*, including *Chlamydia trachomatis* (lymphogranuloma venereum [LGV] and non-LGV strains) and *Chlamydia psittaci*.[21] *Ureaplasma urealyticum* and *Treponema pallidum* are usually resistant. Rifampin has shown synergy with amphotericin B in vitro and in animal models of infection with fungal species such as *Histoplasma capsulatum* and *Aspergillus* species.[22]

Bacteria rapidly develop resistance to rifampin in vitro or in vivo due to mutations altering the β-subunit of the DNA-dependent RNA polymerase. These mutations may occur at many different sites in the RNA polymerase and lead to various degrees of resistance to rifampin.[23] Approximately 1 out of every 10^{10} tubercule bacilli is a resistant mutant. A recent national survey found the incidence of rifampin resistance among previously untreated tuberculous patients to be 0.6 percent as compared with 3.3 percent of patients previously treated for tuberculosis. The rates of isoniazid resistance in this same survey were much higher, 5.3 and 19.3 percent for untreated and previously treated patients, respectively.[19]

The mutation rate to rifampin resistance among other bacteria is higher than that for *M. tuberculosis* (e.g., *Staphylococcus aureus*, 10^{-7}; *Streptococcus* spp., 10^{-7}; *H. influenzae* type B, 10^{-7}; meningococcus, 10^{-7}; and *Escherichia coli*, 10^{-8}).[16,24] Except for short-term meningitis prophylaxis, rifampin should not be used alone because of this rapid development of resistance during monotherapy.

ADVERSE EFFECTS

Short-term meningitis prophylaxis with rifampin has been associated with mild, reversible symptoms in 20–25 percent of recipients as compared with about 10 percent of placebo recipients.[25,26] The symptoms reported most frequently have been dizziness, drowsiness, abdominal pain, diarrhea, nausea, vomiting, headache, visual change, pruritus, and rash. Each of these symptoms usually occurs in less than 5–10 percent of recipients.[26] An orange-red discoloration of urine and permanent staining of soft contact lenses may also occur with such brief regimens.

Chronic daily therapy is associated with a mild, usually self-limited maculopapular rash in up to 5 percent of patients, gastrointestinal complaints in 1–2 percent of patients, asymptomatic elevation of serum enzyme levels in up to 14 percent of adult patients, and overt hepatitis in fewer than 1 percent of patients.[16] More severe rashes such as exfoliative dermatitis and toxic epidermal necrolysis have been rarely reported as being associated with rifampin.[27,28] Of 430 children treated with rifampin and isoniazid for tuberculosis, 14 (3.3 percent) were reported to have hepatotoxic reactions in a recent national survey.[29] In a study of rifampin (15 mg/kg/day) and higher-dose isoniazid (15–20 mg/kg/day) therapy for children with severe tuberculosis, 36 of 44 developed an elevation of hepatic enzyme levels during therapy, and 1 child died of hepatitis.[30] Acute renal failure has been reported during daily therapy and has occasionally required dialysis.[31] The renal failure has been related to a variety of different mechanisms including interstitial nephritis, glomerulonephritis, and massive hemolysis.[32,33] Light-chain proteinuria has been reported to occur in a majority of patients receiving rifampin without apparent ill effect, but in the setting of dehydration these proteins may contribute to development of a cast nephropathy and acute renal failure on this basis.[34,35]

Intermittent administration (less than twice per week) and high individual dosages (greater than or equal to 1200 mg) have been associated with an increased incidence of side effects. A flulike syndrome with fever, chills, and myalgias may develop in up to 20 percent of patients after several months of intermittent therapy and correlates with the presence of anti-rifampin antibodies.[36] These patients may develop eosinophilia, interstitial nephritis, acute tubular necrosis, thrombocytopenia, hemolytic anemia, and even shock.[37] Acute massive hemolysis is rarely associated with such flulike reactions after intermittent therapy, in which case nausea, vomiting, flank pain, and brown turbid urine may be observed; most patients with massive hemolysis develop acute renal failure.[38]

Various effects of rifampin on the central nervous system have been reported, including rare cases of organic brain syndrome. Pseudomembranous colitis has been observed in animal models after rifampin administration to animals colonized with a rifampin-resistant strain of *C. difficile*. One patient has also been reported with pseudomembranous colitis that developed with a rifampin-resistant *C. difficile* during rifampin therapy. This appears to be a very rare side effect with only a few reports of such an association despite widespread chronic use of rifampin in antituberculous chemotherapy.[39] Pancreatitis has been reported in rare cases. Patients have survived overdoses of up to 12 g, turning "lobster red" for several days; facial or periorbital edema, pruritus of the head, and vomiting each occur in a majority of cases of the "red man syndrome" after an overdose.[40]

Rifampin causes an increase in serum bile acid levels and may cause slight elevations of serum bilirubin concentrations that return to normal during the first week of therapy in the absence of hepatitis. Rifampin causes a reduction in 25-hydroxycholecalciferol levels without changing the levels of 1,25-dihydroxycholecalciferol or parathyroid hormone, and osteomalacia has been mentioned as a possible side effect with long-term treatment. It causes increased deiodination and biliary clearance of thyroxine and lowers the serum concentration of thryoxine. The serum concentration of triiodothyronine remains normal.

Immunosuppression has been an alleged side effect of rifampin therapy. Contradictory studies have found diminished or normal antibody responses to various antigens such as sheep red blood cells, pneumococcal vaccine, and tetanus toxoid. Some workers have suggested blunted cell-mediated immunity with a diminished response to phytohemagglutinin in vitro, whereas others have shown no change in response to phytohemagglutinin, concanavalin A, pokeweed mitogen, or purified protein derivative (PPD). Skin tests with PPD have not been consistently altered by rifampin therapy, and no ill effect from this possible immunosuppression in the form of opportunistic infection or an inability to heal tuberculosis has been reported.[41]

Rifampin readily crosses the placenta and has caused teratogenic effects in rodents treated with high doses; such effects have not been observed in humans, except in patients with severe tuberculosis, but rifampin should only be used for severe tuberculous infections during pregnancy.[42]

DRUG INTERACTIONS

Rifampin competitively inhibits the hepatic uptake of several compounds such as cholecystografin and sulfobromophthalein. The addition of isoniazid to rifampin increases the risk of hepatitis slightly, but the combination is usually safe in the absence of prior liver disease.[43] Rifampin is one of the most potent inducing agents for hepatic microsomal enzymes[44] and leads to a decreased half-life for a number of compounds including prednisone, norethisterone, digitoxin, quinidine, ketoconazole, and the sulfonylureas (Table 2).[45–49] These effects have been reported to cause decreased efficacy of oral contraceptive agents, relapse of arrhythmias during quinidine therapy, decompensation of heart failure during digoxin or digitoxin therapy, and exacerbation of diabetes during oral hypoglycemic therapy. Rifampin also reduces the efficacy of warfarin by causing a reduction in prothrombin time in patients anticoagulated with this drug. Patients receiving glucocorticoid therapy for Addison's disease or asthma have relapsed, and transplant patients receiving cyclosporine therapy have developed acute rejection when given rifampin. Hypothyroid patients receiving replacement L-thyroxine may require an increased dosage.[48]

THERAPEUTIC USES

Mycobacterial Infections

The unique pharmacology and bactericidal activity of rifampin have revolutionized chemotherapy for pulmonary tuberculosis, with rifampin-containing treatment courses of 6–9 months yielding cure rates equal to those achieved with 18 months of regimens without rifampin.[50] The regimen of choice for uncomplicated pulmonary or extrapulmonary tuberculosis is now 6 months of daily rifampin (15 mg/kg/day; maximum, 600 mg) and isoniazid (10 mg/kg/day; maximum, 300 mg), with daily pyrazinamide being added for the first 2 months. Additional regimens include isoniazid and rifampin daily for 9 months or twice-weekly, supervised adminstration of isoniazid and rifampin for 9 months in noncompliant patients.[51] It should be emphasized that rifampin monotherapy is contraindicated in mycobacterial

TABLE 2. Medications for Which the Half-Life Is Reduced through Enhancement of Hepatic Metabolism by Rifampin

Barbituates	Ketoconazole
Chloramphenicol	Metaprolol
Cimetidine	Methadone
Clofibrate	Phenytoin
Contraceptives, oral	Propranolol
Cyclosporine	Sulfonylureas
Dapsone	Theophylline
Digitoxin	Thyroxine
Digoxin	Verapamil
Estrogens	Warfarin

disease, as illustrated by one study in which 5 out of 11 tuberculous patients developed rifampin-resistant isolates within 3 months when receiving rifampin alone.[52] The American Thoracic Society has recommended the use of rifampin alone or in conjunction with isoniazid or ethambutol as prophylactic therapy for infected contacts of persons with known isoniazid-resistant tuberculosis. Data regarding the efficacy of such prophylaxis are not available, however, and one failure of rifampin monoprophylaxis in such an instance has been reported in an alcoholic with questionable compliançe.[53]

Rifampin-containing regimens have proved useful in therapy for *M. avium-intracellulare*,[54,55] *Mycobacterium kansasii*,[56] *Mycobacterium xenopi*,[57] *Mycobacterium marinum*,[58] and Calmette-Guérin bacillus (BCG) infections.[59,60]

Rifampin kills *Mycobacterium leprae* faster than do the sulfones. If used in patients with lepromatous leprosy, however, it should be combined with dapsone to prevent the development of resistance. Monthly rifampin doses may be added to daily dapsone therapy without producing the flulike side effects frequently seen with intermittent rifampin administration.[61,62]

Meningitis Prophylaxis

Rifampin has been approved by the Food and Drug Administration (FDA) as prophylaxis for close contacts of patients with meningococcal meningitis at a daily dose of 10 mg/kg (600 mg maximum) for 4 days. The Centers for Disease Control (CDC) recommends 600 mg every 12 hours for 2 days for adults and 10 mg/kg every 12 hours for 2 days for children. Rifampin has been shown to eradicate meningococci from the nasopharynx in approximately 90 percent of carriers.[63–66] Sulfadiazine was formerly recommended for meningococcal prophylaxis, but up to 70 percent of recent meningococcal isolates are resistant to sulfa. Minocycline is also an effective prophylactic agent, but it is associated with a higher incidence of side effects, especially vestibular symptoms.[67] Recent studies have suggested the efficacy of oral ciprofloxacin (4–10 doses) and also of a single intramuscular injection of ceftriaxone (250 mg for adults, 125 mg for children less than 15 years old).[68,69]

Epidemiologic studies of *H. influenzae* type B meningitis have shown a high incidence of secondary disease among preschool contacts.[70] Secondary disease attack rates for this group have been approximately one percent, which yields a relative risk approximately 600 times that of the general population.[71] Rifampin at a single daily dose of 20 mg/kg (up to a maximum dose of 600 mg) for 4 days has been shown to eradicate *H. influenzae* from the nasopharynx in over 90 percent of carriers and to significantly reduce the risk of secondary infection.[25] It has been recommended that families with young children exposed to another member of the household with invasive *H. influenzae* type B disease (e.g., meningitis, epiglottitis, or pneumonia) take rifampin prophylaxis.[71–73] The age below which child household contacts and their families should receive prophylaxis has been debated. All agree that prophylaxis should be given when there are children younger than two years, and some recommend prophylaxis when there are children under 4 years (see Chapter 200).[71,73] Pregnant family members should not take rifampin prophylaxis. Day care center staff (excluding pregnant women) and day care classmates of a child with such disease have also been advised to take rifampin prophylaxis if any of the exposed classmates are younger than 2 years old. Some authorities recommend prophylaxis after a single case in a day care center, while others have advocated instituting prophylaxis only if a second case occurs within 60 days.[73,74] Failure to provide simultaneous rifampin prophylaxis to all day care center contacts including those who have received *Haemophilus* b polysaccharide vaccine has been associated with persistent colonization of children in the center and subsequent cases of disease.[75] The prophylaxis should be given as rapidly as possible after identification of the index case to provide maximal benefit since a majority of secondary cases appear to occur in the week after the onset of the index case. Index cases with invasive *H. influenzae* disease should also be given the same rifampin regimen before hospital discharge because of the 1 percent rate of recurrent systemic disease in index cases after therapy and also the risk of exposing other children to the organism.[76] Attempts to eradicate nasopharyngeal carriage with other drugs active against *H. influenzae*, including ampicillin and trimethoprim-sulfamethoxazole, have been less successful; data regarding the efficacy of quinolones and third-generation cephalosporins for this indication are not yet available.

Endocarditis

The use of rifampin in the treatment of staphylococcal endocarditis remains an unsettled and controversial issue.[77] Rifampin was shown to be superior to therapy with vancomycin, gentamicin, or β-lactams in an experimental model of *S. epidermidis* endocarditis in rabbits.[78] In another rabbit model of *S. epidermidis* endocarditis, rifampin plus teicoplanin proved more effective therapy than either agent alone.[79] A retrospective series of 75 cases of prosthetic valve endocarditis due to *S. epidermidis*, the most common cause of prosthetic valve endocarditis, suggested a trend toward higher survival ($p = .10$) in patients receiving rifampin (900–1200 mg/day) or an aminoglycoside plus vancomycin as opposed to vancomycin alone.[80] The only randomized trial of rifampin therapy in endocarditis compared patients with prosthetic valve endocarditis due to methicillin-resistant *S. epidermidis* who were treated with vancomycin (30 mg/kg/day) and rifampin (300 mg q8h) or with vancomycin and rifampin (same doses) plus gentamicin (3 mg/kg/day). The cure rate was 77 percent with the two-drug regimen and 85 percent with the three-drug regimen. Rifampin resistance developed in six patients receiving the two-drug regimen as compared with none receiving the three-drug regimen.[81] A separate study identified three patients in whom rifampin resistance developed during therapy for prosthetic valve *S. epidermidis* endocarditis with rifampin plus vancomycin.[82]

Several patients with endocarditis due to *S. aureus* have been reported to respond only after the addition of rifampin to nafcillin or vancomycin.[16,83,84] Rifampin therapy for experimental endocarditis due to *S. aureus* in rabbits has been examined by Sande et al.[13,85] In one study, the combination of rifampin with penicillin was antagonistic in vitro against a strain of *S. aureus*, and there was a trend toward slower sterilization of vegetations with the rifampin combination than with penicillin alone. Sterilization of renal abscesses, however, occurred faster in the group receiving the rifampin combination than in the group receiving penicillin alone despite in vitro antagonism. It was suggested that this was due to rifampin's unique ability to penetrate and sterilize abscess fluid and living polymorphonuclear neutrophil (PMN) leukocytes.

In a subsequent study using the same animal model and a methicillin-sensitive strain of *S. aureus* it was found that rifampin plus cloxacillin was additive or synergistic in four of five different regimens studied; the only regimen showing antagonism combined a high dose of cloxacillin (100 mg/kg) with a low dose of rifampin (2 mg/kg).[85] Sande and associates have concluded that rational treatment of staphylococcal endocarditis might involve initial therapy with a β-lactam or vancomycin alone or in combination with an aminoglycoside, which should result in rapid elimination of organisms from vegetations. He suggests the addition of rifampin for cases in which myocardial or metastastic abscesses are detected, while emphasizing the necessity of surgical drainage of abscesses.[86] Adding rifampin after several days of effective therapy with nafcillin or vancomycin plus gentamicin might be less likely to result in the development of rifampin resistance because the titer of organisms exposed to rifampin should then be lower.

The problem of methicillin-resistant *S. aureus* (MRSA) endocarditis has been studied in a rabbit model by Bayer et al., who found that a combination of rifampin (20 mg/kg/day) plus vancomycin (30 mg/kg/day) was significantly more effective than was either drug alone in eliminating organisms from the valve and curing the animal. Rifampin resistance developed in 2 of 4 animals that were sacrificed after treatment with rifampin alone but was not found in any of the 21 animals given the combination.[87] One retrospective study of treatment of MRSA endocarditis in drug addicts did not demonstrate a higher cure rate for rifampin-containing regimens than for vancomycin alone, but such studies are likely to be biased with only the more severely ill patients receiving rifampin. Randomized trials are needed to accurately assess the efficacy of rifampin for endocarditis due to MRSA.

The problem of rifampin resistance developing during therapy for endocarditis that has been noted with methicillin-resistant *S. epidermidis* has also been observed with MRSA during treatment with rifampin and vancomycin.[88,89] Acar and colleagues reported that two of three patients with *S. aureus* endocarditis who had failed therapy with another regimen developed rifampin resistance when rifampin was added to either vancomycin or pristinamycin.[84] It has been suggested by the results of one study that, although rifampin resistance may develop in the presence of a β-lactam such as nafcillin in vitro, the rate of developing such resistance is lower with this combination than with rifampin alone; by contrast, this study found that vancomycin did not suppress the emergence of rifampin resistance when incubated with rifampin in vitro.[90] The results of other studies, however, have suggested that incubation of vancomycin with rifampin in vitro can suppress the emergence of rifampin resistance.[91,92]

The efficacy of rifampin in *S. aureus* endocarditis will have to be proved by randomized controlled trials. In the meantime, it would appear reasonable to consider using rifampin in cases with renal, myocardial, splenic, or cerebral abscess formation or because of failure of conventional therapy. If rifampin were to be added, an optimal regimen would probably include at least two other drugs such as gentamicin and either nafcillin or vancomycin to minimize the probability of developing rifampin resistance during therapy.

The value of serum bactericidal titers and of in vitro synergy studies of antibiotic combinations including rifampin are of unclear value. Serum bactericidal titers have not been clearly demonstrated to predict the clinical outcome in patients with endocarditis,[93] and in vitro studies of rifampin and vancomycin or nafcillin with large batteries of staphylococcal isolates have produced inconsistent results in different laboratories, with most studies finding indifference for a majority of isolates.[94–101] Synergy studies performed with the same strain of *S. aureus* and the same concentrations of antibiotics have yielded directly contradictory results using checkerboard and time-kill methods.[94,97,102] Faster sterilization of renal abscesses has been shown in one animal model when a combination of rifampin and penicillin was administered despite in vitro evidence of antagonism.[13]

One theme that has emerged from several synergy studies is that lower ratios of the concentration of rifampin to the concentration of oxacillin appear to be less bactericidal in vitro. Since highest peak concentrations and AUC values are achieved by administering a single large daily dose of rifampin (e.g., ≥600 mg for an adult),[5] this approach may be more effective than smaller divided doses would be.

Rifampin (300 mg po bid) has also been recommended in combination with vancomycin and gentamicin for the treatment of endocarditis due to *Corynebacterium* spp.[103] One case of endocarditis due to psittacosis was refractory to several other antibiotics but subsequently responsive to rifampin.[104]

Tolerant Staphylococci

Staphylococci with an antibiotic minimal bactericidal concentration (MBC) much greater than the minimal inhibitory concentration (MIC) (MBC equal to or greater than 32 × MIC) are said to be tolerant to the antibiotic in question. Tolerance to nafcillin and/or vancomycin has been described in several cases of persistent staphylococcal infection. The addition of rifampin has led to improved serum bactericidal levels and the successful treatment of such infections in several cases.[105,106] No randomized trials of such therapy for this indication are available.

Staphylococcal Carriage and Furunculosis

Rifampin has been shown to reduce the rate of staphylococcal nasal colonization markedly,[107–109] whereas systemic penicillinase-resistant penicillins or intranasal gentamicin cream has not eradicated nasal carriage.[110] Mandell and Sande (unpublished data) have used cloxacillin plus rifampin to eradicate nasal carriage and interrupt the course of recurrent furunculosis. Methicillin-resistant staphylococcal nasal carriage in nosocomial epidemics has been successfully eradicated by using a combination of rifampin plus either vancomycin or trimethoprim-sulfamethoxazole.[110–113]

Methicillin-Resistant Staphylococcal Infection

Methicillin-resistant infections should be treated with vancomycin, to which they are uniformly sensitive. There are no data to support the routine addition of rifampin to vancomycin, but if there is inadequate response to vancomycin alone, then the addition of gentamicin, rifampin, or both should be considered. The development of rifampin resistance has been reported during therapy for MRSA infections with vancomycin plus rifampin,[84,89] and the addition of gentamicin to the regimen may help prevent the development of rifampin resistance.[81]

Streptococcal Carriage

Chronic pharyngeal carriage of *Streptococcus pyogenes* in children has sometimes resulted in multiple courses of antibiotic therapy for apparent streptococcal pharyngitis with each new cold because of continuing positive cultures after completion of each course of therapy, and even in tonsillectomy. Eradication of carriage is not usually medically indicated for chronic carriers, but when carriage eradication is desired, rifampin, 10 mg po bid for 4 days, plus benzathine penicillin has been shown to eradicate *S. pyogenes* in 93 percent of cases.[114] Such therapy for the eradication of *S. pyogenes* has been tried in patients with psoriasis, with apparent benefit to their skin disease.[115]

Group B streptococci are the leading cause of sepsis and meningitis in neonates, and efforts to eradicate colonization are now being studied. A recent study of treatment of experimentally exposed infant rats showed that rifampin plus penicillin eradicated group B streptococci for 80 percent of the animals, a significantly higher rate than for either drug alone.[116] Clinical data are not available.

Osteomyelitis and Septic Arthritis

Experimental animal data suggest that rifampin combined with another antistaphylococcal drug such as nafcillin or vancomycin provides better results than does single drug therapy for chronic staphylococcal osteomyelitis, even when the drug combination is antagonistic in vitro.[117] Controlled trials are necessary to confirm these data in human infection, however. The only randomized trial evaluating a rifampin-containing regimen in chronic staphylococcal osteomyelitis was halted after the enrollment of 18 patients: there was a trend toward a higher rate of favorable response in the group receiving rifampin and nafcillin (8 of 10) as compared with the group receiving nafcillin alone (4 of 8). The difference was not statistically significant ($p = .2$), but the statistical power was only 40 percent for detecting significance in the 30 percent higher rate of response that was observed because of the small sample size.[118]

Rifampin is not part of the usual regimen for staphylococcal arthritis, but it has been added with success in occasional patients initially refractory to nafcillin alone[119]; however, rifampin resistance has developed in one patient due to MRSA treated with vancomycin and rifampin.[90]

Legionella

Both *L. pneumophila* and *L. micdadei* are sensitive to rifampin. It has been suggested that rifampin be added to erythromycin for patients with legionnaires' disease when the illness does not respond to erythromycin alone, but data from randomized trials are lacking.

Brucellosis

Rifampin has been shown to be superior to tetracycline in therapy for experimental brucellosis in rodents, and there have been several case reports of successful therapy for human infections. In one uncontrolled study, relapses occurred after rifampin monotherapy, thus suggesting the need for combination therapy if rifampin is used.[120] A randomized trial comparing tetracycline (or doxycycline) regimens containing either rifampin or streptomycin found that all patients responded to both regimens but a significantly higher proportion of the rifampin recipients relapsed (39 percent) as compared with streptomycin recipients (7 percent).[121] Rifampin resistance has also developed during such therapy and has been documented during clinical relapse. Several studies of rifampin and doxycycline therapy for patients with neurobrucellosis have suggested a high rate of efficacy, with relapse rates between 0 and 10 percent.[122]

Infection Occurring in Patients with Chronic Granulomatous Disease of Childhood

Rifampin has been shown to kill living intracellular staphylococci in neutrophils from healthy people and from patients with chronic granulomatous disease.[123] One patient with an axillary staphylococcal abscess responded dramatically to the addition of rifampin after months of unsuccessful therapy with vancomycin, nafcillin, and gentamicin.[124]

Infected Cerebrospinal Fluid Shunts and Vascular Grafts

Cerebrospinal fluid shunt infections have responded to the addition of rifampin in several cases after an initial failure with multiple-drug therapy excluding rifampin.[125–127] Data from controlled trials are lacking.

Therapy with rifampin plus clinadamycin for aortic Dacron grafts experimentally infected with *S. aureus* was found to cure the infection in seven of seven dogs as compared with five of seven dogs cured with cefazolin therapy.[128] Data from clinical trials are not available.

Cutaneous Leishmaniasis

When a patient with *Leishmania mexicana amazonensis* refractory to previous antileishmanial therapy was treated with rifampin and isoniazid for intercurrent mycobacterial infection, the cutaneous leishmaniasis improved.[129] Several uncontrolled series have suggested that rifampin may be efficacious for this disease,[130] but controlled trials are still needed.[131]

Urinary Tract Infections

A number of studies have been conducted that show the efficacy of rifampin in the treatment of urinary tract infections. Rifampin resistance has arisen with monotherapy, but combination therapy with trimethoprim has resulted in cure rates that are comparable to those of trimethoprim-sulfamethoxazole.[132] Rifampin combined with trimethoprim has been used with success in eradicating persistent, relapsing infections of the kidney or prostate.[132] Rifampin combinations are not the drug of choice for infections of the urinary tract but may be considered when conventional therapy fails.

Urethritis

Although not a first-line drug for gonococcal urethritis, rifampin (900 mg) plus erythromycin (1 g) as a single oral dose has been shown to cure 95 percent of patients with gonorrhea, with equivalent efficacy against penicillinase-producing *Neisseria gonorrhoeae* (PPNG) strains.[133,134] Despite excellent activity against chlamydia in vitro, a single dose of rifampin in combination with erythromycin showed poor efficacy in the treatment of chlamydial urethritis.[134]

Chancroid

Rifampin has good activity against *Haemophilus ducreyi*, the causative agent of chancroid, and has been shown effective in treatment,[135] but intramuscular ceftriaxone and oral erythromycin are the treatments of choice.[136]

Infections Due to Multiply Resistant Pseudomonas aeruginosa

Most isolates of *Pseudomonas aeruginosa* are relatively resistant to rifampin, with MICs ranging from 32 to 64 μg/ml. Occasional isolates of *P. aeruginosa*, however, are also resistant to available β-lactams, aminoglycosides, or both. In vitro data have suggested synergy of ticarcillin, tobramycin, and rifampin against such resistant strains,[137] and case reports of patients refractory to conventional therapy who responded dramatically after the addition of rifampin to their regimen suggest that rifampin may be of value in combination therapy for such infections.[138] Rifampin combined with imipenem has also shown in vitro syngery against *P. aeruginosa* and *Enterobacter* spp. and an additive effect against *Serratia marcescens*; in vitro synergy was also shown for the combination of rifampin, imipenem, and ciprofloxacin against each of these three species.[139] Data from clinical trials are needed on the use of rifampin in such combination therapy.

Anaerobic Infections

Data from experimental animal models suggest that rifampin is as effective as metronidazole in the prevention of abscess formation and eradication of *Bacteriodes fragilis* after intraperitoneal injection of the organism. Clinical data are not available.[140,141]

Rifampin is highly active against *C. difficile* and has been used in combination with vancomycin to successfully interrupt relapsing pseudomembranous colitis in one series.[142]

Meningitis

Rifampin has been used successfully in the therapy for several cases of meningitis refractory to other available antibiotics. *Flavobacterium meningosepticum* is a rare cause of meningitis and occurs primarily in neonates but sometimes in adults after surgery as well. Most strains are susceptible to trimethoprim-sulfamethoxazole, imipenem, vancomycin, and rifampin. Rifampin has been used successfully as part of combination therapy with one or more of these other agents in curing such patients.[131,143] Randomized trials of such therapy are not available.

Rifampin was also added to the regimen of a patient with *H. influenzae* meningitis who had not responded clinically to therapy with chloramphenicol or subsequently with ampicillin and trimethoprim-sulfamethoxazole. The patient responded dramatically after the addition of rifampin.[144]

Rifapentine

Rifapentine is a new cyclopentyl rifamycin with antibacterial[145,146] and antimycobacterial[147,148] activity similar to that of rifampin but has a longer half-life of approximately 14 to 18 hours in animals (rat, mouse, and rabbit).[149] Sixty-five percent of an oral dose of 10 mg/kg is absorbed by such animals; its hepatic metabolism, biliary excretion, and wide distribution throughout body tissues are each similar to that of rifampin, as is its marked induction of hepatic microsomal oxidase activity.[150] This drug appears to be several times more active against *M. tuberculosis* and *M. leprae* than rifampin is, and its longer half-life may facilitate therapy by allowing less frequent administration. Data from clinical trials are not yet available.

Rifabutin

Rifabutin (ansamycin, LM 427) is a semisynthetic spiropiperidyl derivative of rifamycin S that shows good activity against most species of mycobacteria including all rifampin-sensitive *M. tuberculosis* strains and about one-third of rifampin-resistant strains; strains highly resistant to rifampin are usually resistant to rifabutin. Rifabutin shows better activity against the *M. avium-intracellulere* complex (MAC) of organisms than do other rifamycins; it inhibits 81 percent of MAC strains at a concentration of 1.0 mg/ml as compared with only 6 percent being inhibited by rifampin at this concentration.[151]

Rifabutin is absorbed from the gastrointestinal tract with a peak level of 0.49 mg/ml about 4 hours after ingestion of 300 mg in an adult. The serum half-life is 16 hours, and protein binding is 20 percent. The drug is taken up by all tissues and especially concentrated in the lungs, where levels may be 10-fold higher than in serum. Both hepatic and renal clearance occur as with other rifamycins, and although animal models suggest less of an effect on hepatic microsomal enzyme activity than rifampin has, several reports have suggested that rifabutin may increase corticosteroid metabolism in patients. The rates and types of side effects from rifabutin appear to be comparable to rifampin from initial reports, but better quantification of these reactions is needed from controlled clinical trials.[151]

Rifabutin has been used in open trials for the treatment of MAC disease in patients with acquired immunodeficiency syndrome (AIDS) without dramatic benefit,[152,153] but it may prove more useful in the treatment of pulmonary MAC disease in non-AIDS patients because of higher concentrations in lung tissue and a better immune system.

Randomized clinical trials of rifabutin therapy for patients with newly diagnosed pulmonary tuberculosis, MAC pulmonary disease, and drug-resistant tuberculosis are needed.

REFERENCES

1. Sensi P. History of the development of rifampin. Rev Infect Dis. 1983;5(Suppl):402.
2. Sensi P, Maggi N, Furesz S, et al. Chemical modifications and biological properties of rifamycins. Antimicrob Agents Chemother. 1966;6:699.
3. Mandell GL. Interaction of intraleukocytic bacteria and antibiotics. J Clin Invest. 1973;52:1673.
4. Wehrli W, Knusel F, Schmid K, et al. Interaction of rifamycin with bacterial RNA polymerase. Proc Natl Acad Sci USA. 1968;61:667.
5. Acocella G. Pharmacokinetics and metabolism of rifampin in humans. Rev Infect Dis. 1983;5(Suppl):428.
6. Krukenberg CC, Mischler PG, Massad EN, et al. Stability of 1% rifampin suspensions prepared in five syrups. Am J Hosp Pharm. 1986;43:2225–8.
7. Purohit SD, Gupta ML, Gupta PR. Dietary constituents and rifampicin absorption. Tubercle. 1987;68:151.
8. Advenier C, Gobert C, Houin G, et al. Pharmacokinetic studies of rifampicin in the elderly. Ther Drug Monit. 1983;5:61–5.
9. Koup JR, Williams-Warren J, Viswanathan CT, et al. Pharmacokinetics of rifampin in children II. Oral bioavailability. Ther Drug Monit. 1986;8:17–22.
10. Koup JR, Williams-Warren J, Weber A, et al. Pharmacokinetics of rifampin in children I. Multiple dose intravenous infusion. Ther Drug Monit. 1986;8:11–6.
11. Furesz S. Chemical and biological properties of rifampicin. Antibiot Chemother. 1970;16:316.
12. Solberg CO, Halstensen A, Digranes A, et al. Penetration of antibiotics into human leukocytes and dermal suction blisters. Rev Infect Dis. 5:S468, 1983.
13. Sande MA, Johnson ML. Antimicrobial therapy of experimental endocarditis caused by *Staphylococcus aureus*. J Infect Dis. 1975;131:367.
14. Mandell GL, Vest TK. Killing of intraleukocytic *Staphylococcus aureus* by refampin: In vitro and in vivo studies. J Infect Dis. 1972;125:486.
15. Mandell GL. The antimicrobial activity of rifampin: Emphasis on the relation to phagocytes. Rev Infect Dis. 1983;5(Suppl):463.
16. Farr B, Mandell GL. Rifampin. Med Clin North Am. 1982;66:157.
17. Thornsberry C, Hill BC, Swenson JM, et al. Rifampin: Spectrum of antibacterial activity. Rev Infect Dis. 1983;5(Suppl):412.
18. Collins CH, Yates MD. Low incidence of rifampin resistant tubercle bacilli. Thorax. 1982;37:526.
19. Cauthen GM, Kilburn JO, Kelly GD, et al. Resistance to anti-tuberculosis drugs in patients with and without prior treatment: Survey of 31 state and large city laboratories, 1982–1986. Am Rev Respir Dis. 1988;137:260.
20. Woodley CL, Kilburn JO. In vitro susceptibility of *Mycobacterium avium* complex and *Mycobacterium tuberculosis* strains to a spiro-piperidyl rifamycin. Am Rev Respir Dis. 1982;126:586.
21. Schachter J. Rifampin in chalmydial infections. Rev Infec Dis. 1983;5(Suppl):562.
22. Medoff G. Antifungal action of rifampin. Rev Infect Dis. 1983;5(Suppl):614.
23. Wehrli W. Rifampin: Mechanisms of action and resistance. Rev Infec Dis. 1983;5(Suppl):407.
24. Yogev R, Melick C, Glogowski W. In vitro development of rifampin resistance in clinical isolates of *Haemophilus* influenzae type B. Antimicrob Agents Chemother. 1982;21:387.
25. Band JD, Fraser DW, Ajello G, et al. Prevention of *Hemophilus* influenzae type b disease. JAMA. 1984;251:2381–6.
26. Band JD, Fraser DW. Adverse effects of two rifampicin dosage regimens for the prevention of meningococcal infection. Lancet. 1984;1:101.
27. Goldin HM, Schweitzer WJ, Bronson DM. Rifampin and exfoliative dermatitis. Ann Intern Med. 1987;107:789.
28. Okano M, Kitano Y, Igarashi T. Toxic epidermal necrolysis due to rifampicin. J Am Acad Dermatol. 1987;17:303.
29. O'Brien RJ, Long MW, Cross FS, et al. Hepatotoxicity from isoniazid and rifampin among children treated for tuberculosis. Pediatrics. 1983; 72:491–9.
30. Tsagaropoulou-Stinga H, Mataki-Emmanouilidou T, Karida-Kavalioti S, et al. Hepatotoxic reactions in children with severe tuberculosis treated with isoniazid-rifampin. Pediatr Infect Dis. 1985;4:270–3.
31. Qunibi WY, Godwin J, Eknoyan G. Toxic nephropathy during continuous rifampin therapy. South Med J. 1980;73:791.
32. Grosset J, Leventis S. Adverse effects of rifampin. Rev Infect Dis. 1983;5(Suppl):440.
33. Murray AN, Cassidy MJD, Templecamp C. Rapidly progressive glomerulonephritis associated with rifampicin therapy for pulmonary tuberculosis. Nephron. 1987;46:373.
34. Soffer O, Nassar VH, Campbell WG Jr. Light chain cast nephropathy and acute renal failure associated with rifampin therapy. Am J Med. 1987;82:1052.
35. Winter RJD, Banks RA, Collins CMP, et al. Rifampicin induced light chain proteinuria and renal failure. Thorax. 1984;39:952.
36. Poole G, Stradling P, Worlledge S. Potentially serious side-effects of high dose twice weekly rifampicin. Postgrad Med J. 1971;47:742–7.
37. Girling DJ, Hitze HL. Adverse reactions to rifampicin. Bull WHO. 1979;57:45.
38. Tahan SR, Diamond JR, Blank JM, et al. Aute hemolysis and renal failure with rifampicin-dependent antibodies after discontinuous administration. Transfusion. 1985;25:124–7.
39. Fekety R, O'Connor R, Silva J. Rifampin and pseudomembranous colitis. Rev Infect Dis. 1983;5(Suppl):524–7.
40. Bolan G, Laurie RE, Broome CV. Red man syndrome: Inadvertent administration of an excessive dose of rifampin to children in a day-care center. Pediatrics. 77:633, 1986.
41. Humber DP, Nsanzumuhire H, Aluoch HA, et al. Controlled double-blind study of the effect of rifampin on humoral and cellular immune responses in patients with pulmonary tuberculosis and in tuberculosis contacts. Am Rev Respir Dis. 1980;122:425.
42. Snider DE Jr, Layde PM, Johnson MW, et al. Treatment of tuberculosis during pregnancy. Am Rev Respir Dis. 1980;122:65.
43. Mandell GL, Sande MA. Drugs used in the chemotherapy of tuberculosis and leprosy. In: Goodman AG, Goodman LS, Gilman A, eds. The Pharmacological Basis of Therapeutics. 6th ed. New York: Macmillan; 1980:1203–6.
44. Ohnhaus EE, Kirchhof B, Peheim E. Effect of enzyme induction on plasma lipids using antipyrine, phenobarbital, and rifampicin. Clin Pharmacol Ther. 1979;25:591.

45. Twum-Barima Y, Carruthers SG. Quinidine-rifampin interaction. N Engl J Med. 1981;304:1466.
46. Brass C, Galgiani JN, Blaschke TF, et al. Disposition of ketoconazole, an oral antifungal, in humans. Antimicrob Agents Chemother. 1982;21:151.
47. Baciewicz AM, Self TH, Bekemeyer WB. Update on rifampin drug interactions. Arch Intern Med. 1987;147:565.
48. Baciewicz AM, Self TH. Rifampin drug interactions. Arch Intern Med. 1984;144:1667–71.
49. Isley WL. Effect of rifampin therapy on thyroid function tests in a hypothyroid patient on replacement L-thyroxine. Ann Intern Med. 1987;107:517.
50. British Thoracic Association: A controlled trial of six months chemotherapy in pulmonary tuberculosis. Second report: Results during the 24 months after the end of chemotherapy. Am Rev Respir Dis. 1982;126:460.
51. Anonymous. Drugs for tuberculosis. Med Lett 1988;30:43.
52. Baronti A, Lukinovich N. A pilot trial of rifampicin in tuberculosis. Tubercle. 1968;49:180.
53. Livengood JR, Sigler TG, Foster LR, et al. Isoniazid resistant tuberculosis: A community outbreak and report of a rifampin prophylaxis failure. JAMA. 1985;253:2847–9.
54. Hunter AM, Campbell IA, Jenkins PA, et al. Treatment of pulmonary infections caused by mycobacteria of the *Mycobacterium avium-intracellulare* complex. Thorax. 1981;36:326.
55. Baron EJ, Young LS. Amikacin, ethambutol, and rifampin for treatment of disseminated *Mycobacterium avium-intracellulare* infections in patients with acquired immune deficiency syndrome. Diagn Microbiol Infect Dis. 1986;5:215–20.
56. Ahn CH, Lowell JR, Ahn SS, et al. Chemotherapy for pulmonary disease due to *Mycobcterium kansasii*: Efficacies of some individual drugs. Rev Infect Dis. 1981;3:1028.
57. Bogaerts Y, Elinck W, van Renterghem D, et al. Pulmonary disease due to *Mycobacterium xenopi*: Report of two cases. Eur J Respir Dis. 1982;63:298.
58. Donta ST, Smith PW, Levitz RE, et al. Therapy of *Mycobacterium marinum* infections. Arch Intern Med. 1986;146:902–4.
59. Kallenius G, Moller E, Ringden O, et al. The first infant to survive a generalized BCG infection. Acta Paediatr Scand. 1982;71:161.
60. Izumi AK, Matsunaga J. BCG vaccine-induced lupus vulgaris. Arch Dermatol. 1982;118:171.
61. Yawalkar SJ, McDougall AC, Longuillon J, et al. Once monthly rifampicin plus daily dapsone in initial treatment of lepromatous leprosy. Lancet. 1982;1:1119.
62. Bullock WE. Rifampin in the treatment of leprosy. Rev Infect Dis. 1983;5(Suppl):606–13.
63. Deal WB, Sanders E. Efficacy of rifampin in treatment of meningococcal carriers. N Engl J Med. 1969;281:641–5.
64. Devine LF, Rhode SL, Pierce WE. Rifampin: Effect of two-day treatment on the meningococcal carrier state and the relationship to the levels of drug in sera and saliva. Am J Med Sci. 1971;261:79–83.
65. Weidmer CE, Dunkel TB, Pettyjohn FS, et al. Effectiveness of rifampin in eradicating the meningococcal carrier state in a relatively closed population: Emergence of resistant strains. J Infect Dis. 1971;124:172–8.
66. Beaty HN. Rifampin and minocycline in meningococcal disease. Rev Infect Dis. 1983;5(Suppl):451–8.
67. Jacobson JA, Daniel B. Vestibular reactions associated with minocycline. Antimicrob Agents Chemother. 1975;8:453–6.
68. Schwartz B, Al-Ruwais A, A'Ashi J, et al. Comparative efficacy of ceftriaxone and rifampicin in eradicating pharyngeal carriage of group A *Neisseria meningitidis*. Lancet. 1988;1:1239–42.
69. Pugsley MP, Dworzack DL, Horowitz EA, et al. Efficacy of ciprofloxacin in the treatment of nasopharyngeal carriers of *Neisseria meningitidis*. J Infect Dis. 1987;156:211–3.
70. Broome CV, Mortimer EA, Katz SL, et al. Use of chemoprophylaxis to prevent the spread of *Hemophilus enfluenzae* B in day-care facilities. N Engl J Med. 1987;316:1226–8.
71. Anonymons. Update: Prevention of *Haemophilus influenzae* type b disease. MMWR. 1986;35:170–80.
72. Respiratory and Special Pathogens Epidemiology Branch (CDC): Prevention of secondary cases of *Haemophilus influenzae* type B disease. MMWR. 1982;31:672.
73. Brunnel PA, Bass JW, Daum RS, et al. Revision of recommendation for use of rifampin prophylaxis of contacts of patients with *Haemophilus influenzae* infection. Pediatrics. 1984;74:301–2.
74. Dashefsky B, Wald E, Li K. Management of contacts of children in day care with invasive *Haemophilus influenzae* type b disease. Pediatrics. 1986;78:939–40.
75. Wilde J, Adler SP. Molecular epidemiology of *Haemophilus influenzae* type B: failure of rifampin prophylaxis in a day care center. Pediatr Infect Dis. 1986;5:505–8.
76. Cates KL, Krause PJ, Murphy TV, et al. Second episodes of *Haemophilus influenzae* type b disease following rifampin prophylaxis of the index patients. Pediatr Infect Dis J. 1987;6:512–5.
77. Sande MA. The use of rifampin in treatment of nontuberculous infections. Rev Infect Dis. 1983;5(Suppl):399.
78. Vazquez GJ, Archer GL. Antibiotic thrapy of experimental *Staphylococcus epidermidis* endocarditis. Antimicrob Agents Chemother. 1980;17:280–5.
79. Tuazon CU, Washburn D. Teicoplanin and rifampicin singly and in combination in the treatment of experimental *Staphylococcus epidermidis* endocarditis in the rabbit model. J Antimicrob Chemother. 1987;20:233–7.
80. Karchmer AW, Archer GL, Dismukes WE. *Staphylococcus epidermis* causing prosthetic valve endocarditis: Microbiological and clinical observations as guides to therapy. Ann Intern Med. 1983;48:447.
81. Karchmer AW, Archer GA. Methicillin-resistant *Staphylococcus epidermidis* (SE) prosthetic valve (PV) endocarditis (E): A therapeutic trial (Abstract 476). Program and Abstracts of the Twenty-fourth Interscience Conference on Antimicrobial Agents and Chemotherapy. October 8–10, 1984.
82. Chamovitz B, Bryant RE, Gilbert D, et al. Prosthetic valve endocarditis caused by *Staphylococcus epidermidis*. JAMA. 1985;253:2867–8.
83. Swanberg L, Tuazon CU. Rifampin in the treatment of serious staphylococcal infections. Am J Med Sci. 1984;287:49–54.
84. Acar JF, Goldstein FW, Duval J. Use of rifampin for the treatment of serious staphylococcal and gram-negative bacillary infections. Rev Infect Dis. 1983;5(Suppl):502–6.
85. Zak O, Scheld M, Sande M. Rifampin in experimental endocarditis due to *Staphylococcus aureus* in rabbits. Rev Infect Dis. 1983;5(Suppl):481–90.
86. Kapusnik JE, Parenti F, Sande M. The use of rifampicin in staphyloccal infections—a review. J Antimicrob Chemother. 1984;13:61–6.
87. Bayer AS, Lam K. Efficacy of vancomycin plus rifampin in experimental aortic-valve endocarditis due to methicillin-resistant *Staphyloccus aureus*: In vitro–in vivo correlations. J Infect Dis. 1985;151:157–65.
88. Eng RHK, Smith SM, Tillem M, et al. Rifampin resistance. Development during the therapy of methicillin-resistant *Staphylococcus aureus* infection. Arch Intern Med. 1985;145:146–8.
89. Simon GL, Smith RH, Sande MA. Emergence of rifampin-resistant strains of *Staphylococcus aureus* during combination therapy with vancomycin and rifampin: A report of two cases. Rev Infect Dis. 1983;5(Suppl):507–8.
90. Eng RHK, Smith SM, Buccini FJ, et al. Differences in ability of cell-wall antibiotics to suppress emergence of rifampicin resistance in *Staphylococcus aureus*. J Antimicrob Chemother. 1985;15:201–7.
91. Hackbarth CJ, Chambers HF, Sande MA. Serum bactericidal activity of rifampin in combination with other antimicrobial agents against *Staphylococcus aureus*. Antimicrob Agents Chemother. 1986;29:611–3.
92. Foldes M, Munro R, Sorrell TC, et al. In-vitro effects of vancomycin, rifampicin, and fusidic acid, alone and in combination, against methicillin-resistant *Staphylococcus aureus*. J Antimicrob Chemother. 1983;11:21–6.
93. Coleman DL, Horwitz RI, Andriole VT. Association between serum inhibitory and bactericidal concentrations and therapeutic outcome in bacterial endocarditis. Am J Med. 1982;73:260–7.
94. Traczewski MM, Goldmann DA, Murphy P. In vitro activity of rifampin in combination with oxacillin against *Staphylococcus aureus*. Antimicrob Agents Chemother. 1983;23:571.
95. Watanakunakorn C, Guerriero JC. Interaction between vancomycin and rifampin against *Staphylococcus aureus*. Antimicrob Agents Chemother. 1981;19:1089.
96. Walsh TJ, Auger F, Tatem BA, et al. Novobiocin and rifampicin in combination against methicillin-resistant *Staphylococcus aureus*: An in-vitro comparison with vancomycin plus rifampicin. J Antimicrob Chemother. 1986;17:75–82.
97. Varaldo PE, Debbia E, Schito GC. In vitro activity of teichomycin and vancomycin alone and in combination with rifampin. Antimicrob Agents Chemother. 1983;23:402–6.
98. Zinner SH, Lagast H, Klastersky J. Antistaphylococcal activity of rifampin with other antibiotics. J Infect Dis. 1981;144:365–71.
99. Van der Auwera P, Klastersky J. In vitro study of the combination of rifampin with oxacillin against *Staphylococcus aureus*. Rev Infect Dis. 1983;5(Suppl):509–14.
100. Van der Auwera P, Klastersky J. Bactericidal activity and killing rate of serum in volunteers receiving teicoplanin alone or in combination with oral or intravenous rifampin. Antimicrob Agents Chemother. 1987;31:1002–5.
101. Ho JL, Klempner MS. In vitro evaluation of clindamycin in combination with oxacillin rifampin or vancomycin against *Staphylococcus aureus*. Diagn Microbiol Infect Dis. 1986;4:133.
102. Bayer AS, Morrison JO. Disparity between timed-kill and checkerboard methods for determination of in vitro bactericidal interactions of vancomycin plus rifampin versus methicillin-susceptible and resistant *Staphylococcus aureus*. Antimicrob Agents Chemother. 1984;26:220–3.
103. Sande MA, Scheld WM. Combination antibiotic therapy of bacterial endocarditis. Ann Intern Med. 1980;92:390.
104. Jariwalla AG, Davies BH, White J. Infective endocarditis complicating psittacosis: Response to rifampicin. Br Med J. 1980;280:155.
105. Faville RJ, Zaske DE, Kaplan EL, et al. *Staphylococcus aureus* endocarditis: Combined therapy with vancomycin and rifampin. JAMA. 1978;240:1963.
106. Simmons NA. Synergy and rifampicin. J Antimicrob Chemother. 1977;3:109.
107. Wheat LJ, Kohler RB, White AL, et al. Effect of rifampin on nasal carriers of coagulase-positive staphylococci. J Infect Dis. 1981;144:177.
108. Wheat LJ, Kohler RB, Luft FC, et al. Long term studies of the effect of rifampin on nasal carriage of coagulase-positive staphylococci. Rev Infect Dis. 1983;5(Suppl):459–62.
109. McNally TP, Lewis MR, Brown DR. Effect of rifampin and bacitracin on nasal carriers of *Staphylococcus aureus*. Antimicrob Agents Chemother. 1984;25:422–6.
110. Locksley RM, Cohen ML, Quinn TC, et al. Multiply antibiotic-resistant *Staphylococcus aureus*: Introduction, transmission, and evolution of nosocomial infection. Ann Intern Med. 1982;97:317.
111. Ward TT, Winn RE, Hartstein AI, et al. Observations relating to an inter-

hospital outbreak of methicillin resistant *Staphylococcus aureus*: Role of anticrobial therapy in infection control. Infect Control. 1981;2:453.
112. Ellison H, Judson FN, Peterson LC, et al. Oral rifampin trimethoprim-sulfamethoxazole therapy in symptomatic carriers of methicillin-resistant *Staphylococcus aureus* infections. West J Med. 1984;140:735–40.
113. Pearson JW, Christiansen KJ, Annear DI, et al. Control of methicillin-resistant *Staphylococcus aureus* (MRSA) in an Australian metropolitan teaching hospital complex. Med J Aust. 1985;142:103–8.
114. Tanz RR, Shulman ST, Barthel MJ, et al. Penicillin plus rifampin eradicates pharyngeal carriage of group A streptococci. J Pediatr. 1985;106:876–80.
115. Rosenberg EW, Noah PW, Zanolli MD, et al. Use of rifampin with penicillin and erythromycin in the treatment of psoriasis. J Am Acad Dermatol. 1986;14:761–4.
116. Millard DD, Shulman ST, Yogev R. Rifampin and penicillin for the elimination of group B streptococci in nasally colonized infant rats. Pediatr Res. 1985;19:1183–6.
117. Norden CW, Shaffer M. Treatment of experimental chronic osteomyelitis due to *Staphylococcus aureus* with vancomycin and rifampin. J Infect Dis. 1983;147:352.
118. Norden CW, Bryant R, Palmer D, et al. Chronic osteomyelitis caused by *Staphylococcus aureus*: Controlled clinical trial of nafcillin therapy and nafcillin-rifampin therapy. South Med J. 1986;79:947–51.
119. Beam TR. Sequestration of *Staphylococcus aureus* at an inaccessible focus. Lancet. 1979;2:227.
120. LLoren-Terol J, Busquets RM. Brucellosis treated with rifampicin. Arch Dis Child. 1980;55:486.
121. Ariza J, Gudiol F, Pallares R, et al. Comparative trial of rifampin-doxycycline versus tetracycline-streptomycin in the therapy of human brucellosis. Antimicrob Agents Chemother. 1985;28:548–51.
122. Perez MAH, Rodriguez BA, Garcia AF, et al. Treatment of nervous system brucellosis with rifampin and doxcycline (Letter). Neurology. 1986;36:1408–9.
123. Ezer G, Soothill JF. Intracellular bactericidal effect of rifampicin in both normal and chronic granulomatous disease polymorphs. Arch Dis Child. 1974;49:463.
124. Lorber B. Rifampin in chronic granulomatous disease. N Engl J Med. 1980;303:111.
125. Archer G. Tenenbaum JM, Haywood HB. Rifampin therapy of *S. epidermidis*: Use in infections from indwelling artificial devices. JAMA. 1978;240:751.
126. Bolton WK, Sande MA, Normansell DE, et al. Ventriculojugular shunt nephritis with *Corynebacterium bovis*. Am J Med. 1975;59:417.
127. Ring JC, Cates KL, Belani KK, et al. Rifampin for CSF shunt infections caused by coagulase-negative staphylococci. J Pediatr. 1979;95:317.
128. Wakefield TW, Schaberg DR, Pierson CL, et al. Treatment of established prosthetic vascular graft infection with antibiotics preferentially concentrated in leukocytes. Surgery. 1987;102:8–14.
129. Peters W, Shaw JJ, Lainson R, et al. Potentiating action of rifampicin and isoniazid against *Leishmania mexicana amazonensis*. Lancet. 1981;1:1122.
130. Even-Paz Z, Weinrauch L, Livshin R, et al. Rifampicin treatment of cutaneous leishmaniasis. Int J Dermatol. 1982;21:110.
131. Conti R, Parenti F. Rifampin therapy for brucellosis, *Flavobacterium meningitis*, and cutaneous leishmaniasis. Rev Infect Dis. 1983;5(Suppl):600–5.
132. Brumfitt W, Dixson S, Hamilton-Miller JMT. Use of rifampin for the treatment of urinary tract infections. Rev Infect Dis. 1983;5(Suppl):573–82.
133. Desudchit P, Nunthapisud P, Rukjutitum S, et al. Rifampicin-erythromycin combination for the treatment of gonococcal urethritis in men. Southeast Asian J Trop Med Public Health. 1984;15:360–3.
134. Oriel JD, Ridway GL, Goldmeir D, et al. Treatment of gonococcal urethritis in men with a rifampicin-erythromycin combination. Sex Transm Dis. 1982;9:208–11.
135. Plummer FA, Nsanze H, D'Costa LJ, et al. Short-course and single-dose antimicrobial therapy for chancroid in Kenya: Studies with rifampin alone and in combination with trimethoprim. Rev Infect Dis. 1983;5(Suppl):565–72.
136. Treatment of sexually transmitted diseases. Med Lett. 1988;30:5–10.
137. Zuravleff JJ, Yu VL, Yee RB. Ticarcillin-tobramycin-rifampin: In vitro synergy of the triplet combination against *Pseudomonas aeruginosa*. J Lab Clin Med. 1983;101:896–902.
138. Yu VL, Zuravleff JJ, Peacock JE, et al. Addition of rifampin to carboxypenicillin-aminoglycoside combination for the treatment of *Pseudomonas aerugionosa* infection: Clinical experience with four patients. Antimicrob Agents Chemother. 1984;26:575–7.
139. Chin NX, Heu HC. Synergy of imipenen, a novel carbapenem, and rifampin and ciprofloxacin against *Pseudomonas aeruginosa*, *Serratis marcescens* and *Enterobacter* species. Chemotherapy. 1987;33:183–8.
140. Fu KP, Lasinski ER, Zoganas HC, et al. Therapeutic efficacy and pharmacokinetic properties of rifampicin in a *Bacteroides fragilis* intra-abdominal abscess. J Antimicrob Chemother. 1984;14:633–40.
141. Fu KP, Lasinski ER, Zoganas HC, et al. Efficacy of rifampicin in experimental *Bacteroides fragilis* and *Pseudomonas aeruginosa* mixed infections. J Antimicrob Chemother. 1985;15:579–85.
142. Buggy BP, Fekety R, Silva J Jr. Therapy of relapsing *Clostridium difficile*-associtaed diarrhea and colitis with the combination of vancomycin and rifampin. J Clin Gastroenterol. 1987;9:155–9.
143. Hirsh BE, Wong B, Kiehn TE, et al. A case of *Flavobacterium meningoseptcum* bacteremia in an adult with acute leukemia. Use of rifampin to clear persistent infection. Diagn Microbiol Infect Dis. 1986;4:65–9.
144. Lewis MA, Priestley BL. Addition of rifampicin in persistent *Haemophilus influenzae* type B meningitis. 1986;292:448–9.
145. Varaldo PE, Debbia E, Schito GC. In vitro activities of rifapentine and rifampin, alone and in combination with six other antibiotics, against methicillin-susceptible and methicillin-resistant staphylococci of different species. Antimicrob Agents Chemother. 1985;27:615–8.
146. Korvic J, Yu VL, Sharp JA. Interaction of rifampicin or rifapentine with other agents against *Pseudomonas aerugionosa*. J Antimicrob Chemother. 1987;19:847–8.
147. Dickinson JM, Mitchison DA. In vitro properties of rifapentine (MDL473) relevant to its use in intermittent chemotherapy of tuberculosis. Tubercle. 1987;68:113–8.
148. Bermudez LEM, Wu M, Young LS. Intracellular killing of *Mycobacterium avium* complex by rifapentine and liposome-encapsulated amikacin. J Infect Dis. 1987;156:510–3.
149. Assandri A, Ratti B, Cristina T. Pharmacokinetics of rifapentine, a new long lasting rifamycin, in the rat, the mouse and the rabbit. J Antibiot (Tokyo). 1984;37:1066–73.
150. Durand DV, Hampden C, Boobis AR, et al. Induction of mixed function oxidase activity in man by rifapentine (MDL473), a long-acting rifamycin derivative. Br J Clin Pharmacol. 1986;21:1–7.
151. O'Brien RJ, Lyle MA, Snider DE. Rifabutin (ansamycin LM 427): A new rifamycin-S derivative for the treatment of mycobacterial diseases. Rev Infect Dis. 1987;9:519–30.
152. Hawkins CC, Gold JWM, Whimbey E, et al. *Mycobacterium avium* complex infections in patients with the acquired immunodeficiency syndrome. Ann Intern Med. 1986;105:184–8.
153. Masur H, Tuazon C, Gill V, et al. Effect of combined clofazimine and ansamycin therapy on *Mycobacterium avium–Mycobacterium intracellulare* bacteremia in patients with AIDS. J Infect Dis. 1987;155:126–29.

25. METRONIDAZOLE

SYDNEY M. FINEGOLD
GLENN E. MATHISEN

DESCRIPTION

Metronidazole was introduced in 1959 for the treatment of *Trichomonas vaginalis* infections. It is now known to be effective against most infections involving anaerobic bacteria and against certain other parasitic infections. Metronidazole diffuses well into all tissues including the central nervous system. It is well tolerated and has the best bactericidal activity of all drugs active against anaerobic bacteria.

Metronidazole is a nitroimidazole drug with the chemical formula 1-(2-hydroxyethyl)-2-methyl-5-nitroimidazole. It has a low molecular weight, 171.

SPECTRUM OF ACTIVITY, RESISTANCE

Table 1 from Sutter[1] summarizes the activity of metronidazole against 793 strains of anaerobic and microaerophilic bacteria. Note that virtually all of the organisms tested were inhibited by 16 μg/ml or less except for one-third of gram-positive non-spore-forming bacilli and 7 percent of *Capnocytophaga* sp. Metabolites are found in serum and urine, and Sutter found that the hydroxy metabolite of metronidazole was slightly less active than was the parent compound against many anaerobes but had equivalent or better activity against some. The acid metabolite has poor activity against anaerobes. In general, studies by other workers have given comparable results in terms of the in vitro activity of metronidazole. Wüst[2] found that seven strains of *Propionibacterium acnes* required 100 μg/ml for inhibition. Werner et al.[3] also noted that the hydroxy metabolite of metronidazole was roughly comparable in activity to the parent compound. We found that only about 25 percent of the strains of *Actinomyces* and *Arachnia* are susceptible to metronidazole at achievable levels. In a recent study, Rosenblatt and Edson[4]

TABLE 1. Activity of Metronidazole against Anaerobic and Microaerophilic Bacteria

Bacteria	No. Strains	Cumulative Percentage Susceptible to Indicated Concentration (μg/ml) 4	8	16	32
Bacteroides fragilis[a]	161	90	99	100	—
B. melaninogenicus[b]	60	98	100	—	—
Other bacteroides and *Selenomonas* sp.	154	95	98	100	—
Fusobacterium sp.	65	100	—	—	—
Anaerobic gram-negative cocci	24	92	96	100	—
Anaerobic gram-positive cocci	124	98	—	—	—
Clostridium perfringens	18	94	100	—	—
Other *Clostridium* sp.	73	97	99	—	100
Gram-positive nonsporulating bacilli	87	57	60	62	66
Capnocytophaga sp.	27	52	70	93	—

[a] Includes all species of the *B. fragilis* group.
[b] Includes *B. melaninogenicus* and *B. asaccharolyticus* ssp.
(From Sutter,[1] with permission.)

noted somewhat less activity against anaerobic gram-positive cocci (a minimum inhibitory concentration for 70 percent of strains [MIC_{70}] of 6.25 and MIC_{90} of >25 μg/ml). *Propionibacterium acnes* was highly resistant. The study by Chow et al.[5] found significantly more resistance among anaerobes to metronidazole than was indicated by the studies previously cited.

Also sensitive to metronidazole are *Treponema pallidum,* oral spirochetes, *Campylobacter fetus,* and *Gardnerella vaginalis.* In certain animal models, *Escherichia coli* may be inhibited by metronidazole when it is present together in a mixture with *Bacteroides fragilis.* However, in another animal model[6] there was no activity against *E. coli.* We have noted decreased counts of *E. coli* initially present together with anaerobes in the bypassed loop of patients with ileal bypass for obesity who were treated with metronidazole for "bypass enteropathy."

Resistance to metronidazole develops rarely. Resistant strains identified include one strain each of *Bacteroides fragilis, Bacteroides distasonis,* what was originally described as *Bacteroides melaninogenicus* ss *melaninogenicus* and *Bacteroides bivius.* Phillips et al.[7] note that they have seen occasional marginally resistant isolates of *B. bivius, Bacteroides ureolyticus,* and perhaps *B. melaninogenicus.* Tally et al.[8] studied a metronidazole-resistant strain of *B. fragilis.* They found that the uptake of metronidazole by cells was slower than in a sensitive strain. Also, the rate of reduction of metronidazole was four times less than with a sensitive control strain, possibly due to decreased nitroreductase activity. Although rare, case reports suggest that resistant organisms may develop in patients receiving therapy, and this could lead to a clinical relapse of infection.[9,10] *Trichomonas vaginalis* may become resistant to metronidazole, and several case reports have described recalcitrant vaginal trichomoniasis secondary to resistant strains.[11–13]

MODE OF ACTION

Mechanism of Action

It is convenient to think of the action as occurring in four successive steps[14]: (*1*) entry of the drug into the bacterial cell, (*2*) reductive activation, (*3*) toxic effect of the reduced intermediate product(s), and (*4*) release of inactive end products. A key feature is reduction of the nitro group of the drug; the drug acts as a preferential electron acceptor, being reduced by low–redox potential electron transport proteins (ferredoxin-like and flavodoxin-like). Reduction of the drug decreases the intracellular concentration of unchanged drug, thus maintaining a gradient that drives the uptake and generates compounds that are toxic to the cell. The toxicity is due to short-lived intermediate compounds or free radicals that produce damage by interaction with DNA and possibly other macromolecules. The cytotoxic intermediates decompose into nontoxic and inactive end products, including acetamide and 2-hydroxethyl oxamic acid.

Metabolic Products

As noted before, the hydroxy derivation of metronidazole has significant antianaerobic activity; it is more active than metronidazole is on *G. vaginalis.* The acid derivative of metronidazole has relatively little activity, less than one-tenth as much as metronidazole against *B. fragilis* and *Trichomonas.*[14] The drug is also conjugated; the glucuronide has no activity on *Trichomonas* and is not taken up.[14]

Bactericidal Activity

Metronidazole is a potent bactericidal agent. It typically kills organisms at the same concentration or within one twofold dilution of that required for inhibition.[15] Under reduced conditions, metronidazole has a rapid onset of bactericidal activity. Killing rates are not affected by inoculum size, nutritional requirements, or growth rate.[16,17]

Bartlett et al.[18] found metronidazole to be the most effective drug in a *B. fragilis* subcutaneous abscess model in mice even when treatment was delayed for 8–120 hours after challenge.

PHARMACOLOGY

When given orally, metronidazole is absorbed rapidly and almost completely. Serum levels are similar during the elimination phase after equivalent doses by the intravenous and oral routes. Blood levels are proportional to the administered dose. The standard intravenous dosage regimen that has been used in the United States consists of a loading dose of 15 mg/kg of body weight followed by 7.5 mg/kg every 6 hours. This results in peak and trough steady-state plasma levels averaging 25 μg/ml and 18 μg/ml, respectively. There is very little protein binding of metronidazole. The half-life is 8 hours. Absorption of metronidazole is not affected by ingestion of food, but peak levels may be markedly delayed. Metronidazole is absorbed after vaginal administration, but peak serum levels (mean, 1.2 μg/ml) and bioavailability (20 percent) are lower than by oral or intravenous administration.[19] Absorption after rectal administration is quite good, although peak serum levels occur approximately 3 hours after insertion. Metronidazole is rapidly transferred across the placenta; peak serum levels in the fetus are equivalent to maternal levels after intravenous administration to pregnant women.[20]

There is a large apparent volume of distribution of metronidazole that is equivalent to about 80 percent of body weight; it reaches all tissues and fluids. Therapeutic levels are achieved in amniotic fluid, the unobstructed biliary tract, alveolar bone, cerebrospinal fluid and brain abscess contents, cord blood, pleural empyema fluid, hepatic abscesses, middle ear discharge, middle ear mucosa, breast milk, pelvic tissues (concentrations attained in the myometrium and fallopian tubes are nearly the same as concomitant serum levels), saliva, seminal fluid, and vaginal secretions. Levels achieved in the aqueous humor were between one-third and one-half those attained in the serum.[21]

During metabolization of metronidazole, five major products are formed. The most important one is the hydroxy derivative. In addition, there is an acid metabolite, acetylmetronidazole, metronidazole glucuronide, and the glucuronide conjugate of hydroxy metronidazole. A sulfate conjugate may also be found on occasion. Metronidazole and its metabolites are eliminated primarily in the urine (60–80 percent of the dose). From 6 to 15 percent is excreted in the feces.

The elimination half-life of metronidazole in patients with no renal function is the same as in healthy people. However, the hydroxy metabolite may accumulate in patients with absent renal function, and although dosage adjustment is usually not considered necessary in the absence of hepatic disease, consideration might be given to dosage adjustment in patients initially receiving large doses. Metronidazole and its metabolites are rapidly removed by hemodialysis; the elimination half-life of metronidazole is reduced to 2.6 hours. Dose reduction is generally not necessary in patients undergoing chronic ambulatory peritoneal dialysis.[22] In patients with impaired hepatic function, even without concomitant renal function impairment, the plasma clearance of metronidazole is delayed. Although data are limited, pharmacokinetic studies in patients with significant liver disease suggest that doses should be reduced by at least 50 percent in this patient population.[23,24]

ADMINISTRATION AND DOSAGE

Table 2 gives dosage recommendations and routes of administration for the major indications for metronidazole therapy. The intravenous route is recommended initially for seriously ill patients. Since oral therapy gives blood levels comparable to those achieved by the intravenous route, we may switch when conditions warrant.

As noted, the standard regimen in the United States for intravenous administration has been a loading dose of 15 mg/kg of body weight followed by a maintenance schedule of 7.5 mg/kg every 6 hours. Clearly, the half-life of the drug would warrant administration at longer intervals such as every 8 or even every 12 hours. The manufacturer recommends that intravenous infusions be administered over a period of 1 hour. However, a number of foreign investigators have administered the drug in as little as 20 minutes without any apparent adverse effects. The maximum daily dose recommended is 4 g.

After reconstitution, metronidazole hydrochloride should be diluted with intravenous fluid to a concentration not exceeding 8 mg/ml and should be neutralized to pH 6.0–7.0 with sodium bicarbonate before administration. There is also a metronidazole intravenous solution (Flagyl IV RTU), a ready-to-use isotonic solution that does not require dilution or buffering before infusion.

The duration of therapy will vary according to the entity being treated. Certain recommendations are made in Table 2. For serious infections, however, we may often need to treat the patient for 2–4 weeks or longer.

Comments regarding dosage in patients with impaired renal and/or hepatic function have been noted in the earlier section on pharmacology.

ADVERSE REACTIONS, PRECAUTIONS

In general, metronidazole is well tolerated. The more commonly encountered major and minor adverse reactions are listed in Table 3. There may also be furring of the tongue, glossitis, stomatitis, dry mouth, headache, fever, dizziness, syncope, and occasionally overgrowth of *Candida* in the oral cavity or vagina. Thrombophlebitis has been reported with intravenous infusion but is seldom seen now with proper buffering of the preparation. Gastrointestinal side effects include nausea, epigastric distress, anorexia, and less commonly, vomiting or diarrhea. Although pseudomembranous colitis has been reported rarely with metronidazole therapy, the drug has proved effective therapeutically for this condition and is comparable to vancomycin in effectiveness. The most serious adverse effects are those involving the central nervous system. These are rare unless large doses and/or prolonged therapy is used. If abnormal neurologic symptoms are observed, treatment with the drug must be discontinued immediately. Metronidazole should be used with caution in people with a history of seizures or other central nervous system disorders. The peripheral neuropathy may take a considerable period of time to resolve.

There has been concern about mutagenicity in the Ames *Salmonella* mutant system and carcinogenicity of metronidazole. Reduction of the nitro group of the compound is necessary for both antibacterial activity and mutagenic activity. Mutagenic activity has been detected in the urine of patients receiving 750 mg/day of metronidazole. When a mutant *Salmonella* that did not possess nitroreductase was used in the mutagenic testing system, metronidazole could not be demonstrated to be a mutagen. Thus, the drug itself is not mutagenic, but rather it is one or more reduction products of it. Some protozoa, bacteria (including facultative anaerobes), and fungi possess nitroreductase activity. Eukaryotic tissues have very little nitroreductase activity. It has been suggested that during metronidazole therapy some reduction products of the drug might escape from the bacterial cells and serve as mutagens to the host's mammalian tissue. However, these active derivatives are very short-lived and either promptly bind to macromolecules within the bacterial cell or are promptly reduced to compounds that are not mutagenic or carcinogenic. The drug has been studied specifically for mutagenic potential in eukaryotic test systems (human lymphocytes in vitro and lymphocytes of patients receiving metronidazole therapy). No chromosomal aberrations or sister chromatid exchanges could be detected in vitro with metronidazole or its metabolites in concentrations of 1000–10,000 μg/ml. No lymphocyte abnormalities were noted in patients receiving a short course of metronidazole therapy.[25,26] Metronidazole has shown tumorigenic activity in several studies in mice involving lifetime (or almost lifetime) oral administration. Female rats given metronidazole over long periods (sometimes for life) had a significant increase in neoplasms, especially mammary tumors, as compared with controls. Interestingly, in one study drug-fed rats lived longer than did controls. Two lifetime studies in hamsters were negative (see Finegold[27]). It should be noted that acetamide has been found in the urine of patients

TABLE 2. Major Indications for Metronidazole: Administration and Dosage

Indication	*Route of Administration*	*Dosage*
Susceptible anaerobic infections	iv	Loading dose of 15 mg/kg, then 7.5 mg/kg q6h
	po	1–2 g/day in 2–4 doses q6–12h
Nonspecific vaginitis	po	500 mg bid for 7 days
Trichomonas vaginitis	po	250 mg tid for 7 days *or* 5000 mg bid for 5 days *or* 2 g in single dose
Amebiasis (intestinal or extraintestinal)	iv or po	750 mg tid for 10 days
Giardiasis	po	250 mg bid or tid for 5–7 days *or* 2 g/day for 3 days

TABLE 3. Adverse Effects Related to Metronidazole Therapy

Major adverse reactions (rare)
Seizures, encephalopathy
Cerebellar dysfunction, ataxia
Peripheral neuropathy
Disulfiram reaction with alcohol
Potentiation of effects of warfarin
Pseudomembranous colitis
Pancreatitis
Minor adverse reactions
Minor gastrointestinal disturbances
Reversible neutropenia
Metallic taste
Dark or red-brown urine
Maculopapular rash, urticaria
Urethral, vaginal burning
Gynecomastia

receiving metronidazole and prolonged feeding of high doses of this compound to rats has produced hepatocarcinomas.[28] A study in rats[29] using the dimethylhydrazine (DMH) model for colon neoplasia noted that the addition of metronidazole on a long-term basis had an apparent cocarcinogenic effect. As Condon notes in the discussion of this paper, the DMH tumor model is relatively specific and may not readily be extrapolated to humans.[29] Indeed, in another study looking at bile salt–induced colorectal cancer in rats, metronidazole administration appeared to reduce the carcinogenic effect of sodium deoxycholate.[30]

Long-term follow-up of a cohort of 771 women who received metronidazole therapy for the treatment of vaginal trichomoniasis during the 1960s has not shown an increased incidence of malignancy.[31] It should be recognized that these patients received relatively low doses of the drug for brief periods of time (7–10 days). A recent report raises the possibility of carcinogenicity in three patients with Crohn's disease who had received prolonged therapy with metronidazole[32]; these observations remain anecdotal, and further studies are clearly needed. Although metronidazole appears to be safe, the long-term effects of high-dose prolonged therapy are not completely known, and such usage should be avoided if other alternatives are available.

Metronidazole crosses the placental barrier, and concerns have been raised about possible teratogenic effects in light of the evidence for mutagenicity in bacterial systems. To date, there has been little evidence for this in animal models, although one study has raised the possibility of fetal "genotoxicity" in pregnant golden Syrian hamsters fed high doses of metronidazole.[33] Studies in pregnant women who had received metronidazole during pregnancy for the treatment of vaginal trichomoniasis have not shown an increased incidence of stillbirths, small-for-age infants, premature infants, or teratogenicity.[34] Although there is one paper that raises the possibility of a metronidazole-induced teratogenic effect,[35] again, this may well be a coincidence and is not supported by other human or animal studies; nevertheless, the use of metronidazole during pregnancy should be reserved for situations in which it is clearly needed. Metronidazole during the first trimester should be avoided.

Because metronidazole is excreted into breast milk, nursing should be discontinued during and for 2 days after therapy with metronidazole.

Drug Interactions, Interference with Laboratory Tests

In patients ingesting alcohol, metronidazole may cause reactions similar to those produced by disulfiram. Patients should be advised not to drink alcohol when taking this drug. Metronidazole inhibits the metabolism of warfarin and other oral coumarin-type anticoagulants. Therefore, if concomitant use must be carried out, the dosage of the anticoagulant should be reduced to maintain the desired prothrombin time.

Metronidazole interferes with certain chemical analyses for the serum enzyme glutamic oxaloacetic transaminase, which results in falsely low or negative values.

EFFECT ON NORMAL FECAL FLORA

In subjects who have a healthy gastrointestinal tract and are not receiving other drugs, metronidazole has very little effect on the fecal flora.[36] This is thought to be due to the drug being rapidly reduced by the bowel flora under the usual anaerobic conditions in the colon. Why this would not have an impact on the organisms carrying out the reduction, as it does in the course of treating infections, is not at all clear. In patients on high-dosage regimens, in patients with diarrhea, and in patients receiving certain other antimicrobial agents concurrently, there may be a significant impact of metronidazole on the fecal flora. For example, when oral neomycin or kanamycin (active primary against nonanaerobes) is given with metronidazole, there is a significant impact on both the anaerobic and aerobic flora. Thus, it has been feasible to use metronidazole for therapy in certain conditions such as ileal bypass enteropathy and for preoperative "bowel preparation" along with an oral aminoglycoside.

CLINICAL USES

Parasitic Infections

Metronidazole has been used successfully for therapy for *Trichomonas* vaginitis for many years. It is also an effective agent for therapy of amebic liver abscess and has been used with generally good results in intestinal amebiasis. The drug is also effective against giardiasis, being at least as active as quinacrine for this purpose.

Some workers have felt that metronidazole has been effective in *Balantidium coli* infection and in infection due to *Dracunculus medinensis,* but these indications are certainly not well established. Metronidazole has been used in the treatment of cutaneous leishmaniasis, although it appears to be less effective than are other available agents.[37]

Anaerobic Infections

As is suggested by the spectrum of activity of metronidazole, this drug is useful for the vast majority of anaerobic infections. Certainly actinomycosis is one notable exception, and infections with *P. acnes,* which are quite rare, would be another. There is one other setting in which metronidazole may represent less than optimum therapy—anaerobic infections of the lower respiratory tract. Data from Sanders et al.[38] show a relatively high rate of suboptimal response. Most treatment failures had mixed infections with aerobic bacteria as well as anaerobes. The addition of penicillin G or ampicillin for mixed infections involving streptococci, pneumococci, or *Haemophilus influenzae* or the addition of erythromycin in the case of a penicillin-allergic patient would likely provide an excellent regimen. In the case of aspiration pneumonia involving aerobic and/or facultative gram-negative bacilli and/or *Staphylococcus aureus,* other appropriate therapy to cover these agents would be needed along with metronidazole. Many anaerobic infections are mixed with aerobic or facultative bacteria, of course, and particularly in sicker patients, therapy aimed at both categories of organisms is desirable.

The excellent distribution of metronidazole throughout the body, including the central nervous system, and the impressive bactericidal activity of this compound, even against organisms that are not actively multiplying, make it an excellent choice for a number of serious infections, including brain abscess and other central nervous system infections involving anaerobes, endocarditis due to anaerobic bacteria, and perhaps, any anaerobic infection of serious nature in patients who are immunocompromised.

The *B. fragilis* group of organisms is the one most commonly encountered in anaerobic infections overall. Until recently, there were only three drugs that were consistently active against this group—metronidazole, chloramphenicol, and clindamycin. Recently, a number of centers have been encountering varying degrees of resistance of the *B. fragilis* group to clindamycin. Thus, metronidazole may become an even more important part of our armamentarium for the management of anaerobic infections. It should be noted, however, that in intra-abdominal infections, in which *B. fragilis* is almost always involved, comparative studies[16] failed to show any significant difference among metronidazole, clindamycin, chloramphenicol, ticarcillin, or cefoxitin; most of these were used together with an aminoglycoside.

The resistance of a number of clostridia other than *Clostrid-*

ium perfringens to cefoxitin and clindamycin again suggests that metronidazole might have an advantage in selected intra-abdominal and obstetric and gynecologic infections. However, there are no specific data to back up this point.

Metronidazole has been useful against other types of anaerobic infections including bacteremia, infections of bones and joints, soft tissue infections, oral and dental infections, and head and neck infections. Metronidazole has also provided good results in the therapy for nonspecific vaginitis, a condition in which various anaerobes, *G. vaginalis,* or both may be important.[39] As noted elsewhere, it has been effective in the management of pseudomembranous colitis due to *Clostridium difficile*. Limited studies have shown that fecal levels of metronidazole (up to 1,212 μg/g dry weight and 24.2 μg/g wet weight feces) may be attained by using either an oral or parenteral route in patients with active colitis.[40,41] The parenteral route may be especially useful in patients who have *C. difficile*–induced toxic megacolon and are unable to take oral medications. A recent clinical study suggests that metronidazole may be more effective than penicillin is for antimicrobial therapy for tetanus.[42] Metronidazole is not a suitable alternative to penicillin for syphilis.

Other Therapeutic Uses

Metronidazole has been used experimentally in very high doses as a hypoxic cell sensitizer in radiotherapy for malignancy.

Metronidazole has been useful in a number of types of bowel bacterial overgrowth syndromes such as complications of jejunoileal bypass for obesity[43] and dysfunction of the continent ileostomy,[44] and for the prevention of intrahepatic cholestasis associated with total parenteral nutrition.[45] Although not everyone agrees, it appears that metronidazole has had a beneficial effect in Crohn's disease by producing a lessening of diarrhea (in patients with colonic involvement) and promoting the healing of perianal lesions and erythema nodosum.[46] The prolonged use of the drug, however, may result in a significant incidence of metronidazole-induced peripheral neuropathy,[47] and concerns have been raised about possible carcinogenic effects of the drug.[32]

Metronidazole is said to be beneficial in the treatment of acne rosacea whether used orally or topically.[48]

An intriguing report[49] notes striking decreases in serum cholesterol and triglyceride levels in patients receiving metronidazole for other indications. Only short courses of therapy were used. There is no information as to the mechanism of this effect.

Prophylactic Use

Several groups have carried out prospective controlled studies of metronidazole, alone or in combination with other agents, for prophylaxis in patients undergoing elective colonic surgery, gynecologic surgery, or emergency appendectomy. In the case of appendectomy, a perforated appendix is an indication for therapy rather than prophylaxis, and in uncomplicated appendicitis, the frequency of postoperative infection is quite low. In general, however, in these studies metronidazole has appeared to be as effective as other effective prophylactic agents. It should be kept in mind, however, that the prophylactic use of metronidazole is not an approved indication for the drug in the United States at present. Finally, it should be appreciated that not all of the prophylactic trials have found metronidazole effective. Metronidazole was not effective prophylactically in one study of hysterectomy[50] and in one study of appendectomy for nonperforated appendictis.[51]

REFERENCES

1. Sutter VL. In vitro susceptibility of anaerobic and microaerophilic bacteria to metronidazole and its hydroxy metabolite. In: Finegold SM, George WL, Rolfe RD, eds. Proceedings of the First United States Metronidazole Conference. Tarpon Springs, FL, February 1982. New York: Biomedical Information Corp; 1982:61.
2. Wüst J. Susceptibility of anaerobic bacteria to metronidazole, ornidazole, and tinidazole and routine susceptibility testing by standardized methods. Antimicrob Agents Chemother. 1977;11:631.
3. Werner H, Schädler G, Krasemann C. In vitro activity of azlocillin, metronidazole and its hydroxy metabolite against anaerobes. Arzneimittelforsch Drug Res. 1983;33:574.
4. Rosenblatt JE, Edson RS. Metronidazole. Mayo Clin Proc. 1983;58:154.
5. Chow AW, Bednorz D, Guze LB. Susceptibility of obligate anaerobes to metronidazole: An extended study of 1,054 clinical isolates. In: Finegold SM, McFadzean JA, Roe FJC, eds. Metronidazole. Proceedings of the International Metronidazole Conference, Montreal, May 1976. Princeton, NJ: Excerpta Medica; 1977:286.
6. Reznikov M, McDonald PJ. Effect of metronidazole on *Escherichia coli* in the presence of *Bacteroides fragilis:* An investigation in mice. Chemotherapy. 1983;29:225.
7. Phillips I, Warren C, Taylor E, et al. The antimicrobial susceptibility of anaerobic bacteria in a London teaching hospital. J Antimicrob Chemother. 1981;8:17.
8. Tally FP, Snydman DR, Shimell MJ, et al. Mechanisms of antimicrobial resistance of *Bacteroides fragilis*. In: Phillips I, Collier J, eds. Metronidazole. Proceedings of the Second International Symposium on Anaerobic Infections, Geneva, April 1979. London: The Royal Society of Medicine and Academic Press, New York: Grune & Stratton, 1979:19.
9. Ingham HR, Eaton S, Venables CW, et al. *Bacteroides fragilis* resistant to metronidazole after long-term therapy. Lancet. 1978;1:214.
10. Sprott MS, Ingham HR, Hickman JE, et al. Metronidazole-resistant anaerobes. Lancet. 1983;1:1220.
11. Krajden S, Lossick JG, Wilk E, et al. Persistent *Trichomonas vaginalis* infection due to a metronidazole-resistant strain. Can Med Assoc J. 1986;134:1373–4.
12. Müller M, Meingassner JG, Miller WA, et al. Three metronidazole-resistant strains of *Trichomonas vaginalis* from the United States. Am J Obstet Gynecol. 1980;138:808–12.
13. Dombrowski MP, Sokol RJ, Bronsteen RA. Intravenous therapy of metronidazole-resistant *Trichomonas vaginalis*. Obstet Gynecol. 1987;69:524–5.
14. Müller M. Mode of action of metronidazole on anaerobic bacteria and protozoa. In: Rhône-Poulenc Pharma Inc, Montreal. Proceedings of the North American Metronidazole Symposium on Anaerobic Infections, Scottsdale, AZ, October 1981. Surgery. 1983;93:165.
15. Nastro LJ, Finegold SM. Bactericidal activity of five antimicrobial agents against *Bacteroides fragilis*. J Infect Dis. 1972;126:104.
16. Tally FP, Sullivan CE. Metronidazole: In vitro activity, pharmacology and efficacy in anaerobic bacterial infections. Pharmacotherapy. 1981;1:28.
17. Corrodi P, Busch DF, Sutter VL, et al. Factors affecting the in vitro antibacterial activity of metronidazole In: Finegold SM, McFadzean JA, Roe FJC, eds. Metronidazole. Proceedings of the International Metronidazole Conference, Montreal, May 1976. Princeton, NJ: Excerpta Medica; 1977:299.
18. Bartlett JG, Dezfulian M, Joiner K. Relative efficacy and critical interval of antimicrobial agents in experimental infections involving *Bacteroides fragilis*. Arch Surg. 1983;118:181.
19. Fredricsson B, Hagström B, Nord C-E, et al. Systemic concentrations of metronidazole and its main metabolites after intravenous, oral and vaginal administration. Gynecol Obstet Invest. 1987;24:200–7.
20. Visser AA, Hundt HKL. The pharmacokinetics of a single intravenous dose of metronidazole in pregnant patients. J Antimicrob Chemother. 1984;13:279–83.
21. Mattila J, Nerdrum K, Rouhiainen H, et al. Penetration of metronidazole and tinidazole into the aqueous humor in man. Chemotherapy. 1983;29:188.
22. Guay DR, Meatherall RC, Baxter H, et al. Pharmacokinetics of metronidazole in patients undergoing continuous ambulatory peritoneal dialysis. Antimicrob Agents Chemother. 1984;25:306–10.
23. Lau AH, Evans R, Chang C-W, et al. Pharmacokinetics of metronidazole in patients with alcoholic liver disease. Antimicrob Agents Chemother. 1987;31:1662–4.
24. Loft S, Sonne J, Dossing M, et al. Metronidazole pharmacokinetics in patients with hepatic encephalopathy. Scand J Gastroenterol. 1987;22:117–23.
25. Lambert B, Lindblad A, Lindsten J, et al. Genotoxic effects of metronidazole in human lymphocytes in vitro and in vivo. In: Phillips I, Collier J, eds. Metronidazole. Proceedings of the Second International Symposium on Anaerobic Infections, Geneva, April 1979. London: The Royal Society of Medicine and Academic Press; New York: Grune & Stratton; 1979:229.
26. Hartley-Asp B. Chromosomal studies on human lymphocytes exposed to metronidazole in vivo and in vitro. In: Phillips I, Collier J, eds: Metronidazole. Proceedings of the Second International Symposium on Anaerobic Infections, Geneva, April 1979. London: The Royal Society of Medicine and Academic Press; New York: Grune & Stratton; 1979:237.
27. Finegold SM. Metronidazole. Ann Intern Med. 1980;93:585.
28. Koch RL, Chrystal EJT, Beaulieu BB, et al. Acetamide—a metabolite of metronidazole formed by the intestinal flora. Biochem Pharmacol. 1979;28:3611.
29. Sloan DA, Fleiszer DM, Richards GK, et al. Increased incidence of experimental colon cancer associated with long-term metronidazole therapy. Am J Surg. 1983;145:66.
30. Rainey JB, Maeda M, Williams C, et al. The cocarcinogenic effect of intra-

rectal deoxycholate in rats is reduced by oral metronidazole. Br J Cancer. 1984;49:631–6.
31. Beard CM, Noller KL, O'Fallon WM, et al. Cancer after exposure to metronidazole. Mayo Clin Proc. 1988;63:147–53.
32. Krause JR, Ayuyang HQ, Ellis LD. Occurrence of three cases of carcinoma in individuals with Crohn's disease treated with metronidazole. Am J Gastroenterol. 1985;80:978–82.
33. Garry VF, Nelson RL. Host-mediated transformation: Metronidazole. Mutat Res. 1987;190:289–95.
34. Robbie MO, Sweet RL. Metronidazole use in obstetrics and gynecology: A review. Am J Obstet Gynecol. 1983;145:865–81.
35. Cantú JM, Garcia-Cruz D. Midline facial defect as a teratogenic effect of metronidazole. March Dimes Birth Defect Fdn 1982;18:85–8.
36. Lewis RP, Wideman P, Sutter VL, et al. The effect of metronidazole on human fecal flora. In. Finegold SM, McFadzean JA, Roe FJC, eds. Metronidazole. Proceedings of the International Metronidazole Conference, Montreal, May 1976. Princeton, NJ: Excerpta Medica; 1977:307.
37. Chong H. Oriental sore. A look at trends in and approaches to the treatment of leishmaniasis. Int J Dermatol. 1986;25:615–23.
38. Sanders CV, Hanna BJ, Lewis AC, et al. The use of metronidazole in the treatment of anaerobic pleuropulmonary infections. In: Phillips I, Collier J, eds. Metronidazole. Proceedings of the Second International Symposium on Anaerobic Infections, Geneva, April 1979. London: The Royal Society of Medicine and Academic Press; New York: Grune & Stratton, 1979:83.
39. Swedberg J, Steiner JF, Deiss F, et al. Comparison of single-dose vs one-week course of metronidazole for symptomatic bacterial vaginosis. JAMA. 1985;254:1046–9.
40. Kleinfeld DI, Sharpe RJ, Donta ST. Parenteral therapy for antibiotic-associated pseudomembranous colitis. J Infect Dis. 1988;157:389.
41. Bolton RP, Culshaw MA. Faecal metronidazole concentrations during oral and intravenous therapy for antibiotic associated colitis due to *Clostridium difficile*. Gut. 1986;27:1169–72.
42. Ahmadsyah I, Salim A. Treatment of tetanus: An open study to compare the efficacy of procaine penicillin and metronidazole. Br Med J. 1985;291:648–50.
43. Drenick EJ. Extraintestinal complications of jejunoileal bypass for obesity. In: Finegold SM, George WL, Rolfe RD, eds. Proceedings of the First United States Metronidazole Conference, Tarpon Springs, FL, February 1982. New York: Biomedical Information Corp; 1982:371.
44. Kelly DG, Phillips SF, Kelly KA, et al. Dysfunction of the continent ileostomy: Clinical features and bacteriology. Gut. 1983;24:193.
45. Capron J-P, Herve M-A, Gineston J-L, et al. Metronidazole in prevention of cholestasis associated with total parenteral nutrition. Lancet. 1983;1:446.
46. Gilat T. Metronidazole in Crohn's disease (Editorial). Gastroenterology. 1982;83:702.
47. Duffy LF, Daum F, Fisher SE, et al. Peripheral neuropathy in Crohn's disease patients treated with metronidazole. Gastroenterology. 1985;88:681–4.
48. Nielsen PG. Metronidazole treatment in rosacea. Int J Dermatol. 1988;27:1–5.
49. Davis JL, Schultz TA, Mosley CA. Metronidazole lowers serum lipids. Ann Intern Med. 1983;99:43.
50. Vincelette J, Finkelstein F, Aoki FY, et al. Double-blind trial of perioperative intravenous metronidazole prophylaxis for abdominal and vaginal hysterectomy. In: Rhône-Poulenc Pharma Inc, Montreal. Proceedings of the North American Metronidazole Symposium on Anaerobic Infections, Scottsdale, AZ, October 1981. Surgery. 1983;93:185.
51. Keiser TA, MacKenzie RL, Feld R, et al. Prophylactic metronidazole in appendectomy: A double-blind controlled trial. In: Rhône-Poulenc Pharma Inc, Montreal. Proceedings of the North American Metronidazole Symposium on Anaerobic Infections, Scottsdale, AZ, October 1981. Surgery. 1983;93:201.

BIBLIOGRAPHY

Finegold SM, McFadzean JA, Roe FJC, eds. Metronidazole. Proceedings of the International Metronidazole Conference, Montreal, May 1976. Princeton, NJ: Excerpta Medica; 1977.
Finegold SM. Metronidazole. Ann Intern Med. 1980;93:585.
Finegold SM, George WL, Rolfe RD, eds. Proceedings of the First United States Metronidazole Conference, Tarpon Springs, FL, February 1982. New York: Biomedical Information Corp; 1982.
Kucers A, Bennett N McK, Kemp RJ, eds. Metronidazole. In: The Use of Antibiotics. Philadelphia: JB Lippincott; 1987.
May & Baker, Ltd. "Flagyl" (Metronidazole) in Anaerobic Infections. Essex, England: May & Baker, Ltd; 1979.
Phillips I, Collier J, eds. Metronidazole. Proceedings of the Second International Symposium on Anaerobic Infections, Geneva, April 1979. London: The Royal Society of Medicine and Academic Press; New York: Grune & Stratton 1979.
Rhône-Poulenc Pharma Inc., Montreal. Proceedings of the North American Metronidazole Symposium on Anaerobic Infections, Scottsdale, AZ, October 1981. Surgery. 1983;93:123.
Rosenblatt JE, Edson RS. Metronidazole. Mayo Clin Proc. 1987;62:1013–17.
Stranz MH, Bradley WE. Metronidazole (Flagyl IV, Searle). Drug Intell Clin Pharm. 1981;15:838.

26. ERYTHROMYCIN, LINCOMYCIN, AND CLINDAMYCIN

NEAL H. STEIGBIGEL

Erythromycin and the lincosamide antibiotics, lincomycin and clindamycin, are chemically unrelated but possess similar biologic properties in terms of mechanisms of action and resistance, antimicrobial activity, and clinical pharmacology. Erythromycin, currently the most important of the macrolide antibiotics, has a few primary indications in therapy and is often useful as an alternative to penicillin G. It is one of the safest antibiotics in clinical use. Clindamycin has been restricted in use by its potential gastrointestinal toxicity but remains particularly important in the treatment of certain anaerobic infections. Lincomycin is now mainly of historic interest.

ERYTHROMYCIN

Derivation, Chemistry, and Preparations

Erythromycin was derived in 1952 from a strain of *Streptomyces erythreus* obtained from soil from the Philippines. The structure (Fig. 1) consists of a 14-membered macrocyclic lactone ring, therefore the class name *macrolide*, attached to two sugar moities. Erythromycin base is poorly soluble in water, has a pK of 8.8, is rapidly inactivated by gastric acid, and is often inconsistently absorbed after oral administration. Pharmaceutical preparations for oral use have been made with an aim to diminish destruction by gastric acid and to promote better absorption. Six preparations for oral use are available: enteric-coated tablets (Ilotycin, E-mycin, Ery-Tab, Robimycin, and generics), enteric-coated pellets in capsules (Eryc), and "film"-coated (Filmtab, Abbott) tablets of the base; stearate salt (formed in association with the amino group on desosamine) and available as film-coated tablets (Erythrocin, Bristamycin, other brand names, and generics); ethylsuccinate ester (formed with the hydroxyl group on desosamine), available in tablet, chewable, and liquid forms (Erythrocin, Eryped, EES, Pediamycin); and lauryl sulfate salt of the propionyl ester (the estolate), available in tablet, capsule, or liquid forms (Ilosone). There are two water-soluble salts of erythromycin prepared for intravenous use, erythromycin gluceptate (Ilotycin gluceptate) and erythromycin lactobionate (Erythrocin lactobionate). The drug is not given intramuscularly because of pain on injection. Erythromycin base is also available in 1.5 and 2 percent topical solutions, gels, and creams for treatment of acne vulgaris and in an ophthalmic ointment for treatment of bacterial conjunc-

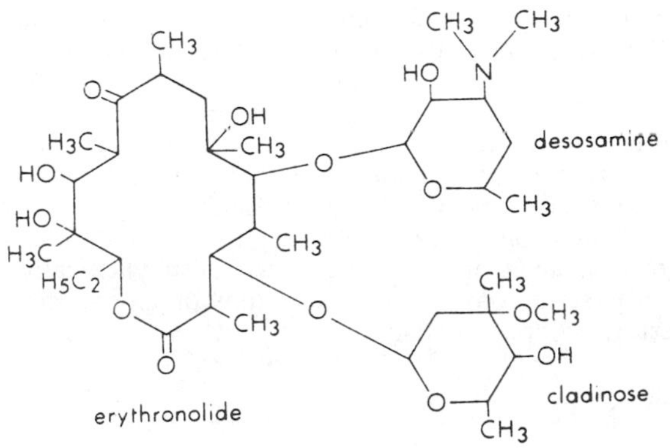

FIG. 1. Erythromycin base.

tivitis and prevention of neonatal gonococcal and chlamydial conjunctivitis.

Mechanisms of Action

Erythromycin inhibits RNA-dependent protein synthesis at the step of chain elongation in susceptible prokaryotic organisms. A single molecule of the antibiotic reversibly binds to the 50S ribosomal subunit, resulting in blockage of the transpeptidation and/or translocation reactions.[1–3] In some bacteria erythromycin interferes with the ribosomal binding of other macrolides, lincomycin, and chloramphenicol, suggesting common or overlapping binding sites for these antibiotics.

Antimicrobial Activity and Mechanisms of Resistance

The antimicrobial activity of erythromycin is broad in spectrum, being exhibited against gram-positive and gram-negative bacteria, including actinomycetes and mycobacteria, as well as against treponemes, mycoplasmas, *Chlamydia*, and rickettsia. Depending on the drug concentration, bacterial species, phase of growth, and density of the inoculum, erythromycin may be primarily bacteriostatic or bactericidal. Bacterial killing is favored by higher antibiotic concentrations, lower bacterial density, and rapid growth.[4] The activity of erythromycin, which is a weak base, increases markedly with increasing pH over the range 5.5–8.5, for both gram-positive and gram-negative bacteria,[5,6] possibly reflecting increased entry into the bacterial cell of the un-ionized drug that is more plentiful at the higher pH.

The in vitro susceptibilities of potential pathogens to erythromycin are listed in Table 1.[7–13] Erythromycin shows high activity against pneumococci and group A streptococci, although occasional resistant clinical isolates have been encountered, especially from patient populations recently exposed to erythromycin or lincomycin.[14,15] Of 200 strains of *Streptococcus pneumoniae* isolated from patients with pneumococcal disease in a survey conducted in Spain, 5 were found to be highly resistant to erythromycin and clindamycin.[16] In a study in Japan, 60 percent of strains of group A streptococci isolated from infected children were highly resistant to erythromycin and lincomycin.[17] Almost all of these resistant strains were of type 12, and erythromcyin had been widely used to treat respiratory infections in Japan in the several years before the study. A survey of 474 group A streptococcal strains isolated from patients in Oklahoma in 1980 indicated that 5 percent had minimal inhibitory concentrations (MIC) to erythromycin by microtiter broth dilution ≥ 1 μg/ml.[18] The emergence of resistance to erythromycin encountered in clinical isolates of these organisms from patient populations treated with this antibiotic is consistent with in vitro studies with pneumococci and streptococci subcultured sequentially in the presence of erythromycin, demonstrating the selection of erythromycin resistance and often cross-resistance to other macrolides and lincomycin. Similar in vitro results are obtained with staphylococci.[19] Although resistance to erythromycin by *Staphylococcus aureus* may be selected by its use in hospitals,[20] most clinical isolates are presently sensitive, to this agent. However, there is always a potential for the emergence, during treatment in an individual patient, of erythromycin resistance by *S. aureus*.[7,19,21,22] These strains may demonstrate the emergence of one-step high-level resistance to erythromycin alone or may show cross-resistance to other macrolides and to lincomycin and clindamycin. In addition, staphylococci isolated from patients treated with erythromycin may exhibit a phenomenon called *dissociated resistance* by Garrod.[23] Only a small proportion of the population of such staphylococcal isolates exhibit resistance when grown in large concentrations of erythromycin; however, in the presence of lower concentrations of erythromycin almost the entire population demonstrates resistance to erythromycin, to other macrolides, and to the lincosamide antibiotics. In the absence of erythromycin these organisms appear sensitive to these antibiotics.

TABLE 1. In Vitro Susceptibilities to Erythromycin

	Minimum Inhibitory Concentration (μg/ml)	
Organism	Range	Median
S. pneumoniae	0.001–0.2[a]	0.05
S. pyogenes	0.005–0.2[a]	0.04
S. "viridans"	0.02–3.1[a]	0.06
Enterococcus	0.1–>100	1.5
S. aureus	0.005–>100	0.4
S. epidermidis	0.2–>100	0.6
C. diphtheriae	0.006–3.1[a]	0.02
C. perfringens	0.1–6[a]	0.8
L. monocytogenes	0.1–0.3	0.2
B. pertussis	0.02–1.6	0.3
N. gonorrhoeae	0.005–0.4[a]	0.1
N. meningitidis	0.1–1.6	0.4
H. influenzae	0.1–6	3.1
C. jejuni	0.05–>50	0.2
B. fragilis	0.1–>100	≤0.25
L. pneumophila	0.06–0.5	0.1
M. pneumoniae	0.001–0.02	0.005
C. trachomatis	0.1–0.5	0.1
B. catarrhalis	0.03–0.125	0.07

[a] Occasional clinical isolates are more resistant.

The majority of strains of the "viridans" group of streptococci, *Listeria monocytogenes*, and *Corynebacterium diphtheriae* show appreciable susceptibility to erthromycin. Many strains of *Clostridium perfringens* may be only moderately sensitive.[24] Appreciable in vitro activity has been demonstrated against *Actinomyces israelii*, *Mycobacterium scrofulaceum*, and *Mycobacterium kansasii*,[25] and against *Nocardia asteroides* when combined with ampicillin.[26]

With gram-negative bacteria, erythromycin displays consistent and useful activity against *Neisseria meningitidis*, *Neisseria gonorrhoeae*, and *Bordetella pertussis*[8] and somewhat lower activity against *Haemophilus influenzae*.[27] High bacteriostatic and bactericidal activity is demonstrated against over 90 percent of strains of *Campylobacter jejuni*.[10] Erythromycin has activity against some species of gram-negative anaerobes, but *Bacteroides fragilis* strains are usually resistant.[28] The Enterobacteriaceae are usually resistant, except as the pH rises to 8.5.[6]

The extensive spectrum of activity of erythromycin is also demonstrated by its clinically useful activity against such diverse organisms as *Treponema pallidium*, *Legionella pneumophila*,[9] *Mycoplasma pneumoniae*, *Ureaplasma urealyticum*, some strains of *Rickettsia*, and *Chlamydia trachomatis*. Erythromycin is about 50 times more potent against *M. pneumoniae* than tetracycline.[29] Erythromycin-resistant variants of *M. pneumoniae* have been isolated in the laboratory and from a patient.[30]

Resistance to erythromycin may be the result of the following: (*1*) Decreased permeability of the cell envelope to the drug is exhibited by the Enterobacteriaceae; cell-free systems and protoplasts of these organisms are susceptible to the drug.[31,32] Plasmid-mediated erythromycin resistance in *S. epidermidis* due to decreased permeability to the drug has also been described.[33] (*2*) Alteration in a single 50S ribosomal protein of the receptor site confers resistance to erythromycin and often to other macrolides, lincomycin, and clindamycin; in some but not all strains this is associated with a decreased binding affinity for erythromycin.[2] This one-step high-level resistance is the result of chromosomal mutation, has been demonstrated in some strains of *Bacillus subtilis*, *Streptococcus pyogenes*, and *Escherichia coli* and probably occurs in *S. aureus*. (*3*) Alteration in the 23S ribosomal RNA of the 50S ribosomal subunit by methylation of adenine.[34–37] This is associated with resistance to erythromycin and often to other macrolides (M), lincocasamides (L, lincomycin and clindamycin), and streptogramin type B (S_B); this pattern of resistance is referred to as the MLS_B

phenotype. The resistance is due to decreased binding of the antibiotics to their targets on the ribosome and is usually mediated by a plasmid. It can be exhibited by strains of *S. aureus*, streptococci (including *S. pneumoniae*), *C. diphtheriae, B. fragilis, C. perfringens*, *Listeria* species, and *Legionella* species.[38] This phenomenon may be constitutive or inducible by subinhibitory concentrations of erythromycin that bring about induction of the methylating enzyme. The inducible mechanism seems to explain the phenomenon of dissociated resistance already described. Several determinants of MLS_B resistance have been defined,[39,40] including the erm A, erm B, and erm C genes, which occupy plasmids in *S. aureus*. The nucleotide sequence of erm A has been determined.[41] (*4*) Inactivation of erythromycin by enzymatic hydrolysis brought about by strains of Enterobacteriaceae with high-level resistance has been demonstrated.[42] These organisms possess an erythromycin esterase encoded by a plasmid-mediated determinant.[43]

Clinical Pharmacology

The peak serum levels obtained after single doses of various erythromycin preparations are given in Table 2.[7,8,28,44,45] Erythromycin base is subject to destruction by gastric acid, and preparations of the base have been made with an acid-resistant coating to delay drug dissolution until it reaches the small bowel. The esters and ester salts of erythromycin are more acid stabile, form a stable suspension in water, and are tasteless. These characteristics are used in the liquid suspensions for children. Erythromycin base (absorbed intact), stearate (absorbed as the base), and ethylsuccinate (absorbed both as the intact ester and as the free base after hydrolysis in the intestine) are usually absorbed more completely in the fasting state, although one study demonstrated increased absorption of a stearate preparation when taken with a meal.[45] After absorption, about 45 percent of the ethylsuccinate preparation is present in the serum as the inactive ester and about 55 percent as the active base. Average serum levels achieved under fasting conditions with these preparations are similar; however, results with the base may be erratic. Erythromycin base has become available in a capsule containing enteric-coated granules; this preparation is promoted as giving more uniform absorption,[46,48] but some enteric-coated tablets may provide similar blood levels.[47] The absorption of the estolate is not affected by food, and the resulting peak serum level consists of both free base (20–30 percent) (active form) and estolate (70–80 percent) (much less active); the level of base thus achieved is similar to that achieved by the other oral preparations taken in comparable doses in the fasting state. The clinical significance of the much less active esterified form of the drug that is present in serum in appreciable concentration is controversial. It would seem that in treatment of infections of only moderate severity by organisms highly sensitive to erythromycin (*S. pneumoniae*, *S. pyogenes*, *M. pneumoniae*), differences in therapeutic results using the various oral preparations will be insignificant. Limited clinical comparisons confirm that suspicion.[49] However, in the treatment of group A streptococcal pharyngitis in children, substantially higher rates of bacteriologic eradication and lower rates of gastrointestinal side effects have been reported with the estolate preparation in comparison with the ethylsuccinate formulation.[50] Intravenous preparations of erythromycin achieve appreciably higher serum levels and should be used to treat serious infections requiring erythromycin.

Erythromycin is distributed through total body water.[51] Values given for protein binding vary from 40 to 90 percent; however, the significance of such binding is speculative.[52] The drug persists in tissues longer than in the blood. The ratios of tissue or body fluid concentrations to simultaneous serum concentrations (usually at peak) are for aqueous humor, 0.3; ascites, 0.4; bile, 28; middle ear exudate in otitis media, 0.3–0.7; pleural fluid, 0.7; prostatic fluid, 0.4; cerebrospinal fluid without meningitis, 0–0.02, with meningitis, 0.05–0.1; infected maxillary paranasal sinus, 0.4–0.8; tonsil, 0.3. Concentrations achieved in the middle ear in otitis media are adequate to treat pneumococcal and group A streptococcal infections but are not adequate to eradicate consistently *H. influenzae*.[53,54] High concentrations of erythromycin are achieved in alveolar macrophages[55] and polymorphonuclear leukocytes[56] compared to those in extracellular fluid.

There are very limited data on concentrations of erythromycin achieved in the cerebrospinal fluid of patients with meningitis, which suggest that large parenteral doses may be effective against meningeal infection by highly susceptible organisms such as *S. pneumoniae*.[57] Limited data from patients with septic arthritis suggest poor penetration of synovial fluid. Erythromycin is transferred across the placenta; fetal serum concentrations are about 2 percent of those in maternal serum, but higher concentrations accumulate in fetal tissue and amniotic fluid.[58] The drug is excreted in breast milk.

Up to 4.5 percent of an oral dose and 15 percent of a parenteral dose of erythromycin are recoverable in the urine.[7,8] Urine concentrations after oral doses are often high, but quite variable. Erythromycin is concentrated by the liver and excreted into the bile in high concentrations; however, only about 1.5 percent of the dose of the base and 0.2 percent of the ester can be recovered in bile in the first 8 hours, and some of this is reabsorbed from the intestine.[59] The higher serum levels achieved by the estolate have been attributed to both better absorption and lower biliary excretion. After an oral dose, large concentrations of the antibiotic are found in feces, probably representing ingested drug that was never absorbed as well as some that was excreted in bile. A large proportion of absorbed drug cannot be accounted for by urinary or biliary excretion or by tissue binding and may be inactivated in the liver by demethylation.[60]

The normal serum half-life of erythromycin is 1.4 hours, and appreciable serum levels are maintained for 6 hours. In anuric patients, the half-life is only prolonged to about 5 hours, and dosage reduction in patients with renal failure is generally therefore not necessary.[61] Erythromycin is not removed by peritoneal dialysis or hemodialysis.

TABLE 2. Serum Levels of Erythromycin in Adults

			Peak Serum Level	
Preparation	*Dose (mg)*	*Route*	*Hours After Dose*	*μg/ml*
Base	250	Oral	4	0.3–1.0[a]
	500			0.3–1.9
Stearate	250 (fasting)	Oral	3	0.2–1.3
	500 (fasting)		3	0.4–1.8
	500 (after food)		3	0.1–0.4[b]
Ethylsuccinate	500	Oral	0.5–2.5	1.5[c] (0.6[d])
Estolate	250	Oral	2–4	1.4–1.7
	500		3.5–4	4.2[c] (1.1[d])
Lactobionate	200	Intravenous	Immediately	3–4
	500		1	9.9
Gluceptate	250	Intravenous	Immediately	3.5–10.7
	1000		1	9.9

[a] Somewhat higher levels reported with some enteric-coated preparations after repeated doses.[46,47]
[b] One study demonstrated higher levels (to 2.8 μg/ml) with dose taken during a meal.[45]
[c] Total drug (inactive ester and free base).
[d] Free base.

ADVERSE REACTIONS

Erythromycin is one of the safest antibiotics in clinical use. Untoward reactions except for pseudomembranous colitis are not life threatening and, with the exception of the irritative reactions, are rare.

1. Irritative reactions are as follows:

a. Dose-related abdominal cramps, nausea, vomiting, and diarrhea occur more commonly in children and young adults than in older individuals and may be associated with intravenous as well as oral administration. These side effects appear to be due to a gastrointestinal motility-stimulating effect of the 14-membered ring macrolides.[62,63]
b. Thrombophlebitis with intravenous use can be decreased by appropriate dilution of the dose in at least 250 ml of solution and by avoiding rapid bolus infusions (infuse over about 45–60 minutes).

2. Allergic reactions include skin rash, fever, and eosinophilia.
3. Cholestatic hepatitis occurs rarely[64] and almost always with the estolate preparation and chiefly in adults.[65] The syndrome typically begins after 10 days of therapy, but more rapidly in those previously treated, and consists of nausea, vomiting, and abdominal pain followed by jaundice, fever, and abnormal liver function tests consistent with cholestatic hepatitis. These findings are sometimes accompanied by rash, leukocytosis, and eosinophilia. The abnormalities generally clear within days to a few weeks after stopping the drug but may return rapidly on rechallenge. The syndrome appears to represent a hypersensitivity reaction to the specific structure of the estolate compound.[66] However, hepatocyte toxicity induced by the drug or its metabolites, as well as allergy to altered hepatocyte components, may be contributory.[67] Milder forms of the syndrome occur with the estolate and may be more common in pregnant women.[68] It must be distinguished from false-positive serum glutamic-oxaloacetic transaminase (SGOT) elevations that occur in patients taking the estolate.[69] The latter may be found when SGOT is determined by colorimetric procedures rather than by an enzymatic method and seems to result from an interfering substance present in the blood in association with estolate administration. Reversible hepatotoxicity has occurred with the stearate salt and the ethylsuccinate ester of erythromycin.[70,71]
4. Transient hearing loss has been reported very rarely in association with the use of large intravenous doses of erythromycin lactobionate or large doses of oral erythromycin.[72,73] This may occur more commonly in elderly patients with renal insufficiency.[74–76]
5. Hypertrophic pyloric stenosis developed in five infants during administration of erythromycin estolate.[77]
6. Superinfection, especially of the gastrointestinal tract or vagina, with *Candida* species or gram-negative bacilli may occur, as with other antibiotics.
7. Psudomembranous colitis caused by overgrowth of toxin-producing *Clostridium difficile* occurs rarely with the use of erythromycin.[78,79]

Drug Interactions

Incompatibility during administration between intravenous preparations of erythromycin and other drugs has been reported; the latter include vitamin B complex and vitamin C, cephalothin, tetracycline, chloramphenicol, colistin, heparin, metraminol, and diphenylhydantoin. Erythromycin may produce interactions with other drugs by interfering with their hepatic metabolism through the cytochrome P-450 enzyme system.[80] When oral theophylline and oral erythromycin are used concurrently, increased blood levels of theophylline and potential theophylline toxicity may result.[81] By the same mechanism, erythromycin can increase the anticoagulant effect of warfarin[82] and interfere with the metabolism of methylprednisolone,[83] carbamazapine,[84] and cyclosporine,[85] sometimes leading to toxicity with the latter two drugs. Erythromycin can increase the bioavailability of digoxin by interfering with its inactivation by gut flora.[80] Erythromycin may inhibit the assay organism used in some determinations of serum folic acid. Sequential use of erythromycin and clindamycin should be avoided when possible because of the potential for the development of cross or "dissociated" resistance.

Uses of Erythromycin

Erythromycin has a few indications for use as the drug of choice and a larger number of important applications as an alternative drug to penicillin G (Table 3).[86] When used in adults by the oral route, preparations other than the estolate are generally preferable because they have less risk of cholestatic hepatitis. Absorption, particularly with the enteric-coated base, stearate, or ethylsuccinate preparations taken in the fasting state or before meals, is usually adequate. The estolate preparation should be particularly avoided during pregnancy, when hepatotoxicity may be more common.[68] When higher serum levels are needed in more severe infections requiring erythromycin therapy, the drug should be given intravenously.

Treatment of *M. pneumoniae* infection with erythromycin, as with tetracycline, shortens the clinical course of the infection; radiologic clearing of pulmonary lesions occurs earlier with erythromycin.[87] Clinical experience and studies in vitro and in guinea pigs suggest that erythromycin is the most active available agent in treating pneumonia caused by L. pneumophila or *L. micdadei*.[9,88,89] Erythromycin treatment of patients with gastroenteritis caused by *C. jejuni* hastens the eradication of the organism from the feces, but it does not appear to alter the clinical course of uncomplicated infection when therapy begins 4 days or more after the onset of symptoms.[90] However, earlier treatment of young children with acute dysentery associated with *C. jejuni* has recently been shown to shorten the course of diarrhea and fecal excretion of the organism.[91] Nevertheless, in an institutional setting in Thailand where *C. jejuni* strains were frequently resistant to erythromycin in vitro, early treatment of infants with diarrhea due to this organism was not beneficial.[92] Treatment of infants with erythromycin for pneumonia due to *C. trachomatis* appears to speed recovery and eradication of the shedding of organisms.[93] Erythromycin is preferable to tetracycline in treating chlamydial pelvic infection during pregnancy.[86] Erythromycin base given orally together with neomycin on the day before colorectal surgery and combined with vigorous purgation is about as effective as parenteral cephalosporin administration just before surgery in decreasing the incidence of septic complications.[94] However, in the presence of bowel obstruction or when there is need for emergency surgery, the parenteral antibiotic regimen should be used.[86] The results of treating syphilis with erythromycin during pregnancy must be considered uncertain at best; fetal syphilis may not be eradicated, and therefore convincing evidence of potentially dangerous penicillin allergy should be obtained before this type of therapy is used.[95] When erythromycin is used to treat syphilis in pregnancy, the infant should be treated with penicillin at birth. Erythromycin may occasionally be useful in treating urinary tract infections due to gram-negative bacilli that might otherwise require the use of more toxic agents.[96] Urine pH must generally be raised to 8.0 or above to achieve effective activity at urinary concentrations against the gram-negative bacilli. Erythromycin may be used as an alternative antibiotic in the treatment of anthrax and in infections by *B. catarrhalis, E. corrodens,* and *L. monocytogenes*. Erythromycin is not consistently effective in treatment of infections due to *H. influenzae*,[53,54] and in vitro studies suggest resistance by some strains of *C. perfringens*.[24] In view of the availability of more effective alternative drugs, erythromycin should not be used alone in the treatment of deep-seated staphylococcal infections because of the potential for the emergence of resistant strains during therapy.[19,21,22] Experimental studies and limited clinical data suggest that erythromycin combined with a penicillin may demonstrate synergy[21,97] against S. aureus; further studies are needed to exploit the potential in therapy.

TABLE 3. Major Uses of Erythromycin

Indication	*Doses of Erythromycin for Adults*	*Alternative Drug*
Infection in which erythromycin is the drug of first choice		
M. pneumoniae infections	0.5 g tid-qid po[a]	Tetracycline
Legionella pneumonia	0.5–1.0 g qid po[a]	Rifampin + erythromycin
Diphtheria[b]	Carrier state: 500 mg qid po for 10 days	Penicillin G
	Disease:[a] followed by oral for 10 days	Penicillin G
Pertussis	0.5 g qid po	Ampicillin
Chl. trachomatis pneumonia or conjunctivitis	10 mg/kg qid po[a]	Trimethoprim-sulfamethoxazole
Chlamydial pelvic infection in pregnancy	0.5–1.0 g qid po[a,c]	Sulfisoxazole
C. jejuni gastroenteritis	250 mg qid po	Ciprofloxacin
Prevention of infection after colorectal surgery	1 g po each of neomycin and erythromycin base at 1, 2, and 11 P.M. on the day before surgery combined with vigorous purgation over the 2 days before surgery	Parenteral cephalosporin
Infections in which erythromycin is an important alternative drug		*Drug of first choice*
Groups A, C, C, G streptococcal infection	250–500 mg qid po[a,d]	Penicillin G
S. pneumoniae infection	250–500 mg qid po[a]	Penicillin G
Rheumatic fever prophylaxis	250 mg bid po	Penicillin G
Prevention of bacterial endocarditis (in dental procedures)	1.0 g po 2 hr before procedure, then 500 mg 6 hr later	Penicillin V
Lymphogranuloma venereum	500 mg qid po for 21 days	Tetracycline
Chancroid	500 mg qid po for 7 days	Ceftriaxone
Nongonococcal urethritis	500 mg qid po for 7 days	Tetracycline
Syphilis 1°, 2°, latent (<1 yr) in pregnancy	500 mg qid po for 15 days[e]	Penicillin G
latent (>1 yr) in pregnancy	500 mg qid po for 30 days[e]	Penicillin G
Bronchopulmonary anaerobic infections	0.5 gm qid po	Penicillin G; clindamycin
Acne vulgaris	250 mg qid po or topical preparation	Tetracycline po and a number of topical drugs
Urinary tract infection	500 mg qid po[f]	Many agents

[a] Intravenous therapy (2–4 g/day) should be used in serious illness or when oral therapy is not possible or reliable.
[b] Antitoxin is essential primary therapy for disease.
[c] Severe pelvic inflammatory disease is often polymicrobial in origin; treatment of such cases should include other agents more active against likely facultative and anaerobic enteric bacteria and/or *N. gonorrhoeae*.
[d] Treatment should be continued for 10 days for Group A.
[e] Effectiveness uncertain. Careful follow-up needed when used in pregnancy. Infants should be treated with penicillin at birth.
[f] Urine pH must be raised to greater than 8 with sodium bicarbonate.

Other Macrolides

Trioleandomycin, an ester of the 14-membered ring macrolide oleandomycin, has no advantages over erythromycin and may occasionally cause cholestatic hepatitis. Spiramycin, a 16-membered ring macrolide, has been reported to have some effectiveness in the treatment of diarrhea due to cryptosporidium[98] and in toxoplasmosis,[99] but confirmation of its effectiveness is needed.

Several investigational macrolides are of current interest. Clarithromycin (A-56268) (TE-031) (Abbott Laboratories) is a 6-0-methyl derivative of erythromycin with in vitro antibacterial activity equal to or slightly greater than that of erythromycin.[100] Roxithromycin (RU-28965) (Roussel) is an ether oxime derivative of erythromycin with somewhat less in vitro antibacterial activity than erythromycin, but with a longer half-life, which may allow twice daily oral dosing.[100,101] Azithromycin (CP 62,993) (Pfizer Laboratories) is a 15-membered ring macrolide differing from erythromycin by having a methyl-substituted nitrogen in the macrolide ring. Compared to erythromycin, it is somewhat less active in vitro against gram-positive bacteria, substantially more active against *H. influenzae*, and generally somewhat more active against *B. catarrahalis, N. gonorrhoeae,* and *Campylobacter* species.[100,102] Azithromycin also shows promising activity against *T. gondii* in mouse protection studies involving both intraperitoneal and intracerebral infections.[103] It shows more stability to gastric acid, a longer half-life, and increased concentrations in tissues compared to erythromycin.[104]

LINCOMYCIN AND CLINDAMYCIN

Derivation, Chemistry, and Preparations

Lincomycin was isolated in 1962 from an organism, *Streptomyces lincolnensis*, obtained from soil near Lincoln, Nebraska. Its biologic properties are similar to those of erythromycin, but it is chemically unrelated, consisting of an amino acid linked to an amino sugar (Fig. 2). Chemical modification provided clindamycin (7-chloro-7-deoxy-lincomycin) (Fig. 2) with increased antibacterial potency and absorption after oral administration.[105] Since there are no therapeutic advantages for lincomycin over clindamycin, the discussion will concentrate on the latter, although both are still marketed as pharmaceuticals. Both are weak bases that are readily water soluble when provided as salts.

Lincomycin (Lincocin) is available as the hydrochloride salt in 250- and 500-mg capsules and syrup for oral administration and in solution (300 mg/ml) for parenteral use. Clindamycin (Cleocin) is prepared as the hydrochloride salt of the base in 75- and 150-mg capsules and of the palmitate ester for pediatric suspension. It is supplied as the phosphate ester for intramuscular or intravenous use (150 mg/ml). It is also available in a topical solution for the treatment of acne vulgaris.

Mechanisms of Action

The lincosamide antibiotics have, in susceptible organisms, the same or overlapping 50S ribosomal binding sites as those for the macrolides and chloramphenicol, and they may compete with these drugs for binding.[2,3] Protein synthesis is inhibited primarily in early chain elongation by interference with the transpeptidation reaction.[1,3]

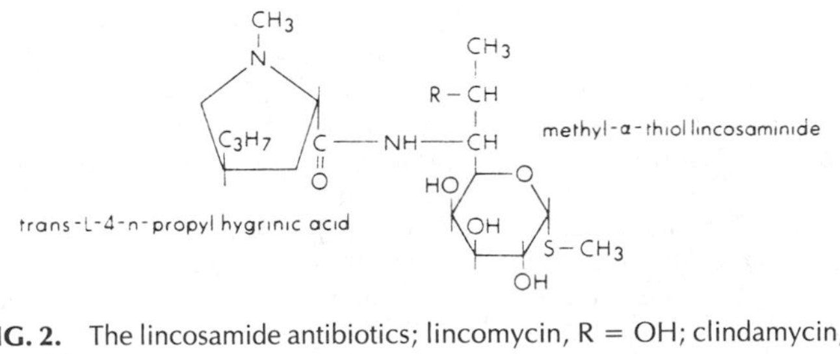

FIG. 2. The lincosamide antibiotics; lincomycin, R = OH; clindamycin, R = Cl.

Antimicrobial Activity and Mechanisms of Resistance

In vitro susceptibilities to clindamycin are given in Table 4.[7,12,105,106] Clindamycin is more potent than lincomycin but similar in degree of activity to erythromycin against staphylococci, pneumococci, *S. pyogenes,* and streptococci of the "viridans" group. However, while erythromycin demonstrates at least moderate activity against the enterococcus, *H. influenzae,* and *N. meningitidis,* clindamycin is generally inactive against these organisms at clinically achievable concentrations. In contrast, clindamycin shows significantly greater activity than erythromycin against most clinically significant anaerobic bacteria, particularly *B. fragilis*[107,108] and some erythromycin-resistant strains of *S. aureus.*[109] Clindamycin is one of the most active antibiotics available against *B. fragilis.* In a survey of nine hospitals in the United States that provided 750 strains of the *B. fragilis* group in 1981, 6 percent of isolates were resistant to clindamycin (MIC > 4 μg/ml by an agar dilution method); this represented 0–13 percent of strains in individual institutions.[12] In a similar survey by the same group involving eight centers and 678 isolates of the *B. fragilis* group collected in 1984 and 1985, 5 percent were resistant to clindamycin, representing 0–10 percent of the strains in individual institutions.[106] Of the species belonging to the *B. fragilis* group, clindamycin resistance was found in 5 percent of *B. fragilis,* 10 percent of *Bacteroides thetaiotaomicron,* 15 percent of *B. vulgatus,* 6 percent of *B. distasonis,* and 7 percent of *B. ovatus.*[106] Resistance to clindamycin by anaerobes also includes 10–20 percent of clostridial species other than *C. perfringens,* about 10 percent of peptococci, and most *Fusobacterium varium* strains.[107,108] All the Enterobacteriaceae are resistant to clindamycin.

There have been occasional reports of clinical isolates of lincosamide-resistant *S. pneumoniae,*[15,16] *S. pyogenes,*[14,17] and "viridans" group streptococci; these strains are usually also resistant to erythromycin. In most hospitals at present, the majority of isolates of *S. aureus* are sensitive to lincomycin or clindamycin[108]; however, resistance occurs in 15–20 percent of strains.[110] Lincomycin resistance has been reported in 20 percent of methicillin-resistant strains[111] and in 50 percent of erythromycin-resistant strains[112] of *S. aureus.* Cross resistance of *S. aureus* between lincomycin and clindamycin is complete. The minimal inhibitory concentrations of clindamycin and erythromycin in vitro are generally similar for *S. aureus* strains that are sensitive to both agents; however, resistance can be selected in vitro by serial subculture in the presence of subinhibitory concentrations of either, and it occurs slowly for clindamycin and more rapidly for erythromycin.[109,113] In contrast, strains that are sensitive to clindamycin and resistant to erythromycin can be rapidly selected for clindamycin resistance by serial subculture on clindamycin. Consistent with these in vitro observations, the emergence of clindamycin-resistant *S. aureus* has been noted in clindamycin-treated patients, in particular when the organisms had demonstrated erythromycin resistance at the onset of treatment.[109] Clindamycin resistance, often crossing to erythromycin, has also emerged from treated patients infected with *S. aureus* that were initially sensitive to erythromycin.[114] Resistance of the "dissociated" type may also emerge during treatment of patients.[113]

TABLE 4. In Vitro Susceptibilities to Clindamycin

Organism	Minimum Inhibitory Concentration (μg/ml) Range	Median
S. pneumoniae	0.002–0.04[a]	0.01
S. pyogenes	0.02–0.1[a]	0.04
S. viridans	0.005–0.04[a]	0.02
Enterococcus	12.5–>100	100
S. aureus	0.04–>100	0.1
S. epidermidis	0.1–>100	0.1
C. perfringens	<0.1–8	0.8
N. gonorrhoeae	0.01–6.3	3.1
N. meningitidis	6.3–25	12.5
H. influenzae	0.4–50	12.5
B. fragilis group	<0.125–>256	0.25
B. melaninogenicus	≤0.1–1	≤0.1
Fusobacterium spp.	≤0.5[a]	≤0.5
Peptococcus spp.	≤0.1–>100	≤0.5
Peptostreptococcus spp.	≤0.1–0.8	≤0.5
M. pneumoniae	1.6–3.1	3.1

[a] Occasional clinical isolates are more resistant.

The antibacterial activity of lincomycin and clindamycin has been shown, in limited in vitro studies, to be bactericidal for *S. pneumoniae, S. pyogenes,* and *S. aureus.* Its killing activity is similar to that of erythromycin and therefore probably varies with the concentration, bacterial species, and inoculum. It is more slowly bactericidal for *S. aureus* than are the penicillins[115] and is inconsistently bactericidal for *B. fragilis.*[116]

Mechanisms of resistance to the lincosamide antibiotics include the following: (*1*) Alteration in a single 50S ribosomal protein of the receptor site confers resistance to erythromycin and often to the lincosamides[2]; this mechanism has already been discussed for erythromycin. (*2*) Alteration in the 23S ribosomal RNA of the 50S ribosomal subunit by methylation of adenine[34–37] has also been discussed. It is usually plasmid mediated and provides the MLS_B type of resistance, which includes that exhibited by some strains of *S. aureus* and *B. fragilis* to clindamycin.[39] (*3*) Inactivation of lincomycin and clindamycin by a few isolates of staphylococci, including *S. aureus,* which possess a 4-lincosamide 0-nucleotidyltransferase that catalyzes the nucleotidylation of the hydroxyl group in position 4 of the antibiotics.[117] This adenylation of the lincosamides is associated with high-level resistance to lincomycin, but clindamycin resistance may not be detected by routine methods. The adenylation of clindamycin is associated with impaired bactericidal activity and decreased activity at high inoculum levels. The nucleotide sequences of the plasmid-mediated genes, lin A and lin A′, which encode for the inactivating enzymes, have been determined.

Clinical Pharmacology

Peak serum levels achieved after oral administration of clindamycin occur earlier and are at least twice as high as those of lincomycin. Absorption of clindamycin is about 90 percent and is slightly delayed, but not decreased, by ingestion of food, whereas that of lincomycin is markedly decreased.[105] Mean peak serum concentrations of clindamycin in adults after single oral doses of 150 and 300 mg occur at 1 hour and are 2.5 and 3.6 μg/ml, respectively; at 6 hours they are 0.7 and 1.1 μg/ml, respectively. The esters, clindamycin palmitate in suspension for oral use and clindamycin phosphate for parenteral use, are absorbed as the inactive ester and rapidly hydrolyzed in the blood to the active base. After intramuscular administration, which causes little pain, mean peak serum levels are reached in 3 hours and are about 6 μg/ml after a 300-mg dose and 9 μg/ml after a 600-mg dose; at 12 hours they are 0.7 and 0.9 μg/ml, respectively.[118] In adult healthy volunteers, immediately following 20–45-minute intravenous infusions of 600, 900, or 1200 mg of clindamycin phosphate, serum levels of base are 10, 11, and 14 μg/ml, respectively. Higher levels after intravenous infusion have been reported in infected patients under treatment.[119] Dose regimens of intravenous clindamycin using 900 mg every 8 hours or 600 mg every 6 hours are considered acceptable.[120]

Limited studies have demonstrated good penetration of most tissues by the lincosamides excepting clinically insignificant entry of clindamycin into the cerebrospinal fluid, even with meningitis.[7,121] The concentration in bone in relationship to serum levels is particularly high.[122] Clindamycin administered to pregnant women readily passes the placental barrier and enters fetal blood and tissues.[58] Clindamycin is actively transported into polymorphonuclear leukocytes and macrophages[123] and is present in relatively high concentrations, compared to peak serum levels, in experimental abscesses.[124]

The normal half-life of clindamycin is 2.4 hours. Most of the absorbed drug is metabolized, probably by the liver, to products with variable antibacterial activity, including *N*-demethyl-clindamycin (more active than the parent compound) and clindamycin sulfoxide (less active), which have been detected in bile and urine but not in serum.[118] High bioactivity is found in bile, mostly as the *N*-demethyl metabolite; this represents a minor route of excretion and accounts for the activity assayed in feces after parenteral administration.[118,125] Clindamycin activity in feces persists for at least 5 days after 48 hours of parenteral administration and is associated with a major reduction in the population of sensitive bacteria in the colon lasting for up to 14 days.[126] Clindamycin concentration in bile is markedly diminished or absent when the common bile duct is obstructed.[127] High clindamycin bioactivity, also mostly in the *N*-demethyl form, is found in the urine and persists for up to 4 days after a single dose, suggesting slow release from tissues.[118] Accurate data on the proportion of absorbed clindamycin that is excreted in the urine are not available because of the variable activity of the metabolites and their unknown proportions in urine.

The half-life of clindamycin is increased from 2.4 to about 6 hours in patients with severe renal failure, and peak blood levels after parenteral administration are about twice those in healthy people.[128] If modified at all, parenteral doses should be halved in such patients. Some prolongation of clindamycin activity in serum is noted in patients with severe liver disease.[129] Appreciable dose modification should be made when there is concomitant severe renal and hepatic disease in the same patient. Neither hemodialysis nor peritoneal dialysis removes significant amounts of clindamycin.

Adverse Reactions

1. Allergic reactions include a variety of rashes, fever, and rare cases of erythema multiforme and anaphylaxis.
2. Diarrhea occurs in up to 20 percent of patients and is more common with oral administration. However, the major toxicity of lincomycin and clindamycin that now appreciably limits their use is the occurrence of pseudomembranous colitis caused by a toxin secreted by *C. difficile* that overgrows in the presence of these antibiotics.[130–132] This has been reported in 0.01–10 percent of clindamycin-treated patients.[108,133] The syndrome may occur in association with administration of other antibiotics but does so less frequently; it is not related to the dose and may occur after oral or parenteral therapy. The variable incidence of colitis in different reports has been ascribed to different diagnostic methods and the variable epidemiology of *C. difficile*.[108,133] It may begin during or as long as several weeks after a course of lincomycin or clindamycin therapy and is characterized by diarrhea, sometimes bloody, with fever and cramps and the appearance of yellow-white plaques on the colonic mucosa, seen by proctoscopy. The toxin of *C. difficile* can be detected in the stool of nearly all patients with antibiotic-associated pseudomembranous colitis and in about 20 percent of patients with antibiotic-associated diarrhea by a cytotoxicity assay using tissue culture cells.[79,132] The cytotoxic effect can be prevented by neutralization of the toxin in the stool extract with *Clostridium sordelli* antitoxin. The syndrome can be protracted and may end fatally. Prompt cessation of the antibiotic is essential. Use of antiperistaltic drugs should be avoided since they may worsen the condition. Vancomycin given by mouth in doses of 125–500 mg qid is the drug of choice for treatment of this type of pseudomembranous colitis, although oral bacitracin and oral metronidazole may be effective as well.[134,135] Relapse after treatment may occur.
3. Hepatotoxicity: Minor reversible elevation of transaminase levels, unassociated with other evidence of liver abnormality, has been commonly observed in patients receiving clindamycin, especially by the parenteral route. Some of these may have been false-positive reactions associated with colorimetric rather than specific enzymatic measurements.[105] However, rare cases of frank hepatotoxicity, including jaundice associated with hepatocellular damage, have been observed.[136]
4. Isolated cases of reversible neutropenia, thrombocytopenia, and agranulocytosis associated with lincomycin or clindamycin therapy have been reported; their relationship to the antibiotic administration was uncertain.
5. Occasional reports of hypotension, ECG changes, and rarely cardiopulmonary arrest have been reported when large intravenous doses of lincomycin were given rapidly. This has not been reported with clindamycin.
6. Local irritative reactions are rare with these drugs. Intramuscular and intravenous administration is generally well tolerated.

Drug Interactions

Clindamycin may block neuromuscular transmission and may enhance the action of other blocking agents.[137] Clindamycin phosphate in solution is physically incompatible with ampicillin, diphenylhydantoin, barbiturates, aminophylline, calcium gluconate, and magnesium sulfate.

Uses of Clindamycin

The higher activity and absorption properties of clindamycin, along with no greater potential for toxicity, compared with lincomycin, favors the former in all indications for use of these antibiotics. The lincosamides have been used in a variety of infections, often with good effect; however, the appreciation of the potential for serious or even fatal toxicity with pseudomembranous colitis and the availability of safer alternative antibiotics should now generally limit the use of clindamycin to a few indications[86]:

1. Infections that are outside of the central nervous system and are likely to involve *B. fragilis* or other penicillin-resistant anaerobic bacteria. These particularly involve polymicrobial intra-abdominal or gynecologic pelvic infections.[108] Clindamycin is likely to be beneficial where there is spillage of fecal flora associated with tissue damage, as in cases involving bowel damage or perforation. In these situations, studies of experimental animal models and patients with infection suggest that clindamycin decreases the likelihood of abscess formation involving fecal organisms, especially *B. fragilis*.[138,139] In these conditions, clindamycin is administered together with an aminoglycoside, because additional activity is required against Enterobacteriaceae. The beneficial effect of clindamycin in preventing or ameliorating morbidity from fecal abscess formation or other infections appears to be superior to that of penicillin, cephalothin, or aminoglycosides.[138,140] However, in comparative trials of therapy for intra-abdominal or pelvic sepsis, clindamycin, cefoxitin, metronidazole, imipenem, and chloramphenicol have shown similar effectiveness.[108,141] In addition, given its excellent in vitro activity against the *B. fragilis* group,[106] regimens including ticarcillin-clavulanic acid can be expected to give similar clinical results.

Clindamycin may offer no advantage over penicillin G in the treatment of anaerobic bronchopulmonary infections,[142] except that it serves as an alternative in patients allergic to penicillin. However, in a prospective randomized study of 39 patients with community-acquired putrid lung abscess, clindamycin was more effective than penicillin in terms of the time until eradication of fever and fetid sputum and the "overall response" to treatment.[143] The study involved small numbers of patients and had some flaws in the analysis;[144] however, the superiority of clindamycin for some patients was demonstrated and may relate to observations that 15–25 percent of anaerobic pulmonary infections involve β-lactamase-producing strains of *B. fragilis*, *B. melaninogenicus*, *B. ruminicola*, and *B. ureolyticus*, which are resistant to penicillin.[108,144] Clindamycin may therefore be preferable for the treatment of this condition, particularly in seriously ill patients or in those who have responded poorly to penicillin.

2. Clindamycin is useful as an alternative to penicillin in treatment of *C. perfringens* infections.
3. Clindamycin may sometimes be useful as an alternative to a penicillin in the treatment of staphylococcal infections. However, its more limited bactericidal rate for staphylococci compared with that of the penicillins, and particularly the real potential for the emergence of clindamycin-resistant strains in treated patients, are disadvantages. The latter problem, noted especially but not only with erythromycin-resistant strains, appreciably limits its effectiveness in the therapy of deep-seated staphylococcal infections, particularly endocarditis.[114,122] Vancomycin or the cephalosporins are usually better alternatives to the penicillins for the latter. Although high concentrations of clindamycin are achieved in bone, an advantage of clindamycin for the treatment of osteomyelitis in patients has not been established.
4. The topical solution of clindamycin may be used to treat acne vulgaris.[145] However, it should be noted that pseudomembranous colitis associated with the use of topical clindamycin has been reported.[146]
5. Clindamycin has been reported to have some success in treating experimental animals and small numbers of patients with toxoplasmosis of the central nervous system.[147,148] These studies require confirmation in controlled clinical trials.
6. Clindamycin has been reported to be effective in the treatment of falciparum malaria,[149] but its relative place in the treatment of this infection compared to that of other regimens has not been established. It has also been reported to be useful in the treatment of babesiosis[86,150]; it is suggested that clindamycin be used together with quinine for such treatment.[86]
7. Several studies have suggested that the coexistence of β-lactamase-producing *S. aureus* or *Bacteroides* species and group A streptococci may be associated with the failure of penicillin to eradicate the latter, resulting in recurrent tonsillitis. These studies suggest lower recurrence rates when clindamycin is used.[151] Most recurrences of streptococcal pharyngitis are reinfections rather than relapses, and widespread use of clindamycin for this common problem will likely lead to a substantial number of cases of pseudomembranous colitis,[152] as well as selection for clindamycin-resistant strains of group A streptococci.

Doses of clindamycin, for adults depend on the site, severity of the infection, and condition of the patient. Oral doses are usually 150–300 mg every 6 hours and parenteral doses, given every 6–12 hours, usually total 600–2700 mg/day, occasionally higher.

REFERENCES

1. Pestka S. Inhibitors of protein synthesis. In: Weissbach H, Pestka S, eds. Molecular Mechanisms of Protein Biosynthesis. New York: Academic Press; 1977:467.
2. Oleinick NL. The erythromycins. In Corcoran JW, Hahn FE, eds. Mechanism of Action of Antimicrobial and Antitumor Agents. New York: Springer-Verlag; 1975:396.
3. Franklin TJ, Snow GA. Biochemistry of Antimicrobial Action. 3rd ed. London: Chapman and Hall; 1981:128.
4. Haight TH, Finland M. Observations on mode of action of erythromycin. Proc Soc Exp Biol Med. 1952;81:188–93.
5. Haight TH, Finland M. The antibacterial action of erythromycin. Proc Soc Exp Biol Med. 1952;81:175–83.
6. Sabath LD, Gerstein DA, Loder PB, et al. Excretion of erythromycin and its enhanced activity in urine against gram-negative bacilli with alkalinization. J Lab Clin Med. 1968;72:916–23.
7. Garrod LP, Lambert HP, O'Grady F. Antibiotic and Chemotherapy. 5th ed. Edinburgh: Churchill Livingstone; 1981:183.
8. Washington JA II, Wilson WR. Erythromycin: A microbial and clinical perspective after 30 years of clinical use. I. Mayo Clin Proc. 1984;60:189–203; II. 1985;60:271–8.
9. Edelstein PM, Meyer RD. Susceptibility of *Legionella pneumophila* to twenty antimicrobial agents. Antimicrob Agents Chemother. 1980;18:403–8.
10. Vanhoff R, Gordts B, Dierickx R, et al. Bacteriostatic and bactericidal activities of 24 antimicrobial agents against *Campylobacter fetus* subsp. jejuni. Antimicrob Agents Chemother. 1980;18:118–21.
11. Kuo C, Wang S, Grayston T. Antimicrobial activity of several antibiotics and a sulfonamide against *Chlamydia trachomitis* organisms in cell culture. Antimicrob Agents Chemother. 1977;12:80–3.
12. Tally FP, Cuchural GJ, Jacobus NV, et al. Susceptibility of the *Bacteroides fragilis* group in the United States in 1981. Antimicrob Agents Chemother. 1983;23:536–40.
13. Ahmad F, McLeod DT, Croughan MJ, et al. Antimicrobial susceptibility of *Branhamella catarrhalis* isolates from bronchopulmonary infections. Antimicrob Agents Chemother. 1984;26:424–5.
14. Sanders E, Foster MT, Scott D. Group A beta-haemolytic streptococci resistant to erythromycin and lincomycin. N Engl J Med. 1968;278:538–40.
15. Dixon JM: Pneumococcus resistant to erythromycin and lincomycin. Lancet. 1967;1:573.
16. Linares J, Garau J, Dominiquez C, et al. Antibiotic resistance and serotypes of *Streptococcus pneumoniae* from patients with community acquired pneumococcal disease. Antimicrob Agents Chemother. 1983;23:545–7.
17. Maruyama S, Yoshioka H, Fujita K, et al. Sensitivity of group A streptococci to antibiotics. Am J Dis Child. 1979;133:1143–5.
18. Istre GR, Welch DF, Marks MI, et al. Susceptibility of group A beta-hemolytic *Streptococcus* isolates to penicillin and erythromycin. Antimicrob Agents Chemother. 1981;20:244–6.
19. Haight TH, Finland M. Resistance of bacteria to erythromycin. Proc Soc Exp Biol Med. 1952;81:183–8.
20. Lepper MH, Dowling HF, Jackson GG, et al. Effect of antibiotic usage in the hospital on the incidence of antibiotic-resistant strains among personnel carrying staphylococci. J Lab Clin Med. 1953;42:832.
21. Griffith RS, Black HR. Erythromycin. Med Clin North Am. 1970;54:1199–215.
22. Haight TH, Finland M. Laboratory and clinical studies on erythromycin. N Engl J Med. 1952;247:227–32.
23. Garrod LP. The erythromycin group of antibiotics. Br Med J. 1957;2:57–63.
24. Sapico FL, Kwok Y, Sutter V, et al. Standardized antimicrobial disc susceptibility testing of anaerobic bacteria: In vitro susceptibility of *Clostridium perfringens* to nine antibiotics. Antimicrob Agents Chemother. 1972;2:320–5.
25. Molavi A, Weinstein L. In vitro activity of erythromycin against atypical mycobacteria. J Infect Dis. 1971;123:216–9.
26. Finland M, Bach MC, Garner C, et al. Synergistic action of ampicillin against *Nocardia asteroides*: Effect of time of incubation. Antimicrob Agents Chemother. 1974;5:344–53.
27. Fernandes PB, Hardy D, Bailer R, et al. Susceptibility testing of macrolide antibiotics against *Hemophilus influenzae* and correlation of in vitro results with in vivo efficacy in a mouse septicemia model. Antimicrob Agents Chemother. 1987;31:1243–50.
28. Kucers A. Chloramphenicol, erythromycin, vancomycin, tetracyclines. Lancet. 1982;ii:425–9.
29. Jao RL, Finland M. Susceptibility of *Mycoplasma pneumoniae* to 21 antibiotics in vitro. Am J Med Sci. 1967;253:639–50.
30. Niitu Y, Hasegawa S, Kubota H. In vitro development of resistance to erythromycin, other macrolide antibiotics, and lincomycin in *Mycoplasma pneumoniae*. Antimicrob Agents Chemother. 1974;5:513–9.
31. Mao JC-H, Putterman M. Accumulation in gram-positive and gram-negative bacteria as a mechanism of resistance to erythromycin. J Bacteriol. 1968;95:1111–7.
32. Taubeneck U. Susceptibility of *Proteus mirabilis* and its stable L-forms to erythromycin and other macrolides. Nature. 1962;196:195–6.
33. Lampson BC, von David W, Parisi JT. Novel mechanism for plasmid-mediated erythromycin resistance by pNE24 from *Staphylococcus epidermidis*. Antimicrob Agents Chemother. 1986;30:653–8.
34. Weisblum B, Siddhikol C, Lai CJ, et al. Erythromycin inducible resistance in *Staphylococcus aureus*: Requirements for induction. J Bacteriol. 1971;106:835–47.
35. Lai CJ, Weisblum B, Fahnestock SR, et al. Alteration of 23S ribosomal RNA and erythromycin-induced resistance to lincomycin and spiramycin in *Staphylococcus aureus*. J Mol Biol. 1973;74:67–72.
36. Fujisawa Y, Weisblum B. A family of *r*-determinants in *Streptomyces* spp. that specifies inducible resistance to macrolide, lincosamide, and streptogramin type B antibiotics. J Bacteriol. 1981;146:621–31.
37. Lai CJ, Weisblum B. Altered methylation of ribosomal RNA in an erythromycin-resistant strain of *Staphylococcus aureus*. Proc Natl Acad Sci USA. 1971;68:856–60.

38. Dowling JN, McDevitt DA, Pasculle WA. Isolation and preliminary characterization of erythromycin-resistant variants of *Legionella micdadei* and *Legionella pneumophila*. Antimicrob Agents Chemother. 1985;27:272–4.
39. Courvalin P, Ounissi H, Arthur M. Multiplicity of macrolide–lincosamide–streptogramin antibiotic resistance determinants. J Antimicrob Chemother. 1985;16(Suppl A):91–100.
40. Weisblum B. Inducible resistance to macrolides, lincosamides and streptogramin type B antibiotics: The resistance phenotype, its bacteriological diversity and structural elements that regulate expression. A review. J Antimicrob Chemother. 16(Suppl A):726–30.
41. Murphy E. Nucleotide sequence of erm A, a macrolide–lincosamide–streptogramin B determinant in *Staphylococcus aureus*. J Bacteriol. 1985;162(2):633–40.
42. Barthelemy P, Autissier D, Gerbaud G, et al. Enzymatic hydrolysis of erythromycin by a strain of *Escherichia coli*. J Antibiot. 1984;37:1692–6.
43. Ounissi H, Courvalin P. Nucleotide sequence of the gene ere A encoding the erythromycin esterase in *Escherichia coli*. Gene. 1985;35:271–8.
44. Bechtol LD, Stephens VC, Pugh CT, et al. Erythromycin esters: Comparative in-vivo hydrolysis and bioavailability. Curr Ther Res. 1976;20:610–22.
45. Malmborg A. Effect of food on absorption of erythromycin. A study of two derivatives, the stearate and the base. J Antimicrob Chemother. 1979;5:591–9.
46. McDonald PJ, Mather LE, Story MJ. Studies on absorption of a newly developed enteric-coated erythromycin base. J Clin Pharmacol. 1977;17:601–6.
47. DiSanto AR, Chodos DJ. Influence of study design in assessing food effects on absorption of erythromycin base and erythromycin stearate. Antimicrob Agents Chemother. 1981;20:190–6.
48. Yakatan GJ, Rasmussen CE, Feis PJ et al. Bioinequivalence of erythromycin ethylsuccinate and enteric-coated erythromycin pellets following multiple oral doses. J Clin Pharmacol. 1985;25:36–42.
49. Janicki RS, Garnham JC, Worland MC, et al. Comparison of erythromycin ethylsuccinate, stearate and estolate treatments of group A streptococcus infections of the upper respiratory tract. Clin Pediatr (Phila). 1975;14:1098–1107.
50. Ginsburg CM, McCracken GH Jr, Crow SD, et al. Erythromycin therapy for group A streptococcal pharyngitis. Results of a comparative study of the estolate and ethylsuccinate formulation. Am J Dis Child. 1984;138:536–9.
51. Osono T, Umezawa H. Pharmacokinetics of macrolides, lincosamides and streptogramins. J Antimicrob Chemother. 1985;16(Suppl A):151–66.
52. Welling PG. The esters of erythromycin. J Antimicrob Chemother. 1979;5:633–4.
53. Bass JW, Steele RW, Wiebe RA, et al. Erythromycin concentrations in middle ear exudates. Pediatrics. 1971;48:417–22.
54. Howard JE, Nelson JD, Clahsen J, et al. Otitis media of infancy and early childhood. Am J Dis Child. 1976;130:965–70.
55. Hand WL, Corwin RW, Steinberg TH, et al. Uptake of antibiotics by human alveolar macrophages. Am Rev Respir Dis. 1984;129(6):933–7.
56. Miller MF, Martin JR, Johnson P, et al. Erythromycin uptake and accumulation by human polymorphonuclear leukocytes and efficacy of erythromycin in killing ingested *Legionella pneumophila*. J Infect Dis. 1984;149(5):714–8.
57. Romansky MJ, Nasou JP, Davis DS, et al. The treatment of 171 patients with erythromycin, including 132 with bacterial pneumonia. Antibiotics Annual. New York: Medical Encyclopedia; 1956, 1955–1956:48.
58. Phillipson A, Sabath LD, Charles D. Transplacental passage of erythromycin and clindamycin. N Engl J Med. 1973;288:1219–21.
59. Hammond JB, Griffith RS. Factors affecting the absorption and biliary excretion of erythromycin and two of its derivatives in humans. Clin Pharmacol Ther. 1961;2:308–12.
60. Mao JC-H, Tardrew PL. Demethylation of erythromycin by rabbit tissues in vitro. Biochem Pharmacol. 1965;14:1049–58.
61. Kunin CM. A guide to use of antibiotics in patients with renal disease. Ann Intern Med. 1967;67:151–8.
62. Itoh Z, Suzuki T, Nakaya M, et al. Gastrointestinal motor-stimulating activity of macrolide antibiotics and analysis of their side effects on the canine gut. Antimicrob Agents Chemother. 1984;26:863–9.
63. Itoh Z, Suzuki T, Nakaya M, et al. Structure–activity relation among macrolide antibiotics in initiation of interdigestive migrating contractions in the canine gastrointestinal tract. Am J Physiol. 1985;11:G320–5.
64. Inman WHW, Rawson NSB. Erythromycin estolate and jaundice. Br Med J. 1983;286:1954–5.
65. Braun P. Hepatotoxicity of erythromycin. J Infect Dis. 1969;119:300–6.
66. Tolman KG, Sannella JJ, Freston JW. Chemical structure of erythromycin and hepatotoxicity. Ann Intern Med. 1974;81:58–60.
67. Pessayre D, Larrey D, Funck-Brentano C, et al. Drug interactions and hepatitis produced by some macrolide antibiotics. J Antimicrob Chemother. 1985;16(Suppl A):181–94.
68. McCormack WM, George H, Donner A, et al. Hepatotoxicity of erythromycin estolate during pregnancy. Antimicrob Agents Chemother. 1977;12:630–5.
69. Sabath LD, Gerstein DA, Finland M. Serum glutamic oxalacetic transaminase: False elevation during administration of erythromycin. N Engl J Med. 1968;279:1137–9.
70. Sullivan D, Csuka ME, Blanchard B. Erythromycin ethylsuccinate hepatotoxicity. JAMA. 1980;243:1074.
71. Auckenthaler RW, Zwahlen A, Waldvogel FA. Macrolides. In: Peterson, PK, Verhoef J, eds. The Antimicrobial Agents Annual. v. 2. Amsterdam: Elsevier; 1987:120.
72. Karmody CS, Weinstein L. Reversible sensorineural hearing loss with intravenous erythromycin lactobionate. Ann Oral Rhinol Laryngol. 1977;86:9–11.
73. Eckman MR, Johnson T, Riess R. Partial deafness after erythromycin (Letter). N Engl J Med. 1975;292:649.
74. Mery JP, Kanfer A. Ototoxicity of erythromycin in patients with renal insufficiency (Letter). N Engl J Med. 1979;301:944.
75. Taylor R, Schofield IS, Ramos JM, et al. Ototoxicity of erythromycin in peritoneal dialysis patients (Letter). Lancet. 1981;2:935–6.
76. Haydon RC, Thaelin JW, Davis WE. Erythromycin ototoxicity: Analysis and conclusions based on 22 case reports. Otolaryngol Head Neck Surg. 1984;92:678–84.
77. Filippo JA. Infantile hypertrophic pyloric stenosis related to ingestions of erythromycin estolate: A report of five cases. J Pediatr Surg. 1976;11:177–80.
78. Gantz NM, Zawacki JK, Dickerson J, et al. Pseudomembranous colitis associated with erythromycin. Ann Intern Med. 1979;91:866–7.
79. Bartlett JG. Antimicrobial agents implicated in *Clostridium difficile* toxin-associated diarrhea or colitis. Johns Hopkins Med J. 1981;149:6–9.
80. Ludden TM. Pharmacokinetic interactions of the macrolide antibiotics. Clin Pharmacokinet. 1985;10:63–79.
81. Reisz G, Pingleton SK, Melethil S, et al. The effect of erythromycin on theophylline pharmacokinetics in chronic bronchitis. Ann Rev Respir Dis. 1983;127:581–4.
82. Bachmann K, Schwartz JI, Forney R Jr, et al. The effect of erythromycin on the desposition kinetics of warfarin. Pharmacology. 1984;28:171–6.
83. LaForce CF, Szefler SJ, Miller ME, et al. Inhibition of methylprednisolone elimination in the presence of erythromycin therapy. J Allergy Clin Immunol. 1983;72:34–9.
84. Wong YY, Lundden TD, Bell RD. Effect of erythromycin on carbamazepine kinetics. Clin Pharmacol Ther. 1983;33:460–4.
85. Martell R, Heinrichs D, Stiller CR, et al. The effects of erythromycin in patients treated with cyclosporine. Ann Intern Med. 1986;104:660–1.
86. Handbook of Antimicrobial Therapy. The Medical Letter on Drugs and Therapeutics. New Rochelle, NY: Medical Letter; 1988.
87. Rasch JR, Mogabgab WJ. Therapeutic effect of erythromycin on *Mycoplasma pneumoniae* pneumonia. Antimicrob Agents Chemother. 1965;5:693–9.
88. Kirby BD, Synder KM, Myer RD, et al. Legionnaires' disease: Report of sixty-five nosocomially acquired cases and review of the literature. Medicine. 1980;59:188–205.
89. Muder RF, Yu VL, Zuravleff MS. Pneumonia due to the Pittsburgh pneumonia agent: New clinical perspective with a review of the literature. Medicine. 1983;62:120–8.
90. Anders BJ, Lauer BA, Paisley JW, et al. Double-blind placebo controlled trial of erythromycin for treatment of *Campylobacter* enteritis. Lancet. 1982;1:131–2.
91. Salazar-Lindo E, Sack B, Chea-Woo E, et al. Early treatment with erythromycin of *Campylobacter jejuni*-associated dysentery in children. J Pediatr. 1986;109:355–60.
92. Taylor DN, Blaser MJ, Escheverria P. Erythromycin-resistant *Campylobacter* infections in Thailand. Antimicrob Agents Chemother. 1987;31:438–42.
93. Beem MD, Saxon E, Tipple MA. Treatment of chlamydial pneumonia of infancy. Pediatrics. 1979;63:198–203.
94. Clarke JS, Condon RE, Fenton LJ, et al. Preoperative oral antibiotics reduce septic complications of colon operations: Results of prospective randomized, double-blind clinical study. Ann Surg. 1977;186:251–9.
95. Fenton LJ, Light IJ. Congenital syphilis after maternal treatment with erythromycin. Obstet Gynecol. 1976;47:492–4.
96. Zinner SK, Sabath LD, Casey JI, et al. Erythromycin and alkalinization of the urine in treatment of urinary tract infections due to gram-negative bacilli. Lancet. 1971;1:1267–8.
97. Steigbigel RT, Greenman RL, Remington JS. Antibiotic combinations in the treatment of experimental *Staphylococcus aureus* infection. J Infect Dis. 1975;131:245–51.
98. Soave R. Cryptosporidiosis and isosporiasis in patients with AIDS. Infectious Dis Clin North Am. 1988;2:485–92.
99. Chang HR, Pechere J-C. In vitro effects of four macrolides (roxithromycin, spiramycin, azithromycin [CP-62,993], and A-56268) on *Toxoplasma gondii*. Antimicrob Agents Chemother. 1988;32:524–9.
100. Barry AL, Jones RN, Thornsberry C. In vitro activities of azithromycin (CP 62,993), clarithromycin (A-56268; TE-031), erythromycin, roxithromycin, and clindamycin. Antimicrob Agents Chemother. 1988;32:752–4.
101. Puri SK, Lassman HB. Roxithromycin: A pharmacokinetic review of a macrolide. J Antimicrob Chemother. 1987;20(Suppl B):89–100.
102. Retsema J, Girard A, Schelkly W, et al. Spectrum and mode of action of azithromycin (CP62,993), a new 15-membered ring macrolide with improved potency against gram-negative organisms. Antimicrob Agents Chemother. 1987;31:1939–47.
103. Araujo FG, Guptill DR, Remington JS. Azithromycin, a macrolide with potent activity against *Toxoplasma gondii*. Antimicrob Agents Chemother. 1988;32:755–7.
104. Girard AE, Girard D, English AR, et al. Pharmacokinetic and in vivo studies with azithromycin (CP 62,993), a new macrolide with an extended half-life

and excellent tissue distribution. Antimicrob Agents Chemother. 1987;31:1948–54.
105. McGehee RF Jr, Smith CB, Wilcox C, et al. Comparative studies of antibacterial activity in vitro and absorption and excretion of lincomycin and clindamycin. Am J Med Sci. 1968;256:279–92.
106. Cuchural GJ Jr, Tally FP, Jacobus NV, et al. Susceptibility of the *Bacteroides fragilis* group in the United States: Analysis by site of isolation. Antimicrob Agents Chemother. 1988;32:717–22.
107. Sutter VL: In vitro susceptibility of anaerobes: Comparison of clindamycin and other antimicrobial agents. J Infect Dis. 1977;135(Suppl):S7–12.
108. Bartlett JG. Anti-anaerobic antibacterial agents. Lancet. 1982;2:478–81.
109. McGehee RF, Barrett FF, Finland M. Resistance of *Staphylococcus aureus* to lincomycin, clindamycin and erythromycin. Antimicrob Agents Chemother. 1969;1968:392–7.
110. Nunnery AW, Riley HD. Clinical and laboratory studies of lincomycin in children. Antimicrob Agents Chemother–1964;1965:142–6.
111. Barrett FF, McGehee RF Jr, Finland M. Methicillin resistance *Staphylococcus aureus* at Boston City Hospital. N Engl J Med. 1968;279:441–8.
112. Desmyter J, Reybrouck G. Lincomycin sensitivity of erythromycin-resistant staphylococci. Chemotherapia. 1964;9:183–9.
113. Duncan IBR. Development of lincomycin resistance by staphylococci. Antimicrob Agents Chemother–1967. 1968:723–9.
114. Watanakunakorn C. Clindamycin therapy of *Staphylococcus aureus* endocarditis. Clinical relapse and development of resistance to clindamycin, lincomycin and erythromycin. Am J Med. 1976;60:419–25.
115. Sande MA, Johnson ML. Antimicrobial therapy of experimental endocarditis caused by *Staphylococcus aureus*. J Infect Dis. 1975;131:367–75.
116. Nastro LJ, Finegold SM. Bactericidal activity of five antimicrobial agents against *Bacteroides fragilis*. J Infect Dis. 1972;126:104–7.
117. Leclercq R, Brisson-Noel A, Duval J, et al. Phenotypic expression and genetic heterogeneity of lincosamide inactivation in *Staphylococcus* spp. Antimicrob Agents Chemother. 1987;31:1887–91.
118. DeHaan RM, Metzler CM, Schellenberg D, et al. Pharmacokinetic studies of clindamycin phosphate. J Clin Pharmacol. 1973;13:190–209.
119. Fass RJ, Salow S. Clindamycin: Clinical and laboratory evaluations of parenteral therapy. Am J Med Sci. 1972;263:369–82.
120. Townsend RJ, Baker RP. Pharmacokinetic comparison of three clindamycin phosphate dosing schedules. Drug Intell Clin Pharmacol. 1987;21:279–81.
121. Panzer JD, Brown DC, Epstein WL, et al. Clindamycin levels in various body tissues and fluids. J Clin Pharmacol. 1972;12:259–62.
122. Nicholas P, Meyers BR, Levy RN. Concentrations of clindamycin in human bone. Antimicrob Agents Chemother. 1975;8:220–1.
123. Prokesch RC, Hand WL. Antibiotic entry into human polymorphonuclear leukocytes. Antimicrob Agents Chemother. 1982;23:373–80.
124. Joiner KA, Lowe BR, Dzink JL, et al. Antibiotic levels in infected and sterile subcutaneous abscesses in mice. J Infect Dis. 1981;143(3):487–94.
125. McCall CE, Steigbigel NH, Finland M. Lincomycin: Activity in vitro and absorption and excretion in normal young men. Am J Med Sci. 1967;254:144–55.
126. Kager L, Liljeqvist L, Malmborg AS, et al. Effect of clindamycin prophylaxis on the colonic microflora in patients undergoing colorectal surgery. Antimicrob Agents Chemother. 1981;20:736–40.
127. Brown RB, Martyak SN, Barza M, et al. Penetration of clindamycin phosphate into the abnormal human biliary tract. Ann Intern Med. 1976;84:168–70.
128. Joshi A, Stein R. Altered serum clearance of intravenously administered clindamycin phosphate in patients with uremia. J Clin Pharmacol. 1974;14:140–4.
129. Williams DN, Crossley K, Hoffman C, et al. Parenteral clindamycin phosphate: Pharmacology with normal and abnormal liver function and effect on nasal staphylococci. Antimicrob Agents Chemother. 1975;7:153–8.
130. Rifkin GD, Fekety FR, Silva J Jr, et al. Antibiotic-induced colitis: Implication of a toxin neutralized by *Clostridium sordellii* antitoxin. Lancet. 1977;11:1103–6.
131. Bartlett JG, Chang TW, Gurwith M, et al. Antibiotic-associated pseudomembranous colitis due to toxin-producing clostridia. N Engl J Med. 1978;298:531–4.
132. Bartlett JG. Antibiotic-associated pseudomembranous colitis. Rev Infect Dis. 1979;1:530–9.
133. Tedesco FJ. Clindamycin and colitis: A review. J Infect Dis. 1977; 135(Suppl):S95–8.
134. George WL, Rolfe RD, Finegold SM. Treatment and prevention of antimicrobial agent-induced colitis and diarrhea. Gastroenterology. 1980;79:366–72.
135. Bartlett JG. Treatment of *Clostridium difficile* colitis. Gastroenterology. 1985;89:1192–5.
136. Elmore M, Rissing JP, Rink L, et al. Clindamycin-associated hepatotoxicity. Am J Med. 1974;57:627–30.
137. Fogdall RP, Miller RD. Prolongation of a pancuronium-induced neuromuscular blockade by clindamycin. Anesthesiology. 1974;41:407–8.
138. Thadepalli H, Gorbach SL, Broido PW, et al. Abdominal trauma, anaerobes, and antibiotics. Surg Gynecol Obstet. 1973;137:270–6.
139. Weinstein WM, Onderdonk AB, Bartlett JG, et al. Antimicrobial therapy of experimental intra-abdominal sepsis. J Infect Dis. 1975;132:282–6.
140. diZerega G, Yonekura L, Roy S, et al. A comparison of clindamycin–gentamicin and penicillin–gentamicin in the treatment of post-cesarean section endometritis. Am J Obstet Gynecol. 1979;134:238–42.
141. Solomkin JS, Fant WK, Rivera JD, et al. Randomized trial of imipenem/cilastatin versus gentamicin and clindamycin in mixed flora infections. Am J Med. 1985;78:85–91.
142. Bartlett JG, Gorbach SL. Treatment of aspiration pneumonia and primary lung abscess: penicillin G vs. clindamycin. JAMA. 1975;234:935–7.
143. Levison ME, Mangura CT, Lorber B, et al. Clindamycin compared with penicillin for the treatment of anaerobic lung abscess. Ann Intern Med. 1983;98:466–71.
144. Bartlett JG, Gorbach SL. Penicillin or clindamycin for primary lung abscess? (Editorial). Ann Intern Med. 1983;98:546–8.
145. Leyden JJ, Shalita AR, Saatjian GD, et al. Erythromycin 2% gel in comparison with clindamycin phosphate 1% solution in acne vulgaris. Am J Am Acad Dermatol. 1987;16:822–7.
146. Parry MF, Rha CK. Pseudomembranous colitis caused by topical clindamycin phosphate. Arch Dermatol. 1986;122:583–4.
147. Hofflin JM, Remington JS. Clindamycin in a murine model of toxoplasmic encephalitis. Antimicrob Agents Chemother. 1987;31:492–6.
148. Israelski DM, Remington JS. Toxoplasmic encephalitis in patients with AIDS. Infect Dis Clin North Am. 1988;2:429–45.
149. el Wakeel ES, Homeida MM, Ali HM, et al. Clindamycin in the treatment of falciparum malaria in Sudan. Am J Trop Med Hyg. 1985;34:1065–8.
150. Wittner M, Rowin KS, Tanowitz HB, et al. Successful chemotherapy of transfusion babesiosis. Ann Intern Med. 1982;96:601–4.
151. Brook I, Hirokawa R. Treatment of patients with a history of recurrent tonsillitis due to group A beta-hemolytic streptococci. A prospective randomized study comparing penicillin, erythromycin and clindamycin. Clin Pediatr. 1985;24:331–6.
152. Hermans P. Lincosamides. In Peterson PK, Verhoef J, eds. The Antimicrobial Agents Annual. v. 2. Amsterdam: Elsevier; 1987:114.

27. VANCOMYCIN AND TEICOPLANIN

ROBERT FEKETY

VANCOMYCIN

Structure

Vancomycin is a complex soluble glycopolypeptide that has a molecular weight of approximately 1450 daltons. While similar to two new glycopeptide antimicrobials, teichomycin and daptomycin (LY 146032), it is unrelated to all other antibiotics. When vancomycin was first introduced, commercial preparations contained as much as 30 percent of another substance of unknown nature that probably contributed to its side effects.[1,2] Current preparations are more pure and appear to be less toxic than the early preparations were.

Derivation and Nomenclature

Vancomycin (Vancocin from Lilly and Vancoled from Lederle) is a narrow-spectrum bactericidal antibiotic obtained from *Streptomyces orientales*. Introduced in 1956 because of its effectiveness against penicillin-resistant staphylococci, it was relegated because of its toxicity to the role of alternate therapy when methicillin became available. With spread of methicillin-resistant staphylococci in the United States in recent years, vancomycin underwent a marked increase in frequency of use and popularity, and it is now the drug of choice for treating infections with this organism. It is also the drug of choice for oral treatment of patients with severe antibiotic-associated colitis caused by *Clostridium difficile*.

Mechanism of Action

Vancomycin inhibits synthesis and assembly of the second stage of cell wall peptidoglycan polymers by complexing with the D-alanyl-D-alanine precursor. In addition, it injures protoplasts by altering the permeability of their cytoplasmic membrane and also impairs RNA synthesis. The multiple mechanisms of its action may contribute to the observed low frequency of the development of resistance. Rapidly and tightly bound to organisms, vancomycin exerts a bactericidal effect without a lag period, but only on multiplying organisms.

Antimicrobial Activity

Both *Staphylococcus aureus* and *Staphylococcus epidermidis* are susceptible to vancomycin. Marked resistance has not been observed. Concentrations of 1–5 μg/ml or less are almost invariably inhibitory, even with isolates resistant to methicillin, and most organisms are killed at about the same concentrations. A small proportion of strains require 10–20 μg/ml for inhibition, and about 20 percent of organisms are deficient in autolysins and relatively tolerant to the bactericidal action of vancomycin.[3,4] Slime biofilms on plastic foreign bodies also may be responsible for the persistence of staphylococci, particularly *S. epidermidis,* and treatment failures.[5] Recently, a coagulase-negative staphylococcus, speciated as *Staphylococcus haemolyticus,* was shown to be relatively resistant to vancomycin (minimum inhibitory and bactericidal concentrations [MIC, MBC] increased fourfold to 8 and 12 μg/ml, and the MBC with heavy inocula was as high as 32 μg/ml) and associated with the failure of treatment until a foreign body was removed. These organisms were also resistant to teicoplanin but were killed at low concentrations of daptomycin.[6] *Streptococcus pygoenes,* group B streptococci, corynebacteria JK, *Streptococcus pneumoniae,* and *Clostridium difficile* are highly susceptible. *Listeria monocytogenes* is usually susceptible. Anaerobic or microaerophilic streptococci, clostridia including *Clostridium perfringens, Bacillus anthracis, Actinomyces,* lactobacilli, diphtheroids, *C. diphtheriae,* corynebacteria CDC-D2, and *Neisseria gonorrheae* are usually susceptible.[7,8] Nutritionally variant streptococci may be killed by vancomycin alone.[9] Viridans streptococci, *Streptococcus agalactiae, Streptococcus bovis,* and *Enterococcus faecalis* (formerly *S. faecalis*) isolates are usually inhibited at concentrations attainable in serum, but few if any *Enterococcus* isolates are killed at concentrations less than 100 μg/ml.[4] A synergistic bactericidal effect is shown by 40–70 percent of *Enterococcus* isolates when vancomycin is combined with streptomycin, and the combinatin of vancomycin plus gentamicin is almost always bactericidal at attainable concentrations[10,11] unless so-called high-level gentamicin-resistant isolates are implicated.[12] Recently, vancomycin-resistant isolates of *Enterococcus faecalis, Enterococcus faecium,*[13] *Enterococcus gallinarum,*[14] and *Leukonostoc* species (which may be misidentified as streptococci)[15] have been detected. The mechanism of resistance is unknown. There is no cross-resistance between vancomycin and other unrelated antibiotics, and significant resistance rarely if ever develops during therapy. Cross-resistance with teicoplanin or daptomycin occurs but is variable. Antibacterial activity varies little between pH 6.5 and 8. Some *Neisseria gonorrhoeae* isolates are susceptible enough to be missed on cultures when vancomycin-containing selective media (Thayer-Martin) are used. *Flavobacterium meningosepticum* is susceptible at attainable concentrations (between 16 and 25 μg/ml), but other gram-negative bacilli, mycobacteria, fungi, and *Bacteroides* are not susceptible.

Pharmacology

Administration. After being dissolved in sterile water, vancomycin should be given intravenously in 100–250 ml of 5% dextrose or 0.9% NaCl over a period of at least 30–60 minutes.[1] It can also be given by continuous intravenous drip, but intermittent infusion is preferred. Rapid or bolus administration is dangerous, especially if 1 g doses are used, because it causes histamine release by basophiles and mast cells,[16] which can cause flushing (the "red-neck syndrome"), anaphylactoid reactions and even cardiac arrest.[9] Antihistamines may help prevent this. Hydrocortisone (20 mg) can be added to the infusion to reduce side effects, but this mixture may precipitate at high concentrations. Heparin and vancomycin also can precipitate at high concentrations, so they should not be infused simultaneously through the same intravenous line.[17] Because of pain on injection, no satisfactory intramuscular preparation is available. Vancomycin is absorbed poorly from the gastrointestinal tract, even when the colon is inflamed, and it is used orally for the treatment of enterocolitis[1,18–20] and for the prevention of infection in cancer patients.[21]

Distribution, Excretion, and Protein Binding. Vancomycin is eliminated from the body almost exclusively by glomerular filtration. Within 24 hours 80–90 percent of an administered dose appears in the urine. A small amount may be eliminated via the liver and biliary tract. The half-life of vancomycin in serum is 6–8 hours in persons with normal renal function. In anuria, it may be prolonged to about 9 days, and it may be detected in serum for as long as 21 days after a single 1 g dose.[22,23] From 10 to 55 percent is protein bound in serum; this is believed to have a negligible effect on clinical results.

Concentrations in Body Fluids and Tissue. Serum levels 1–2 hours after the intravenous administration of a 500 mg dose to adults range from 6 to 10 μg/ml, with an average of 8 μg/ml after repeated dosing. Peak levels of up to 50 μg/ml may be seen. When 1 g is given slowly intravenously, peak and trough levels of 20–50 μg/ml and 5–10 μg/ml, respectively, can be achieved; these are considered desirable and appropriate concentrations. Urinary concentrations range from 100 to 300 μg/ml. When vancomycin (0.5 g q6h) is given orally, levels of 1000–9000 μg/ml are found in stool, but only trace amounts are ordinarily found in serum[7,8,19]; levels as high as therapeutic levels have been found occasionally in the serum of anuric patients given the drug orally to treat colitis.[24] When 125 mg is given orally, stool concentrations have ranged from 100 to 800 μg/ml. When vancomycin is given intravenously, levels of up to 100 μg/ml may be found in stools of some patients, but the drug is undetectable in the stools of most patients.[8] Vancomycin is not found in the cerebrospinal fluid (CSF) of persons without meningitis, but bactericidal levels have been found in the CSF of most but not all patients with meningitis (<1–7 μg/ml). Small supplemental amounts (3–5 mg) may be given intrathecally in meningitis if there is no response after 48 hours of intravenous therapy.[25] A larger intrathecal dose may be needed for less susceptible organisms such as flavobacteria. Vancomycin is irritating when injected into serous or synovial cavities, and peritonitis has been reported after direct instillation.[26] Adequate concentrations are reached in pleural, pericardial, synovial, and ascitic fluids after intravenous administration, and low levels are found in bile.[7]

Since the kidney is the only significant organ of elimination of vancomycin, high and potentially toxic serum levels can be attained in patients with renal insufficiency unless the dosage is reduced appropriately.[21,23,27] It is recommended that a loading dose of 15 mg/kg may be given to all adults, regardless of renal function. To achieve a mean therapeutic concentration of 20 μg/ml in the serum of adults with renal impairment, a simple formula can be used to estimate maintenance dosage: the daily parenteral dose of vancomycin in milligrams is 150 plus 15 times the creatinine clearance in milliliters per minute.[27] Another strategy is to give 1 g every 36 hours when the serum creatinine concentration is 1.5–5 mg/100 ml and 1 g every 10–14 days when it is greater than 5 mg/100 ml. As little as 1 g may yield effective serum concentrations for 7–14 days in anuric patients.[23] There is a nomogram[28] that may be more accurate than the aforementioned simple rules for dosing patients with renal failure. In difficult situations, serum concentrations should be monitored whichever method is used to estimate the dosage. It is designed to provide steady-state concentrations of 15 μg/ml[28] and is probably the most accurate dosing method.[29] Hemodialysis does not remove significant amounts of vancomycin, but peritoneal dialysis can.[21,23,26] Hemofiltration may be very efficient at removing it and useful in managing overdosage in patients with renal failure.[30] Serum levels should be monitored at frequent, regular intervals in dialyzed, uremic, or seriously ill patients to ascertain that safe, yet adequate concentrations are present. Cardiopulmonary bypass is associated with a fall in serum levels because of dilution.[31] A preoperative dose of 15 mg/kg is needed before bypass surgery, and 10 mg/kg should be given after bypass surgery if renal function is normal. Pediatric dosing is discussed in the later section on major uses and doses.

Toxicity and Adverse Reactions

With the purified preparations now available, adverse reactions seem to be much less frequent than when vancomycin was first introduced. The most frequent side effects consist of fever, chills, and phlebitis at the site of the infusion. These are less frequent if the drug is infused slowly in a large volume of fluid. Tingling and flushing of the face, neck, and thorax (the "red-neck syndrome") are frequently experienced, especially if 1 g doses are given [32] and if the drug is infused very rapidly[33]; this is related to histamine release, not to allergic hypersensitivity. Shock has occurred after rapid intravenous infusion of the drug, especially during surgery. Reversible leukopenia or eosinophilia sometimes develop.[34] Maculopapular or diffuse erythomatous rashes, presumably on a hypersensitivity basis, occur in 4–5 percent of patients and may persist for weeks despite discontinuation of vancomycin treatment in patients with marked renal failure. They may respond to steroid or antihistamine therapy. Lacrimation has been reported.[16] One case of antibiotic-induced *C. difficile* colitis has been reported after the intravenous use of vancomycin.[35]

An important adverse reaction to vancomycin is neurotoxicity, which is manifested by auditory nerve damage and hearing loss. This is infrequent if serum concentrations are maintained below 30 μg/ml and is more common with concentrations of 80 μg/ml or more. Tinnitus and high-tone hearing loss are frequently an antecendent to deafness. Hearing occasionally improves when treatment with the drug is discontinued but usually continues to deteriorate and is permanent.[36,37] Nephrotoxicity was relatively common with early impure preparations of vancomycin, especially when given in high doses; it is usually transient or reversible. With appropriate doses selected by monitoring renal function and serum concentrations, nephrotoxicity is now uncommon.[37–39] Though vancomycin is no longer appreciably nephrotoxic, high doses given by the parenteral route should be avoided, and serum levels should be carefully monitored when other nephrotoxic drugs are being given. The risk of nephrotoxicity appears to be enhanced even with safe levels when drugs such as aminoglycosides or ethacrynic acid are given concomitantly.

Drug Interactions

Vancomycin is incompatible with many drugs in intravenous solutions, especially chloramphenicol, adrenal corticosteroids, and methicillin. Heparin (at very high concentrations) may inactivate vancomycin in intravenous solutions and be responsible for persistent bacteremia.[17] Vancomycin is not stable enough for use with certain implantable pumps.[40]

Major Uses and Doses

The usual intravenous dose of vancomycin for adults with normal renal function is 1 g every 12 hours (15 mg/kg) or 500 mg (6.5–8 mg/kg) every 6 hours. In severely ill patients with normal renal function such as those with meningitis, 1 g may be given every 8 hours for 2 or 3 days until the infection is under control. Morbidly obese patients with severe infections may require high doses, which should be based upon total body weight, creatinine clearance, and monitoring serum levels.[41] Various dosage regimens have been proposed for pediatric usage. For newborn infants, 15 mg/kg should be given slowly intravenously every 12 hours during the first week of life or every 8 hours in those 8–30 days of age; 10 mg/kg every 6 hours is recommended for older infants and children and 15 mg/kg every 6 hours for infants and children with staphylococcal central nervous system infections. Monitoring serum levels is desirable, especially in preterm infants.[42] A continuous drip can be used.[43,44] An oral dose of 125–500 mg four times per day has been used to treat adults with *Clostridium difficile* colitis (R. Fekety, J. Silva, C. Kauffman, et al., unpublished observations). In infants and children with *Clostridium difficile* colitis, an oral dose of 500 mg/1.73 m^2 every 6 hours has been recommended.[45] Oral therapy is much more reliable than intravenous therapy is for the treatment of *Clostridium difficile* colitis.

The intravenous dosage must be reduced in patients with renal impairment and monitored to achieve peak serum concentrations no higher than 30–40 μg/ml and troughs ranging from 5 to 10 μg/ml; if a continuous infusion is used, a steady-state concentration of 15 μg/ml seems desirable.[25,26,35,46] Recent evidence indicates that impaired liver function may also delay the elimination of vancomycin and require a dosage modification.[47]

Vancomycin should be used primarily for serious infections. Intravenous vancomycin is the therapy of choice for serious staphylococcal infections in patients with methicillin-, oxacillin-, nafcillin-, or cephalothin-resistant organisms or in patients who cannot be given these primary drugs.[7,38,48–52]

All strains of methicillin-resistant staphylococci have been susceptible to low concentrations of vancomycin, but rare isolates show clinically significant tolerance to its bactericidal action.[4,48,51,53] When treatment of serious infections with vancomycin given alone has failed, the addition of gentamicin, rifampin, or trimethoprim-sulfamethoxazole may be tried. Since antagonism may occur rarely with some of these combinations of antimicrobials,[48] these combinations should not be routine, and serum bacteriostatic and bactericidal levels ideally should be monitored as a guide to therapy when they are used. When vancomycin is used for adults in conjunction with an aminoglycoside, its dosage should rarely exceed 0.5 g every 8 hours.[38] However, methicillin-resistant *S. epidermidis* endocarditis involving a prosthetic valve is best treated with the usual doses of vancomycin for 4 weeks in combination with rifampin plus the addition of an aminoglycoside for the first 2 weeks only.[52]

Vancomycin has a very rapid and potent bactericidal effect, and were it not for its potential toxicity, it might be the preferred drug for treating all serious staphylococcal infections. Survival rates of 60–75 percent have been achieved with vancomycin in patients with staphylococcal endocarditis or bacteremia.[1,7] Survival in patients aged 70 years or older is about 50 percent. The usual duration of therapy is 4–6 weeks. Success rates of 75 percent or greater have been reported in patients with pneumonia, parotitis, or meningitis.

While vancomycin penetrates into the central nervous system in most ill patients in amounts adequate to treat meningitis and shunt infections, this is not always the case,[25] and removal of foreign bodies or supplemental intraventricular or intrathecal instillation of vancomycin may be required in patients with a poor response.[53–55] Cerebrospinal fluid concentrations need not be greater than about 25 μg/ml, so intrathecal doses of 3 mg are usually adequate.

Vancomycin is the treatment of choice in patients with *E. faecalis* (enterococcal) endocarditis who are allergic to penicillin. In this setting it is best given along with an aminoglycoside since vancomycin alone is not dependably bactericidal against these streptotocci.[10,11,56,57] Since bactericidal synergism between gentamicin and vancomycin has been demonstrated with most enterococci (until recently),[12,58] gentamicin is preferable to streptomycin, which is not synergistic with as many as 40 percent of these organisms. Laboratory studies of synergism with the patient's organism or Schlicter tests on their serum may be helpful in determining the best regimen during the course of treatment. A vancomycin dose of 0.5 g every 8 hours iv plus streptomycin, 0.5 g every 12 hours im, or gentamicin, 60–80 mg (1 mg/kg) every 8 hours iv for 1 month, is recommended for adults with normal renal function. More vigorous or prolonged therapy may be needed for complicated cases, as when a prosthetic valve is infected. Patients should be monitored closely for signs of ototoxicity or nephrotoxicity, and drug dosages should be carefully adjusted in renal failure. Viridans streptococcal or *S. bovis* endocarditis may be treated with vancomycin alone if the MBC for the isolate is no more than 10 μg/ml; otherwise it should be combined with streptomycin or another aminoglycoside.[7,38]

Other serious infections with resistant organisms that have been responsive to vancomycin include *Corynebacterium* endocarditis in patients with prosthetic valves and *Flavobacterium meningosepticum* meningitis.[7,25,54]

Vancomycin has been considered the drug of choice for treating acute staphylococcal pseudomembranous enterocolitis, which is now a rare disease. In two series of cases, 67 of 72 patients were cured (93 percent).[18,59] It was usually given orally, 500 mg diluted in water every 6 hours for adults.

Although metronidazole is less expensive and also effective,[61] orally administered vancomycin is considered the drug of choice by most investigators for treating *seriously* ill patients with antibiotic-associated *Clostridium difficile* (pseudomembranous) colitis. This organism is always susceptible to vancomycin, and treatment failures are very rare unless treatment is delayed.[18,19,62,63] Dosages of either 125 or 500 mg four times daily have been effective and the lower and less expensive dose seems as good as the larger one.[63a] Vancomycin is very useful in treating relapses of colitis cause by *C. difficile*.[62] Preferably, vancomycin should be given orally to treat colitis since the drug is needed to inhibit toxin production in the lumen of the bowel and not for inhibition of the organism in tissues.[62] Intravenous vancomycin is not as reliable since adequate concentrations may not be achieved within the lumen when it is given in this way. In patients with ileus, vancomycin should be given orally or by nasogastric tube in 500 mg doses every 6 hours, and both vancomycin (in full parenteral doses) plus metronidazole should be given intravenously. Even though little vancomycin will be absorbed from the intestinal tract, serum levels should be monitored to prevent toxicity when it is used by both routes. When nasogastric tubes are needed for administering vancomycin, they can be clamped for 30–60 minutes after administration. When patients have ileus, the drug has been given by enema or via an ileostomy or colostomy.

Staphylococcal peritonitis occurring during peritoneal dialysis can be treated with intravenous vancomycin alone. The administration of 1 g intravenously will yield peritoneal fluid concentrations greater than 5 μg/ml for a week or more in this setting.[26,42] Others have noted that peritoneal dialysis may remove vancomycin from the blood and have recommended instilling vancomycin into the peritoneal cavity at a concentration of 25 μg/ml in addition to parenteral vancomycin to ensure good levels in peritoneal fluid.[63] In fact, it may be possible to treat staphylococcal peritonitis in chronic peritoneal dialysis patients solely by the intraperitoneal administration of vancomycin at a concentration of 50 μg/ml in the dialysate.[63,64] However, vancomycin given intraperitoneally with some preparations can be irritating[65]; furthermore, organisms protected by a biofilm on the catheter may be clinically tolerant and responsible for a relapse.[5] The addition of rifampin to vancomycin to treat refractory staphylococcal peritonitis in chronic dialysis can be curative.[66]

According to an American Heart Association Advisory Committee,[67,68] vancomycin is useful in the prevention of bacterial endocarditis in patients who are allergic to penicillin and undergoing dental or respiratory tract procedures.[67] The mechanism of prevention may be either by the bactericidal action of vancomycin or by interference with the ability of the organism to adhere to the endocardium. One gram is given slowly intravenously over a period of 60 minutes before the procedure; no repeat dose is necessary. For genitourinary or gastrointestinal surgery or instrumentation, vancomycin can be given as above plus gentamicin, 1.5 mg/kg; these may be repeated once 8–12 hours later.[67] Vancomycin can be used prophylactically for the placement of prosthetic valves, with an initial intravenous dose of 15 mg/ml given over a period of 1 hour just before surgery, followed by 10 mg/kg immediately after bypass surgery (if renal function is normal),[31] and 1.7 mg/kg gentamicin before surgery and 8 hours later. The efficacy of this regimen has not been proved, but it is designed to prevent *S. aureus, S. epidermidis,* and coliform infections of the prosthesis and sternum. Vancomycin is often included in empirical therapy for febrile neutropenic patients, but unless there is good evidence to suggest a staphylococcal infection, its use probably should not be routine.[69]

Vancomycin has been used in prophylactic oral nonabsorbable antibiotic regimens designed to prevent endogenous infections in patients with cancer or leukemia.[21] Such patients seem to experience a lower rate of *C. difficile* colitis complicating their chemotherapy. Otherwise, these regimens are probably of no value unless protective environments and leukocyte transfusions are available and used.

Vancomycin has been used prophylactically in order to prevent staphylococcal infections in patients receiving chronic dialysis, but this has resulted in the emergence of vancomycin-resistant enterococci and serious enterococcal infections.[14]

It is obvious that there has been a resurgence of the use of vancomycin in the last 2 decades. Many new indications for its use have been established, and much new information has been accumulated. An excellent review of newer knowledge about vancomycin has been published.[70]

TEICOPLANIN

Teicoplanin (formerly named teichomycin A) is a new glycopeptide antibiotic derived from the fermentation products of *Actinoplanes teichomyceticus*.[71] While it is widely used in Europe for the treatment of gram-positive infections, it is still investigational in the United States. Teicoplanin is a complex of six analogues having the same linear heptapeptide base and an aglycone containing aromatic amino acids with D-mannose and *N*-acetyl-D-glycosamine as sugars, with a molecular weight ranging from 1562 to 1891. Teicoplanin is chemically similar to vancomycin and ristocetin but with important differences responsible for the unique physical and chemical properties of the complex.[72] It has greater lipophilicity than vancomycin does, which results in excellent tissue penetration. Other consequences are a long elimination half-life, slow release from tissues, and water solubility at physiologic pH. It has few if any inactive metabolites.[73]

Mechanism of Action and Pharmacokinetics

Teicoplanin has an antibacterial spectrum and mechanism of action similar to that of vancomycin. It is bactericidal, although tolerance has been observed to its bactericidal action. The development of resistance during treatment has not been reported. It impairs cell wall synthesis by inhibiting polymerization of peptidoglycan, but at different sites from those inhibited by β-lactams.[74,75] It does this by forming a complex with the terminal D-alanyl-D-alanine precursor, which fits into a "pocket" in the teicoplanin molecule.[76] It has an elimination half-life of 40–70 hours after intravenous administration, a disappearance curve that fits both a two- and a three-compartment model, and a volume of distribution of 0.5–0.8 liter/kg.[77,78] Protein binding is as high as 90 percent,[76] which may account for its slow renal clearance. Because of its long half-life, it can be given intramuscularly or intravenously once per day.[79] It has usually been given in a daily intravenous dose of 2–3 mg/kg after a loading dose of 6 mg/kg (400 mg).[80] When single intravenous injections of 3 or 6 mg/kg were given rapidly (over a period of 5 minutes) to healthy volunteers, peak plasma concentrations of 53 and 112 μg/ml were observed, and concentrations of 2.1 and 4.2 μg/ml were observed at 24 hours. Similar concentrations were seen after intramuscular dosing with 3 mg/kg. When 3 mg/kg was administered to volunteers at a constant rate over a period of 30 minutes, peak concentrations were about 22 μg/ml. After six intramuscular doses of 200 mg (3 mg/kg) over a 5-day period, mean peak levels of 12.1 μg/ml were reached. Trough levels were 5.4–7.3 μg/ml,[78] and the calculated elimination half-life was about 99 hours. Urinary concentrations ranged from 16 to 156 μg/ml from day 1 through day 7. About 80 percent of the drug was eliminated in urine.[79] Teicoplanin was not significantly absorbed from the intestinal tracts of human volunteers.[73] In patients with renal impairment, serum concentrations are related to creatinine clearance, which can be used for adjusting the dosage.[80] Teicoplanin is well tolerated by children. A dose of 10 mg/kg/day has been recommended for children and 6 mg/kg/day for neonates.[81]

ANTIBACTERIAL ACTIVITY

Teicoplanin has excellent bactericidal activity against gram-positive organisms, including *S. pneumoniae, S. pyogenes,* other streptococci, *Enterococcus faecalis, S. aureus* (both penicillinase-producing and methicillin-resistant organisms), *S. epidermidis, Clostridium* species, corynebacteria JK, *Propionibacterium acnes,* and *Listeria monocytogenes.*[82–84] Inhibitory concentrations range from 0.025 to 3.1 μg/ml. Some strains of *S. epidermidis* and *S. haemolyticus* are relatively resistant to teicoplanin but susceptible to vancomycin.[85,86] Against many susceptible organisms, teicoplanin is two to four times as active as vancomycin. Teicoplanin was the most active antimicrobial agent against *E. faecalis,* but like vancomycin, it is rarely bactericidal for this species. Teicoplanin is more active than vancomycin is against *Clostridium difficile,* but it is even more highly bound by cholestyramine.[87] It is not active against gram-negative organisms, mycobacteria, or fungi. Teicoplanin does not give rise to stably resistant mutants in vitro, and it shows no cross-resistance with nonglycopeptide antibiotics. Like vancomycin, teicoplanin can be synergistic with rifampin or aminoglycosides against staphylococci, enterococci, other streptococci, and *Listeria.*[88–92]

Toxicity

Teicoplanin produces only mild pain at the site of injection. After slow intravenous infusion, it has not caused thrombophlebitis[93] or adverse effects on platelet function or coagulation.[94] Studies with 100 human volunteers showed no untoward effects at doses of up to 7.5 mg/kg. When used by rapid intravenous infusion in 310 hospitalized infected patients with infections, significant adverse effects were uncommon (2 percent), and no patient developed flushing or the "red-man syndrome."[95] However, ototoxicity has been reported.[95–97]

Clinical Uses

Teicoplanin is similiar to vancomycin, with the advantage of less frequent dosing and, because of its greater potency and therapeutic ratio, the potential for less nephrotoxicity and ototoxicity. It may be useful for patients who have had neutropenic or allergic reactions to vancomycin.[98]

Clinical cures were seen in 96 percent of 88 patients treated with 200–400 mg teicoplanin once daily for coagulase-negative staphylococcal infections[99,100] and in 79–91 percent of 1781 patients with various gram-positive infections.[97,99] These included methicillin-resistant *S. aureus* (MRSA) infections, pneumonia, endocarditis, septicemia, and joint infections. Some of these patients developed ototoxicity or nephrotoxicity, but many of them had also received an aminoglycoside.[97]

When patients with serious staphylococcal infections were treated with doses of 200 mg/day, only 44 percent were cured.[101] Treatment failure was related to the presence of foreign bodies and poor tissue concentrations. The high degree of protein binding of teicoplanin may have been an important factor in these low-doses treatment failures. Doses of 400 mg/day or more will probably be needed for the successful treatment of severe infections. When used once daily for prophylaxis in cardiac surgery, teicoplanin was associated with higher than expected numbers of sternal wound and urinary tract infections.[102] Other potential indications include shunt infections and treatment of gram-positive peritonitis in chronic dialysis patients.[103,104]

REFERENCES

1. Alexander MR. Review of vancomycin after 15 years of use. Drug Intell Clin Pharm. 1974;8:520.
2. Perkins HR, Nieto M. The chemical basis for the action of the vancomycin group of antibiotics. Ann NY Acad Sci. 1974;235:348.
3. Gopal V, Bisno AL, Silverblatt FJ. Failure of vancomycin treatment in *Staphylococcus aureus* endocarditis. In vivo and in vitro observations. JAMA. 1976;236:1604.
4. Sabath L, Wheeler N, Laverdiere M, et al: A new type of penicillin resistance in *Staphylococcus aureus.* Lancet 1977;1:443.
5. Evans RC, Holmes CJ. Effect of vancomycin hydrochloride on *staphylococcus epidermidis* biofilm associated with silicone elostomen. Antimicrob Agents Chemother. 1987;31:889–94.
6. Schwalke RS, Stapleton JT, Gilligan PH. Emergence of vancomycin resistance in coagulase-negative staphylococci. N Engl J Med. 1987;316:927–31.
7. Geraci JE. Vancomycin. Mayo Clin Proc 1977;52:631.
8. Geraci JE, Heilman FR, Nichols DR, et al. Some laboratory and clinical experiences with a new antibiotic, vancomycin. Proc Staff Meet Mayo Clin. 1956;31:564.
9. Reimer LG. Measurement of serum bactericidal activity and use of vancomycin for treatment of nutritionally variant streptococcal bacteremia. Diagn Microbiol Infect Dis. 1987;6:319–22.
10. Watanakunakorn C, Bakie C. Synergism of vancomycin-gentamicin and vancomycin-streptomycin against enterococci. Antimicrob Agents Chemother. 1973;4:120.
11. Harwick HJ, Kalmanson GM, Guze LB: In vitro activity of ampicillin or vancomycin combined with gentamicin or streptomycin against enterococci. Antimicrob Agents Chemother. 1973;4:383.
12. Mederski-Samoraj BD, Murray BE. High level resistance to enterococci in clinical isolates of staphylococci. J Infect Dis. 1983;147:751–7.
13. Uttley AC, Collins CH, Naidoo J, et al. Vancomycin-resistant enterococci. Lancet 1988;1:57–8.
14. Kaplan AH, Gilligan PH, Facklam RR. Recovery of resistant enterococci during vancomycin prophylaxis. J Clin Microbiol. 1988;26:1216–8.
15. Rubin LG, Velozzi E, Shapiro J, et al. Infection with vancomycin-resistant "streptococci", due to *Leuconostoc* species. J Infect Dis. 1988;157:216.
16. Polk RE, Healy DP, Schwartz LB, et al. Vancomycin and the red-man syndrome: Pharmacodynamics of histamine release. J Infect Dis. 1988;157:502–7.
17. Barg NL, Fekety R, Supena R: Persistant staphylococcal bacteremia in an intravenous drug abuser. Antimicrob Agents Chemother. 1986;29:209–11.
18. Khan MY, Hall WH: Staphylococcal enterocolitis-treatment with oral vancomycin. Ann Intern Med. 1966;65:1.
19. Tedesco F, Markham R, Gurwith M, et al. Oral vancomycin for antibiotic-associated pseudomembranous colitis. Lancet 1978;2:226–8.
20. Silva J, Batts DH, Fekety R, et al. Treatment of *Clostridium difficile* colitis and diarrhea with vancomycin. Am J Med. 1981;71:815–22.
21. Bodey G: Oral antibiotic prophylaxis in protected environment units: Effect of nonabsorbable and absorbable antibiotics on the fecal flora. Antimicrob Agents Chemother. 1972;1:343.
22. Lindholm DD, Murray JS. Persistance of vancomycin in the blood during renal failure and its treatment by hemodialysis. N Engl J Med. 1966;274:1047.
23. Eykyn S, Phillip I, Evans J: Vancomycin for staphylococcal shunt infections in patients on regular hemodialysis. Br Med J. 1970;3:80.
24. Spitzer PC, Eliopoulos GM. Systemic absorption of enteral vancomycin in a patient with pseudomembranous colitis. Ann Intern Med. 1984;100:533–4.
25. Hawley HB, Gump DW. Vancomycin therapy of bacterial meningitis. Am J Dis Child. 1973;126:261.
26. Ayus JC, Enkas JF, Tong TG, et al. Peritoneal clearance and total body elimination of vancomycin during chronic intermittent peritoneal dialysis. Clin Nephrol. 1979;11:129–32.
27. Nielsen HE, Hansen JE, Korsager B, et al. Renal excretion of vancomycin in kidney disease. Acta Med Scand. 1975;197:261.
28. Moellering RC, Krogstad DJ, Greenblatt DJ. Vancomycin therapy in patients with impaired renal function. A nomogram for dosage. Ann Intern Med. 1981;94:343–6.
29. Matzke G, Kovarik JM, Rybak MJ, et al. Evaluation of the vancomycin clearance: Creatinine-clearance relationship for predicting vancomycin dosage. Clinical Pharm 1985;4:311–5.
30. Matzke GR, O'Connell MB, Collins AJ, et al. Disposition of vancomycin during hemofiltration. Clin Pharmacol Ther. 1986;40:425–30.

31. Austin TW, Leake J, Coles JC, et al. Vancomycin blood levels during cardiac surgery. Card J Surg 1981;24:423–5.
32. Healy DP, Polk RE, Garson ML, et al. Comparison of steady-state pharmacokinetics of two dosage regimens of vancomycin in normal volunteers. Antimicrob Agents Chemother. 1987;31:393–7.
33. Newfield P, Roizen MF. Hazards of rapid administration of vancomycin. Ann Intern Med. 1979;91:581.
34. Mordenti J, Ries C, Brooks GF, et al. Vancomycin-induced neutropenia complicating bone marrow recovery in a patient with leukemia. Case report and a review of the literature. Am J Med. 1986;30:333–5.
35. Miller SN, Ringler RP. Vancomycin-induced pseudomembranous colitis. J Clin Gastroenterol. 1987;9:114–5.
36. Traber PG, Levine DP. Vancomycin ototoxicity in a patient with normal renal function. Ann Intern Med. 1981;95:458–60.
37. McHenry MC, Gavan TL. Vancomycin. Pediatr Clin North Am 1983;30:31–47.
38. Geraci JE, Hermans PE. Vancomycin. Mayo Clin Proc. 1983;58:88–91.
39. Appel GB, Neu HC. The nephrotoxicity of antimicrobial agents. N Engl J Med. 1977;296:722.
40. Greenberg RN, Saud AMK, Kennedy DJ, et al: Instability of vancomycin in Infusaid drug pump model 100. Antimicrob Agents Chemother. 1987;31:610–1.
41. Blovin RA, Bauer LA, Miller DD, et al. Vancomycin pharmacokinetics in normal and morbidity obese subjects. Antimicrob Agents Chemother. 1982;21:575–80.
42. Nagvi SH, Kennan WJ, Reichley RM, et al: Vancomycin pharmcokinetics in small, seriously ill infants. Am J Dis Child. 1986;140:107–10.
43. Riley HD. Vancomycin and novobiocin. Med Clin North Am 1970;54:1277.
44. Schaad CVB, McCracken GH, Nelson JD. Clinical pharmacology and efficacy of vancomycin in pediatric patients. J Pediatr. 1980;96:119–26.
45. Batts DH, Martin D, Holmes R, et al. Treatment of antibiotic-associated *Clostridium difficile* diarrhea with oral vancomycin. J Pediatr. 1980;97:151–53.
46. Rotschafer JC, Crossley K, Zaski DE, et al. Pharmacokinetics of vancomycin. Observations in 28 patients and dosage recommendations. Antimicrob Agents Chemother. 1982;22:391–94.
47. Brown N, Ho DHW, Fong KL, et al. Effects of hepatic function on vancomycin clinical pharmacology. Antimicrob Agents Chemother. 1983;23:603–9.
48. Watanakunakorn C. Treatment of infections due to methicillin-resistant *Staphylococcus aureus*. Ann Intern Med. 1982;97:376–8.
49. Myers JP, Linnemann CC. Bacteremia due to methicillin-resistant *Staphylococcus aureus*. J Infect Dis. 1982;4:532–6.
50. Sorrell TC, Packham DR, Shanker S, et al. Vancomycin therapy for methicillin-resistant *Staphylococcus aureus*. Ann Intern Med. 1982;97:344–50.
51. Levine DP, Cushing R, Jim J, et al. Community-acquired methicillin-resistant *Staphylococcus aureus* endocarditis in the Detroit Medical Center. Ann Intern Med. 1982;330–8.
52. Karchmer AW, Archer GL, Dismukes WE. *Staphylococcus epidermidis* causing prosthetic-valve endocarditis. Microbiologic and clinical observations as guides to therapy. Ann Intern Med. 1983;98:447–55.
53. Sutherlan GE, Palitang EG, Marr JJ, et al. Sterilization of Ommaya reservoir by instillation of vancomycin. Am J Med. 1981;71:1068–70.
54. Gump DW. Vancomycin for treatment of bacterial meningitis. Rev Infect Dis. 1981;3(Suppl):289–92.
55. Swayne RS, Rampling A, Newsom SWB. Intraventricular vancomycin for treatment of shunt-associated ventriculitis. J Antimicrob Chemother. 1987;19:249–53.
56. Westenfelder GO, Paterson PY, Reisberg BE, et al. Vancomycin–streptomycin synergism in enterococcal endocarditis. JAMA. 1973;223:37.
57. Harwick HJ, Kalmanson GM, Guze LB. Pyelonephritis. XVII. Comparison of combinations of vancomycin, ampicillin, streptomycin, and gentamicin in the treatment of enterococcal infection in the rat. J Infect Dis. 1974;129:358.
58. Zervos MJ, Kauffman CA, Therasse PM, et al. Nosocomial infection by gentamicin-resistant *Streptococcus faecalis*. Ann Intern Med. 1987;106:687–91.
59. Esposito AL, Gleckman RA: Vancomycin, a second look. JAMA. 1977;238:1756.
60. Teasley DG, Gerding DN, Olson MM, et al. Prospective randomised trial of metronidazole versus vancomycin for *Clostridium difficile*-associated diarrhea and colitis. Lancet 1983;2:1043–6.
61. Fekety R, Silva J, Armstrong J, et al. Treatment of antibiotic-associated enterocolitis with vancomycin. Rev Infect Dis. 1981;3(Suppl):273–81.
62. Tedesco FJ. Treatment of recurrent antibiotic-associated pseudomembranous colitis. Am J Gastroenterol. 1982;77:220–1.
63. Nielsen HE, Sorensen I, Hansen HE. Peritoneal transport of vancomycin during peritoneal dialysis. Nephron. 1979;24:274–7.
63a. Fekety R, Silva J, Kauffman C, et al. Treatment of antibiotic-associated *Clostridium difficile* colitis with oral vancomycin: Comparison of two dosage regimens. Am J Med. 1989;86:15–19.
64. Morse GD, Farolino DF, Apicella MA, et al. Comparative study of intraperitoneal and intravenous vancomycin pharmcokinetics during continuous ambulatory peritoneal dialysis. Antimicrob Agents Chemother. 1987;31:173–7.
65. Piraino B, Bernardini J, Johnston J, et al. Chemical peritonitis due to intraperitoneal vancomycin. Peritoneal Dialysis Bull. 1987;7(Suppl):59.
66. Buggy BP, Schaberg DR, Swartz RD. Intraleukocytic sequestration as a cause of persistent *Staphylococcus aureus* peritonitis in continuous ambulatory peritoneal dialysis. Am J Med. 1984;76:1035–40.
67. Kaye D. Prophylaxis for infective endocarditis: An update. Ann Intern Med. 1986;104:419–23.
68. Kaplan EL, Anthony BF, Bisno A, et al. Prevention of bacterial endocarditis (abstract). Circulation. 1977;56:139–43.
69. Rubin M, Hathorn JW, Marshall D, et al. Gram-positive infections and the use of vancomycin in 550 episodes of fever and neutropenia. Ann Intern Med. 1988;108:30–35.
70. Wise RI, Kory M, ed. Reassessments of vancomycin—a potentially useful antibiotic. Rev Infect Dis. 1981;3(Suppl):199–300.
71. Williams AH, Gruneberg RN. Teicoplanin. J Antimicrob Chemother. 1984;14:441–8.
72. Parenti F. Structure and mechanism of action of teicoplanin. J Hosp Infect. 1986;7(Suppl A):79–83.
73. Neville LD, Baillod R, Grady D, et al. Teicoplanin in patients with chronic renal failure on dialysis: Microbiological and pharmakokinetic aspects. Int J Clin Pharm Res. 1987;7:485–90.
74. Somma S, Gastaldo L. Mechanism of action of teichomycin A_2, a new antibiotic. In: Current Chemotherapy and Immunotherapy, Proceedings of the 12th International Congress of Chemotherapy, Florence, Italy, July 1981:19–24. Project Report, Clinical Investigator Brochure, Merrell Dow Research Institute, Cincinnati, June 1984.
75. Greenwood D. Microbiological properties of teicoplanin. J Antimicrob Agents Chemother. 1988;21(Suppl A):1–13.
76. Parenti F. Glycopeptide antibiotics. J Clin Pharmacol. 1988;28:136–40.
77. McNulty CAM, Garden GMF, Wise R, et al: The pharmacokinetics and tissue penetration of teicoplanin. J Antimicrob Chemother. 1985;16:743–9.
78. Verbist L, Tjandramaga B, Hendrickx B, et al. In vitro activity and human pharmacokinetics of teicoplanin. Antimicrob Agents Chemother. 1984;12:119–28.
79. Buniva G, DelFavero A, Bernareggi A, et al. Pharmacokinetics of ^{14}C-teicoplanin in healthy volunteers. J Antimicrob Chemother. 1988;21(Suppl A):23–8.
80. Bonati M, Traina GL, Rosiva R, et al. Pharmacokinetics of a single intravenous dose of teicoplanin in subjects with various degrees of renal impairment. Antimicrob Agents Chemother. 1988;21(Suppl A):29–37.
81. Tarral E, Jehl F, Tarral A, et al. Pharmacokinetics of teicoplanin in children. J Antimicrob Chemother. 1988;21(Suppl A):47–51.
82. Domart Y, Pierre C, Clair B, et al. Pharmacokinetics of teicoplanin in critically ill patients with various degrees of renal impairment. Antimicrob Agents Chemother. 1987;31:1600–4.
83. Bauernfeind A: Teichomycin and AM-715 activity on staphylococci enterococci in comparison to other antibiotic agents (abstract). In: Proceedings of the 21st Interscience Conference on Antimicrobiol Agents and Chemotherapy. Chicago: American Society for Microbiology; November 1981.
84. Jadeja L, Fainstein V, LeBlanc B, et al. Comparative in vitro activities of teichomycin and other antibiotics against JK diphtheroids. Antimicrob Agents Chemother. 1983;24:145–6.
85. Greenwood D. Microbiological properties of teicoplanin. J Antimicrob Chemother. 1988;21(Suppl A):1–3.
86. Felmingham D, Solomonides K, O'Hare MD, et al. The effect of medium and inoculum on the activity of vancomycin and teicoplanin against coagulase-negative staphylococci. Antimicrob Agents Chemother. 1987;10:609–19.
87. Pantosti A, Luzzi I, Cardine R, et al. Comparison of the in vitro activities of teicoplanin and vancomycin against *Clostridium difficile* and their interactions with cholestyramine. Antimicro Agents Chemother. 1985;28:847–8.
88. Van der Auwera P, Klastersky J. Bactericidal activity and killing rate of serum in volunteers receiving vancomycin or teicoplanin with and without amikacin given intravenously. J Antimicrob Chemother. 1987;19:623–35.
89. Van der Auwera P, Joly P. Comparative in-vitro activities of teicoplanin, vancomycin, coumermycin and ciprofloxacin, alone and in combination with rifampicin or LM427, against *Staphylococcus aureus*. J Antimicrob Chemother. 1987;19:313–20.
90. Watanakunakorn C. In-vitro activity of teicoplanin alone and in combination with rifampicin, gentamicin or tobramycin against coagulase-negative staphylococci. J Antimicrob Chemother. 1987;19:439–43.
91. Tuazon CU, Washburn D. Teicoplanin and rifampicin singly and in combination in the treatment of experimental *Staphylococcus epidermidis* endocarditis in the rabbit model. J Antimicrob Chemother. 1987;20:233–7.
92. Shanson DC, Todayon M. Activity of teicoplanin compared with vancomycin alone, and combined with gentamicin, against penicillin tolerant viridans streptococci and enterococci causing endocarditis. J Hosp Infect. 1986;7(Suppl A):65–72.
93. Williams AH, Gruneberg RN, Webster A, et al. Teicoplanin in the treatment of infection caused by gram-positive organisms. J Hosp Infect. 1986;7(Suppl A):101–3.
94. Agnelli G, Longetti M, Guerciolini R, et al. Effects of the new glycopeptide antibiotic teicoplanin on platelet function and blood coagulation. Antimicrob Agents Chemother. 1987;31:1609–12.
95. Stille W, Sietzen W, Dieterich HA, et al. Clinical efficacy and safety of teicoplanin. J. Antimicrob. Chemother. 1988;21(Suppl A):69–79.
96. Maher ER, Hollman A, Gruneberg RN. Teicoplanin-induced ototoxicity in Down's Syndrome. Lancet. 1986;1:613.
97. Drabu YJ, Walsh B, Blakemore PH, et al. Teicoplanin in infections caused by methicillin-resistant staphylococci. J Antimicrob Chemother. 1988;21(Suppl A):89–92.

98. Schlemmer B, Falkman H, Boudjadja A, et al. Teicoplanin for patients allergic to vancomycin. N Engl J Med. 1988;318:1127–8.
99. Lewis P, Garaud JJ, Parenti F. A multicentre open clinical trial of teicoplanin in infections caused by gram-positive bacteria. J Antimicrob Chemother. 1988;21(Suppl A):61–7.
100. Harding I, Garaud JJ. Teicoplanin in the treatment of infections caused by coagulase-negative staphylococci. J Antimicrob Chemother. 1988;21(Suppl A):93–103.
101. Galanakis N, Giamarellou H, Vlachogiannis N, et al: Poor efficacy of teicoplanin in treatment of deep-seated staphylococcal infections. Eur J Clin Microbiol Infect Dis. 1988;7:130–4.
102. Wilson APR, Treasure T, Gruneberg RN, et al. Antibiotic prophylaxis in cardiac surgery: A prospective comparison of two dosage regimens of teicoplanin with combination of flucloxacillin and tobramycin. J Antimicrob Chemother. 1988;21:213–33.
103. Neville LO, Baillod RA, Brumfitt W, et al. Efficacy and safety of teicoplanin in gram-positive peritonitis in patients on peritoneal dialysis. J Antimicrob Chemother. 1988;21(Suppl A):123–31.
104. Bowley JA, Pickering SJ, Scantlebury AJ, et al. Intraperitoneal teicoplanin in the treatment of peritonitis associated with continuous ambulatory peritoneal dialysis. J Antimicrob Chemother. 1988;21(Suppl A):133–9.

28. POLYMYXINS

ROBERT FEKETY

STRUCTURE

Polymyxin A, B, C, D, and E are related cyclic basic polypeptides characterized by poor diffusibility, a molecular weight of about 1100, an antimicrobial spectrum limited to gram-negative aerobes, and significant toxicity. All but polymyxin B and E are too toxic for therapeutic use in humans.[1] Colistin is identical to polymyxin E; it differs from polymyxin B in only 1 of its 10 amino acids.[2]

DERIVATION AND NOMENCLATURE

Polymyxins are derived from *Bacillus polymyxa*. Polymyxin B sulfate was introduced for clinical use in 1947. It is marketed in units that are only 65–75 percent pure; 1 unit of polymyxin B sulfate is equivalent to 0.1 μg of pure polymyxin base. Colistin (polymyxin E, Coly-Mycin) was introduced clinically in 1961 as the methanesulfonate (colistimethate) derivative. Its advatage is that it is less painful than polymyxin B sulfate is after intramuscular injection.[3] Methanesulfonation of the free amino groups of polymyxins has a (temporarily) detrimental effect on their antibacterial action; colistimethate is essentially inactive until hydrolyzed within the body to the colistin base.[4] Thus, colistimethate may be thought of as a repository form of intramuscular polymyxin.

MECHANISM OF ACTION

The polymyxins act like cationic detergents or surfactants. They disrupt the osmotic integrity of the cell membrane by interacting with its phospholipids and increasing cellular permeability. This effect allows vital intracellular constituents such as nucleic acids and proteins to leak out, with subsequent death of the cell. The polymyxins are bactericidal and kill resting cells without necessarily lysing them. Susceptibility may be related to the phospholipid content of the cell wall–membrane complex.[3] Resistant organisms have cell walls that prevent access of the drug to the membrane. Calcium reduces the antibacterial action of polymyxins by interfering with their attachment to the membrane. Interestingly, polymyxins may also interfere with some of the actions of bacterial endotoxins, but this effect is inhibited by calcium and is of uncertain clinical significance.

ANTIMICROBIAL ACTIVITY

Polymyxin B and colistin (polymyxin E) have identical antibacterial spectra and show complete cross-resistance.[1,3,5] On a weight basis, polymyxin B sulfate is slightly more active and toxic than colistin sulfate is and is much more active than colistin methanesulfonate is.[6] The polymyxins are almost exclusively active against gram-negative bacilli. Their primary clinical usefulness is for *Pseudomonas* infections. *Pseudomonas aeruginosa* isolates are almost always inhibited by concentrations lower than 8 μg/ml. *Escherichia coli, Klebsiella pneumoniae, Enterobacter, Salmonella, Shigella, Vibrio, Haemophilus, Pasteurella, Bordetella*, and the other *Pseudomonas* species are usually susceptible. *Proteus, Providencia, Serratia*, and *Neisseria* isolates are usually resistant, as are gram-positive organisms and obligate anaerobes.[1,5] There is no cross-resistance with other antibiotics, and resistance rarely develops during therapy. Polymyxins have some slight activity against various fungi, but this has had no clinical significance. Rifampin combined with polymyxin B may be synergistic against multiply resistant *Serratia* isolates. Synergism against *Pseudomonas* has been demonstrated in vitro between polymyxins and tetracycline, chloramphenicol, carbenicillin, and trimethoprim/sulfamethoxazole, but the clinical significance of this enhancement for the most part is not known.[1,3,6] The combination of polymyxin and trimethoprim/sulfamethoxazole has been useful in severe *Pseudomonas cepacia* or *maltophilia* infections.

PHARMACOLOGY: ADMINISTRATION AND ABSORPTION

The polymyxins are not absorbed when given orally. They are intended primarily for parenteral use. Polymyxin B sulfate is the only derivative of polymyxin B that is available for treatment. It can be given intravenously, intramuscularly, intrathecally, orally, topically, endobronchially, or by aerosol. Polymyxins are quite painful when given intramuscularly, and the pain may persist for several hours. However, when the drugs are given intravenously, local adverse effects are minimal. Colistin is available as the sulfate for oral use and as the sodium salt of the colistimethate derivative for parenteral use. Colistimethate is less painful than polymyxin B is on intramuscular injection. Colistimethate can be given by slow intravenous infusion, but even when given slowly its intravenous use may result in inadequate serum and tissue antibacterial activity if colistimethate is eliminated from the body by the kidneys before hydrolysis to the active base can take place.[4] (A bioassay of colistimethate in serum after intravenous or intramuscular administration encounters a related problem in that unhydrolyzed drug may become hydrolyzed and therefore may become more active during the assay.)

When a total daily dose of parenteral polymyxin B of 2.5 mg (25,000 units)/kg is infused in 300–500 ml of 5% dextrose in water (D_5W), peak serum concentrations of approximately 5 μg/ml are obtained. Ninety-five percent of *P. aeruginosa* isolates are susceptible to this concentration. These organisms are also susceptible at the serum levels of 5–8 μg/ml that are achieved with intramuscular colistin (2.5–5.0 mg/kg/day). By virtue of the renal excretion of colistimethate, urinary concentrations of 10–160 μg/ml are achieved with it. The serum half-life of colistin is 2–4.5 hours and that of polymyxin B, 6–7 hours. With an intramuscular injection, there may be a delay of several hours before effective urinary levels are achieved with both drugs, but colistimethate, being less bound to kidney tissues, is excreted more rapidly than is polymyxin B.[4] These drugs may be found in the urine for 2–3 days after treatment has been discontinued. Polymyxins do not pass into the cerebrospinal fluid well, even in the presence of inflammation, and in the treatment of meningitis they must be given intrathecally.[3] Nor do they pass readily into pleural, synovial, or brain tissues. Furthermore, they may combine with tissue cell membranes and the constituents of exudates (such as polyphosphates), which may explain why the polymyxins seem to be relatively ineffective in infections of the pleura, synovium, or brain.[3] Polymyxins cross the placental barrier, and concentrations of 1 μg/ml may be found in the fetus.

The excretion of the polymyxins is mostly via the kidneys. They are excreted primarily by glomerular filtration; there is no tubular secretion or reabsorption. Renal insufficiency results in decreased renal excretion of polymyxins, increased serum levels, and a greater likelihood of toxicity. The half-life in serum of polymyxin B or E in anuric patients is 48–72 hours. Doses must be reduced appropriately and renal function monitored carefully to avoid toxicity (Table 1). Urinary concentrations are reduced in the presence of renal failure.[5] Hemodialysis has no appreciable effect on serum concentrations, but peritoneal dialysis removes small amounts (1 mg/hr), and it may be useful in an overdosage.[7]

While orally administered polymyxins are poorly absorbed from the intact gastrointestinal tract of adults, they may be absorbed from the gastrointestinal tract of premature or newborn infants, and their oral use is thus hazardous and contraindicated in this population.[5] After being administered orally, polymyxins are not found in the tissues of the bowel wall in significant amounts, which may account for their ineffectiveness in the treatment of shigellosis.

Polymyxin is often used topically, usually in concentrations of 0.1% polymyxin (1 mg/ml or 1 mg/g), in combination with other antibiotics such as bacitracin or neomycin for the treatment of skin, mucous membrane, eye, and ear infections. Polymyxins are poorly absorbed from these surfaces. Polymyxin B is sometimes used for irrigation of various sites of infection. This can be dangerous since polymyxin B is absorbed well from serous cavities such as the peritoneum and the resultant high serum concentrations may result in the induction of apnea.

The protein binding of polymyxins has not been studied extensively but may be as high as 75 percent. These drugs lose much of their antibacterial activity in the presence of serum.[1]

TOXICITY AND ADVERSE REACTIONS

The two most important side effects of polymyxins are neurotoxicity and nephrotoxicity. Allergic reactions (including fever and skin rashes) are rare after polymyxin administration, but they are histamine releasers, and some patients have developed urticaria or shock after the rapid intravenous infusion of polymyxins. Pain at the site of injection is common. This can be reduced by mixing with a local anesthetic. For example, 50 mg polymyxin B may be mixed with 2 ml of 2% procaine in saline; colistimethate formerly was supplied mixed with dibucaine. When a serum concentration of 1–2 μg/ml or more of polymyxins is achieved, most patients will experience circumoral or stocking-glove paresthesias, sometimes with flushing, dizziness, vertigo, ataxia, slurred speech, drowsiness, or confusion. These are less frequent with lower doses, in children, and when injections are given no more frequently than every 8 hours. These neurotoxic side effects disappear soon after therapy with the drugs has been discontinued. Polymyxins also have a curare-like action on striated muscles and block neuromuscular transmission. High serum concentrations may result in apnea, which can be treated with intravenous calcium chloride.

Dose-related nephrotoxicity is the most important side effect of polymyxins. In general, the more antibacterially active derivative, polymyxin B, is more toxic than colistin is. At therapeutically equivalent doses, they are frequently and equally nephrotoxic,[3,6] and renal function should be carefully monitored during therapy. Renal toxicity probably follows attachment of the antibiotics to the membrane of the renal convoluted tubular epithelium. This may be accentuated or potentiated by aminoglycosides or other nephrotoxic drugs, which should therefore be avoided. At appropriate therapeutic dosages, approximately 20 percent of patients experience nephrotoxicity manifested by a rising serum creatinine level and an abnormal urinary sediment, and 1–2 percent develop acute tubular necrosis. Nitrogen retention, probably related to a reduction in the glomerular filtration rate, frequently increases for a week or so after treatment with these drugs has been discontinued but is usually reversible.[8] Anuria and tubular necrosis with serious renal failure are particularly common in patients who have received excessive doses or in whom the drug therapy is continued in usual doses in the face of impaired renal function. In renal failure, polymyxins should be used only with great care and in reduced doses (Table 1).[3,5,8,9] Patients receiving no more than 2.2 mg/kg daily usually tolerate polymyxin B well even for long periods.

Little diarrhea or disturbance of the gastrointestinal flora results when these drugs are used. Dyspnea may occur after the use of polymyxin by aerosol, and respiratory arrest has been reported.

MAJOR USES AND DOSES

The polymyxins are used infrequently parenterally and almost exclusively for serious, life-threatening *Pseudomonas* or gram-negative bacillary infections caused by organisms resistant to other drugs or in patients with these infections who are intolerant or allergic to the preferred drugs. The usual dose of polymyxin B for adults with normal renal function is 1.5–2.5 mg (15,000–25,000 units)/kg/day given by continuous intravenous infusion. The intramuscular dosage is 2.5–3.0 mg/kg/day given at 4- or 6-hour intervals. Septic infants may receive up to 40,000–45,000 units/kg/day. Adults with normal renal function may be given 2.5–5.0 mg/kg colistimethate/day in two or three divided doses (iv or im). Polymyxin B is preferred to colistimethate for intravenous use since it does not require hydrolysis for activation.[5]

Polymyxins are second-line or alternate drugs since they are relatively ineffective in patients with bacteremia and involvement of deep tissues, and they are especially ineffective in compromised hosts with granulocytopenia.[10] Endocarditis usually cannot be cured with the polymyxins without the aid of surgery or other drugs. When bacteremia is associated with a removable or treatable focus, these drugs may be useful. Best results have been obtained with urinary tract infections or septicemias arising from the urinary tract.[3,7]

The rare patient with meningitis requiring polymyxins should be treated intrathecally. The usual intrathecal dose of polymyxin B is 5–10 mg/day in adults; in children younger than 2 years of age, a dose of 2 mg/day is used. Amounts greater than 10 mg (100,000 units) should never be used intrathecally for meningitis alone. It is believed that nothing is gained by adding intravenous therapy when patients are treated intrathecally. Daily intrathecal therapy should be given for 3–5 days and then every other day for 3 weeks or for 2 weeks after cultures are negative and the cerebrospinal fluid (CSF) glucose level is normal.

Urinary tract infections can be treated with relatively low and

TABLE 1. Reduction in Polymyxin Dosage to Avoid Drug-Induced Renal Injury

	Parenteral Dose (mg/kg Body Weight) When Creatinine Clearance Is			
Drug	Normal, or ≥80% of Normal	80–≥30% of Normal	<30% of Normal	With Anuria
Polymyxin B, sulfate	2.5–3.0 mg/day	1st day, 2.5 mg; daily thereafter at 1.0–1.5 mg	1st day, 2.5 mg; every 2–3 days thereafter, 1.0–1.5 mg	1st day, 2.5 mg; every 5–7 days thereafter, 1.0 mg
Colistimethate (polymyxin E)	3.0–5.0 mg/day	1st day, 3.0 mg; daily thereafter at 1.5–2.5 mg	1st day, 3.0 mg; every 2–3 days thereafter, 1.5–2.5 mg	1st day, 2.5 mg; every 5–7 days thereafter, 1.5 mg

well-tolerated doses of intramuscular colistimethate (2.5 mg/kg/day in divided dosage for 7–10 days). Results are better with acute than with chronic urinary infections, in which relapses are frequent within a few months.

Some investigators believe that the prevention of urinary tract infections in patients requiring indwelling (Foley) catheters for periods up to 2 weeks may be achieved by using triple-lumen catheters and continuous irrigation of the bladder with a solution of neomycin (40 mg/liter) and polymyxin B (20 mg/liter). Usually, no more than 1 liter of irrigant is used per day unless urine flow rates are very high.[11]

Aerosolized polymyxins have been used in the treatment of respiratory infections due to *Pseudomonas* in patients with cystic fibrosis or bronchiectasis and in the prevention of *Pseudomonas* infections in respiratory intensive care units during periods of high risk.[12] Usually, the solution contains 2–10 mg/ml, and 2 ml is aerosolized six to eight times per day. Ultimately, the development of resistant organisms has limited the efficacy of this measure; to delay this, intermittent use of the regimens has been tried. Polymyxin has been combined with neomycin and amphotericin B, other nonabsorbed antimicrobials, via the oral route for infection prophylaxis and selective decontamination of the digestive tract in patients with acute leukemia.[13] The oropharynx and stools of most patients became free of gram-negative bacilli within 1 week.

In creams, sprays, and solutions containing 0.5–3 mg/ml, polymyxins are useful in the prevention and treatment of skin infections and in the treatment of external otitis or corneal ulcers. When administered topically, it is often combined with neomycin and bacitracin. Subconjunctival injection of up to 100,000 units polymyxin B per day may be used in the treatment of *Pseudomonas* infections of the cornea and conjunctivae. A total dose of 200 mg/day should not be exceeded.

Polymyxins may be useful when administered orally to small children with localized gastroenteritis due to enteropathogenic *E. coli*, but they are relatively useless in patients with *Salmonella* or invasive *Shigella* enteritis. An oral dose of colistin sulfate of 15–20 mg/kg/day in three divided doses for 5–20 days has been used with *E. coli* outbreaks, but 3–5 mg/kg/day is the usual oral dose. These drugs should not be used orally in neonates and premature infants.

When polymyxins are combined with sulfamethoxazole and trimethoprim, they are often synergistic and can be useful in the treatment of serious infections with multiply drug-resistant *Serratia* and *Pseudomonas cepacia, P. maltophilia*, or *P. aeruginosa* isolates.[14–16] A combination of polymyxin B and rifampin has also been used successfully in seriously ill patients with drug-resistant nosocomial *Serratia* infections.[17]

REFERENCES

1. Jawetz E. Polymyxin, colistin and bacitracin. Pediatr Clin North Am. 1961;8:1057.
2. Wilkinson S. Identity of colistin and polymyxin E. Lancet. 1963;1:922.
3. Goodwin NJ. Colistin and sodium colistimethate. Med Clin North Am. 1970;54:1267.
4. Barnett M, Bushby SRM, Wilkinson S. Sodium sulphomethyl derivatives of polymyxins. Br J Pharmacol. 1964;23:552.
5. Hoeprich PD. The polymyxins. Med Clin North Am. 1970;54:1257.
6. Nord NM, Hoeprich PD. Polymyxin B and colistin. A critical comparison. N Engl J Med. 1964;270:1030.
7. Goodwin N, Friedman E. The effects of renal impairment, peritoneal dialysis, and hemodialysis on serum sodium colistimethate levels. Ann Intern Med. 1968;68:984.
8. Fekety FR, Norman PS, Cluff LE. The treatment of gram-negative bacillary infections. The toxicity and efficacy of large doses in forty-eight patients. Ann Intern Med. 1962;57:214.
9. Appel GB, Neu HC. The nephrotoxicity of antimicrobial agents. N Engl J Med. 1977;296:663.
10. Whitecar JP, Luna M, Bodey GP. *Pseudomonas* bacteremia in patients with malignant disease. Am J Med Sci. 1970;260:216.
11. Marten CM, Bookrajian EN. Bacteriuria prevention after indwelling urinary catheterization. Arch Intern Med. 1962;110:703.
12. Feeley TW, duMoulin GC, Hedley-Whyte J, et al. Aerosol polymyxin and pneumonia in seriously ill patients. N Engl J Med. 1975;293:471.
13. van der Waaij D, Gaus W, Krieger D, et al. Bacteriological data on a prospective multicenter study of the effect of two different regimens for selective decontamination in patients with acute leukemia. Infection. 1986;14:268–74.
14. Thomas FE, Leonard JM, Alford RH. Sulfamethoxazole-trimethoprim polymyxin therapy of serious multiply drug-resistant *Serratia* infections. Antimicrob Agents Chemother. 1976;9:201.
15. Rosenblatt JE, Stewart PR. Combined activity of sulfamethoxazole, trimethoprim, and polymyxin B against gram-negative bacilli. Antimicrob Agents Chemother. 1974;6:84.
16. Nord C, Wadstrom T, Wretlind B. Synergistic effects of combinations of sulfamethoxazole, trimethoprim and colistin against *Pseudomonas maltophilia* and *P. cepacia*. Antimicrob Agents Chemother. 1974;6:521.
17. Ostenson RC, Fields BT, Nolan CM. Polymyxin B and rifampin: New regimen for multiresistant *Serratia marcescens* infections. Antimicrob Agents Chemother. 1977;12:655.

29. SULFONAMIDES AND TRIMETHOPRIM

STEPHEN H. ZINNER
KENNETH H. MAYER

The modern era of antimicrobial chemotherapy began in 1932 with the first reports by Gerhard Domagk of the protective activity of prontosil against murine streptococcal infections. This drug was an outgrowth of the German dye industry and had been commercially available since the early twentieth century. Prontosil (sulfachrysoidine) exerted its antibacterial activity due to the release in vivo of para-aminobenzenesulfonamide (sulfanilamide). This agent was the first antibacterial used in the United States, in an unsuccessful attempt, in July, 1935, to treat a 10-year-old girl late in the course of meningitis and sepsis due to *Haemophilus influenzae*.[1] During the late 1930s, the basic sulfanilamide compound was modified to remove unpleasant side effects while expanding its spectrum of activity. More recent modifications have resulted in compounds of specific usefulness, for example, in urinary infections (those compounds that are highly soluble), or those nonabsorbable sulfonamides that act only within the gastrointestinal tract.

Trimethoprim is a 2,4-diamino-pyrimidine and, as such, inhibits the enzyme dihydrofolate reductase, resulting in interference in folic acid and subsequent pyrimidine synthesis in the bacterial cell. Trimethoprim is one of several such compounds synthesized and studied by Hitchings and coworkers in the 1950s and 1960s. The use of trimethoprim as a potentiator of sulfonamide activity was introduced by Bushby and Hitchings in 1968.[2] In the subsequent decade the combination of trimethoprim-sulfamethoxazole has been introduced clinically and has found a place in the chemotherapy of many infectious diseases. These agents, available in a fixed drug combination, show true antibacterial synergism against a wide variety of organisms.

SULFONAMIDES

Structure

The clinically useful sulfonamides are derived from sulfanilamide (para-aminobenzenesulfonamide) that is similar in structure to para-aminobenzoic acid (PABA), a factor required by bacteria for folic acid synthesis (Fig. 1).

A free amino group at the 4 position is associated with enhanced activity. Increased activity due to increased PABA inhibition is associated with substitutions at the sulfonyl radical (SO_2)—attached to the 1 carbon, as seen with sulfadiazine, sulfisoxazole, and sulfamethoxazole, all of which are more active than the parent compound, sulfanilamide. The nature of these substitutions determines other pharmacologic properties of the drug such as absorption, solubility, and gastrointestinal

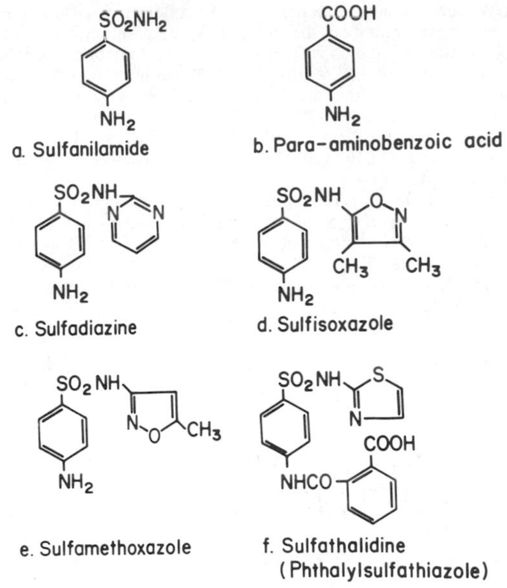

FIG. 1. Structural formulas of selected sulfonamides.

tolerance. Substitutions at the 4-amino group result in decreased absorption from the gastrointestinal tract (e.g., phthalylsulfathiazole).

Derivation and Nomenclature

Since the introduction of sulfonamides into clinical medicine, dozens of compounds have been used. However, relatively few survive today, and they can be classified as (*1*) short- or medium-acting sulfonamides, (*2*) long-acting sulfonamides, (*3*) sulfonamides limited to the gastrointestinal tract, and (*4*) topical sulfonamides.

Short- or Medium-Acting Sulfonamides. Sulfisoxazole *United States Pharmacopeia* (USP) (sulphafurazole *British Pharmacopeia*–BP, 3,4-dimethyl-5-sulfanilamidoisoxazole, Gantrisin, SK-Soxazole) is a highly soluble drug especially useful in urinary tract infections. Sulfamethoxazole USP (5-methyl-3-sulfanilamidoisoxazole; Gantanol) is somewhat less soluble than sulfisoxazole and yields higher blood levels. It is the sulfonamide presently most frequently combined with trimethoprim. Sulfadiazine USP (2-sulfanilamidopyridine) is highly active, attains high blood and cerebrospinal fluid levels, and is associated with low protein binding and lower solubility than the above drugs. Sulfamethizole USP (2-sulfanilamide-5-methyl-1:3:4-thiazole; Microsul, Thiosulfil) is used for urinary tract infections. Sulfadimidine and sulfacarbamide are available in the United Kingdom.

Short-acting sulfonamides are also available in several combinations. Sulfisoxazole, sulfamethoxazole, and sulfamethizole are each combined with phenazopyridine, a urinary analgesic, as Azo Gantrisin, Azo Gantanol, Microsul-A, Sul-Azo, and Thiosulfil-A Forte. Phenazopyridine is also present with sulfamethazole and sulfadiazine in Suladyne. Sulfamethizole is also combined with tetracycline and phenazopyridine in Urobiotic and Azotrex, but these two preparations have been classified by the Food and Drug Administration (FDA) as lacking evidence of effectiveness as a fixed drug combination.

Long-Acting Sulfonamides. Sulfamethoxypyridazine (3-sulfanilamido-6-methoxy-pyridazine) and sulfameter [4-amino-*N*-(5-methoxy-2-pyrimidinyl)] benzene-sulfonamide are no longer available for single daily dose therapy, as they were associated with hypersensitivity reactions such as Stevens-Johnson syndrome. Neither sulfadimethoxine (Madribon) nor any other long-acting sulfonamides other than sulfadoxine are currently available in the United States.

Sulfadoxine, originally known as sulformethoxine [*N'*-(5,6-dimethoxy-4-pyrimidyl) sulfanilamide] is a very long-acting sulfonamide that, combined with pyrimethamine, is available as Fansidar. Sulfadoxine has a half-life of 100–230 hours and reaches a peak serum level of 51–76 μg/ml 2.5–6 hours after an oral dose of 500 mg. Fansidar is active in the treatment and prophylaxis of malaria due to chloroquine-resistant *Plasmodium falciparum*.[3] Due to the unknown teratogenic potential of pyrimethamine, Fansidar should not be recommended for prophylaxis of pregnant women, and its use has been associated with Stevens-Johnson syndrome. Also, some strains of *P. falciparum* from Southeast Asia and South America may be resistant.

Sulfonamides Limited to the Gastrointestinal Tract. Sulfaguanidine (*N'*amidinosulfanilamide), sulfasuxidine (2-(para-succinylsulfanilamido)-thiazole, succinylsulfathiazole), and sulfathalidine [2(para-phthalyl-sulfanilamido)-thiazole] are relatively poorly absorbed from the gastrointestinal tract. They have been used in the past to suppress the susceptible bowel flora before surgery.

Salicylazosulfapyridine (sulfasalazine, Azulfidine) is a sulfonamide derivative used in the treatment of ulcerative colitis. This drug is absorbed in its parent form as sulfapyridine, and significant blood levels of this compound are measurable.

Topical Sulfonamides. Mafenide acetate (para-aminomethylbenzene sulfonamide, Sulfamylon cream) is available for use in the topical therapy of burns. However, its use has been limited by metabolic acidosis due to carbonic anhydrase inhibition. Silver sulfadiazine has fewer side effects and is used extensively for burns.[4] Here the sulfonamide acts primarily as a vehicle for release of silver ions that exert an antibacterial effect. Recent reports of outbreaks of silver-resistant infections in burn units may ultimately limit its usefulness.[5,6] Various combinations of other sulfonamides are available as vaginal creams or suppositories (e.g., Sultrin vaginal cream and tablets, AVC cream and suppositories, Sulfamel, Vagitrol).

There are a variety of ophthalmic ointments and solutions of sulfacetamide sodium USP (a highly soluble sulfonamide) available for use in treating conjunctivitis due to susceptible bacteria and as adjunctive therapy of trachoma (e.g., Bleph, Cetamide, Isoph, Sulamyd).

Mechanisms of Action

Although a wide variety of chemical modifications of the sulfonamides has been synthesized, all basically share the same mechanism of action. The sulfonamides are bacteriostatic in that they inhibit bacterial growth via interference with microbial folic acid synthesis. More specifically, sulfonamides inhibit competitively the incorporation of PABA into tetrahydropteroic acid,[7–9] and they in turn may be incorporated into dihydropteroate.[10] Sulfonamides may have a higher affinity for the microbial enzyme tetrahydropteroic acid synthetase than the natural substrate PABA. Richmond[11] has suggested that sulfonamides may act on bacterial repressor genes or by feedback inhibition to decrease formation of new enzyme. The ultimate result of decreased folic acid synthesis is a decrease in bacterial nucleotides, with subsequent inhibition of bacterial growth.

Antimicrobial Activity In Vitro

Sulfonamides exhibit in vitro inhibitory activity against a broad spectrum of gram-positive and gram-negative bacteria as well as *Actinomyces*, *Chlamydia*, *Plasmodia*, and *Toxoplasma* (Table 1). The in vitro antimicrobial sensitivity of sulfonamides

TABLE 1. In Vitro Activity of Sulfonamides Against Representative Organisms[a]

	Range of MIC[b] *(μg/ml)*
Gram-positive	
Staphylococcus aureus	8–64
Streptococcus pneumoniae	4–128
Streptococcus pyogenes	0.5–16
Enterococcus faecalis	25–250
Corynebacterium diphtheriae	25–75
Listeria monocytogenes	3–75
Bacillus anthracis	12–100
Gram-negative	
Escherichia coli	4–64
Klebsiella spp.	8–128
Proteus mirabilis	8–128
Serratia marcescens	25–>1000
Salmonella sp.	16–128
Shigella sp.	2–32
Haemophilus influenzae	1–16
Neisseria gonorrhoeae	4–32
Neisseria meningitidis	0.25–>10
Pseudomonas aeruginosa	>100–200
Other	
Chlamydia trachomatis	0.1
Nocardia asteroides	2–16

[a] The acquisition of plasmids may increase MICs.
[b] Minimum Inhibitory Concentration. Range is expressed for a variety of sulfonamide compounds.
(Data from Garrod et al.,[27] Bushby,[28] and Bach et al.[23])

is strongly influenced by the size of the inoculum and the composition of the test media. High concentrations of PABA and thymidine inhibit sulfonamide activity.

Antimicrobial Resistance. Resistance to sulfonamides is widespread and may be found in more than 20 percent of community and nosocomial strains of bacteria, including staphylococci, Enterobacteriaceae, *Neisseria meningitidis*, and *Pseudomonas* sp.[12]

Organisms may develop resistance or partial resistance by mutation, resulting in either microbial overproduction of PABA[13] or a structural change in dihydropteroate synthetase, an enzyme that has lowered affinity for sulfonamide.[14] The former mechanism has been implicated in resistant strains of *Neisseria gonorrhoeae* and *Staphylococcus aureus*,[13,15] and the latter has been found in strains of *Escherichia coli*.[16] Resistance also may be mediated by plasmids, episomal-resistance transfer factors (R factors) that may code for the production of drug-resistant enzymes, such as dihydropteroate synthetase,[17] or may result in decreased bacterial cell permeability to sulfonamides.[18] R-factor transfer can occur in the gastrointestinal tract as well as in vitro and has been seen especially with Enterobacteriaceae.[19] More than one resistance mechanism may be operating simultaneously.[20]

Plasmid-mediated sulfonamide resistance has greatly increased in recent years, often in conjunction with trimethoprim resistance. More than one-fourth of the uropathogens and one-half of the clinical *Shigella* isolates studied in Sweden,[21,22] England,[12,23] and the United States[24] were sulfonamide-resistant. *Salmonella* resistance to sulfonamides has also increased in the United States,[25] often in conjunction with resistance to other antibiotic classes. The increase in sulfonamide-resistant *Haemophilus ducreyi* in Asia and Africa has been associated with a plasmid related to those found in Enterobacteriaceae.[26]

Pharmacology

Routes of Administration. Sulfonamides are usually administered orally, although sulfadiazine and sulfisoxazole are available for use as intravenous or subcutaneous preparations. These latter forms are used rarely, if at all. Sulfacetamide is available as ophthalmic preparations, and silver sulfadiazine and mafenide acetate are applied topically in burn patients and are associated with significant absorption of sulfonamide percutaneously. Vaginal preparations are available for topical application.

Absorption. Most of the short- and medium-acting sulfonamides are absorbed rapidly and almost completely in the un-ionized state from the small intestine and stomach. Compounds with *N*-1 substitutions are absorbed poorly, as are more acidic compounds (e.g., phthalylsulfathiazole, Fig. 1f). Long-acting sulfonamides also are absorbed rapidly but have a much slower excretion rate. Topical sulfonamides are absorbed and may result in detectable blood levels.

Distribution. The sulfonamides generally are well distributed throughout the body, entering the cerebrospinal fluid and synovial, pleural, and peritoneal fluids with concentrations approaching 80 percent of serum levels. Blood and tissue levels are related to the degree of protein binding (Table 2) and lipid solubility. Sulfonamides administered in pregnancy readily cross the placenta and are present in the fetal blood and amniotic fluid.[31]

Excretion. Acetylation and glucuronidation occur in the liver, and free and metabolized drug appears in the urine. Glomerular filtration is probably a route of excretion, although partial reabsorption and active tubular secretion also are involved, especially at low creatinine clearance rates. Urinary excretion is more rapid for those sulfonamides with low pKa values (e.g., sulfamethizole, sulfisoxazole), and alkalinization of the urine increases excretion by this route. Plasma half-lives vary widely and are related inversely to lipid solubility and directly to pKa but are not clearly related to the degree of protein binding.[30] Small amounts of sulfonamides are found in bile, human milk, prostatic secretions, saliva, and tears.

Protein Binding and Blood or Tissue Levels. Sulfonamides are bound variably and not irreversibly to plasma albumin, and the bound drug is inactive (Table 2). Levels obtainable in cerebrospinal and other body fluids are inversely related to the degree of protein binding. The amount of free drug in plasma is directly related to pKa.[30]

Use in Renal Insufficiency. Sulfonamides can be used in renal failure, but therapeutic serum levels will persist longer because of reduced excretion, and the dosage must be reduced and the interval between doses extended proportional to the degree of renal impairment. Protein binding of sulfonamides is decreased in severe renal insufficiency.[32] The *N*-4 acetylated metabolite of sulfonamides may accumulate in patients with renal failure, especially during prolonged therapy. This derivative loses its antibacterial effect but still may have toxic properties. Plasma levels of sulfonamide should be measured every 3 days, and peak concentrations of sulfamethoxazole should be less than 120 μg/ml.

TABLE 2. Levels in Blood, Cerebrospinal Fluid, Plasma Half-life, and Protein Binding of Some Sulfonamides

Drug	*Peak Blood Level*[a] *(μg/ml)*	*Serum Level in CSF (%)*	*Plasma Half-life (hours)*	*Protein Binding (%)*
Sulfadiazine	30–60	40–80	17	45
Sulfisoxazole	40–50	30–50	5–6	92
Sulfamethoxazole	80–100	25–30	11	70
Sulfadoxine	50–75	20–30	100–230	80–98

[a] Approximate free sulfonamide level after a 2 g oral dose.
(Data from Anand[30] and Garrod et al.[27])

Toxicity and Adverse Reactions

Sulfonamides may cause nausea, vomiting, diarrhea, rash, fever, headache, depression, jaundice, hepatic necrosis, and a serum sicknesslike syndrome. Earlier, less soluble compounds (sulfadiazine, sulfathiazole) used in excessively high doses were associated with crystalluria and tubular deposits of sulfonamide crystals. These complications could be minimized by the maintenance of high urine flow and alkalinization of the urine. This complication usually is not seen with modern soluble sulfonamides. Tubular necrosis, interstitial nephritis, or necrotizing angiitis may be associated rarely with sulfonamide sensitivity.

More serious adverse reactions due to sulfonamides may include acute hemolytic anemia (sometimes related to a deficiency in erythrocyte glucose-6-phosphate dehydrogenase—G6PD), aplastic anemia, agranulocytosis, thrombocytopenia, and leukopenia. A recent study showed that G6PD-deficient patients who received trimethoprim-sulfamethoxazole did not have hemolytic reactions during therapy.[33]

Sulfonamides should not be administered during the last month of pregnancy because they compete for bilirubin-binding sites on plasma albumin and may increase fetal blood levels of unconjugated bilirubin, increasing the risk of kernicterus. Also, because of the immature fetal acetyl transferase system, blood levels of free sulfonamide may be increased, further adversely affecting the risk of kernicterus.[30]

Finally, significant hypersensitivity reactions may occur due to sulfonamides administered via any route. The most important of these include erythema nodosum, erythema multiforme (including Stevens-Johnson syndrome), drug eruption, vasculitis similar to periarteritis nodosa, and anaphylaxis. Long-acting sulfonamides have been associated with fatal hypersensitivity reactions, especially in children, and this severely limits their use. Locally applied sulfonamides (e.g., to skin) may be associated with any of these adverse reactions.

Drug Interactions

Sulfonamides may displace from albumin-binding sites drugs such as warfarin, thus increasing the effective activity of the displaced drug. Anticoagulant dosage therefore should be reduced during sulfonamide therapy. Sulfonamides also displace methotrexate from its bound protein, thereby increasing methotrexate toxicity. An increased hypoglycemic effect of chlorpropamide and tolbutamide may occur during sulfonamide therapy, possibly due to the same mechanism or to structural similarities. Sulfonamides may potentiate the action of some thiazide diuretics, phenytoin, and uricosuric agents. Conversely, sulfonamides themselves may be displaced from binding sites by indomethacin, phenylbutazone, salicylates, probenecid, and sulfinpyrazone, resulting in increased sulfonamide activity.

The activity of sulfonamides may be decreased by procaine and other local anesthetics derived from PABA. Methenamine compounds should not be used with sulfonamides because of the formation of insoluble urinary precipitates. Intravenous solutions of sulfonamides are physically incompatible with chloramphenicol, aminoglycosides, lincomycin, methicillin, tetracyclines, vancomycin, norepinephrine, insulin, procaine, Ringer lactate solution, and others. Sulfonamides may decrease protein-bound iodine and ^{131}I uptake and may produce false-positive Benedict tests for urine glucose and false-positive sulfosalicylic acid tests for urine proteins.[34–36]

Major Clinical Use

Sulfonamides are primarily used in the treatment of acute urinary tract infections, but increasing resistance has diminished their effectiveness. Most first episodes of infection in the unobstructed urinary tract will be due to *E. coli* that are often sensitive to sulfonamides. Sulfisoxazole is administered orally in a usual dosage of 1 g qid. Since the infecting organism of any urinary tract infection may or may not be sensitive to sulfonamides, the choice of therapy should be based on appropriate sensitivity tests (see Chapter 58).

Sulfonamides are also quite effective in the therapy of infections due to *Nocardia asteroides*. Therapy must include 4–6 g or more daily after a loading dose of 4 g and should be continued for 4–6 months or longer if necessary (see Chapter 94). Sulfonamides may be useful in combination with other antimycobacterial drugs for the management of infections due to rifampin-resistant *Mycobacterium kansasii*.[37]

Sulfonamides are effective in the prophylaxis of patients against recurrent attacks of rheumatic fever associated with group A β-hemolytic streptococcal infections, but they are not effective for therapy for established streptococcal pharyngitis. Sulfonamide prophylaxis of close contacts of patients with meningitis due to *N. meningitidis* is effective if the infecting organism is known to be sulfonamide-sensitive (adult dose for sulfadiazine is 1 g q12h for 2 days). Sulfonamides have been used to treat toxoplasmosis and *P. falciparum* malaria (with pyrimethamine), meliodosis, dermatitis herpetiformis, lymphogranuloma venereum, and chancroid; topical and systemic therapy is effective for trachoma and inclusion conjunctivitis (usually with topical tetracycline). Nongonococcal urethritis due to *Chlamydia*, but not *Ureaplasma urealyticum*, responds well to sulfonamide therapy (see Chapter 94). Sulfasalazine is used in the treatment of inflammatory bowel diseases and has had some success in patients with rheumatoid arthritis and other inflammatory conditions.[38,39] Currently, sulfonamides are used frequently in combination with trimethoprim (see below).

TRIMETHOPRIM

Structure and Derivation

Trimethoprim is a 2,4-diamino-5-(3′,4′,5′-trimethoxybenzyl) pyrimidine (Fig. 2). This drug was synthesized by Hitchings and coworkers as a dihydrofolate reductase inhibitor thought to potentiate the activity of sulfonamides by sequential inhibition of folic acid synthesis.[2] In the United States, trimethoprim is now available as a single agent as well as in combination with sulfamethoxazole (see below). Trimethoprim does have antibacterial activity of its own, and its pharmacology will be reviewed.

Mechanism of Action

Trimethoprim owes its activity to powerful inhibition of bacterial dihydrofolate reductase, which is the enzyme step after the step in folic acid synthesis blocked by sulfonamides. Trimethoprim is 50,000–100,000 times more active against bacterial dihydrofolate reductase than against the human enzyme. Trimethoprim interferes with the conversion of dihydrofolate to tetrahydrofolate, the precursor of folinic acid and ultimately purine and DNA synthesis (Fig. 3). The sequential blockage of the same biosynthetic pathway by sulfonamides and trimethoprim results in a high degree of synergistic activity against a wide spectrum of microorganisms. Humans do not synthesize

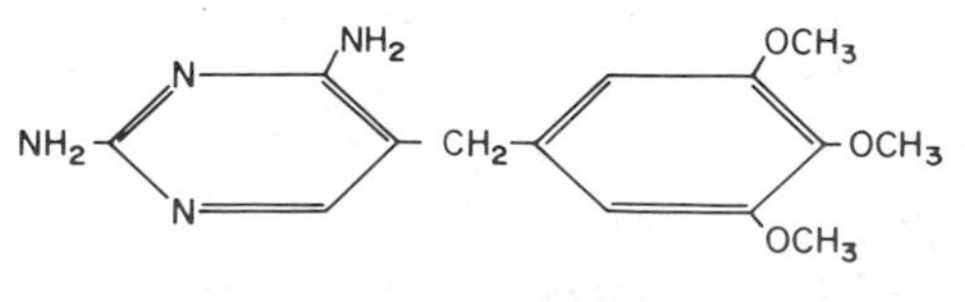

TRIMETHOPRIM
(2,4-diamino-5-(3′,4′,5′-trimethoxybenzyl)pyrimidine)

FIG. 2. Chemical structure of trimethoprim.

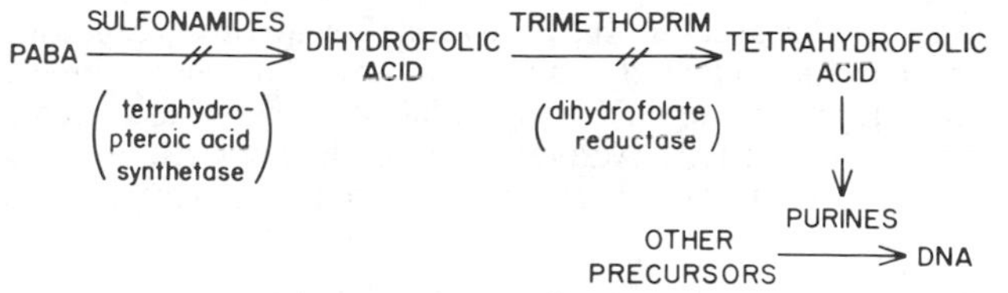

FIG. 3. Action of sulfonamides and trimethoprim on the metabolic pathway of bacterial folic acid synthesis.

folic acid but require it in their diet, and therefore human purine synthesis is not affected significantly by the enzyme inhibition by trimethoprim.[40,41]

Antimicrobial Activity

Trimethoprim is quite active in vitro against many gram-positive cocci and most gram-negative rods except for *Pseudomonas aeruginosa* and *Bacteroides* sp. (Table 3). *Treponema pallidum, Mycobacterium tuberculosis, Mycoplasma* sp., and most anaerobes are resistant. Thymidine will inhibit the in vitro activity of trimethoprim, but the addition of thymidine phosphorylase or 5 percent lysed horse blood to Mueller-Hinton or other sensitivity media removes this inhibition. The minimum inhibitory concentration (MIC) will vary considerably with the media used.[46]

Potentiation of the action of trimethoprim is seen in combination with sulfamethoxazole (see below and Table 3). Antibacterial synergism has been demonstrated in vitro for trimethoprim and polymyxins[47] and for trimethoprim and aminoglycosides against some gram-negative bacilli.[48] The combination of trimethoprim–sulfamethoxazole is active in vitro against many isolates of tested *S. aureus*.[49] *Streptococcus pyogenes, Streptococcus pneumoniae, E. coli, Proteus mirabilis, Shigella* sp., *Salmonella* sp., *Pseudomonas cepacia, Pseudomonas pseudomallei, Yersinia enterocolitica*, and *N. gonorrhoeae*.[50]

Variable bactericidal effects have been noted when enterococci are tested against trimethoprim–sulfamethoxazole.[45,45a] The susceptibility of Enterobacteriaceae may vary greatly between locations and within the same location from year to year, due to the spread of trimethoprim-resistant plasmids and transposons.[50] Almost all strains of *P. aeruginosa* are resistant in vitro to trimethoprim–sulfamethoxazole.[49]

Trimethoprim combined with sulfamethoxazole or dapsone has been effective in the treatment of *Pneumocystis carinii* pneumonia in immunocompromised patients (see below). *Listeria monocytogenes*,[51] *Branhamella catarrhalis*,[52] and atypical mycobacteria[53] have been shown to be susceptible to the combination of trimethoprim and sulfamethoxazole.

The optimal ratio for in vitro synergism of trimethoprim–sulfamethoxazole in combination is 1:20, but this ratio does not always obtain in vivo. The synergism seen with trimethoprim–sulfamethoxazole depends somewhat on the sensitivity of the organism to each drug. In one study[54] over 95 percent of organisms sensitive to both drugs showed synergism, whereas 60 percent of sulfamethoxazole-resistant strains and 45 percent of trimethoprim-resistant strains showed synergism.

Resistance to Trimethoprim. Bacteria may develop trimethoprim resistance by frequent passage in media containing the drug. Clinical resistance has increased. In one hospital in France[50] trimethoprim-resistant Enterobacteriaceae (MIC $\geq$ 4 μg/ml) increased from 18 to 25 percent of isolates. A decrease in the ratio of strains resistant to both sulfamethoxazole and trimethoprim compared with stains resistant only to trimethoprim may reflect an increase in independent trimethoprim resistance, and this might be a useful monitoring parameter in hospitals.[55]

TABLE 3. In Vitro Activity of Trimethoprim Against Representative Organisms

Organism	MIC[a] Alone (μg/ml)	MIC with Sulfamethoxazole (μg/ml, 1:20)[b]
Gram-positive		
Staphylococcus aureus	0.15–2	0.04–1.6
S. epidermidis	0.02	—
Streptococcus pneumoniae	0.004–5	0.05–1.5
S. pyogenes	0.02–1	0.015–0.4
Enterococcus faecalis	0.15–0.5	0.015–0.4[b]
Corynebacterium diphtheriae	0.15–0.5	0.05–0.15
Listeria monocytogenes	0.05–1.5	0.015–0.15
Clostridium perfringens	2–50	—
Propionibacterium acnes	0.07	—
Gram-negative		
Escherichia coli	0.01–>5	0.005–>5
Klebsiella sp.	0.15–5	0.05–3.1
Proteus mirabilis	0.15–1.5	0.05–0.15
Serratia marcescens	0.8–50	0.4–50
Salmonella sp.	0.01–0.4	0.05–0.15
Shigella sp.	0.04–0.8	0.02–0.5
Citrobacter freundii	0.2	—
Vibrio cholera	0.2	—
Haemophilus influenzae	0.1–12.5	0.04–50
Neisseria gonorrhoeae	0.2–128	0.15–3.1
N. meningitidis	3.1–50	0.01–1.6
Pseudomonas aeruginosa	50–1000	3.1–100
P. cepacia	1–2	—
P. maltophilia	>32	>32
Bacteroides fragilis	≥4.0	—
Other		
Nocardia asteroides	3 100	1.5
Chlamydia trachomatis	20	—

[a] MIC vanes with the method, inoculum size, and media used. Acquisition of residence plasmids may increase MIC's.
[b] MBC may be much higher.[45]
(Data from refs. 27–29 and 42–44.)

Trimethoprim resistance may be due to changes in cell permeability, loss of bacterial drug-binding capacity, and overproduction of or alterations in dihydrofolate reductase. However, the clinically most important mechanism is due to plasmid-mediated dihydrofolate reductases that are resistant to trimethoprim.[56–58]

Eleven distinctive dihydrofolate reductases have been described in recent years in Enterobacteriaceae, *P. aeruginosa*, or *S. aureus*.[58,59] They are frequently plasmid-mediated[50,58,59a] and may be disseminated by highly mobile transposons (such as Tn7) with wide host species' ranges.[60] Outbreaks due to trimethoprim-resistant conjugative plasmids have been noted in Europe,[58–62] East Asia,[63,64] South America,[65] and the United States.[65,66] Increases in endemic trimethoprim resistance, particularly among Enterobacteriaceae, have been especially marked in developing countries.[67] With more than one-third of the *E. coli* and *Salmonella* resistant to trimethoprim in several South American and Asian nations, the use of this low-cost agent for the treatment of urinary tract infections and serious enteric infections is imperiled.

Permeability changes may occur in the bacterial cell and result in resistance to both trimethoprim and sulfonamides. Thymine requiring auxotrophs may also account for clinically significant resistance to both drugs. These mutants lack thymidylate synthetase and are probably less virulent than are sensitive strains.[68,69]

Pharmacology

Routes of Administration. Trimethoprim is available as 100 mg tablets for oral use. Trimethoprim is absorbed readily and almost completely from the gastrointestinal tract. Peak serum levels after taking 100 mg appear 1–4 hours after ingestion and approach 1 μg/ml. The coadministration of sulfamethoxazole does not affect the rate of absorption or serum levels of trimethoprim.

Trimethoprim is also available in fixed combination with sulfamethoxazole in a ratio of 1:5 for oral use (trimethoprim, 80 mg; sulfamethoxazole, 400 mg; Bactrim, Septra); double-strength and quarter-strength pediatric tablets are available, as is an oral suspension containing 40 mg trimethoprim and 200 mg sulfamethoxazole per 5 ml. Intravenous trimethoprim (16 mg/ml) plus sulfamethoxazole (80 mg/ml) is available. When administered intravenously, 10 ml or 160 mg trimethoprim (with 800 mg sulfamethoxazole) produces a peak serum trimethoprim concentration of 3.4 μg/ml in 1 hour. After repeated doses, the peak trimethoprim concentration may approach 9 μg/ml.[70] Similar peak levels may be reached with oral therapy, but at 2–4 hours after taking the dose.[71,72]

Distribution. Trimethoprim is widely distributed in tissues and may appear in kidney, lung, and sputum in higher concentrations than in plasma, as well as in bile, saliva, human breast milk, and seminal fluid.[73] Trimethoprim is also found in prostatic fluid at two to three times the serum concentration, but lower levels may be present in patients with chronic prostatitis.[74,75] Cerebrospinal fluid levels are about 40 percent of serum levels.

Metabolism and Excretion. Approximately 60–80 percent of an administered dose of trimethoprim is excreted in the urine via tubular secretion within 24 hours. The remainder of the drug is excreted by the kidney in one of four oxide- or hydroxyl-derivatives. The urinary metabolites are bacteriologically inactive.[70] Trimethoprim is also excreted in the bile. The serum half-life ranges from 9 to 11 hours in healthy subjects and is prolonged in patients with renal insufficiency. Unlike sulfamethoxazole, the excretion rate of trimethoprim is increased with acidification of the urine, and serum protein binding (65–70 percent) does not decrease significantly with increasing degrees of uremia.[32] Urine concentrations in healthy subjects (60–1000 μg/ml) are usually in excess of the MIC of most urinary pathogens.[32] Trimethoprim–sulfamethoxazole can be given in the usual doses to patients with creatinine clearances of 30 ml/min or greater. One-half the usual daily dose can be given to patients with creatinine clearances of 15–30 ml/min, but trimethoprim-sulfamethoxazole is not recommended for use in patients with clearances less than 15 ml/min.[32,76,77] Both trimethoprim and nonacetylated sulfamethoxazole are removed by hemodialysis.[32] Patients needing chronic peritoneal dialysis can receive the equivalent of one double-strength trimethoprim–sulfamethoxazole tablet every 48 hours.

Toxicity and Side Effects

The toxic and undesired effects of trimethoprim–sulfamethoxazole include all those discussed above for sulfonamides. Nausea, vomiting, diarrhea, anorexia, and hypersensitivity reactions are the most frequent.[78,79] Rash has been noted frequently in patients with the acquired immunodeficiency syndrome (AIDS).[80–82] In 2 patients with AIDS, transient pulmonary infiltrates and hypotension developed following reexposure to trimethoprim–sulfamethoxazole.[83] In addition, impaired folate utilization may be seen in humans with prolonged administration. This is usually manifest as a megaloblastic marrow, with hypersegmented polymorphonuclear leukocytes. Also leukopenia, thrombocytopenia, and granulocytopenia may be seen. The administration of folinic acid usually prevents or treats effectively the antifolate effects of trimethoprim, and the latter drug's antibacterial efficacy is not impaired except possibly against enterococci. Pseudomembranous colitis has been described with trimethoprim–sulfamethoxazole but is uncommon.[84] Renal dysfunction may occur in patients with pre-existing renal disease, but this is reversible with dose reduction.[85] Trimethoprim–sulfamethoxazole may cause an increase in measured serum creatinine.[86] Drug-induced hepatitis has been reported infrequently.[81] Active levels of phenytoin may be increased markedly by trimethoprim–sulfamethoxazole.[87]

Trimethoprim Plus Other Antimicrobial Agents

Other sulfonamides, such as sulfamoxole, sulfadiazine, sulfadimidine, and sulfametrol, have been combined with trimethoprim, but more clinical studies are needed to recommend their use over the currently used combination.[88–90] Trimethoprim–sulfadiazine was reported to be less likely to accumulate in the kidneys of elderly patients with impaired renal function than trimethoprim–sulfamethoxazole.[89] Combinations of trimethoprim with other agents such as rifampin[91–93] polymyxin,[47] amikacin,[94] and metronidazole[95] have been suggested or used. Extensive clinical experience with these combinations is lacking. Recent reports suggest that trimethoprim–dapsone is more efficacious for the treatment of *P. carinii* pneumonia than dapsone alone.[80,96,97]

Clinical Use

Urinary Tract Infections. Trimethoprim–sulfamethoxazole is useful in the treatment of recurrent or chronic urinary tract infections due to sensitive organisms. Many Enterobacteriaceae are sensitive to the combined action of these drugs. The combination is also effective in acute pyelonephritis and cystitis (see Chapter 58), although either antibiotic alone could be appropriate for susceptible isolates.

Because trimethoprim accumulates in prostatic secretions, trimethoprim–sulfamethoxazole is often effective in bacterial prostatitis,[75] as well as in orchitis and epididymitis due to susceptible bacteria.

The usual dosage in an adult for the treatment of acute prostate or urinary infection is two tablets every 12 hours or one double-strength tablet every 12 hours. The pediatric dose for urinary tract infection is 150–185 mg/m^2 for trimethoprim and 750–925 mg/m^2 for sulfamethoxazole daily in two divided doses. Single-dose therapy with one or two double-strength tablets may be effective in women with uncomplicated lower urinary tract infection.[98,99] However, in patients with chronic tissue invasive urinary infections, longer-term therapy of up to 6 weeks might be required.[100]

Trimethoprim–sulfamethoxazole has been shown to be useful in the long-term suppressive therapy of adults and children with chronic or recurrent urinary infections, and extremely low doses (one-half to one tablet at bedtime or every other night) are effective.[101,102] Trimethoprim is thought to achieve effective concentrations in the vaginal secretions, and it is believed by some that it exerts its protective effect on reducing the number of recurrent infections in this manner despite the fact that trimethoprim–sulfamethoxazole-resistant organisms may be present in the vaginal and stool flora.[103] Trimethoprim alone is effective therapy for uncomplicated and recurrent urinary infections in women. Usual doses are 100–200 mg bid,[103–105] and nightly doses of 100 mg may be effective suppressive therapy.[105,106] Trimethoprim alone has been felt by some to be preferable to the combination of trimethoprim–sulfamethoxazole for acute urinary tract infections and possibly other infections as well.[107,108] However, trimethoprim-resistant organisms might increase with extended use.

Respiratory Tract Infections. Trimethoprim–sulfamethoxazole is effective in the treatment of acute bronchitis and pneumonitis due to sensitive organisms, although it is not the treatment of choice for any single organism. Trimethoprim–sulfamethoxazole may be as effective as tetracyclines in the reduction of acute exacerbations in patients with chronic bronchitis,[108–110] but full doses should be used. Although not usually considered for use in seriously ill patients with pneumonia, intravenously administered trimethoprim–sulfamethoxazole may be effective in patients with infections due to susceptible gram-negative bacteria.[111]

Consistent with its antibacterial spectrum, trimethoprim–sulfamethoxazole may be as effective as ampicillin for the treatment of sinusitis and otitis media,[112] and ampicillin-resistant strains of *H. influenzae* and *Branhamella catarrhalis* might be susceptible.[52]

Gastrointestinal Infections. Although antibiotics per se prolong the carrier state in acute gastroenteritis due to *Salmonella* sp., trimethoprim–sulfamethoxazole may be effective in eliminating chronic *Salmonella* carriage including carriers of *Salmonella typhi*, especially in patients over 2 years of age. Typhoid fever also may be treated successfully with this combination, although the development of resistant strains has been increasingly reported.[50,67] Trimethoprim–sulfamethoxazole is effective in shigellosis,[113] especially due to ampicillin-resistant strains; however, susceptibility testing is necessary given reports of plasmid-mediated outbreaks of resistant organisms.[114] Intravenous administration may be necessary for patients with some of these infections. Trimethoprim–sulfamethoxazole also may be effective in the treatment of diarrhea due to enteropathogenic *E. coli* and in the treatment and prophylaxis of traveler's diarrhea[115–117] if the prevalence of resistant strains in the area to be visited is low. The combination may be a useful adjunct to fluids in the treatment of cholera[118]; however, plasmid-mediated trimethoprim resistance has been reported in East Asia.[119]

Sexually Transmitted Diseases. Trimethoprim–sulfamethoxazole may be effective in the treatment of uncomplicated gonorrhea when used in several dosage regimens (e.g., 2 tabs po bid for 5 days, 4 tabs bid for 2 days, and a single dose of 8 tabs).[120–122] For pharyngeal gonorrhea, especially that due to penicillinase producing *N. gonorrhoeae*. 9 tablets/day for 5 days has been recommended.[123] However, almost half of the *N. gonorrhoeae* that were chromosomally resistant to penicillin in one study were resistant to trimethoprim–sulfamethoxazole as well.[124] Nongonococcal urethritis due to *Chlamydia trachomatis* may be treatable with the combination, but its activity is due to the sulfonamide.[125] The combination is also effective therapy for chancroid and lymphogranuloma venereum. It is ineffective for syphilis. Trimethoprim plus sulfametrole has been successful as a single-dose regimen for chancroid.[90]

Other Infections. Trimethoprim–sulfamethoxazole is useful against brucellosis (long-term therapy for 6 weeks),[126] biliary tract infections, acute and chronic osteomyelitis,[127,128] periodontal infection,[129] mycetoma due to paracoccidioidomycosis and other fungi,[130] and nocardiosis.[131,132] Individual cases of successful response to combination therapy have been described for melioidosis,[133] *P. cepacia* bacteremia,[134] Whipple's disease,[135] and Wegener's granulomatosis.[135a]

Intravenous trimethoprim–sulfamethoxazole has been useful in treating gram-negative rod bacteremia and staphylococcal bacteremia and endocarditis, although other agents may be preferred.[95,136,137,137a] Trimethoprim–sulfamethoxazole plus extended spectrum β-lactams and/or aminoglycosides provide effective broad-spectrum antimicrobial coverage in the management of febrile neutropenic patients.[138,139] Meningitis due to susceptible organisms may be successfully treated,[139a] but other agents are usually preferred. The combination may be effective in meningitis due to *Listeria monocytogenes*.[51]

Trimethoprim plus sulfalene and trimethoprim–sulfamethoxazole have been used in the treatment of susceptible *P. falciparum* infections, although these combinations are not very active against multiple-resistant strains. In vitro efficacy has been suggested for *Toxoplasma gondii*[140] and *M. kansasii*, *Mycobacterium marinum*, and *Mycobacterium scrofulaceum*, and some clinical successes have been reported.[37,53,141]

PNEUMOCYSTIS CARINII INFECTIONS. Trimethoprim–sulfamethoxazole has been highly efficacious in the treatment of *P. carinii* pneumonia in immunocompromised patients with and without AIDS[80,81,142,143] (see Chapters 110 and 256). The usual daily dose is trimethoprim 20 mg/kg/day; sulfamethoxazole 100 mg/kg/day in up to four divided doses iv, or two to three doses orally. Patients with AIDS frequently respond to therapy but have a higher incidence of toxic reactions, particularly neutropenia and rash.[81] Although the toxicities are different, the efficacy and drug reactions associated with systemic pentamidine are comparable.[144] The recommended duration of therapy is 21 days. Trimethoprim–sulfamethoxazole has been successfully used for the chemoprophylaxis of *P. carinii* pneumonia.[81,145,146]

PROPHYLACTIC THERAPY OF NEUTROPENIC PATIENTS. Several studies have presented evidence of a striking reduction in gram-negative rod bacteremia in neutropenic patients treated prophylactically with trimethoprim–sulfamethoxazole (2 tabs bid or more until stools were free of Enterobacteriaceae) compared with untreated control neutropenic patients.[147–149] Other studies have not universally shown benefit in preventing bacteremia in neutropenic patients with acute myelocytic leukemia.[150] Trimethoprim–sulfamethoxazole may prolong recovery from induction chemotherapy-induced neutropenia, as has been reported in some but not all studies.[151,152]

Trimethoprim Use in Pregnancy. The teratogenicity of trimethoprim in humans is not clearly defined, but this drug is not recommended for use in pregnancy at this time. It is, however, well tolerated in pediatric populations.[153]

REFERENCES

1. Carithers HA. The first use of an antibiotic in America. Am J Dis Child. 1974;128:207–11.
2. Bushby SRM, Hitchings GH. Trimethoprim, a sulphonamide potentiator. Br J Pharmacol Chemother. 1968;33:72–90.
3. Pearson RD, Hewlett EL. Use of pyrimethamine–sulfadoxine (Fansidar) in prophylaxis against chloroquine-resistant *Plasmodium falciparum* and *Pneumocystis carinii*. Ann Intern Med. 1987;106:714–8.
4. Ballin JC. Evaluation of a new topical agent for burn therapy. Silver sulfadiazine (Silvadene). JAMA. 1974;230:1184–5.
5. Mayer KH, Hopkins JD, Gilleece ES, et al. Molecular evolution, species distribution, and clinical consequences of an endemic aminoglycoside resistance plasmid. Antimicrob Agents Chemother. 1986;29:628–33.
6. McHugh G, Moellering RC Jr, Hopkins CC, et al. *Salmonella typhimurium* resistant to silver nitrate, chloramphenicol and ampicillin: a new threat in burn units? Lancet. 1975;1:235–40.
7. Woods DD. Relation of p-aminobenzoic acid to mechanism of action of sulphamilamide. Br J Exp Pathol. 1940;21:74–90.
8. Fildes P. Rational approach to research in chemotherapy. Lancet. 1940;1:955–7.
9. Miller AK, Bruno P, Berglund RM. The effect of sulfathiazol on the in vitro synthesis of certain vitamins by *Escherichia coli*. J Bacteriol. 1947;54:9.
10. Brown GH. The biosynthesis of pteridines. Adv Enzymol. 1971;35:35–77.
11. Richmond MH. Structural analogy and chemical reactivity in the action of antibacterial compounds, In: Biochemical Studies of Antimicrobial Drugs. Proceedings of the Sixteenth Symposium of the Society of General Microbiology. London: Cambridge University Press; 1966:301.
12. Hamilton-Miller JMJ. Mechanisms and distribution of bacterial resistance to diaminopyrimidines and sulphonamides. J Antimicrob Chemother. 1979;5(Suppl B):61–73.
13. Landy M, Larkun NW, Oswald EJ, et al. Increased synthesis of p-aminobenzoic acid associated with the development of resistance in *Staph aureus*. Science. 1943;97:265–67.
14. Wolf B, Hotchkiss RD. Genetically modified folic acid synthesising enzymes in pneumococcus. Biochemistry. 1940;2:145–50.
15. Landy M, Gerstung RB. p-Aminobenzoic acid synthesis by *Neisseria gonorrhoeae* in relation to clinical and cultural sulfonamide resistance. J Bacteriol. 1944;47:448.
16. Swedberg G, Castensson S, Sköld O. Characterization of mutationally altered dihydropteroate synthase and its ability to form a sulfonamide-containing dihydrofolate analog. J Bacteriol. 1979;137:129–36.
17. Sköld O: R-factor mediated resistance to sulfonamides by a plasmid-borne, drug resistant dihydropteroate synthase. Antimicrob Agents Chemother. 1976;9:49–54.

18. Kabins SA, Panse MV, Cohen S. Role of R-factor and bacterial host in sulfonamide resistance mediated by R-factor in *Escherichia coli*. J Infect Dis. 1971;123:158–68.
19. Watanabe T. Infective heredity of multiple drug resistance in bacteria. Bacteriol Rev. 1963;27:87–115.
20. Then RL. Mechanisms of resistance to trimethoprim, the sulfonamides and trimethoprim–sulfamethoxazole. Rev Infect Dis. 1982;4:261–9.
21. Burman LG. Apparent absence of transferable resistance to nalidixic acid in pathogenic gram-negative bacteria. J Antimicrob Chemother. 1977;3:509–14.
22. Hansson HB, Walder M, Juhlin I. Susceptibility of shigellae to mecillinam, nalidixic acid, trimethoprim, and five other antimicrobial agents. Antimicrob Agents Chemother. 1981;19:271–4.
23. Davies JR, Farrant WN, Uttley AHC. Antibiotic resistance of *Shigella sonnei*. Lancet. 1970;2:1157–60.
24. Gordon RC, Thompson TR, Carlson W, et al. Antimicrobial resistance of shigellae isolated in Michigan. JAMA. 1975;231:1159–64.
25. Ryder RW, Blake PA, Murlin AC, et al. Increase in antibiotic resistance among isolates of salmonella in the United States, 1967–1975. J Infect Dis. 1980;142:485–91.
26. Albritton WL, Brunton JL, Slaney L, Maclean I. Plasmid-mediated sulfonamide resistance in *Haemophilus ducreyi*. Antimicrob Agents Chemother. 1982;21:159–66.
27. Garrod LP, Lambert HP, O'Grady F. Antibiotic and Chemotherapy. 4th ed. Edinburgh and London: Churchill Livingstone; 1973.
28. Bushby SRM. Trimethoprim–sulfamethoxazole: in vitro microbiologic aspects. J Infect Dis. 1973;128:S442–62.
29. Bach MC, Finland M, Gold W, et al. Susceptibility of recently isolated pathogenic bacteria to trimethoprim and sulfamethoxazole separately and combined. J Infect Dis. 1973;128:S508–33.
30. Anand N. Sulfonamides and sulfones, In: Corcoran JW, Hahn FE, eds. Antibiotics III: Mechanism of Action of Antimicrobial and Antitumor Agents. Berlin: Springer-Verlag; 1975:668.
31. Sparr RA, Pritchard JA. Maternal and newborn distribution and excretion of sulfamethoxypyridazine (Kynex). Obstet Gynecol. 1958;12:131–4.
32. Craig WA, Kunin CM. Trimethoprim–sulfamethoxazole: pharmacodynamic effects of urinary pH and impaired renal function. Ann Intern Med. 1973;78:491–7.
33. Markowitz N, Saravolatz LD. Use of trimethoprim–sulfamethoxazole in a glucose-6-phosphate dehydrogenase-deficient population. Rev Infect Dis. 1987;9:S218–25.
34. Dunea G, Freedman P. Proteinuria. JAMA. 1968;203:973–84.
35. Hansten PD. Drug Interactions. 2nd ed. Philadelphia: Lea & Febiger; 1973.
36. Griffin JP, D'Arcy PF. A Manual of Adverse Drug Interactions. Bristol: John Wright and Sons; 1975:63.
37. Ahn CH, Wallace RJ Jr, Steel LC, et al. Sulfonamide-containing regimens for disease caused by rifampin-resistant *Mycobacterium kansasii*. Am Rev Respir Dis. 1987;135:10–6.
38. Peppercorn MA. Sulfasalazine: pharmacology, clinical use, toxicity, and related new drug development. Ann Intern Med. 1984;3:377–84.
39. Pullar T, Hunter JA, Capell HA. Sulphasalazine in rheumatoid arthritis: a double-blind comparison of sulphasalazine with placebo and sodium aurothiomalate. Br Med J. 1983;287:1102–6.
40. Burchall JJ. Trimethoprim and pyrimethamine, In: Corcoran JW, Hahn FE, eds. Antibiotics III: Mechanism of Antimicrobial and Antitumor Agents. Berlin: Springer-Verlag; 1975:304.
41. Hitchings GT. The biochemical basis for the antimicrobial activity of septrin. In: Bernstein LS, Salter AJ, eds. Trimethoprim/Sulphamethoxazole in Bacterial Infections. Edinburgh and London: Churchill Livingstone, 1973:7–16.
42. Phillips I, Warren C. Activity of sulfamethoxazole and trimethoprim against *Bacteroides fragilis*. Antimicrob Agents Chemother. 1976;9:736–40.
43. Trehane JD, Day J, Yeo CK, et al. Susceptibility of chlamydiae to chemotherapeutic agents. In Hobsen D, Holmes KK, eds. Nongonococcal Urethritis and Related Infections. Washington, DC: Am Soc Microbiology; 1977:214–22.
44. Moody MR, Young VM. In vitro susceptibility of *Pseudomonas cepacia* and *Pseudomonas maltophilia* to trimethoprin and trimethoprim–sulfamethoxazole. Antimicrob Agents Chemother. 1975;7:836–9.
45. Najjar A, Murray BE. Failure to demonstrate a consistent in vitro bactericidal effect of trimethoprim sulfamethoxazole against enterococci. Antimicrob Agents Chemother. 1987;31:808–10.
45a. Goodhart GL. In vivo versus in vitro susceptibility of enterococcus to trimethoprim-sulfamethoxazole. JAMA. 1984;252:2748–9.
46. Dornbusch K, Moore WB. The effects of different media on the response of bacteria to sulphonamides and trimethoprim using the disc-diffusion method and regression line analysis, In: Bernstein LS, Salter AJ, eds. Trimethoprim/Sulphamethoxazole in Bacterial Infections. Edinburgh and London: Churchill Livingstone; 1973:39–51.
47. Simmons NA. Colistin, sulphamethoxazole and trimethoprim in synergy against gram-negative bacilli. J Clin Pathol. 1970;23:757–64.
48. Parsley TL, Provonchee RB, Glicksman C, et al. Synergistic activity of trimethoprim and amikacin against gram-negative bacilli. Antimicrob Agents Chemother. 1977;12:349–54.
49. Bushby SRM. Sensitivity patterns and use of a combined disc of trimethoprim–sulphamethoxazole, In: Bernstein LS, Salter AJ, eds. Trimethoprim/Sulphamethoxazole in Bacterial Infections. Edinburgh and London: Churchill Livingstone; 1973:31–8.
50. Goldstein FW, Papadopoulou B, Acar JF. The changing of trimethoprim resistance in Paris, with a review of worldwide experience. Rev Infect Dis. 1986;8:725–37.
51. Armstrong RW, Slater B. *Listeria monocytogenes* meningitis treated with trimethoprim–sulfamethoxazole. Pediatr Infect Dis J. 1986;5:712–3.
52. Riley TV, Degiovanni C, Hoyne GF. Susceptibility of *Branhamella catarrhalis* to sulphamethoxazole and trimethoprim. J Antimicrob Chemother. 1987;19:39–43.
53. Wallace RJ Jr, Swanson JM, Silcox VA, et al. Treatment of nonpulmonary infections due to *Mycobacterium fortuitum* and *Mycobacterium chelonei* based on in vitro susceptibility. J Infect Dis. 1985;152:500–14.
54. Bohni E. Vergleichende bakteriologishe untersuchungen mit der Kombination Trimethoprim Sulfamethoxazole in vitro and in vivo. Chemotherapy. 1969;14(Suppl):1–21.
55. O'Brien TF, Acar JF, Altmann G, et al. Laboratory surveillance of synergy between and resistance to trimethoprim and sulfonamides. Rev Infect Dis. 1982;4:351–7.
56. Richards HN, Datta N, Sojka NJ, et al. Trimethoprim resistance plasmids and transposons in Salmonella. Lancet. 1978;2:1194–5.
57. Burchall JJ, Pelwell L, Fling ME. Molecular mechanisms of resistance to trimethoprim. Rev Infect Dis. 1982;4:246–54.
58. Houvinen P. Trimethoprim resistance. Antimicrob Agents Chemother. 1987;31:1451–6.
59. Goldstein FW, Labigne-Roussel A, Gerbaud G, et al. Transferable plasmid-mediated antibiotic resistance in *Acinetobacter*. Plasmid. 1983;10:138–47.
59a. Sundstrom L, Vinayagamoorthy T, Skold O. Novel type of plasmid-borne resistance to trimethoprim. Antimicrob Agents Chemother. 1987;31:60–6.
60. Steen R, Sköld O. Plasmid-borne or chromosomally mediated resistance by Tn7 is the most common response to ubiquitous use of trimethoprim. Antimicrob Agents Chemother. 1985;27:933–7.
61. Fleming MP, Datta N, Grüneberg RN. Trimethoprim resistance determined by R factors. Br Med J. 1972;1:726–8.
62. Saroglou G, Parakevopoulou P, Paniara O, Kontomichalou P. Trimethoprim resistance plasmids from Enterobacteriaceae isolated in Greece. In: Mitsuhashi S, Rosival L, Krcméry V, eds. Antibiotic Resistance. Berlin: Springer-Verlag; 1980:267–71.
63. Agarwal KC, Panhotra BR, Mahanta J, et al. Typhoid fever due to chloramphenicol resistant *Salmonella typhi* associated with R-plasmid. Indian J Med Res. 1981;73:484–8.
64. Goldstein FW, Chumpitaz JC, Guevara JM, et al. Plasmid-mediated resistance to multiple antibiotics in *Salmonella typhi*. J Infect Dis. 1986;153:261–6.
65. O'Brien TF, Hopkins JD, Gilleece ES, et al. Molecular epidemiology of antibiotic resistance in *Salmonella* from animals and human beings in the United States. N Engl J Med. 1982;307:1–6.
66. Mayer KH, Fling ME, Hopkins JD, et al. Trimethoprim resistance in multiple genera of Enterobacteriaceae at a U.S. hospital: spread of the type II dihydrofolate reductase gene by a single plasmid. J Infect Dis. 1985;5:783–9.
67. Murray BE, Alvarado T, Kim K-H, et al. Increasing resistance to trimethoprim–sulfamethoxazole among isolates of *Escherichia coli* in developing countries. J Infect Dis. 1985;152:1107–3.
68. Smith HW, Tucker JF. The virulence of trimethoprim resistant thymine-requiring strains of *Salmonella*. J Hyg (Lond). 1976;76:97–108.
69. Maskell R, Okubadejo OA, Payne RH, et al. Human infections with thymine-requiring bacteria. J Med Microbiol. 1978;11:33–45.
70. Grose WE, Bodey GP, Loo TL. Clinical pharmacology of intravenously administered trimethoprim–sulfamethoxazole. Antimicrob Agents Chemother. 1979;15:447–51.
71. Bach MC, Gold O, Finland M. Absorption and urinary excretion of trimethoprim, sulfamethoxazole, and trimethoprim–sulfamethoxazole: results with single doses in normal young adults and preliminary observations during therapy with trimethoprim–sulfamethoxazole. J Infect Dis. 1973;128:S584–98.
72. Kaplan SA, Weinfeld RE, Abruzzo CW, et al. Pharmacokinetic profile of trimethoprim–sulfamethoxazole in man. J Infect Dis. 1973;128:S547–55.
73. Pater RB, Welling PG. Clinical pharmacokinetics of co-trimoxazole (trimethoprim/sulfamethoxazole). Clin Pharmacokinet. 1980;5:405–23.
74. Winningham DG, Nemoy NJ, Stamey TA. Diffusion of antibiotics from plasma into prostatic fluid. Nature. 1968;219:139–43.
75. Meares EM Jr. Prostatitis: Review of pharmacokinetics and therapy. Rev Infect Dis. 1982;4:475–83.
76. Welling PG, Craig WA, Amidon GL, et al. Pharmacokinetics of trimethoprim and sulfamethoxazole in normal subjects and in patients with renal failure. J Infect Dis. 1973;128(Suppl):556–66.
77. Salter AJ. Trimethoprin sulfamethoxazole: an assessment of more than 12 years of use. Rev Infect Dis. 1982;4:196–236.
78. Jick H. Adverse reactions to trimethoprim–sulfamethoxazole in hospitalized patients. Rev Infect Dis. 1982;4:426–8.
79. Lawson DH, Paice BJ. Adverse reactions to trimethoprim–sulfamethoxazole. Rev Infect Dis. 1982;4:429–33.
80. Masur H, Kovacs JA. Treatment and prophylaxis of *Pneumocystis carinii* pneumonia. In: Moellering RC Jr, ed. Infectious Disease Clinics of North America (Medical Management of AIDS). Philadelphia: WB Saunders; 1988:419–28.
81. Wofsy CB. Use of trimethoprim–sulfamethoxazole in the treatment of *Pneumocystis carinii* pneumonitis in patients with acquired immunodeficiency syndrome. Rev Infect Dis. 1987;9:S184–91.

82. Gordin FM, Simon GL, Wofsy CB, et al. Adverse reactions to trimethoprim-sulfamethoxazole in patients with acquired immunodeficiency syndrome. Ann Intern Med. 1984;100:495–9.
83. Silvestri RC, Jensen WA, Zibrak JD, et al. Pulmonary infiltrates and hypoxemia in patients with the acquired immunodeficiency syndrome re-exposed to trimethoprim–sulfamethoxazole. Am Rev Respir Dis. 1987;136:1003–4.
84. Cameron A, Thomas M. Pseudomembranous colitis and co-trimoxazole. Br Med J. 1977;1:1321.
85. Bailey RR, Little PJ. Deterioration in renal function in association with co-trimoxazole therapy. Med J Aust. 1976;1:914–6.
86. Trollfors B, Wahl, Alestig K. Co-trimoxazole, creatinine and renal function. J Infect. 1980;2:221.
87. Hansen JM, Kampmann JP, Sierbaek-Nielsenk, et al. The effect of different sulfonamides on phenytoin metabolism in man. Acta Med Scand [Suppl] 1979;624:106–10.
88. Bernstein LS. Combination of trimethoprim with sulfonamides other than sulfamethoxazole. Rev Infect Dis. 1982;4:411–8.
89. Bergan T, Allgulander S, Fellner H. Pharmacokinetics of co-trimazine (sulphadiazine plus trimethoprim) in geriatric patients. Chemotherapy. 1986;32:478–85.
90. Dylewski J, D'Costa LJ, Nsanze H, et al. Single dose therapy with trimethoprim—sulfametrole for chancroid in females. Sex Transm Dis. 1986;13:166–8.
91. Brumfitt W, Hamilton-Miller JMT. Rifamprim (rifampicin plus trimethoprim): pharmacokinetics and effects on the normal flora of man. Biopharm Drug Dispos. 1981;2:157–66.
92. Kerry DW, Hamilton-Miller JMT, Brumfitt W. Trimethoprim and rifampicin: in vitro activities separately and in combination. J Antimicrob Chemother. 1975;1:417–27.
93. Alvarez S, DeMaria A Jr, Kulkarni R, et al. Interactions of rifampin and trimethoprim in vitro. Rev Infect Dis. 1982;4:390–401.
94. Zinner SH, Lagast H, Kasry A, et al. Synergism of trimethoprim combined with aminoglycosides in vitro and in serum of volunteers. Eur J Clin Microbiol. 1982;1:144–8.
95. Salter AJ. Trimethoprim–sulfamethoxazole in treatment of severe infections. Rev Infect Dis. 1982;4:338–50.
96. Leoung GS, Mills J, Hopewell PC, et al. Dapsone–trimethoprim for *Pneumocystis carinii* pneumonia in acquired immunodeficiency syndrome. Ann Intern Med. 1986;105:48–54.
97. Mills J, Leoung G, Medina I, et al. Dapsone is ineffective therapy for *Pneumocystis* pneumonia in patients with AIDS (Abstract). Clin Res. 1986;34:101A.
98. Tolkoff-Rubin NE, Weber D, Fang LST, et al. Single dose therapy with trimethoprim–sulfamethoxazole for urinary tract infection in women. Rev Infect Dis. 1982;4:444–8.
99. Counts GW, Stamm WE, McKevitt M, et al. Treatment of cystitis in women with a single dose of trimethoprim–sulfamethoxazole. Rev Infect Dis. 1982;4:484–90.
100. Gleckman R, Crowley M, Natsios GA. Treatment of recurrent invasive urinary-tract infections of men. N Engl J Med. 1979;301:878–80.
101. Harding GKM, Ronald AR, Nicolle LE, et al. Long-term antimicrobial prophylaxis for recurrent urinary tract infection in women. Rev Infect Dis. 1982;4:438–43.
102. Stamey TA. Recurrent urinary tract infections in female patients: an overview of management and treatment. Rev Infect Dis. 1987;9:S195–208.
103. Brumfitt W, Pursell R. Double-blind trial to compare ampicillin, cephalexin, co-trimoxazole and trimethoprim in treatment of urinary infection. Br Med J. 1972;2:673–6.
104. Kasanen A, Toivanen P, Sourander L, et al. Trimethoprim in the treatment of long-term control of urinary tract infection. Scand J Infect Dis. 1974;6:91–6.
105. Iravani A, Richard GA, Baer H. Treatment of uncomplicated urinary tract infection with trimethoprim versus sulfisoxazole with special reference to antibody-coated bacteria and faecal flora. Antimicrob Agents Chemother. 1981;19:842–50.
106. Stamm WE, Counts GW, Wagner KR, et al. Antimicrobial prophylaxis or recurrent urinary tract infections. Ann Intern Med. 1980;92:770–5.
107. Reeves D. Sulphonamides and trimethoprim. Lancet. 1982;2:370–3.
108. Amyes SGB, Doherty CJ, Wonnacott S. Trimethoprim and co-trimoxazole: a comparison of the use in respiratory tract infections. Scand J Infect Dis. 1986;18:561–6.
109. Pandy GJ. Trimethoprim/sulphamethoxazole and doxycycline in acute exacerbations of chronic bronchitis in general practice: a comparative study. Med J Aust. 1979;1:264–6.
110. Pines A. Trimethoprim–sulfamethoxazole in the treatment and prevention of purulent exacerbations of chronic bronchitis. J Infect Dis. 1973;128:S706–9.
111. Schmidt U, Sen P, Kapila R, et al. Clinical evaluation of intravenous trimethoprim sulfamethoxazole for serious infections. Rev Infect Dis. 1982;4:332–7.
112. Shurin PA, Pelton SI, Donner A, et al. Trimethoprim–sulfamethoxazole compared with ampicillin in the treatment of acute otitis media. J Pediatr. 1980;96:1081–87.
113. Nelson JD, Kusmiesz H, Shelton S. Oral or intravenous trimethoprim–sulfamethoxazole therapy for shigellosis. Rev Infect Dis. 1982;4:546–50.
114. Bannatyne RM, Toma S, Cheung R, et al. Resistance to trimethoprim and other antibiotics in Ontario shigellae (Letter). Lancet. 1980;1:425–6.
115. Thoren A, Wolde-Mariam I, Stintzing G, et al. Antibiotics in the treatment of gastroenteritis caused by enteropathogenic *Escherichia coli*. J Infect Dis. 1980;141:27–31.
116. DuPont HL, Evans DG, Rios N, et al. Prevention of travelers' diarrhea with trimethoprim–sulfamethoxazole. Rev Infect Dis. 1982;4:533–9.
117. DuPont HL, Reves RR, Galindo E, et al. Treatment of travelers' diarrhea with trimethoprim-/sulfamethoxazole and with trimethoprim alone. N Engl J Med. 1982;307:841–4.
118. Francis TI, Lewis EA, Oyediran ABOO, et al. Effect of chemotherapy on the duration of diarrhoea, and on vibrio excretion by cholera patients. J Trop Med Hyg. 1971;74:172–6.
119. Threlfall EJ, Rowe B, Huq I. Plasmid-encoded multiple antibiotic resistance in *Vibrio cholerae* El Tor from Bangladesh (Letter). Lancet. 1980;1:1247–8.
120. Svindland HB. Treatment of gonorrhoea with sulphamethoxazole–trimethoprim. Lack of effect on concomitant syphilis. Br J Vener Dis. 1973;49:50–3.
121. Lawrence A, Phillips E, Nicol C. Various regimens of trimethoprim–sulfamethoxazole in the treatment of gonorrhea. J Infect Dis. 1973;128(Suppl):S673–8.
122. Rahim G. Single dose treatment of gonorrhoea with cotrimoxazole. A report on 1,223 cases. Br J Vener Dis. 1975;51:179–82.
123. Centers for Disease Control. 1985 STD treatment guidelines. MMWR [Suppl]. 1985;34:4S.
124. Centers for Disease Control. Chromosomally mediated resistant *Neisseria gonorrhoeae*—United States. MMWR. 1984;33:408–10.
125. Hammerschlag MR. Activity of trimethoprim–sulfamethoxazole against *Chlamydia trachomatis* in vitro. Rev Infect Dis. 1982;4:500–5.
126. Daikos GK, Papapolyzos N, Marketos N, et al. Trimethoprim–sulfamethoxazole in brucellosis. J Infect Dis. 1973;128(Suppl):S731–3.
127. Bajpai J, Chaturvedi Sn, Khanuja SPS. Chemotherapy of acute bone and joint infections. Int Surg. 1977;62:172–4.
128. Millard FJC. Trimethoprim/sulphamethoxazole in the treatment of chronic osteomyelitis. In Bernstein LS, Salter AJ, eds. Trimethoprim–Sulphamethoxazole in Bacterial Infections. Edinburgh: Churchill Livingstone; 1973:195–9.
129. Lakshmanan CDS. Comparative evaluation of cotrimoxazole and demeclocycline in periodontal bacterial infection (Abstract 128). J Dent Res. 1976;55(Special issue D):D137.
130. Mahgoub ES. Medical management of mycetoma. Bull WHO. 1976;54:303.
131. Welsh O, Sauceda E, Gonzalez J, et al. Amikacin alone and in combination with trimethoprim–sulfamethoxazole in the treatment of actinomycotic mycetoma. J Am Acad Dermatol. 1987;17:443–8.
132. Wallace RJ, Septimus EJ, Williams JH, et al. Use of trimethoprim–sulfamethoxazole for the treatment of infections due to *Nocardia*. Rev Infec Dis. 1982;4:315–25.
133. Morrison IM. Chronic melioidosis. Proc R Soc Med. 1970;63:239–49.
134. Neu HC, Garvey GJ, Bleach MP. Successful treatment of *Pseudomonas cepacia* endocarditis in a heroin addict with trimethoprim sulfamethoxazole. J Infect Dis. 1973;128(Suppl):768–70.
135. Viteri AL, Greene JF Jr, Chandler JB Jr. Whipple's disease, successful response to sulfamethoxazole–trimethoprim. Am J Gastroenterol. 1981;75:309–14.
135a. Deremee RA, McDonald TJ, Weiland LH. Wegener's granulomatosis: observations on treatment with antimicrobial agents. Mayo Clin Proc. 1985;60:27–32.
136. Geddes AM, Ball AP, Farrell ID. Co-trimoxazole for the treatment of serious infections. J Antimicrob Chemother. 1979;5(Suppl B):221–30.
137. Quintiliani R, Levitz RE, Nightingale CH. Potential role of trimethoprim–sulfamethoxazole in the treatment of serious hospital-acquired infections. Rev Infect Dis. 1987;9:S160–5.
137a. Sattler FR, Remington JS. Intravenous sulfamethoxazole and trimethoprim for serious gram-negative bacillary infection. Arch Intern Med. 1983; 143:1709–12.
138. Menichetti F, Del Favero A, Guerciolini R, et al. Empiric antimicrobial therapy in febrile granulocytopenic patients. Randomized prospective comparison of amikacin plus piperacillin with and without parenteral trimethoprim sulphamethoxazole. Infection. 1986;14:261–7.
139. Young LS, Hindler J. Use of trimethoprim–sulfamethoxazole singly and in combination with other antibiotics in immunocompromised patients. Rev Infect Dis. 1987;9:S177–81.
139a. Levitz RE, Quintilliani R. Trimethoprim-sulfamethoxazole for bacterial meningitis. Ann Int Med. 1984;100:881–90.
140. Israelski DM, Remington JS. Toxoplasmic encephalitis in patients with AIDS. In: Moellering RC Jr, ed. Infectious Disease Clinics of North America (Medical Management of AIDS). Philadelphia: WB Saunders; 1988:429–45.
141. Wallace RJ, Wissk, Bushby MB, et al. In vitro activity of trimethoprim and sulfamethoxazole against nontuberculosis mycobacteria. Rev Infect Dis. 1982;4:326–31.
142. Sattler RF, Remington JS. Intravenous trimethoprim–sulfamethoxazole therapy for *Pneumocystis carinii* pneumonia. Am J Med. 1981;70:1215–21.
143. Young LS. Trimethoprim–sulfamethoxazole in the treatment of adults with pneumonia due to *Pseumocystis carinii*. Rev Infect Dis. 1982;4:608–13.
144. Wharton JM, Coleman DL, Wofsy CB, et al. Trimethoprim-sulfamethoxa-

zole or pentamidine for *Pneumocystis carinii* pneumonia in the acquired immunodeficiency syndrome, Ann Int Med. 1986;105:37–44.
145. Hughes WT, Smith BL. Intermitten chemoprophylaxis for *Pneumocystis carinii* pneumonia. Antimicrob Agents Chemother. 1983;24:300–5.
146. Fischl MA, Dickinson GM. Trimethoprim–sulfamethoxazole prophylaxis of *Pneumocystis carinii* pneumonia in acquired immunodeficiency syndrome (Abstract 436). In: Program and Abstracts of the 25th Interscience Conference on Antimicrobial Agents and Chemotherapy. Washington, DC: American Society for Microbiology; 1985:230.
147. Gurwith M, Brunton J, Lank B, et al. A prospective controlled investigation of prophylactic trimethoprim/sulfamethoxazole in hospitalized granulocytopenic patients. Am J Med. 1979;66:248–56.
148. Kauffman CA, Liepman MA, Bergman AG, et al. Trimethoprin/sulfamethoxazole prophylaxis in neutropenic patients: reduction of infections and effect on bacterial and fungal flora. Am J Med. 1983;74:599–607.
149. Gualtieri RJ, Donowitz GR, Kaiser DC, et al. Double-blind randomized study of prophylactic trimethoprim/sulfamethoxazole in granulocytopenic patients with hematologic malignancies. Am J Med. 1983;74:934–40.
150. EORTC International Antimicrobial Therapy Project Group. Trimethoprim–sulfamethoxazole in the prevention of infection in neutropenic patients. J Infect Dis. 1984;150:372–9.
151. Wade JC, Schimpff SC, Hargadon MT, et al. A comparison of trimethoprim–sulfamethoxazole plus nystatin with gentamicin plus nystatin in the prevention of infections in acute leukemia. N Engl J Med. 1981;304:1057–62.
152. Wade JC, de Jongh CA, Newman KA, et al. Selective antimicrobial modulation as prophylaxis against infection during granulocytopenia: trimethoprim–sulfamethoxazole vs. nalidixic acid. J Infect Dis. 1983;147:624–34.
153. Overturf GD. Use of trimethoprim–sulfamethoxazole in pediatric infections: relative merits of intravenous administration. Rev Infect Dis. 1987;9:S168–73.

30. QUINOLONES

VINCENT T. ANDRIOLE

Most of the new antimicrobial agents that either have been or will be introduced for clinical use in the near future are the newer 4-quinolone antibacterial agents, particularly the 6-fluorinated piperazinyl quinolones. Nalidixic acid, described by Lescher and colleagues in 1962,[1] was the first in this series of agents. Oxolinic acid and cinoxacin were introduced in the 1970s. Shortly thereafter the development of the newer quinolones progressed rapidly and was spearheaded by the introduction of a fluorine at the 6 position in the basic nucleus. This procedure enhanced and broadened the antibacterial activity of these agents and led to the development of newer 4-quinolones with antibacterial activities 1000 times that of nalidixic acid.[2] The newer quinolones have an extremely broad antibacterial spectrum, unique mechanism of action, good absorption from the gastrointestinal tract after oral administration, excellent tissue distribution, and low incidence of adverse reactions.[3]

CHEMISTRY AND CLASSIFICATION

All of the compounds in the quinolone class of antibacterial agents are structurally similar. Yet, there are some differences in the basic nucleus so that they can be divided into four general groups, i.e., naphthyridines, cinnolines, pyrido-pyrimidines, and quinolones (Fig. 1). The addition of an oxygen at the 4 position in the basic nucleus of each of these groups produces a common skeleton, 4-oxo-1,4-dihydroquinolone, more commonly called *4-quinolone*.[2] The naphthyridines (nalidixic acid and enoxacin) have an additional nitrogen in the 8 position and are 8-aza-4-quinolones. The cinnolines (cinoxacin), with an additional nitrogen in the 2 position, are 2-aza-4-quinolones. The pyrido-pyrimidines (pipemidic and piromidic acids), with additional nitrogens in the 6 and 8 positions, are 6,8-diaza-4-quinolones (Fig. 2). All of the other agents (oxolinic acid, norfloxacin, ciprofloxacin, ofloxacin, pefloxacin, amifloxacin, fleroxacin, flumequine, lomefloxacin, temafloxacin, difloxacin, acrosoxacin [rosoxacin], piroxacin, and irloxacin [pirfloxacin]) are classified simply as 4-quinolones (Fig. 3).[2,3] Numerous additional compounds have been synthesized and are undergoing development.[3]

Structural features common to the 4-quinolones include a carboxyl group at the 3 position and a piperazine ring (except flumequine and oxolinic acid) at the 7 position of the quinolone nucleus. The introduction of a fluorine at the 6 position and substitutions at the 1 and 8 positions of the quinolone or naphthyridine nucleus and the para position of the piperazine ring are responsible for differences in the in vitro activity and pharmacologic properties of these compounds (Figs. 2 and 3).[4]

Nalidixic acid (1-ethyl-7-methyl-1, 8-naphthyridine-4-one-3-carboxylic acid) is one of a series of 1,8-naphthyridine derivatives first described by Lesher and colleagues in 1962.[1] This compound is only slightly soluble in water but is readily soluble in dilute alkali and is stable in urine. Nalidixic acid is marketed as Neggram (Winthrop, 1964). Oxolinic acid (5-ethyl-5,8-dihydro-8-oxo-1,3-dioxolo-[4,5-g]-quinolone-7-carboxylic acid), a quinolone derivative, is a crystalline substance that is a weak organic acid.[5-7] Oxolinic acid is marketed by Utibid (Warner-Lambert, 1975). Cinoxacin [1-ethyl-1,4-dihydro-4-oxo (1,3)dioxolo(4,5-g)cinnoline-3-carboxylic acid] is similar to nalidixic acid.[8] It is a yellow-white crystalline solid with a pKa of 4.7, which is insoluble in water and poorly lipid soluble but is soluble in alkaline solution. Cinoxacin is marketed as Cinobac (Dista/Lilly, 1981). Norfloxacin [1-ethyl-6-fluoro-1,4-dihydro-4-oxo-7-(1-piperazinyl)-3-quinolone carboxylic acid (AM 715 or MK-0366) is similar to nalidixic acid.[9,10] It is a yellow-white crystalline solid only slightly soluble in water. Norfloxacin is marketed as Noroxin (Merck). Ciprofloxacin [1-cyclopropyl-6-fluoro-1,4-dihydro-4-oxo-7-(1-piperazinyl)-3-quinolone carboxylic acid hydrochloride] (Bay 09867) is also a new quinolone derivative similar in structure to nalidixic acid.[11] It is a light yellow crystalline substance slightly soluble in water. Ciprofloxacin is marketed as Cipro (Miles/Bayer). Additional new antibacterial agents that are currently under development and that will most likely be marketed in the near future include enoxacin [1-ethyl-6-fluoro-1,4-dihydro-4-oxo-7-(1-piperazinyl)-1,8-naphthyridine-3-carboxylic acid] (Warner-Lambert); ofloxacin [9-fluoro-2,3-dihydro-3-methyl-10-(4-methyl-1-piperazinyl)-7-oxo-7H-pyrido-[1,2,3,de][1,4]-benzoxacine-6-carboxylic acid] (Ortho); fleroxacin [6,8-difluoro-1-(2-fluoro-ethyl)-1,4-dihydro-7-(4-methyl-1-piperazinyl)-4-oxo-3-quinolone carboxylic acid] (Roche); lomefloxacin [1-ethyl-6-8-difluoro-1,4-dihydro-7-(3-methyl-1-piperazinyl)-4-oxo-3-quinolone carboxylic acid] (Searle); and pefloxacin [1-ethyl-6-fluoro-1,4-dihydro-7-(4-methyl-1-piperazinyl)-4-oxo-3-quinolone carboxylic acid] (Bellon/Dianippon).[3]

Also, acrosoxacin (rosoxacin) [1-ethyl-1,4-dihydro-4-oxo-7-(4-pyridyl)3-quinolone carboxylic acid] (Sterling), amifloxacin [6-fluoro-1,4-dihydro-1-methylamino-7-(4-methyl-1-piperazinyl)-4-oxo-3-quinolone carboxylic acid] (Sterling), flumequine [9-fluoro-6,7-dihydro-5-methyl-1-ozo-1H,5H-benzo-(ij)-2-quinolicine carboxylic acid] (Riker), difloxacin [6-fluoro-1(4-fluoro-phenyl -1,4-dihydro-7- (4-methyl-1-piperazinyl) -4-oxo-3-quinolone carboxylic acid] (Abbott), irloxacin (pirfloxacin) [1-ethyl-6-fluoro-1,4-dihydro-4-oxo-7- (1-pyrrolyl) -3-quinolone carboxylic acid] (Esteve), piroxacin [1-ethyl-1,4-dihydro-4-oxo-7-(1-pyrrolyl)-3-quinolone carboxylic acid] (Esteve), and temafloxacin [6-fluoro-1-(2,4-difluoro-phenyl)-1,4-dihydro-7-(4-methyl-1-piperazinyl)-4-oxo-3-quinolone carboxylic acid] (Abbott) along with a number of other compounds are also new antibacterial quinolones currently under development.[3,4]

MECHANISM OF ACTION

Early studies have shown that nalidixic acid rapidly inhibits DNA synthesis in susceptible bacterial cells, although not in mammalian cells, whereas protein and RNA synthesis continue.[12,13] Inhibition of DNA synthesis by nalidixic acid has

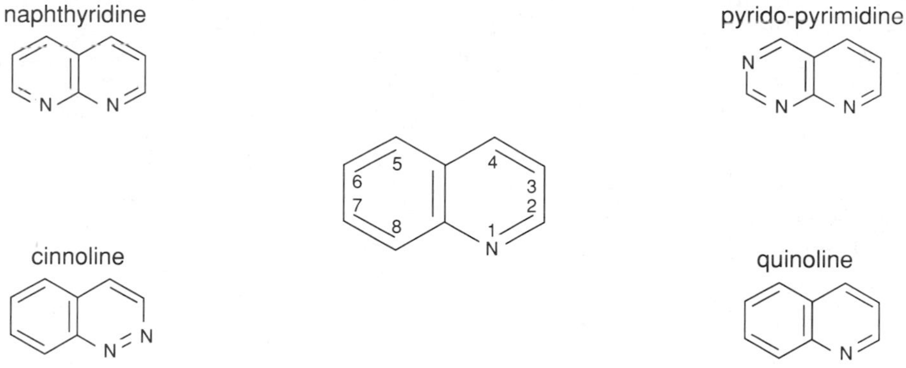

FIG. 1. Chemical structure of the four general groups of the 4-quinolones and its system of ring numbering. (Modified from Smith et al.,[2] with permission.)

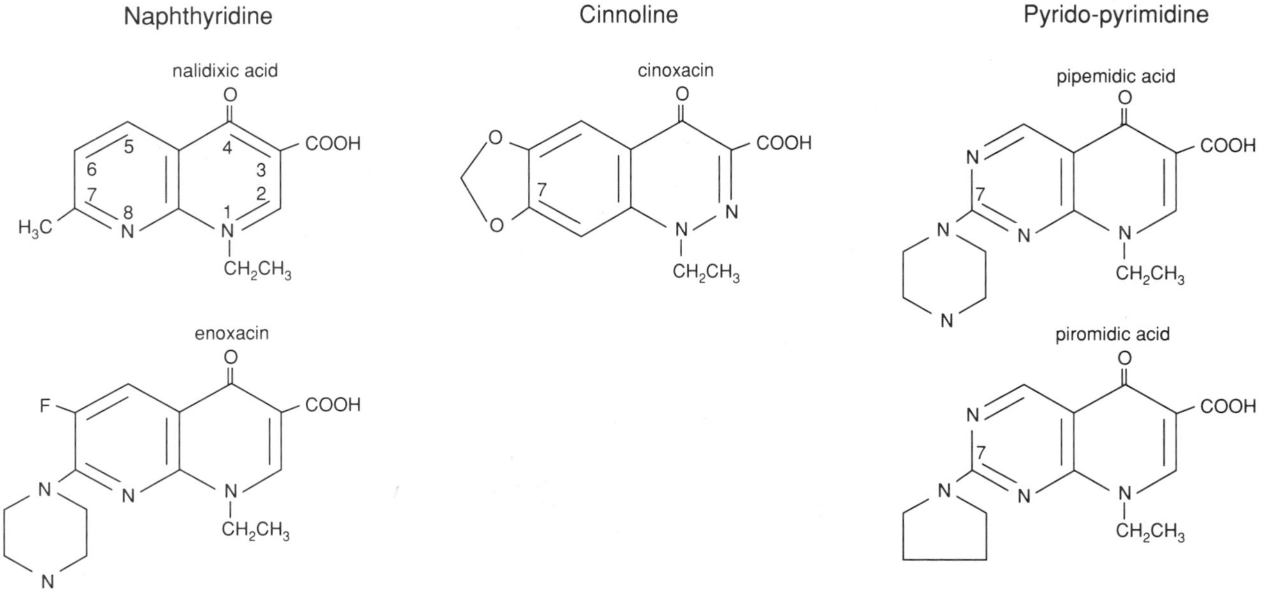

FIG. 2. Structures of naphthyridine, cinnoline, and pyrido-pyrimidine derivatives. (Modified from Smith et al.,[2] with permission.)

been shown to be reversible since bacterial cells exposed to the drug will resume growth when placed in drug-free media.[14] Nalidixic acid does not bind to purified DNA,[15] although recent work suggests that some quinolones may bind to DNA. Nalidixic acid does affect replication at a stage beyond the production of deoxynucleoside triphosphates and inhibits synthesis taking place on the double-stranded DNA template.[16] Recent studies indicate that the bactericidal activity of nalidixic acid as well as 4-quinolones is reduced significantly if RNA or protein synthesis is inhibited.[17] Although all 4-quinolones are bactericidal, these drugs exhibit a single most-bactericidal concentration, so greater or lesser concentrations result in less bacterial death.[2,13] This paradoxical effect of decreased killing at higher concentrations is most likely a dose-dependent inhibition of RNA synthesis.[2,13,14]

Other studies indicate that the mechanism of action of nalidixic acid is by inhibition of DNA topoisomerases (gyrases), of which four subunits (two A monomers and two B monomers) have been defined.[18,19] The topoisomerases, which have been found in every organism examined, are required to supercoil strands of bacterial DNA into the bacterial cell.[20,21] Each chromosomal domain is transiently nicked during supercoiling, which results in single-stranded DNA. When supercoiling is completed, the single-stranded DNA state is abolished by an enzyme that seals the nicked DNA. The sealing action of this enzyme is inhibited specifically by nalidixic acid.[2,13] The same enzyme, identified by Gellert et al.[22] and termed DNA gyrase or topoisomerase II (nicking–closing enzyme), nicks double-stranded chromosomal DNA, introduces supercoils, and seals the nicked DNA.[2,3,22–24] The A subunits are thought to introduce the nicks, the B subunits are thought to cause supercoiling, and then the A subunits seal the nick they produced initially.[2,24] Some of the newer 4-quinolones may act slightly differently from nalidixic acid, which prevents the A subunits from sealing the nicks in chromosomal DNA. The newer 4-quinolones may affect both the A and B subunits of DNA gyrase since mutations that affect the B subunit change the bacterial sensitivity to the 4-quinolones.[2,17,25,26] The identification of DNA gyrase has led to the development of new quinolone compounds that may have increased activity against DNA gyrase.

ANTIMICROBIAL ACTIVITY

Nalidixic acid has greater antimicrobial activity against gram-negative rods than against gram-positive bacteria (Table 1). It is active against most enterobacteriaceae. Approximately 99 percent of the strains of *Escherichia coli*, 98 percent of *Proteus mirabilis*, 75–97 percent of other *Proteus* sp., 92 percent of

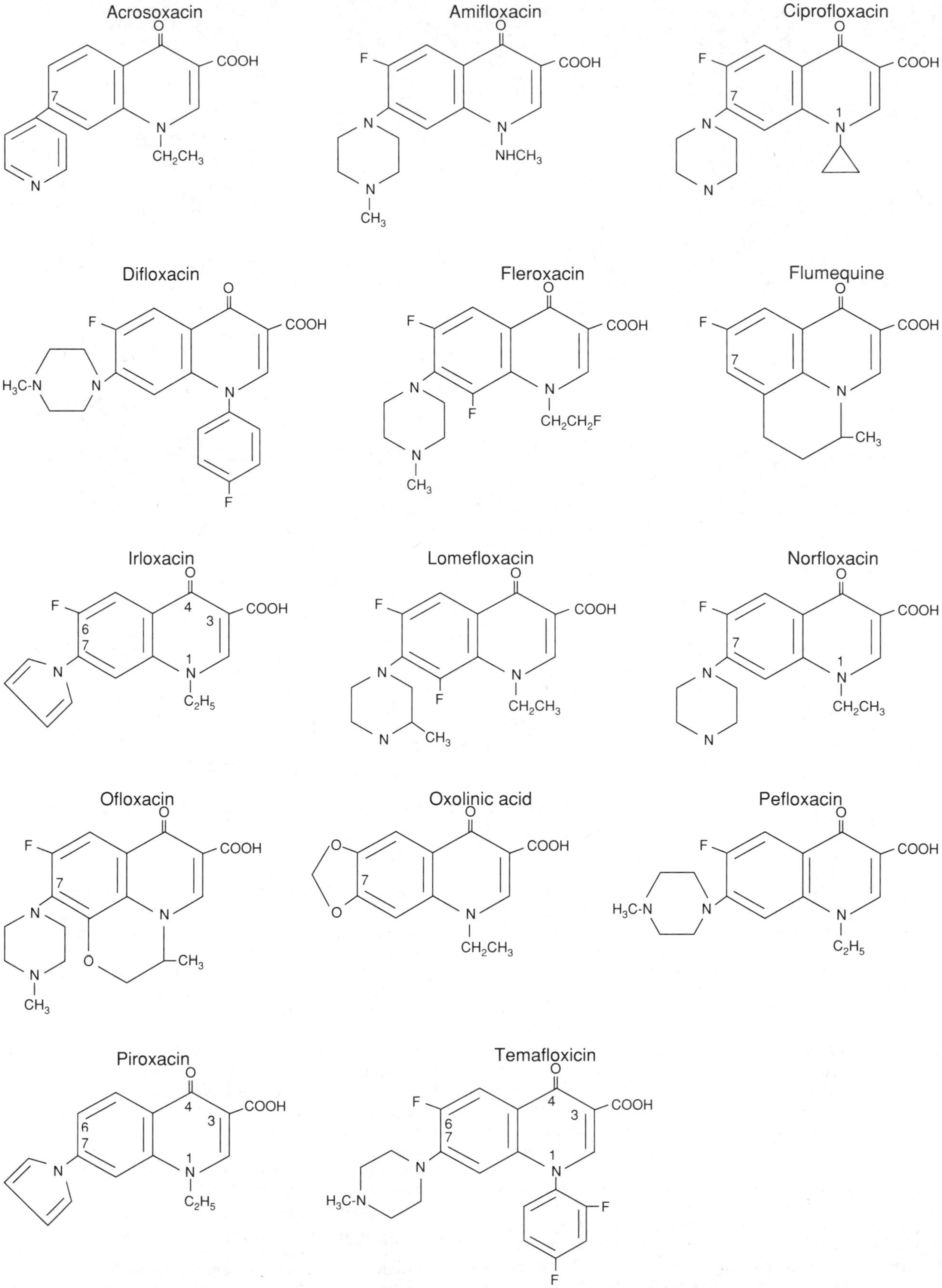

FIG. 3. Chemical structure of the 4-quinolones that are derivatives of the quinoline nucleus.

TABLE 1. In Vitro Activity of Selected 4-Quinolones

Organism	*Nalidixic Acid*	*Ciprofloxacin*	*Enoxacin*	*Norfloxacin*	*Ofloxacin*	*Perfloxacin*
Gram-negative aerobes						
E. coli	8 (4–128)[a]	0.03 (0.015–0.06)	0.5 (0.25–1)	0.125 (0.06–0.5)	0.125 (0.06–0.25)	0.125 (0.125–0.25)
K. pneumoniae	8 (1–128)	0.125 (0.06–0.25)	0.5	0.25 (0.125–1)	0.25	0.5
Enterobacter sp.	32 (4–128)	0.125 (0.03–0.5)	0.5 (0.25–4)	0.5 (0.125–2)	0.5 (0.125–1)	0.5 (0.25–1)
Citrobacter sp.	8 (4–>100)	0.03 (0.03–0.06)	0.5	0.25 (0.125–0.5)	0.5	0.5
S. marcescens	>128 (16–>256)	1 (0.25–2)	2 (0.5–4)	1 (0.5–8)	1 (0.25–2)	1 (0.25–2)
Shigella sp.	4	0.03 (0.015–0.06)	0.125	0.06 (0.03–0.125)	0.125 (0.06–0.125)	0.125
Salmonella sp.	8 (4–8)	0.015 (≤0.015–0.03)	0.25 (0.125–0.25)	0.125 (0.06–0.125)	0.125 (0.06–0.125)	0.125 (0.06–0.25)
P. mirabilis	16 (4–32)	0.06 (0.03–0.125)	0.5 (0.25–1)	0.25 (0.125–0.5)	0.25 (0.25–0.5)	0.5 (0.25–1)
Proteus sp. (indole-positive)	8 (4–16)	0.06	0.25 (0.25–0.5)	0.125 (0.06–0.125)	0.25	0.25
M. morganii	8 (2–8)	0.015 (0.015–0.03)	0.25 (0.25–0.5)	0.125 (0.03–0.25)	0.125 (0.125–0.25)	0.25 (0.25–0.5)
P. aeuruginosa	≥128	0.5 (0.25–1)	4 (2–8)	2 (0.06–8)	4 (2–4)	4 (2–8)
H. influenzae	1 (1–2)	0.015 (0.015–0.03)	0.125 (0.06–0.25)	0.06 (0.03–0.125)	0.03 (0.03–0.06)	0.06 (0.03–0.06)
L. pneumophila	NA	(0.03–0.125)	NA	(0.125–0.5)	NA	NA
N. gonorrhoeae	1 (1–2)	≤0.015	0.03 (0.015–0.06)	0.06 (0.015–0.125)	0.03 (0.015–0.06)	0.06 (0.03–0.06)
N. meningitidis	2	0.004	0.06	0.03	0.015	0.03
Gram-negative anaerobes						
B. fragilis	128 (64–256)	8 (4–32)	32 (16–128)	64 (16–>128)	4 (4–8)	16 (8–16)
Bacteroides sp.	256	16 (16–32)	32 (32–64)	128 (128–256)	NA	NA
Gram-positive aerobes						
S. aureus (MS)	≥128 (32–>128)	0.5 (0.25–1)	2 (1–4)	2 (1–4)	0.5 (0.25–1)	0.5 (0.125–1)
S. aureus (MR)	>64 (32–128)	0.5 (0.5–1)	2	2	0.5 (0.25–0.5)	1 (0.5–1)
S. epidermidis	>64 (64–128)	0.25 (0.125–0.5)	1	2 (1–4)	0.5 (0.25–1)	1 (0.5–2)
S. pneumoniae	≥128 (64–≥256)	1 (0.5–2)	16	16 (4–16)	2 (1–2)	8 (8–16)
S. pyogenes	≥128	1 (0.5–2)	8 (8–16)	16 (8–32)	4	8
S. agalactiae	>128 (>128–512)	1 (0.5–2)	16 (16–32)	16 (8–32)	2 (1–4)	16
Enterococcus	>128 (64–>128)	2 (0.5–2)	8 (8–16)	8 (4–32)	2 (2–4)	4
Gram-positive anaerobes						
Peptococcus	256	2	8	8	4	NA
Peptostreptococcus	≥64	1 (0.5–8)	8	4 (2–4)	2	NA
Clostridium sp.	≥256	16 (8–32)	32 (32–64)	64 (32–128)	16 (8–16)	NA

Abbreviations: NA: not available; MS: methicillin sensitive; MR: methicillin resistant.
[a] Values are means of the minimum 90 percent inhibitory concentration in micrograms per milliliter.
(From Norris et al.,[27] with permission.)

Klebsiella and *Enterobacter* spp., and 80 percent of other coliform bacteria are sensitive to the drug at concentrations that are easily achieved in the urine, that is, 16 μg/ml or lower.[1,28] Some strains of *Salmonella* and *Shigella* are also sensitive, and *Brucella* sp. may be sensitive. *Pseudomonas* sp. and *Serratia* sp. are resistant. Resistance of sensitive gram-negative bacteria to the drug can be induced in vitro by serial passage of these bacteria in increasing concentrations of nalidixic acid.[29] Resistance may also be acquired during treatment of bacteriuria, so repeat urine culture and sensitivity testing are of practical clinical importance.[30] Gram-positive bacteria including *Staphylococcus aureus*, *Streptococcus pneumoniae*, and *Enterococcus faecalis* are resistant to nalidixic acid.[1,18]

The antibacterial spectrum of activity of oxolinic acid is similar to nalidixic acid. It is primarily active against gram-negative bacteria with the exception of *Pseudomonas* sp. Oxolinic acid is significantly more active than nalidixic acid is in vitro and is two to four times more active in vivo.[5,31] Oxolinic acid inhibits 95 percent of the strains of *E. coli*, 92 percent of *P. mirabilis*, 89 percent of other *Proteus* sp., 91 percent of other coliform bacteria, and 64 percent of *Klebsiella–Enterobacter* isolates at concentrations of 1.56 μg/ml or less.[32] Although *Klebsiella–Enterobacter* isolates are less susceptible, 93 percent are inhibited by 6.25 μg/ml, an amount of oxolinic acid easily achieved in urine.[32] *Neisseria gonorrhoeae* and *Neisseria meningitidis* are also inhibited at concentrations of 0.01–0.19 μg/ml of the drug.[5] Except for *S. aureus* strains that are inhibited at concentrations of 6.25 μg/ml, oxolinic acid has no significant activity against other gram-positive bacteria or fungi.[5] Sensitive gram-negative bacteria can acquire resistance to oxolinic acid in a stepwise manner in vitro similar to that observed with nalidixic acid. Cross-resistance between these two agents has been demonstrated, that is, oxolinic acid–resistant strains are also resistant to nalidixic acid and vice versa. Also, resistance is not reversed in vitro even after 10–12 consecutive passages in drug-free media.[6] As with nalidixic acid, resistance to oxolinic acid may also be acquired during treatment of patients with bacteriuria, so follow-up urine culture and sensitivity testing are clinically important.[33]

The antibacterial spectrum of activity of cinoxacin, although similar to that of nalidixic acid, is greater against some bacterial species[8,34] but is less than that of oxolinic acid.[35] Cinoxacin is active against most strains of gram-negative bacteria that cause urinary tract infections at concentrations that are readily attained in the urine. Cinoxacin inhibits more than 90 percent of *E. coli* strains at a concentration of 16 μg/ml. It is active against all *Proteus* sp. and most strains of *Klebsiella*, *Enterobacter*, *Citrobacter*, *Providencia*, and *Serratia* spp. Cinoxacin also demonstrates in vitro activity against *Salmonella, Shigella*, *Alcaligenes*, *Acinetobacter*, *Moraxella*, and *Haemophilus* spp. as well as against *Clostridium perfringens*, *Clostridium tetani*, *N. meningitidis*, and *Pseudomonas pseudomallei*. Cinoxacin has negligible activity against *Pseudomonas aeruginosa* and gram-positive cocci such as *S. aureus*, *Staphylococcus saphrophyticus*, *Streptococcus* sp., and enterococci.[8,34–36] Cross resistance among bacterial isolates develops among cinoxacin, nalidixic acid, and oxolinic acid.[35,37] Resistance to cinoxacin of organisms that are usually susceptible can be induced in vitro and is mediated presumably via chromosomes since there is no evidence that resistance is transferred as an extrachromosomal plasmid.[38]

Norfloxacin is 100 times more active than nalidixic acid is, with a spectrum that includes enterococci and staphylococci as well as *Pseudomonas*.[9] Norfloxacin is active against most strains of gram-negative and gram-positive bacteria that cause urinary tract infections at concentrations that are readily attained in the urine. Norfloxacin inhibits more than 90 percent of strains of *E. coli* at a concentration of 0.2 μg/ml, *Klebsiella* species at 0.4 μg/ml; *Salmonella* and *Shigella* species at 0.1 μg/ml; *Citrobacter* species at 0.4 μg/ml; *Enterobacter cloacae* at 0.2 μg/ml; *Enterobacter aerogenes* at 0.4 μg/ml; *Enterobacter agglomerans* at 0.2 μg/ml; *Proteus mirabilis* at 0.1 μg/ml; *Mor-*

ganella species at 0.2 μg/ml; *Proteus vulgaris* at 0.8 μg/ml; *Proteus rettgeri* at 0.3 μg/ml; *Providencia* species at 1.6 μg/ml; *Pseudomonas aeruginosa*, including gentamicin-resistant strains, at 0.8 μg/ml; *Pseudomonas maltophilia* at 3.1 μg/ml; *Serratia marcescens* at 3.1 μg/ml; *Acinetobacter calcoaceticus* at 8 μg/ml; and *Yersinia*, *Arizona*, *Aeromonas*, and *Campylobacter* at concentrations below 1 μg/ml. Norfloxacin is also active against *Haemophilus influenzae* at concentrations of 0.12 μg/ml; *Neisseria gonorrhoeae*, regardless of β-lactamase activity, at 0.016 μg/ml; and *Branhamella catarrhalis* at 0.25 μg/ml. Norfloxacin is somewhat less active against gram-positive species, with 90 percent of strains of *Staphylococcus aureus* inhibited at concentrations of 2 μg/ml, methicillin-resistant strains of *S. aureus* at 4.0 μg/ml, *S. saprophyticus* at 4 μg/ml, *S. epidermidis* at 1 μg/ml, *Streptococcus pyogenes* at 4–6 μg/ml, *Streptococcus agalactiae* at 8 μg/ml, *Enterococcus faecalis* at 12.5 μg/ml, *Streptococcus pneumoniae* at 16 μg/ml, and *Listeria* species at 3.1 μg/ml. Members of the *Bacteroides fragilis* group of anaerobes are relatively resistant to norfloxacin since they are inhibited at concentrations of 8–128 μg/ml, as are most other anaerobes. Norfloxacin has some activity against *Gardnerella vaginalis*, inhibiting 90 percent of isolates at 16–32 μg/ml, and *Ureaplasma urealyticum* at concentrations of 8 μg/ml.[10,31,39–43]

Ciprofloxacin, although similar in antibacterial activity, is even more potent than norfloxacin is. Ciprofloxacin is active against most strains of gram-negative and gram-positive bacteria that cause infections at concentrations that are easily attained in most tissues and body fluids. Ciprofloxacin inhibits more than 90 percent of strains of *E. coli* at a concentration of 0.06 μg/ml, *Klebsiella* species at 0.25 μg/ml, *Salmonella* and *Shigella* species at 0.015 and 0.008 μg/ml respectively, *Citrobacter diversus* at 0.03 μg/ml, *Citrobacter freundii* at 0.125 μg/ml, *Enterobacter cloacae* at 0.03 μg/ml, *Enterobacter aerogenes* at 0.06 μg/ml, *Proteus mirabilis* at 0.06 μg/ml, *Proteus vulgaris* at 0.06 μg/ml, *Morganella morganii* at 0.016 μg/ml, *Providencia stuartii* at 0.5 μg/ml, *Pseudomonas aeruginosa* at 0.25 μg/ml, *Pseudomonas maltophilia* at 4 μg/ml, *Pseudomonas cepacia* at 8 μg/ml, *Serratia marcescens* at 0.13 μg/ml, *Acinetobacter calcoaceticus* at 0.5 μg/ml, *Yersinia enterocolitica* at 0.06 μg/ml, *Campylobacter jejuni* at 0.12 μg/ml, *Aeromonas hydrophilia* at 0.008 μg/ml, and *Pasteurella multocida* at 0.016 μg/ml. Ciprofloxacin is also active against *H. influenzae* at concentrations of 0.015 μg/ml, *Branhamella catarrhalis* at 0.03 μg/ml, *Gardnerella vaginalis* at 1 μg/ml, and *Neisseria gonorrhoeae*, regardless of β-lactamase activity, at 0.004 μg/ml. In contrast to norfloxacin, ciprofloxacin is more active against *Bacteroides fragilis*, with 90 percent of strains inhibited at concentrations of 4 μg/ml, *Bacteroides melaninogenicus/oralis* group at 4 μg/ml, *Bacteroides urealyticus* at 0.06 μg/ml, *Fusobacteria* sp. at 4 μg/ml, *Mobiluncus* sp. at 1 μg/ml, and *Peptococcus* sp. at 2 μg/ml, *Peptostreptococcus* sp. at 2 μg/ml, and *Clostridia* sp. at 16 μg/ml. Similarly, ciprofloxacin is more active than norfloxacin is against gram-positive bacteria, with 90 percent of strains of *Staphylococcus aureus*, including methicillin-resistant strains, inhibited at concentrations of 0.5 μg/ml; *Staphylococcus epidermis* at 0.25 μg/ml; *Streptococcus pyogenes* at 1 μg/ml; *Streptococcus agalactiae* at 1 μg/ml; *Enterococcus faecalis* at 2 μg/ml; *Streptococcus pneumoniae* at 2 μg/ml; viridans streptococci at 2 μg/ml; *Legionella pneumophila* at 0.03–0.125 μg/ml; *Mycobacterium tuberculosis* at 0.25–1 μg/ml (atypical mycobacteria are less susceptible); and *Listeria monocytogenes* at 1 μg/ml. Compared with norfloxacin, ciprofloxacin has increased activity against all bacterial species studied. Ciprofloxacin has excellent activity against *Chlamydia trachomatis* and inhibits 90 percent of isolates at 1 μg/ml.[11,27,31,44–48]

The antibacterial activity of the newer 4-quinolones under development (listed before) are similar to that of ciprofloxacin, which, with few exceptions, is the most potent of the newer 4-quinolones.[31]

MECHANISMS OF BACTERIAL RESISTANCE

The selection in vitro of bacterial variants with reduced susceptibility to the quinolones has occurred after serial exposure of bacteria to subinhibitory drug concentrations.[27,31] These variants with reduced quinolones susceptibility have been obtained from gram-negative and gram-positive organisms. The resulting strains may exhibit cross-resistance to other quinolones. The mechanism of resistance usually involves either (1) mutations in the gene coding for DNA gyrase so that there is reduced quinolone affinity for the A subunit or (2) mutations that change the outer membrane porins.[27,31,45–51] Relative resistance to antibiotics unrelated to the quinolones has been observed when reduced susceptibility to the quinolones is caused by reduced outer membrane porin F activity.[31,52]

The exact mechanism for the development of bacterial resistance to the quinolones has not been determined. However, recent work suggests that the quinolones are unable to bind to DNA gyrase subunit A if serine, in the 83 position of subunit A, is replaced by tryptophan (L.M. Fisher, personal communication).

Since quinolones interfere with DNA gyrase activity, which is necessary for plasmid replication, plasmid-mediated quinolone resistance was not expected to occur. In fact, quinolones were expected to promote a loss of plasmids and inhibit the transfer of R-factor–mediated resistance.[27,53] However, recent reports suggest that plasmid-mediated resistance may be possible, although rare.[31,54,55]

PHARMACOLOGY

Nalidixic acid is administered by the oral route and is well absorbed (96 percent) from the gastrointestinal tract.[56] It is rapidly metabolized in the liver to hydroxynalidixic acid, which is biologically active, and to antibacterially inactive monoglucuronide conjugates, both of which, along with the parent compound, are rapidly excreted by the kidney into the urine. The biologically active drug in the plasma consists of the hydroxylated metabolite (one-third) and the parent compound (two-thirds), which are 63 and 93 percent, respectively, bound to plasma proteins.[57] Plasma levels of 20–50 μg/ml may be attained 2 hours after a single oral dose of 1 g of the drug.[58] The drug does not accumulate in tissues even after prolonged administration, and the kidney is the only organ in which tissue concentrations may exceed plasma levels.[56] Nalidixic acid does not diffuse into prostatic fluid.[59] It will appear in human milk of lactating mothers and therefore may be harmful to the newborn.[60] Excretion is almost completely via the kidney into the urine. About 85 percent of the drug in the urine is in the conjugated inactive form. Most of the remainder is present as biologically active hydroxynalidixic acid, which is 16 times more active than is the parent compound and is primarily responsible for the therapeutic effect of this drug in the treatment of urinary tract infection.[57] Urine concentrations of the active drug after a 0.5–1.0 g single oral dose in adults range from 25 to 250 μg/ml and remain between 100 and 500 μg/ml with a 1 g oral dose administered every 6 hours.[29,58] Bactericidal levels of the drug are also attained in the urine of patients with moderate or advanced renal failure.[58] The antibacterially active component of the drug does not accumulate in the serum of azotemic patients during continuous therapy[58] as do the inactive monoglucuronides that may also contribute to toxicity.[61] Although increased toxicity has not been observed in patients with advanced renal failure who were given the usual doses of nalidixic acid, the drug should be used cautiously in these patients as well as in patients with liver disease since conjugation of the drug may be impaired in this latter group.

Oxolinic acid is also administered orally, after which active and inactive metabolites are excreted in the urine and eliminated in the feces. Plasma levels of oxolinic acid after oral administration are low to borderline with respect to antimicrobic activity against susceptible bacteria. An effective bactericidal concentration for most susceptible microorganisms is achieved in the urine within 4 hours and is sustained for 12 hours after the recommended oral dose. The concentration of oxolinic acid attained in 24-hour urine collections after an oral dose of 2 g/day averaged 38 μg/ml with a range of 16–64 μg/ml.[62] Although oxolinic acid given to patients with moderate or advanced renal failure did not further impair or damage the kidney or interfere with the drug's renal excretion, it should be used cautiously in patients with severely impaired renal function. Since oxolinic acid is excreted in human milk, it is contraindicated in nursing mothers.

Cinoxacin is also administered orally and is rapidly and almost completely absorbed from the gastrointestinal tract. Peak plasma levels usually occur in 2–3 hours and are in the range of <4–14.8 and 2.8–28 μg/ml after an oral dose of 250 and 500 mg, respectively. Approximately 70 percent of cinoxacin is bound to plasma proteins. It has a serum half-life of approximately 1 hour, which may increase threefold in patients with creatinine clearance of less than 30 ml/min/1.73 m^2. Although concomitant ingestion of food delays the absorption of cinoxacin and causes a 30 percent reduction in mean peak plasma levels, overall recovery of the drug in urine is not affected significantly. Peak urine concentrations (88–925 μg/ml) occur within 4–6 hours and are decreased in patients with impaired renal function. Cinoxacin concentrations in human prostatic tissue range from 0.6 to 6.3 μg/g, whereas concentrations in renal tissue exceed those in serum.[63] Approximately 60 percent of an orally administered dose is excreted into the urine unchanged in patients with normal renal function, and 40 percent is metabolized by the liver. Cinoxacin is metabolized to at least four microbiologically inactive metabolites that represent approximately 30–40 percent of the ingested dose.[64] The renal clearance of cinoxacin exceeds the glomerular filtration rate, and probenecid inhibits cinoxacin excretion by the kidney. Thus, this drug is excreted by both glomerular filtration and tubular secretion.[65] Changes in urinary pH do not influence cinoxacin excretion significantly. It is not known whether cinoxacin is excreted into human milk. Because other drugs in this class are excreted into human milk and because of the potential for serious adverse reactions from cinoxacin in nursing infants, the drug should not be used in nursing women.

Norfloxacin is also administered orally and is readily absorbed from the gastrointestinal tract. Peak plasma levels usually occur 1–2 hours after each dose and are in the range of 0.75, 1.58, 2.41, 3.15, and 3.87 μg/ml for doses of 200, 400, 800, 1200, and 1600 mg, respectively. The half-life of norfloxacin is 3–4.5 hours for all doses studied. Concentrations in urine peak at 1–2 hours after administration. Mean peak values for increasing doses of norfloxacin (200, 400, 800, 1200, and 1600 mg) are 200, 478, 697, 992, and 1045 μg/ml, respectively. Renal clearances approximate 285 ml/min. Approximately 30 percent of each dose is excreted into urine as unmetabolized norfloxacin, with lesser quantities of glucuronide conjugate and six active metabolites with modifications in the piperazine ring being excreted.[27,66–68] Crystals of norfloxacin are occasionally observed during microscopic examination of freshly voided urine collected after the 1200 and 1600 mg doses. However, crystalluria is not encountered at lower doses.[66] Concentrations of norfloxacin in human milk are below the bioassay detection limits.[67]

Ciprofloxacin is also administered orally and is rapidly absorbed from the gastrointestinal tract. Peak plasma levels usually occur in 1–1.5 hours and are approximately 2–3 μg/ml after an oral dose of 500 mg. Approximately 35 percent of ciprofloxacin is bound to plasma proteins. It has a serum half-life 3–4.5 hours. Peak urine concentrations occur within 4 hours. Approximately 20 percent of the administered dose can be recovered as active drug in the urine during the first 4 hours, with a total of 30–60 percent by 24 hours. Renal clearance of ciprofloxacin is 4.9 ml/min/kg or 267 ml/min.[67,68] Approximately 10 percent of ciprofloxacin is excreted into the urine in the form of four different metabolites.[67] Approximately 15 percent of ciprofloxacin is recoverable in feces (10 percent as ciprofloxacin, 5 percent as metabolites); less than 1 percent appears in bile. Ciprofloxacin is the most thoroughly studied quinolone in all respects. Its extravascular penetration into tissues and other body compartments is better than or comparable to other newer quinolones.[67] For example, ciprofloxacin penetrates blister fluid well, with 57 percent of the serum concentration recoverable. Also, the concentration of ciprofloxacin in blister fluid exceeds that in serum about 3 hours after administration.[69] It is not known whether ciprofloxacin is excreted into human milk. A parenteral preparation of ciprofloxacin is also available and is currently under investigation.

The pharmacokinetic properties of some of the newer quinolones are summarized in Table 2. The newer quinolones in general exhibit linear pharmacokinetics. Peak serum concentrations occur 1–3 hours after oral administration. Food delays absorption so that serum peaks appear later and are moderately lower.[67] Absorption is also reduced by concomitant administration of magnesium or aluminum hydroxide antacids, by H-2 blockers (ranitidine), and by other drugs that decrease peristalsis or delay the gastric emptying time.[27,67] None of the newer quinolones is extensively bound (only up to 30 percent) to serum proteins. Their long serum half-life allows twice-daily or once-daily dosing. The newer quinolones undergo renal and hepatic metabolism. Renal elimination is by glomerular filtration and active tubular secretion, which is blocked by probenicid (except fleroxacin). Urinary recovery of the newer quinolones after oral administration ranges from 70 to 85 percent for lomefloxacin and ofloxacin to 5 to 15 percent for pefloxacin and difloxacin,[70] with 62 percent for enoxacin, 50–60 percent for fleroxacin, 31 percent for ciprofloxacin, and 27 percent for norfloxacin.[3,27,67,70] The antibacterial activity of the quinolones is reduced at lower urinary pH values (pH 5.5–6.0 vs. pH 7.4).[3] Hepatic metabolism includes conjugation with glucuronic acid as well as carboxylation, hydroxylation, and demethylation.[71] Pefloxacin and difloxacin undergo extensive hepatic metabolism, followed by enoxacin and, to a lesser degree, norfloxacin, ciprofloxacin, and fleroxacin. Lomefloxacin and ofloxacin undergo the least hepatic metabolism. Biliary concentrations of the quinolones (ciprofloxacin, enoxacin, ofloxacin, and pefloxacin) are two to 8 times the simultaneous serum concentrations.[67]

The quinolones penetrate well into body fluids and into cells and tissues by passive diffusion across capillary membranes. Those quinolones with a longer half-life have smaller penetration ratios.[67] Also, ciprofloxacin and norfloxacin have high intracellular concentrations inside human neutrophils, whereas pefloxacin penetrates poorly into alveolar macrophages and neutrophils.[67] The tissue penetration of some of the newer quinolones is summarized in Table 3.

Intravenous preparations of some of the newer four-quinolones are undergoing clinical investigation. The intravenous preparation of ciprofloxacin will probably be approved and released for clinical use before the parenteral preparations of other newer quinolones; it is prepared as the 0.1 percent excess lactate salt.[71a] The pharmacology of intravenously administered ciprofloxacin has been studied with doses ranging from 25 to 200 mg, though most studies have used either 100 or 200 mg administered by bolus injection. These dose-ranging studies demonstrate a linear increase in the area under the concentration-time curve, and produce a half-life of approximately 4 hours.[71b] Peak serum concentrations of 3.80 ± 0.62 μg/ml are achieved with intravenous infusions of 200 mg. Although renal clearance accounts for two-thirds of the total serum clearance, approximately 75 percent is recovered in the urine as parent compound plus metabolites.[71b] Intravenous ciprofloxacin is excreted into bile unchanged and 14 percent is recovered in feces.

TABLE 2. Pharmacokinetic Properties of Selected Newer Quinolones

Drug	*Dose (mg)*	*C_{max} (mg/L)*	*Half-life (hr)*	*Protein Binding (%)*	*Bioavailability (%)*	*VD (liters)*	*Urinary Excretion (%)*	
							Unchanged	*Metabolites*
Ciprofloxacin	500	2–3	3–4.5	35	85	250	30–60	10
Norfloxacin	400	1.5	3–4.5	15	80	225	20–40	20
Ofloxacin	400	3.5–5.0	5–6	8–30	85–95	100	70–90	5–10
Enoxacin	400	2–3	4–6	43	90	190	50–55	15
Pefloxacin	400	4–5	10–11	25	90	110	5–15	55
Fleroxacin	400	4–6	10	23	96	100	60–70	10
Lomefloxacin	400	3	8	NA	NA	190	70	10
Difloxacin	400	4–5	26	42	NA	140	10	20

Abbreviations: C_{max}: peak serum concentration; VD: volume of distribution; NA: data not available.

TABLE 3. Penetration of Selected Quinolones into Body Fluids and Tissues

Fluid/Tissue	*Ciprofloxacin*	*Norfloxacin*	*Ofloxacin*	*Enoxacin*	*Pefloxacin*	*Fleroxacin*
Blister fluid	++++	++++	++++	++++	+++	++++
Saliva	++	++	+++	+++	+++	+++
Bronchial secretions	++	—	+++	++++	++++	—
Pleural fluid	+++	—	—	—	—	—
Nasal secretions	+++	+++	++++	++++	+++	++++
Tears	++	++	+++	++	+++	+++
Sweat	+	+	++	++	++	++
Cerebrospinal fluid	+	—	++	—	+++	—
Prostatic fluid	+++	++	++++	++	—	++
Ejaculate	+++++	—	++++	++++	—	++++
Lung	++++	—	++++	+++++	++++	—
Kidney	+++++	+++++	+++++	++++	—	—
Bone	++++	—	++	++	++	—
Skin	++++	—	—	++++	—	—
Muscle	++++	—	—	++++	—	—
Fat	++++	—	—	+++	—	—

Abbreviations: +: area under the curve (AUC) ratios or concentration ratios <0.1; ++: AUC ratios or concentration ratios 0.1–0.5; +++: AUC ratios or concentration ratios 0.5–1; ++++: AUC ratios or concentration ratios 1–4; +++++: AUC ratios or concentration ratios >4 of tissue or fluid vs. serum.
(Modified from Sörgel et al.,[68] with permission.)

Also, renal impairment reduces the serum clearance of ciprofloxacin, with a doubling of the half-life in anephric patients; thus, the dose should be reduced by 50 percent in patients with creatinine clearances of 20 to 30 ml/min/1.73m^2.[71b]

DOSAGE ADJUSTMENTS IN RENAL OR HEPATIC INSUFFICIENCY

Dosage adjustments in patients with renal insufficiency (creatinine clearance below 80 ml/min) are recommended for ofloxacin and lomefloxacin since they undergo minimal hepatic metabolism and are excreted predominantly unchanged in the urine.[70] Adjustments in the dose of enoxacin, fleroxacin, and pefloxacin may be necessary in patients with moderate renal insufficiency; this also holds for norfloxacin and ciprofloxacin but only when creatinine clearance is severely impaired.[3,48,67]

Dosage adjustments in patients with hepatic disease may be required for pefloxacin, difloxacin, and possibly enoxacin,[67,70,71] whereas norfloxacin and ciprofloxacin may accumulate only in patients with severe hepatic failure.[27,67]

TOXICITY AND ADVERSE REACTIONS

Oral nalidixic acid is usually well tolerated, although a number of adverse reactions have been reported. Gastrointestinal side effects include nausea, vomiting, diarrhea, and abdominal pain. Dermatologic reactions include pruritus, nonspecific rashes, and urticaria associated with eosinophilia as well as photosensitivity reactions involving skin surfaces exposed to sunlight that are most commonly manifested as a sunburn and rarely as a bullous eruption.[72–74] Patients receiving the drug should be cautioned to avoid excessive exposure to direct sunlight. Ophthalmologic side effects include blurred vision, diplopia, photophobia, abnormal accommodation, and changes in color perception, all of which disappear with cessation of therapy. Central nervous system reactions include headaches, drowsiness, asthenia, giddiness, vertigo, syncope, sensory changes, grand mal seizures, and acute reversible toxic psychosis[75–77] as well as pseudotumor cerebri with intracranial hypertension, papilledema, and bulging fontanelles in infants and young children,[78–81] which reverses after the cessation of therapy. Also, convulsions, hyperglycemia, and glycosuria without abnormal serum ketone levels has been reported in one patient who took an overdose of nalidixic acid.[82] Therefore, the drug should not be given to patients with convulsive disorders, pre-existing mental instability, parkinsonism, or cerebral vascular insufficiency, nor to infants or pregnant women in the first trimester, and it probably should not be used in children.

Nalidixic acid has rarely been associated with blood dyscrasias and hemolytic anemia that sometimes is associated with glucose-6-phosphate dehydrogenase (G6PD)-deficient red blood cells.[60,83] The drug has also rarely been associated with cholestatic jaundice and possibly may precipitate acute respiratory failure in patients with impaired respiratory function.[84]

Oxolinic acid has been associated frequently with excitative central nervous system responses, which include restlessness, insomnia, nervousness, dizziness, headache, and nausea.[56] This potential is increased in elderly patients and is more common with oxolinic acid than with nalidixic acid. Less frequent reactions include abdominal pain, vomiting, anorexia, diarrhea, constipation, pruritus, and weakness. Abnormal liver function test results and reduced leukocyte counts have also been observed. Rare reactions include photophobia, palpitations, swelling of extremities, reduction in hematocrit or hemoglobin values, eosinophilia, urticaria, rash, soreness of mouth and gums, and metallic taste. A seizure occurred in one patient with known epilepsy, and hallucinations and hysteria occurred in one patient who received a larger dose than was recommended. All reactions are reversible with cessation of treatment.

Oral cinoxacin is well tolerated, and adverse reactions occur infrequently (4.4 percent) and are reversible.[65] Gastrointestinal reactions are the most common side effects, and nausea is the most frequent (3 percent of patients), followed by vomiting, anorexia, abdominal cramps, and diarrhea. The frequency of adverse central nervous system reactions is less than 1 percent. These consist of headache, dizziness, insomnia, paresthesias, perineal burning, photophobia, and tinnitus. Hypersensitivity reactions (less than 3 percent) include urticaria, morbilliform rash, pruritus, and edema. Abnormal liver (serum glutamic-oxaloacetic transaminase [SGOT], serum glutamic-pyruvic transaminase [SGPT], and alkaline phosphatase) and renal (blood urea nitrogen [BUN] and serum creatinine) function values have been observed in fewer than 1 percent of patients who have received cinoxacin. This drug should be used with caution in patients with a history of liver disease. Also, the use of cinoxacin in prepubertal children and during pregnancy is not recommended.

The newer fluoroquinolones norfloxacin, ciprofloxacin, ofloxacin, enoxacin, and pefloxacin have similar toxicities and incidences of adverse reactions.[85] Compared with other antimicrobial agents, the newer quinolones can be considered relatively safe agents. Even so, adverse effects have been observed during clinical trials with these agents. Gastrointestinal side effects are the most frequent (0.8–6.8 percent of patients) and include nausea, vomiting, dyspepsia, epigastric/abdominal pain, anorexia, diarrhea, flatulence, and dry mouth.[85] Antibiotic-associated colitis has been seen but only very rarely.[86]

Central nervous system side effects are the next most commonly observed adverse reactions (0.9–1.8 percent of patients) and can be divided into mild reactions and severe neurotoxic side effects that require interruption of therapy. Mild reactions include headache, dizziness, tiredness, insomnia, faintness, agitation, listlessness, restlessness, abnormal vision, and bad dreams. Severe reactions are rare (<0.5 percent) and include hallucinations, depressions, psychotic reactions and grand mal convulsions. In general, these side effects occur after only a few days of treatment and stop when therapy is discontinued.[85,86] The exact mechanism of central nervous system toxicity associated with quinolone therapy has not been defined. Although the quinolones do inhibit the receptor binding of γ-aminobutyric acid (GABA), which is an inhibitory neurotransmitter, the concentrations required for inhibition are higher than can probably be attained clinically.[87,88]

Skin and allergic reactions are the third most commonly observed side effects (0.6–2.4 percent of patients) and include erythema, urticaria, rash, pruritus, and photosensitivity reactions of skin surfaces exposed to sunlight.[85,86] Very rare cases of hypotension, tachycardia, nephrotoxicity (elevations in serum creatinine levels), thrombocytopenia, leukopenia, anemia, and transient elevations in liver enzyme concentrations have been observed.[85,86] Animal toxicology has described testicular toxicity, ocular damage (including subcapsular cataracts, retinal changes, and altered visual acuity), as well as arthropathy, gait abnormalities, and articular cartilage lesions in weight-bearing joints in juvenile animals.[85] Although the significance of these findings in human adults is unclear, there is concern about the effect of the newer quinolones in children and adolescents. Thus, the newer quinolones have not been approved for use in pediatric patients in the United States.

DRUG INTERACTIONS

Nalidixic acid–glucuronide conjugates may produce a false-positive reaction for urine glucose when tested with Benedict solution such as Clinitest, but not with glucose oxidase test strips such as Clinistix. Diabetic patients treated with this drug should be so alerted. Nitrofurantoin interferes with the therapeutic action of nalidixic acid.

The safety of the concomitant use of oxolinic acid and other central nervous system stimulants has not been established. Also, oxolinic acid may enhance the effects of the oral anticoagulants bishydroxycoumarin and warfarin by displacing these drugs from serum albumin binding sites. Nitrofurantoin also interferes with the therapeutic action of oxolinic acid.[89]

Some of the newer quinolones increase significantly the peak and trough serum concentrations of theophylline in patients receiving theophylline therapy. Increases in theophylline plasma concentrations are very significant with enoxacin (111 percent) and, to a much lesser extent, with ciprofloxacin (23 percent), pefloxacin (20 percent), and ofloxacin (12 percent).[90–92] The 4-oxo metabolite of the piperazine ring in these quinolones is thought to compete with theophylline for liver enzymes and interfere with theophylline clearance.[91] Thus, the dose of theophylline probably should be halved in patients also receiving enoxacin, whereas no routine reduction in the theophylline dose is recommended for ciprofloxacin, ofloxacin or pefloxacin. However, monitoring theophylline levels is recommended in patients also receiving one of these quinolones.

Some of the newer quinolones also interfere with the clearance of caffeine. Enoxacin increases the plasma concentration of caffeine by 41 percent and reduces the clearance by 78 percent. Ciprofloxacin increases the half-life of caffeine only modestly (15 percent), and ofloxacin does so only minimally.[93,94]

CLINICAL USES

The newer quinolones have proved to be effective therapies for infection of the urinary tract, respiratory tree, gastrointestinal tract, skin, soft tissue, and bone and for sexually transmitted bacterial diseases.

Urinary Tract Infections

Nalidixic acid, oxolinic acid, cinoxacin, norfloxacin, and ciprofloxacin have established roles in treating urinary tract infections. Nalidixic acid (*adults*: 1 g qid for 1–2 weeks, thereafter 0.5 g qid if needed; *children*: 55 mg/kg/day in four divided doses for 1–2 weeks, thereafter 33 mg/kg/day if needed), oxolinic acid (*adults*: 750 mg bid for 2 weeks; *children*: not recommended), and cinoxacin (*adults*: 250 mg qid 500 mg bid for 1–2 weeks; *children*: not recommended) have been used in acute and recurrent uncomplicated urinary infections due to susceptible organisms. Nalidixic acid has also been used as long-term therapy for frequently recurrent bacteriuria, in adults, and in children with bacteriuria associated with urinary tract abnormalities.[29,95] The follow-up cure rate was disappointingly similar to that observed with other agents, and resistance to nalidixic acid commonly emerged during treatment.[29] In contrast, the rapid emergence of resistant organisms during acute and long-term treatment with cinoxacin has not been observed. The efficacy of cinoxacin prophylaxis for frequently recurrent urinary infections is less clear.[96,97] Nalidixic acid, oxolonic acid, and cinoxacin should not be used in patients with renal carbuncles or perinephric abscesses.

The newer quinolones are also at least as effective as other well established agents for the treatment of *uncomplicated* urinary infections.[3] Single doses of norfloxacin (800 mg), ciprofloxacin (100 or 250 mg), and ofloxacin (200 mg) are highly effective in women with simple cystitis caused by enterobacteriacae but may be less effective against *Staphylococcus saprophyticus*.[3,98] Also, 3–10 days of therapy with norfloxacin, ciprofloxacin, ofloxacin, or enoxacin resulted in excellent bacteriologic cure rates in uncomplicated urinary infections.[3,27,98]

Norfloxacin, ciprofloxacin, ofloxacin, and enoxacin, given for 5–10 days to patients with nosocomial or *complicated* urinary infections, resulted in higher cure rates than did amoxicillin, amoxicillin plus clavulanic acid, trimethoprim-sulfamethoxazole, or parenteral antibiotic therapy.[3,27,98]

The newer quinolones ciprofloxacin (1000 mg/day), ofloxacin

(300–600 mg/day), pefloxacin (800 mg/day), and norfloxacin (800 mg/day), given to patients with either acute or chronic *prostatitis* for 28 (range, 5–84) days, cured 63–92 percent of patients.[3,99–102]

Respiratory Tract Infections

Ciprofloxacin, ofloxacin, enoxacin, and pefloxacin, given for 10 (range, 7–15) days to patients with purulent bronchitis, acute exacerbations of chronic bronchitis, or pneumonia, resulted in clinical cure or improvement (76–91 percent) and bacteriologic cure (68–83 percent) in most patients. However, bacteriologic persistence, relapse, or treatment failure occurred in 49 percent of patients with *Pseudomonas aeruginosa* infections, in 39 percent with *Streptococcus pneumoniae* infections, and in 33 percent with *Staphylococcus aureus* infections.[3,103] Although the newer quinolones are effective for the treatment of bronchitis, they should not be used to treat either community-acquired or aspiration pneumonia because of their reduced activity against *S. pneumoniae* and against those microaerophilic and anaerobic bacteria associated with aspiration pneumonia. In contrast, the newer quinolones may have value for the treatment of hospital-acquired pneumonia caused by aerobic gram-negative bacteria.[3,27] Also, ciprofloxacin (750 mg twice daily) has proved to be a useful alternative to conventional parenteral therapy for cystic fibrosis patients with acute exacerbations of their pulmonary infections, although resistant organisms may emerge.[3,104,1005] Ciprofloxacin may have value also for treating malignant external otitis caused by *Pseudomonas aeruginosa*, which currently requires parenteral combination therapy.

The newer quinolones should not be used for acute sinusitis because of the possible presence of pneumococci and anaerobic streptococci. However, these agents may be useful in specific cases of chronic sinusitis when aerobic gram-negative bacteria susceptible to the newer quinolones are responsible. These agents should not be used for otitis media since they are currently not recommended for use in pediatric patients. Of importance, norfloxacin has not been approved for and should not be used for any type of respiratory tract infection.

Gastrointestinal Infections

The bacterial pathogens causing diarrheal disease, including toxigenic *E. coli*, *Salmonella*, *Shigella*, *Campylobacter* and *Vibrio spp.*, are highly susceptible to the newer quinolones, which also provide high drug concentrations in the lumen of the gut and the mucosa. These factors contribute to the eradication of these pathogens from the intestine within 48 hours of initiating therapy.[106–108] Ciprofloxacin (500 mg bid for 5 days) and norfloxacin (400 mg bid for 5 days) have been studied extensively in patients with either acute bacterial diarrhea or acute traveller's diarrhea. Both of these agents have a greater than 90 percent cure rate and are comparable to trimethoprim-sulfamethoxazole.[3,106–108] Although these newer agents are effective in treating bacterial and traveller's diarrhea, they should not be used as prophylactic agents to prevent acute traveller's diarrhea because this disease responds promptly to treatment once symptoms develop and because of the concern that resistance may develop more rapidly with the indiscriminate use of the newer quinolones. These agents should probably be reserved and used as an alternative for persons with a history of trimethoprim-sulfamethoxazole hypersensitivity or for persons in areas where resistance to trimethoprim-sulfamethoxazole is common.[3,109] Ciprofloxacin, 500 mg twice daily for 2–15 (mean, 13) days, and ofloxacin, 200 mg twice daily for 6–30 days, given to patients with typhoid fever cured all patients; none relapsed or became a chronic carrier.[3] Preliminary reports suggest that ciprofloxacin, 500–750 mg twice daily for 4 weeks, eliminated the chronic *Salmonella* carrier state in 86 percent of patients treated and followed for 10–12 months.[3]

Although the newer quinolones inhibit *Campylobacter pylori*, which has been associated with antral gastritis, these agents have not been effective in the treatment of *C. pylori*–associated gastritis.[3,110] Also, some relapses have been reported in patients with *Brucella* infections who have been treated with the newer quinolones.[3]

Skin and Soft Tissue Infections

Oral therapy with some of the newer quinolones, i.e., ciprofloxacin, ofloxacin, and enoxacin, appear to be as effective as alternative parenteral agents in treating a variety of skin and skin structure infections.[3,27] Patients with bacterial infections of the skin and soft tissue, including patients with cellulitis, subcutaneous abscesses, wound infections, and infected ulcers, generally in diabetic patients, have been treated successfully with the newer oral quinolones, primarily ciprofloxacin.[3,111–114] Most patients received 750 mg ciprofloxacin orally twice daily for 14 days, with clinical cure or improvement observed in 95 percent of patients. Bacteriologic cure rates were lower in patients infected with gram-positive organisms than were observed for infections caused by gram-negative aerobic bacteria.[3,112] Also, therapy failed in 25 percent of anaerobic infections. Ciprofloxacin, 750 mg orally twice daily for 7–28 days, eradicated colonization with methicillin-resistant *Staphylococcus aureus* (MRSA) in 79 percent of evaluable patients.[115] Although ciprofloxacin has the potential to eradicate MRSA colonization, there is the potential for the development of increased resistance to this and other newer quinolones.[3]

Osteomyelitis

Current experience with the newer oral quinolones as monotherapy for osteomyelitis, particularly when caused by gram-negative aerobic pathogens, is very encouraging. Most patients with osteomyelitis who have been treated with one of the newer quinolones received ciprofloxacin orally in a dose of 750 mg twice daily. The mean duration of therapy was 8 weeks (range, 4 days to 6 months). Patients with either acute or chronic osteomyelitis either in native bone or complicating a foreign body were treated. Clinical cure or improvement occurred in approximately 80 percent of patients with adequate follow-up of at least 6 months to more than 1 year. Treatment failures occurred in 15 percent, and a few patients developed recurrence of their infection. The infecting organism developed resistance to the newer quinolone used in therapy in only a small number (0.5 percent) of patients, primarily those with *Pseudomonas aeruginosa* infections.[3,116] Thus, ciprofloxacin has an established efficacy in the treatment of osteomyelitis and should facilitate home therapy for many patients with osteomyelitis.

Sexually Transmitted Diseases

Ciprofloxacin, ofloxacin, difloxacin, amifloxacin, lomefloxacin, norfloxacin, fleroxacin, pefloxacin, and enoxacin are extremely active in vitro against *Neisseria gonorrhoeae*, including penicillinase-producing strains (PPNG), and ciprofloxacin is especially active against *Haemophilus ducreyi*.[3,31] *Chlamydia trachomatis* isolates are susceptible to ciprofloxacin, ofloxacin, and difloxacin but are resistant to enoxacin and norfloxacin.[117,118] *Gardnerella vaginalis* isolates are relatively resistant to these agents, as are *Ureaplasma urealyticum*, although ciprofloxacin is active against the latter about 50 percent of the time.[3,119] Thus, the newer quinolones, on the basis of their in vitro activity, have been used to treat a variety of sexually transmitted diseases.

Gonococcal Infections

In uncomplicated gonococcal infections in both men and women, single oral doses of either 500, 250, or 100 mg of ciprofloxacin, 660, 400, or 200 mg of enoxacin, 400 mg of pefloxacin, 800, 600, 400, or 200 mg of ofloxacin, or 800 mg of norfloxacin cured 95–100 percent of patients, including patients infected with PPNG. Thus, the lowest effective oral single dose of the newer quinolones has been 100 mg of ciprofloxacin, which has cured almost 100 percent of patients with urethral as well as rectal gonorrhea and is probably effective for pharyngeal gonococcal infections. However, there is little experience with these newer agents in the treatment of *disseminated gonococcal* infections.[3]

Chlamydia Urethritis, Postgonococcal Urethritis, Nongonococcal Urethritis

None of the current quinolones is effective as single-dose therapy for *C. trachomatis* urethritis, nor are they able to prevent postgonoccal urethritis (PGU) when used as single-dose therapy in gonococcal infections. Ciprofloxacin, however, in a dose of 750 mg orally twice daily for 4 days eradicated *C. trachomatis* in 60 percent of co-infected patients and reduced the incidence of PGU from 35 percent to 12.8 percent.[3,120] Currently, ciprofloxacin in a dose of 500 mg three times daily and ofloxacin in a dose of 100 mg three times daily for 14 days have cured most patients with nongonococcal urethritis (NGU) caused by *C. trachomatis*, whereas norfloxacin is not effective.[3,120] However, the newer quinolones are less effective than is doxycycline in NGU patients with chlamydial infections alone.[120] Thus, further studies are needed to accurately define the efficacy of the newer quinolones in NGU.

Chancroid

Patients with chancroid and *H. ducreyi* infections have responded successfully to either a 500 mg oral single dose (95 percent cure rate) of ciprofloxacin or 500 mg twice daily for 3 days (100 percent cure rate). Currently the 3-day, six-dose ciprofloxacin regimen, which cured all patients with chancroid, is preferred.[3,121]

Nonspecific Vaginitis

Ciprofloxacin in an oral dose of 500 mg twice daily for 7 days given to women with nonspecific vaginitis caused by *Corynebacterium* spp., *Bacteroides* spp., and *Gardnerella vaginalis* produced clinical and bacteriologic cures in 73 percent of patients. Clinical improvement without bacteriologic eradication occurred in an additional 18 percent, and 9 percent failed to respond,[3,122] Vaginal colonization with *Candida albicans* occurred in 32 percent of these patients, but without clinical signs or symptoms of yeast infection.[3]

Other Infections

Immunocompromised Host. Ciprofloxacin and norfloxacin have been used successfully as *prophylactic* agents in granulocytopenic patients.[3,124–128] Prophylaxis was begun 1–2 days before the initiation of cytotoxic therapy and continued until the granulocyte count rose above 500 cells/mm^3. Ciprofloxacin prevented whereas norfloxacin reduced but did not prevent colonization by gram-negative bacilli, nor did norfloxacin influence the incidence of gram-positive bacteremia.[124] Clinical experience with the newer quinolones in the *treatment* of severe infections in immunocompromised patients is very preliminary.[3,128] Limited experience with ciprofloxacin, ofloxacin, and pefloxacin suggest a potential role for these agents in immunocompromised patients, but further trials are needed to establish their value.

Central Nervous System Infections. Ciprofloxacin, ofloxacin, and pefloxacin do penetrate into cerebrospinal fluid and brain tissue.[3,68,129,130] However, clinical experience with the newer quinolones as therapeutic agents for central nervous system bacterial infections is only anecdotal.[3] These agents should not be used empirically for central nervous system infections but should be reserved for special cases caused by multiantibiotic-resistant aerobic gram-negative bacteria. Of note, in *meningococcal carriers* oral ciprofloxacin in a dose of either 500 mg twice daily for 5 days or 250 mg twice daily for 2 days eradicated the meningococci in 100 and 96 percent, respectively, of nasopharyngeal carriers.[131,132]

The newer quinolones, particularly ciprofloxacin and ofloxacin, inhibit *M. tuberculosis* and *M. avium-intracellulare* and may be useful in drug-resistant mycobacterial infections with these organisms, but clinical studies are needed to define their effectiveness.[3]

REFERENCES

1. Lesher GY, Froelich EJ, Gruett MD, et al. 1,8-naphthyridine derivatives. A new class of chemotherapeutic agents. J Med Pharmacol Chem. 1962; 5:1063.
2. Smith JT, Lewin CS. Chemistry and mechanisms of action of the quinolone antibacterials. In: Andriole VT, ed. The Quinolones. London: Academic Press; 1988;23–81.
3. Andriole VT. Clinical overview of the newer 4-quinolone antibacterial agents. In: Andriole VT, ed. The Quinolones. London: Academic Press; 1988;155–200.
4. Crumplin G. Aspects of chemistry in the development of 4-quinolone antibacterial agents. Rev Infect Dis. 1988;1(Suppl):2–9.
5. Turner FJ, Ringel SM, Martin JF, et al. Oxolinic acid, a new synthetic antimicrobial agent. I. In vitro and in vivo activity. Antimicrob Agents Chemother. 1967;475.
6. Ringel SM, Turner FJ, Lindo FL, et al. Oxolinic acid, a new synthetic antimicrobial agent. II. Bactericidal rate and resistance development. Antimicrob Agents Chemother. 1967;480.
7. Ringel SM, Turner FJ, Roemer S, et al. Oxolonic acid, a new synthetic antimicrobial agent. III. Concentrations in serum, urine, and renal tissue. Antimicrob Agents Chemother. 1967;486.
8. Wick WE, Preston DS, White WA, et al. Compound 64716, a new synthetic antibacterial agent. Antimicrob Agents Chemother. 1973;4:415.
9. Ito A, Hirai K, Inoue M, et al. In vitro antibacterial activity of AM 175, a new nalidixic acid analog. Antimicrob Agents Chemother. 1980;17:103.
10. Downs JT, Andriole VT, Ryan JL. In vitro activity of MK 0366 against clinical urinary pathogens including gentamicin-resistant *Pseudomonas aeruginosa*. Antimicrob Agents Chemother. 1982;21:670.
11. Wise R, Andrew JM, Edwards LJ. In vitro activity of Bay 09867, a new quinolone derivative, compared with those of other antimicrobial agents. Antimicrob Agents Chemother. 1983;23:559.
12. Goss WA, Deitz WH, Cook TM. Mechanism of action of nalidixic acid on *Escherichia coli*. II. Inhibition of deoxyribonucleic acid synthesis. J Bacteriol. 1965;89:1068.
13. Crumplin GC, Smith JT. Nalidixic acid: An antibacterial paradox. Antimicrob Agents Chemother. 1975;8:251–61.
14. Deitz WH, Cook TM, Goss WA. Mechanism of action of nalidixic acid on *Escherichia coli*. III. Conditions required for lethality. J Bacteriol. 1966; 91:768.
15. Bourguignon GJ, Levitt M, Sternglanz R. Studies on the mechanism of action of nalidixic acid. Antimicrob Agents Chemother. 1973;4:479.
16. Pratt WB. The urinary tract antiseptics. In: Pratt WB, ed. Chemotherapy of Infection. New York: Oxford University Press; 1977:215.
17. Smith JT. Awakening the slumbering potential of the 4-quinolone antibacterials. Pharmacol J. 1984;233:299–305.
18. Higgens NP, Peebles CL, Sugino A, et al. Purification of subunits of *Escherichia coli*. DNA gyrase and reconstitution of enzymic activity. Proc Natl Acad Sci USA. 1978;75:1773–7.
19. Pedrini A. Nalidixic acid. In: Hahn FE, ed. Antibiotics. v. 5. Berlin: Springer-Verlag. 1979:154.
20. Wang JC. Interactions between DNAs and enzymes. The effect of superhelical turns. J Mol Biol. 1974;87:797–816.
21. Wang JC. DNA topoisomerases. Annu Rev Biochem. 1985;54:665–7.
22. Gellert M, Mizuuchi K, O'Dea MH, et al. DNA gyrase. An enzyme that introduces superhelical turns into DNA. Proc Natl Acad Sci USA. 1976;73:3872–6.
23. Sugino A, Peebles CL, Krenzer KN, et al. Mechanism of action of nalidixic acid. Purification of *E. coli* Nal A gene production and its relationship to DNA gyrase and a novel nicking–closing enzyme. Proc Natl Acad Sci USA. 1977;74:4767.
24. Gellert M, Mizuuchi K, O'Dea MH, et al. Nalidixic acid resistance. A second genetic character involved in DNA gyrase activity. Proc Natl Acad Sci USA. 1977;74:4772–6.
25. Inoue S, Ohue T, Yamagishi J, et al. Mode of incomplete cross-resistance among pipemidic, piromidic, and nalidixic acids. Antimicrob Agents Chemother. 1978;14:240–5.

26. Yamagishi J, Yoshida H, Yamayoshi M, et al. Nalidixic acid–resistant mutations of the gyr B gene of *Escherichia coli*. Mol Gen Genet. 1986;204:367–73.
27. Norris S, Mandell GL. The quinolones: History and overview. In: Andriole VT, ed. The Quinolones. London: Academic Press; 1988:1–22.
28. Barlow AM. Nalidixic acid in infections of urinary tract. Br Med J. 1963;2:1308.
29. Buchbinder M, Webb JC, Anderson LV, et al. Laboratory studies and clinical pharmacology of nalidixic acid (WIN 18,320). Antimicrob Agents Chemother. 1962;308.
30. Ronald AR, Turck M, Petersdorf RG. A critical evaluation of nalidixic acid in urinary tract infections. N Engl J Med. 1966;275:1081.
31. Phillips I, King A, Shannon K. In vitro properties of the quinolones. In: Andriole VT, ed. The Quinolones. London: Academic Press; 1988:83–117.
32. Cox CE. Oxolinic acid therapy of recurrent urinary tract infections. Del Med J. 1970;42:327.
33. D'Alessio DJ, Olexy VM, Jackson GG. Oxolinic acid treatment of urinary tract infections. Antimicrob Agents Chemother. 1967;490.
34. Mardh PA, Colleen S, Andersson KE. Studies in cinoxacin. I. In vitro activity of cinoxacin as compared to nalidixic acid, against urinary tract pathogens. J Antimicrob Chemother. 1977;3:411.
35. Gordon RG, Stevens LI, Edmiston CE, et al. Comparative in vitro studies of cinoxacin, nalidixic acid, and oxolinic acid. Antimicrob Agents Chemother. 1976;10:918.
36. Jones RN, Fuchs PC. In vitro antimicrobial activity of cinoxacin against 2,968 clinical bacterial isolates. Antimicrob Agents Chemother. 1976;10:146.
37. Goss WA, Deitz WH, Cook TM. Mechanism of action of nalidixic acid on *Escherichia coli*. II. Inhibition of deoxyribonucleic acid synthesis. J Bacteriol. 1965;89:1068.
38. Ott JL, Gordee RS. Inhibition of R-factor transfer by cinoxacin. Current chemotherapy. In: Proceedings of the 10th International Congress on Chemother. Washington, DC: American Society for Microbiology; 1978:688.
39. King A, Warren C, Shannon K, et al. In vitro antibacterial activity of norfloxacin (MK 0366). Antimicrob Agents Chemother. 1982;21:604.
40. Neu HC, Labthavikul P. In vitro activity of norfloxacin, a quinolone-carboxylic acid, compared with that of beta-lactams, aminoglycosides, and trimethoprim. Antimicrob Agents Chemother. 1982;22:23.
41. Norrby SR, Jonsson M. Antibacterial activity of Norfloxacin. Antimicrob Agents Chemother. 1983;23:15.
42. Corrado ML, Cherubin CE, Shulman M. The comparative activity of norfloxacin with other antimicrobial agents against gram-positive and gram-negative bacteria. J Antimicrob Chemother. 1983;11:369.
43. Gadebusch HH, Shungu DL, Weinberg E, et al. Comparison of the antibacterial activity of norfloxacin (MK 0366, AM 715), a new organic acid, with that of other orally absorbed chemotherapeutic agents. Infection. 1982;10:41.
44. Bauernfeind A, Petermuller C. In vitro activity of ciprofloxacin, norfloxacin and nalidixic acid. Eur J Clin Microbiol. 1983;2:111.
45. Muytjens HL, van der Ros–van de Repe J, van Veldhuizen G. Comparative activities of ciprofloxacin (Bay 09867), norfloxacin, pipemidic acid, and nalidixic acid. Antimicrob Agents Chemother. 1983;24:302.
46. Fass RJ. In vitro activity of ciprofloxacin (Bay 09867). Antimicrob Agents Chemother. 1983;24:568.
47. Heessen FWA, Muytjens HL. In vitro activities of ciprofloxacin, norfloxacin, pipemidic acid, cinoxacin, and nalidixic acid against *Chylamydia trachomatis*. Antimicrob Agents Chemother. 1984;25:123.
48. Wolfson JS, Hooper DC. The fluoroquinolones: Structure, mechanisms of action and resistance, and spectra of activity in vitro. Antimicrob Agents Chemother. 1985;28:581–6.
49. Olsson-Lilejequist B, Gezelius L, Svensson SB. Selection of multiple antibiotic resistance by norfloxacin and nalidixic acid in *Klebsiella* and *Enterobacter* (Abstract 106). In: Proceedings of the 25th Interscience Conference on Antimicrobial Agents and Chemotherapy, Minneapolis. Washington, DC: American Society for Microbiology; 1985.
50. Hirai K, Aoyama H, Suzue S, et al. Isolation and characterization of norfloxacin-resistant mutants *Escherichia coli* K-12. Antimicrob Agents Chemother. 1986;30:248–53.
51. Hiraei K, Suzue S, Irikura T, et al. Mutations producing resistance to norfloxacin in *Pseudomonas aeruginosa*. Antimicrob Agents Chemother. 1987;31:582–6.
52. Sanders CC, Sanders WE, Goering RV, et al. Selection of multiple antibiotic resistance by quinolones, beta-lactams, and aminoglycosides with special reference to cross-resistance between unrelated drug classes. Antimicrob Agents Chemother. 1984;26:797–801.
53. Hirai K, Irikura T, Iyobe S, et al. Inhibition of conjugal transfer of R-plasmids by norfloxacin in *Pseudomonas aeruginosa*. Chemotherapy. 1984;32:471–6.
54. Crumplin GC. Plasmid-mediated resistance to nalidixic acid and new 4-quinolones? Lancet. 1987;2:854–5.
55. Munshi MH, Sack DA, Haider K, et al. Plasmid-mediated resistance to nalidixic acid in *Shigella dysenteriae* type I. Lancet. 1987;2:419–21.
56. McChesney EW, Froelich EJ, Lesher GY, et al. Absorption, excretion and metabolism of a new antibacterial agent, nalidixic acid. Toxicol Appl Pharmacol. 1964;6:292.
57. Portmann GA, McChesney EW, Stander H, et al. Pharmacokinetic model for nalidixic acid in man. II. Parameters for absorption, metabolism and elimination. J Pharm Sci. 1966;55:72.
58. Stamey TA, Nemoy NJ, Higgins M. The clinical use of nalidixic acid. A review of some observations. Invest Urol. 1969;6:582.
59. Stamey TA, Meares EM, Winningham DG. Chronic bacterial prostatitis and the diffusion of drugs into prostatic fluid. J Urol. 1970;103:187.
60. Belton EM, Jones RV. Haemolytic anaemia due to nalidixic acid. Lancet. 1965;2:691.
61. Adam WR, Dawborn JK. Plasma levels and urinary excretion of nalidixic acid in patients with renal failure. Aust NZ J Med. 1971;1:126.
62. Atlas E, Clark H, Silverblatt F, et al. Nalidixic acid and oxolinic acid in the treatment of chronic bacteriuria. Ann Intern Med. 1969;70:713.
63. Burt RAP, Morgan T, Payne JP, et al. Cinoxacin concentrations in plasma, urine, and prostatic tissue after oral administration to man. Br J Urol. 1977;49:147.
64. Black HR, Israel KS, Wolen RL, et al. Pharmacology of cinoxacin in humans. Antimicrob Agents Chemother. 1979;15:165.
65. Scavone JM, Gleckman RA, Fraser DG. Cinoxacin: Mechanism of action, spectrum of activity, pharmacokinetics, adverse reactions, and therapeutic indications. Pharmacotherapy. 1982;2:266.
66. Swanson BN, Boppana VK, Vlasses PH, et al. Norfloxacin disposition after sequentially increasing oral doses. Antimicrob Agents Chemother. 1983; 23:284.
67. Bergan T. Pharmacokinetics of fluorinated quinolones. In: Andriole VT, ed. The Quinolones. London: Academic Press; 1988:119–54.
68. Sörgel F, Jaehde U, Naber K, et al. Pharmacokinetic disposition of quinolones in human body fluids and tissues. Clin Pharmacokinet. In press.
69. Crump B, Wise R, Dent J. Pharmacokinetics and tissue penetration of ciprofloxacin. Antimicrob Agents Chemother. 1983;24:784.
70. Lode H, Hoffken G, Olschewski P, et al. Pharmacokinetics of ofloxacin after parenteral and oral administration. Antimicrob Agents Chemother. 1987;31:1338–42.
71. White LO. Metabolism of 4-quinolones. Quinolones Bull. 1987;3:1–4.
71a. Bergan T, Thorsteinsson SB, Solberg R, et al. Pharmacokinetics of ciprofloxacin: intravenous and increasing oral doses. Am J Med. 1987;82(Suppl 4A):97–102.
71b. Drusano GL. An overview of the pharmacology of intravenously administered ciprofloxacin. Am J Med. 1987;82(Suppl 4A):339–345.
72. Zelickson AS. Phototoxic reaction with nalidixic acid. JAMA. 1964; 190:556.
73. Burry JN, Crosby RWL. A case of phototoxicity to nalidixic acid. Med J Aust. 1966;2:698.
74. Mathew TH. Nalidixic acid. Med J Aust. 1966;2:243.
75. Cahal DA. Reactions to nalidixic acid. Br Med J. 1965;2:590.
76. Finegold SM, Miller LG, Posnick D, et al. Nalidixic acid: Clinical and laboratory studies. Antimicrob Agents Chemother. 1966;189.
77. Kremer L, Walton M, Wardle EN. Nalidixic acid and intracranial hypertension. Br Med J. 1967;4:488.
78. Boreus LO, Sundstrom B. Intracranial hypertension in a child during treatment with nalidixic acid. Br Med J. 1967;2:744.
79. Fisher OD. Nalidixic acid and intracranial hypertension. Br Med J. 1967;3:370.
80. Cohen DN. Intracranial hypertension and papilledema associated with nalidixic acid therapy. Am J Ophthalmol. 1973;76:680.
81. Rao KG. Pseudotumor cerebri associated with nalidixic acid. Urology. 1974;4:204.
82. Islam MA, Sreedharan T. Convulsions, hyperglycaemia, and glycosuria from overdose of nalidixic acid. JAMA. 1965;192:1100.
83. Mandal BK, Stevenson J. Haemolytic crisis produced by nalidixic acid. Lancet. 1970;1:614.
84. Today's drugs. Nalidixic acid. Br Med J. 1967;1:741.
85. Stahlmann R, Lode H. Safety overview: Toxicity, adverse effects and drug interactions. In: Andriole VT, ed. The Quinolones. London: Academic Press; 1988:201–33.
86. Adam D, Andrassy K, Christ W, et al. [Arbeitsgemeinschaft "Arzneimittelsicherheit" der Paul-Ehrlich-Gesellschaft fur Chemotherapie]. Vertraglichkeit der Gyrase-Hemmer. Munch Med Wochenschr. 1987;129:45–46.
87. Hori S, Shimada J, Saito A, et al. Effect of new quinolones on gamma-aminobutyric acid receptor binding (Abstract 396). In: Proceedings of the 25th Interscience Conference on Antimicrobial Agents and Chemotherapy, Minneapolis. Washington, DC: American Society for Microbiology; 1985.
88. Hori S, Shimada J, Saito A, et al. Inhibitory effect of quinolones on gamma-aminobutyric acid receptor binding. Structure activity relationship (Abstract 438). In: Proceedings of the 26th Interscience Conference on Antimicrobial Agents and Chemotherapy, New Orleans. Washington, DC: American Society for Microbiology; 1986.
89. Westwood GPC, Hooper WL. Antagonism of oxolinic acid by nitrofurantoin. Lancet. 1975;1:460.
90. Wijnands WJA, van Herwaarden CLA, Vree TB. Enoxacin raises plasma theophylline concentrations (Letter). Lancet. 1984;2:108–9.
91. Wijnands WJA, Vree TB, van Herwaarden CLA. The influence of quinolone derivatives on theophylline clearance. Br J Clin Pharmacol. 1986;22:677–83.
92. Gregoire SL, Grasela ThH Jr, Freer JP, et al. Inhibition of theophylline effects. Antimicrob Agents Chemother. 1987;31:375–378.
93. Staib AH, Harder S, Mieke S, et al. Gyrase-inhibitors impair caffeine elimination in man. Methods Find Exp Clin Pharmacol. 1987;9:193–8.
94. Stille W, Harder S, Mieke S, et al. Decrease of caffeine elimination in man

during co-administration of 4 quinolones. J Antimicrob Chemother. 1987;20:729–734.
95. Kneebone GM. A clinical appraisal of nalidixic acid in urinary tract infections in childhood. Med J Aust. 1965;2:947.
96. Landes RR. Long term dose cinoxacin therapy for the prevention of recurrent urinary tract infections. J Urol. 1980;123:47.
97. Schaeffer AJ, Jones JM, Flynn SS. Prophylactic efficacy of cinoxacin in recurrent urinary tract infection: Biologic effects on the vaginal and fecal flora. J Urol. 1982;127:1118.
98. Malinverni R, Glauser MP. Comparative studies of fluoroquinolones in the treatment of urinary tract infections. Rev Infect Dis. 1988;10(Suppl):153–63.
99. Bologna M, Vaggi L, Flammini D, et al. Norfloxacin in prostatitis: Correlation between HPLC tissue concentrations and clinical results. Drugs Exp Clin Res. 1985;11:95–100.
100. Suzuki K, Tamai H, Naide Y, et al. Laboratory and clinical study of ofloxacin in the treatment of bacterial prostatitis. Hinyokika Kijo. 1984;30:1505–18.
101. Weidner W, Schiefer HG, Dalhoff A. Treatment of chronic bacterial prostatitis with ciprofloxacin. Am J Med. 1987;82(Suppl):280–3.
102. Remy G, Rouger C, Chavanet P, et al. Use of ofloxacin for prostatitis. Rev Infect Dis. 1988;10(Suppl):173–4.
103. Thys JP. Quinolones in the treatment of bronchopulmonary infections. Rev Infect Dis. 1988;10(Suppl):212–7.
104. Bosso JA, Black PG, Matsen JM. Ciprofloxacin versus tobramycin plus azlocillin in pulmonary exacerbations in adult patients with cystic fibrosis. Am J Med. 1987;82(Suppl):180–4.
105. Scully BE, Nakatomi M, Ores C, et al. Ciprofloxacin therapy in cystic fibrosis. Am J Med. 1987;(Suppl):196–201.
106. DuPont HL, Ericsson CD, Robinson A, et al. Current problems in antimicrobial therapy for bacterial enteric infection. Am J Med. 1987;82:324–8.
107. Pichler HET, Diridl G, Stockler K, et al. Clinical efficacy of ciprofloxacin compared with placebo in bacterial diarrhea. Am J Med. 1987;82:329–32.
108. DuPont HL, Corrado ML, Sabbaj J. Use of norfloxacin in the treatment of acute diarrheal disease. Am J Med. 1987;82(Suppl):79–83.
109. Ericsson CD, Johnson PC, DuPont HL, et al. Ciprofloxacin or trimethoprim-sulfamethoxazole as initial therapy for traveler's diarrhea. Ann Intern Med. 1987;106:216–20.
110. Glupczynski Y, Labbe M, Burette A, et al. Treatment failure of ofloxacin in *Campylobacter pylori* infection. Lancet. 1987;2:1096.
111. Fass RJ. Treatment of skin and soft tissue infections with oral ciprofloxacin. J Antimicrob Chemother. 1986;18(Suppl):153–7.
112. Eron LJ. Therapy of skin and skin structure infections with ciprofloxacin. Am J Med. 1987;82(Suppl):244–6.
113. Valainis GT, Pankey GA,, Katner HP, et al. Ciprofloxacin in the treatment of bacterial skin infections. Am J Med. 1987;82(Suppl):230–2.
114. Self PL, Zeluff BA, Sollo D, et al. Use of ciprofloxacin in the treatment of serious skin and skin structure infections. Am J Med. 1987;82(Suppl):239–41.
115. Mulligan ME, Ruane RJ, Johnston L, et al. Ciprofloxacin for eradication of methicillin-resistant *Staphylococcus aureus* colonization. Am J Med. 1987;82(Suppl):215–9.
116. Andriole VT. Treatment of osteomyelitis with quinolones. Quinolones Bull. 1987;3:15–7.
117. Schachter J, Moncada J. In vitro activity of ciprofloxacin against *Chlamydia trachomatis*. Am J Med. 1987;82 (Suppl):42–3.
118. Hartinger A, Hartmut B, Korting HC. In vitro activity of ciprofloxacin and ofloxacin against clinical isolates of *Chylamdia trachomatis*. Rev Infect Dis. 1988;10(Suppl):151–2.
119. Krausse R, Ullmann U. In-vitro-Aktivitat von Enoxazin Ciprofloxacin und Tetracyclin gegenuber *Mycoplasma hominis* und *Ureaplasma urealyticum*. Z Antimikrob Antineoplast Chemother. 1984;2:83–8.
120. Fong IW. Treatment of chlamydial urethritis with ofloxacin or ciprofloxacin. Quinolones Bull. 1986;2:10–1.
121. Naamara W, Plummer FA, Greenblatt RM, et al. Treatment of chancroid with ciprofloxacin. Am J Med. 1987;82(Suppl):317–20.
122. Carmona O, Hernandez-Gonzalez, Kobelt R. Ciprofloxacin in the treatment of nonspecific vaginitis. Am J Med. 1987;82(Suppl):321–3.
123. Neu HC. The quinolones: Prospects. In: Andriole VT, ed. The Quinolones. London: Academic Press; 1988:235–54.
124. Winston DJ, Ho WG, Champlin RE, et al. Norfloxacin for prevention of bacterial infections in granulocytopenic patients. Am J Med. 1987; 82(Suppl):40–6.
125. Winston DJ, Ho WG, Nakao SL, et al. Norfloxacin versus vancomycin/polymyxin for prevention of infections in granulocytopenic patients. Am J Med. 1986;80:884–90.
126. Karp JE, Merz WG, Hendricksen C, et al. Oral norfloxacin for prevention of gram-negative bacterial infections in patients with acute leukemia and granulocytopenia. Ann Intern Med. 1987;106:1–6.
127. Dekker AW, Rozenberg-Arska M, Verhoef J. Infection prophylaxis in acute leukemia: A comparison of ciprofloxacin with trimethoprim-sulfamethoxazole and colistin. Ann Intern Med. 1987;106:7–12.
128. Webster A, Gaya H. Quinolones in the treatment of serious infections. Rev Infect Dis. 1988;10(Suppl):225–33.
129. Norrby SR. 4-Quinolones in the treatment of infections of the central nervous system. Rev Infect Dis. 1988;10(Suppl):253–5.
130. Wolff M, Regnier B, Daldoss C, et al. Penetration of pefloxacin into cerebrospinal fluid of patients with meningitis. Antimicrob Agents Chemother. 1984;26:289–91.
131. Renkonen OV, Sivonen A, Visakorpi R. Effect of ciprofloxacin on carrier rate of *Neisseria meningitidis* in army recruits in Finland. Antimicrob Agents Chemother. 1987;31:962–3.
132. Pugsley MP, Dworzack DL, Horowitz EA, et al. Efficacy of ciprofloxacin on the treatment of nasopharyngeal carriers of *Neisseria meningitidis*. J Infect Dis. 1987;156:211–3.

31. URINARY TRACT AGENTS: NITROFURANTOIN AND METHENAMINE

VINCENT T. ANDRIOLE

Several antibacterial drugs are concentrated primarily in the urinary tract, that is, in the renal tubules with back diffusion into the renal parenchyma, and/or in the urine of the renal pelves and bladder. Since effective plasma concentrations are not obtained with safe doses of these agents, they cannot be used to treat patients with systemic infections and should only be used to treat patients with infections of the urinary tract. For this reason these drugs (nitrofurantoin and methenamine) are known as urinary tract antiseptics.

NITROFURANTOIN

Nitrofurantoin, *O*-(5-nitrofurfurylideneamino)-hydantoin, is one of a series of synthetic nitrofuran compounds that belong to a class of organic substances characterized by a heterocyclic ring consisting of four carbon atoms and one oxygen atom. (Fig. 1). This compound has been available for clinical use in a microcrystalline form since 1953 and is marketed as Furadantin (Eaton). Since nitrofurantoin is of limited solubility in water, a macrocrystalline form of the drug was prepared in 1967 and is marketed as Macrodantin (Eaton).

Mechanism of Action

The precise mechanism of action of nitrofurantoin is not known, although there is evidence that the drug inhibits a variety of enzyme systems in bacteria.[1] Nitrofurans can also enter mammalian cells and have been shown to affect several enzymes in these cells, the most notable of which is to arrest spermatogenesis in animals.[2] Also, at high local concentrations nitrofurantoin immobilizes human sperm.[3]

Antimicrobial Activity

Nitrofurantoin is active against a wide spectrum of gram-positive and gram-negative bacteria and particularly against many strains of the common urinary tract pathogens (Table 1).

Bacterial species with a minimum inhibitory concentration (MIC) of 32 μg/ml or less of nitrofurantoin are considered sensitive since this concentration of the drug can easily be achieved

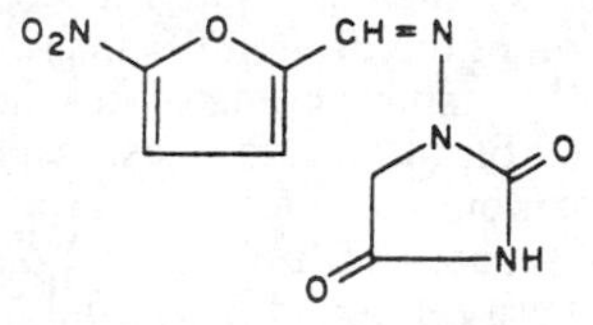

FIG. 1. Structure of nitrofurantoin.

TABLE 1. Nitrofurantoin Antibacterial Spectrum In Vitro

Gram-positive organisms	Gram-negative organisms
Bacillus subtilis	*Enterobacter aerogenes*
Corynebacterium sp. (diphtheroids)	*Alcaligenes faecalis*
Staphylococcus aureus	*Escherichia coli*
Enterococcus faecalis	*Klebsiella pneumoniae*
	Proteus mirabilis
	Proteus morganii
	Proteus rettgeri
	Proteus vulgaris
	Pseudomonas aeruginosa

in the urine with usual therapeutic doses. *Escherichia coli* is very sensitive (96 percent) to nitrofurantoin at this concentration, as are other coliform bacteria (68 percent), whereas *Enterobacter* and *Klebsiella* spp. are less susceptible (36 percent).[4] Most *Proteus* sp. (92 percent) are moderately resistant, and *P. aeruginosa* is almost always resistant.[4] The usual MIC of nitrofurantoin for *E. coli* is 16 μg/ml, whereas *Enterobacter* and *Klebsiella* spp. may require 100 μg/ml and *P. mirabilis*, 200 μg/ml.[4] The drug is also active against staphylococci and enterococci, and the MICs are lower, 4.0 μg/ml for *S. aureus* and 25.0 μg/ml for *Enterococcus faecalis*.[1] Salmonellae, shigellae, and *Neisseria* sp. are also susceptible to nitrofurantoin, as are *S. pyogenes*, *S. pneumoniae*, and *Corynebacterium* spp. including *C. diphtheriae*, but their susceptibility to the drug is of little practical importance.[1] In contrast to nalidixic and oxolonic acid, microorganisms sensitive to nitrofurantoin do not readily become resistant to this drug.

Pharmacology

Nitrofurantoin is usually administered orally and is rapidly and completely absorbed from the gastrointestinal tract. The drug crosses the blood-brain and the placental barrier. Only very low levels of antibacterial activity are attained in serum after usual oral doses of the drug, and nitrofurantoin does not accumulate in the serum of patients with normal renal function when given continuously in recommended doses. Also, therapeutically active concentrations of the drug are not attained in most body tissues. The serum half-life is about 20 minutes in patients with normal renal function because about two-thirds of the drug is rapidly metabolized in tissues, with inactivation apparently occurring in all body tissues, although the liver may play a major role.[5] One-third of the drug is rapidly excreted into the urine by both glomerular filtration and tubular secretion, with significant reabsorption when the urine is acid.[5] Nitrofurantoin acts as a weak acid, so in an aciid urine more of the drug is in the undissociated form, and more of the drug is reabsorbed, with less appearing in the urine. In an alkaline urine, more of the drug is in the dissociated or ionized form, little of the drug is reabsorbed, and more appears in the urine,[6] but the antibacterial efficacy is decreased.[7] Therefore, the urine should not be alkalinized. Nitrofurantoin has been shown to diffuse into the interstitial tissue of the renal medulla[8] and to be present in higher concentrations in the lymphatics draining the medulla than in serum.[9] Since one-third of an orally administered dose of the drug is excreted unchanged (i.e., in a therapeutically active form) into the urine,[5] an average dose of nitrofurantoin yields a urine concentration of approximately 200 (range, 50–250) μg/ml in patients with normal renal function. (Nitrofurantoin may color the urine brown.) However, recovery of the drug from the urine is linearly related to creatinine clearance, so the concentration of the drug in the urine of uremic patients may be insufficient to inhibit common urinary tract pathogens when the glomerular filtration rate is less than 30 ml/min.[10] Furthermore, nitrofurantoin accumulates in the serum of patients with creatinine clearances of less than 60 ml/min,[10] and blood levels may range between 5 and 6.5 μg/ml in severe uremia,[11] which increases the danger of systemic toxicity developing, particularly peripheral neuropathy.[12] Although nitrofurantoin is removed by hemodialysis, it is contraindicated in patients with significant renal impairment as well as in newborn and premature infants, who may also develop toxic blood levels.

The macrocrystalline form of nitrofurantoin (Macrodantin) was introduced to delay absorption from the gastrointestinal tract. Since nitrofurantoin is of limited solubility in water, an increase in size of the drug particles might significantly retard it solution rate in and consequently its absorption from the alimentary tract. Delaying the drug's entrance into body fluids was hoped to lower its peak serum concentration and decrease the incidence and severity of nausea and vomiting without significantly affecting its concentration in the urinary tract.[13] Studies on humans have shown that, although the urinary excretion of the macrocrystals is prolonged, there is no difference between macrocrystals and fine particles in the percentage of dose recovered from the urine. The macrocrystalline form results in maximum urinary concentrations of about 150 μg/ml after a dose of 100 mg and is probably associated with a lower incidence of side effects and better patient tolerance than the microcrystalline form is.[14] The mechanism of action, antimicrobic activity, and pharmacology of the macrocrystalline form is otherwise similar to conventional microcrystalline nitrofurantoin.

Toxicity and Adverse Reactions

Gastrointestinal irritation is the most common side effect of nitrofurantoin therapy, particularly anorexia, nausea, and vomiting, which may be controlled by a reduction in dosage or by the concomitant administration of food or milk, although sometimes it is severe enough to require discontinuation of treatment with the drug. Diarrhea and abdominal pain occur less frequently. Gastrointestinal intolerance appears to occur less frequently in patients receiving nitrofurantoin macrocrystals than in those receiving microcrystalline tablets.[14] The crystalline and macrocrystalline forms are therapeutically equivalent.

Hypersensitivity reactions occur occasionally and may involve the skin, lungs, blood, and liver. Also chills, drug fever, arthralgia, a lupus erythematosis syndrome, and anaphylaxis have been observed.

Dermatologic allergic manifestations include maculopapular, erythematous, or eczematous rashes, urticaria, angioneurotic edema, and pruritus and usually subside when treatment of the drug is stopped.[1] Pulmonary reactions include asthmatic attacks in patients with a history of asthma as well as acute, subacute, or chronic reactions. Acute pneumonitis is commonly manifested by the sudden onset of fever, chills, cough, dyspnea, chest pain, pulmonary infiltration with consolidation or pleural effusion seen on x-ray films, and eosinophilia.[15] This syndrome is more common in elderly patients, and the symptoms usually occur within the first week of treatment but may become evident within hours or days or in some cases after a prolonged period after starting nitrofurantoin therapy. This pneumonitis is probably immunologically mediated and is rapidly reversible with cessation of therapy. Corticosteroid treatment may be beneficial and necessary in severe cases.[16] The syndrome rapidly recurs after rechallenge with the drug,[17] and there is some evidence that cell-mediated immunity is implicated in this type of nitrofurantoin sensitivity.[18] In *subacute* pneumonitis the symptoms are more insidious, fever and eosinophilia are observed less often, and recovery may be slower. *Chronic* pulmonary reactions are rare and usually occur in patients receiving continuous therapy for 6 months or more. An insidious onset of malaise, dyspnea on exertion, cough, altered pulmonary function, and roentgenographic and histologic findings of interstitial fibrosis with or without interstitial pneumonitis are common.[19,20] Fever is rarely prominent. This syndrome may also have an immunologic basis. In some cases improvement occurs with cessation of nitrofurantoin and institution of steroid therapy. However, the severity of this reaction and the degree of resolution appear to be related to the amount of time therapy is continued after the onset of clinical signs and symptoms. Permanently impaired pulmonary function may occur even after treatment with the drug is discontinued, especially when the syndrome is not recognized early.

Hematologic reactions include leukopenia, granulocytopenia, eosinophilia, megaloblastic anemia, and hemolytic anemia. Megaloblastic anemia is rare and appears to be due to folic acid deficiency, particularly when repeated courses of the drug are used.[21] Nitrofurantoin can precipitate an acute hemolytic anemia in patients with glucose-6-phosphate dehydrogenase–deficient red blood cells, which is found in 10 percent of blacks and a small percentage of Mediterranean and Near-Eastern ethnic groups. Also the drug should not be given to infants with immature red cell enzyme systems.

Hepatotoxic reactions are very rare and include cholestatic jaundice with prodromal fever, rash, and eosinophilia[22] and hepatocellular damage.[23]

Neurologic reactions include headache, drowsiness, dizziness, nystagmus, which is readily reversible, and peripheral polyneuropathy. This peripheral neuritis is an ascending sensorimotor neuropathy, which may be progressive if treatment with the drug is continued and is one of the most serious side effects of nitrofurantoin therapy.[24] Although it occurs more commonly in patients with renal failure,[12] it also occurs in patients with normal blood urea nitrogen levels and low creatinine clearances[25] as well as in patients, especially the elderly, with normal renal function who receive prolonged courses of nitrofurantoin. The mechanism is unknown,[26] but demyelination and degeneration of both sensory and motor nerves occur. Treatment with the drug should be stopped at the earliest signs of neuritis such as paresthesias.

Transient alopecia may occur. Also, a 17-month-old infant who received nitrofurantoin for 68 days developed permanent yellow discoloration of those teeth that erupted during therapy.[21]

Drug Interactions

Nitrofurantoin antagonizes the action of nalidixic and oxolinic acids.[28]

METHENAMINE

Methenamine (hexamethylenetetramine, hexamethyleneamine, hexamine) is a tertiary amine and has the properties of a monoacidic base in its salt formation and can be combined with an unlimited number of organic and inorganic compounds. It is a colorless, odorless compound that is readily soluble in water and forms weakly basic solutions of pH 8.0–8.5. Its chemical structure is shown in Figure 2.

Methenamine was introduced by Nicolaier in 1895 for the treatment of urinary infections[29] and is available, as the pure base, in 0.5 g tablets as methenamine, *National Formulary* (NF) (Lilly). Methenamine has also been combined with mandelic acid, apparently because of Rosenheim's observations in 1935[30] that mandelic acid is excreted in the urine unchanged and, when given in large doses, renders the urine bactericidal. The combination of methenamine and mandelic acid is marketed as methenamine mandelate under the trade name Mandelamine (Warner-Chilcott). Methenamine has also been combined with hippuric acid to form the salt methenamine hippurate, and this combination is marketed as Hiprex (Merrell-National) and Urex (Riker).

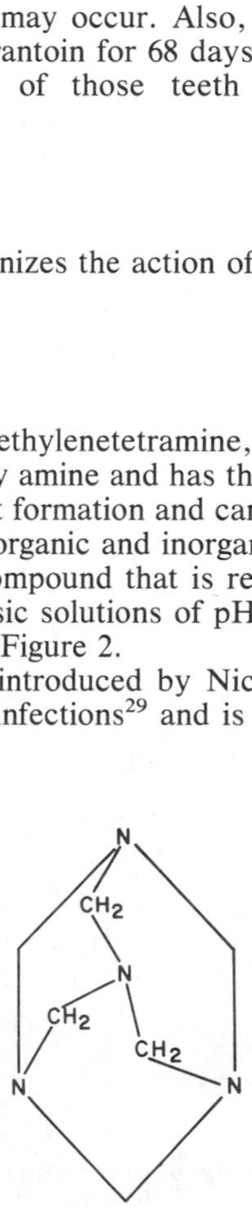

FIG. 2. Structure of methenamine.

Mechanism of Action

Methenamine itself is not bactericidal, nor, regardless of concentration, is it antibacterial in alkaline solutions. Its mechanism of action is due to its hydrolysis, at an acid pH, to ammonia and formaldehyde according to the following reaction:

$$N_4(CH_2)_6 + 6H_2O + 4H^+ \rightleftarrows 4NH_4^+ + 6HCHO$$

Formaldehyde is the active degradation product of methenamine[29] and can only be liberated from methenamine at a pH below 7.0,[31] for example, 6% is yielded at pH 6 and 20% at pH 5. Only two body fluids, gastric juice and urine, are capable of releasing formaldehyde from methenamine.[31–34] Although methenamine has no antimicrobial activity in the presence of alkaline fluids, formaldehyde is equally bactericidal at acid and alkaline pHs.[33] Nevertheless, the degradation of methenamine to formaldehyde is entirely dependent on two factors: proper acidification of the urine and time for hydrolysis of methenamine to occur. Furthermore, the ultimate antibacterial effect of methenamine, that is, through the generation of formaldehyde, is also dependent on the concentration of methenamine in the urine as well as on the urine pH and the time the drug remains in the urine.[35,36] Specifically, at an average urinary methenamine concentration of 0.75 mg/ml and in a quite acid urine (pH 5.0–5.5), at least 1 hour is needed to generate approximately 25 μg/ml of free formaldehyde, 2 hours more reliably produces bactericidal levels of free formaldehyde, and 3 hours is required to reach 90 percent of the final equilibrium.[36] Low concentrations of methenamine in the urine are inadequate to generate bactericidal levels of free formaldehyde regardless of urine pH and time.[36]

Since the proper function of methenamine is dependent on an acid urine, various poorly metabolized acids have been used to acidify the urine putatively during therapy with methenamine. The acids most commonly used are mandelic acid, hippuric acid, ascorbic acid, and acid-producing foods such as cranberry juice. Also, a low pH alone is bacteriostatic, so acidification could possibly serve a double function. Furthermore, mandelic acid and hippuric acid are bacteriostatic in vitro aside from their effect on pH. These organic acids inhibit the metabolism of bacteria by means of their un-ionized molecules.[37] For these reasons, these acids are widely thought to contribute to the lowering of urinary pH as well as to producing an antibacterial effect in urine, which, if true, would be an advantage. However, it is important to emphasize that to achieve this effect, that is, bacteriostasis, in urine it is necessary to administer these acids (mandelic, hippuric, ascorbic, and cranberry juice) in prohibitively large doses, otherwise the urine is not rendered inhibitory. Equally important is that the prepared combinations of the methenamine salts of organic acids, methenamine mandelate and hippurate, when given as currently recommended, contain only a fraction of the dosage of the organic acid (mandelic or hippuric) that is required to either exert an antibacterial effect in the urine or to influence the pH of the urine. Unfortunately, there is little evidence that the acid forms (mandelic or hippuric) of the methenamine salt contribute in any way to the antibacterial activity of methenamine.[38] Fortunately, in most circumstances normal urine, in the absence of diuresis, is sufficiently acid to liberate free formaldehyde from methenamine.[39]

Antimicrobial Activity

Methenamine, through the liberation of free formaldehyde into the urine, is active against all gram-positive and gram-negative bacteria and also against fungi. Almost all bacteria are susceptible to free formaldehyde at about the same concentration, that is, 20 μg/ml.[38] However, urinary tract infections due to urea-splitting organisms such as *Proteus* sp. may not respond to methenamine because it is difficult to acidify the urine in the presence of these infections and free formaldehyde is not liberated. Significant resistance cannot be induced in vitro[40] and is not a problem with methenamine because bacteria and fungi do not become resistant to formaldehyde.

Pharmacology

Methenamine, methenamine mandelate, and hippurate are rapidly absorbed from the gastrointestinal tract, but 10–30 percent is hydrolyzed by the gastric juice in the stomach unless the drug is protected by enteric coating. Because of the ammonia produced, methenamine is contraindicated in patients with hepatic insufficiency. Antimicrobial activity is not achieved in the blood since methenamine does not liberate formaldehyde in serum and mandelic or hippuric acid serum levels are too low to produce any antibacterial effect. Methenamine diffuses widely into body fluids since it is distributed through total body water including that of red blood cells; cerebrospinal, synovial, and pericardial fluids; and both aqueous and vitreous humors of the eye.[31] Only methenamine, not formaldehyde, is present in these body fluids since almost no formaldehyde is generated at physiologic pH, so there is no antibacterial activity in tissues, body fluids, or blood. Methenamine is rapidly excreted into urine. Its clearance from the blood is considerably less than its glomerular filtration rate,[41] and its half-life in blood is quite long. Also, in the presence of an optimally acid urine, only 2–20 percent of the methenamine present is converted to free formaldehyde. Over 90 percent of an administered dose will be excreted into the urine within 24 hours. Although some antibacterial activity may be demonstrated within half an hour, adequate antibacterial activity through the generation of sufficient formaldehyde does not occur, even in a properly acid urine (pH 5.0–5.5), until at least 1 hour and more likely 2 hours after the administration of methenamine. This antibacterial activity is not found in urine from the renal pelvis or ureter but only in bladder urine because the transit time down the renal tubules, calyces, and pelvis into the bladder is too short to allow the generation of significant amounts of formaldehyde.[32,38,42] Exceptions may occur in extremely dehydrated patients with highly acid urine or in those with some degree of obstructive renal residual urine. The antibacterial activity in bladder urine may be maintained for at least 6 hours or until the patient voids, after which hydrolysis of new methenamine will have to occur to render newly formed urine bactericidal.[38] It is probably best not to force fluids on a patient receiving methenamine because a diuretic urine may be more alkaline and diuresis may reduce the concentration of free formaldehyde to a noninhibitory (<20 μg/ml) level. Except for urine, so little methenamine decomposes in body fluids and tissues that it is virtually nontoxic systemically, and renal insufficiency is no contraindication to methenamine alone. Also, since the acidifying ability of the renal tubules functions in azotemia, these patients can convert methenamine to formaldehyde. However, the acid salts are contraindicated, and methenamine mandelate may precipitate crystalluria.

Toxicity

Methenamine is usually well tolerated, as are both the methenamine salts mandelate and hippurate, but some patients develop gastrointestinal side effects such as gastric distress, nausea, vomiting, and diarrhea. Some patients complain of bladder irritation, with dysuria, frequency, albuminuria, and hematuria, particularly with high doses or prolonged administration. Various rashes may also occur. The methenamine salts should be avoided in patients with gout because these drugs may precipitate urate crystals in the urine.

Drug Interactions

Methenamine combines with sulfamethizole and possibly other sulfonamides in the urine, which results in mutual antagonism.

MAJOR USES AND DOSAGE

In addition to the general uses and doses described in Table 2, these urinary tract agents have also been used as prophylactic and suppressive agents in patients with recurrent urinary tract infections as well as in catheterized patients with bacteriuria and in chronically infected patients with neurogenic bladders subjected to long-term indwelling catheter drainage. Nitrofurantoin has also been used for long-term suppressive therapy, particularly during pregnancy and in children with persistent or frequently recurrent bacteriuria, with reasonably good results.[43–45] Bacterial resistance was not a problem with nitrofurantoin. Methenamine has also been used successfully as prophylactic therapy in men with recurrent bacteriuria[46] as well as in patients with recurrent bacteriuria caused by multiply antibiotic-resistant gram-negative bacilli or by yeasts because these pathogens are susceptible to formaldehyde.[7,41,47,48] In addition, it has been successfully used as a prophylactic agent in otherwise healthy girls and women who have recurring urinary tract infection in the absence of structural abnormalities of the urinary tract,[47,49] although it does not appear to be as effective as trimethoprim sulfamethoxazole administered once daily in these patients.[49] In short, nitrofurantoin, methenamine, or trimethoprim-sulfamethoxazole appear to be the reasonable

TABLE 2. Urinary Tract Agents

Agent	*Dosage*	*Use*
Nitrofurantoin	Adults: 50 or 100 mg qid for 1–2 wk Children: 1.25–1.75 mg/kg qid for 1–2 wk	Acute and recurrent uncomplicated urinary tract infections due to susceptible organisms or long-term suppressive therapy for frequently recurrent bacteriuria (single dose of 50–100 mg in adults or 1 mg/kg bid in children). Do not use in patients with renal insufficiency, renal carbuncle, perinephric abscess, or in infants.
Methenamine	Adults: 0.5–2 g (usually 1 g) qid or bid Children: 15 mg/kg qid	Chronic suppressive treatment of urinary tract infections when urine pH is 5.5 or less. Not a primary drug for acute urinary tract infections.
Methenamine mandelate	Adults: 1 g qid Children: 15 mg/kg qid	Chronic suppressive treatment of urinary tract infections when urine pH is 5.5 or less. Not a primary drug for acute urinary tract infections.[a]
Methenamine hippurate	Adults: 1 g bid Children age 6–12 yr: 0.5–1 g bid	Chronic suppressive treatment of urinary tract infections when urine pH is 5.5 or less. Not a primary drug for acute urinary tract infections.[a]

[a] One gram of methenamine mandelate or hippuric acid contains only 480 mg of methenamine and 520 mg of mandelic or hippuric acid. These combinations contain an amount of acid that is unlikely to contribute significant antibacterial activity to the urine. Also, there is little evidence that these acid forms contribute to the antibacterial activity of methenamine.

agents for the prophylaxis of frequently recurrent urinary tract infections.

Methenamine has also been used regularly to treat patients with chronic bacteriuria in the presence of indwelling bladder catheters or patients who are receiving intermittent bladder catheterization as well as patients with neurogenic bladders with indwelling catheters. There is little evidence that methenamine, when given as methenamine mandelate or hippurate, prevents the acquisition of or eradicates bacteriuria in patients with suprapubic or indwelling Foley catheters.[50,51] This is understandable since the mechanism of action of methenamine requires the generation of formaldehyde, which takes a minimum of 1 hour to be made in sufficient antibacterial concentrations. It is unlikely that urine remains in the bladder long enough for this reaction to occur in patients with constant bladder drainage. On the other hand, methenamine could potentially be effective in patients with neurogenic bladders who are receiving intermittent catheterization since urine would remain in the bladder for sufficient periods of time. However, recent observations indicate that methenamine, when given as the mandelic acid salt methenamine mandelate, was ineffective as either a suppressive or prophylactic agent in patients undergoing intermittent catheterization.[51] It is important to emphasize that the methenamine used in all these studies was combined with mandelic or hippuric acid as methenamine mandelate or hippurate. The actual amount of methenamine in these combinations is less than half of the total dose administered, which may have provided inadequate urine concentrations of methenamine for the generation of sufficient formaldehyde.

In summary, the urinary tract agents discussed in this chapter seem to be effective in treating acute, uncomplicated symptomatic bacteriuria of the lower urinary tract. Nitrofurantoin is effective in treating upper tract infection and frequent bacteriuria as well as a long-term suppressive agent in children and pregnant women. Methenamine, used properly, is also effective in women with uncomplicated recurrent bacteriuria, including those that are multiply antibiotic resistant, and as a prophylactic agent in men with recurrent infection. There is little convincing evidence that methenamine combined with mandelic or hippuric acid has any advantage over the use of methenamine alone. In fact, there is a strong possibility that, when these salts are used in the doses currently recommended, insufficient methenamine is delivered to the urine to generate adequate concentrations of formaldehyde.

REFERENCES

1. Kucers A, Bennett NM. Nitrofurans. In: Kucers A, Bennett NM, eds. The Use of Antibiotics. Philadelphia: JB Lippincott; 1979:749.
2. Paul HE, Paul MF. The nitrofurans—chemotherapeutic properties. In: Schnitzer RJ, Hawking F, eds. Experimental Chemotherapy. New York; Academic Press; 1966:521.
3. Albert PS, Mininberg DJ, Davis JE. Nitrofurans: Sperm-immobilizing agents. Their tissue toxicity and clinical application. Urology. 1974;4:307.
4. Turck M, Ronald AR, Petersdorf RG. Susceptibility of Enterobacteriaceae to nitrofurantoin correlated with eradication of bacteriuria. Antimicrob Agents Chemother. 1966;446.
5. Reckendorf HK, Castringius RG, Spingler HK. Comparative pharmacodynamics, urinary excretion, and half-life determinations of nitrofurantoin sodium. Antimicrob Agents Chemother. 1962:531, 1963.
6. Andriole VT. Factors affecting antibiotic concentrations in urine and kidney tissue. In: Proceedings of the Fourth International Congress on Nephrology Stockholm. Basel: S. Karger; 1969:338.
7. Pratt WB. The urinary tract antiseptics. In: Pratt WB, ed. Chemotherapy of Infection. New York: Oxford University Press; 1977:215.
8. Currie GA, Little PJ, McDonald SJ. The localization of cephaloridine and nitrofurantoin in the kidney. Nephron. 1966;3:282.
9. Katz YJ, Cockett ATK, Moore RS. Renal lymph and antibacterial levels in the treatment of pyelonephritis. Life Sci. 1964;3:1249.
10. Sachs J, Greer T, Noell P, et al. Effect of renal function on urinary recovery of orally administered nitrofurantoin. N Engl J Med. 1968;278:1032.
11. Loughridge L. Peripheral neuropathy due to nitrofurantoin. Lancet. 1962; 2:1133.
12. Felts JH, Hayes DM, Gergen JA, et al. Neural, hematologic and bacteriologic effects of nitrofurantoin in renal insufficiency. Am J Med. 1971;51:331.
13. Hailey FJ, Glascock HW. Gastrointestinal tolerance to a new macrocrystalline form of nitrofurantoin: A collaborative study. Curr Ther Res. 1967;9:600.
14. Kalowski S, Radford N, Kincaid-Smith P. Crystalline and macrocrystalline nitrofurantoin in the treatment of urinary tract infection. N Engl J Med. 1974;290:385.
15. Dawson RB. Pulmonary reactions to nitrofurantoin. N Engl J Med. 1966; 274:522.
16. Morgan LK. Nitrofurantoin pulmonary hypersensitivity. Med J Aust. 1970; 2:136.
17. Murray MJ, Kronenberg R. Pulmonary reactions simulating cardiac pulmonary edema caused by nitrofurantoin. N Engl J Med. 1965;273:1185.
18. Pearsall HR, Ewalt J, Tsoi MS, et al. Nitrofurantoin lung sensitivity: Report of a case with prolonged nitrofurantoin lymphocyte sensitivity and interaction of methenamine-stimulated lymphocytes with alveolar cells. J Lab Clin Med. 1974;83:728.
19. Rosenow EC, DeRemee RA, Dines DE. Chronic nitrofurantoin pulmonary reaction: Report of five cases. N Engl J Med. 1968;279:1258.
20. Holmberg L, Boman G, Bottiger LE, et al. Adverse reactions to nitrofurantoin. Analysis of 921 reports. Am J Med. 1980;69:733.
21. Bass BH: Megaloblastic anaemia due to nitrofurantoin. Lancet. 963;1:530.
22. Ernaelsteen D, Williams R. Jaundice due to nitrofurantoin. Gastroenterology. 1961;41:590.
23. Bhagwat AG, Warren RE. Hepatic reaction to nitrofurantoin. Lancet. 1969; 2:1369.
24. Ellis FG. Acute polyneuritis aftter nitrofurantoin therapy. Lancet. 1962; 2:1136.
25. Craven RS. Furadantin neuropathy. Aust NZ J Med. 1971;1:246.
26. Toole JF, Parrish ML. Nitrofurantoin polyneuropathy. Neurology (NY). 1973;23:554.
27. Ball JS, Ferguson AW. Permanent discoloration of primary definition by nitrofurantoin. Br Med J. 1962;2:1103.
28. Westwood GPC, Hooper WL. Antagonism of oxolonic acid by nitrofurantoin. Lancet. 1975;1:460.
29. Nicolaier A. Ueber die therapeutische verwendung des Urotropin (Hexamethylente tramin). Dtsch Med Wochenschr. 1895;21:541.
30. Rosenheim ML. Mandelic acid in the treatment of urinary infections. Lancet. 1935;1:1032.
31. Hanzlik PJ, Collins AB. Hexamethylenamine: The liberation of formaldehyde and the antiseptic efficiency under different chemical and biological conditions. Arch Intern Med. 1913;12:578.
32. Levy LH, Strauss A. A clinical and bacteriological study of hexamethylenamin as a urinary antiseptic. Arch Intern Med. 1914;14:730.
33. Shohl AT, Deming CL. Hexamethylenamin: Its quantitative factors in therapy. J Urol 1920;4:419.
34. De Eds F. Fate of hexamethylenamin in the body and its bearing on systemic antisepsis. Arch Intern Med. 1924;34:511.
35. Heathcote RSA. Hexamine as an urinary antiseptic. 1. Its rate of hydrolysis at different hydrogen ion concentrations. II. Its antiseptic power against various bacteria in urine. Br J Urol. 1935;7:9.
36. Jackson J, Stamey TA. The Riker method for determining formaldehyde in the presence of methenamine. Invest Urol. 1971;9:124.
37. Draskoczy P, Weiner N. Effect of organic acids on oxidative metabolism of *Escherichia coli*. Fed Proc. 1960;19:140.
38. Stamey TA. General and specific principles of therapy. In: Stamey TA, ed. Urinary Infections. Baltimore: Williams & Wilkins; 1972:253.
39. Elliot JS, Sharpe RF, Lewis L. Urinary pH. J Urol. 1959;81:339.
40. Duca CJ, Scudi JV. Some antibacterial properties of Mandelamine (methenamine mandelate). Proc Soc Exp Biol Med. 1947;66:123.
41. Scudi JV, Reinhard JF. Absorption, distribution and renal excretion of mandelamine (methenamine mandelate). J. Lab Clin Med. 1948;33:1304.
42. Hinman F. An experimental study of the antiseptic value in the urine of the internal use of hexamethylenamin. JAMA. 1913;61:1601.
43. Marshall M, Johnson SH. Use of nitrofurantoin in chronic and recurrent urinary tract infections in children. JAMA 1959;169:919.
44. Normand ICS, Smellie JM. Prolonged maintenance chemotherapy in the management of urinary infection in childhood. Br Med J. 1965;1:1023.
45. Brumfitt W, Smith GW, Hamilton-Miller JMT, et al. A clinical comparison between macrodantin and trimethoprim for prophylaxis in women with recurrent urinary infection. J Antimicrob Agents Chemother. 1985;16:111–120
46. Freeman RB, Smith WM, Richardson JA, et al. Long-term therapy for chronic bacteriuria in men: U.S. Public Health Service cooperative study. Ann Intern Med. 1975;83:133.
47. Holland NH, West CD. Prevention of recurrent urinary tract infections in girls. Am J Dis Child. 1963;105:560.
48. Brumfitt W, Hamilton-Miller JMT, Gargon RA, et al. Long-term prophylaxis of urinary infections in woman: Comparative trial of trimethoprim, methenamine hippurate, and topical povidone-iodine. J Urol. 1983;130:1110–4.
49. Harding GK, Roland AR. A controlled study of antimicrobial prophylaxis of recurrent urinary infection in women. N Engl J Med. 1974;291:597.
50. Gerstein AR, Okun R, Gonick HC, et al. The prolonged use of methenamine hippurate in the treatment of chronic urinary tract infections. J. Urol. 1968;100:767.
51. Vainrub B, Musher DM. Lack of effect of methenamine in suppression of, or prophylaxis against, chronic urinary infection. Antimicrob Agents Chemother. 1977;12:625.

32. ANTIMYCOBACTERIAL AGENTS

ROBERT H. ALFORD

Drugs for mycobacterial infections will be categorized under three headings: those primarily for *Mycobacterium tuberculosis,* drugs for "atypical" mycobacterial infections, and agents principally for the treatment of leprosy. Traditionally, antimicrobials for tuberculosis have been classified further as "first-line drugs" having superior efficacy with acceptable toxicity and "second-line" drugs either having less efficacy, greater toxicity, or both.[1–4]

Antituberculous drugs vary according to bactericidal function and site of action in tuberculous lesions.[4] All of the first-line agents are bactericidal except for ethambutol. The bactericidal action of pyrazinamide (PZA) against actively metabolizing tubercle bacilli was overlooked initially because infections in PZA-treated animals relapsed due to metabolically inactive organisms ("persisters") that regrew.

In site of action, drugs may exert their effects against mycobacteria either within cavities, intracellularly, or intermittently replicating in closed caseous lesions: (*1*) four agents have activity against the large, actively dividing extracellular populations in cavities—isoniazid (INH), rifampin, streptomycin, and ethambutol. Pyrazinamide is inactive at the neutral or slightly alkaline pH encountered in such areas. (*2*)Against intracellular mycobacteria, isoniazid, rifampin, and pyrazinamide are active, whereas streptomycin, other aminoglycosides, and capreomycin lose their activity at acidic pH. (*3*) Slowly replicating organisms in caseous lesions are killed only by rifampin and, somewhat less readily, by INH. Thus, the combination of INH and rifampin is bactericidal for all three populations in tuberculous lesions. (*4*) A fourth population of dormant organisms may be particularly difficult to eradicate. These principles are especially important in designing "short-course" chemotherapy and for resistant or relapsing infections.[4,5]

FIRST-LINE ANTITUBERCULOSIS DRUGS

Isoniazid

Derivation and Structure. Isoniazid, isonicotinic acid hydrazide (INH), a synthetic agent, was demonstrated in 1952 to be effective in the treatment of human tuberculosis.[6] Its structure is indicated in Figure 1.

Mechanism of Action. Isoniazid, bactericidal against growing *Mycobacterium tuberculosis* in vitro, is static against "resting" organisms. It acts primarily by inhibition of the synthesis of mycolic acid,[3] an important component of mycobacterial cell walls. Against certain "atypical" mycobacteria, INH in higher concentration also affects energy-requiring metabolic pathways.[7]

Antimicrobial Activity. Against *M. tuberculosis,* 0.025–0.05 μg/ml of INH is inhibitory. Isoniazid can kill intracellular organisms provided they are replicating. Tubercle bacilli become resistant to INH administered alone. Initially susceptible isolates will become INH-resistant in 71 percent of cases treated for 3 months with INH alone.[6] Resistance results from selection under the antimicrobic pressure of less susceptible variants of *M. tuberculosis* that initially number 1 in 10^6 bacilli among untreated mycobacterial populations. Surviving bacilli exhibit decreased INH uptake. Large populations like the 10^9–10^{10} bacilli in open pulmonary cavities are especially likely to contain significant numbers of resistant mycobacteria that subsequently overgrow and lead to secondary resistance. Emergence of resistance depends on the type and duration of prior therapy.[8] Significant primary resistance to INH in untreated cases occurs in approximately 6 percent of isolates in the United States and should be anticipated, particularly in immigrants from regions having high levels of endemic drug resistance. Primary resistance has been documented in 43 percent of Korean isolates of *M. tuberculosis.*[9]

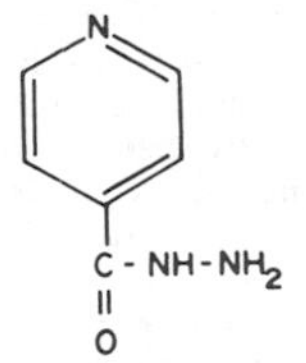

FIG. 1. Structure of isoniazid.

Pharmacology. Isoniazid, well absorbed orally or intramuscularly, is subsequently distributed throughout the body including the cerebrospinal fluid. CSF levels are usually about 20 percent of plasma levels but in the presence of meningeal inflammation may equal plasma concentrations.

Metabolism of INH is initially by liver *N*-acetyl transferase. Its rate of acetylation is determined genetically, with slow acetylation inherited as an autosomal recessive trait[3] that varies from 5 percent in Canadian eskimos to 83 percent in Egyptians; 10–15 percent of Orientals are slow acetylators, as are 58 percent of American whites.[3] Six hours after a 4 mg/kg oral dose, slow acetylators have INH serum levels of >0.8 μg/ml and rapid acetylators, <0.2 μg/ml.[1] The striking bimodal distribution of serum half-lives caused by acetylation status is depicted in Figure 2. Acetylator status does not affect outcome with daily therapy because plasma levels are well above inhibitory concentrations. However, weekly intermittent therapy may be adversely affected, with rapid acetylators faring less well. Primarily excreted as metabolically altered drug in the urine, some unaltered INH appears there as well. Dosage modification in hepatic or renal failure is not usually necessary, but in the presence of severe hepatic insufficiency, a reduction in dosage by one-half is recommended, and with significant renal failure, a dosage reduction to 150–200 mg/day is recommended for slow acetylators.[10] Table 1 indicates antituberculous drugs requiring dosage modification in hepatic or renal failure.

Adverse Reactions. Isoniazid has infrequent major toxicities that include hepatitis. Approximately 15 percent of INH recipients will have some elevation in serum glutamic-oxaloacetic transaminase (SGOT) levels that resolves with continued therapy. Although fatal INH hepatitis had been clearly documented by 1970,[11] early reports infrequently recognized it. Documen-

TABLE 1. Dosage Modification Requirement for Antituberculous Drugs Used in Hepatic or Renal Failure

Antimicrobial	*Hepatic Failure*	*Renal Failure*
Ethionamide	Yes	No
Isoniazid	Yes	Minor
Pyrazinamide	Yes	Yes[a]
Rifampin	Yes	No
Thiacetazone	Yes	Minor
Amikacin	No	Yes
Capreomycin	No	Yes
Cycloserine	No	Yes
Ethambutol	No	Yes
Kanamycin	No	Yes
Para-aminosalicylic acid	No	Yes
Streptomycin	No	Yes
Viomycin	No	Yes

[a] Accumulation of toxic metabolites.

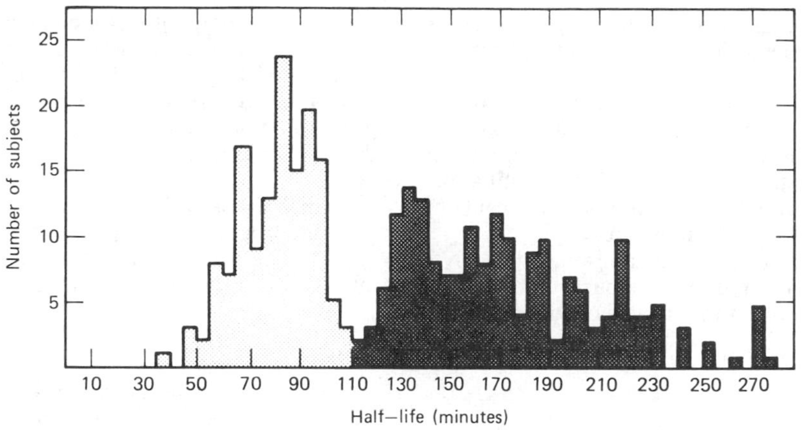

FIG. 2. Bimodal distribution of isoniazid half-lives as related to acetylation status. Patients received 5 mg/kg intravenously. Light bars indicate rapid acetylators and dark bars, slow acetylators. (From Pratt,[3] with permission.)

tation of the incidence of major INH hepatotoxicity awaited a large prophylactic trial reported in 1972 in which 19 of 2321 recipients developed serious hepatitis and 2 died.[12] Hepatotoxicity occurs at any time but is most likely to occur 4–8 weeks after the onset of treatment. Isoniazid hepatotoxicity is clearly correlated with age, as is indicated in Table 2, presumably due to the diminished capacity for repair of INH hepatocellular damage in the elderly. Hepatotoxicity is also more likely to occur in alcoholics with pre-existing liver damage.[12,14] Hepatocellular damage is usually evident histologically, while toxic cholestasis is infrequent. Chronic infection caused by hepatitis B is not a contraindication to the prophylactic use of INH.[15] Isoniazid hepatotoxicity was initially thought to reflect acetylator status, with increased risk for toxicity in rapid acetylators because of an acetylhydrazine metabolite. Subsequent studies have demonstrated that INH hydrolase induced by rifampin apparently increased the production of hepatotoxic hydrazine in *slow* acetylators treated daily with INH and rifampin.[16] Monitoring of concentrations of hepatic enzymes in plasma is generally unnecessary except in the elderly. Patients should be advised to discontinue INH therapy at the onset of symptoms consistent with beginning hepatitis.

Appreciation of the frequency of INH hepatotoxicity has not significantly limited therapeutic indications but has had a major impact on "chemoprophylactic" usage. No longer is "routine" INH chemoprophylaxis of adult purified protein derivative (PPD) skin test converters recommended, with special caution indicated in people over the age of 35.[13]

Neurotoxicity. Peripheral neuropathy occurs in 17 percent of those receiving 6 mg/kg/day of INH but less frequently with a conventional dosage. Neuropathy is especially likely in people with poor nutrition or underlying neuropathy resulting from alcoholism, diabetes, or uremia and is more frequent in slow acetylators who have higher serum levels of unaltered drug. Increased pyridoxine excretion is caused by INH administration. Pyridoxine replacement does not affect INH antimicrobial action[3] but does ameliorate the neuropathy.

TABLE 2. Age-Related Incidence of Isoniazid Hepatotoxicity

Age (yr)	*Serious Hepatotoxicity (% Patients)*
<20	"Rare"
20–34	0.3
35–49	1.2
50>	2.3

(From Centers for Disease Control.[13])

Central nervous system (CNS) INH toxicity may cause aberrations ranging from memory loss to psychosis or seizures. Particular caution should be exercised when administering INH to people with convulsive disorders. Optic neuropathy has been reported. Toxic CNS reactions are not related directly to pyridoxine deficiency for certain but have responded to its administration.[1]

Hypersensitivity Reactions. Fever that may be sustained or "spiking," skin eruptions, or hematologic abnormalities may occur. A substantial number of INH recipients develop positive antinuclear antibody (ANA) reactions, and some will manifest an INH-induced lupuslike syndrome that is usually reversible upon discontinuation of treatment with the drug.

Other Reactions. Arthritic disorders associated with INH administration have included Dupuytren's contracture and the "shoulder–hand" syndrome. Pellagra may occur in malnourished recipients of INH.[1,3] Pyridoxine deficiency–related anemia can occur.

Significant Drug Interactions. Phenytoin (Dilantin) toxicity is potentiated by INH. Mental changes, nystagmus, and ataxic gait can result, especially in slow acetylators in whom high INH levels inhibit phenytoin metabolism. Combined INH and rifampin therapy predisposes to elevation of serum hepatic enzyme levels in up to 29 percent of recipients of that combination. Plasma INH levels are increased by concurrent para-aminosalicylic acid (PAS) because of interference with acetylation.

Usage. Isoniazid is indicated for all forms of tuberculosis. In 1952, pulmonary disease was found to respond favorably to INH.[6] Tuberculous meningitis was almost always fatal before the advent of chemotherapy. Isoniazid-containing regimens yielded 83 percent survival rates as compared with 45 percent with streptomycin plus PAS.[17] Survival in miliary disease reached 77 percent with INH as compared with 22 percent with streptomycin plus PAS.[18] Therapeutic regimens include one or more companion drugs to discourage emergence of INH-resistant bacilli. Indications for INH include preventive therapy or "chemoprophylaxis" of selected PPD skin test converters.

Availability and Dosage. Isoniazid is available as INH, Nydrazid, Hyzyd, and Niconyl, for example. Dosage forms include 100 and 300 mg tablets, syrup containing 10 mg/ml, and a 100 mg/ml solution for parenteral injection. The usual dosage is 5–10 mg/kg/day (preferably 300 mg as a single daily dose), with the lower dosage range used routinely in adults for most therapy or "prophylaxis." Higher dosage schedules may be used for serious infections and for infants and children. Divided doses result in plasma concentrations below recommended therapeutic levels.

Intermittent therapy such as twice-weekly high-dose INH (15 mg/kg orally) combined with streptomycin (25–30 mg/kg im), ethambutol (50 mg/kg po), low-dose rifampin (600 mg po), or pyrazinamide is being used more frequently after an initial period of daily drug administration.[19] Such intermittent regimens are less expensive and encourage compliance.

Although not recommended for intravenous infusion, INH for injection has been administered intravenously[10] and can be given in this way cautiously when other routes of administration are contraindicated.

Ethambutol

Derivation and Structure. Ethambutol was discovered in 1961 among synthetic compounds being screened for antituberculous activity. Its structure is indicated in Figure 3.

Mechanism of Action. Ethambutol is tuberculostatic. Its precise mechanism of action is not known, although it is probably an antimetabolite affecting RNA synthesis.

Pharmacology. Ethambutol administered orally is 75–80 percent absorbed and yields peak plasma levels of 5 μg/ml after a dose of 25 mg/kg. It is distributed throughout the body, including the CSF. Although little ethambutol crosses normal meninges, levels 10–50 percent of those in serum appear in CSF with meningeal inflammation. After conversion of approximately 15 percent of absorbed ethambutol to inactive metabolites, 80 percent of the parent and metabolized drug is excreted in the urine. Thus, it becomes necessary to modify the dosage in significant renal failure.

Antimicrobial Activity. Ethambutol is bacteriostatic in vitro and also within macrophages[20] at concentrations of approximately 1 μg/ml against most strains of *M. tuberculosis*, even those that are INH-resistant. Resistance of a stepwise nature occurs when ethambutol is administered without companion drugs. Primary resistance has been reported only occasionally, and cross-resistance with other antimycobacterial drugs is unusual. Thus, ethambutol's principal role is as a "companion" drug to retard emergence of resistance.

Adverse Reactions. The major toxicity of ethambutol is neuropathic. Peripheral neuropathy may occur, but more common is the retrobulbar neuritis that is reported regularly with a dosage of 50 mg/kg/day. Characteristically, impairment of visual acuity or color vision develops, and there may be constriction of visual fields. More likely in association with high-dose or prolonged ethambutol administration, retrobulbar neuritis is usually reversible. Blindness has occurred in the elderly with as little as 15 mg/kg/day. Consequently, patients receiving ethambutol should be instructed to report optic symptoms, and visual acuity and color perception should be tested every 4–6 weeks. Gastrointestinal intolerance is infrequent. Hyperuricemia occurs secondary to decreased urinary uric acid excretion. Infrequent hypersensitivity reactions include dermatitis, arthralgias, and fever.

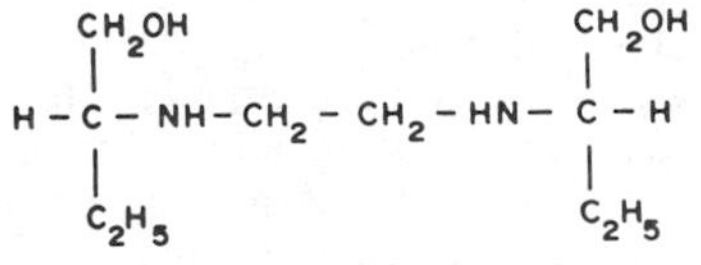

FIG. 3. Structure of ethambutol.

Usage. Ethambutol is indicated for infections due to *M. tuberculosis*. With combined therapy, resistance develops slowly. Because of its greater activity, lower incidence of side effects, and better record of compliance, ethambutol has largely replaced PAS in the United States as a bacteriostatic companion drug for isoniazid.

Availability and Dosage. Ethambutol is available as ethambutol hydrochloride (Myambutol) supplied in 100 and 400 mg tablets. The usual dosage is 15–25 mg/kg/day initially, followed after 60 days by 15 mg/kg/day as a single daily dose.

Rifampin

Derivation and Structure. Rifampin (termed rifampicin in the United Kingdom) is a semisynthetic derivative of a complex macrocyclic antibiotic, rifamycin B, produced by *Streptomyces mediterranei*. In 1967, it was introduced for clinical trials against mycobacterial infections. Its complex macrocyclic structure is indicated in Figure 4.

Mechanism of Action. Rifampin inhibits mycobacterial DNA-dependent RNA polymerase. Human RNA polymerase is insensitive to rifampin's action. It is bactericidal against *M. tuberculosis* at 0.005–0.2 μg/ml. Rifampin's lipid solubility enhances intracellular penetration.

Unlike any other combination, rifampin and INH have consistently sterilized tissue in experimental murine tuberculosis.

Pharmacology. Rifampin is well absorbed orally and yields peak levels of 7–8 μg/ml after 600 mg po. It is widely distributed throughout the body, including cerebrospinal fluid. CSF levels have ranged from undetectable to 0.5 μg/ml in healthy people and reach 50 percent of the plasma concentration with meningeal irritation. Rifampin is deacetylated to an active form that undergoes biliary excretion and enterohepatic recirculation. Due to autoinduction of rifampin's metabolizing enzymes (cytochrome P-450–coupled), biliary excretion increases with continued therapy. Excretion is primarily into the gastrointestinal tract, with lesser excretion in the urine. Both serum concentrations and urinary excretion increase in the presence of hepatic failure.[21] Probenecid causes decreased excretion by blocking hepatic uptake. In liver failure, some dosage reduction is indicated, but a full dosage can be administered in renal failure.

Antimicrobial Activity. Rifampin is active against *M. tuberculosis* to a degree comparable with INH. It affects intracellular, slowly replicating bacilli in caseous foci or intracavitary organisms as noted previously. In vitro, rapid, one-step resistance emerges with a low frequency, which precludes rifampin's use alone. Low-frequency resistance has been reported among clinical isolates of *M. tuberculosis*.[22]

Hepatotoxicity. Adverse reactions are rather frequent with

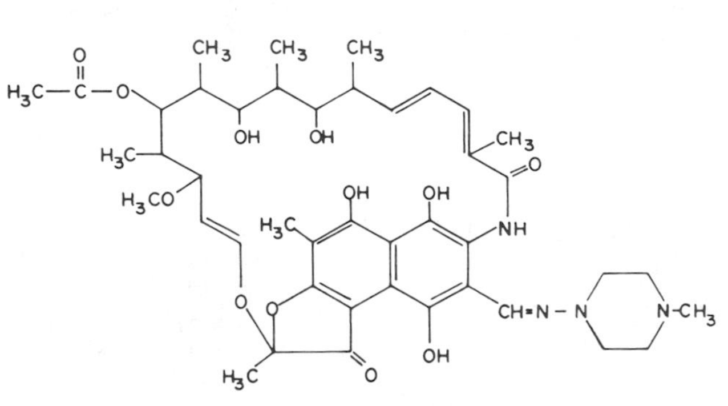

FIG. 4. Structure of rifampin.

rifampin, but only 6 of 372 patients taking the drug for 20 weeks had to discontinue therapy because of adverse effects.[23] The major adverse effect is hepatotoxicity, which has caused 16 deaths in 500,000 rifampin recipients.[1]

Minimal abnormalities in liver function test findings are common in people receiving rifampin and usually resolve even with continuation of the drug. Characteristically, elevations of bilirubin and alkaline phosphatase levels are noted, whereas elevations of hepatocellular enzymes such as SGOT can result from rifampin, INH, or both. Rifampin-induced toxic liver changes occur earlier and produce a patchier cellular abnormality with less marked periportal inflammation than does the hepatitis caused by INH.[24] Alcoholics with pre-existing liver damage appear to be especially prone to serious rifampin-induced liver toxicity. Concomitant INH appears to increase the risk of rifampin-related hepatotoxicity. It has been suggested that rifampin not be given to alcoholics with underlying liver damage "unless other drug combinations are contraindicated."[24] Such advice is hard to follow since alcoholism also predisposes to INH hepatitis and because alternatives such as PZA, PAS, and ethionamide also may be hepatotoxic. Children appear to be at an increased risk of serious rifampin-associated hepatotoxicity, perhaps in part because of relatively higher doses. Jaundice has been frequent (27 percent) in children with tuberculous meningitis who were receiving rifampin in combination regimens but could have been potentiated by phenytoin or other seizure medications.[25]

Effects on Immune Parameters. The effects of rifampin on humoral and cell-mediated immunity appear to be extensive but are of uncertain significance. Light-chain proteinuria occurs in 85 percent of those receiving rifampin.[26] It inhibits blastic transformation of phytohemagglutinin-stimulated lymphocytes and interferes with cutaneous reactivity to intradermal tuberculin.[27]

Hypersensitivity Reactions. Flushing, fever, pruritus without a rash, urticaria, eosinophilia, hemolysis, and renal failure due to interstitial nephritis[28] may occur after rifampin administration. A systemic flulike syndrome, at times associated with thrombocytopenia, appears to have an immunologic basis and has been described most often with intermittent high-dose rifampin. However, regimens employing 600 mg of rifampin twice weekly have recently produced the flulike syndrome very infrequently.[29]

Other Side Effects. The widespread systemic distribution of rifampin is reflected in the orange color appearing in urine, feces, saliva, sputum, pleural fluid, tears, soft contact lenses, sweat, semen, and CSF of people receiving the drug. Patients should be appropriately forewarned. With overdosage, a "red-man" syndrome caused from drug discoloration has occurred. Infrequently, gastrointestinal intolerance may result.

Significant Drug Interactions. By potentiating hepatic microsomal cytochrome P-450–related enzymatic reactions, rifampin induces increased hepatic excretion of a number of drugs and other compounds metabolized by the liver. A list of many of this expanding number of substances is given in Table 3. Several of these interactions appear clinically significant.[30,31] In this manner, it causes decreased activity of the coumarin-type anticoagulants that persists 5–7 days after rifampin therapy is discontinued. Menstrual irregularities and decreased efficacy of oral contraceptives have been reported due to potentiation of steroid hormone metabolism. On the other hand, competition for excretion with contrast materials used in cholecystography may result in a failure to visualize the gallbladder. Rifampin crosses the placenta readily and is not approved for use in pregnancy. There is interference with gastrointestinal absorption of rifampin by PAS. Probenecid administration causes increased plasma rifampin concentrations.

TABLE 3. Compounds Having Rifampin-Induced Reduction in Plasma Levels[a]

Barbiturates	Ketoconazole
Bile acids	Methadone
Chloramphenicol	Metoprolol
Clofibrate	Phenytoin
Cyclosporine	Prednisone—glucocorticoids
Digoxin	Propranolol
Digitoxin	Sulfonylureas
Estrogens	Theophylline
Itraconazole	Verapamil

[a] Reviewed in Baciewicz et al.[30]

Usage. Rifampin's efficacy is indicated in pulmonary tuberculosis by sputum conversion 2 weeks earlier with rifampin than with non-rifampin-containing regimens.[23] Because of rifampin's potent antimycobacterial action, combination regimens with it have yielded gratifying results in short-duration therapy and in retreatment of drug-resistant tuberculosis. Rifampin in combination with INH has been recommended for extrapulmonary tuberculous infections including tuberculous meningitis.

Availability and Dosage. Rifampin is available in the United States as Rifadin and Rimactane, supplied as 300 mg capsules. The usual dose is 600 mg once daily for adults and 10–20 mg/kg/day for children (not to exceed 600 mg/day). Twice weekly 1200 and 900 mg dosage regimens have largely been abandoned due to unacceptably high numbers of toxic reactions. A 600 mg twice-weekly regimen has been generally well tolerated. Rifampin capsules can be opened and the drug suspended in simple or flavored sugar syrup for pediatric administration. The suspension can be refrigerated for up to 2 weeks.

Rifabutin

Several other spiropiperidyl rifamycins have a high degree of activity against mycobacteria including *M. tuberculosis, M. avium-intracellulare* complex, and *M. fortuitum.*[32] Rifabutin (ansamycin, LM-427), a derivative of rifamycin-S is more active in vitro and effective in experimental murine tuberculosis than is rifampin, even against some rifampin-resistant strains.[33–35] Characterized by a long half-life (16 hours) in humans and marked tissue tropism producing tissue concentrations 5- to 10-fold greater than in plasma, rifabutin in animals is no more toxic than is rifampin. Clinical investigations are underway to define rifabutin's role in the treatment of tuberculosis and *M. avium-intracellulare* infections.

Streptomycin

Derivation and Structure. Streptomycin, an aminoglycoside antimicrobic introduced in the 1940s, was the first drug to reduce tuberculosis mortality. Its structure, mechanism of action, and pharmacology are given in Chapter 22. Briefly, the drug is administered intramuscularly and yields serum levels of 25–30 μg/ml after a 1 g injection. It is practically excluded from the CNS. Streptomycin's toxicities are similar to other aminoglycoside antibiotics but has less nephrotoxicity and greater vestibular toxicity than do most aminoglycosides.

Antimicrobial Activity. In vitro, streptomycin is bactericidal for *M. tuberculosis,* but in animals it can be only suppressive and is inactive against intracellular tubercle bacilli. Concentrations of 0.4–10 μg/ml are inhibitory. Rapid emergence of resistance has long been recognized as a hazard of single-drug therapy with streptomycin. Approximately 1 bacterium in 10^6 is primarily resistant to streptomycin. Such high concentrations of tubercle bacilli most often reside in cavitary pulmonary lesions. Primarily occurring cross-resistance to streptomycin is found most often among patient populations having a high incidence of INH resistance. Among other aminoglycosides, amikacin and dibukacin appear to possess superior activity to streptomycin against *M. tuberculosis*.[36] However, familiarity, low toxicity, and reasonable price cause streptomycin to remain the aminoglycoside of choice for tuberculosis.

Usage. Streptomycin is indicated in multiple-drug therapy for tuberculosis. Caution must be exercised with a prolonged dosage of greater than 1 g/day and with administration to the elderly or persons with impaired renal function. Care must also be taken if streptomycin is used in combination with other nephrotoxic or ototoxic antibiotics.

Availability and Dosage. Streptomycin sulfate for injection is provided in 0.5 g/ml single-injection vials and mulidose vials. The customary dose in adults ranges from 2 g daily to 1 g twice weekly (most often 500 mg to 1 g daily). Higher dosage schedules are indicated for initial short-term (2–4 weeks) therapy, with subsequent reduction to 1 g/day or less. Children should receive 20–40 mg/kg/day in two divided doses q12h.

Pyrazinamide

Derivation. Pyrazinamide (PZA) is a synthetic analog of nicotinamide that has been elevated to first-line usage for "short-course" therapy regimens because of its bactericidal action[4] plus acceptable toxicity at relatively low doses. Its structure is indicated in Figure 5

Mechanism of Action. Pyrazinamide is bactericidal for the tubercle bacillus at 12.5 μg/ml. Its maximal activity in vitro is at an acid pH, like that existing intracellularly in tuberculous lesions. Its precise action is unknown. Despite good activity at an acid pH in vitro and inhibitory concentrations within mononuclear cells,[20] PZA is barely active in macrophages pretreated with the drug, which leaves unanswered the mechanism of its apparently selective intracellular action.[37] Resistance evolves rapidly when PZA is used alone. Metabolically inactive tubercle bacilli are resistant to PZA, thus rendering it inappropriate for long-term therapy.[4] Primary resistance is less than 1 percent.

Pharmacology. Well absorbed orally, PZA is widely distributed throughout the body in concentrations exceeding inhibitory levels for the tubercle bacillus. Peak plasma concentrations are approximately 50 μg/ml. A half-life of 12–24 hours lends itself to once-daily dosing. Pyrazinamide crosses inflamed meninges. It is metabolized by the liver, and its metabolic products, including principally pyrazinoic acid, are excreted mainly in the urine, so it is best avoided in renal failure.

Toxicity. Hepatotoxicity occurring in up to 15 percent of people receiving pyrazinamide in initial trials long ago discouraged its use. Early trials of PZA employed dosages of 40–50 mg/kg/day for prolonged periods. Currently recommended regimens of 20–35 mg/kg/day appear to be much safer.[38,39] Patients with pre-existing liver disease probably should not receive the drug; symptoms and hepatic function tests should be monitored in those receiving PZA. Other side effects include urate retention in 56 percent of PZA recipients.[39] Photosensitivity and rash have been reported.

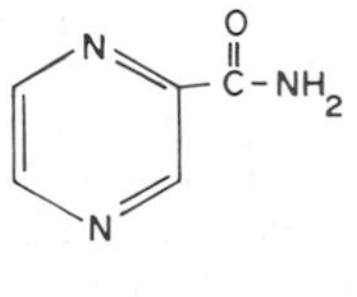

FIG. 5. Structure of pyrazinamide.

Usage. Because of a fear of hepatotoxicity, PZA has been reserved in the United States for the treatment of patients with drug-resistant infections. In other nations, it has played a role in initial therapy, particularly in areas of high primary resistance. Low in price, it can be administered once weekly, thus favoring its usage in developing nations. Now PZA is receiving attention worldwide as a component of multidrug short-course chemotherapy.[4,29,39]

Availability and Dosage. Pyrazinamide is available in 500 mg tablets. The usual dose is 20–35 mg/kg/day orally in two to four spaced doses equivalent to 1.5–2.0 g daily. Apparently it has been well tolerated in a twice-weekly dosage of 50 mg/kg, not to exceed 3 g/day, for short-course regimens. It has even been administered in a 90 mg/kg dose once weekly with little overt hepatotoxicity.

SECOND-LINE ANTITUBERCULOUS DRUGS

Para-aminosalicylic Acid

This synthetic compound, supplied as a sodium or calcium salt or resin, inhibits the growth of mycobacteria by impairment of folate synthesis. Para-aminosalicylic acid is incompletely absorbed orally. A 4 g oral dose yields plasma concentrations of 7–8 μg/ml. Eighty-five percent of absorbed PAS is excreted in the urine in the form of various degradation products.

Toxicity. Chief among side effects of PAS is gastrointestinal intolerance, which may be severe and thus often causes poor patient compliance with treatment regimens. Para-aminosalicylic acid can cause a reversible drug-induced lupus-like syndrome or can produce lymphoid hyperplasia. Recipients can develop a mononucleosis-like syndrome with fever, rash, lymphadenopathy, hepatosplenomegaly, and occasionally toxic hepatitis. Hypersensitivity to PAS is frequent, occurring in 5–10 percent. Further, it seems to cross-sensitize to streptomycin and INH in patients who are receiving multidrug regimens. Readministration of any of the components in a combination regimen after PAS hypersensitivity may subsequently result in reaction to the companion drug. Increased toxicity of INH in association with para-aminosalicylate may result from PAS inhibition of INH acetylation.

Usage. Para-aminosalicylic acid was once included in standard combination therapy for *M. tuberculosis*. In the United States, it has, to a large extent, been supplanted by ethambutol. Due to its low cost, PAS retains a place in multidrug therapy in developing countries but is becoming less favored because of poor compliance.

Availability and Dosage. Para-aminosalicylic acid is provided as acid salts (Pamisyl), as a sodium-potassium-free ascorbate (Pascorbic), and as a resin (Resipas). Dosage forms include 500 mg tablets and 4 g resin packets. The customary dose is 10–12 g/day in three to four divided doses for adults (6–8 g/day of the sodium-potassium–free ascorbate) and, in children, 200–300 mg/kg/day in divided doses.

Cycloserine

Derivation. Initially produced by fermentation, cycloserine is now synthesized. By virtue of inhibition of cell wall synthesis, cycloserine possesses antimicrobial activity against a broad range of prokaryotic microorganisms including mycobacteria. Five to 20 μg/ml inhibits *M. tuberculosis*.

Pharmacology. Cycloserine is readily absorbed orally, with peak serum levels of 20–50 μg/ml. Widely distributed among tissues, no blood-brain barrier exists to cycloserine.[1] Approximately two-thirds of the drug is excreted unchanged in urine, and the remainder is metabolized to inactive forms.

Side Effects. Peripheral neuropathy or CNS dysfunction can be caused by cycloserine. Behavioral alterations or seizures can result. In patients with latent seizures, treatment with the drug is contraindicated.

Usage. Cycloserine is one of several agents to choose from for retreatment or treatment of primarily resistant *M. tuberculosis*.

Availability and Dosage. Cycloserine is provided as Seromycin in 250 mg capsules. The usual dose is 500–1000 mg/day in two divided doses, with 500 mg daily used most frequently.

Ethionamide

Derivation. Ethionamide, a derivative of isonicotinic acid, was synthesized in 1956. It is tuberculostatic at 0.6–2.5 μg/ml against susceptible strains.

Pharmacology. Ethionamide is absorbed well orally and yields peak plasma concentrations of 20 μg/ml. It is widely distributed and penetrates both normal and inflamed meninges to yield CSF concentrations approximately the same as in serum. The drug is metabolized by the liver, with metabolites excreted mainly in the urine. Ethionamide interferes with INH acetylation.

Side Effects. Most people taking ethionamide will experience gastrointestinal irritation with nausea and, frequently, vomiting. Various neurologic disorders can be caused by ethionamide, including peripheral neuropathy or psychiatric disturbances that may require discontinuation of therapy with the drug and reportedly are alleviated by pyridoxine and nicotinamide. Reversible hepatotoxicity, heralded by increasing SGOT values, may occur in approximately 5 percent of ethionamide recipients. Hypersensitivity-type rash or poor diabetic control are infrequent complications.

Usage. Ethionamide is among the choices of agents for treatment of primarily or secondarily resistant tuberculosis.

Availability and Dosage. Ethionamide is available as Trecator-SC in 250 mg tablets. The usual initial dosage is 250 mg twice daily (or as a single dose on retiring) and is increased by 125 mg/day until 1 g/day is reached. Commonly, 500–750 mg becomes the maximum dose because of gastrointestinal intolerance.

Kanamycin, Viomycin, Capreomycin, Amikacin

These agents are considered as a group because all must be administered by intramuscular injection, have similar pharmacokinetics and toxicities, and are excreted by the kidneys. The first three have been employed principally as alternative agents in retreatment regimens for resistant tuberculosis. These agents have additive ototoxicity and nephrotoxicity and should not be given, as a rule, in combination with each other, streptomycin, or another aminoglycoside.

Kanamycin. Kanamycin is an aminoglycoside antibiotic described in Chapter 19 to which some resistant tubercle bacilli are susceptible. Except for lower price, kanamycin has no advantages over amikacin as an alternative in treatment schedules. (See ''Amikacin.'')

AVAILABILITY AND DOSAGE. Kanamycin sulfate is supplied as Kantrex, 0.5 g/2 ml, 1 g/3 ml, or 75 mg/2 ml (pediatric dose form), for intramuscular injection. The usual dose is 15 mg/kg/day, which for practical purposes is 1 g/day in most adults.

Viomycin. Viomycin is a complex basic polypeptide antibiotic for injection.[2] Certain resistant *M. tuberculosis* strains are susceptible. Cross-resistance to viomycin and capreomycin occurs regularly and is seen less consistently between viomycin and kanamycin.[40] Susceptible strains of *M. tuberculosis* are inhibited by 1–10 μg/ml.

AVAILABILITY AND DOSAGE. Viomycin sulfate for injection is supplied as Viocin in 1 and 5 g vials. The usual dosage is 2 g twice weekly, administered as 1 g every 12 hours on the days of injection. One to 2 g daily has been used for periods of not longer than 1 to 2 weeks.

Capreomycin. Capreomycin is a polypeptide antibiotic produced by *Streptomyces capreolus*. Susceptible *M. tuberculosis* strains are susceptible to 1–50 μg/ml (usually 10 μg/ml), depending on the culture medium. Average peak serum concentrations of 30 μg/ml are achieved. Cross-resistance occurs chiefly between capreomycin and viomycin but also between capreomycin and kanamycin. According to some authorities, capreomycin is less toxic than viomycin is and especially less toxic than is kanamycin.[40] Capreomycin may be employed in the retreatment of resistant tuberculosis as one component of a multiple-drug regimen.

AVAILABILITY AND DOSAGE. Capreomycin sulfate is supplied as Capastat. The dosage is 1 g intramuscularly daily for 2–4 months and is reduced to 1 g two to three times weekly thereafter.

Amikacin. In vitro and in animal trials amikacin is among the most active if not the most active aminoglycoside against *M. tuberculosis*.[36] It has not been used extensively in human tuberculosis. Due to expense and toxicity, it should not supplant streptomycin as the first-line aminoglycoside for the initial treatment of susceptible tuberculosis. Except for cost it probably would replace its congener kanamycin since both have similar pharmacokinetics and toxicities. In renal failure, amikacin might be chosen because assays for it are more generally available.

USAGE. Amikacin appears to have merit as an alternative drug for the retreatment of resistant *M. tuberculosis* infections.

Amithiozone

Amithiozone (thiacetazone), a thiosemicarbazole, is quite active against most strains of *M. tuberculosis*. Susceptible strains are inhibited by 1 μg/ml.[1,2] Peak serum concentrations are 1–2 μg/ml. Resistance to amithiozone readily develops with single-drug therapy and necessitates combination regimens. Toxicity (gastrointestinal irritation and marrow suppression) has precluded use of this agent in Europe and the United States. (The drug is unavailable in the United States.) Gastrointestinal toxicity is comparable to that of PAS. Additionally, hepatic damage has occurred, usually in patients receiving INH concomitantly. Apparently there is a lower incidence of untoward effects in African populations. Consequently, because of its low price, amithiozone has been used as a ''first-line'' drug particularly in East African developing nations.[2] Amithiozone (Panthrone, Tibione) is administered orally in a dose of 150 mg/day or 450 mg twice weekly.

β-Lactams

Most mycobacteria produce β-lactamases, and several β-lactamase–resistant β-lactam antibiotics or combinations with β-lactamase inhibitors such as clavulanic acid are active in vitro against *M. tuberculosis*[41] and various atypical mycobacteria. The activity of β-lactam agents on intracellular mycobacterial replication is greatly diminished. Ceforanide, active in vitro in the macrophage model in concentrations as high as 50 μg/ml is unable to retard the tubercle bacillus.[20] Similarly, cefotaxime, ceftizoxime, or cefoperazone lack intracellular activity against *M. avium-intracellulare* strains that were susceptible in vitro.[42] However, cefoxitin has proved efficacious in susceptible *M. fortuitum* infections,[43] which gives hope that stable β-lactams sufficiently active against problem mycobacteria may be forthcoming.

DRUGS FOR THE TREATMENT OF ATYPICAL MYCOBACTERIAL INFECTIONS

"Atypical" (i.e., nontuberculous) mycobacteria vary greatly in susceptibility to antimicrobics. Some are susceptible to agents used principally for the treatment of tuberculosis; other atypicals respond to various antibiotics used more commonly for treating pyogenic bacterial infections; and still others, especially among the *M. avium-intracellulare* group, are frequently broadly resistant. Mycobacteria of the *M. avium-intracellulare* complex often contain plasmids that contribute to their broad antimicrobial resistance.[44] Choosing appropriate therapy for atypicals is further confounded because methodology for susceptibility testing varies. Standardization of atypical mycobacterial identification and susceptibility testing methods is in progress.[45] Rational chemotherapy for atypical mycobacterial infections that is based on susceptibility results has become feasible.[46] Regardless of therapy with combinations of drugs active in vitro against *M. avium-intracellulare,* outcomes in the acquired immunodeficiency syndrome (AIDS) are poor.[47]

ANTITUBERCULOUS DRUGS USED FOR THE TREATMENT OF ATYPICAL MYCOBACTERIA

Isoniazid

Agents used principally for the treatment of *M. tuberculosis* were evaluated years ago for activity against "atypical" mycobacteria.[48] Isoniazid inhibits nearly 40 percent of the strains of *M. kansasii* at a concentration of 1–5 μg/ml, as contrasted with only 10–30 percent of *M. avium-intracellulare* strains that are inhibited by that concentration. Some authorities include INH in multidrug regimens for the treatment of many atypical mycobacterial infections even in the face of in vitro INH resistance. Because of borderline susceptibilities of most atypical mycobacteria, doses of INH up to 10–15 mg/kg/day have been used with accompanying increased toxicity.

Rifampin, Rifabutin

Rifampin is used for the treatment of many atypical mycobacterial infections. In vitro, 93–100 percent of *M. kansasii* strains are inhibited by 0.25–1 μg/ml, and virtually all *M. marinum* are susceptible.[49,50] About one-half of *M. scrofulaceum* or *M. avium-intracellulare* strains are inhibited in vitro by 4–16 μg/ml of rifampin. The *M. fortuitum* complex is universally resistant to rifampin, although *M. ulcerans* bacilli are generally susceptible. The response of *M. marinum* infections to rifampin has been particularly encouraging. Synergy of rifampin and other agents is often demonstrable in vitro. Its role as a single agent is discouraged to prevent the emergence of resistance. Rifabutin (ansamycin, LM-427) is inhibitory against all strains of *M. avium-intracellulare* in a concentration of <2 μg/ml.[33–35] It is concentrated severalfold in tissue and apparently has no greater toxicity than rifampin. Controlled clinical trials are underway.

Aminoglycosides

Aminoglycosides have been extensively used for the treatment of atypical mycobacterial infections. Of *M. kansasii* strains, 86 percent are streptomycin susceptible, as are 93 percent of *M. scrofulaceum*. Forty-four percent of strains of *M. avium-intracellulare* have been streptomycin sensitive. The *M. fortuitum* complex is generally resistant, whereas *M. ulcerans* strains demonstrate universal susceptibility to streptomycin in vitro.[51] Despite in vitro susceptibility, streptomycin has not been effective in *M. ulcerans* infections, probably because of inactivity against bacilli located intracellularly, and indeed, surgical excision of Buruli ulcers remains the only effective treatment. Kanamycin is not active in vitro against most *M. kansasii* strains, whereas most *M. scrofulaceum* isolates are kanamycin susceptible, and *M. avium-intracellulare* and *M. fortuitum* are not predictably kanamycin sensitive.

Amikacin and dibekacin,[52] congeners of kanamycin, appear to have greater activity against atypical mycobacteria than the parent compound does. Many atypicals are susceptible to 12.5 μg/ml of amikacin.[36] However, marked variability exists between mycobacteria in susceptibility to amikacin. Virtually all *M. marinum* strains are susceptible to 3 μg/ml of amikacin,[50] but only 50 percent of the *M. fortuitum* group are susceptible to 12.5 μg/ml,[53] whereas other aminoglycosides are even less active.[54] Susceptibility of *M. avium-intracellulare* varies.

Ethambutol, ethionamide, and cycloserine possess variable activity against *M. avium-intracellulare* and have been employed in combination for infections caused by that group. Capreomycin frequently is the only antituberculous drug showing activity against *M. fortuitum*.

MISCELLANEOUS ANTIMICROBIALS FOR THE TREATMENT OF ATYPICAL MYCOBACTERIA

Erythromycin

Nearly all strains of *M. kansasii* and *M. scrofulaceum* and some of those of *M. avium-intracellulare* are susceptible to concentrations of erythromycin that can be achieved in plasma by conventional therapy.[55] Erythromycin has been effective in susceptible *M. chelonae* infections.[43]

Tetracyclines

Some strains included in the *M. fortuitum-chelonae* complex are tetracycline susceptible. Although extensive in vitro testing has not been performed, encouraging clinical results have occurred with tetracyclines, especially minocycline (Minocin) in *M. marinum* infections.[49]

Sulfonamides

Sulfamethoxazole is active against *M. fortuitum*. Localized infections have been cured with sulfamethoxazole alone or in combination with trimethoprim.[43]

M. marinum infections have responded to therapy with trimethoprim-sulfa, but most strains are resistant to concentrations in vitro.[50]

Clofazimine

Discussed more fully under antileprosy drugs, clofazimine (Lamprene) has shown promising in vitro activity against *M. avium-intracellulare*. Most strains tested are inhibited by 1.6–2.0 μg/ml.[32,56] However, trials of clofazimine in combination therapy against *M. avium-intracellulare* in persons having AIDS yielded disappointing results.[48]

Other Antimicrobics

Active chemotherapeutic agents for serious *M. fortuitum* and *M. avium-intracellulare* infections are greatly needed. Cefoxitin (Mefoxin), cefmetazole, and imipenem-cilastatin (Primaxin), apparently because of resistance to *M. fortuitum* β-lactamase, are active in vitro against approximately 80 percent of *M. fortuitum* strains at achievable plasma concentrations.[57] Ciprofloxacin (Cipro) is active against most *M. avium-intracellulare* strains in vitro and consequently deserves further study.[58]

A summary of in vitro susceptibility data of atypical mycobacteria is supplied in Table 4. The table serves as a guide only. It is a compilation of data from a number of laboratories, some using nonstandard methodology or testing a small number of strains. Furthermore, in vitro susceptibility of atypical mycobacteria to an antimicrobial agent fails to guarantee therapeutic efficacy. The earlier cited failure of clofazimine in *M. avium-intracellulare* infections and of streptomycin against *M. ulcerans* indicates the limitations of extrapolating in vitro data to clinical experience. As a rule, good therapeutic outcomes are more likely when agents are used to which atypical mycobacteria are susceptible in vitro, and poor outcomes can be anticipated when there is in vitro resistance. Especially for more resistant atypical mycobacterial infections like those caused by *M. avium-intracellulare* or the *M. fortuitum* complex, well-designed clinical trials with active antimicrobials are needed. Readily available analyses of plasma levels of the antimycobacterial agents are also needed to assess the efficacy and toxicity of drug regimens. The polypharmacy of atypical mycobacterial infections without confirmatory susceptibility testing and plasma concentrations continues to foster unnecessary toxicity and expense.

DRUGS FOR THE TREATMENT OF LEPROSY

Background

The special parasite–host relationship of *Mycobacterium leprae* (Hansen's bacillus), which is characterized by persistence of the organism in tissue for years, has mandated prolonged chemotherapy to prevent relapses. Thus bacillary persistance has long been the major consideration in designing therapy for leprosy (Hansen's disease). Now the second factor is resistance.

Chemotherapy for leprosy for years has consisted, for practical purposes, of dapsone alone. This produced gratifying clinical results and was affordable. Because of monotherapy, however, resistance of leprosy bacilli, both secondary and now primary, has emerged as a worldwide concern[63] and has led to the long overdue use of multidrug therapeutic regimens for leprosy.[64]

Dapsone and Other Sulfones

Derivation and Structure. Diaminodiphenyl sulfone (dapsone, DDS), a synthetic compound, was demonstrated to be effective against rat leprosy in 1941 and soon thereafter was used successfully in human trials. Its structure is indicated in Figure 6.

Mechanism of Action. Sulfones are bacteriostatic presumably by the same mechanism by which sulfonamides interfere with folate synthesis.

Antimicrobial Activity. By mouse footpad inoculation, as little as 0.003 μg/ml of dapsone inhibits *Mycobacterium leprae*.[65] Dapsone appears "weakly bactericidal" for most leprosy bacilli. It has been estimated that 99.9 percent of bacillary populations are killed after 3–4 months of therapy with dapsone.[64] However, despite initial susceptibility, "persister" bacilli apparently exist for years. Secondary dapsone resistance is evident, principally in lepromatous (multibacillary) patients in whom resistance has emerged 5–24 years after commencing therapy.[66] The incidence of secondary resistance varies widely between geographic regions and occurs in up to 19 percent of cases. Fully resistant *M. leprae* should be suspected when patients supervised on 100 mg dapsone daily relapse during treatment.[63] Apparently because of the spread of infection from secondarily resistant cases, primary dapsone resistance is now encountered as frequently as is secondary resistance. Partial (usual) to fully developed (infrequent) primary dapsone resistance varies in frequency, depending on geographic area.

Pharmacology. Oral dapsone is well absorbed. Distributed throughout body fluids, tissue levels are approximately 2 μg/ml. The serum half-life of dapsone is 21–44 hours, with some drug retention for up to 3 weeks. Dapsone is acetylated, with 70–80 percent being excreted as metabolites in the urine. The dosage thus should be reduced in significant renal failure.

Side Effects and Adverse Reactions. Dapsone, an oxidant drug, can produce minor hemolysis in patients receiving 200–300 mg/day. Insignificant hemolysis occurs at doses under 100 mg/day in healthy people or at doses of 50 mg/day or less in people with glucose-6-phosphate dehydrogenase (G6PD) deficiency. Methemaglobinemia is common. Gastrointestinal intolerance occurs and is manifested by anorexia with occasional

TABLE 4. Antimicrobials for "Atypical" Mycobacteria: Likelihood of In Vitro Susceptibilities Being within Range of Achievable Serum Concentrations

Category	*Runyon Group*	*Mycobacterial Species*	*Likelihood of Susceptibility to Antimicrobial*[a]
Photochromogens	I	*M. kansasii*	Erythromycin (4+), rifampin (4+), streptomycin (4+), ethionamide (4+), amikacin (3+), cycloserine (3+), ethambutol (3+), viomycin (3+), INH (2+)
		M. marinum	Rifampin (4+), amikacin (4+), kanamycin (4+), minocycline (3+)
Scotochromogens	II	*M. scrofulaceum*	Amikacin (4+), erythromycin (4+), kanamycin (4+), streptomycin (4+), rifampin (3+), ethionamide (2+), INH (1+)
Nonchromogens	III	*M. avium-intracellulare*	Amikacin (4+), rifabutin (4+), clofazimine (3+), ethionamide (2+), rifampin (2+), streptomycin (2+), cycloserine (2+), kanamycin (1+), INH (1+), ethambutol (1+), viomycin (1+), erythromycin (1+)
Rapid growers	IV	*M. fortuitum*	Cefoxitin (4+), cefmetazole (3+), imipenem-cilastatin (3+), amikacin (3+), minocycline (2+), capreomycin (2+), kanamycin (2+), ethionamide (1+), gentamicin (1+), viomycin (1+)
		M. chelonae ssp. *chelonae*	Amikacin (3+), kanamycin (3+), erythromycin (2+)
		M. chelonae ssp. *abscessus*	Cefoxitin (4+), amikacin (3+), kanamycin (3+), erythromycin (2+)
Other		*M. ulcerans*	Rifampin (4+), streptomycin (4+), clofazimine (2+)

[a] Compilation of data from published sources ranked according to the percentage of tested strains that were found susceptible to achievable serum concentrations of the antimicrobials: 81–100% = (4+), 61–80% = (3+), 41–60% = 2+, 21–40% = (1+).
(Data from references 32, 34–37, 42–44, 47–51, 52–62.)

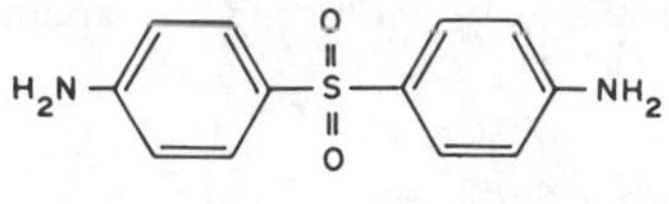

FIG. 6. Structure of dapsone.

nausea and vomiting. Hematuria, fever, pruritus, and skin rashes can occur.

Reactions encountered with dapsone or other sulfones may be difficult to extricate from the reactions that occur because of the disease itself.[67] A *sulfone syndrome* has been reported 5–6 weeks after initiation of therapy and is characterized by fever, jaundice, dermatitis, and lymphadenopathy—a picture somewhat like infectious mononucleosis.[68] Its likelihood is diminished by a gradual increase in dapsone doses until a full therapeutic dosage is attained. Also, during dapsone administration, erythema nodosum leprosum (ENL, type 2) reactions commonly become manifested in persons with multibacillary disease. In borderline or intermediate cases, reactional states (lepra, type 1, upgrade or downgrade) may be accentuated by dapsone therapy.[67] Although apparently infrequent, hypersensitivity reactions to dapsone may thus be difficult to recognize due to the complexity of the illness.

Usage. Dapsone continues to be the basic therapeutic agent for *M. leprae* infections, often as a component of multidrug programs.

Availability and Dosage. Dapsone is available as Alvosulfon tablets of 25 or 100 mg. To avoid untoward reactions, it is begun in a dose of one 25 mg tablet per week with a gradual increase by one tablet per week or so until a full therapeutic dose is reached—usually 100 mg/day. An appropriately reduced dosage is given to children.

Acedapsone

Derivation. Acedapsone (4,4′-diacetyldiaminodiphenylsulfone) is a long-acting repository derivative of dapsone.

Pharmacology. Slow absorption of acedapsone occurs from injection sites, with peak concentrations occurring between 22 and 35 days later. The parent compound has little activity against *M. leprae* but is converted into active dapsone. Its half-life is 46 days and 43 days for the derived dapsone.[69] Because of its long half-life, injections only five times yearly have been used. A 300 mg im dose maintained dapsone levels in volunteers above the inhibitory concentration for *M. leprae,* which was measured in mice for approximately 100 days.

Usage. This repository drug has been employed in *M. leprae* infections with promising results. Microbiologic and clinical responses are somewhat slower than with daily dapsone, which raises the concern that resistance may become a problem. Long-term studies with acedapsone by injection five times yearly have yielded encouraging results indicated by the fact that 91 percent of patients improved or "healed" after 6 years.[70] Acedapsone shows promise, especially in areas where other routes of therapy are not feasible. Trials incorporating widely spaced doses of rifampin plus acedapsone are in progress with the hope of reducing the burden of *M. leprae* more rapidly, thus lessening the likelihood of acedapsone—dapsone resistance.

Sulfoxone

Less well absorbed and more expensive, the disubstituted sulfone sulfoxone is sometimes better tolerated by the gastrointestinal tract than is dapsone. It is formulated in 165 mg enteric-coated tablets with a usual daily dose of 330 mg.[1]

Rifampin

Mechanism of Action and Resistance. The mechanism of action of rifampin against *M. leprae* is presumed to be by inhibition of DNA-dependent RNA polymerase, which produces a relatively rapid bactericidal effect. The inhibitory concentration of rifampin for human strains of *M. leprae* tested in mice is 0.3 μg/ml. A tabulation of the relative activity of antileprosy drugs in clearing tissue of viable bacilli is shown in Table 5.

Usage. Clinical trials of rifampin have indicated that rifampin differs by several orders of magnitude in its initial effectiveness as compared with other antileprosy drugs. Demonstration by skin biopsy that a single dose of 1500 mg of rifampin can reduce the viability of leprosy bacilli to undetectable levels by 3–5 days is truly remarkable. However, limitations of biopsy evaluations are inherent since the method can only account for a decrease to about 10^8 total leprosy bacilli.[71] Prolonged therapy for multibacillary lepromatous disease with 600 mg of rifampin daily has failed to eradicate large bacterial populations. Evidently, in leprosy as in other infections rifampin as a solitary therapeutic agent promotes bacterial resistance. Despite generally satisfactory clinical results with rifampin alone, relapses have occurred.[64]

Although it causes a rapid decrease in *M. leprae* populations, rifampin should be used with another, preferably two, companion drugs, including dapsone for multibacillary disease. The high cost of rifampin has discouraged its use in economically deprived areas. However, once-monthly therapy with 600–1200 mg of rifampin in combination-drug regimens has produced satisfactory clinical responses without adverse reactions.[64,72] Lepra and ENL reactions with rifampin have been comparable or less severe than with sulfones.

Rifabutin (ansamycin) and rifapentine, two investigational substituted rifamycins, have activity against *M. leprae*. In mice, these compounds are even more active than rifampin,[73] which raises interest in human therapeutic trials.

Clofazimine (B-663)

Derivation and Structure. The structure of clofazimine, a phenazine dye, is indicated in Figure 7.

Mechanism of Action and Antimicrobial Activity. Clofazimine's precise mechanism of action is not known. Highly lipophilic and binding to mycobacterial DNA, clofazimine is weakly bactericidal against *M. leprae*. Its action may relate to iron chelation with resulting production of nascent oxygen radicals intracellularly.[74] The inhibitory concentration of clofazimine in mouse tissue is between 0.1 and 1 mg/kg.[75] A delay of some 50 days ensues before tissue antimicrobic activity can be demonstrated in humans.

TABLE 5. Efficacy of Antileprosy Agents in Rendering Tissue Free of Bacilli[a]

Antimicrobial	Adult Human Dosage	Time until Tissue Negative by Mouse Footpad Assay (Days) Range	Median
Rifampin	1500 mg once	<3–<5	<3
Rifampin	600 mg/day	3–<14	<7
Dapsone	50 mg/day[a]	21–>134	61
Clofazimine	200 mg/day[b]	94–138	113
Acedapsone	225 mg/q 75 days	44–>306	214

[a] Dosage raised to 50 mg/day over a period of 4 weeks.
[b] Dosage decreased to 100 mg/day in some patients having excessive skin pigmentation.
(Modified from Shepard et al.,[71] with permission.)

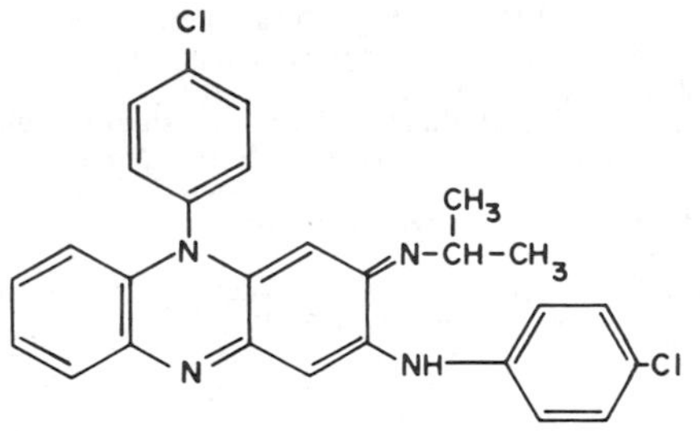

FIG. 7. Structure of clofazimine.

Pharmacology. Clofazimine's pharmacokinetics are complex. Absorption is quite variable, with 9–74 percent of an administered dose appearing in feces. The route of administration is oral and results in plasma concentrations of 0.4–3 μg/ml with a half-life of approximately 70 days. Clofazimine is widely distributed through reticuloendothelial tissues, especially in the liver, spleen, lung, adrenals, adipose tissue, and skin lesions. Red-orange crystals of clofazimine can be observed microscopically in phagocytic reticuloendothelial cells. Precise concentrations in tissues can only be estimated because of the very uneven distribution of the drug. It is largely unmetabolized and subsequently excreted slowly, with less than 1 percent of a dose appearing in urine. Biliary excretion appears to be the major route of disposition of clofazimine. Excretion also occurs in breast milk. A dosage of 100 mg/day has been calculated to eventually result in total accumulation of at least 10 g of drug in human tissue.[75]

Adverse Reactions. Gastrointestinal intolerance may occur. Skin pigmentation is the major side effect from drug accumulation and results in red-brown to almost black skin discoloration in susceptible people. Other side effects are negligible.

Usage. Clofazimine is expensive. Its principal role has been as therapy for sulfone-resistant infections and for people who are sulfone intolerant, usually because of severe sulfone-associated ENL or lepra reactions. These reactions occur much less frequently with clofazimine than with dapsone,[76] possibly promoted by the anti-inflammatory properties of clofazimine.

Availability and Dosage. Clofazimine is available as Lamprene in 100 mg capsules. For monotherapy, its dose has ranged from 300 mg monthly to 600 mg daily and has usually been 100–300 mg/day. The administration of clofazimine alone once weekly or less frequently has resulted in diminished efficacy.[76] In combination therapeutic regimens for multibacillary disease, the recommended dosage has been either 300 mg monthly or 50–100 mg daily.

ADDITIONAL DRUGS FOR THE TREATMENT OF MULTIBACILLARY LEPROSY

Amithiozone (Thiacetazone)

Derivation, structure, pharmacokinetics, untoward reactions, and dosage of this thiosemicarbazone are described under second-line drugs for tuberculosis.

Usage. Amithiozone's efficacy is greater in tuberculoid than in lepromatous (multibacillary) disease. The drug can be administered when sulfones cannot be tolerated. Considerable cross-resistance occurs with sulfones. Amithiozone is not available in the United States.

Long-Acting Sulfonamides

Hypersensitivity reactions including erythema multiforme (Stevens-Johnson syndrome) can result from long-acting sulfonamides. Used with varying degrees of success for the treatment of leprosy, they have no particular advantage over sulfones, share cross-resistance with them, and consequently have been supplanted by the sulfones.

Ethionamide and Prothionamide

Ethionamide has been described under second-line agents for tuberculosis. It and its congener prothionamide possess similar pharmacokinetics and dosing and provide alternatives to clofazimine in multidrug regimens for multibacillary disease, principally in people who are unable to tolerate or who will not accept clofazimine due to skin pigmentation. Ethionamide and prothionamide are apparently weakly bactericidal for *M. leprae*. Both drugs are available as 125 or 250 mg tablets. The dosage with either is 375–500 mg daily.[64] Both agents are expensive, cause a considerable degree of gastrointestinal intolerance, and rarely cause drug-induced hepatitis.

CHEMOTHERAPY-ASSOCIATED REACTIONS IN LEPROSY

Febrile reactions in people with leprosy can be treated with acetylsalicylic acid (aspirin) in conventional dosages. Chloroquine phosphate (Aralen, Avloclor, Resochin) in a dose of 250–500 mg of diphosphate daily has been used in some centers for treatment-associated reactions. Methylprednisolone, 60 mg daily initially, followed by tapering of the dosage, has been reasonably efficacious.[77] Thalidomide in an initial dosage of 400 mg daily has been used to lessen therapy-associated reactions. Thalidomide therapy should not be abruptly discontinued due to exacerbations of reactions. Consequently, a gradually tapering dosage and even maintenance with 50 mg/day has been recommended.[78] Because of teratogenic potential, thalidomide should never be administered to pregnant women or those of childbearing age. Patients who manifest puzzling severe reactions are best managed by a specialist.[67]

REFERENCES

1. Mandell GL, Sande MA. Drugs used in the chemotherapy of tuberculosis and leprosy. In: Gilman AS, Goodman LS, Rall TW, et al., eds. The Pharmacological Basis of Therapeutics. ed. 7. New York: MacMillan Publishing Co, 1985:199–1218.
2. Kucers A, Bennett NM. Drugs Mainly for Tuberculosis. Part III. In: *The Use of Antibiotics*. 4th ed. Philadelphia: JB Lippincott, 1987:1351–437.
3. Pratt WB. Chemotherapy of tuberculosis. In: Chemotherapy of Infection. New York: Oxford University Press; 1977:231–62.
4. Stead WW, Dutt AK. Chemotherapy for tuberculosis today. Am Rev Respir Dis. 1982;125(suppl 3):94–101.
5. National ACCP Consensus Conference on Tuberculosis. Standard therapy for tuberculosis 1985. Chest. 1985;87(suppl 2):117–24.
6. Tuberculosis Chemotherapy Trials Committee. Interim report to the Medical Research Council; the treatment of pulmonary tuberculosis with isoniazid. Br Med J. 1952;2:735–46.
7. Herman, RP, Weber MM. site of action of isoniazid on the electron transport chain and its relationship to nicotinamide adenine dinucleotide regulation in *Mycobacterium phlei*. Antimicrob Agents Chemother. 1980;17:450–4.
8. Costello HD, Caras GJ, Snider DE. Drug resistance among previously treated tuberculosis patients: A brief report. Am Rev Respir Dis. 1980;121:313–6.
9. Carpenter JL, Covelli HD, Avant ME, et al. Drug resistant *Mycobacterium tuberculosis* in Korean isolates. Am Rev Respir Dis. 1982;126:1092–5.
10. Bowersox DW, Winterbauer RH, Steward GL, et al. Isoniazid doses in patients with renal failure. N Engl J Med. 1973;289:84–7.
11. Grossman LA, Kaplan HJ, Brittingham TE. Jaundice and death from isoniazid. J Tenn Med Assoc. 1970;63:23–8.
12. Kopanoff DE, Snider DE, Caras GJ. Isoniazid-related hepatitis. Am Rev Respir Dis. 1978;117:991–1001.
13. Centers for Disease Control. National Consensus Conference on Tuberculosis. Preventive treatment of tuberculosis. Chest. 1985;87(suppl 2):128–32.
14. Gronhagen-Riska C, Hellstrom PE, Froseth B. Predisposing factors in hepatitis induced by isoniazid-rifampin treatment of tuberculosis. Am Rev Respir Dis. 1978;118:461–6.

15. McGlynn KA, Lustabader ED, Sharrar, RG, et al. Isoniazid prophylaxis in hepatitis B carriers. Am Rev Respir Dis. 1986;134:666–8.
16. Gangadharam PRJ. Isoniazid, rifampin, and hepatotoxicity. Am Rev Respir Dis. 1986;133:963–5.
17. Falk A. US Veterans Administration–Armed Forces cooperative study on the chemotherapy of tuberculosis. XIII. Tuberculous meningitis in adults with special reference to survival, neurologic residuals, and work status. Am Rev Respir Dis. 1965;91:823–31.
18. Falk A. US Veterans Administration–Armed Forces cooperative study on the chemotherapy of tuberculosis. XII. Results of treatment in miliary tuberculosis: A followup study of 570 adult patients. Am Rev Respir Dis. 1965;91:6–12.
19. American Thoracic Society. Intermittent therapy for adults with tuberculosis. Am Rev Respir Dis. 1974;110:374–6.
20. Crowle AJ. Studies of antituberculosis chemotherapy with an in vitro model of human tuberculosis. Semin Respir Infect. 1986;1:262–4.
21. Acocella G, Bonollo M, Garimoldi M, et al. Kinetics of rifampicin and isoniazid administered alone and in combination to normal subjects and patients with liver disease. Gut. 1972;13:47–53.
22. Stottmeier KD. Emergence of rifampin-resistant *Mycobacterium tuberculosis* in Massachusetts. J Infect Dis. 1976;133:88–90.
23. Newman R, Doster BE, Murray FJ, et al. Rifampin in initial treatment of pulmonary tuberculosis. A US Public Health Service tuberculosis therapy trial. Am Rev Respir Dis. 1974;109:216–32.
24. Thompson JE. The effect of rifampicin on liver morphology in tuberculous alcoholics. Aust NZ J Med. 1976;6:111–6.
25. Rahajoe NN, Rahajoe N, Boediman I, et al. The treatment of tuberculous meningitis in children with a combination of isoniazid, rifampicin, and streptomycin—preliminary report. Tubercle. 1979;60:245–50.
26. Braber CD, Jebaily J, Galphin RL, et al. Light chain proteinuria and humoral immunocompetence in tuberculosis patients treated with rifampin. Am Rev Respir Dis. 1973;107:713–7.
27. Grassi GG, Pozzi E. Effect of rifampin on delayed hypersensitivity reactions. J Infect Dis. 1972;126:542–4.
28. Flynn CT, Rainford DJ, Hope E. Acute renal failure and rifampin: Danger of unsuspected intermittent dosage. Br Med J. 1974;2:482.
29. Dutt AK, Stead WW. Present chemotherapy for tuberculosis. J Infect Dis. 1982;146:698–704.
30. Baciewicz AM, Self TH, Bekemeyer WB. Update on rifampin drug interactions. Arch Intern Med. 1987;147:565–8.
31. Langhof E, Madsen S. Rapid metabolism of cyclosporin and prednisone in kidney transplant patient receiving tuberculostatic treatment. Lancet. 1983;2:1031.
32. Greene JB, Sidhu GS, Lewin S, et al. *Mycobacterium avium intracellulare:* A cause of disseminated life-threatening infection in homosexuals and drug abusers. Ann Intern Med. 1982;97:539–46.
33. Heifets LB, Iseman MD, Lindholm-Levy PJ, et al. Determination of ansamycin MICs for *Mycobacterium avium* complex in liquid medium by radiometric and conventional methods. Antimicrob Agents Chemother. 1985;28:570–5.
34. Masur H, Tuazon C, Gill V, et al. Effect of combined clofazimine and ansamycin therapy on *Mycobacterium avium–Mycobacterium intracellulare* bacteremia in patients with AIDS. J Infect Dis. 1987;155:127–9.
35. O'Brien RJ, Lyle MA, Snider DE Jr. Rifabutin (ansamycin LM 427): A new rifamycin-S derivative for the treatment of mycobacterial diseases. Rev Infect Dis. 1987;9:519–30.
36. Sanders WE Jr, Cacciatore R, Valdez J, et al. Activity of amikacin against mycobacteria in vitro and in experimental infections with *M. tuberculosis.* Am Rev Respir Dis. 1976;113(suppl 4):59.
37. Nalin R, Potar M, David HL. Pyrazinamide is not effective against intracellularly growing *Mycobacterium tuberculosis*. Antimicrob Agents Chemother. 1987;31:287.
38. Girling DJ. The hepatic toxicity of antituberculous regiments containing isoniazid, rifampicin, and pyrazinamide. Tubercle. 1978;59:13–32.
39. Zierski M, Bek E. Side effects of drug regimens used in short-course chemotherapy for pulmonary tuberculosis. A controlled clinical study. Tubercle. 1980;61:41–9.
40. McClatchy JK, Kanes W, Davidson PT, et al. Cross-resistance in *M. tuberculosis* to kenamycin, capreomycin, and viomycin. Tubercle. 1977;58:29–34.
41. Cynamon MH, Palmer GS. In vitro activity of amoxicillin in combination with clavulanic acid against *Mycobacterium tuberculosis*. Antimicrob Agents Chemother 1983;24:429–31.
42. Nozawa RT, Kato H, Yokota T, et al. Susceptibility of intra- and extracellular *Mycobacterium avium-intracellulare* to cephem antibiotics. Antimicrob Agents Chemother. 1985;27:132–134.
43. Wallace RJ Jr, Swenson JM, Silcox VA, et al. Treatment of nonpulmonary infections due to *Mycobacterium fortuitum* and *Mycobacterium chelonei* on the basis of in vitro susceptibilities. J Infect Dis. 1985;152:500–14.
44. Crawford JT, Bates JH. Isolation of plasmids from mycobacteria. Infect Immun. 1979;24:979–81.
45. Sommers HM, McClatchy JK. Laboratory diagnoses of the mycobacterioses. Cumitech 16. In: Morello JA, ed. Cumulative Techniques and Procedures in Microbiology. Washington, DC: American Society for Microbiology; 1983.
46. Irwin RS, Pratter MR, Corwin RW, et al. Pulmonary infection with *Mycobacterium chelonei:* Successful treatment with one drug based on disk diffusion susceptibility data. J Infect Dis. 1981;145:772.
47. Hawkins CC, Gold JWM, Whimbey E, et al. *Mycobacterium avium* complex infections in patients with the acquired immunodeficiency syndrome. Ann Intern Med. 1986;105:184–8.
48. Hobby GL, Redmond WB, Runyon EH, et al. A study on pulmonary disease associated with mycobacteria other than *Mycobacterium tuberculosis:* Identification and characterization of the mycobacteria. XVIII. A report of the Veterans Administration–Armed Forces cooperative study. Am Rev Respir Dis. 1967;95:954–71.
49. Rynearson TK, Shronts JS, Wolinsky E. Rifampin: In vitro effect on atypical mycobacteria. Am Rev Respir Dis. 1971;104:272–74.
50. Sanders WJ, Wolinsky E. In vitro susceptibility of *Mycobacterium marinum* to eight antimicrobial agents. Antimicrob Agents Chemother. 1980;18:529–31.
51. Leach RH, Fenner F. Studies on *Mycobacterium ulcerans* and *Mycobacterium balnei*. III. Growth in semisynthetic culture media of Dubos and drug sensitivity in vitro and in vivo. Aust J Exp Biol Med Sci. 1954;32:835–52.
52. Nozawa RT, Kato H, Yokota T. Intra- and extracellular susceptibility of *Mycobacterium avium-intracellulare* complex to aminoglycoside antibiotics. Antimicrob Agents Chemother. 1984;26:841–4.
53. Sanders WE Jr, Hartwig EC, Schneider NJ, et al. Susceptibility of organisms in the *Mycobacterium fortuitum* complex to antituberculous and other antimicrobial agents. Antimicrob Agents Chemother. 1977;12:295–7.
54. Clegg HW, Foster MT, Sanders WE Jr, et al. Infection due to organisms of the *Mycobacterium fortuitum* complex after augmentation mammoplasty: Clinical and epidemiologic features. J Infect Dis. 1983;147:427–33.
55. Molavi A, Weinstein L. In vitro activity of erythromycin against atypical mycobacteria. J Infect Dis. 1971;123:216–9.
56. Gangadharam PRJ, Candler ER. Activity of some antileprosy compounds against *Mycobacterium intracellulare* in vitro. Am Rev Respir Dis. 1977;115:705–8.
57. Cynamon MH, Palmer GS. In vitro susceptibility of *Mycobacterium fortuitum* to *N*-formidoyl thienamycin and several cephamycins. Antimicrob Agents Chemother. 1982;22:1079–81.
58. Swenson JM, Thornsberry C, Silcox VA. Rapidly growing mycobacteria: Testing of susceptibility to 34 antimicrobial agents by broth microdilution. Antimicrob Agents Chemother. 1982;22:186–92.
59. Loria PR. Minocycline hydrochloride treatment for atypical acid-fast infection. Arch Dermatol. 1976;112:517–9.
60. Donta ST, Smith PW, Levitz RE, et al. Therapy of *Mycobacterium marinum* infections. Use of tetracyclines vs rifampin. Arch Intern Med. 1986;146:902–4.
61. Yajdo DM, Nassos PS, Hadley WK. Therapeutic implication of inhibition versus killing of *Mycobacterium avium* complex by antimicrobial agents. Antimicrob Agents Chemother. 1987;31:117–20.
62. Brown TH. The rapidly growing mycobacteria—*Mycobacterium fortuitum* and *Mycobacterium chelonei*. Infect Control. 1985;6:283–7.
63. US Public Health Service Centers for Disease Control. Increase in prevalence of leprosy caused by dapsone-resistant *Mycobacterium leprae*. MMWR. 1982;30:637–8.
64. WHO Study Group. Chemotherapy of Leprosy for Control Programmes. Geneva: World Health Organization; 1982.
65. Levy L, Peters JH. Susceptibility of *Mycobacterium leprae* to dapsone as a determinant of patient response to acedapsone. Antimicrob Agents Chemother. 1976;9:102–12.
66. Pearson JMH, Rees RJW, Waters MFR. Sulphone resistance in leprosy. A review of one hundred proven clinical cases. Lancet. 1975;2:69–72.
67. Case records of the Massachusetts General Hospital. Weekly clinicopathological exercises. Case 49-1985. Erythema nodosum leprosum reaction in patient with lepromatous leprosy. N Engl J Med. 1985;313:1464–72.
68. Adverse reactions to dapsone (editorial). Lancet. 1981;2:184–5.
69. Peters JH, Murray JF, Gordon GR, et al. Acedapsone treatment of leprosy patients: Response versus drug disposition. Am J Trop Med Hyg. 1977;26:127–36.
70. Russell DA, Shepard CC, McRae DH, et al. Acedapsone (DADDS) treatment of leprosy patients in the Karimui of Papua New Guinea: Status at six years. Am J Trop Med Hyg. 1975;24:485–95.
71. Shepard CC, Levy L, Fasal P. Further experience with the rapid bactericidal effect of rifampin on *Mycobacterium leprae*. Am J Trop Med Hyg. 1974;23:1120–4.
72. Yawalkar SJ, Languillon J, Hajra SK, et al. Once-monthly rifampicin plus dapsone in initial treatment of lepromatous leprosy. Lancet. 1982;1:1199–202.
73. Pattyn SR. Rifabutin and rifapentime compared with rifampin against *Mycobacterium leprae* in mice. Antimicrob Agents Chemother. 1987;31:134.
74. Niwa Y, Sakance T, Miyachi Y, et al. Oxygen metabolism in phagocytes of leprotic patients: Enhanced endogenous superoxide dismutase activity and hydroxyl radical generation by clofazimine. J Clin Microbiol. 1984;20:837–42.
75. Levy L. Pharmacologic studies of clofazimine. Am J Trop Med Hyg. 1974;23:1097–109.
76. US Leprosy Panel. Spaced clofazimine therapy of lepromatous leprosy. Am J Trop Med Hyg. 1976;25:437–44.
77. Grove DI, Warren KS, Mahmoud AAF. Algorithms in the diagnosis and management of exotic diseases. XV. Leprosy. 1976;134:205–10.
78. Convit J, Browne SG, Languillon J, et al. Therapy of leprosy. Bull WHO. 1970;42:667–72.

33. ANTIFUNGAL AGENTS

JOHN E. BENNETT

The broad array of topical agents already available and the gratifying number of systemic agents now entering clinical trial have necessitated that this chapter be limited to major drugs either now on the market or likely to be marketed in the near future.

TOPICAL AGENTS

Topical Agents for Cutaneous Use

Use of topical agents is confined to infections of the epidermis, hair, nails, and cornea. This form of application is not effective in deeper cutaneous infections, such as sporotrichosis, blastomycosis, or chromomycosis. The choice between treating superficial infections with a topical or systemic agent depends on the fungus and on the site and extent of the lesion. For example, topical therapy is rarely used for ringworm of the scalp, nails, or extensive *Trichophyton rubrum* lesions of the trunk. The efficacy of topical agents in ringworm of the beard or in chronic noninflammatory sole and palm lesions also tends to be poor. Among the topical agents, the choice of formulation is important. Creams or solutions are preferred for fissured or inflamed intertriginous areas such as on the toe webs, groin, or scrotum. Use of powder, whether administered by a shake container or aerosol, is confined to mild lesions in those same areas or to preventive therapy in patients with repeated relapses of tinea pedis. Sprays are not recommended for the face. None of the preparations for cutaneous use should be applied to the vagina or eye. Secondary bacterial infection requires ancillary measures. Despite some antibacterial effect of the imidazoles in vitro, none of the antifungals included here have useful antibacterial activity.

The plethora of agents used for topical application necessitates that older agents with limited indications, such as iodine, sulfur, and gentian violet, not be discussed. Undecylenic acid and its salts, while widely used in nonprescription formulations, has too little efficacy to warrant further comment. While a list of nonprescription drugs would also include tolnaftate and miconazole, other agents can be expected to be added. Changes are also frequent as to which formulations of antifungal agents are marketed in combination with corticosteroids or antibacterial agents.

Details of the treatment of cutaneous mycoses are beyond the scope of this chapter, except to note that the agents listed below are generally applied twice daily and do not differ substantially in the duration of therapy necessary for cure.

Salicylic and Benzoic Acids (Whitfield's ointment). Salicylic acid is widely used in topical preparations as a keratolytic agent, often combined with other agents. The ointment marketed for nonprescription use in ringworm usually contains 3% salicylic acid and 6% benzoic acid. Although Whitfield's ointment can be used in mild tinea pedis, occlusive effects of the ointment and mild irritation of the salicylic acid make the undiluted preparation inappropriate for inflamed or macerated toe webs or scrotal infections. Except for its low cost, there is little to recommend the use of Whitfield's ointment in ringworm.

The most commonly used topical preparations for cutaneous use are given in Table 1. *Ciclopirox olamine* (Loprox), *haloprigin* (Halotex), and *naftifine* (Naftin) creams are all active against both ringworm, tinea versicolor, and candidiasis. *Tolnaftate* (Tinactin, Aftate, Zeasorb-AF) is active against ringworm and tinea versicolor but not against candidiasis.

TABLE 1. Topical Antifungals for Cutaneous Application

	Preparations Available in the United States			
Agent	*Cream*	*Solution*	*Ointment*	*Powder*
Polyenes				
Nystatin	X		X	X
Amphotericin	X		X	
Imidazoles and triazoles				
Clotrimazole	X	X	X	
Econazole	X			
Ketoconazole	X			
Miconazole	X			
Other agents				
Ciclopirox	X			
Haloprigin	X	X		
Naftifine	X			
Tolnaftate	X	X		X

Polyenes. A large number of macrolide polyene antibiotics are known and have broad-spectrum antifungal activity in vitro.[1] Topically, they are useful only against *Candida*, not ringworm. The hypertrophic skin lesions of chronic mucocutaneous candidiasis do not respond to these antibiotics, although macerated or intertriginous lesions typically respond well. These polyenes are derived by biosynthesis from aerobic actinomycetes, are poorly soluble in water, and share a common mechanism of action. The antifungal activity depends upon binding to the cytoplasmic membrane sterols such as ergosterol and thereby increasing membrane permeability.[2] Other pharmacologic properties are discussed later. Only *nystatin* and *amphotericin B* are readily available for topical use in the United States. *Natamycin* (pimaricin, Natacyn) is available from the manufacturer (Alcon) as a 5% suspension for ophthalmic use in fungal keratitis.

Imidazoles. These synthetic compounds and the triazoles, a closely related class, remain the object of active drug development. Lists of these agents rapidly become outdated. A current list of compounds marketed in the United States and their commercial names includes *clotrimazole* (Lotrimin, Mycelex), *econazole* nitrate (Spectazole), and *ketoconazole* (Nizoral). *Bifonazole* and *tioconazole*, both imidazoles, and *terconazole*, a triazole, have been effective in clinical trials, and some are available overseas. Others are available only for vaginal use, as will be discussed later. The structural formulas of the most commonly used agents are included in Figure 1. These compounds all share the same mechanism of action and the same indications for use. As will be discussed later in this chapter, in systemic use the compounds differ in solubility, human metabolism, and side effects. The imidazoles and triazoles inhibit fungal cytochrome P-450-dependent 14-α-demethylase, blocking the conversion of lanosterol and other 14-methylsterols to ergosterol.[3] The abnormal sterols interfere with membrane permeability. At the high concentrations that might be achieved topically, these agents directly damage the cytoplasmic membrane. The antifungal spectrum is extremely broad in vitro but fungistatic. Clinical efficacy has been demonstrated in ringworm of the body, foot, hand, and perineum, as well as in cutaneous candidiasis and tinea versicolor.[4]

Topical Agents for Vaginal Use

Vulvovaginal candidiasis is a common disease that can cause substantial chronic discomfort. Except for ineffective nostrums, all the agents are available by prescription only. Both tablets and creams are marketed for once-a-day use, preferably at bedtime to facilitate retention. If candidiasis has extended onto the vulva or perineum, creams that can be applied topically as well as vaginally may have an advantage over tablets. Cream dispensers are designed to administer 5 g per use. The differences between creams and vaginal troches are less important

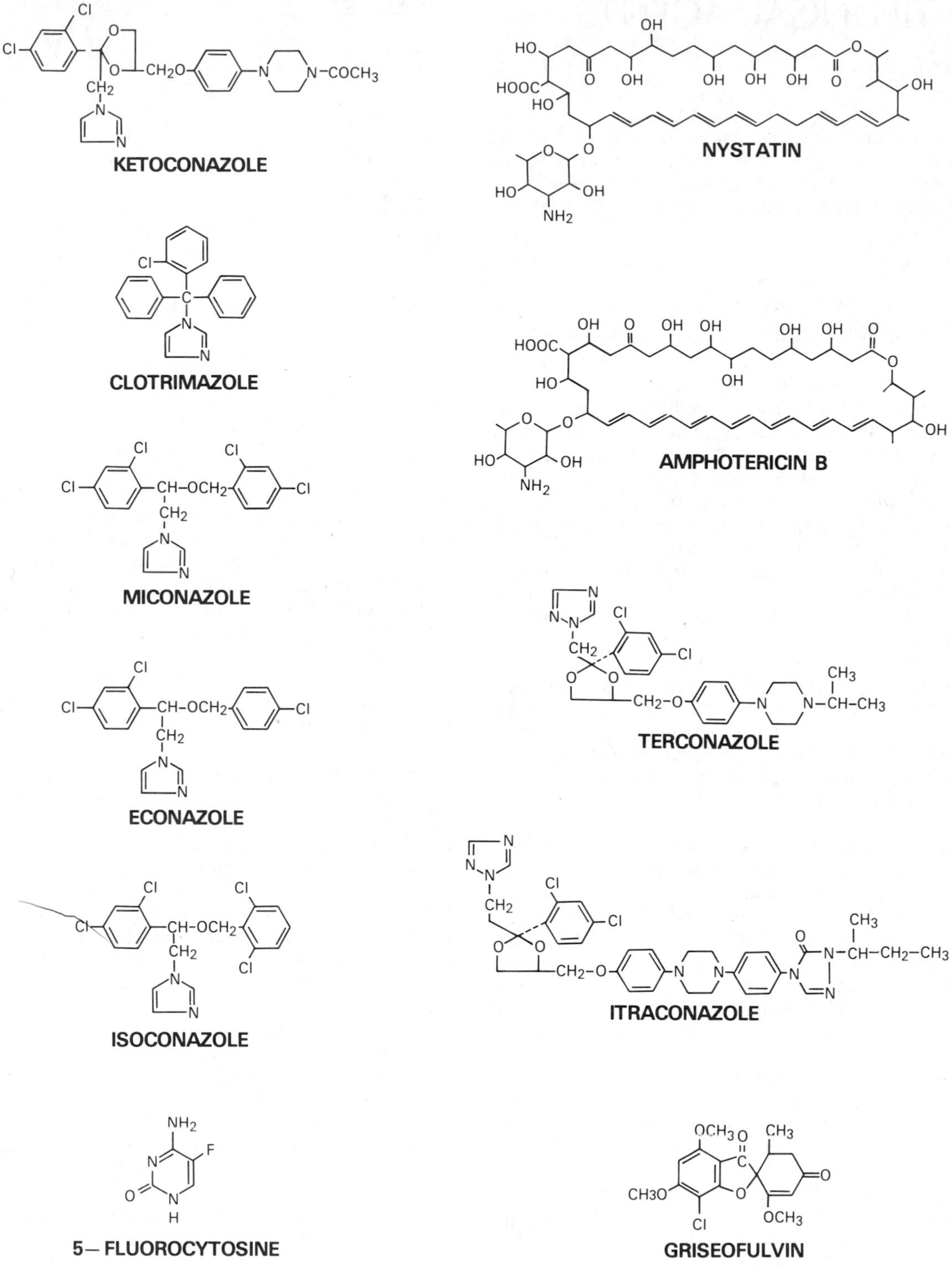

FIG. 1. Structures of the major antifungal agents.

than correct insertion deep in the vagina. Some preparations have a patient package insert with a clear set of instructions. The duration of therapy is longer for polyene troches than for the imidazoles, leading to increasing use of the latter class. The duration of therapy for the imidazoles, as stated in the literature or in the package insert, seems more dependent on the design of the original clinical studies than on the efficacy of the product. Most of the studies of imidazoles have shown short-term efficacy of roughly 80–90 percent if high-risk patients are excluded, such as patients relapsing from recent treatment.[5–8] Data on late relapse after treatment with these drug are hard to find, although relapse is acknowledged to be common. Ingestion of nystatin tablets to decrease the fecal *Candida* concentration has been recommended to aid treatment and prevent relapse of vulvovaginal candidiasis, but the evidence of efficacy remains unconvincing. Although a fecal reservoir for relapse appears likely, the reduction in fecal colony counts by oral nystatin is small. Even the massive doses of oral nystatin used in laminar flow units usually have not eradicated *Candida* from the feces.

Adverse effects of vaginal therapy are few. Allergy to any

one imidazole probably precludes the use of other imidazoles, Local irritation or burning, rarely a serious problem, does vary among preparations. Some systemic absorption, generally less than 10 percent of the dose, has been documented for many of the vaginal imidazoles and may be a general phenomenon. This is of theoretical interest in that it might cause birth defects during the first trimester of pregnancy or alter the metabolism of other medications taken by the patient. However, none of these consequences has been observed. Systemic absorption of vaginal polyenes probably does not occur. A list of agents currently available for vaginal use is given in Table 2. Compounds available in Canada, such as *econazole* (Ecostatin), or only overseas, such as isoconazole, are not listed. *Butoconazole* (Femstat), *miconazole* (Monistat 3 and Monistat 7), and econazole are formulated as the nitrate for vaginal use. The triazole *terconazole* (Terazol 3 and Terazol 7) and *clotrimazole* (Gync-Lotrimin and Mycelex-G) are marketed as the base, not as a salt. Trade names differ in Canada.

ORAL THERAPY FOR SUPERFICIAL MYCOSES

Agents for the Treatment of Oral Candidiasis (Thrush)

Nystatin (Mycostatin, Nilstat, and generic), named for New York State, is produced by *Streptomyces noursei*. The drug is available as an oral suspension of 100,000 units/ml. Adults should swish 5–10 ml around in the mouth three times a day. Swallowing the suspension rather than expectorating it may help to treat subclinical esophageal candidiasis in immunosuppressed patients. Nystatin suspension is not absorbed from the gastrointestinal tract and, except for its bitter taste, is remarkably free from adverse effects. Vaginal tablets of nystatin can be held in the mouth and used as troches, but these are bitter and not designed for this use. A better alternative is the use of *clotrimazole* troches. These pleasant-tasting 10-mg tablets are effective in oral thrush when used five times a day.[9] Each tablet should not be chewed but kept in the mouth until it dissolves. Although some absorption occurs after the drug is swallowed, no adverse effects or systemic efficacy occurs. Oral ketoconazole, 200–400 mg/day, is also effective in oral candidiasis and may the drug of choice when concomitant esophagitis is present.[10–12] Unfortunately, none of the above regimens is very effective for oral or esophageal candidiasis in severely neutropenic patients. Intravenous amphotericin B may be necessary in such patients.

Oral Therapy of Superficial Cutaneous Infections

Systemic therapy of ringworm of the scalp, beard, and nails of the hand is preferred to topical therapy. Chronic noninflammatory ringworm of the soles and palms, as well as extensive ringworm of the trunk or groin, may also require systemic therapy. The preferred drug for these indications is griseofulvin because of its efficacy and low incidence of adverse effects. Although ketoconazole can be used for griseofulvin-resistant ringworm, the chance of serious side effects indicates that readily remedial causes of griseofulvin failures should be sought: erratic drug ingestion, too low a dose, and incorrect diagnosis. Candidiasis of the nail or skin, particularly of the groin, can resemble ringworm closely and does not respond to griseofulvin. None of the currently available topical or systemic agents is very effective against ringworm of the toenail. White superficial onychomycosis, while rare, is more responsive to griseofulvin. In young adult women who are concerned about the cosmetic problem, a 12- to 18-month course of griseofulvin may be worth a trial. Duration of therapy depends on the rate of nail growth, which may be slower than normal.

Griseofulvin. This agent, derived from a species of *Penicillium*, is active against ringworm but not against *Candida* or tinea versicolor. It is poorly active topically but reaches the skin and hair after ingestion. Absorption is favored by reducing the particle size and perhaps by ingestion with a fatty meal. A microcrystalline form (generic, Fulvicin-U/F, Grifulvin V and Grisactin) is available as 125-, 250-, and 500-mg tablets, plus a pediatric suspension of 125 mg/5 ml. The ultramicrocrystalline form (Fulvicin-P/G, Gris-PEG, and Grisactin Ultra) comes in 125-, 165-, 250-, and 330-mg tablets. The two forms have comparable efficacy. Griseofulvin is metabolized in the liver with a serum half life of 24–36 hours. Blood levels can be depressed by phenobarbital therapy and may require increasing the griseofulvin dose. Conversely, metabolism of warfarin anticoagulants is increased by griseofulvin. Adverse reactions to griseofulvin are uncommon. Headache may be observed early in therapy but usually disappears with continued use. Allergic reactions can occur, apparently unrelated to penicillin allergy. Hepatotoxic reactions have been observed in patients with acute intermittent porphyria. A variety of other side effects have also been observed, but a causal relationship is much less clear. Safety during pregnancy has not been established.

The usual daily dose is 500, 750, or 1000 mg daily for the microcrystalline drug, with children receiving 10 mg/kg. The 500 mg/day dose is reserved for mild infections and small adults. A dose of 330 mg daily is recommended for the ultramicrocrystalline form. Either preparation can be given once daily at the end of a meal, but dividing the dose into twice daily administration may help maintain therapeutic levels in the epidermis and is recommended for refractory infections.

Ketoconazole. The pharmacologic properties of this synthetic agent will be discussed later. Of relevance here is that the drug readily reaches the skin surface from the blood, most prominently by the way of apocrine sweat. Ketoconazole has definite activity against ringworm, chronic mucocutaneous candidiasis, and tinea versicolor.[13] At least in part because ketoconazole is reserved for griseofulvin failures, the efficacy of ketoconazole may not be striking. Certainly, the poor efficacy and potential toxicity of ketoconazole contraindicate its use in onychomycosis. In contrast, ketoconazole is the drug of choice for patients with chronic mucocutaneous candidiasis.[10] For tinea versicolor, topical therapy with selenium sufide shampoo or one of the many other agents is preferred. However, oral ketoconazole can be a very effective and useful drug for patients with extensive relapsing tinea versicolor.

Terbinafine. This oral agent, an allylamine structurally related to naftifine, has been evaluated in Europe for treatment of ringworm. In early short-term studies, the agent appeared to be comparable to griseofulvin. Evidence that the drug and its

TABLE 2. Topical Agents for Vaginal Candidiasis

Agent	Formulation[a]	Days of Therapy
Polyene		
Nystatin (generic, Korostatin, Mycostatin, Nilstat)	100,000 unit tablet	14
Imidazole/Triazole		
Butoconazole (Femstat)	2% cream	3[b] 6[c]
Clotrimazole (Gyne-Lotrimin, Mycelex-G)	100-mg tablet	7 for 1 tablet/day 3 for 2 tablets/day[b]
	500-mg tablet	1
	1% cream	7–14
Miconazole (Monistat)	100-mg suppository	7
	200-mg suppository	3
	2% cream	7
Terconazole (Terazol)	0.4% cream	7
	80-mg suppository	3

[a] All formulations are designed to be used once a day, preferably at bedtime. The creams are dispensed in 5 gs per use, irrespective of concentration. Tablets are for vaginal use.
[b] Recommendation for nonpregnant women.
[c] Recommendation for pregnant women.

metabolites accumulate substantially during long-term administration may limit its use in onychomycosis.

Systemic Therapy of Candida Vulvovaginitis

Ketoconazole. The efficacy of oral ketoconazole in *Candida* vulvovaginitis is comparable to that of the topical imidazoles and triazoles. Ketoconazole is given as 400 mg/day for 5 days. However, the drug is contraindicated during pregnancy because of its potential teratogenicity and during breast-feeding because of its secretion into breast milk. Hepatotoxic and other adverse reactions also overweigh the convenience of oral administration and the possibility of use during menstruation. Perhaps for the woman with smear-positive chronic relapsing vaginal candidiasis, prophylactic courses could be considered, as recommended by Sobel.[14]

TREATMENT OF DEEP MYCOSIS

Oral iodides are useful only in cutaneous sporotrichosis and possibly in *Basidiobolus* infections, and therefore will not be included here. The of hydroxystilbamidine in blastomycosis has been eclipsed by better drugs and is also omitted.

Amphotericin B

Structure and Mechanism of Action. Amphotericin B is produced by *Streptomyces nodosus*. The major mechanism of antifungal effect appears to be combination of the drug with ergosterol, fungisterol, or similar sterols in the fungal cytoplasmic membrane, altering membrane permeability.[2] Drug-resistant strains in usually susceptible species remain a rarity. Other proposed mechanisms of chemotherapeutic effect include oxidative damage[15] and immunomodulation. Although the seven conjugated double bonds (Fig. 1) are essential for activity, alteration of the carboxyl primary amino group or the internal lactam linkage has also decreased activity. The negligible aqueous solubility of this drug at neutral pH has led to several formulations for intravenous use.

Desoxycholate Formulation. The commercially available intravenous formulation is a colloidal complex of amphotericin B, 50 mg, and desoxycholate, 41 mg, together with 25.2 mg sodium phosphate buffer. When the desoxycholate-amphotericin B powder is dissolved in 5% dextrose in water, a clear yellow colloidal solution results. Although low ionic strength additives such as hydrocortisone or heparin may be added, the solution becomes cloudy due to aggregation of the colloid if sodium or potassium salts are added to the bottle. The likelihood that cloudy solutions give lower blood levels has led to the recommendation that cloudy solutions be discarded. The colloidal solution is stable at room temperature under normal illumination for the usual infusion intervals. The older recommendation that infusion bottles be covered with foil to protect them from light has been convincingly demonstrated to be wrong.[16] Infusion bottles can also be stored for 24–48 hours under refrigeration before use. Another incorrect assertion has been that hydrocortisone added to the bottle inactivates amphotericin B. An important precaution is that 0.22-μm filters should not be placed in the infusion line because some drug may be removed. Filters with 0.45-μm-diameter pores do not remove drug.

Other Formulations. Alternative solutions to the problem of intravenous infusion have been proposed because of the toxicity of the desoxycholate complex. Esterification of the carboxyl group and N-acylation result in water-soluble micellar preparations but have reduced antifungal activity. Various salts of the methyl ester were given to animals and a small group of patients and seemed to cause less nephrotoxicity. Leukoencephalopathy with this derivative has halted further clinical studies.[17] None of the N-acyl derivatives have reached clinical trial.

Currently, interest has centered on liposomal encapsulated preparations of amphotericin B. In these preparations amphotericin B is intercalated into the phospholipid bilayer membrane, rather than included in the enclosed aqueous phase. Two entirely different formulations have reached early clinical trial. One preparation is 5 mol% amphotericin B in a 7:3 mixture of dimyristoylphosphatidylcholine:dimyristoylphosphatidyl glycerol (DMPC:DMPG). This preparation is quite heterogeneous in size and shape on scanning electron microscopy, containing both sheets and multilamellar spherical liposomes, the former containing more amphotericin B than the latter. The size of the sheets and spheres ranges from roughly 0.5 to 6 μm,[18] which is considerably larger than the micelles of the desoxycholate complex. Although little data on toxicity and pharmacology have been reported, more than 30 patients have received doses of 1 mg/kg or more, apparently with little toxicity. Blood levels with comparable preparations have been too low to be measured readily at these doses. The majority of the drug appears to be cleared by macrophages in the lung, liver, and spleen. Chemotherapeutic activity in experimental murine infections was not lost, although larger doses were necessary for an effect equivalent to that of the desoxycholate complex. Future clinical studies are planned with 30 mol% amphotericin B in the same phospholipid, a formulation that provides only sheets and ribbons, not spherical particles.[19] A different approach to liposomal amphotericin B has been to create unilamellar liposomes less than 0.2 μm in diameter. The two unilamellar preparations given to humans thus far both used a fatty acid with a longer chain length than DMPC:DMPG (i.e., stearic acid rather than myristic acid) and differed in net charge and the presence of cholesterol. Pharmacologic studies on one of these preparations have found blood levels at least as high as with the desoxycholate complex, but with much less toxicity.[20] No data on the efficacy of the unilamellar preparations in humans have been reported to date, although efficacy in experimental murine candidiasis and cryptococcosis has been reported.

Pharmacology. Concentrations of amphotericin B in biologic fluids have usually been measured by bioassay,[21] but high-pressure liquid chromatography,[22] ^{86}Rb release,[23] and radiometric respirometry[24] have been described. Despite the proliferation of methods, routine determination of amphotericin B serum, urine, or cerebrospinal fluid concentrations has no definite clinical value. Nonetheless, amphotericin B assays have revealed some remarkable pharmacologic properties of this drug. When colloidal amphotericin B is admixed in serum, desoxycholate separates from amphotericin B,[25] and more than 95 percent of the latter binds to serum proteins,[26] principally to β-lipoprotein.[27] Presumably the drug is bound to the cholesterol carried on this protein. The majority of the drug leaves the circulation promptly, perhaps bound to cholesterol-containing cytoplasmic membranes. Amphotericin B is stored in the liver and other organs; the drug appears to reenter the circulation slowly.[28] Most of the drug is degraded in situ with only a small percentage being excreted in urine[21,28] or bile.[29] Blood levels are uninfluenced by hepatic or renal failure.[26,29] Hemodialysis does not alter blood levels, except for an occasional patient with lipemic plasma who may be losing drug by adherence to the dialysis membrane.[26] Concentrations of amphotericin B in fluids from inflamed areas, such as pleura, peritoneum, joint, vitreous humor,[30] and aqueous humor, are roughly two-thirds of the trough serum level. Cord blood from one infant contained an amphotericin B concentration of 0.37 μg/ml, half the simultaneous maternal trough blood level. Amphotericin B penetrates poorly into either normal or inflamed meninges, vitreous humor, or normal amniotic fluid. Urine concentrations are similar to serum concentrations. Peak serum concentrations with conventional intravenous doses are roughly 0.5–2.0 μg/ml but fall rapidly initially to slowly approach a plateau of roughly 0.2–0.5 μg/ml.[21,31,32]

Clinical Use. Toxicity of intravenous amphotericin B is formidable, but nearly all patients can complete a conventional course of therapy. Therapy is best begun with a small test dose, such as 1 mg in adults, to assess the patient's febrile response. This dose can be given in 20 ml of 5% dextrose over 10–20 minutes. The patient's temperature, pulse and respiration rates, and blood pressure are recorded every 30 minutes for 4 hours.

Acute reactions due to amphotericin B follow a distinctive time course. The onset, often associated with a rigor, begins about 30–90 minutes after the start of the infusion and rarely lasts for more than 2–4 hours. Hypoxemia and hypotension or hypertension may occur during the rigor. These reactions are less marked in patients who are already receiving therapeutic doses of adrenal corticosteroids or who are given hydrocortisone, 25–50 mg, with amphotericin B. Giving hydrocortisone by intravenous bolus before amphotericin B may be preferable to administering the two drugs together when reactions occur early in the infusion, before much hydrocortisone has been received. Infants and young children also seem less prone to acute reactions. Intravenous meperidine has been advocated to ameliorate a rigor once it has begun, but the rigor usually lasts for only 15–45 minutes. Meperidine given when the rigor is about to end anyway makes little sense. Acetaminophen premedication may be used to replace hydrocortisone when reactions are mild. The rapidity of the dose escalation during initiation of therapy depends upon the severity of the acute reactions, the patient's ability to tolerate the reaction, and the rate of progression of the mycosis.

A patient with a rapidly progressing infection, with good cardiopulmonary status, and with a mild reaction to the test dose can for the next dose be given amphotericin B, 0.3 mg/kg, with hydrocortisone hemisuccinate, approximately 0.7 mg/kg. Patients already receiving supraphysiologic doses of adrenal corticosteroids receive little or no benefit from additional steroid in the infusion. A smaller second dose is appropriate for fragile patients with marked reactions to the test dose. Therapy for indolent mycoses may also be initiated slowly and without the addition of hydrocortisone. Tolerance to the febrile reactions develops with time, allowing diminution and eventual discontinuance of the hydrocortisone. The amphotericin B dose is advanced progressively to about 0.5 mg/kg/day by the third to fifth day in patients with prior normal renal function. This dose is maintained or advanced slowly to 0.6 mg/kg/day or, at most, 0.7 mg/kg/day while biweekly determinations of blood creatinine, hematocrit, potassium, and bicarbonate levels are observed. Each infusion is given over 2–3 hours in 500 ml of 5% dextrose in water. I prefer to add heparin, 1000 units, to this infusion, although there is no proof that this decreases phlebitis.

Azotemia is a normal concomitant of amphotericin B therapy.[33] The azotemia reaches a plateau during therapy at a level commensurate with the daily dose. Other nephrotoxic drugs, including cyclosporine,[34] increase azotemia. Salt repletion can improve renal function in the sodium-depleted patient.[35,36] A therapeutic course of amphotericin B is usually followed by a permanent reduction in glomerular filtration rate. This reduction is unrelated to the azotemia during therapy but is correlated with the total dose.[33] Dosage reduction during therapy to keep the serum creatinine level below 3.5 mg/dl is recommended only to help keep nausea and vomiting from causing dehydration and cachexia. Adequate oral intake of high-potassium foods, such as certain fruits and meat, can help prevent hypokalemia.

During an average course of therapy, the patient's serum creatinine level rises to 2.0–3.0 mg/dl, cyllindruria occurs, the hematocrit falls to 20–30 percent and, in one-fourth of the patients, hypokalemia necessitates oral potassium supplements. Weight loss of 15 lb is common. Renal tubular acidosis may occur but rarely requires treatment.[37] Headache and phlebitis are common. Rare side effects include thrombocytopenia, mild leukopenia, anaphylaxis, and burning sensations on the soles of the feet. Neither rash nor hepatotoxicity has been clearly documented. Side effects disappear in the first 3 months after therapy. The slow disappearance of side effects perhaps reflects the slow catabolism of the drug, which can be found in serum and urine up to 6 weeks after a course of therapy.[21,31] Several pregnant patients have received intravenous amphotericin B during the second or third trimester without fetal damage. However, safety in pregnancy is not clearly established.

Mechanisms for the toxic reactions are not fully understood. Amphotericin B-induced cell permeability probably accounts for the loss of intracellular potassium into the blood and excreted with the urine. Ventricular tachycardia in experimental animals given rapid injections of 5 mg/kg may also result from membrane damage. Renal damage morphologically is primarily injury to both proximal and distal tubular cells.[38] Glomerular damage is subtle or absent. Conceivably, nephrotoxicity in humans results from renal vascular constriction, such as occurs in dogs.[39] Anemia is normocytic, normochromic, and accompanied by a normal-appearing bone marrow. Erythrocyte survival is normal.[40] The serum erythropoietin level is abnormally low for the degree of anemia.[41] Acute respiratory deterioration was thought to have occurred in one institution when amphotericin B was given during or right after leukocyte transfusion.[42] Aggregation of leukocytes by amphotericin B[43] with trapping in the lung has been proposed. The rarity of this phenomenon has raised consideration of a third factor, perhaps bacterial endotoxin, necessary to create the syndrome. Febrile reactions to amphotericin B are usual and may be mediated by an entirely different process than renal toxicity. In vitro, the drug causes release of interleukin-1 and tumor necrosis factor from human peripheral blood monocytes.[44] Both mediators can cause fever.

Administration of amphotericin B on alternate days rather than daily does not reduce nephrotoxicity if the alternate-day dose is doubled. The number of venipunctures is decreased, and ambulation is facilitated by an alternate-day double-dose schedule, but more febrile reactions may be encountered. The therapeutic effects of both regimens are indistinguishable. Adequate hydration and salt replacement remain the best measures to minimize azotemia.

Mycoses with a useful response to amphotericin B include blastomycosis, candidiasis, histoplasmosis, cryptococcosis, paracoccidioidomycosis, coccidioidomycosis, aspergillosis, mucormycosis, and extracutaneous sporotrichosis. Doses range from 0.4 to 0.6 mg/kg/day, depending on the mycosis. Lower doses (−0.3 mg/kg) have been used largely in situations in which spontaneous recovery is a good possibility, such as esophagitis due to *Candida*. The duration of therapy in systemic mycoses is 6–12 weeks in most patients. Esophagitis due to *Candida* is often treated for only 5–7 days.

Localized injections of amphotericin B may be useful. Sporotrichosis or coccidioidomycosis of joints may benefit by intra-articular injections of 5–15 mg, depending on joint size. Intrathecal amphotericin B is essential in coccidioidal meningitis. After test doses of 0.05 and 0.1 mg, doses of 0.2–0.5 mg are given from one to three times per week into the lumbar, cisternal, or ventricular cerebrospinal fluid. Hydrocortisone, 5–15 mg, in the injection helps to decrease the resulting fever, headache, and nausea. Lumbar injections may cause temporary radicular pain and loss of motor function in the legs, rectum, and bladder.[45] Use of 10% glucose as a diluent and positioning the patient during injection to permit hyperbaric flow toward the brain may decrease local myelopathy.[46] Injections into the lateral cerebral ventricle through a subcutaneous siliconized rubber reservoir are useful, but the complication rate is high.[47] Bladder irrigations with amphotericin B, 50 μg/ml, in distilled water have been used in *Candida*-induced cystitis.[48] Corneal baths with 1 mg/ml are irritating but beneficial in keratomycosis.

Amphotericin B in Combination with Other Drugs

Under certain conditions, the antifungal activity of amphotericin B can be enhanced with flucytosine, rifampin, or tetracycline. Use of the amphotericin B–flucytosine combination will be discussed in the section dealing with the latter drug. Rifampin, which is not antifungal when used alone, decreases the in vitro concentration of amphotericin B necessary to inhibit the growth of *Candida*,[49] *Histoplasma*,[50] *Cryptococcus*,[51] and *Aspergillus* spp.[52] The amount of reduction is roughly from twofold to fourfold. In experimental mouse infections with *Histoplasma*,[53] *Blastomyces*,[53] and *Aspergillus*,[54] but not *Coccidioides*[55] or *Candida*,[56] rifampin therapy resulted in a significant decrease in the dose of amphotericin B necessary to prolong life. Perhaps significant is the fact that the combination did not result in a therapeutic effect superior to that obtainable with optimum doses of amphotericin B alone. This would suggest an amphotericin-B-sparing rather than amphotericin-B-enhancing effect. Anecdotal clinical experiences with this combination have revealed neither a noticeable improvement in therapeutic efficacy nor a definite synergistic toxicity.

Tetracycline provided an amphotericin-B-sparing effect in experimental murine coccidioidomycosis.[57] In vitro, minocycline decreased the concentration of amphotericin B necessary to inhibit many strains of *Candida* and *Cryptococcus*.[58] This combination has attracted little clinical attention thus far because of all the potential toxic interactions between tetracyclines and amphotericin B.

Combinations of amphotericin B with antitumor agents have received clinical trial based on favorable experience in experimental animals.[59]

Amphotericin B combined with ketoconazole has not appeared particularly promising in vitro or in vivo. The effect in vitro is very method dependent.[60] Under some conditions, antagonism can be demonstrated.[61] In experimentally infected mice, the effect of the combination in candidiasis,[62] histoplasmosis,[63] and cryptococcosis[62,63] was not superior to that of the better single drug.

FLUCYTOSINE

Flucytosine (5-fluorocytosine [5-FC], Ancobon) is the fluorine analogue of a normal body constituent, cytosine (Fig. 1). The drug was synthesized as a potential antitumor agent, but that property was lacking. Routine screening discovered the antifungal effect, which became the sole use of this drug.[64] Flucytosine is a white powder, moderately soluble in water, very stable on dry storage, and marketed as 250- and 500-mg capsules. Absorption from the gastrointestinal tract is rapid and complete. Approximately 90 percent is excreted unchanged in the urine. Protein binding is barely measurable.[26] Cerebrospinal fluid concentrations approximate 74 percent of simultaneous serum concentrations. The drug is readily cleared by hemodialysis.[26,65] Peritoneal dialysis also removes flucytosine from the body.

The half-life of the drug in the serum of patients with normal renal function is 3–5 hours.[66] Abnormal hepatic function has no influence, but decreased renal function can prolong the half-life to beyond 24 hours.

Mechanism of flucytosine's antifungal action appears to be by deamination to 5-fluorouracil (5-FU) and then conversion through several steps to 5-fluorodeoxyuridylic acid monophosphate, a noncompetitive inhibitor of thymidylate synthetase.[67] This interferes with DNA synthesis. Additional mechanisms of action may also be operative.[68]

Flucytosine is usually given as 150 mg/kg/day in four divided doses. Patients with a serum creatinine level of 1.7 mg/dl or greater usually require dose reduction. As an approximation, the total daily dose should be reduced to 75 mg/kg, with a creatinine clearance of 26–50 ml/min, and to 37 mg/kg when the creatinine clearance is 13–25 ml/min.[69] Ideally, the blood level should be measured in azotemic patients 2 hours after the last dose and immediately before the next dose. These values should range between 50 and 100 μg/ml. Patients receiving hemodialysis may be given a single postdialysis dose of 37.5 mg/kg. Further doses are adjusted by blood level. Reliable biologic,[70] enzymatic,[71] and physical[72] methods are available to assay flucytosine, even in the presence of amphotericin B.

Flucytosine given alone to patients with normal renal, hematologic, and gastrointestinal function is associated with very infrequent adverse effects. These include rash, diarrhea, and, in about 5 percent, hepatic dysfunction. In the presence of azotemia or concomitant amphotericin B, leukopenia, thrombocytopenia, and enterocolitis may appear and can be fatal. These complications seem to be far more frequent among patients whose flucytosine blood levels exceed 100–125 μg/ml.[69] Patients receiving flucytosine should have their leukocyte count and platelet count determined twice a week. Serum alkaline phosphatase and transaminase levels should be followed weekly. Appearance of loose stools or dull abdominal pain should prompt withholding of the drug to evaluate the progression of symptoms. Patients with bone marrow and gastrointestinal toxicity from flucytosine often tolerate the drug at reduced dosages. Patients with rash or hepatotoxicity have not been rechallenged. Flucytosine is teratogenic for rats and is contraindicated in pregnancy.

Conversion of flucytosine to 5-FU within the human body occurs in sufficient degree to be a possible explanation for toxicity to bone marrow and gastrointestinal tract.[73] It is possible that secretion of the drug into the colon occurs, where flucytosine becomes deaminated by intestinal bacteria and is reabsorbed as 5-FU.[74]

Flucytosine has a beneficial effect in cryptococcosis, candidiasis, and chromomycosis. It is not the drug of choice for any infection except chromomycosis because the clinical efficacy in the first two mycoses is inferior to that of amphotericin B and because secondary drug resistance is common in all three infections. Although the frequency and clinical significance of primary drug resistance are debatable, drug resistance arising during therapy is usually profound and accompanied by clinical deterioration. Mechanisms for the drug resistance may include loss of deaminase and decreased permeability to the drug. This problem has been significant enough to cause flucytosine to be used largely in combination with amphotericin B.

Flucytosine in Combination with Amphotericin B

Flucytosine and amphotericin B are at least additive in their effects in vitro and in mice experimentally infected with doubly sensitive isolates of *Candida* and *Cryptococcus*.[75,76] Results with *Aspergillus* are contradictory.[52,63] In animals, the combination has never been better than an optimum dose of amphotericin B alone. Flucytosine permitted a lower dose of amphotericin B to be used to gain the same therapeutic effect, and amphotericin B prevented the emergence of secondary drug resistance. These same advantages have been confirmed in two large multicenter studies of cryptococal meningitis.[77,78] Experience with candidiasis remains limited, but the combination has been recommended in *Candida* meningitis[79] and arthritis.

Physicians not familiar with the combination are more likely to encounter serious toxicity than with amphotericin B alone. This is particularly true in patients with rapidly changing azotemia or poor bone marrow reserve. Leukopenia and diarrhea are common and difficult to manage in patients with the acquired immunodeficiency syndrome (AIDS). Oral flucytosine may not be reliably ingested by patients who are confused or vomiting. Intravenous flucytosine has to be obtained directly from the manufacturer but is used at the same dose as the capsule formulation. There is no less diarrhea or leukopenia with intravenous administration.

Combination regimens with amphotericin B doses in excess of 0.3 mg/kg/day or 0.6 mg/kg every other day cause sufficient azotemia to make the safe administration of flucytosine difficult. The amphotericin-B-sparing function of flucytosine in this setting is lost. At present, there are no clear indications for adding flucytosine to amphotericin B regimens containing these higher doses.

Flucytosine resistance has occurred, albeit uncommonly, during combination therapy. Use of the combination in such patients incurs the risk of toxicity without evidence that flucytosine adds to the therapeutic effect. Whenever flucytosine is used to treat a patient who has received that drug before, the isolate should be tested for susceptibility. In most laboratories, a minimum inhibitory concentration (MIC) of 15 μg/ml or less is considered sensitive.

IMIDAZOLES

The imidazole ring (Fig. 1) confers antifungal activity upon a variety of synthetic organic compounds. Unlike the 5-nitroimidazoles such as metronidazole, activity against bacteria and protozoa, although measurable, has not been clinically significant. Most of the imidazoles reaching clinical trials have had similar in vitro activity, encompassing a broad range of superficial and deep pathogens.[13,80] Determination of activity in vitro has shown a marked dependence of the result upon inoculum size, pH, culture medium, and incubation time.[80,81] There are no widely accepted methods for measuring in vitro activity, and no firm indications for performing such tests can be offered. Secondary drug resistance has been encountered but is extremely rare.[82]

N-substitution of imidazoles has created a family of drugs called *triazoles* that have the same antifungal spectrum and mechanism of action as imidazoles but less effect upon human sterol metabolism. Both imidazoles and triazoles inhibit 14-α-demethylation of lanosterol in fungi by binding to one of the cytochrome P-450 (cyt. P-450) enzymes.[3] This leads to accumulation of 14-α-methylsterols and reduced concentrations of ergosterol, a sterol essential for a normal fungal cytoplasmic membrane. Inhibition of cyt. P-450 also decreases the synthesis of testosterone and cortisol in mammals. By studying cyt. P-450 inhibition in vitro, new drugs can be selected that are more active in inhibiting fungal ergosterol synthesis and less active in mammalian sterol synthesis. For example, in vitro study of itraconazole found that 14-α-demethylation of lanosterol in *Candida albicans* was inhibited at 100-fold lower concentrations than those required to inhibit mammalian sterol synthesis.[3] It is not surprising, then, that the newer triazoles, such as itraconazole and fluconazole, have not caused decreased cortisol and testosterone levels in patients, as was seen with ketoconazole.

Many of the newer triazoles have properties that may allow them to replace ketoconazole—not only less hormonal inhibition but also fewer drug interactions, a parenteral formulation, better distribution into body fluids, less gastrointestinal distress, and less hepatotoxicity. N-substitution of the imidazole ring is thought to confer greater metabolic stability on the triazoles and to offer the potential for slower elimination. Both itraconazole and fluconazole have longer serum half-lives than ketoconazole.

Ketoconazole

This synthetic agent differs from its closely related congener, miconazole, in its solubility at pH less than 3. Solubility in acidic aqueous solutions is conferred in large part by the basic piperazine ring.

The pharmacology of ketoconazole has been reviewed.[13,83] The drug is metabolized in the liver and excreted as inactive drug in the bile and, to a small extent, in the urine. Very little biologically active drug appears in urine. Serum protein binding exceeds 90 percent. The drug is not removed significantly by hemodialysis or peritoneal dialysis. Decreased renal or hepatic function does not alter plasma drug levels. Based on studies of oral ingestion by volunteers, the initial half-life is approximately 2 hours, with a β-phase half-life of about 9 hours commencing 8–12 hours after ingestion.

Oral absorption of ketoconazole varies among different individuals. Serious gastrointestinal disease, such as the graft-versus-host reaction,[84] may lead to low blood levels. H_2-receptor blocking agents, such as ranitidine, famotidine, or cimetidine, should not be given to patients taking ketoconazole because blood levels of the latter drug are drastically reduced. Although oral ingestion of hydrochloric acid along with ketoconazole has been said to reverse this effect in volunteers, acid administration would be contraindicated in patients requiring H_2-blocking agents. Citric acid does not seem acidic enough to overcome the effect of H_2-blocking agents.[83] Antacids can be given to patients taking ketoconazole but should be separated in time. Rifampin causes a substantial lowering of ketoconazole blood levels, probably by accelerating metabolism. Isoniazid possibly has the same effect. Occasional patients have had elevated phenytoin or oral anticoagulant levels while taking ketoconazole. Cyclosporine blood levels should be monitored during ketoconazole therapy because these levels sometimes increase, causing nephrotoxicity.[85] Penetration into the cerebrospinal fluid is very poor, even in the presence of inflammation.[86] Low concentrations are found in vaginal secretions,[87] saliva, and breast milk.

Ketconazole is presently available only as scored 200-mg tablets. Used as two tablets daily (400 mg), the drug is effective in nonmeningeal histoplasmosis and blastomycosis of the non-immunosuppressed host.[88] Therapy is continued for 6–12 months. Improvement may require 2–4 weeks to be evident. Although the dose can be advanced to 600 or 800 mg daily in patients not responding to therapy, there is more evidence of increased toxicity than increased efficacy.[86,88] Both disseminated and chronic pulmonary histoplasmosis respond to ketoconazole therapy. Histoplasmosis in AIDS responds too poorly to risk the use of this drug for acute therapy, although long-term ketoconazole has been used to prevent relapse after amphotericin B treatment.[89] Paracoccidioidomycosis responds well to ketoconazole.[90] Disseminated nonmeningeal coccidioidomycosis may be partially and temporarily controlled by ketoconazole.[91] Among patients with disseminated coccidioidomycosis who respond well, relapse is usual if the drug is stopped. With all these mycoses, patients with grave, rapidly progressing infection should receive amphotericin B. The slow therapeutic response and variable absorption of ketoconazole make it a poor choice in such patients. If the mycosis involves the meninges, ketoconazole is too ineffective to warrant trial.

Ketoconazole is of no value in cryptococcosis. There is no evidence that it accelerates the normal resolution of pulmonary lesions or prevents spread to the central nervous system. Patients who have been treated with amphotericin B for cryptococcal meningitis have relapsed while taking ketoconazole. The response is also negligible in chromomycosis and extracutaneous sporotrichosis. Although the response in cutaneous sporotrichosis also tends to be poor, a dose of 400 mg/day may be tried in patients with allergic reactions to iodide, the drug of choice. As will be mentioned later, itraconazole may be a better choice. Ketoconazole has been used in Old World leishmaniasis and was useful in *Leishmania major* but not in *L. tropica or L. aethiopica* infections (see Chapter 252). Studies on New World leishmaniasis are still inconclusive but not encouraging.

Aspergillosis does not respond to ketoconazole. Additionally, there is concern, based upon experience with mice, that subsequent use of amphotericin B may be antagonized.[92] The agents of mucormycosis have all been resistant to imidazoles and triazoles in vitro, discouraging clinical use for that indication.

The most frequent toxic effects of ketoconazole are anorexia, nausea, and vomiting. These reactions occurred in 17 percent of 71 patients taking 400 mg/day and in 29 percent of those receiving 800 mg/day.[88] Gastrointestinal distress is most common when the drug is first begun and can be partially controlled by taking the tablets with food. Dividing doses above 400 mg/day has not been recommended because hormonal suppression is prolonged. Ketoconazole causes a dose-dependent depression of serum testosterone and adrenocorticotropic hormone (ACTH)-stimulated cortisol response.[93,94] While this effect is quite modest at the recommended dose of 400 mg/day, doses of 800–1,200 mg/day cause a profound enough effect to have prompted trials in the treatment of ACTH-secreting tumors and prostatic cancer. Hypertension has been seen in a few of these high-dose patients in association with increased deoxycorticosterone, corticosterone, and 11-deoxycortisol levels. Gynecomastia, impotence, decreased libido, oligospermia, and azospermia in men and menstrual irregularities in women may also be seen during prolonged therapy.[88,93] Allergic rash has been seen in 10 percent of patients.[88] Pruritus occurs with equal frequency, sometimes associated with a complaint of dry skin. Perhaps the most grave complication of ketoconazole therapy is hepatitis.[95] Fortunately, this complication is quite rare, estimated to appear in 1 in 15,000 exposed individuals. Asymptomatic slight elevation of transaminases is not rare and is generally transient. This event is distinguished from the potentially lethal hepatitis by the presence of symptoms and the progressive course. Ketoconazole hepatitis begins as anorexia, malaise, nausea, and vomiting. Abnormalities of either or both serum transaminase and alkaline phosphatase become increasingly profound, soon accompanied by jaundice. Eighty percent of cases occur within the first 3 months, but the onset can occur at any time. Progression can be surprisingly swift. Patients should be instructed to discontinue ketoconazole if they experience the above symptoms and told to call their physician. If hepatotoxicity is suspected, serum transaminase and alkaline phosphatase should be measured within a day or two of discontinuing therapy. Symptomatic patients with abnormal liver function should not be rechallenged with ketoconazole. Of course, if serum chemistries are normal, the drug can be reinstituted. Some authorities have recommended that liver function be measured periodically.[95] This procedure does not protect the patient who has a rapid onset of hepatitis in the interval between tests but does require that all patients with abnormalities be contacted in order to inquire about symptoms and arrange for repeat testing.

Itraconazole

Despite its marked structural similarity to ketoconazole, itraconazole differs in several respects. Peak blood levels are lower than with ketoconazole, but tissue levels are higher. Antifungal activity is better in both susceptibility testing and in in vitro systems measuring the inhibition of *C. albicans* cyt. P-450.[3] Ingesting this lipophilic drug with meals substantially enhances absorption. With 200 mg once daily taken with breakfast, peak blood levels by day 15 were 1.07 μg/ml, as measured by high-pressure liquid chromatography.[96] Elimination from serum is triexponential, making calculations of half-life somewhat variable, being reported as roughly 20–36 hours.[96] Itraconazole is extensively metabolized in the liver, but neither renal dysfunction, hemodialysis, nor continuous peritoneal dialysis alters metabolism.[97] About 99 percent of serum itraconazole is protein bound. Drug concentrations are negligible in the urine and cerebrospinal fluid. At the doses used to date, there has been no effect on serum testosterone or ACTH-stimulated cortisol concentrations. Rifampin can reduce itraconazole levels. Interactions with H_2-receptor blocking agents, oral anticoagulants, and phenytoin have not yet been studied. The ability of itraconazole to elevate blood levels of cyclosporine has been reported in some patients[98,99] but not in others.[100] Dose-related nausea has been the most common adverse effect. Headache, hypertension, or edema has been noted in a few patients, but the relationship to itraconazole is not firmly established. Early indications are that hepatotoxicity is less common than with ketoconazole.

Conclusions about clinical utility are based upon the reactions of only small numbers of patients but suggest that primary indications for itraconazole will be the same as those for ketoconazole (i.e., coccidioidomycosis, paracoccidioidomycosis, blastomycosis, histoplasmosis, mucocutaneous candidiasis, and refractory cases of tinea versicolor or tinea corporis).[101–103] Itraconazole is given only by the oral route. The dose in systemic mycoses has been 200–400 mg/day, or half the dose of ketoconazole. A few reports of responses in cutaneous sporotrichosis[104] and invasive aspergillosis[105] have encouraged further study of these mycoses and may be evidence of an expanded spectrum of activity.

Fluconazole

This low molecular weight, fluorine-substituted bis-triazole has pharmacologic properties that differ strikingly from those of ketoconazole and itraconazole. The drug is water soluble, essentially completely absorbed from the gastrointestinal tract, administered by oral or intravenous routes, excreted unchanged in the urine, only 11 percent bound to serum proteins, and distributed throughout the body.[106,107] Penetration into cerebrospinal fluid is excellent, cerebrospinal fluid levels being about 70 percent of serum levels. The elimination half-life from serum is about 25 hours.[106,108] There does not appear to be any inhibition of testosterone[109] or cortisol synthesis at the doses used so far. Little is known about drug interactions. Oral absorption is not dependent upon gastric acid, as with ketoconazole. A major issue yet to be resolved is the necessity of obtaining blood levels when fluconazole is administered to azotemic patients. Although the drug clearly accumulates in azotemic patients, no dose-related toxicity has yet been reported. Nomograms for adjusting the dose in azotemic patients are available, but determination of blood levels is preferred.

Efficacy has been reported so far in oral thrush of AIDS patients,[110] in denture stomatitis,[111] and in one patient with *Candida* endocarditis.[112] Of greater interest are the anecdotes about responses in cryptococcal meningitis.[113–115] Some patients with cryptococcal meningitis, mostly AIDS patients, have clearly improved during fluconazole therapy. A multicenter study is in progress to determine whether the drug, given orally, can decrease the incidence of relapse in AIDS patients whose cryptococcal meningitis has been treated with amphotericin B.

REFERENCES

1. Hamilton-Miller JMT. Chemistry and biology of the polyene macrolide antibiotics. Bacteriol Rev. 1973;37:166.
2. Kerridge D, Whelan WL. The polyene macrolide antibiotics and 5-fluorocytosine: Molecular actions and interactions. In: Trinci APJ, Riley JF, eds. Mode of Action of Antifungal Agents. London: British Mycological Society; 1984:343–75.
3. Vandem Bossche H, Bellens D, Cools W, et al. Cytochrome P-450: Target for itraconazole. Drug Dev Res. 1986;8:287–98.
4. Fromtling RA. Imidazoles as medically important antifungal agents: An overview. Drugs Today. 1984;20:325–49.
5. Stern GE, Gurwith D, Mummaw N, et al. Single dose tioconazole compared with 3-day clotrimazole treatment in vulvovaginal candidiasis. Antimicrob Agents Chemother. 1986;29:969–71.
6. Gabriel G, Thin RNT. Clotrimazole and econazole in the treatment of vaginal candidosis. Br J Vener Dis. 1983;59:56–8.
7. Svendsen E, Lie S, Gunderson TH, et al. Comparative evaluation of miconazole, clotrimazole and nystatin in the treatment of *Candida* vulvo-vaginitis. Curr Ther Res. 1978;23:666.

8. Franklin R. Seven day clotrimazole therapy for vulvovaginal candidiasis. South Med J. 1978;71:141.
9. Shechtman LB, Funaro L, Robin T, et al. Clotrimazole treatment of oral candidiasis in patients with neoplastic disease. Am J Med. 1984;76:91.
10. Horsbaugh CR, Kirkpatrick CH. Long-term therapy of chronic mucocutaneous candidiasis with ketoconazole: Experience with twenty-one patients. Am J Med. 1983;74:23.
11. Fazio RA, Wickremesinghe PC, Arsure EL. Ketoconazole treatment of *Candida* esophagitis; a prospective study of 12 cases. Am J Gastroenterol. 1983;78:261.
12. Hughes WT, Bartley DL, Patterson GG, et al. Ketoconazole and candidiasis: A controlled study. J Infect Dis. 1983;147:1060.
13. Heel RC, Brogden RN, Carmine A, et al. Ketoconazole: A review of its therapeutic efficacy in superficial and systemic fungal infections. Drugs. 1982;23:1.
14. Sobel JD. Recurrent vulvovaginal candidiasis. A prospective study of the efficacy of maintenance ketoconazole therapy. N Engl J Med. 1986;315:1455–8.
15. Sokol-Anderson ML, Brajtburg, Medoff G. Amphotericin B-induced oxidative damage and killing of *Candida albicans*. J Infect Dis. 1986;154:76–83.
16. Block ER, Bennett JE. Stability of amphotericin B in the infusion bottle. Antimicrob Agents Chemother. 1973;4:648.
17. Ellis WG, Sobel RA, Nielsen SL. Leukoencephalopathy in patients treated with amphotericin B methyl ester. J Infect Dis. 1982;146:125.
18. Lopez-Berestein G, Fainstein V, Hopfer R, et al. Liposomal amphotericin B for the treatment of systemic fungal infections in patients with cancer: A preliminary study. J Infect Dis. 1985;151:704–10.
19. Janoff AS, Boni LT, Popescu MC, et al. Unusual lipid structures selectively reduce the toxicity of amphotericin B. Proc Natl Acad Sci USA. 1988;85:6122–6.
20. Sculier JP, Coune A, Meunier F, et al. Pilot study of amphotericin B entrapped in sonicated liposomes in cancer patients with fungal infections. Eur J Cancer Clin Oncol. 1988;24:527–38.
21. Bindschadler DD, Bennett JE. A pharmacologic guide to the clinical use of amphotericin B. J Infect Dis. 1969;120:427.
22. Mayhew JW, Fiore C, Murray T, et al. An internally standardized assay for amphotericin B in tissues and plasma. J Chromatog. 1983;274:271.
23. Cosgrove RF, Fairbrother JE. Bioassay method for polyene antibiotics based on the measurement of rubidium efflux from rubidium-loaded yeast cells. Antimicrob Agents Chemother. 1977;11:31.
24. Merz WG, Fay D, Thumar B, et al. Susceptibility testing of filamentous fungi to amphotericin B by a rapid radiometric method. J Clin Microbiol. 1984;19:54.
25. Jagdis FA, Monji N, Lawrence RM, et al. Distribution of radiolabeled amphotercin B methyl ester and amphotericin B in nonhuman primates. Sixteenth Interscience Conference of Antimicrobial Agents and Chemotherapy. Washington, DC: American Society of Microbiology; 1976:abstract 305.
26. Block ER, Bennett JE, Livoti LG, et al. Flucytosine and amphotericin B: Hemodialysis effects on the plasma concentration and clearance. Ann Intern Med. 1974;80:613.
27. Bennett JE. Amphotericin B binding to serum betalipoprotein. In Iwata K, ed. Recent Advances in Medical and Veterinary Mycology. Tokyo: University of Tokyo Press; 1977:107.
28. Atkinson AJ, Bennett JE. Amphotericin B pharmacokinetics in humans. Antimicrob Agents Chemother. 1978;13:271.
29. Craven PC, Ludden TM, Drutz DJ, et al. Excretion pathways of amphotericin B. J Infect Dis. 1979;140:329.
30. Fisher JF, Taylor AT, Clark J, et al. Penetration of amphotericin B into the human eye. J Infect Dis. 1983;147:164.
31. Christiansen KJ, Bernard EM, Gold JWM, et al. Distribution and activity of amphotericin B in humans. J Infect Dis. 1985;152:1037–43.
32. Starke JR, Mason EO, Kramer WG, et al. Pharmacokinetics of amphotericin B in infants and children. J Infect Dis. 1987;155:766–74.
33. Butler WT, Bennett JE, Alling DW, et al. Nephrotoxicity of amphotericin B. Early and late effects in 81 patients. Ann Intern Med. 1964;61:175.
34. Kennedy MS, Deeg HJ, Siegel M, et al. Acute renal toxicity with combined use of amphotericin B and cyclosporine after marrow transplantation. Transplantation. 1982;35:211.
35. Heidemann HT, Gerkens JF, Spickard WA, et al. Amphotericin B nephrotoxicity in humans decreased by salt repletion. Am J Med. 1983;75:475.
36. Branch RA. Prevention of amphotericin B-induced renal impairment. Arch Intern Med. 1988;148:2389–94.
37. McCurdy DK, Frederic M, Elkinton JR. Renal acidosis due to amphotericin B. N Engl J Med. 1968;278:124.
38. Utz JP, Bennett JE, Brandriss MW, et al. Amphotericin B toxicity. Ann Intern Med. 1964;61:334.
39. Gerkens JF, Heidemann HT, Jackson EK, et al. Effect of aminophylline on amphotericin B nephrotoxicity in the dog. J Pharmacol Exp Ther. 1983;224:609.
40. Brandriss M, Wolff S, Moores R, et al. Anemia induced by amphotericin B. JAMA. 1964;189:663.
41. MacGregor RR, Bennett JE, Erslev AJ. Erythropoietin concentration in amphotericin B-induced anemia. Antimicrob Agents Chemother. 1978;14:270.
42. Wright DG, Robichaud KJ, Pizzo PA, et al. Lethal pulmonary reactions associated with the combined use of amphotericin B and leukocyte transfusions. N Engl J Med. 1981;304:1185.
43. Boxer LA, Ingraham LM, Allen J, et al. Amphotericin-B promotes leukocyte aggregation of nylon-wool-fiber-treated polymorphonuclear leukocytes. Blood. 1981;58:518.
44. Gelfand JA, Kimball K, Burke JF, et al. Amphotericin B treatment of human mononuclear cells in vitro results in secretion of tumor necrosis factor and interleukin-1. Clin Res. 1988;36:456A.
45. Carnevale NT, Galgiani JN, Stevens DA, et al. Amphotericin B-induced myelopathy. Arch Intern Med. 1980;140:1189.
46. Alazraki NP, Fierer J, Halpern SE, et al. Use of a hyperbaric solution for administration of intrathecal amphotericin B. N Engl J Med. 1974;290:641.
47. Diamond RD, Bennett JE. A subcutaneous reservoir for intrathecal therapy of fungal meningitis. N Engl J Med. 1973;288:186.
48. Wise GJ, Wainstein S, Goldberg P, et al. *Candida* cystitis. Management by continuous bladder irrigation with amphotericin B. JAMA. 1973;224:1636.
49. Edwards JE, Morrison J, Henderson DK, et al. Combined effect of amphotericin B and rifampin on *Candida* species. Antimicrob Agents Chemother. 1980;17:484.
50. Kobayashi GS, Medoff G, Schlessinger D, et al. Amphotericin B potentiation of rifampicin as an antifungal agent against the yeast phase of *Histoplasma capsulatum*. Science. 1972;177:709.
51. Fujita NK, Edwards JE: Combined in vitro effect of amphotericin B and rifampin on *Cryptoccus neoformans*. Antimicrob Agents Chemother. 1981;19:196.
52. Kitahara M, Seth UK, Medoff G, et al. Activity of amphotericin B, 5-fluorocytosine and rifampin against six clinical isolates of *Aspergillus*. Antimicrob Agents Chemother. 1976;9:915.
53. Kitahara M, Kobayashi GS, Medoff G. Enhanced efficacy of amphotericin B and rifampicin in treatment of murine histoplasmosis and blastomycosis. J Infect Dis. 1976;133:663.
54. Arroyo J, Medoff G, Kobayashi GS. Therapy of murine aspergillosis with amphotericin B in combination with rafampin or 5-fluorocytosine. Antimicrob Agents Chemother. 1977;11:21.
55. Huppert M, Pappagianis D, Sun SH, et al. Effect of amphotericin B and rifampin against *Coccidioides immitis* in vitro and in vivo. Antimicrob Agents Chemother. 1976;9:406.
56. Graybill JR, Ahrens J. Interaction of rifampin with other antifungal agents in experimental murine candidiasis. Rev Infect Dis. 1983;5:S620.
57. Huppert M, Sun SH, Vukovich KR. Combined amphotericin B-tetracycline therapy for experimental coccidioidomycosis. Antimicrob Agents Chemother. 1974;5:473.
58. Lew M, Beckett KM, Levin MJ. Combined activity of minocycline and amphotericin B in vitro against medically important yeasts. Antimicrob Agents Chemother. 1978;14:465.
59. Presant CA, Klahr C, Santala R. Amphotericin B induction of sensitivity to adriamycin, 1,3-*bis* (2-chloroethyl)-1-nitrosourea (BCNU) plus cyclophosphamide in human neoplasia. Ann Intern Med. 1977;86:47.
60. Brajtburg J, Kobayashi D, Medoff G, et al. Antifungal action of amphotericin B in combination with other polyene or imidazole antibiotics. J Infect Dis. 1982;146:138.
61. Sud IJ, Feingold DS. Effect of ketoconazole on the fungicidal action of amphotericin B in *Candida albicans*. Antimicrob Agents Chemother. 1983;23:185.
62. Graybill JR, Williams DM, Cutsem EV, et al: Combination therapy of experimental histoplasmosis and cryptococcosis with amphotericin B and ketoconazole. Rev Infect Dis. 1980;2:551.
63. Polak A, Scholer HJ, Wall M. Combination therapy of experimental candidiasis and aspergillosis in mice. Chemotherapy. 1982;28:461.
64. Bennett JE: Flucytosine. Ann Intern Med. 1977;86:319.
65. Ittel TH, Legler UF, Polak A, et al. 5-Fluorocytosine kinetics in patients with acute renal failure undergoing continuous hemofiltration. Chemotherapy. 1987;33:77–84.
66. Cutler RE, Balir AD, Kelly MR. Flucytosine kinetics in subjects with normal renal function. Clin Pharmacol Ther. 1978;24:333.
67. Diasio RB, Bennett JE, Myers CE: Mode of action of 5-fluorocytosine. Biochem Pharmacol. 1978;27:703.
68. Oliver SO, Williamson DH. The molecular events involved in the induction of petite yeast mutants by fluorinated pyrimidines. Mol Gen Genet. 1976;146:253.
69. Stamm AM, Diasio RB, Dismukes WE, et al. Toxicity of amphotericin B plus flucytosine in 194 patients with cryptococcal meningitis. Am J Med. 1987;83:236–42.
70. Kaspar RL, Drutz DJ. Rapid, simple bioassay for 5-Fluorocytosine in the presence of amphotericin B. Antimicrob Agents Chemother. 1975;7:462.
71. Huang CM, Kroll MH, Ruddel M, et al. An enzymatic method for 5-fluorocytosine. Clin Chem. 1988;34:59–62.
72. Harding SA, Johnson GF, Solomon HM. Gas chromatographic determination of 5-fluorocytosine in human serum. Clin Chem. 1976;22:772.
73. Diasio RB, Lakings DE, Bennett JE. Evidence for conversion of 5-fluorocytosine to 5-fluorouracil in humans. Possible factor in 5-fluorocytosine clinical toxicity. Antimicrob Agents Chemother. 1978;14:903.
74. Harris BE, Manning BW, Federle TW, et al. Conversion of 5-fluorocytosine to 5-fluorouracil by human intestinal microflora. Antimicrob Agents Chemother. 1986;29:44–8.
75. Medoff G, Comfort M, Kobayashi GS. Synergistic action of amphotericin

B and 5-fluorocytosine against yeast-like organisms. Proc Soc Exp Biol Med. 1971;138:571.
76. Polak A. Synergism of polyene antibiotics with 5-fluorocytosine. Chemotherapy. 1978;24:2.
77. Dismukes WE, Cloud GC, Gallis HA, et al. Treatment of cryptococcal meningitis with combination amphotericin B and flucytosine for four as compared with six weeks. N Engl J Med. 1987;317:334–41.
79. Smego RA, Perfect JR, Durack DT. Combined therapy with amphotericin B and 5-fluorocytosine for *Candida* meningitis. Rev Infect Dis. 1984;6:791–801.
80. Custem JV. The antifungal activity of ketoconazole. Am J Med. 1983;74(Suppl):9.
81. Galgiani JN. Antifungal susceptibility tests. Antimicrob Agents Chemother. 1987;31:1867–70.
82. Ryley JF, Wilson RG, Barrett-Bee KJ. Azole resistance in *Candida albicans*. Sabouraudia. 1984;22:53.
83. Daneshmend TK, Warnock DW. Clinical pharmacokinetics of ketoconazole. Clin Pharmacokinet. 1988;14:13–34.
84. Van HV, Piens MA, Archimbaud E, et al. Serum levels of ketoconazole in bone marrow transplanted patients. Nouv Rev Fr Hematol. 1983;25:241–4.
85. Schroeder TJ, Melvin DB, Clardy CW, et al. Use of cyclosporine and ketoconazole without nephrotoxicity in two heart transplant recipients. J Heart Transplant. 1987;6:84–9.
86. Sugar AM, Alsip SG, Galgiani JN, et al. Pharmacology and toxicity of high-dose ketoconazole. Antimicrob Agents Chemother. 1987;31:1874–8.
87. Nusch W, Plempel M. Microbiological determination of bay N 7133 and ketoconazole after oral application in cervical and vaginal smears of patients. Mykosen. 1983;26:12.
88. NIAID Mycoses Study Group. Treatment of blastomycosis and histoplasmosis with ketoconazole. Results of a prospective randomized clinical trial. Ann Intern Med. 1985;103:861–72.
89. Johnson PC, Khardori N, Najjar AF, et al. Progressive disseminated histoplasmosis in patients with acquired immunodeficiency syndrome. Am J Med. 1988;85:152–8.
90. Restrepo A, Gomez I, Cano LE, et al. Post-therapy status of paracoccidioidomycosis treated with ketoconazole. Am J Med. 1983;74:53.
91. Galgiani JN, Stevens DA, Graybill JR, et al. Ketoconazole therapy of progressive coccidioidomycosis. Comparison of 400 and 800 mg doses and observations at higher doses. Am J Med. 1988;84:603–10.
92. Schaffner A, Frick PG. The effect of ketoconazole on amphotericin B in a model of disseminated aspergillosis. J Infect Dis. 1985;151:902–10.
93. Pont A, Graybill JR, Craven PC, et al. High-dose ketoconazole therapy and adrenal and testicular function in humans. Arch Intern Med. 1984;144:2150–3.
94. De Coster R, Caers R, Haelterman C, et al. Effect of a single administration of ketoconazole on total and physiologically free plasma testosterone and 17-beta-oestradiol levels in healthy male volunteers. Eur J Clin Pharmacol. 1985;29:489–93.
95. Lewis JH, Zimmerman HJ, Benson GD, et al. Hepatic injury associated with ketoconazole therapy. Gastroenterology. 1984;86:503–13.
96. Hardin TC, Graybill JR, Fetchick R, et al. Pharmacokinetics of itraconazole following oral administration to normal volunteers. Antimicrob Agents Chemother. 1988;32:1310–13.
97. Boelaert J, Schurgers M, Matthys E, et al. Itraconazole pharmacokinetics in patients with renal dysfunction. Antimicrob Agents Chemother. 1988;32:1595–7.
98. Kwan JTC, Foxall PJD, Davidson DGC, et al. Interaction of cyclosporin and itraconazole. Lancet. 1987;2:282.
99. Trenk D, Brett W, Jahnchen E, et al. Time course of cyclosporin/itraconazole interaction. Lancet. 1987;2:1335–6.
100. Novakova I, Donnelly P, de Witte T, et al. Itraconazole and cyclosporin nephrotoxicity. Lancet. 1987;2:920–1.
101. Phillips P, Fetchick R, Weisman I, et al. Tolerance to and efficacy of itraconazole in treatment of systemic mycoses: Preliminary results. Rev Infect Dis. 1987;9(Suppl 1):S87–S93.
102. Lavalle P, Suchil P, de Ovando F, et al. Itraconazole for deep mycoses: Preliminary experience in Mexico. Rev Infect Dis. 1987;9(Suppl 1):S64–S70.
103. Borelli D. A clinical trial of itraconazole in the treatment of deep mycoses and leishmaniasis. Rev Infect Dis. 1987;9(Suppl 1):S57–S63.
104. Restrepo A, Robledo J, Gomez I, et al. Itraconazole therapy in lymphangitic and cutaneous sporotrichosis. Arch Dermatol. 1986;122:413–7.
105. Viviani MA, Tortorano AM, Woenstenborghs R, et al. Experience with itraconazole in deep mycoses in northern Italy. Mykosen. 1987;30:233–44.
106. Dismukes WE. Azole antifungal drugs: Old and new. Ann Intern Med. 1988;109:177–9.
107. Farrow PR, Faulkner JK, Brammer KW. The pharmacokinetics and tissue penetration of fluconazole in man. Rev Infect Dis. In press.
108. Tucker RM, Williams PI, Arathoon EG, et al. Pharmacokinetics of fluconazole in cerebrospinal fluid and serum in human coccidioidal meningitis. Antimicrob Agents Chemother. 1988:32:369–73.
109. Hanger DP, Jevons S, Shaw JTB. Fluconazole and testosterone: In vivo and in vitro studies. Antimicrob Agents Chemother. 1988;32:646–8.
110. Dupont B, Drouhet E. Fluconazole in the management of oropharyngeal candidosis in a predominantly HIV antibody-positive group of patients. J Med Vet Mycol. 1988;26:67–71.
111. Budtz-Jorgensen E, Holmstrup P, Krogh P. Fluconazole in the treatment of *Candida*-associated denture stomatitis. Antimicrob Agents Chemother. 1988;32:1859–63.
112. Isalska BJ, Stanbridge TN. Fluconazole in the treatment of candidal prosthetic valve endocarditis. Br Med J. 1988;297:178–9.
113. Byrne WR, Wajszczuk CP. Cryptococcal meningitis in the acquired immunodeficiency syndrome (AIDS): Successful treatment with fluconazole after failure of amphotericin B. Ann Intern Med. 1988;108:384–5.
114. Stern JJ, Hartman BH, Sharkey P, et al. Oral fluconazole therapy for patients with acquired immunodeficiency syndrome and cryptococcosis: Experience with 22 patients. Am J Med. 1988;85:477–80.
115. Sugar AM, Saunders C. Oral fluconazole as suppressive therapy of disseminated cryptococcosis in patients with acquired immunodeficiency syndrome. Am J Med. 1988;85:481–9.

34. ANTIVIRAL AGENTS

FREDERICK G. HAYDEN
R. GORDON DOUGLAS, JR.

Antiviral drugs with proven therapeutic (Table 1) and prophylactic effectiveness are currently available for a number of common and, in some instances, clinically severe viral infections. In part as a response to acquired immunodeficiency syndrome (AIDS) and its sequelae, the search for new antiviral agents and therapeutic approaches for managing viral diseases has become increasingly intense. Recently licensed agents include zidovudine for human immunodeficiency virus (HIV)-1 infections, aerosolized ribavirin for respiratory syncytial virus (RSV) infections in infants, and intralesional recombinant α-interferon for genital papilloma. Ganciclovir and foscarnet have shown impressive activity against cytomegalovirus (CMV) infections. A number of antiretroviral and antiherpes agents are currently in various stages of development.

MECHANISMS OF ACTION

Chemotherapeutic agents for viral infections can be categorized into three broad groups: agents that directly inactivate intact viruses (virucidal), those that inhibit viral replication at the cellular level (antiviral), and those that augment or modify the host response to infection (immunomodulating). Virucidal agents may cause direct inactivation in a single step, such as with detergents, organic solvents like ether or chloroform, and ultraviolet light, or in multiple steps, as with photodynamic inactivation. However, such agents have not proved clinically useful in the treatment of established mucocutaneous herpes simplex virus (HSV) infections. Treatments that destroy both host tissues and virus simultaneously, such as cryotherapy, cautery, or podophyllin treatment of warts, are useful only in discrete mucocutaneous infections. One potential use of virucidal agents may be in preventing transmission of certain viral infections.

Antivirals

Since viral replication depends primarily on host cell metabolic functions, the challenge has been to identify agents that inhibit virus-specific events such as attachment to the cell, uncoating of the viral genome, or assembly of progeny virions, or that preferentially inhibit virus-directed, as contrasted to host cell-directed, macromolecular synthesis. While many compounds exist that exhibit antiviral activity in vitro, most affect some host cell function and are associated with low therapeutic ratios or unacceptable toxicity in humans.[1]

Currently useful antivirals selectively inhibit specific events in viral replication and, consequently, most have a restricted spectrum of antiviral activity. Similarly, since these agents inhibit ongoing replication at the host cell level, they are not effective in elimination of nonreplicating or latent viruses.

TABLE 1. Viral Infections in Which Antiviral Agents Have Proved Therapeutic Efficacy

Type of Infection	*Antiviral Drug*	*Route of Administration*	*Usual Dosage*
Herpes simplex virus (HSV) encephalitis	Acyclovir[a]	IV	10 mg/kg/8 hr in constant 1 hr infusion for 14–21 days
	Vidarabine	IV	15 mg/kg/day for 14–21 days. Less effective than acyclovir
Neonatal HSV	Acyclovir[a]	IV	10 mg/kg/8 hr in constant 1 hr infusion for 10–14 days
	Vidarabine[a]	IV	30 mg/kg/day for 10–14 days; constant infusion over 12–24 hours
Genital HSV			
Primary	Acyclovir	IV	5 mg/kg/8 hr for 5 days; constant infusion over 1 hr; indicated in severe initial infections
	Acyclovir	Oral	1,000 mg/day in five divided doses for 10 days
	Acyclovir	Topical	4–6 applications/day for 7–14 days; ½ in. ribbon of 5% ointment per 4 square in. applied with gloved finger
Recurrent	Acyclovir	Oral	1,000 mg/day in five divided doses for 5 days; see text regarding long-term suppression
HSV keratoconjunctivitis[b]	Idoxuridine	Topical	One drop of 0.1% solution every 1 hr while awake and every 2 hr at night; instillation of 0.5% ointment 5 times/day
	Vidarabine	Topical	½ in. ribbon of 3% ointment 5 times/day
	Trifluridine	Topical	One drop of 1% solution every 2 hr (up to 9 drops/day)
	Acyclovir[a]	Topical	½ in. ribbon of 3% ophthalmic ointment 5 times/day
Mucocutaneous HSV Immunocompromised host	Acyclovir	IV	250 mg/m²/8 hr for 7–10 days; dosage of 5 mg/kg/8 hr effective in adults
	Acyclovir	PO	2,000–4,000 mg/day in five divided doses for 10 days
	Acyclovir	Topical	Six applications/day for 7 days; ½ in. ribbon of 5% ointment per 4 square in. applied with gloved finger; useful only in limited, non-life-threatening infections
Herpes zoster	Acyclovir[a]	IV	500 mg/m²/8 hr for 7 days[d]; constant infusion over 1 hr; oral route of administration under study
Immunocompromised hosts[c]	Vidarabine[a]	IV	10 mg/kg/day for 5–7 days; constant infusion over 12–24 hr
Normal hosts	Acyclovir[a,e]	PO	4,000 mg/day in five divided doses for 5–7 days
Varicella Immunocompromised hosts	Acyclovir[a]	IV	500 mg/m²/8 hr for 7 days[d]
	Vidarabine[a]	IV	10 mg/kg/day for 5–7 days; constant infusion over 12–24 hr
Cytomegalovirus retinitis[h]	Ganciclovir[a,g]	IV	5.0 mg/kg/12 hr or 2.5 mg/kg/8 hr in 1 hr infusion for 14–21 days; see text regarding long-term suppression
Influenza A virus[f]	Amantadine	Oral	200 mg/day for 5–7 days; 4.4 mg/kg/day in children 1–9 yr to maximum of 150 mg; see text regarding prophylactic administration
	Rimantadine[a]	Oral	200–300 mg/day for 5–7 days; optimal dosage under study
RSV bronchiolitis/pneumonia	Ribavirin	Aerosol	Requires small particle aerosol generator; exposure 18–22 hr/day for 3–5 days at reservoir conc. 20 mg/ml, the delivered dose 0.8–1.8 mg/kg/hr depending on age
HIV-1 disease	Zidovudine	Oral	200 mg every 4 hr; alternative dose schedules under study
Genital papilloma (refractory)	Interferon (rIFN-α2b)	Intralesional	1 × 10⁶ units intralesional injection (0.1 ml) in up to 5 warts three times per week on alternate days for 3 weeks

[a] Not currently approved by the Food and Drug administration for this indication (January, 1989).
[b] Treatment of HSV ocular infections should be supervised by an ophthamologist. Duration of therapy and dosage depends on response.
[c] Antiviral therapy is most effective in localized herpes zoster ≤3 days duration.
[d] Dosage recommendations are those used in studies that showed efficacy in this condition. Acyclovir dosage of 250 mg/m² is approximately 6.2 mg/kg, and 500 mg/m² is approximately 12.4 mg/kg in a 70 kg adult. Dosage of 10 mg/kg/8 hr for 5–10 days recommended for VZV infection by some authorities.
[e] Efficacy established in older adults treated within 1–2 days of rash onset and in ophthalmic zoster.
[f] Efficacy documented only in uncomplicated influenza ≤48 hr duration.
[g] Currently available on compassionate use basis from Syntex Corp., Palo Alto, CA.
[h] See text regarding efficacy of the investigational drug foscarnet.

Drug Resistance

A related problem, which may limit the effectiveness of an antiviral drug, is the development of viral resistance to the inhibitory action of the drug. A well documented laboratory phenomenon for a variety of antiviral agents, in vivo development of drug resistance has been found during use of idoxuridine in HSV keratitis, acyclovir therapy of mucocutaneous HSV infection,[2–7] rimantadine treatment of influenza,[8–10] and recently ganciclovir treatment of CMV disease in AIDS patients.[11]

Host Immune Response

Since antivirals are virustatic or inhibitory in their activity, viral infection may resume when the compound is removed. Intact host immunologic responses remain essential for recovery from virus infections. Immunosuppression due to transplantation, cancer chemotherapy, or AIDS has been associated with high rates of recrudescent or chronic viral infections. Responses to antiviral treatment may be delayed and the risk of selecting drug-resistant viruses higher in such patients. Antivirals that impair host responses to infection, such as cytosine arabinoside in herpes zoster, may actually prolong the course of infection. Even effective antiviral agents, like acyclovir in primary HSV infections, may alter humoral and cellular immune responses, possibly by reducing viral antigen exposure.[12–16] Factors other than inhibition of viral replication alone are important in healing certain viral diseases, particularly mucocutaneous HSV infections, in which it has been possible to demonstrate antiviral effects without clinical benefit.

Combination Chemotherapy

The combined use of antiviral agents with different mechanisms of action has been investigated as a means of increasing antiviral activity, reducing the risk of toxicity, and preventing the development of drug-resistant virus. Combination therapy has been used successfully in experimental infections due to enteroviruses, influenza, HIV, and various herpesviruses.[17–22] Combined treatment with vidarabine and human leukocyte interferon has been reported to be clinically useful in chronic hepatitis B virus infections but is also associated with an increased risk of toxicity.[23,24] Combinations of vidarabine and acyclovir are expected to undergo testing in life-threatening HSV infections,[25] and alternating use of toxic agents, such as zidovudine and dideoxycytidine in AIDS, is being explored.[26]

Immunomodulation

Immunomodulating agents used for treating viral infections include those that supplement deficient host immune responses, such as exogenous antibody in chronic echovirus infection or interferon in herpes zoster of immunocompromised hosts. Intravenous immunoglobulin in combination with ganciclovir has been shown to be effective in CMV pneumonitis in bone marrow recipients.[27,28] Administration of transfer factor from persons recovering from chickenpox was shown to transfer cell-mediated immune (CMI) responses and to protect susceptible leukemic children from varicella, whereas a subsequent study in seropositive bone marrow was negative.[29] Chemical agents that appear to augment CMI responses, such as levamisole or inosiplex, have been used with variable success; all of these agents remain investigational.[29]

Drug Administration

Prophylaxis vs. Therapy. Prophylactic administration, as in amantadine hydrochloride for influenza A virus infection or methisazone in smallpox, is generally more effective than therapeutic administration. Since most antivirals probably serve to protect uninvolved cells and limit the spread of infection, rapid etiologic diagnosis and early administration of antiviral drugs are necessary for therapeutic efficacy.

Clinical and Laboratory Evaluation. Clinical efficacy depends on achieving effective antiviral concentrations at the site of infection, and specifically, adequate intracellular concentrations of an antiviral agent or its active metabolites. Pharmacokinetic studies that define absorption, stability in body fluids, tissue distribution, and metabolic fate of antiviral drugs are important in selecting proper dosage. Unfortunately, no standardized or generally accepted correlations exist between in vitro inhibitory concentrations, achievable blood or body fluid concentrations of antiviral agents, and clinical response.[1,30] Animal models are useful in testing antiviral agents, but may differ from the corresponding human infection in regard to pathogenesis, drug sensitivity of the virus, and drug pharmacology or toxicity.

Topical Administration. Topical application of antivirals to the cornea, skin, mucous membranes, or respiratory tract attempts to provide high concentrations at the site of infection and to avoid the possible toxicity of systemic administration. Topically applied drugs must be able to penetrate such barriers as stratified epithelium or local secretions to reach the site of active viral replication. For example, although beneificial in the treatment of HSV keratitis, topically applied vidarabine and its monophosphate derivative are ineffective in recurrent genital or labial HSV infections, except when applied by iontophoresis.[31,32]

Delivery of antiviral drugs to the respiratory tract in the form of small particle aerosols has been used with some benefit in influenza A, influenza B, and particularly RSV infections,[33–39] and the use of intranasally administered interferon has been shown to be protective in rhinovirus colds.[40]

ANTIVIRALS OF PROVEN EFFECTIVENESS

Acyclovir (Acycloguanosine, ACV, Zovirax)

Spectrum. Acyclovir (9-[2-hydroxyethoxymethyl]guanine) is a guanosine analogue that has an acyclic side chain, instead of the cyclic sugar moiety of natural nucleosides (Fig. 1). Its antiviral activity is limited to herpesviruses, including HSV types 1 and 2, varicella zoster virus (VZV), and Epstein-Barr virus.[41–45] Depending on the type of cell culture, acyclovir concentrations causing 50 percent reduction in plaque formation average 0.02–0.2 μg/ml for type 1 HSV, 0.03–0.5 μ/ml for type 2 HSV, and 0.8–1.2 μg/ml for VZV. Concentrations of approximately 1.6 μg/ml inhibit the replication of Epstein-Barr virus DNA in productively infected cells, but higher concentrations do not affect latent or persistent infection.[44] CMV plaque formation is inhibited by concentrations of 22.7 μg/ml and greater.[45] Acyclovir has shown antiviral activity in various animal models of HSV infection when administered topically, parenterally, or orally and in simian varicella when given systemically.[46–48] In HSV-induced skin infections of mice, early topical application prevents both lesions and the development of latent infection in sensory ganglia.

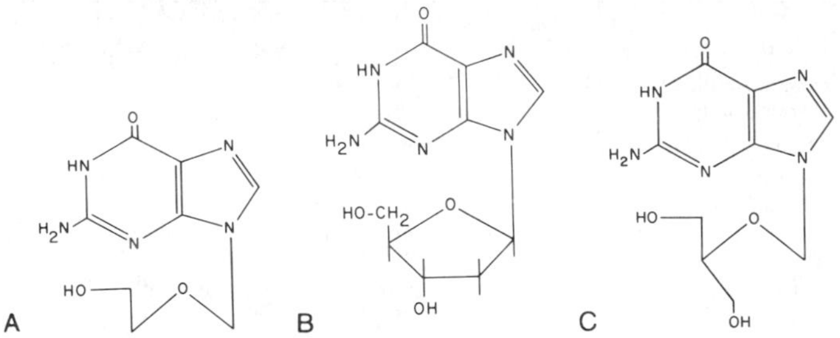

FIG. 1. Chemical structures of acyclovir **(A)**, the nucleoside deoxyguanosine **(B)**, and ganciclovir **(C)**.

Uninfected mammalian cells are generally unaffected by acyclovir concentrations ≤70 μg/ml. Acyclovir (20 μg/ml) does not alter cell-mediated immune responses of human peripheral blood leukocytes (PBL)[49] or affect human granulocyte progenitor cell growth[50] in vitro. Other studies have found that concentrations of 6.4–22.7 μg/ml inhibited the proliferative responses of human PBL to mitogens or herpesvirus antigens.[51,52]

Enhanced antiherpesvirus activity has been reported in combination with different agents[18,21,22] under laboratory conditions, and acyclovir potentiates the in vitro inhibition of HIV-1 by zidovudine.[53]

Mechanism of Action. The antiviral mechanism of action of acyclovir involves inhibition of viral DNA synthesis. It is the prototype of a group of antiviral agents that are activated by thymidine kinase to become inhibitors of viral polymerases.[41,54] Acyclovir uptake and intracellular phosphorylation to the monophosphate derivative are facilitated by HSV-induced thymidine kinase.[54] Cellular enzymes convert the monophosphate to acyclovir triphosphate, which is present in 40- to 100-fold higher concentrations in HSV-infected than in uninfected cells. The triphosphate form selectively inhibits viral DNA polymerase, and to a much smaller extent cellular DNA polymerases, and competes with guanosine triphosphate as a substrate for this enzyme.[55] Acyclovir triphosphate is also incorporated into viral DNA, where it acts as a chain terminator, because of the lack of a 3′-hydroxyl group.[56] Formation of a complex between the terminated DNA template containing acyclovir and the enzyme may lead to irreversible inactivation of the DNA polymerase.[57] The DNA polymerases of various herpesviruses differ in their degree of inhibition by acyclovir triphosphate; the polymerase of Epstein-Barr virus appears to be especially sensitive to its inhibitory action.[58]

Resistance. Alterations in either the viral thymidine kinase (TK) or DNA polymerase can cause acyclovir resistance in vitro.[59,60] Such mutants usually require acyclovir concentrations ≥3 μg/ml for inhibition. Most clinical acyclovir-resistant isolates have been TK-deficient ones recovered from immunocompromised patients receiving multiple courses of therapy. In animal models, acyclovir-resistant mutants with deficient TK activity appear to be less virulent and less likely to cause latent central nervous system (CNS) infection than wild-type strains, but some of these strains cause progressive mucocutaneous disease in highly immunocompromised hosts.[59,61,62] Clinical isolates that are acyclovir-resistant because of an altered TK substrate specificity or because of altered DNA polymerase also have been rarely recovered from treated patients.[59,63] One study found that 40 percent of HSV strains from untreated patients contained acyclovir-resistant virus, accounting for at least one percent of the total virus population.[6,7] Acyclovir-resistant strains of HSV with diminished TK activity have been isolated from immunocompromised patients given intravenous acyclovir for mucocutaneous HSV infections[2–5] and from patients with genital HSV infections before and after therapy.[64] One study of bone marrow transplant patients treated with intravenous acyclovir for recurrent mucocutaneous HSV infections recovered acyclovir-resistant virus in 1 of 52 first-treatment courses and 2 of 22 second courses.[5] Breakthrough isolates recovered during oral suppressive therapy include both resistant and sensitive phenotypes.[65,66] Lack of response to acyclovir associated with the presence of acyclovir-resistant mutants has been a particular problem in AIDS patients with mucocutaneous HSV infections.[11] Although documented,[59] VZV resistance has not yet been recognized as a clinical problem.[67] TK mutants remain sensitive to drugs like vidarabine and phosphonoformate that are not phosphorylated by the viral enzyme,[68] and these agents, particularly foscarnet, may be useful in such patients.

Pharmacology. The bioavailability of oral acyclovir is low (15 to 30 percent) and decreases with increasing doses.[69,70] Peak concentrations of 0.3–0.9 μg/ml occur at about 1.5 hours after 200 mg oral doses taken every 4 hours,[71] and peak levels average 1.8 μg/ml with 800 mg doses.[72] Bioavailability is lower in transplant patients, in whom doses of 400 mg five times daily provide peak levels of 0.7–0.9 μg/ml.[73] A liquid suspension has somewhat lower oral bioavailability; peak plasma concentrations average 1.0 μg/ml in children receiving 600 mg/m^2 doses.[74] An acyclovir prodrug, desciclovir or 6-deoxyacyclovir, is rapidly absorbed and converted to acyclovir by xanthine oxidase and provides blood levels comparable to those following intravenous dosing.[75,76]

Peak and trough plasma concentrations at the end of a 1-hour acyclovir infusion average 9.8 μg/ml and 0.7 μg/ml after 5 mg/kg/8 hr and 20.7 and 2.3 after 10 mg/kg/8 hr, respectively.[69] The volume of distribution corresponds to total body water. Cerebrospinal fluid concentrations are approximately one-half of plasma values.[69] After oral administration, salivary concentrations average 13 percent of simultaneous plasma concentrations, but vaginal secretion concentrations range from 15 to 170 percent of plasma values.[71] Zoster vesicular fluid levels are similar to those in plasma.[75] Aqueous humor levels average 37 percent of concurrent plasma values.[77] Breast milk concentrations average over threefold higher than those in serum.[78] Percutaneous absorption of acyclovir after topical administration appears to be low; plasma concentrations ranging from <0.01 to 0.3 μg/ml have been detected in herpes zoster patients treated topically. In patients with genital HSV infections treated with topical acyclovir, concentrations in genital lesions at 4 to 12 hours after application range widely (0.002–38 μg/ml), and no detectable acyclovir is present in cervicovaginal secretions.[64]

The plasma elimination $T_{1/2}$ of systemic acyclovir averages about 3 hours (range 1.5–6.3 hours) in adults with normal renal function, but is slightly longer (mean 3.8 hours) in neonates and increases to 19.5 hours in anuric patients.[69,79,80] Renal excretion of unmetabolized acyclovir by glomerular filtration and tubular secretion accounts for 60 to 91 percent of an administered dose, while less than 15 percent is excreted as 9-carboxymethoxymethylguanine or minor metabolites.[81,82] By competing for the organic acid secretory pathway, acyclovir may decrease the renal clearance of other drugs eliminated by active renal secretion, such as methothexate.[70] Dosage reductions are indicated in patients with creatinine clearances less than 50 ml/min/1.73 m^2 (see Table 2). Acyclovir is readily hemodialyzable, and 60 percent of the drug in the body will be removed during a 6-hour hemodialysis.[80,83] Peritoneal dialysis is severalfold less efficient in removing acyclovir, so that dosing supplementation is not needed during CAPD. An intravenous dose of 2.5 mg/kg/day has been proposed in CAPD patients.[84]

Toxicity. Acyclovir has shown mutagenic activity in some in vitro assays at high concentrations. No significant immunosuppressive activity, carcinogenicity, or teratogenicity has been noted in animal studies,[85] but safety in the pregnant human has not been established. High doses decrease spermatogenesis and causes testicular atrophy in animals.

Topical acyclovir may cause transient burning when applied to genital lesions, more commonly in first episodes and in female patients.[64] The polyethylene glycol base of topical acyclovir may cause mucosal irritation and is not approved for intravaginal use.

Intravenous acyclovir is generally well tolerated,[86] although inflammation, phlebitis, and rarely vesicular eruption[81] may occur at the injection site following extravasation of the alkaline solution (pH 9–11). Uncommonly reported side effects include rash, diaphoresis, hematuria, hypotention, headache, and nausea.[70] Approximately 1 percent of patients receiving intravenous acyclovir have manifested encephalopathic changes characterized by lethargy, obtundation, tremors, confusion, hallucinations, delerium, seizures, or coma.[86,88–91] Neurotoxicity is associated with renal insufficiency and unexpectedly high serum acyclovir concentrations.[91] Concurrent interferon administration or intrathecal methotrexate may be risk factors. One study found that 4 percent of bone marrow transplant recipients developed one or more neurotoxic symptoms after 2 to 18 days of intravenous acyclovir therapy (750–3,000 mg/m^2/day) for herpesvirus infection.[89] Most had diffuse electroencephalogram (EEG) abnormalities and increased cerebrospinal fluid concentrations of myelin basic protein. Improvement or resolution of symptoms occurred within 1 to 2 weeks after stopping treatment with acyclovir, but two patients developed neurologic symptoms again after reinstitution of therapy.

Reversible renal dysfunction has been observed in approximately 5 percent of patients treated with intravenous acyclovir at a dosage of 5 mg/kg/8 hr. In animals acyclovir can cause a crystalline nephropathy. Acyclovir solubility decreases to 2.5 mg/ml at 37°C, and crystalluria has been described in several adult and pediatric patients.[92,93] Bolus infusion, dehydration, pre-existing renal insufficiency, and high dose appear to be associated risk factors. Obstructive nephropathology related to high intravenous doses may be manifested by nausea, emesis, flank pain, and azotemia in patients without other risk factors.[93]

TABLE 2. Acyclovir Dosage Adjustments Suggested for Patients with Impaired Renal Function

Creatinine Clearance (ml/min/1.73 m²)	*Standard Dose (%)*	*Dosing Interval (hours)*
>50	100	8
25–50	100	12
10–25	100	24
0–10[a,b,c]	50	24

[a] An alternative in patients with end-stage renal disease is administration of 14 percent of standard dose every 8 hr after loading with 37 percent of the standard dose.[80]
[b] Posthemodialysis administration of 60–100 percent of standard dose.[83]
[c] Oral acyclovir dose adjustments are needed for severe renal insufficiency; suggested dosage is 200 mg every 12 hr at creatinine clearance <10 ml/min/1.73 m^2.
(Recommendations taken from Blum et al.[69] and Lanskin et al.[80])

One study found that one-half of adults receiving 500 mg/m²/dose for treatment of herpes zoster had reversible increases in serum creatinine of at least 25 percent,[94] although a subsequent study at the same dose found renal dysfunction in only 6 percent of acyclovir recipients.[95] Adverse symptoms and renal dysfunction have been related to high acyclovir plasma levels (>25 μg/ml) following intravenous use.[90]

Oral acyclovir has been associated infrequently with nausea, emesis, and headache. During long-term suppression of genital herpes, no effects on sperm motility or morphology have been recognized.[96]

No serious adverse drug interactions have been documented. Probenecid decreases the renal clearance and prolongs the plasma $T_{1/2}$.

Clinical Studies. Extensive clinical testing has established acyclovir as the treatment of choice in many types of HSV and VZV infections (Table 1). Comparative trials with vidarabine have found acyclovir to be superior in regard to efficacy and/or toxicity in HSV encephalitis[97,98] and in varicella[99] or herpes zoster[100] of immunocompromised patients, whereas comparable activity has been found in neonatal HSV infections.[101] Ease of administration has also led many physicians to prefer acyclovir.

A number of placebo-controlled, double-blind clinical trials have demonstrated the therapeutic efficacy of acyclovir in primary genital HSV infections.[102–107] Topical acyclovir is associated with therapeutic and antiviral effects of smaller magnitude than oral or intravenous administration (see Table 3), and does not influence the frequency of new lesion formation after initiation of treatment. Because some patients treated with topical acyclovir develop new lesions and/or increased symptoms after stopping therapy, longer durations of application (10–14 days) have been advocated.[64,105] Topical acyclovir has minimal clinical efficacy in patients with pre-existing HSV antibodies (nonprimary initial infection), such as individuals with a history of orofacial HSV infection, and although associated with an antiviral affect, topical acyclovir offers no significant clinical benefit in recurrent genital HSV infections.[105,108,109]

Intravenous acyclovir has been shown to reduce markedly the duration of viral shedding, time to healing, and duration of symptoms in patients hospitalized with severe primary genital HSV infections.[103] Similarly, in outpatients with initial genital HSV infections, oral acyclovir (200 mg 5 times daily for 10 days) has been associated with significant reductions in virus shedding, symptoms, and time to healing, as well as prevention of new vesicle formation compared with placebo.[103,107] Oral acyclovir has become the best outpatient regimen for initial genital HSV infections at the present time. None of these regimens has been associated with consistent reductions in the risk of recurrent genital lesions. Higher oral doses (400 mg five times daily for 10 days) provides similar benefit in first-episode HSV proctitis.[110] Acyclovir therapy decreases the humoral and cellular immune response to HSV following first-episode genital herpes.[15,16]

TABLE 3. Relative Effectiveness of Different Acyclovir Formulations in Treating First-Episode or Recurrent Genital Herpes Simplex Virus

	Percent Reduction Compared with Placebo		
	Duration of Viral Shedding	*Duration of Pain*	*Duration of Lesions*
First episode			
Intravenous	85	57	57
Oral	80	44	35
Ointment	55	26	29
Recurrent[a]			
Oral	46	12	21
Ointment	45[b]	0	0

[a] Patient-initiated therapy.
[b] Women only; no effect in males.
(Data from refs. 109, 111, and 113.)

Controlled clinical trials have also shown that oral acyclovir is associated with antiviral activity and statistically significant but modest clinical affects (Table 3) in recurrent genital HSV infections.[107,111] One study found that when therapy was initiated by patients during the prodrome or at the first sign of lesions, oral acyclovir was associated with significant but modest reductions in the durations of shedding (mean 2.1 vs. 3.9 days), time to healing (5.7 vs. 7.2 days), and frequency of new lesion formation (7 vs. 22 percent), but no difference in the duration of pain.[111]

In patients with frequently recurring genital herpes, chronic oral acyclovir (400–1,000 mg/day in divided doses) reduces the frequency of recurrences (~90 percent reduction) and protects 65–85 percent of patients from recurrence during a 4-month period.[65,102,112,113] Doses of 400 mg twice daily are well-tolerated and associated with 85 percent reduced frequency of recurrences over 2 years' use.[114] A dose regimen of 200 mg three times daily may be as effective and less costly. Ingestion of 800 mg doses once daily appears efficacious, but weekend only use is unsuccessful.[115,116] Asymptomatic shedding may occur during suppression, and occasional cases of transmission to sexual partners have been documented.[117] Following completion of acyclovir administration, patients generally return to their previous pattern of recurrent infection. Guidelines for this expensive intervention have been published.[102,113] Chronic suppression may be useful in other patients with disabling recurrences of herpes whitlow or HSV-related erythema multiforme.

In recurrent orolabial HSV infections, topical acyclovir reduces the duration of virus shedding in patients treated within hours of symptom onset but is not associated with clinical benefit compared with placebo.[119] Topical application of 5% acyclovir in a cream formulation, not currently available in the United States, has been reported to be therapeutically effective in both recurrent labial and genital HSV infections,[118] which suggests that penetration of intact skin is the crucial factor in effectiveness. Oral acyclovir (200–400 mg five times daily for 5 days) provides modest clinical benefit in recurrent orolabial herpes and cannot be routinely recommended.[119] In patients with a history of sun-induced recurrences, short-term prophylaxis (400 mg twice daily for 1 week) reduces the risk of recurrence by 75 percent in a high-risk setting.[120]

Systemic acyclovir in various regimens has been used successfully for both the prevention and treatment of mucocutaneous HSV infections in immunosuppressed patients.[111–127] Prophylactic intravenous acyclovir (250 mg/m²/8 to 12 hours), begun prior to transplantation and continuing for several weeks, is highly effective in reducing the incidence of HSV disease in seropositive bone marrow transplant recipients,[121,122] but patients may develop mild or asymptomatic HSV infections after acyclovir therapy is discontinued, and no effect on CMV infections is found. Once daily administration is inadequate. In patients who can tolerate oral medications, oral acyclovir (400 mg five times daily for 5 weeks) is also effective in preventing HSV relapses in marrow transplant patients.[73,123] Low doses of oral acyclovir (200 mg/8 hr for 30 days) appear to be effective in renal transplant patients.[124] In marrow transplant patients, long-term oral acyclovir (400 mg three times daily for 6 months) also reduces the risk of herpes zoster.[122] No immunosuppressive effects or adverse effects on marrow engraftment have been found. High-dose intravenous acyclovir (500 mg/m²/8 hr) beginning 5 days before bone marrow transplantation and continuing for 30 days afterwards is associated with delayed CMV excretion, 50 percent lower risk of CMV disease, and significantly improved survival compared with placebo in CMV-seropositive patients.[125] Chronic oral acyclovir (200 mg/6 hr) reduces the frequency of recurrent mucocutaneous HSV infections in immunosuppressed hosts[126] and during intense periods of leukemia chemotherapy.[127]

In therapeutic trials in immunocompromised patients with established mucocutaneous HSV infection, intravenous acyclovir (250 mg/m^2/8 hr for 7 days) shortens the median healing time by 25–65 percent, duration of pain and local symptoms by 30–60 percent, and the period of virus shedding by 60–80 percent when compared with placebo,[113,128] but recurrences are common after cessation of therapy. Oral acyclovir (800 mg five times per day) is also effective in marrow transplant patients.[129] Topical acyclovir theapy for labial or facial HSV infections in immunocompromised patients diminishes the duration of virus shedding and may shorten the time to loss of pain and healing of lesions.[130] However, topical acyclovir should be used only in limited extraoral mucocutaneous HSV infections in such patients.

The clinical usefulness of acyclovir in varicella zoster virus infections is established in immunocompromised patients but less clear in othewise healthy adults and children. In immunocompetent older adults, several studies have found that intravenous acyclovir is associated with significant reductions in the time to healing of skin lesions and the duration of pain during the acute phase of herpes zoster, if administered within 72–96 hours of the onset of symptoms.[94,131] In one study, acyclovir therapy (500 mg/m^2/8 hr for 5 days) significantly shortened the duration of virus shedding (2 vs. 5 days), duration of pain (2 vs. 5 days), duration of new lesion formation (2 vs. 4 days), and time to 50 percent healing (7 vs. 14 days) compared with placebo.[94] Because of the lower acyclovir sensitivity of VZV relative to HSV and acyclovir's low bioavailability, high oral doses are needed in treating VZV infections. Oral acyclovir (600–800 mg five times daily for 7–10 days) reduces acute pain, new lesion formation, and healing time in older adults, if treatment can be initiated within 1–2 days of rash onset.[72,132–135] Lower doses and later initiation of therapy are ineffective. Reductions in ocular complications (keratopathy, stromal keratitis, anterior uveitis) have been reported with oral acyclovir treatment of zoster ophthalmicus, even in patients treated after 72 hours of rash onset.[133] Unfortunately, no consistent effect on the incidence or severity of postherpetic neuralgia has been found with intravenous or oral acyclovir in herpes zoster, although one trial found a lower incidence of chronic pain (4 vs. 17 percent) during the first three months after oral treatment.[132] The combined use of oral prednisolone and acyclovir does not decrease the likelihood of postherpetic neuralgia compared to acyclovir alone.[135a] Patients with ophthalmic zoster and older adults ($\geq$60 years) with zoster of short duration appear to be appropriate candidates for this expensive treatment. Topical application of opthalmic acyclovir is more effective than topical corticosteroids in reducing ocular relapses of zoster ophthalmicus.[136] In varicella of previously healthy adults, intravenous acyclovir was associated with reductions in fever and vesicle duration but not in local symptoms.[137] Anecdotal reports suggest efficacy in varicella pneumonia or encephalitis.[138–140] Studies of oral acyclovir in childhood varicella are in progress.

In immunocompromised patients, intravenous acyclovir (500 mg/m^2/8 hr for 7 days) reduced the frequency of cutaneous dissemination (4 vs. 21 percent) and visceral complications (0 vs. 8 percent) compared with placebo.[95] Similar trends were seen in patients who had disseminated zoster at the time of initiating therapy, but no significant differences were observed in resolution of lesions or pain. One trial in severely compromised patients found that intravenous acyclovir reduced the duration of new lesion formation (3 vs. 6 days), time to complete healing (17 vs. 20 days), and risk of cutaneous dissemination (0 vs. 50 percent) compared with vidarabine,[100] whereas another comparative trial found no differences in efficacy between the drugs.[141] In immunosuppressed children with varicella, intravenous acyclovir (500 mg/m^2/8 hr for 5–7 days) is associated with a lower frequency of visceral complications (0 vs. 45 percent), compared with placebo,[142] and about 1-day reductions in the duration of vesicle formation and time to full crusting.[143] Early relapses of infection may occur following cessation of therapy, and treatment may be ineffective in established visceral disease.[144]

Intravenous acyclovir has been shown to be more effective and less toxic than vidarabine in treating HSV encephalitis.[97,98] The proportion of patients surviving at 6 months is increased from 46 to 50 percent with vidarabine to 81 percent with acyclovir. In neonates, immunosuppressed patients, and rarely in apparently healthy adults, early relapses of encephalitis may follow initial acyclovir therapy,[12–14,145] such that longer courses of treatment may be warranted. Progressive neurologic deterioration in infants has been managed with chronic suppressive oral acyclovir.[13]

Trials of intravenous acyclovir in established CMV infections have shown no consistent clinical benefit, although reductions in viremia and viral titers in the urine have been observed in some patients.[88,146,147] In an uncontrolled study of bone marrow transplant recipients with pneumonia, high-dose acyclovir was associated with possible bone marrow and neurologic toxicity but no clinical benefit.[88]

In infectious mononucleosis of normal hosts, intravenous or oral acyclovir is associated with transient suppression of virus excretion in the saliva and possibly slight reductions in upper respiratory symptoms but no effects on other disease parameters.[148,149] In one case of Epstein-Barr virus-related post-transplant lymphoma, acyclovir therapy appeared to suppress orofacial shedding of virus and induced transient remissions, although the patient ultimately died from a polyclonal B cell lymphoma.[150] Some but not all cases of severe Epstein-Barr virus infections have apparently responded to acyclovir.[150–152] Epstein-Barr virus-related oral hairy leukoplakia responds to oral acyclovir.[153] Acyclovir is ineffective in controlled studies in patients with chronic fatigue syndrome.[154]

Intravenous acyclovir has been reported to inhibit hepatitis B virus replication and enhance the effect of interferon in chronic infection,[155] but intravenous therapy for 4 weeks was of no significant benefit in a controlled trial in chronic hepatitis B patients.[156]

Amantadine (Symmetrel)

Spectrum. Amantadine (1-adamantanamine hydrochloride) is a symmetrical tricyclic amine (Fig. 2) that specifically inhibits the replication of influenza A viruses at low concentrations ($\leq$1.0 μg/ml).[157] By plaque assay, the 50 percent inhibitory concentrations of amantadine range from 0.2 to 0.4 μg/ml for human influenza A viruses including H1N1, H2N2, and H3N2 subtypes.[158,159] Clinical isolates vary in their susceptibility to amantadine,[160] but the significance of such differences is not defined. Higher concentrations (25–50 μg/ml) have variable in vitro inhibitory activity against some influenza B, rubella, paramyxo-, and arenaviruses,[157,161] but these concentrations are too high to be clinically relevant. Such amantadine concentrations may also be cytotoxic and can inhibit lymphocyte transformation responses to mitogen and specific antigens.

Both prophylactic and therapeutic activity has been demonstrated in experimental influenza A virus infection of ani-

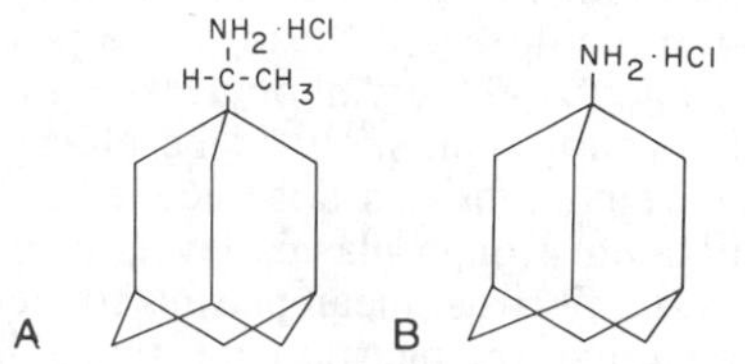

FIG. 2. Chemical structures of **(A)** rimantadine hydrochloride and amantadine hydrochloride **(B)**.

mals.[162] In animals, aerosol delivery of amantadine directly to the respiratory tract has greater efficacy than systemic administration.[19] Amantadine and ribavirin combinations show enhanced antiviral and therapeutic effects in vitro and in experimental murine influenza.[163]

Mechanism of Action. The exact mechanism of action of amantadine is undefined, but it appears to inhibit an early stage in viral replication, possibly uncoating of the viral genome in lysosomes.[157,164–167] Attachment and penetration of influenza virus appear to proceed normally in the presence of amantadine, and no direct effect on virus-associated RNA-dependent RNA polymerase activity has been found. Amantadine is readily concentrated and retained in the lysosomal fraction of mammalian cells, but its antiviral effect is quickly lost upon its removal from surrounding medium.[164] These findings indicate that most of the cell-associated amantadine may not contribute to its anti-influenza action and that amantadine mediating antiviral action may be taken up from the extracellular fluid with the virus.[165] Amantadine-mediated increases in lysosomal pH may inhibit virus-induced membrane fusion events and account for its broad antiviral spectrum at higher concentrations.[157,168] Effects on late replicative steps with impaired assembly of virions has been found for certain avian influenza viruses.[167]

Genetic reassortment studies indicate that amantadine sensitivity is primarily influenced by gene segment 7 coding for the M proteins, although the gene coding for the hemagglutinin may influence the sensitivity of certain strains.[167] Sensitivity of human isolates to low concentrations (1 μg/ml) of amantadine is a property conferred by the M2 protein, which is incorporated into the plasma membranes of influenza A, but not influenza B, virus-infected cells and into the virion.[8,167] Single amino acid changes in a critical transmembrane region of the M2 protein are associated with drug resistance, which indicates that this domain is the prime target of action.

Resistance. Resistance to amantadine is readily achieved in the laboratory by serial passage of influenza A virus strains in the presence of amantadine in vitro or in animals. Such isolates are cross-resistant to rimantadine. When amantadine treatment is given to birds infected with a highly pathogenic avian influenza virus, drug-resistant virus may emerge and cause death in the treated animals.[169] Furthermore, under conditions stimulating natural transmission, contact birds receiving amantadine prophylaxis frequently develop severe disease due to virulent drug-resistant virus after exposure to treated birds.[170] Administration of vaccine and amantadine together, but not vaccine alone, is protective for contact birds. Amantadine-resistant virus generated in the avian influenza model are virulent, genetically stable, and able to compete for infection with wild-type virus, such that transmission of drug-resistant virus may occur after cessaton of amantadine use.[171] Drug-resistant strains have been isolated from untreated patients[160] and recently from pediatric patients treated with rimantadine.[8–10,172] More studies are needed to define the clinical importance of such viruses.

Pharmacology. Amantadine is well absorbed after oral administration of capsule, tablet, or syrup forms.[173–176] The time to peak plasma level averages 2–4 hours but varies widely. Peak plasma concentrations average 0.2–0.4 μg/ml after administration of single 100 mg doses.[174] Steady-state peak plasma concentrations average 0.5–0.8 μg/ml on a 100 mg twice daily regimen in healthy young adults.[173,174] The elderly require only one-half of the weight-adjusted dose needed for young adults to achieve equivalent trough plasma levels of 0.3 μg/ml.[175] In children with cystic fibrosis, mean plasma concentrations were 0.6 μg/ml during long-term ingestion of 6 mg/kg/day, which suggests that such children require relatively large doses. Disproportionate increases in plasma concentrations as a function of dose may explain the high rates of neurotoxicity, including seizures, observed in one study employing 6.6 mg/kg/day doses in mentally handicapped patients.[176] Although some evidence suggests that amantadine is concentrated in pulmonary tissues,[177] nasal secretion and salivary levels of amantadine approximate those found in the serum.[174] Cerebrospinal fluid levels are about one-half of those in plasma, and amantadine is excreted in breast milk. After intermittent small-particle aerosol administration, nasal wash concentrations range from 2 to 19 μg/ml,[33] and the drug readily appears in the urine, indicating rapid absorption.

Amantadine is excreted unmetabolized in the urine through glomerular filtration and probably tubular secretion.[178] The plasma elimination $T_{1/2}$ is about 12–18 hours but ranges widely in apparently healthy young adults. Because of age-related declines in renal function, plasma $T_{1/2}$ increases up to twofold in the elderly,[174] and even more in patients with impaired renal function, in whom plasma concentrations from 1.0 to 5.0 μg/ml have been associated with confusion, delerium, hallucinations, seizures, and other signs of neurotoxicity.[178] In patients with creatinine clearance less than 10 ml/min/1.73 m^2, the $T_{1/2}$ may be as long as 30 days. Dosage guidelines for patients with renal insufficiency are summarized in Table 4. Amantadine is poorly excreted in hemodiaysis patients, and the amount removed by a single dialysis is only a small portion of the total body stores.[178,179] Monitoring of plasma concentrations in such patients is desirable but impractical.

Toxicity. In preclinical testing, amantadine lacked anti-inflammatory, antipyretic, or anticholinergic effects, but clinical observations of dry mouth, pupillary dilation, toxic psychosis, and urinary retention in acute overdose suggest that anticholinergic activity is present in humans.[173] Amantadine demonstrates indirect activity on the adrenergic nervous system by affecting accumulation, release, and reuptake of catecholamines in the central and peripheral nervous systems. The dopamine-enhancing effects of amantadine are probably the basis for its beneficial effects in parkinsonian patients. Ventricular irritability occurs in animals given high doses of intravenous or oral amantadine, and one case of malignant ventricular arrhythmia after amantadine overdose has been described in humans.[180] Amantadine is teratogenic in rodents, and its safety has not been established during pregnancy or lactation.

Orally administered amantadine is generally well tolerated, and no serious renal, hepatic, or hematopoetic toxicity has been documented. Long-term amantadine ingestion has been associated with livido reticularis, peripheral edema, orthostatic hypotension, and in isolated cases congestive heart failure, vision loss, and urinary retention. Patients with pre-existing seizure disorders have been reported to develop an increased frequency of major motor seizures during relatively high-dose amantadine

TABLE 4. Amantadine Dosage Regimens for Prophylaxis and Alterations in Renal Failure

	Suggested Dosage
No renal insufficiency	
Children, 1–9 yr	4.4 mg/kg/day once daily or in divided doses, up to 150 mg/day
Ages 10–64 yr	200 mg once daily or in divided doses
Ages ≥65 yr	100 mg/day
Creatinine clearance (ml/min/1.73 m^2)	
≥80[a]	200 mg once daily or in divided doses
60–80	200 mg/100 mg alternate days
40–60	100 mg daily
30–40	200 mg twice weekly
20–30	100 mg three times a week
10–20	200 mg/100 mg alternating every 7 days

[a] Based on adult dosage of 200 mg per day.
(Data from Horadan et al.[178] and Advisory Committee on Immunization Practices.[195])

ingestion,[181] but amantadine has also been used to treat refractory childhood epilepsy.[182] Psychiatric side effects in parkinsonian patients and psychotic exacerbations in schizophrenic patients have occurred with addition of amantadine.[183]

The most common side effects related to amantadine ingestion are minor gastrointestinal and central nervous system complaints. These include nervousness, lightheadedness, difficulty concentrating, insomnia, and loss of appetite or nausea.[173,184] Amantadine-associated side effects are related to dosage and duration of administration. Although higher doses have been used in the treatment of parkinsonian symptoms, dosages of 300 mg/day are poorly tolerated by healthy working adults and are also associated with significantly decreased performance on psychomotor tests designed to measure sustained attention and problem-solving ability.[185] In contrast, dosages of 200 mg/day has not been associated with consistent changes in psychomotor or academic performance in healthy adults.[185–188] When used for long-term influenza prophylaxis at dosages of 200 mg/day, adverse complaints have occurred in 5–33 percent of subjects and excess withdrawals because of drug side effects in 6–11 percent, relative to placebo.[173,184,188,189] Complaints typically develop within the first week of administration, often resolve despite continued ingestion, and are promptly reversible on discontinuation of the drug. During repeated dosing, trough steady-state plasma concentrations >0.45 μg/ml or peak concentrations >1.0 μg/ml are associated with an increased risk of CNS side effects.[190,191] Serious neurotoxic reactions may be transiently reversed by physostigmine administration.

The potential of CNS adverse effects appears to be increased by concomitant ingestion of antihistamines or anticholinergic drugs. Coadministration with anticholinergics in elderly patients may cause toxic delirum and visual hallucinations including lilliputian (small) and colored human figures. A diuretic combination of triamterene and hydrochlorothiazide was associated with CNS toxicity and a 50 percent increase in plasma amantadine concentration due to decreased renal clearance in one case.[192]

Clinical Studies. The clinical usefulness of amantadine as an antiviral agent is limited to the prevention and treatment of influenza A virus infections.[173,193] Early studies showed that amantadine was ineffective in the prophylaxis of influenza B or experimentally induced measles virus infections. A number of placebo-controlled, blinded studies have documented the prophylactic efficacy of amantadine at a dosage of 200 mg/day against the development of clinical illness in experimentally induced and naturally occurring influenza A virus infections.[173,184] The efficacy of amantadine in preventing illness documented to be secondary to influenza infection has ranged from 50 to over 90 percent, rates comparable to those obtained with inactivated influenza A virus vaccines. Prophylactic efficacy has been demonstrated in preventing nosocomial influenza and possibly in curtailing established nosocomial outbreaks.[181,182] Postexposure prophylaxis in family contacts has been associated with inconsistent protection.[173] Dosages of 100 mg/day have been shown to be protective against influenza A infection in semiclosed populations of teenaged students,[194] and studies to assess the efficacy of nontoxic lower doses are in progress.

Seasonal prophylaxis with amantadine is an alternative in high-risk patients, if the influenza vaccine cannot be administered because of toxicity or allergy, may be ineffective because the epidemic strain differs substantially from the antigens represented in the vaccine, or is unlikely to induce an adequate immune response, as in patients with primary or acquired immunodeficiency.[195] Because of the additive effect of antibody-associated protection and that provided by amantadine, the combined use of preseason vaccine and chemoprophylaxis during an outbreak provides optimal protection for particularly high-risk patients. To prevent the spread of influenza to high-risk patients, amantadine prophylaxis can be used in unimmunized health care workers and household members who have regular contact. Prophylaxis should be begun as soon as influenza is identified in a community or region and should be continued throughout the period of risk (usually 4–8 weeks), since any beneficial effects diminish rapidly after discontinuation of the drug. Alternatively, since amantadine does not interfere with the response to inactivated vaccine, the drug can be started in conjunction with immunization and continued for 2 weeks until protective antibody develops.

A series of controlled trials has demonstrated that amantadine is also an effective therapeutic agent in naturally occurring influenza A virus infection of previously healthy young adults.[173,90,196,197] When begun within 1–2 days of onset of symptoms, a dosage of 200 mg/day has been shown to reduce the duration of fever and systemic complaints by 1–2 days and in some studies to decrease the duration of virus shedding compared with placebo. One study found that amantadine-treated students were able to return to class more rapidly compared with placebo recipients.[196] One study comparing the efficacy of aspirin and amantadine treatment of naturally occurring H1N1 subtype influenza found that aspirin-treated patients defervesced more rapidly but experienced significantly higher rates of drug-related side effects and slower symptomatic improvement than amantadine recipients.[197] Other studies of adults with infection due to H3N2 subtype influenza viruses have found that certain abnormalities of peripheral airway function, but not airway hyperreactivity, resolve more quickly in amantadine-treated patients. However, trials to date have not determined whether amantadine prevents the pulmonary complications of influenza in high-risk patients or whether it is therapeutically useful in patients with established pulmonary complications. Therapeutic efficacy in children has received little study. Intermittent aerosol administration of amantadine has also proven therapeutically active in uncomplicated, naturally occurring influenza.[33] An injectable formulation is currently not available.

Ganciclovir (DHPG, 2′-NDG, BIOLF-62, B759U, Cytovene)

Spectrum. Ganciclovir (9-[1,3-dihydroxy-2-propoxymethyl]guanine) is an acyclic nucleoside analogue of guanine that differs from acyclovir in having an additional hydroxymethyl group on the side chain (Fig. 1). This agent has in vitro activity against all herpesviruses, but its unique characteristic is potent inhibition of CMV replication.[198–203] In plaque reduction assays, strains of HSV-1 and HSV-2 are inhibited by 0.05–0.6 μg/ml ganciclovir, CMV by 0.2–2.8 μg/ml, and VZV by 0.4–10 μ/ml. Thus, 50 percent inhibitory concentrations are similar to acyclovir against HSV and VZV but 10- to 50-fold lower against human CMV strains. Concentrations of 1–5 μg/ml also inhibit Epstein-Barr virus-mediated transformation of cord blood lymphocytes.[198] Systemic ganciclovir is effective at relatively low dosages (5–10 mg/kg/day) in rodent models of CMV[201] and HSV[198,199] infections. Effective doses in HSV encephalitis in mice are lower than those of acyclovir. Topically applied ganciclovir is active in models of HSV keratitis[204] and CMV pneumonia.[205] The combination of ganciclovir and β-interferon is synergistic in simian varicella.[206]

Although high concentrations are needed to inhibit the growth of uninfected cells, the 50 percent inhibitory concentrations for human bone marrow progenitor cells are about 0.6 μg/ml ganciclovir, compared with >25 μg/ml acyclovir.[207] In vitro, significant inhibition of human lymphocyte proliferative responses to mitogen and antigen occurs at 5–10 μg/ml ganciclovir.[208] Immune reactions that require active DNA synthesis may be depressed at therapeutic ganciclovir concentrations.

Mechanism of Action. Ganciclovir is an inhibitor of viral DNA synthesis. Intracellular ganciclovir is phosphorylated to the monophosphate derivative by infection-induced kinases, the viral thymidine kinase during HSV infection, and possibly a cellular deoxyguanosine kinase during CMV infection.[198,201,209,210] Ganciclovir di- and triphosphates are formed through the action of cellular enzymes. At least 10-fold higher concentrations of the triphosphate are present in CMV-infected cells compared with uninfected cells exposed to ganciclovir.[201] Intracellular ganciclovir triphosphate concentrations are also over 10-fold higher than those of acyclovir triphosphate in CMV-infected cells exposed to the drugs under similar conditions, and ganciclovir triphosphate levels decline much more slowly after drug removal.[209,210] These differences may account in part for ganciclovir's greater anti-CMV activity and explain how single daily doses are effective in suppressing human CMV infections.

Ganciclovir triphosphate is a competitive inhibitor of dGPT incorporation into DNA and preferentially inhibits viral rather than host cellular DNA polymerase.[211,212] Incorporation of ganciclovir triphosphate into viral DNA causes a slowing and subsequent cessation of viral DNA chain elongation.[213] Because of the two hydroxyl groups on the acyclic side chain, ganciclovir is incorporated internally into both host cell and viral DNA.[211]

Resistance. Ganciclovir is over 40-fold less active against acyclovir-resistant, thymidine kinase-deficient HSV strains.[198,199] HSV strains resistant to ganciclovir because of DNA polymerase mutation have been demonstrated in the laboratory, although some HSV strains resistant to gancyclovir because of DNA polymerase mutations retain sensitivity to ganciclovir.[212,214] A CMV strain resistant to ganciclovir because of reduced intracellular accumulation of ganciclovir triphosphate has been produced in the laboratory.[215] Ganciclovir-resistant strains of CMV have been uncommonly isolated from immunocompromised patients who remain culture-positive despite receiving the drug.[11,216,217]

Pharmacology. The oral bioavailability of ganciclovir in humans is very low (<5 percent of the administered dose),[218] and, consequently, almost all clinical trials have used intravenous administration. Peak and 6-hour trough plasma levels average 0.7–0.8 μg/ml and 0.2–0.3 μg/ml, respectively, after 20 mg/kg oral doses.[218] Oral doses of 1 gm three times daily are associated with greater bioavailability, perhaps related to gradual absorption, and peak plasma concentrations of 3–4 μg/ml. Prodrugs that are converted to ganciclovir and that have greater oral bioavailability are under development. The peak plasma concentrations at the end of a 1-hour 5 mg/kg or 2.5 mg/kg intravenous infusion average 8–11 μg/ml and 4–6 μg/ml, respectively.[217,219,220] Eight-hour trough concentrations after 2.5 mg/kg are 0.4–0.6 μg/ml. Following intravenous dosing, limited evidence suggests that aqueous and subretinal fluid levels are similar to those in serum and may persist longer.[221,222] Cerebrospinal fluid levels average 24–70 percent and brain tissue 38 percent of those in plasma.[217,220] After intravitreal injection of 200 μg ganciclovir, levels of about 1.2 μg/ml (51 hours) and 0.1 μg/ml (97 hours) have been found.[223]

The plasma elimination $T_{1/2}$ averages 3–4 hours in patients with normal renal function. In patients with mild renal insufficiency (serum creatinine (SCr) 1.4–2.5 mg/dl), plasma elimination $T_{1/2}$ averages 5.3 hours and increases to 9.7 hours in those with moderate (SCr 2.5–4.5) and to 28.5 hours in those with severe renal insufficiency (SCr >4.5).[224] Dose-independent kinetics are observed over the usual dose range, and twice daily administration of 5 mg/kg intravenously does not result in accumulation of ganciclovir in the plasma. Because ganciclovir is eliminated unmetabolized by renal excretion (>90 percent of dose), the clearance of ganciclovir correlates with creatinine (CrCl) clearance, and dose reductions are necessary in patients with renal impairment (CrCl <50 ml/min). A hemodialysis run reduces the plasma levels of ganciclovir by approximately 50 percent.

Toxicity. Ganciclovir is teratogenic in rabbits and is mutagenic in several different systems.[224] Systemic ganciclovir in mice and dogs causes significant toxicity involving the male and female reproductive, hematopoietic, and gastrointestinal systems. Testicular atrophy and bone marrow hypocellularity have been observed in animals at ganciclovir dosages comparable to those used in humans. Ganciclovir has carcinogenic potential in animals.

Evaluation of ganciclovir toxicity in humans has been difficult, because its use is restricted to severely ill patients with various concurrent illnesses and medications. The most common adverse events have been leukopenia, specifically neutropenia (<1,000 cells/mm^3) occurring in 40 percent or more of patients and thrombocytopenia (<50,000 platelets/mm^3) in up to 20 percent.[219,224–231] Neutropenia is most commonly observed during the second week of treatment, but may begin months later, and has been reversible in most patients, although persistent neutropenia complicated by fatal infections has been reported. The risk of neutropenia is higher in AIDS patients and is greatly enhanced by concurrent zidovudine therapy.[232] It may also be higher with tid dosing. Central nervous system side effects ranging in severity from headache to behavioral changes and psychosis to convulsions and coma have been described in 5–15 percent of treated patients. About one-third of patients receiving ganciclovir treatment have had to interrupt or prematurely stop therapy because of bone marrow or CNS toxicity. Frequent monitoring of blood counts for leukopenia is necessary to adjust doses, and treatment should be temporarily discontinued if the absolute neutrophil count falls below 500 cells/mm^3.

Anemia, rash, fever, liver function test abnormalities, azotemia, nausea or vomiting, and eosinophilia have also been reported. Phlebitis at the infusion site may be due to the alkaline pH of the solution. In the event of massive overdosage, hemodialysis and hydration may be effective in reducing plasma ganciclovir levels. Limited studies have found that about one-third of AIDS patients treated with long-term ganciclovir have greater than 50 percent increases in blood follicle-stimulating hormone (FSH), luteinizing hormone (LH), and testosterone values, perhaps related to gonadal toxicity.[231] Oral ganciclovir is associated with nausea.

Clinical Studies. Because of its toxicity, ganciclovir use has been limited to patients with life- or sight-threatening CMV infections. Compassionate use studies began in 1984 in AIDS patients and others with various immunodeficiency states related to transplantation or chemotherapy. The lack of placebo-controlled studies involving significant patient numbers and the use of various treatment regimens have compromised the interpretation of the results. The typical initial or induction treatment dosages have been 7.5–10 mg/kg/day in two or three divided doses given for 10 to 21 days. The largest experience and the clearest clinical responses have been in AIDS patients with CMV retinitis, over 85 percent of whom have improved or stabilized their disease with the initial treatment course.[219,227,232–235] Fundoscopic improvement is usually evident by 10–14 days. Historical controls indicate that over 90 percent of untreated AIDS patients will have progressive retinal disease leading to blindness, whereas retinitis in transplant patients may resolve spontaneously with reduction in immunosuppression. Approximately 90 percent of treated patients have a conversion of urine, blood, and throat cultures to negative or at least a greater than 100-fold reduction in viral titers. The median time to virologic response at these sites ranges from 3 to 8 days. Among AIDS patients who have responded to initial ganciclovir treatment, almost all have relapsed at a median of 2–5 weeks after cessation of therapy.[219,224,227] High doses of ganciclovir (25 to

35 mg/kg/week given once daily on 5 days/week), but not low doses (10–20 mg/kg/week), are effective suppressive therapy and increase the proportion of subjects free of relapse at 120 days from less than 15 percent to nearly 60 percent. Retinal detachments are common during long-term follow-up.[236] Ganciclovir-treated AIDS patients maintained on long-term suppressive therapy appear to have improved survival compared with historical controls.[231] Optimal dose schedules for initial and suppressive therapy have not been established.

Clinical improvement in 65 percent or more of patients and virologic responses have been found in uncontrolled studies of other CMV syndromes in AIDS patients, particularly CMV esophagitis, colitis, wasting syndrome, and possibly pneumonia.[219,226–228] Variable responses have been described in CNS syndromes.[219,229] In bone marrow transplant recipients, virologic responses but no reduction in mortality have been observed in patients with biopsy-proven CMV pneumonia treated with ganciclovir alone[217] or in combination with corticosteroids.[237] The combined use of ganciclovir and anti-CMV immune globulin has been associated with improved survival (43–80 percent) in CMV pneumonia compared with historical controls.[27,28] Uncontrolled studies suggest that renal or heart transplant and other immunosuppressed patients with pneumonia or other CMV syndromes respond to ganciclovir.[230,239,240]

Intravitreal ganciclovir is well tolerated in the rabbit eye[241] and has been used in limited studies for treating CMV retinitis in patients who are unable to tolerate systemic ganciclovir.[223]

Idoxuridine (IDU, IUDR, Stoxil, Herplex, Dendrid)

Idoxuridine (5-iodo-2′-deoxyuridine) is an iodinated thymidine analogue that inhibits the in vitro replication of various DNA viruses, particularly herpesviruses and poxviruses.[242] Plaque production by most clinical isolates of HSV type 1 is inhibited by concentrations of 2–10 μg/ml. Idoxuridine's antivirual mechanism of action is not completely defined, but the phosphorylated derivatives interfere with various enzyme systems, and the triphosphate inhibits viral DNA synthesis and is incorporated into both viral and cellular DNA. Resistance to the antiviral effect of idoxuridine readily develops under laboratory conditions and has occurred in viral isolates recovered from idoxuridine-treated patients with HSV keratitis. In humans, intravenously administered idoxuridine is rapidly metabolized to iodouracil and uracil. Extremely low plasma concentrations of idoxuridine (0.1–0.4 ppm) were detected in about one-half of patients treated topically with 40% idoxuridine in dimethyl sulfoxide. Idoxuridine is teratogenic, mutagenic, and immunosuppressive in certain experimental systems.

Clinical Studies. Parenteral idoxuridine is not useful because of liver function abnormalities and serious bone marrow toxicity.

The therapeutic usefulness of topically applied idoxuridine depends on the site of infection and the vehicle of administration. Idoxuridine in ointment or solution form is ineffective in recurrent herpes labialis, varicella, or localized herpes zoster, whereas frequent application of idoxuridine dissolved in dimethyl sulfoxide (5–40% idoxuridine in 100% DMSO) has been reported to hasten the healing of skin lesions and shorten the duration of pain in localized herpes zoster. Topical application of 30% idoxuridine in DMSO may shorten the duration of viral shedding in recurrent or primary genital HSV infections, but does not reduce the duration of symptoms or healing time.[243] Mild local burning after topical application of DMSO is common, and headache, dizziness, sedation, nausea, and localized and generalized dermatitis have also been reported. DMSO is teratogenic and can cause adverse ocular effects in laboratory animals.

In the United States, idoxuridine is approved by the FDA only for topical treatment of HSV keratitis.[244,245] Controlled trials and extensive clinical experience have indicated greater efficacy in epithelial infections, especially initial episodes, than in stromal infections. Adverse reactions include pain, pruritis, inflammation, or edema involving the eye or lids and rarely allergic reactions.

Ribavirin (Virazole)

The synthetic nucleoside ribavirin (1-beta-D-ribofuranosyl-1,2,4-triazole-3-carboxamide) is a guanosine analogue (Fig. 3), in which both the base and the D-ribose sugar are necessary for antiviral activity.[246] Ribavirin inhibits the in vitro replication of a wide range of RNA and DNA viruses, including myxo-, paramyxo-, arena-, bunya-, RNA tumor, herpes, adeno-, pox-, and retroviruses including HIV-1.[246–250] By plaque assay the ED_{50} concentrations range from 3 to 10 μg/ml for influenza A and B[248] and RSV[241] viruses. Inhibitory concentrations for a particular virus differ markedly in different cell types, and the ability of cells to take up ribavirin and form active metabolites may be important determinants of antiviral activity. Ribavirin is generally not active against viruses with single-stranded RNA genomes that act directly as messenger RNA, such as entero- and rhinoviruses. Relatively high concentrations (30–50 μg/ml) inhibit acute HIV infection of human lymphocytes.[249] Ribavirin antagonizes the anti-HIV-1 effects of zidovudine but enhances the activity of purine dideoxynucleosides.[250]

Low concentrations of ribavirin (2–10 μg/ml) reversibly inhibit macromolecular synthesis and the proliferation of certain rapidly dividing, uninfected mammalian cells.[248] Ribavirin suppresses nucleic acid synthesis in quiescent and mitogen-stimulated human peripheal blood lymphocytes in vitro,[252] but does not adversely affect polymorphonuclear leukocyte functions.[253] Inhibition of mast cell secretory responses occurs after in vitro ribavirin exposure.[254]

Aerosol administration has greater therapeutic activity than the parenteral route in animal models of influenza[19] and RSV infection.[255] Brief aerosol exposures (4 hr/day) employing threefold higher reservoir concentrations are also effective in models of influenza and RSV infection.[256] Parenterally administered ribarivin has antiviral and therapeutic activity in animal models of lassavirus, other arenaviruses, and bunyavirus infections,[251,257–259] but late deaths due to central nervous system infection may occur despite ribavirin therapy.[258] Enhanced therapeutic efficacy occurs in certain animal models when ribavirin is administered in liposomes or in combination with other antivirals or immune modulators.[163,259–261] Parenteral immunoglobulin potentiates the antiviral activity of aerosol ribavirin in the cotton rat model of RSV infection,[261] and increased anti-influenza activity is seen with combinations of ribavirin and amantadine or rimantadine.[163]

Mechanism of Action. The antiviral mechanism of action of ribavirin is not fully defined but relates to alteration of cellular nucleotide pools and of viral messenger RNA formation.[246] Intracellular phosphorylation to the mono-, di-, and triphosphate

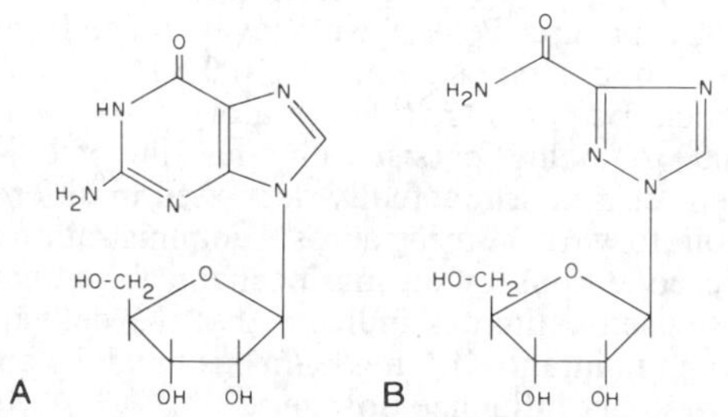

FIG. 3. Chemical structures of the nucleoside guanosine (**A**) and ribavirin (**B**).

derivatives is mediated by host cell enzymes. In both uninfected and RSV-infected cells, the predominant derivative (>80 percent) is the triphosphate, which is rapidly degraded ($T_{1/2}$ <2 hours) after removal of drug from the surrounding medium.[262] Ribavirin monophosphate competitively inhibits inosine-5′-phosphate dehydrogenase (IMPDH) and interferes with the synthesis of guanosine triphosphate (GTP) and thus nucleic acid synthesis. However, inhibition of this normal cellular enzyme would not fully account for a selective antiviral action, although inhibition of IMPDH and resultant decreased concentrations of competing guanosine could potentiate other antiviral effects. Ribavirin triphosphate has been reported to selectively inhibit influenza virus RNA polymerase activity and to be a competitive inhibitor of the GTP-dependent 5′-capping of viral messenger RNA. Ribavirin triphosphate appears to inhibit the initiation and particularly the elongation of capped mRNA primer fragments by the influenza virus polymerase complex,[263] which in turn causes inhibition of viral protein synthesis.

Ribavirin has biologic activities beyond its antiviral and cytotoxic effects. In rodents, parenteral ribavirin inhibits the serum antibody but not cellular immune responses to inactivated influenza vaccine and diminishes in vivo primary antibody responses and memory cell generation to T-dependent and T-independent antigens.[264] In experimental animals, ribavirin has therapeutic activity against transplantable virus-induced tumors and autoimmune diseases.

Resistance. In contrast to other synthetic antiviral agents, resistance to ribavirin has not been produced under experimental conditions, except for the recent description of ribavirin-resistant sindbis virus mutants.[265] No ribavirin-resistant RSV have been detected during aerosol therapy of children.[36]

Pharmacology. Following oral administration, bioavailability averages 45 percent.[266] Following single oral doses of 600, 1200, or 2400 mg, peak plasma concentrations occur at 1–2 hours and average 1.3, 2.5, and 3.2 μg/ml, respectively. Tenfold higher peak plasma levels occur 0.5 hours after intravenous administration of equivalent doses.[266] Ribavirin accumulates during prolonged oral dosing, such that trough plasma levels average 1.3 and 3.3 μg/ml during the second week of treatment with 200 and 400 mg every 8 hours, respectively.[267] Plasma concentrations average approximately 24 μg/ml and 17 μg/ml after intravenous doses of 1000 and 500 mg, respectively, in Lassa fever patients.[268] During chronic oral administration of 300 mg twice daily cerebrospinal fluid levels average more than two-thirds of those in plasma (1.5–3 μg/ml).[269]

The disposition of ribavirin is complex. The β-phase $T_{1/2}$ is about 2.0 hours, but a prolonged terminal (γ)-phase $T_{1/2}$ of 36 hours occurs after single doses.[266] Ribavirin triphosphate concentrates in erythrocytes (~3 percent of dose), and RBC levels gradually decrease, with an apparent $T_{1/2}$ of about 40 days.[270] With chronic administration and RBC accumulation of ribavirin, the terminal plasma $T_{1/2}$ increases to 1–2 weeks.[267] Renal excretion accounts for approximately one-third of the drug's clearance, but hepatic metabolism is the major route of elimination.

With aerosol administration, plasma levels increase with the duration of exposure. Peak plasma levels range from 0.5 to 2.2 μg/ml after 8 hours exposure and from 0.8 to 3.3 μg/ml after 20 hours in pediatric patients.[268] Respiratory secretion levels often exceed 1000 μg/ml and persist with a half-life of 1.4–2.5 hours. The amount of ribavirin actually deposited in different regions of the respiratory tract during aerosol administration in different pathologic conditions or during mechanical ventilation is not certain. Revised estimates indicate that the delivered dose is twice as high in infants (1.8 mg/kg/hr) as in adults and that various other factors influence dosage.[270]

Toxicity. Ribavirin has been found to have cell-transforming, mutagenic, tumor-promoting, and possibly gonadotoxic activities in preclinical testing. Ribavirin is teratogenic and embryotoxic in small mammals[271] and is consequently contraindicated in pregnancy.

Prolonged administration causes a dose-dependent, macrocytic anemia in animals and humans,[271] and increased reticulocyte counts occur in ribavirin-treated patients after cessation of oral therapy.[272] Systemic ribavirin causes dose-related anemia due to extravascular hemolysis[267] and, at higher doses, suppression of bone marrow release of erythroid elements. Reversible increases of serum bilirubin in up to one-quarter of recipients, serum iron, and uric acid concentrations occur during short-term administration of oral ribavirin.[271,272] Chronic oral therapy is also associated with dose-related gastrointestinal and central nervous system complaints, including headache, lethargy, insomnia, and mood alteration in HIV-infected patients.[267]

Aerosolized ribavirin has been well tolerated except for mild conjunctival irritation and rash, transient wheezing, and occasional reversible deterioration in pulmonary function.[36,39,274] No adverse hematologic effects have been associated with aerosol ribavirin. One study did not find evidence of ribavirin absorption in health care providers working in the environment of aerosol-treated infants,[275] but another detected environmental contamination and ribavirin absorption in one nurse.[275a] When used in conjunction with mechanical ventilation, in-line filters, modified circuitry, and frequent monitoring are required to prevent plugging of ventilator valves and tubing with precipitates of ribavirin.[276–279] The possible effects of such modifications on drug delivery to the lower respiratory tract are undefined.

Clinical Studies. Ribavirin aerosol is approved by the Food and Drug Administration for treatment of RSV bronchiolitis and pneumonia in children.[279] A special aerosol generator utilizing a modified Collison nebulizer is needed to produce particles of proper aerodynamic size to reach the lower respiratory tract (SPAG-2, Viratek Corp). In infants less than 1 year old, the estimated delivered dose is 1.8 mg/kg/hr of aerosol exposure, when the reservoir concentration is 20 mg/ml ribavirin.[270] An initial controlled trial found that aerosolized ribavirin (20 hours exposure/day for 3–6 days) shortened the duration of virus shedding and improved certain clinical measures, including arterial oxygen saturation, in infants hospitalized with RSV pneumonia.[36] Similar studies of infants with RSV disease found that aerosolized ribavirin (12–22 hr/day for 3–5 days) was associated with some reductions in illness severity but not in duration of hospitalization or virus shedding.[37–39,276] More rapid improvements in illness severity and oxygenation have been documented in high-risk subjects with bronchopulmonary dysplasia or congenital heart disease.[38,39] Expert opinion varies about the overall clinical value, indications for use, and optimal length of aerosol ribavirin therapy in RSV infections.[279–282] Trials to date have not determined whether this costly intervention reduces the likelihood of intubation or death, shortens hospitalization time, or provides long-term benefit. Decreased RSV-specific serum neutralizing antibody titers, as well as diminished nasopharyngeal secretion RSV-specific IgE and IgA responses, may occur in ribavirin treated children compared with placebo,[37,283] but the clinical significance of these findings is uncertain.

Anecdotal reports also suggest efficacy of aerosol ribavirin in severe influenza and parainfluenza virus infection.[284] Ribavirin aerosol treatment for an average of 12–18 hours per day for 3 days was associated with reductions in viral titers, fever, and systemic illness compared with placebo in young adults with uncomplicated influenza A or B virus infection in some but not all studies.[284,285] The relative therapeutic activity of aerosolized ribavirin and oral amantadine or rimantadine in influenza A virus infections and the value of aerosolized or intravenous ribavirin in high-risk groups, such as infants or adults hospitalized with influenza, are undetermined. Oral doses of 1000 mg/day had no clinical or antiviral activity in naturally occurring influenza A virus infection of adults.[272] An oral regimen with loading doses (3.6 mg over 3 hours) may provide clinical benefit in uncomplicated influenza.[286]

In Lassa fever patients at high risk of death because of elevated serum asparate aminotransferase levels or high-titer viremia, intravenous (4 gm/day) or oral ribavirin significantly reduced mortality, especially when therapy was initiated during the first 6 days of illness.[287] High-dose intravenous therapy has also been associated with reduced mortality in Korean hemorrhagic fever[288] and with antiviral effects in Argentine hemorrhagic fever.[289] Uncontrolled studies of chronic oral ribavirin 600 mg/day have found acceptable tolerance and possible antiviral effects in AIDS and ARC patients, but no consistent effects on T4 counts, viral isolation, or serum p24 antigen levels have been documented.[267,290] A placebo-controlled trial reported that ribavirin 800 mg/day reduced the risk of progression from lymphadenopathy syndrome to AIDS.[291] Oral ribavirin has also been reported to provide clinical benefit in measles, acute hepatitis, and mucocutaneous herpes virus infections,[292–294] but confirmation of such observations is needed.

Rimantadine Hydrochloride (Flumadine)

Spectrum. Rimantadine (alpha-methyl-1-adamantane methylamine hydrochloride) is a structural analogue of amantadine (Fig. 2) and shares its antiviral spectrum and mechanism of action. In yield reduction assays, most clinical isolates of influenza A virus are inhibited by ≤ 1 μg/ml, and concentrations of 0.1–0.4 μg/ml inhibit plaque formation by 50 percent or more.[158,159] In ferret tracheal organ culture, rimantadine has comparable antiviral activity to amantadine at four- to eightfold lower concentrations.[295] Concentrations of 10 μg/ml and higher are inhibitory for other enveloped viruses, including parainfluenza, influenza B, rubella, and dengue.[296] Such concentrations are also toxic to ciliated epithelium[295] and inhibitory to lymphocyte blastogenic responses in vitro.

Orally or parenterally administered rimantadine is effective in the prevention and treatment of influenza in various animal models, in which it appears to be more effective than amantadine on a weight basis. Treatment of infected mice limits the extent of virus replication and reduces the risk of transmission to exposed, uninfected animals. In mice, small particle aerosol delivery of rimantadine appears to be associated with greater antiviral and clinical effects than does intraperitoneal administration of comparable doses. Rimantadine exhibits enhanced antiviral activity in combination with ribavirin, interferon, or protease inhibitors.[163,297]

Mechanism of Action. Rimantadine inhibits an early step in the influenza virus replicative cycle, probably viral uncoating at the lysosomal stage.[298,299] Some studies suggest that rimantadine inhibits hemagglutinin-mediated fusion of the viral envelope and lysosomal membrane through increases in lysosomal pH.[300] Such an effect may account for the nonselective inhibitory effect of higher concentrations. However, interference with the removal of M protein from influenza viral ribonucleoproteins has been described,[299] and genetic studies have found that rimantadine's specific effect on human influenza A virus replication at low concentrations relates to gene 7 and its product the M2 protein.[8,167] Single amino acid changes at one of four or five sites in a critical hydrophobic transmembrane region of the M2 protein are associated with drug resistance.

Resistance. Rimantadine-resistant strains of influenza A virus may be readily recovered after passage of the virus in cell culture (frequency 10^{-3}–10^{-4}) or in animals in the presence of the compound.[8,170] Such isolates are cross-resistant to amantadine. In an avian model of influenza, treatment of infected birds is associated with the excretion of rimantadine-resistant virus within several days, and such viruses are capable of infecting and causing severe disease in contact animals receiving rimantadine prophylaxis.[170]

Young children treated with oral rimantadine for established influenza A virus infections may excrete drug-resistant virus by days 4–6 of therapy.[8,9] Transmission of drug-resistant influenza viruses to household contacts receiving rimantadine prophylaxis has also been found in families.[172] The clinical significance of these observations requires further study, but the finding raises questions about the routine use of these drugs in treating pediatric patients, who tend to shed virus longer and in higher titers than adults.

Pharmacology. Rimantadine in tablet form is well but slowly absorbed, and oral absorption does not appear to be decreased by the presence of food.[174,304] A syrup formulation, intended for pediatric use, has oral bioavailability slightly lower than the tablet.[305] The mean time to maximum plasma concentration averages 2–6 hours after administration. With multiple doses of 100 mg twice daily, the steady-state peak and trough plasma concentrations in healthy adults are approximately 0.4–0.5 μg/ml and 0.2–0.4 μg/ml, respectively.[306] In infants receiving doses of 3 mg/kg each day, steady-state peak serum levels range from 0.1 to 0.6 μg/ml.[307] No important age-related changes in plasma levels or pharmacokinetics have been found in healthy elderly adults or in children.[174,308,309] However, steady-state plasma concentrations in elderly nursing home residents receiving 100 mg twice daily averaged over twofold higher (mean, 1.2 μg/ml) than those observed in healthy adults,[303] which indicates the need for dose reductions in such patients. Rimantadine has an exceedingly large volume of distribution, and concentrations in nasal mucus average 50 percent higher than those in plasma.[174,309] Concentration of rimantadine in respiratory secretions could in part account for its efficacy despite lower plasma concentrations than with amantadine.

In contrast to amantadine, rimantadine is extensively metabolized following oral administration. Less than 15 percent of the dose is excreted unchanged in the urine, and approximately 20 percent of the dose is excreted in the urine as hydroxylated metabolites.[174,310] The remaining metabolites have not been fully identified. The plasma elimination $T_{1/2}$ of rimantadine averages 24–36 hours, approximately twofold longer than that of amantadine. In patients with chronic liver disease, without significant hepatocellular dysfunction, no clinically important differences in single-dose pharmacokinetics were found in one study.[311] In hemodialysis patients with severe renal failure, the clearance of rimantadine is decreased by 40 percent, and the elimination $T_{1/2}$ is about 55 percent longer.[310] Guidelines for dose adjustment in less severe renal insufficiency are being developed. Hemodialysis removes only a small amount of rimantadine, so that supplemental doses are not required.[310]

Toxicity. In animals given 5–20 times the recommended human doses, central nervous system (tremors, convulsions) and gastrointestinal side effects, as well as renal glomerular changes at very high doses, are observed during long-term administration. Rimantadine is not mutagenic in vitro and does not appear to cause teratogenic effects in rabbits or rats. However, safety in pregnancy has not been established.

Rimantadine administration is associated with dose-related, reversible side effects qualitatively similar to those observed with amantadine.[173] However, central nervous system side effects are significantly less frequent with rimantadine at dosages of 200 or 300 mg per day.[184,185,196] Rimantadine 300 mg/day is associated with significantly higher rates of gastrointestinal complaints, but not central nervous system or sleep disturbances compared with placebo.[185] Unlike amantadine, it is not associated with alterations of psychomotor test performance at this dosage. Most studies in adults and children have found excess withdrawal rates of less than 5 percent compared with placebo.[301,302] However, conventional 200 mg per day doses are associated with higher plasma levels and side effect rates in elderly nursing home residents.[303] The wider therapeutic margin of rimantadine, relative to amantadine, relates to differences in pharmacokinetics between the drugs.[190] Similar rates of CNS side effects are observed at comparable plasma concentrations. Rimantadine use has been anecdotally associated with exacerbations of seizures.

No clinically important laboratory abnormalities have been described, except for slight (less than threefold) elevations in transaminases in small numbers of subjects, and no serious end organ toxicity of rimantadine is recognized.[302] Drug interactions with rimantadine have not been studied, but patients receiving it concurrently with drugs affecting CNS function (e.g., antihistamines, antidepressants, and minor tranquilizers) should be watched for increased evidence of side effects.

Clinical Studies. Placebo-controlled, double-blind trials have shown that rimantadine is effective in preventing either experimentally induced or naturally occurring influenza virus infection.[173,184,193,312–314] Daily dosages of 200 mg in adults and of 5 mg/kg/day in children[313] have proven effective in preventing illness due to various influenza A subtypes during seasonal prophylaxis. One 6-week field trial comparing equivalent 200 mg/day dosages of rimantadine and amantadine found that the drugs were 85 and 91 percent effective, respectively, in preventing laboratory-documented influenza A illness.[184] In immunized nursing home patients, rimantadine (100 mg bid) had 75 percent efficacy in preventing influenza A illness compared with placebo during a community epidemic.[193] During a 5-week household-based study, rimantadine (5 mg/kg/day) administration to school-aged children decreased the risk of influenza A illness in recipients (100 percent efficacy) and possibly in their family contacts.[313] Studies to determine the minimally effective dose for long-term prophylaxis in healthy and high-risk elderly adults and the utility of postexposure prophylaxis in the family setting are currently in progress.

Therapeutic use of rimantadine is effective in uncomplicated influenza A virus infections, if treatment is begun within 48 hours of illness onset.[173,196,314,315] Oral rimantadine (300 mg/day) has therapeutic effects in uncomplicated, naturally occurring influenza A virus infection comparable to those of amantadine (200 mg/day). One study employing equivalent 100 mg bid dosing found that amantadine-treated patients tended to improve more rapidly than rimantadine-treated patients over the first 24 hours, but that by 48 hours after initiating therapy, both groups had significantly less fever, greater symptomatic improvement, and lower frequencies of virus shedding than placebo-treated patients.[196] Similar therapeutic benefit has been found in elderly influenza patients treated with rimantadine.[314] Because of rimantadine's slow absorption, low initial plasma levels, and long elimination half-life, therapeutic regimens using larger doses (400–600 mg in divided doses) over the first 24 hours of treatment may provide greater antiviral and clinical effects.[315] The possible value of rimantadine in treating acute influenza in high-risk patients to prevent complications and in treating severe influenza in hospitalized patients is currently under study. Aerosolized rimantadine has received limited study.[316]

In children with influenza A/H3N2 subtype infection, rimantadine treatment (6 mg/kg/day, up to 150 mg for those <9 years) for 5 days was associated with lower symptom burden, fever, and viral titers during the first 2 days of treatment compared with acetaminophen administration, but rimantadine-treated children had more prolonged shedding of influenza virus.[8,9] A similar study involving children with milder H1N1 subtype infection found reductions in viral shedding on the first and second days of treatment but no significant clinical benefit of rimantadine compared with acetaminophen.[10] No effects on antibody responses have been found when rimantadine is used for treatment of established influenza, but effects on other host responses to infection have not been critically evaluated. The optimal dose and duration of therapy have not been established in children, and the problem of rapid emergence of drug-resistant virus[8,10] may limit its therapeutic application in this age group.

Trifluridine (5-trifluoromethyl-2′-deoxyuridine, trifluorothymidine, Viroptic)

Trifluridine is a fluorinated pyrimidine nucleoside that has in vitro inhibitory activity against HSV types 1 and 2, cytomegalovirus, vaccinia, and some strains of adenovirus.[242,317] Its antiviral mechanism of action is undefined but involves inhibition of viral DNA synthesis. It also inhibits cellular DNA synthesis at relatively low concentrations. The triphosphate derivative is incorporated into viral, and to a lesser extent cellular DNA, in competition with deoxythymidine triphosphate. Trifluridine is active against thymidine kinase-negative strains of HSV, which indicates that this enzyme is not essential to its action. It also exhibits mutagenic, teratogenic, and antineoplastic activities in experimental systems.

Its use as an antiviral agent is currently limited to topical therapy of ocular HSV infections, in which it is approved by the Food and Drug Administration for treatment of primary keratoconjuctivitis and recurrent epithelial keratitis due to HSV types 1 and 2.[244,245] Topical trifluridine has been found to be more active than idoxuridine, but trials comparing its efficacy with that of topical vidarabine have generally found no significant differences.[318] Topical trifluridine has been effective in some patients who have not responded clinically to idoxuridine or vidarabine. Adverse reactions include discomfort upon instillation, palpebral edema, and, uncommonly, hypersensitivity reactions, irritation, superficial punctate, or epithelial keratopathy.

Vidarabine (ara-A, adenine arabinoside, Vira-A)

Spectrum. Vidarabine (9-beta-D-ribofuranosyladenine) is an analogue of adenine deoxyriboside (Fig. 4), which has in vitro antiviral activity against HSV types 1 and 2, VZV, Epstein-Barr virus, animal herpesviruses, vaccinia and variola viruses, and rhabdo and some RNA tumor viruses. Vidarabine also inhibits the in vitro replication of idoxuridine or acyclovir-resistant HSV strains and acyclovir-resistant VZV strains, but has variable activity against cytomegalovirus.[319–321] Plaque formation by most HSV and VZV strains is completely inhibited by 3.0 μg/ml or less of vidarabine. This concentration does not inhibit mytogen-or antigen-induced lymphocyte blastogenesis or lymphocyte cytotoxicity to herpesvirus-infected target cells in vitro.

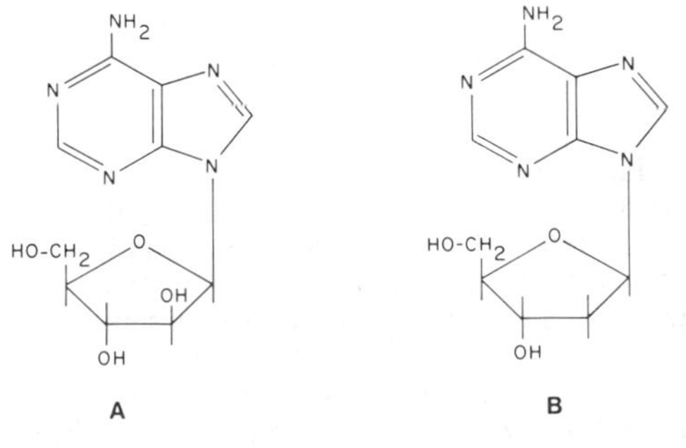

FIG. 4. Chemical structures of vidarabine (**A**) and the nucleoside deoxyadenosine (**B**).

Mechanism of Action. The antiviral mechanisms of vidarabine are not completely understood but it is an inhibitor of HSV DNA synthesis. Vidarabine is phosphorylated by cellular enzymes to the triphosphate derivative, which competitively inhibits HSV, and, to a lesser extent, cellular DNA polymerase activity. Vidarabine triphosphate is incorporated into both cellular and viral DNA, where it may act as a chain terminator for newly synthesized HSV nucleic acid.[322] The principal metabolite in vivo and in cell culture is hypoxanthine arabinoside (ara-Hx), a compound with 30- to 50-fold less antiviral activity than vidarabine.[320] However, ara-Hx appears to enhance the antiviral activity of vidarabine both in vitro and in specimens from patients receiving vidarabine. The carbocyclic analogue of vidarabine (cyclaradine) is resistant to the action of adenosine deaminase and retains comparable antiviral activity in vitro and in animal models.[323,324]

Vidarabine triphosphate inhibits other enzyme systems, including ribonucleoside reductase, RNA polyadenylation, and S-adenosylhomocysteine hydrolase, an enzyme involved in transmethylation reactions, both in vitro and in RBC collected from treated patients.[54,325,326] This effect continues for over 1 week following cessation of therapy and may contribute to the antiviral and toxic effects of vidarabine. In mice, vidarabine administration augments humoral immune responses and delayed hypersensitivity reactions and prolongs survival in cryptococcal infection, perhaps mediated through interference with normal suppressor cell function.[327] Changes in the viral DNA polymerase can cause drug resistance, but it is not a recognized clinical problem.

Pharmacology. Following intravenous infusion, vidarabine is rapidly deaminated to ara-Hx by adenosine deaminase.[328] This enzyme is widely distributed through body tissues but in animals is present in relatively low concentrations in blood and brain. Samples for measurement of vidarabine levels need to be collected in the presence of an inhibitor of adenosine deaminase, such as 2-deoxycorformicin, and quickly frozen to prevent in vitro deamination. During a constant 12-hour infusion (10 mg/kg/12 hr), plasma ara-Hx concentrations peak at 3–6 μg/ml, but no or minimal concentrations of vidarabine (0.2–0.4 μg/ml) are detectable in adults by HPLC assay.[328,329] Ara-Hx is present in CSF at concentrations averaging 35 percent of plasma values, although CSF/plasma ratios over 90 percent have been found in infants.[330] Another study found that peak ara-Hx concentrations averaged 3.7 μg/ml in full-term infants and 8.5 μg/ml in preterm infants at a dosage of 15 mg/kg/12 hr[330] indicating that higher weight-adjusted dosages may be required in full-term infants.

The primary route of clearance is renal, and 40–53 percent of the total of the daily dose is recovered in the urine as ara-Hx and 1–3 percent as the parent drug.[228] The serum half-life of ara-Hx is approximately 3.5 hours in adults. Studies with labeled vidarabine have found accumulation of radioactivity in RBC over 5–7 days and lasting up to 3 weeks. In patients with impaired renal function, plasma ara-Hx concentrations rise and may be associated with neurologic or other side effects.[331] A dosage reduction of 25 percent has been recommended for patients with severe renal insufficiency,[331] but guidelines of proven value have not been established. Ara-Hx is readily cleared during hemodialysis (50 percent over 6 hours), so that dosages should be given after dialysis.[331]

Toxicity. Vidarabine has been shown to be mutagenic, teratogenic, and oncogenic in experimental systems, and its use should be restricted to serious infections. During human use, dose-related gastrointestinal toxicity is common with vidarabine and may be manifested by anorexia, nausea, vomiting, diarrhea, and/or weight loss.[328] The principal difficulty encountered during systemic administration of vidarabine relates to its poor solubility (≤0.45 mg/ml) and the consequent infusion of large fluid volumes, often 1.5–2.5 liters at a dosage of 15 mg/kg/day.

At dosages higher than normally used (20 mg/kg/day), vidarabine is associated with megaloblastic bone marrow changes and sometimes with anemia, leukopenia, or thrombocytopenia. Infusion-related thrombophlebitis, weakness, hypokalemia, rash, and the syndrome of inappropriate secretion of antidiuretic hormone (SIADH) have been described, but controlled trials in serious herpes virus infections at dosages of 10–15 mg/kg/day have not documented serious bone marrow, liver, or renal toxicity.

A variety of neurologic side effects have been reported during vidarabine therapy. High dosages, concurrent interferon or possibly allopurinol therapy, acute leukemia and its treatment, and the presence of pre-existing hepatic or renal insufficiency have been predisposing risk factors.[332–335] The reported neurotoxicities include pain syndromes, usually in the extremities and sometimes lasting up to 6 months after cessation of therapy; tremor, often accentuated by intention and at times associated with facial grimacing, myoclonus, ataxia, or dysgraphia; and alterations in behavior or mentation, including disorientation, depression, aphasia, akinetic mutism, agitation, hallucinations, and, rarely, coma or seizures. Electroencephalograms have shown diffuse changes consistent with metabolic encephalopathy in some cases, but may not correlate with clinical manifestations. In several patients, an unusual brain pathology consisting of chromatolysis and neuronal degeneration has been described.[335] Monitoring of ara-Hx concentrations in patients with hepatic or renal insufficency is desirable, but not available in most laboratories.

Clinical Studies. The most notable successes with vidarabine have been observed in patients with HSV and VZV infections, but acyclovir has replaced it for most indications. The efficacy of vidarabine administered topically in HSV keratoconjunctivitis is well established and is superior to idoxuridine, in that topical vidarabine is effective in patients who cannot receive idoxuridine because of allergy, toxicity, or clinical drug resistance. Vidarabine (15 mg/kg/day for 10 days) increases survival in biopsy-proven HSV encephalitis to 46–61 percent at 6 months, but recent comparative studies have found intravenous acyclovir to be superior in efficacy.[97,98,336] Trials using combinations of acyclovir and vidarabine are planned. Vidarabine treatment reduces the mortality of neonatal HSV infection complicated by visceral dissemination or CNS involvement to 38–40 percent, compared with 74 percent in placebo recipients.[337] A trial comparing the efficacy of acyclovir and vidarabine (30 mg/kg/day) for neonatal infection did not find differences in survival between these treatments.[101] Development of disseminated HSV infection in a neonate has occurred despite vidarabine prophylaxis.[338] Vidarabine (10 mg/kg/day for 7 days) is of limited usefulness in mucocutaneous HSV infections of immunocompromised hosts.[339] Clinically modest reductions in the durations of pain, fever, and shedding of HSV type 1 are observed in vidarabine recipients,[339] but it is an alternative in patients with acyclovir-resistant HSV infections.

In immunocompromised patients with localized herpes zoster of less than 72-hour duration, vidarabine (10 mg/kg/day for 7 days) decreases the frequency of cutaneous dissemination (8 vs. 24 percent), visceral complications (5 vs. 19 percent), time to healing, and total duration of postherpetic neuralgia.[340] A comparative trial with acyclovir in disseminating zoster is in progress. In immunocompromized patients with varicella, vidarabine accelerated the resolution of new vesicle formation and fever and reduced the risk of varicella-related complications.[341] However, a comparative trial in varicella of immunocompromised children was stopped because of neurotoxicity, which occurred in 16 percent of vidarabine recipients.[335]

No therapeutic benefit has been observed in smallpox, despite use of high vidarabine doses (20 mg/kg/day for 7 days), or in patients with advanced progressive multifocal leukoencephalopathy. Uncontrolled studies in patients with congenital CMV infection or the CMV mononucleosis syndrome found transient suppression of virus excretion in the urine during vidarabine therapy. A randomized study of bone marrow transplant recipients found that intermittent administration of low vidarabine doses (5 mg/kg/day) did not reduce the frequency of interstitial pneumonia or CMV isolations. Administration of higher doses (10 mg/kg/day) to renal transplant patients with CMV-associated illness was associated not only with no therapeutic effect compared to placebo, but also with neurologic toxicity in 29 percent of recipients.[334]

In chronic hepatitis B virus infection, vidarabine is associated with reductions in plasma HBV-specific DNA polymerase activity and titers of HBsAg and HBeAg in some patients.[342] The phosphorylated ester of vidarabine, ara-AMP or vidarabine phosphate, is much more water soluble than the parent drug and can be administered intravenously or intramuscularly in chronic hepatitis.[343] The antiviral activity and the pharmacokinetics, metabolism, and toxicities of ara-AMP in man are similar to those of vidarabine.[343–345] Bone marrow toxicity and severe pain syndromes, typically involving lower extremity muscles and sometimes lasting more than 3 months after therapy, have been described in vidarabine phosphate recipients.[345] However, double-blind, placebo-controlled studies found that vidarabine phosphate alone or alternating with human leukocyte interferon does not provide long-term benefit to patients with chronic active or persistent hepatitis B.[346,347] Corticosteroid pretreatment followed by chronic vidarabine or vidarabine phosphate may increase response rates in chronic hepatitis B,[348,349] but steroid withdrawal can be associated with hepatic failure.[350] Vidarabine phosphate conjugated with lactosaminated human serum albumin, which selectively enters hepatocytes, is effective in inhibiting HBV replication at three- to sixfold lower doses than the free phosphate and is well tolerated during short-term administration.[351]

Zidovudine [azidothymidine, AZT, Retrovir]

Spectrum. Zidovudine (3′-azido-3′-deoxythymidine) is a thymidine analog in which the 3′ hydroxyl has been replaced by an azido ($-N_3$) group (Fig. 5). Zidovudine has antiviral activity against HIV-1 and other mammalian retroviruses.[53,352–355] Concentrations of 0.013 μg/ml produce a 50 percent decrease in supernatant reverse transcriptase activity in either HIV-1-infected human T-cell lines or peripheral blood lymphocytes.[352] Depending on the assay method and cell type, zidovudine 0.02–1.3 μg/ml is inhibitory for HIV-1 replication and cytopathology during exogenous infection of various cell types, whereas much higher concentrations are required to block replication in chronically infected cells.[355–361] High concentrations do not inhibit the spread of HIV through giant cell formation in cocultivation studies,[362] and viral replication may proceed in T-cell lines despite the presence of inhibitory concentrations of zidovudine.[363] Zidovudine appears to have minimal phosphorylation and negligible antiviral activity (>20 μg/ml) in human monocyte-derived macrophages, which may serve as a reservoir for HIV replication in vivo.[364] Anti-HIV-1 activity is potentiated by acyclovir, interferon, mismatched double-stranded RNA (ampligen), granulocyte–macrophage colony stimulating factor, and neutralizing antibody, but is antagonized by thymidine or ribavirin in vitro.[53,352,357–360] Zidovudine is inhibitory for HTLV-I,[365] but it appears to be less active against HIV-2.[361] Zidovudine 1.4–2.7 μg/ml is also inhibitory for Epstein-Barr virus replication but not for HSV or VZV. Many Enterobacteriaceae and *Vibrio* strains are inhibited at low concentrations of zidovudine (0.03–1.0 μg/ml), but bacterial resistance to zidovudine develops rapidly.[366] Inhibition of *G. lambia* but not other protozoans has also been described.[367]

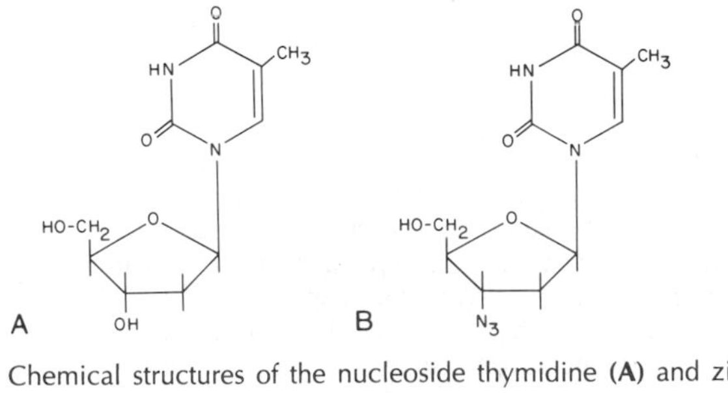

FIG. 5. Chemical structures of the nucleoside thymidine (**A**) and zidovudine (**B**).

Zidovudine concentrations that inhibit the growth of human cell lines are generally >50 μg/ml,[367] although one T-cell line was inhibited by 5 μg/ml. Human myeloid and erythroid progenitor cells are inhibited by low concentrations (0.3–0.6 μg/ml, respectively).[207,368] Uridine partially reverses zidovudine's hematopoietic toxicity for human granulocyte–macrophage progenitor cells without impairing its anti-HIV-1 activity in mononuclear cells.[368] Partial inhibition of mitogen-induced blastogenesis of peripheral blood mononuclear cells is observed at concentrations of ≥2.7 μg/ml.[352]

In animal models of retroviral infection, zidovudine administration after virus exposure can suppress or prevent the development of infection,[353,369,370] which suggests possible usefulness in postexposure prophylaxis. Administration during gestation to pregnant females delays the onset of virus-induced CNS infection in offspring infected in utero in a murine model of retroviral infection.[369]

Mechanism of Action. Zidovudine's primary antiviral mechanism of action is inhibition of viral RNA-dependent DNA polymerase (reverse transcriptase).[371–373] Phosphorylation by cellular kinases results in high intracellular levels of the monophosphate, but low levels of the di- and triphosphates.[371] Concentrations of the phosphorylated forms of zidovudine are similar in uninfected and infected cells. Zidovudine triphosphate competitively inhibits the viral reverse transcriptase and is also inhibitory for cellular α-DNA polymerase at 100-fold higher concentrations. Thus, the antiviral selectivity of zidovudine is due to its greater affinity for HIV reverse transcriptase than for human DNA polymerases. In T-lymphocytic cell lines, triphosphate levels peak at 5 hours but then decline during further incubation with zidovudine.[355] The monophosphate is a competitive inhibitor of cellular thymidylate kinase, which leads to reduced intracellular levels of thymidine triphosphate.[371] Because thymidine triphosphate competes for the HIV reverse transcriptase, reduced levels may enhance the inhibition of the enzyme by zidovudine. Reduced levels of normal pyrimidines may also contribute to bone marrow toxicity.[372] The triphosphate is also incorporated into the growing DNA chain by reverse transcriptase. Because the 3′-azido groups prevents the formation of 5′-3′phosphodiester linkages, zidovudine acts as a chain terminator of DNA synthesis.

Resistance. Selection of zidovudine-resistant HIV mutants is difficult in the laboratory. Gene transfer studies employing site-specific mutagenesis have enabled the construction of zidovudine-resistant HIV-1 reverse transcriptases. Recent evidence indicates that zidovudine-resistant HIV strains may be recovered from patients who remain virus-positive on long-term therapy.[373] The frequency and clinical significance of such isolates and their mechanisms of resistance and possible sensitivity to other agents are under study.

Pharmacology. The oral bioavailability of zidovudine is approximately 60–65 percent.[374] Zidovudine is rapidly absorbed from the gastrointestinal tract, with peak serum concentrations occurring at 0.5–1.5 hours, although some patients may have poor or delayed absorption.[375] Following chronic oral administration of 250 mg every 4 hours, the steady-state peak (1.5 hours postdose) and trough plasma concentrations average 0.6–1.0 μg/ml and 0.1–0.2 μg/ml, respectively, although the range of observed concentrations is very broad.[367,375] Mean peak and trough levels of 0.4 to 0.5 and 0.1 μ/ml, respectively, have been found in those receiving 100 mg q4h.[376] Oral doses of 80–120 mg/m^2 give peak plasma concentrations of 1.1–1.4 μg/ml in children. No plasma drug accumulation occurs during prolonged dosing in those with normal renal function. Cerebrospinal fluid concentrations average 24–100 percent of those in plasma, which indicates significant penetration into the central nervous system.[367,374–378] Semen concentrations are 1.3- to 20-fold higher than serum,[375] which suggests sequestration due to the low pH of prostatic secretions. Zidovudine plasma protein binding is only 34–38 percent.

The plasma elimination $T_{1/2}$ is approximately 1 hour (0.8–1.9 hours). Zidovudine is rapidly metabolized to the 5′-glucuronide derivative, (GAZT) which has a similar elimination $T_{1/2}$ but lacks the HIV inhibitory activity of the parent compound. Following oral administration, the urinary recovery of zidovudine and GAZT averages 14 percent and 74 percent, respectively, of the dose. Renal clearance involves both glomerular filtration and tubular secretion. Definitive guidelines for dose adjustments of zidovudine in patients with impaired renal or hepatic function are not available at present. Accumulation of GAZT, but not zidovudine, occurs in renal failure but without obvious toxicity. Concomitant acyclovir does not affect zidovudine pharmacokinetics.[376]

Toxicity. Zidovudine causes transformation of mammalian cells in vitro at ≥0.5 μg/ml and chromosome abnormalities in cultured human lymphocytes at ≥3 μg/ml. In monkeys treated for 3–6 months, dose-related anemia and bone marrow suppression occur. The potential carcinogenicity and teratogenicity of the compound have not been fully studied.

The major toxicities of zidovudine recognized in clinical trials are granulocytopenia and anemia, which occur in up to 45 percent of recipients during relatively short-term administration.[367,379,380] The risk of hematologic toxicities is inversely related to the pretreatment T4 lymphocyte, hemoglobin, and granulocyte values and is directly related to the zidovudine dose and duration of therapy. Patients with more advanced disease or vitamin B_{12} deficiency are also at greater risk of marrow toxicity. The risk of significant granulocytopenia (<750/mm^3) is 19 percent in those with initial T4 counts >100/mm^3 and 51 percent in those with counts ≤100/mm^3.[379] During prolonged treatment the incidence of granulocytopenia remains relatively constant. Anemia associated with erythroid hypoplasia or megaloblastic bone marrow changes may occur as early as 2–4 weeks, but most commonly after the first 6 weeks of therapy,[381] whereas granulocytopenia usually occurs after 6–8 weeks. Macrocytosis is common but does not predict transfusion-requiring anemia. Pancytopenia related to partially reversible bone marrow failure has occurred at 14–17 weeks after starting therapy in up to 5 percent of patients.[382] Careful hematologic monitoring is required. Anemia can be managed by transfusion support, which is required by about 30 percent of patients, whereas zidovudine-induced erythroid hypoplasia, granulocytopenia (≤750/mm^3), or thrombocytopenia may require dose interruption or reduction.

Significantly higher rates of severe headache, nausea, insomnia, and myalgia occur in zidovudine recipients compared with placebo.[379] These symptoms sometimes require dose adjustment or discontinuation but may resolve despite continued zidovudine use. Severe neurotoxicity with seizures, as early as 48 hours after starting therapy,[383,384] Wernicke's encephalopathy, and a polymyositislike syndrome occurring at 6–17 months of therapy have been reported.[385] Late-onset progressive wasting with proximal muscle weakness, reduced exercise tolerance, and myalgia or less commonly acute rhabdomyolisis with muscle tenderness and high CPK levels have been described. After recovery, resumption of zidovudine can cause recurrence. Progressive nail pigmentation may occur in black patients.[386] A variety of other clinical adverse events have been reported in zidovudine-treated patients but at rates similar to those observed in placebo-treated.

Drugs that inhibit glucuronidation and/or renal excretion of zidovudine (e.g., probenicid) may increase the risks of marrow toxicity. Acetaminophen, which may increase plasma levels by inhibiting zidovudine metabolism, has been specifically associated with an increased frequency of leukopenia in one study.[379] Coadministration with drugs that are nephrotoxic or cytotoxic may increase the risk of hematologic toxicity. Concurrent ganciclovir markedly increases the risk of myelosuppression, and interferon of neutropenia and hepatotoxicity. Concomitant dapsone has been associated with severe anemia. Zidovudine therapy may alter plasma diphenylhydantion levels. Several cases of neurotoxicity (lethargy, convulsion) have been described during concomitant use of zidovudine and acyclovir, but subsequent studies have not documented an excessive risk. Acute overdose of zidovudine causes CNS depression but apparently no severe marrow toxicity.[387]

Clinical Studies. An initial 6-week dose escalating study of intravenous and oral zidovudine found that 79 percent of patients showed increased circulating T4 lymphocyte counts and that over 30 percent of anergic patients recovered cutaneous delayed-type hypersensitivity to at least one antigen.[380] In 1986 a randomized, double-blind, placebo-controlled, multicenter trial[378,388] established the efficacy of zidovudine therapy in adult AIDS patients with recently documented *Pneumocystis carini* pneumonia (PCP) and in symptomatic HIV-infected patients, the majority of whom had T4 counts ≤200 cells/mm^3. Treatment (250 mg q4h) over a mean period of 17 weeks was associated with a 91 percent efficacy in reducing mortality at 24 weeks and 56 percent in preventing opportunistic infections acquired after the first 6 weeks of treatment. Significant increases in T4 counts (transient in AIDS patients), return of cutaneous DTH reactivity in 29 percent of patients, weight gain, and stabilization of functional status also occurred. However, over one-third of patients required dose reduction or discontinuation because of hematologic toxicity. After 36 weeks of follow-up, zidovudine treatment was associated with a sixfold decrease in mortality compared with placebo, and the estimated mortality of the zidovudine group followed for 72 weeks was about 30 percent.[388,388a] Those with higher performance status, hemoglobin >12 g/dl, or with treatment initiated <90 days after PCP diagnosis have better prognosis. Concurrent prophylaxis for PCP is associated with much lower mortality during maintenance zidovidine (8 percent vs. 39 percent without prophylaxis at 1 year).[389] Chronic oral zidovudine is also associated with significant decreases in serum HIV p24 core antigen levels as early as 4 weeks.[391] However, zidovudine does not significantly reduce the rate of virus recovery from peripheral blood samples, and treated-patients must be regarded as infections.[388]

The minimally effective dosage of zidovudine for long-term use is currently undefined for different target groups. Dose schedules involving less frequent administration (250 mg or 500 mg q6h or 500 mg q12h) appear to be effective in reducing p24 antigenemia and increasing T4 cell counts in a majority of asymptomatic HIV-infected patients.[391] Studies in small numbers of AIDS or ARC patients found that full-dose zidovudine treatment (200–250 q4h) is associated with 90 percent or greater decreases in circulating p24 antigenemia in those with high antigen levels (>100 pg/ml), but that increases may be observed with lower doses (100 q4h or 250 q8h).[392] The addition of acyclovir to zidovudine does not appear to increase anti-HIV activity or toxicity during short-term use,[376,391] but may reduce

TABLE 5. Selected Antiviral Agents of Investigative Interest

Drug [Ref. No.]	*Mechanism of Action*	*Toxicities*	*Comments/Clinical Use*
Dideoxycytidine (DDC) [407]	Reverse transcriptase inhibition.	Skin rash, stomatitis, arthritis, fever. Dose-related painful peripheral neuropathy after several months.	Oral bioavailability 70–80%. Dose-related reductions in p24 antigenemia. Proposed use is to alternate monthly or weekly with zidovudine.
Dextran sulfate [408]	Blocks attachment of virus to CD4 receptor; inhibits syncytia formation.	Oral use: gastrointestinal upset, possibly CNS effects, abnormal LFT.	Synergistic in vitro with zidovudine. Efficacy and oral bioavailability not established.
Ampligen (mismatched, double-stranded RNA) [409]	Uncertain, interferon-like effects.	Myalgia, fever, chills, hypotension after IV administration.	Antiviral effects in initial clinical tests.
Suramin [409]	Reverse transcriptase inhibition.	Fever, rash, malaise, CNS, bone marrow, proteinuria, abnormal LFT.	No clinical or immune benefit in AIDS/ARC found to date.
Antimoniotungstate (HPA-23) [409]	Reverse transcriptase inhibition.	Thrombocytopenia, renal dysfunction, abnormal LFT.	No clinical or immune benefit in AIDS/ARC found to date.
CD4 receptor protein [410]	Inhibition of attachment/penetration.	Not defined.	Clinical trials with soluble recombinant CD4 molecules in progress. Peptide fragments and conjugates under development.

severe opportunistic infections and mortality to a greater extent than zidovudine alone during chronic administration in AIDS patients.[389]

Uncontrolled studies suggest a beneficial effect on HIV-associated neurologic disease.[377,378,393] Objective improvements in dementia and peripheral neuropathy are apparent within 8 weeks, and up to one-half of patients show sustained neurologic improvement 5–10 months after starting therapy.[378] Recent controlled studies indicate that AIDS patients show significantly improved sustained attention, memory, and visual-motor skills at 8 and 16 weeks of therapy.[390] Continuous intravenous infusion has improved neurodevelopmental abnormalities in encephalopathic children and IQ scores in children without overt encephalopathy.[377] Rebounds in serum and CSF p24 antigen levels and development of acute, self-limited meningoencephalitis have occurred shortly after zidovudine dose reductions.[394] Zidovudine treatment may benefit HIV-associated thrombocytopenia, psoriasis, and lymphocytic interstitial pneumonia.[367,395] The clinical value of zidovudine in pediatric infections, in patients with less severe manifestations of HIV infection (e.g., asymptomatic seropositivity, persistent generalized lymphodenopathy), in postexposure prophylaxis (e.g., needlestick exposure in health care workers), and the efficacy and toxicity of various combination regimens (zidovudine plus interferon, dideoxycitidine, or immunomodulators) are subjects of ongoing controlled clinical trials.

Foscarnet (PFA)

Foscarnet (trisodium phosphonoformate hexahydrate) is a simple inorganic pyrophosphate analogue that inhibits herpesvirus DNA polymerase and retroviral reverse transcriptase. It is active in vitro against most herpes viruses, including cytomegalovirus, hepadna viruses and human immunodeficiency virus. Unlike zidovudine, it also enters macrophages and inhibits HIV in these cells.[396] Resistance due to altered viral DNA polymerase can be generated in the laboratory but has not been observed in clinical isolates.

The drug is nephrotoxic, causing tubular trophy in animals, and other side effects have been noted in humans.[397,398] The drug increases urinary output and fluid intake. It has been associated with malaise, nausea, vomiting, fatigue, and headache. Anemia is common, but granulocytopenia does not occur. Tremor, seizures, irritability, and hallucinosis have been associated with high plasma concentrations. Phlebitis, hypo- and hypercalcemia, hyperphosphatemia, and abnormal transaminase values may also develop. Hypocalcemia may be enhanced by simultaneous administration of pentamidine.

Foscarnet is usually given by the intravenous route, often as a bolus of 20 mg/kg over 30 minutes followed by a continuous infusion of 230 mg/kg/24 h for 2–3 weeks.[399] Alternative dosing regimens to avoid continuous infusions include 60 mg/kg 3 times daily for 2 weeks, followed by a single dose 5 to 7 days per week for maintenance therapy.[400,401] Oral absorption is low. Intermittent infusions of 60 mg/kg/8 hours give peak plasma concentrations averaging 150 μg/ml.[400] The initial plasma T 1/2 averages 3–6 hours. Foscarnet penetrates into the CSF and the eye. Its disposition is complex, and bone deposition accounts for up to 20 percent of the administered dose. The drug is excreted by the kidney, and, because of its nephrotoxicity, the dose must be reduced if serum creatinine levels rise. It is suggested that the infusion be reduced by 20 mg/kg/24 hr for each 20 μmol/liter increase in the serum creatinine above 70 μmol/liter.[399]

Foscarnet has been used primarily to treat cytomegalovirus and HIV infections. In CMV retinitis in patients with AIDS, clinical responses appear to be similar to those observed with ganciclovir.[399,401,402] However, foscarnet has been less well studied. The problem of relapse after discontinuation of foscarnet is similar to that observed with ganciclovir. In a study of patients with AIDS and ARC treated with intravenous foscarnet for 3 weeks, eight patients converted from virus-positive to virus-negative during the study period, and six remained virus-free during 3 months of follow-up.[403] In another study, 15 patients with AIDS were treated for 14 days. No effect on HIV cultures was observed, but p24 antigen disappeared in five of eight patients, only to reappear 4–23 weeks later.[397] Interestingly, CMV culture positivity fell from 46 percent before treatment to 17 percent during treatment, and returned to 37 percent after foscarnet treatment. Other studies have confirmed the effect on p24 antigen.[404]

Foscarnet thus offers a major advantage over ganciclovir for the treatment of CMV infection in persons with AIDS, in that it does not affect granulocyte numbers. However, optimal dose schedules for initial treatment and chronic suppression have not been defined. It also appears to be a useful agent in severe acyclovir-resistant HSV infections.[405] Topical application of 3% foscarnet cream provides marginal clinical benefits in recurrent mucocutaneous HSV infections.[398,406] If the problem of renal toxicity can be overcome, it could become a useful agent.

For information on other antiretroviral agents of investigative interest, see Table 5.

REFERENCES

1. Newton AA. Tissue culture methods for assessing antivirals and their harmful effects. In: Field HJ, ed. Antiviral Agents: the Development and Assessment of Antiviral Chemotherapy. v. 1. Boca Raton, FL: CRC Press; 1988:23–67.
2. Crumpacker CS, Schnipper LE, Marlowe SI, et al. Resistance to antiviral drugs of herpes simplex virus isolated from patients treated with acyclovir. N Engl J Med. 1982;306:343–6.
3. Burns WH, Saral R, Santos GW, et al. Isolation and characterization of

resistant herpes simplex virus after acyclovir therapy. Lancet. 1982;1:421–3.

4. Sibrack CD, Gutman LT, Wilfert CM, et al. Pathogenicity of acyclovir-resistant herpes simplex virus type 1 from an immunodeficient child. J Infect Dis. 1982;146:673–82.
5. Wade JC, McLaren C, Myers JD. Frequency and significance of acyclovir-resistant herpes simplex virus isolated from marrow transplant patients receiving multiple courses of treatment with acyclovir. J Infect Dis. 1983;148:1077–82.
6. Parris DS, Harrington JE. Herpes simplex virus variants resistant to high concentrations of acyclovir exist in clinical isolates. Antimicrob Agents Chemother. 1982;22:71–7.
7. Smith KO, Kennell WL, Poirier RH, et al. In vitro and in vivo resistance of herpes simplex virus to 9-(2-hydroxyethoxymethyl)guanine (acycloguanosine). Antimicrob Agents Chemother. 1980;17:144–50.
8. Belshe RB, Smith MH, Hall CB, et al. Genetic basis of resistance to rimantadine emerging during treatment of influenza virus infection. J Virol. 1988;62:1508–12.
9. Hall CB, Dolin R, Gala CL, et al. Children with influenza A infection: treatment with rimantadine. Pediatrics. 1987;80:275–82.
10. Thompson J, Fleet W, Lawrence E, et al. A comparison of acetaminophen and rimantadine in the treatment of influenza A infection in children. J Med Virol. 1987;249–55.
11. Erice A, Chou S, Biron KK, et al. Progressive disease due to ganciclovir-resistant cytomegalovirus in immunocompromised patients. N Eng J Med. 1989;320:289–93.
12. Yeager AS. Genital herpes simplex infections: effect of asymptomatic shedding and latency on management of infections in pregnant women and neonates. J Invest Dermatol. 1984;83:053s–6s.
13. Gutman LT, Wilfert CM, Eppes S. Herpes simplex virus encephalitis in children: analysis of cerebrospinal fluid and progressive neurodevelopmental deterioration. J Infect Dis. 1986;154:415–21.
14. Brown ZA, Ashley R, Douglas J, et al. Neonatal herpes simplex virus infection: relapse after initial therapy and transmission from a mother with an asymptomatic genital herpes infection and erythema multiforme. Pediatr Infect Dis J. 1987;6:1057–61.
15. Bernstein DI, Lovett MA, Bryson YJ. The effects of acyclovir on antibody response to herpes simplex virus in primary genital infections. J Infect Dis. 1984;150:7–13.
16. Lafferty WE, Brewer LA, Corey L. Alteration of lymphocyte transformation response to herpes simplex virus infection by acyclovir therapy. Antimicrob Agents Chemother. 1984;26:887–91.
17. Hirsch MS. Antiviral drug development for the treatment of human immunodeficiency virus infections. Am J Med. 1988;85(Suppl 2A):182–85.
18. Hall MJ, Duncan IB. Antiviral drugs and interferon combinations. In: Field HJ, ed. Antiviral Agents: The Development and Assessment of Antiviral Chemotherapy. v. 1. Boca Raton, FL: CRC Press; 1988;29–85.
19. Wilson SZ, Knight V, Wyde PR, et al. Amantadine and ribavirin aerosol treatment of influenza A and B infection in mice. Antimicrob Agents Chemother. 1980;17:642–8.
20. Hayden FG, Douglas RG, Jr, Simons R. Enhancement of activity against influenza viruses by combinations of antiviral agents. Antimicrob Agents Chemother. 1980;18:536–41.
21. Stanwick TL, Schinazi RF, Campbell DE, et al. Combined antiviral effect of interferon and acyclovir on herpes simplex virus types 1 and 2. Antimicrob Agents Chemother. 1981;19:672–4.
22. Schinazi RF, Peters J, Williams CC, et al. Effect of combinations of acyclovir with vidarabine or its 5′-monophosphate on herpes simplex viruses in cell culture and in mice. Antimicrob Agents Chemother. 1982;22:499–507.
23. Sacks SL, Scullard GH, Pollard RB, et al. Antiviral treatment of chronic hepatitis B virus infection: pharmacokinetics and side effects of interferon and adenine arabinoside alone and in combination. Antimicrob Agents Chemother. 1982;21:93–100.
24. Smith CI, Kitchen LW, Scullard GH, et al. Vidarabine monophosphate and human leukocyte interferon in chronic hepatitis B infection. JAMA. 1982;247:2261–5.
25. Besser R, Krämer G, Rambow A, et al. Combined therapy with acyclovir and adenosine arabinoside in herpes simplex encephalitis. Eur Neurol. 1987;27:197–200.
26. Yarchoan R, Thomas RV, Allain J-P, et al. Phase I studies of 2′,3′-dideoxycytidine in severe human immunodeficiency virus infection as a single agent and alternating with zidovudine (AZT). Lancet. 1988;1:76–80.
27. Schmidt GM, Forman SJ, Zaia JA, et al. Treatment of cytomegalovirus associated pneumonitis with ganciclovir (DHPG) and immunoglobin following allogeneic bone marrow transplantation: antiviral and therapeutic response. Clin Res. 1988;36:470A.
28. Reed EC, Bowden RA, Dandliker PS, et al. Treatment of cytomegalovirus pneumonia with ganciclovir and intravenous cytomegalovirus immunoglobin in patients with bone marrow transplants. Ann Intern Med. 1988;109:783–8.
29. Steele RW, Charlton RK. Immune modulators as antiviral agents. In: Drew WL, ed. Clinics in Laboratory Medicine. v. 7. Philadelphia: WB Saunders; 1987:911–24.
30. Hayden FG, Laskin OL, Douglas RG Jr. Antiviral agents. In: Lourian V, ed. Antibiotics in Laboratory Medicine, 2nd ed. Baltimore: Williams & Wilkins; 1986:359–80.
31. Hatcher VA, Friedman-Kien AE, Marcus EL, et al. Arabinosyladenine monophosphate in genital herpes: a double-blind, placebo-controlled study. Antiviral Res. 1982;2:283–90.
32. Gangarosa LP, Hill JM, Thompson BL, et al. Iontophoresis of vidarabine monophosphate for herpes orolabialis. J Infect Dis. 1986;154:930–4.
33. Hayden FG, Hall WJ, Douglas RG, Jr. Therapeutic effects of aerosolized amantadine in naturally acquired infection due to influenza A virus. J Infect Dis. 1980;141:535–42.
34. Knight V, Wilson SZ, Quarles JM, et al. Ribavirin small-particle aerosol treatment of influenza. Lancet. 1981;2:945–9.
35. McClung HW, Knight V, Gilbert BE, et al. Ribavirin aerosol treatment of influenza B virus infection. JAMA. 1983;249:2671–4.
36. Hall CB, McBride JT, Walsh EE, et al. Aerosolized ribavirin treatment of infants with respiratory syncytial viral infection. N Engl J Med. 1983;308:1443–47.
37. Taber LH, Knight V, Gilbert BE, et al. Ribavirin aerosol treatment of bronchiolitis associated with respiratory syncytial virus infection in infants. Pediatrics. 1983;72:613–18.
38. Hall CB, McBride JT, Gala CL, et al. Ribavirin treatment of respiratory syncytial virus infection in infants with underlying cardiopulmonary disease. JAMA. 1985;254:3047–51.
39. Rodriguez WJ, Kim HW, Brandt CD, et al. Aerosolized ribavirin in the treatment of patients with respiratory syncytial virus disease. Pediatr Infect Dis J. 1987;6:159–63.
40. Hayden FG. Intranasal interferons for control of respiratory viral infections. In: Revel M, ed. Clinical Aspects of Interferons. Boston: Kluwer Academic Publishers; 1988;3–16.
41. Dorsky DI, Crumpacker CS. Drugs five years later: acyclovir. Ann Intern Med. 1987;107:859–74.
42. Biron KK, Elion GB. In vitro susceptibility of varicella-zoster virus to acyclovir. Antimicrob Agents Chemother. 1980;18:443–7.
43. Colby BM, Shaw JE, Elion GB, et al. Effect of acyclovir [9-(2-hydroxyethoxymethyl)guanine] on Epstein-Barr virus DNA replication. J Virol. 1980;34:560–8.
44. Lin J-C. Smith MC, Cheng YC, et al. Epstein-Barr virus: inhibition of replication by three new drugs. Science. 1983;221:578–9.
45. Lang DJ, Cheung K-S. Effectiveness of acycloguanosine and trifluorothymidine as inhibitors of cytomegalovirus infection in vitro. Am J Med. 1982;73(Suppl):49–53.
46. Kern ER. Acyclovir treatment of experimental genital herpes simplex virus infections. Am J Med. 1982;73(Suppl):100–8.
47. Collins P, Oliver NM. Acyclovir treatment of cutaneous herpes in guinea pigs and herpes encephalitis in mice. Am J Med. 1982;73(Suppl):96–9.
48. Soike KF, Gerone PJ, Acyclovir in the treatment of simian varicella virus infection of the African green monkey. Am J Med. 1982;73(Suppl):112–7.
49. Steele RW, Marmer DJ, Keeney RE. Comparative in vitro immunotoxicology of acyclovir and other antiviral agents. Infect Immun. 1980;28:957–62.
50. McGuffin RW, Shiota FM, Meyers JD. Lack of toxicity of acyclovir to granulocyte progenitor cells in vitro. Antimicrob Agents Chemother. 1980;10:471–3.
51. Levin MJ, Leary PL, Arbeit RD. Effect of acyclovir on the proliferation of human fibroblasts and peripheral blood mononuclear cells. Antimicrob Agents Chemother. 1980;17:947–53.
52. Wingard JR, Hess AD, Stuart RK, et al. Effect of several antiviral agents on human lymphocyte functions and marrow progenitor cell proliferation. Antimicrob Agents Chemother. 1983;23:593–7.
53. Mitsuya H, Broder S. Strategies for antiviral therapy in AIDS. Nature. 1987;325:773–8.
54. Elion GB. History, mechanism of action, spectrum and selectivity of nucleoside analogs. In: Mills J, Corey L, eds. Antiviral Chemotherapy: New Directions for Clinical Application and Research. New York: Elsevier; 1986;118–37.
55. Derse D, Cheng Y-C, Furman PA, et al. Inhibition of purified human and herpes simplex virus-induced DNA polymerases by 9-(2-hydroxyethoxymethyl)granine triphosphate. J Biol Chem. 1981;256:11447–51.
56. McGuirt PV, Furman PA. Acyclovir inhibition of viral DNA chain elongation in herpes simplex virus-infected cells. Am J Med. 1982;73(Suppl):67–71.
57. Furman PA, St. Clair MH, Spector T. Acyclovir triphosphate is a suicidal inactivator of the herpes simplex virus DNA polymerase. J Biol Chem. 1984;259:9575–9.
58. Pagano JS, Datta AK. Perspectives on interactions of acyclovir with Epstein-Barr and other herpes viruses. Am J Med. 1982;73(Suppl):18–26.
59. Collins P. Viral sensitivity following the introduction of acyclovir. Am J Med. 1988;85(Suppl 2A):129–34.
60. Coen D, Schaffer PA. Two distinct loci confer resistance to acycloguanosine in herpes simplex virus type 1. Am J Med. 1982;73(Suppl):2265–9.
61. Norris SA, Kessler HA, Fife KH. Severe, progressive herpetic whitlow caused by an acyclovir-resistant virus in a patient with AIDS. J Infect Dis. 1988;157:209–10.
62. Erlich KS, Mills J, Chatis P, et al. Acyclovir-resistant herpes simplex virus infections in patients with the acquired immunodeficiency syndrome. N Engl J Med. 1989;320:293–6.
63. Ellis MN, Keller PM, Fyfe JA, et al. Clinical isolate of herpes simplex virus type 2 that induces a thymidine kinase with altered substrate specificity. Antimicrob Agents Chemother. 1987;31:1117–25.
64. Corey L, Holmes KK. Genital herpes simplex virus infections: current concepts in diagnosis, therapy, and prevention. Ann Intern Med. 1983;98:973–83.

65. Straus SE, Takiff HE, Seidlin M, et al. Suppression of frequently recurring genital herpes. N Engl J Med. 1984;310:1545–50.
66. Lehrman SN, Douglas JM, Corey L, et al. Recurrent genital herpes and suppressive oral acyclovir therapy. Ann Intern Med. 1986;104:786–90.
67. Cole NL, Balfour HH Jr. Varicella-zoster virus does not become more resistant to acyclovir during therapy. J Infect Dis. 1986;153:605–8.
68. Larder BA, Darby G. Susceptibility to other antiherpes drugs of pathogenic variants of herpes simplex virus selected for resistance to acyclovir. Antimicrob Agents Chemother. 1986;29:894–9.
69. Blum RM, Liao SHT, de Miranda P. Overview of acyclovir pharmacokinetic disposition in adults and children. Am J Med. 1982;73(Suppl):186–92.
70. Laskin OL. Clinical pharmacokinetics of acyclovir. Clin Pharmocokinet. 1983;8:187–201.
71. Van Dyke RB, Connor JD, Wyborny C, et al. Pharmacokinetics of orally adminsitered acyclovir in patients with herpes progenitalis. Am J Med. 1982;73(Suppl):172–5.
72. McKindrick MW, McGill JI, White JE, et al. Oral acyclovir in acute herpes zoster. Br Med J. 1986;293:1529–32.
73. Wade JC, Newton B, Flournoy N, et al. Oral acyclovir for prevention of herpes simplex virus reactivation after bone marrow transplantation. Ann Intern Med. 1984;100:823–8.
74. Sullender WM, Arvin AM, Diaz PS, et al. Pharmacokinetics of acyclovir suspension in infants and children. Antimicrob Agents Chemother. 1987;31:1722–6.
75. Peterslund NA, Esmann V, Geil JP, et al. Open study of 2-amino-9-(hydroxyethoxymethyl)-9H-purine (desciclovir) in the treatment of herpes zoster. J Antimicrob Chemother. 1987;20:743–51.
76. Petty BG, Whitley RJ, Liao S, et al. Pharmacokinetics and tolerance of desciclovir, a prodrug of acyclovir, in healthy human volunteers. Antimicrob Agents Chemother. 1987;31:1317–22.
77. Hung SO, Patterson A, Rees PJ. Pharmacokinetics of oral acyclovir (Zovirax) in the eye. Br J Ophthamol. 1984;68:192–5.
78. Meyer LJ, de Miranda P, Sheth N, et al. Acyclovir in human breast milk. Am J Obstet Gynecol. 1988;158:586–8.
79. Hintz M, Connor JD, Spector SA, et al. Neonatal acyclovir pharmacokinetics in patients with herpes virus infections. Am J Med. 1982;72(Suppl):210–4.
80. Laskin OL, Longstreth, Whelton A, et al. Effect of renal failure on the pharmacokinetics of acyclovir. Am J Med. 1982;73(Suppl):197–201.
81. DeMiranda P, Good SS, Laskin OL, et al. Disposition of intravenous radioactive acyclovir. Clin Pharmacol Ther. 1981;30:662.
82. De Miranda P, Good SS, Krasny HC, et al. Metabolic fate of radioactive acyclovir in humans. Am J Med. 1982;73(Suppl):215–20.
83. Krasny HC, Liao SHT, de Miranda P, et al. Influence of hemodialysis on acyclovir pharmacokinetics in patients with chronic renal failure. Am J Med. 1982;73(Suppl):202–4.
84. Boelaert J, Schurgers M, Daneels R, et al. Multiple dose pharmacokinetics of intravenous acyclovir in patients on continuous ambulatory peritoneal dialysis. J Antimicrob Chemother. 1987;20:69–76.
85. Quinn RP, Wolberg G, Medzihradsky J, et al. Effect of acyclovir on various murine in vivo and in vitro immunologic assay systems. Am J Med. 1982;73(Suppl):62–6.
86. Keeney RE, Kirk LE, Bridgen D. Acyclovir tolerance in humans. Am J Med. 1982;73(Suppl):176–81.
87. Sylvester RK, Ogden WB, Draxler CA, et al. Vesicular eruption. JAMA. 1986;255:385–6.
88. Wade JC, Hintz M, McGuffin RW, et al. Treatment of cytomegalovirus pneumonia with high-dose acyclovir. Am J Med. 1982;73(Suppl):249–56.
89. Wade JC, Meyers JD. Neurologic symptoms associated with parenteral acyclovir treatment after marrow transplantation. Ann Intern Med. 1983;98:921–5.
90. Bean B, Aeppli D. Adverse effects of high-dose intravenous acyclovir in ambulatory patients with acute herpes zoster. J Infect Dis. 1985;151:362–4.
91. Feldman S, Rodman J, Gregory B. Excessive serum concentrations of acyclovir and neurotoxicity. J Infect Dis. 1988;157:385–8.
92. Potter JL, Krill CE. Acyclovir crystalluria. Pediatr Infect Dis. 1986;5:710–2.
93. Sawyer MH, Webb DE, Balow JE, et al. Acyclovir-induced renal failure: clinical course and histology. Am J Med. 1988;84:1067–71.
94. Bean B, Braun C, Balfour HH Jr. Acyclovir therapy for acute herpes zoster. Lancet. 1982;2:118–21.
95. Balfour HH Jr, Bean B, Laskin OL, et al. Acyclovir halts progression of herpes zoster in immunocompromised patients. N Engl J Med. 1983;308:1448–53.
96. Douglas JM Jr, Davis LG, Remington ML, et al. A double-blind, placebo-controlled trial of chronically administered oral acyclovir on sperm production in men with frequently occurring genital herpes. J Infect Dis. 1988;157:588–93.
97. Whitley RJ, Alford CA, Hirsch MS, et al. Vidarabine versus acyclovir therapy in herpes simplex encephalitis. N Engl J Med. 1986;314:144–9.
98. Sköldenberg B, Alestig K, Burman L, et al. Acyclovir versus vidarabine in herpes simplex encephalitis. Lancet. 1984;2:706–11.
99. Feldman S, Lott L. Varicella in children with cancer: impact of antiviral therapy and prophylaxis. Pediatrics. 1987;80:465–72.
100. Shepp DH, Dandliker PS, Meyers JD. Treatment of varicella-zoster virus infection in severely immunocompromised patients. N Engl J Med. 1986;314:208–12.
101. Whitley RJ, Arvin A, Corey L, et al. Vidarabine versus acyclovir therapy of neonatal herpes simplex virus, HSV, infection (Abstract #986). Pediatr Res. 1986;20:323A.
102. Mertz GJ. Diagnosis and treatment of genital herpes infections. In: Knight V, Gilbert BE, eds. Infectious Disease Clinics of North America, Philadelphia: WB Saunders; 1987;341–66.
103. Corey L, Fife KH, Benedetti JK, et al. Intravenous acyclovir for the treatment of primary genital herpes. Ann Intern Med. 1983;98:914–21.
104. Bryson YJ, Dillon M, Lovett M, et al. Treatment of first episodes of genital herpes simplex virus infection with oral acyclovir. N Engl J Med. 1983;308:916–21.
105. Corey L, Nahmias AJ, Guinan ME, et al. A trial of topical acyclovir in genital herpes simplex virus infections. N Engl J Med. 1982;306:1313–9.
106. Mindel A, Adler MW. Intravenous acyclovir treatment for primary genital herpes. Lancet. 1982;1:697–700.
107. Nilsen AE, Aasen T. Efficacy of oral acyclovir in the treatment of initial and recurrent genital herpes. Lancet. 1982;2:571–3.
108. Reichman RC, Badger GJ, Guinan ME, et al. Topically administered acyclovir in the treatment of recurrent herpes simplex genitalis: a controlled trial. J Infect Dis. 1983;147:336–40.
109. Luby JP, Gnann JW Jr, Alexander WJ, et al. A collaborative study of patient-initiated treatment of recurrent genital herpes with topical acyclovir or placebo. J Infect Dis. 1984;150:1–6.
110. Rompalo AM, Mertz GJ, Davis LG, et al. Oral acyclovir for treatment of first-episode herpes simplex virus proctitis. JAMA. 1988;259:2879–81.
111. Reichman RC, Badger GJ, Mertz GJ, et al. Patient-initiated therapy of recurrent herpes simplex genitalis with orally administered acyclovir. JAMA. 1984;251:2103–07.
112. Douglas JM, Critchlow C, Benedetti J, et al. A double-blind study of oral acyclovir for suppression of recurrences of genital herpes simplex virus infection. N Engl J Med. 1984;310:1551–6.
113. Gold D, Corey L. Acyclovir prophylaxis for herpes simplex virus infections. Antimicrob Agents Chemother. 1987;31:361–7.
114. Mertz GJ, Eron L, Kaufman R, et al. prolonged continuous versus intermittent oral acyclovir treatment in normal adults with frequently recurring genital herpes simplex virus infection. Am J Med. 1988;85(Suppl 2A):14–19.
115. Mostow SR, Mayfield JL, Marr JJ, Drucker JL. Suppression of recurrent genital herpes by single daily dosages of acyclovir. Am J Med. 1988;85(Suppl 2A):30–3.
116. Straus SE, Seidlin M, Takiff HE, et al. Double-blind comparison of weekend and daily regimens of oral acyclovir for suppression of recurrent genital herpes. Antiviral Res. 1986;6:151–9.
117. Rooney JF, Felser JM, Ostrove JM, et al. Acquisition of genital herpes from an asymptomatic sexual partner. N Engl J Med. 1986;314:1561–4.
118. Kinghorn GR, Turner EB, Barton IG, et al. Efficacy of topical acyclovir cream in first and recurrent episodes of genital herpes. Antiviral Res. 1983;3:291–301.
119. Raborn GW, McGaw WT, Grace M, et al. Treatment of herpes labialis with acyclovir: review of three clinical trials. Am J Med. 1988;85(Suppl 2A):39–42.
120. Spruance S, Hamill M, Hoge W, et al. Suppression of herpes simplex labialis at ski resorts with oral acyclovir (Abstract #1182). Programs and Abstracts of the Twenty-sixth International Conference on Antimicrobial Agents and Chemotherapy. 1986:312.
121. Saral R, Burns WH, Laskin OL, et al. Acyclovir prophylaxis of herpes-simplex-virus infections. N Engl J Med. 1981;305:63–7.
122. Lundgren G, Wilczek H, Lonnqvist B, et al. Acyclovir prophylaxis in bone marrow transplant recipients. Scand J Infect Dis. 1985;47:137–44.
123. Gluckman E, Devergie A, Melo R, et al. Prophylaxis of herpes infections after bone marrow transplantation by oral acyclovir. Lancet. 1983;2:706–8.
124. Seale L, Jones CJ, Kathpalia S, et al. Prevention of herpesvirus infections in renal allograft recipients by low-dose oral acyclovir. JAMA. 1985;254:3435–8.
125. Meyers JD, Reed EC, Shepp DH, et al. Acyclovir for prevention of cytomegalovirus infection and disease after allogeneic marrow transplantation. N Engl J Med. 1988;318:70–5.
126. Straus S, Seidlin M, Takiff H, et al. Oral acyclovir to suppress recurrent herpes simplex virus infections in immunodeficient patients. Ann Intern Med. 1984;100:522–24.
127. Saral R, Ambinder RF, Burns WH, et al. Acyclovir prophylaxis against herpes simplex virus infection in patients with leukemia. Ann Intern Med. 1983;99:773–76.
128. Wade JC, Newton B, McLaren C, et al. Intravenous acyclovir to treat mucocutaneous herpes simplex infection after marrow transplantation. Ann Intern Med. 1982;96:265–69.
129. Shepp DH, Newton BA, Dandliker PS, et al. Oral acyclovir therapy for mucocutaneous herpes simplex infections in immunocompromised marrow transplant recipients. Ann Intern Med. 1985;102:783–5.
130. Whitley R, Barton N, Collins E, et al. Mucocutaneous herpes simplex virus infections in immunocompromised patients. Am J Med. 1982;73(Suppl):236–40.
131. Peterslund NA, Ipsen J, Schonheyder H, et al. Acyclovir in herpes zoster. Lancet. 1981;2:827–30.
132. Huff JC, Bean B, Balfour HH Jr, et al. Therapy of herpes zoster with oral acyclovir. Am J Med. 1988;85(Suppl 2A):84–9.
133. Cobo M. Reduction of the ocular complications of herpes zoster ophthalmicus by oral acyclovir. Am J Med. 1988;85(Suppl 2A):90–3.

134. Wassilew SW, Reimlinger S, Nasemann T, Jones D. Oral acyclovir for herpes zoster: a double-blind controlled trial in normal subjects. Br J Dermatol. 1987;117:495–501.
135. Wood MJ, Ogan PH, McKendrick MW, et al. Efficacy of oral acyclovir treatment of acute herpes zoster. Am J Med. 1988;85(Suppl 2A):79–83.
135a. Esmann V, Kroon S, Peterslund NA, et al. Prednisolone does not prevent post-herpetic neuralgia. Lancet. 1987;2:126–9.
136. McGill J, Chapman C. A comparison of topical acyclovir with steroids in the treatment of herpes zoster keratouveitis. Br J Ophthalmol. 1983;67:46–50.
137. Al-Nakib W, Al-Kandari S, El-Khalik DMA, et al. A randomised controlled study of intravenous acyclovir (Zovirax) against placebo in adults with chickenpox. J Infect. 1983;6:49–56.
138. Schlossberg D, Littman M. Varicella pneumonia. Arch Intern Med. 1988;148:1630–2.
139. Boyd K, Walker E. Use of acyclovir to treat chickenpox in pregnancy. Br Med J. 1988;296:393–4.
140. Johns DR, Gress DR. Rapid response to acyclovir in herpes zoster-associated encephalitis. Am J Med. 1987;82:560–2.
141. Vilde JL, Bricaire F, Leport C, et al. Comparative trial of acyclovir and vidarabine in disseminated varicella-zoster virus infections in immunocompromised patients. J Med Virol. 1986;20:127–34.
142. Prober CG, Kirk LE, Keeney RE. Acyclovir therapy of chickenpox in immunosuppressed children—a collaborative study. J Pediatr. 1982;101:622–5.
143. Nyerges G, Meszner Z, Gyarmati E, et al. Acyclovir prevents dissemination of varicella in immunocompromised children. J Infect Dis. 1988;157:309–13.
144. Balfour HH Jr. Intravenous acyclovir therapy for varicella in immunocompromised children. J Pediatr. 1984;104:134–6.
145. VanLandingham KE, Marsteller HB, Ross GW, et al. Relapse of herpes simplex encephalitis after conventional acyclovir therapy. JAMA. 1988;259:1051–3.
146. Balfour HH Jr, Bean B, Mitchell CD, et al. Acyclovir in immunocompromised patients with cytomegalovirus disease. Am J Med. 1982;73(Suppl):241–248.
147. Plotkin SA, Starr SE, Bryan CK. In vitro and in vivo responses of cytomegalovirus to acyclovir. Am J Med. 1982;73(Suppl):257–261.
148. Andersson J, Britton S, Ernberg I, et al. Effect of acyclovir on infectious mononucleosis: a double-blind, placebo-controlled study. J Infect Dis. 1986;153:283–90.
149. Andersson J, Skoldenberg B, Henle W, et al. Acyclovir treatment in infectious mononucleosis: a clinical and virological study. Infection. 1987;15:S14–20.
150. Hanto DW, Frizzera G, Gajl-Peczalska KJ, et al. Epstein-Barr virus-induced B-cell lymphoma after renal transplantation. N Engl J Med. 1982;306:913–8.
151. Sullivan JL, Bryon KS, Brewster FE, et al. Treatment of life-threatening Epstein-Barr virus infections with acyclovir. Am J Med. 1982;73(Suppl):262–6.
152. Schooley RT, Carey RW, Miller G, et al. Chronic Epstein-Barr virus infection associated with fever and interstitial pneumonitis. Ann Intern Med. 1986;104:636–43.
153. Resnick L, Herbst JS, Ablashi DV, et al. Regression of oral hairy leukoplakia after orally administered acyclovir therapy. JAMA. 1988;259:384–8.
154. Straus SE, Dale JK, Tobi M, et al: Acyclovir treatment of the chronic fatigue syndrome: lack of efficacy in a placebo-controlled trial. N Engl J Med. 1988;319:1692–8.
155. Schalm SW, VanBuuren HR, Heytink RA, DeMan RA. Acyclovir enhances the antiviral effect of interferon in chronic hepatitis B. Lancet. 1985;2:358–60.
156. Alexander GJM, Fagan EA, Hegarty JE, Yeo J, Eddleston ALWF, Williams R. Controlled clinical trial of acyclovir in chronic hepatitis B virus infection. J Med Virol. 1987;21:81–7.
157. Couch RB, Six HR. The antiviral spectrum and mechanism of action of amantadine and rimantadine. In: Mills J, Corey L, eds. Antiviral Chemotherapy: New Directions for Clinical Application and Research, New York: Elsevier; 1986;50–57.
158. Hayden FG, Cote KM, Douglas RG, Jr. Plaque inhibition assay for drug susceptibility testing of influenza viruses. Antimicrob Agents Chemother. 1980;17:865–70.
159. Browne MJ, Moss MY, Boyd MR. Comparative activity of amantadine and ribavirin against influenza virus in vitro: possible clinical relevance. Antimicrob Agents Chemother. 1983;23:503–5.
160. Pemberton RM, Jennings R, Potter CW, Oxford JS. Amantadine resistance in clinical influenza A (H3N2) and (H1N1) virus isolates. J Antimicrob Chemother. 1986;18(Suppl B):135–40.
161. Koff WC, Elm JL, Jr., Halstead SB. Inhibition of dengue virus replication by amantadine hydrochloride. Antimicrob Agents Chemother. 1980;18:125–9.
162. Hayden FG. Animal models of influenza virus infection for evaluation of antiviral agents. In: Zak O, Sande MA, eds. Experimental Models in Antiviral Chemotherapy. v. 3. London: Academic Press; 1986;353–71.
163. Hayden FG. Combinations of antiviral agents for treatment of influenza virus infections. J Antimicrob Chemother. 1986;18(Suppl B):177–83.
164. Richman DD, Yazaki P, Hostetler KY. The intracellular distribution and antiviral activity of amantadine. Virology. 1981;112:81–90.
165. Richman DD, Hostetler KY, Yazaki PJ, Clark S. Fate of influenza A virion proteins after entry into subcellular fractions of LLC cells and the effect of amantadine. Virology. 1986;151:200–10.
166. Oxford JS, Galbraith A. Antiviral activity of amantadine: a review of laboratory and clinical data. Pharmacol Ther. 1980;11:181.
167. Hay AJ, Zambon MC, Wolstenholme AJ, Skehel JJ, Smith MH. Molecular basis of resistance of influenza A viruses to amantadine. J Antimicrob Chemother. 1986;18(Suppl B):19–29.
168. Beyer WEP, Ruigrok RWH, van Driel H, Masurel N. Influenza virus strains with a fusion threshold of pH 5.5 or lower are inhibited by amantadine. Arch Virol. 1986;90:173–81.
169. Beard CW, Brugh M, Webster RG. Emergence of amantadine-resistant H5N2 avian influenza virus during a simulated layer flock treatment program. Avian Dis. 1987;31:533–7.
170. Webster RG, Kawaoka Y, Bean WJ, Beard CW, Brugh M. Chemotherapy and vaccination: a possible strategy for the control of highly virulent influenza virus. J Virol. 1985;55:173–6.
171. Bean WJ, Webster RG. Biological properties of amantadine-resistant influenza virus mutants. Antiviral Res. 1988;9:128.
172. Belshe RB, Tomlinson DL, Burk B, Pizzuti D. Occurrence and transmission of amantadine/rimantadine resistant influenza A virus (Abstract). Intersci Conf Antimicrob Agents Chemother. 1988;no. 99:127.
173. Tominack RL, Hayden FG. Rimantadine hydrochloride and amantadine hydrochloride use in influenza A virus infections. In: Moellering RC, Knight V, Gilbert BE, eds: Infectious Disease Clinics of North America. Philadelphia: WB Saunders; 1987;1:459–78.
174. Hayden FG, Minocha A, Spyker DA, Hoffman HE. Comparative single-dose pharmacokinetics of amantadine hydrochloride and rimantadine hydrochloride in young and elderly adults. Antimicrob Agents Chemother. 1985;28:216–21.
175. Aoki FY, Sitar DS. Amantadine kinetics in healthy elderly men: implications for influenza prevention. Clin Pharmacol Ther. 1985;37:137–44.
176. Aoki FY, Sitar DS. Clinical pharmacokinetics of amantadine hydrochloride. Clin Pharmacokinet. 1988;14:35–51.
177. Fishaut M, Mostow S. Amantadine for severe influenza A pneumonia in infancy. Am J Dis Child. 1980;134:321–23.
178. Horadam VW, Sharp JG, Smilack JD, et al. Pharmacokinetics and amantadine hydrochloride in subjects with normal and impaired renal function. Ann Intern Med. 1981;94:454–8.
179. Soung L-S, Ing TS, Daugirdas JT, et al. Amantadine hydrochloride pharmacokinetics in hemodialysis patients. Ann Intern Med. 1980;93:46–9.
180. Sartori M, Pratt CM, Young JB. Malignant cardiac arrhythmia induced by amantadine poisoning. Am J Med. 1984;77:388–91.
181. Atkinson WL, Arden NH, Patriarca PA, Leslie N, Lui K-J, Gohd R. Amantadine prophylaxis during an institutional outbreak of type A (H1N1) influenza. Arch Intern Med. 1986;146:1751–6.
182. Shields WD, Lake JL, Chugani HT. Amantadine in the treatment of refractory epilepsy in childhood: an open trial in 10 patients. Neurology. 1985;35:579–81.
183. Nestelbaum Z, Siris SG, Rifkin A, Klar H, Reardon GT. Exacerbation of schizophrenia associated with amantadine. Am J Psychiatry 1986;143:1170–1.
184. Dolin R, Reichman RC, Madore HP, et al. A controlled trial of amantadine and rimantadine in the prophylaxis of influenza A infection. N Engl J Med. 1982;307:580–4.
185. Hayden FG, Gwaltney JM Jr, Van de Castle RL, et al. Comparative toxicity of amantadine hydrochloride and rimantadine hydrochloride in healthy adults. Antimicrob Agents Chemother. 1981;19:226–33.
186. Millet VM, Dreisbach M, Bryson YJ. Double-blind controlled study of central nervous system side effects of amantadine, rimantadine, and chlorpheniramine. Antimicrob Agents Chemother. 1982;21:1–4.
187. Kantor RJ, Stevens D, Potts DW, et al. Prevention of influenza A/USSR/77 (H1N1): an evaluation of the side effects and efficacy of amantadine in recruits at Fort Sam Houston. Milit Med. May, 1980;312–5.
188. Bryson YJ, Monahan C, Pollack M, et al. A prospective double-blind study of side effects associated with the administration of amantadine for influenza A virus prophylaxis. J Infect Dis. 1980;141:543–47.
189. Pettersson RF, Hellström P-E, Penttinen K, et al. Evaluation of amantadine in the prophylaxis of influenza A (H1N1) virus infection: a controlled field trial among young adults and high-risk patients. J Infect Dis. 1980;142:377–83.
190. Hayden FG, Hoffman HE, Spyker DA. Differences in side effects of amantadine hydrochloride and rimantadine hydrochloride relate to differences in pharmacokinetics. Antimicrob Agents Chemother. 1983;23:458–64.
191. Arden NH, Patriarca PA, Fasano MB, et al. The roles of vaccination and amantadine prophylaxis in controlling an outbreak of influenza A (H3N2) in a nursing home. Arch Intern Med. 1988;148:865–8.
192. Wilson TW, Rajput AH. Amantadine-dyazide interaction. Can Med Assoc J. 1983;129:974–5.
193. World Health Organization. Current status of amantadine and rimantadine as anti-influenza-A agents. Bull WHO. 1985;63:51–56.
194. Payler DK, Purdham PA. Influenza A prophylaxis with amantadine in a boarding school. Lancet. 1984;1:502–4.
195. Advisory Committee on Immunization Practices. Prevention and control of influenza. MMWR. 1988;37:361–73.
196. Van Voris LP, Betts RF, Hayden FG, et al. Successful treatment of naturally occurring influenza A/USSR/77 H1N1. JAMA. 1981;245:1128–31.
197. Younkin SW, Betts RF, Roth FK, et al. Reduction in fever and symptoms

in young adults with influenza A/Brazil/78 H1N1 infection after treatment with aspirin or amantadine. Antimicrob Agents Chemother. 1983;23:577–82.
198. Field AK, Davies ME, DeWitt C, et al. 9-[2-hydroxy-1-(hydroxymethyl)ethoxy]methyl guanine: A selective inhibitor of herpes group virus replication. Proc Natl Acad Sci USA. 1983;80:4139–43.
199. Smee DF, Martin JC, Verheyden JPH, Matthews TR. Antiherpesvirus activity of the acyclic nucleoside 9-(1,3-dihydroxy-2-propoxymethyl)guanine. Antimicrob Agents Chemother. 1983;23:676–82.
200. Mar E-C, Cheng Y-C, Huang E-S. Effect of 9-(1,3-dihydroxy-2-propoxymethyl)guanine on human cytomegalovirus replication in vitro. Antimicrob Agents Chemother. 1983;24:518–21.
201. Freitas VR, Smee DF, Chernow M, Boehme R, Matthews TR. Activity of 9-(1,3-dihydroxy-2-propoxymethyl)guanine compared with that of acyclovir against human, monkey, and rodent cytomegaloviruses. Antimicrob Agents Chemother. 1985;28:240–5.
202. Baba M, Konno K, Shigeta S, deClercq E. Inhibitory effects of selected antiviral compounds on newly isolated clinical varicella-zoster virus strains. Tohoku J Exp Med. 1986;148:275–83.
203. Plotkin SA, Drew WL, Felsenstein D, Hirsch MS. Sensitivity of clinical isolates of human cytomegalovirus to 9-(1,3-dihydroxy-2-propoxymethyl)guanine. J Infect Dis. 1985;152:833–4.
204. Shiota H, Naito T, Mimura Y. Anti-herpes simplex virus (HSV) effect of 9-(1,3-dihydroxy-2-propoxymethyl)guanine (DHPG) in rabbit cornea. Curr Eye Res. 1987;6:241–5.
205. Debs RJ, Montgomery AB, Brunette EN, deBruin M, Stanley JD. Aerososl administration of antiviral agents to treat lung infection due to murine cytomegalovirus. J Infect Dis. 1988;157:327–31.
206. Soike KF, Eppstein DA, Gloff CA, Cantrell C, Chou T-C, Gerone PJ. Effect of 9-(1,3-dihydroxy-2-propoxymethyl)-guanine and recombinant human beta interferon alone and in combination on simian varicella virus infection in monkeys. J Infect Dis. 1987;156:607–14.
207. Sommadossi J-P, Carlisle R. Toxicity of 3′-azido-3′-deoxythymidine and 9-(1,3-dihydroxy-2-propoxymethyl)guanine for normal human hematopoietic progenitor cells in vitro. Antimicrob Agents Chemother. 1987;31: 452–4.
208. Bowden RA, Digel J, Reed EC, Meyers JD. Immunosuppressive effects of ganciclovir on in vitro lymphocyte responses. J Infect Dis. 1987;156:899–903.
209. Biron KK, Stanat SC, Sorrell JB, et al. Metabolic activation of the nucleoside analog 9-[2-hydroxy-1-(hydroxy-methyl)ethoxy]methyl guanine in human diploid fibroblasts infected with human cytomegalovirus. Proc Natl Acad Sci USA. 1985;82:2473–7.
210. Smee DF, Boehme R, Chernow M, Binko B, Mathhews TR. Intracellular metabolism and enzymatic phosphorylation of 9-(1,3-dihydroxy-2-propoxymethyl)guanine and acyclovir in herpes simplex virus-infected and uninfected cells. Biochem Pharmacol. 1985;34:1049–56.
211. Frank KB, Chiou J-F, Cheng Y. Interaction of herpes simplex virus-induced DNA polymerase with 9-(1,3-dihydroxy-2-propoxymethyl)guanine triphosphate. J Biol Chem. 1984;259:1566–9.
212. St Clair MH, Miller WH, Miller RL, Lambe CU, Furman PA. Inhibition of cellular alpha DNA polymerase and herpes simplex virus-induced DNA polymerases by the triphosphate of BW759U. Antimicrob Agents Chemother. 1984;25:191–4.
213. Reid R, Mar E-C, Huang E-S, Topal MD. Insertion and extension of acyclic, dideoxy, and ara nucleotides by herpesviridae, human a and human b polymerases. J Biol Chem. 1988;263:3898–904.
214. Crumpacker CS, Kowalsky PN, Oliver SA, Schnipper LE, Field AK. Resistance of herpes simplex virus to 9-[2-hydroxy-1-(hydroxymethyl)ethoxy]methyl guanine: Physical mapping of drug synergism within the viral DNA polymerase locus. Proc Natl Acad Sci USA. 1984;81:1556–60.
215. Biron KK, Fyfe JA, Stanat SC, et al. A human cytomegalovirus mutant resistant to the nucleoside analog. 9-[(2-hydroxy-1-(hydroxymethyl)ethoxy)methyl]guanine (BW B759U), induces reduced levels of BW B759U-triphosphate. Proc Natl Acad Sci USA. 1986;83:8769–73.
216. Cole NL, Balfour HH Jr. In vitro susceptibility of cytomegalovirus isolates from immunocompromised patients to acyclovir and ganciclovir. Diagn Microbiol Infect Dis. 1987;6:255–61.
217. Shepp DH, Dandliker DH, deMiranda P, et al. Activity of 9-[(2-hydroxy-1-(hydroxymethyl)ethoxymethyl)]guanine in the treatment of cytomegalovirus pneumonia. Ann Intern Med. 1984;103:368–73.
218. Jacobson MA, deMiranda P, Cederberg DM, et al. Human pharmacokinetics and tolerance of oral ganciclovir. Antimicrob Agents Chemother. 1987;31:1251–4.
219. Laskin OL, Cederberg DM, Mills J, Eron LJ, Mildvan D, Spector SA. Ganciclovir for the treatment and suppression of serious infections caused by cytomegalovirus. Am J Med. 1987;83:201–7.
220. Fletcher C, Sawchuk R, Chinnock B, deMiranda P, Balfour HH Jr. Human pharmacokinetics of the antiviral drug DHPG. Clin Pharmacol Ther. 1986;40:281–6.
221. Jabs DA, Newman C, deBustros S, Polk F. Treatment of cytomegalovirus retinitis with ganciclovir. Ophthalmology. 1987;94:824–30.
222. Jabs DA, Wingard JR, deBustros S, deMiranda, Saral R. BW B759U for cytomegalovirus retinitis: intraocular drug penetration. Arch Ophthalmol. 1986;104:1436–7.
223. Henry K, Cantrill H, Fletcher C, Chinnock BJ, Balfour HH Jr. Use of intravitreal ganciclovir (dihydroxy propoxy methyl guanine) for cytomegalovirus retinitis in a patient with AIDS. Am J Ophthamol. 1987;103:17–23.
224. Investigator's Monograph. Ganciclovir [9-(1,3-dihydroxy-2-propoxymethyl)guanine]. 5th ed. Palo Alto, CA: Syntex Inc., December, 1987.
225. Collaborative DHPG Treatment Study Group. Treatment of serious cytomegalovirus infections with 9-(1,3-dihydroxy-2-propoxymethyl)guanine in patients with AIDS and other immunodeficiencies. N Engl J Med. 1986;314:801–5.
226. Mills J. 9-(1,3-dihydroxy-2-propoxymethyl)guanine (DHPG) for treatment of cytomegalovirus infections. In: Mills J, Corey L, eds. Antiviral Chemotherapy: New Directions for Clinical Application and Research. New York: Elsevier; 1986:195–203.
227. Jacobson MA, Mills J. Serious cytomegalovirus disease in the acquired immunodeficiency syndrome (AIDS). Ann Intern Med. 1988;108:585–94.
228. Chachoua A, Dieterich D, Krasinski K, et al. 9-(1,3-2-propoxymethyl)guanine (ganciclovir) in the treatment of cytomegalovirus gastrointestinal disease with the acquired immunodeficiency syndrome. Ann Intern Med. 1987;107:133–7.
229. Fiala M, Cone LA, Cohen N, et al. Responses to neurologic complications of AIDS to 3′-azido-3′-deoxythymidine and 9-(1,3-dihydroxy-2-propoxymethyl) guanine. I. Clinical features. Rev Infect Dis. 1988;10:250–6.
230. Erice A, Jordan C, Chace BA, Fletcher C, Chinnock BJ, Balfour HH Jr. Ganciclovir treatment of cytomegalovirus disease in transplant recipients and other immunocompromised hosts. JAMA. 1987;257:3082–7.
231. Kotler DP, Culpepper-Morgan JA, Tierney AR, Klein EB. Treatment of disseminated cytomegalovirus infection with 9-(1,3 dihydroxy-2-propoxymethyl)guanine: evidence of prolonged survival in patients with the acquired immunodeficiency syndrome. AIDS Res. 1986;2:299–308.
232. Jacobson MA, DeMiranda P, Gordon SM, et al. Prolonged pancytopenia due to combined ganciclovir and zidovudine therapy. J Infect Dis. 1988;158:489–90.
233. Henderly DE, Freeman WR, Causey DM, Rao NA. Cytomegalovirus retinitis and response to therapy with ganciclovir. Ophthalmology. 1987;94:425–34.
234. Holland GN, Sidikaro Y, Kreiger AE, et al. Treatment of cytomegalovirus retinopathy with ganciclovir. Ophthalmology. 1987;94:815–23.
235. Orellana J, Teich SA, Friedman AH, Lerebours F, Winterkorn J, Mildvan D. Combined short- and long-term therapy for the treatment of cytomegalovirus retinitis using ganciclovir (BW B759U). Ophthalmology. 1987;94:831–8.
236. Freeman WR, Henderly DE, Wan WL, et al. Prevalence, pathophysiology, and treatment of rhegmatogenous retinal detachment in treated cytomegalovirus retinitis. Am J Ophthalmol. 1987;103:527–36.
237. Reed EC, Dandliker PS, Meyers JD. Treatment of cytomegalovirus pneumonia with 9-[2-hydroxy-1-(hydroxymethyl)ethoxymethyl]guanine and high-dose corticosteroids. Ann Intern Med. 1986;105:214–5.
238. Emanuel D, Cunningham I, Jules-Elysee K, et al. Cytomegalovirus pneumonia after bone marrow transplantation successfully treated with the combination of ganciclovir and high-dose intravenous immune globulin. Ann Intern Med. 1988;109:777–82.
239. Hecht DW, Snydman DR, Crumpacker CS, Werner BG, Heinze-Lacey B, the Boston Renal Transplant CVM Study Group. Ganciclovir for treatment of renal transplant-associated primary cytomegalovirus pneumonia. J Infect Dis. 1988;157:187–90.
240. Keay S, Bissett J, Merigan TC. Ganciclovir treatment of cytomegalovirus infections in iatrogenically immunocompromised patients. J Infect Dis. 1987;156:1016–21.
241. Pulido J, Peyman GA, Lesar T, Vernot J. Intravitreal toxicity to hydroxyacyclovir (BW-B759U), a new antiviral agent. Arch Ophthalmol. 1985;103:840–1.
242. Prusoff WH. Idoxuridine or how it all began. In: DeClercq E, ed. Clinical Use of Antiviral Drugs. Norwell: Martinus Nijhoff; 1988:15–24.
243. Silvestri DL, Corey L, Holmes KK. Ineffectiveness of topcial idoxuridine in dimethyl sulfoxide for therapy of genital herpes. JAMA. 1982;248:953–59.
244. Kaufman HE. The treatment of herpetic eye infections with trifluridine and other antivirals. In: DeClercq E, ed. Clinical Use of Antiviral Drugs. Norwell: Martinus Nijhoff; 1988:25–38.
245. Pavan-Langston DR. Ocular viral diseases. In: Galasso GJ, Merigan TC, Buchanan RA, eds. Antiviral Agents and Viral Diseases of Man. 2nd ed. New York: Raven Press; 1984:207–45.
246. Gilbert BE, Knight V. Minireview: biochemistry and clinical applications of ribavirin. Antimicrob Agents Chemother. 1986;30:201–5.
247. Hruska JF, Bernstein JM, Douglas RG Jr, et al. Effects of ribavirin on respiratory syncytial virus in vitro. Pharmacol Ther. 1980;6:770–75.
248. Browne MJ. Comparative inhibition of influenza and parainfluenza virus replication by ribavirin in MDCK cells. Antimicrob Agents Chemother. 1981;19:712–15.
249. McCormick JB, Mitchell SW, Getchell JP, Hicks DR. Ribavirin suppresses replication of lymphadenopathy-associated virus in cultures of human adult T lymphocytes. Lancet. 1984;2:1367–9.
250. Baba M, Pauwels R, Balzarini J, Herdewijn P, DeClercq E, Desmyter J. Ribavirin antagonizes inhibitory effects of pyrimidine 2′,3′-dideoxynucleosides but enhances inhibitory effects of purine 2′,3′-dideoxynucleosides on replication of human immunodeficiency virus in vitro. Antimicrob Agents Chemother. 1987;31:1613–7.
251. Stephen EL, Jones DE, Peters CJ, et al. Ribavirin treatment of toga-, arena-

and bunyavirus infections in subhuman primates and other laboratory animal species. In: Smith RE, Kirkpatric W, eds. Ribavirin: Broad Spectrum Antiviral Agent. New York: Academic Press; 1980:169.
252. Peavy DL, Koff WC, Hyman DS, et al. Inhibition of lymphocyte proliferative responses by ribavirin. Infect Immun. 1980;29:583–89.
253. Steele RW, Crosby DL, Steele RW, Pilkington NS Jr, Charlton RK. Effects of ribavirin on neutrophil function. Am J Med Sci. 1988;295:503–6.
254. Marquardt DL, Gruber HE, Walker LL. Ribavirin inhibits mast cell mediator release. J Pharmacol Exp Ther. 1987;240:145–9.
255. Hruska JF, Morrow PE, Suffin SC, et al. In vivo inhibition of respiratory syncytial virus by ribavirin. Antimicrob Agents Chemother. 1982;21:125–30.
256. Wyde PR, Wilson SZ, Patrella R, Gilbert BE. Efficacy of high dose-short duration ribavirin aerosol in the treatment of respiratory syncytial virus infected cotton rats and influenza B virus infected mice. Antiviral Res. 1987;7:211–20.
257. Jahrling PB, Hesse RA, Eddy GA, et al. Lassa virus infection of rhesus monkeys: pathogenesis and treatment with ribavirin. J Infect Dis. 1980;141:580–89.
258. Weissenbacher MC, Calello MA, Merani MS, McCormick JB, Rodriguez M. Therapeutic effect of the antiviral agent ribavirin in junin virus infection of primates. J Med Virol. 1986;20:261–7.
259. Kende M, Lupton HW, Rill WL, Levy HB, Canonico PG. Enhanced therapeutic efficacy of poly(ICLC) and ribavirin combinations against Rift Valley Fever virus infection in mice. Antimicrob Agents Chemother. 1987;31:986–90.
260. Gangemi JD, Nachtigal M, Barnhart D, Krech L, Jani P. Therapeutic efficacy of liposome-encapsulated ribavirin and muramyl tripeptide in experimental infection with influenza or herpes simplex virus. J Infect Dis. 1987;155:510–7.
261. Gruber WC, Wilson SZ, Throop BJ, Wyde PR. Immunoglobulin administration and ribavirin therapy: efficacy in respiratory syncytial virus infection of the cotton rat. Pediatr Res. 1987;21:270–4.
262. Smee DF, Mathews TR. Metabolism of ribavirin in respiratory syncytial virus-infected and uninfected cells. Antimicrob Agents Chemother. 1986;30:117–21.
263. Wray SK, Gilbert BE, Knight V. Effect of ribavirin triphosphate on primer generation and elongation during influenza virus transcription in vitro. Antiviral Res. 1985;5:39–48.
264. Peavy DL, Powers CN, Knight V. Inhibition of murine plaque-forming cell responses in vivo by ribavirin. J Immunol. 1981;126:861–64.
265. Scheidel LM, Durbin RK, Stollar V. Sindbis virus mutants resistant to mycophenolic acid and ribavirin. Virology. 1987;158:1–7.
266. Laskin OL, Longstreth JA, Hart CC, et al. Ribavirin disposition in high-risk patients for acquired immunodeficiency syndrome. Clin Pharmacol Ther. 1987;41:546–55.
267. Roberts RB, Laskin OL, Laurence J, et al. Ribavirin pharmacodynamics in high-risk patients for acquired immunodeficiency syndrome. Clin Pharmacol Ther. 1987;42:365–73.
268. Connor JD, Hintz M, Van Dyke R, McCormick JB, McIntosh K. Ribavirin pharmacokinetics in children and adults during therapeutic trials. In: Smith RA, Knight V, Smith JAD, eds. Clinical Applications of Ribavirin. Orlando: Academic Press; 1984:107–23.
269. Crumpacker C, Bubley G, Lucey D, Hussey S, Connor J. Ribavirin enters cerebrospinal fluid. Lancet. 1986;2:45–6.
270. Knight V, Yu CP, Gilbert BE, Divine GW. Estimating the dosage of ribavirin aerosol according to age and other variables. J Infect Dis. 1988;158:443–8.
271. Hillyared IW. The preclinical toxicology and safety of ribavirin. In: Smith RA, Kirkpatric W, eds. Ribavirin: A Broad Spectrum Antiviral Agent. New York: Academic Press; 1980:59.
272. Smith CB, Charette RP, Fox JP, et al. Lack of effect of oral ribavirin in naturally occurring influenza A virus (H1N1) infection. J Infect Dis. 1980;141:548–54.
273. Minkoff DI, Connor DJ. Clinical use of ribavirin and the treatment of herpes zoster in otherwise normal adults. In: Smith RA, Kirkpatric W, eds. Ribavirin: A Broad Spectrum Antiviral Agent. New York: Academic Press; 1980:185–99.
274. Light B, Aoki FY, Serrette C. Tolerance of ribavirin aerosol inhaled by normal volunteers and patients with asthma or chronic obstructive airway disease. In: Smith RA, Knight V, Smith JAD, eds. Clinical Applications of Ribavirin. New York: Academic Press; 1984:97–105.
275. Rodriguez WJ, Dang Bui RH, Connor JD, et al. Environmental exposure of primary care personnel to ribavirin aerosol when supervising treatment of infants with respiratory syncytial virus infections. Antimicrob Agents Chemother. 1987;31:1143–6.
275a. Harrison RJ, Bellows JD. Reproductive risk to health care workers administering ribavirin aerosol (Abstract). Intersci Conf Antimicrob Agents Chemother. 1988;no. 96:126.
276. Conrad DA, Christenson JC, Waner JL, Marks MI. Aerosolized ribavirin treatment of respiratory syncytial virus infection in infants hospitalized during an epidemic. Pediatr Infect Dis J. 1987;6:152–8.
277. Frankel LR, Wilson CW, Demers RR, et al. A technique for the administration of ribavirin to mechanically ventilated infants with severe respiratory syncytial virus infection. Crit Care Med. 1987;15:1051–4.
278. Outwater KM, Meissner C, Peterson MB. Ribavirin administration to infants receiving mechanical ventilation. Am J Dis Child. 1988;142:512–5.
279. Rodriguez WJ, Parrott RH. Ribavirin aerosol treatment of serious respiratory syncytial virus infection in infants. In: Moellering RC, ed. Infectious Disease Clinics of North America, Antiviral Chemotherapy. Philadelphia: WB Saunders; 1987:425–39.
280. American Academy of Pediatrics. Policy statement: ribavirin therapy of respiratory syncytial virus. AAP News. December, 1986.
281. Wald ER, Dashefsky B, Green M. In re ribavirin: a case of premature adjudication? J Pediatr. 1988;1:155–8.
282. McIntosh K. Chemotherapy of respiratory syncytial virus infections. In: Mills J, Corey L, eds. Antiviral Chemotherapy: New Directions for Clinical Application and Research. New York: Elsevier; 1986:83–8.
283. Rosner IK, Welliver RC, Edelson PJ, Geraci-Ciardullo K, Sun M. Effect of ribavirin therapy on respiratory syncytial virus-specific IgE and IgA responses after infection. J Infect Dis. 1987;155:1043–7.
284. Knight V, Gilbert BE. Ribavirin aerosol treatment of influenza. In: Moellering RC, ed. Infectious Disease Clinics of North America, Antiviral Chemotherapy. Philadelphia: WB Saunders; 1987;441–57.
285. Bernstein DI, Reuman PD, Sherwood JR, Young EC, Schiff GM. Ribavirin small-particle-aerosol treatment of influenza B virus infection. Antimicrob Agents Chemother. 1988;32:761–4.
286. Stein DS, Creticos CM, Jackson GG, et al. Oral ribavirin treatment of influenza A and B. Antimicrob Agents Chemother. 1987;31:1285–7.
287. McCormick JB, King IJ, Webb PA, et al. Lassa fever: effective therapy with ribavirin. N Engl J Med. 1986;314:20–6.
288. Canonico PG. Efficacy of ribavirin against viral hemorrhagic fevers and other exotic RNA viral infections. Programs and Abstracts of the International Symposium: Basic and Clinical Approaches to Virus Chemotherapy, June 19–22, 1988, Helsinki, Finland. Final Programme Antivirals 88, p. 68.
289. Enria DA, Briggiler AM, Levis S, Vallejos D, Maiztegui JI, Canonico PG. Preliminary report, tolerance and antiviral effect of ribavirin in patients with Argentine hemorrhagic fever. Antiviral Res. 1987;7:353–9.
290. Crumpacker C, Heagy W, Bubley G, et al. Ribavirin treatment of acquired immunodeficiency syndrome (AIDS) and the acquired-immunodeficiency-syndrome-related complex (ARC). Ann Intern Med. 1987;107:664–74.
291. Mansell PW, Haseltine PN, Roberts RB, Dickinson GM, Leeder JM. Ribavirin delays progression of lymphadenopathy syndrome (LAS) to the acquired immune deficiency syndrome (AIDS) (Abstract). In: Abstracts Volume: III International Conference on AIDS. Washington, DC: National Institutes of Health and the World Health Organization; 1987:58.
292. Palmieri G, Ambrosi G, Ferrano G, Agrati AM, Palazzini E. Clinical and immunological evaluation of oral ribavirin administration in recurrent herpes simplex infections. J Internat Med Res. 1987;15:264–75.
293. Patki SA, Gupta P. Evaluation of ribavirin in the treatment of acute hepatitis. Chemotherapy. 1982;28:298–303.
294. Bierman SM, Kirkpatric W, Fernandez H. Clinical efficacy of ribavirin in the treatment of genital herpes simplex virus infection. Chemotherapy. 1981;27:139–45.
295. Burlington DB, Meiklejohn G, Mostow SR. Anti-influenza A virus activity of amantadine hydrochloride and rimantadine hydrochloride in ferret tracheal ciliated epithelium. Antimicrob Agents Chemother. 1982;21:794–9.
296. Koff WC, Elm JL Jr, Halstead SB. Suppression of dengue virus replication in vitro by rimantadine hydrochloride. Am J Trop Med Hyg. 1981;30:184–9.
297. Zhirnov OP. High protection of animals lethally infected with influenza virus by aprotinin-rimantadine combination. J Med Virol. 1987;21:161–7.
298. Bukrinskaya AG, Vorkunova NK, Kornilayeva GV, Narmanbetova RA, Vorkunova GK. Influenza virus uncoating in infected cells and effect of rimantadine. J Gen Virol. 1982;60:49–59.
299. Bukrinskaya AG, Vorkunova NK, Pushkarskaya NL. Uncoating of a rimantadine-resistant variant of influenza virus in the presence of rimantadine. J Gen Virol. 1982;60:61–6.
300. Donath E, Herrmann A, Coakley WT, Groth T, Egger M, Teager M. The influence of the antiviral drugs amantadine and rimantadine on erythrocyte and platelet membranes and its comparison with that of tetracaine. Biochem Pharmacol. 1987;36:481–7.
301. Levin M. Experience with amantadine and rimantadine in children. J Respir Dis. 1987;8(Suppl 11A):S60–6.
302. Reele SB. Adverse drug experiences during rimantadine trials. J Respir Dis. 1987;8(Suppl 11A):S81–6.
303. Patriarca PA, Kater NA, Kendal AP, Bregman DJ, Smith JD, Sikes RK. Safety of prolonged administration of rimantadine hydrochloride in the prophylaxis of influenza A infections in nursing homes. Antimicrob Agents Chemother. 1984;26:101–3.
304. Wills RJ, Rodriguez LC, Choma N, Oakes M. Influence of a meal on the bioavailability of rimantadine HCl. J Clin Pharmacol. 1987;27:821–3.
305. Wills RJ, Choma N, Buonpane G, Lin A, Keigher N. Relative bioavailability of rimantadine HCl tablet and syrup formulations in healthy subjects. J Pharm Sci. 1987;76:886–8.
306. Wills RJ, Farolino DA, Choma N, Keigher N. Rimantadine pharmacokinetics after single and multiple doses. Antimicrob Agents Chemother. 1987;31:826–8.
307. Nahata MC, Brady MT. Serum concentrations and safety of rimantadine in paediatric patients. Eur J Clin Pharmacol. 1986;30:719–22.
308. Anderson EL, Van Voris LP, Bartram J, Hoffman HE, Belshe RB. Pharmacokinetics of a single dose of rimantadine in young adults and children. Antimicrob Agents Chemother. 1987;31:1140–2.
309. Tominack RL, Wills RJ, Gustavson LE, Hayden FG. Multiple-dose phar-

macokinetics of rimantadine in elderly adults. Antimicrob Agents Chemother. 1988;32:1813–19.
310. Capparelli EV, Stevens RC, Chow MSS, Izard M, Wills RJ. Rimantadine pharmacokinetics in healthy subjects and patients with end stage renal failure. Clin Pharmacol Ther. 1988;43:536–41.
311. Wills RJ, Belshe R, Tomlinsin D, et al. Pharmacokinetics of rimantadine hydrochloride in patients with chronic liver disease. Clin Pharmacol Ther. 1987;42:449–54.
312. Zlydnikov DM, Kubar OI, Kovaleva TP, et al. Study of rimantadine in the USSR: a review of the literature. Rev Infect Dis. 1981;3:408–21.
313. Clover RD, Crawford SA, Abell TD, Ramsey CN Jr, Glezen WP, Couch RB. Effectiveness of rimantadine prophylaxis of children within families. Am J Dis Child. 1986;140:706–9.
314. Betts RF, Treanor JJ, Graman PS, Bentley DW, Dolin R. Antiviral agents to prevent or treat influenza in the elderly. J Respir Dis. 1987;8(Suppl 11A):S56–9.
315. Hayden FG, Monto AS. Oral rimantadine hydrochloride therapy of influenza A virus H3N2 subtype infection in adults. Antimicrob Agents Chemother. 1986;29:339–41.
316. Hayden FG, Zylidnikov DM, Iljenko VI, et al. Comparative therapeutic effect of aerosolized and oral rimantadine HCl in experimental human influenza A virus infection. Antiviral Res. 1982;2:147–53.
317. Spector SA, Tyndall M, Kelly E. Inhibition of human cytomegalovirus by trifluorothymidine. Antimicrob Agents Chemother. 1983;23:113–18.
318. Van Bijsterveld OP, Post H. Trifluorothymidine versus adenine arabinoside in the treatment of herpes simplex keratitis. Br J Ophthalmol. 1980;64:33–6.
319. Field H, McMillan A, Darby G. The sensitivity of acyclovir-resistant mutants of herpes simplex virus to other antiviral drugs. J Infect Dis. 1981;143:281–4.
320. Gephart JF, Lerner AM. Comparison of the effects of arabinosyladenine, arabinosylhypoxanthine, and arabinosyladenine 5′-monophosphate against herpes simplex virus, varicella-zoster virus, and cytomegalovirus with their effects on cellular deoxyribonucleic acid synthesis. Antimicrob Agents Chemother. 1981;19:170–8.
321. Biron KK, Fyfe JA, Noblin JE, et al. Selection and primary characterization of acyclovir-resistant mutants of varicella zoster virus. Am J Med. 1982;73(Suppl):383–6.
322. Pelling JC, Drach JC, Shipman C, Jr. Internucleotide incorporation of arabinosyladenine into herpes simplex virus and mammalian cell dna. Virology. 1981;109:323–35.
323. Shannon WM, Westbrook L, Arrett G, et al. Comparison of the efficacy of vidarabine, its carbocyclic analog (cyclaradine), and cyclaradine-5′-methoxy-acetate in the treatment of herpes simplex type 1 encephalitis in mice. Antimicrob Agents Chemother. 1983;24:538–43.
324. Vince R, Dalarge S, Lee H, et al. Carbocyclic arabinofuranosyladenine (cyclaradine): efficacy against genital herpes in guinea pigs. Science. 1983;221:1405–6.
325. Sacks SL, Merigan TC, Kaminska J, et al. Inactivation of S-adenosylhomocysteine hydrolase during adenine arabinoside therapy. J Clin Invest. 1982;69:226–30.
326. Cantoni GL, Aksamit RR, Kim I-K. Methionine biosynthesis and vidarabine therapy. N Engl J Med. 1982;307:1079.
327. Hinrichs J, Kitz D, Kobayashi G, et al. Immune enhancement in mice by ARA-A. J Immunol. 1983;130:829–33.
328. Whitley R, Alford C, Hess F, et al. Vidarabine: a preliminary review of its pharmacological properties and therapeutic use. Drugs. 1980;20:267–82.
329. Buchanan RA, Kinkel AW, Alford CA Jr, et al. Plasma levels and urinary excretion of vidarabine after repeat dosing. Clin Pharmacol Ther. 1980;27:690–6.
330. Shope TC, Kauffman RE, Bowman D, et al. Pharmacokinetics of vidarabine in infants and children treated for herpes infection. J Infect Dis. 1983;148:721–25.
331. Aronoff GR, Szwed JJ, Nelson RL, et al. Hypoxanthine-arabinoside pharmacokinetics after adenine arabinoside administration to a patient with renal failure. Antimicrob Agents Chemother. 1980;18:212–4.
332. Friedman HM, Grasela T. Adenine arabinoside and allopurinol—possible adverse drug interaction. N Engl J Med. 1981;304:423.
333. Etta LV, Brown J, Mastri A, et al. Fatal vidarabine toxicity in a patient with normal renal function. JAMA. 1981;246:1703–5.
334. Marker SC, Howard RJ, Groth KE, et al. A trial of vidarabine for cytomegalovirus infection in renal transplant patients. Arch Intern Med. 1980;140:1441–4
335. Feldman S, Robertson PK, Lott L, Thornton D. Neurotoxicity due to adenine arabinoside therapy during varicella-zoster virus infections in immunocompromised children. J Infect Dis. 1986;154:889–93.
336. Whitley RJ, Soong S-J, Hirsch MS, et al. Herpes simplex encephalitis, vidarabine therapy and diagnostic problems. N Engl J Med. 1981;304:313–8.
337. Whitley RJ, Yeager A, Kartus P, et al. Neonatal herpes simplex virus infection: follow-up evaluation of vidarabine therapy. Pediatrics. 1983;72:778–85.
338. Feder HM Jr. Disseminated herpes simplex infection in a neonate during prophylaxis with vidarabine. JAMA. 1988;259:1054–5.
339. Whitley RJ, Spruance S, Hayden F, et al. Vidarabine therapy of mucocutaneous herpes simplex virus infections in the immunocompromised host. J Infect Dis. 1984;149:1–8.
340. Whitley RJ, Soong S-J, Dolin R, et al. Early vidarabine therapy to control the complications of herpes zoster in immunosuppressed patients. N Engl J Med. 1982;307:971–5.
341. Whitley R, Hilty M, Haynes R, et al. Vidarabine therapy of varicella in immunosuppressed patients. J Pediatr. 1982;101:125–31.
342. Bassendine MF, Chadwick RG, Salmeron J, et al. Adenine arabinoside therapy in HBsAg-positive chronic liver disease: a controlled study. Gastroenterology. 1981;80:1016–22.
343. Weller IVD, Bassendine MF, Murray AK, et al. HBsAg-positive chronic liver disease: inhibition of viral replication by highly soluble adenine arabinoside 5′-monophosphate (ARA-AMP). Gastroenterology. 1980;79:1129.
344. Whitley RJ, Tucker BC, Kinkel AW, et al. Pharmacology, tolerance, and antiviral activity of vidarabine monophosphate in humans. Antimicrob Agents Chemother. 1980;18:709–15.
345. Preiksaitis JK, Lank B, Ng PK, et al. Effect of liver disease on pharmacokinetics and toxicity of 9-b-D-arabinofuranosyladenine-5′-phosphate. J Infect Dis. 1981;144:358–64.
346. Garcia G, Smith CI, Weissberg JI, et al. Adenine arabinoside monophosphate (vidarabine phosphate) in combination with human leukocyte interferon in the treatment of chronic hepatitis B. Ann Intern Med. 1987;107:278–85.
347. Hoofnagle JG, Hanson RG, Minuk GY, et al. Randomized controlled trial of adenine arabinoside monophosphate for chronic type B hepatitis. Gastroenterology. 1984;86:150–7.
348. Perrillo RP, Regenstein FG, Bodicky CJ, Campbell CR, Sanders GE, Sunwoo YC. Comparative efficacy of adenine arabinoside 5′ monophosphate and prednisone withdrawal followed by adenine arabinoside 5′ monophosphate in the treatment of chronic active hepatitis type B. Gastroenterology. 1985;88:780–6.
349. Yokosuka O, Omata M, Imazeki F, et al. Combination of short-term prednisolone and adenine arabinoside in the treatment of chronic hepatitis B. Gastroenterology. 1985;89:246–51.
350. Perrillo RP. Severe hepatic failure after ARA-A-prednisolone for chronic type B hepatitis (Reply to letter). Gastroenterology. 1987;274–5.
351. Fiume L, Bonino F, Mattioli A, et al. Inhibition of hepatitis B virus replication by vidarabine monophosphate conjugated with lactosaminated serum albumin. Lancet. 1988;2:13–15.
352. Mitsuya H, Weinhold KJ, Furman PA, et al. 3′-azido-3′-deoxythymidine (BW A509U): an antiviral agent that inhibits the infectivity and cytopathic effect of human T-lymphotropic virus type III/lymphadenopathy-associated virus in vitro. Proc Natl Acad Sci USA. 1985;82:7096–100.
353. Ruprecht RM, O'Brien LG, Rossoni LD, Nusinoff-Lehrman S. Suppression of mouse viraemia and retroviral disease by 3′-azido-3′-deoxythymidine. Nature. 1986;323:467–9.
354. Dahlberg JE, Mitsuya H, Balm SB, Broder S, Aaronson SA. Broad spectrum antiretroviral activity of 2′,3′-dideoxy-nucleosides. Proc Natl Acad Sci USA. 1987;84:2469–73.
355. Balzarini J, Pauwels R, Baba M, et al. The *in vitro* and *in vivo* anti-retrovirus activity, and intracellular metabolism of 3′-azido-2′,3′-dideoxythymidine and 2′,3′-dideoxycytidine are highly dependent on the cell species. Biochem Pharmacol. 1988;37:897–906.
356. Nakashima H, Matsui T, Harada S, et al. Inhibition of replication and cytopathic effect of human T cell lymphotropic virus type III/lymphadenopathy-associated virus by 3′-azido-3′-deoxythymidine in vitro. Antimicrob Agents Chemother. 1986;30:933–7.
357. Hartshorn KL, Vogt MW, Chou T-C, et al. Synergistic inhibition of human immunodeficiency virus in vitro by azidothymidine and recombinant alpha A interferon. Antimicrob Agents Chemother. 1987;31:168–72.
358. Vogt MW, Hartshorn KL, Furman PA, et al. Ribavirin antagonizes the effect of azidothymidine on HIV replication. Science. 1987;235:1276–9.
359. Mitchell WM, Montefiori DC, Robinson WE Jr, Strayer DR, Carter WA. Mismatched double-stranded RNA (ampligen) reduces concentration of zidovudine (azidothymidien) required for in-vitro inhibition of human immunodeficiency virus. Lancet. 1987;1:890–2.
360. Hammer SM, Gillis JM. Synergistic activity of granulocyte-macrophage colony-stimulating factor and 3′-azido-3′-deoxythymidine against human immunodeficiency virus in vitro. Antimicrob Agents Chemother. 1987;31:1046–50.
361. Richman DD. Dideoxynucleosides are less inhibitory in vitro against human immunodeficiency virus type 2 (HIV-2) than against HIV-1. Antimicrob Agents Chemother. 1987;31:1879–81.
362. Nakashima H, Tochikura T, Kobayashi N, Matsuda A, Ueda T, Yamamoto N. Effect of 3′-azido-2′,3′-dideoxythymidine (AZT) and neutralizing antibody on human immunodeficiency virus (HIV)-induced cytopathic effects: implication of giant cell formation for the spread of virus in vivo. Virology. 1987;159:169–73.
363. Smith MS, Brian EL, Pagano JS. Resumption of virus production after human immunodeficiency virus infection of T lymphocytes in the presence of azidothymidine. J Virol. 1987;61:3769–73.
364. Richman DD, Kornbluth RS, Carson DA. Failure of dideoxynucleosides to inhibit human immunodeficiency virus replication in cultured human macrophages. J Exp Med. 1987;166:1144–9.
365. Matsushita S, Mitsuya H, Reitz MS, Broder S. Pharmacological inhibition of in vitro infectivity of human T lymphotropic virus type 1. J Clin Invest. 1987;80:394–400.
366. Elwell LP, Ferone R, Freeman GA, et al. Antibacterial activity and mechanism of action of 3′-azido-3′-deoxythymidine (BW A5509U). Antimicrob Agents Chemother. 1987;31:274–80.

367. Hirsch MS. AIDS commentary—azidothymidine. J Infect Dis. 1988;157:427–31.
368. Sommadossi J-P, Carlisle R, Schinazi RJ, Zhou Z. Uridine reverses the toxicity of 3′-azido-3′-deoxythymidine in normal human granulocyte-macrophage progenitor cells in vitro without impairment of antiretroviral activity. Antimicrob Agents Chemother. 1988;32:997–1001.
369. Sharpe AH, Jaenisch R, Ruprecht RM. Retroviruses and mouse embryos: a rapid model for neurovirulence and transplacental antiviral therapy. Science. 1987;236:1671–4.
370. Tavares L, Roneker C, Johnston K, Nusinoff-Lehrman S, deNoronha F. 3′-azido-3′-deoxythymidine in feline leukemia virus-infected cats: a model for therapy and prophylaxis of AIDS. Cancer Res. 1987;4:3190–4.
371. Furman PA, Fyfe JA, St Clair MH, et al. Phosphorylation of 3′-azido-3′-deoxythymidine and selective interaction of the 5′-triphosphate with human immunodeficiency virus reverse transcriptase. Proc Natl Acad Sci USA. 1986;83:8333–7.
372. Yarchoan R, Broder S. Development of antiretroviral therapy for the acquired immunodeficiency syndrome and related disorders. N Engl J Med. 1987;316:557–64.
373. Larder BA, Darby G, Richman DD. HIV with reduced sensitivity to zidovudine (AZT) isolated during prolonged therapy. Science. 1989;243:1731–4.
374. Klecker RW Jr, Collins JM, Yarchoan R, et al. Plasma and cerebrospinal fluid pharmacokinetics of 3′-azido-3′-deoxythymidine: a novel pyrimidine analog with potential application for the treatment of patients with AIDS and related diseases. Clin Pharmacol Ther. 1987;41:407–12.
375. Henry K, Chinnock BJ, Quinn RP, Fletcher CV, deMiranda P, Balfour JJ Jr. Concurrent zidovudine levels in semen and serum determined by radioimmunoassay in patients with AIDS or AIDS-related complex. JAMA. 1988;259:3023–3026.
376. Surbone A, Yarchoan R, McAtee N, et al. Treatment of the acquired immunodeficiency syndrome (AIDS) and AIDS-related complex with a regimen of 3′-azido-2′,3′-dideoxythymidine (Azidothymidine or Zidovudine) and acyclovir. Ann Intern Med. 1988;108:534–40.
377. Pizzo PA, Eddy J, Falloon J, et al. Effect of continuous intravenous infusion of zidovudine (AZT) in children with symptomatic HIV infection. N Engl J Med. 1988;319:889–96.
378. Yarchoan R, Thomas RV, Grafman J, et al. Long-term administration of 3′-azido-2′,3′-dideoxythymidine to patients with AIDS-related neurological disease. Ann Neurol. 1988;23:S82–7.
379. Richman DD, Fischl MA, Grieco NH, et al. The toxicity of azidothymidine (AZT) in the treatment of patients with AIDS and AIDS-related complex. N Engl J Med. 1987;317:192–7.
380. Yarchoan R, Weinhold KJ, Lyerly HK, et al. Administration of 3′-azido-3′-deoxythymidine, an inhibitor of HTLV-III/LAV replication, to patients with AIDS or AIDS-related complex. Lancet. 1986;1:575–80.
381. Walker RE, Parker RI, Kovacs JA, et al. Anemia and erythropoiesis in patients with the acquired immunodeficiency syndrome (AIDS) and Kaposi sarcoma treated with zidovudine. Ann Intern Med. 1988;108:372–6.
382. Gill PS, Rarick M, Brynes RK, Causey D, Loureiro C, Levine AM. Azidothymidine associated with bone marrow failure in the acquired immunodeficiency syndrome (AIDS). Ann Intern Med. 1987;107:502–5.
383. Hagler DN, Frame PT. Azidothymidine neurotoxicity (Letter). Lancet. 1986;2:1392–3.
384. Davtyan DG, Vinters HV. Wernicke's encephalopathy in AIDS patient treated with zidovudine. Lancet. 1987;1:919–20.
385. Bessen LJ, Greene JB, Louie E, Seitzman P, Weinberg H. Severe polymyositis-like syndrome associated with zidovudine therapy of AIDS and ARC (Letter). N Engl J Med. 1988;318:708.
386. Furth PA, Kazakis AM. Nail pigmentation changes associated with azidothymidine (zidovudine). Ann Intern Med. 1987;107:350.
387. Pickus OB. Overdose of zidovudine. N Engl J Med. 1988;318:1206.
388. Fischl MA, Richman DD, Grieco MH, et al. The efficacy of azidothymidine (AZT) in the treatment of patients with AIDS and AIDS-related complex. N Engl J Med. 1987;317:185–91.
388a. Richman D, Andrews J, and the AZT Collaborative Working Group. Results of continued monitoring of participants in the placebo-controlled trial of zidovudine for serious human immunodeficiency virus infection. Am J Med. 1988;85(Suppl 2A):208–13.
389. Fiddian AP. Clinical experience with anti-HIV agents. Presented at the International Symposium: Basic and Clinical Approaches to Virus Chemotherapy, June 19–22, 1988, Helsinki, Finland. Final Program Antivirals 88, p. 65.
390. Schmitt FA, Bigley JW, McKinnis R, et al. Neuropsychological outcome of zidovudine (AZT) treatment of patients with AIDS and AIDS-related complex. N Engl J Med. 1988;319:1573–8.
391. de Wolf F, Goudsmit J, de Gans J, et al. Effect of zidovudine on serum human immunodeficiency virus antigen levels in symptom-free subjects. Lancet. 1988;1:373–6.
392. Jackson GG, Paul DA, Falk LA, et al. Human immunodeficiency virus (HIV) antigenemic (p24) in the acquired immunodeficiency syndrome (AIDS) and the effect of treatment with zidovudine (AZT). Ann Intern Med. 1988;108:175–80.
393. Dalakas MC, Yarchoan R, Spitzer R, Elder G, Sever JL. Treatment of human immunodeficiency virus-related polyneuropathy with 3′-azido-2′,3′-dideoxythymidine. Ann Neurol. 1988;23:S92–4.
394. Helbert M, Peddle B, Kocsis A, et al. Acute meningo-encephalitis on dose reduction of zidovudine. Lancet. 1988;1:1249–52.
395. Greisman SE, Johnston CA. The effect of azidothymidine on HIV-related thrombocytopenia. N Engl J Med. 1988;318:516–7.
396. Crowe S, Kirihara J, McGrath M, et al. Contrasting antiretroviral efficacy of zidovudine (AZT) and phosphonoformate (PFT) in HIV-infected macrophages. Fourth International Conference on AIDS, Stockholm, 1988, #3132.
397. Gaub J, Pederson C, Poulsen A-G, et al. The effect of focarnet (phosphonoformate) on human immunodeficiency virus isolation, T-cell subsets and lymphocyte function in AIDS patients. AIDS. 1987;1:27–33.
398. Öberg B, Behrnetz S, Eriksson B, et al. Clinical use of foscarnet (phosphonoformate). In: DeClercq E, ed. Clinical Use of Antiviral Drugs. Martinus Nijoff Publishing; 1988;223–40.
399. Walmsley SL, Chew E, Read SE, et al. Treatment of cytomegalovirus retinitis with trisodium phosphonoformate hexahydrate (foscarnet). J Infect Dis. 1988;157:569–572.
400. Jacobson MA, Crowe S, Levy J, et al. Effect of foscarnet therapy on infection with human immunodeficiency virus in patients with AIDS. J Infect Dis. 1988;158:862–5.
401. Singer DRJ, Fallon TJ, Schulenburg WE, et al. Foscarnet for cytomegalovirus retinitis (Letter). Ann Intern Med. 1985;103:962.
402. Bloom JN, Palestine AG. The diagnosis of cytomegalovirus retinitis. Ann Intern Med. 1988;109:963–9.
403. Farthing CF, Dalgleish AG, Clark A, et al. Phosphonoformate (foscarnet): a pilot study in AIDS and AIDS related complex. AIDS. 1987;1:21–25.
404. Bergdahl S, Sonnerborg A, Larsson A, Strannegard O. Declining levels of HIV p24 antigen in serum during treatment with foscarnet (Letter). Lancet. 1988;1:1052.
405. Chatis PA, Miller CH, Schrager LE, et al. Successful treatment with foscarnet of an acyclovir-resistant mucocutaneous infection with herpes simplex virus in a patient with acquired immunodeficiency syndrome. N Engl J Med. 1989;320:297–300.
406. Lawee D, Rosenthal D, Aoki FY, et al. Efficacy and safety of foscarnet for recurrent orolabial herpes: a multicenter randomized double-blind study. CMAJ. 1988;138:329–33.
407. Merigan TC, Skowron G, Bozzette SA, et al. Circulating p24 antigen levels and response to dideoxycytidine in human immunodeficiency virus (HIV) infections: a phase I and II study. Ann Intern Med. 1989;110:189–94.
408. Abrams DI, Kuno S, Wong R, et al. Oral dextran sulfate (UA001) in the treatment of the acquired immunodeficiency syndrome (AIDS) and AIDS-related complex. Ann Intern Med. 1989;110:183–8.
409. Clumeck N, Hermans P. Antiviral drugs other that zidovudine and immunomodulating therapies in human immunodeficiency virus infection. Am J Med. 1988;85(Suppl 2A):165–72.
410. Öberg B. Antiviral therapy. J Acq Imm Def Syn. 1988;1:257–66.

35. INTERFERONS

FREDERICK G. HAYDEN

Since their discovery in 1957 as mediators of the phenomenon of viral interference, that is, inhibition of the growth of one virus by another, interferons (IFNs) have become recognized as potent cytokines that are associated with complex antiviral, immunomodulating, and antiproliferative actions.[1] Interferons can be broadly defined as proteins or glycoproteins that are synthesized by host cells in response to various inducers and that in turn cause biochemical changes leading to a nonselective antiviral state in exposed cells of the same species. Production of IFN requires both de novo RNA and protein synthesis. Inducers include viruses, particularly double-stranded RNA viruses; various organisms capable of intracellular growth; bacterial endotoxins; polyanions; and certain low-molecular-weight organic compounds. Interferon activity is usually measured in terms of antiviral effects in cell culture. Typically, 1 unit of IFN activity is the amount present in a sample dilution that causes a 50 percent reduction in virus replication or expression in certain cell lines and is generally expressed as international units (IU) relative to National Institutes of Health (NIH) or World Health Organization (WHO) reference standards.

Early investigations of the possible clinical usefulness of IFNs were largely dependent on the use of inducers and limited quantities of human leukocyte IFN. Since the early 1980s, the availability of purified IFNs produced by recombinant DNA technology has allowed extensive study of these proteins in viral infections, malignancies, and certain other disorders. Parenteral IFN is currently approved for use in hairy cell leukemia, selected patients with Kaposi sarcoma, and intralesionally in refractory condyloma acuminata.

CLASSIFICATION

Formally designated on the basis of the cell types from which they were derived, three major classes of human IFNs are currently recognized (Table 1). Each type is immunologically distinct and has a fixed pattern of species specificity in addition to differing physiochemical characteristics.[1,3] Interferon-α and -β may be produced by nearly all cells in response to viral infection, whereas IFN-γ is restricted to T lymphocytes responding to mitogens or antigenic stimuli. The principal antiviral interferons, IFN-α and -β, are approximately 30 percent homologous at the amino acid level, whereas IFN-γ shares less than 20 percent homology. Human IFN-α actually comprises a family of over two dozen species that share a high degree of amino acid sequence homology (>50 percent) but have differing in vitro antiproliferative and antiviral effects on human cells. Human leukocyte- or lymphoblastoid-derived IFN preparations contain at least 18 distinct subtypes of IFN-α, as well as small amounts of IFN-β. Recombinant IFNs in clinical testing are over 95 percent pure and have very high specific activities (1 to 4×10^8 IU/mg protein).

Interferon-γ has a different spectrum of antiviral and immunomodulating properties from the other IFNs, with which it shows synergistic antiviral effects in certain test systems.[5,6] Interferon-γ is a potent macrophage-activating factor, and consequently, it is being evaluated in human infections associated with cellular parasites and/or defective macrophage function, including lepromatous leprosy[7] and human immunodeficiency virus (HIV) infection[8] (see Chapter 8). It also activates polymorphonuclear leukocytes (see Chapter 7).

MECHANISMS OF ACTION

Antiviral Effects

A wide range of different RNA and DNA animal viruses are sensitive to the antiviral actions of IFNs, although considerable differences exist for different viruses and assay systems.[4,9] Synergistic antiviral effects have been seen with combinations of IFN-γ and IFN-α or -β. Also, IFNs exhibit additive or synergistic antiviral activity with various synthetic antivirals against herpes, influenza, picorna-, retro-, and arboviruses under laboratory conditions.[6]

Interferons are not directly antiviral but cause biochemical changes in exposed cells that lead to viral resistance. The initial step involves IFN binding to specific cell surface receptors, which are shared between IFN-α and -β, but are different for IFN-γ.[1] The onset of IFN antiviral action is rapid, and alterations in cellular mRNA occur within minutes. Depending on the virus and cell type, IFN's antiviral effects are mediated through the inhibition of viral penetration or uncoating (e.g., papovaviruses), synthesis or methylation of messenger RNA, translation of viral proteins, or viral assembly and release (e.g., retroviruses).[9] For most viruses the principal replicative step inhibited by IFN is viral protein synthesis. After IFN exposure, cells produce a series of proteins, usually including a unique 2′,5′-oligoadenylate synthetase and a protein kinase, either of which can inhibit protein synthesis in the presence of double-stranded RNA. The 2′,5′-oligoadenylate synthetase produces adenylate oligomers that activate a latent cellular endoribonuclease (RNase L) in the presence of double-stranded RNA to cleave both cellular and viral RNAs. The protein kinase selectively phosphorylates two proteins involved in protein synthesis, eukaryotic initiation factor 2 (eIF-2) and a ribosome-associated one called P_1. Interferon may also block mRNA capping by inhibiting transmethylation reactions. Interferon induction of a phosphodiesterase, which cleaves a portion of transfer RNA and thus prevents peptide elongation, also contributes to the inhibition of protein synthesis. However, except possibly for the Mx protein in influenza virus infections, no consistent correlations exist between induction of a particular enzyme or protein and resistance to specific viruses across a range of cell types.[1,4,9] The specific effects important in inhibiting a particular virus are likely to be different for the different groups of viruses. Interferon exposure may also reduce the expression of certain cellular genes, including selected oncogenes and those involved in collagen synthesis.

The assay of IFN in clinical specimens has received study as a means of viral diagnosis.[10] Similarly, elevated levels of 2′,5′-oligoadenylate synthetase activity in peripheral white blood cells have been used for a marker for IFN exposure or endogenous release in different conditions.

TABLE 1. Nomenclature and Classification of Human Interferons

	Class		
Characteristics	α	β	γ
Former designations	Type I, leukocyte	Type I, fibroblast	Type II, immune
No. species	>24	1[a]	1
No. amino acids	165–166	166	143
Apparent MW[b]	16,000–27,000	20,000	15,500–25,000
Disulphide bonds	2	1	0
Glycosylation	Variable[c]	Yes	Yes
Acid stability (pH 2)	Yes[d]	Yes	No
Chromosome coding for IFN[e]	9	9	12

[a] Interferon-β_2 (designated interleukin-6) has negligible antiviral effects and functions primarily as a β-cell differentiation factor (BSF-2). It has minimal sequence homology with classic IFN-β and is encoded by a different chromosome.[2] Its classification as an IFN is unsettled.
[b] The molecular weight (MW) range relates to post-translation modifications including the formation of dimers, glycosylation, and protein binding. The MW of nonglycosylated recombinant IFN-$\alpha_2$is approximately 19,500.
[c] Generally not, but several species are glycosylated.
[d] Acid-labile IFN-α occur in certain pathologic states.
[e] The action of IFNs are mediated through chromosome 21, which encodes a glycoprotein receptor for IFN-α and -β. The IFN-γ receptor is encoded on human chromosome 6.
(Data from Zoon[3] and Greenberg.[4])

Non-antiviral Actions

The non-antiviral effects of IFN include inhibiting delayed-type hypersensitivity responses and lymphocyte blastogenesis and prolonging survival of allogeneic grafts, enhancing (low concentration) or suppressing (high concentration) antibody formation, increasing natural killer cell activity and antibody-dependent cellular cytotoxicity, enhancing phagocytic and cytolytic activity of macrophages, inhibiting macrophage migration, increasing the expression of major histocompatibility (MHC) antigens on cell surfaces, inhibiting the growth of intracellular parasites, augmenting IgE-mediated histamine release, increasing the expression of Fc receptors on lymphocytes and accessory cells, interfering with the attachment of hormones and certain toxins to ganglioside receptors on the cell membrane, priming for (low concentration) or inhibiting (high concentration) IFN production; inhibiting the growth of rapidly dividing cells; and enhancing (low concentration) or inhibiting the differentiation (high concentration) of cells.[1,3,5]

Interferon-γ generally has more potent immunoregulatory effects than IFN-α or -β does, particularly with respect to macrophage function, expression of class II MHC antigens, and mediation of local inflammatory responses.[11] Interferon-γ is also approximately 1000-fold more active than IFN-α is in inhibiting the hepatic schizogony of *Plasmodium falciparum* in human hepatocyte cultures[12] (see Chapter 8).

The pleomorphic effects of IFN on immune functions suggests that immunoregulation may be one of its major functions in the host. Complex interactions exist between IFNs and other parts of the immune system. For example, IFN-γ enhances the expression of interleukin-2 (IL-2) receptors on T lymphocytes, and IL-2 appears to modulate IFN-γ production, probably through effects on cellular cyclic guanosine monophosphate (cGMP) levels. The induction of cytotoxic T-lymphocyte responses appears to require both IL-2 and IFN-γ. Interferon-α is both produced by macrophages and can modify macrophage functions by increasing phagocytosis and cytolytic activity. The antiviral action of tumor necrosis factor appears to be mediated by IFN-β.[2]

Role in Viral Infections

Interferons may ameliorate viral infections by exerting antiviral effects and by modifying the immune response to infection. For example, IFN-induced expression of MHC antigens may contribute to the antiviral actions of IFN by enhancing the lytic effects of cytotoxic T lymphocytes. Many observations suggest that IFN titers generally appear at the sites of viral replication at the time of or just after peak titers of virus and before humoral antibody responses. High IFN titers are usually followed by a reduction in virus titer, although persistently elevated IFN titers have been recognized in certain chronic and acute (e.g., hemorrhagic fevers) viral infections. Interferon and its inducers are effective in preventing a variety of viral infections when administered before virus exposure. In animal models, the severity of viral infections is increased by administering antisera to species-specific IFN. In humans, the lack of endogenous IFN responses has been observed in severe viral infections including herpes zoster in immunocompromised hosts, fatal influenza viral pneumonia, chronic hepatitis B virus (HBV) infection, and in HIV infection complicated by opportunistic infections.

In contrast to resolution of viral infection, IFN production may be involved in immunologically mediated tissue damage in various viral diseases.[13] Interferon elaboration has been associated with disease in lymphocytic choriomeningitis virus infection of newborn mice and visna virus infection of sheep. Unusual acid-labile IFN-α has been observed in patients with certain autoimmune disorders and the acquired immunodeficiency syndrome (AIDS), where its presence appears to predict disease progression.[8] In more general terms, IFNs may mediate some of the systemic symptoms associated with viral infections.

HUMAN PHARMACOKINETICS

The pharmacokinetics of IFN are not well characterized. These molecules appear to behave like other small circulating plasma proteins such that after systemic administration low levels of IFN are detected in respiratory secretions, cerebrospinal fluid, eye, and brain.[4] Interferon-α is relatively stable in most body fluids, whereas IFN-β and -γ appear to readily lose activity. However, it is unknown whether measurable IFN levels at a particular site accurately reflect its antiviral or other biologic activities.

Oral administration does not result in detectable serum levels and is not used clinically. After the intramuscular or subcutaneous injection of IFN-α, plasma levels are dose related, peak at 4–8 hours, and return to baseline by 18–36 hours. Accumulation occurs with repetitive dosing. In contrast, intramuscular or subcutaneous injections of IFN-β or -γ results in negligible plasma levels, although increases in peripheral blood leukocyte 2′,5′-oligoadenylate synthetase levels may occur. Peak serum levels average 400–500 units/ml after intramuscular IFN-α doses of approximately 18×10^6 units.

Levels of 2′,5′-oligoadenylate synthetase have been considered to be an index of biologic responsiveness to IFN. After a single intramuscular injection (18×10^6 units of IFN-α), peripheral blood mononuclear cells show increases in their 2′-5′-oligoadenylate synthetase activity beginning at 6 hours and lasting through 4 days and an antiviral state in the same cells starting at 1 hour, peaking at 24 hours, and slowly decreasing to baseline by 6 days after injection.[14] Thus the biologic effects of IFN last days longer than do detectable serum levels. Similarly, after intranasal administration, an antiviral effect lasts at least 18 hours in exposed respiratory mucosa.

After intravenous dosing, both IFN-α and -β are cleared rapidly in a biphasic fashion. Leukocyte and recombinant IFN-α species have an elimination half-life ($T_{1/2}$) of approximately 2 hours in the circulation. The clearance of IFN includes inactivation by various body fluids and metabolism by different organs, primarily the kidney and to some extent the liver, heart and skeletal muscle, and lung. The rate of IFN clearance is less than 2 percent of the glomerular infiltration rate, and negligible biologically active IFN is excreted in the urine.

TOXICITY

Both purified natural and recombinant IFNs are associated with dose-related toxicities that limit their clinical use. With systemic administration, an influenza-like syndrome consisting of fever, chills, headache, myalgia, and occasionally nausea, vomiting, or diarrhea is expected within several hours after initiating doses of 10^4–10^5 units/kg. A systemic dose of approximately 1×10^6 IU/day is generally well tolerated by most patients. Temperatures may range over 40°C, but the fever usually resolves within 12 hours after intramuscular administration.

Up to one-half of patients receiving intralesional therapy for genital warts experience the flulike illness, although symptoms usually decrease during the first week of therapy. The febrile responses are mediated through the production of hypothalamic prostaglandins[15] and can be moderated by pretreatment with various antipyretics.

Major toxicities that limit parenteral therapy are bone marrow suppression with granulocytopenia and thrombocytopenia; neurotoxicity manifested by somnolence, confusion, behavioral disturbance, electroencephalogram (EEG) changes, and rarely seizures[16]; reversible neurasthenia with profound fatigue and anorexia, weight loss, and myalgia during long-term use; and possibly cardiotoxicity with hypotension, arrhythmias, and congestive cardiomyopathy. Leukopenia tends to be most marked by the second week of therapy. Elevations in hepatic enzyme and triglyceride levels are common, and renal insufficiency may occur. Interferon prophylaxis has been associated with severe leukoencephalopathy in bone marrow transplant recipients[17] and with acute steroid-resistant rejection and nephrotic syndrome in kidney transplant recipients. Interferon and its inducers reduce the metabolism of various drugs by the hepatic cytochrome P-450–dependent mixed-function oxidase system and significantly increase plasma half-lives and levels of drugs like theophylline.[18] The development of serum neutralizing antibodies to exogenous IFNs varies with the IFN type, dose, and route of administration but may be associated with a loss of clinical responsiveness.[19,20] Antibodies directed against recombinant IFN-α may or may not cross react with natural IFN-α or other recombinant species, and patients with neutralizing antibodies against recombinant IFN-α subtypes may respond to natural IFN-α.

Local reactions consisting of tenderness and erythema occur after subcutaneous injection. Intranasal administration avoids systemic side effects but is associated with mucosal friability and ulceration and complaints of nasal dryness, stuffiness, and bleeding in up to 50 percent of recipients, depending on the dose and duration of administration.[21] Clinical irritation is preceded by marked histopathologic changes consisting of infiltration by lymphocytic cells in the nasal submucosa.

Interferon is an abortifacient in monkeys at high doses, and its safety during pregnancy is not established.

CLINICAL STUDIES

Extensive clinical testing has been done with various IFN formulations and routes of administration to assess IFN's possible value in the treatment and prevention of viral infections.[4,22] Clinical use of IFNs has been limited by its relative lack of potency, dose-limiting side effects, and the availability of competing antiviral agents. Although various trials have established that IFN is clearly superior to placebo in certain situations (Table 2), convincing clinical benefit has been demonstrated in very few viral diseases. Therapeutic use has generally been limited to the treatment of select chronic viral infections or acute ones associated with the failure of endogenous IFN responses.

Herpes Viruses

Several controlled studies have documented some clinical and virologic efficacy with IFN in the prevention or treatment of herpesvirus infections (Table 2). Although some trials have reported beneficial effects, no consistent reductions in symptoms and lesion duration have been observed with topical or parenteral IFN treatment of recurrent or initial genital herpes.[4,22–25] In such studies, parenteral IFN has been frequently associated with febrile responses and often with reversible neutropenia. The magnitude of the clinical benefit when used for the treatment or suppression of recurrent genital herpes is less than that seen with oral acyclovir.[23] In localized herpes zoster of cancer patients, early treatment with high-dose (approximately 36×10^6 units/day for 5–7 days) intramuscular leukocyte-derived IFN reduces progression of the primary dermatome, the risk of cutaneous or visceral dissemination, and the severity of post-herpetic neuralgia.[22] Lower doses or shorter durations of therapy are less effective. A 69 percent lower rate of cutaneous dissemination of localized zoster was found in cancer patients treated with recombinant IFN-α 36 MU/day for 7 days, as compared with placebo, but side effects were common in IFN recipients.[26] Parenteral IFN-α is also effective in reducing the risk of visceral dissemination in varicella of immunocompromised children, but alternative treatments, acyclovir and vidarabine, are available. In cytomegalovirus (CMV) infections, long-term administration reduces the risk of CMV disease in seropositive renal allograft recipients, but systemic IFN is not effective in preventing CMV infection or improving survival in bone marrow recipients when begun after marrow allografting.[17] Interferon is also ineffective in treating established CMV infections.[22]

In superficial herpes simplex virus (HSV) keratitis, the combined administration of topical IFN-α with trifluridine or acyclovir appears to be more effective than single-agent therapy is.[4]

TABLE 2. Viral Infections in which Interferons Have Efficacy

Systemic administration	
	Chronic hepatitis B
	Chronic non-A, non-B hepatitis
	Suppression of CMV infections (renal transplantation)
	Herpes zoster in immunocompromised hosts
	Varicella in immunocompromised hosts
	Prevention of orofacial HSV after trigeminal surgery
	Condyloma acuminatum
	Juvenile laryngeal papillomatosis
Intralesional	
	Condyloma acuminata, verucca vulgaris
Topical application	
	Herpes simplex keratoconjunctivitis
	Prevention of rhinovirus colds

Hepatitis

Chronic hepatitis B virus (HBV) infections have also shown responsiveness to parenterally administered leukocyte and recombinant IFN-α.[27–29] In addition to acute reductions in serum HBV DNA concentrations and Dane particle markers, interferon administration on a long-term basis (up to 6 months) is associated with the permanent loss of DNA polymerase activity in the serum with or without the loss of hepatitis B surface antigen (HBsAg) in up to one-third of patients. DNA polymerase activity declines to 15–35 percent of pretreatment values within 48 hours of initiating therapy with intramuscular IFN (3–20×10^6 units/day). One trial employing 6 months' treatment with lymphoblastoid IFN-α found a 26 percent seroconversion rate to antibody to hepatitis B e antigen (HBeAg) that was associated with a hepatitis-like illness in the third month of therapy and later with clearance of HBsAg.[27] Clearance of serum HBeAg is often associated with symptomatic improvement and normalization of aminotransferase levels. Another study using recombinant IFN-α (2.5–10×10^6 units/m^2 intramuscularly three times per week) for 3–6 months found that 70 percent of Chinese patients had undetectable serum HBV DNA levels at the end of therapy but that 47 percent experienced reactivation of HBV infection and only 15 percent had sustained clearance of HBeAg 12 months after the end of therapy.[29] Female patients appear to be more responsive than males are, and Caucasian carriers more responsive than Chinese, most of whom are infected from birth.[29,29a] Concurrent steroid administration or HIV infection are associated with reduced response rates. The combined results of various trials indicate that relatively low doses of parenteral IFN (2.5–5×10^6 units/day) are as effective as higher doses in inhibiting HBV replication and are better tolerated, that prolonged administration (2–4 months) is needed to increase the likelihood of a lasting response, but that overall rates of seroconversion from HBeAg to anti-HBe are below 50 percent with single-agent IFN therapy.[27,29a] Optimal dose schedules and possible effects on long-term sequelae remain under study.

Despite evidence indicating short-term enhancement of antiviral effects by combinations of systemic IFN-α with vidarabine, acyclovir, or corticosteroid pretreatment, no dual therapies have yet emerged that provide greater long-term benefit or reductions in toxicity compared with IFN above.[29a,29b] The combination of vidarabine monophosphate and interferons has been disappointing.[30] Suppression of DNA polymerase activity has also been observed with recombinant IFN-β–serine (IFN-β_{ser}) during short-term use, but the addition of IFN-γ to IFN-β_{ser} did not improve responsiveness and may have been associated with additive toxicity in one short-term study.[31] A recent trial found that a 6-week tapered regimen of prednisone followed by 90 days' treatment with subcutaneous recombinant IFN-α (5×10^6 IU/day) was associated with clearing of HBV DNA markers and the normalization of aminotransferase values in 50 percent and the disappearance of HBsAg in 22 percent of treated subjects.[32]

Long-term, low-dose IFN-α therapy may be effective in reducing serum aminotransferase levels and improving hepatic histology in some patients with chronic non-A, non-B hepatitis.[33] Sustained biochemical and some hepatic histologic improvements have been observed in some patients with chronic non-A, non-B hepatitis treated with recombinant IFN-α at doses as low as 1×10^6 IU three times per week.[33] Controlled trials are in progress.

Papillomavirus

Responses in condylomata acuminata have been observed with various IFN preparations administered topically, intralesionally, and parenterally.[4,34] Intralesional IFN has been demonstrated to be a clinically useful intervention in refractory condylomata acuminata.[34–38] In one trial employing recombinant IFN-α_2 (1×10^6 IU per lesion three times weekly for 3 weeks), complete resolution of injected warts occurred in 36 percent of patients by 13 weeks follow-up, but no effects on untreated lesions were observed.[35] In a study of purified leukocyte-derived IFN-α ($2.5–5.5 \times 10^5$ IU/25 mm^2 of lesion twice weekly for 8 weeks), complete responses occurred in 62 percent of patients.[38] Response rates are two- to threefold higher than those observed in placebo recipients, and further complete responses occur with a second course of therapy. No differences in response rates have been found in lymphoblastoid IFN-α, recombinant IFN-α, and fibroblast-derived IFN-β.[37] Responding lesions generally show involution within 4 weeks and maximal decreases at 4–12 weeks after initiating therapy. Intralesional therapy does not benefit uninjected warts and may miss asymptomatic areas of infection, but complete responders appear to have relatively low relapse rates (21–33 percent) during short-term follow-up. Efficacy has been demonstrated in patients previously failing conventional therapies, but responsiveness is poor in HIV-infected patients.[35] Mild to moderate systemic side effects (8–10 percent dropout rate), discomfort at the injection site, and leukopenia (up to 30 percent) are common with intralesional IFN. Thus, intralesional therapy for discreet lesions appears to be effective and reasonably tolerated, although the cost-effectiveness of this intervention relative to ablative therapies like cryosurgery has not been determined.

In extensive disease, intramuscular or subcutaneous administration has been advocated but may be associated with greater toxicity than is observed with intralesional dosing,[34,39,40] Parenteral doses of 1×10^6 IU/mm^2/day for 14 days followed by three doses per week for 1 monthe are well tolerated but associated with complete resolution of lesions in a minority of patients.[40a] Intramuscular recombinant IFN-γ is also associated with therapeutic activity in refractory genital papillomavirus infections, including those involving the cervix.[41] Multimodality treatments involving systemic IFN have not yet documented greater response rates than with topical podophyllin or with laser therapy used above.[40a] Interferon use should be currently reserved for patients with recalcitrant disease, those who have repeatedly failed conventional therapy, or those who have such extensive involvement that conventional therapy is impractical.[39] The possible usefulness of IFN in managing human papillomavirus (HPV)-induced cervical dysplasia has not been critically evaluated, but one trial employing an IFN gel was unsuccessful.[42]

Plantar warts appear to be substantially less responsive to intramuscular recombinant IFN-α than are genital warts.[36] Limited evidence suggests that verruca vulgaris may respond to intralesional IFN-α.[43] Responses to intralesional and systemic IFN have also been observed in the rare HPV-related condition of epidermodysplasia verruciformis.[34]

In juvenile laryngeal papillomatosis (JLP), most of the children have some initial decrease in lesions in response to systemic IFN.[4,34] However, HPV DNA persists despite lesion regression such that recurrence rates are high after the cessation of therapy. The long-term response to parenteral IFN-α in recurrent JLP is quite variable.[44] One recent trial employing intramuscular leukocyte-derived IFN, 2 MU/m^2 three times per week for 12 months, found significant reductions in papilloma growth rates during the first 6 months and in the need for urgent surgical procedures but no long-term benefits when compared with laser therapy alone.[45] Adult-onset laryngeal disease appears to be more responsive than that in children. Optimal dose schedules have not been determined in laryngeal papillomatosis, and multicenter controlled trials in conjunction with carbon dioxide laser therapy are in progress.

Respiratory Viruses

Except for adenovirus, IFN has broad-spectrum antiviral activity against respiratory viruses in vitro. In experimentally induced infections in humans, the intranasal administration of leukocyte or recombinant IFN-α has been found to be protective against rhinovirus, coronavirus, and to a lesser extent influenza virus infections.[21] However, during long-term daily use under natural conditions, prophylactic intranasal IFN-α is protective only against rhinovirus colds, and chronic use is limited by the occurrence of local nasal side effects. Studies to date have failed to determine an IFN type and dosage that is both protective against rhinovirus infections and well tolerated during long-term use. When used for postcontact prophylaxis in the family setting, intranasal recombinant IFN-α_2 (5×10^6 units once daily for 7 days) is associated with approximately 40 percent reductions in secondary respiratory illnesses and nearly 90 percent protection against rhinovirus colds during the period of use.[46,47] However, protection against other respiratory viral infections has not been observed in such studies, and intranasal IFN-α_2 is therapeutically ineffective in established rhinovirus colds.[48]

Human Immunodeficiency Virus

The interaction of the IFN system with HIV infection is complex, and it is currently difficult to predict the clinical usefulness of exogenous IFNs. Unusual IFN species and IFN inactivators are frequently present in the sera of AIDS patients.[49] Interferons have dose-related inhibitory activity against HIV in T-lymphocyte cultures.[8] High doses of IFN-α induce 10–50 percent response rates in Kaposi sarcoma patients without benefiting concurrent herpesvirus infections or immune function.[8,50] Recent open trials of prolonged IFN-α_2 therapy (up to 36×10^6 IU/day) have found that responding KS patients have higher pretreatment T4 lymphocyte counts and may experience T4 count increases, falls in p24 antigen levels, and fewer opportunistic infections compared with nonresponders.[51,52] Initial clinical trials with high doses of IFN-α or -γ have found some antiviral effects but no significant immune reconstitution in patients with advanced AIDS. One controlled study of IFN found no survival benefit in such patients.[53] Studies of lower-dose regimens and combination therapy with other cytokines are in progress. In vitro synergy between IFN and zidovudine, phosphonoformate, or ribavirin has led to clinical testing of drug combinations.

REFERENCES

1. Pestka S, Langer JA, Zoon KC, et al. Interferons and their actions. Annu Rev Biochem. 1987;56:727–77.
2. Reis LFL, Le J, Hirano T, et al. Antiviral action of tumor necrosis factor in human fibroblasts is not mediated by B cell stimulatory factor 2/IFN-beta$_2$, and is inhibited by specific antibodies to IFN-beta. J Immunol. 1988; 140:1566–70.
3. Zoon KC. Human interferons: Structure and function. In: Interferon 9, London: Academic Press; 1987:1–12.
4. Greenberg SB. Human interferon in viral diseases. Infect Dis Clin North Am. 1987;1:383–423.
5. Johnson HM. Interferon-mediated modulation of the immune system. In: Pfeffer LM, ed. Mechanisms of Interferon Actions. v. 2. Boca Raton, FL: CRC Press; 1987:59–77.
6. Hall MJ, Duncan IB. Antiviral drug and interferon combinations. In: Field JH, ed. Antiviral Agents: The Development and Assessment of Antiviral Chemotherapy. v. 2. Boca Raton, FL: CRC Press; 1988:29–84.
7. Nathan CF, Kaplan G, Levis WR, et al. Local and systemic effects of intradermal recombinant interferon-gamma in patients with lepromatous leprosy. N Engl J Med. 1986;315:6–15.
8. Pomerantz RJ, Hirsch MS. Interferon and human immunodeficiency virus infection. In: Interferon 9. London: Academic Press; 1987:113–27.
9. Whitaker-Dowling P, Youngner JS. Antiviral effects of interferon in different virus–host cell systems. In: Pfeffer LM, ed. Mechanisms of Interferon Actions. v. 1. Boca Raton, FL: CRC Press; 1987:83–98.
10. Skidmore SJ, Jarlow MJ. Interferon assay as a viral diagnostic test. J Virol Methods. 1987;16:155–8.
11. Heremans H, Dijkmans R, Sobis H, et al. Regulation by interferons of the local inflammatory response to bacterial lipopolysaccharide. J Immunol. 1987;138:4175–9.
12. Mellouk S, Maheshwari RK, Rhodes-Feuillette A, et al. Inhibitory activity of interferons and interleukin 1 on the development of *Plasmodium falciparum* in human hepatocyte cultures. J Immunol. 1987;139:4192–5.

13. Hooks JJ, Detrick B. The interferon system and disease. In: Pfeffer LM, ed. Mechanisms of Interferon Actions. v. 2. Boca Raton, FL: CRC Press; 1987:113–328.
14. Barouki FM, Witter FR, Griffin DE, et al. Time course of interferon levels, antiviral state, 2′,5′-oligoadenylate synthetase and side effects in healthy men. J Interferon Res. 1987;7:29–39.
15. Dinarello CA, Cannon JG, Wolff SM. New concepts on the pathogenesis of fever. Rev Infect Dis. 1988;10:168–89.
16. McDonald EM, Mann AH, Thomas HC. Interferons as mediators of psychiatric morbidity. Lancet. 1987;2:1175–8.
17. Meyers JD, Flournoy N, Sanders JE, et al. Prophylactic use of human leukocyte interferon after allogeneic marrow transplantation. Ann Intern Med. 1987;107:809–16.
18. Williams SJ, Baird-Lambert JA, Farrell GC. Inhibition of theophylline metabolism by interferon. Lancet. 1987;2:939–41.
19. Steis RG, Smith JW II, Urba WJ, et al. Resistance to recombinant interferon alfa-2a in hairy-cell leukemia associated with neutralizing anti-interferon antibodies. N Engl J Med. 1988;318:1409–13.
20. Spiegel RJ, Spicehandler JR, Jacobs SL, et al. Low incidence of serum neutralizing factors in patients receiving recombinant alfa-2b interferon (Intron A). Am J Med. 1986;80:223–8.
21. Hayden FG. Intranasal interferons for control of the common cold. In: Revel M, ed. Clinical Aspects of Interferon. Boston: Kluwer Academic Publishers; 1988:3–16.
22. Ho M. Interferon for the treatment of infections. Annu Rev Med. 1987;38:51–9.
23. Kuhls TL, Sacher J, Pineda E, et al. Suppression of recurrent genital herpes simplex virus infection with recombinant alfa2 interferon. J Infect Dis. 1986;154:437–42.
24. Pazin GJ, Harger JH, Armstrong JA, et al. Leukocyte interferon for treating first episodes of genital herpes in women. J Infect Dis. 1987;156:891–8.
25. Eron LJ, Toy C, Salsitz B, et al. Therapy of genital herpes with topically applied interferon. Antimicrob Agents Chemother 1987;31:1137–9.
26. Winston DJ, Eron LJ, Ho M, et al. Recombinant interferon alpha-2a for treatment of herpes zoster in immunosuppressed patients with cancer. Am J Med. 1988;85:147–51.
27. Davis GL, Hoofnagle JH. Interferon in viral hepatitis: Role in pathogenesis and treatment. Hepatology. 1986;6:1038–41.
28. Alexander GJM, Fagan EA, Daniels HM, et al. Loss of HBsAg with interferon therapy in chronic hepatitis B virus infection. Lancet. 1987;2:66–9.
29. Lok ASF, Wu P-C, Lai C-L, et al. Long-term follow-up in a randomised controlled trial of recombinant alpha$_2$-interferon in Chinese patients with chronic hepatitis B infection. Lancet. 1988;2:298–302.
29a. Thomas HC. Hepatitis B viral infection. Am J Med. 1988;85(Suppl 2A):135–40.
29b. DeMan RA, Schalm SW, Heijtink RA, et al. Long-term follow-up of antiviral combination therapy in chronic hepatitis B. Am J Med. 1988;85(Suppl 2A):150–54.
30. Garcia G, Smith CI, Weissberg JI, et al. Adenine arabinoside monophosphate (vidarabine phosphate) in combination with human leukocyte interferon in the treatment of chronic hepatitis B. Ann Intern Med. 1987;107:278–85.
31. Bissett J, Eisenberg M, Gregory P, et al. Recombinant fibroblast interferon and immune interferon for treating chronic hepatitis B virus infection: Patients' tolerance and the effect on viral markers. J Infect Dis. 1988;157:1076–80.
32. Perrillo RP, Regenstein FG, Peters MG, et al. Prednisone withdrawal followed by recombinant alpha interferon in the treatment of chronic type B hepatitis. Ann Intern Med. 1988;109:95–100.
33. Hoofnagle JH, Mullen KD, Jones DB, et al. Treatment of chronic non-A, non-B hepatitis with recombinant human alpha interferon. N Engl J Med. 1986;315:1575–8.
34. Weck PK, Brandsma JL, Whisnant JK. Interferons in the treatment of human papillomavirus diseases. Cancer Metastasis Rev. 1986;5:139–65.
35. Eron LJ, Judson F, Tucker S, et al. Interferon therapy for condylomata acuminata. N Engl J Med. 1986;315:1059–64.
36. Vance JC, Bart BJ, Hansen RC, et al. Intralesional recombinant alpha-2 interferon for the treatment of patients with condyloma acuminatum or verruca plantaris. Arch Dermatol. 1986;122:272–7.
37. Reichman RC, Oakes D, Bonnez W, et al. Treatment of condyloma acuminatum with three different interferons administered intralesionally. Ann Intern Med. 1988;108:675–9.
38. Friedman-Kien AE, Eron LJ, Conant M, et al. Natural interferon alfa for treatment of condylomata acuminata. JAMA. 1988;259:533–8.
39. Trofatter KF Jr. Interferon. Obstet Gynecol Clin North Am. 1987;14:569–79.
40. Gall SA, Hughes CE, Mounts P, et al. Efficacy of human lymphoblastoid interferon in the therapy of resistant condyloma acuminata. Obstet Gynecol. 1986;67:643–51.
40a. Weck PK, Buddin DA, Whisnaut JK. Interferons in the treatment of genital papillomavirus infections. Am J Med. 1988;85(Suppl 2A):159–164.
41. Kirby PK, Kiviat N, Beckman A, et al. Tolerance and efficacy of recombinant human interferon gamma in the treatment of refractory genital warts. Am J Med. 1988;85:183–8.
42. Byrne MA, Moller BR, Tayor-Robinson D, et al. The effect of interferon on human papillomaviruses associated with cervical intraepithelial neoplasia. Br J Obstet Gynecol. 1986;93:1136–44.
43. Berman B, Davis-Reed L, Silverstein L, et al. Treatment of verrucae vulgaris with alfa2 interferon. J Infect Dis. 1986;154:328–30.
44. Lusk RP, McCabe BF, Mixon JH. Three-year experience of treating recurrent respiratory papilloma with interferon. Ann Otol Rhinol Laryngol. 1987; 19:158–62.
45. Healy GB, Gelber RD, Trowbridge AL, et al. Treatment of recurrent respiratory papillomatosis with human leukocyte interferon. N Engl J Med. 1988;319:401–7.
46. Hayden FG, Albrecht JK, Kaiser DL, et al. Prevention of natural colds by contact prophylaxis with intranasal alpha2-interferon. N Engl J Med. 1986; 314:71–5.
47. Douglas RB, Moore BW, Miles HB, et al. Prophylactic efficacy of intranasal alpha2-interferon against rhinovirus infections in the family setting. N Engl J Med. 1986;314:65–70.
48. Hayden FG, Kaiser DL, Albrecht JK. Intranasal recombinant alfa-2b interferon treatment of naturally occurring common colds. Antimicrob Agents Chemother. 1988;32:224–30.
49. Ikossi-O'Connor MG, Chadha KC, Lillie MA, et al. Interferon inactivator(s) in patients with AIDS and AIDS-related Kaposi''s sarcoma. Am J Med. 1986;81:783–5.
50. Krown SE. The role of interferon in the therapy of epidemic Kaposi's sarcoma. Semin Oncol. 1987;14:27–33.
51. Lane HC, Feinberg J, Davey V, et al. Anti-retroviral efects of interferon-α in AIDS-associated Kaposi sarcoma. Lancet. 1988;2:1218–1222.
52. DeWit R, Boucher CAB, Veenhof KHN, et al. Clinical and virological effects of high-dose recombinant interferon-α in disseminated AIDS-related Kaposi sarcoma. Lancet. 1988;2:1214–1217.
53. Friedland GH, Landesman SH, Crumpocker CS, et al. A clinical trial of recombinant α-IFN in patients with AIDS. III International Conference on AIDS. Washington DC, June 1987;165.

36. ANTIPARASITIC AGENTS

DAVID E. VAN REKEN
RICHARD D. PEARSON

A comprehensive discussion of antiparasitic chemotherapy must take into account the large number of parasites that can infect humans, the complexity of their life cycles, differences in their metabolism, and the wide array of drugs that have been developed to treat them. Taxonomically, parasites are divided into protozoa and helminths.[1–4] The protozoa often have complex life cycles but are unicellular. Helminths, on the other hand, have highly developed neuromuscular systems, digestive tracts, reproductive organs, and integuments. It is not surprising that most drugs effective against the helminths are not active against protozoa, and vice versa.

The susceptibility of the parasites to chemotherapeutic agents correlates to a high degree with taxonomy and metabolism (Table 1). The parasites can be grouped along these two parameters. The protozoa that inhabit the gastrointestinal lumen and vagina form one group. Although they arise from several taxonomic classes,[1] they share a common microenvironment and in many instances have similar metabolic adaptations. Included in this group are the various amoebae of the superclass Rhizopodia, the luminal flagellates of the class Zoomastigophorea, and *Balantidium coli* of the class Ciliata. The second major group includes members of the phylum Apicomplexa. These protozoa are important causes of morbidity and mortality worldwide. Included are *Plasmodium* spp., which cause malaria, *Babesia* spp., *Toxoplasma gondii*, *Cryptosporidium* spp., and *Isospora belli*. The latter three "coccidians" have emerged as important pathogens in persons with acquired immunodeficiency syndrome (AIDS). *Pneumocystis carinii*, which has not yet been classified, shares with members of the Apicomplexa the propensity to cause severe disease in the setting of AIDS and susceptibility to certain drugs. The third group of protozoan pathogens include flagellates of the class Zoomastigophorea, family Trypanosomidiae. They are arthropod borne and produce leishmaniasis, Chagas disease, and African sleeping sickness.

The susceptibility of helminths also correlates relatively closely with taxonomy. The helminths can be divided into ne-

TABLE 1. Spectrum of Activity of the Major Antiparasitic Drugs Licensed for Use in the United States, Available in the United States Only from the Manufacturer (*), Available from the CDC Drug Service, Centers for Disease Control (**), or Not Currently Available in the United States (***)

Drug	*Indications*
Amoebae, intestinal and vaginal Flagellates, and *Balantidium coli*	
Metronidazole	*Entamoeba histolytica* (invasive disease) *Entamoeba polecki* *Trichomonas vaginalis* *Blastocystis hominis* *Giardia lamblia* *Balantidium coli* (alternative)
Emetine, dehydroemetine**	*Entamoeba histolytica* (invasive disease)
Iodoquinol	*Entamoeba histolytica* (luminal infection) *Dientamoeba fragilis* *Blastocystis hominis* *Balantidium coli* (alternative)
Diloxanide furoate**	*Entamoeba histolytica* (asymptomatic luminal infection) *Entamoeba polecki* (luminal infection)
Paromomycin	*Entamoeba histolytica* (asymptomatic luminal infection) *Dientamoeba fragilis*
Quinacrine	*Giardia lamblia*
Furazolidone	*Giardia lamblia* (alternative)
Tetracycline	*Balantidium coli* *Dientamoeba fragilis*
Amphotericin B	*Naegleria* spp. (used with miconazole and rifampin)
Apicomplexa and *Pneumocystis carinii*	
Chloroquine	Suppressive prophylaxis and treatment of the asexual erythrocytic phase of *Plasmodium vivax, P. ovale, P. malariae,* and susceptible *P. falciparum*.
Primaquine	Radical cure of the exoerythrocytic hypnozoites of *P. vivax* and *P. ovale*.
Quinine	Treatment of chloroquine-resistant *P. falciparum*; effective against asexual erythrocytic phase of other *Plasmodium* spp.
Quinidine	Treatment of chloroquine-resistant *P. falciparum* when parenteral therapy is required; effective against asexual erythrocytic phase.
Mefloquine***	Prophylaxis and treatment of chloroquine-resistant *P. falciparum*; effective against asexual erythrocytic phase of other *Plasmodium* spp.
Tetracyclines	
Tetracycline	Used with quinine to treat asexual erythrocytic state of chloroquine-resistant *P. falciparum* in Southeast Asia.
Doxycycline	Used alone or with chloroquine for suppressive prophylaxis in Southeast Asia in areas where there is endemic chloroquine-resistant *P. falciparum*.
Dihydrofolate reductase inhibitors and sulfonamides	
Pyrimethamine/short-acting sulfonamides	Used with quinine to treat asexual erythrocytic phase of chloroquine-resistant *P. falciparum* acquired in areas other than Southeast Asia. *Toxoplasma gondii* (when treatment is indicated).
Pyrimethamine-sulfadoxime (Fansidar)	Presumptive treatment of chloroquine-resistant *P. falciparum* in areas where isolates remain sensitive; occasionally used for suppressive prophylaxis of chloroquine-resistant *P. falciparum* in persons at high risk.
Trimethoprim-sulfamethoxazole (cotrimoxazole)	*Pneumocystis carinii* *Isospora belli*
Proguanil***[a]	Used with chloroquine for suppressive prophylaxis in areas of East Africa where there is chloroquine-resistant *Plasmodium falciparum*
Macrolide antibiotics	
Clindamycin	Used with steroids for treatment of ocular *Toxoplasma gondii* in immunocompetent hosts; used with pyrimethamine for *T. gondii* encephalitis in persons with AIDS who cannot tolerate sulfonamides. Used with quinine for treatment of *Babesia* spp.
Spiramycin***[b]	*Toxoplasma gondii* during pregnancy and in the neonate *Cryptosporidium* species (efficacy uncertain)
Pentamidine isethionate	Treatment and prophylaxis of *Pneumocystis carinii* (alternative when given parenterally; aerosolized administration may become prophylaxis of choice in persons with AIDS)
Members of the Family Trypanosomatidae	
Suramin**	*Trypanosoma brucei gambiense* and *Trypanosoma brucei rhodesiense* (hemolymphatic stage)
Melarsoprol B**	*Trypanosoma brucei gambiense* and *Trypanosoma brucei rhodesiense* (late disease with central nervous system involvement)
Eflornithine*	*Trypanosoma brucei gambiense* (both stages; still considered investigational but will likely emerge as the treatment of choice)
Nifurtimox**	*Trypanosoma cruzi*
Benznidazole***	*Trypanosoma cruzi* (alternative)
Stibogluconate sodium**	*Leishmania* spp.
Meglumine antimoniate***	*Leishmania* spp.

(*Continued*)

TABLE 1. *(Continued)*

Drug	*Indications*
Members of the Family Trypanosomatidae *continued*	
Amphotericin B	*Leishmania* spp. (alternative)
Pentamidine isethionate	*Leishmania* spp. (alternative)
	Trypanosoma brucei gambiense (alternative for use in the hemolymphatic stage)
Helminthic diseases: Nematodes (roundworms)	
Benzimidazoles	
Mebendazole	*Ascaris lumbricoides*
	Hookworm
	Trichuris trichiura
	Enterobius vermicularis
	Capillaria philippinensis
	Gnathostoma spinigerum (surgical removal is an alternative)
	Mansonella perstans
	Angiostrongylus cantonensis
	Trichinella spiralis (recommended by some; used with steroids)
	Visceral larva migrans (alternative)
	Echinococcus granulosus and *Echinococcus multilocularis* (investigational; for treatment of inoperable lesions)
Albendazole*	*Echinococcus granulosus* and *Echinococcus multilocularis* (investigational; probably the best choice for treatment of inoperable lesions)
	Intestinal nematodes (alternative; investigational)
Thiabendazole	*Strongyloides stercoralis*
	Cutaneous larva migrans
	Visceral larva migrans
	Trichostrongylus spp.
	Angiostrongylus costaricensis (surgical intervention is the alternative)
	Dracunculus medinensis (alternative)
	Capillaria philippensis (alternative)
	Trichinella spiralis (used with steroids; some recommend mebendazole)
Piperazine citrate	*Ascaris lumbricoides* (alternative)
Pyrantel pamoate	*Enterobius vermicularis*
	Ascaris lumbricoides
	Hookworm
	Trichostrongylus spp. (alternative)
Diethylcarbamazine	*Wuchereria bancrofti*
	Brugia malayi
	Mansonella ozzardi
	Loa loa
	Tropical eosinophilia
	Visceral larva migrans
	Onchocerca volvulus (alternative; usually followed by suramin to kill adult worms; ivermectin is now the drug of choice)
Ivermectin*	*Onchocerca volvulus*
	Broad range of nematodes and blood sucking arthropods (use for these indications is investigational)
Metronidazole	*Dracunculus medinensis*
Helminthic diseases: Trematodes (flukes) and Cestodes (tapeworms)	
Praziquantel	*Schistosoma* spp.
	Clonorchis sinensis
	Opisthorchis viverrini
	Paragonimus westermani
	Fasciolopsis buski
	Heterophyes heterophyes
	Metagonimus yokogawai
	Diphyllobothrium latum (alternative)
	Taenia solium (adult worm and cysticercosis)
	Taenia saginata (alternative)
	Dipylidium caninum (alternative)
	Hymenolepis nana
Metrifonate	*Schistosoma haematobium* (alternative)
Oxamniquine	*Schistosoma mansoni* (alternative)
Bithionol	*Fasciola hepatica*
	Paragonimus westermani (alternative)
Niclosamide	*Diphyllobothrium latum*
	Taenia saginata
	Taenia solium
	Dipylidium caninum
	Hymenolepis nana (alternative)
	Fasciolopsis buski

[a] Can be purchased over the counter in London and major cities in East Africa (e.g., Nairobi, Kenya).
[b] Can be used with the approval of the FDA.

matodes (roundworms),[2] which are subdivided into those that live in the lumen of the intestine and those that reside in tissue; trematodes (flukes); and cestodes (tapeworms).[3,4] Chemotherapeutic agents are often active against multiple genera within these groups. Major advances have been made in the treatment of helminthic diseases during the past decade. Specifically, praziquantel has revolutionized the treatment of trematode infections, including schistosomiasis, as well as cerebral cysticercosis, and ivermectin the treatment of onchocerciasis.

The discussion of antiparasitic drugs that follows is arranged according to these groups. The approach is imperfect in that some drugs are active against pathogens in more than one group. This is particularly true for praziquantel, which is active against a broad spectrum of trematodes and cestodes, and two investigational drugs, albendazole, with activity against nematodes and cestodes, and ivermectin, with activity against nematodes and blood-sucking arthropods. Nonetheless, the approach taken provides a logical framework in which to organize the data. Drugs that have broad spectrums of activity are discussed in the context of their primary indications.

The dosage and duration of therapy for specific parasitic diseases are provided in Tables 2–4.[5] Not all of these drugs are available through pharmacies in the United States. Some can be obtained only from the manufacturer (indicated by *). Others have not been licensed in the United States but are available only from the CDC Drug Service (**), Centers for Disease Control, Atlanta, Georgia 30333. Some cannot be obtained in the United States (***), but they are discussed because they are used elsewhere or hold promise for the future.

DRUGS ACTIVE AGAINST LUMINAL PROTOZOA: AMEBAE, INTESTINAL AND VAGINAL FLAGELLATES, AND THE CILIATE BALANTIDIUM COLI

Metronidazole and Other Nitroimidazoles

Metronidazole (Fig. 1), tinidazole,*** and ornidazole*** have selective toxicity against numerous anaerobic and microaerophilic organisms. Only metronidazole, 2-methyl-5-nitroimidazole-1-ethanol, has been licensed in the United States. It is highly effective in the treatment of symptomatic *Entamoeba histolytica*[6,7] and *E. polecki* infections,[8] enteritis due to *Giardia lamblia*,[9,10] and vaginitis due to *Trichomonas vaginalis*.[11,12] It is also considered an alternative drug for the treatment of two other enteric pathogens, *Blastocystis hominis*[13] and *B. coli*.[14] Metronidazole is active against trophozoites of *Entamoeba* species, but it does not invariably eradicate the cysts.[15] A luminally active agent is required for this purpose and to treat asymptomatic cyst passers. Metronidazole has also been advocated as empiric therapy for presumptive protozoal enterocolitis in areas of the world where laboratory facilities are insufficient to provide a specific diagnosis.[16] Finally, metronidazole is recommended for the treatment of the guinea worm, *Dracunculus medinensis*,[17] but its clinical effects are related to a reduction in inflammation rather than to a lethal effect on the worm. The use of metronidazole against anaerobic bacterial pathogens is summarized in Chapter 25.

Metronidazole has Food and Drug Administration (FDA) approval for the treatment of amebiasis and trichomoniasis, but not giardiasis. This does not prevent physicians from using metronidazole for diseases like giardiasis, in which data support its efficacy.[18] The cure rate with the doses of metronidazole recommended for giardiasis (Table 2) is slightly lower than with quinacrine,[9,10,16] but metronidazole is generally better tolerated and many physicians prefer it over quinacrine.

Metronidazole is available as 250- and 500-mg tablets for oral use and in vials with 500 mg lyophilized powder for parenteral administration. When it is administered orally, 90–95 percent is absorbed[19,20]; peak serum levels are reached within 1 hour. It is widely distributed throughout the body and penetrates well into tissues, abscesses, fluid compartments, vaginal secretions, bone, the central nervous system, and breast milk.[21] Only 1–11 percent of the drug is bound to protein. The elimination half-life is 6.2–11.5 hours.[21] Approximately 80 percent of metronidazole and its metabolites are excreted via the kidney. The principal metabolites result from oxidation of side chains and glucuronide formation. Although renal failure prolongs the half-life of these metabolites, the hepatic metabolism is such that the drug dosage need not be modified during renal failure, but it should be adjusted in liver failure. The metabolites are removed by dialysis.

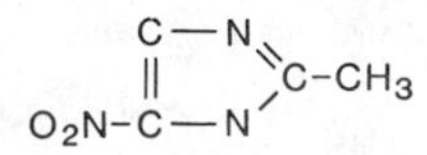

FIG. 1. Metronidazole.

Metronidazole is activated in anaerobic organisms by reduction of the 5-nitro group through a sequence of intermediate steps involving microbial electron transport proteins of low redox potential.[22] This results in a concentration gradient across the membrane of the parasite and permits accumulation of high concentrations of the reduced compound within the cell. Metronidazole acts as an electron sink, depriving the anaerobe of reducing equivalents. Furthermore, the reduced form of metronidazole causes loss of the helical structure of DNA, strand breakage, and impaired template function.[23,24]

Side effects are seldom severe enough to cause discontinuation of the drug. Gastrointestinal side effects include nausea, vomiting, diarrhea, and a metallic aftertaste. They are less common with the low doses (250 mg tid) recommended for giardiasis than with the high doses (750 mg tid) used for amebiasis. Other less frequent side effects include headache, dizziness, rash, urethral burning, vaginal or oral candidiasis, and reversible neutropenia.[25] The urine of some persons may become red or brown due to the presence of metabolites. Metronidazole may potentiate the anticoagulant effects of coumarin.[26] Rarely, patients treated with metronidazole experience sensory neuropathies or central nervous system toxicity with vertigo, ataxia, seizures, or encephalopathy.[27] Pseudomembranous colitis is also rare. Alcohol should be avoided because of the disulfiram (Antabuse)-like effects of metronidazole and the drug–drug interaction that can result in acute psychosis or a confusional state.[28]

The potential role of metronidazole in human carcinogenesis has been the subject of debate. Metronidazole has not been shown to be carcinogenic in humans, but it is mutagenic for certain strains of *Salmonella typhimurium*.[29] Furthermore, human urine contains metabolites that are carcinogenic in rodents.[30] However, 10-year follow-up of patients who received metronidazole for trichomoniasis has revealed no increase in the prevalence of cancer.[31,32]

Tinidazole and ornidazole, two other 5-nitroimidazole derivatives, have amebicidal and trichomonicidal activity similar to that of metronidazole, but fewer side effects.[7,33] A single 2-gr dose of tinidazole has been used successfully to treat giardiasis. Both tinidazole and ornidazole are well absorbed orally, have good tissue penetration, and are widely distributed in the body. Tinidazole and ornidazole have half-lives of 14 and 12–13 hours, respectively.[34] They are excreted primarily in urine, 50 percent of tinidazole and 96 percent of ornidazole in the form of metabolites.[35] These drugs have a favorable side effects profile in comparison to metronidazole. Reported side effects include anorexia, headache, and dizziness.

Emetine and Dehydroemetine**

Emetine, for many years the drug of choice for invasive amebiasis, is a tissue-active amebicide prepared from ipecac, which comes from the root of *Cephaëlis ipecacuanha*. The root is still used as a traditional medicine for the treatment of bloody diarrhea in some rural areas of South and Central America. Emetine and dehydroemetine have appreciable toxicity. They are reserved for persons with extraintestinal amebiasis, usually amebic liver abscesses,[36] who do not respond to metronidazole or for the rare person in whom metronidazole cannot be used. They are often given concomitantly with choroquine, which at high doses is a tissue active amebicide.[37] Iodoquinol or another luminally active agent is necessary to eradicate amebic cysts from the gastrointestinal tract.

TABLE 2. Drugs for Treatment of Parasitic Infections

Infection	*Drug*	*Adult Dosage**	*Pediatric Dosage**
Amebiasis (*Entamoeba histolytica*)			
Asymptomatic			
Drug of choice:	Iodoquinol[1]	650 mg tid × 20d	30–40 mg/kg/d in 3 doses × 20d
Alternatives:	Diloxanide furoate[2]	500 mg tid × 10d	20 mg/kg/d in 3 doses × 10d
	Paromomycin	25–30 mg/kg/d in 3 doses × 7d	25–30 mg/kg/d in 3 doses × 7d
Mild to moderate intestinal disease			
Drugs of choice:	Metronidazole[3,4]	750 mg tid × 10d	35–50 mg/kg/d in 3 doses × 10d
	followed by iodoquinol[1]	650 mg tid × 20d	30–40 mg/kg/d in 3 doses × 20d
Alternative:	Paromomycin	25–30 mg/kg/d in 3 doses × 7d	25–30 mg/kg/d in 3 doses × 7d
Severe intestinal disease			
Drugs of choice:	Metronidazole[3,4]	750 mg tid × 10d	35–50 mg/kg/d in 3 doses × 10d
	followed by iodoquinol[1]	650 mg tid × 20d	30–40 mg/kg/d in 3 doses × 20d
Alternatives:	Dehydroemetine[2,5]	1 to 1.5 mg/kg/d (max. 90 mg/d) im for up to 5d	1 to 1.5 mg/kg/d (max. 90 mg/d) im in 2 doses for up to 5d
	followed by iodoquinol[1]	650 mg tid × 20d	30–40 mg/kg/d in 3 doses × 20d
OR	Emetine[5]	1 mg/kg/d (max. 60 mg/d) im for up to 5d	1 mg/kg/d in 2 doses (max. 60 mg/d) im for up to 5d
	followed by iodoquinol[1]	650 mg tid × 20d	30–40 mg/kg/d in 3 doses × 20d
Hepatic abscess			
Drugs of choice:	Metronidazole[3,4]	750 mg tid × 10d	35–50 mg/kg/d in 3 doses × 10d
	followed by iodoquinol[1]	650 mg tid × 20d	30–40 mg/kg/d in 3 doses × 20d
Alternatives:	Dehydroemetine[2,5]	1 to 1.5 mg/kg/d (max. 90 mg/d) im for up to 5d	1 to 1.5 mg/kg/d (max. 90 mg/d) im in 2 doses for up to 5d
	folllowed by chloroquine phosphate	600 mg base (1 gram)/d × 2d, then 300 mg base (500 mg)/d × 2–3 wks	10 mg base/kg (max. 300 mg base)/d × 2–3 wks
	plus iodoquinol[1]	650 mg tid × 20d	30–40 mg/kg/d in 3 doses × 20d
OR	Emetine[5]	1 mg/kg/d (max. 60 mg/d) im for up to 5d	1 mg/kg/d (max. 60 mg/d) im in 2 doses for up to 5d
	followed by chloroquine phosphate	600 mg base (1 gram)/d × 2d, then 300 mg base (500 mg)/d × 2–3 wks	10 mg base/kg (max. 300 mg base)/d × 2–3 wks
	plus iodoquinol[1]	650 mg tid × 20d	30–40 mg/kg/d in 3 doses × 20d
Amebic meningoencephalitis, primary			
Naegleria spp.			
Drug of choice:	Amphotericin B[6,7]	1 mg/kg/d iv, uncertain duration	1 mg/kg/d iv, uncertain duration
Acanthamoeba spp.			
Drug of choice:	see footnote 8		
Ancylostoma duodenale, see Hookworm			
Angiostrongyliasis			
Angiostrongylus cantonensis			
Drug of choice:	Mebendazole[7,9,10]	100 mg bid × 5d	100 mg bid × 5d for children >2 years
Angiostrongylus costaricensis			
Drug of choice:	Thiabendazole[7,9]	25 mg/kg tid × 3d[11] (max. 3 grams/day)	25 mg/kg tid × 3d[11] (max. 3 grams/day)
OR	surgical intervention		
Anisakiasis (*Anisakis* spp.)			
Treatment of choice:	Surgical removal		
Ascariasis (*Ascaris lumbricoides*, roundworm)			
Drug of choice:	Mebendazole	100 mg bid × 3d	100 mg bid × 3d for children >2 years
OR	Pyrantel pamoate	11 mg/kg once (max. 1 gram)	11 mg/kg once (max. 1 gram)
Alternative:	Piperazine citrate	75 mg/kg (max. 3.5 grams)/d × 2d	75 mg/kg (max. 3.5 grams)/d × 2d
Babesiosis (*Babesia* spp.)			
Drugs of choice:[12]	Clindamycin[7]	1.2 grams bid parenteral or 600 mg tid oral × 7d	20–40 mg/kg/d in 3 doses × 7d
	plus quinine	650 mg tid oral × 7d	25 mg/kg/d in 3 doses × 7d
Balantidiasis (*Balantidium coli*)			
Drug of choice:	Tetracycline[7]	500 mg qid × 10d	10 mg/kg qid × 10d (max. 2 grams/d)
Alternatives:	Iodoquinol[1,7]	650 mg tid × 20d	40 mg/kg/d in 3 doses × 20d
	Metronidazole[3,7]	750 mg tid × 5d	35–50 mg/kg/d in 3 doses × 5d
Blastocystis hominis infection			
Drug of choice:	Iodoquinol[1]	650 mg tid × 20d	30–40 mg/kg/d in 3 doses × 20d
OR	Metronidazole[3,7]	750 mg tid × 10d	35–50 mg/kg/d in 3 doses × 10d
Capillariasis (*Capillaria philippinensis*)			
Drug of choice:	Mebendazole[7]	200 mg bid × 20d	200 mg bid × 20d
Alternative:	Thiabendazole[7]	25 mg/kg/d × 30d	25 mg/kg/d × 30d
Chagas disease, see Trypanosomiasis			
Clonorchis sinensis, see Fluke infection			

(*Continued*)

* The letter d indicates day.

[1] Dosage and duration of administration should not be exceeded because of possibility of causing optic neuritis; maximum dosage is 2 grams/day.

[2] In the USA, this drug is available from the CDC Drug Service, Centers for Disease Control, Atlanta, Georgia 30333; telephone: 404-639-3670 (evenings, weekends, and holidays: 404-639-2888).

[3] Metronidazole is carcinogenic in rodents and mutagenic in bacteria; it should generally not be given to pregnant women, particularly in the first trimester.

[4] Outside the USA, ornidazole and tinidazole are also used.

[5] Dehydroemetine is probably as effective and probably less toxic than emetine. Because of its toxic effects on the heart, patients receiving emetine should have electrocardiographic monitoring and should remain sedentary during therapy.

[6] One patient with a *Naegleria* infection was successfully treated with amphotericin B, micronazole, and rifampin (JS Seidel et al, N Engl J Med, 306:346, 1982).

[7] Considered an investigational drug for this condition by the U.S. Food and Drug Administration.

[8] Experimental infections with *Acanthamoeba* spp. have been reported to respond to sulfadiazine (CG Culbertson, Annu Rev Microbiol, 25:231, 1971). Amebic keratitis due to *Acanthamoeba* sp. has been reported to respond to topical miconazole, propamidine isethionate, and antibiotics (MB Moore et al, Am J Ophthalmol, 100:396, 1985).

[9] Effectiveness documented only in animals.

[10] Analgesics, corticosteroids, and careful removal of CSF at frequent intervals can relieve symptoms. Albendazole and ivermectin have been used successfully in animals.

[11] This dose is likely to be toxic and may have to be decreased.

TABLE 2. *(Continued)*

Infection	*Drug*	*Adult Dosage**	*Pediatric Dosage**
Cryptosporidiosis (*Cryptosporidium* spp.)			
Drug of choice:[13]	Spiramycin	1 gram tid PO × 14d or more	
Cutaneous larva migrans (creeping eruption)			
Drug of choice:	Thiabendazole	25 mg/kg bid (max. 3 grams/d) × 2–5d and/ or topically	25 mg/kg bid (max. 3 grams/d) × 2–5d and/ or topically
Cysticercosis, see Tapeworm infection			
Dientamoeba fragilis infection			
Drug of choice:	Iodoquinol[1]	650 mg tid × 20d	40 mg/kg/d in 3 doses × 20d
OR	Tetracycline[7]	500 mg qid × 10d	10 mg/kg qid × 10d (max. 2 grams/d)
OR	Paromomycin	25–30 mg/kg/d in 3 doses × 7d	25–30 mg/kg/d in 3 doses × 7d
Diphyllobothrium latum, see Tapeworm infection			
Dracunculus medinensis (guinea worm) infection			
Drug of choice:	Metronidazole[3,7]	250 mg tid × 10d	25 mg/kg/d (max. 750 mg/d) in 3 doses × 10d
Alternative:	Thiabendazole[7]	25–37.5 mg/kg bid × 3d[11]	25–37.5 mg/kg bid × 3d[11]
Echinococcus, see Tapeworm infection			
Entamoeba histolytica, see Amebiasis			
Entamoeba polecki infection			
Drugs of choice:	Metronidazole[3,7]	750 mg tid × 10d	35–50 mg/kg/d in 3 doses × 10d
	followed by diloxanide furoate[2]	500 mg tid × 10d	20 mg/kg/d in 3 doses × 10d
Enterobius vermicularis (pinworm) infection			
Drug of choice:	Pyrantel pamoate	A single dose of 11 mg/kg (max. 1 gram); repeat after 2 weeks	A single dose of 11 mg/kg (max. 1 gram); repeat after 2 weeks
OR	Mebendazole	A single dose of 100 mg; repeat after 2 weeks	A single dose of 100 mg for children >2 years; repeat after 2 weeks
Fasciola hepatica, see Fluke infection			
Filariasis			
Wuchereria bancrofti, Brugia (W.) malayi, Mansonella ozzardi, Loa loa			
Drug of choice:[14]	Diethylcarbamazine[15]	Day 1: 50 mg, oral, p.c. Day 2: 50 mg tid Day 3: 100 mg tid Days 4 through 21: 2 mg/kg tid	Day 1: 25–50 mg Day 2: 25–50 mg tid Day 3: 50–100 mg tid Days 4 through 21: 2 mg/kg tid
Mansonella perstans			
Drug of choice:[16]	Mebendazole[7]	100 mg bid × 30d	
Tropical eosinophilia			
Drug of choice:	Diethylcarbamazine	2 mg/kg tid × 7–10d	2 mg/kg tid × 7–10d
Onchocerca volvulus			
Drug of choice:	Ivermectin[7,17]	150 μg/kg PO once, repeated every 6 to 12 months	150 μg/kg PO once
Alternatives:	Diethylcarbamazine[15]	25 mg/d × 3d, then 50 mg/d × 5d, then 100 mg/d × 3d, then 150 mg/d × 12d	0.5 mg/kg tid × 3d (max. 25 mg/d), then 1.0 mg/kg tid × 3–4d (max. 50 mg/d), then 1.5 mg/kg tid × 3–4d (max. 100 mg/d), then 2.0 mg/kg tid × 2–3 wks
	followed by suramin[2,18]	100–200 mg (test dose) iv, then 1 gram iv at weekly intervals × 5 wks	10–20 mg (test dose) iv, then 20 mg/kg iv at weekly intervals × 5 wks
Fluke, hermaphroditic, infection			
Clonorchis sinensis (Chinese liver fluke)			
Drug of choice:	Praziquantel[7]	25 mg/kg tid × 2d	25 mg/kg tid × 2d
Fasciola hepatica (sheep liver fluke)			
Drug of choice:[19]	Bithionol[2]	30–50 mg/kg on alternate days × 10–15 doses	30–50 mg/kg on alternate days × 10–15 doses
Fasciolopsis buski (intestinal fluke)			
Drug of choice:	Praziquantel[7]	25 mg/kg tid × 1d	25 mg/kg tid × 1d
OR	Niclosamide[7]	a single dose of 4 tablets (2 g) chewed thoroughly	11–34 kg: a single dose of 2 tablets (1 g) >34 kg: a single dose of 3 tablets (1.5 g)
Alternative:	Tetrachloroethylene[20]	0.1 ml/kg (max. 5 ml)	0.1 ml/kg (max. 5 ml)
Heterophyes heterophyes (intestinal fluke)			
Drug of choice:	Praziquantel[7]	25 mg/kg tid × 1d	25 mg/kg tid × 1d
Metagonimus yokogawai (intestinal fluke)			
Drug of choice:	Praziquantel[7]	25 mg/kg tid × 1d	25 mg/kg tid × 1d
Opisthorchis viverrini (liver fluke)			
Drug of choice:	Praziquantel[7]	25 mg/kg tid × 1d	25 mg/kg tid × 1d
Paragonimus westermani (lung fluke)			
Drug of choice:	Praziquantel[7]	25 mg/kg tid × 2d	25 mg/kg tid × 2d
Alternative:	Bithionol[2]	30–50 mg/kg on alternate days × 10–15 doses	30–50 mg/kg on alternate days × 10–15 doses

(Continued)

* The letter d indicates day.

12 Concurrent use of pentamidine and trimethoprim-sulfamethoxazole has been reported to cure an infection with *B. divergens* (D Raoult et al, Ann Intern Med, 107:944, 1987).

13 Limited clinical results suggest a decrease in diarrhea with therapy. Prospective studies of efficacy are ongoing. Infection is self-limiting in immunocompetent patients.

14 Several reports indicate that ivermectin may be effective for treatment of *W. bancrofti* (S Diallo et al, Lancet, 1:1030, 1987) and *M. ozzardi* (TB Nutman et al, J Infect Dis, 156:662, 1987).

15 Diethylcarbamazine should be administered with special caution in heavy infections with *Loa loa* because it can provoke ocular problems or an encephalopathy. Antihistamines or corticosteroids may be required to decrease allergic reactions due to disintegration of microfilariae in treatment of all filarial infections, especially those caused by *Onchocerca* and *Loa loa*. Surgical excision of subcutaneous *Onchocerca* nodules is recommended by some authorities before starting drug therapy.

16 Ivermectin may also be effective.

TABLE 2. *(Continued)*

Infection	*Drug*	*Adult Dosage**	*Pediatric Dosage**
Giardiasis (*Giardia lamblia*)			
Drug of choice:	Quinacrine HCl	100 mg tid p.c. × 5d	2 mg/kg tid p.c. × 5d (max. 300 mg/d)
Alternatives:	Metronidazole[3,4,7]	250 mg tid × 5d	5 mg/kg tid × 5d
	Furazolidone	100 mg qid × 7–10d	1.25 mg/kg qid × 7–10d
Gnathostomiasis (*Gnathostoma spinigerum*)			
Treatment of choice:	Surgical removal		
OR	Mebendazole[7,21]	200 mg q3h × 6d	
Hookworm infection (*Ancylostoma duodenale, Necator americanus*)			
Drug of choice:[22]	Mebendazole	100 mg bid × 3d	100 mg bid × 3d for children >2 years
OR	Pyrantel pamoate[7]	11 mg/kg (max. 1 gram) × 3d	11 mg/kg (max. 1 gram) × 3d
Hydatid cyst, see Tapeworm infection			
Hymenolepis nana, see Tapeworm infection			
Isosporiasis (*Isospora belli*)			
Drug of choice:	Trimethoprim-sulfamethoxazole[7,23]	160 mg TMP, 800 mg SMX qid × 10d, then bid × 3 wks	
Leishmaniasis			
L. braziliensis, L. mexicana (American cutaneous and mucocutaneous leishmaniasis)			
Drug of choice:[24]	Stibogluconate sodium[2]	20 mg/kg/d (max. 800 mg/d) iv or im × 20d may be repeated or continued until there is a response	20 mg/kg/d im or iv (max. 800 mg/d) × 20d
Alternative:	Amphotericin B[7]	0.25 to 1 mg/kg by slow infusion daily or every 2d for up to 8 wks	0.25 to 1 mg/kg by slow infusion daily or every 2d for up to 8 wks
L. donovani (kala azar, visceral leishmaniasis)			
Drug of choice:	Stibogluconate sodium[2,25]	20 mg/kg/d (max. 800 mg/d) im or iv × 20d (may be repeated)	20 mg/kg/d im or iv (max. 800 mg/d) × 20d
Alternative:	Pentamidine isethionate	2–4 mg/kg/d im for up to 15 doses	2–4 mg/kg/d im for up to 15 doses
L. tropica. L. maior (oriental sore, cutaneous leishmaniasis)			
Drug of choice:	Stibogluconate sodium[2,26]	10 mg/kg/d (max. 600 mg/d) im or iv × 6–10d (may be repeated)	10 mg/kg/d im or iv (max. 600 mg/d) × 6–10d
Alternative:	Topical treatment[27]		
Lice infestation (*Pediculus humanus, capitis, Phthirus pubis*)[28]			
Drug of choice:	1% Permethrin[29]	Topically	Topically
Alternatives:	Pyrethrins with piperonyl butoxide	Topically[30]	Topically[30]
	Lindane	Topically[30]	Topically[30]
Loa loa, see Filariasis			
Malaria, see Tables 3 and 4			
Mites, see Scabies			
Naegleria spp., see Amebic meningoencephalitis, primary			
Necator americanus, see Hookworm infection			
Onchocerca volvulus, see Filariasis			
Opisthorchis viverrini, see Fluke infection			
Paragonimus westermani, see Fluke infection			
Pediculus capitis, humanus, Phthirus pubis, see Lice			
Pinworm, see *Enterobius*			
Pneumocysts carinii pneumonia[31]			
Drug of choice:	Trimethoprim-sulfamethoxazole	TMP 20 mg/kg/d, SMX 100 mg/kg/d oral or iv in 4 doses × 14d	TMP 20 mg/kg/d, SMX 100 mg/kg/d oral or iv in 4 doses × 14d
Alternative:	Pentamidine isethionate	4 mg/kg/d im × 14d	4 mg/kg/d im × 14d
Roundworm, see Ascariasis			
Scabies (*Sarcoptes scabiei*)			
Drug of choice:[32]	Lindane	Topically once	Topically
Alternatives:	Sulfur in petrolatum	Topically	Topically
	10% Crotamiton	Topically	Topically
Schistosomiasis			
S. haematobium			
Drug of choice:	Praziquantel	20 mg/kg tid × 1d	20 mg/kg tid × 1d
S. japonicum			
Drug of choice:	Praziquantel	20 mg/kg tid × 1d	20 mg/kg tid × 1d
S. mansoni			
Drug of choice:	Praziquantel	20 mg/kg tid × 1d	20 mg/kg tid × 1d
Alternative:	Oxamniquine	15 mg/kg once[33]	10 mg/kg bid × 1d[33]

(Continued)

* The letter d indicates day.

17 Ivermectin in a dose of 200 μg/kg has been reported to be as effective as diethylcarbamazine in decreasing the number of microfilaria and causes fewer adverse ophthalmologic reactions (BM Greene et al, N Engl J Med, 313:133, 1985; AT White et al, J Infect Dis, 156:463, 1987). Semiannual to annual prophylaxis appears to be effective in keeping microfilarial counts at low levels.

18 Some Medical Letter consultants use suramin only if ocular microfilariae persist after diethylcarbamazine therapy and nodulectomy.

19 Unlike infections with other flukes, *Fasciola hepatica* infections may not respond to praziquantel. Limited data indicate that albendazole may be effective in this condition.

20 Given on empty stomach. Although approved for human use, it is available currently only as a veterinary product. No alcoholic beverage should be consumed before or for 12 hours after therapy. Keep patient at bedrest for 4 hours after treatment.

21 In felines, ancylol (2, 6, diodo-4-nitrophenol) by subcutaneous injection has been effective against migrating larvae.

22 Albendazole is also effective (RNG Pugh, Ann Trop Med Parasitol, 80:565, 1986).

23 Shorter courses of trimethoprim-sulfamethoxazole may be equally effective. Preliminary studies suggest that a 7–10 day initial course of trimethoprim-sulfamethoxazole may be as effective as a 4.5 week course and that recurrences may be prevented by weekly doses of pyrimethamine-sulfadoxine (R Soave and WD Johnson, Jr, J Infect Dis, 157:225, 1988). In sulfonamide-sensitive patients, such as some patients with AIDS, pyrimethamine 50–75 mg daily has been effective. In immunocompromised patients, it may be necessary to continue therapy indefinitely.

24 Limited data indicate that ketoconazole, 400 to 600 mg daily for 28 days, may be effective for treatment of *L. panamensis* and *L. mexicana* (cutaneous).

TABLE 2. *(Continued)*

Infection	*Drug*	*Adult Dosage**	*Pediatric Dosage**
S. mekongi			
Drug of choice:	Praziquantel	20 mg/kg tid × 1d	20 mg/kg tid × 1d
Sleeping sickness, see Trypanosomiasis			
Strongyloidiasis (*Strongyloides stercoralis*)			
Drug of choice:[34]	Thiabendazole	25 mg/kg bid (max. 3 grams/d) × 2d[35]	25 mg/kg bid (max. 3 grams/d) × 2d[35]
Tapeworm infection, adult or intestinal stage			
Diphyllobothrium latum (fish), *Taenia saginata* (beef), *Taenia solium* (pork),[36] *Dipylidium caninum* (dog)			
Drug of choice:	Niclosamide	A single dose of 4 tablets (2 grams) chewed thoroughly	11–34 kg: a single dose of 2 tablets (1 gram); >34 kg: a single dose of 3 tablets (1.5 grams)
OR	Praziquantel[7]	10–20 mg/kg once	10–20 mg/kg once
Hymenolepsis nana (dwarf tapeworm)			
Drug of choice:	Praziquantel[7]	25 mg/kg once	25 mg/kg once
Alternative:	Niclosamide	A single daily dose of 4 tablets (2 grams) chewed thoroughly, then 2 tablets daily × 6d	11–34 kg: a single dose of 2 tablets (1 gram) × 1d, then 1 tablet (0.5 g)/d × 6d; >34 kg: a single dose of 3 tablets (1.5 grams) × 1d, then 2 tablets (1 gram)/d × 6d
Tapeworm infection, larval or tissue stage			
Echinococcus granulosus			
Drug of choice:	See footnote 37		
Echinococcus multilocularis[38]	See footnote 38		
Cysticercus cellulosae (cysticercosis)			
Drug of choice:[39]	Praziquantel[7]	50 mg/kg/d in 3 divided doses × 14d	50 mg/kg/d in 3 divided doses × 14d
Alternative:	Surgery		
Toxocariasis, see Visceral larva migrans			
Toxoplasmosis (*Toxoplasma gondii*)[40]			
Drugs of choice:	Pyrimethamine[41]	25 mg/d × 3–4 wks	2 mg/kg/d × 3d, then 1 mg/kg/d[42] (max. 25 mg/d) × 4 wks
	plus		
	trisulfapyrimidines	2–6 grams/d × 3–4 wks	100–200 mg/kg/d × 3–4 wks
Alternative:	Spiramycin	2–4 grams/d × 3–4 wks	50–100 mg/kg/d × 3–4 wks
Trichinosis (*Trichinella spiralis*)			
Drugs of choice:	Steroids for severe symptoms		
	plus thiabendazole or mebendazole[43]	25 mg/kg bid × 5d (max. 3 grams/d)	25 mg/kg bid × 5d
Trichomoniasis (*Trichomonas vaginalis*)			
Drug of choice:[44]	Metronidazole[3]	2 grams once or 250 mg tid orally × 7d	15 mg/kg/d orally in 3 doses × 7d
Trichostrongylus infection			
Drug of choice:	Thiabendazole[7]	25 mg/kg bid × 2d (max. 3 grams/d)	25 mg/kg bid × 2d
Alternative:	Pyrantel pamoate[7]	11 mg/kg once (max. 1 gram)	11 mg/kg once (max. 1 gram)
Trichuriasis (*Trichuris trichiura, whipworm*)			
Drug of choice:	Mebendazole	100 mg bid × 3d	100 mg bid × 3d for children >2 yrs
Trypanosomiasis			
T. cruzi (South American trypanosomiasis, Chagas' disease)			
Drug of choice:	Nifurtimox[2]	8–10 mg/kg/d orally in 4 divided doses × 120d	1–10 yrs: 15–20 mg/kg/d in 4 divided doses × 90d; 11–16 yrs: 12.5–15 mg/kg/d in 4 divided doses × 90d
Alternative:	Benznidazole[45]	5–7 mg/kg × 30–120d	

(Continued)

* The letter d indicates day.

[25] For the African form of visceral leishmaniasis, therapy may have to be extended to at least 30 days and may have to be repeated.

[26] Ketoconazole, 400 mg daily for four to eight weeks, has also been reported to be effective (J Viallet et al, Am J Trop Med Hyg, 35:491, 1986).

[27] Application of heat 39° to 42°C directly to the lesion for 20 to 32 hours over a period of 10 to 12 days has been reported to be effective in *L. tropica* (FA Neva et al, Am J Trop Med Hyg, 33:800, 1984).

[28] For infestation of eyelashes with crab lice, use petrolatum.

[29] FDA-approved for head lice only.

[30] Some consultants recommend a second application one week later to kill hatching progeny.

[31] AIDS patients may need longer duration of therapy. For AIDS patients who develop hypersensitivity or resistance to both TMP/SMX and pentamidine, trimetrexate with leucovorin rescue or a combination of dapsone and trimethoprim may be effective. Aerosolized pentamidine has been tried for both treatment and prophylaxis (Medical Letter, 29:103, 1987).

[32] 5% permethrin, not yet marketed in the USA, could prove to be the drug of choice when it becomes available.

[33] In East Africa, the dose should be increased to 30 mg/kg/d, and in Egypt and South Africa, 30 mg/kg/d × 2d. Neuropsychiatric disturbances and seizures have been reported in some patients (H Stokvis et al, Am J Trop Med Hyg, 35:330, 1986).

[34] Albendazole or ivermectin have also been effective.

[35] In disseminated strongyloidiasis, thiabendazole therapy should be continued for at least five days. In immunocompromised patients it may be necessary to continue therapy or use other agents (see footnote 34).

[36] Niclosamide is effective for the treatment of *T. solium* but, since it causes disintegration of segments and release of viable eggs, its use creates a theoretical risk of causing cysticercosis. It should therefore be followed in three or four hours by a purge. Quinacrine is preferred by some clinicians because it expels *T. solium* intact. Others prefer praziquantel, which also kills larvae.

[37] Surgical resection of cysts is the treatment of choice. When surgery is contraindicated, or cysts rupture spontaneously during surgery, mebendazole (experimental for this purpose in the USA) can be tried (JF Wilson and RL Rausch, Ann Trop Med Parasitol, 76:165, 1982; ADM Bryceson et al, Trans R Soc Trop Med Hyg, 76:510, 1982). Albendazole has also been reported to be effective (DL Morris et al, JAMA, 253:2053, 1985). Flubendazole has also been used with some success (E Tellez-Giron et al, Am J Trop Med Hyg, 33:627, 1984). Praziquantel and albendazole will kill protoscolices and may be useful in case of spill during surgery.

[38] Surgical excision is the only reliable means of treatment although recent reports have been encouraging about use of albendazole or mebendazole (JF Wilson et al, Am J Trop Med Hyg, 37:162, 1987; A Davis et al, Bull WHO, 64:383, 1986.)

[39] Corticosteroids should be given for two to three days before and during praziquantel therapy. Praziquantel should not be used for ocular or spinal cord cysticercosis. Albendazole, 15 mg/kg × 30d, which can be repeated, has been used successfully (F Escobedo et al, Arch Intern Med, 147:738, 1987).

[40] In ocular toxoplasmosis, corticosteroids should also be used for anti-inflammatory effect on the eyes.

[41] Pyrimethamine is teratogenic in animals. To prevent hematological toxicity from pyrimethamine, it is advisable to give leucovorin (folinic acid), about 10 mg/day, either by injection or orally. Pyrimethamine alone 50–75 mg daily has been used to treat CNS toxoplasmosis after sulfonamide sensitivity develops. Pyrimethamine 25 mg/d plus clindamycin 1.2 to 2.4 gm/d in divided doses has also been used. In AIDS patients treatment should continue indefinitely.

[42] Every two to three days for infants. Most authorities would treat congenitally infected newborns for about one year.

[43] The efficacy of thiabendazole for trichinosis is not clearly established; it appears to be effective during the intestinal phase but its effect on larvae that have migrated is questionable. In the tissue phase, mebendazole 200–400 mg tid × 3 days, then 400–500 mg tid × 10 days, may be effective. Albendazole may also be effective for this indication.

[44] Sexual partners should be treated simultaneously. Outside the USA, ornidazole and tinidazole have been used for this condition. Metronidazole-resistant strains have been reported; higher doses of metronidazole for longer periods of time are sometimes effective against these strains.

TABLE 2. *(Continued)*

Infection	*Drug*	*Adult Dosage**	*Pediatric Dosage**
T. gambiense, T. rhodesiense (African trypanosomiasis, sleeping sickness)			
Hemolymphatic stage			
Drug of choice:[46]	Suramin[2]	100–200 mg (test dose) iv, then 1 gram iv on days 1, 3, 7, 14, and 21	20 mg/kg on days 1, 3, 7, 14 and 21
Alternative:	Pentamidine isethionate	4 mg/kg/d im × 10d	4 mg/kg/d im × 10d
Late disease with CNS involvement			
Drug of choice:[46]	Melarsoprol[2,47]	2–3.6 mg/kg/d iv × 3 doses; after 1 wk 3.6 mg/kg/d iv × 3 doses; repeat again after 10–21 days	18–25 mg/kg total over 1 mo. Initial dose of 0.36 mg/kg iv, increasing gradually to max. 3.6 mg/kg at intervals of 1–5d for total of 9–10 doses
Alternatives:	Tryparsamide	One injection of 30 mg/kg iv every 5d to total of 12 injections; may be repeated after 1 mo.	Unknown
	plus suramin[2]	One injection of 10 mg/kg iv every 5d to total of 12 injections; may be repeated after 1 mo.	
Visceral larva migrans[48]			
Drug of choice:[49]	Diethylcarbamazine[7]	2 mg/kg tid × 7–10d	2 mg/kg tid × 7–10d
OR	Thiabendazole	25 mg/kg bid × 5d (max. 3 grams/d)	25 mg/kg bid × 5d (max. 3 g/d)
Alternative:	Mebendazole[7]	200–400 mg/d × 5d[50]	
Whipworm, see Trichuriasis			
Wuchereria bancrofti, see Filariasis			

* The letter d indicates day.
[45] Limited data.
[46] In drug-resistant cases of *T. gambiense* infections, elflornithine (difluoromethylornithine, Merrell Dow) has been used successfully; field trials are now underway (H Taelman et al, Am J Med, 82:607, 1987; F Doua et al, Am J Trop Med Hyg 37:525, 1987; J Pepin et al, Lancet, 2:1431, 1987). It is highly effective in both CNS and non-CNS infections with *T. gambiense*.
[47] In frail patients, begin with as little as 18 mg and increase the dose progressively. Pretreatment with suramin has been advocated for debilitated patients.
[48] For severe symptoms or eye involvement, corticosteroids can be used in addition.
[49] Ivermectin and albendazole have been effective in some animal studies.
[50] One report of a cure using 1 gram tid for 21 days has been published (A Bekhti, Ann Intern Med, 100:463, 1984).
(From Ref. 5, with permission.)

Emetine is administered by deep intramuscular injection; oral administration is prevented by severe gastrointestinal irritation. Emetine is well absorbed from muscle and is excreted very slowly.[38] It can be detected in the urine for 1–2 months after completion of treatment. It is distributed to the spleen, kidney, and lung, but the highest concentrations are found in the liver, which enhances its activity in the treatment of amebic liver abscesses.[38] Negligible amounts are detected in the blood. Emetine acts by inhibiting protein synthesis in eukaryotic cells.[38,39]

Emetine is responsible for toxicity in multiple organs. Diarrhea, nausea, and vomiting are frequent. Muscle weakness, aching, tenderness, and stiffness are experienced by the majority of persons who receive a cumulative dose of 1300 mg.[40] The most serious untoward effects are cardiovascular. These include precordial pain, weakness, arrhythmias, hypotension, tachycardia, congestive heart failure, and occasionally death.[41] Electrocardiographic (ECG) changes are characterized by a prolonged Q-T interval, T-wave inversion, and S-T depression. The ECG tends to return to normal 1–2 weeks after cessation of therapy.[42] Emetine has direct toxic effects on skeletal and cardiac muscles.[43] Local toxicity at the site of injection includes muscle pain, tenderness, and stiffness. Less common are urticarial reactions. Persons receiving emetine require hospitalization and careful monitoring for signs of toxicity. Emetine is contraindicated in persons with cardiac and renal disease and is relatively contraindicated in children and pregnant women.

Dehydroemetine has a shorter half-life than emetine, as well as diminished frequency and severity of side effects.[56] It is also less potent then emetine, and higher doses must be used to obtain the desired therapeutic effect.

Iodoquinol

Iodoquinol (diiodohydroxyquin), a halogenated oxyquinoline (5,7-diiodo-8-quinolinol), is a luminally active agent used to eradicate cysts in persons with asymptomatic *E. histolytica* infection or after metronidazole administration in persons with invasive intestinal or extraintestinal disease. Iodoquinol is also recommended for the treatment of *Dientamoeba fragilis* and *B. hominis*, and it is used as an alternative drug for the treatment of *B. coli*.

Iodoquinol is available in 210- and 250-mg tablets. It is poorly absorbed and best tolerated if given with meals. The mechanism of action is not known. Reported side effects include headache, diarrhea, nausea, vomiting and abdominal pain, fever, and itching. Occasionally, the drug is associated with iodine dermatitis (iodine toxicoderma). The high iodine content (63 percent) can interfere with the results of thyroid function tests for months after completion of therapy. Iodoquinol is contraindicated in persons with iodine intolerance.

A related compound, iodochlorhydroxyquin***, which is better absorbed than iodoquinol, gained notoriety as a cause of subacute myelo-optic neuropathy. This syndrome and its relationship to iodochlorhydroxyquin were first described in Japan, where the syndrome occurred in near-epidemic proportions. The discontinuation of iodochlorhydroxyquin led to an almost immediate reduction in the number of cases of subacute myelo-optic neuropathy.[44] Optic nerve damage or inflammation and a peripheral neuropathy may occur with prolonged high doses of iodoquinol as well. The dosage regimen recommended for amebic disease (Table 2) avoids these complications, but the recommended doses and duration of therapy should never be exceeded.[21]

Diloxanide Furoate**

Diloxanide furoate, a substituted acetanilide, 4-(*N*-methyl-2,2-dichloroacetamido)phenyl-2-furoate, is a luminally active agent used for the treatment of asymptomatic *E. histolytica* infection.[45–48] It is also used to eradicate cysts of *E. polecki* after treatment with metronidazole. It is ineffective in the treatment of extraintestinal amebiasis. Diloxanide furoate is hydrolyzed by intestinal esterases releasing diloxanide, the absorbed form of the amebicide. Delayed or reduced absorption of the ester results in higher concentrations in the large intestine and the desired luminal effect.

Diloxanide furoate is formulated in 500-mg tablets. In experimental animals, 60–90 percent of the drug is excreted in the urine within 48 hours.[41] Excretion in the feces accounts for 4–9 percent. Diloxanide is amebicidal at low concentrations, but the mechanism of action is unknown. There are rarely serious side effects at the recommended dosage. The most common untoward effect is flatulence.[48] Mild gastrointestinal complaints may also occur. The low cost of the drug makes it an excellent alternative for the treatment of asymptomtic intestinal amebic infections in developing countries.

Paromomycin

Paromomycin, an aminoglycoside, is a luminally active, poorly absorbed durg that is used for the treatment of asymptomatic intestinal amebiasis.[49,50] It acts directly on amebae and has antibacterial activity in the colon.

Paromomycin is available in 250-mg capsules. Side effects are primarily gastrointestinal and include nausea, vomiting, abdominal cramps, and diarrhea in some patients. Paromomycin, like other aminoglycosides, is potentially ototoxic and nephrotoxic when administered parenterally. Very little is adsorbed from the gastrointestinal tract, but it is contraindicated in persons with renal failure. Paromomycin also has some activity against human tapeworms,[51] but it is rarely used for that purpose.

Quinacrine

Quinacrine (Fig. 2), 3-chloro-7-methoxy-9-(1-methyl-4-diethylaminobutylamino)acridine, a yellow dye with a 4-aminoquinoline radical linked to a benzene ring, is widely used for the treatment of giardiasis.[9,10,52–54] Many experts in the United States consider it the drug of choice for this disease (Table 2). The cure rate in adults is approximately 90 percent,[9] but it may be lower in children.[53] It is the least expensive of the three drugs that are commonly used to treat *G. lamblia*. Quinacrine is also active against adult tapeworms but has largely been replaced by niclosamide, which is less toxic. During World War II, quinacrine was used for malaria prophylaxis and treatment.

Quinacrine is available in 100-mg tablets. It is well absorbed from the gastrointestinal tract and is widely distributed throughout the body. Quinacrine can intercalate into DNA and inhibit nucleic acid synthesis.[55] Whether this relates to its antiparasitic activity is unknown. Quinacrine has strong tissue-binding properties and can be detected in urine for up to 2 months after cessation of therapy.

Data on toxicity were accumulated during the widespread use of quinacrine as an antimalarial.[56] Quinacrine has a bitter, unpleasant taste and can induce nausea and vomiting, especially in children. Other common side effects include headache and dizziness. At high doses, quinacrine can turn the skin and urine yellow. This effect is seen in 4–5 percent of persons treated for giardiasis.[10,57] The sclerae are usually spared. A bright yellow-green fluorescence under Wood's light confirms that the discoloration is due to quinacrine and not bilirubin. The yellow skin discoloration lasts for periods ranging from a few weeks to several months.

Uncommon side effects of quinacrine include skin rashes, fever, and reversible acute, toxic psychosis. The last occurs in 0.1–1.5 percent of persons receiving the drug and usually lasts for 2–4 weeks.[58] The mechanism is unknown. Quinacrine is contraindicated in patients with a history of psychosis. Very rarely, blood dyscrasias have been reported to follow treatment. Quinacrine is also contraindicated in pregnancy, since it readily crosses the placental barrier. Patients with psoriasis occasionally develop extensive exfoliative dermatitis and should not receive the drug.

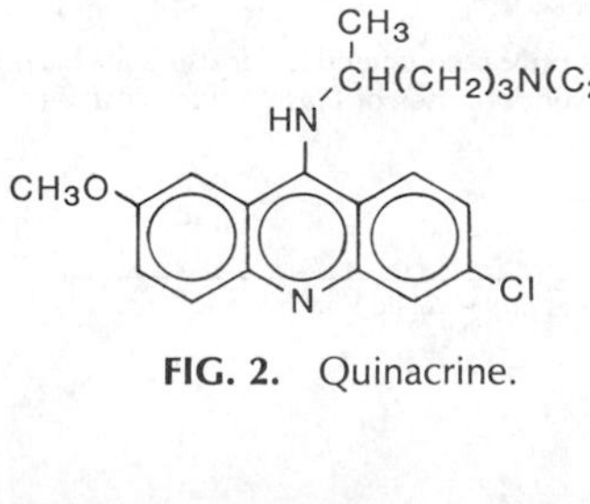

FIG. 2. Quinacrine.

There are two important potential drug interactions with quinacrine. First, like metronidazole, quinacrine has a disulfiram-like effect. Adult patients should be warned not to drink alcohol, and children taking quinacrine should not be given ethanol-containing medications. Second, quinacrine interferes with the metabolism of primaquine and may result in toxic levels of primaquine. The inhibitory effect on primaquine metabolism may last for up to 3 months after the last dose of quinacrine is administered.

Furazolidone

Furazolidone, 3-[(5-Nitro-2furanyl)methylene)-amino]-2-oxazolidinone, is a nitrofuran derivative. Like other nitrofurans, it acts by damaging DNA. It is the only anti-*Giardia* drug available as a liquid, and it is commonly used for the treatment of giardiasis in children.[53,59,60] Furazolidone also has some activity against *I. belli* and a variety of bacteria.[61]

Furazolidone is available as a suspension containing 25 mg/5 ml and 100-mg tablets. It is largely unabsorbed after oral administration.[61] Common side effects include nausea, vomiting, diarrhea, and fever. Some of the metabolites are brown and may discolor the urine. Other rare side effects are hypotension, urticaria, serum sickness, and hypersensitivity reactions. A mild to moderate hemolysis may occur in patients with glucose-6-phosphate dehydrogenase (G6PD) deficiency. As with metronidazole and quinacrine, alcohol should not be ingested because furazolidone has disulfiram-like activity. It is also a monoamine oxidase inhibitor. Furazolidone should not be administered to mothers who are breast-feeding their infants or given to neonates, since hemolytic anemia due to glutathione instability may occur.

DRUGS USED AGAINST MEMBERS OF THE PHYLUM APICOMPLEXA AND PNEUMOCYSTIS CARINII

Members of the phylum Apicomplexa pose substantial risks to people throughout the world. *Plasmodium* spp. continue to cause morbidity and mortality throughout the tropics. Attempts to eradicate malaria by mass residual insecticide spraying have failed, and there has been a resurgence of malaria in some areas.[62] Increasing resistance of *Plasmodium* spp. to prophylactic and therapeutic regimens has further complicated the situation. The four *Plasmodium* spp. that infect humans are responsible for 100–125 million estimated cases of malaria worldwide each year. It is estimated that between 0.7 and 1 million deaths annually in sub-Saharan Africa alone are due to malaria. As of 1984, 56 percent of the world's population lived in areas where malaria is a serious problem.[63]

As travel has increased, so has the exposure of nonimmune hosts to malaria. Every year approximately 1 million Americans travel to tropical or subtropical areas where they are at risk of acquiring malaria. Prophylaxis is effective, but the evolution of drug resistance among *Plasmodium falciparum* continues to pose problems.[64] The erythrocytic stage of malaria is the most sensitive to chemotherapy. The exoerythrocytic stage is difficult to treat, and the sporozoite stage is resistant to all known forms of chemotherapy.

Toxoplasma gondii infects people throughout the world.[65] It is an important cause of birth defects, and it has emerged as the most frequent opportunistic pathogen causing encephalitis in persons with AIDS.[66] *Cryptosporidium* spp. and *I. belli* are other coccidians that have emerged as important pathogens among persons with AIDS. They produce chronic diarrhea with weight loss in that setting. *Cryptosporidium* has increasingly been recognized as a cause of self-limited diarrhea in immunologically normal hosts as well.[67]

Another pathogen, *P. carinii*, which causes pneumonia in over 60 percent of persons with AIDS, has not yet been classified taxonomically.[68,69] Recent evidence suggests that it may be a fungus.[69a] Although not in the phyla Apicomplexa, its chemotherapy will be discussed here, since several drugs active against *P. carinii* are active against organisms within the Apicomplexa.

Aminoquinolines Used for the Prophylaxis and Treatment of Malaria

Chloroquine. Chloroquine (Fig. 3), 7-chloro-4-(4-diethylamino-1-methylbutylamino)-quinoline, the best known of the 4-aminoquinolines, has been the mainstay of antimalarial chemotherapy and prophylaxis (Tables 3 and 4). It is active against the erythrocytic stages of *Plasmodium vivax, Pl. ovale, Pl. malaria*, and, in a decreasing number of regions, *Pl. falciparum*.[62,70] The emergence of resistant strains of *Pl. falciparum* has been increasing steadily over the past 20 years.[71] The majority of strains in East Africa, Southeast Asia, and areas of South America are now chloroquine resistant. Since 1980 chloroquine resistance has become frequent in Central Africa, and reports of chloroquine resistance have come from West Africa.[72,73]

Chloroquine has also been used for the treatment of amebic liver abscess concurrently with emetine and for rheumatoid arthritis and systemic lupus erythematosus (SLE). It was once recommended for persons with *Babesia* infection, but it was found to be ineffective.[74]

Chloroquine phosphate is available as a bitter white medication, which is dispensed in tablets containing 250 or 500 mg (150 and 300-mg base, respectively). Chloroquine is rapidly absorbed after oral ingestion and is slowly excreted. The therapeutic blood concentration is reached within 2 or 3 hours. Chloroquine is widely distributed throughout the body but is relatively concentrated in the liver, spleen, kidneys, and erythrocytes. It is metabolized by alkylation in the liver, but approximately 50 percent of the drug is excreted in the urine. The half-life is 4 days, which allows for once-a-week prophylaxis.[75,76] Approximately 50 percent of chloroquine is protein bound. The renal status of the patient does not affect the amount used for acute malaria, but prophylactic doses need to be reduced for those with reduced renal function.[76]

Chloroquine is concentrated in parasitized erythrocytes 100-fold more than in nonparasitized ones.[77] In erythrocytes with schizonts, the concentration of chloroquine is 600-fold greater than in plasma. Chloroquine is toxic for the asexual erythrocytic stages of *Plasmodium* spp. It has a marked and rapid effect on the hemoglobin-containing digestive vesicles of intraerythrocytic parasites. After therapy, there is fusion of adjacent vesicles, followed by sequestration of the fused vesicles and their malaria pigment into a large autophagic vacuole.[78,79] Chloroquine binds with high affinity to ferriprotoporphyrin IX, which is a product of hemoglobin degradation by the parasite, and to its oxo-dimer. Complexing of chloroquine to this metabolite of hemoglobin may prevent it from being detoxified, and the complex is known to damage membranes. This complex may be responsible for the killing of intraerythrocytic parasites, but the hypothesis has not been proven. At high concentrations, chloroquine also intercalates into DNA, but it is doubtful that this is the mechanism of its antimalarial activity. It can also inhibit ornithine decarboxylase.[80]

Recently, attention has focused on the concentration of chloroquine in the acid-vesicle system of susceptible *Pl. falciparum*.[81,82] It is thought that chloroquine may thus interfere with the endocytosis and proteolysis of hemoglobin and the intracellular targeting of lysosomal enzymes. Resistant parasites transport chloroquine out of intraparasitic compartments more rapidly than susceptible strains and maintain lower chloroquine concentrations in their acid vesicles.[82] There is experimental

TABLE 3. Drugs Used in the Prophylaxis and Presumptive Treatment of Malaria

Drug	Prophylaxis: Adult Dose	Prophylaxis: Pediatric Dose	Presumptive Treatment for Travelers to Areas of Chloroquine Resistance
Chloroquine phosphate (Aralen[a])	300 mg base (500 mg salt) orally, once/week	5 mg/kg base (8.3 mg/kg salt) orally, once/week, up to maximum adult dose of 300 mg base	Chloroquine is not recommended for the presumptive treatment of malaria acquired in areas of known chloroquine resistance.
Hydroxychloroquine sulfate (Plaquenil[a])	310 mg base (400 mg salt) orally, once/week	5 mg/kg base (6.5 mg/kg salt) orally, once/week, up to maximum adult dose of 310 mg base	Hydroxychloroquine is not recommended for the presumptive treatment of malaria acquired in areas of known chloroquine resistance.
Doxycycline	100 mg orally, once/day	>8 years of age: 2 mg/kg of body weight orally, once/day up to adult dose of 100 mg/day	Tetracyclines are not recommended for the presumptive treatment of malaria.
Proguanil (Paludrine[a])	200 mg orally, once/day, in combination with weekly chloroquine	<2 yrs: 50 mg/day 2–6 yrs: 100 mg/day 7–10 yrs: 150 mg/day >10 yrs: 200 mg/day	Proguanil is not recommended for the presumptive treatment of malaria.
Pyrimethamine-sulfadoxine[b] (Fansidar[a])	1 tablet (25 mg pyrimethamine and 500 mg sulfadoxine) orally, once/week	2–11 mos: ⅛ tab/wk 1–3 yrs: ¼ tab/wk 4–8 yrs: ½ tab/wk 9–14 yrs: ¾ tab/wk >14 yrs: 1 tab/wk	*Adult Dose*: 3 tablets (75 mg pyrimethamine and 1,500 mg sulfadoxine), orally, as a single dose *Pediatric Dose*: 2–11 mos: ¼ tab; 1–3 yrs: ½ tab; 4–8 yrs: 1 tab; 9–14 yrs: 2 tabs; >14 yrs: 3 tabs as a single dose
Primaquine	15 mg base (26.3 mg salt) orally, once/day for 14 days, or 45 mg base (79 mg salt) orally, once/week for 8 weeks	0.3 mg/kg base (0.5 mg/kg salt) orally, once/day for 14 days, or 0.9 mg/kg base (1.5 mg/kg salt) orally, once/week for 8 weeks	Primaquine is only recommended for use after leaving an endemic area to prevent relapses of *Plasmodium vivax* and *P. ovale*.

[a] Use of trade names is for identification only and does not imply endorsement by the U.S. Department of Health and Human Services or the Public Health Service.
[b] Not usually recommended for prophylaxis. See text.
(From Centers for Disease Control.[115])

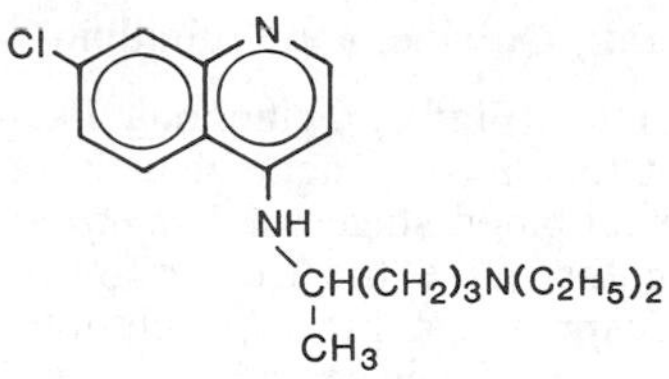

FIG. 3. Chloroquine.

evidence that this can be reversed with calcium channel blockers, raising the theoretical possibility that chloroquine plus an additional agent that blocks the efflux of chloroquine might be effective against chloroquine-resistant strains.[83]

Chloroquine is a relatively safe chemoprophylactic and therapeutic drug when used at the recommended doses for malaria. Oral administration is preferred. Occasional temporary side effects include headache, nausea, vomiting, blurred vision, dizziness, fatigue, and confusion.[70,76] Some Africans experience pruritis, which responds to an antihistamine. Rare side effects include depigmentation of the hair, corneal opacities, weight loss, insomnia, leukopenia, myalgias and exacerbation of psoriasis, and eczema or other exfoliative dermatoses. Extremely rare reactions include blood dyscrasias, toxic psychosis, and photophobia. Permanent retinal damage is rarely associated with malaria prophylaxis and treatment but has occurred with long-term, high-dose therapy given to persons with collagen vascular diseases.[84] Chloroquine is contraindicated in persons with retinal disease, psoriasis, or porphyria.

Chloroquine can also be given by intravenous infusion, but it must be administered slowly and with great caution.[70,85] Respiratory depression, hypotension, cardiovascular collapse, and seizures can follow excessively rapid parenteral administration. These are apparently due to toxic levels of chloroquine in the circulation. Heart block and cardiac arrest are thought to be due to a direct toxic effect on the myocardium at high plasma concentrations. It is recommended that oral administration be substituted for parenteral administration as soon as possible.[70] Deaths from chloroquine toxicity also occur in accidental ingestion by children, in adults who habitually self-medicate, and in those who attempt suicide. The ingestion of 5 g of chloroquine is fatal unless treatment is initiated immediately with mechanical ventilation, diazepam, and epinephrine.[86]

Chloroquine has been implicated in severe cochleovestibular abnormalities in the fetus of a mother taking high doses for the treatment of SLE.[87] There has been no such association between chloroquine administered in antimalarial doses and fetal abnormalities.[76]

Amodiaquine*.** Amodiaquine is another 4-aminoquinolone, which has been used for more than 40 years. Its mechanism of action is thought to be the same as that of chloroquine, although it has activity against some strains of *Pl. falciparum*

TABLE 4. Treatment of Malaria

Drug		*Adult Dosage*	*Pediatric Dosage*
All *Plasmodium* except chloroquine-resisttant *P. falciparum*			
Oral			
Drug of choice:	Chloroquine phosphate[1,2]	600 mg base (1 gram), then 300 mg base (500 mg) 6 hrs later, then 300 mg base (500 mg)/d × 2d	10 mg base/kg (max. 600 mg base), then 5 mg base/kg 6 hrs later, then 5 mg base/kg/d × 2d
Parenteral			
Drug of choice:	Quinine dihydrochloride[3]	600 mg in 300 ml normal saline iv over 2 to 4 hrs; repeat q8h until oral therapy can be started (max. 1800 mg/d)	25 mg/kg/d; give ⅓ of daily dose over 2 to 4 hrs; repeat q8h until oral therapy can be started (max. 1800 mg/d)
OR	Quinidine gluconate[4,5]		
Alternative:	Chloroquine HCl[2]	200 mg base (250 mg) im q6h if oral therapy cannot be started	Not recommended
Chloroquine-resistant *P. falciparum*			
Oral			
Drugs of choice:	Quinine sulfate[6,7]	650 mg tid × 3–7d	25 mg/kg/d in 3 doses × 3d
	plus pyrimethamine	25 mg bid × 3d	<10 kg: 6.25 mg/d × 3d 10–20 kg: 12.5 mg/d × 3d 20–40 kg: 25 mg/d × 3d
	plus sulfadiazine	500 mg qid × 5d	100–200 mg/kg/d in 4 doses × 5d (max. 2 grams/d)
Alternatives:	Quinine sulfate[7,8]	650 mg tid × 7d	25 mg/kg/d in 3 doses × 3d
	plus tetracycline	250 mg qid × 7d	5 mg/kg qid × 7d
Parenteral			
Drug of choice:	Quinine dihydrochloride[3]	same as above	same as above
OR	Quinidine gluconate[4,5]		
Prevention of relapses: *P. vivax and P. ovale* only			
Drug of choice:	Primaquine phosphate[9]	15 mg base (26.3 mg)/d × 14d or 45 mg base (79 mg)/wk × 8 wks	0.3 mg base/kg/d × 14d

[1] If chloroquine phosphate is not available, hydroxychloroquine sulfate is as effective; 400 mg of hydroxychloroquine sulfate is equivalent to 500 mg of chloroquine phosphate.
[2] In *P. falciparum* malaria, if the patient has not shown a response to conventional doses of chloroquine in 48–72 hours, parasitic resistance to this drug should be considered. Intramuscular injection of chloroquine is painful and can cause abscesses.
[3] Available in the USA only from the Centers for Disease Control, telephone 404-488-4046 (nights, weekends, or holidays call 404-639-2888). *P. falciparum* infections from Southeast Asia may require a loading dose of 20 mg/kg (NJ White et al, Am J Trop Med Hyg, 32:1, 1983).
[4] Considered an investigational drug for this condition by the U.S. Food and Drug Administration.
[5] Optimal dosage for treatment of malaria is currently under investigation. For up-to-date information, telephone the Centers for Disease Control (daytime 404-488-4046; nights, weekends, holidays 404-639-2888). ECG monitoring is necessary to detect arrhythmias. Some experts consider quinidine more effective than quinine.
[6] Quinine alone will usually control an attack of resistant *P. falciparum* but, in a substantial number of infections, particularly with strains from Southeast Asia, it fails to prevent recurrence; addition of pyrimethamine and sulfadiazine or tetracycline lowers the rate of recurrence. The duration of quinine sulfate therapy depends on the geographic site.
[7] For treatment of *P. falciparum* infections acquired in Thailand, quinine should be given for seven days instead of three, combined with seven days of tetracycline. Ref. 5 recommends quinine sulfate for 3 days.
[8] Quinine plus tetracycline may be the regimen of choice in areas such as Thailand where resistance to pyrimethamine plus sulfonamides is common.
[9] Primaquine phosphate can cause hemolytic anemia, especially in patients whose red cells are deficient in glucose-6-phosphate dehydrogenase. This deficiency is most common in Blacks, Orientals, and Mediterranean peoples. Patients should be screened for G-6-PD deficiency before treatment. Primaquine should not be used during pregnancy.
(From Ref. 5, with permission.)

resistant to chloroquine. Amodiaquine is not available in the United States. It was briefly recommended for travelers to areas with chloroquine-resistant *Pl. falciparum*, but that recommendation was quickly withdrawn when reports of fatal agranulocytosis appeared in persons taking it as weekly antimalarial prophylaxis.[88,89] Amodiaquine is no longer recommended for malaria prophylaxis or therapy.

Primaquine. Primaquine (Fig. 4) is an 8-aminoquinoline, 8-(4-amino-1-methylbutylamino)-6-methoxyquinoline. It is the only drug available that is effective in eradicating the exoerythrocytic, hypnozoite forms of *Pl. vivax* and *Pl. ovale* in the liver.[90] It has some activity against the asexual blood stages of *Pl. vivax*, but this action is not sufficient to allow it to be used alone for suppressive prophylaxis. The 8-aminoquinolines also have gametocytocidal activity against all four *Plasmodium* spp. that infect humans, but this is not of clinical significance. Primaquine is used after chloroquine to provide a radical cure for persons with acute *Pl. vivax* or *Pl. ovale* malaria or after chloroquine prophylaxis in persons exposed to these forms of malaria.[91] The relapse rate of persons infected with *Pl. vivax* is low after primaquine therapy, except for those with some strains of *Pl. vivax* from the southwestern Pacific, such as the Chesson strain, which requires higher doses given either daily or at weekly intervals.[92,93]

Primaquine phosphate is supplied in tablets containing 26.3 mg of the salt, which is equivalent to 15 mg of the base. It has a bitter taste, and may be crushed and added to sweet liquid or fruit to make it more palatable. The dosage is usually expressed in terms of the base. Primaquine is readily absorbed when taken orally. Plasma concentrations reach a peak at 6 hours and decline to undetectable levels by 24 hours.

Primaquine interferes with the mitochondrial function of *Plasmodium*. It is fully active only after metabolism by the host, but the nature of the active metabolites is not clear. Based on studies with pamoquine***, the first of this series of drugs, the metabolites are thought to affect both the mitochondrial electron transport chain and pyrimidine synthesis.[78]

The major toxicity with primaquine is hemolysis in persons with G6PD deficiency.[94,95] G6PD deficiency is rare in whites, but there are more than 100 million people worldwide with this deficiency (1 percent of males in the Middle East, 5 percent of Chinese males, and 10 percent of black males). Persons from these groups should be tested for G6PD deficiency before primaquine is prescribed. Similarly, the administration of primaquine should be discontinued if darkening of the urine or a fall in hematocrit is noted. For persons with the more mild African form of G6PD deficiency, a dose of 45 mg (base) weekly for 8 weeks has been used.[92] For patients with the more severe Mediterranean variety, 30 mg weekly for 30 weeks has been recommended.[95]

Apart from the potential for hemolysis, primaquine is usually well tolerated.[76] Abdominal cramps, epigastric distress, and nausea occur in some patients. Mild anemia, cyanosis (methemoglobinemia), and leukocytosis are observed in some persons given higher doses. Rare complications include granulocytopenia or agranulocytosis, hypertension, and arrhythmia.

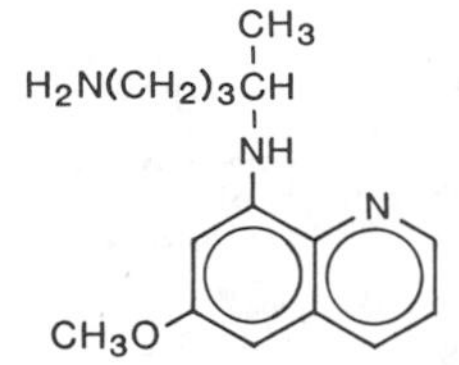

FIG. 4. Primaquine.

Cinchona Alkaloids, Quinine, and Quinidine

Quinine. Quinine (Fig. 5), a cinchona alkaloid, was the first successful agent for the treatment of malaria.[70] It is effective against the asexual blood stages of *Plasmodium* spp. With the introduction of chloroquine, the use of quinine fell dramatically, but with the widespread emergence of chloroquine-resistant *Pl. falciparum*, quinine has once again become widely used.[70] Only in Thailand has progressively decreased sensitivity to quinine been a problem. Quinine acts rapidly against asexual erythrocytic stages of all four *Plasmodium* spp. that infect humans.

Quinine sulfate is supplied as 260- and 325-mg tablets and in capsules of 130, 200, 260, 300, and 325 mg. The tablets have a very bitter taste. Quinine is rapidly absorbed after oral administration and reaches peak levels in 1–3 hours. Peak serum concentrations after a dose of 10 mg/kg are 7–17 μg/ml; side effects can be seen at concentrations above 10 μg/ml.[76] Quinine is formulated for parenteral use as quinine hydrochloride** in 2-ml ampules containing 300 mg/ml. The parenteral preparation is available in the United States only through the Centers for Disease Control. Intravenous quinidine, its dextrostereoisomer, is effective and available in virtually all hospitals, It is usually used instead.

Quinine is metabolized in the liver and excreted in the urine, mainly as metabolites.[96] Only 20 percent of the drug is excreted unchanged.[97] It is not as avidly bound to tissues as chloroquine and has a shorter half-life of 5–15 hours. Monitoring blood levels is recommended for persons with impaired renal or hepatic function, and dose reduction is necessary in severe renal failure.[98]

The exact mechanism of action as an antimalarial is unknown, but quinine, like chloroquine, appears to act at the level of the hemoglobin-containing digestive vesicles of the intraerythrocytic parasite. Quinine is a competitive inhibitor of pigment clumping by chloroquine,[78] and malaria pigment first becomes translucent and then disappears with therapy. Quinine also intercalates into DNA, but this does not appear to be its primary mode of action.

Quinine has the poorest therapeutic-to-toxic ratio of all of the antimalarial drugs.[99] The side effects of quinine are collectively referred to as *cinchonism* and include tinnitis, decreased hearing, headache, dysphoria, nausea, vomiting, and mild visual disturbances.[70,99] These alterations are dose related and reversible. Other less common side effects include skin rashes, including urticaria, angioedema of the face, pruritis, agranulocytosis, and, rarely, massive hemolysis in persons with falciparum malaria (blackwater fever). Quinine can cause respiratory depression in patients with myasthenia gravis. It has a curare-like effect on skeletal muscle and has been useful in the treatment of painful nocturnal leg cramps. Other potential adverse reactions include hypoglycemia in patients with high *Pl. falciparum* parasitemia. This is due to the parasites' consumption of glucose and the release of insulin from the pancreas by quinine.[100] It responds to the administration of intravenous glucose. Quinine causes hemolysis in patients with G6PD deficiency. It can stimulate uterine contractions and may produce abortion if given in high doses. However, quinine has been used

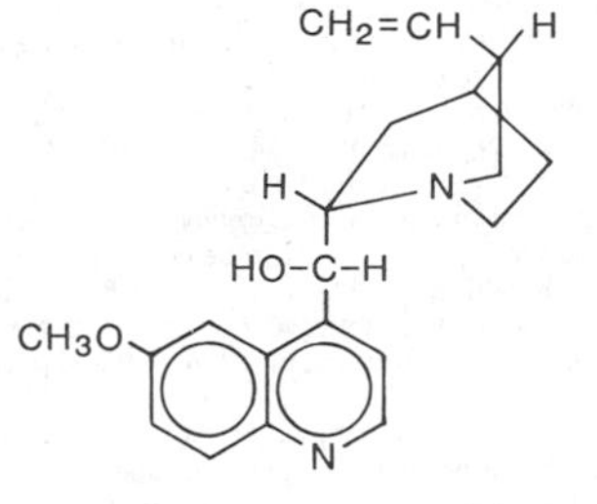

FIG. 5. Quinine.

successfully to treat seriously ill women with malaria in the third trimester of pregnancy.[101] Quinine must be used cautiously by the intravenous route, since rapid intravenous infusion may cause shock due to myocardial depression and peripheral vasodilatation. Overdoses are associated with convulsions, coma, delirium, depressed respiration, circulatory collapse, and death.

Quinidine. Quinidine is the dextrostereoisomer of quinine. It is used in the United States on an investigational basis for the parenteral treatment of chloroquine-resistant falciparum malaria in persons who cannot take oral quinine. A major advantage of parenteral quinidine over parenteral quinine is that quinidine is available in virtually every hospital because of its role in the treatment of cardiac arrhythmias. Quinidine gluconate has been successfully used to treat severe malaria in children and adults unable to take oral medications.[102,103]

Quinidine gluconate is available for intravenous administration. The half-life of quinidine is 12.8 hours. ECG changes including prolonged Q-Tc intervals are common, but life-threatening arrhythmias are rare if proper doses are used. Hypotension may occur if the infusion is too rapid. The rate of infusion, blood pressure, and ECGs of persons receiving intravenous quinidine should be monitored closely.[104]

4-Quinoline-Carbinolamines (Quinoline Methanols): Mefloquine***

Mefloquine (Fig. 6) is a quinolone-methanol derived chemically from quinine. Mefloquine was the result of a search for a new antimalarial drug by researchers at the Walter Reed Army Institute of Research.[70,71] Like quinine and chloroquine, mefloquine is a blood schizontocidal drug and has no effect on exoerythrocytic schizonts or gametocytes.[77] Used as a single dose, it has been effective against all *Plasmodium* spp., including chloroquine-resistant and pyrimethamine-sulfadoxime-resistant isolates of *Pl. falciparum*.[105–108] West African strains of *Pl. falciparum* appear less susceptible to mefloquine in vitro than Southeast Asian strains.[109] A unified effort has been made to restrict its use for treatment and prophylaxis to areas with chloroquine-resistant *Pl. falciparum*. It has not yet been licensed for use in the United States.

Mefloquine is available only for oral administration. Administered in tablet form, it is slowly and incompletely absorbed.[110] Mefloquine is widely distributed in the body, and 99 percent of the drug is protein bound. It has a long half-life in humans, ranging from 6 to 23 days, with a mean of 14 days. It is extensively metabolized and excreted through bile and feces. Mefloquine concentrates on red blood cell membranes and seems to interfere with the food vacuoles of *Plasmodium* in a manner similar to that of quinine.[111] It has been administered as a suspension via a nasogastric tube to unconscious patients with cerebral malaria. Absorption was rapid, with an absorption half-life of 1.5 hours. Plasma mefloquine levels were over 200 ng/ml within 3 hours.[112] While intravenous quinidine is usually the drug of choice for severe malaria in patients who cannot take oral medications, mefloquine through a nasogastic tube is necessary in areas where quinine resistance is encountered (e.g., Thailand).[112] Mefloquine cannot be administered parenterally because it causes intense local irritation.

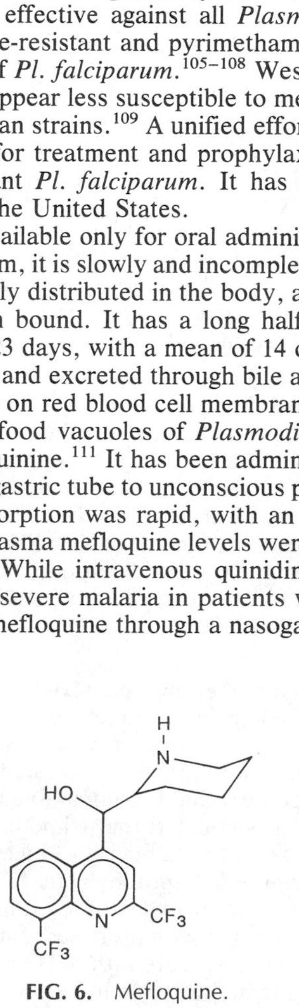

FIG. 6. Mefloquine.

Mefloquine is generally well tolerated. Large amounts can produce nausea and dizziness. Sinus bradycardia has been observed in approximately 7 percent of persons treated with this drug. The heart rate returns to normal within 2 weeks. Patients have been asymptomatic, and ECGs have revealed no sign of myocardial damage.[113] Repeated high doses have caused histologic abnormalities in the retinas of experimental animals.

Tetracycline and Doxycycline

Tetracycline has been used with quinine to treat acute falciparum malaria in areas such as Thailand where *Pl. falciparum* is resistant to pyrimethamine, sulfonamides, and chloroquine and has decreased susceptibility to quinine.[114] Doxycycline, a long-acting tetracycline, has been used prophylactically in these regions. It has not been as thoroughly evaluated as other prophylactic drugs. The Centers for Disease Control recommend the use of daily doxycycline alone[115]; others advise using doxycycline with weekly chloroquine to provide optimal protection against *Pl. vivax*.[5]

Tetracyclines are well absorbed orally. Their pharmacology is discussed in Chapter 23. They inhibit protein synthesis in prokaryotic ribosomes, and it is likely that they affect parasite protein synthesis as well.[78] The most common untoward effects are gastrointestinal. Photosensitivity occurs in approximately 3 percent of recipients and is a potential problem for travelers to the tropics. Candida vaginitis can also complicate tetracycline use. Finally, the tetracyclines are not recommended during pregnancy or for children less than 8 years of age because they are concentrated in bone and teeth and may cause dental staining, hypoplasia of dental enamel, and impaired bone growth in young children.

Artemisinine (Qinghaosu)***

Artemisinine is a sesquiterpene lactone derived from the wormwood plant *Artemisia annua*.[70,77] It has been used as a traditional medication by the Chinese for the treatment of malaria and has activity against chloroquine-resistant *Pl. falciparum* in humans.

The mode of action is poorly understood but appears to be unique to this group of drugs. Artemisinine is thought to act primarily on the integrity of the parasite's membrane. The first biochemical effect, cessation of protein synthesis, is observed within an hour of exposure. Resistance to artemisinine in *Plasmodium yoelii* has been produced in mice.[77] Troublesome was the observation that artemisinine-resistant parasites also displayed marked cross-resistance to chloroquine, quinine, and mefloquine, possibly due to a modification of the membrane composition of the parasite. The use of artemisinine or related compounds for the treatment of chloroquine-resistant falciparum malaria is still investigational.

Dihydrofolate Reductase Inhibitors and Sulfonamides

The diaminopyrimidine dihydrofolate reductase inhibitors, pyrimethamine and trimethoprim, have been used alone or, more commonly, in conjunction with sulfonamides for the prevention and treatment of malaria,[78,116] *I. belli*,[117] *P. carinii* pneumonia,[68,69,118–120] and toxoplasmosis.[121–125] They act at sequential steps in the folic acid cycle. *Plasmodium* spp. and presumably other sensitive parasites carry out pyrimidine synthesis de novo, in which reduced folic acid derivatives are essential cofactors. Unlike mammalian cells, these parasites cannot use preformed pyrimidines obtained through salvage pathways. Pyrimethamine is more active than trimethoprim in inhibiting the dihydrofolate reductases of *Plasmodium* spp. and *T. gondii*.

Conversely, trimethoprim has greater activity against bacteria and has been widely used for the treatment of *P. carinii* and *I. belli*. Both of these drugs can inhibit mammalian dihydrofolate reductase when used at high concentrations. This is more of a problem with pyrimethamine than with trimethoprim. In most instances, a sulfonamide is administered concurrently to inhibit a second step in the folic acid metabolic pathway.

Recent studies indicate that trimetrexate, a low molecular weight, lipid-soluble dihydrofolate reductase inhibitor, is active against *P. carinii*[126] and *T. gondii*.[127] Folinic acid has been used with trimetrexate to minimize its inhibitory effects on bone marrow. Development of new dihydrofolate reductase inhibitors that are preferentially active against protozoal enzymes is now underway.

Pyrimethamine and Short-Acting Sulfonamides. Pyrimethamine (Fig. 7), a 2,4-diaminopyrimidine, has been used on a weekly basis for malaria prophylaxis and with sulfadiazine and quinine for the treatment of chloroquine-resistant *Pl. falciparum*.[5] The usefulness of pyrimethamine with a sulfonamide has been limited by the emergence of resistant *Pl. falciparum* and *Pl. vivax*. Pyrimethamine and sulfadiazine or trisulfapyrimidines are the treatment of choice for toxoplasmosis. The majority of persons who acquire toxoplasmosis have self-limited disease and do not require treatment. In immunocompromised persons, including those with AIDS, toxoplasmic encephalitis is life-threatening. Therapy with high doses of pyrimethamine and sulfonamides is recommended for prolonged periods of time.[121,123] Congenital toxoplasmosis is also treated with pyrimethamine and sulfonamides.[124,125] The optimal treatment for acute toxoplasmosis during pregnancy is uncertain; pyrimethamine is contraindicated, at least for the first trimester, and sulfonamides cannot be used close to the time of delivery because they displace bilirubin from binding sites on albumin. Spiramycin is an alternative, but it is available in the United States only with special approval from the FDA.[128]

Pyrimethamine is well absorbed orally; the half-life is 4–6 days.[129] It is extensively metabolized; less than 3 percent of the drug is excreted unchanged in the urine in 24 hours. Pyrimethamine acts preferentially to inhibit the parasite's dihydrofolate reductase. It mimics dihydrofolate, competing with this metabolite to inhibit the enzyme. Pyrimethamine is approximately 1000-fold more active against the parasite than the host's dihydrofolate reductase.[130]

Pyrimethamine is very well tolerated at a dose of 25 mg/week, which has been used for malaria prophylaxis. Blood dyscrasias, rash, vomiting, seizures, and shock are all rare side effects.[76] Bone marrow suppression with neutropenia, anemia, and thrombocytopenia are seen with the higher doses used for the treatment of toxoplasmosis (25 mg/day). Careful follow-up with complete blood counts is necessary, but concurrent administration of folinic acid usually prevents these complications. Pyrimethamine is teratogenic in animals and is contraindicated during the first 16 weeks of pregnancy.[131,132] It has been used to treat pregnant women with primary toxoplasmosis after this period, but concern remains about its safety. Some experts have argued that there has not been unequivocal documentation of pyrimethamine-associated birth defects at the dose levels used for malaria prophylaxis.[133,134]

Sulfonamides decrease the activity of dihydropteroate synthetase and reduce the binding of *p*-aminobenzoic acid (PABA)

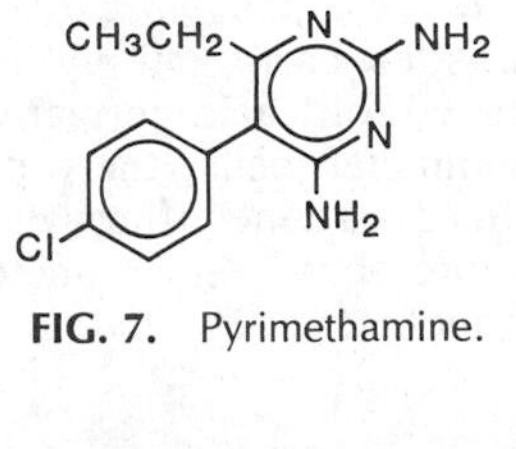

FIG. 7. Pyrimethamine.

to this enzyme in several members of the Apicomplexa. The sulfonamides are described in detail in Chapter 29. They are well absorbed orally. The most common untoward effects are allergic reactions and gastrointestinal complaints. Allergic reactions include fever and rash. Less common are toxic epidermal necrolysis, erythema multiforme, Stevens-Johnson syndrome, hepatitis, pneumonitis, bone marrow depression, and serum sickness.[135]

Untoward effects are encountered in 60 percent of persons with AIDS treated for toxoplasmic encephalitis[122] with pyrimethamine and a sulfonamide. These effects include fever, skin rashes, bone marrow suppression, and hepatotoxicity. When these effects occur, pyrimethamine or an alternative investigational drug such as trimetrexate or spiramycin has been used as a single agent, but their effectiveness has not been well documented.

Fansidar (Pyrimethamine and Sulfadoxine). Fansidar, which consists of pyrimethamine 25 mg and sulfadoxine 500 mg, was previously recommended as prophylaxis for travelers to areas with chloroquine-resistant *Pl. falciparium*.[116] It is seldom indicated for prophylaxis now because it has been associated with life-threatening allergic reactions. In addition, Fansidar resistance has emerged in many areas. Fansidar has been administered to prevent *P. carinii* pneumonia in patients with AIDS, but the risk of serious untoward allergic reactions has limited its acceptance.[136]

Sulfadoxine, like pyrimethamine, is well absorbed from the gastrointestinal tract. Its half-life is 5–9 days.[129] The severe reactions observed with Fansidar have been attributed to sulfadoxine. Fatalities with prophylactic Fansidar have occurred in 1 in 11,000 to 1 in 26,000 users.[137,138] In 1984, American travelers who took Fansidar as weekly malaria prophylaxis in Kenya were as likely to die from Fansidar toxicity as from malaria. Most of the severe cutaneous reactions, including toxic epidermal necrolysis, erythema multiforme, and the Stevens-Johnson syndrome, have occurred soon after the start of prophylaxis, usually within the first 5 weeks of therapy.[137,138] Other serious but unusual side effects with sulfadoxine include serum sickness, bone marrow suppression, hepatitis, hepatic granuloma, and pneumonitis.[116] No fatal reactions have yet been reported when Fansidar (three tablets in a single dose) has been used for the treatment of chloroquine-resistant falciparum malaria. It is still prescribed as empiric treatment for persons who develop symptoms of malaria abroad and cannot promptly obtain medical evaluation.[5]

Pyrimethamine-Sulfadoxime-Mefloquine (Fansimef).*** The combination of pyrimethamine, sulfadoxine, and mefloquine has been used for the treatment of chloroquine-resistant *Pl. falciparum*.[107,114,139,140] The goal is to reduce the likelihood of developing further resistance. This combination, formulated as Fansimef[140] (pyrimethamine 25 mg, sulfadoxime 500 mg, and mefloquine 250 mg), has also been used prophylactically, but has the potential for the severe allergic cutaneous reactions observed with sulfadoxime.

Trimethoprim-Sulfamethoxazole (Cotrimoxazole). The combination of trimethoprim-sulfamethoxazole, formulated at a ratio of 1:5, is the treatment of choice for *P. carinii*.[68,69,118–120,141] The response rate of patients treated for *P. carinii* pneumonia is 80–85 percent and is comparable to that with pentamidine. It has been postulated that trimethoprim-sulfamethoxazole has a static rather than a microbicidal effect on *P. carinii*.[142] Daily[143] or intermittent[144] prophylactic trimethoprim-sulfamethoxazole has been shown to decrease the incidence of *P. carinii* infection among immunocompromised children and has been proposed for use with patients with AIDS who tolerate the drug. Trimethoprim-sulfamethoxazole has also been used effectively to treat *I. belli* infection in AIDS patients, but relapses are common even after high-dose, prolonged therapy.[117]

Both trimethoprim and sulfamethoxazole are well absorbed when administered orally. Peak blood levels are reached in 1–4 hours. The half-lives are similar: 10–12 hours for trimethoprim and 9–11 hours for sulfamethoxazole.[135] Excretion is through the kidney; renal failure prolongs the half-lives of both drugs. Trimethoprim has greater lipid solubility than sulfamethoxazole, and its apparent volume of distribution is five to six times greater. As a result, the drugs are formulated at a trimethoprim/sulfamethoxazole ratio of 1:5. Single-strength tablets contain 80 mg trimethoprim and 400 mg sulfamethoxazole; double-strength tablets have 160 mg trimethoprim and 800 mg sulfamethoxazole. It is also available in suspension for oral use containing 40 mg trimethoprim and 200 mg sulfamethoxazole per 5 ml for children. For intravenous use, trimethoprim-sulfamethoxazole is available as a solution containing 16 mg trimethoprim and 80 mg sulfamethoxazole per milliliter.

In patients without AIDS, common side effects include gastrointestinal upset (4 percent) and skin reactions (3 percent).[145] Rare adverse reactions include agranulocytosis, aplastic anemia, acute interstitial nephritis, Stevens-Johnson syndrome, jaundice, headaches, depression, and hallucinations.[146] Malnourished individuals on prolonged therapy may require concomitant therapy with folinic acid to prevent megaloblastic anemia. The drug combination is not recommended during pregnancy.[135]

For unknown reasons, patients with AIDS have an unusually high incidence of severe adverse reactions when given trimethoprim-sulfamethoxazole.[69] Approximately 65 percent of AIDS patients experience significant drug-related symptoms, half of which are severe enough to result in discontinuation of therapy.[68,69,147–149] These adverse reactions include neutropenia, fever, and rashes in one-third of these patients and thrombocytopenia, intolerable gastrointestinal effects, and hepatitis in one-tenth.[148,149] Prophylaxis against *P. carinii* is likely to be effective in this group but is often impossible because of the frequency of side effects.

Dapsone and Pyrimethamine or Trimethoprim. Dapsone, a sulfone that has been widely used in the treatment of leprosy, is used outside the United States in combination with pyrimethamine as prophylaxis against malaria. Maloprim, a combination of pyrimethamine 25 mg and dapsone 100 mg, has been used weekly for malaria prophylaxis. More recently, dapsone has been used with trimethoprim for the treatment of *P. carinii* pneumonia[150,151] and for its prevention.[152] When used with trimethoprim for the treatment of nonmoribund AIDS patients with *P. carinii*, the combination appears as effective as and less toxic than trimethoprim-sulfamethoxazole.[150,151]

Like the sulfonamides, dapsone interferes with folic acid metabolism by competitively inhibiting the enzyme dihydropteroate synthetase. Dapsone is available in 25-mg and 500-mg tablets. It is well absorbed after oral administration and is widely distributed in body tissues.[153] About 70–80 percent of the drug is bound to plasma protein. After acetylation and deacetylation, the drug is excreted in the urine as glucuronide or sulfate conjugates. The half-life is variable but averages 25–27 hours.[154] Serious side effects of dapsone include hemolytic anemia, methemoglobinemia, and bone marrow suppression. Very rarely, when maloprim has been used in high doses, the agranulocytosis has been fatal.[155] Uncommon side effects include peripheral neuropathy, anorexia, vomiting, vertigo, blurred vision, tinnitis, fever, headache, pruritis, psychosis, hematuria, and skin rash. Severe skin rashes occur in some AIDS patients given dapsone and trimethoprim; some resolve after the trimethoprim dose is reduced. Trimethoprim is contraindicated in patients with G6PD deficiency or known hypersensitivity to sulfonamides. Complete blood counts should be performed at least weekly on patients receiving dapsone.

Proguanil.*** Proguanil, also known as *chloroquanide*, was the first agent found to inhibit plasmodial dihydrofolate reductase. The elucidation of its mechanism of action led to the synthesis of the diaminopyrimidines, pyrimethamine and trimethoprim.[156] Proguanil has been used for prophylaxis against *Pl. falciparum* and *Pl. vivax*. It acts too slowly to be employed for the treatment of acute malaria. Proguanil is currently used with chloroquine as prophylaxis in travelers to East Africa.[5] It provides protection against chloroquine-resistant strains of *Pl. falciparum* there[157]; chloroquine is administered concurrently because of the potential resistance of *Pl. vivax* to proguanil. The use of proguanil outside of East Africa has been limited by the resistance of *Pl. falciparum*. Proguanil is not available in the United States but can be purchased in Canada, England, and pharmacies in East Africa.

Proguanil is formulated in 100-mg tablets. It is slowly absorbed after oral administration. It reaches peak serum concentrations in 2–4 hours, and the serum levels decline to practically zero by 24 hours.[76] It must be taken daily to provide effective prophylaxis. The concentration of proguanil in erythrocytes is six times that in plasma. Approximately 40–60 percent is excreted in the urine and 10 percent in the feces. It is the metabolite 2,4-diamino-1-*p*-chlorophenyl-1,6-dihydro-6,6-dimethyl-1,3,5-triazine that inhibits parasite dihydrofolate reductase.[76]

Proguanil is thought to be innocuous at the daily dose levels used for malaria prophylaxis. At higher levels, it can produce nausea, vomiting, abdominal pain, and diarrhea. Excessive amounts have been associated with hematuria, proteinuria, and casts in the urine.

Lipid-Soluble Antifolates: Trimetrexate* and Piritrexin***.** Trimetrexate (2,4-diamino 5-methyl-6-[3,4,5-trimethyl-oxyanilino) methyl] quinazoline) is a low molecular weight dihydrofolate reductase inhibitor. It was developed as a myelosuppressive agent but was found to have antiparasitic activity. In preliminary studies, trimetrexate has been effective for the treatment of *P. carinii*[126] and *T. gondii*.[127] It is 1500 times more potent in inhibiting protozoal dihydrofolate reductase than trimethoprim. Trimetrexate is lipid soluble and readily enters host cells as well as protozoa. It has been used effectively with sulfadiazine to treat experimental murine toxoplasmosis.[127] When it was used without a sulfonamide or sulfone to treat *P. carinii* in persons with AIDS, the frequent allergic side effects seen with those compounds were avoided. Folinic acid (leucovorin) was administered concurrently to prevent bone marrow suppression. Adverse effects in patients receiving trimetrexate and leucovorin include leukopenia, rash, elevated aminotransferase levels, and reversible peripheral neuropathy, but they are usually mild. Piritrexin is another lipid-soluble dihydrofolate reductase inhibitor, which in combination with sulfadiazine has been shown to have activity against *T. gondii* in the murine model.[158]

Macrolide Antibiotics Active against Apicomplexa

Clindamycin. Clindamycin, a macrolide antibiotic, has been used along with prednisone for the treatment of ocular toxoplasmosis in immunocompetent patients.[159,160] It has relatively good penetration into the eye and inhibits replication of *T. gondii*. Although the outcome of therapy has been good, there are no prospective studies comparing clindamycin with the combination of pyrimethamine and a sulfonamide. Clindamycin also is of potential use with quinine in the treatment of malaria, and this combination is the treatment of choice for symptomatic human babesiosis.[161]

The pharmacokinetics and untoward effects of clindamycin are discussed in Chapter 26. The major concern is the development of pseudomembranous colitis, a side effect that increases in incidence with age.

Spiramycin* (Available by Special Request from the FDA) and Roxithromycin.***** Spiramycin, another macrolide antibiotic, is widely used as an additive in animal feeds. It is active against *T. gondii*, but it has not yet been licensed for use in the United States. Spiramycin has been used to treat primary toxoplasmosis acquired during pregnancy. In a recent study, only 3.7 percent of fetuses became infected in mothers who acquired toxoplasmosis during the first 16 weeks of pregnancy when they received spiramycin.[128] Spiramycin has been reported to be effective in a few persons with AIDS and *Cryptosporidium* infection. Prospective studies of its efficacy are ongoing. Spiramycin is dispensed in 500-mg capsules.

Roxithromycin, an ether oxime derivative of erythromycin, has shown activity against *T. gondii* in mice.[162,163] It acts synergistically with interferon-γ in the murine model of toxoplasmosis.

Pentamidine

Pentamidine isethionate (Fig. 8) is a diamidine that has been used as an alternative drug for the treatment of *P. carinii* pneumonia,[68,69,118,120] the hemolymphatic stage of *Trypanosoma brucei gambiense* infection,[164] and some forms of leishmaniasis.[165–167] Approximately 80–85 percent of patients with *P. carinii* pneumonia respond to intravenously administered pentamidine isethionate, but 50 percent or more suffer ontoward effects with the drug.[68,69,118,120] Parenteral pentamidine is usually reserved for patients who cannot tolerate trimethoprim-sulfamethoxazole. The concurrent use of pentamidine with trimethoprim-sulfamethoxazole has not increased the response rate but may increase the toxicity.[168] Recent studies indicate that aerosolized pentamidine is effective for the prevention of *P. carinii* pneumonia and possibly for its treatment.[169–171b] The effectiveness of therapy is dependent on the nebulization system and the size of the particles.

Pentamidine isethionate is a white powder that is water soluble; each 1.74 mg contains 1 mg of pentamidine base.[172] It is available in 300-mg ampules for intramuscular or intravenous administration. Intramuscular injections are frequently complicated by pain, swelling, and sterile abscesses at the administration site. Pentamidine is now most commonly given intravenously after being diluted in 100–250 ml of 5% dextrose in water. It must be administered slowly over 1–2 hours.[173] Pentamidine is highly tissue bound and excreted slowly over an extended period of time. It does not penetrate the central nervous system.

The mechanism of action has not yet been defined. Pentamidine is known to bind to DNA in a nonintercalative manner.[174] It interacts selectively with trypanosomal kinetoplast DNA, resulting in swelling and loss of structure of the kinetoplast.[175] Pentamidine also inhibits RNA polymerase,[176] ribosomal function,[177] nucleic acid, protein, and phospholipid synthesis,[178] and polyamine synthesis.[179] It can inhibit folic acid synthesis,[180] but this does not appear to be its mode of action. It can also inhibit trypsin and related proteases.[181] At a high concentration, pentamidine impairs oxygen consumption.[182]

The administration of pentamidine isethionate, either by the intravenous or intramuscular routes, is associated with toxicity in 50 percent of persons.[183] Adverse effects include tachycardia, nausea, vomiting, dizziness, rash, facial flushing, breathlessness, and a metallic taste. Severe hypotension may result after an intramuscular injection or after rapid intravenous infusion.[173]

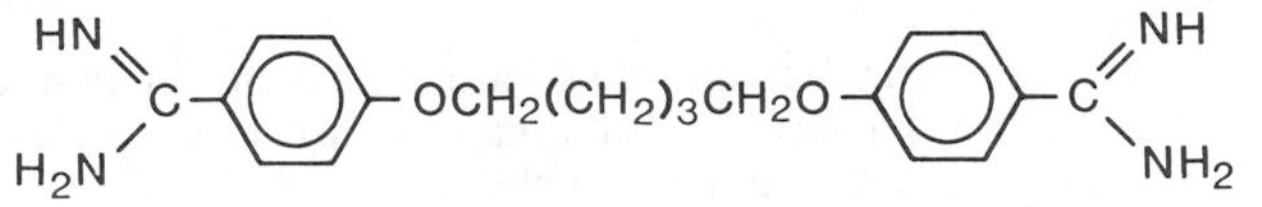

FIG. 8. Pentamidine.

Hypoglycemia has been reported during therapy in 6–9 percent of persons treated in the United States.[183,184] It can be severe and life-threatening, and may even occur after the completion of therapy. It is probably due to a direct toxic effect of pentamidine on pancreatic β cells.[185,186] The hypoglycemia may be followed by the development of insulin-dependent diabetes mellitus. Severe hypoglycemia may be controlled with diazoxide,[187] but it is not known if this will prevent the subsequent development of diabetes mellitus. Reversible renal failure occurs in approximately 25 percent of persons who receive pentamidine.[184] Although severe renal failure has been reported in a few patients, it has been impossible to attribute the renal toxicity solely to pentamidine because of the concurrent administration of other nephrotoxic agents. Other adverse effects of pentamidine include leukopenia and thrombocytopenia, elevated transaminases, fever, hypocalcemia, confusion, hallucinations, and, rarely, cardiac arrhythmias. Rare cases of fatal pancreatitis have been reported in patients with AIDS who received pentamidine.

In preliminary studies, aerosolized pentamidine seems to have been much better tolerated.[170,171] Only a small amount of drug reaches the systemic circulation.[171] Untoward effects include bronchospasm, particularly in patients with a history of asthma or chronic obstructive pulmonary disease, pharyngeal irritation, and a metallic taste. Pretreatment with inhaled bronchodilators may prevent bronchospasm. If subsequent studies confirm the efficacy and safety of inhaled pentamidine, it may replace parenterally administered pentamidine and trimethoprim-sulfamethoxazole for the prevention of *P. carinii* in persons with AIDS.

DRUGS FOR TREATMENT OF TRYPANOSOMATIDAE

Members of the genera *Trypanosoma* and *Leishmania* are important pathogens. *Trypanosoma brucei gambiense* and *Tr. brucei rhodesience* cause African sleeping sickness. The early hemolymphatic stage of disease has traditionally been treated with suramin or pentamidine isethionate.[5] Neither of these compounds reaches therapeutic levels in the central nervous system. Once central nervous system involvement is documented, melarsoprol B, a highly toxic trivalent arsenical, has been the treatment of choice. In recent studies, eflornithine, an inhibitor of ornithine decarboxylase, has been shown to be effective even in patients with far advanced central nervous system involvement with *Tr. brucei gambiense*.[188–190] It has not been associated with serious toxicity. Although still experimental, eflornithine will probably emerge as the treatment of choice for *Tr. brucei gambiense*. The therapeutic situation is worse with *Trypanosoma cruzi*, the cause of Chagas disease in Central and South America.[191] The drug currently available, nifurtimox, is variably effective and frequently associated with sufficiently severe toxicity to necessitate discontinuation of therapy.[191] The alternative, benznidazole, seems to offer no advantage. Efforts continue to identify more effective, less toxic compounds.

The various *Leishmania* spp. produce cutaneous, mucosal, or visceral disease on every continent except Antarctica and Australia. The pentavalent antimonials, stibogluconate sodium, and meglumine antimoniate, are widely used for the treatment of leishmaniasis, but some *Leishmania* spp. (e.g., *Leishmania ethiopica*) and persons with syndromes such as mucosal leishmaniasis or diffuse cutaneous leishmaniasis respond poorly.[192] Pentamidine isethionate[166–168] and amphotericin B serve as alternative drugs. Several new compounds are currently under study.[192]

Suramin**

Suramin is a nonmetallic compound that is used for the treatment of the hemolymphatic stage of African trypanosomiasis.

It has also been used on occasion as chemoprophylaxis against *Tr. brucei gambiense* in persons working in highly endemic regions.[5] Suramin is also active against adult *Onchocerca volvulus*. When used to treat onchocerciasis, it is administered after a course of diethylcarbamazine, which kills microfilariae.

Suramin sodium is a white microcrystalline powder that is readily soluble in water.[193] It is dispensed in 1.0-g vials for parenteral administration. It cannot be given orally. Suramin binds to plasma proteins and persists at low levels in the serum for up to 3 months after infusion. There seems to be negligible metabolism of the drug. Suramin does not penetrate the central nervous system, which limits its usefulness to the hemolymphatic stage of African trypanosomiasis.

Its mechanism of action is uncertain, but at low concentrations suramin is known to inhibit multiple enzymes. It is a polyanion and forms firm complexes with proteins. The antitrypanosomal activity of suramin correlates with its inhibition of glycerol-3-phosphate oxidase and glycerol-3-phosphate dehydrogenase, parasitic enzymes involved in energy metabolism.[194]

Suramin causes a variety of untoward effects.[195] Immediate reactions include nausea, vomiting, shock, loss of consciousness, and occasionally death. Fever and urticaria may also occur. Later reactions, which appear up to 24 hours after administration, include fever, papular rash, exfoliative dermatitis, stomatitis, paresthesias of the palms and soles, photophobia, lacrimation, palpebral edema, and hyperesthesia. These may be followed by renal dysfunction with albuminuria, hematuria, and renal casts. Other reactions include chronic diarrhea and severe prostration. Jaundice, hemolytic anemia, and agranulocytosis are rare. The frequency and severity of side effects are more severe in malnourished hosts.[193] Suramin is relatively contraindicated in persons with pre-existing kidney or liver disease.

In persons treated for onchocerciasis, additional side effects occur, apparently due to the release of worm antigens. These include the formation of abscesses around the adult worms, papular eruptions and desquamation, and aggravation of ocular inflammation.

Melarsoprol**

Melarsoprol, or Mel B, is a trivalent arsenical used for the treatment of central nervous system trypanosomiasis. It is effective in some but not all cases. Melarsoprol is also potentially effective in treatment of the hemolymphatic phase, but it is too toxic to be recommended in that setting.

Melarsoprol is only slightly soluble in water, but it is readily soluble in propylene glycol, in which it is dispensed as a 3.6% weight/volume solution.[193] Melarsoprol is administered intravenously. A small but sufficient amount of the drug penetrates the central nervous system, where it can have a lethal effect on trypanosomes. Arsenicals react avidly with sulfhydryl groups. They thereby interact with a number of proteins and inactivate enzymes. This is the most likely mechanism of action against trypanosomes, as well as the cause of melarsoprol's pronounced toxicity. There is evidence to suggest that melarsoprol acts differentially on parasite pyruvate kinase, which is a terminal glycolytic enzyme.[196] Melarsoprol is oxidized to a nontoxic or less toxic pentavalent metabolite that is excreted.

Melarsoprol is a highly toxic drug.[197] Febrile reactions are common and may be accompanied by hypertension, abdominal pain, vomiting, and arthralgia. Reactive encephalopathy is the most serious side effect and results in death in approximately 6 percent of recipients.[198] It usually appears in the first 3 or 4 days of therapy. The clinical manifestations include headache, dizziness, mental dullness, confusion, and ataxia with progression to obtundation and seizures. Less common untoward effects include hemorrhagic encephalopathy and agranulocytosis. Allergic reactions including rashes may complicate subsequent courses of therapy. On occasion, the appearance of numerous casts in the urine or evidence of hepatotoxicity necessitates a modification of therapy. Severe hemolysis can occur in patients with G6PD deficiency. The gastrointestinal side effects can be reduced by administering the drug slowly to fasting patients. Melarsoprol therapy may precipitate erythema nodosum in patients who have leprosy.

Eflornithine*

Eflornithine (DL-α-difluoromethylornithine) has proven to be highly effective in the treatment of African sleeping sickness due to *Tr. brucei gambiense*, even in patients with advanced central nervous system disease.[188–190] Eflornithine has also been effective in 35–40 percent of patients with *P. carinii* pneumonia refractory to pentamidine and/or trimethoprim-sulfamethoxazole.[199–201]

Eflornithine hydrochloride can be administered intravenously or orally; 80 percent of the drug is excreted unchanged in the urine.[202] Serum levels during administration of 20 g/day by intravenous infusion approach 1200 nmol/ml; oral administration of 5 g every 4 hours produces levels of approximately 500 nmol/ml.[188] The ratio of cerebrospinal fluid to serum concentration ranges from 0.09 to 0.45.[188] The highest cerebrospinal fluid levels have been found in persons with the most severe central nervous system involvement. Eflornithine is an enzyme-activated, irreversible inhibitor of the enzyme ornithine decarboxylase, which is involved in the first step in the polyamine pathway. Polyamines play an essential role in the growth, differentiation, and replication of the trypanosomatids.[202–205]

Eflornithine is well tolerated. Adverse effects are usually mild and reversible. They include anemia, thrombocytopenia, leukopenia, nausea, vomiting, diarrhea, and transient hearing loss. Eflornithine is a much safer drug than either pentamidine, suramin, or melarsoprol, all of which it is likely to replace for the treatment of *Tr. brucei gambiense*. Further studies are needed to document its efficacy and to establish the optimal dose and duration of therapy.

Nifurtimox**

Nifurtimox, 4-[(5-Nitrofurfurylidene)amino]-3-methylthiomorpholine-1,1-dioxide, a nitrofuran, is the most widely used drug for the treatment of acute Chagas disease.[191,206] It can reduce the duration of symptoms of acute disease, and it decreases mortality due to myocarditis and meningoencephalitis. The level and duration of parasitemia are also reduced. However, in the clinical trials done to date, there have been significant numbers of treatment failures. There also seems to be geographic variation in responsiveness. Treatment has been found to be most effective in Argentina and Chile; therapy in Brazil and in some other countries has been less successful. Prolonged therapy for 120 days is recommended,[5] and it is not unusual for a treatment course to be terminated prematurely because of drug toxicity. The effectiveness of nifurtimox in the treatment of patients with the indeterminant phase or chronic Chagas disease has not been documented.

Nifurtimox is formulated as 100-mg tablets. It is well absorbed orally. Biotransformation occurs rapidly, and only low concentrations are found in blood and tissue.[193] Nifurtimox is active against both the trypomastigote and amastigote forms of *T. cruzi*. The trypanocidal action relates to the ability of nifurtimox to form reactive oxygen radicals that are toxic to the parasite.[206]

Toxicity is experienced by 40–70 percent of persons who receive nifurtimox. This is probably due, at least in part, to free radical formation and oxidative damage to host tissues.[207] Most of the symptoms are related to the gastrointestinal tract and the central and peripheral nervous systems.[193] Nifurtimox seems to be better tolerated by children than adults. Nausea, vomiting, abdominal pain, anorexia, and weight loss are common and may require premature termination of therapy. Neurologic sequelae include restlessness, disorientation, insomnia, twitching, paresthesias, polyneuritis, weakness, and stiffness. Convulsions may occur. Rashes, neutropenia, and decreased sperm counts have also been reported. The side effects are usually reversible with discontinuation of the drug, but they frequently pose a therapeutic dilemma given the prolonged course of therapy that is necessary. More effective, less toxic agents are clearly needed for the treatment of Chagas disease.

Benznidazole***

Benznidazole, a nitroimidazole derivative, is another relatively toxic drug that has been used for the treatment of Chagas disease.[191,208] It has not been studied as extensively as nifurtimox, but it seems to be of relatively similar efficacy.[209] Benznidazole is administered orally, usually for several weeks. Therapy is often limited by peripheral neuropathy, rash, or bone marrow suppression. It is not available for use in the United States.

Pentavalent Antimony; Stibogluconate Sodium** and Meglumine Antimoniate***

The leishmaniases are a group of clinical syndromes caused by multiple *Leishmania* spp. The manifestations of infection and the response to chemotherapy depend on the immune responses of the host, as well as the susceptibility of the causative organism to antimicrobial agents. The pentavalent antimonials, stibogluconate sodium and meglumine antimoniate, have been widely used for the treatment of leishmaniasis.[192] The compounds are thought to be of comparable efficacy and toxicity. Stibogluconate is the only pentavalent antimonial available in the United States. It has been the most extensively studied and is used in Africa and India.[210–212] Meglumine antimoniate is used in francophone countries, as well as in Central and South America.

The efficacy of the pentavalent antimonials varies with the leishmanial syndrome and the causative *Leishmania* sp. (see Chapter 252). Good responses are observed in the majority of persons with visceral leishmaniasis. Responses in persons with cutaneous leishmaniasis depend on the causative *Leishmania* sp. Pentamidine isethionate and amphotericin B have been used as alternative drugs when the antimonials fail. Efforts continue to develop new drugs active against the *Leishmania*. spp. Attention has focused on the pyrazolopyrimidines, allopurinol and allopurinol ribonucleoside[213–215]; on ketaconazole,[216] which appears to be effective in the treatment of some forms of New World leishmaniasis; on topical paromomycin with methylbenzethonium chloride for *Leishmania major* infection[217]; and on several other drugs.

Sodium stibogluconate is available in sterile aqueous solution for parenteral administration. It is supplied in 10-ml bottles; each milliliter contains 330 mg of drug, which is equivalent to 100 mg of pentavalent antimony. Meglumine antimoniate is available in 5-ml bottles, with 85 mg of antimony per milliliter. These drugs are prescribed on the basis of their antimony content. They can be administered intramuscularly but are usually given intravenously, either undiluted over a 5-minute period or diluted in 50 ml of 5% dextrose in water or saline and administered over 20 minutes. The antimony concentration in blood is best described by a three-compartment model, with a short initial distribution phase followed by biexponential elimination, primarily through the kidney.[218–220] The mean half-lives for the elimination phases have been reported to be 1.7 and 33 hours after intravenous administration and 2 and 766 hours after the drug is given intramuscularly. The slow terminal elimination phase may be due to conversion of pentavalent to trivalent antimony. The latter may be responsible for the toxicity seen with long-term, high-dose therapy. The mechanism of action is uncertain. Pentavalent antimony is concentrated in cells of reticuloendothelial origin, where the drug is thought to affect parasite metabolism.

The pentavalent antimonials are relatively well tolerated.[192,210,211,219,220] Most of the data on toxicity have come from studies of children or adolescents. Common adverse effects include abdominal pain, nausea, vomiting, malaise, headache, elevated transaminase levels, nephrotoxicity, weakness, myalgias, arthralgias, fever, skin rash, cough, and pneumonitis, but these seldom prevent completion of the treatment course. Dose-related changes are observed in the ECG. The most common are ST-T wave changes and prolonged Q-T intervals. Rarer but more serious effects are atrial and ventricular arrhythmias; sudden death has been associated with high-dose therapy. The use of pentavalent antimonials is relatively contraindicated in patients with myocarditis, hepatitis, and nephritis.

Pyrazolopyrimidines (Allopurinol and Allopurinol Ribonucleoside***)

Allopurinol, allopurinol riboside, and other purine analogues can inhibit the growth of *Leishmania* spp.[213–215] and *Tr. cruzi*.[191,221] The metabolism of purines in the kinetoplastids differs significantly from that in humans. The trypanosomatids rely on salvage pathways to obtain purine analogues, whereas humans synthesize purines de novo. Allopurinol, a pyrazolopyrimidine, inhibits *Leishmania* spp. and *Tr. cruzi* in vitro and in animal models. Allopurinol has been shown to be effective when administered with stibogluconate sodium to persons with visceral leishmaniasis who failed to respond to stibogluconate sodium alone.[215] The usefulness of allopurinol in humans has been limited by its rapid metabolism by xanthine oxidase. Allopurinol ribonucleoside, an inosine analogue, also is active against *Leishmania* spp. and some strains of *Tr. cruzi*. It is not metabolized as rapidly as allopurinol in humans and is currently being evaluated. Some other purine analogues, such as formycin B, are also lethal for these organisms but are too toxic to be used in humans.[221]

Amphotericin B and Ketaconazole

Amphotericin B has been used as an alternative drug in the treatment of visceral and mucocutaneous leishmaniasis.[222,223] The precise mechanism of its antiparasitic activity is uncertain, but it probably affects the parasite's surface membrane. Its use in the treatment of leishmaniasis is limited by its apprecible toxicity, the requirement for intravenous administration, and the prolonged course of therapy. Amphotericin B has also been used with miconazole and rifampin to treat amebic encephalitis due to *Naegleria* spp.[5] The pharmacokinetics and toxicity are detailed in Chapter 33.

Preliminary studies suggest that ketaconazole may be effective for the treatment of cutaneous leishmaniasis due to *Leishmania mexicana*.[216] Prospective, randomized, controlled studies are needed to document its efficacy, since the natural course of infection is self-resolution.

DRUGS FOR TREATMENT OF INTESTINAL NEMATODES (ROUNDWORMS)

The intestinal nematodes remain prevalent in areas of the world where sanitation is poor. As many as 80 percent of rural inhabitants in developing areas may be infected with one or more spp. In the United States, intestinal helminths are most likely to be encountered among immigrants from endemic areas or occasionally in returning travelers who have had intense rural exposure. Transmission of intestinal nematodes continues to occur in some areas of North America.

Mebendazole

Mebendazmole (Fig. 9), a synthetic benzimidazole, methyl 5-benzoylbenzimidazole-2 carbamate, is widely used for treat-

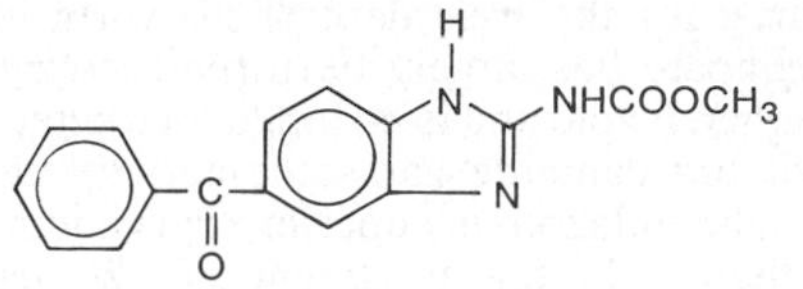

FIG. 9. Mebendazole.

ment of intestinal nematodes.[224] It is highly effective against *Ascaris lumbricoides*,[225] *Necator americanus* and *Ancylostoma duodenale*,[226] and *Trichuris trichiura*[225,227] at doses of 100 mg twice a day for 3 days. It is also effective in persons infected with more than one of these nematodes, which is the norm in impoverished areas.[226] Treatment over several days is often more effective than a single larger dose of mebendazole for these organisms. In contrast, *Enterobius vermicularis* responds to a single dose of 100 mg with a repeat dose given after 2 weeks.[227] The effect of mebendazole on *Strongyloides stercoralis* has been variable[228–231]; thiabendazole remains the drug of choice.[5] Mebendazole has been used at higher doses, 200 mg twice a day for 20 days, for the treatment of *Capillaria philippinensis*, an uncommon cause of chronic malabsorption in Southeast Asia.[224]

Mebendazole has been used at very high doses, 40 mg/kg body weight per day, for prolonged periods of time to treat inoperable cysts of *Echinococcus granulosus* and *E. multilocularis*.[232–235] Although usually not curative, mebendazole prevents progression of the primary lesion and suppresses or prevents metastasis. In general, mebendazole seems to be more effective against *E. multilocularis*. Mebendazole has also been used in the perioperative period to decrease the likelihood of peritoneal implants in case cyst contents are accidentally spilled at surgery.[236,237] Recent studies indicate that anthelmintic metabolites of albendazole attain higher serum and cyst concentrations than those of mebendazole. Albendazole will likely replace mebendazole for the treatment of inoperable echinococcosis.[238–241]

Mebendazole is active against adult *Trichinella spiralis* and appears to have some activity against invading larvae.[242,243] No comparative data are available for humans, but mebendazole has been relatively effective in the treatment of experimental trichinosis in animals and is much less toxic than thiabendazole. Some recommend it for human trichinosis. Mebendazole has activity against two filaria spp., *Loa loa* and *Mansonella perstans*.[244,245] It is considered the drug of choice, 100 mg twice a day for 30 days, for *M. perstans*,[244] against which diethylcarbamazine is not active. Diethylcarbamazine remains the treatment of choice for *L. loa*.

Mebendazole is dispensed in 100-mg tablets. It is only slightly soluble in water and is poorly absorbed from the gastrointestinal tract.[246] This contributes to its low frequency of side effects but limits its usefulness in treating tissue larvae. Up to 10 percent of an orally administered dose of mebendazole is recovered within 48 hours in the urine. Most of the drug excreted by the kidney is the decarboxylated metabolite. Mebendazole selectively blocks glucose uptake by nematodes without affecting blood glucose levels in the host.[246] It selectively blocks microtubule assembly in helminths.[247] Parasite immobilization and death follow, but it can take several days for susceptible nematodes to be cleared from the gastrointestinal tract. Mebendazole also inhibits the development of the ova of hookworms and *Trichuris*.

Side effects are uncommon when mebendazole is used at low doses (100 mg twice a day for 3 days) for the treatment of the common intestinal helminths.[224,246] Transient abdominal pain and diarrhea occur in a small number of persons, usually those with massive parasite burdens. Migration of adult *A. lumbricoides* to the nose or mouth occurs occasionally. Mebendazole produce embryotoxicity and teratogenicity in pregnant rats after a single oral dose of 10 mg/kg; it is therefore contraindicated in pregnant women.[248]

At the high doses (40 mg/kg/day) used for the treatment of inoperable echinococcal cysts, systemic side effects such as alopecia, liver enzyme abnormalities, and transient bone marrow suppression with severe but reversible neutopenia have been observed.[224,249,250] The white blood cell count should be followed closely after initiation of high-dose therapy, since neutropenia is usually observed within the first 30 days.

Albendazole* and Flubendazole***

Neither of these benzimidazole compounds is licensed for use in the United States. Albendazole, methyl (5-(propylthio)-1H-benzimidazol-2-yl) carbamate, has a broad spectrum of activity. It is highly effective when used in a single dose of 400 mg for oral treatment of intestinal helminth infections including *A. lumbricoides, Tri. trichiura*, and the hookworms.[251–255] It is thus ideally suited for mass treatment programs. Albendazole at high doses (10 mg/kg body weight per day for 28 days, followed by a 2-week rest period, then repeated for up to five cycles) appears to be more effective against inoperable echinococcal cysts than mebendazole.[238–240] Albendazole may also be effective in preventing postsurgical recurrence of echinococcal cysts, as demonstrated by animal and, less conclusively, human data.[241] Albendazole has activity against tapeworms in the human intestine, but it is less active than niclosamidc.[253] Finally, albendazole (15 mg/kg for 1 month) has recently been shown to be effective in the treatment of a small group of patients with parenchymal neurocysticercosis.[256]

Albendazole is dispensed as 200-mg tablets or as a 2% solution for oral administration. It is not well absorbed. It is metabolized to albendazole sulfoxide in the liver. This metabolite is scolicidal and achieves relatively high levels in serum and within echinococcal cysts. Albendazole is well tolerated when used in single-dose regimens for intestinal helminths. High-dose, prolonged therapy for echinococcal disease has occasionally been complicated by hepatitis and obstructive jaundice.[257] The liver toxicity has reversed after discontinuation of the drug.

Flubendazole is the parafluoro analogue of mebendazole. It has a spectrum of activity against intestinal helminths that is similar to that of mebendazole. Flubendazole is not as well absorbed. Initially, flubendazole was thought to lack teratogenicity, but recent animal studies suggest that it is teratogenic when administered by gavage.[258] Flubendazole has also led to clinical improvement in a small group of persons with neurocysticercosis, but given its poor absorption, it is unlikely to replace praziquantel for the treatment of cysticercosis.[259]

Thiabendazole

Thiabendazole, 2-(4′-thiazolyl)-1H-benzimidazole, is among the most potent anthelmintic drugs,[260] but its use has been limited by the high frequency of untoward effects. Thiabendazole is active against a number of adult nematodes that infect the gastrointestinal tract and against larvae in tissues. It is much better absorbed then mebendazole. The most common indication for thiabendazole is the treatment of *S. stercoralis*[5,261,262] or *S. fuelleborni*[263] infection. It is also used for *Trichostrongylus* infections,[264] cutaneous larvae migrans,[265] visceral larva migrans,[261] and trichinosis.[5,266,267] Some cases of human trichinosis have shown marked clinical improvement with thiabendazole. Anti-inflammatory, antipyretic, and analgesic effects of thiabendazole may have contributed to the clinical response. Studies in animals experimentally infected with *Trich. spiralis* suggested that some but not all larvae are killed by thiabendazole. Although thiabendazole is active against the hookworms, *A. lumbricoides, Ent. vermicularis*, and, to a lesser extent, *Tri. trichiura*,[261] mebendazole in general has higher response rates and is far less toxic.

Thiabendazole is available in 500-mg tablets and as an oral suspension of 500 mg/5 ml. It is rapidly absorbed after oral administration; peak concentrations occur in plasma about 1 hour after treatment.[246] It is recommended that the drug be given with meals. Unfortunately, no parenteral preparation is available, which poses a problem for some patients with disseminated *S. stercoralis* infection. Most of the drug is excreted in urine within 24 hours as 5-hydroxythiabendazole conjugated as the glucuronide or as the sulfate. The precise mechanism of action is not known. Thiabendazole inhibits the fumarate reductase of susceptible helminths, and this may prevent them from eliminating reducing equivalents such as succinic acid.[268–270] Recent studies suggest that thiabendazole, like mebendazole, may interfere with microtubule assembly.[271]

Approximately half of the persons who receive thiabendazole experience one or more side effects. Most frequent are nausea, anorexia, vomiting, and dizziness.[246] Less common are diarrhea, epigastric pain, pruritus, drowsiness, giddiness, and headache. Rare side effects include tinnitus, abnormal sensation in the eyes, numbness, decreased pulse and blood pressure, elevated liver enzymes, and progressive bile duct injury.[246,272] Seizures have been reported in a child with Down syndrome.[273] Transient neutropenia has been observed in some patients. Allergic manifestations such as fever, facial flush, angioneurotic edema, lymphadenopathy, perianal rash, and skin rashes are also observed; some or all of these may be due to the release of parasite antigens or the underlying disease process. Thiabendazole can give urine an asparagus-like odor, and crystalluria has been observed. Because of the central nervous system effects, activities requiring alertness should be avoided during therapy. The drug should be used with caution in persons with hepatic disease or decreased hepatic function. Thiabendazole has been found to be genotoxic in in vitro and in vivo assays,[274] and it is relatively contraindicated in pregnancy.

Pyrantel Pamoate

Pyrantel pamoate is recommended for the treatment of *Ent. vermicularis, A. lumbricoides, N. americanus*, and *Ancylostoma duodenale*.[275,276] It is considered an alternative drug for *Trichostrongylus* infection. It is not active against the whipworm, *Tri. trichura*. Oxantel***, an m-oxyphenol derivative that has not been licensed in the United States, is effective against *Tri. trichura*.

Pyrantel is available as a suspension (250 mg of pyrantel base/5 ml). It is poorly absorbed; less than 15 percent is excreted in the urine as the parent drug or metabolite.[277–279] Pyrantel and its analogues are depolarizing neuromuscular blocking agents. The resulting nicotinic activation results in spastic paralysis of the worm. Pyrantel also inhibits acetylcholinesterases. There is depolarization and increased spike discharge frequency in muscle cells of susceptible nematodes.

Pyrantel pamoate has minimal toxicity at the oral doses used to treat intestinal helminths. Mild, transient gastrointestinal symptoms, headache, drowsiness or insomnia, and dizziness are occasionally encountered. The nitrosated metabolites of pyrantel pamoate are mutagenic in bacteria. Pyrantel pamoate has not been studied in pregnancy, and it is not recommended for pregnant women or children under 1 year of age. Pyrantel and piperazine, which produces hyperpolarization with a reduction in spike wave activity in helminthic muscle cells, appear to be mutually antagonistic and should not be used together.[277–278]

Pyrvinium pamoate***

Pyrvinium pamoate, a cyanide dye, is an alternative drug for the treatment of *Ent. vermicularis*.[280,281] It is still considered an alternative drug for the treatment of pinworm infections, but pyrvinium pamoate has largely been replaced by pyrantel pamoate and mebendazole and is no longer marketed in the United States. Pyrvinium pamoate has some activity against *S. stercoralis*, but thiabendazole is superior. Pyrvinium pamoate has not been effective in the treatment of *Tri. trichura* or *N. americanus*.

Pyrvinium pamoate is a deep red crystalline solid that is insoluble in water.[279] It is available in tablets containing 50 mg of pyrvinium base and as a suspension containing the equivalent of 10 mg of pyrvinium base per milliliter. Its anthelmintic activity is thought to be associated with inhibition of respiration in aerobic organisms and with interference with the absorption of exogenous glucose in intestinal helminths.

Pyrvinium pamoate is generally well tolerated. Side effects, which occur in a minority of recipients, include nausea, vomiting, and abdominal cramping. Emesis has been associated with the suspension. It is recommended that the tablets be swallowed without chewing. Patients should be told that the drug will color stools bright red and that the suspension will stain if spilled. Pyrvinium pamoate is genotoxic in *Saccharomyces cerevisiae*, but little if any of it is absorbed after oral administration, and human and animal studies have not demonstrated mutagenic metabolites in the urine after a single therapeutic dose.[282]

Piperazine

Piperazine citrate is effective in the treatment of *A. lumbricoides*. It has largely been replaced in the United States by mebendazole, which is less toxic, but piperazine is less expensive and is still used in some developing areas. Piperazine also has activity against *Ent. vermicularis*. Piperazine derivatives have a broad range of pharmacologic activity. Some substituted piperazines are central serotonin agonists; others depress monosynaptic spinal cord excitation, block chloride channels, have antioxidant effects, display antiarrhythmic activity, or act as vasodilators. One, diethylcarbamazine, is effective against filariae.

Piperazine salts are available as tablets containing 250 mg and as syrups and suspensions containing 100 per milliliter.[246] Piperazine is well absorbed orally. Some of the drug is metabolized; the remainder is excreted in the urine. Piperazine causes flaccid paralysis of susceptible intestinal helminths. It acts as a low-potency agonist at extrasynaptic γ-aminobutyric acid (GABA) receptors on the bag region of *Ascaris suum*.[283] Activation of these receptors gives rise to an increase in chloride conductance. There is also hyperpolarization and suppression of spontaneous action potentials.[284] Worms are excreted alive, usually without migrating.

Piperazine is generally well tolerated. On occasion, there are gastrointestinal symptoms, transient neurologic side effects, or urticarial reactions. Lethal overdoses are associated with convulsions and respiratory depression. Epileptic activity may be exaggerated, and piperazine is contraindicated in persons with a history of seizures.[285] Neurotoxicity has also been observed in persons with impaired renal function. Visual disturbances, ataxia, and hypotonia occur rarely.[286] The drug has been used during pregnancy without apparent adverse effects, but it has not been thoroughly evaluated in this setting. Although adverse dermatologic reactions are rare, they have been reported in persons sensitized to topical ethylenediamine.[287]

DRUGS FOR TREATMENT OF SYSTEMIC NEMATODES

Diethylcarbamazine*

Diethylcarbamazine (Fig. 10) is a piperazine derivative, *N,N*-diethyl-4-methyl-1-piperazinecarboxamide dihydrogen citrate. It results in the rapid destruction of microfilariae of *Wuchereria*

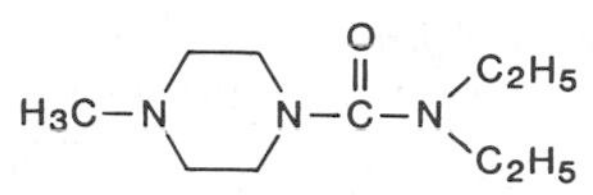

FIG. 10. Diethylcarbamazine.

bancrofti, Brugia malayi, and *B. timori*, the three lymphatic-dwelling filariae infecting humans.[288,289] There is presumptive evidence that it kills the adult worms of these species, and it currently is the drug of choice for each of them. It has been successfully used in community-based mass treatment programs.[290] Diethylcarbamazine is also the treatment of choice for *L. loa*[5,291] and has been recommended for *Mansonella ozzardi*,[5] but the results have been variable.[292,293] It has been used successfully to treat persons with pulmonary infiltrates with eosinophilia in the tropics,[294] presumably because this syndrome is in many instances caused by microfilariae in the lungs. Diethylcarbamazine has also been used as an alternative mode of therapy for visceral larva migrans, with variable success.[295]

Diethylcarbamazine rapidly kills microfilariae of *Onchocerca volvulus* in the skin and eye, but the resulting inflammatory reaction can cause severe damage.[296–298] Prednisone and antihistamines have been administered concomitantly to limit inflammation. Diethylcarbamazine does not affect adult *O. volvulus*, and microfilariae reaccumulate after completion of therapy[299] unless suramin (see above under "Drugs for Treatment of Trypanosomatidae") is administered concurrently to kill adult worms. Ivermectin, which has not yet been licensed in the United States, has emerged as the drug of choice for the treatment of onchocerciasis.

Diethlycarbamazine is available in 50-mg tablets.[246] It is readily absorbed from the gastrointestinal tract. Peak blood levels are reached in 1–2 hours; the serum half-life is approximately 8 hours.[300] The parent compound and its metabolites are cleared through the kidney.[301,302] Diethylcarbamazine is distributed equally throughout all body compartments except adipose tissue, and there is little accumulation even after repeated doses are given. The drug seems to have two types of effects on microfilariae. First, it is associated with a decrease in muscle activity, leading eventually to immobilization of the worm.[303] The piperazine moiety may result in hyperpolarization, resulting in the observed paralysis.[246] Second, the drug appears to alter the surface membranes of microfilariae, resulting in enhanced killing by the host's immune system.[304,305] Diethylcarbamazine has also been shown to enhance the adherence properties of eosinophils and polymorphonuclear leukocytes,[306] and there is evidence to suggest that platelets may mediate the action on microfilariae.[307] Untoward effects include those produced directly by the drug and inflammatory reactions that follow the release of filarial antigens. Common reactions include headache, malaise, weakness, arthralgia, anorexia, nausea, and vomiting. The gastrointestinal effects are usually dose related. Acute psychotic reactions have been reported but are rare.

During treatment of onchocerciasis with diethylcarbamazine, systemic reactions include severe pruritus, edema of the skin, fever, hypotension, heightened eosinophilia, lymphadenopathy, splenomegaly, and proteinuria.[308,309] Ocular complications may result in permanent sequelae and include visual field constriction, optic nerve pallor, chorioretinitis, anterior uveitis, and punctate keratitis.[296–299,308–311] These systemic and ocular reactions are apparently due to the release of filarial antigens and generally correlate with the degree of microfilaremia in the skin and eye. They follow the onset of therapy and may be severe. The acute effects usually last for only 3–7 days. The elicitation of such reactions by even low doses of diethylcarbamazine is the basis for the Mazzotti test,[312] which has been used to diagnose onchocerciasis. Steroids are usually administered to patients with ocular involvement who receive diethlycarbamazine. Ivermectin also is microfilaricidal, but kills slowly and is much less toxic. It has replaced diethylcarbamazine for the treatment of persons with ocular onchocerciasis. In *W. bancrofti* and *B. malayi* infections, localized swellings or nodules may develop along lymphatics, and there may be accompanying lymphadenitis.[309] Transient hydrocele formation or lymphedema may be observed. Encephalopathy has occurred rarely in persons treated for *L. loa*.

Ivermectin*

Ivermectin is the 22,23-dihydro derivative of avermectin B1, a macrocyclic lactone produced by the actinomycete *Streptomyces avermitilis*.[313] It is active at low doses against a broad spectrum of nematodes and blood-sucking arthropod parasites of animals. One of the major recent advances in anthelmintic therapy has been the introduction of ivermectin for treatment of human onchocerciasis.[296–299,313–315] Ivermectin kills microfilariae in the skin as well as in the eye, but the local inflammatory responses are less severe than with diethylcarbamazine. This is particularly important in the eye, where microfilariae disappear slowly after ivermectin therapy. Ivermectin does not kill adult *O. volvulus*, but it does inhibit oviposition. It is active against other filarial pathogens such as *W. bancrofti*.[316] Ivermectin has an extremely broad spectrum of antinematodal activity.[313] It is now widely used in veterinary practice for control and treatment of helminthic and arthropod infestations.

Ivermectin is odorless and colorless, and has been effective when administered as a single oral or parenteral dose. It is concentrated in the liver and adipose tissues. Only a small percentage of the drug is excreted in the urine; the rest is excreted in the stool. Ivermectin acts by blocking signal transmission from interneurons to excitatory motor neurons. GABA is the neurotransmitter that is blocked, but ivermectin does not appear to compete with GABA for binding and does not bind directly to the GABA binding site.[313] In animals, GABA-mediated nerves are present only in the central nervous systems, whereas they are found in peripheral muscle in susceptible invertebrates. Ivermectin is usually well tolerated. The initiation of therapy in persons with onchocerciasis may be complicated by fever, pruritus, headache, and cutaneous edema, but the side effects are less frequent and less severe than those of diethylcarbamazine or suramin.[296–299,313–315] In cattle, 30 times the recommended dose was tolerated without signs of toxicity, but death was reported at 40 times the recommended dose. No teratogenicity has been reported in animals.

DRUGS FOR TREATMENT OF PLATHYHELMINTHS: TREMATODES (FLUKES) AND CESTODES (TAPEWORMS)

Praziquantel

The most important recent addition to the therapeutic armamentarium against helminths has been praziquantel (Fig. 11), 2-(cyclohexylcarbonyl-(1,2,3,6,7,11b)-hexyahydro-4H-pyrazino(2,1-*a*)isoquinoline-4-one), a compound that has a broad spectrum of activity against tematodes and cestodes, is well absorbed orally, is given in several doses in 1 or a few days, and has mild untoward effects.[18,317–320] Praziquantel is highly

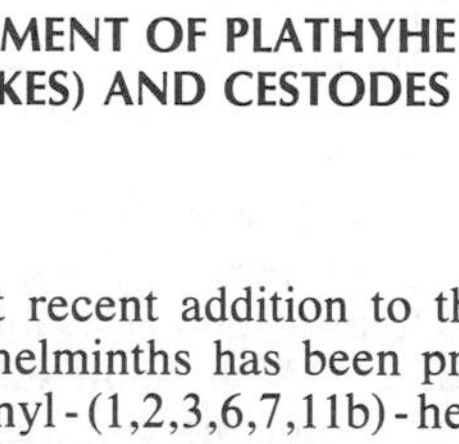

FIG. 11. Praziquantel.

effective against all of the *Schistosoma* spp. that infect humans,[317–330] includin *S. japonicum*, against which there was previously no good form of chemotherapy. It has even been effective in the treatment of *S. japonicum* infection of the central nervous system.[331] Praziquantel is also the drug of choice for the liver flukes *Clonorchis sinensis* and *Opisthorchis viverrini*,[317–320,332–334] the lung flukes *Paragonimus westermani, P. kellicoti*, and other *Paragonimus* spp.[317–320,335–338] and the intestinal flukes *Heterophyes heterophyes, Fasciolopsis buski*, and *Metagonimus yokogawai*.[317–320] Only against the liver fluke, *Fasciola hepatica*, have praziquantel failures been frequent.[339,340]

Praziquantel is also highly active against adult and larval forms of the cestodes.[317–319] Although double-blind, placebo-controlled studies have not been performed, the cumulative experience indicates that praziquantel is the drug of choice for the treatment of neurocysticercosis due to *Taenia solium*.[341–349] It is very effective in the treatment of parenchymal disease. Praziquantel is less effective when there is subarachnoid involvement and is ineffective against cysts in the ventricular system[349] or eye.[350,351] Some prefer praziquantel for the treatment of intestinal *Ta. solium* infestation.[352] It is highly effective against adult *Ta. saginata, Diphyllobothrium latum*, and *D. pacificum*,[352] but niclosamide is equally effective, less expensive, has fewer side effects, and is therefore more widely used against those organisms. In the case of *Hymenolepis nana*, praziquantel may be preferable to niclosamide; praziquantel can be given as a single dose, whereas niclosamide must be given daily for 6 days. Unfortunately, praziquantel is unlikely to be effective in the treatment of human hydatid disease. It is active against adult *Echinococcus* spp. in the canine gastrointestinal tract and damages protoscolices in hydatids, but the germinal layer of the hydatid is not destroyed.[353–357]

Praziquantel is a heterocyclic pyrazino-isoquinoline derivative with an unusually broad range of anthelmintic activity. It is dispensed as 600-mg tablets. The drug is crystalline and nearly colorless.[318,319] It is nearly insoluble in water. A peak serum concentration of 1 μm/ml is reached 1–2 hours after an oral dose of 50 mg/kg body weight is administered. Praziquantel is approximately 80 percent protein bound. There is pronounced first pass metabolism.[358] Approximately 80 percent of praziquantel is excreted in the urine in 4 days; 90 percent of that amount is excreted within the first 24 hours. The remainder is excreted in the feces. The pharmacokinetics of the drug were not significantly altered in one patient undergoing hemodialysis. The concentration of praziquantel in the cerebrospinal fluid is approximately 14–20 percent of the concentration of free plus protein-bound drug in the plasma.[359,360] Plasma levels have been decreased in patients with neurocysticercosis receiving dexamethasone simultaneously.

Praziquantel is rapidly taken up by flukes and tapeworms. It is uniformly distributed in these organisms but is not metabolized. Praziquantel increases the permeability of the flukes' tegument to calcium ions.[361–364] In adult schistosomes, an influx of calcium is followed by tetanic contraction and paralysis of the musculature. The initial effects are very rapid, and intense vacuolation of the tegument is observed.[361] Adult worms are then swept to the liver, where they are attacked by phagocytes. Praziquantel also results in increased exposure of parasite antigens on the surface of adult schistosomes.[365] In the tapeworm *Hymenolepis diminuta*, praziquantel causes calcium release from endogenous stores, and the worm suffers massive contraction.[366] Expulsion from the gastrointestinal tract follows. The tegument of the neck of the tapeworm develops blebs, but the scolex and proglottids appear to be unaffected.

Praziquantel is generally well tolerated.[317–320] Reactions are common, but are usually mild and transient. The most frequent ones are nausea, vomiting, abdominal pain, dizziness, headache, and lassitude. Only rarely is vomiting severe. In some instances, adverse effects may be due to allergic responses that follow the release of worm antigens. For example, urticarial reactions have been observed during the treatment of paragonimiasis.[367] Intense abdominal pain and bloody diarrhea have on occasion occurred in patients heavily infected with *Schistosoma mansoni*.[368–370] Finally, increased intracranial pressure, cerebral edema, and inflammation have been observed during the treatment of neurocysticercosis, and corticosteroids are now used concomitantly in this setting.[371,372] There has been no evidence of mutagenicity or teratogenicity in vitro, but there is an increase in the abortion rate in rats given three times the single human therapeutic dose. Praziquantel is also excreted in breast milk, and it is recommended that women not nurse on the day that praziquantel is given or during the subsequent 72 hours.

Metrifonate***

Metrifonate, an organophosphate that is metabolized in humans to dichlorvos,[373] is an alternative to praziquantel for the treatment of *Schistosoma hematobium*. Metrifonate is less expensive than praziquantel and of comparable efficacy, and it has been used in mass treatment programs.[374,375]

Metrifonate is an organophosphorus inhibitor of acetylcholinesterase.[376] It is well absorbed after oral ingestion.[377] When given to humans, metrifonate causes a decrease of 95 percent in plasma cholinesterase activity within 6 hours of administration. This activity usually returns to normal relatively quickly. Erythrocyte cholinesterase is inhibited to approximately 50 percent of pretreatment values but takes 2 or 2.5 months to return to normal levels.[377] Persons treated with metrifonate should not receive neuromuscular blocking agents or be exposed to insecticides with anticholineserase effects for at least 48 hours. Although the drug is usually well tolerated, mild vertigo, lassitude, nausea, vomiting, and occasionally bronchospasm have been reported. One limitation in large-scale treatment programs is that metrifonate must be given at intervals of 2 weeks, whereas praziquantel is administered in 1 day.

Oxamniquine

Oxamniquine, a tetrahydroquinoline, provides an alternative to praziquantel for the treatment of *S. mansoni* infections.[378–381] It seems to be more effective against strains of *S. mansoni* found in the New World, and it is less expensive than praziquantel. Oxamniquine has been used in mass treatment programs; a large-scale control program based on community therapy has been quite successful in Brazil.[382]

Oxamniquine is dispensed in 250-mg capsules. It is well absorbed orally, and the parent drug and its metabolites are excreted in the urine. It is given as a single dose. Side effects include dizziness, which may occur in 40 percent of the treated population, and drowsiness. Convulsions have occasionally been reported, and oxamniquine should not be used in persons with epilepsy. Orange to red discoloration of the urine has been associated with treatment.

Niridazole***

Niridazole, a nitrothiazole derivative, 1-(5-nitro-2-thiazolyl)-2-imidazolidinone, once widely used for the treatment of schistosomiasis,[383,384] is now seldom if ever indicated. It is far more toxic than praziquantel, metrifonate, and oxamniquine and offers no advantage in efficacy. In addition to schistosomiasis, it is effective in the treatment of dracunculiasis (guinea worm disease), where it acts by reducing swelling and pain and permitting relatively easy extraction of the adult worm.[383]

Niridazole is absorbed orally over several hours and is largely metabolized in the liver.[383] It can cause agitation, confusion, hallucinations, seizures, and electroencephalographic changes, particularly in persons with impaired hepatic function due to hepatosplenic schistosomiasis. It should not be used in persons with hepatic dysfunction or neuropsychiatric disorders.[385] Niridzole can also produce electrocardiographic changes, as well as transitory decreases in fertility. Other side effects include nausea, vomiting, diarrhea, loss of appetite, and headache. Less commonly encountered are insomnia, skin rash, and paresthesis. Niridazole can initiate hemolysis in persons with G6PD deficiency.[386]

Oltipaz***

Oltipaz is a new antischistosomal compound that has been studied in human schistosomiasis. Although it appears to be effective in the treatment of *S. mansoni* infection,[387] it offers no advantage over praziquantel.

Bithionol**

Bithionol is the drug of choice for treatment of *F. hepatica*[5] and is an alternative to praziquantel for the treatment of paragonimiasis.[388] Bithionol is administered orally, usually on alternate days, for 10–15 doses. It has been associated with urticaria, photosensitivity reactions, and gastrointestinal complaints. These allergic reactions may be due, in part or solely, to the release of worm antigens.

Niclosamide

Niclosamide (Fig. 12), *N*-(2′-chloro-4′-nitrophenyl)-5-chlorosalicylamide, given as a single dose, is the drug of choice for *Ta. saginata*, the beef tapeworm, *D. latum*, the fish tapeworm, and *Dipylidium caninum*, the dog tapeworm.[389] It is poorly absorbed, less expensive and less toxic than praziquantel, and highly effective against adult cestodes in he gastrointestinal tract. In the case of *Taenia solium*, treatment with niclosamide is usually followed by a purge to reduce the theoretical risk of autoinfection. Niclosamide results in disintegration of the adult tapeworm. Some physicians prefer to use quinacrine (see above under "Drugs Active Against Luminal Protozoa") for *Ta. solium*, since it causes the expulsion of the adult worm intact. Others prefer praziquantel, which is active against larval as well as adult forms, and might prevent cysticercosis if autoinfection occurred. Niclosamide is as active against *H. nana*, the dwarf tapeworm, as is praziquantel, but a single dose of praziquantel is effective, whereas niclosamide must be administered daily for 6 days.[5]

Niclosamide is very poorly absorbed and nontoxic. It is supplied in 500-mg vanilla-flavored tablets, which should be chewed thoroughly and then washed down with water. The anthelminthic mechanisms of niclosamide are not completely understood. The drug appears to uncouple oxidative phosphorylation in the scolex and proximal segments of the adult tapeworm and to stimulate adenosine triphosphatase activity of mitochondria, resulting in death of the worm and rapid disintegration of the scolex.[390] Niclosamide is remarkably free of toxicity, except for occasional mild gastrointestinal complaints, light-headedness, and, rarely, rash. Information on side effects has been collected in an uncontrolled manner, and it is uncertain whether a placebo group would differ significantly in respect to these symptoms.[391] When expulsion of the worm is delayed, neither the scolex nor the proglottids may be identifiable in the stool.

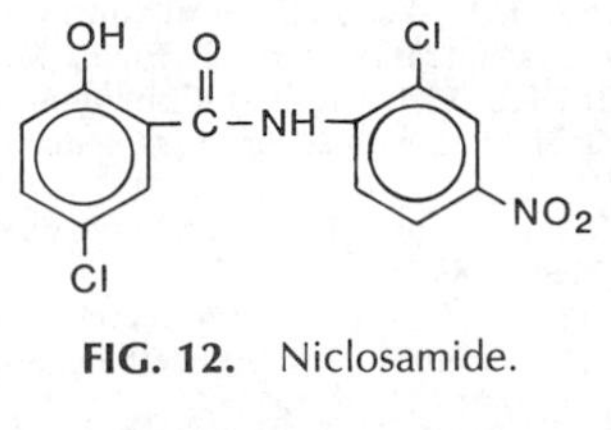

FIG. 12. Niclosamide.

REFERENCES

1. Lee JJ, Hutner SH, Bovee EC. An Illustrated Guide to the Protozoa. Lawrence, Kans.: Society of Protozoologists; 1985.
2. Levine ND. Nematode Parasites of Domestic Animals and of Man. Minneapolis: Burgess; 1968.
3. Burt DRR. Platyhelminthes and Parasitism. An Introduction to Parasitology. New York: American Elsevier; 1970.
4. Erasmus DA. The Biology of Trematodes. New York: Crane, Russak; 1972.
5. Drugs for parasitic infections. Med Lett Drugs Ther. 1988;30:15–22.
6. Powell SJ, Wilmot AJ, Elsdon-Dew R. Further trials of metronidazole in amoebic dysentery and amoebic liver abscess. Ann Trop Med Parasitol. 1967;61:511–4.
7. Welsh JS, Rowsell BJ, Freeman C. Treatment of intestinal amoebiasis and giardiasis: Efficacy of metronidazole and tinidazole compared. Med J Aust. 1978;1:469–71.
8. Salaki JS, Shirey JL, Strickland GT. Successful treatment of symptomatic *Entamoeba polecki* infection. Am J Trop Med Hyg. 1979;28:190–3.
9. Wolfe MS. Giardiasis. N Engl J Med. 1978;298:319–21.
10. Lerman SJ, Walker RA. Treatment of giardiasis. Literature review and recommendations. Clin Pediatr. 1982;21:409–14.
11. Lossick JG. Treatment of *Trichomonas vaginalis* infections. Rev Infect Dis. 1982;4(Suppl):S801–18.
12. Rein MF. Current therapy of vulvovaginitis. Sex Transm Dis. 1981;8:316–20.
13. Wolfe MS. *Blastocystis hominis* infection. In: Strickland GT, ed. Hunter's Tropical Medicine. 6th ed. Philadelphia: Saunders; 1984:513.
14. Walzer PD, Judson FN, Murphy KB, et al. Balantidiasis outbreak in Truk. Am J Trop Med Hyg. 1973;22:33–41.
15. Spillman R, Ayala SC, DeSanchez CE. Double blind test of metronidazole and tinidazole in the treatment of asymptomatic *Entamoeba histolytica* and *Entamoeba hartmanni* carriers. Am J Trop Med Hyg. 1976;25:549–51.
16. Dupont HL, Sullivan PS. Giardiasis: The clinical spectrum, diagnosis and therapy. Pediatr Infect Dis. 1986;5:S131–8.
17. Sharma VP, Rathore HS, Sharma MM. Efficacy of metronidazole in dracunculiasis: A clinical trial. Am J Trop Med Hyg. 1979;28:658–60.
18. Weniger BG, Schantz PM. Praziquantel and refugee health. JAMA. 1984;251:2391–2.
19. Houghton GW, Smith J, Thorpe PS, et al. The pharmacokinetics or oral and intravenous metronidazole in man. J Antimicrob Chemother. 1979;5:621–3.
20. McGilveray IJ, Midha KK, Loo JCK, et al. The bioavailability of commercial metronidazole formulations. Int J Clin Pharmacol. 1978;16:110–5.
21. Norris SM, Ravdin JI. The pharmacology of antiamebic drugs. In: Ravdin JI, ed. Amebiasis: Human Infection by *Entamoeba histolytica*. New York: Wiley; 1988:734–40.
22. Lindmark DG, Müller M. Antitrichomonad action, mutagenicity, and reduction of metronidazole and other nitroimidazoles. Antimicrob Agents Chemother. 1976;10:476–82.
23. Knight RC, Skolimowski IM, Edwards DI. The interaction of reduced metronidazole with DNA. Biochem Pharmacol. 1978;27:2089–93.
24. LaRusso NF, Tomasx M, Müller M, et al. Interaction of metronidazole with nucleic acids in vitro. Mol Pharmacol. 1977;13:872–82.
25. Lefebver Y, Hesseltine HC. The peripheral white blood cells and metronidazole. JAMA. 1965;194:15–8.
26. Kazmier FJ. A significant interaction between metronidazole and warfarin. Mayo Clin Proc. 1976;51:782–4.
27. Kusumi RK, Plouffe JF, Wyatt RH, et al. Central nervous system toxicity associated with metronidazole therapy. Ann Intern Med. 1980;93:59–60.
28. Rothstein E, Clancy DD. Toxicity of disulfiram combined with metronidazole. N Engl J Med. 1969;280:1006–7.
29. Rosenkranz HS, Speck WT. Studies on the significance of the mutagenicity of metronidazole for *Salmonella typhimurium*. In: Finegold SM, ed. Metronidazole, Proceedings of the International Metronidazole Conference, Montreal, Quebec, Canada, May 26–28, 1976. Princeton, N.J.: Excerpta Medica; 1977:119–25.
30. Koch RL, Beaulieu BB Jr, Chrystal EJT, et al. A metronidazole metabolite in human urine and its risk. Science. 1981;211:398–400.
31. Beard CM, Noller KL, O'Fallon WM, et al. Lack of evidence for cancer due to use of metronidazole. N Engl J Med. 1979;301:519–22.
32. Friedman GD, Cancer after metronidazole (Letter). N Engl J Med. 1980;302:519.
33. Bassily S, Farid Z, El-Masry NA, et al. Treatment of intestinal *E. histolytica* and *G. lamblia* with metronidazole, tinidazole and ornidazole: A comparative study. J Trop Med Hyg. 1987;90:9–12.
34. Goldman P. The development of 5-nitroimidazoles for the treatment and prophylaxis of anaerobic bacterial infections. J Antimicrob Chemother. 1982;10(Suppl A):23–33.
35. Rossignol JF, Maisonneuve H, Cho YW. Nitroimidazoles in the treatment of trichomoniasis, giardiasis, and amebiasis. Int J Clin Pharmacol Ther Toxicol. 1984;22:63–72.
36. Powell SJ, Wilmot AJ, MacLeod IN, et al. A comparative trial of dehydroemetine and emetine hydrochloride in identical dosage in amoebic liver abscess. Ann Trop Med Parasitol. 1967;61:26–8.

37. Scragg JN, Powell SJ. Emetine hydrochloride and dehydroemetine combined with chloroquine in the treatment of children with amoebic liver abscess. Arch Dis Child. 1968;43:121–3.
38. Yang WCT, Dubick M. Mechanism of emetine cardiotoxicity. Pharmacol Ther. 1980;10:15–26.
39. Grollman AP. Inhibitors of protein synthesis. V. Effects of emetine on protein and nucleic acid biosynthesis in HELA cells. J Biol Chem. 1968;243:4089–94.
40. Klatskin G, Friedman H. Emetine toxicity in man: Studies on the nature of early toxic manifestations, their relation to the dose level, and their significance in determining safe dosage. Ann Intern Med. 1948;28:892–915.
41. Webster LT Jr. Drugs used in the chemotherapy of protozoal infections: Amebiasis, giardiasis, and trichomoniasis. In: Gilman AG, Goodman LS, Rall TW, et al, eds. The Pharmacological Basis of Therapeutics. 7th ed. New York: Macmillan; 1985:1049–57.
42. Kent L, Kingsland RC. Effects of emetine hydrochloride on the electrocardiogram in man. Am Heart J. 1950;39:576–87.
43. Bradley WG, Fewings JD, Harris JB, et al. Emetine myopathy in the rat. Br J Pharmacol. 1976;57:29–41.
44. Oakley GP Jr. The neurotoxicity of the halogenated hydroxyquinolines. JAMA. 1973;225:395–7.
45. Wolfe MS. The treatment of intestinal protozoal infections. Med Clin North Am. 1982;66:707–20.
46. Krogstad DJ, Spencer HC Jr, Healy GR. Amebiasis. N Engl J Med. 1978;298:262–5.
47. Pehrson P, Bengtsson E. Treatment of non-invasive amoebiasis. A comparison between tinidazole alone and in combination with diloxanide furoate. Trans R Soc Trop Med Hyg. 1983;77:845–6.
48. Wolfe MS. Nondysenteric intestinal amebiasis: Treatment with diloxanide furoate. JAMA. 1973;224:1601–4.
49. Simon M, Shookhoff HB, Terner H, et al. Paromomycin in the treatment of intestinal amebiasis: A short course of therapy. Am J Gastroenterol. 1967;48:504–11.
50. Soderman WA Jr. Amebiasis (clinical seminar). Am J Dig Dis. 1971;16:51–60.
51. Botero D. Paromomycin as effective treatment of *Taenia* infections. Am J Trop Med. 1970;19:234–7.
52. Smith JW, Wolfe MS. Giardiasis. Ann Rev Med. 1980;31:373–83.
53. Craft JC, Murphy T, Nelson JD. Furizolidone and quinacrine. Comparative study of therapy for giardiasis in children. Am J Dis Child. 1981;135:164–6.
54. Bassily S, Farid Z, Mikhail JW, et al. The treatment of *Giardia lamblia* infection with mepacrine, metronidazole and furazolidone. J Trop Med Hyg. 1970;73:15–8.
55. Rollo IM. Miscellaneous drugs used in the treatment of protozoal infections. In: Gilman AG, Goodman LS. Gilman A, eds. The Pharmacological Basis of Therapeutics. 6th ed. New York: Macmillan; 1980:1070–9.
56. Findlay GM. Recent Advances in Chemotherapy. v. II. 3rd ed. London: J & A Churchill; 1951:341–68.
57. Sokol RJ, Lichtenstein PK, Farrell MK. Quinacrine hydrochloride-induced yellow discoloration of the skin in children. Pediatrics. 1982;69:232–3.
58. Lindenmayer JP, Vargas P. Toxic psychosis following use of quinacrine. J Clin Psychiatry. 1981;42:162–4.
59. Wolfe MS. Giardiasis. JAMA. 1975;233:1362–5.
60. Pratt WB, Fekety R. Chemotherapy in protozoal diseases. In: The Antimicrobial Drugs. New York: Oxford University Press; 1986:385–413.
61. Levi GC, de Avila CA, Neto VA. Efficacy of various drugs for treatment of giardiasis. A comparative study. Am J Trop Med Hyg. 1977;26:564–5.
62. Wyler DJ. Malaria—resurgence, resistance, and research. N Engl J Med. 1983;308:875–8, 934–40.
63. Hilton D. Malaria: A new battle plan. Contact. 1987;95:1–5.
64. Lobel HO, Campbell CC, Pappaioanou M, et al. Use of prophylaxis for malaria by American travelers to Africa and Haiti. JAMA. 1987;257:2626–7.
65. Remington JS, Desmonts G. Toxoplasmosis. In: Remington JS, Klein JO, eds. Infectious Diseases of the Fetus and Newborn Infant. 2nd ed. Philadelphia: Saunders; 1983:143–263.
66. Wong B, Gold JWM, Brown AE, et al. Central-nervous-system toxoplasmosis in homosexual men and parenteral drug abusers. Ann Intern Med. 1984;100:36–42.
67. Current WL, Reese NC, Ernst JV, et al. Human cryptosporidiosis in immunocompetent and immunodeficient persons: Studies of an outbreak and experimental transmission. N Engl J Med. 1983;308:1252–7.
68. Kaufman DL. *Pneumocystis carinii* pneumonia. Adv Exp Med Biol. 1986;202:153–69.
69. Kovacs JA, Hiemenz JW, Macher AM, et al. *Pneumocystis carinii* pneumonia: A comparison between patients with the acquired immunodeficiency syndrome and patients with other immunodeficiencies. Ann Intern Med. 1984;100:663–71.
69a. Edman JC, Kovacs JA, Mazur H, et al. Ribosomal RNA sequence shows *Pneumocystis carinii* to be a member of the fungi. Nature. 1988;334:519–22.
70. Krogstad DJ, Herwaldt BL, Schlesinger PH. Antimalarial agents: Specific treatment regimens. Antimicrob Agents Chemother. 1988;32:957–61.
71. Development of mefloquine as an antimalarial drug. *Bull WHO*. 1983;61:169–78.
72. Chloroquine-resistant *Plasmodium falciparum* malaria in West Africa. JAMA. 1987;257:2556–9.
73. LeBras J, Hatin I, Bouree P, et al. Chloroquine-resistant falciparum malaria in Benin. Lancet. 1986;2:1043–4.
74. Miller LH, Neva FA, Gill F. Failure of chloroquine in human babesiosis (*Babesia microti*): Case report and chemotherapeutic trial in hamsters. Ann Intern Med. 1978;88:200–2.
75. Brohult J, Rombo L, Sirleaf V, et al. The concentration of chloroquine in serum during short and long term malaria prophylaxis with standard and "double" dosage in non-immunes: Clinical implications. Ann Trop Med Parasitol. 1979;73:401–5.
76. Webster LT Jr. Drugs used in the chemotherapy of protozoal infections: Malaria. In: Gilman AG, Goodman LS, Rall TW, et al, eds. The Pharmacological Basis of Therapeutics. 7th ed. New York: Macmillan; 1985:1029–48.
77. Andrews P, Haberkorn A, Thomas H. Antiparasitic drugs: Mechanisms of action, pharmacokinetics, and in vitro and in vivo assays of drug activity. In: Lorian V, ed. Antibiotics in Laboratory Medicine. 2nd ed. Baltimore: Williams & Wilkins; 1986;282–345.
78. Warhurst DC. Antimalarial drugs: Mode of action and resistance. J Antimicrob Chemother. 1986;18(Suppl B):51–9.
79. Warhurst DC, Homewood CA, Baffaley VC. The chemotherapy of rodent mlaria. XX. Autophagic vacuole formation in *Plasmodium berghei* in vitro. Ann Trop Med Parasitol. 1974;68:265–81.
80. Konigk E, Putfarken B. Inhibition of ornithine decarboxylase in vitro cultured *Plasmodium falciparum* by chloroquine. Tropenmed Parasitol. 1983;34:1–3.
81. Krogstad DJ, Schlesinger PH. The basis of antimalarial action: Non-weak base effects of chloroquine on acid vesicle pH. *Am J Trop Med Hyg*. 1987;36:213–20.
82. Krogstad DJ, Schlesinger PH. Acid-vesicle function, intracellular pathogens and the action of chloroquine against *Plasmodium falciparum*. N Engl J Med. 1987;317:542–9.
83. Martin SK, Oduola AMJ, Milhous WK. Reversal of chloroquine resistance in *Plasmodium falciparum* by verapamil. Science. 1987;235:899–901.
84. Marks JS. Chloroquine retinopathy: Is there a safe daily dose? Ann Rheum Dis. 1982;41:52–8.
85. White NJ, Watt G, Bergvist Y, et al. Parenteral chloroquine for treating falciparum malaria. J Infect Dis. 1987;155:192–201.
86. Riou B, Barriot P, Rimailho A, et al. Treatment of severe chloroquine poisoning. N Engl J Med. 1988;318:1–6.
87. Hart CW, Naunton RF. The ototoxicity of chloroquine phosphate. Arch Otolaryngol. 1964;80:407–12.
88. Hatton CSR, Peto TEA, Bunch C, et al. Frequency of severe neutropenia associated with amodiaquine prophylaxis against malaria. Lancet. 1986;1:411–4.
89. Cook GC. *Plasmodium falciparum* infection: Problems in prophylaxis and treatment in 1986. Q J Med. 1986;61:1091–115.
90. Saxena AK, Saxena M. Advances in chemotherapy of malaria. Prog Drug Res. 1986;30:221–80.
91. Looareesuwan S, White NJ, Chittamas S, et al. High rate of *Plasmodium vivax* relapse following treatment of falciparum malaria in Thailand. Lancet. 1987;2:1052–5.
92. Alving AS, Johnson CF, Tarlov AR, et al. Mitigation of the haemolytic effect of primaquine and enhancement of its action against exoerythrocytic forms of the Chesson strain of *Plasmodium vivax* by intermittent regimens of drug administration: A preliminary report. Bull WHO. 1960;22:621–31.
93. Clyde DF, McCarthy VC. Radical cure of Chesson strain vivax malaria in man by 7, not 14, days of treatment with primaquine. Am J Trop Med Hyg. 1977;26:562–3.
94. Kellermeyer RW, Tarlov AR, Brewer GJ, et al. Hemolytic effect of therapeutic drugs: Clinical considerations of the primaquine-type hemolysis. JAMA. 1962;180:388–94.
95. Clyde DF. Clinical problems associated with the use of primaquine as a tissue schizontocidal and gametocytocidal drug. Bull WHO. 1981;59:391–5.
96. Brodie BB, Baer JE, Craig LC. Metabolic products of the cinchona alkaloids in human urine. J Biol Chem. 1951;188:567–81.
97. White NJ, Looareesuwan S, Warrell DA, et al. Quinine pharmacokinetics and toxicity in cerebral and uncomplicated falciparum malaria. Am J Med. 1982;73:564–72.
98. Canfield CJ, Miller LH, Bartelloni PJ, et al. Acute renal failure in *Plasmodium falciparum* malaria. Arch Intern Med. 1968;122:199–203.
99. Pratt WB, Fekety R. Chemotherapy of malaria. In: The Antimicrobial Drugs. New York: Oxford University Press; 1986:355–84.
100. White JN, Warrell DA, Chanthavanich P, et al. Severe hypoglycemia and hyperinsulinemia in falciparum malaria. N Engl J Med. 1983;309:61–6.
101. Phillips RE, Looareesunwan S, White NJ, et al. Quinine pharmacokinetics and toxicity in pregnant and lactating women with falciparum malaria. Br J Clin Pharmacol. 1986;21:677–83.
102. Phillips RE, Warrell DA, White NJ, et al. Intravenous quinidine for the treatment of severe falciparum malaria. N Engl J Med. 1985;312:1273–8.
103. Rudnitsky G, Miller KD, Padua T, et al. Continuous-infusion quinidine gluconate for treating children with severe *Plasmodium falciparum* malaria. J Infect Dis. 1987;155:1040–3.
104. Swerdlow CD, Yu JO, Jacobsen E, et al. Safety and efficacy of intravenous quinidine. Am J Med. 1983;75:36–42.
105. Botero D, Restrepo M, Montoya A. Prospective double-blind trial of two different doses of mefloquine plus pyrimethamine-sulfadoxine compared

with pyrimethamine-sulfadoxine alone in the treatment of falciparum malaria. Bull WHO. 1985;63:731–7.
106. De Sousa JM, Sheth UK, Oliveira RMG, et al. An open, randomized, phase III clinical trial of mefloquine and of quinine plus sulfadoxime-pyrimethamine in the treatment of symptomatic falciparum malaria in Brazil. Bull WHO. 1985;63:603–9.
107. Tin F, Hlaing N, Tun T, et al. Falciparum malaria treated with a fixed combination of mefloquine, sulfadoxine and pyrimethamine: A field study in adults in Burma. Bull WHO. 1985;63:727–30.
108. Chongsuphajaisiddhi T, Sabchareon A, Chantavanich P, et al. A phase-III clinical trial of mefloquine in children with chloroquine-resistant falciparum malaria in Thailand. Bull WHO. 1987;65:223–6.
109. Oduola AMJ, Milhous WK, Salako LA, et al. Reduced in-vitro susceptibility to mefloquine in West African isolates of *Plasmodium falciparum*. Lancet. 1987;2:1304–5.
110. Desjardins RW, Pamplin CL III, von Bredow J, et al. Kinetics of a new antimalarial, mefloquine. Clin Pharmacol Ther. 1979;26:372–9.
111. Jacobs GH, Aikawa M, Milhous WK, et al. An ultrastructural study of the effects of mefloquine on malaria parasite. Am J Trop Med Hyg. 1987;36:9–14.
112. Chanthavanich P, Looareesuwan S, White NJ, et al. Intragastic mefloquine is absorbed rapidly in patients with cerebral malaria. Am J Trop Med Hyg. 1985;34:1028–36.
113. Harinasuta T, Bunnag D, Wensdorfer WH. A phase II clinical trial of mefloquine in patients with chloroquine-resistant falciparum malaria in Thailand. Bull WHO. 1983;61:299–305.
114. Meek SR, Doberstyn EB, Gaürzère BA, et al. Treatment of falciparum malaria with quinine and tetracycline or combined mefloquine/sulfadoxine/pyrimethamine on the Thai–Kampuchean border. Am J Trop Med Hyg. 1986;35:246–50.
115. Centers for Diease Control. Recommendations for the prevention of malaria in travelers. MMWR. 1988;37:277–84.
116. Pearson RD, Hewlett EL. Use of pyrimethamine-sulfadoxine (Fansidar) in prophylaxis against chloroquine-resistant *Plasmodium falciparum* and *Pneumocystis carinii*. Ann Intern Med. 1987;106:714–18.
117. DeHovitz JA, Pape JW, Boncy M, et al. Clinical manifestations and therapy of *Isospora belli* infection in patients with the acquired immunodeficiency syndrome. N Engl J Med. 1986;315:87–90.
118. Hughes WT, Feldman S, Chaudhary SC, et al. Comparison of pentamidine isethionate and trimethoprim-sulfamethoxazole in the treatment of *Pneumocystis carinii* pneumonia. J Pediatr. 1978;92:285–91.
119. Young LS. Trimethoprim-sulfamethoxazole in the treatment of adults with pneumonia due to *Pneumocystis carinii*. Rev Infect Dis. 1982;4:608–13.
120. Siegel SE, Wolff LJ, Baehner RL, et al. Treatment of *Pneumocystis carinii* pneumonitis: A comparative trial of sulfamethoxazole-trimethoprim v. pentamidine in pediatric patients with cancer: Report from Childrens Cancer Study Group. Am J Dis Child. 1984;138:1051–4.
121. Luft BJ, Conley F, Remington JS. Outbreak of central-nervous-system toxoplasmosis in Western Europe and North America. Lancet. 1983;1:781–4.
122. Haverkos HW. Assessment of therapy for toxoplasma encephalitis. The TE study group. Am J Med. 1987;82:907–14.
123. Luft BJ, Remington JS. Toxoplasmic encephalitis. J Infect Dis. 1988;157:1–6.
124. Wilson CB, Remington JS. Toxoplasmosis. In: Feigin RD, Cherry JD, eds. Textbook of Pediatric Infectious Diseases. 2nd ed. Philadelphia: Saunders; 1987:2067–78.
125. McCabe R, Remington JS. Toxoplasmosis: The time has come. N Engl J Med. 1988;318:313–5.
126. Allegra CJ, Chabner BA, Tuazon CU, et al. Trimetrexate for the treatment of *Pneumocytis carinii* pneumonia in patients with the acquired immunodeficiency syndrome. N Engl J Med. 1987;317:978–85.
127. Kovacs JA, Allegra CJ, Chabner BA, et al. Potent effect of trimetrexate, a lipid-soluble antifolate, on *Toxoplasma gondii*. J Infect Dis. 1987;155:1027–32.
128. Daffos F, Forestier F, Capella-Pavlovsky M, et al. Prenatal management of 746 pregnancies at risk for congenital toxoplasmosis. N Engl J Med. 1988;318:271–5.
129. Weidekamm E, Plozza-Nottebrock H, Forgo I, et al. Plasma concentrations of pyrimethamine and sulfadoxine and evaluation of pharmacokinetic data by computerized curve fitting. Bull WHO. 1982;60:115–22.
130. Jaffe JJ. Dihydrofolate reductase in parasitic protozoa and helminths. In: Van den Bossche H, ed. Biochemistry of Parasites. London: Academic Press: 1972;219–33.
131. Hayama T, Kokue E. Use of the Goettingen miniature pig for studying pyrimethamine teratogenesis. CRC Crit Rev Toxicol. 1985;14:403–21.
132. Petter C, Bourbon J. Foetal red cell macrocytosis induced by pyrimethamine; its teratogenic role. Experientia. 1975;31:369–70.
133. Pyrimethamine combinations in pregnancy. Lancet. 1983;2:1005–7.
134. Harpey, JP, Darbois Y, LeFèbvre G. Teratogenicity of pyrimethamine (Letter). Lancet. 1983;2:399.
135. Mandell GL, Sande MA. Antimicrobial agents: Sulfonamides, trimethoprim-sulfamethoxazole, and urinary tract antiseptics. In: Gilman AG, Goodman LS, Rall TW, et al, eds. The Pharmacological Basis of Therapeutics. 7th ed. New York: Macmillian; 1985:1095–1114.
136. Navin TR, Miller KD, Satriale RF, et al. Adverse reactions associated with pyrimethamine-sulfadoxine prophylaxis for *Pneumocystis carinii* infections in AIDS (Letter). Lancet. 1985;1:1332.
137. Miller KD, Lobel HO, Satriale RF, et al. Severe cutaneous reactions among American travelers using pyrimethamine-sulfadoxine (Fansidar) for malaria prophylaxis. Am J Trop Med Hyg. 1986;35:451–8.
138. Rombo L, Stenbeck J, Lobel HO, et al. Does chloroquine contribute to the risk of serious adverse reactions to Fansidar? Lancet. 1985;2:1298–9.
139. Karbwang J, Bunnag D, Breckenridge AM, et al. The pharmacokinetics of mefloquine when given alone or in combination with sulphadoxine and pyrimethamine in Thai male and female subjects. Eur J Clin Pharmacol. 1987;32:173–7.
140. De Sousa JM, Sheth UK, Oliveira RMG, et al. A phase I clinical trial of Fansimef (mefloquine plus sulfadoxine-pyrimethamine) in Brazilian male subjects. Bull WHO. 1985;63:611–5.
141. Young LS. Treatment and prevention of *Pneumocystis carinii* infection. In: Young LS, ed. *Pneumocystis carinii* Pneumonia: Pathogenesis, Diagnosis, Treatment. New York: Marcel Dekker; 1984:175–94.
142. Wharton JM, Coleman DL, Wolfsy CB, et al. Trimethoprim-sulfamethoxazole or pentamidine for *Pneumocystis carinii* pneumonia in the acquired immunodeficiency syndrome. Ann Intern Med. 1986;105:37–44.
143. Hughes WT. Five year absence of *Pneumocystis carinii* pneumonitis in a pediatric oncology center. J Infect Dis. 1984;150:305–6.
144. Hughes WT, Rivera GK, Schell MJ, et al. Successful intermittent chemoprophylaxis for *Pneumocystis carinii* pneumonitis. N Engl J Med. 1987;316:1627–32.
145. Jick H. Adverse reactions to trimethoprim-sulfamethoxazole in hospitalized patients. Rev Infect Dis. 1982;4:426–8.
146. Pratt WB, Fekety R. The antimetabolites. In: The Antimicrobical Drugs, New York: Oxford University Press; 1986:229–51.
147. Kaufman DL. *Pneumocystis carinii* pneumonia. Adv Exp Med Biol. 1986;202:153–69.
148. Gordin FM, Simon GL, Wofsy CB, et al. Adverse reactions to trimethoprim-sulfamethoxazole in patients with the acquired immunodeficiency syndrome. Ann Intern Med. 1984;100:495–9.
149. Small CB, Harris CA, Friedland GH, et al. The treatment of *Pneumocystis carinii* pneumonia in the acquired immunodeficiency syndrome. Arch Intern Med. 1985;145:837–40.
150. Leoung GS, Mills J, Hopewell PC, et al. Dapsone-trimethoprim for *Pneumocystis carinii* pneumonia in the acquired immunodeficiency syndrome. Ann Intern Med. 1986;105:45–8.
151. Medina I, Leoung G, Mills J, et al. Oral therapy for *Pneumocystis carinii* pneumonia in AIDS: A randomized double blind trial for trimethoprim-sulfamethoxazole versus dapsone-trimethoprim for first episode (abstract). Third International Conference on AIDS, Washington, D.C., June 1–5, 1987.
152. Metroka CE, Lange R, Braun N, et al. Successful chemoprophylaxis for *Pneumocystis carinii* pneumonia with dapsone in patients with AIDS and ARC (abstract). Third International Conference on AIDS, Washington, D.C., June 1–5, 1987.
153. Mandell GL, Sande MA. Antimicrobial agents: Drugs used in the chemotherapy of tuberculosis and leprosy. In: Gilman AG, Goodman LS, Rall TW, et al, eds. *The Pharmacological Basis of Therapeutics*. 7th ed. New York: Macmillan; 1985:1199–218.
154. Pratt WB, Fekety R. Drugs that act on mycobacteria: Isoniazid, rifampin, ethambutol, and streptomycin; the minor antituberculosis drugs; drugs effective against leprosy. In: Pratt WB, Fekety R, eds. The Antimicrobial Drugs. New York: Oxford University Press; 1986:277–314.
155. Cook GC. Prevention and treatment of malaria. Lancet. 1988:1:32–7.
156. Rollo IM. The mode of action of sulphonamides, Proguanil and pyrimethamine on *Plasmodium gallinaceum*. Br J Pharmacol Chemother. 1955;10:208–14.
157. Fogh S, Schapira A, Bygbjerg IC, et al. Malaria chemoprophylaxis in travellers to East Africa: A comparative prospective study of chloroquine plus proguanil with chloroquine plus sulfadoxine-pyrimethamine. Br Med J. 1988;296:820–2.
158. Araujo FG, Guptill DR, Remington JS. In vivo activity of piritrexin against *Toxoplasma gondii*. J Infect Dis. 1987;156:828–30.
159. Lakhanpal V, Schocket SS, Nirankari VS. Clindamycin in the treatment of toxoplasmic retinochoroiditis. Am J Ophthalmol. 1983;95:605–13.
160. Ferguson JG Jr. Clindamycin therapy for toxoplasmosis. Ann Ophthalmol. 1981;13:95–100.
161. Clindamycin and quinine treatment for *Babesia microti* infections. MMWR. 1983;32;65–6.
162. Chan J, Luft BJ, Activity of roxithromycin (RU28965), a macrolide, against *Toxoplasma gondii* infection in mice. Antimicrob Agents Chemother. 1986;30:323–4.
163. Hofflin JM, Remington JS. In vivo synergism of roxithromycin (RU965) and interferon against *Toxoplasma gondii*. Antimicrob Agents Chemother. 1987;31:346–8.
164. King H, Lourie EM, York W. Studies in chemotherapy XIX: Further report on new trypanocidal substances. Ann Trop Med Parasitol. 1938;32:117–92.
165. Kager PA, Rees PH, Manguyu FM, et al. Clinical, haematological and parasitological response to treatment of visceral leishmaniasis in Kenya: A study of 64 patients. Trop Geogr Med. 1984;36:21–35.
166. Jha TK. Evaluation of diamidine compound (pentamidine isethionate) in the treatment of resistant cases of kala-azar occurring in North Bihar, India. Trans R Soc Trop Med Hyg. 1983;77:167–70.
167. Thakur CP. Epidemiological, clinical and therapeutic features of Bihar kala-azar (including post kala-azar dermal leishmaniasis). Trans R Soc Trop Med Hyg. 1984;78:391–8.

168. Kluge RM, Spaulding DM, Spain AJ. Combination of pentamidine and trimethoprim-sulfamethoxazole in the therapy of *Pneumocystis carinii* pneumonia in rats. Antimicrob Agents Chemother. 1978;13:975–8.
169. Montgomery AB, Debs JR, Luce JM, et al. Aerosolised pentamidine as sole therapy for *Pneumocystis carinii* pneumonia in patients with acquired immunodeficiency syndrome. Lancet. 1987;2:480–3.
170. Conte JE Jr, Hollander H, Golden JA. Inhaled or reduced-dose intravenous pentamidine for *Pneumocystis carinii* pneumonia. Ann Intern Med. 1987;107:495–8.
171. Bernard E, Schmitt H, Pagel L, et al. Safety and effectiveness of aerosol pentamidine for prevention of PCP in patients with AIDS (abstract). 27th Interscience Conference on Antimicrobial Chemotherapy. New York: 1987.
171a. Corkery KJ, Luse JM, Montgomery AB. Aerosolized pentamidine for treatment and prophylaxis of *Pneumocystis carinii* pneumonia: An update. Respiratory Care. 1988;33:676–85.
172. Pearson RD, Hewlett EL. Pentamidine for the treatment of *Pneumocystis carinii* pneumonia and other protozoal diseases. Ann Intern Med. 1985;103:782–6.
173. Navin TR, Fontaine RE. Intravenous versus intramuscular administration of pentamidine (Letter). N Engl J Med. 1984;311:1701–2.
174. Williamson J. Effects of trypanosides on the fine structure of target organisms. Pharmacol Ther. 1979;7:445–512.
175. Croft SL, Brazil RP. Effect of pentamidine isethionate on the ultrastructure and morphology of *Leishmania mexicana amazonensis* in vitro. Ann Trop Med Parasitol. 1982;76:37–43.
176. Waring MJ. The effects of antimicrobial agents on ribonucleic acid polymerase. Mol Pharmacol. 1965;1:1–13.
177. Wallis OC. The effect of pentamidine on ribosomes of the parasitic flagellate *Crithidia* (*Strigomonas*) *oncopelti*. J Protozool. 1966;13:234–9.
178. Gutteridge WE. Some effects of pentamidine di-isethionate on *Crithidia fasciculata*. J Protozool. 1969;16:306–11.
179. Bachrach U, Brem S, Wertman SB, et al. *Leishmania* spp: Effect of inhibitors on growth and on polyamine and macromolecular syntheses. Exp Parasitol. 1979;48:464–70.
180. Waalkes TP, Makulu DR. Pharmcologic aspects of pentamidine. Natl Cancer Inst Monogr. 1976;43:171–7.
181. Geratz JD. Inhibitory effect of aromatic diamidines on trypsin and enterokinase. Experientia. 1969;25:1254–5.
182. Hill GC, Hutner SH. Effect of trypanocidal drugs on terminal respiration of *Crithidia fasciculata*. Exp Parasitol. 1968;22;207–12.
183. Walzer PD, Perl DP, Krogstad DJ, et al. *Pneumocystis carinii* pneumonia in the United States: Epidemiologic, diagnostic, and clinical features. Ann Intern Med. 1974;80:83–93.
184. Western KA, Perera DR, Schultz MG. Pentamidine isethionate in the treatment of *Pneumocystis carinii* pneumonia. Ann Intern Med. 1970;73:695–702.
185. Bouchard P, Sai P, Reach G, et al. Diabetes mellitus following pentamidine-induced hypoglycemia in humans. Diabetes. 1982;31:40–5.
186. Osei K, Falko JM, Nelson KP, et al. Diabetogenic effect of pentamidine: In vitro and in vivo studies in a patient with malignant insulinoma. Am J Med. 1984;77:41–6.
187. Fitzgerald DB, Young IS. Reversal of pentamidine-induced hypoglycemia with oral diazoxide. J Trop Med Hyg. 1984;87:15–9.
188. Taelman H, Schechter PJ, Marcelis L, et al. Difluoromethylornithine, an effective new treatment of Gambian trypanosomiasis. Am J Med. 1987;82:607–14.
189. Di Bari C, Pastore G, Roscigno G, et al. Late-stage African trypanosomiasis and eflornithine (Letter). Ann Intern Med. 1986;105:803–4.
190. Van Nieuwenhove S, Schechter PJ, Declercq J, et al. Treatment of gambiense sleeping sickness in the Sudan with oral DFMO (DL-α-difluoromethylornithine), an inhibitor of ornithine decarbopxylase; first field trial. Trans R Soc Trop Med Hyg. 1985;79:692–8.
191. Marr JJ, Docampo R. Chemotherapy for Chagas' disease: A perspective of current therapy and considerations for future research. Rev Infect Dis. 1986;8:884–903.
192. Pearson RD, Navin TR, Sousa AQ, et al. Leishmaniasis. In: Kass EH, Platt R, eds. Current Therapy in Infectious Diseases. Toronto: BC Decker; 1989, in press.
193. Webster LT Jr. Drugs used in the chemotherapy of protozoal infections: Leishmaniasis, trypanosomiasis and other protozoal infections. In: Gilman AG, Goodman LS, Rall TW, et al, eds. The Pharmacological Basis of Therapeutics. 7th ed. New York: Macmillan; 1985:1058–65.
194. Fairlamb AH, Bowman IB. *Trypanosoma brucei*: Suramin and other trypanocidal compounds: Effects on sn-glycerol-3 phosphate oxidase. Exp Parasitol. 1977;43:353–61.
195. Fuglsang H, Anderson J. Side effects of suramin. In: Research and Control of Onchocerciasis in the Western Hemisphere. Pan American Health Organization, Scientific Publication No 298:54–7.
196. Flynn IW, Bowman IBR. Further studies on the mode of arsenicals on trypanosome pyruvate kinase (Abstract). Trans R Soc Trop Med Hyg. 1969;63:121.
197. Robertson DHH. Chemotherapy of African trypanosomes. Practitioner. 1962;188:80–3.
198. Arrox JOL. Melarsoprol and reactive encephalopathy in *Trypanosoma brucei rhodesiense*. Trans R Soc Trop Med Hyg. 1987;81:192.
199. Golden JA, Sjoerdsma A, Santi DV. *Pneumocystis carinii* pneumonia treated with alpha-difluoromethylornithine. West J Med. 1984;141:613–23.
200. Gilman TM, Paulson YJ, Boylen CT, et al. Eflornithine treatment of *Pneumocystis carinii* pneumonia in AIDS. JAMA. 1986;256:2197–8.
201. McLess BD, Barlow JLR, Kuzma RJ, et al. Studies on successful eflornithine treatment of *Pneumocystis carinii* pneumonia in AIDS patients failing conventional therapy (Abstract). Third International Conference on AIDS, Washington, D.C., June 1–5, 1987.
202. Bacchi CJ. Content, synthesis, and function of polyamines in trypanosomatids: Relationship to chemotherapy. J Protozool. 1981;28:20–7.
203. Sjoerdsma A, Schechter PJ. Chemotherapeutic implications of polyamine biosynthesis inhibition. Clin Pharmacol Ther. 1984;35:287–300.
204. Brener Z. Present status of chemotherapy and chemoprophylaxis of human trypanosomiasis in the Western Hemisphere. Pharmacol Ther. 1979;7:71–90.
205. Haegele KD, Alken RG, Grove J, et al. Kinetics of alpha-difluromethylornithine: An irreversible inhibitor of ornithine decarboxylase. Clin Pharmacol Ther. 1981;30:210–7.
206. Docampo R, Morena SNJ. Free radical metabolites in the mode of action of chemotherapeutic agents and phagocytic cells on *Trypanosoma cruzi*. Rev Infect Dis. 1984;6:223–38.
207. Moreno SNJ, Palmero DJ, de Palmero KE, et al. Stimulation of lipid peroxidation and ultrastructural alternations by nifurtimox in mammalian tissues. Medicina (B Aires). 1980;40:553–9.
208. Apt W, Arribada A, Arab F, et al. Clinical trial of benznidazole and an immunopotentiator against Chagas' disease in Chile (Letter). Trans R Soc Trop Med Hyg. 1986;80:1010.
209. Andrade SG, Magalhaes JB, Pontes AL. Evaluation of chemotherapy with benznidazole and nifurtimox in mice infected with *Trypanosoma cruzi* strains of different types. Bull WHO. 1985;63:721–6.
210. Anabwani GM, Ngira JA, Dimiti G, et al. Comparison of two dosage schedules of sodium stibogluconate in the treatment of visceral leishmaniasis in Kenya. Lancet. 1983;1;210–2.
211. Report of a WHO Expert Committee. The leishmaniases. Geneva: WHO Technical Report Series 701; 1984.
212. Ballou WR, McClain JB, Gordon DM, et al. Safety and efficacy of high-dose sodium stibogluconate therapy of American cutaneous leishmaniasis. Lancet. 1987;2:13–6.
213. Marr JJ, Berens RL. Pyrazolopyrimidine metabolism in the pathogenic trypanosomatides. Mol Biochem Parasitol. 1983;7:339–56.
214. Neal RA, Croft SL, Nelson DJ. Anti-leishmanial effect of allopurinol ribonucleoside and the related compounds, allopurinol, thiopurinol, thiopurinol ribonucleoside, and of formycin B, sinefungin and the lepidine WR 6026. Trans R Soc Trop Med Hyg. 1985;79:122–8.
215. Kager PA, Rees PH, Wellde BT, et al. Allopurinol in the treatment of visceral leishmaniasis. Trans R Soc Trop Med Hyg. 1981;75:556–9.
216. Weinrauch L, Livshin R, El-On J. Cutaneous leishmaniasis: Treatment with ketaconazole. Cutis. 1983;32:288–9, 294.
217. El-On J, Weinrauch L, Livshin R, et al. Topical treatment of recurrent cutaneous leishmaniasis in ointment containing paromomycin and methylbenzethionium chloride. Br Med J. 1985;291:704–5.
218. Chulay JD, Fleckenstein L, Smith DH. Pharmacokinetics of antimony during treatment of visceral leishmaniasis with sodium stibogluconate or meglumine antimoniate. Trans R Soc Trop Med Hyg. 1988;82:69–72.
219. Information material for physicians—Pentostam (sodium antimony gluconate), HHS, PHS, CDC protocol. Provided by the Centers for Disease Control to physicians administering Pentostam in the United States.
220. Berman JD. Chemotherapy for leishmaniasis: Biochemical mechanisms, clinical efficacy, and future strategies. Rev Infect Dis. 1988;10:560–86.
221. Croft SL, Neal RA. The effect of allopurinol ribonucleoside and formycin B on *Trypanosoma cruzi* infections in mice. Trans R Soc Trop Med Hyg. 1985;79:517–8.
222. Sampaio SAP, Godoy JT, Paiva L, et al. The treatment of American (mucocutaneous) leishmaniasis with amphotericin B. Arch Dermatol. 1960;82:627–35.
223. Crofts MAJ. Use of amphotericin B in mucocutaneous leishmaniasis. J Trop Med Hyg. 1976;79:111–3.
224. Keystone JS, Murdoch JK. Mebendazole. Ann Intern Med. 1979;91:582–6.
225. Wolfe MS, Wershing JM. Mebendazole. Treatment of trichuriasis and ascariasis in Bahamian children. JAMA 1974;230:1408–11.
226. Partono F, Purnomo, Tangkilisan A. The use of mebendazole in the treatment of polyparasitism. Southeast Asian J Trop Med Public Health. 1974;5:258–64.
227. Miller MJ, Krupp IM, Little MD, et al. Mebendazole: An effective anthelmintic for trichuriasis and enterobiasis. JAMA. 1974;230:1412–4.
228. Abadi K. Single dose mebendazole therapy for soil-transmitted nematodes. Am J Trop Med Hyg. 1985;34:129–33.
229. Islam N, Chowdhury NA. Mebendazole and pyrantel pamoate as broad-spectrum anthelmintics. Southeast Asian J Trop Med Public Health. 1976;7:81–4.
230. Pelletier LL Jr, Baker CB. Treatment failures following mebendazole therapy for chronic strongyloidiasis. J Infect Dis. 1987;156:532–3.
231. Wilson KH, Kauffman CA. Persistent *Strongyloides stercoralis* in a blind loop of the bowel. Successful treatment with mebendazole. Arch Intern Med. 1983;143:357–8.
232. Witassek F, Bircher J. Chemotherapy of larval echinococcosis with mebendazole: Microsomal liver function and cholestasis as determinants of plasma drug level. Eur J Clin Pharmacol. 1983;25:85–90.
233. Luder J, Witassek F, Weigand K, et al. Treatment of cystic echinococcosis

(*Echinococcus granulosus*) with mebendazole: Assessment of bound and free drug levels in cyst fluid and of parasite vitality in operative specimens. Eur J Clin Pharmacol. 1985;28:279–85.
234. Rudwan MA, Mousa A-RM, Muhtaseb SA. Abdominal hydatid disease: Follow-up of mebendazole therapy by CT and ultrasonography. Int Surg. 1986;71:22–6.
235. Rausch RL, Wilson JF, McMahon BJ, et al. Consequences of continuous mebendazole therapy in alveolar hydatid disease—with a summary of a ten-year clinical trial. Ann Trop Med Parasitol. 1986;80:403–19.
236. Smego DR, Smego RA Jr. Hydatid cyst: Preoperative sterilization with mebendazole. South Med J. 1986;79:900–1.
237. Sayek I, Cakmakci M. The effect of prophylactic mebendazole in experimental peritoneal hydatidosis. Surg Gynecol Obstet. 1986;163:351–3.
238. Wilson JF, Rausch RL, McMahon BJ, et al. Albendazole therapy in alveolar hydatid disease: A report of favorable results in two patients after short-term therapy. Am J Trop Med Hyg. 1987;37:162–8.
239. Mansueto S, Di Rosa S, Farinella E, et al. Albendazole in the treatment of hydatid disease: More than a hope (Letter). Trans R Soc Trop Med Hyg. 1987;81:168.
240. Okelo GBA. Hydatid disease: Research and control in Turkana, III. Albendazole in the treatment of inoperable hydatid disease in Kenya—a report on 12 cases. Trans R Soc Trop Med Hyg. 1986;80:193–5.
241. Morris DL. Pre-operative albendazole therapy for hydatid cyst. Br J Surg. 1987;74:805–6.
242. Levin ML. Treatment of trichinosis with mebendazole. Am J Trop Med Hyg. 1983;32;980–3.
243. Hess JA, Chandrasekar PH, Mortiere M, et al. Comparative efficacy of ketoconazole and mebendazole in experimental trichinosis. *Antimicrob Agents Chemother*. 1986;30:953–4.
244. Van Hoegaerden M, Ivanoff B, Flocard F, et al. The use of mebendazole in the treatment of filariasis due to *Loa loa* and *Mansonella perstans*. Ann Trop Med Parasitol. 1987;81:275–82.
245. Van Hoegaerden M, Flocard F. Mebendazole treatment of loiasis (Letter). Lancet. 1985;1:1278.
246. Webster LT Jr. Drugs used in the chemotherapy of helminthiasis. In: Gilman AG, Goodman LS, Rall TW, et al, eds. The Pharmacologic Basis of Therapeutics. 7th ed. New York: Macmillan; 1985:1009–28.
247. Howells RE, Delves CJ. A simple method for the identification of compounds which inhibit tubulin polymerization in filarial worms. Ann Trop Med Parasitol. 1985;79:507–12.
248. Official Product Monographs, Vermox Tablets. Raritan, NJ: Ortho Pharmaceutical Corp; June 11, 1978 (cited in Ref. 224).
249. Levin MH, Weinstein RA, Axelrod JL, et al. Severe, reversible neutropenia during high-dose mebendazole therapy for echinococcosis. JAMA. 1983;249:2929–31.
250. Fernández-Bañares F, González-Huix F, Xiol X, et al. Marrow aplasia during high dose mebendazole treatment. Am J Trop Med Hyg. 1986;35:350–1.
251. Rossignol JF, Maisonneuve H. Benzimidazoles in the treatment of trichuriasis: A review. Ann Trop Med Parasitol. 1984;78:135–44.
252. Bassily S, El-Masry NA, Trabolsi B, et al. Treatment of ancyclostomiasis and ascariasis with albendazole. Ann Trop Med Parasitol. 1984;78:81–2.
253. Hui-lan Z, Wei-ji C, Rossignol JF, et al. Albendazole in nematode, cestode, trematode and protozoan (giardia) infections. Chin Med J. (Engl.) 1986;99:912–5.
254. Jagota SC. Albendazole, a broad-spectrum anthelmintic, in the treatment of intestinal nematode and cestode infections: A multicenter study in 480 patients. Clin Ther. 1986;8:226–31.
255. Pugh RNH, Teesdale CH, Burnham GM. Albendazole in children with hookworm infection. Ann Trop Med Parasitol. 1986;80:565–7.
256. Escobedo F, Penagos P, Rodriguez J, et al. Albendazole therapy for neurocysticercosis. Arch Intern Med. 1987;147:738–41.
257. Morris DL, Smith PG. Albendazole in hydatid disease—hepatocellular toxicity. Trans R Soc Trop Med Hyg. 1987;81:343–4.
258. Yoshimura H. Teratogenicity of flubendazole in rats. Toxicology. 1987;43:133–8.
259. Téllez-Girón E, Ramos MC, Dufour L, et al. Treatment of neurocysticercosis with flubendazole. Am J Trop Med Hyg. 1984;33:627–31.
260. Brown HD, Matzuk AR, Ilves IR, et al. Antiparasitic drugs. IV. 2-(4′-Thiazolyl)-benzimidazole; a new anthelmintic (Letter). J Am Chem Soc. 1961;83:1764–5.
261. Campbell WC, Cuckler AC. Thiabendazole in the treatment and control of parasitic infections in man. Tex Rep Biol Med. 1969;27 (Suppl 2):665–92.
262. Berk SL, Verghese A, Alvarez S, et al. Clinical and epidemiological features of strongyloidiasis—a prospective study in rural Tennessee. Arch Intern Med. 1987;147:1257–61.
263. Barnish G, Barker J. An intervention study using thiabendazole suspension against *Strongyloides fulleborni*-like infections in Papua, New Guinea. Trans R Soc Trop Med Hyg. 1987;81:60–3.
264. Gordon H McL. Thiabendazole: A highly effective anthelmintic for sheep. Nature. 1961;191:1409–10.
265. Stone OJ. Systemic and topical thiabendazole for creeping eruption. Tex Rep Biol Med. 1969;27(Suppl 2):659–63.
266. Campbell WC, Denham DA. Chemotherapy. In: Campbell WC, ed. *Trichinella* and Trichinosis. New York: Plenum Press; 1983:335–66.
267. Hennekeuser HH, Pabst K, Poeplau W, et al. Thiabendazole for the treatment of trichinosis in humans. Tex Rep Biol Med. 1969;27(Suppl 2):581–96.
268. Criado Fornelio A, Rodriguez Caabeiro F, Jimenez Gonzalez A. The mode of action of some benzimidazole drugs on *Trichinella spiralis*. Parasitology. 1987;95:61–70.
269. Robinson HJ, Silber R, Graessle OE. Thiabendazole: Toxicological, pharmacological and antifungal properties. Tex Rep Biol Med. 1969;27(Suppl 2):537–60.
270. Köhler P, Bachmann R. The effects of the antiparasitic drugs levamisole, thiabendazole, praziquantel, and chloroquine on mitochondrial electron transport in muscle tissue from *Ascaris suum*. Mol Pharmacol. 1978;14:155–63.
271. Watts SDM, Rapson EB, Atkins AM, et al. Inhibition of acetylcholinesterase secretion from *Nippostrongylus brasiliensis* by benzimidazole anthelmintics. Biochem Pharmacol. 1982;31:3035–40.
272. Manivel JC, Bloomer JR, Snover DC. Progressive bile duct injury after thiabendazole administration. Gastroenterology. 1987;93:245–9.
273. Tchao P, Templeton T. Thiabendazole-associated grand mal seizures in a patient with Down syndrome. J Pediatr. 1983;102:317–8.
274. De Pargament MDM, de Vinuesa ML, Larripa I. Mutagenic bioassay of certain pharmacological drugs. I. Thiabendazole (TBZ). Mutat Res. 1987;188:1–6.
275. Austin WC, Courtney W, Danilewicz JC, et al. Pyrantel tartrate, a new anthelmintic effective against infections of domestic animals. Nature. 1966;212:1273–4.
276. Bumbalo TS, Fugazzoto DJ, Wyczalek JV. Treatment of enterobiasis with pyrantel pamoate. Am J Trop Med Hyg. 1969;18:50–2.
277. Aubry ML, Cowell P, Davey MJ, et al. Aspects of the pharmacology of a new anthelminthic: Pyrantel. Br J Pharmacol. 1970;38:332–44.
278. Eyre P. Some pharmacodynamic effects of the nematocides: Methyridine, tetramisole and pyrantel. J Pharm Pharmacol. 1970;22:26–36.
279. Rollo IM. Drugs used in the chemotherapy of helminthiasis. In: Gilman AG, Goodman LS, Gilman A, eds. The Pharmacological Basis of Therapeutics. 6th ed. New York: Macmillan; 1980:1013–37.
280. Royer A. Preliminary report on a new antioxyuritic Poquil. Can Med Assoc J. 1956;74:297.
281. Sawitz WG, Karpinski FE Jr. Treatment of oxyuriasis with pyrrovinyquinium chloride (Poquil). Am J Trop Med Hyg. 1956;5:538–43.
282. Hennig UGG, Galindo-Prince OC, Cortinas da Nava, C, et al. A comparison of the genetic activity of pyrvinium pamoate with that of several other anthelmintic drugs in *Saccharomyces cerevisiae*. Mutat Res. 1987;187:79–89.
283. Martin RJ. γ-Aminobutyric acid- and piperazine-activated single-channel currents from *scaris suum* body muscle. Br J Pharmacol. 1985;84:445–61.
284. Saz HJ, Bueding E. Relationships between anthelmintic effects and biochemical and physiological mechanisms. Pharmacol Rev. 1966;18:871–94.
285. Nickey LN. Possible precipitation of petit mal seizures with piperazine citrate. JAMA. 1966;195:1069–70.
286. Parsons AC. Piperazine neurotoxicity: "Worm wobble." Br Med J. 1971;4:792.
287. Wright S, Harman RRM. Ethylenediamine and piperazine sensitivity. Br Med J. 1983;287:463–4.
288. Ottesen EA. Efficacy of diethylcarbamazine in eradicating infection with lymphatic-dwelling filariae in humans. Rev Infect Dis. 1985;7:341–56.
289. Partono F. Treatment of elephantiasis in a community with timorian filariasis. Trans R Soc Trop Med Hyg. 1985;79:44–6.
290. Kim JS, No BU, Lee WY. Brugian filariasis: 10-year follow-up study on the effectiveness of selective chemotherapy with diethylcarbamazine on Che Ju island, Republic of Korea. Bull WHO. 1987;65:67–75.
291. Hawking F. Chemotherapy of filariasis. Antibiot Chemother. 1980;30:135–62.
292. Montestruc E, Blanche R, Laborde R. Action du 1-diethylcarbamyl 4-methylpiperazine sur *Filaria ozzardi*. Bull Soc Pathol Exot. 1950;43:275–8 (cited in Ref. 293).
293. Bartholomew CF, Nathan MD, Tikasingh ES. The failure of diethylcarbamazine in the treatment of *Mansonella ozzardi* infections. Trans R Soc Trop Med Hyg. 1978;72:423–4.
294. Nesarajah MS. Pulmonary function in tropical eosinophilia before and after treatment with diethylcarbamazine. Thorax. 1975;30:574–7.
295. Wiseman RA, Woodruff AW, Pettitt LE. The treatment of toxocaral infection: Some experimental and clinical observations. Trans R Soc Trop Med Hyg. 1971;65:591–8.
296. Taylor HR. Recent developments in the treatment of onchocerciasis. Bull WHO. 1984;62:509–15.
297. Lariviere M, Vingtain P, Aziz M, et al. Double-blind study of ivermectin and diethylcarbamazine in African onchocerciasis patients with ocular involvement. Lancet. 1985;2:174–7.
298. Diallo S, Aziz MA, Lariviere M, et al. A double-blind comparison of the efficacy and safety of ivermectin and diethylcarbamazine in a placebo controlled study of Senegalese patients with onchocerciasis. Trans R Soc Trop Med Hyg. 1986;80:927–34.
299. Dadzie KY, Bird AC, Awadzi K, et al. Ocular findings in a double-blind study of ivermectin versus diethylcarbamazine versus placebo in the treatment of onchocerciasis. Br. J Ophthalmol. 1987;71:78–85.
300. Hawking F. Chemotherapy of filariasis. In: Schnitzer RJ, Hawking F, eds. Experimental Chemotherapy. v. 1. New York: Academic Press; 1963:893–912.
301. Rée GH, Hall AP, Hutchinson DBA, et al. Plasma levels of diethylcarbamazine in man. Trans R Soc Trop Med Hyg. 1978;71:542–3.
302. Faulkner JK, Smith KJ. Dealkylation and N-oxidation in the metabolism of

1-diethyl-carbamyl-4-methylpiperazine in the rat. Xenobiotica. 1972;2:59–68.

303. Langham ME, Kramer TR. The in vitro effect of diethylcarbamazine on the motility and survival of *Onchocerca volvulus* microfilariae. Tropemed Parasitol. 1980;31:59–66.
304. Hawking F. Diethylcarbamazine and new compounds for the treatment of filariasis. Adv Pharmacol Chemother. 1979;16:129–94.
305. Van den Bossche H. A look at the mode of action of some old and new antifilarial compounds. Ann Soc Belg Med Trop. 1981;16;287–96 (cited in Ref. 264).
306. King CH, Greene BM, Spagnuolo PJ. Diethylcarbamazine citrate, an antifilarial drug, stimulates human granulocyte adherence. Antimicrob Agents Chemother 1983;24:453–6.
307. Cesbron J-V, Capron A, Vargaftig BB, et al. Platelets mediate the action of diethylcarbamazine on microfilariae. Nature. 1987;325:533–6.
308. Greene BM, Taylor HR, Brown EJ, et al. Ocular and systemic complications of diethylcarbamazine therapy for onchocerciasis: Association with circulating immune complexes. J Infect Dis. 1983;147:890–7.
309. Ottesen EA. Description, mechanisms and control of reactions to treatment in the human filariases. Ciba Found Symp. 1987;127:265–83.
310. Rivas-Alcala AR, Greene BM, Taylor HR, et al. Chemotherapy of onchocerciasis: A controlled comparison of mebendazole, levamisole, and diethylcarbamazine. Lancet. 1981;2:485–90.
311. Dominguez-Varquez A, Taylor HR, Greene BM, et al. Comparison of flubendazole and diethylcarbamazine in treatment of onchocerciasis. Lancet. 1983;1:139–43.
312. Francis H, Awadzi K, Ottesen EA. The Mazzotti reaction following treatment of onchocerciasis with diethylcarbamazine: Clinical severity as a function of infection intensity. Am J Trop Med Hyg. 1985;34:529–36.
313. Campbell WC, Fisher MH, Stapley EO, et al. Ivermectin: A potent new antiparasitic agent. Science. 1983;221:823–8.
314. Coulaud JP, Lariviere M, Aziz MA, et al. Ivermectin in onchocerciasis (Letter). Lancet. 1984;2:526–7.
315. Aziz MA, Diallo S, Diop IM, et al. Efficacy and tolerance of ivermectin in human onchocerciasis. Lancet. 1982;2:171–3.
316. Kumaraswami V, Ottesen EA, Vijayasekaran V, et al. Ivermectin for the treatment of *Wuchereria bancrofti* filariasis: Efficacy and adverse reactions. JAMA. 1988;259:3150–3.
317. Mahmoud AAF. Praziquantel for the treatment of helminthic infections. Adv Intern Med. 1987;32:193–206.
318. Pearson RD, Guerrant RL. Praziquantel: A major advance in anthelminthic therapy. Ann Intern Med. 1983;99:195–8.
319. Pearson RD, Wilson ME. Role of praziquantel in the treatment of helminthic diseases. Int Med Specialist. 1986;7:183–204.
320. Wegner DHG. The profile of the trematodicidal compound praziquantel. Arzneim Forsch. 1984;34:1132–6.
321. Davis A, Biles JE, Ulrich A-M. Initial experience with praziquantel in the treatment of human infections due to *Schistosoma haematobium*. Bull WHO. 1979;57:773–9.
322. Katz N, Rocha RS, Chaves A. Preliminary trials with praziquantel in human infections due to *Schistosoma mansoni*. Bull WHO. 1979;57:781–5.
323. Da Silva LC, Sette H Jr, Christo CH, et al. Praziquantel in the treatment of the hepatosplenic form of schistosomiasis mansoni. Arzneim Forsch. 1981;31:601–3.
324. Coutinho A, Domingues ALC, Neves J, et al. Treatment of hepatosplenic schistosomiasis mansoni with praziquantel. Preliminary report on tolerance and efficacy. Arzneim Forsch. 1983;33:787–91.
325. Bassily S, Farid Z, Dunn M, et al. Praziquantel for treatment of schistosomiasis in patients with advanced hepatosplenomegaly. Ann Trop Med Parasitol. 1985;79:629–34.
326. Santos AT, Blas BL, Noseñas JS, et al. Preliminary clinical trials with praziquantel in *Schistosoma japonicum* infections in the Philippines. Bull WHO. 1979;57:793–9.
327. Santos AT, Blas BL, Portillo G, et al. Phase III clinical trials with praziquantel in *S. japonicum* infections in the Philippines. Arzneim Forsch. 1984;34:1221–3.
328. Fu F-Y, Zheng JS, Chen W-Q, et al. Further experience with praziquantel in schistosoma japonicum infections. Chin Med J (Engl). 1984;97:47–52.
329. Nash TE, Hofstetter M, Cheever AW, et al. Treatment of *Schistosoma mekongi* with praziquantel: A double-blind study. Am J Trop Med Hyg. 1982;31:977–82.
330. Keittivuti B, Keittivuti A, O'Rourke T, et al. Treatment of *Schistosoma mekongi* with praziquantel in Cambodian refugees in holding centers in Prachinburi Province, Thailand. Trans R Soc Trop Med Hyg. 1984;78:477–9.
331. Watt G, Adapon B, Long GW, et al. Praziquantel in treatment of cerebral schistosomiasis. Lancet. 1986;2:529–32.
332. Rim H-J, Lyu K-S, Lee J-S, et al. Clinical evaluation of the therapeutic efficacy of praziquantel (Embay 8440) against *Clonorchis sinensis* infection in man. Ann Trop Med Parasitol. 1981;75:27–33.
333. Liu Y-H, Qiu Z-D, Wang X-G, et al. Praziquantel in clonorchiasis sinensis: A further evaluation of 100 cases. Chin Med J (Engl). 1982;95:89–94.
334. Bunnag D, Harinasuta T. Studies on the chemotherapy of human opisthorchiasis in Thailand: I. Clinical trial of praziquantel. Southeast Asian J Trop Med Public Health. 1980;11:528–31.
335. Spitalny KC, Senft AW, Meglio FD, et al. Treatment of pulmonary paragonimiasis with a new broad-spectrum antihelminthic, praziquantel. J Pediatr. 1982;101:144–6.
336. Rim H-J, Chang Y-S. Chemotherapeutic effect of niclofolan and praziquantel in the treatment of paragonimiasis. Korean Univ Med J. 1980;17:113–28.
337. Knobloch J, Paz G, Feldmeier H, et al. Serum antibody levels in human paragonimiasis before and after therapy with praziquantel. Trans R Soc Trop Med Hyg. 1984;78:835–6.
338. Pachucki CT, Levandowski RA, Brown VA, et al. American paragonimiasis treated with praziquantel. N Engl J Med. 1984;311:582–3.
339. Farid Z, Trabolsi B, Boctor F, et al. Unsuccessful use of praziquantel to treat acute fascioliasis in children (Letter). J Infect Dis. 1986;154:920–1.
340. Farag HF, Ragab M, Salem A, et al. A short note on praziquantel in human fascioliasis. J Trop Med Hyg. 1986;89:79–80.
341. Botero D, Castano S. Treatment of cysticercosis with praziquantel in Columbia. Am J Trop Med Hyg. 1982;31:811–21.
342. Gomez JG, Sanchez E, Pardo R. Treatment of cysticercosis with praziquantel (Letter). Arch Neurol. 1984;41:1022.
343. De Ghetaldi LD, Norman RM, Douville AW Jr. Cerebral cysticercosis treated biphasically with dexamethasone and praziquantel. Ann Intern Med. 1983;99:179–81.
344. Biller J, Azar-Kia B, O'Keefe P. Cysticercosis and praziquantel therapy (Letter). Neurology. 1984;34:1621–2.
345. Sotelo J, Torres B, Rubio-Donnadieu F, et al. Praziquantel in the treatment of neurocysticercosis: Long-term follow-up. Neurology. 1985;35:752–5.
346. Robles C, Sedano AM, Vargas-Tentori N, et al. Long-term results of praziquantel therapy in neurocysticercosis. J Neurosurg. 1987;66:359–63.
347. Leblanc R, Knowles KF, Melanson D, et al. Neurocysticercosis: Surgical and medical management with praziquantel. Neurosurgery. 1986;18:419–27.
348. Norman RM, Kapadia C. Cerebral cysticercosis: Treatment with praziquantel. Pediatrics. 1986;78:291–4.
349. Vasconcelos D, Cruz-Segura H, Mateos-Gomez H, et al. Selective indications for the use of praziquantel in the treatment of brain cysticercosis. J Neurol Neurosurg Psychiatry. 1987;50:383–8.
350. Santos R, Chavarria M, Aguirre AE. Failure of medical treatment in two cases of intraocular cysticercosis. Am J Ophthalmol. 1984;97:249–50.
351. Kestelyn P, Taelman H. Effect of praziquantel on intraocular cysticercosis: A case report. Br J Ophthalmol. 1985;69:788–90.
352. Groll E. Praziquantel for cestode infections in man. Acta Trop (Basel). 1980;37:293–6.
353. Gemmell MA, Johnstone PD, Oudemans G. The effect of praziquantel on *Echinococcus granulosus, Taenia hydatigena*, and *Taenia ovis* infections in dog. Res Vet Sci. 1977;23:121–3.
354. Morris DL, Richards KS, Chinnery JB. Protoscolicidal effect of praziquantel—in vitro and electron microscopical studies of *Echinococcus granulosus*. J Antimicrob Chemother. 1986;18:687–91.
355. Heath DD, Lawrence SB. The effect of mebendazole and praziquantel on the cysts of *Echinococcus granulosus, Taenia hydatigena*, and *T. ovis* in sheep. NZ Vet J. 1978;26:11–5.
356. Thomas H, Gonnert R. Zur Wirksamkeit von Praziquantel bei der experimentellen Cysticercose und Hydatidose. Z Parasitenkd. 1978;55:165–79.
357. Marshall I, Edwards GT. The effects of sustained release praziquantel on the survival of protoscolices of *Echinococcus granulosus equinus* in laboratory mice. Ann Trop Med Parasitol. 1982;76:649–51.
358. Leopold G, Ungethum W, Groll E, et al. Clinical pharmacology in normal volunteers of praziquantel, a new drug against schistosomes and cestodes: An example of a complex study covering both tolerance and pharmacokinetics. Eur J Clin Pharmacol. 1978;14:281–91.
359. Andrews P. Pharmakokinetische Tieruntersuchungen mit Droncit unter Verwendurg einer biologischen Prufmethode. Vet Med Nachr. 1976;2:154–6.
360. Thomas H, Andrews P, Mehlhorn H. New results on the effect of praziquantel in experimental cysticercosis. Am J Trop Med Hyg. 1982;31:803–10.
361. Andrews P. Praziquantel: Mechanisms of anti-schistosomal activity. Pharmacol Ther. 1985;29:129–56.
362. Xiao S-H, Friedman PA, Catto BA, et al. Praziquantel-induced vesicle formation in the tegument of male *Schistosoma mansoni* is calcium dependent. J Parasitol. 1984;70:177–9.
363. Gardner DR, Brezden BL. The sites of action of praziquantel in smooth muscle of *Lymnaea stagnalis*. Can J Physiol Pharmacol. 1984;62:282–7.
364. Ruenwongsa P, Hutadilok N, Yuthavong Y. Stimulation of Ca^{2+} uptake in the liver fluke *Opisthorchis viverrini* by praziquantel. Life Sci. 1983;32:2529–34.
365. Harnett W, Kusel JR. Increased exposure of parasite antigens at the surface of adult *Schistosoma mansoni* exposed to praziquantel in vitro. Parasitology. 1986;93:401–5.
366. Prichard RK, Bachmann R, Hutchinson GW, et al. The effect of praziquantel on calcium in *Hymenolepis diminuta*. Mol Biochem Parasitol. 1982;5:297–308.
367. Johnson RJ, Jong EC, Dunning SB, et al. Paragonimiasis: Diagnosis and the use of praziquantel in treatment. Rev Infect Dis. 1985;7:200–6.
368. Polderman AM, Gryseels B, Gerold JL, et al. Side effects of praziquantel in the treatment of *Schistosoma mansoni* in Maniema, Zaire. Trans R Soc Trop Med Hyg. 1984;78:752–4.

369. Farid Z, Wallace CK. Schistosomiasis and praziquantel (Letter). Ann Intern Med. 1983;99:883.
370. Watt G, Baldovino PC, Castro JT, et al. Bloody diarrhoea after praziquantel therapy (Letter). Trans R Soc Trop Med Hyg. 1986;80:345–6.
371. Markwalder K, Hess K, Valavanis A, et al. Cerebral cysticercosis: Treatment with praziquantel. Am J Trop Med Hyg. 1984;33:273–80.
372. Sotelo J, Escobedo F, Rodriguez-Carbajal J, et al. Therapy of parenchymal brain cysticercosis with praziquantel. N Engl J Med. 1984;310:1001–7.
373. Davis A, Bailey DR. Metrifonate in urinary schistosomiasis. Bull WHO. 1969;41:209–24.
374. Omer AHS, Teesdale CH. Metrifonate trial in the treatment of various presentations of *Schistosoma haematobium* and *S. mansoni* infections in the Sudan. Ann Trop Med Parasitol. 1978;72:145–50.
375. Feldmeier H, Doehring E, Daffala AA, et al. Efficacy of metrifonate in urinary schistosomiasis: Comparison of reduction of *Schistosoma haematobium* and *S. mansoni* eggs. Am J Trop Med Hyg. 1982;31:1188–94.
376. Reiner K, Krauthacker B, Simeon V, et al. Mechanism of inhibition in vitro of mammalian acetylcholinesterase and cholinesterase in solutions of 0,0-dimethyl 2,2,2-trichloro-1-hydroxyethyl phosphonate (Trichlorphon). Biochem Pharmacol. 1975;24:717–22.
377. Nordgren I, Bengtsson E, Holmstedt B, et al. Levels of metrifonate and dichlorvos in plasma and erythrocytes during treatment of schistosomiasis with Bilarcil. Acta Pharmacol Toxicol. 1981;49 (Suppl V):79–86.
378. Katz N, Zicker F, Pereira JP. Field trials with oxamniquine in a schistosomiasis mansoni-endemic area. Am J Trop Med Hyg. 1977;26:234–7.
379. Katz N. Chemotherapy of schistosomiasis mansoni. Adv Pharmacol Chemother. 1977;14:1–70.
380. Omer AHS. Oxamniquine for treating *Schistosoma mansoni* infection in Sudan. Br Med J. 1978;2:163–5.
381. Kilpatrick ME, Farid Z, Bassily S, et al. Treatment of schistosomiasis mansoni with oxamniquine—five years' experience. Am J Trop Med Hyg. 1981;30:1219–22.
382. Machado PA. The Brazilian program for schistosomiasis control, 1975–1979. Am J Trop Med Hyg. 1982;31:76–86.
383. Goble FC, ed. The pharmacological and chemotherapeutic properties of niridazole and other antischistosomal compounds. Ann NY Acad Sci. 1969;160:423–946.
384. Farid Z, Bassily S, Lehman JS Jr, et al. A comparative evaluation of the treatment of *Schistosoma mansoni* with niridazole and potassium antimony tartrate. Trans R Soc Trop Med Hyg. 1972;66:119–24.
385. Davidson JC. Neuropsychiatric effects and EEG changes in niridazole therapy. Trans R Soc Trop Med Hyg. 1969;63:579–81.
386. Sonnet J, Doyen A. Effects of niridazole on erythropoiesis of Congolese treated for schistosomiasis and amoebiasis. Ann NY Acad Sci. 1969; 160:786–98.
387. De Carvalho SA, Neto V, Zeitune JM, et al. Avaliaco terapeutica do oltipraz na infeccao humana pelo *S. mansoni*. Rev Inst Med Trop Sao Paulo. 1986;28:271–7.
388. Kim JS. Treatment of *Paragonimus westermani* infections with bithionol. Am J Trop Med Hyg. 1970;19:940–2.
389. Pearson RD, Hewlett EL. Niclosamide therapy for tapeworm infections. Ann Intern Med. 1985;102:550–1.
390. Hecht VG, Gloxhuber C. Experimentelle Untersuchungen mit N-(2′-Chlor-4′-Nitrophenyl)-5-Chlorsalicylamid, einem neuen Bandwurmmittel: 2. Mitteilung: toxikologische Untersuchungen. Arzneim Forsch. 1960;10:884–5.
391. Perera DR, Western KA, Schultz MG. Nicclosamide treatment of cestodiasis: Clinical trials in the United States. Am J Trop Med Hyg. 1970; 19:610–2.

37. PROBLEMS IN ANTIBIOTIC USAGE

CALVIN M. KUNIN

The general problem of appropriate use of drugs has existed for a long time. Osler could assume a position of therapeutic nihilism in the early 1900s since there were few effective agents available to him. The antibiotic era, which began less than 45 years ago, is much more complex. There are a wealth of excellent agents from which to choose, each with its own special benefits and economic, toxic, and ecologic costs. We now have the luxury of debating the value of using antibiotics to prevent complications of relatively simple problems such as the common cold or a sore throat, and we can more readily deal with serious surgical and life-threatening infections.

Soon after antibiotics were introduced, it was recognized that they were being overused and misused. A review of the subject by Jawetz in 1956[1] eloquently stated the problems of the attractiveness of new antibiotics to physicians, exaggerated claims, and the enormous impact of promotion by the drug companies on medical practice. The following year, based on a nationwide study, Welch et al.[2] described the relatively high frequency of severe reactions to antibiotics. In 1959, Finland et al.[3] documented the increasing occurrence of serious bacterial infections since the introduction of antibacterial agents. Reimann and D'Ambola[4] conducted one of the earliest surveys on the appropriate use of antibiotics in 1966 and clearly demonstrated that antibiotics were often used inappropriately. In 1974, Lockwood[5] described the syndrome of compulsive antibiotic prescribing and advocated the formation of an organization called Antibiotics Anonymous to deal with the problem. More recently, the Alliance for Prudent Use of Antibiotics has been formed to monitor the problem worldwide. It is therefore appropriate that a chapter appear in this book on infectious disease to examine the problem and explore potential solutions.

MAGNITUDE OF ANTIMICROBIAL USE IN THE UNITED STATES

Antimicrobial drugs are the second most commonly used class of drugs, second only to cardiovascular agents. According to data from the *U.S. Industrial Outlook,* published by the Department of Commerce, the value of pharmaceutical industry shipments was 27.1 billion dollars in 1986. It is estimated that about 12–15 percent, or about 3–4 billion dollars, was for anti-infective agents. These figures do not include costs of markup or administration of the agents, which could readily double the expenditure. About 45 percent of the expenditure for anti-infective drugs was for outpatient use. The remainder, consisting mostly of the more expensive parenteral agents, was used in hospitals and long-term care facilities. According to the Food and Drug Administration (FDA), 196 million outpatient prescriptions for anti-infective agents were filled in 1984. This accounted for 13.1 percent of all prescriptions. Much of this expenditure is for treatment of conditions such as sinusitis, bronchitis, and respiratory infecions. Since most of these are caused by viruses, much of this expenditure is wasted.[6]

In hospitals, antimicrobial agents are given to 20–40 percent of patients and account for about 25 percent of total drug acquisition costs.[7] We will later show that much of this antimicrobial use is not only unnecessary but also a waste of resources and is potentially harmful to the patient and society.

REASONS FOR CONCERN ABOUT APPROPRIATE USE OF ANTIMICROBIAL AGENTS

Selection of Resistant Bacteria

The development of resistant organisms was recognized by Paul Ehrlich as a potential problem during his early studies of organic arsenicals almost 100 years ago. The overall problem of the emergence of resistant strains is discussed in Chapter 16 and is a persistent theme throughout the sections on antimicrobial chemotherapy. Multiple-drug-resistant organisms derived through the transfer of plasmids or through transduction by bacteriophages have amplified the problem. At first, the focus was on the emergence of resistant bacteria in hospitals, where antimicrobial agents are used most heavily. A causal relationship between antibiotic usage and resistance of organisms in hospitals has been established on the basis of evidence of consistent associations of the emergence of resistant strains with concurrent variations in use in populations over time.[8] More recently, common virulent organisms resistant to previously effective agents have been encountered in office practice as well; this problem is particularly troublesome in developing nations, which can least afford it. This phenomenon has forced physicians to alter their cost/benefit equation and to use expensive and potentially toxic drugs for the treatment of infections due to staphylococci, gonococci, *Haemophilus influenzae, Shigella,* and the pneumococci in focal outbreaks.

Three approaches to the problem of emerging resistant strains are being explored. The simplest and least costly measure is to decrease the selective pressure exerted by antibiotics. Several groups have presented evidence that control of usage will result in reversion of the bacterial population to sensitive organisms.[9,10] A second approach is to develop immunogens that can enhance host resistance to virulent organisms. Development of a polyvalent pneumococcal vaccine is an example of this approach. The major difficulty with the use of vaccines is the complex problems of effective delivery to the target high-risk population and the multiplicity of immunogens needed to deal with an expanding number of microorganisms for which vaccines are being developed. The third and most costly approach is to develop and exploit new antimicrobial agents or alter the chemical structure of older agents to circumvent mechanisms of resistance developed by the microorganisms. This has been the major path taken by the pharmaceutical industry and is most accepted by the medical community.

Rising Costs of Medical Care: Emergence of the "Drugs of Fear"

A new antimicrobial era emerged during the 1970s, the era of the "drugs of fear,"[11] a term that refers to fear on the part of physicians of failing to provide patients with the very best drug for a presumed infection. Although many lives have been saved by these drugs, the underlying conditions that precipitate infection with "difficult hospital bacteria" have not been resolved, and therefore in many cases, the drugs have been used without effect or have simply delayed death. Widespread use of these agents ensures their own phased obsolescence as new resistant organisms emerge, and it also increases the costs of medical care. We can expect costs to increase with only modest improvement in therapeutic efficacy.

Adverse Reactions to Antimicrobial Agents

Untoward toxic effects of antibiotics are well known; they range from death from anaphylaxis or aplastic anemia with penicillin and chloramphenicol, respectively, to severe diarrhea from lincosamides, rash from ampicillin, nephrotoxicity and ototoxicity from the aminoglycosides, and bleeding disorders with some of the new β-lactam antibiotics. Cluff[12] and Seidl et al.[13] reported that approximately 5 percent of the hospitalized patients who are given an antibiotic will experience some adverse reaction to the drug and about 20 percent of patients requiring medical care have a history of adverse reaction(s) to an antibiotic.

EVIDENCE OF INAPPROPRIATE USE OF ANTIMICROBIAL AGENTS

Office Practice

Drug prescribing was examined in a careful epidemiologic study by Stolley et al.[14] They reported that market research data indicated that about 95 percent of physicians will issue one or more prescriptions to a patient whom they diagnose as having the "common cold." Almost 60 percent of these prescriptions are for antibiotics, with the tetracyclines and penicillins being the most popular choices. In their own study in a U.S. community, they found that antibiotics were the most commonly dispensed drugs (15.3 percent of all prescriptions). Another analysis by the same group of investigators[15] showed that prescribing patterns are largely determined by educational experiences. Higher ratings for appropriate drug use and lower frequency of chloramphenicol use in particular were found among more recently trained physicians who had more postgraduate training. Currently amoxicillin, erythromycin, and penicillins are among the 10 most commonly used antibiotics in office practice. Trimethoprim combinations and cephalexin are among the top 30 agents (National Center for Health Statistics advance data, 1987). It is only a matter of time before impact is felt of the use of the orally absorbed quinolones.

We can roughly estimate the magnitude of overuse. Approximately 750 million dollars is spent annually on prescriptions for sinusitis, bronchitis, and respiratory infections. If 60 percent of these prescriptions are for antimicrobial agents,[14] the cost for these drugs is 450 million dollars. Assuming that at least one-half of the prescriptions are inappropriate, about 225 million dollars are wasted each year.

It has been argued that antibiotics should be used more often to treat the bacterial complications of upper respiratory infections,[16] but carefully conducted clinical studies have clearly demonstrated the lack of efficacy with this approach in otherwise healthy adults.[17] It has also been argued that the major reason for the marked decrease in rheumatic fever may be due to the widespread use of antibiotics in office practice, but Stollerman[18] has presented forceful arguments that this is more closely associated with changes in the pathogenetic characteristics of the group A streptococci. There is still considerable disagreement among practitioners of various specialities concerning the proper use of antibiotics to treat respiratory infections.[19] In one study of usage in an emergency room,[20] 31 percent of infections encountered were respiratory. Antibiotic prescribing was appropriate in 78 percent of the cases.

The problem of antibiotics overusage in office practice has been compounded in recent years by the promotion of new high-cost proprietary agents such as oral cephalosporins, new derivatives of ampicillin, and the new quinolones. These agents rarely cure more patients, but do cost more.

Despite the widespread use of new antibiotics in office practice, there are still practitioners who continue to prescribe chloramphenicol, mostly for upper respiratory infections, and tetracycline to children under the age of 8 years, despite repeated recommendations against this practice by the Committee on Drugs of the American Academy of Pediatrics. According to the studies of Ray et al.,[21,22] a small group of physicians located in rural, primary care settings account for most of these inappropriate prescriptions. The most alarming finding is that physicians who recently finished training also take part in these poor practices.

Hospital Practice

There are now numerous studies in representative hospital populations that document that antimicrobial agents are used for unjustifiable reasons or that the wrong drug, dose, or duration of therapy is selected *about half the time* (Table 1). One of the remarkable findings of all these studies is that even though criteria for justified or acceptable usage may differ the results are generally the same.

Virtually all the studies identify the same reasons for overuse and excessive costs of antimicrobial agents in hospitals. These are (*1*) inappropriate use of agents for prophylaxis of surgical infections and (*2*) high cost of parenteral agents, particularly the cephalosporin and aminoglycoside antibiotics, which account for 70 percent of the total antibiotic costs.[7,26,30,31]

In recent years the proportion of costs for cephalosporins has increased because of the introduction of many new expensive agents. They have tended to replace the portion of usage occupied by aminoglycosides. The most representative study of the use of antimicrobial drugs in general hospitals in the United States was conducted by Shapiro et al.[32] They studied 20 short-stay general hospitals in Pennsylvania selected by a stratified random-sampling technique. Approximately 30 percent of the

TABLE 1. Summary of Studies Evaluating Appropriate Use of Antimicrobial Agents in Hospitals

Hospitals	*Investigators*	*No. Patients*	*Findings*	
Community (7 hospitals surveyed)	Scheckler and Bennett[23]	2094	62% of patients treated had no evidence of infection	
Community	Roberts and Visconti[24]	340	13% rational, 21% questionable, 66% irrational	
Pediatric	Gibbs et al.[25]	167	32% rational, 49% questionable, 19% irrational	
University	Kunin et al.[11]	500	52% inappropriate[a]	
University	Castle et al.[26]	50	64% inappropriate[a]	
University	Petrello et al.[27 b]	65	42.6% rational, 48% irrational, 9.3% insufficient data	
University	Maki and Schuna[28]	549	41% inappropriate	
VA	Jones et al.[29] Before	145	64% inappropriate	NS
	After[c]	200	51% inappropriate	
Community	Achong et al.[30] Before	219	42%[d] 50%[e] irrational	0.02[f]
	After	240	24%[d] 25%[e] irrational	

[a] Judged inappropriate according to criteria in Table 3.
[b] Use of clindamycin only.
[c] Education program in appropriate use of antimicrobial agents.
[d] Surgical service.
[e] Gynecologic service.
[f] Degree of significant difference.

patients received an antimicrobial drug during hospitalization, and about 30 percent received the drugs for prophylaxis in operations or invasive nonsurgical procedures. Despite indications that prophylaxis, when useful at all, is effective only when given concurrently with and for 24–48 hours after an operation, it was usually continued throughout hospitalization. Almost 80 percent of prophylactic antimicrobial agents were administered at least 48 hours after an operation or procedure (Fig. 1). It is apparent that most of the costs were for periods when the drugs would not be helpful to the patient. Similar results were obtained in a survey of 27 hospitals in Minnesota.[33] Savings of 18–50 percent could be achieved by limiting the duration of drug administration. A benefit/cost analysis of antimicrobial prophylaxis in abdominal and vaginal hysterectomy demonstrated that using three doses of cefazolin would markedly reduce costs.[34] The benefits would be eroded by use of newer, more expensive cephalosporins.

Self-Administration

It is quite common to learn from patients that they often treat themselves with drugs prescribed in the past or given to them by friends or relatives. Chretien et al.,[35] in a study of students going to a university health service, have reported that this is a frequent practice, especially for the treatment of respiratory symptoms.

Usage in Other Countries

Misuse of antibiotics is a major problem all over the world. In many Asian and South American countries, potent antibiotics are sold without prescription. A review of antibiotics marketed in Central America[36] revealed that in most countries more than 200 different antibiotic drug products were sold. At least one-third of these were drug combinations of questionable value. Most of the drugs used in the Third World originate from the major Western pharmaceutical companies that promote agents unacceptable in their own countries. Large-scale epidemics of typhoid fever, gonorrhea, and meningococcal meningitis may be traced to resistant strains originating in Third World countries in which antibiotic use is poorly controlled, self-prescribing is common,[37] and physicians often use antibiotics inappropriately.[38] A study in Israel[39] revealed that 30 percent of pharmacy costs could be accounted for by antibiotics (as in the United States), but that Israeli physicians tend to use less expensive agents such as ampicillin more widely than cephalosporins. In the United Kingdom, a study of antibiotic usage for prophylaxis in surgery revealed enormous variation among London teaching hospitals in regard to choice of drug, dose, and timing of administration.[40] In a district general hospital in Londin, ampicillin, cloxacillin, and other penicillins accounted for 61 percent of all antibiotic usage.[41] This is quite different from the United States, in which much more expensive agents are used. Nevertheless, most of the patients were treated without bacteriologic evidence of the infecting agent, and only 7 percent of antibiotics prescribed for surgical prophylaxis fulfilled reasonable criteria for their use. Similar results were obtained in a National Prevalence Survey conducted in 43 hospitals in England.[42] Although oral agents were most commonly used, parenteral agents accounted for 72 percent of the costs.

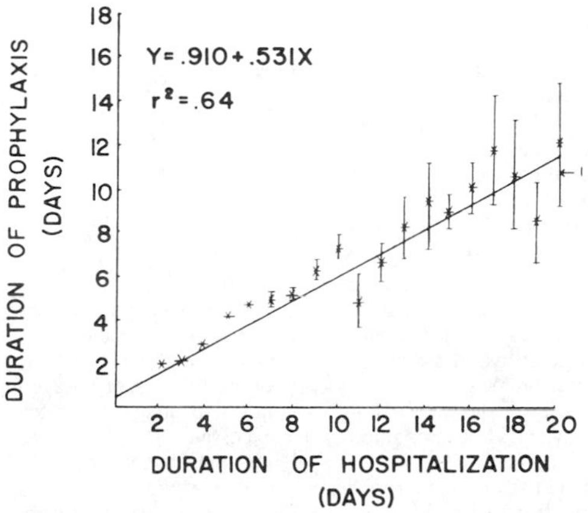

FIG. 1. Duration of antimicrobial prophylaxis in relation to duration of hospitalization. (From Shapiro et al.,[32] with permission.)

Antibiotic Use in Animals

Antibiotics are commonly used in farm animals for growth promotion and for therapeutic and prophylactic purposes. The magnitude of use in the world is highly variable. It is somewhat less in Europe than in the United States and is more sporadic and uncontrolled in Third World countries. The major fear is that plasmid-mediated, multiply resistant strains originating in farm animals will spread to the human population. The issues of control of the use of antibiotics in animals as they relate to human health are complex and controversial. Not all animal pathogens cause disease in humans. For example, staphylococci in cattle, poultry, and dogs are distinct from those that present a problem in humans. In contrast, *Salmonella* and some strains of *Campylobacter* infect humans as well as animals. *Escherichia coli* is a rich source of R plasmids that are potentially transferable in the human gut. Outbreaks of food-borne *Salmonella* infections due to multiply resistant strains may present a major problem, particularly when they produce invasive disease in compromised hosts. In one carefully studied outbreak of infection due to multiple-antibiotic-resistant *Salmonella newport*, the organisms could be traced to meat distributed from beef cattle fed subtherapeutic amounts of antimicrobial agents. Most of the infected patients had been taking penicillin derivatives, before the onset of salmonellosis.[43]

There is very little evidence that the major problem of antibiotic resistance observed in hospitals can be attributed to use in animals, but rather it is the result of excessive use of therapeutic or prophylactic antibiotics in humans. Experts agree, however, that antibiotics important for treating human infections should not be used for animals.[44]

Methods to Define the Problem and Evaluate Appropriate Usage

As awareness of the excessive use of antimicrobial agents increases, demands for accountability will require the development of clear-cut methods to evaluate the problem.

Because of control over the use of medical care services, physicians have a unique fiduciary responsibility to patients and the public. If this is perceived to be misused, the freedom enjoyed by physicians to prescribe whatever drugs they choose will be limited by action of the government or third-party payers. We are beginning to witness this in implementation of diagnostic related groups (DRGs) by Medicare and by the powerful forces in the community that seek to reduce care costs. This also offers an opportunity for implementing programs to improve prescribing as the financial emphasis in hospitals shifts from billing for all goods and services to fixed reimbursement.[45–47] An exciting development in this regard is the enormous cost savings that can be obtained by the use of long-acting parenteral antibiotics in outpatient or home therapy.[48–50] Cost savings are achieved by eliminating the need for prolonged hospital stay and by less frequent dosage intervals. Under these circumstances even the most expensive agents can be used with considerable cost-effectiveness.

Most of the studies reported in the literature use different criteria for appropriateness of use. This makes it difficult to compare data gathered in different institutions. Broad categories of surveillance methods are presented in Table 2 together with a brief list of the advantages and disadvantages of each. The simplest and least expensive method is to obtain gross utilization data from hospital pharmacies. This method can often identify a special problem such as overuse of chloramphenicol or a newly introduced agent. Attention can then be focused on individual services, particularly on patterns of use in a major problem area such as surgical prophylaxis. Drug orders can also be audited in relation to specific indications such as the use of antibiotics for upper respiratory infections. Case reviews can be conducted by using broad judgmental criteria established by specialists in the field. Examples of evaluation categories proposed by Kunin et al.[11] and modified by Jones and his group[29] are presented in Table 3.

An advisory committee on infectious disease to the Veterans Administration (VA) established specific guidelines and audits for antibiotic use to aid individual hospital staffs in conducting their own programs of surveillance.[51] The Infectious Diseases Society of America has developed a set of guidelines for control of the use of antimicrobial agents in hospitals.[52] It is recommended that the guidelines be implemented by a team delegated with this responsibility by the Pharmacy and Therapeutics and Infection Control Committees. The teams consist of a physician knowledgeable in infectious diseases, an infection control practioner, a clinical pharmacist, and a clinical microbiologist. The savings to the hospital in costs and potential reduction of resistant organisms should more than offset the support needed for the team.

Several groups have experimented with methods to evaluate appropriate use of antimicrobial agents in ambulatory practice. Useful data are being gathered by the Kaiser-Permanente group in California and by others. Ray et al.[21,22] have reported that Medicaid data can be used as a surveillance method of individual practitioners. The major advantage is the ability to detect a small group of aberrant physicians who appear to account for most of the inappropriate usage.

CONSTRAINTS OF MEDICAL PRACTICE THAT LEAD TO INAPPROPRIATE USAGE

To solve the problem of inappropriate usage, we must understand the constraints under which physicians work and the pressures that are exerted on them to prescribe drugs. An overall scheme of the elements that motivate the patient to seek help and to comply with the physician and the forces that lead the physician to prescribe drugs are outlined in Figure 2. Each of

TABLE 2. Methods of Surveillance of Antimicrobial Agent Usage in Hospitals

Gross use data based on pharmacy records
Inexpensive; provides secular trends on usage of individual agents and costs; may be used for interhospital comparisons when adjusted for patient hospital days; may identify unusual practices that may lead to more detailed studies
Utilization by services
Inexpensive if pharmacy record system is on unit dose system or can identify shipment to specific wards; will provide data on problems of use by different groups of physicians and may lead to detailed studies of potential problem areas; will refine gross utilization for more appropriate interhospital coomparisons
Survey of routine orders for prophylaxis in surgery
Requires chart review of all cases for specific operations; provides data on actual practices of individual surgeons; permits comparison of practices in different hospitals; identifies unusual practices and can be used for feedback to the surgical service
Survey of orders for specific infectious diseases
Based on discharge diagnosis such as pneumonia, bronchitis, urinary tract infection; provides data on actual practices of individual physicians; permits comparison of practice according to specialty groups and can be used for feedback in education programs
Case review by independent experts
Requires establishment of strict criteria to avoid subjective or varying standards; requires establishment of feedback loops to practicing physicians; may identify specific problems of individual physicians
Guidelines audit
Hospital staffs establish standards of practice and guidelines based on national criteria; audit is used to evaluate compliance with self-imposed standards; enables peer pressure to provide checks and balances; mutes external judgmental evaluations; must be altered as new knowledge of new agents is introduced; may be used for interhospital comparisons

TABLE 3. Suggested Categories for Determining Appropriate Use of Antimicrobial Agents by Peer Review

Categories	
Kunin et al.	*Jones et al.*
Appropriate use	
Agree with the use of antimicrobial therapy/prophylaxis	Appropriate
	Probably appropriate
Agree with the use of antimicrobial therapy/prophylaxis, but a potentially fatal bacterial infection cannot be ruled out or prophylaxis is probably appropriate; advantages derived remain controversial	
Inappropriate use	
Agree with the use of antimicrobial therapy/prophylaxis, but a different (usually less expensive or toxic) antimicrobial is preferred	More effective drug recommended
	Less expensive/toxic drug recommended
	Improper dosage or dosage interval
Agree with the use of antimicrobial therapy/prophylaxis, but a modified dose is recommended	Unjustified, length of treatment excessive
	Unjustified, use of any antimicrobial not indicated
Disagree with the use of antimicrobial therapy/prophylaxis; administration is unjustified	Records insufficient for categorization

(Data from Kunin et al.[11] and Jones et al.[29])

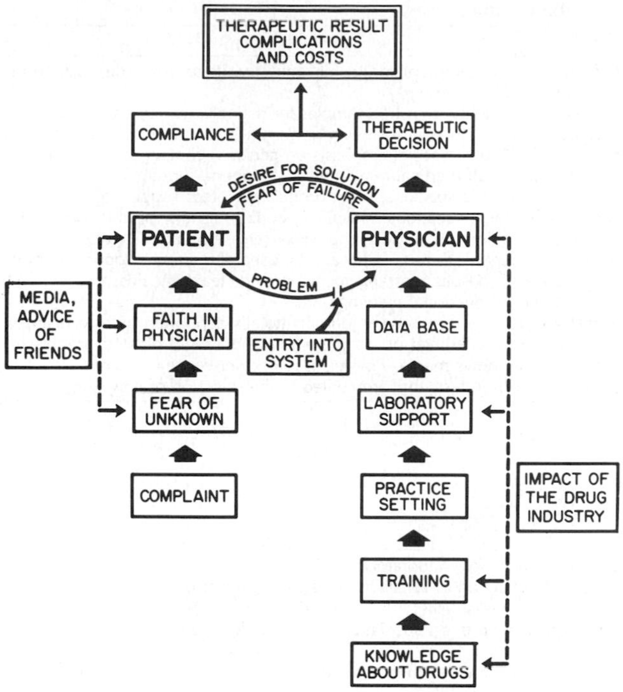

FIG. 2. Outline of the elements and complex interrelationships that influence the patient to use drugs.

the factors leading to misuse of antimicrobial agents is described in Table 4. They begin with the desire of physicians to help their patients and end with the ready solution offered by the pharmaceutical manufacturers to satisfy these needs.

The pharmaceutical manufacturers are keenly aware of the needs of the practicing physician. Dr. Donald Kennedy, a former FDA commissioner, estimated that in 1977 the industry spent $4000 per physician on direct drug advertising. IMS America, Limited, reported that advertising by U.S. drug companies in 1984 cost almost 1.4 billion dollars and was rising at a rate of about 8 percent per year. This does not include funds spent for premarketing evaluation of new drugs by clinical investigators. It is apparent that enormous pressure is exerted on the physician. Not all these funds are spent directly on individual physicians but are often invested in medical education programs. Some of the methods of promotional attack and their objectives are presented in Table 5. We must realize that every step in the medical educational process, beginning with the undergraduate years and upward, is subjected to heavy pharmaceutical promotion, including pressure on academic physicians who tend to set standards of practice.[53]

PROPOSALS FOR IMPROVEMENT OF ANTIBIOTIC USE

Methods to improve the use of antibiotics have been proposed in several editorials and reviews. Most emphasize the need for improved education of physicians in the diagnosis and treatment of infectious diseases. Some institutions have developed effective programs by requiring consultation for high-cost oral cephalosporins,[54] compulsory prospective antibiotic control,[55] antibiotic prescription forms that justify the reason for antibiotic use,[56] or routine surveillance.[57] The efficacy of each of the proposed methods to control the misuse of antibiotics (Table 6) depends on whether they meet the needs of the practicing physician.

The first method is education.[58] Neu and Howrey[59] demonstrated that there were major deficiencies in the physician's knowledge of antibiotic use, and they emphasized the need for further postgraduate education in this field. However, even though continued medical education is expanding in the United States, there is no concrete evidence that it improves actual practice. One study evaluating the effect of education was conducted by Jones et al.[29] The staff at a VA hospital did not show improvement in antibiotic use after an intensive educational program (Table 1). Gilbert and Jackson[60] reported success in improving antibiotic use by targeting their campaign for one drug, gentamicin. Achong et al.[30] reported remarkable success that in large part was attributable to improved use of antibiotics in surgical prophylaxis.

Another method, control of contact between pharmaceutical representatives and staff physicians, is only sporadically successful in a few institutions. The representative is usually visualized as a helpful colleague who provides quick information and favors and is properly obsequious. Entry is aided by advertising gimmicks and gifts, provision of funds for education, guest speakers, and funds for research or fellowship training.

TABLE 4. Factors That Lead to Inappropriate Use of Antimicrobial Agents

Motivation of the physician to give the best treatment	Desire to provide the patient with the very best drug available without regard to outside influences such as cost; fear of failure to provide the patient with the most appropriate drugs; desire to prevent infection before it may occur
Belief that if a small amount of drug will be effective, higher and more prolonged usage might be better	For example, the use of high dose intravenous penicillin for pneumococcal infections rather than equally effective smaller doses of procaine penicillin
Use of multiple antimicrobial agents or broad-spectrum agents to cover unusual organisms	Often appropriate in patients with severe leukopenia, but usually used as a substitute for diagnostic judgment
Inappropriate use of resources of clinical microbiology laboratory	Failure to obtain appropriate cultures; delay in transport of specimens and receiving needed information; poor interpersonal relations with the diagnostic laboratory; lack of explanation of results of tests by the laboratory; resistance of the laboratory to use simple culture methods in wards and clinics; need for consultant for interpretation of stained specimens; availability of rapid tests such as penicillinase production, Quellung reactions, tube dilution sensitivities, serum bactericidal levels; inappropriate sensitivity testing of ineffective agents (e.g., nitrofurantoin for systemic gram-negative infection)
Pressure from the patient to be treated with an antimicrobial agent	Desire to get rid of infection as soon as possible to avoid interference with life-style; concern of parents about febrile illness in their child; enhanced expectation for a solution of problems by drugs; fear of the unknown
Cost and availability of radiographic studies and diagnostic tests in relation to ready solution offered by drugs	Depends on practice setting, availability and costs of radiographic studies and diagnostic tests, policy of third-party payors, and distribution of physicians and other health care providers
Adequacy of the physician's knowledge of diagnostic procedures and management of patients with infectious disease	Depends on the extent of exposure to these disciplines in medical school and during postgraduate training; number of years since graduation, medical discipline, continuing education, self-instruction from literature, source(s) of information, experience in caring for patients with simple vs. complicated infectious disease
Malpractice considerations	Have forced physicians to practice defensive medicine by ordering excessive tests and using drugs to solve anticipated problems; explain in part, the overuse of oral cephalosporins in the hope that these new, more expensive, but relatively safe drugs will prevent embarrassment later; the threat of malpractice tends to decrease the usage of more toxic agents such as aminoglycoside antibiotics
Solution provided by pharmaceutical manufacturers	Take advantage of the above concerns and problems by offering often expensive and inappropriate panaceas and using heavy promotion; exploitation of the fear of failure by the physician to help his patient and of the concept that "if it might do some good and probably will do little harm, why not try it?"

TABLE 5. Methods Used by the Pharmaceutical Industry to Influence Physician Prescribing Habits

Group	*Objectives*	*Methods*
Medical students	Develop confidence in industry	Gifts of books, equipment, drugs for family; visits to plant; distribution of learning aids
House staff and fellows	Develop confidence in specific products	Same as for students, plus free samples for patients; advice on products by representatives; support for travel to meetings, throw-away journals
Practicing physicians	Create image of common goal of the physician and industry	Same as above plus special emphasis on personal contact with firm representatives; small medical-related gifts, stationery, forms
Hospital and medical societies	Create general goodwill for entry of representatives of the firm	Support for outside speakers, often product-oriented; support of meetings, entertainment, educational aids films, books—usually product oriented
General media	Raise public expectation for new drugs	News releases timed with development or release of a new agent
Academic physicians	Influence leaders to introduce new drugs to students and physicians	Support of directed studies of new agents; general research support; support for trainees; consultant arrangements, provide teaching aids; travel to national and international meetings
Medical media	Increase awareness of new products; blunt attack of critics	Direct advertising; throw-away journals (totally supported by advertising), published proceedings of symposia on new drugs; planted articles in throw-away news media, *Physicians' Desk Reference*
Diagnostic laboratories	Increase awareness of new agents	Special diagnostic tests that are related to the selection of new drugs

TABLE 6. Methods Used to Control the Use of Antimicrobial Agents in Hospitals

Education programs on the use of antimicrobial agents
- Staff conferences
- Lectures by outside authorities
- Audiovisual programs
- Clinical pharmacist consultants
- Hospital–Pharmacy Committee newsletters
- Independent sources of information (medical letter, AMA drug evaluations)

Control of contact between pharmaceutical representatives and staff physicians
- Registration in the pharmacy
- Visits to staff physicians by appointment only
- Policy concerning entry of salesmen to patient care areas
- Restricted time and place of displays
- Policy on free samples, gifts
- Policy on sponsoring speakers, distribution of literature, and advertising note paper

Hospital formulary
- Restriction of formulary to minimum number of agents needed for most effective therapy
- Elimination of duplicative agents
- Substitution rules for least expensive, most effective agent among a given class of agents
- Generic terminology required for all orders and labels

Diagnostic microbiology laboratory sensitivity tests
- Appropriate selection of sensitivity tests for organism and site
- Use of generic class disks
- Restriction of reports on specialized agents unless specifically requested or indicated
- Print own resort forms with generic terminology

Automatic stop orders for specific high-cost agents

Written justification for high-cost agents
- In cases where alternative, equally effective, less expensive or toxic agents may be used (e.g., oral cephalosporins, new parenteral aminoglycosides, and cephalosporins, lincosamides, chloramphenicol)

Required consultation
- This is to be done after first 3 doses of specific high-cost agents are ordered (e.g., aminoglycosides, parenteral cephalosporins, carbenicillin-ticarcillin, lincosamides)

Controlled agents
- Release of specific agents that may alter the ecology of hospital flora requires approval by infectious disease consultants (e.g., amikacin, carbenicillin-ticarcillin)

Guidelines and audits of antimicrobial usage
- These permit the hospital staff to set standards of use based on local needs and judgments, guided by independent criteria. An audit is based on compliance with these standards but requires a well-structured, authoritative feedback loop.

It is extremely difficult even for the academic physician to restrict these people since the information they bring is often valuable and the companies do develop many excellent antimicrobial agents. However, I believe that contact with drug representatives should be limited and restricted only to providing new information in a physician- and hospital-controlled setting. Some have proposed that ''counterdetailing'' by clinical pharmacists may help.[61] Schaffner et al.[62] have shown that visits to office-based practitioners by physician counselors was the most effective method to reduce the prescribing of overused antibiotics.

The hospital formulary committee can be extremely useful in examining the claims and need for new agents. It is in this area that the clinical pharmacist may be of greatest help by advising the committee on the relative benefits of adding or deleting agents from the formulary.

In many ways, the diagnostic laboratory also plays a key role in the selection of antimicrobial agents by physicians. So it is exceedingly important that antibiotic sensitivity tests results be reported by generic name and class and be tailored to the best agents according to the organism and site of infection.[63]

Several imaginative methods have been developed to control antibiotic usage. These include automatic ''stop'' orders for specific high-cost agents, the use of single daily doses of long-acting agents that can also be given intramuscularly,[48–50] prospective monitoring of use, computer surveillance,[64–66] and cost sharing by outpatients.[67] A rational approach described by Quintiliani et al. is to ''streamline'' the sequence of therapy.[68] A modification of this approach is shown in Table 7. The physician can move rapidly from presumptive therapy in stage I to definitive therapy in stage II by the early use of rapid diagnostic procedures such as examination of wounds and body fluids with Gram stains and specific antibodies.

Written justification for the use of antibiotics on the prescription is an effective method to decrease inappropriate usage. This forces physicians to explain their actions, and the requirement to write even a brief justification tends to blunt unnecessary prescribing. McGowan and Finland[69] have demonstrated that the removal of this requirement has been followed by increased use of these agents.

Required consultations and control of high-cost or toxic agents by experts have been shown to work well in an institution in which there is an active training program in infectious disease and a strong infectious disease group interested in antimicrobial therapy. However, these measures are not applicable at this time to many hospitals in the United States. Nevertheless, the results of these two approaches are instructive. They clearly demonstrate that most antibiotic usage is wasteful and unnecessary. For example, we have been able to reduce overusage markedly by generating an automatic consultation through the hospital pharmacy once the first three doses of an expensive, potentially toxic agent are ordered. This avoids denying the

TABLE 7. Three Typical Stages of Antibiotic Therapy in Hospital-Associated Infections

Stage	*Patient's Condition*	*Diagnosis/Treatment*
Initial	Presumed to have an infectious process	Blood cultures, aspiration of wound or body fluid, gram or other specific stain Specific, established agents may be used effectively
I (days 1–3)	Clinically unstable; uncertain of cause or site of infection	Empirical therapy, β-lactam and aminoglycoside or extended-spectrum β-lactam
II (days 4–6)	Begins to stabilize; causative agent identified	Specific therapy often with single, long-acting, narrow spectrum; parenteral or even oral agent may be used
III (days 7 and beyond)	Clinically stable, completion of therapy	Oral therapy or long-acting parenteral agent administered as outpatient or at home

(Modified from Quintiliani et al.,[68] with permission.)

patient a needed drug but permits early appraisal of the appropriateness of the antibiotic. As the program continues, less consultation is required since physicians soon become aware that their practice will be reviewed with them. Cephalosporin antibiotic use fell dramatically during the period of control. In most cases, a less expensive agent such as penicillin G was used instead, or postsurgical use of a cephalosporin was curtailed. Evaluation of patient records revealed that no patient was denied adequate therapy during the control period. The difference between the use of this class of drugs before and after control measures indicates the amount of this drug unnecessarily prescribed in the hospital.

Since most hospital staffs must function without the aid of experts in antimicrobial therapy, independent guidelines for appropriate use are needed. These guidelines need to be updated continuously. They potentially offer a basis for local discussion of the issues and modifications that best suit the judgment and needs of the practicing physicians. The most critical guidelines are for prophylaxis in surgery and for the use of oral and parenteral cephalosporin antibiotics. It is in these areas that the highest cost and greatest waste occurs. The guidelines are not excessively restrictive since they are based on the best available data from the surgical literature that emphasize short perioperative courses of the most effective agents. This auditing function measures compliance with local standards and provides feedback to the hospital staff who fail to adhere to guidelines accepted by their peers. The report of success in controlling overuse by Achong et al.[30] supports the idea that a well-informed and concerned staff can reduce the inappropriate use of antibiotics.

SUMMATION AND COMMENTARY

This chapter has described the problem of overuse of antibiotics. It is part of a larger problem of overuse of medical care facilities, diagnostic tests, and other drugs. The problem and its solution depend on knowledge of the constraints in medical practice that tend to lead the physician to overprescribe antibiotics. Instruction in infectious disease and antimicrobial therapy has been severely curtailed recently in most medical schools. This error, in my view, must be redressed by greater rather than less formal instruction. The problem, however, extends well beyond the formative years of the physician's education and cannot be solved by a punitive approach to the pharmaceutical industry. The industry simply exploits the constraints of medical practice to sell its products.

The overuse of antibiotics is not simply an economic problem, even though it is easily measured by these standards, nor is it just poor practice because of the heavy price paid for ecologic changes with new, resistant microbial strains. Most importantly, in my view, it reveals how effectively we as physicians use scientific technology to help our patients. The solution to the problem rests on our willingness to use this technology wisely.

REFERENCES

1. Jawetz E. Antimicrobial chemotherapy. Annu Rev Microbiol. 1956;10:85.
2. Welch H, Lewis CN, Weinstein HI, et al. Severe reactions to antibiotics: A nationwide survey. Antibiot Med Chem Ther. 1957;4:800.
3. Finland M, Jones WF, Barnes MW. Occurrence of serious bacterial infections since introduction of antibacterial agents. JAMA. 1959;170:84.
4. Reimann HA, D'Ambola J. The use and cost of antimicrobics in hospitals. Arch Environ Health. 1966;13:631.
5. Lockwood, WR. Antibiotics anonymous. N Engl J Med. 1974;290:465.
6. Simmons HE, Stolley PD. This is medical progress? Trends and consequences of antibiotic use in the United States. JAMA. 1974;227:1023.
7. Craig WA, Sarver KP. Antimicrobial usage in the USA. In: Williams JD, Geddes AM, eds. Chemotherapy, v. 4. New York: Plenum; 1976:293.
8. McGowan JE Jr. Antimicrobial resistance in hospital organisms and its relation to antibiotic use. Rev Infect Dis. 1983;5:1033.
9. Sogaard H, Zimmerman-Nielsen C, Sibioni K. Antibioticresistant gram-negative bacilli in a urological ward for male patients during a 9-year period: Relationship to antibiotic consumption. J Infect Dis. 1974;130:646.
10. Bulger RJ, Sherris JC. Decreased incidence of antibiotic resistance among *Staphylococcus aureus*. A study in a university hospital over a 9-year period. Ann Intern Med. 1968;69:1099.
11. Kunin CM, Tupasi T, Craig WA. Use of antibiotics: A brief exposition of the problem and some tentative solutions. Ann Intern Med. 1973;79:555.
12. Cluff LE. The prescribing habits of physicians. Hosp Pract. 1967;2:100.
13. Seidl LG, Thornder GF, Smith SW, et al. Studies on epidemiology of adverse drug reactions. III. Reactions in patients on general medical service. Bull Johns Hopkins Hosp. 1966;119:299.
14. Stolley PD, Becker MH, McEvilla JB, et al. Drug prescribing and use in an American community. Ann Intern Med. 1972;76:537.
15. Becker MH, Stolley PD, Lasagna L, et al. Differential education concerning therapeutics and resultant physician prescribing patterns. J Med Educ. 1972;47:118.
16. Antibiotics for common colds? (Editorial). Lancet. 1976;1:132.
17. Stott NCH, West RR. Randomized controlled trial of antibiotics in patients with cough and purulent sputum. Lancet. 1976;2:556.
18. Stollerman GH: The relative rheumatogenicity of strains of group A streptococci. Mod Concepts Cardiovasc Dis. 1975;44:35.
19. Greenberg RA, Wagner EH, Wolf SH, et al. Physician opinions on the use of antibiotics in respiratory infections. JAMA. 1978;240:650.
20. Bernstein LR, Barriere SL, Conte JE. Utilization of antibiotics: Analysis of appropriateness of use. Ann Emerg Med. 1982;11:400.
21. Ray WA, Federspiel CF, Schaffner W. Prescribing of chloramphenicol in ambulatory practice. An epidemiologic study among Tennessee Medicaid recipients. Ann Intern Med. 1976;84:266.
22. Ray WA, Federspiel CF, Schaffner W. Prescribing of tetracycline to children less than 8 years old. JAMA. 1977;237:2069.
23. Scheckler WE, Bennett JV. Antibiotic usage in seven community hospitals. JAMA. 1970;213:264.
24. Roberts AW, Visconti JA. The relational and irrational use of systemic antimicrobial drugs. Am J Hosp Pharm. 1972;29:1054.
25. Gibbs CW Jr, Gibson JT, Newton DS. Drug utilization review of actual versus preferred pediatric antibiotic therapy. Am J Hosp Pharm. 1973;30:892.
26. Castle M, Wilfert CM, Cate TR, et al. Antibiotic use at Duke University Medical Center. JAMA. 1977;237:2819.
27. Petrello MA, Linkewich JA, Gluckman SJ, et al. Clindamycin prescribing patterns in a university hospital. Am J Hosp Pharm. 1975;32:1111.
28. Maki DG, Schuna AA. A study of antimicrobial misuse in a university hospital. Am J Med Sci. 1978;275:271.
29. Jones SR, Bratton T, McRee E. The effect of an educational program upon hospital use. Am J Med Sci. 1977;273:79085.
30. Achong MR, Theal HK, Wood J, et al. Changes in hospital antibiotic therapy after a quality-of-use study. Lancet. 1977;2:1118.
31. McGowan JE Jr, Finland M. Effects of minitoring the use of antibiotics: An interhospital comparison. South Med J. 1976;69:193.
32. Shapiro M, Townsend TR, Rosner B, et al. Use of antimicrobial drugs in general hospitals. N Engl J Med. 1979;301:351.
33. Crossley K, Gardner LC. Antimicrobial prophylaxis in surgical patients. JAMA. 1981;245:722.

34. Shapiro M, Schoenbaum SC, Tager IB, et al. Benefit–cost analysis of antimicrobial prophylaxis in abdominal and vaginal hysterectomy. JAMA. 1983;249:1290.
35. Chretien JH, McGarvey M, de Stowlinski A, et al. Abuse of antibiotics, a study of patients attending a university clinic. Arch Intern Med. 1975;135:1063.
36. Gustafsson LL, Wide K. Marketing of obsolete antibiotics in Central America. Lancet. 1981;1:31.
37. Tomson G, Sterky G. Self-prescribing by way of pharmacies in three Asian developing countries. Lancet. 1986;2:620–1.
38. Kunin CM, Lipton HL, Tupasi T, et al. Social, behavior, and practical factors affecting antibiotic use worldwide: Report of task force 4. Rev Infect Dis. 1987;9(Suppl):270.
39. Levy M, Nir I, Superstine E, et al. Antimicrobial therapy in patients hospitalized in a medical ward. A report from the Boston collaborative drug surveillance program. Isr J Med Sci. 1975;11:322.
40. Study group in the use of antimicrobial drugs: Prophylactic antimicrobial drug therapy at five London teaching hospitals. Lancet. 1977;1:1351.
41. Cook D, Salter AJ, Phillips I: Antimicrobial misuse, antibiotic policies and information responses. J Antimicrob Chemother. 1980;6:435.
42. Leigh DA. Antimicrobial usage in forty-three hospitals in England. J Antimicrob Chemother. 1982;9:75.
43. Holmberg SD, Osterholm MT, Senger KA, et al. Drug-resistant *Salmonella* from animal fed antimicrobials. N Engl J Med. 1984;311:617.
44. DuPont HL, Steele JH. Use of antimicrobial agents in animal feeds: Implications for human health. Rev Infect Dis. 1987;9:447.
45. Kunin CM. The responsibility of the infectious disease community for the optimal use of antimicrobial agents. J Infect Dis. 1985;151:388.
46. Gitch DW. New ways of managing under prospective payment and their impact on the principles and practice of infectious diseases. Rev Infect Dis. 1986;8:494.
47. Iannini PB. DRGs and outpatient antibiotics. Infect Control. 1986;7:289.
48. Poretz DM, Eron LJ, Goldenberg RI, et al. Home intravenous antibiotic therapy: A team approach. JAMA. 1982;248:336.
49. Smego RA Jr. Home intravenous antibiotic therapy. Arch Intern Med. 1985;145:1001.
50. Eisenberg JM, Kitz DS. Savings from outpatient antibiotic therapy for osteomyelitis. Economic analysis of a therapeutic strategy. JAMA. 1986;255:1584.
51. Kunin CM. Guidelines and audits for use of antimicrobial agents in hospitals. J Infect Dis. 1977;135:335.
52. Marr JJ, Moffet HL, Kunin CM. Guidelines for improving use of antimicrobial agents in hospitals: A statement of the Infectious Diseases Society of America. J Infect Dis. 1988;157:869.
53. Musher DM. Antibiotics: The medium is the message (Letter). Rev Infect Dis. 1983;5:809.
54. Seligman SJ. Reduction in antibiotic costs by restricting use of an oral cephalosporin. Am J Med. 1981;71:941.
55. Recco RA, Gladstone JL, Friedman SA, et al. Antibiotic control in a municipal hospital. JAMA. 1979;241:2283.
56. Durbin WA, Lapidas B, Goldmann DA. Improved antibiotic usage following introduction of a novel prescription system. JAMA. 1981;246:1796.
57. Feldman L, Lamson M, Gallelli JF, et al. Surveillance of nosocomial infections by antibiotic monitoring. JAMA. 1979;241:2806.
58. Counts GW. Review and control of antimicrobial usage. JAMA. 1977;238:2170.
59. Neu HC, Howrey SP. Testing the physician's knowledge of antibiotic use: Self-assessment and learning via videotape. N Engl J Med. 1975;293:1291.
60. Gilbert DN, Jackson J. Effect of an education program on the proper use of gentamicin in a community hospital (Abstract). Clin Res. 1976;24:112.
61. Hendeles L. Need for "counter-detailing" antibiotics. Am J Hosp Pharm. 1976;33:918.
62. Schaffner W, Ray WA, Federspiel CF, et al: Improving antibiotic prescribing in office practice. A controlled trial of three educational methods. JAMA. 1983;250:1728.
63. Kunin CM. Antibiotic sensitivity tests: How to get the most out of them. Wis Med J. 1971;70:206.
64. Williams RR, Gross PA, Levin JF. Cost containment of the second-generation cephalosporins by prospective monitoring at a community teaching hospital. Arch Intern Med. 1985;145:1978.
65. Evans RS, Larsen RA, Burke JP, et al. Computer surveillance of hospital-acquired infections and antibiotic use. JAMA. 1986;256:1007.
66. Heineman HS, Watt VS. All-inclusive concurrent antibiotic usage review: A way to reduce misuse without formal controls. Infect Control. 1986;7:168.
67. Foxman B, Valdez RB, Lohr KN, et al. The effect of cost sharing on the use of antibiotics in ambulatory care: Results from a population-based randomized controlled trial. J Chronic Dis. 1987;40:429.
68. Quintiliani R, Cooper BW, Briceland LL, et al. Economic impact of streamlining antibiotic administration. Am J Med. 1987;82(Suppl 4A):391.
69. McGowan JE Jr, Finland M. Usage of antibiotics in a general hospital: Effect of requiring justification. J Infect Dis. 1974;130:165.
70. Kunin CM, Efron HY. Audits of antimicrobial guidelines for peer review. JAMA.. 1977;237:1001, 1003, 1134, 1241, 1243, 1366, 1367, 1481, 1482, 1605, 1607, 1723, 1724, 1725, 1859, 1860, 1967, 1968, 1969.

38. TABLES OF ANTIMICROBIAL AGENT PHARMACOLOGY

SANDRA NORRIS
CHARLES H. NIGHTINGALE
GERALD L. MANDELL

The selection of an appropriate dose of an antimicrobial agent is based on information such as the site of infection, the identity and known or presumed antibiotic susceptibility of the infecting organism, dose-related drug toxicity, and the patient's ability to eliminate the drug. This chapter serves as a centralized source of pharmacologic information frequently sought for antimicrobial agents. For more detailed information about specific agents, see the appropriate chapter.

Generic and trade name tables for antimicrobial agents are provided. The antimicrobial "family" classification is also included to help the reader locate specific information in subsequent tables.

DOSING GUIDELINES

Generally, *dosage* selections from the upper end of the dosage range are recommended for severe, life-threatening infections (sepsis, meningitis). The lowest dosages are used for urinary tract infections. A sizable range in dosing *intervals* exists for some antimicrobial agents, with the longer duration between doses appropriate for less severe infections in which a critical threshold level in serum or other site of infection (e.g., central nervous system) is not mandatory or the drug concentrates significantly at the site of infection (urine, bile).

Dosing recommendations for the following drugs result from preliminary, premarketing clinical trials and at the time of publication have not been officially approved by the U.S. Food and Drug Administration: apalcillin, carumonam, cefepime, cefmenoxime, cefotiam, cefpiramide, cefpirome, cefsulodin, clarithromycin, enoxacin, fleroxacin, fluconazole, ganciclovir, itraconazole, lomefloxacin, ofloxacin, pefloxacin, rimantadine, roxithromycin, teicoplanin, temafloxacin, and temocillin. To prevent dosing errors, these recommendations should be checked with recent package inserts or current reference sources.

DOSAGE ADJUSTMENT FOR RENAL IMPAIRMENT

Drug half-life in *adults* with impaired renal function and changes related to dialysis procedures (HD: hemodialysis, PD: peritoneal dialysis) are summarized for the user. An alternative to the elongation of the interval between doses is reduction of the daily dose given at the "usual" dosing interval (Bennett et al.). Antimicrobial serum levels should be determined and patient-specific dosage adjustments made on the basis of these determinations.

Unless otherwise stated, the doses indicated for hemodialysis should supplement "anuric doses." The "usual adult dose" is for parenteral therapy unless designated oral (po).

With the increasing use of chronic ambulatory peritoneal dialysis (CAPD), drug addition to the dialysate solution with direct instillation into the peritoneal cavity is becoming a widely used method of drug delivery. Generally, one adds an amount of drug to dialysate solution to mimic the target serum concentration. For example, add 5 mg gentamicin per liter of dialysate solution for a desired serum level of 5 μg/ml.

BODY FLUID CONCENTRATIONS

In determining the appropriateness of a particular antibiotic for a given site of infection, the ultimate concentration of a drug as compared with the minimum inhibitory concentration for the infecting organism is critical rather than percent penetration as compared with serum. For example, the aminoglycosides are ineffective therapy for meningitis although they penetrate into the cerebrospinal fluid to a higher degree than does penicillin G, which is effective therapy for certain organisms. Percent penetration (relationship between peak concentration in a specific body fluid to serum) is, however, a valuable tool for comparisons among similar agents.

GENERIC-TRADE NAMES

Generic	Trade	Family
Acyclovir	Zovirax	Antiviral agents
Amantadine	Symmetrel	Antiviral agents
Amdinocillin	Coactin	Penicillins
Amikacin	Amikin	Aminoglycosides
Aminosalicylic acid	PAS Para Parasal Rexipas	Antimycobacterial agents Antimycobacterial agents Antimycobacterial agents Antimycobacterial agents
Amoxicillin	Amoxil Larotid Polymox Robamox Trimox	Penicillins Penicillins Penicillins Penicillins Penicillins
Amphotericin B	Fungizone	Antifungal agents
Ampicillin	Ampen Amcill Omnipen Omnipen N PenA Penbritin Pensyn Polycillin Polycillin N Principen Probampacin Supen Totacillin	Penicillins Penicillins Penicillins Penicillins Penicillins Penicillins Penicillins Penicillins Penicillins Penicillins Penicillins Penicillins Penicillins
Ampicillin probenecid	Polycillin-PRB Trojacillin-Plus	Penicillins Penicillins
Ansamycin	—	Antimycobacterial agents
Apalcillin	—	Penicillins
Azlocillin	Azlin	Penicillins
Aztreonam	Azactam	Other β-lactams
Bacampicillin	Spectrobid	Penicillins
Benzathine penicillin	Bicillin Permapen	Penicillins Penicillins
Bithionol	Bitin	Antiparasitic agents
Capreomycin	Capastat	Antimycobacterial agents
Carbenicillin	Geopen Pyopen	Penicillins Penicillins
Carbenicillin indanyl sodium	Geocillin	Penicillins
Cefaclor	Ceclor	Cephalosporins
Cefadroxil	Duricef	Cephalosporins
Cefamandole	Mandol	Cephalosporins
Cefazolin	Ancef Kefzol	Cephalosporins Cephalosporins
Cefmenoxime	Cefmax	Cephalosporins
Cefonicid	Monocid	Cephalosporins
Cefoperazone	Cefobid	Cephalosporins
Ceforanide	Precef	Cephalosporins
Cefotaxime	Claforan	Cephalosporins
Cefotetan	Cefotan	Cephalosporins
Cefotiam	—	Cephalosporins
Cefoxitin	Mefoxin	Cephalosporins
Cefsulodin	Cefomonil	Cephalosporins
Ceftazidime	Fortaz Tazicef Tazidime	Cephalosporins
Ceftizoxime	Cefizox	Cephalosporins
Ceftriaxone	Rocephin	Cephalosporins
Cefuroxime	Zinacef	Cephalosporins
Cephalexin	Keflex	Cephalosporins
Cephaloglycine	Kafocin	Cephalosporins
Cephaloridine	Loridine	Cephalosporins
Cephalothin	Keflin	Cephalosporins
Cephapirin	Cefadyl	Cephalosporins
Cephradine	Anspor Velosef	Cephalosporins Cephalosporins
Chloramphenicol	Chloromycetin	Chloramphenicol
Chloroquine	Aralen	Antiparasitic agents
Chlortetracycline	Aureomycin	Tetracyclines
Cinoxacin	Cinobac	Other urinary tract agents
Ciprofloxacin	Cipro	Quinolones
Clavulanate + amoxicillin	Augmentin	β-Lactamase inhibitors
Clavulanate + ticarcillin	Timentin	β-Lactamase inhibitors
Clindamycin	Cleocin	Lincosamides
Clofazimine	Lamprene	Antimycobacterial agents
Clotrimazole	Mycelex Lotrimin	Antifungal agents Antifungal agents
Cloxacillin	Tegopen	Penicillins
Colistimethate	Colymycin M	Polymyxins
Colistin	Colymycin S	Polymyxins
Cotrimoxazole	Bactrim Septra	Sulfonamides + trimethoprim
Cyclacillin	Cyclapen	Penicillins
Cycloserine	Oxamycin Seromycin	Antimycobacterial agents Antimycobacterial agents
Dapsone	Avlosulfon	Antimycobacterial agents
Demeclocycline	Declomycin	Tetracyclines
Dicloxacillin	Dycill Dynapen Pathocil Veracillin	Penicillins Penicillins Penicillins Penicillins
Diethylcarbamazine	Hetrazan	Antiparasitic agents

(Continued)

GENERIC-TRADE NAMES *(Continued)*

Generic	Trade	Family
Diiodohydroxyquin	Panaquin	Antiparasitic agents
Diloxanide furoate	Furamide	Antiparasitic agents
Doxycycline	Doxy II Doxychel Vibramycin	Tetracyclines Tetracyclines Tetracyclines
Emetine	—	Antiparasitic agents
Enoxacin	Comprecin	Quinolones
Erythromycin	E-mycin Erypar Ethril Ilotycin Kesso-mycin Robimycin	Erythromycins Erythromycins Erythromycins Erythromycins Erythromycins Erythromycins
Erythromycin estolate	Ilosone	Erythromycins
Erythromycin ethylsuccinate	E.E.S. Pediamycin	Erythromycins Erythromycins
Erythromycin ethylsuccinate plus sulfisoxazole	Pediazole	
Erythromycin stearate	Bristamycin Erythrocin Pfizer-E	Erythromycins Erythromycins Erythromycins
Ethambutol	Myambutol	Antimycobacterial agents
Ethionamide	Trecator-SC	Antimycobacterial agents
Flucytosine	Ancobon	Antifungal agents
Furazolidone	Furoxone	Antiparasitic agents
Fusidic acid	—	Fusidic acid
Ganciclovir	Cytovene	Antivirals
Gentamicin	Garamycin	Aminoglycosides
Griseofulvin	Fulvicin P-G Fulvicin U F Grifulvin V Gris-PEG Grisactin	Antifungal agents Antifungal agents Antifungal agents Antifungal agents Antifungal agents
Hetacillin	Versapen Versapen K	Penicillins Penicillins
Idoxuridine	Dendrid Herplex Stoxil	Antiviral agents Antiviral agents Antiviral agents
Imipenem + cilastatin	Primaxin	Other β-lactams
Iodoquinol (diiodohydroxyquin)	Yodoxin	Antiparasitic agents
Isoniazid	Hyzyd INH Niadox Niconyl Nydrazid	Antimycobacterial agents Antimycobacterial agents Antimycobacterial agents Antimycobacterial agents Antimycobacterial agents
Itraconazole	Sporanox	Antifungal agents
Kanamycin	Kantrex	Aminoglycosides
Ketoconazole	Nizoral	Antifungal agents
Lincomycin	Lincocin	Lincosamides
Mafenide	Sulfamylon	Sulfonamides + trimethoprim
Mebendazole	Vermox	Antiparasitic agents
Melarsoprol	Arsobal Mel B	Antiparasitic agents Antiparasitic agents
Methacycline	Rondomycin	Tetracyclines
Methenamine hippurate	Hiprex Urex	Other urinary tract agents Other urinary tract agents
Methenamine mandelate	Mandelamine	Other urinary tract agents
Methicillin	Celbenin Dimocillin RT Staphcillin	Penicillins Penicillins Penicillins
Metrifonate	Bilarcil	Antiparasitic agents
Metronidazole	Flagyl	Metronidazole
Mezlocillin	Mezlin	Penicillins
Miconazole	Micatin Monistat	Antifungal agents Antifungal agents
Minocycline	Minocin Vectrin	Tetracyclines Tetracyclines
Moxalactam	Moxam	Cephalosporins
Nafcillin	Nafcil Unipen	Penicillins Penicillins
Nalidixic acid	Cybis NegGram	Quinolones Quinolones
Neomycin	Mycifradin	Aminoglycosides
Netilmicin	Netromycin	Aminoglycosides
Niclosamide	Niclocide Yomesan	Antiparasitic agents Antiparasitic agents
Nifurtimox	Lampit	Antiparasitic agents
Niridazole	Ambilhar	Antiparasitic agents
Nitrofurantoin	Cyantin Furadantin Macrodantin Trantoin	Other urinary tract agents Other urinary tract agents Other urinary tract agents Other urinary tract agents
Norfloxacin	Noraxin	Other urinary tract agents
Novobiocin	Albamycin	—
Nystatin	Mycostatin Nilstat	Antifungal agents Antifungal agents
Oxacillin	Bactocill Prostaphlin Resistopen	Penicillins Penicillins Penicillins
Oxamniquine	Vansil	Antiparasitic agents
Oxolinic acid	Utibid	Quinolones
Oxytetracycline	Terramycin Uri-Tet	Tetracyclines Tetracyclines
Para-aminosalicylic acid, *see* aminosalicylic acid		
Paromomycin	Humatin	Antiparasitic agents
Penicillin G	Pentids Pfizerpen	Penicillins Penicillins
Penicillin G procaine	Crysticillin Duracillin AS Wycillin	Penicillins Penicillins Penicillins
Penicillin G sodium + penicillin G procaine	Duracillin FA	Penicillins
Penicillin G + phenoxymethyl penicillin	Kesso-pen	Penicillins
Penicillin V potassium (phenoxymethyl penicillin)	Betopen VK Ledercillin VK Penapar VK Pen Vee K Robicillin VK Uticillin VK V-Cillin K Veetids	Penicillins Penicillins Penicillins Penicillins Penicillins Penicillins Penicillins Penicillins
Pentamidine	Pentam 300 Lomidine	Antiparasitic agents Antiparasitic agents
Phenazopyridine	Azo Gantrisin	—
Phenethicillin	Darcil Maxipen Synicillin	Penicillins Penicillins Penicillins
Piperacillin	Pipracil	Penicillins
Piperazine	Antepar	Antiparasitic agents
Pivmecillinam	Selexid	Penicillins
Pivmecilliam sulfamicillin		Penicillins
Polymyxin B	Aerosporin	Polymyxins
Praziquantel	Biltricide	Antiparasitic agents
Primaquine phosphate	Primaquine	Antiparasitic agents
Pyrantel pamoate	Antiminth	Antiparasitic agents
Pyrazinamide	—	Antimycobacterial agents
Pyrimethamine	Daraprim	Antiparasitic agents
Pyrimethamine-sulfadoxine	Fansidar	Antiparasitic agents
Pyrivinium pamoate	Povan	Antiparasitic agents
Quinacrine	Atabrine	Antiparasitic agents
Quinine sulfate	—	Antiparasitic agents
Ribavirin	Virazole	Antiviral agents

(Continued)

GENERIC-TRADE NAMES *(Continued)*

Generic	*Trade*	*Family*
Rifampin	Rifadin Rimactane	Antimycobacterial agents Antimycobacterial agents
Rifampin-isoniazid	Rifamate	Antimycobacterial agents
Rimantadine	Flumadine	Antiviral agents
Silver sulfadiazine	Silvadine	Sulfonamides + trimethoprim
Spectinomycin	Trobicin	Aminoglycosides
Stibogluconate	Pentostam	Antiparasitic agent
Succinylsulfathiazole	Rolsul Sulfasuxidine	Sulfonamides + trimethoprim Sulfonamides + trimethoprim
Sulbactam + ampicillin	Unasyn	β-Lactamase inhibitors
Sulbactam + cefoperazone	—	β-Lactamase inhibitors
Sulfacetamide	Bleph Isopto cetamide Sulamyd sodium	Sulfonamides + trimethoprim Sulfonamides + trimethoprim Sulfonamides + trimethoprim
Sulfachlorpyridazine	Sonilyn	Sulfonamides + trimethoprim
Sulfacytine	Renoquid	Sulfonamides + trimethoprim
Sulfadiazine	Sulfadyne	Sulfonamides + trimethoprim
Sulfadoxine	Fansidar	Sulfonamides + trimethoprim
Sulfamethizole	Thiosulfil Urifon	Sulfonamides + trimethoprim Sulfonamides + trimethoprim Sulfonamides + trimethoprim
Sulfamethoxazole	Gantanol	Sulfonamides + trimethoprim
Sulfasalazine	Azulfidine	Sulfonamides + trimethoprim
Sulfisoxazole	Gantrisin	Sulfonamides + trimethoprim
Sultamicillin	—	β-Lactamase inhibitors
Suramin	Germanin	Antiparasitic agents
Teichomycin	—	—
Temocillin	—	Penicillins
Tetracycline	Achromycin Kesso-tetra Panmycin Polycycline Robitet Steclin Sumycin Tetracyn Tetrex	Tetracyclines Tetracyclines Tetracyclines Tetracyclines Tetracyclines Tetracyclines Tetracyclines Tetracyclines Tetracyclines
Thiabendazole	Mintezol	Antiparasitic agents
Ticarcillin	Ticar	Penicillins
Tobramycin	Nebcin	Aminoglycosides
Tolnaftate	Tinactin	Antifungal agents
Trifluridine	Viroptic	Antiviral agents
Trimethoprim	Proloprim Trimpex	Sulfonamides + trimethoprim Sulfonamides + trimethoprim
Trimethoprim-sulfamethoxazole	Bactrim Septra	Sulfonamides + trimethoprim Sulfonamides + trimethoprim
Trisulfapyrimidines	Terfonyl	Sulfonamides + trimethoprim
Troleandomycin	TAO	—
Vancomycin	Vancocin	Vancomycin
Vidarabine	Vira-A	Antiviral agents
Viomycin	Vinactane Viocin	Antimycobacterial agents Antimycobacterial agents
Zidovudine (AZT)	Retrovir	Antiviral agents

TRADE-GENERIC NAMES

Trade	*Generic*	*Family*
Achromycin	Tetracycline	Tetracyclines
Aerosporin	Polymyxin B	Polymyxins
Albamycin	Novobiocin	—
Ampen	Ampicillin	Penicillins
Ambilhar	Niridazole	Antiparasitic agents
Amcill	Ampicillin	Penicillins
Amikin	Amikacin	Aminoglycosides
Amoxil	Amoxicillin	Penicillins
Ancef	Cefazolin	Cephalosporins
Ancobon	Flucytosine	Antifungal agents
Anspor	Cephradine	Cephalosporins
Antepar	Piperazine citrate	Antiparasitic agents
Antiminth	Pyrantel pamoate	Antiparasitic agents
Apace	Cefotetan	Cephalosporins
Aralen	Chloroquine	Antiparasitic agents
Arsobal	Melarsoprol	Antiparasitic agents
Atabrine	Quinacrine	Antiparasitic agents
Augmentin	Clavulanate + amoxicillin	β-Lactamase inhibitors
Aureomycin	Chlortetracycline	Tetracyclines
Avlosulfon	Dapsone	Antimycobacterial agents
Azactam	Aztreonam	Other β-lactams
Azlin	Azlocillin	Penicillins
Azo Gantrisin	Phenazopyridine	—
Azulfidine	Sulfasalazine	Sulfonamides + trimethoprim
Bactocill	Oxacillin	Penicillins
Bactrim	Trimethoprim-sulfamethoxazole	Sulfonamides + trimethoprim
Betopen VK	Penicillin V potassium	Penicillins
Bicillin	Benzathine penicillin G	Penicillins
Bilarcil	Metrifonate	Antiparasitic agents
Biltricide	Praziquantel	Antiparasitic agents
Bitin	Bithionol	Antiparasitic agents
Bleph	Sulfacetamide	Sulfonamides + trimethoprim
Bristamycin	Erythromycin stearate	Erythromycins
Canesten	Clotrimazole	Antifungal agents
Capastat	Capreomycin	Antimycobacterial agents
Ceclor	Cefaclor	Cephalosporins
Cefadyl	Cephapirin	Cephalosporins
Cefizox	Ceftizoxime	Cephalosporins
Cefmax	Cefmenoxime	Cephalosporins
Cefobid	Cefoperazone	Cephalosporins
Cefomonil	Cefsulodin	Cephalosporins
Celbenin	Methicillin	Penicillins
Chloromycetin	Chloramphenicol	Chloramphenicol
Cinobac	Cinoxacin	Other urinary tract agents
Cipro	Ciprofloxacin	Quinolones
Claforan	Cefotaxime	Cephalosporins
Cleocin	Clindamycin	Lincosamides
Coactin	Amdinocillin	Penicillins
Colymycin M	Colistimethate	Polymyxins
Colymycin S	Colistin	Polymyxins

(*Continued*)

Trade	Generic	Family
Compresin	Enoxacin	Quinolones
Crysticillin	Penicillin G procaine	Penicillins
Cyantin	Nitrofurantoin	Other urinary tract agents
Cybis	Nalidixic acid	Quinolones
Cyclapen	Cyclacillin	Penicillins
Cytovene	Ganciclovir	Antivirals
Daraprim	Pyrimethamine	Antiparasitic agents
Darcil	Phenethicillin	Penicillins
Declomycin	Demeclocycline	Tetracyclines
Dendrid	Idoxuridine	Antiviral agents
Dimocillin RT	Methicillin	Penicillins
Doxy II	Doxycycline	Tetracyclines
Doxychel	Doxycycline	Tetracyclines
Duracillin AS	Penicillin G procaine	Penicillins
Duracillin FA	Penicillin G sodium + penicillin G procaine	Penicillins
Duricef	Cefadroxil	Cephalosporins
Dycill	Dicloxacillin	Penicillins
Dynapen	Dicloxacillin	Penicillins
E-mycin	Erythromycin	Erythromycins
E.E.S.	Erythromycin ethylsuccinate	Erythromycins
Erypar	Erythromycin	Erythromycins
Erythrocin	Erythromycin stearate	Erythromycins
Ethril	Erythromycin	Erythromycins
Fansidar	Pyrimethamine-sulfadoxine	Antiparasitic agents
Flagyl	Metronidazole	Metronidazole
Flumadine	Rimantadine	Antiviral agents
Fortaz	Ceftazidime	Cephalosporins
Fulvicin P-G	Griseofulvin	Antifungal agents
Fulvicin U-F	Griseofulvin	Antifungal agents
Fungizone	Amphotericin B	Antifungal agents
Furadantin	Nitrofurantoin	Other urinary tract agents
Furamide	Diloxanide furoate	Antiparasitic agents
Furoxone	Furazolidone	Antiparasitic agents
Gantanol	Sulfamethoxazole	Sulfonamides + trimethoprim
Gantrisin	Sulfisoxazole	Sulfonamides + trimethoprim
Garamycin	Gentamicin	Aminoglycosides
Geocillin	Carbenicillin indanyl sodium	Penicillins
Geopen	Carbenicillin	Penicillins
Germanin	Suramin	Antiparasitic agents
Grifulvin V	Griseofulvin	Antifungal agents
Gris-PEG	Griseofulvin	Antifungal agents
Grisactin	Griseofulvin	Antifungal agents
Herplex	Idoxuridine	Antiviral agents
Hetrazan	Diethylcarbamazine	Antiparasitic agents
Hiprex	Methenamine hippurate	Other urinary tract agents
Humatin	Paromomycin	Antiparasitic agents
Hyzyd	Isoniazid	Antimycobacterial agents
Ilosone	Erythromycin estolate	Erythromycins
Ilotycin	Erythromycin	Erythromycins
INH	Isoniazid	Antimycobacterial agents
Isopto cetamide	Sulfacetamide	Sulfonamides + trimethoprim
Kafocin	Cephaloglycine	Cephalosporins
Kantrex	Kanamycin	Aminoglycosides
Keflex	Cephalexin	Cephalosporins
Keflin	Cephalothin	Cephalosporins
Kefzol	Cefazolin	Cephalosporins

Trade	Generic	Family
Kesso-mycin	Erythromycin	Erythromycins
Kesso-pen	Penicillin G + phenoxymethyl penicillin	Penicillins
Kesso-tetra	Tetracycline	Tetracyclines
Lampit	Nifurtimox	Antiparasitic agents
Lamprene	Clofazimine	Antimycobacterial agents
Larotid	Amoxicillin	Penicillins
Ledercillin VK	Penicillin V potassium	Penicillins
Lincocin	Lincomycin	Lincosamides
Lomidine	Pentamidine	Antiparasitic agents
Loridine	Cephaloridine	Cephalosporins
Lotrimin	Clotrimazole	Antifungal agents
Macrodantin	Nitrofurantoin	Other urinary tract agents
Mandelamine	Methenamine mandelate	Other urinary tract agents
Mandol	Cefamandole	Cephalosporins
Maxipen	Phenethicillin	Penicillins
Mefoxin	Cefoxitin	Cephalosporins
Mel B	Melarsoprol	Antiparasitic agents
Mezlin	Mezlocillin	Penicillins
Micatin	Miconazole	Antifungal agents
Minocin	Minocycline	Tetracyclines
Mintezol	Thiabendazole	Antiparasitic agents
Monocid	Cefonicid	Cephalosporins
Monistat	Miconazole	Antifungal agents
Moxam	Moxalactam	Cephalosporins
Myambutol	Ethambutol	Antimycobacterial agents
Mycifradin	Neomycin	Aminoglycosides
Mycostatin	Nystatin	Antifungal agents
Nafcil	Nafcillin	Penicillins
Nebcin	Tobramycin	Aminoglycosides
NegGram	Nalidixic acid	Quinolones
Netromycin	Netilmicin	Aminoglycosides
Niadox	Isoniazid	Antimycobacterial agents
Niclocide	Niclosamide	Antiparasitic agents
Niconyl	Isoniazid	Antimycobacterial agents
Nilstat	Nystatin	Antifungal agents
Nizoral	Ketoconazole	Antifungal agents
Noraxin	Norfloxacin	Other urinary tract agents
Nydrazid	Isoniazid	Antimycobacterial agents
Omnipen	Ampicillin	Penicillins
Omnipen-N	Ampicillin	Penicillins
Oxamycin	Cycloserine	Antimycobacterial agents
PAS	Aminosalicylic acid	Antimycobacterial agents
Panaquin	Diiodohydroxyquin	Antiparasitic agents
Panmycin	Tetracycline	Tetracyclines
Para	Aminosalicylic acid	Antimycobacterial agents
Parasal	Aminosalicylic acid	Antimycobacterial agents
Pathocil	Dicloxacillin	Penicillins
Pediamycin	Erythromycin ethylsuccinate	Erythromycins
Pediazole	Erythromycin ethylsuccinate plus sulfisoxazole	Erythromycins
Pen Vee K	Penicillin V potassium	Penicillins
PenA	Ampicillin	Penicillins
Penapar VK	Penicillin V potassium	Penicillins
Penbritin	Ampicillin	Penicillins
Pensyn	Ampicillin	Penicillins
Pentam 300	Pentamidine	Antiparasitic agents
Pentids	Penicillin G	Penicillins
Pentostam	Stibogluconate	Antiparasitic agents

(Continued)

Trade	*Generic*	*Family*
Permapen	Benzathine penicillin G	Penicillins
Pfizer-E	Erythromycin stearate	Erythromycins
Pfizerpen	Penicillin G	Penicillins
Pipracil	Piperacillin	Penicillins
Polycillin	Ampicillin	Penicillins
Polycillin-N	Ampicillin	Penicillins
Polycillin-PRB	Ampicillin probenecid	Penicillins
Polycycline	Tetracycline	Tetracyclines
Polymox	Amoxicillin	Penicillins
Povan	Pyrivinium pamoate	Antiparasitic agents
Precef	Ceforanide	Cephalosporins
Primaquine	Primaquine phosphate	Antiparasitic agents
Primaxin	Imipenem + cilastatin	Other β-lactams
Principen	Ampicillin	Penicillins
Probampacin	Ampicillin	Penicillins
Proloprim	Trimethoprim	Sulfonamides + trimethoprim
Prostaphlin	Oxacillin	Penicillins
Pyopen	Carbenicillin	Penicillins
Renoquid	Sulfacytine	Sulfonamides + trimethoprim
Resistopen	Oxacillin	Penicillins
Retrovir	Zidovudine (AZT)	Antiviral agents
Rezipas	Aminosalicylic acid	Antimycobacterial agents
Rifadin	Rifampin	Antimycobacterial agents
Rifamate	Rifampin-isoniazid	Antimycobacterial agents
Rimactane	Rifampin	Antimycobacterial agents
Robamox	Amoxicillin	Penicillins
Robicillin VK	Penicillin V potassium	Penicillins
Robimycin	Erythromycin	Erythromycins
Robitet	Tetracycline	Tetracyclines
Rocephin	Ceftriaxone	Cephalosporins
Rolsul	Succinylsulfathiazole	Sulfonamides + trimethoprim
Rondomycin	Methacycline	Tetracyclines
Selexid	Pivmecillinam	Penicillins
Septra	Trimethoprim-sulfamethoxazole	Sulfonamides + trimethoprim
Seromycin	Cycloserine	Antimycobacterial agents
Silvadine	Silver sulfadiazine	Sulfonamides + trimethoprim
Sonilyn	Sulfachlorpyridazine	Sulfonamides + trimethoprim
Spectrobid	Bacampicillin	Penicillins
Sporanox	Itraconazole	Antifungal agents
Staphcillin	Methicillin	Penicillins
Steclin	Tetracycline	Tetracyclines
Stoxil	Idoxuridine	Antiviral agents
Sulamyd sodium	Sulfacetamide	Sulfonamides + trimethoprim
Sulfadyne	Sulfadiazine	Sulfonamides + trimethoprim
Sulfamylon	Mafenide	Sulfonamides + trimethoprim
Sulfasuxidine	Succinylsulfathiazole	Sulfonamides + trimethoprim
Sumycin	Tetracycline	Tetracyclines
Supen	Ampicillin	Penicillins
Symmetrel	Amantadine	Antiviral agents
Synicillin	Phenethicillin	Penicillins
TAO	Troleandomycin	—
Tazicef	Ceftazidime	Cephalosporins
Tazidime	Ceftazidime	Cephalosporins
Tegopen	Cloxacillin	Penicillins
Terfonyl	Trisulfapyrimidines	Sulfonamides + trimethoprim
Terramycin	Oxytetracycline	Tetracyclines
Tetracyn	Tetracycline	Tetracyclines
Tetrex	Tetracycline	Tetracyclines
Thiosulfil	Sulfamethizole	Sulfonamides + trimethoprim
Ticar	Ticarcillin	Penicillins
Timentin	Clavulanate + ticarcillin	β-Lactamase inhibitors
Tinactin	Tolnaftate	Antifungal agents
Totacillin	Ampicillin	Penicillins
Trantoin	Nitrofurantoin	Other urinary tract agents
Trecator-SC	Ethionamide	Antimycobacterial agents
Trimox	Amoxicillin	Penicillins
Trimpex	Trimethoprim	Sulfonamides + trimethoprim
Trobicin	Spectinomycin	Aminoglycosides
Trojacillin-Plus	Ampicillin probenecid	Penicillins
Unasyn	Ampicillin + Sulbactam	β-Lactamase inhibitors
Unipen	Nafcillin	Penicillins
Urex	Methenamine hippurate	Other urinary tract agents
Uri-tet	Oxytetracycline	Tetracyclines
Urifon	Sulfamethizole	Sulfonamides + trimethoprim
Utibid	Oxolinic acid	Quinolones
Uticillin VK	Penicillin V potassium	Penicillins
V-Cillin K	Penicillin V potassium	Penicillins
Vancocin	Vancomycin	Vancomycin
Vansil	Oxamniquine	Antiparasitic agents
Vectrin	Minocycline	Tetracyclines
Veetids	Penicillin V potassium	Penicillins
Velosef	Cephradine	Cephalosporins
Veracillin	Dicloxacillin	Penicillins
Vermox	Mebendazole	Antiparasitic agents
Versapen	Hetacillin	Penicillins
Versapen-K	Hetacillin	Penicillins
Vibramycin	Doxycycline	Tetracyclines
Vinactane	Viomycin	Antimycobacterial agents
Viocin	Viomycin	Antimycobacterial agents
Vira-A	Vidarabine	Antiviral agents
Virazole	Ribavirin	Antiviral agents
Viroptic	Trifluridine	Antiviral agents
Wycillin	Penicillin G procaine	Penicillins
Yodoxin	Iodoquinol	Antiparasitic agents
Yomesan	Niclosamide	Antiparasitic agents
Zinacef	Cefuroxime	Cephalosporins
Zovirax	Acyclovir	Antiviral agents

ANTIMICROBIAL AGENT PHARMACOLOGY: PENICILLINS

Drug (Oral Absorption, %)	Serum and Urine Concentration for Selected Doses			Dosage Recommendations						
				Adults			Children		Newborn (Parenteral)	
	Dose (g)	Peak Serum (μg/ml)	Peak or Range, Urine (μg/ml)	Oral (Dose/Interval)	Parenteral (Dose/Interval)	Maximum Daily Dose (g)	Oral (Dose/Interval)	Parenteral (Dose/Interval)	Up to 1 wk (Dose/Interval)	1–4 wk (Dose/Interval)
Amdinocillin	10 mg/kg[c]	50	1260		10 mg/kg q4–6h			10 mg/kg q4–6h (not approved)		
Amoxicillin (89)	0.25 po[d] 0.5 po[d]	4.7 (avg) 7.5 (avg)	 600–2000	0.25–0.5 g q8h		3	6.6–13.3 mg/kg q8h		Not recommended	
Ampicillin (50 avg)	0.25 po[d] 0.5 po[d] 1 po[d] 0.5 IV 0.5 IM 1 IV	1.8–2.9 2.5–4 2–6 2.9–7.1 8 40	90 100–700 100–1450 130–610 500–1000	0.5–1 g q6h	1–2 g q4–6h[e]	12	12.5–25 mg/kg q6h	25–50 mg/kg q6h[f]	50–100 mg/kg/day q12h	150–200 mg/kg/day q6–8h
Apalcillin	0.5 IM 1 IV[i,j] 2 IV[j]	28–37 47–58 208	 835							
Azlocillin[k] (minimal)	2 IV[c] 2 IV[j] 3 IV[c] 3 IV[j]	300 165 350 214	2200–8100		2–4 g q4–6h[l]	24		50 mg/kg q4h or 75 mg/kg q6h[m] (not approved)	Not recommended	
Bacampicillin[n] (60–90)	0.4 po 0.8 po	6–8 11–14		0.4–0.8 g q12h		1.6	12.5–25 mg/kg q12h			
Carbenicillin (minimal)	1 IM 2 IM 1 IV 1 g/hr IV 3 IV[c]	15–20 47 45–71 160 278	 2500 1000 4165		5–6.5 g q4–6h[o]	40		25–100 mg/kg q4–6h	200–300 mg/kg/day q8h	400 mg/kg/day q6–8h
Carbenicillin indanyl sodium (30–50)	0.382 po (1 tablet)	6.5	1130	1–2 tablets q6h		3	7.5–12.5 mg/kg q6h			
Cloxacillin (50)	0.5 po	7–14	410–1080	0.5–1 g q6h		4	12.5–25 mg/kg q6h		Not recommended	
Cyclacillin	0.25 po 0.5 po	6–7 11–12		0.25–0.5 g q6h		2	12.5–25 mg/kg q6h		Not recommended	
Dicloxacillin (37–74)	0.5 po	15–18		0.25–0.5 g q6h		4	3.125–6.25 mg/kg q6h		Not recommended	
Hetacillin[p]	0.225 po 0.45 po	1.7–2.1 2.5–2.7		0.225–0.45 g q6h			5.6–11.25 mg/kg q6h			
Methicillin (minimal)	1 IV[c] 1 IM 2 IV[j]	60 18 80			1–2 g q4–6h	12		25–33.3 mg/kg q4–6h	25 mg/kg q8–12h[q]	25 mg/kg q6–8h[r]
Mezlocillin[k] (minimal)	1 IM 2 IV[c] 3 IV[c] 3 IV[j]	15 199 310 263	 >4000		3–4 g q4–6h	24		50 mg/kg q4–6h	150 mg/kg/day q12h	300 mg/kg/day q6h[s]
Nafcillin (10–20 erratic)	0.5 IV[j]	11		0.5–1 g q6h	0.5–1.5 g q4–6h	9	12.5–25 mg/kg q6h	150 mg/kg/day q4–6h	25 mg/kg q12h	25 mg/kg q8h
Oxacillin (33)	0.5 po 0.5 IM	5–6 11	 200–2000	0.5–1 g q6h	0.5–2 g q4–6h	12	12.5–25 mg/kg q6h	37.5–50 mg/kg q6h	50–75 mg/kg/day q8–12h	100–150 mg/kg/day q6–8h
Penicillin G (15–30)	0.25 po 0.5 po 3 IV[j] (4.8 × 10^6 U) 12 g/day IV (19.2 × 10^6 U)[t]	0.6 1.5–2.7 400 16	85	0.5–1 g q6h	1.2–24 × 10^6 U/day q2–12h[u]	24 × 10^6 U	6.25–12.5 mg/kg q6h	100,000–250,000 U/kg/day q2–12h[u]	50,000–150,000 U/kg/day q8–12h	75,000–250,000 U/kg/day q6–8h
Penicillin V (60) (phenoxymethyl penicillin)	0.5 po	3–5		0.25–0.5 g q6h		4	6.25–12.5 mg/kg q6h		Not recommended	
Procaine penicillin G	600,000 U IM	1			0.3–4.8 × 10^6 U/day IM			25,000 U/kg q12–24h		
Penicillin G benzathine	1.2 × 10^6 U IM	0.12 U/ml	20 U/ml		2.4 × 10^6 U IM[w]	2.4 × 10^6 U IM		50,000 U/kg IM	50,000 U/kg IM	50,000 U/kg IM
Piperacillin[k] (minimal)	2 IV[c] 4 IV[j] 4 IV[c]	220 244 412	 1,000–8,500		3–4 g q4–6h	24		50 mg/kg q4–6h (Not approved)		
Ticarcillin (minimal)	1 IM 3 IV 5 IV	35 190 327	2000		3 g q4–6h	24–30		50 mg/kg q4–6h	150–225 mg/kg/day q8–12h[x]	225–300 mg/kg/day q6–8h[x]
Temocillin (minimal)	0.5 IV[c] 1 IV[c] 2 IV[c]	78 160 236	100–500		0.5–1 g q12h					

[a] Penicillins penetrate minimally across uninflamed meninges into the CSF.
[b] Penicillins do not appear in sufficient quantities to treat infections in the infant but do appear in quantities that could lead to allergic sensitization.
[c] IV push (over 2–5 min).
[d] Fasting.
[e] Meningitis should be treated q4h.
[f] Up to 400 mg/kg/day for *Haemophilus influenzae* type b meningitis in children.
[g] Mean concentration.
[h] Candidiasis and diarrhea in infants may result from ampicillin administration to nursing mothers. (*Pharm J.* 1976;217:219.)
[i] Remarkable differences in peak serum levels measured immediately after a 2-minute bolus (1 g: 825 μg/ml) as compared with a 2-hour infusion.
[j] Infusion (over 15–30 minutes).
[k] Dose-dependent pharmacokinetics.
[l] For severe, life-threatening infections: 4 g q4h.

Serum Half-life (hr): For Creatinine Clearance (ml/min) >80	<10	With Dialysis: HD	PD	Usual Adult Dose and Interval Adjustment For Creatinine Clearance (ml/min): Dose	>80	80–50	50–10	<10 (Anuric)	Dosage for Dialysis: Dose after HD Supplemental to Anuric	Daily Dose during PD	CSF/Serum (%) Inflamed Meninges[a]	Newborn Serum/Maternal Serum (%)	Breast Milk/Maternal Serum[b] (%)	Bile/Serum (%)	Aqueous Humor/Serum (%)
0.8–1	3.4–5.6	1.8		10 mg/kg	4 hr	4 hr	6–8 hr	8 hr	10 mg/kg					400	
1	16	2.2–4.5		0.25–0.5 g po	8 hr	8 hr	12 hr	12–24 hr	0.25 g		5–10	100	5		
0.5–1	8–20	2–5	10.9	1–2 g	4–6 hr	6 hr	8 hr	12 hr	0.5 g		8–13[g]	100	11[h]	100–1000	2–8
1.5–2															
1	5	1.5–2.6	Minimal	2–4 g	4–6 hr	4–6 hr	8 hr	12 hr	3 g		13.3[g]				
1	8–20	2–5		0.4–0.8 g po	12 hr	12 hr	12 hr	24 hr				65–75	1.7–3.6	17	
0.5–1	12.5	6	4.2–7.4	5–6.5 g	4–6 hr	6 hr	2–3 g q6–8h	2 g q12h	2 g	2 g q6h	9.4[g]	50–100	0.4	50–75	Up to 3
0.5	0.8	Minimal	Minimal	0.5–1 g po	6 hr	6 hr	6 hr	6 hr							
0.5	3.5			0.25–0.5 g po	6 hr	6 hr	12–24 h	24 h							
0.7	1–2	1.6	Minimal	0.25–0.5 g po	6 hr	6 hr	6 hr	6 hr			Minimal	0–10		5–8	
0.3			0.225–0.45 g po	6 hr											
0.5	4	Minimal	Minimal	1–2 g	4–6 hr	6 hr	8 hr	12 hr	2 g		3–12	50–100		20–50	1–2
1.1[i]	1.6–2.6	1.2–1.4	Minimal	3–4 g	4–6 hr	4–6 hr	6–8 hr	8–12 hr	2–3 g	Anuric dosage	14[g]	100		1000	
0.5	1.2	Minimal	Minimal	0.5–1.5 g	4–6 hr	4–6 hr	4–6 hr	4–6 hr			9–20	10–15		4000	1–2
0.5	2	Minimal	1.4	0.5–2 g	4–6 hr	4–6 hr	4–6 hr	4–6 hr				10–15	≤3.5	20–40	0–20
0.5	7–10	5		1.2–24 × 10^6 U/day	2–12 hr	2–12 hr	2–12 hr	$\frac{1}{3}$–$\frac{1}{2}$ maximum daily dose[v]	0.5 × 10^6 U		2–6	100	6 avg	200–800	
1	4			0.25–0.5 g po	6 hr	6 hr	8 hr	12 hr	0.25 g						
1.3–1.5	2.1–5	1.2–2.4	3.6	3–4 g	4–6 hr	4–6 hr	6–12 hr	12 hr	2 g q8h + 1 g after HD		15.7[g]		1	1000	
1–1.5	13	6	Minimal	3 g	4–6 hr	4–6 hr	2–3 g q6–8h	2 g q12h	3 g	3 g q12h	9.5[g]				
4.5–5	18–27	4.5		0.5–1 g	12 hr	12 hr	12–24 hr	36–48 hr	0.5 g						

[m] Up to 450 mg/kg/day for patients with cystic fibrosis.
[n] 100% of a dose of bacampicillin is metabolized to ampicillin.
[o] 4–8 g/day usually sufficient for urinary tract infections.
[p] The antibiotic activity of hetacillin is provided by its rapid conversion to ampicillin.
[q] For meningitis, 50 mg/kg q8–12h.
[r] For meningitis, 50 mg/kg q6–8h.
[s] For infants weighing less than 2000 g, 75 mg/kg q8h.
[t] By continuous infusion.
[u] The interval between parenteral doses is variable: it can be as frequent as every 2 hours for initial therapy of meningococcemia or as long as 12 hours between IM doses of procaine penicillin G.
[v] Patients on low daily doses usually tolerate full dosage. Upper dosage limit approximation: dose (10^6 U/day) = 3.2 + (CLCR/7). (*Ann Intern Med.* 1975;82:194).
[w] Patients with latent syphilis of more than 1 year's duration should be treated with penicillin G benzathine, 2.4 million units weekly for 4 weeks.
[x] For infants <2000 g: 75 mg/kg q12h for first week and 75 mg/kg q8h for 1–4 weeks old. Those >2000 g: 75 mg/kg q8h for the first week and 100 mg/kg q8h for 1–4 weeks old.

ANTIMICROBIAL AGENT PHARMACOLOGY: CEPHALOSPORINS

Drug (Oral Absorption, %)	Serum and Urine Concentration for Selected Doses: Dose (g)	Peak Serum (μg/ml)	Peak or Range, Urine (μg/ml)	Dosage Recommendations: Adults, Oral (Dose/Interval)	Adults, Parenteral (Dose/Interval)	Maximum Daily Dose (g)	Children, Oral (Dose/Interval)	Children, Parenteral (Dose/Interval)	Newborn (Parenteral), Up to 1 wk (Dose/Interval)	Newborn (Parenteral), 1–4 wk (Dose/Interval)
First generation										
Cefadroxil[c] (90–100)	0.25 po 0.5 po 1 po	9 18 28–34	1200–1800	1–2 g/day q12–24h		2	15 mg/kg q12h			
Cefazolin	0.5 IM 1 IM 1 IV	40 59–68 188	2460 4010		0.5–1.5 g q6–8h	6		8.3–25 mg/kg q6–8h	15–20 mg/kg q12h	15–20 mg/kg q8–12h
Cephalexin[c] (80–100)	0.25 po[f] 0.50 po[f]	8 15–18	1000–2300	0.25–1 g q6h		4	6.25–25 mg/kg q6h		Not recommended	
Cephalothin	1 IV[g] 1 IM 2 IV[g]	40–60 20 80 100	2500		0.5–2 g q4–6h	12		75–160 mg/kg/day q4–6h	40 mg/kg/day q8–12h	60–80 mg/kg/day q6–8h
Cephapirin	1 IV[j] 2 IV[k] 1 IM	70 129 9.4	2560 1280		0.5–2 g q4–6h	12		10–20 mg/kg q6h		
Cephradine Oral (90–100)	0.5 po[f] 1 IM	15–19 10–14	1000	0.25–1 g q6–12h		4	6.25–12.5 mg/kg q6–12h			
Parenteral	1 IV	60–86	1975		0.5–2 g q6h	8		12.5–25 mg/kg q6h	Not recommended	
Second generation										
Cefaclor[c,d]	0.25 po 0.5 po 1 po	5–7 15 35	600 900	0.25–0.5 g q8h		4	6.6–13.3 mg/kg q8h			
Cefamandole	1 IM 1 IV[g] 2 IV	20–35 90 165	 5000		0.5–2 g q4–6h	12		50–150 mg/kg/day q4–8h		
Cefonicid	7.5 mg/kg IV[k] 0.5 IM 1 IV[g] 1 IV[k]	95–155 40–60 150 221–261	500		0.5–2 g q24h	2				
Cefotetan	0.5 IM 1 IV[k] 2 IV[j]	35 142–180 200	1000 1400–2000 3500–4000		1–2 g q12h	6		20–30 mg/kg q12h		
Cefotiam	1 IV[g] 2 IV[g]	50 135			1–2 g q12h					
Cefoxitin	1 IM 1 IV[g]	20 110–125	450 3000	1–2 g q4–6h or 3 g q6h	12		20–26.6 mg/kg q4–6h			30 mg/kg q8h
Cefuroxime	0.5 IM 1 IM 1 IV[k] 1.5 IV[g]	25 40 100 65	 5000–7000		0.75–1.5 g q8h[m]	9		50–240 mg/kg/day[n] q6–8h	Not recommended	30–50 mg/kg/day q8–12h
Cefuroxime axetil (30–40)	0.25 po 0.5 1	4.1 7.0 13.6		0.125–0.5 g q12h			0.125–0.5 g q12h			
Third generation										
Cefepime	0.5 IV[g]	34								
Cefixime (50)	0.2 po 0.4 po	1.7–1.9 2.7–3.0	52 84	0.4 g/day q12–24h			8 mg/kg/day q12–24h			
Cefmenoxime	1 IV[g] 1 IM 2 IV[g]	40 15 95	1740 3620		0.5–2 g q4–6h	12		10–20 mg/kg q6h	Not recommended	
Cefoperazone	1 IV[j] 2 IV	100–125 200	1600 2000		1–4 g q8h or 0.5–3 g q6h	12 16 by continuous infusion in immunocompromized patient		25–100 mg/kg q12h		
Cefotaxime (desacetyl cefotaxime)	1 IM 1 IV[j] 2 IV[j] 1 IV[k] 2 IV[k]	20 40 80–90 102 9.8	2010		1–2 g q4–12h	12		50–180 mg/kg/day q4–6h	25–50 mg/kg q12h	25–50 mg/kg q8h
Cefpiramide	1IV[k] 2 IV[g]	303 320	1087							
Cefpirome	1 IM 1 IV	28.6 97.1								

Serum Half-life (hr)				Usual Adult Dose and Interval Adjustment					Dosage for Dialysis						
For Creatinine Clearance (ml/min)		With Dialysis			For Creatinine Clearance (ml/min)										
>80	<10	HD	PD	Dose	>80	80–50	50–10	<10 (Anuric)	Dose after HD Supple-mental to Anuric	Daily Dose during PD	CSF/Serum (%) In-flamed Menin-ges[a]	New-born Serum/Maternal Serum (%)	Breast Milk/Maternal Serum[b] (%)	Bile/Serum (%)	Aqueous Humor/Serum (%)
1.2–1.6[d]	20–25	2.5–3.4		1 g po	12–24 hr	12–24 hr	25–50: q12h 10–25: q24h	36–48 hr	0.5–1 g			50	0.9–1.9	22	
1.5–2	20–70	6.5–9.0	20–46[e]	0.5–1.5 g	6–8 hr	8 hr	0.5–1 g q8–12h	0.5–1 g q24h	0.25–0.5 g		1–4	35–69	3	29–300	<1.7
0.5–1.2	11–20	4.5–6		0.25–1 g po	6 hr	6 hr	500 mg 8–12 hr	250 mg q12–24h	0.25–1 g		Minimal	60	2	216	11
0.5–1	3–18[h]	2.5–3	5.1	0.5–2 g	4–6 hr	6 hr	8 hr	0.5 g q6–8h	Supplemental dose	No supple-mental dose[i]	1.2–5.6	16–41	7–26[j]	22–172	4
0.5–1	1.5–2.4	1.8		0.5–2 g	4–6 hr	6 hr	8 hr	12 hr	7.5–15 mg/kg before dialysis			60	7		
0.75–1.5	8–15			1–2 g	6 hr[l]	6 hr	8 h or 250–500 mg q6h	250 mg q12–24 hr	1–2 g	500 mg q6h for CAPD	≤1	9–22	14–20	10–400	5–9
0.5–1	2–3	1.5–2		0.25–0.5 g po	8 hr	8 hr	8 hr (50–100% usual dose)	8 hr (25–33% usual dose)	Repeat dose after HD				2	≥60	1–3
0.5–1	11	6.6	7.2	0.5–2 g	4–6 hr	1–2 g q6h	1–2 g q8h	0.5–1 g q12h	Supplemental dose	No supple-mental dose	0.5–20		2.4	300–400	1.5
4.4	50–100	70		0.5–2 g	24 hr	0.5–1.5 g q24h	0.25–1 g q24–48h	0.25–1 g q3–5 days	No extra dose				<1	<10	<1
3–4.6	12–35.1	5.6–7.5	5–9% removed	1–2 g	12 hr	12 hr	24 hr	48 hr	Supplemental dose		0.8–3.6		2.3	1000	
0.7–1		2.4						Reduce the dose by 25%			10	75–130	0–trace	20–25	
0.75–1	10–22	4	Minimal (7.8 with CAPD)	1–3 g	4–6 hr	1–2 g q8h	1–2 g q12h	0.5–1 g q12–24h	1–2 g		<1–77	33–50	up to 3	280	4–7
1–2	15	3.75	5.4–13.6[o]	0.75–1.5 g	8 hr	8 hr	8–12 hr	24 hr	Supplemental dose	No supple-mental dose	11–56	20–33	up to 3	35–80	10–14
1.2–1.3															
2															
3.3–4.0	11.1	8.2	14.9 (CAPD)					0.2 g q24h[s]	No supplemental dose						
0.8–1.2	8			0.5–2 g	4–6 hr	6–8 hr	12–24 hr	24h	30–50% main-tenance dose		3	30	<25	81–526	2.6–5
1.6–2.6	2.5	2.2		1–4 g	6–8 hr	6–8 hr	6–8 hr	6–8 hr[p]	Schedule the dose after dialysis		1.8–3.1	20–50	Up to 1.5	800–1200	1–6
0.9–1.1	2.5–3.4	1.6	2.9	1–2 g	4–8 hr	4–8 hr	6–12 hr	12 hr	Maintenance dose × 50%		10–25	25[q]	Up to 3–8	59	0.5–4
1.3	10–15	3.16												493	
4.4–5.4	8.3														
2															

ANTIMICROBIAL AGENT PHARMACOLOGY: CEPHALOSPORINS *(Continued)*

Drug (Oral Absorption, %)	Serum and Urine Concentration for Selected Doses			Dosage Recommendations						
				Adults			Children		Newborn (Parenteral)	
	Dose (g)	Peak Serum (μg/ml)	Peak or Range, Urine (μg/ml)	Oral (Dose/Interval)	Parenteral (Dose/Interval)	Maximum Daily Dose (g)	Oral (Dose/Interval)	Parenteral (Dose/Interval)	Up to 1 wk (Dose/Interval)	1–4 wk (Dose/Interval)
Cefsulodin	1 IM 1 IV[g] 2 IV[g]	20 65 140	 1500–3500		1–2 g q6–8h	12		15–25 mg/kg q6h		
Ceftazidime	1 IV[g] 1 IM 2 IV[g]	70–80 38–43 170–180	4000–6000		0.5–2 g q8–12h	6		30–50 mg/kg q8h	60–100 mg/kg/ day q8–12h	60–150 mg/kg/ day q8–12h
Ceftizoxime	0.5 IM 1 IV[g] 2 IV[g]	13.3 60–90 120–130	1120		1–4 g q8–12h	12		50 mg/kg q6–8h		
Ceftriaxone[t]	0.5 IM 1 IV[g] 2 IV[g]	50 150 270	 995 2700		0.5–2 g q12–24h[u]	4[v]		50–100 mg/kg/ day q12–24h[w]	50 mg/kg/day	50–75 mg/kg/day
Moxalactam	0.5 IV[j] 1 IV[g] 2 IV[k] 1 IM	57 60–100 150–200 27	446 2100 4200		0.5–4 g q8–12h[y]	12[y]		50 mg/kg q6–8h[y,z]	50 mg/kg q12h[y,z]	50 mg/kg q8h[y,z]

[a] Cephalosporins penetrate minimally across uninflamed meninges into the CSF.
[b] Cephalosporins do not appear in sufficient systemic quantities via breast milk to treat infections in the infant but could theoretically sensitize the newborn.
[c] Oral.
[d] Dose-dependent pharmacokinetics.
[e] Only two patients studied.
[f] Fasting.
[g] Infusion (over a period of 30 minutes).
[h] Biphasic elimination.
[i] Peritoneal dialysis is reported to diminish the mean peak concentration of cephalothin by 24 percent as well as reducing the subsequent cephalothin levels by as much as 50 percent from baseline. Despite this enhanced elimination during peritoneal dialysis, the cephalothin serum level persisted above 16 μg/ml for 12 hours. (*Am J Med Sci*. 1969;257:116.)
[j] Data from rabbits.
[k] Intravenous push (over a period of 2–5 minutes).
[l] Parenteral doses can be divided q4–6h.
[m] Up to 3 g every 8 hours for meningitis.
[n] Up to 240 mg/kg/day divided every 6–8 hours for meningitis.

ANTIMICROBIAL AGENT PHARMACOLOGY: OTHER β LACTAMS AND β-LACTAMASE INHIBITORS

Drug (Oral Absorption, %)	Serum and Urine Concentration for Selected Doses			Dosage Recommendations						
				Adults			Children		Newborn (Parenteral)	
	Dose (g)	Peak Serum (μg/ml)	Peak or Range, Urine (μg/ml)	Oral (Dose/Interval)	Parenteral (Dose/Interval)	Maximum Daily Dose (g)	Oral (Dose/Interval)	Parenteral (Dose/Interval)	Up to 1 wk (Dose/Interval)	1–4 wk (Dose/Interval)
Other β-lactams										
Aztreonam (minimal)	0.5 IV[a] 0.5 IM 1 IV[a] 1 IM 2 IV[a]	54 22 90 47 205	1400 3000 6500		0.5–2 g q6–12h	8		18.75–37.5 mg/kg q6h (not approved)		
Carumonam	1 2	190 300			0.5–2 g q8h					
Impenem (minimal)	0.25 IV 0.5 IV 1 IV	22 43 68–78	50 100[c] > or = 100		0.5–1 g q6–8h	4		15–25 mg/kg q6h[d]	16.6–33.3 mg/kg q8h (preliminary)	
β lactamase inhibitors										
Clavulanate (50)	0.125 po 0.25 po 0.2 IV[a]	4 6 13.4	380 680	0.25–0.5 g q8h[e]	3.1 g q4–6h[f]		6.7–13.3 mg/kg q8h[g]			
Sulbactam (60–80)	0.5 IV[l] 1 IV[i] 0.25 po[j] 0.5 po	30 60 3.6 4.4–5.1	 480		1.5–3 g q6–8h[k]	4 g[l]		37.5 mg/kg q6h or 50 mg/kg q8h[k]	75 mg/kg q12h[k]	112.5 mg/kg q8h[k]

[a] IV infusion over 30 minutes.
[b] Animal data.
[c] Urine concentrations are obtained with concomitant administration of dehydropeptidase inhibitor, cilastatin.
[d] For children 3 years of age or less: 25 mg/kg/dose; for children over 3 years: 15 mg/kg/dose to a maximum of 3 g/day.
[e] As Augmentin: 250 mg and 500 mg tablets contain 250 mg and 500 mg, respectively, of amoxicillin and 125 mg and 250 mg, respectively, of clavulanate (2:1 ratio).
[f] As Timentin: 3 g ticarcillin plus 0.1 g clavulanate.

Serum Half-life (hr)				Usual Adult Dose and Interval Adjustment					Dosage for Dialysis		CSF/Serum (%) Inflamed Meninges[a]	Newborn Serum/Maternal Serum (%)	Breast Milk/Maternal Serum[b] (%)	Bile/Serum (%)	Aqueous Humor/Serum (%)
For Creatinine Clearance (ml/min)		With Dialysis			For Creatinine Clearance (ml/min)										
>80	<10	HD	PD	Dose	>80	80–50	50–10	<10 (Anuric)	Dose after HD Supplemental to Anuric	Daily Dose during PD					
1.6–1.9	10–13	2.1–3.3	8.9	0.5–3 g	6 hr	8 hr	0.25–1.5 g q6h or 1 g q12h	0.5 g q12h or 1 g q24h	0.25 g	1 g q18–24h	11		1		16
1.8	16.1–25	2.8	8.7	0.5–2 g	8–12 hr	8–12 hr	1–1.5 g q12–24h	0.5–0.75 g q24–48h	1 g loading 1 g post dialysis	1 g then 0.5 g q24h	21.5		7	33	3–12
1.7	25–36	4–4.9	10.2–12 (CAPD)	1–4 g	8–12 hr	0.5–1.5 g q8h	0.25–1 g q12h	0.25–1 g q24–48h	Give scheduled dose after dialysis	3 g q48h	21–22	28–33	1–6	34–82	3.6–6
8[d]	11.9–15.4	16.1	12.2 (CAPD)	0.5–1 g	12–24 hr	12–24 hr	12–24 hr	12–24 h[x]	No supplemental dose		7–11	18–25	4	Up to 1000	
2.5	5–22	4	16.7	0.5–4 g	8–12 hr	0.5–3 g q8h	0.25–2 g q8h or 0.25–3 g q12h	0.25 g q12h to 1 g q24h	1–2 g	1 g q36–48h or 0.5g q18–24h	4–55[aa]	30–40	2.7	152–224	1–16

[o] The bioavailability of cefuroxime axetil is variable depending on the presence of food in the GI tract. In general, the degree of absorption increases when given with or shortly after food (f = 52%) compared with fasting state (f = 37%).
[p] From manufacturer's data: "When hepatic function is essentially normal, cefoperazone generally does not require adjustment of usual dosages in cases of renal impairment, including end-stage renal failure." Antibiotic serum concentrations are recommended, however, to assess the drug accumulation for patients with renal compromise receiving greater than 4 g/day.
[q] From fetal samples after abortion.
[r] From investigator's brochure: fetal rat data.
[s] Dose for CrCl < 20 ml/min.
[t] Nonlinear kinetics; 35 μg/ml at 12 hours and 15 μg/ml at 24 hours.
[u] For the treatment of uncomplicated gonococcal infections, 0.125 to 0.25 g as a single intramuscular dose is effective.
[v] The maximum recommended daily dose is currently 2 g; however, data for adult meningitis are incomplete.
[w] For gram-negative meningitis in children, the manufacturer recommends initial loading dose of 75 mg/kg.
[x] Serum levels of ceftriaxone should be monitored in patients with severe renal impairment or concomitant renal and hepatic compromise.
[y] Bleeding time should be monitored in patients receiving more than 4 g/day for more than 3 days. Prophylactic vitamin K, 10 mg/wk, should be given to patients treated with moxalactam.
[z] For gram negative meningitis in children, the manufacturer recommends an initial loading dose of 100 mg/kg.
[aa] Data from clinical studies have reported CSF penetration up to 40 percent.

Serum Half-life (hr)				Usual Adult Dose and Interval Adjustment					Dosage for Dialysis		CSF/Serum (%) Inflamed Meninges	Newborn Serum/Maternal Serum (%)	Breast Milk Maternal Serum (%)	Bile/Serum (%)	Aqueous Humor/Serum (%)
For Creatinine Clearance (ml/min)		With Dialysis			For Creatinine Clearance (ml/min)										
>80	<10	HD	PD	Dose	>80	80–50	50–10	<10 (Anuric)	Dose after HD Supplemental to Anuric	Daily Dose during PD					
1.7–2	6–8.7	2.7	3–7.1	0.5–2 g	6–12 hr	8–12 hr	12–24 hr	24–36 hr	15 mg/kg	30 mg/kg q24h	8[b]		Minimal	60–100	5–14
1.3–1.7	11.3			0.5–2 g	8hr	8–12 hr	12–24 hr	0.25–1 g q 24 hr							
1	4	2.5		0.5–1 g	6–8 hr	0.5 g q6–8 h	0.5 g q6–12 h	0.25–0.5 g q24h	2 g/day max and one dose after HD		20–30			Minimal	3
0.7–1.4	3.8	1.2		0.25–0.5 g po 3.1 g[f]	8 hr 4–6 hr	8 hr 4–6 hr	12 hr 2 g q4–8h	12–24 hr 2 g q12h	3.1 g[f]	3.1 g q12h[f]	8.4	100	Minimal	50[h]	
1	20	2.4		1.5–3 g[k]	q6–8h	q6–8h	q8–12h	q24h			2–20	100	Minimal	33	

[g] Based on the amoxicillin component.
[h] Data obtained 1 hour after a dose of oral Augmentin (amoxicillin plus clavulanic acid).
[i] Administered as Unasyn (2:1 ratio of ampicillin and sulbactam) over a period of 15 minutes.
[j] As sultamicillin, a double ester of ampicillin and the β-lactamase inhibitor sulbactam.
[k] As Unasyn: ampicillin plus sulbactam in 2:1 combination; 1 g + 0.5 g and 2 g + 1 g, respectively.
[l] Expressed as the sulbactam component.

ANTIMICROBIAL AGENT PHARMACOLOGY: AMINOGLYCOSIDES

	Serum and Urine Concentration for Selected Doses			Dosage Recommendations						
				Adults			Children		Newborn (Parenteral)	
		Peak Serum	Peak or Range, Urine	Oral	Parenteral	Maximum Daily Dose	Oral	Parenteral	Up to 1 wk	1–4 wk
Drug (Oral Absorption, %)	Dose (g)	(μg/ml)		Dose/Interval		(g)	Dose/Interval			
Amikacin	5 mg/kg IM 7.5 mg/kg IM 7.5 mg/kg IV	16 21 38	830 700		5 mg/kg q8h or 7.5 mg/kg q12h	1.5 g		5 mg/kg q8h or 7.5 mg/kg q12h	7.5–10 mg/kg q12h	7.5–10 mg/kg q8h
Gentamicin (minimal)	1.25 mg/kg IM	5–7	5–100		1–1.7 mg/kg q8h[f]	5 mg/kg		1–2.5 mg/kg q8h[f]	2.5 mg/kg q12h	2.5 mg/kg q8h
Kanamycin	0.5 g IM	14–29	140–250		5 mg/kg q8h or 7.5 mg/kg q12h	1.5 g	150–250 mg/kg/day q1–6h	5–10 mg/kg q8h	7.5–10 mg/kg q12h	7.5–10 mg/kg q8h
Neomycin (minimal)	4.0 g po[j]	4		6.6 mg/kg q4h ≤3 days[k]		3 g po	12.5–25 mg/kg q6h			
Netilmicin	2 mg/kg IM 2.5 mg/kg IM	6 7.5			1.5–3.25 mg/kg q12h or 1.3–2.2 mg/kg q8h	6.5 mg/kg		1–2.5 mg/kg q8h	2.5 mg/kg q12h	2.5 mg/kg q8h
Spectinomycin	2 g IM 4 g IM	74 199	9000		2 g once[l]	4 g		40 mg/kg once IM	Not recommended	
Streptomycin	0.5 g IM 1 g IM	6–42 25–50	300–400 1000		0.5–1 g q12h	2 g		10–15 mg/kg q12h	Not recommended	
Tobramycin	1 mg/kg IM 2 mg/kg IV	4 3.1–14	75–100 320		1–1.7 mg/kg q8h	5 mg/kg		1–2 mg/kg q8h[f]	2 mg/kg q12h	2 mg/kg q8h

[a] The dosing strategy for aminoglycosides involves the use of ideal (lean) body weight (IBW) for dosage calculation. In obese patients, this approach would result in serum antibiotic concentrations less than expected. Alternative dosing recommendations have been proposed that account for the change in drug distribution volume with obesity:
(1) Lean body weight + 40 percent of the excess weight, defined as total body weight (TBW) minus ideal body weight (IBW). (*J Infec Dis*. 138:499–505, 1978;138:499–505.)
(2) IBW + 58 percent of excess weight (TBW-IBW). (*Clin Pharmacol Ther*. 1979;26:508.)
(3) IBW + 38 percent of excess weight (TBW-IBW). (*Am J Hosp Pharm*. 1980;37:519–22.)

[b] Or calculate the dosage interval in hours as nine times the serum creatinine concentration in mg/100 ml (amikacin, kanamycin) or eight times the serum creatinine concentration in mg/100 ml (gentamicin, netilmicin, tobramycin). Alternatively, refer to nomogram in F.A. Sarubbi, Jr., et al., *Ann Intern Med*. 1978;89:612–18. The simplicity of these predictive methods makes them useful for establishing initial dosing schedules, but serum antimicrobial concentrations should be determined subsequently to ensure therapeutic, nontoxic blood levels.

[c] Mean percentage penetration into CSF of aminoglycoside antibiotics in normal rabbits has been reported to be less than 10 percent.

[d] Aminoglycosides do not penetrate the biliary tree in the presence of obstruction.

ANTIMICROBIAL AGENT PHARMACOLOGY: TETRACYCLINES

	Serum and Urine Concentration for Selected Doses			Dosage Recommendations						
				Adults			Children		Newborn (Parenteral)	
		Peak Serum	Peak or Range, Urine	Oral	Parenteral	Maximum Daily Dose	Oral	Parenteral	Up to 1 wk	1–4 wk
Drug (Oral Absorption, %)	Dose (g)	(μg/ml)		Dose/Interval		(g)	Dose/Interval			
Chlortetracycline (30)	0.25 po 0.5 po	1.5–2.5 7	320	See tetracycline			See tetracycline		Not recommended	
Demeclocycline (66)	0.3 po	1.5–1.7		0.15 g q6h or 0.3 g q12h		1.2	6.6–13.2 mg/kg/day q6–12h		Not recommended	
Doxycycline (90–100[g])	0.1 po[f] 0.1 IV[g] 0.2 po 0.2 IV[g]	1.8–2.9 2.5 3.7–6.7 4	100–200 200–300	0.1 g q12–24h	0.1 g q12–24h	0.2	2.2 mg/kg q12–24h	2.2 mg/kg q12–24h	Not recommended	
Methacycline (58)	0.15 po 0.3 po	1.3 2.4		0.15 g q6h or 0.3 g q12h		1.2	6.6–13.2 mg/kg/day q6–12h		Not recommended	
Minocycline (95–100[g])	0.2 po 0.2 IV	2–3 4.2–6.6	15[h]	0.2 g once then 0.1 g q12h	0.2 g once then 0.1 g q12h	0.4	4 mg/kg once then 2 mg/kg q12h	4 mg/kg once then 2 mg/kg q12h	Not recommended	
Oxytetracycline (59)	0.25 po 0.5 po	1.3–1.4 4–4.2	300	See tetracycline	0.25–0.5 g q12h	4	See tetracycline	6 mg/kg q12h	Not recommended	
Tetracycline (75[g])	0.25 po 0.5 po 0.5 IV[f]	1.5–2.2 3–4.3 8	300	0.25–0.5 g q6h	0.125–0.5 g q6–12h	2	25–50 mg/kg/day q6–12h	10–20 mg/kg/day q6–12h	Not recommended	

[a] The tetracyclines cause a brown discoloration of the teeth and may retard the growth of bone in the human fetus and children. They are not recommended for use in patients younger than 12 years of age.

[b] Patients in the convalescent stage of poliomyelitis.

[c] Not detected at a dose of 300 mg/day.

[d] Biliary levels determined after an IV injection of 500 mg of the antibiotic.

[e] Serum levels of doxycycline are reduced by 20 percent if given with food, whereas serum levels of tetracycline are reduced up to 50 percent. The oral absorption of minocycline is not significantly impaired by food or milk.

Serum Half-life (hr)				Usual Adult Dose and Interval Adjustment					Dosage for Dialysis						
For Creatinine Clearance (ml/min)		With Dialysis			For Creatinine Clearance (ml/min)						CSF/ Serum (%) Inflamed Meninges	Newborn Serum/ Maternal Serum (%)	Breast Milk Maternal Serum (%)	Bile/ Serum (%)	Aqueous Humor/ Serum (%)
>80	<10	HD	PD	Dose	>80	80–50	50–10	<10 (Anuric)	Dose after HD Supplemental to Anuric	Daily Dose during PD					
2–2.5	44–86[e]	3.75–5.6	17.9–29	5–7.5 mg/kg	8–12 hr	12 hr	24–36 hr	36–48 hr	2.5–3.75 mg/kg	3–4 mg/2 liters dialysate removed	15–24	20		30	0–4
2–3	48–72	8–10	5–15[g]	1.5 mg/kg	8 hr	8–12 hr	12–24 hr	24–48 hr	1–1.5 mg/kg	1 mg/2 liters dialysate removed	10–30	30–40		30–60	<8
2.2–3	30–80[h]	4.9	5[f]	5–7.5 mg/kg	8–12 hr	24 hr	24–72 hr	72–96 hr	5 mg/kg	3.75 mg/kg qd	43	50	35	100	
3				6.6 mg/kg po	4 hr										
2.2–2.5	33	5.5		1.3–2.2 mg kg	8 hr	8–12 hr	12–24 hr	24–48 hr	2 mg/kg		21–26				
1.7	18.5–29.3			2 g once[f]											
2–3	100–110			0.5–1 g	12 hr	24 hr	24–72 hr	72–96 hr	5 mg/kg		20	10–40	<25	40–300	
2–2.75	50–70	2.9–10	12–16	1.5 mg/kg	8 hr	8–12 hr	12–24 hr	24–48 hr	1 mg/kg	1 mg/2 liters dialysate removed	14–23	50		10–20	18

[e] Half-life of 86.5 h in anephric patients and 44.3 h in patients with minimal residual kidney function.
[f] For meningitis, aminoglycosides may be administered intraventricularly in single, supplemental daily doses until CSF cultures are negative. (Gentamicin and tobramycin dose: 5–10 mg for adults; 1–2 mg for infants; not recommended for the newborn). Up to 10 mg/kg/day may be administered parenterally for cystic fibrosis.
[g] In the absence of an inflammatory response, peritoneal clearance is diminished, and the half-life is reported as approximately 29 hours. The elimination half-life during CAPD is 36 hours.
[h] The serum half-life of kanamycin in severely uremic patients may be prolonged to 70–80 hours.
[i] As dialysis continues, removal of drug is slower, and the half-life is reportedly prolonged to 48 hours.
[j] Although neomycin is classified as nonabsorbable, some absorption from the GI tract does occur. A review of neomycin-induced deafness has identified ototoxicity as a consequence of all modes of administration—parenteral, aerosol, oral, wound and bowel irrigation, and cutaneous.
[k] The recommended dosage schedule for bowel evacuation; as adjunctive therapy for hepatic coma; 25 mg/kg q6h for 24 hours, then 12.5 mg/kg q6h thereafter.
[l] For disseminated gonoccocal infections, spectinomycin may be administered at 2 g every 12 hours for 3 days.

Serum Half-life (hr)				Usual Adult Dose and Interval Adjustment					Dosage for Dialysis						
For Creatinine Clearance (ml/min)		With Dialysis			For Creatinine Clearance (ml/min)						CSF/ Serum (%) Inflamed Meninges	Newborn Serum/ Maternal Serum (%)	Breast Milk Maternal Serum (%)	Bile/ Serum (%)	Aqueous Humor/ Serum (%)
>80	<10	HD	PD	Dose	>80	80–50	50–10	<10 (Anuric)	Dose after HD Supplemental to Anuric	Daily Dose during PD					
5.6	6.8–11	Minimal		0.25–0.5 g po	6 hr	Not recommended					2–6[b]		40	333	
10–16				0.15–0.3 g po	6–12 hr	Not recommended							70[c]	2000[d]	10–30
18.5	19.5–25	18.8		0.1 g po	12–24 hr	12–24 hr	12–24 hr	12–24 hr	No supplemental dose		12–20		30–40	300–2000	10–13
7–15	Up to 44 hr			0.15–0.3 g po	6–12 hr	Not recommended									
11–26	12–30[i]			0.1 g po	12–24 hr	Not recommended						77	8–26	3000	17
9	48–66	24	Minimal	0.25–0.5 g po	6 hr	Not recommended					0–6.7		20–140	400–1000	
8.5	57–108	j		0.25–0.5 g po	6 hr	Not recommended					10–25	60–70	25–150	500–1000	9–11

[f] Infused over 60 min.
[g] Infused over 30 min.
[h] Urine concentration of minocycline approximates 5–10 times the serum concentration (lowest of the tetracyclines).
[i] Little accumulation in renal failure but aggravation of uremia reported even with a reduced dosage.
[j] Tetracycline plasma level decreased by 14–27 percent with hemodialysis.

ANTIMICROBIAL AGENT PHARMACOLOGY: ERYTHROMYCIN, LINCOSAMIDES, CHLORAMPHENICOL, AND METRONIDAZOLE

	Serum and Urine Concentration for Selected Doses			Dosage Recommendations						
				Adults			Children		Newborn (Parenteral)	
		Peak Serum	Peak or Range, Urine	Oral	Parenteral	Maximum Daily Dose	Oral	Parenteral	Up to 1 wk	1–4 wk
Drug (Oral Absorption, %)	Dose (g)	(μg/ml)		Dose/Interval		(g)	Dose/Interval			
Clarithromycin 14-OH metabolite	0.5 g po	2.4 1.0		0.25–0.5 g q12h			7.5 mg/kg q12h			
Erythromycin (18–45[a])				0.25–0.5 g q6h	0.25–1 g q6h	4	7.5–12.5 mg/kg q6h	3.75–12.5 mg/kg q6h	Not recommended	
base stearate ethyl succinate[d]	0.25 po[b] 0.5 po[b] 0.5 po	0.3–1 0.4–1.9 1.5 (0.6)	13–46[c] 30	0.333 g q8h or 0.25–0.5 g q6–12h 0.4 g q6–12h						
lactobionate	0.5 IV	9.9			0.25–0.5 g IV q6h			30–50 mg/kg/day q6h IM		
gluceptate	1 IV	9.9			0.25–0.5 g IV q6h			30–50 mg/kg/day q6h IM		
estolate	0.5 po	4.2[e]		0.25–0.5 g q6–12h			40 mg/kg/day q6–12h			
Clindamycin (approx. 90[f])	0.15 po 0.3 IM 0.6 IV[g]	1.9–3.9 4.8–6 10	3–4	0.15–0.45 g q6h	0.15–0.9 g q6–8h	8	2–8 mg/kg q6–8h	2.5–10 mg/kg q6h[h]	5 mg/kg q6–8h	
Lincomycin (20–30)	0.6 IV[j] 0.5 po 0.6 IM	19 2.6 9.5	 13–259	0.5 g q6–8h	0.6–1 g q8–12h	8	10–15 mg/kg q6–8h	2.5–5 mg/kg q6h[h]	Not recommended	
Chloramphenicol (75–90)	0.5 po 1 po[u] 1 IV	3–4 11.2–18.4 5–12[l]	70–150[m] 200	12.5–25 mg/kg q6h	12.5–25 mg/kg q6h	4.8	12.5–25 mg/kg q6h	12.5–25 mg/kg q6h	25 mg/kg q24h[n]	25 mg/kg q12–24h[n]
Metronidazole[o] (95[p]) (67–82 rectal[q]) (19 vaginal)	0.25 po 0.5 po 0.5 IV 0.5 rectal suppository 0.5 vaginal	5 10 10[g] 20–25[k] 5.1 1.2–1.8	50–390	7.5 mg/kg q6h[r]	7.5 mg/kg q6h[r]	4	7.5 mg/kg q6h	7.5 mg/kg q6h	15 mg/kg once, then 7.5 mg/kg q12h	15 mg/kg once, then 7.5 mg/kg q8–12h
Roxithromycin (72–85)	0.15 g po 0.3 g po	5.4–7.9 10.4	17.4 37.7	0.15 g q12h or 0.3 g q24h			2.5–5 mg/kg q12h			

[a] The extent of gastrointestinal absorption of erythromycin formulations relates to the chemical structure and its susceptibility to gastric acid, the protective enteric coating, and the concomitant presence of food. (*Am J Hosp Pharm*. 1980;37:1119–205.)
[b] Fasting.
[c] Alkalinization of the urine pH to 8 increases the amount of nonionized drug that remains in the urine and enhances the local antibacterial activity.
[d] Absorption of the ethylsuccinate preparation is enhanced by food. After absorption, 45 percent of the ethylsuccinate preparation is present in serum as the inactive ester and 55 percent as the active base; 1.5 μg/ml total (0.6 μg/ml free base).
[e] Erythromycin estolate total drug concentration with 500 mg dosing is 4.2 μg/ml (ester plus base) or 1.1 μg/ml free base.
[f] Absorption is not decreased by food.
[g] IV infusion (over 30 minutes).
[h] Total daily dose may be divided every 8 hours
[i] Dose modification should be made with coexisting renal and hepatic disease.
[j] IV infusion over 2 h.
[k] Multiple dose (500 mg q8h).

ANTIMICROBIAL AGENT PHARMACOLOGY: POLYMYXINS, VANCOMYCIN, AND FUSIDIC ACID

	Serum and Urine Concentration for Selected Doses			Dosage Recommendations						
				Adults			Children		Newborn (Parenteral)	
		Peak Serum	Peak or Range, Urine	Oral	Parenteral	Maximum Daily Dose	Oral	Parenteral	Up to 1 wk	1–4 wk
Drug (Oral Absorption, %)	Dose	(μg/ml)		Dose/Interal		(g)	Dose/Interval			
Colistimethate (minimal)	75 mg IM 150 mg IM 150 mg IV	1–2 6–8 10–13	50 200–270		0.8 1.7 mg/kg q8h	5 mg/kg		1.7–2.3 mg/kg q8h	Not recommended	
Polymyxin B (minimal[d])	50 mg IM 2.5 mg/kg IV (infused in 0.3–0.5 liters)	2–8 5			1.5–2.5 mg/kg/day continuous IV infusion[e]	2.5 mg/kg		up to 4–4.5 mg/kg/day continuous IV infusion[f]	Not recommended	
Vancomycin (minimal)	0.5 g IV 1 g IV 0.125 g q6h po	6–10 20–50 <1[h]	 100–300	0.125–0.5 g q6h	15 mg/kg q12h or 6.5–8 mg/kg q6h[i]	2g	12.5 mg/kg q6h	10 mg/kg q6h[i]	15 mg/kg q12h	15 mg/kg q8h

Serum Half-life (hr): For Creatinine Clearance (ml/min) >80	<10	With Dialysis: HD	PD	Usual Adult Dose and Interval Adjustment: Dose	For Creatinine Clearance (ml/min) >80	80–50	50–10	<10 (Anuric)
6.7	21.6							
1.4	4–6	No change	No change	0.25–1 g	6 hr	6 hr	6 hr	6 hr
2.4	3.4–6	1.9–6	4.6	0.15–0.9 g	6–8 hr	6–8 hr	6–8 hr	6–8 hr[i]
4–6	10–13		10.3–15.4	0.5 g po	6 hr	6 hr	12 hr	24 hr or 25–50% dose
1.5–3.5	3.2–4.3	0.8–2.7	3.8	12.5–25 mg/kg	6 hr	6 hr	6 hr	6 hr
6–14[s]	8–15[t]	2.6	5.6–10.9	7.5 mg/kg	6 hr[r]	6 hr	6 hr	6 hr
8.3–13	16–17.9							

Serum Half-life >80	Dosage for Dialysis: Dose after HD Supplemental to Anuric	Daily Dose during PD	CSF/Serum (%) Inflamed Meninges	Newborn Serum/Maternal Serum (%)	Breast Milk Maternal Serum (%)	Bile/Serum (%)	Aqueous Humor/Serum (%)
6.7			Minimal		30	7000	
1.4	None	No change	6–10	5–25	50	400–2800	25–30
2.4	None	No change	Minimal	6–46	38–50	250–300	
4–6	None	No change	1–7	25–36	13	250–400	8–75
1.5–3.5	Schedule the dose after dialysis	No change	45–99	30–106	51–61	100–200	
6–14[s]	No change	No change	43–100	97	60–100	100	33–50
8.3–13			Minimal	30–40	0.05		50–200

[l] Intramuscular administration may produce a plasma level of active drug that is but one-half that achieved with a comparable oral dose and is therefore not recommended. The intravenous preparation (succinate ester) produces serum chloramphenicol levels 30–50 percent less than those achieved with a comparable oral dose.
[m] The urine concentration of unmetabolized chloramphenicol is inversely correlated with the renal function. When the creatinine clearance is below 20 ml/min, less than 1 percent of the dose is excreted in the active form as compared with 5–10 precent in patients with normal renal function.
[n] Initial dosage. Subsequent dosage should be based on the determination of serum concentrations (10 to 25 μg/ml, desired). For premature infants throughout the first month of life, the initial dosage is 25 mg/kg/day.
[o] Dosage for anaerobic bacterial infections. The first dose (loading dose) should be 15 mg/kg. The dosage shuld be reduced with severe hepatic disease.
[p] Absorption of metronidazole is not significantly decreased by food.
[q] Rectal absorption is inversely dependent on the dose.
[r] Clinical work with metronidazole completed outside the United States supports the use of an 8-hour dosing interval.
[s] Patients with alcoholic liver disease eliminate metronidazole more slowly, a half-life of 18.3 hours, than do subjects with normal liver function and may therefore require dosage modification to avoid accumulation of metronidazole and its metabolites. (*Antimicrob Agents Chemother.* 1987;31:1662–4.)
[t] The hydroxy metabolite may accumulate in anuric patients.
[u] Multiple dose (1 g q6h).

Serum Half-life (hr): For Creatinine Clearance (ml/min) >80	<10	With Dialysis: HD	PD	Usual Adult Dose and Interval Adjustment: Dose	For Creatinine Clearance (ml/min) >80	80–50	50–10	<10 (Anuric)
2–3	10–20	1.5	Poor	0.8–1.7 mg/kg	8 hr	2.5 mg/kg on day 1, then 1–1.5 mg/kg q24h	2.5 mg/kg on day 1, then 1–1.5 mg/kg q24–72h	2.5 mg/kg on day 1, then 1–1.5 mg/kg q48–72h[a]
6	48–72			1.5–2.5 mg/kg/day	24 hr	3 mg/kg on day 1, then 1.5–2.5 mg/kg q24h	3 mg/kg on day 1, then 1.5–2.5 mg/kg q24–72h	3 mg/kg on day 1, then 1.5–2.5 mg/kg q48–72h[a]
4–6[k]	240	Negligible effect	18	15 mg/kg q12h or 6.5–8 mg/kg q6h	6–12 hr	See the nomogram, Chapter 27 or *Antimicrob Agents Chemother.* 1984;25:433		

Serum Half-life >80	Dosage for Dialysis: Dose after HD Supplemental to Anuric	Daily Dose during PD	CSF/Serum (%) Inflamed Meninges	Newborn Serum/Maternal Serum (%)	Breast Milk/Maternal Serum (%)	Bile/Serum (%)	Aqueous Humor/Serum (%)
2–3	[b]	[c]	Minimal	50	18	Not detectable	25–30
6			Minimal[g]			Not detectable	
4–6[k]	No change	[l]	7–21	20[m]	33–66[n]	50	Minimal

Drug (Oral Absorption, %)	Serum and Urine Concentration for Selected Doses: Dose	Peak Serum (μg/ml)	Peak or Range, Urine (μg/ml)	Dosage Recommendations: Adults Oral (Dose/Interal)	Adults Parenteral (Dose/Interal)	Maximum Daily Dose (g)	Children Oral (Dose/Interval)	Children Parenteral (Dose/Interval)	Newborn (Parenteral) Up to 1 wk	Newborn (Parenteral) 1–4 wk
Teichoplanin	3 mg/kg IV[q] 6 mg/kg IV[q]	53 112			0.2–0.4 g q24h			10 mg/kg q24h	6 mg/kg q24h (preliminary)	
Fusidic acid	0.5 g po	14–38[o]	<1	0.5–1 g q8h	580 mg q8h IV[p]		6.6–16.6 mg/kg q8h	6.6 mg/kg q8h		

[a] The interval is extended to every 5–7 days for the anuric patient.
[b] The rate of removal of colistimethate by hermodialysis or peritoneal dialysis remains controversial. Studies using a Koiff twin coil dialyzer demonstrate no removal (*N Engl J Med.* 1964;270:394–7; *Ann Intern Med.* 1968;68:984–94.), whereas studies using the Kiil type dialyzer recommend the dose be adjusted so that the patient receives a 2–3 mg/kg dose after dialysis. (*Br Med J.* 1968;1:484–5; *Antimicrob Agents Chemother.* 1964;373–8.)
[c] Small quantities of colistimethate are removed by PD with clearance rates ranging from 5.8–11.3 ml/min. Supplemental doses may be considered on the basis of the duration of dialysis and the need to maintain target serum levels.
[d] The only significant absorption from the gastrointestinal tract has been observed in newborn animals and small infants.
[e] Although not recommended, the IM dosage of polymyxin B for adults is 2.5–3.0 mg/kg/day given in 4–6 divided doses.
[f] Although not recommended, the daily dose may be divided and given by the IM route.
[g] Although rarely used, the daily intrathecal dose of polymyxin B is 5–10 mg for adults and 2 mg for children over 2 years of age. Intrathecal therapy should be administered on a daily basis for the first 3–5 days and then every other day for 3 weeks or for 2 weeks after negative CSF cultures and a normal CSF glucose concentration.

ANTIMICROBIAL AGENT PHARMACOLOGY: SULFONAMIDES AND TRIMETHOPRIM

Drug (Oral Absorption, %)	Serum and Urine Concentration for Selected Doses: Dose (%)	Peak Serum (μg/ml)	Peak or Range, Urine (μg/ml)	Dosage Recommendations: Adults Oral (Dose/Interal)	Adults Parenteral (Dose/Interal)	Maximum Daily Dose (g)	Children Oral (Dose/Interval)	Children Parenteral (Dose/Interval)	Newborn (Parenteral) Up to 1 wk	Newborn (Parenteral) 1–4 wk
Trimethoprim-sulfamethoxazole (TMP-SMX) (85–90)	0.16/0.8 po 0.16/0.8 IV[a]	2/40 3.4/47.3	120/300[b]	2 tablets q12h or 1 tablet q6h[c]	4–5 mg/kg q6–12h (as TMP)[c]	4 tablets orally or 1.2 g TMP, 6 g SMX intravenously (usual)	4–5 mg/kg q6–12h (as TMP)[c]	4–5 mg/kg q6–12h (as TMP)[c]	Not recommended[d]	
Trimethoprim (80)	0.32 po 0.1 po	5.5 1	30–160[f]	0.1 g q12h		0.2	2 mg/kg q12h (not approved in children less than 12 years old)			
Sulfonamides (70–90)										
Sulfisoxazole	2 po	40–50 (free)		0.5–1 g q6h[g]	25 mg/kg q6h[g]	8	120–150 mg/kg/day q4–6h	100 mg/kg/day q6–8h[g]	Not recommended	
Sulfamethoxazole	2 po	80–100 (free)		1 g q8–12h[i]		3	25–30 mg/kg q12h[j]		Not recommended	
Sulfamethizole	2 po	60		0.5–1 g q6–8h		6	7.5–11.25 mg/kg q6h		Not recommended	
Sulfacytine	0.25 po	17	420	0.5 g initial dose, then 0.25 g q6h		1	Not recommended		Not recommended	
Sulfadiazine	0.5 po	20–40		2–4 g initial dose, then 0.5–1 g q4–6h	Not recommended	6	120–750 mg/kg/day q4–6h[g]		Not recommended	
Sulfadoxine[l]	2 po	50–75 (free)		1 tablet every wk or 2 tablets every other wk[m]		1.5	By age[n]		Not recommended	
Sulfasalazine (10–15)	2 po	14 sulfasalazine 21 sulfapyridine (total)		0.5–1 g q4–6h		4[n]	30–60 mg/kg/day q4–8h		Not recommended	
Sulfaphenazole	2 po	100–150		2–3 g, then 1 g q12h		2	66 mg/kg, then 33 mg/kg q12h		Not recommended	

[a] Infused over 60 minutes.
[b] The urine concentrations of the drugs depend on the urine flow rate, urine pH, and the time of collection. The approximate urine concentration for trimethoprim is 100 times the plasma concentration; for sulfamethoxazole the level is 5 times the concentration in plasma. Alkalinization of the urine increases the renal excretion of sulfonamides. See footnote f.
[c] Each tablet contains 80 mg trimethoprim and 400 mg sulfamethoxazole. Double-strength tablets are also available and are usually administered at one tablet q12h. The suspension contains 40 mg trimethoprim and 200 mg sulfamethoxazole per 5 ml. Parenteral dosage ranges from 8 to 20 mg/kg/day trimethoprim and 40 to 100 mg/kg/day sulfamethoxazole.
[d] Unsuitable for the newborn because the appropriate dosage requires a ratio of trimethoprim: sulfamethoxazole of 1:3 and the only formulation available is a 1:5 combination. (*J Pediatr.* 1982;100:647–50.)
[e] Nonacetylated SMX.
[f] Renal clearance of trimethoprim is increased with acidification of the urine.

Serum Half-life (hr)				Usual Adult Dose and Interval Adjustment					Dosage for Dialysis						
For Creatinine Clearance (ml/min)		With Dialysis			For Creatinine Clearance (ml/min)										
>80	<10	HD	PD	Dose	>80	80–50	50–10	<10 (Anuric)	Dose after HD Supplemental to Anuric	Daily Dose during PD	CSF/ Serum (%) Inflamed Meninges	Newborn Serum/ Maternal Serum (%)	Breast Milk/ Maternal Serum (%)	Bile/ Serum (%)	Aqueous Humor/ Serum (%)
40–70	125	163		0.4 g	24 hr	0.2 g q24h or 0.4 g q48h	0.2 g q24h or 0.4 g q48h	0.13 g q24 or 0.4 g q72h							
				0.5–1 g po	8 hr	8 hr	8 hr	8 hr							

[h] The stool concentration ranges from 100 to 800 μg/ml.
[i] The incidence of "red-man syndrome" may be decreased by using a 500 mg dose instead of 1 g (*Antimicrob Agents Chemother*. 1987;31:393–7.)
[j] Doses as high as 60 mg/kg/day may be necessary for staphylococcal CNS infections.
[k] The elimination half-life of vancomycin varies with age: 5.9–9.8 hours in newborns, 4.1 hours in older infants, 2.2–3 hours in children.
[l] Conflicting opinion exists with regard to the dosage alteration of vancomycin during PD. The regimen chosen will depend upon the frequency and duration of dialysis as well as the nature of the infection being treated. Serum concentrations should be measured and the dosage regimen adjusted accordingly.
[m] Data from animals (rabbits).
[n] Data from animals (cats).
[o] Accumulation occurs with multiple doses of 0.5 g given every 8 hours; a mean serum level of 71 μg/ml has been reported after 96 hours of therapy.
[p] Diethanolamine fusidate, 580 mg = 500 mg sodium fusidate.
[q] IV infusion over a period of 5 minutes.

Serum Half-life (hr)				Usual Adult Dose and Interval Adjustment					Dosage for Dialysis						
For Creatinine Clearance (ml/min)		With Dialysis			For Creatinine Clearance (ml/min)										
>80	<10	HD	PD	Dose	>80	80–50	50–10	<10 (Anuric)	Dose after HD Supplemental to Anuric	Daily Dose during PD	CSF/Serum (%) Inflamed Meninges	Newborn Serum/ Maternal Serum (%)	Breast Milk/ Maternal Serum (%)	Bile/ Serum (%)	Aqueous Humor/ Serum (%)
11/9	25/27	9.4/11.7[e]		4–5 mg/kg (as TMP)	6–12 hr	12 hr	18 hr	24–48 hr	4–5 mg/kg (as TMP)	0.16/0.8 q48h[f]	30–50/25–30	100/70–90	125/10	100–200/ 40–70	10–45/ 20–30
7.5	14–46	9.4		0.1 g po	12 hr	12 hr	24 hr	24–48 hr			30–50	70–100	100	100	10
											30–80	70–90	10	40–70	20–30
4–6[h]	12			0.5–1 g po	6 hr	6–8 hr	8–12 hr	12–24 hr			30–50				
10–12[k]	22–50			1 g po	8–12 hr						25–30				
2	58			0.5–1 g po	6–8 hr										
4				0.25 g po	6 hr										
10–12	34			0.5–1 g po	4–6 hr						50–80				
150–200				0.5 g po or 1 g po	every wk every other wk										
7.6				0.5–1 g po	4–6 hr										
				1 g po	12 hr										

[g] Administer one-half of the daily dose as the initial dose.
[h] Under normal conditions the half-life of elimination was determined as 6 hours, whereas under alkaline conditions the half-life approached 4 hours.
[i] Administer a 2 g loading dose: 4 regular strength tablets or 2 double-strength tablets.
[j] Administer a 50–60 mg/kg loading dose. The maximum dose for children should not exceed 75 mg/kg/24 h.
[k] Under acidic conditions, the half-life of elimination is slightly longer (11 hours) than under alkaline conditions (9 h).
[l] For malaria prophylaxis. The first dose should be given 1–2 days before departure to an endemic area and the course continued throughout the stay and 4–6 weeks thereafter.
[m] One tablet = 500 mg sulfadoxine and 25 mg pyrimethamine.
[n] Under 4 years: $\frac{1}{4}$ tablet weekly or $\frac{1}{2}$ tablet every other week; 4–8 years: $\frac{1}{2}$ tablet weekly or 1 tablet every other week; 9–14 years: $\frac{3}{4}$ tablet weekly or $1\frac{1}{2}$ tablet every other week.
[o] Although doses up to 12 g have been administered, a daily dosage exceeding 4 g is associated with an increased incidence of adverse effects.

ANTIMICROBIAL AGENT PHARMACOLOGY: QUINOLONES AND OTHER URINARY TRACT AGENTS

Drug (Oral Absorption, %)	Serum and Urine Concentration for Selected Doses: Dose	Peak Serum (μg/ml)	Peak or Range, Urine (μg/ml)	Dosage Recommendations: Adults, Oral (Dose/Interal)	Adults, Parenteral (Dose/Interal)	Maximum Daily Dose	Children, Oral (Dose/Interval)	Children, Parenteral (Dose/Interval)	Newborn (Parenteral), Up to 1 wk (Dose/Interval)	Newborn (Parenteral), 1–4 wk (Dose/Interval)
Quinolones										
Cinoxacin (97)	0.25 po 0.5 po	8 16	400	0.25 g q6h or 0.5 g q12h[a]		1	Not recommended			
Ciprofloxacin (69–85)	0.5 po 0.75 po 0.2 IV[d]	2.9 4 3.8	300–450 550–700	0.25–0.75 g q12h	0.2–0.3 g q12h		Not recommended			
Enoxacin (80–90)	0.4 po 0.6 po 0.2 IV	2.8–3.6 4 1.8	250–300 337	0.4 g q12h	0.4 g q12h		Not recommended			
Fleroxacin (99)	0.4 po 0.1 IV	4.4 2.85	210	0.4 g q12–24h (preliminary)			Not recommended			
Lomefloxacin	0.2 po 0.4 po	2.1 3–4.7	170	0.4 g q12–24h (preliminary)			Not recommended			
Nalidixic acid (96)	1 po	25–35	150–400	1 g q6h[a]		4	Not recommended		Not recommended	
Norfloxacin (30–40)	0.2 po 0.4 po 0.8 po	0.75 1.6 2.4	200 480 700	0.2–0.4 g q12h[a]		0.8				
Ofloxacin (85–90)	0.2 po 0.4 po 0.6 po	2.6 8.6 11	218	0.2–0.4 g q12h			Not recommended			
Oxolinic acid (poor)	0.75 po	0.9–3.6	45–100 avg	0.75 q12h[a]		2	Not recommended		Not recommended	
Pefloxacin (98)	0.4 po 0.4 IV[g]	3.8–5.6 5.8	100–115	0.4 g q12–24h			Not recommended			
Temafloxacin (100)	0.2 po 0.4 po 0.6 po	2 3.7 7		0.2–1.2 g/day q12–24h						
Other urinary tract agents										
Indanyl carbenicillin (30–40)	0.382 po (1 tablet) 1 po	6.5 6–17	1130	1–2 tablets q6h[a]		3	7.5–12.5 mg/kg q6h[a]			
Methenamine mandelate[h] (70[i])	1 po		40 (formaldehyde)	1 g q6h[a]		4	12.5–18.75 mg/kg q6h[a]		Not recommended	
Methenamine hippurate[h] (100)	1	70–100 μmol/liter[k]	1100–1500 (methenamine) approx 50 (formaldehyde)	1 g q12h[a]		4	12.5–25 mg/kg q12h[a]		Not recommended	
Nitrofurantoin (good but variable)	0.1 po	<1	150[l]	0.05–0.1 g q6h[a]		0.4	1.25–1.75 mg/kg q6h[a]		Not recommended	

[a] Used primarily for the treatment of urinary tract infections.
[b] Use during pregnancy not recommended.
[c] Animal pharmacology studies indicate the presence of drug in the milk of lactating rats receiving oral doses of cinoxacin. Human data are currently unavailable.
[d] Infused over a period of 30 minutes.
[e] Ineffective urinary concentrations expected with compromised renal function.
[f] Breast milk percentage extrapolated from data indicating 4 μg/ml breast milk concentration in four patients (*Lancet*. 1965;2:691). Hemolytic anemia has been described in one nursing infant whose mother received nalidixic acid.
[g] Infused over a period of 60 minutes.
[h] Usually coadministered with an acidifying agent to convert the methenamine salts in urine to ammonia and bactericidal formaldehyde (pH < OR = 5.5). Mandelic and hippuric acids are mildly antiseptic and contribute to urine acidification.

ANTIMICROBIAL AGENT PHARMACOLOGY: ANTIMYCOBACTERIAL AGENTS

Drug (Oral Absorption, %)	Serum and Urine Concentration for Selected Doses: Dose	Peak Serum (μg/ml)	Peak or Range, Urine (μg/ml)	Dosage Recommendations: Adults, Oral (Dose/Interal)	Adults, Parenteral (Dose/Interal)	Maximum Daily Dose	Children, Oral (Dose/Interval)	Children, Parenteral (Dose/Interval)	Newborn (Parenteral), Up to 1 wk (Dose/Interval)	Newborn (Parenteral), 1–4 wk (Dose/Interval)
Ansamycin	0.075–0.3 g	0.2–0.5		0.15–0.3 g/day		0.3 g				
Capreomycin[a] (minimal)	1 g	30	1685		0.75–1 g q24h 15–20 mg/kg/day IM[b]	20 mg/kg/day		15–30 mg/kg/day IM (not approved)		
Clofazimine				0.1 g/day[c]		0.6 g				
Cycloserine (70–90)	0.25 g po 0.5 g po	10	55–340	0.25–0.5 g q12h		1 g	3.5–5 mg/kg q12h (not approved)			

Serum Half-life (hr): For Creatinine Clearance (ml/min) >80	Serum Half-life (hr): For Creatinine Clearance (ml/min) <10	Serum Half-life (hr): With Dialysis HD	Serum Half-life (hr): With Dialysis PD	Usual Adult Dose and Interval Adjustment: Dose	For Creatinine Clearance (ml/min): >80	80–50	50–10	<10 (Anuric)	Dosage for Dialysis: Dose after HD Supplemental to Anuric	Dosage for Dialysis: Daily Dose during PD	CSF/Serum (%) Inflamed Meninges	Newborn Serum/Maternal Serum (%)	Breast Milk/Maternal Serum (%)	Bile/Serum (%)	Aqueous Humor/Serum (%)
1.5	8.4	3–4.4		0.25–0.5 g po	6–12 hr	0.25 g q8h	0.25 g q12–24h	Not recommended				[b]	<100 (18–78)[c]		
3–5	5–10			0.25–0.75	12 hr	12 hr	0.25–0.5 g 12–18 hr	0.25–0.5 g 24 hr	Give dose after dialysis		15–40			500–1000	3–22
5–7	40	9.8									67			900	
9–12	30														
7–8.5	21													700	
1.5	21			1 g po	6 hr	6 hr	6 hr	Not recommended[e]					13[f]	100	
3–4	5–10			0.2–0.4 g po	12 hr	12 hr	12–24 hr	24 hr				Nil	Nil	300–700	
5–8	25–50	10		0.2	12 hr	12 hr	24–48 hr	48 hr	None			60–90	15–75	250	
6–7				0.75 g po	12 hr		Not recommended[e]	Not recommended[e]					Not recommended	200–300	
8–12	11–15										45–60			200–600	
7.7															
0.5–1	12.5			1–2 tablets po	6 hr	6 hr	6 hr	Not recommended[e]							
3–6				1 g po	6 hr	6 hr	Not recommended[e]	Not recommended[e]			[j]			[j]	[j]
4				1 g po	12 hr	12 hr	Not recommended[l]	Not recommended[l]			[j]	50	70–100	[j]	[j]
0.3	1			0.05–0.1 g po	6 hr	6 hr	Not recommended[e,m]	Not recommended[e,m]				100	<25[n]	200–400	

[i] Oral absorption is decreased 30 percent by enteric coating.
[j] Methenamine penetrates a number of body fluids, including bile and cerebrospinal fluid. This penetration proves clinically inconsequential since negligible amounts of formaldehyde are generated at physiologic pH (see Chapter 31).
[k] The serum concentration of methenamine has no clinical significance.
[l] Alkaline conditions reduce tubular reabsorption, which yields higher nitrofurantoin concentrations in urine.
[m] Nitrofurantoin accumulates in the serum of patients with a creatinine clearance <60 ml/min, which leads to systemic toxicity.
[n] Although only small amounts of nitrofurantoin have been detected in breast milk, the drug could cause hemolytic anemia in a glucose-6-phosphate dehydrogenase–deficient infant exposed in this manner.

Serum Half-life (hr): For Creatinine Clearance (ml/min) >80	Serum Half-life (hr): For Creatinine Clearance (ml/min) <10	Serum Half-life (hr): With Dialysis HD	Serum Half-life (hr): With Dialysis PD	Usual Adult Dose and Interval Adjustment: Dose	For Creatinine Clearance (ml/min): >80	80–50	50–10	<10 (Anuric)	Dosage for Dialysis: Dose after HD Supplemental to Anuric	Dosage for Dialysis: Daily Dose during PD	CSF/Serum (%) Inflamed Meninges	Newborn Serum/Maternal Serum (%)	Breast Milk/Maternal Serum (%)	Bile/Serum (%)	Aqueous Humor/Serum (%)
				0.15–0.3 g po	24 hr	24 hr	0.15 g q24h	0.075 g q72h							
				0.75–1 g	24 hr									Minimal	
70 days				0.1 g po	24 hr										
				0.25–0.5 g po	12 hr						100	100	72		

ANTIMICROBIAL AGENT PHARMACOLOGY: ANTIMYCOBACTERIAL AGENTS *(Continued)*

	Serum and Urine Concentration for Selected Doses			Dosage Recommendations						
				Adults			Children		Newborn (Parenteral)	
		Peak Serum	Peak or Range, Urine	Oral	Parenteral	Maximum	Oral	Parenteral	Up to 1 wk	1–4 wk
Drug (Oral Absorption, %)	Dose	(μg/ml)		Dose/Interal		Daily Dose	Dose/Interval			
Ethambutol (80)	25 mg/kg po	2–5		15 mg/kg/day[d]		15 mg/kg/day[d]	15 mg/kg/day (not approved)			
Ethionamide	1 g po	20		0.25–0.5 g q12h		1 g	5–10 mg/kg q12h (not approved)			
Isoniazid[e]	0.3 g po	7		5 mg/kg/day (0.3 g)[f]	5 mg/kg/day IM	0.6 g	10–20 mg/kg/day q12–24h[g]	10–20 mg/kg/day q12–24h IM		
Para-amino salicylic acid	4 g po (free acid)	75 7–8		3 g q6–8h		12 g	66.6–75 mg/kg q6–8h			
Pyrazinamide	1 g po	45	60	15–30 mg/kg/day[k]		3 g	15–30 mg/kg/day q12–24h			
Rifampin (100)	0.6 g po (fasting)	10[l]	240	0.6 g/24 hr[m]		1.2 g[m]	10–20 mg/kg/day q12–24h			
Streptomycin	1 g IM	25–50	1000		15 mg/kg/day IM[o]	2 g		10–15 mg/kg q12h IM		
Viomycin					1 g q12h twice weekly	2 g				

[a] Pharmacokinetics similar to streptomycin.
[b] The dosage is 1 g IM daily for 2–4 months and is reduced to 1 g two to three times weekly thereafter.
[c] In combination therapeutic regimens, 300 mg monthly to 50–100 mg daily is recommended.
[d] Doses as high as 25 mg/kg/day are occasionally administered during the first 2–3 months of therapy. Intermittent therapy consists of 50 mg/kg/day administered twice weekly.
[e] To minimize the risk of polyneuritis from isoniazid-induced pyridoxine deficiency, pyridoxine (15–50 mg) is often given concurrently.
[f] For noncompliant patients, 15 mg/kg can be given twice weekly under supervision. For prophylaxis, isoniazid is usually given for a year in a daily dose of 300 mg for adults and 10 mg/kg (up to 300 mg maximum for children.
[g] In children with tuberculosis meningitis, some clinicians use 30 mg/kg/day for the first few weeks.
[h] Specific elimination kinetics of isoniazid depend on the acetylator phenotype of the individual; the half-life for rapid acetylators is 0.5–1.5 hours and for slow acetylators, 2–4 hours.

ANTIMICROBIAL AGENT PHARMACOLOGY: ANTIFUNGAL AGENTS

	Serum and Urine Concentration for Selected Doses			Dosage Recommendations						
				Adults			Children		Newborn (Parenteral)	
		Peak Serum	Peak or Range Urine	Oral	Parenteral	Maximum	Oral	Parenteral	Up to 1 wk	1–4 wk
Drug (Oral Absorption, %)	Dose	(μg/ml)		Dose/Interval		Daily Dose	Dose/Interval			
Amphotericin (poor)	0.1–1 mg/kg	0.5–5.5	≤5		0.25–1 mg/kg q24h[a]	1 mg/kg[b]		0.25–1 mg/kg q24h[a]	0.1–1 mg/kg/day[a]	0.1–1 mg/kg/day[a]
Fluconazole	0.1 po 0.2 po	4.5–8 10	50	0.2–0.4 g q24h	0.2–0.4 g q24h	0.4 g				
Flucytosine (90)	150 mg/kg/day po	50–80	5800	37.5 mg/kg q6h	37.5 mg/kg q6h	150 mg/kg	37.5 mg/kg q6h		Not recommended	
Giseofulvin (50[d])	1 g po	1–2.8[e]	Minimal	0.5–1 g/day in single or 2–4 doses[d]		2 g	10 mg/kg/day[d]			
Itraconazole	0.2 po	0.6	Not detected	0.2–0.4 g q24h		0.4 g				
Ketoconazole[f]	0.2 g po 0.4 g po	3–4.5 7	Minimal	0.2–0.4 g q24h		0.8 g	5–10 mg/kg/day q12–24h[g]			
Miconazole (25–30)	0.5 g IV[i]	2–9			0.066–1.2 g q8h[i]	3.6 g		6.6–13.3 mg/kg q8h		
Nystatin (minimal)[m]	All doses	Minimal		400,000–600,000 units q6h (4–6 ml)		4 × 10^4 units	250,000–500,000 units q6h (2.5–5 ml)		100,000 units q6h (0.25 ml) (po)	100,000 units q6h (0.25 ml) (po)

[a] A test dose of 1 mg infused over 15 minutes is often given to assess febrile reactions prior to proceeding to higher doses.
[b] Or up to 1.5 mg/kg every other day.
[c] Data from rabbits.
[d] Dose for conventional microsize griseofulvin. Significant interindividual variation exists with griseofulvin absorption. Bioavailability studies have demonstrated a 150 percent greater absorption of ultramicrosize products (Fulvicin P-G, Gris-PEG). Dosing guidelines for ultramicrosize griseofulvin are 330–660 mg daily for adults and 7.25 mg/kg/day for children (*J Pharmokinet Biopharm.* 1980;8:347–62).
[e] The serum level is increased with a high-fat meal.
[f] Oral absorption is variable and is decreased during simultaneous administration of H_2 antagonists or antacids.

Serum Half-life (hr)				Usual Adult Dose and Interval Adjustment					Dosage for Dialysis						
For Creatinine Clearance (ml/min)		With Dialysis			For Creatinine Clearance (ml/min)						CSF/Serum (%) Inflamed Meninges	Newborn Serum/Maternal Serum (%)	Breast Milk/Maternal Serum (%)	Bile/Serum (%)	Aqueous Humor/Serum (%)
>80	<10	HD	PD	Dose	>80	80–50	50–10	<10 (Anuric)	Dose after HD Supplemental to Anuric	Daily Dose during PD					
4–6	7–32			15 mg/kg/day po	15 mg/kg/day	15 mg/kg/day	7.5 mg/kg/day	5 mg/kg/day	15 mg/kg/day on dialysis day	15 mg/kg/day during PD	25–50	~100			
2–4				0.25–0.5 g po	12 hr						100				
0.5–4[h]	8 (avg)	3.4		5 mg/kg po	24 hr	24 hr	24 hr	24 hr[j]	5 mg/kg	[j]	100	High	100		
1	23			3 g po	6–8 hr						Poor				
9–10				25 mg/kg/day po	6–12 hr						100				
2.5–5[n]	2–5	Minimal	Minimal	0.6 g po	24 hr	24 hr	24 hr	24 hr	No supplemental dose	No supplemental dose	10–30	33	20–60	10,000	
2–3	100–110			15 mg/kg/day	24 hr	24 hr	24–72 hr	72–96 hr	5 mg/kg		20	10–40	<25	40–300	
				1 g	12 hr twice weekly						Poor				

[i] For slow acetylators (at least one-half of white Americans), the daily dose should be reduced to 200 mg.
[j] In cases where peritoneal dialysis has been used for the management of acute isoniazid intoxication, the procedure decreased INH serum concentration by 68% over 24 hours (*N Engl J Med* 269:852–3 1963).
[k] When given intermittently, the adult dosage is 50 mg/kg twice weekly. The daily dosage is divided in two to four equally spaced doses.
[l] An increase in dose results in a disproportionate increase in peak serum concentration: after 300, 600, and 1200 mg doses, the peak serum levels reached 4, 10, and over 30 μg/ml, respectively.
[m] For noncompliant patients, supervised therapy with 600 mg rifampin twice a week can be given. The dose for the prophylaxis of meningococcal meningitis is 600 mg twice daily for 2 days.
[n] The serum half-life increases with the dose: 2.5, 3, and 5 hours after doses of 300, 600, and 900 mg, respectively.
[o] An alternative dosage schedule is 25–30 mg/kg twice weekly.

Serum Half-life (hr)				Usual Adult Dose and Interval Adjustment					Dosage for Dialysis						
For Creatinine Clearance (ml/min)		With Dialysis			For Creatinine Clearance (ml/min)						CSF/Serum (%) Inflamed Meninges	Newborn Serum/Maternal Serum (%)	Breast Milk/Maternal Serum (%)	Bile/Serum (%)	Aqueous Humor/Serum (%)
>80	<10	HD	PD	Dose	>80	80–50	50–10	<10 (Anuric)	Dose after HD Supplemental to Anuric	Daily Dose during PD					
24 or more	24 or more	Minimal		0.25–1 mg/kg IV	24 hr	24 hr	24 hr	24 hr	No change		2–3	50			25
24	48			0.2–0.4 g po	24 hr	24 hr	48 hr	≥72 hr			50–90				64[c]
4–6	30–70	5–6		37.5 mg/kg po	6 hr	6 hr	12–24 hr	15–25 mg/kg q24h or by plasma level of 50–75	20–37.5 mg/kg		70				
20	20			0.5–1 g po	24 hr	24 hr	24 hr	24 hr				80			
18–36	18–36	18–36	18–36	0.2–0.4 g po	24 hr	24 hr	24 hr	24 hr			Not detected				43[c]
6.5–9.6[h]		Minimal	Minimal	0.2–0.4 g po	24 hr	24 hr	24 hr	24 hr			Minimal			Minimal	~10
2.1/24.1[k]	24[l]	Minimal	Minimal	0.066–1.2 g IV	8 hr	8 hr	8 hr	8 hr			Minimal				
				400,000–600,000 units po	6 hr	6 hr	6 hr	6 hr							

[g] Less than 20 kg: 50 mg; 20–40 kg: 100 mg; greater than 40 kg: 200 mg.
[h] Ketoconazole has a dose-dependent elimination with half-lives of 6.5, 8.1, and 9.6 hours after doses of 100, 200, and 400 mg, respectively.
[i] Over a period of 15 minutes.
[j] The manufacturer recommends an initial test dose of 200 mg.
[k] Triphasic half-life with a 0.4-hour absorption half-life and 2.1- and 24-hour elimination half-lives.
[l] Neither renal impairment nor hemodialysis affects elimination, although plasma concentrations are greater in patients with azotemia due to decreased distribution volume.
[m] Dosage for oral candidiasis. Nystatin suspension = 100,000 units/ml.

ANTIMICROBIAL AGENT PHARMACOLOGY: ANTIVIRAL AGENTS

Drug (Oral Absorption, %)	Serum and Urine Concentration for Selected Doses: Dose	Peak Serum (μg/ml)	Peak or Range Urine (μg/ml)	Dosage Recommendations: Adults Oral (Dose/Interval)	Adults Parenteral (Dose/Interval)	Maximum Daily Dose	Children Oral (Dose/Interval)	Children Parenteral (Dose/Interval)	Newborn (Parenteral) Up to 1 wk (Dose/Interval)	Newborn (Parenteral) 1–4 wk (Dose/Interval)
Acyclovir (15–20)	2.5 mg/kg[a] 5 mg/kg[a] 0.2 po q4h	6.8 9.8 0.3–0.9		0.2–0.8 g q4h (5 doses/day)	5–10 mg/kg q8h[a]	30 mg/kg		5–15 mg/kg q8h	5–15 mg/kg q8h	5–15 mg/kg q8h
Amantadine (85–90)	0.1 po	0.3–0.4		0.1 g q12h or 0.2 g q24h[c]		0.2 g	2.2–4.4 mg/kg q12h[d]			
Ganciclovir (DHPG) (<5%)	2.5 mg/kg	4.8–6.2			2.5–5 mg/kg q8–12h[a]					
Ribavirin (50)	Aerosol over 20 hr 0.6 po 1.2 po	0.8–3.3 μg/ml 1.3 μg/ml 2.5 μg/ml		0.3–1.2 g q12h[g] (preliminary)			Aerosol 190 μg/liter of air at 12.5 liter/min over 12–18 hr/day			
Rimantidine (>90)	0.1 po	0.44–0.86 μg/ml		0.1–0.15 g q12h[f]			3 mg/kg q12h			
Vidarabine	10–15 mg/kg/day (12 h)	0.2 vidarabine 6–8 arahypoxanthine			10–15 mg/kg/day over 12 h	15 mg/kg		10–15 mg/kg/day over 12 hours	15–30 mg/kg/day over 12 hours	15–30 mg/kg/day over 12 hours
Zidovudine (63–95)	0.1 q4h po	0.4–0.5 μg/ml		0.2 g q4h (around the clock)						

[a] Intravenous infusion over a period of 1 hour.
[b] Data from manufacturer's product information using animals.
[c] Decrease to 0.1 g q24h for patients older than 65 years or with active seizure disorder.
[d] The dose for children 1–9 years old should not exceed 150 mg/day.
[e]

Creatinine Clearance (ml/min · 1.73 meter^2)	Suggested Maintenance Regimen
50	100 mg daily
40	100 mg daily
30	200 mg twice weekly
20	100 mg thrice weekly
10	200 mg/100 mg alternating every 7 days

(From *Ann Intern Med.* 1981;94:454.)

ADVERSE DRUG INTERACTION INVOLVING ANTIMICROBIAL AGENTS

Interacting Drugs	*Adverse Effect*	*Probable Mechanism*
Acyclovir with		
Narcotics	Increased meperidine effect	Decreased renal excretion
Probenecid	Possible increased acyclovir toxicity	Decreased renal excretion
Amantadine with		
Anticholinergics	Hallucinations, confusion, nightmares	Mechanism not established
Aminoglycoside antibiotics with		
Amphotericin B	Nephrotoxocity	Synergism
Bumetanide	Increased ototoxicity	Additive
Cephalosporins	Increased nephrotoxicity	Mechanism not established
Cisplatin	Increased nephrotoxicity	Mechanism not established
Cyclosporine	Increased renal toxicity	Possibly additive or synergism
Digoxin	Probable decreased digoxin effect with oral gentamicin or neomycin	Decreased absorption
Ethacrynic acid	Increased ototoxicity	Additive
Furosemide	Increased ototoxicity and nephrotoxicity	Additive
Magnesium sulfate	Increased neuromuscular blockade	Additive
Methotrexate	Possible increased methotrexate toxicity with kanamycin	Mechanism not established
	Possible decreased methotrexate effect with oral aminoglycosides	Decreased absorption
Miconazole	Possible decreased tobramycin concentration	Mechanism not established
Neuromuscular blocking agents	Neuromuscular blockade	Additive
Nonsteroidal anti-inflammatory drugs	Possible aminoglycoside toxicity in preterm infants with indomethacin given for patent ductus closure	Decreased renal clearance
Penicillins	Decreased aminoglycoside effect with high concentrations of carbenicillin or ticarcillin	Inactivation
Polymyxins	Increased nephrotoxicity; neuromuscular blockade	Additive
Vancomycin	Possible increased nephrotoxicity and ototoxicity	Additive
Aminosalicylic acid (PAS) with		
Probenecid	Increased PAS toxicity	Decreased renal excretion
Rifampin	Rifampin effectiveness may be decreased; separate doses by 8–12 hr	Decreased GI absorption due to excipient bentonite

(*Continued*)

Serum Half-life (hr)				Usual Adult Dose and Interval Adjustment					Dosage for Dialysis						
For Creatinine Clearance (ml/min)		With Dialysis			For Creatinine Clearance (ml/min)						CSF/Serum (%) Inflamed Meninges	Newborn Serum/Maternal Serum (%)	Breast Milk/Maternal Serum (%)	Bile/Serum (%)	Aqueous Humor/Serum (%)
>80	<10	HD	PD	Dose	>80	80–50	50–10	<10 (Anuric)	Dose after HD Supplemental to Anuric	Daily Dose during PD					
2.2–5	20	5.7		5 mg/kg	8 hr	8 hr	12–24 hr	2.5 mg/kg q24h	Give daily dose after HD		50	100[b]	300		37
12–17	Up to 30 days	Minimal		200 mg q24h or 100 mg q12h po	12 hr	100 mg q12–24h	200 mg/day alternate days to alternating q7days[e]		None		50–60				
2–3	29								[f]		24–67				
24–72[h]									[i]		67–115				
25–36	44	Minimal effect							None						
1.5	Decreased			10–15 mg/kg/day	10–15 mg/kg/day	10–15 mg/kg/day	10–15 mg/kg/day	7.5–15 mg/kg/day	Give daily dose after HD		35 to >90				
1											50–100				

[f] Hemodialysis reduces the ganciclovir plasma concentration by approximately 50 percent.
[g] Respiratory syncytial virus bronchiolitis/pneumonia requires a small-particle aerosol generator. After exposure 18–22 hours per day for 3–5 days at a reservoir concentration of 20 mg/ml, the delivered dose is 0.8–1.4 mg/kg/hr depending on age.
[h] Ribavirin accumulates in RBCs with chronic administration and prolongs the terminal plasma half-life up to 2 weeks.
[i] A dosage reduction may be necessary in the elderly, whose plasma levels exceed by twofold those observed in healthy, young adults receiving equivalent doses.

ADVERSE DRUG INTERACTION INVOLVING ANTIMICROBIAL AGENTS *(Continued)*

Interacting Drugs	*Adverse Effect*	*Probable Mechanism*
Amphotericin B with		
Aminoglycoside antibiotics	Nephrotoxicity	Synergism
Cyclosporine	Increased renal toxicity	Possible synergism
Digitalis glycosides	Increased digitalis toxicity	Hypokalemia
Neuromuscular blocking agents	Increased neuromuscular blocking effect	Hypokalemia
Cephalosporins with		
Alcohol	Disulfiram-like effect with cefamandole, cefoperazone, and moxalactam	Inhibition of intermediary metabolism of alcohol
Aminoglycoside antibiotics	Increased nephrotoxicity	Mechanism not established
Anticoagulants, oral	Possible increased anticoagulant effect with moxalactam or cefamandole	Mechanism not established
Aspirin	Possible increased bleeding risk with moxalactam	Additive
Ethacrynic acid	Increased nephrotoxicity	Mechanism not established
Furosemide	Increased nephrotoxicity	Mechanism not established
Heparin	Possible increased bleeding risk with moxalactam	Additive
Penicillins	Possible increased cefotaxime toxicity with azlocillin in patients with renal impairment	Decreased excretion
Vancomycin	Increased nephrotoxicity	Additive
Chloramphenicol with		
Acetaminophen	Possible decreased chloramphenicol effect	Increased metabolism
Anticoagulants (oral)	Increased dicumarol effect	Decreased metabolism
Barbiturates	Increased barbiturate effect; decreased chloramphenicol effect	Decreased metabolism Increased metabolism
Cimetidine	Aplastic anemia	Possibly additive or synergism
Etomidate	Prolonged anesthesia	Decreased metabolism
Hypoglycemics, sulfonylurea	Increased hypoglycemic effect	Mechanism not established
Phenytoin	Increased phenytoin toxicity Possible increased chloramphenicol toxicity	Decreased metabolism Mechanism not established
Rifampin	Decreased chloramphenicol effect	Increased metabolism
Clindamycin with		
Neuromuscular blocking agents	Increased neuromuscular blockade	Additive

(*Continued*)

ADVERSE DRUG INTERACTION INVOLVING ANTIMICROBIAL AGENTS *(Continued)*

Interacting Drugs	*Adverse Effect*	*Probable Mechanism*
Colistimethate, same as polymyxin B		
Cycloserine with		
Alcohol	Increased alcohol effect or convulsions	Mechanism not established
Isoniazid	CNS effects, dizziness, drowsiness	Mechanism not established
Erythromycins with		
Anticoagulant, oral	Hypoprothrombinemia potentiated	Possible decreased metabolism
Carbamazepine	Increased carbamazepine toxicity	Possibly decreased metabolism
Corticosteroids	Increased effect and possible toxicity of methylprednisolone	Decreased excretion
Cyclosporine	Increased cyclosporine toxicity	Probably decreased metabolism
Digoxin	Increased digoxin effect	Decreased gut metabolism and increased absorption
Ergot alkaloids	Increased ergot toxicity	Mechanism not established
Phenytoin	Possible increased or decreased effect	Altered metabolism
Theophyline	Increased theophylline effect and possible toxicity	Decreased metabolism
Fluoroquinolones with		
Antacids	Decreased fluoroquinolone effect with aluminum or magnesium antacids	Decreased absorption
Theophyllines	Possible theophylline toxicity	Decreased metabolism
Griseofulvin with		
Anticoagulants, oral	Decreased anticoagulant effect	Mechanism not established
Contraceptives, oral	Decreased contraceptive effect	Increased metabolism
Hydroxychloroquine with		
Digoxin	Increased digoxin effect	Mechanism not established
Isoniazid with		
Alcohol	Increased incidence of hepatitis	Mechanism not established
	Decreased isoniazid effect in some alcoholic patients	Increased metabolism
Aluminum antacids	Decreased isoniazid effect	Decreased absorption
Anticoagulants, oral	Possible increased anticoagulant effect	Decreased metabolism
Benzodiazepines	Pharmacologic effects of benzodiazepines may be increased; documented with diazepam and triazolam	Decreased metabolism
Carbamazepine	Increased toxicity of both drugs	Altered metabolism
Cycloserine	CNS effects, dizziness, drowsiness	Mechanism not established
Disulfiram	Psychotic episodes, ataxia	Altered dopamine metabolism
Enflurane	Possible nephrotoxicity	Increased metabolism of enflurane caused increased fluoride concentration
Ketoconazole	Decreased ketoconazole effect	Decreased concentration
Phenytoin	Increased phenytoin toxicity	Decreased metabolism
Rifampin	Possible increased isoniazid hepatotoxicity	Possible increased toxic metabolites
Ketoconazole with		
Alcohol	Possible disulfiram-like reaction	Mechanism not established
Antacids	Decreased ketoconazole effect	Decreased absorption
Anticoagulants, oral	Increased anticoagulant effect	Mechanism not established
Corticosteroids	Increased methylprednisolone effect	Decreased metabolism
Cyclosporine	Increased concentration of cyclosporine in blood	Mechanism not established
H_2 antagonists	Possible decreased antifungal effect	Decreased absorption
Isoniazid	Decreased ketoconazole effect	Decreased blood concentrations
Phenytoin	Altered effects of one or both drugs	Altered metabolism
Rifampin	Decreased rifampin and ketoconazole effects	Decreased blood concentrations
Lincomycin with		
Kaolin-pectin	Decreased lincomycin effect	Decreased absorption
Neuromuscular blocking agents	Increased neuromuscular blockade	Additive
Metronidazole with		
Alcohol	Mild disulfiram-like symptoms	Possible inhibition of intermediary metabolism of alcohol
Anticoagulants, oral	Increased anticoagulant effect	Decreased metabolism
Barbiturates	Decreased metronidazole effect with phenobarbital	Probably increased metabolism
Cimetidine	Possible increased metronidazole toxicity	Decreased metabolism
Disulfiram	Organic brain syndrome	Mechanism not established
Lithium	Lithium toxicity	Mechanism not established
Miconazole with		
Aminoglycosides	Possible decreased tobramycin concentration	Mechanism not established
Anticoagulants, oral	Increased anticoagulant effect	Mechanism not established
Hypoglycemics, sulfonylurea	Severe hypoglycemia	Mechanism not established
Phenytoin	Increased phenytoin toxicity	Decreased metabolism
Nalidixic acid with		
Anticoagulants, oral	Increased anticoagulant effect	Displacement from binding sites
Nitrofurantoin with		
Antacids	Possible decreased nitrofurantoin effect	Decreased absorption
Para-aminosalicylic acid, *see* aminosalicylic acid		
Penicillins with		
Allopurinol	Increased incidence of rash with ampicillin	Mechanism not established
Aminoglycosides	Decreased aminoglycoside effect with high concentrations of carbenicillin or ticarcillin	Inactivation
Anticoagulants, oral	Decreased anticoagulant effect with nafcillin and didoxacillin	Increased metabolism
β-Adrenergic blockers	Possible decreased atenolol effect with ampicillin	Decreased absorption
Cephalosporins	Possible increased cefotaxime toxicity with azlocillin in patients with renal impairment	Decreased excretion

(*Continued*)

Interacting Drugs	Adverse Effect	Probable Mechanism
Contraceptives, oral	Decreased contraceptive effect with ampicillin or oxacillin	Decreased enterohepatic circulation of estrogen
Lithium	Hypernatremia with ticarcillin	Large sodium load from ticarcillin and decreased renal excretion
Methotrexate	Possible increased methotrexate toxicity	Decreased excretion
Polymyxin B with		
Aminoglycoside antibiotics	Increased nephrotoxicity; increased neuromuscular blockade	Additive
Neuromuscular blocking agents	Increased neuromuscular blockade	Additive
Vancomycin	Increased nephrotoxicity	Additive
Rifampin with		
Aminosalicylic acid	Rifampin effectiveness may be decreased; separate doses by 8–12 h	Decreased GI absorption due to excipient bentonite
Anticoagulants, oral	Decreased anticoagulant effect	Increased metabolism
Barbiturates	Decreased barbiturate effect	Increased metabolism
Benzodiazepines	Possible decreased oral and IV diazepam effect	Increased metabolism
β-Adrenergic blockers	Decreased β-blocker effect	Increased metabolism
Chloramphenicol	Decreased chloramphenicol effect	Increased metabolism
Clofibrate	Pharmacologic effects of clofibrate may be decreased	Increased metabolism–enzyme induction
Contraceptives, oral	Decreased contraceptive effect	Increased metabolism
Corticosteroids	Decreased corticosteroid effect	Increased metabolism
Cyclosporine	Decreased cyclosporine effect	Increased metabolism
Digitalis	Decreased digitoxin and digoxin effect	Increased metabolism
Disopyramide	Decreased disopyramide effect	Probably increased metabolism
Hypoglycemics, sulfonylurea	Decreased hypoglycemic effect	Increased metabolism
Isoniazid	Possible increased hepatotoxicity	Possible increased toxic metabolites
Ketoconazole	Decreased effect of both drugs	Increased metabolism
Methadone	Methadone withdrawal symptoms	Increased metabolism
Mexiletene	Decreased antiarrhythmic effect	Increased metabolism
Phenytoin	Decreased phenytoin effect	Increased metabolism
Progestins	Decreased norethindrone effect	Increased metabolism
Quinidine	Decreased quinidine effect	Increased metabolism
Theophyllines	Decreased theophylline effect	Increased metabolism
Verapamil	Decreased verapamil effect	Increased metabolism
Spectinomycin with		
Lithium	Increased lithium toxicity	Decreased renal excretion
Sulfonamides with		
Anticoagulants, oral	Increased anticoagulant effect	Decreased metabolism and displacement from binding sites
Barbiturates	Increased thiopental effect	Decreased albumin binding
Cyclosporine	Decreased cyclosporine effect with sulfamethazine	Possibly increased metabolism
Digoxin	Possible decreased digoxin effect with sulfasalazine	Decreased digoxin absorption
Hypoglycemics, sulfonylurea	Increased hypoglycemic effect	Mechanism not established
Methotrexate	Possible increased methotrexate toxicity	Decreased renal clearance and displacement from binding
Monoamine oxidase inhibitors	Possible increased phenelzine toxicity with sulfisoxazole	Decreased metabolism
Phenytoin	Increased phenytoin effect, except possibly with sulfisoxazole	Decreased metabolism
Tetracyclines with		
Alcohol	Decreased doxycycline effect in alcoholics	Increased metabolism
Antacids, oral	Decreased oral tetracycline effects	Decreased tetracycline absorption
Anticoagulants, oral	Increased anticoagulant effect	Mechanism not established
Antidepressants, tricyclic	Localized hemosiderosis with amitriptyline and minocycline	Possible synergism
Barbiturates	Decreased doxycycline effect	Increased metabolism
Bismuth subsalicylate	Decreased tetracycline effect	Decreased absorption
Carbamazepine	Decreased doxycycline effect	Increased metabolism
Contraceptives, oral	Decreased contraceptive effect	Possible decreased enterohepatic circulation of estrogen
Digoxin	Increased digoxin effect	Decreased gut metabolism and increased absorption
Iron, oral	Decreased tetracycline effect, but not with doxycycline	Decreased absorption
	Decreased iron effect	Decreased absorption
Lithium	Increased lithium toxicity	Decreased renal excretion
Methotrexate	Possible increased toxicity	Displacement from binding
Molindone	Decreased tetracycline effect	Calcium as an excipient inhibits absorption
Phenformin	Increased lactic acidosis	Possible decreased phenformin excretion
Phenytoin	Decreased doxycycline effect	Increased metabolism
Rifampin	Possible decreased doxycycline effect	Increased metabolism
Theophyllines	Possible theophylline toxicity	Mechanism not established
Zinc sulfate	Decreased tetracycline effect	Decreased absorption
Thiabendazole with		
Theophyllines	Increased theophylline toxicity	Decreased metabolism
Trimethoprim with		
Amiloride	Trimethoprim may potentiate hyponatremia caused by the concomitant use of amiloride with thiazide diuretics	Additive
Azathioprine	Leukopenia	Mechanism not established
Cyclosporine	Increased nephrotoxicity	Synergism
Digoxin	Possible increased digoxin effect	Decreased renal excretion and possibly decreased metabolism
Thiazide diuretics	Trimethoprim may potentiate hyponatremia caused by the concomitant use of amiloride with thiazide diuretics	Additive

(Continued)

ADVERSE DRUG INTERACTION INVOLVING ANTIMICROBIAL AGENTS *(Continued)*

Interacting Drugs	*Adverse Effect*	*Probable Mechanism*
Trimethoprim-sulfamethoxazole with		
Anticoagulants, oral	Increased anticoagulant effect	Decreased metabolism
Antidepressants, tricyclic	Recurrence of depression	Mechanism not established
Lidocaine	Methemoglobinemia	Probably additive
Mercaptopurine	Decreased antileukemic effect	Mechanism not established
Methotrexate	Megaloblastic anemia	Additive inhibition of folate metabolism
Phenytoin	Increased phenytoin toxicity	Probably decreased metabolism
Pimozide	Decreased pimozide effect	Mechanism not established
Vancomycin with		
Aminoglycosides	Possible increased nephrotoxicity and ototoxicity	Possibly additive
Cephalosporins	Increased nephrotoxicity	Additive
Digoxin	Possible decreased digoxin effect	Possibly decreased absorption
Paromomycin	Increased nephrotoxicity	Additive
Polymyxins	Increased nephrotoxicity	Additive
Vidarabine with		
Allopurinol	Increased neurotoxicity	Decreased metabolism
Theophyllines	Increased theophylline effect	Decreased metabolism
Zidovudine with		
Acetaminophen	Granulocytopenia	Mechanism not established
Acyclovir	Neurotoxicity	Mechanism not established

(Data from Rizack et al.)

BIBLIOGRAPHY

Abramowicz M. Handbook of Antimicrobial Therapy. revised ed. New York: Medical Letter; 1986.

Anderson PO. Drugs and breast feeding: A review. Drug Intell Clin Pharm. 1977;11:208–23.

Bennett WM. Update on drugs in renal failure. In Advances in Nephrology. Chicago: Year Book Medical Publishers; 1986.

Bennett WM, Aronoff GR, Morrison G, et al. Drug prescribing in renal failure; dosing guidelines for adults. Am J Kidney Dis. 1983;3:155–93.

Biller JA, Yeager AM. The Harriet Lane Handbook. 9th ed. Chicago: Year Book Medical Publishers; 1981.

Brigss GG, Freeman RK, Yaffe SJ. Drugs in Pregnancy and Lactation. 2nd ed. Baltimore: Williams & Wilkins; 1986.

Keller F, Offerman G, Lode H. Supplementary dose after hemodialysis. Nephron. 1982;30:220–7.

Kucers A, Bennet NM. The Use of Antibiotics. 4th ed. London: William Heinemann; 1987.

Lorian V. Antibiotics in Laboratory Medicine. 2nd ed. Baltimore: Williams & Wilkins; 1986.

Manuel MA, Paton TW, Cornish WR. Drugs and peritoneal dialysis. Peritoneal Dialysis Bull 1983;117–25.

Matsuda SL. Transfer of antibiotics into maternal milk. Biol Res Preg. 1984;5:57–60.

McCracken GH, Nelson JD. Antimicrobial Therapy for Newborns. 2nd ed. New York: Grune & Stratton; 1983.

Nelson JD. 1987–1988 Pocketbook of Pediatric Antimicrobial Therapy. Baltimore: Williams & Wilkins; 1987.

Paton TW, Cornish WR, Manuel MA, et al. Drug therapy in patients undergoing peritoneal dialysis. Clin Pharmacokinet. 1985;10:404–26.

Peterson PK, Matzke G, Keane WF. Current concepts in the management of peritonitis in patients undergoing continuous ambulatory peritoneal dialysis. Rev Infec Dis. 1987;9:604–12.

Platzker ACD, Lew CD, Steward D. Drug administration via breast milk. Hosp Pract. 1980;15:111–22.

Reynolds JE, Prasad AB. Martindale The Extra Pharmacopoeia. 28th ed. London: Pharmaceutical Press; 1982.

Richards ML, Prince RA, Kenaley KA, et al. Antimicrobial penetration into cerebrospinal fluid. Drug Intell Clin Pharm. 1981;15:341–68.

Rizack MA, Hillman CDM: The Medical Letter Handbook of Adverse Drug Interactions. New York: Medical Letter; 1989:5–143.

Rollins DE, Klaassen DC. Biliary excretion of drugs in man. Clin Pharmacokinet. 1979;4:368–79.

Sanford JP. Guide to Antimicrobial Therapy United States of America. J.P. Sanford, M.D., 1988.

Schonfeld H, ed. Pharmacokinetics. Antibiot Chemother. 1978;25:1–320.

Schonfeld H, ed. Pharmacokinetics II. Antibiot Chemother. 1982;31:1–224.

Wilson JT, Brown RD, Cherek DR, et al. Drug excretion in human breast milk: Principles, pharmacokinetics and projected consequences. Clin Pharmacokinet. 1980;5:1–65.

MAJOR CLINICAL SYNDROMES

PART II

SECTION A. FEVER

39. PATHOGENESIS OF FEVER

CHARLES A. DINARELLO
SHELDON M. WOLFF

Fever is an elevation of temperature above the normal daily variation. Infections are most commonly associated with fever, but noninfectious causes such as inflammatory, neoplastic, and immunologically mediated diseases may also have fever as their primary clinical presentation. Fever is best understood at the hypothalamic level. The thermoregulatory center located in the anterior region of the hypothalamus regulates interal temperature at about 37°C (98.6°F) primarily by its ability to balance heat loss from the periphery with heat production from tissues, particularly the liver and muscles. During fever, the balance is adjusted to increase the internal temperature.

Individuals maintain body temperature at about 37°C despite wide variations in environmental temperatures. For some individuals, normal body temperature can be below or above 37°C without constituting a pathologic process. During a 24-hour period, body temperature varies from a low point in the early morning to the highest levels at 4–6 PM. The amplitude of this daily variation, also called the circadian temperature rhythm, is about 0.6°C (1°F), and individuals retain their circadian rhythm throughout life despite intervening bouts of prolonged illness. During fever, the morning low and evening high temperature pattern can still be observed. In the occasional situation in which elevated temperature is really hyperthermia (see below), this rhythm is absent.

Endogenous pyrogens are polypeptides produced by the host in response to infection, injury, inflammation, or antigenic challenge. These polypeptides cause fever by their ability to trigger biochemical changes in the hypothalamus, particularly prostaglandin synthesis. The first endogenous pyrogen described has now been identified as interleukin-1 (IL-1). Recombinant human IL-1s produce fever in experimental animals at doses of 100 ng/kg. Interferons (IFNs), produced as a consequence of viral infection, are also endogenous pyrogens. Recombinant human IFN-α produces chills and fever in humans. Two other endogenous pyrogens are tumor necrosis factor (TNF) and IL-6.

PYROGENS

Pyrogens are substances that cause fever and may be exogenous or endogenous.[1] Exogenous pyrogens are derived from outside the host, and the vast majority of exogenous pyrogens are microbial products, toxins, or the microbes themselves. The best studied of an exogenous pyrogen is the lipopolysaccharide produced by all gram-negative bacteria and commonly called "endotoxin." Endotoxins are large molecules (>300,000 daltons). Another group of bacterial substances that are potent pyrogens are produced by gram-positive organisms. There are the enterotoxins of *Staphylococcus aureus* and the group A streptococcal erythrogenic toxins. A staphylococcal toxin of clinical importance is the toxic shock syndrome toxin associated with strains of *S. aureus* isolated from patients with the toxic shock syndrome. The gram-positive exotoxins are polypeptides in the 20,000–30,000 dalton range. Like the endotoxins from gram-negative bacteria, the toxins produced by staphylococci and streptococci produce fever in experimental animals when injected intravenously in the submicrogram per kilogram range. Of considerable importance is the fact that endotoxin is a highly pyrogenic molecule in humans since 2–3 ng/kg produces fever and generalized symptoms in volunteers.[2]

ENDOGENOUS PYROGENS

In contradistinction to exogenous pyrogens, endogenous pyrogens are polypeptides produced by various host cells, particularly the monocyte/macrophage. They initiate fever by their ability to trigger the hypothalamic thermoregulatory center. Early concepts of the pathogenesis of fever proposed that exogenous pyrogens produced fever by their ability to act directly on the brain. This was later shown to be an unlikely explanation since there was a requirement for an intermediate role for leukocytes. It was subsequently shown that exogenous pyrogens produce fever by first inducing the release of endogenous pyrogens. Endogenous pyrogens then gain entrance to the circulation, either directly or through the lymph, and reach the hypothalamus. There they initiate a cascade of changes in arachidonic acid metabolites, neurotransmitters, and ions that raise the set-point.

It was originally believed that there was a single endogenous pyrogen characterized by its ability to produce fever in rabbits and other experimental animals. After the injection of endogenous pyrogen-containing leukocyte supernatants, there is a rapid rise in body temperature, usually within 5–10 minutes, whereas exogenous pyrogens cause a more delayed onset of fever. In addition, the fever-inducing property of endogenous pyrogens is destroyed by mild heat (70°C), whereas most exogenous pyrogens are more heat resistant.

Initial characterization of human endogenous pyrogen revealed two polypeptides with molecular weights of 14,000–15,000 daltons and two isoelectric points of 6.8 and 5.1. These have been subsequently respectively renamed IL-1β and IL-1α. The two IL-1s have been cloned,[3,4] their entire amino acid sequences are known, and recombinant IL-1s produce typical endogenous pyrogen fever when injected into animals. In rabbits, 50–100 ng/kg induces a peak rise of 0.5–0.8°C within 50 minutes.[1]

Other molecules have been cloned, and the recombinant forms have produced fever when injected into animals or humans. These are tumor necrosis factor (TNF-α),[5] lymphotoxin (TNF-β), IL-6,[6] and IFN-α.[1] Together with IL-1β and IL-1α, these substances can be classified as endogenous pyrogens or as endogenous *pyrogenic cytokines*. The term *cytokine* refers to polypepides produced by a variety of cells that induce biochemical changes in other cells. Each pyrogenic cytokine is a product of a separate gene; elevated plasma levels of some pyrogenic cytokines are found in humans during fever (discussed below).

Interleukin-1, TNF, IL-6, and IFN possess other biologic properties in addition to producing fever (discussed in the section on acute-phase responses). A wide spectrum of exogenous pyrogens induce the synthesis and release of these pyrogenic cytokines. These are listed in Table 1. Most of the exogenous pyrogenic substances can be recognized by their association with febrile diseases. In addition, there are substances produced by the host that cause fever because they stimulate the synthesis and release of the endogenous pyrogenic cytokines. For example, antigen–antibody complexes derived from blood incom-

TABLE 1. Organisms and Substances Inducing Pyrogenic Cytokines[a]

Viruses (influenza, Newcastle disease virus, cytomegalic disease virus)
Bacteria (whole cells, *Staphylococcus epidermidis, Borrelia burgdorferi*)
Peptidoglycans (cell walls of all bacteria)
Muramyl peptides (naturally occurring breakdown products of peptidoglycans)
Endotoxins (lipopolysaccharides of gram-negative bacteria)
Enterotoxins (A, B, C, D from *Staphylococcus aureus*)
Toxic shock syndrome toxin-1 (from toxic shock syndrome-associated *Staphylococcus aureus*)
Erythrogenic toxins (from group A streptococci)
Capsular polysaccharides (from *Cryptococcus neoformans*)
Yeasts (whole cells of *Candida albicans*, other yeasts)
Tuberculin (from mycobacteria in sensitive individuals)
Antigen–antibody complexes (requires the activation of complement)
Complement components (C5a, C3a)
Lymphocyte products (IL-2, interferons-γ^b)
Polynucleic acids (poly I:C)
Pyrogenic steroids (etiocholanolone, bile salts)
Drugs (via the production of lymphocyte products in sensitized individuals, for example, penicillin)
Pyrogenic cytokines (IL-1, TNF)
Drugs (bleomycin)

[a] Data are derived from both in vitro and in vivo studies.
[b] Interferon-α augments the production of pyrogenic cytokines induced by microbial products.

patibility are pyrogens because they induce the production of IL-1 and TNF.

THE HYPOTHALAMIC CONTROL OF CORE TEMPERATURE

The control of body temperature in humans takes place at the hypothalamic level. Clusters of neurons located in both the preoptic anterior and posterior portions of the hypothalamus receive two kinds of signals: one pathway is from other neurons with connections in the periphery to cold and warm receptors. The other signal is provided by the temperature of the blood bathing the hypothalamic region. These signals are integrated by both "warm" and "cold" neurons whose discharge rate varies with the blood temperature and levels of several neurotransmitters. Together, the area is called the "thermoregulatory center." In health, this center maintains the body temperature of the internal organs between 37° and 38°C. This is the core temperature, and it is best measured in the esophagus close to the great vessels.

Parts of the brain and the liver can have a higher temperature, about 38°C, and the skin is maintained at a lower temperature. The lower temperature of the skin varies with the state of vasoconstriction and the distance to large arteries. Therefore, the axillary temperature tends to be about 1° lower (36°C) than the core temperature is. Oral and rectal temperatures reflect core temperature. Oral readings are probably lower because of mouth breathing, which is particularly important in patients with respiratory infections and rapid breathing. Freshly voided urine temperatures also can reflect the core temperature. In general, with the exception of young children, a correct measurement of the oral temperature is a very good approximation of the true core temperature in most clinical settings.

Using vasoconstriction, vasodilation, sweating, and at times, shivering, the body maintains its temperature in the face of moderate environmental cold or heat. However, these physiologic manipulations cannot overcome severe temperature differences in the environment. Thus the hypothalamic thermoregulatory center also sends signals to the cerebral cortex where behavioral changes such as seeking less severe environmental temperatures, special posturing, or the use of special clothing to help maintain normal body temperature are initiated. The metabolic rate of humans is constantly producing more heat than is necessary to maintain the core body temperature at 37°C; therefore, hypothalamic temperature control is often regulating the amount of heat loss by vasodilation and evaporation. In severe cold, the hypothalamus triggers rapid muscle contractions (shivering) to produce more heat.

Hyperthermia

Despite physiologic and behavioral control of body temperature, excessive heat production or the inability to lose heat may result in elevated core temperatures; this is called hyperthermia. For example, overinsulating clothing can result in elevated core temperatures. Thus, although most patients with elevated body temperatures have fever, there are instances in which an elevated temperature is not fever but hyperthermia.

Hyperthermia is an elevation of the core temperature at a time when the hypothalamic set-point is at normothermic levels. In hyperthermia, elevation of the core temperature occurs because heat loss mechanisms are inhibited or are not adequate. These include heat stroke syndromes in which excessive heat is produced by work or environmental conditions (such as high humidity) that prevent adequate heat loss. Certain metabolic diseases such as hyperthyroidism can result in mild elevations of core temperature. Some pharmacologic agents that interfere with thermoregulation by blocking sweating or vasodilation can also produce an elevation of the core temperature. Once again, these syndromes represent hyperthermia because they take place in the presence of a normal hypothalamic set-point. Hyperthermia characteristically does not respond to antipyretics. Even overinsulation of children can elevate the core temperature, which appears to be fever but is, in fact, hyperthermia.

In some patients the hypothalamic set-point is elevated owing to local trauma, hemorrhage, tumor, or intrinsic hypothalamic malfunction. The term *hypothalamic fever* is sometimes used to describe elevated temperatures caused by abnormal hypothalamic function. However, most patients with hypothalamic damage have *hypo*thermia or do not respond properly to mild environmental temperature changes. In those few patients in whom hypothalamic fever is suspected, a diagnosis depends on demonstrating other abnormal hypothalamic functions such as the production of hypothalamic releasing factors, an abnormal response to cold, and an absence of circadian temperature and hormonal rhythms. Hyperthermia can also occur when certain anesthetics produce a rapid uncoupling of oxidative phosphorylation in susceptible individuals. This is known as malignant hyperthermia[7] and is often fatal. Another form of hyperthermia is seen in patients taking certain neuroleptic drugs.[8]

There is no way to rapidly differentiate fever from hyperthermia. Clinical history usually plays an important role. However, in addition to the clinical history of the patient, there are aspects of some forms of hyperthermia that may alert the clinician; for example, in heat stroke syndromes and in patients taking drugs that block sweating, the skin is very hot but dry. Antipyretics do not reduce the elevated temperature in hyperthermia, whereas there is usually some decrease in body temperature in febrile patients after adequate doses of either aspirin or acetaminophen.

The Febrile Response

Fever is due to an upward shift of the set-point in the hypothalamus to febrile levels. In fever, the hypothalamic set-point is raised, and this triggers the vasomotor center to commence vasoconstriction. Blood is shunted from the periphery, essentially decreasing the usual heat loss and resulting in an increase in blood temperature. For most fevers, this is sufficient to raise body temperatures 2–3°C. Shivering is also triggered at this time in order to increase heat production from the muscles, but shivering is frequently not required if heat conservation mechanisms raise the blood temperature to the required level.

The processes of heat conservation and heat production continue until the temperature of the blood bathing the hypothalamic neurons matches the new setting. At that point, the hypothalamus maintains the new febrile temperature just as it does at normothermic levels. In fact, studies have shown that the mechanisms of heat balance in fever are the same as in the afebrile state, the only difference being that, in fever, the body temperature is maintained at the higher level.

When the hypothalamic set-point is reset downward, the processes of heat loss through vasodilation and sweating are initiated. Behavioral changes are also triggered at this time, and the removal of insulating clothing or bedding takes place.

Persistent fevers are sometimes classified as "intermittent" or "remittent"; intermittent fevers are characterized as daily fever spikes followed by a return to normal body temperature, whereas remittent fevers do not return to normal body temperatures. The biochemical or neurologic basis for these different fever patterns in some infectious diseases remains unknown.

Some hypothalamic substances have been reported to reduce fever; these include various neuropeptides such as somatostatin, arginine vasopressin,[9] and α-melanocyte–stimulating factor.[10] These substances appear to be produced in greater amounts during fever. In animal models, they suppress fever at the hypothalamic level and can be considered to function as intrinsic central antipyretics. For example, arginine vasopressin is thought to prevent fever in pregnant animals immediately before and after birth. In the pre-antibiotic era, fever due to a variety of infectious diseases rarely exceeded 106°F, and there has been speculation that this natural "thermal ceiling" is mediated by these neuropeptides functioning as central antipyretics. It is possible that an absence of the production of these natural antipyretics may account for the failure of some febrile patients to return to baseline body temperature.

Effect of Endogenous Pyrogenic Cytokines on the Hypothalamus

Each endogenous pyrogenic cytokine is a product of a separate gene. Interleukin-1β and IL-1α both recognize the IL-1 receptor, and TNF-α and TNF-β also share a common receptor. Receptors for these pyrogenic cytokines have been observed to be distributed in several areas in the brain, including the hypothalamus. There does not appear to be a particular concentration of cytokine receptors in the hypothalamus, but rather they appear throughout the brain.

During fever, hypothalamic tissue and third cerebral ventricle levels of prostaglandin E_2 (PGE_2) are elevated.[11] The highest concentrations of PGE_2 are near the circumventricular vascular organs (organum vasculosum lamina terminalis), which are networks of enlarged capillaries. Destruction of these organs reduces the ability of pyrogens to produce fever. Experiments have not been able to show, however, that pyrogenic cytokines pass from the circulation into the brain substance. Thus, it appears that endogenous pyrogens interact with the endothelium of these capillaries, which is probably the first step in initiating fever.

The interaction of endogenous pyrogens with the hypothalamic circumventricular vascular organs is poorly understood; however, cultured endothelial cells produce PGE when stimulated with IL-1 or TNF. In addition, these pyrogenic cytokines induce a variety of other changes in endothelial cells including increased adhesion of leukocytes, the release of platelet-activating factor, and the synthesis of plasminogen activator inhibitor.[1,12]

Figure 1 illustrates the key events in the generation of fever. Infections and toxins produced by many microorganisms stimulate the monocyte/macrophage to synthesize and release the various endogenous pyrogenic cytokines. As shown, other cells have the potential to produce these endogenous pyrogens. The pyrogenic cytokines cause fever by their ability to initiate metabolic changes in the hypothalamic thermoregulatory center. Of these, the synthesis of PGE_2 appears to play a critical role. The ability of systemic drugs such as aspirin to inhibit the synthesis of prostaglandins at the hypothalamic level accounts for their antipyretic effect. The elevation in the hypothalamic temperature set-point that is brought about by elevated prostaglandin levels triggers the brain centers controlling heat production and peripheral vascular tone. Neuronal transmission delivers this information to the periphery, and the core temperature begins to rise.

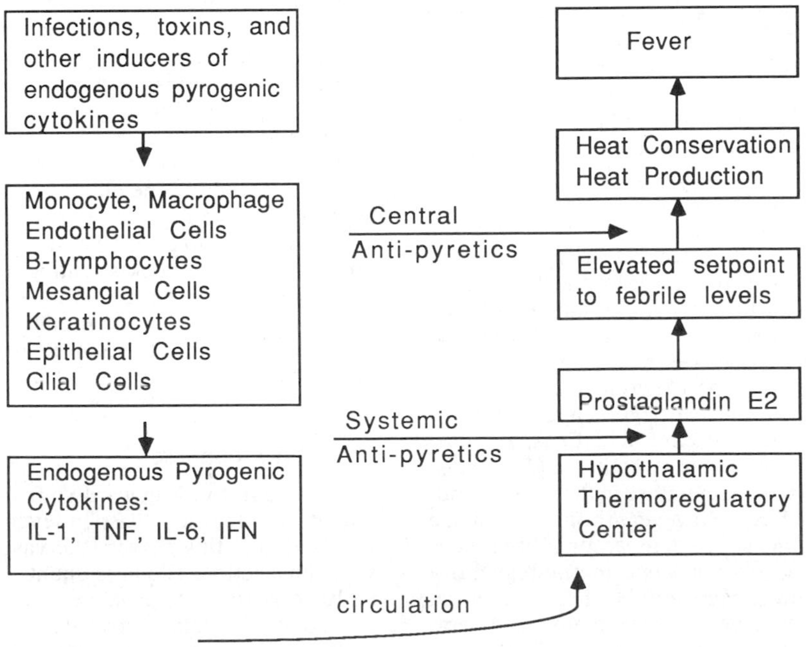

FIG. 1. Scheme for the pathogenesis of fever.

FEVER THERAPY

Throughout history, fever therapy has been used to treat a variety of diseases, both physical and psychological. Sometimes these therapies have been quite successful, for example, the treatment of tertiary syphilis with malarial fever, which brought its inventor a Nobel prize. Most often, however, fever therapies have been replaced with drugs for specific infections. Nevertheless, there is continued interest and investigation into fever therapy. One problem in interpreting the data of such studies is the need to differentiate fever therapy in which a pyrogen or infection induces a fever from what occurs in hyperthermic therapy in which the core temperature is elevated directly by applying heat or preventing its removal. The use of hyperthermia in the treatment of various malignancies is being used today with some success. In these situations, microwave energy is delivered to the patient, and the core temperature can be raised under controlled conditions. Hyperthermia is particularly successful when combined with chemotherapy or radiation. However, hyperthermia treatment should not be equated with fever therapy. In fever therapy, the inducing agent causes a febrile response, but in addition, a variety of pyrogenic and nonpyrogenic cytokines are produced that can affect the host defense.

ANTIPYRETIC THERAPY

There is a continuing debate on whether physicians should recommend reducing the elevated temperature that occurs in a variety of infectious diseases. A decision not to treat the fever may be based on evidence that the elevated temperature may offer the patient a benefit because under some experimental conditions host defense mechanisms are enhanced by an elevated temperature. Is this evidence sufficient to advise patients not to take antipyretics? Unfortunately, there are few human studies, and these do not show a dramatic difference in recovery from viral upper respiratory infections between groups taking or not taking antipyretics. There are, on the other hand, limited animal data and more extensive in vitro data that support the concept that certain host defense functions are enhanced by elevated temperatures. Temperatures of 39°C augment T- and B-cell responses, the generation of cytolytic T cells, B-cell activity, and immunoglobulin synthesis.[13,14] For example, in vitro microbial growth is suppressed at elevated temperatures, and lymphocyte activation and antibody formation are increased. But there are no studies showing that patients not taking antipyretics eliminate their viral infections faster or produce more antibodies. Witholding aspirin from children with viral-like illnesses appears warranted on the basis that this is a risk factor for the development of Reye syndrome. Children with fever, particularly those at risk for a febrile seizure, can be treated with acetaminophen.

An extraordinarily high fever (>41.5°C) is often called hyperpyrexia. Hyperpyrexia can be observed in patients with severe infections, but it most common occurs in patients with central nervous system hemorrhages. Antipyretics reduce the fever but because of the dangerously high temperatures, cooling blankets and water–alcohol bathing are employed to accelerate peripheral heat losses. There are effective means of reducing elevated temperatures, but in the absence of antipyretics that lower the hypothalamic set-point, peripheral cooling can be counterproductive since cold receptors in the skin send signals to the spinal cord and brain for reactive vasoconstriction, thus reducing heat loss mechanisms. Similarly, drugs such as atropine and other muscarinics block sweating and make heat loss more difficult.

Studies in patients receiving controlled hyperthermia treatment for various neoplasms have shown that temperatures as high as 42°C can be tolerated for 4 hours without irreversible organ damage. Nevertheless, fever increases the demand for oxygen and can aggravate pre-existing cardiac or pulmonary insufficiency. For every increase of 1°C over 37°C, there is a 13 percent increase in O_2 consumption. In addition, elevated temperatures can induce mental changes in patients with organic brain disease. Therefore, treatment of fever in some patient groups is recommended.

Children with previous febrile or nonfebrile seizures also should be aggressively treated to reduce fever. However, it is unclear what triggers the febrile seizure since there is no absolute correlation between the temperature elevation and the onset of a febrile seizure in susceptible children.

Antipyretics and the Treatment of Fever

The ability of the pyrogenic cytokines to induce PGE_2 synthesis is an important event in the production of fever. Numerous experiments have shown that the inhibitors of the cyclooxygenase enzyme system are potent antipyretics. There is a direct correlation of the antipyretic potency of various drugs and the inhibition of brain cyclooxygenase.[15] Acetaminophen is a poor cyclooxygenase inhibitor in peripheral tissue and is without noteworthy anti-inflammatory activity; however, in the brain acetaminophen is oxidized, and the oxidized form inhibits cyclooxygenase activity.[16,17] This oxidation explains the potent antipyretic effect of acetaminophen.

Studies have shown that there is no difference between oral aspirin and acetaminophen in reducing fever in humans. Nonsteroidal anti-inflammatory agents (indomethacin, ibuprofen, etc.) are also antipyretics and can be used for this purpose. Chronic high-dose antipyretic therapy such as aspirin or nonsteroidal anti-inflammatory agents used in arthritis does not reduce the normal core body temperature. Thus, there appears to be no role of PGE_2 in normal thermoregulation. There is some evidence in rats that the increase in body temperature that takes place during the day is, in part, due to cytokine release as a result of physical activity and is reducible by antipyretics. However, there are no similar studies in humans, and the evidence suggests that circadian variation in humans is unaffected by antipyretics.

Corticosteroids are also effective antipyretics. However, they act at two levels: (*1*) similar to the cyclooxygenase inhibitors, corticosteroids reduce PGE_2 synthesis by inhibiting the activity of phospholipase A_2, and (*2*) unlike the cyclooxygenase inhibitors, corticosteroids block the transcription of the mRNA for the pyrogenic cytokines. Drugs that interfere with vasoconstriction (phenothiazines, for example) can also act as antipyretics, as can drugs that block muscle contractions. However, these are not true antipyretics because they can also reduce the core temperature independently of hypothalamic control.

MEASUREMENT OF CIRCULATING PYROGENIC CYTOKINES

Radioimmunoassays (RIAs) and enzyme-linked immunosorbent assay (ELISA) kits for each pyrogenic cytokine are available commercially. Because the pyrogenic cytokines are products of blood leukocytes that are affected by the clotting process, the collection of freshly obtained plasma in the presence of protease inhibitors is preferred.[18] Although there are relatively few comprehensive studies on febrile patients, a pattern appears to be emerging: the height of temperature elevation does not correlate with the concentration of the cytokine in the circulation. For example, in human volunteers given an injection of endotoxin, the peak of the fever occurs 4 hours after intravenous injection, but the peak elevation in circulating TNF occurs after 90 minutes.[19] In these same studies, IL-1β concentrations in the plasma increase slowly and reach peak elevation after 180 minutes, whereas maximal IL-6 levels occur at 120 minutes.

In studies of septic patients, there is no correlation between the level of IL-1β and TNF in the same sample. This is supported by evidence showing that the genes for these two cytokines are independently regulated and are on two difference chromosomes. In patients receiving high-dose IL-2 therapy, plasma TNF, IL-1β, and IL-6 concentrations are elevated, but once again, these are not similarly elevated among the patients, and peak plasma levels do not correlate with the peak of the fever. Deficiencies in cytokine production in vitro from blood leukocytes have been described in various disease states.

Despite no overt evidence of fever or illness, some healthy individuals have elevated plasma TNF, IL-1, or IL-6 levels. Studies do show that some of the pyrogenic cytokines are elevated in burns, sepsis, malaria, exacerbations of rheumatoid arthritis,[20] and renal allograft rejection. They are also elevated after strenuous exercise and ovulation.[21]

Pyrogenic cytokines may be present in the circulation but bound to carrier molecules that reduce or prevent interaction with the capillary network in the hypothalamic thermoregulatory center. There is evidence to support this concept since IL-1β requires extraction from plasma proteins such as α_2-macroglobulin before being assayed.[18] The concentration of cytokine-binding proteins appears to increase in chronic diseases and may be due to an increased production of hepatic acute-phase proteins.

Aspirin and nonsteroidal anti-inflammatory agents prevent fever but do not prevent the synthesis and release of pyrogenic cytokines. In fact, the in vitro production of the pyrogenic cytokines from blood leukocytes from human subjects taking oral cyclooxygenase inhibitors is enhanced. Hence, it is possible to measure elevated plasma cytokine levels in individuals who are afebrile because of antipyretic therapy. There are no studies on plasma pyrogenic cytokine levels as a function of diurnal temperature variation; however, preprandial and postprandial levels of IL-1β are within the coefficient of variation.

ACUTE PHASE CHANGES

Infections, trauma, inflammatory processes, and some malignant diseases induce a constellation of host responses that are collectively referred to as the "acute-phase response." This response is associated with characteristic metabolic changes in liver protein synthesis, but on closer examination, changes also occur in several other systems including the hematologic, endocrinologic, neurologic, and immunologic. These changes are called acute because most are observed within hours or days after the onset of infection or injury. The full spectrum of the response includes dramatic increases in the synthesis of several unique hepatic proteins that are not produced in health. One of these, C-reactive protein, is a marker of the acute-phase response and can be used as an indicator of disease. The increased plasma concentrations of acute-phase hepatic proteins, glycoproteins, and globulins are responsible for elevated erythrocyte sedimentation rates. Increases in gluconeogenesis, energy expenditure, and muscle proteolysis occur and contribute to the weight loss. Increased sleep and lethargy are frequent clinical complaints. Thyroid dysfunction can be present, and there is often abnormal glucose tolerance and lipid metabolism. In addition, anemia develops despite adequate stores of iron. This may be due to the suppressive effect of TNF on hematopoiesis. The hypergammaglobulinemia that is often a component of the acute-phase response may be mediated by IL-6. This pyrogenic cytokine induces hepatic acute-phase protein synthesis.[22] and is a potent B-lymphocyte growth and differentiation factor.

Although the most striking changes in the acute-phase response is observed in patients with bacterial infections, burns, or multiple injuries, clinicians also encounter acute-phase changes in patients with occult infections or chronic illnesses such as rheumatoid arthritis, Crohn's disease, and several autoimmune diseases. The presence of acute-phase changes can also serve as an indicator of silent cancers, particularly renal cell carcinoma and Hodgkin's disease. The various components of the response are remarkably consistent despite the considerable variety of pathologic processes that induce it. For example, plasma levels of several acute-phase proteins are elevated after myocardial infarction, a bone fracture, or bacterial pneumonia.

The pyrogenic cytokines IL-1,[23,24] TNF,[25] IL-6,[22] and to a lesser extent, INF-α can induce, in part, many of the acute-phase changes in animals that are observed in humans. Interferon-α is produced primarily during viral infections. Although it shares with IL-1, TNF, and IL-6 the ability to produce fever, sleep, and lethargy, IFN-α does not induce hepatic acute-phase protein synthesis. Thus, elevated erythrocyte sedimentation rates and neutrophilia are not commonly observed during viral infections. Interferon-γ, produced during immunologic reactions such as organ transplant rejection and drug fever, induces some hepatic acute-phase proteins in vitro but, like IFN-α, is a weak inducer of acute-phase changes in the liver. Table 2 compares the multiple biologic effects of the different cytokines involved in acute-phase responses.

The patient with a localized bacterial infection represents an excellent example of the development of the acute-phase response. At the onset of the infection, blood monocytes and tissue macrophages become activated either by phagocytosis of the invading microbe or by exposure to its products or toxins; the process results in the synthesis and release of the pyrogenic cytokines. These mediators enter the circulation and reach the brain where they initiate fever. Although fever is clearly one of the most obvious signs of the acute-phase response, other components of the response can be present without apparent clinical manifestations. One of the most sensitive measures of the acute-phase response is an increase in the number and immaturity of circulating neutrophils. The release of neutrophils is due to the direct action of IL-1 on the bone marrow neutrophil stores. In addition, IL-1 stimulates stem cells to become more responsive to various colony-stimulating factors. In human subjects injected with small doses of endotoxin, marked neutrophilia can be measured in the absence of fever. Serum zinc and iron levels are depressed. Low serum iron levels associated with anemia in the face of adequate iron stores is characteristic of the acute-phase response. A decreased serum iron content probably plays an important role in protecting the host against various bacteria. For example, the reduction in serum iron concentration can suppress the growth rate of several microorganisms and certain tumor cells that have a strict requirement for iron as a growth factor.

Within 8–12 hours after the onset of infection or trauma, the liver increases the synthetic rate of the so-called acute-phase proteins. The response includes increases in protein levels nor-

TABLE 2. Biologic Properties of IL-1, TNF, and IL-6

Biological Property	*IL-1*[a]	*TNF*[b]	*IL-6*
Endogenous pyrogen	+	+	+
Hepatic acute-phase proteins	+	+	+
Decreased albumin synthesis	+	+	+
Fibroblast proliferation	+	+	+
B-lymphocyte activation	+	+	+
T-lymphocyte activation	+	+	+
B-lymphocyte immunoglobulin synthesis	+	+	+
Hematopoietic stem cell activation	+	−	+
Nonspecific resistance to infection	+	+	+
Radioprotection	+	+	−
Endothelial cell activation	+	+	−
Synovial cell stimulation	+	+	−
Bone resorption	+	+	−
Induction of IL-1 and TNF	+	+	−
Induction of IL-6	+	+	−

[a] Data derived from recombinant IL-1β or IL-1α.
[b] Similar data obtained using either TNF-α or TNF-β (lymphotoxin).

mally found in health as well as the appearance of new proteins that serve as markers of a pathologic event.[26] Several normal plasma proteins increase severalfold during the acute-phase response. These include haptoglobin, certain protease inhibitors, complement components, ceruloplasmin, and fibrinogen. However, true acute-phase reactants increase several hundredfold. These include serum amyloid A protein (a precursor of the amyloid fibril in secondary amyloidosis) and C-reactive protein. C-reactive protein was named for its ability to interact with the C-polysaccharide of pneumococci and was the first acute-phase protein described. Albumin and cytochrome synthesis is depressed during acute-phase responses.[26]

Of all the acute-phase proteins, C-reactive protein and serum amyloid A protein are clinically the most important because their presence serves as an indicator of disease. These proteins are structurally related. C-reactive protein is particularly useful as a marker of the hepatic acute-phase protein response and can be measured easily in most clinical laboratories.

Despite the anabolic processes of the liver, the acute-phase response is accompanied by a pronounced catabolism of muscle protein that is associated with a loss of body weight and an overall negative nitrogen balance.[27] Fever increases oxygen and caloric demands, and a negative nitrogen balance can result from the oxidation of amino acids from skeletal muscle, which contributes to wasting. These amino acids are largely used for gluconeogenesis. In addition, there can be demineralization of bone. Although the metabolic demands of elevated temperature contribute to the increased need for energy substrates, the host also requires a large supply of amino acids for the synthesis of new protein at a time when food intake may be severely impaired or appetite reduced. Amino acids are required for immunologic and reparative processes such as the clonal expansion of lymphocytes and the proliferation of fibroblasts. Also, they are needed for the synthesis of hepatic acute-phase proteins, immunoglobulins, and collagen. The mechanism of providing ample amino acids for these cellular functions seems to be well orchestrated during the acute-phase response. The catabolism during infection and inflammation differs from that of starvation. Unlike starvation, in which large amounts of ketones are spilled into the urine, a septic individual excretes protein with small amounts of ketones. Interleukin-1 and TNF inhibit lipoprotein lipase and hence interfere with lipid metabolism.

In addition to the biochemical changes during acute-phase responses, appetite is depressed. In fact, a depressed appetite may play a greater role in the negative nitrogen balance of chronic disease than the mobilization of tissue does. Interleukin-1 and TNF are potent suppressors of appetite in animals.

The presence of certain acute-phase changes in an otherwise healthy individual can alert the physician to hidden disease. Measuring the levels of adrenocorticotropic hormone (ACTH), cortisol, growth hormone, and vasopressin is not particularly useful, although they are elevated during acute-phase responses. Measurement of C-reactive protein can assist the physician in determining the presence of disease in patients with vague, constitutional complaints. C-reactive protein levels are usually less than 100 μg/liter but increase within hours 10- to 1000-fold. In severe bacterial infections, the serum level can rise from undetectable to over 100 mg/liter in 48 hours. The presence of elevated levels of C-reactive protein or serum amyloid A protein, even in the absence of fever or neutrophilia, may indicate occult infection or malignant change. Increases in C-reactive protein and serum amyloid A protein occur in patients of any age and also in immunocompromised patients with opportunistic infections.

Not all inflammatory diseases are associated with elevated C-reactive protein levels. Patients with scleroderma, ulcerative colitis, and lupus erythematosus may not show rises in C-reactive protein levels. A failure to develop hepatic protein changes and the neutrophilia of the acute-phase response seems to be related to the presence of circulating inhibitors of IL-1 and TNF.

The role of acute-phase proteins in host defense and repair is not entirely clear. Studies suggest that the major role of C-reactive protein is to bind serum lipids or opsonize pneumococci, whereas serum amyloid A is thought to be immunosuppressive. Ceruloplasmin scavenges toxic free oxygen radicals that are injurious to many tissues. What is clear, however, is that the production and physical structure of these acute-phase proteins have been conserved through 400 million years of evolution, and therefore they have presumably been useful to the host. This argues that the acute-phase response, like fever, is a positive aspect of the host defense against infection.

REFERENCES

1. Dinarello CA, Cannon JG, Wolff SM. New concepts on the pathogenesis of fever. Rev Infect Dis. 1988;10:168–89.
2. Wolff SM. Biological effects of bacterial endotoxins in man. J Infect Dis. 1973;128(Suppl):733.
3. Auron PE, Webb AC, Rosenwasser LJ, et al. Nucleotide sequence of human monocyte interleukin-1 precursor cDNA. Proc Natl Acad Sci USA. 1984;81:7907.
4. Lomedico PT, Gubler U, Hellmann CP, et al. Cloning and expression of murine interleukin-1 cDNA. Nature. 1984;312:458.
5. Dinarello CA, Cannon JG, Wolff SM, et al. Tumor necrosis factor (cachectin) is an endogenous pyrogen and induces interleukin-1. J Exp Med. 1986;163:1433–50.
6. Helle M, Brakenhoff JP, DeGroot ER, et al. Interleukin-6 is involved in interleukin-1–induced activities. Eur J Immunol. 1988;18:957.
7. Smith RJ. Malignant hyperthermia. Preoperative assessment of the risk factors. Br J Anaesth. 1988;60:317.
8. Allsop P, Twigley AJ. The neuroleptic malignant syndrome. Case report with a review of the literature. Anesthesia. 1987;42:49.
9. Naylor AM, Ruwe WD, Veale WL. Antipyretic action of centrally administered arginine vasopressin but not oxytocin in the cat. Brain Res. 1986;385:156.
10. Lipton JM, Clark WG. Neurotransmitters in temperature control. Annu Rev Physiol. 1986;48:613.
11. Coceani F, Lees J, Bishai I. Further evidence implicating prostaglandin E_2 in the genesis of pyrogen fever. Am J Physiol. 254:R463, 1988;254:463.
12. Dejana E, Breviario F, Erroi A, et al. Modulation of endothelial cell function by different molecular species of interleukin-1. Blood. 1987;69:695–9.
13. Duff GW, Durum SK. Fever and immunoregulation: Hyperthermia, interleukin-1 and 2, and T-cell proliferation. Yale J Biol Med. 1982;55:437.
14. Hanson DF, Murphy PA, Silicano R, et al. The effect of temperature on the activation of thymocytes by interleukin-1 and interleukin-2. J Immunol. 1983;130:216.
15. Flower R, Vane JR. Inhibition of prostaglandin synthetase in brain explains the anti-pyretic activity of paracetamol. Nature. 1972;240:410.
16. Peterson RG. Consequences associated with nonnarcotic analgesics in the fetus and newborn. Fed Proc. 1985;44:2309.
17. Harvison PJ, Egan RW, Gale PH, et al. Acetaminophen and analogs as co-substrates and inhibitors of prostaglandin H synthetase. Chem Biol Interact. 1988;64:251.
18. Cannon JG, Van der Meer JWM, Kwiatkowski D, et al. Interleukin-1β in human plasma: Optimization of blood collection, plasma extraction and radioimmunoassay. Lymphokine Res. 1988;7:457–67.
19. Michie HR, Manogue KR, Spriggs DR, et al. Detection of circulating tumor necrosis factor after endotoxin administration. N Engl J Med. 1988;318:1481–6.
20. Eastgate JA, Symons JA, Wood NC, et al. Correlation of plasma interleukin-1 levels with disease activity in rheumatoid arthritis. Lancet. 1988;2:706.
21. Cannon JG, Dinarello CA. Increased plasma interleukin-1 activity in women after ovulation. Science. 1985;227:1247–49.
22. Gauldie J, Richards C, Harnish D, et al. Interferon beta-2/B-cell stimulating factor type 2 shares identity with monocyte-derived hepatocyte stimulating factor and regulates the major acute phase protein response in liver cells. Proc Natl Acad Sci USA. 1987;84:7251.
23. Dinarello CA. The biology of interleukin-1. FASEB J. 1988;2:108.
24. Ramadori G, Sipe JD, Dinarello CA, et al. Pretranslational modulation of acute phase hepatic protein synthesis by murine recombinant interleukin-1 and purified human IL-1. J Exp Med. 1985;162:930–42.
25. Perlmutter DH, Dinarello CA, Punsal PI, et al. Cachectin/tumor necrosis factor regulates hepatic acute-phase gene expression. J Clin Invest. 1986;78:1349–54.
26. Pepys MB, Baltz ML. Acute phase proteins with special reference to C-reactive protein and related proteins (pentaxins) and serum amyloid A protein. In: Dixon FJ, Kunkel HG, eds. Advances in Immunology. v. 34. New York: Academic Press; 1983:141–211.
27. Beisel WR. Magnitude of the host nutritional responses to infection. Am J Clin Nutr. 1977;30:1236–47.

40. FEVER OF UNKNOWN ORIGIN

CHARLES A. DINARELLO
SHELDON M. WOLFF

Fever is such a common manifestation of illness that it is not surprising to find accurate descriptions of the febrile patient in early recorded history. There is evidence that the symbol of a flaming brazier was used by the ancient Sumerians to denote fever and that cuneiform inscriptions of the sixth century BC had adapted this symbol into a single ideogram for fever and inflammation.[1] By the time of Hippocrates and later during the Roman Empire, physicians were so well acquainted with the signs and symptoms of febrile diseases that their detailed descriptions of typhoid and malarial fevers can still be used as examples of these protracted fevers. However, only some fevers of prolonged nature can be diagnosed from descriptive histories, and most patients with long-standing fevers require a careful and thorough investigation. Today, the physician charged with the problem of determining the cause of a prolonged fever must consider the spectrum of febrile diseases, which, through the years, has changed under the influence of nutritional, hygienic, and environmental effects. In addition, age, geographic location, and iatrogenic involvement are also important factors that play a role in determining the cause of prolonged fever.

In most patients with fever lasting 1 or 2 weeks, the underlying cause is soon discovered or the patient recovers spontaneously. In the latter case, a protracted viral illness is usually presumed to be the source of the fever. In other patients, however, fever continues for 2 or 3 weeks during which time physical examination, chest x-ray films, blood tests, and routine cultures do not reveal the cause of fever. In these patients a provisional diagnosis of fever of unknown origin (FUO) is made. Some physicians, for the purpose of retrospective studies, have set strict criteria for undiagnosed, febrile illness to be classified as a FUO. In general, a patient may be considered to have a FUO if a cause of the fever cannot be found after 2 to 3 weeks despite thorough physical examination and related laboratory tests. Although a provisional diagnosis of FUO is made after 2 weeks of fever, many patients with FUO have fever for months and some more than a year. In the latter situation, the fever is often present for varying periods of time, disappears, and returns again.

In some studies, FUO has been defined as a daily elevation in oral temperature of 100.2°F (38°C) or higher for 3 weeks without an identified cause. Since the daily rhythm in core temperature varies from individual to individual, we believe that an FUO is best defined when considering the normal temperature rhythm for the patient and the presence of an associated pathologic change. Chronic fatigue syndrome, previously called chronic Epstein-Barr infection, has attracted considerable attention recently; one of the major clinical complaints of this syndrome is recurrent "feverish feelings."[2] Most patients are afebrile, and even those with fever have temperatures generally below 101°F.

There are no shortcuts in determining the cause of a FUO. Only a well-organized systematic approach that is carried out with an awareness of the multiple causes of fever shortens the duration of the investigation. In this regard, reports on patients with FUOs have been helpful, since they call attention to both the varied causes and incidence of long-standing fevers. From these studies several general conclusions can be made. It is best to divide patients into three age groups: under 6 years; 6–14 years; and over 14 years. Patients under 6 years of age have a high incidence of infection, primarily upper respiratory or urinary tract and systemic-viral, while collagen–vascular diseases and inflammatory bowel disease are the most prevalent causes in the 6–to 16-year age group (Table 1). Rheumatic fever as a cause of FUO in American children has decreased in the last 2 decades, although recent reports suggest that the incidence of rheumatic fever in the USA may be rising again. On the other hand, the incidence of tuberculosis as a cause of FUO in children has dropped less sharply.

In adults, infections are also the most common cause of FUO. Using studies made in the antibiotic era only, Table 2 indicates that infection predominates as the most frequently diagnosed source of persistent fever. However, it can be generally stated that as the duration of fever increases, the likelihood of an infectious cause decreases. This statement has been substantiated by studies of patients with FUOs lasting for longer than 1 year in which infections were the third most common cause of the FUO.[12] Following infections, malignancies compose the next most frequent source of FUO in adults. Recent studies on large groups of patients with FUOs have been reported.[13–16] In general, infectious causes of FUO are still as common, but malignancies are increasingly identified as the cause of FUOs. This is not the case, however, in children. Nevertheless, in both adults and children with neoplastic disease as a source of fever, lymphomas and leukemias are the most prevalent. The third most common diagnosis in adult patients with FUO is collagen–vascular disease. The actual incidence of collagen–vascular disease in patients with FUO is possibly higher than is shown in Table 2, since some studies limit this diagnosis to systemic lupus erythematosus, rheumatoid arthritis, and systemic vasculitis. It may be better to classify these diseases as autoimmune rather than collagen–vascular. It is useful then to consider the three major causes of FUO, i.e., infection, malignancy, and autoimmune disease, since more than 70 percent of patients fall into one of these three groups. However, there are many diseases that have been grouped in studies as "miscellaneous," and in adults these include drug fever,[17] erythema multiforme, granulomatous hepatitis, regional enteritis, pulmonary embolism, sarcoidosis, familial Mediterranean fever, Fabry's disease, hypertriglyceridemia, alcoholic hepatitis, and factitious fever.[18–20] In children, miscellaneous causes of FUO have been milk allergy, Behçet syndrome, and heavy metal intoxication. Although fever can be the presenting sign of the initial infection with human immunodeficiency virus (HIV), most FUOs in these patients are due to other infectious agents. Because of the high incidence of unusual infections in HIV-infected patients, any patient from a high-risk group seeking medical attention for an FUO requires a test for the presence of HIV antibodies.

Other important factors in determining the causes of FUO are the type of institution in which the patient is evaluated. A tertiary care facility may see more unusual illness because of the nature of their referral patterns. Inner city hospitals may have much higher incidence of infectious disease since patients may lack proper evaluation or therapy before being seen in the hospital. In the same type of hospital, adult patients may be older and thus more likely to have a malignant neoplasm as a cause of their FUO. Thus, other factors such as economics, race, geography, and so forth may determine the distribution of diagnoses in a given report.

In patients in whom fever persists for longer than 6 months without an identifiable source, the spectrum of diagnoses is different. In these patients a high incidence of granulomatous disease has been seen as well as the adult manifestation of Still's disease.[21] The diagnoses in these patients are shown in Table 3. In all studies, there is a group of patients in whom diagnosis cannot be made after years of fever, and the diagnosis remains FUO. A few of these patients may have abnormal hypothalamic thermoregulation, but in most patients this diagnosis remains speculative. Factitious fevers are consistently reported in studies on FUO, and these include adults and children. Also in-

TABLE 1. Fever of Unknown Origin in Children

References	Dates of Study	No. of Cases	Established Causes (%) Infections	Collagen–Vascular Disease	Neoplasms	Miscellaneous	Undiagnosed
McClung[3]	1959–69	99	29	11	8	19	32
Pizzo, Lovejoy, and Smith[4]	1966–72	100	52	20	6	10	12
Lohr and Hendley[5]	1967–74	54	33	18	13	15	19

TABLE 2. Fever of Unknown Origin in Adults

References	Dates of Study	No. of Cases	Established Causes (%) Infections	Collagen–Vascular Disease	Neoplasms	Miscellaneous	Undiagnosed
Petersdorf and Beeson[6]	1952–57	100	36	13	19	25	7
Sheon and Van Ommen[7]	1959–60	60	21	13	6	20	40
Deal[8]	1970	34	35	15	20	9	20
Frayha and Uwaydah[9]	1967–70	49	43	14	27	6	10
Howard, Hahn, Palmer, and Hardin[10]	1969–76	100	37	19	31	8	5
Larson, Featherstone, and Petersdorf[11]	1970–80	105	30	16	31	10	12

TABLE 3. Prolonged Fever of Unknown Origin[a]

	Percentage of Cases
No fever[b]	27
FUO	19
Miscellaneous	13
Factitious	9
Granulomatous hepatitis	8
Neoplasm	7
Still's disease	6
Infections	6
Colagen–vascular disease	4
Familial Mediterranean fever	3

[a] Evaluation of 347 patients studied from 1961 to 1977 at the National Institutes of Health.[2] Fever was present for more than 1 year in 75 percent of the cases (mean = 4 years).[3]
[b] Includes patients with exaggerated circadian temperature rhythm.

cluded in the diagnosis of a factitious fever are patients who inject themselves with contaminated materials.[22]

Searching for the underlying cause of prolonged fever requires an open mind and a carefully organized approach by the physician. Since most patients who receive a provisional diagnosis of FUO have no obvious source of fever, we recommend an investigation that includes certain clinical tests that can be considered "routine" for these patients. The work-up may be divided into the following categories: (*1*) observation of temperature pattern, (*2*) historical aspects, (*3*) physical examinations, (*4*) laboratory tests, (*5*) noninvasive procedures, and (*6*) invasive procedures.

TEMPERATURE PATTERN

It is important to establish that the patient with a presumptive diagnosis of FUO is, in fact, having fever. There are a few patients who seek medical assistance with a chief complaint of persistent fever and, on closer investigation, do not have fever but rather an exaggerated circadian temperature rhythm. This conclusion can be reached by measuring the daily temperature at approximately 6 AM and 6 PM.[23] In the absence of associated symptoms like sweating, chills, and elevated pulse rate and in the absence of abnormal laboratory, radiologic, or physical findings, these patients can be considered to be normal. In a large series of patients referred to us at the National Institutes of Health with a presumptive diagnosis of FUO for longer than 6 months, 27 percent failed to manifest evidence of ongoing disease during the 2–3 weeks of inpatient observation.[12] In fact, many patients with so-called benign fever of unknown origin probably belong in this category.[24] It is not uncommon for children of overly concerned parents or from troubled families to seek medical work-up for nonexistent fever that they consider "low grade."

Fever patterns have been classified as continuous, remittent, and intermittent; however, observation and characterization of fever patterns have little or no significance in the diagnosis of prolonged fevers. There are two notable exceptions: malaria and cyclic neutropenia. To a lesser extent the fever associated with Hodgkin's disease (Pel-Ebstein) may be helpful in making this diagnosis. The well-synchronized malarial paroxysm can be used to help to make a diagnosis of malaria, although demonstration of the malarial parasite in blood smears is required for diagnostic confirmation. In nonendemic areas, well-synchronized malarial fevers are rarely seen, and this diagnosis is usually suspected on learning of recent travel to malaria-infested areas.[25] Patients with tertian malaria (fever every other day) and quartan malaria (fever on day 1 and day 4 and so forth) can have low-grade fever in between the paroxyms, and most new malarial infections take 1–2 weeks before the paroxyms are synchronized.

The other fever pattern that is most suggestive of a specific diagnosis consists of a 21-day cycle. This fever accompanies cyclic neutropenia in which the peripheral neutrophil count falls to very low levels every 21 days.[26] It is common for these patients to have concurrent ulcers of the mucous membranes.

Other fevers that have been previously considered to be periodic are those of familial Mediterranean fever and Hodgkin's disease. Although such fevers can occur at regular intervals, patients with these diseases do not have a strict periodicity to their fevers like those of malaria or cyclic neutropenia but rather periods of no fevers or irregular fevers.

HISTORICAL ASPECTS

Clues to the diagnosis of certain febrile diseases may be obtained from historical characteristics and symptoms; examples include transient skin rashes in patients with autoimmune and collagen–vascular disease, the injection of medications in patients with drug fever, and hematuria in patients with renal cell carcinoma. Since patients with FUO often have atypical manifestations of their diseases, many symptoms are present only transiently and are not easily recalled during routine questioning. History of other symptoms such as myalgias, malaise, rigors, sweating, and weight loss may be nonspecific in that they are characteristic of elevated body temperature due to a diversity of causes.

Travel and exposure to certain agents or animals is critical information needed to make a diagnosis of several febrile diseases. For example, in the period from 1970 to 1975 there was a threefold increase in the number of civilian cases of malaria imported into the United States.[25] Clearly, knowledge of travel to regions where malaria is indigenous can be key in suspecting this disease. Knowledge of tick bites is often absent in some cases of tick-transmitted diseases, but awareness of the endemic tick-infested areas is valuable even when the patient denies a tick bite. Certain parts of the United States are endemic areas for *Coccidioides, Histoplasma,* and *Blastomyces,* and the diagnosis of disease due to these organisms can be aided by a history of travel to such areas. Occupational hazards are important aspects of an accurate history. For example, exposure to beryllium can lead to a febrile illness, and knowledge of such exposure should expedite the diagnostic work-up of patients with berylliosis.

PHYSICAL EXAMINATION

There is no substitute for a complete physical examination in evaluating a patient with FUO. Furthermore, these patients require repeated physical examinations on a regular basis during investigation into their disease. Such patients may develop skin lesions, fundoscopic changes, organomegaly, and masses late in the course of their disease. All too often patients receive a thorough physical examination at the time of initial medical evaluation for persistent fever, and subsequently the caring physician focuses on laboratory and other diagnostic procedures, never returning to the bedside to repeat the entire physical examination. There are some areas in particular that require almost daily inspection, and these include examination of the skin, eyes, nail beds, lymph nodes, and abdomen, and auscultation of the heart. The rashes of Still's disease are usually faint and fade quickly, the skin lesions of patients with systemic vasculidites who have an FUO may appear late in the disease and in very few numbers. Atypical areas, for example under the scrotal and breast folds, must be inspected for a complete examination of the skin. To make a diagnosis of vasculitis, the involved skin lesion must be located and a biopsy must be done.

Regular inspection of the peripheral lymph nodes is necessary. Many febrile diseases involving the lymph nodes that manifest as FUO may involve only a single node. Illnesses such as Hodgkin's disease, toxoplasmosis, or infectious mononucleosis can manifest atypically with a single node enlargement.[27] Draining lymph nodes of the head and neck, breast, and pelvic regions can be involved in neoplastic and infectious processes in these areas.

The importance of a complete eye examination in patients with FUO cannot be overstated. Because many FUOs manifest with no apparent localizing symptoms and because the eye is often involved in systemic disease, proper examination of the eye is indicated in every patient with prolonged fevers even in the absence of ophthalmalogic symptoms. Examination of the eye can be divided into the orbit, cornea, conjunctiva, uveal tract, and retina. Proptosis due to orbital involvement can be seen in isolated lymphomas of the orbit, retrorbital granulomatous disease such as Wegener's granulomatosis, neurofibromas, and metastatic disease to the orbit.

Band keratopathy can be seen in children with Still's disease and sarcoidosis. Punctate epithelial loss associated with tear deficiency and dry eyes is a striking finding of rheumatoid arthritis and can be an initial sign of lupus erythematosus and other collagen–vascular diseases. Marginal ulceration of the cornea can be observed in arteritides as an early manifestation of these diseases.[28]

Conjunctival lesions can be present in several systemic infections, especially viral and chlamydial infections.[29] Frank conjunctivitis can accompany tuberculosis, syphilis, tularemia, fungal infections (particularly histoplasmosis), cat-scratch fever, erythema multiforme, and erythema nodosum. Petechial hemorrhages associated with bacterial endocarditis are often observed in conjunctival as well as in retinal vessels.

The uveal tract is often involved in granulomatous as well as nongranulomatous diseases. The latter include lupus erythematosus, vasculidites, serum sickness, and other hypersensitivity diseases. Sarcoidosis, toxoplasmosis, syphilis, tuberculosis, and Still's disease can result in significant uveitis. Thus, a slit-lamp examination is desirable in the evaluation of a patient with FUO, even in the absence of ocular complaints. Ophthalmoscopy will reveal diseases that involve the optic nerve, retinal vessels, and choroidal tissues. Many systemic febrile diseases can have retinal as well as uveal manifestations.

LABORATORY TESTS

Cultures, antibody titers, complete blood counts, urine analyses, and direct examination of blood and other body fluids are mandatory procedures used in the evaluation of unexplained fevers. Most patients who are given a presumptive diagnosis of FUO have already had some or many laboratory investigations without revealing a specific cause. Some tests need to be repeated at regular intervals during a work-up of a patient with FUO, and these include serum samples for rising antibody titers and, most importantly, repeated cultures of blood and other body fluids for infectious agents. It should be emphasized that in both adults and children, the most often encountered cause of unexplained fever is infection. The importance of multiple blood cultures (e.g., up to six over a period of time) cannot be overstressed in uncovering many infections, especially endocarditis and osteomyelitis. The failure in diagnosing these and other infections sometimes lies with insufficient numbers of blood cultures and to a lesser extent in the inadequacy of cultures taken during concurrent antibiotic therapy. Polymicrobial sepsis often indicates self-induced infection.[22] Multiple urine cultures are also necessary, particularly in the absence of urinary tract symptoms and pyuria. In children, although urine cultures may be difficult to obtain, these are important. Silent urinary tract infections are common in the pediatric age group. In smaller children, direct bladder needle aspiration should be considered if routine procedures fail to yield adequate samples. Urine cultures are also important for the diagnosis of tuberculosis in children and adults. Other body fluids and tissues that may require multiple cultures include sputum, CSF, stool, and bone marrow. Morning gastric contents can also be cultured for mycobacteria. It is critical to culture tissues such as liver or lymph nodes that are removed during biopsy. Sputa, CSF, bone marrow, liver, and lymph nodes are cultured for aerobic and anaerobic bacteria, mycobacteria, and fungi. Viral cultures and inoculation of material into embryonated chick eggs, mice, and guinea pigs should also be considered. It is sometimes easier to isolate and to identify some infectious agents using animal and yolk sac inoculation. The recognition of the cause of the legionnaires' disease outbreak of 1976 illustrates an example of the usefulness of such procedures.[30]

Direct examination of the blood is necessary to confirm a diagnosis of malaria, trypanosomiasis, and relapsing fever. Thick and thin smears of blood stained with Giemsa or Wright stain require careful examination, particularly in light infections. Demonstration of *Borrelia* may require multiple smears. Wet mounts using phase contrast microscopy are also useful in the detection of spirochetes. Direct examination of spinal fluid sediment with India ink remains a fast and reliable method for detecting cryptococci. In the latter infection, large amounts of spinal fluid and repeated cultures are sometimes needed to make a diagnosis. Direct examination of stool samples is still the preferred method for demonstrating several parasitic infections. Although schistosomiasis and amebic abscess of the liver can both manifest as FUO, the diagnosis is much more likely to be made by means other than stool examination.

Rising antibody titers can be diagnostic in many infectious diseases, and it behooves the clinician who is working up a patient for FUO to obtain serum samples from the patient at regular intervals. It is advisable to freeze and to retain a portion of each sample in the event it is necessary to demonstrate a rising antibody titer to an agent isolated or suspected subsequently. Lyme disease is a good example, although some patients with Lyme disease fail to manifest antibodies to the spirochete. This is particularly true of viral and other infectious agents that are difficult to culture on artificial media.

Each antibody determination has its limitations as to specificity in that there are sometimes more false-positive than false-negative results. In addition, some antibody titers may reveal a recent infection with an organism that is not responsible for the prolonged fever. Newer and more specific immunologic methods are constantly being developed, and it is the responsibility of the physician to be aware of these while considering which immunologic test is most specific in uncovering the underlying cause of an FUO.

Patients with FUO often have elevated serum levels of "acute-phase reactants." These may include fibrinogen, haptoglobin, ceruloplasmin, C-reactive protein, and other α_2-globulins. These are part of the nonspecific changes often measurable and elevated with fever. Other nonspecific changes that accompany fever that are frequently found in patients with FUO include elevations in the erythrocyte sedimentation rate, increased ability of neutrophils to reduce nitroblue tetrazolium, low serum iron and zinc concentrations, and an increased peripheral neutrophil count. To what degree these determinations are useful in working up a patient with FUO depends on the characteristics of certain disease processes. In general, they are nonspecific and are of little value (see chapter 39). However, the erythrocyte sedimentation rate, for example, is usually markedly high in patients with temporal arteritis and Still's disease. It must be pointed out, however, that certain acute changes may be absent in some patients with FUO, and that these changes are by themselves not indicative of a specific diagnosis. Levels of etiocholanolone do not correlate with fever, and this substance plays no role in causing fever.[31]

NONINVASIVE PROCEDURES

The technical advances in diagnostic radiology, radionuclide scanning, and other methods have reduced the need for invasive procedures in evaluating a patient with FUO. These include plain film contrast studies, tomography, selective cinearteriography, radionuclide scans, computerized tomographic scanning, ultrasonography, and magnetic resonance imaging. There are advantages to using each procedure depending on the pathologic process. Some radiologic procedures should be considered "routine" in working up patients with FUO and include chest x-ray films, upper gastrointestinal contrast study with small-bowel follow-through, and barium enema. Chest x-ray films should be repeated periodically, and any radiologic study should be repeated if symptoms arise pertaining to a specific area. There are a large number of pulmonary diseases that cause prolonged fever and, in rare patients, show no demonstrable involvement on chest x-ray films; for example, in sarcoidosis, mycoses, tuberculosis, many of the pneumoconioses, and infiltrative lung disease, chest x-ray films may be normal in the presence of biopsy-proven disease.[32]

Radionuclide scanning procedures using technetium (Tc) 99m sulfur colloid, gallium (Ga) citrate or indium-III are available for the evaluation of many infectious, inflammatory, or neoplastic processes. Success in localizing a process using these radiopharmaceuticals depends on the pathogenic process. ^{67}Ga was initially used to detect bone tumors, but it now has been shown that the radionuclide concentrates in many neoplastic and inflammatory tissues. The mechanism by which ^{67}Ga localizes in inflammatory tissue is thought to be related to the presence of sequestered leukocytes.[33] Whole body gallium citrate (^{67}Ga) scans are often used as a screening procedure in patients with FUO and can localize abscesses, lymphomas, and infectious and other neoplastic processes.[34] However, there are known false-positive and false-negative results with this procedure. Technetium 99m sulfur colloid is also used in scanning and seems to be especially useful in the early diagnosis of osteomyelitis. Radiographic abnormalities develop late in this disease, and scanning techniques are able to localize the disease early, probably because of increased blood flow. To reduce false-positive results, it is advisable to use radionuclide scanning techniques in combination with computed tomography and ultrasonography.[35] Recently, it was reported that indium-111 granulocyte scintigraphy in FUO patients might be useful in diagnosing those with infections.[36]

Computed tomography (CT) scanning is one of the more important noninvasive diagnostic methods available in evaluation of patients with FUO. It appears that CT scanning of the head can detect intracranial lesions early and is superior to angiography for demonstrating cerebral abscesses. CT scanning is also useful in detecting epidural abscesses, retrobulbar masses, and diseases involving the sinus and nasopharynx.[37] Although intracranial tumors, hemorrhages, and hydrocephalus are not common causes of FUO, the usefulness of CT scanning for localizing these processes in the hypothalamus and, in particular, for hypothalamic tumors, has been documented.[38] The efficacy of whole body CT scanning in working up a patient with FUO depends on the extent and location of the disease.[39] For example, CT scanning is effective in delineating intra-abdominal abscesses and retroperitoneal, retrosternal, and mesenteric lymph nodes that may be the causes of FUO. The procedure can also detect defects in the spleen, liver, kidney, adrenals, pancreas, heart, mediastinum, and pelvis, but radionuclide scanning and ultrasonography are also efficacious in demonstrating disease in these organs and regions. For some patients, more than one noninvasive method may be necessary to demonstrate and to confirm abnormalities. Greater use of CT scanning has reduced the need for invasive procedures.[40]

Ultrasonography has been helpful in demonstrating the presence of cardiac abnormalities that may be a cause of fever. Echocardiography can detect valvular vegetations[41] and atrial tumors; it should be included as a "screening" procedure in patients with FUO. Ultrasonography is particularly useful in diagnosing abnormalities in the pancreas, gallbladder, liver, spleen, pelvis, and abdomen.[42–44]

Lymphangiography is a well-established method for demonstrating retroperitoneal, iliac, and periaortic lymph nodes. The involvement of these nodes in patients with lymphomas and Hodgkin's disease that manifest as FUO has been noted in several studies. With the advent of CT scanning, lymphangiography is infrequently used.

SKIN TESTING

With a few exceptions, such as the purified protein derivative (PPD) test for tuberculosis, most skin tests are of limited value in the diagnosis of FUO. Nevertheless, it is important to test for reactivity to tuberculin in patients with FUO. It is necessary at the same time to test for reactivity to other antigens such as mumps, streptodornasestreptokinase, or *Candida*. The lack of sensitivity to these latter antigens often suggests diseases like miliary tuberculosis or Hodgkin's disease. However, patients with FUO, particularly debilitated patients, may have depressed immunologic reactions secondary to nutritional factors.

INVASIVE PROCEDURES

Biopsy of liver and bone marrow should be considered routine in the work-up of FUO if the studies mentioned above are unrevealing. Other biopsy sites may include skin, pleura, lymph nodes, kidney, muscle, nerve, intestine or any tissue that may be involved either on physical examination, scans, or radiographs. Bronchoscopy, peritonoscopy, and other endoscopies are used for both inspection and obtaining tissues and fluids. Proper disposition of the biopsy material requires an organized plan to divide the tissue for maximal information. This is particularly true with needle biopsy material. Bacterial, viral, fungal, and mycobacterial cultures must be done on appropriate tissue. Reports of unusual organisms cultured from the biopsy material of many patients with FUO underscore the importance of this procedure. There is no substitute for a positive culture in uncovering the cause of fever. Microscopic examination also requires advanced organization. Proper staining may be critical to identification of organisms in tissues as well as in certain tissue and intracellular deposits. For example, formalin-fixed tissue should be stained with Brown–Brenn or Brown–Hopps for bacteria, Ziehl–Neelsen for mycobacteria, methenamine silver and periodic acid–Schiff for fungi, and the Dieterle silver-impregnation method for other bacteria and organisms. If possible, a section of the tissue block should always be retained for further sections or stains. Frozen sections can also be used for immunologic procedures. Using anti-IgG, anti-IgM, other anti-immunologlobin and anticomplement sera coupled to fluorescein dyes, these proteins can be identified in certain tissues of patients with autoimmune and collagen–vascular diseases.

With the increasing specificity and safety of noninvasive diagnostic methods, the need for diagnostic laparotomy in patients with FUO has markedly decreased. A diagnostic laparotomy may be indicated in patients with FUO and abdominal pain when the approaches outlined above have failed.[45] Percutaneous liver biopsy is a highly valuable procedure and should be performed on all patients with prolonged FUO.[18,46] Liver biopsy provides tissues for microscopic and microbiologic studies and is safe for most patients. A normal finding on liver biopsy is also helpful in that it is reassuring in those cases in which no diagnosis can be made.[46]

CAUSES OF FEVER OF UNKNOWN ORIGIN

Bacterial Infections

Any bacterial infection can be the source of prolonged fever, especially those that produce little or no obvious inflammation. In these situations localizing symptoms that would indicate the site of infection are missing.

Abscesses. Abscesses are frequently encountered as causes of FUO, and intra-abdominal sites are the most common. Liver and subphrenic abscesses are often seen in patients who have had previous abdominal surgery or in whom intestinal disease had resulted in a small perforation with intestinal leakage. Abdominal abscesses are potential complications in patients undergoing colonoscopy or sigmoidoscopy. Similarly, abdominal abscesses can occur in women following certain gynecologic procedures such as culdoscopy or curetage. Abscesses also can occur following ruptured ovarian cysts. Dental and brain abscesses are less common than an abdominal site as causes of unexplained fever because localizing symptoms are usually present early in the disease; nevertheless, these should be considered as possible causes of a FUO.

Osteomyelitis. Osteomyelitis is a common cause of FUO since symptoms are often masked or are interpreted as nervous or muscular in origin. For example, patients with osteomyelitis of the vertebral bodies or the leg may have symptoms of nerve root compression. Osteomyelitis of the mandible or maxilla can manifest as headache or toothache. Thus, osteomyelitis of any bone can be a cause of FUO because inflammation and pain may occur later in such patients. In this regard, sinusitis can cause prolonged fever without local symptoms except for mild headache.[47]

Subacute Bacterial Endocarditis. Another bacterial source for an FUO in which there may be no localizing symptoms is subacute bacterial endocarditis. This disease is sometimes a cause of FUO because it may not be diagnosed early due to either insufficient or negative blood cultures or to the absence of characteristic physical findings. There have been reports of culture–negative bacterial endocarditis in the past, but modern bacteriologic techniques appear to have reduced this number substantially. Drug addicts and the occasional user of intravenous contaminated materials are at increased risk of developing tricuspid valve infections, which are sometimes abacteremic. Another cause of negative blood cultures in bacterial endocarditis is concomitant antimicrobial therapy, since small doses of antibiotics can render blood cultures negative. For this reason, blood cultures should be repeated several days following cessation of antibiotics. The presence of bacterial endocarditis in the absence of an audible murmur is rare, but some murmurs, particularly in very young and elderly patients, are mistaken as physiologic. In these circumstances, bacterial endocarditis is not considered as a cause of fever, and hence these patients are given a diagnosis of FUO.

Biliary System Infections. Bacterial infections of the biliary system include ascending cholangitis, cholecystitis, frank empyema of the gallbladder, and infection of the pancreatic duct. The organisms gain entrance from the duodenum, and in the majority of cases there is a pre-existing disease like pancreatitis or cholelithiasis. However, patients with bacterial infections of the biliary system who have been diagnosed as having FUO have little or no right upper quandrant discomfort that would indicate the site of infection. Patients with suppurative biliary tract infection had no localizing physical findings or tenderness before laparotomy.[6,48,49] Furthermore, in these patients liver function tests had been normal and hence the diagnosis had been made primarily at laparotomy. Newer methods such as computerized scanning and sonography have lessened the need for such operations in these patients.

Urinary Tract Infections. Urinary tract infections due to bacteria are infrequently encountered as causes of FUO because positive urine cultures make this diagnosis early in a febrile illness. Thus, patients with urinary tract infections that manifest as FUO have negative or intermittently positive urine cultures. Perinephric abscesses may spill bacteria into the urine inconsistently, and some urinary tract infections have such a low titer of bacteria (1000–5000 organisms/ml) that the culture results do not suggest the urinary tract as a source of the fever. In children, particularly in girls with bladder reflux and in boys with posterior urethral valves, urinary tract infections are common causes of FUO. Obtaining urine for culture in small children is difficult, and contaminating organisms are often misleading. Bladder aspiration is indicated in such children with bacteriuria to rule out urinary tract infection as a cause of FUO. When urinary tract infections are a cause of prolonged fever, there usually is absence of symptoms like dysuria, frequency, or lower back pain.

Tuberculosis. *Mycobacterium tuberculosis* is perhaps the single most often cultured organism as a cause of FUO. Although its incidence in producing disease has been markedly reduced, *M. tuberculosis,* nevertheless, continues as a cause of prolonged, unexplained fevers. This is particularly true in patients with certain immunologic deficiency states as well as in those patients with acquired increased susceptibility to infection due to immunosuppressive therapy. There are some patients in whom fever is the only symptom and whose chest x-ray films appear normal. Extrapulmonary tuberculosis is probably the most common manifestation of this infection as a FUO.[50] Miliary tuberculosis including tuberculosis of the spleen, liver, bone, kidney, meninges, peritoneum, and pericardium have all been reported as causes of prolonged fever. Even in cases of overwhelming miliary tuberculosis, the lung fields and other organ sites do not always show signs of involvement until weeks following the onset of fever,[51] and hence diagnosis may be delayed. In addition, the diagnosis of tuberculosis as a cause of fever may not be apparent, since cultures may not become positive before 4–6 weeks. Furthermore, a negative skin test may be due to disseminated disease, and when such is the case, the clinician is often misled by the absence of a positive reaction. Although atypical mycobacteria cause disease, they usually do not manifest as FUO.

Miscellaneous Infections. Intestinal bacterial infections rarely manifest as prolonged fever in the absence of other symptoms. The notable exception to this is salmonellosis, in which fever may be the only abnormality. The causative agent in Whipple's disease (intestinal lipodystrophy) is thought to be bacterial in nature, and this disease has been encountered as a cause of prolonged fever.[48,52] The vast majority of bacterial infections causing prolonged, unexplained fever are confined to specific sites, that is, abscess in organs or infection in certain spaces. There are also a few bacterial infections that may cause prolonged fevers and in which the causative organism is disseminated, residing primarily in the reticuloendothelial and lymphatic systems. These include brucellosis, bartonellosis, and listeriosis. Of these diseases, brucellosis is clearly most frequently encountered as an FUO. Diagnosis rests, as in all bacterial infections, on positive bacterial cultures as well as on the presence of increasing serum antibody titers.

Spirochetal Infections

Relapsing fever. Of the three medically important genera of spirochetes, *Treponema, Leptospira,* and *Borrelia,* only the last is often associated with prolonged fever and is sometimes called "relapsing fever" because the fever characteristically occurs in paroxysms separated by afebrile intervals. Although louse-borne relapsing fever due to infections of *Borrelia recurrentis* occurs worldwide, it is most prevalent in times of war or famine; the tick-borne form of this disease caused by *B. pakeri, B. hermsii,* or *B. turicatae* has been reported in the western and southwestern United States and frequently manifests as a FUO.[53,54] Louse-borne relapsing fever usually occurs in epidemics, and diagnosis is made during the initial febrile episodes. However, tick-borne relapsing fever affects campers and hikers in a sporadic fashion, and patients often are given a provisional diagnosis of FUO until careful direct examination of the blood for the presence of spirochetes or culture in chick embryos suggests the etiology of the infection. The patient may be unaware of a recent tick bite, and during the second or third fever relapse the disease may be overlooked as having an infectious etiology. The initial clinical manifestations of louse-borne relapsing fever can be confused with those caused by tick-borne rickettsiae, but subsequent attacks of relapsing fever may manifest with only fever and no localizing signs.

Leptospirosis. Leptospirosis is a spirochetal infection that can manifest as an FUO, although illness is usually acute and self-limited. During the first phases of leptospirosis, the organisms can be cultured from the blood, but during the second and third phases ("immune phases"), organisms may be absent from body fluids and fever may be the only manifestation. In these cases the cause of prolonged fever may be ascertained by serologic tests.[55]

Rat-Bite Fever. *Spirillum minor,* the spirochete that causes rat-bite fever, cannot be cultured on artificial media, but inoculation of the patient's blood into mice confirms a diagnosis in 10 days to 2 weeks. The history of a rat bite should alert the physician to the diagnostic possibility. Rarely, mouse bites have also been shown to cause the disease. Darkfield microscopy of blood may demonstrate the organism; however, in patients with spirochetal infection who appear to have an FUO, the organism may be absent from body fluids, and diagnosis depends on the presence of specific antibody titers.

Rickettsial Infections In the preantibiotic era, it was not uncommon for typhus to be the cause of undiagnosed fevers. Although rickettsial infections are often associated with high fevers that in untreated cases may last up to 20 days, these diseases are rarely encountered as FUOs today. Clinical manifestations such as the cutaneous exanthem and severe headache, which are present in almost all cases,[56] and the specificity of serologic tests alert physicians to the cause of fever early in the disease.

Chlamydial Infections Psittacosis caused by *Chlamydia psittaci* can occur in the absence of cough and respiratory symptoms and with normal chest x-ray findings. In these situations, fever may be the sole symptom of the disease and splenomegaly the only physical finding. Because fever in psittacosis may be prolonged as long as 3 months, psittacosis has been reported as an infectious cause of FUO in several studies. Isolation of the organism may be difficult in these cases, but diagnosis can be made from a rising titer of complement-fixing antibody. Other chlamydial diseases such as trachoma as well as genital tract infections are usually not associated with fever. Lymphogranuloma venereum, although usually diagnosed without difficulty, may manifest as an FUO.

Viral Infections Viruses can cause prolonged fever in some patients. This is particularly true in children, and the spectrum of infectious causes of FUO in young children includes more viral etiologies than in adults. The proof of a viral agent causing prolonged, unexplained fever rests with two criteria: isolation of the agent and immunologic evidence of infection. Problems arise when the patient does not have a typical immunologic response to the agent and when associated signs and symptoms such as skin rashes and lymphadenopathy are missing or have gone unnoticed. This is particularly true of some viral infections in children. Infectious mononucleosis is perhaps the most commonly encountered viral disease producing prolonged fever without appropriate immunologic response. For example, not all patients develop significant titers of heterophile antibody early in the course of the disease. The disease can thus often be diagnosed by the presence of antibody to Epstein-Barr virus-associated antigens. Rarely, the development of both heterophile and Epstein-Barr virus antibodies is delayed several weeks and diagnosis is difficult. Other viral illnesses associated with FUO include hepatitis, cat-scratch fever, and cytomegalovirus infections.

Fungal Diseases

There is little question that the incidence of fungal diseases, particularly deep mycoses, has increased as a result of the use of antibiotics and immunosuppressive therapy. Many fungal diseases, for example, histoplasmosis, blastomycosis, and coccidiomycosis, manifest primarily as pulmonary infections and are detected early in the disease process. Other fungal diseases, notably cryptococcosis and disseminated histoplasmosis, are less easily detected, and fever may be the major manifestation.

Histoplasmosis involving the reticuloendothelial and lymphatic system may manifest as prolonged, unexplained fever. The clinical manifestations of this form of histoplasmosis are not unlike that of disseminated tuberculosis. Cryptococcal meningitis is often undiagnosed for several weeks and may manifest as an FUO. Headaches and behavioral changes usually lead to an examination of the spinal fluid. With increasing use of antibiotics, particularly in patients being treated with immunosuppressive agents, some of the indigenous fungi, for example, *Candida albicans,* have caused disseminated disease and fever.

Parasitic Disease

Malaria. In endemic areas, malaria is seldom a cause of unexplained fever, but in nonendemic areas, this infection has the potential to go undetected. This may be due to several factors, including the failure of travelers to use prophylactic antimalarials properly, resistant forms, nonsynchronized febrile paroxysms, and the physician's unawareness of travel to endemic areas by the patient. In fact, most reports of malaria as a cause of FUO are due to failure to suspect malaria early in the disease. Blood transfusion as a cause of malarial transmission occurs rarely but increases during periods of war in malarious areas.

Toxoplasmosis. Toxoplasmosis can manifest as FUO and is often discovered in patients with lymph node enlargement during lymph node biopsy. A few patients have minimal lymph node swelling and may have fever as the predominant symptom. Rising antibody titers can detect the disease when it is suspected.

Trypanosomiasis. Trypanosomiasis due to *Trypanosoma rhodesiense* is carried by the tsetse fly vector in East and Central Africa, and visitors to these areas, even for periods as brief as an overnight flight stop, can contract the disease. The disease is rather acute, accompanied by prominent erythematous rash, central nervous system alterations, and high fever. Trypanosomes can be detected in routine blood smears during the disease. *Trypanosoma gambiense* is found in West and Central Africa and produces a more subtle form of onset. Fever begins irregularly and is accompanied by an evanescent rash, splenomegaly, and lymphadenopathy. The disease is less acute than that caused by *T. rhodesiense* and may be present for months as an FUO before blood smears are examined. Visitors to Africa or natives arriving in the United States from endemic areas can have delayed onset of disease.

Other Parasitic Diseases. Leishmaniasis, trichinosis, and amebic liver abscess are parasitic diseases that can have prominent febrile manifestations and, because of their relative infrequency in the United States, may be missed as a cause of unexplained fever.

NEOPLASTIC DISEASES

Unexplained fever is a common manifestation of many malignancies (Table 4). All solid tumors have the potential to cause obstruction and subsequent infection; hence, malignancy and fever may coexist. In these situations, the neoplastic process indirectly causes the fever. However, even in the absence of infection, certain neoplasms are particularly associated with fever, and when these are treated the fever may disappear. In these cases, the neoplasm is thought to be a direct source of the fever.

The mechanism by which a neoplastic process causes fever may be related to its ability either to produce endogenous pyrogens itself or to induce the production of endogenous pyrogens from normal leukocytes. Tissue obtained from patients with Hodgkin's disease, histiocytic lymphomas, and renal cell carcinoma liberate endogenous pyrogens spontaneously in vitro,[57–60] and it is likely that the same process takes place in vivo. In addition to some tumors producing their own endogenous pyrogens, others undergo necrosis as a result of rapid growth, and necrotic debris induces the infiltration of leukocytes in the inflammatory response.[61] Endogenous pyrogens can be the products of inflammatory leukocytes and may be produced in association with tumor necrosis.

TABLE 4. Malignancies Commonly Manifesting as FUO

Hodgkin's disease
Non-Hodgkin's lymphoma
Leukemia (including aleukemia and preleukemia)
Renal cell carcinoma
Hepatoma
Atrial myxomas

Certain neoplasms have a high incidence of manifestation as FUO, and some patients with these malignancies seek medical attention primarily because of recurrent fevers. These neoplasms include lymphoma and other reticuloses, renal cell carcinoma, atrial myxoma, hepatoma, and carcinoma of the intestinal tract. Disseminated carcinomatosis is also a cause of FUO. Nonmalignant neoplasms that are associated with prolonged fever are giant lymph node hyperplasia[62,63] and infantile cortical hyperostosis.[64] It should be pointed out, however, that these benign neoplasms may have an infectious or inflammatory etiology, athough no agent has yet been isolated. Angiomyolipoma is a benign renal tumor that occurs almost exclusively in patients with tuberous sclerosis and can manifest as an FUO.[65]

Lymphomas and Leukemias. Of all the lymphomas, Hodgkin's disease is most commonly associated with recurrent fever, although non-Hodgkin's lymphoma may cause FUO. The likelihood of fever as an initial symptom in Hodgkin's disease increases with the number of lymph nodes involved, and fever is a prominent symptom when disease is present in retroperitoneal nodes. In these latter instances, routine studies to detect a cause of the persistent fever fail, and patients require more specific investigation to uncover the source of fever. Lymphomas that primarily involve the spleen have a high incidence of fever and can manifest along with anorexia, malaise, and weight loss as an FUO.[66] When present, a Pel-Ebstein pattern of fever (3- to 10-day cycles of febrile and afebrile periods) is highly suggestive of Hodgkin's disease.

Acute leukemias may be associated with fever, and sometimes this occurs in the presence of a normal peripheral blood smear, as seen in aleukemic leukemia and preleukemia. In such patients diagnosis is often delayed. Bone marrow aspiration may uncover the aleukemic phase, but in preleukemic forms, fever may persist, and bone marrow aspirates remain nondiagnostic for very long periods.[67] The incidence of fever in the preleukemic form of monocytic leukemia is high and, in general, the number of preleukemias, including myelogenous leukemia, that manifest as FUO varies from 10 to 30 percent in different studies.[67–69]

Renal Cell Carcinoma. Carcinoma of the kidney is often insidious, and many patients do not have hematuria but rather fever as the major symptom.[70] Two large series put the incidence of persistent fever as a manifesting symptom at 11 percent and 12 percent[71] of the cases. There also seems to be a high incidence of a sedimentation rate greater than 100 mm/hr in patients with fever and renal cell carcinoma.[72] In many cases there are no metastases but rather a well-encepsulated neoplasm. Removal of the tumor almost always results in the cessation of fever. Of interest is the fact that investigators have found that the tumor cells synthesize and release endogenous pyrogens spontaneously in vitro, while renal tumor cells taken from patient's who did not have fever did not release endogenous pyrogen.[73]

Tumors of the Liver. There is a greater incidence of metastatic adenocarcinoma to the liver than primary hepatomas, but the latter tumor is often considered as a likely cause of an FUO. Some patients with hepatomas seek medical help because of persistent fever,[74] and several reports of FUO have listed hepatoma as the final diagnosis. Primary or metastatic tumors to the liver that are associated with prolonged fever are not diagnostic problems when accompanied by jaundice or abnormal liver function tests. However, patients with normal liver functions and only fever are admitted to hospitals with the diagnosis of FUO.

Atrial Myxomas. Although myxomas of the atria are very rare neoplasms, they have a high association of fever and manifest as FUO.[75,76] The mechanism of producing fever is not understood but may be related to embolic phenomena or the production of interleukin-6. Murmurs may not be present.

Other Tumors. The list of other tumors that can manifest as FUO is varied. Adenocarcinoma of the large intestine, bronchogenic carcinoma, and adenocarcinoma of the breast particularly when they metastisize can cause a FUO. Children tend to have a different spectrum of neoplasms that manifest as FUO. Acute leukemias are most prevalent in children and can manifest as unexplained fever. Solid tumors in children that may manifest as FUO include neuroblastoma and central nervous system tumors.

Hypersensitivity and Autoimmune Diseases There is a sizable group of diseases that manifest as FUO and that fall into the general categories of hypersensitivity, autoimmune, rheumatic, or collagen–vascular diseases (Table 5). Patients with these diseases may have prolonged, unexplained fever as the prominent symptom of disease, while other clinical manifestations such as cutaneous lesions and joint involvement are either absent or go undetected. Similarly, laboratory tests that would ordinarily alert the physician to the diagnosis are normal. For example, patients with systemic lupus erythematosus (LE) may have fever as a predominant symptom and a negative LE preparation. In several series, 12, 18, and 20 percent of the patients with an unequivocal diagnosis of systemic lupus erythematosus had negative LE preparations.[77,78] Using immunofluorescence, antinuclear antibodies can be found in more than 90 percent of the patients.[78] Fever can be the initial manifestation of the disease in 5 percent of the cases,[78] and such patients are considered to have FUO when they have only fever and no serologic evidence of lupus. Later, additional clinical manifestations may appear such as arthritis, and serologic tests may become positive, which assures a diagnosis of lupus erythematosus.

Patients with various forms of vasculitis can initially have fever as a prominent sign, and cutaneous manifestations may not occur. Biopsy of affected areas, when they appear, confirms the diagnosis. Drug-induced vasculitis is often associated with fever and can manifest as FUO.[79] Drugs that are often associated with hypersensitivity vasculitis include penicillin, sulfonamides, isoniazid, and propylthiouracil, but any drug can cause hypersensitivity vasculitis.

Rheumatoid arthritis can be associated with persistent fever, but in adults, joint involvement usually indicates the proper diagnosis. In children, however, joint involvement may be minimal or absent, and many patients have an FUO. In fact, of all the autoimmune diseases that manifest as FUO in the pediatric age group, juvenile rheumatoid arthritis is undoubtedly the most common.[80,81] Still's disease is the diagnosis given to those children who have primarily systemic manifestations in the absence of arthritis. A complex of high fever, evanescent rash, lymphadenopathy, and splenomegaly with varying degrees of arthralgias and myalgias is typical for Still's disease. Because of its acute onset, it may stimulate other diseases and may pose diagnostic difficulties.

Adults with FUO may also have Still's disease. Onset of the adult form of Still's disease occurs most often between ages 20 and 30, but in some patients onset occurs in childhood and is followed by asymptomatic intervals that may be as long as 10 years. The clinical manifestation in adults is almost identical to that in children. However, adults often have other associated symptoms such as sore throat during febrile episodes.[82] Radiologic evidence of joint changes are often absent in the adult form of Still's disease, and there is no rheumatoid factor present. An elevated white blood cell count with an increase in polymorphonuclear leukocytes and an elevated erythrocyte sedimentation rate are characteristic. The diagnosis of Still's disease as the cause of unexplained fever in adults rests with the presence of its symptom complex in the absence of other diseases.[82,83]

TABLE 5. Hypersensitivity and Autoimmune Diseases Causing FUO

Systemic lupus erythematosus	Polyarteritis nodosa
Still's disease	Erythema multiforme
Polymyalgia rheumatica	Mixed connective tissue disease
Drug fever	Serum sickness
Hypersensitivity vasculitis	Rheumatic fever
Idiopathic vasculitis	

Although rare in the United States, rheumatic fever can manifest as FUO, but in such patients, the classic criteria as established by Jones,[84] are not all present.[15] Although more prevalent in children, acute rheumatic fever in the adult may manifest with less than the full constellation of signs. Rheumatic fever must be differentiated from bacterial endocarditis, rheumatoid arthritis, and systemic lupus erythematosus.

There are also patients in whom a diagnosis of an autoimmune or collagen–vascular disease is almost certain, but its classification is difficult. Although these patients may have fever as the prominent symptom, other symptoms and laboratory data suggest unclassified collagen–vascular disease. Mixed connective tissue disease can manifest as FUO, and in such patients elevated titers of extractable nuclear antigen will confirm the diagnosis. Erythema multiforme with fever may be found in this group of illnesses.

Fever may be the only manifestation of hypersensitivity to drugs, including propriety preparations. Some drugs can cause fever in the absence of an immunologically based hypersensitivity reaction; these include atropine, lyseric acid, some antidepressants, amphotericin B, and bleomycin. The mechanism for atropine and central nervous system-acting drugs causing elevated temperature is through interference with heat regulatory mechanisms, and, as such, the elevated temperature is not fever but rather hyperthermia (see Chapter 39). True drug fever is an immunologically based disease in which, either through previous exposure or recent administration, sensitization takes place to the drug as a foreign antigen. It has been proposed that sensitized T lymphocytes release endogenous pyrogen-inducing substances that cause the fever. Removal of the antigen usually brings about a decrease in the fever within 48 hours.

Fever due to first use of amphotericin B or bleomycin is not due to hypersensitivity reactions but rather to the direct ability of these drugs to stimulate production of endogenous pyrogenic cytokines. In some cases, these drugs, which are given parenterally, may contain endotoxins as contaminants.

In a study published in 1964, cutaneous manifestations were present in a majority of the cases of drug fever.[85] In a large study of 148 episodes of drug fever in 142 patients, cutaneous manifestations were present in only 18 percent of patients, and less than half of these were urticarial in nature.[86]

The most common manifestation of drug fever is seen in the patient being treated with antibiotics and in whom the protracted fever is due to drug hypersensitivity and not to the infection. Withdrawing the drug usually results in disappearance of the fever. For this reason, the patient's history is critical in establishing a diagnosis of drug fever. Some patients suddenly develop fever to common drugs like INH or other agents that have been taken for years without evidence of any hypersensitivity. The variety of agents that have been reported to be the source of FUO is broad. Some agents, however, tend to be particularly associated with fever in the absence of other clinical manifestations and include salicylates, thiouracil, diphenylhydantoin (Dilantin), iodides, isoniazid, methyldopa, and penicillin.

Thyroiditis is usually associated with local pain and fever, and does not manifest as FUO. However, a small number of patients with subacute thyroiditis may be unaware of local tenderness and may have persistent fever. Examination of the thyroid gland reveals local tenderness even when there is limited involvement,[61] and appropriate thyroid function tests and serologic measurements assure the diagnosis.

Granulomatous Diseases

The four major types of granulomatous diseases that produce prolonged, unexplained fevers are: granulomatous hepatitis, sarcoidosis, inflammatory bowel disease, and temporal arteritis. In general, granulomatous disease can go undetected for many months and yet be the cause of high fevers. In fact, in patients with FUO lasting for longer than 1 year, granulomatous causes were more numerous than neoplasms or autoimmune diseases.[12,21] When the patient has a FUO, localizing symptoms are often absent, while diagnosis requires identification of granulomas in biopsy material or radiologic evidence of lesions typical of the process (e.g., Crohn's disease).

Granulomatous Hepatitis. Granulomatous hepatitis of unknown etiology accounts for a large number of cases of prolonged FUO. Granulomas in the liver represent a pathologic response to injury in that they are induced by many infectious diseases. Some of the diseases that are commonly associated with hepatic granulomas include tuberculosis and other mycobacterial infections, histoplasmosis, syphilis, some parasitic diseases, sarcoidosis, and neoplasms.[21,87–89] It is essential to rule out these and other underlying diseases. However, there is a group of patients with FUO and granulomas in the liver in whom no specific underlying process can be found.[88] The disease is usually associated with high fever intermittently present for periods of months to years and occurs most often during the fifth or sixth decade of life. The only laboratory data that suggest granulomatous hepatitis are mildly elevated alkaline phosphatase levels in many patients and elevated serum transaminase determinations in even fewer. However, these may be normal in a small number of patients, and only liver biopsy confirms the diagnosis.

Sarcoidosis. Sarcoidosis is a systemic granulomatous disease that commonly manifests with pulmonary, skin, or lymphoid involvement. However, a small percentage of patients with sarcoidosis have fever, weight loss, and weakness as initial symptoms without localizing signs or symptoms. In fact, some patients with sarcoidosis have a daily temperature elevation greater than 101°F for months, and in these patients granulomas usually can be found in the liver, while the lung fields remain clear. Fever in sarcoidosis is sometimes associated with erythema nodosum.

Inflammatory Bowel Disease. Crohn's disease or granulomatous colitis are granulomatous processes primarily involving the terminal ileum and colon, and nearly one-third of the patients have fever. A small percentage of these patients can have no gastrointestinal symptoms and only high fevers.[21,90–92] This is particularly true of young adults in whom fever can be present for months or years without symptoms referable to the gastrointestinal tract. For this reason, it is important to obtain a detailed small bowel contrast study in patients with FUO. Of all gastrointestinal diseases that cause fever, Crohn's disease is the most likely to be a cause of FUO. Ulcerative colitis, although not a granulomatous disease, rarely manifests as a FUO. There have been reports, however, of patients with high fevers and no intestinal symptoms who later have sigmoidoscopic evidence of this disease.[61,92,93]

Temporal Arteritis. Giant cell arteritis with polymyalgia rheumatica affects patients usually in the sixth and seventh decades of life and may manifest as FUO. The symptom complex includes headache, visual disturbances, and myalgias and arthralgias. It should be pointed out, however, that none of these symptoms need be present for temporal arteritis to cause prolonged fever. Patients with unexplained recurrent fevers and mild headaches or visual disturbance should be considered for temporal artery biopsy, particularly in the sixth and seventh decades of life.[21] Associated laboratory findings are anemia and very high sedimentation rates. Biopsy specimens of the temporal artery reveal granulomas even in cases in which no temporal artery tenderness was demonstrated. In one series, 44 percent of the patients with biopsy-proven temporal arteritis had no tenderness to palpation,[94] and hence it is important to consider this disease in the absence of clinical signs or symptoms in patients with FUO. Takayasu's disease can also manifest as a FUO.[95]

Inherited Disorders

There are at least four inherited diseases that are associated with intermittent fever, sometimes unexplained for years. These are familial Mediterranean fever, which is inherited in about one-half of the patients as an autosomal recessive trait[96]; Fabry's disease or angiokeratoma corporis difusum, an X-linked disorder[97]; hypertriglyceridemia; and a syndrome of deafness, urticaria and progressive amyloidosis that is familial or associated with chromosomal aberration.[98,99]

Familial Mediterranean Fever. Familial Mediterranean fever (FMF) is always associated with unexplained intermittent fever, usually beginning in childhood. Besides fever, FMF has distinct clinical signs and symptoms and laboratory data that, although nonspecific, together suggest this diagnosis in the absence of other disease.[100] These are fever, evidence of serosal inflammation—usually peritoneal or pleural, distinctive skin lesions (painful erythematous swellings), occasional joint pains, and headache. FMF is not periodic but rather a disease characterized by intermittent attacks of fever and serosal pain. In some patients, the attacks may be separated by a number of years, while in others they may occur weekly or more frequently. Spontaneous remissions and recurrence are typical of the disease. Attacks are associated with leukocytosis, elevated sedimentation rate, and elevated levels of several acute phase reactants. Admittedly nonspecific, these usually return to normal following the attacks. Although rarely seen in the United States, amyloidosis is often diagnosed in patients with FMF in the Middle East.

Familial Mediterranean fever is initially diagnosed as FUO because of the misconception that this disease is found only in Sephardic Jews, Armenians, and Arabs. Although there is unquestionably a much higher incidence of this disease in such patients, FMF occurs in patients of other extractions such as western Europeans.[100] The expression of the disease also seems milder in those patients living in the United States in that the skin lesions, joint involvement, and the development of amyloidosis are rarely encountered. Most patients primarily have recurrent bouts of abdominal or chest pain with fever. The fever in FMF may be high during some attacks, and during others, the temperature may be only minimally elevated. After a careful diagnostic work-up in which no evidence of infectious, hypersensitive, or autoimmune disease can be found in patients with symptoms and signs of FMF, this diagnosis can be made. A diagnosis of FMF is usually made after years of recurrent attacks. Prophylactic oral colchicine therapy has been shown to prevent attacks of FMF.[101]

Fabry's Disease. Fabry's disease is an X-linked inborn error of glycosphingolipid metabolism resulting from the deficient activity of a specific alphaglactosidase.[97] There is a systemic accumulation of the glycosphingolipid substrate trihexosyl ceramide, and this results in vascular and renal insufficiency and death in the third or fourth decade. Clinically, the disease is recognized by punctate skin lesions that are most numerous around the genitals and buttocks. Patients have unexplained attacks of fever and pain and also have severe acroparethesias. The recurrent fever can manifest as an FUO, particularly when the characteristic lesions are missed. The enzymatic defect can be detected in plasma, urine, and leukocytes.[97]

Hypertriglyceridemia. Hypertriglyceridemia associated with recurrent fever and abdominal pain can present as FUO, and reduction of saturated fat intake results in the disappearance of the fever and pain.[21] Hyperlipidemia type V may be associated with recurrent bouts of abdominal pain, with evidence of pancreatitis, with elevated amylase levels and may manifest as FUO.

Deafness, Urticaria, and Amyloidosis. The syndrome of deafness, urticaria, and amyloidosis has been described as a heredofamilial disease that is associated with bouts of high-spiking fever and a nonitching urticarial exanthem.[98,99] Progressive deafness is usually present since early childhood, and the febrile episodes begin in adolescence. Amyloidosis with renal failure occurs later. During the second decade of life this syndrome can manifest as FUO.

Central Nervous System Causes of FUO

The term *central* fever has been used to describe fever that is due to pathologic processes in or near the thermoregulatory center of the hypothalamus. There are several diseases that can affect the region of the thermoregulatory center, and these include metastatic tumor, primary CNS tumors, hemorrhage, degenerative diseases, vascular abnormalities, metabolic disorders, and infectious processes. In addition, such lesions more commonly produce endocrine disturbances. It should be pointed out, however, that lesions in or near the hypothalamus that affect thermoregulation are more likely to produce persistent hypothermia rather than hyperthermia. For example, sarcoid granulomas, degenerative processes,[102] tumor invasion,[103] hemorrhage into the third cerebral ventricle,[104] Wernicke's encephalopathy with hypothalamic hemorrhages,[105] and other hypothalamic lesions[106] are most often associated with hypothermia. Nevertheless, a few patients with hypothalamic disturbances may have persistent or intermittently elevated body temperature.[21,106–108] These patients with fever, like the patients with hypothermia, do not have normal mechanisms of thermoregulation and may exhibit poikilothermia.[107] In addition, these patients may lose their daily temperature rhythm.[109] Patients with local infectious processes, like encephalitis, may have an FUO and minimal changes in the CSF.

Children with central nervous system disease are more likely to develop hyperthermia than are adults. Diencephalic seizure disorders, degenerative brain diseases, chronic heavy metal intoxication, and central nervous system tumors, including CNS leukemia, are often associated with fever.[3–5] Nevertheless, hypothalamic lesions or disorders that are thought to be a cause of persistent unexplained fevers are extremely rare.

Factitious Illness

Careful observation of the daily temperature pattern can often lead to a diagnosis of factitious fever, since the circadian temperature rhythm may be absent; in some, the temperature may always be elevated. In addition to abnormal circadian temperature rhythms in patients with factitious fevers, evidence of vasoconstriction, sweating, or increased pulse rate are usually absent despite thermometer readings in excess of 39°C. The use of numbered and electronic thermometers and the simultaneous measurement of urine and body temperature are methods that help in making a diagnosis of factitious fevers.[110,111] Factitious fevers are usually suspected late in the work-up of patients with FUO,[22] but awareness of these methods can alert the attending physician before institution of a costly investigation. Most of these patients have false fevers, and the methods by which they manipulate thermometers is varied and often very ingenious. Others may inject pyrogenic materials or bacteria and induce real fever. Whatever the method used, diagnosis can be difficult, and many patients undergo extensive investigation before the factitious source of their illness is uncovered. There is a high incidence of patients with factitious illness in the health professions, particularly young women.[21] Once the factitious nature of the illness is discovered and the patient is confronted, psychiatric therapy often proves to be very beneficial. In patients with prolonged FUO, usually longer than 6 months, factitious illness accounts for 9 percent of the cases.[12] In addition, there is a higher incidence of association of self-mutilation in those patients with FUO lasting for prolonged periods. Repeated recovery of multiple and unusual organisms from blood and other cultures also suggests factitious illness.

Miscellaneous Causes of FUO

Postoperative fever due to halothane sensitization can persist and can manifest as FUO, although this is usually a self-limited febrile disease.[112] In general, cardiac surgical procedures, particularly those using pump-bypass, are most often followed by prolonged or recurrent fevers that may continue into the second or third postoperative week. In these patients, no infectious cause can be found, although approximately 6 percent have a postpericardiotomy syndrome.[113] The pathogenetic mechanisms proposed for these persistent fevers include exacerbation of pre-existing rheumatic fever, inflammatory response to blood in the pericardial cavity, and autoimmune response to traumatized cardiac tissue.[113] Neurosurgical procedures are also commonly associated with postoperative fever, and this may be related to the presence of blood in the third cerebral ventricle. A low-grade, aseptic meningitis can manifest as persistent fever after the excision of certain tumors from the CNS.[114] Septic thrombophlebitis, particularly of the pelvic veins, and small pulmonary embolization can manifest as FUO.[115] Inflammation resulting from radiation therapy may cause fever.[116] Pheochromocytomas can manifest as FUO years before the tumor is detected.[117] Laennec's cirrhosis is frequently accompanied by fever and is present in over one-third of the patients.[118] Fever due to cirrhosis is moderate but prolonged, and patients with cirrhosis have laboratory and pathologic evidence of active hepatic disease. However, these patients may be diagnosed as FUO only when the evidence of hepatic disease is undetected. The diagnosis of alcoholic hepatitis is frequently made in patients who are admitted to community hospitals with FUOs.

The only true cyclic or periodic cause of fever is cyclic neutropenia, in which the neutrophils are low or absent from the peripheral blood at 21-day intervals.[26] During this time, patients are susceptible to infection. Fever may be prominent during the neutropenic phase, and these patients are considered to have periodic fever before the correct diagnosis is made.

Many patients with the acquired immunodeficiency syndrome (AIDS) initially have an FUO. In the majority, the fever is due to an infection that is often relatively easy to diagnose. Thus, as in all FUO patients, AIDS patients should be evaluated thoroughly, with particular attention to the wide variety of infectious agents that may cause fever.

Exaggerated Circadian Temperature Rhythm

A large number of young children of both sexes, as well as young female adolescents, have been evaluated because of

FUO. These persons have often had a previous acute, self-limited febrile illness of infectious origin. The patient or the family then becomes involved in the frequent monitoring of temperature. Following recovery from this illness, it is noted that the temperature (usually in the early evening) never returns to "normal." These persons seem to have exaggerated daily swings, and their normal evening temperature may be 99–100°F.[109] After a minimal work-up, which is completely normal, we observe such persons and encourage them to not take their temperature unless they are ill. Unfortunately, many of these persons have been subjected to unnecessarily expensive, painful, and often dangerous procedures when, in fact, they are normal. Many years of follow-up have substantiated that these patients were not ill but merely had this exaggerated daily swing in temperature brought to their attention by a routine, self-limited infectious illness.

MANAGEMENT

There are a few general principles in approaching the patient with prolonged fever in whom no underlying source can be determined. A significant number of patients with undiagnosed fevers have good prognoses in that they eventually recover. Another group have intermittent bouts of fever for years but are otherwise well. These groups require no therapy, and mortality in the undiagnosed groups has been found in several studies to be low.[21] Nonspecific therapy for those patients with persistent fever and debilitating nutritional and physiologic imbalances may be instituted with caution. Clinical and laboratory evidence suggest that processes of amino acid oxidation contribute to the negative nitrogen balance of chronic fevers and that this may be partially reversed by cyclooxygenase inhibitors. The approach to empiric therapy in a patient with FUO must first consider whether the risk of the therapy outweighs potential benefit. Thus, there are few, if any indications for empiric antibiotic or cytotoxic chemotherapy. Our approach is to use antipyretics such as acetylsalicylic acid or acetaminophen first. These are given in maximum dosages, and if the patient improves, they are continued for varying periods of time. If these drugs fail, then other prostaglandin synthetase inhibitors such as indomethacin or ibuprofen are tried. If these agents prove ineffective and the patient continues to be ill, then adenal corticosteroid therapy should be considered if the physician is convinced that the underlying cause of the FUO is not infectious. Initially, we give prednisone around the clock and at a reasonable anti-inflammatory dosage (e.g., 10 mg every 6 hours). If improvement occurs and signs of inflammation recede, then we switch the patient to a single daily dose and eventually to alternate-day therapy. The latter is done to minimize undersirable side effects.

It must be emphasized that if the source of the fever defies diagnosis despite a thorough work-up as outlined then, depending on the severity of the illness, reevaluation must be done at reasonable intervals. Most empiric therapy is nonspecific, and the patient may have a relapse after treatment. With such patients or with therapeutic failures, it may be necessary to perform another complete evaluation as often as every 4–6 months, since in rare patients abnormalities may become apparent only after prolonged periods.

REFERENCES

1. Atkins E, Bodel P. Clinical fever: its history, manifestations and pathogenesis. Fed Proc. 1979;38:57.
2. Holmes GP, Kaplan JE, Grant NM, et al. Chronic fatigue syndrome: a working case definition. Ann Intern Med. 1988;108:387–9.
3. McClung HJ. Prolonged fever of unknown origin in children. Am J Dis Child. 1972;124:544.
4. Pizzo PA, Lovejoy FH, Smith DH. Prolonged fever in children: Review of 100 cases. Pediatrics. 1975;55:486.
5. Lohr JA, Hendley JO. Prolonged fever of unknown origin: a record of experiences with 54 childhood patients. Clin Pediatr. 1977;16:768.
6. Petersdorf RG, Beeson PB. Fever of unexplained origin. Medicine. 1961;40:1.
7. Shoen RP, Van Ommen RA. Fever of obscure origin. Am J Med. 1963;34:486.
8. Deal WB. Fever of unknown origin. Postgrad Med. 1971;50:182.
9. Frayha R, Uwaydah M. Fever of unknown origin. Leb Med J. 1973;26:49.
10. Howard P Jr, Hahn HH, Palmer PL, et al. Fever of unknown origin: a prospective study of 100 patients. Tex Med. 1977;73:56.
11. Larson EB, Featherstone HJ, Petersdorf RG. Fever of undetermined origin: diagnosis and follow up of 105 cases, 1970–80. Medicine. 1982;61:269.
12. Aduan R, Fauci A, Dale D, et al. Prolonged fever of unknown origin. Clin Res. 1978;26:558A.
13. Brusch JL, Weinstein L. Fever of unknown origin. Med Clin North Am. 1988;72:1247–61.
14. Petersdorf RG. FUO: how it has changed in 20 years. Hosp Pract. 1985;20:84I–84M, 84P, 84T–84V passim.
15. Barbado FJ, Vazquez JJ, Pena JM, et al. Fever of unknown origin: a survey on 133 patients. J Med. 1984;15:185–92.
16. Kerttula Y, Hirvonen P, Pettersson T. Fever of unknown origin: a follow-up investigation of 34 patients. Scand J Infect Dis. 1983;15:185–7.
17. Young EJ, Feinstein V, Mosher DM. Drug-induced fever: cases seen in the evaluation of unexplained fever in a general hospital population. Rev Infect Dis. 1982;4:69.
18. Jacoby GA, Swartz MN. Fever of undetermined origin. N Engl J Med. 1973;289:1407.
19. Gleckman R, Crowley M, Esposito A. Fever of unknown origin: a view from the community hospital. Am J Med Sci. 1977;274:21.
20. Oppel TW, Bernstein CA. The differential diagnosis of fevers. Med Clin North Am. 1954;38:891.
21. Wolff SM, Fauci AS, Dale DC. Unusual etiologies of fever and their evaluation. Annu Rev Med. 1975;26:277.
22. Aduan R, Fauci A, Dale D, et al. Factitious fever and self-induced infection. Ann Intern Med. 1979;90:230.
23. Dinarello C, Wolff, SM. Pathogenesis of fever in man. N Engl J Med. 1978;298:607.
24. Weinstein L. Clinically benign fever of unknown origin: a personal retrospective. Rev Infect Dis. 1985;7:692–9.
25. Reilly PC, Reilly MC. High-risk travel and malaria. N Engl J Med. 1977;296:1536.
26. Wright DG, Dale DC, Fauci AS, et al. Human cyclic neutropenia: clinical review and long term follow-up of patients. Medicine. 1981;60:1.
27. Krick JA, Remington JA. Toxoplasmosis in the adult—an overview. N Engl J Med. 1978;298:550.
28. Thoft RA. Corneal disease. N Engl J Med. 1978;298:1239.
29. Schacter J. Chlamydial infection. N Engl J Med. 1978;298:428.
30. McDade JE, Shepard CC, Fraser DW, et al. Legionnaires' disease. N Engl J Med. 1977;297:1197.
31. Wolff SM, Kimball HR, Perry S, et al: The biological properties of etiocholanolone. Ann Intern Med. 1967;67:1268.
32. Epler GR, McLoud TC, Graensler EA, et al. Normal chest roentgenograms in chronic diffuse infiltrative lung disease. N. Engl J Med. 1978;298:934.
33. Blain DC, Carroll M, Carr EA, et al. ^{67}Ga citrate for scanning experimental staphylococcal abscesses. J Nucl Med. 1973;14:99.
34. Habibian MR, Staab EV, Matthews HA. Gallium citrate Ga 67 scans in febrile patients. JAMA. 1975;233:1073.
35. McNeil BJ, Sanders R, Alderson PO, et al. A prospective study of computed tomography, ultrasound, and gallium imaging in patients with fever. Radiology. 1981;139:647.
36. Schmidt KG, Rasmussen JW, Sorensen PG, et al. Indium-111 granulocyte scintigraphy in the evaluation of patients with fever of undetermined origin. Scand J Infect Dis. 1987;19:339.
37. Abrams HL, McNeil BJ. Medical implications of computed tomography. N Engl J Med. 1978;298:255.
38. Spiegel AM, DiChiro G, Gordon P, et al. Diagnosis of radiosensitive hypothalamic tumors without craniotomy. Ann Intern Med. 1976;85:290.
39. Abrams HL, McNeil BJ. Medical implications of computed tomography. N Engl J Med. 1978;298:310.
40. Rowland MD, Del Bene VE. Use of body computed tomography to evaluate fever of unknown origin. J Infect Dis. 1987;156:408.
41. Nomeir AM. Bacterial endocarditis: echocardiographic and clinical evaluation during therapy. J Clin Ultrasound. 1976;4:23.
42. DiMagno EP, Malagelada JR, Taylor WF, et al. A prospective comparison of current diagnostic tests for pancreatic cancer. N Engl J Med. 1977;297:737.
43. Ulrich PC, Sanders RC. Ultrasonic characteristics of pelvic inflammatory masses. J Clin Ultrasound. 1976;4:199.
44. Rau J. Ultrasonic or radiologic cholecystography. N Engl J Med. 1977;297:62.
45. Rothman DL, Schwartz SI, Adams JT. Diagnositic laparotomy for fever or abdominal pain of unknown origin. Am J Surg. 1977;133:273.
46. Mitchell DP, Hanes TE, Hoyumpa AM, et al. Fever of unknown origin. Arch Intern Med. 1977;137:1001.
47. Katz P, Fauci AS. *Nocardia asteroides* sinusitis. JAMA. 1977;238:2397.
48. Geraci JE, Weed LA, Nichols DR. Fever of obscure origin. The value of abdominal exploration in diagnosis. JAMA. 1959;169:1302.

49. Fisher HC, White MH Jr. Biliary tract disease in the aged. Arch Surg. 1951;63:536.
50. Fung WO, Ong SC, Lee YS. Splenic tuberculosis presenting as pyrexia of unknown origin. Med J Aust. 1973;1:446.
51. Boettinger LE, Nordenstam HH, Wester PO. Disseminated tuberculosis as a cause of fever of obscure origin. Lancet. 1962;1:19.
52. Maizel H, Ruffin JM, Dobbins WO III. Whipple's disease: a review of 19 patients from one hospital and a review of the literature since 1950. Medicine. 1970;49:175.
53. Smith L. Relapsing fever: a case history. Calif Med. 1969;110:322.
54. Southern PM Jr, Sanford JP. Relapsing fever. Medicine. 1969;48:129.
55. Sundahragiati B, Kasemsuvan P, Harinasuta C, et al. Leptospirosis as a cause of pyrexia of unknown origin in Thailand. Ann Trop Med Parasitol. 1966;60:247.
56. Hattwick MA, O'Brien RJ, Hanson BF. Rocky Mountain spotted fever: epidemiology of an increasing problem. Ann Intern Med. 1976;84:732.
57. Cranston WI, Luff RH, Owen D, et al. Studies on the pathogenesis of fever in renal carcinoma. Clin Sci Mol Med. 1973;45:459.
58. Bodel P. Pyrogen release *in vitro* by lymphoid tissue from patients with Hodgkin's disease. Yale J Biol Med. 1974;47:101.
59. Bodel P. Generalized perturbations in the host physiology caused by localized tumors. Tumors and fever. Ann NY Acad Sci. 1974;230:6.
60. Bodel P. Spontaneous pyrogen production by mouse histiocytic and myelomonocytic tumor cell lines in vitro. J Exp Med. 1978;147:1503.
61. Molavi A, Weinstein L. Persistent perplexing pyrexia: some comments on etiology and diagnosis. Med Clin North Am. 1970;54:379.
62. Lee SL, Rosner F, Rivero I, et al. Refractory anemia with abnormal iron metabolism. N Engl J Med. 1965;272:761.
63. Miller JS, Miller JJ. Benign giant lymph node hyperplasia presenting as fever of unknown origin. J Pediatr. 1975;87:237.
64. Padfield R, Hicken P. Cortical hyperostosis in infants: a radiological study of sixteen patients. Br J Radiol. 1970;43:231.
65. Campbell EW, Brantley R, Harrold M, et al. Angiomyolipoma presenting as fever of unknown origin. Am J Med. 1974;57:843.
66. Ahmann DL, Kiely JM, Harrison EG, et al. Malignant lymphoma of the spleen. Cancer. 1966;19:461.
67. Zanger B, Dorsey HN. Fever: a manifestation of preleukemia. JAMA. 1976;236:1266.
68. Meachan GC, Weisberger AS. Early atypical manifestations of leukemia. Ann Intern Med. 1954;41:780.
69. Kumar S, Bhargava M. Preleukemia acute myelogenous leukemia. Acta Haematol. 1970;43:21.
70. Bowman HS, Martinez E. Fever, anemia and hyperhaptoglobinemia. Ann Intern Med. 1968;68:613.
71. Boettiger LE. Fever of unknown origin: IV. Fever in carcinoma of the kidney. Acta Med Scand. 1957;156:477.
72. Gordon DA. The extra-renal manifestations of hypernephroma. Can Med Assoc J. 1963;88:61.
73. Rawlins MD, Luff RH, Cranston WI. Pyrexia in renal carcinoma. Lancet. 1970;1:1371.
74. Berman C. Primary carcinoma of the liver. In: Greenstein JP, Haddow H (eds). Advances in Cancer Research 5. New York: Academic Press; 1958:67.
75. Goodwin JF, Stanfield CA, Steiner RE. Clinical features of left atrial myxoma. Thorax. 1962;17:91.
76. Petersdorf RG. Fever of unknown origin. Ann Intern Med. 1969;70:864.
77. Rothfield N, Phythin JM, McEwen C, et al. The role of antinuclear reactions in the diagnosis of systemic lupus erythematosus: a study of 53 cases. Arthritis Rheum. 1961;4:223.
78. Estes D, Christian CL. The natural history of systemic lupus erythematosus by prospective analysis. Medicine. 1971;50:85.
79. Fauci AS, Haynes B, Katz P. The spectrum of vasculitis. Ann Intern Med. 1978;89:660.
80. Calabro JJ, Marchesano JM. Fever associated with juvenile rheumatoid arthritis. N Engl J Med. 1967;276:11.
81. Calabro JJ, Marchesano JM. Juvenile rheumatoid arthritis. N Engl J Med. 1967;277:696.
82. Bujak JS, Aptekar RG, Decker JL, et al. Juvenile rheumatoid arthritis presenting in the adult as fever of unknown origin. Medicine. 1973;52:431.
83. Fabricant MS, Chandor SB, Friou GJ. Still's disease in adults. JAMA. 1973;225:273.
84. Jones TD. The diagnosis of rheumatic fever. JAMA. 1944;126:481.
85. Cluff LE, Johnson JE III. Drug fever. Prog Allergy. 1964;8:149.
86. Mackowiak PA. Southwestern Internal Medicine Conference. Drug fever: mechanisms, maxims, and misconceptions. Am J Med Sci. 1987;294:275–86.
87. Wolff SM, Simon HB. Granulomatous hepatitis and prolonged fever of unknown origin. Trans Am Climatol Assoc. 1973;84:149.
88. Simon HB, Wolff SM. Granulomatous hepatitis and prolonged fever of unknown origin: a study of 13 patients. Medicine. 1973;52:1.
89. Fauci AS, Wolff SM. Granulomatous hepatitis. Prog Liver Dis. 1976;5:609.
90. Crohn BB, Yarnis H. Regional Ileitis. 2nd ed. New York: Grune & Stratton; 1958.
91. Lee FI, Davies DM. Crohn's disease presenting as pyrexia of unknown origin. Lancet. 1961;1:1205.
92. Tumen HJ. Fever as a symptom of gastrointestinal disease. Am J Dig Dis. 1964;9:314.
93. Fransen H, Boettiger LE. Fever of more than two weeks' duration. Acta Med Scand. 1966;179:147.
94. Fauchald P, Rygvold O, Oipstese B. Temporal arteritis and polymyalgia rheumatica. Ann Intern Med. 1972;77:845.
95. Roberts WC, MacGregor RR, DeBlanc HJ, et al. The prepulseless phase of pulseless disease, or pulseless disease with pulses. Am J Med. 1969;46:313.
96. Sohar E, Prass M, Heller J, et al. Genetics of familial Mediterranean fever (FMF). Arch Intern Med. 1961;107:529.
97. Desnick RJ, Allen KV, Desnick SJ, et al. Fabry's disease: enzymatic diagnosis of hemizygotes and heterozygotes. J Lab Clin Med. 1973;81:157.
98. Andersen V, Buch NH, Jensen MK, et al. Deafness, urticaria and amyloidosis. Am J Med. 1967;42:449.
99. Muckle TJ, Wells M. Urticaria, deafness and amyloidosis. A new heredofamilial syndrome. Q J Med. 1962;31:325.
100. Wolff SM. Familial Mediterranean fever. In: Wintrobe MM, Isselbacher KJ, Petersdorf RG, et al., eds. Harrison's Principles of Internal Medicine. 11th ed. New York: McGraw-Hill; 1987:1450.
101. Dinarello CA, Wolff SM, Goldfinger SE, et al. Colchicine therapy for familial Mediterranean fever. N Engl J Med. 1974;291:934.
102. Bauer HG. Endocrine and other clinical manifestations of hypothalamic disease: a survey of 60 cases with autopsies. J Clin Endocrinol. 1954;14:13.
103. Fox RH, Davies TW, Marsh FP, et al. Hypothermia in a young man with an anterior hypothalamic lesion. Lancet. 1970;2:185.
104. Hey EN. Thermal regulation in the newborn. Br J Hosp Med. 1972;8:51.
105. Philip G, Smith JF. Hypothermia and Wernicke's encephalopathy. Lancet. 1973;2:122.
106. Johnson RH, Spalding JMK. Disorders of the Autonomic Nervous System. Philadelphia: FA Davis; 1974:153.
107. Wolff SM, Adler RC, Buskirk ER, et al. A syndrome of periodic hypothalamic discharge. Am J Med. 1964;36:956.
108. Simon HB. Extreme pyrexia. JAMA. 1976;236:2419.
109. Dinarello CA, Wolff SM. Molecular basis of fever in humans. Am J Med. 1982;72:799.
110. Kleinman M. Letter to editor. N Engl J Med. 1977;296:886.
111. Murray H, Tuazon C, Guerero IC, et al. Urinary temperature. N Engl J Med. 1977;296:23.
112. Dykes MHM. Unexplained postoperative fever. JAMA. 1971;216:641.
113. Ross DF, Rose MR, Rapaport FT. Febrile responses associated with cardiac surgery. J Thorac Cardiovasc Surg. 1974;67:251.
114. Cantu RC, Moses JM, Kjellberg RN, et al. An unusual cause of aseptic postoperative fever in a neurosurgical patient. Clin Pediatr. 1966;5:747.
115. Dunn LJ, Van Voorhis LW. Enigmatic fever and pelvic thrombophletitis. N Engl J Med. 1967;276:262.
116. Van Herik M. Fever as a complication of radiation therapy for carcinoma of the cervix. Am J Roentgenol Rad Ther Nucl Med. 1965;93:104.
117. Wallberg AV. Operat phaeochromocytoin med lycklig utgang. Nord Med. 1949;41:470.
118. Tisdale WA, Klatskin G. The fever of Laennec's cirrhosis. Yale J Biol Med. 1960;33:94.

41. THE ACUTELY ILL PATIENT WITH FEVER AND RASH

DAVID J. WEBER
WALTER R. GAMMON
MYRON S. COHEN

A recognizable rash can lead to immediate diagnosis and appropriate therapy. Material isolated from involved skin, when properly handled, can confirm a specific diagnosis. Unfortunately, rashes are often quite bewildering. Dermatologists, who are generally more comfortable with evaluation of the skin, are not always available for immediate consultation. Furthermore, not infrequently, dermatologists and infectious disease specialists differ in their approach to the patient with a rash.

In this chapter we will provide a framework emphasizing the following: (*1*) diagnostic approach to patients with fever and rash, (*2*) categories of skin lesions, and (*3*) brief description of the most important febrile illnesses characterized by a rash.

APPROACH TO THE PATIENT

In the initial evaluation of patients with fever and rash three problems are critical. First, whether the patient is well enough to provide further history, or immediate cardiorespiratory support is required. Second, whether the nature of the rash (in the context of presentation) demands institution of isolation precautions. Isolation is required primarily for patients whose illnesses allow airborne spread of the pathogen and includes both viral and bacterial diseases. Hospital isolation guidelines should be employed with urgency. All patients with undiagnosed infectious diseases should be treated with caution by personnel who should avoid intimate contact with secretions and employ universal blood and body fluid precautions.[1] Third, a skin lesion consistent with meningococcal disease (see below) requires emergent antibacterial therapy. Similar urgency may be warranted when lesions suggest bacterial septic shock since appropriate use of antibiotics may improve survival.[2]

The history obtained from the patient should elicit the following information:

1. Drug ingestion within the past 30 days
2. Travel outside of the local area
3. Occupational exposures
4. Sun exposure
5. Immunizations
6. Sexually transmitted disease exposure including risk factors for infection with human immunodeficiency virus (HIV)
7. Immunologic status including chemotherapy, steroid use, hematologic malignancy, and functional or anatomic asplenia
8. Valvular heart disease
9. Prior illnesses including a history of drug and/or antibiotic allergies
10. Exposure to febrile or ill individuals within the recent past
11. Exposure to wild or rural habitats and wild animals
12. Pets and habits

The clinician should pay particular attention to the season of the year, which dramatically affects the epidemiology of febrile rashes. Physical examination should focus on the following:

1. Vital signs
2. General appearance
3. Signs of toxicity
4. Presence and location of adenopathy
5. Presence of genital, mucosal, and/or conjunctival lesions
6. Detection of hepatosplenomegaly
7. Arthritis
8. Signs of nuchal rigidity, meningismus, or neurologic dysfunction

Key ingredients in arriving at a correct diagnosis include (*1*) dermatologic classification of the rash[3–5] (Table 1),[5–10] (*2*) distribution of the rash, (*3*) pattern of progression, and (*4*) timing of the development of rash (relative to the onset of illness and fever) (Table 2). Rashes may be classified by histologic or pathophysiologic criteria,[11] which is generally not of immediate benefit to the clinician. It must be emphasized that noninfectious processes often include skin rash and fever and should be considered strongly during the initial evaluation. Drug reactions, which occur with about 1 in 20 courses of drug therapy, should be considered in any patient presenting with a rash.[12]

TABLE 1. Systemic Infections with Prominent Cutaneous Manifestations

Organism (Disease)	*Macules, Papules*	*Vesicles, Bullae*	*Petechia, Purpura*
Viruses			
Human immunodeficiency (HIV-1) virus	X		
Echoviruses	X	X	X
Coxsackieviruses	X	X	X
Rubeola (measles)	X		
Atypical measles	X		X
Adenovirus	X		X
Lymphocytic choriomeningitis virus	X		
Dengue virus	X		X
Viral hemorrhagic fevers			X
Rubella (German measles)	X		X
Arboviruses	X		
Colorado tick fever	X		
Yellow fever			X
Varicella-zoster (disseminated)		X	
Herpes simplex (disseminated)		X	
Varicella (Chickenpox)		X	
Vaccinia		X	
Cytomegalovirus	X		
Congenital cytomegalovirus			X
Epstein-Barr virus	X		X
Hepatitis B	X		
Parvovirus (erythema infectiosum)	X		
Bacteria			
Chlamydia psittaci	X		
Mycoplasma pneumoniae	X	X	
Rickettsia			
R. rickettsia (Rocky Mountain spotted fever)	X		X
R. akari (rickettsialpox)	X	X	
R. prowazekii (epidemic/louse-borne typhus)	X		X
R. typhi (endemic/murine typhus)	X		
R. tsutsugamushi (scrub typhus)	X		
Salmonella typhi	X		
Francisella tularensis	X		
Streptobacillus moniliformis (rat-bite fever)	X		X
Treponema pallidum (secondary)	X		
Neisseria gonorrhoeae			X
Neisseria meningitidis			X
Leptospira sp.	X		
Borrelia sp. (relapsing fever)	X		X
Borrelia burgdorfii (Lyme)	X (annular)		
Spirillum minor (rat-bite fever)	X		
Staphylococcal aureus	X		X
Streptococci–Group A (scarlet fever)	X		
Fungi (disseminated)			
Candida sp.	X		
Cryptococcus neoformans	X		
Histoplama capsulatum	X		
Blastomyces dermatitidis	X		
Coccidioidomycosis immitis	X		
Protozoal			
Toxoplasma gondii	X		
Plasmodium falciparum (malaria)			X

(Data from references 5–10.)

HOST DEFENSE PROPERTIES OF SKIN

The skin is a relatively inhospitable environment for the growth of most pathogenic microorganisms. The hostility of that environment is mainly attributed to two factors. The relative dryness of most cutaneous surfaces provides an insufficient amount of moisture to support significant growth of pathogens, and colonization with strains of bacteria and yeast (normal resident flora), generally regarded as nonpathogenic, appears to exclude more pathogenic species.[13–15] Resident flora may actually produce metabolites that are inhibitory to the growth of more pathogenic species. Examples include bacterial lipases that liberate from sebum free fatty acids that inhibit various strains of *Streptococcus pyogenes* and antibiotic metabolites derived from *S. epidermidis* that kill strains of *Micrococcus* and *Streptococcus*.[16–18] Eradication of resident flora greatly enhances the survival of *S. aureus* and the subsequent development of infection.[19]

Normal skin is an impenetrable barrier to microorganisms. The barrier to penetration is the outermost layer of skin known as the stratum corneum. The stratum corneum is composed of corneified envelopes of dead keratinocytes joined by a relatively impermeable intercellular substance. Together, the cell envelopes and intercellular substance form a physical barrier approximately 10–15 μm thick.[20] The skin is richly supplied with both endogenous and exogenous cellular and humoral mediators of inflammation that subserve host defense functions.[21]

Epidermis and dermis are home to several cell types that may

TABLE 2. Skin Lesions and Systemic Infections

Lesion	*Common Pathogens*	*Histologic Findings*	*Smears Positive for Pathogens*	*Time of Appearance (After Onset of Illness)*
Symmetric peripheral gangrene, acrocyanosis	Noninfectious or gram-negative bacteria	Bleeding in skin, vascular thrombosis, perivascular infiltration	No	12–36 hr
Multiple purpuric lesions in seriously ill patients	*Neisseria meningitidis, Rickettsia,* other gram-negative bacteria	Vascular thrombosis, perivascular hemorrhage	Yes[a]	12–36 hr[b]
Ecthyma gangrenosum, erythema multiforme, bullous lesions	*Pseudomonas*, other gram-negative bacteria	Veins mainly involved, intima spared, inflammatory reaction	Yes	Several days
Macronodular lesions	*Candida*	Hyphae, mononuclear perivascular reaction	No	Several days
Delayed-onset rash with nonsymmetrical scattered maculopapular or vesicular lesions	*Neisseria gonorrhoeae, N. meningitidis*	Perivascular mononuclear infiltrate, immune complex	Occasionally (few bacteria only)	3–10 days
Polymorphous lesions	*N. meningitidis, N. gonorrhoeae, Salmonella*			
Rose spots	*Salmonella*, various bacteria	Perivascular mononuclear inflammation	No	5–10 days
Toxic erythema	*S. aureus, Streptococcus*	Dilation and perivascular edema	No	At presenation

[a] Except for Rocky Mountain spotted fever, in which biopsy and immunofluorescent staining are important for early diagnosis.
[b] In Rocky Mountain spotted fever, 1–7 days.
(From Kingston et al.,[11] with permission.)

generate soluble factors that initiate and amplify the inflammatory response. Those cells include the keratinocyte, fibroblast, mast cell, Langerhans cell, endothelial cell, and monocyte/macrophage. Recent studies show that keratinocytes are capable of synthesizing a number of proinflammatory and immunostimulatory cytokines (the interleukins IL-1, IL-3, and IL-6; tumor necrosis factor-α; and granulocyte-macrophage colony-stimulating factor), complement proteins and arachidonate metabolites including prostaglandins and leukotrienes.[22,23] The mast cells that reside around dermal vessels can be stimulated by a variety of factors including those derived from microorganisms to make and release promotors of inflammation such as histamine, arachidonate metabolites, proteinases, and factors that can recruit and activate leukocytes.[24] The skin may play an active role in the initiation, development, and expression of specific immune responses to microorganism through a system of skin-associated lymphoid tissues and keratinocytes.[25,26]

PATHOGENESIS OF SKIN RASH

Skin rash with fever can result from a local infectious process due to virtually any class of microbe that has been allowed to penetrate the stratum corneum and multiply locally. However, exanthems are more cogent to this discussion. An exanthem is a cutaneous eruption due to the systemic effects of a microorganism on the skin. An enanthem is an eruption of similar etiology involving the mucus membranes.

Microorganisms produce eruptions by (*1*) multiplication in the skin (e.g., herpesviruses); (*2*) release of toxins that act on skin structures (e.g., scarlet fever, *Pseudomonas aeruginosa*); (*3*) evoking an inflammatory response involving phagocytes and lymphocytes (in this case the microbicidal/tumorcidal metabolism of host defense cells is directed at the skin); and (*4*) via effects on vasculature, including vaso-occlusion and necrosis and/or vasodilation with edema and hyperemia. Obviously, for many eruptions several mechanisms can play a role.

DIFFERENTIAL DIAGNOSIS AND SKIN RASH

There are two ways to approach the investigation of infectious rash, either by the type of lesion visualized or by knowledge of individual pathogens and the rashes they produce. Unfortunately, neither system is inclusive. Accordingly, both approaches are taken in this section.

Characteristics of the Lesion

Morphologic types of skin lesions include macules, papules, plaques, nodules, vesicles, bullae, and pustules. Macules are flat, nonpalpable lesions in the plane of the skin. Papules are small palpable lesions elevated above the plane of the skin. Large papules are referred to as nodules. Vesicles and bullae are small and large blisters, respectively, and pustules are palpable lesions filled with pus. Plaques are large flat lesions that are palpable. In addition to morphology, lesions are characterized by their color and particularly by the presence or absence of hemorrhage. Lesions may be skin colored, hyperpigmented or hypopigmented, or one of several other colors of which redness is the most common. Blanching erythematous lesions are those in which erythema is due to vasodilation, while nonblanching erythemas may be due to extravasation of blood. Purpuric lesions are those in which there is hemorrhage into the skin and may be small, petechial or large, ecchymotic. We have divided our discussion into rashes that are maculopapular (a rash characterized by flat and elevated lesions), nodular, vesiculobullous, erythematous, and purpuric.

Maculopapular Eruptions

Maculopapular eruptions are usually seen in viral illnesses and immune-mediated syndromes. Common viral etiologies include the classic childhood viral diseases such as measles, rubella, erythema infectiosum, and roseola.[27] Other viral agents that often produce a rash are atypical measles, coxsackieviruses, echoviruses, cytomegalovirus, and hepatitis B.[28] Erythema multiforme is considered a special category of maculopapular rash. Erythema infectiosum (fifth disease) is now known to be caused by parvovirus B19. Besides erytherma infectiosum, other disease manifestations of infection with parvovirus B19 include aplastic crisis in patients with sickle cell anemia, arthritis, and, most recently, fetal death and hydrops fetalis. Erythema infectiosum is characterized by a three-stage rash. The initial stage is that of an erythematous, warm but nontender "slapped cheek" facial rash. Simultaneously up to four days later, a variable rash appears on the extremities, which has a morbilliform, confluent, or annular appearance. Later the rash may remit and recur with stress, exercise, sunlight, or bathing. The rash usually disappears within one to two weeks.[27a]

Lesions of erythema multiforme usually begin as round to oval macules and papules that vary in size from less than a centimeter up to 1–2 cm in diameter. Typical lesions have central erythema surrounded by a narrow ring of normal-appearing skin that is in turn surrounded by another thin ring of erythema to form target lesions. The central area may be dark red, blue, or dusky grey in color and may develop into a blister (bullous erythema multiforme). Lesions are typically symmetrically distributed on the trunk and extremities and may show a predilection for knees, elbows, palms, and soles. Mucosal involvement is usually present and painful. The degree of mucosal involvement varies from oral blisters and erosions to a hemorrhagic conjunctivitis and stomatitis. When the latter are present with fever, the term *Stevens-Johnson syndrome* is applied. The distribution, symmetry, tendency to iris formation, and bulla should allow proper identification. Most cases of erythema multiforme are idiopathic. In children and adults infections are a leading etiology, but in adults many cases are idiopathic or due to drug exposure. Infectious diseases linked to erythema multiforme are summarized in Table 3. Atypical rashes suggestive of erythema multiforme may occur in chronic meningococcemia, bacterial endocarditis, secondary syphilis, staphylococcal scalded skin syndrome, Kawasaki disease, toxic shock syndrome, Rocky Mountain spotted fever, collagen vascular disease, and a variety of viral disorders.

Several life-threatening infections may present with blanching erythematous maculopapular lesions before evolving into petechiae. These include meningococcemia, Rocky Mountain spotted fever, and dengue fever. Although rheumatic fever has as one of its diagnostic findings a configurate, migrating erythema known as erythema marginatum, it may also be associated with a maculopapular eruption and subcutaneous nodules. Patients with enteric fever due to *Salmonella* may develop "rose spots," a transient scattering of rose-colored macules over the abdomen.

Secondary syphilis is often accompanied by a rash with highly variable morphology. Lesions may be macular, maculopapular, papulosquamous, or pustular. Occasionally all types of lesions may occur in the same individual.

Nodular Lesions

A nodule is a palpable, solid round or ellipsoidal lesion, usually resulting from disease in the dermis. Nonerythematous nodules may suggest candidal sepsis (see below), but other fungal disease including blastomycosis, histoplasmosis, coccidioidomycosis, sporotrichosis, and histoplasmosis may produce skin nodules. Bacteria such as *Nocardia* and atypical mycobacteria may also cause nodular lesions. Lesions consistent with ecthyma gangrenosum suggest *Pseudomonas* sepsis. A skin biopsy specimen with appropriate stains and cultures will define the diagnosis.

The lesions of erythema nodosum are characterized by tender, erythematous nodules that vary in diameter from less than a centimeter to several centimeters. They are usually multiple and located on the anterior portions of the legs but may be solitary and occur on the upper part of the body. They typically do not suppurate but rarely may do so. The lesions will often develop in crops and usually heal in days to a few weeks without scarring. Infectious agents are a prominant cause of this lesion (Table 4).

TABLE 3. Differential Diagnosis of Erythema Multiforme

Noninfectious
Drugs
X-ray therapy
Infectious
Herpes simplex infections
Epstein-Barr virus
Adenovirus
Coxsackie B5
Vaccinia (smallpox innoculation)
Mycoplasma pneumoniae
Chlamydia (psitticosis, lymphagranuloma venereum)
Cat scratch (?)
Salmonella typhi
Yersinia
Mycobacterium tuberculosis
Histoplasma capsulatum
Coccidioides immitis

TABLE 4. Differential Diagnosis of Erythema Nodosum

Noninfectious
Systemic lupus erythematosus
Sarcoidosis
Ulcerative colitis
Crohn's colitis
Behçet's disease
Drugs
Pregnancy
Infectious
Streptococcal infection
Mycobacterium tuberculosis
Mycobacterium leprae
Chlamydia trachomatus (lymphagranuloma venereum)
Yersinia infection
Histoplasma capsulatum
Blastomyces dermatitidis
Coccidioides immitis

Diffuse Erythema

Diffuse erythema, especially if desquamation or peeling is present, should lead to consideration of scarlet fever, toxic shock syndrome, mucocutaneous lymph node syndrome (Kawasaki disease), staphylococcal scalded skin syndrome, Stevens-Johnson syndrome, and toxic epidermal necrolysis. Desquamation may occur late in all of these syndromes, and its absence early in the disease course should not be considered a reason for excluding any disease process. Most of these disorders can be easily differentiated by the patient's history and appropriate diagnostic tests.

Vesiculobullous Eruptions

A vesicle is a circumscribed, elevated lesion containing free fluid. A vesicular lesion larger than 0.5 cm is termed a bulla. Most vesiculobullous eruptions are immunologic or primarily dermatologic. Infectious diseases to be considered include varicella, disseminated herpes simplex, eczema herpeticum, enteroviruses, and coxsackieviruses (includes A16, the cause of hand, foot, and mouth disease). Tzanck smear of a scraping from a blister may allow determination of a herpes infection, either zoster or varicella. Vesicles can be confused with pustules. A pustule is an elevation of the skin enclosing a purulent exudate. Vesicular lesions may become pustules, but diffuse pustular diseases usually represent a dermatologic illness (e.g., pustular psoriasis) or a cutaneous infection (e.g., pustular *Pseudomonas* lesions after the use of contaminated hot tubs or staphylococcal folliculitis). Pustular skin lesions associated with arthralgias should lead to a consideration of gonoccemia, *Moraxella* bacteremia, chronic meningococcemia, subacute bacterial endocarditis, coxsackie infection, and Behçet syndrome.

Petechial Purpuric Eruptions

Petechiae are lesions less than 3 mm in diameter containing extravascated red blood cells or hemoglobin. Larger lesions are termed ecchymoses. Diffuse petechial lesions should always prompt emergent investigation. In critically ill patients these lesions are often associated with symmetric peripheral gangrene, consumptive coagulopathy, and shock. The most common infectious etiologies include gram-negative organisms, especially *N. meningitidis* and *Rickettsia*. Less commonly *Listeria monocytogenes* or staphylocci may be associated with a similar clinical picture. Asplenic patients are at an increased risk of overwhelming sepsis, which may be accompanied by symmetric peripheral gangrene.[29–36] About half of the infections are due to *S. pneumoniae*.[29,31,36]

Viral illnesses associated with petechial rashes include coxsachie A9, echovirus 9, Epstein-Barr virus, cytomegalovirus, atypical measles and the viral hemorrhagic fevers (see Chapter 142). Children with coxsackievirus and echovirus infections may appear very ill, and differential diagnosis from meningococcemia is difficult.

Rashes are a prominent characteristic of rickettsial disease except for Q fever. Although Rocky Mountain spotted fever is the most common rickettsial disease in the United States, endemic typhus has been noted on the Gulf Coast and epidemic typhus among immigrants and in the mid-Atlantic states. Lesions caused by rickettsiae are usually generalized and symmetric. An eschar (tache noire) characteristically develops at the site of inoculation in the following rickettsial infections: African tick typhus (*R. conorii*), North Asian tick-borne rickettsiosis (*R. siberica*), Queensland tick typhus (*R. australis*), rickettsialpox (*R. akari*), and scrub- or chigger-borne typhus (*R. tsutsugamushi*).

In patients with an appropriate travel history, infection with *P. falciparum* must be considered. Heavy parasitization may lead to severe hemolysis, renal failure, central nervous system findings, and petechiae secondary to thrombocytopenia.

The most important causes of noninfectious petechiae are thrombocytopenia, large and small vessel necrotizing vasculitis, and pigmented purpuric eruptions.

Enanthem

While attempting to classify the exanthem, it is critical that a thorough search (including the mouth, conjunctiva, vagina, rectum, and glans penis) be made for enanthems. In allergic reactions the mucous membranes are frequently involved. Koplick spots, diagnostic of rubeola, are blue-grey spots on red—a grain of sand on the buccal mucosa opposite the end molar. A strawberry tongue suggests Kawasaki disease, toxic shock syndrome, or scarlet fever. Petechiae of the palate are common in scarlet fever, and with infectious mononucleosis petechiae of the hard and soft palate are common. Oral ulcers occur in a variety of immunologic diseases presenting with exanthems and also with coxsackie A16.

PATHOGENS OR INFECTIOUS CONDITIONS STRONGLY ASSOCIATED WITH RASH

Having outlined the general categories by which skin lesions due to infectious agents should be divided, it is worth describing in more detail the spectrum of skin lesions associated with discrete pathogens or pathogenic processes.

Septicemia

Kingston and Mackey have classified the skin lesions associated with septicemia into five pathogenic processes[11] (major infectious etiologies): (*1*) disseminated intravascular coagulation (DIC) and coagulopathy (*Neisseria meningitidis, Streptococcus* sp., enteric gram-negative bacilli); (*2*) direct vascular invasion and occlusion by bacteria and fungi (*N. meningitidis, P. aeruginosa, Candida* sp., *Aspergillus* sp., *Rickettsia* sp.); (*3*) immune vasculitis and immune complex formation (*N. meningitidis, N. gonorrhoeae, Salmonella typhi*); (*4*) emboli from endocarditis (*S. aureus, Streptococcus* sp.); and (*5*) vascular effects of toxins (staphylococcal scalded skin syndrome, toxic shock syndrome, scarlet fever). A variety of bacteria may spread to the skin, generally producing discrete lesions from which bacteria can be isolated or recognized on biopsy.

Cutaneous manifestations of DIC include symmetric peripheral gangrene, purpura fulminans, localized gangrene, acrocyanosis, purpura, ecchymosis, bleeding from wound and venipuncture sites, and subcutaneous hematoma.[11,37] Symmetric peripheral gangrene is defined as ischemic necrosis simultaneously involving the distal portions of two or more extremities without proximal arterial obstruction.[38] Etiologies include cardiogenic shock and other low flow states, disorders that induce severe vasospasm such as ergot poisoning and Raynaud syndrome, disorders that lead to obstruction of small blood vessels such as cold agglutinins or primary polycythemia, snake bites, and infectious agents.[38–40] *Neisseria meningitidis* is the organism most commonly responsible for symmetric peripheral gangrene, but is may occur due to *S. pneumoniae, S. aureus, Streptococcus* sp., *E. coli, Klebsiella* sp., *Proteus* sp., *Aeromonas hydrophila, Aspergillus,* and other gram-negative organisms.[37,39,41] Symmetric peripheral gangrene is preceded by bleeding into the skin, ecchymosis, purpura, and acrocyanosis (a grayish cyanosis that does not blanch on pressure and occurs on the lips, legs, nose, ear lobes, and genitalia). Subsequently the ecchymotic lesions become confluent, blister and necrose, and develop into eschars.[11] The histology reveals a Shwartzman-like reaction in the skin with diffuse and extensive hemorrhages, perivascular cuffing, and intravascular thrombosis. Bacteria are usually absent from smears of the lesions. Shock rather than DIC appears to be the major factor in the pathogenesis of symmetric peripheral gangrene.

The term *purpura fulminans* has been used synonymously with symmetric peripheral gangrene and in a more restricted sense to describe symmetric bleeding into the skin and subsequent necrosis after a benign infection.[11] This latter syndrome is best described in children and usually follows by several days pharyngitis or a viral exanthem.[39,42,43] Common agents include varicella, measles, or streptococci. Histologically, it resembles an Arthus reaction or localized Shwartzman reaction[44] with deposition of antigen–antibody complexes in tissues.

Infections Due to Neisseria Species

N. meningitidis. Purpuric skin lesions have been noted in 80–90 percent of patients with fulminant meningococcemia.[44–46] The lesions characteristically are petechial but may blanch early in the course of infection and resemble a viral exanthem. The petechiae are irregular, small, and often raised with pale centers. Lesions most commonly occur on the extremities and truck but may also be found on the head, palms, soles, and mucous membranes. Symmetric peripheral gangrene may occur, often in association with DIC. Histology reveals diffuse endothelial damage, fibrin thrombi, necrosis of the vessel walls, and perivascular hemorrhage in the involved skin.[46,47] Aspirates of the involved areas frequently will reveal organisms when Gram stained.[45,48] Meningococcal endotoxin is a potent producer of the dermal Shwartzman reaction in mice and probably plays an important role in the frequency of hemorrhagic cutaneous manifestations in meningococcal infections.[49] Skin lesions and bacteremia are rarely seen in patients with meningococcal pneumonia.[50]

Chronic meningococcemia is a rare disease. The classic clinical constellation of symptoms includes intermittent or sustained fevers; recurring maculopapular, nodular, or petechial eruptions; and migratory arthritis or arthralgias with little systemic toxicity.[51,52] Skin lesions were noted to occur in 93 percent of 148 patients.[52] A variety of skin lesions may occur in chronic meningococcemia. The most frequently reported lesions are pale to pink-colored macular and papular lesions, which occur in over 40 percent of cases. Nodular lesions, mostly on the lower extremities, may occur. These lesions may be distinguished from those of erythema nodosum by their tendency to be less painful and lack the bluish border characteristic of erythema nodosum. Petechiae of variable size may occur with vesicular or pustular centers. Small, irregularly round, subcutaneous hemorrhages with a bluish gray center containing pus cells are a distinctive lesion of this syndrome. Ecchymotic areas or hemorrhagic tender nodules that are located deep in the dermis may also occur. Lesions associated with chronic meningococcemia tend to appear in showers in association with the onset of fever. In contrast to the lesions associated with fulminant meningococcemia, the lesions associated with chronic meningococcemia rarely include organisms demonstrable by Gram-stained smear or biopsy.[53]

Neisseria gonorrhoeae. Disseminated gonococcal infection (DGI) follows untreated mucosal infection in about 0.5–3 percent of patients.[54,55] Skin lesions are the most common manifestation of DGI and occur in 50–70 percent of patients.[56] The eruption typically appears during the first day of symptoms and may recur with each bout of fever.[57] The skin lesions associated with DGI begin as tiny red papules or petechiae 1–5 mm in diameter, many of which evolve rapidly through vesicular or pustular stages to develop a grey necrotic center, often on a hemorrhagic base.[57,58] Papules, bullae, pustules, and hemorrhagic lesions may all be present simultaneously. The lesions tend to be scanty but widely distributed. The distal portions of the extremities are most commonly involved, with sparing of the scalp, face, trunk, and oral mucous membranes. Histologic examination will reveal local vasculitis, fibrin deposition, necrosis, and neutrophil infiltration.[59] Gram-stained smears of material from skin lesions infrequently reveal organisms, although most smears are positive for gonococci when examined by immunofluorescence techniques. Circulating immune complexes may play a role in the pathogenesis of DGI-associated skin lesions.[60]

Pseudomonas Infection

Skin lesions have been reported to accompany *P. aeruginosa* sepsis in 13–39 percent of patients.[61–63] The dermatologic manifestations of *P. aeruginosa* sepsis include ecthyma gangrenosum,[62,63–71] subcutaneous nodules,[62,72–76] vesicular lesions,[62] gangrenous cellulitis,[62,63] small papules resembling the rose spots of typhoid fever,[77] and grouped petechiae.[70] Ecthyma gangrenosum, the most characteristic skin lesion caused by *P. aeruginosa,* has generally been reported to occur in 1.3–2.8 percent of septic patients,[61,78,79] but one report noted ecthyma gangrenosum in 28 percent of patients with *Pseudomonas* bacteremia.[63]

Ecthyma gangrenosum lesions begin as a painless round erythematous macule with or without an adherent vesicle that soon becomes indurated and progresses to a hemorrhagic bluish bulla. Later the lesion sloughs to form a gangrenous ulcer with a gray-black eschar and a surrounding erythematous halo. The process evolves rapidly over a period of 12–24 hours. Lesions may be discrete or multiple and are usually found in the groin, axilla, or perianal areas but may occur anywhere on the body. Although most commonly associated with *P. aeruginosa* sepsis, ecthyma gangrenosum has also been reported in sepsis with other pseudomonal species,[80] *A. hydrophila,*[81,82] *Candida* sp.,[83] *Serratia marcescens,*[65] *S. aureus,*[65] *Aspergillus* sp.,[65] and *Mucur* sp.[65] It may also result from vasculitis or malignant infiltration.[84] Rarely ecthyma gangrenosum due to *P. aeruginosa* may occur in the absence of sepsis.[71,85,86]

Histologically ecthyma gangrenosum is characterized by three features: bacterial invasion of the media and adventitia of vein walls deep in the dermis, sparing of the intima and lumen, and minimal inflammation.[67,69,81,84] Bacterial invasion results in marked fibrin exudation and frank hemorrhage, followed by ballooning of the upper dermis with resulting bullous formation. Finally, necrosis of the exudated dermis occurs. Bacteria are readily visible in biopsy samples and can be demonstrated in Gram-stained material scraped from the base of the lesion.[66]

Subcutaneous nodules may result from *P. aeruginosa* bacteremia. Characteristically, the nodules are erythematous and warm and may be either fluctuant or nonfluctuant and either tender or nontender. Despite prolonged antibiotic therapy, these lesions may contain viable bacteria weeks after the blood has been cleared of infection. The absence of fluctuance may be due to either the lack of pus in neutropenic patients and/or the deep location of the abscess. Although therapy may require incision and drainage,[74,75] prolonged therapy with drainage may result in a cure.[72,76]

Subacute Bacterial Endocarditis

Skin lesions have been reported to accompany bacterial endocarditis in 15–50 percent of cases in recent series.[87–90] Skin lesions include Osler nodes, Janeway lesions, and petechiae.

Osler nodes occur in about 5–15 percent of patients with subacute bacterial endocarditis. They are tender, indurated, erythematous nodules with a pale center about 1.0–1.5 mm in diameter.[91,92] Osler nodes most commonly occur on the pads of the fingers or toes but may occur on the thenar and hypothenar eminences and over the arms. Pain may be elicited by palpating the tips of the digits. They tend to occur in crops, are rarely numerous, and tend to be transient. The lesions usually resolve without necrosis or suppuration 1–3 days after antibiotic therapy. Histologically, Osler nodes show microabscesses with microemboli in adjacent arterioles. Osler nodes are most commonly associated with subacute bacterial endocarditis due to infection with streptococci but may occur in endocarditis due to fungi and gram-negative bacilli[92] or in systemic lupus erythematosus, typhoid, and gonococcemia.[11] Osler nodes probably represent microemboli leading to vascular occlusion with localized vasculitis.

Janeway lesions consist of small erythematous macules or less commonly small nodular hemorrhages in the palms and soles. Although they may be seen in subacute bacterial endocarditis, they are more common in acute endocarditis, especially that due to *S. aureus*. Unlike Osler nodes, they are painless. Histologically they show microabscesses with neutrophil infiltration of capillaries.

Petechiae are the most common skin and mucous membrane lesions in endocarditis and occur in about 50 percent of patients. The lesions are small, flat, reddish brown lesions that do not blanch on pressure. Mucous membrane involvement is common. Petechiae frequently occur in small crops. Lesions usually are transient.

Infections Due to Staphylococcus aureus

Staphylococcus aureus is responsible for a variety of infectious syndromes that may produce local or diffuse skin lesions.[93–97] Mechanisms of diffuse skin lesions include (*1*) production of toxins (staphylococcal scalded skin syndrome, toxic shock syndrome), (*2*) as a consequence of shock, and (*3*) due to vascular invasion often in association with endocarditis.

Staphylococcal scalded skin syndrome. *Staphyloccus aureus* belonging to phage group II (types 3A, 3B, 3C, 55, 71) may produce exfoliative toxins. These toxins are capable of causing a clinical spectrum of disease that includes bullous impetigo, a generalized scarlatiniform eruption without exfoliation, and exfoliative disease (staphylococcal scalded skin syndrome [SSSS]).[95,97,98–101] Bullous impetigo, the most limited variant that results from toxin-producing *S. aureus,* is characterized by discrete, flaccid bullae containing clear or cloudy yellow fluid. Lesions are frequently localized to the umbilicus or axillae, and the surrounding skin is normal or mildly erythematous. The bullae rapidly rupture and leave raw, denuded areas that re-epithelialize in 5–7 days. Affected infants are afebrile and lack constitutional signs.

SSSS usually occurs in neonates (Ritter's disease) or young children but may occur in older children or rarely in adults. Most cases in adults occur in association with renal impairment or immunosuppression.[102–104] Unlike bullous impetigo where the staphylococcal infection is in the skin at the site of the lesion, in SSSS the infection is often at a distant site or not on the skin at all. SSSS begins abruptly with a diffuse, blanchable erythema in association with marked skin tenderness, fever, and irritability. Light stroking of the ill-defined bullae will cause rupture and separation of the upper portion of the epidermis (Nikolsky sign). Generalized desquamation usually occurs. Unless secondary infection intervenes, the skin heals within 10–14 days. A skin biopsy (or a frozen section for presumptive diagnosis) may be employed to distinguish between SSSS and toxic epidermal necrolysis (TEN). In SSSS the cleavage plane of the early intraepidermal bulla is just beneath the granular cell layer, whereas in TEN the bulla is subepidermal and is seen at the basement membrane zone. Early distinction between these two diseases is important because the therapy for SSSS includes antistaphylococcal antibiotics whereas in TEN discontinuation of treatment with the offending drug may be lifesaving.

A mild form of SSSS is characterized by a generalized scarlatiniform eruption with exfoliation (staphylococcal scarlet fever). The skin has a sandpaper roughness and Pastia's lines are present, but the strawberry tongue and palatal enanthem of streptococcal scarlet fever are not present.

Toxic shock syndrome. Toxic shock syndrome (TSS) is an acute febrile illness characterized by a generalized erythematous eruption almost certainly due to in vivo production of a toxin at the site of localized, often relatively asymptomatic or unnoticed infection caused by *S. aureus* capable of toxin production.[95] The putative toxin, TSS toxin 1, has been shown to be identical[105] to enterotoxin F[106] and exotoxin C.[107] TSS toxin 1 has been demonstrated to be a potent, nonspecific inducer of IL-1 production; to be a potent, nonspecific T-cell mitogen; and to induce the suppression of a number of immune responses. The exact pathogenesis of TSS is still unclear.[108] Recently, TSS Toxin-1-producing coagulase-negative staphylococci have been linked to TSS.[109] Most cases of TSS have occurred in menstruating females, often in association with tampon use.[110,111] Nonmenstrual TSS has been associated with a variety of infections including postoperative, cutaneous, and burn infections and postpartum complications.[112–114] More recently TSS has been linked to *S. aureus* respiratory infection, often after viral influenza.[115–118]

TSS may vary from a relatively mild disease, often misdiagnosed as a viral syndrome, to a severe life-threatening illness. The most common symptoms include a temperature greater than 40°C, hypotension, and diffuse erythroderma with desquamation 1–2 weeks after the onset of illness. Additional early features include conjunctival, oropharyngeal, and/or vaginal hyperemia; vomiting and diarrhea; and myalgias.[119–122] Most patients have abnormalities in three or more organ systems: (*1*) muscular—rhabdomyolysis; (*2*) central nervous system—toxic encephalopathy; (*3*) renal—azotemia; (*4*) liver—abnormal transaminases; and (*5*) hematologic—thrombocytopenia. The rash of TSS is almost always present within the first 24 hours of illness. Desquamation occurs after 7–10 days, most prominently on the hands and feet. Histologically, the epidermis exhibits cleavage in the basilar layers, which differentiates TSS from SSSS and from viral and drug eruptions.[123]

Staphylococcus aureus septicemia may be associated with erythematous, petechial, or pustular lesions.[124] In addition, lesions associated with endocarditis such as Osler nodes, Janeway lesions, and splinter hemorrhages may occur. Such skin lesions have been reported in 10–64 percent of patients with staphylococcal septicemia.[125] Purpuric lesions may at times be so extensive as to mimic meningococcemia or Rocky Mountain spotted fever.[126–129] Gram-stained smears of the material in these lesions will usually reveal gram-positive cocci.

Rickettsial Infections

Rickettsiae are obligate intracellular parasites whose primary target in humans appears to be the endothelial cell.[130] After parasitization of the endothelial cell, necrosis of the media and intima results in thrombosis, microinfarcts, and extravasation of blood. The end result is increased vascular permeability and vasculitis.

Rash is a hallmark of Rocky Mountain spotted fever,[131–135] the most common rickettsial disease in the United States. Initially, the patient develops a maculopapular rash that may not be appreciated by the patient or the physician. Subsequently, the rash becomes more definite and petechial. Characteristically, the rash appear between the second and sixth days of illness (average, 4 days). However, the rash may be absent in 5–17 percent of patients, and in up to 50 percent it may not appear within the first 3 days of illness.[131,132,134,136,137] Most commonly, the rash begins on the extremities, often around the wrists and ankles, and spreads centripetally to the trunk, with relative sparing of the face. However, the rash may begin on the trunk (10 percent) or have a diffuse onset (10 percent). Characteristically, the rash involves the palms and/or soles in the later stages of infection. Over time, the rash, which begins as maculopapular lesions, may progress to become petechial or ecchymotic. Rarely, the rash may be urticarial or pruritic. Since the mortality of infection may be decreased from 15 to 3 percent[132] with appropriate therapy, antibiotics should never be delayed by the absence of rash.

Candidiasis

The incidence and relative frequency of *Candida* as a nosocomial pathogen appear to be increasing.[138–141] Disseminated candidiasis is frequently fatal and is a major cause of death in immunocompromised patients.[142,143] Predisposing factors are malignancy with cytotoxic therapy, neutropenia, antimicrobial therapy, hyperalimentation, severe burn injuries, very low weight neonates, intravenous catheters, systemic adrenocortical steroids, and gastrointestinal surgery.[142,143]

Disseminated candidiasis may be accompanied by a characteristic macronodular skin rash in up to 13 percent of patients.[143] The lesions are discrete, firm, nontender, subcutaneous raised erythematous areas or nodules.[144–146] Nodules may have a pale center, and some may become hemorrhagic. Often the lesions are diffuse, but they may be localized to a small area. The face is usually spared. Histologically the middle and lower dermis are involved and show vessels distended by fungal pseudohyphae, platelet aggregates, and fibrin. Scant lymphocytic perivenular infiltrate may be present.

The diagnosis of disseminated candidiasis may be established by biopsy and culture of these lesions. However, the diagnosis may be missed unless multiple sections of the subcutaneous tissue are carefully examined.

Chronic mucocutaneous candidiasis results from impaired function of the T-lymphocyte system and may be a manifestation of a variety of cutaneous syndromes.[147]

Many other fungi produce nodular lesions identical to *Candida* and must be considered in the immunocompromised host. In patients with the acquired immunodeficiency syndrome (AIDS), cryptococci may cause umbilicated nodules that look like molluscum contagiosum.

Immunocompromised Patients

The diagnosis of skin lesions in the immunocompromised patient is complex because of the wide range of potential microbial pathogens that may occur in patients with abnormal immune responses.[148,149] Cutaneous lesions of suspected infectious etiology should undergo biopsy. Biopsy samples should be processed by using the most rapid and sensitive methods for detecting microbes both histologically and immunologically, and appropriate stains and cultures should be obtained to optimize the chance for identifying the pathogen. Biopsy samples should be divided into two portions: the first should be sent to histology for evaluation by routine and special stains to detect fungi, mycobacteria, and bacteria. The second portion should be sent to microbiology and cultured for aerobic and anaerobic bacteria, mycobacteria, and fungi. Direct fungal touch preparations and Gram, acid-fast, and modified acid-fast stains should be performed. Viral culture should be considered when herpesviruses are considered.

Human Immunodeficiency Virus

HIV infection commonly results in dermatologic disorders.[150–153] After initial exposure to HIV many patients appear to develop a "seroconversion" disease that is clinically similar to mononucleosis. Manifestations may include transient fevers, myalgias, headache, urticaria, aseptic meningitis and rash.[150,154–161] The rash is maculopapular and usually confined to the trunk.

Kaposi sarcoma in the patient with HIV infection usually begins as multiple reddish to salmon-colored round or oval macules with a halo of surrounding pallor. Lesions are usually multiple, symmetric, and widely distributed over the body, but occasionally only one or a few lesions will develop, usually on the head, neck, or distal parts of the extremities. About 50 percent of patients will develop lesions in the mouth or sites within the gastrointestinal tract. The lesions slowly enlarge and rapidly develop nodularity and a deep red-blue color. Lesions vary in size from a few millimeters to a centimeter in diameter. The lesions are usually asymptomatic and rarely show evidence of necrosis. The diagnosis is made by biopsy.

Well-described primary dermatologic disorders of HIV infection patients include seborrheic dermatitis,[150,151,153,162] ichthyosis,[150,162–164] infectious eczemoid dermatitis,[150,162] yellow nail syndrome,[162] papular eruption,[162] vitiligo,[165] telangiectasias of the anterior portion of the chest,[166] and alopecia.[150,162,167] Several patients with HIV have developed an eosinophilic pustular rash responsive to ultraviolet therapy.[168]

Oral manifestations of HIV infection include oral candidiasis, hairy leukoplakia, herpes infection, and Kaposi sarcoma.[150,169] Oral candidiasis occurs in greater than 50 percent of HIV patients and takes the following forms: (*1*) overt thrush with pseudomembranous patches on the tongue and/or buccal mucosa; (*2*) erythematous, atrophic patches on the hard mucosa; or (*3*) a hypertrophic coating on the dorsum of the tongue.

Cutaneous lesions in HIV-infected persons may be caused by a variety of microorganisms, even when the classic target organs for a particular infectious agent do not include the skin.[170–172] Also, common cutaneous infections may occur in florid or unusual forms in AIDS patients. Herpes zoster occurs with a higher than expected frequency in HIV-infected persons.[150,152,162] Chronic varicella-zoster infection has been reported.[171,173] Severe, chronic herpes simplex lesions have been reported.[162] These ulcers are frequently perianal in homosexual men but may also involve the lips and perioral area. Secondary syphilis may produce a diffuse, erythematous, nonpruritic, maculopapular skin eruption.[174] In patients with AIDS, typical serologic tests (i.e., VDRL and fluorescent treponemal antibody absorption test [FTA-ABS]) for syphilis may be unreliable, and a biopsy of the skin lesion with silver staining to show the spirochetes may be required for diagnosis. Cytomegalovirus,[170] disseminated candidiasis, *C. neoformans*, [170,175] *H. capsulatum*,[170] *C. immitis*,[176] *Acanthamoeba castellani*,[173] and *M. avium-intracellulare* infection[173] may involve the skin. Skin lesions may yield multiple pathogens.[177,178] Recently several groups have reported AIDS patients with papules and nodules histologically identified as epithelioid angiomatosis that may be mistaken for Kaposi sarcoma. A microorganism consistent with the cat-scratch bacillus has been identified in these lesions by use of the Warthin-Starry stain.[179,180]

Drug reactions are common in patients with AIDS. Up to 50 percent of patients treated with trimethoprim-sulfamethoxazole will develop a rash, usually an erythematous, maculopapular rash involving the entire body[181,182] that is commonly associated with fever. Stevens-Johnson syndrome may develop. Rash may also accompany pentamadine therapy[181] or dapsone-trimethoprim.[183]

Dermatologic signs that have been suggested as early evidence of HIV infection include the following: macular exanthematous rash, especially in conjunction with a mononucleosis-like illness; seborreic dermatitis, extensive folliculitis; herpes zoster in young persons; oral candidiasis in patients not recently treated with antibiotics; prolonged herpes eruption; explosive new psoriasis; and oral hairy leukoplakia.

REFERENCES

1. Centers for Disease Control. Recommendations for prevention of HIV transmission in the health-care setting. MMWR. 1987;36(Suppl 2):3–18.
2. Kreger BE, Craven DE, McCabe WR. Gram-negative bacteremia. IV. Reevaluation of clinical features and treatment in 612 patients. Am J Med. 1980;68:344–55.
3. Valman HB. Common rashes. Br Med J. 1981;283:970–1.
4. Fitzpatrick TB, Bernhard JD. The structure of skin lesions and fundamentals of diagnosis. In: Jeffers JD, Scott E, White J, eds. Dermatology in General Medicine. Textbook and Atlas. 3rd ed. New York: McGraw-Hill; 1987:20–49.
5. Lazarus GS, Goldsmith LA, Tharp MD. Diagnosis of skin disease. Philadelphia: FA Davis; 1980
6. Fitzpatrick TB, Johnson RA. Differential diagnosis of rashes in the acutely ill febrile patient and in life-threatening diseases. In: Jeffers JD, Scott E, White J, eds. Dermatology in General Medicine. Textbook and Atlas. 3rd ed. New York: McGraw-Hill; 1987:21–2.
7. Johnson M-L. Dermatologic problems. In: Samily AH, ed. Textbook of Diagnostic Medicine. Philadelphia: Lea & Febiger; 1987:768–89.
8. Corey L, Kirby P. Rash and fever. In: Braunwald E, Isselbacher KJ, Petersdorf RG, et al., eds. Harrison's Principles of Internal Medicine. 11th ed. New York: McGraw-Hill; 1987:240–4.
9. Oblinger MJ, Sande MA. Fever and Rash. In: Stein JH, ed. Internal Medicine. Boston: Little, Brown; 1983:1173–8.
10. Kline PP. Fever and rash. Emerg Decisions. 1988;April:27–37.
11. Kingston ME, Mackey D. Skin clues in the diagnosis of life-threatening infections. Rev Infect Dis. 1986;8:1–11.
12. Swinyer LJ. Drug eruptions in an emergency department setting. Emerg Med Clin North Am. 1985;3:717–35.
13. Fitzpatrick TB, Bernhard JD, Soter NA. Correlation of pathophysiology of skin. In: Jeffers JD, Scott E, White J, eds. Dermatology in General Medicine. Textbook and Atlas. 3rd ed. New York: McGraw-Hill; 1987:69–73.
14. Kligman AM, Leyden JJ, McGinley KJ. Bacteriology. J Invest Dermatol. 1976;67:160–8.
15. Leyden JJ, McGinley KJ, Nordstrom KM, et al. Skin microflora. J Invest Dermatol. 1987;88(Suppl):65–72.
16. Aly R, Maiback HI, Strauss WG, et al. Survival of microorganisms on human skin. J Invest Dermatol. 1972;58:205–10.
17. Selwyn S, Ellis H. Skin bacteria and skin disinfection reconsidered. Br Med J. 1972;1:136–40.
18. Milyani RM, Selwyn S. Quantitative studies on competitive activities of skin bacteria growing on solid media. J Med Microbiol. 1977;11:379–86.
19. Singh G, Marples RR, Kligman AM. Staphylococcus infections in humans. J Invest Dermatol. 1971;57:149–62.
20. Blank IH. The skin as an organ of protection. In: Fitzpatrick TB, Eisen AZ, Wolff K, et al., eds. Dermatology in General Medicine. 3rd ed. New York: McGraw-Hill; 1987:337–42.
21. Ray TL, Wuepper KD. Experimental cutaneous candidiasis in rodents. Arch Dermatol. 1978;114:539–43.
22. Sauder DN, Wong D, McKenzie R, et al. The pluripotent keratinocyte: Molecular characterization of epidermal cytokines (abstract). Clin Res. 1988;36:692.
23. Grabbe J, Rosenback T, Czarnetzki BM. Production of LTB4-like chemotactic arachidonate metabolities from human keratinocytes. J Invest Dermatol. 1985;85:527–30.
24. Siraganian RP. Mast cells and basophils. In: Gallin JI, Goldstein IM, Snyderman R, eds. Inflammation, Basic Principles and Clinical Correlates. New York: Raven Press; 1988:513–42.

25. Streilein JW. Circuits and signals of the skin-associated lymphoid tissues (SALT). J Invest Dermatol. 1985;85(Suppl):10–13.
26. Morhenn VB, Nickoloff BJ, Mansbridge JN. Induction of the synthesis of triton-soluble proteins in human keratinocytes by gamma interferon. J Invest Dermatol. 1985;85(Suppl):27–9.
27. Valman HB. Infectious diseases. Br Med J. 1981;283:1038–9.
27a. Thurn J. Human parvovirus B19: Historical and clinical review. Rev Infect Dis. 1988;10:1005–11.
28. Cohen MS. Relationship between host defense defects and infectious disease. Infect Med. 1986;3:182–88.
29. Baccarani M, Fiacchini M, Galieni P, et al. Meningitis and septicaemia in adults splenectomized for Hodgkin's disease. Scand J Haematol. 1986;36:492–8.
30. Scully RE, Mark EJ, McNeely BU, eds. Case records of the Massachusetts General Hospital. Case 29-1986. N Engl J Med. 1986;315:241–9.
31. Scully RE, Mark EJ, McNelly BU, eds. Case records of the Massachusetts General Hospital. Case 20-1983. N Engl J Med. 1983;308:1212–8.
32. O'Neal BJ, McDonald JC. The risk of sepsis in the asplenic adult. Ann Surg. 1981;194:775–8.
33. Sekikawa T, Shatney CH. Septic sequelae after splenectomy for trauma in adults. Am J Surg. 1983;145:667–73.
34. Zarrabi MH, Rosner F. Serious infections in adults following splenectomy for trauma. Arch Intern Med. 1984;144:1421–4.
35. Green JB, Shackford, SR, Sise MJ, et al. Late septic complications in adults following spenectomy for trauma: A prospective analysis in 144 patients. J Trauma 1986;26:999–1004.
36. Evans D. Postsplenectomy sepsis 10 years or more after operation. J Clin Pathol. 1985;38:309–11.
37. Robboy SJ, Mihm MC, Colman RW, et al. The skin in disseminated intravascular coagulation. Prospective analysis of thirty-six cases. Br J Dermatol. 1973;88:221–9.
38. Goodwin JN, Berne TV. Symmetrical peripheral gangrene. Arch Surg. 1974;108:780–4.
39. Chu DZJ, Blaisdell FW: Purpura fulminans. Am J Surg. 1982;143:356–62.
40. McGouran RCM, Emmerson GA. Symmetrical peripheral gangrene. Br Heart J. 1977;39:569–72.
41. Thisyakorn U, Ningsanond V. Purpura fulminans produced by *Aeromonas hydrophila:* A case report. Southeast Asian J Trop Med. 1985;16:532–3.
42. Dudgeon DL, Kellogg DR, Gilchrist GS, et al. Purpura fulminans. Arch Surg. 1971;103:351–8.
43. Hjort PF, Rapaport SI, Jorgensen L. Purpura fulminans. Report of a case successfully treated with heparin and hydrocortisone. Review of 50 cases from the literature. Scand J Haematol. 1964;1:169–92.
44. Hjort PF, Rapaport SI. The Shwartzman reaction: Pathogenetic mechanisms and clinical manifestations. Annu Rev Med. 1965;16:135–69.
45. Hill WR, Kinney TD. The cutaneous lesions in meningococcemia: A clinical and pathologic study JAMA. 1947;134:513–8.
46. DeVoe IW. The meningococcus and mechanisms of pathogenicity. Microbiol Rev. 1982;46:162–90.
47. Sotto MN, Langer B, Hoshino-Shimizu S, et al. Pathogenesis of cutaneous lesions in acute meningococcemia in humans: Light, immunofluorescent, and electron microscopic studies of skin biopsy specimens. J Infect Dis. 1976;133:506–14.
48. Bernhard WG, Jordan AC. Purpuric lesions in meningococcic infections. 1944;29:273–81.
49. Davis CE, Arnold K. Role of meningococcal endotoxin in meningococcal purpura. J Exp Med. 1974;140:159–71.
50. Koppes GM, Ellenbogen C, Gebhart RJ. Group Y meningococcal disease in United States Air Force recruits. Am J Med. 1977;62:661–6.
51. Leibel RL, Fangman JJ. Chronic meningococcemia in childhood. Am J Dis Child. 1974;127:94–8.
52. Benoit FL. Chronic meningococcemia. Am J Med. 1963;35:103–12.
53. Ognibene AJ, Dito WR. Chronic meningococcemia. Arch Intern Med 1964;114:29–32.
54. Barr J, Danielsson D. Septic gonococcal dermatitis. Br Med J. 1971;1:482–5.
55. Holmes KK, Weisner PJ, Pederson AHB, et al. The gonococcal arthritis–dermatitis syndrome. Ann Intern Med. 1971;75:470–1.
56. Handsfield HH. Disseminated gonococcal infection. Clin Obstet Gynecol. 1975;18:131–42.
57. Abu-Nassar H, Hill N, Fred HL, et al. Cutaneous manifestations of gonococcemia. Arch Intern Med. 1963;112:731–7.
58. Holmes KK, Counts GW, Beaty HN. Disseminated gonococcal infection. Ann Intern Med. 1971;74:979–93.
59. Tronca E, Handsfield HH, Wiesner PJ, et al. Demonstration of *Neisseria gonorrhoeae* with fluorescent antibody in patients with disseminated gonococcal infection. J Infect Dis. 1974;129:583–6.
60. Walker LC, Ahlin TD, Tung KSK, et al. Circulating immune complexes in disseminated gonorrheal infection. Ann Intern Med. 1978;89:28–33.
61. Flick MR, Cluff LE. *Pseudomonas* bacteremia. Am J Med. 1976;60:501–8.
62. Forkner CE, Frei E, Edgcomb JH, et al. *Pseudomonas* septicemia. Am J Med. 1958;25:877–89.
63. Whitecar JP, Luna M, Bodey GP. *Pseudomonas* bacteremia in patients with malignant diseases. Am J Med Sci. 1970;260:216–23.
64. Anderson MG. *Pseudomonas* septicaemia and ecthyma gangrenosum. S Afr Med J. 1979;55:504–9.
65. Bodey GP, Bolivar R, Fainstein V, et al. Infections caused by *Pseudomonas aeruginosa*. Rev Infect Dis. 1983;5:279–313.
66. Curtin JA, Petersdorf RG, Bennett IL. *Pseudomonas* bacteremia: Review of ninety-one cases. Ann Intern Med. 1961;54:1077–107.
67. Dorff GJ, Geimer NF, Rosenthal DR, et al. *Pseudomonas* septicemia. Arch Intern Med. 1971;128:591–5.
68. Fast M, Woerner S, Bowman W, et al. Ecthyma gangrenosum. Can Med Assoc J. 1979;120:332–4.
69. Greene SL, Su WPD, Muller SA. Ecthyma gangrenosum: Report of clinical, histopathologic, and bacteriologic aspects of eight cases. J Am Acad Dermatol. 1984;11:781–7.
70. Hall JH, Callaway JL, Tindall JP, et al. *Pseudomonas aeruginosa* in dermatology. Arch Dermatol. 1968;97:312–24.
71. van den Broek PJ, van der Meer JWM, Kunst MW. The pathogenesis of ecthyma gangrenosum. J Infect. 1979;1:263–7.
72. Bagel J, Grossman ME. Subcutaneous nodules in *Pseudomonas* sepsis. Am J Med. 1986;80:528–9.
73. Llistosella E, Revella A, Moreno A, et al. Panniculitis in *Pseudomonas aeruginosa* septicemia. Acta Derm Venereol (Stockh) 1984;64:447–9.
74. Picou KA, Jarratt MT. Persistent subcutaneous abscesses following *Pseudomonas* sepsis. Arch Dermatol. 1979;115:459–60.
75. Reed RK, Larter WE, Sieber OF, et al. Peripheral nodular lesions in *Pseudomonas* sepsis: The importance of incisions and drainage. J Pediatr. 1976;88:977–9.
76. Schlossberg D. Multiple erythematous nodules as a manifestation of *Pseudomonas aeruginosa* septicemia. Arch Dermatol. 1980;116:446–7.
77. Stanley MM. Bacillus pyocyaneus infections. Am J Med. 1947;9:253–367.
78. Baltch AL, Griffin PE. *Pseudomonas aeruginosa* bacteremia: A clinical study of 75 patients. Am J Med Sci. 1977;274:119–29.
79. Bodey GP, Jadeja L, Elting L. *Pseudomonas* bacteremia. Arch Intern Med. 1985;145:1621–9.
80. Mandell IN, Feiner HD, Price NM, et al. *Pseudomonas cepacia* endocarditis and ecthyma gangrenosum. Arch Dermatol. 1977;113:199–202.
81. Ketover BP, Young LS, Armstrong D. Septicemia due to *Aeromonas hydrophila:* Clinical and immunologic aspects. J Infect Dis. 1973;127:284–90.
82. Shackelford PG, Ratzan SA, Shearer WT. Ecthyma gangrenosum produced by *Aeromonas hydrophilia*. J Pediatr. 1973;83:100–1.
83. Fine JD, Miller JA, Harrist TJ, et al. Cutaneous lesions in disseminated candidiasis mimicking ecthyma gangrenosum. Am J Med 1981;70:1133–5.
84. Musher DM. Cutaneous and soft-tissue manifestations of sepsis due to gram-negative enteric bacilli. Rev Infect Dis. 1980;2:854–66.
85. El Baze P, Ortonne J-P. Ecthyma gangrenosum. J Am Acad Dermatol. 1985;13:299–300.
86. Huminer D, Siegman-Igra Y, Morduchowicz G, et al. Ecthyma gangrenosum without bacteremia. Arch Intern Med. 1987;147:299–310.
87. Von Reyn CF, Levy BS, Arbeit RD, et al. Infective endocarditis: An analysis based on strict case definitions. Ann Intern Med. 1981;94:505–18.
88. Venezio FR, Westenfelder GO, Cook FV, et al. Infective endocarditis in a community hospital. Arch Intern Med. 1982;142:789–92.
89. Terpenning MS, Buggy BP, Kauffman CA. Infective endocarditis: Clinical features in young and elderly patients. Am J Med. 1987;83:626–34.
90. King K, Harkness JL. Infective endocarditis in the 1980s. Part 1. Aetiology and diagnosis. Med J Aust. 1986;144:536–40.
91. Alpert JS, Krous HF, Dalen JE, et al. Pathogenesis of Osler's nodes. Ann Intern Med. 1976;85:471–3.
92. Yee J, McAllister CK. Osler's nodes and the recognition of infective endocarditis: A lesion of diagnostic importance. South Med J. 1987;80:753–7.
93. Harvey D. Staphylococcal infections. J Antimicrob Chemother. 1979;5(suppl. A):21–26.
94. Sheagren JN. *Staphylococcus aureus*. The persistent pathogen (first of two parts). N Engl J Med. 1984;310:1368–73.
95. Sheagren JN. *Staphylococcus aureus*. The persistent pathogen (second of two parts). N Engl J Med. 1984;310:1437–42.
96. Sheagren JN. Staphylococcal infections of the skin and skin structures. Cutis. 1985;361:2–6.
97. Wickboldt LG, Fenske NA. Streptococcal and staphylococcal infections of the skin. Hosp Pract. 1986;21:41–7.
98. Dowsett EG. The staphylococcal scalded skin syndrome. J Hosp Infect. 1984;5:347–54.
99. Elias PM, Fritsch P, Epstein EH. Staphylococcal scalded skin syndrome. Arch Dermatol. 1977;113:207–19.
100. Hebert AA, Esterly NB. Bacterial and candidal cutaneous infections in the neonate. Dermatol Clin. 1986;4:3–21.
101. Melish ME, Glasgow LA. Staphylococcal scalded skin syndrome: The expanded clinical syndrome. J Pediatr. 1971;78:958–67.
102. Borchers SL, Gomez EC, Isseroff RR. Generalized staphylococcal scalded skin syndrome in anephric boy undergoing hemodialysis. Arch Dermatol. 1984;120:912–8.
103. O'Keefe R, Dagg JH, MacKie RM. The staphylococcal scalded skin syndrome in two elderly immunocompromised patients. Br Med J. 1987;295:179–80.
104. Richard M, Mathieu-Serra A. Staphylococcal scalded skin syndrome in a homosexual adult. J Am Acad Dermatol. 1986;15:385–9.
105. Igarashi H, Fujikawa H, Usami H, et al. Purification and characterization of *Staphylococcus aureus* FRI 1169 and 587 toxic shock syndrome exotoxins. Infect Immun. 1984;44:175–81.

106. Bergdoll MS, Crass BA, Reiser RF, et al. A new *Staphylococcus* enterotoxin, enterotoxin F, associated with toxic-shock-syndrome *Staphylococcus aureus* isolates. Lancet. 1981;1:1017–21.
107. Schlievert PM, Shands KN, Dan BB, et al. Identification and characterization of an exotoxin from *Staphylococcus aureus* associated with toxic-shock syndrome. J Infect Dis. 1981;143:509–16.
108. Kass EH. The toxic shock syndrome revisited. Postgrad Med J. 1985;61(Suppl 1):45–48.
109. Crass BA, Bergdoll MS. Involvement of coagulase-negative staphylococci in toxic shock syndrome. J Clin Microbiol 1986;23:43–5.
110. Davis JP, Chesney PJ, Wand PJ, et al. Toxic shock syndrome. Epidemiologic features, recurrence, risk factors, and prevention. N Engl J Med. 1980;303:1429–35.
111. Fisher RF, Goodpasture HC, Peterie JD, et al. Toxic shock syndrome in menstruating women. Ann Intern Med. 1981;94:156–63.
112. Holt PA, Armstrong AM, Norfolk GA, et al. Toxic-shock syndrome due to staphylococcal infection of a burn. Br J Clin Pract. 1987;41:582–83.
113. Reingold AL, Dan BB, Shands KN, et al. Toxic-shock syndrome not associated with menstruation. Lancet. 1982;1:1–4.
114. Reingold AL, Hargrett NT, Dan BB, et al. Nonmenstrual toxic shock syndrome. A review of 130 cases. Ann Intern Med. 1982;96:871–4.
115. Bates I. Characteristic rash associated with staphylococcal pneumonia. Lancet. 1987;2:1026–7.
116. Center for Disease Control. Toxic shock syndrome associated with influenza-Minnesota. MMWR. 1986;35:143–4.
117. Center for Disease Control. Toxic shock syndrome following influenza-Oregon; Update on influenza activity—United States. MMWR. 1987;36:64–5.
118. Wilkins EGL, Ney F, Roberts C, et al. Probable toxic shock syndrome with primary staphylococcal pneumonia. J Infect. 1985;11:231–2.
119. Finch R, Whitby M: Toxic shock syndrome. J R Coll Physicians Lond. 1985;19:219–23.
120. Tofte RW, Williams DN. Clinical and laboratory manifestations of toxic shock syndrome. Ann Intern Med. 1982;96:843–7.
121. Tofte RW, Williams DN. Toxic shock syndrome: Clinical and laboratory features in 15 patients. Ann Intern Med. 1981;94:149–56.
122. Tofte RW, Williams DN. Toxic shock syndrome. Recognition and management of a diverse disease. Postgrad Med. 1983;73:275–88.
123. Todd J, Fishuat M, Kapral F, et al. Toxic-shock syndrome associated with phage-group-1 staphylococci. Lancet. 1978;2:1116–7.
124. Plaut MD. Staphylococcal septicemia and pustular purpura. Arch Dermatol 1969;99:82–5.
125. Musher DM, McKenzie SO. Infections due to *Staphylococcus aureus*. Medicine (Baltimore). 1977;56:383–409.
126. Aach R, Kissane J, eds. A thirty-eight year old woman with overwhelming sepsis. Am J Med. 1972;53:233–41.
127. Murray HW, Tuazon CU, Sheagren JN. Staphylococcal septicemia and disseminated intravascular coagulation. Arch Intern Med. 1977;137:844–47.
128. Milunski MR, Gallis HA, Fulkerson WJ. *Staphylococcus aureus* septicemia mimicking fulminant Rocky Mountain spotted fever. Am J Med. 1987;83:801–3.
129. Rahal JJ, MacMahon E, Weinstein L. Thrombocytopenia and symmetrical peripheral gangrene associated with staphylococcal and streptococcal bacteremia. Ann Intern Med. 1968;69:35–43.
130. Walker DH. Rickettsial disease: An update. In: Majno G, Cotran RS, Kaufman N, eds. Current Topics in Inflammation and Infection. Baltimore: Wiliams & Wilkins; 1982:188–204.
131. Current trends. Rocky Mountain spotted fever—United States, 1986. MMWR. 1987;36:314–5.
132. Helmick CG, Bernard KW, D'Angelo LJ. Rocky Mountain spotted fever: Clinical, laboratory, and epidemiological features of 262 cases. J Infect Dis. 1984;150:480–8.
133. Hazard GW, Ganz RN, Nevin RW, et al. Rocky Mountain spotted fever in the Eastern United States. N Engl J Med. 1969;280:57–62.
134. Kaplowitz LG, Fischer JJ, Sparling PF. Rocky Mountain spotted fever: A clinical dilemma. In: Remington JS, Swartz MN: Current Clinical Topics in Infectious Diseases. New York: McGraw-Hill; 1981:89–108.
135. Sexton DJ, Burgdorder W. Clinical and epidemiologic features of Rocky Mountain spotted fever in Mississippi, 1933–1973. South Med J. 1975;68:1529–35.
136. Cohen JI, Corson AP, Corey GR. Late appearance of skin rash in Rocky Mountain spotted fever. South Med J. 1983;76:1457–8.
137. Ramsey PG, Press OW. Successful treatment of Rocky Mountain 'spotless' fever. West J Med. 1984;140:94–6.
138. Centers for Disease Control. Nosocomial infection surveillance. MMWR. 1984;35(Suppl):17–29.
139. Drutz DJ, Jarvis WR, de Repentigny L, et al. Severe nosocomial yeast infections. Conversations Infect Control. 1985;6:1–12.
140. Morrison AJ, Freer CV, Searcy MA, et al. Nosocomial bloodstream infections: Secular trends in a statewide surveillance program in Virginia (abstract 452). In: Proceedings of the 25th Interscience Conference on Antimicrobial Agents and Chemotherapy. Minneapolis: American Society for Microbiology, 1985.
141. Weber DJ, Rutala WA. Epidemiology of nosocomial fungal infections. In: McGinnis MR, ed. Current Topics in Medical Mycology. v. 2. New York: Springer Publishing; 1988:305–37.
142. Bodey GP. Fungal infection and fever of unknown origin in neutropenic patients. Am J Med. 1986;80:112–9.
143. Maksymiuk AW, Thongprasert S, Hopfer R, et al. Systemic candidiasis in cancer patients. Am J Med. 1984;77(Suppl):20–7.
144. Bodey GP. Candidiasis in cancer patients. Am J Med. 1984;77(Suppl):13–9.
145. Balandran L, Rothschild H, Pugh N, et al. A cutaneous manifestation of systemic candidiasis. Ann Intern Med. 1973;78:400–3.
146. Jacobs MI, Magid MS, Jarowski CI. Disseminated candidiasis. Arch Dermatol. 1980;116:1277–9.
147. Kirkpatrick CH. Host factors in defense against fungal infections. Am J Med. 1984;77(Suppl):1–12.
148. Dreizen S, McCredie KB, Bodey GP, et al. Unusual mucocutaneous infections. Postgrad Med. 1986;79:287–94.
149. Wolfson JS, Sober AJ. Dermatologic manifestations of infection in the compromised host. In: Rubin RH, Young LS, eds. Clinical Approach to Infection in the Compromised Host. New York: Plenum; 1988:115–30.
150. Valle S. Dermatologic findings related to human immunodeficiency virus infection in high-risk individuals. J Am Acad Dermatol. 1987;17:951–61.
151. Triana AF, Shapiro RS, Polk BF, et al. Mucocutaneous findings in acquired immunodeficiency syndrome/AIDS-related complex patients. J Am Acad Dermatol. 1987;16:888–9.
152. Koslow RA, Phair JP, Friedman HB, et al. Infection with the human immunodeficiency virus: Clinical manifestations and their relationship to immune deficiency. Ann Intern Med. 1987;107:474–80.
153. Matis WL, Triana A, Shapiro R, et al. Dermatologic findings associated with immunodeficiency virus infection. J Am Acad Dermatol. 1987;17:746–51.
154. Calabrese LH, Proffitt MR, Levin KH, et al. Acute infection with the human immunodeficiency virus (HIV) associated with acute brachial neuritis and exanthematous rash. Ann Intern Med. 1987;107:849–51.
155. Denning DW, Amos A, Wall RA. Oral and cutaneous features of acute human immunodeficiency virus infection. Cutis. 1987;40:171–5.
156. Ho DD, Sarngadharan MG, Resnick L, et al. Primary human T-lymphotrophic virus type III infection. Ann Intern Med. 1985;103:880–3.
157. Kessler HA, Blaauw B, Spear J, et al. Diagnosis of human immunodeficiency virus infection in seronegative homosexuals presenting with an acute viral syndrome. JAMA. 1987;258:1196–9.
158. Ruutu P, Suni J, Oksanen K, et al. Primary infection with HIV in a severely immunosuppressed patient with acute leukemia. Scand J Infect Dis. 1987;19:369–72.
159. Valle S-L. Febrile pharyngitis as the primary sign of HIV infection in a cluster of cases linked by sexual contact. Scand J Infect Dis. 1987;19:13–7.
160. Biggs B, Newton-John HF. Acute HTLV-III infection. Med J Aust. 1986;144:545–7.
161. Boyko WJ, Schechter MT, Craib KJP, et al. The Vancouver lymphadenopathy-AIDS study: 7. Clinical and laboratory features of 87 cases of primary HIV infection. Can Med Assoc J. 1987;137:109–13.
162. Goodman DS, Teplitz ED, Wishner A, et al. Prevalence of cutaneous disease in patients with acquired immunodeficiency syndrome (AIDS) or AIDS-related complex. J Am Acad Dermatol. 1987;17:210–20.
163. Brenner S. Acquired ichthyosis in AIDS. Cutis. 1987;39:421–6.
164. Young L, Steinman HK. Acquired ichthyosis in a patient with acquired immunodeficiency syndrome and Kaposi's sarcoma. J Am Acad Dermatol. 1987;16:395–6.
165. Duvic M, Rapini R, Hoots WK, et al. Human immunodeficiency virus–associated vitiligo: Expression of autoimmunity with immunodeficiency? J Am Acad Dermatol. 1987;17:656–62.
166. Fallon R, Abell E, Kingsley L, et al. Telangiectasias of the anterior chest in homosexual man. Ann Intern Med. 1986;105:679–82.
167. Schonwetter RS, Nelson EB: Alopecia areata and the acquired-immunodeficiency-syndrome–related complex. Ann Intern Med. 1986;104:287.
168. Buchness MR, Lim HW, Hatcher VA, et al. Eosinophilic pustular folliculitis in the acquired immunodeficiency syndrome. N Engl J Med. 1988;318:1183–6.
169. Cohen PR, Kurzrock R. Tongue lesions in the acquired immunodeficiency syndrome. Cutis. 1987;40:406–9.
170. Penneys NS, Hicks B. Unusual cutaneous lesions associated with acquired immunodeficiency syndrome. J Am Acad Dermatol. 1985;13:847–52.
171. Kaplan MH, Sadick N, McNutt NS, et al. Dermatologic findings and manifestations of acquired immunodeficiency syndrome (AIDS). J Am Acad Dermatol. 1987;16:485–506.
172. Laurence J. Dermatologic manifestations of HIV infection. Infections in Surgery. 1987;6:488–95.
173. Janier M, Hillion B, Baccard M, et al. Chronic varicella zoster infection in acquired immunodeficiency syndrome. J Am Acad Dermatol. 1988;18:584–5.
174. Hicks CB, Benson PM, Lupton GP, et al. Seronegative secondary syphilis in a patient infected with the human immunodeficiency virus (HIV) with Kaposi sarcoma. Ann Intern Med. 1987;107:492–5.
175. Libow LF, Dobert D, Sibulkin D. Co-existent cutaneous cryptococcosis and Kaposi's sarcoma in a patient with the acquired immunodeficiency syndrome. Cutis. 1988;41:159–64.
176. Pichard JG, Sorotzkin RA, James RE III. Cutaneous manifestations of disseminated coccidioidomycosis in the acquired immunodeficiency syndrome. Cutis. 1987;39:203–5.
177. Gretzula J, Penneys NS. Complex viral and fungal skin lesions of patients with acquired immunodeficiency syndrome. J Am Acad Dermatol. 1987;16:1151–4.
178. Kwan TH, Kaufman HW. Acid-fast bacilli with cytomegalovirus and her-

pesvirus inclusions in the skin of an AIDS patient. Am J Clin Pathol. 1986;85:236–8.
179. Angritt P, Tuur SM, Macher AM, et al. Epithelioid angiomatosis in HIV infection: Neoplasm or cat-scratch disease? Lancet. 1988;1:996.
180. LeBoit PE, Berger TG, Egbert BM, et al. Epitheloid haemangioma-like vascular proliferation in AIDS: Manifestation of cat scratch disease bacillus infection? Lancet 1988;1:960–3.
181. Gordin FM, Simon GL, Wofsy CB, et al. Adverse reactions to trimethoprim-sulfamethoxazole in patients with the acquired immunodeficiency syndrome. Ann Intern Med. 1984;100:495–9.
182. Wofsy CB. Use of trimethoprim-sulfamethoxazole in the treatment of *Pneumocystis carinii* pneumonitis in patients with acquired immunodeficiency syndrome. Rev Infect Dis. 1987;9(Suppl 2):184–94.
183. Leoung GS, Mills J, Hopewell PC, et al. Dapsone-trimethoprim for *Pneumocystis carinii* pneumonia in the acquired immunodeficiency syndrome. Ann Intern Med. 1986;105:45–8.

SECTION B. UPPER RESPIRATORY INFECTIONS

42. THE COMMON COLD

JACK M. GWALTNEY, JR.

While the designation "the common cold" is a time-honored phrase used by both physician and lay persons alike for the identification of acute minor respiratory illness, current scientific knowledge discloses that there is no basis for the concept of a single entity implied by the use of such a term. Instead, "the common cold" is a group of diseases caused, for the most part, by members of five families of viruses. The viruses in these families have distinctive biochemical properties that govern their differing pathogenic and epidemiologic behavior. In addition, the immunotypes of the different viral families have antigenic variations that are of biologic importance to the immune system of their human host. The problem of controlling acute respiratory disease presents a complex challenge that will require specific approaches suitable for the properties of the individual virus groups. Thus the hope for the development of a single "cure for the common cold" is an unrealistic expectation, which has historically led to the diversion of resources into attempts at simplistic and unrealistic solutions.

As a clinical entity, the common cold is a mild, self-limited, catarrhal syndrome that is the leading cause of acute morbidity and of visits to a physician in the United States. It is also a major cause of industrial and school absenteeism.[1] A small proportion of colds is complicated by bacterial infections of the paranasal sinuses and the middle ear, which require antimicrobial therapy.

Based on early observations of their contagious nature, colds have long been thought to be due to infectious agents. It was not until the isolation of a number of new respiratory viruses in tissue culture in the 1950s that the specific etiology of colds was known. The first of these, a parainfluenza virus, was shown to cause acute respiratory disease in 1955.[2] In 1956, the first of the rhinoviruses was isolated from adults with common colds.[3,4] The following year, respiratory syncytial virus was related to acute respiratory illness in infants,[5] and, in 1958, one of the enteroviruses, coxsackievirus A21, was recovered from military recruits with mild respiratory disease.[6] The latest group of common cold viruses to be discovered, the coronaviruses, was first reported in the 1960s.[7,8] Since that time no new cold viruses have been found, although the specific cause of some colds remains unknown. Other respiratory viruses, such as influenza virus and adenovirus, produce the common cold syndrome but are characteristically associated with a more severe illness, which often involves the lower respiratory tract. The discovery of the large number of cold viruses revealed for the first time the complexity of the problem and indicated that it will be a difficult one to control.

ETIOLOGY

The major respiratory viruses causing colds and similar upper respiratory illnesses are found in the myxovirus, paramyxovirus, adenovirus, picornavirus, and coronavirus groups (Table 1).[9–12] Within these groups of viruses are many different antigenic types. The rhinovirus group, which accounts for approximately 30 percent of colds in adults, has 100 antigenically different types. The percentage of colds caused by the coronavirus group and the number of serologic types of this virus have not been fully determined, but it is believed that these viruses are an important cause of colds. The three parainfluenza viruses and the respiratory syncytial virus each account for a proportion of colds on an annual basis. Influenza virus and adenovirus produce a spectrum of illness that overlaps the common cold syndrome. Some of the enteroviruses produce coryza, as do some viruses that usually produce more characteristic findings, such as exanthem. Because mild streptococcal pharyngitis cannot be differentiated from viral pharyngitis on clinical grounds, it also is included as a cause of "colds." The etiology of approximately 35 percent of colds in adults remains unknown. Some undiagnosed illnesses may result from the insensitivity of methods currently used for detecting known viruses, and others may be due to undiscovered agents. Colds in children are caused by the same viruses in roughly the same proportion, but the total number of colds that can be diagnosed in children is significantly lower. In some studies, as high as 70 percent of acute respiratory illnesses in children could not be assigned an etiology.

Colds are a frequent illness because of the large number of different causative viruses and also because reinfections may

TABLE 1. Viruses Associated with the Common Cold

	Antigenic Types	*Percentage of Cases*[a]
Rhinoviruses	100 types and 1 subtype	30–35
Coronavirus	3 or more types	≥10
Parainfluenza virus	4 types	10–15
Respiratory syncytial virus	1 type	
Influenza virus	3 types	
Adenovirus	33 types	
Other viruses (enterovirus, rubeola, rubella, varicella)		5
Presumed undiscovered viruses		30–35
Group A β-hemolytic streptococci[b]		5–10

[a] Estimated percentage of colds annually.
[b] Included because differentiation of streptococcal and viral pharyngitis is not possible by clinical means.

occur with the same virus type. Second infections probably occur with members of all the viral groups; with some, such as coronavirus, reinfections appear to be particularly common. Up to 80 percent of persons infected with coronavirus OC43 have had prior neutralizing antibody to the virus.[13]

SEASONAL INCIDENCE

The respiratory viruses have a worldwide distribution. Annual epidemics of upper respiratory tract disease occur in the colder months in temperate areas and during the rainy season in the tropics. In the United States the respiratory disease season begins in late August to mid-September.[14,15] Respiratory illness rates rise sharply over a few weeks and then remain elevated until spring. During March, April, and May, rates decline to the low summer level.

The events controlling the seasonal variation in attack rates of acute respiratory disease are not well understood. Adding to the complexity of the problem has been the discovery that some of the virus groups have their own seasonal pattern within the overall respiratory disease season. Rhinovirus outbreaks occur in the early fall and in mid- to late-spring,[15] and coronaviruses are most prominent in the winter.[13] Studies with a specific virus, rhinovirus type 15, showed that chilling of volunteers did not increase their susceptibility to infection and illness.[16] Thus the effect of thermal cold per se on the host does not appear to be the explanation for the seasonal outbreaks of colds.

Undoubtedly, among the responsible variables for seasonal fluctuations in colds are the bringing together of children during school periods and the increased crowding indoors of populations during colder months.[17] Also, seasonal changes in relative humidity may be an important variable controlling prevalence of the different virus families because of the effect of differing relative humidities on virus survival. In general, enveloped viruses survive better under conditions of low relative humidity, as found in colder months of the year, while the converse is true for nonenveloped viruses.

ATTACK RATES

During peak months in the respiratory disease season in the United States, adults average six to eight colds per 1000 persons per day.[15] In the summer, rates fall to two to three colds per 1000 per day. Overall, adults in the United States average two to four colds per year and children six to eight.[14,15] In one 10-year study of illness in families, young children in nursery school averaged up to nine colds for the period of September through May! Illness rates decline in older children and reach adult levels in adolescence. Men have slightly more colds than women up to the age of adolescence, but after that the incidence is slightly higher in women, perhaps reflecting their exposure to young children. Adults with children in the home have more colds than those without this exposure.[14,18] Tonsillectomy does not reduce the incidence of colds.[14] Cigarette smokers have the same incidence of colds as nonsmokers, but the severity of their illness is greater.[15,19]

TRANSMISSION

The main reservoir of respiratory viruses is in young children. Spread of colds takes place most commonly in the home[14,18] and school.[20] Children acquire new viral strains from their schoolmates, which they then bring home and pass to other family members. Two- to five-day intervals occur between cases. Secondary attack rates of family members vary, depending on age, position in the family, and prior immunity to the virus. Age and immunity are related risk factors. Young children and mothers have high secondary attack rates as a result of close and prolonged exposure to school children in the family. The secondary attack rate of fathers is relatively low.

The mechanism(s) for the spread of cold viruses has not been well established. Possible means of transmission include (*1*) direct contact with infectious secretions on skin and environmental surfaces, (*2*) large particles of respiratory secretions that are briefly transported in air, (*3*) infectious droplet nuclei suspended in air, and (*4*) combinations of these methods.[21] For some viruses, such as rhinovirus, close physical contact appears necessary for efficient spread. Infectious rhinovirus is produced primarily in the nose and is shed in highest concentrations in nasal secretions. Peak viral titers in nasal mucus occur on the second to fourth day of experimental infection and coincide with the period of maximum communicability.[21] A high proportion of persons with natural and experimental rhinovirus colds have recoverable virus on their hands. With experimental rhinovirus infection, brief hand contact permits ready transfer of virus-contaminated nasal secretions from the hands of infected subjects to the hands of susceptible subjects. When the contaminated fingers of the susceptible subjects are then placed in contact with the nasal and conjunctival mucosa, infection results in a high percentage of cases.[22] In a recent study, which has not been confirmed, treatment of the fingers with a virucidal solution reduced the rate of infection in mothers exposed to other family members with fresh colds.[23] This latter study provides the only direct evidence on the mechanisms of common cold transmission under natural conditions and suggests that a proportion of colds are spread by a hand contamination/self-inoculation route.

Another rhinovirus transmission model has been developed in which virus is reliably transmitted through the air in large-and/or small-particle aerosol.[24] This model demonstrates the feasibility of the aerosol route of spread but does not prove that it occurs under natural conditions. Studies conducted in the field with intervention techniques specific for aerosol transmission are needed to address that question. There is epidemiologic evidence that influenza and adenovirus may spread, at least in part, by small airborne droplets. Thus, all the respiratory viruses may not behave in the same way, and further studies are necessary to determine which route or routes of transmission are important in the natural dissemination of all these viruses.

PATHOGENESIS

Viral invasion of the upper respiratory tract is the basic mechanism in the pathogenesis of colds, but the specific events leading to clinical illness are not well understood. Infection with common cold viruses is characteristically of short duration and self-limited. For example, maximum rhinovirus shedding lasts 3 weeks or less in young adults with experimental colds,[25,26] and coronavirus excretion has been detected for only 1–4 days.[13] Cold viruses are not usually present in asymptomatic persons,[27] although subclinical infections do occur and viral carriage may be somewhat prolonged in children.[28]

Characteristic changes have been described in sloughed columnar epithelial cells in nasal secretions of persons with natural colds of unknown etiology.[29] Cells with persistent ciliary activity have been found in nasal secretions in the first through the third day of illness. Also, some exfoliated cells show degenerative changes characterized by progressive nuclear pyknosis and the formation of apparent inclusion bodies. More recently ciliated epithelial cells containing viral antigen have been found in the nasal mucus of volunteers with experimental rhinovirus colds.[30]

Attempts to demonstrate specific histopathologic changes in nasal biopsy specimens of volunteers with rhinovirus colds[31] or in rhinovirus-infected nasal polyp cultures[32] have not been successful. A subsequent study by light and electron microscopy of nasal biopsy specimens from young adults with natural colds confirmed the absence of destruction of the nasal epithelium.[33] In this study there was a significant increase in the number of neutrophils in the epithelium and in the lamina propria. The number of epithelial mast cells was not increased. The findings with rhinovirus contrast with the destructive changes to the respiratory epithelium that are seen with influenza virus infection.

With rhinovirus colds, the period of maximum viral excretion in nasal secretions coincides with the peak of clinical illness[34] and of appearance of ciliated epithelial cells in nasal mucus.[30] At that time, large quantities of protein, including immunoglobulins, are present in nasal secretions. In addition to any direct destructive effect that the virus may have on the respiratory mucous membrane, it is possible that immunologic mechanisms and chemical mediators may play a role in the pathogenesis of the common cold. In this regard, high concentrations of bradykinin and lysylbradykinin have been measured in nasal secretions of volunteers with experimental rhinovirus colds.[35] Pathogenic mechanisms for the various respiratory viruses are undoubtedly somewhat different.

The self-limited cold virus infection may lead to pathogenic events that affect the resident bacterial flora of the upper respiratory tract and result in secondary bacterial infection. Bacteria become able to invade normally sterile areas such as the sinuses, middle ear, and perhaps the tracheobronchial tree. The variables involved in triggering invasive bacterial infection are unknown but probably include viral damage to the mucociliary cleansing mechanism of the upper respiratory tract. It is currently unknown whether direct viral invasion of the sinus, middle ear, and tracheobronchial tree is necessary for subsequent bacterial infection to occur or whether the viral involvement can remain localized to the nasal and pharyngeal mucous membrane. However, respiratory viruses have been recovered from sinus[36] and middle ear[9] aspirates obtained by direct puncture from patients with acute infections at these sites. Abnormalities in eustachian tube function and middle ear pressures have been consistently observed in volunteers with experimental rhinovirus infection.[37] During colds, increases have also been noted in titers of resident bacterial populations of the upper airways, but the significance of this is unknown.[38,39]

CLINICAL CHARACTERISTICS

The incubation period of the common cold varies somewhat with the different viruses but is usually between 48 and 72 hours. The cardinal symptoms are nasal discharge, nasal obstruction, sneezing, sore or "scratchy" throat, and cough.[14,19] Slight fever may be found, but temperature elevation of more than a degree is distinctly uncommon in the adult. Infants and young children may have more frequent temperature elevation. The early symptoms may be minimal with only mild malaise and nasal complaints. With rhinovirus infection, sneezing, nasal discharge, and nasal obstruction usually begin simultaneously on the first day of illness and rapidly increase to maximum severity by the second or third day. Paralleling the nasal symptoms are sore, dry, or "scratchy" throat. Cough and hoarseness may also begin early in the course of illness and, when present, tend to persist until the end of the first week of symptoms by which time nasal and pharyngeal complaints have usually subsided. Limited information is available suggesting that symptom patterns are similar with coronavirus colds.[13]

The median duration of rhinovirus colds is 1 week, but in approximately one-quarter the illnesses last up to 2 weeks. In cigarette smokers with rhinovirus colds, cough is increased and prolonged. Other complaints include mild burning of the eyes; true conjunctivitis is not seen except in some adenovirus and enterovirus infections. There may also be loss of sense of smell and taste and a feeling of pressure in the ears or sinuses due to obstruction and/or mucosal swelling. The voice may have a nasal quality. Painful maceration of the skin around the nostrils is often bothersome when rhinorrhea has been profuse and persistent.

On physical examination the findings may be few despite the subjective discomfort of the patient. A red nose and a dripping nasal discharge are the characteristic features of the cold sufferer, but many patients have minimal outward manifestations of the infection. The nasal mucous membrane may have a glassy appearance due to the exudation of serum proteins and increased mucus secretions. It is difficult to judge accurately the presence of increased erythema of the mucous membrane of the nose and throat due to normal variations in the color of these structures. Marked pharyngeal erythema and exudate are not seen with rhinovirus and coronavirus infections, but they do occur with pharyngoconjunctival fever of adenovirus infection. Examination of the chest may reveal the presence of rhonchi.

The clinical picture of the common cold is similar in children and adults. However, in young children parainfluenza virus and respiratory syncytial virus infection may lead to viral pneumonia, croup, and bronchiolitis, while in adults these viruses usually cause only colds. In both adults and children the upper airway manifestations of rhinovirus, coronavirus, parainfluenza virus, and respiratory syncytial virus infections are indistinguishable in the individual patient.

DIAGNOSIS

The manifestations of the common cold are so typical that self-diagnosis by the patient is usually correct. Hay fever and vasomotor rhinitis may give similar nasal symptoms, but the recurrent and chronic nature of these diseases is soon recognized by the patient and easily diagnosed by the physician from the patient's history. Diagnosis of the specific virus involved is usually not possible on the basis of clinical observation. Some acute respiratory infections, such as influenza and pharyngoconjunctival fever, when seen in a typical epidemiologic setting, can be recognized without benefit of viral culture or serologic tests. Knowledge of the characteristic seasonal patterns for the different virus groups may also aid in the identification of a particular virus.

The main challenge to the physician is to distinguish the uncomplicated cold from the approximately 0.5 percent of cases with secondary bacterial sinusitis and the 2 percent with otitis media.[14] This is not easy because of the lack of inexpensive and noninvasive diagnostic tests for these infections. A complete examination should be performed on the pharynx, nasal cavity, ears, and sinuses. In the pharynx, marked injection or exudate should raise suspicion of streptococcal or adenovirus infection, Vincent's angina, mononucleosis, or diphtheria. Occasionally, patients have small vesicles on the palate due to coxsackievirus A infections. The presence of nasal polyps is suggestive of an underlying allergic problem. In children, a foreign body may lead to persistent nasal discharge. Examination of the ears is directed at finding changes in the appearance of the tympanum, indicating infection (see Chapter 46). The use of the pneumatic otoscope is helpful in determining if fluid is present behind the ear drum. The sinuses should be examined by transillumination under optimal conditions (see Chapter 47).

Sinus radiography is a sensitive diagnostic test for infection of the sinuses, but the expense of the procedure has prevented its widespread use. The most valuable laboratory test in patients with pharyngeal complaints is rapid antigen detection for group A β-hemolytic streptococci. Many of the respiratory viruses can be isolated in cell culture, although specific virologic diagnosis is not usually available in clinical practice. Rhinoviruses grow in human embryonic lung cells (WI-38), myxo- and paramyxoviruses in primary Rhesus monkey kidney cells, and respiratory syncytial virus in Hep 2 cells. Isolation of coronavirus in cell culture has proved difficult with currently available techniques. The sensitivity of the tests for isolating viruses can vary widely with changes in the sensitivity of the cell cultures.

The serologic diagnosis of influenza, parainfluenza, respiratory syncytial, and adenovirus infection is available in some state health department laboratories. Serum specimens should be obtained in the acute phase of illness and approximately 3 weeks later and tested simultaneously. A fourfold or greater rise in antibody titer is indicative of infection. Serologic diagnosis of rhinovirus infection is not practical because of the many different antigenic types. Rapid techniques using fluorescent antibody or other immunodiagnostic procedures on respiratory secretions may become practical in the future and would be useful if antiviral chemotherapy becomes available.

TREATMENT

Only symptomatic treatment is available for the uncomplicated common cold. Individual measures directed at controlling nasal and pharyngeal complaints and cough are more effective than all-inclusive cold remedies found in tablets and capsules. Direct application to the nasal membrane of vasoconstrictors such as 0.5 or 0.25% phenylephrine or 1% ephedrine drops or sprays are recommended to provide symptomatic relief of nasal obstructions and to promote drainage of nasal secretions. Patients should be instructed to place themselves in a head down position when administering decongestants to achieve penetration of the drug to inaccessible areas of the nasal cavity. An interval of approximately 1 minute should be allowed between three separate applications of drops or spray. Decongestants should be used every 4 hours on a regular basis. Patients should be cautioned on the rebound effect that results if decongestants are used continuously for more than 3 or 4 days. Recently, it has been shown that intranasal application of a topically active parasympatholygic, ipratropium, was effective in reducing nasal secretions.[40]

Sore throat is relieved by warm saline gargles and cough by liquids or cough drops containing dextromethorphan. Cough suppression in the severe case is best achieved with preparations containing codeine. The regular application of an ointment containing a petrolatum base is useful in controlling painful maceration of the nares. Aspirin and bed rest are of value when headache and constitutional symptoms are prominent. The patient should restrict his activities during the height of the illness, at which time he is most contagious to others. Regular handwashing and care to avoid contamination of the environment with nasal secretions may also help to prevent spread.

Antibiotics have no place in the treatment of uncomplicated colds, and antihistamines have only a minimal effect in reducing nasal secretions.[41] Until truly effective and specific treatment becomes available, there will continue to be fads in the use of unproven cold remedies. The ingestion of large doses of vitamin C has been widely used as a preventive or therapeutic measure for colds. In some instances, controlled studies have shown a modest beneficial effect of vitamin C for colds. However, a careful analysis of the studies has indicated that a placebo effect could not be ruled out. Many participants correctly surmised from the taste of the contents of the capsules used whether they were receiving vitamin C or a placebo.[42] In volunteers experimentally infected with rhinovirus, vitamin C in doses of 3 g/day was not effective in preventing infection and illness.[43,44]

PROSPECTS FOR CONTROL

Vaccine development has reached an impasse because of the discovery of the many different cold viruses, particularly the 100 rhinoviruses. Unless ways are found to combine large numbers of viral antigens effectively or to take advantage of minor antigenic cross-relationships that exist, prospects for common cold vaccines are not good. A number of chemical compounds have inhibitory activity against respiratory viruses in tissue culture systems, and attempts are being made to develop antiviral agents for clinical use. The activity of such compounds tends to be relatively group-specific, but some have shown activity against most of the rhinoviruses.

The most promising approach to control of colds has come through the development of interferon. Topically applied intranasal recombinant human interferon-α_2 has a highly effective prophylactic activity against experimental rhinovirus infection.[45–47] When given therapeutically in the same manner, interferon has reduced viral excretion, but its effect on development of illness has been of only minimal to moderate benefit.[48] In addition, topically applied intranasal interferon, when used longer than approximately 1 week, is associated with local side effects in the nose, such as stuffiness, dryness, discomfort, and pinpoint areas of ulceration.[49–51] To avoid these problems associated with the biologic properties of interferon, a strategy has been proposed and tested that employs short-term contact prophylaxis by family members exposed to individuals with colds of recent onset. Using this approach, two field studies have observed an approximately 40 percent reduction of total colds and a virtual elimination of rhinovirus-specific infections in exposed individuals.[52,53] Side effects were avoided by the short duration of application of the interferon. The success of these studies is a cause for optimism, although topical interferon-α_2 apparently failed to prevent colds due to viruses other than those in the rhinovirus group. The failure of a "broad spectrum" antiviral agent, such as interferon, to be effective for all cold viruses emphasizes the reality of the need to develop individual approaches for the different virus groups.

Another approach under investigation is to develop ways to interrupt the transmission of colds. Since spread of some viruses may occur by direct hand contact/self-inoculation, handwashing and avoiding finger-to-nose and finger-to-eye contact should be practiced, particularly with exposure to a cold sufferer. It may be possible to develop virucidal preparations for use on the hands that interrupt transmission of infection.[23] Also, covering coughs and sneezes with disposable nasal tissues is recommended as a means of controlling aerosol transmission.

REFERENCES

1. Rice DP, Feldman JJ, White KL. The current burden of illness in the United States. Occasional Papers of the Institute of Medicine. Washington, DC: National Academy of Sciences; 1976:1.
2. Chanock RM. Association of a new type of cytopathogenic myxovirus with infantile croup. J Exp Med. 1956;104:55.
3. Pelon W, Mogabgab WJ, Phillips IA, et al. A cytopathogenic agent isolated from naval recruits with mild respiratory illness. Proc Soc. Exp Biol Med. 1957;94:262.
4. Price WH. The isolation of a new virus associated with respiratory clinical disease in humans. Proc Natl Acad Sci USA. 1956;43:892.
5. Chanock RM, Roizman B, Myers R. Recovery from infants with respiratory illness of a virus related to Chimpanzee Coryza Agent (CCA). I. Isolation, properties, and characterization. Am J Hyg. 1957;66:281.
6. Lennette EH, Fox VL, Schmidt NJ, et al: The COE virus: an apparently new virus recovered from patients with mild respiratory disease. Am J Hyg. 1958;68:272.
7. Tyrrell DAJ, Bynoe ML. Cultivation of a novel type of common-cold virus in organ cultures. Br Med J. 1965;1:1467.
8. Hamre D, Procknow JJ: A new virus isolated from the human respiratory tract. Proc Soc Exp Biol Med. 1966;121:190.
9. Gwaltney JM Jr. Virology of middle ear. Ann Otol Rhinol Laryngol 1971;80:365.
10. Stuart-Harris CH, Andrewes C, Andrews BE, et al. A collaborative study of the aetiology of acute respiratory infection in Britain 1961–4. A report of the Medical Research Council working party on acute respiratory virus infections. Br Med J. 1965;2:319.
11. Hamre D, Connelly AP Jr, Procknow JJ. Virologic studies of acute respiratory disease in young adults. IV. Virus isolations during four years of surveillance. Am J Epidemiol. 1966;83:238.
12. Monto AS, Ullman BM. Acute respiratory illness in an American community; the Tecumseh study. JAMA. 1974;227:164.
13. Monto AS. Coronaviruses. In Evans AS, ed. Viral Infections of Humans: Epidemiology and Control. New York: Plenum; 1982:151.
14. Dingle JH, Badger GF, Jordan WS Jr. Illness in the Home: Study of 25,000 Illnesses in a Group of Cleveland Families. Cleveland: The Press of Western Reserve University; 1964:1.
15. Gwaltney JM Jr, Hendley JO, Simon G, et al. Rhinovirus infections in an industrial population. I. The occurrence of illness. N Engl J Med. 1966;275:1261.
16. Douglas RG Jr, Lindgren KM, Couch RB. Exposure to cold environment and

rhinovirus common cold: failure to demonstrate effect. N Engl J Med. 1968;279:743.
17. Gwaltney JM Jr. The Jeremiah Metzger Lecture. Climatology and the common cold. Trans Am Clin Climatol Assoc. 1984;96:159.
18. Hendley JO, Gwaltney JM Jr, Jordan WS Jr. Rhinovirus infections in an industrial population. IV. Infections within families of employees during two fall peaks of respiratory illness. Am J Epidemiol. 1969;89:184.
19. Gwaltney JM Jr, Hendley JO, Simon G, et al. Rhinovirus infections in an industrial population. II. Characteristics of illness and antibody response. JAMA. 1967;202:494.
20. Beem MO. Acute respiratory illness in nursery school children: a longitudinal study of the occurrence of illness and respiratory viruses. Am J Epidemiol. 1969;90:30.
21. Gwaltney JM Jr. Epidemiology of the common cold. Ann NY Acad Sci. 1980;353:54.
22. Gwaltney JM Jr, Moskalski PB, Hendley JO. Hand-to-hand transmission of rhinovirus colds. Ann Intern Med. 1978;88:463.
23. Hendley JO, Gwaltney JM Jr. Mechanisms of transmission of rhinovirus infections. Epidemiol Rev. 1988;10:242.
24. Dick EC, Jennings LC, Mink KA, et al. Aerosol transmission of rhinovirus colds. J Infect Dis. 1987;156:442.
25. Cate TR, Couch RB, Johnson KM. Studies with rhinoviruses in volunteers: production of illness, effect of naturally acquired antibody, and demonstration of a protective effect not associated with serum antibody. J Clin Invest. 1964;43:56.
26. Winther B, Gwaltney JM Jr, Mygind N, et al. Sites of rhinovirus recovery after point inoculation of the upper airway. JAMA. 1986;256:1763.
27. Hamre D, Rhinoviruses. In: Melnick JL, ed. Monographs in Virology 1. Basel: Karger;1968:1.
28. Frank AL, Taber LH, Wells CR, et al. Patterns of shedding of myxoviruses in children. J Infect Dis. 1981;144:433.
29. Bryan WTK, Bryan MP, Smith CA. Human ciliated epithelial cells in nasal secretions. Transactions of the 85th Annual Meeting of the American Laryngological Association. 1964:145.
30. Turner RB, Hendley JO, Gwaltney JM Jr. Shedding of infected ciliated epithelial cells in rhinovirus colds. J Infect Dis. 1982;145:849.
31. Douglas RG, Jr, Alford BR, Couch RB. Atraumatic nasal biopsy for studies of respiratory virus infection in volunteers. Antimicrob Agents Chemother. 1968;8:340.
32. Hamory BH, Hendley JO, Gwaltney JM Jr. Rhinovirus growth in nasal polyp organ culture. Proc Soc Exp Biol Med. 1977;155:577.
33. Winther B, Brofeldt S, Christensen B, Mygind N. Light and scanning electron microscopy of nasal biopsies from patients with naturally acquired common colds. Acta Otolarungol. 1984;97:309.
34. Douglas RG Jr, Cate TR, Gerone PJ, et al. Quantitative rhinovirus shedding patterns in volunteers. Am Rev Respir Dis. 1966;94:159.
35. Naclerio RM, Proud D, Lichtenstein LM, et al. Kinins are generated during experimental rhinovirus colds. J Infect Dis. 1988;157:133.
36. Evans FO Jr, Sydnor JB, Moore WEC, et al. Sinusitis of the maxillary antrum. N Engl J Med. 1975;293:735.
37. Doyle WJ, McBride TP, Skoner DP, et al. A double blind placebo-controlled clinical trial of the effect of chlorpheniramine on the response of the nasal airway, middle ear and eustachian tube to provocative rhinovirus challenge. Pediatr Infect Dis J. 1988;7:222.
38. Straker E, Hill AB, Lovell RA. A study of the nasopharyngeal bacterial flora of different groups of persons observed in London and south-east England during the years 1930 to 1937. Reports on Public Health and Medical Subjects, no. 90. London: His Majesty's Stationery Office; 1939:7.
39. Brimblecombe FSW, Cruickshank R, Master P, et al. Family studies of respiratory infections. Br Med J. 1958;1:119.
40. Borum P, Olsen L, Winther B, and Mygind N. Ipratropium nasal spray: a new treatment for rhinorrhea in the common cold. Am Rev Respir Dis. 1981;123:418.
41. Howard JC Jr, Kantner TR, Lilienfield LS, et al. Efféctiveness of antihistamines in the symptomatic management of the common cold. JAMA. 1979;242:2414.
42. Chalmers TC. Effects of ascorbic acid on the common cold. An evaluation of the evidence. Am J Med. 1975;58:532.
43. Walker GH, Bynoe ML, Tyrrell DAJ. Trial of ascorbic acid in prevention of colds. Br Med J. 1967;1:603.
44. Schwartz AR, Togo Y, Hornick RB, et al. Evaluation of the efficacy of ascorbic acid in prophylaxis of induced rhinovirus 44 infection in man. J Infect Dis. 1973;128:500.
45. Scott GM, Phillpotts RJ, Wallace J, et al. Purified interferon as protection against rhinovirus infections. Br Med J. 1982;284:1822.
46. Hayden FG, Gwaltney JM Jr. Intranasal interferon-alpha$_2$ for prevention of rhinovirus infection and illness. J Infect Dis. 1983;148:543.
47. Samo T-C, Greenberg SB, Couch RB Jr, et al. Evaluations of efficacy and tolerance to intranasally applied recombinant leukocyte A interferon in normal volunteers. J Infect Dis. 1983;148:535.
48. Hayden FG, Gwaltney JM Jr. Intranasal interferon-α_2 treatment of experimental rhinoviral colds. J Infect Dis. 1984;150:174.
49. Farr BM, Gwaltney JM Jr, Adams KF, et al. Intranasal interferon-α_2 for prevention of natural rhinovirus colds. Antimicrob Agents Chemother. 1984;26:31.
50. Douglas RM, Albrecht JK, Miles HB, et al. Intranasal interferon-α_2 prophylaxis of natural respiratory virus infection. J Infect Dis. 1985;151:731.
51. Hayden FG, Gwaltney JM Jr, Johns ME. Prophylactic efficacy and tolerance of low-dose intranasal interferon-alpha$_2$ in natural respiratory viral infections. Antiviral Res. 1985;5:11.
52. Hayden FG, Albrecht JK, Kaiser DL, et al. Prevention of natural colds by contact prophylaxis with intranasal alpha$_2$-interferon. New Engl J Med. 1986;314:71.
53. Douglas RM, Moore BW, Miles HB, et al. Prophylactic efficacy of intranasal alpha$_2$-interferon against rhinovirus infections in the family setting. N Engl J Med. 1986;314:65.

43. PHARYNGITIS

JACK M. GWALTNEY, JR.

Acute pharyngitis is an inflammatory syndrome of the pharynx caused by several different groups of microorganisms. Most cases are of viral etiology and occur as part of common ccold and influenzal syndromes. The most important of the bacterial infections is due to the group A β-hemolytic streptoccoccus (*Streptococcus pyogenes*). It is important to differentiate streptococcal from viral pharyngitis because of the response of streptococcal infection to penicillin therapy and the ineffectiveness of antibiotic therapy in the viral infections. Also streptococcal pharyngitis may be complicated by acute rheumatic fever and acute glomerulonephritis. There are other uncommon or rare types of pharyngitis that are of clinical importance, and the list of these conditions continues to grow as new etiologic associations are established.

ETIOLOGY

The known microbial causes of pharyngitis are shown in Table 1. The relative importance of the different agents is not fully defined, and it is still not possible to determine the cause of a sizable proportion of cases. The results of epidemiologic investigations are influenced by the season of the year, the age of the population, the severity of illness, and the diagnostic methods used in the various studies. The importance of the various agents listed in Table 1 are known to cause acute respiratory illness[1–4] and on the results of specific studies of the cause of pharyngitis.[5,6] A large amount of mild pharyngitis is associated with rhinovirus and coronavirus colds. Adenovirus and herpes simplex virus pharyngitis, although less common, are important because of their clinical severity. Others of the known respiratory viruses each account for a small proportion of cases. Primary human immunodeficiency syndrome (HIV) infection has joined the list of viral infections associated with acute pharyngitis.[7]

Approximately 15 percent of all cases of pharyngitis are due to *S. pyogenes*. In children with sore throat, *S. pyogenes* may cause up to half of the cases during some periods. The importance of non-group A β-hemolytic streptococci as a cause of pharyngitis is not entirely clear. While non-group A β-hemolytic streptococci, especially strains in groups C and G, have been associated with food-borne outbreaks of pharyngitis,[8,9] non-group A strains have not been clearly implicated in the nonepidemic setting.[10–12] Mixed anaerobic bacterial infection (Vincent's angina) causes an occasional case of acute pharyngitis as does *Corynebacterium diphtheriae, Corynebacterium hemolyticum, Yersinia entero colitica*, and *Neisseria gonorrhoeae*.

Mycoplasma pneumoniae has been associated with pharyngitis since the late 1950s,[13] but in epidemiologic studies of unselected patients, *M. pneumoniae* has not been an important cause of the disease.[5,6,10,11,14] The role of chlamydial infections in pharyngitis is under continuing investigation. A report of an association with *C. trachomatis*[15] was not confirmed,[11,16,17] but

TABLE 1. Microbial Causes of Acute Pharyngitis

	Syndrome/Disease	Estimated Importance[a]
Viral		
Rhinovirus (89 types and 1 subtype)	Common cold	20
Coronavirus (4 or more types)	Common cold	≥5
Adenovirus (types 3, 4, 7, 14, 21)	Pharyngoconjunctival fever, ARD	5
Herpes simplex virus (types 1 and 2)	Gingivitis, stomatitis, pharyngitis	4
Parainfluenza virus (types 1–4)	Common cold, croup	2
Influenza virus (types A and B)	Influenza	2
Coxsackievirus A (types 2, 4–6, 8, 10)	Herpangina	<1
Epstein-Barr virus	Infectious mononucleosis	<1
Cytomegalovirus	Infectious mononucleosis	<1
Human immunodeficiency virus	Primary HIV infection	<1
Bacterial		
Streptococcus pyogenes (group A β-hemolytic streptococcus)	Pharyngitis/tonsillitis, scarlet fever	15–30
Mixed anaerobic infection	Gingivitis, pharyngitis (Vincent's angina)	<1
	Peritonsillitis/peritonsillar abscess (quinsy)	<1
Neisseria gonorrhoeae	Pharyngitis	<1
Corynebacterium diphtheriae	Diphtheria	≥1
Corynebacterium ulcerans	Pharyngitis, diphtheria	<1
Corynebacterium hemolyticum (*Arcanobacterium hemolyticum*)	Pharyngitis, scarlatiniform rash	<1
Yersinia enterocolitica	Pharyngitis, enterocolitis	<1
Treponema pallidum	Secondary syphilis	<1
Chlamydial		
Chlamydia psittaci	ARD, pneumonia	Unknown
Mycoplasmal		
Mycoplasma pneumoniae	Pneumonia/bronchitis/pharyngitis	<1
M. hominis (type 1)	Pharyngitis in volunteers	Unknown
Unknown		40

[a] Estimated percentage of cases of pharyngitis due to indicated organism in civilians of all ages.

the TWAR strain of *C. psittaci* has recently been isolated from patients who have pharyngitis associated with febrile bronchitis and pneumonia.[18]

EPIDEMIOLOGY

Most pharyngitis occurs during the colder months of the year, during the respiratory disease season. Viral agents such as rhinoviruses tend to have annual periods of peak prevalence, which are most important in the fall and spring; coronaviruses have been found most often in the winter. Influenza appears in epidemics, which in the United States usually occur between December and April. In military recruits adenoviruses cause the syndrome acute respiratory disease (ARD) during the colder months. In civilians wintertime ARD occurs as well as epidemics of pharyngoconjunctival fever in the summer. Streptococcal pharyngitis occurs during the respiratory disease season, with peak rates of infection in late winter and early spring. The reservoir for the agents that cause pharyngitis is in humans. For details on the epidemiologic behavior of these organisms, the reader is referred to the chapters dealing with each.

PATHOGENESIS

Symptoms of sore or scratchy throat occur in approximately 50 percent of people with rhinovirus colds[19] and in 20–70 percent of people with respiratory illness due to coronavirus.[20,21] Pharyngeal complaints are present in up to 80 percent of people with parainfluenza virus illness[22] and in approximately 50 percent of people with type A influenza[19] and adenovirus illness.[22] Other viral respiratory illnesses with pharyngitis occur with coxsackievirus A21, echoviruses 6 and 20,[22] herpes simplex virus,[23] Epstein-Barr (EB) virus, and cytomegalovirus infections.

The pathogenic mechanisms are undoubtedly different for the various organisms. Nasal epithelial biopsies obtained from volunteers with experimental rhinovirus infections have shown little or no evidence of viral cytopathic effect.[24,25] However, it has recently been discovered that bradykinin and lysylbradykinin are generated in the nasal passages of persons with experimental rhinovirus colds.[26] These inflammatory mediators are potent stimulators of pain nerve endings. Also, volunteers given experimental intranasal challenge with bradykinin have developed symptoms of sore throat.[27] With other respiratory virus infections, such as adenovirus and coxsackievirus, there is evidence that direct invasion of pharyngeal mucosa occurs.

The events leading to invasive streptococcal infection of the pharynx and tonsil are also not well understood. Pharyngeal carriage of *S. pyogenes* is commonly observed in asymptomatic people. Factors that influence the balance between colonization and invasive infection may include natural and acquired host immunity and interference among the bacteria present in the oropharynx. *Streptococcus pyogenes* elaborates a number of extracellular factors, including erythrogenic toxin, hemolysins, streptokinase, deoxyribonuclease, proteinase, and hyaluronidase, which are of known or possible pathogenic importance.

The usual pathologic changes occurring in viral pharyngitis are edema and hyperemia of the tonsils and the pharyngeal mucous membrane. An inflammatory exudate may be present with adenovirus and EB virus infections; with the latter, nasopharyngeal lymphoid hyperplasia also occurs. Vesiculation and mucosal ulceration may occur with herpes simplex virus and some coxsackievirus A infections. With streptococcal pharyngitis there is an intense, inflammatory response in the pharyngeal membrane, and there may be exudate and hemorrhage of the tonsils and pharyngeal walls. With diphtheria a fibrous pseudomembrane containing necrotic epithelium, leukocytes, and bacterial colonies develops on the epithelial surface.

CLINICAL PRESENTATION

Pharyngitis with the Common Cold

Mild-to-moderate pharyngeal discomfort is frequently present during a cold but is often not the primary complaint. The symptom is characterized as soreness, scratchiness, or irritation. Severe pharyngeal pain and dysphagia are not characteristic of this type of pharyngitis. Nasal symptoms and cough are also usually present. Systemic complaints of feverishness, chilliness, malaise, and myalgia are not prominent, and a temperature elevation is unusual in adults and older children. On examination, the pharynx may appear normal or show a mild amount of edema and erythema. Rhinorrhea and postnasal discharge are usually present, but pharyngeal and tonsillar exudates and painful lymphadenopathy are not seen. Pharyngeal complaints usually subside over 3 or 4 days, and most patients have recovered by the end of a week (see Chapter 42).

Pharyngitis with Influenza

Sore throat is a major complaint in some patients with influenza. It is usually associated with other manifestations of the disease, such as myalgia, headache, and cough.[10,19] Coryzal symptoms and hoarseness may also be present. Temperature elevations are common in both adults and children, reaching levels of 38.3°C or higher. Edema and erythema of the pharyngeal mucosa may be present but are not marked. Pharyngeal exudates and painful cervical adenopathy are not present. Defervescence occurs in 3–4 days on the average, but in some uncomplicated cases fever may last up to a week (see Chapter 142).

Pharyngoconjunctival Fever

The clinical presentation of adenoviral pharyngitis is usually more severe than pharyngitis associated with the common cold. Malaise, myalgia, headache, chills, and dizziness often accompany adenovirus infections. Temperature elevations persist for 5–6 days in studies of recognized cases. Sore throat is often marked. On examination, pharyngeal erythema and exudate may be present, mimicking streptococcal pharyngitis. A distinguishing feature of adenovirus pharyngitis, when present, is conjunctivitis, which occurs in one-third to one-half of cases. The conjunctivitis is of the follicular type and is bilateral in about one-fourth of the cases when it occurs. Cough, hoarseness, and substernal pain occur in ARD in military recruits but are usually not prominent features of pharyngoconjunctival fever (see Chapter 122).

Acute Herpetic Pharyngitis

Primary infection with herpes simplex virus may present as an acute pharyngitis. Mild cases are indistinguishable from those caused by other respiratory viruses. In severe cases of herpetic pharyngitis, the presence of inflammation and exudate may mimic full-blown streptococcal pharyngitis. Vesicles and shallow ulcers of the palate are characteristic of herpetic infection and when present are helpful in the differential diagnosis. Tender cervical adenopathy and fever are seen in some cases. Vesicles or ulcers are present on the labial and buccal mucosa when there is an associated gingivostomatitis. Acute primary herpetic infection should be distinguished from chronic mucocutaneous infection of the oropharynx due to herpes simplex virus. The chronic form of the disease is seen exclusively in patients with impaired immunity and is characterized by large shallow, painful ulcers that slowly progress unless the patient's immune status improves or antiviral therapy is given (see Chapter 118).

Herpangina

This uncommon type of pharyngitis caused by coxsackieviruses is distinguished by the presence of small vesicles (1–2 mm) on the soft palate, uvula, and anterior tonsillar pillars. The lesions rupture to become small white ulcers. Herpangina has been recognized primarily in children, in whom it may manifest as a severe febrile illness with marked sore throat and dysphagia. In some cases anorexia and abdominal pain mimic acute appendicitis (see Chapter 150).

Infectious Mononucleosis

Exudative tonsillitis or pharyngitis occurs in approximately one half the cases of infectious mononucleosis due to the EB virus. Fever and cervical adenopathy are usually present. The pharyngeal complaints of mononucleosis are usually associated with other characteristic features of the disease, such as headache and persistent malaise and fatigue. Generalized adenopathy may be present, and there is enlargement of the spleen in approximately half the cases. The mononucleosis syndrome is also associated with cytomegalovirus infection. Some patients with cytomegalovirus mononucleosis have pharyngeal soreness, but examination of the pharynx is usually unremarkable (see Chapters 120 and 121).

HIV Infection

Febrile pharyngitis is a characteristic feature of primary infection with human immunodeficiency virus (HIV).[12,28] Following an incubation period of 3–5 weeks, patients have developed fever and pharyngitis associated with varying amounts of myalgia, arthralgia, lethargy, and in some cases nonpruritic maculopapular rash. This has been followed in approximately 1 week by the development of lymphadenopathy. Pharyngeal hyperemia, sometimes marked, has been noted as well as mucosal ulcerations, but exudate has not been described (see Chapter 108).

Streptococcal Pharyngitis

The severity of illness associated with *S. pyogenes* infection of the pharynx varies greatly. In a severe case, there is marked pharyngeal pain, dysphagia, and a temperature of 39.4°C or greater. The pharyngeal membrane is a fiery red, and a thick exudate covers the posterior pharynx and tonsillar area. Edema of the uvula is often pronounced. Tender, enlarged cervical nodes and a leukocyte count of over 12,000/mm^3 complete the picture of an acute suppurative bacterial infection. At the other extreme are those streptococcal infections that are so mild as to go unrecognized by the patient or that are indistinguishable from pharyngitis caused by the common respiratory viruses. Infection with strains of *S. pyogenes* that produce erythrogenic toxin results in the characteristic erythematous rash of scarlet fever (see Chapter 176).

The clinical features of pharyngeal infection with strains of groups C and G streptococci are similar to those of *S. pyogenes*, including the occurrence of purulent exudates.[14] Most identified cases occur in the setting of a common source food epidemic; cold hard-boiled eggs are recognized as an important vehicle.

Anaerobic Pharyngitis (Vincent's Angina) / Peritonsillitis/Peritonsillar Abscess (Quinsy)

Pharyngeal and tonsillar infection with a mixture of anaerobic bacteria and spirochetes, while uncommon, still occurs. *Streptococcus pyogenes* and *Staphylococcus aureus* may play a role in some cases. With this infection, a purulent exudate coats the membrane, and there may be a foul odor to the breath. Postanginal septicemia (Lemierre's disease) is a specific form of the condition caused by *Fusobacterium necrophorum*.[29] It is associated with jugular vein septic thrombophlebitis and metastatic infection to the lung and other sites. The disease is most common in adolescents and young adults. Exudative tonsillitis or peritonsillar abscess may be present but in some patients will have subsided by the time the patient is seen. With jugular vein thrombophelebitis, there is pain, swelling, neck stiffness, and dysphagia.

With development of an abscess, pharyngeal pain is usually severe, and dysphagia and low grade fever are common. On examination, there is inflammation and swelling of the peritonsillar area with medial displacement of the tonsil. The infection is usually limited to one side, but when the condition is bilateral, partial obstruction of the pharynx occurs. Rarely, there is extension of the infection along the carotid sheath and into the mediastinum.[30] (see Chapter 49).

Gonorrheal Pharyngitis

The incidence of gonococcal infections of the pharynx has increased in recent years. Most infections are asymptomatic, but gonorrheal infection may be responsible for an occasional case of mild pharyngitis[190] (see Chapter 190).

Diphtheria

Although uncommon today, diphtheria still occurs in unvaccinated populations in the United States. The disease characteristically has a slow onset, and pharyngeal discomfort is usually not marked. Temperature elevation is present but is low grade. The characteristic tonsillar or pharyngeal membrane varies from light to dark gray and is firmly adherent to the tonsil and pharyngeal mucosa. Human infection with *Corynebacterium ulcerans* is a rare cause of human pharyngeal infection. It is associated with the consumption of raw milk and has presented as mild pharyngitis but in one case presented as serious diphtheria[32] (see Chapter 183).

Corynebacterium hemolyticum has been increasingly identified as a cause of exudative pharyngitis.[33–35] Characteristically, the infection has been recognized in adolescents and young adults and is associated with a diffuse, sometimes pruritic, erythematous maculopapular skin rash on the extremities and trunk. Cases of *C. hemolyticum* with membranous pharyngitis that mimics diphtheria[36] and with peritonsillar abscess[37] have also been reported.

Yersinial Pharyngitis

Yersinia enterocolitica causes exudative pharyngitis, which in adults may occur without the typical enterocolitis seen in children. Fever, prominent cervical lymphadenopathy, and abdominal pain with or without diarrhea have been reported.[38] A fulminant course with high mortality has been associated with reported cases of yersinial pharyngitis, making recognition important.

Mycoplasmal Pharyngitis

Epidemiologic studies of pharyngitis have associated some cases with *Mycoplasma pneumoniae* infection. The illnesses observed have been relatively mild and have had no distinguishing clinical features. *Mycoplasma pneumoniae* characteristically causes bronchitis and primary atypical pneumonia (see Chapter 162).

Noninfectious Pharyngitis

Occasional cases presenting as an inflammatory pharyngitis may have noninfectious causes. These include conditions such as bullous pemphigoid, systemic lupus erythematosis, Behçet's disease, and paraquat ingestion. Kawasaki syndrome may present as a febrile sore throat without exudate. It occurs in children and is associated with characteristic findings of the lips, tongue, and skin.

DIAGNOSIS

The primary objectives in the diagnosis of acute pharyngitis are to distinguish cases of common viral etiology from those due to *S. pyogenes* and to detect and identify the occasional case due to an unusual or rare cause. In the majority of cases, an etiologic diagnosis is not possible on clinical grounds alone. The presence of pharyngeal or tonsillar exudates, skin rash, or conjunctivitis aids in the differential diagnosis, but these findings are not present with sufficient frequency to be helpful in most cases.

The list of etiologic agents associated with the presence of pharyngeal exudate include groups A, C, and G streptococci; the anaerobic bacteria; *C. diphtheriae; C. hemolyticum; Y. enterocolitica*; adenovirus; herpes simplex virus; and EB virus. However, pharyngeal exudate is not always present with these infections so that its absence does not exclude them from consideration. On the other hand, exudate is rarely, if ever, seen in the large group of cases of pharyngitis due to the common cold viruses and influenza. The presence of skin rash suggests the possibility of infection with *S. pyogenes, C. hemolyticum,* HIV, and EB virus. Toxic shock syndrome should also be considered. The presence of conjunctivitis suggests adenovirus infection.

The development of rapid antigen detection tests, using a specimen collected by throat swab, has been a significant advance in the diagnosis of streptococcal pharyngitis. Tests employing a latex agglutination system are highly specific (95–99%) and moderately sensitive (70–90%), compared with throat culture.[39–41] Also, newer solid phase enzyme immunoassay tests, which give similar results, are becoming available.[42] The performance characteristics of the antigen detection tests have dictated a strategy in which a positive test establishes the diagnosis of streptococcal pharyngitis, while a negative test should be followed by a standard throat culture on sheep blood agar. Among the advantages of routinely performing an antigen detection test and/or culture in patients with pharyngitis are that the test results may influence the management of family members and other close contacts who subsequently become ill, and a negative test should prompt consideration of the more unusual, and sometimes serious, causes of pharyngeal infection, especially in patients with fever and exudative disease.

The patient's history and a consideration of epidemiologic factors may be helpful in suggesting a specific etiologic diagnosis in cases in which the antigen detection test is negative. Other family members frequently have common colds and influenzal illnesses. The season of the year and the occurrence of known epidemics may provide clues of diagnosis. Rhinovirus infections predominate in the fall and spring and coronavirus infections in the winter. The occurrence of an influenza epidemic in the community is usually known to the physician. Patients with pharyngoconjunctival fever, a summer illness, may give a history of swimming, and they or a family member may have conjunctivitis. The diagnosis of infectious mononucleosis, primary HIV infection, and diphtheria may be suggested by the nonpharyngeal manifestations of these infections.

Examination of the structures of the pharynx should be thorough and should include mirror examination of the nasopharynx and larynx when diphtheria is suspected. In children under the age of 3 years, the presence of an exudate is a less reliable indicator of streptococcal infection than it is in older children and adults. Diphtheria produces a pseudomembrane that may be mistaken for an exudate. The presence of small vesicles or ulcers suggests herpes simplex virus infection or herpangina. The mucosal lesions of herpangina are less numerous and more confined to the area of the palate than those of herpes simplex virus, which may involve the entire oropharynx. Aphthous stomatitis, a benign condition of unknown cause, produces small painful mucosal ulcers that are sometimes confused with those of herpetic infection. Aphthosis tends to be recurrent, in contrast to acute herpetic pharyngitis, and with the usual case of aphthosis there are fewer lesions, which are usually located in the anterior part of the mouth.

Medial displacement of one or both tonsils is seen with peritonsillitis or peritonsillar abscess, and dysphagia may be present. Patients with postanginal septicemia with jugular vein thrombophlebitis will have malaise, fever, and chills, suggestive of serious illness. Also pain, tenderness, and swelling at the angle of the jaw and stiff neck are characteristic, but these findings may be subtle. Patients with infectious mononucleosis usually have generalized adenopathy and may have enlargement of the spleen. Severe sore throat and odynophagia in an adult in the absence of findings in the pharynx should suggest epiglottitis (Chapter 48).

Laboratory tests are available to help in the diagnosis of some of the above-mentioned infections. *Neisseria gonorrhea* may be detected on Thayer-Martin or other suitable media. Vincent's angina is diagnosed by a crystal violet stained smear of the pharyngeal or tonsillar exudate showing the presence of numerous fusobacteria and spirochetes. Blood cultures should be obtained in cases of suspected postanginal septicemia, and radiographic examination of the lungs, bones, and large joint may detect metastatic infection. A throat culture using Loeffler's medium should be obtained on all suspected cases of diphtheria (see Chapter 182). The hemolysis associated with *C. hemolyticum* becomes maximal at 48–72 hours and is more prominent on rabbit and human blood agar than sheep blood agar; thus this organism may be missed on standard throat culture.[34] The diagnosis of infectious mononucleosis can be confirmed by specific serologic tests (see Chapter 121). Serum antigen has been detected in cases of pharyngitis due to primary HIV infection.[28] Also, suspected cases of this infection should be followed for appearance of serum antibody to HIV (see Chapter 108). Cultures and serologic tests for influenza virus, adenovirus, herpes simplex virus, cytomegalovirus, and *M. pneumoniae* are now available in some large laboratories. Acute and convalescent (3-week) serum specimens are necessary for serologic tests for these agents. Laboratory tests for the common cold viruses are not readily available.

Pharyngitis due to noninfectious causes may sometimes present a diagnostic problem. Pemphigus, bullous pemphigoid, and systemic lupus erythematosus are among the diseases that can cause pharyngeal inflammation and discomfort. Also drug reactions are sometimes manifest by pharyngeal soreness, as is agranulocytosis. The presence of other manifestations of these diseases, particularly involvement of the skin, is helpful in leading to the diagnosis.

TREATMENT AND PREVENTION

Antimicrobial Therapy

Streptococcal Pharyngitis. Patients with pharyngitis due to *S. pyogenes* should receive a 10-day course of penicillin or an equivalent antibiotic if the patient is allergic to penicillin. The recommended oral dose of penicillin V in adults is 200,000 or 250,000 units every 6–8 hours and in children 50,000 units/kg/24 hours divided into three or four equal doses. An injection of long-acting benzathine penicillin is an excellent, although painful, form of therapy because it does not require patient compliance. The adult dose of benzathine penicillin is 1.2 million units. In patients who are allergic to penicillin, a 10-day course of erythromycin is recommended. The availability of rapid antigen detection tests for *S. pyogenes* has reduced, but not eliminated, the dilemma of when to begin antimicrobial therapy in the suspected case. In patients with a positive antigen test, treatment should be started immediately, with the goals of providing maximal symptomatic relief for the acute illness, eradicating or suppressing the infection to prevent transmission, and preventing suppurative and nonsuppurative complications.[43–47] In patients with a negative test in which the clinical diagnosis of streptococcal pharyngitis is still entertained, either of two strategies is recommended. One strategy is to await the results of throat culture before starting treatment; the other is to begin therapy when the patient is originally seen and to discontinue treatment if the culture is negative. Both of these approaches have advantages and disadvantages. Withholding treatment until culture results are known limits the immediate therapeutic benefit of antimicrobial therapy but reduces unnecessary drug use. Beginning treatment before the results of culture are known provides maximal therapeutic benefit but exposes many patients to an antimicrobial drug unnecessarily. Initiation of treatment within 1 week of the onset of streptococcal pharyngitis will prevent subsequent acute rheumatic fever,[48] and either of the two approaches will achieve this goal (see Chapter 177).

Reports of therapeutic failure with penicillin therapy as manifested by recurrent symptomatic illness[49,50] do not warrant the abandonment of penicillin as the drug of choice for streptococcal pharyngitis at the present time.[47] It has long been known that a 10-day course of penicillin does not necessarily eradicate carriage of the organism from the pharynx. However, the clinical importance of these bacteriologic failures in asymptomatic persons has not been established. Patients with recurrent clinical illness associated with the documented presence of *S. pyogenes* in the pharynx require antimicrobial therapy. It is unavoidable that some "cases" of streptococcal pharyngitis, initial or recurrent, which are diagnosed by currently available means in reality represent persons with viral pharyngitis who are merely colonized with *S. pyogenes*.

Because the incidence of acute rheumatic fever declined to a low level in the United States, the need for *any* antimicrobial treatment of streptococcal pharyngitis has been questioned. However, the recent resurgence of rheumatic fever in some areas of the United States[51–53] and its continuing prevalence in other areas of the world are sufficient reasons not to abandon the general policy of using antimicrobials in the treatment of streptococcal pharyngitis. Discounting the benefit in rheumatic fever prevention and in reduction of acute morbidity, treatment is still important for prevention of suppurative complications of streptococcal pharyngitis, which include sinusitis, otitis media, mastoiditis, lateral sinus thrombosis, bacteremia, and pneumonia.

Anaerobic Pharyngitis/Peritonsillitis/Peritonsillar Abscess. Oral penicillin in the doses recommended for streptococcal pharyngitis has been successfully used in the treatment of anaerobic pharyngitis and peritonsillitis. The use of early antimicrobial therapy has reduced but not eliminated the cases that require surgical drainage of an abscess. Suspected cases of postanginal septicemia require hospitalization and appropriate diagnostic evaluation.[29] Parenteral treatment with high doses of penicillin or another antimicrobial with activity against *F. necrophorum* should be given for a prolonged course.

Diphtheria. The treatment of diphtheria is described in Chapter 183. *Corynebacterium hemolyticum* pharyngitis has been reported not to respond to a standard 10-day course of penicillin V but did respond to one injection of benzathine penicillin or a course of oral erythromycin.[33,34]

Yersinial Pharyngitis. *Yersinia enterocolitica* is usually susceptible to aminoglycosides, trimethoprim-sulfamethoxazole, and third-generation cephalosporins but resistant to penicillin (see Chapter 207).

Gonorrheal Pharyngitis. The treatment of gonococcal infections is described in Chapter 190.

Mycoplasmal Pharyngitis. The treatment of *M. pneumoniae* is described in Chapter 162.

Viral Pharyngitis. Amantadine, if given early in the course of illness, has a therapeutic effect for type A influenza. It is recommended for cases of presumed influenzal pharyngitis occurring during a known influenza type A epidemic (see Chapter 34). Chronic oropharyngeal herpetic infection in an immunosuppressed patient should be treated with acyclovir. Acyclovir is not recommended for acute herpetic pharyngitis in otherwise healthy people (see Chapter 34).

Symptomatic Therapy

Treatment is directed at relieving pharyngeal discomfort and associated systemic or respiratory symptoms. Warm saline gargles and supportive measures such as rest, aspirin, and liquids are sufficient in most cases of viral pharyngitis. Symptomatic therapy is also helpful in relieving symptoms of streptococcal pharyngitis. Patients with severe streptococcal pharyngitis or peritonsillitis may be in extreme discomfort and require liberal use of analgesics during the early course of illness. Hospitalization is rarely necessary unless supportive care is unavailable or dehydration results from diminished fluid intake.

Prevention

Tonsillectomy has been shown to reduce the incidence of throat infections in children who were severely affected with recurrent pharyngitis.[54] However, it is not recommended as a routine practice.[55] Active immunization is available for types A and B influenza and for diphtheria (see Chapters 142, 296). The prophylactic administration of amantadine is also effective against type A influenza. Liver adenovirus vaccines have been used successfully in military populations but are not available for civilian use (see Chapter 122). There has been work on experimental vaccines for a number of the agents that cause pharyngitis, including *S. pyogenes*, but these vaccines are still in the experimental stage of development.

REFERENCES

1. Stuart-Harris CH, Andrewes C, Andrews BE, et al. A collaborative study of the aetiology of acute respiratory infection in Britain 1961–4. A report of the Medical Research Council working party on acute respiratory virus infections. Br Med J 1965;2:319.
2. Gwaltney JM Jr. Virology of middle ear. Ann Otol Rhinol Laryngol. 1971;80:365.
3. Hamre D, Connelly AP Jr, Procknow JJ. Virologic studies of acute respiratory disease in young adults. IV. Virus isolations during four years of surveillance. Am J Epidemiol. 1966;83:238.
4. Monto AS, Ullman BM: Acute respiratory illness in an American community: The Tecumseh study. JAMA 1974;227:164.
5. Evans AS, Dick EC. Acute pharyngitis and tonsillitis in University of Wisconsin students. JAMA. 1964;190:699.
6. Glezen WP, Clyde WA Jr, Senior RJ, et al. Group A streptococci, mycoplasmas, and viruses associated with acute pharyngitis. JAMA 1967;202:455.
7. Valle, S-L. Febrile pharyngitis as the primary sign of HIV infection in a cluster of cases linked by sexual contact. Scand J Infect Dis. 1987;19:13–17.
8. Stryker WS, Fraser DW, Facklam RR. Foodborne outbreak of group G streptococcal pharyngitis. Am J Epidemiol. 1982;116:533–40.
9. Cohen D, Ferne M, Rouach T, et al. Foodborne outbreak of group G streptococcal sore throat in an Israeli military base. Epidemiol Infect. 1987;99:249–55.
10. McMillan JA, Sandstrom C, Weiner LB, et al. Viral and bacterial organisms associated with acute pharyngitis in a school-aged population. J Pediatr. 1986;109:747–52.
11. Reed BD, Huck W, Lutz LJ, et al. Prevalence of *Chlamydia trachomatis* and *Mycoplasma pneumoniae* in children with and without pharyngitis. J Fam Prac. 1988;26:387–92.
12. Hofkosh D, Wald ER, Chiponis DM. Prevalence of non-group-A β-hemolytic streptococci in childhood pharyngitis. South Med J. 1988;81:329–31.
13. Denny FW. Current problems in managing streptococcal pharyngitis. J Pediat. 1987;111:797–806.
14. Gwaltney JM Jr, Hendley JO, Simon G, et al. Rhinovirus infections in an industrial population. I. The occurrence of illness. N Engl J Med. 1966;275:1261.
15. Komaroff AL, Aronson MD, Pass TM, et al: Serologic evidence of chlamydial and mycoplasmal phyaryngitis in adults. Science. 1983;222:927–9.
16. Gerber MA, Ryan RW, Tilton RC, et al. Role of *Chlamydia trachomatis* in acute pharyngitis in adults. J Clin Microbiol. 1984;20:993–4.
17. Huss H, Jungkind D, Amadio P, et al. Frequency of *Chlamydia trachomatis* as the cause of pharyngitis. J Clin Microbiol. 1985;22:858–60.
18. Grayston JT, Kuo C-C, Wang S.-P, et al. A new *Chlamydia psittaci* strain, TWAR, isolated in acute respiratory tract infections. N Engl J Med. 1986;315:161–8.
19. Gwaltney JM Jr. Rhinoviruses. In: Evans AS, ed. Viral Infections of Humans: Epidemiology and Control. New York: Plenum; 1982:491.
20. Hendley JO, Fishburne HB, Gwaltney JM Jr. Coronavirus infections in working adults. Am Rev Respir Dis. 1972;105:805.
21. Wenzel RP, Hendley JO, Davies JA, et al. Coronavirus infections in military recruits. Three-year study with coronavirus strains OC43 and 229E. Am Rev Respir Dis 1974;109:621.
22. Tyrrell DAJ: Common Colds and Related Diseases. Baltimore: Williams & Wilkins; 1965.
23. Glezen WP, Fernald GW, Lohr JA. Acute respiratory disease of university students with special reference to the etiologic role of herpesvirus hominis. Am J Epidemiol. 1975;101:111.
24. Douglas RG Jr, Alford BR, Couch RB: Atraumatic nasal biopsy studies of respiratory virus infections in volunteers. Antimicrob Agents Chemother. 1968;8:340–2.
25. Winther B, Farr B, Turner RB, et al. Histopathologic examination and enumeration of polymorphonuclear leukocytes in the nasal mucosa during experimental rhinovirus colds. Acta Otolaryngol [Suppl] (Stockh) 1984;413:19–24.
26. Naclerio RM, Proud D, Lichtenstein, et al. Kinins are generated during experimental rhinovirus colds. J Infect Dis. 1988;157:133–142.
27. Proud D, Reynolds CJ, Lacapra S, et al. Nasal provocation with bradykinin induces symptoms of rhinitis and a sore throat. Am Rev Respir Dis. 1988;137:613–16.
28. Kessler HA, Blaauw B, Spear J, et al. Diagnosis of human immunodeficiency virus infection in seronegative homosexuals presenting with an acute viral syndrome. JAMA. 1987;258:1196–9.
29. Seidenfeld SM, Sutker WL, Luby JP. *Fusobacterium necrophorum* septicemia following oropharyngeal infection. JAMA. 1982;248:1348.
30. Scully RE, Galdabini JJ, McNeely BU: Case records of the Massachusetts General Hospital. N Engl J Med. 1978;298:894.
31. Hutt DM, Judson FN. Epidemiology and treatment of oropharyngeal gonorrhea. Ann Intern Med. 1986;104:655.
32. Hart RJC. *Corynebacterium ulcerans* in humans and cattle in North Devon. J Hyg Camb. 1984;92:161–4.
33. Banck G, Nyman M. Tonsillitis and rash associated with *Corynebacterium haemolyticum*. J Infect Dis. 1986;154:1037–40.
34. Miller RA, Brancato F, Holmes KK. *Corynebacterium hemolyticum* as a cause of phyaryngitis and scalatiniform rash in young adults. Ann Intern Med. 1986;105:867–72.
35. Greenman JL. *Corynebacterium hemolyticum* and pharyngitis. Ann Intern Med. 1987;106:633.
36. Green SL, LaPeter KS. Pseudodiphtheritic membranous pharyngitis caused by *Corynebacterium hemolyticum*. JAMA. 1981;245:2330.
37. Kovatch AL, Schuit KE, Michaels RH. *Corynebacterium hemolyticum* peritonsillar abscess mimicking diphtheria. JAMA. 1983;249:1757.
38. Rose FB, Camp CJ, Antes EJ. Family outbreak of fatal *Yersinia enterocolitica* pharyngitis. Am J Med. 1987;82:636–7.
39. Berkowitz CD, Anthony BF, Kaplan EL, et al. Cooperative study of latex agglutination to identify group A streptococcal antigen on throat swabs in patients with acute pharyngitis. J Pediatr. 1985;107:89.
40. Schwartz RH, Hayden GF, McCoy P, et al. Rapid diagnosis of streptococcal pharyngitis in two pediatric offices using a latex agglutination kit. Pediatr Infect Dis. 1985;4:647.
41. Roddy OF, Clegg HW, Clardy LT, et al. Comparison of a latex agglutination kit and four culture methods for identification of group A streptococci in a pediatric office laboratory. J Pediatr. 1986;108:347.
42. Radetsky M, Solomon JA, Todd JK. Identification of streptococcal pharyngitis in the office laboratory: reassessment of new technology. Pediatr Infect Dis J. 1987;6:556.
43. Nelson JD. The effect of penicillin therapy on the symptoms and signs of streptococcal pharyngitis. Pediatr Infect Dis. 1984;3:10.
44. Krober MS, Bass JW, Michels GN. Streptococcal pharyngitis. Placebo-controlled double-blind evaluation of clinical response to penicillin therapy. JAMA. 1985;253:1271.
45. Randolph MF, Gerber MA, DeMeo KK, et al. The effect of antibiotic therapy on the clinical course of streptococcal pharyngitis. J Pediatr. 1985;106:870.
46. Denny FW. Effect of treatment on streptococcal pharyngitis: is the issue really settled? Pediatr Infect Dis. 1985;4:352.
47. McCracken GH Jr. Diagnosis and management of children with streptococcal pharyngitis. Pediatr Infect Dis. 1986;5:754.
48. Caranzaro FJ, Stetson CA, Morris AJ, et al: The role of the streptococcus in the pathogenesis of rheumatic fever. Am J Med. 1954;17:749.
49. Brook I. The role of beta-lactamase-producing bacteria in the persistence of streptococcal tonsillar infection. Rev Infect Dis. 1984;6:601.
50. Gastanaduy AS, Kaplan EL, Hume BB, et al. Failure of penicillin to eradicate Group A streptococci during an outbreak of pharyngitis. Lancet. 1980;2:498.
51. Wald ER, Dashefsky B, Feidt C, et al. Acute rheumatic fever in western Pennsylvania and the tristate area. Pediatrics. 1987;80:371.
52. Congeni B, Rizzo C, Congeni J, et al. Outbreak of acute rheumatic fever in northeast Ohio. J Pediatr. 1987;111:176.
53. Papadimos T, Escamilla J. Acute rheumatic fever at a Navy training center—San Diego, California. Leads from the MMWR. JAMA. 1988;259:1782.
54. Paradise JL, Bluestone CD, Bachman RZ, et al. Efficacy of tonsillectomy for recurrent throat infection in severely affected children. Results of parallel randomized and nonrandomized clinical trials. New Engl J Med. 1984;310:674.
55. Hendley JO. Tonsillectomy: justified but not mandated in special patients. New Engl J Med. 1984;310:717.

44. ACUTE LARYNGITIS

JACK M. GWALTNEY, JR.

Acute laryngitis usually occurs in association with the common cold and influenzal syndromes. Lowering of the normal pitch of the voice, hoarseness, and occasionally aphonia are the characteristic complaints[1,2]; obstruction of the airway is rare in adults. In young children, airway obstruction due to infection of the larynx and tracheobronchial tree is more common, and acute laryngitis must be distinguished from acute bacterial supraglottitis (epiglottitis) (see Chapter 48). Acute supraglottitis has been recognized with increasing frequency in adults, but is still unusual.

Hoarseness is present in 20 percent of cases of common respiratory illness.[3] It occurs most frequently with midwinter illnesses and correlates with the occurrence of cough and, to a lesser extent, sore throat. All the major respiratory viruses have been reported to cause hoarseness (Table 1).[3–6] Influenza virus, rhinovirus, and adenovirus have most often been the cause of laryngitis in reported studies. The role of secondary bacterial invasion in acute laryngitis is not clear; however, *Branhamella catarrhalis* has been recovered from the nasopharynx of 50 to 55 percent of adults with acute laryngitis compared with 6 to 14 percent of controls.[7,8] Hoarseness was also reported by approximately 10 percent of adults with streptococcal pharyngitis.[4] Unusual causes of laryngitis include syphilis, tuberculosis,[9] herpes zoster,[10] histoplasmosis, blastomycosis, and candidiasis. Candidal laryngitis has been recognized chiefly in patients with impaired immunity.[11,12]

Diagnosis of acute laryngitis is usually apparent from the history and clinical characteristics of the illness. Eighty-seven percent of patients with laryngitis reporting to an otolaryngology clinic had preceding upper respiratory tract infection symptoms, and 13 percent reported prior voice abuse.[8] Examination of the larynx reveals hyperemia, edema, or vascular injection of the vocal cords, and there may be superficial mucosal ulcerations. The presence of an exudate or membrane on the pharyngeal or laryngeal mucosa should arouse the suspicion of streptococcal infection, mononucleosis, or diphtheria. In acute epiglottitis, the epiglottis is characteristically intensely red and greatly swollen. Patients with traumatic aphonia usually give a history of excessive use of the voice.

Treatment consists primarily of resting the voice until hoarseness and aphonia have subsided. Inhalation of moistened air on a regular basis may also give relief. A recent double-blind study failed to show a beneficial effect of penicillin V in the treatment of adults with acute laryngitis.[8] Until there is evidence for the value of antimicrobials in the treatment of acute laryngitis, they are not recommended for what is usually a benign self-limited disease. Diphtheritic laryngitis and acute bacterial epiglottitis require specific antimicrobial therapy. Patients with hoarseness persisting longer than 10 days to 2 weeks should have a laryngoscopic examination to exclude tumors and other chronic diseases of the larynx.

TABLE 1. Occurrence of Hoarseness with Acute Respiratory Infections

Infectious Agent	*Percentage of Cases*
Viruses	
Influenza virus	22–37 (3,4)[a]
Rhinovirus	10–25 (4,5)
Adenovirus	6–25 (5,6)
Parainfluenza virus	2–18 (5)
Respiratory syncytial virus	10 (5)
Coxsackievirus A21	9 (5)
Coronavirus	Not determined[b]
Bacteria	
Streptococcus pyogenes	10 (4)

[a] Reference numbers.
[b] In one small study of hospitalized Marine recruits, hoarseness was present in 7 of 11 patients with coronavirus infection diagnosed by seroconversion to coronavirus OC43.[13]

REFERENCES

1. Proctor DF: The upper airways. II. The larynx and trachea. Am Rev Respir Dis. 1977;115:315.
2. Vaughan CW. Current concepts in otolaryngology. Diagnosis and treatment of organic voice disorders. N Engl J Med. 1982;307:863.
3. Dingle JH, Badger GF, Jordan WS Jr: Illness in the Home. A study of 25,000 Illnesses in a Group of Cleveland Families. Cleveland: The Press of Western Reserve University; 1964:66.
4. Gwaltney JM Jr: Rhinoviruses. In: Evans, AS, Ed. Viral Infections of Humans: Epidemiology and Control. 2nd ed. New York: Plenum; 1982:507.
5. Tyrrell DAJ: *Common Colds and Related Diseases*. Baltimore: Williams & Wilkins; 1965:95.
6. McNamara MJ, Pierce WE, Crawford YE, et al. Patterns of adenovirus infection in the respiratory diseases of naval recruits. A longitudinal study of two companies of naval recruits. Am Rev Respir Dis. 1962;86:485.
7. Schalén L, Christensen P, Kamme C, et al. High isolation rate of *Branhamella catarrhalis* from the nasopharynx in adults with acute laryngitis. Scand J Infect Dis. 1980;12:277.
8. Schalen L, Christensen P, Eliasson I, et al. Inefficacy of penicillin V in acute laryngitis in adults. Evaluation from results of double-blind study. Ann Otol Laryngol. 1985;94:14.
9. Bachman AL, Zizmor J, Noyek AM. Tuberculosis of the larynx. Semin Roentgenol. 1979;14:325.
10. Lederer FJ, Soboroff BJ. Medical problems related to diseases of the larynx. Otolaryngol Clin North Am. 1970;3:599.
11. Lawson R, Bodey G, Luna M. *Candida* infection presenting as laryngitis. Am J Med Sci. 1980;280:173.
12. Dudley JP, Byrne WJ, Kobayashi R, et al. *Candida* laryngitis in chronic mucocutaneous candidiasis. Its association with *Candida* esophagitis. Ann Otol Rhinol Laryngol. 1980;89:574.
13. Wenzel RP, Hendley JO, Davies JA, et al. Coronavirus infections in military recruits. Three-year study with coronavirus strains OC43 and 229E. Am Rev Respir Dis. 1974;109:621.

45. ACUTE LARYNGOTRACHEOBRONCHITIS (CROUP)

CAROLINE BREESE HALL

. . . the sharp stridulous voice which I can resemble to nothing more nearly than the crowing of a cock . . . is the true diagnostic sign of the disease.—Francis Home, 1765[1]

Croup or acute laryngotracheobronchitis is an age-specific viral infection of the upper and lower respiratory tract that produces inflammation in the subglottic area and results in the striking picture of dyspnea accompanied on inspiration by the characteristic stridulous notes of croup. Croup demonstrates perhaps best the piquant interaction of host and microorganism. Age, sex, an undefined predisposition of the child, and the type of virus all appear to influence the susceptibility and severity of the infection.

Francis Home of Edinburgh first introduced the word *croup* in his famous treatise "An Inquiry into the Nature, Causes and Cure of the Croup" in which he describes 12 patients with croup.[1] Croup was derived from the old Scottish term *roup*, which meant "to cry out in a shrill voice."

Croup at that time and for the next century was the term often applied to a number of disease entities including diphtheria. John Cheyne, however, appeared to describe not only diphtheria, cynanche trachealis, but also croup that appeared most similar to the viral laryngotracheobronchitis of today.[2] Bretonneau in 1859 argued that diphtheria was a separate and specific disease.[3] However, the confusion between "membranous," or "true croup," and "spasmodic," or "false croup," continued. Differentiation awaited Klebs' discovery of *Corynebacterium diphtheriae* in 1883. In 1948 Rabe[4] classified the forms of infectious croup according to etiology—bacterial or nonbacterial—and suggested that the latter, larger group might be viral in origin. In only 15 percent of his 347 patients was he able to identify a pathogen, namely, *C. diphtheriae* or *Haemophilus influenzae* type b.

INCIDENCE

Croup occurs mostly in children between the ages of 3 months and 3 years, with a peak occurrence in the second year of life.[5–8] In a Seattle prepaid group practice the annual incidence of croup per 1000 children under 6 years of age was 7.[5] In the first 6 months of life the rate was 5.2, and in the second 6 months of life, the rate was 11. The peak incidence was 14.9 in the second year of life, and fell to half that rate in the third year of life. In a group practice in North Carolina, the incidence was about three to five times higher, with a peak of 47 per 1000 each year for children in the second year of life.[8] Even in the first 6 months of life the incidence was 24, and after 6 years of age it was 4.6. In series of hospitalized or outpatient cases of croup, boys predominate, although the attack rates of upper respiratory illnesses by these same viral agents show no sex preference.[5,7–11]

ETIOLOGY

Acute laryngotracheobronchitis may be caused by a variety of viral agents and occasionally by *Mycoplasma pneumoniae* (Table 1).[5,6,8–14] Parainfluenza type 1 virus is the most common cause of croup in the United States and Great Britain (Table 1). Parainfluenza type 3 virus is usually the second most frequently associated agent. In infants this virus more commonly tends to cause bronchiolitis and pneumonia. However, the more frequent manifestation in children 2–3 years of age is croup, and in older children it is tracheobronchitis.[9] Influenza A virus is also a major cause of croup, but its annual incidence varies because of its unpredictable nature and fluctuating seasonal occurrence. Although croup caused by influenza A virus may be less frequent than that from the parainfluenza viruses, some studies have reported it to be more severe,[15–17] while others have not.[8] Influenza A virus may produce croup in a broader age range of children and sometimes with a higher frequency of hospitalization. In Washington, D.C., between 1957 and 1976, 14.3 percent of the croup patients had influenza A or B viral infection.[12] Influenza A more commonly caused croup than did influenza B virus, and interestingly, the frequency of croup appeared to be related to the particular strain of influenza. Croup was more frequently observed in H3N2 than in H2N2 epidemics.[17]

Only a small proportion (approximately 5 percent) of respiratory syncytial viral infections result in croup, but anywhere from 1 to 11 percent of the reported croup cases have been associated with this virus (Table 1). Similarly, croup is an unusual manifestation of adenoviral infection, but these viruses may contribute a small proportion of cases. In contrast, croup is the characteristic manifestation of parainfluenza type 2 viral infection. The total proportion of croup cases produced by parainfluenza type 2 virus is, however, less than that associated with its relatives, types 1 and 3. This is because type 2 virus tends to be a less frequent visitor to a community and sizable outbreaks of infection with parainfluenza type 2 virus are unusual in comparison to outbreaks with type 1.[7–9] Rhinoviruses, enteroviruses, and *M. pneumoniae* all contribute a small, but variable proportion of cases. At all ages the parainfluenza viruses are the major agents. Respiratory syncytial virus (RSV), however, rarely causes croup in children older than 5 years, and the influenza viruses and *M. pneumoniae* predominately cause croup in this older age group.[8]

Of all these agents, only parainfluenza type 1 virus, influenza viruses, and sometimes RSV and parainfluenza type 2 virus occur in epidemics and have a great enough predilection for causing croup as to produce an appreciable rise in the occurrence of croup cases when they are prevalent in a community.[5,8,11,17,18] An appreciable proportion of parainfluenza type 3 infections are also manifested as croup, but this virus is usually more sporadic in its appearance.[8] When epidemic, however, parainfluenza type 3 virus may also cause a discernable increase in the number of croup cases observed.[5,8,11]

EPIDEMIOLOGY

The epidemiologic patterns of croup mainly reflect the seasonal personalities of the major agents. Since parainfluenza type 1 virus causes the largest proportion of croup cases, the major peak of cases occurs when this virus is prevalent in the community. In recent years parainfluenza type 1 virus has tended to cause outbreaks of infection every other year in the fall.[7,9,11] Outbreaks of croup that occur in the winter to early spring are most apt to be related to influenza A viral activity and, to a lesser extent, to respiratory syncytial viral activity.[7–9,18] Sporadic cases of croup are commonly associated with parainfluenza type 3 virus. This virus had been isolated throughout much of the year, but more recently has been observed to have swells

TABLE 1. Percentage of Croup Cases Associated with Various Agents

	Reported Series								
Agent	*Cramblett 1977[12] (%)*	*Parrott et al. 1962[13] (%)*	*Loda et al. 1968[14] (%)*	*Glezen et al. 1971[9] (%)*	*Foy et al. 1973[5] (%)*		*Buchan et al. 1974[11] (%)*	*Downham et al. 1974[6] (%)*	*Denny et al. 1983[8] (%)*
Parainfluenza virus									
Type 1	8	21	39	21	13[a]	6.4[b]	25	26	18
Type 2	6	8	1.6	4	1.4	7.3	1.7	6	3
Type 3	14	10	1.6	9	3	13	8	10	6.6
Influenza A	6	} 8		2	1	3.7	10	6	1.4
Influenza B				1	1	2			1.2
Respiratory syncytial		8	11.4	6	1	9	1.7	6	3.8
Adenovirus	4	9	3	1	4	4.6	1.7	3	
Rhinovirus				0.6	2		1	6	
Enterovirus	12			1	1		1		
Other viruses							5		2
Mycoplasma pneumoniae			5	1.4	0.5	2		1	1.4
Total percentage of cases with identified agent	50	64	62	47	56		54	64	37.6

[a] Identified by isolation of agent.
[b] Identified by serology.

of activity during the warmer months of late spring and summer.[6,9,11] Sporadic cases of croup may also be caused by any of the less common agents such as the adenoviruses, rhinoviruses, and *M. pneumoniae*, which may be prevalent through many months of the year. Croup from enteroviruses, although uncommon, tends to occur in the summer and early fall. Parainfluenza type 2 virus tends to produce smaller outbreaks of infection at less predictable intervals, commonly in the fall and early winter.[6–8,11]

PATHOPHYSIOLOGY

The viral infection initially affects the upper respiratory tract, usually producing inflammation of the nasal passages and nasopharynx. Subsequently the infection spreads downward to involve essentially all levels of the respiratory tract. The classic signs of croup—the stridor, hoarseness, and cough—arise mostly from the inflammation occurring in the larynx and trachea. However, involvement of the lower respiratory tract is also present in most cases requiring hospitalization.[19] The inflammation and obstruction are greatest at the subglottic level. This is because it is the least distensible part of the airway since it is encircled by the cricoid cartilage with the narrow anterior ring and the larger posterior quadrangular lamina.

Inflammation at the subglottic level results in the characteristic obstruction observed in viral croup. The impeded flow of air through this narrowed area produces the classic high-pitched vibratory sounds, or stridor. This is most apparent on inspiration since the negative pressure tends to narrow the extrathoracic airway further, much as sucking on a partially occluded paper straw causes it to collapse inwardly. This is enhanced in young children since their airway walls are relatively compliant.[20] In 1836 Ley[21] descriptively expressed this as

> The shrill sonorous inspiration so characteristic of this complaint, marks very unequivocally its seat. . . . From some cause there is an unusual approximation of the sides of the glottis . . . the influence being very analogous to that produced by too strong compression of the reed against the mouthpiece of the clarionet by the lips of one who has made no great proficiency in that instrument, when a harsh, squeaking sound is produced abundantly discordant and grating to the ear.

In histologic sections, inflammatory changes may be seen in the epithelium, the mucosa, and the submucosa of the larynx, trachea, and the linings of the bronchi, bronchioles, and even the alveoli.[22] Small areas of atelectasis may also be present.

Why children in the second year of life are particularly prone to develop croup is not entirely clear. However, this may be partly explained by the fact that most of these children are experiencing primary infection with the viral agent, which is more likely to be manifested by spread of the virus to involve the lower respiratory tract and also by the anatomy. The diameters of the larynx and glottis are relatively smaller in the young child, and inflammation of the membranes lining these passages causes a relatively greater degree of obstruction. Airway resistance is highly sensitive to even small changes in the diameter of the airway. In fact, the resistance to airflow is inversely related to the fourth power of the radius of the airway. Furthermore, the mucous membrane is relatively looser and more vascular and the cartilage ring less rigid. Also, nasal obstruction and crying can aggravate the dynamic narrowing of the child's airway.

Immunologic mechanisms may also be involved in the pathogenesis of croup. Urquhart and colleagues[23] have suggested that the pathogenesis of croup may be different in children with abrupt vs. gradual onset. Noting a different serologic response in such children, they hypothesized that croup of sudden onset resulted from a hypersensitivity reaction to parainfluenza type 1 virus in children with previous infection with a closely related paramyxovirus such as parainfluenza type 3. In the children with a more gradual onset of prodromal upper respiratory tract symptoms for more than 1 day, antibody to the parainfluenza viruses in the acute-phase serum was less often present and in lower titers than in the acute sera of patients with a sudden onset of croup.

Greater concentrations of IgE antibody to parainfluenza viral antigen and histamine have been detected in children with parainfluenza viral infections whose illness was manifested as croup, wheezing, or both in comparison to those with only upper respiratory tract illness.[24] Furthermore, the lymphoproliferative responses of peripheral blood lymphocytes from children with parainfluenza viral croup were significantly greater than those from children with upper respiratory tract illness, and their histamine-induced suppression of the lymphoproliferative response was diminished.[25] From these findings, Welliver et al.[24,25] have suggested that a defect in immunoregulation, similar to that found in atopic subjects, contributes to the pathogenesis of croup.

Physiologic Correlations

When the infection produces obstruction at the subglottic level, the child's tidal volume initially declines. This, however, is compensated by an increase in the respiratory rate to maintain adequate alveolar ventilation (Fig. 1). If, however, the degree of obstruction increases, the work of breathing may increase such that the child tires and can no longer maintain the necessary compensatory respiratory effort. The tidal volume may then further decrease, and as the respiratory rate declines, hy-

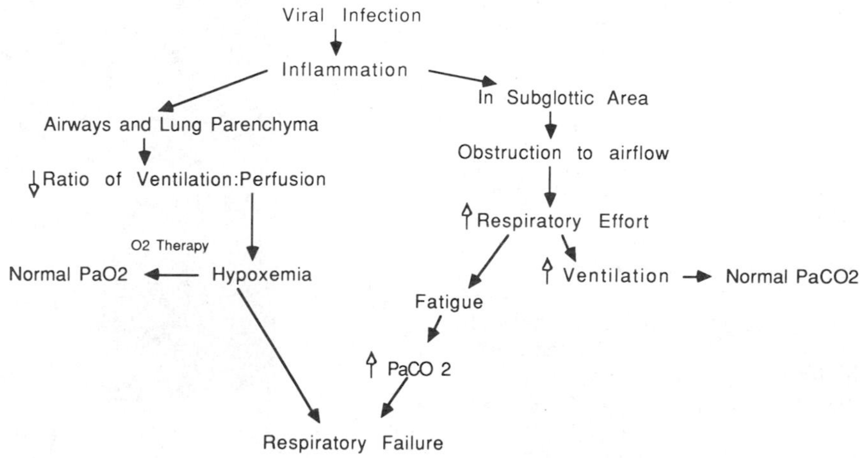

FIG. 1. Physiologic abnormalities in croup.

percarbia and secondary hypoxemia ensue. The subglottic obstruction does not result in hypoxemia until this stage, when respiratory failure occurs.

Hypoxemia, however, occurs in 80 percent of the children hospitalized with croup.[19] The hypoxemia arises from the inflammation in the lung parenchyma, which results in an abnormally low ratio of ventilation to perfusion and an increased alveolar-to-arterial gradient (Fig. 1).

CLINICAL MANIFESTATIONS

> The disease generally comes on in the evening after the little patient has been exposed to the weather during the day and often after a slight catarrh of some days' standing. At first his voice is observed to be hoarse and pulling . . . he awakens with a most unusual cough, rough and stridulous. And now his breathing is laborious, each inspiration being accompanied by a harsh, shrill noise."—John Cheyne, 1814[2]

Most children with croup have a history of an upper respiratory tract infection for 1 to several days previously. Commonly the child has had rhinorrhea, a sore throat, and mild cough. Most children have fever, either initially during the upper respiratory tract infection or at the onset of croup. Children with croup from influenza A and parainfluenza viruses commonly have fevers with temperatures ranging from 38–40°C.[26] Fever with respiratory syncytial viral infection tends not to be as high.

The onset of croup is commonly heralded by hoarseness and a deepening cough. The cough is usually not productive but has the striking brassy tone that has earned it the sobriquet "seal's bark." The child may awaken at night with this distinctive cough, tachypnea, and the characteristic inspiratory stridor. In 1836, Ley[21] described the stridor as "the crowing of a cock, the yelping of a fox, the barking of a dog, the braying of an ass, or a ringing sound, as if the voice came from a brazen tube." The child may sit forward in bed and appear apprehensive. Commonly accompanying the stridor are retractions of the chest wall, usually most marked in the supraclavicular and suprasternal area.

In children who are more severely affected, auscultation of the chest commonly reveals not only the inspiratory stridor but also rales, rhonchi, and/or wheezing. Occasionally, a markedly distressed child will have stridor on expiration as well as inspiration. The respiratory rate is commonly elevated to 35–45/min. However, respiratory rates much above 50/min are uncommon in children with croup, in contrast to the marked tachypnea often evident in bronchiolitis. With progression of the disease, auscultation of the chest may reveal poor exchange of air with diminished breath sounds.

One of the hallmarks of croup is its fluctuating course. A child may clinically appear to worsen or improve within an hour. In milder cases of croup, children commonly improve in the morning, only to worsen again at night. In most children the course of croup is 3–4 days, although the cough may persist for a longer period.

LABORATORY FINDINGS

In most cases of croup the white blood cell and differential counts are not particularly abnormal or helpful. In the more severely stressed child the white blood cell count may be somewhat elevated, and if hypoxemia is present, an increase in the proportion of immature polymorphonuclear cells may be observed.

Hypoxemia (PaO_2 <85 mmHg) occurs in most hospitalized children, and hypercapnea is present in over half.[19] In the study of Newth et al.,[19] most children hospitalized with croup had PaO_2 values between 50 and 80 mmHg, and about half had $PaCO_2$ values in the normal range below 40 mmHg. The rest had $PaCO_2$ levels between 40 and 50 mmHg. Only 1 of the 35 children manifested hypercarbia of greater then 50 mmHg. Few other pulmonary function studies have been obtained in children with croup, but in five out of six children in one study the functional residual capacity was found to be increased.[27]

DIAGNOSIS

The diagnosis of croup is usually based on the characteristic clinical picture. However, differentiation from noninfectious causes of stidor such as foreign body aspiration or an allergic reaction, and from *H. influenzae*-induced epiglottis usually may be made on the basis of both the history and the anterior–posterior and lateral roentgenograms of the neck.[28]

Characteristically the course of epiglottitis is much more rapidly progressive, and the children appear to be in a more toxic state. The history of an upper respiratory tract infection with rhinorrhea and laryngitis is usually not present in epiglottitis. The absence of the distinctive cough or "seal's bark" and the presence of marked dysphagia with drooling are often two of the more helpful differentiating clinical signs. In viral laryngotracheobronchitis the anterior–posterior view of the neck (Fig. 2) shows the characteristic subglottic swelling, sometimes described as the "hourglass" or "steeple" sign. In epiglottitis, the lateral neck view may show the edematous epiglottis without subglottic narrowing (see Chapter 48). The roentgenographic picture may not, however, always be diagnostic for croup or epiglottitis, and controversy exists about their reliability and usefulness in the acute situation.[29–31]

Identification of the specific viral agent may be accomplished by isolation in tissue culture or by one of the newer techniques of rapid viral diagnosis.[32] Serologic diagnosis generally may be made only retrospectively, and for some of the major agents of croup serologic rises are variable and unreliable. With parainfluenza viral infections, heterotypic antibody rises are frequent among the various types of the parainfluenza viruses and the related viruses such as mumps.[13,33] Furthermore, during reinfection no measurable antibody response may occur.[33]

In reported series the cause has been determined in approximately one-third to two-thirds of the cases of croup (Table 1), which is higher than that generally reported for other respiratory tract syndromes. Viral isolation has usually been accomplished from throat, tracheal, and nasal wash specimens.[5,6,8,9,11,14,26] Rapid diagnostic techniques, mostly the enzyme-linked im-

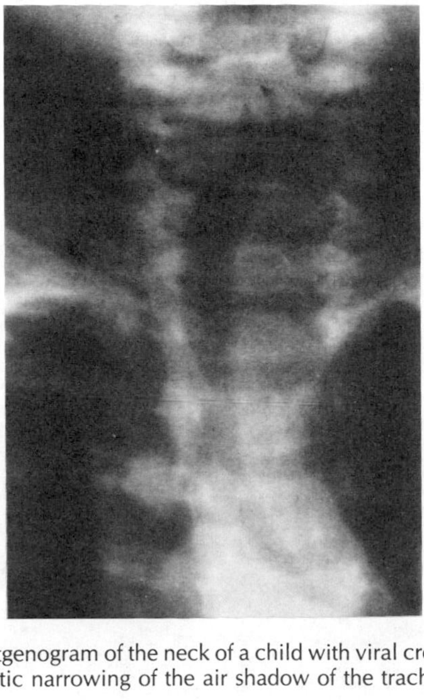

FIG. 2. Roentgenogram of the neck of a child with viral croup that shows the characteristic narrowing of the air shadow of the trachea in the subglottic area.

munosorbent assay (ELISA) and immunofluorescent techniques, have also been successfully used.[6,32,34–38]

COMPLICATIONS

The severity of croup appears to be influenced by both virus and host factors. Some children appear predisposed to croup, with repetitive episodes from a variety of agents. John Cheyne[2] noted ". . . the first attack establishes a predisposition to the disease. I have observed, that after the first attack, a slighter cause will produce Croup a second time than is required originally."

Children with repeated episodes of croup are sometimes diagnosed as having *spasmodic croup*.[39] An allergic diathesis or hyperreactivity of the airway may contribute to the illness in these children since positive intradermal skin tests and family members with allergy have been frequently seen in children with recurrent versus single episodes of croup.[40–42] A tendency toward lower serum IgA levels has also been noted in children with recurrent croup.[43] Nevertheless, a viral infection initiates the croup even in these children, and the disease cannot be distinguished clinically.

Boys are particularly prone to develop croup for reasons that are not entirely clear.[7–9,11,40,44] However, recently Taussig[45] has shown that young girls had significantly larger flow rates than did boys. This suggests that there are differences anatomically or in intrinsic airway resistance that are related to sex, which might in part explain why young boys tend to develop lower respiratory tract disease more frequently or more severely than do young girls.

Severe croup has sometimes been reported as more frequent with influenza A viral infection than with the other viral agents.[15,16] In the study of Howard et al.[15] made during an outbreak of influenza A infection, 10 out of 25 infants hospitalized with croup required tracheotomy. This complication has been estimated to occur in about 5–12 percent of the cases of croup.[44,46,47] In Adair and coworkers'[46] review of reported cases of laryngotracheobronchitis, the percentage requiring tracheotomy varied between 0 and 13 percent. The associated mortality rate in these series ranged from 0 to 2.7 percent. Of the major acute complications, respiratory failure necessitating such airway intervention is the most frequent. Subglottic stenosis after intubation occasionally occurs in children with complicated and prolonged courses.[44,46–49]

Pneumonia cannot truly be considered a complication of croup but should rather be thought of as a part of the disease. Parenchymal involvement, as evidenced by hypoxemia, is present in most hospitalized children, whether it is visible on the chest roentgenogram or not. Less common complications include pneumothorax, pulmonary edema, and aspiration pneumonia. Aspiration of gastric contents is most likely to occur during emergency intubation. Transient pulmonary edema without evidence of cardiac enlargement has been described in children with croup.[49–51] The mechanism leading to this complication is not completely understood, but it may arise from a neurogenic effect on the pulmonary vasculature, as a direct result of alveolar hypoxia, or possibly from an increased alveolar–capillary gradient causing a leakage of intravascular fluids.

Whether long-term complications can follow croup is currently speculative. The disease is self-limited, and recovery appears clinically to be complete. However, several follow-up studies of children with croup early in life have shown an increased frequency of hyperreactivity of the airways and altered pulmonary function that, in some children, may be clinically occult.[27,47,52,53] In one study of 12-year-old children who had a history of hospitalization for croup, elevated residual volumes and significant reductions in forced vital capacity (FVC), forced expiratory volume in 1 second (FEV_1), and maximal expiratory flow between 25 and 75 percent of vital capacity ($FEF_{25-75\%}$) were found.[53] Hyperreactivity of the airways has been observed in each of these follow-up studies of children with croup.[27,47,52,53]

THERAPY

Despite a Pandora's box of home therapies for croup, none has proved to be consistently effective. The natural fluctuations in the course of croup make evaluation of many therapies difficult. Vaporizers and other means of producing steam or mist in the home have long been advised. The beneficial effects of these devices have not actually been proved, and in one small controlled trial humidification provided no benefit.[54] These methods certainly provide humidification of the upper airway, but the droplet size produced is generally too large to reach the lower respiratory tract. The advantages of such home humidification devices must be balanced against the discomfort or fear they may produce in the child. Crying and lack of rest may aggravate the condition.

In hospitalized patients, the essence of successful management is close observation and good supportive care based on a thorough understanding of the physiologic changes associated with croup. Clinical estimation of the severity of croup is difficult. Cyanosis may not be present despite compromising degrees of hypoxemia.[55] Of the clinical signs, an increasing respiratory rate is often the best indication of hypoxemia. The severity of the stridor and retractions reflect more the degree of subglottic obstruction and are not indicative of the arterial oxygen saturation. Hence, in all children ill enough to require hospitalization the objective criteria of determining arterial blood gases should be used initially in the management. Capillary as well as arterial blood gases may be used, but oximetry offers a simple, noninvasive means of following the child's arterial oxygen saturation.[56]

In children with hypoxemia, supplemental oxygen becomes the mainstay of therapy.[48,57,58] Children with PaO_2 values of less than 60 mmHg will benefit from supplemental oxygen. Since the hypoxemia in children without marked hypercarbia results from an abnormal ratio of ventilation to perfusion, the hypoxemia will respond to oxygen therapy, usually at relatively low concentrations (Fig. 1).

Humidification of the airway may be administered by an ultrasonic nebulizer fitted to a mask or an oxygen tent. Although humidification of the lower airway theoretically may be achieved by this means, the value of such therapy has not been proved.

In one of the few animal studies of croup, cold-dry, cold-moist, and dry air were more effective in the dog model in decreasing airway resistance.[59] All of these types of air contain little humidification as compared with warm-moist air, which was least effective.

A variety of pharmacologic agents have been evaluated in the treatment of croup. The only one that currently appears to be of possible benefit is racemic epinephrine. L-Epinephrine has also been suggested as being as efficient since it contains only the active isomer.[60] The reported results with racemic epinephrine, however, have not been consistent.[61–65] Gardner and colleagues in a controlled double-blind study administered nebulized racemic epinephrine by face mask to croup patients and evaluated their response clinically.[62] The racemic epinephrine proved to be no more effective than the saline. In a subsequent double-blind study by Westley and coworkers,[63] racemic epinephrine was delivered by intermittent positive-pressure breathing and resulted in significant clinical improvement. In both of these studies the response was evaluated clinically. Taussig and colleagues,[64] however, evaluated the effect of racemic epinephrine by intermittent positive-pressure breathing clinically and with concurrent determinations of the blood gases. The racemic epinephrine resulted in clinical improvement in terms of stridor and retractions but did not alter the arterial PO_2. It would appear, therefore, that such therapy may have benefit by providing clinical improvement and thus deterring fatigue. Such therapy should, however, be used with the understanding that the amelioration of clinical signs is transient, continued observation is necessary, and despite the clinical appearance, the degree of hypoxemia is unchanged.

Corticosteroid therapy generally has not been shown to be beneficial and remains controversial.[61,66–68] The many studies evaluating steroid use in croup have been recently reviewed, and most all have been noted to have faults in their design or methods.[66] Despite this, some continue to recommend steroids for selected cases of severe croup.[44] Antibiotic therapy in viral croup is not indicated, and secondary bacterial infection is uncommon.

A few children, despite adequate supportive therapy, may fatigue and develop respiratory failure, demonstrated by a climbing $PaCO_2$ level. If a mechanical airway becomes necessary, nasotracheal intubation is the preferred method, provided personnel skilled in this technique are available.[47–49] Complications with nasotracheal intubation are less than with tracheostomies. In Schuller and Birck's[47] 8-year follow-up study of children receiving nasotracheal intubation for croup and epiglottitis, the rate of immediate and reversible complications was 7 percent, and for the delayed, irreversible complications the rate was 1.6 percent. The average period of intubation for the children with croup was 88 hours as compared with 55 hours for those with epiglottitis.

BACTERIAL TRACHEITIS

Recently, an atypical form of croup has been described and designated as *bacterial tracheitis*.[69–72] This uncommon entity tends to affect somewhat older children but may affect any age and produce a dramatic, acute onset marked by high fever, stridor, and dyspnea with copious amounts of purulent sputum. The clinical picture may resemble epiglottitis and progress rapidly, requiring endotracheal intubation or tracheotomy. The area of inflammation and obstruction, however, is subglottic and is covered with a thick exudate. The lateral soft tissue roentgenogram of the neck characteristically reveals a normal epitlottis with subglottic narrowing within which a shaggy membrane may sometimes be visible.

The organisms most commonly recovered from this exudate are *Staphylococcus aureus*, group A β-hemolytic streptococci, and *H. influenzae* type b.[69–72] The pathogenesis of this entity, nevertheless, is not clear. The syndrome appears to develop in children who are predisposed by previous conditions, especially those associated with injury to the trachea. Children who have been recently intubated and sometimes those with a preceding viral infection appear to be at risk. In one reported case *Chlamydia trachomatis* was isolated from the tracheal exudate along with *S. aureus*.[72]

The rapidly progressive course of this disease demands its prompt diagnosis and differentiation from viral croup by its clinical and roentgenographic picture. Direct laryngoscopy can confirm the diagnosis and provide specimens of the localized exudate for culture. Initial antibiotic therapy should be broad enough to cover the associated major pathogens.

REFERENCES

1. Home F. An Inquiry into the Nature, Cause and Cure of Croup. Edinburgh, 1765.
2. Cheyne J. Essays on the Diseases of Children, with Cases and Dissections. Philadelphia 1802–1808. Philadelphia: Anthony Finley Merritt; 1814:20.
3. Semple RH. Memoirs on diphtheria. From the Writings of Bretonneau, Guersant, Trousseau, Bouchut, Empis, Daviot. London: New Sydenham Society Publications; 1859:5.
4. Rabe EF. Infectious croup: I. Etiology. Pediatrics. 1948;2:255–65.
5. Foy HM, Cooney MK, Maletzky AJ, et al. Incidence and etiology of pneumonia, croup and bronchiolitis in pre-school children belonging to a prepaid medical care group over a four year period. Am J Epidemiol. 1973;97:80–92.
6. Downham MAPS, McQuillan J, Gardner PS. Diagnosis and clinical significance of parainfluenza virus infections in children. Arch Dis Child. 1974; 49:8–15.
7. Glezen WP, Denny FW. Epidemiology of acute lower respiratory disease in children. N Engl J Med. 1973;288:498–505.
8. Denny FW, Murphy TF, Clyde WA Jr, et al. Croup: An 11 year study in a pediatric practice. Pediatrics. 1983;71:871–6.
9. Glezen WP, Loda FA, Clyde WA Jr, et al. Epidemiogical patterns of acute lower respiratory disease of children in a pediatric group practice. J Pediatr. 1971;78:397–406.
10. Loda FA, Glezen WP, Clyde WA Jr. Respiratory disease in group day care. Pediatrics. 1972;49:428–37.
11. Buchan KA, Marten KW, Kennedy DH. Aetiology and epidemiology of viral croup in Glasgow, 1966–72. J Hyg (Camb). 1974;73:143–50.
12. Cramblett HG. Croup (epiglottitis, laryngitis, laryngotracheobronchitis). In: Kendig EL Jr, Chernick V, eds. Disorders of the Respiratory Tract in Children. 3rd ed. Philadelphia: WB Saunders; 1977:353.
13. Parrott RH, Vargosko AJ, Kim HW, et al. Acute respiratory diseases of viral etiology. III. Myxoviruses: Parainfluenza. Am J Public Health. 1962;52:907–17.
14. Loda FA, Clyde WA Jr, Glezen WP, et al. Studies of the role of viruses, bacteria, and *M. pneumoniae* as causes of lower respiratory tract infections in children. J Pediatr. 1968;72:161–76.
15. Howard JB, McCracken GH Jr, Luby JP. Influenza A 2 virus as a cause of croup requiring tracheotomy. J Pediatr. 1972;81:1148–50.
16. Eller JJ, Fulginiti VA, Plunket DC, et al. Attack rates for hospitalized croup in children in a military population: Importance of A_2 influenza infection. Pediatr Res. 1972;6:126.
17. Kim HW, Brandt CD, Chanock RM, et al. Influenza A and B virus infection in infants and young children during the years 1957–1976. Am J Epidemiol. 1979;109:464–79.
18. Hall CB, Douglas RG Jr. Respiratory syncytial virus and influenza: Practical community surveillance. Am J Dis Child. 1976;130:615–20.
19. Newth CJ, Levison H, Bryan AC. The respiratory status of children with croup. J Pediatr. 1972;81:1068–73.
20. McBride JT. Stridor in childhood. J Fam Pract. 1984;19:782–90.
21. Ley H. An Essay on the Laryngismus Stridulus or Croup-like Inspiration of Infants. London: Churchill; 1836:6.
22. Szpunar J, Glowacki J, Laskowski A, et al. Fibrinous laryngotracheobronchitis in children. Arch Otolaryngol. 1971;93:173–8.
23. Urquhart GED, Kennedy DH, Ariyawansa JP. Croup associated with parainfluenza type 1 virus: Two subpopulations. Br Med J. 1979;1:1604.
24. Welliver RC, Wong DT, Middleton E Jr, et al. Role of parainfluenza virus-specific IgE in pathogenesis of croup and wheezing subsequent to infection. J Pediatr. 1982;101:889–96.
25. Welliver RC, Sun M, Rinaldo D. Defective regulation of immune responses in croup due to parainfluenza virus. Pediatr Res. 1985;19:716–20.
26. Hall CB, Geiman JM, Breese BB, et al. Parainfluenza viral infections in children: Correlation of shedding with clinical manifestations. J Pediatr. 1977;91:194–8.
27. Loughlin G, Taussig LM. Pulmonary function in children with a history of laryngotracheobronchitis. J Pediatr. 1979;94:365–9.
28. Rapkin RH. The diagnosis of epiglottitis: Simplicity and reliability of radiographs of the neck in the differential diagnosis of the croup syndrome. J Pediatr. 1972;80:96–8.
29. Currarino G, Williams B. Lateral inspiration and expiration radiographs of the neck in children with laryngotracheobronchitis (croup). Radiology. 1982;195:365–6.
30. Jones JL. False positives in lateral neck radiographs used to diagnose epiglottitis (Letter). Ann Emerg Med. 1983;12:797.
31. Stankiewicz JA, Bowes AK. Croup and epiglottitis: A radiologic study. Laryngoscope. 1985;95:1159–60.
32. Richman D, Schmidt N, Plotkin S, et al. Summary of a workshop on new and useful methods in rapid viral diagnosis. J Infect Dis. 1984;150:941–51.
33. Bloom HH, Johnson KM, Jacobsen R, et al. Recovery of parainfluenza viruses from adults with upper respiratory illness. Am J Hyg. 1961;74:50–9.
34. McIntosh K, Wilfert C, Chernesky M, et al. Summary of a workshop on new and useful techniques in rapid viral diagnosis. J Infect Dis. 1980;142:793–802.
35. Grauballe PC, Johnsen NJ, Hornsleth A. Rapid diagnosis by immunofluorescence of viral infections associated with the croup syndrome in children. Acta Pathol Microbiol Scand [B]. 1974;82:41–7.
36. Gardner PS, McQuillin J, McGuckin R, et al. Observations on clinical and immunofluorescent diagnosis of parainfluenza virus infections. Br Med J. 1971;2:7–12.
37. Gardner PS, McGuckin R, McQuillin J. Adenovirus demonstrated by immunofluorescence. Br Med J. 1972;3:175.
38. Marks MI, Nagahama H, Eller JJ. Parainfluenza virus immunofluorescence. In vitro and clinical application of the direct method. Pediatrics. 1971; 48:73–8.
39. McLain LG. Croup syndrome. Am Fam Physician. 1987;36:207–14.
40. Hide DW, Guyer BM. Recurrent croup. Arch Dis Child. 1985;60:585–6.
41. Laufer P. The relationship of respiratory allergies to croup. J Asthma. 1986;23:9–10.
42. Zach M, Erban A, Olinsky A. Croup, recurrent croup, allergy, and airways hyper-reactivity. Arch Dis Child. 1981;56:336–41.
43. Zach M. Serum IgA in recurrent croup. Am J Dis Child. 1983;137:184–5.

44. Postma DS, Jones RD, Pillsbury HC III. Severe hospitalized croup: Treatment trends and prognosis. Laryngoscope. 1984;94:1170–5.
45. Taussig LM. Maximal expiratory flows at functional residual capacity: A test of lung function for young children. Am Rev Respir Dis. 1977;116:1031–8.
46. Adair JC, Ring WH, Jordan WS, et al. Ten year experience with IPPB in the treatment of acute laryngotracheobronchitis. Anesth Analg (Cleve). 1971;50:649–55.
47. Schuller DE, Birck HG. The safety of intubation in croup and epiglottitis: An eight-year follow-up. Laryngoscope. 1975;85:33–46.
48. Hen J Jr. Current management of upper airway obstruction. Pediatr Ann. 1986;15:274–94.
49. Kilham H, Gillies J, Benjamin B. Severe upper airway obstruction. Pediatr Clin North Am. 1987;34:1–14.
50. Broniatowski M. Croup. Ear Nost Throat J. 1985;64:12–21.
51. Travis KW, Todres ID, Shannon DC. Pulmonary edema associated with croup and epiglottitis. Pediatrics. 1977;59:695–8.
52. Zach MS, Schnall RP, Landau LI. Upper and lower airway hyperreactivity in recurrent croup. Am Rev Respir Dis. 1980;121:979–83.
53. Gurwitz D, Corey M, Levison H. Pulmonary function and bronchial reactivity in children after croup. Am Rev Respir Dis. 1980;122:95–9.
54. Bourchier D, Dawson KP, Fergusson DM. Humidification in viral croup: A controlled trial. Aust Paediatr J. 1984;20:289–91.
55. Hall CB, Hall WJ, Speers DM. Clinical and physiological manifestations of bronchiolitis and pneumonia: Outcome of respiratory syncytial virus. Am J Dis Child. 1979;133:798–802.
56. Gussack GS, Tacchi EJ. Pulse oximetry in the management of pediatric airway disorders. South Med J. 1987;80:1381–4.
57. Barker GA. Current management of croup and epiglottitis. Pediatr Clin North Am. 1979;26:565–79.
58. Newth CJL, Levison H. Diagnosing and managing croup and epiglottitis. J Respir Dis. 1981;2:22–41.
59. Wolfsdorf J, Swift DL. An animal model simulating acute infective upper airway obstruction of childhood and its use in the investigation of croup therapy. Pediatr Res. 1978;12:1062–5.
60. Davis HW, Gartner JC, Galvis AG, et al. Acute airway obstruction: Croup and epiglottitis. Pediatr Clin North Am. 1981;28:859–80.
61. Cherry JD. The treatment of croup: Continued controversy due to failure of recognition of historic, ecologic, etiologic, and clinical perspectives. J Pediatr. 1979;94:352.
62. Gardner HG, Powell KR, Roden VJ, et al. The evaluation of racemic epinephrine in the treatment of infectious croup. Pediatrics. 1973;52:52–5.
63. Westley CR, Cotton EK, Brooks JG. Nebulized racemic epinephrine by IPPB for the treatment of croup: A double-blind study. Am J Dis Child. 1978;132:484–87.
64. Taussig LM, Castro O, Beaudry PH, et al. Treatment of laryngotracheobronchitis (croup). Use of intermittent positive-pressure breathing and racemic epinephrine. Am J Dis Child. 1975;129:790–3.
65. Bass JW, Bruhn FW, Merrit WT. Corticosteroids and racemic epinephrine with IPPB in the treatment of croup. J Pediatr. 1980;96:173–4.
66. Tunnessen WW Jr, Feinstein AR. The steroid-croup controversy: An analytic review of methodologic problems. J Pediatr. 1980;96:751–6.
67. Asher MI, Beaudry PH. Croup and corticosteroid therapy. J Pediatr. 1981;97:506–7.
68. Leipzig B, Oski FA, Cummings CW, et al. A prospective randomized study to determine the efficacy of steroids in treatment of croup. J Pediatr. 1979;94:194–6.
69. Jones R, Santos JI, Overall JC. Bacterial tracheitis. JAMA. 1979;242:721–6.
70. Liston SL, Gehrz RC, Jarvis CW. Bacterial tracheitis. Arch Otolaryngol. 1981;107:561–4.
71. Davidson S, Barzilay Z, Yahav J, et al. Bacterial tracheitis: A true entity? J Laryngol Otol. 1982;96:173–5.
72. Miller BP, Arthur JD, Parry WH, et al. Atypical croup and chlamydia trachomatis (Letter). Lancet. 1982;1:1022.

46. OTITIS EXTERNA, OTITIS MEDIA, MASTOIDITIS

JEROME O. KLEIN

OTITIS EXTERNA

Infection of the external auditory canal (otitis externa) is similar to infection of skin and soft tissue elsewhere. Unique problems occur because the canal is narrow and tortuous; fluid and foreign objects enter, are trapped and cause irritation and maceration of the superficial tissues. The pain and itching that results may be severe because of the limited space for expansion of the inflamed tissue. Infections of the external canal may be subdivided into four categories: acute localized otitis externa, acute diffuse otitis externa, chronic otitis externa, and malignant otitis externa. Recent reviews by Senturia et al.[1] and Bergstrom[2] provide more complete information.

Pathogenesis

The external auditory canal is approximately 2.5 cm long from the concha of the auricle to the tympanic membrane. The lateral half of the canal is cartilaginous; the medial half tunnels through the temporal bone. A constriction, the isthmus, present at the juncture of the osseous and cartilaginous portions, limits entry of wax and foreign bodies to the area near the tympanic membrane. The skin of the canal is thicker in the cartilaginous portion and includes a well-developed dermis and subcutaneous layer. The skin lining the osseous portion is thinner and firmly attached to the periosteum and lacks a subcutaneous layer. Hair follicles are numerous in the outer third and sparse in the inner two-thirds of the canal.

The microbial flora of the external canal is similar to the flora of skin elsewhere. There is a predominance of *Staphylococcus epidermidis, S. aureus*, diphtheroids, and to a lesser extent, anaerobic bacteria such as *Propionibacterium acnes*.[3–5] Pathogens responsible for infection of the middle ear, *Streptococcus pneumoniae, Haemophilus influenzae*, or *Branhamella (Moraxella) catarrhalis*, are uncommonly found in cultures of the external auditory canal when the tympanic membrane is intact.

The epithelium absorbs moisture from the environment. Desquamation and denuding of the superficial layers of the epithelium may follow. In this warm, moist environment, the organisms in the canal may flourish and invade the macerated skin. Inflammation and suppuration follow. Invasive organisms include those of the normal skin flora and gram-negative bacilli, particularly *Pseudomonas aeruginosa*. Malignant otitis media is a necrotizing infection frequently associated with *P. aeruginosa*. The organism gains access to the deeper tissues of the ear canal and causes a localized vaculitis, thrombosis, and necrosis of tissues. Diabetic microangiopathy of the skin overlying the temporal bone results in poor local perfusion and a milieu for invasion by *P. aeruginosa*.[6]

Clinical Manifestations and Management

Acute localized otitis externa may occur as a pustule or furuncle associated with hair follicles; it is due to *Staphylococcus aureus*. Erysipelas caused by group A *Streptococcus* may involve the concha and the canal. Pain may be severe. Bluish, red hemorrhagic bullae may be present on the osseous canal walls and also on the tympanic membrane. Adenopathy in the lymphatic drainage areas is often present. Local heat and systemic antibiotics are usually curative. Incision and drainage may be necessary to relieve severe pain.

Acute diffuse otitis externa (swimmer's ear) occurs mainly in hot, humid weather. The ear itches and becomes increasingly painful. The skin of the canal is edematous and red. Gram-negative bacilli, mainly *P. aeruginosa*, may play a significant role. A severe hemorrhagic external otitis due to *P. aeruginosa* was associated with mobile redwood hot tub systems.[7] Gentle cleansing to remove debris including irrigation with hypertonic saline (3%) and cleansing with mixtures of alcohol (70–95%) and acetic acid should be used initially. Hydrophilic solutions such as 50% Burrow solutions may be used for 1–2 days to reduce inflammation. Ear drops of topical antibiotics (including neomycin and polymyxin) combined with a steroid in an acid vehicle serve to diminish local inflammation and infection. Systemic antibiotics may be necessary if there is significant tissue infection.

Chronic otitis externa is due to irritation of drainage from the middle ear in patients with chronic suppurative otitis media. Itching may be severe. Management is directed to treatment of the middle ear disorder. Rare causes of chronic otitis externa include tuberculosis, syphilis, yaws, leprosy, and sarcoidosis.

Malignant otitis externa is a severe, necrotizing infection that spreads to adjacent areas of soft tissue, cartilage, and bone. Severe pain and tenderness of the tissues around the ear and mastoid is accompanied by drainage of pus from the canal. The elderly, diabetic, and debilitated patient is at particular risk. Life-threatening disease may result from spread to the sigmoid sinus, jugular bulb, base of the skull, meninges, and brain. Permanent facial paralysis is frequent. Diagnostic tests for underlying disease should be instituted. The canal should be cleansed, devitalized tissue removed, and ear drops with antipseudomonal antibiotics combined with steroid instilled. Systemic therapy with antimicrobial regimens including coverage for *Pseudomonas* sp. (such as gentamicin and/or ticarcillin or piperacillin) should be used for 4–6 weeks.

Fungal otitis may be part of a general or local fungal infection. *Aspergillus* sp. are responsible for most cases of fungal otitis. *Candida albicans* is a frequent cause of external otitis in children with chronic mucocutaneous candidiasis.

OTITIS MEDIA

Otitis media, or inflammation of the middle ear, is defined by the presence of fluid in the middle ear accompanied by signs or symptoms of illness. A survey of the office practice of physicians who provided medical care to children showed that otitis media was the most frequent diagnosis recorded for illness.[8] The peak incidence occurs in the first 3 years of life. The disease is less common in the school-age child, adolescent, and adult. Nevertheless, infection of the middle ear may be the cause of fever, significant pain, and impaired hearing in these age groups. In addition, adults suffer from the sequelae of otitis media of childhood: hearing loss, cholesteatoma, adhesive otitis media, and chronic perforation of the tympanic membrane. A comprehensive review of otitis media is included in a recent text, *Otitis Media in Infants and Children*.[9]

Epidemiology

By 3 years of age, more than two-thirds of children have had one or more episodes of acute otitis media, and one-third have had three or more episodes.[10] The highest incidence of acute otitis media occurs between 6 and 24 months of age. Subsequently, the incidence declines with age except for a limited reversal of the downward trend between 5 and 6 years of age, the time of school entry. Although considered uncommon in adults, a survey identified almost 4 million visits to physicians by adults each year for middle ear infection.

Some racial groups such as American Indians and Canadian and Alaskan Eskimos have high rates of infection and severe middle ear disease. Poverty with its accompanying factors of crowding, poor sanitation, and inadequate medical facilities is common to these groups. Whether other factors specifically related to race or culture are involved remains unknown. Other epidemiologic factors of importance identified in a recent study of Boston children[10] include the following: age at first episode is an important predictor of recurrent otitis media in that infants who have otitis media during the first year of life are at increased risk of recurrent disease, males have more episodes of acute otitis media and are at increased risk for recurrent disease, breast-feeding is associated with decreased risk for recurrent otitis media during the first year of life, and recurrent otitis media in a sibling is an important risk feature. Children in group and day care are more likely than are children cared for at home to experience recurrent episodes of acute otitis media.[11]

Pathogenesis

The middle ear is part of a continuous system that includes, medially and anteriorly, the nares, nasopharynx, and eustachian tube and, posteriorly, the mastoid air cells. These structures are lined with a respiratory epithelium that contains ciliated cells, mucus-secreting goblet cells, and cells capable of secreting local immunoglobulins.

Anatomic or physiologic dysfunction of the eustachian tube appears to play a critical role in the development of otitis media. The eustachian tube has at least three physiologic functions with respect to the middle ear: protection of the ear from nasopharyngeal secretions, drainage into the nasopharynx of secretions produced within the middle ear, and ventilation of the middle ear to equilibrate air pressure with that in the external ear canal. When one or more of these functions is compromised, the results may be development of fluid and infection in the middle ear. Congestion of the mucosa of the eustachian tube may result in obstruction. Secretions that are constantly formed by the mucosa of the middle ear accumulate behind the obstruction, and if a bacterial pathogen is present, a suppurative otitis media may result.

Microbiology

Bacteria. The microbiology of otitis media has been documented by appropriate cultures of middle ear effusions obtained by needle aspiration. Many studies of the bacteriology of acute otitis media have been performed. The results are remarkably consistent in demonstrating the importance of *S. pneumoniae* and *H. influenzae* in all age groups[9] (Table 1).

Streptococcus pneumoniae is the most important bacterial cause of otitis media. Relatively few types are responsible for most disease. The most common types in order of decreasing frequencies are 19, 23, 6, 14, 3, and 18.[11–13] All are included in the currently available 23-type pneumococcal polysaccharide vaccine.

Otitis media due to *H. influenzae* is associated with nontypable strains in the vast majority of patients. In approximately 10 percent, the otitis is due to type b; some of these patients appear to be in a very toxic state, and about one-quarter have concomitant bacteremia or meningitis.[14] Until recently, *H. influenzae* appeared to be limited in importance to preschool children; however, recent studies indicate that *H. influenzae* is a significant cause of otitis media in older children, adolescents, and adults.

Recent studies indicate an increasing importance of *B. catarrhalis*.[15,16] The organism was isolated from the middle ear fluids of 19 percent of 200 middle ear specimens from 146 Pittsburgh children with acute otitis media.[16] Prior to 1970 almost all strains of *B. catarrhalis* were sensitive to penicillin. Today most strains produce β-lactamase and are resistant to penicillin G, ampicillin, and amoxicillin.

Viruses. Virologic and epidemiologic data suggest that viral infection is frequently associated with acute otitis media.[17–19]

TABLE 1. Bacterial Pathogens Isolated from Middle Ear Fluid in 4675 Children with Acute Otitis Media[a]

Microorganism	*Mean Percentage of Children with Pathogen*
Streptococcus pneumoniae	33
Haemophilus influenzae	21
Streptococcus, group A	8
Staphylococcus aureus	2
Branhamella catarrhalis	3
Gram-negative enteric bacilli	1
Miscellaneous bacteria	1
None or nonpathogens	31

[a] Twelve reports from centers in the United States, Finland, and Sweden, 1952–1981.[9]

In a study of children attending a day care program, isolation of viruses from the upper respiratory tract was correlated with a clinical diagnosis of otitis media. Virus outbreaks coincided with epidemics of otitis media. Recent studies identify respiratory viruses[17] or viral antigens[18] in approximately one-quarter of middle ear fluids of children with acute otitis media. Respiratory syncytial virus, influenza virus, enteroviruses, and rhinoviruses were the most common viruses found in middle ear fluids.

Mycoplasma, Chlamydia, and Unusual Organisms. *Mycoplasma pneumoniae* was responsible for hemorrhagic bullous myringitis in a study of nonimmune volunteers inoculated with the organism.[20] However, the middle ear fluid of a large number of patients (771) has been studied, and *M. pneumoniae* was isolated in only one case.[21,22] Although mycoplasmas do not appear to play a significant role in acute otitis media, some patients with lower respiratory tract disease due to *M. pneumoniae* may have concomitant otitis media.

Chlamydia trachomatis is associated with acute respiratory infections in infants under age 6 months and is a cause of acute infection of the middle ear in this age group. The organism has been isolated from middle ear fluid of infants with acute infection.[23]

Uncommon forms of otitis include diphtheritic otitis, tuberculous otitis, otogenous tetanus, and otitis due to *Ascaris lumbricoides*.

Immunology

The middle ear is the site of a secretory immune system similar to those of other areas of the respiratory tract. Local and systemic immune responses occur in patients with acute or chronic otitis media with effusion. In the middle ear, immunologically active antigen interacts with immunocompetent cells in the lamina propria to produce a local immune response. The middle ear effusion that results from acute or chronic infection contains all the major classes of immunoglobulins, complement, cells, immune complexes of antigen and antibody, and various chemical mediators of inflammation. The role of these substances in the course of otitis media is uncertain. The immune response to various antigens may prevent subsequent infection, assist in clearance of fluid during the acute episode, or contribute to the accumulation and persistence of fluid in the middle ear cavity.

Diagnosis and Clinical Course

Acute otitis media is defined by the presence of fluid in the middle ear along with signs or symptoms of acute illness. Signs and symptoms may be specific, such as ear pain, ear drainage, or hearing loss, or may be nonspecific, such as fever, lethargy, or irritability. Vertigo, nystagmus, and tinnitus may occur. Redness of the tympanic membrane is an early sign of otitis media, but erythema alone is not diagnostic of middle ear infection since it may be caused by inflammation of the mucosa throughout the upper respiratory tract.

The presence of fluid in the middle ear is determined by the use of pneumatic otoscopy, a technique that permits an assessment of the mobility of the tympanic membrane. The motion of the tympanic membrane is proportional to the pressure applied by gently squeezing and then releasing the rubber bulb attached to the head of the otoscope. Normal mobility is apparent when positive pressure is applied and the tympanic membrane moves rapidly inward; with release of the bulb and the resulting negative pressure, the membrane moves outward. Fluid or high negative pressure in the middle ear dampens the mobility of the tympanic membrane. Tympanometry uses an electroacoustic impedance bridge to record compliance of the tympanic membrane and middle ear pressure. This technique presents objective evidence of the status of the middle ear and the presence or absence of fluid.

Fluid persists in the middle ear for prolonged periods after the onset of acute otitis media even though symptoms usually resolve within a few days after initiation of antimicrobial therapy. About 70 percent of children with otitis media have fluid in the middle ear 2 weeks after the onset of disease, 40 percent still have fluid 1 month after onset, and 10 percent still have fluid 3 months after the first signs of middle ear infection.[10]

Patients with middle ear effusion suffer from hearing loss of variable severity. On average, a patient with fluid in the middle ear has a 25 db (pure tone average) loss.[24] Since development is dynamic during infancy when the incidence of acute otitis media is highest, there is concern that any impediment to reception or interpretation of auditory stimuli might have an adverse effect. Recent studies suggest that children with histories of recurrent episodes of acute otitis media score lower in tests of speech, language, and cognitive abilities than do their disease-free peers.[25–26]

The results of microbiologic studies of middle ear effusions in patients with otitis media are so consistent that the choice of antimicrobial agents may be based on knowledge of the bacteriology acquired from the many investigations rather than the results of cultures from other sites such as the throat or nasopharynx (Table 1). If the patient is toxic or has focal infection elsewhere, culture of the blood and culture of the focus are warranted. Needle aspiration of the middle ear effusion (tympanocentesis) to define the microbiology should be considered in selected patients: the patient who is critically ill at the onset, the patient who has not responded to initial antimicrobial therapy in 48–72 hours and is toxic, and the patient with altered host defenses (e.g., immunologic defect, including the newborn infant).

Management

Acute Otitis Media. ANTIMICROBIAL AGENTS. The preferred antimicrobial agent for the patient with otitis media must be active against *S. pneumoniae, H. influenzae*, and in some areas, *B. catarrhalis*. Group A streptococci and *S. aureus* are infrequent causes of acute otitis media and need not be considered in initial therapeutic decisions. Gram-negative enteric bacilli must be considered when otitis media occurs in the newborn infant, in the patient with a depressed immune response, and in the patient with suppurative complications of chronic otitis media. Amoxicillin or ampicillin are the current drugs of choice for initial treatment since they are effective against the two major pathogens and are less expensive than alternative regimens are. The current incidence of ampicillin-resistance *H. influenzae* and *B. catarrhalis* is not high enough to require a change in initial therapy. Other drugs that are satisfactory include amoxicillin-clavulanate, cefuroxime-axetil, trimethoprim-sulfamethoxazole (TMP-SMZ), the fixed combination preparation of erythromycin and sulfisoxazole, cefaclor, and combinations of a sulfonamide and penicillin G (administered by mouth or as a single intramuscular dose of the benzathine salt), penicillin V, or erythromycin. Trimethoprim-sulfamethoxazole, cefaclor, or the combination of erythromycin and a sulfonamide provide antimicrobial coverage for *H. influenzae* and *S. pneumoniae* and are acceptable regimens for the child with an allergy to penicillin. If the child has had a major reaction to a penicillin (an immediate or accelerated reaction with urticaria, bronchospasm, or hypotension), cross-reactivity of penicillins and cephalosporins must be considered possible, and the use of a cephalosporin should be avoided.

Some children with acute otitis media due to a bacterial pathogen improve without the use of antimicrobial agents. Clinical resolution may occur because the contents of the middle ear are discharged through the eustachian tube or after spontaneous perforation of the tympanic membrane. The cases of spontaneous resolution of acute otitis media are important to the investigator who must consider this factor in an analysis of the results of new therapeutic regimens, but they do not weigh against the use of appropriate antimicrobial agents for the treatment of acute otitis media to uniformly resolve the clinical signs and prevent suppurative complications.

With appropriate antimicrobial therapy, most children with acute otitis media are significantly improved within 48–72 hours. If there is no improvement, the patient should be examined. Toxicity with persistent or recurrent fever or otalgia should prompt consideration of tympanocentesis to identify the causative organism; the appropriate antimicrobial agent may then be chosen on the basis of results of Gram staining and culture of the middle ear fluid. If signs persist but the child is not toxic and aspiration is not performed, the initial antimicrobial regimen should be changed to one that is effective for less common organisms, including β-lactamase–producing *H. influenzae* and *B. catarrhalis*. If ampicillin or amoxicillin was given initially, then amoxicillin-clavulanate, TMP-SMZ, erythromycin-sulfisoxazole, or cefaclor should be administered.

DECONGESTANTS AND ANTIHISTAMINES. Nasal and oral decongestants, administered either alone or in combination with an antihistamine, are used extensively for treatment of otitis media with effusion. The use of the drugs is based on the consideration that they reduce congestion of the respiratory mucosa and relieve the obstruction of the eustachian tube that results from inflammation caused by respiratory infection. The results of clinical trials, however, indicate no significant evidence of efficacy of any of these preparations, used alone or in combination, for relief of signs of disease or decrease in time spent with middle ear effusion.[27] A recent symposium reviewed the efficacy and safety of antihistamines in the treatment of upper respiratory tract infections.[28]

Chronic Otitis Media. The term *chronic otitis media* includes recurrent episodes of acute infection and prolonged duration of middle ear effusion usually resulting from a previous episode of acute infection. For the prevention of recurrent episodes of acute otitis media, management includes the consideration of chemoprophylaxis (the use of antimicrobial agents) and immunoprophylaxis (the use of pneumococcal vaccine). For the management of persistent middle ear efflusions, three surgical methods are considered: myringotomy, adenoidectomy, and placement of tympanostomy tubes.

Chemoprophylaxis has been shown to be of value in the prevention of acute illness in children who have suffered from recurrences of middle ear infections.[29–31] Although the results are inadequate to provide conclusive evidence of the efficacy of chemoprophylaxis, they are persuasive in that a reduction of episodes of acute febrile illnesses due to otitis media occurred. On the basis of available information,[31] a protocol has been suggested that uses a once-a-day regimen of amoxicillin or sulfisoxazole during winter and spring, the periods of high incidence of infections of the respiratory tract. Chemoprophylaxis may suppress symptoms of otitis media, but middle ear effusion may persist (though without apparent symptoms). The physician who chooses to use chemoprophylaxis to prevent acute recurrent disease must examine the patient at approximately 1-month intervals for middle ear effusion.

Pneumococcal vaccines have been evaluated for the prevention of recurrences of acute otitis media in children.[32–34] As in previous studies, children less than 2 years of age had unsatisfactory responses to single-dose regimens. The vaccine reduced the number of episodes of acute otitis media due to types of *S. pneumoniae* present in the vaccine, but the reduction was not sufficient to alter the experience of the children with middle ear infections. The basis for failure of the vaccine was due to the poor immunologic response to the polysaccharide antigens in the young infants enrolled in the trials. The data suggested that the vaccine was likely to be more effective in children over the age of 2 years.[34]

Surgical management of the persistent effusion of the middle ear includes the use of myringotomy, adenoidectomy, and the placement of tympanostomy tubes. Myringotomy, or incision of the tympanic membrane, is a method of draining middle ear fluid. Before the introduction of antimicrobial agents, myringotomy was the major method of managing suppurative otitis media. Today, the use of myringotomy is limited to the relief of intractable ear pain, hastening resolution of mastoid infection, and drainage of persistent middle ear effusion that is unresponsive to medical therapy.

Enlarged adenoids may obstruct the orifice of the eustachian tube in the posterior portion of the nasopharynx and interfere with adequate ventilation and drainage of the middle ear. Recent studies of the use of adenoidectomy in children with prolonged effusions in the middle ear identify in selected children a beneficial effect in reducing time spent with effusion.[35,36]

Tympanostomy tubes resemble small collar buttons. They are placed through an incision in the tympanic membrane to provide drainage of fluid and ventilation of the middle ear. The placement of these tubes is now one of the most common surgical procedures in children. The criteria for the placement of tubes include persistent middle ear effusions unresponsive to adequate medical treatment over a period of 3 months and persistent negative pressure. Hearing improves dramatically after placement of the ventilating tubes. The tubes have also been of value in patients who have difficulty maintaining ambient pressure in the middle ear such as would occur due to barotrauma in airline personnel. The liabilities of the placement of tubes include those of anesthesia associated with the procedure, persistent perforation, scarring of the tympanic membrane, development of cholesteatoma, and otitis media caused by swimming with ventilating tubes in place, but these occur infrequently.

MASTOIDITIS

The proximity of the mastoid to the middle ear cleft suggests that most cases of suppurative otitis media are associated with inflammation of the mastoid air cells (Fig. 1). The incidence of clinically significant mastoiditis, however, is low since the introduction of antimicrobial agents. Nevertheless, acute and chronic disease still occurs and may be responsible for significant morbidity and life-threatening disease.

Pathogenesis

At birth, the mastoid consists of a single cell, the antrum, connected to the middle ear by a small channel. Pneumatization of the mastoid bone takes place soon after birth and is extensive by 2 years of age. The clinical importance of the mastoid is related to contiguous structures including the posterior cranial fossa, the middle cranial fossa, the sigmoid and lateral sinuses, the canal of the facial nerve, the semicircular canals, and the petrous tip of the temporal bone. The mastoid air cells are lined with modified respiratory mucosa, and all are connected with the antrum.

Infection in the mastoid follows middle ear infection. Initially, there is hyperemia and edema of the mucosal lining of the air cells. Serous, then purulent exudate collects in the cells. Necrosis of bone due to pressure of the purulent exudate on the thin bony septa follows. Coalescence of pus in contiguous areas results in abscess cavities.

Clinical Manifestations

Acute mastoiditis is usually accompanied by acute infection in the middle ear. During early stages, the signs are those of acute otitis media with hearing loss, otalgia, and fever. Subsequently,

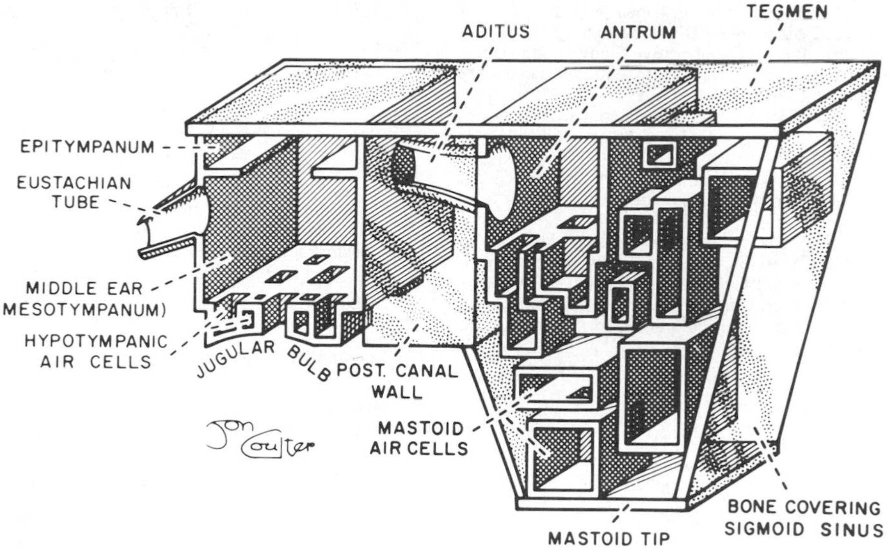

FIG. 1 Diagrammatic representation of the anatomy of the middle and mastoid air cell system showing the narrow connection (aditus and antrum) between the two.

swelling, redness, and tenderness is present over the mastoid bone. The pinna is displaced outward and downward. A purulent discharge may emerge through a perforation in the tympanic membrane.

Diagnosis

Roentgenographs of the mastoid area may show a loss of sharpness of the shadows of cellular walls due to demineralization of bony septa and cloudiness of areas of pneumatization due to inflammatory swelling of the air cells.

Cultures for bacteria from ear drainage fluid must be taken with care to distinguish fresh drainage fluid from material in the external canal. The canal must be cleaned and fresh pus obtained as it exudes from the tympanic membrane. If the tympanic membrane is not perforated, tympanocentesis should be performed to obtain material from the middle ear.

Management

The antimicrobial drugs of choice for acute infection are similar to those for acute otitis media: antibiotics with activity against *S. pneumoniae* and *H. influenzae*. If the disease in the mastoid has had a prolonged course, coverage for *S. aureus* and gram-negative enteric bacilli may be considered for initial therapy until the results of cultures become available.

A mastoidectomy is performed when an abscess has formed in the mastoid bone. The procedure should be performed at a time when sepsis has been controlled by antimicrobial agents.

References

1. Senturia BH, Marcus MD, Lucente FE. Diseases of the External Ear. An OtologicDermatologic Manual. 2nd ed. New York: Grune & Stratton; 1980.
2. Bergstrom L. Diseases of the external ear. In Bluestone CD, Stool SE eds. Pediatric Otolaryngology, Philadelphia, WB Saunders, 1983;347.
3. Riding KH, Bluestone CD, Michaels RH, et al. Microbiology of recurrent and chronic otitis media with effusion. J Pediatr 1978;93:739–43.
4. Pelton SI, Teele DW, Shurin PA, et al. Disparate cultures of middle ear fluids. Am J Dis Child. 134:951–953, 1980;134:951–3.
5. Brook I, Schwartz R. Anaerobic bacteria in acute otitis media. Acta Otolaryngol. 1981;91:111–4.
6. Otitis due to *Pseudomonas aeruginosa* serotype 0:10 associated with mobile redwood hot tub system—North Carolina. MMWR. 1982;31:541–2.
7. Doroghazi RM, Nadol JB, Hyslop NE, et al. Invasive external otitis. Am J Med. 1981;71:603–13.
8. Koch H, Dennison NJ. Office visits to pediatricians. National Ambulatory Medical Care Services, National Center for Health Statistics, 1974.
9. Bluestone CD, Klein JO, eds. Otitis Media in Infants and Children. Philadelphia: WB Saunders; 1987.
10. Wald ER, Dashefsky B, Byers C, et al. Frequency and severity of infections in day care. J Pediatr. 1968;112:540–6.
11. Kamme C, Ageberg M, Lundgren K. Distribution of *Diplococcus pneumoniae* types in acute otitis media in children and influence of the types on the clinical course in penicillin V therapy. Scand J Infect Dis. 1970;2:183–90.
12. Austrian R, Howie VM, Ploussard JH. The bacteriology of pneumococcal otitis media. Johns Hopkins Med J. 1977;141:104–11.
13. Gray BM, Converse GM, Dillion, HC. Serotypes of *Streptococcus pneumoniae* causing disease. J Infect Dis. 1979;140:979–83.
14. Harding AL, Anderson P, Howie VM, et al. *Haemophilus influenzae* isolated from children with otitis media. In: Sell SHW, Karzon DT, eds. *Haemophilus influenzae*. Nashville: Vanderbilt University Press; 1973:21.
15. Van Hare GF, Shurin PA, Marchant CD, et al. Acute otitis media caused by *Branhamella catarrhalis*: Biology and therapy. Rev Infect Dis 1987;9:16–27.
16. Kovatch AL, Wald ER, Michaels RH: β-Lactamase–producing *Branhamella catarrhalis* causing otitis media in children. J Pediatr. 1983;102:261–4.
17. Chonmaitree T, Howie VM, Truant AL. Presence of respiratory viruses in middle ear fluids and nasal wash specimens from children with acute otitis media. Pediatrics. 1986;77:698–702.
18. Klein BS, Dallette ER, Volken RH. The role of respiratory syncytial virus and other viral pathogens in acute otitis media. J Pediatr. 1982;101:16–20.
19. Henderson FW, Collier AM, Sanyal MA, et al. A longitudinal study of respiratory viruses and bacteria in the etiology of acute otitis media with effusion. N Engl J Med. 1982;306:1377.
20. Rifkind DR, Chanock RM, Kravetz H, et al. Ear involvement (myringitis) and primary atypical pneumonia following inoculation of volunteers with Eaton agent. Am Rev Respir Dis. 1962;85:479–89.
21. Klein JO, Teele DW. Isolation of viruses and mycoplasma from middle ear effusions: A review. Ann Otol Rhinol Laryngol. 1976;85:140–44.
22. Sobeslavsky O, Syrucek L, Bruckoya M, et al. The etiological role of *Mycoplasma pneumoniae* in otitis media in children. Pediatrics. 1965;35:652–7.
23. Tipple MA, Beem MO, Saxon EM. Clinical characteristics of the afebrile pneumonia associated with *Chlamydia trachomatis* infection in infants less than 6 months of age. Pediatrcs. 1979;63:192–7.
24. Fria TJ, Cantekin EI, Eichler JA. Hearing acuity of children with effusion. Arch Otolaryngol. 1985;111:10–6.
25. Holm VA, Kunze LH: Effects of chronic otitis media on language and speech development. Pediatrics. 1969;43:833–9.
26. Teele DW, Klein JO, Rosner BA. Otitis media with effusion during the first three years of life and development of speech and language. Pediatrics. 1984;74:282–7.
27. Cantekin EI, Mandel EM, Bluestone CD. Lack of efficacy of a decongestant–antihistamine combination for otitis media with effusion ("secretory" otitis media) in children. N Engl J Med. 1983;308:297–301.
28. Bluestone CD, Connell JT, Doyle WJ, et al. Symposium: Questioning the efficacy and safety of antihistamines in the treatment of upper respiratory infection. Pediatr Infect Dis J. 1988;7:15–42.
29. Perrin JM, Charney E, MacWhinney JB, et al. Sulfisoxazole as chemoprophylaxis for recurrent otitis media: A double-blind crossover study in pediatric practice. N Engl J Med. 1974;291:664–7.
30. Maynard JE, Fleshman JK, Tschopp CF. Otitis media in Alaskan Eskimo children: Prospective evaluation of chemoprophylaxis. JAMA. 1972;219:597–9.

31. Klein JO, Bluestone CD. Acute otitis media: Management of pediatric infectious diseases in office practice. Pediatr Infect Dis. 1982;1:66–73.
32. Teele DW, Klein JO, the Greater Boston Collaborative Study Group Use of pneumococcal vaccine for prevention of recurrent acute otitis media in infants in Boston. Rev Infect Dis. 1981;3 (Suppl):113.
33. Sloyer JL, Ploussard JH, Howie VM. Efficacy of pneumococcal polysaccharide vaccine in preventing acute otitis media in infants in Huntsville, Alabama. Rev Infect Dis. 1981;3(Suppl):119.
34. Makela PH, Leinonen M, Pukander J, et al. A study of the pneumococcal vaccine in prevention of clinically acute attacks of recurrent otitis media. Rev Infect Dis. 1981;3(Suppl):124.
35. Paradise JL, Bluestone CD, Rogers KD, et al. Efficacy of adenoidectomy in recurrent otitis media: Historical overview and preliminary results from a randomized, controlled trial. Ann Otol Rhinol Laryngol. 1980;89:319–21.
36. Gates GA, Avery CA, Prihoda TJ, et al. Effectiveness of adenoidectomy and tympanostomy tubes in the treatment of chronic otitis media with effusion. N Engl J Med. 1987;317:1444–51.

47. SINUSITIS

JACK M. GWALTNEY, JR.

Acute sinusitis is an infection of one or more of the paranasal sinuses that usually complicates a common cold or other viral infection of the upper respiratory tract. A minor proportion of cases are associated with dental infection. Acute sinusitis may also occur in patients with allergic rhinitis or anatomic abnormalities of the nose that interfere with normal mucociliary function in the sinus cavity. Sinusitis in turn may be complicated by serious intracranial infections such as bacterial meningitis, epidural and subdural abscess, and brain abscess.

ETIOLOGY

The infectious agents responsible for most cases of acute maxillary sinusitis are listed in Table 1. The information is from studies in which specimens for culture were obtained by direct sinus puncture and aspiration to avoid contamination by nasopharyngeal flora.[1,2,5–10] *Streptococcus pneumoniae* and unencapsulated strains of *Haemophilus influenzae* accounted for approximately one-half of all cases. Mixtures of anaerobic bacteria were associated with 6 percent of infections in adults. Sinusitis due to anaerobic bacteria was usually found in patients with associated dental disease. *Staphylococcus aureus, Streptococcus pyogenes, Branhamella catarrhalis*, and other gram-negative bacteria were each associated with a proportion of the total cases. α-Hemolytic streptococci have also been recovered in pure culture in high titers from aspirates of acute infected sinuses. In children, anaerobic infections were not seen, presumably due to less frequent dental infections, and *B. catarrhalis* was recovered almost as frequently as *H. influenzae*.[10]

Rhinovirus, influenza virus, and parainfluenza virus were recovered alone or in combination with bacteria in approximately one-fifth of the adult cases. Whether the sequence was for the viral infection to precede the bacterial infection or for a simultaneous invasion by both organisms was not clear.

Nosocomial sinusitis has been most often associated with *Pseudomonas aeruginosa, Klebsiella pneumoniae, Enterobacter* sp. and *Proteus mirabilis* and was often polymicrobic.[3] *Pseudomonas aeruginosa* was also the most frequent isolate in sinus aspirates from patients with cystic fibrosis.[11]

A small proportion of sinus disease results from fungal infections. The list of fungal infections associated with sinus disease continues to grow and includes aspergillosis.[12,13] phaeohyphomycosis,[14,15] mucormycosis, pseudallescheriasis, and many other mycoses.[16–18] Whereas acute fungal sinusitis occurs in patients with serious underlying diseases, most patients with chronic fungal sinusitis are otherwise healthy.

TABLE 1. The Microbial Etiology of Acute Community-Acquired Antral Sinusitis

	Percent of Cases Mean (Range)	
Microbial Agent	*Adults*	*Children*
Bacteria		
S. pneumoniae	31 (20–35)	36
H. influenza (unencapsulated)	21 (6–26)	23
S. pneumoniae and *H. influenzae*	5 (1–9)	—
Anaerobic bacteria (*Bacteroides, Peptostreptococcus, Fusobacterium* sp., and so forth)	6 (0–10)	—
S. aureus	4 (0–8)	—
S. pyogenes	2 (1–3)	2
B. catarrhalis	2	19
Gram-negative bacteria[a]	9 (0–24)	2
Viruses		
Rhinovirus	15	—
Influenza virus	5	—
Parainfluenza virus	3	2
Adenovirus	—	2

[a] One study had a 24 percent isolation of gram-negative bacteria, but in four other studies the recovery rate was not over 5 percent. Gram-negative bacteria recovered included *P. aeruginosa, K. pneumoniae*, and *E. coli*.

EPIDEMIOLOGY

Approximately 0.5 percent of common upper respiratory infections are complicated by acute sinusitis.[19] The incidence of sinusitis parallels the incidence of acute infections of the upper respiratory tract, being most prevalent during the fall, winter, and spring months. Sinus infection in the summer is often associated with swimming. Sinusitis is more common in adults than in children. Full development of the maxillary, frontal, and sphenoidal sinuses is not reached until adolescence. Some physicians have the clinical impression that the incidence of acute sinusitis is increased in cigarette smokers, but studies of this risk factor are not available.

PATHOGENESIS

Most acute sinusitis is thought to be a bacterial complication of viral colds. This idea is supported by studies in which viruses were recovered from sinus aspirates of patients with maxillary sinusitis.[1,2] The exact pathogenic mechanisms involved are unknown. The sinuses are normally sterile as a result of continuous mucociliary cleansing of particulate matter that enters the sinus cavity. However, respiratory viruses are efficient in eluding the protection provided by the mucous blanket of normal respiratory epithelium and in initiating infection. When viral infection occurs in a sinus there is presumed disruption of the normal cleansing mechanism, opening the way for secondary bacterial invasion. From 5 to 10 percent of the cases of acute maxillary sinusitis result from infection originating from a dental source. The floor of the maxillary sinus is close to the roots of the molars and bicuspids, and infection at these sites may spread to the sinus cavity.

During acute sinusitis, the sinus mucosal lining is characteristically inflamed and swollen. Mucosal erosion may occur with some viral infections, such as influenza, but pathologic descriptions of the findings in specific infections are not available. An exudate develops in the sinus cavity containing polymorphonuclear leukocytes that are usually present in concentrations greater than 5000 cells/mm^3.[1] The bacterial titers in exudates from acutely infected sinuses are usually greater than 10^5 cfu/ml and may reach levels of 10^8 cfu/ml.

Noninfectious conditions that predispose to acute sinusitis include anatomic abnormalities such as congenital choanal atresia, septal deviation, foreign bodies, and tumors. Allergic reactions in the nose cause mucosal swelling and polyp formation that also may lead to infection. Recently, attention has been called to nosocomial sinusitis in hospitalized patients, resulting from indwelling nasal tubes of various types, or nasal packing.[3]

Prolonged and repeated episodes of infection in untreated or inadequately treated patients probably lead to irreversible changes in the mucosal lining of the sinus, resulting in chronic sinusitis. The normal ciliated epithelium is replaced by stratified squamous epithelium that may eventually fill the sinus lumen. Sterility is no longer maintained in the sinus cavity. Cultures of surgical specimens obtained aseptically from patients with chronic sinus disease have grown a wide variety of gram-positive and gram-negative bacteria.[4] Anaerobic bacteria, *Staphylococcus aureus*, and *Streptococcus* of the *viridans* group were recovered most often. The ongoing bacterial growth is secondary to the structural damage, which leads to a loss of the sinus membranes' capacity for self-cleansing. Thus, infection is not thought to be the basic problem in chronic sinusitis, although acute infectious exacerbations due to organisms such as *Streptococcus pneumoniae* and *H. influenzae* sometimes occur.

CLINICAL PRESENTATION

Acute sinusitis usually develops during the course of a common cold or influenzal illness. Facial pain and purulent nasal discharge are the most constant features of the disease. Other complaints include headache, nasal obstruction, disorders of smell, and a nasal quality to the voice. A purulent nasal and/or postnasal discharge is usually present; with maxillary sinusitis pus is characteristically observed in the middle meatus on examination of the nose. In a small proportion of cases, erythema and tenderness are present over the involved sinus, but the absence of such external manifestations of inflammation should not exclude the diagnosis of acute sinusitis. Edema of the eyelids and excessive tearing occur with ethmoid sinusitis. Appearance of chemosis, proptosis, or limited extraocular movement should suggest the possibility of orbital extension from the ethmoidal infection. In maxillary sinusitis of dental origin, the findings of caries and signs of associated dental infection may be present. Temperature elevation has been reported in only approximately one-half of adults and children with acute maxillary sinusitis diagnosed by sinus puncture. In children, cough was the most common complaint; also fetid breath was a frequent sign.[10] In both children and adults the clinical features of acute sinusitis are often difficult to distinguish from those of a prolonged cold. In some studies, patients with acute sinusitis have become asymptomatic despite the persistence of pus and active infection in the sinus cavity as determined by sinus puncture.[1]

Maxillary sinusitis frequently occurs alone. Infection of the other sinuses is more often associated with concomitant infection of another sinus. Patients who develop intracranial extension of infection, such as meningitis and brain abscess, usually show the characteristic signs of these infections. It may be difficult to determine when acute frontal sinusitis has progressed to a frontal lobe abscess of the brain. Inflammation and tenderness over the frontal sinus is often lacking with this infection. Patients may become apathetic and have a minimum of complaints because of destruction of the frontal lobe cortex (Fig. 1).

Osteomyelitis of the frontal bone may occur by spread from the frontal or ethmoid sinuses. Pus may collect under the periosteum of the frontal bone causing swelling and edema over the forehead, a condition known as Pott puffy tumor.[20]

Nosocomial sinusitis resulting from indwelling nasal tubes has occurred most often during the second week of hospitalization.[3] Unilateral maxillary sinusitis was most common, followed by bilateral maxillary disease and pansinusitis. Fever and leukocytosis were common. Unexplained fever in patients with indwelling nasal tubes is an indication for evaluation for sinus infection.

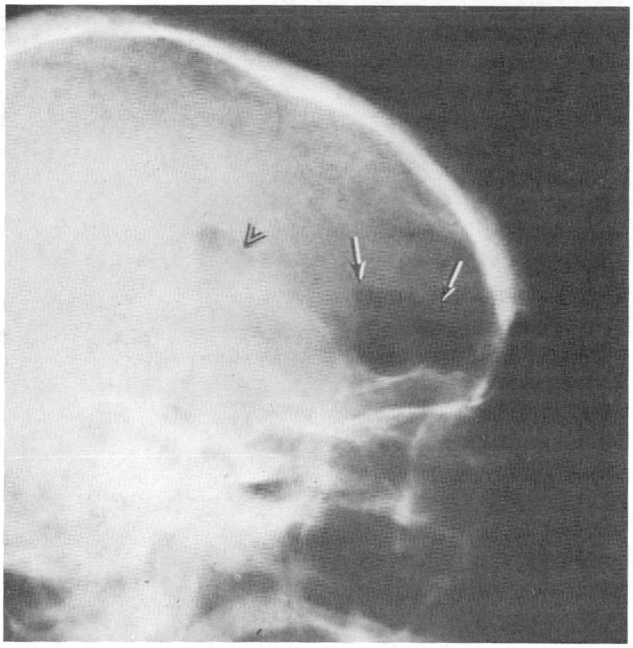

FIGURE 1. Lateral sinus roentgenogram of a patient with acute frontal sinusitis complicated by abscess of the frontal lobe of the brain. Destruction of the posterior wall of the frontal sinus resulted in air in the abscess cavity (→) and in the lateral ventricle (⩔). The infection was caused by *S. aureus*.

DIAGNOSIS

Diagnostic evaluation should include a history and an examination of the pharynx, nose, ears, sinuses, and teeth. Information should be obtained on the occurrence of coryzal and influenzal illness and of respiratory allergies. Because the "typical" complaints of acute sinusitis frequently overlap those of a prolonged but uncomplicated common cold, it is not possible to make a diagnosis of sinusitis on history and physical examination alone in many patients.

Valuable information may be obtained from transillumination of the maxillary and frontal sinuses although this method is less used than in the past. Transillumination should be performed in a completely darkened room. In patients with previously normal sinuses, the finding of complete opacity of the sinus on transillumination is strong evidence for the presence of active infection.[1] Conversely, the finding of normal light transmission is equally good evidence that no infection is present. The finding of diminished light tránsmission, "dullness" but not complete opacity, is less helpful. Approximately one-quarter of the patients with this finding were found to have active infection as determined by sinus puncture, while the remaining three-quarters were normal. It should be emphasized that sinus transillumination is less helpful in patients with chronic sinusitis in whom absent or reduced light transmission may be a persistent finding.

The most sensitive routine test for the diagnosis of acute sinusitis in adults and children over 1 year of age is radiologic examination of the sinuses. The presence of radiologic opacity, an air–fluid level, or of mucosal thickening is strong evidence for the presence of active infection (Fig. 2)[1,2,21,22] In children under 1 year of age, sinus radiographs appear to be of limited utility.[22] Also, the value of sinus radiology in diagnosing active infection is limited in patients with chronic sinusitis because of persistent radiologic abnormalities in such patients.

While not practical for routine diagnosis of community-acquired sinusitis, (computed tomography (CT)) and magnetic resonance imaging (MRI) provide very sensitive methods for evaluating abnormalities of the paranasal sinuses. These techniques

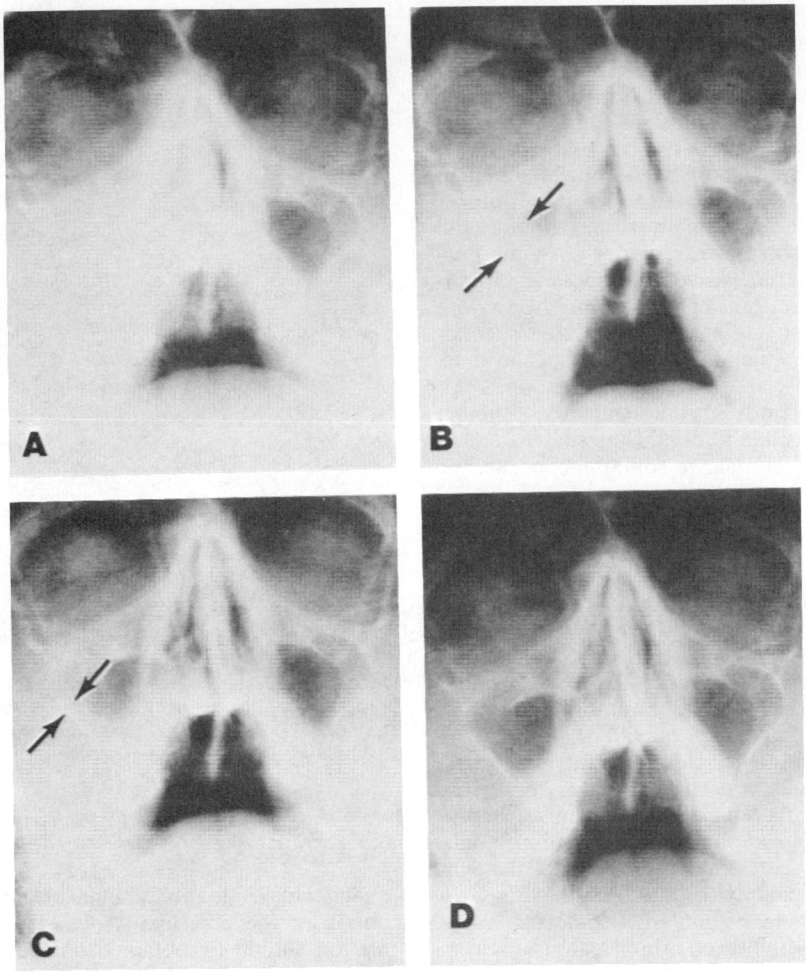

FIGURE 2. Serial roentgenograms of a patient with acute infection of the right maxillary antrum (occipitomental views). **(A)** February 18, complete opacity of the antrum. Culture of sinus aspirate yielded *H. influenzae* in a titer of 10^6 cfu/ml. **(B)** February 25, marked thickening of the mucosal lining. **(C)** March 4, diminished thickening of the mucosal lining. **(D)** March 18, normal. The patient received ampicillin from February 18 to February 26.

are particularly useful for examination of the ethmoid and sphenoid sinuses, since conventional radiography lacks optimal sensitivity here. CT or MRI is also useful whenever orbital extension of ethmoid sinusitis is expected.

The specific microbial etiology of acute sinusitis can be determined only by culture of an exudate or a rinse obtained directly from the sinus by puncture and aspiration. Cultures of nasal pus or of sinus exudates obtained by rinsing through the natural sinus ostium give unreliable information because of contamination with resident bacterial flora in the nose. Since the microbial etiology of acute sinusitis has been well described in studies using direct puncture,[1–3,5–10] there is no indication for using sinus puncture in the management of the average case of acute sinusitis. However, sinus puncture should be performed for bacterial diagnosis in patients with unusually severe sinusitis, particularly if intracranial extension of the infection is suspected. Also, sinus puncture is of value in patients who have not responded to empiric antimicrobial therapy, those with severe immunosuppression, and those with nosocomial sinusitis when it is not possible to predict the identity and antimicrobial sensitivity of the causative agent.

The antral sinus is punctured below the inferior turbinate of the nose and the frontal sinus below the infraorbital rim of the eye. Thorough cleansing of the puncture site with an antiseptic solution such as povidone–iodine is important to prevent contamination of the specimen with surface bacteria. Specimens for culture should be aspirated through the puncture needle or through a plastic catheter and should not be obtained by collecting material that has been rinsed through the natural sinus ostium. When free fluid cannot be obtained from the sinus cavity, 1 ml of antibiotic-free normal saline or Ringer's lactate solution can be instilled and aspirated to provide a specimen. The syringe containing the specimen should be transported to the laboratory for examination by gram stain and aerobic and anaerobic bacterial culture. When available, quantitative culture of the specimen is useful to help to detect bacterial contaminants accidentally introduced into the specimen. Most bacteria causing active sinus infection are present in titers of $\geq 10^5$ cfu/ml, while titers of contaminants in a freshly processed specimen are usually less.

In patients with acute sinusitis in whom intracranial complications, such as bacterial meningitis and brain abscess, are suspected appropriate diagnostic evaluations should be conducted promptly (see Chapters 66 and 70).

Noninfectious causes of persistent sinus disease which enter the differential diagnosis of sinusitis include Wegener's granulomatosis, lethal midline granuloma, and its variant polymorphic reticulosis.

TREATMENT

Antimicrobial Therapy

Although viruses may play a role in the initiation of acute sinusitis, the disease should be treated as a bacterial infection. The

TABLE 2. Antimicrobials Effective in the Therapy of Acute Sinusitis

Antimicrobial Agent	*Recommended Oral Dose in Adults*
Ampicillin	500 mg q6h
Amoxicillin	500 mg q8h
Cyclacillin	500 mg q8h
Bacampicillin	800 mg bid
Trimethoprim-sulfamethoxazole (80 mg/400 mg)	2 tablets bid
Cefaclor	500 mg q6h
Cefuroxime axetil	250 mg q12h

efficacy of antimicrobials for treating acute sinusitis has been established in studies employing pre- and posttreatment sinus aspirations.[23,24] Antimicrobial therapy must be selected on an empiric basis since in the usual case, sinus puncture to determine a specific microbial diagnosis is not indicated. Therapy should ideally cover all the bacteria listed in Table 1, but primarily it should be effective for both *S. pneumoniae* and *H. influenzae*. Antimicrobials shown to be effective in acute sinusitis in studies employing pre- and posttreatment sinus aspirations[24–27] and the doses recommended are listed in Table 2. A 10-day course of therapy is recommended based on findings in the sinus puncture studies. Ampicillin or amoxicillin is recommended for the initial treatment of uncomplicated community-acquired sinusitis. In evaluating the response to these drugs, it should be remembered that they are not effective against β-lactamase-producing bacteria. For the penicillin-allergic patient, trimethoprim-sulfamethoxazole is an alternative that provides adequate coverage against both *S. pneumoniae* and *H. influenzae*. Sinusitis due to penicillin-resistant strains of bacteria requires treatment with a penicillinase-resistant antimicrobial agent. In areas where *Haemophilus* and *Branhamella* isolates are often β-lactamase producers, a third-generation cephalosporin may be an appropriate choice when parenteral therapy is indicated.

Supportive Therapy

Nasal decongestants should be used in the supportive treatment of acute sinusitis. Phenylephrine nose drops, 0.25 or 0.5%, are recommended for use on a regular basis as described in Chapter 42. If pain is severe, codeine may be required. Most patients with acute sinusitis can be successfully treated as outpatients. For patients with severe infection and for those in whom intracranial extension of infection is a consideration, hospitalization is advisable for parenteral antimicrobial therapy, close observation and prompt initiation of diagnostic tests when needed. Antihistamines may thicken purulent sinus fluid and impair drainage. Their use for acute sinusitis is to be discouraged.

Surgical Therapy

Patients with severe sinus infection or those suspected of developing intracranial or orbital complications should be evaluated with computerized tomography for emergency or early surgical drainage. Infection of the orbit frontal[28] and sphenoid[29] sinuses should be recognized as conditions in which surgical intervention may be required.

SUBACUTE AND CHRONIC SINUSITIS

Sinus lavage has been used traditionally for the treatment of patients with acute sinusitis in whom complaints have persisted. A series of irrigations of the affected sinus appears to be beneficial. When lavage is performed via direct sinus puncture, a sample of the sinus contents should be aspirated and cultured quantitatively for bacterial identification and antibiotic sensitivities.

Once sinusitis has reached a chronic state, there is no evidence that it is primarily an infectious problem, although patients with permanent mucosal damage of the sinuses may have acute infectious exacerbations. Infectious exacerbations, which are recognized in patients with chronic sinus disease, should be treated in the same way as described above for the treatment of an acute infection. Surgical procedures, such as creation of an artificial ostium to facilitate sinus drainage and submucous resection, are used in the treatment of patients with chronic sinusitis.

Measures to Prevent Acute or Chronic Sinusitis

There are no proven ways to prevent acute sinusitis. When control of colds and influenzal illness becomes practical, the incidence of sinusitis should decline. For the present, prompt and regular use of vasoconstrictors in nasal drops or sprays for the treatment of colds may help to reduce the incidence of secondary bacterial infection of the sinuses, but this is unproven. Control of nasal allergies and corrective surgery for nasal abnormalities may promote normal sinus drainage and thus lessen the risk of sinus infection. Good dental hygiene and prompt treatment of tooth root infection may help reduce the incidence of acute infection of the maxillary sinus secondary to dental disease.

Effective antimicrobial therapy for patients with acute sinusitis may help to reduce the incidence of chronic sinus disease, although this is not established. The diversity of bacteria responsible for acute sinusitis limits the choice of antimicrobials that have an adequate spectrum of activity, particularly for both *S. pneumoniae* and *H. influenzae*. Penicillin, tetracyclines, and cephalosporins, which have been widely used in the past to treat acute sinusitis, do not provide optimum coverage for both these organisms. Undoubtedly, many patients with acute sinusitis who were given one of these drugs did not receive effective treatment. This may have resulted in the infection causing permanent damage to the sinus and may have been a preventable cause of chronic sinusitis.

REFERENCES

1. Evans FO, Sydnor JB, Moore WEC, et al. Sinusitis of maxillary antrum. N Engl J Med. 1975;293:735.
2. Hamory BH, Sande MA, Sydnor A Jr, et al. Etiology and antimicrobial therapy of acute maxillary sinusitis. J Infect Dis. 1979;139:197.
3. Caplan ES, Hoyt NJ. Nosocomial sinusitis. JAMA. 1982;247:639.
4. Frederick J, Braude AI. Anaerobic infection of the paranasal sinuses. N Engl J Med 1974;290:135.
5. Urdal K, Berdal P. The microbial flora in 81 cases of maxillary sinusitis. Acta Otolaryngol. 1949;37:20.
6. Björkwall T. Bacteriologic examinations in maxillary sinusitis: bacterial flora of the maillary antrum. Acta Otolaryngol. 1950;83(Suppl):33.
7. Lystad A, Berdal P, Lung-Iversen L. The bacterial flora of sinusitis with in vitro study of the bacterial resistance to antibiotics. Acta Otolaryngol. 1964;188(Suppl):390.
8. Rantanen T, Arvilommi H. Double-blind trial of doxycycline in acute maxillary sinusitis; a clinical and bacteriological study. Acta Otolaryngol. 1973; 76:58.
9. Axelsson A, Broson JE. The correlation and maxillary sinus in acute maxillary sinusitis. Laryngoscope. 1973;83:2003.
10. Wald ER, Milmoe GJ, Bowen A'D, et al. Acute maxillary sinusitis in children. N Engl J Med. 1981;304:749.
11. Shapiro ED, Milmoe, Wald ER, et al. Bacteriology of the maxillary sinuses in patients with cystic fibrosis. J Infect Dis. 1982;146:589.
12. McGuirt WF, Harril JA. Paranasal sinus aspergillosis. Laryngoscope. 1979;89:1563.
13. Rinaldi MG. Invasive aspergillosis. Rev Infect Dis. 1983;5:1061.
14. Padhye AA, Ajello L, Wieden MA, et al. Phaeohyphomycosis of the nasal sinuses caused by a new species of *Exserohilum*. J Clin Microbiol. 1986;24:245.
15. MacMillan RH III, Cooper PH, Body BA, et al. Allergic fungal sinusitis due to *Curvularia lunata*. Hum Pathol. 1987;18:960.
16. Parfrey NA. Improved diagnosis and prognosis of mucormycosis. A clinicopathologic study of 33 cases. Medicine 1986;65:113.

17. Kern ME, Uecker FA. Maxillary sinus infection caused by the homobasidiomycetous fungus *Schizophyllum commune*. J Clin Microbiol. 1986;23:1001.
18. Washburn RG, Kennedy AW, Begley MG, et al. Chronic fungal sinusitis in apparently normal hosts. Medicine. 1988;67:231–47.
19. Dingle JH, Badger GF, Jordan WS Jr. Illness in the Home. A Study of 25,000 Illnesses in a Group of Cleveland Families. Cleveland: The Press of Western Reserve University; 1964;292.
20. Wells RG, Sty JR, Landers AD. Radiological evaluation of Pott puffy tumor. JAMA. 1986;255:1331–1333.
21. Lusted LB, Keats TE. Atlas of Roentgenographic Measurement. 4th ed. Chicago: Year Book Medical Publishers; 1978.
22. Kovatch AL, Wald ER, Ledesma-Medina J, et al. Maxillary sinus radiographs in children with non-respiratory complaints. Pediatrics. 1984;73:306.
23. Carenfelt C, Eneroth C-M, Lundberg C, et al. Evaluation of the antibiotic effect of treatment of maxillary sinusitis. Scand J Infect Dis. 1984;73:306.
24. Gwaltney JM Jr, Sydnor A Jr, Sande MA. Etiology and antimicrobial treatment of acute sinusitis. Ann Otol Rhinol Laryngol. 1981;90:68.
25. Farr B, Scheld M, Gwaltney JM Jr, et al: Bacampicillin HCl in the treatment of acute maxillary sinusitis. Bull NY Acad Med. 1983;59:477.
26. Scheld WM, Sydnor A Jr, Farr B, et al. Comparison of cyclacillin and amoxicillin for therapy of acute maxillary sinusitis. Antimicrob Agents Chemother. 1986;30:250.
27. Sydnor A Jr, Gwaltney JM Jr, Scheld WM. Cefuroxime axetil vs. cefaclor therapy of acute maxillary sinusitis. Presented at the 28th Interscience Conference on Antimicrobial Agents and Chemotherapy, Los Angeles, October 24, 1988.
28. Middleton WG, Briant TDR, Fenton RS. Frontal sinusitis—a 10 year experience. J Otolaryngol. 1985;14:197.
29. Lew D, Southwick FS, Montogomery WW, et al. Sphenoid sinusitis. A review of 30 cases. N Engl J Med. 1983;309:1149.

48. EPIGLOTTITIS

JAMES E. BURNS
J. OWEN HENDLEY

Acute epiglottitis (supraglottitis) is a rapidly progressive cellulitis of the epiglottis and adjacent structures that has the potential for causing abrupt, complete airway obstruction.

The typical patient is a 2- to 4-year-old boy having at any time of the year a 6- to 12-hour history of fever and dysphagia. Sore throat is the most prominent symptom in older children and adults. At the time medical attention is sought, varying degrees of respiratory distress may be evident. The patient usually prefers to sit leaning forward while drooling oral secretions. Respirations tend to be tentative and careful without marked tachypnea. Tachycardia is usually commensurate with fever but may be related to hypoxia and be out of proportion to fever.[1] Inspiratory stridor and hoarseness occur frequently, but the barking cough and aphonia that may occur in croup syndrome are rare. The diagnosis is established by finding an edematous "cherry red" epiglottis. The course of acute epiglottitis may be fulminating, as emphasized by the report of a patient who progressed from being completely asymptomatic to having complete airway obstruction in 30 minutes.[2] The course may be more languid in adults, but the disease is potentially no less serious.[3]

Laboratory data include moderate leukocytosis with a "shift to the left," positive cultures of blood and the epiglottis, and evidence of pneumonia on chest x-ray films in up to 25 percent of cases.[4,5] A roentgenogram of the lateral neck may show an enlarged epiglottis, ballooning of the hypopharynx, and normal subglottic structures (Fig. 1).[6] However, the use of x-ray films in the diagnosis of epiglottitis is questionable both because of the delay in securing an airway while the films are being obtained and the poor sensitivity (as low as 31 percent) and specifity (as low as 44 percent) of this procedure.[3,7,8] The epiglottis should be visualized directly, even if the x-ray findings are negative, in those patients in whom there is a strong suspicion of epiglottitis. This examination should be performed only when prepared to immediately secure the airway. In adults, examination of the epiglottis may be safer than in children.[3] *Haemophilus influenzae* type b is isolated from cultures of blood and/or epiglottis in most pediatric and up to 26 percent of adult patients with epiglottitis,[9] an association first demonstrated by Le Mierre and associates in 1936.[10] Other agents occasionally implicated are pneumococci, staphylococci, streptococci, and *H. paraphrophilus*.[2,11,12] The role of viruses in epiglottitis is not established.

H. influenzae bacteremia occurs in up to 100 percent of children with epiglottitis.[1,13] Significantly, this bacteremia has been associated with only a small number of metastatic infections such as meningitis and arthritis.[1,4,14,15]

DIFFERENTIAL DIAGNOSIS

The croup syndrome is the most frequent differential consideration in epiglottitis. Although the barking cough typical of croup is an infrequent feature of epiglottitis, differentiation from croup is sometimes difficult unless the epiglottis is visualized. In contrast to epiglottitis, croup is frequently preceded by an upper respiratory infection, has a more gradual onset, involves somewhat younger children (aged 3 months to 3 years), and may last up to a week. The etiology is usually viral, and the area of obstruction is subglottic while the epiglottis is normal. Children with croup are more likely to prefer to lie supine and do not have the dysphagia and drooling that are characteristic of epiglottitis. In croup, x-ray films of the lateral aspect of the neck are more likely to reveal a normal epiglottis and may show the airway narrowed in the sublottic region (Fig. 1),[6] but they may have up to a 24 percent false-positive rate for readings consistent with epiglottitis.[7]

Diphtheria can be differentiated from epiglottitis by the presence of a pseudomembrane in the respiratory tract and the presence of typical organisms on direct smear and culture of the membrane. Allergic laryngeal edema (angioneurotic edema) and foreign body aspiration lack the toxic manifestations of epiglottitis and often have a history that is helpful in suspecting the correct diagnosis. Retropharyngeal abscess, peritonsillar abscess, and lingual tonsillitis are other rare causes of upper airway obstruction; these can usually be differentiated from epiglottitis on physical examination.

THERAPY

Maintenance of an adequate airway should be the primary concern as soon as the diagnosis of epiglottitis is even suspected in a child or an adult.

There has been discussion over the years about whether all patients with epiglottitis should have an artificial airway (tracheostomy or endotracheal tube) inserted as soon as the diagnosis is made or whether a period of observation before insertion of an airway is justifiable. In recent years there has been agreement among most authors that provision of an airway immediately is the safest course.[2,3,16–20] Observation of a child with epiglottitis for signs of airway obstruction cannot be recommended since the mortality is up to 6–25 percent in those observed and 33–80 percent in those in whom obstruction occurs.[2,21]

The use of an endotracheal tube rather than a tracheostomy for provision of the artificial airway is preferred as therapy for acute epiglottitis by most authors.[5,17–19,22] In spite of theoretic difficulties with insertion of an endotracheal tube through the region of the inflamed epiglottis, this has not proved to be a problem. An advantage to the use of an endotracheal tube is the ease of its removal after the 36–48 hours required for the inflammation and edema to subside after institution of appropriate antimicrobial therapy.

Because of the potential for rapid deterioration to complete respiratory obstruction, patients even suspected of having acute epiglottitis should be handled as a medical emergency. Patients

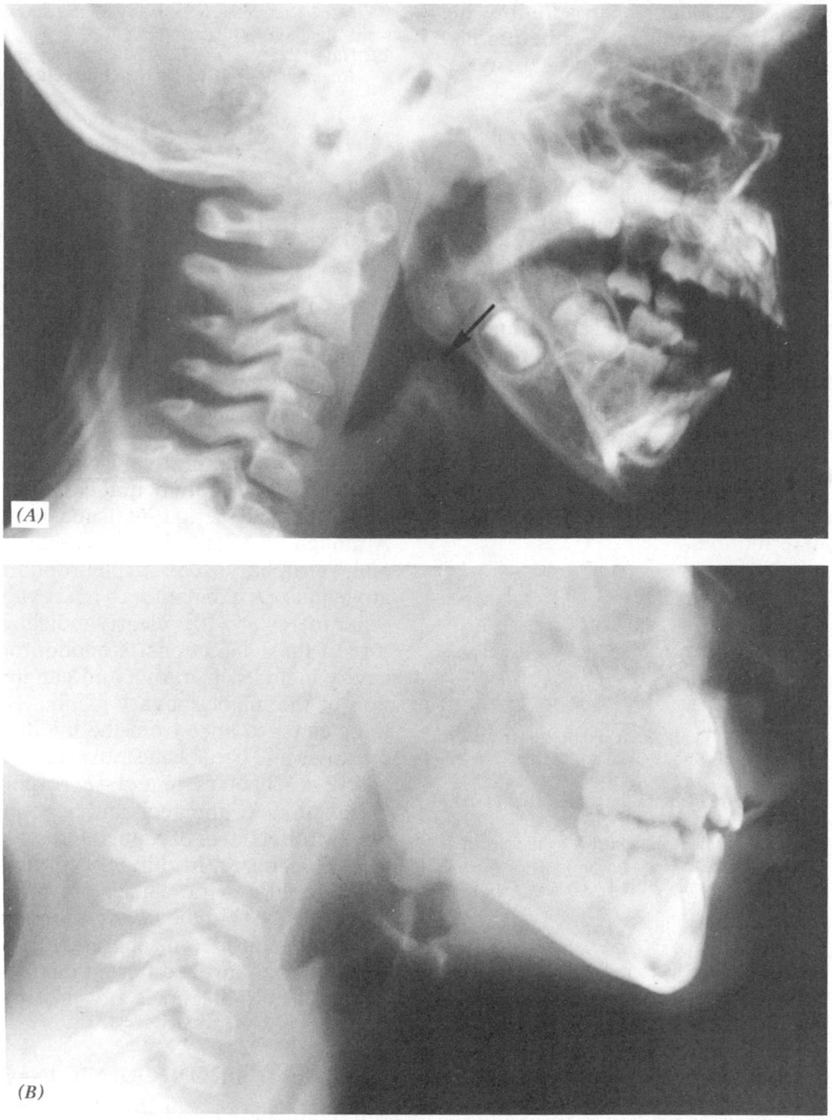

Fig. 1. Lateral neck roentgenograms. **(A)** Enlarged epiglottis—the thumb sign[6]—in a patient with acute epiglottitis. Arrows indicate epiglottitis. **(B)** Normal epiglottis—the little finger sign—in a patient with croup syndrome. (Courtesy of Dr. Caroline B. Hall, University of Rochester School of Medicine, Rochester, NY.)

being transported between medical facilities and within such facilities must be accompanied by personnel capable of securing the airway should obstruction occur.

The epiglottis can be visualized in most patients by depressing the tongue with a depressor placed as far posteriorly as the tonsillar pillars. However, it is unwise to examine the epiglottis of a pediatric patient suspected of having epiglottitis because of the possibility of precipitating complete airway obstruction or vagally mediated cardiopulmonary arrest. It is also unwise to restrain pediatric patients in the supine position because this may also lead to airway obstruction.[20] As a consequence, it is safer to transfer a patient thought to have acute epiglottitis to an operating room and then visualize the epiglottis with a laryngoscope or bronchoscope after all is in readiness for insertion of an artificial airway under controlled conditions. As soon as the diagnosis is made, by visualization of the "cherry red" epiglottis, an uncuffed endotracheal tube should be inserted or a tracheostomy performed. If the epiglottis is normal, the patient may be managed in a manner appropriate for croup or laryngotracheobronchitis. If difficulty is encountered or if obstruction occurs while trying to establish the airway, the possibility of ventilating the apneic patient by bag and mask or mouth-to-mouth ventilation should not be overlooked.[16,17]

After establishment of an airway, samples of blood and the epiglottis should be cultured, and the patient should be administered intravenous antibiotic therapy directed at *H. influenzae*. In view of the risk of infection with ampicillin-resistant *H. influenzae,* ampicillin, 200 mg/kg/day, and chloramphenicol, 75–100 mg/kg/day, both in four divided doses intravenously, have been conventional therapy.[23] At present, intravenous cefuroxime (100–200 mg/kg/day in three divided doses) or a third-generation cephalosporin such as cefotaxime (100–150 mg/kg/day in four doses) may be used for initial therapy.

Patients with acute epiglottitis are usually improved 36–48 hours after initiation of appropriate antibiotic therapy. Depending on the patient's progress, the artificial airway can usually be removed in 48 hours. Before extubation the patient should be afebrile and alert with either a leak around the endotrachael tube or evidence of resolution by direct visualization with a fiber-optic laryngoscope.[19,24] Antibiotics should be continued for 7–10 days. The route by which the antibiotic is administered after extubation should be dictated by the clinical response and status of the patient.

If the patient with epiglottitis has household contacts who are younger than 4 years old, rifampin prophylaxis given once daily for 4 days in a dose of 20 mg/kg/day (maximum of 600 mg/day) is recommended for all household contacts.[25] In addition, the patient should receive rifampin in the same dosage before discharge to prevent reintroduction of the organism into the household (see Chapter 184).

IMMUNITY

An episode of *H. influenzae* epiglottis usually results in high levels of serum antibody to capsular polysaccharide.[26] This response appears to provide immunity since second cases of epiglottitis are extremely rare. The presence of maternally derived serum antibody at birth explains the infrequent occurrence of *H. influenzae* infections in infants. After the disappearance of this maternal antibody there is an inverse relationship between rising levels of naturally acquired antibody and the declining incidence of epiglottitis.[27]

Widespread use of *H. influenzae* type b polysaccharide vaccine should decrease the incidence of epiglottitis.[28] However, since approximately one-third of cases occur in children under 18 months of age, the disease will not disappear with the current conjugated vaccine given at 18 months.[29]

REFERENCES

1. Sendi K, Crysdale WS. Acute epiglottitis: Decade of change—a 10-year experience with 242 children. J Otolaryngol. 1987;16:196–202.
2. Bass JW, Steele RW, Wiebe RA. Acute epiglottitis: A surgical emergency. JAMA. 1974;229:671–5.
3. MayoSmith MF, Hirsch PJ, Wodzinski SF, et al. Acute epiglottitis in adults: An eight-year experience in the state of Rhode Island. N Engl J Med. 1986;314:1133–9.
4. Molteni RA. Epiglottitis: Incidence of extraepiglottic infection: Report of 72 cases and review of the literature. Pediatrics. 1976;58:526–31.
5. Battaglia JD, Lockhart CH. Management of acute epiglottitis by nasotracheal intubation. Am J Dis Child. 1975;129:334–6.
6. Podgore JK, Bass JW. The "thumb sign" and "little finger sign" in acute epiglottitis. J Pediatr. 1976;88:154–5.
7. Stankiewicz JA, Bowes AK. Croup and epiglottitis: A radiologic study. Laryngoscope. 1985;95:1159–60.
8. Jones JL, Holland P. False positives in lateral neck radiographs used to diagnose epiglottitis. Ann Emerg Med. 1983;12:797.
9. Mustoe T, Strome M. Adult epiglottitis. Am J Otolaryngol. 1983;4:393–9.
10. Le Mierre A, Meyer A, Laplane R. Les septicemies a bacille de pfeiffer. Ann Med. 1936;39:97–119.
11. Berenberg W, Kevy S. Acute epiglottitis in childhood. N Engl J Med. 1958;258:870–4.
12. Jones RN, Slepack J, Bigelow J. Ampicillin-resistant *Haemophilus paraphrophilus* laryno-epiglottitis. J Clin Microbiol. 1976;4:405–7.
13. Alexander HE, Ellis C, Leidy G. Treatment of type-specific hemophilus infections in infancy and childhood. J Pediatr. 1942;20:673–98.
14. Dajani AD, Asmar BI, Thirumoorthia MC. Systemic *Haemophilus influenzae* disease: An overview. J Pediatr. 1979;94:355–64.
15. Branfors-Helander P, Jeppsson P-H. Acute epiglottitis: A clinical, bacteriological, and serological study. Scand J Infect Dis. 1975;7:103–11.
16. Adair JC, Ring WH. Management of epiglottitis in children. Anesth Analg. 1975;54:622–5.
17. Blanc VF, Weber ML, Ludec C, et al. Acute epiglottitis in children: Management of 27 consecutive cases with nasotrachael intubation with special emphasis on anaesthetic considerations. Can Anaesth Soc J. 1977;24:1–11.
18. Rapkin RH. Nasotrachael intubation in epiglottitis. Pediatrics. 1975;56:110–2.
19. Baines DB, Wark H, Overton JH. Acute epiglottitis in children. Anaesth Intensive Care. 1984;13:25–8.
20. Bass JW, Fajardo JE, Brien JH, et al. Sudden death due to acute epiglottitis. Pediatr Infect Dis. 1985;4:447–9.
21. Rapkin RH. Tracheostomy in epiglottitis. Pediatrics. 1973;52:426–9.
22. Schuller DE, Brick HG. The safety of intubation in croup and epiglottitis: An eight year follow-up. Laryngoscope. 1975;85:33–46.
23. McCracken GH Jr. Commentary. J Pediatr. 1979;94:987.
24. Gonzalez C, Reilly JS, Kenna MA, et al. Duration of intubation in children with acute epiglottitis. Otolaryngol Head Neck Surg. 1986;95:477–81.
25. Committee on Infectious Diseases, American Academy of Pediatrics. In Peter G, ed. Report of the Committee on Infectious Diseases. Evanston, IL: American Academy of Pediatrics; 1986:169–74.
26. Whisnant JK, Rogentine GN, Gralnick MA, et al. Host factors and antibody response in *Haemophilus influenzae* type b meningitis and epiglottitis. J Infect Dis. 1976;133:448–55.
27. Schneerson R, Rodrigues LP, Parke JC Jr, et al. Immunity to disease caused by *Hemophilus influenzae* type b. J Immunol. 1971;107:1081–9.
28. Petola H, Käyhty H, Virtanen M, et al. Prevention of *Hemophilus influenzae* type b bacteremic infections with the capsular polysaccharide vaccine. N Engl J Med. 1984;310:1561–6.
29. Hay JW, Daum RS. Cost-benefit analysis of two strategies for prevention of *Haemophilus influenzae* type b infections. Pediatrics. 1987;80:319–29.

49. INFECTIONS OF THE ORAL CAVITY, NECK, AND HEAD

ANTHONY W. CHOW

Infections of the oral cavity most commonly are odontogenic in origin and include dental caries, pulpitis, periapical abscess, gingivitis, and periodontal and deep fascial space infections. Although rare, such life-threatening complications as intracranial, retropharyngeal, or pleuropulmonary extension and hematogenous dissemination to heart valves, prosthetic device, and other metastatic foci clearly indicate the potentially serious nature of these infections. Nonodontogenic infections of the oral cavity include ulcerative and gangrenous stomatitis and infection of the major salivary glands. Suppurative orofacial infections can also arise from the middle ear, oronasopharynx, and mastoids and paranasal sinuses; these have been discussed elsewhere in Chapters 46 and 47, respectively.

Infections of the neck and head in the adult most commonly result from human or animal bites, trauma, irradiation, and surgical procedures. In children, cervical adenitis or thyroiditis due to bacterial or viral causes are more common. Rarely do embryologic cysts in the neck region become secondarily infected. These are considered separately from oral infections since they frequently involve a different microflora and require alternative approaches to diagnosis and therapy.

OROFACIAL ODONTOGENIC INFECTIONS

Microbiologic Considerations

The microbiota associated with odontogenic infections is complex and generally reflects the indigenous oral flora. Despite this complexity, recent evidence strongly supports a causative role of specific microorganisms in different forms of odontogenic infections. This emerging concept of specific microbial cause has created considerable dilemma in our traditional approach to the diagnosis and management of such infections. Since the microflora associated with these infections is typically polymicrobial, it does not necessarily follow that each component of this complex flora has equal pathogenic potential or that the numerically predominant cultivable microflora are the most important. Furthermore, it may not be necessary to eradicate the complete microflora for effective therapy. An appreciation of the indigenous oral flora and the host factors that may modify its composition and knowledge of the specific microorganisms implicated in different odontogenic infections should therefore greatly assist in a more rational approach to such infections arising from the oral cavity.

Indigenous Oral Flora. The oral cavity cannot be regarded as a single, uniform environment. Although representative species of microorganisms can be isolated from most areas of the mouth, certain sites such as the tongue, tooth surface, gingival crevice, and saliva tend to favor colonization by specific organisms[1–3] (Table 1). Quantitative studies indicate that obligate anaerobes constitute a large and important part of the

TABLE 1. Predominant Cultivable Bacteria from Various Sites of the Oral Cavity

		Total Viable Count (Mean %)			
Type	*Predominant Genus or Family*	*Gingival Crevice*	*Dental Plaque*	*Tongue*	*Saliva*
Facultative					
Gram-positive cocci	*Streptococcus*	28.8	28.2	44.8	46.2
	S. mutans	(0–30)	(0–50)	(0–1)	(0–1)
	S. sanguis	(10–20)	(40–60)	(10–20)	(10–30)
	S. mitior	(10–30)	(20–40)	(10–30)	(30–50)
	S. salivarius	(0–1)	(0–1)	(40–60)	(40–60)
Gram-positive rods	*Lactobacillus* *Corynebacterium*	15.3	23.8	13.0	11.8
Gram-negative cocci	*Branhamella*	0.4	0.4	3.4	1.2
Gram-negative rods	Enterobacteriaceae	1.2	ND	3.2	2.3
Anaerobic					
Gram-positive cocci	*Peptostreptococcus*	7.4	12.6	4.2	13.0
Gram-positive rods	*Actinomyces* *Eubacterium* *Lactobacillus* *Leptotrichia*	20.2	18.4	8.2	4.8
Gram-negative cocci	*Veillonella*	10.7	6.4	16.0	15.9
Gram-negative rods		16.1	10.4	8.2	4.8
	Fusobacterium	1.9	4.1	0.7	0.3
	Bacteroides, pigmented	4.7	ND	0.2	ND
	Bacteroides, nonpigmented	5.6	4.8	5.1	2.4
	Campylobacter	3.8	1.3	2.2	2.1
Spirochetes	*Treponema*	1.0	ND	ND	ND

Abbreviations: ND: not detected.
(Data from Chow et al.,[1] Hardie,[2] and Hamada et al.[3])

residential oral flora. In the gingival crevice of healthy adults, for example, the total microscopic counts averaged 2.7×10^{11} microorganisms per gram wet weight.[4] The total cultivable anaerobic bacteria averaged 1.8×10^{11} microorganisms per gram, whereas facultative bacteria averaged 2.2×10^{10} microorganisms per gram, an eightfold difference. Overall, *Streptococcus, Peptostreptococcus, Veillonella, Lactobacillus, Corynebacterium*, and *Actinomyces* account for more than 80 percent of the total cultivable oral flora. Facultative gram-negative rods are uncommon in healthy adults but may be more prominent in seriously ill, hospitalized, and elderly patients.[5,6] Unique ecologic niches are observed. For example, *Streptococcus sanguis, S. mutans*, and *S. mitis* as well as *Actinomyces viscosus* preferentially colonize the tooth surface.[7] In contrast, *S. salivarius* and *Veillonella* sp. have a predilection for the tongue and buccal mucosa.[2] *Fusobacterium*, pigmented *Bacteroides*, and anaerobic spirochetes appear concentrated in the gingival crevice.[2] Factors that appear to govern these localization patterns include selective adherence characteristics of certain bacteria for various types of cells, local environmental conditions such as oxygen tension, oxidation–reduction potential (Eh) and pH, interbacterial coaggregation, and microbial inhibition.[2,8,9] Apart from anatomic considerations, numerous factors such as age, diet and nutrition, eruption of deciduous dentition, oral hygiene, smoking habits, the presence of dental caries or periodontal disease, antimicrobial therapy, hospitalization, pregnancy, as well as genetic and racial factors may influence the composition of the oral flora.[2,7–9]

Microbial Specificity in Odontogenic Infections. Although it had been recognized for some time that odontogenic infections are initiated by microorganisms through the establishment of dental plaques, the microbial specificity of these infections was not fully appreciated until recently. This breakthrough was brought about by technological advances in sampling and anaerobic culture of specimens as well as by improved methods for species identification and taxonomy. Important differences in bacterial compositions have been noted for dental caries, gingivitis, and different forms of periodontitis when compared with cultures from healthy tissues.[10–12] An etiologic association of *S. mutans* in dental caries has been firmly established.[13,14] *Streptococcus mutans* is the only organism consistently isolated from all decayed dental fissures and is the only organism consistently found in greater numbers in carious teeth as compared with noncarious teeth. The infectious and transmissable nature of this organism in dental caries has been demonstrated in both experimental animals and longitudinal studies in humans. Similarly, in gingivitis and periodontitis, a unique and specific bacterial composition of the subgingival plaque has been identified. In the healthy periodontium, the microflora is sparse and consists mainly of gram-positive organisms such as *S. sanguis* and *Actinomyces* sp. In the presence of gingivitis, the predominant subgingival flora shifts to a greater proportion of anaerobic gram-negative rods, and *Bacteroides intermedius* is most commonly isolated.[11,12,15] With established periodontitis, the flora further increases in complexity with a preponderance of anaerobic gram-negative and motile organisms. *Bacteroides gingivalis* (formerly *B. asaccharolyticus* and *B. melaninogenicus* ssp. *asaccharolyticus*) is most commonly isolated. In juvenile periodontitis, a clinical variant seen primarily in adolescents, the subgingival plaque mainly consists of saccharolytic organisms, with *Actinobacillus actinomycetemcomitans* and *Capnocytophaga* sp. as the most common identifiable species. *Bacteroides gingivalis* is rarely found in this condition.[12,16] In suppurative odontogenic infections such as periapical abscesses or deep fascial space infections, a polymicrobial flora is usually present, with *Fusobacterium nucleatum*, pigmented *Bacteroides, Peptostreptococcus, Actinomyces*, and *Streptococcus* as the most predominant isolates.[1,17] Except in selected patients with serious underlying illnesses, facultative gram-negative bacilli and *Staphylococcus aureus* are uncommonly isolated.[18,19]

This microbial specificity demonstrated for different odontogenic infections probably reflects the acquisition of a unique microflora during the development of a supragingival dental plaque and its progression to a subgingival dental plaque.[20] Plaques that accumulate above the gingival margin are composed mainly of gram-positive facultative and microaerophilic cocci and rods; plaques that accumulate below the gingival margin are composed mainly of gram-negative anaerobic rods and motile forms including spirochetes (Fig. 1). Microorganisms residing within the supragingival plaque are characterized by their ability to adhere to the tooth surface and by their saccharolytic activity. Microorganisms in the subgingival plaque are frequently asaccharolytic and need not be adherent.

Pathogenetic Mechanisms

Suppurative orofacial infections are usually preceded by dental caries or periodontal disease. The pathogenetic mechanisms of cariogenesis remain poorly defined. The most universally accepted theory is that originated by W. D. Miller in 1882, which proposes that bacterial action on carbohydrates produces acidic substances that cause demineralization and dissolution of the hard tissues of the tooth.[21,22] In order for dental caries to develop three factors need to be present: (*1*) a susceptible tooth surface (host factors), (*2*) acidogenic (acid-producing) and aciduric (able to grow at low pH) bacteria within a dental plaque (microbial factors), and (*3*) carbohydrates and simple sugars (dietary factors). In the healthy host, at least three mechanisms serve to protect the tooth from carious decay: (*1*) the cleaning action of the tongue and buccal membranes which acts to re-

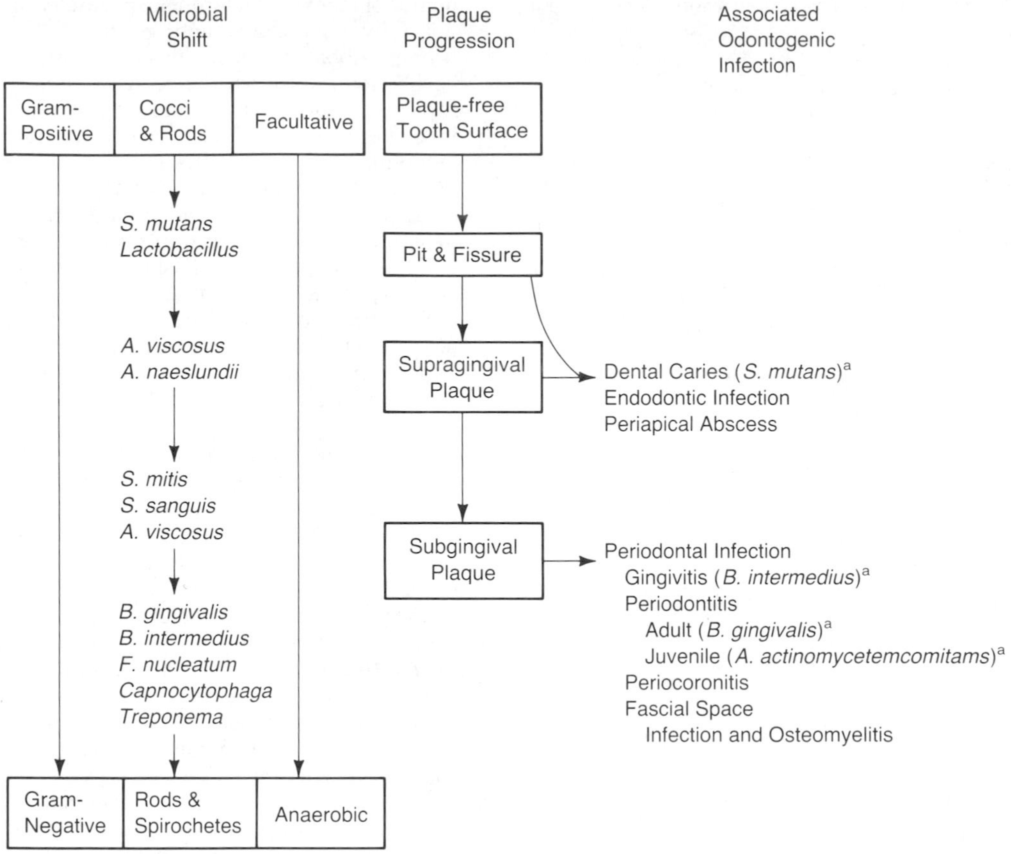

FIG. 1. Microbial specificity in odontogenic infections. A unifying hypothesis demonstrating a microbial shift from a plaque-free tooth surface and progression to supragingival and subgingival plaque organisms. (From Chow,[21] with permission.)

move any food particles from the proximity of the tooth; (*2*) the buffering effect of saliva, which has a neutral pH, washes away bacterial acids, and provides essential substrates for remineralization and repair of damaged tooth surfaces; and (*3*) the protective effect of an acellular bacteria-free coating of salivary origin on the tooth surface, known as the acquired pellicle, which acts as a surface barrier to most dietary and bacterial acids and other proteolytic substances. In the absence of tooth brushing and flossing, the acquired pellicle becomes rapidly colonized and is replaced by the bacterial plaque. It is not surprising, therefore, that carious lesions occur most often in areas inaccessible to the self-cleaning mechanisms of the mouth and on the occlusal surfaces and interproximal sites that are protected from the reaches of the toothbrush.

Unlike dental caries, diet does not appear to have a significant role in the pathogenesis of periodontal disease. The periodontal microflora associated with the subgingival plaque elicits an inflammatory host response that ultimately results in destruction of the periodontium.[11,16,20,22] Two major predisposing factors are poor oral hygiene and increasing age. Other factors include hormonal effects, with exacerbation of disease activity during puberty, menstruation, and pregnancy. Diabetes causes an increased incidence, particularly in juvenile diabetics. Finally, various genetic disorders are associated with an increased incidence of periodontal disease. In particular, those with neutrophil defects (such as Chédiak-Higashi syndrome, agranulocytosis, cyclic neutropenia, and Down syndrome) have a higher incidence of periodontal disease.[22]

It is a tribute to the local defenses in the healthy host that infections within the oral cavity are not more common. Establishment of the normal resident flora appears to be particularly important in providing a strong mucosal defense against colonization and invasion by potential pathogens ("colonization resistance").[23,24] Other nonspecific local defenses include the continuous cell shedding and turnover of the mucosal epithelium and the constant flow of saliva containing lysozyme, lactoferrin, β-lysin, lactoperoxidase, and other antimicrobial systems.[23] Various salivary glycoproteins and histidine-rich polypeptides have been reported to inhibit bacteria and fungi and may prevent infection by the inhibition of microbial attachment to oral epithelium by way of competition for cellular receptor sites or clumping of microorganisms. The epithelial barrier may be affected by radiation therapy, cancer chemotherapy, or trauma. A reduced turnover rate of the epithelial cells will allow retention of adherent organisms. A reduction in saliva volume will also have significant effects on the oral environment and predispose to microbial invasion. In addition to nonspecific host defenses, specific humoral and cellular immune mechanisms are also important. Specific antibodies are present in saliva, with secretory IgA as the predominant immunoglobulin.[25] Salivary antibodies may affect the oral flora by aggregation of organisms and prevention of their attachment to mucosal epithelium. Cell-mediated immunity is important in oral defense against intracellular pathogens including viruses, fungi, and bacteria. In the severely immunocompromised patient, a reactivation of viral infection involving the oral cavity is common, often with potentially life-threatening complications.[26] In addition to humoral and cellular immunity, various phagocytic cells in the oral mucosa also appear important. Phagocytic cells such as lymphocytes, granulocytes, and macrophages are abundant in the lamina propria and presumably contribute to the removal of foreign matter that has breached the epithelial barrier. Unique defects in host defenses have been identified in periodontal infections.[20] For example, impairment of neutrophil chemotaxis has been demonstrated in patients with juvenile periodontitis.[27,28] A number of oral anaerobes and streptococci implicated in periodontitis including *B. gingivalis, B. intermedius, B. melaninogenicus, Capnocytophaga* sp., *S. sanguis*, and *S. mitis* are found to secrete IgA proteases.[29,30] The pathogenic significance of this finding is uncertain at present; it has been suggested that cleavage of IgA by microbial IgA proteases may impair local mucosal immunity of the host. It remains to be seen if similar or other defects of host resistance can be identified in different forms of destructive odontogenic infections.

Anatomic Considerations

Soft tissue infections of odontogenic origin tend to spread along planes of least resistance from the supporting structures of the affected tooth to various potential spaces in the vicinity. Accumulated pus, therefore, must generally perforate bone at the site where it is thinnest and weakest before it extends into the periapical areas or deeper fascial spaces. In the mandible, this is usually in the region of the molar teeth on the lingual aspect and more anterior on the buccal aspect.[31,32] In the maxilla, the bone is weakest on the buccal aspect throughout and relatively thicker on the palatal aspect. If pus perforates through either the maxillary or mandibular buccal plate, it will present intraorally if inside the attachment of the buccinator muscle to the maxilla or mandible and extraorally if outside this muscle attachment (Fig. 2). When a mandibular infection perforates lingually, it presents in the sublingual space if the apices of the involved teeth lie above the attachment of the mylohyoid muscle (e.g., mandibular incisor, canines, premolars, and first molars) and in the submandibular space if below the attachment of this muscle (e.g., second and third molars) (Fig. 2). Thus, these local anatomic barriers of bone, muscle, and fascia predetermine the routes of spread, extent, and clinical manifestations of many orofacial infections of odontogenic origin. The clinically important "fascial spaces" most often involved are illustrated in Figures 3 and 4. These are potential spaces between layers of fascia normally bound together by loose connective tissue. The breakdown of these attachments by a spreading infective process results in a fascial space infection. These spaces intercommunicate with one another to varying degrees, and the potential pathways of extension from one space to another are illustrated in Figure 5. A thorough understanding of the potential *anatomic routes* of infection will not only provide valuable information on the nature and extent of infection but will also suggest the optimum surgical approach for effective drainage.

Clinical Presentations

Odontogenic infections originate in either the dental pulp or the periodontium. The most common site is the dental pulp and results in dentoalveolar infections.

Dentoalveolar Infections. Pulpal infection most frequently results from carious exposure, rarely from physical or chemical injury. The carious process most frequently begins in pits and fissures on the occlusal surfaces of molars and premolars, which encourage food retention. Interproximal sites and the gingival margin are the next most common. Demineralization of the enamel results in discoloration, the first visible evidence of carious involvement. Destruction of the enamel and dentin and invasion of the pulp produce either a localized or generalized pulpitis. If drainage from the pulp is obstructed, a rapid progression with pulpal necrosis and proliferation of endodontic microorganisms leads to invasion of the periapical areas (periapical abscess) and alveolar bone (acute alveolar abscess).

Clinically, the tooth is sensitive to percussion and to both heat and cold during early or reversible pulpitis, although the painful response will stop abruptly when the stimulus is withdrawn. During late or irreversible pulpitis, the tooth is exquisitely painful to a hot stimulus, with prompt relief by the application of cold. If drainage is established through the tooth before extension into the periapical region, chronic irritation from the necrotic pulp may result in periapical granuloma or cyst formation that may be relatively asymptomatic. Dental radiographs are particularly helpful for the detection of silent lesions, particularly those caused by interproximal caries, which are difficult to detect clinically.

The principles of treatment in dentoalveolar infections include prompt elimination of the infected pulp, deep periodontal scaling, or extraction of the affected tooth. Dentoalveolar abscess should be surgically drained at the same time. Other supportive measures include hydration, a soft diet, analgesics, and oral hygiene. Antibiotic therapy is indicated primarily if drainage cannot be adequately established or when infection has perforated the cortex and spread into surrounding soft tissue.

Gingivitis and Periodontal Infections. *Periodontal disease* is a general term that refers to all diseases involving the supporting structures of the teeth (periodontium), which include the gingiva, periodontal ligament, alveolar bone, and cementum. In the early phase of periodontal disease, infection is confined to the gingiva (gingivitis). Later, the underlying supporting tissues are affected (periodontitis), ultimately leading to complete destruction of the periodontium and a permanent loss of teeth. Periodontal infections tend to localize in intraoral soft tissues and seldom spread into deeper structures of the face or neck.

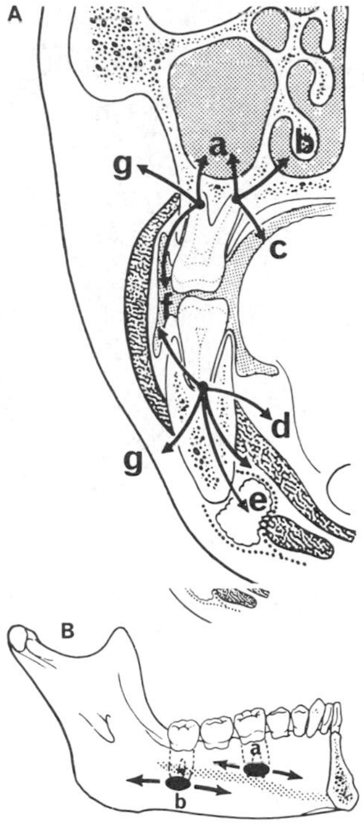

FIG. 2. Routes of spread of odontogenic orofacial infections along planes of least resistance. **(A)** Coronal section in the region of the first molar teeth: a: maxillary antrum; b: nasal cavity; c: palatal plate; d: sublingual space (above the mylohyoid muscle); e: submandibular space (below the mylohyoid muscle); f: intraoral presentation with infection spreading through the buccal plates inside the attachment of the buccinator muscle; g: extraoral presentation to buccal space with infection spreading through the buccal plates outside the attachment of the buccinator muscle. **(B)** Lingual aspect of the mandible: a: apices of the involved tooth above the mylohyoid muscle, with spread of infection to the sublingual space; b: apices of involved tooth below the mylohyoid muscle, with spread of infection into the submandibular space. (From Chow et al.,[1] with permission.)

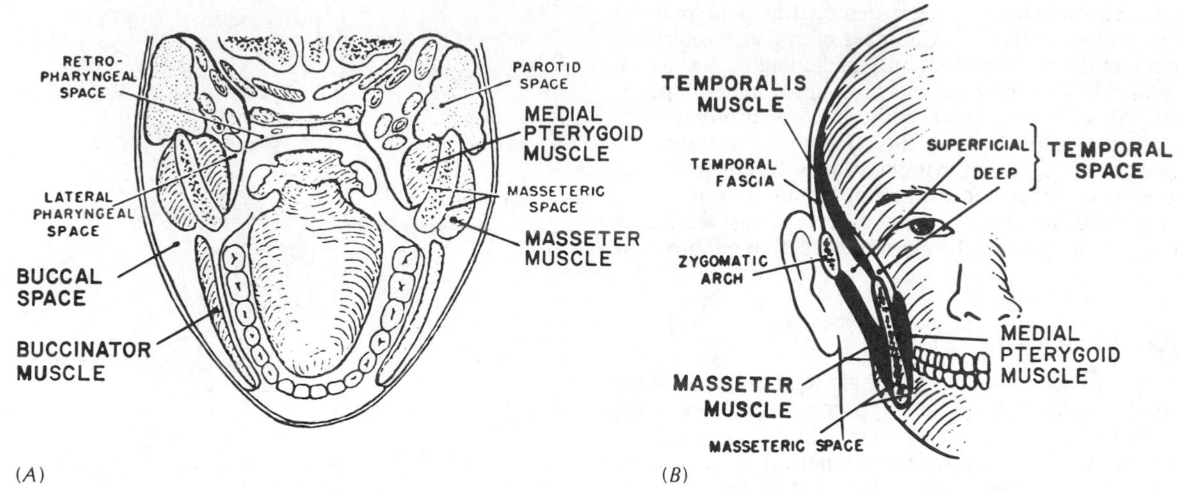

FIG. 3. Fascial spaces around the mouth and face. **(A)** Horizontal section at the level of the occlusal surface of the mandibular teeth. **(B)** Frontal view of the face. (From Chow et al.,[1] with permission.)

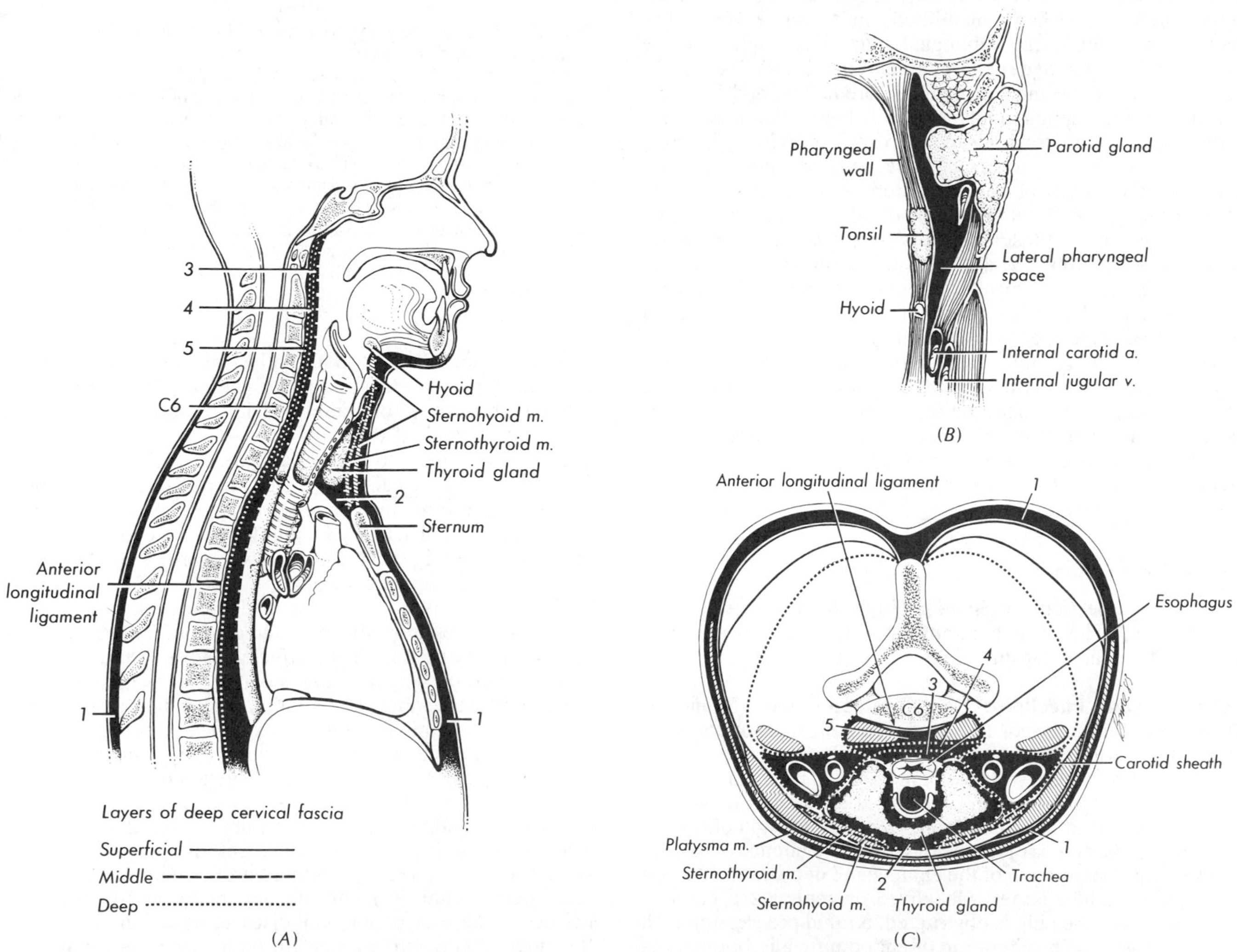

FIG. 4. Relation of lateral pharyngeal, retropharyngeal, and prevertebral spaces to the posterior and anterior layers of the deep cervical fascia (DCF). 1: Superficial space; 2: pretracheal space; 3: retropharyngeal space; 4: "danger" space; 5: prevertebral space. **(A)** Midsagittal section of the head and neck. **(B)** Coronal section in the suprahyoid region of the neck. **(C)** Cross section of the neck at the level of the thyroid isthmus.

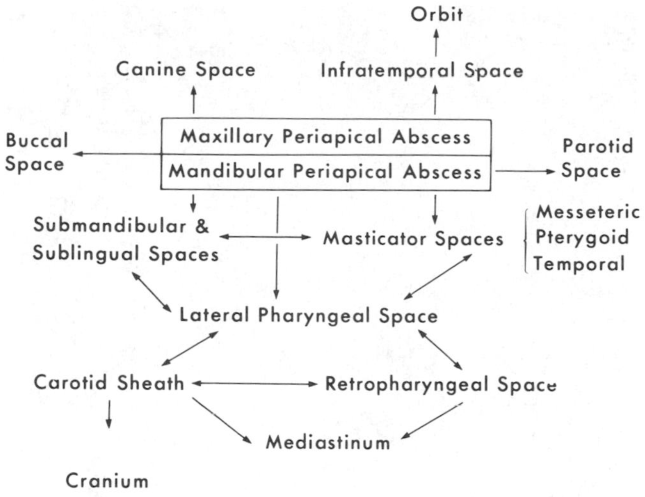

FIG. 5. Potential pathways of extension in deep fascial space infections.

GINGIVITIS. Acute and chronic inflammation of the gingiva is initiated by local irritation and microbial invasion.[11,16,22] Subgingival plaque is always present. In simple gingivitis, there is a bluish red discoloration, with swelling and thickening of the free gingival margin. A tendency for bleeding of the gums after eating or toothbrushing may be one of the earliest findings. There is usually no pain, but a mild fetor oris may be noticed. In acute necrotizing ulcerative gingivitis (Vincent's disease, or trench mouth), the patient typically experiences a sudden onset of pain in the gingiva that interferes with normal mastication. Necrosis of the gingiva occurs mainly in the interdental papilla and results in a marginated, punched-out, and eroded appearance. A superficial grayish pseudomembrane is formed, and a characteristic halitosis with altered taste sensation is present. There is usually associated fever, malaise, and regional lymphadenopathy. Treatment includes local débridement and lavage with oxidizing agents, which usually brings relief from pain within 24 hours. Antibiotic therapy with penicillin or metronidazole is indicated and is highly effective.[33,34]

PERIODONTITIS. Chronic inflammation of the periodontium is the major cause of tooth loss in adults. The destructive process proceeds insidiously, usually beginning in early adulthood. Subgingival plaque is always present, and both supragingival and subgingival calculi are usually abundant. Unlike pulpal infection in which drainage is frequently obstructed, periodontal infections drain freely, and patients experience little or no discomfort. Associated sensations include pressure and an itchy feeling in the gums and between the teeth, a bad taste in the mouth, hot and cold sensitivity, and vague pains in the jaws. The gingiva is inflamed and discolored, bleeds readily, and presents as periodontal pockets around the affected teeth. Frank pus can be readily expressed by digital pressure or may exude freely from the pockets. As periodontitis advances, the supporting tissues are destroyed, ultimately leading to loosening and exfoliation of teeth. Localized juvenile periodontitis is a particularly destructive form of periodontitis seen in adolescents and is characterized by rapid vertical bone loss affecting the first molar and incisor teeth. Plaque is usually minimal, and calculus is absent. A specific defect with impaired neutrophil chemotaxis has been demonstrated in this condition. Recent experience suggests excellent therapeutic results with systemic tetracycline or metronidazole combined with local periodontal treatment involving root débridement and surgical resection of inflamed periodontal tissues.[20,35–37]

PERIODONTAL ABSCESS. Periodontal abscesses may be focal or diffuse and present as red, fluctuant swelling of the gingiva, which is extremely tender to palpation. These abscesses are always in communication with a periodontal pocket from which pus can be readily expressed after probing. Treatment is surgical and aimed at drainage of loculated pus.

PERICORONITIS. Pericoronitis is an acute localized infection associated with gum flaps overlying a partially erupted or impacted wisdom tooth. Food debris and microorganisms become entrapped under the affected gingival tissues. If drainage is interrupted due to sudden swelling or trauma, infection extends along fascial planes of least resistance into adjacent soft tissues. The underlying alveolar bone is usually not involved. Clinically, the pericoronal tissues are erythematous and swollen. Digital pressure will produce a small amount of exudate from under the infected flap. Since the masticator spaces are often involved, marked trismus secondary to irritation of the masseter or medial pterygoid muscle is a prominent presenting feature. Treatment of pericoronitis includes gentle débridement and irrigation under the tissue flap. The use of antibiotics and incision and drainage may be necessary if cellulitis of fascial planes occurs. Excision of the operculum or extraction of the involved tooth may also be considered.

Deep Fascial Space Infections. Infections of either odontogenic or oropharyngeal origin may extend to potential fascial spaces of the lower part of the head and upper portion of the neck. These "space infections" can be conveniently divided into those around the face (masticator, buccal, canine, and parotid spaces), those in the suprahyoid region (submandibular, sublingual, and lateral pharyngeal spaces), and those involving the infrahyoid region or the total neck (retropharyngeal, "danger," and pretracheal spaces).[19,31,32]

MASTICATOR SPACES. Masticator spaces consist of the masseteric, pterygoid, and temporal spaces, all of which are well differentiated but intercommunicate with each other as well as with the buccal, submandibular, and lateral pharyngeal spaces (Fig. 3). Infection of the masticator spaces occurs most frequently from molar teeth, particularly the third molars (wisdom teeth). Clinically, the hallmark of masticator space infection is trismus and pain in the area of the body or ramus of the mandible. Swelling may not be a prominent finding, especially in the masseteric compartment, since infection exists deep in large muscle masses, which obscures or prevents clinically apparent swelling. When present, swelling tends to be brawny and indurated, which suggests the possibility of cervicofacial actinomycosis or mandibular osteomyelitis. If infection extends internally, it can involve an area close to the lateral pharyngeal wall and result in dysphagia. A true lateral pharyngeal space infection, however, is accompanied by displacement of the lateral pharyngeal wall toward the midline, a finding not present in masticator space infections. Infection of the deep temporal space usually originates from involvement of the posterior maxillary molar teeth. Very little external swelling is observed early in the course; if present, it usually affects the preauricular region and an area over the zygomatic arch. As infection progresses, the cheek, eyelids, and whole side of the face may be involved (Fig. 6). Infection may extend directly into the orbit via the inferior orbital fissure and produce proptosis, optic neuritis, and abducens nerve palsy.

BUCCAL, CANINE, AND PAROTID SPACES. As noted previously, infections arising from mandibular or maxillary bicuspid and molar teeth tend to extend in a lateral or buccal direction. The relation of the root apices to the origins of the buccinator muscle determines whether infection will exit intraorally into the buccal vestibule or extraorally into the buccal space (Fig. 2). Infection of the buccal space is readily diagnosed because of marked cheek swelling with minimal trismus and systemic symptoms. There is a great tendency to resolution with antibiotic therapy alone. Drainage, if required, is superficial and should be performed extraorally. Involvement of the maxillary incisors and canines may result in a canine space infection, which presents as dramatic swelling of the upper lip, canine fossa, and frequently the periorbital tissues. Pain is usually moderate, and

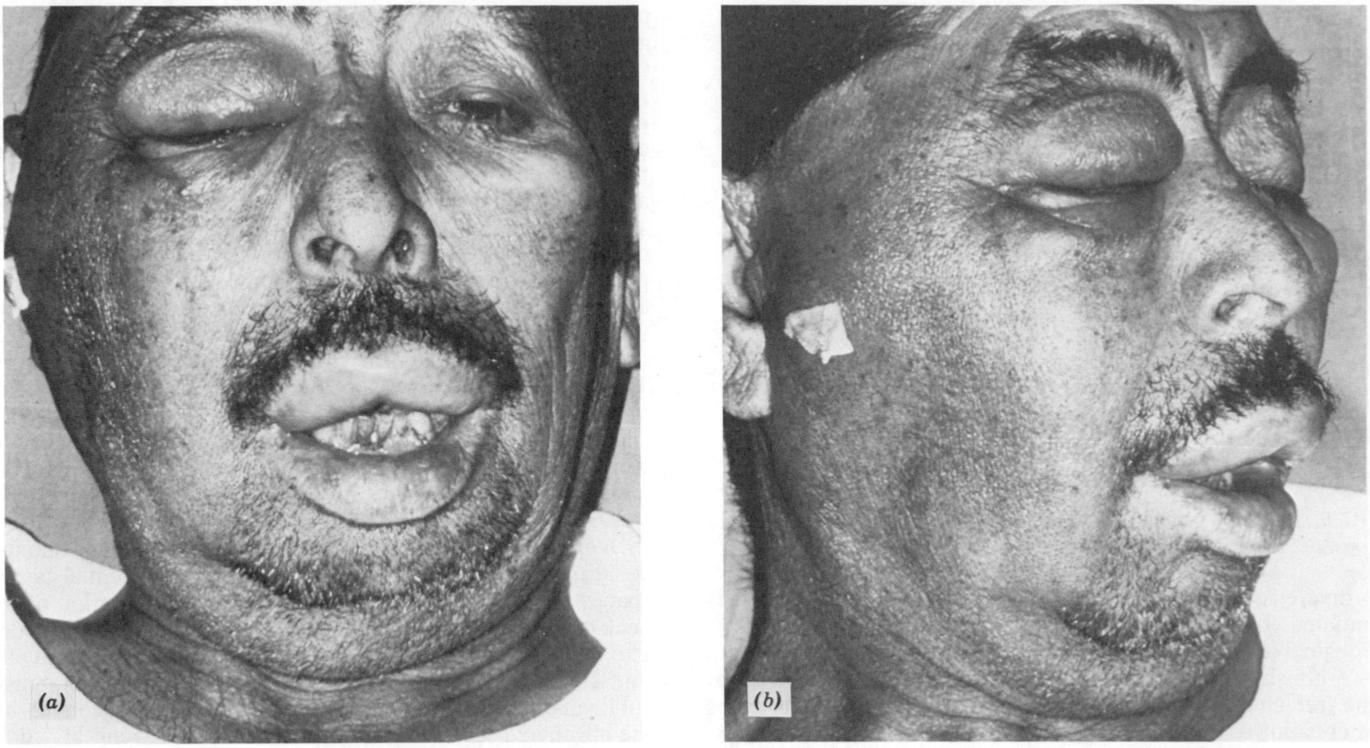

FIG. 6. Deep temporal space infection with spread to the right parotid space and the orbit. This patient developed right optic neuritis with permanent loss of vision in that eye. **(A)** Frontal view. **(B)** Lateral view. (From Chow, et al.,[1] with permission.)

systemic signs are minimal. Occasionally, a purulent maxillary sinusitis may result due to direct extension of infection into the adjoining antrum. Treatment consists of antibiotics and drainage, which can be accomplished intraorally. Parotid space infection from an odontogenic cause generally represents secondary spread from a masseteric space infection in the area of the ramus of the mandible (Fig. 3). There is marked swelling of the angle of the jaw without associated trismus. Pain may be intense and accompanied by high fever and chills. Because of its close relationship with the posterior aspect of the lateral pharyngeal space, a parotid space infection carries the potential risk of direct extension into the "danger" and visceral spaces and hence to the posterior mediastinum (Fig. 4).

SUBMANDIBULAR AND SUBLINGUAL SPACES. These two spaces are separated by the mylohyoid muscle (Fig. 2), and the submandibular space is further divided into the submaxillary and submental spaces. Infection in these spaces usually arises from the second and third mandibular molar teeth since their root apices lie inferior to the mylohyoid muscle. There is typical swelling, although much less trismus in contradistinction to masseteric space infection since the major muscles of mastication are usually not involved. Submandibular odontogenic infection should be distinguished from submandibular sialadenitis and lymphadenitis that are due to other causes. Therapy includes antibiotics, dental extraction, and extraoral surgical drainage. Infection of the sublingual space generally arises from mandibular incisors since their root apices lie above the mylohyoid muscle. Clinically, this space infection presents as a brawny, erythematous, tender swelling of the floor of the mouth that begins close to the mandible and spreads toward the midline or beyond. Some elevation of the tongue may be noted in late states. Surgical drainage of the sublingual space should be performed intraorally by an incision through the mucosa parallel to Wharton's duct. If the submandibular space is also to be drained, both spaces can be reached through a submandibular approach.

The term *Ludwig's angina* has been loosely applied to a heterogenous array of infections involving the sublingual, submaxillary, and submandibular spaces.[38] However, for therapeutic and prognostic purposes, it is desirable to restrict this diagnosis to cases that conform to the following classic description: (*1*) the infection is always bilateral, (*2*) both the submandibular and sublingual spaces are involved, (*3*) the infection is a rapidly spreading indurated cellulitis without abscess formation of lymphatic involvement, and (*4*) the infection begins in the floor of the mouth. A dental source of infection has been found in 50–90 percent of reported cases. The second and third mandibular molars are most commonly involved. Clinically, patients present with a brawny boardlike swelling in the submandibular spaces that does not pit on pressure (Fig. 7). The mouth is usually held open and the floor elevated, which pushes the tongue to the roof of the mouth. Eating and swallowing are difficult, and respiration may be impaired by obstruction from the tongue. A rapid progression of the infection will result in edema of the neck and glottis and may precipitate asphyxiation. Fever and systemic toxicity are usually present and may be severe. Treatment requires high doses of parenteral antibiotics, airway monitoring, early intubation or tracheostomy when required, soft tissue decompression, and surgical drainage.

LATERAL PHARYNGEAL SPACE. The lateral pharyngeal space (also known as the pharyngomaxillary space) in the lateral aspect of the neck is shaped like an inverted cone, with its base at the skull and its apex at the hyoid bone (Fig. 4). Its medial wall is contiguous with the carotid sheath, and it lies deep to the pharyngeal constrictor muscle. Infection of the lateral pharyngeal space may result from pharyngitis, tonsillitis, parotitis, otitis, mastoiditis, as well as odontogenic infection, especially if the masticator spaces are primarily involved. If the anterior compartment is infected, the patient will exhibit fever, chills, marked pain, trismus, swelling below the angle of the mandible, dysphagia, and medial displacement of the lateral pharyngeal wall. Although not prominent, dyspnea can occur. Posterior compartment infection is characterized by septicemia with little pain or trismus. Swelling is usually internal and deep and can often be missed because it is behind the palatopharyngeal arch.

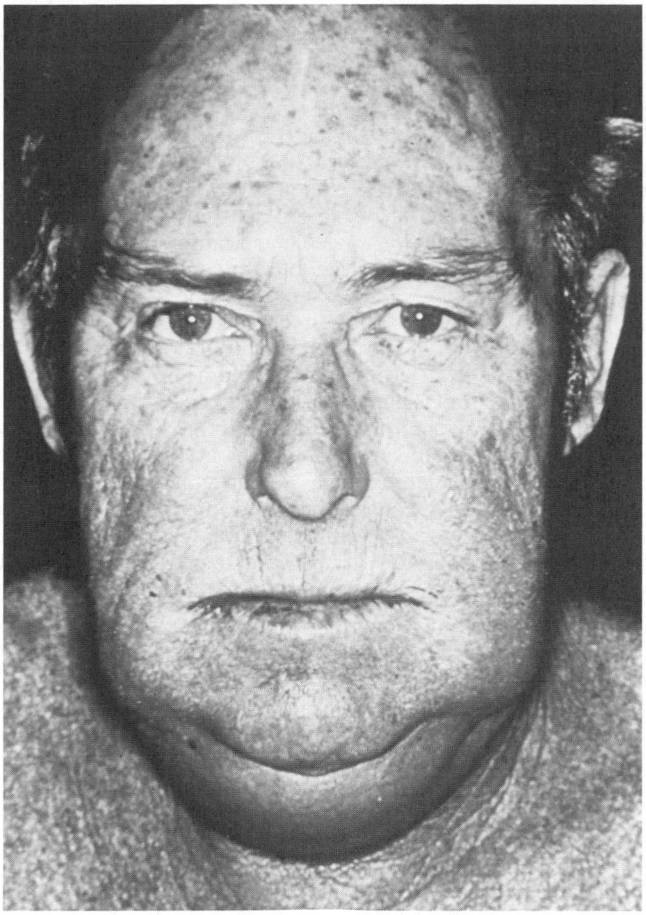

FIG. 7. Early appearance of a patient with Ludwig's angina with a brawny boardlike swelling in the submandibular spaces (arrows). (From Chow et al.,[1] with permission.)

Complications, particularly if the posterior compartment is involved, include respiratory obstruction from edema of the larynx, thrombosis of the internal jugular vein, and erosion of the internal carotid artery. Because respiratory obstruction from laryngeal edema can occur suddenly, the patient must be closely observed, and prophylactic tracheostomy may be required. Treatment includes high levels of antibiotics and surgical drainage. It is usually prudent to wait for the infection to localize before drainage is attempted unless respiratory obstruction or hemorrhage necessitates early surgical intervention.

RETROPHARYNGEAL, DANGER, AND PRETRACHEAL SPACES. The retropharyngeal space comprises the posterior part of the visceral compartment in which the esophagus, trachea, and thyroid glands are enclosed by the middle layer of deep cervical fascia (Fig. 4). It lies behind the hypopharynx and the esophagus and extends inferiorly into the superior mediastinum to about the level from T1 to T2. Posterior to this compartment lies the "danger" space, which descends directly into the posterior mediastinum to the level of the diaphragm. Infection of the retropharyngeal space may result from contiguous infection of the lateral pharyngeal space or from lymphatic spread from more distant sites to involve the retropharyngeal lymph nodes. Dysphagia, dyspnea, nuchal rigidity, esophageal regurgitation, as well as high fever and chills may be present. Bulging of the posterior pharyngeal wall may be observed. Lateral soft tissue radiographs of the neck may reveal marked widening of the retropharyngeal space. Infection of the retropharyngeal space is potentially life-threatening and requires prompt surgical drainage. Complications include hemorrhage and spontaneous rupture into the airway with asphyxiation, laryngeal spasm, bronchial erosion, and thrombosis of the jugular vein. The pretracheal space comprises the anterior portion of the visceral compartment and completely surrounds the trachea. Most commonly, infections reach this space through perforations of the anterior esophageal wall, occasionally through contiguous extension from a retropharyngeal space infection. The clinical presentation is characterized by severe dyspnea, but hoarseness may be the first complaint. Swallowing is difficult, and regurgitation of fluids through the nose may occur. A pretracheal space infection is always serious because of possible extension into the mediastinum, and prompt surgical drainage is critically important.

Complications of Odontogenic Infections

Complications of odontogenic infections can occur either by hematogenous spread or by direct extension. Transient bacteremia is common during or after various dental procedures, especially extraction of infected teeth.[39] The temporal relationship between these procedures and subsequent bacterial endocarditis and cardiovascular prosthetic infections is well documented.[10] Reports of infected total hip replacements after dental procedures add further concern.[22,40] Prophylactic antibiotic treatment during dental procedures, although frequently used, remains a controversial issue, especially in the absence of pre-existing valvular heart disease. Complications of odontogenic infections secondary to direct extension include mediastinal spread,[41] intracranial suppuration (especially cavernous sinus thrombosis),[42] suppurative jugular thrombophlebitis, carotid artery erosion,[43] maxillary sinusitis,[1] and osteomyelitis.[44] Acute mediastinitis and intracranial suppuration secondary to odontogenic infections are relatively uncommon in the postantibiotic era.

Suppurative Jugular Thrombophlebitis and Carotid Artery Erosion. These are uncommon complications of oropharyngeal or odontogenic infections in the postantibiotic era. Extension of infection to the carotid sheath, which encloses both the internal jugular vein and the internal carotid artery, usually arises from the lateral pharyngeal space.[43] Since the carotid sheath space in this area is relatively compact with little areolar connective tissue, there is little tendency of spread up and down this vascular sheath, with the exception of possible retrograde thrombophlebitis and intracranial extension. The major concern is protracted septicemia and erosion of the carotid artery or one of its branches.

The onset of suppurative jugular thrombophlebitis is acute, with shaking chills, spiking fevers, and profound prostration. Localizing signs of pain and swelling at the angle of the jaw, tenderness and induration along the sternocleidomastoid muscle, and swelling of the lateral pharyngeal wall with dysphagia and neck ridigity are usually present. However, these findings may be subtle, and their clinical significance may not be fully recognized until postmortem. Systemic evidence of infection such as septic pulmonary emboli and metastatic abscesses to the brain, lungs, kidneys, and joints is not infrequent. The usual recommended treatment consists of external drainage of the lateral pharyngeal space and ligation of the internal jugular vein. *Fusobacterium necrophorum* has been the organism most frequently isolated from blood cultures,[45,46] and mortality remains high. Important warning signals that may herald major hemorrhage due to erosion of the carotid artery include multiple episodes of minor bleeding from the oral cavity or ear and ecchymosis of oral and cervical tissue. With the onset of major hemorrhage, primary considerations are maintenance and protection of the airway because death may occur more rapidly from asphyxiation than from hemorrhagic shock. Appropriate treatment consists of emergency carotid ligation after the restoration of blood volume and pressure. Hemorrhage is controlled by local compression until ligation can be attempted.

The mortality for emergency ligation ranges from 30 to 50 percent. Cerebrovascular accident is a significant complication in survivors.

Septic Cavernous Sinus Thrombosis. This dreaded complication is fortunately rare in the postantibiotic era. Facial furuncles and purulent paranasal sinusitis were the major predisposing conditions. Infection of the maxillary teeth was the most common dental cause. Eagleton[47] described six criteria for the diagnosis of septic cavernous sinus thrombosis to help distinguish it from other less lethal infections, particularly those of the ethmoid sinus and the orbit: (*1*) a known site of infection; (*2*) evidence of blood stream invasion; (*3*) early signs of venous obstruction in the retina, conjunctiva, and eyelid; (*4*) paresis of the third, fourth, and sixth cranial nerves resulting from inflammatory edema; (*5*) abscess formation in neighboring soft tissue; and (*6*) evidence of meningeal irritation. Before the antibiotic era, septic cavernous sinus thrombosis was virtually always fatal. Mortality since 1970 has been markedly reduced to 15–30 percent.[43,48,49] Treatment requires early recognition, high-dose intravenous antibiotics, and surgical decompression of the underlying predisposing infection. Anticoagulation and steroids are not indicated.

Maxillary Sinusitis. In many people, the roots of the maxillary molars lie proximate to the maxillary antrum. At times, congenital bony defects occur, with the root adjacent to the sinus membrane. In these cases, sinusitis can result from direct extension of an odontogenic infection or from perforation of the sinus floor during extraction of a maxillary tooth.[1] The clinical presentation of secondary sinus involvement is similar to that of primary sinus disease.

Osteomyelitis of the Jaws. The mandible is much more susceptible to osteomyelitis than is the maxilla, mainly because the cortical plates of the latter are thin and its medullary tissues are relatively poor in vascular supply.[44] In view of the large number of odontogenic infections and the intimate relationship of teeth to the medullary cavity, it is surprising that osteomyelitis of the jaws is not more frequent. When osteomyelitis occurs, there is usually a predisposing condition that affects host resistance such as a compound fracture, previous irradiation, osteopetrosis, Paget's disease, diabetes mellitis, or steroid therapy. With initiation of infection, the intramedullary pressure markedly increases, further compromising blood supply and leading to bone necrosis. Pus travels through the haversian and perforating canals, accumulates beneath the periosteum, and elevates it from the cortex. If pus continues to accumulate, the periosteum is eventually penetrated, and mucosal and cutaneous abscesses and fistulas may develop. As the inflammatory process becomes more chronic, granulation tissue is formed. Spicules of necrotic and nonviable bone may become either totally isolated (sequestrum) or encased in a sheath of new bone (involucrum). Severe mandibular pain is a common symptom and may be accompanied by anesthesia or hypoesthesia on the affected side. In protracted cases, mandibular trismus may develop. A clinical variant is chronic sclerosing osteomyelitis associated with a proliferative periostitis. Clinically, it is characterized by a localized, hard, nontender swelling over the mandible. Actinomycosis and radiation necrosis are two common causes of this form of osteomyelitis of the jaws.

Treatment of osteomyelitis of the jaws is complicated by the presence of teeth and persistent exposure to the oral environment. Antibiotic therapy needs to be prolonged, often requiring weeks to months. Adjunctive therapy with hyperbaric oxygen may prove beneficial in hastening the healing process, particularly for the chronic sclerosing variety.[44,50] Surgical management including sequestrectomy, saucerization, decortication, and closed-wound suction irrigation may occasionally be necessary. Rarely, in advanced cases the entire segment of the infected jaw may have to be resected.

Diagnostic Approaches

Specimen Collection and Processing. It is imperative that the normal resident oral flora be excluded during specimen collection in order that culture results be appropriately interpreted. For closed-space infections, needle aspiration of loculated pus by an extraoral approach is desirable, and specimens should be transported immediately to the laboratory under anaerobic conditions. For intraoral lesions, direct microscopic examination of stained smears often provides more useful information than do culture results from surface swabs. Gram and acid-fast stains for bacteria and potassium hydroxide preparations for fungi should be routinely performed. Tissue biopsy specimens examined for typical histopathology and the presence of microbial antigens by immunofluorescence are particularly useful in suspected mycobacterial, fungal, and viral infections. In chronic osteomyelitis, soft tissue swelling and draining fistulas are frequently present. Aspirates from the adjacent soft tissue swellings may be valuable, but cultures from the sinus tracts may be misleading since these sinus tracts are often colonized by organisms that do not reflect what is actually occurring within the infected bone.[51] Bone biopsies for histopathology and culture are often required for a definitive diagnosis.

Imaging Techniques for the Localization of Infection. Ultrasonography, radionuclide scanning, and computed tomography (CT) are particularly useful for the localization of deep fascial space infections of the head and neck.[52,53] A lateral radiograph of the neck may demonstrate compression or deviation of the tracheal air column or the presence of gas within necrotic soft tissues.[54] In retropharyngeal infections, lateral radiographs of the cervical spine or CT scanning can help determine whether the infection is in the retropharyngeal space or the prevertebral space.[55] The former suggests an odontogenic source, whereas the latter suggests involvement of the cervical spine. Technetium bone scanning used in combination with gallium- or indium-labeled white blood cells is particularly useful for the diagnosis of acute or chronic osteomyelitis and for the differentiation of infection or trauma from malignancy. In acute osteomyelitis, both the bone scan and gallium scan are likely to have positive findings. In chronic osteomyelitis, the gallium or indium scans may be negative, but the technetium may be positive. Similarly, both scans may be positive during infection and trauma, while neoplasms in the bone may be associated only with a positive bone scan but negative gallium or indium scan results.

Therapeutic Considerations

Dental Caries and Periodontitis. For both caries prevention and treatment of periodontitis, the clinical goal must continue to be control of the supragingival and subgingival plaques. With the emerging concept of microbial specificity in these infections, the prospect of specific antimicrobial therapy appears increasingly promising.[10,20,37,56] In localized juvenile periodontitis, for example, systemic tetracycline therapy directed against *A. actinomycetemcomitans* and combined with local periodontal treatment has yielded excellent results.[35,36] Unfortunately, the administration of tetracycline to children under 5 years of age can cause staining of the permanent dentition and is not generally recommended. Similarly, in advanced periodontitis, several double-blind studies have indicated that systemic metronidazole plus mechanical débridement of the root surfaces is more effective than placebo treatment plus mechanical débridement.[37] The successful treatment of acute necrotizing ulcerative gingivitis with metronidazole has been well documented, and in fact such treatment by Shinn et al.[33] led to the discovery of metronidazole as a unique anaerobicidal agent.

Several topical agents appear to have cariostatic effects in humans. By far the most effective is fluoride. Fluoride forms a complex with the apatite crystals in dentin by replacing the hydroxyl group, thereby lending strength to the entire structure.[10] Further, fluoride promotes remineralization of the carious lesions and also exerts a bacteriostatic effect. Topical chlorhexidine is another compound with useful anticariogenic properties. It acts as a cationic detergent killing a wide range of bacteria and is retained on the oral surfaces for prolonged periods to prevent plaque advancement.[22] Unfortunately, it has a bitter taste and stains the enamel and tongue. Prolonged application may also promote the emergence of resistant microorganisms. Among the antibiotics, although both penicillin and tetracycline have cariostatic effects in animal models, only topical application of vancomycin has been shown to reduce dental caries with some degree of success in humans.[10] Other important approaches to caries and periodontitis prevention include the adoption of improved oral hygiene through more effective educational programs,[13] a reduction of cariogenic oral flora by diet modification with sucrose substitutes, and active immunization against caries by the use of vaccines prepared from *S. mutans*.[57–59]

Suppurative Odontogenic Infections. The most important therapeutic modality for pyogenic odontogenic infections is surgical drainage and removal of necrotic tissue. Needle aspiration by the extraoral route can be particularly helpful both for microbiologic sampling and for evacuation of pus. The need for definitive restoration or extraction of the infected tooth, the primary source of infection, is readily apparent. Deep periodontal scaling and endodontic treatments with root filling may be required in most instances. Effective surgical management requires a thorough understanding of the most likely anatomic routes of spread. The neighboring potential fascial spaces should be carefully and systematically surveyed. The optimum timing for incision and drainage is equally important. Premature incision into an unlocalized cellulitis in an ill-conceived search for pus can disrupt the normal physiologic barriers and cause further diffusion and extension of infection.

Antibiotic therapy is important in halting the local spread of infection and in preventing hematogenous dissemination. Antimicrobial agents are generally indicated if fever and regional lymphadenitis are present or when infection has perforated the bony cortex and spread into surrounding soft tissue. Severely immunocompromised patients are particularly at risk for unhalted and spreading orofacial infections, and empirical broad-spectrum antimicrobial therapy in these patients is warranted.[60,61] The choice of specific antibiotics for the treatment of odontogenic infections requires not so much the results of bacterial culture and sensitivity as knowledge of the indigenous organisms that colonize the teeth, gums, and mucous membranes. By far most of these organisms, including both anaerobes and aerobes, are sensitive to penicillin.[60–63] Thus, penicillin monotherapy in doses appropriate for the severity of infection remains a good choice. The problem of β-lactamase production and penicillin resistance among *Bacteroides* sp., particularly B. *melaninogenicus*, has been increasingly recognized, and treatment failure with penicillin in odontogenic infections due to such β-lactamase–producing strains has been reported.[64–66] Thus, in patients with life-threatening deep fascial space infections and in patients who have had an unfavorable or delayed response to penicillin, alternative therapy with a broader spectrum against anaerobes as well as facultative gram-negative bacilli may be considered. Penicillin-allergic patients may be treated with either clindamycin or cefoxitin. Ambulatory patients with less serious odontogenic infections may be treated with amoxicillin, ampicillin, or doxycycline. Erythromycin and tetracycline are not preferred in orofacial odontogenic infections because of emergence of resistance among oropharyngeal anaerobes and some strains of streptococci.[60] Metronidazole, although highly active against anaerobic gram-negative bacilli and spirochetes, is only moderately active against anaerobic cocci and is not active against aerobes, including streptococci.[1,61,67] Except in acute necrotizing gingivitis and in advanced periodontitis,[33,34,37] it should not be used as a single agent in odontogenic infections. In the compromised host such as the patient with leukemia and severe neutropenia after chemotherapy, it is prudent to cover for facultative gram-negative bacilli as well, and agents with broad-spectrum activity against both aerobes and anaerobes are desirable (Table 2).

TABLE 2. Empirical Antibiotic Regimens for Odontogenic Soft Tissue Infections

Normal host
Penicillin G, 1–4 million units iv q4–6h
Clindamycin, 600 mg iv q6–8h
Cefoxitin, 1–2 g iv q6h
Compromised host (each of following ± an aminoglycoside)
Piperacillin, 3 g iv q4h
Cefoxitin, 1–2 g iv q6h
Cefotetan, 2 g iv q12h
Imipenem/cilastatin, 500 mg iv q6h
Ticarcillin/clavulanate, 3.0 g/0.1 g iv q4–6h

OROFACIAL NONODONTOGENIC INFECTIONS

Nonodontogenic infections of the oral cavity most frequently occur secondary to chemical, thermal, or traumatic injury. Virtually all infectious microorganisms can present with intraoral manifestations, particularly sexually transmitted agents and childhood viral enanthems. Cancer patients with mucositis from cytotoxic drugs are especially prone to acute and chronic opportunistic infections of the oral cavity, particularly candidiasis, aspergillosis, mucormycosis, herpetic gingivostomatitis, and mixed gram-negative infections.[68,69] In this section, some of the conditions affecting primarily the oral mucosa and salivary glands in which an infectious cause is either proved or suspected will be briefly discussed.

Infections of the Oral Mucosa

Noma, or Gangrenous Stomatitis. Noma, or gangrenous stomatitis, also known as cancrum oris, is an acute, fulminating, and gangrenous infection of the oral and facial tissues. It usually occurs in the presence of severe debilitation and malnutrition, and children are most often affected. The earliest lesion is a small, painful, red spot or vesicle on the attached gingiva in the premolar or molar regions of the mandible. A necrotic ulcer rapidly develops and undermines the deeper tissue. Painful cellulitis of the lips and cheeks is observed as the lesion extends outward in a conelike fashion. Within a short period, sloughing of necrotic soft tissues occurs and exposes underlying bone, teeth, and deeper tissues.

Fusospirochetal organisms such as *Borrelia vincentii* and *Fusobacterium nucleatum* are consistently cultured from noma lesions. *Bacteroides melaninogenicus* may also be present. Biopsy specimens of tissue from the advancing lesion show a mat of predominantly gram-negative threadlike bacteria that cannot be positively identified.[70] Thus, this lesion bears a similarity to acute necrotizing ulcerative gingivitis in several respects but appears to be more focal and destructive, involving deeper tissues beyond the gingiva. Treatment of noma requires high doses of intravenous penicillin. Every effort should be directed to correct the dehydration and underlying malnutrition and debility. Loose teeth and sequestra may be removed, but saucerization should be avoided. Healing is by secondary intention. Serious mutilation and facial deformity may require subsequent cosmetic surgery.

Apthous Stomatitis. Aphthous ulcers are the most common cause of recurrent oral lesions. This entity must be distinguished from oral ulceration due to herpes simplex, coxsackievirus, agranulocytosis, and Behçet's and other diseases. Three major clinical variants are recognized: (*1*) minor aphthous ulcers, (*2*) major aphthous ulcers, and (*3*) herpetiform aphthous ulcers.[71] The true cause of aphthous ulcerations is not known, although a number of infectious agents including viruses have been implicated. The most prevailing hypothesis suggests that the mechanism causing the ulceration is autoimmune in nature. Circulating humoral antibodies and sensitized T lymphocytes active against oral mucosa have been demonstrated in patients with aphthous ulcers.[71] Furthermore, the active T lymphocytes undergo a phase of rapid proliferation just before the onset of ulceration. The origin of the autoantibodies is not clear, and no common antigenic factor between oral epithelium and the indigenous microflora has been demonstrated.

In their most characteristic form, minor aphthous ulcers appear as a number of small ulcers on the buccal and labial mucosa, the floor of the mouth, or the tongue. The palatal soft tissues are rarely involved. Moreover, the ulcers are concentrated in the anterior part of the oral cavity, whereas the pharynx and tonsillar fauces are rarely implicated. A prodromal stage is usually present. The ulcers appear gray-yellow, often with a raised and erythematous margin, and are exquisitely painful. Lymph node enlargement is seen only with secondary bacterial infection. The course of ulceration varies from a few days to a little over 2 weeks and is followed by spontaneous healing. Major aphthous ulcers are more protracted and last up to several months. All areas of the oral cavity including the soft palate and tonsillar areas may be involved. Long periods of remission may be followed by intervals of intense ulcer activity. Herpetiform aphthous ulcers are small and multiple and characteristically affect the lateral margins and tip of the tongue. The ulcers are gray, without a delineating erythematous border, and are extremely painful, which makes eating and speaking difficult. Despite its name, there is little clinical resemblance to an acute herpetic gingivostomatitis. Although intranuclear inclusions have been demonstrated in herpetiform aphthous ulcers, there is no evidence to suggest that these inclusions bear any relationship to presence of viruses.

The treatment of aphthous ulcers is primarily symptomatic. Strict oral hygiene should be maintained, and the use of antiseptic mouthwashes may be helpful in temporarily reducing secondary infection. Local anaesthetic lozenges or gels may be used as a last resort for brief periods of pain relief. Topical or systemic steroids may be beneficial in selected people with extensive disease, but caution must be exercised in their administration.

Mucositis and Stomatitis in the Severely Immunocompromised. Much of what is known about management of oromucosal infections has been studied in cancer patients being treated with radiotherapy, chemotherapy, and bone marrow transplantation.[68,72] Other patient groups that develop oromucosal complications include those undergoing solid organ transplantation, patients with the acquired immunodeficiency syndrome (AIDS),[73] and those with autoimmune diseases associated with xerostomia and systemic immunosuppression. The underlying mechanism appears to be a breakdown of the mucosal epithelium that leads to mucositis, secondary bacterial or fungal infection, or reactivation of latent viral infection. Oral candidiasis, herpes simplex, varicella-zoster, and cytomegalovirus infections are the most common manifestations. Mucositis that complicates radiation or chemotherapy most commonly involves the nonkeratinized oral epithelium, including the buccal and labial mucosa, soft palate, oropharynx, floor of the mouth, and ventral and lateral surfaces of the tongue. Ulceration and pseudomembrane formation are evident usually between 4 and 7 days after the initiation of chemotherapy when the rate of destruction of the basal epithelium exceeds that of proliferation of new cells. The clinical manifestations may be quite variable. The lesions are often protracted in duration and may not be associated with an inflammatory reaction, thereby masking the usual signs and symptoms. Pain or tenderness may be the only abnormal finding. Since the etiologic agents of infection cannot be readily predicted on clinical grounds alone in such patients, specific microbiologic diagnosis by culture, histopathology or antigen detection techniques is critical for appropriate treatment. Topical as well as systemic antimicrobial agents may be indicated along with antiseptic (e.g., chlorhexidine) and anesthetic (e.g., benzydamine, viscous lidocaine, etc.) applications.[74] Frequent saline rinses may reduce mucosal irritation, remove thickened secretions or debris, and increase moisture in the mouth.[68] Coating agents such as milk of magnesia or aluminum hydroxide gel (Amphojel) have been useful for the symptomatic relief of painful oral lesions. Topical or oral cytoprotective agents (e.g., sucralfate) or nonsteroidal anti-inflammatory analgesics (e.g., benzydamine, salicylates, etc.) may provide additional benefit, but further controlled clinical trials are required to assess their appropriate indications and efficacy.[74,75] Meticulous oral and dental hygiene, effective management of xerostomia, selective suppression of oropharyngeal microbial colonization, and early control of reactivation by latent viral infections appear to be the critical steps to prevent and reduce the overall morbidity of oromucosal infections in the severely immunocompromised.[68,76]

Infections of the Salivary Gland

Sialadenitis, or infection of salivary tissue, is a relatively common disease. Sialolithiasis in elderly patients leads to ductal obstruction and secondarily to suppuration of the salivary gland and appears to be a major predisposing condition. In this regard, stones of Wharton's duct are much more common than are those of Stensen's duct, and obstructive sialadenitis is much more frequent with the submandibular than the parotid gland.[77] Other predisposing factors for sialadenitis include dehydration, general debility, sialogogic drugs, and trauma.

Suppurative Parotitis. Acute bacterial parotitis is a specific clinical entity primarily affecting the elderly, malnourished, dehydrated, or postoperative patient. Clinically, there is a sudden onset of firm, erythematous swelling of the pre- and postauricular areas that extends to the angle of the mandible. This is associated with exquisite local pain and tenderness. Systemic findings of high fevers, chills, and marked toxicity are generally present. Progression of the infection may lead to massive swelling of the neck, respiratory obstruction, septicemia, and osteomyelitis of the adjacent facial bones. Staphylococci have been the predominant isolates, and antibiotic therapy should include an antistaphylococcal agent. Early surgical drainage and decompression of the gland are generally required since spontaneous drainage is uncommon.

Chronic Bacterial Parotitis. In this condition, parotitis is recurrent with intermittent acute exacerbations. There is chronic, low-grade, bacterial infection resulting in functional destruction of the salivary gland. Pus, when obtained directly from the gland, usually reveals the growth of staphylococci or mixed oral aerobes and anaerobes. Sialography during remission may reveal a sialectatic pattern of pooling of contrast medium that suggests multiple cystic cavities in place of the normal acinar pattern. Chronic parotitis may be confused with Sjögren syndrome, a noninfectious illness characterized by the triad of xerostomia, keratoconjunctivitis, and systemic autoimmune disease such as rheumatoid arthritis, lupus erythematosus, scleroderma, periarteritis nodosa, and polymyositis. The presence of associated temporomandibular arthritis or arthralgia should strongly suggest Sjögren syndrome rather than chronic bacterial parotitis.

Therapy for chronic parotitis should initially be conservative and consist of systemic antibiotics and ductal saline or antibiotic irrigations. Parotidectomy may eventually be required for people with long-standing infection.

Viral Parotitis. Mumps parotitis is characterized by the rapid, painful swelling of one or both parotid glands within 2–3 weeks after exposure. A prodromal phase of preauricular pain, fever, chills, and headache may be present. Other viral causes of parotitis include influenza and enteroviruses, and specific neutralizing antibody titers may be required for distinguishing these from true mumps. Mumps parotitis usually resolves spontaneously in 5–10 days. Symptomatic relief of pain and fever is necessary, and prevention of dehydration and secondary bacterial infection is essential.

MISCELLANEOUS INFECTIONS OF THE NECK AND HEAD

In the antibiotic era, dental causes have surpassed oropharyngeal and tonsillar sources of deep neck infections.[78] Other miscellaneous infections of the neck and head include suppurative cervical adenitis, infected embryologic cysts of the neck, various infections secondary to human and animal bites, maxillofacial trauma, irradiation, and surgical procedures of the head and neck.

Cervical Adenitis

Cervical adenitis, which presents unilaterally in association with warm, tender, enlarged, and fluctuant lymph nodes, is usually due to pyogenic infections. Its anatomic location in relationship to major cervical landmarks will provide the clinical clues to the primary source of infection.[31,79] Bilateral acute cervical adenitis generally suggests a nonspecific or viral cause, toxoplasmosis, or group A streptotoccal infection. A more chronic or recurrent cervical adenitis should suggest the possibility of typical or atypical mycobacteriosis, human immunodeficiency virus infection, Epstein-Barr virus or cytomegalovirus mononucleosis, cat-scratch fever, actinomycosis, sarcoidosis, as well as lymphoproliferative and neoplastic disorders.

Infected Embryologic Cysts

Three distinct embryologic abnormalities can present with infection in the neck. They are (*1*) cystic hygroma or lymphangioma, (*2*) pharyngeal and bronchial cleft cysts, and (*3*) thyroglossal duct cysts.[78,79] Cystic hygroma is associated with a diffuse tumor mass usually evident within the first 2 years of life. It commonly involves the lower aspect of the neck, but it can appear anywhere in the cervical region. It is probably an abnormal development of lymphatic vessels from the jugular lymphatic sacs. Sudden enlargement by infection or hemorrhage into a lymphangioma may cause obstruction of the upper airways. Pharyngeal cleft cysts can develop from the first, second, or third pharyngeal clefts, although the second is most common. They usually present in childhood as fistulas or masses just posterior to the angle of the mandible along the anterior border of the sternocleidomastoid muscle. The mass can fluctuate in size, and enlargement can be associated with upper respiratory infection. Thyroglossal duct cysts originate from the foramen cecum of the tongue and descend through the body of the hyoid bone into the anterior portion of the neck. Any residual secretory lining may give rise to a thyroglossal duct cyst that is midline in location. It can cause respiratory obstruction or fistula formation if secondarily infected. Treatment of these congenital abnormalities during secondary bacterial infection requires broad-spectrum antibiotics such as a cephalosporin. Definitive surgical excision to prevent recurrence should be performed after complete resolution of the acute process.

Suppurative Thyroiditis

Although infections of the thyroid gland are rare, they are potentially life-threatening. Such infections may arise by a variety of pathways including hematogenous dissemination, direct spread from an adjacent deep fascial space infection, an infected thyroglossal fistula, or anterior perforation of the esophagus. Pre-existing diseases of the thyroid gland such as a goiter or adenoma are frequently present.[80,81] Acute suppurative thyroiditis is characterized by fever, local pain, tenderness, warmth, erythema, and symptoms of dysphagia, dysphonia, hoarseness, or pharyngitis. The infection may involve single or both lobes, and fluctuance may not be apparent until late in the course. Subacute thyroiditis may have similar local findings, but systemic manifestations are not as severe and tend to be more self-limiting. Laboratory investigation of thyroid infections should include ultrasonography, radionuclide scanning, and lateral radiographs or CT scanning of the neck for evidence of peritracheal extension; thyroid function tests; and diagnostic needle aspiration for microbiologic diagnosis. *Staphylococcus aureus, S. pyogenes*, and *S. pneumoniae* are most frequently isolated. Other pathogens include *H. influenzae*, viridans streptococci, *Eikonella corrodens, Bacteroides, Peptostreptococcus*, and *Actinomyces* species. Treatment requires specific antimicrobial agents and appropriate surgical drainage.

Infections from Bites, Maxillofacial Trauma, Irradiation, and Surgical Wounds

Human and Animal Bites. Human and animal bite wounds to the head and neck are relatively common. Although they may look innocuous initially, serious complications can occur. For this reason, empirical antibiotic therapy is recommended when the bite wound involves the face, head, or neck. Recent studies that used adequate anaerobic culture techniques indicate indigenous oral flora rather than the skin flora to be the major source of bite wound infections.[82] Streptococci, *Eikenella corrodens*, and *S. aureus* are the most prevalent facultative organisms, and *Bacteriodes*, and *Peptostreptococcus* are the most common anaerobic isolates. Penicillin-resistant gram-negative rods are infrequent. *Eikenella corrodens* is unique in that it is susceptible to penicillin and ampicillin but resistant to oxacillin, methicillin, nafcillin, and clindamycin.[63] In animal bite wounds, *Pasteurella multocida* has been a common cause of infection.[83] It is susceptible to penicillin. In view of these findings, penicillin remains the antibiotic of choice for initial therapy for both human and animal bite wounds.

Maxillofacial Trauma. Automobile and motorcycle accidents cause the most severe maxillofacial trauma. Particular attention should be paid to fractures that may traverse sinus cavities and teeth-bearing areas of the maxilla or mandible since secondary infection rates at these sites are particularly high. Treatment is aimed not only at correcting the fracture but also at prevention of infection and subsequent osteomyelitis. Early stabilization of the fracture and the jaws is generally required to protect the airway. Tracheostomy with use of inflated, cuffed endotracheal tubes may prevent aspiration of blood and other foreign materials. The occurrence of otorrhea or rhinorrhea with a persistent cerebrospinal fluid leak should be carefully observed.

Irradiation and Postsurgical Wounds. Malignancies of the head and neck are frequently treated with a combination of irradiation, chemotherapeutic agents, and surgical resection. Infectious complications are particularly common after such procedures. Pharyngocutaneous fistulas, osteonecrosis of the mandible, or radionecrosis of the laryngeal cartilage may occur. *Staphylococcus aureus* and *Pseudomonas aeruginosa* are frequent pathogens. Prolonged courses of intravenous antibiotics selected according to culture and sensitivity data as well as frequent wound débridement and cleansing are indicated. Although some controversy still exists, immunocompromised patients undergoing oropharyngeal surgery for cancer should receive perioperative antibiotics since they are at particular high risk for infection.[78,83,84] A broad-spectrum antibiotic such as cefazolin, cefuroxime, or cefoxitin appears appropriate in this setting.[18,84,85]

REFERENCES

1. Chow AW, Roser SM, Brady FA. Orofacial odontogenic infections. Ann Intern Med. 1978;88:392.
2. Hardie J. Microbial flora of the oral cavity. In: Schuster GS, ed. Oral Microbiology and Infectious Disease. Baltimore: Williams & Wilkins; 1983:162.
3. Hamada S, Slade HD. Biology, immunology and cariogenicity of *Streptococcus mutans*. Microbiol Rev. 1980;44:331.
4. Gordon DF, Stutman M, Loesche WJ. Improved isolation of anaerobic bacteria from the gingival crevice area of man. Appl Microbiol. 1971;21:1046.
5. Valenti WM, Trudell RB, Bentley DW. Factors predisposing to oropharyngeal colonization with gram-negative bacilli in the aged. N Engl J Med. 1978; 298:1108.
6. Rosenthal S, Tager IB. Relevance of gram-negative rods in the normal pharyngeal flora. Ann Intern Med. 1975;83:355.
7. Schuster GS, Burnett GW. The microbiology of oral and maxillofacial infections. In: Topazian RG, Goldberg MH, eds. Management of Infections of the Oral and Maxillofacial Regions. Philadelphia: WB Saunders; 1981:39.
8. Hardie JM, Bowden GH. The normal microbial flora of the mouth. In: Skinner FA, Carr JG, eds. The Normal Microbial Flora of the Mouth. London: Academic Press; 1974:47.
9. Geddes DAM, Jenkins GN. Intrinsic and extrinsic factors influencing the flora of the mouth. In: Skinner FA, Carr JG, eds. The Normal Microbial Flora of the Mouth. London: Academic Press; 1974:85.
10. Schachtele CF. Dental caries. In: Schuster GS, ed. Oral Microbiology and Infectious Diseases. Baltimore: Williams & Wilkins; 1983:197.
11. Patters MR. Periodontal disease. In: Schuster GS, ed. Oral Microbiology and Infectious Diseases. Baltimore: Williams & Wilkins; 1983:234.
12. Van Palenstein, Helderman WH. Microbial etiology of periodontal disease. J Clin Periodont. 1981;8:261.
13. Shaw JH. Causes and control of dental caries. N Engl J Med. 1987;317:996.
14. Loesche WJ. Role of *Streptococcus mutans* in human dental decay. Microbiol Rev. 1986;50:353.
15. Moore WEC, Holdeman LV, Smibert RM, et al. Bacteriology of experimental gingivitis in young adult humans. Infect Immun. 1982;38:651.
16. Socransky SS, Tan ACR, Haffajee AD, et al. Present status of studies on the microbial etiology of periodontal disease. In: Genco RJ, Mergenhagen SE, eds. Host–Parasite Interactions in Periodontal Diseases. Washington DC: American Society for Microbiology; 1982:1.
17. Willams BL, McCann GF, Schoenknecht FD. Bacteriology of dental abscesses of endodontic origin. J Clin Microbiol. 1983;18:770.
18. Greenberg RN, James RB, Marier RL, et al. Microbiologic and antibiotic aspects of infections in the oral and maxillofacial region. J Oral Surg. 1979;37:873.
19. Baker AS, Montgomery WW. Oropharyngeal space infections. Curr Clin Top Infect Dis. 1987;8:227.
20. Newman MG. Anaerobic oral and dental infection. Rev Infect Dis. 1984;6:107.
21. Chow AW. Odontogenic infections. In: Schlossberg D, ed. Infections of the Head and Neck. New York: Springer Publishing; 1987:148.
22. Kureishi K, Chow AW. The tender tooth—dentoalveolar, pericoronal, and periodontal infections. Infect Dis Clin North Am. 1988;2:163.
23. Roscoe DL, Chow AW. Normal flora and mucosal immunity of the head and neck. Infect Dis Clin North Am. 1988;2:1.
24. Sutter VL. Anaerobes as normal oral flora. Rev Infect Dis. 1984;6(Suppl):62.
25. McGhee JR, Michalek SM. Immunobiology of dental caries—microbial aspects and local immunity. Annu Rev Microbiol. 1981;35:595.
26. Saral R, Ambinder RF, Burns WH, et al. Acyclovir prophylaxis against recrudescent herpes simplex virus infections in leukemia patients. A randomized double-blind placebo controlled study. Ann Intern Med. 1983;99:773.
27. Van Dyke TE, Horoszewicz HU, Cianciola LJ, et al. Neutrophil chemotaxis dysfunction in human periodontitis. Infect Immun. 1980;27:124.
28. Cianciola LJ, Genco RJ, Patters MR, et al. Defective polymorphonuclear leukocyte function in human periodontal disease. Nature. 1977;265:445.
29. Genco RJ, Plaut AG, Moellering RC Jr. Evaluation of human oral organisms and pathogenic *Streptococcus* for production of IgA protease. J Infect Dis. 1975;131(Suppl):17.
30. Kilian M. Degradation of immunoglobulins A1, A2, and G by suspected principal periodontal pathogens. Infect Immun. 1981;34:757.
31. Goldberg MH, Topazian RG. Odontogenic infections and deep fascial space infections of dental origin. In: Topazian RG, Goldberg MH, eds. Management of Infections of the Oral and Maxillofacial Regions. Philadelphia: WB Saunders; 1981:173.
32. Thadepalli H, Mandal AK. Anatomic basis of head and neck infections. Infect Dis Clin North Am. 1988;2:21.
33. Shinn DLS, Squires S, McFadzean JA. The treatment of Vincent's disease with metronidazole. Dent Pract. 1965;15:275.
34. Stephen KW, McLatchie MF, Mason DK, et al. Treatment of acute ulcerative gingivitis (Vincent's type). Br Dent J. 1966;121:313.
35. Lindhe J. Treatment of localized juvenile periodontitis. In: Genco RJ, Mergenhagen SE, eds. Host–Parasite Interactions in Periodontal Disease. Washington DC: American Society for Microbiology; 1982:382.
36. Slots J, Reynolds HS, Genco RJ. *Actinobacillus actinomycetemcomitans* in human periodontal disease: A cross-sectional microbiological investigation. Infect Immun. 1980;29:1013.
37. Loesche WJ. The therapeutic use of antimicrobial agents in patients with periodontal disease. Scand J Infect Dis Suppl. 1985;46:106.
38. Finch RG, Snider GE, Sprinkle PM. Ludwig's angina. JAMA. 1980;243:1171.
39. Crawford JJ, Sconyers JR, Moriarty JD, et al. Bacteremia after tooth extractions studied with the aid of prereduced anaerobically sterilized culture media. Appl Microbiol. 1974;27:927.
40. Rubin R, Solvate EA, Lewis R. Infected total hip replacement after dental procedures. Oral Surg. 1976;41:18.
41. McCurdy JA, MacInnis EL, Hays LL. Fatal mediastinitis after a dental infection. J Oral Surg. 1977;35:726.
42. Yoshikawa TT, Quinn W. The aching head—intracranial suppuration due to head and neck infections. Infect Dis Clin North Am. 1988;2:265.
43. Blomquist IK, Bayer AS. Life-threatening deep fascial space infections of the head and neck. Infect Dis Clin North Am. 1988;2:237.
44. Topazian RG. Osteomyelitis of the jaws. In: Topazian RG, Goldberg MH, eds. Management of Infections of the Oral and Maxillofacial Regions. Philadelphia: WB Saunders; 1981:232.
45. Chow AW, Guze LB. Bacteroidaceae bacteremia—clinical experience with 112 patients. Medicine (Baltimore). 1974;53:93.
46. Vogel LC, Boyer KM. Metastatic complications of *Fusobacterium necrophorum* sepsis: Two cases of Lemierre's postanginal septicemia. Am J Dis Child. 1980;134:356.
47. Eagleton WP. Cavernous Sinus Thrombophlebitis and Allied Septic and Traumatic Lesions of the Basal Venous Sinuses. A Clinical Study of Blood Stream Infection. New York: Macmillan; 1926.
48. Harbour RC, Trobe JD, Ballinger WE. Septic cavernous sinus thrombosis associated with gingivitis and parapharyngeal abscess. Arch Ophthalmol. 1984;102:94.
49. Yarington CT Jr. Cavernous sinus thrombosis revisited. Proc R Soc Med. 1977;70:456.
50. Sanders B. Current concepts in the management of osteomyelitis of the mandible. J Oral Med. 1978;33:40.
51. Mackowiak PA, Jones SR, Smith JW. Diagnostic value of sinus-tract cultures in chronic osteomyelitis. JAMA. 1978;239:2772.
52. Salit IE. Diagnostic approaches to head and neck infections. Infect Dis Clin North Am. 1988;2:35.
53. Holt GR, McManus K, Newman RK, et al. Computed tomography in the diagnosis of deep-neck infections. Arch Otolaryngol. 1982;108:693.
54. Wholey MH, Bruwer AJ, Baker HL. The lateral roentgenogram of the neck. Radiology. 1958;71:350.
55. Bryan CS, King BG Jr, Bryant RE. Retropharyngeal infection in adults. Arch Intern Med. 1974;134:127.
56. Loe H, Kornman K. Strategies in the use of antibacterial agents in periodontal disease. In: Genco RJ, Mergenhagen SE, eds. Host–Parasite Interactions in Periodontal Disease. Washington DC: American Society for Microbiology; 1982:376.
57. Danish Medical Research Council Consensus Report. Prevention and control of dental caries. Dan Med Bull. 1986;33:199.
58. Gregory RL, Filler SJ. Protective secretory immunoglobulin A antibodies in humans following oral immunization with *Streptococcus mutans*. Infect Immun. 1987;55:2409.
59. Russell RRB, Johnson NW. The prospects of vaccination against dental caries. Br Dent J. 1987;162:29.
60. Heimdahl A, Nord CE. Treatment of orofacial infections of odontogenic origin. Scand J Infect Dis Suppl. 1985;46:101.
61. Hill MK, Sanders CV. Principles of antimicrobial therapy for head and neck infections. Infect Dis Clin North Am. 1988;2:57.
62. Busch DF, Kureshi LA, Sutter VL, et al. Susceptibility of respiratory tract anaerobes to orally administered penicillins and cephalosporins. Antimicrob Agents Chemother. 1976;10:713.
63. Tami TA, Parker GS. *Eikenella corrodens*—an emerging pathogen in head and neck infections. Arch Otolaryngol. 1984;110:752.
64. Edson RS, Rosenblatt JE, Lee DT, et al. Recent experience with antimicrobial susceptibility of anaerobic bacteria—increasing resistance to penicillin. Mayo Clin Proc. 1982;57:737.

65. Heimdahl A, von Konow L, Nord CE. Isolation of β-lactamase producing *Bacteroides* strains associated with clinical failures with penicillin treatment of human orofacial infections. Arch Oral Biol. 1980;25:687.
66. Murray PR, Rosenblatt JE. Penicillin resistance and penicillinase production in clinical isolates of *Bacteroides melaninogenicus*. Antimicrob Agents Chemother. 1977;11:605.
67. Hood FJC. The place of metronidazole in the treatment of acute orofacial infection. Antimicrob Agents Chemother. 1978;15:71.
68. Epstein JB. The painful mouth—mucositis, gingivitis and stomatitis. Infect Dis Clin North Am. 1988;2:183.
69. Barrett AP. A long-term prospective clinical study of oral complications during conventional chemotherapy for acute leukemia. Oral Surg. 1987;63:313.
70. Topazian RG. Uncommon infections of the oral and maxillofacial regions. In: Topazian RG, Goldberg MH, eds. Management of Infections of the Oral and Maxillofacial Regions. Philadelphia: WB Saunders; 1981:293.
71. Tyldesley WR, ed. Recurrent oral ulcerations. In: Oral Medicine. Oxford: Oxford University Press; 1981:49.
72. Epstein JB, Gangbar SJ. Oral mucosal lesions in patients undergoing treatment for leukemia. J Oral Med. 1987;42:132.
73. Lee PL, Kiviat N, Truelove EL, et al. Oral manifestations in patients with AIDS or AIDS-related disorders. J Dent Res. 1987;66:183.
74. Epstein JB, Stevenson-Moore P. Benzydamine hydrochloride in prevention and management of pain in oral mucositis associated with radiation therapy. Oral Surg. 1986;62:145.
75. Adams S, Toth B, Dudley BS. Evaluation of sucralfate as a compounded oral suspension for the treatment of stomatitis. Clin Pharmacol Ther. 1985;2:178.
76. Epstein JB, Schubert MM. Synergistic effects of sialogogues in management of xerostomia following radiation therapy. Oral Surg. 1987;64:179.
77. Goldberg MH. Infections of the salivary glands. In: Topazian RG, Goldberg MH, eds. Management of Infections of the Oral and Maxillary Regions. Philadelphia: WB Saunders; 1981:293.
78. Adams GL. Infections of the head and neck. In: Simmons RL, Hoeard RF, eds. Surgical Infectious Diseases. New York: Appleton-Century-Crofts; 1982:593.
79. Brook I. The swollen neck—cervical lymphadenitis, parotitis, thyroiditis and infected cysts. Infect Dis Clin North Am. 1988;2:221.
80. Berger SA, Zonszein J, Villanema P, et al. Infectious diseases of the thyroid gland. Rev Infect Dis. 1983;5:108.
81. Freidig EE, McClure SP, Wilson WR, et al. Clinical-histologic-microbiologic analysis of 419 lymph node biopsy specimens. Rev Infect Dis. 1986;8:322.
82. Goldstein EJC, Citron DW, Wield B, et al. Bacteriology of human and animal bite wounds. J Clin Microbiol. 1978;8:667.
83. Herzon FS. The prophylactic use of antibiotics in head and neck surgery. Otolaryngol Clin North Am. 1976;9:781.
84. Seagle MB, Duberstein LE, Gross CW, et al. Efficacy of cefazolin as a prophylactic antibiotic in head and neck surgery. Otolaryngology. 1978;86:568.
85. Zide MF, Sanders CV, Marier RL, et al. Cefuroxime therapy for maxillofacial infections. Curr Ther Res. 1986;40:278.

SECTION C. PLEUROPULMONARY AND BRONCHIAL INFECTIONS

50. ACUTE BRONCHITIS

JACK M. GWALTNEY, JR.

Acute bronchitis is an inflammatory condition of the tracheobronchial tree that is usually associated with a generalized respiratory infection. It occurs most commonly during the winter months when acute respiratory tract infections are prevalent. Patients seen in general practices in Great Britian had annual attack rates of acute bronchitis that varied between 40 and 54 percent 100,000.[1] Weekly attack rates peaked (117–171/100,000) in January and February and fell to trough levels (26–42/100,000) in August. The diagnosis was made most often in children under 5 years of age.

The syndrome of acute bronchitis is associated with infection with both common cold viruses, such as rhinovirus and coronavirus, and lower respiratory tract pathogens, such as influenza virus, adenovirus, and *Mycoplasma pneumoniae*. Secondary bacterial invasion may play a role in the etiology of the syndrome, but this is not well established.

ETIOLOGY

Cough occurs in approximately 50 percent of the cases of common respiratory illness in persons of all ages.[2] Cough is the localizing symptom in the respiratory tract that is most frequently associated with fever and is also highly associated with the occurrence of hoarseness. Infection with members of all the major respiratory virus groups causes cough (Table 1).[2–9] Cases of acute bronchitis are particularly common during influenza epidemics. While rhinovirus infections do not produce as severe an involvement of the tracheobronchial tree as influenza, rhinovirus infections, because of their frequency, are an important cause of acute bronchitis. In populations of military recruits, adenovirus infections are a major cause of acute bronchitis. Among the other respiratory viruses that cause acute bronchitis, measles virus has been recognized as causing a particularly severe form of the disease.

A small proportion of cases are of known nonviral etiology. *Mycoplasma pneumoniae* and *Bordetella pertussis* are among the nonviral causes of acute bronchitis. Recently, a new *Chlamydia psittaci* strain, TWAR, has been associated with acute respiratory tract infections that include cases with the clinical features of acute bronchitis.[10,11] The etiologic role of *Streptococcus pneumoniae* and *Haemophilus influenzae* in acute bronchitis is not clear. Since these bacteria are carried in the resident flora of the upper respiratory tract of normal persons, it is difficult to evaluate studies in which expectorated sputum specimens have been cultured. To examine the role of secondary bacterial infection in the pathogenesis of acute bronchitis, it is

TABLE 1. Cough Associated with Acute Viral Infections of the Respiratory Tract

Virus	Percent of Cases with Cough (References)
Influenza	75–93 (2, 3)
Adenovirus	45–90 (4, 6)
Rhinovirus	32–60 (3, 5)
Coronavirus	10–50 (7, 8)
Parainfluenza virus	2–45 (5)
Respiratory syncytial virus	61 (9)
Coxsackievirus A21	26 (5)
Miscellaneous (rubeola, rubella, and so forth)	—

necessary to conduct studies in which samples are collected from the tracheobronchial tree without contamination from nasopharyngeal flora.

PATHOGENESIS

The pathogenesis of acute bronchitis has not been investigated for all the causative agents. During acute bronchial infection, the mucous membrane of the tracheobronchial tree is hyperemic and edematous, and there are increased bronchial secretions. Destruction of respiratory epithelium may be extensive in some infections, such as influenza,[12] but appears to be minimal in others, such as rhinovirus colds.[13,14] Bronchial mucociliary function may be diminished in infections in which overt mucosal damage is limited.[15] With *M. pneumoniae* infection, bronchial irritation results from the attachment of the organism to the respiratory mucosa, with eventual sloughing of affected cells.[16]

It is also possible that severity of attacks of acute bronchitis may be increased by exposure to cigarette smoke and air pollutants. These substances, in association with recurrent acute bronchial infection, may result in permanent injury to the bronchial tree. Epidemiologic studies support the idea that acute respiratory infections play a role in the pathogenesis of chronic obstructive lung disease.[17,18] Also, studies of pulmonary function in previously healthy adults with acute infection due to some viruses, such as respiratory syncytial virus, have shown prolonged abnormalities in airway resistance and reactivity.[19]

There has been recent interest in examining the relationship between acute bronchitis and heightened airway reactivity. Mild bronchial asthma was found to be increased in patients with a history of recurrent acute bronchitis over that seen in the general population.[20] Also, in a case control study, patients with acute bronchitis were more likely to have a previous history of asthma and a history, or diagnosis, of atopic disease.[21] These findings have raised the question of the possible role of bronchospasm in some cases of prolonged cough associated with acute respiratory infection.

CLINICAL PPRESENTATION

Cough begins early in the course of many acute respiratory infections and tends to become more prominent as the illness progresses (Fig. 1). In the usual cold and influenzal illness, nasal and pharyngeal complaints subside after 3 or 4 days, while the cough tends to persist and to achieve greater prominence.[3] Persons presenting for medical care who are diagnosed as having acute bronchitis probably represent a subset of all patients with acute respiratory infection. In one prospective study of such patients, 45 percent were still coughing 2 weeks after presentation and 25 percent were still coughing after 3 weeks.[22] With a variety of different respiratory virus infections, sputum production was reported in approximately one-half of the cases in which cough was occurring.[4,5] An initially dry cough may later result in mucoid sputum, which characteristically develops a more purulent character in the later stages of illness. A study of natural rhinovirus infections in young adults has shown that the frequency and duration of cough is prolonged in cigarette smokers.[22]

With pronounced tracheal involvement, there may be burning substernal pain associated with respiration and coughing. Dyspnea and cyanosis are not seen in adults unless the patient has underlying chronic obstructive pulmonary disease or other conditions that impair lung function. Rhonchi and coarse rales may be heard on examination of the chest. Signs of consolidation and alveolar involvement are not present in uncomplicated bronchitis. The frequency with which fever occurs depends on the specific infectious agent involved and the age of the patient. In adults, influenza virus, adenovirus, and *M. pneumoniae* infections are commonly associated with temperature elevations.

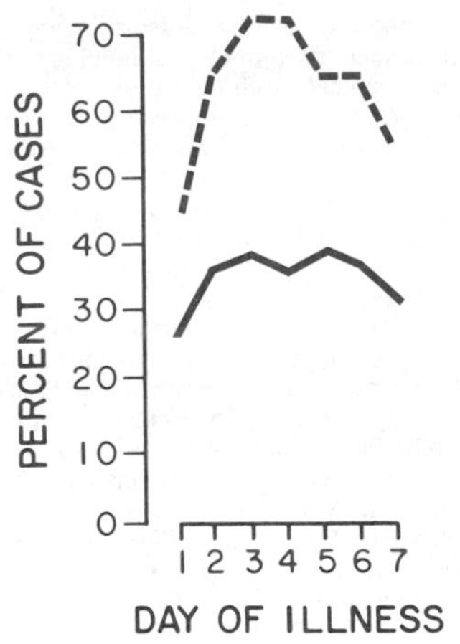

FIG. 1. Occurrence of cough in rhinovirus colds (139 cases) (solid line) and type A_2 influenza (33 cases) (broken line) in young adults. (Modified from Gwaltney,[3] with permission.)

Fever is unusual in adults with bronchitis associated with cold viruses, like rhinovirus and coronavirus.

DIAGNOSIS

Bronchitis may be suspected in the patient with an acute respiratory infection with cough, but because a large number of more serious diseases of the lower respiratory tract cause cough, bronchitis must be considered a diagnosis of exclusion. A complete history should be obtained, including information on exposure to toxic substances and cigarette use. Complaints involving other organ systems should be sought. Epidemiologic considerations and vaccination history may aid in the diagnosis of specific causes of bronchitis, such as influenza, *M. pneumoniae*, and whooping cough.

Included in a complete physical examination should be a careful evaluation of the chest for evidence of pneumonia and signs of cardiovascular and thromboembolic diseases. Radiologic examination of the chest may be required in the occasional patient in whom the question of parenchymal disease of the lung remains after the physical examination. Cultures of respiratory secretions for influenza virus, *M. pneumoniae*, and *B. pertussis* should be obtained when these diseases are suspected. Cultures for the common cold viruses are usually not available. Bacterial cultures of expectorated sputum are not helpful because of the sampling problem of avoiding nasopharyngeal flora and because of the unknown importance of bacterial infection in the etiology of acute bronchitis. Patients in whom cough persists beyond the expected duration of the acute illness should have further diagnostic examinations, including chest x-ray films, sputum cytology, and bronchoscopy to exclude foreign body aspiration, tuberculosis, tumors, and other chronic diseases of the tracheobronchial tree and lungs.

TREATMENT

Treatment of acute bronchitis is symptomatic and is directed primarily at the control of cough. Otherwise, healthy patients do not require hospitalization except in cases of unusual severity. Patients with underlying chronic cardiopulmonary diseases who contract influenzal bronchitis may develop serious ventilatory abnormalities that require hospitalization with ventilatory assistance and oxygen therapy. In the average case, cough suppressants such as dextromethorphan 15 mg po every 6 hours are the main form of treatment required. With severe cough, preparations containing codeine are most useful.[23] The value of expectorants is not well established,[24] and in patients with a good cough reflex, maintaining hydration is probably the most effective way to prevent drying of bronchial secretions. Aspirin and bed rest are beneficial in influenzal syndromes in which malaise and fever are prominent.

The value of antibiotics in the treatment of unselected patients with acute bronchitis is uncertain, and the use of these agents is not recommended as a general practice. Controlled trials[25–29] have given conflicting results, which could result from a number of variables, including type of antibiotic and dosage schedule used, duration of follow-up, season of the year (reflecting prevalence of different pathogens), and adequacy of subject blinding related to drug side effects. *Mycoplasma pneumoniae* infection should be treated with erythromycin or tetracycline (see Chapter 162) and *B. pertussis* infection with erythromycin (see Chapter 208). During epidemics known to be due to influenza A virus, treatment with amantadine (100 mg po bid) is recommended for patients with suspected influenza if the illness is less than 48 hours in duration. Also annual immunization with influenza vaccine or prophylaxis with amantadine is recommended in patients with chronic cardiopulmonary problems (see Chapter 142). Children should receive pertussis vaccine as part of their routine immunizations. It is particularly important to discourage cigarette smoking in patients in whom acute respiratory tract infections are associated with protracted cough and sputum production.

REFERENCES

1. Ayres JG. Seasonal pattern of acute bronchitis in general practice in the United Kingdom 1976–83. Thorax. 1986;41:107–110.
2. Dingle JH, Badger GF, Jordon WS Jr. Illness in the Home: A Study of 25,000 Illnesses in a Group of Cleveland Families. Cleveland: The Press of Western Reserve University; 1964;68.
3. Gwaltney JM Jr. Rhinoviruses. In: Evans AS, ed. Viral Infections of Humans: Epidemiology and Control. 2nd ed. New York: Plenum; 1982:507.
4. Dascomb HE, Hilleman MR. Clinical laboratory studies in patients with respiratory disease caused by adenovirus (RI-APC-ARD agents). Am J Med. 1956;21:161.
5. Tyrrell DAJ. Common Colds and Related Diseases. Baltimore: Williams & Wilkins; 1965.
6. Bloom HH, Forsyth BR, Johnson KM, et al. Patterns of adenovirus infections in Marine Crops personnel. I. A 42-month survey in recruit and nonrecruit populations. Am J Hyg. 1964;80:328.
7. Kaye HS, Marsh HB, Dowdle WR. Seroepidemiologic survey of coronavirus (strain OC43) related infections in a children's population. Am J Epidemiol. 1971;94:43.
8. Hendley JO, Fishburne HB, Gwaltney JM Jr. Coronavirus infections in working adults, Eight-year study with 229E and OC43. Am Rev Respir Dis 1972;105:805.
9. Knight V, Kapikian AZ, Kravetz MH, et al. Ecology of a newly recognized common respiratory agent RS-virus. Ann Intern Med. 1961;55:507.
10. Grayston JT, Kuo C-C, Wang S-P, et al. A new *Chlamydia psittaci* strain, TWAR, isolated in acute respiratory tract infections. N Engl J Med. 1986;315:161–168.
11. Grayston JT, Kuo C-C, Wang S-P, et al. Clinical findings in TWAR respiratory tract infections. In: Oriel JD, Ridgway G, Schacter J, et al. eds. Chlamydial Infections. Cambridge: Cambridge University Press; 1986;337–340.
12. Loosli CG, Stinson SF, Ryan DP, et al. The destruction of type 2 pneumocytes by airborne influenza PR8-A virus: its effect on surfactant and lecithin content of the pneumonic lesions of mice. Chest. 1975;67(Suppl):7S.
13. Douglas RG Jr, Alford BR, Cough RB: Atraumatic nasal biopsy for studies of respiratory virus infection in volunteers. Antimicrob Agents Chemother. 1968;8:340.
14. Winther B, Farr B, Turner RB, et al. Histopathologic examination and enumeration of polymorphonuclear leukocytes in the nasal mucosa during experimental rhinovirus colds. Acta Otoaryngol [Suppl] (Stockh) 1984;413:19–24.
15. Sasaki Y, Togo Y, Wagner NH Jr, et al. Mucociliary function during experimentally induced rhinovirus infection in man. Ann Otol. 1973;82:203.
16. Powell DA, Hu PC, Wilson M, et al. Attachment of *Mycoplasma pneumoniae* to respiratory epithelium. Infect Immun 1976;13:959.
17. Lebowitz MD, Burrows B. The relationship of acute respiratory illness history to the prevalence and incidence of obstructive lung disorders. Am J Epidemiol. 1977;105:544.
18. Monto AS, Ross HW. The Tecumseh study of respiratory illness. X. Relation of acute infections to smoking, lung function and chronic symptoms. Am J Epidemiol. 1978;107:57.
19. Hall WJ, Hall CB, Speers DM. Respiratory syncytial virus infection in adults. Clinical, virologic, and serial pulmonary function studies. Ann Intern Med. 1978;88:203.
20. Hallett JS, Jacobs RL. Recurrent acute bronchitis: the association with undiagnosed bronchial asthma. Ann Allergy. 1985;55:568–570.
21. Williamson HA, Jr, Schultz P. An association between acute bronchitis and asthma. J Fam Prac. 1987;24:35–38.
22. Gwaltney JM Jr, Hendley JO, Simon G, et al. Rhinovirus infections in an industrial population. II. Characteristics of illness and antibody response. JAMA. 1967;202:494.
23. Eddy NB. Codeine and its alternates for pain and cough relief. Ann Intern Med. 1969;71:1209.
24. Kuhn JJ, Hendley JO, Adams KF, Antitussive effect of guaifenesin in young adults with natural colds. Objective and subjective assessment. Chest. 1982;82:713.
25. Stott NC, and West RR. Randomized controlled trial of antibiotics in patients with cough and purulent sputum. Br Med J. 1976;2:556.
26. Franks P, Gleiner JA. The treatment of acute bronchitis with trimethoprim and sulfamethoxazole. J Fam Prac. 1984;19:185–190.
27. Williamson HA Jr. A randomized, controlled trial of doxycycline in the treatment of acute bronchitis. J Fam Pract. 1984;19:481–486.
28. Brickfield FX, Carter WH, Johnson RE. Erythromycin in the treatment of acute bronchitis in a community practice. J Fam Pract. 1986;23:119–122.
29. Dunlay J, Reinhardt R, Roi LD. A placebo-controlled, double-blind trial of erythromycin in adults with acute bronchitis. J Fam Prac 1987;25:137–141.

51. CHRONIC BRONCHITIS AND ACUTE INFECTIOUS EXACERBATIONS

HERBERT Y. REYNOLDS

Chronic bronchitis is a condition in which cough and excessive secretion of mucus are present in the tracheobronchial tree that are not due to other specific diseases such as bronchiectasis, asthma, or tuberculosis. The label "chronic bronchitic" is often loosely applied to patients and is very much a clinical diagnosis. By definition, the diagnosis is given to patients who report to have coughed up sputum on most days during at least 3 consecutive months for more than 2 successive years.[1,2] Some clinical surveys have added to the definition the occurrence of attacks of cough with sputum in the previous 2 years that have prevented the patient from working for a total of at least 3 weeks. If wheezing and bronchospasm occur with the disease, the designation chronic or recurrent asthmatic bronchitis may be used. Emphysema often complicates the clinical presentation. Although the precise diagnosis of emphysema is a morbid and anatomic one, its coexistence is usually inferred. The two diagnoses are usually lumped together and used to identify patients as having "chronic obstructive lung disease with bronchitis and emphysema."

ETIOLOGY AND PATHOLOGY

Although the causes of chronic bronchitis have not been elucidated completely, three factors seem to be of particular importance: cigarette smoking, infection, and inhalation of dust or fumes in the workplace environment. Chronic bronchitis is common and affects about 10–25 percent of the adult population. Bronchitis is more common in men than in women and more common after the age of 40 than before. Smoking, cigarette smoking in particular, is the most important factor associated with the disease. Related diseases that impair mucociliary transport in the lung may be important in susceptible people. The clinician must be alert for the possibility that recurrent respiratory infections and persistent chronic bronchitis might signal that the patient has an immunodeficiency syndrome. This association may become evident in teenagers or young adults and not in young children as generally expected.[3] Investigation for cystic fibrosis, an intrinsic defect in the structure of epithelial cilia, immunoglobulin deficiency involving IgA or selective IgG subclasses,[4,5] and rarely abnormal polymorphonuclear (PMN) granulocyte function should be considered.

Cigarette smoking is a significant airway irritant for most patients. Not all patients with chronic bronchitis, however, have a history of smoking; an average of 6–10 percent of nonsmoking men will have persistent cough and phlegm production. In light-to-moderate smokers (20 or fewer cigarettes per day), the frequency of chronic bronchitis is approximately 25 percent; for heavy smokers (greater than a 40–60 pack-year history) it increases to almost 50 percent. The frequency is less in ex-smokers. Investigators who have performed bronchoalveolar lavage to obtain respiratory cells from human lungs have uniformly found a tremendous increase in the recovery of alveolar macrophages from cigarette smokers as compared with nonsmokers.[6] "Normal" smokers usually yield a small percentage of inflammatory cells (PMN granulocytes) as well. A modest degree of smoking (2–5 pack-years) induces cellular and lavage fluid immunoglobulin changes similar to those found in heavy smokers. Postmortem examination of lungs obtained from young accident victims showed evidence of inflammation involving respiratory bronchioles in smokers but not in nonsmokers. The lesion consisted of clusters of pigmented macrophages in association with edema, fibrosis, and epithelial hyperplasia of the bronchiolar and aveolar walls.[7] Thus, cigarette users, even those who smoke minimally, initiate irritative stimuli that may insidiously culminate years later as chronic bronchitis and possibly other forms of degenerative lung diseases. The realization that cigarette smoke can inactivate the antiprotease function of α_1-antitrypsin in lung secretions further supports this sequence of destructive lung disease.[8,9]

One striking change noted in the lungs of patients with chronic bronchitis is the increase in the number of goblet (mucus-secreting) cells in the surface epithelium of major and smaller bronchi. Whereas goblet cells normally account for one-fourth of the epithelial cells lining the larger bronchi and are virtually absent from the smaller ones, particularly bronchioles,[10] in chronic bronchitis the epithelium may consist almost entirely of such cells. In addition, mucous glands in the walls of the larger bronchi undergo hypertrophy. Normally, the ratio of the mucous glands compared with the bronchial wall (the latter measured from the surface of the epithelium to the inner surface of the cartilaginous plates) is about 0.3, but with enlargement of the mucous glands, as found in chronic bronchitis, the ratio is greater and on the order of 0.6 (Reid index).[11] Besides mucous gland enlargement, chronic bronchitics have irritation of the airway mucosa and more mucus in their peripheral airways. The irritated airways respond by producing extra secretions, exposing sensitive stretch receptors (which aggravates cough), and developing bronchospasm. Inflammation of the mucosa gives rise to swelling and edema, infiltration of PMNs, hyperplasia of goblet cells, and enlargement of bronchial mucus glands as observed in the pathology. However, mechanisms that produce these changes have only been investigated recently.[12]

Explants of human airways (2–10 mm in diameter from the second- to fifth-generation bronchi) can be established and cultured for 2–3 days. Such explants contain normal-appearing mucosal surfaces and goblet cells and intact submucosal glands.[13] In this in vitro system, secretion of mucous glycoproteins can be stimulated with a variety of factors: histamine, slow-reacting substance of anaphylaxis (leukotrienes C, D, and E), IgE antibody, and methacholine. Products of mast cell degranulation and pharmacologic agents can enhance the output of mucous glycoproteins as well as neuropeptides that stimulate cyclic guanosine monophosphate (GMP). Other products of arachidonic acid metabolism can also stimulate these explants to produce mucus.[14] In addition, human blood monocytes and alveolar macrophages produce a mucus secretagogue, after a phagocytic stimulus, that causes the release of mucous glycoprotein from cultured human airways.[15,16]

CLINICAL PRESENTATION

Incessant cough marks most advanced bronchitics. The patient may clear his throat frequently, and during conversation, an outburst of laughter or animated speech can precipitate a loud, raspy, coughing episode. Many patients expectorate sputum throughout the day, but most cough up the largest amount in the morning on arising. Sputum may be tenacious and sticky and vary in appearance from mucoid or whitish to yellowish green and obviously purulent. Many patients have associated nasal problems and often complain of a postnasal drip or sinus congestion. A bad taste in the mouth and halitosis are frequent complaints. Most patients with chronic bronchitis are not incapacitated by their respiratory disorder unless an acute infection or some other illness occurs.

As mentioned, emphysema is often present, and some patients with advanced chronic bronchitis have complications that are determined for the most part by the degree and type of associated emphysema. The use of descriptive terms to separate patients with chronic obstructive lung disease into groups such as "blue bloaters" (or type B) and "pink puffers" (or type A) is often an oversimplification.[17] However, the separation may be useful in understanding the clinical course of the patient with chronic bronchitis and recurrent respiratory infections.

The blue bloater is characterized by severe obstructive lung disease with serious and persistent blood gas abnormalities and an impaired air flow that is worse than predicted from the forced expiratory volume of the first second (FEV_1). Frequent tracheobronchial infections (bacterial and viral) occur and occasionally lead to bronchopneumonia. Dyspnea, although a prominent symptom, is less intense than in the pink puffer. As a consequence of the blood gas derangements, a number of associated features may follow. Somnolence and lethargy can develop. Pulmonary vasospasm induced by the combination of hypoxemia and respiratory acidosis increases pulmonary vascular resistance, which in turn increases the work load of the right ventricle of the heart. Cor pulmonale with peripheral edema and its other attendant consequences may occur. Patients often cough up copious amounts of sputum and do not show radiologic evidence of emphysema. These patients are thought primarily to be severe bronchitics with little evidence of emphysema. In contrast, pink puffers, despite severe airway obstruction, maintain relatively normal blood gases because of high minute ventilation. These patients, frequently underweight and barrel chested, do not appear cyanotic or plethoric and do not develop cor pumonale except terminally. Radiologically emphysema is present. These are considered patients with severe emphysema and little bronchitis. It is now apparent that the clinical distinction between these two syndromes is not clear-cut and that many patients (perhaps the majority) have features of both.

The bronchitic maintains normal body weight and tends to be obese. Normal vesicular breath sounds are diminished, and inspiratory and expiratory rales, rhonchi, and mild wheezing may be heard instead. The chest is noisy rather than quiet, as is observed with emphysema. If pulmonary artery pressure is elevated, cardiac signs may reflect it. With advanced bronchitis and emphysema, the patient may have acrocyanosis, plethoric complexion, and manifestations of overt heart failure. Digital clubbing is not a finding in the uncomplicated bronchitic.

Evidence of an Acute Infectious Exacerbation

Objective signs that bronchitis has worsened in temporal relationship to a documented infection are not always evident. Reliance is placed on the patient's observation that his sputum has changed in color and consistency or has increased in amount. In some patients the development of an increased amount of noneosinophilic purulent sputum is presumptive evidence of infection. However, other patients consistently produce purulent sputum without other evidence of infection. Patients may note increasing cough and dyspnea, but during an acute illness, most will not have symptoms suggesting systemic toxicity such as chills and fever, nor will they develop a blood leukocytosis. Patients often experience chest tightness and increased fatigue. No uniform definition for an acute exacerbation of chronic bronchitis exists.

Sputum Analysis

Cellular analysis[18,19] of a fresh sputum specimen (early morning sample) is necessary in the evaluation of every patient with chronic bronchitis. Continual bronchial irritation is indicated by the presence of many PMN granulocytes, even during quiescent periods of the disease. It is important to determine the number of eosinophils. Ciliated epithelial cells can be recognized, and their number correlates reasonably well with the degree of vigorous coughing that was needed to produce the sputum specimen. A few alveolar macrophages may be identified that in the cigarette smoker characteristically contain yellowish brown cytoplasmic inclusions. Gram stain will often show a mixture of gram-positive and gram-negative bacteria that is consistent with contamination by normal mouth flora or with tracheal colonization by *Haemophilus influenzae* and *Streptococcus pneumoniae*.

The mucus secreted in chronic bronchitis contains various glycoproteins, mucopolysaccharide acids, and albumin. Small amounts of a number of immunoglobulin species are present including secretory IgA, IgG, occasionally IgM and IgE, or proteolytic fragments derived from them. Other proteins present include transferrin, complement components, and enzyme inhibitors such as α_1-antiprotease. With high degrees of bronchial irritation and inflammation, any of the intravascular proteins may be identified in purulent mucus; however, the protein is likely to be fragmented or denatured because of the effect of pH or the action of lysosomal enzymes and other degradative substances in sputum.[20,21] Immunologic analysis of IgA in sputum may help in diagnosing the presence of infection in patients with a flare-up of chronic bronchitis. With active infection, the content of 7S IgA is increased, and free-secretory component is all used; without infection, 11S IgA is increased, and excess secretory component exists.[22]

Radiologic Evidence

Standard chest films contribute little to the definitive diagnosis of chronic bronchitis, but they serve the essential purpose of excluding other diseases that may mimic or contribute to chronic bronchitis. The chest film can appear normal in chronic bronchitis and may not undergo change during infectious exacerbations; therefore, it is not a very sensitive or helpful way of following most patients.

RELATIONSHIP OF INFECTION TO ACUTE EXACERBATIONS

The most enigmatic problem in chronic bronchitis is the role of bacterial infection. Although its exact place is uncertain, bacterial infection does not appear to initiate the disease except possibly in the patient with a history of frequent childhood respiratory infections.[23] However, bacteria are probably significant in perpetuating the disease and may be critical in producing the characteristic exacerbations.

It is generally accepted that the bronchi of nonbronchitics who are free of other lung diseases are almost always sterile, although methods of culture are not perfect and may not exclude oral flora.[24–26] Pathogenic bacteria can be cultured from the bronchi in up to 82 percent of chronic bronchitics. Pathogenic organisms have also been cultured from the airways of nonbronchitics who have carcinoma of the lung or tuberculosis or after radiation to the lung. Thus, various forms of damage to the lung may predispose to bacterial infection. Routine sputum cultures from patients with chronic bronchitis commonly contain nonencapsulated *H. influenzae, S. pneumoniae,* and other oropharyngeal commensal flora. In most clinical series, one or both of these species is recovered from approximately 30–50 percent of the sputum specimens and rightfully can be considered as the baseline microbial flora of many patients with chronic bronchitis. Anaerobic bacteria could be recovered in only 17 percent of transtracheal aspirate specimens.[27] However, sputum carriage of *H. influenzae* and pneumococci does seem to be of particular significance. These bacteria tend to persist in sputum during quiescent intervals, and the frequency of recovery is not greatly increased during acute infectious episodes. The development of purulent sputum is not correlated specifically with the presence of one or the other of these bacteria. However, evidence suggests that purulence is associated with a quantitative increase in the number of pneumococci cultured from sputum.[28] *Mycoplasma pneumoniae* does not seem to be of great importance, for some studies[28,29] attribute only 1–10 percent of acute infections to this organism.

As mentioned, it is often impossible to judge when an acute infection has supervened, microbiologically as well as clinically. This is particularly true of patients who always experience symptoms of cough and produce sputum that is purulent. One study[28] that monitored infectious episodes on the basis of changes in monthly serum antibody titers to a large number of microorganisms indicated that infection could occur frequently without a clinical exacerbation of bronchitis. This was especially true of viral infections. Of those viral infections documented to have occurred by significant changes in serum antibody titers, 40 percent were not associated with a clinical exacerbation.

The following statements summarize the relationship between causative agents[30] and acute flare-ups of infection in chronic bronchitis: (*1*) Chronic colonization of the airways and sputum with unencapsulated strains of *H. influenzae* and with pneumococci occurs in at least one-half of the affected patients. Microbiologically, it is difficult to incriminate one or both these bacteria as the specific cause of an acute infection. However, many physicians usually attribute acute infectious exacerbation to one of these bacteria, and antibiotic selection is often based on this probability. (2) Other bacteria such as hemolytic species of streptococci, *Staphylococcus aureus,* and gram-negative enteric bacilli are infrequent causes of acute infection in chronic bronchitis. Only 5–10 percent of the sputum specimens will contain significant numbers of these other bacteria. Since sputum may be contaminated by oropharyngeal flora, it is uncertain whether these bacteria originate in the lower airways. Other sampling methods such as transtracheal aspiration may be necessary to make this distinction.[27] (*3*) *Mycoplasma pneumoniae* infections can be sporadic and may be responsible for some acute exacerbations. (*4*) Viruses are frequent causes of acute infection. Fully 25–50 percent of acute exacerbations are related to these agents, including influenza, parainfluenza, respiratory syncytial virus, rhinovirus, and coronavirus. Viral infections are seasonal and occur more frequently in winter.

MANAGEMENT

General Considerations

Attempts should be made to have the patient stop smoking or at least reduce the amount of smoking. During the patient's initial evaluation, analysis of the cellular content of a sputum specimen is indicated; if eosinophils are among the inflammatory cells present, an allergic component to the illness should be investigated. Some asthmatics cough instead of wheeze, so it is not infrequent to encounter an asthmatic who has symptoms of chronic cough rather than audible wheezing.[31] Since excessive mucus secretion is common to both asthma and bronchitis, eosinophils in the sputum and in the peripheral blood can be a diagnostic clue. Initial pulmonary function tests to assess expiratory airflow should also include tests performed after the aerosol administration of a bronchodilator, unless a contraindication exists. It is useful to establish whether the patient has a reversible component of bronchospasm to the airway obstruction. Appropriate bronchodilator therapy may improve breathing and may improve exercise tolerance. Patients who develop wheezing during acute infectious exacerbation may profit from a bronchodilator as well. Consultation with an ear, nose, and throat specialist and x-ray films of the sinuses may help to identify a deviated nasal septum, nasal polyps, or chronic sinusitis. A program of weight reduction and a suitable exercise regimen can be considered. Patients should receive a yearly immunization with the current influenza vaccine. Indications for the use of pneumococcal vaccine need individual consideration.

The accumulation and clearance of secretions can be a real problem for some patients, and postural drainage maneuvers are indicated, especially during acute infections. The yield of secretions from postural drainage can sometimes be improved by the addition of two procedures: (*1*) the initial use of an aerosol bronchodilator to achieve maximum dilatation and opening of the airways and then (*2*) humidification or wetting of respiratory secretions. Patients who are plagued with copious secretions and gain benefit from postural drainage ought to receive instruction in the technique from a qualified respiratory therapist. Other therapy aimed at liquifying respiratory secretions or controlling cough are not of particular value. Mucolytic agents designed to loosen and dissolve tenacious secretions are often irritative and actually may serve to increase mucus production. Cough-suppressant drugs are rarely indicated. The effect of sedatives contained in many preparations is generally not desirable, especially for patients with chronic obstructive lung disease. Cough is an efficient way of removing secretions. The use of an intermittent positive-pressure breathing device is rarely justified; if aerosol administration of medications is deemed necessary, a hand-held or motorized nebulizer will provide adequate drug distribution in the airways.

Spirometry and expiratory airflow values may not improve even though the patient has achieved a quiescent and "infection-free" stage. Actually, bronchiolar inflammation and airway resistance may have decreased, but the routine pulmonary tests are generally insensitive to this improvement.

Since most chronic bronchitics continue to be cigarette smokers, they remain in a group that is statistically at increased risk to develop primary lung cancer. Early detection of cancer that is still localized provides the best hope for cure. Therefore, periodic sputum specimens for cytology and chest films are indicated.

Finally, the use of corticosteroid therapy should be mentioned. At some point the bronchitic patient will not rebound from an acute infection despite a vigorous and optimal treatment regimen that includes antibiotics and other ancillary drugs in maximal doses. In such a circumstance, a trial of corticosteroids may be indicated with moderate doses of the drug (20–30 mg/day equivalent of prednisone, for example). Current preference still favors the use of a systemically administered drug instead of a topical aerolized preparation. Because mucus plugging and diffuse areas of obstruction are present in the airways, a systemically absorbed steroid will achieve more even distribution throughout the lung tissue. The steroid effect is often not immediate, so a drug course of 3–6 weeks may be necessary. For many patients with chronic obstructive lung disease, a trial of corticosteroids and inhaled β_2-agonist drugs is worthwhile and may improve dyspnea and the FEV_1 value.[32] Moreover, the use of inhaled atropine can be helpful also, not only for bronchospasm but also to inhibit the formation of mucus and secretions.

Antimicrobial Therapy

Prophylactic treatment with tetracycline decreased the number of exacerbations in patients who had many episodes, but it did nothing for those who ordinarily had few exacerbations. Antibiotic treatment did not alter the rate of decline in pulmonary function.[33] Prophylactic antibiotic therapy may have some usefulness in highly selected patients who experience frequent exacerbations. Either tetracycline (250–500 mg qid po), ampicillin (250–500 mg qid po), amoxicillin (500 mg qid po), or erythromycin (250 mg qid or 500 mg bid po) is an acceptable drug. Trimethoprim-sulfamethoxazole is also effective. Because bacteria such as *Haemophilus influenzae* can inactivate β-lactam antibiotics by secreting β-lactamases, inhibitors such as clavulanate have been combined with amoxicillin. The use of such a combination is appropriate if β-lactamase–producing bacteria are causing infection. Several different strategies appear to be effective. Patients may receive antibiotics daily during the winter months, 4 days/wk during the winter, or a 7-day course at the first sign of a "chest cold."

The effectiveness of the short-term use of antibiotics for acute exacerbations is difficult to assess.[28,29,34,35,36] Infection can cause acute decompensation and is the most common identifiable cause of death in these patients. The usual strategy is to institute a course of antimicrobial therapy for a 7- to 10–day period and hope that the acute flare-up subsides; an objective end point for success is usually lacking. Erythromycin may be prescribed as an alternative on the assumption that it (like tetracycline) is effective for *Mycoplasma* infection. The oral administration of antibiotics is sufficient for most of the acute bacterial flare-ups. Questions exist about the overall benefit of antimicrobial therapy in exacerbations of chronic bronchitis, although they may improve symptoms and reduce disability.

REFERENCES

1. Ciba Guest Symposium. Terminology, definitions and classification of chronic pulmonary emphysema and related conditions. Thorax. 1959;14:286.
2. Medical Research Council. Definition and classification of chronic bronchitis for clinical and epidemiological purposes. A report to the Medical Research Council by their committee on the etiology of chronic bronchitis. Lancet. 1965;1:775.
3. Reynolds HY. Respiratory infections may reflect deficiencies in host defense mechanisms. DM. 1985;31:1–98.
4. Beck GS, Heiner DC. Selective immunoglobulin G4 deficiency and recurrent infections of the respiratory tract. Am Rev Respir Dis. 1981;124:94.
5. Reynolds HY. Immunoglobulin G and its function in the human respiratory tract. Mayo Clin Proc. 1988;63:161–74.
6. Reynolds HY, Merrill WW. Airway changes in young smokers that may antedate chronic obstructive lung disease. Med Clin North Am. 1981;65:667–89.
7. Nieworehner DE, Kleinerman J, Rice DB. Pathologic changes in the peripheral airways of young cigarette smokers. N Engl J Med. 1974;291:755.
8. Gadek JE, Fellis GA, Crystal RG. Cigarette smoking induces functional antiprotease deficiency in the lower respiratory tract of humans. Science. 1979;206:1315.
9. Carp H, Miller F, Hoidal J, et al. Alpha 1-proteinase inhibitor purified from lungs of cigarette smokers contains oxidized methionine and has decreased elastase inhibitory capacity. Proc Natl Acad Sci USA. 1982;779:2041–5.
10. Gail DB, Lenfant CJM. Cells of the lung: Biology and clinical implications. Am Rev Respir Dis. 1983;127:366–87.
11. Reid L. Measurement of the bronchial mucous gland layer: A diagnostic yardstick in chronic bronchitis. Thorax. 1960;15:132.
12. Reynolds HY. Lung Inflammation: Normal host defense or a complication of some diseases? Annu Rev Med. 1987;38:295–323.
13. Shelhamer JH, Marom Z, Kaliner M. Immunologic and neuropharmacologic stimulation of mucous glycoprotein release from human airways in vitro. J Clin Invest. 1980;66:1400–6.
14. Marom Z, Shelhamer JH, Bach NK, et al. Slow-reacting substances (LTC_4 and LTD_4) increase the release of mucus from human airways in vitro. Am Rev Respir Dis. 1982;126:449–51.
15. Marom Z, Shelhamer JH, Kaliner M. Human pulmonary macrophage-derived mucus secretagogue. J Exp Med. 1984;159:844–60.
16. Marom Z, Shelhamer JH, Kaliner M. Human monocyte-derived mucus secretagogue. J Clin Invest. 1985;75:191–98.
17. Burrows B, Niden AH, Fletcher CM, et al. Clinical types of chronic obstructive lung disease in London and Chicago. Am Rev Respir Dis. 1964;90:14.
18. Chodosh S. Examination of sputum cells. N Engl J Med. 1970;282:854.

19. Baigelman W, Chodosh S. Sputum "wet preps": Window on the airways. J Respir Dis 1984;59–70.
20. Wiggins J, Hill SL, Stockley RA. The secretory IgA system of lung secretions in chronic obstructive bronchitis: Comparison of sputum with secretions obtained during fiberoptic bronchoscopy. Thorax. 1984;39:517–23.
21. Niederman MS, Merrill WW, Polomski LM, et al. Influence of sputum IgA and elastase on tracheal cell bacterial adherence. Am Rev Respir Dis. 1986;133:255.
22. Stockley RA, Afford SC, Burnett D. Assessment of 7S and 11S immunoglobulin A in sputum. Am Rev Respir Dis. 1980;122:956.
23. Leeder SR. Role of infection in the cause and course of chronic bronchitis and emphysema. J Infect Dis. 1975;131:731.
24. Laurenzi GG, Potter RT, Kass EH. Bacterial flora of the lower respiratory tract. N Engl J Med. 1961;265:1273.
25. Potter RT, Totman F, Fernandez R, et al. The bacteriology of the lower respiratory tract. Bronchoscopic study of 100 clinical cases. Am Rev Respir Dis. 1968;97:1051.
26. Halperin SA, Suratt PM, Gwaltney JM Jr, et al. Bacterial cultures of the lower respiratory tract in normal volunteers with and without experimental rhinovirus infection using a plugged double catheter system. Am Rev Respir Dis. 1982;125:678.
27. Hass H, Morris JF, Samson S, et al. Bacterial flora of the respiratory tract in chronic bronchitis: Comparison of transtracheal, fiber-bronchoscopic and oropharyngeal sampling methods. Am Rev Respir Dis. 1977;116:41.
28. Gump DW, Phillips CA, Forsyth BR, et al. Role of infection in chronic bronchitis. Am Rev Respir Dis. 1976;113:465.
29. Tager I, Speizer FE. Role of infection in chronic bronchitis. N Engl J Med. 1975;292:583.
30. Reynolds HY. Bacterial adherence to respiratory tract mucosa—a dynamic interaction leading to colonization. Semin Respir Infect. 1987;2:8–19.
31. Corrao WM, Bramen SS, Irwin RS. Chronic cough as the sole presenting manifestation of bronchial asthma. N Engl J Med. 1979;300:633.
32. Mendella LA, Manfreda J, Warren CPW, et al. Steroid response in stable chronic obstructive lung disease. Ann Intern Med. 1982;96:17.
33. Fletcher CM, Oldham PD. Value of chemoprophylaxis and chemotherapy in early chronic bronchitis. A report to the medical research council by their working party on trials of chemotherapy in early chronic bronchitis. Br Med J. 1966;1:1317.
34. Nicotra MB, Rivera M, Awe RJ. Antibiotic therapy of acute exacerbations of chronic bronchitis. Ann Intern Med. 1982;97:18.
35. Bates JH. The role of infection during exacerbations of chronic bronchitis. Ann Intern Med. 1982;97:130.
36. Anthonisen NR, Manfreda J, Warren CPW, et al. Antiobiotic therapy in exacerbations of chronic obstructive pulmonary disease. Ann Intern Med. 1987;106:196.

52. BRONCHIOLITIS

CAROLINE BREESE HALL
WILLIAM J. HALL

In bronchiolitis we must now contend
with both the disease of the "now" and the "then";
For many such infants a mold has been cast,
perhaps by their unborn and unknown past,
which destines that they shall in time wheeze again.
For them this disease
is the distant, boding knell
Of vulnerable lungs
to a microbe's mystic spell.

C.B.H.

Bronchiolitis is an acute viral lower respiratory tract illness occurring within the first 2 years of life. The characteristic clinical findings include an acute onset of wheezing and hyperaeration, most commonly associated with cough, rhinorrhea, tachypnea, and respiratory distress. The entity "bronchiolitis" appears to have been born from a long lineage of confusing sobriquets, including acute catarrhal bronchitis, interstitial bronchopneumonia, spastic bronchopneumonia, capillary or obstructive bronchiolitis, and asthmatic bronchiolitis.[1] Bronchiolitis, however, did not become recognized as a separate entity until the 1940s.[2]

ETIOLOGY

Although bronchiolitis was initially thought to be caused by bacteria, viruses and occasionally *Mycoplasma pneumoniae* are now known to be the instigators of bronchiolitis. Respiratory syncytial virus (RSV) is clearly the major cause, with the parainfluenza viruses being the second most commonly isolated agent (Table 1, Fig. 1).[3–11] A long-term study of respiratory illnesses associated with wheezing in children from a private practice in Chapel Hill, North Carolina, showed that RSV, parainfluenza viruses type 1 and type 3, adenoviruses, rhinoviruses, and *Mycoplasma pneumoniae* make up 87 percent of the isolates obtained from children of all ages.[3] Within the first 2 years of life, RSV accounted for 44 percent of the isolates, with the parainfluenza viruses type 1 and type 3 and adenoviruses each accounting for about 13 percent. Similarly, RSV was in 55 percent of the isolates obtained from children with bronchiolitis from two group practices in Rochester, New York, over a 6-year period.[12] The second most frequently identified agent was parainfluenza type 3, accounting for 11 percent of the cases. The proportion of these agents may change, depending on the population and whether the cases occur as part of an epidemic. In hospitalized cases, the contribution of RSV is even higher, as demonstrated by the Newcastle-upon-Tyne studies in which 74 percent of the infants hospitalized with bronchiolitis had infection with this agent.[10]

EPIDEMIOLOGY

Bronchiolitis shows a definite seasonal pattern in temperate climates, with a yearly upsurge of cases in winter to early spring.[3,7–10,12,13] This pattern mirrors that of its prime agent, RSV. Lesser swells of activity are seen during the fall and spring when the parainfluenza viruses are active.

Bronchiolitis is a common illness during the first year of life, with the peak attack rate occurring between 2 and 10 months of age.[3,5,10,13–16] In the Chapel Hill studies, the incidence of bronchiolitis was about 11 cases per hundred children for both the first and second 6 months of life.[3,13] In the second year of life the incidence fell to approximately one-half. A much higher incidence, however, has been reported[16] in long-term studies of children in a day care center who were examined regularly. Since even the mildest cases were detected, the rate rose to 115 cases per 100 children aged 6 months or less per year. By the second year of life this rate had declined to 32 cases per 100 children per year.

An appreciable proportion of hospital admissions for infants within the first year of life are caused by bronchiolitis, especially that resulting from RSV. In the review by Breese et al.[17] of their group practice, 4 percent of their patients of all ages requiring hospitalization for medical illnesses were bronchiolitis cases. In the Seattle prepaid medical care group, the rate of infants hospitalized with bronchiolitis during the first 6 months of life was 6 per 1000 children per year.[5] Bronchiolitis is more

TABLE 1. Agents Causing Bronchiolitis

Agent	*Cases (%)*	*Epidemiology*
Respiratory syncytial virus	45–75	Yearly epidemics winter to spring
Parainfluenza viruses		
Type 3	8–15	Predominantly spring to fall
Type 1	5–12	Epidemics in the fall every other year
Type 2	1–5	Fall
Rhinoviruses	3–8	Endemic, all seasons
Adenoviruses	3–10	Endemic, all seasons
Influenza viruses	5–8	Epidemic, winter to spring
Mycoplasma pneumoniae	1–7	Endemic, all seasons
Enteroviruses	1–5	Summer to fall

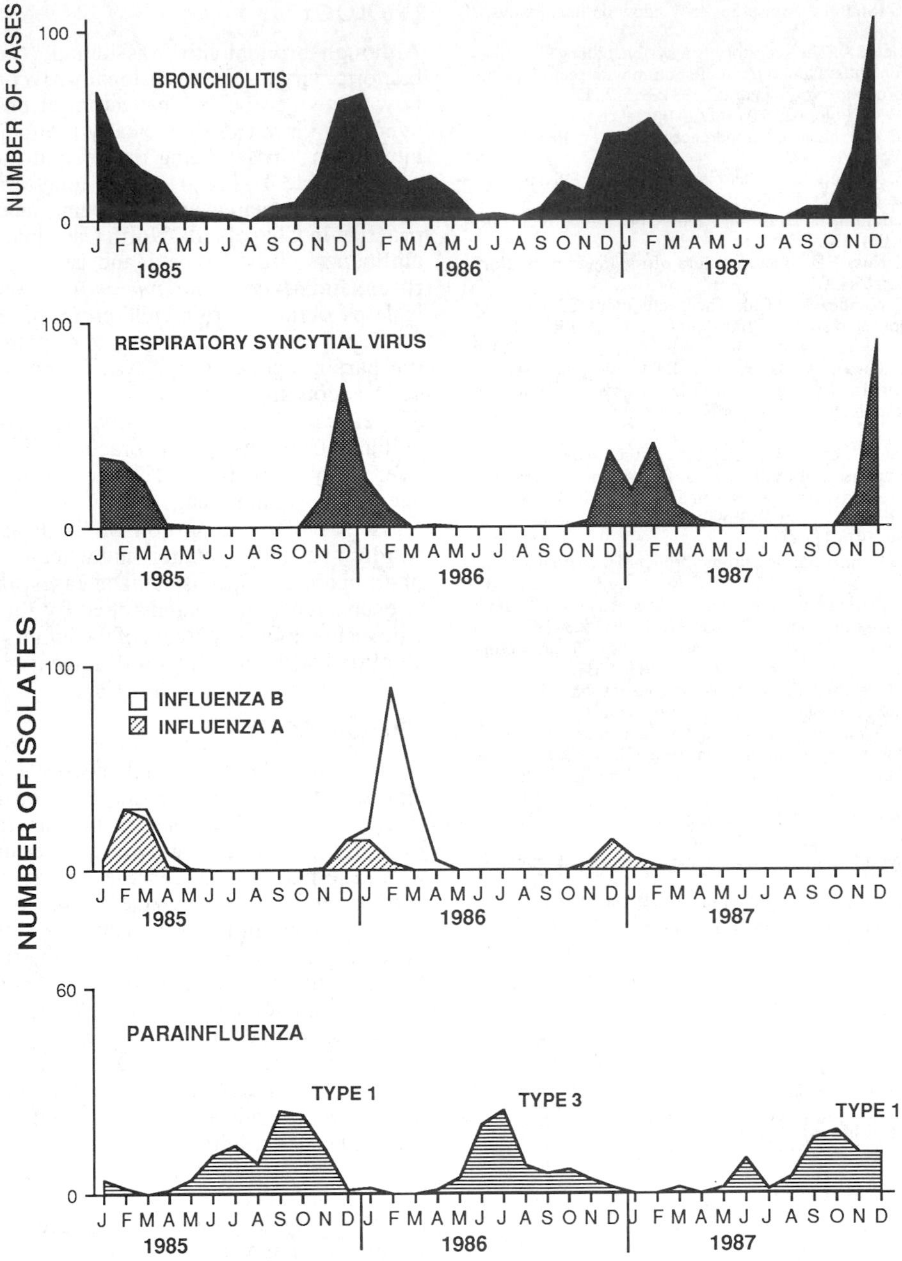

FIG. 1. Patterns of reported cases of bronchiolitis shown in relation to the activity of the major respiratory viruses in Monroe County, New York. Data are obtained from a weekly community surveillance program for infectious diseases.

common in boys, especially in those requiring hospitalization, with a ratio of about 1.5 to 1.[3,15,18]

PATHOPHYSIOLOGY

Engle and Newns[2] in 1940 carefully described the pathologic findings of bronchiolitis, which have subsequently been expanded and further delineated.[1,19–22] The characteristic initial findings are inflammation and necrosis of the respiratory epithelium. Subsequently, the epithelium may proliferate and demonstrate cuboidal cells without cilia. Peribronchiolar infiltration, mostly with mononuclear cells, and edema of the submucosa and adventitia are observed. Necrosis of the bronchiolar epithelium and sloughing subsequently results (Figs. 2 and 3).

Inflammation of the small bronchi and bronchioles is generalized but of varying severity. Since resistance to the flow of air is inversely related to the cube of the radius, this inflammation and edema make the small lumens of an infant particularly vulnerable to obstruction. Plugs of necrotic material and fibrin may completely or partially obstruct the small airways. Smooth muscle constriction does not appear to be important in the obstruction.[22] In areas peripheral to sites of partial obstruction, air becomes trapped by a process similar to a "ball–valve" mechanism. The negative intrapleural pressure during inspiration allows air to flow beyond the point of partial obstruction. However, on expiration, the size of the lumen decreases with the positive pressure, thereby resulting in increased obstruction and hyperinflation. Thus, although airflow is impeded during both inspiration and expiration, the latter is more affected and prolonged. In areas peripheral to complete obstruction, the trapped air eventually becomes absorbed, which results in multiple areas of focal atelectasis. The degree of atelectasis or hy-

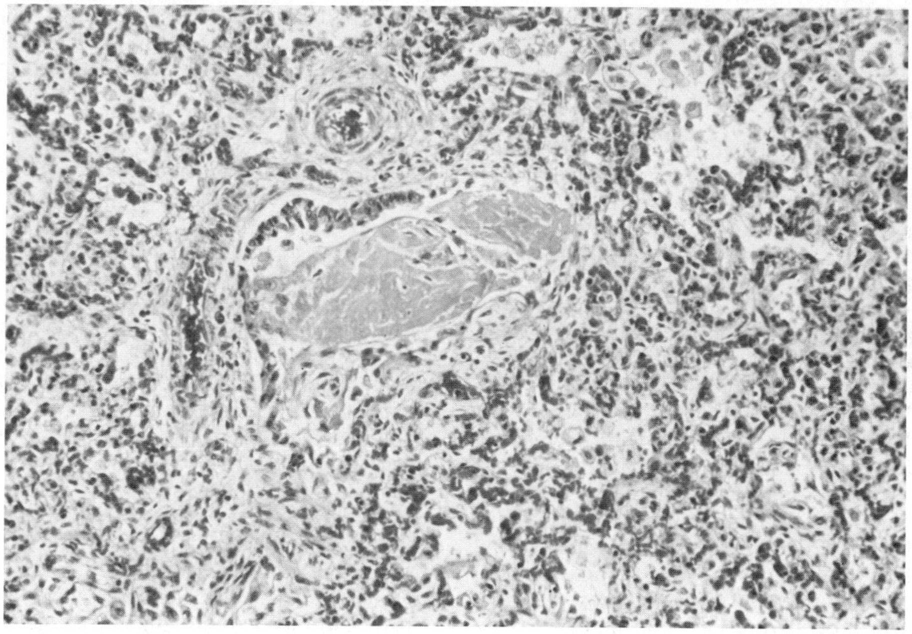

FIG. 2. Inflammation and necrosis in bronchiolitis resulting in obliteration of the bronchiolar lumen.

perinflation that develops is related to the amount of collateral ventilation present.

The physiologic correlates of this resistance to air flow are dyspnea, tachypnea, and a diminished tidal volume. The distribution of ventilation within the infant's lung is also markedly altered. The low ratio of ventilation to perfusion of the lung parenchyma produces arterial hypoxemia. With progression of the disease, hypercarbia ensues. The pathologic process may progress to involve the alveolar walls and spaces and produce an interstitial pneumonitis. Recovery tends to be slow, requiring several weeks.

An abnormal immune response may contribute to the pathogenesis of bronchiolitis and to the subsequent hyperreactivity of the airways that is frequently seen in children who have been hospitalized with bronchiolitis. In infants infected with RSV, specific IgE antibody and histamine have been found to be present in the nasopharyngeal secretions more frequently and in higher titer in those patients whose illness was associated with wheezing.[23,24] Furthermore, the amount of specific IgE antibody and histamine in the secretions correlated with severity of illness as determined by the degree of hypoxia. Infants with RSV-induced wheezing also tended to demonstrate higher degrees of whole blood lymphocyte transformation to RSV.[25] The number of suppressor cells (OKT8 antigen–positive cells) has also been reported to be diminished in convalescing bronchiolitis patients and was associated with higher titers of specific IgE antibody in the secretions.[24] In patients with infection from one of the parainfluenza viruses, similar correlations have been made between illness manifested by wheezing and increased titers of virus-specific IgE antibody in the secretions

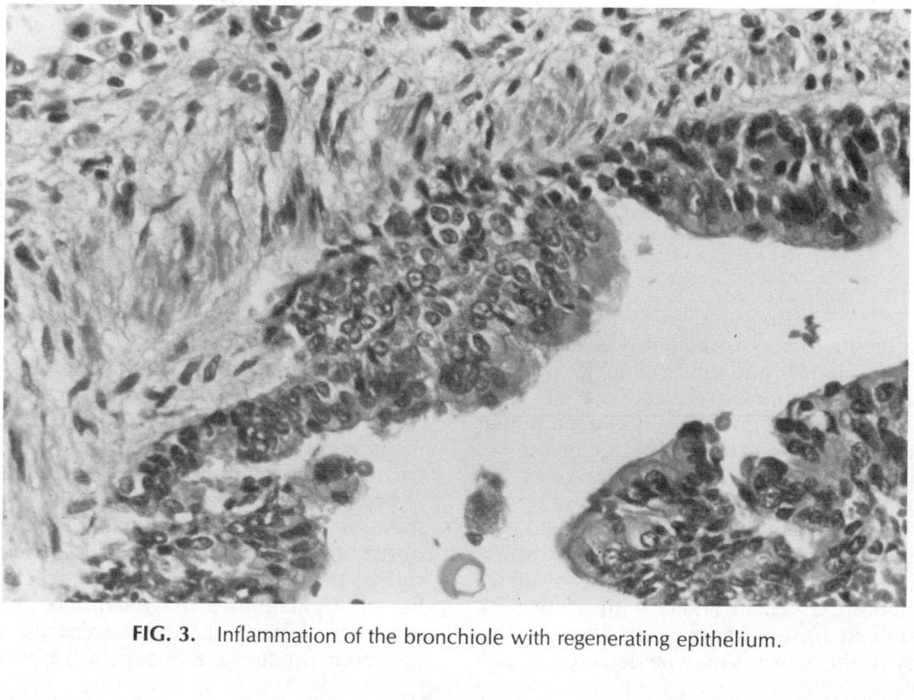

FIG. 3. Inflammation of the bronchiole with regenerating epithelium.

and an increased lymphocyte transformation response to parainfluenza virus.[26]

CLINICAL MANIFESTATIONS

Upper respiratory tract signs, especially coryza and cough, usually herald the onset of bronchiolitis. During a prodromal period of 1–7 days mild fever is common. Lower respiratory tract involvement may appear relatively acute with deepening cough, an increased respiratory rate, and restlessness. With progression, the tachypnea and tachycardia may be marked, although fever may no longer be present. Retractions of the chest wall, flaring of the nasal alae, and grunting are evidence of the increased work of breathing. Cyanosis is rarely evident even though moderate to severe hypoxemia may be present.[22,27] Auscultation, which may vary from hour to hour, reveals wheezing with or without crackles. Increasing dyspnea with decreasing auscultatory findings and movement of air may indicate progressive obstruction and impending respiratory failure.

Dehydration is a common accompaniment of bronchiolitis that results from paroxysms of coughing that may trigger vomiting and from a poor oral intake related to the respiratory distress and lethargy. The tachypnea further increases the fluid requirements. Otitis media, occurring in 10–30 percent of infants, mild conjunctivitis, and occasionally diarrhea may also be present.

For most infants the acute course lasts 3–7 days. Most show improvement within 3–4 days, with a gradual recovery period of 1–2 weeks, but in some it may be prolonged.[27,28]

LABORATORY FINDINGS

The total white blood cell count is usually within the normal range or slightly elevated.[28,29] In hospitalized infants, however, who are more seriously ill and hypoxemic, the white blood cell count may be elevated, and the differential may show a left shift.[27,29] Almost all hospitalized infants with bronchiolitis are hypoxemic, but the degree of hypoxemia is difficult to assess clinically.[27] The degree of wheezing and retractions also cannot be assumed to be indicative of the level of oxygenation. An inverse correlation, however, appears to exist between the respiratory rate and the arterial oxygen saturation.[27,30] Only the most severely ill children develop hypercarbia because most are able to compensate for the increased work of breathing with an elevated respiratory rate.[27,30,31]

The classic findings on chest roentgenogram films are those of hyperinflation, depressed diaphragms, hyperlucency of the parenchyma, and decreased costophrenic angles.[32–35] The bronchovascular markings are usually prominent, with linear densities radiating out from the hila.[36] Multiple areas of atelectasis of varying degrees are also commonly present and difficult to differentiate from the infiltrates of pneumonia. Indeed, both bronchiolitis and pneumonia are frequently present, especially with RSV infection.

DIAGNOSIS

The diagnosis of bronchiolitis is most frequently made on the basis of the characteristic clinical and epidemiologic findings. However, considerable confusion exists over the exact definition of bronchiolitis.[37] A variety of entities may cause a similar picture of dyspnea and wheezing in the infant. Asthma is not easily differentiated, particularly if it is the infant's first episode. Furthermore, the two diseases may be combined. An appreciable proportion of wheezing episodes occurring in a child with an atopic diathesis may arise from viral infections.[38] Respiratory syncytial virus in particular has a propensity to induce wheezing in young children. Even in adults with acute RSV infection clinically manifested as an upper respiratory tract infection, hyperreactivity of the airways may be detected by pulmonary function testing, which lasts for 1 or 2 months.[39] Children who first wheeze during an epidemic of RSV infection may therefore be less likely to have an atopic predisposition than do children who appear to develop bronchiolitis during nonepidemic periods.[40]

Gastric reflux may also produce a picture that is clinically indistinguishable from acute bronchiolitis. Other considerations include obstruction of the airway from a foreign body, vascular rings, retropharyngeal abscess, and even enlarged adenoids. Congestive heart failure may also occasionally cause a similar picture in young infants.

A specific diagnosis of the agent of acute bronchiolitis can be made in an appreciable proportion of infants by viral isolation from respiratory secretions, preferably from a nasal wash.[3,5–10,41] In most cases the viruses associated with bronchiolitis may be identified in tissue culture within 3–7 days. Newer rapid viral diagnostic techniques are available, especially for RSV, that allow identification of the viral antigen in the respiratory secretions within hours to 1 day.[42–44] Serologic determination of the etiologic agent is rarely helpful. Not only does the time required to obtain a convalescent serum preclude its being of help in the clinical management, but also maternally acquired antibody to many of the viral agents of bronchiolitis will be present in these young infants.

THERAPY

Over 2 decades ago Reynolds and Cook[45] noted that "oxygen is vitally important in bronchiolitis, and there is little convincing evidence that any other therapy is consistently or even occasionally useful." Today the mainstay of therapy remains oxygen administration with careful supportive care.[1] Although mist therapy is also commonly employed, its use has not been proved beneficial, and chest physiotherapy has been shown to be of no help.[46]

A variable but sometimes high proportion of infants, especially those with RSV infection, who are admitted to the hospital may require mechanical ventilation,[47,48] which has necessitated high tidal volumes with high peak inspiratory pressures and low respiratory rates to achieve a high minute ventilation.[47] Even though infants with bronchiolitis generally have hyperexpanded lungs, most benefit from positive end-expiratory pressure.

Specific therapy has recently become available for bronchiolitis caused by RSV with ribavirin (1-β-D-ribafuranysol-1,2,4-triazole-3-carboxamide), a synthetic nucleoside.[49] This broad-spectrum antiviral agent has only been approved for infants hospitalized with RSV infections and is administered as a small particle aerosol for 12–18 hours each day, usually for 2–5 days.[50–59] In all of the controlled studies thus far reported, clinical benefit has been demonstrated, with a faster rate of improvement in the severity of illness and the arterial blood gases and with no evidence of toxicity.[49–59] Ribavirin administered via a ventilator, however, requires careful monitoring. The drug can precipitate in the lines of the ventilator, which could cause obstruction of the expiratory valve. The use of one-way valves and filters in the inspiratory and expiratory lines will prevent this potential complication. The aerosolized drug does not appear in these infants to aggravate the wheezing or any airway hyperreactivity as evidenced by the improvement in the arterial blood gases and, second, by serial pulmonary function testing, including carbachol challenge, of RSV-infected volunteers treated with ribavirin or placebo.[60]

Bronchodilator therapy for infants with bronchiolitis is controversial. In most young infants the major cause of the airway obstruction is the inflammation caused by the viral infection rather than smooth muscle contraction.[1,22] Bronchodilators have been administered by a variety of routes and usually have not been successful.[1,61] β-Adrenergic agents in most studies have not produced a beneficial response, as documented by pulmonary function studies,[62–66] and may even produce a detrimental effect.[67]

A few infants, however, may appear to improve with careful bronchodilator therapy.[22,68] A trial of aerosolized or parenteral bronchodilators, therefore, has been recommended by some for those infants who require hospitalization and who may be carefully monitored.[68,69]

Several studies have evaluated the use of steroids in bronchiolitis but have generally not found them to be of benefit.[70–73] The Committee of Drugs of the American Academy of Pediatrics has thus advised against the use of steroids in bronchiolitis. However, a recent study showed a beneficial effect of nebulized beclomethasone dipropionate in infants who, after bronchiolitis, had persistent wheezing.[74] Antibiotics should not be routinely administered to infants with bronchiolitis since bacteria have no role in the etiology. Furthermore, secondary bacterial infection is rarely observed after bronchiolitis.[75]

COMPLICATIONS

With the currently available methods of respiratory support, the mortality from bronchiolitis is very low. The most severe and complicated courses tend to occur in children with underlying conditions such as cardiopulmonary diseases and prematurity.[22,47] Even previously healthy infants, however, tend to have prolonged pulmonary function abnormalities despite clinical improvement.[27,76] Apnea may complicate the course of bronchiolitis, especially in very young infants with RSV infection.[27,77–79]

The long-term effects of bronchiolitis on the immature and developing lung have not been entirely clarified.[22,80] Infants who have been hospitalized with bronchiolitis do, however, appear to be at risk for recurrent wheezing and long-term pulmonary function abnormalities.[81–88] Children who had milder bronchiolitis not requiring hospitalization do not appear to be at the same degree of risk.[81,89] Abnormalities in function of the small airways appear to persist for years but may be clinically silent. The pathogenesis of these long-term effects is not clear. A variety of factors in different studies have been associated with increasing the infant's risk of later pulmonary abnormalities, including passive smoking, lack of breast-feeding, prematurity, crowded homes, and young age at time of the initial respiratory infections.[81,83,84,86–88,90] Controversy exists as to the relative roles of a genetic predisposition toward atopy or hyperreactivity of the lung vs. the direct effect of the virus on the lung during critical stages of development that result in subsequent functional abnormalities.[1,81,90]

BRONCHIOLITIS OBLITERANS

Rarely, a chronic type of bronchiolitis, bronchiolitis obliterans, may develop in infants and young children initially having acute bronchiolitis. This unusual disease appears to develop most commonly after infections with adenovirus, in infants with a certain undefined genetic predisposition, and in bone marrow transplant patients with graft-vs.-host diseases.[22,91–94] The disease has appeared to be particularly prevalent in Indian populations in central Canada and in Polynesians in New Zealand.[91–93] Such infants commonly have bronchopneumonia along with the signs of bronchiolitis that continue for weeks to months with fluctuating severity. Approximately 60 percent of these children develop chronic disease with atelectasis, bronchiectasis, intermittent pneumonia, and hyperinflation. These sequelae are accompanied by severe pathologic abnormalities involving the occlusion and destruction of the bronchi and bronchioles.

REFERENCES

1. Wohl MEB, Chernick V. Bronchiolitis. Am Rev Respir Dis. 1978;118:759–81.
2. Engle S, Newns GH. Proliferative mural bronchiolitis. Arch Dis Child. 1940;15:219–29.
3. Henderson FW, Clyde WA Jr, Collier AM, et al. The etiologic and epidemiologic spectrum of bronchiolitis in pediatric practice. J Pediatr. 1979;95:183–90.
4. Chanock R, Chambon L, Chang W, et al. WHO respiratory disease survey in children. A serologic study. Bull WHO. 1967;37:363–9.
5. Foy HM, Cooney MK, Maletzky AJ, et al. Incidence and etiology of pneumonia, croup and bronchiolitis in preschool children belonging to a prepaid medical care group over a four year period. Am J Epidemiol. 1973;97:80–92.
6. Glezen WP, Loda FA, Clyde WA Jr, et al. Epidemiologic patterns of acute lower respiratory tract disease of children in a pediatric group practice. J Pediatr. 1971;78:397–406.
7. Kim HW, Arrobio JO, Brandt CD, et al. Epidemiology of respiratory syncytial virus infection in Washington, D.C. I. Importance of the virus in different respiratory disease syndromes and temporal distribution of infection. Am J Epidemiol. 1973;98:216–25.
8. Loda FA, Glezen WP, Clyde WA Jr. Respiratory disease in group day care. Pediatrics. 1972;49:428–37.
9. Macasaet FF, Kidd PA, Bolano CR, et al. The etiology of acute respiratory infections. II. The role of viruses and bacteria. J Pediatr. 1968;72:829–39.
10. Gardner PS. How etiologic, pathologic, and clinical diagnosis can be made in a correlated fashion. Pediatr Res. 1977;11:254–61.
11. Chang Tzu-ching, Wang Chih-liang, Han Hsu-lau. Etiologic and clinical investigation of bronchiolitis. Chinese Med J. 1978;4:135–41.
12. Hall CB. Infectious Diseases Newsletter. 1983;31:1 and 1982;29:1.
13. Denny FW, Clyde WA Jr. Acute lower respiratory tract infections in nonhospitalized children. J Pediatr. 1986;108:635–46.
14. Glezen WP. Pathogenesis of bronchiolitis. Epidemiologic considerations. Pediatr Res. 1977;11:239–43.
15. Parrott RH, Kim HW, Arrobio JO, et al. Epidemiology of respiratory syncytial virus infection in Washington, D.C. II. Infection and disease with respect to age, immunologic status, race and sex. Am J Epidemiol. 1973;98:289–300.
16. Denny FW, Collier AM, Henderson FW, et al. The epidemiology of bronchiolitis. Pediatr Res. 1977;11:234–6.
17. Breese BB, Disney FA, Talpey W. The nature of a small pediatric group practice, Part I. Pediatrics. 1966;38:264–77.
18. Kravits H. Sex distribution of hospitalized children with acute respiratory diseases, gastroenteritis and meningitis. Clin Pediatr (Phila). 1965;4:484–91.
19. Aherne W, Bird T, Court SDM, et al. Pathological changes in virus infections of the lower respiratory tract in children. J Clin Pathol. 1970;23:7–18.
20. McLean KH. The pathology of bronchiolitis. A study of its evolution. I. The exudative phase. Aust Ann Med. 1956;5:254.
21. McLean KH. The pathology of bronchiolitis. A study of its evolution. II. The repair phase. Aust Ann Med. 1957;6:29.
22. Wohl MEB. Bronchiolitis. Pediatr Ann. 1986;15:307–13.
23. Welliver RC, Wong DT, Sun M, et al. The development of respiratory syncytial virus specific IgE and the release of histamine in nasopharyngeal secretions after infection. N Engl J Med. 1981;305:841–6.
24. Welliver RC, Kaul TN, Sun M, et al: Defective regulation of immune responses in respiratory syncytial virus infection. J Immunol. 1984;133:1925–30.
25. Welliver RC, Kaul A, Ogra PL. Cell-mediated immune response to respiratory syncytial virus infection: Relationship to the development of reactive airway disease. J Pediatr. 1979;94:370–5.
26. Welliver RC, Wong DT, Sun M, et al. Parainfluenza virus bronchiolitis: Epidemiology and pathogenesis. Am J Dis Child. 1986;14:34–40.
27. Hall CB, Hall WJ, Speers DM. Clinical and physiologic manifestations of bronchiolitis and pneumonia. Am J Dis Child. 1979;133:798–802.
28. Ackerman BD. Acute bronchiolitis: A study of 207 cases. Clin Pediatr (Phila). 1962;1:75–81.
29. Portnoy B, Haynes B, Salvatore MA, et al. The peripheral white blood count in respirovirus infection. J Pediatr. 1966;68:181–8.
30. Reynolds EOR. Arterial blood gas tensions of babies with bronchiolitis. Br Med J. 1963;1:1192–5.
31. Downes JJ, Wood DW, Striker TW, et al. Acute respiratory failure in infants with bronchiolitis. Anesthesiology. 1968;29:426–34.
32. Simpson W, Hacking PM, Court SDM, et al. The radiological findings in respiratory syncytial virus infection in children. Pediatr Radiol. 1974;2:97–100.
33. Simpson W, Hacking PM, Court SDM, et al. The radiological findings in respiratory syncytial virus infection in children. Part II. The correlation of radiological categories with clinical and virological findings. Pediatr Radiol. 1974;2:155–60.
34. Rice RP, Loda F. A roentgenographic analysis of respiratory syncytial virus pneumonia in infants. Radiology. 1966;87:1021–7.
35. Koch DA. Roentgenologic considerations of capillary bronchiolitis. Am J Roentgenol Rad Ther Nucl Med. 1959;82:433–6.
36. Khamapirad T, Glezen WP. Clinical and radiographic assessment of acute lower respiratory tract disease in infants and children. Semin Respir Infect. 1987;2:130–44.
37. McConnochie K. Bronchiolitis: What's in the name? Am J Dis Child. 1983;137:11–3.
38. McIntosh K, Ellis EF, Hoffman LS, et al. The association of viral and bacterial respiratory infections with exacerbations of wheezing in young asthmatic children. J Pediatr. 1973;82:578–90.

39. Hall WJ, Hall CB, Speers DM. Respiratory syncytial virus infections in adults: Clinical, virologic and serial pulmonary function studies. Ann Intern Med. 1978;88:203–5.
40. Polmar SH, Robinson LD Jr, Minnefor AB. Immunoglobulin E in bronchiolitis. Pediatrics. 1972;50:279–84.
41. Hall CB, Douglas RG Jr. Clinically useful method for the isolation of respiratory syncytial virus. J Infect Dis. 1975;131:1–5.
42. Richman D, Schmidt N, Plotkin S, et al: Summary of a workshop on new and useful methods in rapid viral diagnosis. J Infect Dis. 1984;150:941–51.
43. Chonmaitree T, Bessette-Henderson BJ, Hepler RE, et al. Comparison of three rapid diagnostic techniques for detection of respiratory syncytial virus from nasal wash specimens. J Clin Microbiol. 1987;25:746–7.
44. Anestad G, Breivik N, Thoressen T. Rapid diagnosis of RSV and influenza A virus infections by immunofluorescence: Experience with a simplified procedure for the preparation of cell smears from nasopharyngeal secretions. Acta Pathol Microbiol Immunol Scand. 1983;91:267–71.
45. Reynolds EOR, Cook CD. The treatment of bronchiolitis. J Pediatr. 1963;63:1205–7.
46. Webb MSC, Martin GA, Cartlidge PHT, et al. Chest physiotherapy in acute bronchiolitis. Arch Dis Child. 1985;60:1078–9.
47. Frankel LR, Lewiston NJ, Smith DW, et al. Clinical observations on mechanical ventilation for respiratory failure in bronchiolitis. Pediatr Pulmonol. 1986;2:307–11.
48. Outwater KM, Crone RK. Management of respiratory failure in infants with acute viral bronchiolitis. Am J Dis Child. 1984;138:1071–5.
49. Knight V, Gilbert BE. Chemotherapy of respiratory viruses. Adv Intern Med. 1986;31:95–118.
50. Hall CB, McBride JT, Walsh EE, et al. Aerosolized ribavirin treatment of infants with respiratory syncytial virus infection: A randomized double-blind study. N Engl J Med. 1983;308:1443–7.
51. Taber LH, Knight V, Gilbert BE, et al. Ribavirin aerosol treatment of bronchiolitis due to respiratory syncytial virus infection in infants. Pediatrics. 1983;72:613–8.
52. Hall CB, Walsh EE, Hruska JF, et al. Ribavirin aerosol treatment of experimental respiratory syncytial viral infection in young adults: A controlled double-blind study. JAMA. 1983;249:2666–70.
53. Rodriquez WJ, Kim HW, Brandt CD, et al. Aerosolized ribavirin in the treatment of patients with respiratory syncytial virus disease. Pediatr Infect Dis J. 1987;6:159–63.
54. Conrad DA, Christenson JC, Waner JL, et al. Aerosolized ribavirin treatment of respiratory syncytial virus infection in infants hospitalized during an epidemic. Pediatr Infect Dis J. 1987;6:152–8.
55. Caramia G, Palazzini E. Efficacy of ribavirin aerosol treatment for respiratory syncytial virus bronchiolitis in infants. J Int Med Res. 1987;15:227–33.
56. Barry W, Cockburn F, Cornall R, et al. Ribavirin aerosol for acute bronchiolitis. Arch Dis Child. 1986;61:593–4.
57. Frankel LR, Wilson CW, Demers RR, et al. A technique for the administration of ribavirin to mechanically ventilated infants with severe respiratory syncytial virus. Crit Care Med. 1987;15:1051–4.
58. Demers RR, Parker J, Frankel LR, et al. Administration of ribavirin to neonatal and pediatric during mechanical ventilation. Respir Care. 1986;31:1188–96.
59. Outwater KM, Meissner C, Peterson MB. Ribavirin administration to infants receiving mechanical ventilation. Am J Dis Child. 1988;142:512–5.
60. Hall CB, Walsh EE, Hruska JF, et al. Ribavirin treatment of experimental respiratory syncytial virus infection in young adults: A controlled double blind study. JAMA. 1983;249:2666–70.
61. Silverman M. Bronchodilators for wheezy infants? Arch Dis Child. 1984;59:84–7.
62. Phelan PD, Williams HE. Sympathomimetic drugs in acute viral bronchiolitis. Their effect on pulmonary resistance. Pediatrics. 1969;44:493–7.
63. Rutter N, Milner AD, Hiller EJ. Effect of bronchodilators on respiratory resistance in infants and young children with bronchiolitis and wheezy bronchitis. Arch Dis Child. 1975;50:719–22.
64. Henry RL, Milner AD, Stokes GM. Ineffectiveness of ipratropium bromide in acute bronchiolitis. Arch Dis Child. 1983;58:925–6.
65. Lenney W, Milner AD. Alpha and beta adrenergic stimulants in bronchiolitis and wheezy bronchitis in children under 18 months of age. Arch Dis Child. 1978;53:707–9.
66. Radford M. Effect of salbutamol in infants with wheezy bronchitis. Arch Dis Child. 1975;50:535–8.
67. Hughes DM, Lesouef PN, Landau LI. Effect of salbutamol on respiratory mechanics in bronchiolitis. Pediatr Res. 1987;22:83–6.
68. Soto M, Sly PD, Uren E, et al. Bronchodilator response in acute viral bronchiolitis. Pediatr Pulmonol. 1985;2:85–90.
69. Ellis EF. Therapy of acute bronchiolitis. Pediatr Res. 1977;11:263–4.
70. Stecenko MA. Treatment of viral bronchiolitis: Do steroids make sense? Contemp Pediatr 1987;April:121–30.
71. Connolly JH, Field CMB, Glasgow JFT, et al. A double blind trial of prednisolone in epidemic bronchiolitis due to respiratory syncytial virus. Acta Paediatr Scand 1969;58:116.
72. Leer JA, Green JL, Heimlich EM, et al. Corticosteroid treatment in bronchiolitis. A controlled collaborative study in 297 infants and children. Am J Dis Child. 1969;117:495–503.
73. Yaffe SJ, Weiss CF, Cann HM, et al. Should steroids be used in treating bronchiolitis? Pediatrics. 1970;46:640–642.
74. Maayan C, Itzhaki T, Bar-Yishay E, et al. The functional response of infants with persistent wheezing to nebulized beclamethasone dipropionate. Pediatr Pulmonol. 1986;2:9–14.
75. Hall CB, Powell KR, Schnabel KC, et al. The risk of secondary bacterial infection in infants hospitalized with respiratory syncytial viral infection. J Pediatr. 1988;113:266–71.
76. Wohl MEB, Stigol LC, Mead J. Resistance of the total respiratory system in healthy infants and infants with bronchiolitis. Pediatrics. 1969;43:495–509.
77. Bruhn FW, Mokrohisky ST, McIntosh K. Apnea associated with respiratory syncytial virus infection in young infants. J Pediatr. 1977;90:382–6.
78. Anas N, Boettrich C, Hall CB, et al. The association of apnea and respiratory syncytial virus in infants. J Pediatr. 1982;101:65–8.
79. Church NR, Anas NG, Hall CB, et al. Respiratory syncytial virus related apnea in infants: Demographics and outcome. Am J Dis Child. 1984;138:247–50.
80. Workshop on bronchiolitis, sponsored by the National Heart, Blood and Lung Institute Division of Lung Diseases, National Institutes of Health. Pediatr Res. 1977;11:209–70.
81. Twiggs JT, Larson LA, O'Connell EJ, et al. Respiratory syncytial virus infection: Ten-year follow up. Clin Pediatr (Phila). 1981;20:187–90.
82. Kattan M, Keens TG, Lapierre JG, et al. Pulmonary function abnormalities in symptom free children after bronchiolitis. Pediatrics. 1977;59:683–8.
83. Sims DG, Gardner PS, Weightman D, et al. Atopy does not predispose to RSV bronchiolitis or postbronchiolitic wheezing. Br Med J. 1981;282:2086–8.
84. McConnochie KM, Roughman KJ. Bronchiolitis as a possible cause of wheezing in childhood: New evidence. Pediatrics. 1984;74:1–10.
85. Duiverman EJ, Neijens HJ, van Strik R, et al. Lung function and bronchial responsiveness in children who had infantile bronchiolitis. Pediatr Pulmonol. 1987;3:38–44.
86. Hall CB, Hall WJ, Gala CL, et al. A long term prospective study of children following respiratory syncytial virus infection. J Pediatr. 1984;105:358–64.
87. Carlsen KH, Larsen S, Bjerve O, et al. Acute bronchiolitis: Predisposing factors and characterization of infants at risk. Pediatr Pulmonol. 1987;3:153–60.
88. Webb MSC, Henry RL, Milner AD, et al. Continuing respiratory problems three and a half years after acute viral bronchiolitis. Arch Dis Child. 1985;60:1064–7.
89. McConnochie KM, Mark JD, McBride JT, et al. Normal pulmonary function measurements and airway reactivity in childhood after mild bronchiolitis. J Pediatr. 1985;107:54–8.
90. McConnochie KM, Roughman KJ. Breast feeding and maternal smoking as predictors of wheezing in children age 6 to 10 years. Pediatr Pulmonol. 1986;2:260–7.
91. Lang WR, Howden CW, Lars J, et al. Bronchopneumonia with serious sequelae in children with evidence of adenovirus type 21 infections. Br Med J. 1969;1:73–9.
92. Chernick V, Macpherson RI. Respiratory syncytial and adenovirus infections of the lower respiratory tract in infancy. Clin Notes Respir Dis. 1971;10:3.
93. Gold R, Wilt JC, Adhikari PK, et al. Adenoviral pneumonia and its complications in infancy and childhood. J Can Assoc Radiol. 1969;20:218–24.
94. Ralph DD, Springmeyer SC, Sullivan KM, et al: Rapidly progressive airflow obstruction in marrow transplant recipients. Am Rev Respir Dis. 1984;129:641–4.

53. ACUTE PNEUMONIA

GERALD R. DONOWITZ
GERALD L. MANDELL

In 1901, Sir William Osler noted in the fourth edition of his book *The Principles and Practice of Medicine* that "the most widespread and fatal of all acute diseases, pneumonia, is now Captain of the Men of Death."[1] Almost 90 years later, the prominence of pneumonia as a clinical entity remains. It is the sixth most common cause of death in the United States and the most common cause of infection-related mortality.[2] The challenge confronting most clinicians is not in detecting the presence of the disease but rather in identifying its etiology. Since a wide array of microbial agents may cause acute pneumonia (Table 1), and since no single antimicrobial regimen can be expected to cover all the possibilities, specific diagnosis remains a prerequisite for proper therapy. To this end, the pathogenesis of the disease should be understood and information from the his-

TABLE 1. Etiologic Agents of Acute Pneumonia

- Bacterial
  - Common
    - *Streptococcus pneumoniae*
    - *Staphylococcus aureus*
    - *Haemophilus influenzae*
    - Mixed anaerobic bacteria (aspiration)
      - *Bacteroides* spp.
      - *Fusobacterium* spp.
      - *Peptostreptococcus* spp.
      - *Peptococcus* spp.
    - Enterobacteriaceae
      - *Escherichia coli*
      - *Klebsiella pneumoniae*
      - *Enterobacter* spp.
      - *Serratia* spp.
    - *Pseudomonas aeruginosa*
    - *Legionella* spp. (including *L. pneumophila* and *L. micdadei*)
  - Uncommon
    - *Acinetobacter* var. *anitratus*
    - *Actinomyces* and *Arachnia* spp.
    - *Aeromonas hydrophilia*
    - *Bacillus* spp.
    - *Branhamella catarrhalis*
    - *Campylobacter fetus*
    - *Eikenella corrodens*
    - *Francisella tularensis*
    - *Neisseria meningitidis*
    - *Nocardia* spp.
    - *Pasteurella multocida*
    - *Proteus* spp.
    - *Pseudomonas pseudomallei*
    - *Salmonella* spp.
    - *Enterococcus faecalis*
    - *Streptococcus pyogenes*
    - *Yersinia pestis*
- Viral
  - Children
    - Common
      - Respiratory syncytial virus
      - Parainfluenza virus types 1, 2, 3
      - Influenza A virus
    - Uncommon
      - Adenovirus types 1, 2, 3, 5
      - Influenza B virus
      - Rhinovirus
      - Coxsackievirus
      - Echovirus
      - Measles virus
  - Adults
    - Common
      - Influenza A virus
      - Influenza B virus
      - Adenovirus types 4 and 7 (in military recruits)
    - Uncommon
      - Rhinovirus
      - Adenovirus types 1, 2, 3, 5
      - Enteroviruses
        - Echovirus
        - Coxsackievirus
        - Poliovirus
      - Epstein-Barr virus
      - Cytomegalovirus
      - Respiratory syncytial virus
      - Varicella-zoster virus
      - Parainfluenza virus
      - Measles virus
      - Herpes simplex virus
- Fungal
  - *Aspergillus* spp.
  - *Candida* spp.
  - *Coccidioides immitis*
  - *Cryptococcus neoformans*
  - *Histoplasma capsulatum*
  - Agents of mucormycosis
    - *Rhizopus* spp.
    - *Absidia* spp.
    - *Mucor* spp.
- Rickettsial
  - *Coxiella burnetii*
  - *Rickettsia rickettsiae*
- Bacteria-like agents
  - *Mycoplasma pneumoniae*
  - *Chlamydia* spp.
    - *C. psittaci*
    - *C. trachomatis*
    - TWAR
- Mycobacterial
  - *Mycobacterium tuberculosis*
- Parasitic
  - *Ascaris lumbricoides*
  - *Pneumocystis carinii*
  - *Strongyloides stercoralis*
  - *Toxoplasma gondii*
  - *Paragonimus westermani*

tory and physical examination, as well as from the microbiology laboratory, must be used.

PATHOGENESIS

In the absence of disease, normal pulmonary defense mechanisms maintain essentially sterile infralaryngeal airways and parenchyma. The development of acute pulmonary infection indicates either a defect in host defenses, challenge by a particularly virulent microorganism, or an overwhelming inoculum. Infectious agents gain entry to the lower respiratory tract through inhalation of aerosolized material or aspiration of upper airway resident flora. Less frequently, pneumonia results from metastatic seeding of the lungs from the blood stream.

Lung defense mechanisms important in the prevention of infection include (*1*) filtration and humidification of inspired air in the upper airways, (*2*) intact epiglottic and cough reflexes, (*3*) tracheobronchial secretions (the mucous blanket) and mucociliary transport via the ciliated epithelium, (*4*) cell-mediated immunity (alveolar macrophages, T lymphocytes), (*5*) humoral immunity (B lymphocytes, immunoglobulin, complement), and (*6*) polymorphonuclear neutrophils.[3,4]

A number of factors are known to interfere with normal host defenses and to predispose to infection.[3] Alterations in the level of consciousness from any cause (stroke, seizures, drug intoxication, anesthesia, alcohol abuse, and even normal sleep) can compromise epiglottic closure and lead to aspiration of oropharyngeal flora into the lower respiratory tract.[5,6] Cigarette smoke, perhaps the most common agent involved in compromising natural pulmonary defense mechanisms, disrupts both mucociliary function and macrophage activity.[7] Other factors that impair pulmonary clearance of pathogens include hypoxemia,[8] acidosis, alcohol,[9] toxic inhalations,[10,11] pulmonary edema,[12] uremia, malnutrition, corticosteroids,[9] immunosuppressive agents,[13] viral infection,[14] and mechanical obstruction.[4]

Recurrent episodes of bacterial pneumonia suggest the presence of specific predisposing factors,[15,16] which have been categorized by Roth and Gleckman according to the age of the patient.[16] In children and young adults, recurrent pneumonias are associated with congenital defects in host defenses, including leukocyte function[17] and immunoglobulins.[17–20] Congenital defects in cilia activity including the immotile-cilia syndrome,[21] Kartagener syndrome[22] (ciliary dysfunction, situs inversus, sinusitis, bronchiectasis), Young syndrome (azospermia, sinusitis, pneumonia),[23] and cystic fibrosis are other clinical entities associated with recurrent pneumonia in the young. Structural lung abnormalities such as bronchiectasis and pulmonary sequestration[24] are also important predisposing factors for both younger and older patient populations.

In adults, factors predisposing to recurrent pneumonia include acquired defects in host defenses (chronic lymphocytic leukemia, myeloma, hypogammaglobulinemia, the acquired immunodeficiency syndrome [AIDS]), bronchial obstruction due to intrinsic compression (adenomas, carcinomas) or extrinsic compression (lymph node enlargement due to sarcoid or malignancy), and esophageal abnormalities (reflux, stricture).[25] Episodes of altered mental states due to alcohol, trauma, or neurologic disorders are also important factors predisposing to recurrent pneumonia.

CLINICAL EVALUATION

History

The history should attempt to define (*1*) the clinical setting in which the pneumonia is taking place, (*2*) defects in host resistance that could predispose to the development of pneumonia, and (*3*) possible exposure to specific pathogens. Although age and race are usually of little diagnostic value, it should be remembered that mycoplasma pneumonia occurs more often in younger people,[26,27] that gram-negative pneumonia tends to occur in the elderly,[28] and that tuberculosis appears to be more prevalent in nonwhite populations.[29]

Pneumonia has been noted to occur with increased frequency in patients with a variety of underlying disorders such as congestive heart failure, diabetes, alcoholism, and chronic obstructive pulmonary disease.[28,30,31] In one series of 292 patients with pneumonia, only 18 percent were found to have no underlying disease.[28] A history of upper respiratory tract infection has been elicited in 36–50 percent of patients with acute pneumonia, especially in those with pneumococcal disease.[30,32] Recent dental manipulations, sedative overdoses, seizures, alcoholism, or loss of consciousness for any reason should raise the suspicion of anaerobic infection due to aspiration of oral contents.[5]

Specific etiologic agents of pneumonia have been associated with certain underlying diseases. An increased incidence of staphylococcal pneumonia has been noted during epidemics of influenza.[33] Patients with chronic obstructive pulmonary disease are frequently colonized with *Streptococcus pneumoniae* and *Haemophilus influenzae* and are at increased risk for the development of pneumonia caused by these agents.[34] Cystic fibrosis is associated with pseudomonas and staphylococcal pulmonary infection.[35] Pulmonary alveolar proteinosis has been associated with *Nocardia* infection.[36] Patients with AIDS are at high risk for the development of pneumonia caused by *Pneumocystis carinii,* cytomegalovirus, and mycobacteria, as well as more common pulmonary pathogens.[37–39] Pneumonia developing in hospitalized patients often involves enteric gram-negative bacilli, *Pseudomonas aeruginosa,* and *Staphylococcus aureus,* agents that are unusual in nonhospitalized populations.[40] Similarly, pneumonia in the elderly, especially those living in nursing homes or extended care facilities, is more often associated with gram-negative bacilli than is pneumonia in younger populations.[40–42]

Occupational history, history of exposure to animals, travel history, and sexual history are all important in suggesting specific potential infectious agents (Table 2). The presence of noninfectious pulmonary disease such as tumors or pulmonary emboli, which may masquerade as pneumonia, may also be suggested by a careful history.

Physical Examination

Fever is usually present and may be sustained, remittent, or at times hectic. Fever patterns per se, however, are not useful for establishing a specific diagnosis. The temperature should be taken rectally to reduce error due to rapid mouth breathing. Recording of postural changes in blood pressure and pulse rate is useful in assessing hydration and intravascular fluid volume. The pulse usually increases by 10 beats/min for every degree (C) of temperature elevation. A pulse temperature deficit (i.e., a relative bradycardia for the amount of fever) should suggest viral infection, mycoplasmal infection, chlamydial infection, tularemia, or infection with *Legionella* spp. Cyanosis, rapid respiratory rate, the use of accessory muscles of respiration, sternal retraction, and nasal flaring suggest serious respiratory compromise.

Furuncles are rarely secondary to staphylococcal pneumonia acquired by the respiratory route but may signal a source of bacteremia with subsequent hematogenous pneumonia. Herpes labialis is seen in up to 40 percent of the patients with pneumococcal pneumonia.[43] Bullous myringitis is an infrequent although significant finding in mycoplasmal pneumonia.[27] The presence of poor dentition should suggest a mixed infection due to aspiration of anaerobes and aerobes that colonize the oropharynx. While edentulous people may develop anaerobic pneumonia due to aspiration, it is uncommon.[44]

Examination of the thorax may reveal "splinting" or an inspiratory lag on the side of the lesion that is suggestive of bacterial pneumonia. Early in the disease process, definite signs of pulmonary involvement may be lacking or may be manifest only as fine, crackling rales. Chest examination may reveal these early signs of pneumonia even though the chest film is normal. Evidence of consolidation (dullness on percussion, bronchial breath sounds, and E to A changes) is highly suggestive of bacterial infection. Patients with mycoplasmal or viral infection may exhibit few abnormalities on physical examination despite the presence of impressive infiltrates on the chest film.

TABLE 2. Important Environmental Factors in Pneumonia

Pneumonia Associated with	*Environmental History*
Anthrax	Exposure to cattle, swine, horses, goat hair, wool, hides
Brucellosis	Exposure to cattle, goats, pigs; employment as abattoir worker or veterinarian
Melioidosis	Travel to W. Indies, Australia, Guam, S.E. Asia, South and Central America
Plague	Exposure to ground squirrels, chipmunks, rabbits, prairie dogs, rats
Tularemia	Exposure to tissue or body fluids of infected animals (rabbits, hares, foxes, squirrels) or to bites of an infected arthropod (flies, ticks) Handling or ingesting poorly cooked meat from an infected animal
Psittacosis	Exposure to birds (parrots, budgerigars, cockatoos, pigeons, turkeys)
Leptospirosis	Exposure to wild rodents, dogs, cats, pigs, cattle, horses, or exposure to water contaminated with animal urine
Coccidioidomycosis	Travel to San Joaquin Valley, S. California, S.W. Texas, S. Arizona, New Mexico
Histoplasmosis	Exposure to bat droppings or dust from soil enriched with bird droppings
Q fever	Exposure to infected goats, cattle, sheep and their secretions (milk, amniotic fluid, placenta, feces)
Legionnaires' disease	Exposure to contaminated aerosols (e.g., air coolers, hospital water supply)

SPUTUM EXAMINATION

Microscopic examination and culture of expectorated sputum remain the mainstays of the laboratory evaluation of pneumonia despite ongoing controversy concerning their sensitivity and specificity.[45–48] Procurement of expectorated sputum is a noninvasive technique that can be carried out at no risk to the patient, provides samples of lower respiratory tract secretions for immediate evaluation, and in the majority of cases allows the clinician to make a presumptive diagnosis.

Examination of the sputum should include observation of the color, amount, consistency, and odor of the specimen. Mucopurulent sputum is most commonly found with bacterial pneumonia or bronchitis. Sputum of similar nature has been described in one-third to one-half of patients with mycoplasma[27] or adenovirus infections.[49,50] However, scant or watery sputum is more often noted with these and other atypical pneumonias. "Rusty" sputum suggests alveolar involvement and has been most commonly (although not solely) associated with pneumococcal pneumonia.[51] Dark red, mucoid sputum (currant-jelly sputum) suggests Friedlander's pneumonia caused by encapsulated *Klebsiella pneumoniae*.[52] Foul-smelling sputum is associated with mixed anaerobic infections most commonly seen with aspiration.[44]

Where possible, frankly purulent material should be selected for microscopic examination. In all cases of acute pneumonia, a Gram stain of the sputum should be prepared. In order to maximize the diagnostic yield of the sputum examination, only samples free of oropharyngeal contamination should be reviewed. As a guide, the number of neutrophils and epithelial cells should be quantitated under low power (100×), with further examination reserved for samples containing ≥25 neutrophils and ≤10 epithelial cells. Such samples contain minimal oropharyngeal contamination.[53] Samples with more epithelial cells and fewer neutrophils are nondiagnostic and should be discarded. The morphologic and staining characteristics of any bacteria seen should be recorded and an estimate made of the predominant organisms (Figs. 1–4). Where no bacterial predominance exists, this should be noted as well.

In the appropriate clinical setting, a predominance of gram-positive, lancet-shaped diplococci should suggest pneumococ-

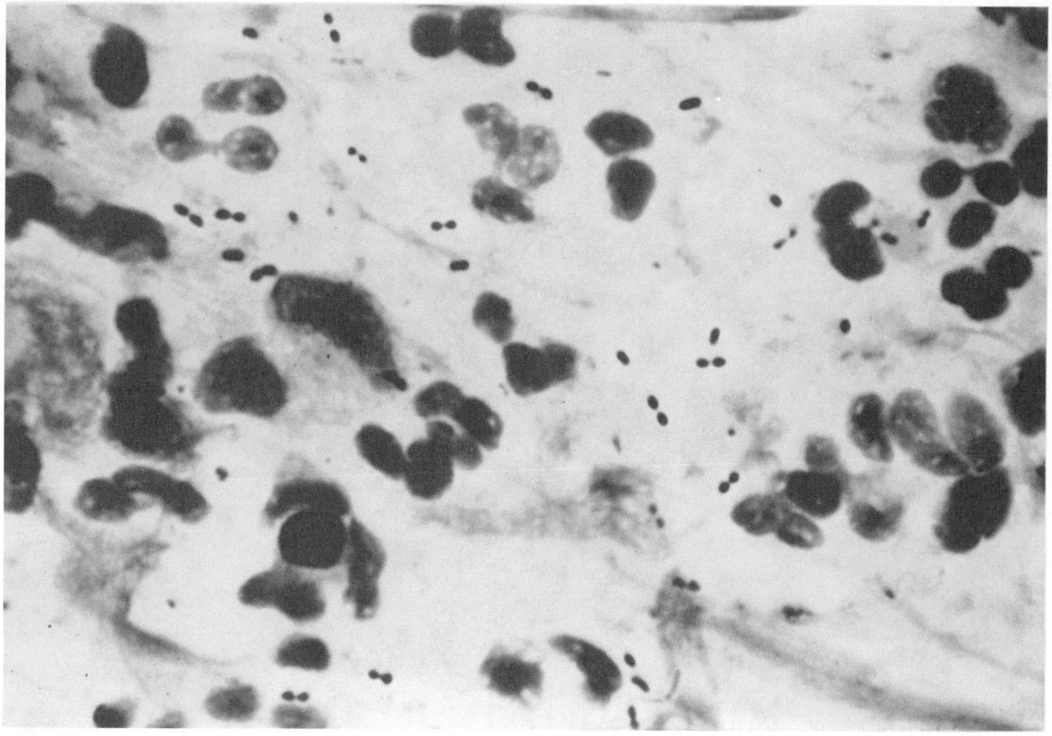

FIG. 1. Expectorated sputum with gram-positive, lancet-shaped diplococci from a patient with pneumococcal pneumonia.

cal infection (Fig. 1). When strict criteria for Gram stain positivity are used (predominant flora and/or more than 10 gram-positive, lancet-shaped diplococci per oil immersion field [100×]), the specificity of the Gram stain for identifying pneumococci has been shown to be 85 percent, with a sensitivity of 62 percent.[54] The diagnostic yield of the sputum examination for pneumococci can be maximized by the use of the quellung reaction. Anticapsular antiserum reacts with capsular polysaccharide, and this may be seen as a distinctly outlined capsule. Rare false-positive results may occur with α-hemolytic streptococci. Occasional false-negative results may occur as well. An 89 percent correlation between pneumococcal isolation by culture and a positive sputum quellung test has been demonstrated.[46]

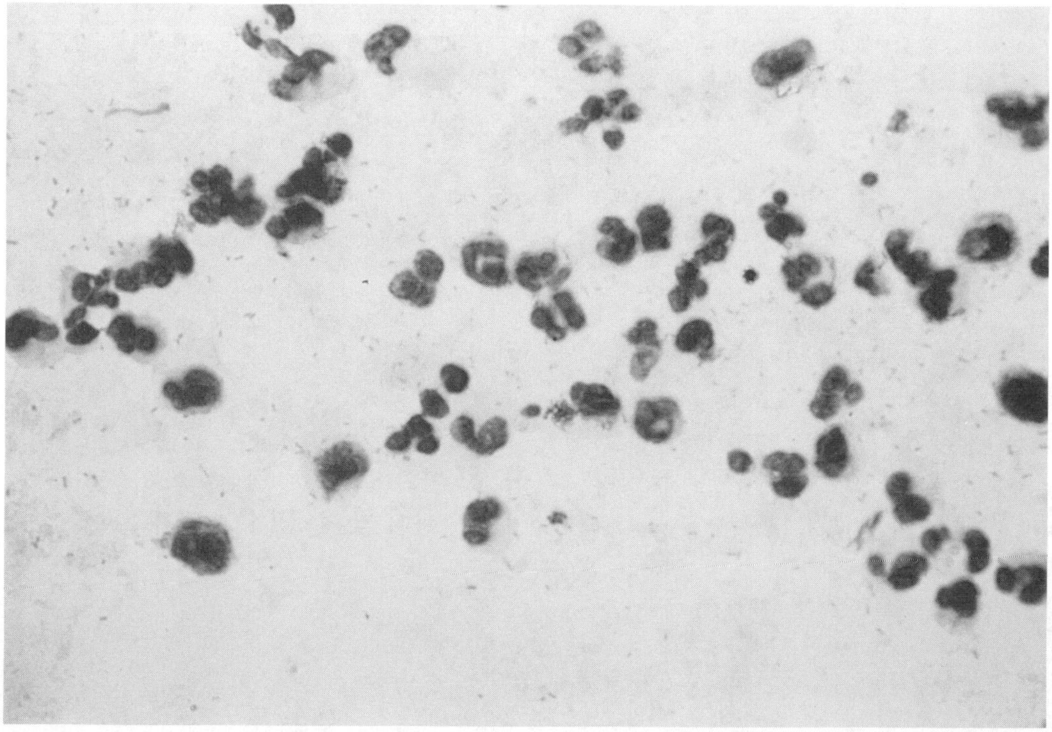

FIG. 2. Expectorated sputum with gram-negative coccobacillary forms from a patient with *Haemophilus influenzae* pneumonia.

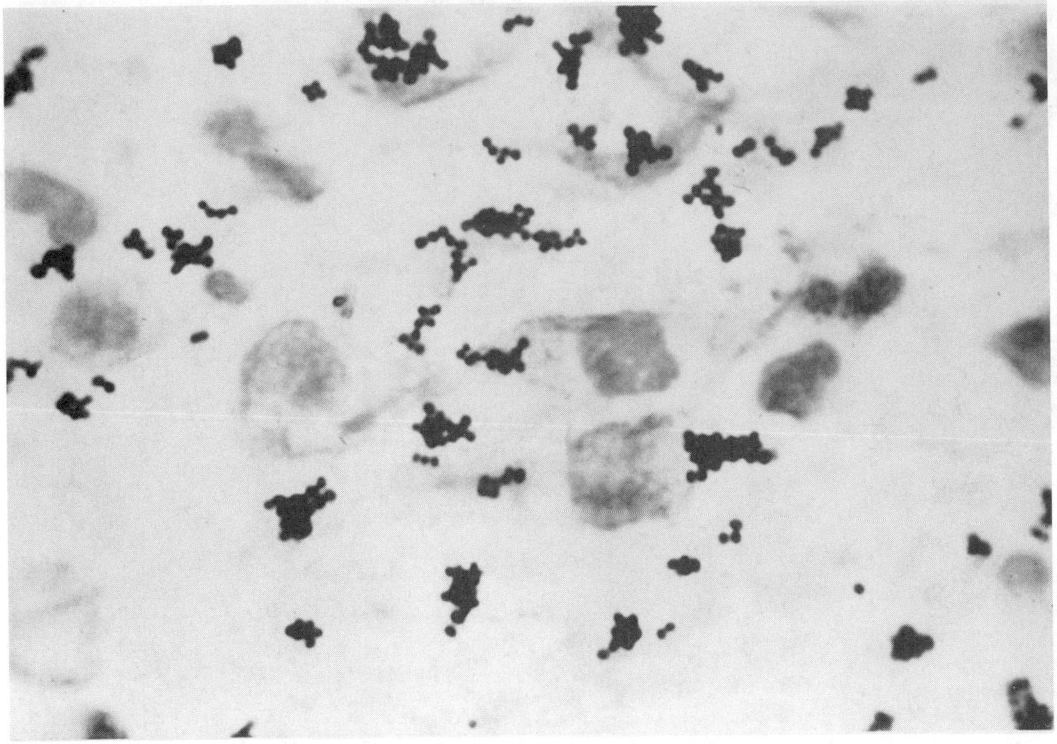

FIG. 3. Expectorated sputum with gram-positive cocci in clumps from a patient with staphylococcal pneumonia.

Since pneumococci may be part of the nasopharyngeal flora in up to 50 percent of healthy adults and may colonize the lower airways in patients with chronic bronchitis, identification of the organism does not always mean that it is the cause of disease.[55–57] However, it is our belief that the large number of pneumococci necessary to produce a positive Gram stain or quellung reaction is unusual in carriers.

The sputum Gram stain is helpful to identify organisms other than the pneumococcus. Small gram-negative coccobacillary organisms are characteristic of *H. influenzae* (Fig. 2). Staphylococci appear as gram-positive cocci in tetrads and grapelike clusters (Fig. 3). Organisms of mixed morphology are characteristic of anaerobic infection. Few bacteria are seen with legionnaires' disease, mycoplasma pneumonia, and viral pneumonia. Sputum examination has been a useful means of diagnosing *P. carinii* pneumonia in patients with AIDS. Use of

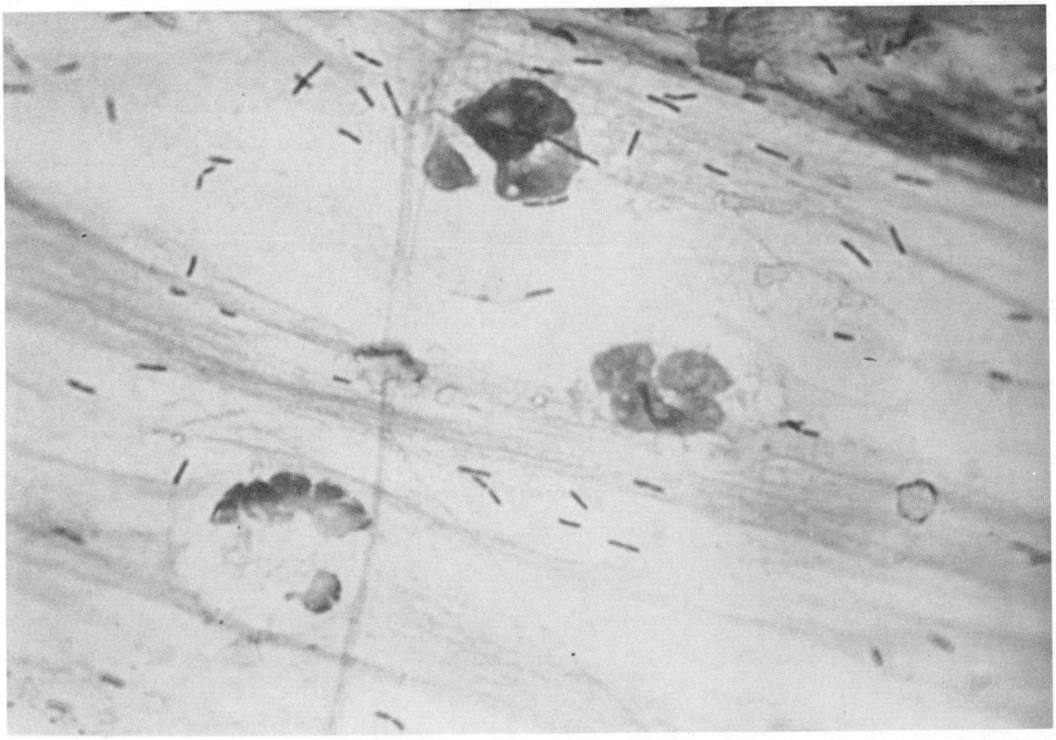

FIG. 4. Expectorated sputum with gram-negative rods in a patient with *Escherichia coli* pneumonia.

the Giemsa or Gomori methanamine silver stain has led to a diagnosis in over 50 percent of cases, making more aggressive diagnostic procedures unnecessary.[58,59]

A variety of diagnostic techniques have been recently introduced that provide the potential for more accurate and rapid identification of the etiologic agents of pneumonia. Nucleic acid hybridization techniques have been used to detect herpes simplex virus, cytomegalovirus, mycoplasma, *Legionella* spp., *Mycobacterium tuberculosis,* and nontuberculosis mycobacterium. Monoclonal antibodies in the immunofluorescence assay and the enzyme-linked immunosorbent assay (ELISA) have been used to rapidly detect a variety of viruses and *Legionella* spp. in respiratory secretions.[60–62] While many of these techniques are of great interest, their general applicability has yet to be determined.

The utility of the sputum culture as a means of diagnosing pneumonia has been questioned. Patients with bacteremic pneumococcal pneumonia have been reported to have negative sputum cultures in 45–50 percent of cases, even when large numbers of organisms have been noted on Gram stain.[63,64] Similarly, 34–47 percent of sputum cultures are negative with proven *H. influenzae* pneumonia.[65,66] Further, sputum cultures have frequently been shown to yield more bacterial species than more invasive methods of obtaining respiratory tract secretions.[67,68] Contamination with gram-negative bacilli from the oropharynx has been noted in 32 percent of sputum cultures.[69]

Several key parameters have been identified in efforts to maximize the diagnostic yield from sputum culture. Procurement of adequate sputum samples is an essential first step. Where fewer than 10 epithelial cells and more than 25 neutrophils per low-power field are noted, oropharyngeal contamination is minimal and sputum samples are comparable to transtracheal aspirates in terms of the number of bacterial species isolated.[53] With increasing numbers of epithelial cells and decreasing numbers of neutrophils, an increased amount of oropharyngeal contamination is present, as indicated by the isolation of more bacterial species.

The presence of alveolar macrophages does not alter the bacteriologic findings when substantial numbers of epithelial cells are present, indicating that otherwise adequate samples of sputum can be contaminated with oropharyngeal contents and thereby rendered nondiagnostic. This type of initial screening has proven helpful in differentiating adequate sputum samples from saliva, thereby increasing the diagnostic yield of sputum culture.

When culture of sputum is delayed, isolation of pneumococci is less likely due to overgrowth of the organism by oropharyngeal flora. Rapid processing of samples is therefore another important factor leading to higher diagnostic yields.

Laboratory techniques for maximizing the useful information from sputum cultures have included quantitative cultures, washing of samples to remove contaminating mouth flora, and the use of mucolytic agents. The varying results noted have not warranted the increased efforts required. Further, washing samples does not guarantee that adequate samples of lower respiratory tract secretions are present.[70] Some reports suggest that with adequate sputum samples and prompt culture of specimens, the diagnostic yield of the sputum culture may approach 100 percent.[45,71,72]

TRANSTRACHEAL ASPIRATION

Although the sputum examination should always be included in the initial evaluation of patients with pneumonia, it may be inadequate for a presumptive diagnosis. In cases in which either (*1*) no sputum is produced, (*2*) no clear predominance of a potential pathogen exists on sputum Gram stain or culture, (*3*) there has been a poor response to antibiotics chosen on the basis of expectorated sputum, (*4*) gram-negative rods or yeast forms are found in the sputum, or (*5*) the possibility of superinfection exists, a more direct method of obtaining lower respiratory tract secretions may be necessary. Transtracheal aspiration should be considered, although this is a potentially dangerous procedure and is now uncommonly performed in patients with acute pneumonia.

Comparative studies have shown that less oropharyngeal contamination occurs in sputum obtained by transtracheal aspiration as compared with expectorated sputum.[67,69,73,74] In patients with chronic obstructive pulmonary disease, fewer yeast forms and fewer species of bacteria (especially anaerobes) were noted in cultures of transtracheal aspirates as compared with cultures of aspirates from fiberoptic bronchoscopy.[75] Furthermore, if anaerobes are to be isolated from the lower respiratory tract, the oropharynx, with its abundant resident flora of anaerobes, must be bypassed.[76] Several authors have reported the clinical usefulness of transtracheal aspiration in defining the etiology of acute bacterial pneumonia.[68,74,77]

False-negative results of cultures of transtracheal aspirate have been reported in 11 percent of samples. Theoretically, false-negative transtracheal aspirates can occur if infection involves the periphery of the lung only or if the involved bronchi are obstructed. In practice, false-negative aspirates seem to be most common in patients treated with antibiotics before the procedure. A false-positive rate of approximately 21 percent has been noted and is thought to be due to oropharyngeal contamination or tracheobronchial colonization, especially in patients with chronic lung disease.[77]

Transtracheal aspiration is carried out by having the patient lie with a pillow under the shoulders so that the neck is hyperextended. The cricothyroid membrane at the base of the thyroid cartilage is located, and the area is prepared and draped (Fig. 5A). After local anesthesia is applied to the skin over the cricothyroid membrane, a large-bore needle containing a 17- or 18-gauge indwelling catheter is inserted through the cricothyroid space in the midline with the needles angled downward toward the coccyx (Fig. 5B). After the trachea has been entered (Fig. 5C), the catheter is advanced several inches and the needle is removed, leaving the catheter in place. With a syringe attached to the catheter, the sputum is aspirated (Fig. 5D). If no material is obtained, 2–3 ml of sterile saline (without antibacterial additives) is injected and aspiration is again attempted. Once the material is obtained, the catheter is removed and firm pressure is applied to the puncture site. Material obtained from transtracheal aspiration should be Gram stained and cultured anaerobically and aerobically.

Transtracheal aspiration is not without risk. Significant hemoptysis,[69,74,78] subcutaneous and mediastinal emphysema,[69,74] aspiration of oral contents,[79] soft tissue infection,[80,81] and pneumothoraces[82] have occurred in association with the procedure. Bradycardia, thought to be due to stimulation of the vagus nerve in the presence of hypoxia and hypercapnia, has been observed and has been associated with cardiorespiratory arrest.[79] Coagulation abnormalities (especially thrombocytopenia) and significant hypoxemia or hypercapnia should be contraindications for the procedure. Patients who are coughing violently are probably at greater risk for mediastinal emphysema. In patients who cannot cooperate, the procedure should be carried out with great care, if at all.

FIBEROPTIC BRONCHOSCOPY

Initial studies concerning the usefulness of fiberoptic bronchoscopy for the diagnosis of bacterial pneumonia demonstrated that the procedure was limited by contamination of specimens by oropharyngeal flora. Cultures obtained via the bronchoscope averaged two to three more bacterial isolates than samples from paired transtracheal aspirates.[75] In patients without lower respiratory tract infections, cultures of aspirates obtained at bronchoscopy produced an average of five different

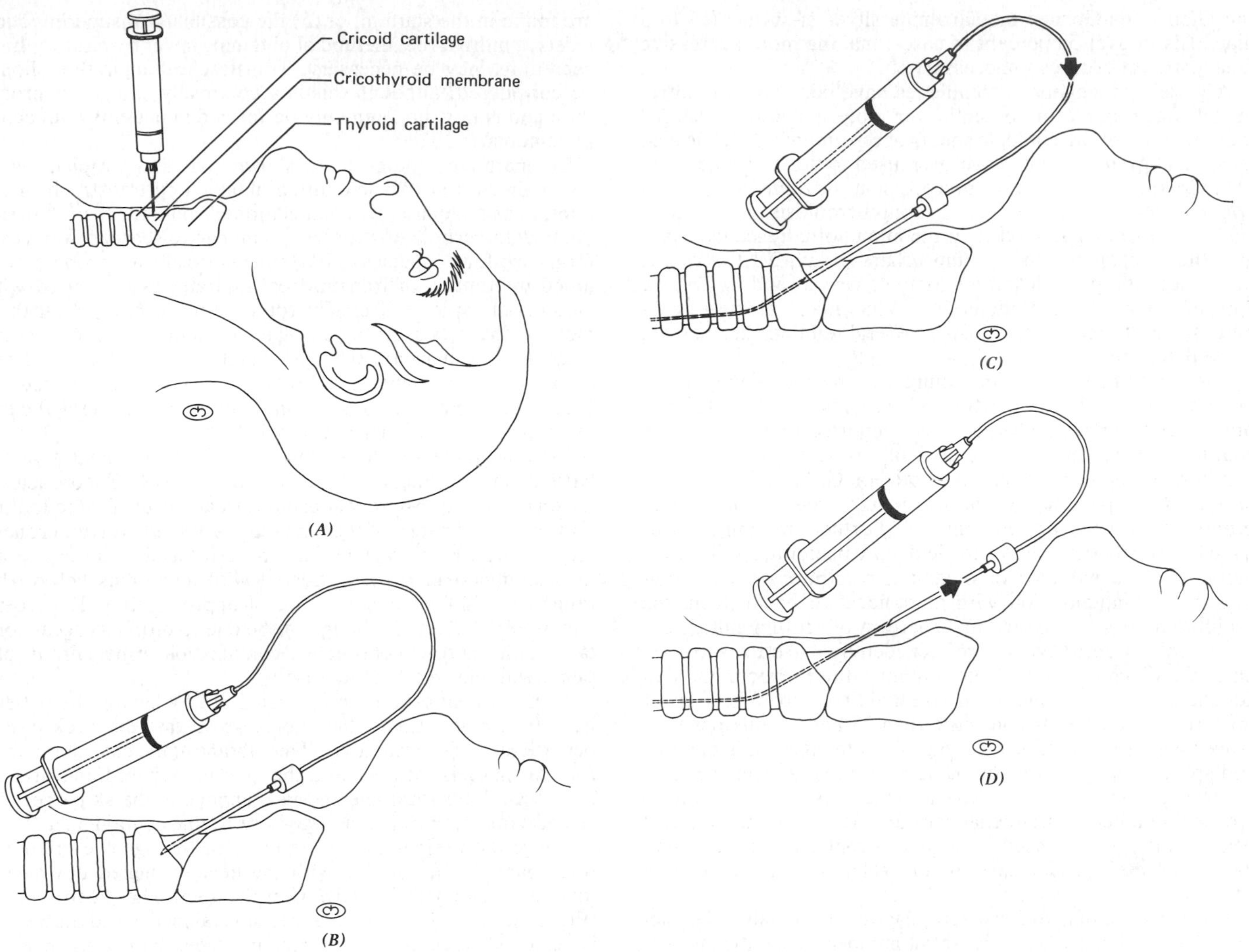

FIG. 5. Transtracheal aspiration. **(A)** The patient's neck is hyperextended, and local anesthesia is applied to the area over the cricothyroid membrane. **(B)** A large-bore needle with an indwelling catheter is inserted through the cricothyroid membrane into the trachea. **(C)** The catheter is advanced several inches into the trachea. **(D)** The needle is carefully withdrawn. Secretions are obtained by aspiration.

bacterial strains.[83] The development of the protected brush catheter (a brush within two catheters sealed at the end with a polyethylene glycol plug) has significantly decreased but not eliminated this problem[84,85] Quantitative culturing has been used to differentiate contaminants from true infecting agents.[84,86,87] Using $\geq 10^3$ colony-forming units per milliliter as a "breakpoint" for determination of the clinical significance of an isolate, studies employing the protected brush catheter have proven experimentally and clinically to be both sensitive (70–97 percent) and specific (95–100 percent) for the diagnosis of bacterial pneumonia.[86–89] However, not all series using this technique have produced impressive results,[90–92] and in some patient groups this technique is not useful. One group consists of patients receiving prior antibiotics, and another includes patients with underlying structural disease, in whom over 50 percent of bronchoscopic specimens yield significant numbers of organisms even in the absence of pneumonia.[86,89] Detection of the antibody coating of organisms found at bronchoscopy has been used in an attempt to differentiate colonization from true infection. Experience has been limited and results have been mixed, with a high false-positive rate noted in patients with chronic bronchitis.[93,94]

Bronchoalveolar lavage, in which a segment of lung is "washed" with sterile fluid, has proved to be an excellent means of diagnosing *P. carinii* and cytomegalovirus pneumonia. In patients with AIDS, the sensitivity of the procedure for detecting these pathogens ranges from 89 to 98 percent.[95,96] By using immunofluorescent monoclonal antibodies to viral antigens or centrifuging lavage material onto tissue culture preparations, the diagnosis of cytomegalovirus pneumonia may be made within hours.[97,98] While bronchoalveolar lavage may detect other pathogens (fungi, mycobacteria) in patients with AIDS, and may be useful in defining the etiology of pneumonia in other immunosuppressed patients, lower sensitivities than those noted above have been observed.[99,100]

By using cytologic screening and microbiologic quantitation of bronchoalveolar lavage fluid, bacterial etiologies of pneumonia have been identified. Criteria of <1 percent squamous epithelial cells and $>10^5$ colony-forming units of a bacterial isolate have been used to diagnose bacterial pneumonias with sensitivities of up to 86 percent and specificities of up to 100 percent.[101,102] Most series have involved patients who were immunocompromised; the applicability of this procedure to general patient populations has not yet been thoroughly evaluated.

LUNG BIOPSY

Direct means of obtaining diagnostic material in patients with pneumonia include percutaneous lung aspiration, transbronchial lung biopsy, thoracoscopy, and open lung biopsy.[103] These procedures are usually reserved for cases of pneumonia in pediatric populations, in which sputum is not routinely available and transtracheal aspiration is dangerous, or in patients who are immunosuppressed, in whom routine diagnostic procedures are often unsuccessful in providing a diagnosis and where unusual pathogens may be present. Biopsy procedures are rarely indicated in the normal person with acute pneumonia. The indications and usefulness of these invasive procedures remain controversial. Lung aspiration has provided a diagnostic yield of 30–82 percent in adults and children, though false-negative rates of up to 18 percent have been reported.[104–107] Bleeding and pneumothorax have been reported as the major complications in 5–39 percent of procedures.[107–109] The use of transbronchial biopsy in the diagnosis of pneumonia has been reviewed recently, revealing similar diagnostic yields though somewhat lower complication rates.[110]

Thoracoscopy, in which the pleura and underlying lung are visualized through a thorascope before biopsy, has been used in several series of children and adults with pneumonia. Despite a diagnostic yield of over 90 percent and low complication rates, there has not been extensive experience with this procedure.[111,112]

Open lung biopsy remains the definitive invasive procedure for making an etiologic diagnosis of pneumonia in immunosuppressed patients.[109,110,113] Review of the recent literature has noted diagnostic yields of 60–100 percent. The incidence of pneumothorax and bleeding is usually less than 10 percent, even in patients who are thrombocytopenic.[110] Some have questioned whether open lung biopsy provides meaningful information that significantly affects patients' clinical outcome.[114,115]

Examination of Pleural Effusions

The characteristics of pleural effusions and their importance in the differential diagnosis of pulmonary disease are discussed in Chapter 54. It should be noted that the incidence of pleural effusions associated with pneumonia varies with the etiologic agent, from approximately 10 percent with pneumococci to 50–70 percent with gram-negative bacilli to up to 95 percent with group A streptococcal disease.[51,116,117] Pleural fluid cultures, when positive, are specific for the etiology of the underlying pneumonia. Furthermore, analysis of pleural fluid may play a major role in differentiating other causes of pulmonary infiltrates that may mimic pneumonia, including tuberculosis, tumors, pulmonary emboli, and collagen vascular diseases. Pleural biopsy specimens from patients with acute bacterial pneumonia are nonspecific and are therefore of little use in the differential diagnosis. Analysis of pleural fluid may be of prognostic significance. A pleural fluid pH of less than 7.0 or a pleural fluid glucose level below 40 mg/100 ml has been associated with the presence of a complicated parapneumonic effusion and the need for a tube thoracostomy.[118]

Blood Culture, Serologic Studies, and Antigen Detection

Approximately 20–30 percent of patients with bacterial pneumonia are bacteremic. Positive blood cultures offer definitive proof of the etiology of an associated pneumonia, and blood should be cultured from all patients suspected of having bacterial pneumonia.

Since the demonstration by Dorff et al. that pneumococcal capsular antigen could be detected by counterimmunoelectrophoresis (CIE),[119] a variety of techniques have been used to identify antigen in urine, serum, and plural fluid. None, including CIE, latex agglutination, and ELISA, have proven to be definitive. Sensitivities vary from 20 to 90 percent, and false-positive rates vary from 8 to 20 percent.[120–123] In a small number of cases, CIE of pleural fluid has been helpful in defining the etiology of empyema in patients with previous antibiotic therapy and negative pleural fluid cultures.[124]

CIE of sputum in patients with bacteremic pneumococcal pneumonia has been positive in 75–100 percent of cases but appears to be less sensitive than either the quellung reaction or culture.[125–127] This test is less helpful in detecting disease caused by pneumococcal types 7 and 14, which contain neutral polysaccharides not easily detected by CIE.[128] Further, although a positive sputum CIE will detect the presence of pneumococcal antigen, it cannot distinguish colonization from true infection.[129,130]

CIE and latex agglutination techniques have been used for the detection of *H. influenzae* and pseudomonas antigens in patients with pneumonia, though clinical experience has been limited and the results disappointing.[131]

Serologic tests have been used to diagnose a variety of other pulmonary pathogens, including *Legionella pneumophila, Legionella micdadei, Mycoplasma pneumoniae, Chlamydia* spp., and *Coxiella burnetii*.[132] The sensitivity and specificity of these assays are variable, and many assays have not been completely standardized. Since many of these tests are not routinely done, their usefulness in making a rapid diagnosis is limited. They are of more help in confirming a clinical diagnosis.

RADIOLOGIC EXAMINATION

The chest film most frequently shows a bronchopneumonia pattern that is not very helpful in making a specific etiologic diagnosis (Fig. 6). However, certain features may be of some diagnostic aid. Lobar consolidation, cavitation, and large pleural effusions support a bacterial etiology (Fig. 7). In cases in which bilateral diffuse involvement is noted, *P. carinii* pneumonia, *Legionella* pneumonia, or a primary viral pneumonia should be suspected. Staphylococcal pneumonia may result from infection metastasizing from a primary focus unrelated to the lung. In these cases, multiple nodular infiltrates throughout the lung may be seen. Staphylococci may cause marked necrosis of lung tissue with ill-defined thin-walled cavities (pneumatoceles), bronchopleural fistulas, and empyema, especially in children[133–135] (Fig. 8). Although pneumatoceles are diagnostically significant findings in staphylococcal pneumonia, they may be seen in pneumonias of other etiologies, including

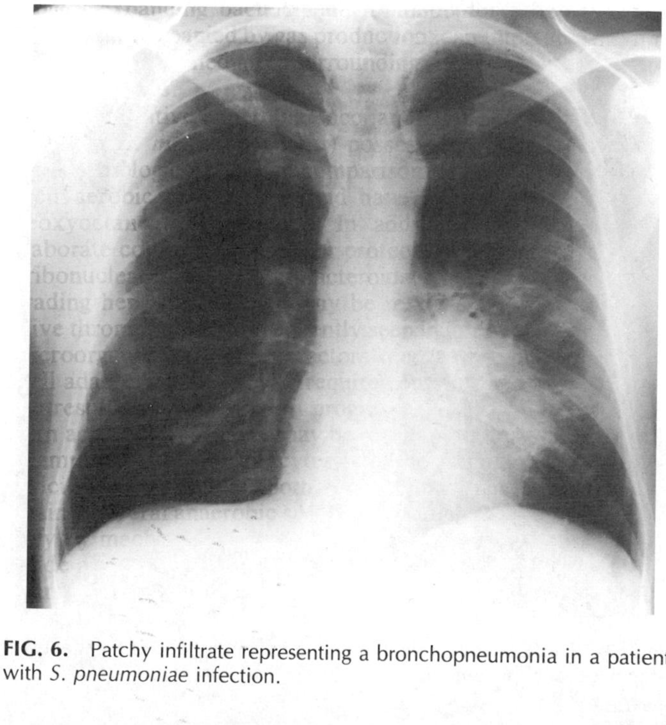

FIG. 6. Patchy infiltrate representing a bronchopneumonia in a patient with *S. pneumoniae* infection.

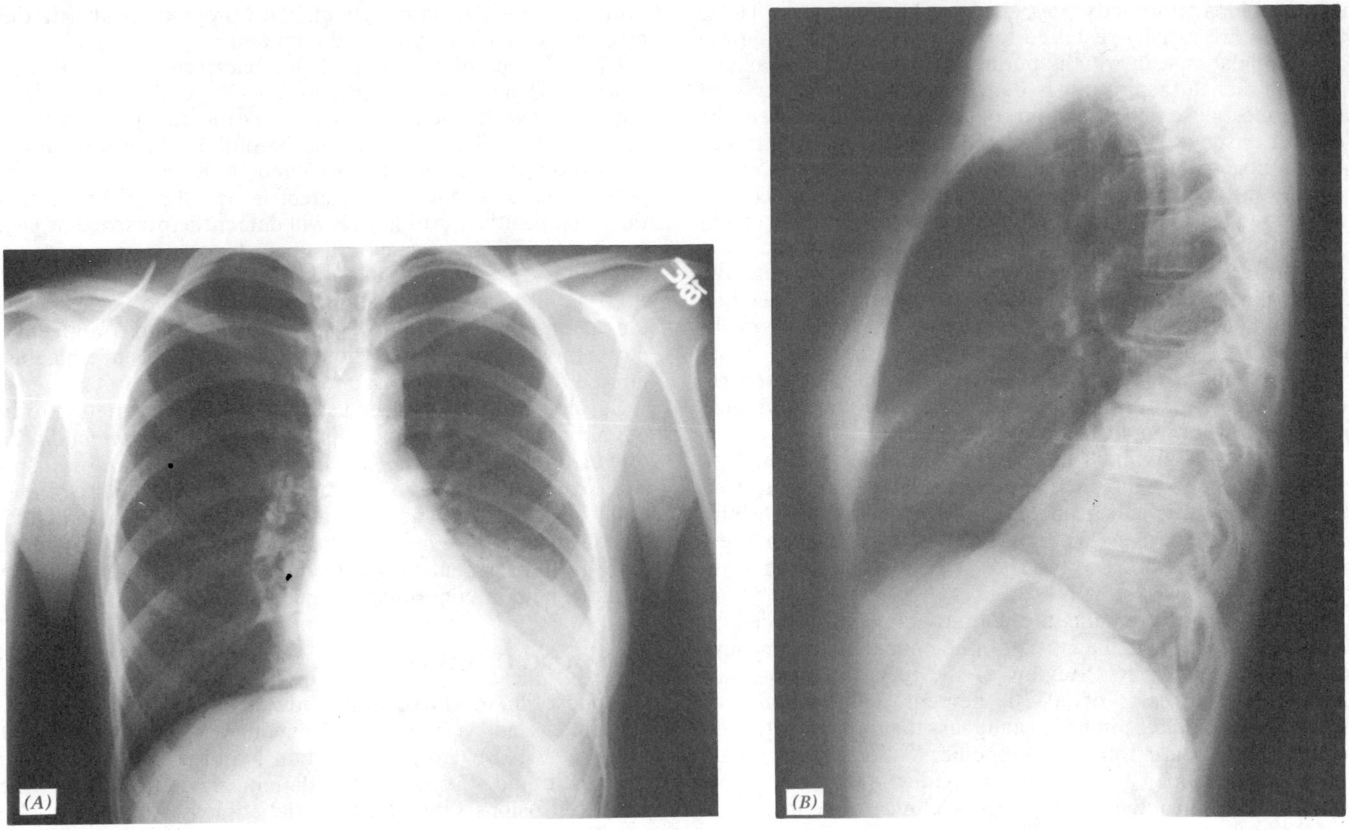

FIG. 7. **(A)** Posteroanterior film showing dense left lower lobe consolidation consistent with a bacterial pneumonia, in this case caused by *S. pneumoniae*. **(B)** Lateral film of patient with left lower lobe pneumococcal pneumonia.

K. pneumoniae, H. influenzae, S. pneumoniae, and, more rarely, *P. carinii.*[136–138] Pulmonary infections due to *Pseudomonas* have a marked tendency toward cavitation. Although its initial manifestation is that of patchy bronchopneumonia, microabscesses form quickly and coalesce to form one or several large abscesses. *Pseudomonas* and other gram-negative bacilli cause lower lobe pneumonia most commonly.[139]

Aspiration pneumonia should be considered along with gram-negative and staphylococcal pneumonias as a source of necrotizing pneumonia, cavitation, and empyema. Aspiration pneumonia commonly involves either the superior segment or the basilar segment of either lower lobe or the posterior segment of the upper lobes, depending on whether aspiration occurred in the dependent or upright position.[140] Chronic aspiration most commonly results in a bilateral lower lobe pneumonia, although it often may appear to involve one side more than the other.[139]

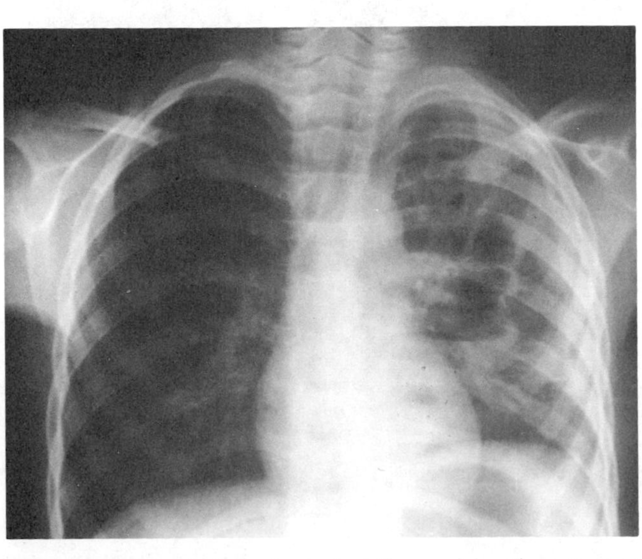

FIG. 8. Pneumatocele formation in the left upper lobe of a patient with staphylococcal pneumonia.

Many viral pneumonias produce generalized destruction of ciliated epithelium with little radiologic distinction between the various viral etiologies. Initially, ciliated epithelial cells, goblet cells, and bronchial mucous gland cells are destroyed. Subsequent involvement may include terminal bronchioles and alveoli. Diffuse hemorrhagic congestion of alveolar septa with red blood cells and inflammatory edema fluid may be seen, especially with primary influenza pneumonia.[141] The x-ray film concomitants of these pathologic findings are varied and may be confusing if a secondary bacterial infection complicates the initial process. Diffuse and localized involvement with both interstitial and alveolar patterns have been noted[142] (Fig. 9). Peribronchial involvement with nodular infiltrates is a pattern often seen with varicella.

Mycoplasmal pneumonia often manifests with an interstitial pattern in a peribronchial distribution. As more edema fluid is elaborated, there may be rapid progression to lobar or sublobar consolidation. Once this consolidation stage is reached, radiologic differentiation between bacterial and myocplasmal pneumonia is difficult. *Mycoplasma* is usually associated with lower lobe disease. Cavitation is rare, although pleural effusion may be seen in 20 percent of the cases.[143]

Legionnaires' disease may initially present with an x-ray picture similar to that of mycoplasmal pneumonia. A patchy interstitial or finely nodular pattern is seen in the lower lobes.[144] However, unlike mycoplasmal pneumonia, pneumonia with more than two-lobe involvement is commonly seen. Rapid progression and pleural effusions are also common.[145] Pneumonia

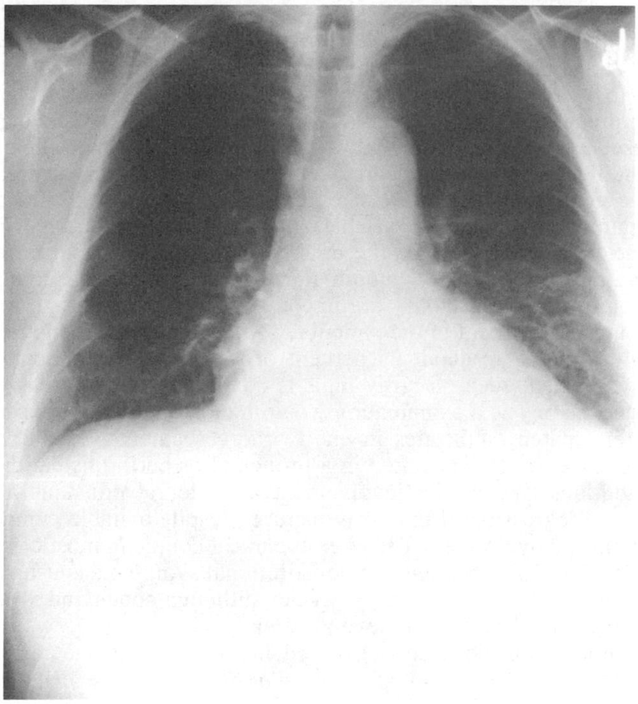

FIG. 9. Bilateral involvement with a mixed interstitial-alveolar pattern in a patient with viral pneumonia.

caused by *L. micdadei* (Pittsburgh pneumonia agent) may present with pulmonary nodules, either single or multiple, as well as with segmental infiltrates. As in pneumonia caused by *L. pneumophila,* rapid radiologic progression of the disease is characteristic.[146]

It must be recognized that x-ray films are most helpful in conjunction with the clinical history and physical examination. This point was clearly shown by Tew et al.,[147] who evaluated readings of x-ray films of patients with pneumonia made without clinical information. Pneumonia was correctly identified as bacterial only 67 percent of the time and as viral only 65 percent of the time. Mycoplasmal pneumonia was incorrectly identified as bacterial 81 percent of the time.

PNEUMONIA SYNDROMES

Acute Community-Acquired Pneumonia

Review of large numbers of patients with community-acquired pneumonia have provided an epidemiologic and clinical profile of this syndrome.[28,30,31,148–150] Typically, patients are in their mid-50s to 60s and usually become ill in midwinter or early spring. Although the onset of pneumonia symptoms is acute and represents a marked change from their usual health, most patients have one or more chronic underlying diseases, including chronic obstructive lung disease, cardiovascular disease, diabetes, or alcoholism.

The onset of disease is usually marked by a sudden chill. Sustained temperature elevations to approximately 40°C, pleuritic chest pain, and cough productive of mucopurulent sputum usually follow.

Physical examination reveals fever, tachypnea, and tachycardia. Localized pulmonary findings with rales are noted early in the disease, and signs of lobar consolidation are noted as the disease progresses. Laboratory evaluation is significant. Most commonly, the white blood cell count is in the range of 15–35,000/mm^3, and the differential cell count reveals an increased number of juvenile forms.[151] Leukopenia may be noted and is a poor prognostic sign.[152] The hematocrit and the red blood cell indices are usually normal. Examination of the sputum reveals thick, purulent material that may be rust colored. The sputum Gram stain reveals numerous neutrophils and bacteria, usually with a single organism predominating. Chest films reveal areas of parenchymal involvement, usually in a bronchopneumonic pattern. Arterial blood gas determinations reveal a moderate degree of hypoxemia due to ventilation perfusion abnormalities.

With the diagnostic tests presently available, a microbiologic diagnosis may be made in 50–70 percent of cases of pneumonia.[150,151] In the past, 50–90 percent of the cases of acute community-acquired pneumonia were caused by *S. pneumoniae*.[30,31,153] More recently, the relative importance of this pneumococcus has decreased. At present, it causes 25–60 percent of the cases of acute community-acquired pneumonia.[149,150,154–156] Advanced age, cigarette smoking, institutionalization, dementia, seizures, and the presence of chronic illnesses such as chronic obstructive pulmonary disease, congestive heart failure, and cerebrovascular disease have been identified as significant risk factors for the development of pneumococcal pneumonia.[157] Severe pneumococcal infections, including pneumonia, have been associated with splenectomy due to trauma or staging for Hodgkin's disease.[158,159]

An estimated 4–15 percent of the cases of acute community-acquired pneumonia are caused by *H. influenzae*.[28,31,150,154–156,160,161] The true incidence of this organism is obscured by the difficulty in isolating it from sputum and identifying it in sputum Gram stain, and by the failure of early studies to differentiate colonization from true infection. *Staphylococcus aureus* accounts for 2–10 percent of acute community-acquired pneumonia,[162] and takes on increased importance as a cause of pneumonia in the elderly and in patients recovering from influenza.[163,164] Patients developing postinfluenza pneumonia are usually younger and have less underlying disease than most other patients with community-acquired pneumonia. Clinical signs and symptoms of influenza are present but appear to resolve over several days. After a variable period of time ranging from 2 to 14 days, symptoms suddenly reappear, with the onset of shaking chills, pleuritic chest pain, and cough productive of purulent sputum. An elevated white blood cell count with a shift to the left, physical signs of pulmonary consolidation and radiographic evidence of focal parenchymal disease appear. The sputum Gram stain is consistent with bacterial pneumonia. Although the pneumococcus still represents the most common etiologic agent, staphylococcal disease occurs with a higher frequency than that noted in non-influenza-related, community-acquired pneumonia.[163,164]

Aerobic gram-negative bacteria, exclusive of *H. influenzae,* and mixed aerobic and anaerobic infections cause most of the remaining cases of acute community-acquired pneumonia. Gram-negative rods may cause 7–18 percent of pneumonia[154–156] and are particularly important pathogens in the elderly. The importance of *Legionella* spp. in causing pneumonia varies greatly in different geographic areas. While incidences as high as 17–22.5 percent have been reported,[153,165] many centers report significantly lower rates[155,156] Recently, *Branhamella catarrhalis* has been identified as a cause of pneumonia.[166–168] The overall incidence of disease due to this bacterium is low, but it is an important pathogen in elderly patients with chronic obstructive pulmonary disease and various forms of immunosuppression. In contrast to disease patterns in adults, viruses are the most important cause of pneumonia in young children. Respiratory syncytial virus and parainfluenza virus type 3 are the major pathogens. Other parainfluenza viruses and low-numbered adenovirus serotypes are also important.

Two clinical entities differ significantly from the above description of community-acquired pneumonia and therefore deserve special mention. Pneumonia in the elderly is a major cause of morbidity and mortality and in some series represents the leading cause of death[169] (see Chapter 295). The clinical presentation may be more subtle than in younger populations, with less frequent complaints of chills and rigor and less fever.[41,170] Bacteremia, metastatic foci of infection, and death are more frequent in older populations.[28,41,152] While the etiologies of pneumonia in the elderly follow the general pattern noted in younger patients, aerobic gram-negative bacilli and *Staph. aureus* play a more important role, especially in patients in nursing homes and extended care facilities.[170–174] Of the gram-negative organisms, *K. pneumoniae* and *H. influenzae,* including non-typable strains, appear especially important. The elderly also appear to be at high risk of infection from organisms such as group B streptococci and *B. catarrhalis*.[42,166–168] Increased oropharyngeal colonization with aerobic gram-negative bacilli has been documented in the elderly, with an increase in colonization paralleling the level of care needed by the patient.[175] Other factors that have been associated with increased colonization include prior use of antibiotics, serious underlying disease, and decreased activity.[171,175]

The etiology of community-acquired pneumonia in patients with AIDS is also different from that noted in other populations. *Pneumocystis carinii* pneumonia occurs in approximately 85 percent of patients at some time during their course.[176,177] In addition to the more common bacterial agents usually associated with community-acquired pneumonia, cytomegalovirus, *Mycobacterium tuberculosis,* and *Cryptococcus neoformans* also play important roles as etiologic agents (see Chapter 108).

Pneumonia in the Setting of Aspiration

The clinical setting in which aspiration occurs involves any disease state in which consciousness is altered and the normal gag and swallowing reflexes are abnormal.

Three major syndromes are recognized as a consequence of aspiration: chemical pneumonitis, bronchial obstruction secondary to aspiration of particulate matter, and bacterial aspiration pneumonia.[178,179] Although chemical pneumonitis and mechanical obstruction usually cause acute symptoms, aspiration pneumonia is more insidious, with symptoms usually occurring gradually several days after the initial episode of aspiration. Pneumonitis, necrotizing pneumonia, abscess, and empyema are common. Symptoms often include fever, weight loss, and productive cough. Putrid sputum is produced in 50 percent of the cases.[44,140] Anemia and an elevated white blood cell count are frequently associated findings. The bacteriologic findings in aspiration pneumonia reflect the flora of the oropharynx, and the importance of periodontal disease in this regard has been noted. Anaerobic bacteria, alone (45–58 percent of the cases) or in combination with aerobes (41–46 percent), are most commonly seen when adequate culture techniques are used.[5,44]

Bacteroides melaninogenicus. *Fusobacterium* spp., and anaerobic gram-positive cocci are the predominant anaerobes isolated. In community-acquired aspiration pneumonia, *Streptococcus* spp. are the most common aerobic isolates.[179,180] In contrast, gram-negative bacilli, and *Staph. aureus* are the most commonly isolated aerobes from nosocomial aspiration pneumonia.[179,180]

Atypical Pneumonia Syndrome

The atypical pneumonia syndrome is a symptom complex representing disease caused most commonly by *Myocplasma pneumoniae*. The older child (>5 years of age), the adolescent, or the young adult is at greatest risk of developing the disease. Increased incidence of disease and true epidemics have been documented in relatively enclosed populations of young adults at military bases, colleges, and boarding schools.[181–183] Mycoplasmal infection occurs throughout the year, although a relative increase in incidence is noted in the late summer and fall. In contrast, adenovirus infection, another cause of atypical pneumonia, most commonly occurs between January and April, outbreaks occurring primarily in military recruit camps.[181,183,184]

The course of the atypical pneumonias is characterized by a 3- to 4-day history of symptoms. Constitutional symptoms seem to predominate over specific respiratory findings. Fever, malaise, coryza, headache, and cough represent the major clinical findings. Pleuritic chest pain, splinting, and respiratory distress are not usually seen. Moist or crepitant rales may be heard. Sputum production is variable, and although it is purulent in one-third to one-half of the cases, Gram stain and culture of sputum usually reveal mouth flora. White blood cell counts greater than 10,000/mm^3 are uncommon, occurring in approximately 20 percent of the patients.[50] An elevated sedimentation rate is noted in about 25 percent of the cases.[185] Pulmonary involvement seen on x-ray films is commonly more extensive than the physical examination would indicate. Unilateral or bilateral patchy infiltrates in one or more segments, usually in the lower lobes, are noted in a bronchial or peribronchial distribution. Upper lobe involvement and pleural effusions are rare. Progression of the x-ray picture, despite a stable clinical picture, may be seen. The overall clinical course in most cases is benign. Disappearance of constitutional symptoms is usually noted in the first and second weeks, although cough and x-ray changes may persist for several weeks.

Other etiologic agents involved in the atypical pneumonia syndrome include TWAR, *Coxiella burnetti* (Q fever), and *Chlamydia psittaci* (psittacosis). Chlamydia trachomatis has been described as a pulmonary pathogen in immunocompromised as well as healthy hosts.[186,187] Productive cough, myalgias, and fever associated with diffuse nonsegmental infiltrates appear most commonly. The agent has also been associated with chronic pneumonia in neonates and infants. Onset occurs at 2–3 weeks of age and is associated with tachypnea, a staccato cough with periods of cyanosis and emesis, lack of fever, and diffuse interstitial and patchy alveolar infiltrates on chest films. Elevated IgG and IgM levels and absolute eosinophilia have also been noted.

The TWAR strain of *Chlamydia* has been identified by culture and serology as the cause of pneumonia presenting both as an atypical pneumonia as well as an acute community-acquired pneumonia.[190,191] Mild to moderate illness with prolonged symptoms and frequent relapses have been characteristic (see Chapter 160).

Of the viral agents associated with atypical pneumonia in adults, influenza A and B and adenovirus types 3, 4, and 7, especially in military recruits, are the most common. Reports of other viral agents causing pneumonia are scant but have included rhinovirus,[192] enterovirus,[193] parainfluenza virus,[194] and respiratory syncytial virus.[195]

Respiratory syncytial virus, the predominant respiratory pathogen in infants and children, is now recognized as an etiology of pneumonia in adults.[195–197] While the number of cases is small, groups at particular risk appear to be the elderly and patients who are immunosuppressed.

Legionnaires' disease may present as either an acute, community-acquired pneumonia or an atypical pneumonia. Although early symptoms of malaise, muscle aches, headache, and nonproductive cough resemble the onset of a "viral syndrome," the rapid progression of pulmonary symptoms is noteworthy. Abdominal pain and gastrointestinal symptoms, especially diarrhea, have been noted. Physical examination reveals only rales; x-ray films show patchy interstitial or nodular infiltrates that may progress rapidly to more widespread consolidation. Approximately 50 percent of cases have bilateral involvement. Transient impairment of renal function, abnormally low serum phosphorus levels, and elevated serum creatinine phosphokinase levels have been described.[144,145,198,199] For the most part, it is not possible to clinically distinguish legionnaires' disease from other bacterial pneumonias.[165]

Pulmonary Infiltrates with Eosinophilia

Pulmonary infiltrates with eosinophilia (PIE) is a syndrome associated with a variety of clinical entities, only some of which are infectious in etiology.[200] Pulmonary eosinophilia with transient, peripheral pulmonary infiltrates and minimal symptoms has been associated with *Ascaris* and *Strongyloides* infections. Prolonged pulmonary eosinophilia associated with weight loss, fever, cough, and dyspnea may be due to tuberculosis, brucellosis, psittacosis, coccidioidomycosis, and parasitic infections including ascariasis, strongyloidiasis, paragonomiasis, echinococcosis, visceral larva migrans, cutaneous larva migrans, *Schistosoma Dirofilaria immitus, Entamoeba histolytica* and infection with *Ancylostoma* spp. Noninfectious etiologies include drug allergy, sarcoidosis, eosinophilic leukemia, and hypersensitivity pneumonitis (i.e., pigeon breeders' disease).[200,201]

It has recently been suggested that chronic eosinophilic pneumonia may represent a unique clinical entity that is a form of collagen-vascular disease or an infection in a hyperimmune patient.[202–204] Interstitial infiltrates, focal interstitial fibrosis, bronchiolitis obliterans, microabscesses, and sarcoid-like granulomas are characteristic pathologic features. A rapid response to steroids has been reported.[204]

Tropical eosinophilia consists of myalgia, fatigue, weight loss, and anorexia associated with cough, frequently with nocturnal exacerbations, dyspnea, and peripheral eosinophilia in patients who have lived in or visited the tropics. X-ray film changes are distinctive and include increased interstitial markings with 2- to 4-mm nodules throughout the lungs with preferential involvement of the bases. Most cases represent microfilarial infection and can be treated with diethylcarbamazine.

Nosocomial Pneumonia and Pneumonia in the Immunosuppressed Host

Nosocomial pneumonia accounts for approximately 10–20 percent of all nosocomial infections and is the leading cause of infection-related mortality in hospitalized patients.[205,206] Important risk factors for the development of disease include advanced age, severity of underlying disease, intubation, use of respiratory equipment, surgery, and previous use of antibiotics.[207–209] Use of antacids and histamine type 2 blockers that raise the gastric pH have been shown to increase stomach colonization with aerobic gram-negative rods and may be another risk factor for the development of pulmonary infection.[210–212]. Approximately 60 percent of cases of nosocomial pneumonia are caused by aerobic gram-negative bacilli, with members of the family Enterobacteriaceae (*K. pneumoniae, E. coli, Serratia marcescens, Enterobacter* spp.) and *Pseudomonas* spp. accounting for the majority of these. *Staphylococcus aureus* causes approximately 13 percent of nosocomial pneumonia, with *S. pneumoniae* causing only 8 percent.[40]

Pneumonia in the immunosuppressed host represents an important subset of nosocomial pneumonia and deserves special emphasis.[213] In patients with nonlymphocytic leukemia, 25 percent of all documented infections are pulmonary.[214] In patients with acute leukemia, 64 percent of fatal bacteremias of known cause originate in the lung, the majority of episodes caused by enteric gram-negative bacilli.[214] Approximately one-fourth of renal transplant recipients,[216,217] as well as one-half of bone marrow transplant patients,[218] will develop pneumonia at some time during their course. Again, the most common bacterial pathogens are gram-negative bacilli. As with other nosocomial pneumonias, pneumonias in the compromised host are most commonly caused by *K. pneumoniae, E. coli,* or *Pseudomonas aeruginosa*. In some series these organisms cause 50 percent of all infections, with mixed gram-negative infections accounting for another 20 percent.[219,220]

In addition to bacterial pathogens, a variety of nonbacterial agents are of etiologic importance. These include fungi (*Aspergillus* spp., agents of mucormycosis, *Candida* spp.), protozoa (*Pneumocystis carinii, Toxoplasma gondii*), parasites (*Strongyloides*), and viruses (herpes zoster virus, cytomegalovirus). Chapter 280 and Part IV, Section B discuss more fully nosocomial pneumonia and infections in the compromised host, respectively.

THERAPY FOR PNEUMONIA

Once the etiologic agent is identified, selection of appropriate therapy is relatively straightforward. (In-depth discussions are provided in the sections dealing with specific antibiotics and etiologic agents.) The choice of antibiotics becomes more difficult when sputum cannot be obtained or when the sputum examination is nondiagnostic. In these cases, empiric therapy should be designed to treat the most likely and/or the most potentially lethal possibilities.

Patients with a mild illness, no history of cigarette abuse, and a nondiagnostic sputum test who present with a sudden onset of fever, a pulmonary infiltrate, and leukocytosis are likely to have pneumococcal pneumonia and may be treated empirically with penicillin. When an atypical pneumonia presentation is noted, empiric use of erythromycin will provide adequate therapy against the pneumococcus as well as against *M. pneumoniae,* the most likely cause of atypical pneumonia. Where *H. influenzae* is suspected, cefuroxime axetil (Ceftin), trimethoprimsulfamethoxazole (Bactrim, Septra) or amoxicillin/clavulanic acid (Augmentin) are appropriate oral regimens.

A seriously ill patient with acute community-acquired pneumonia and a nondiagnostic sputum examination should be treated for the most likely pathogens. Therapy should include coverage for *S. pneumoniae, H. influenzae, Staph. aureus,* and, in some cases, *L. pneumophila*. Selection of antibiotics should take into account the possibility of ampicillin-resistant *H. influenzae* unless it is known that no such resistant organisms have been isolated from the community. While third-generation cephalosporins and broad-spectrum penicillins are not usually needed for therapy of community-acquired pneumonia, they are indicated for therapy of life-threatening disease when gram-negative aerobes are suspected.[221] Erythromycin is the drug of choice for *Legionella* pneumonia and should be added to the above regimens if the diagnosis is suspected.

The therapy for aspiration pneumonia is dependent on whether the episode of aspiration occurs in the community or in the hospital. Penicillin is effective for most cases of community-acquired aspiration pneumonia, since the predominant organisms are usually penicillin sensitive.[222] However, an increased incidence of in vitro penicillin resistance has been observed in several *Bacteroides* spp.[223–226] Clindamycin[227,228] or other agents with potent antianaerobic plus aerobic activity may be used for seriously ill patients and those who do not respond promptly to penicillin. Therapy for nosocomial pneumonia is discussed in Chapter 280.

REFERENCES

1. Osler W. The Principles and Practice of Medicine. 4th ed. New York: D. Appleton; 1901:108.
2. Statistical Abstract of the United States, 104th ed. Washington, DC: US Government Printing Office, 1984.
3. Johanson WG Jr, Gould KG Jr. Lung defense mechanisms. Basics of RD. 1977;6:(2)1–6.
4. Green G. In defense of the lung. Am Rev Respir Dis. 1970;102:691–703.
5. Bartlett J, Gorbach S, Finegold S. The bacteriology of aspiration pneumonia. Am J Med. 1974;56:202–7.
6. Huxley EJ, Viroslav J, Gray WR, et al. Pharyngeal aspiration in normal adults and patients with depressed consciousness. Am J Med. 1978;64: 564–8.
7. Green GM, Carolin D. The depressant effect of cigarette smoke on the in

vitro antibacterial activity of alveolar macrophages. N Engl J Med. 1967;276:421–7.
8. Green GM, Kass EH. The influence of bacterial species on pulmonary resistance to infection in mice subjected to hypoxia, cold stress and ethanolic intoxication. Br J Exp Pathol. 1965;46:360–6.
9. Green GM, Kass EH. The role of the alveolar macrophage in the clearance of bacteria from the lung. J Exp Med. 1964;119:167–76.
10. Coffin DL, Gardner DE, Holzman RS, et al. Influence of ozone on pulmonary cells. Arch Environ Health. 1968;16:633–6.
11. Ehrlich R, Henry MC. Chronic toxicity of nitrogen dioxide. I. Effect on resistance to bacterial pneumonia. Arch Environ Health. 1968;17:860–5.
12. LaForce FM, Mullane JF, Boehme RF, et al. The effect of pulmonary edema on antibacterial defenses of the lung. J Lab Clin Med. 1973;82:634–48.
13. Huber GL, LaForce FM, Mason RJ, et al. Impairment of pulmonary bacterial defense mechanisms by immunosuppressive agents. Surg Forum. 1970;21:285–6.
14. Warshauer D, Goldstein E, Akers T, et al. Effect of influenza viral infection on the ingestion and killing of bacteria by alveolar macrophages. Am Rev Respir Dis. 1977;115:269–77.
15. Winterbauer RH, Bedon GA, Bal WC Jr. Recurrent pneumonia: Predisposing illness and clinical patterns in 158 patients. Ann Intern Med. 1969;70:689–700.
16. Roth RM, Gleckman RA. Recurrent bacterial pneumonia: A contemporary perspective. South Med J. 1985;78:573–9.
17. Donowitz GR, Mandell GL. Clinical presentation and unusual infections. In: Advances in Host Defense Mechanisms. v. 3. Gallin JI, Fauci AS, eds. New York: Raven Press; 1983;55–75.
18. Donabedian H, Gallin JI. The hyperimmunoglobulin E recurrent infection (Jobs) syndrome. Medicine. 1983;62:195–208.
19. Beck S, Heiner DC. Selective immunoglobulin G_4 deficiency and recurrent infections of the respiratory tract. Am Rev Respir Dis. 1981;124:94–96.
20. Ammann AJ, Hong R. Selective IgA deficiency: Presentation of 30 cases and a review of the literature. Medicine. 1971;50:223–36.
21. Eliasson R, Mossberg B, Camner P, et al. The immotile-cilia syndrome. N Engl J Med. 1977;297:1–6.
22. Kartagener M. Zur Pathologie der Bronchiektasien: Bronkiectasien lei situs inversus. Beitr Klin Tuberk. 1933;83:489–501.
23. Handelsman DJ, Conway AJ, Boylan LM, et al. Young's syndrome: Obstructive azospermia and chronic sinopulmonary infections. N Engl J Med. 1984;310:3–9.
24. Savic B, Birtel FJ, Tholen W, et al. Lung sequestration: Report of seven cases and review of 540 published cases. Thorax. 1979;34:96–101.
25. Iverson LIG, May IA, Samson PC. Pulmonary complications in benign esophageal disease. Am J Surg. 1973;126:223–8.
26. Grayston JT, Alexander ER, Kenny GE, et al. Mycoplasma pneumoniae infections: Clinical and epidemiological studies. JAMA. 1965;191:369–74.
27. Murray HW, Masur H, Senterfit L, et al. The protean manifestations of mycoplasma pneumoniae infection in adults. Am J Med. 1975;58:229–42.
28. Dorff GJ, Rytel MW, Farmer SG, et al. Etiologies and characteristic features of pneumonias in a municipal hospital. Am J Med Sci. 1973;266:349–58.
29. MacGregor RR. A year's experience with tuberculosis in a private urban teaching hospital in the postsanitorium era. Am J Med. 1975;58:221–8.
30. Fekety FR, Caldwell J, Grump D, et al. Bacteria, viruses, and mycoplasmas in acute pneumonia in adults. Am Rev Respir Dis. 1971;104:499–507.
31. Sullivan RJ, Dowdle WR, Marine WM, et al. Adult pneumonia in a general hospital: Etiology and host risk factors. Arch Intern Med. 1972;129:935–42.
32. Lepow ML, Balassanian N, Emmerich J, et al. Interrelationships of viral, mycoplasmal and bacterial agents in uncomplicated pneumonia. Am Rev Respir Dis. 1968;97:533–45.
33. Martin CM, Kunin CM, Gottlieb LS, et al. Asian influenza A in Boston, 1957–1958. II. Severe staphylococcal pneumonia complicating influenza. Arch Intern Med. 1959;103:532–42.
34. Sprunt K. Infection in chronic lung disease. Bull NY Acad Med. 1972;48:698–703.
35. Hoiby N. Epidemiological investigations of the respiratory tract bacteriology in patients with cystic fibrosis. Acta Pathol Microbiol Scand B. 1974;82:541–50.
36. Burbank B, Morrione TG, Cutler SS. Pulmonary alveolar proteinosis and nocardiosis. Am J Med. 1960;28:1002–7.
37. Murray JF, Felton CP, Garay SM, et al. Pulmonary complications of the acquired immunodeficiency syndrome: Report of a National Heart Lung and Blood Institute Workshop. New Engl J Med 1984;310:1682–8.
38. Stover DE, White DA, Romano PA, et al. Spectrum of pulmonary diseases associated with the acquired immunodeficiency syndrome. Am J Med. 1985;78:429–37.
39. Witt DJ, Craven DE, McCabe WR. Bacterial infections in adult patients with the acquired immune deficiency syndrome (AIDS) and AIDS-related complex. Am J Med. 1987;82:900–6.
40. Gross PA. Epidemiology of hospital-acquired pneumonia. Semin in Respir Infect. 1987;2:2–7.
41. Marrie TJ, Haldane EV, Faulkner RS, et al. Community acquired pneumonia requiring hospitalization: Is it different in the elderly? J Am Geriatr Soc. 1985;33:671–80.
42. Verghese A, Berk SL, Boelen LJ, et al. Group B streptococcal pneumonia in the elderly. Arch Intern Med. 1982;142:1642–5.
43. Heffron R. Pneumonia. New York: Commonwealth Fund; 1939:505.
44. Bartlett JG, Finegold SM. Anaerobic infections of the lung and pleural space. Am Rev Respir Dis. 1974;110:56–77.
45. Thorsteinsson SB, Musher DM, Fagan T. The diagnostic value of sputum culture in acute pneumonia. JAMA. 1975;233:894–5.
46. Merrill C, Gwaltney JM, Hendley JO, et al. Rapid identification of pneumococci. N Engl J Med. 1973;288:510–2.
47. Drew WL. Value of sputum culture in diagnosis of pneumococcal pneumonia. J Clin Microbiol. 1977;6:62–5.
48. Bartlett RC, Melnick A. Usefulness of Gram stain and routine and quantitative culture of sputum in patients with and without acute respiratory infection. Conn Med. 1970;34:347–51.
49. Bryant RE, Rhoades ER. Clinical feature of adenoviral pneumonia in Air Force recruits. Am Rev Respir Dis. 1967;96:717–23.
50. George RB, Ziskind MM, Rasch JR, et al. Mycoplasma and adenovirus pneumonias—comparison with other atypical pneumonias in a military population. Ann Intern Med. 1966;65:931–42.
51. Reimann H. The Pneumonias. Philadelphia: WB Saunders; 1938:67.
52. Solomon S. Primary Friedlander pneumonia. JAMA. 1937;108:937–47.
53. Murray PR, Washington JA III. Microscopic and bacteriologic analysis of expectorated sputum. Mayo Clin Proc. 1975;50:339–44.
54. Rein MF, Gwaltney JM, O'Brien WM, et al. Accuracy of the Gram's stain in identifying pneumococci in sputum. JAMA. 1978;239:2671–3.
55. Hendley JO, Sande MA, Stewart PM, et al. Spread of *Streptococcus pneumoniae* in families. I. Carriage rates and distribution of types. J Infect Dis. 1975;132:55–61.
56. Finland M. Recent advances in the epidemiology of pneumococcal infections. Medicine. 1942;21:307–44.
57. Lees AW, McNaught W. Bacteriology of lower-respiratory tract secretions, sputum and upper-respiratory tract secretions in "normals" and "chronic bronchitis." Lancet. 1959;2:1112–5.
58. Bigby TD, Margolskee D, Curtis JL, et al. The usefulness of induced sputum in the diagnosis of *Pneumocystis carinii* pneumonia in patients with the acquired immunodeficiency syndrome. Am Rev Respir Dis. 1986;133:515–8.
59. Pitchenik AE, Ganjei P, Torres A, et al. Sputum examination for the diagnosis of *Pneumocystis carinii* pneumonia in the acquired immunodeficiency syndrome. Am Rev Respir Dis. 1986;133:226–9.
60. Tenover FC. Diagnostic deoxyribonucleic acid probes for infection. Dis Clin Microbiol Rev. 1988;1:82–101.
61. Peterson LR, Shanholtzer CJ. Using the microbiology laboratory in the diagnosis of pneumonia. Semin Respir Infect. 1988;3:106–12.
62. Sullivan CJ, Joran ML. Diagnosis of viral pneumonia. Semin Respir Infect. 1988;3:148–61.
63. Barrett-Connor E. The non-value of sputum culture in the diagnosis of pneumococcal pneumonia. Am Rev Respir Dis. 1971;103:845–8.
64. Rathburn HK, Govani I. Mouse inoculation as means of identifying pneumococci in the sputum. Johns Hopkins Med J. 1967;120:46–8.
65. Wallace RJ, Musher DM, Martin RR. *Hemophilus influenzae* pneumonia in adults. Am J Med. 1978;64:87–93.
66. Levin D, Schwarz M, Matthay R, et al. Bacteremic *Hemophilus influenzae* pneumonia in adults. A report of 24 cases and a review of the literature. Am J Med. 1977;62:219–24.
67. Davidson M, Tempest B, Palmer DL, Bacteriologic diagnosis of acute pneumonia, comparison of sputum, transtracheal aspirates, and lung aspirates. JAMA. 1976;235:158–63.
68. Geckeler RW, Gremillion DH, McAllister CK, et al. Microscopic and bacteriological comparison of paired sputa and transtracheal aspirates. J Clin Microbiol. 1977;6:396–9.
69. Kalinske RW, Parker RH, Brandt D, et al. Diagnostic usefulness and safety of transtracheal aspiration. N Engl J Med. 1967;276:604–8.
70. Hoeprich PD. Etiologic diagnosis of lower respiratory tract infections. Calif Med. 1970;112:1.
71. Tillotson JR, Lerner AM. Pneumonias caused by gram negative bacilli. Medicine. 1966;45:65–76.
72. Saadah HA, Nasr FL, Shagoury ME. Washed sputum gram stain and culture in pneumonia. J Okla State Med Assoc. 1980;73:354–9.
73. Ries K, Levison ME, Kaye D. Transtracheal aspiration in pulmonary infection. Arch Intern Med. 1974;133:453–8.
74. Hahn HH, Beaty HN. Transtracheal aspiration in the evaluation of patients with pneumonia. Ann Intern Med. 1970;72:183–7.
75. Jordan GW, Wong GA, Hoeprich PD. Bacteriology of the lower respiratory tract as determined by fiber-optic bronchoscopy and transtracheal aspiration. J Infect Dis. 1976;134:428–35.
76. Bartlett JG, Rosenblatt JE, Finegold SM. Percutaneous transtracheal aspiration in the diagnosis of anaerobic pulmonary infection. Ann Intern Med. 1973;79:535–40.
77. Bartlett JG. Diagnostic accuracy of transtracheal aspiration bacteriologic studies. Am Rev Respir Dis. 1977;115:777–82.
78. Schillaci RF, Iacovoni VE, Conte RS. Transtracheal aspiration complicated by fatal endotracheal hemorrhage. N Engl J Med. 1976;295:488–90.
79. Spencer CD, Beaty HN. Complications of transtracheal aspiration. N Engl J Med. 1972;286:304–6.
80. Lourie B, McKinnon B, Kibler L. Transtracheal aspiration and anaerobic abscess. Ann Intern Med. 1974;80:417–8.
81. Deresinski SC, Steven DA. Anterior cervical infections: Complications of transtracheal aspirations. Am Rev Respir Dis. 1974;110:354–6.

82. Parsons GH, Price JE, Auston PW. Bilateral pneumothorax complicating transtracheal aspiration. West J Med. 1976;125:73–5.
83. Bartlett JG, Alexander J, Mayhew J, et al. Should fiberoptic bronchoscopy aspirates be cultured? Am Rev Respir Dis. 1976;114:73–8.
84. Wimberly N, Faling LJ, Bartlett JG. A fiberoptic bronchoscopy technique to obtain uncontaminated lower airway secretions for bacterial cultures. Am Rev Respir Dis. 1979;119:337–42.
85. Meden G, Hall GS, Ahmad M. Retrieval of microbiological specimens through the fiberoptic bronchoscope. Cleve Clin Q. 1985;52:495–502.
86. Wimberly NW, Bass JB, Boyd BW, et al. Use of a bronchoscopic protected catheter brush for the diagnosis of pulmonary infections. Chest. 1982; 81:556–82.
87. Hays DA, McCarthy LC, Friedman M. Evaluation of two bronchofiberscopic methods of culturing the lower respiratory tract. Am Rev Respir Dis. 1980;122:319–23.
88. Higuchi JH, Coalson JJ, Johanson, WG. Bacteriologic diagnosis of nosocomial pneumonia in primates. Am Rev Respir Dis. 1982;125:53–7.
89. Pollock HM, Hawkins EL, Bonner JR, et al. Diagnosis of bacterial pulmonary infections with quantitative protected cathether cultures obtained during bronchoscopy. J Clin Microbiol. 1983;17:255–9.
90. Halperin SA, Suratt PM, Gwaltney JM, et al. Bacterial cultures of the lower respiratory tract in normal volunteers with and without experimental rhinovirus infection using a plugged double catheter system. Am Rev Respir Dis. 1982;125:678–80.
91. Bordelon JY Jr, Legrand P, Gewin WL, et al. The telescoping plugged catheter in suspected anaerobic infections: A controlled series. Am Rev Respir Dis. 1983;128:465–8.
92. Wimberly NW, Bass JR Jr, Boyd DW, et al. Bronchial brush specimens from patients with stable chronic bronchitis. Chest. 1986;90:534–6.
93. Winterbauer RH, Hutchinson JF, Reinhardt GN, et al. The use of quantitative culture and antibody coating of bacteria to diagnose bacterial pneumonia by fiberoptic bronchoscopy. Am Rev Respir Dis. 1983;128: 98–103.
94. Vereen L, Smart LM, George RB. Antibody coating and quantitative cultures of bacteria in sputum and bronchial brush specimens from patients with stable chronic bronchitis. Chest. 1986;90:534–6.
95. Broaddus C, Dake MD, Stulburg MS, et al. Bronchoalveolar lavage and transbronchial biopsy for the diagnosis of pulmonary infections in the acquired immunodeficiency syndrome. Ann Intern Med. 1986;102:747–52.
96. Orenstein M, Webber CA, Cash M, et al. Value of bronchoalveolar lavage in the diagnosis of pulmonary infection in acquired immune deficiency syndrome. Thorax. 1986;41:345–9.
97. Crawford SW, Bowden RA, Hackman RC, et al. Rapid detection of cytomegalovirus pulmonary infection by bronchoalveolar lavage and centrifugation culture. Ann Intern Med. 1988;108:180–5.
98. Emmanuel D, Peppard J, Stover D, et al. Rapid diagnosis of cytomegalovirus pneumonia by bronchoalveolar lavage using human and murine monoclonal antibodies. Ann Intern Med. 1986;104:476–81.
99. Stover DE, Zaman MB, Hajdu SI, et al. Bronchoalveolar lavage in the diagnosis of diffuse pulmonary infiltrates in the immunosuppressed host. Ann Intern Med. 1984;101:1–7.
100. Martin WJ, Smith TF, Sanderson DR, et al. Role of bronchoalveolar lavage in the assessment of opportunistic pulmonary infections: Utility and complications. Mayo Clin Proc. 1987;62:549–57.
101. Kahn FW, Jones JM. Diagnosing bacterial respiratory infection by bronchoalveolar lavage. J Infect Dis. 1987;155:862–9.
102. Thorpe JE, Baughman RP, Frame PT, et al. Bronchoalveolar lavage for diagnosing acute bacterial pneumonia. J Infect Dis. 1987;155:855–61.
103. Busk MF, Rosenow EC III, Wilson WR. Invasive procedures in the diagnosis of pneumonia. Semin Respir Infect. 1988;3:113–22.
104. Mimica I, Donoso E, Howard JE, et al. Lung puncture in the etiological diagnosis of pneumonia. Am J Dis Child. 1971;122:278–82.
105. Klein JO. Diagnostic lung puncture in the pneumonias of infants and children. Pediatrics. 1969;44:486–92.
106. Bartlett JG. Invasive diagnostic techniques in respiratory infections. In: Pennington JE, ed. Respiratory Infections: Diagnosis and Management. New York: Raven Press; 1983:55–77.
107. Palmer DL, Davidson M, Lusk R. Needle aspiration of the lung in complex pneumonias. Chest. 1980;78:16–21.
108. Bandt PD, Blank N, Castellino RA. Needle diagnosis of pneumonitis, value in high risk patients. JAMA. 1972;220:1578–80.
109. Greenman RL, Goodall PT, King D. Lung biopsy in immune compromised hosts. Am J Med. 1975;59:488–96.
110. Cockerill FR III, Wilson WR, Carpenter HA, et al. Open lung biopsy in immunocompromised patients. Arch Intern Med. 1985;145:1398–1404.
111. Dijkman JH, van der Meer JWM, Bakker W, et al. Transpleural lung biopsy by the thoracoscopic route in patients with diffuse interstitial pulmonary disease. Chest. 1982;82:76–83.
112. Rodgers BM. Thoracoscopy in children. Poumon-Coeur. 1981;37:301–6.
113. Springmeyer SC, Silvestri RC, Sale GE, et al. The role of transbronchial biopsy for the diagnosis of diffuse pneumonias in immunocompromised marrow transplant recipients. Am Rev Respir Dis. 1982;116:763–5.
114. McCabe RE, Brooks RG, Mark JBD, et al. Open lung biopsy in patients with acute leukemia. Am J Med. 1985;78:609–16.
115. McKenna RJ, Mountain CF, McMurtrey MJ. Open lung biopsy in immunocompromised patients. Chest. 1984;86:671–4.
116. Lowell JR. Pleural Effusions—A Comprehensive Review. Baltimore: University Park Press; 1977:96.
117. Unger JD, Rose HD, Unger GF. Gram-negative pneumonia. Diagn Radiol. 1973;107:283–91.
118. Light RN, Girard WM, Jenkinson SG, et al. Parapneumonic effusions. Am J Med. 1970;69:507–12.
119. Dorff GJ, Coonrod JD, Rytel MW. Detection by immunoelectrophoresis of antigen in sera of patients with pneumococcal bacteremia. Lancet. 1971;1:578–9.
120. Cerosalette KM, Roghmann MC, Bentley DW. Comparison of latex agglutination and counterimmunoelectrophoresis for the detection of pneumococcal antigen in elderly pneumonia patients. J Clin Microbiol. 1985; 22:553–7.
121. Ajello GW, Bolan GA, Hayes PS, et al. Commercial latex agglutination tests for detection of *Haemophilus influenzae* Type B and *Streptococcus pneumoniae* antigen in patients with bacteremic pneumonia. J Clin Microbiol. 1987;25:1388–91.
122. Palmer DL, Jones CC. Diagnosis of pneumococcal pneumonia. Semin Respir Infect. 1988;3:131–9.
123. Perlino CA. Laboratory diagnosis of pneumonia due to *Streptococcus pneumoniae*. J Infect Dis. 1985;150:139–144.
124. Coonrod JD, Wilson HD. Etiologic diagnosis of intrapleural empyema by counterimmunoelectrophoresis. Am Rev Respir Dis. 1976;113:637–41.
125. Krook A, Homberg H. Pneumococcal antigens in sputa: ELISA for the detection of pneumococcal C-polysaccharide in sputa from pneumonia patients. Diagn Microbiol Infect Dis. 1987;7:73–5.
126. Sands RL, Green ID. The diagnosis of pneumococcal chest infection by counter-current immunoelectrophoresis. J Appl Bacteriol. 1980;49:471–8.
127. Tugwell P, Greenwood BM. Pneumococcal antigen in lobar pneumonia. J Clin Pathol. 1975;28:118–23.
128. Congeni BL, Nankervis GA. Diagnosis of pneumonia by counterimmunoelectrophoresis of respiratory secretions. Am J Dis Child. 1978;132:684–7.
129. Downes BA, Ellner PD. Comparison of sputum counterimmunoelectrophoresis and culture in diagnosis of pneumococcal pneumonia. J Clin Microbiol. 1979;10:662–5.
130. Schmid RE, Anhalt JP, Wold AD, et al. II. Sputum counterimmunoelectrophoresis in the diagnosis of pneumococcal pneumonia. Am Rev Respir Dis. 1979;119:345–8.
131. Martin SJ, Hogansan DA, Thomas ET. Detection of *Streptococcus pneumoniae* and *Haemophilus influenzae* Type B antigens in acute nonbacteremic pneumonia. J Clin Microbiol. 1987;25:248–50.
132. Campbell JF, Spika JS. The serodiagnosis of nonpneumococcal bacterial pneumonia. Semin Respir Infect. 1988;3:123–30.
133. Lerner AM, Jankauskas K. The classic bacterial pneumonias. Disease-A-Month. Feb 1975:1–46.
134. Willman VL, Lewis JE, Hanlon CR. Staphylococcal pneumonia—surgical considerations in cases in infants and children. Arch Surg. 1961;83:93–7.
135. Highman JH. Staphylococcal pneumonia and empyema in childhood. Am J Roentgenol. 1969;106:103–8.
136. Dines DE. Diagnostic significance of pneumatocoeles of the lung. JAMA. 1968;204:1169–72.
137. Warner JO, Gordon I. Pneumatocoeles following *Haemophilus influenzae* pneumonia. Clin Radiol. 1981;32:99–105.
138. Luddy RE, Champion LA, Schwartz AD. *Pneumocystis carinii* pneumonia with pneumatocele formation. Am J Dis Child. 1977;131:470.
139. Scanlon GT, Unger JD. The radiology of bacterial and viral pneumonias. Radiol Clin North Am. 1973;11:317–38.
140. Bartlett JG, Finegold SM. Anaerobic pleuropulmonary infections. Medicine. 1972;51:413–50.
141. Lindsay MI, Morrow GW. Primary influenzal pneumonia. Postgrad Med. 1971;49:173–8.
142. Conte P, Heitzman ER, Markarian B. Viral pneumonia. Roentgen pathological correlations. Radiology. 1970;95:267–72.
143. Fine NL, Smith LR, Sheedy PF. Frequency of pleural effusions of mycoplasma and viral pneumonias. N Engl J Med. 1970;283:790–3.
144. Fraser DW, Tsai TR, Orenstein W, et al. Legionnaire's disease. Description of an epidemic of pneumonia. N Engl J Med. 1977;297:1189–97.
145. Kirby BD, Snyder KM, Meyer RD, et al. Legionnaire's disease—A cluster of cases (Abstract). Clin Res. 1978;26:A399.
146. Pope TL, Armstrong P, Thompson R, et al. Pittsburgh pneumonia agent chest film manifestations. AJR. 1982;138:237–41.
147. Tew J, Calenoff L, Berlin BS. Bacterial or nonbacterial pneumonia: Accuracy of radiographic diagnosis. Radiology. 1977;124:607–12.
148. Pennington JE. Community-acquired Pneumonia and Acute Bronchitis in Respiratory Infections: Diagnosis and Management. New York: Raven Press; 1973:125–34.
149. Garibaldi RA. Epidemiology of community acquired respiratory tract infections in adults: Incidence, etiology, and impact. Am J Med. 1985;78(Suppl 6B):32–7.
150. Kerttula Y, Leinonen M, Koskela M, et al. The aetiology of pneumonia. Application of bacterial serology and basic laboratory methods. J Infect. 1987;14:21–30.
151. Chatard JA. The leukocytes in acute lobar pneumonia. Johns Hopkins Hosp Rep. 1910;15:89–98.
152. Austrian R, Gold J. Pneumococcal bacteremia with especial reference to bacteremic pneumococcal pneumonia. Ann Intern Med. 1964;60:759–76.

153. MacFarlane JT, Finch RG, Ward MJ, et al. Hospital study of adult community acquired pneumonia. Lancet. 1982;2:255–8.
154. Klimek JJ, Ajemian E, Fontecchio S, et al. Community acquired bacterial pneumonia requiring admission to hospital. Am J Infect Cont. 1983;11:79–82.
155. Levy M, Dromer F, Brion N, et al. Community-acquired pneumonia: Importance of initial non-invasive bacteriologic and radiographic investigations. Chest. 1988;92:43–8.
156. Stratton CW. Bacterial pneumonia. An overview with emphasis on pathogenesis, diagnosis and treatment. Heart Lung. 1986;15:226–44.
157. Lipsky BA, Boyko EJ, Inui TS, et al. Risk factors for acquiring pneumococcal infections. Arch Intern Med. 1986;146:2179–85.
158. Rosner F, Zarrabi MH. Late infections following splenectomy in Hodgkin's disease. Cancer Invest. 1983;1:57–65.
159. Zarrabi MH, Rosner F. Serious infections in adults following splenectomy for trauma. Arch Intern Med. 1984;144:1421–4.
160. Crofton J. The chemotherapy of bacterial respiratory infections. Am Rev Respir Dis. 1970;101:841–59.
161. Hirschmann JV, Everett ED. *Haemophilus influenzae* infections in adults: Report of nine cases and a review of literature. Medicine. 1979;58:80–94.
162. Hausmann W, Karlish AJ. Staphylococcal pneumonia in adults. Br Med J. 1956;2:845–7.
163. Schwarzmann SW, Adler JL, Sullivan RJ, et al. Bacterial pneumonia during the Hong Kong influenza epidemic of 1968–1969. Experience in a city-county hospital. Arch Intern Med. 1971;127:1037–41.
164. Louria DB, Blumenfeld HL, Ellis JT, et al. Studies on influenza. J Clin Invest. 1959;38:213–65.
165. Yu VL, Kroboth FJ, Shonnard J, et al. Legionnaire's disease: New clinical perspective from a prospective pneumonia study. Am J Med. 1982;73:357–61.
166. Nicotra B, Rivera M, Luman I, et al. *Branhamella catarrhalis* as a lower respiratory tract pathogen in patients with chronic lung disease. Arch Intern Med. 1986;146:890–3.
167. Slevin NJ, Aitken J, Thornleg PE. Clinical and microbiological features of *Branhamella catarrhalis* bronchopulmonary infections. Lancet. 1987;1:782–3.
168. Wallace RJ Jr, Musher DM. In honor of Dr. Sarah Branham. A star is born: The realization of *Branhamella catarrhalis* as a respiratory pathogen. Chest. 1986;90:447–50.
169. Gross JS, Neufeld RR, Libon LS, et al. Autopsy study of the elderly institutionalized patients: Review of 234 autopsies. Arch Intern Med. 1988;148:173–6.
170. Verghese A, Berk SL. Bacterial pneumonia in the elderly. Medicine. 1983;62:271–85.
171. Garb JL, Brown RB, Garb JR, et al. Differences in etiology of pneumonias in nursing home and community patients. JAMA. 1978;240:2169–72.
172. Ebright JR, Rytel MW. Bacterial pneumonia in the elderly. J Am Geriatr Soc. 1980;28:220–3.
173. Gleckman RA, Esposito AL. Bacterial pneumonia in the elderly: A reappraisal of conventional therapy with a note on cefamandole. J Am Geriatr Soc. 1979;27:345–7.
174. Berk KC, Holtsdan SA, Wiener SL, et al. Nontypeable *Haemophilus influenzae* in the elderly. Arch Intern Med. 1982;142:532–9.
175. Valenti WM, Trudell RG, Bentley DW. Factors predisposing to oropharyngeal colonization with gram-negative bacilli in the aged. N Engl J Med. 1978;298:1108–11.
176. Murray JF, Felton CP, Garay SM, et al. Pulmonary complications of the acquired immunodeficiency syndrome. Report of a National Heart, Lung and Blood Institute Workshop. N Engl J Med. 1984;310:1682–8.
177. Stover DE, White DA, Romano PA, et al. Spectrum of pulmonary diseases associated with the acquired immune deficiency syndrome. Am J Med. 1985;78:429–37.
178. Bartlett JG, Gorbach SL. The triple threat of aspiration pneumonia. Chest. 1979;68:560–6.
179. Wynne JW, Modell JH. Respiratory aspiration of stomach contents. Ann Intern Med. 1977;87:466–74.
180. Lorber B, Swenson RM. Bacteriology of aspiration pneumonia. A prospective study of community and hospital-acquired cases. Ann Intern Med. 1974;81:329–31.
181. Mogabgab WJ. *Mycoplasma pneumoniae* and adenovirus respiratory illness in military and university personnel 1959–1966. Am Rev Respir Dis. 1968;97:345–58.
182. Forsyth BR, Bloom HH, Johnson KM, et al. Etiology of primary atypical pneumonia in a military population. JAMA. 1965;191:364–8.
183. Wenzel RP, McCormick DP, Smith EP, et al. Acute respiratory disease: Clinical and epidemiologic observations of military trainees. Military Med. 1971;136:873–80.
184. Grayston JT, Kenny GE, Foy HM, et al. Epidemiological studies of *Mycoplasma pneumoniae* infections in civilians. Ann NY Acad Sci. 1967;143:436–46.
185. Mufson MA, Manko MA, Kingston JR, et al. Eaton agent pneumonia—clinical features. JAMA. 1961;178:369–74.
186. Tack KJ, Peterson PK, Rasp FL, et al. Isolation of *Chlamydia trachomatis* from the lower respiratory tracts of adults. Lancet. 1980;1:116–20.
187. Komaroff AL, Aronson MD, Schachter J. *Chlamydia trachomatis* infections in adults with community acquired pneumonia. JAMA. 1981;245:1319–22.
188. Beem MO, Saxon EM. Respiratory tract colonization and a distinctive pneumonia syndrome in infants infected with *Chlamydia trachomatis*. N Engl J Med. 1977;296:306–10.
189. Frommell GT, Bruhn FW, Schwartzman JD. Isolation of *Chlamydia trachomatis* from infant lung tissue. N Engl J Med. 1977;296:1150–2.
190. Cranston JT, Juo C, Wang S, et al. A new *Chlamydia psittaci* strain, TWAR, isolated in acute respiratory tract infection. N Engl J Med. 1986;315:161–8.
191. Marrie TJ, Grayston JT, Wang S, et al. Pneumonia associated with the TWAR strain of *Chlamydia*. Ann Intern Med. 1987;106:507–11.
192. George RB, Mogabgab WJ. Atypical pneumonia with rhinovirus infections. Ann Intern Med. 1969;71:1073–8.
193. Jahn CL, Felton OL, Cherry JD. Coxsackie B1 pneumonia in an adult. JAMA. 1964;189:236–7.
194. Wenzel RP, McCormick DP, Beam WE Jr. Parainfluenza pneumonia in adults. JAMA. 1972;221:294–5.
195. Respiratory syncytial virus—Missouri. Morbid Mortal Wkly Rep. 1977; 26:351.
196. Sorvillo FJ, Huie SF, Strassburg MA, et al. An outbreak of respiratory syncytial virus pneumonia in a nursing home for the elderly. J Infect. 1984;9:252–6.
197. Kasupski GJ, Leers WD. Presumed respiratory syncytial virus pneumonia in three immunocompromised adults. Am J Med Sci. 1983;285:28–33.
198. Legionnaire's disease: Diagnosis and management. Ann Intern Med. 1978;88:363–5.
199. Helms CM, Viner JP, Sturm RH. Comparative features of pneumococcal, mycoplasmal, and legionnaire's disease pneumonias. Ann Intern Med. 1979;90:543–7.
200. Ludmerer KM, Kissare JM. Pulmonary infiltrates and eosinophilia in a young man. Am J Med. 1986;81:533–40.
201. Schatz M, Wasserman S, Patterson R. Eosinophils and immunologic lung disease. Med Clin North Am. 1981;65:1055–71.
202. Citro LA, Gordon ME, Miller WT. Eosinophilic lung disease (or how to slice P.I.E.). Am J Roentgenol. 1973;117:787–97.
203. Liebow AA, Carrington CB. The eosinophilic pneumonias. Medicine. 1969;48:251–85.
204. Jederlinic PJ, Sicilian L, Graensler EA. Chronic eosinophilic pneumonia. Medicine. 1988;67:154–62.
205. Haley RW, Culver DH, White JW, et al. The nationwide nosocomial infection rate: A new need for vital statistics. Am J Epidemiol. 1985;121:159–67.
206. Simmons BP, Wong ES. CDC guidelines for the prevention and control of nosocomial infections: Guideline for prevention of nosocomial pneumonia. Am J Infect Control. 1983;11:230–3.
207. Haley RN, Hooton TM, Culver DH, et al. Nosocomial infections in U.S. hospitals 1975–1976. Am J Med. 1981;70:947–59.
208. Toews GB. Nosocomial pneumonia. Clin Chest Med. 1987;8:467–79.
209. Hooten TM, Haley RW, Culver DH, et al. The joint association of multiple role factors with the occurrence of nosocomial infection. Am J Med. 1981;70:960–70.
210. Donowitz LG, Page MC, Mileur BL, et al. Alteration of normal gastric flora in critical care patients receiving antacid and cimetidine therapy. Infect Control. 1986;7:23–6.
211. Snepar R, Poporad GA, Romano JM, et al. Effect of cimetidine and antacid on gastric microbial flora. Infect Immun. 1982;36:518–24.
212. Driks MR, Craven DE, Celli BR, et al. Nosocomial pneumonia in intubated patients given sucralfate as compared with antacids or histamine type-2 blockers. The role of gastric colonization. N Engl J Med. 1987;317:1376–82.
213. Wilson WR, Cockerill FR, Rosenow EC III. Pulmonary disease in the immunocompromised host. Mayo Clin Proc. 1985;60:610–31.
214. Schimpff SC, Young VM, Greene WH, et al. Origin of infection in acute nonlymphocytic leukemia: Significance of hospital acquisition of potential pathogens. Ann Intern Med. 1972;77:707–14.
215. Chang HY, Rodriguez V, Narboni G, et al. Causes of death in adults with acute leukemia. Medicine. 1976;55:259–68.
216. Peterson PK, Ferguson R, Fryd DS, et al. Infectious disease in hospitalized renal transplant recipients: A prospective study of a complex and evolving problem. Medicine. 1982;61:360–72.
217. Ramsey PG, Rubin RH, Tolkoff-Rubin NE, et al. The renal transplant patient with fever and pulmonary infiltrates: Etiology, clinical manifestations and management. Medicine. 1980;59:206–22.
218. Winston DJ, Gale RP, Meyer DV, et al. Infectious complications of human bone marrow transplantation. Medicine. 1979;58:1–31.
219. Valdivieso M, Gil-Extremera G, Zoronoza J, et al. Gram-negative bacillary pneumonia in the compromised host. Medicine. 1977;56:241–4.
220. Sickles EA, Young VM, Greene WH, et al. Pneumonia in acute leukemia. Ann Intern Med. 1973;79:528–34.
221. Donowitz GR, Mandell GR. Beta-lactam antibiotics (parts 1 and 2). N Engl J Med. 1988;318:419–26, 490–500.
222. Finegold SM, Wexler HM. Therapeutic implications of bacteriologic findings in mixed aerobic-anaerobic infections. Antimicrob Agents Chemother. 1988;32:611–16.
223. Murray PR, Rosenblatt JE. Penicillin resistance and penicillinase production in clinical isolates of *Bacteroides melaninogenicus*. Antimicrob Agents Chemother. 1977;11:605–8.
224. Kirby BD, George WL, Sutter VL, et al. Gram-negative anerobic bacilli: Their role in infection and patterns of susceptibility to antimicrobial agents. I. Little known *Bacteroides* species. Rev Infect Dis. 1980;2:914–51.

225. Bawdon RE, Crane LR, Palchaudhuri S. Antibiotic resistance in anaerobic bacteria: Molecular biology and clinical aspects. Rev Infect Dis. 1982; 4:1075–95.
226. Aldridge KE, Sanders CV, Janney A, et al. Comparison of the activities of penicillin G and new beta-lactam antibiotics against clinical isolates of *Bacteroides* species. Antimicrob Agents Chemother. 1984;26:410–3.
227. Levison ME, Mangura CT, Lorber B, et al. Clindamycin compared with penicillin for the treatment of anaerobic lung abscess. Ann Intern Med. 1983;98:466–71.
228. Bartlett JG, Gorbach SL. Penicillin or clindamycin for primary lung abscess. Ann Intern Med. 1983;98:546–8.

54. PLEURAL EFFUSION AND EMPYEMA

RICHARD E. BRYANT

Although the clinical course and need for surgical drainage of pleural empyema were known to Hippocrates, most of the changes in its recognition and treatment are of recent origin.[1,2] Microbial contamination of the pleural space is usually secondary to pneumonia but may arise from extrapulmonic infection and complicate neoplasm, collagen vascular disease, trauma, or medical or surgical procedures involving the pleura.[2] The mode of presentation is modified by the origin of the infection, the infecting microorganisms, and the patient's underlying disease(s).

ETIOLOGY

Medical and societal changes have modified the types of organisms causing empyema.[3–5] In 1935 acute bacterial empyema at the Boston City Hospital was caused by *Streptococcus pneumoniae* (46 percent), hemolytic streptococci (18 percent), *Staphylococcus aureus* (9 percent), gram-negative bacilli (3 percent), mixed aerobes (6 percent), and anaerobes (13 percent).[3] The cause of bacterial empyema from that institution in 1965 was *S. pneumoniae* (12 percent), hemolytic streptococci (5 percent), *Staph. aureus* (15 percent), gram-negative bacilli (25 percent), mixed aerobes (14 percent), and anaerobes (24 percent).[3] A report from Iowa described a 4-fold fall in the frequency of pneumococcal empyema and a 1.5- and 5-fold increase in staphylococcal and gram-negative bacillary empyema, respectively, in a comparable period.[4] These changes in microbial etiology may be explained by the changes in the types of patients developing empyema. In otherwise healthy patients with pneumonia, the most common causes of pleural empyema may still be *Staph. aureus, S. pneumoniae*, and *Streptococcus pyogenes*.[5] Staphylococcal empyema is especially common in children.

The recent increase in recognition of anaerobic empyema is due to improved microbiologic techniques and recognition of anaerobic infection associated with aspiration pneumonia, putrid lung abscess, and pleural infection arising from oropharyngeal or gastrointestinal sites.[6,7] Bartlett and coworkers found that pleural empyema was caused by aerobic bacteria in 24 percent, anaerobic bacteria in 35 percent, and both aerobic and anaerobic bacteria in 41 percent of 83 medical service patients without prior antibiotic therapy or surgical procedures.[6] Empyema secondary to subdiaphragmatic disease is often polymicrobial and anaerobic in origin.[8]

There is a high frequency of *Staph. aureus* and aerobic gram-negative bacillary infection in patients with post-traumatic or nosocomial empyema.[5,9] Empyema complicating hemothorax is often staphylococcal, while that associated with pneumothorax or serous effusion is often caused by gram-negative aerobic bacilli.[9] Immunocompromised patients have a higher frequency of empyema caused by fungi and gram-negative bacilli.[10] Organ transplant recipients and patients with the acquired immunodeficiency syndrome may reactivate pleural foci of mycobacterial or fungal infection but will rarely present with empyema without disseminated disease. Unsuccessful resection of cavitary coccidioidomycosis may be complicated by empyema from that organism. The association of fistulous tracts from the pleura suggests the possibility of actinomycosis, nocardiosis, or tuberculosis. Less common causes of empyema include extension of extrapulmonic infection caused by salmonella, clostridia, or *Entamoeba histolytica*.

PATHOGENESIS

Pleural effusions are caused by altered oncotic or capillary pressure from renal, cardiac, hepatic, or metabolic diseases. Pleural effusions may occur in 40–50 percent of patients with pneumonia.[2] However, only a small percentage (≈5 percent) of parapneumonic effusions become exudates with the associated microbiologic, chemical, and physical features of empyema.[2,11] Microorganisms gain access to the pleura by direct extension from the lung; from blood or lymphatics; by extension from subdiaphragmatic, mediastinal, pericardial, or cervical infection; and by transthoracic entry from trauma, surgery, or manipulative procedures. Patients with trauma to the esophagus, mediastinum, or heart or those who have had surgery in those areas are at increased risk of infection extending to the pleura. Similarly, patients with retropharyngeal or paravertebral suppurative disease may present with pleural empyema. As the efficiency of trauma rescue programs increase, the frequency of empyema associated with chest and head trauma will increase.[9,10]

Empyema fluid is deficient in opsonins and complement needed for optimal phagocytic function and ultimately develops extremes of hypoxia and acidity that further impair local neutrophil activity.[12,13] Endotoxins and other toxic factors elaborated by bacteria suppress the leukocyte host defense function and permit the growth of bacteria to concentrations of 10^8 bacteria per milliliter of empyema fluid.[14]

Inflammatory exudates may become loculated in a relatively small area or may extend to involve virtually the entire hemithorax, leading to ventilatory dysfunction and to the signs and symptoms of overwhelming sepsis and multiple organ failure. The exuberant inflammatory response can on occasion lead to erosion of the chest wall and to spontaneous drainage of the empyema.

Empyema fluid inhibits antimicrobial efficacy by a number of means. Aminoglycoside activity is suppressed by acid pH (minimum inhibitory concentration [MIC] is increased ≥64-fold by a 1-unit drop in pH), hypoxia (membrane transport of aminoglycosides is an oxygen-dependent step), increased concentrations of divalent cations, and binding of aminoglycosides to the DNA present in pleural pus.[14,15] β-Lactamase from microorganisms can degrade β-lactamase-susceptible β-lactam antibiotics, and chloramphenicol may be degraded by microbial enzymes in pus.[14] Moreover, late in the course of the disease, the growth of organisms within empyema fluid is suppressed to the extent that bacteria become refractory to antibiotic therapy.

By convention, the phases of empyema formation are divided into the *exudate phase*, during which leukocytes increase until pus is formed; the *fibropurulent phase*, during which fibrin formation begins to limit expansion of the lung; and the *organizing phase*, during which fibroblast formation and scarring produce a thick, leathery encasement that traps the lung.[16]

Microbe specific factors affect the pathophysiology of pleural space infection. Induction of experimental empyema in guinea pigs requires inoculation of $>10^6$ organisms per milliliter of

Escherichia coli, or *Staph. aureus* plus *Bacteroides fragilis*, in order to infect >50 percent of animals.[17] Use of umbilical tape as a foreign body does not increase lethality, but addition of blood greatly enhances the lethality of challenge with *E. coli* and *B. fragilis* mixtures.[17]

CLINICAL PRESENTATION

The clinical presentation of empyema is largely nonspecific and reflects the findings of the underlying disease. Patients may have chest pain, dyspnea, weight loss, chills, fever, or night sweats.[4] Development or persistence of fever and leukocytosis in a patient at risk of having a pleural empyema is frequently a clue to its presence. Physical examination often reveals signs of an effusion, but may be unchanged except for altered vital signs. A high index of suspicion and recognition of factors that predispose patients to the development of pleural empyema are the keys to its recognition.

Pleural effusion is demonstrated radiologically when at least 300–500 cc of fluid causes blunting of the costophrenic angles[11]

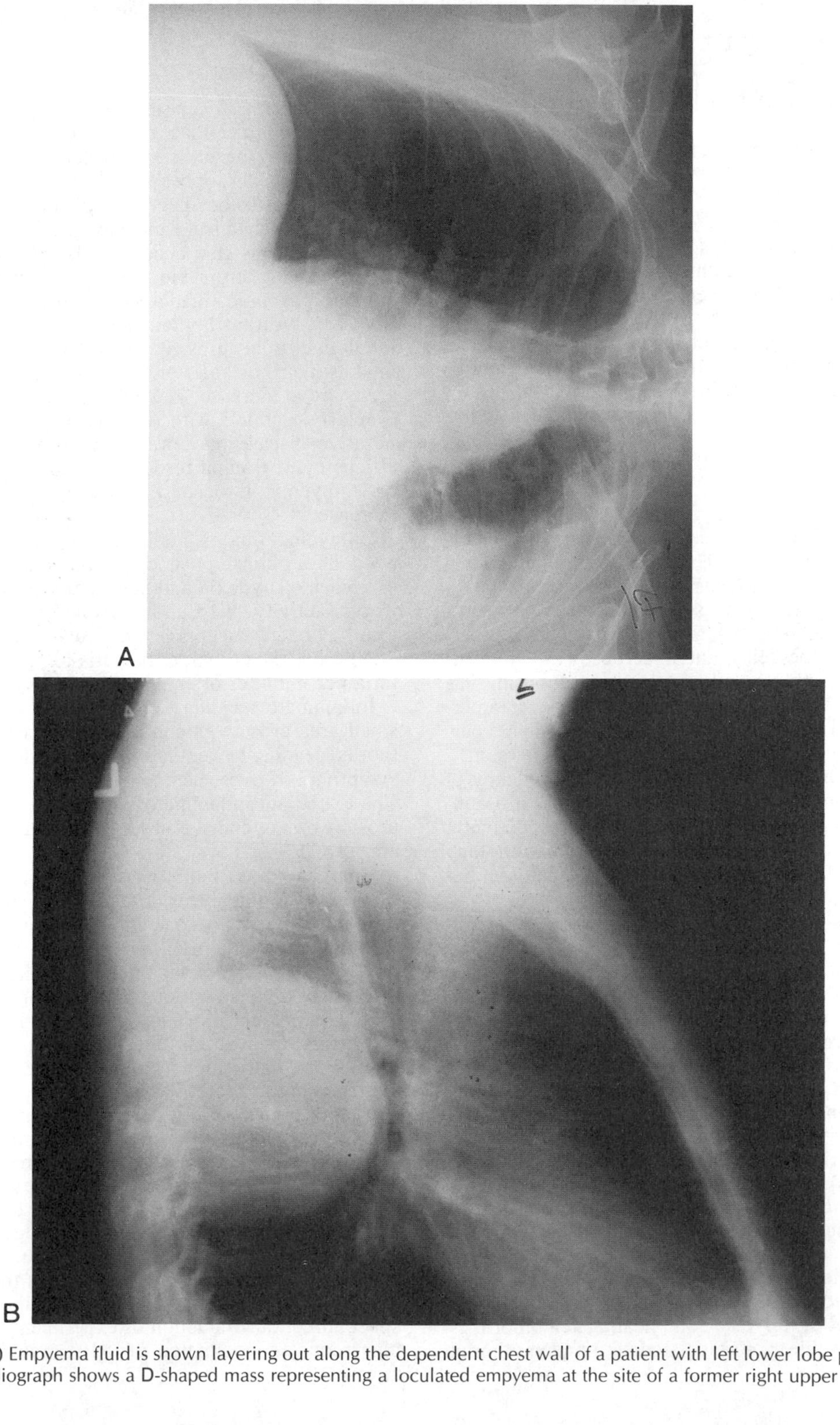

FIG. 1 **(A)** Empyema fluid is shown layering out along the dependent chest wall of a patient with left lower lobe pneumonia. **(B)** The radiograph shows a D-shaped mass representing a loculated empyema at the site of a former right upper lobectomy.

(Fig. 1). Lateral views often show a fluid meniscus and loss of distinct margins of the diaphragm. Lateral decubitus views permit detection of smaller volumes of fluid (100–200 cc) and verify the absence of loculation as fluid "layers out" along the dependent chest wall.[11] Conventional x-ray films may not distinguish effusions developing in interlobar or subpulmonic spaces. Similarly, loculated empyema with a bronchopleural fistula may resemble a lung abscess.

Empyema complicating extensive pneumonia may be difficult to recognize when the lung densities and pleural fluid overlap. Similarly, small volumes of pleural fluid may not be apparent on conventional x-ray films. Fortunately, both ultrasound and computer tomography provide more sensitive techniques for pleural fluid detection.[18,19] Pleural fluid aspiration under ultrasound guidance provides an accurate and safe means of obtaining infected pleural fluid and is especially helpful when fluid volumes are small or loculated.[20,21] However, it is not necessary to tap all parapneumonic effusions if the volume of fluid is small (less than 1 cm in depth on lateral decubitus films), the patient is doing well, and the x-ray picture is improving.[11,22,23]

Computed tomography (CT) is especially helpful for demonstrating pleural fluid accumulation due to extension from mediastinal or subdiaphragmatic disease[19,20] (Fig. 2). This technology can also distinguish between loculated pleural effusions

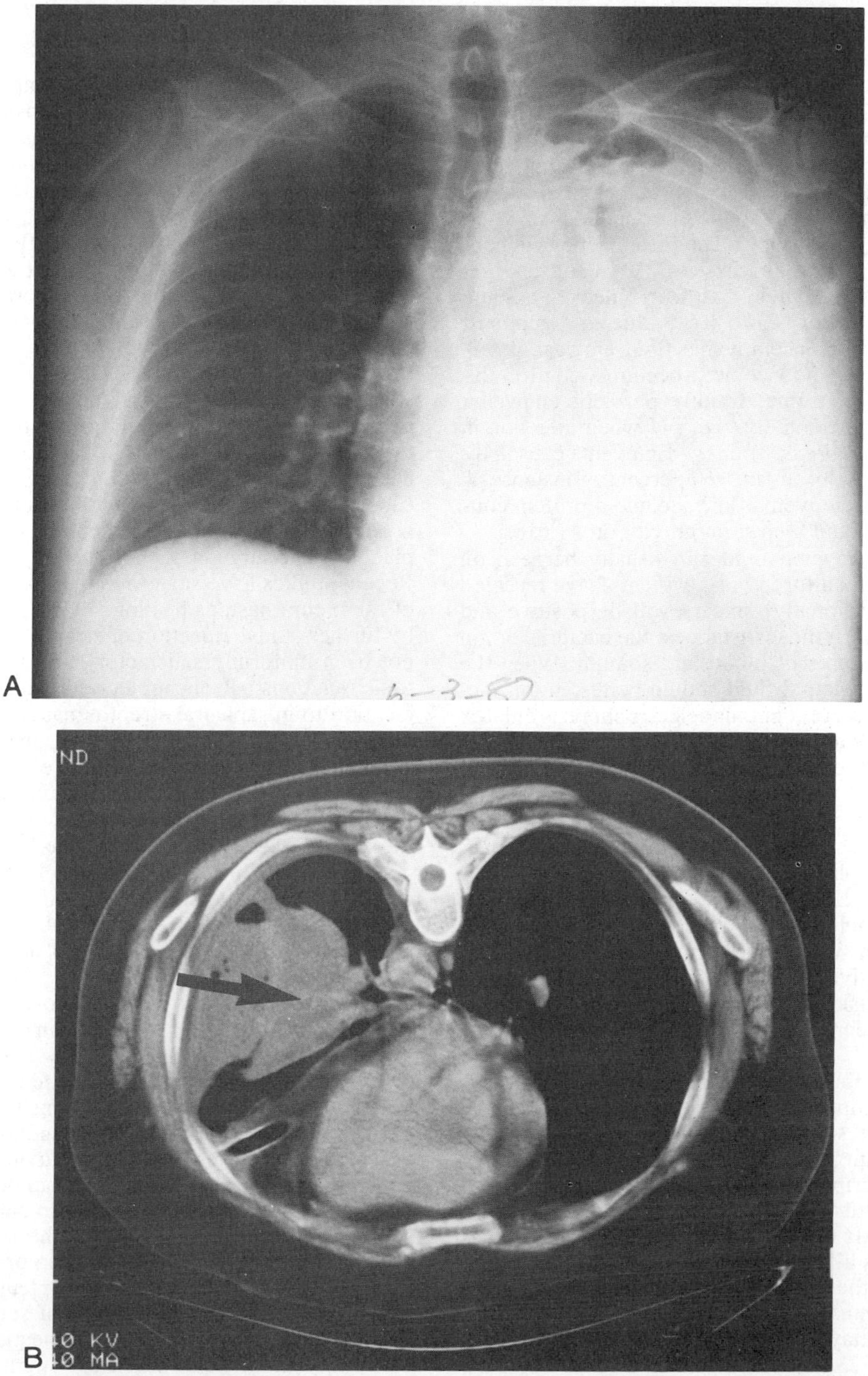

FIG. 2 **(A)** The patient's empyema progressed despite percutaneous drainage and appropriate antibiotic therapy. **(B)** Computed tomography showed malposition of chest tubes, but all attempts at tube drainage failed. The arrow designates the loculated empyema. The patient responded promptly to surgical decortication.

with bronchopleural fistulas and lung abscesses. CT has largely replaced the need for bronchograms to demonstrate bronchopleural fistulas. However, bronchoscopy and bronchography may be needed to define the cause of pleural empyema in patients in whom the etiology of infection is unexplained.[1]

Empyema is documented by finding pus and/or high concentrations of microorganisms in exudative pleural fluid obtained by thoracentesis. The character of the fluid depends on the type and duration of the infection and the associated trauma, surgery, malignancy, or other underlying disease. Initially, the fluid is thin and serous, but it becomes thick and purulent as neutrophil accumulation occurs. The poor correlation between the white blood cell counts in empyema fluid and the clinical features of infection may be due to lysis of neutrophils in pus. However, the status of the infection can be assessed by measuring pleural fluid pH, glucose, and lactic dehydrogenase.[11,22] Empyema fluid characteristically has a pH of less than 7.2, glucose less than 40 mg/dl, and lactic dehydrogenase activity of ≥600–1000 mg/dl.[11,22] Demonstration of these features or the presence of large numbers of bacteria on Gram stain suggests that drainage procedures are necessary. The pH of empyema fluid has the best correlation with the extent of the inflammatory process. Acid pH is primarily metabolic in origin and is caused secondarily by local CO_2 retention.[23] The mean lactic acid concentration of pus from human abscesses is 30 mg/dl, and pH values may be as low as 5.5. Thus, it is not prudent to assume that an empyema fluid pH of 6.0 to 6.5 is due to a ruptured esophagus unless tests like an empyema fluid amylase determination and radiologic or endoscopic procedures confirm the diagnosis. At the other extreme, frankly purulent empyema fluid can have a disproportionately high pH when infection is caused by urea-splitting *Proteus* strains.[24] Empyema caused by anaerobic bacteria is malodorous in ≈60 percent of instances.[6] Less specific findings of empyema fluid include a protein concentration of >3.0 mg/dl and a specific gravity of >1.018.[2]

Microorganisms in empyema fluid can usually be seen on Gram stain and grown in culture unless patients have received antibiotic therapy. Occasionally, smears will be positive and cultures will be negative. In those instances, the bacterial origin should be sought by cultures of blood and sputum. When the diagnosis is in question, pleural fluid should be tested for bacterial antigen by countercurrent immunoelectrophoresis or latex agglutination studies. In addition, fluid should be tested for *Legionella* by direct fluorescent antibody stains and culture because that organism will not be seen on conventional Gram stains. Empyema fluid devoid of microorganisms should also be examined for anaerobes, fungi, mycobacteria, and amoebae. Patients thought to have pleural or pulmonary amebiasis should have serologic tests for *E. histolytica*. Patients at risk of developing nocardiosis should have modified acid-fast stains. Acridine orange may permit visualization of organisms in abscess fluid that is smear negative by Gram stain. It should be noted that chylous pleural effusions may resemble purulent material, but lack white cells or microorganisms and remain opaque after centrifugation.[2]

Potts and coworkers found no bacteria on microscopic examination of 4 of 10 empyema fluids.[23] Two were sterile by culture. Smear-negative sterile empyema fluid has been reported in 6 to 15 percent[1,25] of patients, and culture-negative empyema has been described in up to 37 percent of patients.[25] Although improper culture technique, fastidious microorganisms, and prior antibiotic therapy may account for many cases of sterile empyema. It is likely that certain organisms are killed in pus. However, by the time bacterial empyemas become frankly purulent, they must be drained, whether sterile or not.

Pleural tuberculosis may be diagnosed by pleural fluid cultures or stains in 18 to 23 percent of patients or by cultures, stains, and histologic examination of pleural biopsy specimens in up to 95 percent of patients.[26] Liquid culture media are preferable to solid culture media, and it is rarely necessary to culture more than a single biopsy specimen. Radiometric culture detection methods may increase the speed of diagnosis in patients with pleural tuberculosis. A history of exposure, skin test conversion, or symptoms of weight loss, night sweats, and fever are helpful clues to the diagnosis of tuberculosis. However, patients may be both afebrile and anergic.

The pleural fluid of patients with rheumatoid arthritis, pancreatitis, or malignancy will occasionally have features suggestive of empyema.[2] The rare malignant effusion with a pH of <7.0 is readily diagnosed by cytologic examination and is associated with a worse prognosis than that of alkaline pleural fluid.[22] Exudates of rheumatoid or pancreatic origin only rarely have a pH of <7.2 and can be identified by serologic tests or increased pleural fluid amylase levels, respectively.[2]

TREATMENT

The goals for treatment of pleural empyema are eradication of infection, drainage of pus, and expansion of the lung. The primary treatment of empyema is drainage and will be necessary for patients with pleural fluid containing gross pus, a heavy growth of organisms visible by microscopy, a pH <7.2, glucose <40 mg/dl, and lactic dehydrogenase >1000 mg/dl.[11,22] Those with smear-negative serous pleural fluid with a pH ≥7.2 and intermediate lactic dehydrogenase and glucose levels may be treated with antibiotics and repeat thoracentesis in 12–18 hours to reassess the need for drainage procedures.[11] Those with improving pleural fluid parameters may be followed and reassessed.[11,22]

Repeated thoracentesis is rarely adequate unless the empyema fluid is quite thin and present in small volume. Percutaneous drainage of thin or serous fluid with small-bore catheters early in the course of empyema has been successful. Closed chest tube drainage with an underwater-sealed system is successful in two-thirds of patients, and the system can be placed by the surgeon, the radiologist, or the pulmonologist.[27,28] Recent studies have suggested that thoracoscopy and irrigation of the pleura hastens healing.[29] This needs to be substantiated by further study. Injection of streptokinase into the pleura has not been uniformly satisfactory and has been associated with toxic reactions.[2] Bronchopleural fistula is an absolute contraindication to intrapleural streptokinase.

The need for continued vacuum or water-sealed drainage is assessed by measuring the volume of fluid drained daily and by the size of the residual pleural cavity. Tubes can usually be withdrawn gradually when drainage is less than 50 ml/day and the cavity is less than 50 ml in size.[1,28]

Drainage of thick pleural pus is largely the province of the chest surgeon, who should be involved early in the course of such patients.[28–34] Closed chest tube drainage fails in approximately one-third of patients, who often have more extensive disease or prior chest surgery.[9,10,28] In addition, immunocompromised patients may require more extensive drainage procedures, including early rib resection and open drainage.[10] Management of open drainage tubes with daily irrigation and convalescence for 3–4 months is a tedious and time-consuming but time-honored method. In young adults who are otherwise healthy and are good operative candidates, decortication may be preferable.[27] This procedure provides more rapid recovery and more complete restoration of pulmonary function in adults but may be needed less frequently in children.[1,27] Decortication is traditionally advocated during the second or third week or after the sixth week of the disease in order to minimize the risk of tearing the poorly demarcated pleural peel during the 3–6 weeks of illness. The importance of surgical timing for the decortication procedure has been questioned.[31] Although small bronchopleural fistulas may close spontaneously, many are difficult to treat and require surgical closure. There is considerable variation in the frequency with which surgeons at different centers use rib resection, decortication, or empyectomy to manage empyema.[1,10,32,33] Similarly, several methods are used to treat chronic empyema or empyema that occurs after pneumonectomy. These operative approaches are selected on the basis of expected benefits and risks. Tube drainage has the fewest side effects, is tried first, and is rarely successful in that setting. Alternatives include permanent drainage, obliteration of the empyema space by muscle flaps, sterilization by instillation of antibiotics, and thoracoplasty.[34] The open window thoracostomy procedure devised by Eloesser was adapted to manage postpneumonectomy empyema. It can be used as permanent therapy for patients unable to undergo more extensive surgery.[31,32,34] Patients with bronchopleural fistulas that do not close with tube drainage are often treated successfully with muscle flap transposition by suturing the muscle directly to the bronchus or adjacent to the closed bronchial stump and using the muscle mass to obliterate the empyema cavity.[34] Patients with empyema and residual lung but without bronchopleural fistulas may respond to decortication or, if that fails, to myoplasty. Those without residual lung may respond to placement or irrigation with 0.25% neomycin in the closed chest cavity.[34] However, the risk of noemycin toxicity is substantial and makes this approach less desirable. Thoracoplasty is usually the procedure of last resort.[34]

Tuberculous pleural effusions rarely require more than antibiotic therapy unless a bronchopleural fistula is present. Special care should be taken not to introduce a secondary bacterial infection while performing a diagnostic or therapeutic thoracentesis of a tuberculosis pleural effusion.

The guidelines for optimal antibiotic therapy of bacterial empyema differ little from the recommendations for treatment of suppurative disease at other sites. Antibiotics are selected on the basis of their activity against microorganisms causing or presumed to be causing infection. There is virtually no problem in achieving adequate levels of antibiotics in empyema fluid with parenteral agents.[35] However if the empyema is caused by β-lactamase-producing organisms, β-lactamase-susceptible antibiotics should not be used. β-Lactam antibiotics should be used in high doses for prolonged periods, i.e., usually 2–4 weeks for bacterial infection. Patients with nocardiosis, actinomycosis, tuberculosis, or fungal empyema require even more prolonged therapy. In addition, patients with long-standing bacterial empyema may require prolonged therapy. Aminoglycosides should not be used as single-drug therapy of bacterial empyemas because they are toxic drugs with poor activity in the abscess milieu.[13] However, aminoglycosides may be combined with β-lactam antibiotics to achieve synergistic activity against empyema caused by *Pseudomonas aeruginosa, Enterobacter cloacae, Acinetobacter calcoaceticus*, and *Serratia marcescens*. Ciprofloxacin will probably play a major role in the long-term treatment of gram-negative empyema because it is a potent drug that can be given orally. At present, experience with this agent is too limited to permit it to be recommended as an initial drug of choice for therapy of empyema.

Anaerobic pleural empyema can be treated adequately with clindamycin, β-lactamase-stable β-lactams, or combinations of β-lactam and β-lactamase inhibitors. Although metronidazole is an excellent agent for anaerobic infection, it may be ineffective in anaerobic lung abscesses or partially drained empyemas because the drug is not reduced to its active metabolite in a partially oxygenated environment. Chloramphenicol or tetracycline should not be used to treat empyema caused by anaerobes.

PROGNOSIS

The mortality rate of pleural empyema is affected by the type and severity of infection, the patient's health or associated underlying diseases, and the adequacy of antibiotic therapy and drainage. The complexity of this picture is shown by the fact that the mortality due to empyema at Boston City Hospital rose from 38 percent in 1935 to 49 percent in 1965 despite the availability of antibiotics during the latter year.[3] Although mortality rates of 8 to 15 percent have been reported in otherwise healthy young patients,[27,33] rates of 40 to 70 percent have been reported in the elderly and in groups with severe underlying disease.[10,27] Mortality is increased in patients with nosocomial infection or empyema caused by polymicrobial or resistant gram-negative bacteria.[4] Patients with inadequately drained empyemas often die.[6] There are no criteria validating the superiority of a single technique, but in general, the more fragile or compromised patient may need more rapid achievement of adequate drainage by rib resection, lysis of adhesions, and use of a large-bore drainage tube earlier in the illness because such patients are more vulnerable to the serious sequelae of malnutrition, chronic sepsis, and multiple organ failure associated with delayed drainage of pus.[10] Post-traumatic empyema has a worse prognosis and should be considered for early decortication if (*1*) sepsis is not contained despite adequate antibiotic therapy, (*2*) fluid levels persist, (*3*) ventilatory function is compromised by inadequate lung expansion, or (*4*) pleural drainage is inadequate after 2 weeks of therapy.[9,10] An infected hemothorax rarely responds to tube drainage alone because clots obstruct the tube. Polymicrobial or nosocomial infection carries a worse prognosis because such patients have multiple underlying diseases and poor host defense.[4,5,32] In addition, these patients have an increased frequency of colonization and infection with multiply resistant gram-negative bacilli.[5] Thus, the sickest and most infirm patients often have pus that is hard to drain and organisms that are difficult to treat.

REFERENCES

1. Sherman MM, Subramanian V, Berger RL. Management of thoracic empyema. Am J Surg. 1977;133:474–9.
2. Light RW. Clinical manifestations and useful tests. In: Light RW, ed. Pleural Diseases. Philadelphia: Lea & Febiger; 1983:33–60.
3. Finland M, Barnes MW. Changing ecology of acute bacterial empyema. J Infect Dis. 1978;137:274–91.
4. Weese WC, Shindler ER, Smith IM, et al. Empyema of the thorax then and now. Arch Intern Med. 1973;131:516–20.
5. Vianna NJ. Nontuberculous bacterial empyema in patients with and without underlying disease. JAMA. 1971;215:69–71.
6. Bartlett JG, Finegold SM. Anaerobic infections of the lung and pleural space. Am Rev Resp Dis. 1974;110:56–77.
7. Barlett JG, Thadepalli H, Gorbach SL, et al. Bacteriology of empyema. Lancet. 1974;1:338–40.
8. Ballantyne KC, Sethia B, Reece IJ, et al. Empyema following intra-abdominal sepsis. Br J Surg. 1984;71:723–5.
9. Caplan ES, Hoyt NJ, Rodriguez A, et al. Empyema occurring in the multiply traumatized patient. J Trauma. 1984;24:785–98.
10. Lemmer JH, Botham MJ, Orringer MD. Modern management of adult thoracic empyema. J Thorac Cardiovasc Surg. 1985;90:849–55.
11. Light RW. Parapneumonic effusions and infections of the pleural space. In: Light RW, ed. Pleural Diseases. Philadelphia: Lea & Febiger; 1983:101–18.
12. Lew P, Zubler R, Vaudauz P. Decreased heat-labile opsonic activity and complement levels associated with evidence of C3 breakdown products in infected pleural effusions. J Clin Invest. 1979;63:326–34.
13. Bryant RE. Pus: Friend or foe? In: Root RK, Trunkey D, Sande MD, eds. Contemporary Issues in Infectious Diseases. v. V: New Surgical and Medical Approaches. New York: Churchill Livingstone, 1987;31–48.
14. Bryant RE. Effect of the suppurative environment on antibiotic activity. In: Root RK, Sand MD, eds. Contemporary Issues in Infectious Diseases. v. 1: New Dimensions in Antimicrobial Therapy. New York: Churchill Livingstone, 1984;313–37.
15. Vaudaux P, Waldvogel FA. Gentamicin inactivation in purulent exudates; role of cell lysis. J Infect Dis. 1980;142:586–93.
16. Andrews NC, Parker EF, Shaw RP, et al. Management of nontuberculous empyema. Am Rev Respir Dis. 1963;3:935–6.
17. Mavroudis C, Ganzel BL, Cox SK, et al. Experimental aerobic-anaerobic thoracic empyema in the guinea pig. Ann Thorac Surg. 1987;43:298–302.
18. O'Moore PV, Mueller PR, Simeone JF. Sonographic guidance in diagnostic and therapeutic interventions in the pleural space. AJR. 1987;149:1–5.
19. Mirvis SE, Tobin KD, Kostrubiak I, et al. Thoracic CT in detecting occult disease in critically ill patients. AJR. 1987;148:685–9.
20. Van Sonnenberg E, Nakamoto SK, Mueller PR, et al. CT and ultrasound guided catheter drainage of empyemas after chest-tube failure. Radiology. 1984;151:349–53.
21. Webb WB, La Berge JM. Radiographic recognition of chest tube malposition in the major fissure. Chest. 1984;85:81–3.

22. Good JA, Taryle DA, Maulitz RM, et al. The diagnostic value of pleural fluid pH. Chest. 1980;78:55–9.
23. Potts DE, Levin DC, Sahn SA. Pleural fluid pH in parapneumonic effusions. Chest. 1976;70:328–31.
24. Pine JR, Hollman JL. Elevated pleural fluid pH in *Proteus mirabilis* empyema. Chest. 1983;84:99–111.
25. Yeh TJ, Hall DP, Ellison RG. Empyema thoracis: A review. Am Rev Respir Dis. 1963;88:785–90.
26. Levine H, Metzger W, Lacera D, et al. Diagnosis of tuberculous pleurisy by culture of pleural biopsy specimen. Arch Intern Med. 1970;126:269–71.
27. Mandal AK, Thadepalli H. Treatment of spontaneous bacterial empyema thoracis. J Thorac Cardiovasc Surg. 1987;94:414–8.
28. Miller KS, Sahn SA. Chest tubes. Chest. 1987;91:258–64.
29. Hutter JA, Harari D, Braimbridge MV. The management of empyema thoracis by thoracoscopy and irrigation. Ann Thorac Surg. 1985;39:517–20.
30. Mittapalli MR. Successful treatment of empyema with thoracenteses and intrapleural antibiotics. South Med J. 1980;73:533–4.
31. Hoover EL, Ross MJ, Webb H, et al. Reappraisal of empyema thoracis. Chest. 1986;90:511–5.
32. Grant DR, Finley RJ. Empyema: Analysis of treatment techniques. Can J Surg. 1985;28:449–52.
33. Mayo P. Early thoracotomy and decortication for nontuberculous empyema in adults with and without underlying diseases. Am Surg. 1985;4:230–6.
34. Le Roux BT, Mohlala ML, Odell JA, et al. Suppurative diseases of the lung and pleural space. Part 1: Empyema thoracis and lung abscess. Curr Probl Surg. 1986;23:4–38.
35. Taryle DA, Good JT, Morgan EJ, et al. Antibiotic concentrations in human parapneumonic effusions. Antimicrob Chemother. 1981;7:171–7.

55. LUNG ABSCESS

SYDNEY M. FINEGOLD

Lung abscess is a suppurative pulmonary infection involving the destruction of lung parenchyma to produce one or more large cavities with an air–fluid level. A similar process with multiple small cavitations (less than 2 cm in diameter) has been designated *necrotizing pneumonia* by some clinicians. The distinction is arbitrary since lung abscess and necrotizing pneumonia are different expressions of the same fundamental pathologic process. The earliest manifestation of this type of problem is pneumonia without excavation or abscess formation. In the absence of effective therapy, the disease may progress to lung abscess or to necrotizing pneumonia, with or without pleural empyema. Generally, the specific infecting organisms and the predisposing conditions do not influence the type of clinical disease that results. However, the size of the inoculum of organisms and the defense mechanisms of the host are likely to influence the outcome. Most often lung abscess follows aspiration, and anaerobic bacteria are the major organisms involved.

PREDISPOSING CAUSES

By far the most important background factor for abscess of the lung is aspiration,[1] usually related to altered consciousness. Common causes of altered consciousness in such patients are alcoholism, cerebral vascular accident, general anesthesia, drug overdose or addiction, seizure disorder, diabetic coma, shock, and other serious illness. Other factors in aspiration include dysphagia due to either esophageal disease or neurologic disease, intestinal obstruction, and tonsillectomy or tooth extraction. A study by Huxley et al.[2] using a sensitive radioactive tracer technique determined that 70 percent of patients with depressed consciousness and 45 percent of healthy subjects in deep sleep aspirated. Aspiration occurred more frequently and extensively in patients with depressed consciousness. Impairment of normal clearance mechanisms or the overwhelming of such mechanisms by large volumes of aspirated secretions may result in pulmonary infection. Alcoholics and patients who are acutely or chronically ill (whether or not they are hospitalized or in a nursing home) often demonstrate oropharyngeal colonization with gram-negative bacilli, particularly if they undergo endotracheal intubation and especially if they also receive histamine type 2 blockers or antacids.[3,4]

Next to aspiration, the most important factor predisposing to lung abscess or to necrotizing pneumonia is periodontal disease or gingivitis. Lung abscess is rare in an edentulous person and suggests the possibility of an associated bronchogenic carcinoma.[5] Other underlying processes include bronchiectasis, secondary infection of a bland pulmonary embolus with infarction, septic embolization, bacteremia, inhalation of bacteria-containing aerosols, and intra-abdominal infection. Suppurative inflammation behind an obstruction in a bronchus is another important mechanism. Patients receiving immunosuppressive therapy may develop multiple lung abscesses due to *Nocardia* or other organisms.

PATHOGENESIS AND PATHOLOGIC CHARACTERISTICS

Lung abscess is primarily of endogenous origin. Most of the bacteria involved are elements of the normal flora of the upper respiratory tract. Infections involving *Staphylococcus aureus, Klebsiella,* and other organisms may be of nosocomial origin.

The primary site of lung abscess is the posterior segment of the right upper lobe, with the same segment on the left less commonly affected. Next in frequency of involvement are the apical segments of the lower lobes. These segments are dependent in location when the subject is in a horizontal position, and the distribution relates to the fact that aspiration or inhalation is the primary background factor. Normally, aspirated material is handled effectively by ciliary action, cough, and alveolar macrophages. If the protective mechanisms are not effective, as with ethanol ingestion or viral disease, infection may result. Endotracheal tubes impair coughing, impede pulmonary clearance mechanisms, and allow leakage of oropharyngeal secretions into the tracheobronchial tree. Thick or particulate matter and foreign bodies are not easily removed and thus may lead to bronchial obstruction and atelectasis. With aspiration, gastric acid and enzymes may be the primary offending agents.

Subdiaphragmatic infection may extend to the lung or to the pleural space by way of lymphatics, directly through the diaphragm or defects in it, or by way of the blood stream. Most amebic lung abscesses are located in the right lower lobe adjacent to the diaphragm since they typically arise by direct extension of hepatic abscesses through the diaphragm.

Infection may arise in or behind an obstruction (neoplasm, foreign body, or enlarged mediastinal lymph node). Septic emboli from bacterial endocarditis of the right side of the heart or from pelvic or other deep vein thrombophlebitis may result in a metastatic lung abscess.

Although the virulence of the infecting organism(s) may be a factor determining the nature and extent of the infectious process, this is not usually important in the case of the anaerobes except for *Fusobacterium necrophorum*. However, the number of organisms aspirated may well be an important factor. With certain of the nonanaerobes such as *Klebsiella, Staphylococcus,* and group A *Streptococcus,* virulence may play an important role.

The pathologic characteristic is essentially that of necrosis supervened on inflammation with cavitation and abscess formation. The abscess cavity may become partially lined with regenerated epithelium, and localized bronchiectasis and emphysema may develop. There is usually no significant vascular involvement in lung abscess. However, a septic or bland pulmonary embolus may be the initial event. Once underway, the infection itself may give rise to pulmonary arteritis as in infection caused by *Pseudomonas aeruginosa*.

CLINICAL MANIFESTATIONS

Anaerobic Lung Abscess

In patients with lung abscess admitted to a hospital, symptoms have generally been present for at least 2 weeks. At times the patient will have had several weeks or even months of malaise, low-grade fever, and productive cough before seeking medical attention. Weight loss and anemia are common and confirm that the infection is indolent. Often the patient runs a low-grade fever; that is, a temperature about 101–102°F. Sputum production is usually copious. Foul-smelling sputum or empyema fluid occurs in only about one-half of the patients.[1,5,6]

In patients in whom the course of the infection has been followed radiologically, pneumonia appears first and cavitation subsequently. The earliest time of appearance of a cavity is about 7 days after aspiration; the average is about 12 days. Mediastinal adenopathy occasionally accompanies the parenchymal disease in patients with lung abscess or with other types of anaerobic pulmonary infection.[6] There may be a history of a period of unconsciousness, evidence of alcoholism, diseased gums, absence of the gag reflex, or other indications of the predisposing condition.

The physical findings are those of a pneumonia, with or without pleural effusion, early in the course of the illness. Later there may be amphoric or cavernous breath sounds. Clubbing of the fingers is noted on occasion.

Anaerobic Necrotizing Pneumonia

Usually anaerobic necrotizing pneumonia is confined primarily to one pulmonary segment or lobe. However, it may extend to involve an entire lung or even both lungs (Fig. 1). This type of anaerobic pulmonary infection is the most severe of all. There may be an associated empyema. The disease often spreads rapidly and produces destruction that is characterized by ragged, greenish discoloration of the lung and large putrid sloughs of tissue. This process culminates in "pulmonary gangrene."[5–7]

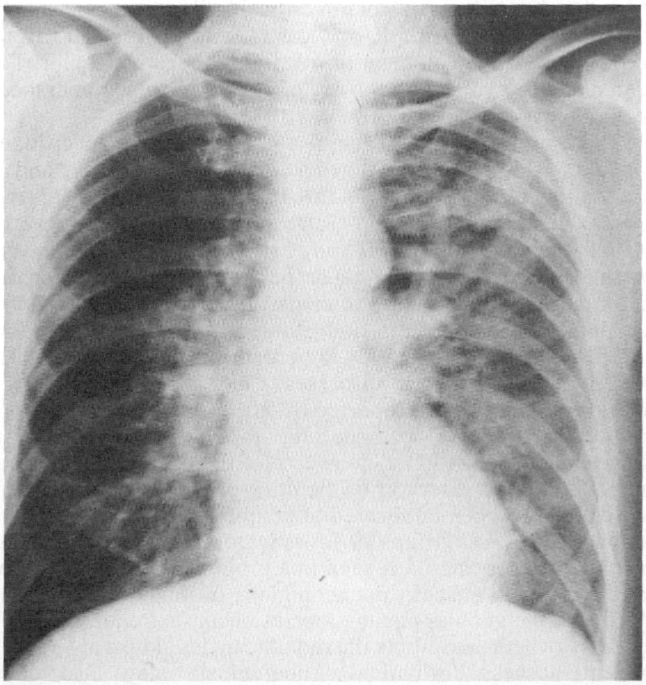

FIG. 1. Posterior–anterior (PA) chest film, anaerobic necrotizing pneumonia, and empyema. There is major involvement of the left lung, less involvement of the right. Note the multiple small excavations and one larger cavity in the left lung and blunting of the left costophrenic angle.

The patients are generally quite ill, with a temperature of 102–103°F. Leukocytosis is usually pronounced; for example, more than 20,000/mm^3. Most of these patients have putrid sputum or empyema fluid when first seen.

Pulmonary actinomycosis may be manifested as a necrotizing pneumonia; a number of cases will be complicated by extension of the process to the pleural space and to the chest wall.

Nonanaerobic Lung Abscess and Necrotizing Pneumonia

In primary infections due to organisms such as *S. aureus, Streptococcus pyogenes, Nocardia,* or *Klebsiella pneumoniae,* the symptoms are those of a severe pneumonia.

Secondary Lung Abscess and Necrotizing Pneumonia

In cases of secondary lung abscess, the basic process (bacteremia, endocarditis, septic thrombophlebitis, subphrenic infection, and so forth) will usually be evident in addition to the pulmonary process. The most characteristic hematogenous lung abscess is seen in staphylococcal bacteremia, especially in children. These abscesses are commonly multiple and peripheral in location. Empyema is frequently seen in this situation (Fig. 2). Repeated septic emboli should be suspected when multiple lesions appear over an extended period.

Less than 5 percent of bland pulmonary infarcts become secondarily infected. Secondary infection of infarcts should be suspected if fever is persistent, if the temperature rises above 103°F for more than 48 hours, or if the white blood cell count rises to more than 20,000 cells/mm^3. Abscess formation may occur within a necrotic pulmonary tumor or behind an obstructing tumor.

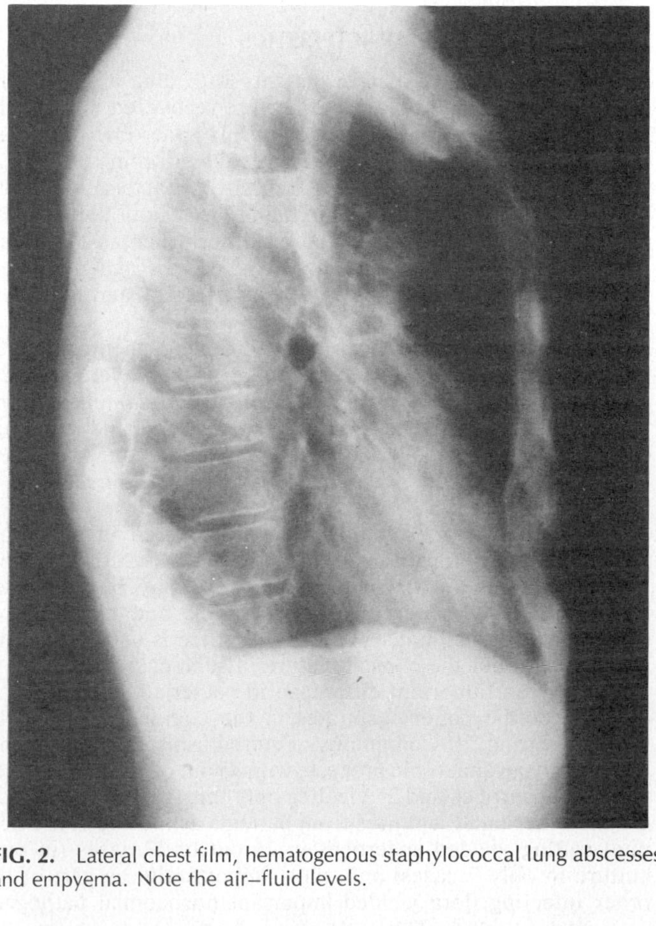

FIG. 2. Lateral chest film, hematogenous staphylococcal lung abscesses and empyema. Note the air–fluid levels.

The syndrome of tonsillitis or pharyngitis (Vincent's angina) with septicemia due to *F. necrophorum,* followed by widespread metastatic disease involving the lungs and other organs, is not commonly seen any longer, probably as a result of early antibiotic therapy for upper respiratory tract infections. However, it is important to be aware of this serious illness that occurs in children and young adults.

Amebic Lung Abscess

In patients with amebic lung abscess, the symptoms of the associated liver abscess will often have been present before the rupture through the diaphragm. After perforation of the liver abscess into the lung, there is a gradually developing cough and expectoration of a peculiar chocolaty or anchovy saucelike sputum. There is no odor to the sputum. The development of a pulmonary amebic abscess varies from a very insidious phenomenon to a dramatic onset with a sudden attack of severe cough productive of a large amount of brownish red sputum.[8] There may be a history of diarrhea, and an appropriate travel history may be elicited.

Complications

Approximately one-third of lung abscesses are complicated by empyema. This may be seen with or without bronchopleural fistulas. Brain abscess (via vertebral veins as a rule) may also be a complication in patients not receiving appropriate therapy early. A brain abscess is typically solitary. There is virtually never dissemination to other organs. Localized bronchiectasis may occur. Amyloidosis is no longer seen.

Complications of amebic abscess[9] include spontaneous perforation creating a cutaneous sinus, hepatobronchial fistula, empyema, secondary bacterial infection, and amebic abscess of the brain.

MICROBIOLOGIC CHARACTERISTICS

In a prospective study of 26 patients with lung abscesses by Bartlett et al.,[1] anaerobic bacteria were recovered in 24 of the 26 transtracheal aspirate specimens. Only anaerobes (including microaerophilic streptococci) were recovered from 16 of the 24 patients, whereas aerobic or facultative bacteria were recovered along with anaerobes in the other 8. Four patients had a single anaerobe recovered in pure culture, whereas 20 patients had multiple isolates, averaging 3.1 bacteria (2.6 anaerobes) per patient. The most commonly encountered anaerobes were gram-negative rods and gram-positive cocci.

Among 28 cases of anaerobic necrotizing pneumonia,[5] 20 yielded only anaerobes. Overall, there was an average of 2.3 anaerobes and 0.4 aerobes per case. *Fusobacterium nucleatum,* pigmented and other *Bacteroides,* and anaerobic and microaerophilic streptococci and cocci predominated among the anaerobes. Another distinctive cause of necrotizing pneumonia is actinomycosis.

The anaerobes most commonly encountered in anaerobic pleuropulmonary infection are listed in Table 1. Although clostridia, including *Clostridium perfringens,* may be recovered from patients with necrotizing pneumonia and empyema or other anaerobic pulmonary infections, there is usually nothing distinctive about the clinical picture in such cases.

There is an important difference in bacterial cause in terms of whether the patient aspirates in the community or in the hospital setting.[6,12] Community-acquired aspiration pneumonia is primarily an anaerobic process, with 35 out of 38 cases studied yielding anaerobes and 25 yielding only this type of organism.[12] On the other hand, cultures from patients aspirating in the hospital setting yielded anaerobes in 26 out of 32 cases (in pure culture in only 7 cases) and, most importantly, as part of the other infecting flora yielded important nosocomial pathogens such as *S. aureus* and various aerobic and facultative gram-negative bacilli such as *Klebsiella, Pseudomonas,* and *Proteus.*

TABLE 1. Anaerobes Most Commonly Encountered in Pleuropulmonary Infection

Gram-negative bacilli
Pigmented *Bacteroides* or *Porphyromonas*
Bacteroides oralis
B. buccae
B. ureolyticus group (especially *B. gracilis*)
B. bivius
B. oralis group
B. fragilis group
Fusobacterium nucleatum
F. necrophorum
F. naviforme
F. gonidiaformans
Gram-positive cocci
Peptostreptococcus (especially *P. anaerobius, P. magnus, P. asaccharolyticus, P. prevotii, P. intermedius*[a], *P. micros*)
Microaerophilic streptococci
Gram-positive spore-forming bacilli
Clostridium perfringens, C. ramosum
Gram-positive non-spore-forming bacilli
Actinomyces sp.
Arachnia sp.
Bifidobacterium dentium (*eriksonii*)

[a] This organism officially belongs in the genus *Streptococcus.*
(Data from Kirby et al.,[10] George et al.,[11] Sutter et al.[20])

Nichols and Smith[13] have shown that patients with bleeding or obstructing duodenal ulcers or with gastric ulcers or malignancy commonly have a much more profuse microflora in the stomach than do people without such pathologic conditions. This flora includes various organisms from the oral flora such as streptococci and anaerobes of various types but also coliform bacilli and, on occasion, *B. fragilis.* Thus, aspiration of gastric contents in people with the aforementioned pathologic conditions would carry with it a greater risk of bacterial infection, and the infecting flora might be different from what would ordinarily be expected. Histamine type 2 blockers or antacids have commonly been used to prevent upper gastrointestinal bleeding due to stress ulcers in critically ill patients. This leads to an elevated gastric pH and gastric and pharyngeal (by the retrograde route) colonization with gram-negative bacilli. This can likely be avoided by the use of sucralfate in lieu of antacids or H2 blockers.[3]

There are also several major aerobic causes of necrotizing pneumonia: *S. aureus, S. pyogenes, K. pneumoniae,* and *P. aeruginosa.* It is said that, on rare occasion, pneumococci (type 3) may cause a lung abscess. Infrequently, other gram-negative bacilli such as *Escherichia coli, Legionella pneumophila,* and perhaps *Proteus* sp. may cause pulmonary necrosis. Uncommon but important causes of cavitating pneumonia are *Nocardia* infection, melioidosis, and glanders. In acute Friedländer's (*Klebsiella*) pneumonia, 25–50 percent of the patients will develop one or more lung abscesses. Lung abscess due to *Pseudomonas cepacia* was reported by Poe et al.[14] The patient was a diabetic and developed the lung abscess after therapy with ultrasonic nebulization. The source of the organism was determined to be the reservoir of the ultrasonic nebulizer. Such nebulizers have been implicated in gram-negative bacillary pneumonia by several groups of investigators. However, although necrotizing pneumonia is seen in a proportion of these groups, a solitary lung abscess is uncommon. In infants with staphylococcal pneumonia, pneumatoceles occur as frequently as abscesses, whereas in adults the radiolucencies almost always represent abscess formation. Tuberculosis may also cause necrotizing pneumonia, and fungal infection (particularly histoplasmosis, coccidioidomycosis, and aspergillosis) sometimes produces this lesion.

Three major groups of bacteria are involved in hematogenous spread to the lungs: gram-positive cocci, notably staphylococci;

gram-negative enteric bacilli; and anaerobic bacteria. Multiple abscesses are likely to be of hematogenous origin, either as a result of bacteremia or of septic embolization. The most characteristic hematogenous lung abscess is seen in staphylococcal bacteremia. Hematogenous pulmonary infection with gram-negative enteric bacilli occurs in association with urinary tract infection or manipulation, after bowel surgery, after septic abortion, or as a nosocomial infection (usually in relation to vascular or urinary tract catheterization). Anaerobic or microaerophilic streptococci and gram-negative anaerobic bacilli may also produce hematogenous necrotizing pulmonary infection secondary to intra-abdominal or pelvic infections. In all of these anaerobic infections, there may be only bacteremia or else a septic thrombophlebitis that results in septic embolization. Uncommon hematogenous necrotizing pulmonary processes are those seen with anthrax, plague, and *Salmonella choleraesuis* infection.

Metastatic lung abscess may occur as a result of septic emboli from bacterial endocarditis of the right side of the heart (*S. aureus* is the major pathogen in this setting) or from pelvic or other deep vein thrombophlebitis. Various anaerobic bacteria and also pyogenic cocci such as *S. aureus* and streptococci not infrequently cause septic thrombophlebitis. As noted earlier, the anaerobes may be involved in this type of process in association with pelvic or intra-abdominal infection or, uncommonly now, with jugular vein thrombophlebitis in association with tonsillopharyngeal infections. Thrombophlebitis of the cavernous sinus most often involves *S. aureus* or streptococci. *Staphylococcus aureus* may also produce septic thrombophlebitis in association with superficial skin or soft tissue infections or in relation to intravenous catheters. The latter setting also may lead to septic thrombophlebitis involving gram-negative bacilli. Various organisms may be involved in secondary infection of bland pulmonary infarcts including staphylococci, streptococci, pneumococci, gram-negative enteric bacilli, and anaerobes of various types. Infection within a necrotic pulmonary tumor or behind an obstructing tumor may lead to abscess formation. Anaerobic bacteria of various types are commonly involved in such infections, but various other infecting organisms including *Mycobacterium tuberculosis* and fungi as well as a variety of bacteria may also be involved.

Unusual organisms may be involved in immunocompromised patients. Thus, there is a report[15] of a lung abscess due to *Rhodococcus* (*Corynebacterium*) *equi* in a renal transplant recipient.

DIAGNOSIS

The typical lung abscess can be suspected on clinical grounds. Most diagnoses are made from the chest roentgenogram, specifically from the presence of a cavity with an air–fluid level or pneumonitis with multiple small excavations located in a dependent segment. Diagnosis of the specific cause as well as differentiation from similar lesions depends on definitive bacteriologic studies. Because of the presence of large numbers of anaerobes as indigenous flora in the mouth and the common presence in hospitalized people of potential pathogens such as *S. aureus* and *K. pneumoniae* as colonizers in the mouth or the upper respiratory tract, it is necessary to obtain a specimen other than expectorated sputum for bacteriologic diagnosis. Empyema fluid, if available, provides an excellent specimen. On occasion, particularly with a mestatic lung abscess, blood cultures may be positive; however, blood cultures may reveal only part of the infecting flora. In the absence of the aforementioned sources of specimens for diagnosis, percutaneous transtracheal aspiration is an easy, safe, and dependable way of establishing the specific cause of the lung abscess or necrotizing pneumonia in patients who are able to cooperate.[16] This procedure should not be used in people with a significant bleeding tendency or in those in whom it is difficult to provide adequate oxygenation. Subcutaneous emphysema is an occasional complication of transtracheal aspiration, usually in patients with a severe cough, and may dissect into the mediastinum. Percutaneous transthoracic aspiration may be useful, particularly in children, but provides a smaller, less satisfactory specimen. Obtaining specimens during fiber-optic bronchoscopy by means of a bronchial brush within a plugged double-lumen catheter has been recommended.[17] It is absolutely essential that the techniques as outlined in detail by Broughton et al.[18] be used exactly as described and that cultures be done quantitatively. Growth at a 10^{-3} dilution is considered significant. The amount of the secretions collected by the brush is 0.001–0.01 ml, so the 10^{-3} dilution represents 10^5–10^6 organisms/ml of lower respiratory tract secretions. The small volume of material obtained and the difficulty one would encounter to arrange for anaerobic transport are a concern; nevertheless, good results appear to have been obtained in a small number of cases of anaerobic pulmonary infection. Recently quantitative culture of fluid obtained by bronchoalveolar lavage (during bronchoscopy) has been stated to provide reliable results in bacterial pneumonia.[19] Studies to date are limited, not fully controlled, and did not include anaerobic cultures but appear promising.

It is essential that material obtained for culture be placed under anaerobic conditions promptly before transport to the laboratory. It is usually desirable to aspirate the material to be cultured into a syringe, to expel all bubbles of air or gas from the syringe and needle, and then to transfer the specimen to a tube that has been gassed out with oxygen-free gas for transport to the laboratory.[20]

Demonstration of the usual underlying liver abscess is basic to the diagnosis of amebic lung abscess, but one may be able to demonstrate *Entamoeba histolytica* in the patient's sputum. Charcot-Leyden crystals in the sputum are suggestive of amebic infection. The usual procedures for the diagnosis of intestinal or hepatic amebiasis should be undertaken. The vast majority of patients with extraintestinal amebiasis will have high titers of hemagglutinating or complement-fixing antibodies.

Differential Diagnosis

Factors that would suggest a cavitating carcinoma rather than lung abscess include the absence of predisposing factors for an aspiration abscess (including an edentulous patient), location of an abscess in a nondependent segment, irregular abscess wall, and failure to respond to antibacterial therapy. Tuberculosis may also simulate a lung abscess or necrotizing pneumonia. Patients with infected lung cysts typically lack the systemic symptoms that may be seen in lung abscess, the cavity wall is thin, and there is no surrounding pneumonitis.

THERAPY AND PROGNOSIS

The primary mode of therapy is the administration of antimicrobial agents. Treatment may need to be continued for 2–4 months to achieve cure without relapse.

The anaerobes involved in lung abscess or in necrotizing pneumonia are increasingly resistant to penicillin G. Reports have appeared of less than optimum response or even frank failure to cure anaerobic lung abscesses or necrotizing pneumonia with penicillin therapy,[21,22] primarily because of β-lactamase producing *Bacteroides*. Metronidazole, or clindamycin, supplemented with penicillin G, represents the treatment of choice for serious anaerobic pulmonary infections. Thus, penicillin G (or penicillin V, ampicillin, or amoxicillin) is no longer used by the author as the sole initial therapy for patients with a suspected or proven anaerobic lung abscess or necrotizing pneumonia who are seriously ill. Penicillin is still favored as the initial therapy for patients who are mildly to moderately ill. Since some of the anaerobic cocci may require 8 units/ml or more of penicillin G for inhibition, one should use large doses of this agent (10–20 million units/day intravenously). After there has been a good clinical response, the regimen can usually be changed to a lower dosage. Patients who are not very ill may be treated satisfactorily with one of the aforementioned oral penicillins. Other penicillins are often considerably less active than is penicillin G. Oral cephalosporins such as cephalexin or cephradine may be used with good effect in patients who are not very ill.

A significant percentage of strains of most anaerobes are resistant to tetracyclines. Accordingly, these compounds should be used only when susceptibility data are available or when the patient's illness is minor so that a therapeutic trial in the patient can be undertaken safely. Clindamycin is active against most anaerobes with the exception of some strains of *Peptostreptococcus, Bacteroides gracilis, Fusobacterium varium,* and some strains of clostridia other than *C. perfringens*; 20 percent of the *B. fragilis* group are resistant in some centers. The addition of penicillin G would increase the spectrum of coverage except for the *B. fragilis* group and *B. gracilis*. Metronidazole is active against all gram-negative anaerobes including the *Bacteroides fragilis* group and other β-lactamase producers. It is also always active against all clostridia. Some anaerobic cocci and most microaerophilic streptococci, *Actinomyces,* and *Arachnia* are resistant. For this reason, metronidazole should ordinarily be used together with penicillin G (or erythromycin) in the treatment of anaerobic pulmonary infections. Certain β-lactam agents are quite active against the *B. fragilis* group and other β-lactamase-producing *Bacteroides* and most other anaerobes, although increasing resistance has been encountered in some centers. Included are cefoxitin, the carboxy penicillins (carbenicillin and ticarcillin), and the piperazine and ureidopenicillins (piperacillin and mezlocillin). Cefoxitin is inactive against one-third of clostridia other than *C. perfringens*. These agents, especially the piperazine and ureidopenicillins and cefoxitin, also have significant activity against various Enterobacteriaceae. Cefoxitin is also active against *S. aureus*, and the penicillins mentioned have activity against *P. aeruginosa*. The third-generation cephalosporins and related new compounds all have less activity against anaerobes, especially the *B. fragilis* group, than do cefoxitin and the broad-spectrum penicillins just discussed. One exception is imipenem, which is active against essentially all anaerobes. Combinations of β-lactam drugs and β-lactamase inhibitors such as ticarcillin plus clavulanic acid and ampicillin plus sulbactam are active against essentially all anaerobes and have good activity vs. *S. aureus* and many gram-negative bacilli. Chloramphenicol is active against essentially all anaerobes of all types and represents another option in a seriously ill patient with necrotizing pneumonia or lung abscess in whom β-lactamase-producing anaerobes may be present.

For staphylococcal infections, a penicillinase-resistant penicillin is preferable, but one of the parenteral cephalosporins or vancomycin may be used in the event of significant allergy. Vancomycin is the drug of choice for methicillin-resistant *S. aureus*. Penicillin G is the drug of choice for group A streptococcal infection. For infections due to *K. pneumoniae* or other facultative or aerobic gram-negative bacilli that may be involved in the type of pulmonary infection under discussion, one of the aminoglycosides would represent a drug of choice, but the extended-spectrum penicillins and combinations of β-lactam drugs and β-lactamase inhibitors have very good activity against some of these organisms. This is also true of imipenem. Gentamicin is ordinarily suitable, but in certain hospitals significant numbers of gram-negative bacilli are resistant to gentamicin; amikacin would then be the drug of choice. In seriously ill patients, particularly those who may be immunosuppressed, the use of appropriate β-lactam agents along with the aminoglycoside is desirable.

Postural drainage is an important aspect of the therapy for a lung abscess. Bronchoscopy may be helpful in effecting drainage and for removal of foreign bodies and biopsy diagnosis of tumors. Surgical resection of lung abscesses is rarely required unless there is a coexisting malignant process. Indeed, surgery is contraindicated because of the hazard of the spread of infection or asphyxiation from spillage of abscess contents. Surgical drainage of a lung abscess through the chest wall is rarely indicated.

Prognosis

The prognosis varies with the type of underlying or predisposing pathologic process, if any, and in the case of acute severe necrotizing pneumonias, the speed with which appropriate therapy is instituted. The mortality in anaerobic lung abscess is 15 percent or less. In anaerobic necrotizing pneumonia it is 25 percent. The mortality may be significantly higher in acute pneumonias caused by *S. aureus, K. pneumoniae,* and other facultative or aerobic gram-negative bacilli. The prognosis in amebic lung abscess is good when the diagnosis and treatment are prompt. Nocardiosis often has a relatively poor prognosis, especially when it complicates a serious underlying disease.

REFERENCES

1. Bartlett JG, Gorbach SL, Tally FP, et al. Bacteriology and treatment of primary lung abscess. Am Rev Respir Dis. 1974;109:510.
2. Huxley EJ, Viroslav J, Gray WR, et al. Pharyngeal aspiration in normal adults and patients with depressed consciousness. Am J Med. 1978;64:564.
3. Driks MR, Craven DE, Celli BR, et al. Nosocomial pneumonia in intubated patients given sucralfate as compared with antacids or histamine type 2 blockers. N Engl J Med. 1987;317:1376–82.
4. Tryba M. Risk of acute stress bleeding and nosocomial pneumonia in ventilated intensive care unit patients: Sucralfate versus antacids. Am J Med. 1987;83(Suppl 3B):117–24.
5. Bartlett JG, Finegold SM. Anaerobic infections of the lung and pleural space. Am Rev Respir Dis. 1974;110:56.
6. Finegold SM. Anaerobic Bacteria in Human Disease. New York: Academic Press; 1977.
7. Bartlett JG, Finegold SM. Anaerobic pleuropulmonary infections. Medicine (Baltimore). 1972;51:413.
8. Craig DF. The Etiology, Diagnosis and Treatment of Amebiasis. Baltimore: Williams & Wilkins; 1944.
9. Ochsner A, DeBakey ME. Pleuropulmonary complications of amebiasis: An analysis of 153 collected and 15 personal cases. J Thorac Surg. 1936;5:225.
10. Kirby BD, George WL, Sutter VL, et al. Gram-negative anaerobic bacilli: Their role in infection and patterns of susceptibility to antimicrobial agents. I. Little-known *Bacteroides* species. Rev Infect Dis. 1980;2:914.
11. George WL, Kirby BD, Sutter VL, et al. Gram-negative anaerobic bacilli: Their role in infection and patterns of susceptibility to antimicrobial agents. II. Little-known *Fusobacterium* species and miscellaneous genera. Rev Infect Dis. 1981;3:599.
12. Bartlett JG, Gorbach SL, Finegold SM. The bacteriology of aspiration pneumonia. Am J Med. 1974;56:202.
13. Nichols RL, Smith JW. Intragastric microbial colonization in common disease states of the stomach and duodenum. Ann Surg. 1975;182:557.
14. Poe RH, Marcus HR, Emerson GL. Lung abscess due to *Pseudomonas cepacia*. Am Rev Respir Dis. 1977;115:861.
15. Savdie E, Pigott P, Jennis F. Lung abscess due to *Corynebacterium equi* in a renal transplant recipient. Med J Aust. 1977;1:817.
16. Bartlett JG, Rosenblatt JE, Finegold SM. Percutaneous transtracheal aspiration in the diagnosis of anaerobic pulmonary infection. Ann Intern Med. 1973;79:535.
17. Wimberly NW, Bass JB Jr, Boyd BW, et al. Use of a bronchoscopic protected catheter brush for the diagnosis of pulmonary infections. Chest. 1982;81:556.
18. Broughton WA, Bass JB, Kirkpatrick MB. The technique of protected brush catheter bronchoscopy. J Crit Ill. 1987;2:63–70.
19. Kahn FW, Jones JM. Diagnosing bacterial respiratory infection by bronchoalveolar lavage. J Infect Dis. 1987;155:862–9.
20. Sutter VL, Citron DM, Edelstein MAC, et al. Wadsworth Anaerobic Bacteriology Manual. 4th ed. Belmont, CA: Star Publishing; 1985.
21. Levison ME, Mangura CT, Lorber B, et al. Clindamycin compared with penicillin for the treatment of anaerobic lung abscess. Ann Intern Med. 1983;98:466.
22. Panwalker AP. Failure of penicillin in anaerobic necrotizing pneumonia. Chest. 1982;82:500.

56. CHRONIC PNEUMONIA

WILLIAM E. DISMUKES

For purposes of this chapter, chronic pneumonia syndrome is defined as a pulmonary parenchymal process that may be caused by either an infectious or a noninfectious agent, has been present for weeks to months rather than for days, and is manifested by abnormal chest x-ray findings and by chronic or progressive pulmonary symptoms. The abnormal chest film, which may reveal any one of several radiologic patterns, is probably the most important criterion. In many patients, the diagnosis of chronic pneumonia may be based more on the pulmonary roentgenographic findings than on the pulmonary symptoms. However, asymptomatic patients who have abnormal chest x-ray findings, for example, a solitary nodule, on routine evaluation should not be considered to have chronic pneumonia.

The major emphasis in this chapter will be on the chronic pneumonias caused by infectious agents; however, it is important to keep in mind that there are noninfectious causes of chronic pneumonia, including collagen-vascular diseases, neoplasia, drugs, radiation, bronchiolitis obliterans organizing pneumonia,[1] and the various types of interstitial fibrosis.

ETIOLOGY

The infectious causes of chronic pneumonia can be divided into two main groups: (*1*) infectious agents that typically cause acute pneumonia and uncommonly cause chronic pneumonia and (*2*) infectious agents that typically cause chronic pneumonia. Among the agents that typically cause acute pneumonia, the anaerobes, *Staphylococcus,* the Enterobacteriaceae, and *Pseudomonas aeruginosa* are the organisms most likely to produce a persistent chronic pneumonia infection. This is usually a necrotizing process that most commonly occurs in patients with underlying disease such as alcoholism, diabetes mellitus, or chronic obstructive lung disease or in hospitalized patients.[2,3] Acute pneumonias caused by *Streptococcus pneumoniae, Mycoplasma pneumoniae, Legionella* sp., *Coxiella burnetii,* or most viruses rarely progress to a chronic pulmonary illness.

Table 1 shows the various causes of chronic pneumonia. In the normal host, tuberculosis,[4] other mycobacterial infections,[5] histoplasmosis,[6] coccidioidomycosis (in the appropriate geographic area),[7] mixed aerobic–anaerobic bacterial infection,[8] actinomycosis,[9] blastomycosis,[10] cryptococcosis,[11] and sporotrichosis[12] are the infections deserving prime consideration. Adiaspiromycosis, caused by *Emmonsia,* is a rare occurrence.[13] In the compromised host, chronic pneumonia should raise the possibility of tuberculosis, nocardiosis, cryptococcosis, and in the appropriate geographic areas, coccidioidomycosis and histoplasmosis.[14,15] In persons with acquired immunodeficiency syndrome (AIDS), a special immunocompromised population, these same infections are frequently seen. In addition, in these individuals, chronic pneumonia may be associated with atypical mycobacteria, *Pneumocystis carinii,* and cytomegalovirus plus noninfectious disorders such as Kaposi sarcoma, lymphoma, and nonspecific interstitial pneumonitis.[16–19] The protozoa and worms listed in Table 1 are uncommon causes of chronic pneumonia disease among people living in the United States, but the diseases caused by these organisms are important considerations in patients who live in or have traveled in areas in which these agents are endemic.

No studies have been done to determine the approximate frequency of the various causes of chronic pneumonia in a large series of patients. This lack of perspective on the incidence of the various etiologies of chronic pneumonia is in contrast to our better overall understanding of the *acute* pneumonia syndrome. In addition, since the introduction of antibiotics in the 1940s, the overall spectrum of pneumonia has changed; new pathogens have emerged, organisms that were previously considered harmless commensals now cause disease, and powerful immunosuppressive therapies render some patients more susceptible to certain microorganisms. Consequently, in considering the differential diagnosis in an individual patient, emphasis on specific entities must, in general, be based less on statistical likelihood and more on a thorough and methodic analysis of all available clinical, epidemiologic, and laboratory data.

TABLE 1. Etiology of Chronic Pneumonia Syndrome

- Infectious agents that *typically* cause chronic pneumonia
  - Bacteria and actinomycetes
    - Mixed aerobic–anaerobic bacteria
    - *Actinomyces* sp.
    - *Arachnia propionica*
    - *Nocardia* sp.
    - *Pseudomonas pseudomallei*
  - Mycobacteria
    - *M. tuberculosis*
    - *M. kansasii*
    - *M. avium-intracellulare* complex
  - Fungi
    - *Blastomyces dermatitidis*
    - *Coccidioides immitis*
    - *Cryptococcus neoformans*
    - *Emmonsia*
    - *Histoplasma capsulatum*
    - *Sporothrix schenckii*
    - *Paracoccidioides brasiliensis*
  - Protozoa
    - *Entamoeba histolytica*
  - Worms
    - *Echinococcus granulosus*
    - Schistosomes—*S. hematobium, S. japonicum, S. mansoni*
    - *Paragonimus westermani*
- Noninfectious causes
  - Neoplasia
    - Carcinoma (primary or metastatic)
    - Lymphoma
  - Lymphomatoid granulomatosis
  - Sarcoidosis
  - Vasculitis
    - Systemic lupus erythematosus
    - Polyarteritis nodosa
    - Allergic angiitis and granulomatosis (Churg-Strauss syndrome)
    - Progressive systemic sclerosis
    - Rheumatoid arthritis
    - Mixed connective tissue syndrome
    - Wegener's granulomatosis
  - Chemicals, drugs, or inhalation
  - Radiation
  - Recurrent pulmonary infarction
  - Pulmonary infiltration with eosinophilia (PIE) syndrome
    - Löffler syndrome—usually transient
    - Tropical eosinophilia
    - Pneumonia plus asthma, e.g., allergic bronchopulmonary aspergillosis
    - Vasculitis
    - Eosinophilic pneumonia—chronic
  - Pneumoconiosis
  - Chronic form of extrinsic allergic alveolitis or hypersensitivity pneumonitis
  - Other lung disease—unknown cause
    - Bronchiolitis obliterans organizing pneumonia
    - Interstitial pneumonia (fibrosing alveolitis, idiopathic pulmonary fibrosis)
      - Usual interstitial pneumonia (UIP)
      - Desquamative interstitial pneumonia (DIP)
      - Lymphoid interstitial pneumonia (LIP)
      - Giant cell interstitial pneumonia (GIP)
    - Eosinophilic granuloma
    - Lymphangioleiomyomatosis
    - Goodpasture syndrome
    - Pulmonary alveolar proteinosis (phospholipidosis)
    - Pulmonary alveolar microlithiasis
    - Idiopathic pulmonary hemosiderosis

EPIDEMIOLOGY

Age, Sex, Race

Although pulmonary tuberculosis over the past several decades has changed from a disease of the young to a disease of the middle-aged and elderly,[20] the significance of the age and sex of a particular patient usually relates more in an indirect manner to other epidemiologic factors. For example, an elderly patient is at higher risk of having a cerebrovascular accident, which in turn might predispose to an aspiration episode and subsequent pneumonia and abscess. Likewise, older, debilitated patients are at higher risk of developing chronic gram-negative necrotizing pneumonia. In a similar manner, the sex of a given patient is more likely to determine occupation or avocation and, ultimately, the likelihood of exposure to certain infectious agents or other etiologic vehicles. The race of the patient may be a more important factor. For example, pulmonary tuberculosis should be the presumptive diagnosis in a black patient with bilateral upper lobe cavitary disease[21]; coccidioidomycosis is more likely to be severe in dark-skinned persons, including blacks and Filipinos, who have lived or have traveled in the southwestern United States, the endemic area for the disease,[7] and chronic cavitary histoplasmosis is less likely to occur in the black population.[6]

Occupation and Avocation

Certain occupations or hobbies should arouse the suspicion of certain diseases. Despite the presence of *Cryptococcus neoformans* in pigeon droppings, the vast majority of patients with pulmonary cryptococcosis have no unusual exposure to pigeons. Occupational exposure to plant materials predisposes to cutaneous and, according to some authorities, pulmonary sporotrichosis.[22] Examples of occupationally or avocationally related conditions include coccidioidomycosis among rock collectors, archeologists conducting excavations, construction workers, or others exposed to desert dust in the endemic area[23,24]; histoplasmosis among persons who are exposed to starling roosts,[25] who clean out old chicken houses with dirt floors,[26] who cut and clear fallen oak trees,[27] or who explore caves inhabited by bats[28]; echinococcosis in those who tend sheep[29]; the pneumoconioses, for example, silicosis and asbestosis, among sandblasters and shipyard workers[30]; and chronic as well as acute pulmonary disease resulting from repeated occupational exposure to agents of allergic alveolitis or to irritant gases such as phosgene, ammonia, ozone, and nitrogen dioxide.[31]

Travel

Since the initial exposure to the agents of many chronic and indolent infectious diseases may have occurred months or years before disease, it is necessary to inquire whether a patient has lived in or has traveled to another part of the United States or the world at any time. For example, a patient with bilateral upper lobe infiltrates with or without cavitation who has never traveled or lived in Central America, Mexico, South America, or west of the Mississippi River is unlikely to have coccidioidomycosis. The exceptions include the occasional worker handling dusty material from the endemic area such as cotton bales. On the other hand, if the patient has lived in the Central, Southeast or mid-Atlantic area of the United States, chronic pulmonary histoplasmosis should be considered since histoplasmosis is endemic in these locations. Paracoccidioidomycosis is acquired only during residence in Mexico and in South or Central America. In addition to identifying a state or country visited, there may be a need for detailed questioning about rural or urban exposure, type of lodging, source of drinking water, exposure to native foods, and so forth. For example, any person who has lived or traveled extensively in Southeast Asia, particularly in low-lying or rice-growing areas, and who subsequently develops chronic pneumonia with pulmonary roentgenographic abnormalities resembling tuberculosis or the respiratory mycoses should be suspected of having melioidosis.[32] Similarly, a businessperson who makes frequent trips to Japan and the Philippines, who admits to eating raw or partly cooked crayfish, and who has chronic pulmonary symptoms plus dense, nodular lung opacities and ring shadows should be suspected of having pulmonary paragonimiasis.[33]

Contacts, Habits, and Drugs

In patients in whom tuberculosis is suspected, contacts among friends or relatives with tuberculosis should be sought. Inquiry should be made into the patient's smoking and drinking history as well as other personal habits. The likelihood of cancer of the lung in a patient with coal worker's pneumoconiosis is greater in a smoker than in a nonsmoker. Aspiration pneumonia, chronic gram-negative bacillary pneumonia, and tuberculosis are more likely to occur in an alcoholic than in a nondrinker. Intravenous drug users who inject heroin or similar agents are not only at risk of developing infection with human immunodeficiency virus (HIV) and subsequently AIDS but also acute pulmonary edema,[34] septic pulmonary emboli followed by necrotizing pneumonia and single or multiple abscesses, or an interstitial granulomatous reaction with pulmonary hypertension.[35] Similarly, frequent use of free-base cocaine has been reported to cause bronchiolitis obliterans organizing pneumonia.[36]

Certain drugs may cause acute and chronic pulmonary symptoms as well as radiographic abnormalities.[37] Early in the course of drug-induced pulmonary disease, the chest roentgenogram findings may be normal; later, an interstitial, nodular, and/or alveolar pattern may be present. Still later, the chest x-ray film may reveal only a fibrotic pulmonary process. The drugs that are more likely to cause chronic pulmonary disease include cytotoxic agents such as bleomycin, busulfan, chlorambucil, methotrexate, and mitomycin and noncytotoxic agents such as amiodarone, gold salts, nitrofurantoin, and penicillamine. Since drug-induced pulmonary disease may develop after drug therapy has been discontinued, the physician should inquire not only about all drugs the patient is presently taking but also about those taken in the recent past.

Similarly, important questions arise in regard to any previous or current antimicrobial therapy. Did the antimicrobial result in roentgenographic or clinical improvement? If not, was the antimicrobial used in sufficient quantity to cure the suspected process or alter its course? Was the appropriate agent used? What effect does the antimicrobial have on the results of cultures? Is the report of "normal flora" on the sputum culture the result of antimicrobial therapy eliminating a specific pathogen?

Underlying Disease

Pulmonary complications including both acute and chronic or refractory pneumonia are especially common in persons with AIDS (see Chapter 108). Patients with diabetes mellitus or preexisting chronic obstructive pulmonary disease are at high risk for developing chronic or persistent bacterial pneumonia. Similarly, chronic obstructive lung disease commonly precedes fibrocavitary histoplasmosis or *M. intracellulare* infection. Recurrent or persistent pneumonia in the same area of the lung raises the suspicion of a local endobronchial lesion that may not be apparent on routine chest x-ray films. Since aspiration may predispose to chronic pneumonia, inquiry should be made into any history of recent dental problems or manipulation, sinusitis with chronic postnasal drip, disorders of swallowing resulting from neurologic or esophageal disease, seizure disorders, recent anesthesia, quantity and effect of alcohol, or any illness leading to an unconscious state. Finally, is the chronic pneumonia community or hospital acquired?

CLINICAL FEATURES

Symptoms

Since there are multiple causes of chronic pneumonia, no single symptom complex is common to all causes. Often, constitutional symptoms including fever, chills, and malaise are present initially. A history of progressive anorexia and weight loss usually indicates chronic illness. Pulmonary symptoms may be present early but frequently appear later in the course of the illness. Any patient with a prolonged illness and nonspecific constitutional complaints plus pulmonary symptoms including a new or persistent cough, sputum production, hemoptysis, chest pain (especially pleuritic pain), or dyspnea deserves medical evaluation, including a chest x-ray.

Inquiries should be made to determine whether there is involvement of extrapulmonary organs. For example, skin lesions might suggest coccidioidomycosis, cryptococcosis, blastomycosis, nocardiosis, or Kaposi sarcoma, whereas mucous membrane lesions would suggest histoplasmosis, paracoccidioidomycosis, or Kaposi sarcoma. Mono- or polyarticular arthritis, polyarthralgias, or localized bone tenderness or pain might indicate a collagen-vascular disease. A history of persistent headache together with the documentation of an abnormal cerebrospinal fluid should raise the suspicion of tuberculosis, cryptococcosis, or coccidioidomycosis involving both the lungs and central nervous system. The presence of focal neurologic symptoms and signs argues strongly for a space-occupying lesion in the central nervous system; such findings in a patient with a cavitary infiltrate seen on a chest film suggest the possibility of a brain abscess associated with chronic suppurative lung disease or pulmonary nocardiosis.

Signs

Although the findings on physical examination of the chest are usually not helpful in differentiating specific causes of chronic pneumonia, the presence of generalized wheezing or other signs of bronchospasm, in the absence of underlying lung disease, indicates an asthmatic component to the pulmonary illness and raises the possibility of a disorder causing both pneumonia and asthma such as extrinsic allergic alveolitis, allergic bronchopulmonary aspergillosis, or allergic granulomatosis and angiitis (Churg-Strauss syndrome). Similarly, localized wheezes suggest the presence of an endobronchial obstructing lesion. The findings of tachycardia, cardiomegaly, gallop rhythm, and ankle edema provide evidence of cardiac disease and suggest that the pulmonary symptoms and signs are at least in part due to cardiovascular causes. The presence of skin lesions, clubbing, cyanosis, or phlebitis are not specific for any single pulmonary disorder but may help to narrow the differential diagnosis, especially when considered along with other clinical and epidemiologic information. Similarly, the findings of jaundice, adenopathy, hepatomegaly, splenomegaly, or ascites suggest that a systemic disorder involving multiple organs is the cause.

DIAGNOSTIC PROCEDURES

Initial Laboratory Studies

Routine laboratory studies may provide some important clues to diagnosis. Pancytopenia may suggest miliary tuberculosis, disseminated histoplasmosis, or metastatic tumor in the bone marrow. Anemia alone is consistent with too many disorders to suggest a cause. A normal white blood cell count does not exclude infection. In particular, mycotic chronic pneumonia is usually associated with a normal or minimally elevated white blood cell count. Leukopenia and/or lymphopenia should raise the suspicion of infection with HIV. In addition, leukopenia should suggest sarcoidosis, systemic lupus erythematosus, tuberculosis, histoplasmosis, or tumor. A leukemoid reaction may be seen in disseminated mycobacteriosis. Leukocytosis is suggestive of but not specific for a bacterial cause.

Laboratory tests that measure the function of other organs may provide more helpful information. Liver function studies including bilirubin, alkaline phosphatase, and serum aspartate aminotransferase determinations and prothrombin time should be obtained in all patients. Urinalysis, with particular attention to the urinary sediment, plus tests of renal function including measure of the blood urea nitrogen and creatinine should also be done. Abnormalities of either liver function, especially elevated enzyme levels, kidney function, or both, should raise the suspicion of disorders that are not limited to the lung but are known to involve multiple organs including lung, liver, and kidney. Such disorders include disseminated histoplasmosis and disseminated mycobacteriosis as well as the collagen-vascular diseases, sarcoidosis, and certain neoplastic diseases, especially the lymphoproliferative types.

An elevated serum globulin level is usually nonspecific and indicates chronic inflammation, although it may indicate an underlying myeloma or another gammopathy predisposing to chronic or recurrent infection. If myeloma is suspected, immunoelectrophoresis of urine and serum is indicated. Similarly, in a patient with an abnormally low serum globulin level, a quantitative serum immunoglobulin determination should be obtained to evaluate the patient for hypogammaglobulinemia.

Studies to Establish an Etiology

A basic core of studies should usually be performed on all patients with chronic pneumonia, regardless of suspected etiology, but there should be flexibility in choosing additional tests or procedures to confirm a specific diagnosis. The orderly sequence of diagnostic studies that is given below necessarily results in oversimplification and consequently overlooks the unique aspects of a given patient's illness.

Chest X-ray Studies. The chest roentgenogram, including a posteroanterior and a lateral film, is probably the single most important diagnostic study. Because of the singular importance of the chest x-ray, Table 2 is provided to emphasize the major radiologic patterns that may be seen. In Table 2 the disorders have been grouped according to the type of radiologic abnormality that is characteristic of the disease. Because there are some disorders in which there is a spectrum of radiologic manifestations, these disorders appear more than once in the table. In selected patients, a computed tomographic examination of the chest may provide additional useful information, especially about the presence and extent of mediastinal, hilar, and pleural disease. For example, documentation of *anterior* mediastinal involvement argues strongly in favor of neoplasia including lymphoma and metastatic carcinoma as the etiology of chronic pneumonia syndrome and argues against an infectious cause.

Tuberculosis and nontuberculous mycobacterial diseases, histoplasmosis, coccidioidomycosis, sporotrichosis, melioidosis, paragonimiasis, and the pneumoconioses, especially silicosis, characteristically produce fibrocavitary disease—a contracted area of lung with linear fibrosis, nodular or rounded densities, and cavitation. In addition, mycobacterial diseases, histoplasmosis, and silicosis characteristically involve the upper lobes. A thin-walled cavity is suggestive of coccidioidomycosis, sporotrichosis, and paragonimiasis, whereas a thick-walled cavity surrounded by an area of pneumonitis is more typical of tuberculosis, nontuberculous mycobacterial diseases, histoplasmosis, melioidosis, nocardiosis, actinomycosis, and pyogenic lung abscess. Cavitation is less common in blastomycosis and cryptococcosis. Ecchinococcal lung lesions occasionally show a crescent of air between the pericyst and endocyst or a collapsed membrane floating on cyst fluid (water

TABLE 2. Radiologic Patterns of Diseases That Commonly Cause Chronic Pneumonia Syndrome

Disease	*Radiologic Characteristics*
Diseases that cause patchy infiltrates and/or bronchopneumonia or lobar consolidation	
Infectious	
Aspiration pneumonia secondary to mixed aerobic and anaerobic infection	Usually dependent portions: superior or basilar segments of lower lobes or posterior segments of upper lobes Pleural involvement with empyema common
Necrotizing pneumonia secondary to Enterobacteriaceae, *P. aeruginosa*, or *S. aureus*	Any lobe or segment Chronic *Klebsiella* pneumonia commonly involves upper lobes May be multiple sites of pulmonary infection secondary to septic embolization
Actinomycosis	Commonly involves lower lobes Cavitation frequently present Pleural involvement with empyema common
Nocardiosis	No distinctive pattern May involve single or multiple lobes Cavitation may be present Pleural involvement may occur
Tuberulous exudative pneumonia	Not restricted to upper lobes Often bilateral with perihilar distribution
Blastomycosis	Often a dense area of lobar or segmental consoliation Cavitation infrequent
Cryptococcosis	Single or multiple patchy infiltrates; less commonly, lobar consolidation Occasionally, single or diffuse nodular lesions
Paracoccidioidomycosis	Asymptomatic bilateral fluffy infiltrates May be extremely indolent
Noninfectious	
Chronic eosinophilic pneumonia	Rapidly progressive, dense infiltrates Usually peripheral (reverse pattern of pulmonary edema)
Bronchiolitis obliterans organizing pneumonia	Focal, patchy ground glass densities
Diseases that cause pulmonary cavitation	
Infectious	
Pyogenic lung abscess	
Complicating aspiration pneumonia	Usually single cavity Location—same as aspiration pneumonia Air–fluid level common
Complicating necrotizing pneumonia	May involve any lobe Often multiple and bilateral, depending on route of acquisition of pneumonia
Tuberculosis—reactivation or adult type	Usually upper lobes Often bilateral May be multiple Fibrosis and calcification common
Atypical mycobacterial disease	Radiologically indistringuishable from tuberculosis, except that cavitation may be more frequent
Melioidosis	Simulates tuberculosis, but may involve any lobe
Histoplasmosis, chronic cavitary	Mimics tuberculosis Upper lobes frequently involved but can involve any lobe Unilateral or bilateral
Coccidioidomycosis	Usually single thin-walled cavity with minimum involvement of surrounding lung Occasionally thick-walled cavity surrounded by extensive parenchymal disease
Sporotrichosis	May mimic tuberculosis but can involve any lobe Cavitation is frequent; thin-walled cavity more likely than thick-walled cavity
Aspergillosis	Single or multiple areas of pneumonia with or without central cavitation Not to be confused with intracavitary fungus ball
Paragonimiasis	Cystlike lesions as well as cavities, usually associated with linear or patchy infiltrates, fibrosis, and/or calcification
Echinococcosis	Single or multiple discrete, sharply defined round lesions (cysts) with little surrounding inflammatory response Cavitation and/or calcification may occur
Noninfectious	
Wegener's granulomatosis and lymphomatoid granulomatosis	Often multiple nodules with cavitation May be unilateral or bilateral
Silicosis	Associated with conglomerate nodular densities, frequently in upper lobes Usually superimposed on background of diffuse nodulation Rarely, eggshell calcification of hilar nodes
Bronchogenic carcinoma	Eccentric cavitation more common in squamous cell type
Lymphoma, especially Hodgkin's disease	Cavitation typically occurs in peripheral parenchymal nodules
Infectious and noninfectious diseases that cause chronic diffuse pulmonary infiltration and fibrosis	
Alveolar cell carcinoma Intrapulmonary bleeding, e.g., Goodpasture syndrome Pulmonary alveolar proteinosis	Alveolar pattern
Sarcoidosis Early asbestosis or berylliosis Bronchiolitis obliterans organizing pneumonia	Ground-glass interstitial pattern

(Continued)

TABLE 2. *(Continued)*

Disease	*Radiologic Characteristics*
Granulomatous infectious diseases, e.g., miliary tuberculosis and disseminated histoplasmosis Sarcoidosis Bronchiolitis obliterans organizing pneumonia Lymphangitic carcinomatosis Wegener's granulomatosis Lymphomatoid granulomatosis Allergic angiitis and granulomatosis Rheumatoid lung disease Pneumoconioses including asbestosis, silicosis, and beryliosis	Nodular interstitial pattern, including miliary spherical nodules
Chronic form of hypersensitivity pneumonitis Idiopathic pulmonary hemosiderosis Radiation injury—chronic Progressive systemic sclerosis Sarcoidosis	Linear interstitial pattern including fine reticular markings and dense fibrosis
Advanced form of fibrosing alveolitis Bronchiectasis Eosinophilic granuloma Sarcoidosis	Honeycombing (coarse reticular pattern with cystic air spaces)

lily sign).[38] Calcification is typical of tuberculosis, histoplasmosis, and coccidioidomycosis but is rare in actinomycosis, nocardiosis, blastomycosis, and cryptococcosis. Abscess of the chest wall or osteomyelitis of a rib adjacent to the pneumonia and/or pleural effusion may be seen in actinomycosis and nocardiosis. Representative x-ray films are shown in Figures 1–15.

Studies in Patients with X-ray Evidence of Localized Infiltrates and/or Cavitation. In all patients with x-ray evidence of localized infiltrates and/or cavitation, examination of the sputum is essential. The specimen of sputum must be a representative sample. If the expectorated sputum is a deep, coughed specimen, of adequate volume, and acceptable after cytologic screening,[39] other procedures to obtain sputum may not be necessary. *Microscopic* examination of sputum should include the following:

1. Gram stains for bacteria and actinomyces
2. Acid-fast or fluorochrome stains for *Mycobacteria* and modified acid-fast stain for *Nocardia*
3. Wet mounts for fungi and eggs of *Paragonimus*
4. Gomori methenamine silver (GMS) stain or periodic acid–Schiff (PAS) stain for fungi.
5. Cytologic preparations for neoplastic cells, eosinophils, fungi

Generous volumes of expectorated sputum (but not 24-hour collections) should also be obtained and sent to the microbiology laboratory for *culture* for bacteria, fungi, and mycobacteria. In addition, it is often diagnostically rewarding if the clinician speaks directly with the personnel in the microbiology laboratory to alert them to specific etiologic considerations. Then the specimens will be inoculated on the most appropriate media, and the microbiologists will be more aware of the suspected pathogens.

In all patients in whom an infectious cause is considered, cultures from sources other than sputum should be obtained. These sources might include the following:

1. Blood
2. Urine
3. Pleural fluid in all patients with pleural effusion. Pleural tissue should also be obtained for culture
4. Cerebrospinal fluid in all patients with central nervous system symptoms or signs
5. Synovial fluid in all patients with joint effusion
6. Skin, mucous membrane, or any tissue obtained at biopsy

To obtain sputum, if adequate sputum cannot be readily produced via spontaneous expectoration by the patient, consider the following:

1. Inducing sputum by the use of hypertonic aerosols or ultrasound, hydration, chest physiotherapy, or postural drainage
2. Bronchoscopy for bronchial washings, transbronchial biopsy, bronchoalveolar lavage, or protected catheter sampling of lower respiratory tract secretions while minimizing upper airway contamination of the sample[40]

Skin tests should be made in all cases in which an infectious cause is considered. The tuberculin skin test is the single most important test. If a patient has never had a tuberculin skin test

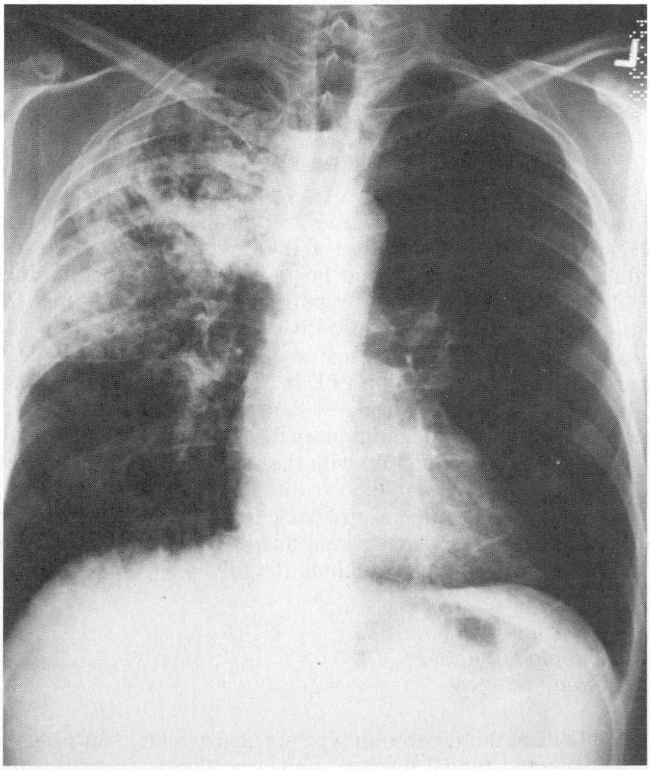

FIG. 1. Mixed aerobic–anaerobic chronic bacterial pneumonia in a 46-year-old alcoholic man with a 3-week history of malaise, nausea, fever, chills, and cough productive of copious amounts of foul-smelling sputum. Note the multiple small cavities throughout the right upper lobe. Long-term penicillin therapy was curative.

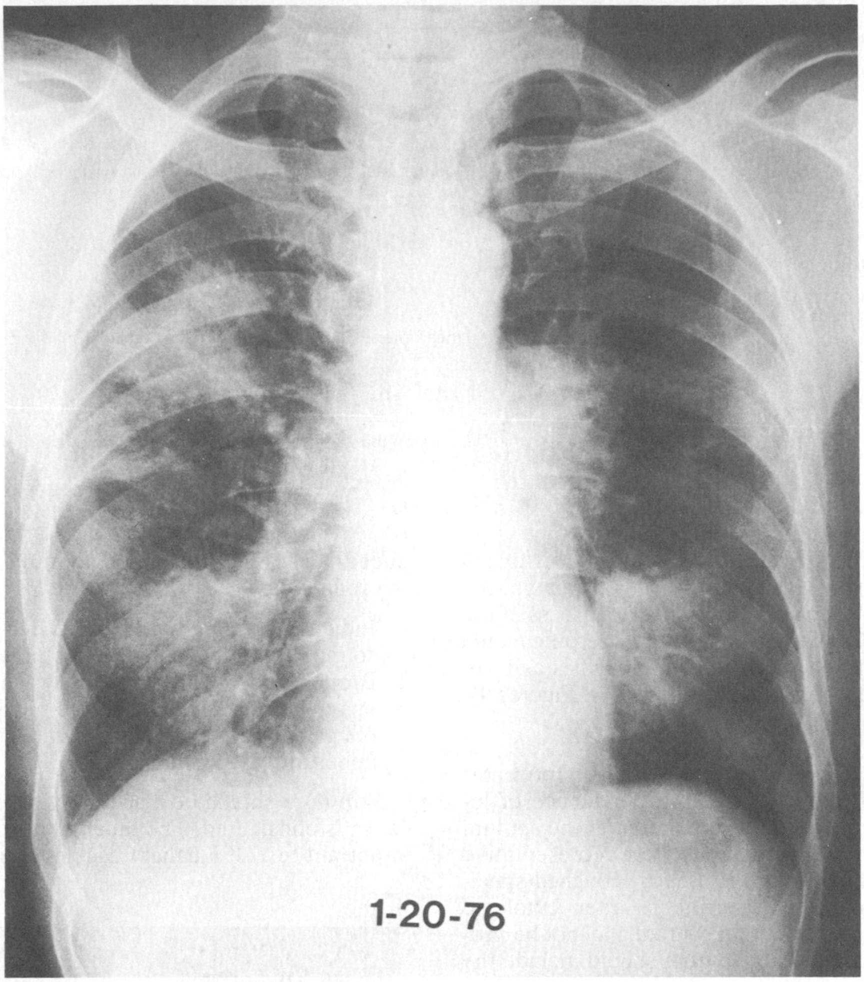

FIG. 2. Pulmonary actinomycosis in a 49-year-old with a 3-month history of chronic productive cough, anorexia, and weight loss. The x-ray film was taken during the initial clinic evaluation. Note the bilateral bronchopneumonia, more marked in the lower lobes. There was no cavitation.

or has had a previously negative response, a 5 tuberculin unit (TU) (intermediate) purified protein derivative (PPD) skin test should be used. If the patient has a history of a positive tuberculin skin response, a TU (first-strength) PPD may be applied. If the intermediate PPD is negative after 48 hours, a 250 TU (second-strength) PPD skin test should then be performed. A nonreactive second-strength PPD in a patient who is shown not to be anergic provides strong evidence against tuberculosis as the cause of the chronic pulmonary disease.[41] Skin test antigens for the detection of infection with the atypical mycobacteria are not commercially available.

Other skin test antigens to check for intact delayed hypersensitivity should be placed simultaneously with a PPD antigen. These "control" antigens include the following:

1. Mumps antigen
2. *Trichophyton* antigen
3. *Candida* antigen

Skin tests of the tuberculin type are also available for patients with suspected fungal disease; however, these are most valuable when used for epidemiologic studies to determine the prevalence of infection in a given population or in a certain geographic area. Like the tuberculin test, fungal skin tests do not distinguish between current and previous infection. Unlike the tuberculin test, a negative result is common with active disease. Hence, fungal skin tests are of little diagnostic value in the individual patient. Of the tests available, the coccidioidin antigen is the best, although a negative response does not exclude coccidioidomycosis. The blastomycin and histoplasmin antigens should not be used for diagnostic purposes in individual patients because of the high incidence of cross-reactions and false-negative results. In addition, histoplasmin may cause a false elevation of serum antibody to the mycelial antigen of *Histoplasma capsulatum*.

Serologic tests for antibodies and antigens are often used when infectious causes, especially fungi, are considered. However, there are problems that include long delays in obtaining results, false-positive results because of cross-reactions to other antigens, and false-negative results. Serologic tests are most helpful in patients when pulmonary mycoses including coccidioidomycosis, cryptococcosis, histoplasmosis, and paracoccidioidomycosis are suspected. Similarly, in patients in whom hypersensitivity pneumonitis is suspected, serum should be examined for precipitating antibodies to various inhalant antigens.

Invasive Procedures. Certain clinical situations dictate that a more aggressive diagnostic approach be used. In patients who are unable to raise sputum spontaneously and in whom attempts to induce sputum production are unsuccessful, invasive procedures may become necessary. Bronchoscopy with a flexible fiber-optic bronchoscope usually is the initial procedure and is diagnostically helpful when accompanied by bronchial washings and transbronchial biopsy with appropriate microbiologic

FIG. 3. X-ray film taken 12 days after that in Figure 2. Note the large loculated pleural effusion on the right.

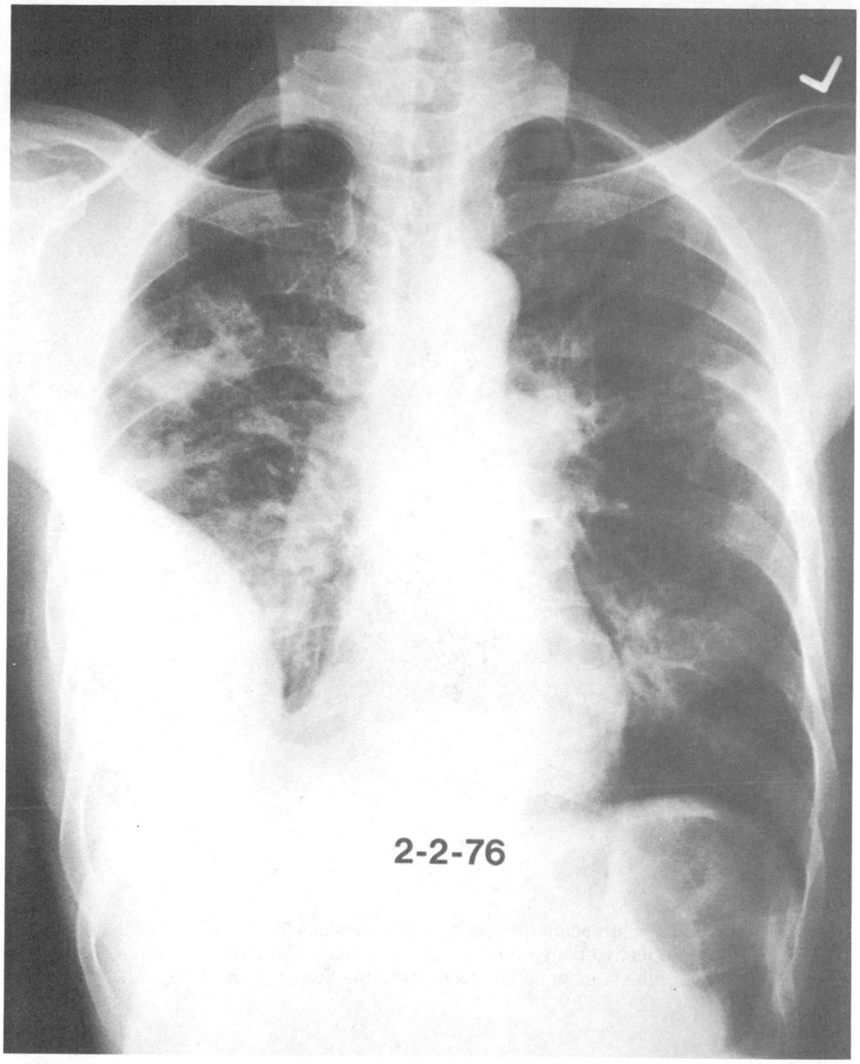

FIG. 4. Pulmonary nocardiosis in a 38-year-old after a renal transplant who was taking corticosteroids and had symptoms of malaise, fever, and a productive cough. Note the extensive consolidation of the right upper lobe with central cavitation.

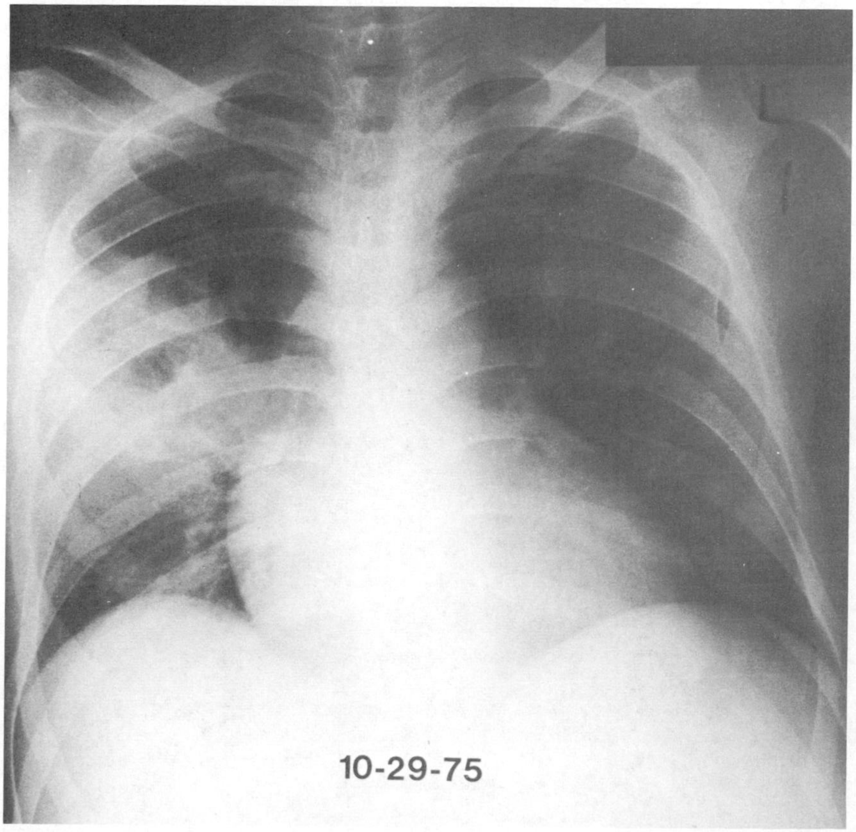

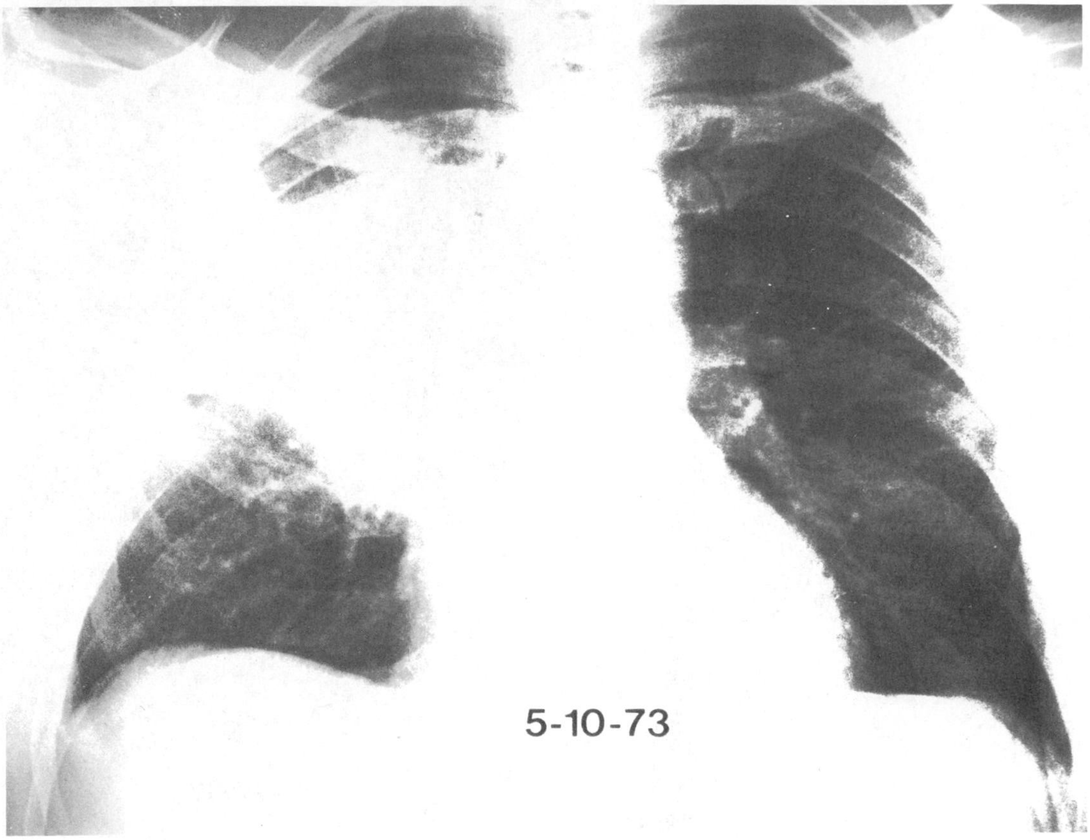

FIG. 5. Chronic pulmonary blastomycosis in a 53-year-old construction worker with a 4-week illness of fever, chills, myalgias, nonproductive cough, anorexia, and weight loss. Note the homogeneous consolidation of the anterior segment of the right upper lobe with some involvement of the apical segment. Right hilar adenopathy is also present.

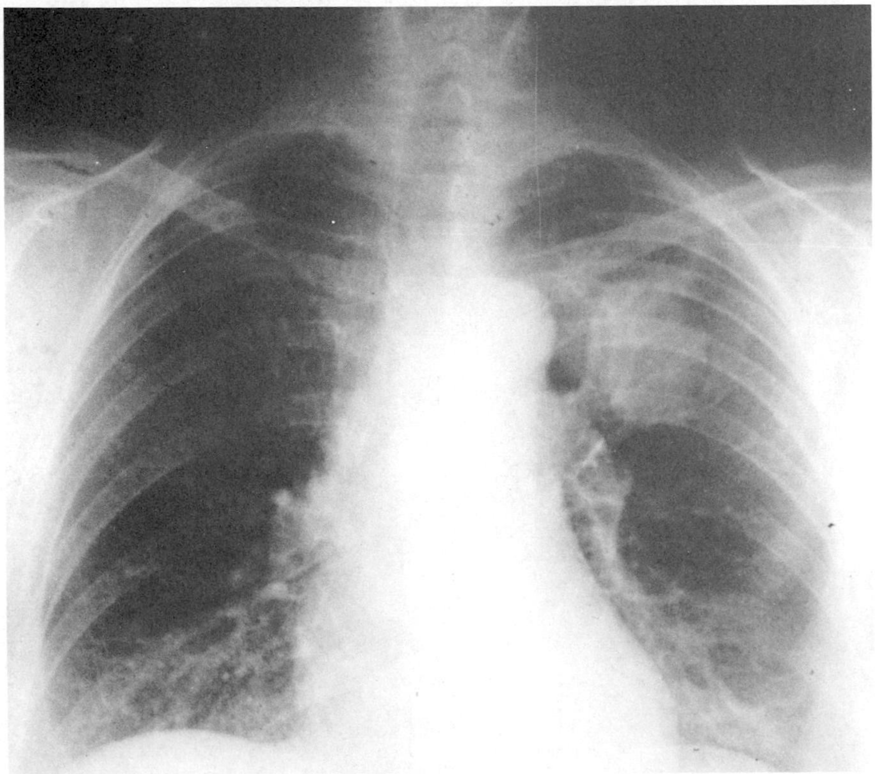

FIG. 6. Pulmonary cryptococcosis in a 54-year-old woman with a 2-month history of headache and chronic cough. Note the large, sharply circumscribed mass in the left upper lobe. She also had culture-proven cryptococcal meningitis.

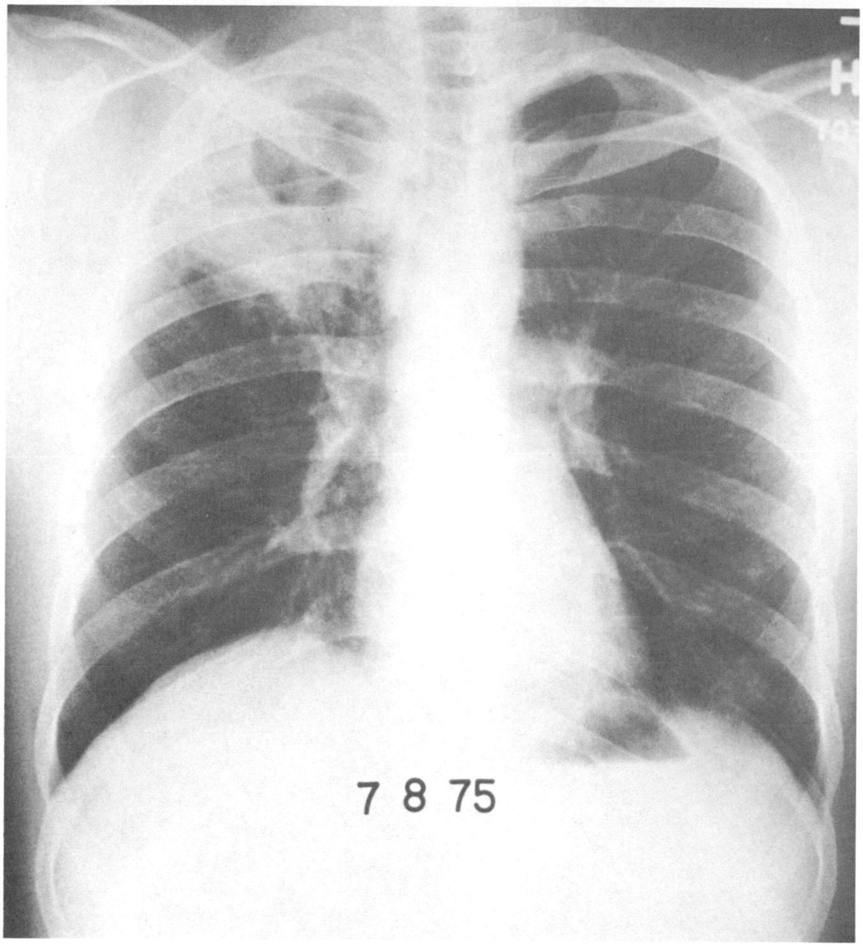

FIG. 7. Cavitary tuberculosis in a 30-year-old man with symptoms of cough, sputum production, and weight loss for 10 months. Note the thick-walled cavity in the right upper lobe with surrounding parenchymal infiltrate. The patient was originally diagnosed as having a nonspecific lung abscess.

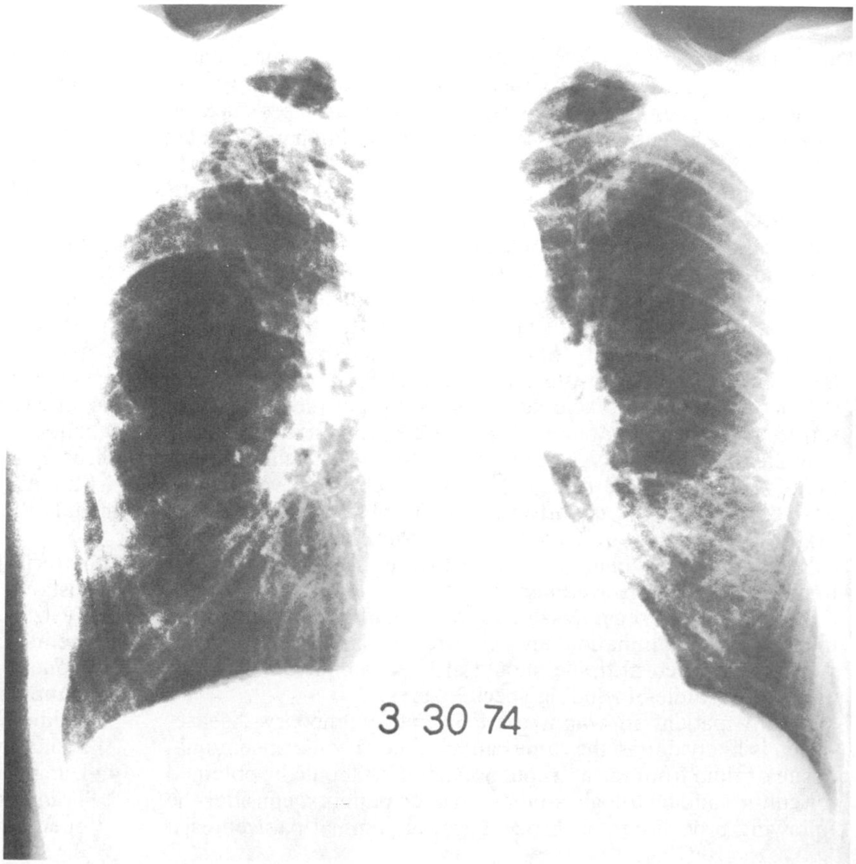

FIG. 8. Atypical tuberculosis caused by *M. avium-intracellulare* in a 68-year-old with chronic obstructive pulmonary disease. At time of this x-ray film, the patient had been symptomatic for 1 year with malaise, anorexia, weight loss, and progressive dyspnea. Note the fibrocavitary appearance of the right upper lung.

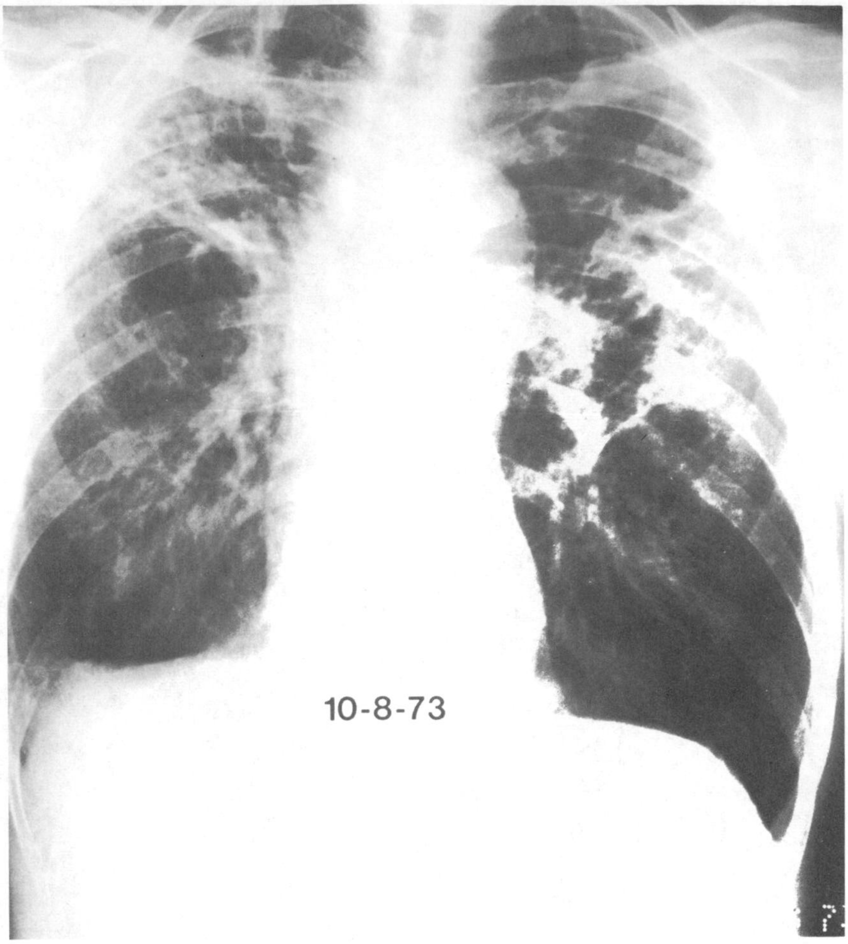

FIG. 9. Chronic cavitary pulmonary histoplasmosis in a 67-year-old with chronic obstructive pulmonary disease and a 4-month history of night sweats, low-grade fever, chronic cough, and weight loss. Note the bilateral fibrocavitary disease primarily involving the upper lobes.

and histologic studies.[42,43] Analysis of bronchoaveloar lavage fluid may increase the diagnostic yield of bronchoscopy, especially in patients with interstitial/alveolar diseases such as sarcoidosis, hypersensitivity pneumonitis, pulmonary alveolar proteinosis, and idiopathic pulmonary fibrosis and in patients with pulmonary complications of AIDS.[44,45] In a patient with extensive pleural involvement, thoracentesis and pleural biopsy may be more helpful diagnostically than bronchoscopy. In some institutions, open lung biopsy is the procedure of choice and performed before bronchoscopy in many immunosuppressed patients with pulmonary disease because of the relatively large piece of tissue obtained, expediency of diagnosis, and safety.[46] By contrast, in other institutions with seasoned operators, percutaneous or transthoracic needle aspiration of the lung is preferred over open lung biopsy and associated with a low risk of complications and a high rate of sensitivity, especially in patients with neoplastic disease.[47,48] Although these various invasive procedures frequently are used to obtain lung tissue for diagnosis, especially in compromised hosts, controversy exists as to whether the benefits exceed the risks and whether the findings lead to improved survival.[49]

All specimens, regardless of source, should be submitted for microscopic examination and culture, as already described. Any lung or pleural tissue should also be submitted for histopathologic studies including special stains.

In any patient in whom there is extrapulmonary disease, which is likely due to the same cause as the chronic pneumonia, tissue or fluid from the extrapulmonary sites should be obtained for culture and histologic studies. In such patients, consider the following procedures: arthrocentesis, abdominal paracentesis, lumbar puncture, bone marrow biopsy, liver biopsy, lymph node biopsy, and skin and muscle biopsy.

Studies in Patients with X-ray Film Evidence of Diffuse Pulmonary Infiltration and Fibrosis. In patients whose x-ray films show a predominately diffuse infiltrative pattern, either of the alveolar or interstitial type (Table 2), pulmonary function studies may be of greater importance. These studies will not only quantitate the degree of pulmonary insufficiency but may help to delineate the disease processes by virtue of the different patterns of pulmonary function impairment. Accordingly, these tests are particularly useful in characterizing those diseases that impair gas transfer and predispose to ventilation—perfusion inequalities, for example, sarcoidosis, interstitial pneumonia, or fibrosing alveolitis.

Studies that may be especially useful in this group of patients include the following:

1. Arterial blood gas studies, including resting and postexercise tests
2. Tests of pulmonary function including spirometric measurements, measurements of lung volume, measurement of pulmonary diffusing capacity and measurement of pulmonary compliance
3. Studies on sputum as previously outlined. Cytologic examination is especially important
4. Lung biopsy to make an accurate morphologic diagnosis. Transbronchial biopsy via the fiberoptic bronchoscope or open lung biopsy are the procedures of choice

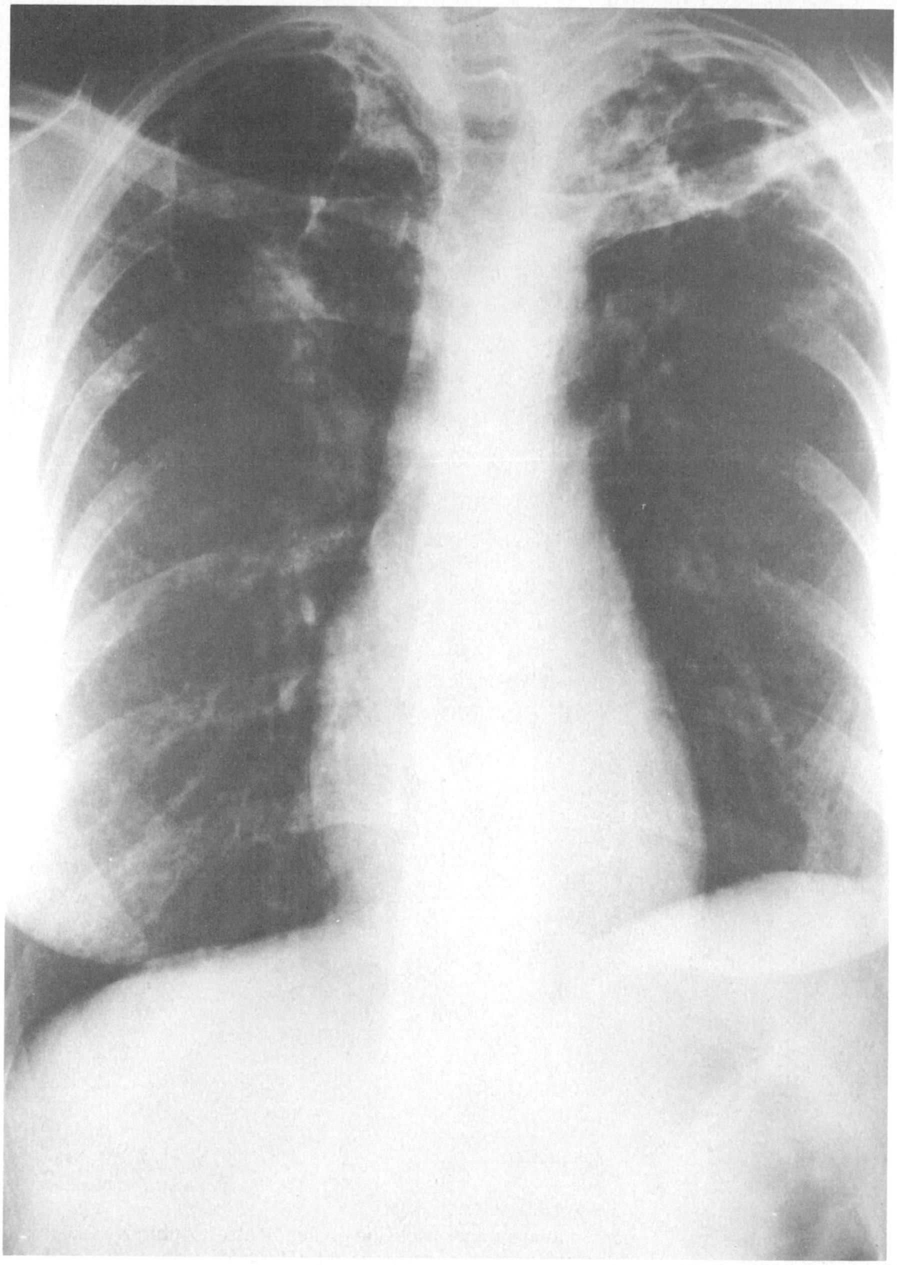

FIG. 10. Cavitary coccidioidomycosis in a 44-year-old woman who had previously lived in El Paso, Texas. She had been previously treated for tuberculosis that was never culture proven. At the time of this x-ray film she complained of hemoptysis. Note the bilateral upper lobe infiltrates with contracted lobes plus large thin-walled cavities as well as smaller thick-walled cavities.

THERAPY

Antimicrobial Agents

If a specific infectious agent is readily identified as the cause of the chronic pneumonia, the appropriate antimicrobial agent(s) should be administered. In many patients, no etiologic agent will be identified on the basis of the initial stains and cultures, and a definitive diagnosis must await the completion of serologic, histologic, and bacteriologic studies as well as other diagnostic tests. In such situations, if immediate empirical therapy is advisable, the choice of antimicrobial agents must be based on the available epidemiologic, clinical, and microbiologic data.

For example, if an otherwise healthy young patient has been ill for a relatively short period (2–3 weeks), the chest x-ray film shows a lobar or patchy pneumonia, especially in the lower lobes, Gram stain of the sputum reveals few-to-moderate polymorphonuclear leukocytes and organisms resembling normal flora, and the patient acquired the infection outside the hospital, the patient may have persistent or chronic pneumonia as a complication of one or more common acute pneumonia syndromes, namely, pneumococcal pneumonia, aspiration pneumonia, *Mycoplasma*-caused pneumonia, or legionnaires' disease. Reasonable empirical therapy in such a patient is erythromycin since this drug, in general, provides effective treatment of these four pneumonias. If, on the other hand, a patient has chronic pneumonia after thoracotomy, initial antimicrobial therapy should provide broad-spectrum coverage against normal mouth flora including anaerobes, *Staphylococcus aureus,* and aerobic gram-negative bacteria. In both of the above cases, once the path-

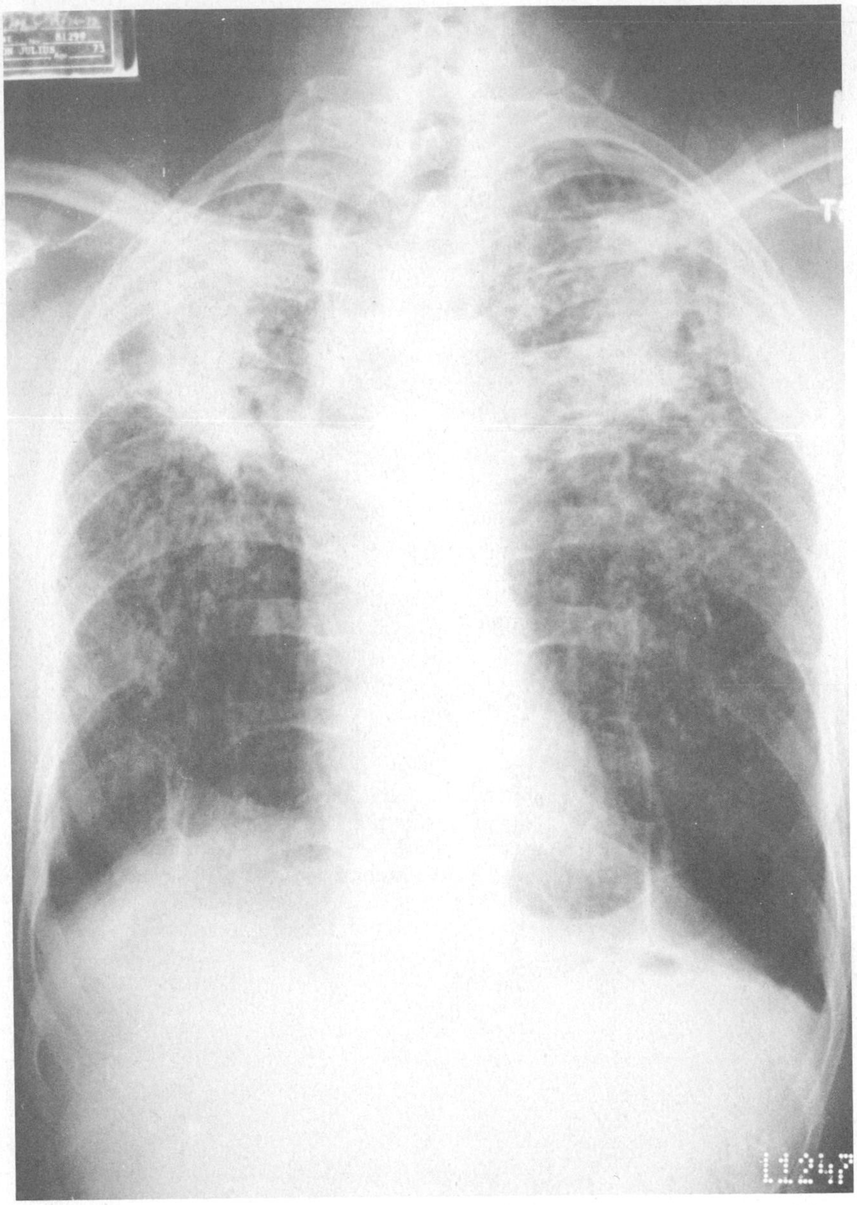

FIG. 11. Conglomerate silicosis in a 73-year-old former miner. Note the nodular masses of fibrous tissue in upper lung fields with upper lobe retraction and cavitation. Tuberculosis was searched for but not found.

ogen(s) has (have) been identified and sensitivity testing completed, appropriate changes in the antibiotic regimen should be made.

If a patient has a more chronic indolent illness, is stable, and does not require immediate empirical therapy, a methodic and thorough diagnostic evaluation is the initial priority. In a patient with bilateral upper lobe cavitary disease in whom the initial microscopic examinations are nonrevealing, the leading considerations include tuberculosis, histoplasmosis, and coccidioidomycosis. In general, in every such patient with a positive tuberculin test response, tuberculosis should be presumed to be the diagnosis until proved otherwise, and antituberculous therapy should be initiated and continued for at least 8 weeks, pending the final results of the mycobacterial cultures. Similarly, disseminated tuberculosis should be strongly suspected in any patient with unexplained fever and a chest film showing a nodular interstitial pattern; prompt institution of antituberculous therapy may be lifesaving in this otherwise fatal condition. In contrast, rarely should antifungal therapy be given empirically to a patient with chronic pneumonia since fungal pulmonary diseases usually progress slowly and the most commonly used agents, amphotericin B and ketoconazole, may be associated with significant toxicity.

Corticosteroids

The question of when to use corticosteroids in the treatment of a patient with chronic pneumonia frequently arises. If the cause of the illness is an infectious agent, particularly a bacterium or a fungus, steroids are usually not indicated. In contrast, corticosteroids may be helpful in chronic pneumonia due to noninfectious causes such as the vasculitidies, sarcoidosis, chronic eosinophilic pneumonia, and many of the fibrotic lung diseases including chronic hypersensitivity pneumonitis (along with avoidance of exposure to the offending antigen).

Supportive Measures

Vigorous measures aimed at good bronchopulmonary hygiene should be instituted. Generous fluid intake and humidified air

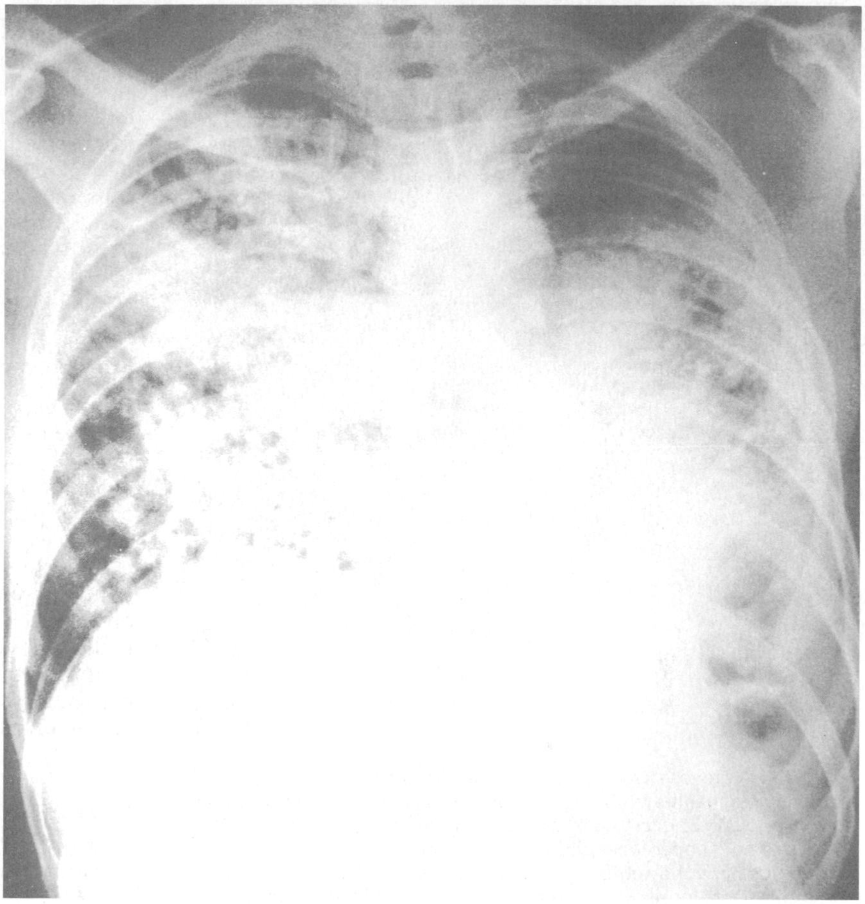

FIG. 12. Alveolar cell carcinoma in a 46-year-old man with a minimal smoking history. His symptoms of 6 months' duration included progressive dyspnea, cough with copious sputum production, and fever. Note the bilateral alveolar filling pattern.

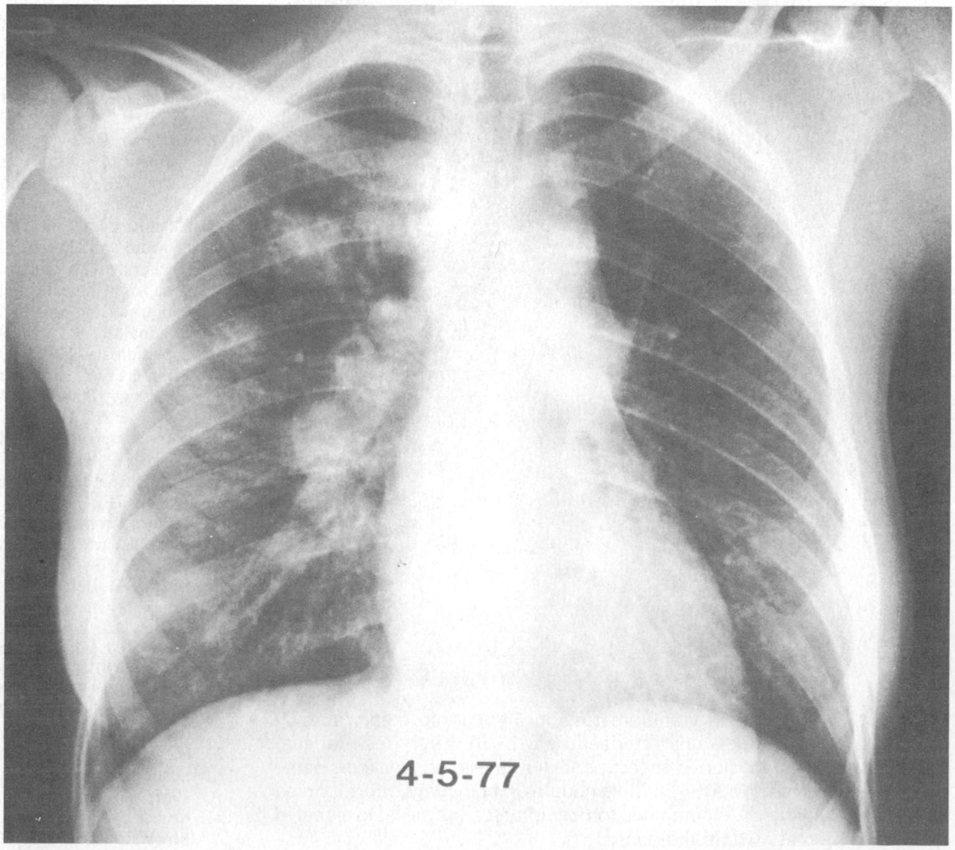

FIG. 13. Pulmonary sarcoidosis in a 22-year-old woman. Note the spherical, nodular opacities in the right lung and prominent right hilar adenopathy.

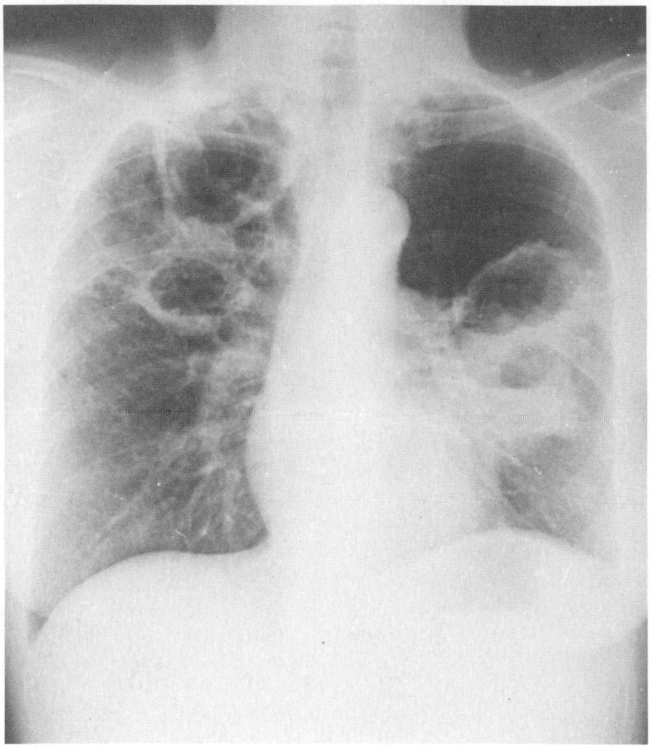

FIG. 14. Wegener's granulomatosis in a 55-year-old woman with a 4-month illness manifested by "sinus" headaches, cough, intermittent hemoptysis, pleuritic chest pain, and a 30 lb weight loss. Note the large cavities in both upper lobes and the subpleural nodule in the right upper lobe. Sinus films showed bilateral ethmoid and maxillary opacification. A pathologic diagnosis was made on tissue obtained at open lung biopsy.

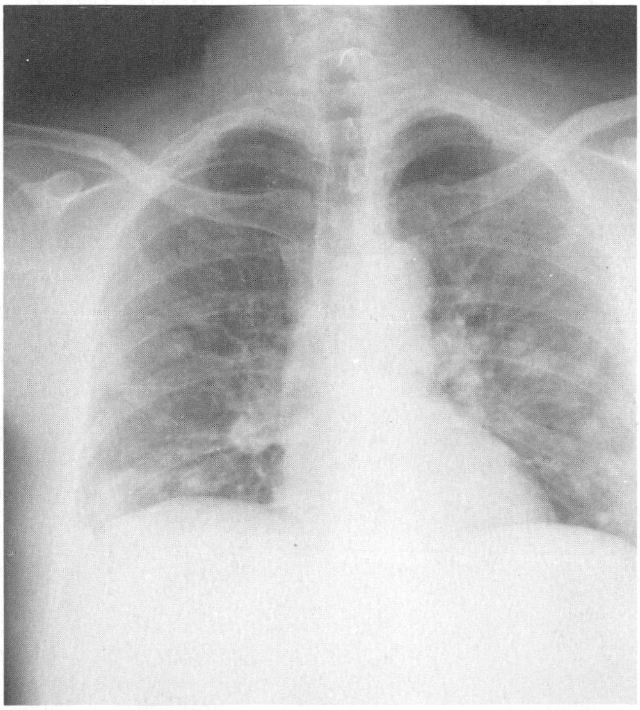

FIG. 15. Lymphomatoid granulomatosis in 54-year-old man with a 2-month progressive illness characterized by a 25 lb weight loss, fatigue, nonproductive cough, slurred speech, and numbness and weakness of the right side of his face. Note the multiple nodules in both lungs, more marked in the lower lung fields. A computed tomography scan of the head revealed an enhancing mass within the pons.

may promote easier expectoration. In patients with chronic cavitary disease or bronchiectasis and in whom there is copious sputum production, postural drainage and chest vibropercussion are important adjuncts. However, these procedures must be carried out with caution in an attempt to prevent infection from spreading to the noninvolved lung. Hypoxia may be a feature of chronic pneumonia; the severity will depend on the cause and the distribution of the pulmonary parenchymal process. Appropriate means of administering oxygen should be used to ensure adequate oxygen supply to the tissues, and alterations in delivery should be made on the basis of sequential arterial blood gas studies.

Bronchoscopy and Surgery

Bronchoscopy may be used as a therapeutic adjunct, especially in patients who have thick tenacious secretions that cannot be raised by noninvasive techniques. In other patients, mucous plugs or foreign bodies may predispose to atelectasis and chronic pneumonia; therapeutic bronchoscopy may be necessary to expand the collapsed lung.

Lobectomy or pneumonectomy should be considered in a patient with chronic destructive pneumonia and multiple macro- or microabscesses involving an entire lobe or lung and a ventilation–perfusion scan indicating nonfunction of the involved lung.[8] Thoracotomy may also be indicated for purposes of decortication of the pleura in patients whose chronic pneumonia has involved the pleura with resulting restrictive lung disease.

REFERENCES

1. Epler GR, Colby TV, McLoud TC, et al. Bronchiolitis obliterans organizing pneumonia. N Engl J Med. 1985;312:152–8.
2. Bartlett JG, Finegold SM. Anaerobic infections of the lung and pleural space. Am Rev Respir Dis. 1974;110:56–77.
3. Lerner AM. The gram-negative bacillary pneumonias. DM. 1980;27:1–56.
4. Khan MA, Kovnat DM, Bachus B, et al. Clinical and roentgenographic spectrum of pulmonary tuberculosis in the adult. Am J Med. 1977;62:31–8.
5. Rosenzweig DU. Pulmonary mycobacterial infections due to *Mycobacterium intracellulare avium* complex—clinical features and course in 100 consecutive cases. Chest. 1979;75:115–9.
6. Goodwin RA, Owens FT, Snell JD, et al. Chronic cavitary histoplasmosis. Medicine (Baltimore). 1976;55:413–52.
7. Bayer AS. Fungal pneumonias; pulmonary coccidioidal syndromes. Part 1 and Part 2. Chest. 1981;79:575–83,686–91.
8. Cameron EWJ, Appelbaum PC, Pudifin D, et al. Characteristics and management of chronic destructive pneumonia. Thorax. 1980;35:340–6.
9. Farrell GE, ed. Actinomycosis of the Thorax. St Louis: Warren H. Green; 1981:1–90.
10. Cush R, Light RW, George RB. Clinical and roentgenographic manifestations of acute and chronic blastomycosis. Chest. 1976;69:345–9.
11. Kerkering TM, Duma RJ, Shadomy S. The evolution of pulmonary cryptococcosis. Clinical implications from a study of 41 patients with and without compromising host factors. Ann Intern Med. 1981;94:611–6.
12. Zvetina JR, Rippon JW, Daum V. Chronic pulmonary sporotrichosis. Mycopathologia. 1978;64:53–7.
13. Emmons CW, Binford CH, Utz JP, et al., eds. Adiaspiromycosis. In: Medical Mycology. Philadelphia: Lea & Febiger; 1977:493–505.
14. Rosenow EC III, Wilson WR, Cockerill FR. Pulmonary disease in the immunocompromised host. Mayo Clin Proc. 1985;60:473–87,610–31.
15. Cairns MR, Durack DT. Fungal pneumonia in the immunocompromised host. Sem Respir Infect 1986;1:166–85.
16. Murray JF, Garay SM, Hopewell PC, et al. Pulmonary complications of the acquired immunodeficiency syndrome: An update. Report of the Second National Heart, Lung and Blood Institute Workshop. Am Rev Respir Dis. 1987;135:504–9.
17. Garay SM, Belenko M, Fazzini E, et al. Pulmonary manifestations of Kaposi's sarcoma. Chest. 1987;91:39–43.
18. Stover DE, White DA, Romano PA, et al. Spectrum of pulmonary diseases associated with the acquired immunodeficiency syndrome. Am J Med. 1985;78:429–37.
19. Suffredini AF, Ognibene FP, Lack EE, et al. Nonspecific interstitial pneumonitis: A common cause of pulmonary disease in the acquired immunodeficiency syndrome. Ann Intern Med. 1987;107:7–13.
20. Stead WW, Lofgren JP, Warren E, et al. Tuberculosis as an endemic and nosocomial infection among the elderly in nursing homes. N Engl J Med. 1985;312:1483–7.
21. Centers for Disease Control. Tuberculosis in minorities—United States. MMWR. 1987;36:77–80.

22. Baum GL, Donnerberg RL, Stewart D, et al. Pulmonary sporotrichosis. N Engl J Med. 1969;280:410–3.
23. Werner SB, Pappagianis D, Heindl I, et al. An epidemic of coccidioidomycosis among archeology students in northern California. N Engl J Med. 1972;286:507–12.
24. Rao S, Biddle M, Balchum OJ, et al. Focal endemic coccidioidomycosis in Los Angeles County. Am Rev Respir Dis. 1972;105:410–6.
25. Latham RH, Kaiser AB, DuPont WD, et al. Chronic pulmonary histoplasmosis following the excavation of a bird roost. Am J Med. 1980;68:504–8.
26. Seward CW. Outbreak of histoplasmosis in Oklahoma. Am Rev Respir Dis. 1970;102:950–8.
27. Ward JI, Weeks M, Allen D, et al. Acute histoplasmosis: Clinical, epidemiologic and serologic findings of an outbreak associated with exposure to a fallen tree. Am J Med. 1979;66:587–95.
28. Hasenclever HF, Shacklette MH, Young RV, et al. The natural occurrence of *H. capsulatum* in a cave. I. Epidemiologic aspects. Am J Epidemiol. 1967;886:238–45.
29. Kahn JB, Spruance C, Harbottle J, et al. Ecchinococcosis in Utah. Am J Trop Med Hyg. 1972;21:185–8.
30. Bristol LJ, Pneumoconioses caused by asbestos and by other siliceous and nonsiliceous dusts. Semin Roentgenol. 1967;2:283–305.
31. Parkes WR, ed. Nonneoplastic disorders due to metallic, chemical and physical agents. In: Occupational Lung Disorders. 2nd ed. London: Butterworths; 1982:454–98.
32. Everett ED, Nelson RA. Pulmonary melioidosis. Am Rev Respir Dis. 1975;112:331–40.
33. Warren KS, Mahmoud AAF. Algorithms in the diagnosis and management of exotic diseases. XXI. Liver, intestinal and lung flukes. J Infect Dis. 1977;135:692–6.
34. Frand UI, Shim CS, Williams MH Jr. Heroin-induced pulmonary edema. Sequential studies of pulmonary function. Ann Intern Med. 1972;77:29–35.
35. Robertson CH, Reynolds RC, Wilson JE. Pulmonary hypertension and foreign body granulomas in intravenous drug abusers. Documentation by cardiac catheterization and lung biopsy. Am J Med. 1976;61:657–64.
36. Patel RC, Dutta D, Schonfeld SA. Free-base cocaine use associated with bronchiolitis obliterans organizing pneumonia. Ann Intern Med. 1987;107:186–7.
37. Cooper JAD, White DA, Matthay RA. Drug-induced pulmonary disease. Part 1: Cytotoxic drugs. Part 2: Noncytotoxic drugs. Am Rev Respir Dis. 1986;133:321–40,488–505.
38. Reeder MM. Radiological Pathological Conference of the Month from Armed Forces Institute of Pathology: Hydatid cyst of the lung. Radiology. 1970;95:429–37.
39. Bartlett JG, Ryan KJ, Smith TF, et al. Cumitech 7A. In: Washington JA II, ed. Laboratory Diagnosis of Lower Respiratory Tract Infections. Washington, DC: American Society for Microbiology; 1987:1–18.
40. Wimberly NW, Bass JB, Boyd BW, et al. Use of bronchoscopic protected catheter brush for the diagnosis of pulmonary infections. Chest. 1982;81:556–62.
41. Stead WW. Second-strength PPD test (Letter). N Engl J Med. 1972;286:844.
42. Fulkerson WJ. Fiberoptic bronchoscopy. N Engl J Med. 1984;311:511–5.
43. Hanson RR, Zavala DC, Rhodes ML, et al. Transbronchial biopsy via flexible fiberoptic bronchoscope: Results in 164 patients. Am Rev Respir Dis. 1976;114:67–72.
44. Crystal RG, Reynolds HY, Kalica AR. Bronchoalveolar lavage: The report of an international conference. Chest. 1986;90:122–31.
45. Stover DE, Zaman MB, Hajdn SI, et al. Bronchoalveolar lavage in the diagnosis of diffuse pulmonary infiltrates in the immunosuppressed host. Ann Intern Med. 1984;101:1–7.
46. Cockerill FR III, Wilson WR, Carpenter HA, et al. Open lung biopsy in immunocompromised patients. Arch Intern Med. 1985;145:1398–1404.
47. Zavala DC, Schoell JE. Ultrathin needle aspiration of the lung in infectious and malignant disease. Am Rev Respir Dis. 1981;123:125–31.
48. Wang KP, Kelly SJ, Britt JE. Percutaneous needle aspiration biopsy of chest lesions: New instrument and new technique. Chest. 1988;93:993–7.
49. Robin ED, Burke CM. Lung biopsy in immunosuppressed patients. Chest. 1986;89:276–8.

57. CYSTIC FIBROSIS

MICHAEL R. KNOWLES
PETER GILLIGAN
RICHARD C. BOUCHER

Because the molecular basis of this genetic disorder is unknown, cystic fibrosis (CF) remains in strict terms a syndrome rather than a disease, and the diagnosis rests on a compatible clinical picture. Diagnostic criteria include chronic obstructive lung disease and/or pancreatic exocrine insufficiency; the presence of characteristic sputum microbiologic flora (i.e., mucoid *Pseudomonas aeruginosa* and *Staphylococcus aureus*); and a family history of CF. The diagnosis is supported by the hallmark laboratory abnormality, an elevated sweat chloride concentration. Although CF is generally regarded as a disease of children, about one-third of currently identified CF patients are adults. It should be noted that the normal range for sweat chloride values in adults is greater than for children. Whereas values must be less than 40 mEq/liter to be clearly normal in children, healthy adults may have values of up to 70 mEq/liter.[1]

CLINICAL MANIFESTATIONS

The clinical manifestations of CF reflect obstruction of organs by viscous secretions and the presence of a chronic bacterial infection in the lung. Although multiple organ systems are involved, chronic airway infection accounts for most disease-related morbidity and mortality. Chronic suppurative airway disease is present in more than 98 percent of adults who have CF, and 95 percent of CF deaths are related to progressive pulmonary insufficiency.[1–3] Most respiratory infections in CF adults are caused by *S. aureus, P. aeruginosa*, and *Haemophilus influenzae*, whereas the incidence of infections with other infectious agents (e.g., *Mycoplasma pneumoniae*, and viruses) is believed to be similar to that of the general population.[4,5]

The clinical picture of CF is dominated by a chronic cough punctuated by episodes of clinical deterioration that are characterized by an increased volume and purulence of sputum, dyspnea, and sometimes anorexia and weight loss. Although adults with CF may exhibit low-grade fever with these exacerbations, high fever is unusual and sepsis or bacteremia is extraordinarily uncommon despite the large number of bacteria in the airways (10^8 organisms per milliliter of sputum). Clinical exacerbations are also associated with modest elevations of white blood cell counts and worsening spirometric values. The chest radiography typically is dominated by cystic bronchiectatic changes and diffuse roentgenographic shadowing that reflects airway wall thickening and retained secretions. Many adult CF patients exhibit an upper lung zone predominance of these roentgenographic abnormalities, which raises the diagnostic possibility of tuberculosis. Hypoxemia and carbon dioxide retention are uncommon in CF adults during acute exacerbations until the forced expired volume in one second (FEV_1) is less than 50 percent of the predicted value. Thus, significant gas exchange abnormalities usually occur only near the terminal stages of the disease and herald a relatively rapid downhill course.

The pulmonary manifestations of CF in adults are frequently complicated by hemoptysis and pneumothorax. Minor hemoptysis occurs in more than 50 percent of CF patients, and massive hemoptysis occurs in 5–10 percent of adult CF patients. Fortunately, medical (nonsurgical) intervention is usually sufficient for the treatment of pulmonary hemorrhage. The presence of CF epithelial defects in the mucosa of the nasal sinuses, and the frequent occurrence of nasal polyps in adults, make symptoms of subacute/chronic sinusitis a major problem in many adult patients. It is important to note that the microbiology of sinusitis is not reflected by the flora identified in expectorated sputum.[6]

Because most CF patients have progressive destruction and loss of pancreatic function, the prevalence of diabetes mellitus in adult CF populations may be as high as 15 percent.[8] The presence of glucose intolerance may add further difficulty to the treatment of pulmonary infection.

PATHOGENESIS

The clinical syndrome of CF reflects an autosomal recessive genetic disorder. Although the CF defect has not been identified in molecular terms, it has been localized to the Cen-q22 region of chromosome 7 with studies using restriction length fragment polymorphisms.[8–10] Linkage analysis allows accurate genetic counseling for the parents of most CF patients.[11]

Two general features characterize the pathogenesis of CF at the cellular level: (*1*) the affected cells in target organs are epithelia; and (*2*) the abnormality in epithelial cells appears to involve regulation of ion transport. The most prevalent defect is abnormal regulation of the activation state of plasma membrane Cl^- channels. Defective Cl^- channel activation has been detected in the epithelia of airways,[12–14] sweat ducts,[15] and the small intestine.[16] In airway epithelia, the Cl^- defect principally reflects abnormalities in cAMP-dependent mechanisms for channel activation.[17,18] A second major defect in ion transport has been detected in CF airway epithelia. The rate of absorption of Na^+ ions from the airway lumen to the interstitium is raised threefold compared to normal.[17] In contrast to the failure of cAMP to activate Cl^- channels in airway epithelia, cAMP further increases the accelerated rate of Na^+ absorption in CF airway epithelia.[17]

Because the ion transport activities of airway epithelia regulate the volume and composition of the liquids (secretions) that line airway surfaces, the ion transport abnormalities that characterize CF affect these liquids. Both accelerated Na^+ absorption and reduced Cl^- channel permeability, by inhibiting Cl^- ion secretion, would be expected to reduce the water content of secretions. The depletion of water, perhaps by changing the viscoelastic properties of secretions and/or the linkage between the mucous component of secretions and cilia, projects reductions in mucociliary and cough clearance. Whether reduced clearance of thickened secretions from the airways is sufficient to lead to persistent staphylococcal and pseudomonal infection is not clear. A role for increased bacterial adherence, perhaps through a change in the $SO_4^=$ content of the airway cell surface glycocalyx, has recently been postulated.[19]

The development of persistent bacterial infection generates a complex series of events that lead to airway wall damage and ultimately to destroyed or bronchiectatic airways. Bacterial exoproducts from both *S. aureus* and *P. aeruginosa* have been implicated in airway destruction. In adults, lipopolysaccharides, exotoxin A, and a cell wall-associated rhamnolipid from *P. aeruginosa* have been implicated as important bacterial toxins.[20] The host inflammatory response appears intact in CF, and the vigorous host response may contribute to airway damage. Chemotactic agents, both bacterial and locally derived (e.g., arachidonic acid metabolites from airway epithelia), attract inflammatory cells into the airway lumen. Polymorphonuclear cell-derived enzymes (e.g., elastase) likely damage airway wall structures. In addition, it has been reported that the chronic antigenic stimulus of persistent airway infections generates immunologically mediated airway wall destruction. The best-documented response of this type is antigen–antibody complex-mediated damage.[21] Eventually, the combination of retained secretions and airway damage deranges gas exchange, perturbs cardiac function, and leads to death.

MICROBIOLOGY

Staphylococcus aureus and *P. aeruginosa* are the primary etiologic agents of pulmonary infection in patients with CF.[22] *Staphylococcus aureus* often colonizes the respiratory tract in the first 2 years of life and can be found in up to 50–60 percent of patients with CF in the United States. Before the advent of effective antistaphylococcal therapy, lung infection due to this organism was the leading cause of death. Antistaphylococcal penicillins such as oxacillin and nafcillin control infections with this organism, and resistance to these agents is very unusual. In patients receiving long-term (>3 months) prophylactic trimethoprim/sulfamethoxazole therapy, approximately 50 percent of *S. aureus* isolated is thymidine dependent.[23] Because thymidine-dependent organisms grow poorly on most commonly used isolation media, and because mucoid *P. aeruginosa* may obscure recognition of its growth, mannitol salts agar must be used to ensure reliable recovery of *S. aureus*.

In childhood or early adolescence, patients with CF become chronically infected with *P. aeruginosa*. Up to 70 percent of patients with CF, primarily adolescents and adults, are infected with this organism. The *P. aeruginosa* isolates recovered from these patients appear to evolve from a smooth, serum-resistant, serotypable organism to a rough, serum-sensitive, nonserotypable one.[24] The latter form of *P. aeruginosa* is characterized by its ability to produce large amounts of an extracellular cell-associated mucoid polysaccharide referred to as *alginate*.[25] Mucoid colonies that result from alginate production are predominant in infected CF patients but are rarely seen in other patients with chronic airway disease.[26] This mucoid variant is believed to be responsible for the formation of microcolonies that are believed to be resistant to both mechanical and immunologic clearance from the airways.

When first isolated, *P. aeruginosa* is usually susceptible to all antipseudomonal β-lactams, imipenem, quinolones, and aminoglycosides. With increasing antimicrobial pressure due to repeated antimicrobial treatment of pulmonary exacerbations, resistance to these agents may develop, especially if each one is used alone. In patients repeatedly treated for *P. aeruginosa*, the organism may remain susceptible only to polymixin b and colistin.

A third organism, *Pseudomonas cepacia*, which has been recovered from up to 20 percent of patients at selected CF centers,[27] has recently been recognized as a potentially important agent in the lung disease of adults with CF. This organism has been associated with significantly increased mortality and presents difficult problems for the clinician. First, *P. cepacia* is usually resistant (>90 percent of isolates) to ticarcillin and aminoglycosides on initial isolation and, after therapy with antipseudomonal β-lactams or trimethoprim/sulfamethoxazole, will often become resistant to them as well. Imipenem and the quinolones are only marginally active against this organism. Second, the organism may be difficult to recover from airway secretions unless specific isolation media[28] are used because the organism grows slowly and may be obscured by other airway flora, particularly mucoid *P. aeruginosa*. Finally, unlike *P. aeruginosa, P. cepacia* produces few easily identifiable virulence factors,[29] making the mechanism by which it produces lung disease obscure.

Other microbes, such as *Haemophilus influenzae, Branhamella catarrhalis, Xanthamonas maltophilia, Achromobacter xylosoxidans*, and Enterobactericeae, may play a role in the pulmonary disease observed in CF patients. Of these organisms, the recovery of *H. influenzae* is particularly difficult because other organisms, particularly *P. aeruginosa*, may overgrow the isolation medium. This obstacle can be overcome by incubating enrichment medium under anaerobic conditions in order to inhibit the growth of *P. aeruginosa*.[30]

Mycobacteria, including *M. tuberculosis, M. avium-intracellulare*, and Runyon group IV mycobacteria, have infrequently been recovered from patients with CF.[31] One of the difficulties in isolating mycobacteria in this population is that proteases present in CF sputa may liquify the Lowestein-Jensen agar slants.

Aspergillus fumigatus may be cultured from CF patients,[32] and elevated titers of IgG antibody may be found in serum from these patients. Unless the patient has pre-existing asthma, he or she does not fulfill the diagnostic criteria for the clinical syndrome of allergic bronchopulmonary aspergillosis.

The exact role of viral infection in pulmonary deterioration of patients with CF has not been clearly defined. In a prospective study, no virus could be recovered from nasopharyngeal washings of symptomatic patients with CF, although some of these patients had serologic evidence of viral infection.[33]

TREATMENT

The goal of therapy is to retard progressive lung damage by controlling bacterial infection with antibiotics, by removing viscous/purulent airway secretions, and by providing proper nutrition for host defense. Antibiotics have played a key role in improved survival, and indications for antimicrobial therapy continue to evolve.[2–5,34]

Broad-spectrum oral antibiotics (amoxicillin, cephalexin, dicloxacillin, tetracycline, trimethoprim/sulfamethoxazole) can provide successful therapy for acute pulmonary exacerbations despite the presence of *P. aeruginosa* that is resistant to these agents. The clinical benefit may reflect antibiotic activity against pathogens that are difficult to culture in the presence of mucoid *P. aeruginosa* (*S. aureus, H. influenzae*) or against airway infection with high concentrations of bacteria ($>10^5$ organisms/per milliliter) that are not typical pathogens.[2] High doses and prolonged therapy (3–4 weeks) are recommended for treatment of acute illnesses (exacerbations) with oral agents. Oral antibiotics are also of benefit in chronic bacterial sinusitis, which results from pathogens that are frequently sensitive to broad-spectrum antimicrobials.[6] The use of oral antibiotics for prophylactic (maintenance) therapy is controversial but may have a useful role in some patients.

Ciprofloxacin is an oral antipseudomonal drug that is useful for intermittent therapy. The emergence of bacterial resistance during monotherapy with this drug limits its usefulness for chronic treatment,[35–37] and the duration of periodic treatment should be limited to 2–4 weeks.[34]

Aggressive parenteral therapy is indicated for clinical exacerbations that do not respond to oral antimicrobials.[2–4,34] Although sterilization of airway secretions rarely occurs and is not the goal of parenteral therapy, the bacterial burden in conducting airways can be reduced[38] and irreversible lung damage presumably retarded. Whereas parenteral therapy should be guided by sputum bacteriology and drug sensitivity, treatment in adult CF patients usually focuses on *P. aeruginosa*. A combination of antibiotics is indicated because thickened airway secretions present a barrier to drug penetration and because aminoglycoside activity can be reduced by suppurative secretions.[39] A combination of antibiotics also protects against the emergence of resistant strains. Therapy usually includes an aminoglycoside (gentamicin, tobramycin, amikacin), plus another agent effective against *P. aeruginosa,* such as antipseudomonal penicillins, cephalosporins (e.g., ceftazidime[40,41]), or imipenem. If *S. aureus* is clinically suspected or cultured from sputum, addition of a specific antistaphylococcal agent should be considered if the antipseudomonal drug therapy is not adequate for *S. aureus*. Increased plasma clearance of almost all effective antibiotics in CF patients dictates the use of large, frequent doses of antimicrobials.[42] For example, CF adults require 6–15/mg/kg/day of gentamicin to achieve desired peak serum levels of 10 μg/ml in a q8h dosing regimen. Aminoglycoside toxicity is uncommon in CF patients, but trough serum levels should be carefully monitored. Parenteral therapy should be continued for a minimum of 10–14 days or until a full clinical and pulmonary functional response has been achieved. Recent experience suggests that effective parenteral antibiotic therapy can be administered on an outpatient basis.[43]

Aerosolized antibiotics can be used for subacute pulmonary exacerbations and to assist in the maintenance of a stable clinical status in some patients.[44] Effective aerosol delivery techniques are essential if this approach is to be successful.[45,46] Colistin is an attractive agent for inhalation therapy.[47] The development of bacterial resistance during prolonged aerosol therapy with colistin does not reduce the response to parenteral alternatives.

Interestingly, despite intensive antibiotic exposure, symptomatic disease with *Clostridium difficile* is uncommon in CF patients despite the presence of the organism in fecal samples.[48,49] The asymptomatic carriage of *C. difficile* may reflect the absence of the capacity of the CF intestinal epithelium to response to *C. difficile*-derived toxins.[16]

The presence of a large bacterial burden in the bronchiectatic airways of patients dictates that airway clearance techniques be combined with antibacterial therapy to achieve optimal results.[3–5] Chest percussion and postural drainage is the time-honored method, but deep breathing, exercise, and voluntary coughing are also effective. Bronchodilators may assist in clearing retained secretions in some patients, but a paradoxical reduction in airflow in some patients,[50] and potential acceleration of abnormal Na^+ transport,[17] suggest that these agents should be used intermittently and with caution in adult CF patients. Anti-inflammatory agents may occasionally be useful in reducing mucosal edema and assisting in airway clearance, but the indications for these agents are poorly defined.[4] There is little role for the use of inhaled mucolytic agents or bronchial lavage.[3]

Chronic malabsorption, coupled with increased caloric requirements due to chronic infection and increased respiratory activity, can induce malnourishment and impaired host–defense mechanisms in CF patients. High caloric intake with supplemental pancreatic digestive enzymes is therefore essential in the treatment of these patients.[51]

Although *A. fumigatus* is frequently cultured from the sputum of CF adults, treatment with systemic corticosteroids is usually not indicated, unless the syndrome of allergic bronchopulmonary aspergillosis is established. The increasing number of adults in the CF patient population is associated with increasing recovery of nontuberculous mycobacteria from sputum cultures.[22] The clinical and radiographic patterns should be monitored for evidence of pathogenic mycobacterial activity.

Annual influenza vaccinations are recommended, but the pneumococcal vaccine is not routinely indicated because of the relative absence of *S. pneumoniae* as a pathogen.

Finally, heart-lung transplants are a novel therapeutic strategy in patients with CF. Of 6 long-term (23 months) surviving patients, 3 had airway infection, 1 with *H. influenzae*, 1 with *P. aeruginosa*, and 1 with *S. aureus* and *P. aeruginosa*.[52]

REFERENCES

1. Davis PB. Cystic fibrosis in adults. In: Lloyd-Still JD, ed. Textbook of Cystic Fibrosis. V. 9. Littleton, Mass: John Wright-PSG; 1983:351–66.
2. Myers MG, Koontz FP, Weinberger M. Lower respiratory infections in patients with cystic fibrosis. In: Lloyd-Still JD, ed. Textbook of Cystic Fibrosis. V. 90. Littleton, Mass: John Wright-PSG; 1983;91–107.
3. Taussig LM, Landau LI, Marks MI. Respiratory system. In: Taussig LM, ed. Cystic Fibrosis. V. 5. New York: Thieme-Stratton; 1984;115–74.
4. Mischler EH. Treatment of pulmonary disease in cystic fibrosis. Semin Respir Med. 1985;6(4):271–84.
5. Thomassen MJ, Demko CA, Doershuk CF. Cystic fibrosis: A review of pulmonary infections and interventions. Pediatr-Pulmonol. 1987;3(5):334–51.
6. Shapiro ED, Milmoe GJ, Wald ER, et al. Bacteriology of the maxillary sinuses in patients with cystic fibrosis. J Infect Dis. 1982;146(5):589–93.
7. Knowles MR, Fernald GW. Diabetes and cystic fibrosis: New questions emerging from increased longevity. J Pediatr. 1988;101:415–16.
8. Egberg H, Mohr J, Schmiegelow K, et al. Linkage relationships of paraoxonase (PON) with other markers: Indication of PON-cystic fibrosis synteny. Clin Genet. 1985;28:265–71.
9. Tsui L-C, Buchwald M, Barker D, et al. Cystic fibrosis locus defined by a genetically linked polymorphic DNA marker. Science. 1985;230:1054–7.
10. Wainwright BJ, et al. Localization of cystic fibrosis locus to human chromosome 7cen-q22. Nature. 1985;318:384–5.
11. Beaudet A, Spence J, O'Brien W, et al. Experience with new DNA markers for the diagnosis of cystic fibrosis. N Engl J Med. 1988;318:50–1.
12. Knowles MR, Stutts MJ, Spock A, et al. Abnormal ion permeation through cystic fibrosis respiratory epithelium. Science. 1983;221:1067–70.
13. Frizzell RA, Rechkemmer G, Shoemaker RL. Altered regulation of airway epithelial cell chloride channels in cystic fibrosis. Science. 1986;233:558–60.

14. Case M. Cl^- impermeability in cystic fibrosis. Nature. 1986;322:407.
15. Quinton PM. Chloride impermeability in cystic fibrosis. Nature. 1983;301:421–2.
16. Berschneider HM, Knowles MR, Azizkhan RG, et al. Altered intestinal chloride transport in cystic fibrosis. FASEB J. 1988;2(10):2625–9.
17. Boucher RC, Stutts MJ, Knowles MR, et al. Na^+ transport in cystic fibrosis respiratory epithelia: Abnormal basal rate and response to adenylate cyclase activation. J Clin Invest. 1986;78:1245–52.
18. Shoumacher RA, Shoemaker RL, Halm DR, et al. Phosphorylation fails to activate chloride channels from cystic fibrosis airway cells. Nature. 1987;330:752–4.
19. Cheng P-W, Boucher RC, Yankaskas JR, et al. Glycoconjugates secreted by cultured human nasal epithelial cells. In: Mastella G, Quinton PM, eds. Cellular and Molecular Basis of Cystic Fibrosis. San Francisco: San Francisco Press; 1988:233–8.
20. Stutts MJ, Schwab JH, Chen MG, et al. Effects of *Pseudomonas aeruginosa* on bronchial epithelial ion transport. Am Rev Respir Dis. 1986;134:17–24.
21. Lewiston NJ, Moss RB. Circulating immune complexes decrease during corticosteroid therapy in cystic fibrosis. Pediatr Res. 1982;16:354.
22. Friend PA. Pulmonary infection in cystic fibrosis. J Infect. 1986;13:55–72.
23. Gilligan PH, Gage PA, Welch DF, et al. Prevalence of thymidine-dependent *Staphylococcus aureus* in patients with cystic fibrosis. J Clin Microbiol. 1987;25:1258–61.
24. Penketh A, Pitt T, Roberts D, et al. The relationship of phenotype changes in *Pseudomonas aeruginosa* to the clinical conditions of patients with cystic fibrosis. Am Rev Respir Dis. 1983;127:605–8.
25. Pier GB. Pulmonary disease associated with *Pseudomonas aeruginosa* in cystic fibrosis: Current status of the host–bacterium interaction. J Infect Dis. 1985;151:575–80.
26. McCarthy VP, Rosenberg G, Rosenstein BJ, et al. Mucoid *Pseudomonas aeruginosa* from a patient without cystic fibrosis: Implications and review of the literature. Pediatr Infect Dis. 1986;5:256–8.
27. Tablan OC, Chorba TH, Schidlow DV, et al. *Pseudomonas cepacia* colonization in patients with cystic fibrosis: Risk factors and clinical outcome. J Pediatr. 1985;107:382–7.
28. Gilligan RH, Gage PA, Bradshaw LM, et al. Isolation medium for the recovery of *Pseudomonas cepacia* from respiratory secretions of patients with cystic fibrosis. J Clin Microbiol. 1985;139:805–8.
29. McKevitt AI, Woods DE. Characterization of *Pseudomonas cepacia* isolates from patients with cystic fibrosis. J Clin Microbiol. 1984;19:291–3.
30. Roberts DE, Cole P. Use of selective media in bacteriological investigation of patients with chronic respiratory infections. Lancet. 1980;1:796–7.
31. Smith MJ, Efthimou J, Hodson ME, et al. Mycobacterial isolations in young adults with cystic fibrosis. Thorax. 1984;39:369–75.
32. Brueton MJ, Ormerod LP, Shah KJ, et al. Allergic bronchopulmonary aspergillosis complicating cystic fibrosis in childhood. Arch Dis Child. 1980;55:348–53.
33. Wang EEH, Prober GC, Munson B, et al. Association of respiratory viral infections with pulmonary deterioration in patients with cystic fibrosis. N Engl J Med 1984;311:1653–8.
34. Michel BC. Antibacterial therapy in cystic fibrosis: A review of the literature published between 1980 and February 1987. Chest. 1988;94(2S):129S–40S.
35. Scully BE, Nakatomi M, Ores C, et al. Ciprofloxacin therapy in cystic fibrosis. Am J Med. 1987;82(4A):196–201.
36. Goldfarb J, Stern RC, Reed MD, et al. Ciprofloxacin monotherapy for acute pulmonary exacerbations of cystic fibrosis. Am J Med. 1987;82(4A):174–9.
37. Stutman HR. Summary of a workshop on ciprofloxacin use in patients with cystic fibrosis. Pediatr Infect Dis J. 1987;6(10):932–5.
38. Smith AL, Redding G, Doershuk C, et al. Sputum changes associated with therapy for endobronchial exacerbation in cystic fibrosis. J Pediatr. 1988;112:547–54.
39. Mendelman PM, Smith AL, Levy J, et al. Aminoglycoside penetration, inactivation, and efficacy in cystic fibrosis sputum. Am Rev Respir Dis. 1985;132:761–5.
40. Blumer JL, Stern RC, Yamashita TS, et al. Cephalosporin therapeutics in cystic fibrosis. J Pediatr. 1986;108(5 Pt 2):854–60.
41. Reed MD, Stern RC, O'Brien CA, et al. Randomized double-blind evaluation of ceftazidime dose ranging in hospitalized patients with cystic fibrosis. Antimicrob Agents Chemother 1987;31(5)698–702.
42. de Groot R, Smith AL. Antibiotic pharmacokinetics in cystic fibrosis: Differences and clinical significance. Clin Pharmacokinet. 1987;13:228–53.
43. Donati MA, Guenette G, Auerbach H. Prospective controlled study of home and hospital therapy of cystic fibrosis pulmonary disease. J Pediatr. 1987;111:28–33.
44. Stead RJ, Hodson ME, Batten JC. Inhaled ceftazidime compared with gentamycin and carbenicillin in older patients with cystic fibrosis infected with *Pseudomonas aeruginosa*. Br J Dis Chest. 1987;81:272–9.
45. Newman SP, Pavia D. Aerosol deposition in man. In: Moren F, Newhouse MT, eds. Aerosols in Medicine: Principles, Diagnosis and Therapy. V. 7. Amsterdam: Elsevier, 1986:193–218.
46. Newman SP, Woodman G, Clarke SW. Deposition of carbenicillin aerosols in cystic fibrosis: Effects of nebulizer system and breathing pattern. Thorax. 1988;43:318–22.
47. Jensen T, Pedersen SS, Garne S, et al. Colistin inhalation therapy in cystic fibrosis patients with chronic Pseudomonas aeruginosa lung infection. J Antimicrob Chemother. 1987;19:831–8.
48. Welkon CJ, Long SS, Thompson CM, et al. *Clostridium difficile* in patients with cystic fibrosis. Am J Dis Child. 1987;139:805–8.
49. Peach SL, Borriello SP, Gaya H, et al. Asymptomatic carriage of *Clostridium difficile* in patients with cystic fibrosis. J Clin Pathol. 1986;39:1013–8.
50. Shapiro GG, Bamman J, Kanarek P, et al. The paradoxical effect of adrenergic and methylxanthine drugs in cystic fibrosis. Pediatrics. 1976;58(5):740–3.
51. Hubbard VS. Nutritional considerations in cystic fibrosis. Semin Respir. Med. 1985;6(4):308–13.
52. Scott J, Higenbottam T, Hutter J, et al. Heart–lung transplantation for cystic fibrosis. Lancet. 1988;2:192–4.

SECTION D.

58. URINARY TRACT INFECTIONS

JACK D. SOBEL
DONALD KAYE

Bacteriuria is a frequently used term and literally means bacteria in the urine. The probability of the presence of infected urine in the bladder can be ascertained by means of quantitating numbers of bacteria in voided urine and in urine obtained via urethral catheterization. *Significant bacteriuria* is a term that has been used to describe the numbers of bacteria in voided urine that exceed the numbers usually due to contamination from the anterior urethra (i.e., $\geq 10^5$ bacteria/ml). The implication is that in the presence of $\geq 10^5$ bacteria/ml urine, infection must be seriously considered. *Asymptomatic bacteriuria* refers to significant bacteriuria in a patient without symptoms.

Urinary tract infection may only involve the lower urinary tract or may involve both the upper and lower tracts. The term *cystitis* has been used to describe the syndrome involving dysuria, frequency, urgency, and occasionally suprapubic tenderness. However, these symptoms may be related to lower tract inflammation without bacterial infection and can be caused by urethritis (for example, gonorrhea or chlamydial urethritis). Furthermore, the presence of symptoms of lower tract infection without upper tract symptoms by no means excludes upper tract infection, which is also often present.

Acute pyelonephritis describes the clinical syndrome characterized by flank pain and/or tenderness and fever, often associated with dysuria, urgency, and frequency. However, these symptoms can occur in the absence of infection (for example, in renal infarction or renal calculus). A more rigorous definition of acute pyelonephritis is the above syndrome accompanied by significant bacteriuria and acute infection in the kidney.

Urinary tract infection may occur de novo or may be a recurrent infection. Recurrences may be either *relapses* or *reinfections*. Relapse of bacteriuria refers to recurrence of bacteriuria with the same infecting microorganism that was present before therapy was started. This is due to persistence of the organism in the urinary tract. Reinfection is a recurrence of bacteriuria with a microorganism different from the original infecting bacterium. It is a new infection. Occasionally reinfection may occur with the same microorganism, which may have persisted in the vagina or feces. This can be mistaken for a relapse.

The term *chronic urinary tract infection* has little meaning in many patients. True chronic infection should really mean persistence of the same organism for months or years with relapses after treatment. Reinfections do not mean chronicity any more than repeated episodes of pneumonia indicate chronic pneumonia. However, in spite of the questionable application of the term, many authorities have grouped patients with relapsing infections and reinfections together as having "chronic infection."

The term *chronic pyelonephritis* is difficult to define and means different things to different authors. To some, chronic pyelonephritis refers to pathologic changes in the kidney due to infection only. However, identical pathologic alterations are found in several other entities such as chronic urinary tract obstruction, analgesic nephropathy, hypokalemic nephropathy, vascular disease, and uric acid nephropathy. Pathologic descriptions do not (and cannot) differentiate between the changes produced by infection versus those produced by these other entities.

Papillary necrosis from infection is an acute complication of pyelonephritis usually in the presence of diabetes mellitis, urinary tract obstruction, sickle cell disease, or analgesic abuse. Papillary necrosis can occur in the absence of infection in some of these conditions. The necrotic renal papillae may slough and cause unilateral or bilateral ureteral obstruction. *Intrarenal abscess* may result from bacteremia or may be a complication of severe pyelonephritis. *Perinephric abscess* occurs when microorganisms from either the renal parenchyma or blood are deposited in the soft tissues surrounding the kidneys.

PATHOLOGIC CHARACTERISTICS

Acute Pyelonephritis

In severe acute pyelonephritis the kidney is somewhat enlarged, and discrete, yellowish, raised abscesses are apparent on the surface (Fig. 1). The pathognomonic histologic feature is suppurative necrosis or abscess formation within the renal substance.[1]

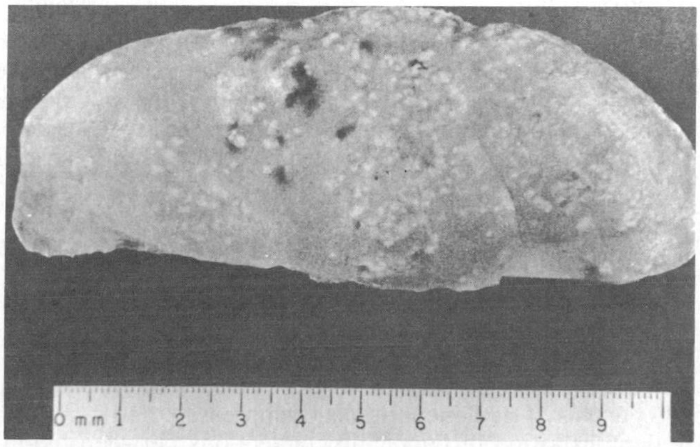

FIG. 1. Acute pyelonephritis in an elderly diabetic man. Note the numerous raised abscesses on the cortical surface. (From Kaye,[340] with permission.

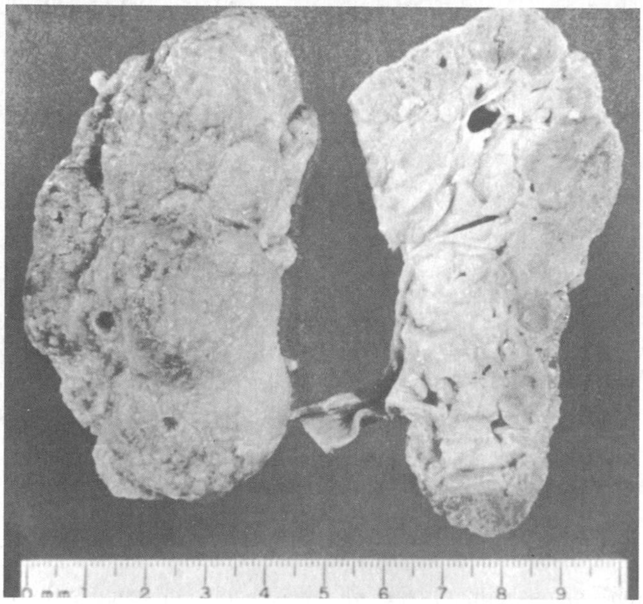

FIG. 2. Chronic pyelonephritis. The kidney is contracted and coarsely scarred, weighing 80 g. Note the thinned cortex and the poorly defined corticomedullary demarcation. (From Kaye,[340] with permission.)

Chronic Pyelonephritis (Chronic Interstitial Nephritis)

The pathologic picture of "chronic pyelonephritis" can be described as follows.[1] One or both kidneys contain gross scars, but even when involvement is bilateral, the kidneys are not equally damaged. This uneven scarring is useful in differentiating chronic pyelonephritis from diseases that cause symmetrical contracted kidneys, for example, chronic glomerulonephritis (Fig. 2). There are inflammatory changes in the pelvic wall with papillary atrophy and blunting. The parenchyma shows interstitial fibrosis with an inflammatory infiltrate of lymphocytes, plasma cells, and occasionally neutrophils (Fig. 3). The tubules are dilated or contracted with atrophy of the lining epithelium. Many of the dilated tubules contain colloid casts, which suggest the appearance of thyroid tissue ("thyroidiza-

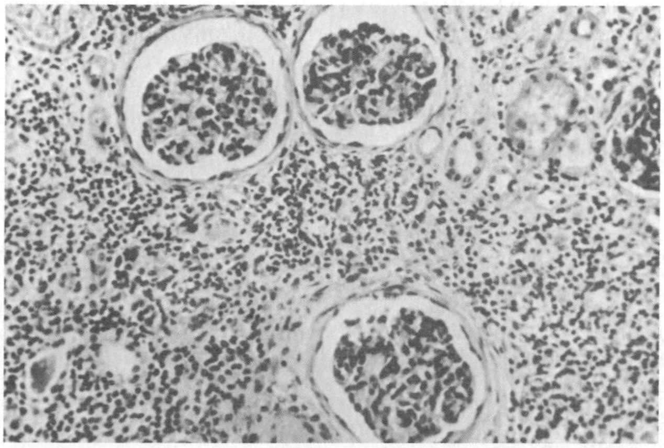

FIG. 3. Chronic pyelonephritis with interstitial and periglomerular fibrosis. Tubules within these scarred areas are atrophic and surrounded by a dense infiltrate of lymphocytes and plasma cells. Glomeruli are well preserved (H&E, ×160). (From Kaye,[340] with permission.)

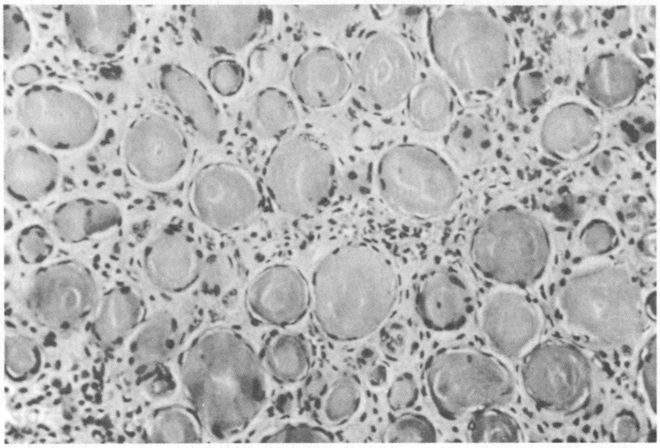

FIG. 4. Chronic pyelonephritis. Tubules are closely packed and filled with eosinophilic casts. Their resemblance to thyroid is striking (H&E, ×160). (From Kaye,[340] with permission.)

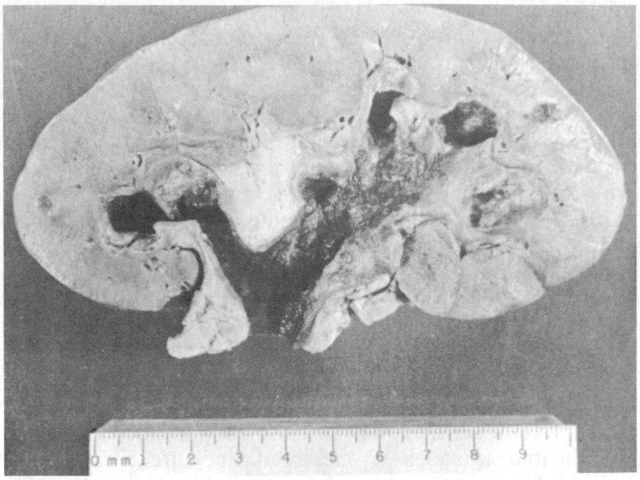

FIG. 5. Papillary necrosis. Necrosis of the renal papillae has resulted in large and irregular defects. The pelvis is hemorrhagic and covered by a granular exudate. (From Kaye,[340] with permission.)

tion'' of the kidney) (Fig. 4). There is also concentric fibrosis about the parietal layer of Bowman capsule (termed *periglomerular fibrosis*) and vascular changes similar to those of benign or malignant arteriolar sclerosis.

Several studies[2–4] have found little correlation between these pathologic findings and evidence for past or present urinary tract infection. Clearly a better term for this pathologic entity would be *chronic interstitial nephritis* to encompass all the clinical states that can cause these changes. To incriminate infection as the sole cause of chronic interstitial nephritis, evidence is required of past or present urinary tract infection and the absence of any other condition that can cause the pathologic picture of chronic interstitial nephritis. These criteria are seldom met, and even if they are, it is frequently impossible to establish whether or not infection is complicating interstitial nephritis of some unrecognized etiology. For example, analgesic nephropathy was not recognized until the 1950s.

Papillary Necrosis Caused by Infection

Frequently both kidneys are affected, and one or more pyramids may be involved[1] (Fig. 5). The pyramids are replaced by wedge-shaped areas of yellow necrotic tissue with the base located at the corticomedullary junction. As the lesion progresses, a portion of the necrotic papilla may break off, producing a calyceal deformity that results in a recognizable radiologic filling defect. The sloughed portion may be voided and in some instances can be recovered from the urine. Microscopically, edema is initially seen of the interstitium. Eventually the lesion resembles an infarct with coagulation necrosis involving the entire pyramid. The collecting tubules are filled with bacteria and polymorphonuclear leukocytes.

PATHOGENESIS OF URINARY TRACT INFECTION

There are three possible routes by which bacteria can invade and spread within the urinary tract. These are the ascending, hematogenous, and lymphatic pathways.

Ascending Route

The urethra is usually colonized with bacteria. Studies[5] using suprapubic puncture techniques have revealed the occasional presence of small numbers of microorganisms in the urine of uninfected persons. Massage of the urethra in women[6] and presumably sexual intercourse[7–11] can force bacteria into the bladder. Furthermore, just one catherization of the bladder will result in urinary tract infection in about 1 percent of ambulatory patients,[12] and infection will develop within 3 or 4 days in essentially all patients with indwelling catheters with open drainage systems.[13] Both the diaphragm in women and condom catheter in men have been shown to predispose to infection.[10,14–18]

The fact that urinary tract infection is much more common in women than men gives support to the importance of the ascending route of infection. The female urethra is short and is in proximity to the warm moist vulvar and perirectal areas, making contamination likely. It has been shown[19] that the organisms that cause urinary tract infection in women colonize the vaginal introitus and periurethral area before urinary infection results. Once within the bladder, bacteria may multiply and then pass up the ureters, especially if vesicoureteral reflux is present, to the renal pelvis and parenchyma. Animal studies[20] have also confirmed the importance of ascending infection. If bladder bacteriuria is established after unilateral ureteral ligation, only the unligated kidney develops pyelonephritis.

Hematogenous Route

Infection of the renal parenchyma by blood-borne organisms clearly occurs in humans. The kidney is frequently the site of abscesses in patients with staphylococcal bacteremia and/or endocarditis.[21] Experimental pyelonephritis can be produced by intravenous injection of several species of bacteria and even *Candida*.[22–26] However, production of experimental pyelonephritis by the intravenous route with gram-negative enteric bacilli, the common pathogens in urinary tract infection, is difficult. Additional manipulations such as creation of ureteral obstruction are often necessary.[24,25,27] It would appear that in humans, infection of the kidney with gram-negative bacilli rarely occurs by the hematogenous route.

Lymphatic Route

Evidence for a significant role for renal lymphatics in the pathogenesis of pyelonephritis is unimpressive and consists of the demonstration of lymphatic connections between the ureters and kidneys in animals, and the fact that increased pressure in the bladder can cause lymphatic flow to be directed toward the kidney.[28,29]

Thus, it would seem at the present level of understanding that the ascending pathway of infection is the most important.

Host Parasite Interaction

The Organism. Although urinary tract infections are caused by many species of microorganisms, most are due to *Escherichia coli*. However, only a few serogroups of *E. coli*—01, 02, 04, 06, 07, 075—cause a high proportion of infections.[30] This has led to the concept of uropathogenic *E. coli*, whereby certain strains of *E. coli* are selected from the fecal flora by the presence of virulence factors that enhance both colonization and invasion of the urinary tract and the capacity to produce disease.[31] Recognized virulence factors include increased adherence to uroepithelial cells,[31] resistance to serum bactericidal activity,[32] higher quantity of K antigen,[30] presence of aerobactin,[33] and hemolysin production.[33] These factors are less frequently observed among serotypes of *E. coli* in the fecal flora that are less likely to produce infection.[31]

In particular, adhesive properties have been suggested to select bacteria capable of reaching and colonizing the normal urinary tract and to influence the level of infection in the urinary tract (i.e., upper versus only lower tract).[31,34] Accordingly, bacteria with enhanced adherence to vaginal and periurethral cells would be selected to colonize the anatomic regions adjacent to the urethral orifice. Human studies and the mouse model of nonobstructive ascending pyelonephritis have confirmed the significance of the adhesive capacity of the urinary pathogen in causing lower and upper tract infection.[35–38] Svanborg-Eden et al. demonstrated that *E. coli* pyelonephritis isolates adhere better than *E. coli* cystitis isolates, and urinary isolates tend to adhere more strongly to uroepithelial cells than random fecal *E. coli* isolates.[38] The major types of surface adhesins on uropathogenic *E. coli* are fimbrial in nature and may be differentiated by the effect of α-methyl-mannoside. The binding of *E. coli* to epithelial cell receptors containing globoseries glycolipid accounts for the attachment of most strains causing kidney infection and is not inhibited by mannose (MR—for mannose-resistant).[39,40] Fimbriae attaching to globoseries receptors are termed *P fimbriae*. The globoseries glycolipid receptors are distributed throughout the urinary tract, particularly in the kidney.[40] Binding of *E. coli* to mannose-containing receptors occurs with most uropathogenic strains. In fact, strains from cystitis patients are more likely to bind than those from pyelonephritis patients.[38] Fimbriae attaching to mannosides are the common type 1 fimbriae (pili), and attachment is inhibited in the presence of mannose (MS—for mannose sensitive). Urinary mucus or slime is rich in mannose residues, and hence *E. coli* possessing MS adhesins adhere avidly to urinary slime.[41] The biologic significance of this phenomenon is unclear. Currently, in addition to type 1 and P fimbriae, a variety of adhesins including S, type 1c and G fimbriae, and M and X adhesins,[42] with differing molecular binding specificities and serologic properties, have been identified on uropathogenic strains of *E. coli* and are expressed in vivo in urine.[42] Adherent bacteria not only persist within the urinary tract but have growth advantages and enhanced toxicity due to restricted diffusion of products secreted by eukaryotic cells.[43]

Currently, a two-phase concept is postulated regarding adherence kinetics in the pathogenesis of urinary tract infection.[34,35] After entry into the lower urinary tract, MS adhesins, present on the majority of Enterobacteriaceae, are thought to be important for colonization of the bladder and lower urinary tract.[44] Mannose-resistant P fimbriae, on the other hand, appear to be critical for the organisms to reach the pelvis and renal parenchyma.[40] There is evidence to suggest that in vivo a urinary pathogen may alter its surface expression or presentation of adhesins so as to ensure survival.[44,45] Type 1 fimbriae increase the susceptibility of *E. coli* to neutrophil phagocytosis.[34] Therefore, not surprisingly, *E. coli* cease to express these fimbriae on reaching the renal parenchyma.[34] This phenomenon is called *phasic variation*. In contrast to type 1 fimbriae, polymorphonuclear leukocytes lack receptors for P fimbriae, and the latter block phagocytosis.[46]

Studies with other species of bacteria have similarly demonstrated the significance of adherence in the pathogenesis of urinary infections. Silverblatt,[45] confirmed the role of fimbriae in *Proteus mirabilis* attachment to the renal pelvic mucosa, and similar observations have been made with *Klebsiella* sp.[47] *Staphylococcus aureus* uncommonly causes cystitis and ascending pyelonephritis; in contrast, *Staphylococcus saprophyticus* is a frequent cause of lower urinary tract infections. *Staphylococcus saprophyticus* adheres significantly better to uroepithelial cells than *S. aureus* or *Staphylococcus epidermidis*.[48] The significance of adherence has been emphasized by inhibition of experimental ascending *E. coli* urinary tract infection by the use of epithelial cell–surface receptor analogues.[49,50] Trimethoprim—sulfamethoxazole, extensively used to prevent urinary infection, at concentrations well below the minimum inhibitory concentration (MIC) reduces synthesis, expression, and adhesive function of type 1 fimbriae.[51]

Evaluation of urinary isolates for virulence characteristics in the presence of underlying structural abnormalities (e.g., severe reflux) frequently fails to demonstrate the typical bacterial virulence factors. Therefore, in complicated urinary tract infections virulence factors are often absent, and a natural selection of uropathogens is not apparent.[34] Similarly, *E. coli* blood isolates obtained from patients with urosepsis following bladder instrumentation lack virulence factors.[52]

The importance of adherence as a virulence factor is not complete without consideration of the role of the host. A difference in receptor density linked to variable susceptibility to infection has been proposed. In women and children with recurrent urinary tract infection, an increased avidity of bacterial attachment has been found to vaginal,[53] periurethral,[54] and uroepithelial[55,56] cells. However, several other authors have failed to corroborate these findings.[57] Thus, the role of receptors as biologic risk factors in uncomplicated urinary tract infections remains unsettled.

Certain other characteristics of bacteria may be important in the production of upper tract infection. Motile bacteria can ascend in the ureter against the flow of urine,[58] and the endotoxins of gram-negative bacilli have been shown to decrease ureteral peristalsis,[59] but contribute to the renal parenchymal inflammatory response by phagocytic cell activation.[60] Production of urease by infecting microorganisms such as *Proteus* species has been related to ability to cause pyelonephritis.[61]

Several experimental studies[23,27] have shown that the greater the number of organisms delivered to the kidneys, the greater the chance of producing infection. The kidney itself is not uniformly susceptible to infection, since very few organisms are needed to infect the medulla, whereas 10,000 times as many are needed to infect the cortex.[22,62] The greater susceptibility of the medulla may be due to the high concentration of ammonia, which may inactivate complement,[63] and to poor chemotaxis of polymorphonuclear leukocytes into an area of high osmolality, low pH, and low blood flow.[64]

The Host. With the exception of urethral mucosa, the normal urinary tract is resistant to colonization by bacteria and for the most part efficiently and rapidly eliminates both pathogenic and nonpathogenic microorganisms that gain access to the bladder. This is achieved by the presence of several lower urinary tract antibacterial defense mechanisms.

Although urine is generally considered to be a good culture medium for most bacteria, it does possess antibacterial activity. Anaerobic bacteria and other fastidious organisms that make up most of the urethral flora generally do not multiply in urine. It has been shown that extremes of osmolality, high urea concentration, and low pH levels are inhibitory for the growth of some of the bacteria that cause urinary tract infection.[65] Furthermore, the pH and osmolality of urine from pregnant women tend to be more suitable for bacterial growth than those of nonpregnant women, which in turn are more suitable for bacterial growth than urine from men.[66] The presence of glucose makes urine a better culture medium, whereas the addition of prostatic fluid to urine inhibits bacterial growth.[66,67] Furthermore, urine has been shown to inhibit the migrating, adhering, aggregating, and killing functions of polymorphonuclear leukocytes.[68]

The flushing mechanism of the bladder apparently exerts a protective effect. When bacteria are introduced into the bladders of humans, there is a tendency for spontaneous clearance.[69] Since "flushing" alone would probably not completely clear the bacteria, there must be additional protective factors. Host factors including bladder catheterization influence susceptibility of uroepithelial cells to attachment by uropathogens, and this in turn increases susceptibility to bacteriuria.[70]

Parsons et al., in a study of bladder defense mechanisms in dogs, demonstrated an active antiadherence mechanism of bladder mucosa.[71] Pretreatment of the bladder with acid was shown to increase bacterial adherence 20- to 50-fold. The increased adherence was independent of the bacterial species employed.[72] Histochemical studies revealed that bacterial adherence was increased by the removal of a surface mucopolysaccharide, glycosaminoglycan, which seems to be responsible for the natural resistance to adherence.[73] Thus, normally small inocula of bacteria are probably unable to adhere, remain suspended in urine, and are removed by voiding. In the presence of a larger bladder inoculum of bacteria, especially with good adhesive qualities, the primary defense of antiadherence may be overcome, colonization can occur, and subsequent bladder infection may result.[74] With the occurence of bladder infection, secondary defense mechanisms such as mobilization of leukocytes, phagocytosis, and bacterial destruction are called on to remove bacteria.[74,75]

Colonization of the vaginal introitus and periurethral region by Enterobacteriaceae is thought by some to be important in the pathogenesis of urinary tract infections in women.[19] Several authors have shown that periurethral colonization with the same organism almost invariably precedes episodes of significant bacteriuria.[19,76,77] Microbiologic studies have demonstrated that the urethra, periurethral region, and vaginal vestibule of women with recurrent urinary tract infections tends to be more commonly colonized with coliform bacteria.[53,54,76] Stamey has postulated that such colonization is often the prelude to new infection[76] and that women with recurrent urinary tract infection have a biologic predisposition to infection. The hypothesis is that these women have defective local perineal and vaginal defense mechanisms that result in increased susceptibility to introital and perineal colonization with urinary pathogens such as coliform bacteria.[76] In a series of studies, the effects of several factors in vaginal secretions on colonization were examined.[53,78–83] It appeared that a low vaginal pH level was the most important factor related to lack of colonization. Furthermore, serogroups of *E. coli* that were more likely to cause urinry tract infection were more resistant to low pH levels than serogroups that did not commonly cause infection. It was also found in these studies that *E. coli* was less susceptible to the inhibitory effects of vaginal fluid than *P. mirabilis* or *Pseudomonas aeruginosa*. Finally, it was noted that *E. coli* adhered more avidly to vaginal epithelial cells of women with recurrent urinary tract infection, and this was attributed to reduced local production of antibodies in vaginal secretions.[53] Kallenius et al. similarly showed that the periurethral cells of young girls prone to recurrent urinary tract infections were more susceptible to bacterial attachment,[54] and other authors found enhanced attachment of *E. coli* to uroepithelial cells of patients with recurrent urinary tract infections.[55,56] Not all authors agree that introital colonization is the most important factor in the pathogenesis of recurrent urinary tract infection.[77,84–87] They point out that introital colonization with Enterobacteriaceae is as common in women not prone to infection. Furthermore, Parsons et al. found no enhanced bacterial adherence to vaginal epithelial cells in women with recurrent urinary tract infection,[57] and Kurdydyk et al. found no difference in IgG and IgA levels in cervicovaginal washings between women prone to infection and those with no past history of urinary tract infection.[88] These studies failed to confirm the hypothesis that women with recurrent bacteriuria possess a local periurethral and vaginal defect in host resistance. Kunin et al.[77] stated the view that all women who do not have a structural or neurologic problem in the voiding mechanism are approximately at the same risk of having a first urinary tract infection. In their view, once established, each infection sets the stage for the next episode, since infection itself may lead to colonization unless periurethral colonization is eradicated by therapy. Antimicrobial therapy per se may alter periurethral flora in favor of colonization with enteric organisms. The longer the interval between infections, the less likelihood there is for recurrences. The antagonists to Stamey's hypothesis have concluded that the decisive factor is not the colonization of the periurethral area per se but rather the ability of these organisms to ascend the urethra including the ability of infecting organisms to adhere to mucosal cells and withstand normal host defense mechanisms.

The role of humoral immunity in the host's defense against infection of the urinary tract, although extensively studied, is poorly understood, as summarized in several reviews.[89–100] During acute pyelonephritis, there is a systemic antibody response. Antibodies against the O antigen and occasionally the K antigen of the infecting strain have been found, and recently antibodies to type 1 and P fimbriae were described.[93,101] IgM antibodies dominate in the response to the first upper tract infection but not to subsequent episodes. Of note is the observation that high levels of IgG antibodies to lipid A correlate with the severity of renal infection and progression of renal parenchyma destruction.[94] An antibody response consisting of IgG and secretory IgA antibodies can be detected in the urine. In contrast to upper tract infection, lower urinary infection is usually associated with a reduced or nondetectable serologic response reflecting the superficial nature of the infection. However, recently Hopkins et al., using a monkey model, reported the production of systemic and urinary IgG and IgA that accompanied experimental cystitis.[102]

In particular, antipili antibodies are absent in the urine in lower tract infection.[99] Systemic serologic response has been used to distinguish between upper and lower urinary tract infection, but is not practical because of too many false-negative and false-positive results. However, local coating of bacteria with antibodies within the kidney (and prostate) has formed the basis of modern localization techniques.

In spite of the impressive systemic and local urinary antibody production that follows acute pyelonephritis, the protective role of these antibodies is unclear. When bacteria persist in the kidney for several months, antigenic drift may occur.[95] Nevertheless, antibodies against several bacterial structures including O and K antigen and more recently fimbrial antigens have been found to protect against hematogenous or ascending pyelonephritis in experimental animals.[92,93,96]

Antibodies may be of value in limiting the damage incurred within the kidney or preventing colonization preceeding recurrence. Svanborg-Eden et al. reported that the urine of patients with pyelonephritis inhibited the adherence of *E. coli* to uroepithelial cells and that this activity was removed by absorption with O antigen.[97] Antibodies have not been shown to protect against bladder infection.[98,99] Cell-mediated immunity has not been shown to play a major role in host defenses against urinary tract infection.[90]

During pyelonephritis, an acute inflammatory exudate consisting predominantly of polymorphonuclear leukocytes is present. Although the inflammatory reaction is directed at limiting bacterial spread and persistence within the kidney, it has been suggested that the infiltrating phagocytic cells may contribute to tissue damage and renal scarring. Using experimental animals, Bille and Glauser were able to reduce parenchymal kidney destruction by inducing neutropenia as well as by interfering with leukocyte migration.[103] The clinical significance of these observations is unclear, since any interference with the normal inflammatory response may possibly contribute to bacteremia.

Several studies[1] have demonstrated persistence of bacterial antigens in kidneys of experimental animals following renal infection. This suggests the possibility of autoimmunity as an explanation for progression of the lesion in "chronic pyelonephritis." An interesting observation is that patients with acute pyelonephritis have increased serum antibody titers against Tamm-Horsfall protein.[104] This protein is formed in the tubular region and is excreted in the urine. It has been speculated that these act as autoantibodies in the renal parenchyma. Cross-reactivity between the Tamm-Horsfall protein and gram-negative bacteria has been reported by Fasth et al., raising the possibility of antibody induced by gram-negative bacilli injuring renal cells containing Tamm-Horsfall protein even after elimination of the bacteria.[100] On the other hand, the highest concentrations of serum IgG and IgA antibodies against Tamm-Horsfall protein were seen in patients with vesicoureteral reflux even in the absence of bacteriuria, suggesting that after tubular–interstitial damage, Tamm-Horsfall antigen could act as an independent antigen unrelated to the presence of bacterial antigens.[100]

Aoki and colleagues,[105] examined kidney tissue from patients with proven pyelonephritis and others with renal scarring suggestive of pyelonephritis who had no history of bacteriuria. Bacterial antigen was found in all patients in the first group and was present in biopsy specimens from most in the second group. They concluded that there might be a group of patients with cryptogenic renal scarring of a pyelonephritic type in whom the pathologic process was related not to the presence of viable bacteria but to an ongoing destructive interaction between bacterial antigen and antibody. Subsequent work[106] has not confirmed the observations of Aoki et al.

There are several abnormalities of the urinary tract that interfere with its natural resistance to infection. Obstruction to urine flow is the most important of these. Extrarenal obstruction can result from congenital anomalies of the ureter or urethra such as valves, stenosis, or bands; calculi; extrinsic ureteral compression from a variety of causes; benign prostatic hypertrophy; and others. Intrarenal obstruction may be produced by entities such as nephrocalcinosis, uric acid nephropathy, analgesic nephropathy, polycystic kidney disease, hypokalemic nephropathy, and the renal lesions of sickle cell trait or disease.[107] Obstruction inhibits the normal flow of urine, and the resulting stasis is probably important in increasing susceptibility to infection.

In animals, obstruction of a ureter markedly increases susceptibility to hematogenous infection.[27] Intrarenal obstruction, experimentally produced by scars in a variety of ways, also increases susceptibility of the kidney to infection. Medullary scars, which produce greater amounts of obstruction than cortical scars, increase the susceptibility of animals to infection more than cortical scars.[108] Furthermore, the intravenous injection of *E. coli* in animals with renal scars from prior staphylococcal pyelonephritis produces pyelonephritis in the regions of intrarenal hydronephrosis caused by the old scars.[109] Men of any age and pregnant women are the most prone to lesions that result in obstruction to the free flow of urine.

Calculi may increase susceptibility to urinary tract infection by producing obstruction. However, not all stones obstruct, and local irritative phenomena may also be important. Furthermore, calculi may develop secondary to infection. It has been observed clinically and experimentally that *Proteus* species and other urea-splitting organisms (e.g., *Klebsiella*) are most likely to produce calculi.[110] Furthermore, bacteria survive deep within the calculi and are extremely difficult to eradicate even by artificial means such as by incubating in solutions containing antibiotics or iodine and alcohol.[111] This may account for the well-known difficulties encountered clinically in trying to cure urinary tract infection in the presence of stones.

Vesicoureteral reflux and urinary tract infection are also intricately related. Reflux due either to a congenital abnormality, bladder overdistension, or unknown etiology, probably contributes to upper tract infection via the ascending route. On the other hand, clinical observations have demonstrated that infection may, in itself, produce reflux especially in children.[112] Reflux tends to perpetuate infection by maintaining a residual pool of infected urine in the bladder after voiding. It is probable that reflux, especially in young children, plays an important role in the production of upper tract infection and subsequent scarring.[113] Patients with incomplete emptying of the bladder for either mechanical reasons (bladder neck obstruction, urethral valves, urethral strictures, prostatic hypertrophy) or neurogenic malfunctions (poliomyelitis, tabes dorsalis, diabetic neuropathy, cord injuries) are prone to frequent urinary tract infections. These patients are subject to bladder overdistension, which may interfere with local defense mechanisms, and, most importantly, frequent instrumentation of the urinary tract.

EPIDEMIOLOGY OF URINARY TRACT INFECTION

Infecting Organisms

There is a great difference between the bacterial flora of the urine in patients with an initial episode of urinary tract infection as compared with the flora from those with frequent recurrences of infection. *Escherichia coli* is by far the most frequent infecting organism in acute infection.[114] In so called "chronic" urinary tract infection, especially in the presence of structural abnormalities of the urinary tract (such as obstructive uropathy, congenital anomalies, neurogenic bladder, and fistulous communication involving the urinary tract), the relative frequency of infection caused by *Proteus, Pseudomonas, Klebsiella Enterobacter* species, and by enterococci and staphylococci increases greatly. In the presence of structural abnormalities, it is also relatively common to isolate multiple organisms from the urine. Since instrumentation and repeated courses of antimicrobial therapy are common in these patients, antibiotic-resistant isolates might be expected.

The hospital environment is an important determinant of the nature of the bacterial flora in urinary tract infection. *Proteus, Klebsiella, Enterobacter, Pseudomonas*, staphylococci, and enterococci are more often isolated from inpatients, as compared with a greater preponderance of *E. coli* in an outpatient population.[115,116] Cross-infections are important in the pathogenesis of hospital-related urinary tract infections, especially with indwelling catheters.[116,117]

Anaerobic organisms are rarely pathogens in the urinary tract.[118] A variety of bacteria may be found in the urine in specific clinical settings. For example, *Salmonella* species are found with *Salmonella* bacteremia.[119] Fungi (particularly *Candida* species) occur in patients with indwelling catheters who are receiving antimicrobial therapy. Coagulase-negative staphylococci are a common cause of urinary tract infection in some reports.[120] *Staphylococcus saprophyticus* tends to cause infection in young, sexually active females.[121,122] Coagulase-positive staphylococci most often invade the kidney from the hematogenous route resulting in intrarenal or perinephric abscesses.[21] Serotyping of *E. coli* has substantially aided in the epidemologic study of urinary tract infection. Using these techniques, it has been demonstrated that only a relatively small number of serologically distinct strains (e.g., 04, 06, 075, and secondarily 01, 02, and 07) are responsible for a major proportion of *E. coli* urinary tract infections.[123,124]

Adenoviruses (particularly type 11) have been strongly implicated as causative agents in hemorrhagic cystitis in pediatric patients, especially boys.[125,126] Cell-wall deficient bacteria have been demonstrated in urine from patients with pyelonephritis, particularly in association with therapy using cell-wall active antibiotics.[127] However, these forms have not been consistently isolated from either urine or renal tissue despite the use of adequate techniques and are probably not of major importance.

Bacteriuria in Children

The problem of urinary tract infection spans all age groups beginning with neonates. The incidence of urinary tract infection in infants up to 6 months is about 2 cases per 1000 live births and is much more common in boys.[128,129] Bacteremia is often present. Autopsy series have also revealed a predominance of infant boys with pyelonephritis.[130]

During the preschool years, urinary tract infection is more common in girls than in boys.[128] When infection occurs in preschool boys it is frequently associated with serious congenital abnormalities. With repeated study over a period of 1 year, the period prevalance of significant bacteriuria in this age group was reported to be 4.5 percent for girls and about 0.5 percent for boys.[131] Infections during this period often are symptomatic, and it is believed that much of the renal damage that occurs from urinary tract infection takes place at this time.[113,132]

Much information on the natural history and epidemiology of urinary tract infection has been gleaned from the studies of Kunin and associates with school children from central Virginia.[133–135] It was found that bacteriuria is common in girls in this population, is often asymptomatic, and frequently recurs. For example, the prevalence of bacteriuria among school girls was about 1.2 percent, and about 5 percent of the girls had significant bacteriuria at some time before leaving high school. About one-third of these patients had some symptom referable to the urinary tract when the bacteriuria was first detected. It was shown that each year about 0.3 to 0.4 percent of the female population (25 percent of those infected) was either cured spontaneously or with antimicrobial agents and was replaced by an equal number who developed bacteriuria. Bacteriuria was rare in school boys (prevalence 0.03 percent).

These studies also provided an opportunity to treat the patients and follow their clinical course. Patients were initially treated for 10 days to 2 weeks. Girls with frequent infections were given longer courses of therapy (1–3 months). Caucasian girls tended to have frequent reinfections, whereas black girls became reinfected less frequently. With each course of therapy, about 20 percent of white girls went into long-term remission. However, when many of these girls were married or became pregnant, bacteriuria recurred at a rate far above that expected for the general population. Over 50 percent developed bacteriuria within 3 months after marriage. Thus, the presence of bacteriuria in childhood defines a population at higher risk for the development of bacteriuria in adulthood.

Bacteriuria in Adults

Once adulthood is reached, the prevalence of bacteriuria increases in the female population. The prevalence of bacteriuria in young nonpregnant women is about 1–3 percent.[136,137] Each year about 25 percent of bacteriuric women clear their bacteriuria and are replaced by an equal number who have become infected (often women who have had urinary infection previously). At least 10–20 percent of the female population experience a symtomatic urinary tract infection at some time during their life.[137,138] Both sexual intercourse and diaphragm use are risk factors for urinary infection in women.[10,14–16,18] The diaphragm can cause urinary obstruction in some women, but its main effect may be a change in vaginal flora.[16]

The prevalence of bacteriuria in adult men is low (0.1 percent or less) until the later years, when it rises. The increase in bacteriuria in older men is probably mainly related to prostatic disease and the resultant instrumentation. Men with bacteriuria frequently have anatomic abnormalities of the urinary tract.

Bacteriuria in the Elderly

At least 10 percent of men and 20 percent of women over 65 have bacteriuria. In contrast to young adults, in whom bacteriuria is 30 times more frequent in women than men, over the age of 65 the ratio alters dramatically, with a progressive decrease in the female–male ratio.[139–141] In both sexes, the prevalance of bateriuria rises substantially. Possible reasons for the high frequency of urinary infection in the elderly include obstructive uropathy from the prostate and loss of bactericidal activity of prostatic secretions in men, poor emptying of the bladder due to prolapse in women, soiling of the perineum from fecal incontinence in demented women, and neuromuscular diseases and increased instrumentation and bladder catheter usage in both sexes.[139,140,142] There is a high rate of spontaneous cure and reinfection in both women and men.[141] The spectrum of microorganisms is unaltered in the elderly.

Bacteriuria in Patients with Other Conditions

Several studies[143,144] have reported a higher prevalence of bacteriuria in hospitalized patients as compared with outpatients. It is stated that the general ill health of hospitalized patients as well as the higher probability of urinary tract instrumentation are the major contributors to these differences.

A single catheterization causes urinary tract infection in only about 1 percent of ambulatory persons.[12] However, after catheterization of hospitalized patients, infection occurs in at least 10 percent.[12] Race apparently does not appreciably affect the prevalence of bacteriuria. However, socioeconomic status is important, with pregnant women from lower socioeconomic groups having a higher prevalence of bacteriuria.[145]

Various underlying diseases have also been associated with an increased frequency of urinary tract infection. While diabetic women have been found to have a higher prevalence of bacteriuria in some studies, others have found no difference in the prevalence between normals and diabetics.[146] The higher prevalence of bacteriuria in diabetics in some series may be attributed, at least in part, to more frequent catheterization.

Black women with sickle cell trait have a higher prevalence of bacteriuria during pregnancy than black women without sickle trait.[147] Other conditions stated to be associated with urinary tract infection (but without documentation) include chronic potassium deficiency, gout, hypertension, and other conditions causing interstitial renal disease.

CLINICAL MANIFESTATIONS

Symptoms

Urinary tract infection in children tends to manifest with different symptoms depending on the age of the child.[128,129,148,149] Symptoms in neonates and children less than 2 years of age are nonspecific.[128,129,148,149] Failure to thrive, vomiting, and fever seem to be the major manifestations. When children over 2 years of age (and more consistently above 5) develop infection, they are more likely to display localizing symptoms such as frequency, dysuria, and abdominal or flank pain.

The manifestations of urinary tract infection in adults are usually easy to recognize. The lower tract symptoms result from bacteria producing irritation of urethral and vesical mucosa causing frequent and painful urination of small amounts of turbid urine. Patients sometimes complain of suprapubic heaviness or pain. Occasionally the urine is grossly bloody or shows a bloody tinge at the end of micturition. Fever tends to be absent in infection limited to the lower tract.

The classic clinical manifestation of upper urinary tract infection includes fever (sometimes with chills), flank pain, and frequently lower tract symptoms (e.g., frequency, urgency, and dysuria). At times the lower tract symptoms antedate the appearance of fever and upper tract symptoms by 1 or 2 days. It should be recognized that the symptoms described, while classic, may vary greatly. In fact, pyelonephritis may show protean clinical manifestations in adults as well as in children. Flank tenderness or discomfort is frequent in upper tract infection in adults and is more intense when there is obstructive disease. Severe pain with radiation into the groin is rare in acute pyelonephritis per se and suggests the presence of a renal calculus. The pain from the kidney is occasionally felt in or near the epigastrium and may radiate to one of the lower quadrants. These manifestations may offer difficulties in differential diagnosis and suggest gallbladder disease or appendicitis.

The vast majority of elderly patients with urinary infection are asymptomatic; in addition, pyuria may be absent.[139,140] Symptoms, when present, are often not diagnostic since noninfected elderly patients often experience frequency, dysuria, hesitancy, and incontinence. Nevertheless, typical symptoms may occur, and less frequently acute pyelonephritis develops, usually necessitating hospitalization. Gleckman et al. found a much higher frequency of bacteremia (61 percent) associated with pyelonephritis in the elderly than is found in the young, and shock commonly supervened.[150] Most of the patients had significant urologic abnormalities. The effect of asymptomatic bacteriuria on the general sense of well-being, appetite, and urinary continence has been studied, and in one investigation no association could be demonstrated.[151]

The clinical manifestations of recurrent or persistent urinary tract infection are more difficult to define. Patients with lower urinary tract involvement tend to have repeated bouts of transient symptomatic or asymptomatic infection. Patients with upper tract infection may have episodes of fever, pain in the renal regions, and dysuria during acute exacerbations or new bouts of infection. However, upper tract infection may result in only lower tract symptoms or no symptoms at all. Patients with urinary tract infection in the presence of an indwelling urinary catheter usually have no lower tract symptoms, but flank pain or fever are common. Urinary tract infection is the most common source of bacteremia produced by gram-negative bacilli. Bacteremia may occur with no urinary symptoms, especially in the presence of an indwelling catheter.

Alterations in Renal Function

In experimentally produced pyelonephritis, the only consistent abnormality of renal function is the inability to concentrate the urine maximally.[152] The mechanism of the concentrating defect is not clear but seems to be related in experimental animals to inflammation and perhaps to increased production of prostaglandins.[153,154] The concentrating defect occurs early in the course of experimental infection and is rapidly reversible with antimicrobial therapy and following the administration of prostaglandin inhibitors.[152,153] The same phenomenon occurs in humans.[155]

Progressive destruction of the kidney (particularly in the presence of obstruction) may occur and give rise to clinical manifestations of renal insufficiency. Bilateral papillary necrosis occasionally can lead to rapidly progressive renal failure.[156]

DIAGNOSIS

Presumptive Diagnosis of Urinary Tract Infection

Microscopic examination of the urine is the first step in laboratory diagnosis of urinary tract infection. A clean-catch midstream urine specimen is centrifuged for 5 minutes at 2000 rpm, and then the sediment is examined under high power. Each leukocyte seen represents about 5–10 cells/mm^3 of urine; 10–50 white cells/mm^3 have been stated to be the upper limit of normal.[157] With this criterion 5–10 leukocytes per high-power field in the sediment from a clean-catch midstream urine specimen is the upper limit of normal, as they represent 50–100 cells/mm^3. Although more elaborate and precise methods for determining the urinary concentration of leukocytes have been evaluated, it is generally not necessary to use these clinically.[157] It should be emphasized that the finding of pyuria is nonspecific, and patients with and without pyuria may or may not have infection.[158] However, the vast majority of patients with symptomatic infection have significant pyuria.[159] Using a stricter definition of pyuria (at least 10 leukocytes per mm^3 of midstream urine by counting chamber), the vast majority of patients with either symptomatic or asymptomatic bacteriuria will have pyuria. However, pyuria without infection remains common.[160]

Microscopic or sometimes gross hematuria is occasionally seen in patients with urinary tract infection (i.e., hemorrhagic cystitis). However, red blood cells may be indicative of other disorders such as calculi, tumor, vasculitis, glomerulonephritis, and renal tuberculosis. White cell casts in the presence of an acute infectious process are strong evidence for pyelonephritis, but the absence of white cell casts does not rule out upper tract infection. White cell casts can also be seen in renal disease in the absence of infection.

Proteinuria is a common although not universal finding in urinary tract infection. Most patients with urinary tract infection excrete less than 2 g of protein in 24 hours; excretion of 3 g or more suggests glomerular disease.

One of the most useful tests for presumptive diagnosis of urinary tract infection is the microscopic examination of a specimen for bacteria. The ability to identify bacteria in the urine depends on whether or not the specimen has been centrifuged and on whether or not it has been stained with Gram or methylene blue stain[161] (Table 1). Smaller numbers of bacteria can be detected microscopically in a stained than in an unstained specimen, and smaller numbers can be detected in a centrifuged than in uncentrifuged urine. Presence of at least one bacterium per oil-immersion field in a midstream, clean-catch, Gram-stained, uncentrifuged urine correlates with $\geq 10^5$ bacteria/ml of urine. As this titer is regarded to represent significant bacteriuria, Gram staining of an uncentrifuged specimen is an easy, rapid, and relatively reliable way to detect significant numbers of organisms. The absence of bacteria in several fields in a stained sedimented specimen indicates the probability of less than 10^4 bacteria/ml.

Several biochemical tests have been devised to detect bacteriuria for presumptive diagnosis. The many variations of the griess test (a diazotization reaction) detect the presence of nitrite in the urine that is formed when bacteria reduce the nitrate that is normally present.[161,162] Bacteria that possess dehydrogenase activity are able to reduce triphenyltetrazolium chloride (TTC), causing a color reaction to occur if these bacteria are present.[161,162] Both tests unfortunately often give false-negative results, but a combination of the two is more accurate. The detection of subnormal urinary glucose in patients with urinary tract infections is another test that has been used with very few false-positive and false-negative results.[163] Because of their general lack of specificity, biochemical tests for bacteriuria should not be routinely used in management of patients with urinary tract infection. Recently, automated rapid screening tests have become available that may be cost-effective for processing large numbers of samples.[164]

TABLE 1. Correlation of Methods of Direct Examination of Urine for Bacteria with Quantitative Cultures

	Unstained	*Stained*
Uncentrifuged	$\geq 10^6 (400\times)$	$\geq 10^5 (1000\times)$
Centrifuged	$\geq 10^5 (400\times)$	$\geq 10^4 (1000\times)$

Diagnosis of Urinary Tract Infection by Culture

Urine in the bladder is normally sterile. Since the urethra and periurethral areas are very difficult to sterilize, even the most carefully collected specimens (including those obtained by catheterization) are frequently contaminated. By quantitating bacteria in midstream, clean-voided urine, it is possible statistically to separate contamination from urinary tract infection. Patients with infection usually have $\geq 10^5$ bacteria/ml in urine in the bladder, and therefore voided urine usually contains $\geq 10^5$ bacteria/ml.[13] Patients without infection have sterile bladder urine and with proper collection, voided urine usually contains $<10^4$ bacteria/ml. However, it is important to remember that about one-third of young women with symptomatic lower tract infection have $<10^5$ bacteria per ml urine (see below under "Urethral Syndrome"). It is likely that a significant proportion of other patients with both symptomatic and asymptomatic infection have $<10^5$ bacteria per ml urine.

Several methods can be employed to quantitate bacteria present in urine. The serial dilution and pour plate method is the most accurate[165] but is cumbersome and not suitable for routine use in a busy clinical laboratory. Calibrated loops serve as a simple inexpensive way to examine quantitatively the bacteriologic characteristics of urine specimens.[166] Platinum loops that deliver 0.01 ml and 0.001 ml are used to streak urine onto agar plates. After incubating at 37°C for 24 hours the number of colony-forming units are counted, and the total number of organisms originally present in the specimen is estimated by multiplying the colony count by 10^2 or 10^3, respectively. A further refinement of the technique involves the use of differential agars to allow isolation from mixed cultures and more rapid identification.

Other methods of quantitative culture include (*1*) the flood plate method, which is similar to the calibrated loop method but involves pipetting a volume of urine onto a plate[165]; (*2*) the filter paper method[165] in which a given volume of urine is absorbed in a piece of filter paper and then put on a plate; and (*3*) the dip inoculum method[167] in which an agar-coated glass slide is dipped into urine. The dip inoculum method and its variants have excellent correlation with pour plate techniques and are available for office use at inexpensive prices.[149]

Acceptable methods for urine collection include (*1*) midstream clean catch, (*2*) catheterization, and (*3*) suprapubic aspiration. The clean-catch method is preferred for routine collection of urine for culture. It avoids the risk of infection inherent in catheterization. The patient must be instructed in the proper technique of obtaining the urine; this is especially important in women. The woman should wash her hands, straddle the commode (facing the back of the commode), wash the vulva from front to back four times with four different sterile gauze pads soaked in green soap or another appropriate cleansing agent and then rinse with two more sponges soaked in sterile distilled water. She should then spread the labia and void, discarding the first portion of urine and collecting the second. The urine should be processed immediately or, if refrigerated at 4°C, can be cultured within 24 hours. In men the prepuce should be retracted, and thereafter the technique is similar. In infants and small children sterile bags have been used for collection of urine, but contamination is common.[168]

In patients unable to cooperate, such as those with an altered sensorium, or those who are unable to void for neurologic or urologic reasons, catheterization may be necessary. When catheterization is performed, scrupulous aseptic technique should be observed.

The suprapubic aspiration method has been established as a safe technique in premature infants, neonates, children, adults, and even pregnant patients.[5,128,149,169] With this method the bladder must be full. The patient refrains from voiding until the bladder can be percussed above the pubic and suprapubic pressure causes the urge to void. After preparation of the skin, the bladder is then punctured above the symphysis pubis with a 22-gauge needle on a syringe (local anesthesia is not required). Following the procedure self-limited hematuria may be observed. Suprapubic aspiration may be indicated in special clinical situations such as in pediatric practice when urine is difficult to obtain. Another situation is the rare adult in whom infection is suspected, results obtained from more routine procedures have been confusing or equivocal, and diagnosis is critical.

If there are more than 10^5 bacteria/ml in a clean-catch urine specimen from an asymptomatic woman, there is an 80 percent probability that this represents true bacteriuria. If two different specimens demonstrate at least 10^5 of the same bacterium per ml, the probability increases to 95 percent. Thus two clean-catch specimens should be obtained in an asymptomatic woman to confirm the diagnosis. When the number of bacteria per ml is between 10^4 and 10^5 in an asymptomatic woman, a confirmatory second specimen will contain $\geq 10^5$ bacteria/ml in only 5 percent of instances. Thus in asymptomatic women 95 percent of the time 10^4–10^5 bacteria/ml represents contamination, with occasional infection manifested by $<10^5$ bacteria per ml urine. In men, in whom contamination is less likely, 10^4 organisms/ml is more suggestive of infection.[170] False-positive cultures are caused by contamination or incubation of urine before processing. False-negative cultures may be due to use of antimicrobial agents, soap from the preparation falling in the urine, total obstruction below the infection, infection with a fastidious organism, renal tuberculosis, and diuresis.[171]

These criteria apply only to the Enterobacteriaceae. Gram-positive organisms, fungi, and bacteria with fastidious growth requirements may not reach titers of 10^5/ml in patients with infection and may be in the 10^4–10^5/ml range.[165] The organism recovered often helps distinguish contamination from true bacteriuria. Samples with counts of less than 10^4 organisms/ml often contain saprophytic skin organisms such as diphtheroids, *Neisseria*, and staphylococci. Pure growth of Enterobacteriaceae is uncommonly found in low-titer specimens but is present in over 90 percent of the urines containing more than 10^5 bacteria/ml. High colony counts containing more than one species of bacteria from urine of asymptomatic persons often represent contamination but may be more significant in the presence of symptoms. Mixed infection occurs in about 5 percent of the cases.

In patients with symptoms of urinary tract infection, one titer of $\geq 10^5$ bacteria per ml urine carries a 95 percent probability of true bacteriuria. With titers of $<10^5$/ml but in the presence of frequency, urgency, and dysuria, women have a one-third chance of having bacterial infection (see "Urethral Syndrome" below). Presence of low numbers of Enterobacteriaceae (i.e., 10^2–10^5/ml) in such women correlates highly with infection. Presence of $<10^2$/ml Enterobacteriaceae is evidence against urinary tract infection.[172]

Samples obtained by catheterization from noninfected patients are less likely to become contaminated enough to demonstrate 10^5 bacteria/ml. For example, one catheterized specimen in an asymptomatic patient that contains 10^5 or more organisms/ml has a 95 percent chance of indicating infection, and counts between 10^4 and 10^5/ml (which are uncommon) are significant at least 50 percent of the time. The contamination is presumably from the urethra. Bladder urine obtained by suprapubic aspiration is either sterile or contains significant growth even if bacterial numbers are below 10^5 ml. The practice of forcing fluids before the procedure tends to reduce titers.[173] In fact, almost 50 percent of such specimens contain $<10^5$ organisms/ml. However, small numbers of bacteria may be found in aspirated urine from presumably noninfected persons.[5] This suggests that bladder urine may be occasionally contaminated from the urethra.

Urethral Syndrome. Most women with acute onset of frequency, urgency, and/or dysuria have urinary tract infection with ≥10^5 bacteria per ml urine (Fig. 6). However, about 40 percent are found to have <10^5 bacteria per ml urine and the term *urethral syndrome* has been used to refer to this entity.[174] Stamm et al.[175] have shown that about one-third of young female patients with the urethral syndrome have bacteria in bladder urine as demonstrated by suprapubic puncture. Thus they have urinary infections that are probably mainly restricted to the lower tract. Furthermore, about a quarter of young women with symptomatic infection localized to the lower urinary tract have <10^5/ml bacteria in urine. Pyuria (defined as ≥8 leukocytes/mm^3 uncentrifuged urine) is found in these patients with bacteria in the bladder but <10^5 ml in voided urine. In a prospective double-blind placebo controlled study such patients were shown to benefit from antimicrobial therapy, confirming the relevance of bacterial pathogens in low titer.[176]

The remaining patients with the urethral syndrome (after excluding those with bacteria in the bladder and those with genital herpes infection or vaginitis) can be divided into two groups: (*1*) those with sterile pyuria from urethritis due to *Chlamydia trachomatis*, less frequently *Neisseria gonorrhoeae* infection, and (*2*) those without pyuria in whom all cultures are negative. The pathogenesis of this symptom complex is unknown, but *Ureaplasma urealyticum* as well as noninfectious factors (traumatic, psychological, allergic, and chemical) have been suggested as causes. Patients with *C. trachomatis* and *N. gonorrhoeae* urethritis respond to antimicrobial therapy. Komaroff et al. reported that vaginitis was a common cause of dysuria, and, accordingly, patients should be questioned regarding vaginal symptoms particularly if the complaint of burning is external, such as pain felt in the inflamed vaginal labia during micturition.[177] Dysuria has also been described in 10 percent of women with initial genital herpes infection.[178]

While symptoms and the clinical setting cannot reliably distinguish between causes of frequency, urgency, and dysruia, they can be suggestive. Bacterial urinary tract infections tend to have a sudden onset of symptoms; suprapubic pain and hematuria may be present. Clinical clues to chlamydial infection include a gradual onset of internal dysuria, a sexually active patient with a recent new sexual partner, and no hematuria.

Strong consideration should be given to performing a pelvic examination in sexually active women with dysuria to evaluate for vaginitis and herpes virus infection. Although the diagnosis of chlamydial infection is best confirmed by culture, chlamydial cultures are expensive and do not give prompt results. Immunofluorescent methods for immediate diagnosis are also expensive. In the absence of a culture or immunofluorescent methods, the findings of pyuria, <10^5/ml bacteria in urine, a negative gonococcal culture, and a negative pelvic examination in a sexually active woman with frequency/dysuria should suggest consideration of therapy for *C. trachomatis* urethritis. Tetracycline would also constitute adequate therapy for the other major possibility—urinary tract infection with <10^5/ml bacteria in urine.

Localization of Site of Infection

Several methods have been used to determine if infection is restricted to the urinary bladder or if the upper tract is also involved. Needle biopsy specimens of the kidney have been cultured.[179] However, this is an unreliable approach because pyelonephritis is a focal disease and specimens obtained by needle biopsy may miss the area of infection.

The most reliable method of localization of infection involves obtaining urine directly from the ureter for quantitative cultures. In one study[170] using this method 95 women and 26 men with bacteriuria were evaluated. Approximately one-half had infection limited to the bladder. History and physical examination were of little value in predicting the site of infection. Turck et al.[180] using similar techniques demonstrated that in women with recurrent urinary tract infection, relapse was associated with upper tract involvement and reinfection with lower tract infection.

Fairley and colleagues[181] devised a technique for assessing ureteral bacteriuria that involves Foley catheterization only. However, results are equivocal in about 10–20 percent of patients.[138,182] As in the ureteral catheterization studies, about 50 percent of the patients have renal infection regardless of signs or symptoms.[182] Methods are also available for localization of bacteria in the prostate gland[183] and are discussed later.

Several studies[184,185] have reported the association of a defect in renal concentrating ability with upper tract infection. As might be expected, patients with unilateral bacteriuria have an ipsilateral defect in concentrating ability.[185] However, there are too many false-positive and false-negative responses to allow the use of concentrating ability for localization of urinary tract infection.

The immune response has been used as a means of localizing the site of infection. The presence of high titers of serum antibody directed against the infecting organism has been correlated with the presence of upper tract infection in patients undergoing ureteral catheterization.[186] Although there is a good

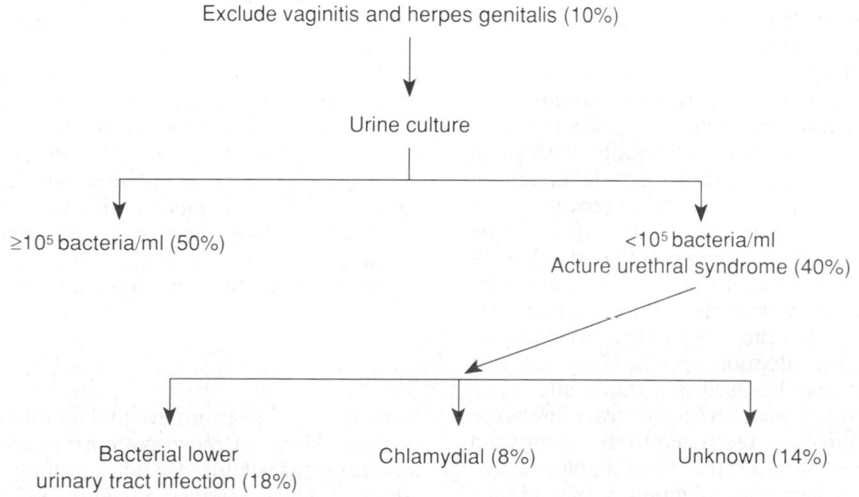

FIG. 6. Relative frequency of causes of acute onset of frequency/dysuria in young women. (Adopted from Stamm et al.,[175] with permission.)

association of high antibody titers and renal infection, there is a high incidence of false-positive and false-negative results (about 20 percent each).

Some investigators have hypothesized that measurement of urinary enzymes may be useful in detection of urinary tract infections and the differentiation of upper versus lower tract involvement. Various enzymes such as lactic dehydrogenase, alkaline phosphatase, β-glucuronidase, catalase, transaminase, leucine amino peptidase, and lysozyme have been evaluated.[187] From these studies, it is apparent that determination of urinary enzyme activity adds little if anything to the diagnostic approach or localization of infection, because a number of inflammatory processes as well as upper or lower tract infection can result in increased enzyme activity.[187,188]

Detection of antibody coating of bacteria (ACB) in urine has been used to localize infection.[189,190] This technique, which uses an immunofluorescent method, appears to be a relatively sensitive, reliable, and noninvasive way of detecting renal bacteriuria. Fluorescein-conjugated anti-human globulin is added to urine containing bacteria, and the bacteria are examined for fluorescence. The sensitivity of the test for ACB has been established collectively by several studies as 88 percent (range 72–100) with a specificity of 76 percent (range 50–100 percent). The predictive value of associating a positive test result for ACB with upper tract infection is 79 percent; the predictive value of associating a negative test result for ACB with bladder bacteriuria is 86 percent.[191] Discrepancies have resulted from lack of standardization of criteria of what constitutes a positive test result. False-negative results occur in 20 percent of patients with early acute pyelonephritis, because it may take several days for adequate antibody titers to develop.[191] An additional cause is the inability of the antibody to combine with certain infecting organisms such as mucoid-coated pseudomonads.[191] False-positive ACB test results occur in approximately 20–30 percent of patients with lower urinary infection. In men, the most important cause of false-positive results is the presence of bacterial prostatitis.[191] In women, false-positive results may be the consequence of contamination of urine samples by small numbers of ACB and yeast from the vaginal vestibule of patients without urinary tract infections. Yeast and pseudomonads may fluoresce even if not coated.[192] Proteinuria, hemorrhagic cystitis—probably because of tissue invasion—bladder tumors, and bladder stones may also be associated with false-positive ACB tests.[191]

Several studies have observed high false-positive and false-negative results in catheterized paraplegics.[191,193] ACB testing has been found to be accurate during pregnancy, and one-half the patients with asymptomatic bacteriuria are ACB-positive.[194,195] Although patients with renal transplants demonstrate an immune response to urinary tract infection, the reliability of ACB testing is as yet unconfirmed.[196]

There has been a major discrepancy in children between ACB localization and direct as well as other indirect localization techniques.[197–199] Difficulty obtaining clean-voided specimens, particularly in small girls, could result in contamination with small numbers of ACB of perineal origin.[197] However, Hellerstein et al.,[198] using catheter-obtained specimens, still observed a high false-positive and false-negative rate. Currently, ACB testing is not widely available to physicians nor is there good evidence to conclude that this assay has a major role in the routine management of patients with urinary tract infections. Its main use is as an epidemiologic tool and in the study of the pathogenesis and treatment of urinary tract infection.

Outcome of therapy can also be used in a crude but useful manner to separate those with upper and lower tract infection. Virtually all patients with infection restricted to the lower tract can be cured with a short course of antimicrobial therapy. However, the relapse rate with upper tract infection is appreciable, even with 7–10 days of therapy.

At present, only ureteral catheterization studies can reliably predict the site of infection in the urinary tract. However, this procedure is not without risk and cannot be justified for routine use. The Fairley bladder washout procedure is also quite reliable but gives equivocal results in about 10–20 percent of the patients. However, it also involves catheterization. The determination of presence of antibody-coated bacteria in the urine is practical and is noninvasive. However, in the clinical management of patients, it is rarely important to localize infection to either the upper tract or the lower tract other than by symptoms.

NATURAL HISTORY OF URINARY TRACT INFECTION

Children

In general, children with urinary tract infections without obstruction or vesicoureteral reflux have a very good prognosis.[113,129,132] In the presence of obstruction (e.g., urethral valves), severe destruction of renal parenchyma can occur.

Reflux is found in 30–50 percent of the children with asymptomatic or symptomatic bacteriuria (Fig. 7).[128,200] Reflux can be caused by obstruction with increased pressure in the bladder, delayed development of the ureterovesical junction, a short intravesical ureter, and/or inflammation of the vesicoureteral junction. Reflux in the presence of infection is associated with the development of scarring detected by intravenous pyelography.[129,132,200] Infants and young children (preschool age group) are at the highest risk for the development of progressive renal scarring.[128,129,132,200–202] These children frequently have severe degrees of reflux with repeated infections, and some develop end-stage renal disease and hypertension. Obstruction (most common in infant boys with congenital anomalies) is likely to be associated with marked reflux.[200–204]

It should be emphasized that the contribution of reflux alone as compared with reflux plus infection in the progression of renal scarring has not been clearly delineated. Reflux alone can apparently lead to renal damage and insufficiency.[188,205,206] Studies in uninfected animals[207] have demonstrated that reflux alone and in particular *intrarenal reflux* can produce "pyelonephritic" scars. It has also been shown that the immature kidneys of infants are more prone to intrarenal reflux.[208] The term *reflux nephropathy*, infected or uninfected, has been suggested to emphasize the primary role of reflux in scarring.[202] However, it is probable that reflux is more likely to lead to severe damage and scarring when infection is also present.[207] It is also clear that infection tends to produce reflux or at least to make it more severe.

After the age of 5, children (predominantly girls) with bacteriuria frequently have renal scars presumably acquired during the preschool years. Many of these children also have reflux. Reflux tends to decrease with elimination of bacteriuria. In addition, mild to moderate degrees of reflux are likely to disappear with the passage of time, probably in relation to maturation of the vesicoureteral junction.[209] Progression of scar already present or development of new ones are uncommon after the age of 5.[135,209–211] In fact, some investigators[212] have questioned the need for detecting and treating bacteriuria in school-aged children. However, it is clear that progression does occur in some of these children, especially in the presence of severe reflux.[209]

Adults

Urinary tract infections are much more common in women than in men. Many of these patients previously had urinary tract infections as children and continue to have infections as adults.[135] Once a woman develops infection, she is more likely to develop subsequent infections than a patient who has had no previous infections.

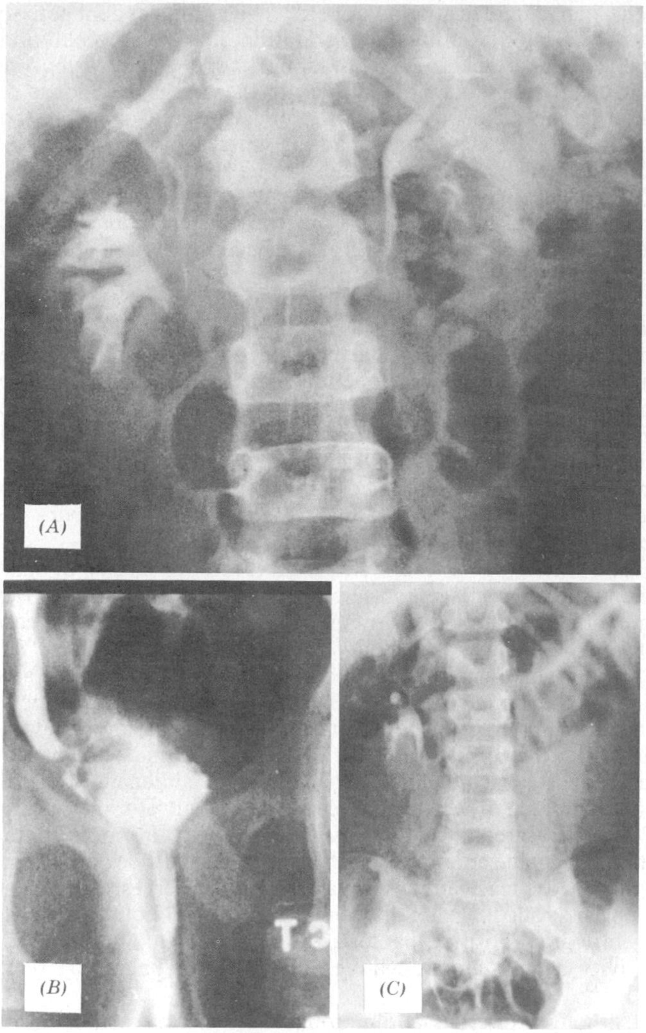

FIG. 7. Vesicoureteral reflux in a 3-year-old girl with recurrent urinary tract infection. (**A**) An intravenous urogram demonstrates duplication of the right renal collecting system with a mild increase in fullness of the right lower renal unit. Although the presence of reflux on the basis of this finding might be suspected, such an inference is not justified since the fullness could be within normal limits. (**B**) A voiding cystourethrogram demonstrates reflux into a dilated right ureter. (**C**) An immediate post-voiding film of the abdomen revealed the reflux to be confined to the lower renal unit on the right. Although in some cases it is possible to suspect the presence of reflux on the basis of the intravenous urogram alone, many cases of reflux are associated with a perfectly normal urogram. (From Kaye,[340] with permission.)

The courses of women with symptomatic recurrent urinary tract infections were described by Kraft and Stamey.[213] However, it was not defined whether these recurrences were reinfections or relapses. Twenty-three patients were followed over a period of 800 months, and each episode of urinary tract infection was treated. The overall attack rate was about 0.2 infections per month. Of interest is that even in these women (i.e., with recurrent urinary tract infections), significant bacteriuria (i.e., $\geq 10^5$ bacteria per ml urine) was present in only 70 percent of symptomatic episodes. Infections tended to occur in clusters with an increased attack rate of 0.5 percent per month. These periods of more frequent infection were followed by a remission or infection-free interval that averaged about 13 months. However, most remissions were followed by further clusters of infection. Thus, in many women it is more correct to use the term *remission* rather than *cure* of urinary tract infection. It may be a simple matter to cure an individual episode, but recurrence is common.

It is clear that urinary tract infection in adults can lead to progressive renal damage in the presence of obstruction.[4] However, recurrent infection in adults in the absence of obstruction rarely, if ever, leads to renal failure.

Autopsy studies[2,214] have shown that it is difficult to implicate infection per se (i.e., in the absence of other renal abnormalities) as an important pathogenetic factor in the production of severe renal disease in adults. One exception might be severe papillary necrosis secondary to infection. In fact, some authors[215] have been unable to find any cases of uncomplicated pyelonephritis that progressed to end-stage renal disease among 173 patients admitted to dialysis programs. In prospective studies,[135,216–221] hundreds of patients have been followed for years with persistent or recurrent infections without documenting progression of renal disease from infection alone.

The role of infection in the progression of clinically or radiographically diagnosed interstitial renal disease has also been examined.[3,222,223] In general, these studies indicate that infection is rarely, if ever, the major factor leading to further renal decompensation. However, infection may occasionally accelerate the progression of the primary underlying disease process.[222] In summary, except for perhaps rare instances there is no evidence to indicate that uncomplicated urinary tract infection alone produces renal failure in adults.[4]

Some studies have demonstrated decreased survival among elderly people with bacteriuria.[224,225] However, other studies have not confirmed this association.[225,226] At present, it is not known if asymptomatic bacteriuria in the elderly has any deleterious effects. Furthermore, there is no evidence to suggest that treatment of asymptomatic bacteriuria in the elderly has any beneficial effects. Therefore, routine treatment of asymptomatic bacteriuria in the elderly is not advocated by most experts.

Hypertension

It is clear that severe renal disease may cause hypertension. The entity of chronic interstitial renal disease (not necessarily related to infection) has also been related to hypertension.[3] It has been suggested that patients with bacteriuria in the absence of other renal disease are more likely to have hypertension, but the data have not shown a clear-cut relationship.[4] No definite cause and effect relationships have been documented.

MANAGEMENT OF URINARY TRACT INFECTION

General Considerations

Ideally antimicrobial agents should only be administered when there is reasonable evidence of infection in the urinary tract. Symptoms are not a reliable indication of infection.[13,175] The diagnosis of infection in the asymptomatic patient should be made on no fewer than two cultures of clean-voided, midstream urine in which the same microorganism is present in significant titers. If the patient is symptomatic, one specimen will suffice, and therapy should be started.

There has been much controversy as to how vigorously chemotherapy should be pursued.[227] A rational approach to the treatment of urinary tract infection depends on an appreciation of the prognosis of the untreated infection and the long-term results to be expected from therapy. The side effects, cost, and inconvenience of different therapeutic regimens must also be considered. As the prognosis of urinary tract infection in nonpregnant adult women seems to be quite good and reinfection is common, therapy probably makes little contribution to the patient's well-being other than eradicating symptoms.

While bacteriuria in the elderly is associated with degenerative and debilitating diseases and in some reports with mortality, there is no convincing evidence for a cause and effect relationship.[225,228] There certainly is no evidence that treatment of the urinary tract infection alters the patient's course. Urinary tract infection serves as a marker for debilitating diseases, which in turn may contribute to mortality. In addition, urinary tract infection is very common in the elderly, and many of these patients become reinfected or relapse after antimicrobial therapy. Furthermore, a higher frequency of side effects from chemotherapy would be expected in an older age group because of pre-existing renal, auditory, and other diseases. Considering the large numbers of patients involved, intensive antimicrobial therapy may lead to an unwarranted financial burden and the danger of drug toxicity and thus may do more harm than good in elderly patients.

In contrast, bacteriuria in preschool children with vesicoureteral reflux (especially if congenital anomalies are present) can result in stunted growth of the kidney, scar formation, and, rarely, renal failure. Bacteriuria in pregnancy may also have serious implications. Treatment of children and pregnant women is most likely to be beneficial. Furthermore, it is feasible to treat all these patients since the prevalence of bacteriuria is relatively low in these groups.

Hospitalized patients with bacteriuria have higher mortality rates than those without bacteriuria.[229,230] This observation may be related to deaths from bacteremia in patients with indwelling urinary catheters.

It is usually necessary to treat all symptomatic patients regardless of age, even when infection is likely to recur. Some patients have such frequent symptomatic episodes (either relapses or reinfections) that they are almost chronically incapacitated. In these patients it may be necessary to give prolonged therapy or prophylaxis to prevent recurrent symptoms.

Nonspecific Therapy

Hydration. Forcing fluids has been advocated in the therapy for urinary tract infection. There is some theoretical support for this modality of treatment. Hydration produces rapid dilution of the bacteria and removal of infected urine by frequent bladder emptying, which in the presence of minimal residual volume may offset the logarithmic growth of gram-negative bacilli. Forcing fluids usually results in a rapid reduction of bacterial counts. Permanent loss of bacteriuria has been reported in a few patients with rapid hydration, but in most patients bacterial counts return to original levels when hydration is stopped (e.g., overnight when urine flow rate and frequency of micturition are reduced).[231]

Medullary hypertonicity tends to inhibit leukocytic migration into the renal medulla, and the high concentration of ammonia tends to inactive complement.[63,64] Abolition of medullary hypertonicity by diuresis would be expected to reverse these effects. In addition, a reduction in bacterial counts in the urine by hydration would enhance the effect of factors otherwise overwhelmed by large numbers of bacteria (e.g., bladder mucosal defenses or the effect of relatively low concentrations of antimicrobial drugs).

Hydration may also have some disadvantages. Increased fluid intake could theoretically result in increased vesicoureteral reflux and possibly cause acute urinary retention in the partially obstructed bladder. The larger urine output results in dilution of antibacterial substances normally present in the urine as well as lower urinary concentrations of antimicrobial agents. Water diuresis also decreases urinary acidification, which enhances the antibacterial activity of urine and certain antimicrobial agents.

As there is no evidence that hydration improves the results of appropriate antimicrobial therapy, and because continuous hydration is inconvenient, we are not in favor of this approach.

Urinary pH. Antibacterial activity of urine results mainly from high urea concentration and osmolality and is pH-dependent, being greater at a lower pH.[65] The pH-dependent activity may be related to a high concentration of various weakly ionizable organic acids, such as hippuric and β-hydroxybutyric acids.[232] The antibacterial activity of these organic acids is related to the concentration of the undissociated molecule that probably penetrates better than the ionized form into the bacterial cell. As these organic acids have a relatively low pKa (the pH at which 50 percent of the molecules are undissociated), the lower the urinary pH, the greater the concentration of undissociated molecules and the greater the antibacterial activity of the organic acid.

Hippuric acid is a common constituent of urine, being the glycine conjugate of dietary benzoic acid, and is bacteriostatic in proportion to the concentration of undissociated molecules.[227] The production of antibacterial activity in urine by ingestion of large volumes of cranberry juice (if the urinary pH level is kept low) results from the appearance in the urine of high concentrations of hippuric acid derived from precursors in the berry. The successful use of mandelic acid, another organic acid, is also dependent on maintenance of a low urinary pH level.

The urinary pH level affects the antibacterial activity of many chemotherapeutic agents used in the treatment of urinary tract infections. The activity of methenamine results from the release of formaldehyde as the urinary pH level is decreased below 5.5. Clinically, methenamine is used in the form of its mandelic acid salt (methenamine mandelate) or its hippuric acid salt (methenamine hippurate). The antibacterial activity of these salts is related to the formation of the unionized organic acid and formaldehyde, which is highly dependent on maintenance of a urinary pH of 5.5 or less. The effectiveness of nitrofurantoin (pKa 7.2) is also greater at low urinary pH level. In contrast, the aminoglycoside antibiotics such as gentamicin, tobramycin, and amikacin are more effective in alkaline urine. Erythromycin and other macrolides, generally considered to be effective primarily against gram-positive bacteria, are known to have increased activity against gram-negative bacilli at an alkaline pH (e.g., 8.5).[233]

Although different antimicrobial agents have maximum effectiveness at different pH levels, most agents exhibit adequate antibacterial activity at usual urinary pH levels. The major exceptions are mandelic and hippuric acids and methenamine. Maintenance of urine at the low pH level required for effective antibacterial activity of organic acids and methenamine can be accomplished by administration of ascorbic acid or methionine. Acidification of the urine can result in precipitation of urate stones, and since oxalate is a metabolite of ascorbic acid, large doses of ascorbic acid can cause formation of oxalate stones.[227]

To acidify the urine, it is often necessary to modify the diet by restriction of agents that tend to alkalinize the urine, for example, milk, fruit juices (except cranberry juice), and sodium bicarbonate. Another major problem with acidification is that patients with renal insufficiency are unable to excrete an acid load and may become systemically acidotic when urinary acidification is attempted. It may be impossible to acidify urine infected with urea-splitting organisms such as *Proteus* species because of production of ammonia from urea. Acidification for long-term antimicrobial therapy should only be used with concomitant use of organic acids or methenamine. Urinary acidification is frequently difficult to achieve[234] and is rarely if ever necessary at present.

Analgesics. Urinary analgesics such as phenazopyridine hydrochloride (Pyridium) have little place in the routine management of symptomatic infections. The dysuria of urinary tract infection usually responds rapidly to antibacterial therapy and requires no local analgesia. If flank pain or dysuria is severe, systemic analgesics can be used. Analgesics such as phenazopyridine hydrochloride may be useful in the management of certain patients with dysuria but without infection.

Principles of Antimicrobial Therapy

Selection of an appropriate antimicrobial agent has become complex because of the increasing number of compounds available, each with its characteristic spectrum and toxic properties. However, in most cases, any of many available agents are perfectly satisfactory. Given two or more drugs with equivalent activity against the infecting microorganism, the agent with the least toxicity should be chosen.

There is no evidence to support any superiority of bactericidal drugs over bacteriostatic agents in urinary tract infection. However, there may be theoretical reasons for using bactericidal drugs in the treatment of relapsing urinary tract infection.

Serum, Tissue, and Urine Concentrations of Antimicrobial Agents. A poor correlation exists between response of bacteriuria and blood levels of antimicrobial agents.[170,235,236] Many oral antimicrobial agents, in the dosages commonly used for urinary tract infection, do not achieve serum levels above the minimal inhibitory concentration for most urinary pathogens.

Disappearance of bacteriuria is closely correlated with the sensitivity of the microorganism to the concentration of the antimicrobial agent achieved in the urine.[170,235,236] Inhibitory urinary concentrations are achieved after oral administration of essentially all commonly used antimicrobial agents. While blood levels do not seem to be important in treatment of urinary tract infection, they may be critical in patients with bacteremia and may be important in the cure of patients with renal parenchymal infection who relapse.

In patients with renal insufficiency, dosage modifications are necessary for agents that are excreted primarily by the kidneys and cannot be cleared by any other mechanism. In renal failure, the kidney may not be able to concentrate an antimicrobial agent in the urine, and difficulty in eradicating bacteriuria may occur. This may be an important factor in failure of therapy for urinary tract infection with aminoglycosides.

In addition, high concentrations of magnesium and calcium as well as a low pH level can raise the minimal inhibitory concentrations of aminoglycosides for gram-negative bacilli to levels above those achievable in the urine of patients with renal failure.[237] In general the penicillins and cephalosporins attain adequate urine concentrations despite severely impaired renal function and are the agents of choice in renal insufficiency.[238]

Response to Therapy. The objective of antimicrobial therapy is to eliminate bacteria from the urinary tract. Symptoms usually abate spontaneously without chemotherapy, even though bacteriuria may persist. Therefore, the results of therapy can only be determined by follow-up urine cultures.

There are four patterns of response of bacteriuria to antimicrobial therapy: cure, persistence, relapse, and reinfection. Quantitative bacterial counts in urine should decrease within 48 hours after initiation of an antimicrobial agent to which the microorganism is sensitive in vitro. If titers do not decrease within this time, the therapy being given will almost invariably be unsuccessful.

Cure is defined as negative urine cultures on chemotherapy and during the follow-up period (usually 1–2 weeks). However, it must be understood that some of these patients will develop reinfection at a later time.

Persistence has been used in two ways to describe response to therapy: (*1*) persistence of significant bacteriuria after 48 hours of treatment and (*2*) persistence of the infecting organism in low numbers in urine after 48 hours. Significant bacteriuria usually persists only if urinary levels of the antimicrobial agent are below the concentration of the drug needed to inhibit the microorganism. This can occur when the infecting strain is resistant to the urinary levels usually attained (i.e., a resistant organism) or because levels are inordinately low (i.e., from not taking the agent, insufficient dosage, poor intestinal absorption, or poor renal excretion as in renal insufficiency). Persistence of the infecting microorganism in low titers in voided urine may mean persistence in the urinary tract or contamination from the urethra or vagina. Bladder puncture cultures would be needed to evaluate the significance of low titers of bacteria obtained on therapy, and we do not routinely recommend this procedure. Also worth noting is the fact that bacteria may persist within the urinary tract during therapy without excretion of organisms in the urine. Sites of persistence within the urinary tract are the renal parenchyma, calculi, and the prostate. The simplest way of determining the significance of persistence of the organism in low titers in the urine is to obtain follow-up urine cultures after therapy has been stopped. Prompt relapse of significant bacteriuria usually follows persistence of the organism in the urinary tract.

Relapse usually occurs within 1–2 weeks after cessation of chemotherapy and is often associated with renal infection, with structural abnormalities of the urinary tract, or with chronic bacterial prostatitis. Relapse indicates that the infecting microorganism has persisted in the urinary tract during therapy. However, an apparent relapse can be related to reinfection (new infection) with the same microorganism. In spite of eradication from the urinary tract, the original infecting organism may still be present in the intestine, vagina, or external urethra and then may cause a new infection. Markedly delayed relapses (more than 1 month after stopping therapy) are much more likely due to this phenomenon or to chronic bacterial prostatitis than to true relapse. Relapses occurring within 1–2 weeks are usually true relapses. One postulated but unsubstantiated mechanism of relapse following treatment with cell-wall active antibiotics (e.g., penicillins and cephalosporins) is persistence of osmotically fragile, cell-wall-deficient forms in the hypertonic renal medulla during therapy, with reversion to normal bacterial forms after therapy is stopped.[127]

After initial sterilization of the urine, *reinfection* may occur during administration of chemotherapy (also called superinfection) or at any time thereafter. Reinfection is easy to identify when there is a change in bacterial species. However, there may be reinfection with a different serotype of the same species (usually *E. coli*) or even the same serotype.

Classification and Antimicrobial Therapy for Different Groups

Symptomatic Urinary Tract Infection. The majority of patients classified as having symptomatic urinary tract infection are women, usually of child-bearing age. The onset of symptoms is frequently related to sexual intercourse. The patient may have upper urinary tract symptoms, lower urinary tract symptoms, or both. As mentioned previously, patients with only lower urinary tract symptoms may also have upper urinary tract infection.

ACUTE PYELONEPHRITIS. Patients who are severely ill with pyelonephritis should be hospitalized. Although mild to moderate illness responds well to orally administered antimicrobial agents, nausea and vomiting may preclude oral treatment, necessitating parenteral therapy. If the patient is reliable, compliant, and tolerates oral therapy, the patient may be treated with a variety of oral antimicrobial agents. At the time of antibiotic selection, a Gram stain of the urine should have indicated the morphology of the infecting organism (e.g., gram-negative bacillus, gram-positive coccus), but the precise identity and antimicrobial susceptibility pattern are usually unknown. Therefore, selection of antimicrobial therapy is usually empiric. When streptococci are seen on Gram stain, ampicillin or amoxicillin is probably the agent of choice. When staphylococci are implicated on Gram stain, cephalosporins (such as cephalexin) are appropriate agents.

Although sulfonamides and ampicillin or amoxicillin have been mainstays of oral therapy for gram-negative bacillus infection for many years, these agents can no longer be recommended as reliable agents, since 25–35 percent of *E. coli* are now resistant.[239] Accordingly, oral antimicrobial agents currently advocated for gram-negative bacillus urinary infection include: trimethoprim, trimethoprim–sulfamethoxazole, cephalexin, amoxicillin–clavulanic acid, and the recently introduced quinolones (norfloxacin and ciprofloxacin). The doses are listed under "Lower Urinary Tract Infection" below. In all patients with symptoms of upper tract infection, therapy should be preceded by culture of a clean-catch midstream urine sample.

In hospitalized patients, particularly those with suspected gram-negative bacillary bacteremia complicating pyelonephritis (high fever, shaking chills, hypotension), parenteral therapy should be used and is directed at the life-threatening bacteremia. In these seriously ill patients the spectrum of antibacterial activity of the initial agents should include all potential pathogens. In seriously ill patients with community-acquired acute pyelonephritis, when the Gram stain reveals gram-negative bacilli, empiric therapy includes a wide selection of antimicrobial agents, e.g., parenteral trimethoprim–sulfamethoxazole, aminoglycosides (e.g., gentamicin 3–5 mg/kg/day), aztreonam 3–6 g/day, ureido-penicillins (mezlocillin, azlocillin, or piperacillin 18 g/day, the ampicillin–sulbactam combination (as 12 g ampicillin/day) or the ticarcillin–clavulanic acid combination (as 18 g ticarcillin/day) and third-generation cephalosporins, e.g., cefotaxime or ceftriaxone, etc. In patients with hospital-acquired gram-negative bacillary infection, particularly when seriously ill, the initial selection of antibiotics should not leave any hiatus in the spectrum of activity and should anticipate the possibility of resistant microorganisms. Under these circumstances ceftazidine (3–6 g/day), ticarcillin–clavulanic acid, aztreonam, or imipenem (2 g/day), often used in combination with aminoglycosides, are recommended. When the susceptibility pattern of the infecting organism is known, therapy can be altered to less expensive single-agent therapy, and oral treatment can be used once response has occurred.

Effective therapy results in a marked decrease in bacterial titers in the urine within 48 hours after onset of treatment. Antimicrobial agents are sometimes effective in vivo even when disk sensitivity tests indicate drug resistance, because most antimicrobials are excreted in the urine in concentrations much higher than tested for by disk sensitivity testing.

If bacteriologic response does not occur by 48 hours, there is no point in continuing the same regimen. Therapy is then changed to an alternate drug on the basis of susceptibility tests (e.g., from the initial isolate). The finding of continuing positive blood cultures or persistent fever and toxicity past the first 3 days suggests the need for investigation to exclude urinary obstruction or intrarenal or perinephric abscess formation. Investigation should include renal ultrasound, computed tomographic scan, and, according to the findings, perhaps an intravenous pyelogram (IVP) examination. The availability of sensitive noninvasive studies has resulted in early diagnosis of intrarenal or perinephric abscess formation that may respond to antibiotic therapy alone. In uncomplicated pyelonephritis after clinical response and defervesence occurs, oral therapy is initiated and should be continued to complete a course of 14 days of antimicrobial therapy.[240] When upper tract infection is complicated by abscesses, more prolonged therapy and perhaps drainage is indicated (see "Perinephric Abscess" and "Intrarenal Abscess" below). All patients with acute pyelonephritis should have at least an ultrasound examination to evaluate for obstruction and/or stones. Follow-up urine cultures are mandatory within 1–2 weeks of completion of therapy in pregnant women, children, and patients with recurrent symptomatic pyelonephritis in whom suppressive maintenance therapy is planned. In the majority of nonpregnant adults who remain asymptomatic, follow-up cultures are optional.

Renal infection is a special problem in adults with hereditary polycystic disease. Although parenchymal infections respond well to appropriate antibiotics, cyst infections frequently fail to improve, and may require lipid-soluble antibiotics, e.g., trimethoprim–sulfamethoxazole[241] or surgical aspiration/drainage. Emphysematous pyelonephritis is most often seen in elderly female diabetics with chronic urinary infections and renal vascular disease. Because of the extraordinary high mortality rate of 70 percent in spite of appropriate antibiotic and supportive therapy, immediate nephrectomy is indicated for this condition[242] (Fig. 8).

LOWER URINARY TRACT INFECTION. *Conventional Therapy.* In the past, 7–10 days of therapy was routinely recommended for patients with lower tract symptoms. However, in recent years it has become apparent that most women with lower tract infection have only a superficial mucosal infection and can be cured with much shorter courses of therapy and in fact with only a single dose of an antimicrobial agent.

Single-Dose Vs. Three-Day Therapy. Single-dose therapy achieves high urinary concentrations that are prolonged for at least 12–24 hours and eliminate infection when confined to the bladder. Cure rates have ranged from 61–100 percent in women with symptoms of lower urinary tract infection.[243–254] In many of these studies methods were used to select patients with infection localized to the lower tract. The regimens used were sulfadoxine 2 g orally, sulfamethoxypyridazine 2 g orally, sulfisoxazole 2 g orally, kanamycin 0.5 g intramuscularly, amoxicillin 3 g orally, trimethoprim–sulfamethoxazole 2 single-strength tablets orally, trimethoprim 400 mg orally, tetracycline 2 g orally, nitrofurantoin 200 mg orally, and cefonicid 1 g intramuscularly. In the studies in which the ACB test was used,

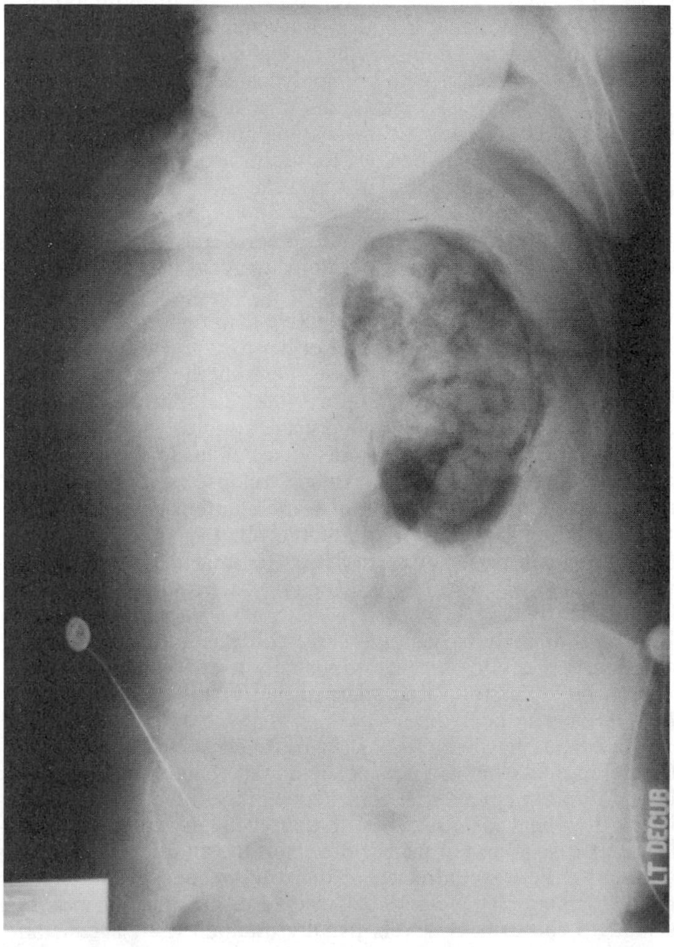

FIG. 8. Flat plate roentgenogram of abdomen showing emphysematous pyelonephritis.

clinical cure was almost always achieved in patients with negative ACB tests.

The advantages of single-dose therapy include lesser expense, assured compliance, fewer side effects, and perhaps less intense selective pressure for emergence of resistant organisms in gut, urinary, or vaginal flora. Possible deleterious effects include a poorer outcome of infections that are actually in the upper tract and are first treated with single-dose therapy, for example, a delay in appropriate therapy may result in more deeply seated infection and impair the response to subsequent more prolonged therapy. Finally, it should not be assumed that every antibiotic administered as a single dose will be effective even with regard to susceptible organisms. Results depend on high sustained urinary concentrations of the antimicrobial agent. For example, a 2 g oral dose of cefaclor resulted in a 57 percent failure rate.[255] Before using single-dose therapy, certain factors should be evaluated, including frequency of attacks, poor response to single-dose therapy in the past, known structural abnormalities, history of childhood infection, symptoms longer than 7 days, pyelonephritis during the past year, diabetes, etc. Any of these factors increases the likelihood of upper tract infection and might mitigate against using single-dose therapy.

A by-product of single-dose therapy is that failure to eradicate a urinary tract infection after a single dose of an agent may indicate in which patient further investigation should be considered. Response to single-dose therapy appears comparable with the ACB test in localizing the site of infection.[256]

Single-dose therapy gives basically 1 day of therapy with regard to antimicrobial activity in the urine. The same results should be achievable with 1 day of standard-dose antimicrobial therapy; however, the data to support this do not exist. Two reviews concluded that 3 days of therapy may be superior to single-dose therapy.[257,258] It is our preference to advocate the concept of short-course therapy, which may constitute single-dose or 3 days of therapy using standard doses. Some of the preferred agents for 3 days of therapy are trimethoprim–sulfamethoxazole (one double-strength tablet twice a day), trimethoprim (100 mg twice a day), cephalexin (250–500 mg four times a day), amoxicillin–clavulanic acid (250–500 mg amoxicillin three times a day), norfloxacin (400 mg twice a day), or ciprofloxacin (500 mg twice a day). With present knowledge, our preference is single-dose trimethoprim–sulfamethoxazole, or trimethoprim alone, or 3 days of these or other agents.

We do not advocate use of sulfonamides, ampicillin, or amoxicillin because of the relatively high frequency of *E. coli* resistant to these agents among community-acquired urinary tract infections.[239]

The approach to management of lower urinary tract infection has evolved to where short-course therapy should become the standard for most female patients with suspected lower tract infection. Preliminary studies in pediatric populations have shown similar good results.[259] Short-course therapy has not been adequately evaluated in men and is not recommended at present. Short-course therapy is not appropriate for women who have a history of previous urinary infection caused by antibiotic-resistant organisms, or more than 7 days of symptoms.[239] In these patients (who have an increased likelihood of upper tract infection) and in males, 7–10 days of therapy are recommended.

If symptoms do not respond or if they recur, a urine culture should be obtained. In pregnant women, children, and patients at high risk for renal damage who remain asymptomatic, follow-up cultures should be obtained 1–2 weeks after discontinuation of therapy to detect relapses.

OFFICE STRATEGY FOR FREQUENCY, URGENCY, AND DYSURIA SYNDROME. When a sexually active woman is first seen with frequency, urgency, and dysuria, urine culture is not mandatory, and the therapeutic decision is based on the clinical presentation and the presence or absence of pyuria. If pyuria (defined as $\geq$ 10 leukocytes/mm^3) is present, antimicrobial therapy is warranted for urinary tract infection. Short-course therapy is a reasonable first approach in adult females except in settings in which occult pyelonephritis is more likely, as described above. An agent likely to be effective against most pathogens (e.g., trimethoprim, trimethoprim–sulfamethoxazole, amoxicillin–clavulanic acid, norfloxacin, ciprofloxacin) should be used. If clinical response does not occur, a culture should be obtained (for the possibility of a resistant organism), and therapy should be changed and directed at chlamydia, with 500 mg tetracycline four times a day for 7 days.

In the nonsexually active female with symptoms of lower tract infection and pyuria, there is a high probability of urinary tract infection; lack of response to therapy probably indicates a resistant organism and mandates a urine culture.

In the absence of pyuria, symptomatic urinary tract infection is unlikely in any patient. Symptomatic response followed by recurrence after therapy is discontinued indicates the probability of upper tract infection and the need for a culture and at least 2 weeks of therapy. Men and children should have a urine culture, and males should receive 7–10 days of treatment.

Asymptomatic Bacteriuria. Most patients with asymptomatic bacteriuria are women and are in the older age groups. Although cure may result following treatment, relapse and especially reinfection are common. The approach to asymptomatic bacteriuria depends on the age of the patient. In children, therapy should be given as described for symptomatic infection. A trial of single-dose or short-course therapy is reasonable. In contrast, therapy for asymptomatic bacteriuria in the adult is by no means mandatory in the absence of obstruction except during pregnancy. Nonpregnant women can be treated providing that a nontoxic antimicrobial agent is used. If the infecting microorganism is resistant to all but toxic agents, then treatment should not be instituted in the nonobstructed patient.

At present, most physicians believe that asymptomatic bacteriuria in the elderly is a benign disease and need not be treated, especially since with vigorous treatment a great many people will be exposed to drug toxicity.

When dealing with asymptomatic bacteriuria, there is no urgency in treating. Therapy should be delayed until two cultures have been obtained for confirmation of presence of bacteriuria. By that time, the identity and antimicrobial susceptibility pattern of the infecting organism will have been determined.

Relapsing Urinary Tract Infection. If the patient relapses after therapy for symptomatic urinary tract infection or for asymptomatic bacteriuria, the most likely possibilities are that the patient has (*1*) renal involvement, (*2*) a structural abnormality of the urinary tract (for example, calculi), or (*3*) chronic bacterial prostatitis.

Relapses, especially in the absence of structural abnormalities, may be related to renal infection that may require a longer duration of therapy. Patients who relapse after a short course or 7–10 days of therapy should be considered for a 2-week course. Turck and colleagues[180] demonstrated that a 6-week course of therapy resulted in a higher cure rate than a 2-week course in patients who relapsed after 2 weeks of therapy.

Structural abnormalities of the urinary tract predispose to relapse. Urinary tract infection in the presence of obstruction is likely to be associated with renal involvement, a tendency for renal functional impairment, and bacteremia. Obstructive lesions can be corrected surgically and should be sought in the evaluation of patients with relapsing infection. Calculi may be a cause of relapse of urinary tract infection. Ultimate success of chemotherapy is dependent on the removal of stones.

Some patients continue to relapse despite surgical correction of urologic abnormalities. In others, surgical correction may not be indicated or feasible, or no abnormalities may be found. In these patients who relapse after 2 weeks of chemotherapy, a repeat course of 2 weeks should be considered. Following another relapse a 4–6-week course should be considered. In men, chronic bacterial prostatitis should first be ruled out.

If relapse occurs after a 6-week course, therapy lasting 6 months or even longer may be considered. Only carefully selected patients, such as children, adults who have continuous symptoms, or adults who are at high risk of developing progressive renal damage (for example, those with obstruction not amenable to surgery), should be considered for 4-week or longer courses of therapy. Asymptomatic adults without obstruction should not receive these longer courses. Some of the agents that can be used for long-term therapy are amoxicillin (250 mg three times a day), cephalexin, trimethoprim–sulfamethoxazole, trimethoprim, norfloxacin, and ciprofloxacin, in usual doses, nitrofurantoin in full dosage for 1 week and then half the usual dose, and carbenicillin indanyl sodium (2 tablets four times daily in adults).

An antimicrobial agent being used for long-term therapy is continued only as long as significant bacteriuria is absent. If bacteriuria persists or relapses during chemotherapy (indicating that the infecting organism is now resistant to that agent), the agent is altered. The aim is to achieve continuous suppression of bacteriuria for the entire course of therapy. If relapse occurs after discontinuation of the antimicrobial agent, therapy is reinstituted with the same or another drug. If deemed necessary, this agent is administered for an additional 6 to 12 months (if bacteriuria remains suppressed). All patients are followed with urine cultures at least monthly while on therapy.

Long-term therapy or even repeated 2-week courses should be reserved for children, symptomatic patients of any age, and patients at high risk of developing progressive renal damage. A creatinine clearance determination and an intravenous pyelogram initially and yearly (or at least every 2 years) should be obtained on patients receiving long-term therapy to determine glomerular filtration rate and structural changes in the kidneys. Blood counts, urinalyses, and liver chemistries (when indicated) are also obtained periodically as tests for drug toxicity.

Reinfection of the Urinary Tract. Patients with reinfection can generally be divided into two groups: (*1*) those who have relatively infrequent reinfections, perhaps only once every 2 or 3 years to several times a year and (*2*) those who develop frequent reinfections. An extreme example of the latter group is patients who become reinfected during or shortly after each course of antimicrobial therapy. With infrequent reinfections, each episode can be approached with therapy as if it were a new episode of either symptomatic or asymptomatic infection. Single-dose or short-course therapy should be used in women with lower tract symptoms. Women with reinfections associated with lower tract symptoms can be managed with self-administration of short-course therapy with onset of symptoms.[260]

Many patients with frequent reinfections after therapy are middle-aged or elderly women in whom infection is limited to the lower urinary tract. Most asymptomatic reinfections in this group should not be treated, because the frequent use of antimicrobial agents in this group is apt to result in toxic side effects, and because progressive destruction of the kidneys is rare. If, however, the episodes are symptomatic or if the likelihood of renal damage is increased, these patients should be treated.

Occasionally patients of any age develop symptomatic reinfection so frequently that they can be incapacitated. In some women, these symptomatic reinfections are associated with sexual activity. Voiding immediately after intercourse may help prevent reinfection. However, single-dose prophylactic chemotherapy taken after sexual intercourse is a more effective method of decreasing episodes.[261]

In other patients with frequent symptomatic reinfections, no precipitating event is apparent; in these patients, when symptoms are severe, long-term chemoprophylaxis may be instituted. Although these courses seem to decrease the frequency of reinfections and symptoms in most patients, it is impossible to prevent completely reinfection in many patients. When reinfection occurs on therapy, the prophylactic agent must be changed.

Long-term chemoprophylaxis should be considered for asymptomatic patients who reinfect frequently and are at risk of developing renal parenchymal damage with each reinfection (for example, young children with vesicoureteral reflux and children and adults with obstructive uropathy). In these groups, keeping the patient abacteriuric helps to protect the kidneys. Several studies in patients with frequent reinfections indicate that such prolonged chemotherapy reduces the frequency of reinfections.

Long-term prophylactic antimicrobial agents have reduced the frequency of symptomatic infections of the urinary tract in older men, women, and children.[262–268] Before prophylaxis is initiated, the patient should receive a course of therapy with an appropriate antimicrobial agent. Trimethoprim–sulfamethoxazole, nitrofurantoin, or trimethoprim alone are particularly useful for long-term prophylaxis, because these drugs are unlikely to allow the emergence of antimicrobial-resistant bacteria with prolonged use.[264,268–270]

Full antimicrobial dosage is not necessary for successful prophylaxis. One 50-mg tablet of nitrofurantoin or one-half tablet of trimethoprim–sulfamethoxazole (40 mg trimethoprim, 200 mg sulfamethoxazole) nightly will suffice. Sulfisoxazole, nalidixic acid, methenamine mandelate, and other agents have been used with good results.[227]

A single dose of an antimicrobial agent immediately before or after coitus can reduce the incidence of urinary tract infection that is related to sexual activity.[261]

Patients receiving long-term prophylaxis should be followed with urine cultures monthly or more often if interim symptomatic episodes develop. Thereapy is continued with the same agent as long as the patient remains abacteriuric. If bacteriuria persists or recurs during administration of an antimicrobial agent, therapy is altered using response of bacteriuria as a parameter of adequacy of therapy. Long-term prophylaxis can be undertaken only if urine cultures are obtained periodically and therapy altered if bacteriuria recurs.

URINARY TRACT INFECTION IN PREGNANCY

Physiologic Alterations in the Urinary Tract

During pregnancy there is dilatation of the ureters and renal pelves with markedly decreased ureteral peristalsis. These changes begin as early as the seventh week of gestation and progress to term.[271] The bladder also decreases in tone so that late in gestation it can contain twice its normal contents without causing discomfort. These changes vary from patient to patient. They are more marked on the right side and are more likely to occur during the first pregnancy or when pregnancies occur in rapid succession (Fig. 9). The urinary tract tends to revert to normal by the second month following delivery.[271,272]

Changes similar to those of pregnancy have been described in the urinary tracts of women taking oral contraceptives.[273] Because of this observation, it has been suggested that the urinary tract alterations may be at least in part related to "hyperestrogenism."[271] Other possible explanations for the alterations are obstruction of the ureters by the gravid uterus and hypertrophy of muscle bundles at the lower end of the ureter.[271] To investigate the effects of estrogens on these changes, Andriole and Cohn[274] treated nonpregnant female and male rats with estrogens and obtained intravenous pyelograms before and during treatment. Hydroureter and marked increased susceptibility to *E. coli* pyelonephritis are observed in both male and female animals.

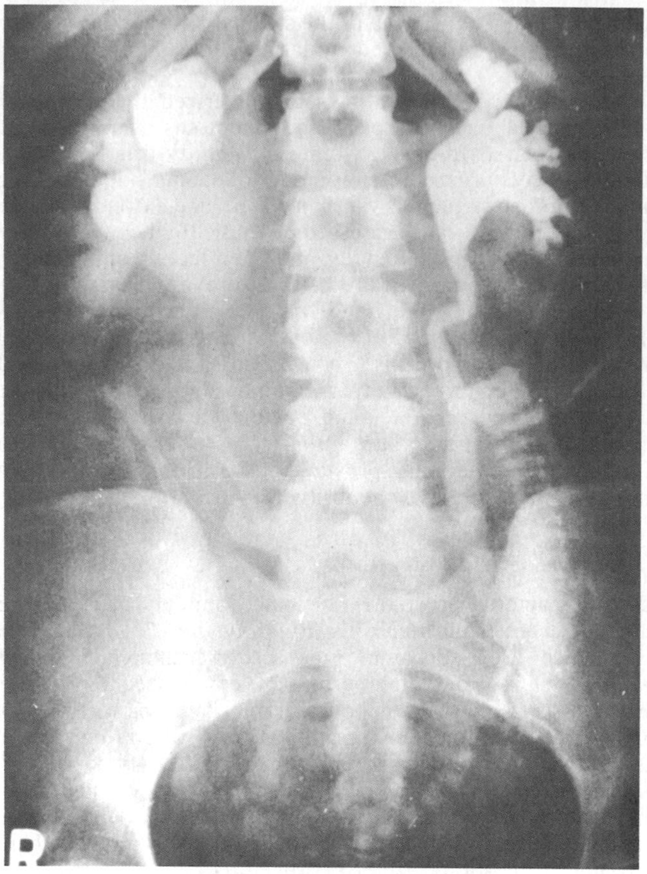

FIG. 9. Urogram in pregnancy. Urography was performed during the seventh month of pregnancy because of severe right-sided pyelonephritis. Although the right hydronephrosis is pronounced, no cause for it other than pregnancy could be found. Following delivery the urogram reverted to normal. Physiologic changes such as these make it difficult to detect superimposed pathologic disorders such as small ureteral calculi when they occur during pregnancy. (From Kaye[340] with permission.)

Epidemiology

The prevalence of asymptomatic bacteriuria in pregnancy ranges from 4 to 7 percent.[275,276] It is unclear if *U. urealyticum* and *Gardnerella vaginalis*, reported by some to be in bladder urine of an additional 10–15 percent of pregnant women, play a significant pathogenic role.[271,277] Pregnant women of higher socioeconomic status have a lower frequency of bacteriuria of pregnancy than women of lower socioeconomic status.[145] The prevalence of bacteriuria also rises with parity and age.[278] For example, in low-income populations, the prevalence of bacteriuria is about 2 percent in primiparas under age 21 as compared with 8–10 percent in grandmultiparas over age 35.[276] Most women who develop bacteriuria during pregnancy have infection at the first prenatal visit. However, 1–1.5 percent of pregnant women or about 25 percent of those with bacteriuria of pregnancy develop infection in the later trimesters.[275,276] The development of symptomatic pyelonephritis late in pregnancy is usually an expression of asymptomatic bacteriuria that was present early in parturition. The marked dilatation of the ureters and pelves during the later stages apparently allows bacteria in the bladder to reach the upper tract and to produce symptomatic pyelonephritis.

About 20–40 percent of the patients with bacteriuria early in gestation develop acute symptomatic pyelonephritis later in pregnancy.[277–280] In contrast, less than 1 percent of patients whose urine is uninfected early in gestation develop acute infection. Therefore, over 75 percent of the cases of acute pyelonephritis can be prevented by eliminating asymptomatic bacteriuria in the early stages of pregnancy.[271,275,276] It has also been noted that those whose bacteriuria fails to respond to treatment are at highest risk of developing symptomatic infection.[281] Lack of cure is probably an indication of upper versus lower tract infection.

An association between acute pyelonephritis of pregnancy and premature delivery was well known in the preantibiotic era.[271] The rate of prematurity can be as high as 20–50 percent. Kass[278] in 1959 reported that there was an association between asymptomatic bacteriuria and prematurity, and that the eradication of bacteriuria significantly reduced the rate of premature delivery. Since then there have been conflicting studies both supporting and denying these observations.[271,276,281] In general, it seems that prematurity is increased in patients with asymptomatic bacteriuria. However, it does not necessarily follow that asymptomatic bacteriuria is a cause of prematurity. It is possible that certain patients are predisposed to both bacteriuria and to deliver premature infants. Some investigators have reported that elimination of bacteriuria decreases the frequency of prematurity.[271,276,281] However, other studies have failed to show a decrease in prematurity or fetal wastage with elimination of asymptomatic bacteriuria.[271,276,281] Neonates of patients refractory to multiple courses of therapy have been reported to have a significantly lower birth weight than infants of those who respond; this phenomenon may be related to the presence of upper tract infection in these patients.[194,281,282] There have been several studies that have attempted to relate asymptomatic bacteriuria to the development of hypertension in pregnancy, but results have been unclear.[276]

Even though the data relating bacteriuria of pregnancy to prematurity are not clear-cut, the relationship of asymptomatic bacteriuria to later development of acute pyelonephritis is indisputable. As acute pyelonephritis has possible serious consequences for both mother and fetus, screening for, and treatment of bacteriuria of pregnancy seems justified. Quantitative urine cultures should be obtained in all pregnant patients at the initial prenatal visit.

Postpartum studies of patients with bacteriuria of pregnancy demonstrate a high frequency of bacteriuria even with treatment during the pregnancy.[283] Postpartum intravenous pyelography of these patients has shown that 10–30 percent have radiologic changes of "chronic pyelonephritis" and other abnormalities.[221,283] These abnormalities are most common in patients in whom renal bacteriuria has been demonstrated or in whom bacteriuria during pregnancy was difficult to eradicate with antimicrobial therapy.[283,284] However, pyelographic abnormalities should not necessarily be attributed to the infection that occurred during the pregnancy. In fact, these abnormalities probably antedate the pregnancy and in most cases are related to childhood infection. Treatment of bacteriuria of pregnancy has little effect on the long-term course of the patient. When patients who had bacteriuria of pregnancy were studied 10–14 years later, there were no differences between those who were treated and those who were not. About 25 percent of the women in each group had bacteriuria at time of follow-up.[221]

Management of Bacteriuria of Pregnancy

Treatment with an appropriate antimicrobial agent is recommended for all pregnant patients found to have significant bacteriuria.[188,271,276,277,280] The goal of therapy is to maintain sterile urine throughout gestation and thereby to avoid the complications associated with urinary tract infection during pregnancy. The administration of a relatively nontoxic drug for 7 days (e.g., a sulfonamide, ampicillin, cephalexin, nitrofurantoin) eradicates bacteriuria in 70–80 percent of patients.[188,271,276] Failure of treatment is most commonly seen in patients with renal infection or radiologic abnormalities of the urinary tract.[188,271,276] Sulfonamides should not be administered in the last few weeks of gestation because of hyperbilirubinemia and kernicterus in the newborn. Tetracyclines should be avoided during pregnancy.

There are relatively few studies evaluating the efficacy of single-dose or 3 days of antimicrobial therapy for asymptomatic bacteriuria during pregnancy. In general, results appear to be inferior to conventional therapy.[271] However, single-dose or 3 days of therapy may be a reasonable first option both in symptomatic and in asymptomatic infection in an attempt to decrease drug administration in pregnancy.

Urine cultures should be obtained 1–2 weeks after discontinuing therapy and at regular intervals (e.g., monthly) for the remainder of gestation. If bacteriuria recurs, therapy should be given for relapse or reinfection, as already discussed. Catheterization should be avoided at the time of delivery. If relapses or multiple reinfections occurred during pregnancy, radiologic evaluation should be considered postpartum.

PROSTATITIS

Bacterial prostatitis can manifest as either an acute or chronic disease. Although the manner by which bacteria reach the prostate is unknown,[285] possibilities include the hematogenous route, ascending infection from the urethra, and lymphatic spread from the rectum. Reflux of infected urine may also play a role in the pathogenesis of bacterial prostatitis.[286] Urethral instrumentation and prostatic surgery are known causes of prostatitis, but many patients have no history of a precipitating event.

Stamey and colleagues[287] have noted that male sex partners of women with vaginal colonization by gram-negative bacilli may develop transient urethral colonization with the same organisms. They postulated that sexual intercourse might play an important role in infection of the prostate.Prostatic fluid normally has substantial antibacterial properties.[67,288] However, the prostatic secretions of some patients with chronic bacterial prostatitis have been shown to lack such activity.[288]

The syndromes of acute and chronic bacterial prostatitis are different and distinct. Acute prostatitis does not usually result in chronic prostatitis, and chronic bacterial prostatitis is not usually antedated by acute prostatitis. Acute prostatitis is an acute infectious disease and is similar to an acute localized infection in any other organ, producing local heat, tenderness, and fever. In contrast, chronic bacterial prostatitis often produces few or no symptoms related to the prostate, which just serves as a nidus of low-grade infection. Some patients with chronic bacterial prostatitis have persistent symptoms such as perineal pressure, low back pain, or difficulty urinating. Symptoms of acute cystitis or pyelonephritis occur when bacteria, which are repeatedly invading the bladder, overcome the defense mechanisms of the bladder.

Bacteria originating in the prostate may be coated with antibody and, therefore, are a cause of a false-positive ACB test.[191,192] Following acute bacterial prostatitis, a serum and local immune response is elicited, with the presence of IgA and IgG bacteria-specific immunoglobulins being detected in prostatic secretions. More prolonged prostatic secretion of IgA is observed in chronic bacterial prostatitis.[289]

Acute Prostatitis

Most cases of acute bacterial prostatitis in the preantibiotic era were caused by *N. gonorrhoeae*. Gram-negative enteric organisms are now the most frequent pathogens.[285] *Neisseria gonorrhoeae* is currently an unusual cause.

Pathologically, acute bacterial prostatitis is characterized by inflammation of part or all of the gland with marked cellular infiltrate (predominantly polymorphonuclear leukocytes), diffuse edema, and hyperemia of the stroma. Microabscesses may occur and may be followed by large, clinically apparent collections of pus.

Acute bacterial prostatitis is characterized by high fever, chills, perineal and back pain, and symptoms of urinary tract infection such as frequency, urgency, and dysuria.[285] The patient may have urinary retention due to bladder outlet obstruction. The prostate gland is warm, swollen, and extremely tender on rectal examination. Expressed prostatic fluid contains many polymorphonuclear leukocytes, and the infecting organism can frequently be seen on Gram stain. However, massage of the acutely infected prostate gland can precipitate bacteremia and should be discouraged. Since most patients also have bacteriuria, the infecting organism can usually be isolated by midstream urine culture. Many antibiotics diffuse well into the acutely inflamed prostate, and acute bacterial prostatitis responds well to appropriate antimicrobial therapy. Complications such as bacteremia, prostatic abscess, epididymitis, seminal vesiculitis, and pyelonephritis may occur.

Chronic Bacterial Prostatitis

Chronic bacterial prostatitis is most commonly caused by *E. coli* (80 percent), but *Klebsiella, Enterobacter, P. mirabilis*, and enterococci are also common causes.[285] Although *S. epidermidis, S. aureus*, and diphtheroids have been frequent isolates in some series,[290] there is considerable doubt as to their real pathogenic role, and most gram-positive bacteria cultured in association with prostatitis represent urethral commensals.[291]

The histologic findings of chronic bacterial prostatitis are focal, nonacute inflammation. similar findings may be noted in patients without evidence of bacterial infection and are therefore not diagnostic of bacterial prostatitis.

Many men with chronic infection of the prostate are totally asymptomatic. However, some have perineal discomfort, low back pain, or dysuria. Symptoms of acute urinary tract infection may appear periodically. In fact, chronic bacterial prostatitis is probably the most common cause of relapsing urinary tract infection in men. Fever, if present, tends to be low grade unless pyelonephritis occurs. The results of rectal examination and intravenous pyelogram are unremarkable unless the patient also has an enlarged prostate gland from benign prostatic hypertrophy or carcinoma.

Because of the focal nature of chronic bacterial prostatitis, needle biopsy of the prostate gland for culture of tissue is unreliable.[292] Demonstration of leukocytes in prostatic fluid is not specific for bacterial prostatitis. Most clinicians agree that >15 leukocytes per high-power field represents an abnormal number of leukocytes in prostatic fluid.[291] Provided that simultaneous urethral and midstream specimens show insignificant pyuria, this finding would indicate prostatic inflammation irrespective of the etiology. Meares and Stamey[183] have described a quantitative localization technique for making the bacteriologic diagnosis. Because bacteria present in the urethra can contaminate prostatic secretions obtained by prostatic massage, accurate diagnosis requires simultaneous quantitative cultures of (*1*) urethral urine (VB_1), (*2*) midstream urine (VB_2), (*3*) prostatic secretions expressed by massage (EPS), and (*4*) the urine voided after massage (VB_3). An ejaculate is probably preferable to the EPS.

The specimens must be cultured immediately after collection, and methods of quantitating small numbers of bacteria must be used. The study should be done at a time the patient does not have significant bacteriuria. If bacteriuria is present, ampicillin, cephalexin, or nitrofurantoin should be given for 2–3 days to sterilize the urine; these agents will not affect bacterial counts in the prostate in chronic bacterial prostatitis. If chronic bacterial prostatitis is present, the number of bacteria in EPS or ejaculate will exceed those in VB_1 or VB_2 urine by at least 10-fold. If no EPS or ejaculate can be obtained, the bacterial counts in the VB_3 specimen should be at least 10-fold higher than the VB_1 or VB_2 samples.

Chronic bacterial prostatitis is very difficult to cure since few antimicrobial agents penetrate well into the noninflamed prostate. Furthermore, the nidus of infection in some patients may be small prostatic calculi or abscesses that presumably are difficult to sterilize. Chronic bacterial prostatitis is therefore likely to persist and cause relapsing urinary tract infection. Unlike classic urinary tract infection, relapses may occur after long periods without bacteriuria (e.g., months). Management may be difficult (see "Therapy," below).

Nonbacterial Prostatitis

This syndrome is the most common type of prostatitis and represents an inflammatory condition of unknown cause.[291] The symptoms are perineal pressure, dysuria, urgency, and/or low back pain, symptoms that can also be caused by chronic bacterial prostatitis. However, bacterial pathogens cannot be demonstrated using sequential quantitative cultures. Urinary tract infection does not occur, although prostatic secretions contain excessive numbers of leukocytes and fat-laden macrophages. The most controversial putative agent of nonbacterial prostatitis is *C. trachomatis*. The problem has been in distinguishing urethral colonization with *Chlamydia* from prostatic infection.[291,293] Similarly, the role of *U. urealyticum* is obscure. The term prostadynia or prostatosis refers to a similar clinical syndrome in the absence of any objective signs of prostatic inflammation. Some feel that the symptoms may be caused by spasm of the pelvic floor musculature.[294] Others feel that there may be a major psychological component. Because the etiology of both entities is unknown, therapy is difficult (see "Therapy," below).

Therapy

A dog model has been used to measure diffusion of antimicrobial agents into the noninflamed prostate.[295] In this system, antimicrobial agents are infused, giving high and constant plasma levels, and prostatic secretions are simultaneously collected. Although the basic macrolides such as erythromycin prenetrated well into prostatic secretions, penicillins, cephalosporins, tetracyclines, nitrofurantoin, and vancomycin did not. The explanation given was that only lipid-soluble and basic compounds are capable of entering the acid milieu of the prostate gland. Trimethroprim has been shown to diffuse into prostatic fluid in high concentrations.[296]

Acute bacterial prostatitis frequently responds dramatically to antibacterial therapy. It is thought that the intense diffuse inflammatory reaction of acute bacterial prostatitis allows the passage of antimicrobial agents from plasma into the prostate.[285] Therefore, in management of acute prostatitis, antimicrobial agents should be given to the patient in doses that achieve therapeutic concentrations in the blood. Measures such as hydration, analgesics, best rest, and stool softeners may be helpful. Urethral instrumentation should be avoided. If acute urinary retention occurs, suprapubic drainage of urine is required through a suprapubic catheter. Prostatic abscess is rarely cured by antimicrobial agents alone and requires surgical drainage. Computed tomography (CT) studies or transrectal ultrasonography are important advances in diagnosis of abscess formation.[297] Drainage can often be achieved by an ultrasound guided needle.

Chronic bacterial prostatitis is very difficult to cure. Partial transurethral prostatectomy is curative only if all the infected tissue is removed; about one-third of the patients are cured by this procedure.[285] However, a higher percentage is cured if a complete transurethral prostatectomy is performed.[291] Complete prostatectomy is contraindicated because of the complications of sexual impotence and incontinence.

The primary approach to chronic bacterial prostatitis is an attempt at cure with antimicrobial therapy. Although occasional cures have been achieved with penicillins, cephalosporins, tetracyclines, or aminoglycosides, the focus of infection in the prostate has usually persisted, resulting in relapse after therapy was discontinued. Better results have been reported in limited trials with trimethoprim–sulfamethoxazole (2 tablets twice a day), oral carbenicillin indanyl sodium, and rifampin in combination with trimethoprim.[298–300] Cure rates have varied from one-third to most of the patients treated with these agents for 1–3 or more months. The sulfonamide component of trimethroprim–sulfamethoxazole probably contributes little, and rifampin may be more suitable than sulfamethoxazole as a partner for trimethroprim. Rifampin has an excellent antibacterial spectrum, but has the unfortunate property of rapid development of resistance. Trimethoprim prevents emergence of resistance to rifampin.[300] Recently preliminary studies with oral quinolones have produced encouraging results.[301] At present, our initial regimen of choice is trimethoprim–sulfamethoxazole, or a quinolone. If therapy fails on these regimens, the patient should be managed either with treatment of acute exacerbations of urinary tract infection or with chronic suppressive therapy using low daily doses (e.g., half-normal doses) of an antimicrobial agent. Nonbacterial prostatitis can be treated empirically with erythromycin or tetracycline relying on clinical response to justify a further trial of therapy. Reassurance is important.

PERINEPHRIC ABSCESS AND INTRARENAL ABSCESS

Perinephric Abscess

Perinephric abscess is an uncommon complication of urinary tract infection.[302] The most common predisposing factors are urinary tract calculi and diabetes mellitus. It usually occurs secondary to obstruction of an infected kidney or calyx or occasionally secondary to bacteremia. It may occur insidiously, and up to one-third of cases may not be diagnosed until autopsy. The infecting bacteria are usually gram-negative enteric bacilli and occasionally gram-positive cocci when the infection is of hematogenous origin.

The patients have a syndrome suggestive of acute pyelonephritis, with fever, abdominal and flank pain (usually unilateral), and often symptoms of lower tract infection. The patient has often been ill for 2 or more weeks. The diagnosis should be strongly considered in any patient with a febrile illness and unilateral flank pain who does not respond to therapy for acute pyelonephritis. A palpable mass may or may not be present. About one-half of the patients have an abnormal plain film of the abdomen (e.g., abdominal mass, a calculus, a poorly defined renal shadow), and 85 percent have abnormal intravenous pyelograms.

Intrarenal Abscess

Intrarenal abscess may occur as a consequence of bacteremia (often caused by coagulase-positive staphylococci). However, these lesions are being recognized with increasing frequency as a complication of classic acute pyelonephritis. The clinical setting is usually that of acute pyelonephritis with high fever, severe flank pain, and tenderness, but with no response or very slow response to appropriate antimicrobial therapy. Most patients with intrarenal abscess respond, although slowly, to antimicrobial therapy, but fever and severe flank pain may persist for days. Occasionally drainage becomes necessary.

Diagnosis and Therapy

The introduction of renal ultrasound and in particular CT scans have added a new dimension of sensitivity and specificity permitting the early diagnosis of intrarenal and perinephric

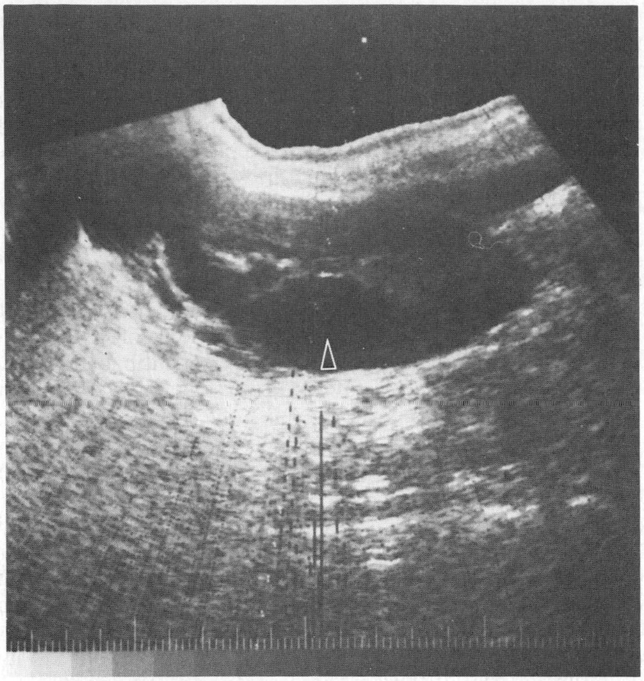

FIG. 10. Ultrasound examination of the kidney showing an intrarenal abscess (arrow). (Courtesy of Dr. George Popky, Philadelphia, PA.)

abscesses[303,304] (Figs. 10 and 11). The most common CT findings include thickening of Gerota's fascia, renal enlargement, focal parenchymal decreased attenuation, and fluid and/or gas in and around the kidney.[305]

In patients with a clinical or radiographic suspicion of perinephric abscess, diagnostic needle aspiration can be safely performed by using ultrasound or CT scan quidance. When an abscess is confirmed, small catheters can be introduced percutaneously via the diagnostic aspiration route to provide immediate decompression as well as continuous and definitive drainage without need for surgery.[303,304] Advantages to guided percutaneous drainage compared with open surgical drainage include earlier diagnosis and treatment, avoidance of general anesthesia and surgery, less expensive therapy, easier nursing

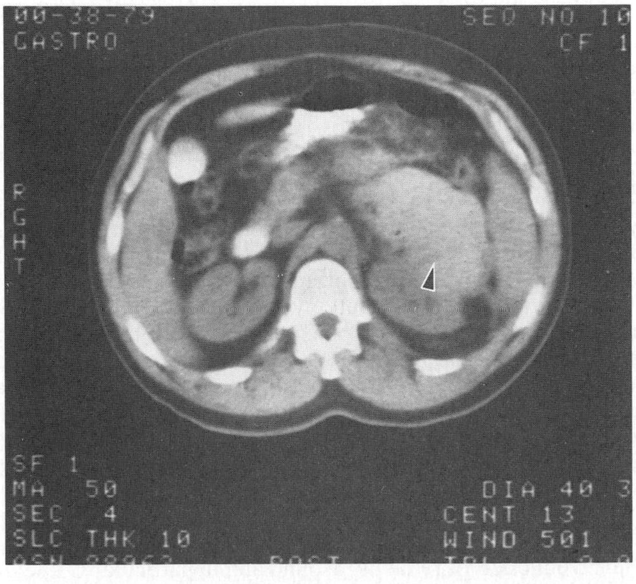

FIG. 11. CT scan showing a perinephric abscess (arrow). (Courtesy of Dr. George Popky, Philadelphia, PA.)

care, and greater patient acceptance of closed drainage. Accordingly, it is now recommended that after starting antimicrobial therapy directed against the most likely pathogens, a trial of percutaneous drainage should be the initial mode of therapy for perinephric abscess. Surgical intervention should be undertaken only when percutaneous drainage fails or is contraindicated. While parenteral antimicrobial therapy directed against the infecting organism isolated from blood or urine should be initiated before drainage, if additional organisms are isolated at the time of surgery, treatment directed against these organisms must be added. Therapy must also be used for the underlying disease (for example, staphylococcal bacteremia or obstructive uropathy).

Percutaneous drainage has been equally effective in drainage of renal abscesses and infected renal cysts, often avoiding the previous approach of open surgical drainage or nephrectomy.[303,306,307]

RADIOLOGIC EVALUATION OF PATIENTS WITH URINARY TRACT INFECTION

Radiologic procedures play an important role in the management of patients with urinary tract infection,[308,309] both in control of complicated episodes of acute pyelonephritis as well as in the investigation of patients of all ages in whom the clinician suspects the presence of underlying structural abnormalities that may be surgically correctable.

Radiologic assessment should commence with a plain film of the abdomen for detection of urinary tract calculi, calcification, soft tissue masses, and abnormal gas collections. In the past, excretory urography in the form of intravenous pyelography was the initial and definitive investigatory study but has been largely replaced by both ultrasonography and CT scans. In general, sonography serves as a rapid, noninvasive, and relatively inexpensive means of evaluating the renal collecting system, parenchyma, and surrounding retroperitoneum.[308] Ultrasound is more sensitive than intravenous pyelography for detecting parenchymal changes associated with renal infection; CT, however, is the most sensitive technique of all. Compared with CT, sonography offers several advantages, including no irradiation, portability, and relative accessibility.[309] Both CT and ultrasound are sensitive in diagnosing intrarenal and perirenal suppuration. Similarly, both these procedures may be used for guidance of percutaneous needle aspiration. Intravenous pyelography remains useful for detecting lesions of the collecting system and ureters. Contrast-enhanced CT provides physiologic information similar to that obtained with IV pyelography, with much better parenchymal delineation but less optimal delineation of the collecting system.[305] All studies requiring parenteral administration of contrast material are associated with some risk of allergy or contrast-induced renal insufficiency. Predisposing factors for renal insufficiency include myeloma, diabetes mellitus, pre-existing renal failure, severe intravascular volume depletion, and recent administration of large doses of iodinated contrast material. Radioisotope studies play only a small role, if any, in the investigation of the urinary tract. Gallium-67 citrate scanning and indium-111-labeled white blood cell studies occasionally prove useful in localizing inflammation or infection to the kidneys in patients with fever of unknown origin and may be of value, after ultrasound or CT scans have identified a solid renal mass, in suggesting the inflammatory nature of the lesion.

Radiologic or ultrasound investigation may be indicated in patients with nonresponsive pyelonephritis (particularly if bacteremic) to identify local complications such as renal and perinephric abscess formation. The most important contribution provided by these modalities is the detection of surgically correctable abnormalities of the urinary tract. Investigation should be considered in patients at greatest risk of having surgically correctable abnormalities. Persons with urinary tract infection included in this high-risk category are all children, men of any age, patients who relapse after therapy, and patients whose infection has been complicated by bacteremia. In the past excretory urography was indicated for all these categories and for adult women only after multiple episodes of urinary tract infection. As mentioned above, given the value of ultrasonography, its availability, and its safety, it is reasonable to study all patients with upper tract infection. Women with bacteriuria of pregnancy in whom eradication of infection is difficult should be evaluated. Whereas ultrasonography can be safely performed during pregnancy, accurate delineation of the urinary tract should be delayed until at least 2 months after delivery, by which time the physiologic alterations of the urinary tract that occur during pregnancy should be reversed.[271,272] Ultrasound examination is also useful in diagnosing lower urinary tract obstruction and detecting residual urine in the bladder. A radionuclide DTPA scan with furosemide to increase urine flow is useful in determining if there is structural as opposed to functional ureteropelvic junction obstruction.

In addition to delineating lesions amenable to surgical correction, urography frequently provides information previously unknown to the patient or physician. For example, unsuspected renal scarring may be seen, suggesting the presence of undiagnosed urinary tract infection in childhood (Fig. 12). Occasionally an unusual or unsuspected type of renal infection such as tuberculosis, papillary necrosis (Figs. 13 and 14), or xanthogranulomatous pyelonephritis may be discovered.[310] The last is a severe and chronic form of kidney inflammation in which areas of renal parenchyma are replaced by an inflammatory granulomatous reaction characterized by lipid-laden macrophages (foam cells).[310] Renal calculi and obstruction are often associated with this lesion.[272] Two major radiologic patterns are seen: that of a localized mass and that of diffuse nodularity. When a mass lesion is present, differentiation from pyogenic abscess, tuberculous abscess, or avascular carcinoma may not be possible.

Excretory urography and voiding cystourethrography are recommended in all boys after the first episode of urinary infection and in preschool girls at least after the second infection.[311] Investigation is indicated since the incidence of vesicoureteral reflux in this population has been reported to be 20–35 percent. Reflux is associated with renal scar formation, and

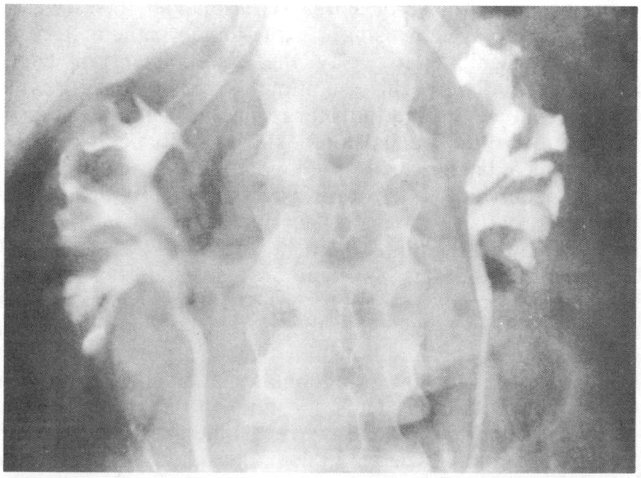

FIG. 12. Bilateral chronic pyelonephritis (retrograde pyelogram). Severe renal insufficiency precluded adequate visualization by excretory urography. Note the severe caliectasis bilaterally with marked left renal atrophy. There is moderate atrophy on the right.

While retrograde pyelography is not infrequently required to demonstrate the collecting system in severely diseased kidneys, it is probably best to avoid the performance of bilateral simultaneous retrograde pyelography in the azotemic patient. (From Kaye,[340] with permission.)

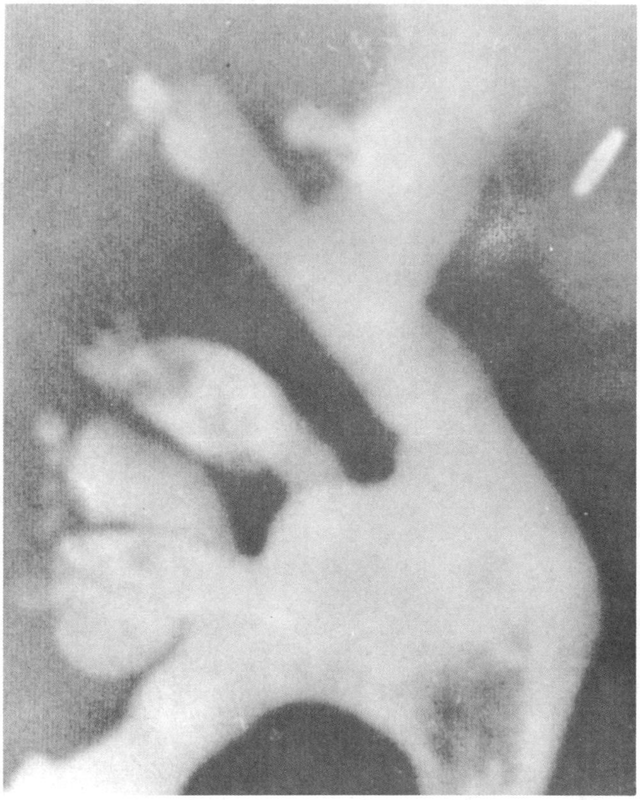

FIG. 13. Renal papillary necrosis (medullary type). Medullary cavities are seen involving almost all the visualized calyces. The cavities tend to be located within the central portion of the medulla rather than at the calyceal fornices. This is the medullary type of papillary necrosis so frequently associated with sickle cell disease, as was the case in this patient. Filling defects within the renal pelvis are attributable to a combination of sloughed papillas, mucus, and pus. (From Kaye,[340] with permission.)

surgery may be indicated in some of these children and infants. There is, however, growing evidence that ultrasonography is as sensitive and may replace intravenous pyelography as the initial study in evaluating children with urinary tract infections[312,313] and detecting children who require corrective surgery.[314,315] In children, intravenous pyelography should be used when other imaging methods show an abnormality and more detailed anatomic visualization of the upper tract is required.[312] As an elective procedure for detection and evaluation of vesicoureteral reflux, conventional cystourethrography or, more commonly, high-resolution radionuclide voiding cystography is still required, especially since reflux with urinary tract dilatation is frequently undetected by ultrasonography and intravenous pyelography. The use of radionuclide cystography involves less irradiation and is better tolerated than conventional contrast material introduced by bladder catheterization.[312] Cystourethrography should be avoided in older children unless intravenous pyelography shows evidence of renal scars. However, even with scars, if serial urographic evaluation demonstrates stability of upper tract lesions, the need for studying the lower tract is questionable. Fairly[316] has suggested that it may be possible to avoid cystourethrography by taking a late roentgenogram (4–6 hours) after intravenous pyelography. By this time the ureters should no longer contain contrast material, but the bladder will be filled. A voiding film taken at this time may then demonstrate presence or absence of reflux. Fairley feels that if no reflux is demonstrated by this method, it is doubtful that cystourethrography will add much in older children and adults. When reflux is found, it should be graded as minimal (grade I) to severe (grade IV), so progression or improvement can be quantitated and decisions on surgery can be made.[200]

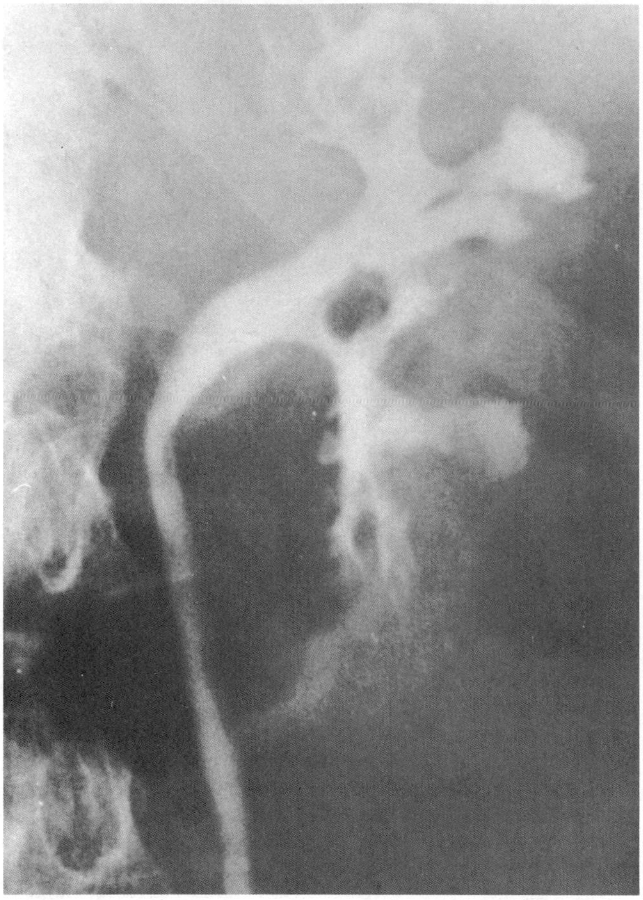

FIG. 14. Renal papillary necrosis (papillary type). The filling defects in the upper calyces represent sloughed papillas that have completely detached from the medulla. This has been referred to as the *ring sign* and indicates the papillary type of renal papillary necrosis. (From Kaye,[340] with permission.)

SURGICAL MANAGEMENT

Surgical therapy in the management of urinary tract infection consists of the elimination of obstructive lesions or calculi and the reimplantation of ureters in the bladder for reflux. An obstruction may be intrinsic (such as renal cysts), or it may be extrinsic anywhere along the urinary conduit from the ureteropelvic junction to the external urethral meatus. Surgical therapy should be directed toward eliminating the obstruction and preserving renal function. After the obstruction is eliminated, the patient should be followed with urine cultures. Urinary tract infection should be treated before surgery to render the urine sterile at the time of surgery; this decreases the possibility of bacteremia occurring in association with the surgery. For management of perinephric or intrarenal abscess see "Perinephric Abscess" and "Intrarenal Abscess," above.

CATHETER-ASSOCIATED URINARY TRACT INFECTION

The urinary tract is one of the most common sites of nosocomial infection, and most of these hospital-acquired infections occur in patients who have undergone urologic manipulation (frequently catheterization).[116] It has been estimated that 10–15 percent of the patients in community hospitals have indwelling urinary catheters. Proper catheter care and management is essential for prevention of infection (see Chapter 281).

Bacteria may enter the bladder at the time of catheterization especially if faulty technique is used. Two pathways have been postulated by which bacteria invade the bladder through indwelling catheters. The most important pathway with open-drainage systems is probably through the catheter lumen via the upward movement of air bubbles, by motility of the bacteria, or by capillary action.[58,317–319] The second route by which bacteria can reach the bladder is through the exudative sheath that surrounds the catheter in the urethra, and this route is probably more important with closed-drainage systems.[320]

The "open system" of indwelling catheters consists of a catheter with two lumens—one for balloon inflation and one for urine that drains into an open receptacle. Fifty percent of the patients with sterile urine before catheterization develop significant bacteriuria within 24 hours with this system; virtually all are infected at 4 days.[13] Furthermore, many of these patients also develop acute pyelonephritis and life-threatening gram-negative bacillary bacteriemia.[321–323]

Bacteria that produce catheter-associated urinary tract infection can be acquired from the patient's fecal flora, or by cross-infection (i.e., transfer of bacteria from patient to patient by hospital personnel).[117]

The incidence of catheter-associated urinary tract infection depends on the method and duration of catheterization. The risk of infection after a single catheterization is about 1 percent,[12] but it is higher in elderly or debilitated patients, in patients with urologic abnormalities, and in pregnant women.[12,324] Patients with indwelling catheters have a much greater risk of infection.

Prevention

Most patients who require indwelling urethral catheters need them for only short periods (less than 1 week).[319] Several systems of bladder drainage have been studied in an attempt to keep bladder urine sterile for this period of time. Administration of systemic antimicrobial agents to patients with open drainage systems does not prevent the development of bacteriuria but does predispose to infection with antibiotic-resistant organisms, such as *Pseudomonas* and *Serratia*.[325] The application of antibiotic ointments to the external urethral meatus, the incorporation of antibiotics into lubricants, and the impregnation of the catheter itself with antibiotics have met with little success in preventing infection with an open drainage system.[317]

In contrast, the use of antibacterial bladder rinses with the open-drainage system using a triple-lumen catheter has been shown to significantly delay the development of bacteriuria.[317,321,322] Several rinse solutions have been used including 0.25 percent acetic acid, nitrofurazone, and neomycin plus polymyxin. All three are capable of substantially delaying the development of bacteriuria (to beyond 10 days in most patients), but the neomycin–polymyxin rinse is probably the most effective. Most patients have sterile urine after catheterization for up to 10 days using this system.[326]

Sterile closed-drainage systems are also capable of preventing bacteriuria in most patients for up to 10 days without the use of antibiotic rinses provided the system is kept closed.[326] Indiscriminant opening and flushing of the sterile closed-catheter system are common causes of contamination and infection. Antibiotic rinses and ointments add little to the protective effect of a closed system.[327–330] However, some studies indicate that there may be an advantage in using systemic antibiotics when the closed system is used for only a few days.[319,327,331]

Closed drainage systems and three-way catheter systems with a neomycin–polymyxin rinse are comparable in preventing infection. However, our preference is for the closed drainage system, because (*1*) it is less expensive; (*2*) it is easier to maintain; and (*3*) if infection occurs, there is a reasonable chance that it will be with an antibiotic-susceptible organism. However, if for some reason frequent irrigation of the catheter is needed, an antibiotic drip is preferable. When catheters are required for many months or permanently, no system prevents infection.

In one study, the outlet tube of the closed urinary drainage set was kept full of 3% hydrogen peroxide at all times, and there was no evidence of bacterial growth in the urine of the collection bag in 92 percent of patients.[332] While this observation is of interest, it does not necessarily mean that there would be a major decrease in infection, as the more important pathway for infection with closed systems is probably via the urethra around the catheter.

Recommendations for urinary catheter care are listed in Table 2.

Treatment

Butler and Kunin,[335] using a closed sterile drainage system, showed that with systemic antimicrobials the initial infecting organism could usually be eradicated even though the catheter remained in place. However, when the catheter remained in place, subsequent reinfection was common, usually with more

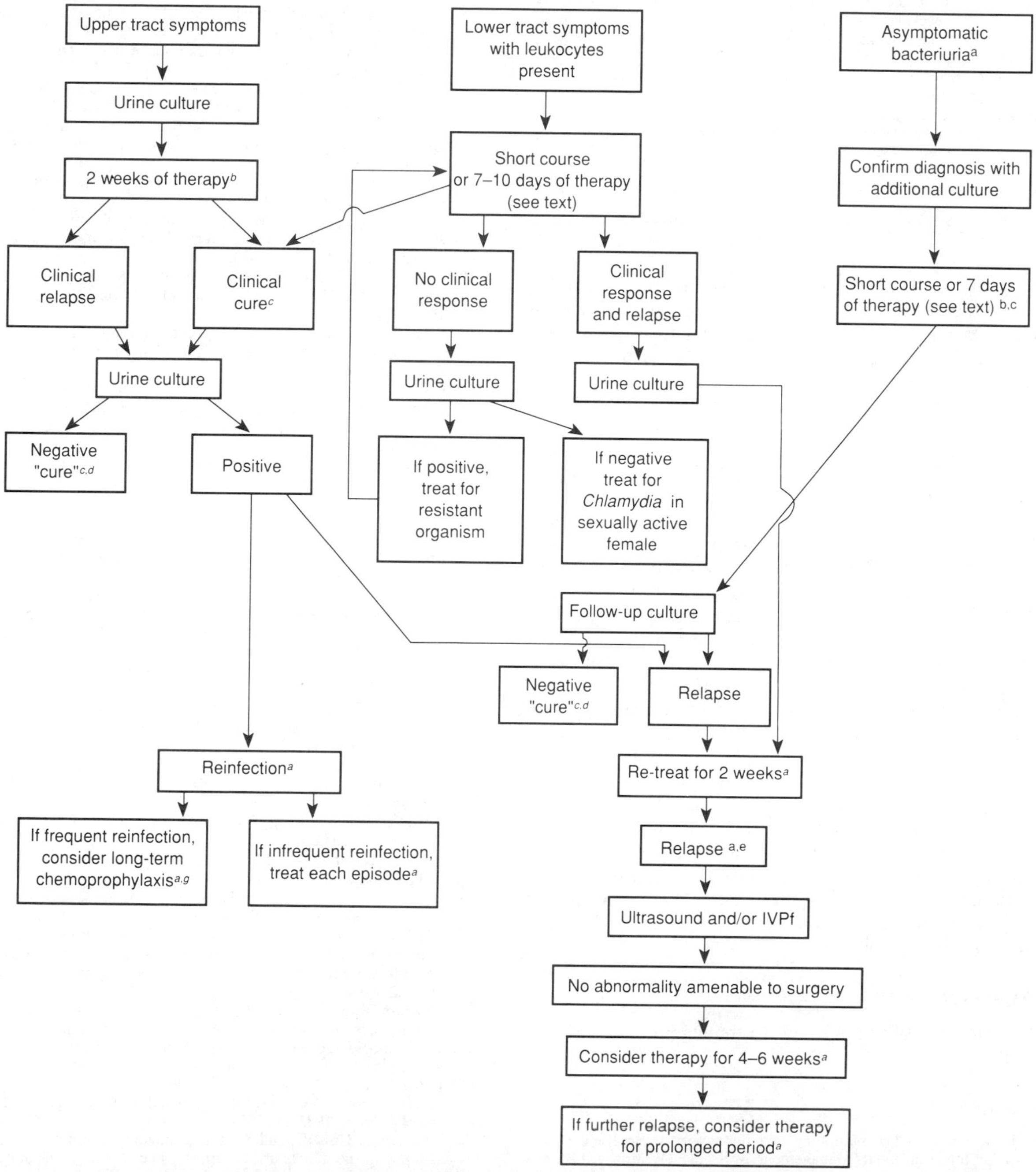

FIG. 15. Management of urinary tract infection.
[a] Consider no therapy in nonpregnant adults without obstructive uropathy or symptoms of urinary tract infection.
[b] Consider ultrasound and/or intravenous pyelogram (IVP) in all children and men with correction of significant lesions.
[c] Follow-up culture required only in pregnancy, in children, and in adults with obstructive uropathy.
[d] Follow-up cultures monthly in pregnant women and at 6 weeks and 6 months in children.
[e] Evaluate men for chronic bacterial prostatitis.
[f] Delay 2 months postpartum in pregnant women.
[g] Consider ultrasound and/or IVP after three to four reinfections in women.

TABLE 2. Guidelines for Indwelling Catheter Care[a]

1. Use only when absolutely necessary—not for convenience. Remove as soon as possible.
2. Catheters should be inserted and maintained by trained personnel only. Catheter teams are preferable.
3. Catheters must be inserted using stringent aseptic technique.
4. Perineal care should be administered twice daily. Antimicrobial ointment can be applied to the meatal-catheter junction.
5. When a sterile closed-drainage system is used, it is mandatory to keep it closed. The catheter and drainage tube must never be disconnected except when irrigation is necessary for obstruction. Sterile technique must be used under these circumstances.
6. Urine for culture should be obtained by aspirating the catheter with a 21-gauge needle after the catheter is prepared with povidone–iodine.
7. "Downhill," nonobstructed flow must be maintained. The catheter should always be below the level of the bladder and the bag should be emptied regularly.
8. Closed sterile drainage systems that have been opened or have leaks must be replaced immediately.
9. Replacement of indwelling catheters is not necessary unless concretions are felt or the system is obstructed.
10. Personnel and patients must be routinely educated on catheter care.
11. Catheterized patients should be separated from each other whenever possible.
12. Postcatheterization urine should be obtained for culture.
13. Patients with cardiac diseases that predispose to bacterial endocarditis should receive prophylactic antibiotics at the time of both catheter insertion and removal.

[a] See Stamm[333] and Fincke et al.[334]

resistant organisms. Although some experts may favor initiating therapy while the catheter is in place, the cost effectiveness of such procedures must be assessed. We prefer to wait until the catheter is removed before treating. While catheter-induced bacteriuria will often spontaneously disappear with removal of the catheter, in those in whom it persists, there is an increased frequency of symptomatic urinary infection during the next year.[319,336] Therefore those who remain bacteriuric 1 week after catheter removal should be treated. If fever, flank pain, or other symptoms of infection occur, therapy must be started even though the catheter remains in place. If the catheter is to remain for months or years, it is our policy to treat only when the patient becomes symptomatic. Some patients who require constant catheter drainage can be managed with intermittent straight catheterization, which may be more likely to avoid infection.[337] Condom catheter drainage in men may avoid infection. However, condom catheter drainage does predispose to infection, especially in uncooperative patients.[17,319]

Candida are occasionally isolated from urine specimens in pure culture but are rarely of clinical significance.[338] Many such specimens were from patients who had had indwelling urethral catheters. Usually these isolates can be ignored; they clear spontaneously when the catheter is removed.[338] However, repeated isolation of pure cultures of yeast from urine may represent urinary tract infection.[26] Under these circumstances, antifungal therapy may become necessary. Irrigation of the bladder with amphotericin B is effective for lower tract fungal infection.[339] Some patients even develop fungus balls, that may obstruct a calyx or the bladder.

SUMMARY FLOW SHEET

Figure 15 summarizes the approach to management of urinary tract infection.

REFERENCES

1. Susin M, Becker EL. The pathology of pyelonephritis. In: Kaye D, ed. Urinary Tract Infection and its Management. St. Louis: CV Mosby; 1972:65–83.
2. Freedman L. Chronic pyelonephritis at autopsy. Ann Intern Med. 1967; 66:697–710.
3. Murray T, Goldberg MD: Etiologies of chronic interstitial nephritis. Ann Intern Med. 1975;82:453–9.
4. Freedman LR. Natural history of urinary tract infection in adults. Kidney Int. 1975;8:S96–S100.
5. Monzon OT, Ory EM, Dobson HL, et al: A comparison of bacterial counts of the urine obtained by needle aspiration of the bladder, catheterization and midstream-voided methods. N Engl J Med. 1958;259:764–7.
6. Bran JL, Levison ME, Kaye D: Entrance of bacteria into the female urinary bladder. N Engl J Med. 1972;286:626–9.
7. Buckley RM, McGuckin M, MacGregor RR. Urine bacterial counts following sexual intercourse. N Engl J Med. 1978;298:321–4.
8. Kelsey MC, Mead MG, Gruneberg RN, et al. Relationship between sexual intercourse and urinary tract infection in women attending a clinic for sexually transmitted diseases. J Med Microbiol. 1979;12:511–2.
9. Nicolle LE, Harding GKM, Preiksaitis J, et al: The association of urinary tract infection with sexual intercourse. J Infect Dis. 1982;146:579–83.
10. Foxman B, Frerichs RR. Epidemiology of urinary tract infection: I. Diaphragm use and sexual intercourse. Am J Public Health. 1985;75:1308–13.
11. Leibovici L, Alpert G, Laor A, et al. Urinary tract infections and sexual activity in young women. Arch Intern Med. 1987;147:345–7.
12. Turck M, Goffe B, Petersdorf RG. The urethral catheter and urinary tract infection. J Urol. 1962;88:834–7.
13. Kass EH. Asymptomatic infections of the urinary tract. Trans Assoc Am Physicians. 1956;69:56–64.
14. Gillespie L. The diaphragm: an accomplice in recurrent urinary tract infections. Urology. 1984;24:25–30.
15. Fihn SD, Latham RH, Roberts P, et al. Association between diaphragm use and urinary tract infection. JAMA. 1985;254:240–5.
16. Fihn SD, Johnson C, Pinkstaff C, et al. Diaphragm use and urinary tract infections: analysis of urodynamic and microbiological factors. J Urol. 1986;136:853–6.
17. Johnson ET. The condom catheter: urinary tract infection and other complications. South Med J. 1983;76:579–82.
18. Strom, BL, Collins, M, West SL, et al. Sexual activity, contraceptive use, and other risk factors for symptomatic and asymptomatic bacteremia. Ann Intern Med. 1987;107:816–23.
19. Stamey TA, Timothy M, Millar M, et al. Recurrent urinary infections in adult women. The role of introital enterobacteria. Calif Med. 1971;115:1–19.
20. Vivaldi E, Cotran R, Zangwill DP, et al. Ascending infection as a mechanism in pathogenesis of experimental non-obstructive pyelonephritis. Proc Soc Exp Biol Med. 1959;102:242–4.
21. Cluff LE, Reynolds RC, Page DL, et al. Staphylococcal bacteremia and altered host resistance. Ann Intern Med. 1968;69:859–73.
22. Freedman LR. Experimental pyelonephritis. VI. Observation on susceptibility of the rabbit kidney to infection by a virulent strain of *Staphylococcus aureus*. Yale J Biol Med. 1960;32:272–9.
23. Guze LB, Goldner BH, Kalmanson GM. Pyelonephritis. I. Observations on the course of chronic non-obstructed enterococcal infection in the kidney of the rat. Yale J Biol Med. 1961;33:372–85.
24. Gorrill RH, DeNavasquez SJ. Experimental pyelonephritis in the mouse produced by *Escherichia coli, Pseudomonas aeruginosa* and *Proteus mirabilis*. J Pathol Bacteriol. 1964;87:79–87.
25. Prat V, Hatala M, Venesova D, et al. Pathogenicity of various strains of *Escherichia coli* for the intact rabbit kidney and the effect of repeated passage on renal tissue. In: Kass EH, ed. Progress in Pyelonephritis. Philadelphia: FA Davis; 1965:135.
26. Louria DB, Finkel G. *Candida* pyelonephritis. In: Kass EH, ed. Progress in Pyelonephritis. Philadelphia: FA Davis; 1965:179.
27. Guze LB, Beeson PB. Experimental pyelonephritis. I. Effect of ureteral ligation on the course of bacterial infection in the kidney of the rat. J Exp Med. 1956;104:803–15.
28. Murphy JJ, Schoenberg HW. The lymphatic system of the urinary tract and pyelonephritis. In: Quinn EL, Kass EH, eds. Biology of Pyelonephritis. Boston: Little, Brown; 1960:89–109.
29. Murphy JJ, Schoenberg HW, Rattner WH, et al. The role of the lymphatic system in pyelonephritis. Surg Forum. 1960;10:880–3.
30. Roberts AP, Phillips R. Bacteria causing symptomatic urinary tract infection or bacteriuria. J Clin Pathol. 1979;32:492–6.
31. Svanborg-Eden C, Hagberg L, Hanson LA, et al. Adhesion of Escherichia coli in urinary tract infection. CIBA Found Symp. 1981;80:161–87.
32. Bjorksten B, Kaijser B. Interaction of human serum and neutrophils with *Escherichia coli* strains: differences between strains isolated from urine of patients with pyelonephritis or asymptomatic bacteriuria. Infect Immun. 1978;22:308–11.
33. Johnson JR, Moseley SL, Roberts PL, et al. Aerobactin and other virulence factor genes among strains of *E. coli*. Infect Immun. 1988;56:405–12.
34. Svanborg-Eden C, Gotschlich EC, Korhonen TK, et al. Aspects of structure and function of pili of uropathogenic *E. coli*. Prog Allergy. 1983;33:189–202.
35. Iwahi T, Abe Y, Nakao M, et al. Role of type 1 fimbriae in the pathogenesis of ascending urinary tract infection induced by *Escherichia coli* in mice. Infect Immun. 1983;39:1307–15.
36. Hagberg L, Hull R, Hull S, et al. Contribution of adhesin to bacterial persistence in the mouse urinary tract. Infect Immun. 1983;40:265–72.
37. Hagberg L, Jodal U, Korhonen TK, et al. Adhesion, haemagglutination and virulence of *Escherichia coli* causing urinary tract infections. Infect Immun. 1981;31:564–70.
38. Svanborg-Eden C, Eriksson B, Hanson LA. Adhesion of *Escherichia coli* to human uroepithelial cells in vitro. Infect Immun. 1977;18:767–74.
39. Kallenius G, Mollby R, Svensson SB, et al. Occurence of P-fimbriated *Escherichia coli* in urinary tract infections. Lancet. 1981;ii:1369–72.
40. Leffler, H, Svanborg-Eden C. Glycolipid receptors for uropathogenic *Escherichia coli* binding to human erythrocytes and uroepithelial cells. Infect Immun. 1981;34:920–9.

41. Orskov I, Ferencz A, Orskov F. Tamm-Horsfall protein or uromucoid is the normal urinary slime that traps type 1 fimbriated *Escherichia coli*. Lancet. 1980;i:887.
42. Pere A, Nawicki B, Saxen H, et al. Expression of P_1 type-1, and type 1c fimbriae of *Escherichia coli* in the urine of patients with acute urinary tract infection. J Infect Dis. 1987;156:567–74.
43. Zafriri D, Gron Y, Eisenstein BI, et al. Growth advantages and enhanced toxicity of *Escherichia coli* adherent to tissue culture cells due to restricted diffusion of products secreted by the cells. J Clin Invest. 1987;79:1210–6.
44. Schaeffer AJ, Schwan WR, Hultgren SJ, et al. Relationship of type 1 pilus expression in *Escherichia coli* to ascending urinary tract infections in mice. Infect Immun. 1987;55:373–80.
45. Silverblatt FS. Host-parasite interaction in the rat renal pelvis: a possible role of pili in the pathogenesis of pyelonephritis. J Exp Med. 1974;140: 1696.
46. Svanborg-Eden C, Bjursten LM, Hull R, et al. Influence of adhesins on the interaction of *Escherichia coli* with human phagocytes. Infect Immun. 1984;44:672–80.
47. Fader RC, Davis CP. Effect of piliation on *Klebsiella pneumoniae* infection in rat bladders. Infect Immun. 1980;30:554–61.
48. Mardh PA, Colleen S, Hovelius B. Attachment of bacteria to exfoliated cells from the urogenital tract. Invest Urol. 1979;16:322–6.
49. Svanborg-Eden C, Freter R, Hagberg L, et al. Inhibition of experimental ascending urinary tract infection by an epithelial cell-surface analogue. Nature. 1982;298:560–2.
50. Aronson M, Medalia O, Schori L, et al. Prevention of colonization of the urinary tract of mice with *Escherichia coli* by blocking of bacterial adherence with methyl-α-D-mannopyranoside. J Infect Dis. 1979;139:329–32.
51. Schifferli DM, Abraham SN, EH Beachey. Influence of trimethoprim and sulfamethoxazole on the synthesis, expression and function of type 1 fimbriae of *Escherichia coli*. J Infect Dis. 1986;154:490–6.
52. Johnson JR, Roberts PL, WE Stamm. P fimbriae and other virulence factors in *Escherichia coli* urosepsis: association with patient's characteristics. J Infect Dis. 1987;156:225–9.
53. Fowler JE, Jr, Stamey TA. Studies of introital colonization in women with recurrent infections. VII. The role of bacterial adherence. J Urol. 1977;117:472–6.
54. Kallenius G, Winberg J. Bacterial adherence to periurethral epithelial cells in girls prone to urinary tract infection. Lancet. 1978;2:540–3.
55. Svanborg-Eden C, Jodal U: Attachment of *Escherichia coli* to urinary sediment epithelial cells from urinary tract infection prone and healthy children. Infect Immun. 1979;26:837–40.
56. Jacobson S, Carstensen A, Kallenius G, et al. Fluorescence-activated cell analysis of P-fimbriae receptor accessibility on uroepithelial cells of patients with renal scarring. Eur J Clin Microbiol. 1986;5:649–54.
57. Parsons CL, Schmidt JD. In vitro bacterial adherence to vaginal cells of normal and cystitis prone women. J Urol. 1980;123:184–7.
58. Weyrauch HM, Bassett JB. Ascending infection in an artificial urinary tract. An experimental study. Stanford Med Bull. 1951;9:25–9.
59. Boyarsky S, Labay P. Ureteral motility. Annu Rev Med. 1969;20:383–94.
60. Svanborg-Eden C, Hagberg L, Hull R, et al. Bacterial virulence versus host resistance in the urinary tracts of mice. Infect Immun. 1987;55:1224–32.
61. Musher DM, Griffith DP, Yawn D, et al. Role of urease in pyelonephritis resulting from urinary tract infection with *Proteus*. J Infect Dis. 1975; 131:177–81.
62. Freedman LR, Beeson PB. Experimental pyelonephritis. IV. Observations on infections resulting from direct inoculation of bacteria in different zones of the kidney. Yale J Biol Med. 1958;30:406–14.
63. Beeson PB, Rowley D. The anticomplimentary effect of kidney tissue. Its association with ammonia production. J Exp Med. 1959;110:685–97.
64. Rocha H, Fekety FR. Acute inflammation in the renal cortex and medulla following thermal injury. J Exp Med. 1964;119:131–8.
65. Kaye D. Antibacterial activity of human urine. J Clin Invest. 1968;47:2374–90.
66. Asscher AW, Sussman M, Weiser R. Bacterial growth in human urine. In: O'Grady F, Brumfitt W, eds. Urinary Tract Infection. London: Oxford University Press; 1968:3–13.
67. Stamey TA, Fair WR, Timothy MM, et al. Antibacterial nature of prostatic fluid. Nature. 1968;218:444–7.
68. Bryant RE, Sutcliffe MC, McGee FA. Human polymorphonuclear leukocyte function in urine. Yale J Biol Med. 1973;46:113–24.
69. Cox CE, Hinman F Jr. Experiments with induced bacteriuria, vesical emptying and bacterial growth on the mechanism of bladder defense to infection. J Urol. 1961;86:739–48.
70. Daifuku R, Stamm WE. Bacterial adherence to bladder uroepithelial cells in catheter associated urinary tract infections. N Engl J Med. 1986;314:1208–13.
71. Parsons CL, Greenspan C, Mulholland SG. The primary antibacterial defense mechanism of the bladder. Invest Urol. 1975;13:72–6.
72. Parsons CL, Schrom SH, Hanno P, et al. Bladder surface mucin: examination of possible mechanism for its antibacterial effect. Invest Urol. 1978;6:196–200.
73. Parsons CL, Mulholland SG, Anwar H. Antibacterial activity of bladder surface mucin duplicated by exogenous glycosaminoglycan (Heparin). Infect Immun. 1979;24:552–7.
74. Mulholland SG. Lower urinry tract antibacterial defense mechanisms. Invest Urol. 1979;17:93–7.
75. Cobbs CG, Kaye D. Antibacterial mechanisms in the urinary bladder. Yale J Biol Med. 1967;40:93–108.
76. Stamey TA. The role of introital enterobacteria in recurrent urinary infections. J Urol. 1973;109:467–72.
77. Kunin CM, Polyak F, Postel E. Periurethral bacterial flora in women. Prolonged intermittent colonization with *Escherichia coli*. JAMA. 1980; 243:134–9.
78. Stamey TA, Timothy MM. Studies of introital colonization in women with recurrent urinary infections. I. The role of vaginal pH. J Urol. 1975;114:261–63.
79. Stamey TA, Kaufman MF. Studies of introital colonization in women with recurrent urinary infections. II. A comparison of growth in normal vaginal fluid of common versus uncommon serogroups of *E. coli*. J Urol. 1975;114:264–7.
80. Stamey TA, Timothy MM. Studies of introital colonization in women with recurrent urinary infections. III. Vaginal glycogen concentrations. J Urol. 1975;114:268–70.
81. Stamey TA, Howell JJ. Studies of introital colonization in women with recurrent urinary infections. IV. The role of local vaginal antibodies. J Urol. 1976;115:413–5.
82. Stamey TA, Mihara G. Studies of introital colonization in women with recurrent urinary infections. V. The inhibitory activity of normal vaginal fluid on *Proteus mirabilis* and *Pseudomonas aeruginosa*. J Urol. 1976;115:416–7.
83. Stamey TA, Mihara G. Studies of introital colonization in women with recurrent urinary infections. VI. Analysis of segmented leukocytes on the vaginal vestibule in relation to enterobacterial colonization. J Urol. 1976;116:72–3.
84. Marsh FP, Murray M, Panchamia P. The relationship between bacterial cultures of the vaginal introitus and urinary infection. Br J Urol. 1972;44:368–75.
85. Elkins IB, Cox CE. Vaginal and urethral bacteriology of young women. I. Incidence of gram negative colonization. J Urol. 1974;111:88–92.
86. Cattell WR, McSherry MA, Northeast A, et al. Periurethral enterobacterial carriage in pathogenesis of recurrent urinary infection. Br Med J. 1974;4:136–9.
87. Brumfitt W, Gargan RA, Hamilton-Miller JMT, Periurethral enterobacterial carriage preceding urinary infection. Lancet. 1987;i:824–6.
88. Kurdydyk LM, Kelly K, Harding GKM, et al. Role of cervicovaginal antibody in the pathogenesis of recurrent urinary tract infection in women. Infect Immun. 1980;29:76–82.
89. Hanson LA. Host parasite relationships in urinary tract infections. J Infect Dis. 1973;127:726–30.
90. Miller TE, North JD. Host response in urinary tract infections. Kidney Internat. 1974;5:179.
91. Hanson LA, Ahlstedt S, Fasth A, et al. Antigens of *Escherichia coli*, human immune response, and the pathogenesis of urinary tract infections. J Infect Dis. 1977;136:S144–9.
92. Kaijser B, Larson P, Olling S, et al. Protection against acute pyelonephritis caused by *Escherichia coli* in rats, using isolated capsular antigen conjugated to bovine serum albumin. Infect Immun. 1983;39:142–6.
93. Hanson LA, Fasth A, Jodal U, et al. Biology and pathology of urinary tract infection. J Clin Pathol. 1981;34:695–700.
94. Mattsby-Baltzer I, Claesson I, Hanson LA, et al. Antibodies to lipid A during urinary tract infection. J Infect Dis. 1981;144:319–28.
95. Mattsby-Baltzer I, Hanson LA, Kaijser B, et al. Experimental *Escherichia coli* ascending pyelonephritis in rats: changes in bacterial properties and the immune response to surface antigens. Infect Immun. 1982;35:639–46.
96. Mattsby-Baltzer I, Hanson LA, Olling S, et al. Experimental *Escherichia coli* ascending infection in rats: active peroral immunization with live *Escherichia coli*. Infect Immun. 1982;35:647–53.
97. Svanborg-Eden C, Svennerholm AM. Secretory immunoglobulin A and G antibodies prevent adhesion of *Escherichia coli* to human urinary tract epithelial cells. Infect Immun. 1978;22:790–7.
98. Rene P, Dinolfo M, Silverblatt FJ. Serum and urogenital antibody response to *Escherichia coli* pili in cystitis. Infect Immun. 1982;38:542–7.
99. Rene P, Silverblatt FJ. Serological response to *Escherichia coli* pili in pyelonephritis. Infect Immun. 1982;37:749–52.
100. Fasth A, Ahlstedt S, Hanson LA, et al. Cross reaction between Tamm-Horsfall glycoprotein and *Escherichia coli*. Int Arch Allergy Appl Immunol. 1980;63:303–11.
101. DeRee JM, Van DenBosch JF. Serological response to the P fimbriae of uropathogenic *Escherichia coli* in pyelonephritis. Infect Immun. 1987; 55:2204–7.
102. Hopkins WJ, Uehling DT, Balish E. Local and systemic antibody responses accompany spontaneous resolution of experimental cystitis in cynomolgus monkeys. Infect Immun. 1987;55:1951–6.
103. Bille J, Glauser MP. Protection against chronic pyelonephritis in rats by suppression of acute suppuration. Effect of colchicine and neutropenia. J Infect Dis. 1982;146:220–6.
104. Hanson LA, Fasth A, Jodal U. Autoantibodies to Tamm-Horsfall protein, a tool for diagnosing the level of urinary-tract infection. Lancet. 1976;1:226–8.
105. Aoki S, Imamura S, Aoki M, et al. Abacterial and bacterial pyelonephritis. Immunofluorescent localization of bacterial antigen. N Engl J Med. 1969; 281:1375–82.
106. Schwartz MM, Cotran RS. Common enterobacterial antigen in human

chronic pyelonephritis and interstitial nephritis. N Engl J Med. 1973; 289:830–5.
107. Rocha H. Pathogenesis and clinical manifestations of urinary tract infection. In: Kaye D, ed. Urinary Tract Infection and Its Management. St. Louis: CV Mosby; 1972:6–27.
108. Rocha H, Guze LB, Freedman LR, et al, Experimental pyelonephritis. III. The influence of localized injury in different parts of the kidney on susceptibility to bacillary infection. Yale J Biol Med. 1958;30:341–54.
109. DeNavasquez SJ. Further studies in experimental pyelonephritis produced by various bacteria, with special reference to renal scarring as a factor in pathogenesis. J Pathol Bacteriol. 1956;71:27–32.
110. Cotran TS, Vivaldi E, Zangwill DP, et al. Retrograde pyelonephritis in rats. Am J Pathol. 1963;43:1–31.
111. Rocha H, Santos LCS. Relapse of urinary infection in the presence of urinary tract calculi: the role of bacteria within the calculi. J Med Microbiol. 1969;2:372–6.
112. Smellie JM, Normand ICS. Experience of followup of children with urinary tract infection. In: O'Grady F, Brumfitt W, eds. Urinary Tract Infection. London: Oxford University Press; 1968:123–38.
113. Smellie JM, Normand ICS. Bacteriuria, reflux, and renal scarring. Arch Dis Child. 1975;50:581–5.
114. Gould JC. The comparative bacteriology of acute and chronic urinary tract infection. In: O'Grady F, Brumfitt W, eds. Urinary Tract Infection. London: Oxford University Press; 1968:43–50.
115. Teles E, Rocha H. Epidemiologia de bacteriuria: prevalencia em pacientes hospitalizados e de ambulatorio. In: Rocha H, ed. Temas de Nefrologia. Salvador: Fundacao Goncalo Moniz, 1967:51.
116. Turck M, Stamm WE. Nosocomial infection of the urinary tract. Am J Med. 1981;70:651–4.
117. Kippax PW. A study of proteus infections in a male urological ward. J Clin Pathol. 1957;10:211–214.
118. Finegold SM, Miller LG, Merrill SL, et al. Significance of anaerobic and capnophilic bacteria isolated from the urinary tract. In: Kass EH, ed. Progress in Pyelonephritis. Philadelphia: FA Davis; 1965:159.
119. Mitchell RG. Urinary tract infections caused by salmonellae. Lancet. 1965;1:1092–3.
120. Paed L, Crump J, Maskell R. Staphylococci as urinary pathogens. J Clin Pathol. 1977;30:427–31.
121. Jordan PA, Iravani A, Richard GA, et al. Urinary tract infection caused by *Staphylococcus saprophyticus*. J Infect Dis. 1980;142:510–5.
122. Hovelius B, Mardh P. *Staphylococcus saprophyticus* as a common cause of urinary tract infections. Rev Infect Dis. 1984;6:328–37.
123. Gruneberg RN, Leigh DA, Brumfitt W. *Escherichia coli* serotypes in urinary tract infection: studies in domicillary, antenatal and hospital practice. In: O'Grady F, Brumfitt W, eds. Urinry Tract Infection. London: Oxford University Press; 1968:68–79.
124. Olling S, Hanson LA, Holmgren J, et al. The bactericidal effect of normal human serum on *E. coli* strains from normals and from patients with urinary tract infections. Infection. 1973;1:24–8.
125. Mufson MA, Zollar IM, Mandad VN, et al. Adenovirus infection in acute hemorrhagic cystitis: a study in 25 children. Am J Dis Child. 1971; 121:281–5.
126. Numazaki YN, Kumasaka T, Yana N, et al. Further study on acute hemorrhagic cystitis due to adenovirus 11. N Engl J Med. 1973;289:344–7.
127. Gutman LT, Turck M, Petersdorf RG, et al. Significance of bacterial variants in urine of patients with chronic bacteriuria. J Clin Invest. 1965;44:1945–2.
128. Boineau, FG, Lewy, JE. Urinary tract infection in children: an overview. Pediatr Ann 1975;4:515–26.
129. McCracken GH. Diagnosis and management of acute urinary tract infections in infants and children. Pediatr Infect Dis. 1987;6:107–12.
130. Neumann CG, Pryles CV. Pyelonephritis in infants and children. Autopsy experience at the Boston City Hospital, 1933–1960. Am J Dis Child. 1962;104:215–29.
131. Randolph MF, Greenfield M. The incidence of asymptomatic bacteriuria and pyuria in infancy. J Pediatr. 1964;65:57–66.
132. Huland H, Busch R. Pyelonephritic scarring in 213 patients with upper and lower urinary tract infections: Long-term followup. J Urol. 1984;132: 936–9.
133. Kunin CM. The natural history of recurrent bacteriuria in school girls. N Engl J Med. 1970;282:1443–8.
134. Kunin CM. Urinary tract infections in children. Hosp Pract. 1976;11:91–8.
135. Gillenwater JY, Harrison RB, Kunin CM. Natural history of bacteriuria in schoolgirls. A long-term case-control study. N Engl J Med. 1979;301: 396–9.
136. Freedman LR, et al. The epidemiology of urinary tract infections in Hiroshima. Yale J Biol Med. 1965;37:262–82.
137. Kass EH, Savage W, Santamarina BAG. The significance of bacteriuria in preventive medicine. In: Kass EH, ed. Progress in Pyelonephritis. Philadelphia: FA Davis; 1965:3.
138. Sanford JP: Urinary tract symptoms and infection. Annu Rev Med. 1975;26:485–98.
139. Kaye D. Urinary tract infection in the elderly. Bull NY Acad Med. 1980;56:209–20.
140. Romano JM, Kaye D. UTI in the elderly: common yet atypical. Geriatrics. 1981;36:113–5.
141. Boscia JA, Kobasa WD, Knight RA, et al. Epidemiology of bacteriuria in an elderly ambulatory population. Am J Med. 1986;80:208–214.
142. Boscia JA, Kaye D. Asymptomatic bacteriuria in the elderly. Infect Dis Clin North Am. Dec, 1987:893–905.
143. Kaitz AL, Williams EJ. Bacteriuria and urinary tract infections in hospitalized patients. N Engl J Med. 1960;262:425.
144. Kass EH. The role of asymptomatic bacteriuria in the pathogenesis of pyelonephritis. In: Quinn EL, Kass EH, eds. Biology of Pyelonephritis. Boston: Little, Brown; 1960:399.
145. Turck M, Goffe B, Petersdorf RG. Bacteriuria of pregnancy. N Engl J Med. 1962;266:857.
146. Forland M, Thomas V, Shelokov A. Urinary tract infections in patients with diabetes mellitus: studies on antibody-coating of bacteria. JAMA. 1977; 238:1924.
147. Whalley PJ, Pritchard JA, Richards JR. Sickle cell trait and pregnancy. JAMA. 1963;186:1132.
148. Govan D. Investigation and management of urinary tract infections in children. Urol Clin North Am. 1974;1:397.
149. Margileth AM, Pedreira FA, Hirschman GH, et al. Urinary tract bacterial infections. Symposium on Pediatric Nephrology. Pediatr Clin North Am. 1976;23:71.
150. Gleckman R, Blagg N, Hibert D, et al. Acute pyelonephritis in the elderly. South Med J. 1982;75:551–4.
151. Boscia JA, Kobasa WB, Abrutyn E, et al. Lack of association between bacteriuria and symptoms in the elderly. Am J Med. 1986;81:979–82.
152. Kaye D, Rocha H. Urinary concentrating ability in early experimental pyelonephritis. J Clin Invest. 1970;49:1427–37.
153. Levison SP, Levison ME. The effect of indomethacin and sodium meclofenamate on the renal concentrating defect in experimental enterococcal pyelonephritis in rats. J Lab Clin Med. 1976;88:958–64.
154. Levison SP, Pitsakis PG, Levison ME. Free water reabsorption during saline diuresis in experimental enterococcal pyelonephritis in rats. J Lab Clin Med. 1982;99:474–80.
155. Norden CW, Tuttle EP. Impairment of urinary concentrating ability in pregnant women with asymptomatic bacteriuria. In: Kass EH, ed. Progress in Pyelonephritis. Philadelphia: FA Davis; 1965:73.
156. Hellebusch AA. Renal papillary necrosis. A urological emergency. JAMA. 1969;210:1098–100.
157. Brumfitt W. Urinary cell counts and their value. J Clin Pathol. 1965;18: 550–5.
158. Thysell H. Evaluation of chemical and microscopical methods for mass detection of bacteriuria. Acta Med Scand. 1969;185:393–400.
159. Brumfitt W, Percival A. Pathogenesis and laboratory diagnosis of non-tuberculous urinary tract infection: a review. J Clin Pathol. 1964;17:482–91.
160. Boscia JA, Levison ME, Abrutyn E, et al. Correlation of pyuria and bacteriuria in elderly ambulatory women. Ann Intern Med. 1989;110:404–5.
161. Cobbs CG. Presumptive tests for urinary tract infections. In: Kaye D, ed. Urinary Tract Infection and Its Management. St. Louis: CV Mosby; 172:43–51.
162. James GP, Paul KL, Fuller JB. Urinary nitrite and urinary tract infection. Am J Clin Pathol. 1978;70:671–8.
163. Fritz H, Kohler L, Schersten B. Assessment of subnormal urinary glucose as an indicator of bacteriuria in population studies. Acta Med Scand. 1969;504(Suppl):256.
164. Pezzlo MT. Automated methods for detection of bacteriuria. Am J Med. 1983;75(1B):71–8.
165. Andriole VT. Diagnosis of urinary tract infection by culture. In: Kaye D, ed. Urinary Tract Infection and Its Management. St. Louis: CV Mosby; 1972:28–42.
166. Hoeprich P. Culture of the urine. J Lab Clin Med. 1960;56:899.
167. Kunin CM. New methods of detecting urinary tract infections. Urol Clin North Am. 1975;2:423–32.
168. Hardy JD, Furnell PM, Brumfitt W. Comparison of sterile bag, clean catch, and suprapubic aspiration in the diagnosis of urinary tract infection in early childhood. Br J Urol. 1976;48:279–83.
169. McFadyen IR, Eykyn SS. Suprapubic aspiration of urine in pregnancy. Lancet. 1968;1:1112–4.
170. Stamey TA, Govan DE, Palmer JM. The localization and treatment of urinary tract infections: the role of bactericidal urine levels as opposed to serum levels. Medicine. 1965;44:1–36.
171. Cattel WR, Sardeson JM, Sutcliffe MB, et al. Kinetics of urinary bacterial response to antibacterial agents. In: O'Grady F, Brumfitt W, eds. Urinary Tract Infection. London: Oxford University Press; 1968:212–26.
172. Stamm WE, Counts GW, Running KR, et al. Diagnosis of coliform infection in acutely dysuric women. N Engl J Med. 1982;307:463–8.
173. Goldberg LM, Vosti KL, Rantz LA. Microflora of the urinary tract examined by voided and aspirated urine culture. In: Kass EH, ed. Progress in Pyelonephritis, Philadelphia: FA Davis; 1965:545.
174. Gallager DJ, Montgomerie JZ, North JD. Acute infections of the urinary tract and the urethral syndrome in general practice. Br Med J. 1965;1:622–6.
175. Stamm WE, Wagner KF, Amsel R, et al. Causes of the acute urethral syndrome in women. N Engl J Med. 1980;303:409–15.
176. Stamm WE, Running K, McKuvitt M, et al. Treatment of the acute urethral syndrome. N Engl J Med. 1981;304:956–8.
177. Komaroff AL, Pass TM, McCue JD, et al. Management strategies for urinary and vaginal infections. Arch Intern Med. 1978;138:1069–73.
178. Stamm WE. Management of the acute urethral syndrome. Drug Ther. 1982;12:155–9, 162–3, 166.

179. Brun C, Raschou F, Eriksen KR. Simultaneous bacteriologic studies or renal biopsies and urine. In: Kass EH, ed. Progress in Pyelonephritis. Philadelphia: FA Davis; 1965:461.
180. Turck M, Ronald AR, Petersdorf RG. Relapse and reinfection in chronic bacteriuria. II. The correlation between site of infection and pattern of recurrence in chronic bacteriuria. N Engl J Med. 1968;278:422–7.
181. Fairley KF, Bond AG, Brown RB, et al. Simple test to determine the site of urinary tract infection. Lancet. 1967;2:427–8.
182. Fairley KF, Carson NE, Gutch RC, et al. Site of infection in acute urinary tract infection in general practice. Lancet. 1971;2:615–8.
183. Meares EM, Stamey TA. Bacteriologic localization patterns in bacterial prostatitis and urethritis. Invest Urol. 1968;5:492–518.
184. Clark H, Ronald AR, Cutler RE, et al. The correlation between site of infection and maximal concentrating ability in bacteriuria. J Infect Dis. 1969;120:47–53.
185. Ronald AR, Cutler RE, Turck M. Effect of bacteriuria on renal concentrating mechanisms. Ann Intern Med. 1969;70:723–30.
186. Reeves DS, Brumfitt W. Localization of urinary tract infection. In: O'Grady F, Brumfitt W, eds. Urinary Tract Infection. London: Oxford University Press; 1968:53–67.
187. Turck M. Localization of the site of recurrent urinary tract infection in women. Urol Clin North Am. 1975;2:433–41.
188. Andriole VT. Advances in the treatment of urinary infections. J Antimicrob Chemother. 1982;(Suppl A):163–72.
189. Thomas V, Shelokov A, Forland M. Antibody-coated bacteria in the urine and the site of urinary tract infection. N Engl J Med. 1974;290:588–90.
190. Jones SR, Smith JW, Sanford JP. Localization of urinary tract infections by detection of antibody-coated bacteria in urine sediment. N Engl J Med. 1974;290:591–3.
191. Thomas VL, Forland M. Antibody coated bacteria in urinary tract infections. Kidney Int. 1982;21:1–7.
192. Jones SR. The current status of urinary tract infection localization by the detection of antibody-coated bacteria in the urinary sediment. In: Gilbert DA, Sanford JP, eds. Infectious Diseases. Current Topics. vol. 1. New York: Grune & Stratton; 1979:97.
193. Merritt JL, Keys TF. Limitations of the antibody-coated bacteria test in patients with neurogenic bladders. JAMA. 1982;247:1723–5.
194. Harris RE, Thomas VL, Shelokov A. Asymptomatic bacteriuria in pregnancy: antibody-coated bacteria, renal function and intrauterine growth retardation. Am J Obstet Gynecol. 1975;126:20–5.
195. Thomas VL, Harris RE, Gilstrap LC III, et al. Antibody-coated bacteria in the urine of obstetrical patients with acute pyelonephritis. J Infect Dis. 1975;131(Suppl):557–61.
196. Riedasch G, Ritz E, Dreikorn K, et al. Antibody-coating of urinary bacteria in transplanted patients. Nephron. 1978;20:267–72.
197. Montplaisir S, Cote P, Martineall B, et al. Localization du site de l'infection urinaire chez l'enfant par la recherche des bacteries recouvretes d'anticorps. Can Med Assoc J. 1976;115:1096–9.
198. Hellerstein S, Kennedy E, Nussbaum L, et al. Localization of the site of urinary tract infections by means of antibody-coated bacteria in the urinary sediment. J Pediatr. 1978;92:188–93.
199. Kwasnik I, Klauber G, Tilton RC. Clinical and laboratory evaluation of the antibody-coated bacteria test in children. J Urol. 1979;121:658–61.
200. Smellie J, Edwards D, Hunter N, et al. Vesico-ureteral reflux and renal scarring. Kidney Int. 1975;8:S65–S72.
201. MacGregor ME, Freeman P. Childhood urinary infection associated with vesicoureteric reflux. Q J Med. 1975;44:481–9.
202. Bailey RR. The relationship of vesico-ureteric reflux to urinary tract infection and chronic pyelonephritis-reflux nephropathy. Clin Nephrol 1973; 1:132–41.
203. Cohen M. The first urinary tract infection in male children. Am J Dis Child. 1976;130:810–3.
204. Siegel SR, Sokoloff B, Siegel B. Asymptomatic and symptomatic urinary tract infection in infancy. Am J Dis Child. 1973;125:45–7.
205. Bakshandeh K, Lynne C, Carrion H. Vesicoureteral reflux and end stage renal disease. J Urol. 1976;557–8.
206. Salfatierra O, Tangaho E. Reflux as a cause of end stage kidney disease. Report of 32 cases. J Urol. 1977;117:441–3.
207. Hodson J, Maling TMJ, McManamon PS, et al. Reflux nephropathy. Kidney Int. 1975;8:S50–8.
208. Rolleston GI, Maling TMJ, Hodson CJ. Intrarenal reflux and the scarred kidney. Arch Dis Child. 1974;49:531–9.
209. Edwards D, Normand ICS, Prescod N, et al. Disappearance of vesicoureteric reflux during long-term prophylaxis of urinary tract infection in children. Br Med J. 1977;2:285–8.
210. Blank E. Caliectasis and renal scars in children. J Urol. 1973;110:225–6.
211. Cardiff-Oxford Bacteriuria Study Group. Sequelae of covert bacteriuria in school-girls. A four year follow-up study. Lancet. 1978;1:889–93.
212. Dodge WF, West EF, Travis LB. Bacteriuria in school children. Am J Dis Child. 1974;127:364–70.
213. Kraft JK, Stamey TA. The natural history of symptomatic recurrent bacteriuria in women. Medicine (Baltimore): 1977;56:55–60.
214. Pawlowski JM, Bloxdorf JW, Kimmelstiel P. Chronic pyelonephritis: a morphologic and bacteriologic study. N Engl J Med. 1963;268:965–9.
215. Schechter H, Leonard CD, Scribner BH. Chronic pyelonephritis as a cause of renal failure in dialysis candidates. JAMA. 1971;216:514–7.
216. Freedman LR, Andriole VA. The long term follow-up of women with urinary tract infections. Proc 5th Int Congr Nephrol (Mexico City) 1974;3:230.
217. Bullen M, Kincaid-Smith P. Asymptomatic pregnancy bacteriuria: a follow-up study 4–7 after years delivery. In: Renal Infection and Renal Scarring. Melbourne: Mercedes Publishing; 1970:33.
218. Gower PE, Haswell B, Sidaway ME, et al. Follow-up of 164 patients with bacteriuria of pregnancy. Lancet. 1968;1:990–4.
219. Asscher AW, Chick S, Radford N, et al. Natural history of asymptomatic bacteriuria in non-pregnant women. In: Brumfitt W, Asscher AW, eds. Urinary Tract Infection. London: University Press; 1973:51.
220. Gaches CGC, Miller KW, Roberts BM, et al. The Bristol pyelonephritis registry: 10 years on. Br J Urol. 1976;47:721–5.
221. Zinner S, Kass EH. Long term (10 to 14 years) follow-up of bacteriuria of pregnancy. N Engl J Med. 1971;285:820–4.
222. Gower PE. A long-term study of renal function in patients with radiological pyelonephritis and other allied radiological lesions. In: Brumfit W, Asscher AW, eds. Urinary Tract Infection. London: Oxford University Press; 1973:74.
223. Johnson CW, Smythe CM. Renal function in patients with chronic bacteriuria. South Med J. 1969;62:81–9.
224. Dontas AS, Kasviki-Charvati P, Panayiotis CL, et al. Bacteriuria and survival in old age. N Engl J Med. 1981;304:939–43.
225. Boscia JA, Abrutyn E, Kaye D. Asymptomatic bacteriuria in elderly persons. Treat or do not treat? Ann Intern Med. 1987;106:764–6.
226. Nordenstam GR, Brandberg CA, Oden AS, et al Bacteriuria and mortality in an elderly population. N Engl J Med. 1986;314:1152–6.
227. Levison ME, Kaye D. Management of urinary tract infection. In: Kaye D, ed. Urinary Tract Infections and Its Management. St Louis: CV Mosby; 1972:188–226.
228. Boscia JA, Kaye D. Asymptomatic bacteriuria in the elderly. Infect Dis Clin North Am. 1987;1893–905.
229. Platt R, Polk BF, Murdock B, et al. Reduction of mortality associated with nosocomial urinary tract infection. Lancet. 1983;i:893–7.
230. Platt R. Adverse consequences of asymptomatic urinary tract infections in adults. Am J Med. 1987;82(Suppl 6B):47–52.
231. O'Grady F, Gauci CL, Watson BW, et al. In vitro models simulating conditions of bacterial growth in the urinary tract. In: O'Grady F, Brumfitt W, eds. Urinary Tract Infection. London: Oxford University Press; 1968:80–92.
232. Kass EH, Zangwill DP. Principles in the long-term management of chronic infection of the urinary tract. In: Quinn EL, Kass EH eds. Biology of Pyelonephritis. Boston: Little, Brown; 1960:663–72.
233. Zinner SH, Sabath LD, Casey JI, et al. Erythromycin plus alkalinization in treatment of urinary infections. Antimicrob Agents Chemother. 1969: 413–6.
234. Vainrub B, Musher DM. Lack of effect of methenamine in suppression of, or prophylaxis against, chronic urinary infection. Antimicrob Agents Chemother. 1977;12:625–9.
235. McCabe WR, Jackson GG. Treatment of pyelonephritis: bacterial drug and host factors in success or failure among 252 patients. N Engl J Med. 1965;272:1037–44.
236. Stamey TA, Fair WR, Timothy MM, et al. Serum versus urinary antimicrobial concentrations in case of urinary tract infections. N Engl J Med. 1974;291:1159–63.
237. Minuth JN, Masher DM, Thorsteinsonn, SB. Inhibition of the antibacterial activity of gentamicin by urine. J Infect Dis. 1976;133:14–21.
238. Kunin CM, Finkelberg Z. Oral cephalexin and ampicillin: antimicrobial activity, recovery in urine, and persistence in blood of uremic patients. Ann Intern Med. 1970;72:349–56.
239. Johnson J, Stamm W, Diagnosis and treatment of acute urinary tract infection. In: Andriole V, ed. Infect Dis Clin North Am. 1987;1:773–91.
240. Stamm WE, McKevitt M, Counts GW. Acute renal infection in women: treatment with trimethoprim-sulfamethoxazole or ampicillin for two or six weeks. A randomized trial. Ann Intern Med. 1987;106:341–5.
241. Schwab SJ, Bander SJ, Klahr S. Renal infection in autosomal dominant polycystic kidney disease. Am J Med. 1987;82:714–8.
242. Michaeli J, Mogle D, Perlberg S, et al. Emphysematous pyelonephritis. J Urol. 1984;131:203–8.
243. Fang LST, Tolokoff-Rubin NE, Rubin RH. Efficacy of single-dose and conventional amoxicillin therapy in urinary-tract infection localized by the antibody-coated bacteria technic. N Engl J Med. 1978;298:413–6.
244. Gruneberg RN, Brumfitt W. Single-dose treatment of acute urinary tract infection. a controlled trial. Br Med J. 1967;3:649–51.
245. Slade N, Crowther ST. Multicenter survey of urinary tract infections in general practice. Br J Urol. 1972;44:105–9.
246. Ronald AR, Boutrous P, Mourtada H. Bacteriuria localization and response to single-dose therapy in women. JAMA. 1976;235:1854–6.
247. Rubin RH, Fang LST, Jones SR, et al. Single-dose amoxicillin therapy for urinary tract infection. JAMA. 1980;244:561–4.
248. Bailey RR, Abbott GD. Treatment of urinary tract infection with a single dose of trimethoprim-sulfamethoxazole. Can Med Assoc J. 1978;118: 551–2.
249. Souney P, Polk BF. Single antimicrobial therapy for urinary tract infections in women. Rev Infect Dis. 1982;4:29–34.
250. Pontzer RE, Krieger RE, Boscia JA, et al. Single-dose cefonicid therapy for urinary tract infections. Antimicrob Agents Chemother. 1983;23:814–6.
251. Rosenstock J, Smith LP, Gurney M, et al. Comparison of single-dose tet-

racycline hydrochloride to conventional therapy of urinary tract infection. Antimicrob Agents Chemother. 1985;27:652–4.
252. Harbord RB, Gruneberg RN. Treatment of urinary tract infection with a single dose of amoxycillin, cotrimoxazole or trimethoprim. Br Med J. 1981;283:1301–2.
253. Grossius G. Single dose nitrofurantoin therapy for urinary tract infections in women. Curr Ther Res 1984;35:925–31.
254. Carlson KJ, Mulley AG. Management of acute dysuria. Ann Intern Med. 1985;102:244–9.
255. Greenberg RN, Sanders CV, Lewis AC. Single-dose therapy for urinary tract infection with cefaclor. Am J Med. 1981;71:841–5.
256. Stamm WE. Single-dose treatment of cystitis. JAMA. 1980;244:591–2.
257. Philbrick JT, Bracikowski JP. Single-dose antibiotic treatment for uncomplicated urinary infections. Less for less? Arch Intern Med. 1985;145: 1672–8.
258. Stamey TA. Recurrent urinary tract infections in female patients: an overview of management and treatment. Rev Infect Dis. 1987;9(Suppl 2):S195–S208.
259. Shapiro ED, Wald ER. Single-dose amoxicillin treatment of urinary tract infection. J Pediatr. 1981;99:989–92.
260. Wong ES, McKevitt M, Running K, et al. Management of recurrent urinary tract infections with patient-administered single-dose therapy. Ann Intern Med 1985;102:302–7.
261. Vosti K. Recurrent urinary tract infection: prevention by prophylactic antibiotics after sexual intercourse. JAMA. 1975;231:934–40.
262. Bailey RR, Roberts AP, Gower PL, et al. Prevention of urinary-tract infection with low-dose nitrofurantoin. Lancet. 1971;2:1112.
263. Freeman RB, Smith WM, Richardson JA, et al. Long-term therapy for chronic bacteriuria in men: U.S. Public Health Service Cooperative Study. Ann Intern Med. 1975;83:133–47.
264. Stamey TA, Condy M, Mihara G. Prophylactic efficacy of nitrofurantoin macrocrystals and trimethoprim-sulfamethoxazole in urinary infection. N Engl J Med. 1977;296:780–3.
265. Smellie JM, Gruneberg RN, Leakey A, et al. Long-term low-dose, co-trimoxazole in prophylaxis of childhood urinary tract infection: Clinical aspects. Br Med J. 1976;2:203–6.
266. Stamm WE, Counts GW, Wagner KF, et al. Antimicrobial prophylaxis of recurrent urinary tract infections. Double-blind placebo control trial. Ann Intern Med. 1980;92:770–5.
267. Harding GKM, Buckwold FJ, Marrie TJ, et al. Prophylaxis of recurrent urinary tract infection in female patients. JAMA. 1979;242:1975–7.
268. Light RB, Ronald AR, Harding GKM, et al. Trimethoprim alone in the treatment and prophylaxis of urinary tract infection. Arch Intern Med. 1981;141:1807–10.
269. Grüneberg RN, Smellie JM, Leaky A, et al. Long-term low-dose, co-trimoxazole in prophylaxis of childhood urinary tract infection: Bacteriologic aspects. Br Med. J. 1976;2:206–8.
270. Brumfitt W, Smith GW, Hamilton-Miller JMT, et al. A clinical comparison between macrodantin and trimethoprim for prophylaxis in women with recurrent urinary infections. J Antimicrob Chemother. 1985;16:111–20.
271. Patterson TF, Andriole VT. Bacteriuria in pregnancy. Infect Dis Clin North Am. 1987;1:807–22.
272. Popky GL, Pollack HW. Radiologic evaluation of patients with urinary tract infection. In: Kaye D, ed. Urinary Tract Infection and Its Management. St. Louis: CV Mosby, 1972:84–123.
273. Guyer PB, Delaney D. Urinary tract dilatation and oral contraceptives. Br Med J. 1970;4:588–90.
274. Andriole VT, Cohen GL. The effect of diethylstilbestrol on the susceptibility of rats to hematogenous pyelonephritis. J Clin Invest 1973;43:1136–45.
275. Norden CW, Kass EH. Bacteriuria of pregnancy: a critical appraisal. Annu Rev Med. 1968;19:431–70.
276. Norden CW. Significance and management of bacteriuria of pregnancy. In: Kaye D, ed. Urinary Tract Infection and Its Management. St. Louis: CV Mosby; 1972:171–87.
277. Pedler SJ, Bint AJ. Management of bacteriuria in pregnancy. Practical Therapeutics. 1987;33:413–21.
278. Kass E. Bacteriuria and pyelonephritis of pregnancy. Trans Assoc Am Physicians. 1959;72:257–64.
279. Kincaid-Smith P, Bullen M. Bacteriuria in pregnancy. Lancet. 1965;1: 395–9.
280. Krieger JN. Complications and treatment of urinary tract infections during pregnancy. Urol Clin North Am. 1986;13:685–93.
281. Condie AP, Williams JD, Reeves DS, et al. Complications of bacteriuria in pregnancy. In: O'Grady F, Brumfitt W, eds. Urinary Tract Infection. London: Oxford University Press; 1968:148–59.
282. Gruneberg R, Leigh D, Brumfitt W. Relation of bacteriuria to acute pyelonephritis, prematurity and fetal mortality. Lancet. 1969;2:1–3.
283. Leigh D, Gruneberg R, Brumfitt W. Long term followup of bacteriuria in pregnancy. Lancet. 1968;1:603–5.
284. Williams JD, Reeves DS, Condie AD, et al. The treatment of bacteriuria in pregnancy. In: O'Grady F, Brumfitt W, eds. Urinary Tract Infection. London: Oxford University Press; 1968:160–9.
285. Meares EM. Prostatitis: a review. Urol Clin North Am. 1975;2:3–27.
286. Kirby RS, Lowe D, Bultitude MI, et al. Intraprostatic urinary reflux: an aetiological factor in abacterial prostatitis. Br J Urol. 1982;54:729–31.
287. Stamey TA. Urinary infections in males. In: Pathogenesis and Treatment of Urinary Tract Infections. Baltimore: Williams & Wilkins; 1980:342–429.
288. Fair WR, Couch J, Wehner N. The purification and assay of the prostatic antibacterial factor (PAF). Biochem Med. 1973;8:329–39.
289. Shortliffe LM, Wehner N. The characterization of bacterial and nonbacterial prostatitis by prostatic immunoglobulins. Medicine. 1986;65:399–414.
290. Drach GW. Prostatitis: man's hidden infection. Urol Clin North Am. 1975;2:499–520.
291. Meares EM Jr. Acute and chronic prostatitis. Infect Dis Clin North Am. 1987;1:855–73.
292. Kohnen PW, Drach GW. Patterns of inflammation in prostatic hyperplasia: a histologic and bacteriologic study. J Urol. 1979;121:755–60.
293. Weidner W, Brunner H, Krause W. Quantitative culture of *Ureaplasma urealyticum* in patients with chronic prostatitis or prostatosis. J Urol. 1980;124:62–7.
294. Segura JW, Opitz J, Green LF. Prostatosis, prostatitis, or pelvic floor tension myalgia? J Urol. 1979;122:168–9.
295. Winningham DF, Nemoy NJ, Stamey TA. Diffusion of antibiotics from plasma into prostatic fluid. Nature 1968;219:139–43.
296. Stamey TA, Bushby SRM, Bragonse J. The concentration of trimethoprim in prostatic fluid: nonionic diffusion or active transport. J Infect Dis. [Suppl] 1973;128:S686–90.
297. Meares EM Jr. Editorial: Prostatic abscess. J Urol. 1986;136:1281–2.
298. Meares EM. Long-term therapy of chronic bacterial prostatitis with trimethoprim-sulfamethoxazole. Can Med Assoc J. 1975:112(spec. no):22–25.
299. Mobley DF. Bacterial prostatitis: treatment with carbenicillin indanyl sodium. Invest Urol. 1981;19:31–3.
300. Giamarellou H, Kosmidis J, Leonidas M, et al. A study of the effectiveness of rifaprim in chronic prostatitis caused mainly by *Staphylococcus aureus*. J Urol. 1982;128:321–4.
301. Weidner W, Schiefer HG, Dalhoff A. Treatment of chronic bacterial prostatitis with ciprofloxacin: results of one year follow-up studies. Am J Med. 1987;82(4):280–3.
302. Thorley JD, Jones SR, Sanford JP. Perinephric abscess. Medicine (Baltimore). 1974;53:441–51.
303. Gerzof SG, Gale ME. Computed tomography and ultrasonography for diagnosis and treatment of renal and retroperitoneal abscesses. Urol Clin North Am. 1982;9:185–93.
304. Rauschkolb EN, Sandler CM, Patel S, et al. Computed tomography of renal inflammatory diseases. J Comp Assist Tomogr. 1982;6:502–6.
305. Bova JG, Potter JL, et al. Renal and perirenal infection. The role of computerized tomography. J Urol. 1985;133:375–8.
306. Costello AJ, Blandy JP, Hately W. Percutaneous aspiration of renal cortical abscess. Urology. 1983;21:201–4.
307. Finn DJ, Palestrant AM, DeWolf WC. Successful percutaneous management of renal abscess. J Urol 1982;127:425–6.
308. Filly R. Ultrasonography. In Friedland GW, Filly R, Goris ML, et al, eds. Uroradiology: An Integrated Approach. New York: Churchill Livingstone; 1983:311.
309. Piccirello M, Rigsby C, Rosenfield AT. Contemporary imaging of renal inflammatory disease. Infect Dis Clin North Am. 1987;1:927–64.
310. Grainger RG, Longstaff AJ. Xanthogranulomatous pyelonephritis: a reappraisal. Lancet. 1982;1:1398–401.
311. Hellerstein S, Wald ER, Winberg J, et al. Consensus: roentgenographic evaluation of children with urinary tract infections. Pediatr Infect Dis. 1984;3:291–3.
312. Honkinen O, Ruuskanen O, Rikalairen H, et al. Ultrasonography as a screening procedure in children with urinary tract infection. Pediatr Infect Dis. 1986;5:633–5.
313. Leonidas JC, McCauley RG, Klauber G, et al. Sonography as substitute for excretory urography in children with urinary tract infection. Am J Roentgenol. 1985;144:815–9.
314. Mason WG Jr. Urinary tract infections in children: renal ultrasound evaluation. Radiology. 1984;153:109–11.
315. Kangarloo H, Gold RH, Fine RN, et al. Urinary tract infection in infants and children evaluated by ultrasound. Radiology. 1985;154:367–73.
316. Fairley KF. The investigation and treatment of urinary tract infection. Med J Aust. 1976;2:305–7.
317. Andriole VT. Care of the indwelling catheter. In: Kaye D, ed. Urinary Tract Infection and Its Management. St. Louis: CV Mosby; 1972:256–66.
318. Gillespie WA, Linton KB, Miller A, et al. The diagnosis, epidemiology and control of urinary infection in urology and gynecology. J Clin Pathol. 1960;13:187–94.
319. Warren JW. Catheter-associated urinary tract infections. Infect Dis Clin North Am. 1987;1:823–54.
320. Garibaldi RA, Burke JP, Britt MR, et al. Meatal colonization and catheter associated bacteriuria. N Engl J Med. 1980;303:316–8.
321. Martin CM, Bookrajian EN. Bacteriuria prevention after indwelling urinary catheterization: a controlled study. Arch Intern Med. 1962;110:703–11.
322. Martin CM, Vaquer F, Meyers MS, et al. Prevention of gram-negative rod bacteremia associated with indwelling urinary tract catheterization. In: Sylvester JC, ed. Antimicrobial Agents and Chemotherapy—1963. Washington, DC: American Society for Microbiology; 1964:617–23.
323. Miller A, Linton KB, Gillespie WA, et al: Catheter drainage and infection in acute retention of urine. Lancet. 1960;1:310–2.

324. Brumfitt W, Davies BL, Rosser E. The urethral catheter as a cause of urinary tract infection in pregnancy and puerperium. Lancet. 1961;2:1059–62.
325. Sanford JP. Hospital-acquired urinary tract infections. Ann Intern Med. 1964;60:903–14.
326. Andriole VT. Hospital acquired urinary tract infections and the indwelling catheter. Urol Clin North Am. 1975;2:451–69.
327. Garibaldi RA, Burke JP, Dickman ML, et al. Factors predisposing to bacteriuria during indwelling urethral catheterization. N Engl J Med. 1974; 291:215–19.
328. Butler HK, Kunin CM. Evaluation of polymyxin catheter lubricant and impregnated catheters. J Urol. 1968;100:560–6.
329. Gladstone JL, Robinson CG. Prevention of bacteriuria resulting from indwelling catheters. J Urol. 1968;99:458–61.
330. Warren JH, Platt R, Thomas RJ, et al. Antibiotic irrigation and catheter-associated urinary tract infection. N Engl J Med. 1978;299:570–73.
331. Platt R, Polk BF, Murdock B, et al. Risk factors for nosocomial urinary tract infection. Am J Epidemiol. 1986;124:977–85.
332. Desautels RE, Chibaro EA, Lang RJ. Maintenance of sterility in urinary drainage bags. SGO. 1982;154:838–40.
333. Stamm WE. Guidelines for prevention of catheter-associated urinary tract infections. Ann Intern Med. 1975;82:386–90.
334. Fincke BG, Friedland G. Prevention and management of infection in the catheterized patient. Urol Clin North Am. 1976;3:313–21.
335. Butler HK, Kunin CM. Evaluation of specific antimicrobial therapy in patients while on closed catheter drainage. J Urol. 1968;100:567–72.
336. Andersen JT, Heisterberg L, Hebjorn S, et al. Suprapubic versus transurethral bladder drainage after colposuspension/vaginal repair. Acta Obstet Gynecol Scand. 1985;64:139–143.
337. Van Den Broek PJ, Dahha TJ, et al. Bladder irrigation with povidone-iodine in prevention of urinary tract infections associated with intermittent urethral catheterization. Lancet. 1985;1:563–5.
338. Thornton GF, Lytton B, Andriole VT. Bacteriuria during indwelling catheter drainage. JAMA. 1966;195:179–183.
339. Dudley MN, Barriere SL. Antimicrobial irrigations in the prevention and treatment of catheter-related urinary tract infections. Am J Hosp Pharm. 1981;38:59–65.
340. Kaye D. Urinary Tract Infection and Its Management. St. Louis: CV Mosby; 1972.

SECTION E

59. GRAM-NEGATIVE SEPSIS

LOWELL S. YOUNG

Bacteremic infections caused by gram-negative bacilli remain one of the major if not the principal infectious disease problem encountered in modern medical centers. These blood stream infections usually represent the most serious extension of a process that initially involves local sites such as the integument, urinary tract, respiratory tract, and mucous membranes of the gastrointestinal tract. While bacteremia can be transient, self-limited, and therefore of little clinical significance (as sometimes occurs spontaneously or with instrumentation of some organs), severe gram-negative rod bacteremia constitutes a medical emergency. It calls for an organized diagnostic approach and aggressive implementation of a therapeutic program directed at terminating blood stream invasion by the infecting microbe and, equally important, correction of the pathophysiologic sequelae to that event.

Gram-negative bacilli are a major component of humans' abundant native microbial flora. Thus it may seem paradoxical that these organisms have assumed such a major role in the modern practice of infectious diseases. There are a number of explanations for this apparent paradox, but one factor seems mainly responsible, namely, microbial opportunism in the face of significant depression of host defenses. This disturbance of the host–parasite relationship assumes many forms, and it would be naive to regard all the major categories of gram-negative bacilli as the cause of only one type of clinical syndrome. Indeed, there are quite clear-cut clinical differences between the fulminating bacteremic infections caused by the plague bacillus or by *Pseudomonas aeruginosa* and the more indolent blood stream infections caused by some *Salmonella* and *Haemophilus* species. The diseases caused by certain important gram-negative organisms are dealt with in individual sections of this book. This chapter will focus on the syndrome of gram-negative rod bacteremia.

HISTORICAL PERSPECTIVE

Diseases such as plague and typhoid fever are caused by well-known organisms, *Yersinia pestis* and *Salmonella typhi*, that are properly classified as gram-negative bacilli. Many of the signs and symptoms of the overwhelming gram-negative rod infections that are seen as nosocomial complications bear similarities to the catastrophic illnesses that have been identified with plague and typhoid that usually affect normal hosts. While the latter are classic examples of gram-negative rod bacteremia, it seems appropriate from an epidemiologic and clinical view to distinguish them from the syndrome of systemic gram-negative bacteremia that appears as a common nosocomial complication of current therapy for medical, surgical, and pediatric disorders.

Clinical descriptions of a "shock" syndrome after infections can be inferred from the work of physicians such as Laennec,[1] but the description of gram-negative rod bacteremia in the form that we appreciate it today is probably most correctly ascribed to work just before the beginning of the present century.[2] In fact, fewer than 100 cases appear to have been reported in the medical literature before 1920.[3] The current upsurge in the problem of gram-negative rod bacteremia is a development that has followed the introduction of antimicrobial agents. Waisbren, in 1951, can be properly credited with the first major report of cases of superinfection caused by gram-negative bacilli after the use of penicillins and tetracyclines to treat gram-positive infection.[4] Since that report many important clinical studies[5–7] have documented the role of gram-negative rods as a cause of bacteremic infection in patients often afflicted with a serious underlying disease. The increase in all types of nosocomial gram-negative bacillary infections that coincides with the introduction of a large number of antibacterial agents need not indicate a causal relationship inasmuch as the availability of new antimicrobial agents can be interpreted as paralleling other advances in medical and surgical practice. Among these developments has been the tendency to use increasingly more immunosuppressive therapy for various disorders and more aggressive surgical intervention. Viewed in this light, gram-negative rod infections can be properly regarded as diseases of medical progress.

INCIDENCE AND EPIDEMIOLOGIC TRENDS

The magnitude of the problem and its economic cost have been difficult to assess. Part of the problem in the United States seems related to the fact that gram-negative rod bacteremia is not an officially reportable disease. The bulk of available data derive from relatively few hospitals that have kept records on infections long enough to discern meaningful trends. The experience of one institution, that of Boston City Hospital, has been unique in that epidemiologic data have been collated by one technique and by one group of observers for a period of almost 40 years, from 1935 to 1972.[8] Bacterimas due to *Escherichia coli* and *Salmonella* species were the only ones that were seen with any frequency before the widespread use of sulfonamides. Between 1957 and 1972 the incidence of *E. coli* bacteremia per 1000 admissions rose fivefold at the Boston City Hospital. Community-acquired cases of *E. coli* bacteremia were usually more common than was hospital-acquired disease, but the case-fatality ratios were higher for the latter group. In 1972 *Klebsiella-Enterobacter* species were the second most common cause of bacteremic gram-negative bacillary infections (after *E. coli*), almost 4 cases/1000 admissions, a higher incidence actually than for *E. coli*. Remarkably, there were no cases of *Klebsiella-Enterobacter* bacteremia (excluding bacteremic Friedländer's pneumonia) identified at this hospital in 1935 and 1941.

Because it is often a complication and the final lethal event in the course of an underlying disease, identification of bacteremia per se may be omitted from an attributable cause of death in a patient with extensive burns or with an advanced hematologic malignancy. Statistical data derived from death certificates probably underestimate the magnitude of the problem, and incidence data from surveys of community or university hospitals, while filling an important gap in present knowledge, have provided little information on the disease-specific incidence of this complication, that is, the frequency in time of gram-negative rod bacteremia associated with underlying disorders such as collagen-vascular disease or lymphoma. It has been shown, for instance, in one cancer treatment center that *P. aeruginosa* represented two-thirds of all gram-negative rod bacteremias and 84 percent of all fatal gram-negative rod bacteremias in patients with acute myelocytic leukemia.[9] *Pseudomonas aeruginosa* has also been shown to be the most lethal bacteremic infection complicating renal, hepatic, cardiac, and bone marrow transplantation.[10–13] There are only limited data, however, on the disease-specific incidence for other gram-negative pathogens.

By extrapolating data obtained at one university hospital, McCabe estimated that as many as 300,000–500,000 cases of systemic gram-negative rod infections had recently occurred each year in the United States and that perhaps one-third to one-half of these cases were fatal.[14] A special task force appointed by the Director of the National Institute of Allergy and Infectious Disease in collaboration with the Centers for Disease Control reviewed much of the reported data on the incidence and mortality from gram-negative rod bacteremia and concluded that the correct figure for incidence in the United States was probably between 100,000 and 300,000 cases per year.[15] Many series have reported that mortality has ranged anywhere from 20 to 50 percent, with a clear-cut increase for those with the most adverse host factors such as neutropenia and immunosuppression (Table 1). However, in recent series this mortality appears to be decreasing.

A major goal of the Centers for Disease Control has been to obtain basic epidemiologic data on the magnitude of this problem and has led to the creation of the National Nosocomial Infections Surveillance.[27,28] The analysis of this information is divided into categories of "primary" and "secondary" bacteremia, the former being those cases in which no source could be identified and the latter being those infections in which the source of infection was secondary to an identifiable source. The 1976 survey[27] indicated that between 49 and 56 percent of all bacteremias were caused by Enterobacteriaceae and *P. aeruginosa*. When fungemias and miscellaneous blood-borne pathogens were deleted from the total, gram-negative rod bacteremia outnumbered all other causes of bacteremic infection. The 1984 survey[28] reflected the overall importance of gram-negative bacilli in nosocomial infections but also underscored the resurgence of gram-positive organisms as causes of bacteremia. Still, the mortality from gram-positive bacteremia has tended to be lower than from gram-negative bacteremia and case fatality ratios for *P. aeruginosa* bacteremia remain high.[29]

RELATIVE FREQUENCY OF GRAM-NEGATIVE BACTERIAL PATHOGENS AND ASSOCIATED MORTALITY

Table 1 summarizes the relative incidence of various aerobic gram-negative pathogens in a number of large series of bacteremic infections that have been reported since 1965.[16–26] This type of information seems valuable only in discerning the broadest trends and associations inasmuch as differences in mortality are likely related to the types of patients cared for at each in-

TABLE 1. Distribution of Gram-Negative Bacteremic Isolates Excluding Polymicrobial Infections

Author	*Period of Observation*	*E. coli*	*Klebsiella*	*Enterobacter*	*Serratia*	*P. aeruginosa*	*Proteus Species*	*Total Episodes/ Mortality*
EORTC[16]	1983–1986	63	9			34		129 (12)
Klastersky[17]	1981–1983	38	8			23		83 (17)
Weinstein[18]	1975–1977	76 (35)[a]	25 (48)			22 (72)		123 (39.8)
Spengler[19]	1968–1974	127 (38.6)	233 (31.8)	67 (35.8)	37 (32.4)	74 (68.9)[b]	30 (36.7)	568 (38.9)
Kreger[20]	1965–1974	189 (19.5)	74 (21.3)	47 (17.0)	11 (18.0)	60 (36.6)	49 (16.3)	430 (22.1)
Singer[21]	1972–1973	86 (17.4)	37 (43.2)		4 (0)	30 (60)	14 (35.7)	171 (31.6)
McHenry[22]	1967–1972	68 (26.4)	72 (26.9)	35 (14.3)	8 (25)	29 (48.3)	11 (27.3)	233 (27.3)
Myerowitz[23]	1968–1969	58 (18)	23 (13)	9 (0)	27 (54)	21 (57)[b]	13 (16)	151 (27.8)
Bryant[24]	1965–1968	83 (21)	57 (33)[b]			45 (71)	19 (16)	204 (34.8)
Dupont[25]	1958–1966	190 (42)	138 (55)[b]			67 (67)[b]	63 (33)	458 (50.7)
Altemeier[26]	1955–1967	93 (48)	68 (66)[b]			39 (77)	42 (67)	242 (61.2)
Usual rank order for frequency		1	2	5[c]	4[c]	3	6[c]	
Usual rank order for mortality		4[c]	2	6[c]	5[c]	1	3[c]	

[a] Values are numbers of isolates; mortality is in parentheses.
[b] Species grouped together.
[c] No significant difference in rank order.

stitution and the time each study was carried out. It has usually been observed that *E. coli* is the most common pathogen and that *K. pneumoniae* is the second most frequent. Some centers have not until recently differentiated among *Klebsiella, Enterobacter*, and *Serratia* species. *Pseudomonas* species are usually the third most common and are often grouped together. When speciated, most of these strains are identified as *aeruginosa*. The relative frequency of *Enterobacter, Serratia*, and *Proteus* bacteremias is probably not significantly different. It is noteworthy that *P. aeruginosa* has been consistently associated with the highest mortality of all bacteremic infections. In all likelihood this is a manifestation of the association of *P. aeruginosa* with neutropenia and clinical conditions like leukemia and extensive burns that have the more adverse clinical prognosis. Systemic *K. pneumoniae* infections appear to be associated with the next highest mortality after *P. aeruginosa*. When the outcome of gram-negative bacteremia is assessed in terms of the nature of underlying disease (such as in leukemia and burns), the mortality associated with specific pathogens (*P. aeruginosa, Klebsiella* species, and so on) appears more similar.

EPIDEMIOLOGY AND GRAM-NEGATIVE BACTEREMIC INFECTIONS

The gastrointestinal tract is the obvious reservoir of gram-negative bacilli, although many other sources of infection exist. Quantitative studies of healthy subjects have indicated that the endogenous fecal flora is predominantly anaerobic and that *E. coli* accounts for the largest proportion of aerobic gram-negative bacilli. Not surprisingly, *E. coli* is often the most common aerobic organism isolated from blood cultures. Additionally, *Bacteroides fragilis* is one of the most common anaerobic constituents of the fecal flora and by analogy is also commonly implicated in anaerobic gram-negative rod bacteremia. Most *E. coli* isolated from healthy people tend to be susceptible to most commonly used antimicrobial agents. Numerous studies, however, have indicated that organisms isolated from the fecal flora of hospitalized patients and those previously receiving antimicrobial therapy tend to have a larger proportion of organisms that are resistant to one or more antimicrobial agents.[30]

The finding that *E. coli* is the most frequently encountered organism in gram-negative rod septicemia seems related to its role in intra-abdominal trauma, postabdominal surgical infections, and pyelonephritis. It is widely accepted that initial fecal contamination of the lower urinary tract is the usual primary event in the pathogenesis of acute pyelonephritis. Thus, it would be expected that *E. coli* is the predominant organism in bacteremic genitourinary infections. Interestingly, *Bacteroides* species are rarely implicated in ascending pyelonephritis, and there must be a significant factor between the ability of aerobes and anaerobes to cause bacteremic infection via the urinary tract.

The dynamic interaction between the native, endogenous fecal flora and sources of gram-negative rods acquired from environmental sources have been the subject of several interesting studies. For instance, with *P. aeruginosa* it is now quite clear from selective microbial sampling surveys of many healthy subjects including medical students and nonhospitalized personnel that the prevalence of fecal carriage, defined as any isolation of *P. aeruginosa* from the stool, is less than 10 percent.[31,32] Fecal carriage increased fivefold with increasing debility or treatment of underlying diseases to neutropenia. Additionally, antimicrobial therapy with broad-spectrum agents predisposes to colonization by *P. aeruginosa*.[33] Careful prospective epidemiologic studies indicate that specific serotypes isolated from stool correlate very well with serotypes of *P. aeruginosa* that are subsequently cultured from blood.[34] Although it is usually possible to define the source of a gram-negative bacteremia, a certain number of intensely immunosuppressed patients may develop bacteremia without an obvious source. It has been postulated that the latter situation represents bacteremia originating from small ulcerations of the gastrointestinal tract. This is supported by some autopsy data and the epidemiologic data indicating a correlation between strains isolated from the blood and the organisms colonizing stool.[35]

It seems plausible that the normal host possesses mechanisms for resisting colonization by these potential pathogens or that the normal flora has an inhibiting effect on some potential pathogens (bacterial interference). Both normal and debilitated subjects are continuously exposed to *P. aeruginosa* from many environmental sources including food and water. Given the setting of the altered host, resistance to colonization by an as yet undefined factor (but perhaps relating to bacterial interference) is lost. Bacteremia ensues after the onset of neutropenia, disruption of mechanical barriers to microbial invasion, development of anatomic obstruction, or a combination of these factors. The evidence for a role of the normal flora in resistance to colonization lies in studies where normal volunteers fed large quantities of *P. aeruginosa* could not be colonized except when oral ampicillin was given concomitantly.[33]

Information on the epidemiology of *P. aeruginosa* infections is relatively more available because this organism can be easily differentiated from *E. coli* in environmental or fecal sampling surveys. Assessment of the epidemiology of *E. coli* bacteremia is more difficult because these organisms are components of the normal fecal flora. Some serotypes of *E. coli* seem more commonly involved in upper urinary tract infections which suggests that there may be some virulence factors that affect bacteremic urinary tract infection.[36] On the other hand, *Klebsiella, Serratia*, and *Proteus* are probably not part of the normal fecal flora of humans, and the same factors promoting *P. aeruginosa* colonization of stool may result in gastrointestinal acquisition. In one study there was a strong correlation between the serotype of *K. pneumoniae* isolated from stool and what appeared in a variety of infected sites including the blood stream.[37] For *Proteus* and *Serratia* infections, less information is available. There are data showing that irrespective of medical therapy the oropharynx of patients with serious underlying diseases becomes readily colonized by gram-negative rods; this parallels the deterioration in overall host status.[38] Thus the oropharynx is another site for colonization by gram-negative rods that precedes other organ involvement or systemic infection. It has been observed that organisms colonization the oropharynx correlate with some bacteremic isolates even when stool cultures are negative for the same organism.[39] This has occurred when some chemotherapeutic agents have caused ulceration of the upper gastrointestinal tract. The gastric mechanisms for elimination or reduction of organisms entering the small and large intestines may be a factor limiting colonization of the lower gastrointestinal tract in these patients.

Besides the gastrointestinal route there are clearly other pathways to invasion of the host. One of the most obvious mechanisms involves acquisition via exposure to contaminated inhalation therapy equipment and by gram-negative rods like *S. marcescens* and *P. aeruginosa*. This can lead to bacteremic gram-negative pneumonia, which has a mortality among the highest observed in gram-negative infections. A wide variety of other sources for gram-negative rods' invasion are possible including indwelling vascular catheters, monitoring devices, urinary tract catheters, drainage tubes, percutaneous reservoirs, contaminated intravenous fluids, and so forth. Instruments used for diagnostic procedures may be contaminated and may introduce infection into a relatively sterile area or may disrupt mucosal barriers in an area with its own microbial flora (like the lower gastrointestinal tract). Decubitus ulcers can be readily colonized by gram-negative rods and can be a source of bacteremic infection.

The plethora of gram-negative bacilli and the wide variety of serogrouping or serotyping systems that are available for organisms such as *E. coli* (more than 160 O types), *K. pneumoniae* (over 80 serotypes), and even *S. marcescens* (almost 20 serotypes) reflects the formidable task involved in defining the epidemiology of certain infections. Within the *E. coli* and *K. pneumoniae* strains there may be certain types that predispose to serious systemic infection. Extensive studies of *K. pneumoniae* infections have indicated that a relatively large proportion of infections are caused by a certain limited number of serotypes.[40] This suggests that certain organisms have selective advantages in some epidemiologic settings.

It is also apparent that antimicrobial usage has a very definite relationship to epidemiologic patterns of gram-negative infections. In immunologically impaired subjects, the bacteremias encountered early in the clinical course tend to be due to *Staphylococcus aureus* or *E. coli*, possibly because of the predominance of these organisms in the native flora. Repeated courses of antimicrobial therapy, such as in the patient receiving antineoplastic therapy, tend to select out for systemic infection due to more antibiotic-resistant bacilli such as *P. aeruginosa*, *Proteus* species, and *Serratia* species. Thus the association of certain organisms with high mortality may reflect the effect of antimicrobial selection rather than intrinsic virulence.

The role of human carriers in the spread of gram-negative rod infections has been described in some situations such as some clusters of *Proteus* infections[41] or *Salmonella* infections. However, the bulk of current information suggests that a carrier situation similar to what has been observed with staphylococci is probably not relevant to the vast majority of gram-negative infections that occur in the hospital setting.

THE CLINICAL SYNDROME: SIGNS AND SYMPTOMS OF GRAM-NEGATIVE ROD BACTEREMIA

There are no specific clinical findings in gram-negative rod bacteremia that distinguish it from systemic infection caused by gram-positive cocci (and for that matter some viral hemorrhagic fevers). Table 2 summarizes some of the clinical findings that suggest the diagnosis and should prompt a careful culture of blood, cultures of likely sources of infection, and possible initiation of therapy. The distinction between primary manifestations and complications is arbitrary; indeed, such complications as hypotension, bleeding, hypoxia, acidosis, and jaundice may be the major clues that first suggest the diagnosis. Although fever and chills are typically encountered, many patients who develop bacteremic infection are debilitated and may not exhibit striking changes in symptomatology early during the course of infection. Paradoxically, hypothermia rather than hyperthermia occasionally can be a manifestation of gram-negative rod infection and is associated with poor prognosis. While neutropenia definitely predisposes to gram-negative bacillary infection, a precipitous decline in the neutrophil count from a normal or an already depressed level is also commonly seen. The clinician should be alert to the possibility that hypotension, a fall in urine output, a decrease in circulating platelet levels, and evidence for bleeding even in the absence of fever and chills could be manifestations of bacteremia.

TABLE 2. Signs and Symptoms Suggesting Gram-Negative Rod Bacteremia

Primary	*Complications*
Fever	Hypotension
Chills	Bleeding
Hyperventilation	Leukopenia
Hypothermia	Thrombocytopenia
Skin lesions	Organ failure
Change in mental status	Lung: cyanosis, acidosis
	Kidney: oliguria, anuria, acidosis
	Liver: jaundice
	Heart: congestive failure

Even before temperature elevation or the onset of chills, bacteremic patients will often begin to hyperventilate. Continuous monitoring of patients in intensive care units has indicated that the earliest clinical finding is apprehension and hyperventilation; thus the earliest metabolic change in septicemia and particularly gram-negative rod infections is a resultant respiratory alkalosis. In the critically ill patient the sudden onset of hyperventilation should lead to drawing blood for culture and to carefully evaluating the patient for the possibility of infection. Change in mental status can be an important clinical clue: while the most common pattern is lethargy or obtundation, an occasional patient may become excited, agitated, or combative or may display bizarre behavior.

Cutaneous manifestations of gram-negative rod bacteremia, usually colorful skin lesions, were described as early as the previous century.[42] Skin lesions have been most commonly associated with *P. aeruginosa* bacteremia. The so-called pathognomonic skin lesion of *P. aeruginosa* bacteremia was described and given the name *ecthyma gangrenosum*.[43] Ecthyma gangrenosum lesions are round or oval, vary from 1 to 5 cm, and have a raised halo or rim of erythema and induration that surround a central are that may begin as vesicle but usually evolves into a necrotic ulcer (Fig. 1). The appearance of these "bull's-eye"–type lesions strongly suggests *P. aeruginosa* infection and has been observed in 5–25 percent of all *Pseudomonas* bacteremias. In the thrombocytopenic patient, the periphery of these lesions may become ecchymotic. Biopsy specimens of the lesions indicate that the underlying process is

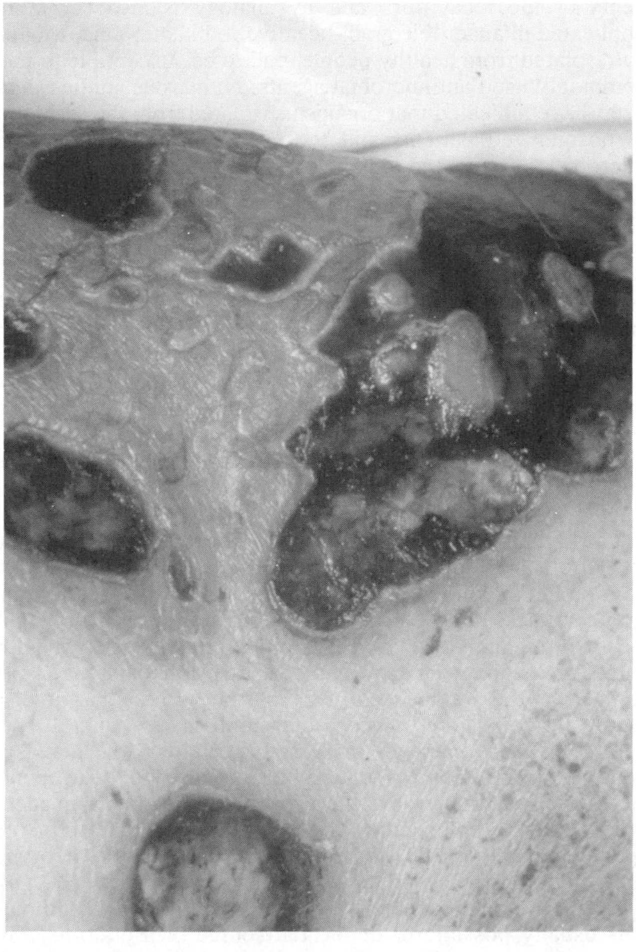

FIG. 1. Ecthyma gangrenosa in a neutropenic patient.

infectious, with direct vascular invasion by bacilli and thrombosis on the venous side of the capillary bed.[43] It seems likely that extracellular products of bacteria such as proteases (elastases) and/or exotoxins are responsible for tissue damage. Nonetheless, there are some reports attributing this phenomenon to local manifestations of Shwartzman reactions in the skin, that is, a localized area of consumption coagulopathy where venous thrombosis triggered perhaps by endotoxin is the initiator of tissue injury. By and large, however, most of these ecthyma lesions appear to be infectious because organisms can be directly aspirated or cultured from these lesions and histopathologic sections reveal organisms invading blood vessel walls. Since bacteria are involved in a demand vasculitis, the presence of ecthyma lesions can be considered tantamount to bacteremia.

It has become clear that, while ecthyma-type lesions are strongly suggestive of *P. aeruginosa* infection, the latter are not the only organisms that can cause this characteristic lesion. *Aeromonas hydrophila* can produce a clinical picture similar to that of *P. aeruginosa* infection, and a large proportion of bacteremic patients have had ecthymalike skin lesions.[44,45] Additionally, cutaneous lesions have been observed in *E. coli*,[46] *Klebsiella, Enterobacter*, and *Serratia* septicemia. Besides ecthyma lesions, colorful vesicular or bullous lesions, cellulitis, diffuse erythematous reactions (similar to scarlet fever), or showers of petechial lesions (not unlike meningococcemia) can be cutaneous manifestations of gram-negative bacteremia.[47] Thus, cutaneous lesions should not lead the clinician to make a specific etiologic diagnosis (although ecthyma-type lesions in the neutropenic patient are most often due to *P. aeruginosa*) but to alert medical personnel to the possibility of a systemic gram-negative bacillary infection, the need for diagnostic measures, and therapeutic intervention. The availability of a lesion from which a biopsy specimen can be obtained and that is easily aspirated, cultured, and processed with Gram stain may provide the basis for an initial microbiologic diagnosis before the isolation and characterization of organisms from blood cultures.

Some patients may have a fulminating bacteremia manifested by shock or rapidly progressing to the stage of shock in a matter of hours. The latter course may be indistinguishable from meningococcemia and is often due to *P. aeruginosa* or *Aeromonas* infection. More typically, however, the onset of shock is slower and follows a period of several hours of hemodynamic instability. A reasonable working definition of shock is hypotension manifested by systolic blood pressures less than 90 mmHg and diastolic pressure less than 60 mm Hg accompanied by tachycardia, peripheral vasoconstriction, and oliguria or anuria. Oliguria is defined by hourly urine outputs of less than 20 ml. The hallmark of shock is tissue hypoperfusion resulting from a decrease in intravascular fluid volume, diminished vascular resistance, or both. Both vasodilatation and increased vascular permeability of some compartments of the circulation may be an initial manifestation of certain pathophysiologic processes (see the section on pathophysiology), and the net effect is a reduction in circulating blood volume.

Many patients may have transient hypotension or oliguria that is quickly ameliorated by prompt corrective measures such as fluid challenge. Others progress from an initial phase of hypotension, tachycardia, and peripheral vasodilatation ("warm shock") to a moribund phase of deep pallor, intense vasoconstriction, and anuria ("cold shock"). The latter state clearly reflects the inability of compensatory mechanisms to maintain perfusion even to vital organs. The onset of shock is seen in perhaps 20–35 percent of the patients with gram-negative rod bacteremia and increases the mortality to perhaps twice that figure.

While clinical findings are likely to reflect the severity and stage of shock rather than a specific microbial etiology, there exists some evidence for hemodynamic differences between shock complicating gram-positive bacteremia and gram-negative bacillemia. Gunnar and colleagues[48] have conducted prospective hemodynamic studies in patients proven to have shock associated with both gram-positive cocci and gram-negative rods. Patients were hospitalized in the intensive care unit of a large municipal hospital, and most had procedures involving urinary tract instrumentation. As shown in Table 3, a number of variables were monitored including heart rate, cardiac index, left ventricular end-diastolic pressure, systemic vascular resistance, and mean arterial pressure. Of these parameters, the cardiac rate and cardiac index (which parallels the former) were significantly lower in patients developing shock secondary to gram-negative bacillary infection. These findings were felt to be consistent with release of a vasodilator substance early during the course of gram-negative bacteremia, but ultimately vasoconstriction was more common in patients with gram-negative infections. Myocardial function also appeared depressed. While both changes in cardiac rate and index reflect decreased tissue perfusion, it should be noted, nonetheless, that the differences were small, with considerable overlap between the two groups. In the individual patient, a single measurement of either heart rate or cardiac index is likely to be of limited value in distinguishing whether the patient has gram-negative or gram-positive infection. For this reason, it still seems prudent in the critically ill patient with septic shock to initiate empirical antimicrobial therapy aimed at both gram-positive and gram-negative causes until the results of cultures are known.

There has been increasing interest focused on pulmonary complications of gram-negative rod bacteremia.[49,50] Some patients, although probably a minority, have bacteremia originating from the lung. These subjects develop infection secondary to aspiration (bronchial embolism) whereby material from the upper respiratory tract that contains gram-negative rods is aspirated into the lung parenchyma and subsequent pneumonitis and bacteremia develops.[51,52] More commonly, however, diffuse pneumonitis can develop secondary to bacteremia and is often of overwhelming severity. The attention of pulmonary physiologists and clinicians has been focused on this complication, which is often referred to as the adult respiratory distress syndrome (ARDS) or "shock lung." It is likely that ARDS reflects a wide variety of pathophysiologic mechanisms and clearly has no single etiology, but gram-negative rod bacteremia is one of them.[49] The mechanism for the diffuse infiltrates may entail direct involvement of the lung by a bacteremic necrotizing pneumonitis or a combination of pulmonary edema (diffuse alveolar/capillary leak) associated with evidence for macro- and microembolization to the lung (consumption coagulopathy).

TABLE 3. Comparison Between Hemodynamic Values during Septic Shock in 19 Patients with Gram-Positive Organisms and 31 Patients with Gram-Negative Organisms Cultured from Blood

	MAP (*mmHg*)	*CVP* (*mmHg*)	*HR* (*per min*)	*CI* (*liter/min/m²*)	*SVR* (*mmHg/liter/min*)	*LVEDP* (*mmHg*)
Gram-positive	57 ± 2[a]	3.5 ± 0.06	119 ± 4	3.8 ± 0.3	8.5 ± 1.1	6.7 ± 1.3
Gram-negative	57 ± 3	5.1 ± 0.7	100 ± 4	2.9 ± 0.2	11.5 ± 0.9	9.8 ± 1.6
p (unpaired)	NS	NS	<.01	<.05	NS	NS

Abbreviations: MAP: mean arterial pressure; CVP: central venous pressure; HR: heat rate; CI: cardiac index; SVR: systemic vascular resistance; LVEDP: left ventricular end-diastolic pressure; NS: not significant.

[a] Mean ± SE.

(From Gunnar et al.,[48] with permission.)

TABLE 4. Factors Affecting the Outcome of Gram-Negative Bacteremia

Underlying disease
Neutropenia
Hypogammaglobulinemia
Diabetes
Alcoholism ± cirrhosis
Renal failure
Respiratory failure
Complications of the bacteremic event at the onset of treatment (e.g., shock, anuria)
Antimicrobial chemotherapy
Grade of severity of bacteremia (polymicrobial bacteremia)
Source of infection
Interval to initiation of treatment
Age

That bacterial products can trigger intrinsic clotting and (pari passu) that the body has mechanisms for resorption of thrombi (activation of the fibrinolytic system) is well known. The complexity of the clinical situation probably relates to the multiple events that are triggered by bacterial invasion of the blood stream and ensuing host responses. Included in this concept is a role for endotoxin-triggered mediators such as tumor necrosis factor (TNF) in the pathophysiologic changes leading to ARDS. The characteristic clinical findings include hypoxia, evidence for a right-to-left shunt, and diffuse pulmonary infiltrates. The most important finding is the relatively normal pulmonary wedge pressure (left ventricular end-diastolic pressure) in the face of a high pulmonary arterial pressure and marked hypoxia (PaO_2 <60 mmHg). This indicates that the diffuse pulmonary capillary leak syndrome and mechanical alterations in lung function are not secondary to left-sided cardiac failure, that is, represent "noncardiogenic" pulmonary edema.

Clearly, it is not the bacteremic event per se but the status of host defense mechanisms and the ability to maintain function of vital organs that are the factors deciding the outcome of any blood stream infection. Table 4 summarizes, in order of estimated importance, some of the factors commonly accepted as affecting prognosis. In addition to underlying disease and complications, other factors can have a significant effect. Although quantitative blood cultures are now less frequently performed, several studies indicate that mortality is greater with high-grade bacteremia and with polymicrobial bacteremia.[28,53] The source of infection may be important because people with leukemia often (with an overall poorer prognosis) have no discernible focus of a primary infection. Age is linked in a biphasic manner to outcome, with poorer survival in the very young and older age groups. The selection of antimicrobial therapy and the urgency with which it is implemented has a definite effect on outcome and will be dealt with later in this chapter.

MICROBIAL PROPERTIES THAT UNDERLIE VIRULENCE AND INVASIVENESS

Despite the extraordinary numbers of organisms with which humans have intimate contact, relatively few types cause significance disease. An important and recurring question is "What are those properties possessed by certain microorganisms that are responsible for their ability to cause disease and that differentiate them from mere saprophytes?" Much of the work in microbial pathogenesis has focused on two areas: first, the characterization of cell wall structures, several of which appear antigenic, that are associated with properties of invasiveness and give the organism some advantage in the face of host defense mechanisms; second, a variety of products that are either released or are closely associated with the microorganism that causes tissue damage such as enzymes, toxins, and metabolic by-products. Some of these microbial properties were recognized in the previous century, but there has been an upsurge of new information on the specific antigenic components of the bacterial cell wall and in the case of certain species, such as species of *Aeromonas* and *Pseudomonas*, new work on the characterization of microbial exotoxins.

Table 5 summarizes some of the implicated mechanisms underlying the ability of certain gram-negative bacilli to cause human disease. Since infection must start at some local site, the property of adherence to a mucosal surface may be important in the initiation of infection such as in the urinary or gastrointestinal tract. Most invasive gram-negative bacilli are serum resistant, that is, not lysed by complement-mediated reactions. Further, some are heavily encapsulated or have surfaces that enable them to resist phagocytosis. Some bacterial cell walls have an antigenic composition similar to host tissue such as blood group substances or sialic acid. As will be discussed, some cell wall constituents are clearly "toxic" and elicit a variety of inflammatory and pyrogenic reactions; there may be differences in the ability of these cell wall constituents to trigger pathophysiologic events. It has been demonstrated that some gram-negative organisms like *Brucella* and the typhoid bacillus survive intracellular and thus can evade host defense mechanisms. Finally, the aforementioned enzymes and toxins can clearly have a deleterious effect on host tissue and an effect on the initiation and propagation of infection as well as "lethal" sequelae.

Figure 2 is a schema of the cell wall antigens of gram-negative bacilli. There are three layers to this cell wall. The so-called outer membrane contains protein, lipid, and carbohydrate, with substantial amounts of the latter arranged in polymeric units or polysaccharides. The heat-stable serologic specificity of gram-negative bacilli, which is the basis for the "O," or somatic, antigen typing scheme, is principally related to the polysaccharide component of the other membrane.[67] The original serologic typing schemata for enteric bacilli proposed by Kauffman[68] and Edwards and Ewing[69] used tube or slide agglutination techniques on antisera produced against boiled organisms. Thus, major antigenic differences were determined by producing antisera (usually in rabbits) against boiled whole cell cultures and the similarities or differences between strains deduced by the pattern of agglutination with test organisms that were similarly boiled. The O antisera produced in this manner react with polysaccharide antigens that are constituents of the outer membrane. In the past, the O antigens of gram-negative organisms have been referred to as synonymous with lipopolysaccharide (LPS) or endotoxin, but as will be discussed subsequently, endotoxic activity appears to be lipid and not polysaccharide associated. The intermediate or murein layer of the gram-negative bacterial cell wall is rigid material composed predominantly of peptidoglycan or mucopeptide. The peptidoglycans of gram-negative bacteria are chemically and antigenically similar if not identical: they are composed of alternating *N*-acetyl glucosamine and *N*-acetyl neuraminic acid residues linked to a tetrapeptide.[70] It is primarily at this site that agents that inhibit cell wall synthesis, such as the penicillins and cephalosporins, have effect and result in osmotically unstable microbial forms, the so-called spheroplasts or L-forms. In that circumstance the structure responsible for retention of the integrity of the microbe is the inner or cytoplasmic membrane. In addition to these basic structures a wide variety of organisms such as *P. aeruginosa* and *E. coli* appear to have one or more flagellar structures that confer properties of motility. Not all

TABLE 5. Probable Mechanisms for "Virulence" of Disease-Causing Gram-Negative Organisms

Mechanisms	*References*
Adherence	54, 55
Serum resistance	56–58
"Antiphagocytic" surfaces	58–60
Have capsular or surface antigens similar to host tissue	61
Capsular or endotoxin type has special trophism	62
Survive intracellularly or are killed slowly	63
Elaborate extracellular factors, e.g., enzymes and toxins	64, 65

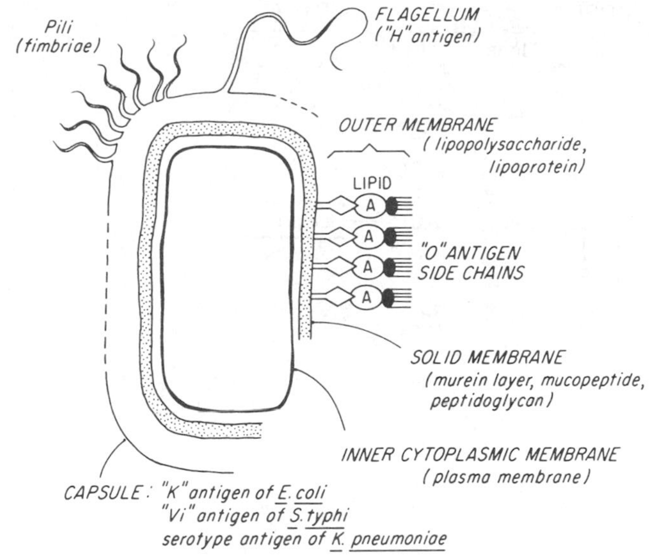

FIG. 2. Major cell wall antigens of gram-negative bacilli. See Figure 3 for details of the outer membrane. (From Young et al.,[66] with permission.)

gram-negative rods are motile or flagellated; *K. pneumoniae* is a notable exception. Additionally, many of these organisms contain structures that lie exterior to the outer membrane. These structures include pili or fimbriae, which are protein in nature and seem important for the attachment or adherence of microbes to mucosal surfaces. Other protein surface structures include porins, literally porelike structures that regulate the entry of nutrients, macromolecules, and antimicrobial agents into the bacterial cell.[71] Finally, a number of organisms, particularly *E. coli* or *Klebsiella* species, have a capsular or envelope antigen, the so-called K antigen, that lies exterior to the O antigen. These antigens are normally highly negatively charged polysaccharides, although a few are protein in nature. Also, *Salmonella typhi* has polysaccharide K-type capsular antigen that has been designated as the so-called Vi antigen.

One of the more confusing aspects of bacterial cell wall composition is the structural interrelationship of previously described components, the assessment of their pathogenic role, and the interaction of these factors with host defense mechanisms. Physicochemical methods for the isolation of cell wall components require large masses of cultured bacteria and result in products that are difficult to purify to homogeneity. Three-dimensional structural analysis of cell wall fractions reveals that there is no clear-cut demarcation between one structure and another, that is, a separation between somatic (O) antigen and capsular (K) antigen. In a broad sense, the schematic representation of Figure 3 can be misleading because it supports the concept of the bacterial cell wall as a multilamellar structure rather than a mosaic of interdigitating antigens that may or may not be exposed on the surface.

One of the greatest areas of confusion is the relationship between the O and K antigens. Originally, K, or capsular, antigens were discovered when it was found that some strains of *E. coli* could not be serotyped by O antiserum unless they were first boiled for approximately an hour.[68] This led to the suggestion that there was a structure exterior to the O antigen that inhibited agglutination; it was inferred that boiling removed or changed the surface characteristics in such a way as to permit reaction with O antiserum. A large series of K antigens of *E. coli* were described in the early work of Kauffman and his coworkers,[68] but more recently, Orskov et al. and have reassessed the concept of the K antigen.[74] These antigens appear to be highly negatively charged acidic polysaccharides whose effect is, indeed, to block agglutination by O antiserum. However, K antigens are not actually destroyed by heating, and the agglutinability that is observed after heating is probably due to rearrangement or alteration of microbial surface structures. Some of the K antigens that were described by Kauffman and his associates do not appear to be acidic polysaccharides but were probably O antigens. Further, the functional definition of the K antigen has now been extended to include some protein structures like the K-88 and K-99 types.[74] The latter protein K antigens have been associated with diarrheal syndromes in animals and appear to facilitate the attachment of these microbes to mucosal surfaces. For the great majority of strains of enteric bacilli, a functional definition of the K antigen encompasses the original concept that K antigen inhibits agglutination by O antiserum. In addition to this, a specific K antigen must be identified as a highly negatively charged surface polysaccharide by biochemical and immunoelectrophoretic techniques.[74] A K antigen may also be a factor promoting adherence to host cells and thus may be responsible for giving an infecting microbe some advantage in the initial contact with the host. Both O (somatic) and K antigens have been associated with the microbial properties of resistance to phagocytosis,[67,75] in effect permitting the microbe to evade engulfment unless specific antibodies are present.

There are several other antigenic structures that have been identified in the gram-negative cell wall. One is an antigen common to Enterobacteriaceae that was originally described by Kunin et al. and Makela and Mayer[76,77] and often referred to as the "common antigen." This appears to be polysaccharide in nature[78] and antigenic. Another antigenic material is lipoprotein in composition and is both covalently linked to the lipid portion of the outer membrane and covalently bound to the murein layer.[79] A large proportion of humans infected by enteric bacilli form antibodies against the "common antigen"[80] and lipoprotein,[81] but it has not been determined whether these antigens are true virulence factors and whether or not the antibody response confers protection against reinfection or death.

From the viewpoint of the pathophysiology of gram-negative rod septicemia, much interest has focused on the "core" region of the outer membrane. As illustrated in Figure 3A, the sequence of constituents from the exterior to the interior of the outer membrane is O antigen, outer "core," and inner "core."[72,73,82] The core region is an acidic hetero-oligosaccharide that in turn is linked to a lipoidal acylated glucosamine disaccharide termed *lipid A*. The innermost constituent of the core region, lipid A, has been chemically characterized[72,73] and exhibits all the hemodynamic, pyrogenic, and inflammatory properties associated with "endotoxicity." The inner "core" linked to lipid A has also been termed *core glycolipid*. Major clues to unraveling of the structure of the outer membrane and its core region and the evidence that lipid A is, indeed, the "toxic" moiety of the gram-negative cell wall have resulted from exhaustive investigative work on both naturally occurring and induced mutants of certain gram-negative bacilli.[67,72,82] Colonies of organisms that have O polysaccharide or somatic antigens tend to be smooth and glistening in their appearance on agar and are often referred to as "smooth." These organisms are often resistant to the killing of complement-mediated bacteriolysis in fresh human serum. Some organisms, however, appear to have a "rough" or coarse irregular appearance in colonial growth, do not grow homogeneously in broth culture media, and tend to autoagglutinate. These so-called rough organisms are hydrophobic because of their lipid content, and immunochemical analysis has revealed that the roughness is associated with a lack of O-specific polysaccharide. A series of mutants have been studied that lack one or more of the sugar moieties normally present in the core region (Fig. 3A). There is progressing roughness associated with cell wall structures that successively lack certain sugar moieties. Because most Enterobacteriaceae have similar inner core regions, a chemotype designation has evolved for identifying the rough mutants that

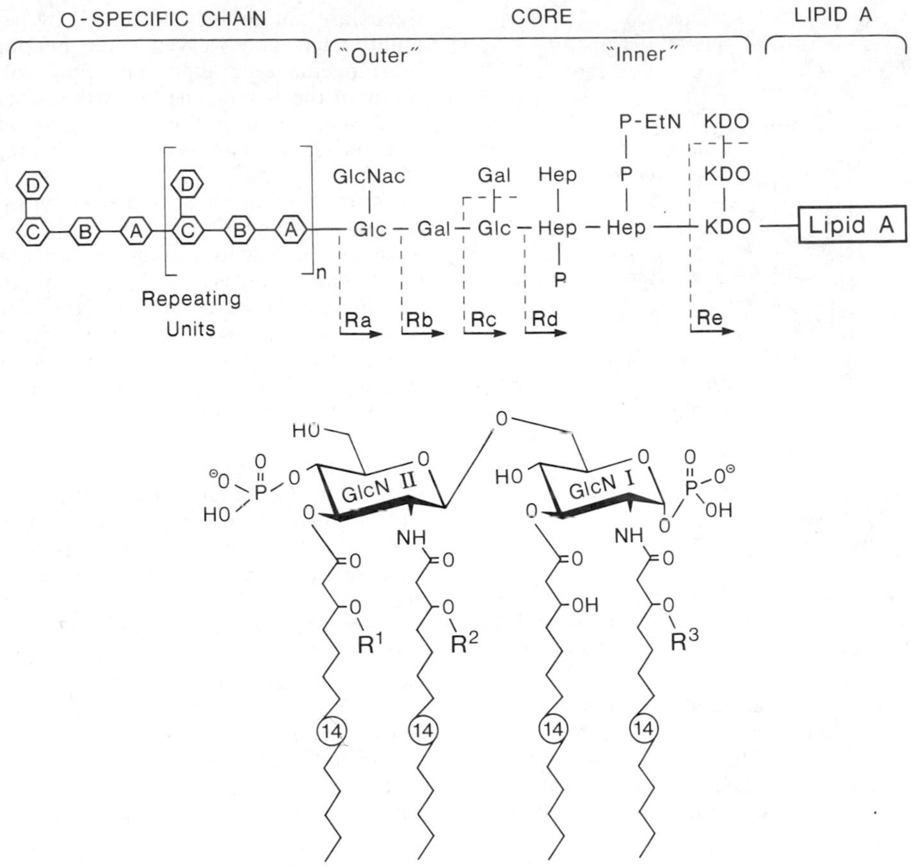

A

Source of Lipid A	Chemical Nature of:		
	R^1	R^2	R^3
E. coli	14:0	12:0	H
S. minnesota	14:0	12:0	H, 16:0
P. mirabilis	14:0	14:0	H, 16:0

B

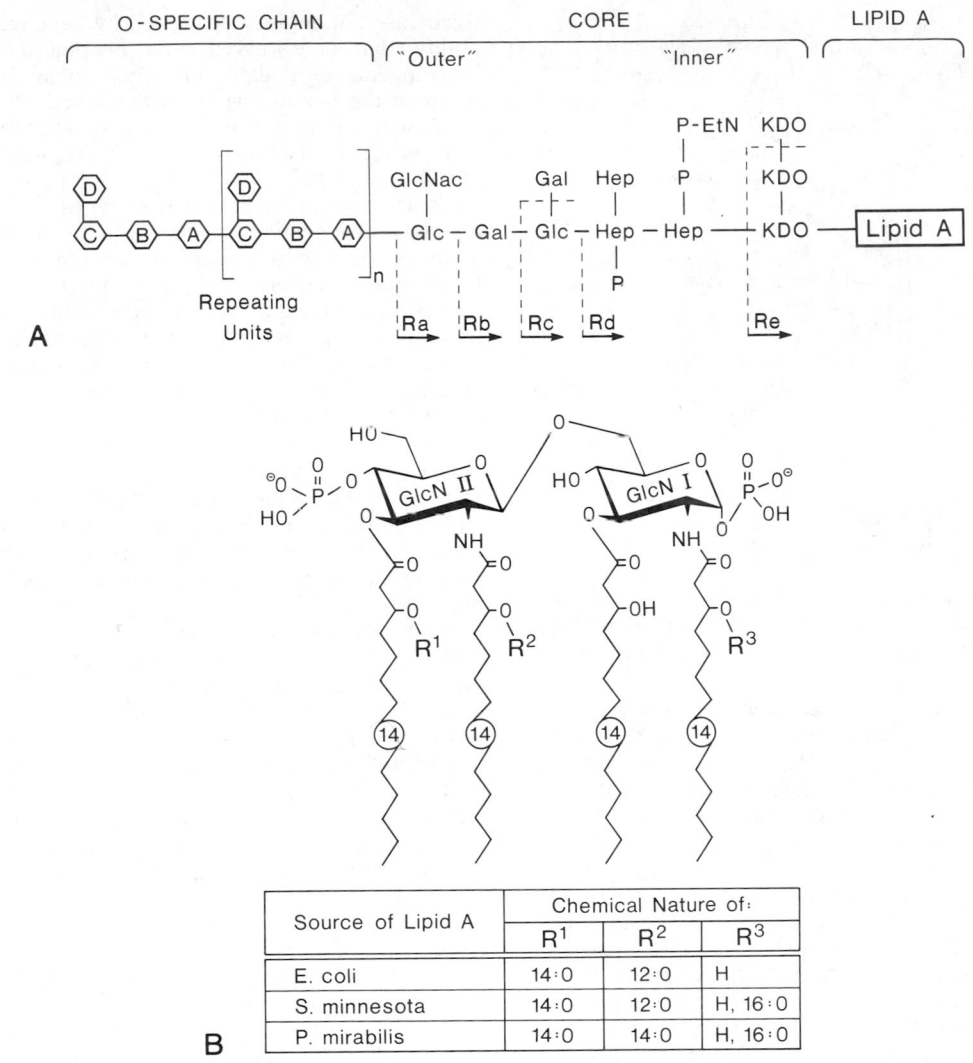

FIG. 3. **(A)** Biochemical structure of the outer membranes (lipopolysaccharides) of enteric bacteria, based primarily on work involving "rough" mutants of *Salmonella* species.[72,73] The "O" antigen side chains of repeating monosaccharide units are linked to lipid A through a "core" structure consisting of *N*-acetylglucosamine (GLcNaC), glucose, (Glu), galactose (gal), heptose (hep), phosphate (P), ethanolamine (ETN), and 2-keto, 3-deoxyoctonate (KDO, also known as manno-octulosonic acid). Chemotype mutants of increasing "roughness" such as "Ra", . . . "Rc" result from the progressive deletion of sugars from the outer to the inner core. The *E. coli* core region contains two KDOs. (Modified from Young et al.,[66] Rietschel et al.,[72] and Brade et al.[73]) **(B)** The chemical structure of the lipid A component of *E. coli, S. minnesota*, and *P. mirabilis* contains two *N*-acetyl glucosamine residues. (Modified from Rietschel et al.[72] and Brade et al.[73]). The numbers in circles indicate the number of carbon atoms in the acyl chains. The distribution of normal fatty acids (with chain lengths of 12 to 16 carbon atoms) at hydroxyl groups (R1, R2, R3) is highly specific and characteristic for the bacterial genus. (Modified from Brade et al.,[73] with permission.)

lack specific, sequential inner core constituents. The "Ra" rough chemotype designates mutants that merely lack attachment to an O-specific antigen, while the designations "Rb, Rc, Rd, and Re" represent mutants containing cell walls with the progressive deletion of individual sugars as one progresses to the inner core. The so-called Re mutants contain only 2-keto, 3-deoxyoctonate (KDO or manno-octulosonic acid) linked to lipid A.

The *E. coli* core region contains two KDOs, while the *Salmonella* core possesses three of these moieties. Lipid A is the most highly conserved component of the aerobic gram-negative LPS structure and appears to be absent in *B. fragilis*.[83] Figure 3B shows the variation in fatty acid composition for lipid A derived from *E. coli, S. minnesota*, and *P. mirabilis*[73]; *Pseudomonas* lipid A also shows differences.[84]

The precise chemical structure of lipid A several biologically active variants and the preparation of a totally synthetic lipid A have been reported in detail.[72,73] Full endotoxicity is expressed by a molecule containing two β-(1-6)D-glucosamine residues, two phosphoryl groups, and five or six fatty acids. Slight modifications in lipid A architecture result in significant changes in biologic activity, thus suggesting that endotoxicity is not dependent on a single lipid A constituent but by several factors including three-dimensional conformation. This knowledge may be of critical importance in devising means for competing with lipid A (lipid A is a nontoxic analogue) as a therapeutic or prophylactic approach[85] or as an antimicrobial in blocking lipid A synthesis.

Recent modifications overall, however, in the limulus gelation reaction that are based on spectrophotometric measurements of the process have improved its sensitivity and reliability.[86] This test, however, should not be used as a substitute for blood cultures. Endotoxin or perhaps more appropriately the lipid A of gram-negative bacilli plays a critical role in the pathophysiology of gram-negative rod infections and is an important cause of the clinical manifestations of disease. Some of the evidence supporting this association is summarized in Table 6. It should be recognized, however, that the toxicity attributed to LPS is not unique to gram-negative organisms since certain cell wall antigens of gram-positive bacteria such as hemolytic group A streptococci have an M protein that has similar "toxic" effects.[98] Nonetheless, in primates there do not appear to be significant differences between the cardiovascular and metabolic effects of viable gram-negative bacilli and those of bacterial endotoxin.

With such circumstantial evidence it has been commonly assumed that endotoxin may be circulating in the blood of humans or animals with bacteremic infections caused by gram-negative bacilli. Certain large-molecular-weight polysaccharide antigens of organisms such as *K. pneumoniae* or *S. typhi* have been found circulating in the blood of humans in the acute stages of bacteremia,[99,100] but it has not been possible to demonstrate consistently circulating endotoxin in bacteremic subjects. A number of endotoxin assay systems have been reported, virtually all using some biologic end point such as the epinephrine skin test in rabbits[101] or the limulus gelation reaction.[86,102] The latter is perhaps the most sensitive assay for endotoxin-like activity in vitro and is based on the observation that endotoxin or LPS causes gelation of fluid extracts from the amebocyte of the horseshoe crab *Limulus polyphemus*. The amebocyte has a plateletlike function; hence, what is observed in a positive reaction is coagulation triggered by quantities as small as a nanogram or picogram of endotoxin. Unfortunately, both false-positive and false-negative limulus gelation test results have been well documented in gram-negative bacteremia, and fungal and gram-positive functions have been associated with positive responses.[103,104] There are several explanations for this including (*1*) inherent problems in the biologic variability of reagent materials and maintaining test materials free of contamination by endotoxin, (*2*) demonstration that fresh human serum contains factors that detoxify or inactivate endotoxin,[105,106] and (*3*) the observation that circulating antibodies may bind or complex with endotoxins and thus give a negative test result.[107,108]

Conflicting reports on the feasibility of detecting endotoxin by the limulus gelation or other tests probably do not rule out a role in human bacteremic infections.[109] The presence of exposed antigen on the bacterial cell wall with or without bacteremia might be sufficient to trigger pathophysiologic sequelae that are observed in certain human disease states (see below). Further, experimental animal studies show that the clearance of infused bacteria by reticuloendothelial cells and circulating phagocytes leads to a rapid reduction in the number of microorganisms within minutes. Some 10^6 organisms/ml/min must be infused at a constant rate to yield a sustained bacteremia of 100–1000 circulating organisms per milliliter.[110] By inference, many more organisms may have actually been introduced into the blood stream than are revealed by quantitative blood cultures of venous blood. The significance of this observation is that endotoxemia may be transient, organisms may be rapidly cleared, after which adverse effects on the host are observed, and the sequelae of certain gram-negative infections may be triggered by far greater numbers of bacteria than are present when an attempt is made to actually document bacteremia or endotoxemia. Conversely, it is conceivable that absorption of bacterial toxins (both endotoxins and exotoxins) may occur from local sites of infection in the absence of bacteremia.[109]

TABLE 6. Evidence Implicating a Role for Bacterial Endotoxins in the Pathophysiology of Gram-Negative Septicemia

Evidence	*References*
1. Similarity in clinical manifestations between infection and administration of LPS to humans or animals	87, 88
2. Common pattern of hematologic changes after LPS administration and infection	89, 90
3. Generation of kinins and activation of Hageman factor in clinical infection and after LPS administration to animals	91, 92
4. Consumption of complement (C3 and alternative-pathway factors) in human infection complicated by shock and in animals given LPS	93, 94
5. Antibody against the "core" glycolipid antigens of LPS protects humans and experimental animals against sequelae of shock and death	95, 96
6. Administration of LPS to human volunteers results in the liberation of TNF; TNF mimics all of the pathophysiologic changes seen in gram-negative sepsis and can be detected in body fluids of septic patients	94, 97

Besides endotoxin, attention has been focused on other bacterial products that might be important in pathogenesis. The proteolytic enzymes might be such factors as are suggested by work with the elastases of *P. aeruginosa*. These elastases are dermonecrotic, cornea damaging, and possibly responsible for some of the changes seen in vasculitic lesions.[65] A correlation with proteolytic activity and virulence for mice has been reported for *P. aeruginosa*.[111]

Some of the other extracellular virulence factors that have been studied include the extracellular toxins of *Aeromonas* species[112] and *P. aeruginosa*.[64] The latter species produces a variety of exotoxins, perhaps the best characterized of which is exotoxin A. This toxin is produced by most clinical isolates of *P. aeruginosa*,[113] is lethal for mammalian cells,[114] and being analogous to diphtheria toxin is a potent inhibitor of protein synthesis.[115] In murine test systems toxin-producing strains are considerably more virulent than are nontoxigenic organisms.[116] In humans, high levels of antibodies directed against exotoxin A correlate with recovery from bacteremic *P. aeruginosa* infection.[117]

The tendency of investigators to usually focus on one microbial disease-producing mechanism has probably led to too narrow a view of the pathogenesis of gram-negative bacillary infection. The factors listed in Table 5 are certainly not mutually exclusive. It seems likely that organisms that are adherent, serum resistant, heavily encapsulated, and producers of extracellular proteolytic enzymes are likely to be more virulent than are those that are rough, serum sensitive, poorly adherent, and nonproteolytic. Not to be underestimated is the capacity of the microbe to survive in the environment of the hospital where seriously ill patients are managed. *Serratia marcescens* and *P. aeruginosa* have few nutritional requirements and can persist in a host of environmental reservoirs. Thus, a "unifying view" of the pathogenesis of gram-negative rod infections culminating in bacteremia takes into account a wide variety of epidemiologic, host, and microbial factors. Epidemiologic factors (types of exposure, antimicrobial usage) involve disruption of what might be termed *colonization immunity*. Microbial factors such as adherence and production of enzymes like proteases help to establish infection in local sites. Bacteremia is abetted by microbial properties of serum resistance and resistance to phagocytosis, but host factors such as numbers and function of phagocytic cells and humoral opsonins are likely to be deficient. Persistence of infection may be due to sequestration of infection in sites relatively protected from host defense mechanisms (deep abscesses, renal medulla, bone), and some phagocytic cells may actually become "sanctuaries" for microbes that survive intracellularly. The adverse sequelae of bacteremia—hypotension, shock, and death—may result from endotoxin, exotoxins, or other microbial products that are either directly lethal or can "trigger" pathophysiologic processes through various mediators or enzymatic reactions. The latter will be reviewed in the ensuing section.

PATHOPHYSIOLOGY OF GRAM-NEGATIVE ROD BACTEREMIA

The pathophysiologic events in gram-negative rod bacteremia are complex, and there are major reasons for our current problems in understanding what actually occurs in humans. First, there is the problem in human studies of trying to relate cause and effect, particularly with regard to the complications of gram-negative bacteremia such as septic shock. For instance, the role of complement activation and consumption of certain components is well documented in septic shock,[93,118] but in all likelihood the depression of levels of certain complement components is a result of bacteremia and the activation of the complement system. Whether or not complement activation can be regarded as a cause of septic shock remains speculative, although a large body of experimental evidence suggests that byproducts of complement activation such as anaphylatoxins enhance vascular permeability and thus may affect both the hemodynamic status of the patient[119] and the functional capability of critical organs like the lung.[120]

Shock associated with gram-negative sepsis represents the extreme aspect of the spectrum of disease manifestations that result from a relative excess of systemically absorbed endotoxin. The complex pattern of pathophysiologic events now appears to be the result of activation or release of various mediators rather than direct endotoxin toxicity.

A second major problem in understanding the pathophysiology of gram-negative bacteremia is the fact that many of the changes that are observed either clinically or histopathologically may not be the manifestations of the infection itself but of a primary disease that is complicated by an infection. In the advanced stages of neoplasia or collagen-vascular disease it may be difficult to distinguish between primary or secondary changes. For instance, bleeding is a major potential complication of leukemias and lymphomas, but demonstration of a hemorrhagic diathesis or histologic evidence of bleeding (or clotting) may be difficult to attribute to the underlying disease, to the treatment of that underlying disease, or to a supervening infection. Finally, there is a major problem in translating the results of animal studies to the human clinical setting because of major species differences in the susceptibility of laboratory animals to gram-negative bacillary infections and the marked discrepancy between what has been observed in such common laboratory animals as dogs and rabbits to what has been seen both clinically and histologically in humans.[121]

Based on the administration of small, fairly nonlethal doses of bacterial endotoxin to humans, it appears that humans are one of the most susceptible species to the pyrogenic effects of bacterial endotoxin.[122] The administration of endotoxins to dogs produces some changes that have been uncommonly observed in human disease such as a diarrheal phase and an acute hypotensive phase that can be blocked by antihistamines.[42] Similarly, there has been a tendency to ascribe the changes of repeated endotoxin administration in rabbits to the reaction originally described by Sanarelli and subsequently elaborated on by Shwartzman and Gerber.[123,124] In the "local" Shwartzman reaction, an initial preparatory dose of endotoxin is injected intracutaneously, and hemorrhagic necrosis is produced by a second intravenous dose. The intravenous doses of endotoxin at 24-hour intervals results in bilateral renal cortical necrosis in rabbits. Hemorrhagic necrosis of the skin has been observed as a manifestation of gram-negative rod bacteremia in humans, although organisms have been recovered from such lesions and might reflect the concurrent bacteremia in contrast to circulating endotoxemia. Clinical and histopathologic findings consistent with a generalized Shwartzman reaction in humans has been reported in women with *E. coli* pyelonephritis, but findings of bilateral renal cortical necrosis in human material that is analogous to that observed in rabbits with the generalized Shwartzman reaction have been relatively rare.[125]

Current evidence favors the concept that the damage exerted by endotoxins is the direct result of the release of various mediators (which, although toxic, can by themselves have a role in host defense) and the triggering of humoral enzymatic mechanisms involving the complement, intrinsic clotting, fibrinolytic, and kinin pathways (Fig. 4). The most important set of developments in our understanding the pathophysiology of gram-negative sepsis is the identification of various mediators or cytokines[126] that are synthesized and released by macrophages and other mononuclear cells after exposure to endotoxin.[127] These cytokines include interleukin-1 (IL-1) (endogenous pyrogen), γ-interferon, a variety of colony-stimulating factors, and TNF (also known as cachectin). Of these biochemically defined substances, TNF appears to be an important if not the most

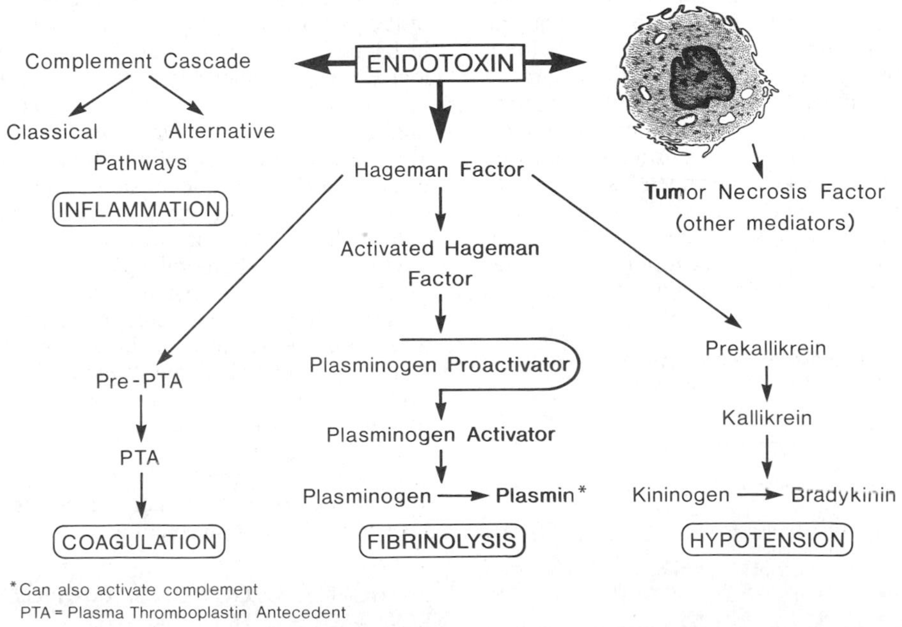

FIG. 4. The biologic effect of gram-negative bacillary endotoxins (lipopolysaccharides) are complex and interrelated. The intravenous administration of tumor necrosis factor (TNF, also known as cachectin) reproduces most of the pathophysiologic events observed in gram-negative sepsis, including the most extreme state, shock. Other mediators (cytokines) and pharmacologically active substances (e.g., prostaglandins) can act in concert with TNF. Lipopolysaccharides have other, diverse biologic effects: they can activate the complement, coagulation, and fibronolytic systems and can trigger a series of enzymatic reactions leading to the release of bradykinins and possibly other vasoactive peptides that cause hypotension.

potent mediator of the pathophysiology of gram-negative sepsis.[128–130] Evidence for this view is derived from studies showing that (*1*) mice that are genetically unresponsive to endotoxin lack the capacity to produce murine TNF from their macrophages[131]; (*2*) the administration of endotoxin to human volunteers results in the liberation of free TNF in plasma accompanied by many symptoms typical of gram-negative infection.[88] Interleukin-1 and γ-interferon were not detected at challenge doses of 4 ng/kg. (*3*) High levels of free TNF in plasma have been associated with morbidity and increased mortality in human meningococcemia[132]; (*4*) the administration of purified recombinant TNF to humans[88,130,133] and animals[134–137] mimics most of the clinical, laboratory, and histopathologic findings seen in gram-negative sepsis and septic shock; and (*5*) antibodies directed against TNF, particularly when given before endotoxin challenge, significantly increased the survival of experimental animals.[128] Protection studies have now employed monoclonal antibodies specific for TNF epitopes.[138] Infusion of anti-TNF murine monoclonal antibodies into primates who were bacteremic abrogated the development of signs of endotoxicity. TNF can also act directly on cellular components of blood and vascular epithelium,[135,139] and it has pyrogenic properties per se.[140] TNF appears to trigger the release of prostaglandins that can act as "second messengers" of systemic toxicity.[141] TNF appears to act synergistically with IL-1[142] or γ-interferon[143] to trigger inflammation and reactions such as the Shwartzman reaction, which have been associated with endotoxemia.[144] An overall conceptual picture would involve an inflammatory cascade of reactions, with TNF as the principal mediatory working synergistically with other biologically active products released by host cells. Clearly, other infectious processes such as parasitic infection can lead to TNF release,[145] so its detection is not specific for gram-negative infection. Furthermore, in some experimental models TNF alone has limited toxicity, but the full range of toxicity seen in clinical infection results from the combined use of TNF and bacterial products[141] (see Table 6). Thus, the identification of TNF as an important mediator of septic shock suggests that the sepsis syndrome is an example of immune system "overresponsiveness" to invading pathogens[137,146] or large doses of provocative antigens (e.g., LPS) in a manner analogous to anaphylaxis.

As shown in Figure 4, gram-negative bacilli and cocci that possess bacterial endotoxins have been shown to activate Hageman factor (factor XII), which in turn directly leads to the activation of the complement, coagulation, fibrinolytic, and bradykinin systems. Not shown in this diagram is the presence, at major stages in these reactions, of inhibitory or regulatory factors such as the inhibitor of the first component of complement, α_2-macroglobulin, and α_1-antitrypsin that can have an important modulating effect on these reactions. What happens in vivo is the result, perhaps quantitatively related, between the stimulus (such as endotoxin or other bacterial factors) and countervening or modulating influences.

Endotoxin can activate the complement system[93,118,147] and it is now appreciated that complement activation may take place through two different mechanisms, the classic and alternative pathways, that appear to have different antibody requirements. To produce thrombocytopenia, experimental studies suggested that activation through the classic pathway is obligatory.[147] There may be both complement-dependent and complement-independent mechanisms that are activated during the course of gram-negative bacteremia.[148] Complement activation results in the release of factors that attract the migration of phagocytic cells into tissue, that is, leukotaxis. Phagocytosis is abetted by activation of C3b and the release of chemotactic factors (C5a); this also leads to the release of anaphylatoxins that increase vascular permeability and enhance or potentiate the inflammatory reaction. It seems important to place this series of events into its proper perspective: complement appears vital for enhancing phagocytosis and lysis of serum-sensitive organisms, thus promoting blood stream clearance of microorganisms. The inflammatory reactions seem beneficial to the host, but excessive complement activation, possibly related to a large bacterial challenge, may well have a deleterious effect.

Activated Hageman factor can initiate the intrinsic clotting cascade through the conversion of plasma thromboplastin antecedent (pre-PTA) to PTA. Eventually, fibrinogen (factor I) is converted to fibrin, and clotting ensues. Uncontrolled activation of coagulation, usually accompanied by shock, will result in thrombosis and consumption of platelets and clotting factors II, V, and VIII. The term *acute disseminated intravascular coagulation* (DIC) has been used synonymously with consumption coagulopathy, defibrination syndrome, and coagulation-fibrinolytic syndrome. In this syndrome the use of coagulation factors II, V, and VIII as well as platelets significantly exceeds production rates and results in levels less than those required for hemostasis. The activation of clotting through an endotoxin-triggered mechanism thus may paradoxically result in clinical bleeding due to the consumption of clotting factors. The end results of disseminated coagulation depend on the target organ. Severe clinical bleeding, thrombosis, tissue ischemia and necrosis, hemolysis, and organ failure (lung, kidney, liver) are common complications.

At the same time as clotting appears to be initiated, countervening mechanisms also appear to be activated by clotting, namely, activation of the fibrinolytic system.[119] Activated Hageman factor appears to effect the conversion of plasminogen proactivator to plasminogen activator. An α_2-macroglobulin influenced by the latter subsequently affects the conversion of plasminogen to plasmin, a potent fibrinolytic substance that mediates clot lysis. The activation of plasmin fibrinolytic systems may thus also contribute to bleeding tendencies. Fibrinolytic mechanisms act to lyse fibrin into soluble peptides called fibrin split products or degradation products, which provide substantial diagnostic evidence for the presence of DIC. Additionally, evidence for a prolonged prothrombin time (PT) and partial thromboplastin time (PTT) is usually present because fibrin split products have anticoagulant activity. It is also of interest that plasmin, the end product of the fibrinolytic system, also has the capacity to initiate the complement cascade, again indicating the interrelationship of the inflammatory reactions that appear to be triggered by a bacterial gram-negative product.

The complication of DIC is not unique to gram-negative infections and has been observed in gram-positive, fungal, and viral infections as well. Furthermore, the pattern of abnormalities in laboratory findings should be assessed rather than relying on one or two laboratory values. Although factor II (prothrombin) is consumed during coagulation, it is a vitamin K dependent factor and can be affected by vitamin K deficiency such as in liver disease. Depression of vitamin K dependent factors with resultant prolongation in PT and PTT have been observed in 25 percent of normotensive septicemic patients without other evidence of DIC.[149] Additionally, patients may develop evidence of thrombocytopenia without DIC. In hypotensive patients, however, prolonged PT and PTT seem to be related to consumption coagulopathy irrespective of the levels of vitamin K dependent factors.[149]

It has been proposed that, in subjects without liver disease, the minimum criteria for the diagnosis of DIC includes thrombocytopnia, detection of fibrin split products, and a reduction in one or more of the coagulation factors II, V, or VII. If hepatic disease is present at the time of infection, reduced factor VIII levels are necessary to confirm the diagnosis of DIC.[149] Table 7 summarizes the general clotting parameters observed in normotensive or hypotensive patients. The levels of factors II, V, and VI may in fact be elevated in patients without hemodynamic alterations. The timing of clotting studies also seems important since levels of some factors and platelets may be initially depressed and then show a "rebound" response.

Demonstration of coagulation defects in conditions such as

TABLE 7. Effect of Bacteremic Infections on Levels of Platelets and Clotting Factors

Condition	Platelets	Factor II	Factor V	Factor VIII	Fibrinogen	Fibrin Split Products
Normotensive	—, ↓	—, ↓	↑	↑	↑	±
Hypotensive	↓	↓	↓	↓	↓	+

Key: —: normal; ↑: elevated; ↓: reduced; +: present.

typhoid fever has not correlated with clinical bleeding; thus, mere detection of laboratory abnormalities is not synonymous with alterations of clinical significance.[150] Further, the pathway via activated Hageman factor is not the only means by which endotoxin or bacterial products may initiate the clotting or bleeding. There are three other mechanisms that have been reported: (*1*) complexes of bacterial antigen with antibody can interact with human leukocytes and result in the release of a procoagulant that can trigger clotting.[151] (*2*) Circulating granulocyte proteases have been detected in gram-negative rod bacteremia, and these substances are capable of digesting clotting proteins in a manner distinct from DIC.[152] (*3*) Endotoxin can cause intimal vascular injury, thereby triggering or aggravating both clotting and bleeding, and this effect is probably mediated by TNF.[135,139]

Renal glomerular microclots as observed in rabbits after injections of endotoxin (generalized Shwartzman-type reaction) appear to be related to endotoxin-activated DIC.[153] Further, this experimental model of DIC suggests a role for both neutrophils and platelets in the initiation or augmentation of the reaction.[144] A reduction in numbers of circulating granulocytes through the use of cytotoxic agents may actually abort the generalized Shwartzman reaction.

The injection of small quantities of bacterial endotoxins into human volunteers indicates that the inflammatory and pyrogenic effects are manifested at low doses such as 5 ng.[87,88,122] The sequence of events appears similar to what has been observed in the monkey with the onset of hypotensive changes within an hour or 2.[154] Similar changes have also been observed after the intravenous injection of bacilli in dogs, although the hypotensive changes observed in the latter animal appear to be biphasic, with the initial phase aborted by the use of antihistamines.[96]

The effect of endotoxin on the kinin system is a direct result of the action of Hageman factor on the conversion of prekallikrein to kallikrein. Kallikrein in turn catalyzes the conversion of kininogen to bradykinin. Bradykinin is a vasoactive peptide whose primary effect is vasodilatation and increased vascular permeability. Tissue damage results from the margination of leukocytes, smooth muscle relaxation, leakage of fluid into the interstitial space, and an "effective" intravascular hypovolemia. Because bradykinin causes decreased peripheral vascular resistance secondary to vasodilatation, hypotension and septic shock ensue, with the result being hypoperfusion of critical organs.

In hypotensive patients with gram-negative bacteremia, Mason and coworkers demonstrated decreased prekallikrein and kallikrein inhibitor levels in blood.[155] Similar studies were also reported by Robinson and associates.[156] These findings were interpreted as indirect evidence for kinin release during severe episodes of infection, presumably by conversion of kininogen to kinins by plasma kallikrein. Infusion of synthetic bradykinin into animals results in hypotension followed by an elevation of cardiac output in response to reduced peripheral vascular resistance.[154] This sequence of events, including an increase in pulmonary vascular resistance, is similar to the circulatory and respiratory responses of humans to sepsis.

In human volunteer studies direct evidence that endotoxin triggers the release of bradykinin was obtained by Kimball and coworkers, who reported elevations of bradykinin levels to as high as 6 ng/ml as measured by radioimmunoassay in subjects given 3 or 5 ng/kg of endotoxin.[91] At these doses, bradykinin reached its maximum level at 1 hour without producing hypotension. These experiments were complicated by the relationship between the formation of angiotensin II and the inactivation of bradykinin since the hypotensive effects of bradykinin may be counteracted by the action of angiotensin II. O'Donnell and colleagues measured the blood prekallikrein levels in human infections and assessed the results with respect to hepatic synthesis since bradykinin is rapidly destroyed by plasma kininases and 90 percent of kinin is removed by single passage through the lung.[157] The highest mortality was observed in groups of patients who were hypotensive and had liver dysfunction. Blood prekallikrein levels were below normal in all groups studied, were significantly less in patients with liver dysfunction, and were reduced proportionally in hypotensive patients to less than 30 percent of the values noted in normotensive groups. These findings suggest that prekallikrein consumption in the hypotensive groups is the result of the process of activating kallikrein and the conversion of kininogen to bradykinin. Circulating kinin levels were elevated in hypotensive patients with or without liver disease.

A further extension of these studies of the kinin-generating system has included human volunteers serially followed after ingestion of 10^5 *Salmonella typhi*.[158] Although none of the clinical illnesses were severe and neither endotoxemia nor hypotension could be documented, the onset of positive blood cultures and fever was accompanied by a fall in platelet count, a reduction in prekallikrein esterase activity, a drop in levels of kallikrein inhibitor, and a rise in high-molecular-weight kininogen clotting activity. These findings plus electrophoretic evidence for the formation of a complex between kallikrein and a C1 esterase inhibitor provide further evidence for activation of the kinin system in gram-negative bacillary infections such as typhoid.

A variety of vasoactive substances including serotonin, endogenous catecholamines, adrenal corticosteroids, lysosomal enzymes, platelet-activating factor (PAF), and endorphins have been found circulating in the blood of animals after endotoxin administration.[121,159,160] In humans with gram-negative bacteremia, alterations in serum lipid profiles[161] and elevations in plasma thromboxane and prostaglandin levels have been observed.[162] These changes may be a result of TNF or a response secondary to bradykinin generation.

If bacteremia is transient, the result may only be a mild fever with little if any hemodynamic changes. The short-lived bacteremia that has been observed after instrumentation of the urinary or gastrointestinal tract indicates that bacteremia can occur without severe sequelae. On the other hand, activation of these inflammatory processes by a substantial inoculum of organisms in the debilitated patient may produce the clinical manifestations observed in severe gram-negative infections, particularly septic shock. Septic shock arises when cardiac output is unable to compensate for a falling blood pressure secondary to vasodilatation, an increased volume of the intravascular bed, and peripheral pooling of blood. The net result of inadequate tissue perfusion is cellular hypoxia and a shift of cellular metabolism from aerobic to anaerobic glycolysis followed by lactic acidosis, lysosomal injury, failure of essential cellular metabolism, and cell death.

The histopathologic changes in gram-negative septicemia include microthromboses of blood vessels on the venous side of the circulation, tissue necrosis, and hemorrhages. With gram-negative infections there appears to be a higher incidence of pulmonary hemorrhages than in other forms of shock,[163] and it is felt that these hemorrhages can aggravate fatal respiratory insufficiency (ARDS). Signs of metastatic pneumonia are found in patients with bacteremia arising from an extrapulmonary source. With a long period of ventilatory support for prolonged hypoxia, evidence of a superimposed aspiration-type pneumonia and hyaline membranes are often observed, but the latter are possibly related to pulmonary oxygen toxicity. Fibrin thrombi in small pulmonary vessels are almost invariably found if the patient dies in shock within 24 hours.[163] Microthrombi are difficult to identify after 48 hours, possibly because of the activation of fibrinolytic systems. After the lungs, the intestine has been most frequently affected, with lesions corresponding to acute ischemic enterocolitis. The liver at necropsy has occasionally shown zonal necrosis, which is not unique to gram-negative infection. Somewhat comparable to the findings in the lung, patients dying early in septic gram-negative shock (within 24 hours) may have fibrin thrombi in the hepatic vasculature. However, extensive necrosis and thrombi are not frequently observed in patients who succumb at longer intervals after the onset of infection.

Much work has been carried out to characterize the renal changes in gram-negative septicemic patients. Evidence for Shwartzman-type reactions has been presented by McKay and associates.[125] Classic lesions of the Shwartzman reaction with cortical necrosis are found infrequently, but other changes have been described that include scattered necrosis, hemorrhage, and tubular necrosis as well.[163]

Adrenal complications of gram-negative septicemia have long been the subject of interest among clinicians and pathologists. Bilateral adrenal cortical hemorrhages are an essential component of the Waterhouse-Friedricksen syndrome associated with meningococcemia, but these changes have been also found in a variety of shock states. They are commonly associated with fibrin thrombi that extend from the cortical sinusoids in the central vein of the adrenals and result in necrosis. Functionally, adrenal cortical necrosis has resulted in increased levels of circulating corticosteroid hormones, and there is little to support the belief that severe meningococcemia or gram-negative rod bacteremia complicated by shock is a functionally hypoadrenal state.

HOST DEFENSES AGAINST GRAM-NEGATIVE BACTERIA

Mechanical barriers are one of the most important factors limiting the systemic invasion of the host by gram-negative bacilli. Because the alimentary canal is clearly the largest reservoir of gram-negative rods in the body, the gastrointestinal mucosa has an important function in restricting entry of these organisms into the blood stream. Bacteremia may result from trauma, penetrating wounds, small surface ulcerations, mechanical obstruction such as caused by tumors, and ischemic necrosis of the bowel. Immunosuppressed people may have multiple small ulcerations of the gastrointestinal mucosa as the apparent source of entry of microorganisms; such ulcerations may be the effect of antineoplastic agents.

Irrespective of whether the organisms are aerobic or anaerobic, the complement-mediated serum bacteriolytic system is an important factor limiting invasion of the host by the great majority of gram-negative organisms that colonize the gastrointestinal tract. Most studies show these colonizing or saprophytic organisms to be serum sensitive, that is, they are killed or lysed by fresh human serum containing functional active components of the classic or alternative complement pathway.[56–58] Nonetheless, it appears that organisms causing bacteremic disease in humans and higher mammals are usually serum resistant or fairly resistant to the native serum bacteriolytic activity. There have been some reports of depressed serum bactericidal activity associated with bacteremic human infection.[164] It is possible that serum-sensitive organisms tend to cause a self-limited bacteremia, and this may well account for the finding that patients who have intermittent portal bacteremia (such as those with ulcerative colitis) or hepatic cirrhosis (where there may be impaired clearance of bacteria) have a wide variety of antibodies against enteric bacteria.[165] The susceptibility of strains to complement-mediated lysis appears to be related to structural defects in the trilamellar cell wall of the organisms rather than to variations in the bacteriolytic power of human serum.[59] Serum resistance seems related to the structural integrity of the LPS and probably quantity of polysaccharide. The amount and structure of capsular (K) antigens may also account for serum resistance.[166] Thus, serum sensitivity is related to microbial structure rather than to a variation in levels of specific antibodies or complement in human serum. While most serum-resistant organisms are "smooth" and most "rough" organisms are serum sensitive, it has been observed that some smooth strains can be used by fresh serum.[167] For some time it has been debated whether or not complement alone can kill serum-sensitive gram-negative bacilli or whether serum bacteriocidal activity has an obligatory requirement for antibodies of the IgG and IgM classes. Since the alternative complement pathway now appears to be activated in the absence of specific antibody, lysis without antibody is possible.[168] However, the presence of antibodies can enhance alternative-pathway activation through the so-called amplification loop.

Complement deficiency states are associated with increased susceptibility to infection, and this has been best documented with genetic deficiencies in certain complement components.[169] Early in life such as in the neonatal period, the alternative pathway is functionally deficient, and this may explain some of the increased susceptibility of newborn infants to gram-negative bacteremia.[170] It has also been reported that functional deficiencies of the alternative pathway are present in such diseases as sickle cell anemia and systemic lupus erythematosus, and this could be a predisposing factor to gram-negative bacillary systemic infections in these conditions.[171,172]

The basis for the presence of "natural" antibodies in normal serum, that is, detection of circulating antibodies against a number of bacteria that have not caused clinical disease, has been the matter of some speculation.[173] Such antibodies could result from low-grade or inapparent infection and would thus be engendered by specific antigenic exposure. Another mechanism by which humans could acquire natural antibodies against specific O or K antigens would be by exposure to organisms that bear similar or identical antigenic determinants but are relatively avirulent.[174] For instance, immunochemical studies now indicate identity between polyribose phosphate, the capsular polysaccharide of *Haemophilus influenzae* type B, and the capsular polysaccharide of *E. coli* K-100.[175] The group-specific B and C polysaccharides of *Neisseria meningitis* are similarly identical to the K-1 and K-92 *E. coli* polysaccharides, respectively.[176,177] *Bacillus pumilis* is an organism with exceedingly low pathogenicity that has cell wall material identical to the group A meningococcal polysaccharide.[178] Only a few scattered cases of group A meningococcal disease have occurred in the United States in the last few decades, yet the majority of the adult population has bactericidal antibody against group A meningococci.[179] Exposure to *B. pumilis* or similar organisms may account for the prevalence of these antibodies in the absence of epidemic meningococcal disease. By analogy, cross-protective immunity against a variety of other bacterial pathogens may derive from antecedent exposure to antigens borne by microorganisms in the human environment with considerbly less pathogenic potential.

Since the great majority of organisms that cause bacteremic disease in humans are resistant to the bactericidal activity of fresh human serum, the burden for clearing organisms from the blood stream must fall to phagocytic cells, whether they are the fixed phagocytes of the reticuloendothelial system or the circulating phagocytes such as the neutrophil or monocyte.[58] There is good correlation between susceptibility to bacterial and in particular gram-negative infections and depressed levels of circulating neutrophils. Since it is commonly observed that bacteremia follows neutropenia,[180] the neutropenic patient might still develop systemic infection in spite of the presence of high levels of antibodies against cell wall antigens. In actual clinical or experimental circumstances antibody levels seem to fall in parallel with levels of circulating phagocytes,[180,181] thus suggesting binding or consumption of antibody before or near the onset of bacteremia.

The humoral opsonic system of humans is complex. Antibodies of both IgG and IgM classes can serve as opsonins, and they are primarily directed against O or K polysaccharide antigens. There is evidence to suggest that K antibodies can be more protective than O antibodies are. Since K antigens lie more exteriorly on the bacterial cell surface than do somatic (O) antigens, K antibodies on a molar basis may be more effective as opsonins than O antibodies are.[182]

Complement activation may play an important role in deciding the pathways to C3b, the critical opsonic protein of the circulating humoral system. Opsonization via the classic complement pathway appears to have an obligatory requirement for specific antibody of either the IgG or IgM type.[183] IgM, in turn, has an obligatory requirement for complement, but IgG may opsonize gram-negative organisms in the absence of complement, although at a slower rate than in the presence of a normally functioning complement system.[184] It has been well demonstrated that phagocytes bind and engulf antibody-coated particles 100 times more efficiently when these particles are also coated with activated complement components.[185] Confirmation of the existence of the properdin or alternative complement pathway has given rise to considerable speculation about the phylogenetic and evolutionary role of this series of enzymatic reactions. Quite logically, the alternative pathway may have preceded the classic pathway since the former seems a more premordial, "nonspecific" mechanism for the recognition of microbial pathogens in the absence of specific antibody.[186] The alternative pathway appears to have an important function in providing nonspecific opsonic support before the availability of the specific antibody.[171] While specific antibody provides the most rapid and efficient opsonization,[187] the myriad numbers of different microbial antigens make it quite unlikely that normal subjects will have natural antibodies to every potential pathogen. Activation of components of the alternative pathway seems to serve an antibody-like function leading toward the activation of C3b. In the initial encounter between host and microbe, the opsonization via the alternative pathway may be important for serum-resistant organisms in the absence of specific antibody. Not all organisms activate the alternative pathway efficiently[75,188,189] and thus require type-specific antibody for efficient opsonization. The absence of type-specific antibody could give rise to relative or absolute deficiencies in the opsonic activity of serum. The finding that some organisms such as *E. coli* or *K. pneumoniae* are not readily phagocytosed in the presence of even normal serum[189] and the further documentation that these strains do not efficiently activate the alternative complement pathway[72] give rise to speculation that the more virulent strains causing human gram-negative rod bacteremia may be restricted in their complement-activating properties.

After gram-negative bacillary infections or immunization with cell wall antigens, specific antibodies of the IgM and IgG classes appear in the circulation; additionally, IgG may be locally secreted. IgM is primarily intravascular, whereas IgG is widely distributed throughout the intra- and extravascular spaces. The relative protective roles of these antibodies have also differed depending on the assay system.[190,191] In in vitro studies using antibodies against *P. aeruginosa* and in opsonophagocytic and bactericidal assays, IgM antibodies were found to be more protective than IgG antibodies.[192] The opposite conclusion was derived from mouse passive protection experiments, that is, IgG antibodies were more protective. This led to the hypothesis that while IgM is more protective in the presence of complement the wider distribution of IgG is the basis for its superior protective activity because such antibodies are present not only in the intravascular space but extravascularly as well. In addition to the aspect of superior tissue distribution, such results may reflect the fact that murine hosts have immature complement systems and actually negligible serum complement activity as compared with nonhuman primates or humans.[193] Such an assay system would tend to overemphasize the activity of IgG antibodies relative to IgM.

Besides passive protection assays, many other techniques have been used to measure antibodies against gram-negative bacillary antigens.[182,190–192] If passive hemagglutination with human or ovine erythrocytes is used, primarily IgM activity is measured. When indirect fluorescent antibody measurements are used, both IgG and IgM antibodies have been associated with protection against shock and death in human infections.[191] It is clear that both IgM and IgG have opsonic and bactericidal activities, particularly in the presence of complement. Fresh serum from healthy patients is efficient in promoting uptake of *P. aeruginosa* by neutrophils. In normal fresh serum, 2-mercaptoethanol reduction, which destroys IgM activity, effectively abolishes the opsonic activity against most bacteremic strains of *P. aeruginosa*.[58]

Whatever the activities of IgM or IgG antibodies as measured by indirect techniques (e.g., hemagglutination, immunofluorescence), functional assays such as opsonophagocytic tests also implicate depressed levels of heat-stable opsonins (humoral factors such as IgG and IgM[55,180] near the onset of bacteremia. Further, there has been some correlation between low levels of these opsonins, the presence of circulating endotoxin-like activity, and poor clinical prognosis.[108]

Antibodies may also play a role on toxin neutralization. Whereas antibodies against O-specific polysaccharide and K antigens appear to have opsonic activity, those directed against the inner "core" regions of the gram-negative cell wall appear to have endotoxin-neutralizing or "antitoxic" capabilities.[94,95] The evidence for this stems from experiments in which the hemodynamic and pathophysiologic effects of injected bacterial endotoxins or live bacilli have been neutralized by antibodies directed against a core glycolipid antigen.[95] Confirmatory studies include the ability of such anti-core antibodies to prevent generalized and local Shwartzman reactions as well as the ability to abort the complications of DIC.[194–196] The protection has been demonstrated both actively and passively. Antibodies against whole bacterial cells (outer cell wall membrane) have the capability of promoting phagocytosis as well as aborting the pathophysiologic sequelae of gram-negative bacteremia.[95] Antibodies against the core regions (Rc, Re structure, lipid A) appear to function mainly by aborting endotoxic activity.

After gram-negative bacillary infection, the bulk of antibody response is directed to somatic (O) antigens, with smaller amounts of antibody directed against core glycolipid antigens.[14] There are many reports that anti-core antibodies appear to protect humans and animals against the sequelae of gram-negative bacteremia and appear to have a broad cross-protective activity.[14,94,95,197–201] In contrast, some investigators have not been able to discern a cross-protective effect for anti-core glycolipid antibodies,[202,203] and even those who find anti-Re antibodies to be protective find little protection with lipid A antibodies.[204] There is evidence from immunization studies in humans that the protective antibody against endotoxin core is IgM rather than IgG.[205] In addition, the failure to observe any cross-protective activity may be related to the nature of the challenge, that is, more heavily encapsulated organisms may not have rough antigenic determinants exposed for neutralization. The failure to find protection with lipid A antisera, even though lipid A appears to be the "toxic" moiety of LPS, suggests that KDO is the immunodominant component of the Re antigen and protective antibodies are best engendered when both KDO and lipid A are linked (as they occur naturally).

How core antibody may exert its cross-protective effect is suggested schematically in Figure 5. Antibody directed against the toxic or core portion of the LPS (e.g., Rc or Re antigen) molecule acts to neutralize a moiety common to most enteric bacilli in a manner analogous to a master key capable of fitting many locks. This protection seems less than type-specific (O antibody) protection and may be considerably less against the more encapsulated bacilli whose core regions are relatively less exposed.

Little information is available on the protective activity of antibodies directed against extracellular toxins such as the exotoxin A of *P. aeruginosa*. It seems clear that antibodies are synthesized in response to infection,[117,206] and in experimental settings such antibodies are protective.[116] Further, the simultaneous presence of antibodies against both exotoxins and somatic antigens may provide enhanced protective activity.[207]

In addition to specific and cross-reactive antibodies, there appear to be a variety of other humoral substances that have endotoxin binding properties, and they may be significant in host defense.[105] These include high-density lipoproteins,[208] serum inactivators of LPS,[106] serum esterases, α-globulins, and transferrin.[209] A specific endotoxin binding protein has been described[210] that has been purified and is protective in animal models. The availability of large quantitites of these materials produced by recombinant techniques may permit an assessment of their relative protective role.

Many patients with serious gram-negative infections, including bacteremia, are neutropenic, and it seems obvious that phagocytic and intraleukocytic microbicidal function is necessary to clear serum-resistant organisms from the blood stream and body fluids.

Except for a few relatively unusual genetic disorders of leukocyte microbicidal activity, impaired killing by phagocytic cells is rare. This does not exclude defects in leukocyte motility (either congenital or drug induced) that predispose to infection, and this has certainly been suggested by several reports.[211,212]

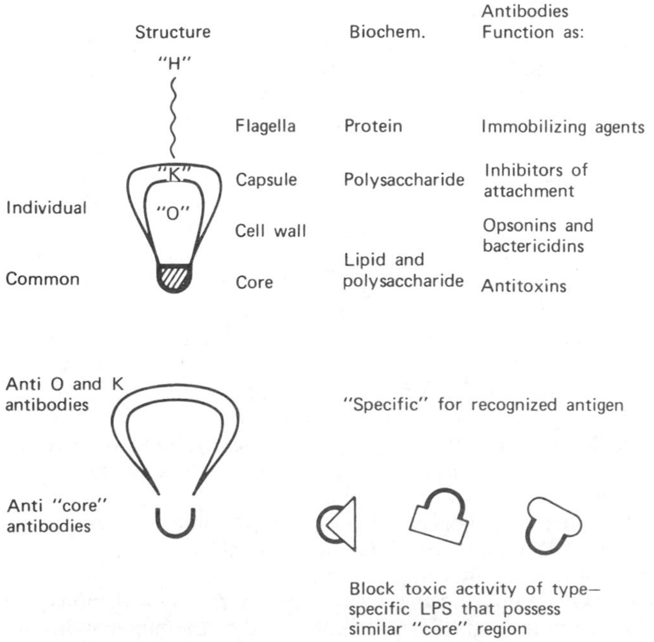

FIG. 5. Schema of the major cell wall antigens of gram-negative bacilli, their biochemical composition, and how antibodies directed against three antigens may function. Multiple functions are possible, that is, opsonin and antitoxin. O and K antibodies have limited specificities, while antibodies directed against the toxic "core" region cross react with most enteric bacilli.

DIAGNOSIS AND ANTIMICROBIAL THERAPY FOR GRAM-NEGATIVE ROD BACTEREMIA

Early clinical suspicion, rigorous diagnostic measures, aggressive initiation of appropriate antimicrobial therapy, comprehensive supportive care, and measures aimed at reversing predisposing causes are the cornerstones of successful management. While diagnostic microbiologic techniques are covered elsewhere in more detail, it is obvious that the clinical suspicion of bacteremia should be promptly confirmed by rapid identification and antimicrobial susceptibility testing of disease-causing organisms. Without confirmation of infection, the clinician will face the dilemma of whether or not to continue therapy with potentially toxic or sensitizing antimicrobial agents. Good liaison between the practicing clinician and the microbiology laboratory may be helpful in selecting methods for the rapid identification of causative organisms and for adjustment of antimicrobial therapy according to some initial biochemical reaction patterns even before the results of in vitro susceptibility tests are available.

In most hospitals it has become a common practice to use commercially available culture systems that aerobic and anaerobic bacterial growth. In untreated patients who are eventually shown to be bacteremic, the very first blood culture set that is taken will be positive more than 75 percent of the time, and the cumulative rate of positivity by the third blood culture set approaches 98 percent.[213] Further, recent analysis of the time interval to positivity of positive blood cultures indicates that for most gram-negative bacilli growth of microorganisms in blood culture bottles or on subcultures is revealed usually by 72 hours of incubation. The use of radiometric or lysis centrifugation techniques may result in even faster results. Thus, three sets of blood cultures and 3 days of careful observation have been sufficient to document of gram-negative bacteremia in more than 90 percent of previously untreated patients who are eventually shown to have blood stream infections.[79] Observation for signs of growth in blood culture bottles for periods of up to 10 days is still recommended for the detection of fastidious organisms or if the patient is receiving antimicrobials when the culture material was obtained.

The rapid isolation of some organisms poses special problems. *Pseudomonas aeruginosa* is an obligate aerobe and may not be rapidly detected just by the conventional technique of examining blood culture bottles for turbidity. One procedure that has been developed to enhance the detection of both aerobic and anaerobic sepsis is that of "blind" subculturing of apparently clear broth culture bottles. After incubation for 24 and 72 hours, blood culture bottles that are not turbid are nonetheless subcultured to aerobic and anaerobic media. The rationale for this approach is that as many as 10^5 organisms can be present and yet a broth suspension may appear to be clear. Particularly for *P. aeruginosa*, the subculture technique is advantagenous because the aerobic environment that the subcultured plates are incubated in supports more rapid, uninhibited growth.

Because of the occurrence of polymicrobial bacteremia in a significant number of cases, the blind subculture technique also permits the identification of variants of bacterial types (two types of the same species such as *E. coli*) as well as mixed cultures before there is overgrowth by one predominant component. In intra-abdominal sepsis, blind subcultures of both aerobic and anaerobic bottles may enhance the yield of multiple pathogens that are likely to be present.

Antimicrobial therapy remains the mainstay of treatment of gram-negative rod bacteremia, but approaches aimed at correcting the predisposition to this complication have a critical bearing on the outcome of the infection. Amelioration of an underlying disease such as achievement of remission in leukemia is usually the major factor determining recovery irrespective of the choice of antimicrobial agents. The removal of foreign bodies that predispose to or potentiate infection, such as intravascular or urinary catheters, may by themselves cause resolution of symptoms and lead to a cure. Transient gram-negative rod bacteremia is a well-documented event, particularly with urinary tract manipulation, and the latter accounts for a number of instances where bacteremic patients have been cured either with inappropriate antibiotics or with no antimicrobial therapy at all.[20,214] A major corollary of the latter observation is that attempts to drain abscesses or to remove obvious sources of infection such as obstructed abdominal viscera are of paramount importance in determining recovery. Antimicrobial sterilization of large abscesses seems futile, although it is possible that small foci of infection could be sterilized by aggressive antimicrobial therapy.

The focus of much of the clinical work in the area of gram-negative sepsis over the last decades has been placed on the evaluation of new antimicrobial agents. There have been relatively few well-controlled, comparative human clinical trials of the efficacy of new antimicrobial regimens as well as definitive studies of the adjunctive measures that have been advocated to support patients during complications of sepsis. Clearly, it is not possible to conduct clinical trials of antibacterial therapy vs. no therapy, but what is lacking are comparisons of the efficacy and toxicity of some of the popular therapeutic regimens.

An analysis of the status of host factors, the severity of underlying disease, and the outcome of gram-negative rod bacteremia has consistently demonstrated increasing mortality in patients with "nonfatal," "ultimately fatal," and "rapidly fatal" diseases.[7,24,66] The classification of underlying disease as proposed by McCabe and Jackson[7] and as modified by others[25] assumes critical importance in attempting to compare treatment results due to the heterogeneity of predisposing or underlying conditions. It is clearly unfair and unscientific to compare therapeutic results in patients with transient bacteremia secondary to a kidney stone (usually these are patients with nonfatal underlying disease) with results in patients developing bacteremia during chemotherapy for acute unremitting leukemia (the usual example of a rapidly fatal disease). Classifying patients with postsurgical or post-traumatic conditions is more difficult, but for the most part intra-abdominal infections complicating surgical procedures or traumatic injury occur in nonimmunosuppressed patients without obvious derangement in host defense mechanisms.

During the 1960s, several major published reports indicated that appropriate antimicrobial therapy (as defined by antimicrobials that inhibited the infecting strain) significantly reduced mortality in patients with nonfatal or ultimately fatal disease.[7,24] It was not possible, however, to show that appropriate antimicrobial therapy significantly improved the chances of recovery in patients with the most adverse host factors, namely, those with rapidly fatal diseases such as acute leukemia in relapse.[24,66] For instance, mortality in three combined series[7,24,215] for patients with rapidly fatal disease who were treated appropriately (the antimicrobial inhibited their infecting strain) was 84 percent vs. 85 percent for patients treated "inappropriately." In contrast, the results of studies carried out since 1968 in patients with cancer and neutropenia have shown a general overall improvement in clinical response rates.[66,216,217] Most of the studies of patients with neutropenia reported since 1968 show survival rates ranging from 40 to 85 percent, especially with some of the most potent modern treatment regimens.[16,17,217,218] There also appears to be some decrease in overall mortality if the series of gram-negative rod bacteremias summarized in Table 1 are viewed chronologically from the oldest to the more recent. Few of these studies, however, assessed the adequacy of therapy by determining whether adequate blood levels of antimicrobial agents were actually achieved in vivo. It should be further recalled that there have been no comparative studies of the relative clinical efficacy of antimicrobial agents available since 1968 and now widely used vs. agents that were commonly used to treat gram-negative infections before that date. The reason for selecting this temporal dividing point is that 1968–1969 marks the beginning (in the United States at least) of the availability of two groups of compounds with activities different from those previously available: both aminoglycosides and β-lactam compounds (broad-spectrum penicillins and cephalosporins) that are active against *P. aeruginosa, Enterobacter* species, indole-positive *Proteus* species, and *Serratia*.

Many factors besides the introduction of new antimicrobial agents could account for the improved therapeutic results observed in certain classes of patients or within the experience of a single institution. These factors would include more aggressive approaches to diagnosis and the initiation of treatment, overall improvements in supportive care, and many of the adjunctive measures detailed in subsequent sections of this chapter. Because of institutional and demographic differences, it seems most fair to assess trends within the experience of a single institution or single observers, and these in selected instances have shown a reduction in mortality.[19,20]

One attitude that has become widely prevalent in the therapeutic approaches to gram-negative rod infection, particularly in the critically ill, has been the willingness to begin empirical broad-spectrum therapy before the results of cultures are obtained.[219] This approach has inherent dangers such as the selection for antimicrobial resistance as well as the risk of drug toxicity. There are some patients with apparently intact host defenses in whom empirical therapy may not be indicated because there is adequate time to obtain material for culture and sensitivity testing. Nonetheless, one definite change in attitude in the last two decades in the approach to the critically ill patient with presumed infection has been to initiate empirical therapy with the intention of making subsequent therapeutic adjustments.

It is only logical that clinicians have used combinations of antimicrobial agents for serious gram-negative rod infections, particularly for those patients with the most adverse prognostic factors. The supporting arguments for combination therapy are multiple and not mutually exclusive: (*1*) Combination therapy makes it possible to cover a broad range of diagnostic possibilities including both gram-positive and gram-negative infection, which may be difficult to distinguish clinically. (*2*) Polymicrobial bacteremia may be present, so rather than being an "either/or" type of choice, the use of two agents may give appropriate therapy for dual infections. (*3*) The use of two agents may prevent the emergence of resistance by eliminating small subpopulations that are resistant to one of the components of the combination. (*4*) Two antimicrobials may interact either additively or synergistically, thus enhancing the sum of antimicrobial activity or (in the case of synergy) permitting a reduction in dosage of one component of the combination such as the agent that is more potentially toxic. While there is no universally accepted definition of antimicrobial synergy and in practice dosage reduction is not usually carried out, there has been considerable investigative interest in determining whether the use of so-called synergistic combinations is associated with improved clinical results in humans.

The role of synergy between antimicrobial agents used to treat bacillary infections has been difficult to assess because of the problems in initiating randomized, prospective human clinical trials comparing the results of synergistic with nonsynergistic combinations. Experimental studies in animals with normal circulating granulocyte counts or in those rendered neutropenic have shown that use of synergistic combinations leads to a more favorable outcome in *P. aeruginosa* infections.[220–222] Several human studies have shown an association between the use of combinations that interact synergistically against infecting strains and improved clinical results.[214,223] In one study, an association was noted between the use of synergistic combinations and improved clinical results in the face of adverse clinical factors such as neutropenia, rapidly fatal underlying disease, and shock.[214] Because multiple agents are usually given on different dosage schedules, it has been difficult to ensure that the drug concentrations that are achieved in vivo reflect test concentrations used in in vitro studies. The finding of serum inhibitory titers by one group equal to or exceeding 1:8 has been associated with favorable clinical outcome.[224] Still, it is possible that good clinical results obtained when using combinations of antimicrobial agents may not be related to synergistic interactions. For instance, with such commonly used agents as aminoglycosides and penicillins, which often interact synergistically in vitro, "peak" blood levels that are used to gauge in vitro susceptibility are actually maintained for rather short periods of time followed by periods of rapid "decay." The use of a broad-spectrum penicillin with an aminoglycoside may merely ensure a more sustained interval of serum inhibitory or bactericidal activity or may avoid too low "trough" levels of such activity. Some investigators believe the latter is a cause of treatment failure and have given continuous infusions of antibiotics to maintain a "constant" blood level.[225] However, it is still unclear whether continuous vs. intermittent administration of antimicrobial agents is superior for a variety of infectious conditions. Factors such as tissue penetration, protein binding, rapidity of killing, and postantibiotic effects are likely to influence the outcome as well as the timing and duration of drug infusion. For critically ill patients with septicemia it is implicit that the administration of all pharmacologic agents should be via the intravenous route.

In selecting antimicrobial therapy, the severity of the underlying disease and the possibility of synergistic interactions are still important considerations. Table 8 summarizes recommendations for initial empirical therapy for presumed gram-negative rod bacteremia. First- and second-generation cephalosporins alone may be justified for community-acquired bacteremia secondary to urinary tract infection in the non-neutropenic host where *E. coli* and *Klebsiella* are the main concerns. For the patient with nosocomial infection, initial therapy should consist of an aminoglycoside initially paired with a β-lactam agent. Preference is expressed for a cephalosporin as the β-lactam agent in the non-neutropenic patient because of the greater likelihood of *Klebsiella* vs. *P. aeruginosa*. The regimen of an aminoglycoside paired with a penicillin or cephalosporin having antipseudomonal activity is preferred for the neutropenic patient, the patient receiving assisted ventilation, or the patient with an extensive burn injury.

Amikacin and netilmicin are semisynthetic aminoglycosides that are less susceptible to attack by bacterial exoenzymes known to inactivate gentamicin and tobramycin.[226] Consideration of these as primary therapy in presumed gram-negative rod bacteremia should be based on the prevalence of resistance to gentamicin or to tobramycin in the institution or on the likelihood of resistance in high-risk patients such as those with neutropenia or thermal injury. If organisms are equally susceptible to all aminoglycosides and adequate therapeutic levels are achieved, the clinical results are likely to be similar. Recommended doses of gentamicin, tobramycin, or netilmicin are 1.7 mg/kg q8h and for amikacin either 5 mg/kg q8h or 7.5 mg/kg q12h. The carbenicillin dose should probably be on the order of 70 mg/kg intravenously q4h with a total dose limited to 36 g/day. More potent semisynthetic penicillins like ticarcillin, mezlocillin, azlocillin, and piperacillin may be given in doses varying from 40 mg/kg q4h to 60 mg/kg q6h.

The third-generation cephalosporins, related β-lactam agents like moxalactam, carbapenems like imipenem, and monobactam agents like aztreonam have markedly augmented activity against enteric bacteria but variable bactericidal effect against *P. aeruginosa*. The potency of cefotaxime, ceftizoxime, and moxalactam against *E coli* and *Klebsiella* (minimum inhibitory concentrations [MICs], often 0.5 μg/ml or less with achievable blood levels 100-fold or more higher) suggests that single-agent therapy directed against those bacteria may be quite successful even in severely compromised hosts. In contrast, resistance among *Pseudomonas, Serratia*, and *Enterobacter* species may emerge rapidly on monotherapy. Ceftazidime and cefsulodin appear most active against *P. aeruginosa*, but the latter is only active against *Pseudomonas*. Clinical trials in which third-generation cephalosporins are combined with an aminoglycoside show results similar to penicillin/aminoglycoside combinations.[227] Monotherapeutic regimens (e.g., ceftazidime, imipenem, or intravenous quinolones) may be effective for fevers of undetermined origin in neutropenic patients and for documented infections due to highly susceptible gram-negative bacteria.[218] However, successful treatment for bacteremic patients with profound persistent neutropenia (e.g., neutrophil counts less than 100/μl) still appears to be linked to the use of two agents that inhibit the infecting strain (irrespective of synergistic interactions.[16,228] In view of excellent responses associated with the initial use of combination therapy it still seems prudent to begin treatment of the critically ill patient with two agents that are likely to be active[216,217] and to modify treatment on the basis of antibiotic susceptibility test results and changes in the status of the host.

There is no evidence that a three-drug regimen, for example, aminoglycoside/penicillin/cephalosporin, is superior to an aminoglycoside/β-lactam combination.[229] Combining bactericidal with bacteristatic agents is generally avoided because some clinical evidence argues against their combined use.

Clinicians should not assume that the administration of apparently adequate doses of antimicrobial agents consistently ensures therapeutic levels. Aminoglycosides have a marrow therapeutic ratio, and there is marked individual variability in the individual peak blood levels of gentamicin.[230] Studies of patients with recurrent or breakthrough bacteremia have indicated an association with subinhibitory blood levels of agents such as gentamicin.[231] In view of the variations in blood pharmacokinetics of aminoglycosides, it would seem prudent in the critically ill patients to monitor blood levels frequently. There is some evidence that such monitoring may also avert potentially toxic complications.[232] The measurement of aminoglycoside blood levels is usually not indicated in patients with bacteremia from the genitourinary tract inasmuch as the levels of many agents excreted in the urine are high. The average duration of treatment in normal hosts experiencing gram-negative sepsis is 10–14 days, but this may be longer if the patient has persistent infection at the source of bacteremia. Treatment of the neutropenic or immunocompromised patient may require an even longer duration. Patients in the latter group should be afebrile for a minimum of 4–7 days and have evidence of resolving infection at the source of bacteremia, and the neutrophil count should be rising and in excess of 500/μl before drug ther-

TABLE 8. Recommended Antimicrobial Regimens for Empirical (Presumptive) Therapy for Gram-Negative Rod Bacteremia

1. Community-acquired infection in the non-neutropenic subject (neutrophil count ≥1000/mm³)
   a. Suspected urinary tract source: ampicillin plus an aminoglycoside
   b. Nonurinary tract source: a third-generation cephalosporin plus/minus an aminoglycoside
2. Hospital-acquired infection, non-neutropenic subject: a third-generation cephalosporin plus an aminoglycoside
3. Neutropenic patient with hospital-acquired infection: antipseudomonal penicillin plus an aminoglycoside or a third-generation cephalosporin plus an aminoglycoside
4. Thermal injury to at least 20 percent of the body surface area: same as 3
5. Pulmonary source associated with inhalation therapy equipment: same as 3
6. Established or suspected gentamicin resistance: use amikacin as the aminoglycoside
7. Nosocomial infection in the setting of resistance to penicillins and cephalosporins: imipenem plus/minus an aminoglycoside

apy is stopped. The exception to this guideline would be patients with marrow failure syndromes who are unlikely to generate white counts as high as 500/μl; in these subjects clinical defervescence alone should suffice.

Oral therapy is ill advised for the bacteremic patient with fever, hemodynamic instability, and factors that might limit absorption of antimicrobial agents from the gut. On the other hand, a change to an effective oral agent (as determined by in vitro testing) is often justified after defervescence if the patient's overall condition is improving. Potentially useful agents include the quinolones, oral cephalosporins or penicillins, and trimethoprim-sulfamethoxazole.

ADJUNCTIVE MEASURES IN THERAPY FOR GRAM-NEGATIVE ROD BACTEREMIA

Maintenance of Adequate Tissue Perfusion with Volume Replacement

Management of fluid and electrolyte balance is a crucial aspect of the care of the patient with gram-negative bacteremia, particularly the person whose course is complicated by shock. Perfusion of vital organs such as the brain and kidney must be maintained. It is clear that the body has an order of priorities that result in distribution of blood preferentially to vital organs; this causes splanchnic vasoconstriction as well as a marked reduction of circulation to the skin. When these compensatory changes are inadequate to maintain adequate perfusion, central arterial pressures will fall. The first goal of management of the patient with bacteremia, particularly in the incipient stages of shock, is adequate monitoring of vital signs so that any hemodynamic changes can be readily counteracted. Insertion of a central venous pressure monitoring device, an arterial catheter, and Swan-Ganz catheters to determine the left atrial end-diastolic pressure are useful measures in the critically ill patient, although it is clear that they present certain infection hazards per se. These monitoring devices are not used to determine optimal therapy but rather the limits of therapy. In other words, normal or low central venous pressure and left atrial end-diastolic pressures (pulmonary wedge pressures) in the presence of a declining systemic arterial blood pressure are an indication for further volume replacement. On the other hand, it is clear that these parameters may rise to dangerously elevated levels without being able to restore adequate arterial perfusion. In the presence of cardiac failure, cautious digitalization with a rapidly acting intravenous digitalis preparation is indicated. Digitalis toxicity may be manifested at relatively lower doses of digitalis in septic shock, and this risk is further enhanced by the administrator of sympathomimetic amines.

There are a number of solutions that can be used to expand intravascular fluid volume and colloid oncotic pressure, including fresh frozen plasma, albumin of the regular type or salt depleted, and various dextran preparations. If the patient is anemic, thrombocytopenic, as well as hypotensive, the transfusion of whole blood in the face of a low central venous pressure is justified. If there is no need for erythrocytes, one of the plasma fractions will suffice. With evidence for bleeding and consumption coagulopathy, the use of fresh frozen plasma may be indicated. There has been a tendency to avoid dextran preparations because of an association with hemorrhagic tendencies. Other authorities have preferred to use crystalloid solutions in preference to colloid.[233]

Use of Sympathomimetic Amines

Sympathomimetic amines have been widely used to treat the hemodynamic complications of shock, but there have been no controlled or comparative studies of the efficacy of different compounds. For many years norepinephrine and epinephrine were the principal agents available. Norepinephrine has intense peripheral vasoconstricting activity, and extravasation around iv infusion sites has led to ischemic necrosis of tissues. There is justifiable concern that its use compromises the perfusion of vital organs. Both norepinephrine and epinephrine increase myocardial irritability. Alternative agents like isoproterenol, dopamine, and dobutamine have largely supplanted norepinephrine. They have an inotropic effect on myocardial function but because of β-adrenergic activity are capable of enhancing peripheral tissue perfusion. Isoproterenol increases the cardiac index but has little effect on mean arterial pressure.[234] Dopamine causes vasodilatation of renal, coronary, and cerebral blood flow while causing an increase in systolic blood pressure and heart rate and an effective reduction in the blood supplied to skeletal muscle. Dobutamine has little chronotropic activity and is otherwise quite similar to dopamine. Presently norepinephrine should be reserved only for those patients in whom it is not possible to support systemic blood pressure and vascular perfusion with dopamine or isoproterenol. Table 9 is a summary of recommended doses and techniques for administering sympathomimetic amines.

Sympathomimetic agents have a wide range of effects, particularly on pulmonary airway passages, regulation of blood sugar, and so forth. None of these considerations is as important as perfusion of vital organs during septic shock. Perhaps the critical factor that is often neglected in the management of patients with sympathomimetic amines is the relationship between fluid therapy and the use of these agents. It is inappropriate to use dopamine and isoproterenol before aggressive volume replacement. If they are used in the presence of a reduced intravascular fluid volume, the vasodilatation secondary to β-adrenergic stimulation can cause a paradoxical decline in blood pressure and decreased tissue perfusion because of the sudden drop in effective intravascular volume. Because of this danger, constant monitoring of central venous pressure and pulmonary wedge pressure is indicated; some authors advocate fluid replacement to the point that either or both of the latter begin to rise to the upper limits of normal. At that juncture it would be appropriate to use an agent such as dopamine, dobutamine, or isoproterenol if the patient remains hypotensive.

In spite of volume replacement, digitalization, and sympathomimetic amine administration, significant metabolic acidosis may ensue. While primary efforts should still be aimed at enhancing tissue perfusion, temporary correction of acidosis may be achieved with infusions of sodium bicarbonate.

Role of Corticosteroids in the Treatment of Gram-Negative Rod Septicemia and Its Complications

Since the clinical availability of corticosteroids, there has been controversy over their effectiveness as adjunctive therapy in the management of infection. Corticosteroids have a variety of metabolic, anti-inflammatory, and immunosuppressive effects, and it is commonly observed that the short-term administration often results in defervescence, thus leading to a clinical impression of improvement. Weitzman and Berger emphasized the

TABLE 9. Sympathomimetic Amines for Support of the Circulation in Septic Shock

Listed in order of preference, to be used after volume replacement and with careful ECG, CVP, and BP monitoring:

1. Dopamine, 2–25 μg/kg/min: increase the rate of infusion (D_5W or saline) q15–20 min until systolic blood pressure exceeds 90 mmHg and the urine output exceeds 30 ml/hr
2. Dobutamine, 2–25 μg/kg/min: titrate as with dopamine
3. Isoproterenol, 5 μg/ml/min: observe the effect within 15–25 min and double the rate of infusion if necessary
4. Norepinephrine: give a test dose of 0.1–0.2 μg/kg and observe the response (usually in minutes). The normal maintenance dose is 0.05 μg/kg/min delivered via a plastic catheter into a large peripheral or central vein

Abbreviations: ECG: electrocardiographic; CVP: central venous pressure; BP: blood pressure; D_5W: 5% dextrose in water.

lack of convincing evidence from controlled studies that corticosteroids accelerate the rate of recovery or lower mortality from sepsis.[235] Nonetheless, there has been widespread belief that corticosteroids are beneficial as adjunctive therapy in gram-negative infections, particularly those complicated by shock. Much of the belief is derived from animal studies wherein healthy experimental subjects of varying susceptibility to the effects of bacterial endotoxin were given large doses of these substances to induce shock. Such doses are questionably associated with the pathogenesis of the complications of shock in humans. Furthermore, the animals used in such studies have almost always been immunologically intact or physiologically normal before the induction of shock.

One of the major issues relating to the efficacy of corticosteroids in human sepsis complicated by shock has been that of dosage. Since relatively low doses (up to 1 mg/kg betamethasone or roughly 25–30 mg/kg equivalent of hydrocortisone) were used in one well-controlled, prospective study[236] and showed no beneficial effect, advocates of corticosteroid therapy have escalated their recommendations so that one study reported a beneficial effect of corticosteroids in doses of 30 mg/kg of methylprednisolone or 2 mg/kg of dexamethasone.[237] Doses in this range were found to improve survival in one controlled clinical trial in patients with typhoid fever.[238] Another comparative study found that large doses of corticosteroids (2 g methylprednisolone for the 70 kg patient) actually reversed septic shock in a significant number of patients. While a transient, "early" effect in increased survival was noted, mortality at the conclusion of the study was similar in both groups, and steroid recipients had a higher incidence of superinfection.[239] Despite these aforementioned studies, however, the largest and most comprehensive, controlled clinical trials in the United States have failed to confirm the beneficial effect of corticosteroids in septic shock. This conclusion was reached in the final report of a multicenter collaborative trial involving the Veterans Administration Hospitals[240] and a multihospital collaborative group[241] involving some of the same investigators who earlier had noted a beneficial effect.[239] Additionally, two other controlled human trials employed similar doses of corticosteroids for ARDS patients and obtained negative results.[242,243] In view of these findings, large doses of prednisone/prednisolone/dexamethasone cannot be recommended as adjunctive therapy for sepsis or shock. Replacement doses of corticosteroids are clearly justified in suspected adrenal insufficiency.

Anticoagulation

The use of anticoagulation, particularly heparinization, to treat septicemic states associated with DIC is logical because there is strong experimental and human clinical evidence that coagulopathy can be terminated by heparinization. At present, however, it is unclear whether anticoagulation has any effect in prolonging survival, however desirable it may be to abolish the sequence of events leading to clotting, consumption of clotting factors, and the onset or aggravation of bleeding. In both human and experimental studies the use of agents such as heparin has failed to significantly decrease the mortality from bacteremic gram-negative infections.[244,245] In human infection the failure to show a difference may be related to the overall poor prognosis of the underlying disease that is complicated by bacteremia. Until it can be shown that a reduction in mortality is consistent, the use of routine anticoagulation in the management of patients with DIC should be avoided. This is particularly true for normotensive people. If bleeding in such patients is associated with depressed levels of platelets or a specific factor, replacement therapy may be required to control the hemorrhage.

For hypotensive septicemic patients, measures aimed at controlling the infection and correcting hemodynamic alterations (volume replacement and sympathomimetic amines) are of primary importance. If the blood pressure responds to such measures (an effect is usually observed within 4 hours), consumption coagulopathy will usually cease. If the patient has bleeding because of the coagulopathy and not from another cause such as an associated gastrointestinal ulcer, replacement therapy is indicated. This should consist of platelet transfusions for thrombocytopenia, cryoprecipitate preparations for hypofibrinogenemia, and fresh frozen plasma for depleted coagulation factors. While this approach theoretically could aggravate coagulopathy by providing additional substrate for clotting, this complication is not commonly observed when replacement therapy is used in conjunction with measures aimed at controlling shock and infection.[149]

For patients with refractory shock and coagulopathy in spite of the preceding measures, heparin therapy may be beneficial in terminating DIC (without evidence that this prolongs life). Other patients who should be considered for anticoagulation are those who appear to have pulmonary embolic phenomena. This includes patients with pelvic thrombophlebitis. Heparin may be given by either intermittent or continuous infusion. The dose for intermittent infusion is 50–100 units/kg of aqueous heparin given by bolus infusion every 4 hours. For continuous infusion the recommended dose of heparin in adult therapy is 10,000 units made up in 500 ml of 5% dextrose in water (D_5W) delivered over a period of approximately 4–6 hours. Since reversal of coagulation tendencies has an immediate effect, it would appear judicious to terminate therapy as soon as possible after the subsidence of fever. Other anticoagulants such as coumadin-type drugs have been shown in experimental model systems to obviate some of the manifestations of endotoxemia such as generalized Shwartzman reaction. On the other hand, there appears to be little indication for coumadin in gram-negative sepsis in view of the slow onset of the defect. Heparin is preferable, and prolonged anticoagulation should be avoided.

Therapeutic Role of Granulocyte Transfusion

Transfusion of granulocytes is a logical strategy to counteract the functional or absolute neutropenia present in many patients who develop gram-negative rod bacteremia. The rationale and techniques for granulocyte transfusion therapy are discussed elsewhere (Chapter 7).

At least four controlled studies have suggested that there may be a benefit for transfused subjects evaluated with regard to short-term survival and resolution of fever.[246–249] Unfortunately, these studies were small, and the nature of both the underlying infection and type of antimicrobial therapy was often unclear. Subsequently, a much larger study randomizing patients with documented gram-negative bacteremia to receive or not to receive neutrophil transfusions showed no difference in recovery rates or survival, even in the subset of patients without evidence of bone marrow recovery.[250] Survival was quite good in the control group as compared with previous studies, and this may have been due to better antimicrobial therapy. The complications of white cell transfusion, particularly viral infections and pulmonary complications, plus the outcome of this more recent study should discourage routine granulocyte transfusions in septicemic, neutropenic patients if appropriate antimicrobial therapy is given. Recent granulocyte transfusion studies have delivered small numbers of neutrophils relative to the normal daily production and the anticipated granulocyte "requirement" in the face of infection.[251] Thus it is conceivable that improvements in techniques for procuring granulocytes so that much larger numbers of cells may be given safely could improve the efficacy of the approach. Presently, it appears that patients who are most likely to benefit from white cell transfusions are those with the potentially reversible defect in granulocyte production such as transient bone marrow aplasia or a neoplastic disorder where there is evidence for an early remission. If appropriate antimicrobial therapy fails in this setting, then granulocyte transfusions might be considered. Candidates least likely to benefit from transfusions are patients who have had multiple courses of unsuccessful therapy for refractory underlying disease such as marrow aplasia or acute leukemia.

Diuretics

Diuretics are commonly used in the management of the early oliguric or anuric phases of bacteremic shock. The use of agents such as furosemide or ethacrynic acid is controversial, however, since there is no controlled study demonstrating that acute renal failure may be avoided by the aggressive use of such agents. The action of potent loop diuretics such as furosemide or ethacrynic acid usually results in a significant increase in the output of dilute urine, but it is unclear whether the aggressive use of diuretics in the early oliguric phases of shock makes the ensuing renal failure less severe. What has been observed is that some of these agents, including both ethacrynic acid and furosemide, may cause deafness and there may be enhanced toxicity when these agents are simultaneously used with agents that can damage eighth nerve or renal function such as aminoglycoside antibiotics. In view of these effects it seems prudent to monitor the patient's vital signs and central venous or left atrial pressure and to use diuretics only when volume expansion is not adequate to maintain urine output.

Other Pharmacologic Agents Used to Treat Patients in Septic Shock

Naloxone, an antagonist of opiates and β-endorphins, has been shown to reverse the course of endotoxic and hypovolemic shock in experimental animals.[252–253] In a small study of humans with prolonged hypotension, an intravenous dose of 0.4–1.2 mg of naloxone resulted in a 45 percent increase in systolic blood pressure that lasted at least 45 minutes.[254] Before naloxone infusion, patients had been treated with fluids, dopamine, and appropriate antibiotics. Nonresponders were subjects who had previously been treated with corticosteroids or phenothiazines. Thus, it appears that naloxone has a transient pressor effect in human shock with the added appeal of no immunosuppressive complications (unlike corticosteroids). However, a small controlled study of naloxone therapy in gram-negative infections complicated by shock failed to demonstrate any benefit.[255]

A wide variety of pharmacologic agents including phenothiazines, antihistamines, anti-inflammatory agents such as indomethacin and phenylbultazone, glucagon, α-adrenergic blocking agents, and vasodilators have been used experimentally as adjunctive therapy for septic shock complicating gram-negative infections. Among the more interesting recent observations is the finding that cyclooxygenase inhibitors can inhibit the effects of TNF.[141,143] Other pharmacologic agents such as pentoxyphylline can inhibit the effect of TNF on neutrophils.[256] However, no controlled studies support the clinical use of any of these pharmacologic agents in humans.

THERAPEUTIC ANTISERUM IN GRAM-NEGATIVE SEPSIS

The use of antiserum to treat bacterial infections antedates the antimicrobial era, but was all but abandoned more than four decades ago. Resurgent interest in the therapeutic applications of antibody stems for the persistently high mortality associated with sepsis often complicated by shock in spite of the use of appropriate antimicrobials. There have been anecdotal reports of the successful use of convalescent serum for *P. aeruginosa* bacteremia[257] or *Pseudomonas* immune globulin in surgical patients,[258] but the latter study was uncontrolled. More recently, Ziegler and associates reported the results of a large multicenter, double-blind trial of therapeutic antiserum prepared by immunizing donors with the "J5" mutant of *E. coli* 0111 (a "rough mutant" with an endotoxin core analogous to an Rc mutant). Mortality was 22 percent in 103 bacteremic recipients of antiserum as opposed to 39 percent in 109 subjects randomized to control serum therapy.[201] An even more significant difference was noted in the ability of antiserum to reverse profound shock. Therapeutic antiserum did not, however, significantly affect survival in patients with cancer and/or neutropenia, and no protective antibody titer or level could be inferred. The encouraging results of Ziegler's group have spurred efforts to prepare human antiserum by active immunization with other core endotoxin antigens,[257] harvest IgG antibodies from high-titer human serum lots and modify them for intravenous use,[260] and produce monoclonal antibodies of murine[199,261] or human origin.[200] A clinical trial of intravenous IgG was unsuccessful, possibly because of low titer or because IgG antibodies are not protective.[205] Murine monoclonals of IgM isotype have been produced that can abrogate the effect of endotoxins and can increase survival above that obtained with antimicrobial therapy.[199,261] Human clinical trials with these antibodies indicate that they are generally well tolerated.[262] It is possible that their benefit may derive from their action on endotoxins liberated during the course of antimicrobial therapy, as has been documented by some investigators.[263] Greater species compatibility and fewer hypersensitivity reactions may be anticipated with the use of human monoclonal antibodies than have been described to date.[200,264] Clinical trials to critically assess these concepts are now underway.

PROPHYLAXIS OF GRAM-NEGATIVE ROD BACTEREMIA

Measures to prevent gram-negative rod bacteremia have ranged from meticulous efforts aimed at limiting the spread of infection within the hospital, the use of prophylactic antimicrobial agents of a topical or systemic form, management of high-risk patients in so-called protective environments, active or passive immunoprophylaxis with type-specific or cross-reactive antibodies, and augmentation of the host granulocyte pool with prophylactic granulocyte transfusions. These measures have been applied to patients with different underlying diseases of varying degrees of severity. The validity of many of these approaches has not been rigorously tested in controlled studies in humans.

It seems reasonable that the simplest and most cost-effective measures for the prophylaxis of gram-negative bacillary infections would involve minimizing the infection hazard associated with such procedures as Foley catheterizations and prolonged intravascular catheterization. The value of antimicrobial prophylaxis of either a topical or systemic nature is highly controversial, but there is emerging evidence that it may be beneficial in certain well-defined circumstances.

Logical applications of antimicrobial prophylaxis include topical application to the skin, the use of an oropharyngeal spray, and orally ingested nonabsorbable antibiotics to suppress the fecal flora. The application of topical agents like silver nitrate, silver sulfadiazine, or sulfamylon to burned skin appears to have significantly reduced the incidence of burn wound sepsis caused by organisms like *P. aeruginosa*[265] The application of a polymyxin spray to the posterior portion of the pharynx appears to have limited gram-negative bacillary colonization of the oropharynx and prevented some cases of nosocomial gram-negative pneumonia.[266] However, such efforts offer the potential hazard of selecting for the emergence of organisms resistant to the prophylactic agent, as has been amply documented with the use of polymyxin sprays.[267]

Since the gastrointestinal tract is a vast reservoir of gram-negative bacilli, an essentially topical approach to prophylaxis is the use of oral nonabsorbable antimicrobial agents. Sterilization of bowel contents is unrealistic, but suppression of the aerobic fecal flora has been achieved to varying degrees with regimens that use polymyxin[268] or gentamicin[269] normally with vancomycin and nystatin. Randomized studies have shown a significant reduction in bacterial sepsis in neutropenic subjects given a polymyxin-containing regimen as compared with placebo.[268] The efficacy of gentamicin-vancomycin-nystatin has been assessed in a three-arm study with management of neutropenic patients in "protected environments" with laminar airflow and under regular ward care.[269] The reduction in infection was similar for both groups receiving oral antimicrobials and was not significantly greater for those additionally managed in laminar airflow rooms.

Regimens containing oral nonabsorbable agents are unpalatable, and patient compliance has been variable. Better-tolerated alternatives include trimethoprim-sulfamethoxazole[270,271] and the newer quinolones. Trimethoprim-sulfamethoxazole has been used to prevent both *Pneumocystis carinii* pneumonia and bacterial infection. Unfortunately, it has no effect against *P. aeruginosa* and may predispose to superinfection with fungi and resistant bacilli. Recent studies suggest a significant reduction in gram-negative infections occurring in neutropenic patients given prophylactic norfloxacin[272] or ciprofloxacin.[273]

AUGMENTATION OF HOST DEFENSES: PROPHYLACTIC GRANULOCYTE TRANSFUSIONS AND IMMUNOPROPHYLAXIS

Patients about to receive intense cytotoxic therapy for leukemia or marrow transplants have been considered candidates for prophylactic white cell transfusions. Although one report was favorable to this approach,[274] a large multicentered study clearly pointed out the dangers associated with prophylactic transfusion.[275] Some studies have shown a reduction in the incidence of gram-negative infections,[274,275] but this was offset by a high incidence of pulmonary complications in the transfused recipients.[275,276] Many of the lung infiltrates were probably due to cytomegalovirus infections. Perhaps most important, there has been no evidence of increased survival in any group receiving daily prophylactic transfusions and having a high incidence of sensitization. In the absence of better methods for reducing complications such as sensitization[277] and transfusion-associated viral infections, there are no indications of prophylactic transfusions outside of an investigative setting.

Augmentation of levels of circulating granulocytes will correct only one component of altered host defenses in the immunosuppressed person. Deficiencies in the levels of circulating immunoglogulins or opsonins might be anticipated in such a person.[55,180] A study of the efficacy of transfused granulocytes demonstrated that therapeutic failures were associated with deficiencies in humoral opsonins.[278] These findings suggest a need to supplement both phagocytes and opsonic factors (including antibody) in the prophylaxis of serious infections in the immunosuppressed host.

With respect to the feasibility of immunoprophylaxis in the prevention of gram-negative bacteremia, the impetus for this approach is the convincing evidence that some bacterial infections can be prevented by active or passive immunization with either cell wall components of certain bacteria or toxoid preparations of extracellular toxins. Particularly with toxoid immunization, as in the case of tetanus, immunity appears to be lifelong. With some of the polysaccharide bacterial vaccines there is evidence that active immunization prevents disease in immunodeficient patients.[279]

Evidence that initial titers of circulating antibodies against either type-specific, cross-reacting, or exotoxin antigens of gram-negative bacilli provide some protection against shock and death in bacteremic human infections raises the possibility that even in states of altered immunity it may be possible to enhance host resistance against certain gram-negative infections.[14,191,207] One of the major obstacles to the development of immunizing preparations has been the multiplicity of somatic antigens of gram-negative organisms. The fact that more than 160 serotypes of *E. coli* and 80 serotypes of *K. pneumoniae* have been identified makes a somatic antigen preparation based on those known antigenic types somewhat akin to trying to develop the vaccine for the common cold. On the other hand, it is true that perhaps 10 serotypes of *E. coli* account for 60 percent of bacteremic coliform infections.[280] It has been demonstrated that with *P. aeruginosa*, one of the most common pathogens in the neutropenic host, approximately seven somatic antigens account for 90 percent of the bacteremic infections.[281] Immunization of experimental animals or healthy people with a *Pseudomonas* LPS vaccine has led to some augmentation of circulating antibody levels against these seven LPS antigens.[180] Some evidence exists, from the study of patients with burn injuries, that this vaccine is protective, but definitive double-blind controlled studies are lacking.[282] Other *Pseudomonas* LPS antigens have been used in controlled studies in burn patients and the results have been significantly in favor of immunization.[283] A randomized, prospective study of *Pseudomonas* immunization in cancer patients showed some overall reduction in *Pseudomonas* infections as well as *Pseudomonas*-associated mortality but no significant reduction in bacteremic *P. aeruginosa* infections.[180] An analysis of the results of that study indicated that many immunosuppressed cancer patients failed to show a significant antibody response to vaccine antigens and that in those who did manifest a significant humoral antibody response elevated antibody titers were short-lived. Most of the *P. aeruginosa* infections that were subsequently documented in the vaccinated or control group were associated not only with neutropenia but also with low levels of circulating opsonizing antibodies against the patient's infecting strains. Thus, it appears that immunization alone is not likely to be successful in the prevention of gram-negative bacteremia in markedly immunosuppressed patients, particularly those who are neutropenic. On the other hand, immunization may provide opsonic support for the function of phagocytic cells, and measures other than active immunization, that is, passive immunization, would be more promising, particularly in those neutropenic subjects who receive granulocyte transfusions. Combined immunization and granulocyte transfusion therapy has been shown to be beneficial in animal model systems.[284] Since infused granulocytes are short-lived and most passive immunization is with IgG preparations (Cohn's fraction II) the administration of passive antibody will require new developments such as stable, nonaggregated immunoglobulins that can be given intravenously.

Interest in the so-called core or cross-reactive antigens of the outer cell wall membrane of enteric bacteria stems from the fact that most Enterobacteriaceae share a common core region that this common core region contains an antigen, lipid A, that is responsible for the properties of "endotoxicity." Evidence from human serologic studies and from experimentally produced infections suggests that antibodies directed against core antigens are protective and that such an immunogen would be more versatile than type-specific antigens.[13,96,191,259]

Antibodies directed against the Re and Rc antigenic determinants would appear to have antitoxin activity (endotoxin neutralizing) and possibly activity as opsonins. From the animal studies, however, one would not anticipate a degree of protection as complete as that observed with O antigen immunization. Baumgartner and colleagues have presented evidence from a controlled clinical trial that J5 antiserum produced in human volunteers (similar to the material studied by Ziegler et al.[201]) prevented gram-negative shock and death.[285] In contrast, the use of a single dose of similar product was ineffective in preventing bacteremic gram-negative infections in patients with prolonged neutropenia.[286] Other prophylactic studies now underway have used pooled immune IgG that has been modified for intravenous use.

The possibility that exposure to "avirulent" organisms that share antigens with disease-causing bacteria might be a feasible technique for engendering active immunity has been assessed experimentally and in healthy people. Human volunteers fed live *E. coli* possessing the K-100 capsular antigen develop circulatory antibodies to the apparently identical *H. influenzae* type B antigen.[287] From the viewpoint of active immunization in the altered host such an approach may face the risk of causing active disease secondary to a live immunogen. It has been shown that there are a number of cross-reactions between antigens contained in the licensed (in the United States) pneumococcal polysaccharide vaccines and the capsular or cell wall antigens of *E. coli* and *Klebsiella*. Antecedent polysaccharide administration has been shown to protect against death from experimental *E. coli* and *Klebsiella* infections, and the administration of the purified antigens could have an effect on the incidence of some gram-negative bacillary infections.[288]

REFERENCES

1. Kwaan HM, Weil MH. Differences in the mechanism of shock caused by bacterial infections. Surg Gynecol Obstet. 1969;128:37.
2. Brill NE, Libman E. Pyocaneus bacillaemia. Am J Med Sci. 1899;118:153.
3. Felty AR, Keefer CS. *Bacillus coli* sepsis. Clinical study of 28 cases of bloodstream invasion by colon bacillus. JAMA. 1924;82:1430.
4. Waisbren BA. Bacteremia due to gram-negative bacilli other than the *Salmonella*. A clinical and therapeutic study. Arch Intern Med. 1951;88:467.
5. Rogers DE. The changing pattern of life-threatening microbial disease. N Engl J Med. 1959;261:677
6. Finland M, Jones WF Jr, Barnes MW. Occurrence of serious bacterial infections since introduction of antibacterial agents. JAMA. 1959;170:2188.
7. McCabe WR, Jackson GG. Gram-negative bacteremia. II. Clinical, laboratory and therapeutic observations. Arch Intern Med. 1962;110:856.
8. McGowan JE, Barnes MW, Finland MW. Bacteremia at Boston City Hospital. Occurrence and mortality during 12 selected years (1935–1972) with special reference to hospital-acquired cases. J Infect Dis. 1975;132:316.
9. Armstrong D, Young LS, Meyer RD, et al. Infectious complications of neoplastic disease. Med Clin North Am. 1971;55:729.
10. Leigh DA. Bacteraemia in patients receiving human cadeveric renal transplants. J Clin Pathol. 1971;24:295.
11. Hill RB, Dahrling BE II, Starzl TE, et al. Death after transplantation: An analysis of sixty cases. Am J Med. 1967;42:327.
12. Montgomery JR, Barrett FF, Williams TW Jr. Infectious complications in cardiac transplant patients. Transplant Proc. 1973;5:1239.
13. Winston DJ, Gale RP, Meyer DV, et al. Infectious complications of human bone marrow transplantation. Medicine Baltimore. 1979;58:1.
14. McCabe WR, Kreger BE, Johns M. Type-specific and cross reactive antibodies in gram-negative bacteremia. N Engl J Med. 1972;287:262.
15. Wolff SM, Bennett JV. Gram-negative rod bacteremia, (Editorial). N Engl J Med. 1974;291:733.
16. EORTC Antimicrobial Therapy Project Group. Ceftazidime combined with a short or long course of amikacin for empirical therapy of gram-negative bacteremia in cancer patients with granulocytopenia. N Engl J Med. 1987;317:1692–98.
17. Klastersky J, Glauser MP, Schimpff SC, et al. Prospective randomized comparison of three antibiotic regimens for empirical therapy of suspected bacteremia infection in febrila granulocytopenic patients. Antimicrobial Agents Chemother. 1986;29:263–70.
18. Weinstein MP, Murphy JR, Reller LB, et al. The clinical significance of positive blood culture: Comprehensive analysis of 500 episodes of bacteremia and fungemia in adults. II. Clinical observations, with special reference to factors influencing prognosis. Rev Infect Dis. 1983;6:54.
19. Spengler RF, Geenough WB III, Stolley PD. A descriptive study of nosocomial bacteremias at The Johns Hopkins Hospital, 1968–1974. Johns Hopkins Med J. 1978;142:77.
20. Kreger BE, Craven DE, Carling P, et al. Gram-negative bacteremia. III. Reassessment of etiology, epidemiology, and ecology in 612 patients. Am J Med. 1980;68:332.
21. Singer C, Kaplan M, Armstrong D. Bacteremia and fungemia complicating neoplastic disease. A study of 364 cases. Am J Med. 1977;62:731.
22. McHenry MC, Gavan TL, Hawk WA, et al. Gram negative bacteremia: variable clinical course and useful prognostic factors. Cleve Clin Q. 1975;42:15.
23. Myerowitz RL, Medeiros AA, O'Brien TF. Recent experience with bacillemia due to gram-negative organisms. J Infect Dis. 1971;124:239.
24. Bryant RE, Hood AF, Hood CE, et al. Factors affecting mortality of gram-negative rod bacteremia. Arch Intern Med. 1971;127:120.
25. DuPont HL, Spink WW. Infections due to gram-negative organisms: An analysis of 860 patients with bacteremia at the University of Minnesota Medical Center, 1958–1966. Medicine Baltimore. 1969;48:307.
26. Altemeier WA, Todd JC, Inge WW. Gram-negative septicemia: A growing threat. Ann Surg. 1967;166:530.
27. Centers for Disease Control. National nosocomial infectious study report, annual summary 1976. February, 1978;1.
28. Centers for Disease Control. Nosocomial infection surveillance, 1984. CDC Surveillance Summary. MMWR. 1986;35:19–29.
29. Young LS. Treatment of infections due to gram-negative bacilli: A perspective of past, present and future. Rev Infect Dis. 1985;7(Suppl 4):572–8.
30. Pollack M, Charache P, Nieman RE, et al. Colonization and antibiotic resistance patterns of gram-negative bacteria in hospitalized patients. Lancet. 1972;2:668
31. Shooter RA, Walter KA, Williams VR, et al. Faecal carriage of *Pseudomonas aeruginosa* in hospital patients. Possible spread from patient to patient. Lancet. 1966;2:1331.
32. Shooter RA, Cooke EM, Gaya H, et al. Food and medicaments as possible sources of hospital strains of *Pseudomonas aeruginosa*. Lancet. 1969;1:1227
33. Buck AC, Cooke EM. The fate of ingested *Pseudomonas aeruginosa* in normal persons. J Med Microbiol. 1969;2:521.
34. Schimpff SC, Young VM, Greene WH, et al. Origin of infection in acute nonlymphocytic leukemia: Significance of hospital acquisition of potential pathogens. Ann Intern Med. 1972;77:707.
35. Young LS. Nosocomial infections in the immunocompromised adult. Am J Med. 1981;70:398–402.
36. Kaijser B. Immunology of *Escherichia coli:* K antigen and its relation to urinary tract infection. J Infect Dis. 1973;127:670.
37. Selden R, Lee S, Wang WL, et al. Nosocomial *Klebsiella* infections. Intestinal colonization as a reservoir. Ann Intern Med. 1971;74:657.
38. Johanson WG, Pierce AK, Sanford JP. Changing pharyngeal bacterial flora of hospitalized patients. Emergency of gram-negative bacilli. N Engl J Med. 1969;281:1137.
39. Schimpff SC, Greene WH, Young VM, et al. *Pseudomonas* septicemia: Incidence, epidemiology, prevention, and therapy in patients with advanced cancer. Eur J Cancer. 1973;9:449.
40. Steinhauer BW, Eickhoff TC, Kislak JW, et al. The *Klebsiella-Enterobacter-Serratia* division: Clinical and epidemiologic characteristics. Ann Intern Med. 1966;65:1180.
41. Burke JP, Ingall D, Klein JO, et al. *Proteus mirabilis* infections in a hospital nursery traced to a human carrier. N Engl J Med. 1971;284:115.
42. Waisbren BA. Gram-negative shock and endotoxin shock. Am J Med. 1964;36:819.
43. Dorff GJ, Geimer NF, Rosenthal DR, et al. *Pseudomonas* speticemia. Arch Intern Med. 1971;128:591.
44. Ketover BP, Young LS, Armstrong D. Septicemia due to *Aeromonas hydrophilia:* Clinical and immunologic aspects. J Infect Dis. 1973;127:284.
45. Davis II WA, Kane JG, Garagusi VF. Human *Aeromonas* infections: A review of the literature and a case report of endocarditis. Medicine (Baltimore). 1978;57:267.
46. Fisher KW, Berger B, Keusch GT. Subepidermal bullae due to *E. coli*. Arch Dermatol. 1974;110:105.
47. Forkner CE, Frei III E, Edgcomb JH, et al. *Pseudomonas* septicemia. Observations on twenty-three cases. Am J Med. 1958;25:877.
48. Gunnar RM, Loeb HS, Winslow EJ, et al. Hemodynamic measurements in bacteremic and septic shock in man. J Infect Dis. 1973;128:287.
49. Hopewell PC, Murray JS. The adult respiratory distress syndrome. Annu Rev Med. 1976;181:343.
50. Rothstein JL, Schreiber H. Synergy between tumor necrosis factor and bacterial products causes hemorrhagic necrosis and lethal shock in normal mice. Proc Natl Acad Sci USA. 1988:85:607–11.
51. Tillotson JR, Lerner AM. Characteristics of nonbacteremic *Pseudomonas* pneumonia. Ann Intern Med. 1968;68:308.
52. Tillotson JR, Lerner AM. Characteristics of pneumonias caused by *Bacillus proteus*. Ann Intern Med. 1968;68:287.
53. Dietzman DE, Fischer GW, Schoenknecht FD. Neonatal *E. coli* septicemia: Bacterial counts in blood. J Pediatr. 1974;85:128.
54. Silverblatt FJ. Host parasite interactions in the rat renal pelvis. A possible role for pili in the pathogenesis of pyelonephritis. J Exp Med. 1974;140:1696.
55. Svanborg-Eden C, Hausson S, Jodal U, et al. Host–parasite interaction in urinary tract. J Infect Dis. 1988;157:421–6.
56. Roantree RJ, Rantz LA. A study of the relationship of the normal bactericidal activity of human serum to bacterial infection. J Clin Invest. 1960;39:72.
57. Fierer J, Finley J, Braude E. A plaque assay on agar for detection of gram-negative bacilli sensitive to complement. J Immunol. 1972;109:1156.
58. Young LS, Armstrong D. Human immunity to *Pseudomonas aeruginosa*. I. In vitro interaction of bacteria, polymorphonuclear leukocytes, and serum factors. J Infect Dis. 1972;126:257.
59. Rowley O: Endotoxins and bacterial virulence. J Infect Dis. 1971;123:317.
60. Sjostedt S. Pathogenicity of certain serological types of *B. coli*. Their mouse toxicity, hemolytic power, capacity for skin necrosis and resistance to phagocytosis and bactericidal faculties of human serum. Acta Pathol Microbiol Scand. 1946;63(Suppl):148.
61. Drach GH, Reed WP, Williams RC Jr. Antigens common to human and bacterial cells. II. *E. coli* 014. The common Enterobacteriacae antigen, blood groups A and B and *E. coli* 086. J Lab Clin Med. 1972;79:38.
62. Davis CE, Arnold K. Role of meningococcal endotoxin in meningococcal purpura. J Exp Med. 1974;140:159.
63. Miller RM, Garbus J, Hornick RB. Lack of enhanced oxygen consumption by polymorphonuclear leukocytes on phagotycosis of virulent *Salmonella typhi*. Science. 1972;175:1010.
64. Liu PV. Extracellular toxins of *Pseudomonas aeruginosa*. J Infect Dis. 1974;130(Suppl):94.
65. Wretlind B, Wadstrom T. Purification and properties of a protease with

elastase activity from *Pseudomonas aeruginosa*. J Gen Microbiol. 1977;103:319.
66. Young LS, Martin WJ, Meyer RD, et al. Gram-negative rod bacteremia: Microbiologic immunologic, and therapeutic considerations. Ann Intern Med. 1977;86:456.
67. Stevens P, Huang S, Welch WD, et al. Restricted complement activity by *Escherichia coli* with the K 1 capsular serotype. J Immunol. 1978;121:2174.
68. Young LS. Role of antibody in infections due to *Pseudomonas aeruginosa*. J Infect Dis. 1974;130(Suppl):111.
69. Zinner SH, McCabe WR. The effects of IgM and IgG antibody in patients with bacteremia due to gram-negative bacilli. J Infect Dis. 1976;133:37.
70. Bjornson AB, Michael JG. Biological activities of rabbit immunoglobulin M and immunoglobulin G antibodies to *Pseudomonas aeruginosa*. Infect Immun.
71. Hancock REW. Role of porins in outer membrane permeability. J Bacteriol. 1987;169:929–33.
72. Rietschel ETH, Wollenweber HW, Russa R, et al. Concepts of the chemical structure of lipid A. Rev Infect Dis. 1986;6:432–8.
73. Brade H, Brade L, Schade U, et al. Structure, endotoxicity, immunogenicity and antigenicity of bacterial lipopolysaccharides (endotoxins, O-antigens). In: Levin J, Buller HR, tenCate JW, et al., eds. Bacterial Endotoxins: Pathophysiological Effects, Clinical Significance, and Pharmacological Control. New York: Alan R Liss; 1988.
74. Orskov I, Orskov F, Jann E, et al. Serology, chemistry and genetics of O and K antigens of *Escherichia coli*. Bacteriol Rev. 1977;41:667
75. Stevens P, Huang S, Welch W, et al. Restricted complement activation by *E. coli* with the K-1 capsular serotype: A possible role in pathogenicity. *J Immunol*. 1978;121:2714.
76. Kunin CM, Beard MV, Halmagyi NE. Evidence for a common hapten associated with endotoxin fractions of *E. coli* and other Enterobacteriaceae. Proc Soc Exp Biol Med. 1962;111:160.
77. Makela PH, Mayer H. Enterobacterial common antigen. Bacteriol Rev. 1976;40:591.
78. Mannel D, Mayer H. Isolation and chemical characterization of the enterobacterial common antigen. Eur J Biochem. 1978;86:361.
79. Braun V, Bosch V, Klumpp ER, et al. Antigenic determinants of murein lipoprotein and its exposure at the surface of Enterobacteriaceae. Eur J Biochem. 1976;62:555.
80. McCabe WR, Johns M, Genio TD. Common enterobacterial antigen. III. Initial titers and antibody response in bacteremia caused by gram-negative bacilli. Infect Immun. 1973;7:393.
81. Griffiths EK, Yoonessi, Neter E. Antibody response to enterobacterial lipoprotein of patients with varied infections due to Enterobacteriacaea. Proc Soc Exp Biol Med. 1977;154:246.
82. Nikaido A, Nikaido K, Subbaiah TV, et al. Rough mutants of *Salmonella typhimurium*. Nature. 1964;201:1298.
83. Kasper DL, Seiler MW. Immunochemical characterization of the outer membrane complex of *Bacteroides fragilis* subspecies *fragilis*. J Infect Dis. 1975;132:440.
84. Meadow P. Wall and membrane structures in the genus *Pseudomonas*. In: Clarke PH, Richmond MH, eds. Genetics and biochemistry of Pseudomonas. London: John Wiley; 1975:6.
85. Golenbock DT, Will JA, Ratez CRH, et al. Lipid X ameliorates pulmonary hypertension and protects sheep from death due to endotoxin. Infect Immun. 1987;55:2471–6.
86. van der Meer JWM, Barza M, Wolff SM, et al. A low dose of recombinant interleukin 1 protects granulocytopenic mice from lethal gram-negative infection. Proc Natl Acad Sci USA. 1988;85:1620–3.
87. Wolff S. Biological effects of bacterial endotoxins in man. J Infect Dis. 1973;128(Suppl):259.
88. Michie HR, Manogue KR, Spriggs DR, et al. Detection of circulating tumor necrosis factor after endotoxin administration. N Engl J Med. 1988;318:1481–6.
89. Corrigan JJ, Walker LR, May N. Changes in the blood coagulation system associated with septicemia. N Engl J Med. 1968;279–851.
90. McKay DG, Shapiro SS. Alterations in the blood coagulation system induced by bacterial endotoxin. I. In vivo (generalized Shwartzman reaction). J Exp Med. 1958;107:353.
91. Kimball HR, Melmon KL, Wolff SM. Endotoxin-induced kinin production in man. Proc Soc Exp Biol Med. 1972;139:1078.
92. Nies AS, Forsyth RP, Williams HE, et al. Contribution of kinins to endotoxin shock in unanesthetized rhesus monkeys. Circ Res. 1968;22:155.
93. Fearon DT, Ruddy S, Schur PH, et al. Activation of the properdin pathway of complement in patients with gram-negative bacteremia. N Engl J Med. 1975;292:937.
94. Ulevitch RJ, Cochran CG, Henson PM, et al. Mediation systems in bacterial lipopolysaccharide-induced hypotension and disseminated intravascular coagulation. I. The role of complement. J Exp Med. 1975;142:1570.
95. Ziegler EJ, Douglas H, Sherman JE, et al. Treatment of *E. coli* and *Klebsiella* bacteremia in agranulocytic animals with antiserum to a UDP-GAL epimerase-deficient mutant. J Immunol. 1973;111:433.
96. Young LS, Ingram J, Stevens P. Functional role of antibody against core glycolipid of Enterobacteriaceae. J Clin Invest. 1975;56:850.
97. Tracey KJ, Wei H, Manogue KR, et al. Cachectin/tumor necrosis factor induces cachexia, anemia, and inflammation. J Exp Med. 1988;167:1211–27.
98. Ginsberg I. Mechanisms of cell and tissue injury induced by group A streptococci: Relation to poststreptococcal sequelae. J Infect Dis. 1972;126:294.
99. Pollack M. Significance of circulating capsular antigen in *Klebsiella* infections. Infect Immun. 1976;13:1543.
100. Dennis EW, Saigh AS. Precipitable typhoid somatic antigen in the serum of typhoid fever patients. Science. 1945;102:208
101. Kass E, Porter P, McGill M, et al. Clinical and experimental observations on the significance of endotoxemia. J Infect Dis. 1973;128(Suppl):299.
102. Levin J, Poore TE, Zauber NP, et al. Detection of endotoxin in the blood of patients with sepsis due to gram-negative bacteria. N Engl J Med. 1970;283:1313.
103. Stumacher RJ, Kovnat MJ, McCabe WR. Limitations of the usefulness of the limulus assay for endotoxin. N Engl J Med. 1973;288:1261.
104. Elin RJ, Hosseini J. Clinical utility of the limulus amebocyte updated test. In: Watson SW, Levin J, Novitsky TJ, eds. Detection of Bacterial Endotoxins with Limulus Amebocyte Lysate Test. New York: Alan R Liss; 1985:307–24.
105. Tesh VL, Vukajlovich SW, Morrison DC. Endotoxin interactions with serum proteins—relationship to biological activity. In: Levin J, Buller HR, tenCate JW, et al., eds. Bacterial Endotoxins: Pathophysiological Effects, Clinical Significance, and Pharmacological Control. New York: Alan R Liss, 1988.
106. Johnson KJ, Ward PA, Goralnick S, et al. Isolation from human serum of an inactivator of bacterial lipopolysaccharide. Am J Pathol. 1977;88:559.
107. Koster F, Levin J, Walter L, et al. Hemolytic uremic syndrome after shigellosis: Relation to endotoxemia and circulating immune complexes. N Engl J Med. 1978;298:927.
108. Young LS. Opsonizing antibodies, host factors, and the limulus assay for endotoxin. Infect Immun. 1975;12:88.
109. Young LS. The complex challenge of bacteremia and endotoxemia. In: Levin J, Buller HR, tenCate JW, et al., eds. Bacterial Endotoxins: Pathophysiological Effects, Clinical Significance, and Pharmacological Control. New York: Alan R Liss; 1988:209–12.
110. Postel J, Schloerb PR, Furtado D. Pathophysiologic alterations during bacterial infusions for the study of bacteremic shock. Surg Gynecol Obstet. 1975;141:683.
111. Muszynski Z. Enzymatic and toxinogenic activity of culture filtrates of high and low virulent strains of *Pseudomonas aeruginosa* on mice. Pathol Microbiol. 1973;39:135.
112. Wretlind B, Mollby R, Wadstrom T. Separation of two hemolysins from *Aeromonas hydrophila* by isoelectric focusing. Infect Immun. 1971;4:503.
113. Pollack M, Taylor NS, Callahan LT III. Exotoxin production by clinical isolates of *Pseudomonas aeruginosa*. Infect Immun. 1977;15:776.
114. Middlebrook JL, Dorland RB. Response of cultured mammalian cells to exotoxins of *Pseudomonas aeruginosa* and *Corynebacterium diphtheriae:* Differential cytotoxicity. Can J Microbiol. 1977;23:183.
115. Iglewski BH, Kabat D. NAD-dependent inhibition of protein synthesis by *Pseudomonas aeruginosa* toxin. Proc Natl Acad Sci USA. 1975;72:2284
116. Pavlovskis OR, Pollack M, Callahan LT III, et al. Passive protection by antitoxin in experimental *Pseudomonas aeruginosa* burn infections. Infect Immun. 1977;18:596.
117. Young LS. Role of exotoxins in the pathogenesis of *Pseudomonas aeruginosa* infections. J Infect Dis. 1980;142:626.
118. McCabe WR. Serum complement levels in bacteremia due to gram-negative organisms. N Engl J Med. 1973;288:21.
119. Schreiber AD, Austen KF. Interrelationships of the fibrinolytic, coagulation, kinin generating, and complement systems. Semin Hematol. 1973;6:4.
120. Jacob HS. Granulocyte-complement interaction. A beneficial antimicrobial mechanism that can cause disease. Arch Intern Med. 1978;138:461.
121. McCabe WR. Gram-negative bacteremia. Adv Intern Med. 1974;19:135.
122. Greisman SE, Hornick RB. Comparative pyrogenic reactivity of rabbit and man to bacterial endotoxin. Proc Soc Exp Biol Med. 1969;131:1154.
123. Sanarelli G: De la pathogenié du choléra (Neuvième mémoirè) Le choléra expérimental. Ann Inst Pasteur Lille. 1924;38:11.
124. Shwartzman G, Gerber LE. Hemorrhagic manifestations of bacterial and virus infections: Experimental studies and pathological interpretations. Ann NY Acad Sci. 1948;49:627.
125. McKay DG, Jewett JF, Reid DE. Endotoxin shock and the general Shwartzman reaction in pregnancy. Am J Obstet Gynecol. 1959;78:546.
126. Dinarello CA, Mier JW. Current Concept: Lymphokines. N Engl J Med. 1987;317:940–5.
127. Morrison DC, Ryan JL. Endotoxins and disease mechanisms. Annu Rev Med. 1987;38:417–32.
128. Beutler B, Milsark IW, Cerami A. Passive immunization with cachectin/tumor necrosis factor (TNF) protects mice from the lethal effects of endotoxin. Nature. 1985;229:869–71.
129. Tracey KJ, Lowry SF, Cerami A. Cachectin: A hormone that triggers acute shock and chronic cachexia. J Infect Dis. 1988;157:413–20.
130. Tracey KJ, Lowry SF, Cerami A. Cachectin/TNF mediates the pathophysiological effects of bacterial endotoxin/lipopolysaccharide (LPS). In: Levin J, Buller HR, tenCate JW, et al., eds. Bacterial Endotoxins: Pathophysiological Effects, Clinical Significance, and Pharmacological Control. New York: Alan R Liss; 1988.
131. Beutler B, Krochin N, Milsark IW, et al. Control of cachectin (tumor necrosis factor) synthesis: Mechanisms of endotoxin resistance. Science. 1986;232:977–80.
132. Waage A, Halstensen A, Espevik T. Association between tumor necrosis factor in serum and fatal outcome in patients with meningococcal disease. Lancet. 1987;1:355–7.

133. Blick M, Sherwin SA, Rosenblum M, et al. Phase I study of recombinant tumor necrosis factor in cancer patients. Cancer Res. 1987;47:2986–9.
134. Mathison JC, Wolfson E, Ulevitch RJ. Participation of tumor necrosis factor in the mediation of gram-negative bacterial lipopolysaccharide-induced injury in rabbits. J Clin Invest. 1988;81:1925–37.
135. Remick DG, Kunkel RG, Larrick JW, et al. Acute in vivo effects of human recombinant tumor necrosis factor. Lab Invest. 1987;56:583–90.
136. Stephens KE, Ishizaka A, Larrick JW, et al. Tumor necrosis factor causes increased pulmonary permeability and edema. Am Rev Respir Dis. 1988;137:1364–70.
137. Tracey KJ, Beutler B, Lowry SF, et al. Shock and tissue injury induced by recombinant human cachectin. Science. 1986;234:470–4.
138. Tracey KJ, Fong Y, Hesse DG, et al. Anti-cachectin/TNF monoclonal antibodies prevent septic shock during lethal bacteremia. Nature. 1987;330:662–4.
139. Nawroth PP, Bank I, Handley D, et al. Tumor necrosis factor/cachectin interacts with endothelial cell receptors to induce release of interleukin-1. J Exp Med. 1986;163:1363–75.
140. Dinarello CA, Cannon JG, Solff SM, et al. Tumor necrosis factor (cachectin) is an endogenous pyrogen and induces production on interleukin 1. J Exp Med. 1986;163:1433–50.
141. Kettelhut IC, Fiers W, Goldberg AL. The toxic effects of tumor necrosis factor in vivo and their preventive by cyclooxygenase inhibitors. Proc Natl Acad Sci USA. 1987;84:4273–7.
142. Okusawa S, Gelfand JA, Ikejima T, et al. Interleukin 1 induces shock-like state in rabbits: Synergism with tumor necrosis factor and the effect of cyclooxygenase inhibition. J Clin Invest. 1988;81:1162–72.
143. Talmadge JE, Bowersox O, Tribble H, et al. Toxicity of tumor necrosis factor is synergistic with gamma-interferon and can be reduced with cyclooxygenase inhibitors. Am J Pathol. 1987;128:410–25.
144. Billiau A. Gamma-interferon: The match that lights the fire? Immunol Today. 1988;9:37–40.
145. Scuderi P, Sterling KE, Lam KS, et al. Raised serum levels of tumor necrosis factor in parasitic infections. Lancet. 1986;2:1364–5.
146. Ulich TR, Kaizhi G, del Castillo J. Rapid communication. Endotoxin-induced cytokine gene expression *in vivo*. I. Expression of tumor necrosis factor mRNA in visceral organs under physiologic conditions and during endotoxemia. Am J Pathol. 1989;134:11–14.
147. Frank MM, May JE, Kane MA. Contributions of the classical alternative complement pathways to the biological effects of endotoxin. J Infect Dis. 1973;128(Suppl):176.
148. Ulevitch RJ, Cochrane CG. Role of complement in lethal bacterial lipopolysaccharide-induced hypotensive and coagulative changes. Infect Immun. 1978;20:204.
149. Corrigan JJ. Heparin therapy in bacterial septicemia. J Pediatr. 1977;91:695.
150. Butler T, Bell WR, Levin J, et al. Studies of blood coagulation, bacteremia, endotoxemia. Arch Intern Med. 1978;138:407.
151. Rothberger H, Zimmerman TS, Spiegelberg HL, et al. Leukocyte procoagulant activity: Enhancement of production in vitro by IgG and antigen–antibody complexes. J Clin Invest. 1977;59:549.
152. Egbring R, Schmidt W, Fuchs G, et al. Demonstration of granulocytic proteases in plasma of patients with acute leukemia and septicemia with coagulation defects. Blood. 1977;49:219.
153. Brown DL, Lachmann PJ. The behaviour of complement and platelets in lethal endotoxin shock in rabbits. Int Arch Allergy. 1973;45:193.
154. Miller RL, Reichgott MJ, Melmon KL. Biochemical mechanisms of generation of bradykinin by endotoxin. J Infect Dis. 1973;128(Suppl):144.
155. Mason JW, Kleeberg U, Dolan P, et al. Plasma kallikrein and Hageman factor in gram-negative bacteremia. Ann Intern Med. 1970;73–545.
156. Robinson JA, Klodnycky ML, Loeb HS, et al. Endotoxin, prekallikrein, complement and systemic vascular resistance: Sequential measurement in man. Am J Med. 1975;59:61.
157. O'Donnell TF, Clowes GHA, Talamo RC, et al. Kinin activation in the blood of patients with sepsis. Surg Gynecol Obstet. 1976;143:539.
158. Colman RW, Edelman R, Scott CF, et al. Plasma kallikrein activation and inhibition during typhoid fever. J Clin Invest. 1978;61:287.
159. Jacobs ER, Bone RC, Wilson JB, et al. Naloxone blockage of endorphins in canine endotoxin shock. Microcirculation. 1982;2:19.
160. Doebber TW, Wu MS, Robbins JC, et al. Platelet activating factor (PAF) involvement in endotoxin-induced hypotension in rats. Biochem Biophys Res Commun. 1985;127:799–808.
161. Gallin JI, Kaye D, O'Leary WM. Serum lipids in infection. N Engl J Med. 1969;281:1081.
162. Reines HD, Halushka PV, Cook JA. Plasma thromboxane concentrations are raised in patients dying with septic. Lancet. 1982;2:174.
163. McGovern VJ. The pathology of shock. In: Sommers S, ed. Pathology Annual. New York: Appleton-Century-Crofts; 1971:279.
164. Waisbren BA, Brown I. A factor in the serum of patients with persisting infection that inhibits the bactericidal activity of normal serum against the organism that is causing the infection. J Immunol. 1966;97:431.
165. Bjornboe M, Prytz H, Orskov F. Antibodies to intestinal microbes in serum of patients with cirrhosis of the liver. Lancet. 1972;1:58.
166. Howard CJ, Glynn AA. The virulence for mice of strains of *Escherichia coli* related to the effects of K antigens on their resistance to phagocytosis and killing by complement. Immunology. 1971;20:767.
167. Vosti KL, Randall E. Sensitivity of serologically classified strains of *Escherichia coli* of human origin to the serum bactericidal system. Am J Med Sci. 1970;259:114.
168. Kierszenbau F, Weinman D. Antibody-independent activation of the alternative complement pathway in human serum by parasitic cells. Immunology. 1977;32:245.
169. Agnello V. Complement deficiency states. Medicine (Baltimore). 1978;57:1.
170. Feinstein PA, Kaplan SR. The alternative pathway of complement activation in the neonate. Pediatr Res. 1975;9:803.
171. Johnston RB, Newman MS, Struth AG. An abnormality of the alternate pathway of complement activation in sickle-cell disease. N Engl J Med. 1973;288:803.
172. Jasin HE, Orozco JH, Ziff M. Serum heat-labile opsonins in systemic lupus erythematosus. J Clin Invest. 1974;53:343.
173. Michael JG, Rosen FS. Association of natural antibodies to gram-negative bacteremia with the gamma macroglobulins. J Exp Med. 1963;118:619.
174. Robbins JB, Myerowitz RL, Whisnant JK, et al. Enteric bacteria cross-reactive with *Neisseria meningitidis* groups A and C and *Diplococcus pneumoniae* types I and III. Infect Immun. 1972;6:651.
175. Schneerson R, Bradshaw M, Whisnant JK, et al. An *Escherichia coli* antigen cross reactive with the capsular polysaccharide of *Hemophilus influenzae* type b. J Immunol. 1972;108:1551.
176. Kasper DL, Winkelhake JL, Zollinger WD, et al. Immunochemical similarity between polysaccharide antigens of *Escherichia coli* 07:K1:NM and group B. *Neisseria meningitidis*. J Immunol. 1973;110:262.
177. Glode MP, Robbins JB, Liu TY, et al. Cross antigenicity and immunogeneicity between capsular polysaccharides of Group C *Neisseria* meningitidis and *Escherichia coli* K 92. J Infect Dis. 1977;135:94.
178. Robbins JB, Gotschlich EC, Liu TY, et al. Bacterial antigens cross-reactive with the capsular polysaccharides of *Hemophilus influenzae* type b, *Neisseria meningitidis* groups A and C, *Diplococcus pneumoniae* types I and III. In: Robbins JB, Horton RE, Krause RM, eds. Proceedings of the Symposium on New Approaches for Inducing Natural Immunity to Pyogenic Organisms. Washington, DC: Department of Health, Education and Welfare; Publication No (NIH) 74–553, 1973:45.
179. Goldschneider I, Gotschlich EC, Artenstein MS. Human immunity to the meningococcus. I. The role of humoral antibodies. J Exp Med. 1969;129:1307.
180. Young LS, Meyer RD, Armstrong D. *Pseudomonas aeruginosa* vaccine in cancer patients. Ann Intern Med. 1973;79:518.
181. Harvath L, Andersen BR. Evaluation of type-specific and nontype-specific pseudomonas vaccine for treatment of pseudomonas sepsis during granulocytopenia. Infect Immun. 1976;13:1139.
182. Kaijser B, Ahlstedt S. Protective capacity of antibodies against *Escherichia coli* O and K antigens. Infect Immun. 1977;17:286.
183. Ruddy S, Gigli I, Austen KF. The complement system of man. N Engl J Med. 1972;287:489.
184. Dossett JH, Williams RC, Quie PG. Studies on interaction of bacteria, serum factors, and polymorphonuclear leukocytes in mothers and newborns. Pediatrics. 1969;44:49.
185. Ehlenberger AG, Nussenzweig V. The role of membrane reception for C_3B and C_3D in phagocytosis. J Exp Med. 1977;145:357.
186. Gotze O, Muller-Eberhard JH. The alternative pathway of complement activation. In: Kunkeland HJ, Dixon FJ, eds. Advances in Immunology. v. 24. New York: Academic Press; 1976:1.
187. Jasin HE. Human heat labile opsonins: Evidence for their mediation via the alternate pathway of complement activation. J Immunol. 1972;109:26.
188. Guckian JC, Christensen WP, Fine DP. Evidence for quantitative variability of bacterial opsonic requirements. Infect Immun. 1978;19:882.
189. Weinstein RJ, Young LS. Neutrophil function in gram-negative rod bacteremia: The interaction between phagocytic cells, infecting organisms, and humoral factors. J Clin Invest. 1976;58:190.
190. Young LS. Role of antibody in infections due to *Pseudomonas aeruginosa*. J Infect Dis. 1974;130(Suppl):111.
191. Zinner SH, McCabe WR. The effects of IgM and IgG antibody in patients with bacteremia due to gram-negative bacilli. J Infect Dis. 1976;133:37.
192. Bjornson AB, Michael JG. Biological activities of rabbit immunoglobulin M and immunoglobulin G antibodies to *Pseudomonas aeruginosa*. Infect Immun. 1970;2:453.
193. Inoue K. Immune bacteriolytic and bactericidal reactions. In: Kwapinski JBG, ed. Research in Immunochemistry and Immunobiology. Baltimore: University Park Press; 1972:177.
194. Young LS. Gram-negative septicemia: Antibody deficiency and specific protection. In: Bayer-Symposium VIII. The Pathogenesis of Bacterial Infections. Berlin: Springer-Verlag; 1985:138–45.
195. Braude A, Douglas H, Davis C. Treatment and prevention of intravascular coagulation with antiserum to endotoxin. J Infect Dis. 1973;128(Suppl):157.
196. Ziegler EJ, Douglas H, Braude A. Human antiserum for prevention of the local Shwartzman reaction and death from bacterial lipopolysaccharides. J Clin Invest. 1973;52:3236.
197. McCabe WR. Immunization with R mutants of *S. minnesota*. I. Protection against challenge with heterologous gram-negative bacilli. J Immunol. 1972;108:601.
198. McCabe WR. Immunoprophylaxis of gram-negative bacillary infections. Annu Rev Med. 1976;27:335.
199. Young LS. Immunoprophylaxis and serotherapy of bacterial infections. Am J Med. 1984;76:664–71.

200. Teng NH, Kaplan HS, Hebert JM, et al. Protection against gram-negative bacteremia and endotoxemia with human monoclonal IgM antibodies. Proc Natl Acad Sci USA. 1985;82:1790–4.
201. Ziegler EJ, McCutchan JA, Fierer J, et al. Treatment of gram-negative bacteremia and shock with human antiserum to a mutant *Escherichia coli*. N Engl J Med. 1982;307:1225.
202. Ng AK, Chen CL, Chang CM, et al. Relationship of structure to function in bacterial endotoxins: Serologically cross-reactive components and their effect on protection of mice against some gram-negative infections. J Gen Microbiol. 1976;94:107.
203. Ziegler EJ. Protective antibody to endotoxin core: The emperor's new clothes? J Infect Dis. 1988;158:286–90.
204. Bruins SC, Stumacher R, Johns MA, et al. Immunization with R mutants of *Salmonella minnesota*. III. Comparison of the protective effect of immunization with lipid A and the Re mutant. Infect Immun. 1977;17:16.
205. McCabe WR, DeMaria A Jr, Berberich H, et al. Immunization with rough mutants of *Salmonella minnesota:* Protective activity of IgM and IgG antibody to the R595 (Re chemotype) mutant. J Infect Dis. 1988;158:291–300.
206. Pollack M, Taylor NS. Serum antibody to *Pseudomonas aeruginosa* exotoxin measured by a passive hemagglutination assay. J Clin Microbiol. 1977;6:58
207. Pollack M, Young LS. Protective activity of antibodies to exotoxin A and lipopolysaccharide at onset of *Pseudomonas aeruginosa* septicemia in man. J Clin Invest. 1979;63:276.
208. Freudenberg MA, Bog-Hansen TC, Back U. Interaction of lipopolysaccharides with plasma high density lipoprotein. Infect Immun. 1980;28:373–80.
209. Berger D, Beger HG. Quantification of the endotoxin-binding capacity of human transferrin. In: Levin J, Buller HR, tenCate JW, et al., eds. Bacterial Endotoxins: Pathophysiological Effects, Clinical Significance, and Pharmacological Control. New York: Alan R Liss; 1988.
210. Ulevitch RJ, Tobias PS. Interactions of bacterial lipopolysaccharides with serum proteins. In: Levin J, Buller HR, tenCate JW, et al., eds. Bacterial Endotoxins: Pathophysiological Effects, Clinical Significance, and Pharmacological Control. New York: Alan R Liss; 1988:309–18.
211. Quie PG, Cates KL. Clinical conditions associated with defective polymorphonuclear leukocyte chemotaxis. Am J Pathol. 1977;88:711.
212. Warden GD, Mason AD, Pruitt BA. Evaluation of leukocyte chemotaxis in vitro in thermally injured patients. J Clin Invest. 1974;54:1001.
213. Washington II JA. Blood cultures: Principles and techniques. Mayo Clin Proc. 1975;50:91.
214. Anderson ET, Young LS, Hewitt WL. Antimicrobial synergism in the therapy of gram-negative bacteremia. Chemotherapy. 1978;24:45.
215. Freid MA, Vosti KL. Importance of underlying disease in patients with gram-negative bacteremia. Arch Intern Med. 1968;121:418.
216. Young LS. Combination or single drug therapy for gram-negative sepsis. In: Remington JS, Swartz MN, eds. Curr Clin Topics Infect Dis. 1982;3:177.
217. Young LS. Empirical antimicrobial therapy in the neutropenic host. N Engl J Med. 1986;315:580.
218. Pizzo PA, Hawthorn JW, Hiemenz J, et al. A randomized trial comparing ceftazidime alone with combination antibiotic therapy in cancer patients with fever and neutropenia. N Engl J Med. 1986;315:552–8.
219. Schimpff S, Satterlee W, Young VM, et al. Therapy with carbenicillin and gentamicin in febrile cancer patients. N Engl J Med. 1971;284:1061.
220. Lumish RM, Norden CW. Therapy of neutropenic rats infected with *Pseudomonas aeruginosa*. J Infect Dis. 1976;133:538.
221. Andriole VT. Synergy of carbenicillin and gentamicin in experimental infection with pseudomonas. J Infect Dis. 1971;124(Suppl):460.
222. Robson HG. Synergistic activity of carbenicillin and gentamicin in experimental pseudomonas bacteremia in neutropenic rats. Antimicrob Agents chemother. 1976;10:646.
223. Klastersky J, Meunier-Carpentier F, Prevost JM. Significance of antimicrobial synergism for the outcome of gram-negative sepsis. Am J Med Sci. 1977;273:157.
224. Sculier JP, Klastersky J. Significance of serum bactericidal activity in gram-negative bacillary bacteremia in patients with and without granulocytopenia. Am J Med. 1984;76:429–35.
225. Feld R, Valdivieso M, Bodey GP, et al. A comparative trial of sisomicin therapy by intermittent versus continuous infusion. Am J Med Sci. 1977;274:179.
226. Price KE, DeFuria MD, Pursiano TA. Amikacin, an aminoglycoside with marked activity against antibiotic-resistant clinical isolates. J Infect Dis. 1976;134(Suppl):249.
227. DeJongh CA, Wade JC, Schimpff SC, et al. Empiric antibiotic therapy for suspected infection in granulocytopenic cancer patients. Am J Med. 1982;73:89.
228. DeJongh CA, Joshi JH, Newman KA, et al. Antibiotic synergism and response in gram-negative bacteremia in granulocytopenic cancer patients. Am J Med. 1986;80:96–100.
229. International Antimicrobial Therapy Project Group of the European Organization for Research and Treatment of Cancer. Combination of amikacin and carbenicillin with or without cefazolin as empirical treatment of febrile neutropenic patients. J Clin Oncol. 1983;1:597–603.
230. Kaye D, Levison ME, Labovitz ED. The unpredictability of serum concentrations of gentamicin. Pharmacolinetics of gentamicin in patients with normal and abnormal renal function. J Infect Dis. 1974;130:150.
231. Anderson ET, Young LS, Hewitt WL. Simultaneous antibiotic levels in "breakthrough" gram-negative rod bacteremia. Am J Med. 1976;61:493.
232. Smith CR, Maxwell RR, Edwards CQ, et al. Nephrotoxicity induced by gentamincin and amikacin. Johns Hopkins Med. J. 1978;142:85.
233. Shine K, Silver M, Young LS, et al. Aspects of the management of shock. Ann Intern Med. 1980;93:723–34.
234. Winslow EJ, Loeb HS, Pahimtoola SH, et al. Hemodynamic studies and results of therapy in 50 patients with bacteremic shock. Am J Med. 1973;54:421.
235. Weitzman S, Berger S. Clinical trial design in studies of corticosteroids for bacterial infections. Ann Intern Med. 1974;81:36.
236. Klastersky J, Cappel R, Debusscher L. Effectiveness of betamethasone in management of severe infections. N Engl J Med. 1971;284:1248.
237. Schumer W. Steroids in the treatment of clinical septic shock. Ann Surg. 1976;184:333.
238. Hotfman SL, Punjabi NH, Kumala S, et al. Reduction of mortality in chloramphenicol-treated severe typhoid fever by high-dose dexamethasone. N Engl J Med. 1981;310:456–7.
239. Sprung CL, Caralis PV, Marcial EH, et al. The effects of high-dose corticosteroids in patients with septic shock: A prospective controlled study. N Engl J Med. 1984;311:1137–43.
240. Veterans Administration Systemic Sepsis Cooperative Study Group. Effect of high dose glucocorticoid therapy on mortality in patients with clinical signs of systemic sepsis. N Engl J Med. 1987;317:659–65.
241. Bone RC, Fisher CJ, Clemmer TP, et al. A controlled clinical trial of high-dose methylprednisolone in the treatment of severe sepsis and septic shock. N Engl J Med. 1987;317:653–8.
242. Bernard GR, Luce JM, Sprungs CL, et al. High-dose corticosteroids in patients with the adult respiratory distress syndrome. N Engl J Med. 1987;317:1565–70.
243. Luce JM, Montgomery AB, Marks JD, et al. Ineffectiveness of high-dose methylprednisolone in preventing parenchymal lung injury and improving mortality in patients with septic shock. Am Rev Respir Dis. 1988;138:62–8.
244. Corrigan JJ Jr, Ray WL, May N. Change in blood coagulation system associated with septicemia. N Engl J Med. 1968;279:851.
245. Corrigan JC, Kiernat JF. Effect of heparin in experimental gram-negative septicemia. J Infect Dis. 1975;131:138.
246. Higby DJ, Yates JW, Henderson ES. Filtration leukopheresis for granulocyte transfusion therapy. N Engl J Med. 1975;292:761.
247. Herzig RH, Herzig GP, Graw RG Jr, et al. Successful granulocyte transfusion therapy for gram-negative septicemia. N Engl J Med. 1977;296:701.
248. Alavi JB, Root RK, Djerassi I, et al. A randomized clinical trial of granulocyte transfusions for infection in acute leukemia. N Engl J Med. 1977;296:706.
249. Vogler WR, Winston EF. A controlled study of the efficacy of granulocyte transfusions in patients with neutropenia. Am J Med. 1977;63:548.
250. Winston DJ, Ho WG, Gale RP. Therapeutic granulocyte transfusions for documented infections. Ann Intern Med. 1982;97:509.
251. Young LS. The role of granulocytes transfusions in treating and preventing infection. Cancer Treat Rep. 1983;67:109.
252. Faden AI, Holaday JW. Experimental endotoxin shock. The pathophysiologic function of endorphins and treatment with opiate antagonists. J Infect Dis. 1980;142:229.
253. Faden AI, Holaday JW. Opiate antagonists: A role in the treatment of hypovolemic shock. Science. 1979;205:317.
254. Peters WP, Johnson MW, Friedman PA, et al. Pressor effect of naloxone in septic shock. Lancet. 1981;1:529.
255. DeMaria A, Craven DE, Heffernan JJ, et al. Naloxone versus placebo in treatment of septic shock. Lancet. 1985;1:1363–5.
256. Sullivan GW, Carper HT, Novick WJ, et al. Inhibition of the inflammatory action of interleukin-1 and tumor necrosis factor (alpha) on neutrophil function by pentoxifylline. Infect Immun. 1988;56:1722–9.
257. Feingold DS, Oski F. *Pseudomonas* infection. Treatment with immune human plasma. Arch Intern Med. 1965;116:326.
258. Jones CE, Alexander JW, Fisher MW. Clinical evaluation of *Pseudomonas* hyperimmune globulin. J Surg Res. 1973;14:87.
259. DeMaria A Jr, Johns MA, Berberich H, et al. Immunization with rough mutants of *Salmonella minnesota:* Initial studies in human subjects. J Infect Dis. 1988;158:301–11.
260. Calandra T, Glauser MP, Schellekens J, et al. Treatment of gram-negative septic shock with human IgG antibody to *Escherichia coli* J5: A prospective, double-blind, randomized trial. J Infect Dis. 1988;158:312–9.
261. Young LS, Gascon R, Alam Soosan, et al. Monoclonal antibodies for treatment of gram-negative infections. Rev Inf Dis. In press.
262. Harkonen S, Scannon P, Mischak RP, et al. Phase I study of a murine monoclonal anti-lipid A antibody in bacteremic and nonbacteremic patients. Antimicrob Agents Chemother. 1988;32:710–6.
263. Shenep JL, Flynn PM, Barrett FF, et al. Serial quantitation of endotoxemia and bacteremia during therapy for gram-negative bacterial sepsis. J Infect Dis. 1988;157:565–8.
264. Pollack M, Ranbitschek, Larrick J. Human monoclonal antibodies that recognize conserved epitopes in the core-lipid A region of lipopolysaccharides. J Clin Invest. 1987;79:1421–30.
265. Lindberg RB, Moncrief JA, Mason AD Jr. Control of experimental and clinical burn wound sepsis by topical application of sulfamylon compounds. Ann NY Acad Sci. 1968;50:950.

266. Greenfield S, Teres D, Bushnell LS, et al. Prevention of gram-negative bacillary pneumonia using aerosol polymixin as prophylaxis. J Clin Invest. 1973;52:2935.
267. Feeley TW, du Moulin GC, Hedley-Whyte J, et al. Aerosol polymixin and pneumonia. N Engl J Med. 1975;293:471.
268. Storring RA, McElwain TJ, Jameson B, et al. Oral non-absorbed antibiotics prevent infection in acute non-lymphoblastic leukaemia. Lancet. 1977;2:837.
269. Schimpff SC, Greene WH, Young VM, et al. Infection prevention in acute nonlymphocytic leukemia. Laminar air flow room reverse isolation with oral, nonabsorbable antibiotics prophylaxis. Ann Intern Med. 1975;82:351.
270. Young LS. Trimethorprim-sulfamethoxazole and bacterial infections during leukemic therapy. Ann Intern Med 1981;95:508.
271. Young LS. Antimicrobial prophylaxis against infection in neutropenic patients. J Infect Dis. 1983;147:611.
272. Karp JE, Merz WG, Hendricksen C, et al. Oral norfloxacin for prevention of gram-negative bacterial infections in patients with acute leukemia and granulocytopenia: A randomized, double-blind, placebo-controlled trial. Ann Intern Med. 1987;106:1–7.
273. Dekker AW, Rozenberg-Arska M, Verhoef J. Infection prophylaxis in acute leukemia: A comparison of ciprofloxacin with trimethoprim sulfamethoxazole and colistin. Ann Intern Med. 1987;106:7–12.
274. Clift RA, Sanders JE, Thomas ED, et al. Granulocyte transfusions for the prevention of infection in patients receiving bone marrow transplants. N Engl J Med. 1978;298:1052.
275. Strauss RG, Connett JE, Gale RP, et al. A controlled trial of prophylactic granulocyte transfusions during initial induction of chemotherapy for acute myelogenous leukemia. N Engl J Med. 1981;305:597.
276. Winston DJ, Ho WG, Young LS, et al. Prophylactic granulocyte transfusions during human bone marrow transplantation. Am J Med. 1980;68:893.
277. Schiffer CA, Aisner J, Daly A, et al. Alloimmunization following prophylactic granulocyte transfusion. Blood. 1979;54:766.
278. Keusch GT, Ambinder EP, Kovacs I, et al. Role of opsonins in clinical response to granulocyte transfusion in granulocytopenic patients. Am J Med. 1982;73:552.
279. Ammann AJ, Addiego J, Wara D, et al. Polyvalent pneumococcal polysaccharide immunization of patients with sickle cell anemia and patient with splenectomy. N Engl J Med. 1977;297:897.
280. Orskov F, Orskov I. *Escherichia coli* O:H serotypes isolated from human blood. Acta Pathol Microbiol Scand LB 1975;83:595.
281. Moody MR, Young VM, Kenton DM, et al. *Pseudomonas aeruginosa* in a center for cancer research. I. Distribution of intraspecies types from human and environmental sources. J Infect Dis. 1972;125:95.
282. Alexander JW, Fisher MW, MacMillan BG. Immunological control of *Pseudomonas* infection in burn patients. A clinical evaluation. Arch Surg. 1971;102:31.
283. Jones RJ, Roe EA, Gupta JL. Low mortality in burned patients in a *Pseudomonas* vaccine trial. Lancet. 1978;2:401.
284. Harvath L, Andersen B, Zander AR, et al. Combined preimmunization and granulocyte transfusion therapy for treatment of *Pseudomonas* septicemia in neutropenic dogs. J Lab Clin Med. 1976;87:840.
285. Baumgartner JD, Glauser MP, McCutchan JA, et al. Prevention of gram-negative shock and death in surgical patients by antibody to endotoxin core glycolipid. Lancet. 1985;1:59–63.
286. McCutchan JA, Wolf JL, Ziegler EF, et al. Ineffectiveness of single-dose human antiserum to core glycolipid (*E. coli* J5) for prophylaxis of bacteremic, gram-negative infections in patients with prolonged neutropenia. Schweiz Med Wochenschr [Suppl] 1983;14:40–5.
287. Schneerson R, Robbins JB. Induction of serum *Haemophilus influenzae* type B capsular antibodies in adult volunteers fed cross-reacting *Escherichia coli* 075:K100:H5. N Engl J Med. 1975;292:1093.
288. Young LS, Stevens P. Cross-protective immunity against gram-negative bacilli: Studies with "core" glycolipid and pneumococcal antigens. J Infect Dis. 1977;136(Suppl):174.

SECTION F

60. PERITONITIS AND OTHER INTRA-ABDOMINAL INFECTIONS

MATTHEW E. LEVISON
LARRY M. BUSH

Intra-abdominal infection may take several forms.[1] Infection may be in the retroperitoneal space or within the peritoneal cavity. Intraperitoneal infection may be diffuse or localized into one or more abscesses. Intraperitoneal abscesses may form in dependent recesses such as the pelvic space or Morison's pouch, in the various perihepatic spaces, within the lesser sac, and along the major routes of communication between intraperitoneal recesses, such as the right paracolic gutter. In addition, infection may be contained within the intra-abdominal viscera, such as hepatic, pancreatic, splenic, tuboovarian, or renal abscesses. Abscesses also frequently form about diseased viscera—pericholecystic, periappendiceal, pericolic, and tuboovarian—and between adjacent loops of bowel, i.e., interloop abscesses.

ANATOMY

The anatomic relationships within the abdomen are important in determining possible sources as well as routes of spread of infection. The peritoneal cavity extends from the undersurface of the diaphragm to the floor of the pelvis. In men the peritoneal cavity is a closed space. In women it is perforated by the free ends of the fallopian tubes. The stomach, jejunum, ileum, cecum, appendix, transverse and sigmoid colons, liver, gallbladder, and spleen lie within the peritoneal cavity, some being suspended by a mesentery.

The peritoneal reflections and mesenteric attachments compartmentalize the intraperitoneal space and route spreading exudate to sites that are often distant from their source (Fig. 1). The transverse mesocolon (14, in Fig. 1) divides the peritoneal cavity horizontally into an upper and a lower space. The greater omentum, extending from the transverse mesocolon and lower border of the stomach, covers the lower peritoneal cavity and further separates the upper from the lower peritoneal cavity (Fig. 2). The small bowel mesentery divides the lower peritoneal space.

The peritoneal cavity has several recesses into which exudate may become loculated. The most dependent recess of the peritoneal cavity in the supine position is in the pelvis. Between the rectum and bladder in men is a pouch of peritoneal cavity that extends slightly below the level of the seminal vesicles. In women, the uterus and fallopian tubes project into the pelvic recess. Between the rectum and body of the uterus is the pouch of Douglas, which lies above the posterior fornix of the vagina. On either side of the rectum and bladder are the pararectal and paravesical fossae. The pelvic recess is continuous with both the right and left paracolic gutters.

The phrenicocolic ligament, which fixes the splenic flexure of the colon to the diaphragm, partially bridges the junction between the left paracolic gutter and the left perihepatic space. In contrast, the right paracolic gutter is continuous with the right subhepatic space and the right subphrenic space. A posterior superior extension of the right subhepatic space, Mori-

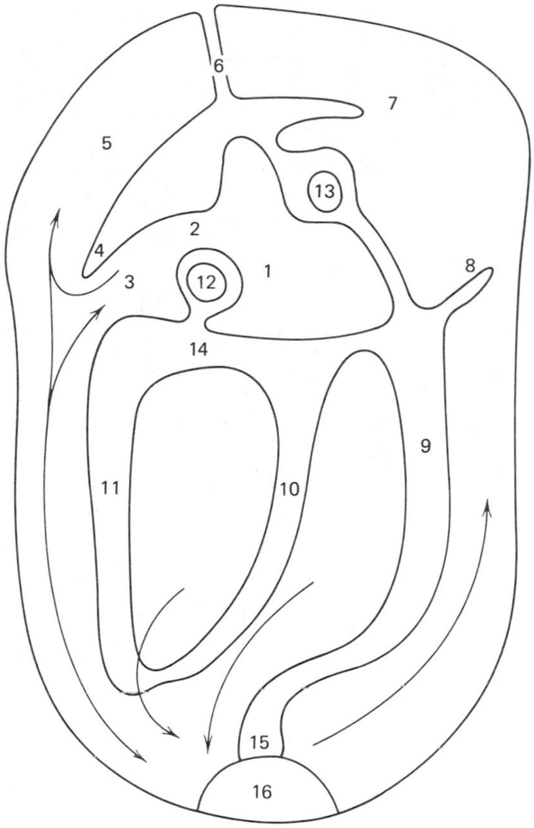

FIG. 1. Schema of the posterior peritoneal reflections and recesses of the peritoneal cavity. 1: Lesser sac; 2: foramen of Winslow; 3: Morison's pouch; 4: right triangular ligament; 5: right subphrenic space; 6: falciform ligament; 7: left subphrenic space; 8: phrenico-colic ligament; 9: bare area of the descending colon; 10: root of the small bowel mesentery; 11: bare area of ascending colon; 12: duodenum; 13: esophagus; 14: root of the transverse mesocolon; 15: bare area of rectum; 16: bladder.

son's pouch, is the most dependent portion in the supine position of the right paravertebral groove and lies just above the beginning of the transverse mesocolon. The horizontal posterior reflection of the serosal surface of the liver onto the diaphragm (the right triangular and coronary ligaments) and vertical reflection (the falciform ligament) divide the right perihepatic space into a right subphrenic and right subhepatic spaces[2] (Figs. 1 and 2A). The left subphrenic and subhepatic spaces communicate freely around the smaller left lobe of the liver and its more superiorly placed left triangular ligament[3,4] (Figs. 1 and 2B). The right and left subphrenic spaces are separated by the falciform ligament, which probably prevents the spread of pus to the opposite side and explains why only about 5–15 percent of subphrenic abscesses are bilateral.[4] The left subhepatic space is divided by the gastrohepatic omentum into an anterior space and the lesser sac (Fig. 2B). Abscesses within the perihepatic spaces become localized by pyogenic membranes. In the right subphrenic space they lie anteriorly or posteriorly and in the subhepatic space superiorly or inferiorly.[3,4] Abscesses of the left perihepatic space are either in the single left subphrenic space or in the lesser sac.[3,4]

The lesser sac, the largest recess of the peritoneal cavity, is connected to the main peritoneal space by the foramen of Winslow, an opening situated between the free border of the gastrohepatic omentum and the posterior parietal peritoneum. The lesser sac is surrounded posteriorly by the pancreas and kidneys, anteriorly by the stomach, and laterally by the liver and spleen. It may also extend to a variable extent between the folds of the greater omentum. Because of the limited communication from the lesser sac to the major cavity via the foramen of Winslow, suppuration in the lesser sac may exist with little or no involvement of the major cavity. Abscesses in the lesser sac lie between the stomach and pancreas but may spread to the right and lie anterior to the right kidney and inferior to the liver.

After intraperitoneal injection of water-soluble contrast material selectively into various intraperitoneal spaces, Meyers has demonstrated that the right paracolic gutter is the main communication between the upper and lower peritoneal cavities.[5] Fluid introduced into the right upper peritoneal space gravitates toward Morison's pouch and then into the right subphrenic space and along the right paracolic gutter into the pelvic recess (Fig. 3). Flow of fluid in the left upper peritoneal space is mainly into the left subphrenic space. The phrenicocolic ligament limits flow inferiorly into the left paracolic gutter. Fluid introduced into the lower peritoneal cavity first gravitates to the pelvic recess and then ascends, whether in the supine or erect position, along the right paracolic gutter into the right subhepatic space, especially into Morison's pouch, and into the right subphrenic space. Ascension of fluid from the pelvic space along the left paracolic gutter is minimal and limited by the phrenicocolic ligament. Although gravity would account for the pooling of fluid in the dependent peritoneal recesses, such as the pelvic recess and Morison's pouch, ascension of fluid from the pelvis to the subphrenic space is probably due to hydrostatic pressure differences between the upper and lower peritoneal cavities created by diaphragmatic motion. Normal intestinal and abdominal wall motion would also account for some spread of intraperitoneal fluid.

The retroperitoneal space lies between the posterior peritoneal membrane and the transversalis fascia, extending from the diaphragm to the pelvic brim. In the anterior retroperitoneal space between the peritoneum and anterior renal fascia lie the ascending and descending colons, duodenum, and pancreas. The kidneys and ureters lie within the posterior retroperitoneal (perinephric) space, between the anterior and posterior renal fasciae. The renal fascia encloses the kidneys and adrenals superiorly and laterally, but not inferiorly, favoring spread of infection in this space inferiorly.[6]

The parietal peritoneum, mainly the anterior portion, is well supplied by somatic afferent nerves and is sensitive to all forms of stimuli. The ability of the anterior parietal peritoneum to sense sharp, well-localized pain in response to local inflammation is of primary importance in diagnosing abdominal infection and may be associated with involuntary abdominal muscle contraction, tenderness, and rebound tenderness. Irritation of the peripheral diaphragmatic peritoneum is felt as pain near the adjacent body wall, and irritation of the central portion is felt as pain referred to the shoulder. Stimulation of the visceral peritoneum, usually due to distension of an organ, causes poorly localized, somewhat dull, pain.

The peritoneal cavity is lined by a serous membrane. The surface area of this membrane approximates that of the skin. The membrane consists of a monolayer of flat polygonal cells beneath which are lymphatics, blood vessels, and nerve endings. Normally, the peritoneal space contains only sufficient fluid to maintain moistness of the surface, facilitating movements of the viscera. Noninflamed serous fluid is clear yellow with a low specific gravity (<1.016) and low protein content (usually <3 g/dl). The protein is predominantly albumin. Fibrinogen is not present and serous fluid will not clot. Solute concentrations are nearly identical to those in plasma. A few leukocytes ($<300/mm^3$), mostly mononuclear cells, and desquamated serosal cells may be found.

The peritoneal membrane is highly permeable. Bidirectional transfer of substances across this membrane is rapid and, because of the large surface area involved, is potentially great in quantity. In fact, the peritoneal surface has been used extensively as a dialyzing membrane for the treatment of uremia and has also been used for the administration of fluid, electrolytes,

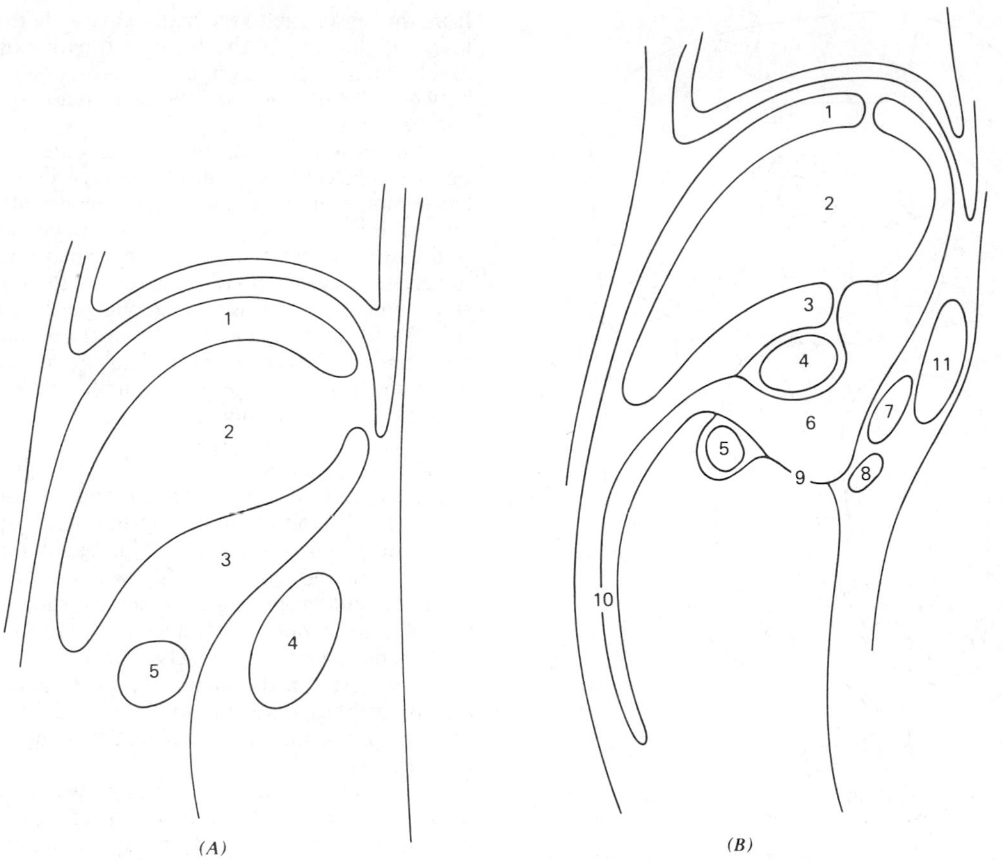

FIG. 2. Schema of a sagittal section of the peritoneal cavity. (**A**) Right upper quadrant. 1: Subphrenic space; 2: liver; 3: subhepatic space; 4: right kidney; 5: transverse colon. (**B**) Left upper quadrant. 1: Subphrenic space; 2: liver—left lobe; 3: subhepatic space; 4: stomach; 5: transverse colon; 6: lesser sac; 7: pancreas; 8: duodenum; 9: transverse mesocolon; 10: omentum; 11: left kidney.

antibiotics, and even blood.[7] The effective serum oncotic pressure and the hydrostatic pressure in the portal veins and lymphatics are major determinants of the rate and direction of fluid movement. The rate of movement of water and solutes between blood and peritoneal fluid is also dependent on concentration gradients between these compartments and has been studied in detail.[8,9] Water and solutes diffuse via blood capillaries and to a lesser extent by lymphatics. Lymphatics are primarily involved in removal of nonirritating colloids and particles into the blood stream. Absorption into lymphatics of particulate matter is thought to take place mostly from the diaphragmatic surface and is aided by the pumping action of diaphragmatic motion.[10] Following infusion of ^{51}Cr-labeled red blood cells into the peritoneal cavity of dogs, Rochlin et al.[11] reported absorption of about 70 percent of the labeled red blood cells by 48–96 hours. This absorption occurred mostly via the lymphatics. In humans, two-thirds of intraperitoneally injected red blood cells in anticoagulated blood have been found in the circulation 8–12 days after infusion.[12] The quantity of resorbed cells was less when no anticoagulant was used with the transfused cells, presumably due to trapping of red blood cells in intraperitoneal clots.[12] Transport of other particulate matter, such as intraperitoneal bacteria, may be similarly impeded because of trapping in fibrinous intraperitoneal exudate.[13]

In addition, there are communications between the peritoneal and pleural cavities that are independent of the blood stream. In patients with Meigs syndrome, for example, radioactive colloidal gold instilled into the peritoneal cavity appears in the pleural space probably as a result of transdiaphragmatic lymphatic transport.[14]

PERITONITIS

Inflammation of the peritoneum may be the result of contamination of the peritoneal cavity with microorganisms, irritating chemicals, or both. There are two major types of infective peritonitis: (*1*) the primary (so-called spontaneous or idiopathic) variety, in which no primary focus of infection is evident, and (*2*) the secondary variety, in which a primary intra-abdominal process such as ruptured appendix or perforated peptic ulcer is evident.

Primary Peritonitis

Etiology. Primary peritonitis is probably not a specific entity with a common cause but represents a group of diseases with different causes having in common only infection of the peritoneal cavity without an evident source. Primary peritonitis occurs at all ages. The prevalence of primary peritonitis in children apparently has been decreasing.[15] In the preantibiotic era, primary peritonitis occurred in about 10 percent of all pediatric abdominal emergencies; it now accounts for less than 1–2 percent.[16,17] The decline has been attributed to widespread use of antibiotics for minor upper respiratory tract illness. Although primary peritonitis may occur in children without predisposing disease,[15] it is known to occur particularly in children with postnecrotic cirrhosis[16,18] and in 2 percent of children with the nephrotic syndrome.[15,19] In one study, it was also frequently associated with urinary tract infections.[16] In some nephrotic children, repeated episodes of peritonitis occur and peritonitis may precede other manifestations of nephrosis.[15]

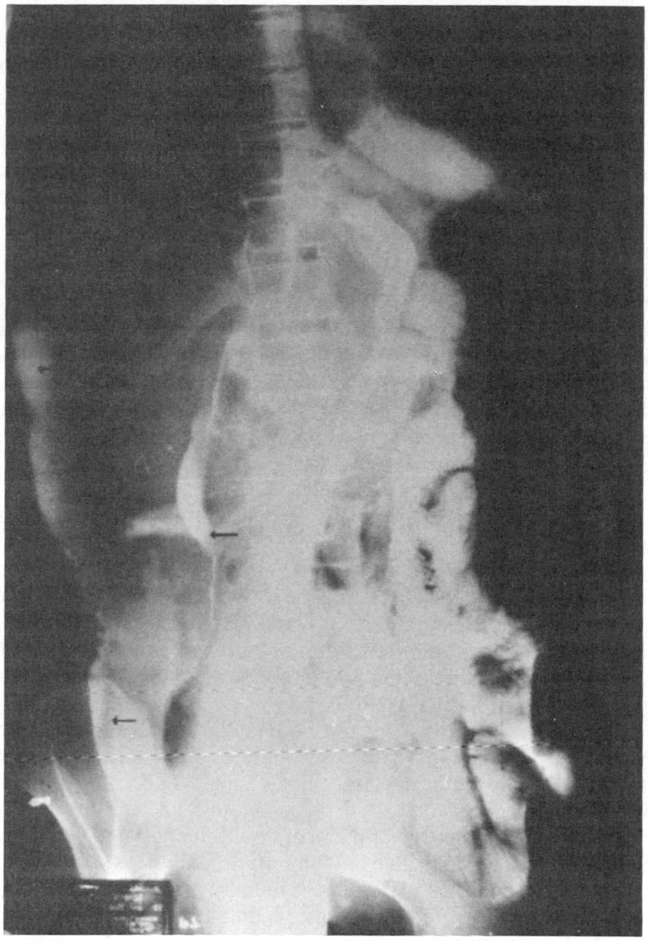

FIG. 3. Abdominal x-ray film (right decubitis) after oral administration of gastrografin to a patient with dehiscence of an esophageal-gastric anastomosis. Radiopaque gastrografin (arrows) can be seen in the subhepatic space, right paracolic gutter, and right subphrenic space, as well as within the lumen of the intestinal tract.

In adults, primary peritonitis usually has been reported in patients with alcoholic cirrhosis and ascites. In 1971 Conn and Fessel summarized their experience with 32 episodes in 28 patients and, in addition, reviewed 46 episodes in 42 patients reported in the literature.[20] Subsequent reports have confirmed and extended their initial findings.[21–28] Primary peritonitis was found to occur in about 10 percent of the patients with alcoholic cirrhosis collected retrospectively.[20,21] Among 63 consecutive patients with cirrhosis and ascites studied prospectively, using optimal aerobic and anaerobic bacteriologic techniques, primary peritonitis was found in 5.[25] Primary peritonitis has also been reported in adults with postnecrotic cirrhosis,[18] chronic active hepatitis,[29] acute viral hepatitis,[30] congestive heart failure,[31] metastatic malignant disease,[32] systemic lupus erythematosus,[33] lymphedema,[34] and, rarely, with no underlying disease.[35] The presence of ascites appears to be the common link among these various conditions.

Bacteriologic Characteristics. Several decades ago, the organisms reported to cause primary peritonitis in children were *Streptococcus pneumoniae* and group A streptococci.[15–17] More recently, the number of nephrotic children with streptococcal peritonitis has declined, and the relative frequency of peritonitis due to gram-negative enteric bacilli[16,17,19] and staphylococci[15,17] apparently has increased.

In cirrhotic patients, microorganisms presumably of enteric origin account for up to 69 percent of the pathogens.[36] *Escherichia coli* is the most frequently recovered pathogen, followed by *Klebsiella pneumoniae, S. pneumoniae*, and other streptococcal species, including enterococci.[20,24,36–38] *Staphylococcus aureus* is an unusual isolate in primary peritonitis, accounting for 2–4 percent of the cases in most series, and has been noted to occur in patients with an erosion of an umbilical hernia.[37] Anaerobes and microaerophilic organisms are infrequently reported.[24,28] Possible explanations include the intrinsic bacteristatic activity of ascites against *Bacteroides* species,[39] the relatively high PO_2 of ascitic fluid,[40] and the lack of optimal anaerobic bacteriologic techniques used to study patients with primary peritonitis in the past. In a review of 126 cases of primary peritonitis in cirrhotic patients recorded in the literature, only 6 percent (eight patients) were due to anaerobic or microaerophilic bacteria, including *Bacteroides* spp., *Bacteroides fragilis, Clostridium perfringens, Peptostreptococcus* spp., *Peptococcus* spp., and *Campylobacter fetus*.[24] Polymicrobial infection was present in four of these eight cirrhotic patients with peritonitis due to anaerobes, in contrast to the relatively low frequency of polymicrobial infection (only 10 of 118 cases of peritonitis) when aerobes alone were involved.

Ascitic fluid with positive cultures but few leukocytes in patients without clinical findings of peritonitis has been noted and called *bacterascites*.[38] This may represent early colonization before a host response.[28] However, patients with a low leukocyte response have the same mortality as those with a greater response.[27] Conversely, several series have identified cases of primary peritonitis with negative ascitic fluid cultures.[20,28] A recent series reported negative cultures in 35 percent of patients with clinical findings consistent with primary peritonitis, ascitic fluid leukocyte counts of $>500/mm^3$, and no evident source of intra-abdominal infection.[41] Blood cultures were positive in one-third of these patients. This variant of primary peritonitis has been termed *culture-negative neutrocytic ascites*.[41] The frequency of culture-negative ascitic fluid may be decreased by inoculating blood culture bottles with ascitic fluid at the bedside.[42]

Bacteremia is present in up to 75 percent of patients with primary peritonitis due to aerobic bacteria,[36] but is rarely found in those with peritonitis due to anaerobes.[24] Usually the same organisms isolated from the peritoneal fluid are recovered from the blood.[20,24]

Occasionally, primary peritonitis may be caused by *Mycobacterium tuberculosis, Neisseria gonorrhoeae,* or *Chlamydia trachomatis*.

Pathogenesis. The route of infection in primary peritonitis is usually not apparent and often it is presumed to be either hematogenous, lymphogenous, transmural migration through an intact gut wall from the intestinal lumen, or, in women, from the vagina via the fallopian tubes. Conn and Fessel[20] have postulated that the hematogenous route is most likely in cirrhotic patients: either (*1*) organisms removed from circulation by the liver may contaminate hepatic lymph and pass through the permeable lymphatic walls into the ascitic fluid or (*2*) portosystemic shunting greatly diminishes hepatic clearance of bacteremia in the portal circulation, which would tend to perpetuate bacteremia and increase the opportunity to cause metastic infection at susceptible sites such as the ascitic collection. The infrequency of primary peritonitis in all forms of ascites except that secondary to liver disease emphasizes the importance of intrahepatic shunting in the pathogenesis of this disease. The hepatic reticuloendothelial system is known to be a major site for removal of bacteria from blood,[43] and animal studies have suggested that destruction of blood-borne bacteria by the reticuloendothelial system is impaired in experimental cirrhosis[44] and in alcoholic liver disease.[45] The decrease in phagocytic activity seen in alcoholic cirrhosis is proportional to the severity of the liver disease.[46] Additionally, alcohol abuse and cirrhosis have been reported to be associated with impaired intracellular killing by monocytes and neutrophils,[47] as well as impaired opsonization[48] and low levels of serum complement.[49] The characteristics of ascitic fluid in nephrosis and cirrhosis predispose to infection. Opsonic activity, as reflected by low levels of complement and immunoglobulins, is reduced in the ascitic fluid of patients with the nephrotic syndrome and cirrhosis.[50,51] Primary bacteremia, usually due to coliforms, is a common complication in cirrhosis,[52] and metastatic infection in the pleural space has also been reported in cirrhotic patients.[53] An increased frequency of gram-negative endocarditis has also been noted in cirrhotics.[54]

Enteric bacteria may also gain access to the peritoneal cavity by directly traversing the intact intestinal wall. This has been demonstrated in animals[55]: Schweinburg et al. demonstrated that in dogs ^{14}C-labeled *E. coli* passed from the bowel into the peritoneal cavity after the introduction of hypertonic solutions into the peritoneum. A similar mechanism may explain the enteric bacterial peritonitis that frequently complicates peritoneal dialysis.[56] The infrequent occurrence of bacteremia and the multiplicity of species in peritoneal fluid when anaerobic bacteria are involved suggest that transmural migration of bacteria is the probable route of infection of ascitic fluid in the majority of these patients.[24] In addition, the occurrence of polymicrobial anaerobic peritonitis in two patients after infusion of vasopressin into the superior mesenteric or gastroduodenal arteries suggests that arterial vasoconstriction decreased the intestinal mucosal barrier and permitted transmural migration of enteric organisms.[22] Colonic microorganisms have been reported to colonize the upper small bowel in cirrhotic patients.[57]

The simultaneous presence of pneumococci in vaginal secretions and peritoneal fluid in girls[58] makes an ascending infection of genital origin likely in these patients. The alkaline vaginal secretions of prepubertal girls may be less inhibitory to bacterial growth than the acidic secretions of postpubertal females. Transfallopian spread is also suggested by the development of primary peritonitis in women with intrauterine devices (IUDs).[59,60] The route of spread in women with gonococcal or chlamydial perihepatitis (Fitz-Hugh-Curtis syndrome) is presumably from the fallopian tubes and paracolic gutters to the subphrenic space, but may also be hematogenous. In the one man with this syndrome, *Neisseria gonorrhoeae* was recovered from a liver biopsy specimen, and the route of spread was presumably via bacteremia.[61]

Although tuberculous peritonitis may result from direct entry into the peritoneal cavity of tubercle bacilli (from the lymph nodes, intestine, or genital tract in patients with active disease of these organs), it is more likely to be disseminated hematogenously from remote foci of tuberculosis, most commonly in the lung. Tuberculous peritonitis may become clinically evident after the initial focus has completely healed.

Clinical Manifestations. Primary peritonitis is an acute febrile illness often confused with acute appendicitis in children. Fever, abdominal pain, nausea, vomiting, and diarrhea are usually present with diffuse abdominal tenderness, rebound tenderness, and hypoactive or absent bowel sounds. In cirrhotic patients with primary peritonitis, preexisting ascites is present. In some patients, the clinical manifestations may be atypical. The onset, for example, may be insidious, and findings of peritoneal irritation may be absent in an abdomen distended with ascites. Fever (>100°F) is the most common presenting sign, occurs in 50–80 percent of cases,[20,27] and may be present without abdominal signs or symptoms or the process may be completely silent. Primary peritonitis in cirrhotic patients is generally associated with other features of end-stage liver disease (hepatorenal syndrome, progressive encephalopathy, and variceal bleeding).

The ascitic fluid protein concentration may be low[20] in abdominal inflammation for the following reasons: (*1*) hypoalbuminemia[62] and (*2*) dilution of ascitic fluid with transudate from the portal system when there is cirrhosis or the portal vein is obstructed.[63] The leukocyte count in peritoneal fluid usually is greater than 300/mm^3 (in 85 percent of cases, >1000/mm^3), with granulocytes predominating in >80 percent of cases.[26] However, the total leukocyte count of some patients with ascites uncomplicated by infection may be similarly elevated.[25] Indeed, an increase in ascites leukocyte counts has been noted during diuresis in patients with chronic liver disease.[64] Recent studies of other parameters of ascitic fluid that may help in diagnosing primary bacterial peritonitis have found the lactate concentration and pH to be useful.[65–67] Ascitic fluid pH <7.35 and lactate >25 mg/dl were more specific but less sensitive than a leukocyte count of >500/mm^3, and using all three parameters together increased the diagnostic accuracy.[66,67] Gram stain of the sediment when positive is diagnostic, but it may be negative in about 60–80 percent of cases with cirrhosis and ascites.[20,26]

Gonococcal perihepatitis (Fitz-Hugh-Curtis syndrome) most often occurs in women. It manifests with sudden onset of pain in the right upper quandrant of the abdomen, at times referred to the right shoulder. There may be low-grade fever, right upper quadrant tenderness, guarding, and a friction rub over the liver.[68] Gonococcal cervicitis and/or salpingitis may or may not be clinically evident. Chlamydial and gonococcal perihepatitis are clinically indistinguishable.

Primary tuberculous peritonitis usually is gradual in onset, with fever, weight loss, malaise, night sweats, and abdominal distension. The abdomen may not be rigid and is often characterized as being "doughy" on palpation. The findings at operation or laparoscopy consist of multiple nodules scattered over the peritoneal surface and omentum. Adhesions and a variable amount of peritoneal fluid are usually present. Ascitic fluid may have an elevated protein concentration (>3 g/dl) and a lymphocytic pleocytosis, but neither may be present, especially in cirrhotic patients.[69] Similarly, *Coccidioides immitis* can cause a granulomatous peritonitis with a variable clinical manifestation.[70]

Diagnosis. The diagnosis of primary peritonitis is one of exclusion of a primary intra-abdominal source of infection and can be made with certainty only after a thorough laparotomy. However, under certain circumstances, laparotomy may be avoided on the basis of findings in peritoneal fluid obtained by paracentesis. For example, if gram-positive organisms are obtained after paracentesis, a diagnosis of primary peritonitis can usually be made and exploratory laparotomy deferred. In children, if gram-negative organisms, a mixed flora, or no organisms are obtained, full exploratory laparotomy is indicated to rule out possible intra-abdominal sources of continuing peritoneal contamination. However, in end-stage cirrhotic patients, exploratory laparotomy may be life-threatening, and the likelihood of finding a primary intra-abdominal focus may be small. Laparotomy performed on cirrhotic patients with sepsis in an attempt to find the source of infection has been reported to have a mortality rate of 80 percent.[71] Surgery in these patients can be deferred while awaiting the response to antimicrobial therapy. Patients with primary peritonitis usually respond within 48 hours to appropriate antimicrobial therapy. The observation of an exponential rate of decline in the number of ascitic fluid leukocytes after the initiation of antimicrobial therapy for primary peritonitis has also been found to help differentiate primary from secondary bacterial peritonitis.[72]

Recovery of pneumococci from peritoneal fluid may not indicate primary peritonitis, as illustrated by a case report of appendicitis and secondary peritonitis due to pneumococci.[73] For this reason, some surgeons have considered the differential diagnosis in children between appendicitis and primary peritonitis too difficult to make without operative examination, even when gram-positive bacteria are identified in peritoneal fluid.[17] Paracentesis for smear and culture is indicated in all cirrhotic patients with ascites and in children with gross proteinuria and abdominal pain, whether or not the diagnosis of nephrotic syndrome was previously established. However, paracentesis is not without hazard, especially in patients with hemorrhagic tendencies or bowel distension. In a retrospective analysis of 242 consecutive diagnostic abdominal paracenteses in patients with liver disease and ascites, major complications were reported in 7, including perforation of the bowel with generalized peritonitis or abdominal wall abscess and serious hemorrhage.[74]

The diagnosis of tuberculous peritonitis can usually be made at operation or laparoscopy and confirmed by the histologic characteristics of the peritoneal biopsy specimen[75] and by bacteriologic examination of the peritoneal biopsy specimen and fluid.[76] The diagnosis of *C. immitis* peritonitis can be made on a wet mount of ascitic fluid, by finding *C. immitis* by culture and by histologic examination.[70]

Prognosis. The treatment of primary peritonitis has been reported to be successful in more than one-half of the cirrhotic patients, but because of the frequency of accompanying end-state cirrhosis, the overall mortality in cirrhotic adults has been as high as 95 percent.[20,23] However, more recent studies have reported lower mortality rates of 70 and 57 percent, with 28 and 40 percent dying from the primary peritonitis, respectively.[26,27] Those patients with the poorest prognosis were found to have renal insufficiency, hypothermia, hyperbilirubinemia, and hypoalbuminemia. The lower mortality rates in these series can perhaps be explained by the less frequent occurrence of hepatic encephalopathy in these later series. Treatment of peritonitis caused by gram-positive organisms, as well as early infections, has been more frequently successful than treatment of gram-negative or late infections. In nephrotic patients with gram-positive infections or in patients who do not have a preterminal underlying illness, the survival rate is over 90 percent.[15]

Treatment. Because the Gram stain is frequently negative in primary bacterial peritonitis, the initial choice of antimicrobial drug is often empiric, based on the most likely pathogens. The antimicrobial regimen can be modified once the results of the culture and susceptibility tests are available.

Some of the third-generation cephalosporin antibiotics have been demonstrated to be as efficacious as the combination of ampicillin plus an aminoglycoside in primary bacterial peritonitis.[77] They also avoid the risk of nephrotoxicity, which is sufficiently frequent in this group of patients to warrant the avoidance of aminoglycosides if an equally effective alternative antimicrobial regimen can be used.[27,78] Other antimicrobial agents such as the broad-spectrum penicillins (e.g., mezlocillin, ticarcillin, piperacillin), carbapenems (e.g., inipenem), and β-lactam antibiotic/β-lactamase inhibitor combinations (e.g., ticarcillin-clavulanate, ampicillin-sulbactam) are potential alternatives.

Primary bacterial peritonitis due either to *S. pneumoniae* or group A streptococci is best treated with penicillin G. Peritonitis suspected of being due to *Staph. aureus* should be treated with a penicillinase-resistant penicillin (e.g., nafcillin) or with a first-generation cephalosporin (e.g., cefazolin). If *Pseudomonas aeruginosa* is isolated, an aminoglycoside antibiotic plus an antipseudomonal penicillin or cephalosporin should be used together. For those situations in which the Gram stain is suggestive of *Bacteroides* or polymicrobial peritonitis is evident, antimicrobials with activity against *B. fragilis* and other anaerobic organisms should be added (e.g., metronidazole, clindamycin).

In those cases where there is a strong clinical suspicion of primary bacterial peritonitis but all cultures are sterile, antimicrobial therapy should be continued. Clinical improvement together with a significant decline in the ascitic fluid leukocyte count should occur after 24 to 48 hours of antimicrobial therapy if the diagnosis is correct.[72,79] The lack of the expected clinical response or the persistence of an elevated ascitic fluid leukocyte count should make other diagnoses a consideration. Antimicrobial therapy should be continued for 10 to 14 days if improvement is noted. The administration of intraperitoneal antimicrobials is not necessary.

Secondary Peritonitis

Etiology. The primary intra-abdominal processes that may give rise to peritonitis are numerous. These include diseases or injuries of the gastrointestinal tract such as perforation of a peptic ulcer; traumatic perforation of the uterus, urinary bladder, stomach, or small or large bowel; spontaneous perforation associated with typhoid, tuberculous,[80] amebic, *Strongyloides*, and cytomegalovirus ulcers; appendicitis, diverticulitis, or intestinal neoplasms; gangrene of the bowel either from strangulation, bowel obstruction, or mesenteric vascular obstruction; suppurative cholecystitis; bile peritonitis; pancreatitis; operative contamination of the peritoneum or disruption of a surgical anastomosis site; lesions of the female genital tract such as septic abortion, puerperal sepsis, postoperative uterine infection, endometritis complicating an IUD,[81] and gonococcal salpingitis or gonococcal vulvovaginitis in children; lesions of the male genital tract such as suppurative prostatitis; and rupture of an intraperitoneal or visceral abscess (e.g., renal or perinephric, tuboovarian, liver, splenic, or pancreatic abscess). Peritonitis is a major hazard of peritoneal dialysis used in the management of renal failure, fluid and electrolytic imbalance, and certain intoxications.[56] Not uncommonly, bacterial peritonitis can occur secondary to the use of peritoneovenous and ventriculoperitoneal shunts.[82,83]

Microbiologic Characteristics. Infrequently, secondary peritonitis is caused by exogenous microorganisms, for example, *Staph. aureus, N. gonorrhoeae*, or *M. tuberculosis*, which have caused infection in intra-abdominal or adjacent viscera and have spread to involve the peritoneum. Most cases of secondary peritonitis, however, are endogenous in origin due to the large number and variety of microorganisms that normally colonize mucous membranes lining certain viscera within the abdominal cavity. Although forming a continuous surface, the mucous membranes of the stomach, upper small bowel, lower small bowel, and large bowel each has a characteristic microflora. The vagina also has a distinct microflora. Normally, invasive activities of indigenous bacteria are controlled by the intact mucosa of the gastrointestinal tract and vagina. Disturbances in this mucosal barrier may occur as a result of spontaneous disease, trauma, or surgical operations that permit escape of indigenous bacteria and may result in infection of the peritoneum, the abdominal viscera, or the retroperitoneal space. The frequency with which various indigenous organisms are recovered from intra-abdominal infection varies according to the site of the primary process and whether the primary process is associated with an alteration of the indigenous microflora.[84]

The stomach normally contains $\leq 10^3$ cfu of microorganisms/ml in the fasting state. If bacteria are present, they are mostly facultative, gram-positive, salivary microorganisms, such as lactobacilli and streptococci. The numbers of these organisms in stomach contents transiently increase after a meal.[85] Gastric flora is more numerous and may be composed of different organisms when there is achlorhydria (e.g., from cimetidine) or blood in the stomach.[85,86] The flora of the upper small intestine is normally sparse and consists of salivary microorganisms.[87] But in the presence of achlorhydria,[85] intestinal obstruction, or other processes affecting motility or absorption, the flora of the small intestine is more profuse and varied. Conditions that favor small bowel stasis include scleroderma, regional enteritis, small bowel strictures, nontropical sprue, tropical sprue, duodenal and jejunal diverticula, presence of an afferent loop of the Billroth II gastrojejunostomy, and intestinal pseudo-obstruction.[88] Large bowel flora has been found in the proximal small bowel of cirrhotic patients.[57] The ileum normally contains *E. coli*, enterococci, and an equal number of microorganisms that are obligately anaerobic, such as *B. fragilis*.[87] It is the colon, however, in which a profuse microflora exists in concentrations of about 10^{11} bacteria/ml of feces, a wet sludge of practically pure bacteria.[89] The colonic flora is predominantly composed of the obligate anaerobes, *B. fragilis*, and *Bifidobacterium* spp., which outnumber facultative microorganisms, primarily *E. coli*, by 10^3–10^4 to 1. Other colonic bacteria are viridans streptococci, enterococci, *Eubacterium* spp., *Klebsiella* spp., *Proteus* spp., *Enterobacter* spp., and *C. perfringens*. The large bowel flora is relatively stable[89] but may be significantly altered by antibiotic therapy.[90]

As would be anticipated from the nature of the gastrointestinal flora, Altemeier[91] reported anaerobes in 96 percent of 100 cases of peritonitis secondary to acute appendicitis with perforation. *Bacteroides melaninogenicus* and anaerobic gram-positive cocci were the most frequent isolates. Recent studies of the bacteriologic characteristics of intra-abdominal infections,[92–94] using modern bacteriologic techniques that provide an anaerobic environment during collection, transport, and incubation, have confirmed the findings of Altemeier that anaerobes play a major role. Finegold reported that in a series of 73 intra-abdominal infections including 16 cases of peritonitis, there were an average of 4.5 isolates per case (range, 1–12 organisms), with 2.5 anaerobes and 2 aerobes or facultatives.[92] The most frequent isolate was *E. coli*, followed by *B. fragilis* (the most common anaerobic isolate), enterococci, other *Bacteroides* spp., *Fusobacterium, C. perfringens*, other clostridia, *Peptococcus, Peptostreptococcus*, and *Eubacterium*. Similar findings have been reported by Gorbach et al. in a series of 43 patients, which included 10 cases of peritonitis, in 93 percent of whom anaerobes or a mixture of anaerobes and facultatives were recovered,[93] and by Swenson et al. in a series of 64 patients, which included 26 cases of peritonitis, in 81 percent of whom anaerobes were recovered.[95]

In these series, bacteremia was reported in about 20–30 percent of patients. Organisms recovered from blood frequently included *B. fragilis* or *E. coli*. In series of patients with *Bacteroides* bacteremia, 14–62 percent had a gastrointestinal source.[101–104]

Together with highly antibiotic-resistant strains of *Serratia* and *Acinetobacter, P. aeruginosa* is more frequently isolated from patients who develop their intra-abdominal infection while in the hospital, after having received broad-spectrum parenteral antimicrobials.[96] However, two recent studies have noted that *P. aeruginosa* comprises a more significant portion of the aerobic isolates in community-acquired intra-abdominal infection[97,98] than had been noted in previous series.[99]

Penetrating injuries to the liver and spleen are rarely followed by infection due to the usual sterility of these organs.[100]

Recent quantitative studies[105–107] in sexually active women during the childbearing period have revealed that the predominant vaginal microflora is composed of five to seven different microorganisms, and that anaerobes are approximately 10 times more numerous than facultative organisms. There are about 10^8–10^9 cfu of anaerobes and about 10^7–10^8 cfu of facultatives per milliliter of vaginal secretions. The most frequent isolates in titers of $\geq 10^5$/ml are obligate or facultative anaerobic lactobacilli, nonenterococcal streptococci, anaerobic gram-positive cocci, Bacteroidaceae other than *B. fragilis* (e.g., *B. melaninogenicus, B. bivius, B. ruminicola*), and a group of unidentified catalase-negative facultative bacilli. Diphtheroids and *S. epidermidis* have also been reported to be frequent vaginal isolates.[107] When specifically looked for, *Gardnerella vaginalis* in high counts has also been found to be only slightly less frequent than lactobacilli in the vaginal secretions of normal women.[105,106] Colonic organisms, such as *B. fragilis*, Enterobacteriaceae, and enterococci are rarely found as predominant components of the normal vaginal flora and probably proliferate at this site only under exceptional circumstances. For example, these organisms have been reported to appear in vaginal secretions in the immediate postoperative periods after vaginal operations,[108] and *C. perfringens* has been reported more frequently in vaginal secretions after difficult labor or abortions.[109] Hite et al.[110] noted the relative infrequency of *Bacteroides* and anaerobic gram-positive cocci in the vagina of normal prenatal women, whereas during the puerperium in both women with postpartum endometritis and noninfected women, these organisms were found to be more prevalent.[110,111] Factors favoring colonization by these anaerobes after surgery and in the puerperium are unknown but are possibly related to blood or necrotic tissue that provides the reduced, enriched environment required by these anaerobes.

Sequential sampling of vaginal secretions during the menstrual cycle has been reported to show constant levels of anaerobes, although recovery of specific organisms varies from specimen to specimen in each woman.[107] By contrast, levels of facultatives decrease 100-fold in the premenstrual week.[107] This variation in microflora may reflect cyclic fluctuation in the vaginal environment due to changes in hormonal activity during the menstrual cycle. Because the vaginal flora varies under certain conditions and members of this flora have differing pathogenicity, the frequency of endogenous intra-abdominal infections of gynecologic origin, as well as the types of pathogens involved, vary accordingly. For example, the frequency of vaginal colonization with group B streptococci increases during pregnancy, and infections due to these organisms are relatively common in the postpartum period.[112] In addition, in women with trichomoniasis, *Bacteroides* species more frequently may be found in vaginal secretions.[106,110] Postpartum infection, presumably due to anaerobes, has been reported to be more frequent in women who have trichomoniasis during pregnancy.[113]

The bacteriologic characteristics of intra-abdominal infection that complicates female genital tract infections is quite similar to secondary peritonitis due to a gastrointestinal source, except for the occurrence of *N. gonorrhoeae* in cul-de-sac aspirates.[114] Data compiled by Swenson et al.,[115] Thadepalli et al.,[116] and Chow et al.[117] indicate that anaerobes were found in 72 percent of 200 gynecologic infections. Anaerobes were especially frequent (92 percent) in closed-space infections such as tuboovarian and pelvic abscesses. *Bacteroides*, in particular *B. fragilis* and *B. melaninogenicus*, and anaerobic gram-positive cocci were the most frequently isolated anaerobes. *Escherichia coli* and streptococci were the most prevalent facultatives. Apparently, even in acute salpingitis, recent bacteriologic studies have demonstrated in the majority of patients the presence of anaerobes, usually gram-positive cocci in cul-de-sac aspirates, despite the recovery of gonococci from the endocervix.[118–120] The data are interpreted as supporting the concept of superinfection with anaerobes after initial infection with *N. gonorrhoeae* late in the course of this disease.[121] In children, gonococcal peritonitis has been rarely reported with gonococcal vulvovaginitis.[122,123]

Intraperitoneal rupture has been reported in 10 percent of the cases of amebic liver abscess and may cause acute generalized peritonitis or a less commonly localized intraperitoneal abscess with a mortality of about 18 percent.[124] Perforation of the colon with bacterial peritonitis due to fulminant amebic colitis is also unusual but often fatal.[125] Similarly, *Strongyloides stercoralis* infestation of the small bowel may rarely cause fatal peritonitis, with or without concurrent bacterial contamination.[126] *Candida* has been isolated from the abdominal fluid in patients undergoing peritoneal dialysis, as has *Staph. aureus*, Enterobacteriaceae, and *P. aeruginosa*.[127] *Candida* peritonitis has also been observed as a complication of gastrointestinal surgery or in perforation of a viscus,[128,129] and its occurrence is related to numerous factors that increase the rate of *Candida* colonization in the gastrointestinal tract. These include immunosuppression, prolonged hospitalization, and antimicrobial and/or antacid therapy. *Candida* is most commonly isolated from the peritoneum after perforation of a gastric or duodenal peptic ulcer, or after spillage of colonic contents into the peritoneum due to trauma, mesenteric artery occlusion, or dehiscence of a surgical anastomosis.

Pathogenesis. The virulence of the bacteria that cause peritonitis is enhanced when certain microorganisms either are combined intraperitoneally with substances such as mucus, enzymes, or hemoglobin or are combined with certain other microorganisms.

Chemical peritonitis can be produced by escape of bile or of gastric or pancreatic secretions into the peritoneal cavity. When gastric acid escapes into the peritoneal cavity, there is an outpouring of serum protein and electrolytes from the blood into the peritoneal cavity. The acidity is quickly neutralized by these buffers and by diffusion of hydrogen ions into the body fluids.[130,131] Widespread necrosis may result from enzymatic digestion after intraperitoneal spillage of potent pancreatic enzymes. Escape of bile into the peritoneal cavity is generally considered to be a very grave, often fatal situation.[132,133] The severity of peritonitis after escape of these intestinal secretions is due in part to subsequent bacterial peritonitis. Indeed, in the dog with experimentally produced partial biliary diversion into the peritoneal cavity, fatal effects were reduced by oral nonabsorbable or parenteral antibiotics.[134] Bacteria may enter the peritoneal cavity with contaminated intestinal secretions through perforations in the gastrointestinal wall, as well as by migration through the wall of the intact gastrointestinal tract, in response to the irritation of bile and possibly other intestinal tract secretions on the serosal surface.[55]

Nemir et al. demonstrated that after experimental strangulation obstruction of a loop of bowel in the dog, the animal usually died within 36 hours, and the peritoneal fluid at first was light pink and eventually became black. When this black fluid was removed and injected into the peritoneal cavity of a normal animal, the recipient also developed a similar fatal peritonitis, but the early peritoneal fluid was nontoxic.[135–137] The toxicity could be largely counteracted by instilling antibiotics into the obstructed loop of intestine or by giving antibiotics simultaneously when the fluid was injected into normal animals.[138,139] Many workers in the past have shown that intraperitoneal injection of large numbers of organisms in pure culture is incapable of producing peritonitis unless some additional factor is present, such as gum tragacanth, talc, mucin, turpentine, or other irritants. It seemed unlikely, therefore, that the toxicity of strangulation obstruction fluid was due to its bacterial content alone. Evidence has been reported that viable bacteria in addition to the presence of free hemoglobin in the peritoneal fluid are necessary to account for the lethality both of bowel strangulation and of the fluid that collects in the peritoneal cavity after bowel strangulation.[140–142] The mechanism by which free hemoglobin enhances peritoneal infection is unknown but perhaps is related to free iron. Iron is required for bacterial metabolism and, in amounts that leave an excess of free iron after having saturated transferrin, may greately enhance infections due to certain microorganisms, such as Enterobacteriaceae and *C. perfringens*.[143] Hau et al. demonstrated that intraperitoneal hemoglobin depresses the influx of granulocytes into the peritoneal cavity in response to intraperitoneal bacteria, and hemoglobin depresses in vitro the chemotactic response of granulocytes and monocytes.[144]

Intraperitoneal fluid and fibrin that enter the peritoneal cavity as a result of the increased vascular permeability due to local trauma or bacterial infection are important components of the inflammatory response and play adjuvant roles. It has been shown that low numbers of *E. coli* in small volumes of saline infused intraperitoneally are innocuous, but these numbers of *E. coli* can become lethal in direct proportion to the increase in the volume of saline infused. This is thought to be related to the resultant dilution of opsonic proteins.[145] Trapping of bacteria beneath layers of fibrin may limit their spread but may also lead to abscess formation and isolation of bacteria from host defense mechanisms.[146]

A number of other substances such as hog gastric mucin, bile salts,[147] and barium sulfate[148,149] have been used as adjuvants in producing lethal intraperitoneal infections. The mechanisms of their respective effects have been the subject of numerous studies. It has been postulated that hog gastric mucin coats bacteria, thus protecting them from intraperitoneal phagocytosis.[150]

Cuevas and Fine[151] have attributed the lethality of bowel strangulation and infectious or chemical irritation of the serosal surface of the bowel to endotoxemia. Endotoxin was thought to escape from the gut lumen, to cross the intact bowel wall into the peritoneal cavity, and then to be absorbed into the systemic circulation. Within minutes after experimental superior mesenteric artery occlusion, endotoxin has been detected in the systemic circulation, before its appearance in the portal vein.[151]

Secondary peritonitis is usually a mixed infection involving predominantly obligate and facultative anaerobes. Obligate anaerobes are sensitive to oxygen in the molecular form and also to bound oxygen, as in organic peroxides. Survival and growth of anaerobes are also dependent on the oxidation-reduction potential, that is, the oxidizing capacity of their environment. Most pathogenic anaerobes require a negative potential of at least -150 mV. Low oxidation-reduction potentials are thought to occur in many abscesses,[152] and oxidation-reduction potentials ≤ -150 mV are measured in abscesses from which anaerobes are recovered.[153] Some anerobic organisms have additional requirements, such as vitamin K, arginine, serum, blood pigments, or bile, before growth is obtained. Thus, establishment of an anaerobic infection requires an environment in which the oxygen tension is very low, the oxidation-reduction potential is low, and abundant nutrients are available to support anaerobic fermentative metabolism. These requirements are usually met by devitalized tissue as a consequence of ischemia, trauma, or neoplastic growth. Once proper conditions are obtained, anaerobic organisms can achieve doubling rates equivalent to those seen with aerobic enteric bacilli. In vivo, the rapidly expanding bacterial and inflammatory cell mass, frequently accompanied by gas production, can interrupt the blood supply to the immediately surrounding tissue and cause further tissue necrosis.

Gram-negative anaerobic cocci and bacilli (including *B. fragilis* and *B. melaninogenicus*) possess endotoxins with much weaker biologic activity in comparison to those extracted from their aerobic counterparts and have low or absent 2-keto-3-deoxyoctanoate content.[153a] In addition, certain anaerobes elaborate collagenase,[155] other proteolytic enzymes, and deoxyribonuclease.[154] Certain Bacteroidaceae are capable of degrading heparin,[156] which may be responsible for the suppurative thrombophlebitis frequently seen in infections due to these microorganisms.[157] These factors tend to provide more areas well adapted to the growth requirements of the anaerobe, with the result that the infection progresses.

In addition, anaerobes may be resistant to host defenses. For example, although leukocytes have been shown to have bactericidal activity under both aerobic and anaerobic conditions against several anaerobic species, including *B. fragilis*, presumably by mechanisms other than those dependent on the superoxide anion O_2^- or H_2O_2,[158] Keusch and Douglas[159] found that granulocytic killing of *C. perfringens* was impaired under anaerobic conditions. Also, a capsule has been demonstrated on *B. fragilis*[160] and *B. asaccharolyticus* (formerly *B. melaninogenicus ss. asaccharolyticus*),[161] which might protect the organisms from phagocytosis and favor abscess formation.[162–164] Some anaerobes, especially *B. fragilis*, may be resistant to the normal bactericidal activity of serum.[158]

Many anaerobic infections appear to be synergistic. Although it is probable that the majority of bacteria isolated in mixed infections are nonpathogenic by themselves, their presence may nevertheless be essential for the pathogenicity of the bacterial mixture. Such examples of bacterial synergism in infection have been demonstrated in periodontal infection by Socransky and Gibbons[165] and in peritonitis by Altemeier.[166]

Facultative organisms in mixed infections may be essential by providing a sufficiently reduced environment for the growth of obligate anaerobic organisms. Another mechanism of bacterial synergy is the generation of a substance by one organism, which is essential for the growth of another, for example, the production of vitamin K (a required growth factor for *B. melaninogenicus*) by diphtheroids. Anaerobes such as *Bacteroides* spp. have also demonstrated the ability to protect aerobic bacteria from phagocytic killing[167,168] and from otherwise effective antibiotic therapy (e.g., via β-lactamase production).[169]

In addition, each component of the pathogenic mixture may contribute in different ways to the clinical picture. After implantation of fecal contents intraperitoneally into rats. Onderdonk et al. observed that *E. coli* initially predominated in the peritoneal exudate.[170] Bacteremia, due to *E. coli* during this phase, was uniformly present and frequently fatal. In rats that survived, indolent intra-abdominal abscesses developed in which *B. fragilis* predominated. Elimination of *E. coli* by early administration of gentamicin reduced early mortality but did not prevent late intra-abdominal abscess due to obligate anaerobes, whereas elimination of obligate anaerobes with clindamycin did not prevent early mortality due to *E. coli* bacteremia but reduced late abscess formation in survivors. These findings indicate that although *E. coli* is responsible for early mortality, anaerobes are responsible for late abscess formation in this model.[171,172]

Pathophysiologic Responses. Whatever the initiating cause of peritonitis, a similar series of reactions takes place, both locally and systemically.

LOCAL RESPONSE. The local inflammatory response of the peritoneum is similar to that in other tissues, but the peritoneal lining presents a large exudative and absorptive surface. At sites of irritation, there is an outpouring of fluid into the peritoneal cavity that, in contrast to normal serous fluid, has a high protein content (>3 g/dl) and many cells, primarily granulocytes, that phagocytize and kill organisms. The exudate contains fibrinogen that polymerizes, and plaques of fibrinous exudate form on the inflamed peritoneal surfaces. This exudate glues adjacent bowel, mesentery, and particularly omentum to each other. Localization is further aided by inhibition of motility in involved intestinal loops. Experimentally, radiopaque medium injected intraperitoneally at one locus can be demonstrated to have spread over much of the greater peritoneal sac within a short time. The extent and rate of intraperitoneal spread of contamination are undoubtedly dependent on the volume and nature of the exudate[13] and on the effectiveness of the localizing processes.

If peritoneal defenses aided by appropriate supportive measures control the inflammatory process, the disease may resolve spontaneously. A second possible outcome is a confined abscess. A third course results when the peritoneal and systemic defense mechanisms are unable to localized the inflammation, which then progresses to spreading diffuse peritonitis. Some of the factors favoring spread of the inflammatory process are (*1*) greater virulence of bacteria, (*2*) greater extent and duration of contamination, or (*3*) impaired host defenses.

SYSTEMIC RESPONSE. Peritonitis leads to changes not only locally in the peritoneal cavity but throughout the body.

Gastrointestinal Tract. Initially in peritonitis there is hypermotility, followed by paralysis of the bowel. Accumulation of fluid and electrolytes in the lumen of the adynamic bowel continues until distension is sufficient to inhibit capillary inflow and secretion ceases.

Cardiovascular. Because of the large surface area of the peritoneum, shifts of fluid into the peritoneal cavity, combined with fluid shifts into the bowel lumen, can produce a profound fall in circulating blood volume and elevation of the hematocrit.[173,174] Fluid and electrolyte loss is further exaggerated by coexistent fever, vomiting, diarrhea, and loss of aspirated gastrointestinal fluid. As the process continues, the decreased venous return to the right side of the heart results in a drop in cardiac output, with resulting hypotension.[174] In addition, the patient may be exposed to the circulatory effects of endotoxin, namely, progressive pooling of blood within tissue capillary beds, producing a further decrease in venous return. Usually, there is evidence of increased adrenergic activity—sweating, tachycardia, and cutaneous vasoconstriction (i.e., cold moist skin, mottled and cyanotic extremities).

With adequate replacement of blood volume, cardiac output may be maintained above normal.[174] Cardiac output of two or even three times normal may be required to satisfy the increased metabolic needs of the body in the presence of infection. Failure to sustain increased cardiac output results in progressive lactic acidosis, oliguria, hypotension, and ultimately death if the infection cannot be controlled.

Respiratory. The intraperitoneal inflammation results in relatively high and fixed diaphragms and considerable pain on respiration. This results in basilar atelectasis with intrapulmonary shunting of blood. Satisfactory compensation is possible only if the increase in energy demands does not exceed the respiratory reserve. Heavy cigarette smoking, chronic bronchitis, emphysema, and obesity compound the problem. With decompensation in respiratory function, hypoxemia is accompanied first by hypocapnia (respiratory alkalosis) and later by hypercapnia (respiratory acidosis). In some patients, pulmonary edema develops, due not to left ventricular failure but perhaps to increased pulmonary capillary leakage as a consequence of hypoalbuminemia or direct effects of bacterial toxins (adult respiratory distress syndrome). In these patients, progressive hypoxemia develops with decreasing pulmonary compliance. This requires volume-cycled ventilatory assistance with increasingly higher concentrations of inspired oxygen and positive end-expiratory pressure.

Renal. Low renal perfusion may be followed by acute tubular necrosis and progressive azotemia.

Metabolic. During the first few days, the excretion of cortisol is increased and subsequently returns to normal.[175] The increased energy demands of infection rapidly deplete body stores of glycogen, followed by catabolism of protein (muscle) and fat, thus accounting for the rapid weight loss of severely infected patients. Prolonged intra-abdominal infection is associated with extreme wasting. Heat production may eventually fail, and body temperature then falls. Exhaustion and death may ensue.

Clinical Manifestations. SYMPTOMS. The early manifestations of peritonitis secondary to disease of abdominal viscera are frequently those of the primary disease process. Moderately severe abdominal pain is almost always the predominant symptom. The pain is aggravated by any motion, even respiration. The progression of abdominal pain is a function of the rate of dissemination of the material producing the pain stimulus. Rupture of a peptic ulcer with massive spillage of gastric contents produces severe epigastric pain that, within minutes, may spread to involve the entire abdomen. In contrast, the spread of pain from a lesion such as a ruptured appendix is much more gradual. Decreased intensity and extent of pain with time usually suggest localization of the inflammatory process.

Anorexia, nausea, and vomiting commonly accompany abdominal pain. Patients may also complain of feverishness, sometimes with chill, thirst, scanty urination, inability to pass feces or flatus, and abdominal distension.

The formation and progression of an intraperitoneal abscess is often gradual: The patient who seemed to be recovering from peritonitis or an abdominal operation stops improving; fever returns, and localizing symptoms may develop.

PHYSICAL FINDINGS. Patients with fully developed peritonitis have a characteristic appearance, the *Hippocratic* facies, including "a sharp nose, hollow eyes, collapsed temples; the ears cold, contracted and their lobes turned out; the skin about the forehead being rough, distended and parched; the color of the whole face being brown, black, livid, lead-colored." Patients with peritonitis characteristically lie quietly in bed, supine, with the knees flexed and with frequent limited intercostal respirations, since any motion intensifies the abdominal pain. Early in the course the patient is alert, restless, and irritable, but later may become apathetic or delerious.

Body temperatures may reach 42°C. Subnormal temperatures in the range of 35°C often seen in the early stages of chemical peritonitis and late in the course of patients with continuing intra-abdominal sepsis or septic shock and are a grave sign.

Increasing tachycardia with weak, thready peripheral pulses reflects decreased effective blood volume. The blood pressure is maintained within normal limits early in the disease process. As peritonitis progresses, the blood pressure lowers to shock levels. Respiration is increasingly rapid and shallow.

Marked abdominal tenderness to palpation is present, usually maximally over the organ in which the process originated. Rebound tenderness, both direct and referred, signifies parietal peritoneal irritation. This finding is sometimes more accurate than direct palpation in locating the point of maximal tenderness as well as in delineating the extent of peritoneal irritation.

Muscular rigidity of the abdominal wall is produced both by voluntary guarding and by reflex muscular spasm. Hyperresonance due to gaseous intestinal distension can usually be demonstrated by percussion. Pneumoperitoneum from a ruptured hollow viscus may produce decreased liver dullness to percussion. Bowel sounds, initially hypoactive, later disappear. Rectal and vaginal examination may reveal tenderness and the presence of a pelvic abscess and may indicate a primary focus in the female pelvic organs.

Abdominal pain and muscle spasm may be deceptively absent in some patients. Those with lax abdominal musculature (e.g., patients in the postpartum period, patients with ascites due to cirrhosis, patients with marked cachexia) may not have abdominal rigidity. Similarly, patients in shock, on glucocorticosteroid therapy, or in whom loculated intra-abdominal abscesses are not in contact with the anterior abdominal wall (e.g., subphrenic, lesser sac, pelvic) may not exhibit marked abdominal pain and spasm. Absent bowel sounds may be the only manifestation of peritonitis in such patients, and a high index of suspicion is necessary.

Diagnostic Studies. The differential diagnosis in patients with symptoms and signs of peritonitis includes pneumonia, sickle cell anemia, herpes zoster, diabetic ketoacidosis, tabes dorsalis, porphyria, familial Mediterranean fever, plumbism, lupus erythematosus, and uremia.

A peripheral blood leukocyte count of 17,000–25,000 white blood cells/mm^3 is usual in acute peritonitis, the differential count showing polymorphonuclear predominance and a moderate to marked shift to the left. However, reliance on the significance of the total white blood cell count may be misleading. Massive peritoneal inflammation may mobilize leukocytes into the diseased area, so there may be, for example, fewer than 5000 white blood cells/mm^3 in the circulating blood, but the differential smear in this situation may show an extreme shift to immature polymorphonuclear forms.

Hemoconcentration and dehydration are reflected by elevated hematocrit and blood urea nitrogen values. Hyperglycemia and glycosuria usually are not present in peritonitis but may be seen in diabetic acidosis and acute pancreatitis, which may manifest with signs suggesting peritonitis. Hematuria and pyuria without bacteriuria may reflect intra-abdominal inflammatory disease such as appendicitis adjacent to the urinary tract. Elevated serum amylase levels may be seen in peritonitis due to almost any cause, but very high levels are only seen in acute pancreatitis. Hyponatremia may be seen in patients given water to replace isotonic fluid losses but is also characteristic of porphyria. Acidosis, both metabolic and respiratory, is present in severe and late peritonitis. Supine, upright, and lateral decubitis x-ray films of the abdomen may reveal distension of both the small intestine and the colon with adynamic loops of bowel or features of mechanical intestinal obstruction, volulus, intussusception, or vascular occlusion. Inflammatory exudate and edema of the intestinal wall produces a widening of the space between adjacent loops. Peritoneal fat lines and psoas shadows may be obliterated. Free air may be visible if there is a ruptured viscus. Chest x-ray films should always be taken to rule out a pulmonary or thoracic problem as the cause of the abdominal distress. The presence of air beneath the diaphragm may be best defined in these pictures. Trapped gas with a fluid level or mottling due to gas may also be visible in intraperitoneal or visceral abscesses. Calcification in the gallbladder or other organs may also be noted on x-ray films.

Needle aspiration of the peritoneal cavity is often helpful. If no fluid can be aspirated, peritoneal lavage with Ringer's lactate solution should be done to obtain fluid for examination. In performing a tap, the region of abdominal scars where bowel may be adherent to the underside of the scar should be avoided. The aspirate is examined grossly for content of blood, pus, bile, or digested fat; chemically, for amylase content; and microscopically, with Gram stain, for bacteria. A positive tap is meaningful; a dry or negative tap is of little significance. Guidance for the tap may be obtained by ultrasound or CT scan.

Prognosis. Survival of a patient with secondary peritonitis depends on many factors, including the age of the patient, the duration of peritoneal contamination, the presence of foreign material (bile or pancreatic secretions, barium), the primary intra-abdominal process, and the microorganisms involved.[176] Altemeier[91] has shown that the more organisms present in peritoneal exudate, the worse the prognosis, although there was no correlation between severity of infection and any particular organism. Mortality increases with more distal gastrointestinal sources of contamination.[177] The age of the patient also influences the mortality from peritonitis. In the very young patient, because of the relatively small omentum, the walling-off process is less effective, so diffuse peritonitis occurs more frequently than in the adult. In the elderly, preexisting conditions such as emphysema, diabetes, or cardiovascular disease reduce the capacity of the patient to meet the demands on the cardiovascular, respiratory, and renal systems during this period of intense metabolic activity.[176] Mortality rates range from 3.5 percent in those with early infection following penetrating abdominal trauma to more than 60 percent in patients with established intra-abdominal infection and secondary organ failure.[178] Persistent peritoneal contamination, leakage of pancreatic enzymes, septicemia, fluid and electrolyte abnormalities, and cardiovascular, renal, and respiratory failure are the principal causes of death.

Treatment. ANTIMICROBIAL THERAPY. Secondary peritonitis is typically polymicrobial, and the pathogens in the majority of patients with secondary peritonitis are derived from the gastrointestinal tract even in patients with a primary gynecologic process. Typically, the facultative microorganisms are *E. coli*, *Klebsiella/Enterobacter* spp., *Proteus* spp., and enterococci, and the obligate anaerobes are *B. fragilis*, *B. melaninogenicus*,

Peptococcus, Peptostreptococcus, Fusobacterium, Eubacterium lentum, and *Clostridium*. Other less commonly isolated pathogens include *Staph. aureus, P. aeruginosa,* and *Candida*.

The role of antimicrobial therapy in the outcome of infection due to anaerobes or due to a mixture of anaerobes and facultative microorganisms is extremely difficult to assess. This is primarily because of the often dramatic response to surgical drainage and débridement alone when there is localized infection. Nevertheless, appropriate antimicrobial therapy has been shown to reduce significantly mortality among patients with bacteremic infections due to Bacteroidaceae or Enterobacteriaceae.[104,179,180] Antimicrobial drugs are expected to control bacteremia and early metastatic foci of infection, to reduce suppurative complications if given early, and to prevent local spread of existing infection. Once suppuration has occurred, it may be difficult to cure the infection if antimicrobial drugs are used without drainage; also, antimicrobial drugs used alone may mask some of the clinical manifestations of abscess formation. Evidence is accumulating, however, that some intra-abdominal abscesses can be treated successfully with antibiotics alone.[181,182]

Antimicrobial therapy should be started immediately after appropriate specimens (e.g., blood and peritoneal fluid) are obtained for culture. This means that antimicrobial therapy is often started before the completion of in vitro antimicrobial sensitivity testing of the specific facultative pathogens. In addition, rapid isolation, identification, and in vitro sensitivity testing of anaerobes, in contrast to testing of facultatives, are often not possible in many community hospitals. Several factors account for the delay in obtaining anaerobic bacteriologic results. For example, infections due to anaerobes are frequently caused by mixtures of five or more microorganisms, and cultures require long periods for growth and isolation. In addition, in vitro sensitivity testing by the conventional disk diffusion technique has not been standardized for anaerobes.[153] Such tests are influenced to a large extent by the growth rate of the bacteria, inoculum size, pH and type of medium, duration of incubation, and CO_2 concentration in the atmosphere.[183,184] In vitro studies of the stability of the β-lactam antibiotics when exposed to reducing agents such as mercaptoamines (cysteine), which are frequently incorporated in media used for the growth of anaerobes, have shown that these compounds are able to open the β-lactam ring and to inactivate penicillins.[185] However, susceptibility of anaerobic organisms can be reliably determined by the broth or agar dilution techniques with appropriate media.[186] Because these tests are generally performed by research laboratories, knowledge of the antimicrobial susceptibility of anaerobes is gained from periodically published reports on anaerobic isolates by centers that specialize in performing these tests. Therefore, initial chemotherapy is usually empiric, based on the use of the most reliable and least toxic antimicrobial agents for the most probable anaerobic and facultative pathogens. In vitro sensitivity reports (usually reliable only for the facultative or aerobic organisms) allows subsequent adjustment of the initial regimen to more specific therapy.

Because these infections are commonly polymicrobial, a broad spectrum of antimicrobial activity is required. Drugs active against anaerobic bacteria may be quite inactive against the accompanying aerobic or facultative pathogens in the mixed infections, and vice versa. For this reason, combinations of usually two or three drugs are used. These combinations of antimicrobial agents are selected for their activity against most of the more virulent pathogens in the infective mixture (e.g., the Enterobacteriaceae and *B. fragilis*). The Enterobacteriaceae in the mixture are significant and frequently cause bacteremia in these patients, as in the rat model of intra-abdominal infection of Onderdonk et al.[170] However, antibiotics need not be active against every pathogen isolated. It is apparent that if only some of the organisms can be eliminated, the synergistic effect may be removed, and the patient's defenses may be able to eradicate the remaining organisms. For example, clindamycin alone (which has no activity against Enterobacteriaceae and enterococci) has been reported to be sufficient treatment for some patients with infections resulting from a mixture of Enterobacteriaceae, enterococci, and anaerobes.[187] Experimental evidence in the rat model of intraperitoneal infection suggests that the enterococcus is not a primary pathogen, although in the presence of anaerobes it may aid in abscess formation.[188] In several clinical studies of anaerobic infections, patients were treated successfully with both gentamicin and clindamycin despite absence of activity of this therapeutic regimen against enterococci.[189,190] However, more recent reviews emphasize the role of the enterococcus in intra-abdominal infections.[191] In some reports, this organism has been noted to emerge as the sole intra-abdominal pathogen, at times associated with enterococcal bacteremia,[192,193] especially if patients with polymicrobial intra-abdominal infection were treated with an antimicrobial agent that lacked activity against the enterococcus.[194,195]

When combinations of antibiotics are used, synergism or antagonism may occur. Chloramphenicol has been shown to impair early bactericidal activity of gentamicin in vitro, and antagonism was demonstrated in mice with experimental *Proteus mirabilis* infection when phagocytic function was impaired (i.e., in neutropenic mice).[196] Two recent studies suggest that clindamycin inhibits early in vitro killing of *E. coli* and *K. pneumoniae* by gentamicin.[197] However, in an in vivo study of aminoglycoside therapy of *E. coli* peritonitis and bacteremia in normal and neutropenic mice, prior or simultaneous administration of clindamycin with the aminoglycoside did not inhibit the therapeutic effect of the aminoglycoside.[198] Clindamycin combined in vitro with gentamicin has been reported to have indifferent or synergistic activity against Enterobacteriaceae after 18 hours of incubation.[199] The activities of various antimicrobial agents against the usual peritoneal pathogens and the results of various clinical trials are discussed in the sections that follow.

Chloramphenicol. At a concentration of 16 μg/ml, chloramphenicol has activity against over 99 percent of the anaerobic pathogens involved in intra-abdominal infection, especially *B. fragilis*.[200] However, resistant strains may inactivate chloramphenicol, so no chloramphenicol is present in abscesses containing these organisms.[201] Up to 15 percent of the strains of *Bacteroides* may require 16 μg/ml for inhibition, a concentration close to the maximum attainable therapeutic serum levels without encountering the dose-related bone marrow suppressive effect.[200] For this reason, chloramphenicol may be difficult to use because of its toxicity for the hematopoietic tissues, especially with the doses and duration of therapy required for severe anaerobic bacterial infection. In addition, patients treated with chloramphenicol have been reported to have persistent bacteremia due to chloramphenicol-sensitive organisms.[202] Chloramphenicol is active against facultative microorganisms involved in polymicrobial anaerobic infections, such as most *E. coli*, other Enterobacteriaceae, and enterococci, but lacks activity against *P. aeruginosa*. The availability of equally effective and potentially less toxic antimicrobial agents to treat anaerobic infections (e.g., clindamycin, metronidazole, imipenem) has all but eliminated the need for chloramphenicol.[203]

Clindamycin. Clindamycin has been reported to inhibit over 95 percent of the anaerobes, including *B. fragilis*, at a concentration of 8 μg/ml.[200] About 15 percent of the strains of *Clostridium* spp. other than *C. perfringens, Peptococci* spp., and rare strains of *Fusobacterium* spp., have been reported to be resistant to clindamycin. Most strains of *B. fragilis* have remained highly susceptible to clindamycin during the past decade.[204,205] Recently, plasmid-mediated, transferable clindamycin resistance in *B. fragilis* has been demonstrated,[204] and clindamycin resistance among *B. fragilis* may have become a problem at certain medical centers. Clindamycin is active against only certain facultative gram-positive cocci, such as

Staph. aureus and *S. pyogenes*, but not *S. faecalis*, and has virtually no activity against Enterobacteriaceae.

Diarrhea is reported to be the most frequent side effect of clindamycin therapy and occurs at an incidence of 2 to 20 percent.[206] The severity of the diarrhea varies but may be associated with pseudomembranous colitis in up to one-half of the patients with diarrhea, as reported in one study.[207] Toxic megacolon, colonic perforation, and death on rare occasions have been reported. The cause has been attributable to an exotoxin produced by clindamycin-resistant strains of *Clostridium difficile*.[206]

Metronidazole. Metronidazole is active against strict anaerobes, inhibits most *B. fragilis. Fusobacterium* spp., and *Clostridium* spp., and has unique bactericidal action against *B. fragilis* and *C. perfringens*.[208] Its in vitro activity, however, is poor against aerobes, microaerophiles, and anaerobes that may become somewhat aerotolerant on subculture (i.e., certain anaerobic gram-positive cocci and sporeless gram-positive rods).[200,209] Despite the poor in vitro activity demonstrated against aerobic and microaerophilic organisms, there is now some in vivo evidence in animal models and humans that metronidazole has activity against *E. coli* and other aerobes in mixed aerobic-anaerobic infections.[210,211] The mechanism for this is poorly understood but may be related to the conversion by *B. fragilis* of metronidazole into active metabolites with activity against *E. coli* and other aerobes.[210] Nonetheless, metronidazole should be used clinically in combination with other antimicrobial agents in the treatment of mixed infections.

Tetracyclines. Sutter et al.[212] noted that while 14 of 15 strains of *B. fragilis* isolated before 1960 were sensitive to tetracycline, only 24 of 63 strains isolated after 1970 were susceptible. Tetracycline similarly has poor activity against many other anaerobes.

Doxycycline and minocycline[213] have been reported to be more active than tetracycline against anaerobic bacteria. However, their activity is relatively poor against *B. fragilis, Clostridum* spp., and anaerobic gram-positive cocci.[213] The large number of resistant anaerobes, especially *B. fragilis*, precludes the use of these drugs as initial therapy.

Cephalosporin. Bacteroides fragilis and other *Bacteroides* species are usually resistant to the so-called first-generation cephalosporins (e.g., cefazolin) and to some second-generation cephalosporins (e.g., cefamandole, cefuroxime). However, cefoxitin is distinctly more active than any of the other second-generation cephalosporins against *Bacteroides* species.[200,214,215] Cefotetan has activity similar to that of cefoxitin, except that it is less active against the *B. fragilis* group (not including *B. fragilis*).[214,215] These first- and second-generation cephalosporins are also active against the majority of the strains of *E. coli*, *P. mirabilis*, and *K. pneumoniae*. The third-generation cephalosporins (e.g., cefotaxime, ceftizoxime, cefoperazone, ceftriaxone, and ceftazidime) have demonstrated significantly better activity against the Enterobacteriaceae, including *Enterobacter* and *Serratia* species. Only ceftazidime, and less so cefoperazone, have activity against *P. aeruginosa*. With a few exceptions, the third-generation cephalosporins have relatively poor activity against *B. fragilis* and other *Bacteroides* species.[216] Moxalactam, an oxacephem with good activity against *B. fragilis*, has been found to be an effective single agent in the treatment of intra-abdominal infections.[217,218] The potential for bleeding secondary to the use of moxalactam has greatly limited its utility.[219] Ceftizoxime is reported to have good in vitro activity against *B. fragilis* and other *Bacteroides* species in some studies,[215,220] but has been found to be inadequate against *Bacteroides* species, including *B. fragilis*, in other in vitro studies.[214,221] Because the activity of ceftizoxime is greatly affected by the inoculum of *Bacteroides* in in vitro studies,[200] this antibiotic would most likely be inadequate in treating severe intra-abdominal infections where the inoculum of organisms is great.

Penicillins. Penicillin G and ampicillin have excellent activity against all anaerobes, with the exception of *Bacteroides* spp. (especially *B. fragilis*) and *Fusobacterium* spp. other than *F. nucleatum*. Ampicillin also is active against 70–80 percent of the strains of *E. coli* and almost all *P. mirabilis*. Although *B. fragilis* has been considered to be resistant to penicillins, in vitro sensitivity testing reveals that over 90 percent of *B. fragilis* isolates may be sensitive to carbenicillin, ticarcillin, mezlocillin, and piperacillin in concentrations of ≤125 μg/ml. In fact, these antibiotics have been reported to be rapidly bactericidal against *B. fragilis*.[222,223] The clinical experience with these broad-spectrum penicillins in the treatment of anaerobic bacterial infection has been reported to be favorable.[224,225] A prospective controlled study has shown that the therapeutic response to ticarcillin was similar to that of clindamycin or chloramphenicol, each in combination with an aminoglycoside in the therapy of intra-abdominal infection.[226]

Because sensitive strains of *B. fragilis* may require up to 125 μg of the broad-spectrum penicillins per milliliter for inhibition, these antibiotics should be used in high dosages (300–500 mg/kg/day) to treat these infections. However, because up to 20 percent of the strains of *B. fragilis* are resistant to concentrations of the broad-spectrum penicillins[227] that can be achieved in serum, use of the broad-spectrum penicillins as the initial therapy for suspected *B. fragilis* infection should be undertaken with caution. In addition, there is some evidence to suggest that penicillin G may fail to achieve concentrations at the site of *B. fragilis* infection, because of both a reduction in penetration of penicillin into infected sites and inactivation of the drug by *B. fragilis*.[228] It is unknown if this is also true for broad-spectrum penicillins. Therapeutic failures despite high doses of penicillin for *B. fragilis* bacteremia have been well documented.[101] Resistance of *B. fragilis* to penicillins is frequently due to production of β-lactamase.[229]

The spectrum of antibacterial activity of the older broad-spectrum penicillins (e.g., carbenicillin, ticarcillin) includes the majority of aerobic gram-negative bacilli (including *P. aeruginosa*) commonly isolated from patients with intra-abdominal infections with the exception of most *Klebsiella* and many *Serratia* spp. However, these penicillins are considerably less active than ampicillin and penicillin G against enterococci. The newer broad-spectrum penicillins (e.g., mezlocillin, azlocillin, piperacillin) are more active than carbenicillin and ticarcillin against the Enterobacteriaceae group, including many strains of *Klebsiella*, and against *P. aeruginosa* and enterococci.[230]

The combination of a β-lactamase inhibitor, such as clavulanic acid or sulbactam, with a penicillin increases the activity of the penicillin against certain β-lactamase producers.[231,232] Ticarcillin-clavulanic acid inhibits 60–80 percent of ticarcillin-resistant strains of Enterobacteriaceae, including most *E. coli* and *Klebsiella* spp., as well as all β-lactamase-producing *Bacteroides* species.[233] However, the combination will not inhibit the inducible β-lactamase produced by *P. aeruginosa, Serratia* spp., *Citrobacter freundii* or *Enterobacter cloacae*.[234] Ampicillin-sulbactam is active against many bacteria resistant to ampicillin, including *E. coli, Klebsiella*, and *Bacteroides* spp.[235,236]

Other β-Lactams. Imipenem, a carbapenem antibiotic, has the broadest antimicrobial spectrum of any current antibiotic,[237] with activity against almost all aerobic and anaerobic bacteria. It is resistant to most β-lactamases except those produced by rare strains of *B. fragilis*.[238] Aztreonam, a monobactam antibiotic, has a spectrum of activity limited to aerobic gram-negative bacilli.[239] It would be necessary to use an antibiotic with anaerobic activity (e.g., clindamycin, metronidazole) along with aztreonam in the treatment of secondary intra-abdominal infections.

Aminoglycosides. Aminoglycosides, except for their excellent spectrum of activity against Enterobacteriaceae and *P. aeruginosa*, do not have much advantage over penicillins or cephalosporins against sensitive strains of these organisms for many reasons. For example, the serum concentrations of gentamicin are unpredictable after a dose based on the body weight, so peak and trough serum levels must be confirmed by any of various assay methods available.[240] In addition, the therapeutic range of peak serum concentrations of 4–8 μg/ml is narrow: levels below 4 μg/ml may likely be below the inhibiting concentration for the pathogen, and levels greater than 10–12 μg/ml may be toxic. Thus, the peak serum levels are either equal to or only slightly greater than the minimum inhibitory concentration (MIC) for the aminoglycoside in vitro.

Aminoglycosides are inactive against obligate anaerobes, and their activity against sensitive pathogens is antagonized by an anaerobic environment.[241] and by reducing substances such as sulfhydryl compounds. Aminoglycosides are also not active in acidic conditions. Both anaerobic and acidic conditions are frequently present in intra-abdominal abscesses. The penicillins and cephalosporins, by contrast, are relatively nontoxic, can be used in concentrations that are many times the MIC for the pathogen, and are active under anaerobic or acidic conditions. For these reasons, the penicillins and cephalosporins are probably more reliable antibiotics than the aminoglycosides against sensitive pathogens. Therefore, if indicated on the basis of in vitro sensitivity testing, penicillins or cephalosporins should be used in preference to aminoglycosides.

Quinolones. The fluoroquinolones (e.g., norfloxacin, ciprofloxacin, enoxacin, ofloxacin) are a new class of antimicrobial agents related to nalidixic acid.[242] They are active against almost all aerobic gram-negative bacilli and most gram-positive cocci, including some enterococci.[243] Their ability to kill bacteria in the stationary phase of growth, along with the lack of development of plasmid-mediated resistance, make the fluoroquinolones potentially valuable antimicrobial agents for the treatment of intra-abdominal infections including abscesses. Current limitations of these agents include the need to administer them orally (though parenteral forms will be available in the future) and the relatively low serum drug concentrations in relation to the potency of some of these agents (e.g., norfloxacin). The addition of an antimicrobial agent active against anaerobic bacteria would be required if the use of a quinolone was considered for secondary intra-abdominal infection.

Controlled Clinical Trials. There is no one antimicrobial regimen applicable to every clinical situation. However, it is clear that for an antimicrobial regimen to be efficacious in the treatment of secondary peritonitis and other intra-abdominal infections, the agents chosen must have significant antibacterial activity against *B. fragilis* and enteric gram-negative bacilli.[244–246] Therapy with an agent with activity against *P. aeruginosa* would be desired if the infectious process developed while in the hospital or after a course of broad-spectrum antibiotics. The need to add specific agents active against the enterococcus remains controversial.[191] Although the results of many antimicrobial trials for treatment of intra-abdominal infections have been published, caution must be exercised when interpreting these studies because of the possibility of inadequate study design and analysis of data.[247] Some of the variables that must be considered are (*1*) differences in patient populations, (*2*) types and severity of underlying illnesses, (*3*) community- vs. hospital-acquired infection, and (*4*) the pathogens isolated.

The standard antimicrobial regimen against which most new regimens are compared is an aminoglycoside in combination with clindamycin.[248–250] The risk of renal toxicity and ototoxicity, along with the need to monitor serum aminoglycoside levels, may limit the use of aminoglycosides as newer agents prove to be useful alternatives.[251] Table 1 lists many of the antimicrobials regimens that have been found to be efficacious for the treatment of intra-abdominal infections in clinical trials. The majority of second- or third-generation cephalosporins have limited activity against the *B. fragilis* group, and their use as single antimicrobial agents for the treatment of intra-abdominal infections has had variable results.[97,262–265] However, combining one of these cephalosporins with clindamycin or metronidazole would likely be an adequate antimicrobial regimen in this setting.[266]

TABLE 1. Comparative Antimicrobial Trials for Treatment of Intra-Abdominal Infections

Regimen	*Reference*
Cefoxitin ± aminoglycoside vs. clindamycin + aminoglycoside	252–254
Moxalactam vs. clindamycin + aminoglycoside	218
Moxalactam vs. cefoxitin + aminoglycoside	255
Ticarcillin + aminoglycoside vs. clindamycin + aminoglycoside	217
Piperacillin vs. cefoxitin	256
Ampicillin-sulbactam vs. clindamycin + aminoglycoside	257
Imipenem vs. clindamycin + aminoglycoside	258–260
Aztreonam + clindamycin vs. clindamycin + aminoglycoside	261

Although the need for treatment is controversial,[267,268] clearly *Candida* species, either as part of a polymicrobial peritoneal infection or as a single isolate, have the potential to cause peritonitis, intraperitoneal abscesses, and subsequent candidemia.[128,269] The dominant clinical view today favors aggressive early therapy of all intra-abdominal isolates of *Candida* species in symptomatic patients with peritonitis, usually with the parenteral administration of at least 375–500 mg amphotericin B over 10–14 days.[270]

The duration of therapy is usually prolonged to prevent relapse because host defenses cannot be relied on to eradicate completely the pathogens from sequestered areas of extensive tissue necrosis and abscess formation. Not all these areas are accessible to adequate surgical drainage. Antibiotic therapy should be given before, during, and after surgery to ensure tissue and blood drug levels that can combat local and metastatic spread of the infection. The dose, the frequency, and usually the route of administration of the antimicrobial agents are maintained to achieve adequate blood and tissue drug concentrations during the entire treatment period and are not necessarily changed as the patient improves.

The intravenous route of antibiotic administration is preferred, especially in shock, when poor perfusion of the gut and muscle preclude use of the oral or intramuscular routes. Blood levels may be less satisfactory after intramuscular administration of certain antibiotics, for example, chloramphenicol. Although some surgeons use antibiotics intraperitoneally at the time of operation in irrigating fluid,[271] others do not.[272] Decreases in the rate of wound infection but not in the rate of intraperitoneal sepsis have been shown with the use of intraperitoneal irrigation.[273] Respiratory arrest may occur after peritoneal absorption of aminoglycosides, and lavage of the peritoneal cavity at the time of surgery with large amounts of saline alone may be sufficient.[274] Also, intravenous or intramuscular antibiotics in adequate doses reach the peritoneum without additional intraperitoneal administration.

The effect of irrigation of the peritoneal cavity with agents such as povidone-iodine has also been studied. In one study, there was a decreased frequency of intra-abdominal abscess formation in the povidone-iodine group compared to that of the saline group.[275] However, povidone-iodine has been shown to be a potent inactivator of such neutrophil functions as chemotaxis and phagocytosis, and thus may have a detrimental effect.[276]

Another technique is to place a plastic catheter through the abdominal wall at the time of the operation so that antibiotics can be injected directly postoperatively into the peritoneal cavity. The method is said to be beneficial clinically,[277] but its superiority over intravenous antibiotics alone has not been proven in clinical peritonitis. Recent comparative studies showed no significant difference in clinical outcome between patients who had irrigation of the peritoneal cavity and those who did not.[278,279] However, when peritoneal dialysis is being done in the presence of peritonitis, antibiotics in therapeutic doses should be included in the dialysis fluid to maintain antibiotic levels in the rapidly exchanged peritoneal fluid.[280] If intraperitoneal antibiotics are used, systemic antibiotics may be necessary as well to maintain adequate blood levels.

HYPERBARIC OXYGEN. Increased oxygen tension attainable with hyperbaric oxygen therapy inhibits and kills *C. perfringens*[281] and reduces the production of *C. perfringens* α-toxin. Hyperbaric oxygenation has been used clinically and experimentally for clostridial myonecrosis, with some reported success.[282] Because *C. perfringens* is a relatively oxygen-tolerant anaerobe in comparison to other obligate anaerobic pathogens, it would be reasonable to assume that hyperbaric oxygen therapy would be at least equally efficacious with anaerobic infections due to these more oxygen-sensitive anaerobes. Except for a few reports[283] almost no clinical or experimental data, however, are available. Hill[284] reported suppression of experimental liver abscesses due to anaerobes in mice treated with hyperbaric oxygen therapy alone. In a more recent study, it appeared that the use of hyperbaric oxygen therapy favorably affected the outcome of experimental sepsis in a rat model, perhaps by enhancing host defense mechanisms.[285] Consideration should also be given to the hazards of hyperbaric oxygen therapy.

GASTROINTESTINAL DRAINAGE. In the presence of peritonitis, the patient should receive nothing by mouth. If no distension is present when treatment is instituted, continuous gastric suction is usually sufficient. For those patients who are distended when treatment is started and for those who become distended in spite of gastric drainage, small intestinal intubation should be instituted.

WATER AND ELECTROLYTE ADMINISTRATION. The type of fluid replacement is determined in large part by the chemical abnormalities found. In general, hypovolemia, dehydration, and metabolic acidosis predominate, so plasma or albumin, Ringer's lactate solution, and 5% dextrose in water usually suffice. The amount to be given in the 2- to 4-hour period before anticipated surgery is determined by watching vital signs, hematocrit values, hourly urinary output, and central venous pressure.

BLOOD AND PLASMA TRANSFUSION. Although many patients recover from an illness satisfactorily with a hemoglobin of 8 or 10 g/dl, some surgeons recommend that the patient be transfused to maintain levels as high as 12–13 g/dl in order to provide a margin of safety should some complication such as septic shock or upper gastrointestinal hemorrhage supervene.

RESPIRATORY SUPPORT. Fluid sequestered in the abdomen and loops of bowel distended by gas may elevate the diaphragm. Inflammation of the parietal peritoneum, including the diaphragmatic surface, leads to guarding and splinting of the muscular wall, which interferes with deep breathing or coughing. A subphrenic abscess may be responsible for splinting of the diaphragm. Retained bronchial secretions may lead to atelectasis and subsequent pneumonitis. These factors that impair the ability to augment respiratory exchange in the face of the increased expenditure of energy required by the inflammatory process produce hypoxemia and respiratory alkalosis. When the patient tires, the combination of metabolic and respiratory acidosis may develop and prove fatal.

Arterial blood gas studies are necessary to detect and quantitate respiratory decompensation. Measures aimed primarily at gastrointestinal decompression, elevation of the head of the bed, and control of the inflammation may sufficiently improve respiration. Administration of oxygen may improve arterial oxygen saturation. If these measures are inadequate, endotracheal intubation or tracheostomy should be done without delay. A volume-cycled respirator should be used and adjusted to give a P_{O_2} of 80–100 mmHg and a normal pH. If the P_{CO_2} is not then normal, metabolic acidosis or alkalosis may need to be treated. As the intra-abdominal process subsides, the patient may be able to breathe spontaneously again and may be weaned from the ventilator. In certain severe cases, positive end-expiratory pressure may also be necessary.

OPERATIVE APPROACH. The aims of an operation for spreading peritonitis are to stop continuing contamination, to remove foreign material from the peritoneal cavity, and to provide drainage of purulent collections. Operation is generally not indicated (*1*) in primary peritonitis, (*2*) in moribund patients who continue to deteriorate despite vigorous supportive therapy, (*3*) in patients in whom the disease process subsides and localizes while they are being prepared for surgery, (*4*) in patients with peritonitis secondary to hemorrhagic pancreatitis, and (*5*) in patients with peritonitis secondary to pelvic inflammatory disease, since this usually responds to nonsurgical therapy.

There is general agreement as to the necessity of (*1*) removing all material, such as necrotic tissue, feces, and blood, from the operative field, since the virulence of peritoneal infections is enhanced by the presence of these substances, (*2*) eliminating any possible anaerobic conditions, and (*3*) reducing the bacterial count to a minimum. Also, in acute diffuse peritonitis, recent studies have clearly shown that copious peritoneal irrigation with isotonic saline or Ringer's lactate solution significantly reduces mortality and morbidity.[274] In localized infection, local drainage alone is adequate because the risk of disseminating infection outweighs any possible benefit of removing foreign material that may have escaped mechanical removal.

Use of multiple drains for drainage of the general peritoneal cavity is physically impossible since exudate and adhesions rapidly isolate and occlude the drains and may increase secondary infections.[286] However, drains are often placed in a dependent point to which fluid can be expected to gravitate or in an area of devitalized tissue that cannot be removed.

Prevention. Prevention of postoperative peritonitis requires avoiding contamination of the peritoneum with gastrointestinal or vaginal secretions. In addition to using good surgical technique, this can be accomplished by early treatment of a primary intra-abdominal infection. For example, Leigh et al. noted that the rate of wound infection in patients with perforated appendix was over 50 percent if no antimicrobial therapy was used and 15 percent in the group given appropriate therapy.[287] Similarly, two studies demonstrate the efficacy of early use of antibiotics in penetrating wounds of the abdomen, especially involving the colon.[288,289] Surgeons have also used various means to reduce the complex gastrointestinal or vaginal flora before clean, contaminated surgery. Mechanical cleansing of the bowel with a low-residue diet and then a liquid diet, cathartics, and enemas can reduce the total fecal mass and coliform count in the colon, although not necessarily the predominant anaerobic flora.[290] The use of oral antibiotics preoperatively to reduce bowel flora is well accepted. *Escherichia coli* in the colonic flora is sensitive to either oral neomycin or kanamycin, whereas *B. fragilis* frequently is sensitive to erythromycin or metronidazole. Thus, combinations such as neomycin-erythromycin base have been shown to be effective in reducing total bowel flora preoperatively and decreasing the incidence of postoperative infection.[291]

Parenteral antibiotics have also been used in gastrointestinal and vaginal surgery prophylactically when there is a chance of contamination with normal microflora at the operative site (clean, contaminated surgery). Up to 30 percent of these types of operations may be complicated by infections. These involve cutting through the large bowel without significant spillage; compromising the blood supply of the large bowel; cutting through stomach or small bowel when there is anticipated intraluminal bacterial overgrowth; appendectomy for appendicitis without rupture; penetrating wounds of the abdomen; gallbladder surgery in the elderly; cesarian section after rupture of the membranes and labor; vaginal hysterectomy in the premenopausal woman; and radical pelvic surgery for gynecologic malignancy.[292] Several studies have shown significant reduction in the frequency of postoperative infection from about 20–30 percent to about 4–8 percent after prophylactic antibiotic use in clean, contaminated surgery.[293,294] The basic principle of antibiotic prophylaxis is to provide adequate tissue levels at the site of contamination and blood levels during the procedure and for possibly up to 24 hours after the procedure.

Peritonitis During Peritoneal Dialysis

Chronic Peritoneal Dialysis. Peritoneal dialysis has been used successfully to treat uremia in patients with end-stage renal disease since the mid-1940s. Peritonitis was a frequently associated side effect that hindered the acceptance of chronic peritoneal dialysis until an improved access catheter was developed by Tenckhoff in 1968. This catheter significantly decreased the incidence of peritonitis, but initial reports of patients undergoing chronic ambulatory peritoneal dialysis (CAPD) with this catheter had peritonitis rates of more than six episodes per patient-year.[295,296] This rate has appeared to decline with the introduction of collapsible plastic bags, improved adapters, and better techniques. However, peritonitis remains the major complication of CAPD today.[297] It occurs at a rate of about one episode per patient a year, with a range from three or more episodes a year to less than one every 2 years. Forty-five percent of CAPD patients develop peritonitis at least once during their initial 6 months on CAPD. This increases to 60–70 percent during the first year.[298–300] Recurrent peritonitis occurs in 20–30 percent of patients and is one of the most common reasons for discontinuation of CAPD.[301] A small proportion of patients seem to have an unusually high frequency of peritonitis.[302] This disparity in the frequency of infection has been attributed, at least in part, to faulty sterile technique on the part of the patient when self-administering CAPD.

The origin of infection in most cases appears to be contamination of the catheter by common skin organisms.[296] Alterations of skin flora in CAPD patients[303] may lead to peritoneal contamination with enteric pathogens. A higher incidence of peritonitis has been reported in dialysis patients who are nasal carriers of *Staph. aureus*.[304] Pathogens may also contaminate the peritoneum from exit-site and subcutaneous-tunnel infections, transient bacteremia, and contamination of the dialysate delivery system during bag exchanges. As mentioned previously, it has been demonstrated that enteric bacteria may also gain access to the peritoneal cavity by transmural migration through an intact intestinal wall after the introduction of hypertonic solutions into the peritoneum.[55] This mechanism may account for enteric bacterial peritonitis in dialysis patients.[56] Polymicrobial infection with fecal organisms suggests perforation of the bowel as a complication of catheter placement.

Alterations in peritoneal defenses may increase the risk of peritonitis in CAPD patients. The antimicrobial function of peritoneal macrophages and polymorphonoclear cells generally requires the presence of opsonins. A reduction in the levels of IgG and C3 has been noted in peritoneal dialysis effluents when compared with serum, and the levels of these crucial opsonizing agents are inversely related to the frequency of peritonitis.[305] The addition of IgG to peritoneal dialysis fluid has been found to have a prophylactic effect.[306] Other important factors that impair host defense mechanisms are the low pH and high osmolality of peritoneal dialysis fluid, both of which can impair polymorphonuclear function and antibiotic efficacy.[307]

Gram-positive organisms compose 60–80 percent of isolates, most commonly *Staph. epidermidis* followed by *Staph. aureus*, *Streptococcus* spp., and diphtheroids. Staphylococcal isolates have been noted to grow on polymer surfaces and frequently produce an extracellular slime substance or biofilm that may protect these bacteria from host defenses.[308] Gram-negative organisms are obtained from 15–30 percent of isolates. *Escherichia coli* is the most common, followed by *Klebsiella/Enterobacter*, *Proteus*, and *Pseudomonas* spp. Less common pathogens include *Acinetobacter* spp., *C. albicans*, and anaerobic bacteria. Rare isolates include *Mycobacterium tuberculosis, Candida parapsilosis, Aspergillus fumigatus, Nocardia asteroides*, and *Fusarium* spp.[302,309–311]

Diagnosis of peritonitis is made when microorganisms and an increased number of leukocytes are present in the dialysate combined with a constellation of clinical findings that include abdominal pain and tenderness (found in 60–80 percent of patients), nausea and vomiting (in 30 percent), fever (in 10–20 percent), and diarrhea (in 10 percent).[296,302,310,311] However, not all these criteria need to be met to fulfill the diagnosis.

The dialysate is almost always cloudy, and microscopic examination reveals a leukocyte count greater than $100/mm^3$, approximately 85 percent being more than $500/mm^3$, with neutrophils predominating.[302] Gram stain of the fluid reveals organisms in 9–50 percent of cases.[296,302] Peripheral leukocytosis has been reported to be a poor indicator for peritonitis in this group of patients.[310] Blood cultures are rarely positive, in contrast to the 30–50 percent positive rate in other types of intra-abdominal infection.

Peritonitis with negative cultures occurs in 5–10 percent of cases. Constant flow of dialysis fluid into and out of the peritoneal cavity dilutes the microbial density and may falsely lower the rate of positive dialysate culture results. Negative cultures may also be due to infection with fastidious organisms, previous antimicrobial treatment, or inadequate culture technique. One method that has been used to improve the yield of dialysate cultures is the filtration method. A 100 ml aliquot of peritoneal fluid is filtered through a 0.45 μm filter. The filter is then washed with sterile saline and incubated in thioglycolate broth.[310] Rubin et al. compared the filtration method with direct inoculation of blood culture bottles and found no significant difference in positive culture rates.[296] Still others found the inoculation of 2–3 ml of dialysate into thioglycolate broth to be the most sensitive culture technique.[310] A recent study comparing direct inoculation of dialysate into a biphasic blood culture system, direct inoculation of dialysate into routine blood culture bottles, and centrifugation of 50 ml of dialysate and culture of the sediment failed to demonstrate a significant difference among these methods in the recovery of a pathogen.[312] All cultures should be performed aerobically. Fungal, mycobacterial, and anaerobic cultures should be performed if clinically indicated (e.g., negative aerobic cultures).

The prognosis of peritonitis in dialysis patients is generally favorable. A recent large series reported less than 1 percent mortality attributed directly to infection.[302] The duration of illness and positive peritoneal fluid cultures after institution of antimicrobial therapy is usually 1–4 days. However, some infections, especially those due to *Staph. aureus, Pseudomonas*, or fungus, resolve more slowly and may cause relapse more frequently.[310]

Adequate levels of antimicrobial agents necessary to treat peritonitis successfully can be obtained in the peritoneal fluid by both systemic and intraperitoneal routes.[302,309,310,313] However, because CAPD peritonitis is a localized infection, the intraperitoneal route is preferred, as no therapeutic advantage of intravenously administered antibiotic has been demonstrated.[314] Although a variety of doses can be found in the literature, the initial doses recommended in Table 2 for intraperitoneal administration result in effective peritoneal fluid drug concentrations. Subsequent dosing is used to maintain these levels. The aim of the dosing regimen is to maintain a concentration of the drug in the peritoneal cavity fluid above the MIC of the offending pathogen for most if not all of the dosing interval. Caution must be exercised when reviewing the MIC and minimum bactericidal concentration (MBC) data, since these concentrations have been demonstrated to be markedly increased when peritoneal dialysis effluent is used as the in vitro growth medium.[315]

Because of the lack of comparative, prospective clinical trials, no one antimicrobial regimen can be called superior to

TABLE 2. Antibiotic Dosage for Peritonitis during Peritoneal Dialysis

Drug	Intraperitoneal Dosage (mg/liter dialysate)	Intraperitoneal Maintenance Dosage (mg/liter dialysate)
Amphotericin B[a]	0.007 mg/kg[b]	0.07 mg/kg
Ampicillin	7 mg/kg	0.7 mg/kg
Cefazolin	5 mg/kg	1.3 mg/kg
Ceftazidime	7 mg/kg	3.5 mg/kg
Clindamycin	4.3 mg/kg	0.7 mg/kg
Gentamicin	0.9 mg/kg	0.5 mg/kg q24h
Piperacillin	14 mg/kg	1.5 mg/kg
Trimethoprim-sulfamethoxazole	80 mg/400 mg/kg	16 mg/80 mg/kg
Vancomycin	9 mg/kg	0.2 mg/kg

[a] A low dose is used initially with progression to a maintenance dose, guided by tolerance to abdominal pain.
[b] Body weight.
(Adapted from Petersen et al.,[311] with permission.)

another. After cultures are obtained, initial antimicrobial therapy should be based on the Gram stain results or the most likely pathogens if the Gram stain is not helpful. A reasonable initial empiric regimen would be vancomycin in combination with an aminoglycoside. Vancomycin is preferable to a cephalosporin because of the frequency of β-lactam resistance (i.e., methicillin resistance) in staphylococci, which predicts resistance to cephalosporins as well. Initial antibiotic choices should be modified, if necessary, after culture results are obtained. The minimum length of therapy needed for dialysis-related peritonitis has not been determined, but the usual duration ranges from 10 days to 3 weeks. Most patients with CAPD peritonitis show clinical improvement within 48–96 hours of the initiation of antimicrobial therapy. If the signs and symptoms of peritonitis persist after 96 hours of therapy, reevaluation is warranted, with consideration given to the possibilities of resistant pathogens, unusual organisms (e.g., mycobacterial, fungal), and other intra-abdominal processes, as recommended by Keane et al.[314]

Fungal peritonitis, usually caused by *C. albicans*, should be treated with amphotericin B.[316–319] If CAPD is continued, amphotericin B should be given intraperitoneally, but it can cause appreciable abdominal pain when given by this route. However, most patients with fungal CAPD infection will fail to respond unless the catheter is removed. Once the catheter is removed, amphotericin B should be given intravenously (30 mg/day). Flucytosine has also been recommended. However, this drug may be difficult to use in end-stage renal disease because of dose-dependent bone marrow toxicity. If this drug is used, serum levels should be monitored closely to prevent the development of toxic levels (>100 μg/ml). There is limited experience with the use of miconazole and ketoconazole in treating fungal peritonitis.[319–322]

Removal of the catheter may be necessary in 10–20 percent of patients. The indications for removal of the catheter include persistent skin exit site or tunnel infection; fungal, fecal, and mycobacterial peritonitis; *P. aeruginosa* peritonitis; persistent peritonitis; recurrent peritonitis with the same organism; and catheter malfunction (e.g., poor flow). The catheter should also be removed in patients with intraperitoneal abscess. Use of oral or intraperitoneal antibiotics has not been shown to be effective in preventing peritonitis during peritoneal dialysis.[56,323]

Acute Peritoneal Dialysis. The incidence of peritonitis during acute peritoneal dialysis has remained stable during the past 20 years. Innovations in technique, which began during the 1960s, reduced the rate of peritonitis from as high as 50 percent to acceptably low levels. These innovations included closed-drainage systems, small-bore catheters, limitation of dialysis to no longer than 48–72 hours, the incorporation of a millipore filter into the tubing, and the development of closed automatic systems. Also, the use of dry-heat incubators to warm the dialysate decreases the risk of contamination that may occur when water baths are used for this purpose.[324]

Some authorities have recommended that cultures of dialysate be obtained every 8–24 hours during acute peritoneal dialysis and at its termination. Culture of dialysate from the last exchange is more useful than culture of the catheter tip at the end of dialysis because of the frequent contamination of the catheter tip at the time of its removal. However, results of such routine cultures, in the absence of symptoms or cloudy fluid, provide a guide of doubtful value for initiation of therapy. More importantly, dialysate samples should be cultured and examined microscopically (cell count, Gram stain) if the dialysate becomes cloudy or the patient develops signs or symptoms of peritonitis (e.g., fever, abdominal pain). Cultures are best obtained by syringe from the port closest to the catheter.

Peritonitis during acute peritoneal dialysis is frequently caused by antibiotic-resistant, hospital-acquired, gram-negative bacilli. Therefore, it is recommended that therapy be initiated with intraperitoneal vancomycin and gentamicin (or tobramycin), with or without concurrent or subsequent addition of the same antibiotics parenterally, depending on the severity of the illness and the response to initial therapy (see Table 2 for dosages). Modification of the antibiotic regimen should be made when the culture results become available.

The clinical manifestations, prognosis, and response to therapy are similar to those described above for peritonitis associated with chronic peritoneal dialysis.

INTRAPERITONEAL ABSCESSES

Etiology

Intraperitoneal abscess may complicate either primary or secondary peritonitis.[325,326] Diseases causing secondary intraperitoneal abscesses include appendicitis, diverticulitis, biliary tract lesions, pancreatitis, perforated peptic ulcers, inflammatory bowel disease, trauma, and abdominal surgery. The relative frequency of abscess formation associated with appendicitis may be declining, and that of trauma and diverticulitis may be increasing.[326,327] The location of an abscess is generally related to the site of primary disease and the direction of dependent peritoneal drainage. For example, appendicitis has been reported to be most commonly associated with right lower quadrant and pelvic abscesses; colonic diverticulitis with left lower quadrant and pelvic abscesses; and pancreatitis with lesser sac abscesses.[325] In one large series[325] of 194 intraperitoneal abscesses, about 44 percent were in the right lower quadrant, 14 percent in the left lower quadrant, and 14 percent in the pelvis, whereas 20 percent were perihepatic. In a more recent series reported by Saini et al.[326] the frequency of various abscess locations had changed somewhat, perhaps reflecting the change in the relative frequency of the various etiologic diseases.

Of the various perihepatic (right subphrenic, right subhepatic, left perihepatic, and lesser sac) abscesses, the most common continues to be in the right subphrenic space, but the difference in numbers between the right and left sides has been falling. In fact, in one large series of 267 cases of intra-abdominal abscesses, about one-half were in the subphrenic space, 60 percent of which were noted in the left perihepatic space.[328] This increased frequency of left perihepatic space abscess has also been noted by Ozeran,[329] Sherman et al.,[330] and Sanders.[331] This is in contrast to the series of Ochsner-DeBakey in 1938[332] when right subphrenic abscesses were the most frequent, due to the numerous ruptured appendices.

In children, appendicitis is still responsible for more than 50 percent of the cases of subphrenic abscesses.[333] In contrast, in adults, perihepatic abscesses currently are seen mainly as postoperative complications[329–331,334] rather than in neglected primary intra-abdominal infections, such as appendicitis or perforated peptic ulcer. This may explain the increasing frequency of subphrenic abscesses, especially on the left, in comparison to other intraperitoneal sites.[328] Usually, the surgery has been in the gastroduodenal and biliary tracts. One group of investigators[335] has noted that abscesses that followed gastric operations were left subphrenic if incidental splenectomy had been performed but right subhepatic if splenectomy had not been done. The subhepatic space is less frequently involved than the subphrenic spaces. Lesser sac abscesses generally follow pancreatitis or perforation of the stomach or duodenum. Multiple perihepatic space abscesses have been reported in 5–26 percent of the patients.[329–331,334,335]

Bacteriologic Findings

These infections are typically polymicrobial. In studies in which bacteriologic techniques permitted isolation of anaerobes, anaerobes were found in 60–70 percent of cases.[325,326,334,336] In one study,[334] anaerobes were recovered in 20 of 24 subphrenic abscesses, and *B. fragilis* was the most common pathogen, with anaerobic cocci and clostridia in 50 percent of the patients. Other bacteria frequently recovered are *E. coli, Klebsiella/Enterobacter* group, *Proteus* spp., *P. aeruginosa, Staph. aureus*, and enterococci.[325,329,330,334]

Pathogenesis

Intraperitoneal abscesses develop as a result of localization of diffuse peritonitis usually in the pelvis, perihepatic spaces, and paracolic gutters. In addition, abscess may develop about diseased organs such as periappendiceal or pericholecystic abscesses, through a penetrating wound (from a stab, gunshot, auto accident, or other trauma), or after a surgical procedure. These abscesses are termed *secondary* and account for the majority of these cases. In contrast, the pathogenesis of primary abscesses is unknown and is presumably similar to that of primary peritonitis.

Clinical Manifestations

An acute course, with a high intermittent fever, shaking chills, abdominal pain, and tenderness over the involved area, is characteristic. The clinical pattern may be that of an acute secondary illness occurring after surgery for primary abdominal disease or a prolonged recuperative course in a patient who has been receiving antibiotics after abdominal surgery. Various authors[330–335] have emphasized the occasional chronicity of subphrenic abscesses and have speculated that the course is often modified by antibiotics. Subphrenic abscesses have been described with 6 months or more of an indolent illness.[337]

Local symptoms and signs vary widely with the location and source of the abscess. Subphrenic abscesses are usually accompanied by chest findings with costal tenderness and pleural or pulmonary involvement, whereas subhepatic abscesses have more dominant signs of upper abdominal or subcostal involvement and fewer pulmonary changes.

Diagnosis

New noninvasive diagnostic procedures including ultrasonography and computed tomography have provided greater sensitivity and specificity than the more traditional methods of radiography and radionuclide scanning.[338,339] However, these older techniques remain useful, and often a combination of diagnostic tests is the optimal approach to confirm the diagnosis of intra-abdominal abscess.[340]

Plain radiographs of the abdomen can suggest the location of abscesses in as many as 50 percent of patients.[341] Radiologic findings associated with a subphrenic abscess may include pleural effusion, elevation of the hemidiaphragm, and/or loss of diaphragmatic movement on fluoroscopy. Routine radiography may also reveal displacement of viscera by an abscess. These findings can be enhanced by contrast radiology. The stomach, for example, may be outlined with barium or air to indicate displacement due to a left perihepatic or lesser sac abscess. The presence of gas, either as a single air-fluid level or mottling within the abscess, may aid localization on routine abdominal radiography.

Combined radionuclide scanning of the lungs and liver with ^{99m}Tc may be especially useful to evaluate the right subphrenic space.[342,343] Normally, the image of the lung and liver blend uniformly in all views. With subphrenic collections, there is a clear separation of the liver from the right lung base. The liver is displaced medially and/or inferiorly, and its superior margins may be locally flattened or indented.[4] Separation of the lung and liver image may also occur in patients with a right pleural effusion or pulmonary perfusion defect or in patients with ascites. These later lesions, however, should not cause defects in the contour of the liver. Subcapsular hematomas and certain hepatic tumors, though, may distort the liver contour and separate the lung from the liver image.

^{67}Ga and ^{111}In-tagged leukocytes are two other radionuclide scans that at times are helpful in detecting intra-abdominal abscesses. Unlike the ^{99m}Tc sulfur colloid liver-spleen scan, which visualizes the entire organ and delineates abnormal areas as "cold" spots due to decreased uptake of the isotope, ^{67}Ga and ^{111}In actually accumulate in areas of inflammation, such as abscesses, and appear as areas of increased radioactivity or "hot" spots[344–347] (Fig. 4). Gallium is excreted into the intestinal tract and can accumulate in any inflammatory process, as well as in certain neoplasms. For these reasons, false-positive scan readings may occur when radioactivity within the lumen of the bowel, within the wall of an inflamed bowel, or within a non-

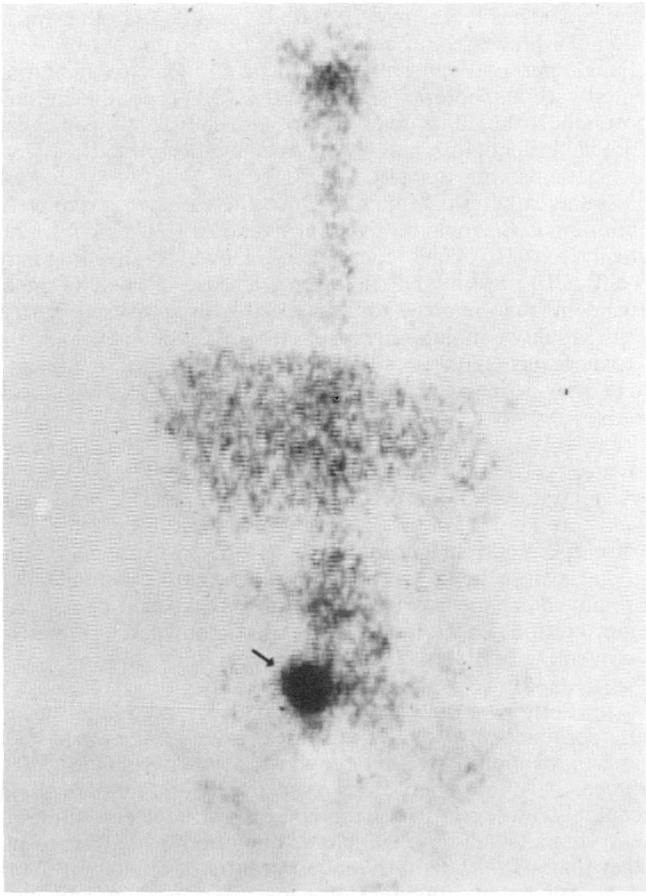

FIG. 4. ^{67}Ga scan in a patient with a regional enteritis and signs of an intra-abdominal abscess. Note the area of increased radioactivity in the right lower quadrant (arrow).

infected operative site in the process of healing is misinterpreted as an intra-abdominal abscess.

^{111}In scans are as sensitive as but more specific than ^{67}Ga scans because the labeled leukocytes tend to concentrate only in areas of inflammation, since, unlike ^{67}Ga, ^{111}In is not secreted into the bowel.[348,349] Approximately one-third of the ^{111}In-labeled leukocytes normally localized in the spleen. For this reason, ^{67}Ga is the preferred agent for detecting left-sided subphrenic abscesses because its less intense splenic uptake allows more accurate discrimination between normal splenic activity and that due to an abscess.

The diagnostic use of ultrasound is a noninvasive technique that is helpful in the determination of the size, shape, consistency, and anatomic relationships of an intra-abdominal mass.[349,351] A pulsed, focused, beam of high-frequency sound is directed into the suspect area of the patient's body by means of a transducer. Echoes are received by the same transducer from skin and tissue planes. The echo pattern is displayed on an oscilloscope as the transducer is moved along the surface of the body. The appearance of abscesses may vary widely from echo-free lesions to highly echo-genic masses, but typically appear as a fluid collection with an irregular wall and the presence of a few internal echoes. Ultrasound images may be obscured by overlying gas-filled viscera and by postoperative wounds and drains.

Computed tomography has proven especially well suited for the diagnosis of intra-abdominal abscess. Definition is unimpeded by intraluminal gas and postoperative changes, except in the presence of surgical metallic clips or residual barium that may disrupt the image. Observed findings consistent with abscess include a low-density tissue mass and a definable capsule. Computed tomography can detect extraluminal gas, a finding highly suggestive of abscess.[339] Contrast material is commonly administered orally, rectally, and intravenously when attempting to diagnose intra-abdominal abscess. The intraluminal contrast material helps to distinguish loops of bowel from abscess cavities, and the parenteral contrast material may enhance a surrounding capsule thus allowing for easier identification.

Magnetic resonance imaging (MRI) has the potential to display normal anatomy and to show abnormal conditions in many of the body's organ systems and anatomic regions.[352,353] However, only a few trials have compared MRI to older radiologic procedures. In one study, MRI demonstrated a clearer delineation of the extent of inflammatory changes than did computed tomography and better distinguished the abscess from the surrounding structures.[354] In addition, the use of MRI does not require the administration of contrast medium and eliminates exposure to radiation, but it may be more costly than other radiologic techniques.

Arteriographic localization has also been helpful.[355] However, overreliance on any one of these techniques is dangerous and should be confirmed by other methods and the clinical findings (Fig. 5).

Prognosis

The period of morbidity is unusually prolonged in patients with intraperitoneal abscesses. Altemeier et al. reported average hospital stays of 21–47 days.[325] The presence of residual or recurrent infection due to inadequate surgical drainage, more common in patients with multiple or bilateral abscesses, is associated with significantly greater mortality.[356]

Treatment

Although conflicts exist in the literature regarding the proper form of drainage of subphrenic abscesses, all agree that the main

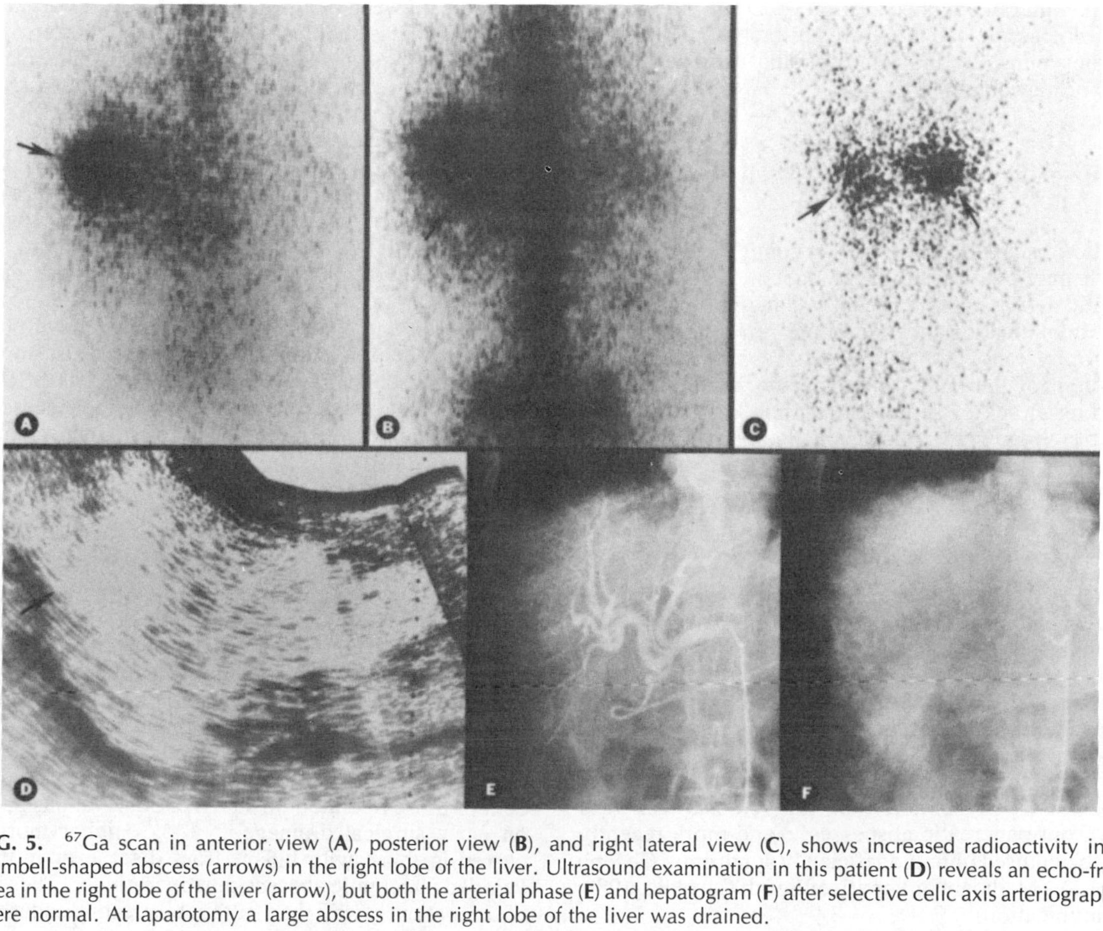

FIG. 5. ^{67}Ga scan in anterior view (**A**), posterior view (**B**), and right lateral view (**C**), shows increased radioactivity in a dumbell-shaped abscess (arrows) in the right lobe of the liver. Ultrasound examination in this patient (**D**) reveals an echo-free area in the right lobe of the liver (arrow), but both the arterial phase (**E**) and hepatogram (**F**) after selective celic axis arteriography were normal. At laparotomy a large abscess in the right lobe of the liver was drained.

therapy for any intraperitoneal abscess is drainage. Effective management is dependent on accurate localization of the abscess, discrimination between single and multiple abscesses, and early and adequate drainage. Conventional therapy for intraperitoneal abscesses has usually included surgical drainage. However, in recent years, successful therapy has been accomplished using percutaneous catheter drainage as an alternative to surgery.[357–359] This method has become possible with the use of refined imaging techniques, especially ultrasonography and computed tomography. The general requirements for percutaneous catheter drainage include (*1*) an abscess that can be adequately approached via a safe percutaneous route; (*2*) an abscess that is unilocular; (*3*) an abscess that is not vascular and the patient has no coagulopathy; (*4*) joint radiologic and surgical evaluation, with surgical backup for any complication or failure; and (*5*) the possibility of dependent drainage via the percutaneously placed catheter. Of the patients who fit these criteria, percutaneous drainage has been successful in 80–90 percent.[359,360] In most series, the frequency of complications ranges from 5 to 15 percent[357,361] and include septicemia, hemorrhage, peritoneal spillage, and fistula formation. In addition, failure may occur due to undrained abscesses or pus too viscid to drain via the catheter. Recent reports indicate that the morbidity and mortality associated with percutaneous drainage may be less than with surgical treatment.[358,362]

Antimicrobial therapy should be started immediately after appropriate specimens (e.g., blood) are obtained for culture, usually this occurs before drainage. Because the pathogens usually are similar to those involved in secondary peritonitis, initial antibiotic therapy is similarly directed at the anaerobes (especially *B. fragilis* and the Enterobacteriaceae. The antimicrobial regimens discussed above in the section on treatment of secondary peritonitis would be appropriate initial therapy. This antibiotic regimen should be adjusted to conform to results of in vitro testing of the infecting organisms isolated from blood or from purulent material obtained at surgery. During the course of a prolonged illness, repeated cultures of blood and purulent collections, when clinically indicated, should provide a basis for change in antimicrobial therapy.

VISCERAL ABSCESS: PANCREATIC ABSCESS

Etiology

Most pancreatic abscesses develop as a complication of pancreatitis, which may be either biliary, alcoholic, postsurgical, or post-traumatic in origin. More recently, pancreatitis has been found to be a complication of endoscopic retrograde cholangiopancreatography (ERCP).[363] Pancreatic abscess occurs in about 1–9 percent of the patients after acute pancreatitis.[364–368] The preceding attack of acute pancreatitis has been noted to be frequently severe.[369,370] Occasionally, penetration of a peptic ulcer or secondary infection of a pancreatic pseudocyst may be the cause of a pancreatic abscess.

Bacteriologic Findings

About one-third to one-half of pancreatic abscesses have been reported to be polymicrobial with mainly enteric facultative microorganisms, such as *E. coli* and other Enterobacteriaceae, enterococci, and viridans streptococci, and occasionally *Staph. aureus*.[366–369] However, since most studies have not used modern anaerobic bacteriologic techniques, it is unknown how frequently anaerobes are involved. More recent series have documented the presence of anaerobic bacteria in pancreatic abscesses.[365,366,371,372] *Mycobacterium tuberculosis* has also been cultured from pancreatic abscesses[373] and more recently in a patient with acquired immunodeficiency syndrome. (Joseph F. John, Jr., M.D., Medical University of South Carolina, 1988: personal communication).

Pathogenesis

The release of enzymes from an acutely damaged pancreas results in pancreatic necrosis. Infection of pancreatic necrosis is most likely a secondary event.[374,375] The mixed enteric bacterial etiology of many pancreatic abscesses suggests that bacteria may reach the pancreas by reflux of contaminated bile. The frequency of bactobilia increases with biliary obstruction and with the patient's age, occurring in approximately 50 percent of those over 70 years of age.[376] The hematogenous route may account for some of the monomicrobial infections, especially those due to *Staph. aureus*.

Clinical Manifestations

The clinical manifestations are varied. The patient may fail to respond to therapy for pancreatitis, or 1–3 weeks after the onset of pancreatitis the patient may suddenly deteriorate after an initial response.[366–369] Abdominal pain that frequently radiates to the back, nausea, and vomiting are present in more than 80–90 percent of patients. Temperature of more than 101°F and abdominal tenderness are usually present, although fever may be absent. Less frequently, jaundice, abdominal distension, or an abdominal mass may be present, or the patient may have generalized peritonitis. The serum amylase level is elevated in 21–66 percent of cases and may remain elevated.

Diagnosis

Radiologic, ultrasonic, radionuclide, and computed tomography studies reveal the lesion in 80–90 percent of the cases. Plain films may show diaphragmatic elevation, pleural effusion, presence of a retrogastric mass, forward displacement of the gastric air shadow on cross-table lateral views of the abdomen, widening of the gastrocolic omentum as seen by an increase in the distance between the gastric and colon gas, or mottling and the presence of gas bubbles in the gastrocolic or retrogastric region. Barium studies may show the visceral displacement (e.g., pressure effects in the posterior gastric wall or displacement and enlargement of the duodenal sweep). Ultrasonography and computed tomography are also useful in the diagnosis of pancreatic abscess.[377,378] Computed tomography appears to be superior to ultrasonography because the images are unaffected by overlying bowel gas and can better demonstrate pancreatic gas collections. It is, however, difficult to discern infected from noninfected pseudocysts by both methods, and diagnostic needle aspiration under ultrasound or CT guidance is often helpful.[377] ^{67}Ga and ^{111}In radionuclide scans have not been found to be very helpful in differentiating pancreatitis or a pseudocyst from an abscess.[379,380] To date, neither has MRI been a very helpful modality in imaging pancreatic abscesses.[381] Spleen scans, angiography, and retrograde duodenoscopic pancreatography may also be useful.[382]

Prognosis

The presence of proteolytic enzymes within the abscess may cause erosion of major blood vessels with intra-abdominal hemorrhage.[368,369] Spread of infection may occur in the retroperitoneum, along the roots of the transverse mesocolon and small bowel mesentery, and may involve suppuration in the lesser sac with extension into the perihepatic spaces. Fistulas may form between the abscess cavity and the stomach, duodenum, or transverse colon. Patients with undrained abscesses seen in surgical practice have a 100 percent mortality.[367] About 53–86 percent of those operated on survive. Survival has been dependent on early surgical drainage.[366,369,371] Higher mortality has occurred in those with biliary tract disease or in those who developed pancreatic abscess postoperatively. These were usually older patients who had ultimately fatal underlying disease.

Death may result from septicemia, peritonitis, pleuropulmonary complications, or hepatic or renal failure.

Treatment

Early surgical drainage is most important. Percutaneous drainage alone appears to be inadequate for the majority of pancreatic abscesses. However, it may do until the patient can be stabilized for surgical drainage.[383,384] Optimal treatment appears to require effective surgical débridement and drainage.[385,386] Also, prompt reoperation is often necessary for persistent infection. The prophylactic use of antibiotics early in the course of pancreatitis has been shown to be ineffective in preventing the subsequent development of pancreatic abscess.[387] Initial antibiotic therapy should have adequate activity against *E. coli*, other Enterobacteriaceae, and anaerobic gram-negative bacilli. The regimens discussed in the section on the treatment of secondary peritonitis would be appropriate choices. Antibiotic therapy should be adjusted according to the results of in vitro sensitivity testing. Routine therapy for pancreatitis should also be used.

VISCERAL ABSCESS: HEPATIC ABSCESS

Etiology

Bacterial abscesses of the liver are relatively uncommon lesions, despite the frequency of cholecystitis, appendicitis, diverticulitis, and peritonitis, which frequently are the source for bacterial infections of the liver. More recently, pyogenic liver abscess has been noted to be one of the infectious complications following liver transplantation,[388] and there is a high frequency of liver abscesses in patients with chronic granulamatous disease.[388] Bacterial abscesses have been reported to be more frequent than amebic liver abscess, especially in the northern United States.[389–392]

Liver abscesses due to *E. histolytica* complicate about 3–9 percent of the cases of amebic colitis.[389] Although there is no sex predominance in bacterial liver abscesses, over 90 percent of amebic liver abscesses occur in men, and patients with amebic liver abscesses are generally younger than those with bacterial abscesses.[389,392] Pyogenic abscesses have been reported in patients with sickle cell anemia.[393] Liver abscesses occur at all ages but are especially rare in children, when they have been noted to follow umbilical vein catheterization in neonates.[394]

Bacteriologic Findings

Pyogenic hepatic abscess is frequently polymicrobial.[392,395–397] Enteric gram-negative bacilli, usually *E. coli*, have been cultured from the majority of pyogenic hepatic abscesses.[392,397,398] The high frequency of "sterile" abscesses, reported in some series to be about 50 percent, is probably due to inadequate anaerobic cultivation.[397,399,400] Recently, as a result of modern anaerobic bacteriologic techniques, anaerobic bacteria have become recognized as a major cause of hepatic abscesses. In reports in which modern anaerobic techniques were used, about 50 percent of all pyogenic liver abscesses were caused by anaerobes, and blood cultures were positive for anaerobes in up to 54 percent of these cases.[399,401] These anaerobes included anaerobic gram-positive cocci, *Bacteroides* spp., *Fusobacterium* spp., and *Actinomyces* spp. Although the frequency of recovery of *Staph. aureus* or group A streptococci from liver abscesses varies among reports, these organisms occur in 20 percent or less of the cases.[389,397,400] *Staph. aureus* is noted to be more frequently isolated in children, primarily in those under 5 years of age[397,402] and is presumably of hematogenous origin.

Staphylococcus aureus microabscesses in the liver may be associated with microabscesses in other organs as part of generalized hematogenous dissemination in children with impaired host defenses (e.g., in acute leukemia).[403]

On rare occasion, *Yersinia enterocolitica* has been isolated from liver abscesses.[404] It most commonly produces an acute gastroenteritis, especially in children, and a right iliac fossa syndrome due to inflammation of the terminal ileum, mesenteric lymphadenitis, or both.

Candida may also invade the liver as part of a systemic infection. However, recently, a marked increase in cases has been observed in which the infection is confined to the liver and/or the spleen.[405,406] Most of these patients have acute leukemia, usually granulocytic, and the microabscesses in the liver are probably secondary to intestinal candida colonization and portal fungemia.[270] The diagnosis is most often delayed because of a nonspecific clinical presentation while the patient is neutropenic. Fever occurs with right upper quadrant abdominal pain and abdominal distension. During this phase of the illness, ultrasound and computed tomography are not helpful, and blood and liver biopsy cultures are usually negative. The diagnosis can be made by histopathologic findings in the liver biopsy. Even when the patient's neutropenia resolves, fever and abdominal pain persist. At this point, ultrasonography or computed tomography may reveal characteristic "bull's-eye" lesions.[406] The response to amphotericin therapy has been noted to be poor, sometimes requiring 2 or 3 months for defervescence.

The specific types of microorganisms that cause hepatic abscess probably vary with the underlying disease. For example, anaerobic abscesses are more frequently cryptogenic or portal in origin, whereas gallbladder disease has been noted in one series in only 2 of 25 patients with anaerobic liver abscesses.[399] Group A streptococcal and *Staph. aureus* abscesses probably result from bacteremia due to these organisms. In the past, it was believed that about 10–20 percent of amebic liver abscesses were secondarily infected with bacteria, usually of enteric origin.[391] However, in more recent series, superinfection was found to have occurred in 0–4 percent of cases.[392] Echinococcal hepatic cysts may also become secondarily infected.

Pathogenesis

The source of infection in the liver may be (*1*) biliary, in which disease of the extrahepatic biliary tract is due to a calculus, stricture, or malignancy and results in ascending cholangitis; (*2*) portal, in which a pathologic process such as appendicitis, diverticulitis,[407] or inflammatory bowel disease[408] is in the bed of the portal venous circulation and may be associated with pylephlebitis (acute suppurative thrombophlebitis in the portal venous system; (*3*) infection in a contiguous structure, such as the gallbladder, which spreads directly to the liver; (*4*) infected foci anywhere in the body via the hepatic artery; (*5*) infection secondary to penetrating wounds and even nonpenetrating trauma to the liver; or (*6*) cryptogenic, in which no source is evident. About one-fourth of the liver abscesses are cryptogenic and are thought to be caused by infection of infarcted portions of the liver.[409] Although a portal venous source, mainly appendicitis, was a common cause of liver diseases in the past, biliary disease in recent series is now the most common source.[397,410]

Pyogenic abscesses may be single or multiple. Multiple abscesses are more apt to be due to biliary tract disease,[400] whereas abscesses arising via the portal vein are usually solitary[400]; the right lobe is more commonly involved than the left. Amebic abscesses are predominantly solitary in the right lobe.

Clinical Manifestations

The predominant symptoms of pyogenic hepatic abscess include fever and chills of several days' to weeks' duration. Char- acteristically, multiple abscesses associated with a cholangitis give rise to spiking temperatures. Right upp rant pain may be dull, and abscesses high in the right lobe may cause respiratory symptoms such as cough and pleuritic pain with radiation to the right shoulder and an associated pleural rub. Tender hepatomegaly is present in 50–70 percent of the patients. Jaundice is not often present unless ascending cholangitis is a cause of the abscesses or there is extensive hepatic involvement usually associated with multiple abscesses.[389,397,399] Either the indolence of the illness in some patients or the minimal physical findings (no hepatomegaly or abdominal tenderness) may account for these patients having a "fever of unknown origin."[397]

Clinical differentiation of an amebic from a pyogenic abscess is difficult; a history of diarrhea, the presence of chest findings, or the lack of spiking temperatures has been reported in some series to be more common in patients with amebic abscesses, but these characteristics have not been especially frequent in other series of patients with amebic abscesses. Pain in the left upper quadrant of the abdomen in patients with amebic abscess is infrequent but may indicate a left lobe abscess that can extend into the pericardium.[124] Swelling may occur over the right chest wall or there may be point tenderness that localizes abscesses due to ameba.[124]

The serum alkaline phosphatase is the most frequently elevated serum liver enzyme test. Blood cultures have been reported in recent studies to be positive in about one-half of the patients with pyogenic abscesses.[399,400] The presence of viridans streptococcus in several blood cultures in patients with an indolent clinical course and elevated hepatic enzymes without evidence of endocarditis may be an important clue to the diagnosis of liver abscess[411] (Fig. 6). Persistent recovery of viridans streptococci from liver also has been reported in the absence of bacteremia in a patient with an indolent clinical course and persistent serum alkaline phosphatase elevation.[412]

Diagnosis

Elevation and limitation of motion of the right diaphragm, basilar atelectasis, right pleural effusion, or gas within the abscess cavity may be noted on plain films of the abdomen or chest.[413] Scintigraphy with either ^{99m}Tc or ^{67}Ga, ultrasonography, computed tomography and MRI are highly sensitive techniques for the detection of liver abscesses.[414] ^{99m}Tc sulfur colloid liver scan is capable of detecting about 85 percent of lesions greater than 2 cm in diameter.[414] Anteroposterior and lateral views should reveal decreased isotope concentration in both pygenic and amebic abscesses (Fig. 6). ^{67}Ga or ^{111}In scans should reveal areas of increased isotope concentration of pyogenic abscesses (Fig. 5). Because the amebic abscess is not really a purulent lesion, it may show decreased central gallium concentration and may be surrounded by a zone of increased activity in the hypervascular abscess rim.[414]

The hepatic angiographic findings in liver abscess are the mass effect with stretching or displacement of blood vessels and an avascular area surrounded by a blush of contrast seen during the capillary-venous phase of the angiogram.[415]

The effectiveness of ultrasonography for the detection of liver abscess is now well documented.[398,410,416] It has proven especially useful for the evaluation of right upper quadrant structures, primarily because of the absence of air-filled viscera that often impede visualization in other areas of the abdomen. As mentioned previously, the appearance of abscesses may vary from echo-free lesions to highly echogenic masses within the liver. Sonography, as opposed to ^{99m}Tc scintigraphy, can often distinguish abscess from tumor and other solid focal lesions. Computed tomography is also a highly sensitive technique for the diagnosis of liver abscess.[398,417,418] Abscesses produce areas of decreased attenuation on computed tomography (Fig. 7). Both ultrasound and CT may be used to guide needle aspiration for diagnostic and therapeutic purposes.[358,418,419] The aspirated material should be cultured aerobically and anaerobically.

Ultrasound- or CT-guided percutaneous aspiration in patients suspected of having amebic abscess has been recommended to rapidly rule out a pyogenic etiology. Aspiration of sterile fluid that is brownish and without a foul odor is characteristic of an amebic abscess. However, fluid in amebic abscesses may frequently be yellow or green, and possibly is secondarily infected with enteric bacteria. Diagnosis is confirmed by finding *E. histolytica* on direct microscopy or culture of the aspirate or wall of the abscess. In endemic areas, aspiration is usually not performed if amebic abscess is suspected clinically because of the favorable response to drug therapy. Serologic tests indicative of past or present amebiasis are positive in over 90 percent of amebic liver abscesses but may be misleading in endemic areas.[392]

Prognosis

The prognosis of pyogenic liver abscesses depends on the rapidity with which the diagnosis is made and treatment is started. High mortality is also associated with advanced age and serious underlying disease. In the past, the mortality from pyogenic abscesses ranged from about 24 to 79 percent,[397,399,400] and un-

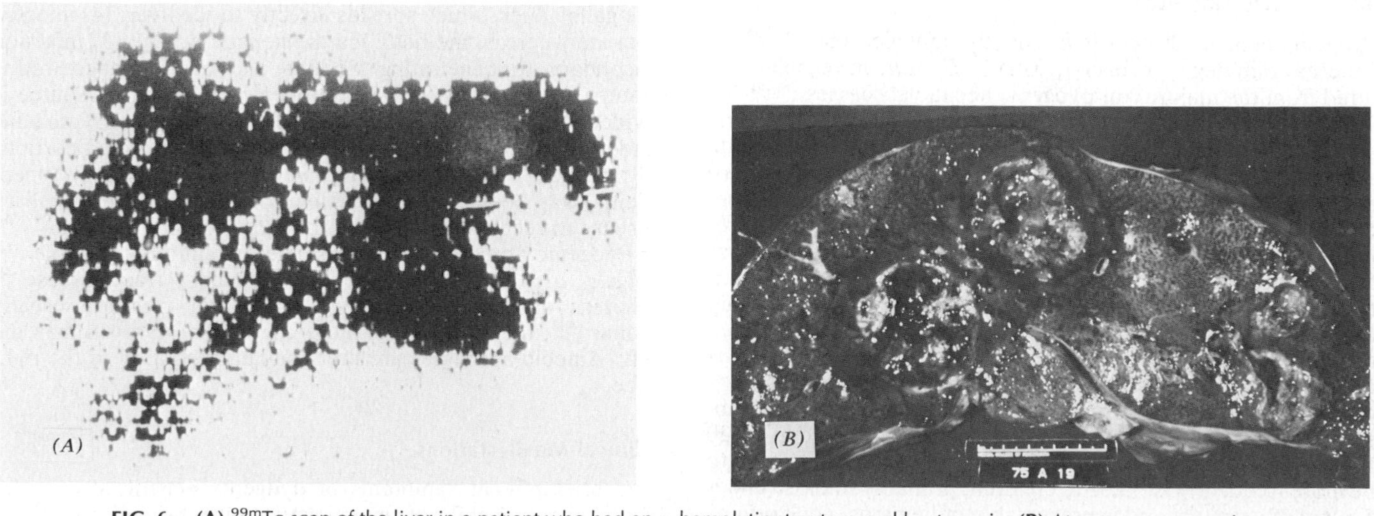

FIG. 6. **(A)** ^{99m}Tc scan of the liver in a patient who had an α-hemolytic streptococcal bacteremia. **(B)** At autopsy, cut section of the liver revealed several large abscesses that corresponded to areas of decreased radionuclide uptake in Figure 6A. At laparotomy, needle aspiration failed to yield pus, perhaps because of its viscosity, as evidenced at necropsy.

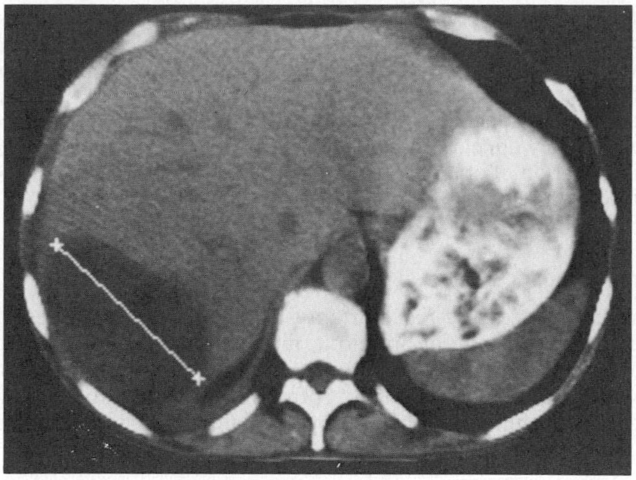

FIG. 7. Abdominal CT scan reveals a liver abscess (arrow) due to a mixture of anaerobic and aerobic pathogens. The abscess developed following drainage of an appendiceal abscess.

drained abscesses had a reported mortality of up to 100 percent.[420,421] Recent series, however, have shown an improvement in prognosis, with cure rates of 88–100 percent.[181,182,419] Traditional therapy for pyogenic liver abscesses has been surgical drainage and antibiotics; however, the recently reported high success rates have occurred in patients treated with either antibiotics plus percutaneous drainage or antibiotics alone. The older series reporting high mortality for undrained abscesses may have included patients who were not candidates for surgical drainage because of poor clinical condition or extensive infection (i.e., multiple small abscesses). The apparent improvement in prognosis during recent years may be related to earlier diagnosis afforded by the use of ultrasonography and computed tomography. Mortality of uncomplicated amebic abscesses is reported to be less than 1 percent in recent series.[124,392] However, amebic abscesses that rupture into the peritoneal or pericardial cavity carry an 18 or 30 percent mortality, respectively, and amebic abscesses that rupture into the bronchi or pleura carry a 6 percent mortality.[124]

Treatment

The treatment of pyogenic liver abscesses has changed during recent years as the use of ultrasonography and computed tomography has become common for diagnosis and therapy. These imaging procedures offer the ability to follow closely the resolution of the abscess during therapy and allow precise placement of percutaneous catheters for single or continuous drainage. Some series have reported high cure rates after antibiotic treatment without concomitant percutaneous drainage.[181,182] However, most other reports have emphasized the necessity of some drainage procedure to ensure a good outcome.[419,420,422,423] Most patients will defervesce within 2 weeks of the start of medical therapy and drainage.[392] However, some patients who are cured by medical and drainage therapy may still take up to 4 weeks to defervescence.[392] It has been recommended that surgery be considered for patients whose fever persists for more than 2 weeks despite percutaneous catheter drainage and appropriate antimicrobial therapy.[392]

The abscess should decrease in size following percutaneous catheter drainage. Should the patient's condition not improve and fever not resolve within 48 hours after catheter drainage, repeat ultrasound or CT scan should be performed to assess for undrained loculations of pus. Surgery is required for hepatic abscesses secondary to biliary obstruction. Loculated or highly viscous abscesses also usually require surgical incision and drainage.

Antibiotic therapy should be started as soon as the diagnosis is suspected and should be directed at the expected pathogens. Because the pathogens usually are similar to those involved in secondary peritonitis, initial antibiotic therapy is similarly directed at the anaerobes (especially *B. fragilis*) and the Enterobacteriaceae. The antimicrobial regimens outlined earlier in the section on treatment of secondary peritonitis would be appropriate initial therapy. At the time of drainage, cultures are taken of the abscess for aerobic and anaerobic incubation, and specific antibiotic therapy is instituted on the basis of the culture results. Therapy should be prolonged, usually for more than 1 month. Up to 4 months of antibiotic therapy for multiple pyogenic abscesses has been recommended to prevent relapses.[399]

Amebic abscess is usually treated with a tissue amebicide, such as metronidazole or parenteral dehydroemetine.[424] Metronidazole has cure rates similar to those of dehydroemetine and has the advantage of being active for both the hepatic and intestinal phase of the disease and of being less toxic. Aspiration of the cavity has been recommended not only for diagnosis but also for therapeutic drainage by some authors.[124] However, others have found aspiration to be unnecessary, except in the occasional patient who responds poorly to medical therapy or in patients with large left lobe abscesses that may rupture into the pericardium and cause death.[392] Aspiration may also be indicated to evacuate an expanding abscess in an attempt to prevent imminent rupture. Repeated aspiration has been recommended if more than 250 ml is obtained initially.[124] If a solitary right lobe abscess occurs in a male, despite the finding of bacteria in the aspirate, additional antiamebic therapy has been recommended initially because of the likelihood of a secondarily infected amebic abscess.

VISCERAL ABSCESS: SPLENIC ABSCESS

Etiology

Splenic abscesses are uncommon lesions and may occur in patients with sickle hemoglobinopathies, trauma, or bacteremia, or in intravenous drug abusers.[425] Usually multiple small abscesses develop as a complication of hematogenous dissemination. One-quarter of these abscesses have been reported to be solitary.[426]

Bacteriologic Characteristics

Splenic abscesses that develop during the course of bacterial endocarditis are usually due to *Staph. aureus* or streptococcus. Enterobacteriaceae (e.g., *Salmonella*) and anaerobic microorganisms have also been recovered.[425–427] In one series, the bacteriology of the abscess was polymicrobial in 25 percent and included anaerobes.[425] The proportion of splenic abscesses reported to have sterile cultures has declined as anaerobic culture techniques have improved. Fungi (mostly *Candida* species) have been isolated from splenic abscesses with greater frequency during the past decade as the population with conditions predisposing to infections with *Candida* has increased (e.g., patients on high-dose corticosteroids or cancer chemotherapy). Fungal splenic abscesses are often part of the syndrome of hepatosplenic candidiasis.[405,407] Blood cultures have been reported to be positive in 70 percent of patients with multiple splenic abscesses but in only 14 percent with solitary abscesses.[425]

Pathogenesis

Splenic abscesses most likely develop as a metastatic process. Some are related to infection in contiguous organs and others from infected traumatic hematomas or infarcts, for example, in patients with sickle hemoglobinopathies.

Manifestations

Left upper quadrant abdominal pain is usual. Irritation of the adjacent diaphragm may result in pain referred to the left shoulder. Splenic enlargement and tenderness are often present, with high, spiking temperatures and perhaps a splenic rub. No clinical findings to suggest splenic involvement may occur in some patients with multiple small splenic abscesses.[425,426]

Diagnosis

Radiographic examination may reveal an elevated left hemidiaphragm, basilar pulmonary infiltrates, atelectasis, or a left pleural effusion. Shift of the colon and stomach down and to the right, and extraintestinal gas, either diffusely mottled or producing an air-fluid level in the left upper quadrant, may also be seen.[425,426] Radionuclide imaging with ^{99m}Tc sulfur colloid may also be helpful. However, ^{67}Ga may have relatively low sensitivity, in part due to the inherent normal splenic uptake of this isotope.[427,428] Ultrasonography, computed tomography, and MRI are the preferred diagnostic techniques for the evaluation of suspected splenic abscess[429,430] (Fig. 8). Computed tomography appears to be somewhat superior to ultrasound for visualization of splenic structure because of adjacent gas-filled viscera and inconstant position in the left upper quadrant.[428]

Treatment

In untreated cases, the mortality rate with splenic abscess is 100 percent.[428] Initial antibiotic therapy should have a broad spectrum of activity. A combination of antibiotics that has activity against streptococci and both aerobic and anaerobic gram-negative bacilli would be appropriate initial antimicrobial ther-

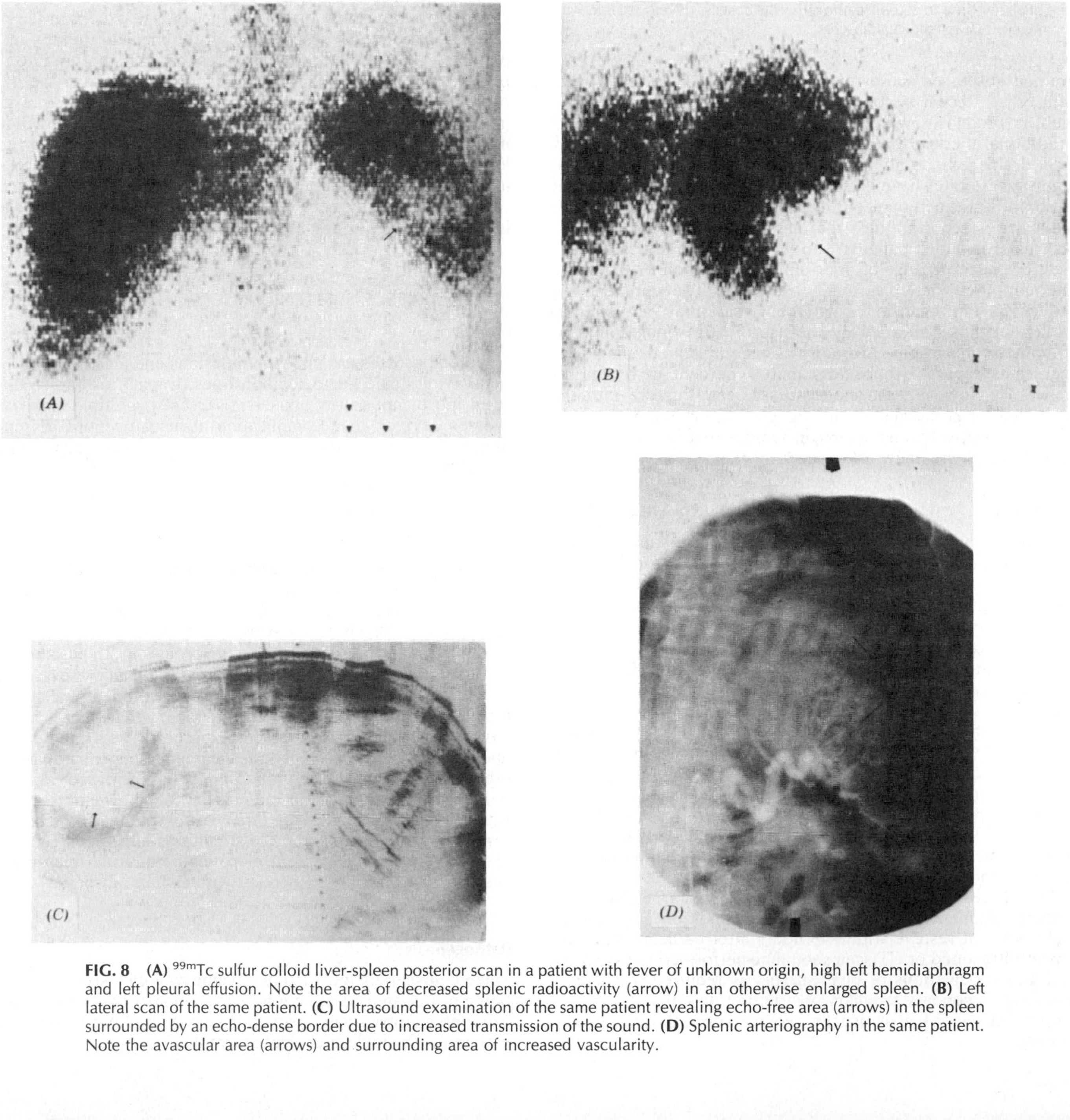

FIG. 8 **(A)** ^{99m}Tc sulfur colloid liver-spleen posterior scan in a patient with fever of unknown origin, high left hemidiaphragm and left pleural effusion. Note the area of decreased splenic radioactivity (arrow) in an otherwise enlarged spleen. **(B)** Left lateral scan of the same patient. **(C)** Ultrasound examination of the same patient revealing echo-free area (arrows) in the spleen surrounded by an echo-dense border due to increased transmission of the sound. **(D)** Splenic arteriography in the same patient. Note the avascular area (arrows) and surrounding area of increased vascularity.

apy. Subsequent modifications of antibiotic therapy may be based on results of blood cultures or cultures of material obtained at the time of surgery. With multiple, small abscesses, and with some large solitary abscesses when feasible, splenectomy is the treatment of choice; otherwise when the spleen is surrounded by extensive adhesions, incision and drainage may be preferred.[425–427,431] Percutaneous drainage was successful in 15 of 22 patients in one series,[425] but its indications, efficacy, and safety remain to be determined.[432]

SPECIFIC SOURCES OF INTRA-ABDOMINAL INFECTION

Acute Appendicitis

Appendicitis manifests as right lower quadrant abdominal pain accompanied by anorexia, nausea, and vomiting. When the inflamed appendix lies in the anterior position, tenderness is often maximal at or near McBurney's point with low-grade fever, rebound tenderness, voluntary guarding at first, and then abdominal rigidity. Variations in the anatomic location of the appendix may result in variations in the location of the pain and physical findings. For example, a retrocecal appendix may cause principally flank or back pain and tenderness; a pelvic appendix may cause suprapubic pain; and on rectal examination pain may be felt locally and suprapubically.

Persistent obstruction of the appendiceal lumen, usually due to a fecalith, leads to gangrene and rupture of the pus-filled organ. During the several hours between onset of acute appendicitis and rupture, adjacent viscera and omentum may wall off and confine the subsequent spill to the periappendiceal area, with development of an inflammatory mass felt in the right lower quadrant. If the walling-off process is incomplete, spreading diffuse peritonitis occurs. The two sites for loculation of intraperitoneal spread are the pelvic recess and the right subhepatic space. Pylephlebitis and liver abscess may complicate the picture. Colonic microflora, namely a mixture of *B. fragilis, B. melaninogenicus*, anaerobic gram-positive cocci, and Enterobacteriaceae, are the primary pathogens in appendicitis and its complications.

The therapy for appendicitis without rupture and for ruptured appendicitis with local or diffuse peritonitis is surgery. If perforation is suspected to have occurred, antibiotic therapy is initiated while the patient is being prepared for surgery. For recommendation of specific antimicrobial agents, see the section on therapy for secondary peritonitis. The severity of appendicitis is related to the development of the rupture of the appendix, which is more common in children and the elderly. Meckel's diverticulitis may manifest in a manner identical to that of acute appendicitis, and the therapeutic approach is similar.

Although not a source of intra-abdominal infection, nonspecific mesenteric lymphadenitis is often confused with appendicitis in children and may account for the symptoms suggestive of appendicitis in up to 20 percent of these patients. It is a self-limited, sometimes recurrent illness in childhood of unknown etiology that primarily involves mesenteric nodes in the right iliac fossa. The nodes are enlarged and discrete. The adjacent bowel and peritoneum are at most mildly inflamed, and a small amount of clear serous peritoneal fluid is frequently present. The patient has fever, poorly localized right lower quadrant tenderness, rebound tenderness, and voluntary guarding, but rarely abdominal rigidity. On occasion, leukocytosis is present.

Since the clinical manifestation of nonspecific mesenteric lymphadenitis is so similar to that of acute appendicitis, the therapeutic approach is surgical to rule out appendicitis. Even though the appendix may appear normal, an appendectomy should be done, since a recurrent episode of mesenteric adenitis may again lead to misinterpretation. An identical clinical picture can be caused by rubeola, infectious mononucleosis, and *Yersinia* spp.

Diverticulitis

Diverticula of the colon are herniations of the mucosa and submucosa through the circular muscular layer. Diverticula are usually located in the sigmoid and descending colons, and usually occur after 35 years of age. Inflammation is the most frequent complication of diverticulosis. The pathogenesis is similar to that of appendicitis. Diverticulitis is more frequent in patients with widespread diverticulosis, and the frequency of the complication increases with age. The inflammation may remain localized to the bowel wall as a simple diverticulitis. Complications such as confined perforation with pericolic abscess to which adjacent viscera and omentum are adherent,[433] fistula formation, or, less commonly, free perforation with spreading peritonitis may occur.[434] The clinical picture of uncomplicated sigmoid diverticulitis resembles that of appendicitis, but with findings on the left side of the abdomen. Urinary symptoms are sometimes present as a result of inflammation close to the bladder or ureter and may be followed by fistulization. Pneumaturia and fecaluria often accompanied by chills and fever indicate fistulization between the colon and urinary tract. Passage of flatus and feces through the vagina indicates fistulas into the uterus or vagina. With uncomplicated diverticulitis, low-grade fever and mild leukocytosis are usually found with tenderness, some rigidity in the left lower quadrant and/or suprapubic area, and normal bowel sounds. Perforation produces clinical findings of an intraperitoneal abscess or of diffuse peritonitis.

It is advisable to defer the barium enema until the process has abated with conservative therapy. Nonoperative therapy should be tried for the first few attacks of acute uncomplicated diverticulitis or for well-localized pericolic abscesses. For confined perforation, conservative treatment may resolve an inflammatory mass sufficiently to permit a one-stage resection of the diseased portion of the colon.[435] Operative therapy for recurrent acute diverticulitis is indicated if the patient does not respond promptly within about 48 hours, if there is free perforation with diffuse peritonitis, and if carcinoma cannot be ruled out. Initial nonoperative treatment consists of parenteral fluids, broad-spectrum antibiotics, and nasogastric suction. Antibiotic recommendations are similar to those discussed in the section on therapy for secondary peritonitis.

Regional Enteritis

The onset of regional enteritis may be acute, especially in the young, and may mimic acute appendicitis. The correct diagnosis of early regional enteritis may be made only at operation, which reveals a thickened bowel wall and mesenteric lymph node involvement. Usually, however, the diagnosis is established by contrast radiography.

Perforation as the result of an ulcer burrowing through the entire thickness of the bowel wall may occur.[436] Usually the perforation is confined and may result in abscesses or internal fistulas. Rarely does the ulcer perforate freely into the peritoneal cavity. Perianal or perirectal abscesses and fistulas are also common manifestations of regional enteritis.

Systemic antibiotics are often of value in the management of suppurative complications (see the section on antimicrobial therapy for secondary peritonitis). Surgery is indicated to drain abdominal abscesses, to correct fistulas, and for free perforation. The principal complications of surgery are enterocutaneous fistula, intraperitoneal or wound sepsis, and prolonged postoperative ileus.

Necrotizing Enterocolitis in Neutropenic Patients (Typhlitis)

Necrotizing enterocolitis occurs in patients who are severely granulocytopenic from any cause, including acute leukemia, aplastic anemia, cyclic neutropenia, Felty's syndrome, and chemotherapy for various neoplasms.[437–439]

Pathologically, the bowel is edematous, with marked thickening of the wall. The luminal surface has discrete areas of punctate ulceration, which at times may coalesce. There is also transmural inflammation with hemorrhagic necrosis and degeneration of the muscularis mucosae. The inflammatory cells found in histologic specimens are almost always mononuclear. It is thought that bacteria found in the normal gut flora opportunistically invade the ulcerations in the bowel during periods of profound neutropenia. Due to the lack of granulocytes, these organisms proliferate and cause local destruction by elaboration of exotoxins.[437]

Initially, the signs and symptoms are similar to those of acute appendicitis. These patients present with a new fever, abdominal pain, rebound tenderness in the right lower quadrant (because of the predominance of cecal involvement), and diarrhea. Rapid progression to the development of an acute abdomen is not uncommon.

Plain radiographs of the abdomen may demonstrate a boggy, thickened cecum and possibly the presence of gas within the wall of the colon.[440]

The mortality rate with neutropenic enterocolitis is greater than 50 percent.[441] Although the management of this disease is somewhat controversial,[442,443] antimicrobial therapy with activity against the aerobic and anaerobic gut bacteria, together with surgical resection of the necrotic bowel, is generally recommended.

Actinomycosis

Actinomycosis is an uncommon suppurative infection produced by the anaerobe *Actinomyces israelii* or one of several closely related species. The cecal area is most frequently the site of abdominal actinomycosis. Typically, the history begins with an attack of acute appendicitis or with recurrent bouts of right lower quadrant pain and fever, which prompts surgery for a presumptive diagnosis of appendicitis. At surgery an indurated pericecal mass is found with sinus tracts. After appendectomy, persistent draining sinuses form. The diagnosis of actinomycosis is made by demonstration of "sulfur granules" in the purulent sinus discharge and by histologic examination of the tissues. Treatment is discussed in Chapter 233.

ACUTE CHOLECYSTITIS

Pathogenesis

In over 90 percent of patients with acute cholecystitis, gallstones are impacted in the cystic duct.[444] Thus, it is generally assumed that a sudden change in the degree of obstruction leads to a sudden increase in intraductal pressures, which produces distension of the gallbladder, compromising the blood supply and lymphatic drainage. This is followed by tissue necrosis and proliferation of bacteria present in calculous gallbladders. Although infection may not be a primary cause of acute cholecystitis, it develops in over half of the cases. Infective complications include empyema or gangrene of the gallbladder, emphysematous cholecystitis, pericholecystic abscess, intraperitoneal abscess, peritonitis, cholangitis, liver abscess, and bacteremia. A detailed schema for the proposed pathogenesis of acute cholecystitis is shown in Figure 9.

Pathologic Findings

Acute cholecystitis is usually superimposed on a histologic picture of chronic cholecystitis. Ninety-five percent of the gallbladders removed for acute cholecystitis exhibit fibrosis, flattening of the mucosa, and clusters of chronic inflammatory cells as sequelae of previous disease. Rokitansky-Aschoff sinuses are present in 56 percent of the cases. These sinuses represent mucosal herniations presumably related to increased hydrostatic pressure during previous episodes of cystic duct obstruction. The early acute changes may be only edema and venous congestion. This is followed by focal necrosis and an influx of neutrophils as secondary bacterial proliferation occurs. This may then be followed by actual gangrene or perforation (Table 3).

Symptoms and Signs

Initial obstruction of the cystic duct may be accompanied by only mild epigastric pain followed by reflex nausea and vomiting. If the obstruction is transient, these symptoms subside within 1–2 hours. With persistent obstruction the findings of acute cholecystitis evolve. Pain shifts to the right upper quad-

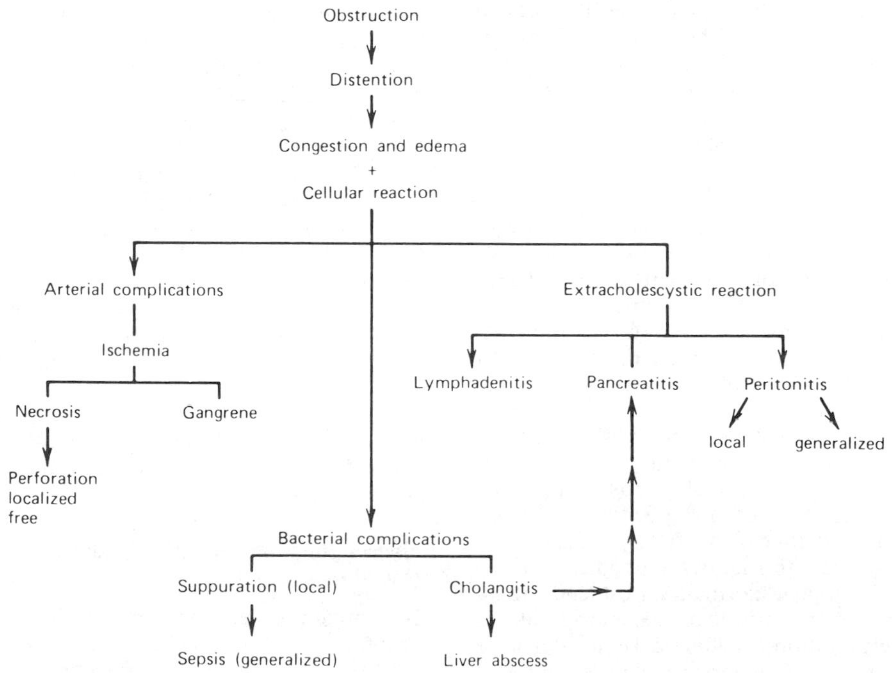

FIG. 9 Pathogenesis of acute cholecystitis.

TABLE 3. Pathologic Classification of Acute Cholecystitis

Edema	
Edema and congestion	
Focal necrosis	
Suppuration	Intramural
	Intraluminal
	Pericholecystic
Gangrene	
Perforation	Localized
	Free

rant and becomes increasingly severe. Signs of peritoneal irritation may be present, and in a small number of patients the pain may radiate to the right shoulder or scapula. The gallbladder is palpable in 30–40 percent of the cases.[445] Moderate temperature elevations and minimal icterus occur in two-thirds of patients. However, repeated chills and fever, jaundice, or hypotension would suggest suppurative cholangitis as a consequence of common duct obstruction (see below under "Bacteriologic Findings"). Most patients with acute cholecystitis have a complete remission within 1–4 days. However, approximately 25–30 percent of patients require surgery or develop some complication.

Laboratory Findings

The laboratory data obtained rarely are required to make the diagnosis of acute obstructive cholecystitis, but they may be indicative of further complications (see the next section). The leukocyte count is usually moderately elevated, with a slight increase in early segmented forms. Fifty percent of the patients have mild hyperbilirubinemia; forty percent have a mild elevation of serum aspartate aminotransferase (AST) levels; twenty-five percent have elevated alkaline phosphatase levels; and only ten percent have mild elevations of serum amylase levels.[446]

Bacteriologic Findings

In the presence of cholecystitis and cholelithiasis, appreciable numbers of various bacteria may be found in the bile and walls of the gallbladder, even in the absence of symptoms. The frequency of bactobilia is higher (*1*) the longer the duration and severity of symptoms, (*2*) in the elderly (>60–70 years of age), (*3*) in the jaundiced patient, (*4*) in acute cholecystitis (up to 94 percent of patients) in comparison to chronic cholecystitis, and (*5*) especially when the common duct is obstructed.[376,447]

The organisms found in the biliary tract are commonly the same as the normal intestinal flora, namely, the enteric gram-negative bacilli, including *E. coli, Klebsiella/Enterobacter*, and *Proteus* spp., as well as the enterococci.[376,448] In addition, recent studies have demonstrated the frequent recovery of anaerobic organisms including *Bacteroides, Clostridia*, and *Fusobacterium* spp.[448] When present, these anaerobes are frequently involved in polymicrobic infections, mixed with other anaerobes and aerobic gram-negative bacilli.[449]

Patients from whom anaerobes have been recovered were reported more likely to have had prior multiple, complex, biliary tract surgical procedures, especially biliary-intestinal anastomoses and common duct manipulations. These patients often have severe symptoms and a high incidence of postoperative infectious complications, especially wound infections.[450]

The source of bactobilia is unknown, but has been assumed to be the duodenum, and spread is assumed to occur via an ascending route.[449] Although the duodenum normally has a sparse flora in the fasting state, higher counts occur transiently after meals and in conditions that allow bacterial overgrowth in the stomach (achlorhydria or gastric obstruction) or in the small bowel (obstruction, diverticula, or blind loops).

Roentgenographic and Related Studies

An upright chest film is of limited value. In two-thirds of the cases the right hemidiaphragm is elevated. Since subdiaphragmatic free air cannot originate in the biliary tract, if present, it indicates another disease process. In only about 10–15 percent of cases are calcified gallstones seen on plain films of the abdomen, but this finding in any case indicates only cholelithiasis. Occasionally, a diffusely calcified gallbladder ("porcelainized gallbladder") may be seen. Since this rarely, if ever, develops into acute cholecystitis, its presence should strongly suggest another diagnosis. The demonstration of gas limited to the gallbladder wall or lumen is diagnostic of emphysematous cholecystitis.

Oral cholecystography is of little value in diagnosing acute cholecystitis because it requires too long a preparation time and is not applicable in jaundiced or vomiting patients. Intravenous cholangiography has been replaced by more sensitive and specific techniques. Recent advances in ultrasonography and nuclear medicine have made these modalities the diagnostic studies of choice for acute cholecystitis. Both imaging modalities are noninvasive, with little reported morbidity, and have been reported to have sensitivity and specificity values of greater than 90 percent. Sonographic findings consistent with acute cholecystitis include the presence of stones, thickened gallbladder wall, dilated lumen of the gallbladder, or a pericholecystic collection.[451,452] Hepatobiliary scanning with one of the ^{99m}Tc-labeled acetanilide iminodiacetic acid derivatives (IDA) is also a sensitive and rapid study for the diagnosis of acute cholecystitis.[451–453] Even in the presence of moderately severe liver dysfunction,[453] the IDA nuclide is concentrated in the liver and excreted into the bile, resulting in visualization of the functioning hepatobiliary system, including the gallbladder and duodenum, within the first hour. In acute cholecystitis, however, since the cystic duct is occluded by a stone or mucosal inflammation, the gallbladder is not visualized, despite common duct and small bowel visualization. During the first hour, nonvisualization of the gallbladder also occurs in more than 50 percent of patients with chronic cholecystitis, but usually the gallbladder is visualized in delayed images obtained up to 4 hours after IDA administration. In chronic cholecystitis and cholelithiasis, a normal cholescintigram may also occur if the cystic duct is patent.

Findings consistent with acute cholecystitis may also be demonstrated with computed tomography, but this technique should not be used for initial screening.[454]

Recently, MRI was found to provide both functional and anatomic information, and was sensitive in detecting gallbladder disease in patients with suspected cholecystitis.[455]

Complications

Perforation occurs in 10–15 percent of the cases. A small percentage of these are acute free perforations into the peritoneal cavity. These cases are readily recognizable, since they have the catastrophic symptoms and signs of diffuse peritonitis. More frequently, the omentum and serosa of contiguous viscera localize the perforation early. In such cases, there is persistent fever, often a palpable mass that may be in a somewhat atypical location, and occasionally a friction rub. Acute emphysematous cholecystitis is seen most commonly in elderly diabetic men. Systemic symptoms are more severe, and the classic x-ray picture of the abdomen reveals gas within the gallbladder lumen, frequently with a gas-fluid level, and gas in a ring along the contours of the gallbladder wall.[456] Cholangitis is described in detail below. Pancreatitis may also complicate cholecystitis.

Here the pain is more midline and may radiate to the back. Urine and serum amylase are often elevated.

Differential Diagnosis

In addition to the complications noted above, the differential diagnosis should include myocardial infarction, perforating ulcer, right lower lobe pneumonia, intestinal obstruction, hepatitis, perihepatitis, and acute disease involving the right kidney. Radiographs of the chest and abdomen, electrocardiograms, and urinalysis can exclude these in the majority of cases.

Antimicrobial Therapy in Acute Obstructive Cholecystitis

Certainly in severely ill or elderly patients or in patients with infectious complications such as emphysematous cholecystitis, perforation with peritonitis or a pericholecystic collection and cholangitis should be treated early for infection possibly due to enteric gram-negative bacilli and anaerobic bacteria, including *B. fragilis*.[367,447,448] An appropriate initial antibiotic regimen includes an aminoglycoside (gentamicin or tobramycin) or a cephalosporin in addition to an agent such as clindamycin or metronidazole, to treat for *B. fragilis*. The antimicrobial regimens discussed in the section on treatment of secondary peritonitis would be appropriate alternatives. A more specific antibiotic regimen should be substituted when results of antimicrobial sensitivity testing of the isolated pathogens become available.

The role of antibiotics for the treatment of uncomplicated acute cholecystitis remains unclear. A large retrospective study has demonstrated that routine antibiotic therapy for acute cholecystitis did not appear to affect the outcome of the attack or to decrease the incidence of local infectious complications such as empyema or pericholecystic abscess formation.[457] These results could be due to the fact that although high concentrations of antibiotics may be present in blood, tissues, and common duct bile, these levels do not appear in the gallbladder bile, blocked by the almost universal presence of cystic duct obstruction in acute cholecystitis, and thus are unable to eradicate bactobilia.

Available evidence suggests that perioperative antibiotics are a helpful adjunct to surgery to prevent postoperative infectious complications.[458] Because wound infection is thought to be due to contamination of the incision with infected bile at the time of operation, prophylactic antibiotics should be given in a manner that will achieve high blood and tissue concentrations at the time of surgery.

Perioperative antibiotics have been recommended in situations in which the frequency of bactobilia is high (such as in the elderly and in those with either a history of jaundice or jaundice at operation, common duct obstruction from stones, chills and fever, or previous biliary tract surgery). Also, it has been recommended that administration of prophylactic antibiotics be dependent on the results of an intraoperative Gram stain of bile.[376] Although ineffective against enterococci and some anaerobes, a cephem antibiotic appears to be a reasonable choice.[458]

Surgery

Immediate surgery is indicated for gangrenous (emphysematous) cholecystitis, perforation with peritonitis, and suspected pericholecystic abscess. In these patients, cholecystectomy with intraoperative cholangiography is the procedure of choice. However, in patients with severe clinical deterioration, a cholecystostomy and removal of cystic duct stones may prove to be a temporizing life-saving measure until a second definitive procedure can be performed,[459,460] provided there is no evidence of suppurative cholangitis (i.e., repeated chills, fever, jaundice, and hypotension), which would require immediate decompression of the common bile duct. Cholecystostomy is not an adequate operation for acute suppurative cholangitis unless the common duct is clearly decompressed through a large patent cystic duct.

The timing of surgery in patients with uncomplicated acute cholecystitis has been controversial. Supporters of delayed surgery after the acute attack has subsided following conservative management feel that morbidity is decreased and that the delay may lower the frequency of unnecessary surgery when the diagnosis is unclear.[461] However, many recent series have supported early surgery reporting that a deceptively benign presentation, especially in the elderly, may actually mask the presence of complications and prompt an inappropriate delay in surgery. Also, no difference in morbidity has been reported between early and delayed surgery, and recent advances in diagnostic studies have markedly decreased the incidence of misdiagnosis.[462,463] The disadvantages of delayed surgery include prolonged hospitalization and a significant incidence of recurrent symptoms that may precipitate urgent surgery under less favorable conditions.

CHOLANGITIS

Cholangitis may be defined as varying degrees of inflammation and/or infection involving hepatic and common bile ducts. Since the mucosa of the gallbladder is continuous with that of the common bile duct via the cystic duct, it is not surprising that varying degrees of choledochitis occur as a limited cholangitis with cholecystitis. In fact, specimens of the common duct taken at the time of cholecystectomy for acute cholecystitis usually show localized edema and inflammation. However, this disease is indistinguishable from uncomplicated acute cholecystitis. In this section, we focus on the more severe entities of ascending cholangitis and acute obstructive suppurative cholangitis.

Pathogenesis

In a manner similar to that described for cholecystitis, obstruction of the common duct results in increased pressure, edema, congestion, and necrosis of the walls of the biliary tree followed by rapid proliferation of bacteria within the biliary tree. In most instances, obstruction is due to gallstones.[464] However, obstruction may be due to prior biliary tract surgery, tumor, chronic calcific pancreatitis, and parasitic infections. Fulminant cholangitis has also been reported as a complication of ERCP.[465]

Pathogenic Findings

Microscopic examination of the common duct reveals marked fibrous thickening and focal areas of chronic inflammation. Superimposed on this is necrosis of the mucosa and dense infiltration of acute inflammatory cells. In the liver, portal inflammation is uniformly seen. Usually, this is a dense neutrophilic infiltrate. In 40 percent of the cases, numerous microabscesses are present. Bile duct dilatation and cholestasis are also present.

Symptoms and Signs

Patients usually have an antecedent history compatible with gallbladder disease. The onset is usually acute, with high fever, chills, and diffuse pain and tenderness over the liver. Jaundice is usually prominent. In some cases, shock and other findings of gram-negative bacteremia may be present; altogether 85 percent of the patients fulfill Charcot's triad of fever, chills, and jaundice.[466]

Laboratory Findings

There is usually marked leukocytosis with an increase in immature forms. The serum bilirubin level is often higher than 4 mg/dl and the serum alkaline phosphatase level is significantly higher than that encountered in acute cholecystitis. Serum AST level is modestly elevated. Biochemical and even clinical evidence of disseminated intravascular coagulation may be present.

Bacteriologic Findings

Little adequate data are available on the bacteriologic findings in cholangitis. Recent studies using detailed aerobic and anaerobic culture techniques suggest that the bacteriologic findings in cholangitis are similar to those in acute obstructive cholecystitis. Gram-negative enteric bacilli and anaerobic bacteria are the most common isolates. Those patients with a stent in their bile duct may harbor resistant flora such as *P. aeruginosa*. Unlike uncomplicated cholecystitis, bacteremia occurs in approximately 50 percent of the cases. *Escherichia coli* (52 percent of the isolates), *B. fragilis* (22 percent), and *C. perfringens* (16 percent) are the most frequent isolates from blood cultures.

Roentgenographic and Related Studies

An upright chest film is of limited value. The right hemidiaphragm is frequently elevated. Other findings are similar to those described above for acute cholecystitis and are nonspecific. Oral cholecystography is of no value. Intravenous cholangiography is usually not helpful since the serum bilirubin level is frequently higher than 4.0 mg/dl and has been replaced by less morbid and more sensitive techniques. Ultrasonography can easily be used to evaluate gallbladder size, the presence of stones, and the degree of bile duct dilatation. Marked bile duct dilatation in a patient with the clinical picture described above corroborates this diagnosis. It is important to note that not all patients with obstructive cholangitis have a grossly dilated biliary tree, and ultrasonography is unlikely to be helpful in these cases. Obstruction of the common bile duct can be diagnosed by hepatobiliary scanning with one of the ^{99m}Tc-labeled derivatives of IDA. In this case, no component of the biliary system or small bowel is visualized, despite adequate hepatic uptake. In obstructive cholangitis, however, ultrasonography is the preferred study due to its ability to visualize dilated ducts and the decreased dependability of IDA scintigraphy in the presence of severe jaundice.[467] Percutaneous transhepatic cholangiography and endoscopic retrograde cholangiography are extremely valuable in evaluating bile duct obstruction. However, it is seldom feasible to use these techniques in the acutely ill patient with cholangitis.

Complications

Bacteremia and shock occur commonly and perhaps are best included as part of the clinical picture of obstructive cholangitis. Perforation of the gallbladder may occur and is described under complications of acute cholecystitis. In some less acute cases, macroscopic hepatic abscesses may develop. This clinical picture may be similar to cholangitis alone. However, ultrasonography, computed tomography, or technetium or gallium scans may visualize multiple defects in the hepatic parenchyma. Finally, pancreatitis may occur as a complication.

Differential Diagnosis

Acute cholecystitis and its complications, hepatic abscess, perforating ulcer, pancreatitis, intestinal obstruction, right lower lobe pneumonia, acute disease involving the right kidney, and bacteremic shock related to another focus of infection should all be considered in the differential diagnosis. In acute cholecystitis the patient is usually less ill; in addition, the serum bilirubin level is usually less than 4.0 mg/dl, the serum alkaline phosphatase level is not markedly elevated, and ultrasonography of cholescintigraphy usually demonstrate a patent, nondilated hepatic and common duct. Patients with hepatic abscesses not due to obstructive cholangitis are usually not as acutely ill; hepatic tenderness, when present, is also not as severe, and liver function tests may be only minimally abnormal. Diagnostic studies usually detect a macroscopic parenchymal defect. In pancreatitis, the pain and tenderness are more midline and may radiate to the back. Serum and urine amylase levels are significantly elevated, but liver function tests are not markedly abnormal. Finally, radiographs of the chest and abdomen and urinalysis exclude the majority of other possibilities.

Antimicrobial Therapy in Cholangitis

Prompt institution of appropriate antibiotic therapy is mandatory, since these severe infections are frequently complicated by bacteremia and shock. Based on the bacteriologic findings described above and on the known in vitro susceptibilities of these organisms, an appropriate regimen would be clindamycin or metronidazole plus an aminoglycoside or cephalosporin antibiotic. The antimicrobial regimens discussed in the section on treatment of secondary peritonitis would be alternative choices. This antibiotic regimen is directed primarily at the complicating bacteremia, since antibiotics alone will not sterilize the biliary tract in the face of obstruction.[448]

Surgery

Prompt operative intervention with decompression of the common duct is mandatory in all but those few patients who respond promptly to antibiotics.[468] In all patients who undergo surgery, regardless of the procedure, operative cholangiography should be performed. The simplest but least satisfactory procedure is simple cholecystostomy if patency of the cystic duct is assured. However, if at all possible, a cholecystectomy should be performed, followed by common duct exploration and T-tube drainage. In more complicated cases, choledochoduodenostomy or cholecystoduodenostomy may have to be performed.

REFERENCES

1. Altemeier WA, Culbertson WR, Fullen WD. Intra-abdominal sepsis. In: Welch CE, Hardy JD, eds. Advances in Surgery. Chicago: Year Book Medical Publishers; 1971:281–333.
2. Boyd DP. The subphrenic spaces and the emperor's new robes. N Engl J Med. 1966;275:911–7.
3. Whalen JP, Bierny JP. Classification of perihepatic abscesses. Radiology. 1969;92:1427–37.
4. Sanders RC, James AE Jr, Fischer K. Correlation of liver scans and images with abdominal radiographs in perihepatic sepsis. Am J Surg. 1972;124:346–52.
5. Myers MA. The spread and localization of acute intraperitoneal effusions. Radiology. 1970;95:547–54.
6. Altemeier WA, Culbertson WR, Fullen WD, et al. Intra-abdominal abscesses. Am J Surg. 1973;125:70–9.
7. Henderson LW, Nolph KD. Altered permeability of the peritoneal membrane using hypertonic peritoneal dialysis fluid. J Clin Invest. 1969;48:992–1001.
8. Shear L, Swartz C, Shinaberger JA, et al. Kinetics of peritoneal fluid absorption in adult men. N Engl J Med. 1965;272:123–7.
9. Boen ST. Kinetics of peritoneal dialysis: A comparison with artificial kidney. Medicine. 1961;40:243–87.
10. Tsilibury EC, Wissig SL. Absorption from the peritoneal cavity: SEM study of the mesothelium covering the peritoneal surface of the muscular portion of the diaphragm. Am J Anat. 1977;149:127–33.
11. Rochlin DB, Zill H, Blakemore WS. Studies of the resorption of chromium-51 tagged erythrocytes from the peritoneal cavity; the absorption of fluids and particulate matter from the peritoneal cavity. Int Abstr Surg. 1958;107:1–14.
12. Pritchard JA, Adams RH. The fate of blood in the peritoneal cavity. Surg Gynecol Obstet. 1957;105:621–9.

13. Zinsser HH, Pryde AW. Experimental study of physical factors, including fibrin formation, influencing the spread of fluids and small particles within and from the peritoneal cavity of the dog. Ann Surg. 1952;136:818–27.
14. Macbeth RA, Mackenzie WC. The abdominal wali, umbilicus, peritoneum, mesenteries, and retroperitoneum. In: Sabiston DC Jr, ed. Davis-Christopher Textbook of Surgery. 10th ed. Philadelphia: WB Saunders; 1972:773–95.
15. Nohr CW, Marshall DG. Primary peritonitis in children. Can J Surg. 1984;27(2):179–81.
16. McDougal WS, Izant RJ, Zollinger RM Jr. Primary peritonitis in infancy and childhood. Ann Surg. 1975;181:310–3.
17. Golden GT, Shaw A. Primary peritonitis. Surg Gynecol Obstet. 1972;135:513–6.
18. Epstein M, Calia FM, Gabuzda GJ. Pneumococcal peritonitis in patients with postnecrotic cirrhosis. N Engl J Med. 1968;278:69–71.
19. Speck WT, Dresdale SS, McMillan RW. Primary peritonitis and the nephrotic syndrome. Am J Surg. 1974;127:267–9.
20. Conn HO, Fessel JM. Spontaneous bacterial peritonitis in cirrhosis: Variations on a theme. Medicine. 1971;50:161–97.
21. Conn HO. Spontaneous bacterial peritonitis, multiple revisitations. Gastroenterology. 1976;70:455–7.
22. Bar-Meir S, Conn HO. Spontaneous bacterial peritonitis induced by intra-arterial vasopressin therapy. Gastroenterology. 1976;70:418–21.
23. Curry N, McCallum RW, Guth PH. Spontaneous peritonitis in cirrhotic ascites: A decade of experience. Am J Dig Dis. 1974;19:685–92.
24. Targan SR, Chow AW, Guze LB. Role of anaerobic bacteria in spontaneous peritonitis of cirrhosis: Report of two cases and review of the literature. Am J Med. 1977;62:397–403.
25. Kline MM, McCallum RW, Guth PH. The clinical value of ascitic fluid culture and leukocyte count studies in alcoholic cirrhosis. Gastroenterology. 1976;70:408–12.
26. Weinstein MP, Iannini PB, Stratton CW, et al. Spontaneous bacterial peritonitis: A review of 28 cases with emphasis on improved survival and factors influencing prognosis. Am J Med. 1978;64:592–8.
27. Hoefs JC, Canawati HN, Sapico FL, et al. Spontaneous bacterial peritonitis. Hepatology. 1982;2:399–407.
28. Pinzello G, Simonetti R, Craxi A, et al. Spontaneous bacterial peritonitis: A prospective investigation in predominantly nonalcoholic cirrhotic patients. Hepatology. 1983;3:545–9.
29. Conn HO. Cirrhosis. In: Schiff L, Schiff ER, eds. Diseases of the Liver. 5th ed. Philadelphia: JB Lippincott; 1982:847–977.
30. Thomas FB, Fromkes JJ. Spontaneous bacterial peritonitis associated with acute viral hepatitis. J Clin Gastroenterol. 1982;4:259–62.
31. Runyon BA. Spontaneous bacterial peritonitis with cardiac ascites. Am J Gastroenterol. 1984;79:796.
32. Isner J, MacDonald JS, Schein PS. Spontaneous *Streptococcus pneumoniae* peritonitis in a patient with metastatic gastric cancer. Cancer. 1979;39:2306–9.
33. Shesol BF, Rosato EF, Rosato FE. Concomitant acute lupus erythematosus and primary pneumococcal peritonitis. Am J Gastroenterol. 1975;63:324–6.
34. Friedland JA, Harris MN. Primary pneumococcal peritonitis in a young adult. Am J Surg. 1970;119:737–9.
35. Golden GT, Stevenson TR, Ritchie WP Jr. Primary peritonitis in adults. South Med J. 1975;68:413–4.
36. Wilcox CM, Dismukes WE. Spontaneous bacterial peritonitis: A review of pathogenesis, diagnosis and treatment. Medicine. 1987;66:447–56.
37. Correia JP, Conn HO. Spontaneous bacterial peritonitis in cirrhosis: Endemic or epidemic? Med Clin North Am. 1975;59:963–81.
38. Hoefs JC, Runyon BA. Spontaneous bacterial peritonitis. Dis Mon. 1985;31(9):1–48.
39. Fromkes JJ, Thomas FB, Mekhjian HS, et al. Antimicrobial activity of human ascitic fluid. Gastroenterology. 1977;73:668–72.
40. Scheckman P, Onderdonk AB, Bartlett JG. Anaerobes in spontaneous peritonitis. Lancet. 1977;2:1223.
41. Runyon BA, Hoefs JC. Culture-negative neutrocytic ascites: A variant of spontaneous peritonitis. Hepatology. 1984;4:1209–11.
42. Runyon BA, Umland ET, Merlin T. Inoculation of blood culture bottles with ascitic fluid: Improved detection of spontaneous bacterial peritonitis. Arch Intern Med. 1987;147:73–75.
43. Beeson PB, Brannon ES, Warren JU. Observations on the sites of removal of bacteria from the blood in patients with bacterial endocarditis. J Exp Med. 1945;81:9–23.
44. Rutenburg AM, Sonnenblick F, Koven I, et al. Comparative response of normal and cirrhotic rats to intravenously injected bacteria. Proc Soc Exp Biol Med. 1959;101:279–81.
45. Lahnborg G, Friman L, Berghem L. Reticuloendothelial function in patients with alcoholic liver disease. Scand J Gastroenterol. 1981;16:481–9.
46. Rimola A, Soto R, Bory F, et al. Reticuloendothelial system phagocytic activity in cirrhosis and its relation to bacterial infections and prognosis. Hepatology. 1984;4:53–8.
47. Rajkovic IA, Williams R. Abnormalities of neutrophilic phagocytosis, intracellular killing and metabolic activity in alcoholic cirrhosis and hepatitis. Hepatology. 1986;6:252–62.
48. Wyke RJ, Rajkovic IA, Eddleston WF, et al. Defective serum opsonization in patients with chronic liver disease (Abstract). Gut. 1979;20:A931.
49. Yousif-Kadura AGM, Rajkovic IA, Wyke RJ, et al. Defects in serum attractant activity in different types of chronic liver disease. Gut. 1984;25:79–84.
50. Simberkoff MS, Moldover NH, Weiss G. Bactericidal and opsonic activity of cirrhotic ascites and nonascitic peritoneal fluid. J Lab Clin Med. 1978;91:831–9.
51. Runyon BA, Hoefs JC. Ascitic fluid analysis in the differentiation of spontaneous bacterial peritonitis from gastrointestinal performation into ascitic fluid. Hepatology. 1984;4:447–50.
52. Whipple RL Jr, Harris JF. *E. coli* septicemia in Laennec's cirrhosis of the liver. Ann Intern Med. 1950;33:462–9.
53. Murray HW, Marks SJ. Spontaneous bacterial empyema, pericarditis and peritonitis in cirrhosis. Gastroenterology. 1977;72:772–3.
54. Snyder N, Atterbury CE, Correia JP, et al. Increased concurrence of cirrhosis and bacterial endocarditis. Gastroenterology. 1977;73:1107–13.
55. Schweinburg FB, Seligman AM, Fine J. Transmural migration of intestinal bacteria: A study based on the use of radioactive *Escherichia coli*. N Engl J Med. 1950;242:747–51.
56. Schwartz FD, Kallmeyer J, Durea G, et al. Prevention of infection during peritoneal dialysis. JAMA. 1967;199:79–81.
57. Gorbach SL, Lai D, Levitan R. Intestinal microflora in Laennec's cirrhosis. J Clin Invest. 1970;49:36a.
58. McCartney JE, Fraser J. Pneumococcal peritonitis. Br J Surg. 1922;9:479–89.
59. Herbert TJ, Mortimer PP. Recurrent pneumococcal peritonitis associated with an intrauterine contraceptive device. Br J Surg. 1974;61:901–2.
60. Brinson RR, Kolts BE, Monif GRG. Spontaneous bacterial peritonitis associated with an intrauterine device. J Clin Gastroenterol. 1986;8:82–4.
61. Kimball MW, Knee S. Gonococcal perihepatitis in a male. The Fitz-Hugh-Curtis syndrome. N Engl J Med. 1970;282:1082–4.
62. Luetscher JA Jr. Electrophoretic analysis of the proteins of plasma and serous effusions. J Clin Invest. 1941;20:99–106.
63. Witte MH, Witte CL, Davis WM, et al. Peritoneal transudate: A diagnostic clue to portal system obstruction in patients with intra-abdominal neoplasms or peritonitis. JAMA. 1972;221:1380–3.
64. Hoefs JC. Increase in ascites white blood cell and protein concentrations during diuresis in patients with chronic liver disease. Hepatology. 1981;1:249–54.
65. Stassen WN, McCullough AJ, Bacon BR, et al. Immediate diagnostic criteria for bacterial infection of ascitic fluid: Evaluation of ascitic fluid polymorphonuclear leukocyte count, pH, and lactate concentration, alone and in combination. Gastroenterology. 1986;90:1247–54.
66. Garcia-Tsao G, Conn HO, Lerner E. The diagnosis of bacterial peritonitis: Comparison of pH, lactate concentration and leukocyte count. Hepatology. 1985;5:91–6.
67. Yang C-Y, Liaw F, Chu E-M, et al. White count, pH and lactate in ascites in the diagnosis of spontaneous bacterial peritonitis. Hepatology. 1985;5:85–90.
68. Vickers FN, Maloney PJ. Gonococcal perihepatitis: Reports of three cases with comments on diagnosis and treatment. Arch Intern Med. 1964;114:120–3.
69. Burack WR, Hollister RM. Tuberculous peritonitis: A study of forty-seven proved cases encountered by a general medical unit in twenty-five years. Am J Med. 1960;28:510–23.
70. Saw EC, Shields SJ, Comer TP, et al. Granulomatous peritonitis due to *Coccidioides immitis*. Arch Surg. 1974;108:369–71.
71. Harrison RN, Cryer HM, Howard DA, et al. Clarification of risk factors for abdominal operations in patients with hepatic cirrhosis. Ann Surg. 1984;199:648–65.
72. Runyon BA, Hoefs JC. Spontaneous vs. secondary bacterial peritonitis: Differentiation by response of ascitic fluid neutrophil count to antimicrobial therapy. Arch Intern Med. 1986;146:1563–5.
73. Dimond M, Proctor HJ. Concomitant pneumococcal appendicitis, peritonitis and meningitis. Arch Surg. 1976;111:888–9.
74. Mallory A, Schaefer JW. Complications of diagnostic paracentesis in patients with liver disease. JAMA. 1978;239:628–30.
75. Levine H. Needle biopsy of peritoneum in exudative ascites. Arch Intern Med. 1967;120:542–5.
76. Dineen P, Homan WP, Grafe WR. Tuberculous peritonitis: 43 years experience in diagnosis and treatment. Ann Surg. 1976;184(6):717–22.
77. Felisart J, Rimona A, Arroyo V, et al. Cefotaxime is more effective than is ampicillin-tobramycin in cirrhotics with severe infections. Hepatology. 1985;5:457–62.
78. Cabrera J, Arroyo V, Ballesta AM, et al. Aminoglycoside nephrotoxicity in cirrhosis: Value of urinary β_2-microglobulin to discriminate functional renal failure from acute tubular damage. Gastroenterology. 1982;82:97–105.
79. Runyon BA, Hoefs JC. Ascitic fluid chemical analysis before, during and after spontaneous bacterial peritonitis. Hepatology. 1985;5:257–9.
80. Porter JM, Snowe RJ, Silver D. Tuberculous enteritis with perforation and abscess formation in childhood. Surgery. 1972;71:254–7.
81. Rowland TC Jr. Severe peritonitis complicating an intrauterine contraceptive device. Am J Obstet Gynecol. 1971;110:786–7.
82. Prokesch RC, Rimland D. Infectious complications of the peritoneovenous shunt. Am J Gastroenterol. 1983;78:235–40.
83. Reynold M, Sherman JO, Mclone DG. Ventriculoperitoneal shunt infections masquerading as an acute abdomen. J Pediatr Surg. 1983;18:951–4.

84. Nichols RL. Intra-abdominal infections: An overview. Rev Infect Dis. 1985;7(Suppl 4):S709–15.
85. Drasar BS, Shiner M, McLeod GM. Studies on the intestinal flora. I. The bacterial flora of the gastrointestinal tract in healthy and achlorhydric persons. Gastroenterology. 1969;56:71–9.
86. Nichols RL, Smith JW. Intragastric microbial colonization in common disease states of the stomach and duodenum. Ann Surg. 1975;182:557–61.
87. Gorbach SL, Plaut AG, Nahas L, et al. Studies of intestinal microflora. II. Microorganisms of the small intestine and their relations to oral and fecal flora. Gastroenterology. 1967;53:856–67.
88. Drasar BS, Shiner M. Studies on the intestinal flora. Part II. Bacterial flora of the small intestine in patients with gastrointestinal disorders. Gut. 1969;10:812–9.
89. Gorbach SL, Nahas L, Lerner PI, et al. Studies of intestinal microflora. I. Effects of diet, age, and periodic sampling of numbers of fecal microorganisms in man. Gastroenterology. 1967;53:845–55.
90. Finegold SM. Interaction of antimicrobial therapy and intestinal flora. Am J Clin Nutr. 1970;23:1466–71.
91. Altemeier WA. The bacterial flora of acute perforated appendicitis with peritonitis. Ann Surg. 1938;107:517–28.
92. Finegold SM. Abdominal and perineal infections. In: Finegold SM, ed. Anaerobic Bacteria in Human Disease. New York. Academic Press; 1977;257–313.
93. Gorbach SL, Thadepalli H, Norsen J. Anaerobic microorganisms in intraabdominal infections. In: Balows A, de Haan RM, Dowell VR Jr, et al, eds. Anaerobic Bacteria: Role in Disease. Springfield, Ill: Charles C. Thomas; 1974:399–407.
94. Lorber B, Swenson RM. The bacteriology of intra-abdominal infections. Surg Clin North Am. 1975;55:1349–54.
95. Swenson RM, Lorber B, Michaelson TC, et al. The bacteriology of intraabdominal infections. Arch Surg. 1974;109:398–9.
96. Tally FP, McGowan K, Kellum JM, et al. A randomized comparison of cefoxitin with or without amikacin and clindamycin plus amikacin in surgical sepsis. Ann Surg. 1981;193:318–23.
97. Aronoff SC, Olson MM, Gaudierer MWL, et al. *Pseudomonas aeruginosa* as a primary pathogen in children with bacterial peritonitis. J Pediatr Surg. 1987;22:861–4.
98. Heseltine PNR, Yellin AE, Applebaum MD, et al. Perforated and gangrenous appendicitis: An analysis of antibiotic failures. J Infect Dis. 1983;148:322–9.
99. Dunn DL, Simmons RL. The role of anaerobic bacteria in intra-abdominal infections. Rev Infect Dis. 1984;6(Suppl 1):S139–46.
100. Nichols RL, Smith JW, Klein DB, et al. Risk of infection after penetrating abdominal trauma. N Engl J Med. 1984;311:1065–70.
101. Bodner SJ, Koenig MG, Goodman JS. Bacteremic *Bacteroides* infections. Ann Intern Med. 1970;73:537–44.
102. Gelb EF, Seligman SJ. Bacteroidaceae bacteremia. Effect of age and focus of infection upon clinical course. JAMA. 1970;212:1038–41.
103. Fry DE, Garrison RN, Polk HC Jr. Clinical implications in *Bacteroides* bacteremia. Surg Gynecol Obstet. 1979;149:189–92.
104. Chow AW, Guze LB. Bacteroidaceae bacteremia: Clinical experience with 112 patients. Medicine. 1974;53:93–126.
105. Levison ME, Korman LC, Carrington ER, et al. Quantitative microflora of the vagina. Am J Obstet Gynecol. 1977;127:80–5.
106. Levison ME, Trestman I, Quach R, et al. Quantitative bacteriology of the vaginal flora in vaginitis. Am J Obstet Gynecol. 1979;133:139–44.
107. Bartlett JG, Onderdonk AB, Drude E, et al. Quantitative bacteriology of the vaginal flora. J Infect Dis. 1977;136:271–7.
108. Ohm M, Galask RP. The effect of antibiotic prophylaxis on patients undergoing vaginal operations: II. Alteration of microbial flora. Am J Obstet Gynecol. 1975;123:597–604.
109. Ramsay AM. The significance of *C. welchii* in the cervical swab and blood serum in postpartum and postabortum sepsis. J Obstet Gynecol. 1949;56:247–58.
110. Hite KE, Hesseltine HC, Goldstein L. A study of the bacterial flora of the normal and pathologic vagina and uterus. Am J Obstet Gynecol. 1947;53:233–40.
111. Gibbs RS, O'Dell TN, MacGregor RR, et al. Puerperal endometritis: A prospective microbiologic study. Am J Obstet Gynecol. 1975;121:919–25.
112. Baker CJ, Barrett FF, Yow MD. The influence of advancing gestation on group B streptococcal colonization in pregnant women. Am J Obstet Gynecol. 1975;122:820–3.
113. Penza JF. Moniliasis and trichomoniasis. In: Charles D, Finland M, eds. Obstetric and Perinatal Infections. Philadelphia: Lee & Febiger; 1973:209.
114. Finegold SM. Female genital tract infections. In: Finegold SM, ed. Anaerobic Bacteria in Human Disease. New York: Academic Press; 1977: 350–85.
115. Swenson RM, Michaelson TC, Daly MJ, et al. Anaerobic bacterial infections of the female genital tract. Obstet Gynecol. 1973;42:538–41.
116. Thadepalli H, Gorbach SL, Keith L. Anaerobic infections of the female genital tract: Bacteriologic and therapeutic aspects. Am J Obstet Gynecol. 1973;117:1034–40.
117. Chow AW, Marshall JR, Guze LB. Anaerobic infections of the female genital tract: Prospects and perspectives. Obstet Gynecol Surg. 1975;30:477–94.
118. Chow AW, Malkasian KI, Marshall JR, et al. The bacteriology of acute pelvic inflammatory disease. Value of cul-de-sac cultures and relative importance of gonococcal and other aerobic or anaerobic bacteria. Am J Obstet Gynecol. 1975;122:876–9.
119. Eschenbach DA, Buchanon TM, Pollock HM, et al. Polymicrobial etiology of acute pelvic inflammatory disease. N Engl J Med. 1975;293:166–71.
120. Wasserheit JN, Bell TA, Kiviat NB, et al. Microbial causes of proven pelvic inflammatory disease and efficacy of clindamycin and tobramycin. Ann Intern Med. 1986;104:187–93.
121. Monif GRG, Welkos SI, Baer H, et al. Cul-de-sac isolates from patients with endometritis-salpingitis-peritonitis and gonococcal endocervicitis. Am J Obstet Gynecol. 1976;126:158–61.
122. Burry VF. Gonococcal vulvovaginitis and possible peritonitis in prepubertal girls. Am J Dis Child. 1971;121:536–7.
123. Fuld GL. Gonococcal peritonitis in a prepubertal child. Am J Dis Child. 1968;115:621–2.
124. Adams EB, MacLeod IN. Invasive amebiasis. II. Amebic liver abscess and its complications. Medicine. 1977;56:325–34.
125. Turner GR, Millikan M, Carter R, et al. Surgical significance of fulminating amebic colitis. Report of perforation of the colon with peritonitis. Am Surg. 1965;31:759–63.
126. Lintermans JP. Fatal peritonitis, an unusual complication of *Strongyloides stercoralis* infestation. Clin Pediatr. 1975;14:974–5.
127. Eisenberg ES, Leviton I, Soeiro R. Fungal peritonitis in patients receiving peritoneal dialysis: Experience with 11 patients and review of the literature. Rev Infect Dis. 1986;3:309–21.
128. Bayer AS, Blumenkrantz MJ, Montgomerie JZ, et al. Candida peritonitis: Report of 22 cases and review of the English literature. Am J Med. 1976;61:832–40.
129. Solomkin JS, Flohr AB, Quie PG, et al. The role of candida in intraperitoneal infections. Surgery. 1980;88:524–30.
130. Howard JM, Singh LM. Peritoneal fluid pH after perforation of peptic ulcers. Arch Surg. 1963;87:483–4.
131. Mortez WH, Erickson WG. Neutralization of hydrochloric acid in the peritoneal cavity. Arch Surg. 1957;75:834–7.
132. Santschi DR, Huizenga KA, Scudamore HH, et al. Bile ascites. Arch Surg. 1963;87:851–6.
133. Diamonon JS, Barnes JP. Choleperitoneum. Am Surg. 1964;30:331–4.
134. Cohn I, Cotlar AM, Atik M, et al. Bile peritonitis. Ann Surg. 1960;152:827–35.
135. Nemir P Jr, Hawthorne HR, Cohn I, et al. I. The cause of death in strangulation obstruction. An experimental study. Ann Surg. 1949;130:857–73.
136. Nemir P Jr, Hawthorne HR, Cohn I, et al. II. The lethal action of the peritoneal fluid. Ann Surg. 1949;130:874–80.
137. Barnett WO, Hardy JD. Observations concerning the peritoneal fluid in experimental strangulated intestinal obstruction: The effects of removal from the peritoneal cavity. Surgery. 1958;43:440–4.
138. Barnett WO, Doyle RS. The effects of neomycin upon the toxicity of peritoneal fluid resulting from strangulation obstruction. Surgery. 1958;44:442–6.
139. Barnett WO, Messina AJ. The influence of massive antibiotics in experimental strangulation obstruction. Gastroenterology. 1959;36:534–6.
140. Davis JH, Yull AB. A possible toxic factor in abdominal surgery. J Trauma. 1962;2:291–300.
141. Filler RM, Sleeman HK, Hendry WS, et al. Lethal factors in experimental peritonitis. Surgery. 1966;60:671–8.
142. Lee JT Jr, Ahrenholz DN, Nelson RD, et al. Mechanisms of the adjuvant effect of hemoglobin in experimental peritonitis. V. The significance of the coordinated iron component. Surgery. 1979;86:41–8.
143. Weingerg ED. Roles of iron in host–parasite interactions. J Infect Dis. 1971;124:401–10.
144. Hau T, Nelson RD, Fiegel VD, et al. Mechanisms of the adjuvant action of hemoglobin in experimental peritonitis—2. Influence of hemoglobin on human leukocyte chemotaxis in vitro. J Surg Res. 1977;22:174–80.
145. Dunn DL, Barke RA, Ahrenholz DH, et al. The adjuvant effect of peritoneal fluid in experimental peritonitis. Ann Surg. 1984;199:37–43.
146. Rotstein OD, Pruett TL, Simmons RD. Fibrin in peritonitis. V. Fibrin inhibits phagocytic killing of *Escherichia coli* by human polymorphonuclear leukocytes. Ann Surg. 1986;203:413–9.
147. Schneierson SS, Amsterdam D, Perlman E. Enhancement of intraperitoneal staphylococcal virulence for mice with different bile salts. Nature. 1961;190:829–30.
148. Sisel RJ, Donovan AJ, Yellin AE. Experimental fecal peritonitis. Influence of barium sulfate or water-soluble radiographic contrast material on survival. Arch Surg. 1972;104:765–8.
149. Westfall RH, Nelson RH, Musselman MM. Barium peritonitis. Am J Surg. 1966;112:760–3.
150. Olitzki L. Mucin as a resistance-lowering substance. Bacteriol Rev. 1948;12:149–72.
151. Cuevas P, Fine J. Role of intraintestinal endotoxin in death from peritonitis. Surg Gynecol Obstet. 1972;134:953–7.
152. Bieluch VM, Tally FP. Pathophysiology of abscess formation. Clin Obstet Gynecol. 1983;10:93–103.
153. Gorbach SL, Bartlett JG. Anaerobic infections (third of three parts). N Engl J Med. 1974;290:1289–94.
153a. Hofstad T. Endotoxins of anaerobic gram-negative microorganisms. In: Balows A, de Haan RM, Dowell VR Jr., et al., eds. Anaerobic Bacteria: Role in Disease. Springfield, IL: Charles C. Thomas; 1974:295.

154. Bjornson HS. Enzymes associated with the survival and virulence of gram-negative anaerobes. Rev Infect Dis. 1984;6(Suppl 1):S21–4.
155. Gibbons RJ, MacDonald JB. Degradation of collagenous substrates by *Bacteroides melaninogenicus*. J Bacteriol. 1961;81:614–21.
156. Gesner BM, Jenkin CR. Production of heparinase by bacteroides. J Bacteriol. 1961;81:595–604.
157. Bjornson H, Hill EO. Bacteroidaceae in thromboembolic disease. Effects of cell wall components on blood coagulation in vivo and in vitro. Infect Immun. 1974;9:337–41.
158. Casciato DA, Rosenblatt JE, Goldberg LS, et al. In vitro interaction of *Bacteroides fragilis* with polymorphonuclear leukocytes and serum factors. Infect Immun. 1975;11:337–42.
159. Keusch GT, Douglas SD. Intraleukocytic survival of anaerobic bacteria. Clin Res. 1974;22:445A.
160. Kasper DL. The polysaccharide capsule of *Bacteroides fragilis* subspecies fragilis: Immunochemical and morphologic definition. J Infect Dis. 1976;133:79–87.
161. Mansheim BJ, Orderdonk AB, Kasper DL. Immunochemical characterization of surface antigens of *Bacteroides melaninogenicus*. Rev Infect Dis. 1979;1:263–77.
162. Onderdonk AB, Kasper DL, Cisneros RL, et al. The capsular polysaccharide of *Bacteroides fragilis* as a virulence factor: Comparison of the pathogenic potential of encapsulated and unencapsulated strains. J Infect Dis. 1977;136:82–9.
163. Ingham HR, Tharagonnet D, Sisson PR, et al. Inhibition of phagocytosis in vitro by obligate anaerobes. Lanct. 1977;2:1252–4.
164. Simon GL, Klempner MS, Kasper DL, et al. Alterations in opsonophagocytic killing by neutrophils of *Bacteroides fragilis* associated with animal and laboratory passage: Effect of capsular polysaccharide. J Infect Dis. 1982;145:72–7.
165. Socransky SS, Gibbons RJ. Required role of *Bacteroides melaninogenicus* in mixed anaerobic infections. J Infect Dis. 1965;115:247–53.
166. Altemeier WA. The pathogenicity of the bacteria of appendicitis peritonitis. Surgery. 1942;11:374–84.
167. Namavar FA, Verweij MJ, Bal M, et al. Effects of anaerobic bacteria on killing of *Proteus mirabilis* by human polymorphonuclear leukocytes. Infect Immun. 1983;40:930–5.
168. Rotstein OD, Nasmith PE, Grinstein S. The bacteroides by-product succinic acid inhibits neutrophil respiratory burst by reducing intracellular pH. Infect Immun. 1987;55:864–70.
169. Brook I. Anaerobic infections in childhood. Rev Infect Dis. 1984;6(Suppl 1):S187–92.
170. Onderdonk AB, Weinstein WN, Sullivan NM, et al. Experimental intra-abdominal abscess in rats: Quantitative bacteriology of infected animals. Infect Immun. 1974;10:1256–9.
171. Weinstein WM, Onderdonk AB, Bartlett JG, et al. Antimicrobial therapy of experimental intraabdominal sepsis. J Infect Dis. 1975;132:282–6.
172. Onderdonk AB, Bartlett JG, Louie T, et al. Microbial synergy in experimental intra-abdominal abscess. Infect Immun. 1976;13:22–6.
173. Rosoff L. Weil M, Bradely EC, et al. Hemodynamic and metabolic changes associated with bacterial peritonitis. Am J Surg. 1967;114:180–9.
174. MacLean LD, Mulugan WG, McLean APH, et al. Patterns of septic shock in man: A detailed study of 56 patients. Ann Surg. 1967;166:543–62.
175. Davis JH. Current concepts of peritonitis. Am Surg. 1967;33:673–81.
176. Pine RW, Wertz MJ, Lennard ES, et al. Determinants of organ malfunction or death in patients with intra-abdominal sepsis. Arch Surg. 1983;118:242–9.
177. Dellinger EP, Wertz MJ, Meakins JL, et al. Surgical infection stratification system for intra-abdominal infection. Arch Surg. 1985;120:21–9.
178. Meakins JL, Solomkin JS, Allo MD, et al. A proposed classification of intra-abdominal infections. Stratification of etiology and risk for future therapeutic trials. Arch Surg. 1984;119:1372–8.
179. Nobles ER Jr. Bacteroides infections. Ann Surg. 1973;177:601–6.
180. Young LS, Martin WJ, Meyer RD, et al. Gram-negative rod bacteremia. Microbiologic, immunologic and therapeutic considerations. Ann Intern Med. 1977;86:456–71.
181. Maler JA Jr, Reynolds TB, Yellin AE. Successful medical treatment of pyogenic liver abscess. Gastroenterology. 1979;77:618–22.
182. Herbert DA, Fogel DA, Rothman J, et al. Pyogenic liver abscesses: Successful nonsurgical therapy. Lancet. 1982;1:134–36.
183. Stalons DR, Thonsberry C, Dawell VR. Effect of culture medium and carbon dioxide concentration on growth of anaerobic bacteria commonly encountered in clinical specimens. Appl Microbiol. 1974;27:1098 1104.
184. Rosenblatt JE, Schoenknecht F. Effect of several components of anaerobic incubation on antibiotic susceptibility test results. Antimicrob Agents Chemother. 1972;1:433–40.
185. Wagoner ES, Gorman M. The reaction of cysteine and related compounds with penicillins and cephalosporins. J Antibiot. 1971;24:647–58.
186. Wilkins TD, Chalgren S. Medium for use in antibiotic susceptibility testing of anaerobic bacteria. Antimicrob Agents Chemother. 1976;10:926–8.
187. Gorbach SL, Thadepalli H. Clindamycin in pure and mixed anaerobic infections. Arch Intern Med. 1974;134:87–92.
188. Bartlett JG, Louie TJ, Onderdonk AB, et al. Whither the enterococcus? 15th ICACC. Abstract No. 297. Washington, DC; September 24–26, 1975.
189. Fass RJ, Scholand JF, Hodges GR, et al. Clindamycin in the treatment of serious anaerobic infections. Ann Intern Med. 1973;78:853–9.
190. Levison ME, Santoro J, Bran JL, et al. In vitro activity and clinical efficacy of clindamycin in the treatment of infections due to anaerobic bacteria. J Infect Dis. 1977;135:S49–53.
191. Dougherty SH. Role of enterococcus in intra-abdominal sepsis. Am J Surg. 1984;148:303–12.
192. Weinstein MP, Reller LB, Murphy J, et al. The clinical significance of positive blood cultures: A comprehensive analysis of 500 episodes of bacteremia and fungemia in adults. I. Laboratory and epidemiologic observations. Rev Infect Dis. 1983;5:35–53.
193. Shales DM, Levy J, Wolinsky E. Enterococcal bacteremia without endocarditis. Arch Intern Med. 1981;141:578–81.
194. Dougherty SH, Flohr AB, Simmons RL. Breakthrough enterococcal septicemia in surgical patients. Arch Surg. 1983;118:232–7.
195. Salzer W, Pegram PS, McCan CE. Clinical evaluation of moxalactam: Evidence of decreased efficacy in gram-positive aerobic infection. Antimicrob Agents Chemother. 1983;23:565–70.
196. Sande MA, Overton JW. In vivo antagonism between gentamicin and chloramphenicol in neutropenic mice. J Infect Dis. 1973;128:247–50.
197. Zinner SH, Provonchee RB, Elias KS. Effect of clindamycin on the in vitro activity of amikacin and gentamicin against gram negative bacilli. Antimicrob Agents Chemother. 1976;9:661–4.
198. Ekwo E, Peter G. Effect of clindamycin on aminoglycoside activity in murine model of *Escherichia coli* infection. Antimicrob Agents Chemother. 1976;10:893–8.
199. Fass RJ, Rotilie CA, Prior RB. Interaction of clindamycin and gentamicin in vitro. Antimicrob Agents Chemother. 1974;6:582–7.
200. Cuchural GJ Jr, Tally FB, Jacobus NV, et al. Susceptibility of the *Bacteroides fragilis* group in the United States: Analysis by site of isolation. Antimicrob Agents Chemother. 1988;32:717–22.
201. Louis TJ, Bartlett JG, Onderdonk AB, et al. Failure of chloramphenicol therapy of experimental intra-abdominal sepsis. 17th ICAAC. Abstract No. 25. New York; October 12–14, 1977.
202. Thadepalli H, Gorbach SL, Bartlett JG. Apparent failure of chloramphenicol in anaerobic infections. 13th ICAAC. Abstract No. 117. Washington DC; September 19–21, 1973.
203. Van Scoy RE, Wilkowske CJ, O'Fallon WM, et al. Clindamycin versus chloramphenicol in treatment of anaerobic infections: A prospective, randomized double-blind study. Mayo Clin Proc. 1984;59:842–6.
204. Tally FB, Sosa A, Jacobus NV, et al. Clindamycin resistance in *Bacteroides fragilis*. J Antimicrob Chemother. 1981;8(Suppl):43–8.
205. Tally FP, Cuchural GH Jr, Jacobus NV, et al. Nationwide study of the susceptibility of the *Bacteroides fragilis* group in the United States. Antimicrob Agents Chemother. 1985;28:675–7.
206. Wilson WR, Cockerhill FR III. Tetracyclines, chloramphenicol, erythromycin and clindamycin. Mayo Clin Proc. 1987;62:906–15.
207. Tedesco FJ, Barton RW, Alpers DH. Clindamycin associated colitis: A prospective study. Ann Intern Med. 1974;81:429–33.
208. Ralph ED, Kirby WMM. Unique bactericidal action against *Bacteroides fragilis* and *Clostridium perfringens*. Antimicrob Agents Chemother. 1975;8:409–14.
209. Chow AW, Patten V, Guze LB. Susceptibility of anaerobic bacteria to metronidazole: Relative resistance of non-spore-forming gram-positive bacilli. J Infect Dis. 1975;131:182–5.
210. Onderdonk AB, Louie TJ, Tally FP, et al. Activity of metronidazole against *Escherichia coli* in experimental intra-abdominal sepsis. J Antimicrob Chemother. 1979;5:201–10.
211. Bartlett JG, Louie TJ, Gorbach SL, et al. Therapeutic efficacy of 29 antimicrobial regimens in experimental intra-abdominal sepsis. Rev Infect Dis. 1981;3:535–42.
212. Sutter VL, Kwoh Y-Y, Finegold SM. Standardized antimicrobial disc susceptibility testing of anaerobic bacteria. I. Susceptibility of *Bacteroides fragilis* to tetracyclines. Appl Microbiol. 1972;23:268–75.
213. Sutter VL, Finegold SM. Susceptibility of anaerobic bacteria to 23 antimicrobial agents. Antimicrob Agents Chemother. 1976;10:736–52.
214. Wexler HM, Finegold SM. In vitro activity of cefotetan compared with that of other antimicrobial agents against anaerobic bacteria. Antimicrob Agents Chemother. 1988;32:601–4.
215. O'Keefe JP, Vlenezio FR, Divincenzo CA, et al. Activity of newer beta-lactam agents against clinical isolates of *Bacteroides fragilis* and other *Bacteroides* species. Antimicrob Agents Chemother. 1987;31:2002–4.
216. Rolfe RD, Finegold SM. Comparative in vitro activity of new beta-lactam antibiotics against anaerobic bacteria. Antimicrob Agents Chemother. 1981;200:600–9.
217. Tally FP, Kellum JM, Ho TF, et al. Randomized prospective study comparing moxalactam and cefoxitin with or without tobramycin for treatment of serious surgical infections. Antimicrob Agents Chemother. 1986;29:244–9.
218. Schentag JJ, Wells PB, Reitberg DP, et al. A randomized clinical trial of moxalactam alone versus tobramycin plus clindamycin in abdominal sepsis. Ann Surg. 1983;198:35–41.
219. Andrassy K, Bechtold H, Ritz F. Hypoprothrombinemia caused by cephalosporins. J Antimicrob Chemother. 1985;15:133–6.
220. Aldridge KE. Comparison of the activities of penicillin G and new beta-lactam antibiotics against clinical isolates of *Bacteroides* species. Antimicrob Agents Chemother. 1984;26:410–3.
221. Chow AW, Finegold SM. In vitro activity of ceftizoxime against anaerobic bacteria and comparison with other cephalosporins. J Antimicrob Chemother. 1982;10(Suppl c):45–50.

222. Schoutens E, Yourassowsky E. Speed of bactericidal action of penicillin G, ampicillin and carbenicillin on *Bacteroides fragilis*. Antimicrob Agents Chemother. 1974;6:227–31.
223. Trestman I, Kaye D, Levison ME. Activity of semisynthetic penicillins and synergism with mecillinam against *Bacteroides* species. Antimicrob Agents Chemother. 1979;16:283–6.
224. Swenson RM, Lorber B. Clindamycin and carbenicillin in treatment of patients with intra-abdominal and female genital tract infections. J Infect Dis. 1977;135:S40–5.
225. Winston DJ, Murphy W, Young LS, et al. Piperacillin therapy for serious bacterial infections. Am J Med. 1980;69:255–61.
226. Harding GKM, Buckwalk FJ, Ronald AR, et al. Prospective, randomized comparative study of clindamycin, chloramphenicol, and ticarcillin, each in combination with gentamicin, for therapy of intra-abdominal and female genital tract sepsis. J Infect Dis. 1980;142:384–93.
227. Levison ME, Trestman I, Egert J, et al. Evaluation of ticarcillin in anaerobic infections. 17th ICAAC. Abstract No. 176. New York; October 12–14, 1977.
228. O'Keefe JP, Tally FP, Barza M, et al. Inactivation of penicillin G during experimental infection with *Bacteroides fragilis*. J Infect Dis. 1978;137:437–42.
229. Sykes RB, Squibb Institute for Medical Research. The classification and terminology of enzymes that hydrolyze beta-lactam antibiotics. J Infect Dis. 1982;145:762–5.
230. Eliopoulos GM, Moellering RC Jr. Azlocillin, mezlocillin and piperacillin: New broad-spectrum penicillins. Ann Intern Med. 1982;97:755–60.
231. Gould IM, Wise R. Beta-lactamase inhibitors. In: Peterson PK, Verhoef J, Amsterdam BV, eds. The Antimicrobial Agents Annual. 2nd ed. New York: Elsevier; 1987:58–69.
232. Wise R, Andrews JM, Bedford KA. Clavulanic acid and CP-45, 899: A comparison of their in vitro activity in combination with penicillins. J Antimicrob Chemother. 1980;6:197–206.
233. Donowitz GR, Mandell GL. Beta-lactam antibiotics (first of two parts). N Engl J Med. 1988;313:419–26.
234. Bansal MB, Chuah SK, Thadepalli H. In vitro activity and in vivo evaluation of ticarcillin plus clavulanic acid against aerobic and anaerobic bacteria. Am J Med. 1985;79(Suppl 5B):33–8.
235. Retsema JA, English AR, Girard A, et al. Sulbactam/ampicillin: In vitro spectrum, potency and activity in models of acute infection. Rev Infect Dis. 1986;8(Suppl 5):S528–42.
236. Reinhardt JF, Johnston L, Ruane P, et al. A randomized double blind comparison of sulbactam/ampicillin and clindamycin for the treatment of aerobic and aerobic-anaerobic infections. Rev Infect Dis. 1986;8(Suppl 5): S569–75.
237. Jones RN. Review of the in vitro spectrum of activity of imipenem. Am J Med. 1985;78(Suppl 6A):22–32.
238. Yotsuji A, Minami S, Inoue M, et al. Properties of a novel beta-lactamase produced by *Bacteroides fragilis*. Antimicrob Agents Chemother. 1983;24:925–9.
239. Jacobus NV, Ferreira MC, Barza M. In vitro activity of aztreonam, a monobactam antibiotic. Antimicrob Agents Chemother. 1982;22:832–8.
240. Kaye D, Levison ME, Labovitz ED. The unpredictability of serum concentrations of gentamicin: Pharmacokinetics of gentamicin in patients with normal and abnormal renal function. J Infect Dis. 1974;130:150–4.
241. Verklin RM Jr, Mandell GL. Alteration of effectiveness of antibiotics by anaerobiosis. J Lab Clin Med. 1977;89:65–71.
242. Wolfson JS, Hooper DC. The fluoroquinolones: Structures, mechanisms of action and resistance, and spectra of activity in vitro. Antimicrob Agents Chemother. 1985;28:581–86.
243. Neu HE. New antibiotics: Areas of appropriate use. J Infect Dis. 1987;155:403–17.
244. Finegold SM, Wexler HM. Therapeutic implications of bacteriologic findings in mixed aerobic-anaerobic infections. Antimicrob Agents Chemother. 1988;32:611–6.
245. David IB, Buck JR, Filler RM. Rational use of antibiotics for perforated appendicitis in childhood. J Pediatr Surg. 1982;17:494–500.
246. Norwegian Study Group for Colorectal Surgery. Should antimicrobial prophylaxis in colorectal surgery include agents effective against both anaerobic and aerobic microorganisms? A double blind multicenter study. Surgery. 1984;97:402–7.
247. Solomkin JS, Meakins JC, Allo MD, et al. Antibiotic trials in intra-abdominal infections. A critical evaluation of study design and outcome reporting. Ann Surg. 1984;200:29–39.
248. Stone HH. Metronidazole in the treatment of surgical infections. Surgery. 1983;93(2):230–4.
249. Aoki FY, Biron S, Doris PJ, et al. Prospective, randomized comparison of metronidazole and clindamycin, each with gentamicin, for the treatment of serious intra-abdominal infection. Surgery. 1983;93(2):217–20.
250. Canadian Metronidazole-Clindamycin Study Group: Prospective, randomized comparison of metronidazole and clindamycin, each with gentamicin, for the treatment of serious intra-abdominal infections. Surgery. 1983;93:221–9.
251. Ho JL, Barza M. Role of aminoglycoside antibiotics in the treatment of intra-abdominal infection. Antimicrob Agents Chemother. 1987;31:485–91.
252. Drusano GL, Warren WJ, Saah AJ, et al. A prospective randomized controlled trial of cefoxitin versus clindamycin-aminoglycoside in mixed aerobic-anaerobic infections. Surg Gynecol Obstet. 1982;154:715–20.
253. Tally FP, McGowan K, Kellum JM, et al. A randomized comparison of cefoxitin with or without amikacin and clindamycin plus amikacin in surgical sepsis. Ann Surg. 1981;193:318–23.
254. Nichols RL, Smith JW, Klein DB, et al. Risk of infection after penetrating abdominal trauma. N Engl J Med. 1984;311:1065–70.
255. Harding GKM, Buckwold FJ, Ronald AR, et al. Prospective, randomized, comparative study of clindamycin, chloramphenicol, and ticarcillin, each in combination with gentamicin, in therapy for intra-abdominal and female genital tract sepsis. J Infect Dis. 1980;142:384–93.
256. Najem AZ, Kaminski CR, Spiller CR, et al. Comparative study of parenteral piperacillin and cefoxitin in the treatment of surgical infections of the abdomen. Surgery. 1983;157:423–5.
257. Study Group of Intra-Abdominal Infections: A randomized controlled trial of ampicillin plus sulbactam vs gentamicin plus clindamycin in the treatment of intra-abdominal infections. Rev Infect Dis. 1986;8(Suppl 5):S533–88.
258. Scandinavian Study Group. Imipenem-cilastatin versus gentamicin-clindamycin for treatment of serious bacterial infections. Lancet. 1983;1:868–71.
259. Solomkin JS, Fant WK, Rivera JO, et al. Randomized trial of imipenem-cilastatin versus gentamicin and clindamycin in mixed flora infections. Am J Med. 1985;78(Suppl 6A):85–91.
260. Guerra JG, Casaline GE, Plomina JC, et al. Imipenem-cilastatin versus gentamicin-clindamycin for treatment of moderate to severe infections in hospitalized patients. Rev Infect Dis. 1985;7(Suppl 3):463–70.
261. Birolini D, Moraes MF, Soare de Souza O. Aztreonam plus clindamycin vs tobramycin plus clindamycin for the treatment of intra-abdominal infections. Rev Infect Dis. 1985;7(Suppl 4):S724–8.
262. Harding GJ, Vincelette A, Rachlis I, et al. A preliminary report on the use of ceftizoxime vs clindamycin/tobramycin for the therapy of intra-abdominal and pelvic infections. J Antimicrob Chemother. 1982;10(Suppl C):191–2.
263. Lou MA, Chen DF, Bansal M, et al. Evaluation of ceftizoxime in acute peritonitis. J Antimicrob Chemother. 1982;(Suppl C):183–9.
264. Berne TV, Yellin AW, Applebaum MC, et al. Antibiotic management of surgically treated or perforated appendicitis: Comparison of gentamicin and clindamycin versus cefamandole versus cefoperazone. Am J Surg. 1982;144:8–12.
265. Lau WY, Fan ST, Chu KW, et al. Randomized, prospective and double-blind trial of new beta-lactams in the treatment of appendicitis. Antimicrob Agents Chemother. 1985;28:639–42.
266. Saurio IH, Aruilommi C, Silvola H. Comparison of cefuroxime and gentamicin in combination with metronidazole in the treatment of peritonitis due to perforation of the appendix. Acta Chir Scand. 1983;149:423–6.
267. Peoples JB. *Candida* and perforated peptic ulcers. Surgery. 1986;100:758–64.
268. Rutledge R, Mandel SR, Wilde RE. *Candida* species. Insignificant contaminant or pathogenic species? Am Surg. 1986;52:299–302.
269. Marsh PK, Tally FP, Kellum J, et al. *Candida* infections in surgical patients. Ann Surg. 1983;198:42–7.
270. Sobel JD. *Candida* infections in the intensive care unit. Crit Care Clin North Am. 1988;4:325–44.
271. Hau T, Nishilawa R, Phuangsab A. Irrigation of the peritoneal cavity and antibiotics in the treatment of peritonitis. Surg Gynecol Obstet. 1983;156:25–30.
272. Rambo WM. Irrigation of the peritoneal cavity with cephalothin. Am J Surg. 1972;123:192–5.
273. Nichols RL. Management of intra-abdominal sepsis. Am J Med. 1985;80(Suppl 6B):204–9.
274. Hudspeth AS. Radical surgical debridement in the treatment of advanced generalized bacterial peritonitis. Arch Surg. 1975;110:1233–6.
275. Sindelar WF, Mason GR. Intraperitoneal irrigation with povidone-iodine solution for the prevention of intra-abdominal abscess in the bacterially contaminated abdomen. Surg Gynecol Obstet. 1979;148:409–11.
276. Ahrenholz DH, Simmons RL. Povidone-iodine in peritonitis. I. Adverse effects of local instillation in experimental *E. coli* peritonitis. J Surg Res. 1979;26:458–63.
277. Bhushan C, Mital VK, Elhence IP. Continuous postoperative peritoneal lavage in diffuse peritonitis using balanced saline antibiotic solution. Int Surg. 1975;60:526–8.
278. Hallerback B, Anderson C, Englund N, et al. A prospective randomized study of continuous peritoneal lavage postoperatively in the treatment of purulent peritonitis. Surg Gynecol Obstet. 1986;163:433–6.
279. Leiboff AR, Soroff HS. The treatment of generalized peritonitis by closed postoperative peritoneal lavage: A critical review of the literature. Arch Surg. 1987;122:1005–10.
280. Smithivas T, Hyams PJ, Matalon R, et al. The use of gentamicin in peritoneal dialysis. I. Pharmacologic results. J Infect Dis. 1971;124:S77–83.
281. Hill GB, Osterhout S. Experimental effects of hyperbaric oxygen on selected clostridial species. In vitro studies. J Infect Dis. 1972;125:17–25.
282. Holland JA, Hill GB, Wolfe WG, et al. Experimental and clinical experience with hyperbaric oxygen in the treatment of clostridial myonecrosis. Surgery. 1975;77:75–85.
283. Schreiner A, Tonjum S, Digranes A. Hyperbaric oxygen therapy in bacteroides infections. Acta Chir Scand. 1974;140:73–6.
284. Hill GB. Hyperbaric oxygen exposures for intrahepatic abscesses produced in mice by nonsporeforming anaerobic bacteria. Antimicrob Agents Chemother. 1976;9:312–7.
285. Thom SR, Lavermann MW, Hart GB. Intermittent hyperbaric oxygen therapy for reduction of mortality in experimental polymicrobial sepsis. J Infect Dis. 1986;154:504–10.

286. Haller JA Jr, Shaker IJ, Donahoo JS, et al. Peritoneal drainage versus non-drainage for generalized peritonitis from ruptured appendicitis in children: A prospective study. Ann Surg. 1973;177:595–600.
287. Leigh DA, Simmons K, Norman E. Bacterial flora of the appendix fossa in appendicitis and postoperative wound infection. J Clin Pathol. 1974;27:997–1000.
288. Follen WD, Hunt J, Altemeier WA. Prophylactic antibiotics in penetrating wounds of the abdomen. J Trauma. 1972;12:282–8.
289. Fabian TC, Boldreghini SJ. Antibiotics in penetrating abdominal trauma. Comparison of ticarcillin plus clavulanic acid with gentamicin plus clindamycin. Am J Med. 1985;79(Suppl 5B):157–60.
290. Nichols RL, Gorbach SL, Condon RE. Alteration of intestinal microflora following preoperative mechanical preparation of the colon. Dis Colon Rectum. 1971;14:123–7.
291. Condon RE, Bartlett JG, Greenlee H, et al. Efficacy of oral and systemic antibiotic prophylaxis in colorectal operations. Arch Surg. 1983;118:496–502.
292. Kaiser AB. Antibiotic prophylaxis in surgery. N Engl J Med. 1986;315:1129–38
293. Baum ML, Anish Ds, Chalmers TC, et al. A survey of clinical trials of antibiotic prophylaxis in colon surgery: Evidence against further use of non-treatment controls. N Engl J Med. 1981;305:795–9.
294. Guglielmo BJ, Hohn DC, Koo PJ, et al. Antibiotic prophylaxis in surgical procedures: A critical analysis of the literature. Arch Surg. 1983;118:943–55.
295. Holph KD, Sorkin M, Rubin J, et al. Continuous ambulatory peritoneal dialysis: Three-year experience at one center. Ann Intern Med. 1980;92:609–13.
296. Rubin J, Rogers WA, Taylor HM, et al. Peritonitis during continuous ambulatory peritoneal dialysis. Ann Intern Med. 1980;92:7–13.
297. Fenton SSA, Pei Y, Delmore T, et al. The CAPD peritonitis rate is not improving with time. Trans Am Soc Artif Intern Organs. 1986;32:546–9.
298. Vas SL. 2. Peritonitis of peritoneal dialysis patients: Pathogenesis and treatment. Med Microbiol. 1986;5:21–63.
299. Peterson PK, Matzke GR, Keane WF. Current concepts in the management of peritonitis in continuous ambulatory peritoneal dialysis patients. Rev Infect Dis. 1987;9(3):604–12.
300. Everett ED. Diagnosis, prevention and treatment of peritonitis. Perit Dialy Bull. 1984;4(Suppl):139–42.
301. Steinberg SM, Cutler SJ, Novak JK, et al. Report of the national CAPD registry of the National Institutes of Health: Characteristics of participants and selected outcome measures for the period January 1, 1981 through August 31, 1984. In: National CAPD Registry of the National Institute of Arthritis, Diabetes, and Digestive and Kidney Diseases. Washington, DC: US Public Health Services; 1985.
302. Kraus ES, Spector DA. Characteristics and sequelae of peritonitis in diabetics and non-diabetics receiving chronic intermittent peritoneal dialysis. Medicine. 1983;62:52–7.
303. Fenton S, Wu G, Cattran D, et al. Clinical aspects of peritonitis in patients on CAPD. Perit Dialy Bull. 1981;1(Suppl):4–8.
304. Sewell CM, Clarridge J, Lacke C, et al. Staphylococcal nasal carriage and subsequent infection in peritoneal dialysis patients. JAMA. 1982;248:1493–5.
305. Keane WJ, Comty CM, Verbrugh HA, et al. Opsonic deficiency of peritoneal dialysis effluent in CAPD. Kidney Int. 1984;25:539–43.
306. Lamperi S, Carozzi S, Nasini MG. Intraperitoneal immunoglobulin treatment in prophylaxis of bacterial peritonitis in CAPD. In: Khanna R, Nolph KD, Provant B, et al, eds. Advances in CAPD. Toronto: University of Toronto Press; 1986:110.
307. Duwe AK, Vas SI, Weatherhead IW. Effects of composition of peritoneal dialysis fluid on chemiluminescence, phagocytosis and bacterial activity in vitro. Infect Immun. 1981;33:130 – 5.
308. Marrie TJ, Noble MA, Costerton JW. Examination of the morphology of bacteria adhering to peritoneal dialysis catheters by scanning and transmission electron microscopy. J Clin Microbiol. 1983;18:1388–98.
309. Arfania D, Everett ED, Nolph KD, et al. Uncommon causes of peritonitis in patients undergoing peritoneal dialysis. Arch Intern Med. 1981;141:61–4.
310. Vas SI. Microbiologic aspects of chronic ambulatory dialysis. Kidney Int. 1983;23:83–92.
311. Peterson PK, Keane WF. Infections in chronic peritoneal dialysis patients. In: Remington JS, Swartz MN, eds. Current Clinical Topics in Infectious Diseases. New York: McGraw-Hill; 1985:239–60.
312. Woods GL, Washington JA II. Comparison of methods for processing dialysate in suspected continuous ambulatory peritoneal dialysis-associated peritonitis. Diagn Microbiol Infect Dis. 1987;7:155–7.
313. Gokal R, Ramos JM, Francis DM, et al. Peritonitis in continuous ambulatory peritoneal dialysis: Laboratory and clinical studies. Lancet. 1982;2:1388–91.
314. Keane WF, Everett ED, Fine RN, et al. CAPD related peritonitis management and antibiotic therapy recommendations: Travenol Peritonitis Management Advisory Committee. Perit Dialy Bull. 1987;7:55–68.
315. Verbrogh HA, Keane WF, Conroy WE, et al. Bacterial growth and killing in chronic ambulatory peritoneal dialysis fluids. J Clin Microbiol. 1984;20:199–203.
316. Eisenberg ES, Leviton I, Soeiro R. Fungal peritonitis in patients receiving peritoneal dialysis: Experience with 11 patients and review of the literature. Rev Infect Dis. 1986;8:309–21.
317. Rubin J, Kirchner K, Walsh D, et al. Fungal peritonitis during continuous ambulatory peritoneal dialysis: A report of 12 cases. Am J Kidney Dis. 1987;10:361–8.
318. Kerr CM, Perfect JR, Craven PC, et al. Fungal peritonitis in patients on continuous ambulatory peritoneal dialysis. Ann Intern Med. 1983;99:334–7.
319. Vargemezis V, Papadopoulov ZL, Llamos H, et al. Management of fungal peritonitis during continuous ambulatory peritoneal dialysis (CAPD). Perit Dialy Bull. 1986;6:17–20.
320. McNeely DJ, Vas SI, Dambros N, et al. *Fusarium* peritonitis: An uncommon complication of continuous ambulatory peritoneal dialysis. Perit Dialy Bull. 1981;1:94–6.
321. Chapman JR, Warnock DW. Ketoconazole and fungal CAPD peritonitis. Lancet. 1983;2:510–1.
322. McGuire NM, Port FK, Kauffman CA. Ketoconazole pharmacokinetics in continuous peritoneal dialysis. Perit Dialy Bull. 1984:4:199–201.
323. Axelrod J, Meyers BR, Hirschman SZ, et al. Prophylaxis with cephalothin in peritoneal dialysis. Arch Intern Med. 1973;132:368–71.
324. Abrutyn E, Goodhart GL, Roos K, et al. *Acinetobacter calcoaceticus* outbreak associated with peritoneal dialysis. Am J Epidemiol. 1978;107:328–35.
325. Altemeir WA, Culbertson WR, Fullen WD, et al. Intra-abdominal abscesses. Am J Surg. 1973;125:70–9.
326. Saini S, Kellum JM, O'Leary MP, et al. Improved localization and survival in patients with intra-abdominal abscesses. Am J Surg. 1983;145:136–42.
327. Gibson DM, Feliciano DV, Mattox KL, et al. Intra-abdominal abscess after penetrating abdominal trauma. Am J Surg. 1981;142:699–703.
328. Patterson HC. Left subphrenic abscesses. Am Surg. 1977;43:430–3.
329. Ozeran RS. Subdiaphragmatic abscess: Diagnosis and treatment. Am Surg. 1967;33:64–7.
330. Sherman NJ, Davis JR, Jesseph JE. Subphrenic abscess: A continuing hazard. Am J Surg. 1969;117:117–23.
331. Sanders RC. The changing epidemiology of subphrenic abscess and its clinical and radiological consequences. Br J Surg. 1970;57:449–55.
332. Ochsner A, DeBakey M. Subphrenic abscess. Collective review of 3608 collected and personal cases. Surg Gynecol Obstet. 1939;66:426.
333. Mackenzie M, Fordyle J, Young DG. Subphrenic abscess in children. Br J Surg. 1975;62:305–8.
334. Wang SMS, Wilson SE. Subphrenic abscess. The new epidemiology. Arch Surg. 1977;112:934–6.
335. DeCosse JJ, Poulin TL, Fox PS, et al. Subphrenic abscess. Surg Gynecol Obstet. 1974;138:841–6.
336. Gorbach SL. Treatment of intra-abdominal infection. Am J Med. 1984;76(Suppl 5A):107–10.
337. Milne GAC, Geere IIW. Chronic subphrenic abscess: The missed diagnosis. Can J Surg. 1977;20:162–5.
338. Mueller PR, Simeone JF. Intra-abdominal abscesses: Diagnosis by sonography and computed tomography. Radiol Clin North Am. 1983;21:425–43.
339. Ferrucci JT Jr, Van Sonnenberg E. Role of ultrasound and computed tomography in the diagnosis and treatment of intraabdominal abscess. In: Remington JS, Swartz MN, eds. Current Clinical Topics in Infectious Diseases. New York: McGraw-Hill; 1982:136–59.
340. Kerlan RK Jr, Pogany AC, Jeffrey RB, et al. Radiologic management of abdominal abscesses. AJR. 1985;144:145–9.
341. Connell TR, Stephens DH, Carlson HC, et al. Upper abdominal abscess: A continuing and deadly problem. AJR. 1980;134:759–65.
342. Middleton HM, Patton DD, Hoyumpa AM, et al. Liver-lung scan in the diagnosis of right subphrenic abscess. Dig Dis Sci. 1976;21:215–22.
343. Gold RP, Johnson PM. Efficacy of combined liver-lung scintillation imaging. Radiology. 1975;117:105–11.
344. Caffee HH, Watts G, Mena I. Gallium 67 citrate scanning in the diagnosis of intra-abdominal abscess. Am J Surg. 1977;133:665–9.
345. Tsan M. Mechanism of gallium 67 accumulation in inflammatory lesions. J Nucl Med. 1985;26:88–92.
346. Disbro M, Datz F, Cook P, et al. Indium-111 labeled leukocytes: Clinical utility and accuracy. Clin Nucl Med. 1982;7:44–6.
347. Froelich JW, Krasicky GA. Radionuclide imaging of abdominal infections. Curr Concepts Diag Nucl Med. 1985;2:12–6.
348. Coleman RE, Brack RE, Welch DM, et al. Indium-111 labeled leukocytes in the evaluation of suspected abdominal abscess. Am J Surg. 1980;139:99–104.
349. Sfakianakis GN, A-Sheitch W, Heal A, et al. Comparisons of scintigraphy with In-111 leukocytes and Ga^{67} in the diagnosis of occult sepsis. J Nucl Med. 1982;23:618–26.
350. Hill BA, Yamaguchi K, Flynn JJ, et al. Diagnostic sonography in general surgery. Arch Surg. 1975;110:1089–94.
351. Goudie E, Andrew WK. The role of diagnostic ultrasound in the assessment of masses in the left upper quadrant of the abdomen. S Afr Med J. 1976;50:1391–4.
352. Baker HL Jr, Berquist TN, Kispert DB, et al. Magnetic resonance imaging in a routine clinical setting. Mayo Clin Proc. 1985;60:75–90.
353. Cammoun D, Hendee WR, Davis KA. Clinical applications of magnetic resonance imaging—current status. West J Med. 1985;143:793–803.
354. Wall SD, Fisher MR, Amparo EG, et al. Magnetic resonance imaging in the evaluation of abscesses. AJR. 1985;144:1217–21.
355. Jacobs JB, Hammond WG, Poppman JL. Arteriographic localization of suprahepatic abscesses. Radiology. 1969;93:1299–300.
356. Halasz NA. Subphrenic abscess: Myths and facts. JAMA. 1970;214:724–6.

357. Gerzof SG, Robbins AH, Johnson WC. Percutaneous catheter drainage of abdominal abscesses. N Engl J Med. 1981;305:653–7.
358. Mandel SR, Boyd D, Jaques PF, et al. Drainage of hepatic, intra-abdominal and mediastinal abscesses guided by computerized axial tomography: Successful alternative to open drainage. Am J Surg. 1983;145:120–5.
359. Pruett TL, Simmons RL. Status of percutaneous catheter drainage of abscesses. Surg Clin North Am. 1988;68:89–105.
360. Brolin RE, Nosher JL, Leiman S, et al. Percutaneous catheter versus open surgical drainage in the treatment of abdominal abscesses. Am Surg. 1984;50:102–8.
361. Van Sonnenberg E, Ferruci JT Jr, Mueller PR, et al. Percutaneous drainage citrate in acute pancreatitis. Appl Radiol. 1978;1:163–5. diology. 1982;142:1–10.
362. Olak J, Christov NV, Stein LA, et al. Operative vs percutaneous drainage of intra-abdominal abscesses. Arch Surg. 1986;121:141–6.
363. Hurley JE, Vargish T. Early diagnosis and outcome of pancreatic abscesses in pancreatitis. Am Surg. 1987;53:29–33.
364. Kodesch R, DuPont HL. Infectious complications of acute pancreatitis. Surg Gynecol Obstet. 1973;136:763–8.
365. Becker JM, Pemberton JH, Diamgno EP, et al. Prognostic factors in pancreatic abscess. Surgery. 1984;96:455–60.
366. Shi ECP, Yeo BW, Ham JM. Pancreatic abscesses. Br J Surg. 1984;71:689–91.
367. Altemeier WA, Alexander JW. Pancreatic abscess. A study of 32 cases. Arch Surg. 1963;87:80–9.
368. Holden JL, Berne TV, Rosoff LSR. Pancreatic abscess following acute pancreatitis. Arch Surg. 1976;111:858–61.
369. Miller TA, Lindenauer SM, Frey CF, et al. Pancreatic abscess. Arch Surg. 1974;108:545–51.
370. Ransom JHC, Balthazar E, Caccavale R, et al. Computed tomography and the prediction of pancreatic abscess in acute pancreatitis. Ann Surg. 1985;201:656–63.
371. Aranha GU, Prinz RA, Greenlee HB. Pancreatic abscess: An unresolved surgical problem. Am J Surg. 1982;144:534–8.
372. Bradley EL, Fulenwider JT. Open treatment of pancreatic abscess. Surg Gynecol Obstet. 1984;159:509–13.
373. Stambler JB, Klibaner MI. Tuberculous abscess of the pancreas. Gastroenterology. 1982;83:922–5.
374. Sostre CF, Flournoy JG, Bova P, et al. Pancreatic phegmon: Clinical features and course. Dig Dis Sci. 1985;30:918–27.
375. Berger HG, Krautzberger W, Bittner R, et al. Results of surgical treatment of necrotizing pancreatitis. World J Surg. 1985;9:972–9.
376. Keighley MRB, Drysdale RB, Quoraiski AH, et al. Antibiotic treatment of biliary sepsis. Surg Clin North Am. 1975;55:1379–90.
377. Crass RA, Meyer AA, Jeffrey RB, et al. Pancreatic abscess: Impact of computerized tomography on early diagnosis and surgery. Am J Surg. 1985;150:127–31.
378. Williford ME, Foster WL Jr, Halversen RA, et al. Pancreatic pseudocyst: Comparative evaluation of sonography and computed tomography. Am J Roentgenol. 1983;140:53–7.
379. Bicknell TA, Kohatsu S, Goodwin DA. Use of indium-111 labeled autologus leukocytes in differentiating pancreatic abscess from pseudocyst. Am J Surg. 1981;142:312–6.
380. Tanaka T, Miskin FS, Buozas DJ, et al. Pancreatic uptake of gallium-67 citrate in acute pancreatitis. Appl Radiol. 1978;1:163–5.
381. Paushter DM, Modic MT, Borkowski GP, et al. magnetic resonance: Principles and applications. Med Clin North Am. 1984;68:1393–1421.
382. Weiss HD, Anacker H, Kramann B, et al. The diagnosis of necrotizing pancreatic lesions by means of duodenoscopic pancreatography. Its value for the surgical procedure. Am J Gastroenterol. 1975;64:26–33.
383. Karlson KB, Martia EC, Fankochen EL, et al. Percutaneous drainage of pancreatic pseudocysts and abscesses. Radiology. 1982;142:619–24.
384. Pruett TC, Rotstein OD, Crass J, et al. Percutaneous aspiration and drainage for selected abdominal infections. Surgery. 1984;96:731–7.
385. Ranson JH, Spencer FC. Prevention, diagnosis and treatment of pancreatic abscess. Surgery. 1977;82:99–106.
386. Warshaw AL, Jin G. Improved survival in 45 patients with pancreatic abscess. Ann Surg. 1985;202:408–15.
387. Finch WT, Sawyers JL, Schenker S. A prospective study to determine the efficacy of antibiotics in acute pancreatitis. Ann Surg. 1976;183:667–71.
388. Kusne S, Dummer JS, Singh N, et al. Infections after liver transplantation. An analysis of 101 consecutive cases. Medicine. 1988;67:132–43.
389. Barbour GL, Juniper K Jr. A clinical comparison of amebic and pyogenic abscesses of the liver in sixty-six patients. Am J Med. 1972;53:323–34.
390. Dietrich RB. Experience with liver abscess. Am J Surg. 1984;147:288–91.
391. Ribaudo JM, Ochsner A. Intrahepatic abscesses: Amebic and pyogenic. Am J Surg. 1973;125:570–4.
392. Barnes PF, DeLock KM, Reynolds TN, et al. A comparison of amebic and pyogenic abscess of the liver. Medicine. 1987;66:472–83.
393. Shulman ST, Beem MO. A unique presentation of sickle cell disease. Pyogenic hepatic abscess. Pediatrics. 1971;47:1019–22.
394. Williams JW, Rittenberry A, Dillard R, et al. Liver abscess in newborn: Complications of umbilical vein catheterization. Am J Dis Child. 1973;125:111–3.
395. Gyorffy EJ, Frey CF, Silva J Jr, et al. Pyogenic liver abscess. Diagnostic and therapeutic strategies. Ann Surg. 1987;206:699–705.
396. Sabbaj J, Anaerobes in liver abscess. Rev Infect Dis. 1984;6(Suppl 1):152–5.
397. Rubin RH, Swartz MN, Malt R. Hepatic abscess: Changes in clinical, bacteriologic and therapeutic aspects. Am J Med. 1974;57:601–10.
398. McDonald MI, Corey GR, Gallis HA, et al. Single and multiple pyogenic liver abscesses. Medicine. 1984;63:291–302.
399. Sabbaj J, Sutter VL, Finegold SM. Anaerobic pyogenic liver abscess. Ann Intern Med. 1972;77:629–38.
400. Lazarchick J, de Souza E, Silva NA, et al. Pyogenic liver abscess. Mayo Clin Proc. 1973;48:349–55.
401. Perera MR, Kirk A, Noone P. Presentation, diagnosis and management of liver abscess. Lancet. 1980;2:629–32.
402. Loh R, Wallace G, Thong Y. Successful non-surgical management of pyogenic liver abscess. Scand J Infect Dis. 1987;19:137–40.
403. Kaplan SL. Pyogenic liver abscess. In: Feigin RD, Cherry JD, eds. Textbook of Pediatric Infectious Disease. Philadelphia: Saunders; 1981:537–40.
404. Rabson AR, Koornhof HJ, Notman J, et al. Hepatosplenic abscesses due to *Yersinia enterocolitica*. Br Med J. 1972;4:341.
405. Haron E, Feld R, Tuffnell P, et al. Hepatitic candidiasis: An increasing problem in immunocompromised patients. Am J Med. 1987;83:17–26.
406. Thaler M, Pastakia B, Shawker T, et al. Hepatic candidiasis in cancer patients: The evolving picture of the syndrome. Ann Intern Med. 1988;108:88–100.
407. Wallack MK, Brown AS, Austrian R, et al. Pyogenic liver abscess secondary to asymptomatic sigmoid diverticulitis. Ann Surg. 1976;184:241–3.
408. Sparberg M, Gottschalk A, Kirsner JB. Liver abscess complicating regional enteritis: Report of two cases. Gastroenterology. 1965;49:548–51.
409. Lee JF, Block GE. The changing clinical pattern of hepatic abscesses. Arch Surg. 1972;104:465–70.
410. Miedema BW, Dineen P. The diagnosis and treatment of pyogenic liver abscesses. Ann Surg. 1984;200:328–35.
411. Williams RA, Finegold SM. Pyogenic and amebic liver abscess and splenic abscess. In: Wilson SE, Finegold SM, Williams RA, eds. Intra-Abdominal Infection. New York: McGraw-Hill; 1982:139–56.
412. Weinstein L. Bacterial hepatitis: A case report on an unrecognized cause of fever of unknown origin. N Engl J Med. 1978;299:1052–4.
413. Foster SC, Schneider B, Seaman WB. Gas-containing pyogenic intra-hepatic abscesses. Radiology. 1970;94:613–8.
414. Stenson WF, Eckert T. Pyogenic liver abscess. Arch Intern Med. 1983;143:126–8.
415. Madayag MA, LeFleur RS, Braunstein P, et al. Radiology of hepatic abscesses. NY State J Med. 1975;75:1417–23.
416. Reynolds TB. Medical treatment of pyogenic liver abscesses. Ann Intern Med. 1982;96:373–4.
417. Callen PW. Computed tomographic evaluation of abdominal and pelvic abscesses. Radiology. 1979;131:171–5.
418. Koehler PR, Moss AA, Diagnosis of intraabdominal and pelvic abscesses by computerized tomography. JAMA. 1980;244:49–52.
419. Gerzof SG, Johnson WC, Robbins AH, et al. Intrahepatic pyogenic abscesses: Treatment by percutaneous drainage. Am J Surg. 1985;149:487–94.
420. Altemeier WA, Schowenserdt CG, Whiteby DH. Abscesses of the liver: Surgical consideration. Arch Surg. 1970;101:258–66.
421. DeBakey ME, Jordan GL Jr. Hepatic abscesses, both intra- and extra-hepatic. Surg Clin North Am. 1977;57:325–37.
422. Attar B, Levendoglu H, Cuasay N. CT-guided percutaneous aspiration and catheter drainage of pyogenic liver abscesses. Am J Gastroenterol. 1986;81:550–5.
423. McCorkell SJ, Niles NC. Pyogenic liver abscess: Another look at medical management. Lancet. 1985;1:803–6.
424. Drugs for parasitic infections. Med Let. 1988;30:15–24.
425. Nelken N, Isnatius J, Skinner M, et al. Changing clinical spectrum of splenic abscess. A multicenter study and review of the literature. Am J Surg. 1987;154:27–34.
426. Gadacz T, Way LW, Dunphy JE. Changing clinical spectrum of splenic abscess. Am J Surg. 1974;128:182–7.
427. Chun CH, Raff MJ, Contreras L, et al. Splenic abscess. Medicine. 1980;59:50–63.
428. Linos DA, Nagorney DM, McIlrath DC. Splenic abscess: The importance of early diagnosis. Mayo Clin Proc. 1983;58:261–4.
429. Grant E, Mertens MA, Mascatello VJ. Splenic abscess: Comparison of four imaging methods. AJR. 1979;132:465–6.
430. Pawar S, Kay CJ, Gonzalez R, et al. Sonography of splenic abscess. AJR. 1982;138:259–62.
431. Sarr MG, Zuidema GD. Splenic abscess: Presentation, diagnosis and treatment. Surgery. 1982;92:480–5.
432. Quinn SF, von Sonnenberg E, Casola G, et al. Interventional radiology in the spleen. Radiology. 1986;161:289–91.
433. Byrne RV. Localized perforated diverticulitis. Arch Surg. 1964;88:552–5.
434. Lozon AA, Duff JH. Acute perforation of the colon. Can J Surg. 1976;19:48–51.
435. Rodkey GV, Welch CE. Colonic diverticular disease with surgical treatment. A study of 338 cases. Surg Clin North Am. 1974;54:655–74.
436. Tugwell P, Southcott D, Walmesley P. Free perforation of the colon in Crohn's disease. Br J Clin Pract. 1972;26:44–5.
437. Prolla JC, Kirsner JB. The gastrointestinal lesions and complications of the leukemias. Ann Intern Med. 1964;61:1084–1103.

438. Pokorney BH, Jones JM, Skaikh BS, et al. Typhlitis: A treatable cause of recurrent septicemia. JAMA. 1980;243:682–3.
439. Mulholland MW, Delaney JP. Neutropenic colitis and aplastic anemia: A new association. Ann Surg. 1983;197:84–90.
440. Archibald RG. Nelson JA. Necrotizing enterocolitis in acute leukemia: Radiographic findings. Gastrointest Radiol. 1987;3:63–5.
441. Alt B, Glass NR, Sallinger H. Neutropenic enterocolitis in adults: Review of the literature and assessment of surgical intervention. Am J Surg. 1985;149:405–8.
442. Shaked A, Shinar E, Freund H. Neutropenic typhlitis: A plea for conservatism. Dis Colon Rectum. 1983;26:351–2.
443. Varki AP, Armitage JO, Feagler JR. Typhlitis in acute leukemias: Successful treatment by early surgical intervention. Cancer. 1979;43:695–7.
444. Berk JE, Zinbers SS. Acute Cholecystitis: Medical Aspects. In: Berk JE, Haubrich WS, Kalser MH, et al, eds. 4th ed. Gastroenterology. Philadelphia: WB Saunders; 1985;6:3597–3616.
445. Bailey HA, Thrush LB. Consideration of acute cholecystitis: An analysis of seventy-six cases. Am J Surg. 1951;82:328–33.
446. Schein CJ. Acute Cholecystitis. New York: Harper & Row; 1972:63–5.
447. Truedson H, Elmros T, Holm S. The incidence of bacteria in gallbladder bile at acute and elective cholecystectomy. Acta Chir Scand. 1983;149:307–13.
448. Pitt HA, Postier RG, Cameron JC. Biliary bacteria: Significance and alteration after antibiotic therapy. Arch Surg. 1982;117:445–9.
449. Finegold S. Anaerobes in biliary tract infection. Arch Intern Med. 1979;139:1338–9.
450. Bourgalt AM, England DM, Rosenblatt JE, et al. Clinical characteristics of anaerobic bactibilia. Arch Intern Med. 1979;139:1346–9.
451. Samuels BI, Freitas JE, Bree RL, et al. A comparison of radionuclide hepatobiliary imaging and real-time ultrasound for the detection of acute cholecystitis. Radiology. 1983;147:207–10.
452. Gill PT, Dillon E, Leahy AL, et al. Ultrasonography, HIDA scintigraphy or both in the diagnosis of acute cholecystitis? Br J Surg. 1985;72:267–8.
453. Johnson DG, Coleman RE. New techniques in radionuclide imaging of the alimentary system. Radiol Clin North Am. 1982;20:635–51.
454. Kane RA, Costello P, Duszlak E. Computed tomography in acute cholecystitis: New observations. AJR. 1983;141:697–701.
455. McCarthy S, Hricak H, Cohen M, et al. Cholecystitis: Detection with MR imaging. Radiology. 1986;158:333–6.
456. Mentzer RM, Golden CT, Chandler JG, et al. A comparative appraisal of emphysematous cholecystitis. Am J Surg. 1975;125:10–5.
457. Kune GA, Burdon JGW. Are antibiotics necessary in acute cholecystitis? Med J Aust. 1975;2:627–30.
458. Hirschmann JV, Inui TS. Antimicrobial prophylaxis: A critique of recent trials. Rev Infect Dis. 1980;2:1–23.
459. Bulow S, Dronberg O, Lung-Kristenson K. Reappraisal of surgery for suppurative cholecystitis. Arch Surg. 1977;112:282–4.
460. Moore EE, Kelly GL, Driver T, et al. Reassessment of simple cholecystostomy. Arch Surg. 1979;114:515–8.
461. Naitove A. When cholecystectomy? Hosp Pract. 1978;13:121–8.
462. Jarvinen HJ, Hastbacka J. Early cholecystectomy for acute cholecystitis: A prospective randomized study. Ann Surg. 1980;191:501–5.
463. Morrow DJ, Thompson J, Wilson SE. Acute cholecystitis in the elderly: A surgical emergency. Arch Surg. 1979;113:1149–52.
464. Thompson JE Jr, Tompkins RK, Longmire WP Jr. Factors in the management of acute cholangitis. Ann Surg. 1982;117:437–44.
465. Bilboa MK, Dotter CT, Lee TG, et al. Complications of endoscopic retrograde cholangiopancreatography. A study of 10,000 cases. Gastroenterology. 1976;70:314–20.
466. Hinshaw DB. Acute obstructive cholangitis. Surg Clin North Am. 1973;53:1089–94.
467. Ralls PW, Colletti PM, Halls JM, et al. Prospective evaluation of ^{99m}TC-IDA cholescintigraphy and gray-scale ultrasound in the diagnosis of acute cholecystitis. Radiology. 1982;144:369–71.
468. Welch JP, Donaldson G. The urgency of diagnosis and surgical treatment of suppurative cholangitis. Am J Surg. 1976;131:527–32.

SECTION G. CARDIOVASCULAR INFECTIONS

61. ENDOCARDITIS AND INTRAVASCULAR INFECTIONS

W. MICHAEL SCHELD
MERLE A. SANDE

INFECTIVE ENDOCARDITIS

The term *infective endocarditis* (IE) denotes infection of the endocardial surface of the heart and implies the physical presence of microorganisms in the lesion. Although the heart valves are most commonly affected, the disease may also occur on septal defects or on the mural endocardium. Infection of arteriovenous shunts, arterioarterial shunts (patent ductus arteriosus), and coarctation of the aorta are also included under this heading since the clinical manifestations are similar. The term *infective endocarditis,* first used by Thayer in the Gibson lectures of 1930 and later popularized by Lerner and Weinstein,[1,2] is preferable to the old term *bacterial endocarditis* since chlamydiae, rickettsiae, fungi, and perhaps even viruses may be responsible for the syndrome.

In the past, the disease has been classified as "acute" or "subacute." This was based on the usual progression of the untreated disease and is mainly of historic interest. The acute form follows a fulminant course, usually with high fever, systemic toxicity, and leukocytosis, with death occurring in several days to less than 6 weeks. It is classically associated with infection caused by *Staphylococcus aureus, Streptococcus pyogenes, Streptococcus pneumoniae,* and *Neisseria gonorhoeae.* The subacute (death in 6 weeks to 3 months) and "chronic" (death in greater than 3 months) forms are usually considered together. They commonly occur in the setting of prior valvular disease and are characterized by a slow, indolent course with a low-grade fever, night sweats, weight loss, and vague systemic complaints. This form of the disease is classically caused by the viridans streptococci. Although useful conceptually, this classification ignores the nonbacterial forms of IE and the frequent overlap in manifestations by individual organisms such as the enterococci. A classification based on the etiologic agent responsible is preferable since it has implications for the course usually followed, the likelihood of pre-existing heart disease, and the appropriate antimicrobial agent(s) to employ.

Although relatively uncommon, IE has received considerable attention by both clinicians and scientists for the past century. The clinical manifestations of the disease are so varied that they may be encountered in any of the medical subspecialities. Successful management is dependent on the close cooperation of medical and surgical disciplines. This collaboration has markedly improved the outlook of a disease that was universally fatal 45 years ago. The disease has attracted considerable investigative interest. Although the factors that influence its development are now more clearly identified, many questions remain about the unique aspects of this infection. For example, (*1*) why do organisms lodge specifically on the cardiac valves rather than elsewhere in the vascular tree; (*2*) what enables the microorganisms to survive on the valve surface after colonization; (*3*) why do only a relatively small number of strains of bacteria produce the vast majority of cases of endocarditis, while many others produce only bacteremia; (*4*) what factors are responsible for the marked variations in the manifestation of the disease; and (*5*) why is the infection so difficult to eradicate with antibiotics even though the infecting organisms are often exquisitely sensitive to the drugs in vitro? These questions will be discussed in detail in the following sections.

Epidemiology

The incidence of IE is difficult to determine since the criteria for diagnosis and the methods of reporting vary with different series.[3] An analysis based on strict case definitions often reveals that only a small proportion (≈20 percent) of clinically diagnosed cases are categorized as definite. Nevertheless, IE accounted for approximately 1 case/1000 hospital admissions with a range of 0.16–5.4 cases/1000 admissions in a review of 10 large surveys.[3,4] This incidence has not changed in the past 30 years.[5] The mean annual incidence was 3.8/100,000 person-years in Olmstead County, Minnesota, from 1950 to 1981 with no significant change during this interval.[6] A similar figure of 1.7/100,000 person-years was reported from a prospective survey in Louisiana[7] and is analogous to results from the United Kingdom.[8] In an autopsy study[9] there was no change in the yearly number of cases of IE in the United Kingdom from 1939 to 1967. The proportion of acute cases has increased from approximately 20 percent in the pre-antibiotic era to 33 percent.[4,5] Despite these changes in the disease spectrum, IE remains a prevalent disease with a significant mortality in the antibiotic era.[10]

The mean age of patients with IE has gradually increased in the antibiotic era. In 1926, the median age was less than 30 years;[11] this had increased to 39 years by 1943, and currently over 50 percent of the patients are older than 50 years.[5,12,13] At the present time, 54 percent (range, 41–69 percent) of the cases occur in patients aged 31–60, 26 percent (range, 12–40 percent) in patients less than 30 years of age, and 21 percent (range, 8–38 percent) in people older than 60 years.[2] The mean age of patients with IE caused by group D streptococci is even higher: 61–67 years.[14] The disease remains uncommon in children. The mean age for men is 6–7 years older than that for women, and men are more commonly affected (54–69 percent of the cases, the mean male:female ratio is 1.7:1 with a range of 1.2–3.0:1 in 17 large series). In patients under the age of 35, more cases occur in women. A number of factors may relate to this shift in age distribution. First, there has been a change in the substrate of the underlying heart disease due to a decline in the incidence of acute rheumatic fever and rheumatic heart disease countered by the increasing importance of degenerative heart disease in elderly patients. Second, the age of the population has been steadily increasing, and people with rheumatic or congenital heart disease are surviving longer. A new form of the disease (nosocomial endocarditis) secondary to new therapeutic modalities (intravenous catheters, hyperalimentation lines, pacemakers, dialysis shunts, and so forth) has emerged.[3] Of 125 cases of endocarditis recently reviewed in Seattle, 35 were nosocomial in origin (28 percent).[15] Although nosocomial endocarditis accounted for only 14.3 percent of cases in another recent study, 64 percent of patients were over 60 years of age, and mortality was high.[16] It is interesting, however, that the age-adjusted incidence for the most common organisms (viridans streptococci) has not appreciably changed.[17]

The heart valve involved by the infection varies considerably with the proportion of acute cases reported in each series. The distribution ranges from 28 to 45 percent for the mitral valve alone, 5 to 36 percent for the aortic valve alone, and 0 to 35 percent for the aortic and mitral valves combined. The tricuspid valve is rarely involved (0–6 percent), and the pulmonary valve even less (<1 percent).[12,14,15,18] Both right- and left-sided disease is present in 0–4 percent.[2] Involvement of the aortic valve alone is increasing in frequency and correlates with the increase in acute cases; the incidence was 5 percent in 1938 and rose to 39 percent by 1978.[12] The aortic valve is involved in 61 percent of the male cases but in only 31 percent of the female cases.[15]

Almost any type of structural heart disease may predispose to IE, especially when the defect results in turbulence of blood flow. Rheumatic heart disease has been the underlying lesion in 37–76 percent of the infections in the past, and the mitral valve is involved in more than 85 percent of these cases.[4] If the mitral valve is solely involved, women outnumber men by 2:1. The aortic valve is affected in approximately 50 percent of these cases, and if involved alone, men outnumber women by 4:1. Right-sided endocarditis is a rare and accounts for fewer than 10 percent of all cases occurring in patients with rheumatic heart disease. The proportion of cases related to rheumatic heart disease has continued to decline to ≤25 percent in the past two decades.[19]

Congenital heart disease (especially patent ductus arteriosus, ventricular septal defect, coarctation of the aorta, bicuspid aortic valve, tetralogy of Fallot, and pulmonic stenosis) is responsible in 6–24 percent of the cases.[4] Endocarditis is uncommon in the secundum atrial septal defects, probably because this lesion results in a low-pressure shunt with little turbulence. The congenitally bicuspid aortic valve, erroneously attributed to rheumatic carditis in the past,[20] is now recognized as an important condition in elderly patients (especially men), is the underlying lesion in over 20 percent of the cases occurring over the age of 60, and is associated with a poor prognosis despite rapid valve replacement.[21] Marfan's syndrome, when associated with aortic insufficiency, has also been associated with IE.

The "degenerative" cardiac lesions (calcified mitral annulus, calcific nodular lesions secondary to arteriosclerotic cardiovascular disease, post-myocardial infarction thrombus, and so forth) assume the greatest importance in the 30–40 percent of the patients without any demonstrable underlying valvular disease. The actual contribution made by these lesions is unknown, but they occur with an increased incidence in the elderly. In one series, degenerative lesions were present in 50 percent of patients over 60 years old with native valve endocarditis.[22] The contribution of these degenerative cardiac lesions to the development of IE is apparent in an analysis of 148 patients treated in London since 1970.[23,24] The underlying structural cardiac defects were as follows: rheumatic heart disease, 39; congenital defects, 13; and normal or degenerate valves, 65. Similarly, only 31 percent of patients with IE in a recent series[25] had known cardiac disease. Although a calcified mitral annulus is fairly frequent in elderly women, this lesion is rarely complicated by IE (only 3 of 80 in one report).[26] When acute cases of IE are considered separately, over 50 percent have no recognized underlying cardiac disease.

Many other conditions such as luetic heart disease, arterioarterial fistulas, hemodialysis shunts or fistulas, intracardiac pacemaker wires, and intracardiac prostheses may predispose to endocarditis. Prosthetic valve endocarditis is rising in incidence in proportion to other forms of endocarditis and is discussed in Chapter 62. Infective endocarditis also occurs more frequently in seriously ill hospitalized patients who are compromised hosts and who are subjected to invasive intravascular access procedures (intravenous catheters including central venous pressure monitoring lines, hyperalimentation lines, intracardiac pacemaker wires, and so on).[12] Another group with an increased risk of IE are intravenous ("mainlining") drug abusers. (This group will be considered in detail in a later section.)

Although idiopathic hypertrophic subaortic stenosis (IHSS) or asymetric hypertrophy of the interventricular septum has not classically been recognized as a condition leading to bacterial endocarditis, by 1982, 32 such cases had been reported in the literature.[27–29] In seven cases examined histologically the infection was found on the aortic valve in three cases, mitral valve in two, both valves in one, and the subaortic endocardium in one. This distribution is likely related to the associated mitral regurgitation due to the displacement of the anterior leaflet by the abnormal ventricular architecture and by the turbulence of the jet stream affecting the aortic valve distal to the intraventricular obstruction. The age of patients developing endocarditis ranged from 20 to 66 years, and in most cases (70 percent) the disease was produced by viridans streptococci. Approximately 5 percent of patients with IHSS develop IE.[29] Infective endocarditis is more common in the subset of patients with IHSS who have hemodynamically severe forms of the disease manifested by a higher peak systolic pressure gradient and a high prevalence of symptoms. New murmurs develop in 36 percent of patients with IHSS complicated by IE, and this new physical finding correlates with a higher mortality rate.[29]

The association of the mitral prolapse syndrome and endocarditis has also been only recently recognized. Of 87 consecutive cases of IE reported from Stanford University, 10 (11 percent) occurred in patients with well-documented mitral valve prolapse.[30] These 10 cases represented over one-third of the 28 cases in which isolated mitral regurgitation was the predisposing condition. Four additional cases occurred in patients who were not studied by echocardiography or angiography but who had clinical evidence of the mitral prolapse syndrome. Thus, 40–50 percent of the cases of IE associated with isolated insufficient mitral valves probably occurred in patients with the mitral prolapse syndrome. In a recent series[22] of 63 cases of native valve endocarditis diagnosed in Memphis from 1980 to 1984, mitral valve prolapse was the most common underlying lesion (29 percent). In another study,[31] 5 of 58 patients with mitral valve prolapse followed prospectively for 9–22 years developed endocarditis. This syndrome should be suspected in patients with midsystolic clicks with or without a late systolic murmur. The condition is common and has been recognized in 0.5–20 percent of otherwise healthy people, especially young women. It has become apparent that mitral valve prolapse is only one component of a developmental syndrome. This lesion is often associated with a distinct habitus in women,[32] von Willebrand's disease, or ophthalmoplegia. Some of these characteristics may be useful in identifying patients at high risk for IE. It is important to emphasize that all 25 patients who developed IE on a prolapsing mitral valve had a holosystolic murmur, and none had the isolated click without a murmur.[30] The risk of IE appears to be increased in the subset of patients with mitral valve prolapse who exhibit valvular redundancy.[22] Nevertheless, the risk of IE is clearly higher in patients with mitral valve prolapse. In a careful retrospective epidemiologic matched case control analysis, the odds ratio (8.2; 95 percent confidence interval, 2.4–28.4) indicates a substantially higher risk for the development of IE in these patients when compared with controls.[33] It appears that once IE develops in people with mitral valve prolapse, the symptoms and signs are more subtle and the mortality rate less when compared with left-sided IE of other types.[34]

Pathogenesis

In vitro observations and studies in experimental animals have demonstrated that the development of IE most likely requires the simultaneous occurrence of several independent events, each of which may be influenced by a host of separate factors. The valve surface must first be altered to produce a suitable site for bacterial attachment and colonization. Surface changes may be produced by various local and systemic stresses, including blood turbulence. These alterations result in the deposition of platelets and fibrin and in the formation of so-called nonbacterial thrombotic endocarditis (NBTE). Bacteria must then reach this site and adhere to the NBTE to produce colonization. Certain strains appear to have a selective advantage in adhering to platelets and/or fibrin and thus produce the disease with a lower inoculum. After colonization, the surface is rapidly covered with a protective sheath of fibrin and platelets to produce an environment conducive to further bacterial multiplication and vegetation growth. The interaction of these events is depicted in Figure 1. In the following sections, these factors will be considered independently (see Scheld[35] and Freedman[36] for in-depth discussions).

Nonbacterial Thrombotic Endocarditis. Luschka, in 1852, first suggested that endocarditis resulted when septic coronary emboli lodged in the vessels of the cardiac valve.[37] This hypothesis was discarded since cardiac valves are poorly vascularized and only in the proximal portion, which does not coincide with the area of infection.[38–40] It is now clear that the initial colonization occurs on the endothelial surface of the valve. In experimental animals it is nearly impossible to produce IE with intravenous injections of bacteria unless the valvular surface is first damaged or otherwise altered. When a polyethylene catheter is passed across the aortic valve of a rabbit, endocarditis is readily produced with intravenously injected bacteria or fungi.[41,42] Microscopic examination of this early lesion demonstrates the organisms intimately adherent to fibrin–platelet deposits overlying interstitial edema and mild cellular distortion that have formed in areas of valvular trauma.[43] Scanning electron micrographs of the damaged valvular surface confirm the adhesion of microorganisms to these areas of fibrin–platelet deposition early in the disease course.[44] The organisms are rapidly covered by fibrin.[45] Opossums and pigs are the only animals known to develop endocarditis readily without experimentally induced valvular alteration.[46] The stress of captivity is apparently sufficient in these animals to produce subtle valvular changes that lead to both spontaneous endocarditis and a markedly increased susceptibility to the disease after the intravenous injection of bacteria. In other animals and probably in humans, alteration of the valve surface is a prerequisite for bacterial colonization. Angrist first recognized the importance of these deposits as the critical factor in allowing bacterial colonization of

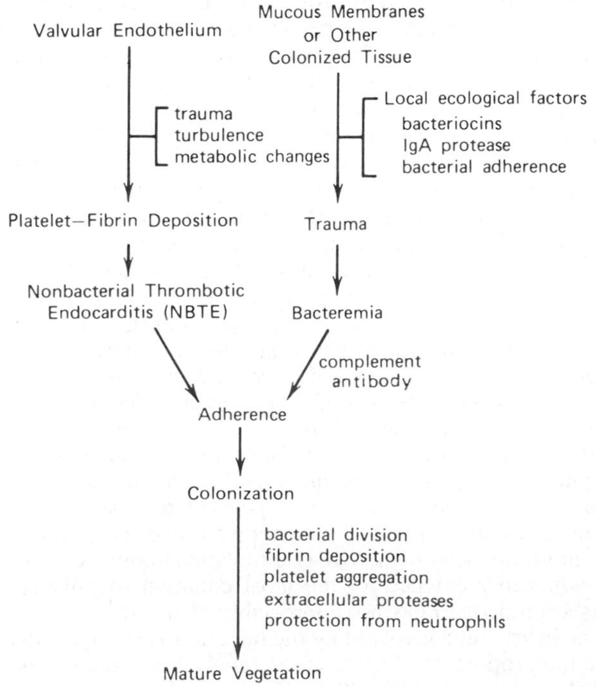

FIG. 1. Proposed scheme for the pathogenesis of infective endocarditis.

valve surfaces and suggested the term *nonbacterial thrombotic endocarditis*. Many forms of exogenous stress produce these lesions experimentally including infection, hypersensitivity states, cold exposure, simulated high altitude, high cardiac output states, cardiac lymphatic obstruction, and hormonal manipulations.[47] These procedures all increase the susceptibility of the animals to IE.

Nonbacterial thrombotic endocarditis has been found in patients with malignancy (particularly pancreatic, gastric, or lung carcinoma) or other chronic wasting diseases, rheumatic or congenital heart disease,[39] uremia, connective tissue diseases such as systemic lupus erythematosus, after the placement of intracardiac catheters (e.g., Swan-Ganz), and even after a self-limited acute illness. In a careful analysis performed in Japan, NBTE was found in 2.4 percent of 3404 autopsies, especially in elderly people with chronic wasting disease.[48] Importantly, NBTE was most frequent on the low-pressure side of the cardiac valves along the line of closure, precisely the site most often involved in IE. Whether this lesion is always essential for the development of endocarditis in humans is unknown.

Hemodynamic Factors. Infective endocarditis characteristically occurs on the atrial surface of the mitral valve and the ventricular surface of the aortic valve when associated with valvular insufficiency. Rodbard[49] showed that this localization is related to a decrease in lateral pressure (presumably with decreased perfusion of the intima) immediately "downstream" from the regurgitant flow. Lesions with high degrees of turbulence (small ventricular septal defect with a jet lesion, valvular stenosis < insufficient valves) readily create conditions that lead to bacterial colonization, whereas defects with a large surface area (large ventricular septal defect), low flow (ostium secundum atrial septal defect), or attenuation of turbulence (chronic congestive heart failure with atrial fibrillation) are rarely implicated in IE. Cures of IE achieved with ligation alone of an arteriovenous fistula or patent ductus arteriosus also stress the importance of hemodynamic factors. A hyperdynamic circulation itself, such as that created after experimentally induced arteriovenous fistulas in dogs or fistulas and shunts in hemodialysis patients, indirectly may lead to IE by producing NBTE.[38]

The degree of mechanical stress exerted on the valve also affects the location of the endocarditis.[50] In 1024 autopsy cases of IE reviewed through 1952, the incidence of valvular lesions was as follows: mitral, 86 percent; aortic, 55 percent; tricuspid, 19.6 percent; and pulmonic, 1.1 percent. This correlates with the pressure resting on the closed valve: 116, 72, 24, and 5 mmHg, respectively.

Transient Bacteremia. In the setting of pre-existent NBTE, transient bacteremia may result in the colonization of these lesions and to the development of IE.[51] Transient bacteremia occurs whenever a mucosal surface heavily colonized with bacteria is traumatized, such as with dental extractions and other dental procedures and gastrointestinal, urologic, and gynecologic procedures[51,52] (Table 1). The degree of bacteremia is proportional to the trauma produced by the procedure and to the number of organisms inhabiting the surface, and the organisms isolated reflect the resident microbial flora. The bacteremia is usually low grade (≤10 colony-forming units [cfu]/ml) and transient; the blood stream is usually sterile in less than 15–30 minutes. It is noteworthy that in two studies where blood cultures were drawn from patients with severe gingival disease before the dental procedure, spontaneous bacteremia was identified in 9–11 percent. Other studies have demonstrated an even higher frequency of spontaneous bacteremia. Of the blood cultured from healthy people, 60–80 percent were positive when filters and anaerobic techniques were used.[53] The degree of bacteremia, however, was low, with only 2–10 cfu/5 ml of blood isolated. "Nonpathogenic" organisms such as *Propionibacterium acnes, Actinomyces viscosus, Staphylococcus epidermidis,* and other *Actinomyces* or streptococcal species were responsible. Frequent episodes of silent bacteremia are also suggested by the identification of circulating humoral antibodies to the resident oral flora and by the noted increase in sensitized peripheral T cells to the flora of dental plaque.

TABLE 1. Incidence of Bacteremia after Various Procedures

Procedure/Manipulation	*Percentage of Positive Blood Cultures*
Dental	
Dental extraction	18–85
Periodontal surgery	32–88
Chewing candy or paraffin	17–51
Tooth brushing	0–26
Oral irrigation device	27–50
Upper airway	
Bronchoscopy (rigid scope)	15
Tonsillectomy	28–38
Nasotracheal suctioning/intubation	16
Gastrointestinal	
Upper GI endoscopy	8–12
Sigmoidoscopy/colonoscopy	0–9.5
Barium enema	11
Percutaneous needle biopsy of liver	3–13
Urologic	
Urethral dilatation	18–33
Urethral catheterization	8
Cystoscopy	0–17
Transurethral prostatic resection	12–46
Obstetric/Gynecologic	
Normal vaginal delivery	0–11
Punch biopsy of the cervix	0
Removal/insertion of an IUD	0

(From Everett et al.,[52] with permission.)

Another factor of critical importance during the transient bacteremia stage is susceptibility of the potential pathogen to complement-mediated bactericidal activity. Only "serum-resistant" gram-negative aerobic bacilli (e.g., *Escherichia coli, Pseudomonas aeruginosa, Serratia marcescens*) reliably produce experimental IE in rabbits,[54,55] and this property is found in all isolates from human cases of IE. Although experimental IE can be induced in rats with "serum-sensitive" *E. coli,* the organisms are eliminated rapidly upon catheter removal.[55]

Microorganism–Nonbacterial Thrombotic Endocarditis Interaction. The ability of certain organisms to adhere to NBTE is a critical early step in the development of endocarditis. Gould et al[56] showed that organisms frequently associated with IE (enterococci, viridans streptococci, *Staphylococcus aureus, S. epidermidis, P. aeruginosa*) adhered more avidly to normal canine aortic leaflets in vitro than did organisms uncommon in IE (*Klebsiella pneumoniae, E. coli*). In addition, *S. aureus* and the viridans streptococci produce IE more readily than does *E. coli* in the rabbit model of IE.[57] This observation correlates with the relative frequency with which these organisms produce the disease in humans. The rarity of IE due to gram-negative aerobic bacilli may also be related to their "serum sensitivity," as above.

Recent studies with an elegant experimental model of IE after dental extraction in rats with periodontitis, which closely resembles the presumed pathogenetic sequence in humans, also suggest an important role for bacterial adhesion to NBTE in the early events. Although viridans streptococci were much more commonly isolated than were group G streptococci in blood cultures obtained 1 minute postextraction, the latter strains caused 83 percent of the IE episodes in this rat model.[58,59] This propensity to cause IE was associated with an increased adhesion of group G streptococci to fibrin–platelet matrices in vitro.[59]

The adherence of oral streptococci to NBTE may depend on

the production of a complex extracellular polysaccharide, dextran. This polymer plays an essential role in the pathogenesis of dental caries by *Streptococcus mutans*.[60] It allows the organism to adhere tightly to the surface of dental enamel. The enhanced ability to adhere to inert surfaces may also be important in IE. In an analysis of 719 cases of streptococcal infections in the United Kingdom, 317 cases of IE were found.[61] The most common etiologic agents were *S. sanguis* (16.4 percent of the cases), previously called "streptococcus SBE," and *S. mutans* (14.2 percent). When a ratio denoting endocarditis to nonendocarditis bacteremia was derived (Table 2), the relative propensity for a particular organism to cause endocarditis could be predicted. The ratios range from 14.2:1 for *S. mutans* to a reversed ratio of 1:32 for *S. pyogenes*. Only the first four organisms listed in Table 2 (all with ratios greater than 3:1) produce extracellular dextran. This suggests that dextran production may also be a virulence factor in the pathogenesis of IE.

The role of dextran in the adherence of oral streptococci to NBTE has also been studied in vitro by using artificial fibrin–platelet matrices (simulating NBTE). The amount of dextran produced by the organism in broth correlated with adherence and was increased by incubating the organism in sucrose (which stimulates dextran production) and was decreased by the addition of dextranase (which removes the dextran from the cell surface). The addition of exogenous dextran to *S. sanguis* grown in sucrose-free media increased adherence. Dextran production also correlated directly with the ability of these organisms to produce endocarditis in vivo in the rabbit model.[62] The strain of *S. sanguis* produced endocarditis less readily when incubated in dextranase than did control strains, and a strain that produced large quantities of dextran produced endocarditis more easily than did a strain that produced relatively small quantities of dextran. Dextran production also increases the adherence of *S. mutans* to traumatized canine aortic valves in vitro,[63] an effect dependent on polymers of higher molecular weight.[64] Thus, dextran formation by oral streptococci may be a virulence factor for the production of IE by these organisms.[65] It is clear, however, that non-dextran-producing streptococci may produce endocarditis in humans and adhere to artificial fibrin–platelet surfaces in vitro,[66] which suggests that other microbial surface characteristics are instrumental for this early event. Whatever the role of the extracellular glycocalyx in microbial adhesion, its presence may retard antimicrobial therapy for streptococcal endocarditis[67] (see below).

A similar important role of adhesion to NBTE in the pathogenesis of IE has also been shown for yeasts. *Candida albicans* adheres readily to NBTE in vitro and produces IE in rabbits more readily than does *C. krusei,* a nonadherent yeast rarely implicated in IE in humans.[68] Although microbial adhesion is a crucial early event in the pathogenesis of IE, the precise intracardiac loci are unknown and may differ among organisms.

TABLE 2. Ratio of Infective Endocarditis Cases to Nonendocarditis Bacteremia for Various Streptococci

Bacteria	*Endocarditis: Nonendocarditis*
S. mutans	14.2:1
S. bovis I	5.9:1
DX + *S. mitior*[a]	3.3:1
S. sanguis	3.0:1
S. mitior	1.8:1
Unclassified "viridans"	1.4:1
Enterococcus faecalis	1:1.2
Miscellaneous streptococci	1:1.3
S. bovis II	1:1.7
S. anginosus	1:2.6
Group G streptococci	1:2.9
Group B streptococci	1:7.4
Group A streptococci	1:32.0

[a] DS +: dextran-positive.
(Modified from Parker et al.,[61] with permission.)

Most organisms probably adhere initially to a constituent of NBTE; some evidence implicates fibronectin as the host receptor within NBTE.[69] Other normal constituents of damaged endothelium or NBTE (e.g., fibrinogen, laminin, type 4 collagen, etc.[70]) may also serve to bind circulating bacteria. Other organisms may bind directly to, or become ingested by endothelial cells as the initial event[71–73]; this sequence appears important in the initiation of IE by *S. aureus* on "normal" cardiac valves. Although the specific microbial surface–host receptor ligand relationship remain obscure, this is an active area of investigation because inhibition of these events may provide novel prophylactic strategies.

The importance of adherence characteristics in the development of endocarditis has also been examined by using preincubation of organisms with antibiotics. Many classes of drugs, after incubation even at subinhibitory concentrations, decrease the adhesion of streptococcal species to fibrin–platelet matrices and damaged canine valves in vitro.[74] Several elegant studies in animal models have verified the significance of this in vitro observation since preincubation of the organism in subinhibitory antibiotic concentrations prevents the development of endocarditis in vivo.[75,76] This has direct relevance to the chemoprophylactic prevention of IE (see Chapter 63). In one study, subinhibitory concentrations of penicillin were found to result in a loss of streptococcal lipoteichoic acid with reduced adhesion to NBTE and an impaired ability to produce IE in vivo.[77] Thus, antibiotics may prevent IE by at least two mechanisms: (*1*) bacterial killing and (*2*) inhibition of adhesion to NBTE.[78]

Since platelets are (with fibrin) the major constituents of NBTE, the role of the platelet in the pathogenesis of endocarditis has also been studied. Some strains of bacteria have been found to be potent stimulators of platelet aggregation and the release reaction.[79] Endocarditis-producing strains of staphylococci and streptococci more actively aggregate platelets than do other bacteria that less frequently produce IE. Platelet–bacterial aggregates have been found in the peripheral blood in patients with bacteremia. The importance of these bacterial–platelet aggregates in the formation of the vegetation or, conversely, in the effect of the aggregation on the rate of removal of organisms from the circulation is unknown. Even small numbers of platelets greatly increased the adherence of oral streptococci to fibrin in vitro.[62] Recent studies[80] have shown that *S. sanguis,* an important cause of IE, aggregates platelets and adheres to these blood components by protease-sensitive components, not dextrans. A platelet receptor for ligands on certain strains of *S. sanguis* was suggested. This platelet aggregation by viridans streptococci, however, requires both direct platelet binding and plasma components.[81] Recent experiments implicate IgG in this specific streptococcal–platelet interaction and suggest that platelet activation is mediated through the platelet surface, 40,000 molecular weight Fc receptor.[82]

Once the colonization of the valve occurs and a critical mass of adherent bacteria develops, the vegetation enlarges by further platelet–fibrin deposition and continued bacterial proliferation. The bacterial colonies are found beneath the surface of the vegetation (variable, depending on the intracardiac location[83]), and infiltration by phagocyte cells is minimal; hence the vegetation creates an environment of impaired host resistance. These conditions allow for unimpaired bacterial growth resulting in extremely high colony counts of 10^9–10^{10} bacteria/g of tissue. Bacteria deep within the fibrin matrix have been shown by autoradiography to reach a state of reduced metabolic activity.[84] Recent studies by Freedman and others suggest that impairment of host defenses (e.g., neutropenia, corticosteroids) potentiates progression of the disease when the tricuspid but not the aortic valve is involved[85,86] but is largely dependent on the intracardiac location of the vegetation.[87] The role of granulocytes within the vegetation is unsettled. When vegetation formation is retarded with anticoagulants in experimental animals with IE, the organisms appear to divide on the surface, total bacterial titers are lower, and the clinical disease is more explosive.[68,69] In addition, it has been suggested that phagocytosis of microorganisms by monocytes on or within the vegetation generates tissue thromboplastin formation that then acts as a stimulant to fibrin deposition and growth of the vegetation.[90] The best evidence, however, suggests that coagulation activation initiated by tissue factor,[91] with subsequent local thrombus formation, is responsible for the initiation of vegetation growth and persistence on the cardiac valve. It appears that some organisms (i.e., *S. aureus*) induce tissue factor production by endothelium without the necessity for host cytokines.[92]

Immunopathologic Factors. Infective endocarditis causes the stimulation of both humoral and cellular immunity as manifested by hypergammaglobulinemia, splenomegaly, and the presence of macrophages in the peripheral blood. The possibility that preformed antibody increased the likelihood of the development of IE was suggested by the spontaneous occurrence of IE in animals receiving repeated immunizations with live pneumococci.[93] It was suggested that these antibodies produced bacterial agglutination in vivo that increased the chances of valvular colonization. Recent studies in animals have suggested a protective role for circulating antibody. Rabbits preimmunized with heat-killed streptococci plus Freund's adjuvant had a significantly higher median infective dose (ID_{50}) than did nonimmunized controls after aortic valve trauma.[94] Others have found similar results with *S. sanguis, S. mutans,* and *S. pneumoniae*.[95] In other experiments, we demonstrated that antibody directed against cell surface components (including mannan) reduced the adhesion of *Candida albicans* to fibrin and platelets in vitro and endocarditis production in vivo.[96] This effect may be dependent on the infecting organism, however, since antibody to *Staphylococcus epidermidis* and *Staphylococcus aureus* does not prevent the development of endocarditis in immunized animals or result in reduced bacterial concentrations in infected vegetations or kidneys,[97] perhaps due to the inability of immune sera to enhance opsonophagocytosis of staphylococci. Therefore, the role of preformed antibody in the pathogenesis of IE remains unclear. Intravascular agglutination of bacteria may, in fact, decrease the frequency of endocarditis by reducing the actual number of circulating organisms.

Rheumatoid factor (anti-IgG IgM antibody) develops in about 50 percent of patients with IE of greater than 6 weeks' duration.[98] Rheumatoid factors have been found at the time of admission in 24 percent of the patients with acute staphylococcal endocarditis (less than 6 weeks' duration), and the frequency increased to 40 percent if fever persisted for 2 weeks after the initiation of antibiotic therapy.[99] Over two-thirds of the patients became seronegative after 6 weeks of therapy, and two patients with a second episode of acute IE promptly redeveloped positive rheumatoid factors. The titers correlate with the level of hypergammaglobulinemia and decrease with therapy. Rheumatoid factor may play a role in the disease process by blocking IgG opsonic activity (by reacting with the Fc fragment), stimulating phagocytosis, and/or accelerating microvascular damage. Rheumatoid factor (IgM) has not been eluted from the immune complex glomerulonephritis associated with IE.[100] Antinuclear antibodies also occur in IE and may contribute to the musculoskeletal manifestations, low-grade fever, or pleuritic pain.[101]

Infective endocarditis, like malaria, schistosomiasis, syphilis, kala-azar, and leprosy, is associated with a constant intravascular antigenic challenge; therefore, the development of several classes of circulating antibody is not unexpected. Opsonic (IgG), agglutinating (IgG, IgM), and complement-fixing (IgG, IgM) antibodies, cryoglobulins (IgG, IgM, IgA, C3, fibrinogen), and macroglobulins have all been described in IE.[102,103] By using the sensitive Raji cell or Clq deviation techniques, circulating immune complexes have been found in high titer in virtually all patients with IE.[104] Circulating immune complexes are found with increased frequency in connection with a long duration of illness, extravalvular manifestations, hypocomplementemia, and right-sided IE. Levels fall and become undetectable with successful therapy. Patients with IE and circulating immune complexes may develop a diffuse glomerulonephritis that is analogous to the nephritis seen with infected ventriculoatrial shunts.[105] Immune complexes plus complement are deposited subepithelially along the glomerular basement membrane to form a "lumpy-bumpy" pattern. Immunoglobulin eluted from these lesions has been shown to cross react with bacterial antigens.[106] In addition, bacterial antigens have actually been demonstrated within circulating immune complexes.[107] Some of the peripheral manifestations of IE, such as Osler nodes, may also result from a deposition of circulating immune complexes. Pathologically these lesions resemble an acute Arthus reaction. However, the finding of positive culture aspirates in Osler nodes[108] suggests that they may in fact be due to septic emboli rather than immune complex deposition. In some diffuse purpuric lesions in IE, immune complex deposits (IgG, IgM, and complement) have been demonstrated in the dermal blood vessels by immunofluorescence.[109] Quantitative determinations of serum immune complex concentrations are useful in gauging the response to therapy. Effective treatment leads to a prompt decrease, with eventual disappearance of circulating immune complexes.[110] Conversely, therapeutic failures or relapses are characterized by rising titers or a reappearance of circulating immune complexes.[111]

Pathologic Changes

Heart. The classic vegetation of IE is usually located along the line of closure of a valve leaflet on the atrial surface for atrioventricular valves or the ventricular surface for semilunar valves. Vegetations may be single or multiple, are a few millimeters to several centimeters in size, and vary in color, consistency, and gross appearance. Microscopically, the lesion consists primarily of fibrin, platelet aggregates, and bacterial masses; neutrophils and red blood cells are rare. Destruction of the underlying valve may coexist. With treatment, healing occurs by fibrosis and occasionally calcification. The vegetation in acute cases is larger, softer, and more friable and may be associated with suppuration, more necrosis, and less healing than in subacute cases.[37,112] This infection may lead to perforation of the valve leaflet, rupture of the chordae tendinae, interventricular septum, or papillary muscle. Staphylococcal endocarditis frequently results in valve ring abscesses[113] with fistula formation into areas of the myocardium or pericardial sac. Aneurysms of the valve leaflet or sinus of Valsalva are also common. Valvular stenosis may result from large vegetations. Myocarditis, myocardial infarction, and pericarditis[112,113] are frequently found at autopsy. Myocardial abscesses are found in 20 percent of the autopsy cases and are associated primarily with acute staphylococcal endocarditis with hectic fever, a rapid onset of congestive heart failure, and conduction disturbances. Myocardial infarcts are found in as many as 40–60 percent of the autopsied cases, often without diagnostic changes in the electrocardiogram. Pericarditis is much more common in acute IE.

Embolic phenomena are common in IE. In the pre-antibiotic era, 70–95 percent of the patients had clinically demonstrable embolic events, but this has decreased to 15–35 percent today. Pathologic evidence of embolization is still detected in 45–65 percent of autopsies, most frequently involving the renal, splenic, coronary, or cerebral circulation. Emboli and immune complex deposition contribute to the extracardiac manifestations of IE and may involve virtually any organ system. When large emboli occlude major vessels, fungal endocarditis, marantic endocarditis, or an intracardiac myxoma should be suspected.

Kidney. Three pathologic processes may be found in the kidney in IE: abscess, infarction, or glomerulonephritis. Abscesses are infrequent, but infarctions have been seen in 56 percent of the autopsy cases.[1] The kidney is usually normal in size but may be slightly swollen, and petechiae may be found in the capsule. When renal biopsies are done during active IE, the renal architecture is abnormal in *all* cases,[114] even in the absence of clinical or biochemical evidence of renal disease. "Focal" glomerulonephritis is found in 48–88 percent of the cases but is rare in acute IE. It is a focal, local, and segmental process characterized by endothelial and mesangial proliferation, hemorrhage, neutrophilic infiltration, fibrinoid necrosis, crescent formation, and healing by fibrosis. Diffuse glomerulonephritis is found in 17–80 percent of the cases and consists of generalized cellular hyperplasia in all glomerular tufts. A less common condition called membranoproliferative glomerulonephritis is associated with endocarditis due to *S. epidermidis* and characterized by marked mesangial proliferation and by splitting of the glomerular basement membrane. Renal interstitial cellular infiltration is common.[114]

Of the patients with IE, 10–15 percent will exhibit an immune complex glomerulonephritis similar to that seen in lupus erythematosus.[105,106,110,111] The evidence for immune complex deposition rather than recurrent embolic phenomenon as the primary pathogenic mechanism includes the following:

1. Bacteria are rarely if ever seen in the lesions.
2. Glomerulonephritis occurs with right-sided IE.
3. Glomerulonephritis is rare in acute IE even though large, friable vegetations result in widespread metastatic abscess formation.
4. Immunofluorescent staining with anti-immunoglobulin antibody reveals the typical lumpy-bumpy distribution seen in other forms of immune complex nephritis.
5. In diffuse glomerulonephritis, subepithelial electron-dense deposits are seen by electron microscopy, with IgG, IgM, IgA, and/or complement demonstrated in these deposits by immunofluorescence.
6. Specific antibacterial antibody can be eluted from the lesions.[106]
7. Anti-glomerular basement membrane antibody has been found in a single case of IE with nephritis.
8. The glomerulonephritis is often accompanied by hypocomplementemia and a positive rheumatoid factor in serum.
9. All these abnormalities usually resolve with successful antimicrobial therapy as the concentration of circulating immune complexes declines.

Mycotic Aneurysms. Mycotic aneurysms usually develop during active IE but are occasionally detected months or years after successful treatment. They are more common with viridans streptococcal infections and are found in 10–15 percent of the autopsied cases. They may arise by any of the following mechanisms: (*1*) direct bacterial invasion of the arterial wall with subsequent abscess formation and/or rupture, (*2*) septic or bland embolic occlusion of the vasa vasorum, or (*3*) immune complex deposition with resultant injury to the arterial wall. The aneurysms tend to occur at bifurcation points. They are found in the cerebral vessels (primarily the peripheral branches of the middle cerebral artery), but they also occur in the abdominal aorta, sinus of Valsalva, a ligated patent ductus arteriosus, and the splenic, coronary, pulmonary, and superior mesenteric arteries. Myoctic aneurysms are usually clinically silent until rupture occurs; consequently, their true incidence in active IE is unknown.[115]

Central Nervous System. Cerebral emboli occur in at least one-third of all cases[37] and most commonly affect the middle cerebral artery and its branches. Three percent of the cerebral emboli from all causes are secondary to IE. Cerebral infarction, arteritis, abscesses, mycotic aneurysms, intracerebral or subarachnoid hemorrhage, encephalomalacia, cerebritis, and meningitis have all been reported.[116] True acute purulent meningitis is rare except in pneumococcal endocarditis, but multiple microabscesses (cerebritis) are relatively common in acute staphylococcal endocarditis.

Spleen. Spenic infarctions have been reported in 44 percent of the autopsy cases but are rarely detected clinically.[37] Abscess formation and rupture have been described but are uncommon. Splenic enlargement is common, and virtually all cases are associated with hyperplasia of the lymphoid follicles, an increase in secondary follicles, proliferation of reticuloendothelial cells, and scattered focal necrosis.[112]

Lung. When right-sided IE is present, pulmonary emboli with or without infarction, acute pneumonia, pleural effusion, or empyema are common and are due to septic or bland emboli.

Skin. Petechiae are found in 20–40 percent of the cases (Fig. 2) (see below). Osler nodes microscopically consist of arteriolar intimal proliferation with extension to venules and capillaries and may be accompanied by thrombosis and necrosis. A diffuse perivascular infiltrate consisting of neutrophils and monocytes surrounds the dermal vessels. Immune complexes have been demonstrated in the dermal vessels. Janeway lesions consist of bacteria, neutrophilic infiltration, necrosis, and subcutaneous hemorrhage (Fig. 3). Janeway lesions are due to septic emboli and reveal subcutaneous abscesses on histologic examination.[117]

Eye. "Roth spots" consist microscopically of lymphocytes surrounded by edema and hemorrhage in the nerve fiber layer of the retina (Fig. 4).[118]

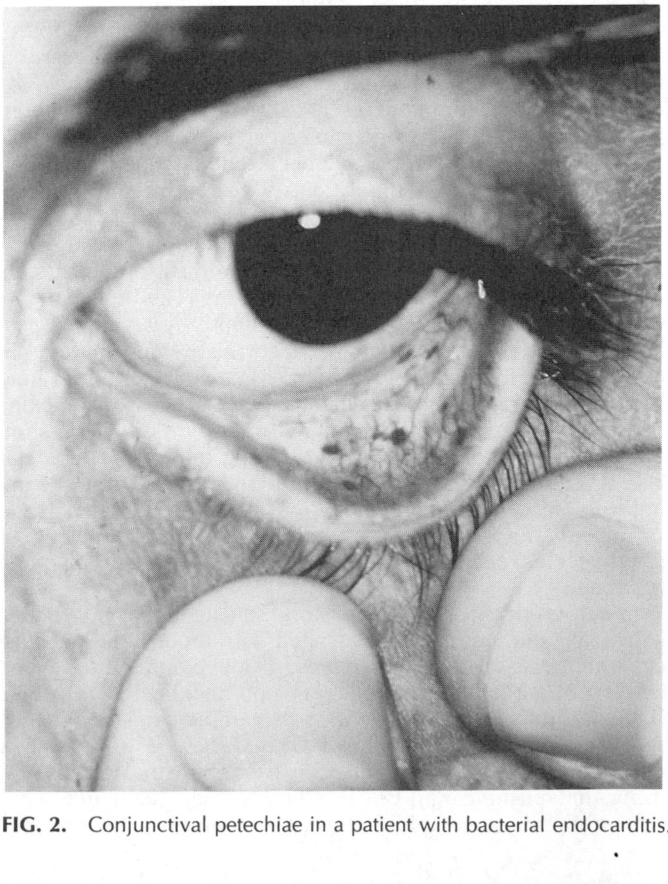

FIG. 2. Conjunctival petechiae in a patient with bacterial endocarditis.

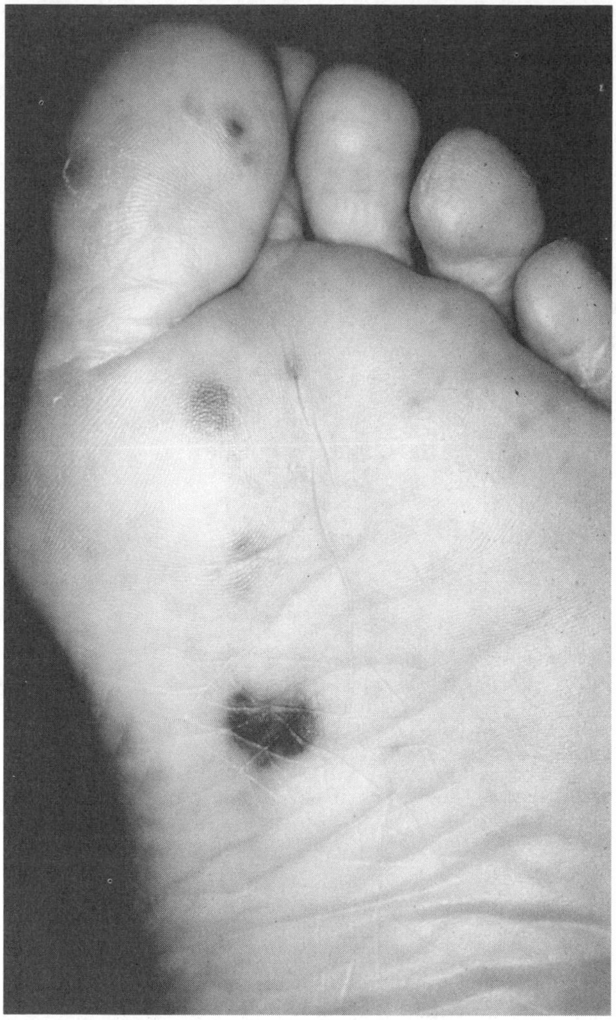

FIG. 3. Janeway lesions in a patient with Staphylococcus aureus endocarditis. (From Hook et al.,[483] with permission.)

Clinical Manifestations

The interval between an event likely to produce bacteremia (e.g., dental extraction) and the onset of symptoms of IE, contrary to older estimates, is actually quite short. The so-called "incubation period" in 84 percent of 76 cases of streptococcal endocarditis was less than 2 weeks.[119] However, the time from the onset of symptoms to diagnosis in the subacute form of IE is quite long, with a median interval of approximately 5 weeks.

The symptoms and signs (Table 3) are protean, and essentially any organ system may be involved. Four processes contribute to the clinical picture[37]: (*1*) the infectious process on the valve including the local intracardiac complications; (*2*) bland or septic embolization to virtually any organ; (*3*) constant bacteremia, often with metastatic foci of infection; and (*4*) circulating immune complexes and other immunopathologic factors.[36,121] As a result, the clinical presentation of patients with IE is highly variable and the differential diagnosis often broad.[122]

Fever is common but may be absent (5 percent of the cases), especially in the setting of congestive heart failure (CHF), renal failure, a terminal disease, old age,[123] or previous antibiotic therapy. The fever pattern is usually remittent, and the patient's temperature rarely exceeds 103°F except in acute IE.[120] Nonspecific symptoms such as anorexia, weight loss, malaise, fatigue, chills, weakness, nausea, vomiting, and night sweats are common, especially in subacute cases.[15] These nonspecific symptoms often result in an incorrect diagnosis of malignancy,

TABLE 3. Clinical Manifestations of Infective Endocarditis

Symptoms	*Percentage*	*Physical Findings*	*Percentage*
Fever	80	Fever	90
Chills	40	Heart murmur	85
Weakness	40	Changing murmur	5–10
Dyspnea	40	New murmur	3–5
Sweats	25	Embolic phenomenon	>50
Anorexia	25	Skin manifestations	18–50
Weight loss	25	Osler nodes	10–23
Malaise	25	Splinter hemorrhages	15
Cough	25	Petechiae	20–40
Skin lesions	20	Janeway lesion	<10
Stroke	20	Splenomegaly	20–57
Nausea/vomiting	20	Septic complications	20
Headache	15	(pneumonia,	
Myalgia/arthralgia	15	meningitis, etc.)	
Edema	15	Mycotic aneurysms	20
Chest pain	15	Clubbing	12–52
Abdominal pain	10–15	Retinal lesion	2–10
Delirium/coma	10	Signs of renal failure	10–15
Hemoptysis	10		
Back pain	10		

(Data from Lerner et al.,[1] Pelletier et al.,[15] Venezio et al.,[25] and Weinstein et al.[120])

collagen vascular disease, tuberculosis, or other chronic diseases.

Heart murmurs occur in over 85 percent of the cases but may be absent with right-sided or mural infection. The classic "changing murmur" and the development of a new murmur (usually aortic insufficiency) are uncommon and occur in 5–10 percent and in 3–5 percent of the cases, respectively. When present, these are diagnostically useful signs and usually complicate acute staphylococcal disease. New or changing murmurs are less common in the elderly and often lead to diagnostic confusion.[123,124] Over 90 percent of patients who demonstrate a new regurgitant murmur will develop CHF. The incidence of CHF appears to be increasing (approximately 25 percent in 1966 and 67 percent in 1972)[15] and is now the leading cause of death in IE. Pericarditis is rare but, when present, is usually accompanied by myocardial abscess formation as a complication of staphylococcal infection.

The classic peripheral manifestations are found in up to one-half of the cases but the prevalence has decreased in recent years. Clubbing is present in 10–20 percent, especially if the disease is of long duration, and may recede with therapy. The complete syndrome of hypertrophic osteoarthropathy is rare. Splinter hemorrhages are linear red to brown streaks in the fingernails or toenails and are commonly found in IE. They are a nonspecific finding and are often seen in the elderly or in people experiencing occupation-related trauma. These lesions are most suggestive of IE when located proximally in the nail bed. Petechiae are found in 20–40 percent of the cases, particularly after a prolonged course, and usually appear in crops on the conjunctivae (Fig. 2), buccal mucosa, palate, and extremities. These lesions are initially red and nonblanching but become brown and barely visible in 2–3 days. Petechiae may result from either local vasculitis or emboli. Osler nodes are small, painful, nodular lesions usually found in the pads of fingers or toes and occasionally in the thenar eminence. They are 2–15 mm in size and are frequently multiple and evanescent, disappearing in hours to days. Osler nodes are rare in acute cases of IE but occur in 10–25 percent of all the cases. They are not specific for IE since they may be seen in systemic lupus erythematosus, marantic endocarditis, hemolytic anemia, and gonococcal infections and in extremities with cannulated radial arteries. Janeway lesions (Fig. 3) are hemorrhagic, macular, painless plaques with a predilection for the palms or soles. They persist for several days and are thought to be embolic in origin and occur with greater frequency in staphylococcal endocarditis. Roth spots (Fig. 4) are oval, pale, retinal lesions surrounded by hemorrhage and are usually located near the optic disk. They occur in less than 5 percent of the cases of IE and may also be found in

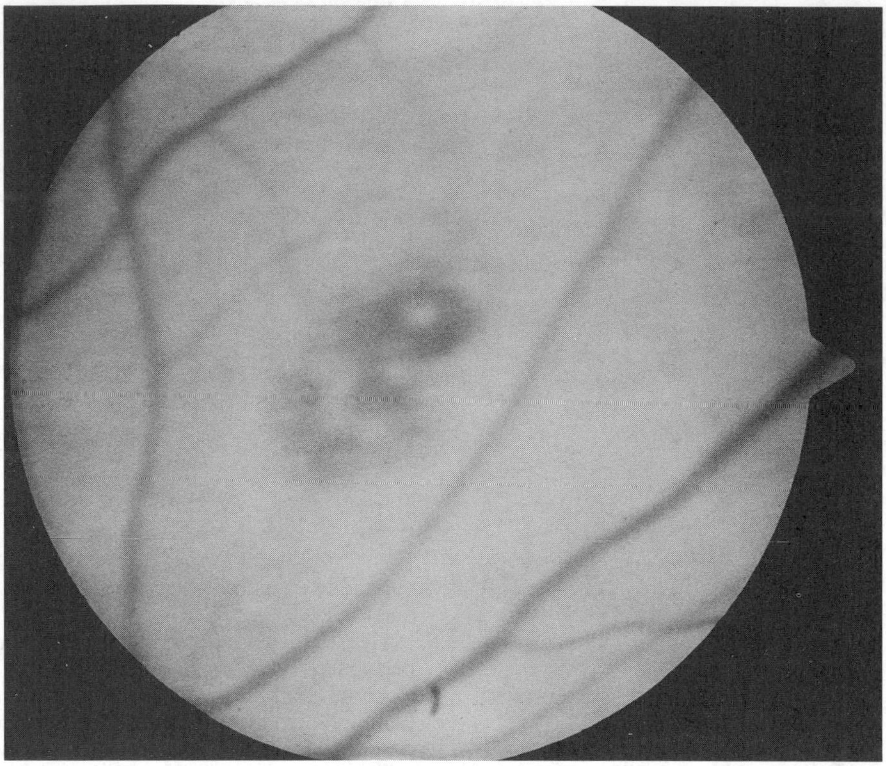

FIG. 4. Retina from a patient with viridans streptococcal endocarditis showing Roth spots. (From Hook et al.,[483] with permission.)

anemia, leukemia, and connective tissue disorders such as systemic lupus erythematosus.

Splenomegaly has been reported in 25–60 percent of all the cases and is more common in patients with endocarditis of prolonged duration. The incidence of splenomegaly appears to be progressively decreasing since the advent of antibiotics.

Musculoskeletal manifestations are common in IE. In a review of 192 cases,[125] 44 percent of the patients had musculoskeletal symptoms. These symptoms usually occur early in the disease and were the only initial complaint in 15 percent of the cases. They included proximal oligo- or monoarticular arthralgias (38 percent), lower extremity mono- or oligoarticular arthritis (31 percent), low back pain (23 percent), and diffuse myalgias (19 percent). These findings may mimic rheumatic disease and result in a diagnostic delay.

Major embolic episodes, as a group, are second only to congestive heart failure as a complication of IE and occur in at least one-third of cases. Splenic artery emboli with infarction may result in left upper quadrant abdominal pain with radiation to the left shoulder, a splenic or pleural rub, or a left pleural effusion. Renal infarctions may be associated with microscopic or gross hematura, but renal failure, hypertension, and edema are uncommon. Retinal artery emboli are rare (fewer than 2 percent of the cases) and may be manifested by a sudden complete loss of vision. A panophthalmitis has been reported with pneumococcal endocarditis. Pulmonary emboli arising from right-sided endocarditis is a common feature in narcotic addicts (see below). Coronary artery emboli usually arise from the aortic valve and may cause myocarditis with arrythmias or myocardial infarction. Major vessel emboli (femoral, brachial, popliteal, or radial arteries) are more frequent in fungal endocarditis.

Neurologic manifestations occur in 20–40 percent of the cases and may dominate the clinical picture, especially in staphylococcal endocarditis. A sudden neurologic event in a young person should suggest IE. Major cerebral emboli afflict 10–30 percent of the patients and may result in hemiplegia, sensory loss, ataxia, aphasia, or an alteration in mental status.[116,126] Mycotic aneurysms of the cerebral circulation occur in 2–10 percent of the cases. They are usually single, small, and peripheral and may lead to devastating subarachnoid hemorrhage. Other features include seizures, severe headache, visual changes, choreoathetoid movements, mononeuropathy, and cranial nerve palsies. A toxic encephalopathy with symptoms ranging from a mild change in personality to frank psychosis may occur, especially in elderly patients.

Patients with IE may have symptoms of uremia. In the preantibiotic era, renal failure developed in 25–35 percent of the cases, but presently fewer than 10 percent are affected. When uremia does develop, diffuse glomerulonephritis with hypocomplementia is usually found, but focal glomerulonephritis has also been implicated. Renal failure is more common with longstanding disease but usually subsides with appropriate antimicrobial treatment alone. IE may be confused with thrombotic thrombocytopenic purpura when neurologic signs, fever, renal failure, anemia, and thrombocytopenia are present.[127]

Infective Endocarditis in Drug Addicts. Acute infection accounts for ≈60 percent of hospital admissions among intravenous drug abusers; IE is implicated in 5–8 percent of these episodes.[128] It has proved difficult to accurately predict the presence of IE in the febrile drug addict,[129] although cocaine use by the intravenous drug user should heighten the suspicion of IE.[130] Cocaine use was strongly associated with the presence of IE in 102 intravenous drug users in San Francisco when analyzed by logistic regression analysis in comparison with febrile addicts from other causes. Although may of the aforementioned clinical manifestations are seen in addicts with endocarditis, several distinctions are worthy of emphasis. In this group of patients, two-thirds have no clinical evidence of underlying heart disease, and there is a predilection for the infection to affect the tricuspid valve. Only 35 percent of addicts ultimately proven to have IE demonstrate heart murmurs on admission.[128] The frequency of valvular involvement is as follows: tricuspid alone or in combination with others, 52.2 percent; aortic alone, 18.5 percent; mitral alone, 10.8 percent; and aortic plus mitral, 12.5 percent.[2] Of these patients with tricuspid valve infection, 30 percent have pleuritic chest pain, pulmonary findings may dominate the clinical picture, and the chest roentgenogram will document abnormalities (infiltrates, effusion, etc.) in 75–85 percent of patients.[131] Roentgenographic evidence of septic pulmonary emboli is eventually present in 87 percent of cases.[132] Signs of tricuspid insufficiency (gallop rhythm, systolic regurgitant murmur louder with inspiration, large V waves, or a pulsatile liver) are present in only one-third of the cases. Most of these patients are 20–40 years old (80 percent), and men predominate 4–6:1. The course of acute staphylococcal endocarditis in the addict tends to be less severe than in nonaddicts.[131] Almost two-thirds of these patients have extravalvular sites of infection that are helpful in the diagnosis.[131–133]

Laboratory Findings

Hematologic parameters are often abnormal in IE, but none are diagnostic. Anemia is nearly always present (70–90 percent of the cases) and has the characteristics of the anemia of chronic disease with normochromic, normocytic indices, a low serum iron concentration, and a low iron-binding capacity. The anemia tends to worsen with the duration of the illness. Thrombocytopenia occurs in 5–15 percent of the cases but is common in neonatal IE. Leukocytosis is present in 20–30 percent of cases but is rare in the subacute variety, whereas counts of 15,000–25,000/mm^3 are not uncommon in acute IE. The differential count is usually normal, but there may be a slight shift to the left. Leukopenia is uncommon (5–15 percent) and, when present, is usually associated with splenomegaly. Large mononuclear cells can be detected in the peripheral blood in approximately 25 percent of the patients, but the yield is higher in blood taken from an earlobe puncture. This finding is nonspecific since similar cells have been found in malaria, typhus, typhoid fever, and tuberculosis.

The erythrocyte sedimentation rate (ESR) is nearly always (90–100 percent) elevated, with a mean value of 57 mm/hr found in one large series.[15] In the absence of renal failure, congestive heart failure, or disseminated intravascular coagulation, a normal ESR is evidence against a diagnosis of IE. Hypergammaglobulinemia is detected in 20–30 percent of the cases and may be accompanied by a plasmacytosis in the bone marrow aspirate. A positive rheumatoid factor is found in 40–50 percent of the cases, especially when the duration of the illness is greater than 6 weeks.[98] Hypocomplementemia (5–15 percent) parallels the incidence of abnormal renal function test results (elevated creatinine level in 5–15 percent). A false-positive Venereal Disease Research Laboratory (VDRL) test is uncommon (0.2 percent).

The urinalysis is frequently abnormal; proteinuria occurs in 50–65 percent of the cases and microscopic hematuria in 30–50 percent. Red cell casts may be seen in as many as 12 percent of the cases[15]; gross hematura, pyuria, white cell casts, and bacteriuria may also be found.

Circulating immune complexes can be detected in most cases of IE but are also found in 32 percent of the patients with septicemia but without endocarditis, in 10 percent of the healthy controls, and in 40 percent of noninfected narcotic addicts.[98] However, levels greater than 100 μg of aggregated human γ-globulin equivalent per milliliter were found only in IE (35 percent of the cases). Detection of high levels of immune complexes may be useful in the diagnosis of right-sided IE in narcotic addicts or in culture-negative cases. In addition, since the levels fall with appropriate treatment, serial measurement of immune complexes may assist in management of the disease.[110,111] Mixed-type cryoglobulins are detectable in 84–95 percent of the patients with IE but are also a nonspecific finding. Although nonspecific and virtually always elevated in IE, serial determination of the serum C-reactive protein concentration may be useful to monitor therapy and detect intercurrent complications or infections.[134]

The detection of vegetations by ^{67}Ga myocardial imaging initially appeared to be a useful diagnostic tool. Of 11 patients in one study,[135] 7 had infected vegetations localized by scans including one culture-negative case that was confirmed at autopsy. Further studies are needed to determine the potential value of noninvasive imaging of cardiac vegetations by using a radiolabeled compound, for example, ^{99m}Tc-labeled antibacterial antibody[136] or ^{111}In-labeled platelets[137] because both have shown promise in experimental endocarditis. At present, these techniques must be considered investigational. Radiographic techniques are occasionally useful in the diagnosis or decisions regarding surgical intervention. For example, computed tomography (CT) of the abdomen detected splenic infarcts in 6 of 25 (24 percent) consecutive patients with IE in one series[138]: 2 of 6 were asymptomatic.

The blood culture is the single most important laboratory test performed in a diagnostic work-up of IE. The bacteremia is usually continuous and low grade (80 percent of the cases have less than 100 cfu/ml of blood).[139] In approximately two-thirds of the cases, all the blood cultures drawn will be positive.[15] When bacteremia is present, the first two blood cultures will yield the etiologic agent more than 90 percent of the time. In a review of 206 cases of IE seen over a 15-year period at The New York Hospital,[140] 95 percent of the blood cultures were positive. In streptococcal endocarditis, the first blood culture was positive in 96 percent of cases, and one of the first two cultures was positive in 98 percent. When antibiotics had been administered in the previous 2 weeks, the rate of positive cultures declined from 97 to 91 percent ($p < .02$). The influence of outpatient antibiotic administration on blood culture positivity was more significant in another retrospective analysis;[141] 64 percent of 88 cultures were positive in 17 patients receiving antibiotics before hospitalization vs. 100 percent in 15 patients without antibiotic exposure. In nonstreptococcal endocarditis, the first blood culture was positive in 86 percent of the cases and when two cultures were taken, in 100 percent. Most blood cultures contained only a few organisms; over 50 percent of the cultures contained 1–30 bacteria/ml. Only 17 percent of the cultures yielded more than 100 bacteria/ml. The bacteremia was also constant with little variation in quantitative culture determinations in any individual patient. The sensitivity of blood cultures for the detection of streptococci is particularly susceptible to prior antibiotic therapy and/or the media employed.[142]

On the basis of these studies, the following procedures for culturing blood are recommended. At least three blood culture sets (no more than two bottles per venipuncture) should be obtained in the first 24 hours. More cultures may be necessary if the patient has received antibiotics in the preceding 2 weeks. At least 10 ml of blood (where feasible) should be injected into both trypticase soy (or brain–heart infusion) and thioglycollate broth.[143,144] Trypticase soy bottles should be transiently "vented." Pour plates may be made at the bedside for an estimate of the degree of bacteremia. Supplementation with 15% sucrose (in an attempt to isolate cell wall-deficient forms) or the use of prereduced anaerobic media is unrewarding.[145] The newer commercial media are also effective, but comparative data are few. In general, culture of arterial blood offers no advantage over venous blood. Inspection for macroscopic growth should be performed daily and routine subcultures done on days 1 and 3. The cultures should be held for at least 3 weeks. When gram-positive cocci grow on the initial isolation but fail to grow on subculture, nutritionally variant (thiol-dependent) streptococci should be suspected.[146] In this event, subculture should be onto media supplemented with either 0.05–0.1% L-cysteine or 0.001% pyridoxal phosphate.

Intraleukocytic bacteria have been visualized in peripheral blood in approximately 50 percent of the cases[147] by a simple "monolayer" technique. This may be helpful in culture-negative cases or when patients have been receiving antibiotics.[148]

Ribitol teichoic acids are major constituents of the cell wall of staphylococci. Gel diffusion and counterimmunoelectrophoresis techniques have been used to detect teichoic acid antibodies in the serum of patients suspected of having *Staphylococcus aureus* endocarditis. Teichoic acid antibodies can be detected by counterimmunoelectrophoresis in over 95 percent of the patients,[149] but the rate of false-positive tests may exceed 10 percent. Serial titrations of serum by using the double-agar diffusion technique can be used to detect the low titers found in some healthy people. Antibody titers $\geq$1:4 are indicative of disseminated staphylococcal disease (endocarditis, multiple metastatic abscesses, or hematogenous osteomyelitis). Since these conditions all require prolonged antimicrobial therapy, this test may be of practical value if the results are positive. The value of a negative result is controversial; some authorities suggest that a short course of antimicrobial therapy is justified in this instance,[150] while others find a negative test response helpful only if all clinical signs are indicative of "benign" (i.e., superficial) staphylococcal bacteremia.[151] This issue is unresolved; we view this test as confirmatory of clinical suspicions only. The detection of other circulating staphylococcal antigens (e.g., capsular polysaccharide by enzyme-linked immunosorbent assay [ELISA]) has been documented in experimental animal models of IE,[152] but experience in humans in scant.

Special Diagnostic Tests. These tests are not routinely used (with the exception of echocardiography) in all cases of IE but may be useful in two situations: (*1*) in the diagnostic approach to culture-negative IE and (*2*) in decisions about surgical intervention during active infection.

The incidence of so-called blood culture-negative endocarditis has varied from 2.5 to 31 percent in published series.[153] If the patients have not received previous antibiotic therapy and the blood cultures are obtained as outlined, these cases should represent fewer than 5 percent of the total. Some of the aforementioned tests (rheumatoid factor, teichoic acid antibodies, earlobe histiocytes, monolayer technique for intraleukocytic bacteria) may be helpful in identifying such cases, but other procedures are often necessary. If the patient has received antibiotics, blood cultures in hypertonic media may allow detection of cell wall-defective organisms. Supplementation of media with vitamin B_6 or with cysteine may assist the recovery of nutritionally variant streptococci. The lysis–centrifugation blood culture technique assists in the detection of staphylococci and fungi, but nutritionally variant streptococci do not survive this procedure, and yields of pneumococci and anaerobes are decreased.[155] Routine use of this technique is not indicated, but it may be helpful in suspected culture-negative cases of IE. Since some anaerobes, *Brucella* sp., and members of the HACEK group (see below) are slow-growing organisms, holding cultures for 4 weeks may increase the recovery rate. Cultures of bone marrow or urine may rarely be positive when blood cultures are negative. Serologic studies are necessary for the diagnosis of Q fever, murine typhus,[156] or psittacosis endocarditis. Special culture techniques (e.g., for *Legionella* sp.[157]) are indicated in patients with suspected prosthetic valve endocarditis when initial cultures are "negative" (Chapter 62). Other tests to exclude collagen vascular diseases are usually necessary in patients undergoing evaluation for culture-negative, native-valve IE.[158]

Blood cultures are negative in over 50 percent of the cases of fungal endocarditis.[159] The lysis–centrifugation method of blood culture is also useful in detecting fungi. This disease is increasing in frequency and usually affects narcotic addicts, patients with prosthetic valves, or hospitalized patients receiving antibiotics and/or hyperalimentation. Use of the Castaneda principle (a culture of blood in a bottle containing both agar and liquid broth) has been shown to increase the yield of fungal cultures.[145] Blastospores and pseudohyphae have been found in Wright-stained peripheral blood in at least one case of *Candida*-induced endocarditis.[160] Various serologic procedures have been used in an attempt to substantiate a diagnosis of fungal endocarditis. Tests for the determination of antifungal antibody are poorly standardized, variably sensitive, often nonspecific, and difficult to interpret.[161] In a rabbit moddel of *Candida*-induced endocarditis, both precipitating and agglutinating antibodies were detected after 12 days of active infection, and titers rose progressively until death of the animals.[162] In contrast, animals without endocarditis developed only a transient rise in antibody titers after a single intravenous injection of viable *Candida albicans*. Newer tests for detecting fungal antigen in serum are more promising as indicators of invasive fungal disease. Tests for mannan antigenemia (a constituent of the cell wall of *Candida*) by hemagglutination inhibition, by gas–liquid chromatography, or by the ELISA method[163,164] have been reported as helpful in the diagnosis of disseminated candidiasis. In addition, a reliable radioimmunoassay for the detection of *Aspergillus* antigenemia is currently under investigation. When embolism to major vessels occurs, an embolectomy should be performed, and the material should be examined by both special fungal stains and culture. Identification of the fungus by either technique is diagnostic of fungal endocarditis even when blood cultures are sterile.

The use of echocardiography in the diagnosis of IE was first reported in 1973.[165] To date, echocardiograms have correctly identified vegetations on all valves. Most reports have focused on left-sided disease. The sensitivity and specificity of this technique is uncertain; however, two studies correctly identified 33 of 52 vegetations documented surgically or at autopsy.[166,167] The characteristic finding is a shaggy dense band of irregular echoes in a nonuniform distribution on one or more leaflets with full unrestricted motion of the valve. The smallest vegetation detected was approximately 2 mm, but the acoustic impedance of the mass relative to the surrounding structures is a more important factor than size is in identifying the vegetation. The use of two-dimensional cross-sectional real-time techniques improves the diagnostic accuracy over M-mode methods.[168] If the vegetation is calcified (which may occur early and independent of the healing process), the sensitivity of echocardiography may be increased. Echocardiography has correctly localized vegetations in culture-negative cases. Echocardiography may be of special value in the detection of the large friable vegetations characteristic of fungal endocarditis. However, its use with prosthetic heart valves has been disappointing because of the difficulty in resolution around the prosthetic device. Many reports have appeared[169] that have evaluated the role of echocardiography in the diagnosis and management of suspected IE and were summarized in a cogent analysis.[170] These studies suggest the following: (*1*) variable sensitivity for the detection of vegetations (<50 to >90 percent positive), and therefore a negative study does not exclude IE; (*2*) the echocardiogram is useless in excluding IE; (*3*) false-positive results are extremely rare; (*4*) only technically adequate studies are really valuable, a characteristic heavily dependent on the experience of the person performing the examination; (*5*) echocardiography is extremely valuable in assessing local complications of IE, especially surrounding the aortic valve; (*6*) patients with a "vegetation" identified by echocardiography are at an increased risk for subsequent systemic emboli, congestive heart failure, the need for emergency surgery, and death, especially with aortic valve involvement. This influence on prognosis has hastened earlier surgery in some cases,[171] but this point remains controversial.[172] A positive echocardiogram in a patient with IE should serve as an adjunctive piece of evidence, together with clinical parameters, in indicating surgical intervention. Visualization of vegetations by echocardiography is not sufficient alone to prompt early surgery.[173] Serial echocardiograms often reveal the persistence of vegetations after successful therapy, but sequential studies may be useful in the timing of surgical intervention. Esophageal lead echocardiograms have been especially useful in detecting vegetations. Short-term changes in vegetation size during therapy do not correlate well with clinical outcome.[174] However, a new technique, digital image processing of two-dimensional echocardiograms, may differentiate active from healed lesions.[175] If substantiated, this method may be useful in "culture-negative" cases (particularly with suspected recurrent IE) or when the response to therapy is suboptimal or inconclusive.

In conjunction with the physical examination, phonocardiography, and electrocardiography, the echocardiogram may play an important role in assessing the severity of acute aortic insufficiency in cases of active IE.[176] In this setting, classic physical findings such as a wide pulse pressure and bounding pulses are often absent; however, there is usually a reduction in intensity of the first heart sound and Austin Flint murmurs may be audible. The chest roentgenogram and electrocardiogram may be normal. The degree of mitral valve preclosure (as determined by echocardiography) correlates with the elevation of the left ventricular end-diastolic pressure. If this event occurs before the Q wave on the electrocardiogram, rapid surgical intervention is recommended.

Cardiac catheterization with quantitative blood cultures proximal and distal to suspected sites of infection has been useful in the localization of vegetations in both right-sided and left-sided IE.[177] Multiple specimens from identical sites are necessary since minor fluctuations in bacteremia do occur. However, this technique is potentially dangerous and has been associated with rapid clinical deterioration when used in the setting of acute aortic insufficiency complicated by progressive congestive heart failure.[177] Cardiac catheterization does provide valuable hemodynamic and anatomic information in patients with IE when considering surgical intervention.[133] Properly performed, the procedure is safe as demonstrated by the lack of postcatheterization emboli or hemodynamic deterioration in 35 consecutive patients in one series.[178]

Cineangiography is the definitive procedure in determining the anatomic alterations resulting from the infection. If is of value in determining the degree of aortic regurgitation, in assessing the contribution of left ventricular dysfunction in congestive heart failure, in visualizing ventricular and aortic aneurysms, and in gauging the patency of the coronary arteries. This information may be critically important in determining a surgical approach, especially if multivalvular involvement is documented. The additional information gained from obtaining right- and left-heart pressures with complete cardiac catheterization are not useful in decisions on therapy in acute IE.[177]

Etiologic Agents

Streptococci. A plethora of microorganisms have been implicated in IE, but streptococci and staphylococci account for 80–90 percent of the cases in which identification is made. The most common etiologic agents are outlined in Table 4. The streptococci still cause most of the cases of IE,[25] especially in the community hospital setting. The disease usually runs a classic subacute course with multiple nonspecific symptoms as outlined in Table 3. Over 80 percent of these patients have underlying heart disease. Infective endocarditis in a young woman with isolated mitral valve involvement is almost universally caused by streptococci. Approximately 20 percent of the cases are seen because of embolic phenomena. With modern medical and surgical management, the cure rate should exceed 90 percent in cases of nonenterococcal streptococcal endocarditis, although complications may ensue in more than 30 percent of cases.[179]

TABLE 4. Etiologic Agents in Infective Endocarditis

Agent	*Percentage of Cases*
Streptococci	60–80
Viridans streptococci	30–40
Enterococci	5–18
Other streptococci	15–25
Staphylococci	20–35
Coagulase-positive	10–27
Coagulase-negative	1–3
Gram-negative aerobic bacilli	1.5–13
Fungi	2–4
Miscellaneous bacteria	<5
Mixed infections	1–2
"Culture negative"	<5–24

The nomenclature of the streptococci is confusing, and various authors differ in terminology used. Streptococci of the viridans group (not a true species) are α-hemolytic and usually nontypeable by the Lancefield system. The most common streptococci isolated from cases of endocarditis are *S. sanguis, S. bovis, S. mutans,* and *S. mitior*.[61] In a series of 317 cases of streptococcal endocarditis, the breakdown was as follows: α-hemolytic, 45 percent; nonhemolytic, nongroup D, 21 percent; group D, 25 percent; pyogenic (groups A, B, C, G), 5 percent; miscellaneous, 3 percent; and aerococci, 1.3 percent. The α-hemolytic strains included *S. sanguis* (16.4 percent of all cases of IE), non-dextran-producing *S. mitior* (13.2 percent), dextran-positive *S. mitior* (7.3 percent), and an unclassified group (7.9 percent). Some isolates of *S. sanguis,* formerly called "streptococcus SBE," are in Lancefield group H, however, most are nontypeable. *Streptococcus mutans* (14.2 percent), *S. anginosus* (5.4 percent), and *S. salivarius* (1.3 percent) comprised the nonhemolytic, non-group D strains. Group D organisms included the enterococci (8 percent) and *S. bovis* (17 percent). In another analysis,[180] viridans streptococci caused 58 percent of cases of IE at the New York Hospital from 1970 to 1978. The various responsible species were as follows: *S. mitior,* 31 percent; *S. bovis,* 27 percent; *S. sanguis,* 24 percent; *S. mutans,* 7 percent; vitamin B_6 dependent *S. mitior,* 5 percent; *S. anginosus,* 4 percent; and others, 2 percent—all of which are slightly different from the experience in the United Kingdom. A similar species distribution was observed in 48 patients (with 51 episodes of IE) reported from Washington, D.C.[181] There appears to be no correlation, however, between the clinical outcome and the species involved[179,181] with the exception of nutritionally deficient strains (see below). Viridans streptococci remain the most commonly isolated pathogens in IE cases associated with mitral valve prolapse.[182] The relative role of each species overall is problematic, however, since species designations of identical strains among laboratories are often disparate.[179]

Streptococcus mutans, the etiologic agent in 14.2 percent of the cases in the review of Parker and Ball,[61] is microaerophilic, pleomorphic, and fastidious. Two-thirds of strains will hydrolyze bile-esculin,[183] a test used to identify group D organisms, and thus may be confused with enterococci. Other characteristics of *S. mutans* include the absence of group D antigen (some strains are positive for group E), production of acid from mannitol, a failure to hydrolyze hippurate, and the formation of gelatinous deposits (dextran) in media containing 5% sucrose. This organism may be difficult to isolate and to identify. It often requires over 3 days for primary isolation, grows best on horse blood agar in 5–10% CO_2 on subculture, and is very pleomorphic, resulting in confusion with diphtheroids. *Streptococcus mutans* was first isolated in 1924 by Clark from dental caries lesions of humans and was first reported in 1928 to cause IE.

The central importance of this organism in dental caries has been amply documented.

Streptococcus bovis is a normal inhabitant of the gastrointestinal tract of humans and many animal species. It is important to separate this organism from the other members of group D (the enterococci) because their respective therapeutic approaches are different (see below). Group D organisms are presumptively identified by bile-esculin hydrolysis.[184,185] However, only the enterococci (*E. faecalis* and its varieties *zymogenes* and *liquifaciens, E. faecium, E. durans*) grow in 6.5% NaCl whereas *S. bovis* and *S. equinus* (a very rare cause of IE) are salt sensitive. Seventy-five percent of strains of *S. bovis* are heat tolerant, and they may also grow and produce acid in "*E. faecalis* broth"; therefore, these methods are unreliable for separation.[186] Arginine hydrolysis by enterococci and starch hydrolysis by *S. bovis* are other means for reliable separation. The association of bacteremia due to *S. bovis* with carcinoma of the colon and other lesions of the gastrointestinal tract suggests that colonoscopy and/or a barium enema be performed when this organism is isolated from blood cultures.[187,188]

Enterococci are normal inhabitants of the gastrointestinal tract and occasionally the anterior urethra or mouth. All enterococci are in Lancefield's group D; are catalase-negative and nonmotile; and may exhibit α-, β-, or γ-hemolysis on blood agar. They grow well in sodium azide ("SF broth"), 40% bile, 6.5% NaCl, and 0.1% methylene blue and can survive at 56°C for 30 minutes or at a pH of 9.6.[189] They should be separated from *S. bovis*. The enterococcus group is responsible for 5–18 percent of the cases of IE, and the incidence appears to be increasing,[190] especially in intravenous drug addicts. The disease usually runs a subacute course and affects older (mean age, 59) men after genitourinary manipulation or younger (mean age, 37) women after obstetric procedures. The mean duration of nonspecific symptoms such as malaise, fatigue, anorexia, and weight loss was 140 days in one review. Over 40 percent of the patients have no underlying heart disease although >95 percent develop a heart murmur during the course of the illness. Classic peripheral manifestations are uncommon (fewer than 25 percent of the cases). Bacteriuria with enterococci is a helpful diagnostic clue and was found in 4 of 15 patients[189] in one study. Cure is difficult because of resistance to antibiotics, and a high mortality persists in this disease. With the increasing usage of third-generation cephalosporins and other factors, recent reports[191–193] emphasize an alarming increase in enterococcal bacteremias during the past two decades. Most enterococcal bacteremias are nosocomial in origin, often polymicrobial (42 percent in one large series[193]) and are associated with serious underlying disorders. Factors that suggest IE in patients with enterococcal bacteremia include (*1*) community acquisition, (*2*) pre-existent valvular heart disease, (*3*) a cryptogenic source, and (*4*) the absence of polymicrobial bacteremia.[193] Antibiotic usage patterns, the aging of the population, and more invasive procedures in hospitalized adults all portend a continued increase in serious enterococcal infections, including IE, in the future.

Before 1945, *S. pneumoniae* was responsible for approximately 10 percent of cases of IE, but this has decreased to approximately 1–3 percent currently.[120] The course is usually fulminant and is often (in approximately one-third of cases) associated with perivalvular abscess formation and/or pericarditis. Left-sided involvement is the rule, and there is a predilection for the aortic valve (≈70 percent). Many patients with pneumococcal endocarditis are alcoholics (≈40 percent), and concurrent meningitis is present in ≈70 percent of cases.[194,195] The overall mortality remains at approximately 50 percent, usually due to rapid valvular destruction and hemodynamic compromise.

Nutritionally variant streptococci (usually *S. mitior*) may cause difficulties in isolation and were implicated in 5.4 percent of the cases of streptococcal endocarditis at The New York Hospital.[196] The organisms do not grow on subculture unless L-cysteine or pyridoxal (vitamin B_6) is supplemented. Infective endocarditis due to nutritionally deficient streptococci is virtually always indolent in onset and associated with prior heart disease.[197] Therapy remains difficult because systemic embolization, relapse, and death are not infrequent (17–27 percent of cases). A closely related species, *S. mitis,* although not nutritionally deficient, also causes serious infections, including IE, in adults[198] and has emerged as an important causative agent of IE among drug addicts in some areas (i.e., New York City[199]). Group B streptococci (*S. agalactiae*) are normal inhabitants of the mouth, vagina, and anterior urethra in 5–12 percent of the general population. In 149 patients with group B streptococcal infections, the serotypes isolated were Ia in 46 percent, II in 22 percent, and III in 11 percent.[200] Although long recognized as a cause of bacteremia and meningitis in neonates, serious *S. agalactiae* infections in adults have been emphasized recently.[201] Risk factors for group B streptococcal sepsis and IE in adults include diabetes mellitus, carcinoma, alcoholism, hepatic failure, and intravenous drug use.[201–203] Like *S. bovis,* occasional cases occur in association with villous adenomas of the colon.[204] Over 70 cases of group B streptococcal IE have been reported.[202,203] Underlying heart disease is common, the male-to-female ratio is 1.4:1, the mean age is approximately 54 years, and left-sided involvement predominates. The overall mortality is nearly 50 percent. The organism does not produce fibrinolysin, which may be responsible for the large crumbling vegetations and frequent major systemic emboli. A similar clinical picture with a destructive process, left-sided predominance, frequent complications, and high mortality (≈40 percent) has been observed in the 47 cases of group G streptococcal endocarditis reported in the literature.[205,206]

Streptococcus anginosus is a rare cause of IE (≈6–7 percent of cases) but is unusual among these streptococci in that it has a predilection for suppurative complications including brain, liver, perinephric and other abscesses, cholangitis, peritonitis, and empyema,[207] although evidence for pathogenicity in these infections is circumstantial. Some of these complications occur during IE with this organism and may require surgical attention. Approximately 50 percent of *S. anginosus* strains carry the group F antigen,[208] but most strains are nongroupable, and the nomenclature is confusing,[209] with substantial differences between American and British classification schemes. Although some strains display α- or β-hemolysis, most isolates (≈60 percent) are nonhemolytic. Many previously reported cases of *S. intermedius* or *S. milleri* infections are now considered in the *S. anginosus* group.[209] Infective endocarditis caused by *S. anginosus* may result in "virulent" intracardiac complications (e.g., myocardial abscess, purulent pericarditis) more typical of *S. aureus* infections.[210]

Infective endocarditis due to *Gemella haemolysans* was recognized recently.[211] This organism is now placed in genus V of the family Streptococcaceae. *Gemella* should be suspected if blood cultures reveal a variable morphology (resembling diphtheroids) and an indeterminate Gram stain. The antimicrobial susceptibility of *Gemella* sp. is similar to that of the viridans streptococci.

Staphylococci. Staphylococci cause 20–30 percent of the cases of IE, and 80–90 percent of these are due to coagulase-positive *S. aureus. Staphylococcus aureus* is the causative agent in most cases of acute IE, but only a minority of patients with *S. aureus* bacteremia seen currently have IE.[212,213] The organism attacks normal (no clinically detectable cardiac disease) heart valves in approximately one-third of the patients. The course is frequently fulminant with widespread metastatic infection and results in death in approximately 40 percent of the cases.[214–217]

Myocardial abscesses (with conduction disturbances), purulent pericarditis, and valve ring abscesses are more common in staphylococcal endocarditis than in other forms. Peripheral foci of suppuration (lung, brain, spleen, kidney, and so forth) are common and afflict over 40 percent of these patients.[214,217] These extravascular sites of involvement may offer clues for an early diagnosis, especially in addicts.[131,132] This disease is often unsuspected and therefore not clinically recognized in elderly patients, and mortality rates often exceed 50 percent in patients over 50 years of age, especially when nosocomially acquired.[124,218] The rare entity of neonatal endocarditis is also often caused by *S. aureus*[219]; survival is unusual.

Infective endocarditis in narcotic addicts is often due to *S. aureus,* but the disease tends to be less severe, with mortality rates of 2–6 percent.[131,132] The recent emergence of methicillin-resistant strains (MRSA) in addicts with staphylococcal IE in the Detroit area is disturbing.[128,220] Among 180 bactermic addicts admitted to the Detroit Medical Center in 1 year, 24 percent grew MRSA, and 41 percent of the patients overall had IE. Previous hospitalizations, long-term addiction (particularly in males), and nonprescribed antibiotic use were predictive of MRSA acquisition (odds ratio, 8.6:1[220]).

Staphylococcus epidermidis is an important agent in prosthetic valve endocarditis (see Chapter 62) and in infants with umbilical venous catheters in neonatal intensive care units.[221] Although still rare, recent reports[222–224] have emphasized the importance of coagulase-negative staphylococci in native-valve IE, particularly in patients with mitral valve prolapse.[222] Approximately two-thirds of patients have pre-existent valvular disease. Although indolent in onset, complications of IE were frequent; despite this, medical and/or surgical therapy was usually successful. Separation of IE from uncomplicated bacteremias due to *S. epidermidis* (implicated in ≈50 percent of native-valve coagulase-negative staphylococcal endocarditis) may be difficult, but a solid-phase radioimmunoassay for the detection of IgG antibodies is promising.[225] Extensive laboratory evaluation[226] reveals that most *S. epidermidis* endocarditis isolates are distinct and do not represent common-source outbreaks despite the frequent shift to a small-colony variant by many strains in vivo.[227]

Gram-Negative Bacilli. Gram-negative aerobic bacilli have been reported to cause 1.3–4.8 percent of the cases of IE, but in two reports,[228,229] they accounted for over 10 percent of the cases. In the latter reports, approximately two-thirds of the cases coexisted with or followed serious gram-positive infections. In spite of an increasing incidence of gram-negative bacillary septicemia, IE due to these organisms remains uncommon, but the incidence is increasing. Only 1.7 percent of 452 valvular infections reported in the 1960s were caused by gram-negative organisms vs. 7 percent in more recent series.[230] A total of 56 cases of IE due to gram-negative bacteria were seen at the Mayo Clinic from 1958 to 1975, 35 in the last decade alone.[231] Most cases were due to "fastidious" nonenteric organisms (see below); this group caused 10 percent of the IE cases seen at this institution. Narcotic addicts, prosthetic valve recipients, and patients with cirrhosis[232] appear to be at an increased risk for the development of gram-negative bacillary endocarditis. The duration of illness is usually less than 6 weeks, most patients are aged 40–50 years, and the sex distribution is equal.[233] In gram-negative septicemia, the blood stream is usually cleared readily with appropriate antimicrobial agents. In contrast, in gram-negative bacillary endocarditis persistent bacteremia is common even with high levels of antimicrobial activity. Congestive heart failure is common, and the prognosis is poor. Most series report a mortality approaching 75–83 percent,[15,233] but recent experience indicates a better prognosis[231] with a cure rate of 62 percent in 21 patients infected with aerobic enteric bacilli. A heart murmur noted during an episode of gram-negative sepsis with unexplained anemia or the persistence of positive blood cultures despite adequate antibiotics may indicate endocarditis. In the early postoperative period after prosthetic valve replacement, sustained gram-negative bacillary bacteremia does not necessarily imply IE,[234] and other foci of infection (sternal wound, pneumonia, urinary tract, iv catheters, and so forth) should be carefully sought (see Chapter 62).

Among the Enterobacteriaceae, *Salmonella* sp. were most common in early reports. These organisms have an affinity for abnormal cardiac valves, usually on the left side of the heart.[233,235] Although many serotypes have been implicated, most cases are due to *S. chloraesuis, S. typhimurium,* and *S. enteritidis*. Valvular perforation and/or destruction, atrial thrombi, myocarditis, and pericarditis are common, and the outlook is grave. Salmonellae may also produce endarteritis in aneurysms of major vessels (see below).

In a review of 44 cases of Enterobacteriaceae endocarditis due to species other than *Salmonella,*[233] the following organisms were identified: *E. coli,* 17; *Citrobacter* sp., 1; *Klebsiella-Enterobacter* sp., 9; *Serratia marcescens,* 13; *Proteus* sp., 2; and *Providencia* sp., 2. There were 19 additional cases of endocarditis due to *Serratia marcescens* reported from San Francisco[236]; 17 occurred in narcotic addicts. Two-thirds of these patients had previously normal heart valves, and most of the infections occurred on the aortic and mitral valves. The cases are characterized by large vegetations with near-total occlusion of the valve orifice in the absence of significant underlying valvular destruction. The overall mortality ranges from 68 to 73 percent since a cure of left-sided IE due to the Enterobacteriaceae is uncommon with medical therapy alone. Since 1974, 17 more cases of IE due to *S. marcescens* have been observed in the San Francisco area; 15 occurred in intravenous drug abusers. As above, only 3 of 10 patients with left-sided involvement survived despite antimicrobial combination therapy and high serum bactericidal activity. Valve replacement after ≃7–10 days of antibiotics was recommended for these difficult infections.[237] Approximately a dozen cases of IE due to *Campylobacter fetus* have been reported since the first case in 1955.[238]

The first case of *Pseudomonas*-induced endocarditis was recognized in 1899; over 110 cases have subsequently been reported.[128,220,230,239–241] Most (95 percent) of the patients have abused intravenous drugs.[128,239–241] Males predominate by a ratio of 2.5:1, and the mean age is 30 years. The organism affects normal valves in most cases. Major embolic phenomena and rapidly progressive congestive heart failure are common. Ecthyma gangrenosum, the necrotizing cutaneous lesion characteristic of *Pseudomonas* bacteremia, has occasionally been noted, especially in cases of IE due to *Pseudomonas cepacia*.[242] The disease carries the highest mortality in patients over 30 years of age (73 percent mortality vs. 33 percent in younger patients), when the duration of illness is less than 5 days (raises the mortality from 41 percent to 76 percent), and when there is left-sided cardiac involvement.[240,243] Due to the gloomy outlook and frequent complications,[128] early surgery is recommended by many authorities for *Pseudomonas* endocarditis.[241] Nearly all addicts with *P. aeruginosa* endocarditis in recent reports[128,220,241] have abused pentazocine and tripelennamine ("T's and blues").

Unusual Gram-Negative Bacteria. Endocarditis produced by several other gram-negative species has received recent attention. *Neisseria gonorrhoeae* was responsible for 5–10 percent of the cases of IE before the introduction of penicillin but is now rarely implicated. In the older series, one-half of the patients with gonococcal endocarditis had involvement of the right side of the heart and exhibited the characteristic double quotidian fever pattern. Of the 34 cases of gonococcal endocarditis reported since 1949,[244] 23 occurred in men. Skin manifestations consistent with the gonococcal arthritis–dermatitis syndrome or endocarditis are documented in only 20 percent of cases. Most of the cases of gonococcal endocarditis now follow an indolent course, in contrast to the often fulminant progression in the pre-antibiotic era. Nonpathogenic *Neisseria* sp. (*N. perflava, N. flava, N. pharyngis, N. mucosa, N. sicca, N. flavesceus* and especially *Branhamella [Neisseria] catarrhalis*) are now isolated more frequently in IE than are gonococci, but they usually produce infection on abnormal or prosthetic heart valves.[245,246] *Haemophilus* sp., predominantly *H. paraphrophilus, H. parainfluenzae,* and *H. aphrophilus,* account for 0.8–1.3 percent of all cases of IE.[247–250] This disease usually runs a subacute course and occurs in the setting of pre-existing valvular disease. Emboli to major peripheral arteries were recently found in six of seven cases of *H. parainfluenzae* endocarditis,[247] and major central nervous system complications are relatively frequent.[250] *Haemophilus aphrophilus* produced a similar clinical pattern and has been transmitted from dogs to humans. Single cases of IE due to *H. segnis* and *H. aegyptius* have been reported from Denmark and Israel, respectively.[251,252] A closely related organism, *Actinobaccillus actinomycetemcomitans,* is a rare cause of subacute endocarditis (35 cases reported) with a mortality of 34 percent.[253,254] Infective endocarditis due to *Cardiobacterium hominis*[255] resembles the disease caused by Haemophilus sp.; 26 cases of IE due to this organism were reported by 1983. Only one extravascular infection due to *C. hominis* has been documented (meningitis during IE). At least 28 cases of *Kingella* endocarditis (*K. kingae,* 25; *K. denitrificans,* 2; *K. indologenes,* 1) have been reported.[256] Approximately 50 percent develop complications, including acute stroke in ≈25 percent of cases. A dozen cases of IE due to *Eikenella corrodens* have been reported; intravenous drug use (especially amphetamines) was implicated in five patients.[257] All these organisms (the HACEK group) are fastidious and may require 2–3 weeks for primary isolation. Routine subculturing onto supplemented chocolate agar or incubation in atmospheres of 5–10% CO_2 is necessary for the isolation of these organisms and should be performed in all culture-negative cases of IE. Granular growth in broth is characteristic and should suggest their presence. In addition, the clinical syndrome produced by this group is virtually identical with a subacute course of IE: large friable vegetations, frequent emboli, and the development of congestive heart failure and often eventual valve replacement.[258]

Gram-Positive Bacilli. Infective endocarditis due to various species of corynebacteria (diptheroids) is uncommon and usually occurs on damaged or prosthetic valves,[259] although native-valve infections (e.g., *C. haemolyticum* in an addict) are rarely reported. *Listeria monocytogenes* has been isolated from 44 cases of IE.[260,261] Most cases of IE due to *Listeria* have occurred in patients without any underlying defect in host defenses, although pre-existent heart disease is present in ≈50 percent. The mean age was 51 years and the overall mortality 48 percent.[261] Lactobacilli have also been reported to cause a subacute form of IE and are rare, with only 24 cases reported.[262] Despite an initial response to therapy, relapse of this infection is not unusual (≈40 percent of cases). These organisms also may take several weeks for isolation on blood culture. Over 90 percent of 49 serious infections caused by *Erysipelothrix rhusiopathiae* were characterized as endocarditis.[263] Occupational or vocational animal or fish exposure is a major risk factor, and approximately one-third of patients are alcoholics. Most patients are male, a characteristic erysipeloid skin lesion is present in ≈40 percent of cases, and the organism exhibits significant aortic valve tropsim (involved in 70 percent of patients).[263] The overall mortality was 38 percent. Nearly all cases of *Bacillus* endocarditis involve the tricuspid valve in addicts. *Rothia dentocariosa* is a rare cause of IE (five reported cases) but has led to significant central nervous system complications.[264]

Anaerobic Bacteria. Nonstreptococcal anaerobic bacteria were responsible for 1.3 percent of all the cases of IE in 1970.[265] *Bacteroides fragilis* was the predominant pathogen in a review of 67 cases from the literature.[266] The following organisms were isolated: *B. fragilis,* 35.8 percent; *B. oralis,* 3.0 percent; *B. melaninogenicus,* 3.0 percent; *Fusobacterium necrophorum,* 13.4 percent; *Fusobacterium nucleatum,* 9.0 percent; *Clostridium* sp., 13.4 percent; *Propionibacterium acnes,* 7.5 percent; *Dialister granuliformans,* 1.5 percent; and unidentified, 16.4 percent. Over one-third of the unidentified cases were also thought by the authors to represent *B. fragilis.* Approximately 25 percent of these cases were polymicrobial, usually mixed with anaerobic or microaerophilic streptococci. The portal of entry for *B. fragilis* was most likely the gastrointestinal tract, while *B. oralis, B. melaninogenicus,* or fusobacteria originated from the mouth or upper resiratory tract. Two-thirds of the patients were over 40 years of age and had pre-existing heart disease. The course is usually subacute except for *F. necrophorum,* which characteristically produces a more fulminant disease. These organisms usually cause extensive valve destruction, congestive heart failure, and major systemic emboli (in 60–70 percent of the cases). Thromboembolic episodes are especially common in cases caused by *B. fragilis,* a phenomena that may be related to the heparinase produced by this organism. The mortality in cases of anaerobic endocarditis has ranged from 21 to 46 percent,[266] but one series from California noted no deaths in seven patients with anaerobic or microaerophilic endocarditis,[267] which constituted 10.6 percent of the IE cases seen. This is similar to a 7.7 percent incidence reported by others[3] and suggests that anaerobic endocarditis may be more prevalent now than it was in 1970.[268] Isolation of these organisms may be improved by the newer culture techniques currently in use.

Other Bacteria. Many other genera of bacteria have been described in cases of IE; however, consideration of these organisms separately is beyond the scope of this review. These include *Acinetobacter, Alcaligenes, Bordetella, Flavobacterium, Micrococcus, Moraxella, Paracolon, Streptobacillus, Vibrio,* and *Yersinia. Brucella* sp. continue as important etiologic agents in Spain and in Saudi Arabia where these organisms are responsible for ≈10 percent of IE cases.[269] Aggressive medical therapy with valve replacement is usually necessary for a cure of *Brucella* endocarditis.

Etiology of Infective Endocarditis in Addicts. The organisms responsible for IE in narcotic addicts require separate consideration since the distribution differs from other patients with IE. The frequency of the etiologic agents isolated before 1977 in seven major series were as follows[2]: *S. aureus,* 38 percent; *Pseudomonas aeruginosa,* 14.2 percent; *Candida* sp., 13.8 percent; enterococci, 8.2 percent; viridans streptococci, 6.0 percent; *S. epidermidis*, 1.7 percent; gram-negative aerobic bacilli, 1.7–15 percent; other bacteria, 2.2 percent; mixed infections, 1.3 percent; and culture-negative, 12.9 percent. In addition, there appears to be an unexplained geographic variation in the causal agents of narcotic-associated IE. *Staphylococcus aureus* predominated in New York City, Washington, D.C., Chicago, and Cincinnati; *Pseudomonas aeruginosa* was commonly isolated in Detroit, but methicillin-resistant *S. aureus* now predominates.[128,220] The most recent compilation from Detroit[128] indicates the distribution of causative agents in addicts with IE ($n = 74$) as follows: *S. aureus,* 60.8 percent; streptococci, 16.2 percent; *P. aeruginosa,* 13.5 percent; polymicrobial, 8.1 percent; and *Corynebacterium* JK, 1.4 percent. Although *S. aureus* IE in this population was usually tricuspid, streptococci infected left-sided valves significantly more often than the other pathogens. Biventricular and multiple-valve infections occurred most commonly in *Pseudomonas* endocarditis; all of these addicts abused "T's and blues." There is an increased incidence of enterococcal endocarditis in Cleveland. *Serratia marcescens* was once an important pathogen in San Francisco,[237] but currently *S. aureus* is the most common (≈85 percent) etiologic agent (M. Sande, personal communication). These differences do not correlate with contamination of "street" heroin.[270] The high incidence of staphylococcal endocarditis may be partially explained by an increase in nasal and/or oral carriage of this organism.[271] Heroin usage in the previous week was associated with an *S. aureus* isolation rate of 35 percent from skin, nose, or throat cultures; this declined to 11 percent (not significantly different from controls) if heroin had not been injected in the preceding 2 weeks. This suggests an endogenous source for the infecting organism since *S. aureus* is infrequently (<5 percent) isolated from street heroin or injection paraphernalia. The exact incidence of IE in narcotic addicts is unknown. A conservative estimate is 1.5–2 cases of IE per 1000 addicts at risk per year.[128,272] Moreover, intravenous drug use is the most common risk factor for the development of recurrent native-valve IE; 43 percent of 281 patients surveyed from 1975 to 1986 with this syndrome were addicts.[273]

Fungi. Most of the cases of fungal endocarditis can be grouped into three categories: (*1*) narcotic addicts, (*2*) patients after reconstructive cardiovascular surgery, and (*3*) patients after prolonged intravenous and/or antibiotic therapy. In a review of 24 patients with fungal endocarditis seen at the New York University Medical Center from 1968 to 1973,[159] 11 were heroin addicts, 9 had undergone cardiac surgery, and 5 had other serious illnesses requiring antibiotics or hyperalimentation. Underlying heart disease and a tendency for major systemic embolization were noted in two-thirds of these patients. *Candida parapsilosis* and *C. tropicalis* predominated in the addicts, whereas *C. albicans* and *Aspergillus* sp. caused most cases in nonaddicts. In 23 addicts reviewed, *C. parapsilosis* was responsible in 12 patients (52 percent), and other *Candida* sp. (*C. guillermondii, C. stellatoidea, C. krusei, C. tropicalis*) caused most of the remaining cases. *Candida albicans* was isolated in only 1 of the 23 addicts. In contrast, in 82 patients who developed fungal endocarditis after cardiac surgery, the reported distribution of causative organisms was different. *Candida albicans* and *Aspergillus* sp. each accounted for approximately one-third of the isolates. *Candida parapsilosis* was found in fewer than 10 percent. Fungal endocarditis was documented in 29 patients after prolonged intravenous therapy, and in 17 it developed during the treatment of bacterial endocarditis. One-half of this group of patients was infected with *C. albicans*. The overall cure rate in cases of fungal endocarditis is poor (14.5 percent in cases treated since 1968). The poor prognosis may be due to (*1*) the large bulky vegetations, (*2*) the tendency for fungal invasion of the myocardium, (*3*) widespread systemic septic emboli, (*4*) the poor penetration of antifungal agents into the vegetation,[274] (*5*) the low toxic/therapeutic ratio of the available antifungal agents, and (*6*) the usual lack of fungicidal activity with these compounds. A cure is virtually impossible without surgical intervention (see below). Fatal endocarditis due to *Candida* sp. has also followed Swan-Ganz catheterization.

In a review of 25 cases of *Aspergillus*-induced endocarditis in which cultures were made,[275] the organisms isolated were as follows: *A. fumigatus*, 14; *A. flavus*, 4; *A. niger*, 3; and *A. ustus, A. sydowi, A. terreus,* and *A. glaucus*, 1 each. Only 5 of 34 patients in this series had positive blood cultures, and only 1 patient survived. A few cases, usually fatal, of *Aspergillus* endocarditis after coronary artery bypass surgery have been described. *Aspergillus clavatus* was isolated in one case. Other fungi that have caused IE include *Histoplasma, Blastomyces, Coccidioides, Cryptococcus, Hansenula, Hormodendrum, Mucor, Paecilomyces, Phialophora,* and *Oerskovia*. Fungal endocarditis was unknown before 1945, and the incidence is increasing; currently 1.2–2.6 percent of all cases of IE are due to fungi. Endocarditis has also been caused by higher bacteria such as *Actinomyces, Arachnida, Nocardia,* and *Mycobacterium* species.

Other Microorganisms. Five cases of IE due to *Spirillum minor*, a spirochete, have been reported.[276] This organism is widely distributed in nature, especially in fresh or salt water with organic debris. *Spirillum minor* is the etiologic agent of "rat-bite fever" (sodoku), but rodent transmission was not documented in the cases of endocarditis. Pre-existent heart disease or severe underlying disease (e.g., aplastic anemia) is usually present, although one case occurred in an otherwise healthy person.

Infective endocarditis due to *Coxiella burnetii* (the cause of Q fever) is well documented in the United Kingdom and Australia with over 200 recognized cases and was recently reported in the United States.[277] Ten cases of Q fever endocarditis were recognized in four Dublin teaching hospitals in only 3 years.[278] Q fever is usually a self-limited respiratory illness due to the inhalation of infected aerosols, especially from animal products. The first endocarditis cases were reported in 1959. Males outnumber females by a ratio of 6:1, and 90 percent have pre-existing heart disease. Most cases of IE are chronic with a history of an influenza-like illness occurring 6–12 months previously. Risk factors may include exposure to parturient cats or rabbits. The aortic valve is involved in over 80 percent of the cases. Hematuria is uncommon even though it is frequently observed in acute Q fever. Hepatosplenomegaly and hepatitis, common features in other types of Q fever, are usual in IE caused by this organism. Other important clues are thrombocytopenia (90 percent) and hypergammaglobulinemia. Immune complex-mediated glomerulonephritis develops in ≈25 percent of cases.[278] The rickettsiae were demonstrated histologically in the valve tissue in 62 percent of the cases, and the organism was isolated in 83 percent. The diagnosis is best made serologically; a positive antibody titer by complement fixation to the phase I antigen is indicative of chronic infection, whereas a fourfold rise in titer to the phase II antigen is associated with active current infection. A phase I antibody titer greater than 1:200 is considered virtually diagnostic of Q fever endocarditis. Isolation of *Coxiella burnetii* by inoculation of valve suspensions into a human fetal diploid fibroblast cell line appears to be a promising technique.[279] The prognosis with medical therapy alone is poor, and valve replacement is often necessary for a cure (see below). This agent may also cause endarteritis. A single case of IE due to the causative agent of murine typhus has been reported.[156]

Chlamydia psittaci, the agent of psittacosis, has been implicated in at least 10 well-documented cases of IE.[280] This organism may also cause myocarditis or pericarditis. Most of the cases have been associated with psittacine bird exposure; in one case, chlamydiae were found in the liver of the suspected budgerigar. However, transmission from pet cats has also been proposed. The course is subacute, and the diagnosis is often made retrospectively. Most patients had pre-existing heart disease. A diagnosis can be established with the demonstration of complement-fixing antibodies. Cure usually requires valve replacement and prolonged antibiotic therapy. The mortality in this small group was 40 percent. Two well-documented cases of IE due to *C. trachomatis* have been reported.[281] Microimmunofluorescence tests are necessary for a diagnosis. A single case of IE due to *Mycoplasma pneumoniae* was proposed in a case report, but cultural confirmation was lacking.[282]

The role of viruses in IE is unknown. Experimentally, Coxsackie B virus has been shown to produce valvular and mural endocarditis in mice and cynomologus monkeys.[283] In these studies the viral antigen was demonstrated in the valvular tissue by immunofluorescent techniques. Although the enteroviruses are commonly implicated in cases of myocarditis or pericarditis in humans, there is no proof that viral infections produce IE in the human. Adenoviruses are also capable of producing IE in mice.[284] Persand has described a case of "cytomegalovirus endocarditis," but bacteria were also cultured from a mural lesion.

"Culture-Negative" Endocarditis. As discussed earlier, sterile blood cultures have been noted in 2.5–31 percent of the cases of IE.[153,158,285,286] This may be due to several factors: (*1*) subacute right-sided endocarditis; (*2*) cultures taken toward the end of a chronic course (longer than 3 months); (*3*) if uremia supervenes in a chronic course, a higher percentage of cases may be culture-negative; (*4*) mural endocarditis as in ventricular septal defects, post-myocardial infarction thrombi, or pacemaker wires; (*5*) slow growth of fastidious organisms such as anaerobes, *Haemophilus* sp., *Actinobacillus* sp., *Cardiobacterium* sp., nutritionally variant streptococci, or *Brucella* sp; (*6*) the prior administration of antibiotics[285,286]; (*7*) fungal endocarditis; (*8*) endocarditis caused by obligate intracellular parasites such as rickettsiae, chlamydiae, and perhaps viruses; or (*9*) noninfective endocarditis or an incorrect diagnosis. Attention to the proper collection of blood cultures, serologic tests, and newer diagnostic techniques may reduce the proportion of "culture-negative" cases.

THERAPY FOR INFECTIVE ENDOCARDITIS

The response to antimicrobial therapy for IE is unique among bacterial infections. Although the organisms may be exquisitely sensitive to the antibiotics used, complete eradication takes weeks to achieve, and relapse of disease is not unusual. There are a few possible explanations for these phenomena: (*1*) the infection exists in an area of impaired host resistance and is tightly encased in a fibrin meshwork where the bacterial colonies are free to divide without interference from phagocytic cells, and (*2*) the number of bacteria in these vegetations reaches tremendous population densities (10^9–10^{10} cfu/g). At these high populations, the organisms may exist in a state of reduced metabolic activity and cell division as was suggested by Durack and Beeson in studies of L-alanine incorporation into bacterial cell walls.[84] A similar finding is observed in broth in vitro after 18 hours of incubation. In both situations the bacteria are less susceptible to the bactericidal action of penicillin or other drugs that require cell wall synthesis and division for maximum activity. The relative importance of antimicrobial penetration into vegetations and the response to therapy is unresolved. Although multiple studies have examined antibiotic concentrations in human cardiac valve tissue obtained during surgery,[287] usually in close agreement with concurrent serum concentrations, the relevance of these data to therapy for IE is unknown and has not altered current recommendations. Information on antimicrobial concentration in vegetations, either in experimental models or in humans with IE, is sparse. Agents that are selectively localized in vegetations (vs. normal endocardium), such as porphyrins,[288] may be useful in the diagnosis and/or drug delivery to the site of infection as carriers for other compounds. Studies in animals have confirmed that when vegetation formation is inhibited with anticoagulants the organisms are eradicated more rapidly with penicillin treatment than in control animals with larger vegetations.[88] Furthermore, enzymatic modification of the glycocalyx in the vegetations of experimental streptococcal endocarditis by in vivo dextranase administration facilitates the bactericidal activity of penicillin by more rapid sterilization of the lesion.[289] In contrast, tissue-type plasminogen activator produced a concentration-dependent lysis of fibrin clots or vegetations infected with *S. epidermidis* or *S. sanguis* but did not enhance antimicrobial activity in in vitro models.[290,291]

Certain general principles have been accepted that provide the framework for the current recommendations for treatment of endocarditis. Parenteral antibiotics are recommended over oral drugs because of the importance of sustained antibacterial activity. Erratic absorption makes oral drugs less desirable. Short-term therapy has been associated with relapse of disease, and all current recommendations emphasize extended drug administration. Early studies by the British Medical Research Council[292] first emphasized the necessity for prolonged treatment. Bacteriostatic antibiotics are generally ineffective in the treatment of bacterial endocarditis. Their use has been associated with frequent relapses and/or a failure to control the infection. A symptomatic response to such agents as tetracycline, erythromycin, or in some cases, clindamycin should not be accepted as indicative of successful treatment since once treatment with these agents is discontinued relapse is common. Likewise, antibiotic combinations should produce a rapid bactericidal effect. This is seen with synergistic combinations such as penicillin plus an aminoglycoside against most viridans streptococci or enterococci. In experimental animals it has been shown that the rate of bactericidal action expressed by a drug or combination of drugs in broth is predictive of the relative rate that the organisms will be eradicated from the cardiac vegetations in vivo. Antagonistic combinations such as penicillin plus chloramphenicol, which are less rapidly bactericidal, are less effective in experimental endocarditis than is the single bactericidal drug (penicillin) alone.[293]

Patients with IE may have an associated myocarditis complicated by cardiac arrhythmias and congestive heart failure and require close observation in an intensive care environment with electrocardiographic monitoring. As discussed below, the selection of antibiotics should be based on antimicrobial susceptibility tests and the treatment monitored with periodic determinations of serum bactericidal activity and/or antimicrobial blood levels when indicated. Blood cultures should be obtained during the early phase of therapy to ensure eradication of the bacteremia. The use of anticoagulants during therapy for endocarditis has been associated with fatal subarachnoid hemorrhage and other bleeding complications. Most authorities agree that anticoagulant administration is this setting is contraindicated, but this area remains controversial.

All patients with IE should be managed in facilities with rapid access to cardiothoracic surgery. Although persistent or recurrent fever despite appropriate antimicrobial therapy may be due to pulmonary or systemic emboli or drug hypersensitivity, the most common cause is extensive valve ring or adjacent structure infection.[294] These patients and many others with IE require surgery, often emergently. Close monitoring and early surgical consultation is therefore essential.

Tests Useful for Antimicrobial Treatment Monitoring

Management of IE demands careful considerations of the choice, dose, and duration of antimicrobial therapy. The following laboratory tests can help the physician to monitor treatment and can aid in rational therapeutic decisions. In every case of bacterial endocarditis, the etiologic agent must be isolated in pure culture, and the minimum inhibitory concentration (MIC) and the minimum bactericidal concentration (MBC) must be determined for the usual antibiotics used (see below). Standard disk sensitivity testing is unreliable, and results may be misleading without the quantitative information provided by determining the MICs and MBCs. During therapy the serum can be monitored for bactericidal activity against the offending organism as originally described by Schlicter and MacIlean.[295] The performance of this test varies greatly, and consequently there are disagreements in interpretation. The inoculum size, composition of the broth, timing of samples ("peak" vs. "trough"), methods of dilution and subculture, and criteria for determination of the bactericidal end point are among the important variables. Perhaps because of these problems and the frequent adverse events unrelated to bactericidal effects, the serum bactericidal titer (SBT) often correlates poorly with the clinical outcome in patients with IE. There is still intense disagreement regarding the value of this test in monitoring therapy for IE. A retrospective review[296] of 17 reports published between 1948 and 1980 failed to confirm any correlation between and SBT $\geq$1:8 and therapeutic success.[297] Controversy regarding the usefulness of "peak" vs. "trough" SBTs abounds.[298] When all of these variables are standardized,[299,300] the SBT test may be useful in selected patients with IE. A recent prospective multicenter study[301] evaluated a standardized SBT method in 129 patients with bacterial endocarditis. Peak and trough SBT ratios of ≥1:64 and 1:32 predicted bacteriologic cure in all patients, but specific levels could *not* be used to accurately predict bacteriologic failure or clinical outcome. Although there are problems with this study,[297] recent data[302] support a role for the SBT when standarized and performed in the presence of 50% human serum: all patients with peak SBTs ≥1:32 were cured, whereas 7 of 21 (33 percent) with SBTs ≤1:16 failed treatment.[302] Unless precluded by drug toxicity, it seems reasonable to attempt to achieve this level (1:8–1:16) of activity in patients, although this goal may be unattainable in some forms (e.g., gram-negative bacillary, enterococcal) of IE. Performance of the SBT test is usually unnecessary in patients with viridans streptococcal endocarditis but may be useful when *(1)* the organism is inherently resistant or tolerant to one of the drugs administered or *(2)* the response to therapy is suboptimal.

In some forms of IE, combinations of antibiotics are used routinely.[303] These regimens are based on synergy studies performed in vitro and results obtained in experimental animal models of IE. In difficult cases with a slow therapeutic response or in those due to unusual organisms, a determination of synergistic combinations of antibiotics may be helpful. In these cases, tests for bactericidal synergism may be undertaken by standard techniques such as broth dilution, microtiter "checkerboards," or "time–kill" curves in broth. Proper attention to standardized techniques, especially inoculum size, are critically important for a meaningful interpretation of the results.

When aminoglycosides are used in therapy, the concentration of antibiotic in the serum should be periodically determined. These agents have a low toxic–therapeutic ratio, especially in elderly patients or in those with renal disease. Peak and trough concentrations should be measured, and the dose should be altered accordingly. This method is superior to reliance solely on nomograms for dosage changes. When synergy with another agent is demonstrable, serum concentrations of the aminoglycosides lower than those generally considered "therapeutic" may be adequate, thus lessening the potential for toxicity. Levels can be determined by microbiologic assays using agar well diffusion (±15 percent accuracy), radioimmunoassay, or enzyme assay with equally satisfactory results.

Antimicrobial Therapy

"Penicillin-Sensitive" Streptococcal Endocarditis. Most strains of viridans streptococci, "other" streptococci (including *S. pyogenes*), and nonenterococcal group D streptococci (primarily *S. bovis*) are exquisitely sensitive to penicillins with an MIC of <0.2 μg/ml. However, 15–20 percent of viridans streptococci are "resistant" to this arbitrary concentration of penicillin.[180,196] In addition,[183] approximately 15 percent of the strains of *S. mutans* demonstrate a low MIC to penicillin (<0.1 μg/ml), but the MBC is considerably higher (1.25–50 μg/ml). These organisms should probably be considered "penicillin-tolerant" and should be treated accordingly. Although dependent on the in vitro methodology employed, recent studies suggest that tolerance to penicillin among viridans streptococci is more prevalent than previous reports suggested.[304] For example, 19 percent of viridans streptococci cultured from gingiva and blood after dental procedures were tolerant,[305] especially among *S. mutans* (27 percent) and *S. mitior* (20 percent) isolates. Almost identical figures were reported among blood culture isolates of viridans streptococci,[306] with tolerance defined as a penicillin MBC-to-MIC ratio exceeding 10:1. Nearly all strains of nutritionally dependent streptococci are tolerant to penicillin.[307,308] The influence of the tolerance phenomenon on the response to penicillin therapy in experimental endocarditis is not known; two recent studies yielded conflicting results.[309,310] Data on human infections with tolerant strains and the therapeutic results are unavailable. Except for nutritionally variant streptococci, we do not believe that the demonstration of tolerance by an isolate of viridans streptococci influences therapeutic decisions.

By broth dilution susceptibility tests, the usual MBC for these so-called penicillin-sensitive streptococci is as follows: penicillin, 0.1–1.0 μg/ml; cephalothin, 0.15–1.25 μg/ml; vancomycin, 0.15–0.4 μg/ml; streptomycin, 6.25–50 μg/ml; and gentamicin, 1.56–3.12 μg/ml.[311,312] *Streptococcus bovis* is 10–5000 times more susceptible to penicillin than are the other group D species (enterococci). They are also relatively susceptible to oxacillin, methicillin, and lincomycin, while the enterococci are resistant.[185] Virtually all streptococci in this group demonstrate synergism in vitro between penicillin or vancomycin and streptomycin, gentamicin, or kanamycin[313,314] (see below). The first strains of viridans streptococci with high-level streptomycin resistance (MIC ≥1000 μg/ml) were reported in 1982 from Paris. Although these strains are rare (2–8 percent of isolates in some locales[315]) the documentation of aminoglycoside-modifying enzymes and the lack of penicillin–streptomycin synergy in vitro and in experimental animal models[315,316] is alarming. These penicillin-susceptible strains are killed synergistically by penicillin–gentamicin combinations. Significant antibiotic antagonism has been shown with the combination of clindamycin and gentamicin for *S. mutans*. The in vitro synergism between penicillin and aminoglycosides has been found to correlate with a more rapid rate of eradication of bacteria from cardiac vegetations in vivo in the rabbit endocarditis model[315,317,318] for the common viridans streptococci. All of these studies have been summarized in recent reviews.[179,198,319–321]

The combination of penicillin and streptomycin has been used in over 200 cases at the New York Hospital–Cornell Medical Center since 1959 without a documented relapse.[313] This clinical experience has been confirmed elsewhere,[2] but the overall reported relapse rate is 1.4 percent.[320] This regimen is as follows: aqueous penicillin G, 10–20 million units iv qd, or procaine penicillin G, 1.2 million units im q6h for 4 weeks, combined with streptomycin, 0.5 g im q12h for the first 2 weeks. Studies by Wilson and colleagues at the Mayo Clinic[322,323] demonstrated that a 2-week course of intramuscular procaine penicillin (1.2 million units q6h) and streptomycin (0.5 g q12h) cured ≥99 percent of patients with penicillin-sensitive streptococcal endocarditis. These results are similar to those obtained with therapy consisting of β-lactams alone for a total of 4 weeks[324,325] but significantly better than penicillin alone for 2 weeks; the latter regimen was associated with a 50 percent relapse rate when low doses of penicillin were used and improved to 17 percent with higher penicillin dosages. The 2-week penicillin–streptomycin regimen is the most cost-effective and is the preferred therapy in uncomplicated penicillin-sensitive (MIC ≤0.1 μg/ml) streptococcal endocarditis in young patients. Four weeks of penicillin alone is recommended in patients with impaired renal function or those particularly susceptible to the low risk of streptomycin-induced ototoxicity (the elderly). The "Cornell regimen" of 4 weeks of penicillin plus an initial 2 weeks of streptomycin is recommended in patients with a complicated course, a history of disease exceeding 3 months' duration, or prosthetic valve endocarditis due to these sensitive strains or when susceptibility testing reveals the rare penicillin-resistant streptococci.[326] The preferred regimen for IE due to penicillin-"tolerant" streptococci is unsettled. These concepts have been recently summarized[320,321] and serve as a basis for the recommendations of the American Heart Association on therapy for penicillin-sensitive streptococcal endocarditis.[327] We believe that gentamicin, at a dosage of 1.0 mg/kg (not to exceed 80 mg) im or iv q8h, can be substituted for streptomycin in the aforementioned regimens when combination therapy is deemed advisable. A penicillin–gentamicin regimen is indicated for viridans streptococcal endocarditis if high-level streptomycin resistance is present[315,316] or for strains with a penicillin MIC ≥0.2 and <0.5 μg/ml.[327] Strains with a penicillin MIC >0.5 μg/ml should be treated as for enterococcal endocarditis (see below). Due to the enhanced rate of bacterial killing in animal models[328,329] and the high relapse rates of ≈17 percent,[330] we also believe the "Cornell regimen" should be employed for all patients with IE due to nutritionally variant streptococci. Other regimens for the treatment of this disease (e.g., vancomycin plus rifampin) deserve further study.[330] In the penicillin-allergic patient when a cephalosporin is deemed safe, several regimens are acceptable: cephalothin, 2 g iv q4h, or cefazolin, 1–2 g im or iv q8h for 4 weeks, combined with streptomycin, 0.5 g im q12h, or gentamicin, 1 mg/kg (≤80 mg) im or iv q8h for the initial 2 weeks. Although ceftriazone at a dosage of 2 g daily for 4 weeks has been successfully employed in 49 cases of streptococcal endocarditis (M.P. Glauser, personal communication) and the prolonged half-life of this agent may facilitate outpatient therapy, the first-generation agents are preferred pending further data. When treatment with β-lactams are contraindicated, the regimen of choice is vancomycin, 1 g iv q12h (or 500 mg iv q6h) for 4 weeks; experience with teicoplanin or daptomycin is too preliminary.

"Penicillin-Resistant" Streptococcal Endocarditis (e.g., MIC for penicillin ≥0.5 μg/ml).[327] Infective endocarditis due to the enterococcus is the third most common form of the disease and is the most resistant to therapy. The mortality still approximates 20 percent,[189] and relapses are not uncommon. By broth dilution susceptibility tests, the MIC determinations for most enterococci are as follows: penicillin, 0.4–12.5 μg/ml; ampicillin, <0.4–3.1 μg/ml; cephalothin, 12.5–25 μg/ml; vanomycin, 0.78–3.1 μg/ml; streptomycin, 3.1–>50 μg/ml; and gentamicin, 6.25–25 μg/ml. Ampicillin is approximately twice as active as penicillin by weight. In contrast, the usual MBCs are as follows: penicillin, >6.25 μg/ml (80 percent are >100 μg/ml); cephalothin, >100 μg/ml; streptomycin, >25 μg/ml; vancomycin, >100 μg/ml; and gentamicin, ≤25 μg/ml.[331] *Enteroccus faecium* strains are more resistant to β-lactams than *E. faecalis* strains.[332] Thus, in general these agents are bacteriostatic against the enterococci and should not be administered alone in this disease. This bacteriostatic action of agents known to inhibit cell wall synthesis is due to a defective bacterial autolytic enzyme system.[333,334] As stated before, all β-lactams, including imipenem, are bacteriostatic against enterococci in vitro. However, a new mechanism of penicillin-resistance among *E. faecalis* was described in 1983: plasmid-mediated β-lactamase production. At least two strains have been isolated,[335] both demonstrating, in addition, high-level resistance to all aminoglycosides (see below). β-Lactamase production by *E. faecium* has not been demonstrated to date. Patients with IE due to these strains should receive vancomycin plus an aminoglycoside, although animal experiments with penicillin–β-lactamase inhibitor combinations appear promising.[336]

Cell wall–active antibiotics plus an aminoglycoside are synergistic and produce a bactericidal effect in vitro against most enterococcal strains. Successful treatment of enterococcal endocarditis requires such combinations. Studies in experimental models[337] suggest that "low-dose" streptomycin (peak serum concentrations of 9.1 μg/ml) in combination with penicillin is sufficient to treat streptomycin-susceptible enterococcal endocarditis. "High-level" streptomycin resistance (MIC >2000 μg/ml) is demonstrable in 40 percent of the enterococcal strains. This resistance correlates with an inability to demonstrate in vitro synergism between penicillin and streptomycin.[190,338] These highly resistant strains demonstrate synergism between a penicillin and gentamicin in vitro[339,340] at clinically achievable serum concentrations. Enhanced activity with the penicillin and gentamicin combination was seen in vivo for both streptomycin-resistant and streptomycin-sensitive enterococci in the rabbit model of IE.[341] No differences in results were seen when penicillin was combined with low- vs. high-dose gentamicin (peak serum levels of 3.06 and 8.05 μg/ml, respectively) in the treatment of experimental streptomycin-resistant enterococcal endocarditis.[342] Early reports[343,344] revealed high-level gentamicin resistance among enterococci in up to 14 percent of isolates. This phenomenon has become prevalent in some areas[345,346] among *E. faecalis* strains. Although the strains infrequently cause IE, resistance to multiple aminoglycosides is common. High-level gentamicin (and other aminoglycoside) resistance has been recently documented for clinical isolates of *E. faecium* as well.[347] This resistance mechanism is plasmid mediated through the production of aminoglycoside-modifying enzymes and can be transferred among strains. In addition, penicillin- or vancomycin–aminoglycoside synergy is not apparent against these organisms in vitro. The optimal therapy for IE due to these highly resistant strains has not been established. None of the currently recommended regimens in current use is bactericidal against these isolates, and valve replacement[348] may be necessary for a cure. When these isolates are encountered, all available aminoglycosides must be tested separately because the organism may be susceptible to one while resistent to others. Some isolates are sensitive to quinolones or daptomycin, but these agents have received scant attention in human infections. At this time, we favor long-term therapy (8–12 weeks) with high dosages of penicillin (20–40 million units iv daily in divided doses) or ampicillin (2–3 g iv q4h) for IE due to these multiply aminoglycoside-resistant enterococci, pending further data.

Vancomycin is also bacteriostatic against enterococci and exhibits synergy with the aminoglycosides in vitro. The vancomycin–streptomycin combination synergistically kills 40–80 percent of enterococcal strains, whereas the vancomycin–gentamicin combination demonstrates synergy against 93–98 percent.[349] Vancomycin therapy alone was ineffective in eradicating enterococci from cardiac vegetations in the rabbit model of endocarditis, but the combination of vancomycin plus gentamicin rapidly achieved a bactericidal effect.[341] Vancomycin combined with rifampin has an indifferent effect against enterococci (43/48 strains) in vitro; antagonism is observed rarely.[350] Of some concern, outbreaks of infection due to vancomycin-resistant enterococci have been described recently.[351] The resistance is plasmid mediated (at least for two well-studied strains of *E. faecium*[352]) for glycopeptide antibiotics (e.g., vancomycin and teicoplanin but not LY146032), but the biochemical mechanism is unknown. Enterococci are no longer uniformly susceptible to glycopeptide antibiotics, but the impact of this development on therapy for IE is unclear presently. The cephalosporins are relatively inactive against enterococci, even in combination with an aminoglycoside, and should not be used in this disease. The quinolones (i.e., ciprofloxacin) and daptomycin (LY146032) do not appear promising for the treatment of enterococcal endocarditis.[353,354]

Although controlled trials are lacking, clinical experience would dictate that enterococcal endocarditis be treated with combination antimicrobial therapy for at least 4–6 weeks.[320,321,327] The recommended regimen is as follows: aqueous penicillin G, 20 million units iv qd combined with streptomycin, 0.5 g im q12h, or gentamicin, 1 mg/kg im or iv q8h, for 4–6 weeks. If toxicity (vestibular, aural, or renal) occurs, the streptomycin dose is divided into a q6h regimen. If the streptomycin MIC determined for the infecting strain is ≥2000 μg/ml, gentamicin should be substituted for streptomycin, although relapses or therapeutic failures are unusual with penicillin plus streptomycin. Some authorities recommend penicillin plus gentamicin as the initial therapy. If the peak serum bactericidal level is <1:8, the penicillin dose may be increased, or the aminoglycoside drug may be changed in accordance with in vitro tests. Wilson et al. have recently analyzed the experience at the Mayo Clinic of 56 patients treated for 4 weeks with aqueous penicillin G (20 million units iv qd) combined with either streptomycin, 0.5 g im q12h, for enterococcal IE due to streptomycin-sensitive strains or with gentamicin (1 mg/kg im q8h) for IE due to streptomycin-resistant strains.[355] Relaps rates were high (12.5 percent) for both regimens; however, all patients who relapsed had had symptoms suggestive of IE for longer than 3 months. Relapses also only occurred in patients with mitral valve involvement. All patients who received over 3 mg/kg qd of gentamicin developed reversible nephrotoxicity (defined as a twofold increase in serum creatinine concentration) and 19 percent of patients receiving streptomycin for 4 weeks developed irreversible vestibular toxicity. Although this was not a prospective randomized trial, we believe that selected patients with enterococcal endocarditis may be treated with 4 weeks of combination therapy. The exceptions include mitral valve involvement, symptomatic illness exceeding 3 months, enterococcal prosthetic valve endocarditis (PVE), and patients with a relapse(s) of enterococcal endocarditis.

The penicillin-allergic patient presents the clinician with a difficult therapeutic dilemma. Vancomycin as a single drug at 1 g iv q12h has been used in the treatment of enterococcal endocarditis. However, experience is limited, and because of its lack of bactericidal activity in vitro and poor performance in experimental endocarditis, vancomycin should be combined with streptomycin or gentamicin. Unfortunately, this combination is potentially more nephrotoxic, and clinical proof of the superiority of this regimen over vancomycin alone is not available. The other therapeutic option in the allergic patient is "penicillin desensitization" followed by the administration of penicillin and an aminoglycoside.

Staphylococcal Endocarditis. The mortality in acute staphylococcal endocarditis still approximates 40 percent, and the preferred antibiotic regimen is controversial. Mortality is highest for men, patients over 50 years of age, and patients with left-sided involvement and/or central nervous system manifestations. In addition, narcotic addicts appear to have a lower mortality than do nonaddicts. Most *S. aureus* isolates, whether community or hospital acquired, are now resistant to penicillin G (MIC >0.2 μg/ml). The current recommended regimen includes a penicillinase-resistant penicillin (nafcillin or oxacillin, 1.5–2 g iv q4h) or a cephalosporin (cephalothin, 2 g iv q4h, or cefazolin, 2 g im q8h) given for 4–6 weeks.[214,215,356] The addition of gentamicin produces a synergistic effect against *S. aureus* in vitro and in experimental staphylococcal endocarditis in rabbits.[357] However, the combination did not improve the survival rate (60 percent) over that observed with a penicillin derivative alone in a small group of patients.[217] Combination therapy did not improve the results of therapy for staphylococcal IE in addicts,[358] but the mortality rate is low in this subgroup of patients (≃2–8 percent) with this disease. Combination therapy may permit a shorter duration of therapy in addicts with *S. aureus* endocarditis. Two weeks of nafcillin plus tobramycin (1 mg/kg iv q8h) cured 47 of 50 (94 percent) intravenous drug abusers with right-sided endocarditis[359] without evidence of renal failure, extrapulmonary metastatic infectious complications, aortic or mitral involvement, meningitis, or infection by MRSA. In addition, anecdotal case reports in nonaddicts with staphylococcal endocarditis suggest a beneficial response by the addition of gentamicin in patients failing to respond to nafcillin therapy.[360] This issue was addressed in a multicenter prospective trial comparing nafcillin alone with nafcillin plus gentamicin (for the initial 2 weeks) in the treatment of endocarditis due to *S. aureus*.[361] Although the combination resulted in a more rapid rate of eradication of the bacteremia, the incidence of nephrotoxicity was increased, and no improvement in mortality was achieved. Despite these results, many authorities still use combination therapy for short periods (e.g., 3–5 days), especially in fulminant cases. If the organism is susceptible to penicillin (MIC, <0.1 μg/ml), then this agent in a dose of 20 million units iv qd should be used. The response to treatment may be slow, often with fever and positive blood cultures lasting up to 1 week.[214] In penicillin-allergic patients or if the staphylococcus is "methicillin-resistant," vancomycin, 1 g iv q12h for 6 weeks, is recommended.[327,356,362] Clindamycin has been used to treat over 60 cases of staphylococcal endocarditis but is associated with an unacceptable relapse rate, and its use is not recommended.[363] The optimal therapy for IE due to "tolerant" strains of *S. aureus* is controversial.[364,365] One retrospective study[366] suggested that patients with IE due to these tolerant strains had a more complicated course; however, combination therapy did not appear to be of benefit. Another controversial area is the adjunctive role of rifampin, the most active antibiotic currently available against *S. aureus* in vitro, in therapy for IE. Due to the emergence of resistant strains, this drug is ineffective alone. Unfortunately, in vitro studies on rifampin combinations with either β-lactam agents or vancomycin are frequently contradictory, and the results in experimental IE induced by *S. aureus* are dependent on which drug in the combination exerts the greatest bactericidal activity in vivo.[367] At present, rifampin should be reserved for patients demonstrating poor serum bactericidal activity during therapy with a β-lactam or vancomycin, or in those with suppurative complications (e.g., valve-ring abscesses). Several new agents including teicoplanin, fosfomycin, and quinolones (e.g., ciprofloxacin, enoxacin, difloxacin, etc.) are active against MRSA in vitro and are as rapidly bactericidal as vancomycin in experimental animal models of IE due to MRSA,[368] although resistance to the quinolones has emerged during therapy. Experience with these drugs in humans with *S. aureus* endocarditis is scant.

Some authors[369] have felt that when *S. aureus* bacteremia occurs in a patient with a removable focus of infection the risk of concurrent endocarditis is low, and treatment schedules may be shortened to 2–3 weeks, thus avoiding the high costs, risks of suprainfection, and/or antibiotic reactions associated with prolonged therapy. In another study, 8 of 21 patients with an infected intravenous catheter as the suspected source of *S. aureus* bacteremia developed endocarditis.[370] We concur with the findings of Bayer et al.[371] who identified four parameters predictive of the presence of IE in 72 patients with *S. aureus* bacteremia in a prospective study: (*1*) the absence of a primary site of infection; (*2*) community acquisition of infection; (*3*) metastatic sequelae; and (*4*) valvular vegetations detected by echocardiography. Therefore, short-term therapy should be used only if endocarditis can be reasonably excluded by methods previously discussed.

Staphylococcus epidermidis is the most common etiologic agent in cases of prosthetic valve endocarditis. Most of these strains (87 percent) are methicillin resistant when isolated within 1 year of valve implantation. Recent studies[372] suggest that the optimal antimicrobial therapy of these infections is vancomycin plus rifampin, perhaps with the addition of an aminoglycoside as well. The recent emergence of vancomycin resistance among coagulase-negative staphylococci[373] is cause for concern. These concepts are discussed further in Chapter 62.

Endocarditis Due to Enterobacteriaceae or Pseudomonas Species. Of 125 cases of IE reported from Seattle, 4.8 percent were due to gram-negative aerobic bacilli.[15] These patients had a mortality of 83 percent, and none treated without surgery survived. The prognosis is especially poor with left-sided cardiac involvement. Determination of tube dilution MBCs are necessary to guide therapy. Certain combinations of penicillins or cephalosporins and aminoglycosides have been shown to be synergistic against many of these strains and are usually recommended. For IE due to most strains of *E. coli* or *Proteus mirabilis* a combination of a penicillin, either ampicillin (2 g iv q4h) or penicillin (20 million units iv qd) with an aminoglycoside, usually gentamicin (1.7 mg/kg q8h), is suggested. Third-generation cephalosporins are extremely active against *E. coli* in vitro, and some (e.g., ceftriaxone) have proved effective in experimental animal models of *E. coli* endocarditis,[374] even when long dosing intervals were used. This group of agents deserves further evaluation in humans for IE due to susceptible gram-negative bacilli. A combination of a third generation cephalosporin and an aminoglycoside (either gentamicin or amikacin) is recommended for *Klebsiella* endocarditis. Left-sided IE due to *S. marcescens* is refractory to medical therapy alone; valve replacement is invariably required to effect a cure.[237]

Pseudomonas aeruginosa remains an important pathogen in addicts with IE. Medical therapy may be successful in *P. aeruginosa* endocarditis involving the right side of the heart. If the disease is refractory to antibiotics, tricuspid valvulectomy or "vegetectomy"[375] without valve replacement is indicated.[240,376] Although valve replacement is often necessary for a cure of left-sided IE due to *P. aeruginosa,*[240,377] recent experience[128] with 10 patients (7 with left-sided involvement alone or in combination with tricuspid disease) suggests that medical therapy alone is occasionally curative. Studies in animals with experimental *Pseudomonas* endocarditis[378] offer an explanation for these disparate results: the penetration into vegetations and the time antibiotic concentrations exceeded the MBC were both significantly greater in tricuspid than in aortic vegetations for both ceftazidime and tobramycin.

The optimal antimicrobial regimen for *P. aeruginosa* endocarditis is evolving; the most extensive experience has been at the Detroit Medical Center. Problems have emerged with all potential regimens in animal models of this disease, as extensively studied by Bayer, Levison, and colleagues: (*1*) therapy with β-lactams (e.g., ceftazidime) has failed due to the constitutive hyperproduction of type Id β-lactamase[379]; (*2*) aminoglycoside-resistant isolates due to permeability defects emerge during therapy[380] and (*3*) no postantibiotic effect of β-lactams against *P. aeruginosa* is evident in vivo,[381] thus necessitating frequent (or continuous) drug administration. Treatment failures of *Pseudomonas* endocarditis in humans have been due to the selection of isolates with an enhanced production of type Id β-lactamase.[382] Based on clinical experience,[128,220,239,240] however, the preferred regimen for IE due to *P. aeruginosa* is high-dose tobramycin (8 mg/kg/day iv or im in divided doses q8h) with maintenance of peak and trough concentrations of 15–20 and ≤2 μg/ml, respectively, in combination with an extended-spectrum penicillin (e.g., ticarcillin, piperacillin, azlocillin) or ceftazidime in full doses. The toxicity associated with this regimen is surprisingly low; treatment should be combined for a minimum of 6 weeks. The quinolones are promising for the treatment of *Pseudomonas* endocarditis on the basis of favorable results in animal models[379] and in humans,[383] but the development of stepwise resistance during therapy may limit the efficacy of this class of drugs in the future.

Infective endocarditis due to *Haemophilus* sp. is usually responsive to ampicillin alone[231] administered for 3 weeks. However, therapy for IE due to these (and other) fastidious gram-negative organisms must be individualized on the basis of in vitro susceptibility data; in practice, β-lactam–aminoglycoside combinations are usually employed for approximately 1 month. The role of the newer third-generation cephalosporins in the treatment of IE due to gram-negative bacilli is unknown despite excellent in vitro activity and the potential for the avoidance of aminoglycoside-induced toxicity. It is important to emphasize that the above recommendations offer a rough guide for initial treatment. However, it is imperative that each isolate be subjected to sensitivity testing in vitro to ensure the optimal selection of antibiotics.

Endocarditis Due to Anaerobic Bacilli. Although IE caused by anaerobic bacilli is uncommon, the mortality is high. *Bacteroides fragilis* is isolated in many of these cases and is responsible for most fatalities. Most strains of anaerobic bacilli, with the exception of *B. fragilis,* are sensitive to penicillin in vitro, and this agent, in a dose of 20 million units iv qd, is the recommended therapy.[266,267] In addition, 33 percent of the strains of *B. fragilis* demonstrate an MIC of penicillin that is less than 25 μg/ml, and increasing resistance to penicillin among multiple anaerobic genera is evident. However, penicillin is only bacteriostatic against these strains (MBC invariably greater than 100 μg/ml), and relapse of the disease is common. Although clindamycin, carbenicillin, and chloramphenicol readily inhibit most strains of *B. fragilis,* they lack bactericidal activity, and they are poor therapeutic choices even though several patients have been cured with either high-dose penicillin, chloramphenicol (1 g iv q6h), clindamycin (600 mg iv q6h), or carbenicillin (5 g iv q3h). Due to excellent bactericidal activity in vitro and the serum concentrations attained, metronidazole, ticarcillin plus clavulanic acid, or imipenem are reasonable choices for therapy for anaerobic endocarditis.[268]

Pneumococcal, Gonococcal, and Meningococcal Endocarditis. Infective endocarditis caused by these organisms is now very rare. Pneumococcal endocarditis must be considered in any patient with pneumococcal bacteremia, especially if meningitis is present. Most common in alcoholics, the organism generally attacks the aortic valve and results in valvular insufficiency, often with perivalvular abscess formation and/or pericarditis. Type 12 pneumococci cause over 20 percent of the cases of pneumococcal endocarditis but are a rare (5 percent of the cases) cause of pneumococcal pneumonia. Penicillin, 20 million units iv qd for 4 weeks, is recommended for the treatment of pneumococcal endocarditis.

The gonococci that cause systemic infection are usually susceptible to penicillin.[384] These organisms as well as the meningococci can be effectively treated with the same penicillin regimen recommended for pneumococcal endocarditis. Although endocarditis due to penicillin-resistant gonococci (PPNG or chromosomally mediated) has not been reported, ceftriaxone has been used successfully to treat gonococcal endocarditis.[385]

Fungal Endocarditis. The incidence of IE caused by fungi has undergone a striking increase in the past decade. Fungal endocarditis occurs principally in a setting of narcotic addiction, after cardiac surgery, after the prolonged intravenous administration of drugs (especially "broad-spectrum" antibiotics), and in the compromised host. The overall survival rate in patients treated since 1968 is only 14.5 percent.[159] The preferred mode of therapy is unknown. The use of antifungal agents alone has been almost universally unsuccessful in achieving a cure of this disease. The addition of surgical measures to antifungal therapy may result in an improvement in prognosis, but to date there is insufficient clinical experience. When fungal endocarditis is diagnosed, a combined medical/surgical approach should be undertaken.

The mainstay of antifungal drug therapy is amphotericin B. This agent is toxic and produces multiple side effects including fever, chills, phlebitis, headache, anorexia, anemia, hypokalemia, renal tubular acidosis, nephrotoxicity, nausea, and vomiting. Drug toxicity is frequent and commonly necessitates alterations in the regimen. Dosages and the technique of administration are given in Chapter 33.

After 1–2 weeks of amphotericin B therapy at "full" dosages, surgery should probably be performed. If isolated tricuspid endocarditis is present, as in a narcotic addict, total tricuspid valvulectomy can usually be performed. Rarely, removal of the vegetation alone is curative. Most of these patients tolerate the valvulectomy without the development of significant right-sided heart failure. Valve replacement is necessary for left-sided fungal endocarditis. The duration of antifungal therapy after surgery is empirical, but 6–8 weeks is usually recommended.

It is possible that combination antifungal therapy may improve the poor survival from fungal endocarditis. Some strains of *Candida* sp. and *Cryptococcus neoformans* are inhibited in vitro by concentrations of 5-fluorocytosine achieved with the oral administration of 150 mg/kg/day in six divided doses. Synergism between 5-fluorocytosine and amphotericin B has been documented for these yeasts in vitro and in the treatment of cryptococcal meningitis. This combination was fungicidal and perhaps instrumental in the cure of one case of *Aspergillus* endocarditis. However, in the rabbit model of endocarditis due to *Candida albicans,*[162] the addition of 5-fluorocytosine did not improve the rate of eradication of fungal organisms from the vegetation when compared with amphotericin B alone. Potentiation of amphotericin B activity by rifampin has been noted for virtually all strains tested of *Candida* sp. and for a few isolates of *Histoplasma capsulatum*. The therapeutic advantage of the addition of 5-fluorocytosine or rifampin to amphotericin for fungal endocarditis requires further investigation, but initial results in animal models of disseminated candidiasis are not encouraging.[386] The role of triazoles and imidazoles in the treatment of fungal endocarditis has received scant attention. On the basis of animal model data,[387] high-dose intraconazole may be of value in the treatment of *Aspergillus* endocarditis, but valve replacement will likely remain imperative for a cure.

Q Fever Endocarditis. More than 200 well-documented cases of this form of IE have been reported, and the mortality exceeds 65 percent.[277–279] The only antibiotics effective in acute Q fever, chloramphenicol and the tetracyclines, are rickettsiostatic. In addition, chloramphenicol cannot be administered for the prolonged periods of time necessary in this disease. The mortality with tetracycline therapy alone is at least 70 percent, and the recovery of *Coxiella burnetii* from valve tissue after 4 years of tetracycline therapy[277] both argue against medical therapy alone. Thus, most authorities agree that valve replacement is probably required for cure. Based on in vitro data and anecdotal experience,[279,388,389] the following approach is suggested: doxycycline (100 mg po q12h) or tetracycline (500 mg po q6h) plus trimethoprim-sulfamethoxazole (approximately 480 mg trimethoprim plus 2400 mg sulfisoxazole daily in four divided doses) in combination with valve replacement. The duration of therapy is empirical but should usually exceed 1 year; treatment can be stopped when there is no clinical evidence of infection and phase I antibody titers are <1:128 by complement fixation.[279] Rifampin plus cotrimoxazole is not recommended for Q fever endocarditis. A careful follow-up for recrudescence of infection is essential.

Infective Endocarditis Due to Chlamydiae. Albeit based on limited experience, a combination of valve replacement and prolonged (greater than 3 months) tetracycline therapy seems justified in these cases. Rifampin has cured at least one case of chlamydial IE after therapy with tetracyclines had failed, but exposure to this agent rapidly induces the emergence of rifampin resistance of *C. trachomatis* in tissue culture.[390] The role of combination regimens (e.g., rifampin plus erythromycin or tetracycline) deserves further study.

Culture-Negative Endocarditis. The therapy for this entity is controversial, but the regimen usually used will "cover" the enterococcus and fastidious gram-negative bacilli and consists of a combination of penicillin, 20 million units iv qd in divided doses, or ampicillin, 2 g iv q4h, plus streptomycin, 0.5 g im q12h, or gentamicin, 1.7 mg/kg im or iv q8h. When staphylococcal endocarditis is a strong consideration (narcotic addicts or after cardiac surgery), a penicillinase-resistant penicillin or a cephalosporin in full dosage should be added to this regimen. If clinical improvement occurs, some authorities recommend discontinuation of treatment with the aminoglycoside after 2 weeks. The other agent(s) should be continued for a full 6 weeks of treatment. Continued surveillance for an etiologic agent and careful follow-up are mandatory. An analysis of any correlation between the response to empirical antimicrobial therapy and survival was performed in 52 patients with culture-negative endocarditis[286]: 92 percent of the patients who became afebrile within the first week of therapy survived vs. only 50 percent if fever persisted longer than 7 days. Most deaths were caused by major systemic emboli or uncontrollable congestive heart failure due to valvular insufficiency.

Surgical Therapy

In recent years, valve replacement has become an important adjunct to medical therapy in the management of IE and is now used in ≥25 percent of the cases. The generally accepted indications for surgical intervention during active IE are as follows: (*1*) refractory congestive heart failure; (*2*) more than one serious systemic embolic episode; (*3*) uncontrolled infection; (*4*) valve dysfunction as demonstrated by fluoroscopy; (*5*) ineffective antimicrobial therapy (e.g., fungal endocarditis); (*6*) resection of mycotic aneurysms; (*7*) most cases of prosthetic valve endocarditis; and (*8*) local suppurative complications including perivalvular or myocardial abscesses with conduction system abnormalities, heart block, etc. The major indications in the past have been persistent infection and congestive heart failure.[391–393] For example, congestive heart failure during active IE was the indication for surgery in 86 percent of 108 patients undergoing valve replacement at Stanford from 1963 to 1984.[393]

The most frequent causes of death in IE, in approximate order, are congestive heart failure, embolic phenomena, rupture of a mycotic aneurysm, complications of cardiac surgery, lack of response to antimicrobial therapy, and prosthetic valve endocarditis.[2–15] Failure to make a diagnosis or renal failure are rare causes of death. In a recent review from Seattle,[15] congestive heart failure was present in 91 percent of the patients who died. Overall, two-thirds of the patients in this series of 125 cases developed congestive heart failure, and this complication appears to be increasing in frequency. The overall mortality in this group of patients was 37 percent.

When acute aortic regurgitation complicated by congestive heart failure supervenes in IE, the mortality still exceeds 50 percent. The classic physical findings of chronic aortic regurgitation are often absent in these patients.[176] The current trend is to advise early surgery in this group of patients since nothing is gained by delay. In a series of 28 patients from Birmingham, Alabama, with acute aortic regurgitation, 4 had no congestive heart failure and were treated medically, and all survived. In contrast, 7 of 11 patients with mild congestive heart failure and 7 of 8 with moderate to severe congestive heart failure died during medical therapy, often suddenly and with pathologic evidence of coronary emboli and myocardial infarction. Four of five patients with moderately severe congestive heart failure who underwent surgery survived. This suggests that early surgical intervention may improve the survival statistics in this setting. Similar results were obtained at the Mayo Clinic (3/11 deaths). The hemodynamic status of the patient, not the activity of the infection, is the critical determining factor in the timing of cardiac valve replacement.[394] The hemodynamic severity of the acute aortic regurgitation may be assessed by determining the degree of mitral valve preclosure by echocardiography. If premature closure of the mitral valve occurs before the Q wave of the electrocardiogram, then the left ventricular end-diastolic pressure is very high, and surgical intervention is urgently required. Nothing is gained by temporizing, even if only a few hours of antibiotics can be administered. When congestive heart failure persists despite digoxin, diuretics, and other therapeutic modalities, surgery is also indicated. In 80 patients subjected to aortic valve replacement for IE, the surgical cure rate was 72 percent. There were no instances of subsequent infection of the prosthesis, but 16 percent developed paravalvular regurgitation. This latter complication was usually easily controlled medically. Organisms visible on Gram stain, positive cultures or annular abscesses at the time of surgery are associated with late complications.[393] When left-sided IE is present and the clinical assessment implicates more than one valve or extravalvular extension of the disease, then cardiac angiography is useful in delineating the proper surgical approach (see above).

In contrast to left-sided IE where congestive heart failure is the usual indication for surgical intervention, in right-sided IE persistent infection is the indication for surgery in over 70 percent of the patients. Most of the patients are narcotic addicts, with IE caused by organisms that are difficult to eradicate with antimicrobial therapy alone (e.g., fungi, gram-negative aerobic bacilli). Tricuspid valvulectomy is now the procedure of choice for refractory right-sided IE.[395] Subsequent valve replacement, at a second operation, is advised only when medical management fails to control the hemodynamic manifestations and the patient has ceased using illicit drugs. Combination antimicrobial therapy with optimal serum bactericidal activity should be continued for 4–6 weeks postoperatively. These patients may develop mild to moderate right-sided heart failure, but this is easily tolerated, and the success rate of this approach is over 70 percent. Persistent fever, recurrent pulmonary emboli, or vegetations demonstrable by echocardiography usually do not require tricuspid valvulectomy in this setting.[396] In addition, many surgeons contend that a return to the use of illicit drugs and reinfection of the valve after initial cure is a contraindication to reoperation.[397]

Outstanding reviews on the indications for surgery during therapy for IE are available.[392,398] The rationale for surgical intervention, including major and minor criteria for valve replacement, are discussed in detail. A point system weighting multiple factors has been devised by Alsip and colleagues to assist in decision making concerning surgery in patients with active IE.[398] The value of this system remains to be defined. It has become apparent that virtually all patients with prosthetic valve endocarditis (except those with late disease caused by penicillin-sensitive viridans streptococci) require valve replacement for consistent cures (see Chapter 62).

SUPPURATIVE THROMBOPHLEBITIS

Suppurative thrombophlebitis is an inflammation of the vein wall due to the presence of microorganisms and is frequently associated with thrombosis and bacteremia. Suppuration of the vein wall is usually absent in intravenous catheter-related sepsis and bacteremia secondary to contaminated intravenous fluid and will not be discussed here. Suppurative thrombophlebitis may be classified into four forms: superficial, central (including pelvic), cavernous sinus, and infection of the portal vein (pylephlebitis). The last two conditions have become rare since the introduction of antibiotics. In contrast, superficial suppurative thrombophlebitis has been steadily increasing in incidence since the introduction of the plastic intravenous cannula. Superficial suppurative thrombophlebitis secondary to intravenous fluid therapy was first described in 1947[399] when 93 cases were reported, 43 of which were amenable to surgical therapy.

Epidemiology

In 1973, approximately one of every four hospitalized patients received intravenous therapy for a total of over 10 million patients annually in the United States.[400] Suppurative thrombophlebitis accounts for up to 10 percent of all nosocomial infections and is a particular problem in burned patients where it represents a common cause of death due to infection. In several large series of burned patients,[401–404] suppurative thrombophlebitis developed in 4–8 percent and increased in frequency if cutdowns were performed. Suppurative thrombophlebitis is also found in other hospitalized patients (especially those with cancer and/or those receiving steroid therapy).[405,406] Seven such cases were recognized in a recent 18-month period in Charleston, South Carolina,[407] and 35 cases were identified in 7 years in Louisville, Kentucky. Suppurative thrombophlebitis may also be increasing in frequency. Eight cases were encountered during an 8-month period in Johannesburg; suppurative thrombophlebitis was estimated to represent a minimum incidence of 0.12 percent of all admissions.[408] When using strict criteria, 29 episodes of suppurative thrombophlebitis in 27 patients were identified in a large Air Force hospital within 4 years.[409] Based on data from the National Nosocomial Infection Study, Rhame and associates estimate the overall incidence of suppurative thrombophlebitis as 88 per 100,000 discharges, but this disease is underreported.[410] Suppurative thrombophlebitis is also common in abusers of intravenous drugs.[411] This condition is unusual during childhood[412] but may occur as a complication related to intravenous therapy. Catheter-related sepsis without suppurative thrombophlebitis is more common and affects at least 25,000 patients per year in the United States.[413] The risk of this complication is approximately 40 times higher with plastic cannulas (8 percent) than with steel or ''scalp vein'' cannulas (0.2 percent). Irritation to the vein wall and the subsequent development of suppurative thrombophlebitis is greater with polyethylene catheters when compared with those constructed of Teflon or Silastic materials. Central venous catheterization has been employed for over 30 years for hemodynamic monitoring, total parenteral nutrition (TPN), and infusion of drugs. The exact incidence of suppurative thrombophlebitis of the central veins commonly cannulated (i.e., jugulars, subclavian, venae cavae) is unknown. Catheter-induced thrombosis is relatively common. Autopsy series have revealed central venous thrombosis in 37 percent of catheterized subjects, but this diagnosis is rarely recognized because most patients are asymptomatic. When examined by phlebography at the time of catheter withdrawal, 42 percent of catheters have sleeve thrombi, and another 8 percent revealed veno-occlusive thrombi.[414] In addition, sepsis has been reported in ≈7 percent of patients receiving TPN and other medications by the central route. When thrombosis and bacterial or fungal contamination/sepsis coexist, suppurative thrombophlebitis may intervene. At least 50 cases of suppurative thrombophlebitis of the great thoracic veins have been reported in the literature,[415–417] but this is almost certainly a gross underestimate of the problem. Eight cases in 8 years due to *Candida* sp. alone were observed at the University of Wisconsin.[418] Septic atrial thrombosis, occasionally with a coexistent Budd-Chiari syndrome, has complicated Broviac catheter insertion in infants.[419]

Superficial suppurative thrombophlebitis is a complication of either a dermal infection and/or an indwelling intravenous catheter. Pelvic suppurative thrombophlebitis is associated with parturition, abortion, gynecologic surgery, or a pelvic abscess. Therefore, this is a disease of women of the childbearing age, with most cases occurring between the ages of 15 and 40 years (mean, 20 years). In 123 cases in two reports,[420,421] the predisposing conditions were as follows: vaginal delivery, 39 cases; cesarean section, 19 cases; abortion, 33 cases; and major gynecologic surgery, 32 cases. During a 9-year period in Atlanta, 27 cases of postpartum septic pelvic thrombophlebitis were identified in over 54,000 deliveries.[421] The relative risk for this condition was as follows: parturition, 1/2000 (highest in the inner-city population); septic abortion, 1/200; and major gynecologic surgery, 1/800. The incidence of suppurative thrombophlebitis rises proportionally with the degree of trauma to the pelvic tissues.

Pathogenesis

The pathogenesis of suppurative thrombophlebitis is poorly understood. A thrombus may act as a nidus for local entrapment and colonization of bacteria that gain access to the site from another focus. This is analogous to the proposed role of nonbacterial thrombotic endocarditis in the pathogenesis of IE.

When superficial suppurative thrombophlebitis is associated with intravascular cannulae, the route of infection may be (*1*) migration from the skin between the catheter wall and perivascular tissue, (*2*) from contaminated IV fluid, and (*3*) hematogenous dissemination from an infected focus elsewhere. The relative contribution(s) of these three routes is unknown. The observation that the predominant organism in burn wounds, *Pseudomonas aeruginosa,* is a rare cause of suppurative thrombophlebitis and that suppurative thrombophlebitis usually develops days to weeks after the cutdown incision is healed[402,404] argues against a local cutaneous source in burn patients.

The venous system draining the pelvis includes the intervertebral venous plexus, the lumbar venous plexus, the superficial and deep veins of the abdominal wall, and the hemorrhoidal plexus. Any component of this system may be affected in pelvic suppurative thrombophlebitis, but the veins draining the uterus, including the ovarian veins and the inferior vena cava, are most often involved.[422] Thrombus formation may result from stasis of blood flow due to the gravid uterus and by the hypercoagulable state of parturition. Normal residents of the vaginal or perineal bacterial flora gain access to the thrombus via the blood stream and/or regional lymphatics. There is often an associated endometritis or parametritis. Septic pulmonary emboli and metastatic abscess formation are common.

Pathologic Changes

Regardless of the vein involved, the pathologic changes are similar. The vein is enlarged, tortuous, and thickened. There may be associated perivascular suppuration and/or hemorrhage, and the vein lumen usually contains both pus and thrombus. Microscopically, endothelial damage, fibrinoid necrosis, and thickening of the vein wall are evident. Microabscesses may be present in the vein wall or in the surrounding tissue.[407,423] Gross periphlebitic abscesses are not unusual and may be evident on physical examination. Thrombi frequently extend beyond the area of suppuration. In an autopsy series of peripheral suppurative thrombophlebitis in burned patients, extension of the clot into the great central veins was found in 18 percent of the cases.[402,404] Metastatic abscess formation and septic pulmonary emboli with infarction are found in over 50 percent of the fatal cases. This may result from bacterial liquefaction and fragmentation of affected thrombi within the vein since clot liquefaction is noted commonly in autopsy series.

Clinical Manifestations

Superficial suppurative thrombophlebitis is often difficult to identify since local findings of inflammation may be absent. The disease occurs more frequently when plastic catheters are inserted in the lower extremities, a common practice in burn patients. In 132 cases reported from the burn center at Fort Sam Houston, Texas, the distribution of superficial suppurative thrombophlebitis was as follows: lower extremity (predominantly saphenous system), 100; upper extremity (predominantly antecubital fossa), 32; jugular, 7; and iliac, 4. The mean duration of preceding venous cannulation was 4.81 days, and the latent interval from removal of the catheter to the development of symptoms ranged from 2 to 10 days.[401,403] Fever was present in over 70 percent of the cases, but rigors were rare. Local findings such as warmth, erythema, tenderness, swelling, or lymphangitis were present in only 32 percent of these patients; however, bacteremia with signs of systemic sepsis were found in 84 percent. Septic pulmonary emboli with secondary pneumonia occurred in 44 percent and were often the first diagnostic clue. Thus, pneumonia, sepsis, or metastatic abscess formation was the only manifestation of this disease in two-thirds of the cases. These authors emphasize that the late onset of pneumonia or sepsis in a burned patient demands the careful inspection of all previously cannulated veins since untreated suppurative thrombophlebitis is associated with a high mortality. In these series, fewer than 50 percent of the cases were diagnosed antemortem.[402]

In contrast to the experience with suppurative thrombophlebitis in burn patients, most medical and postoperative patients develop superficial suppurative thrombophlebitis in the upper extremities, and signs of local inflammation are more commonly present (94 percent in one series).[411] Many of these patients are elderly (20/35 over 50 years old) with debilitating diseases and are often receiving antibiotics when superficial suppurative thrombophlebitis intervenes. As above, the duration of intravenous catheterization is an important risk factor; 68 percent of implicated cannulae had been left in place for ≥5 days in patients reported recently.[405,411]

Subperiosteal abscesses of adjacent long bones may complicate superficial suppurative thrombophlebitis in children.[424] The local findings of this condition, including bone tenderness, erythema, warmth, and limitation of motion with occasional extension into the joint space, may overshadow the suppurative thrombophlebitis iself. Septic deep vein thrombosis of the femoral vessels with swollen, tender, and inflamed inguinal areas has been described in intravenous users of heroin and cocaine. Contiguous pelvic bone osteomyelitis is unusual.

Suppurative thrombophlebitis of the thoracic central veins occurs in critically ill patients with central catheters in place, in those receiving TPN, or in patients after long-term cannulation with Broviac, Hickman, and other devices. The systemic findings of sepsis overshadow any local findings of venous occlusion (e.g., superior vena cava syndrome), which are rare in this setting. This syndrome should be suspected in any septic patient when bacteremia and/or fungemia fail to resolve upon removal of the central catheter and institution of appropriate antimicrobial therapy.

Pelvic suppurative thrombophlebitis usually develops 1–2 weeks postpartum or postoperatively and is associated with high fever, chills, anorexia, nausea, vomiting, abdominal pain, and a protracted course.[421] Flank pain may result from ureteral obstruction by enlarged veins. Abdominal tenderness, usually in the right lower quadrant, may be mild to severe. Approximately 80 percent of cases are unilateral on the right side, 14 percent are bilateral, and only 6 percent are unilateral and left sided. This distribution is thought to result from compression of the right ovarian vein at the pelvic brim by the enlarged uterus with retrograde flow on the left and protection from ascending infection. However, the physical examination may be normal. A tender vein can be palpated in 30 percent of the cases on pelvic or abdominal examination.[407] The uterus is usually freely movable. Spread of the process to the femoral vein with edema and tenderness of the lower extremity is unusual. Many of these patients are extremely ill with an acute or chronic course characterized by little or no response to antibiotics and the development of multiple, small, septic pulmonary emboli. Since many of the manifestations are nonspecific, the differential diagnosis is broad and includes acute appendicitis, ureteral obstruction, torsion of an ovarian cyst, pyelonephritis, broad ligament hematoma, parametritis, endometritis, perinephric abscess, pelvic abscess, small bowel volvulus, pelvic inflammatory disease, sickle cell crisis, and ectopic pregnancy.

Laboratory Findings

Bacteremia occurs in 80–90 percent of the cases of superficial suppurative thrombophlebitis. Gross pus within the vein lumen is found in about one-half of the cases, and this finding establishes a diagnosis of suppurative phlebitis. When infection of a venous catheter is suspected, it should be removed and cultured. The results, however, may be misleading since even though bacteria will be isolated in up to 60 percent of the cases a positive culture does not correlate with inflammation.[425] The following semiquantitative culture technique has recently been developed in an attempt to differentiate catheter-related sepsis from suppurative thrombophlebitis. After preparing the skin with alcohol, the catheter is removed with sterile forceps (avoiding skin contact) and is placed in a sterile tube for transport. The catheter is then aseptically cut into 5.7 cm pieces, and each section is rolled across the surface of a 5% sheep blood agar plate. The growth of more than 15 colonies on the plate correlates well[425] with the presence of venous infection. In the few cases of suppurative thrombophlebitis studied by this technique, all catheters have yielded confluent growth. Since the standard 5.7 cm catheter retains approximately 0.7–1.5 mg of moisture on its surface and the plate growth has exceeded 1000 colonies in every case of suppurative thrombophlebitis, bacterial counts must exceed 10^6 organisms/g in the catheter wound. These titers are similar to those found in other types of infected wounds. This technique is simple, rapid, and inexpensive and may prove useful in establishing the need for exploratory venotomy. Simple needle aspiration of the suspected vein may also be diagnostic. ^{111}In-labeled leukocyte imaging studies have detected superficial suppurative thrombophlebitis, but experience is limited.

Other laboratory findings in patients with superficial suppurative thrombophlebitis, for example, leukocytosis, are nonspecific. The chest x-ray film may reveal multiple peripheral densities or a pleural effusion consistent with pulmonary emboli, infarction, abscess, or empyema. The diagnosis of an associated subperiosteal abscess is difficult: bone and gallium scans usually reveal hyperperfusion without definite osteomyelitis, routine x-ray films are virtually always negative, and CT often demonstrates only soft tissue swelling with obliteration of tissue planes. High-resolution CT scans may improve these results.[424] The diagnosis of deep central vein suppurative thrombophlebitis in the thorax is established by venography with the demonstration of thrombi in a patient with positive blood cultures, but CT with contrast enhancement is probably as sensitive and is noninvasive. Experience with magnetic resonance imaging and ^{111}In-labeled leukocytes is meager.

In most cases of pelvic suppurative thrombophlebitis there is a peripheral blood leukocytosis, and the urinalysis is usually normal. The chest x-ray film may reveal multiple septic pulmonary emboli, and abdominal x-ray films may show a pelvic mass. Intravenous pyelography can be useful in disclosing ureteral obstruction. Real-time ultrasonography is very helpful in delineating the location and extent of the thrombus, but the ileus that is often associated with this infection may render interpretation difficult. Computed tomography reveals low attenuation with contrast enhancement in suppurative venous thrombosis and is very sensitive in the diagnosis of pelvic suppurative thrombophlebitis.[426,427] Magnetic resonance imaging may be even more sensitive and can differentiate fresh ($\leq$1 week old) from organizing or subacute thrombosis, but experience is limited.[428] These sensitive and noninvasive techniques may lead to an increased recognition of pelvic suppurative thrombophlebitis, earlier diagnosis, and improved outcome. The role of newer diagnostic techniques such as pelvic venography, transuterine phebography, ^{111}In-labeled leukocyte scanning, and laparoscopy is still undefined. Since bacteremia is demonstrated in only 20–30 percent[420,421,429] of cases of pelvic suppurative thrombophlebitis, negative blood cultures do not exclude the diagnosis.

Etiologic Agents

Staphylococcus aureus was the causative agent of 65–78 percent of the cases of superficial suppurative thrombophlebitis reported before 1968. In recent years, most have been due to the Enterobacteriaceae, especially *Klebsiella-Enterobacter* sp.[405,411] These agents are acquired nosocomially and are often resistant to multiple antibiotics. Nearly all patients with superficial suppurative thrombophlebitis due to gram-negative aerobic bacilli or fungi are receiving broad-spectrum antibiotics at the time the disease becomes manifested. In a review of 86 cases compiled from the literature reported since 1970, the organisms isolated were as follows: *Klebsiella-Enterobacter* sp., 34; *Providencia* sp., 5; *Proteus* sp., 5; *Serratia* sp., 3; *E. coli,* 6; *P. aeruginosa,* 3; *S. aureus,* 15; *C. albicans,* 9; *S. epidermidis,* 4; and enterococci, 2.[405,411] Suppurative thrombophlebitis due to gram-negative pathogens and *E. faecalis* is more common (than *S. aureus*) in patients with significant intra-abdominal pathology.[409] *Staphylococcus aureus,* other gram-positive cocci, and *Candida* sp. were more frequent when this risk factor was absent. Multiple organisms are isolated in up to 14 percent of cases. Anaerobic isolates are extremely rare. An increase in incidence of superficial suppurative thrombophlebitis due to *Candida* sp. was reported recently[430,431]; all patients were receiving antibiotics without hyperalimentation. None were neutropenic or receiving corticosteroids. In one series of seven patients observed in a 15-month interval,[431] all had concomitant or preceding bacterial infections and had received a median of five antibiotics for at least 2 weeks. Preceding candidal colonization at other sites (e.g., sputum, urine) was often present. Although not documented by culture, histopathologic evidence suggests that cytomegalovirus may cause suppurative thrombophlebitis in patients with the acquired immunodeficiency syndrome (AIDS) despite therapy with ganciclovir.[432]

The responsible agents in pelvic suppurative thrombophlebitis are poorly defined since blood cultures are often negative and most investigators did not use adequate anaerobic techniques. The organisms isolated in approximate order of frequency are *Bacteroides* sp., microaerophilic or anaerobic streptococci, *E. coli* and other coliforms, and β-hemolytic streptococci. The predominance of *Bacteroides* sp. may be related to the heparinase produced by this organism. A prolonged latent period (up to 3 weeks) may occur before blood cultures become positive. The more extensive use of anaerobic isolation techniques and the routine culturing of surgical specimens may serve to clarify the role of anaerobic bacteria in this entity.

Presumptive Therapy

Superficial suppurative thrombophlebitis is a lethal iatrogenic disease, and surgery is usually necessary for cure. The first reported successful cure of suppurative thrombophlebitis followed surgical ligation of the vein by John Hunter in 1784.[433] All investigators strongly endorse surgical excision as an integral part of the management. In a review of 24 patients,[402] 14 were treated medically alone, and all died either directly from suppurative thrombophlebitis with persistent bacteremia or secondary to metastatic complications. However, of 10 patients who underwent surgical exploration, 7 survived, and only 1 of the 3 deaths was attributable to suppurative thrombophlebitis. Antibiotics should also be used in the treatment of this disease; initial treatment with a semisynthetic penicillin (e.g., nafcillin, 2 g iv q4–6h) plus an aminoglycoside (e.g., gentamicin, 1.0–1.7 mg/kg iv or im q8h) is recommended since the Enterobacteriaceae and/or staphylococci are the usual etiologic agents. The duration of therapy is unknown and largely empirical. The role of antifungal therapy for superficial suppurative thrombophlebitis due to *Candida albicans* is controversial.[430,431] Although most of these infections can be cured by vein excision, a short course of amphotericin B (approximately 200 mg) is advised postoperatively, pending further data. Antifungal therapy is mandatory in the immunosuppressed patient or if signs of metastatic complications (e.g., endophthalmitis) develop.

When superficial suppurative thrombophlebitis is considered, an exploratory venotomy is necessary. This procedure should be performed proximal to the suspected site; the vein should be ligated and then "milked" in an attempt to express purulent material for inspection by Gram stain and culture. If no pus is apparent, an exploratory venotomy is necessary to establish the diagnosis. Simple ligation was thought to be sufficient 30 years ago, but the rate of relapse with ongoing sepsis was high. Therefore, the segment of vein and all its involved tributaries should be totally excised. Radical surgery from the ankle to the groin may be required in some burn patients. Nevertheless, local or regional anesthesia alone is often sufficient (approximately 90 percent of cases) for vein excision. Backbleeding, indicative of a patent lumen, should be evident at the point of vein transection. Vein excision is usually followed by prompt (≤24 hours) defervescence. If systemic symptoms, bacteremia, and/or marked local findings persist after vein excision, reexploration is necessary with careful attention to total removal of all involved veins and drainage of contiguous (e.g., periphlebitic, subperiosteal) abscesses. It should be stressed, however, that the role of less radical surgery in therapy for superficial suppurative thrombophlebitis has not been addressed adequately. Although the literature supports vein excision, this experience stems largely from burn centers. Despite infection with gram-negative bacilli or *Candia* sp., six of eight children with superficial suppurative thrombophlebitis were cured by local incision and drainage of the involved site plus parenteral antimicrobials.[408] Radical surgery with extensive excision can perhaps be reserved for patients failing these measures. Delayed closure is preferred over primary wound closure. If osteomyelitis is documented in the adjacent long bones, antimicrobial therapy should be continued for a least 6 weeks. Resection of the involved vasculature in most patients with suppurative thrombophlebitis of the great central veins is technically impossible. Fortunately, medical therapy is usually sufficient.[415–418,434] The recommmended approach is catheter removal, full-dose anticoagulation with heparin,[418,434] and parenteral antibiotics. The duration of therapy is unsettled; 2–3 weeks after catheter removal is suggested. The antibiotics employed are the same as for superficial suppurative thrombophlebitis. Experience with more potent agents (e.g., third-generation cephalosporins) for suppurative thrombophlebitis due to gram-negative bacilli is scant, but trials are indicated. Because heparin may precipitate vancomycin with a partial loss of antibacterial activity at concentrations present in intravenous lines,[435] these drugs should not be administered simultaneously by the same intravenous access when MRSA, *S. epidermidis, E. faecalis,* etc., are suspected or grown. Unlike *Candida* IE, suppurative thrombophlebitis of the great central veins due to *Candida* sp. is curable medically, but antifungal regimens must be continued longer than those usually adequate for superficial suppurative thrombophlebitis. Based on limited data,[418] amphotericin B at a daily dose of 0.7 mg/kg to a total dosage ≥22 mg/kg plus 5-fluorocytosine (100–150 mg/kg/day in four divided doses, if tolerable) is recommended after catheter removal. Surgery may, however, be essential in patients with suppurative thrombophlebitis of the thoracic or neck veins when perivascular collections are present.[418]

The optimal therapy for pelvic suppurative thrombophlebitis is still controversial. Because anaerobic streptococci and *Bacteroides* sp. predominante, the initial antibiotics of choice are aqueous penicillin G, 20 million units iv qd, plus either clindamycin, 450–600 mg iv q6h, metronidazole, 500–750 mg iv q8h, or chloramphenicol, 1 g iv q6h. The use of heparin is debated. The addition of heparin after several days of unsuccessful treatment with antibiotics may itself produce an antipyretic effect.[429] In one series of 46 patients with pelvic suppurative thrombophlebitis[421] including 7 with massive ovarian vein involvement and 15 with septic pulmonary emboli, 42 patients become afebrile within 7 days (mean, 2.5 days) while receiving penicillin, chloramphenicol, and heparin. Four patients required exploratory laparotomy, and pelvic abscesses were found in three. These results argue strongly that medical therapy alone is often effective, but no controlled studies on the use of heparin have been done. When medical therapy is unsatisfactory, surgery with drainage of abscesses and usually ligation of the implicated venous system must be performed. Some authorities[422] feel that inferior vena cava and/or ovarian vein ligation should be performed in all these cases, but the evidence for this approach is inconclusive.

Prevention

The incidence of superficial suppurative thrombophlebitis can be reduced by the same preventive procedures that are used for intravenous cannulae in general. These include the use of "scalp vein" cannulae whenever possible, the avoidance of lower extremity cannulations, insertion under aseptic conditions, secure anchoring of the cannula, and frequent replacement (at least every 48–72 hours) of intravenous fluid bottles, cannulae, and connecting tubing. Although neomycin-polymixin B-bacitracin ointment is effective in reducing the incidence of cutdown infections,[436] this modality has not demonstrated consistent benefit with intravenous cannulae.[437] When clinical signs of bacteremia occur in a patient receiving intravenous fluids, the following steps should be taken: (*1*) blood cultures should be obtained, (*2*) intravenous administration should be discontinued and all cannulae removed, (*3*) the intravenous fluid itself should be cultured, (*4*) the cannula should be cultured semiquantitatively on blood agar as described by Maki et al.,[425] and (*5*) appropriate antibiotic therapy should be initiated. If clinical signs of sepsis and bactermia persist despite appropriate antibiotic therapy, then an intravascular focus (including suppurative thrombophlebitis at a previously cannulated vein) should be sought as discussed above.

INFECTIVE ENDARTERITIS AND "MYCOTIC ANEURYSMS"

The term "mycotic aneurysm" was coined by Osler in the Gulstonian lectures of 1885, to describe a mushroom-shaped aneurysm that developed in a patient with subacute bacterial endocarditis. At that time mycotic was used to refer to all microorganisms. Presently, the use of myocotic has been restricted specifically to fungal infections, but the term mycotic aneurysm is still used for all extra- (or intra-) cardiac aneurysms of infectious etiology except for syphilitic aortitis. Unfortunately, this term has also been used to describe pre-existing aneurysms secondarily infected from contiguous or distant foci or pseudoaneurysms arising from trauma or iatrogenic causes. "Endarteritis" refers to inflammation of the arterial wall, which may occur with or without coexistent aneurysmal dilatation. Unless an aneurysm or coarctation of the aorta is present, infective endarteritis is usually a postmortem diagnosis. Since infected aneurysms differ in their pathogenesis, the various classifications, given in Table 5, will be examined separately.[438] Infections of arterial prosthetic devices are dealt with in detail in Chapter 62 and are not considered here.

Epidemiology

Although incidence figures are unavailable, a localized suppurative process of the arterial wall is rare. Estimates derived

TABLE 5. Classification of "Mycotic Aneurysms"

Pre-existent Arterial Status	Source of Infection
Normal	Intravascular
Atherosclerotic	Embolism
Aneurysm	Bacteremia with "seeding"
Arterial prosthesis	Extension from adjacent endocardial focus or erosion
	Extravascular
	Contiguous site of infection
	Iatrogenic

from autopsy series of aortic aneurysms are available but ignore infections at other locations in the arterial tree. In a review of over 22,000 autopsies performed at the Boston City Hospital from 1902 to 1951,[439] aortic aneurysms were found in 1.5 percent. However, mycotic aneurysms constituted only 2.6 percent of these lesions. In another review of 178 aneurysms found among more than 20,000 autopsies at the Mayo Clinic from 1925 to 1954,[440] only 6 were felt to be of infectious origin. In the preantibiotic era, infected aneurysms were predominantly confined to patients with IE; in a series of 217 cases reported in 1923,[441] 86 percent were associated with IE. With the advent of antibiotics, mycotic aneurysms in IE have become less prevalent, and hematogenous seeding of a previously damaged arteriosclerotic vessel constitutes the most common mechanism. There is also evidence to suggest that this entity is increasing in frequency. In reviewing four large series,[115,442–444] 78 lesions of this type were discovered from 1946 to 1975. Only eight of these were reported before 1957. Because most of these lesions arise in areas of severe atherosclerosis, males predominate by a ratio of 3:1, and the average age has been 65 years. The mean age for mycotic aneurysms that occur with IE is younger (approximately 40 years), and the sex distribution is nearly equal. Estimates of the incidence of mycotic aneurysms in patients with IE range up to 15 percent.[115,445] Approximately 3–4 percent of IE patients develop intracranial mycotic aneurysms.[446] These lesions remain a significant cause of morbidity and mortality due to intracerebral and subarachnoid hemorrhage, especially in young people in developing countries where acute rheumatic fever, rheumatic heart disease, and resultant IE are still prevalent.[447] Nine intracranial mycotic aneurysms associated with IE were treated in one neurosurgical unit in South Africa in a recent 18-month period, with five deaths.[447]

Pathogenesis

Four different mechanisms have been postulated to produce infection of the arterial wall: (*1*) embolomycotic aneurysms secondary to septic microemboli to the vasa vasorum, (*2*) extension from a contiguous infected focus, (*3*) hematogenous seeding of the intima during bacteremia originating from a distant infection, and (*4*) trauma to the arterial wall with direct contamination.[448] Embolomycotic aneurysms usually occur in patients with active IE, and the incidence of this type has declined in the antibiotic era. The source of infection is the cardiac vegetation with production of arterial emboli that lodge in the vasa vasorum, often at points of bifurcation of the affected artery. Contiguous foci of infection such as a caseous tuberculous lymph node or pyogenic vertebral osteomyelitis may extend directly to major vessels with subsequent aneurysm formation. The normal arterial intima is very resistant to infection. However, when this lining is altered by congenital malformations (e.g., coarctation of the aorta) or acquired disease (especially atherosclerotic plagues and/or ulcers), resistance to infection is lowered, and the surface may become colonized by blood-borne organisms. This hypothesis is analogous to the central role of nonbacterial thrombotic endocarditis in the pathogenesis of IE. An intraluminal thrombus associated with an atherosclerotic vessel may also serve as a nidus for colonization. Atherosclerosis accounts for over 74 percent of secondarily infected aneurysms. Luetic arteritis and cystic medical necrosis have also been associated with secondary infection.[442] Trauma to the arterial wall with subsequent infection has been associated with narcotic addicts due to needle trauma[449] as well as with gunshot wounds, vascular surgery, cardiac catheterization, and even puncture of a femoral artery for analysis of arterial blood gases.[438] These events, if associated with contamination, usually lead to pseudoaneurysm formation in a peripheral artery and a contiguous abscess in extravasated blood.

Pathologic Changes

Infection of the arterial tree has been recognized by pathologists for more than a century. Virchow first demonstrated local dilatation of the arterial wall at the site of a septic embolus in 1847. Infection superimposed on an atherosclerotic aorta was first reported by Koch in 1851. Stengel and Wolfroth[441] collected 217 cases of mycotic aneurysms in 1923. Since these lesions are probably underreported, pathologic material has been scant in recent years.

Most mycotic aneurysms that develop during the course of IE are situated in the sinus of Valsalva or in the supravalvular proximal thoracic aorta (>70 percent develop proximal to the aortic arch). Aneurysms are more frequent in the right and/or posterior sinus and may be complicated by acquired shunts (rupture into the right ventricle is most common site), tamponade, coronary artery occlusion, or an atrioventricular conduction block.[450] Less commonly major visceral, intracranial, and peripheral arteries are involved. Fewer than 10 percent are found in the upper extremities, but these arteries are usually not examined adequately by pathologic or radiologic techniques. Multiple lesions are identified in many IE patients with mycotic aneurysms.[451] Saccular forms appear to be more common than fusiform ones are.[440] The aneurysms vary in size from 1 mm to more than 10 cm. As mentioned before, many of these aneurysms arise from emboli to the vasa vasorum, and occasionally the embolus can be demonstrated grossly and microscopically. Acute and chronic inflammation is found diffusely through the arterial wall; necrosis, hemorrhage, abscess formation, and bacterial colonies may all be present in the sections. The elastica and muscularis layers are usually obliterated, but the intima is often intact. Rupture with surrounding hemorrhage and infection may be present.

Secondary infection of a pre-existing aneurysm is most commonly found in the abdominal aorta (70 percent of the cases) since this is the area most frequently and severely damaged by atherosclerosis. Ascending and descending aortic aneurysms each account for about 15 percent of the cases. The primary bacteremia most commonly originates from distal infections in soft tissue, lung, bone, or joint. The arterial infection usually begins in the distal abdominal aorta or iliac arteries as a focus of inflammation on an ulcerated atheromatous plaque. The wall of the aneurysm is thinned, and there is focal acute and chronic inflammation that may lead to arterial rupture. Even "bland" aortic aneurysms commonly have some mild inflammation (predominantly lymphocytes and mononuclear cells) in the wall; however, infected atherosclerotic aneurysms are characterized by acute polymorphonuclear inflammation, necrosis, abscess formation, hemorrhage, and visible bacterial colonies. This lesion is probably underreported since the focal suppuration may be limited in extent and overlooked unless routine culture and histologic sections are examined on every aortic aneurysm specimen. Erosion and rupture may be present without aneurysmal dilatation. Lumbar or thoracic osteomyelitis is present in up to one-third of the cases[442] and may either precede the aneurysm or develop secondary to contiguous spread from the vascular infection.

When contamination accompanies arterial injury, an infected pseudoaneurysm may result. These lesions are located in the extremities in over 80 percent of the cases and are characterized by more extensive local tissue inflammation than are the two types mentioned previously. Infection as a cause of pseudoaneurysm formation is increasing; 17 of 57 (30 percent) such lesions seen in the past decade[452] were infected.

Of special interest are mycotic aneurysms in renal transplant patients. In 640 renal transplants performed at the University of Minnesota over a period of 8 years, perinephric infections developed in 28 patients, and 8 of these developed mycotic aneurysms.[453] These lesions were evident clinically $1\frac{1}{2}$–4 months post-transplant. Six were located in the external iliac artery, with one each in the internal iliac artery and aorta. All these lesions were secondary to contiguous foci of infection in the deep tissues of the transplant wound.[453,454]

Clinical Manifestations

When mycotic aneurysms occur during the course of IE, manifestations of the underlying disease may be evident. Peripheral middle cerebral artery aneurysms constitute 2.5–6.2 percent of all intracranial aneurysms[445–447,455] and are usually secondary to infection. Intracranial mycotic aneurysms are usually clinically silent. When hemorrhage occurs, a sudden onset of severe headache with rapid deterioration in the level of consciousness is noted. The time interval from the diagnosis of IE to the onset of hemorrhage is variable (0–35 days) with a mean of 18 days.[446] Some of these lesions produce premonitory or "herald" neurologic findings including focal deficits and seizures. Unfortunately, these symptoms are relatively common in patients with IE without intracranial aneurysms, and the differential diagnosis as well as decisions regarding arteriography are difficult.[456] A sudden focal deficit consistent with embolism is seen in ≈23 percent of patients and should prompt arteriography.[456] Mycotic aneurysms tend to occur more commonly in females of a younger age than does IE in general. They must be differentiated from aneurysms secondary to tumor emboli (especially choriocarcinoma or atrial myxoma), trauma, arteritis, or moyamoya disease and from congenital aneurysms. Visceral artery aneurysms are uncommon but, when present, are almost uniformly due to infection[448] or polyarteritis nodosa. The most common location is in the superior mesenteric artery. Although superior mesenteric artery aneurysms account for only 8 percent of visceral artery aneurysms overall, most are of infectious etiology.[457] Symptoms include an acute onset of colicky abdominal pain, but the presentation is variable. Hepatic artery aneurysms may produce colicky right upper quadrant pain, fever, jaundice, and gastrointestinal hemorrhage.[458] There are over 190 cases of this entity reported in the literature; 75 percent were extrahepatic and 25 percent intrahepatic. When the external iliac artery is involved, a triad of clinical signs may be present: pain in the lower extremity (especially the anterior aspect of the thigh) with quadriceps muscle wasting and a depressed knee jerk, arterial insufficiency of the extremity with coolness, pallor, and depressed pulses, and bacteremia.[459] Distal aneurysms (e.g., femoral) occasionally present with unusual manifestations including arthritis and purpura in the affected limb.

When more peripheral arteries are involved (usually with a pseudoaneurysm), a tender diffusely indurated mass is present in 92 percent of cases. The mass is pulsatile with an associated bruit in 50–60 percent of patients, and approximately 20–30 percent are associated with decreased peripheral pulses, skin changes, or even frank gangrene.[454] Local suppuration, petechiae, and purpura are often present, and the lesion may be confused with localized cellulitis or an abscess without consideration of vascular involvement. In abusers of illicit drugs, 80 percent of mycotic aneurysms occur in the lower extremity, with the remainder in the radial, brachial, or occasionally carotid arteries. Only 50 percent of these patients are febrile on admission. A superimposed septic arthritis may also be present.[460]

Although most infected aortic atherosclerotic aneurysms occur in elderly men, there are no pathognomonic findings to separate these patients from those with bland uninfected aneurysms. Fever is a helpful differentiating sign (present in over 70 percent of the patients) since it is uncommon in patients with bland aneurysms. Back pain or abdominal pain each occur in about one-third of the cases. A draining cutaneous sinus may be present. Separation of an infected aneurysm from the entity of inflammatory abdominal aortic aneurysms may be difficult. Inflammatory abdominal aortic aneurysms were first described in 1935 and account for 5–10 percent of abdominal aortic aneurysms; the lesions are usually infrarenal and often lead to ureteral obstruction due to the densely adherent fibrotic mass surrounding the vessel.[461] In a large series of 2816 patients undergoing repair of abdominal aortic aneurysms, 127 (4.5 percent) had inflammatory abdominal aortic aneurysms.[462] Most patients (123/127) were men and heavy smokers. Inflammatory abdominal aortic aneurysms are associated with an elevated erythrocyte sedimentation rate (73 percent), weight loss, symptoms (back and/or abdominal pain in 30–50 percent), and a higher operative mortality. Continuing bacteremia despite "appropriate" antimicrobial therapy in an elderly (especially diabetic) patient with no signs of IE is suggestive of an infected intravascular site. The aneurysm is palpable in 50–60 percent of the cases.[444,448] In most cases, the onset is insidious, and a low-grade fever may be present for several months before diagnosis. The nonspecificity of the clinical manifestations is reflected by the 75 percent preoperative rupture rate for this entity. Rupture may occur into the retroperitoneal space or peritoneal cavity (56 percent), pleural cavity (9 percent), duodenum (12 percent), esophagus (6 percent), mediastinum (3 percent), or the pericardium (3 percent). The most common site of aortoenteric fistulas is between the aorta and the third portion of the duodenum. Short periods of "herald" bleeding are common warning signs before exsanguinating hemorrhage occurs.[463] Severe pain and the rapid onset of shock usually accompany rupture of the aneurysm.

Laboratory Findings

There are no characteristic laboratory abnormalities in this group of diseases. When mycotic aneurysms occur with IE, alterations suggesting the underlying disease may be present. Patients with infected aortic aneurysms usually demonstrate a leukocytosis (65–83 percent), but this is nonspecific and may be present when the aneurysm is bland. Bacteremia is found in 53 to >90 percent of the cases, is continuous, and usually does not clear with antibiotic therapy alone. Evidence for a primary source of bacteremia (e.g., pneumonia, osteomyelitis) may be evident but is absent in up to 46 percent of the cases.[442] The abdominal aorta is noted to be calcified on abdominal x-ray films in 47 percent,[444] and anterior vertebral body erosion has been demonstrated in 18 percent. A lack of calcification is suggestive of infection since 70–80 percent of bland aneurysms demonstrate this finding on abdominal x-ray films. Certain procedures (e.g., intravenous pyelography, sonography, computed tomography) may reveal the presence of an aneurysm but are often not satisfactory for preoperative detail. The absence of intimal calcification, an associated perianeurysmal fluid collection or osteomyelitis, or the sudden appearance of an aneurysm in a septic patient are all suggestive features of an infected abdominal aortic aneurysm by computed tomography.[464] Gas in the aortic wall is diagnostic, but rare. Although the sensitivity is unknown, ^{67}Ga and ^{111}In leukocyte imaging have been used to localize intra-arterial infections.[465] Nevertheless, preoperative angiography is often preferred to precisely delineate the extent of aneurysmal involvement.[466] This information may alter the operative approach and may minimize the complications. Two-dimensional or M-mode echocardiography is a very useful noninvasive technique for documenting mycotic aneurysms in the vicinity of the aortic valve, (e.g., sinus of Valsalva, supravalvular, subvalvular), and this technique is adjunctive to aortic root angiography preoperatively.[467] Intraoperative epicardial echocardiography has also been used to facilitate the surgical approach. When a hepatic aneurysm is suspected, liver scans and ultrasonography may be helpful before angiography.[458]

Etiologic Agents

Before the antibiotic era, mycotic aneurysms associated with IE were usually due to the more "virulent" organisms such as the β-hemolytic group A streptococci, pneumococci, or *H. influenzae*. With the decline of these organisms as causal agents in IE, most of these lesions are now due to streptococci or staphylococci and follow the incidence patterns outlined in Table 4 for the underlying disease.

When bacteria "seed" a pre-existing atherosclerotic vessel, the etiologic agents are markedly different from those found in mycotic aneurysms associated with IE. Gram-positive organisms cause approximately 60 percent of these lesions, but gram-negative (chiefly *Salmonella*) bacilli are isolated in 35 percent. Staphylococci are implicated in 40 percent of the cases overall,[444] and over two-thirds of these are *S. aureus*. Salmonellae cause 20 percent of the cases and involve, in order of frequency, the aorta and femoral and iliac arteries. Only 1 of 24 cases reported before 1974 was above the renal arteries.[468] Lumbar osteomyelitis due to *Salmonella* was present in one-third of cases. The presumed portal of entry is the gastrointestinal tract. *Salmonella enteritidis* strains are isolated in 40 percent of cases, which is proportional to their overall rate of isolation in the United States. *Salmonella chloreaesuis,* an uncommon clinical isolate, appears to be particularly pathogenic for this condition since this species was isolated in 32 percent of the cases.[469] *Salmonella typhi* is very rarely implicated in this disorder (one case report). *Salmonella* infections of aortic aneurysms were first reported in 1948. The predilection for involvement by this organism is not understood, but *Salmonella* organisms tend to "seed" abnormal tissues during bacteremia, e.g., hematomas, malignant tumors, cysts, gallstones, bone infarcts, and altered endothelium (aortic aneurysms). It has been estimated that 25 percent of patients over 50 years of age with *Salmonella* bacteremia have an intravascular focus of infection.[470] *Arizona* species (especially *A. hinshawii*) are closely related to *Salmonella* sp., cause similar clinical syndromes, and also infect aortic aneurysms in elderly diabetic males.[471] The following organisms also produce infection in atherosclerotic aneurysms: *E. coli, P. aeruginosa, Proteus* sp., *Citrobacter freundii, Klebsiella-Enterobacter* sp., *S. marcescens, Campylobacter fetus,*[472] *Listeria monocytogenes, Bacteroides fragilis,* gonococci, group A or C streptococci, diphtheroids, enterococci, and pneumococci. Fungal mycotic aneurysms are rare in the intracranial compartment, with only 13 definite cases reported by 1981.[473] The most common etiologic agents are *Aspergillus* sp., agents of mucormycoses, and *Candida* sp. The first two agents may involve intracranial arteries by direct extension from foci of sinusitis. One case of multiple intracranial aneurysms due to *Coccidioides immitis* that occurred during therapy for basilar meningitis has been described. Fungal mycotic aneurysms tend to involve larger, more proximal vessels at the base of the brain (11/18 [61 percent] carotid or basilar) than do bacterial causes with IE.[474] Tuberculous aneurysms are now uncommon and when present are due to contiguous foci of infection.

Pseudoaneurysms resulting from intra-arterial or perivascular injection of illicit street drugs, often in addicts with sclerosed veins due to repeated intravenous inoculation, are associated with contiguous abscesses. The causative agents are *S. aureus* (76 percent), *P. aeruginosa* (18 percent), and many others.[449]

Therapy

No uniformly acceptable approach has been devised for the treatment of mycotic aneurysms in IE. The treatment of intracranial mycotic aneurysms is particularly controversial. Some of these lesions appear to resolve with antimicrobial therapy alone. In a review of 56 aneurysms occurring in 45 patients,[475] 3 of 20 patients died when treated with antibiotics alone. Mild to moderate neurologic deficits were observed in 8 of the 17 survivors. Likewise, 6 of 25 patients treated with both antibiotics and surgery died, and 9 of 19 survivors were left with mild to moderate neurologic deficits. Others report a different experience with a higher mortality in the nonsurgical group,[446] but patients were selected only after subarachnoid hemorrhage had occurred. For example, in a review of 13 intracranial mycotic aneurysms,[446] 6/8 patients treated with antibiotics alone died, and no deaths were observed in the surgically treated group. In a review of 85 cases treated between 1954 and 1978, 20 of 38 patients treated solely with antibiotics died vs. 8 of 30 operated upon.[445] The distal location of most intracranial mycotic aneurysms associated with IE may permit ligation and excision with fewer complications when compared with surgery for berry aneurysms in the circle of Willis. Interestingly, the mortality rate was low in patients with multiple aneurysms (4/15) treated with antibiotics alone. In one series, the mortality was 29 percent after rupture of an intracranial mycotic aneurysm. The use of serial angiography may be useful in following these patients since the aneurysm(s) may change in size or new lesions may develop. In 21 patients subjected to serial angiography, the mycotic aneurysm increased in size in 5, did not change in 1, became smaller in 6, and completely resolved in 11, and new aneurysms developed in 2. Therefore, over 50 percent of these peripheral intracranial aneurysms resolved with antibiotic therapy alone during the treatment of IE.[475] Surgery is indicated for aneurysms increasing in size on repeat angiography[476,477] but may be deferred for 4–6 weeks for those remaining the same size (if the patient is an acceptable medical risk). The definitive treatment for aneurysms decreasing in size on repeat serial angiography every 2 weeks is unclear. Computed tomograpy is not helpful in localizing the aneurysm but provides important information if hematomas, infarcts, or abscesses develop. The antibiotics used are governed by the etiologic agent of the IE (see above).

Peripheral vessels are usually involved when arterial trauma (narcotic addict, gunshot wound, iatrogenic) results in pseudoaneurysm formation with infection. Therapy with antibiotics, proximal ligation of the vessel, resection of the pseudoaneurysm, and appropriate drainage result in cures in 75 percent of the cases. Vascular reconstruction through uninfected tissue planes with autogenous grafts is necessary when limb viability is dependent on the affected vessel. This is encountered more frequently in the lower extremity. For example, severe ischemia developed in 9 of 28 patients after excision of mycotic aneurysms of the common femoral artery[449] in one series of 52 cases. Amputation was required in only 11 percent of a large series of 54 aneurysms among drug addicts recently seen at the Henry Ford Hospital; there were no deaths.[478]

The mortality for patients with infected atherosclerotic aneurysms still exceeds 90 percent; approximately 40-long-term survivors have been reported since 1962.[469,479,482] A high index of suspicion is necessary to intervene surgically before rupture occurs since this complication is uniformly fatal and occurs in about 80 percent of the cases. When gram-negative bacilli are the cause of the infection, "early" (e.g., within 2 weeks after the first positive blood culture) rupture occurs much more frequently (84 percent) than if gram-positive bacteria are isolated (10 percent). Survival after surgery is also more common (75 percent) for patients with aneurysms infected with gram-positive cocci than for those with gram-negative bacilli (25 percent). Antibiotics should be used in this disease; but even if the lesion is sterilized (only one reported case), the aneurysm may still continue to enlarge and rupture, so therefore surgery is required. At surgery, the aneurysm and any intraluminal thrombus must be sectioned, Gram stained, and cultured. If infection is present, all aneurysmal tissue and surrounding inflammation must be resected before grafting. Basic principles of grafting in this situation include the use of autogenous rather than synthetic grafts and insertion only in clean noninfected tissue planes. If the graft is placed in the infected area, then continued infection, leakage, thrombus formation, abscess formation, and rupture usually result. Although some authorities have achieved a successful result by restoration of vascular continuity in situ after radical débridement,[479,481] this approach is not recommended in most cases. In a review of 24 patients with abdominal aortic aneurysms infected with *Salmonella* sp., 10 died after rupture without surgery, and another 7 patients survived grafting only to succumb to continued leakage from the anastomosis (only 5 were long-term survivors). If a graft is inserted in situ and persistent fever and bacteremia or emboli to the lower extremities ensue, reoperation with extra-anatomic grafting is mandatory. Since the resected area is contaminated, special bypass techniques (especially thoracoiliac, transpubic, or axillofemoral) are usually required. When an axillofemoral approach is used, a single graft should be inserted for both lower extremities since long-term patency is prolonged under these circumstances.[480,482] Bactericidal antibiotics should be continued for 6–8 weeks postoperatively, and peak serum bactericidal levels of at least 1:8 should be achieved. The actual agents used are dependent on the isolated organism (or the morphologic characteristics of the organisms in the surgical specimen) and on the results of in vitro susceptibility testing.

REFERENCES

1. Lerner PI, Weinstein L. Infective endocarditis in the antibiotic era. N Engl J Med. 1966;274:199.
2. Watanakunakorn C. Changing epidemiology and newer aspects of infective endocarditis. Adv Intern Med. 1977;22:21.
3. Von Reym CF, Levy BS, Arbeit RD, et al. Infective endocarditis: An analysis based on strict case definitions. Ann Intern Med. 1982;94:505.
4. Kaye D. Definitions and demographic characteristics. In: Kaye D, ed. Infective Endocarditis. Baltimore: University Park Press; 1976:1.
5. Durack DT, Petersdorf RG. Changes in the epidemiology of endocarditis. In: Kaplan EL, Taranta AV, eds. Infective Endocarditis. An American Heart Association Symposium. Dallas: American Heart Association; 1977:3.
6. Griffin MR, Wilson WR, Edwards WD, et al. Infective endocarditis. Olmsted County, Minnesota, 1950 through 1981. JAMA. 1985;254:1199–202.
7. King JW, Nguyen VQ, Conrad SA. Results of a prospective statewide reporting system for infective endocarditis. Am J Med Sci. 1988;295:517–27.
8. Shulman ST. Infective endocarditis: 1986. Pediatr Infect Dis. 1986;5:691–4.
9. Hayward GW. Infective endocarditis: A changing disease. Br Med J. 1973;2:706.
10. Anonymous (Editorial). Infective endocarditis. Br Med J. 1981;1:677.
11. Thayer WS. Studies on bacterial (infective) endocarditis. Johns Hopkins Hosp Rep. 1926;22:1.
12. Garvey GJ, Neu HC. Infective endocarditis: An evolving disease. Medicine (Baltimore). 1978;57:105.
13. Lien EA, Solberg CO, Kalager T. Infective endocarditis 1973–1984 at the Bergen University Hospital: Clinical feature, treatment and prognosis. Scand J Infect Dis. 1988;20:239–46.
14. Come PC. Infective endocarditis: Current perspectives. Compr Ther. 1982;8:57.
15. Pelletier LL, Petersdorf RG. Infective endocarditis: A review of 125 cases from the University of Washington Hospitals, 1963–72. Medicine (Baltimore). 1977;56:287.
16. Terpenning MS, Buggy BP, Kaufmann CA. Hospital-acquired infective endocarditis. Arch Intern Med. 1988;148:1601–3.
17. Cherubin CE, Neu HC. Infective endocarditis at the Presbyterian Hospital in New York City from 1938–1967. Am J Med. 1971;51:83.
18. Roberts WC, Buchbinder NA. Right-sided valvular infective endocarditis. A clinicopathologic study of 12 necropsy patients. Am J Med. 1972;53:7.
19. Kaye D. Changing pattern of infective endocarditis. Am J Med. 1985;78(Suppl 6B):157–62.
20. Roberts WC, Perloff JK, Constantin T. Severe valvular aortic stenosis in patients over 65 years of age. Am J Cardiol. 1971;27:497.
21. Delahaye JP, Loire R, Milon H, et al. Infective endocarditis on stenotic aortic valves. Eur Heart J. 1988;9(Suppl E):43–9.
22. McKinsey DS, Ratts TE, Bisno AL. Underlying cardiac lesions in adults with infective endocarditis. The changing spectrum. Am J Med. 1987;82:681–8.
23. Lowes JA, Hamer J, Williams G, et al. Ten years of infective endocarditis at St. Bartholomew's hospital: Analysis of clinical features and treatment in relation to prognosis and mortality. Lancet. 1980;1:133.
24. Moulsdale MT, Eykyn SJ, Phillips I. Infective endocarditis, 1970–1979. A study of culture-positive cases in St. Thomas' Hospital. Q J Med. 1980;49:315.
25. Venezio FR, Westenfelder GO, Cook FV, et al. Infective endocarditis in a community hospital. Arch Intern Med. 1982;142:789.
26. Fulkerson PK, Beaver BM, Avseon JC, et al. Calcification of the mitral annulus: Etiology, clinical associations, complications and therapy. Am J Med. 1979;66:967.
27. Cardelia JV, Befeler B, Hildner FJ, et al. Hypertrophic subaortic stenosis complicated by aortic insufficiency and subacute bacterial endocarditis. Am Heart J. 1971;81:543.
28. Wang K, Gobel FL, Gleason DF. Bacterial endocarditis in idiopathic hypertrophic subaortic stenosis, Am Heart J. 1975;89:359.
29. Chagnac A, Rudniki C, Loebel H, et al. Infectious endocarditis in idiopathic hypertrophic subaortic stenosis. Report of three cases and review of the literature. Chest. 1982;81:346.
30. Corrigan D, Bolen J, Hancock EW, et al. Mitral valve prolapse and infective endocarditis. Am J Med. 1977;63:215.
31. Jeresaty RM. Mitral valve prolapse—click syndrome. Prog Cardiovasc Dis. 1973;15:623.
32. Schutte JE, Gaffney FA, Blend L, et al. Distinctive anthropometric characteristics of women with mitral valve prolapse. Am J Med. 1981;71:533.
33. Clemens JD, Horwitz RI, Jaffe CC, et al. A controlled evaluation of the risk of bacterial endocarditis in persons with mitral-valve prolapse. N Engl J Med. 1982;307:776.
34. Nolan CM, Kane JJ, Grunow WA. Infective endocarditis and mitral prolapse. A comparison with other types of endocarditis. Arch Intern Med. 1981;141:447.
35. Scheld WM. Pathogenesis and pathophysiology of infective endocarditis. In: Sande MA, Kaye D, Root RK, eds. Endocarditis. v. 1. Contemporary Issues in Infectious Diseases. London: Churchill Livingston; 1984:1–32.
36. Freedman LR. The pathogenesis of infective endocarditis. J Antimicrob Chemother. 1987;20(Suppl A):1–6.
37. Weinstein L, Schlesinger JJ. Pathoanatomic, pathophysiologic, and clinical correlations in endocarditis (first of two parts). N Engl J Med. 1974;291:832.
38. Levison ME. Pathogenesis of infective endocarditis. In: Kaye D, ed. Infective Endocarditis. Baltimore: University Park Press; 1976:29.
39. Angrist AA, Oka M. Pathogenesis of bacterial endocarditis. JAMA. 1963;183:249.
40. Durack DT, Beeson PB. Pathogenesis of infective endocarditis. In: Rahimtoola SH, ed. Infective Endocarditis. New York: Grune & Stratton, 1978:1.
41. Durack DT, Beeson PB. Experimental bacterial endocarditis. I. Colonization of a sterile vegetation. Br J Exp Pathol. 1972;53:44.
42. Durack DT, Beeson PB, Petersdorf RG. Experimental endocarditis. III. Production and progress of the disease in rabbits. Br J Exp Pathol. 1973;54:142.
43. Durack DT. Experimental bacterial endocarditis. IV. Structure and function of very early lesions. J Pathol. 1975;115:81.
44. McGowan DA, Gillett R. Scanning electron microscopic observations of the surface of the initial lesion in experimental streptococcal endocarditis in the rabbit. Br J Exp Pathol. 1980;61:164.
45. Ferguson DJP, McColm AA, Ryan DM, et al. Experimental staphylococcal endocarditis and aortitis. Morphology of the initial colonization. Virchows Arch [A] 1986;410:43–8.
46. Sherwood BF, Rowlands DT, Vakilzadeh J, et al. Experimental bacterial endocarditis in the opossum (*Didelphis virginiana*). Am J Pathol. 1971;64:513.
47. Sande MA: Experimental endocarditis. In: Kaye D, ed. Infective Endocarditis. Baltimore: University Park Press; 1976:11.
48. Chino F, Kodama A, Otake M, et al: Nonbacterial thrombotic endocarditis in a Japanese autopsy sample. A review of 80 cases. Am Heart J. 1975;90:190.
49. Rodbard S. Blood velocity and endocarditis. Circulation. 1963;27:18.
50. Lepeschkin E. On the relation between the site of valvular involvement in endocarditis and the blood pressure resting on the valve. Am J Med Sci. 1952;224:318.
51. Okell CC, Elliott SD. Bacteraemia and oral sepsis. With special reference to the aetiology of subacute endocarditis. Lancet. 1935;2:869.
52. Everett ED, Hirschmann JV. Transient bacteremia and endocarditis prophylaxis: A review. Medicine (Baltimore). 1977;56:61.
53. Loesche WJ. Indigenous human flora and bacteremia. In: Kaplan EL, Taranta AV, eds. Infective Endocarditis. An American Heart Association Symposium. Dallas: American Heart Association; 1977:40.
54. Durack DT, Beeson PB. Protective role of complement in experimental *Escherichia coli* endocarditis. Infect Immun. 1977;16:213.
55. Yersin B, Glauser M-P, Guze L, et al. Experimental *Escherichia coli* endocarditis in rats: Roles of serum bactericidal activity and duration of catheter placement. Infect Immun. 1988;56:1273–80.
56. Gould K, Ramirez-Ronda CH, Holmes RK, et al. Adherence of bacteria to heart valves in vitro. J Clin Invest. 1975;56:1364.
57. Freedman LR, Valone J Jr. Experimental infective endocarditis. Prog Cardiovasc Dis. 1979;22:169.
58. Overholser CD, Moreillon P, Glauser MP. Experimental bacterial endocarditis after dental extractions in rats with periodontitis. J Infect Dis. 1987;155:107–12.
59. Moreillon P, Overholser CD, Malinverni R, et al. Predictors of endocarditis in isolates from cultures of blood following dentral extractions in rats with periodontal disease. J Infect Dis. 1988;157:990–5.
60. Gibbons RJ, Nygaard M. Synthesis of insoluble dextran and its significance in the formation of gelatinous deposits by plaque-forming streptococci. Arch Oral Biol. 1968;13:1249.
61. Parker MT, Ball LC. Streptococci and aerococci associated with systemic infection in man. J Med Microbiol. 1976;9:275.
62. Scheld WM, Valone JA, Sande MA. Bacterial adherence in the pathogenesis

of endocarditis. Interaction of bacterial dextran, platelets, and fibrin. J Clin Invest. 1978;61:1394.
63. Ramirez-Ronda CH. Adherence of glucan-positive and glucan-negative streptococcal strains to normal and damaged heart valves. J Clin Invest. 1978;62:805.
64. Ramirez-Ronda CH. Effects of molecular weight of dextran on the adherence of *Streptococcus sanguis* to damaged heart valves. Infect Immun. 1980;29:1.
65. Pelletier LL Jr, Coyle M, Petersdorf R. Dextran production as a possible virulence factor in streptococcal endocarditis. Proc Soc Exp Biol Med. 1978;158:415.
66. Crawford I, Russell C. Comparative adhesion of seven species of streptococci isolated from the blood of patients with subacute bacterial endocarditis to fibrin-platelet clots in vitro. J Appl Bacteriol. 1986;60:127–33.
67. Dall L, Barnes WG, Lane JW, et al. Enzymatic modification of glycocalyx in the treatment of experimental endocarditis due to viridans streptococci. J Infect Dis. 1987;156:736–40.
68. Scheld WM, Calderone RA, Alliegro GM, et al. Yeast adherence in the pathogenesis of *Candida* endocarditis. Proc Soc Exp Biol Med. 1981;168:208.
69. Scheld WM, Strunk RW, Balian G, et al. Microbial adhesion to fibronectin in vitro correlates with production of endocarditis in rabbits. Proc Soc Exp Biol Med. 1985;180:474–82.
70. Becker RC, DiBello PM, Lucas FV. Bacterial tissue tropism: An in vitro model for infective endocarditis. Cardiovasc Res. 1987;21:813–20.
71. Vercellotti G, Lussenhop D, Peterson PK, et al. Bacterial adherence to fibronectin and endothelial cells: A possible mechanism for bacterial tissue tropism. J Lab Clin Med. 1984;103:34–43.
72. Ogawa SK, Yurberg ER, Hatcher VB, et al. Bacterial adherence to human endothelial cells in vitro. Infect Immun. 1985;50:218–24.
73. Hamill RJ, Vann JM, Proctor RA. Phagocytosis of *Staphylococcus aureus* by cultured bovine aortic-endothelial cells: Model for post adherence events in endovascular infections. Infect Immun. 1986;54:833–6.
74. Scheld WM, Zak O, Vosbeck K, et al. Bacterial adhesion in the pathogenesis of endocarditis. Effect of subinhibitory antibiotic concentrations on streptococcal adhesion in vitro and the development of endocarditis in rabbits. J Clin Invest. 1981;68:1381.
75. Bernard J-P, Francioli P, Glauser MP, et al. Vancomycin prophylaxis of experimental *Streptococcus sanguis* endocarditis: Inhibition of bacterial adherence rather than bacterial killing. J Clin Invest. 1981;68:1113.
76. Glauser MP, Francioli P. Successful prophylaxis against experimental streptococcal endocarditis with bacteriostatic antibiotics. J Infect Dis. 1982;146:806.
77. Lowry FD, Chang DS, Neuhaus EG, et al. Effect of penicillin on the adherence of *Streptococcus sanguis* in vitro and in the rabbit model of endocarditis. J Clin Invest. 1983;71:668.
78. Glauser MP, Bernard JP, Moreillon P, et al. Successful single-dose amoxicillin prophylaxis against experimental streptococcal endocarditis. Evidence for two mechanisms of protection. J Infect Dis. 1983;147:568.
79. Clawson CC, Rao Gunda HR, White JG. Platelet interaction with bacteria. IV. Stimulation of the release reaction. Am J Pathol. 1975;81:411.
80. Herzberg MC, Brintzenhofe KL, Clawson CC. Aggregation of human platelets and adhesion of *Streptococcus sanguis*. Infect Immun. 1983;39:1457.
81. Sullam PM, Valone FH, Mills J. Mechanisms of platelet aggregation by viridans group streptococci. Infect Immun. 1987;55:1743–50.
82. Sullam PM, Jarvis GA, Valone FH. Role of immunoglobulin G in platelet aggregation by viridans group streptococci. Infect Immun. 1988;56:2907–11.
83. Ferguson DJP, McColm AA, Ryan DM, et al. A morphological study of experimental staphylococcal endocarditis and aortitis II. Inter-relationship of bacteria, vegetation and cardiovasculature in established infections. Br J Exp Pathol. 1986;67:679–86.
84. Durack DT, Beeson PB. Experimental bacterial endocarditis. II. Survival of bacteria in endocardial vegetations. Br J Exp Pathol. 1972;53:50.
85. Yersin BR, Glauser MP, Freedman LR. Effect of nitrogen mustard on natural history of right-sided streptococcal endocarditis: Role of cellular host defenses. Infect Immun. 1982;35:320.
86. Meddens MJM, Thompson J, Eulderink F, et al. Role of granulocytes in experimental *Streptococcus sanguis* endocarditis. Infect Immun. 1982;36:325.
87. Meddens MJM, Thompson J, Mattie H, et al. Role of granulocytes in the prevention and therapy of experimental *Streptococcus sanguis* endocarditis in rabbits. Antimicrob Agents Chemother. 1984;25:263–7.
88. Hook EW III, Sande MA. Role of the vegetation in experimental *Streptococcus viridans* endocarditis. Infect Immun. 1974;10:1433.
89. Thorig L, Thompson J, Eulderink F, et al. Effects of monocytopenia and anticoagulation in experimental *Streptococcus sanguis* endocarditis. Br J Exp Pathol. 1980;61:108.
90. van Ginkel CJW, Thorig L, Thompson J, et al. Enhancement of generation of monocyte tissue thromboplastin by bacterial phagocytosis: Possible pathway for fibrin formation on infected vegetations in bacterial endocarditis. Infect Immun. 1979;25:388.
91. Drake TA, Rodgers GM, Sande MA. Tissue factor is a major stimulus for vegetation formation in enterococcal endocarditis in rabbits. J Clin Invest. 1984;73:1750–3.
92. Drake TA, Pang M. *Staphylococcus aureus* induces tissue factor expression in cultured human cardiac valve endothelium. J Infect Dis. 1988;157:749–56.
93. Mair W. Pneumococcal endocarditis in rabbits. J Pathol Bacteriol. 1923;26:426.
94. Scheld WM, Thomas JH, Sande MA. Influence of preformed antibody on experimental *Streptococcus sanguis* endocarditis. Infect Immun. 1979; 25:781.
95. Durack DT, Gilliland BC, Petersdorf RG. Effect of immunization on susceptibility to experimental *Streptococcus mutans* and *Streptococcus sanguis* endocarditis. Infect Immun. 1978;22:52.
96. Scheld WM, Calderone RA, Brodeur JP, et al. Influence of preformed antibody on the pathogenesis of experimental *Candida albicans* endocarditis. Infect Immun. 1983;40:950.
97. Greenberg DP, Ward JI, Bayer AS. Influence of *Staphylococcus aureus* antibody on experimental endocarditis in rabbits. Infect Immun. 1987; 55:3030–4.
98. Williams RC, Kunkel HG. Rheumatoid factors and their disappearance following therapy in patients with SBE. Arthritis Rheum. 1962;5:126.
99. Sheagren JN, Tuazon CV, Griffin C, et al. Rheumatoid factor in acute bacterial endocarditis. Arthritis Rheum. 1976;19:887.
100. Phair JP, Clarke J. Immunology of infective endocarditis. Prog Cardiovasc Dis. 1979;22:137.
101. Bacon PA, Davidson C, Smith B. Antibodies to *Candida* and autoantibodies in subacute bacterial endocarditis. Q J Med. 1974;43:537.
102. Laxdal T, Messner RP, Williams RC. Opsonic, agglutinating, and complement-fixing antibodies in patients with subacute bacterial endocarditis. J Lab Clin Med. 1968;71:638.
103. Horwitz D, Quismorio FP, Friou GJ. Cryoglobulinemia in patients with infectious endocarditis. Clin Exp Immunol. 1975;19:131.
104. Bayer AS, Theofilopoulos AN, Eisenberg R, et al. Circulating immune complexes in infective endocarditis. N Engl J Med. 1976;295:1500.
105. Gutman RA, Striker GE, Gilliland BC, et al. The immune complex glomerulonephritis of bacterial endocarditis. Medicine (Baltimore). 1972;51:1.
106. Levy RL, Hong R. The immune nature of subacute bacterial endocarditis (SBE) nephritis. Am J Med. 1973;54:645.
107. Inman RD, Redecha PB, Knechtle SJ, et al. Identification of bacterial antigens in circulating immune complexes of infective endocarditis. J Clin Invest. 1982;70:271.
108. Alpert JS, Krous HF, Dalen JE, et al. Pathogenesis of Osler's nodes. Ann Intern Med. 1976;85:471.
109. Lowenstein MB, Urman JD, Abeles M, et al. Skin immunofluorescence in infective endocarditis. JAMA. 1977;238:1163.
110. Cabane J, Godeau P, Herreman G, et al. Fate of circulating immune complexes in infective endocarditis. Am J Med. 1979;66:277.
111. Kauffman RH, Thompson J, Valentijn RM, et al. The clinical implications and the pathogenetic significance of circulating immune complexes in infective endocarditis. Am J Med. 1981;71:17.
112. Krause JR, Levison SP. Pathology of infective endocarditis. In: Kaye D, ed. Infective Endocarditis. Baltimore: University Park Press; 1976:55.
113. Roberts WC. Characteristics and consequences of infective endocarditis (active or healed or both) learned from morphologic studies. In: Rahimtoola SH, ed. Infective Endocarditis. New York: Grune & Stratton: 1978;55.
114. Morel-Maroger L, Sraer JD, Herreman G, et al. Kidney in subacute endocarditis. Pathological and immunofluorescence findings. Arch Pathol. 1913;94:205.
115. Anderson CB, Butcher HR, Ballinger WF. Mycotic aneurysms. Arch Surg. 1974;109:712.
116. Greenlee JE, Mandell GL. Neurological manifestations of infective endocarditis: A review. Stroke. 1973;4:958.
117. Kerr A Jr, Tan JS. Biopsies of the Janeway lesion of infective endocarditis. J Cutan pathol. 1979;6:124.
118. Silverberg HH. Roth spots. Mt Sinai J Med. 1970;37:77.
119. Starkebaum M, Durack D, Beeson P. The "incubation period" of subacute bacterial endocarditis. Yale J Biol Med. 1977;50:49.
120. Weinstein L, Rubin RH. infective endocarditis—1973. Progr Cardiovasc Dis. 1973;16:239.
121. Freedman LR. Infective endocarditis and other intravascular infections. In: Braude AI, David CE, Fierer J, eds. Medical Microbiology and Infectious Diseases. Philadelphia: WB Saunders; 1981:1511.
122. Hermans PE. The clinical manifestations of infective endocarditis. Mayo Clin Proc. 1982;57:15.
123. Terpenning MS, Buggy BP, Kauffman CA. Infective endocarditis: Clinical features in young and elderly patients. Am J Med. 1987;83:626–34.
124. Espersen F, Frimodt-Moller N. *Staphylococcus aureus* endocarditis. A review of 119 cases. Arch Intern Med. 1986;146:1118–21.
125. Churchill MA, Geraci JE, Hunder GG. Musculoskeletal manifestations of bacterial endocarditis. Ann Intern Med. 1977;87:754.
126. Lerner PI. Neurologic complications of infective endocarditis. Med Clin North Am. 1985;69:385–98.
127. Bayer AS, Theofilopaulos AN, Eisenberg R, et al. Thrombotic thrombocytopenic purpura-like syndrome associated with infective endocarditis. A possible immune complex disorder. JAMA. 1977;238:408.
128. Levine DP, Crane LR, Zervos MJ. Bacteremia in narcotic addicts at the Detroit Medical Center II. Infectious endocarditis: A prospective comparative study. Rev Infect Dis. 1986;8:374–96.
129. Marantz PR, Linzer M, Feiner CJ, et al. Inability to predict diagnosis in febrile intravenous drug abusers. Ann Intern Med. 1987;106:823–8.

130. Chambers HF, Morris DL, Tauber MG, et al. Cocaine use and the risk for endocarditis in intravenous drug users. Ann Intern Med. 1987;106:833–6.
131. Chambers HF, Korzeniowski OM, Sande MA, et al. *Staphylococcus aureus* endocarditis: Clinical manifestations in addicts and nonaddicts. Medicine (Baltimore). 1983;62:170.
132. Sklaver AR, Hoffman TA, Greenman RL. Staphylococcal endocarditis in addicts. South Med J. 1978;71:638.
133. Thadepalli H, Francis CK. Diagnostic clues in metastatic lesions of endocarditis in addicts. West J Med. 1978;128:1.
134. McCartney AC, Orange GV, Pringle SD, et al. Serum C reactive protein in infective endocarditis. J Clin Pathol. 1988;41:44–8.
135. Wiseman J, Rouleau J, Rigo P, et al. Gallium-67 myocardial imaging for the detection of bacterial endocarditis. Radiology. 1976;120:135.
136. Wong DW, Dhawan VK, Tanaka T, et al. Imaging endocarditis with technitium 99m-labeled antibody—an experimental study: Concise communication. J Nucl Med. 1982;23:229.
137. Riba AL, Thakur ML, Gottschalk A, et al. Imaging experimental infective endocarditis with indium-111-labeled blood cellular components. Circulation. 1979;59:336.
138. Haft JI, Altieri J, Smight LG, et al. Computed tomography of the abdomen in the diagnosis of splenic emboli. Arch Intern Med. 1988;148:193–7.
139. Beeson PB, Brannon ES, Warren JV. Observations on the sites of removal of bacteria from the blood of patients with bacterial endocarditis. J Exp Med. 1945;81:9–23.
140. Werner AS, Cobbs CG, Kaye D, et al. Studies on the bacteremia of bacterial endocarditis. JAMA. 1967;202:199.
141. Pazin GJ, Saul S, Thompson ME. Blood culture positivity. Suppression by outpatient antibiotic therapy in patients with bacterial endocarditis. Arch Intern Med. 1982;142:263.
142. McKenzie R, Reimer LG. Effect of antimicrobials on blood cultures in endocarditis. Diagn Microbiol Infect Dis. 1987;8:165–72.
143. Aronson MD, Bos DH. Blood cultures. Ann Intern Med. 1987;106:246–53.
144. Washington JA II, Ilstrup DM. Blood cultures: Issues and controversies. Rev Infect Dis. 1986;8:792–802.
145. Washington JA II. The role of the microbiology laboratory in the diagnosis and antimicrobial treatment of infective endocarditis. Mayo Clin Proc. 1982;57:22.
146. Carey RB, Gross KC, Roberts RB. Vitamin-B_6–dependent *Streptococcus mitior* (*mitis*) isolated from patients with systemic infections. J Infect Dis. 1975;131:722.
147. Powers DL, Mandell GL. Intraleucocytic bacteria in endocarditis patients. JAMA. 1974;227:313.
148. Whitcomb DC. Bugs in the blood: Acute staphylococcal septicemia and endocarditis diagnosed by staining the buffy coat. NC Med J. 1986;47:293–5.
149. Tuazon CU, Sheagren JW. Teichoic acid antibodies in the diagnosis of serious infections with *Staphylococcus aureus*. Ann Intern Med. 1976;84:543.
150. Bayer AS, Tillman DB, Concepcion M, et al. Clinical value of teichoic acid antibody titers in the diagnosis and management of staphylococcemias. West J Med. 1980;132:294.
151. Kaplan JE, Palmer DL, Tung KSK. Teichoic acid antibody and circulating immune complexes in the management of *Staphylococcus aureus* bacteremia. Am J Med. 1981;70:769.
152. Arbeit RD, Nelles MJ. Capsular polysaccharide antigenemia in rats with experimental endocarditis due to *Staphylococcus aureus*. J Infect Dis. 1987;155:242–6.
153. Cannady PB, Sanford JP. Negative blood cultures in infective endocarditis. A review. South Med J. 1976;69:1420.
154. Walker RC, Henry NK, Washington JA II, et al. Lysis-centrifugation blood culture technique. Clinical impact in *Staphylococcus aureus* bacteremia. Arch Intern Med. 1986;146:2341–3.
155. Washington JA II. The microbiological diagnosis of infective endocarditis. J Antimicrob Chemother. 1987;20(Suppl A):29–36.
156. Austin SM, Smith SM, Co B, et al. Case report: Serologic evidence of acute murine typhus infection in a patient with culture-negative endocarditis. Am J Med Sci. 1987;293:320–3.
157. Tompkins LS, Roessler BJ, Redd SC, et al. *Legionella* prosthetic-valve endocarditis. N Engl J Med. 1988;318:530–5.
158. Walterspiel JN, Kaplan SL. Incidence and clinical characteristics of "culture-negative" infective endocarditis in a pediatric population. Pediatr Infect Dis. 1986;5:328–32.
159. Rubenstein E, Noreiga ER, Simberkoff MS, et al. Fungal endocarditis: Analysis of 24 cases and review of the literature. Medicine (Baltimore). 1975;54:331.
160. Kobza K, Steenblock U. Demonstration of candida in blood smears. Br Med J. 1977;1:1640.
161. Merz WG, Evans GL, Shadomy S, et al. Laboratory evaluation of serological tests for systemic candidiasis: A cooperative study. J Clin Microbiol. 1977;5:596.
162. Sande MA, Bowman CR, Calderone RA. Experimental *Candida albicans* endocarditis: Characterization of the disease and response to therapy. Infect Immun. 1977;17:140.
163. Warren RC, Bartlett A, Bidwell DE, et al. Diagnosis of invasive candidosis by enzyme immunoassay of serum antigen. Br Med J. 1977;1:1183.
164. Scheld WM, Brown RS Jr, Harding SA, et al. Detection of circulating antigen in experimental *Candida albicans* endocarditis by an enzyme-linked immunosorbent assay. J Clin Microbiol. 1980;12:679.
165. Dillan JC, Feigenbaum H, Konecke LL, et al. Echocardiographic manifestations of valvular vegetations. Am Heart J. 1973;86:698.
166. Boucher CA, Fallion JT, Myers GS, et al. The value and limitations of echocardiography in recording mitral valve vegetations. Am Heart J. 1977;94:37.
167. Thomson KR, Nanda NC, Gramiak R. The reliability of echocardiography in the diagnosis of infective endocarditis. Radiology. 1977;125:473.
168. Melvin ET, Berger M, Lutzker LG, et al. Noninvasive methods for detection of valve vegetations in infective endocarditis. Am J Cardiol. 1981;47:271.
169. Mintz GS, Kotler MN. Clinical value and limitations of echocardiography. Its use in the study of patients with infectious endocarditis. Arch Intern Med. 1980;140:1022.
170. Popp RL. Echocardiography and infectious endocarditis. In: Remington JS, Swartz MN, eds. Current Clinical Topics in Infectious Diseases. v. 4. New York: McGraw-Hill; 1983:98.
171. Davis RS, Strom JA, Frishman W, et al. The demonstration of vegetations by echocardiography in bacterial endocarditis. An indication for early surgical intervention. Am J Med. 1980;57:69.
172. Martin RP, Mettzer RS, Chia EL, et al. Clinical utility of two-dimensional echocardiography in infective endocarditis. Am J Cardiol. 1980;46:379.
173. Bayer AS, Blomquist IK, Bello E, et al. Tricuspid valve endocarditis due to *Staphylococcus aureus*. Correlation of two-dimensional echocardiography with clinical outcome. Chest. 1988;93:247–53.
174. Manolis AS, Melita H. Echocardiographic and clinical correlates in drug addicts with infective endocarditis. Implications of vegetation size. Arch Intern Med. 1988;148:2461–5.
175. Tak T, Rahimtoola SH, Kumar A, et al. Value of digital image processing of two-dimensional echocardiograms in differentiating active from chronic vegetations of infective endocarditis. Circulation. 1988;78:116–23.
176. Mann T, McLaurin L, Grossman W, et al. Assessing the hemodynamic severity of acute aortic regurgitation due to infective endocarditis. N Engl J Med. 1975;293:108.
177. Mills J, Abbott J, Utley JR, et al. Role of cardiac catheterization in infective endocarditis. Chest. 1977;72;576.
178. Welton DE, Young JB, Raizner AE, et al. Value and safety of cardiac catheterization during active infective endocarditis. Am J Cardiol. 1979;44:1306.
179. Sussman JI, Baron EJ, Tenenbaum MJ, et al. Viridans streptococcal endocarditis: Clinical, microbiological, and echocardiographic correlations. J Infect Dis. 1986;154:597–603.
180. Roberts RB, Krieger AG, Schiller NL, et al. Viridans streptococcal endocarditis: The role of various species, including pyridoxal-dependent streptococci. Rev Infect Dis. 1979;1:955.
181. Tuazon CV, Gill V, Gill F. Streptococcal endocarditis: Single vs. combination antibiotic therapy and the role of various species. Rev Infect Dis. 1986;8:54–60.
182. Baddour LM, Bisno AL. Infective endocarditis complicating mitral valve prolapse: Epidemiologic, clinical, and microbiologic aspects. Rev Infect Dis. 1986;8:117–37.
183. Harder EJ, Wilkowske CJ, Washington JA, et al. *Streptococcus mutans* endocarditis. Ann Intern Med. 1974;80:364.
184. Watanakunakorn C. *Streptococcus bovis* endocarditis. Am J Med. 1974;56:256.
185. Moellering RC, Watson BK, Kunz LJ. Endocarditis due to group D streptococci. Comparison of disease caused by *Streptococcus bovis* with that produced by the enterococci. Am J Med. 1974;57:239.
186. Hoppes WL, Lerner PI. Nonenterococcal group D streptococcal endocarditis caused by *Streptococcus bovis*. Ann Intern Med. 1974;81:588.
187. Klein RS, Reuco RA, Catalano MT, et al. Association of *Streptococcus bovis* with carcinoma of the colon. N Engl J Med. 1977;297:800.
188. Steinberg D, Naggar CZ. *Streptococcus bovis* endocarditis with carcinoma of the colon. N Engl J Med. 1977;297:1354.
189. Mandell GL, Kaye D, Levison ME, et al. Enterococcal endocarditis: An analysis of 38 patients observed at the New York Hospital–Cornell Medical Center. Arch Intern Med. 1970;125:258.
190. Serra P, Brandimarte C, Martino P, et al. Synergistic treatment of enterococcal endocarditis. Arch Intern Med. 1977;137:1562.
191. Malone DA, Wagner RA, Myers JP, et al. Enterococcal bacteremia in two large community teaching hospitals. Am J Med. 1986;81:601–6.
192. Hoffmann SA, Moellering RC Jr. The enterococcus: "Putting the bug in our ears." Ann Intern Med. 1987;106:757–61.
193. Maki DG, Agger WA. Enterococcal bacteremia: Clinical features, the risk of endocarditis, and management. Medicine (Baltimore).1988;67:248–69.
194. Ugolini V, Pacifico A, Smitherman TC, et al. Pneumococcal endocarditis update: Analysis of 10 cases diagnosed between 1974 and 1984. Am Heart J. 1986;112:813–19.
195. Powderly WG, Stanley SL Jr, Medoff G. Pneumococcal endocarditis: Report of a series and review of the literature. Rev Infect Dis. 1986;8:786–91.
196. Carey RB, Brause BD, Roberts RB: Antimicrobial therapy of vitamin B_6-dependent streptococcal endocarditis. Ann Intern Med. 1977;87:150.
197. Stein DS, Nelson KE. Endocarditis due to nutritionally deficient streptococci: Therapeutic dilemna. Rev Infect Dis. 1987;9:908–16.
198. Catto BA, Jacobs MR, Shlaes DM. *Streptococcus mitis*. A cause of serious infection in adults. Arch Intern Med. 1987;147:885–8.
199. Rapeport KB, Giron JA, Rosner F. *Streptococcus mitis* endocarditis. Report of 17 cases. Arch Intern Med. 1986;146:2361–3.
200. Hager WD, Speck EL, Mathew PK, et al. Endocarditis with myocardial

abscesses and pericarditis in an adult. Group B streptococcus as a cause. Arch Intern Med. 1977;137:1725.
201. Opal SM, Cross A, Palmer M, et al. Group B streptococcal sepsis in adults and infants. Contrasts and comparisons. Arch Intern Med. 1988;148:641–5.
202. Gallagher PG, Watanakunakorn C. Group B streptococcal endocarditis: Report of seven cases and review of the literature, 1962–1985. Rev Infect Dis. 1986;8:175–88.
203. Scully BE, Spriggs D, Neu HC. *Streptococcus agalactiae* (Group B) endocarditis—a description of twelve cases and review of the literature. Infection. 1987;15:169–76.
204. Wiseman A, Rene P, Crelinsten GL. *Streptococcus agalactiae* endocarditis: An association with villous adenonas of the large intestine. Ann Intern Med. 1985;103:893–4.
205. Venezio FR, Gullberg RM, Westenfelder GO, et al. Group G streptococcal endocarditis and bacteremia. Am J Med. 1986;81:29–34.
206. Smyth EG, Pallett AP, Davidson RN. Group G streptococcal endocarditis: Two case reports, a review of the literature and recommendations for treatment. J Infect. 1988;16:169–76.
207. Murray HW, Gross KC, Masur H, et al. Serious infections caused by *Streptococcus milleri*. Am J Med. 1978;64:759.
208. Shlaes DM, Lerner PI, Wolinsky E, et al. Infections due to Lancefield group F and related streptococci (*S. milleri, S. anginosus*). Medicine (Baltimore). 1981;60:197.
209. Gossling J. Occurence and pathogenicity of the *Streptococcus milleri* group. Rev Infect Dis. 1988;10:257–85.
210. Hosea SW: Virulent *Streptococcus viridans* bacterial endocarditis. Am Heart J. 1981;101:174.
211. Buu-Joi A, Sapoetra A, Branger C, et al. Antimicrobial susceptibility of *Gemella haemolysans* isolated from patients with subacute endocarditis. Eur J Clin Microbiol. 1982;1:102.
212. Mylotte JM, McDermott C, Spooner JA. Prospective study of 114 consecutive episodes of *Staphylococcus aureus* bacteremia. Rev Infect Dis. 1987;9:891–908.
213. Eykyn SJ. Staphylococcal sepsis. The changing pattern of disease and therapy. Lancet. 1988;1:100–4.
214. Watanakunakorn C, Tan JS, Phair JP. Some salient features of *Staphylococcus aureus* endocarditis. Am J Med. 1973;54:473.
215. Musher DM, McKenzie SO. infection due to *Staphylococcus aureus*. Medicine (Baltimore). 1977;56:383.
216. Bayer AS. Staphylococcal bacteremia and endocarditis. State of the art. Arch Intern Med. 1982;142:1169.
217. Thompson RL. Staphylococcal infective endocarditis. Mayo Clin Proc. 1982;57:106.
218. Julander I. Unfavourable prognostic factors in *Staphylococcus aureus* septicemia and endocarditis. Scand J Infect Dis. 1985;17:179–87.
219. O'Callaghan C, McDougall P. Infective endocarditis in neonates. Arch Dis Child. 1988;63:53–7.
220. Crane LR, Levine DP, Zervos MJ, et al. Bacteremia in narcotic addicts at the Detroit Medical Center. I. Microbiology, epidemiology, risk factors, and empiric therapy. Rev Infect Dis. 1986;8:364–73.
221. Noel GJ, O'Loughlin JE, Edelson PJ. Neonatal *Staphylococcus epidermidis* right-sided endocarditis: Description of five catheterized infants. Pediatrics. 1988;82:234–9.
222. Baddour LM, Phillips TN, Bisno AL. Coagulase-negative staphylococcal endocarditis. Occurrence in patients with mitral valve prolapse. Arch Intern Med. 1986;146:119–21.
223. Harris LF, O'Shields H. Coagulase-negative staphylococcal endocarditis: A view from the community hospital. South Med J. 1986;79:1379–86.
224. Caputo GM, Archer GL, Calderwood SB, et al. Native valve endocarditis due to coagulase-negative staphylococci. Clinical and microbiologic features. Am J Med. 1987;83:619–25.
225. Espersen F, Wheat LJ, Bemis AT, et al. Solid-phase radio-immunoassay for IgG antibodies to *Staphylococcus epidermidis:* Use in serious coagulase-negative staphylococcal infections. Arch Intern Med. 1987;147:689–93.
226. Etienne J, Brun Y, El Solh N, et al. Characterization of clinically significant isolates of *Staphylococcus epidermidis* from patients with endocarditis. J Clin Microbiol. 1988;26:613–7.
227. Baddour LM, Simpson WA, Weems JJ Jr, et al. Phenotypic selection of small-colony variant forms of *Staphylococcus epidermidis* in a rat model of endocarditis. J Infect Dis. 1988;157:757–63.
228. Finland M, Barnes MW. Changing etiology of bacterial endocarditis in the antibacterial era. Experiences at Boston City Hospital 1933–1965. Ann Intern Med. 1970;72:341.
229. Pedersen FK, Petersen EA. Bacterial endocarditis of Blegdamshospitalet in Copenhagen 1944–1973. Scand J Infect Dis. 1976;8:99.
230. Cohen PS, Maquire JH, Weinstein L. Infective endocarditis caused by gram-negative bacteria: A review of the literature, 1945–1977. Prog Cardiovasc Dis. 1980;22:205.
231. Geraci JE, Wilson WR. Endocarditis due to gram-negative bacteria. Report of 56 cases. Mayo Clin Proc. 1982;57:145.
232. Snyder N, Atterbury CE, Correia JP, et al. Increased occurrence of cirrhosis and bacterial endocarditis. Gastroenterology. 1977;73:1107.
233. Carruthers M. Endocarditis due to enteric bacilli other than salmonellae: Case reports and literature review. Am J Med Sci. 1977;273:203.
234. Sande MA, Johnson WD, Hook EW, et al. Sustained bacteremia in patients with prosthetic cardiac valves. N Engl J Med. 1972;286:1067.
235. Schneider PJ, Nernoff J, Gold JA. Acute salmonella endocarditis. Report of a case and review. Arch Intern Med. 1967;120:478.
236. Mills J, Drew D. *Serratia marcescens* endocarditis. Ann Intern Med. 1976;85:397.
237. Cooper R, Mills J. *Serratia* endocarditis. A follow-up report. Arch Intern Med. 1980;140:199.
238. Caramelli B, Mansur AJ, Grinberg M, et al. *Campylobacter fetus* endocarditis on a prosthetic heart valve. South Med J. 1988;81:802–3.
239. Reyes MP, Brown WJ, Lerner AM. Treatment of patients with *Pseudomonas* endocarditis with high dose aminoglycoside and carbenicillin therapy. Medicine (Baltimore). 1978;57:57.
240. Reyes MP, Lerner AM. Current problems in the treatment of infective endocarditis due to *Pseudomonas aeruginosa*. Rev Infect Dis. 1983;5:314.
241. Wieland M, Lederman MM, Kline-King C, et al. Left-sided endocarditis due to *Pseudomonas aeruginosa*. A report of 10 cases and review of the literature. Medicine (Baltimore). 1986;65:180–9.
242. Noriega ER, Rubinstein E, Simberkoff M, et al. Subacute and acute endocarditis due to *Pseudomonas cepacia* in heroin addicts. Am J Med. 1975;59:29.
243. Reyes MP, Palutke WA, Wylin RF, et al. *Pseudomonas* endocarditis in the Detroit Medical Center 1969–1972. Medicine (Baltimore). 1973;52:173.
244. Jurica JV, Bomzer CA, England AC III. Gonococcal endocarditis: A case report and review of the literature. Sex Trans Dis. 1987;14:231–3.
245. Dover D, Danzinger Y, Pinkhaus J. *Neisseria catarrhalis* endocarditis. Ann Intern Med. 1977;86:116.
246. Davis CL, Towns M, Henrich WL, et al. *Neisseria mucosus* endocarditis following durg abuse. Case report and review of the literature. Arch Intern Med. 1983;143:583.
247. Chunn CJ, Jones SR, McCutchan JA, et al. *Haemophilus parainfluenzae* infective endocarditis. Medicine (Baltimore). 1977;56:99.
248. Lynn DJ, Kane JG, Parker RH. *Haemophilus parainfluenzae* and influenzae endocarditis: A review of forty cases. Medicine (Baltimore). 1977;56:115.
249. Geraci JE, Wilkowske CJ, Wilson WR, et al. *Haemophilus* endocarditis. Report of 14 cases. Mayo Clin Proc. 1977;52:209.
250. Parker SW, Apicella MA, Fuller CM. *Hemophilus* endocarditis. Two patients with complications. Arch Intern Med. 1983;143:48.
251. Bangsborg JM, Tuede M, Skinhoj P. *Haemophilus seguis* endocarditis. J Infect. 1988;16:81–5.
252. Porath A, Wanderman K, Simu A, et al. Case report: Endocarditis caused by *Haemophilus aegyptius*. Am J Med Sci. 1986;292:110–11.
253. Vandepitte J, DeGeest H, Jousten P. Subacute bacterial endocarditis due to *Actinobacillus actinomycetemcomitans*. Report of a case with a review of the literature. J Clin Pathol. 1977;30:842.
254. AhFat LNC, Patel BR, Pickens S. *Actinobacillus actinomycetemcomitans* endocarditis in hypertrophic obstructive cardiomyopathy. J Infect Dis. 1983;6:81.
255. Lane T, MacGregor RR, Wright D, et al. *Cardiobacterium hominis:* An elusive cause of endocarditis. J Infect. 1983;6:75.
256. Jenny DB, Letendre PW, Iverson G. Endocarditis due to *Kingella* species. Rev Infect Dis. 1988;10:1065–6.
257. Decker MD, Graham BS, Hunter EB, et al. Endocarditis and infections of intravascular devices due to *Eikinella corrodens*. Am J Med Sci. 1986;292:209–12.
258. Ellner JJ, Rosenthal MS, Lerner PI, et al. Infective endocarditis caused by slow-growing, fastidious, gram-negative bacteria. Medicine (Baltimore). 1979;58:145.
259. Gerry JL, Greenough WB. Diptheroid endocarditis: Report of nine cases and review of the literature. Johns Hopkins Med J. 1976;139:61.
260. Bayer AS, Chow AW, Guze LB. *Listeria monocytogenes* endocarditis: Report of a case and review of the literature. Am J Med Sci. 1977; 273:319.
261. Carvajal A, Frederiksen W. Fatal endocarditis due to *Listeria monocytogenes*. Rev Infect Dis. 1988;10:616–23.
262. Sussman JI, Baron EJ, Goldberg SM, et al. Clinical manifestations and therapy of *Lactobacillus* endocarditis: Report of a case and review of the literature. Rev Infect Dis. 1986;8:771–6.
263. Gorby GL, Peacock JE Jr. *Erysipelothrix rhusiopathiae* endocarditis: Microbiologic, epidemiologic, and clinical features of an occupational disease. Rev Infect Dis. 1988;10:317–25.
264. Shands JW Jr. *Rothia dentocariosa* endocarditis. Am J Med. 1988;85:280–1.
265. Felner JM, Dowell UR. Anaerobic bacterial endocarditis. N Engl J Med. 1970;283:1188.
266. Nastro LJ, Finegold SM. Endocarditis due to anaerobic gram-negative bacilli. Am J Med. 1973;54:482.
267. Nastro FL, Sarma RJ. Infective endocarditis due to anaerobic and microaerophilic bacteria. West J Med. 1982;137:18.
268. Jackson RT, Dopp AC. *Bacteroides fragilis* endocarditis. South Med J. 1988;81:781–2.
269. Al-Kasab S, Fagih MR, Al-Yousef S, et al. *Brucella* infective endocarditis. Successful combined medical and surgical therapy. J Thorac Cardiovasc Surg. 1988;95:862–7.
270. Tuazon CW, Hill R, Sheagren JW. Microbiologic study of street heroin and injection paraphenalia. J Infect Dis. 1974;129:327.
271. Tuazon CW, Sheagren JW. Increased rate of carriage of *Staphylococcus aureus* among narcotic addicts. J Infect Dis. 1974;129:725.

272. Reisberg BE. Infective endocarditis in the narcotic addict. Prog Cardiovasc Dis. 1979;22:193.
273. Baddour LM. Twelve-year review of recurrent native-valve infective endocarditis: A disease of the modern antibiotic era. Rev Infect Dis. 1988;10:1163–70.
274. Rubenstein E, Noreiga ER, Simberkoff MS, et al. Tissue penetration of amphotericin B in *Candida* endocarditis. Chest. 1974;66:376.
275. Carrizosa J, Levison ME, Lawrence T, et al. Cure of *Aspergillus ustus* endocarditis of prosthetic valve. Arch Intern Med. 1974;133:486.
276. McIntosh CS, Nickers PJ, Isaqacs AJ. *Spirillum* endocarditis. Postgrad Med J. 1975;51:645.
277. Applefield MM, Billingsley LJ, Tucker HJ, et al. Q fever endocarditis—a case occurring in the United States. Am Heart J. 1977;93:669.
278. Tobin MJ, Cahill N, Gearty G, et al. Q fever endocarditis. Am J Med. 1982;72:396.
279. Fernandez-Guerrero ML, Muelas JM, Aquado JM. Q fever endocarditis on porcine bioprosthetic valves. Ann Intern Med. 1988;108:209–13.
280. Jones RB, Priest JB, Kuo C-C. Subacute chlamydial endocarditis. JAMA. 1982;247:655.
281. Brearley BF, Hutchinson DN. Endocarditis associated with *Chlamydia trachomatis* infection. Br Heart J. 1981;46:220.
282. Popat K, Barnardo D, Webb-Peploe M. *Mycoplasma pneumoniae* endocarditis. Br Heart J. 1980;44:111.
283. Burch GE, Tsui CY. Evolution of coxsackie viral valvular and mural endocarditis in mice. Br J Exp Pathol. 1971;52:360.
284. Persand V. Two unusual cases of mural endocarditis with a review of the literature. Am J Clin Pathol. 1970;53:832.
285. Van Scoy RE. Culture-negative endocarditis. Mayo Clin Proc. 1982;57:149.
286. Pesanti EL, Smith IM. Infective endocarditis with negative blood cultures. An analysis of 52 cases. Am J Med. 1979;66:43.
287. Daschner FD, Frank V. Antimicrobial drugs in human cardiac valves and endocarditis lesions. J Antimicrob Chemother. 1988;12:776–82.
288. Spokojny AM, Sinclair IN, Schnitt S, et al. Uptake of hematoporphyrin derivative by valvular vegetations in experimental infective endocarditis. Circulation 1985;72:1087–91.
289. Dall L, Barnes WG, Lane JW, et al. Enzymatic modification of glycocalyx in the treatment of experimental endocarditis due to viridans streptococci. J Infect Dis. 1987;156:736–40.
290. Buiting AGM, Thompson J, Emeis JJ, et al. Effects of tissue-type plasminogen activator on *Staphylococcus epidermidis*–infected plasma clots as a model of infected endocardial vegetations. J Antimicrob Chemother. 1987;19:771–80.
291. Buiting AG, Thompson J, Emeis JJ, et al. Effects of tissue-type plasminogen activator (t-PA) on *Streptococcus sanguis*–infected endocardial vegetations in vitro. J Antimicrob Chemother. 1988;21:609–20.
292. Cates JE, Christie RV. Subacute bacterial endocarditis. Q J Med. 1951;20:93.
293. Carrizosa J, Kobasa WD, Kaye D. Antagonism between chloramphenicol and penicillin in streptococcal endocarditis in rabbits. J Lab Clin Med. 1975;85:307.
294. Douglas A, Moore-Gillon J, Eykyn S. Fever during treatment of infective endocarditis. Lancet. 1986;1:1341–3.
295. Schlicter JG, MacIlean H. A method of determining the effective therapeutic level in the treatment of subacute bacterial endocarditis with penicillin. Am Heart J. 1947;34:209.
296. Coleman DL, Horwitz RI, Andriole VT. Association between serum inhibitory and bactericidal concentrations and therapeutic outcome in bacterial endocarditis. Am J Med. 1982;73:260.
297. Mellors JW, Coleman DL, Andriole VT. Value of serum bactericidal test in management of patients with bacterial endocarditis. Eur J Clin Microbiol. 1986;5:67–70.
298. Rahal JJ, Chan Y-K, Johnson G. Relationship of staphylococcal tolerance, teichoic acid antibody, and serum bactericidal activity to therapeutic outcome in *Staphylococcus aureus* bacteremia. Am J Med. 1986; 81:43–52.
299. Wolfson JS, Swartz MN. Serum bactericidal activity as a monitor of antibiotic therapy. N Engl J Med. 1985;312:968–75.
300. Reller LB. The serum bactericidal test. Rev Infect Dis. 1986;8:803–8.
301. Weinstein MP, Stratton CW, Ackley A, et al. Multicenter collaborative evaluation of a standardized serum bactericidal test as a prognostic indicator in infective endocarditis. Am J Med. 1985;78:262–9.
302. Stratton CW. The role of the microbiology laboratory in the treatment of infective endocarditis. J Antimicrob Chemother. 1987;20(Suppl A):41–9.
303. Sande MA, Scheld WM. Combination antibiotic therapy of bacterial endocarditis. Ann Intern Med. 1980;92:390.
304. Meylan PR, Francioloi P, Glauser MP. Discrepancies between MBC and actual killing by viridans group streptococci by cell-wall-active antibiotics. Antimicrob Agents Chemother. 1986;29:418–23.
305. Holloway Y, Pankert J, Hess J. Penicillin tolerance and bacterial endocarditis. Lancet. 1980;1:589.
306. Pulliam L, Inokuchi S, Hadley WK, et al. Penicillin tolerance in experimental streptococcal endocarditis. Lancet. 1979;2:957.
307. Gephart JF, Washington JA II. Antimicrobial susceptibilities of nutritionally variant streptococci. J Infect Dis. 1982;146:536.
308. Holloway Y, Dankert J. Penicillin tolerance in nutritionally variant streptococci. Antimicrob Agents Chemother. 1982;22:1073.
309. Lowry FD, Neuhas EG, Chang DS, et al. Penicillin therapy of experimental endocarditis caused by tolerant *Streptococcus sanguis* and nontolerant *Streptococcus mitis*. Antimicrob Agents Chemother. 1983;23:67.
310. Brennan RO, Durack DT. Therapeutic significance of penicillin tolerance in experimental streptococcal endocarditis. Antimicrob Agents Chemother. 1983;23:273.
311. Baker CW, Thornsberry C. Antimicrobial susceptibility of *Streptococcus mutans* isolated from patients with endocarditis. Antimicrob Agents Chemother. 1974;5:268.
312. Thornsberry C, Baker CN, Facklam RR. Antibiotic susceptibility of *Streptococcus bovis* and other group D streptococci causing endocarditis. Antimicrob Agents Chemother. 1974;5:228.
313. Wolfe JC, Johnson WD. Penicillin-sensitive streptococcal endocarditis. In vitro and clinical observations on penicillin-streptomycin therapy. Ann Intern Med. 1974;81:178.
314. Watanakunakorn C, Glotzbecker C. Synergism with aminoglycosides of penicillin, ampicillin, and vancomycin against nonenterococcal group D streptococci and viridans streptococci. J Med Microbiol. 1977;10:133.
315. Enzler MJ, Rouse MS, Henry NK, et al. In vitro and in vivo studies of streptomycin-resistant, penicillin-susceptible streptococci from patients with infective endocarditis. J Infect Dis. 1987;155:954–8.
316. Farber BF, Yee Y. High-level aminoglycoside resistance mediated by aminoglycoside-modifying enzymes among viridans streptococci: Implications for the therapy of endocarditis. J Infect Dis. 1987;155:948–53.
317. Sande MA, Irvin RG. Penicillin-aminoglycoside synergy in experimental *Streptococcus viridans* endocarditis. J Infect Dis. 1974;129:572.
318. Durack DT, Pelletier LL, Petersdorf RG. Chemotherapy of experimental streptococcal endocarditis. II. Synergism between penicillin and streptomycin against penicillin-sensitive streptococci. J Clin Invest. 1974; 53:929.
319. Drake TA, Sande MA. Studies of the chemotherapy of endocarditis: Correlation of in vitro, animal model, and clinical studies. Rev Infect Dis. 1983;5(Suppl):345.
320. Wilson WR, Geraci JE. Treatment of streptococcal infective endocarditis. Am J Med. 1985;78(Suppl 6B):128–137.
321. Scheld WM. Therapy of streptococcal endocarditis: Correlation of animal model and clinical studies. J Antimicrob Chemother. 1987;20(Suppl A):71–85.
322. Wilson WR, Geraci JE, Wilkowske CJ, et al. Short-term intramuscular therapy with procaine penicillin plus streptomycin for infective endocarditis due to viridans streptococci. Circulation. 1978;57:1158.
323. Wilson WR, Thompson RL, Wilkowske CJ, et al. Short-term therapy for streptococcal infective endocarditis. Combined intramuscular administration of penicillin and streptomycin. JAMA. 1981;245:360.
324. Karchmer AW, Mollering RC Jr, Maki DG, et al. Single antibiotic therapy for streptococcal endocarditis. JAMA. 1979;241:1801.
325. Malacoff RF, Frank E, Andriole VT. Streptococcal endocarditis (nonenterococcal, non-group A). Single vs. combination therapy. JAMA. 1979; 241:1807.
326. Parillo JE, Borst GC, Mazur MH, et al. Endocarditis due to resistant viridans streptococci during oral penicillin chemoprophylaxis. N Engl J Med. 1979;300:296.
327. Bisno AL, Dismukes WE, Durack DT, et al. Antimicrobial treatment of infective endocarditis due to viridans streptococci, enterococci, and staphylococci. JAMA. 1989;261:1471–7.
328. Bouvet A, Cremieux AC, Contrepois A, et al. Comparison of penicillin and vancomycin, individually and in combination with gentamicin and amikacin, in the treatment of experimental endocarditis induced by nutritionally variant steptococci. Antimicrob Agents Chemother. 1985;28:607–11.
329. Henry NK, Wilson WR, Roberts RB, et al. Antimicrobial therapy of experimental endocarditis caused by nutritionally variant viridans group streptococci. Antimicrob Agents Chemother. 1986;30:465–7.
330. Stein DS, Nelson KE. Endocarditis due to nutritionally deficient streptococci: Therapeutic dilemma. Rev Infect Dis. 1987;9:908–16.
331. Watanakunakorn C. Penicillin combined with gentamicin or streptomycin: Synergism against enterococci. J Infect Dis. 1971;124:581.
332. Moellering RC Jr, Korzeniowski OM, Sande MA, et al. Species-specific resistance to antimicrobial synergism in *Streptococcus faecium* and *Streptococcus faecalis*. J Infect Dis. 1979;140:203.
333. Krogstad DJ, Parquette AR. Defective killing of enterococci: A common property of antimicrobial agents acting on the cell wall. Antimicrob Agents Chemother. 1980;17:965.
334. Storch GA, Krogstad DA, Parquette AR. Antibiotic-induced lysis of enterococci. J Clin Invest. 1981;68:639.
335. Murray BE, Church DA, Wanger A, et al. Comparison of two β-lactamase–producing strains of *Streptococcus faecalis*. Antimicrob Agents Chemother. 1986;30:861–4.
336. Ingerman M, Pitsakis PG, Rosenberg A, et al. β-Lactamase production in experimental endocarditis due to aminoglycoside-resistant *Streptococcus faecalis*. J Infect Dis. 1987;155:1226–32.
337. Henry NK, Wilson WR, Geraci JE. Treatment of streptomycin-susceptible enterococcal experimental endocarditis with combinations of penicillin and low- or high-dose streptomycin. Antimicrob Agents Chemother. 1986;30:725–8.
338. Harwick HJ, Kalmanson GM, Guze LB. In vitro activity of ampicillin or vancomycin combined with gentamicin or streptomycin against enterococci. Antimicrob Agents Chemother. 1973;4:383.

339. Weinstein AJ, Moellering RC. Penicillin and gentamicin therapy for enterococcal infections. JAMA. 1973;223:1030.
340. Moellering RC, Wennersten C, Weinberg AW. Synergy of penicillin and gentamicin against enterococci. J Infect Dis. 1971;124(Suppl):207.
391. Hook EW III, Roberts RB, Sande MA. Antimicrobial therapy of experimental enterococcal endocarditis. Antimicrob Agents Chemother. 1975;8:564.
392. Wright AJ, Wilson WR, Matsumoto JY, et al. Influence of gentamicin dose size on the efficacies of combinations of gentamicin and penicillin in experimental streptomycin-resistant enterococcal endocarditis. Antimicrob Agents Chemother. 1982;22:972.
343. Murray BE, Tsao J, Panida J. Enterococci from Bangkok, Thailand, with high-level resistance to currently available aminoglycosides. Antimicrob Agents Chemother. 1983;23:799.
344. Mederski-Samoraj BD, Murray BE. High-level resistance to gentamicin in clinical isolates of enterococci. J Infect Dis. 1983;147:751.
345. Zervos MJ, Dembinski S, Mikesell T, et al. High-level resistance to gentamicin in *Streptococcus faecalis:* Risk factors and evidence for exogenous acquisition of infection. J Infect Dis. 1986;153:1075–83.
346. Zervos MJ, Terpenning MS, Schaberg DR, et al. High-level aminoglycoside-resistant enterococci. Arch Intern Med. 1987;147:1591–4.
347. Eliopoulos GM, Wennersten C, Zighelboim-Daum S, et al. High-level resistance to gentamicin in clinical isolates of *Streptococcus* (*Enterococcus*) *faecium*. Antimicrob Agents Chemother. 1988;32:1528–32.
348. Fernandez-Guerrero ML, Barros C, Rodriquez Tudela JL, et al. Aortic endocarditis caused by genamicin-resistant *Enterococcus faecalis*. Eur J Clin Microbiol. 1988;7:525–7.
349. Watanakunakorn C, Bakie C. Synergism of vancomycin-gentamicin and vancomycin-streptomycin against enterococci. Antimicrob Agents Chemother. 1973;4:120.
350. Watanakunakorn C, Tisone JC. Effects of a vancomycin-rifampin combination on enterococci. Antimicrob Agents Chemother. 1982;22:915.
351. Uttley AH, Collins CH, Naidoo J, et al. Vancomycin-resistant enterococci. Lancet. 1988;1:57–8.
352. Leclercq R, Derlot E, Dural J, et al. Plasmid-mediated resistance to vancomycin and teichoplanin in *Enterococcus faecium*. N Engl J Med. 1988;319:157–61.
353. Fernandez-Guerrero M, Rouse MS, Henry NK, et al. In vitro and in vivo activity of ciprofloxacin against enterococci isolated from patients with infective endocarditis. Antimicrob Agents Chemother. 1987;31:430–3.
354. Bush LM, Boscia JA, Kaye D. Daptomycin (LY146032) treatment of experimental enterococcal endocarditis. Antimicrob Agents Chemother. 1988;32:877–81.
355. Wilson WR, Wilkowski CJ, Wright AJ, et al. Treatment of streptomycin-susceptible and streptomycin-resistant enterococcal endocarditis. Ann Intern Med. 1984;100:816–23.
356. Karchmer AW. Staphylococcal endocarditis. Laboratory and clinical basis for antibiotic therapy. Am J Med. 1985;78(Suppl B):116–27.
357. Sande MA, Courtney KB. Nafcillin-gentamicin synergism in experimental staphylococcal endocarditis. J Lab Clin Med. 1976;88:118.
358. Abrams B, Sklaver A, Hoffman T, et al. Single or combination therapy of staphylococcal endocarditis in intravenous drug abusers. Ann Intern Med. 1979;90:789.
359. Chambers HF, Miller RT, Newman MD. Right-sided *Staphylococcus aureus* endocarditis in intravenous drug abusers: Two week combination therapy. Ann Intern Med. 1988;109:619–24.
360. Murray HW, Wigley FM, Mann JJ, et al. Combination antibiotic therapy in staphylococcal endocarditis: The use of methicillin sodium–gentamicin sulfate therapy. Arch Intern Med. 1976;136:480.
361. Korzeniowski OM, Sande MA, The National Collaborative Endocarditis Study Group. Combination antimicrobial therapy for *Staphylococcus aureus* endocarditis in patients addicted to parenteral drugs and in nonaddicts. A prospective study. Ann Intern Med. 1982;97:496.
362. Craven DE, Kollisch MR, Hsieh CR, et al. Vancomycin treatment of bacteremia caused by oxacillin-resistant *Staphylococcus aureus:* Comparison with β-lactam antibiotic treatment of bacteremia caused by oxacillin-sensitive *Staphylococcus aureus*. J Infect Dis. 1983;147:137.
363. Watanakunakorn C. Clindamycin therapy of *Staphylococcus aureus* endocarditis. Clinical relapse and development of resistance to clindamycin, lincomycin, and erythromycin. Am J Med. 1976;60:419.
364. Kaye D. The clinical significance of tolerance of *Staphylococcus aureus*. Ann Intern Med. 1980;93:924.
365. Jackson MA, Hicks RA. Vancomycin failure in staphylococcal endocarditis. Pediatr Infect Dis J. 1987;6:750–2.
366. Rajashekaraiah KR, Rice T, Rao VS, et al. Clinical significance of tolerant strains of *Staphylococcus aureus* in patients with endocarditis. Ann Intern Med. 1980;93:796.
367. Zak O, Scheld WM, Sande MA. Rifampin in experimental endocarditis due to *Staphylococcus aureus* in rabbits. Rev Infect Dis. 1983;5(Suppl):481.
368. Fernandez-Guerrero M, Rouse M, Henry N, et al. Ciprofloxacin therapy of experimental endocarditis caused by methicillin-susceptible or methicillin-resistant *Staphylococcus aureus*. Antimicrob Agents Chemother. 1988;32:747–51.
369. Iannini PB, Crossley K. Therapy of *Staphylococcus aureus* bacteremia associated with a removable focus of infection. Ann Intern Med. 1976;84:558.
370. Watanakunakorn C, Baird IM. *Staphylococcus aureus* bacteremia and endocarditis associated with a removable infected intravenous device. Am J Med. 1977;63:253.
371. Bayer AS, Lam K, Ginzton L, *Staphylococcus aureus* bacteremia. Clinical, serologic, and echocardiographic findings in patients with and without endocarditis. Arch Intern Med. 1987;147:757–62.
372. Karchmer AW, Archer GL, Dismukes WE. *Staphylococcus epidermidis* causing prosthetic valve endocarditis: Microbiologic and clinical observations as guides to therapy. Ann Intern Med. 1983;98:447.
373. Schwalbe RS, Stapleton JT, Gilligan PH. Emergence of vancomycin resistance in coagulase-negative staphylococci. N Engl J Med. 1987;316:927–31.
374. Joly V, Parigon B, Vallois J-M, et al. Value of antibiotic levels in serum and cardiac vegetations for predicting antibacterial effect of ceftriaxone in experimental *Escherichia coli* endocarditis. Antimicrob Agents Chemother. 1987;31:1632–9.
375. Hughes CF, Noble N. Vegetectomy: An alternative surgical treatment for infective endocarditis of the atrioventricular valves in drug addicts. J Thorac Cardiovasc Surg. 1988;95:857–61.
376. Arbulu A, Thomas NW, Chiscano A, et al. Total tricuspid valvulectomy without replacement in the treatment of *Pseudomonas* endocarditis. Surg Forum. 1971;22:162.
377. Mammana RB, Levitsky S, Sernaque D, et al. Valve replacement for left-sided endocarditis in drug addicts. Ann Thorac Surg. 1983;35:436.
378. Bayer AS, Crowell DJ, Yih J, et al. Comparative pharmacokinetics and pharmacodynamics of amikacin and ceftazidine in tricuspid and aortic vegetations in experimental *Pseudomonas* endocarditis. J Infect Dis. 1988;158:355–9.
379. Bayer AS, Hirano L, Yih J. Development of β-lactam resistance and increased quinolone MIC's during therapy of experimental *Pseudomonas aeruginosa* endocarditis. Antimicrob Agents Chemother. 1988;32:231–5.
380. Parr TR Jr, Bayer AS. Mechanisms of aminoglycoside resistance in variants of *Pseudomonas aeruginosa* isolated during treatment of experimental endocarditis in rabbits. J Infect Dis. 1988;158:1003–10.
381. Hessen MT, Pitsakis PG, Levison ME. Absence of a post-antibiotic effect in experimental *Pseudomonas* endocarditis treated with imipenem, with or without gentamicin. J Infect Dis. 1988;158:542–8.
382. Jimenez-Lucho VE, Saravolatz LD, Medeiros AA, et al. Failure of therapy in *Pseudomonas* endocarditis: Selection of resistant mutants. J Infect Dis. 1986;154:64–8.
383. Daikos GL, Kathopalia SB, Lolans VT, et al. Long-term oral ciprofloxacin: Experience in the treatment of incurable infective endocarditis. Am J Med. 1988;84:786–90.
384. Weisner PJ, Handsfield HH, Holmes KK. Low antibiotic resistance of gonococci causing disseminated infection. N Engl J Med. 1973;288:1221.
385. Black JR, Brint JM, Reichart CA. Successful treatment of gonococcal endocarditis with ceftriaxone. J Infect Dis. 1988;157:1281–2.
386. Ernst JD, Rusmak M, Sande MA. Combination antifungal chemotherapy for experimental disseminated candidiasis: Lack of correlation between in vitro and in vivo observations with amphotericin B and rifampin. Rev Infect Dis. 1983;5(Suppl):626.
387. Longman LP, Martin MV. A comparison of the efficacy of intraconazole, amphotericin B and 5-fluorocytosine in the treatment of *Aspergillus fumigatus* endocarditis in the rabbit. J Antimicrob Chemother. 1987;20:719–24.
388. Haldane EV, Marrie TJ, Faulkner RS, et al. Endocarditis due to Q fever in Nova Scotia: Experience with five patients in 1981–1982. J Infect Dis. 1983;148:978–85.
389. Street AC, Durack DT. Experience with trimethoprim-sulfamethoxazole in treatment of infective endocarditis. Rev Infect Dis. 1988;10:915–22.
390. Jones JB, Ridgeway GL, Boulding S, et al. In vitro activity of rifamycins alone and in combination with other antibiotics against *Chlamydia trachomatis*. Rev Infect Dis. 1983;5(Suppl):556.
391. McAnulty JH, Rahimtoola SH. Surgery for infective endocarditis. JAMA. 1979;242:77.
392. Dinubile MJ. Surgery in active endocarditis. Ann Intern Med. 1980;96:650.
393. D'Agostino RS, Miller DC, Stinson EB, et al. Valve replacement in patients with native valve endocarditis: What really determines operative outcome? Ann Thorac Surg. 1985;40:429–38.
394. Wilson WR, Danielson GK, Giuliani ER, et al. Valve replacement in patients with active infective endocarditis. Circulation. 1978;58:585.
395. Arbulu A, Asfaw I. Tricuspid valvulectomy without prosthetic replacement. Ten years of clinical experience. J Thorac Cardiovasc Surg. 1981;82:684.
396. DiNubile M. Surgery for addiction-related tricuspid valve endocarditis: Caveat emptor. Am J Med. 1987;82:811–3.
397. Arbulu A, Asfaw I. Management of infective endocarditis: Seventeen years' experience. Ann Thorac Surg. 1987;43:144–9.
398. Alsip SG, Blackstone EH, Kirklin JW, et al. Indications for cardiac surgery in patients with active infective endocarditis. Am J Med. 1985;78(Suppl 6B):138–48.
399. Neuhof H, Seley GP. Acute suppurative phlebitis complicated by septicemia. Surgery. 1947;21:831.
400. Goldman DA, Maki DG, Rhame FS, et al. Guidelines for infection control in intravenous therapy. Ann Intern Med. 1973;79:848.
401. O'Neill JA, Pruitt BA, Foley FD, et al. Suppurative thrombophlebitis—a lethal complication of intravenous therapy. J Trauma. 1968;8:256.
402. Stein JM, Pruitt BA. Suppurative thrombophlebitis: A lethal iatrogenic disease. N Engl J Med. 1970;282:1452.
403. Pruitt BA, Stein JM, Foley FD, et al. Intravenous therapy in burn patients.

Suppurative thrombophlebitis and other life-threatening complications. Arch Surg. 1970;100:399.
404. Pruitt BA, McManus WF, Kim SH, et al. Diagnosis and treatment of cannularelated intravenous sepsis in burn patients. Ann Surg. 1980;191:546.
405. Garrison RN, Richardson JD, Fry DE. Catheter-associated septic thrombophlebitis. South Med J. 1982;75:917.
406. Sacks-Berg A, Strampfer MJ, Cunha BA. Suppurative thrombophlebitis caused by intravenous line sepsis. Heart Lung. 1987;16:318–20.
407. Munster AM. Septic thrombophlebitis. A surgical disorder. JAMA. 1974;230:1010.
408. Berkowitz FE, Argent AC, Baise T. Suppurative thrombophlebitis: A serious nosocomial infection. Pediatr Infect Dis J. 1987;6:64–7.
409. Johnson RA, Zajac RA, Evans ME. Suppurative thrombophlebitis: Correlation between pathogen and underlying disease. Infect Control. 1986;7:582–5.
410. Rhame FS, Maki DG, Bennett JV. Intravenous cannula-associated infections. In: Bennett JV, Brachman PS, eds. Hospital Infections. Boston: Little, Brown; 1979:433–42.
411. Baker CC, Peterson SR, Sheldon GF. Septic phlebitis: A neglected disease. Am J Surg. 1979;138:97.
412. Sears N, Grosfeld JL, Weber TR, et al. Suppurative thrombophlebitis in childhood. Pediatrics. 1981;68:630.
413. Zinner MJ, Zuidema GD, Lowery BD. Septic nonsuppurative thrombophlebitis. Arch Surg. 1976;111:122.
414. Brismar B, Hardstedt C, Jacobson S. Diagnosis of thrombosis by catheter phlebography after prolonged central venous catheterization. Ann Surg. 1981;194:779–83.
415. Slagle DC, Gates RH Jr. Unusual case of central vein thrombosis and sepsis. Am J Med. 1986;81:351–4.
416. Kaufman J, Demas C, Stark K, et al. Catheter-related septic central venous thrombosis—current therapeutic options. West J Med. 1986;145:200–3.
417. Veghese A, Widrich WC, Arbeit RD. Central venous septic thrombophlebitis—the role of medical therapy. Medicine (Baltimore). 1985;64:394–400.
418. Strinden WD, Helgerson RB, Maki DG. *Candida* septic thrombosis of the great central veins associated with central catheters. Clinical features and management. Ann Surg. 1985;202:653–8.
419. Haddad W, Idowu J, Georgeson K, et al. Septic atrial thrombosis: A potentially lethal complication of Broviac catheters in infants. Am J Dis Child. 1986;140:778–80.
420. Collins CG, MacCallum EA, Nelson EW, et al. Suppurative pelvic thrombophlebitis. I. Incidence, pathology, and etiology. Surgery. 1951;30:298.
421. Josey WE, Staggers SR. Heparin therapy in septic pelvic thrombophlebitis: A study of 46 cases. Am J Obstet Gynecol. 1974;120:228.
422. Collins CG. Suppurative pelvic thrombophlebitis. A study of 202 cases in which the disease was treated by ligation of the vena cava and ovarian vein. Am J Obstet Gynecol. 1970;108:681.
423. Barenholtz L, Kaminsky NI, Palmer DL. Venous intramural microabscesses: A cause of protracted sepsis with intravenous cannulas. Am J Med Sci. 1973;265:335.
424. Jupiter JB, Ehrlich MG, Novelline RA, et al. The association of septic thrombophlebitis with subperiosteal abscesses in children. J Pediatr. 1982;101:690.
425. Maki DG, Weise CE, Sarafin HW. A semiquantitative culture method for identifying intravenous-catheter-related infection. N Engl J Med. 1977;296:1305.
426. Angel JL, Knuppel RA. Computed tomography in diagnosis of puerperal ovarian vein thrombosis. Obstet Gynecol. 1984;63:61–4.
427. Isada NB, Landy HJ, Larson JW Jr. Postabortal septic pelvic thrombophlebitis diagnosed with computed tomography. J Reprod Med. 1987;32:866–8.
428. Martin B, Molopulos GP, Bryan PJ. MRI of puerperal ovarian vein thrombosis. AJR. 1986;147:291–2.
429. Josey WE, Cook CC. Septic pelvic thrombophlebitis. Report of 17 patients treated with heparin. Obstet Gynecol. 1970;35:891.
430. Torres-Rojas JR, Stratton CW, Sanders CV, et al. Candidal suppurative peripheral thrombophlebitis. Ann Intern Med. 1982;96:431.
431. Walsh TJ, Bustamente CI, Vlahov D, et al. Candidal suppurative peripheral thrombophlebitis: Recognition, prevention, and management. Infect Control. 1986;7:16–22.
432. Peterson P, Stahl-Bayliss CM. Cytomegalovirus thrombophlebitis after successful DHPG therapy. Ann Intern Med. 1987;106:632–3.
433. Miller CJ. Ligation and excision of pelvic veins in treatment of puerperal pyaemia. Surg Gynecol Obstet. 1917;25:431.
434. Topiel MS, Bryan RT, Kessler CM, et al. Treatment of Silastic catheter-induced central vein septic thrombophlebitis. Am J Med Sci. 1986;291:425–8.
435. Barg NL, Supena RB, Fekety R. Persistent staphylococcal bacteremia in an intravenous drug abuser. Antimicrob Agents Chemother. 1986;29:209–11.
436. Moran JM, Atwood RP, Rowe MI. A clinical and bacteriologic study of infections associated with venous cutdowns. N Engl J Med. 1965;272:554.
437. Norden CW. Application of antibiotic ointment to the site of venous catheterization—a controlled trial. J Infect Dis. 1969;120:611.
438. Patel S, Johnston KW. Classification and management of mycotic aneurysms. Surg Gynecol Obstet. 1977;144:691.
439. Parkhurst GF, Decker JP. Bacterial aortitis and mycotic aneurysms of the aorta. A report of 12 cases. Am J Pathol. 1955;31:821.
440. Sommerville RL, Allen EV, Edwards JE. Bland and infected arteriosclerotic abdominal aortic aneurysms: A clinicopathologic study. Medicine (Baltimore). 1959;38:207.
441. Stengel A, Wolfroth CC. Mycotic (bacterial) aneurysms of intravascular origin. Arch Intern Med. 1923;31:527.
442. Bennett DE, Cherry JK. Bacterial infection of aortic aneurysms. A clinicopathologic study. Am J Surg. 1967;113:321.
443. Cliff MM, Soulen RL, Firestone AJ. Mycotic aneurysms: A challenge and a clue. Arch Intern Med. 1970;126:977.
444. Jarrett F, Darling C, Mundth ED, et al. Experience with infected aneurysms of the abdominal aorta. Arch Surg. 1975;110:1281.
445. Bohmfalk GL, Story JL, Wissenger JP, et al. Bacterial intracranial aneurysm. J Neurosurg. 1978;48:369.
446. Frazee JG, Cahan LD, Winter J. Bacterial intracranial aneurysms. J Neurosurg. 1980;53:633.
447. Bullock R, Van Dellen JR, Van den Heever CM. Intracranial mycotic aneurysms. A review of 9 cases. S Afr Med J. 1981;60:970.
448. Jarrett F, Darling RC, Mundth ED, et al. The management of infected arterial aneurysms. J Cardiovasc Surg. 1977;18:361.
449. Johnson JR, Ledgerwood AM, Lucas CE. Mycotic aneurysm. New concepts in therapy. Arch Surg. 1983;118:577.
450. Feigl D, Feigl A, Edwards JE. Mycotic aneurysms of the aortic root. A pathologic study of 20 cases. Chest. 1986;90:553–7.
451. Dean RH, Mecham PW, Weaver FA, et al. Mycotic embolism and embolomycotic aneurysms. Neglected lessons of the past. Ann Surg. 1986;204:300–7.
452. Sedwitz MM, Hye RJ, Stabile BE. The changing epidemiology of pseudoaneurysm. Therapeutic implications. Arch Surg. 1988;123:473–6.
453. Kyriakides GK, Simmons RL, Najarian JS. Mycotic aneurysms in transplant patients. Arch Surg. 1976;111:472.
454. Smith EJ, Milligan SL, Filo RS. *Salmonella* mycotic aneurysms after renal transplantation. South Med J. 1981;74:1399.
455. Olmsted WW, McGee TP. The pathogenesis of peripheral aneurysms of the central nervous system: A subject review from the AFIP. Radiology. 1977;123:661.
456. Salgado AV, Furlan AJ, Keys TF. Mycotic aneurysm, Subarachnoid hemorrhage, and indications for cerebral angiography in infective endocarditis. Stroke. 1987;18:1057–60.
457. Friedman SG, Pogo GJ, Moccio CG. Mycotic aneurysm of the superior mesenteric artery. J Vasc Surg. 1987;6:87–90.
458. Sukerkar AN, Dulay CC, Anandappa E, et al. Mycotic aneurysm of the hepatic artery. Radiology. 1977;124:444.
459. Feinsod FM, Norfleet RG, Hoehn JL. Mycotic aneurysm of the external iliac artery. A triad of clinical signs facilitating early diagnosis. JAMA. 1977;238:245.
460. Merry M, Dunn J, Weissmann R, et al. Popliteal mycotic aneurysm presenting as septic arthritis and purpura. JAMA. 1972;221:58.
461. Plate G, Forsley N, Stigsson L, et al. Management of inflammatory abdominal aortic aneurysm. Acta Chir Scand. 1988;154:19–24.
462. Pennell RC, Hollier LH, Lie JT, et al. Inflammatory abdominal aortic aneurysms: A thirty year review. J Vasc Surg. 1985;2:859–69.
463. Morrow C, Safi H, Beall AC Jr. Primary aortoduodenal fistula caused by *Salmonella* aortitis. J Vasc Surg. 1987;6:415–8.
464. Vogelzang RL, Sohaey R. Infected aortic aneurysms: CT appearance. J Comput Assist Tomogr. 1988;12:109–12.
465. Rivera JV, Blanco G, Perez M, et al. Gallium-67 localization in a mycotic aneurysm of the thoracic aorta. Clin Nucl Med. 1985;10:814–6.
466. Brewster DC, Retana A, Waltman AC, et al. Angiography in the management of aneurysms of the abdominal aorta. N Engl J Med. 1972;292:822.
467. Griffiths BE, Petch MC, English TAH. Echocardiographic detection of subvalvular aortic root aneurysm extending to mitral valve annulus as complication of aortic valve endocarditis. Br Heart J. 1982;47:392.
468. Kanwar YS, Malhotra U, Anderson BR, et al. Salmonellosis associated with abdominal aortic aneurysm. Arch Intern Med. 1974;134:1095.
469. Cohen JI, Bartlett JA, Corey GR. Extra-intestinal manifestations of *Salmonella* infections. Medicine (Baltimore). 1987;66:349–88.
470. Cohen OS, O'Brien TF, Schoenbaum SC, et al. The risk of endothelial infection in adults with *Salmonella* bacteremia. Ann Intern Med. 1978;89:931.
471. McIntyre KE Jr, Malone JM, Richards E. Mycotic aortic pseudoaneurysm with aortoenteric fistula caused by *Arizona hinshawii*. Surgery. 1982;91:173.
472. Anolik JR, Mildvan D, Winter JW, et al. Mycotic aortic aneurysm. A complication of *Campylobacter fetus* septicemia. Arch Intern Med. 1983;143:609.
473. Mielke B, Weir B, Oldring D, et al. Fungal aneurysm: Case report and review of the literature. Neurosurgery. 1981;9:578.
474. Hadley MN, Martin NA, Spetzler RF, et al. Multiple intracranial aneurysms due to *Coccidioides immitis* infection. J Neurosurg. 1987;66:453–6.
475. Bingham WF: Treatment of mycotic intracranial aneurysms. J Neurosurg. 1977;46:428.
476. Leipzig MJ, Brown FD. Treatment of mycotic aneurysms. Surg Neurol. 1985;23:403–7.
477. Rodesch G, Noterman J, Thys JP, et al. Treatment of intracranial mycotic aneurysm: Surgery or not. Acta Neurochir. 1987;85:63–8.
478. Reddy DJ, Smith RF, Elliott JP Jr, et al. Infected femoral artery false aneurysms in drug addicts: Evolution of selective vascular reconstruction. J Vasc Surg. 1986;3:718–24.
479. Johansen K, Devin J. Mycotic aortic aneurysms. A reappraisal. Arch Surg. 1983;118:583.

480. Parsons R, Gregory J, Palmer DL. *Salmonella* infections of the abdominal aorta. Rev Infect Dis. 1983;5:227.
481. Bitseff EJ, Edwards WH, Mulherin JL Jr, et al. Infected abdominal aortic aneurysms. South Med J. 1987;80:309–12.
482. Taylor LM Jr, Deitz DM, McConnell DB, et al. Treatment of infected abdominal aneurysms by extra anatomic bypass, aneurysm excision, and drainage. Am J Surg. 1988;155:655–8.
483. Sande MA, Strausbaugh LJ. Infective endocarditis. In: Hook EW, Mandell GL, Gwaltney JM Jr, Sande MA, eds. Current Concepts of Infectious Diseases. New York: John Wiley & Sons; 1977;55–68.

62. INFECTIOUS DISORDERS OF PROSTHETIC VALVES AND INTRAVASCULAR DEVICES

MICHAEL G. THRELKELD
C. GLENN COBBS

PROSTHETIC VALVE ENDOCARDITIS

Infection of the intracardiac prosthesis is a serious complication of valve replacement surgery. The intravascular foreign body is inherently more susceptible to bacterial colonization than is native valve tissue, and established infection on a prosthetic device is often difficult to eradicate. Although clinical outcome has improved during the past decade, prosthetic valve endocarditis (PVE) remains a significant cause of morbidity and mortality.

Epidemiology

Early and Late Prosthetic Valve Endocarditis. By convention, PVE occurring within 60 days of valve insertion has been termed "early PVE" and endocarditis occurring more than 60 days after valve replacement, "late PVE." However, illness characteristic of early disease may not always become apparent until 6 months or more after the operation. Some investigators have therefore recommended that the time limit for early disease be extended to 6 months or even 1 year.[1,2]

Incidence. A number of authors have described their experiences with PVE during the past two decades.[1–22] Among 25,923 patients undergoing valve replacement, 740 episodes of PVE were observed (an incidence of 2.9 percent). If one uses the traditional 60-day time limit, approximately 37 percent of reported episodes represented "early PVE," while 63 percent were "late PVE." Of the 459 patients identified by sex, 64 percent were male.

Valves in the aortic position were once believed to be more susceptible to infection than are valves in the mitral position. However, more recent studies have failed to confirm this finding.[21] Of 603 reported cases of PVE, 55 percent involved an aortic prosthesis; 32 percent, a mitral prosthesis; and 12 percent, other valves or combinations of valves.[3,4,6–14,18,19,21,22] These differences presumably reflect the frequency of surgery at the different sites.

Types of Prostheses Involved. There are currently more than two dozen varieties of artificial valves in use.[23] They can be classified as mechanical valves (including ball valves, disk valves, hinged leaflet valves, and tilting disk valves) and bioprosthetic tissue valves (including homografts and porcine heterografts). Based on data from several recent series, the incidence of PVE in patients receiving porcine heterografts is 3.1 percent, and the incidence for mechanical valve recipients is 3.8 percent.[2,19,20]

Microorganisms Responsible. Table 1 lists the microbial etiology of PVE in 272 patients with early infection and 429 patients with late.[4–7,13,19,21,22,24] The most common etiologic microorganism was *Staphylococcus epidermidis,* which accounted for 29 percent of episodes. Viridans streptococci accounted for 17 percent and *Staphylococcus aureus* for 14 percent. These frequencies vary substantially from those seen in native valve endocarditis (NVE), in which the viridans streptococci and *S. aureus* account for approximately 50 and 20 percent of episodes, respectively. Aerobic gram-negative bacilli and fungi (especially *Candida* sp. and *Aspergillus* sp.), uncommon in NVE, are important causes of early PVE.

Diphtheroids, a term used to describe corynebacteria other than *Corynebacterium diphtheriae,* are important causes of early PVE.[25] Recognition of their role in PVE has served to emphasize the pathologic potential of these usually avirulent bacteria. Group JK corynebacteria, in particular, are important pathogens of prosthetic devices. A wide variety of other bacterial and fungal species has been reported in individual patients with PVE.

Pathogenesis of Early Prosthetic Valve Endocarditis

Staphylococcus epidermidis is the most common cause of early PVE. Of 16 patients with *S. epidermidis* PVE seen at one center, 11 became ill within 6 months of surgery, with a median time of onset of 2 months.[2] These data suggest that *S. epidermidis* PVE may result from valve contamination occurring in the perioperative period. Several studies have emphasized the potential role of intraoperative contamination in the pathogenesis of early PVE. Kluge et al.[26] during an investigation of microbial contamination occurring during open heart surgery found tissue surfaces and the valvular prostheses to be the most common sites from which microorganisms could be recovered. An important observation was the frequent recovery of *S. epidermidis* and diphtheroids, presumably shed from the skin of the patient or operating room personnel. Another possible mode of contamination was suggested by Blakemore et al.,[27] who found bacteria contaminating blood in the bypass pump. Identical microorganisms were isolated from the air in the operating room, which suggests that suctioning devices used in the operative field inoculated microorganisms into the blood.

TABLE 1. Microorganisms Responsible for Prosthetic Valve Endocarditis

Organism	*Early PVE*[a] *(%)*	*Late PVE (%)*	*Overall (%)*
Staphylococci			
S. epidermidis	35	26	29
S. aureus	17	12	14
Streptococci			
Group D streptococci (including enterococci)	3	9	7
S. pneumoniae	1	<1	1
Other (including viridans streptococci)	4	25	17
Gram-negative bacilli	16	12	13
Diphtheroids	10	4	7
Other bacteria	1	2	2
Candida	8	4	5
Aspergillus	2	1	1
Other fungi	1	<1	1
Culture-negative	1	4	3
Total number			
Microorganisms	292	445	737
Patients	272	429	701

[a] Occurring less than 2 months after surgery.
(Data from Refs. 4–7, 13, 19, 21, 22, and 24.)

In the immediate postoperative period, the prosthetic valve and sewing ring are not yet endothelialized and are apparently quite susceptible to microbial colonization. Bacteria or fungi originating from infected intravascular catheters, cardiac pacemakers, or pressure monitoring devices may seed the prosthesis. One study of patients undergoing open heart surgery demonstrated that 29 percent of intravenous catheters were contaminated.[28] This rate was reduced to 12 percent when catheters were removed sooner. Another study suggested that *S. epidermidis* is readily introduced into the blood stream during thermodilution cardiac output determinations unless careful aseptic technique is practiced.[29] Bacteremia may also result from postoperative infections at extracardiac sites. Dismukes et al.[3] noted pneumonia, wound infection, or contaminated intravascular catheters in 12 patients who subsequently developed early PVE. Another potential (but uncommon) source of infection is contamination of the prosthesis before implantation such as the contamination of glutaraldehyde-fixed porcine prosthetic valves by *Mycobacterium chelonae*.[30,31]

Pathogenesis of Late Prosthetic Valve Endocarditis

The pathogenesis of late PVE appears similar to that of NVE, with microorganisms from a source of transient bacteremia localizing on a prosthesis or area of damaged endocardium. This is reflected in the much higher incidence of infection due to viridans streptococci in late disease. Late PVE caused by *S. epidermidis* or other organisms that typically cause early PVE may result from a delayed onset of the infection acquired in the perioperative period.

Pathology of Prosthetic Valve Endocarditis

Valve ring abscess is a serious complication of PVE in both mechanical and bioprosthetic valves.[3,6,12,32,33] Valve ring abscesses occur when infection involves the sutures used to secure the sewing ring to the periannular tissue; this may result in dehiscence of the valve (Fig. 1). The clinical finding of a paravalvular leak in a patient with PVE is presumptive evidence of a valve ring abscess. Arnett and Roberts described the precise pathologic findings in 22 patients with valve ring abscess. The infectious process involved the entire valve circumference in 14 patients; there was partial involvement in the other 8.[33] Extension of the abscess beyond the valve ring may result in myocardial abscess formation, septal perforation, or purulent pericarditis. In addition to sewing ring abscesses, PVE of bioprostheses may cause leaflet destruction with resulting valvular incompetence.[14,34] Large vegetations occasionally obstruct blood flow and lead to functional valvular stenosis or a combination of stenosis and insufficiency. This complication appears to be more common in mitral PVE than in aortic disease.[14,33,35]

Extracardiac pathologic features classically associated with NVE may also be seen in PVE. Embolic events are common in patients with PVE. Septic emboli to the carotid circulation may lead to a brain infarct, brain abscess, mycotic aneurysm, or hemorrhagic infarct (especially in patients who are excessively anticoagulated). LePort et al. noted that 7 of 17 deaths from their series of patient with late PVE were due to neurologic complications.[36] Peripheral emboli may lead to deep tissue abscesses and mycotic aneurysms.

Immune complex–mediated glomerulonephritis manifested by abnormal urinalysis with or without elevations of serum creatinine levels has been described in patients with PVE.[37–39] Renal pathologic findings are variable but often mimic the diffuse proliferative changes found in poststreptococcal glomerulonephritis. Immunoglobulin and complement deposits can frequently be demonstrated along the glomercular basement membrane (by immunofluorescent staining).

Diagnosis of Prosthetic Valve Endocarditis

Clinical Manifestations. The symptoms and signs of PVE are protean.[6,11,40–42] As shown in Table 2, fever is the most common

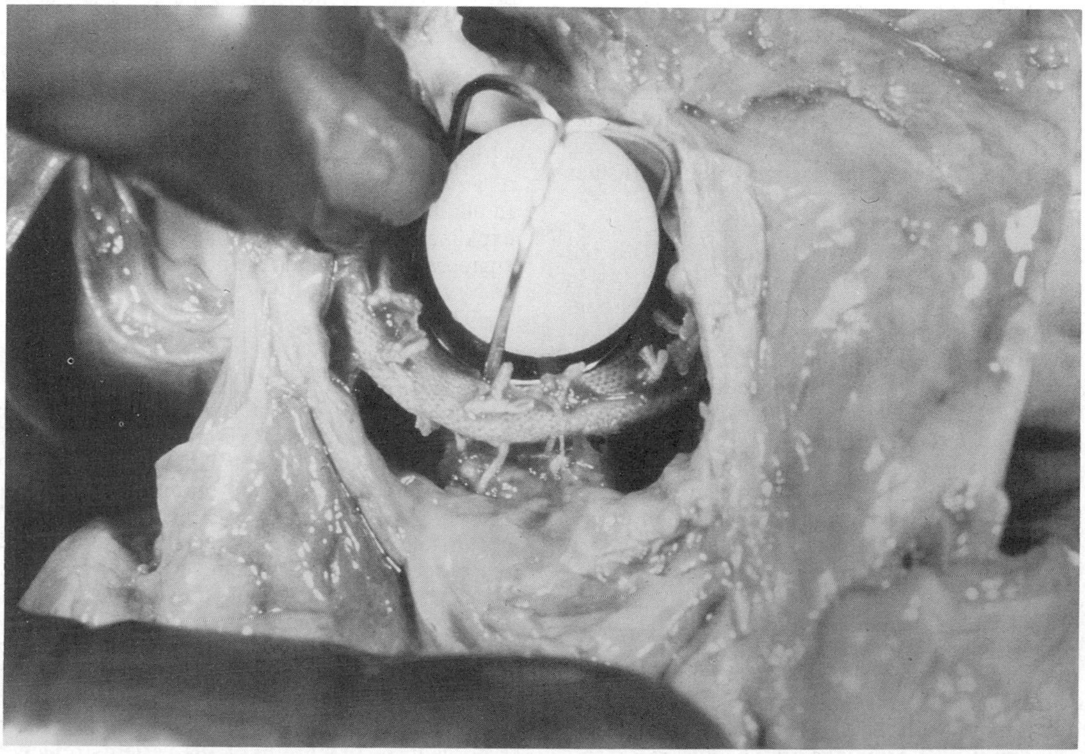

FIG. 1. Autopsy specimen demonstrates valve dehiscence complicating prosthetic valve endocarditis.

TABLE 2. Clinical Findings in Prosthetic Valve Endocarditis (228 Patients)

Finding	%
Fever	97
New or changing murmur	56
Systemic embolus	40
Petechiae	39
Splenomegaly	32
Peripheral signs (Osler nodes, Janeway lesions, Roth spots)	15
Anemia (Hct <35)	74
Hematuria	57
Leukocytosis (WBC >12,000)	54

(Data from Refs. 6, 11, 40, and 42.)

sign and occurs in almost all patients. Clinical evidence of systemic embolization has been reported in 40 percent of patients. The frequency of various organ system involvement by emboli is similar to NVE. Embolization to the central nervous system (CNS) commonly presents as an acute focal neurologic deficit. Splenomegaly is reported in one-third of patients and may be more common in late PVE, presumably reflecting more prolonged antigenemia. Petechiae have been noted in 39 percent, but other peripheral signs due to small emboli or small vessel vasculitis (Osler nodes, Janeway lesions, Roth spots) are less frequently encountered.

New or changing cardiac murmurs have been reported in 56 percent of patients with PVE. Regurgitant murmurs reflect the hemodynamic consequences of valvular insufficiency due to a paravalvular leak, while muffling of heart sounds or stenosis murmurs result from occlusion or malfunction of the prosthetic valve. Although cardiac murmurs may frequently suggest the diagnosis of PVE, in general it is difficult to accurately predict the extent of valvular pathology by auscultation alone.

Laboratory Findings. Anemia is present in many patients with PVE. In late PVE, the degree of anemia is probably a function of the duration of infection. The packed cell volume is a less useful finding in the diagnosis of early PVE. Leukocytosis occurs in only 50 percent of the patients; it may be more frequently seen in those with early PVE. Hematuria (secondary to glomerulonephritis) can be a helpful diagnostic sign in the patient with suspected late PVE but is difficult to interpret in a postoperative patient who may have recently required urethral catheterization. A number of investigators have reported elevated levels of circulating immune complexes in patients with PVE, but their utility for diagnosis or prognosis requires further evaluation.[37,38]

Blood Cultures. The cornerstone of diagnosing PVE is the isolation of an etiologic microorganism from the blood. As in the case of NVE, the bacteremia associated with PVE is continuous. Ninety percent of blood cultures obtained in such patients should reveal the infecting pathogen.[43] Negative blood cultures in a patient who has not received antibiotics is quite unusual in PVE unless the infection is caused by organisms such as *Legionella, Mycobacterium, Rickettsia, Histoplasma capsulatum,* or *Aspergillus* species, which do not grow readily in routine blood cultures. Fastidious microorganisms such as *Haemophilis* species may require prolonged incubation before appearing in blood cultures; therefore, all blood cultures from patients with suspected PVE should be held for a minimum of 3 weeks.

On the other hand, not all instances of bacteremia occurring after valve replacement indicate PVE.[44] Infected wounds and contaminated intravascular catheters may lead to transient bacteremia. Prosthetic valves seem relatively resistant to colonization by gram-negative bacilli, and PVE is rare after transient gram-negative bacteremia. If gram-negative bacteremia clears after the extracardiac source is removed, patients who have no other manifestations of PVE can usually be treated with 2 weeks of intravenous antibiotics.[45] If bacteremia fails to clear or the source of infection is not apparent, the patient should be assumed to have PVE and be treated accordingly. Because gram-positive bacteria are more adherent, their presence in blood cultures usually reflects colonization of the prosthetic device. However, if there is doubt about the significance of a positive blood culture (e.g., a single blood culture growing *S. epidermidis* in the absence of clinical manifestations), antimicrobial therapy may reasonably be withheld while additional cultures are obtained.

Special Studies. Myocardial damage from ischemia, an abscess, or pericarditis may cause a variety of arrhythmias or conduction defects in patients with PVE. In one series, atrioventricular conduction defects occurred in 44 percent of patients with prosthetic aortic valve infection due to extension of the abscess into the conduction system.[41] Serial electrocardiograms or continuous cardiac monitoring may be important for some patients.

Standard echocardiography, which is useful in the management of patients with NVE, has been less helpful in patients with PVE. Echoes generated by the prosthesis are intense, and subtle abnormalities such as small vegetations may be obscured. Bioprosthetic valves are more easily assessed by two-dimensional echocardiography than are mechanical valves.[46] In contrast, Doppler echocardiography does appear to be a valuable technique for the assessment of valvular dysfunction of mechanical as well as bioprosthetic valves. In one series, Doppler echocardiography correctly identified significant regurgitation or obstruction in 15 of 17 patients with malfunctioning prosthetic valves.[47]

Cardiac cinefluoroscopy is a useful procedure for detecting prosthetic valve instability due to loosening of the sewing ring.[6,48] A thrombus or vegetation on the prosthesis may also be suggested by impaired motion of a radiopaque poppet. Cardiac catheterization is often unnecessary in the evaluation of patients with PVE, even when surgical intervention is anticipated. In some circumstances, however, catheterization can provide valuable information including an estimation of the degree of valvular dysfunction, the location of the fistula, an evaluation of left ventricular function, delineation of coronary artery anatomy, or an assessment of possible multiple valve involvement.[49]

Computed tomography of the head is indicated in all patients with PVE and neurologic symptoms. Infarction, hemorrhage, or an abscess can usually be differentiated by this technique. In addition, all patients with neurologic symptoms not readily explained by computed tomography should undergo cerebral angiography to exclude the possibility of an intracranial mycotic aneurysm.[50]

Mortality of Prosthetic Valve Endocarditis

The mortality of patients with PVE remains high. Dismukes analyzed 105 cases of PVE treated between 1976 and 1979 at the Massachusetts General Hospital and the University of Alabama Medical Center and reported an overall mortality of 29 percent. The mortality was 41 percent in early PVE and 21 percent in late disease.[51] More recently, Calderwood et al. reported the outcomes of 116 patients with PVE; in-hospital mortality was 23 percent. The authors applied logistic regression analysis and found that "complicated" infection (defined as persistent fever while receiving antibiotics, changing murmurs heard on physical examination, worsening heart failure, or new conduction abnormalities) was the best predictor of death.[1]

The mortality of PVE varies somewhat with the etiologic microorganism. In a group of 184 patients reviewed by Wilson et al.[52] significantly higher mortality was seen in PVE caused by fungi, gram-negative bacilli, or staphylococci.

Management of Prosthetic Valve Endocarditis

General Principles. Successful management of patients with PVE depends on the same principles used in treating patients with NVE. All patients should be hospitalized, confined to bed during the acute phase of the illness, and monitored carefully for hemodynamic deterioration and arrhythmias. Patients should undergo careful daily physical examination to detect heart failure, changes in murmurs, or evidence of embolization or a mycotic aneurysm.

Antibiotic Therapy. Antimicrobial therapy is based on laboratory identification of the etiologic microorganism and in vitro susceptibility testing; bactericidal antibiotics are necessary. In an effort to enhance in vivo activity, combinations of antibiotics that demonstrate synergistic killing of the pathogen in vitro are often used. Whenever possible, intravenous medications should be administered via scalp vein needles rather than indwelling intravenous catheters to reduce the risk of bacteremia from a contaminated intravascular device. Recommended antibiotic regimens are shown in Table 3.

The combination of aqueous penicillin G plus gentamicin[53,54] is recommended to treat patients with PVE caused by penicillin-susceptible streptococci (minimum inhibitory concentration [MIC] ≤0.1 μg/ml). Streptomycin may be used in place of gentamicin if the MIC for streptomycin is less than 1000 μg/ml. The combination of penicillin G (or ampicillin) and gentamicin is the preferred regimen for PVE due to enterococci[54,55] or other resistant streptococci. The aminoglycoside susceptibility of enterococci should be routinely determined since some strains are highly resistant to all aminoglycosides (MIC, ≥2000 μg/ml).[54,56] There is currently no proven satisfactory treatment regimen for endocarditis caused by aminoglycoside-resistant enterococci (see Chapter 179).

For PVE caused by *S. aureus*, penicillin G is the treatment of choice if the isolate is penicillinase-negative and the MIC for penicillin G is 0.1 μg/ml or less. If penicillinase is produced, a semisynthetic antistaphylococcal penicillin (e.g., nafcillin) should be used instead. Because in vitro studies have demonstrated enhanced killing of *S. aureus* by certain antibiotic combinations, many authorities advocate the addition of gentamicin for the first 2 weeks of therapy. Prosthetic valve endocarditis caused by methicillin-resistant isolates of *S. aureus* must be treated with vancomycin plus gentamicin.

In one study, approximately 80 percent of *S. epidermidis* isolates from patients with PVE were resistant to methicillin.[57] Resistance is not due to β-lactamase production but to alterations in penicillin-binding proteins. Resistance of *S. epidermidis* to methicillin or cephalosporins may not always be apparent by routine in vitro susceptibility testing. Consequently, the use of β-lactam antibiotics alone to treat *S. epidermidis* PVE has resulted in high failure rates.[58] On the basis of currently available data, the combination of vancomycin and rifampin with gentamicin added for the first 2 weeks of therapy appears to be the most effective regimen for *S. epidermidis* PVE.[54,59]

Selection of an antimicrobial regimen for the treatment of diphtheroid PVE is somewhat controversial. If the diphtheroid strain is susceptible to penicillin and gentamicin, therapy with this combination is recommended. The clinical efficacy of penicillin plus gentamicin has also been demonstrated even when the diphtheroid isolate is penicillin resistant,[25] although some would recommend vancomycin in this circumstance. Vancomycin is the therapy of choice for PVE caused by diphtheroid strains (such as group JK corynebacteria) which are resistant to both penicillin and gentamicin.

The design of an antibiotic regimen for PVE caused by aerobic gram-negative bacilli must be based on identification of the organism and careful in vitro susceptibility and synergy studies. Therapy will usually include a β-lactam antibiotic (penicillin, cephalosporin, carbapenem, or monobactam) plus an amino-

TABLE 3. Antimicrobial Therapy for Patients with Bacterial Infections of Prosthetic Valves

Organism	*Regimen*	*Duration of Therapy (wk)*	*Regimen in Penicillin-Allergic Patients*[a,b]
Susceptible streptococci (MIC <0.1 μg/ml Pen G)	Aqueous Pen G[c] plus gentamicin[d,e]	4–6 2	Vancomycin[f] plus gentamicin[d,e] or Cephalothin[g] plus gentamicin[d,e]
Resistant streptococci (MIC >0.1 μg/ml Pen G), enterococci	Aqueous Pen G[c] or ampicillin[h] plus gentamicin[d]	6–8 6–8	Vancomycin[f] plus gentamicin[d]
Staphylococcus aureus			
Methcillin susceptible	Nafcillin[i] plus gentamicin[d]	6–8 2	Cephalothin[g] plus gentamicin[d]
Methcillin resistant	Vancomycin[f] plus gentamicin[d]	6–8 2	Not applicable
Staphylococcus epidermidis	Vancomycin[f] plus rifampin[j] and gentamicin[d]	6–8 6–8 2	Not applicable
Diphtheroids	Aqueous Pen G[c] plus gentamicin[d] or Vancomycin[f,k]	6 6	Vancomycin[f,k] Not applicable
Aerobic gram-negative bacilli	β-Lactam[l] plus aminoglycoside—based on in vitro data	6–8 6–8	Consider aztreonam[l] plus aminoglycoside
Empirical regimen, bacteria not identified	Vancomycin[f] plus gentamicin[d]		Not applicable

[a] The duration of therapy is similar to that recommended for non-penicillin-allergic patients.
[b] Cephalosporins are contraindicated when there is history of penicillin anaphylaxis.
[c] Aqueous penicillin G, 24 million units daily in divided doses q4h.
[d] Gentamicin, 1 mg/kg iv q8h.
[e] Streptomycin may be used for sensitive organisms (MIC <1000 μg/ml).
[f] Vancomycin, 0.5 g iv q6h.
[g] Cephalothin, 2 g iv q4h (or equivalent cephalosporin).
[h] Ampicillin, 2 g iv q4h.
[i] Nafcillin, 2 g iv q4h.
[j] Rifampin, 300 mg po q8h.
[k] Preferred agent for gentamicin-resistant strains.
[l] For strains resistant to all β-lactams, consider ciprofloxacin as a single agent.

glycoside. Newer quinolones may be useful in therapy for resistant organisms, but their efficacy in endocarditis has not yet been established in large-scale clinical trials.[60,61]

Fungal PVE is a very serious disorder that requires combined medical and surgical therapy. For *Candida* endocarditis, high doses of intravenous amphotericin B (up to 1 mg/kg/day) is given in combination with oral flucytosine (dose adjusted for renal function). A preoperative induction course of amphotericin B does not seem to improve outcome; prompt valve replacement is mandatory.[62]

When PVE seems clinically apparent but blood cultures are not yet positive, therapy with vancomycin plus gentamicin should be initiated. For patients in whom infection has been demonstrated at an extracardiac site (e.g., wound infection, pneumonia, urinary tract infection), initial antimicrobial therapy should include drugs active against the microorganism present at that site as well. When PVE is considered but the level of clinical suspicion is low, three or four blood cultures should be obtained by separate venipunctures and the patient observed. If valve replacement is imminent, it is reasonable to initiate empirical antimicrobial therapy with vancomycin and gentamicin. The diagnosis of PVE can usually be confirmed or excluded at the time of surgery.

Serum bactericidal activity should be measured during the first few days of therapy to demonstrate the in vivo activity of the antimicrobial regimen being used. Controversy exists regarding the usefulness of the test, the best method of testing, the optimal antimicrobial activity desired, and the timing of testing (peak vs. trough). In general, a serum bactericidal titer of greater than 1:32 against the infecting bacteria (measured at the time of peak antibiotic concentration) appears to correlate with a more favorable clinical response.[63,64] If a titer of at least 1:8 is not achieved, an increase in dosage or change in antibiotics should be considered, particularly if the patient is not responding clinically.

After the initiation of antimicrobial therapy, blood cultures should be obtained daily for the first 3–4 days and weekly thereafter until the completion of therapy. Usually blood cultures will be sterile within 3–5 days of initiating appropriate antimicrobial therapy. After the completion of therapy, blood cultures should be obtained weekly for 1 month. A relapse necessitates reinstitution of antimicrobial therapy, retesting of the microorganism for antimicrobial susceptibility, and strong consideration of valve replacement. Occasionally, a relapse may be due to persistent infection at an extracardiac site; careful consideration should be given to the possibility of an occult abscess or mycotic aneurysm.

Surgical Therapy. Several general observations can be made regarding the increasingly important role of surgery in the management of PVE. First, the mortality of patients with PVE who undergo valve replacement during active infection is no greater (and may be less) than is the mortality of patients who receive medical therapy alone. Mortality statistics may underestimate the value of surgical intervention in the management of PVE since many of the patients in the medical–surgical treatment group were critically ill and underwent surgery only after failing medical therapy. Second, the risk of recurrent PVE after the surgical removal of an infected prosthesis is real but usually acceptable. The incidence in published series has ranged from 0 to 15 percent, and the microorganisms causing PVE after valve replacement for NVE are usually different from those infecting the native valve.[2,12,65] This perhaps reflects the more complex techniques necessary for repair in these patients. Third, when valve replacement is clinically indicated, there is little to be gained by delaying surgery despite an incomplete course of antibiotic therapy. A delay only increases the chances for serious complications such as refractory heart failure, renal failure, or emboli.[2,12,66]

The objectives of cardiac surgery in PVE are to remove infected tissues and materials and to restore hemodynamic integrity.[67] Other goals include the repair of acquired defects (such as abscesses) and elimination of sources of emboli.[63,68] The decision to proceed with cardiac surgery in the seriously ill patient with PVE is seldom an easy one. To provide some guidelines for physicians and surgeons caring for these patients, we have used a point system to assess the need for valve replacement. If assessment of a patient results in the accumulation of five or more points by the system described in Table 4, we would recommend surgery—emergent surgery in the case of severe heart failure and urgent surgery in the case of other complications.

TABLE 4. Indications for Valve Replacement during Active Prosthetic Valve Endocarditis

Disorder	Point Rating[a]
Heart failure due to valve dysfunction	
Severe	5
Moderate	5
Mild	2
Acute valve obstruction	5
Fungal etiology	5
Persistent bacteremia	5
Organism other than penicillin-susceptible *Streptoccus*	2
Relapse after appropriate therapy	3
One major embolus	2
Two or more emboli	4
Vegetations by echocardiogram	1
Heart block	3
Ruptured ventricular septal defect or sinus of Valsalva	4
Early PVE (<60 days)	2
Unstable prosthesis by fluoroscopy	5
Paravalvular leak	2
Prior prosthetic valve replacement	−2

[a] The accumulation of 5 or more points suggests the need for valve replacement.
(From Alsip et al.,[69] with permission.)

The severity of heart failure is a leading prognostic factor in patients with PVE. In patients with moderate to severe heart failure secondary to valvular dysfunction, emergency valve replacement may be lifesaving. Two large series reported by Richardson et al.[12] and Karchmer et al.[13] contain a total of 52 PVE patients with moderate to severe heart failure. The mortality in the medical therapy group was 100 percent, while the combined medical–surgical therapy group had a 49 percent mortality. Valve replacement is therefore recommended in all PVE patients with moderate to severe heart failure. Emergency valve replacement is also required in patients who develop acute prosthetic obstruction due to large vegetations. Hemodynamically stable patients who may later require valve replacement for mild heart failure or a paravalvular leak should receive a full course of antimicrobial therapy before elective surgery.

Valve replacement within 48–72 hours is recommended in cases of fungal PVE because of the poor response to medical therapy and high frequency of major emboli.[62] In patients with bacterial PVE, valve replacement should be considered whenever bacteremia persists for more than a few days after the initiation of the best antimicrobial therapy.

Anticoagulation. Most patients with mechanical heart valves require long-term anticoagulation to prevent thromboembolic complications. However, the theoretic risks of bleeding at the site of a mycotic aneurysm or embolic infarction raises important questions about the use of anticoagulants in patients with active PVE. Carpenter et al. described 14 patients who received anticoagulants during therapy for PVE. Thirty-six percent had symptomatic episodes of CNS hemorrhage.[70] In contrast, Wilson et al. noted a higher frequency of neurologic complications in PVE patients who did not receive adequate anticoagulation.[71] Although the proper use of anticoagulants remains controversial, most authorities do continue anticoagulation in patients with PVE. However, it may be prudent to monitor patients closely and maintain clotting parameters at the lower end of the therapeutic range.

Prophylaxis

Although there have been no adequate placebo-controlled trials to assess the value of prophylactic antibiotics in valve replacement surgery, they are routinely employed. Prophylaxis, usually with a first-generation cephalosporin, is directed at the prevention of wound infection and PVE due to staphylococci and streptococci; the duration of administration should not exceed 2 days. Vancomycin is an appropriate alternative drug. After discharge from the hospital, the patient should be aware of the importance of prophylactic antimicrobial agents before any procedure likely to cause transient bacteremia (see Chapter 63).

INDWELLING RIGHT ATRIAL CATHETERS

Broviac and Hickman catheters are silicone elastomer intravenous devices designed to permit long-term vascular access for hyperalimentation, drug or blood product administration, and blood sampling[72,73] (see Chapters 61 and 279). The catheters are similar in design, but the Hickman device has a larger diameter, which facilitates aspiration of blood samples. The distal, intravascular portion of the catheter is inserted into the superior vena cava or right atrium via the external jugular or cephalic vein. The extravascular portion, with a Dacron felt cuff in place, is drawn through a subcutaneous chest wall tunnel that exits between the nipple and sternum. The Dacron cuff is designed to permit fibroblast ingrowth to anchor the catheter and prevent microorganisms from tracking along the outside.

Four varieties of infectious complication of Broviac or Hickman catheters include (*1*) exit site infections, (*2*) tunnel infectoins, (*3*) septic thrombophlebitis, and (*4*) isolated bacteremia or fungemia. Press et al. reviewed the courses of 992 oncology patients with a total of 1088 Hickman catheter placements. One hundred forty-three catheter infections were documented (incidence, 0.14 infections/100 catheter days). Exit site infections, isolated bacteremia, tunnel infections, and septic thrombophlebitis accounted for 46, 31, 20, and 4 percent of all infections, respectively.[74]

Microbiology

Presently, gram-positive cocci are responsible for most silicone elastomer catheter infections in the United States.[74–79] *Staphylococcus epidermidis* accounted for 54.1 percent and *Staphylococcus aureus* for 20 percent of the clinical isolates in the review of 143 catheter infections by Press et al. Gram-negative bacilli, gram-positive bacilli, and fungi such as *Candida albicans* respectively accounted for 9, 5, and 7 percent of all clinical isolates.[74]

Pathogenesis

The precise pathogenesis of catheter-related infections is unclear. However, the frequency with which *S. epidermidis* is isolated suggests that microorganisms may track along the catheter from the skin or perhaps are introduced at the time of catheter placement. The risk of hematogenous seeding of the catheter during bacteremia from a distant focus appears to be low.[74]

Clinical Manifestations

The clinical manifestations of catheter infections vary with the sites of involvement. (*1*) Exit site infections are characterized by local warmth, erythema, and tenderness at the site where the catheter exits from the skin. Purulent drainage around the catheter may or may not be evident. (*2*) Tunnel infections may resemble exit site infections, but tenderness and erythema extend up the chest along the subcutaneous tract of the proximal portion of the catheter. Both exit site and tunnel infections may be complicated by the presence of concomitant bacteremia (three of four and three of eight patients, respectively, in one series.[74] (*3*) The manifestations of septic thrombophlebitis reflect bacterial invasion and subsequent thrombosis of the vein that the catheter enters. Patients are almost always bacteremic, and there are local signs of venous insufficiency such as edema of the upper extremity. (*4*) Finally, patients may be bacteremic in the absence of localizing signs or symptoms. This type of infection may be particularly important in neutropenic individuals who are unable to mount a local inflammatory response to infection.

Diagnosis

The early diagnosis of catheter-related infections requires regular examination of the catheter exit site and the skin overlying the tunnel for signs of tenderness and erythema. If infection is suspected, Gram stain and culture should be performed on any purulent material expressed from around the catheter. In addition, blood cultures should be routinely obtained. Cultures drawn through the catheter will occasionally be positive even though peripheral blood cultures are negative.

Therapy

Therapy for indwelling right atrial catheter infections has changed significantly in the 1980s. Previously, clinicians believed that all infected catheters required removal, especially if bacteremia was documented. Many catheters can now be salvaged. Exit site infections with or without associated bacteremia are the type most responsive to antibiotic therapy, with cure rates as high as 85 percent in one series.[74] Bacteremia without evidence of localized catheter infection may also be successfully managed with parenteral antibiotics (see Chapter 61 and 280). Tunnel infections and septic thrombophlebitis are more difficult to eradicate and usually require catheter removal. Similarly, catheters infected with resistant organisms such as gram-negative bacilli or fungi are difficult to salvage. In any case, catheter removal should be considered whenever patients fail to respond to antibiotics as indicated by persistent fever or continued positive blood cultures while receiving therapy. The empirical treatment of catheter-related infections should generally include vancomycin and gentamicin to treat *S. epidermidis*. The therapeutic regimen can be altered on the basis of the antimicrobial susceptibility patterns of organisms isolated. All cases other than mild exit site infections should be treated with approximately 14 days of parenteral antibiotics. Some investigators have advocated the instillation of fibrinolytic agents (streptokinase or urokinase) into the catheter if there is evidence of partial occlusion by a clot. Shuman et al. reported a 90 percent catheter salvage rate when using local fibrinolytic therapy and systemic antimicrobial agents in 28 episodes of bacteremia occuring in 24 patients with indwelling right atrial catheters.[80]

INFECTION OF VASCULAR GRAFTS

Incidence

The reported incidence of vascular prosthesis infection ranges from less than 1 percent to more than 5 percent and varies with the site of graft placement.[81–83] Grafts implanted in the inguinal area (e.g., aortofemoral or femoropopliteal grafts) have a higher rate of infection than do grafts that lie entirely within the abdomen. In one series of 3652 patients receiving primarily aortic, aortoiliac, or aortofemoral grafts, a groin incision was associated with a threefold increase in the incidence of graft infection (1.34 vs. 0.43 percent).[84] Infection rates for grafts in the upper extremities and other sites are less well documented.

Pathogenesis

The mechanisms by which microorganisms colonize vascular grafts include (*1*) contamination at the time of surgery, (*2*) direct extension from an adjacent tissue site, and (*3*) hematogenous seeding during an episode of bacteremia.

Lower extremity grafts are at greatest risk for infection, which may reflect higher rates of perioperative contamination with microorganisms from the skin at the relatively superficial lower extremity graft site. Preoperative extremity infections, postoperative wound infections, and underlying disorders, such as diabetes mellitus may also contribute to the high incidence of infections in femoral and popliteal grafts.

Abdominal aortic grafts have a relatively high incidence of infection with gram-negative enteric bacilli, probably reflecting contamination of the graft by bowel microorganisms. Several investigators have suggested that unsuspected infections in aortic aneurysms may be responsible for some cases of postrepair graft infections. In two recent reports, cultures were obtained from 266 clinically uninfected aneurysmectomy specimens. Bacteria were isolated in 33 instances, with *S. epidermidis* the most common organism.[85,86] However, the incidence of subsequent infections in these individuals was quite low, and the significance of these data remains unclear.

Graft infections may result from bacteremia, but the risk of infection diminishes as the graft becomes incorporated in the host tissue.[87] After an initial inflammatory reaction, fibrous tissue accumulates on the outer surface of the graft, and a pseudointima composed of connective tissue and fibrin begins to form on the inner surface of the graft.[88] A true endothelial lining extends from the native artery but rarely grows more than 10 mm beyond the anastomosis.[89] In animal models, resistance of an implanted graft to blood-borne infection correlates with the degree of pseudointima formation.[90,91]

Microbiology

Table 5 lists by site the etiologic mocroorganisms recovered from 85 patients with graft infections.[82,92,93] *Staphylococcus aureus* and *S. epidermidis* are the most commonly reported causes of graft infections, particularly sites involving the lower extremity.[81,94] Intra-abdominal graft infections are most commonly caused by *E. coli* or other gram-negative enteric bacilli. Data from several large series show that two or more microorganisms were isolated from 37 percent of graft infections; multiple isolates were found in 60 percent of abdominal graft infections and 23 percent of groin infections.[82,92,93,95] Polymicrobial infections most often included a staphylococcus and a gram-negative bacillus or combinations of gram-negative bacilli.

TABLE 5. Microbial Etiology of Vascular Graft Infections

	Anatomic Location of Infection			
Organism	*Abdominal (%)*	*Groin (%)*	*Popliteal (%)*	*Overall (%)*
S. aureus	14	40	33	33
S. epidermidis	7	13	17	12
Streptococci	14	8	25	11
E. coli	42	9	0	16
Proteus sp.	3	11	0	8
Other aerobic gram-negative bacilli	0	8	17	7
Other bacteria	10	5	0	6
Candida sp.	3	1	0	1
Unknown	7	5	8	6
Total number				
Microorganisms	29	85	12	126
Patients	17	60	8	85

(Data from Szilagyi et al.,[82] Becker et al.,[92] and Hoffert et al.[93])

Clinical Features

The local and systemic manifestations of graft infections vary with the location of the prosthesis. Over 70 percent of infections involving groin and popliteal vascular prostheses develop within 2 months of surgery, whereas 70 percent of intra-abdominal graft infections do not become clinically apparent until more than 1 year after surgery.[92,96] The most common presentations of graft infection in the groin or leg are the formation of a localized abscess or draining sinus, the formation of a false aneurysm (which may be associated with pain and a new bruit), thrombosis of the graft, or septic emboli to the distal extremity.[96] Erythema, warmth, or tenderness at a graft site is highly suggestive of infection. Rapid swelling over an area of vascular repair of a hemorrhage from a graft site suggests disruption of the suture line with bleeding or false aneurysm formation. Ischemic changes and a loss of pulses in the distal part of the extremity indicate thrombosis of the arterial implant. Exteriorization of the graft due to a breakdown of overlying tissues is pathognomonic of infection.

The presentation of intra-abdominal graft infections may be subtle. Fever is usually present but may be low grade. Specific findings in aortic graft infections can include abdominal tenderness, retroperitoneal hemorrhage, an abdominal mass due to a false aneurysm, graft thrombosis, ureteral obstruction with hydronephrosis, and septic emboli.[97] Petechiae and spinter hemorrhages similar to those in endocarditis may also occur. Aortoenteric fistula formation due to erosion of the graft into the bowel occurred in 0.36 percent of patients in one series.[84] In 80 percent of cases of aortoenteric fistula, the proximal anastomosis erodes into the third portion of the duodenum[98] A breakdown of the suture line results in upper or lower gastrointestinal bleeding that may be massive. Melena or hematemesis in a patient with an aortic graft should immediately arouse suspicion of a developing aortoenteric fistula.[92,99]

Diagnosis

A variety of diagnostic techniques are useful in evaluating patients with suspected vascular graft infection. If a draining sinus is present, a careful sinogram may reveal the extent of an underlying infectious process. Abscesses and aneurysms may also be demonstrated by noninvasive techniques such as sonography and computerized tomography. Magnetic resonance imaging may prove to be a sensitive technique for diagnosing graft infections. In one report of three patients, magnetic resonance imaging clearly delineated the extent of perigraft infection. Abscesses have a high signal intensity that contrasts strongly with the signal of flowing blood.[100] Gallium scanning has not generally been found to be useful; indium-labeled leukocyte scanning may be a sensitive diagnostic technique, but its specificity appears to be low, at least in the perioperative period.[101] Arteriography is the most precise method for documenting false aneurysm formation, suture line leakage, or graft thrombosis.

Cultures and Gram stains should be obtained on all draining wounds, although cultures obtained at the time of surgical inspection provide more reliable microbiologic data. Routine venous blood cultures should also be obtained. No good estimation of the frequency of positive blood cultures is available, but negative blood cultures do occur in an appreciable number of cases when infection has not yet extended to the graft lumen. Material removed at embolectomy, however, should always be cultured.

Morbidity and Mortality

Morbidity and mortality vary with the position of the graft. In a review of 84 patients with vascular graft infection, O'Hara et al. found an overall 30-day mortality rate of 28 percent. The same authors reported a 1-year mortality rate among the 43 patients who received grafts since 1980 of 46 percent.[84] In another series of infected aortobifemoral prostheses, mortality was 23 percent.[102] Mortality rates are lower for distal graft infections (14 percent[96] in one series of femoropopliteal grafts), largely due to the ease of earlier diagnosis and the decreased severity of bleeding relative to proximal grafts.

The major morbidity associated with graft infection is loss of the extremity supplied by the prosthesis. In one recent review, the amputation rate among 13 patients with aortofemoral infections was 38 percent.[102]

Management

Successful treatment usually requires a combination of systemic antibiotic administration and surgery. Removal of the entire graft and débridement of infected tissue is almost always necessary for cure. Most attempts to treat graft infection with antibiotics and local wound care alone are unsuccessful. Infections occurring at midpoints of long grafts (e.g., axillofemoral) may be temporarily managed by drainage and antibiotics, but graft removal will ultimately be required for a successful outcome. The viability of distal structures depends upon the adequacy of collateral vessels and the feasibility of additional bypass procedures. If the extremity or organ is totally dependent upon flow through the graft, some form of revascularization that bypasses the site of infection should be attempted. For example, axillofemoral grafts may be used to bypass an infected aortic bifurcation graft. If a new graft must be placed in the infected field, some authors have recommended use of autogenous artery or vein grafts, which may be less suceptible to infection than are grafts made of synthetic materials. The only common situation in which removal of a portion of the graft is acceptable occurs when infection involves the distal anastamosis of one branch of an aortofemoral graft; the infected limb may sometimes be removed and the opposite limb preserved. Identification of the infecting microorganism and in vitro susceptibility testing are also essential for successful therapy. Some graft infections may be temporarily managed by drainage and antibiotics, but graft removal will ultimately be required for a successful outcome. Recommended initial antimicrobial regimens for graft infections are generally the same as those recommended for PVE (Table 3). Antibiotics should be administered parenterally for 4 weeks after the prosthetic device is removed.

Prevention

Strict adherence to principles of asepsis, vigorous preoperative skin decontamination, and meticulous surgical technique are the most important factors in preventing wound and graft infections. Simultaneous procedures that could result in bacteremia or wound contamination should be avoided.

Prophylactic antibiotics are routinely employed in vascular operations. A double-blind study of cefazolin vs. placebo demonstrated a significantly lower rate of postoperative wound and graft infections in patients who receive cefazolin.[103] Some surgeons routinely instill antibiotic solutions into the wound before closure, but the value of this practice is unproved.[104] Grafts containing antibiotics incorporated into the material have been developed but remain investigational.[105]

Little information is available to assess the value of prophylactic antibiotics in patients with vascular grafts who undergo manipulations likely to result in bacteremia. Graft infection resulting from such bacteremia appears to be rare, but some authors have recommended that prophylactic antibiotics be given before dental, genitourinary, or other procedures.[106,107] This may have the greatest value in the first few months after graft placement.[108]

INFECTIONS OF DIALYSIS-ACCESS ARTERIOVENOUS FISTULAS

Because of lower rates of infection and thrombosis, surgically created subcutaneous arteriovenous fistulas (AVFs) have generally replaced external arteriovenous cannulas for vascular access in chronic dialysis patients.[109,110] An AVF may be created by direct artery-to-vein anastomosis (native AVF) or by implantation of a prosthetic conduit. Expanded polytetrafluoroethylene is the most commonly used material.

Infectious complications of native vessel AVFs appear to be uncommon. The incidence of infection has averaged less than 2 percent in several recent studies with follow-ups as long as 5 years.[111,112] Infection occurs more frequently in prosthetic AVFs. In three recent studies, infections developed in 11, 23, and 25 percent of patients receiving expanded polytetrafluoroethylene grafts.[111–113]

Microbiology

Staphylococcus aureus is the most common etiologic microorganism and accounts for 60–90 percent of access site infections.[109,110,114–116] Gram-negative bacilli, especially *Pseudomonas aeruginosa* are also commonly encountered.[110,114,116] A prosthetic AVF may become infected through a variety of mechanisms. Contamination may occur at the time of implantation, or a relatively superficial wound infection may extend to involve the graft. In addition, access sites are subjected to multiple needle punctures during dialysis, which may result in direct inoculation of the prosthesis. Hematomas or false aneurysms occurring at puncture sites may also become infected. Bacteremia is a possible but apparently uncommon source of AVF infection.

Clinical Manifestations

Arteriovenous fistula infections may present with local pain, tenderness, erythema, abscess formation, or bacteremia. However, as many as a third of AVF infections have no clinically apparent local findings.[114,117] As with other types of vascular graft infections, involvement of the suture line may result in disruption of the anastomosis and subsequent hemorrhage. Approximately 30 percent of AVF infections are associated with bacteremia. Metastatic infections such as endocarditis or septic pulmonary thromboembolism may occur, especially with staphylococcal AVF infections.[109,117]

Therapy

Management of infected AVFs almost always necessitates the combination of antibiotic administration and surgery. However, there are reports of graft salvage when antimicrobial therapy and surgical débridement are combined. This may be more effective when the infectious process involves only a localized site distant from suture lines.[118] Infection involving native vessel AVFs may respond to antimicrobial therapy alone.[94,114]

Initial empirical antimicrobial therapy for an infected AVF should include agents active against staphylococci and aerobic gram-negative bacilli (e.g., vancomycin, an antipseudomonal β-lactam, and an aminoglycoside). Subsequent therapy must be based upon the susceptibility pattern(s) of the isolated pathogen(s). The doses of all agents must be carefully adjusted for the patient's renal function.

PERMANENT PACEMAKER INFECTIONS

Infection is second only to problems with pacing or sensing as a complication of permanent pacemaker insertion. In one series of 457 patients, the reported incidence of pacemaker infections was 3.6 and 2 percent for epicardial and transvenous devices, respectively.[119] Pacemaker infections may involve any portion of the implanted hardware from the generator box to the pacing electrode. Concomitant bacteremia or endocarditis may also be present.

The most common location for pacemaker infections is the subcutaneous pocket containing the generator box. Most such infections present soon after surgery but may not become evident for 2 years or more. Staphylococci are the most common causes of generator box infections. In one large review, *S. epidermidis* was responsible for 44 percent of pacemaker infections while *S. aureus* was isolated from 29 percent.[120] The most likely pathogenesis of generator box infections is contamination of the device by skin flora at the time of implantation. Wound infection or erosion of the box through the overlying skin may also lead to microbial contamination.

The other major category of pacemaker infection is involvement of the epicardial or transvenous electrodes. This usually results from the direct spread of microorganism along the wires from an infected generator box, but hematogenous seeding occasionally occurs.[121]

The clinical manifestations of pacemaker infection depends upon the site of involvement. Generator box infections typically present with fever and local warmth, erythema, and tenderness over the generator pocket. Isolated lead infections are less common but may present similarly to bacterial endocarditis with fever and positive blood cultures. A definite diagnosis of pacemaker infection depends upon the isolation of an etiologic microorganism from the pacemaker pocket or the blood stream.

Treatment of pacemaker infections remains controversial. All hardware should be removed in both generator box and electrode infections, particularly when these disorders are accompanied by bacteremia. Occasional cures have been reported in generator box infections with parenteral antibiotics and local irrigation alone. Parenteral antimicrobial agents must be chosen carefully on the basis of the identification and susceptibility of the isolated pathogen. The proper duration of therapy is not well established. If any foreign material is left in place, antibiotic administration should be continued for at least 6 weeks, perhaps followed by long-term suppressive therapy. Antimicrobial therapy should continue for approximately 4 weeks after the hardware is removed if bacteremia is documented. Two weeks of antimicrobial therapy may be adequate for nonbacteremic infection if the device is removed.

REFERENCES

1. Calderwood SB, Swinski LA, Karchmer AW, et al. Prosthetic valve endocarditis: Analysis of factors affecting outcome of therapy. J Thorac Cardiovasc Surg. 1986;92:776–83.
2. Ivert TSA, Dismukes WE, Cobbs CG, et al. Prosthetic valve endocarditis. Circulation. 1984;69:223.
3. Dismukes WE, Karchmer AW, Buckley MJ, et al. Prosthetic valve endocarditis: Analysis of 38 cases. Circulation. 1973;48:365.
4. Rossiter SJ, Stinson EB, Oyer PE, et al. Prosthetic valve endocarditis: Comparison of heterograft tissue valves and mechanical valves. J Thorac Cardiovasc Surg. 1978;76:795.
5. Grignon A, Spencer H, Robson HG, et al. Prosthetic valve infections. Can J Surg. 1981;24:615.
6. Masur H, Johnson WD Jr. Prosthetic valve endocarditis. J Thorac Cardiovasc Surg. 1980;80:31.
7. Auger P, Marquis G, Dyrda I, et al. Infective endocarditis update: Experience from a heart hospital. Acta Cardiol. 1981;36:105.
8. Aintablian A, Hilsenrath J, Hamby RJ, et al. Endocarditis in prosthetic valves. NY State J Med. 1976;76:673.
9. Wilson WR, Jaumin PM, Danielson GK, et al. Prosthetic valve endocarditis. Ann Intern Med. 1975;82:751.
10. Slaughter L, Morris JE, Starr A. Prosthetic valvular endocarditis: A 12-year review. Circulation. 1973;47:1319.
11. Petheram IS, Boyce JMH. Prosthetic valve endocarditis: A reiew of 24 cases. Thorax. 1977;32:478.
12. Richardson JV, Karp RB, Kirklin JW, et al. Treatment of infective endocarditis: A 10 year comparative analysis. Circulation. 1978;58:589.
13. Karchmer AW, Dismukes WE, Buckley MJ, et al. Late prosthetic valve endocarditis: Clinical features influencing therapy. Am J Med. 1978;64:199.
14. Bortotti U, Thiene G, Milano A, et al. Pathological study of infective endocarditis on Hancock porcine bioprostheses. J Thorac Cardiovasc Surg. 1981;81:934.
15. Magilligan DJ, Quinn EL, Davila JC. Bacteremia, endocarditis, and the Hancock valve. Ann Thorac Surg. 1977;24:508.
16. Isom OW, Spencer FC, Glassman E, et al. Long-term results in 1375 patients undergoing valve replacement with the Starr-Edwards cloth-covered steel ball prosthesis. Ann Surg. 1977;186:310.
17. Downham WH, Rhoades ER. Endocarditis associated with porcine valve xenografts. Arch Intern Med. 1979;139:1350.
18. Gallo JI, Ruiz B, Carrion MF, et al. Heart valve replacement with the Hancock bioprosthesis: A 6-year review. Ann Thorac Surg. 1981;31:444.
19. Rutledge R, Kim BJ, Applebaum RE. Actuarial analysis of the risk of prosthetic valve endocarditis in 1,598 patients with mechanical and bioprosthetic valves. Arch Surg. 1985;120:469.
20. Hammond GL, Geha AS, Kopf GS, et al. Biological versus mechanical valves: Analysis of 1,116 valves inserted in 1,012 adult patients with a 4,818 patient-year and a 5,327 valve-year follow-up. J Thorac Cardiovasc Surg. 1987;93:182.
21. Calderwood SB, Swinski LA, Waternaux CM, et al. Risk factors for the development of prosthetic valve endocarditis. Circulation. 1985;72:31.
22. Horstkotte D, Korfer R, Loogen F, et al. Prosthetic valve endocarditis: Clinical findings and management. Eur Heart J. 1984;5:17.
23. Chun PKC, Nelson WP. Common cardiac prosthetic valves: Radiologic identification and associated complications. JAMA. 1977;238:401.
24. Delgado DG, Cobbs CG. Infections of prosthetic valves and intravascular devices. In: Mandell GL, Douglas RG Jr, Bennett JE, eds. Principles and Practice of Infectious Diseases. New York: Churchill Livingstone; 1979;690.
25. Murray BE, Karchmer AW, Moellering RC Jr. Diphtheroid prosthetic valve endocarditis: A study of clinical features and infecting organisms. Am J Med. 1980;69:838.
26. Kluge RM, Calia FM, McLaughlin JS, et al. Sources of contamination in open heart surgery. JAMA. 1974;230:1415.
27. Blakemore WS, McGarrity GJ, Thurer RJ, et al. Infection by airborne bacteria with cardiopulmonary bypass. Surgery. 1971;70:830.
28. Freeman R, King B. Analysis of results of catheter tip cultures in open-heart surgery patients. Thorax. 1975;30:26.
29. Stiles GM, Singh L, Imazaki G, et al. Thermodilution cardiac output studies as a cause of prosthetic valve bacterial endocarditis. J Cardiovasc Surg. 1984;88:1035.
30. Centers for Disease Conttrol. Follow-up on mycobacterial contamination of porcine heart valve prostheses—United States. MMWR. 1978;27:92.
31. Rumisek JD, Albus RA, Clarke JS. Late *Mycobacterium chelonei* bioprosthetic valve endocarditis: Activation of implanted contaminant? Ann Thorac Surg. 1985;39:277.
32. Anderson DJ, Bulkley BH, Hutchins GM. A clinicopathologic study of prosthetic valve endocarditis in 22 patients: Morphologic basis for diagnosis and therapy. Am Heart J. 1977;94:325.
33. Arnett EN, Roberts WC. Prosthetic valve endocarditis: Clinicopathologic analysis of 22 necropsy patients with comparison of observations in 74 necropsy patients with active infective endocarditis involving natural left-sided cardiac valves. Am J Cardiol. 1976;38:281.
34. Ferrans VJ, Boyce SW, Billingham ME, et al. Infection of glutaraldehyde-preserved porcine valve heterografts. Am J Cardiol. 1979;43:1123.
35. Karchmer AW, Stinson EB. The role of surgery in infective endocarditis. In Swartz M, Remington J, eds. Current Clinical Topics in Infectious Diseases. McGraw-Hill, New York: 1980:124.
36. Leport C, Vilde JL, Bricaire F, et al. Fifty cases of late prosthetic valve endocarditis: Improvement in prognosis over a 15 year period. Br Heart J. 1987;58:66.
37. Hooper DC, Bayer AS, Karchmer AW, et al. Circulating immune complexes in prosthetic valve endocarditis. Arch Intern Med. 1983;143:2081.
38. Kauffmann RH, Thompson J, Valentijn RM, et al. The clinical implications and the pathogenetic significance of circulating immune complexes in infective endocarditis. Am J Med. 1981;71:17.
39. Neugarten J, Baldwin DS. Glomerulonephritis in bacterial endocarditis. Am J Med. 1984;77:297.
40. Watanakunakorn C. Prosthetic valve infective endocarditis: A review. Prog Cardiovasc Dis. 1979;22:181.
41. Madison J, Wang K, Gobel FI, et al. Prosthetic aortic valvular endocarditis. Circulation. 1975;51:940.
42. Quenzer RW, Edwards LD, Levin S. A comprehensive study of 48 host valve and 24 prosthetic valve endocarditis cases. Am Heart J. 1976;92:15.
43. Washington JA II. The role of the microbiology laboratory in the diagnosis and antimicrobial treatment of infective endocarditis. Mayo Clin Proc. 1982;57:22.
44. Sande MA, Johnson WD Jr, Hook EW, et al. Sustained bacteremia in patients with prosthetic cardiac valves. N Engl J Med. 1972;286:1067.
45. Dismukes WE, Karchmer AW. The diagnosis of infected prosthetic heart valves: Bacteremia versus endocarditis. In Duma RJ, ed. Infections of Prosthetic Heart Valves and Vascular Grafts. Baltimore, University Park Press; 1977:61.
46. Martin RP, French JW, Popp RL. Clinical utility of two-dimensional echocardiography in patients with bioprosthetic valves. Adv Cardiol. 1980;27:294.
47. Panidis IP, Ross J, Mintz GS. Normal and abnormal prosthetic valve func-

tion as assessed by Doppler echocardiography. J Am Coll Cardiol. 1986;8:317.
48. Ellis K, Jaffe C, Malm JR, et al. Infective endocarditis: Roentgenographic considerations. Radiol Clin North Am. 1973;11:415.
49. Welton DE, Young JB, Raizner AE, et al. Value and safety of cardiac catheterization during active infective endocarditis. Am J Cardiol. 1979;44:1306.
50. Dean RH, Waterhouse G, Meacham PW, et al. Mycotic embolism and emolomycotic aneurysms: Neglected lessons of the past. Ann Surg. 1986;204:300.
51. Dismukes WE. Prosthetic valve endocarditis: Factors influencing outcome and recommendations for therapy. In Bisno AL, ed. Treatment of Infective Endocarditis. New York: Grune & Stratton; 1981:67.
52. Wilson WR, Danielson GK, Giuliani ER, et al. Prosthetic valve endocarditis. Mayo Clin Proc. 1982;57:155.
53. Bisno AL, Dismukes WE, Durack DT, et al. Treatment of infective endocarditis due to viridans streptococci. JAMA. 1989;261:1471.
54. Bisno AL, Dismukes WE, Durack DT, et al. Antimicrobial treatment of infectious endocarditis due to viridans streptococci, enterococci, and staphylococci. Submitted for publication.
55. Carrizosa J, Kaye D. Antibiotic synergism in enterococcal endocarditis. J Lab Clin Med. 1976;88:132.
56. Mederski-Samoraj BD, Murray BE. High-level resistance to gentamicin in clinical isolates of enterococci. J Infect Dis. 1983;147:751.
57. Archer GL. Antimicrobial susceptibility and selection of resistance among *Staphylococcus epidermidis* isolates recovered from patients with infections of indwelling foreign devices. Antimicrob Agents Chemother. 1978;14:353.
58. Karchmer AW, Archer GL, Dismukes WE. *Staphylococcus epidermidis* causing prosthetic valve endocarditis: Microbiologic and clinical observations as guides to therapy. Ann Intern Med. 1983;98:447.
59. Karchmer AW, Archer GL, Dismukes WE. *Staphylococcus epidermidis* causing prosthetic valve endocarditis: Microbiologic and clinical observations as guides to therapy. Ann Intern Med. 1983;98:447.
60. Sande MA, Brooks-Fournier RA, Gerberding JL. Efficacy of ciprofloxacin in animal models of infection: Endocarditis, meningitis, and pneumonia. Am J Med. 1987;82:63.
61. Fernandez-Guerrero M, Rouse M, Henry N, et al. Ciprofloxacin therapy of experimental endocarditis caused by methicillin-susceptible or methicillin-resistant *Staphylococcus aureus*. Antimicrob Agents Chemother. 1988;32:747.
62. McLeod R, Remington JS. Fungal endocarditis. In: Rahimtoola SH, ed. Infective Endocarditis. New York: Grune & Stratton; 1978:211.
63. Reller LB. The serum bactericidal test. Rev Infect Dis. 1986;8:803.
64. Weinstein MP. Am J Med. 1985;78:262.
65. Baumgartner WA, Miller DC, Reitz BA, et al. Surgical treatment of prosthetic valve endocarditis. Ann Thorac Surg. 1983;35:87.
66. Mayer KH, Schoenbaum SC. Evaluation and management of prosthetic valve endocarditis. Prog Cardiovasc Dis. 1982;25:48.
67. Dinubile MJ. Surgery in active endocarditis. Ann Intern Med. 1982;96:650.
68. Karp RB. Role of surgery in infective endocarditis. Cardiovasc Clin. 1981;12:157.
69. Alsip SG, Blackstone EH, Kirklin JW, et al. Indications for cardiac surgery in patients with infective endocarditis. Am J Med. 1985;78:138.
70. Carpenter JL, McAllister CK, US Army Collaborative Group. Anticoagulation in prosthetic valve endocarditis. South Med J. 1983;76:1372.
71. Wilson WR, Geraci JE, Danielson GK, et al. Anticoagulant therapy and central nervous system complications in patients with prosthetic valve endocarditis. Circulation. 1978;57:1004.
72. Broviac JW, Cole JJ, Scribner BH. A silicone rubber atrial catheter for prolonged parenteral alimentation. Surg Gynecol Obstet. 1973;136:602.
73. Hickman RO, Buckner CD, Cliff RA, et al. A modified right atrial catheter for access to the venous system in marrow transplant recipients. Surg Gynecol Obstet. 1979;148:871.
74. Press OW, Ramsey PG, Larson EB, et al. Hickman catheter infections in patients with malignancies. Medicine (Baltimore). 1984;63:189.
75. Begala JE, Maher K, Cherry JD. Risk of infection associated with the use of Broviac and Hickman catheters. Am J Infect Control. 1982;10:17.
76. Wade JC, Newman KA, Schimpff SC, et al. Two methods for improved venous access in acute leukemia patients. JAMA. 1981;246:140.
77. Abrahm JL. A prospective study of prolonged central venous access in leukemia. JAMA. 1982;248:2868.
78. Thomas JH, MacArthur RI, Pierce GE, et al. Hickman-Broviac catheters: Indications and results. Am J Surg. 1980;140:791.
79. Lowder JN, Lazarus HM, Herzig RH. Bacteremias and fungemias in oncologic patients with central venous catheters. Arch Intern Med. 1982;142:1456.
80. Schuman ES, Winters V, Gross GF, et al. Management of Hickman catheter sepsis. Am J Surg. 1985;149:627.
81. Liekweg WG, Greenfield LJ. Vascular prosthetic infections: Collected experience and results of treatment. Surgery. 1977;81:335.
82. Szilagyi DE, Smith RF, Elliott JP, et al. Infection in arterial reconstruction with synthetic grafts. Ann Surg. 1972;176:321.
83. Goldstone J, Moore WS. Infection in vascular prostheses: Clinical manifestations and surgical management. Am J Surg. 1974;128:225.
84. O'Hara PJ, Hertzer NR, Beven EG, et al. Surgical management of infected abdominal aortic grafts: Review of a 25-year experience. J Vasc Surg. 1986;3:725.
85. Ilsenfritz FM, Jordan FT. Microbiological monitoring of aortic aneurysm wall and contents during aneurysmectomy. Arch Surg. 1988;123:506.
86. Schwartz JA, Powell TW, Burnham SJ, et al. Culture of abdominal aortic aneurysm contents. An additional series. Arch Surg. 1987;122:777.
87. Moore WS, Malone JM, Keown K. Prosthetic arterial graft material: Influence on neointimal healing and bacteremic infectibility. Arch Surg. 1980;115:1379.
88. DeBakey ME, Jordan GL Jr, Abbott JP, et al. The fate of Dacron vascular grafts. Arch Surg. 1964;89:757.
89. Berger K, Sauvage LR, Rao AM, et al. Healing of arterial prostheses in man: Its incompleteness. Ann Surg. 1972;175:118.
90. Malone JM, Moore WS, Campagna G, et al. Bacteremic infectibility of vascular grafts: The influence of pseudointimal integrity and duration of graft function. Surgery. 1975;78:211.
91. Roon AJ, Malone JM, Moore WS, et al. Bacteremic infectibility: A function of vascular graft material and design. J Surg Res. 1977;22:489.
92. Becker RM, Blundell PE. Infected aortic bifurcation grafts: Experience with 14 patients. Surgery. 1976;80:544.
93. Hoffert PW, Gensler S, Haimovici H. Infection complicating arterial grafts: Personal experience with 12 cases and review of the literature. Arch Surg. 1965;90:427.
94. Wilson SE, Van Wagenen P, Passaro E Jr. Arterial infection. Curr Probl Surg. 1978;15:1.
95. Casali RE, Tucker WE, Thompson BW, et al. Infected prosthetic grafts. Arch Surg. 1980;115:577.
96. Liekweg WG Jr, Levinson SA, Greenfield LJ. Infections of vascular grafts: Incidence, anatomic location, etiologic agents, morbidity, and mortality. In: Duma RJ, ed. Infections of Prosthetic Heart Valves and Vascular Grafts. Baltimore: University Park Press; 1977:239.
97. Rich NM, Collins GJ Jr, Andersen CA. Infected grafts: Clinical presentation and diagnosis. In Duma RJ, ed. Infections of Prosthetic Heart Valves and Vascular Grafts. Baltimore: University Park Press; 1977:253.
98. Elliott JP Jr, Smith RF, Szilagyi DE. Aortoenteric and paraprostheticenteric fistulas. Arch Surg. 1974;108:479.
99. Willwerth BM, Waldhausen JA. Infection of arterial prostheses. Surg Gynecol Obstet. 1974;139:446.
100. Justich E, Amparo EG, Hricak H, et al. Infected aortoiliofemoral grafts: Magnetic resonance imaging. Radiology. 1985;154:133.
101. Sedwitz MM, Davies RJ, Pretorius HT, et al. Indium 111-labeled white blood cell scans after vascular prosthetic reconstruction. J Vasc Surg. 1987;6:476.
102. Schellack J, Stewart MT, Smith RB III, et al. Infected aortobifemoral prosthesis—a dreaded complication. Am Surg. 1988;54:137.
103. Kaiser AB, Clayson KR, Mulherin JL, et al. Antibiotic prophylaxis in vascular surgery. Ann Surg. 1978;188:283.
104. Pitt HA, Postier RG, MacGowan WA, et al. Prophylactic antibiotics in vascular surgery: Topical, systemic, or both? Ann Surg. 1980;192:356.
105. Moore WS, Chvapil M, Seiffert G, et al. Development of an infection-resistant vascular prosthesis. Arch Surg. 1981;116:1403.
106. Moore WS, Malone JM. Vascular infection. In: Simmons RL, Howard RJ, eds. Surgical Infectious Diseases. New York: Appleton-Century-Crofts; 1982:777.
107. Sweeney TF, Kerstein MD. Management of peripheral vascular infections. In: Kerstein MD, ed. Management of Surgical Infections. New York: Futura; 1980:117.
108. Threlkeld MG, Cobbs CG: Questions and Answers: Arterial graft infections—Is antibiotic prophylaxis necessary? JAMA. 1988;259:2608.
109. Ralston AJ, Harlow GR, Jones DM, et al. Infections of Scribner and Brescia arteriovenous shunts. Br Med J. 1971;3:408.
110. Kuruvila KC, Beven EG. Arteriovenous shunts and fistulas for hemodialysis. Surg Clin North Am. 1971;51:1219.
111. Winsett OE, Wolma FJ. Complications of vascular access for hemodialysis. South Med J. 1985;78:513.
112. Kheriakian GM, Roedersheimer LR, Arbaugh JJ. Comparison of autogenous fistula versus expanded polytetrafluoroethylene graft fistula for angioaccess in hemodialysis. Am J Surg. 1986;152:238.
113. Munda R, First MR, Alexander JW, et al. Polytetrafluoroethylene graft survival in hemodialysis. JAMA. 1983;249:219.
114. Dobkin JF, Miller MH, Steigbigel NH. Septicemia in patients on chronic hemodialysis. Ann Intern Med. 1978;88:28.
115. Nsouli KA, Lazarus M, Schoenbaum SC, et al. Bacteremic infection in hemodialysis. Arch Intern Med. 1979;139:1255.
116. Kaslow RA, Zellner SR. Infection in patients on maintenance hemodialysis. Lancet. 1972;2:117.
117. Cross AS, Steigbigel RT. Infective endocarditis and access site infections in patients with hemodialysis. Medicine (Baltimore). 1978;55:453.
118. Bhat DJ, Tellis VA, Kohlberg WI, et al. Management of sepsis involving expanded polytetrafluoroethylene grafts for hemodialysis access. Surgery. 1980;87:445.
119. Oldershaw PJ, Sutton MG, Ward D, et al. Ten-year experience of 359 epicardial pacemaker systems: complications and results. Clin Cardiol. 5:515, 1982.
120. Bluhm G. Pacemaker infections: A clinical study with special reference to prophylactic use of some isoxazolyl penicillins. Acta Med Scand Suppl. 1985;699:1.
121. Wade JS, Cobbs CG. Infections in cardiac pacemakers. In: Remington JS, Swartz MN, eds. Current Clinical Topics in Infectious Diseases. v. 9. New York: McGraw-Hill; 1988:44.

63. PROPHYLAXIS OF INFECTIVE ENDOCARDITIS

DAVID T. DURACK

Infective endocarditis is a serious disease. Even though the etiologic organisms usually can be eradicated by antibiotic treatment, they often leave an unwelcome legacy of permanent valvular damage. Only a minority of patients die during the active phase of infection, but many more suffer further complications and have a shortened life span after being "cured." Therefore, prevention of infective endocarditis has universally been accepted as a worthwhile goal.

It is important to appreciate at the outset that only a small proportion (perhaps 15 percent) of all cases of infective endocarditis can be attributed to bacteremias caused by previous medical, surgical, or dental procedures.[1–6] It follows that the proportion of potentially preventable cases is also small.

Attempted prevention of bacterial infections with antibiotics is most likely to succeed when a single antimicrobial drug is directed against a single pathogen and when the disease occurs with fairly high frequency in the absence of prophylaxis.[5,6] Prevention of endocarditis does not meet these ideals because a variety of antibiotics are used against a variety of organisms and because the disease occurs rarely even if prophylactic antibiotics are not given.

Developments in this field have been hampered by a serious lack of information on which to base recommendations. For example, reliable data are not available to answer even these basic questions: what is the risk of developing infective endocarditis after procedures that cause bacteremia? What procedures and operations should be covered by antibiotics? Is antibiotic prophylaxis effective? If so, which prophylactic antibiotic regimens give the best results? Thus, this area is characterized by uncertainties and controversy.

It is doubtful that sufficient epidemiologic data will ever be accumulated to answer these questions definitively. Random bacteremias occur commonly, probably daily[7,8]; thus patients with underlying heart disease are continually at some risk of developing endocarditis, and it is not possible to determine with certainty which one of many bacteremias, including those caused by health care practitioners, is responsible for an episode of endocarditis.

Clinical investigations of the prophylactic efficacy of antibiotics are also unlikely to provide the answers because an excessively large number of patients would be required to reach a significant conclusion, as the following example illustrates. Let us make the following assumptions: that the risk of acquiring bacterial endocarditis after dental extraction is approximately 1 in 500,[9] that approval for a randomized trial of antibiotic vs. placebo could be obtained from an ethics review committee, and that an antibiotic regimen 100 percent effective in preventing endocarditis is available. An imaginary clinical trial under these admittedly arbitrary conditions might yield the following figures:

Treatment Group		*Number of Patients*	*Cases of Endocarditis*
Placebo		3000	6
Antibiotic		3000	0
	Total	6000	$\chi^2 = 4.2$
			$p < .05$

At least 6000 patients with pre-existing valvular heart disease would have to be studied during dental procedures for the results to reach statistical significance. Although these figures are only approximations, it is obvious that it would be difficult or impossible to carry out such a large study. However, it may be possible to demonstrate the efficacy of prophylaxis by selecting subgroups of patients at highest risk for endocarditis. Among patients with prosthetic heart valves undergoing various surgical procedures, it was recently reported that no cases of endocarditis followed 287 procedures for which antibiotic prophylaxis was given, while 6 occurred after 390 procedures for which it was omitted.[10] This interesting result, which needs to be confirmed, just reaches statistical significance.

We must conclude that attempted prevention of infective endocarditis at present remains an empirical practice. Nevertheless, most authorities agree that prophylaxis should be offered to susceptible patients during certain procedures known to be associated with bacteremia.[1,3–6,11–15]

ESTIMATES OF RISK FOR INFECTIVE ENDOCARDITIS

To determine when antibiotic prophylaxis for infective endocarditis should be given, it is necessary to estimate the relative risk of developing endocarditis after certain procedures. Many investigators have reported on the incidence of transient bacteremia after various manipulations.[3 5,7,8,16–25] It should be noted that incidence of bacteremia varies quite widely between studies and that the frequency with which certain species (especially streptococci) enter the blood may correlate better than the overall incidence of bacteremia with risk of endocarditis. Some representative figures from selected studies are presented in Table 1.

Several hundred cases of endocarditis that were attributed to prior dental procedures have been recorded in the literature. In many of these, the first symptoms of endocarditis appeared within less than 2 weeks.[2] Although the incubation period of endocarditis is not known precisely, the onset of symptoms soon after dental operations in these cases makes a causal relationship seem likely. These case reports provide the basis for the belief that dental procedures often cause endocarditis—a belief that is widely but not universally accepted. The risk of developing infective endocarditis due to a dental extraction certainly must be low because bacteremia is common after this operation and endocarditis is relatively rare. It has been variously estimated that the risk is as high as 1 in 533,[9] as low as 1 in 115,500,[26] or even zero.[27] Most authorities would agree that dental operations do indeed pose a significant risk to susceptible patients, but it appears that the risk of acquiring infective endocarditis is probably *less than 1 percent* for each procedure, even if antibiotic prophylaxis is not given.

Similarly, more than 100 case reports provide reasonably good evidence that bacteremias originating from the genitourinary tract may cause endocarditis, especially when urologic or gynecologic operations are carried out in the presence of urinary or pelvic infections.[28] Evidence that other medical and surgical procedures cause infective endocarditis is rather sketchy. For example, only a handful of cases after miscellaneous operations such as drainage of soft tissue infections, abdominal surgery,

TABLE 1. Incidence of Transient Bacteremia after Various Procedures

Extraction of 1 or more teeth	82%
Periodontal surgery	88%
Brushing teeth	40%
Tonsillectomy	38%
Catheter removal after urologic surgery	50%
Prostatectomy (sterile urine)	11%
Prostatectomy (infected urine)	57%
Normal delivery	4–11%
Diagnostic procedures	
Bronchoscopy	0–15%
Barium enema	10%
Liver biopsy	10%
Upper GI endoscopy	4%
Sigmoidoscopy	0–5%
Colonoscopy	5%

(Data from Refs. 7, 16–18, 22–24.)

TABLE 2. Estimate of Risk of Developing Infective Endocarditis after Various Procedures That May Cause Bacteremias

Significant Risk	*Very Low or Negligible Risk*[a]
Dental procedures likely to cause bleeding (e.g., detailed examinations, scaling, extractions)	Minor dental procedures not causing bleeding (e.g., superficial examinations, simple fillings above the gum line, adjustment of orthodontic appliances)
Oral surgery involving teeth and gums	Spontaneous loss of deciduous teeth
Delivery, abortion, insertion or removal of IUD, dilatation and curettage (*in the presence of pelvic infection*)	Normal delivery, therapeutic abortion, insertion or removal of IUD, dilatation and curettage (*in absence of pelvic infection*)
Tonsillectomy, adenoidectomy	Cardiac catheterization
Urinary catheterization, passage of urethral dilators, cystoscopy, prostatectomy (especially with infected urine or bacterial prostatitis)	Insertion of cardiac pacemaker
Drainage of abscesses, operations involving infected soft tissue	Endotracheal intubation
	Diagnostic procedures Endoscopy of upper and lower GI tract Barium meal, barium enema Liver biopsy Bronchoscopy (with flexible bronchoscope)

[a] The risk for some of these procedures may be significant in patients with prosthetic valves.

diagnostic cardiac catheterization, and the use of oral irrigation devices have been recorded.[29,30] The frequency of bacteremia during normal delivery is very low,[31] and very few cases of endocarditis have been recorded in the setting.[32] Although bacteremias may occur during the performance of common diagnostic procedures such as endoscopies, barium enemas, and liver biopsies, very few cases of endocarditis attributable to these common procedures have been reported.[23,24] Some estimates of the risk related to procedures that may cause bacteremia are offered in Table 2.

Underlying Cardiac Conditions

An assessment of risk in relation to the patient's underlying cardiac condition must also be made (Table 3). These estimates are based on the frequency with which various pre-existing cardiac defects are found in patients with infective endocarditis. Certain conditions strongly predispose to endocardial infection; thus a patient with uncorrected patent ductus arteriosus runs approximately a 30 percent risk of developing the disease during his lifetime.[33] Similarly, congenital or acquired aortic valve disease, interventricular septal defects, mitral stenosis or incompetence, and especially prosthetic valves are known to present a relatively high risk of infection.[29,34,35] At the other end of the spectrum, uncomplicated secundum-type atrial septal defects carry such a low risk for infective endocarditis[29] that prophylaxis is probably not indicated for these patients.[13] Mitral valve

TABLE 3. Estimate of Risk of Developing Infective Endocarditis as Related to Underlying Conditions

Relatively High Risk	*Intermediate Risk*	*Very Low or Negligible Risk*
Prosthetic valves	Mitral valve prolapse	Arterioslerotic plaques
Previous infective endocarditis	Tricuspid valve disease	Coronary artery disease
Patent ductus arteriosus	Pulmonary valve disease	Atrial septal defects
Fallot's tetralogy	Asymmetric septal hypertrophy	Cardiac pacemakers
Ventricular septal defect		Surgically corrected lesions (without prosthetic implants)
Coarctation of the aorta		
Aortic valve disease		
Mitral stenosis and/or insufficiency		
Marfan syndrome		
Intra-atrial alimentation catheters		
Arteriovenous fistulas		

prolapse presents a special problem. This condition increases a person's risk for endocarditis by five- to eightfold,[36] and it underlies a significant proportion of cases of subacute bacterial endocarditis.[37–39] The risk appears to be greater for those with a precordial systolic murmur.[38] Nevertheless, because mitral valve prolapse is so common in the general population while endocarditis is relatively uncommon, a prolapse cannot be regarded as a high-risk lesion,[36] even when a murmur is present. Most authorities currently recommend prophylaxis for patients with prolapse, especially those with mitral regurgitation. On the other hand, a study of benefits vs. costs by decision analysis indicates that prophylaxis for prolapse would not be cost-effective.[40] This study also indicated that, because the incidence of endocarditis when a patient with prolapse undergoes a dental procedure without prophylaxis is very low, the years of life lost from anaphylaxis due to parenteral penicillin could exceed the years of life saved by prevention of endocarditis.

What are the implications of the above for prophylaxis? In the author's opinion, patients with prolapse should receive prophylaxis because (for the individual) the costs and risks of taking two oral doses of amoxicillin are very low, and a serious disease may occasionally be prevented. However, the use of antibiotics could be considered optional rather than mandatory in this setting, and parenteral prophylaxis should be avoided.

INDIRECT EVIDENCE OF EFFICACY OF PROPHYLAXIS

In the absence of definitive data, recommendations for the prophylaxis of infective endocarditis must be based on secondary sources of information. These include anecdotal experience with patients, in vitro study of the organisms that cause bacteremia and endocarditis, and evaluation of the prevention of infective endocarditis in experimental animals.

Uncontrolled Clinical Observations

Case reports describing patients who developed endocarditis after a procedure known to cause bacteremia despite the administration of antibiotics provide anecdotal evidence that attempts to prevent endocarditis are not uniformly successful.[4,41] From 1979 to 1982 an American Heart Association committee collected and recorded examples of apparent prevention failures.[39] Among 52 such cases, mitral valve prolapse was the single most common underlying cardiac lesion (33 percent), followed by various congenital abnormalities (29 percent) and rheumatic heart disease (21 percent). Nineteen percent had prosthetic valve endocarditis. Forty-eight cases (92 percent) followed a dental procedure, and 75 percent of cases were caused by viridans streptococci. Symptoms began fairly soon after the procedure suspected to have caused endocarditis: within 2 weeks in 50 percent and within 5 weeks in 79 percent. Most patients received oral penicillin as prophylaxis. Sixty percent of organisms for which antimicrobial susceptibility was known were sensitive to the antibiotic(s) used for prophylaxis. This experience, although anecdotal, indicates that endocarditis prophylaxis failures are not rare and that failures may occur even when the infecting organism is susceptible to the antibiotics used. It confirms that mitral valve prolapse is a common underlying lesion in patients with streptococcal endocarditis.

In Vitro Studies

A variety of organisms may be found in the blood stream after dental, surgical, and diagnostic procedures, including many strains of anaerobes.[8,17] However, only gram-positive cocci such as viridans streptococci, enterococci, and staphylococci commonly cause infective endocarditis in this setting. It is therefore appropriate to focus on the antibiotic susceptibilities of these organisms in attempting to formulate rational prophylactic programs. Most of the bacteria in the oral flora that are likely to cause endocarditis are sensitive to penicillin G.[1,4,42] In fact, it is widely believed that all strains of viridans streptococci are exquisitely sensitive to penicillin. This is not entirely correct; in some series up to one-third of the strains are partially resistant, with minimal bactericidal concentrations (MBC) for penicillin G of 0.1–1.0 μg/ml or more.[43,44] Ampicillin and amoxicillin both possess good in vitro activity against most streptococci associated with endocarditis[42] and provide high serum concentrations.[11] Almost all strains of viridans streptococci, irrespective of their MBCs, are killed more rapidly and completely by a combination of a penicillin and an aminoglycoside than by a penicillin alone.[45] Similarly enterococci, although more likely to be resistant to both penicillins and aminoglycosides, are usually killed synergistically by these drugs in combination, in vitro and in vivo.[46,47]

Experimental Infective Endocarditis

Study of the prevention of experimental infective endocarditis in animal models has provided another secondary source of information. In 1970 Garrison and Freedman[48] reported that placement of a polyethylene catheter in the rabbit heart led to the development of small sterile vegetations at points of contact between the catheter and endocardium. If staphylococci were placed in the lumen of the catheter, staphylococcal endocarditis resulted. Modification of this model by injecting organisms intravenously[49] provided a suitable in vivo system for examining the efficacy of various antibiotic regimens for the prophylaxis of endocarditis.[47,50–53] A similar model in rats has also been used to investigate antibiotic prophylaxis.[56–60] Under experimental conditions, the time of onset of infective endocarditis is known exactly. Another important advantage is that the incidence of infection in untreated animals can be adjusted easily by altering the inoculum size; thus the problem of very low infection rates in patients can be overcome in animals by choosing an inoculum large enough to infect most of the subjects for the organism under investigation. Significant differences among antibiotic regimens can then be demonstrated with manageable numbers of animals in each group.[47,50–60]

Early experiments comparing the success of various antibiotic regimens against viridans streptococci in this model system showed that bacteriostatic antibiotics were usually ineffective, that penicillin in low doses or in high doses of brief duration was often ineffective, that high penicillin concentrations in serum for 12 hours or more were desirable for effective prophylaxis, that the combination of a penicillin plus an aminoglycoside was synergistic against viridans streptococci as well as enterococci, and that vancomycin provided an excellent alternative to regimens using penicillins.[47,50–52,54] Other antibiotics that proved effective under controlled experimental conditions were ampicillin, amoxicillin,[53,59,60] erythromycin,[60] and rifampin.[58]

Further experiments have modified the view that bactericidal antibiotic activity is essential for prophylaxis. Streptomycin proved surprisingly effective in the prevention of experimental infection by some strains of enterococci, even though the serum concentrations of streptomycin were far too low to kill them.[47] Subinhibitory concentrations of certain antibiotics, especially vancomycin, can inhibit the adherence of streptococci to fibrin surfaces in vitro.[61] More recent experiments have demonstrated successful prophylaxis for various streptococci with sublethal doses of vancomycin, clindamycin, erythromycin, and even a tetracycline.[54,55,60] Penicillin was much less effective in the prevention of experimental streptococcal endocarditis if the strain was tolerant to penicillin.[62] However, penicillin exhibited some prophylactic activity even if the strain was so tolerant that bactericidal concentrations of penicillin could not be achieved in serum.[62] All these findings suggest that prevention can sometimes be achieved by antibiotic effects that fall short of total bacterial killing, perhaps by an alteration of surface structures that mediate adherence to fibrin or by other unknown mechanisms. In other words, bactericidal action may be sufficient but not always necessary for prevention. The implications of these findings for humans are uncertain. At present, it still seems prudent to choose bactericidal drugs for the prophylaxis of infective endocarditis whenever possible.

To place these experimental findings in perspective, it is important to emphasize that direct extrapolations to humans should not be made from the extensive experimental data. If the results are applied too literally, stringent prophylactic regimens that are impractical for general use may be recommended. Although in vivo models provide a closer simulation of human endocarditis than any in vitro system could, there are two important differences. First, a foreign body was present throughout many of these experiments because the intracardiac catheter often was left in place. The presence of a foreign body in tissue lowers the inoculum required to initiate infection and then makes infection harder to eradicate. Therefore, the animal models probably simulate patients with prosthetic valves more closely than they do patients with congenital or rheumatic valvular disease. Second, in many of the experiments a high inoculum was chosen deliberately to make statistical comparisons possible with a relatively small number of animals. Both the presence of a foreign body and the use of a high inoculum would tend to make prevention harder to achieve, so any regimen that proved effective under these rigorous experimental conditions should provide a margin of safety in clinical use.

With these reservations in mind, what has been the real contribution of experimental studies of prevention? Animal models provide a convenient in vivo method for *ranking* prophylactic antibiotic regimens in order of efficacy, but they cannot be used to determine whether any particular antibiotic regimen will or will not prevent endocarditis in patients. For example, experimental findings do not exclude the possibility that tetracycline may prevent endocarditis in some patients. They do support the conclusion that one of the optimal regimens such as vancomycin, or penicillin plus streptomycin, should provide a much wider margin of safety than does a lower-ranking regimen such as tetracycline.[52]

CARDIAC SURGERY

Most cardiovascular surgeons believe that the use of prophylactic antibiotics has reduced the incidence of postcardiotomy endocarditis.[35,63] While this is may be true, it should be noted that numerous technical improvements, introduced during the period when the incidence of postoperative endocarditis was falling, also may have contributed significantly. In fact, the efficacy of antibiotics for the prevention of postcardiotomy endocarditis has not yet been subjected to an adequate, critically controlled trial.[63] The clinical impression that antibiotic prophylaxis during cardiac surgery is effective is now so widely accepted that ethical consent to perform a placebo-controlled trial probably could no longer be obtained.[63]

Early-onset postcardiotomy endocarditis may be caused by a wide variety of organisms including staphylococci, gram-negative bacteria, and fungi. No single antibiotic regimen is effective against all these, and the use of broad-spectrum antibiotics may itself predispose to superinfection with resistant organisms. Therefore, attempts to prevent endocarditis with antibiotics during open heart surgery should probably be limited to a short course of an antistaphylococcal agent such as a cephalosporin or vancomycin.[5,13] Many practitioners add an aminoglycoside in the hope of taking advantage of possible synergism.

Diagnostic cardiac catheterizations (including Swan-Ganz catheters), insertion of pacemakers, coronary artery surgery, pericardial surgery, and the use of the aortic balloon pump all appear to present little risk, and the administration of antibiotics specifically for the prevention of infective endocarditis is not usually recommended during these operations. However, it should be noted that in patients with severe burns (who often develop bacteremias) pulmonary artery catheters have been reported to predispose to both nonbacterial and bacterial endocarditis.[64]

Prosthetic Heart Valves

Extensive clinical experience has established that patients with prosthetic heart valves are at a relatively high risk for infective endocarditis.[10,34,35,65] The high mortality and morbidity associated with prosthetic valve endocarditis and the frequent necessity for repeated valve replacement in later years make its prevention of primary importance. Although the incidence of endocarditis after cardiac surgery has fallen steadily since these operations became commonplace, the risk of endocarditis in the first year remains in the region of 1 percent and thereafter approximates 1 percent per year.[34,35,65] For comparison, the incidence of endocarditis is approximately 0.4 percent per year in patients with rheumatic heart disease.[66] It is important to recognize this risk and to take all possible steps to minimize it. Before cardiac surgery, the dental health of every patient should be evaluated. Any necessary dental work should be completed under close observation and with appropriate antibiotic coverage before valve replacement. Healthy teeth should not be extracted, but if advanced dental or periodontal disease is present, extraction of all teeth should be considered. Thereafter, the patient should maintain good oral hygiene. Consultation between the patient's dentist and physician is important to ensure optimal antibiotic coverage during routine dental procedures. Practitioners may choose to administer prophylaxis to cover certain procedures (such as colonoscopy) that present very little risk in patients without prosthetic valves (see Tables 1 and 2).

Late-onset prosthetic valve endocarditis (later than 60 days after the operation) is more likely to be caused by organisms originating in the oral cavity, just as for native valve endocarditis. Attempted prophylaxis for endocarditis in this setting should be directed against streptococci, not staphylococci and gram-negative bacilli.

Many cardiac patients receive anticoagulant therapy, which may alter the choice of prophylactic antibiotics. Intramuscular injections are contraindicated in patients receiving heparin and should be avoided if possible in patients being administered coumadin. For some patients an oral regimen may suffice, but for patients with prosthetic valves, an intravenous regimen should be chosen.

COMMON ERRORS IN ATTEMPTED PREVENTION OF ENDOCARDITIS

Starting Antibiotic Treatment Too Early

Antibiotics should be administered so as to provide the highest serum levels at the time the procedure causing the bacteremia is performed. There is no rationale to support the common practice of beginning antibiotic therapy earlier than is necessary to meet this criterion. Indeed, if antibiotics are given more than a few hours before the procedure, penicillin-sensitive oral flora may be replaced by penicillin-resistant organisms, and endocarditis, should it occur, may be caused by resistant organisms.[41] For most regimens, the administration of antibiotics 30–60 minutes before the procedure is suitable. If the operation is delayed unexpectedly, doses may have to be repeated.

Continuing Antibiotic Therapy Too Long

As with most other forms of antibiotic prophylaxis, a short course is indicated. Experimental studies provide some evidence that even a single dose may be adequate, providing an optimal antibiotic regimen is chosen.[49,50–52,59] However, many practitioners continue prophylaxis for days.[39,67,68] This wastes antibiotic, may lead to the emergence of resistant organisms, and places the patient at an additional risk of adverse reactions. In any case, a patient who is feeling perfectly well is unlikely to adhere to an unnecessarily prolonged regimen.

Use of Low-Dose Antibiotics

Low-dose prophylactic regimens are often used for the prevention of endocarditis, even though both theoretic considerations and experimental studies indicate that a fairly high serum level of antibiotic is advisable.[39,50,52] Oral therapy is not ideal for this purpose since variability of intestinal absorption may result in relatively low and unreliable serum levels. For this reason I prefer to use parenteral prophylaxis when circumstances allow, for example, when the patient is in the hospital. However, it must be accepted that oral regimens will continue to be used in a great majority of cases because they are more convenient for both patient and practitioner. The full dose should always be given.

Prophylaxis for Tooth Extraction but Not for Lesser Dental Procedures

Much of the literature on infective endocarditis after dental procedures has emphasized tooth *extraction*. However, bacteremias may occur after almost any form of dental manipulation.[1,3,7] One reasonable criterion is to use antibiotic prophylaxis for all procedures likely to cause gingival bleeding.[13] This will exclude many routine check-ups, simple fillings above the gum line, and adjustment of orthodontic appliances but will usually include detailed examination, scaling and cleaning of the teeth by a dentist or hygienist, and more extensive dental operations.

Confusion between Prevention of Rheumatic Fever and Prevention of Infective Endocarditis

One frequently hears that antibiotics were not given to a patient with rheumatic heart disease before dental extractions "because he was already receiving penicillin prophylaxis." Whereas the administration of continuous, low-dose penicillin effectively prevents rheumatic fever, it is *inadequate* to prevent infective endocarditis. The incidence of infective endocarditis in children receiving penicillin for the prevention of rheumatic fever is no less than in those with rheumatic heart disease who are not receiving prophylaxis.[66] Because patients taking low-dose oral penicillin for the prevention of rheumatic fever often carry moderately penicillin-resistant streptococci in the mouth, attempted prevention of infective endocarditis with an oral penicillin regimen in these patients is not advisable. They should receive one of the parenteral regimens or an alternative regimen that does not include penicillin (Table 4).

Failure to Use Prophylaxis for Children

Because bacteremia during dental procedures appears to be somewhat less common in children than in adults, it has been suggested that antibiotic prophylaxis for infective endocarditis is unnecessary in children.[69] However, careful studies indicate that bacteremia does indeed occur in a significant proportion of children after dental procedures,[40] and cases of endocarditis following soon after dental extraction have been reported.[71] The present consensus, therefore, is that children should receive antibiotic prophylaxis for infective endocarditis, with appropriate adjustment of dosages.

TABLE 4. Author's Current Recommendations for Prophylaxis of Endocarditis[a]

Standard regimen	For dental procedures; oral or upper respiratory tract surgery; minor GI or GU tract procedures	Amoxicillin, 3.0 g orally 1 hr before, then 1.5 g 6 hr later[b]
Special regimens	Oral regimen for penicillin-allergic patients (oral and respiratory tract only)	Erythromycin, 1.0 g orally 1–2 hr before, then 0.5 g 6 hr later[b]
	Parenteral regimen for high-risk patients; also for GI or GU tract procedures	Ampicillin 2.0 g im or iv, *plus* gentamicin 1.5 mg/kg im or iv, 0.5 hr before[b]
	Parenteral regimen for penicillin-allergic patients	Vancomycin, 1.0 g iv slowly over 1 hr, starting 1 hr before; *add* gentamicin, 1.5 mg/kg im or iv, if GI or GU tract involved[b]
	Cardiac surgery including implantation of prosthetic valves	Cefazolin, 2.0 g iv, at induction of anesthesia, repeated 8 and 16 hr later[b,c] *or* vancomycin, 1.0 g iv slowly over 1 hr starting at induction, then 0.5 g iv 8 and 16 hr later[b,c,d]

[a] These regimens are empirical suggestions; no regimen has been *proved* effective for the prevention of endocarditis, and prevention failures may occur with any regimen. These regimens are not intended to cover all clinical situations; the practitioner should use his own judgment on safety and cost–benefit issues in each individual case. One or two additional doses may be given if the period of risk for bacteremia is prolonged.

[b] Pediatric dosages: ampicillin, 50 mg/kg; cefazolin, 30 mg/kg; erythromycin, 20 mg/kg for first dose, then 10 mg/kg; gentamicin, 2.0 mg/kg; amoxicillin, for children who weigh more than 60 lb, use the same as for adults; for children less than 60 lb, use half the adult dose; vancomycin, 20 mg/kg.

[c] Gentamicin, 1.5 mg/kg iv, may be given with each dose if postoperative gram-negative infections have occurred with significant frequency at that hospital.

[d] This regimen is recommended for units where *Staphylococcus epidermidis* prosthetic valve infection is a problem.

THE MALPRACTICE DILEMMA

The question of professional liability in the prophylaxis of endocarditis has led to allegations of negligence and malpractice suits. In today's litigious social climate, such claims have become increasingly common. It should be obvious that the lack of basic information referred to earlier makes evaluation of such cases exceedingly difficult. For example, it is hard to establish that any single procedure known to cause bacteremia was the "proximate cause" in a case of endocarditis. It is even harder to prove that the failure of a physician or dentist to administer antibiotics was the direct cause of a patient acquiring endocarditis. If a strict demonstration of proximate cause were always required, it is doubtful that any claim based on the failure to administer prophylaxis could succeed, but juries are sometimes capricious in deciding liability in malpractice cases. Another common problem for the defense in claims based on a failure to administer prophylaxis is our ignorance of the precise duration of the incubation period of infective endocarditis. Damages have been claimed when the first symptoms of endocarditis did not appear for 3 months or more after tooth extractions without antibiotic cover. The likelihood of proximate cause here is remote, because review of case reports indicates that the incubation period is 2 weeks or less in most cases.[2]

In the light of present knowledge, the health care professional can reasonably be expected to appreciate the risk that infective endocarditis may occur under certain circumstances. He should question the patient about underlying conditions that may predispose to endocarditis and should inform susceptible patients of the small risk that they may develop the disease. An antibiotic regimen should be administered to these patients before selected dental, surgical, and genitourinary tract manipulations that might cause bacteremia. Indications for prophylaxis outside these areas are less firmly established at present. A failure to use any recognized antibiotic regimen in preference to another should not be construed as negligence because many different regimens have been published over the past 25 years. Although some authorities recognize evidence that certain antibiotic regimens probably provide a wider margin of efficacy than do others,[11–13,44–60] this evidence is not yet firm enough to make the choice of any particular regimen mandatory.

The risks of toxicity from any prophylactic regimen must be considered carefully. Allergic reactions may occur even after low doses of penicillin; this risk is common to all regimens using penicillins as drugs of choice. However, the risk of anaphylaxis to penicillin is higher for parenteral than for oral administration. Other side effects such as ototoxicity and nephrotoxicity from aminoglycosides or vancomycin are extremely unlikely to occur after the very short courses (1 day or less) now used for the prophylaxis of infective endocarditis.

CURRENT RECOMMENDATIONS

The *Medical Letter*[12] and an American Heart Association Committee[13] have published recommendations for the prophylaxis of infective endocarditis. Such recommendations for prophylaxis[12,13,77] are rather lengthy and complex; while widely known, they are not well understood, and they are often ignored in practice.[39,68,73,74] Therefore, an American Heart Association committee and other advisory bodies are presently developing recommendations for simplified regimens in an attempt to improve compliance. My current suggestions are listed in Table 4.

REFERENCES

1. Hood EW, Kaye D. Prophylaxis of bacterial endocarditis. J Chronic Dis. 1963;15:635.
2. Starkebaum M, Durack D, Beeson P. The "incubation period" of subacute bacterial endocarditis. Yale J Biol Med. 1977;50:49.
3. Everett ED, Hirschmann JV. Transient bacteremia and endocarditis prophylaxis. A review. Medicine (Baltimore). 1977;56:61.
4. Bisno AL. Antimicrobial prophylaxis of endocarditis. In: Bisno AL, ed. Treatment of Infective Endocarditis. New York: Grune & Stratton; 1981:281.
5. Sanford JP. Prophylactic use of antibiotics: Basic considerations. South Med J. 70(Suppl) No. 1, p 2, 1977.
6. Freedman LR. Prophylaxis of intravascular infection. In: Infective Endocarditis and Other Intravascular Infections. New York: Plenum; 1982:63.
7. Cobe HM. Transient bacteremias. Oral Surg. 1954;7:609.
8. Loesche WJ. Indigenous human flora and bacteremia in infective endocarditis. Am Heart Assoc Monogr. 1977;52:40.
9. Kelson SR, White PD. Notes on 250 cases of subacute bacterial (streptococcal) endocarditis studied and treated between 1927 and 1939. Ann Intern Med. 1945;22:40.
10. Horstkotte D, Friedrichs W, Pippert H, et al. Benefit of prophylaxis for infectious endocarditis (IE) in patients with prosthetic heart valves. Z Kardiol. 1986;75:8.
11. Shanson DC. The prophylaxis of infective endocarditis. J Antimicrob Chemother. 1978;4:2.
12. Prevention of bacterial endocarditis. Med Let. 1986;28:22.
13. American Heart Association Committee on Rheumatic Fever and Infective Endocarditis. Prevention of bacterial endocarditis (Abstract). Circulation. 1984;70:1123.
14. Kaye D. Prophylaxis for infective endocarditis: An update. Ann Intern Med. 1986;104:419.
15. McGowan DA. A dental view of controversies in the prophylaxis of infective endocarditis. J Antimicrob Chemother. 1987;20(Suppl A):105.
16. Elliott SD. Bacteriaemia and oral sepsis. Proc R Soc Med. 1939;32:747.
17. Rogosa M, Hampp EG, Nevin TA, et al. Blood sampling and cultural studies in the detection of postoperative bacteremias. J Am Dent Assoc. 1960;60:171.
18. Slade N. Bacteriaemia and septicaemia after urologic operations. Proc R Soc Med. 1958;51:331.
19. LeFrock JL, Ellis CA, Turchik JB, et al. Transient bacteremia associated with sigmoidoscopy. N Engl J Med. 1973;289:467.
20. LeFrock JL, Ellis CA, Klainer AS, et al. Transient bacteremia associated with barium enema. Arch Intern Med. 1975;135:835.
21. Hoffman BI, Kobasa W, Kaye D. Bacteremia after rectal examination. Ann Intern Med. 1978;88:658.
22. Creevy CD, Feeney MJ. Routine use of antibiotics in transurethral prostatic resection. A clinical investigation. J Urol. 1954;71:615.
23. Sande MA. Prophylactic antibiotics during diagnostic procedures of the gastrointestinal tract. Am Heart Assoc Monogr. 1977;52:73.
24. Shorvon PJ, Eykyn SJ, Cotton PB. Gastrointestinal instrumentation, bacteraemia, and endocarditis. Gut. 1983;24:1078.
25. Baltch AL, Pressman HL, Schaffer C, et al. Bacteremia in patients undergoing oral procedures. Study following parenteral antimicrobial prophylaxis as rec-

ommended by the American Heart Association, 1977. Arch Intern Med. 1988;148:1084.
26. Pogrel MA, Welsby PD. The dentist and prevention of infective endocarditis. Br Dent J. 1975;139:12.
27. Schwartz SP, Salman I. The effect of oral surgery on the course of patients with diseases of the heart. Am J Orthodont. 1942;28:331.
28. Vosti KL. Special problems in prophylaxis of endocarditis following genitourinary tract and obstetrical and gynecological procedures. Am Heart Assoc Monogr. 1977;52:75.
29. Kerr AJ Jr. Subacute Bacterial Endocarditis. Springfield, Il: Charles C Thomas; 1955.
30. Drapkin MS. Endocarditis after the use of an oral irrigation device. Ann Intern Med. 1977;87:455.
31. Sugrue D, Blake S, Troy P, et al. Antibiotic prophylaxis against infective endocarditis after normal delivery—is it necessary? Br Heart J. 1980;44:499.
32. Seaworth BJ, Durack DT. Infective endocarditis in obstetric and gynecologic practice. Am J Obstet Gynecol. 1986;154:180.
33. Wood P. Diseases of the Heart and Circulation. 3rd ed. London: Eyre & Spottiswoode; 1968:465.
34. Rossiter SJ, Stinson EB, Oyer PE, et al. Prosthetic valve endocarditis. J Thorac Cardiovasc Surg. 1978;76:795.
35. Braimbridge MV, Eykyn SJ. Prosthetic valve endocarditis. J Antimicrob Chemother. 1987;20(Suppl A):173.
36. Clemens JD, Horwitz RI, Jaffee CC, et al. A controlled evaluation of the risk of bacterial endocarditis in persons with mitral valve prolapse. N Engl J Med. 1982;307:776.
37. Nolan CM, Kane JJ, Grunow WA. Infective endocarditis and mitral prolapse. A comparison with other types of endocarditis. Arch Intern Med. 1981;131:477.
38. MacMahon SW, Hickey AJ, Wilcken DEL, et al. Risk of infective endocarditis in mitral valve prolapse with and without precordial systolic murmurs. Am J Cardiol. 1986;58:105.
39. Durack DT, Disno AL, Kaplan EL. Apparent failures of endocarditis prophylaxis: Analysis of 52 cases submitted to a national registry. JAMA. 1983;250:2318.
40. Clemens JD, Ransohoff DF. A quantitative assessment of pre-dental antibiotic prophylaxis for patients with mitral-valve prolapse. J Chronic Dis. 1984;37:531.
41. Garrod LP, Waterworth PM. The risks of dental extraction during penicillin treatment. Br Heart J. 1962;24:39.
42. Basker MJ, Sutherland R. Activity of amoxycillin, alone, and in combination with aminoglycoside antibiotics against streptococci associated with bacterial endocarditis. J Antimicrob Chemother. 1977;3:273.
43. Blount JG. Bacterial endocarditis. Am J Med. 1965;38:909.
44. Wilson WR, Garaci JE, Wilkowske CJ, et al. Short-term intramuscular therapy with procaine penicillin plus streptomycin for infective endocarditis due to viridans streptococci. Circulation. 1978;57:1158.
45. Wolfe JC, Johnson WD. Penicillin-sensitive streptococcal endocarditis. In vitro and clinical observations on penicillin-streptomycin therapy. Ann Int Med. 1974;81:178.
46. Russell EJ, Sutherland R. Activity of amoxicillin against enterococci and synergism with aminoglycoside antibiotics. J Med Microbiol. 1975;8:1.
47. Durack DT, Starkebaum MK, Petersdorf RG. Chemotherapy of experimental streptococcal endocarditis. VI. Prevention of enterococcal endocarditis. J Lab Clin Med. 1977;90:171.
48. Garrison PK, Freedman LR. Experimental endocarditis. 1. Staphylococcal endocarditis in rabbits resulting from placement of a polyethylene catheter in the right side of the heart. Yale J Biol Med. 1970;42:394.
49. Durack DT, Beeson PB, Petersdorf RG. Experimental bacterial endocarditis. III. Production and progress of the disease in rabbits. Br J Exp Pathol. 1973;54:142.
50. Durack DT, Petersdorf RG. Chemotherapy of experimental streptococcal endocarditis. I. Comparison of commonly recommended prophylactic regimens. J Clin Invest. 1973;52:592.
51. Pelletier LL, Durack DT, Petersdorf RG. Chemotherapy of experimental streptococcal endocarditis. IV. Further observations on prophylaxis. J Clin Invest. 1975;56:319.
52. Durack DT. Experience with prevention of experimental endocarditis. Am Heart Assoc Monogr. 1977;52:28.
53. McGowan DA, Nair S, MacFarlane TW, et al. Prophylaxis of experimental endocarditis in rabbits using one or two doses of amoxycillin. Br Dent J. 1983;155:88.
54. Bernard JP, Francioli P, Glauser MP. Vancomycin prophylaxis of experimental *Streptococcus sanguis*; inhibition of bacterial adherence rather than bacterial killing. J Clin Invest. 1981;68:1113.
55. Glauser MP, Francioli P. Successful prophylaxis against experimental streptococcal endocarditis with bacteriostatic antibiotics. J Infect Dis. 1982;146:806.
56. Moreillon P, Francioli P, Overholser D, et al. Mechanisms of successful amoxicillin prophylaxis of experimental endocarditis due to *Streptococcus intermedius*. J Infect Dis. 1986;154:801.
57. Overholser CD, Moreillon P, Glauser MP. Experimental bacterial endocarditis after dental extractions in rats with periodontitis. J Infect Dis. 1987;155:107.
58. Malinverni R, Bille J, Glauser MP. Single-dose rifampin prophylaxis for experimental endocarditis induced by high bacterial inocula of viridans streptococci. J Infect Dis. 1987;156:151.
59. Malinverni R, Francioli PB, Glauser MP. Comparison of single and multiple doses of prophylactic antibiotics in experimental streptococcal endocarditis. Circulation. 1987;76:376.
60. Malinverni R, Overholser CD, Bille J, et al. Antibiotic prophylaxis of experimental endocarditis after dental extractions. Circulation. 1988;77:182.
61. Scheld WM, Zak O, Vosbeck K, et al. Bacterial adhesion in the pathogenesis of infective endocarditis. Effect of subinhibitory antibiotic concentrations on streptococcal adhesion in vitro and the development of endocarditis in rabbits. J Clin Invest. 1981;68:1381.
62. Hess J, Dankert J, Durack DT. Significance of penicillin tolerance in vivo of experimental *Streptococcus sanguis* endocarditis. J Antimicrob Chemother. 1983;11:555.
63. Schaffner W. Antibiotic prophylaxis in valvular replacement surgery. In: Duma RJ, ed. Infections of Prosthetic Heart Valves and Vascular Grafts. Baltimore: University Park Press; 1977:313.
64. Ehrie M, Alfred PM, Moore FD, et al. Endocarditis with the indwelling balloon-tipped pulmonary artery catheter in burn patients. J Trauma. 1978;18:664.
65. Wilson WR. Prosthetic valve endocarditis: Incidence, anatomic location, cause, morbidity and mortality. In: Duma RJ, ed. Infections of Prosthetic Heart Valves and Vascular Grafts. Baltimore: University Park Press; 1977:3.
66. Doyle EF, Spagnuolo M, Taranta A, et al. The risk of bacterial endocarditis during antirheumatic prophylaxis. JAMA. 1967;201:129.
67. Durack DT. Current practice in prevention of bacterial endocarditis. Br Heart J. 1975;37:478.
68. Brooks SL. Survey of compliance with American Heart Association guidelines for prevention of bacterial endocarditis. J Am Dent Assoc. 1980;101:41.
69. Hurwitz GA, Speck WT, Keller GD. Absence of bacteremia in children after prophylaxis. Oral Surg. 1971;32:891.
70. Peterson LJ, Peacock R. The incidence of bacteremia in pediatric patients following tooth extraction. Circulation. 1976;53:676.
71. Johnson DH, Rosenthal A, Nadas AS. A forty-year review of bacterial endocarditis in infancy and childhood. Circulation. 1975;51:581.
72. Working Party of the British Society for Antimicrobial Chemotherapy. The antibiotic prophylaxis of infective endocarditis. Lancet. 1982;2:1323.
73. Murrah VA, Merry JW, Little JW, et al. Compliance with guidelines for management of dental school patients susceptible to infective endocarditis. J Dent Educ. 1987;51:229.
74. Sadowsky D, Kunzel C. Recommendations for prevention of bacterial endocarditis: Compliance by dental general practitioners. Circulation. 1988;77:1316.

64. MYOCARDITIS, PERICARDITIS AND MEDIASTINITIS

MARIA C. SAVOIA
MICHAEL N. OXMAN

Inflammatory processes affecting the heart frequently involve both the myocardium (myocarditis) and the pericardium (pericarditis). However, involvement of one or the other usually predominates, and the syndromes of myocarditis and pericarditis are sufficiently distinct in clinical presentation, etiology, and pathophysiology to warrant separate consideration.

MYOCARDITIS

Myocarditis, literally inflammation of the myocardium, is a protean disease with a wide variety of infectious and noninfectious etiologies. Postmortem examinations reveal evidence of previously unsuspected myocarditis in 2–10 percent of unselected cases,[1,2] with a higher incidence in young persons who have died suddenly.[3,4] The diagnosis of infectious myocarditis is generally considered when unexplained heart failure or arrhythmias occur in the setting of a systemic febrile illness or after symptoms of an upper respiratory tract infection. The inflammatory process may affect myocytes, vascular elements, the conducting system, autonomic nerves, and/or the interstitium. One or more of at least four mechanisms appear to be involved: (*1*) direct damage to cells by an infectious agent; (*2*) cytotoxicity caused by a circulating toxin; (*3*) cytotoxicity caused by infection-induced immune reactions; and (*4*) nonspecific damage to myocytes as a result of the inflammatory process.

Etiologic Agents

Viruses are the most important infectious cause of myocarditis in the United States and Western Europe. Long before the era of modern virology, pericardial and myocardial involvement was recognized during outbreaks of mumps,[5] influenza,[6] measles,[7,8] poliomyelitis,[9] and enterovirus-associated pleurodynia.[10] In modern times, enteroviruses[11,12] and especially group B coxsackieviruses[13,14] have been the major agents implicated. These small, nonenveloped, single-stranded RNA viruses belonging to the picornavirus family attach to specific receptors on myocardial cells.[11] Though uncommon, symptomatic myocarditis or myopericarditis is also observed in persons infected with many other viruses, particularly arboviruses and arenaviruses (Table 1).

Myocardial involvement is the most common cause of death in diphtheria[45]; the toxin produced by *Corynebacterium diphtheriae* severely damages the myocardium and conduction system. The cardiac damage seen in patients with *Clostridium perfringens* may be the result of toxin, metastatic abscess formation, or both.[46,47] The immunologically mediated carditis associated with acute rheumatic fever[48] is discussed in Chapter 177.

Invasion of the blood stream by any bacterial pathogen may result in metastatic foci in the myocardium, and myocarditis has been recognized in the course of meningococcemia,[49] salmonellosis,[50] brucellosis,[51] and streptococcal and staphylococcal bacteremia.[52] More commonly, bacteria invade the myocardium as a complication of endocarditis by contiguous spread from valvular tissue or via septic embolization of the coronary arteries.[72]

Myocarditis has been observed in the course of *Mycoplasma pneumoniae*[53,54] and *Chlamydia psittaci*[55] infections and is commonly seen in rickettsial infections,[56] especially scrub typhus.[44,57,58] Approximately 10 percent of patients with Lyme disease develop cardiac abnormalities, most commonly conduction system disturbances.[59,60] In South America, the principal agent responsible for myocarditis is *Trypanosoma cruzi*, the protozoan that causes Chagas disease. The initial infection is often asymptomatic but it sometimes results in an acute illness complicated by myocarditis.[65] Myocarditis is the principal manifestation of chronic Chagas disease, which occurs in approximately 30% of infected individuals. These patients typically have cardiomegaly, congestive heart failure (often predominantly right-sided), and conduction disturbances.[66,67] *Trypanosoma gambiense* and *rhodesiense*, the agents of African trypanosomiasis, may also affect the heart with similar results, but central nervous system findings usually predominate.[68] Myocarditis is also observed in trichinosis[69,70] and is responsible for the occasional deaths that occur in severe infections.

In immunocompromised patients, myocarditis occurs as a consequence of a number of disseminated infections. Overt myocarditis is common in disseminated toxoplasmosis,[71] and systemic aspergillosis and candidiasis may also involve the heart.[61,62] Cryptococcal myocarditis has been reported in patients with the acquired immunodeficiency syndrome (AIDS).[63,64] Cardiac abnormalities in AIDS are common but are usually clinically silent.[73–76] In a retrospective review, mild focal myocarditis was found at necropsy in 37 of 71 AIDS cases examined.[77] A potential pathogen was identified in only seven. Heart failure with biventricular dilatation was the most common clinical correlate, occurring in 6 percent of patients. Human immune deficiency virus (HIV) has been cultured from endomyocardial biopsies,[78,79] but the effect of the virus on myocytes is not known. Patients with AIDS may also be infected with known cardiotropic viruses.[79] The full spectrum of diseases associated with HIV infection remains to be elucidated.

TABLE 1. Infectious Causes of Myocarditis

Viruses	
Coxsackie A[11–13]	Yellow fever[28]
Coxsackie B[11–14]	Argentina hemorrhagic fever[29]
Echoviruses[15,16]	Bolivian hemorrhagic fever[29]
Polio[9,17,18]	Lymphocytic choriomeningitis[30]
Mumps[5,19,20]	Adenovirus[31,32]
Rubeola[7,8]	Varicella-zoster[33–35]
Influenza A and B[6,21,22]	Cytomegalovirus[36]
Rabies[23]	Epstein-Barr[37,38]
Rubella[24,25]	Vaccinia[39]
Dengue[26,27]	Variola[40]
Chikungunya[27]	Hepatitis B[41–43]
Bacteria and Rickettsia	
Corynebacterium diphtheriae[44,45]	*Staphylococcus aureus*[52]
Clostridium perfringens[46,47]	*Mycoplasma pneumoniae*[53,54]
Streptococcus pyogenes[44,48]	*Chlamydia psittaci*[55]
Neisseria meningitidis[49]	*Rickettsia rickettsii*[56]
Salmonella[50]	*Rickettsia tsutsugamushi*[44,57,58]
Brucella[51]	*Borrelia burgdorferi*[59,60]
Fungi	
Aspergillus[61,62]	*Cryptococcus*[62–64]
Candida[62]	
Parasites	
Trypanosoma cruzi[65–67]	*Trichinella spiralis*[69,70]
Trypanosoma gambiense[68]	*Toxoplasma gondii*[71]
Trypanosoma rhodesiense[68]	

Pathology and Pathogenesis

Myocardial pathology depends upon the infecting agent, the mechanism of pathogenesis, and the duration of the process. The hallmarks of myocarditis are an inflammatory infiltrate and injury to adjacent myocardial cells. Pathologic changes may be acute or chronic and vary markedly in severity, depending upon the nature of the disease and the point in its course at which tissue is obtained. Some agents, like the coxsackie B viruses, infect the myocytes themselves, while agents like varicella-zoster virus and hepatitis B virus appear to injure vascular endothelial cells. Although routine histology may help in the differential diagnosis, it rarely provides definitive information regarding the etiologic agent. Early in many viral infections, scattered hypereosinophilic myofibers, widespread edema, and only a few inflammatory cells may be present. Later, there is loss of striation, nuclear degeneration, and fragmentation of myofibers. The degenerating or partially necrotic myofibers are usually surrounded by lymphocytes, plasma cells, and macrophages.[13] Polymorphonuclear cells are occasionally seen[3] (Fig. 1). The acute process may resolve completely; healing and chronicity are reflected by the development of interstitial fibrosis and loss of myofibers.[80]

Mouse models of myocarditis induced by infection with either coxsackievirus B3 or encephalomyocarditis virus have revealed several possible pathogenetic mechanisms. Susceptibility to coxsackievirus B-induced myocarditis is age-dependent and genetically determined.[81] Mechanisms of injury vary in different mouse strains.[82–85] In susceptible animals acute myocarditis results from direct infection and cytolysis of myocytes.[3] In surviving animals, neutralizing antibody, perhaps in conjunction with macrophages[86,87] and natural killer (NK) cells,[88] appears to terminate virus replication by 7–9 days after infection.[11,89,90] Exercise[3,11] and corticosteroids[91] markedly enhance mortality during the early stages of infection. Nonsteroidal anti-inflammatory agents may also have deleterious effects.[92] Mice surviving the acute replicative phase of the virus infection may go on to develop severe myocarditis in the absence of recoverable virus. This second phase of virus-induced myocardial destruction is dependent upon the presence of cytolytic T cells,[13] which appear as virus replication ceases. Some of these cytolytic T cells recognize and lyse both infected and uninfected myocytes,[93] and their presence correlates with myocardial damage.[94,95] The severity of myocardial damage caused by this im-

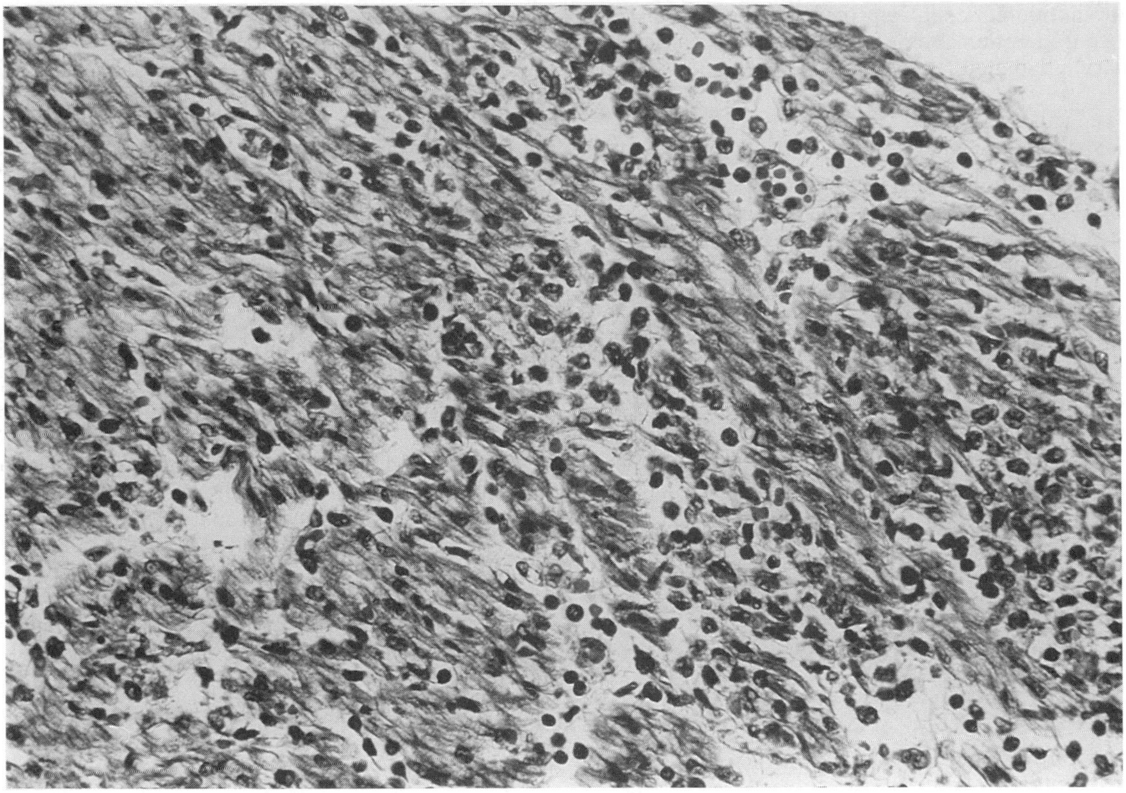

FIG. 1. Coxsackievirus myocarditis with extensive infiltration of mononuclear cells, plasma cells, lymphocytes, and some eosinophils in the interstitial tissue. (×250) (From Bloor,[3] with permission.)

mune mechanism is greatest in male and in pregnant female mice.[96] In some strains of mice less prone to myocarditis, the cytolytic T-cell response appears to be inhibited by suppressor cells.[97] Variants of coxsackievirus B3 that do not evoke cytolytic T cells directed against both infected and uninfected myocytes fail to cause myocarditis even though they are indistinguishable from myocarditic strains in their ability to replicate and stimulate neutralizing antibodies.[98] Mice infected with coxsackievirus B3 also develop heart reactive antibodies,[99,100] which do not cross react with the virus,[101] and these may contribute to myocyte destruction in some strains.[83,102] Certain strains of mice infected with coxsackievirus B3 may go on to develop a picture resembling chronic dilated cardiomyopathy[11,103]—primarily as a result of ongoing immunopathology in the absence of detectable virus. Enterovirus-associated myocarditis in humans appears to present a comparable spectrum of pathogenetic mechanisms and outcomes.

In acute Chagas disease, pathologic examination often reveals parasites within cardiac myocytes. When rupture of the cysts occurs, there is a marked inflammatory infiltrate consisting of lymphocytes, plasma cells, macrophages, and some eosinophils.[65,104] In chronic Chagas disease, the heart is often enlarged and flabby. Aneurysm formation may be present at the apex. The conduction system is often also involved, and this is reflected by a high frequency of rhythm disturbances. Microscopic examination reveals focal mononuclear cell infiltrates and fibrosis.[66,104] In this stage, parasites can only be identified in 25% of patients.[66] The heart, as well as the central nervous system, is often prominently involved in disseminated toxoplasmosis. *Toxoplasma* pseudocysts containing numerous organisms may be readily identified in cardiac tissue, and there is a striking absence of cellular response around them (Fig. 2). Rupture of parasitized fibers is followed by infiltration of neutrophils and eosinophils.[104]

Myocardial microabscesses, affecting both myocytes and the conducting system, may occur in the course of systemic bacterial infections with organisms such as *Staphylococcus aureus*, but heart failure is rarely a direct consequence of such lesions.[72]

Rickettsia and most fungi produce vasculitic lesions with surrounding inflammation. Damage to myocytes may be caused by the adjacent inflammatory process or may reflect anoxia due to occlusion of small blood vessels.

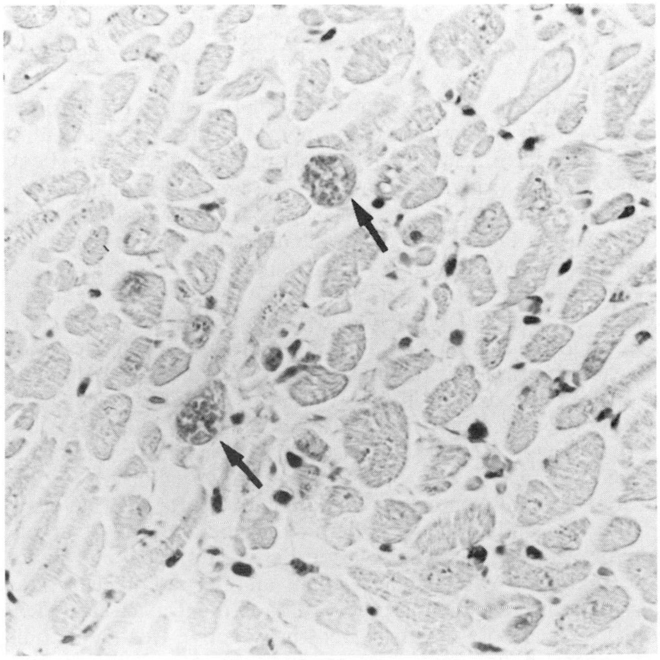

FIG. 2. Cysts of *Toxoplasma gondii* (arrows) are easily visible in the heart of this immunosuppressed patient who died with disseminated toxoplasmosis.

Diphtheria toxin inhibits cellular protein synthesis. This results in hyaline degeneration and necrosis of myocardial fibers, with a secondary inflammatory response.[3,45]

Clinical Manifestations

Patients with myocarditis may be asymptomatic or may have a rapidly progressive fatal disease. The diagnosis of infectious myocarditis is generally considered when a young person develops unexplained heart failure or arrhythmias, or when cardiac abnormalities occur in the course of a recognized systemic infection. Fever, malaise, arthralgias, upper respiratory tract symptoms, and chest pain may precede or accompany coxsackievirus myocarditis,[103,105] but these symptoms are not specific. Supraventricular tachycardia and ventricular extrasystoles are common.[106] Arrhythmias provide early evidence of involvement of the conduction system and are responsible for the occurrence of sudden death in patients with myocarditis. Myocarditis may mimic acute myocardial infarction,[107–110] but care should be taken not to mistake myocardial infarction occurring in a patient with infection for myocarditis.[111] In acute myocarditis, cardiac enzymes may be elevated and remain so for several days.[112] Symptomatic pericarditis may or may not be present.

Diagnosis

In fulminant myocarditis caused by any agent, the diagnosis is usually obvious; signs and symptoms of cardiac dysfunction are plentiful. When findings are more subtle, establishing a firm diagnosis may be difficult. Nonspecific ST- and T-wave abnormalities on the electrocardiogram are frequently cited as presumptive evidence of myocardial involvement, but they may also be seen with fever, hypoxia, electrolyte disturbances, and tachycardia. Failure to reverse T-wave abnormalities with beta blockade has been cited by some as indicative of myocarditis,[112] but physicians should approach the diagnosis of myocarditis based only on the presence of nonspecific ST- and T-wave abnormalities with skepticism,[113] especially in the absence of cardiomegaly on chest radiograph or signs of cardiac failure. Echocardiography may be useful in detecting and quantifying impairment in systolic function.[114,115] Gallium scans may be positive in myocarditis,[116–119] but this technique may lack sensitivity.

At present, the gold standard for the premortem diagnosis of myocarditis is endomyocardial biopsy.[120] Biopsy confirmation of the clinical diagnosis of myocarditis, however, has been highly variable, ranging from 17 to 100 percent in different reports.[120–123] Conversely, in some series, patients undergoing endomyocardial biopsy for the evaluation of congestive cardiomyopathy have shown a surprisingly high incidence of myocarditis,[124–126] while in other series this has not been the case.[127,128] Several factors undoubtedly contribute to this variability and make interpretation of the literature difficult. Most important, perhaps, is the lack of uniform clinical or histologic criteria for the diagnosis of myocarditis.[80] A recent study in which slides from biopsies of 16 patients with dilated cardiomyopathy were submitted to seven experienced pathologists revealed a high degree of interobserver variability.[129] Some question whether sparse focal inflammatory infiltrates have any prognostic significance.[130] Others cite sampling error as an explanation for the poor correlation between clinical and histologic findings.[131] Recent agreement among pathologists on a classification scheme for myocarditis ("the Dallas classification")[130,132] and its use in current prospective treatment trials is a hopeful development. At present, endomyocardial biopsy may be useful in diagnosis, but practitioners should be aware of its limitations. Gallium 57[119] and indium 111-labeled antimyosin antibody scanning[133] may be useful noninvasive tests to screen patients in whom myocarditis is suspected, but experience with these modalities is limited.

Except in neonates, viruses have rarely been isolated from the hearts of patients who have died with myocarditis or from myocardial biopsies.[134] Diagnosis of viral myocarditis is often based on serologic criteria (fourfold or greater rise in antibody titer from acute to convalescent sera) or isolation of the putative agent from other body sites (e.g., stool). At best, such data provide circumstantial evidence for causation of myocardial disease and must be interpreted cautiously, since in a prospective study 26 percent of patients without myocarditis demonstrated serologic evidence of infection with agents known to cause myocarditis.[106] The application of in situ hybridization techniques, which detect virus-specific nucleic acid within cells,[135] and methods that detect or amplify viral nucleic acids[136,137] in biopsy and necropsy specimens may prove useful in the future.

As suggested by data in the mouse model, idiopathic dilated cardiomyopathy may represent the end stage of viral myocarditis.[13,126,138] Serial biopsies have demonstrated progression of fibrosis and scarring in humans,[123,139,140] but the role that viruses play in idiopathic congestive cardiomyopathy remains to be elucidated.[80,141,142]

A wide variety of noninfectious diseases and agents may mimic infectious myocarditis and produce identical clinical syndromes (see Table 2).

Treatment

Treatment of myocarditis should be directed at the specific etiologic agent involved whenever possible. Based on inferences from the murine model of coxsackievirus B3 myocarditis, bed rest remains an important part of therapy. Ensuring adequate oxygenation, avoiding and treating fluid overload if it develops, and monitoring for the development of ventricular arrhythmias constitute usual adjunctive care. In severe cases, cardiac assist devices may be lifesaving.

Most patients with viral myocarditis recover completely[151]; the factors that predispose certain patients to a poor outcome are not clear. Glucocorticoids administered during the acute phase of viral myocarditis have been associated with rapid clinical deterioration, and their deleterious effects have been clearly demonstrated in the acute phase of coxsackievirus infection in mice.[91,152] In some uncontrolled trials, patients with myocarditis on endomyocardial biopsy[119,153] or with positive gallium scans[118] who have been given immunosuppressive agents have shown improvement, but others have not.[127,154] In animal models, early therapy with cyclosporine[155] or anti-inflammatory

TABLE 2. Noninfectious Causes of Myocarditis

Collagen vascular disease[143,144]
Systemic lupus erythematosis
Rheumatoid arthritis
Still's disease
Thyrotoxicosis[143]
Pheochromocytoma[145]
Radiation-induced[146]
Drug-induced (direct toxic)[145]
Cocaine
Alcohol
Emetine
Catecholamines
Arsenic
Cyclophosphamide
Daunorubicin
Adriamycin
Drug-induced (hypersensitivity)[147]
Methyldopa
Sulfonamides
Tetracycline
Scorpion, wasp, and spider stings[145,148]
Agent(s) not yet identified
Kawasaki disease[149]
Giant cell myocarditis[150]

agents[92] increases myocardial damage. Because of the potentially deleterious effects of immunosuppressive therapy, treatment with these agents should await the results of controlled clinical trials now in progress.

PERICARDITIS

Pericarditis may result from either infectious or noninfectious processes. It may be clinically silent or may result in severe hemodynamic compromise and death. In 1892, Sir William Osler called attention to the frequency with which pericarditis was overlooked by the practitioner.[156] In this century the spectrum of organisms causing pericardial inflammation has changed somewhat, and methods of diagnosis have improved. Viral pericarditis appears to predominate and is usually a benign, self-limited disease. Bacterial and tuberculous pericarditis, while now infrequent, still cause significant morbidity and mortality and remain diagnostic challenges.

Etiologic Agents

Because of the difficulties encountered in establishing a specific etiologic diagnosis, most cases of acute self-limited pericarditis are classified as *idiopathic*. Many of these are likely to be caused by viruses.

Most viruses infecting the heart affect both the myocardium and the pericardium (see above). Of the many viruses associated with heart disease, the enteroviruses, especially the coxsackieviruses, are most frequently implicated in pericarditis.[14,157,158] The association of myopericarditis with coxsackieviruses was first recognized in neonates with overwhelming fatal systemic infections.[159] Pericarditis has also been recognized in the setting of epidemic coxsackievirus infection.[160] Coxsackieviruses have been isolated from pericardial fluid[161] infrequently; as with myocarditis, most diagnoses have been based upon the isolation of virus from other body sites (e.g., stool) and/or the demonstration of at least a fourfold rise in antibody titer after the acute illness. Viruses known to cause pericarditis are listed in Table 3.

A wide variety of bacteria can cause pericarditis. In the preantibiotic era, purulent pericarditis occurred primarily as a complication of pneumonia in previously healthy individuals.[172,173,175] Of the 425 cases of purulent pericarditis reported in 1961 by Boyle,[172] 43 percent were associated with pleuropulmonary infections. *Streptococcus pneumoniae* and *Staph. aureus* accounted for more than half of the cases. With the advent of antibiotics, the incidence of purulent pericarditis has decreased markedly. Although staphylococci and streptococci are still etiologic in a substantial number of cases, the incidence of pneumococcal pericarditis has declined substantially, and gram-negative bacilli have assumed a much more important role.[173,175] Patients with purulent pericarditis are now often older and have an underlying predisposing condition. Purulent pericarditis may occur as a complication of meningococcal meningitis or fulminant meningococcemia, but *Neisseria meningitidis*, especially serogroup C, also causes primary pericarditis.[176] *Mycoplasma pneumoniae* can cause pericarditis, and, although uncommon, this manifestation has been observed in nearly 1 percent of patients hospitalized with this infection.[181–183] *Legionella pneumophila* has been isolated from the pericardial fluid,[184,185] and pericarditis has occurred in association with pneumonia[184–186] and endocarditis.[187] Bacterial infections account for proportionately more pericarditis in children, and after *S. aureus, Haemophilus influenzae* is the second most common etiologic agent.[177]

TABLE 3. Infectious Causes of Pericarditis

Viruses	
Coxsackie A[162]	Epstein-Barr[166,167]
Coxsackie B[14,157,158,161]	Varicella-zoster[168]
Echovirus[163]	Cytomegalovirus[169]
Mumps[164]	Herpes simplex[170]
Influenza[165]	Hepatitis B[171]
Bacteria	
Streptococcus pneumoniae[172–174]	*Actinomyces*[180]
Staphylococcus aureus[172,173,175]	*Mycoplasma pneumoniae*[181–183]
Neisseria meningitidis[176]	*Legionella pneumophila*[184–187]
Haemophilus influenzae[172,177,178]	*Mycobacterium tuberculosis*[188–193]
Enteric gram-negative rods[173,179]	*Borrelia burgdorferi*[59,60]
Salmonella[172]	
Fungi	
Histoplasma capsulatum[194,195]	*Cryptococcus neoformans*[198]
Coccidioides immitis[196,197]	*Candida* species[199–201]
Blastomyces dermatitidis[172]	*Aspergillus* species[175,202,203]
Parasites	
Toxoplasma gondii[204,205,211]	Schistosomes[210]
Entamoeba histolytica[206–209]	

Acute or chronic pericarditis is reported to occur in approximately 1 percent of patients with pulmonary tuberculosis.[188] Because of the declining incidence of primary tuberculosis and the use of effective chemotherapy, *Mycobacterium tuberculosis* now accounts for fewer than 5 percent of cases of acute pericarditis.[189,211] Nevertheless, diagnosis is difficult, and mortality remains high.[190] *Mycobacterium tuberculosis* remains an important treatable cause of chronic pericardial effusion and constrictive pericarditis.[191,212]

Fungi are infrequently recognized as a cause of pericarditis. However, in large recent outbreaks, pericarditis occurred in 6 percent of patients with acute symptomatic histoplasmosis.[194] In the majority, it appeared to represent a sterile inflammatory response to infection in adjacent mediastinal lymph nodes, and it resolved spontaneously without specific therapy. In disseminated histoplasmosis the pericardium itself may be infected with *Histoplasma capsulatum*.[195] Pericarditis is rarely recognized in acute coccidioidomycosis. Spontaneously resolving cases resembling those seen in acute histoplasmosis have been described,[196] but most reported cases have occurred in the setting of disseminated coccidioidomycosis and represent *Coccidioides immitis* infection of the heart.[197] Fungal pericarditis, (resulting from direct inoculation or extension of mediastinal infection), is seen with increasing frequency as a complication of cardiothoracic surgery.[175] Pericarditis caused by *Candida* sp., *Aspergillus* sp., *Cryptococcus neoformans*, and other fungi occurs as a consequence of disseminated infection in severely debilitated and immunocompromised patients, especially those with prolonged neutropenia receiving multiple courses of antibiotics.[198–202] The rare parasitic causes of pericarditis are referenced in Table 3.

Pathology, Pathogenesis, and Pathophysiology

The pericardium has two opposing mesothelial surfaces. The parietal pericardium forms a flask-shaped sac that encloses the heart and the origins of the great vessels. It consists of a 1 mm thick layer of dense collagen lined by a single layer of mesothelial cells. The mesothelial cell layer is reflected onto the epicardial surface of the heart to form the visceral pericardium. The parietal pericardium has firm attachments to the sternum, the diaphragm, and the adventitia of the great vessels. The function of the normal pericardium has been a matter of considerable investigation and speculation.[213] It normally contains 15–50 ml of clear fluid, which may act as a lubricant. The pericardium reacts to acute injury by exuding fluid, fibrin, and cells in various combinations.[212] Acute pericarditis may resolve completely or progress to fibrous thickening, with or without constriction.

Cardiotropic viruses generally spread to the myocardium and pericardium hematogenously. Inflammation occurs in both visceral and parietal portions; effusion may develop and be serous, serofibrinous, or serosanguinous. Concomitant myocarditis may or may not be evident. Although most patients with viral pericarditis recover completely, occasional patients have repeated disabling recurrences.[214] The pathophysiology of these recurrences has not been established, but it probably involves immunologic mechanisms and not recurrent or persistent virus replication. Rarely, viral pericarditis leads to constriction as a late complication.[215]

Bacterial pericarditis generally results from (*1*) spread from a contiguous focus of infection within the chest, either de novo or after surgery or trauma; (*2*) spread from a focus of infection within the heart, most commonly from endocarditis; or (*3*) hematogenous infection. The incidence of purulent pericarditis arising from a contiguous pneumonia has steadily decreased and now generally occurs only when there has been significant delay in antibiotic therapy.[173,174] Pericarditis after cardiothoracic or esophageal surgery often occurs in patients with sternal wound infections and/or mediastinitis[175] and may be overlooked. Mortality is high. Pericarditis not infrequently accompanies fatal endocarditis,[72] especially that caused by *S. aureus*.[52] It often results from extension of a perivalvular abcess into the pericardium.[72] However, pericardial effusions in endocarditis may also be hemorrhagic[216] or sympathetic and sterile.[217] The presence of pre-existing nonbacterial pericardial effusion may predispose to the development of purulent pericarditis in bacteremic patients. Although the pericardial fluid may initially be clear,[172,175] it is usually grossly purulent and may be loculated by the time the disease is clinically apparent. Subsequent organization with adhesions, obliteration of the pericardial space, and calcification may occur and result in constrictive pericarditis.

Tuberculous pericarditis may develop from a hematogenous focus present from the time of primary infection, as a result of lymphatic spread from peritracheal, peribronchial, or mediastinal lymph nodes, or by contiguous spread from a focus of infection in lung or pleura. Four pathologic stages in tuberculous pericarditis have been described.[212,218] In the first stage, there is diffuse fibrin deposition, and granulomas with viable mycobacteria are present (Fig. 3). A serous or serosanguinous pericardial effusion then develops, usually quite slowly and often without symptoms. Lymphocytes, monocytes, and plasma cells replace the polymorphonuclear cells present early in infection. In the third stage, the effusion is absorbed, the pericardium thickens, granulomas proliferate, and a thick coat of fibrin is deposited on the parietal pericardium. Acid-fast bacilli become difficult to find as dense fibrous tissue and collagen are deposited. In stage four, which is associated with constriction, the pericardial space is obliterated by dense adhesions, the parietal pericardium is markedly thickened, and many granulomas are replaced by fibrous tissue. This is often followed by the accumulation of cholesterol crystals and calcification. Constrictive pericarditis appears to develop in half of patients with tuberculous pericarditis despite the use of antituberculous chemotherapy.[193,219] Although the incidence of tuberculosis has declined, it remains an important cause of constrictive pericarditis, especially in underdeveloped countries.[212]

Irrespective of etiology, if fluid accumulates rapidly in the pericardium and intrapericardial pressure rises, cardiac tamponade may result. Tamponade implies a progressive limitation of ventricular diastolic filling, with resultant reduction in stroke volume and cardiac output. In a recent series of medical patients with early cardiac tamponade, the etiology was infectious in 12.5 percent, noninfectious in 74 percent, and undetermined in the remainder.[220]

Clinical Manifestations

The presentation of acute pericarditis varies depending on the etiology. In viral or idiopathic pericarditis, chest pain is an important feature. This pain is often retrosternal, radiating to the shoulder and neck, and typically is aggravated by breathing, swallowing, and lying supine. In Smith's review of coxsackievirus B heart disease in adults,[158] 67 percent of patients had chest pain. Fever was present in 59 percent. A concurrent or prodromal flulike illness with malaise, arthralgias, myalgias,

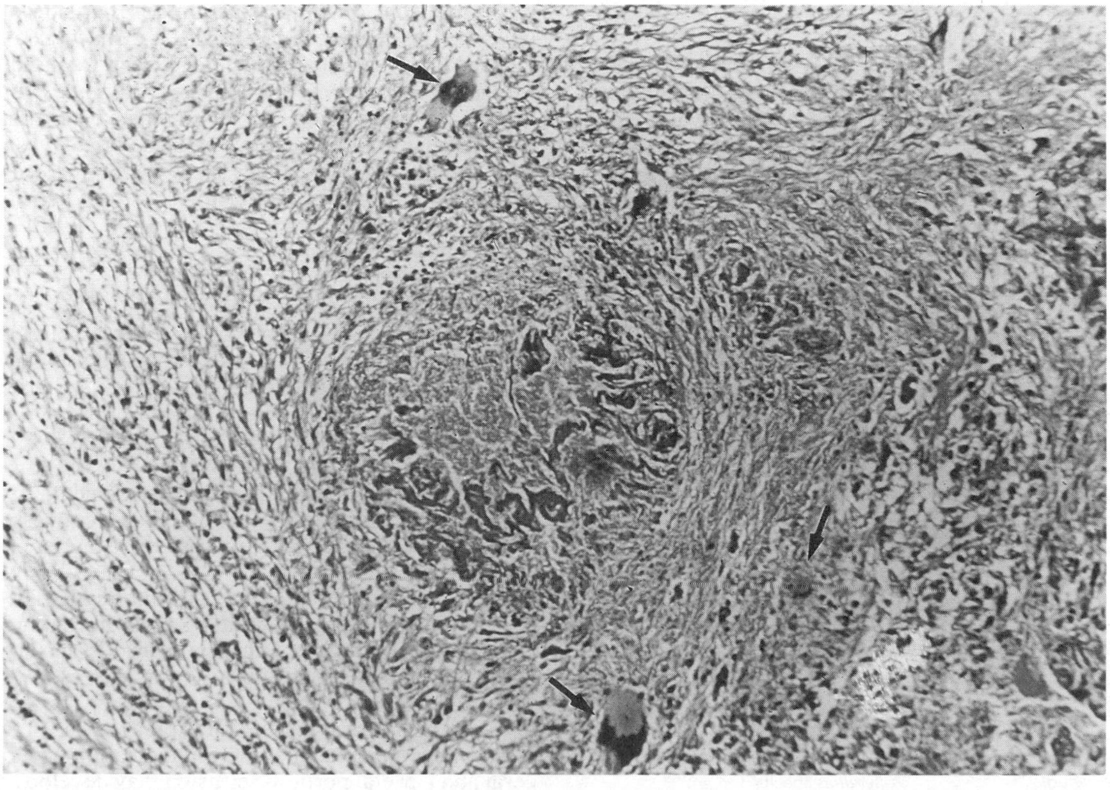

FIG. 3. Tuberculous pericarditis, with a typical granuloma in the pericardium. There is central caseous necrosis with aggregates of epithelioid cells at the periphery. Several multinucleated giant cells (arrows) are present. (×40) (From Bloor,[3] with permission.)

and occasionally cough with sputum was present in 36 percent. Patients with bacterial pericarditis are often acutely ill but frequently do not complain of chest pain.[175] Fever is almost invariably present and dyspnea is common. Bacterial pericarditis is rarely an isolated disease, and the symptoms and signs of the accompanying systemic or local infection may take clinical precedence. Tuberculous pericarditis most often has an insidious onset. Chest pain is present in 39–76 percent[193] but may be vague in nature. Weight loss, night sweats, cough, and dyspnea are common.

The classic physical finding in acute pericarditis is the three-component pericardial friction rub, which reflects cardiac motion during atrial systole, ventricular systole, and rapid ventricular filling in early diastole. This three-component rub was present in 50 percent of patients with acute pericarditis reported by Spodick.[221] The ventricular systolic component is often the loudest and most frequently appreciated. Rubs are often evanescent and may vary in quality; they are characteristically high-pitched, scratching, or grating. In the presence of significant pericardial effusion, there may be jugular venous distension, the most common physical finding in acute cardiac tamponade. Enlargement of the cardiac silhouette usually does not occur until at least 250 ml of fluid have accumulated in the pericardial space[222]; if fluid accumulates rapidly, tamponade may occur without detectable cardiomegaly. A pulsus paradoxus of more than 10 mmHg and a prominent x descent with loss of the y descent in the jugular venous pressure may be present. Dyspnea is common, but signs of left heart failure are usually absent in cardiac tamponade, and clear lung fields may help to differentiate tamponade from cardiogenic shock.

Although the pericardium produces no electrical activity, the electrocardiogram (ECG) is abnormal in 90 percent of patients with acute pericarditis,[222] reflecting diffuse subepicardial inflammation. Characteristic ECG changes are seen in approximately 50 percent of patients.[223] Early in pericarditis, ST segment elevation without change in QRS morphology typically occurs in multiple leads. Several days later, the ST segment returns to baseline, and there is T-wave flattening. During these early stages, there may also be depression of the PR segment. In contrast to myocardial infarction, the T-wave inversions in pericarditis do not generally occur until after the ST segment has returned to baseline. These T-wave inversions may last for weeks or months. Large pericardial effusions may be associated with reduced QRS voltage and electrical alternans. Sinus tachycardia is common, but the presence of other arrhythmias suggests pre-existing underlying heart disease or significant myocardial involvement.[224]

Echocardiography has been proved to be an extremely useful tool for diagnosis of pericardial effusion and should be performed if the situation is not immediately life-threatening. The size of the effusion can be roughly quantitated, and early hemodynamic compromise can often be detected.[222] Computerized tomography has been useful in demonstrating pericardial thickening and, in some cases, in differentiating an uncomplicated transudate from a high-density exudate.[236,237] Magnetic resonance imaging techniques also can easily detect pericardial fluid and thickening[238] but at present have no particular advantage over more conventional methods.

Diagnosis

A wide variety of agents and diseases may cause pericarditis and pericardial effusion (see Tables 3 and 4). Low-grade fever is common to many. A careful history, knowledge of the clinical setting in which the pericarditis occurs, and a search for clues outside the cardiovascular system are helpful in establishing a diagnosis. In a young person without underlying illness who presents with acute pericardial pain, the most likely diagnosis is viral or idiopathic pericarditis. However, establishing a specific viral diagnosis is difficult, costly, and often possible only in retrospect. Virus isolation can be attempted from throat and stool, and acute and convalescent sera can be tested for antibodies to potential pathogens (e.g., the coxsackie B viruses and any other enteroviruses prevalent locally at the time), but these approaches frequently fail to yield a specific diagnosis. Viruses are rarely isolated from pericardial fluid, even in patients in whom the diagnosis of viral myocarditis is highly probable. However, new techniques that permit the detection and identification of minute quantities of viral nucleic acid in the absence of infectious virus may revolutionize the diagnosis of viral and idiopathic pericarditis.

TABLE 4. Major Noninfectious Causes of Acute Pericarditis

Acute myocardial infarction[225]
Uremia[226]
Neoplasia[222]
Primary
Metastatic
Postirradiation[227]
Postcardiac injury
Trauma (penetrating or blunt)[222]
Postmyocardial infarction (Dresslers)[228]
Postpericardiotomy[229]
Dissecting aortic aneurysm[222]
Sarcoidosis[230]
Collagen vascular diseases
Systemic lupus erythematosis[231]
Rheumatoid arthritis[232]
Scleroderma[233]
Rheumatic fever[222]
Drug-induced[222]
Procainamide
Hydralazine
Other
Myxedema[234]

If the clinical suspicion of viral or idiopathic pericarditis is strong in an otherwise healthy patient with uncomplicated pericarditis, pericardiocentesis or other invasive procedures add little diagnostically[211] and carry a small but definite risk.[235] After excluding patients with postpericardiotomy syndrome, myocardial infarction, renal failure, known neoplastic disease, trauma, and irradiation, Permanyer-Miralde et al.[211] prospectively evaluated 231 patients with primary acute pericardial disease. After thorough diagnostic evaluation, 199 were felt to have acute idiopathic pericarditis. Unsuspected neoplastic pericarditis was found in 13, tuberculosis in 9, and collagen vascular disease in 4. Purulent pericarditis, viral pericarditis, and *Toxoplasma gondii* infection were each found in two patients. The diagnostic yield was substantial when pericardiocentesis or pericardiectomy with biopsy were done to relieve cardiac tamponade (39 percent and 54 percent, respectively), but it was only 5 percent when these procedures were done solely for the purpose of diagnosis. The authors concluded that the presence of a pericardial effusion per se is not an indication for an invasive procedure; in patients with pericardial effusion that has persisted for more than 3 weeks, an invasive procedure may be indicated.

Untreated purulent pericarditis is usually rapidly fatal.[175] In acutely ill patients in whom purulent pericarditis is suspected, the diagnosis should be pursued quickly and aggressively. When possible, pericardiotomy with biopsy and drainage is preferable to pericardiocentesis because of greater diagnostic yield and fewer complications.[222] Noninfectious diseases predominate as causes of significant pericardial effusion and cardiac tamponade,[220] but bacterial and tuberculous effusions are more likely to have serious hemodynamic consequences.[235]

Treatment

Bed rest, symptomatic therapy for pain, and careful monitoring for the developmentof hemodynamic compromise are the mainstays of treatment for presumed viral or idiopathic pericarditis. Nonsteroidal anti-inflammatory agents are often successful in relieving symptoms. Because myocarditis often accompanies viral pericarditis and steroids enhance myocardial injury during active virus replication, we believe that steroids should be avoided during the acute illness. Viral or idiopathic pericarditis is generally benign and self-limited, but recurrences[214] and late constriction[215] do occur.

Surgical drainage of the pericardium, in addition to appropriate antibiotic therapy, is essential in almost all patients with purulent pericarditis.[172,175,177] Initial pericardiocentesis may be lifesaving, but fluid often reaccumulates, and constriction can develop rapidly.[175,177] There is little rationale for irrigating the pericardium with antibiotics, because penetration from serum is excellent.[239] With early diagnosis and aggressive therapy, *H. influenzae* pericarditis in young patients has a good prognosis.[177] However, overall mortality in bacterial pericarditis remains high, especially when it develops after surgery or occurs in the course of endocarditis.[175]

The treatment of tuberculous pericarditis remains controversial. Antituberculous therapy has reduced mortality substantially.[240] The addition of steroids to reduce inflammation and avoid late constriction is favored by many, including the authors, but it remains unproved.[190,240,241] Early surgical intervention is advocated in patients with hemodynamic compromise from recurrent effusion or progressive pericardial thickening.[219,240]

MEDIASTINITIS

Infections in the mediastinum may be divided into two categories, acute and chronic, which differ markedly in their microbiology, pathogenesis, presentation, and treatment. Acute mediastinitis is a rare but dreaded disease that complicates oropharyngeal infection,[242,243] perforation of the esophagus,[244] cardiac surgery,[245,246] or infection of contiguous structures. In the preantibiotic era, acute mediastinitis often resulted from infection of the pharynx or the second or third mandibular molars, with dissection downward along anatomic planes. Currently, only a small proportion of cases result from retropharyngeal or odontogenic infections. Rupture of the esophagus is also uncommon; it may occur spontaneously, from erosion with tumor, after sclerotherapy for varicies or esophageal dilatation, or as a postoperative complication. Most cases of acute mediastinitis now occur as a complication of cardiac surgery. The reported incidence of mediastinitis after surgery ranges from 0.4 to 5 percent,[245] with mortality rates from 8.6 to 77 percent.[246] Factors that have been associated with higher rates of infection include serious underlying noncardiovascular diseases, increased complexity of surgery, sternal dehiscence, and emergency reoperation.[246,247]

Patients with acute mediastinitis are often severely ill with fever and tachycardia, and the infection may progress rapidly. There may be crepitus, brawny edema of the neck or chest wall, purulent pleural and/or pericardial effusions, pneumonitis, and mediastinal widening visible on chest radiograph. Postoperative mediastinitis generally occurs within 2 weeks following sternotomy. Patients often first develop fever and bacteremia followed by an abnormal-appearing wound. However, mediastinal widening and sternal instability are infrequent.[246]

The origin of the infection is predictive of its bacteriology. Mouth organisms, especially anaerobes, play an important role in mediastinitis following esophageal perforation and oropharyngeal infection.[248] *Staphylococcus aureus* and gram-negative bacilli, including *Pseudomonas aeruginosa*, are found after surgical procedures. *Staphylococcus epidermidis*, although usually not a pathogen, cannot be ignored in the postsurgical setting if signs of infection are present.[249] Not unexpectedly, pathogens encountered are frequently resistant to the antibiotic used in perioperative prophylaxis.[246]

Computed tomography has proved a very useful aid in the diagnosis of acute mediastinitis and its management.[250,251] Aggressive débridement and drainage in conjunction with appropriate antibiotic therapy are essential, but mortality remains high (24–40 percent).[242,243,246,248]

A more indolent form of mediastinitis, termed fibrosing mediastinitis, may occur as a complication of granulomatous infections such as histoplasmosis or tuberculosis. Fibrosing mediastinitis has been postulated to result from rupture of mediastinal lymph nodes with release of caseous material, which provokes an intense inflammatory reaction. Patients may present with symptoms of occlusion of major mediastinal structures (e.g., superior vena cava syndrome) or with an asymptomatic mass detected on routine chest radiograph. Granulomatous and fibrous mediastinitis may account for up to 10 percent of all primary mediastinal masses and 20 percent of cases of superior vena cava syndrome.[252,253] *Histoplasma capsulatum* is the etiologic agent most commonly implicated.[253] The organism is visible with appropriate staining techniques in from 35 to 73 percent of cases.[254,255] The process is often located near the bifurcation of the trachea or the hilum of the lung. The pathology is variable but generally consists of caseous necrosis with granuloma formation surrounded by dense fibrosis. Organisms are generally not abundant and attempts to grow the organism are usually not successful.[254,256] As the lesions age, the fibrous capsule extends and may invade surrounding tissues, but why this occurs in the individuals so afflicted is a matter of conjecture. Early in disease, surgical resection may be attempted, but during the latter stages, surgery is technically difficult and at best palliative.[253–255]

REFERENCES

1. Saphir O. Myocarditis: a general review with an analysis of two hundred and forty cases. Arch Pathol. 1941;32:1000–51 and 1942;33:88–137.
2. Stevens PJ, Underwood Ground KE. Occurrence and significance of myocarditis in trauma. Aerospace Med. 1970;41:776–80.
3. Bloor CM. Pericarditis and myocarditis. In: Cardiac Pathology. Philadelphia: JB Lippincott; 1978:265–95.
4. Bandt CM, Staley NA, Noren GR. Acute viral myocarditis: clinical and histological changes. Minn Med. 1979;62:234–7.
5. Bengtsson E, Orndahl G. Complications of mumps with special reference to the incidence of myocarditis. Acta Med Scand. 1954;149:381–8.
6. Lucke B, Wight T, Kime E. Pathologic anatomy and bacteriology of influenza: epidemic of autumn 1918. Arch Intern Med. 1919;24:154–237.
7. Degen JA Jr. Visceral pathology in measles; clinicopathologic study of 100 fatal cases. Am J Med Sci. 1937;194:104–11.
8. Lucke B. Postmortem findings in measles bronchopneumonia and other acute infections. JAMA. 1918;70:2006–11.
9. Saphir O, Wile SA. Myocarditis in poliomyelitis. Am J Med Sci. 1942;203:781–8.
10. Sylvest E. Epidemic Myalgia: Bornholm Disease. London: Oxford University Press; 1934.
11. Reyes MP, Lerner AM. Coxsackievirus myocarditis—with special reference to acute and chronic effects. Prog Cardiovasc Dis. 1985;27:373–94.
12. Hirschman SZ, Hammer GS. Coxsackie virus myopericarditis. A microbiological and clinical review. Am J Cardiol. 1974;34:224–32.
13. Woodruff JF. Viral myocarditis. Am J Pathol. 1980;101:427–78.
14. Grist NR, Bell EJ. A six-year study of coxsackievirus B infections in heart disease. J Hyg Camb. 1974;73:165–72.
15. Russell SJM, Bell EJ. Echoviruses and carditis. Lancet. 1970;1:784–5.
16. Bell EJ, Grist NR. ECHO viruses, carditis and acute pleurodynia. Am Heart J. 1971;82:133–8.
17. Jungeblut CW, Edwards JE. Isolation of poliomyelitis virus from the heart in fatal cases. Am J Clin Pathol. 1951;21:601–23.
18. Weinstein L, Shelokov A. Cardiovascular manifestations in acute poliomyelitis. N Engl J Med. 1951;244:281–5.
19. Roberts WC, Fox III SM. Mumps of the heart: clinical and pathological features. Circulation. 1965;32:342–5.
20. Baandrup U, Mortensen SA. Fatal mumps myocarditis. Acta Med Scand. 1984;216:331–3.
21. Hamburger WW. The heart in influenza. Med Clin North Am. 1938;22:111–21.
22. Verel D, Warrack AJN, Potter CW, et al. Observations on the A2 England influenza epidemic. A clinicopathological study. Am Heart J. 1976;92:290–6.
23. Ross E, Armentrout SA. Myocarditis associated with rabies. Report of a case. N Engl J Med. 1962;266:1087–9.
24. Ainger LE, Lawyer NG, Fitch CW. Neonatal rubella myocarditis. Br Heart J. 1966;28:691–7.

25. Kriseman T. Rubella myocarditis in a 9 year old patient. Clin Pediatr. 1984;23:240–1.
26. Chuah SK. Transient ventricular arrhythmia as a cardiac manifestation in dengue haemorrhagic fever—a case report. Singapore Med J. 1987;28:569–72.
27. Obeyesekere I, Hermon Y. Myocarditis and cardiomyopathy after arbovirus infections (dengue and chikingunya fever). Br Heart J. 1972;34:821–7.
28. Cannell DE. Myocardial degenerations in yellow fever. Am J Pathol. 1928;4:431–43.
29. Milei J, Bolomo NJ. Myocardial damage in viral hemorrhagic fevers. Am Heart J. 1982;104:1385–91.
30. Thiede WH. Cardiac involvement in lymphocytic choriomeningitis. Arch Intern Med. 1962;109:50–4.
31. Henson D, Mufson MA. Myocarditis and pneumonitis with type 21 adenovirus infection: association with fatal myocarditis and pneumonitis. Am J Dis Child. 1971;121:334–6.
32. Karjalainen J, Heikkila J, Nieminen MS, et al. Etiology of mild acute infectious myocarditis. Relation to clinical features. Acta Med Scand. 1983;213:65–73.
33. Hackel DB. Myocarditis in association with varicella. Am J Pathol. 1953;29:369–79.
34. Woolf PK, Chung T-S, Stewart J, et al. Life-threatening dysrhythmias in varicella myocarditis. Clin Pediatr. 1987;26:480–2.
35. Coppack SW, Doshi R, Ghose AR. Fatal varicella in a healthy young adult. Postgrad Med J. 1985;61:529–31.
36. Tiula E, Leinikki P. Fatal cytomegalovirus infection in a previously healthy boy with myocarditis and consumption coagulopathy as presenting signs. Scand J Infect Dis. 1972;4:57–60.
37. Webster BH. Cardiac complications of infectious mononucleosis: a review of the literature and report of five cases. Am J Med Sci. 1957;234:62–70.
38. Hudgins JM. Infectious mononucleosis complicated by myocarditis and pericarditis. JAMA. 1976;235:2626–7.
39. Matthews AW, Griffiths ID. Post vaccinal pericarditis and myocarditis. Br Heart J. 1974;36:1043–5.
40. Anderson T, Foulis MA, Grist NR, et al. Clinical and laboratory observations in a smallpox outbreak. Lancet. 1951;1:1248–52.
41. Mahapatra RK, Ellis GH. Myocarditis and hepatitis B virus. Angiology. 1985;36:116–9.
42. Bell H. Cardiac manifestations of viral hepatitis. JAMA. 1971;218:387–91.
43. Ursell PC, Habib A, Sharma P, et al. Hepatitis B virus and myocarditis. Hum Pathol. 1984;15:481–4.
44. Gore I, Saphir O. Myocarditis. A classification of 1402 cases. Am Heart J. 1947;34:827–30.
45. Gore I. Myocardial changes in fatal diphtheria; summary of observations in 221 cases. Am J Med Sci. 1948;215:257–66.
46. Roberts WC, Berard CW. Gas gangrene of the heart in clostridial septicemia. Am Heart J. 1967;74:482–8.
47. Guneratne F. Gas gangrene (abscess) of heart. NY State J Med. 1975;75:1766.
48. Joshi MK, Kandoth PW, Barve RJ, et al. Rheumatic fever: clinical profile of 339 cases with long term follow up. Indian Pediatr. 1983;20:849–53.
49. Brasier AR, Macklis JD, Vaughan D, et al. Myopericarditis as an initial presentation of meningococcemia. Unusual manifestation of infection with serotype W135. Am J Med. 1987;82:641–4.
50. Cohen JI, Bartlett JA, Corey GR. Extra-intestinal manifestations of *Salmonella* infections. Medicine. 1987;66:349–88.
51. Lubani M, Sharda D, Helin I. Cardiac manifestations in brucellosis. Arch Dis Child. 1986;61:569–72.
52. Watanakunakorn C, Tan JS, Phair JP. Some salient features of *Staphylococcus aureus* endocarditis. Am J Med. 1973;54:473–81.
53. Chen S-C, Tsai CC, Nouri S. Carditis associated with *Mycoplasma pneumoniae* infection. AJDC. 1986;140:471–2.
54. Lind K. Manifestation and complications of *Mycoplasme pneumoniae* disease: a review. Yale J Biol Med. 1983;56:461–8.
55. Dymock IW, Lawson JM, MacLennan WJ, et al. Myocarditis associated with psittacosis. Br J Clin Pract. 1971;25:240–2.
56. Marin-Garcia J, Mirvis DM. Myocardial disease in Rocky Mountain spotted fever: clinical, functional, and pathologic findings. Pediatr Cardiol. 1984;5:149–54.
57. Brown GW, Shirai A, Jegathesan M, et al. Febrile illness in Malaysia—an analysis of 1629 hospitalized patients. Am J Trop Med Hyg. 1984;33:311–5.
58. Ognibene AJ, O'Leary DS, Czarnecki SW, et al. Myocarditis and disseminated intravascular coagulation in scrub typhus. Am J Med Sci. 1971;262:233–9.
59. Steere AC, Batsford WP, Weinberg M, et al. Lyme carditis: cardiac abnormalities of Lyme disease. Ann Intern Med. 1980;93:8–16.
60. McAlister HF, Klementowicz PT, Andrews C, et al. Lyme carditis: an important cause of reversible heart block. Ann Intern Med. 1989;110:339–45.
61. Williams AH. *Aspergillus* myocarditis. Am J Clin Pathol. 1974;61:247–56.
62. Atkinson JB, Connor DH, Robinowitz M, et al. Cardiac fungal infections: review of autopsy findings in 60 patients. Hum Pathol. 1984;15:935–42.
63. Lewis W, Lipsick J, Cammarosano C. Cryptococcal myocarditis in acquired immune deficiency syndrome. Am J Cardiol. 1985;9:1240.
64. Lafont A, Wolff M, Marche C, et al. Overwhelming myocarditis due to *Cryptococcus neoformans* in an AIDS patient. Lancet. 1987;2:1145–6.
65. Rosenbaum MB. Chagasic myocardiopathy. Prog Cardiovasc Dis. 1964;7:199–255.
66. Mott KE, Hagstrom JWC. The pathologic lesions of the cardiac autonomic nervous system in chronic Chagas' myocarditis. Circulation. 1965;31:273–86.
67. Mendoza I, Camardo J, Moleiro F, et al. Sustained ventricular tachycardia in chronic Chagasic myocarditis. Am J Cardiol. 1986;57:423–7.
68. Poltera AA, Owor R, Cox JN. Pathological aspects of human African trypanosomiasis in Uganda. Virchows Arch [A] 1977;373:249–65.
69. Barr R. Human trichinosis: report of 4 cases with emphasis on central nervous system involvement and a survey of 500 consecutive autopsies at the Ottawa Civic Hospital. Can Med Assoc J. 1966;95:912–7.
70. Grey DF, Morse BS, Phillips WF. Trichinosis with neurologic and cardiac involvement. Review of the literature and report of three cases. Ann Intern Med. 1962;57:230–44.
71. Yermakov V, Rashid RK, Vuletin JC, et al. Disseminated toxoplasmosis. Case report and review of the literature. Arch Pathol Lab Med. 1982;106:524–8.
72. Buchbinder NA, Roberts WC. Left-sided valvular active infective endocarditis. A study of 45 necropsy patients. Am J Med. 1972;53:20–35.
73. Welch K, Finkbeiner W, Alpers CE, et al. Autopsy findings in the acquired immune deficiency syndrome. JAMA. 1984;252:1152–9.
74. Baroldi G, Carallo S, Moroni M, et al. Focal lymphocytic myocarditis in acquired immunodeficiency syndrome (AIDS): a correlative morphologic and clinical study in 26 consecutive fatal cases. J Am Coll Cardiol. 1988;12:463–9.
75. Cammarosano C, Lewis W. Cardiac lesions in acquired immune deficiency syndrome (AIDS). J Am Coll Cardiol. 1985;5:703–6.
76. Fink L, Reichek N, St. John Sutton MG. Cardiac abnormalities in acquired immune deficiency syndrome. Am J Cardiol. 1984;54:1161–3.
77. Anderson DW, Virmani R, Reilly JM, et al. Prevalent myocarditis at necropsy in the acquired immunodeficiency syndrome. J Am Coll Cardiol. 1988;11:792–9.
78. Calabrese LH, Proffitt MR, Yen-Lieberman B, et al. Congestive cardiomyopathy and illness related to the acquired immunodeficiency syndrome (AIDS) associated with isolation of retrovirus from myocardium. Ann Intern Med. 1987;107:691–2.
79. Dittrich H, Chow L, Denaro F, et al. Human immunodeficiency virus, coxsackievirus, and cardiomyopathy. (Letter) Ann Intern Med. 1988;108:308–9.
80. Edwards WD. Myocarditis and endomyocardial biopsy. Cardiol Clin. 1984;2:647–56.
81. Lyden D, Olszewski J, Huber S. Variation in susceptibility of BALB/c mice to coxsackievirus group B type 3-induced myocarditis with age. Cell Immunol. 1987;105:332–9.
82. Herskowitz A, Wolfgram LJ, Rose NR, et al. Coxsackievirus B_3 murine myocarditis: a pathologic spectrum of myocarditis in genetically defined inbred strains. J Am Coll Cardiol. 1987;9:1311–9.
83. Huber SA, Lodge PA. Coxsackievirus B-3 myocarditis. Identification of different pathogenic mechanisms in DBA/2 and BALB/c mice. Am J Pathol. 1986;122:284–91.
84. Wolfgram LJ, Beisel KW, Herskowitz A, et al. Variations in the susceptibility to Coxsackievirus B_3-induced myocarditis among different strains of mice. J Immunol. 1986;136:1846–52.
85. Khatib R, Probert A, Reyes MP, et al. Mouse strain-related variation as a factor in the pathogenesis of coxsackievirus B3 murine myocarditis. J Gen Virol. 1987;68:2981–8.
86. Rager-Zisman B, Allison AC. The role of antibody and host cells in the resistance of mice against infection by coxsackie B-3 virus. J Gen Virol. 1973;19:329–38.
87. Woodruff JF. Lack of correlation between neutralizing antibody production and suppression of coxsackievirus B-3 replication in target organs: evidence for involvement of mononuclear inflammatory cells in host defense. J Immunol. 1979;123:31–6.
88. Godeny EK, Gauntt CJ. *In situ* immune autoradiographic identification of cells in heart tissue of mice with coxsackievirus B3-induced myocarditis. Am J Pathol. 1987;129:267–76.
89. Godeny EK, Gauntt CJ. Murine natural killer cells limit coxsackievirus B3 replication. J Immunol. 1987;139:913–8.
90. Godeny EK, Gauntt CJ. Involvement of natural killer cells in coxsackievirus B3-induced murine myocarditis. J Immunol. 1986;137:1695–702.
91. Kilbourne ED, Wilson CB, Perrier D. The induction of gross myocardial lesions by a coxsackie (pleurodynia) virus and cortisone. J Clin Invest. 1956;35:362–70.
92. Rezkalla S, Khatib G, Khatib R. Coxsackievirus B3 murine myocarditis: deleterious effects of nonsteroidal anti-inflammatory agents. J Lab Clin Med. 1986;107:393–5.
93. Huber SA, Lodge PA. Coxsackievirus B-3 myocarditis in BALB/c mice. Evidence for autoimmunity to myocyte antigens. Am J Pathol. 1984;116:21–9.
94. Guthrie M, Lodge PA, Huber SA. Cardiac injury in myocarditis induced by coxsackievirus group B, type 3 in BALB/c mice is mediated by Lyt 2^+ cytolytic lymphocytes. Cell Immunol. 1984;88:558–67.
95. Kishimoto C, Kuribayashi K, Masuda T, et al. Immunologic behavior of lymphocytes in experimental viral myocarditis: significance of T lymphocytes in the severity of myocarditis and silent myocarditis in BALB/c-nu/nu mice. Circulation. 1985;71:1247–54.
96. Lyden DC, Huber SA. Aggravation of coxsackievirus, group B, type 3-induced myocarditis and increase in cellular immunity to myocyte antigens

in pregnant BALB/c mice and animals treated with progesterone. Cell Immunol. 1984;87:462–72.
97. Job LP, Lyden DC, Huber SA. Demonstration of suppressor cells in coxsackievirus group B, type 3 infected female BALB/c mice which prevent myocarditis. Cell Immunol. 1986;98:104–13.
98. Huber SA, Job LP. Differences in cytolytic T cell response of BALB/c mice infected with myocarditic and non-myocarditic strains of coxsackievirus group B, type 3. Infect Immun. 1983;39:1419–27.
99. Wolfgram LJ, Beisel KW, Rose NR. Heart-specific autoantibodies following murine coxsackievirus B_3 myocarditis. J Exp Med. 1985;161:1112–21.
100. Neu N, Beisel KW, Traystman MD, et al. Autoantibodies specific for the cardiac myosin isoform are found in mice susceptible to coxsackievirus B_3-induced myocarditis. J Immunol. 1987;138:2488–92.
101. Neu N, Craig SW, Rose NR, et al. Coxsackievirus induced myocarditis in mice: cardiac myosin autoantibodies do not cross-react with the virus. Clin Exp Immunol. 1987;69:566–74.
102. Neu N, Rose NR, Beisel KW, et al. Cardiac myosin induces myocarditis in genetically predisposed mice. J Immunol. 1987;139:3630–6.
103. Kishimoto C, Tomioka N, Kawai C. Clinical findings in acute viral myocarditis. With special attention to experimental and immunological evidence. Herz. 1985;10:15–20.
104. Bloor CM. Protozoal, helminthic and fungal heart disease. In: Cardiac Pathology. Philadelphia: JB Lippincott; 1978:335–366.
105. Abelmann WH. Virus and the heart. Circulation. 1971;44:950–6.
106. Vikerfors T, Stjerna A, Olcen P, et al. Acute myocarditis. Serologic diagnosis, clinical findings and follow-up. Acta Med Scand. 1988;223:45–52.
107. Stratmann HG. Acute myocarditis versus myocardial infarction: evaluation and management of the young patient with prolonged chest pain-case reports. Angiology. 1988;39:253–8.
108. Miklozek CL, Crumpacker CS, Royal HD, et al. Myocarditis presenting as acute myocardial infarction. Am Heart J. 1988;115:768–76.
109. Spodick DH. Infection and infarction. Acute viral (and other) infection in the onset, pathogenesis, and mimicry of acute myocardial infarction. Am J Med. 1986;81:661–8.
110. Beaufils P, Slama R. Myocarditis confirmed by biopsy presenting as acute myocardial infarction. Br Heart J. 1986;4:420.
111. Griffiths PD, Hannington G, Booth JC. Coxsackie B virus infections and myocardial infarction. Results from a prospective, epidemiologically controlled study. Lancet. 1980;1:1387–9.
112. Heikkila J, Karjalainen J. Evaluation of mild acute infectious myocarditis. Br Heart J. 1982;47:381–91.
113. Scott LP III, Gutelius MF, Parrott RH. Children with acute respiratory tract infections. An electrocardiographic survey. Am J Dis Child. 1970;119:111–3.
114. Weinhouse E, Wanderman KL, Sofer S, et al. Viral myocarditis simulating dilated cardiomyopathy in early childhood: evaluation by serial echocardiography. Br Heart J. 1986;56:94–7.
115. Nieminen MS, Heikkila J, Karjalainen J. Echocardiography in acute infectious myocarditis: relation to clinical and electrocardiographic findings. Am J Cardiol. 1984;53:1331–7.
116. Alpert LI, Welch P, Fisher N. Gallium-positive Lyme disease myocarditis. Clin Nucl Med. 1985;9:617.
117. Shulkin BL, Wahl RL. SPECT imaging of myocarditis. Clin Nucl Med. 1987;12:841–2.
118. Robinson JA, O'Connell J, Henkin RE, et al. Gallium-67 imaging in cardiomyopathy. Ann Intern Med. 1979;90:198–9.
119. O'Connell JB, Robinson JA, Henkin RE, et al. Immunosuppressive therapy in patients with congestive cardiomyopathy and myocardial uptake of gallium-67. Circulation. 1981;64:780–6.
120. Fowles RE, Mason JW. Endomyocardial biopsy. Ann Intern Med. 1982;97:885–94.
121. Nippoldt TB, Edwards WD, Holms DR, et al. Right ventricular endomyocardial biopsy. Clinicopathologic correlates in 100 consecutive patients. Mayo Clin Proc. 1982;57:407–18.
122. Parrillo JE, Aretz HT, Palacios I, et al. The results of transvenous endomyocardial biopsy can frequently be used to diagnose myocardial diseases in patients with idiopathic heart failure. Endomyocardial biopsies in 100 consecutive patients revealed a substantial incidence of myocarditis. Circulation. 1984;69:93–101.
123. Takahashi O, Kamiya T, Echigo S, et al. Myocarditis in children—clinical findings and myocardial biopsy findings. Jpn Circ J. 1983;47:1298–303.
124. Dec GW, Palacios IF, Fallon JT, et al. Active myocarditis in the spectrum of acute dilated cardiomyopathies. Clinical features, histologic correlates, and clinical outcome. N Engl J Med. 1985;312:885–90.
125. Zee-Cheng C-S, Tsai CC, Palmer DC, et al. High incidence of myocarditis by endomyocardial biopsy in patients with idiopathic congestive cardiomyopathy. J Am Coll Cardiol. 1984;3:63–70.
126. Fenoglio JJ, Ursell PC, Kellogg CF, et al. Diagnosis and classification of myocarditis by endomyocardial biopsy. N Engl J Med. 1983;308:12–8.
127. Mason JW, Billingham ME, Ricci DR. Treatment of acute inflammatory myocarditis assisted by endomyocardial biopsy. Am J Cardiol. 1980;45:1037–44.
128. Chow LC, Dittrich HC, Shabetai R. Endomyocardial biopsy in patients with unexplained congestive heart failure. Ann Intern Med. 1988;109:535.
129. Shanes JG, Ghali J, Billingham ME, et al. Interobserver variability in the pathologic interpretation of endomyocardial biopsy results. Circulation. 1987;75:401–5.
130. Billingham M. Acute myocarditis: a diagnostic dilemma. Br Heart J. 1987;58:6–8.
131. Kereiakes DJ, Parmley WW. Myocarditis and cardiomyopathy. Am Heart J. 1984;108:1318–26.
132. Aretz HT, Billingham ME, Edwards WD, et al. Myocarditis, a histopathologic definition and classification. Am J Cardiovasc Pathol. 1987;1:3–14.
133. Yasuda T, Palacios IF, Dec GW, et al. Indium 111-monoclonal antimyosin antibody imaging in the diagnosis of acute myocarditis. Circulation. 1987;76:306–11.
134. Weinstein C, Fenoglio JJ. Myocarditis. Hum Pathol. 1987;18:613–8.
135. Easton AJ, Eglin RP. The detection of coxsackievirus RNA in cardiac tissue by *in situ* hybridization. J Gen Virol. 1988;69:285–91.
136. Rotbart HA, Eastman PS, Ruth JL, et al. Nonisotopic oligomeric probes for the human enteroviruses. J Clin Microbiol. 1988;26:2669–71.
137. Erlich HA, Gelfand DH, Saiki RK. Specific DNA amplification. Nature. 1988;331:461–2.
138. Kawai C, Matsumori A, Fujiwara H. Myocarditis and dilated cardiomyopathy. Annu Rev Med. 1987;38:221–39.
139. Lowry PJ, Edwards CW, Nagle RE. Herpes-like virus particles in myocardium of patient progressing to congestive cardiomyopathy. Br Heart J. 1982;48:501–3.
140. Daly K, Richardson PJ, Olsen EGJ, et al. Acute myocarditis. Role of histological and virological examination in the diagnosis and assessment of immunosuppressive treatment. Br Heart J. 1984;51:30–5.
141. Kopecky SL, Gersh BJ. Dilated cardiomyopathy and myocarditis: natural history, etiology, clinical manifestations, and management. In: O'Rourke RA, Crawford MH, eds. Current Problems in Cardiology. Chicago: Year Book Medical Publishers, Inc.; 1987:569–647.
142. Lowry BS. Viruses and heart disease: a problem in pathogenesis. Ann Clin Lab Sci. 1986;16:358–64.
143. Fowler NO. The secondary cardiomyopathies. In: Fowler NO. Myocardial Disease. New York: Grune & Stratton; 1973:337–59.
144. Bank I, Marboe CC, Redberg RF, et al. Myocarditis in adult Still's disease. Arthritis Rheum. 1985;28:452–4.
145. Myocarditis. In: Braunwald E, ed. Heart Disease, a Textbook of Cardiovascular Medicine. 3rd ed. Philadelphia: WB Saunders; 1988:1440–69.
146. Ikaheimo MJ, Niemela KO, Linnaluoto MM, et al. Early cardiac changes related to radiation therapy. Am J Cardiol. 1988;56:943–6.
147. Taliercio CP, Olney BA, Lie JT. Myocarditis related to drug hypersensitivity. Mayo Clin Proc. 1985;60:463–8.
148. Brand A, Keren A, Kerem E, et al. Myocardial damage after a scorpion sting: long-term echocardiographic follow-up. Pediatr Cardiol. 1988;9:59–61.
149. Matsuura H, Ishikita T, Yamamoto S, et al. Gallium-67 myocardial imaging for the detection of myocarditis in the acute phase of Kawasaki disease (mucocutaneous lymph node syndrome): the usefulness of single photon emission computed tomography. Br Heart J. 1987;58:385–92.
150. Humbert P, Faivre R, Fellman D, et al. Giant cell myocarditis: an autoimmune disease? Am Heart J. 1988;115:485–7.
151. Hayakawa M, Inoh T, Yokota Y, et al. A long-term follow-up study of acute viral and idiopathic myocarditis. Jpn Circ J. 1983;47:1304–9.
152. Tomioka N, Kishimoto C, Matsumori A, et al. Effects of prednisolone on acute viral myocarditis in mice. J Am Coll Cardiol. 1986;7:868–72.
153. Ettinger J, Feucht H, Gartner R, et al. Cyclosporine A (CyA) for successful treatment of myocarditis (Letter). Eur Heart J. 1986;7:452.
154. Hosenpud JD, McAnulty JH, Niles NR. Lack of objective improvement in ventricular systolic function in patients with myocarditis treated with azathioprine and prednisone. J Am Coll Cardiol. 1985;6:797–801.
155. Monrad ES, Matsumori A, Murphy JC, et al. Therapy with cyclosporine in experimental murine myocarditis with encephalomyocarditis virus. Circulation. 1986;73:1058–64.
156. Osler, W. The Principles and Practice of Medicine. New York: D Appleton; 1892.
157. Koontz CH, Ray CG. The role of coxsackie group B virus infections in sporadic myopericarditis. Am Heart J. 1971;82:750–8.
158. Smith WG. Coxsackie B myopericarditis in adults. Am Heart J. 1970;80:34–46.
159. Montgomery J, Gear JHS, Prinslou FR, et al. Myocarditis of the newborn. An outbreak in a maternity home in Southern Rhodesia associated with coxsackie group-B virus infection. S Afr Med J. 1955;29:608–12.
160. Helin M, Savola J, Lapinleimu K. Cardiac manifestations during a coxsackie B5 epidemic. Br Med J. 1968;2:97–9.
161. Brodie HR, Marchessault V. Acute benign pericarditis caused by coxsackie virus group B. N Engl J Med. 1960;262:1278–80.
162. Grist NR, Bell EJ. Coxsackie viruses and the heart. Am Heart J. 1969;77:295–300.
163. Russell SJM, Bell EJ. Echoviruses and carditis. Lancet. 1970;1:784–5.
164. Kleinfeld M, Milles S, Lidsky M. Mumps pericarditis: review of the literature and report of a case. Am Heart J. 1958;55:153–6.
165. Proby Cm, Hacket D, Gupta S, et al. Acute myopericarditis in influenza A infection. Q J Med. 1986;60:887–92.
166. Cheng TC. Severe chest pain due to infectious mononucleosis. Postgrad Med. 1983;73:149–52.
167. Shugoll GI. Pericarditis associated with infectious mononucleosis. Arch Intern Med. 1957;100:630–4.
168. Williams AJ, Freemont AJ, Barnett DB. Pericarditis and arthritis complicating chickenpox. Br J Clin Pract. 1983;37:226–7.

169. Kassab A, Demoulin JC, Vanlancker MA, et al. Cytomegalovirus hemopericarditis. Report of 1 case with histologic confirmation. Acta Cardiol. 1987;42:69–72.
170. Freedberg RS, Gindea AJ, Dieterich DT, et al. Herpes simplex pericarditis in AIDS. NY State J Med. 1987;87:304–6.
171. Adler R, Takahashi M, Wright, Jr. HT. Acute pericarditis associated with hepatitis B infection. Pediatrics. 1978;61:716–9.
172. Boyle JD, Pearce ML, Guze LB. Purulent pericarditis: review of literature and report of eleven cases. Medicine. 1961;40:119–44.
173. Klacsmann PG, Bulkley BH, Hutchins GM. The changed spectrum of purulent pericarditis. An 86 year autopsy experience in 200 patients. Am J Med. 1977;63:666–73.
174. Kauffman CA, Watanakunakorn C, Phair JP. Purulent pneumococcal pericarditis. A continuing problem in the antibiotic era. Am J Med. 1973;54:743–50.
175. Rubin RH, Moellering RC. Clinical, microbiologic and therapeutic aspects of purulent pericarditis. Am J Med. 1975;59:68–78.
176. Blaser MJ, Reingold AL, Alsever RN, et al. Primary meningococcal pericarditis: a disease of adults associated with serogroup C *Neisseria meningitidis*. Rev Infect Dis. 1984;6:625–32.
177. Fyfe DA, Hagler DJ, Puga FJ, et al. Clinical and therapeutic aspects of *Haemophilus influenzae* pericarditis in pediatric patients. Mayo Clin Proc. 1984;59:415–22.
178. Schwartz KV, Guercio CA, Katz A. *Haemophilus influenza* pericarditis. Conn Med. 1987;51:423–4.
179. Corachan M, Poore P, Hadley GP, et al. Purulent pericarditis in Papua New Guinea: report of 12 cases and review of the literature in a tropical environment. Trans R Soc Trop Med Hyg. 1983;77:341–3.
180. Ramsdale DR, Gautam PC, Perera B, et al. Cardiac tamponade due to actinomycosis. Thorax. 1984;39:473–4.
181. Linz DH, Tolle SW, Elliot DL. *Mycoplasma pneumoniae* pneumonia. Experience at a referral center. West J Med. 1984;140:895–900.
182. Ponka A. The occurrence and clinical picture of serologically verified *Mycoplasma pneumoniae* infections with emphases on central nervous system, cardiac and joint manifestations. Ann Clin Res. 1979;24:1–60.
183. Sands MJ, Satz JE, Turner WE Jr, et al. Pericarditis and perimyocarditis associated with active *Mycoplasma pneumoniae* infection. Ann Intern Med. 1977;86:544–8.
184. Maycock R, Skale B, Kohler RB. *Legionella pneumophila* pericarditis proved by culture of pericardial fluid. Am J Med. 1983;75:534–6.
185. Reyes RR, Noble RC. Legionnaires' pericarditis. J Ky Med Assoc. 1983;81:757–8.
186. Svendsen JH, Jonsson V, Niebuhr U. Combined pericarditis and pneumonia caused by *Legionella* infection. Br Heart J 1987;58:663–4.
187. Friedland L, Snydman DR, Weingarden AS, et al. Ocular and pericardial involvement in Legionnaires' disease. Am J Med 1984;77:1105–7.
188. Larrieu AJ, Tyers GFO, Williams EH, et al. Recent experience with tuberculous pericarditis. Ann Thorac Surg. 1980;29:464–468.
189. Sagrista-Sauleda J, Permanyer-Miralda G, Soler-Soler J. Tuberculous pericarditis: ten year experience with a prospective protocol for diagnosis and treatment. J Am Coll Cardiol. 1988;11:724–8.
190. Rooney JJ, Crocco JA, Lyons HA. Tuberculous pericarditis. Ann Intern Med. 1970;72:73–8.
191. Desai HN. Tuberculous pericarditis. A review of 100 cases. S Afr Med J. 1979;55:877–80.
192. Dalli E, Quesada A, Juan G, et al. Tuberculous pericarditis as the first manifestation of acquired immunodeficiency syndrome. Am Heart J. 1987;114:905–6.
193. Ortbals DW, Avioli LV. Tuberculous pericarditis. Arch Intern Med. 1979;139:231–4.
194. Wheat LJ, Stein L, Corya BC, et al. Pericarditis as a manifestation of histoplasmosis during two large urban outbreaks. Medicine. 1983;62:110–9.
195. Young EJ, Vainrub B, Musher DM. Pericarditis due to histoplasmosis. JAMA. 1978;240:1750.
196. Larson R, Scherb RI. Coccidioidal pericarditis. Circulation. 1953;7:211–7.
197. Chapman MG, Kaplan L. Cardiac involvement in coccidioidomycosis. Am J Med. 1957;23:87–98.
198. Duvall CP, Carbone PP. *Cryptococcus neoformans* pericarditis associated with Hodgkin's diseases. Ann Intern Med. 1966;64:850–6.
199. Kraus WE, Valenstein PN, Corey GR. Purulent pericarditis caused by *Candida:* report of three cases and identification of high-risk populations as an aid to early diagnosis. Rev Infect Dis. 1988;10:34–41.
200. Eng RHK, Sen P, Browne K, et al. Candida pericarditis. Am J Med. 1981;70:867–9.
201. Kaufman LD, Seifert FC, Eilbott DJ, et al. *Candida* pericarditis and tamponade in a patient with systemic lupus erythematosus. Arch Intern Med. 1988;148:715–7.
202. Walsh TJ, Bulkley BH. *Aspergillus* pericarditis: clinical and pathologic features in the immunocompromised patient. Cancer. 1982;49:48–54.
203. Cooper JAD, Weinbaum DL, Aldrich TK, et al. Invasive aspergillosis of the lung and pericardium in a nonimmunocompromised 33 year old man. Am J Med. 1981;71:903–7.
204. Theologides A, Kennedy BJ. Editorial: Toxoplasmic myocarditis and pericarditis. Am J Med. 1969;47:169–74.
205. Sagrista-Sauleda J, Permanyer-Miralda G, Juste-Sanchez C, et al. Huge chronic pericardial effusion caused by *Toxoplasma gondii*. Circulation. 1982;66:895–7.
206. Ibarra-Perez C, Green LS, Calvello-Juarez M, et al. Diagnosis and treatment of rupture of amebic abscess of the liver into the pericardium. J Thorac Cardiovasc Surg. 1972;64:11–7.
207. Rab SW, Alam N, Hoda AN, et al. Amoebic liver abscess. Some unique presentations. Am J Med. 1967;43:811–6.
208. Baid CS, Varma AR, Lakhotia M. A case of subacute effusive constrictive pericarditis with a probable amoebic aetiology. Br Heart J. 1987;58:296–8.
209. Strang JIG. Two-dimensional echocardiography in the diagnosis of amoebic pericarditis. A case report. S Afr Med J. 1987;71:328–9.
210. Van der Horst R. Schistosomiasis of the pericardium. J R Soc Trop Med Hygiene. 1979;73:243–4.
211. Permanyer-Miralda G, Sagrista-Sauleda J, Soler-Soler J. Primary acute pericardial disease: a prospective series of 231 consecutive patients. Am J Cardiol 1985;56:623–30.
212. Roberts WC, Spray TL. Clinical and morphologic spectrum of pericardial heart disease. Curr Probl Cardiol. 1977;2:1–71.
213. Shabetai R. Function of the pericardium. In: Fowler NO, ed. The Pericardium in Health and Disease. Mount Kisco, NY: Futura; 1985:19–50.
214. Fowler NO, Harbin AD. Recurrent acute pericarditis: follow-up study of 31 patients. J Am Coll Cardiol. 1986;7:300–5.
215. Matthews JD, Cameron SJ, George M. Constrictive pericarditis following coxsackie virus infection. Thorax. 1970;25:624–6.
216. Utley JR, Mills J. Annular erosion and pericarditis. Complications of endocarditis of the aortic root. J Thorac Cardiovasc Surg. 1972;64:76–81.
217. Ribeiro P, Shapiro L, Nihoyannopoulos P, et al. Pericarditis in infective endocarditis. Eur Heart J. 1985;6:975–8.
218. Peel AAF. Tuberculous pericarditis. Br Heart J. 1948;10:195–207.
219. Carson TJ, Murray GF, Wilcox BR, et al. The role of surgery in tuberculous pericarditis. Ann Thorac Surg. 1974;17:163–7.
220. Guberman BA, Fowler NO, Engel PJ, et al. Cardiac tamponade in medical patients. Circulation. 1981;64:633–40.
221. Spodick DH. Pericardial rub: prospective multiple observer investigation of pericardial friction rub in 100 patients. Am J Cardiol. 1975;35:357–62.
222. Lorell BH, Braunwald E. Pericardial disease. In: Braunwald E, ed: A Textbook of Cardiovascular Medicine. 3rd ed. Philadelphia: WB Saunders; 1988:1484–534.
223. Spodick DH. Electrocardiogram in acute pericarditis. Distributions of morphologic and axial changes by stages. Am J Cardiol. 1974;33:470–4.
224. Spodick DH. Frequency of arrhythmias in acute pericarditis determined by holter monitoring. Am J Cardiol. 1984;53:842–5.
225. Krainin FM, Flessas AP, Spodick DH. Infarction associated pericarditis. Rarity of diagnostic electrocardiogram. N Engl J Med. 1984;311:1211–4.
226. Renfrew R, Buselmeier TJ, Kjeilstrand CM. Pericarditis and renal failure. Annu Rev Med. 1980;31:345–60.
227. Brosius FC, Waller BF, Roberts WC. Radiation heart disease. Am J Med. 1981;70:519–30.
228. Dressler W. Post-myocardial infarction syndrome. JAMA. 1956;160:1379–83.
229. Engle MA, Gay WA Jr, Zabriskie JB, et al. The post pericardiotomy syndrome: 25 years experience. J Carijovasc Med. 1984;4:321–32.
230. Silverman KJ, Hutchins GM, Bulkley BH. Cardiac sarcoid: a clinicopathologic study of 84 unselected cases with systemic sarcoidosis. Circulation. 1978;58:1204–11.
231. Ansari A, Larson PH, Bates HD. Cardiovascular manifestations of systemic lupus erythematosis: current perspective. Prog Cardiovasc Dis. 1985;27:421–34.
232. Lebowitz WB. The heart in rheumatoid arthritis (rheumatoid disease). A clinical and pathological study of sixty-two cases. Ann Intern Med. 1963;58:102–23.
233. McWhorter JE, LeRoy RC. Pericardial disease in scleroderma (systemic sclerosis). Am J Med. 1974;57:566–75.
234. Zimmerman J, Yahalom J, Bar-On H. Clinical spectrum of pericardial effusion as the presenting feature of hypothyroidism. Am Heart J. 1983;106:770–1.
235. Krikorian JG, Hancock EW. Pericardiocentesis. Am J Med. 1978;65:808–14.
236. Isner JM, Carter BL, Bankoff MS, et al. Computed tomography in the diagnosis of pericardial heart disease. Ann Intern Med. 1982;97:473–9.
237. Tomoda H, Hoshiai M, Furuya H, et al. Evaluation of pericardial effusion with computed tomography. Am Heart J. 1980;99:701–6.
238. Sechtem U, Tscholakoff D, Higgins CB. MRI of the abnormal pericardium. AJR. 1986;147:245–52.
239. Tan JS, Holmes JC, Fowler NO, et al. Antibiotic levels in pericardial fluid. J Clin Invest. 1974;53:7–12.
240. Quale JM, Lipschik GY, Heurich AE. Management of tuberculous pericarditis. Ann Thorac Surg. 1987;43:653–5.
241. Strang JIG, Kakaza HHS, Gibson DG, et al. Controlled trial of prednisolone as adjuvant in treatment of tuberculous constrictive pericarditis in Transkei. Lancet. 1987;11:1418–22.
242. Levine TM, Wurster CF, Krespi YP. Mediastinitis occurring as a complication of odontogenic infections. Laryngoscope. 1986;96:747–50.
243. Estrera AS, Landay MJ, Grisham JM, et al: Descending necrotizing mediastinitis. Surg Gynecol Obstet. 1983;157:545–52.
244. Bennett DJ, Deveridge RJ, Wright JS. Spontaneous rupture of the esophagus: a review with reports of six cases. Surgery 1970;68:766–70.
245. Sarr MG, Gott VL, Townsend TR. Mediastinal infection after cardiac surgery. Ann Thorac Surg. 1984;38:415–23.

246. Bor DH, Rose RM, Modlin JF, et al. Mediastinitis after cardiovascular surgery. Rev Infect Dis. 1983;5:885–97.
247. Ottino G, De Paulis R, Pansini S, et al. Major sternal wound infection after open-heart surgery: a multivariate analysis of risk factors in 2,579 consecutive operative procedures. Ann Thorac Surg. 1987;44:173–9.
248. Murray PM, Finegold SM. Anaerobic mediastinitis. Rev Infect Dis. 1984;6:S123–7.
249. Kauffman CA, Sheagren JN, Quie PG. *Staphylococcus epidermis* mediastinitis and disseminated intravascular coagulation. Ann Intern Med. 1984;100:60–1.
250. Breatnach E, Nath PH, Delany DJ. The role of computed tomography in acute and subacute mediastinitis. Clin Radiol. 1986;37:139–45.
251. Kay HR, Goodman LR, Teplick SK, et al. Use of computed tomography to assess mediastinal complications after median sternotomy. Ann Thorac Surg. 1983;36:706–14.
252. Schowengerdt CG, Suyemoto R, Beachley Main F. Granulomatous and fibrous mediastinitis. A review and analysis of 180 cases. J Thorac Cardiovasc Surg. 1969;57:365–79.
253. Wieder S, Rabinowitz JG. Fibrous mediastinitis: a late manifestation of mediastinal histoplasmosis. Radiology. 1977;125:305–12.
254. Hewlett TH, Steer A, Thomas DE. Progressive fibrosing mediastinitis. Ann Thorac Surg. 1966;2:345–57.
255. Gryboski WA, Crutcher RR, Holloway JB, et al. Surgical aspects of histoplasmosis. Arch Surg. 1963;87:590–9.
256. Scully RE, Galdabini JJ, McNeely BU. Case records of the Massachusetts General Hospital. Weekly clinicopathological exercises. N Engl J Med. 1976;295:381–8.

SECTION H. CENTRAL NERVOUS SYSTEM INFECTIONS

65. ANATOMIC CONSIDERATIONS IN CENTRAL NERVOUS SYSTEM INFECTIONS

JOHN E. GREENLEE

The pathogenesis and course of central nervous system infections are greatly influenced by the anatomy of the brain and spinal cord and by the relationships of brain and cord to vessels, cranial nerves, spinal nerve roots, meninges, and overlying skeletal structure.

ANATOMIC RELATIONSHIPS OF THE BRAIN AND SPINAL CORD

Relationships of Brain, Meninges, and Skull

The brain is suspended in cerebrospinal fluid (CSF) and is surrounded by three layers of meninges: the pia mater and arachnoid, which constitute the leptomeninges, and the dura mater or pachymeninges (Fig. 1).[1] The pia mater is continuous with the external surface of the brain and cord, forming a cuff of meningeal tissue around penetrating vessels and merging with the ependymal lining of the fourth ventricle at the foramina of Luschka and Magendie. The arachnoid encloses the brain more loosely, and between the pia and arachnoid, completely surrounding the brain and cord and communicating with the fourth ventricle, is the CSF-filled subarachnoid space. The outward pressure of brain and CSF holds the arachnoid in contact with the most superficial layer of meninges, the dura mater. The dura mater is adherent to the periosteum and skull except where it invaginates into the cranial cavity to form four rigid septa: the falx cerebri, falx cerebelli, tentorium cerebelli, and diaphragma selli.

Under normal conditions, the only meningeal compartment within the skull is the subarachnoid space. Infection within this space may involve the entire surface of the leptomeninges around the brain and cord and may also cross the foramina of Luschka and Magendie to produce ventriculitis.[2] During leptomeningitis, intracranial pressure may rise markedly, but this increase in pressure, even if severe, tends to be transmitted to the entire subarachnoid space around the brain and cord (Fig. 1). Unless concomitant abscess or empyema is present, or unless severe edema has developed, there is little displacement of cerebral structures and little risk of brain herniation after lumbar puncture.[2] Infection may also develop between the arachnoid and dura or between the dura and skull by dissecting along tissue planes. Because the arachnoid and dura are attached at only a few points, subdural infection will spread rapidly over the surface of one hemisphere to produce a subdural empyema. Infection outside the dura, on the other hand, will be contained by the attachment of dura to periosteum and bone to form a more localized epidural abscess. Both subdural empyema and epidural abscess behave as mass lesions, and lumbar puncture may precipitate brain herniation.[3]

Relationship of Brain and Meninges to Cranial Structures

The undersurface of the brain rests within the anterior, middle, and posterior cranial fossae. Each fossa abuts on structures from which infection may spread (Fig. 2). The anterior fossa forms the roof of the frontal and ethmoidal sinuses. Infection within either sinus may produce a frontal epidural abscess, subdural empyema over the frontal lobes or falx, or a frontal lobe brain abscess.[3–5] The sella turcica, located between the left and right middle fossae, forms the roof of the sphenoid sinuses. Infection within these sinuses can spread centrally to cause not only epidural abscess and subdural empyema but also palsies of extraocular muscles, optic neuritis, and cavernous sinus thrombophlebitis.[6]

Infections of the middle ear or mastoid within the petrous bone may extend into the middle fossa to involve the temporal lobe or may extend into the posterior fossa to involve the cerebellum or brain stem.[4,5] Rarely, infection within the maxillary sinus may cause temporal lobe abscess.

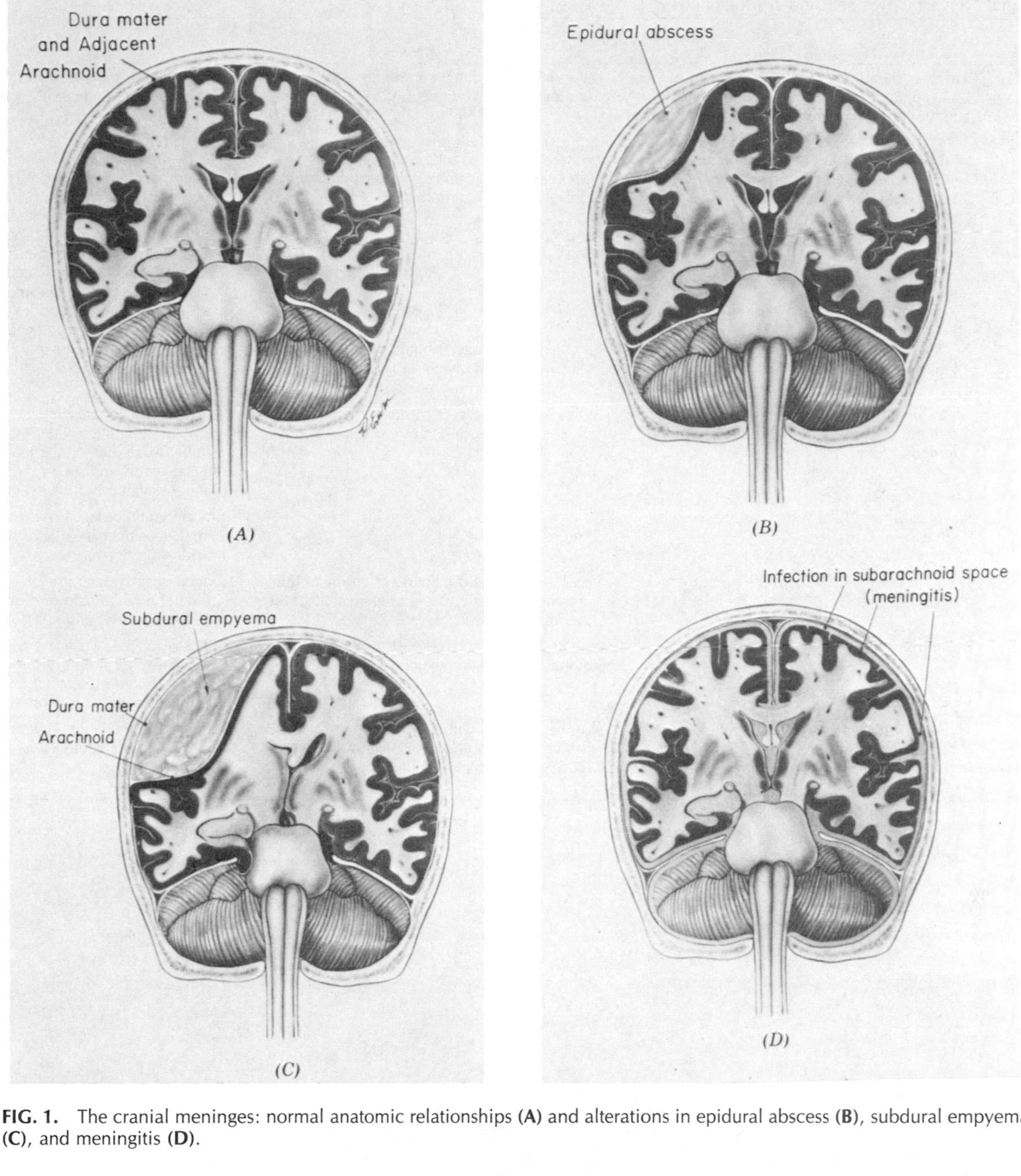

FIG. 1. The cranial meninges: normal anatomic relationships **(A)** and alterations in epidural abscess **(B)**, subdural empyema **(C)**, and meningitis **(D)**.

Injury to Cranial Nerves During Infections

All 12 cranial nerves exit through the meninges at the base of the brain and may be injured during meningitis. Cranial nerve deficits are particularly common in chronic infections of the basilar meninges such as those caused by *Mycobacterium tuberculosis*, *Cryptococcus neoformans*, or sarcoidosis.[7–9] Cranial nerves VII and VIII are most often affected, followed by cranial nerves III, IV, VI, IX, and X. Cranial nerve II may also be involved. If meningeal infection is protracted, multiple cranial nerve deficits may develop and may fluctuate during the course of the illness.[10]

Several of the cranial nerves have anatomic characteristics that predispose them to damage during infections or during states of increased intracranial pressure (see Table 1). Of particular importance is the close relationship of cranial nerve III to the tentorium: compression of the third nerve by the uncus of the temporal lobe is often the initial indication of transtentorial herniation. Cranial nerve VI has the longest intracranial course of any cranial nerve. An isolated paresis of the sixth

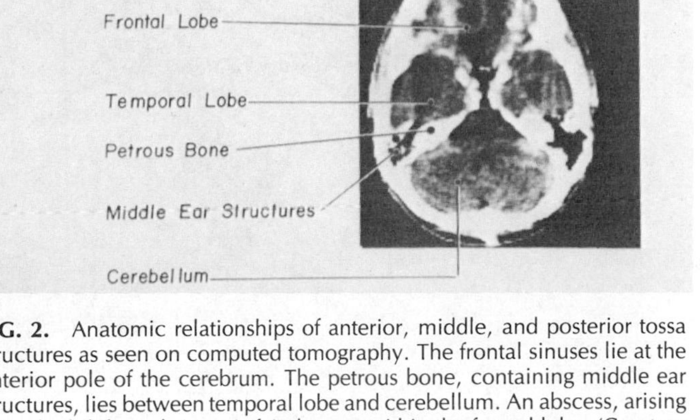

FIG. 2. Anatomic relationships of anterior, middle, and posterior tossa structures as seen on computed tomography. The frontal sinuses lie at the anterior pole of the cerebrum. The petrous bone, containing middle ear structures, lies between temporal lobe and cerebellum. An abscess, arising from the left frontal sinus, is faintly seen within the frontal lobe. (Courtesy of Dr. Frederick Vines, Jacksonville, FL.)

TABLE 1. Cranial Nerve Involvement in CNS Infections

Cranial Nerve or Nerves	*Anatomic Features*	*Significance*	*Consequence*
I	Traverses dura mater and ethmoid bone, surrounded by a cuff of arachnoid; terminates in free nerve endings within the nasal mucosa and nasopharynx.	Is the only cranial nerve in direct contact with the external environment.	May provide a route of direct CNS inoculation for neurotropic viruses.
II	1. Develops as a part of the brain and is contained within the subarachnoid space up to its point of entry into the eye.	1. Increased intracranial pressure causes papilledema. Chronic increased pressure results in optic atrophy.	1. Early signs are retinal vascular engorgement, followed by blurring of the optic disk, with hemorrhages appearing later. Initial visual change is enlargement of the physiologic blind spot. If intracranial hypertension persists, transient visual blurring and concentric constriction of visual fields occur. Chronic papilledema progresses to optic atrophy and blindness. Central scotomas may occur but are rare.
	2. Myelin sheath is composed of central myelin.	2. May be the target of immune response against central myelin in postinfectious encephalitis or encephalomyelitis.	2. Visual field deficit (usually central or centrocecal scotoma).
III	Passes directly beneath the edge of the tentorium cerebelli below the uncus of the temporal lobe.	Is almost always the first structure compressed by the uncus during transtentorial herniation.	Paresis of CN III parasympathetic fibers causes pupillary dilatation. Interruption of nerve supply to all extraocular muscles except lateral rectus and superior oblique causes lateral deviation of the eye and ptosis.
III, IV, V, VI	Travel together in the wall of the cavernous sinus.	All may be affected by cavernous sinus thrombosis.	Total ophthalmoplegia, mid-position fixed pupil, loss of corneal reflex and ipsilateral facial sensation.
V, VI	Travel in close proximity to the tip of the petrous bone.	May be injured in the course of chronic otitis media, especially where osteomyelitis of the petrous tip has developed.	Abducens palsy (lateral rectus weakness) and ipsilateral facial pain or sensory loss (Gradenigo's syndrome).
IX–XI	Exit from skull through jugular foramen.	May be injured by thrombosis of the internal jugular vein at the jugular foramen.	Ipsilateral palatal weakness and diminished gag reflex; weakness of trapezius and sternomastoid muscles on the involved side (jugular foramen syndrome).
III–XII	Myelin sheaths composed of peripheral myelin.	May be involved with peripheral nerves and spinal nerve roots in postinfectious polyneuritis (Landry-Guillain-Barré syndrome).	Deficits of any cranial nerve except I or II may occur. Cranial nerve VII is most often involved.

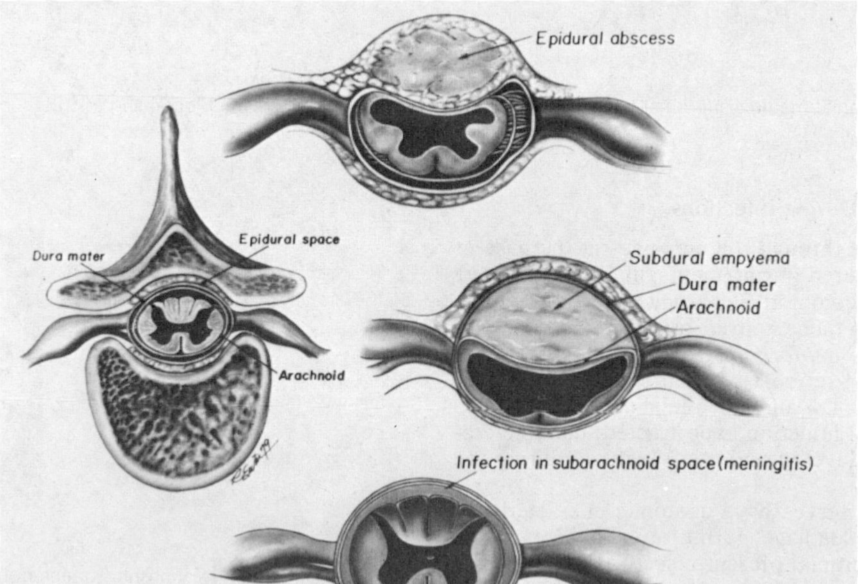

FIG. 3. The spinal meninges and epidural space: normal anatomic relationships and alterations in epidural abscess, subdural empyema, and meningitis.

nerve may indicate either direct involvement of the nerve anywhere along its length or compression due to elevated intracranial pressure.

Anatomic Relationships of the Spinal Cord

The spinal cord extends from the foramen magnum to the level of the L1-L2 intervertebral disk.[11] Below L2 the spinal canal contains the nerve roots, which form the cauda equina. Unlike the cerebral hemispheres, where gray matter is most external, the spinal cord has a central core of gray matter and an external layer of white matter containing ascending and descending nerve tracts. Lesions developing within the cord (intramedullary lesions) often produce neuronal injury at one or more spinal cord segments early in their course and only later expand laterally to involve motor and sensory nerve tracts. Lesions external to the cord, on the other hand, (extramedullary lesions) produce symptoms of nerve root irritation early in their course, followed by long tract signs; injury to central gray matter occurs only later.

The relationships of pia mater, arachnoid, and dura are essentially the same for the spinal cord as for the brain (Fig. 3), and the interface between spinal arachnoid and dura, like its intracranial counterpart, provides a plane along which infection can easily dissect. In contrast to the close adherence of the dura mater to the cranial periosteum and skull, however, the spinal dura and periosteum diverge at the foramen magnum, and by the level of the seventh cervical vertebra are separated by a fat-filled epidural space that offers little resistance to the longitudinal spread of infection. Both spinal subdural empyema and spinal epidural abscess may thus extend over many vertebral segments. Both are usually posterior to the cord and may be inadvertently entered during lumbar puncture (see Fig. 3).

ROLE OF THE INTRACRANIAL CIRCULATION IN CENTRAL NERVOUS SYSTEM INFECTIONS

Vascular Anatomy

Arteries. The brain is supplied by two internal carotid arteries and two vertebral arteries that join to form the basilar artery (Fig. 4).[12–14] Each internal carotid supplies the retina via the ophthalmic artery and bifurcates into an anterior cerebral artery that supplies the medial surface of the cerebrum and a middle cerebral artery that supplies the frontal, parietal, and temporal lobes over the cerebral convexity. The vertebrobasilar system supplies the rostral spinal cord, the brain stem, and the cerebellum before terminating in two posterior cerebral arteries. These angle sharply backward over the tentorium cerebelli to supply the occipital lobes, the posterior parietal lobes, and the posterior and mesial portions of temporal lobes. Because the ophthalmic artery is a branch of the internal carotid, emboli within the anterior circulation may produce monocular visual loss or retinal lesions visible by ophthalmoscopy and may give indirect evidence of an embolic source of central nervous system infection.

The major intracranial arteries differ in both caliber and volume of flow. The middle cerebral arteries receive the greatest volume of blood, followed by the anterior cerebrals and vertebrobasilar system. The likelihood of septic embolization, with resultant brain abscess or mycotic aneurysm, is thus greatest in the branches of the middle cerebral and least in the smaller branches of the posterior circulation.[15] The choroid plexuses also receive a large volume of blood.[16]

The major arteries of the brain are connected at the circle of Willis by anterior and posterior communicating branches and are also connected by smaller anastomotic vessels at the meningeal surface. The intracranial circulation communicates with the external carotid system through anastomoses between the

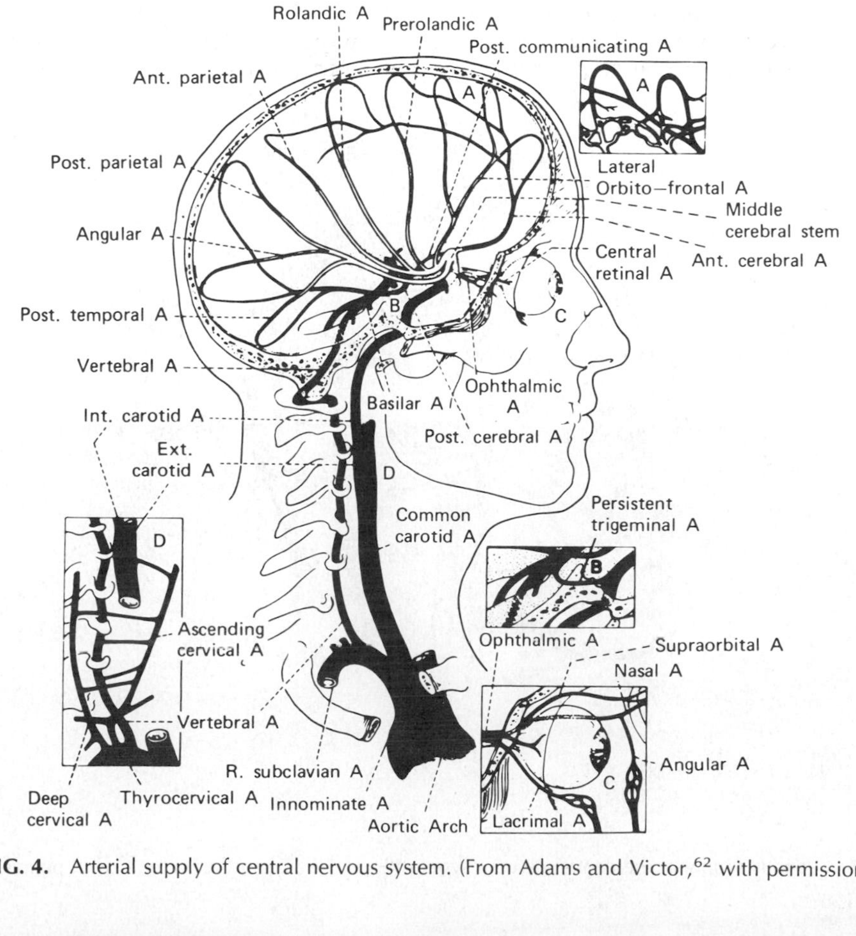

FIG. 4. Arterial supply of central nervous system. (From Adams and Victor,[62] with permission.)

ophthalmic and maxillary arteries and between branches of the vertebrals and the occipital arteries. There is also extensive communication with the meningeal branches of the external carotid via the rete mirabile, a network of small vessels that cross the meninges and anastomose with arteries on the surface of the brain.[12–14] Despite this collateral circulation, however, certain parts of the brain are arterial border zones or "watershed areas," receiving their arterial supply from terminal branches of two or more vessels. The most important of these watershed areas lies between middle and posterior cerebral arteries at the junction of parietal, occipital, and temporal lobes. Similar watershed areas exist on the medial surface of the hemispheres, within the internal capsule, and over the cerebellum. These areas, particularly in the elderly patient with extensive vascular disease, are particularly vulnerable to ischemic injury if any of their supplying vessels becomes compromised. The signs and symptoms produced by watershed infarcts often extend beyond the usual distribution of the vessel involved. Cerebral white matter also forms a watershed area, receiving terminal arterial flow from both penetrating cortical and ventricular vessels. For this reason, white matter is more easily rendered ischemic than is gray matter, and abscesses arising within devitalized brain are most common in white matter or at the gray-white junction.[17]

Veins. The intracranial venous system is composed of three groups of vessels: superficial veins that drain the external portions of cerebrum and brain stem; deep veins that drain central white matter, basal ganglia, and thalamus; and venous sinuses within the dura mater (Fig. 5).[14] The superficial veins of the cerebrum are divided about a watershed area above the Sylvian fissure into veins that empty upward into the superior sagittal sinus and veins emptying downward into the basilar venous sinuses.[18] The superficial and deep cerebral veins are extensively interconnected, and anastomoses exist as well among the venous sinuses. There is also communication of superficial veins and venous sinuses with the extracranial venous system via numerous emissary veins that cross the skull and meninges. Neither intracranial veins nor venous sinuses have valves, so the direction of venous flow may reverse in response to hemodynamic changes. Because of these extensive anastomoses, cortical vein thrombosis or even occlusion of a venous sinus may at times be silent or may produce only transient neurologic abnormalities. If infarction results, clinical findings often evolve slowly and in fluctuating fashion as the thrombotic process involves increasing numbers of venous collaterals. Venous infarcts are frequently hemorrhagic, with irregular borders that are determined by remaining collateral venous drainage.[19] Thrombosis of the posterior portion of the superior sagittal sinus may produce cortical venous thrombosis of both hemispheres, causing bilateral lower extremity weakness. Cortical blindness may be present if both occipital lobes are involved. Because the hand area on the cerebral convexity has two routes of venous drainage, neurologic deficits referable to this area in venous thrombosis frequently resolve.

The cerebral venous sinuses not only drain venous blood but also reabsorb CSF through arachnoid villi, most of which are located along the anterior third of the superior sagittal sinus. Thrombosis of the superior sagittal sinus may block CSF reabsorption and produce communicating hydrocephalus, at times without other symptoms. Impairment of CSF reabsorption may also occur if venous outflow from the superior sagittal sinus is blocked by occlusion of both lateral sinuses or of one lateral sinus where the other is hypoplastic.[14,19]

Capillaries. The capillaries of the brain and cord, except for those of the pituitary, the choroid plexuses, and several circumventricular structures within the brain stem, differ from capillaries elsewhere in the body in that they do not have fenestrations or intercellular clefts.[20] Molecules thus cross cerebral capillaries less by diffusion than on the basis of lipid solubility or by active transport. This relative impermeability of brain capillaries is the basis of the barrier systems that sequester brain and CSF from the extracranial environment and is a major factor in the selection of antibiotics for intracranial infections (see below).

Vascular Supply of the Spinal Cord

The posterior columns and horns of the spinal cord are supplied by an irregular posterior arterial plexus that is virtually never

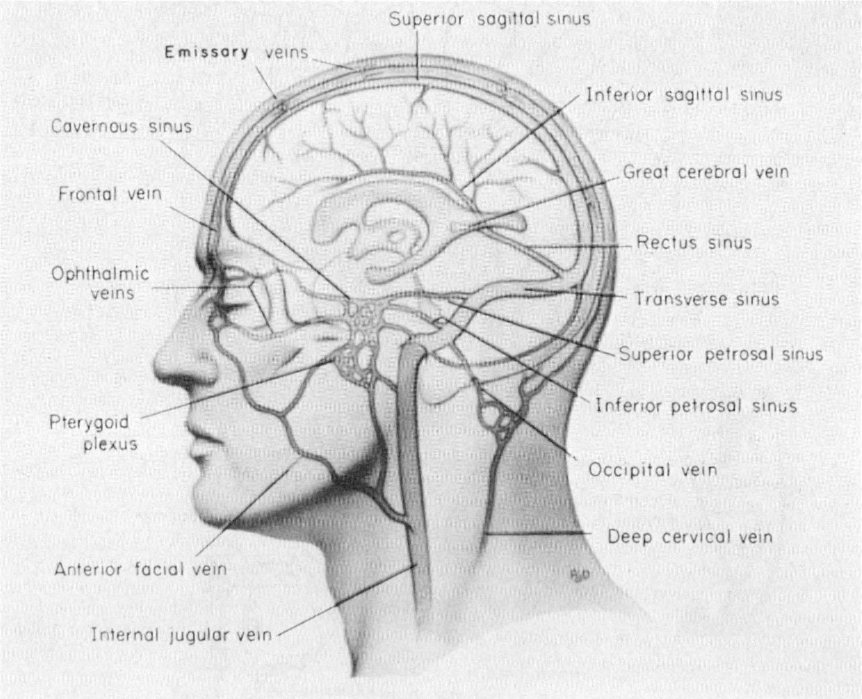

FIG. 5. Venous supply of the central nervous system. (From Truax and Carpenter,[59] with permission.)

involved in infections. The remainder of the cord is supplied by the anterior spinal artery system, which arises from the vertebrals and receives contributory branches from cervical and intercostal arteries and from the descending aorta.[21] In many but not all patients there is a predominant tributary vessel from the aorta, the artery of Adamkiewicz, which joins the anterior spinal artery between cord segments T8 and L4. The thoracic cord above the artery of Adamkiewicz, particularly in the region around T4, may act as a watershed area much like those within the brain and may suffer ischemic injury during systemic hypotension or if vessels above or below it are occluded. The veins of the spinal cord are roughly similar in distribution to the spinal arteries.

Role of Central Nervous System Vessels in Infections

The vessels of the central nervous system provide the most frequent route by which infection reaches the meninges, brain, or cord (see below). In addition, involvement of the vessels themselves may produce ischemic or hemorrhagic injury to the brain or cord, with or without accompanying suppuration. Arteries may be occluded by septic emboli. If the embolus breaks up before irreversible ischemia has occurred, it may produce symptoms of a transient ischemic attack; more protracted ischemia results in infarction. Arterial thrombosis may occur if the vessel wall becomes involved by meningeal inflammation, as in tuberculous meningitis.[7] Multiplication of organisms within vascular endothelial cells, as in Rocky Mountain spotted fever, may cause thrombosis of small vessels.[22] Vasculitis and thrombosis of vessels may also occur as a complication of hepatitis B antigenemia[23,24] and is responsible for the syndrome of ipsilateral cerebral infarction occasionally seen during ophthalmic herpes zoster infections.[25] Similar but more chronic virus-induced vasculitis may be the major pathogenetic mechanism in progressive rubella encephalitis.[26] Occasionally, in bacterial endocarditis or other states of prolonged bacteremia, hyperplasia of vascular endothelial cells or obliterative endarteritis may occur and may occlude the vessel lumen.[27–29] In addition to causing vascular occlusion, arteritis may produce necrosis of the vessel wall and/or formation of a mycotic aneurysm. Rupture of the affected vessel with intracranial hemorrhage may occur during or even after successful therapy for the infection.[15] Spontaneous resolution of mycotic aneurysms may occur,[30] but the likelihood of rupture or spontaneous resolution cannot be predicted in a given case.

The veins of the central nervous system may also thrombose in response to internal or extramural inflammation and may provide a source of sterile or septic emboli to other parts of the nervous system or to the lungs. The infarcted tissue produced by either arterial or venous occlusion may become the site of single or multiple abscesses.

Injury to central nervous capillaries may allow escape of organisms into ischemic brain and may produce transudation of fluid from the vascular compartment and cerebral edema (see below). Loss of integrity of the blood-brain barrier also permits radioisotopes or radiological contrast media to leak into involved brain, allowing localization of lesions by radionuclide, computed tomography (CT), or magnetic resonance (MR) scans (Figs. 2 and 6). Antibiotics normally unable to cross cerebral or meningeal capillaries penetrate the brain or CSF across such injured vessels. As inflammation subsides, capillary integrity is restored, edema resolves, and CSF antibiotic concentrations fall, even if no alteration is made in antibiotic dose or route of administration.

Spinal vessels are rarely involved by infection. Spinal artery occlusion may occur during bacterial endocarditis, Rocky Mountain spotted fever, or tertiary syphilis. Spinal veins may be involved by epidural abscess or subdural empyema and may produce cord injury more extensive than would be expected on the basis of compression alone.

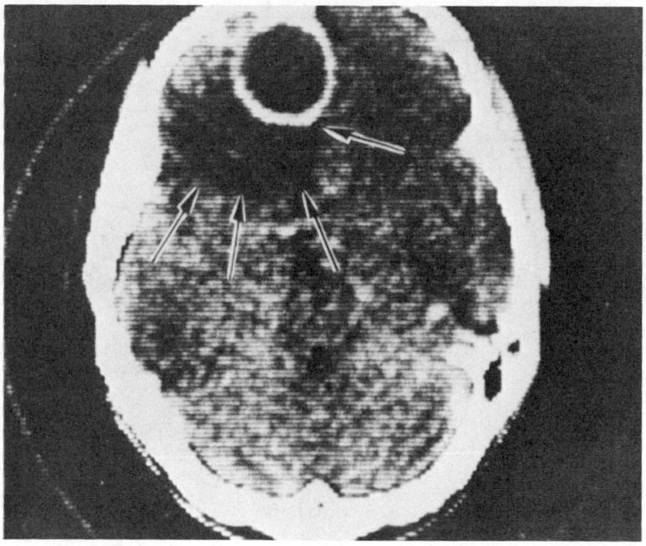

FIG. 6. Brain abscess as seen on computed tomography. The arrows outline an area of cerebral edema equal in size to the abscess itself. This is a more rostral view of the abscess faintly seen in Figure 2. (Courtesy of Dr. Frederick Vines, Jacksonville, FL.)

CEREBROSPINAL FLUID CIRCULATION IN NERVOUS SYSTEM INFECTIONS

Eighty-five percent of the CSF is produced within the lateral, third, and fourth ventricles by the choroid plexuses (see Fig. 7), the remainder forming by diffusion across the meninges.[31] The choroid plexuses resemble renal tubules histologically and produce CSF by secretion rather than passive diffusion. Like renal tubules, the choroid plexuses also contain probenecid-sensitive and other transport mechanisms and are capable of removing weak organic acids including penicillin and gentamicin from the CSF against a concentration gradient.[31] The direction of the CSF circulation is outward through the foramina of Luschka and Magendie into the subarachnoid space, where it circulates around the brain and cord by bulk flow. Reabsorption of CSF occurs by vesicular transport through cells of the arachnoid villi along the superior sagittal sinus. A small amount of CSF may be absorbed directly across the meninges. Complete exchange of CSF occurs every 3 to 4 hours.

The CSF circulation is important in the diagnosis, treatment, and complications of central nervous system infections. Chemical and cellular changes in CSF may provide accurate information about infections within the subarachnoid space and, in extensive leptomeningeal infections, may contain the infectious agent in large numbers.[32] However, lumbar CSF may not always give precise information in chronic basilar or other localized meningeal infections and, unless very large volumes of lumbar CSF are studied,[33,34] may not allow recovery of the infectious agent or contain diagnostic antigens at a time when the causative agent may be isolated by high cervical or cisternal puncture.[34,35] In subdural or epidural infection or in brain abscess, where infection occurs outside the subarachnoid space, the CSF may be normal or may reveal only a mild, nonspecific lymphocytosis, with a slight elevation of the protein concentration and a normal sugar level; organisms are only rarely present.[4,36]

The physiology of the CSF circulation is important in the treatment of ventriculitis with aminoglycosides or other antibiotics that penetrate into CSF poorly. Although it is possible, under experimental conditions, to produce high ventricular levels of agents by the instillation of large volumes,[37] intrathecal administration of antibiotics in conventional volumes produces

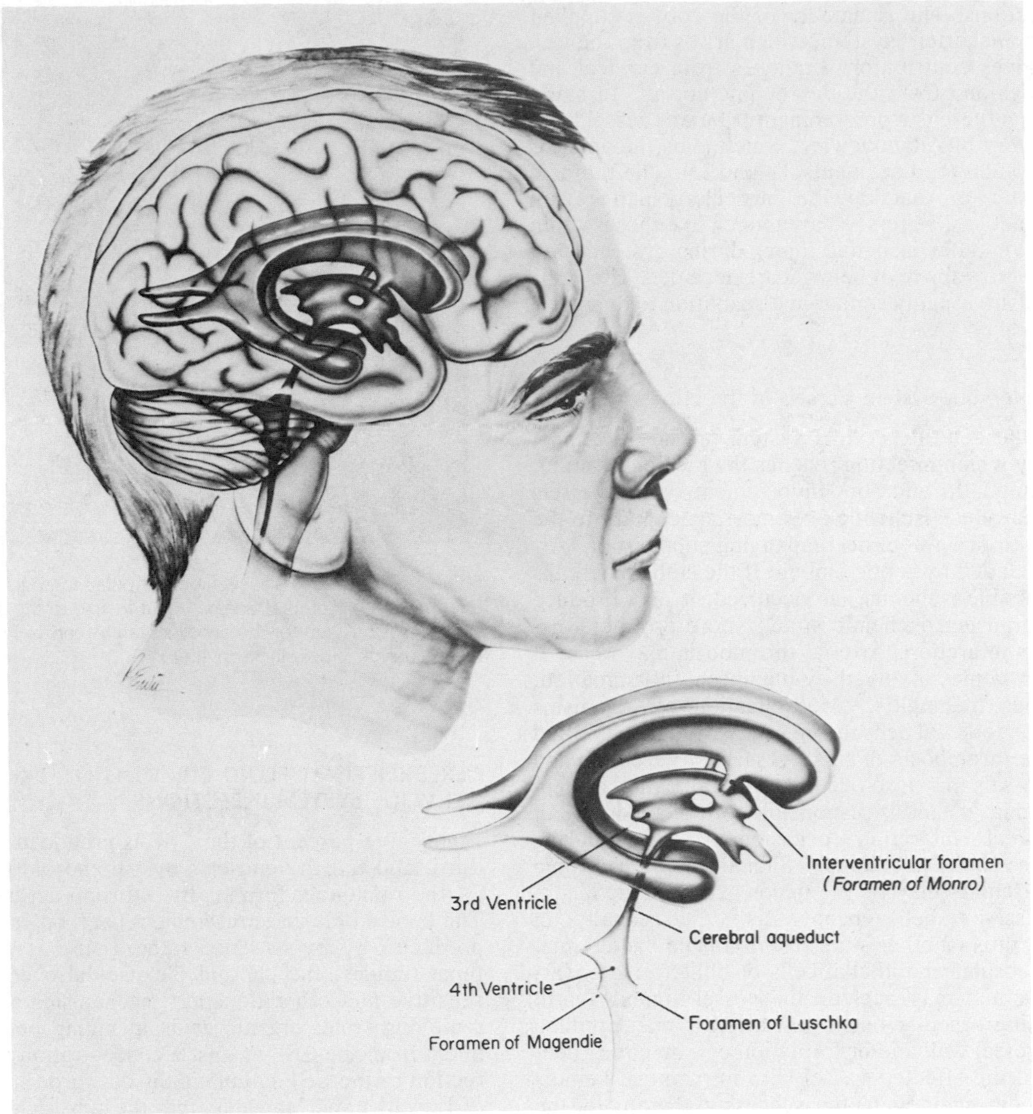

FIG. 7. The cerebral ventricles. The ventricular system is narrowest and hence most easily obstructed at the foramen of Monro, the cerebral aqueduct (aqueduct of Sylvius), and the foramina of Luschka and Magendie.

unreliable ventricular concentrations, and lumbar administration does not allow measurement of the ventricular concentrations achieved.[38] Because of these factors, therapy for ventriculitis with agents that must be instilled directly into the CSF requires direct administration into the ventricles through a subcutaneous reservoir.[38–40]

Infections involving the nervous system may produce communicating or obstructive hydrocephalus. Communicating hydrocephalus follows impairment of CSF reabsorption across the arachnoid villi and may be due to blood within the subarachnoid space, chronic meningitis, or occlusion of the superior sagittal or lateral sinuses. In communicating hydrocephalus, although ventricular dilatation occurs, the increase in pressure is distributed equally throughout the subarachnoid space and ventricular system. Obstructive hydrocephalus develops when there is compromise of CSF circulation within the ventricles and most often represents occlusion of the ventricular system at its narrowest points: the foramina of Luschka and Magendie, the aqueduct of Sylvius, or, rarely, the foramina of Monro. Occlusion may be due to inflammation within the ventricular system or subarachnoid space or to external compression by abscess, mass, or hemorrhage. In obstructive hydrocephalus, ventricular dilatation occurs rostral to the point of obstruction, and the trapped CSF behaves as a mass lesion. Brain herniation may occur and may be precipitated by lumbar puncture. Although lumbar puncture may theoretically be safely used to lower intracranial pressure in communicating hydrocephalus, both communicating and obstructive components are frequently present in central nervous system infections. For this reason, lumbar puncture in the face of papilledema, suspected space-occupying lesion, or increase in ventricular size must be approached with great caution.[41]

ROUTES OF CENTRAL NERVOUS SYSTEM INVOLVEMENT BY INFECTIOUS AGENTS

Most infectious agents reach the central nervous system by hematogenous spread from extracranial foci or by retrograde propagation of infected thrombi within emissary veins. Possible sites for invasion of the CNS by blood-borne bacteria or viruses include vessels within the choroid plexuses, meninges, and brain parenchyma.[26,42,43] Tuberculous meningitis develops by seeding of the cerebrospinal fluid space from subependymal or submeningeal granulomas.[44] Intracranial epidural or subdural infection is usually of venous origin but may occasionally follow spread of organisms through bone. Spinal subdural and epidural infections more often follow bacteremia with or without accompanying osteomyelitis. Brain abscess may be of arterial or venous origin.

The central nervous system itself has no lymphatic system, but lymphatics are present within the spinal epidural space and form a route by which infections of the retropharyngeal, posterior mediastinal, or retroperitoneal spaces may produce spinal epidural abscess. Under experimental conditions, organisms can be shown to enter the subarachnoid space from lymphatics within peripheral nerves, but the spread of infection by this route has never been documented clinically.[26]

Because viruses have been shown experimentally to replicate in Schwann cells surrounding nerves or to ascend within nerves at a rate equal to reverse axoplasmic flow, infection of the nervous system by neurotropic spread of viruses has received a great deal of attention. In clinical situations, however, neurotropism has been shown to be important only for herpes simplex and zoster, which produce latent infection of sensory ganglia, and rabies, which may bind to or near acetylcholine receptors at the neuromuscular junction[45] and reaches the central nervous system by spread within axons. Rare cases of rabies have been reported after exposure to infected aerosols.[26,46] In these instances, the virus is believed to have penetrated free olfactory nerve endings within the nasal cavity, with rapid entry into the central nervous system[26] (see Table 1). Infection of the nervous system via cranial nerve I has also been postulated in herpes simplex encephalitis, because of the frequent involvement of olfactory brain, but has never been proven.

RESPONSE OF THE CENTRAL NERVOUS SYSTEM TO INFECTION

The central nervous system is unlike other organs in its unique cellular composition, its sequestration from the rest of the body by physiologic barriers, and its close confinement within rigid skeletal structures. These properties greatly influence the course of infection.[17] Widespread infection of the brain, involving all tissue elements, is characteristic of many viral encephalitides and of the diffuse cortical inflammation that accompanies bacterial meningitis. The functional specialization of different cell populations and of specific neuroanatomic regions, however, enables infections that involve specific cell types or anatomic areas to produce characteristic neurologic syndromes. Cellular specificity is seen in poliomyelitis, in which infection of motor neurons within spinal cord and medulla produces flaccid paralysis; in rabies, which is almost exclusively an infection of neurons; and in progressive multifocal leukoencephalopathy, in which destruction of oligodendrocytes results in multifocal, scattered areas of demyelination. Predilection for particular anatomic areas is seen in herpes simplex encephalitis, in which involvement of the temporal lobes may produce psychosis, impairment of recent memory, and uncinate seizures. Focal infection may also be seen in the localized encephalitis that precedes brain abscess, in brain abscess itself, or in granulomatous infections of tuberculous, fungal, or other origins. Certain viral agents, such as rabies virus, produce severe neurologic dysfunction in the absence of extensive necrosis or other pathologic changes. The ability of rabies virus to bind to the acetylcholine receptor has been discussed above. Work by Tsiang has shown that acetylcholine binding in brain is progressively impaired during experimental rabies.[47] These observations suggest that rabies virus may produce its clinical effects by interfering with neurotransmitter function. Central nervous system infection by human immune deficiency virus (HIV) in human acquired immunodeficiency syndrome (AIDS) has been associated with a progressive encephalopathy (AIDS-related dementia), a vacuolar myelopathy, and a subacute meningitis. HIV genomic material within brains has been identified predominantly in macrophages. It is not yet known whether neurologic injury by HIV is the result of viral replication per se or is due to virus-induced perturbations of neuronal metabolic activities or neurotransmitter function.[48,49]

Organisms producing acute infection, such as most bacteria, elicit a polymorphonuclear inflammatory response. Subacute or chronic infections such as those caused by *M. tuberculosis*, fungi, or viruses result in a predominantly lymphocytic infiltrate, although large numbers of polymorphonuclear cells may be present if tissue destruction is extensive. Subacute and chronic inflammatory infiltrates often contain plasma cells, and antibody production may occur at the site of infection. The inflammatory response within the brain or spinal cord differs from that in other organs in that it may be less intense and includes infiltration by microglial cells and proliferation of astrocytes. Although abscesses within the brain develop in much the same way that they do in other organs, encapsulation of brain abscesses occurs for the most part not by fibrosis but by the slower, less complete process of gliosis. When the brain has suffered previous ischemic injury, the inflammatory response may be minimal, and reactive gliosis may fail to occur.

Recovery from central nervous system infection involves antibody, cell-mediated immunity, and complement. Antibody is normally excluded from the central nervous system. The presence of antibody in brain or spinal fluid thus indicates diffusion of immunoglobulin molecules across an injured blood-brain barrier or local synthesis of antibody by immunocompetent cells that have gained entry into brain parenchyma.[50] Antibody produced within the central nervous system is oligoclonal, suggesting that the plasma cells responsible for local antibody synthesis are derived from a limited number of B cells.[26] Systemic humoral immunity plays a major protective role against bacterial infections of the central nervous system and may play a role in determining survival in bacterial meningitis.[51] Demonstration of a rise in antibody titers between acute and convalescent sera is an important retrospective means of identifying infections caused by viruses or other agents that are poorly recovered by culture techniques. Determination of CSF antibody titers to specific agents is of more limited value. Because the blood-CSF barrier is poorly permeable to immunoglobulins, the serum:CSF antibody ratio is normally above 200.[52] Injury to the blood-brain barrier can lower this ratio nonspecifically, and intrathecal synthesis of antibody directed against a particular infectious agent may selectively alter the ratio for that agent. Detection of CSF antibody or proof of intrathecal antibody synthesis has proved useful in the diagnosis of chronic or slow infections such as Lyme disease, subacute sclerosing panencephalitis, or progressive rubella encephalitis.[26,53] Investigation of CSF antibody titers has also been employed in epidemiologic studies of central nervous system involvement by HIV.[54] Penetration of antibody across the blood-brain barrier and intrathecal antibody synthesis develop over time, however, and are not reliable initial diagnostic tests in acute infections such as herpes simplex virus encephalitis.[55,56] Cell-mediated immunity comprises the major defense of the central nervous system against infections due to fungi or to intracellular parasites such as viruses, *M. tuberculosis, Listeria monocytogenes*, and *Toxoplasma gondii*. Where cell-mediated immunity is impaired, these organisms are particularly likely to involve the central nervous system and may cause fatal disease despite extremely high titers of specific antibody. Humoral and cell-mediated immune responses are closely related, and severe compromise of T-cell-mediated immune response, as in AIDS, may be accompanied by blunting of humoral immune response.[57] Complement has a number of functions, including the ability to lyse infectious agents or cells expressing viral or other foreign antigens on their surfaces. Complement may thus serve as an important mechanism of host defense against infection, but, in experimental circumstances at least, the action of complement on infected cells may be a major cause of neurologic injury.[58]

In certain infections due to virus or *Mycoplasma* or after immunization, the host may develop an immune response not only against the causative agent but also against the basic protein of peripheral or central myelin. Reaction against peripheral myelin produces segmental demyelination and at times axonal loss within nerve roots and peripheral nerves, causing an ascending motor paralysis (Landry-Guillain-Barre syndrome). Reaction to central myelin results in a monophasic illness characterized by perivascular inflammation and multifocal demyelination of brain, spinal cord, and optic nerve.[26] In severe cases, necrosis and/or hemorrhage of white matter may occur.

The Role of Edema and Brain Herniation in Central Nervous System Infections

Infection and inflammation produce not only local injury to nervous system parenchyma but also loss of capillary integrity with transudation of intravascular fluid into brain or cord.[60] The resultant edema is an almost invariable part of infection of the central nervous system, occurring not only around brain abscess (Fig. 6) but also in viral encephalitis, as a part of the diffuse cortical encephalitis that accompanies bacterial meningitis and as a complication of both infarction and hemorrhage. In meningitis, encephalitis, or ischemia, additional brain swelling may result from entry of extracellular water into injured cells. Interstitial edema of periventricular structures may develop in hydrocephalus. Although a small amount of edema may be asymptomatic, larger amounts frequently act as a space-occupying lesion.

Inflammation, hemorrhage, hydrocephalus, and edema may all produce displacement of brain or cord. In infections of the nervous system any or all of these conditions may be present simultaneously. Although the nervous system is able to deform greatly beneath gradual compression, both brain and spinal cord are poorly compliant beneath rapidly expanding lesions and, within the rigid confines of the skull or spinal column, have little room in which to be displaced before significant compression occurs. Displacement of one cerebral hemisphere will force brain tissue beneath the falx cerebri and over the tentorium cerebelli (Fig. 8).[61] Herniation beneath the falx is usually asymptomatic. Herniation of the temporal lobe over the tentorium, however, initially produces paresis of cranial nerve III and may cause corticospinal tract signs ipsilateral to the lesion as the contralateral cerebral peduncle is compressed against the tentorium (Fig. 8). Coma follows, and there is progressive loss of brain stem reflexes culminating in respiratory arrest as the medullary respiratory centers are affected. The characteristic neurologic syndromes that result at successively lower levels of brain stem function are described in detail in the monograph by Plum and Posner[61] and an understanding of these syndromes is crucial to the management of the patient with central nervous system infection. It should be kept in mind, however, that posterior fossa mass lesions such as a cerebellar abscess or hemorrhage may produce rapid compression of the medulla and pons without antecedent midbrain signs. Compressive lesions may also occur within the spinal column. Because of the narrow diameter of the spinal canal, even a small intrinsic or extrinsic lesion may rapidly progress to cord necrosis and effective cord transection.

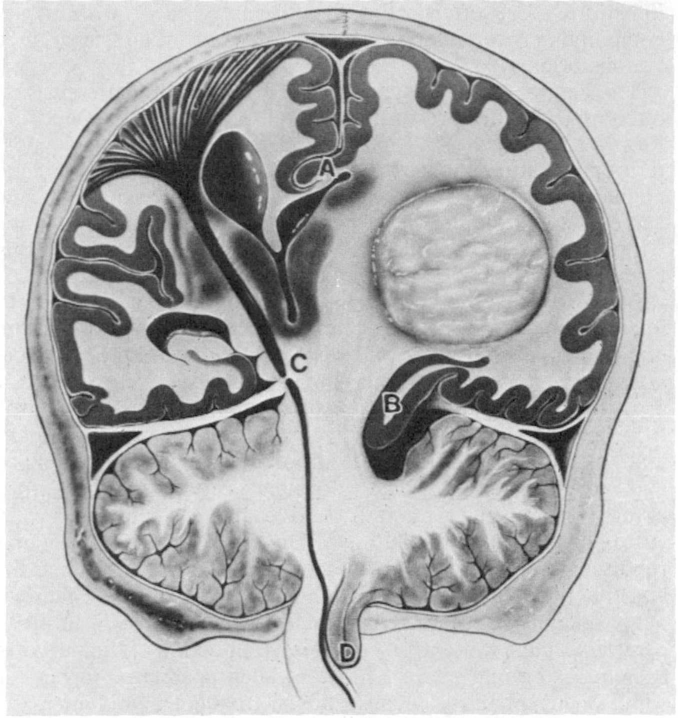

FIG. 8. Consequences of brain displacement by a mass lesion: herniation of cingulate gyrus beneath the falx cerebri (*A*); herniation of the uncus of the temporal lobe over the tentorium cerebelli (*B*), with compression of the contralateral corticospinal tract against the tentorium (*C*) and development of false localizing signs; herniation of the cerebellar tonsils through the foramen magnum (*D*).

The treatment of mass lesions within the skull or spinal canal requires prompt therapy in addition to antibiotics and is of particular urgency in patients with lesions of the posterior fossa or spinal canal because of the rapidity with which brain stem or cord compression may develop. Treatment of cerebral edema should be begun as soon as suspected (see Table 2).[60] Osmotic agents are effective in all types of edema but are most useful acutely since their continued administration may cause a rebound in intracranial pressure. Dexamethasone is effective in brain abscess[60] but is of less certain value in meningitis, encephalitis, or ischemia. The benefits of corticosteroids in edema due to infection must always be weighed against their possible

TABLE 2. Short-Term Therapy for Cerebral Edema[a]

Therapy	*Mechanism of Action*	*Dosage or Therapeutic End-Point*	*Remarks*
Hyperventilation	Decreases intracranial vascular volume	PCO_2 should be lowered to 25–30 torr	Produces almost immediate fall in intracranial pressure (ICP) but requires intubation and mechanical ventilation unless the patient is spontaneously hyperventilating.
Mannitol	Hyperosmolar effect	Give as a 20% solution IV 1–1.5 g/kg over 10 min and a total of 2.5–3 g/kg over 1–1.5 hours	Produces rapid fall in ICP. Rebound of ICP may occur due to diffusion of mannitol into brain tissue but may be minimized by fluid restriction or diuretic therapy with furosemide or ethacrynic acid. Patient should undergo urinary catheterization at initiation of therapy. Mannitol produces transient intravascular hypervolemia and may precipitate congestive heart failure. Protracted use of mannitol necessitates measurement of intake and output, serum electrolytes, and serum osmolality.
Corticosteroids	Mechanism uncertain	Dexamethasone, 10 mg IV followed by 4 mg IV at 6-hour intervals	Produces fall in intracranial pressure over several hours, without rebound. Most effective in edema associated with brain abscess. Efficacy in meningitis or ischemic infarction is less well established.

[a] Medical therapy of increased intracranial pressure is never a substitute for evacuation of loculated infection or relief of hydrocephalus. Intracranial pressure monitoring may be essential in assessing efficacy of treatment. Other less proven measures have been employed when the therapeutic measures listed above have been unsuccessful.[60]

deleterious effects on host immune response. At no time is medical treatment of cerebral edema a substitute for evacuation of a surgically approachable abscess, empyema, or hemorrhage, nor does it obviate the need for shunting in the presence of hydrocephalus. Appropriate neuroradiologic studies should be begun as soon as a mass lesion is suspected, and plans should be made for immediate surgery if indicated.

ACKNOWLEDGMENTS

Work on this chapter was supported in part by the Veterans Administration.

REFERENCES

1. Bargmann W, Oksche A, Fix JD, et al. Meninges, choroid plexuses, ependyma, and their reactions. In: Haymaker W, Adams RD, eds. Histology and Histopathology of the Nervous System. Springfield, IL: Charles C Thomas; 1982:560–714.
2. Schwartz MN, Dodge PR. Bacterial meningitis—a review of selected aspects. N Engl J Med. 1965;272:725.
3. Kaufman DM, Litman N, Miller MH. Sinusitis: induced empyema. Neurology. 1983;33:123.
4. Kaplan RJ. Neurological complications of infections of the head and neck. Otol Clin N Am. 1976;9:729.
5. Beckhuis GJ, Taylor M. Ear and sinus aspects of intracranial suppurative disease. In: Gurdjian ES, ed. Cranial and Intracranial Suppuration. Springfield, IL: Charles C Thomas; 1969:42–58.
6. Dale BAB, Mackenzie J. The complications of sphenoid sinusitis. J Laryngol Otol. 1983;97:661–70.
7. Tandon PN. Tuberculous meningitis. In: Vinken PJ, Bruyn GW, Klawans HL, eds. Handbook of Clinical Neurology. Part 1. Amsterdam: North Holland; 1978:195–262.
8. Lewis JL, Rabinovich S. The wide spectrum of cryptococcal infections. Am J Med. 1972;53:315.
9. Delaney P. Neurologic manifestations in sarcoidosis. Review of the literature with a report of 23 cases. Ann Intern Med. 1977;87:336.
10. Symonds C. Recurrent multiple cranial nerve palsies. J Neurol Neurosurg Psychiatr. 1959;21:95.
11. DeMyer W. Anatomy and clinical neurology of the spinal cord. In: Baker AB, Joynt RJ, eds. Clinical Neurology. v. 3. Philadelphia: Harper & Row; 1987:1–24.
12. Toole JF. Applied anatomy of the brain arteries. In: Toole JF, ed. Cerebrovascular Disorders. 3rd ed. New York: McGraw-Hill; 1984:1–18.
13. Dudley AW. Cerebrospinal blood vessels normal and diseases. In: Haymaker W, Adams RD, eds. Histology and Histopathology of the Nervous System. Springfield, IL: Charles C Thomas; 1982:714–97.
14. Stehbens WE. Pathology of the cerebral blood vessels. In: Anatomy of the Blood Vessels of the Brain and Spinal Cord. St Louis: CV Mosby; 1972:1–59.
15. Roach MR, Drake CG. Ruptured cerebral aneurysms caused by microorganisms. N Engl J Med. 1956;273:240.
16. Csaky TZ. Choroid plexus. In Lajtha A, ed. Handbook of Neurochemistry. v. 2. London: Plenum; 1969:49–69.
17. Slager UT. Infections and parainfectious inflammations. In: Basic Neuropathology. Baltimore: Williams & Wilkins; 1970:89–135.
18. Merwarth HR. The syndrome of the rolandic vein. Am J Surg. 1942;56:526.
19. Toole JF. Anatomy and diseases of the venous system. In: Cerebrovascular Disorders. 3rd ed. New York: McGraw-Hill; 1984:391–404.
20. Oldendorf WH. Permeability of the blood-brain barrier. In: Tower DB, ed. The Nervous System. v. 1. New York: Raven Press; 1975:279–89.
21. Moossy J. Vascular diseases of the spinal cord. In: Baker AB, Joynt RJ, eds. Clinical Neurology. v. 3. Philadelphia: Harper & Row; 1987:1–19.
22. Miller JQ, Price TR. The nervous system in Rocky Mountain spotted fever. Neurology. 1972;22:561.
23. Duffy J, Lidsky M, Sharp JT, et al. Polyarthritis, polyarteritis, and hepatitis B. Medicine. 1976;55:19.
24. Sergent JS, Lockshin MD, Christian CL, et al. Vasculitis with hepatitis B antigenemia. Medicine. 1976;55:1.
25. Reshef E, Greenberg SB, Jankovic J. Herpes zoster ophthalmicus followed by contralateral hemiparesis: report of two cases and review of the literature. J Neurol Neurosurg Psychiatr. 1985;48:122–7.
26. Johnson RT. Viral Infections of the Nervous System. New York: Raven Press; 1982.
27. Winkelman NW, Eckel JL. Productive endarteritis of the small cortical vessels in severe toxemias. Brain. 1927;50:608.
28. Winkelman NW, Eckle JL. The brain in bacterial endocarditis. Arch Neurol Psychiatr. 1930;23:1161.
29. Woollam DHM, Miller JW. Vascular tissues in the central nervous system. In: Minckler J, ed. Pathology of the Nervous System. v. 1. New York: McGraw-Hill; 1968:486–98.
30. Moskowit MA, Rosenbaum AE, Tyler HR. Angiographically monitored resolution of cerebral mycotic aneurysms. Neurology. 1974;24:1103.
31. Fishman RA. Cerebrospinal Fluid in Diseases of the Nervous System. Philadelphia: WB Saunders; 1980.
32. DeJong RN. Spinal puncture and the examination of the cerebrospinal fluid. In: The Neurological Examination. 4th ed. Hagerstown: Harper & Row; 1976:741.
33. Ellner JJ, Bennett JE. Chronic meningitis. Medicine. 1976;55:341.
34. Gonyea EF. Cisternal puncture and cryptococcal meningitis. Arch Neurol. 1973;28:200.
35. Berger MP, Paz. Diagnosis of cryptococcal meningitis. JAMA. 1976;236:2517.
36. Samson DS, Clark K. A current review of brain abscess. Am J Med. 1973;54:201.
37. Rieselback RE, DiChiro G, Freireich EJ, et al. Subarachnoid distribution of drugs after lumbar injection. N Engl J Med. 1962;267:1273.
38. Kaiser AB, McGee ZA. Aminoglycoside therapy of gram-negative bacillary meningitis. N Engl J Med. 1975;293:1215.
39. McCracken GH, Mize SG. A controlled study of intrathecal antibiotic therapy in gram-negative enteric meningitis of infancy. J Pediatr. 1976;89:66.
40. Salmon JH. Ventriculitis complicating meningitis. Am J Dis Child. 1972;124:35.
41. Duffy GP. Lumbar puncture in the presence of raised intracranial pressure. Br Med J. 1969;1:407.
42. Netsky MG, Shuangshoti S. The choroid plexus in health and disease. In: Inflammatory Disorders of the Chroid Plexus and Ependyma. Charlottesville: University of Virginia Press; 1975:249–64.
43. Moxon ER, Smith AL, Averill DR, et al. *Haemophilus influenzae* meningitis in infant rats after intranasal inoculation. J Infect Dis. 1974;129:154.
44. Rich AR, McCordock HA. The pathogenesis of tuberculous meningitis. Bull Johns Hopkins Hosp. 1933;52:5.
45. Rupprecht CE, Dietzschold B. Perspectives on rabies virus pathogenesis. Lab Invest. 1987;57:603.
46. Winkler WG, Fashinell TR, Leffingwell L, et al. Airborne rabies transmission in a laboratory worker. JAMA. 1973;266:1219.
47. Tsiang H. Neuronal function impairment in rabies-infected rat brain. J Gen Virol. 1982;61:277.
48. McArthur JC. Neurologic manifestations of AIDS. Medicine. 1987;66:407.
49. Pert CB, Smith CC, Ruff MR, et al. AIDS and its dementia as a neuropeptide disorder: role of VIP receptor blockade by human immunodeficiency virus envelope. Ann Neurol. 1987;32(Suppl):S71.
50. Greenlee JE, Johnson RT. Virology and neurological disease. In: Swash M, Kennard C, eds. The Scientific Basis of Clinical Neurology. London: Churchill Livingstone; 1985:619.
51. Oppenheimer SI, O'Toole RD, Petersdorf RG. Bacterial meningitis. In: Goldensohn ES, Appel SH, eds. Scientific Approaches to Clinical Neurology. v. 1. Philadelphia: Lea & Febiger; 1977:434–51.
52. Tourtellotte W. On cerebrospinal fluid immunoglobulin-G (IgG) quotients in multiple sclerosis and other diseases. J Neurol Sci. 1970;10:279.
53. Finkel MF. Lyme disease and its neurological complications. Arch Neurol. 1988;45:99–104.
54. McArthur JC, Cohen BA, Farzedegan, et al. Cerebrospinal fluid abnormalities in homosexual men with and without neuropsychiatric findings. Ann Neurol. 1988;32(Suppl):S34.
55. Nahmias AJ, Whitley RJ, Visintine AN, et al. Herpes simplex encephalitis: laboratory evaluations and their diagnostic significance. J Infect Dis. 1982;145:829.
56. Koskiniemi M, Vaheri A, Taskinen E. Cerebrospinal fluid alterations in herpes simplex virus encephalitis. Rev Infect Dis. 1984;6:608.
57. Bowen DL, Lane HC, Fauci AS. Immunopathogenesis of the acquired immunodeficiency syndrome. Ann Intern Med. 1985;103:704.
58. Hirsch RL, Griffin DE, Winkelstein JA. The effect of complement depletion on the course of Sindbis virus infection in mice. J Immunol. 1978;121:1276.
59. Truax RC, Carpenter MB. Human Neuroanatomy. 6th ed. Baltimore: Williams & Wilkins; 1969.
60. Ropper AH, Kennedy SK, Zervas NT. Neurological and Neurosurgical Intensive Care. Baltimore: University Park Press; 1982.
61. Plum F, Posner JB. The Diagnosis of Stupor and Coma. 3rd ed. Philadelphia: FA Davis; 1980.
62. Adams RD, Victor M. Principles of Neurology. 2nd ed. New York: McGraw-Hill; 1981:532.

66. ACUTE MENINGITIS

ZELL A. McGEE
J. RICHARD BARINGER

Acute meningitis is a medical emergency that requires the utmost in diagnostic and therapeutic skills. The death rate, about 30 percent, has changed little in the last 25 years. To lower the death rate further will require: (*1*) earlier recognition of meningitis, (*2*) more rapid determination of the most likely etiologic agent, (*3*) more rapid initiation of appropriate antimicrobial therapy (within 30 minutes in acutely ill patients), (*4*) earlier recognition of those conditions in which cerebrospinal fluid (CSF) bacterial cultures are negative (aseptic meningitis syndrome) but in which antimicrobial therapy is required, and (*5*) earlier recognition and treatment of the consequences (e.g., acidosis, disseminated intravascular coagulation) of the septicemia that frequently accompanies bacterial meningitis. This chapter, in addition to providing information about specific types of meningitis, focuses on how the physician can most easily recognize meningitis and can best approach the patient with known or suspected meningitis to minimize the risk of neurologic damage or death.

EPIDEMIOLOGY

In bacterial meningitis caused by *Streptococcus pneumoniae*, *Neisseria meningitidis*, and *Haemophilus influenzae*, the immediate source of the invading pathogen is usually the bacterial flora that colonizes the nasopharynx. Although there is great variability in the duration of colonization before invasion, the greatest risk of meningitis seems to be in patients who have recently been colonized. Approximately 25 percent of healthy people acquire new strains of pneumococci each year[1] and 6 percent acquire new strains of meningococci.[2] *Haemophilus influenzae* colonization, which occurs in less than 3 percent of normal infants and seldom in adults,[3] occurs much more frequently in case contacts (in about 50 percent of children <5 years old and in about 20 percent of adults and children 5 years or older.[4] Pneumococci and meningococci usually require several weeks to spread among a family unit following the initial nasopharyngeal acquisition by one family member.[1,2] Colonization and secondary cases of meningococcal meningitis and *H. influenzae* meningitis usually follow close contact (sleeping together, eating together, kissing, and so on).[5] However, acquisition of one of these meningeal pathogens usually results in the asymptomatic carrier state. Although asymptomatic carriers can spread meningeal pathogens, the likelihood of spread of a particular pathogen may vary with the presence or absence of disease, the type of disease, and probably other factors. For instance, colonization rates of *H. influenzae* in children younger than 5 years old are 20 percent if the index case has epiglottitis versus 55 percent if the index case has meningitis.[4] The epidemiology of other types of bacterial meningitis as well as viral, fungal, and amebic meningitis are discussed below in sections dealing with these specific agents.

PATHOPHYSIOLOGY

The pathogenesis of most cases of meningitis almost certainly involves at least six steps. These steps include (*1*) attachment to epithelial cells of nasopharyngeal and oropharyngeal mucosa, (*2*) transgression of the mucosal barrier, (*3*) survival in the bloodstream (avoiding phagocytic cells and bacteriolytic activity), (*4*) entry into the CSF, (*5*) survival in the CSF, and (*6*) production of disease in the meninges and brain.

It seems likely that in meningitis at least some of the damage to the meninges and brain is effected by various cytokines, which are biologic mediators that can cause severe tissue damage and death.[6] Although Waage et al.[7] did not show that cytokines per se produce brain damage in meningitis, they did demonstrate in patients with meningococcal meningitis, septicemia, or both that the serum concentration of tumor necrosis factor, a potent cytokine elicited by lipopolysaccharide (endotoxin)[6] correlates directly with the likelihood of death.[7]

The bacteria that most frequently cause meningitis are capable of doing so because they have a variety of virulence mechanisms, each one of which may play a unique role in one or more of the successive steps of the pathogenic process. Our knowledge of these mechanisms is incomplete but is best worked out for *N. meningitidis*.

The bacteria that cause meningitis usually attach to and colonize host mucosal surfaces in the nasopharynx. Both *H. influenzae* and *N. meningitidis* have pili that appear to mediate attachment.[8,9] Host cell-surface receptors for meningococcal pili appear to be concentrated on certain cells in the oro- and nasopharynx.[9–11] The distribution of these receptors appears to determine the sites of meningococcal colonization.

Meningococci are ingested by certain epithelial cells of the nasopharyngeal mucosa.[10] Whether meningococci and other meningeal pathogens are passed through such cells to the subepithelial tissues where they have access to the bloodstream is not yet known. However, such a mechanism results in transgression of mucosal barriers by other human pathogens.[11]

Once in the bloodstream, the most frequently successful meningeal pathogens appear to avoid phagocytosis by polymorphonuclear leukocytes and cells of the reticuloendothelial system by virtue of having antiphagocytic capsules.[12,13] The available pneumococcal and meningococcal vaccines probably intervene in this pathogenesis by eliciting antibodies that neutralize the antiphagocytic capsules and enhance phagocytosis. Gram-negative meningeal pathogens may avoid being killed by antibody and complement by having special lipopolysaccharides on their surfaces or by having outer membrane proteins that deter bacteriolysis or combine with blocking IgA antibodies.[14,15]

How bacteria cross from the bloodstream into the CSF is not known. Many bacteria, encapsulated and unencapsulated, from the oropharynx and other sites cause bacteremia but not meningitis.[16] The possible role of polysaccharides is suggested by the observation that only certain capsular types of pneumococci, meningococci, *H. influenzae*, *Escherichia coli*, and group B streptococci have a particular predilection for causing meningitis.[12,13]

Bacteria probably enter the CSF space from the blood via the choroid plexuses of the lateral ventricles and then spread to the extracerebral CSF space along normal paths of CSF flow.[17–20] They also may enter the CSF space directly through defects of congenital or traumatic origin or from parameningeal suppurative foci. The CSF is generally devoid of sufficient humoral factors or phagocytic cells to repel successfully the initial invasion of pathogens.[20,21] The ingress of antibody, complement, and phagocytic cells that occurs during the course of meningitis may ablate infections with some bacterial strains but may be ineffective in halting the lethal progression of infection with other strains.

Meningeal pathogens are generally limited to the subarachnoid space.[22,23] Thus, the disordered function of the nervous system in meningitis is likely to result from occlusion of blood vessels traversing the subarachnoid space and from the intense inflammatory process with attendant necrosis of nerve roots, cerebral edema, cerebral ischemia and possible hydrocephalus.

If there are defects in host defenses, bacteria that do not ordinarily have the virulence factors necessary to complete all steps of the pathogenic process may do so and cause meningitis, or bacteria that can complete all steps may do so more easily and more often. Lack of humoral immunity, the presence of complement defects, loss of integrity of the CSF space, and other, less well-defined factors, such as the stress of boot camp and viral infections, all predispose to meningitis.[24–26]

In viral meningitis and meningoencephalitis, the etiologic agents reach the nervous system by one or more of three major routes: neural pathways, the olfactory tract, and the blood stream. Most viruses causing meningitis use the hematogenous route after undergoing multiplication of the site of entry or in regional lymph nodes draining the entry site. The precise mechanisms by which most viruses enter the CSF and produce neurologic damage are still under investigation.[27]

The mechanisms of pathogenicity in fungal infections are less well studied but seem to be similar to those in bacterial meningitis.

SPECIFIC CAUSES OF MENINGITIS AND THEIR TREATMENT

The specific causes of meningitis (Table 1) can be divided into two major diagnostic groups, bacterial meningitis and the aseptic meningitis syndrome. Bacterial meningitis, which may have an acute presentation (symptoms of less than 24 hours' duration) or a subacute presentation (symptoms of 1–7 days' duration), can generally be diagnosed quickly by examining a Gram stain of the sediment of the CSF. Those patients with negative Gram stains and negative bacterial cultures may be considered to have the aseptic meningitis syndrome. However, the absence of bacteria on Gram strain and negative bacterial cultures do not exclude an etiologic role for bacteria or other treatable agents.

Bacterial Meningitis

Pneumococcal Meningitis. In adults *Streptococcus pneumoniae* is the most frequent bacterial species causing meningitis. Pneumococcal meningitis occurs in the very young, the old, and those of any age with a predisposing factor. Pneumonia, sinusitis, endocarditis, old or recent head trauma, CSF leak, splenectomy, sickle hemoglobinopathy, bone marrow transplantation, and alcoholism predispose to or accompany meningitis caused by pneumococci more often than meningitis caused by meningococci or *H. influenzae*.[26,28–30] Also, patients with pneumococcal meningitis are somewhat more likely to have alterations of consciousness or focal neurologic defects than are patients with meningococcal or *H. influenzae* meningitis. The most critical element in therapy appears to be early administration of adequate amounts of the optimal antimicrobial (i.e., crystalline penicillin G, 70,000 units/kg iv q8h for neonates and 50,000 units/kg iv q4th in adults). In penicillin-allergic patients, chloramphenicol (25 mg/kg iv q6h in adults) is the best alternative to penicillin. The mortality is 30–60 percent. Some patients die despite apparently optimal antimicrobial therapy with sterilization of the CSF and other body fluids. In those who survive, residual defects of hearing, convulsions, hemiparesis, or other more selective nerve deficits may persist. Although penicillin is the drug of choice, it may not provide adequate therapy for meningitis caused by the approximately 2 percent of pneumococcal strains that are relatively resistant to penicillin (MIC ≥ 0.1 μg/ml). Therefore the Centers for Disease Control now recommend that all clinically significant pneumococcal isolates be screened for penicillin susceptibility with oxacillin disks.[31]

TABLE 1. Conditions Presenting as Acute Meningitis

Infectious diseases
Bacteria and spirochetes
Streptococcus pneumoniae
Neisseria meningitidis
Haemophilus influenzae
Streptococcus (particularly group B)
Listeria monocytogenes
Treponema pallidum
Leptospires
Staphylococcus aureus
Pseudomonas aeruginosa
Enteric gram-negative bacilli
Staphylococcus epidermidis
Propionibacterium acnes
Viruses
Echovirus
Coxsackievirus types A and B
Enterovirus
Mumps virus
Herpes simplex virus types 1 and 2
Epstein-Barr virus
Human Immunodeficiency virus
Herpes zoster virus
Cytomegalovirus
California encephalitis virus
St. Louis encephalitis virus
Colorado tick fever virus
Lymphocytic choriomeningitis virus
Poliovirus
Parasites
Naegleria
Angiostrongylus
Strongyloides stercoralis (hyperinfection syndrome)
Infections resembling acute meningitis
Rickettsiosis and ehrlichiosis
Brain abscess (see Chapter 70)
Epidural or subdural abscess (see Chapter 71 and 72)
Tuberculosis, cryptococcosis, and other forms of chronic meningitis (see Chapter 67)
Viral and other causes of encephalitis (see Chapter 68)
Noninfectious causes of acute meningitis syndrome
Mollaret's meningitis
Drug-induced meningitis
Epidermoid cyst of the meninges

Meningococcal Meningitis. In contrast to pneumococcal meningitis, meningococcal meningitis is primarily a disease of children and young adults; less than 10 percent of the cases occur in patients over age 45.[32] A majority of cases occur in the winter or spring, a time when viral meningitis is relatively infrequent. Four meningococcal serogroups are responsible for a majority of the disease: serogroups A and C are most often associated with epidemics of meningococcal meningitis; serogroup B is the primary cause of sporadic cases; and serogroup Y causes sporadic cases of pneumonia, sometimes associated with meningitis.[33] Meningococcal meningitis may be rapidly progressive. Approximately 50 percent of those hospitalized within the first 24 hours of their illness subsequently die, some within a few hours of the onset of symptoms.[30,34] Thus, early suspicion, performance of a lumbar tap, and prompt therapy are critical. The presence of petechiae in a patient with meningitis most likely indicates the presence of meningococcemia, although petechiae are sometimes seen in meningitis due to echovirus type 9, in pneumococcal meningitis in asplenic patients, or with concomitant endocarditis caused by pneumococci or staphylococci.[32,35] About half the patients with meningococcal meningitis have petechiae, purpuric lesions, or both.[30,34] Subclinical or clinical disseminated intravascular coagulation, which frequently accompanies meningococcemia, may progress to hemorrhagic infarction of the adrenal glands, renal cortical necrosis, widespread pulmonary microvascular thrombosis, shock, and death. Therefore early antimicrobial therapy (crystalline penicillin G, 50,000 units/kg iv q4h) must be accompanied by efforts to control acidosis, tissue hypoxia, shock, adrenal insufficiency, and disseminated intravascular coagulation if these complications occur (Ch. 189). An approach to prevention of meningococcal meningitis in contacts of cases is discussed in the last section of this chapter.

Haemophilus Influenzae Meningitis. *Haemophilus influenzae* type b is the most common bacterial cause of meningitis between the neonatal period and age 6 years.[34] The occurrence of *H. influenzae* meningitis in older patients should prompt efforts to exclude the presence of otitis media, other parameningeal foci of infection, CSF leak, or an immunodeficiency disease, since these often accompany *H. influenzae* meningitis in older patients. Pharyngitis and otitis media are associated with *H. influenzae* meningitis in one-half and two-thirds of the cases, respectively.[30] In contrast to meningococcal meningitis, petechiae rarely occur in *H. influenzae* meningitis. A substantial proportion of *H. influenzae* isolates are resistant to ampicillin. Most of these strains are infected with a plasmid (Ch. 201) that mediates production of β-lactamase, an enzyme that destroys penicillins and some cephalosporins. Because approximately 20 percent of the cases of *H. influenzae* meningitis are caused by these ampicillin-resistant strains, ampicillin plus chloramphenicol is currently recommended by some authorities as therapy for meningitis known or likely to be caused by *H. influenzae*.

The chloramphenicol is stopped if the organism is ampicillin susceptible. The third-generation cephalosporins are very active against β-lactamase producing and nonproducing strains and are considered by many to be the drugs of choice for serious ampicillin-resistant *H. influenzae* infections (see Chapter 201).[36,37] The continuation or recurrence of decreased mentation or fever after antimicrobial therapy may indicate the presence of subdural effusions, a relatively frequent complication in *H. influenzae* meningitis. The death rate is approximately 3–8 percent.[34] Intelligence testing has revealed mental deficits in 30–50 percent of the children who have had *H. influenzae* meningitis, and this infection is thought to be the leading cause of acquired mental retardation in the United States.[3] The evidence that *H. influenzae* meningitis occurs in clusters and that chemoprophylaxis may stop contact spread is reviewed in the section on prevention of meningitis.

Gram-Negative Bacillary Meningitis. Whereas pneumococci, meningococci, and *H. influenzae* combined have continued to cause approximately 40 percent of the cases of bacterial meningitis in adults over the last 20 years, the proportion of cases of meningitis caused by gram-negative bacilli (exluding neonatal meningitis and that caused by *H. influenzae*) has increased significantly, and the proportion caused by staphylococci and streptococci has decreased.[38,39] This trend is not surprising since gram-negative bacillary meningitis is usually hospital acquired, and the proportion of hospital-acquired infections caused by gram-negative bacilli remains substantial.

Approximately 30 percent of the cases of gram-negative bacillary meningitis occur in conjunction with head trauma (especially in association with CSF rhinorrhea), about 50 percent of cases occur after neurosurgical procedures, and 20 percent are "medical" (e.g., in patients with accompanying gram-negative sepsis, ruptured brain abscess, impaired host defenses, or strongyloidiasis).[39,40] The most likely gram-negative bacilli causing meningitis at any time after the neonatal period are *Klebsiella* (approximately 40 percent of the cases), *E. coli* (15–30 percent), and *Pseudomonas* (10–20 percent).[39,41] However, the flora causing this type of meningitis may vary somewhat from hospital to hospital.

The presence of meningitis is less likely to be suspected in patients with gram-negative bacillary meningitis because most of them have had head trauma or a neurosurgical procedure and already have altered consciousness, signs of meningeal irritation, and an elevated CSF protein or WBC count. Thus, the presence of fever, the readiness of the physician to do a spinal tap, and a low CSF glucose concentration may be the most useful keys to the diagnosis. Although it is important to start therapy early, initial Gram stains may be negative in up to 50 percent of the patients.[41] In these patients the CSF lactic acid determination and the limulus lysate assay[42,43] may be useful.

The third-generation cephalosporins have provided a significant advance in the therapy of gram-negative bacillary meningitis. Although older cephalosporins were usually not effective in treating bacterial meningitis of any etiology owing to inadequate CSF concentrations, intravenous therapy with the third-generation cephalosporins usually results in CSF concentrations many times the MBC for the most frequently infecting bacteria. For example, CSF concentrations of cefotaxime (at 12 g/day iv) for therapy of *E. coli* meningitis usually exceeds the MBC for the infecting organism by 50- to 60-fold.[37,44] This high ratio of CSF drug concentration to the MBC is similar to that seen during high-dose penicillin therapy of pneumococcal meningitis. Use of third-generation cephalosporins is discussed further in a separate section below.

The optimal antimicrobial, route of administration, and duration of therapy of gram-negative bacillary meningitis have never been defined in a systematic trial. If the patient is not severely ill, therapy for meningitis can be begun with a third-generation cephalosporin in high doses (e.g., cefotaxime, 50 mg/kg iv q6h or ceftazidime 2 g q8h) plus a systemic aminoglycoside (e.g., amikacin 5 mg/kg iv q8h). With *Pseudomonas aeruginosa* meningitis, ceftazidime plus an aminoglycoside might be selected (see below). Use of an aminoglycoside is largely to aid in treatment of extracerebral manifestations. If the organism is initially resistant or becomes resistant to the third-generation cephalosporin during therapy, the physician should consider intraventricular administration of an aminoglycoside given with systemic aminoglycoside plus systemic ticarcillin or piperacillin (75 mg/kg iv q6h).[45–49] If there is reason to belive that the infection may be limited to the extracerebral CSF space (e.g., meningitis associated with spinal surgery), a trial of intralumbar aminoglycoside—0.03 mg of tobramycin or gentamicin per ml of estimated CSF volume or 0.1 mg of amikacin per ml of estimated CSF volume every 24 hours—may be warranted. The total CSF volume in individuals without hydrocephalus has been estimated to be 40–60 ml in infants and 60–100 ml in young children; for older children and adults of average build, estimate 1 ml of CSF per pound body weight.[20,49] If there is no reason to suspect that the infection is limited to the extracerebral CSF space, most data suggest that intraventricular aminoglycoside offers a better chance of cure than lumbar intrathecal drug.

Intravenous trimethoprim-sulfamethoxazole has been used occasionally in gram-negative bacillary meningitis.[50] Its use in *Listeria* meningitis will be discussed later.

If the patient is critically ill—has an altered sensorium or is in a coma—and there is no reason to suspect that the gram-negative bacilli present are unlikely to respond to third-generation cephalosporins, these are the drugs of choice. If, however, epidemiologic, cultural, or susceptibility data suggest that the organism is unlikely to respond to third-generation cephalosporins an Ommaya or Rickham reservoir should be put in place immediately, and intraventricular and systemic therapy should be begun in the operating room with gentamicin, tobramycin, or amikacin along with systemic ticarcillin or piperacillin in the doses suggested above. As soon after emplacement of the reservoir as possible, computed axial tomography or simple injection of a bolus of air through the catheter with subsequent skull x-ray films should be performed to ensure that the catheter is actually in the cerebral ventricles. The reservoir and catheter can be used immediately after their emplacement. After the first dose of aminoglycoside into the ventricle, the concentration should be monitored in the lumbar CSF to ensure adequate distribution of the drug throughout the CSF space. In addition, ventricular levels of aminoglycoside should be measured just before the next intraventricular dose every 2 or 3 days, and the dose altered to maintain this "trough" level in an approximate range of 2–10 μg/ml.

Regardless of the drug chosen for treatment of the meningitis per se, the patient should also be treated intravenously with antimicrobials appropriate for gram-negative bacteremia that is present in 70 percent or more of the patients with gram-negative meningitis.[51] Therapy for the meningitis should be maintained for 10 days after cultures of the CSF become sterile. Spinal fluid cultures may be positive for 10 days or more on a regimen that will eventually result in a cure. During this time colony counts of organisms in the CSF, which are performed every 2 to 3 days, should show a progressive decrease in the number of organisms if therapy is effective.

Meningeal irritation with radiculitis occasionally occurs with intralumbar and intraventricular administration of aminoglycosides, but ototoxicity has not been a problem. In seven patients observed by one of the authors, serial audiograms have been normal despite CSF concentrations of aminoglycosides as high as 200 μg/ml.

Third-Generation Cephalosporins. Some of the third-generation cephalosporins, particularly cefotaxime and ceftazidime, have become the drugs of choice for meningitis caused by most aerobic gram-negative bacilli. Response rates of 80–90 percent have been reported for meningitis caused by *E. coli*, *Klebsiella pneumoniae*, and *Serratia* sp.[52,53] Somewhat lower responses have been reported for *Enterobacter* and *Salmonella*. In every case, the patient's isolate must be tested for susceptibility to the third-generation caphalosporin to be used. Drug resistance arising during therapy has also been encountered.[54] With *P. aeruginosa*, activity of third-generation cephalosporins is quite variable. Cefotaxime, ceftizoxime, moxalactam, and ceftriaxone are not indicated in meningitis caused by *Ps. aeruginosa*. Some of the cephalosporins that have antipseudomonal activity in vitro, such as cefoperazone, are not sufficiently active to be used in meningitis. With ceftazidime, the rate of response has been reported to be as high as 80 percent in *Ps. aeruginosa* meningitis.[55] However, drug resistance arising during therapy is a problem of sufficient magnitude that we believe that the preferred therapy is intraventricular and systemic aminoglycoside in conjunction with systemic ticarcillin or piperacillin.[45–49] Also notable is that a substantial portion of patients with gram-negative bacillary meningitis have recently had neurosurgical procedures. The bleeding tendency induced by moxalactam, cefoperaxone, and other cephalosporins with a methyltetrazolethiol group raises concern about the use of these drugs in such patients. Activity of third-generation cephalosporins against gram-positive cocci is variable. Moxalactam has too little activity against gram-positive cocci and should not be used for meningitis caused by gram-positive cocci, including pneumococcus or streptococcus. With *S. aureus*, none of the third-generation cephalosporins would be the drug of choice for meningitis. Patients with staphylococcal meningitis who are allergic to penicillin and therefore cannot be given nafcillin, oxacillin, or methicillin can be treated with vancomycin.

Against the usual pathogens of acute bacterial meningitis of childhood, *H. influenzae*, *N. meningitidis* and *S. pneumoniae*, cefotaxime and ceftazidime have given rates of cure that are comparable but not superior to those of other regimens.[56,57] However, experience is still small compared with that with older agents, and the ability to prevent the long-term sequelae such as deafness or mental retardation will take time to assess. Penicillin G remains the drug of choice for meningitis caused by *N. meningitidis* and susceptible strains of *S. pneumoniae*. Activity of the third-generation cephalosporins against *Enterococcus* and *Listeria* is poor. None of these drugs should be used as sole agents in initial therapy of meningitis when one of these pathogens is suspect, such as in neonatal meningitis.

Use of Corticosteroids in Acute Bacterial Meningitis. A recent placebo-controlled study of 200 infants and older children with bacterial meningitis evaluated the efficacy of dexamethasone, 0.15 mg/kg every 6 hours for the first 4 days of therapy.[58] The antibacterial antibiotic was changed from cefuroxime to ceftriaxone during the study. Aside from the expected effects on fever and spinal fluid analysis (protein, glucose, and lactate), the only statistically significant benefit of dexamethasone was on deafness. Of the children not receiving dexamethasone, 15.5 percent lost auditory acuity, while only 3.3 percent of dexamethasone recipients experienced hearing loss. Follow-up of these children for assessment of long-term neurologic sequelae is needed to see whether other differences may appear. Additionally, too few patients with meningitis caused by organisms other than *H. influenzae* were included to determine how these results apply more generally to bacterial meningitis of childhood. At present, no firm recommendation for dexamethasone can be made for children with meningitis due to organisms other than *H. influenzae* or for adults.

Group B Streptococcal Meningitis. Group B streptococci seldom cause meningitis in adults except in conjunction with endocarditis. The features of neonatal meningitis caused by group B streptococci are discussed later in this chapter.

Listeria Meningitis. *Listeria monocytogenes* can cause meningitis in normal adults[59] but most often causes meningitis in neonates, in the aged, or in immunosuppressed patients.[59,60] In some centers *Listeria* is the primary cause of meningitis in renal transplant patients.[60] In neonates the source of *Listeria* is the genital tract or subclinical infection of the mother, which is transferred to the baby during birth; the source in adults is probably other adults, food,[61] or the patient's own flora. Gram stains of the CSF are often negative, but the cultures are positive. The organisms, which are gram-positive rods, may be mistaken for diphtheroids and considered skin contaminants unless the physician is alert to this possibility and asks the laboratory to make a special effort to test for *Listeria*. β-hemolysis (clear) on blood agar and motility of such organisms strongly suggests *Listeria*. The therapy of choice is ampicillin (100 mg/kg iv q8h in neonates, 200 mg/kg per day divided into doses every 4 hours for adults). An aminoglycoside is usually added. However, a number of therapeutic successes with trimethoprim-sulfamethoxazole[62] suggest that this drug combination may be as effective or more effective than ampicillin plus an aminoglycoside. Therapy should be continued for 3 weeks or longer as indicated clinically.

Other Causes of Bacterial Meningitis. *Staphylococcus aureus* may cause meningitis, especially in conjunction with brain abscesses, paranasal sinusitis, endocarditis, or severe staphylococcal septicemia. The drug of choice is nafcillin or oxacillin, 2 g iv q4h. Infection with *S. aureus* or *S. epidermidis* in conjunction with CSF shunts presents special problems dealt with in a subsequent section of this chapter. A wide variety of other bacteria occasionally cause meningitis.[30,34]

Partially Treated Bacterial Meningitis. At the time the diagnosis of bacterial meningitis is considered and a lumbar puncture is obtained, 25–50 percent of the patients already will have received antimicrobial therapy.[63,64] The Gram stains and cultures of CSF from such patients are more often negative than those of untreated patients,[65] so an erroneous diagnosis of viral meningitis may be made. However, the CSF white cell and differential counts and the protein and glucose levels are generally not significantly altered by prior therapy; several days are required to decrease the number of polymorphonuclear leukocytes and to reverse the high-protein and low-glucose levels of bacterial meningitis. Counterimmunoelectrophoresis (CIE) and latex agglutination tests are routinely used in many hospitals and may detect antigens of pneumococci, meningococci, *H. influenzae* and group B streptococci in spinal fluid when Gram stain and culture have been rendered negative by prior therapy.[43,66] These tests are not sensitive enough to exclude a bacterial etiology when a negative result is obtained. Other tests such as the limulus lysate assay or lactic acid concentration may also point to a bacterial etiology in this situation.[42,43] If a search for a bacterial etiology is negative, the physician should not necessarily conclude that the meningitis is "partially treated" and initiate antibacterial therapy. Work-up of other causes of the aseptic meningitis syndrome, such as brain abscess, tuberculous meningitis, and cryptococcal meningitis (Table 1), should be initiated even if a decision to begin antibacterial therapy is made. When no treatment is given, a repeat lumbar puncture in 8–12 hours may be useful.

Other Causes of the Syndrome

Parameningeal Suppurative Foci. Suppurative foci adjacent to the meninges may cause signs of meningeal irritation and CSF abnormalities indistinguishable from those observed in the aseptic meningitis syndrome when it is caused by viruses. If not misinterpreted, the finding of the aseptic meningitis syndrome can be a valuable clue to the presence of a focus of life-threatening infection that may require antimicrobials, surgery, or both. All patients with meningitis should have sinus and mastoid x-ray studies; this is of particular importance if there is a history of sinusitis, mastoiditis, of middle ear infection. The finding of abnormalities on these x-ray studies, the finding of alterations of mentation, focal nerve deficits (excluding ophthalmoplegias), or the presence of diseases that predispose to brain abscess such as endocarditis or lung abscess should prompt the performance of a computed axial tomography (CAT) scan or magnetic resonance imaging to detect a brain abscess (see Chapter 70). Especially in the setting of a recent superficial staphylococcal infection, the finding of localized back pain and peripheral nerve abnormalities should suggest spinal epidural abscess and prompt consideration of a spinal CAT scan or magnetic resonance imaging.[67,68] Foci of dermal sinus infection (Fig. 1), cranial osteomyelitis, mastoiditis, and middle ear or paranasal sinus infection may also be detectable by a thorough physical examination. Other suppurative foci, such as subdural empyema or suppurative intracranial phlebitis, require special diagnostic procedures (see Chapters 71, 72).

Tuberculous Meningitis. Although tuberculous meningitis is more often subacute or chronic (see Chapter 229), it may have a rapid onset and progression, especially in immunosuppressed hosts. It usually occurs in the course of miliary tuberculosis or with rupture of a subependymal tubercle. Thus, x-ray and other signs of tuberculosis may or may not be present. In this acute form, the WBCs in the CSF may be primarily polymorphonuclear leukocytes. Other features of the laboratory diagnosis are discussed later in the chapter.

Amebic Meningitis. Free-living amebas of the genus *Naegleria*, which are widely distributed in water, soil, air, and decomposing organic matter, occasionally cause acute, purulent meningoencephalitis in humans. Most patients give a history of swimming in a warm, freshwater lake or indoor swimming pool and of severe, persistent frontal headache.[69,70] The diagnosis can be made by observing motility of the amebas (often mistaken for macrophages) on wet mount or hanging drop suspensions of CSF. Since centrifugation or refrigeration destroys the amebas, the tests should be performed on fresh, uncentrifuged CSF. The organisms can be cultured on a lawn of *E. coli* on agar or observed histologically in cytologic studies of CSF.[69] Although progression to death is the rule, high doses of amphotericin B administered systemically and intraventricularly[71] have been associated with recovery.[72]

Syphilitic Meningitis. Acute meningitis is an infrequent manifestation of syphilis (Chapter 213). It can mimic completely other causes of the aseptic meningitis syndrome; but papilledema may occur in conjunction with hydrocephalus. Cranial or peripheral nerve signs, mental deterioration, and convulsions occur more frequently in syphilitic than in viral meningitis.[73,74] Meningitis may occur months to years after primary infection, but a majority of cases occur within the first year, probably in conjunction with the dissemination of spirochetes that occurs in the secondary stage of syphilis. Central nervous system invasion is now known to be more common than appreciated previously. In one study, 30 percent of 40 patients with untreated primary or secondary syphilis had *Treponema pallidum* isolated from their CSF.[75] In 25 percent of the patients with acute syphilitic meningitis, the meningitis is the first manifestation of infection with *T. pallidum*.[73] Thus, serum and CSF serologic testing are most important in evaluating the possibility of syphilis in a patient with the aseptic meningitis syndrome. Intramuscular penicillin regimens for neurosyphilis and syphilitic meningitis may be inadequate; optimal therapy is aqueous penicillin G, 3.5 million units iv q4h for 2 weeks.

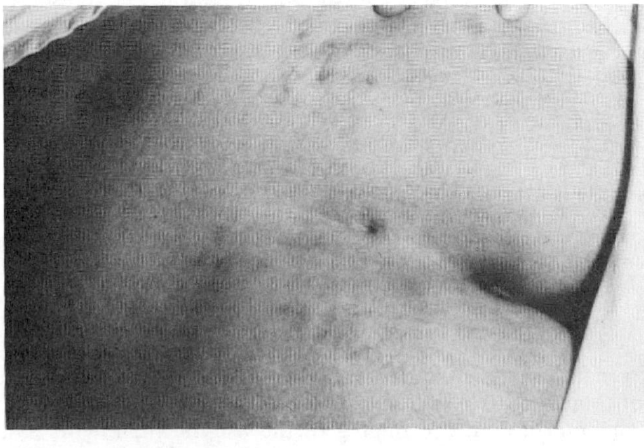

FIG. 1. Midline dermal sinus in the coccygeal area of a patient with recurrent gram-negative bacillary meningitis.

Viral Meningitis. Patients with viral meningitis have rapid onset of headache, low-grade fever, stiff neck, and photophobia. Despite their obvious discomfort, they are usually alert and oriented. Most are children or young adults. Patients with encephalitis have early onset of lethargy, obtundation, confusion, seizures, and focal neurologic signs.

Distinction between viral and bacterial meningitis is best made by lumbar puncture. In viral meningitis, the CSF usually contains 50 to 500 leukocytes/mm^3, predominantly lymphocytes. Early in the course of the disease, the CSF may have a predominance of neutrophils, but rarely exceeding 90 percent, as is seen in bacterial meningitis. Repeat lumbar puncture in 12 to 24 hours can be helpful in borderline cases by showing a shift to lymphocyte predominance in viral meningitis. CSF glucose is above 40 mg/dl in viral meningitis, with the exception of some patients with mumps, herpes simplex, or lymphocytic choriomeningitis virus. Protein is elevated but rarely beyond 200 mg/dl. Cultures of CSF and blood for bacteria should be obtained in every case. Early in the course of enteroviral meningitis, the virus may be recovered from the CSF, but yields are low. If a viral diagnosis is to be pursued, throat washings and stool should be tested as well as CSF. Both acute and convalescent serum should be obtained for serology. These studies may be useful in outbreaks but not facilitate the management of individual cases.

The etiology of viral meningitis varies with the season of the year, the age of the patient, and the geographic location. In the United States, about 70 percent of cases are due to enteroviruses, especially echovirus types 4, 6, 9, 11, 16, and 30 and coxsackievirus types A7, A9, and B2-5. Most of these cases occur in children in the late summer and early fall, but a few cases may continue to occur well into the winter months. Arbovirus meningitis also occurs in the summer months, contributing to the frequency of viral meningitis during the months of July, August, and September.

Mumps virus, in contrast, tends to be more frequent in the late winter and early spring. The herpesvirus and human immunodeficiency virus infections[76] occur sporadically year round. Poliovirus and lymphocytic choriomeningitis virus cause remarkably few cases of viral meningitis in the United States but remain important causes worldwide. Viral meningitis caused by adenovirus and cytomegalovirus may be seen in immunocompromised patients.

Meningitis of subacute or chronic onset may be considered acute if the early symptoms are not elicited or understood by the clinician. In this way, tuberculous, cryptococcal, and carcinomatous meningitis appear in the differential diagnosis of acute meningitis. Acid-fast smear of centrifuged CSF should be done when tuberculosis is a possibility, in addition to culturing several milliliters of CSF for mycobacteria. Rapid diagnosis of cryptococcal meningitis can be afforded by testing CSF and serum for cryptococcal antigen and by India ink smear of centrifuged CSF sediment. Confirmation of the diagnosis requires recovery of *Cryptococcus neoformans* from CSF. The best test for carcinomatous meningitis is CSF cytology.

Imaging by CAT or magnetic resonace imaging (MRI) can be helpful in detecting parameningeal infection, brain abscess, intracerebral neoplasm, epidural or subdural abscess, and herpes simplex virus encephalitis. Patients who are severely ill with fever, peripheral leukocytosis, polymorphonuclear predominance in the CSF, altered consciousness, papilledema, or focal neurologic signs deserve aggressive investigation and use of these imaging techniques. Antibacterial antibiotic therapy may be required in such patients, even in the absence of a firm diagnosis. However, many patients with the typical features of viral meningitis are not very ill and can be observed in the hospital. Improvement often begins in 24 to 72 hours.

Leptospiral Meningitis. Leptospires have been implicated in about 5 percent of cases of the aseptic meningitis syndrome.[77] About half the patients with leptospirosis have meningeal signs, and over 80 percent have abnormal CSF findings.[78] In leptospirosis an acute septicemic phase, characterized by the rapid onset of fever, chills, nausea and vomiting, myalgia, conjunctival suffusion, headache, and meningismus, either blends with or is followed in a few days by a phase in which rash, renal and hepatic damage, and meningitis may dominate the clinical picture.[78,79] In many cases the disease is mild, and the patient has a vague history of flulike prodromal illness followed by the septic meningitis syndome. The meningitis is occasionally accompanied by varying degrees of encephalitis or spinal involvement.[78] Thus, the illness may be indistinguishable from viral meningitis, including the early predominance of polymorphonuclear leukocytes in the CSF and CSF glucose concentrations seldom less than 40 mg/100 ml. There are two major clues to the specific etiology: (*1*) the history of contact with water frequented by domestic animals or rodents and (*2*) the occurrence of meningitis in conjunction with the clinical illness like that described for leptospirosis. The diagnosis is confirmed by documenting a fourfold or greater rise in agglutination titers. Although the disease is usually self-limited and does not require therapy, some authors suggest using 10 million units of penicillin per day in especially severe cases.

Neoplastic Meningitis. The presence in the CSF of tumor cells from a variety of neoplasms can produce the aseptic meningitis syndrome. Among patients with the syndrome, the usually modest elevation of cells and protein, at times in association with marked hypoglycorrhachia, should suggest the diagnosis, which can be confirmed by cytologic examination of the CSF.[34]

Cyst-Related Meningitis. Cells and other debris released from dermoid or epidermoid cysts into the subarachnoid space can cause meningitis, which tends to be recurrent.[34,80]

Chemical Meningitis. The onset of the aseptic meningitis syndrome in temporal proximity to spinal anesthesia or to diagnostic radiologic studies that involve the subarachnoid space (e.g., myelograms or pneumoencephalograms) should suggest not only bacterial meningitis but also chemical meningitis. The chemicals implicated include procaine and various soaps or disinfections in which syrings or needles are treated. Chemical meningitis may produce marked hypoglycorrhachia—glucose level less than 1 mg/dl.[81]

Drug-Induced Meningitis. A variety of pharmaceutical products that are administered orally or intravenously are capable of causing meningitis. To compound the problem, the settings in which the offending products are given are frequently ones in which the host is immunocompromised so that a microbial etiology of the meningitis is likely to be suspected and antibiotic or antiviral therapy given unnecessarily.

Drug-induced meningitis has clinical and laboratory features that suggest an acute aseptic meningitis syndrome, in that no bacteria or fungi are detected by culture, by microscopic examination of the centrifuged CSF sediment, or by antigen detection tests. Nevertheless, the patients often appear acutely ill, with a stiff neck, temperature over 103°F (39.4°C), and CSF findings that suggest a bacterial etiology because the CSF leukocyte counts frequently exceed $1000/mm^3$, of which over 80 percent are polymorphonuclear neutrophils. The protein concentration in the CSF is usually over 150 mg/dl, but the glucose concentration is usually within the normal range.

Co-trimoxazole (trimethoprim-sulfamethoxazole [TMP-SMX]) can cause aseptic meningitis.[82,83] It is not clear which of the two components is the major offender; the syndrome has been reproduced by readministration of the drugs, but only in combination.[82,83] Drug-induced meningitis can occur during TMP-SMX treatment of *Pneumocystis carinii* pneumonia in AIDS patients and simulate either AIDS meningitis or an opportunistic infection of the central nervous system. Such an event might necessitate switching the therapy of the pneumocystis infection from TMP-SMX to pentamidine.

A recently marketed murine monoclonal antibody preparation, Orthoclone OKT3, which is often given for acute kidney allograft rejection, has also been associated with an aseptic meningitis syndrome that usually comes on within 72 hours of administration and resolves with cessation of administration of the product.[84]

Another drug that immunocompromises a host, azathioprine, can also cause acute aseptic meningitis. In one of the reported cases the patient had papilledema in addition to headache, meningismus, and CSF pleocytosis.[85] Because papilledema rarely occurs in acute meningitis, the findings in this patient might have suggested chronic meningitis or a space-occupying lesion (e.g., a tumor or brain abscess). Whereas in a patient with papilledema the need to exclude space occupying lesions is not obviated by getting a history of their taking azathioprine, the possibility that azathioprine is causing the meningitis must be considered and administration of the drug discontinued if no alternative cause of the papilledema and meningitis is found.

The nonsteroidal anti-inflammatory agents ibuprofen,[86,87] tolmetin,[88] naproxen,[89] and sulindac have also been reported to cause an aseptic meningitis syndrome; ibuprofen-associated meningitis has occurred primarily in patients with systemic lupus erythematosus or mixed connective tissue disease. Although a number of the patients have developed meningitis on first exposure to the drugs, the circumstances of the reported cases favor a hypersensitivity etiology of the meningitis.

A careful drug history and chart review in a patient with the aseptic meningitis syndrome may identify recent exposure to one of the drugs discussed above and, in conjunction with laboratory tests which fail to indicate the presence of a microbial agent in the CSF, may help avoid unnecessary antibiotic or antiviral therapy.

Other Nonantimicrobial-Requiring Causes of Meningitis. Mollaret's meningitis is characterized by recurrent febrile episodes in which signs and symptoms of meningitis begin abruptly, reach maximal intensity within 12 hours, and diminish over 1–4 days without therapy. The CSF usually shows a polymorphonuclear pleocytosis; mononuclear cells and large "epithelial cells" may also be seen. The patients are free of symptoms between episodies.[90] A variety of other conditions that may produce apparently noninfectious, often recurrent meningitis include Behçet syndrome, Vogt-Koyanagi-Harada syndrome, sarcoidosis, and systemic lupus erythematosus.[34]

STRATEGY FOR DIAGNOSIS AND THERAPY

Recognition of Meningitis

Some patients seek medical attention early in the course of their infection and have only subtle signs of meningitis; these are the patients who have the best chance of recovery if the diagnosis is made promptly and therapy is instituted early. Carpenter and Petersdorf[30] comment on the recognition of meningitis as follows:

> Meningeal infection should be considered in every patient with a history of infection of the upper respiratory tract interrupted by one of the ''meningeal'' symptoms—vomiting, headache, lethargy, confusion or stiff neck. When first seen, some of the patients present a rather unimpressive picture with no more than low-grade fever, mild headache or occasional vomiting. Nevertheless, the possibility of meningeal infection must be carefully considered.

In neonates, infants, and the aged, the signs and symptoms of meningitis may be especially subtle. There may be no more to suggest meningitis than the presence of fever plus irritability, lassitude, confusion, poor feeding, unstable or low temperature, or the occurrence of seizures. Stiff neck or full fontanelles may be relatively late signs of meningitis in infants. Whereas clinical judgment is certainly called for, the adage ''If you think of doing a spinal tap, do one'' still holds. The diagnostic value of a lumbar puncture far outweights the small risk of harm.[91]

Acute Versus Subacute Presentation of Meningitis

Most patients with meningitis have some clear-cut signs and symptoms of meningitis when they are first seen by a physician. There is often fever, heahache, vomiting, photophobia, and mental dysfunction ranging from lethargy to coma. Seizures and cranial nerve deficits are not uncommon, but papilledema oc-

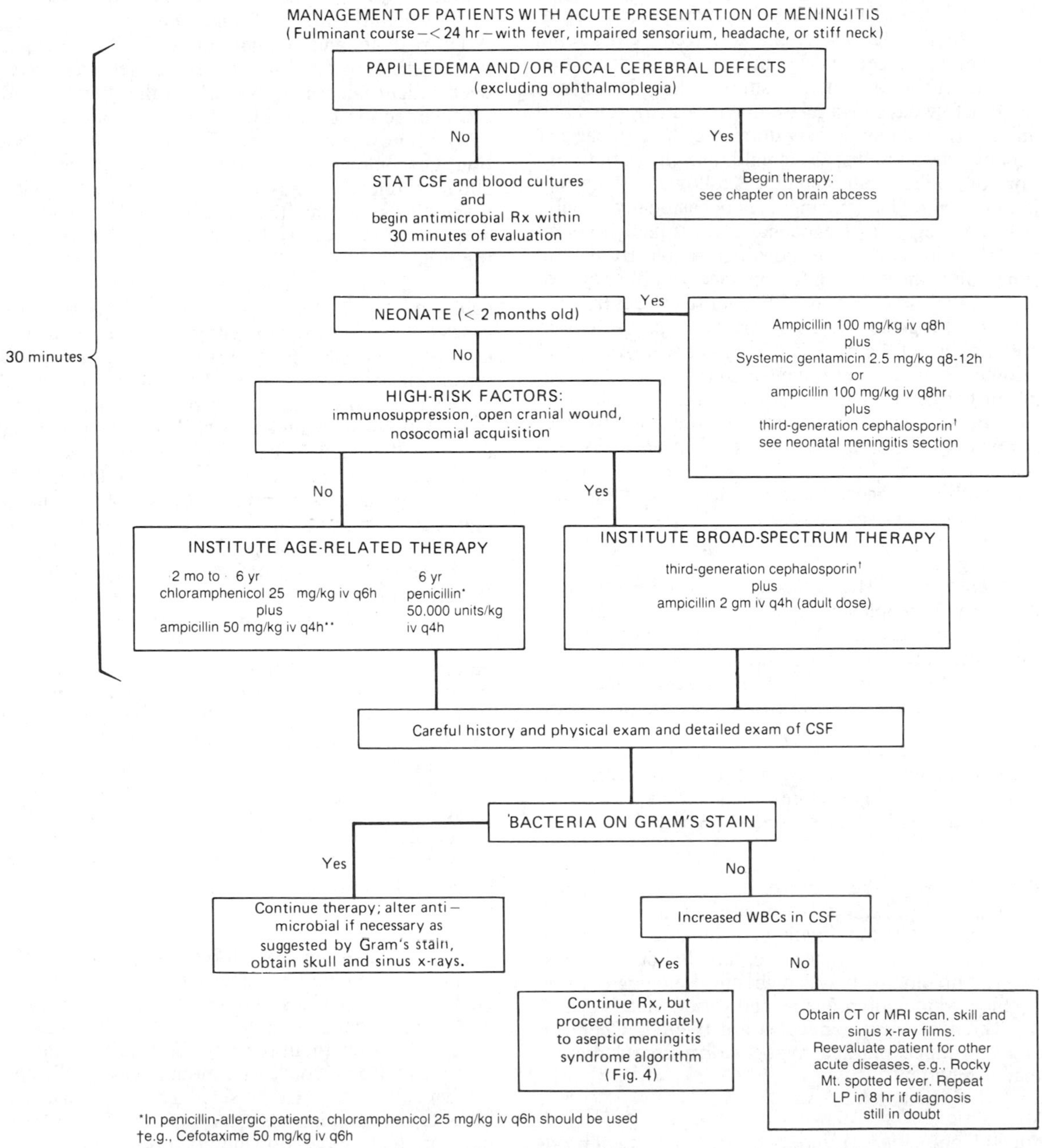

*In penicillin-allergic patients, chloramphenicol 25 mg/kg iv q6h should be used
†e.g., Cefotaxime 50 mg/kg iv q6h
**Third generation cephalosporin is an alternative to chloramphenicol-ampicillin.

FIG. 2. Algorithm for management of patients with acute presentation of meningitis.

curs so infrequently that its presence should prompt a search for a mass lesion such as a brain abscess.[34,91] In patients with such clear-cut signs of meningitis, the examining physician should immediately make the determination of whether the patient has an *acute* or a *subacute* presentation of meningitis. The signs and symptoms may be similar in the two groups. However, in the *acute presentation* (Fig. 2), signs and symptoms have been present less than 24 hours and are rapidly progressive; the most likely etiology is pyogenic bacteria (Table 1); and the death rate is approximately 50 percent. An acute presentation of meningitis will be seen in approximately 10 percent of the patients with infectious meningitis. In the *subacute presentation* (Fig. 3), signs and symptoms have usually been present for 1–7 days before evaluation; there are a number of possible etiologic agents or conditions (e.g., viruses, pyogenic bacteria, leptospires, tubercle bacilli, fungi, parameningeal foci); and the death rate, even in the presence of pyogenic bacterial meningitis, is less than half that of the acute presentation. Almost all patients with viral meningitis and 75 percent of the patients with bacterial meningitis exhibit a subacute presentation of meningitis.[30,34,92]

The first consideration in a patient with the acute presentation of meningitis is therapy, not specific diagnosis, as outlined in Figure 2. The brief physical examination before lumbar puncture should include a check for papilledema or focal neurologic defects (excluding ophthalmoplegia); these findings are a contraindication to a lumbar puncture until a CAT or MRI scan has excluded a mass lesion because of the increased risk of uncal herniation. In this situation, cultures of blood and other appropriate sites should be obtained and therapy initiated immediately thereafter, before getting the CAT scan. If papilledema is not present, blood cultures and CSF are obtained and intravenous antimicrobial therapy is begun with 30 minutes of encountering the patient. Examination of a Gram stain of the CSF before giving therapy would be a waste of potentially valuable therapeutic time. Only the most elementary data are necessary to make an adequate choice of an antimicrobial regimen. (Fig. 21). The need for prompt antimicrobial therapy is emphasized by the occurrence of death within hours of the onset of symptoms in some patients. Especially in acutely ill patients, the goal of therapy is to treat before the pathologic processes of the meningitis are irrevocably committed to lethal progression.

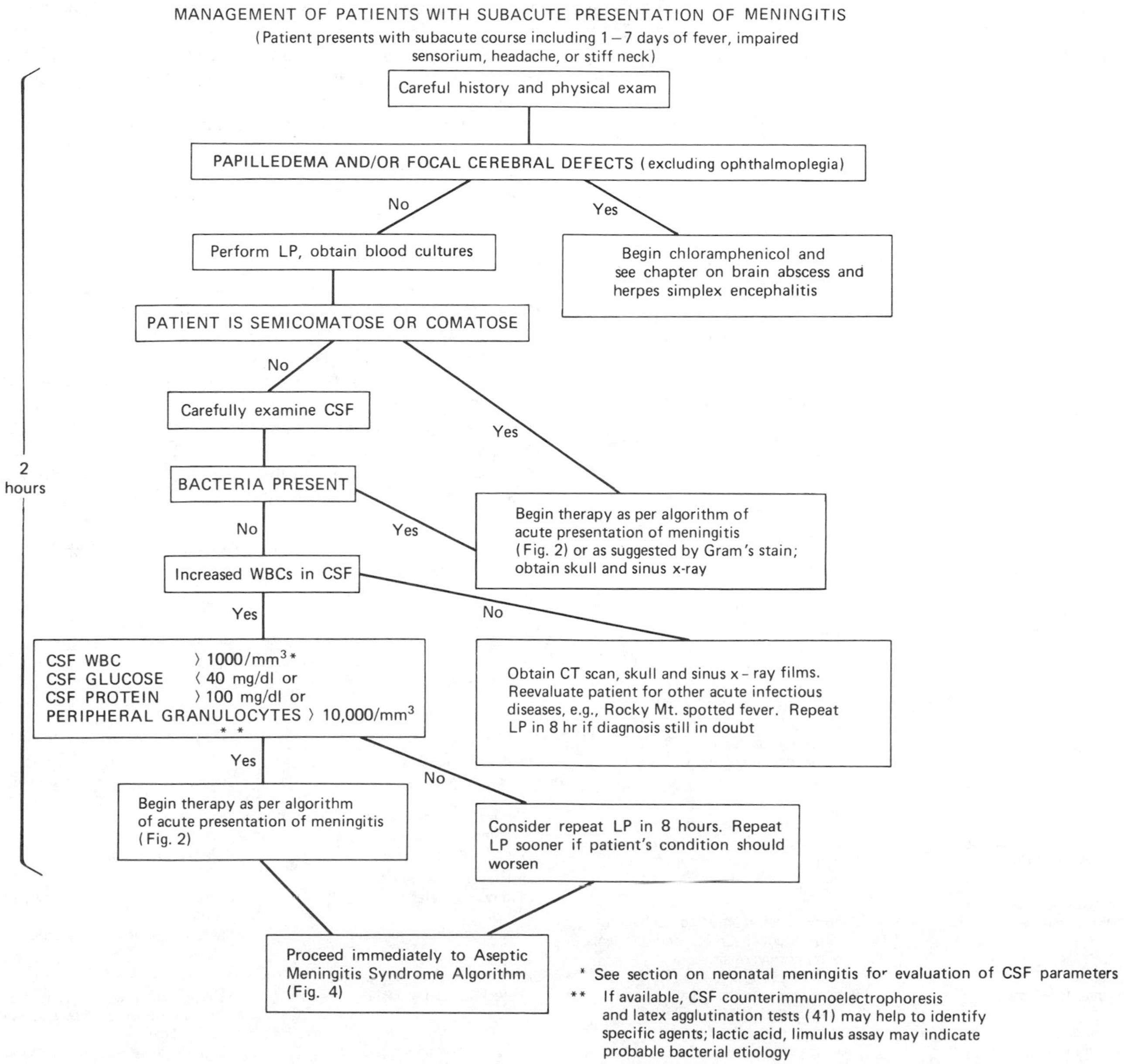

FIG. 3. Algorithm for management of patients with subacute presentation of meningitis.

In a patient with the subacute presentation of meningitis early emphasis is on diagnosis (Fig. 3).

Diagnosis. Once therapy has been initiated in patients with an acute presentation of meningitis (Fig. 2), or once it has been determined that a patient has a subacute presentation of meningitis (Fig. 3), attention should be focused on determining the most likely organism. A decision on the need for a change of therapy in the former group or on the design of optimal therapy in the latter group should be made within 2 hours of first seeing the patient. This generally provides ample time for performing history and physical examinations, for obtaining cultures of blood and CSF, for a complete examination of the CSF (cell count, differential count, protein and glucose level determinations, and special stains), and, if necessary, for tests to detect antigens of specific meningeal pathogens.[43]

As noted in Table 1, the etiologic agent may be bacterial, viral, fungal, protozoan, parasitic, neoplastic, or chemical. Despite this variety of potential causes, the physician who uses an organized approach to the problem can rapidly and correctly predict the etiology agent in a majority of patients. Thus, there are elements of the history (e.g., the season of the year, previous skull fracture) and the physical examination (e.g., a search for midline dermal sinuses [Fig. 1]) that should be systematically considered because they may point to or away from specific microorganisms (Table 2). The physical examination may not only provide clues to the etiology but also may indicate the need for surgery to provide adequate primary therapy or to prevent relapse (Table 3). In addition, the physical examination provides important baseline data to serve as a reference for any changes in the patient's condition. *There is no substitute for the same physician performing a complete initial neurologic examination and carefully reexamining the patient periodically for changes in the neurologic status.*

To decide the most likely etiologic agent, the CSF cell count, differential count, and protein and glucose level determinations may be of limited value. If the cell count is over 1000/mm^3, the protein concentration is over 150 mg/dl, and the glucose concentration less than 30 mg/dl, a bacterial etiology is likely and tuberculous or viral meningitis is quite unlikely (an exception is mumps or lymphocytic choriomengitis).[92] However, for each of these parameters there are 30–40 percent of the cases of bacterial meningitis that overlap the range of values for tuberculous, fungal, and viral meningitis. Although the differential count is more likely to show a predominance of polymorphonuclear leukocytes (PMNs) in bacterial meningitis and a predominance of lymphocytes in nonbacterial meningitis, there is overlap of these groups (e.g., one-third of the cases of tuberculous and viral meningitis have a predominance of PMNs, and about 10 percent of the cases of bacterial meningitis have greater than 80 percent lymphocytes).[92] Therefore the physician is seldom justified in excluding bacterial meningitis and deciding not to treat for it solely on the basis of the CSF cell count and protein and glucose concentrations.

After the history has been taken and the physical examination has been performed (Tables 2 and 3), attention should be focused on performing in a logical sequence those laboratory tests that indicate a specific microbial agent or group of agents (Table 4). Of first priority is a thorough examination of the Gram stained sediment of centrifuged CSF. In 80–90 percent of the patients whose bacterial cultures are positive, the organisms are seen on the Gram stain.[92] This rate is about 60 percent if the patient has had prior antimicrobial therapy.[34,65]

In patients who have bacterial meningitis but for whom the results of the initial Gram stain of the CSF are negative, the history, physical examination, and the characteristics of the CSF can be most helpful. Since therapy cannot await the results of culture, other nonspecific tests suggesting a bacterial etiology (e.g., CSF lactic acid), as well as specific tests for certain bacterial agents (e.g., CIE, limulus lysate assay, and latex agglutination tests,[43,66] should be performed if they are available.

TABLE 2. Historical and Other Data Suggesting Specific Etiologic Agents

Historical Data	*Microorganisms*
Age	
Neonates	*E. coli*, group B streptococci, *Listeria*, herpes simplex 2
Infants <2 months	Group B streptococci, *Listeria*, *E. coli*
Children <10 years	Viruses, *H. influenzae*, pneumococci, meningococci
Young adults	Viruses, meningococci
Adults	Pneumococci, meningococci
Elderly	Pneumococci, gram-negative bacilli, *Listeria*
Epidemiology	
Summer and fall	Coxsackievirus or echovirus, leptospires
Hospital acquired	Gram-negative bacilli, staphylococci, *Candida*
Sibling with meningitis	Meningococci, *H. influenzae*
Swimming in freshwater lake	Amebas
Handling hamsters or mice	Lymphocytic choriomeningitis
Contact with water frequented by rodents or domestic animals	Leptospires
Exposure to tuberculosis	*M. tuberculosis*
Prior meningitis	Pneumococci
Associated infection	
Upper respiratory infection	Viruses, *H. influenzae*, pneumococci, meningococci
Pneumonia	Pneumococci, meningococci
Sinusitis	Pneumococci, *H. influenzae*, anaerobic bacteria
Otitis	Pneumococci, *H. influenzae*, anaerobic bacteria
Cellulitis	Streptococci, staphylococci
Brain abscess	Anaerobes
Trauma	
Closed skull fracture	Pneumococci, gram-negative bacilli
Open skull fracture or craniotomy	Gram-negative bacilli, staphylococci
CSF otorrhea and rhinorrhea	Pneumococci, gram-negative bacilli, staphylococci, *H. influenzae*
Underlying Condition	
Diabetes mellitus	Pneumococci, gram-negative bacilli, staphylococci, *Cryptococcus*, agents of mucormycosis
Alcoholism	Pneumococci
Leukemia, lymphoma	Pneumococci, gram-negative bacilli, *Cryptococcus*, *M. tuberculosis*
Steroid therapy	*Cryptococcus*, *M. tuberculosis*
Acquired immunodeficiency syndrome	HIV, *Cryptococcus*

TABLE 3. Physical Findings of Importance in Patients With Suspected Meningitis

Abnormal Physical Findings	*Clinical and Etiologic Interpretation*
Neurologic	
Impaired higher integrative function	Severe infection, probably pyogenic bacteria; rule out viral encephalitis
Focal cerebral signs	Severe, uncomplicated pyogenic meningitis; rule out brain abscess, herpes encephalitis
Late onset of focal cerebral signs	Delayed thrombosis of cortical veins
Head, eyes, ears, neck, and throat	
Neck stiffness	Suggests infection of subarachnoid space
Sinusitis, otitis, CSF otorrhea or rhinorrhea, skull fracture	See Table 2
Early papilledema	Rule out brain abscess
Cardiac–respiratory	
Pulmonary rales	Pneumococci, meningococci, *H. influenzae*
Pathologic heart murmur	Bacterial endocarditis—pneumococci, *S. aureus*
Skin	
Petechiae and/or rashes	Meningococci, echovirus type 9, leptospires, *S. aureus*, *Haemophilus aegyptius*
Midline dermal sinuses	Gram-negative bacilli, staphylococci
Herpes progenitalis or labialis	Herpes simplex 2

The designation "aseptic meningitis syndrome" is helpful because it circumscribes a number of specific causes of meningitis that should be pursued by the examining physician. It is critical to note that even if the routine bacterial cultures are, or are likely to be, negative, *many of the causes of the aseptic meningitis syndrome require antimicrobial therapy, surgical intervention, or both.* Although the initiation of specific therapy in such patients may be delayed for a few hours pending appropriate diagnostic procedures, complete failure to administer such therapy may result in death or severe morbidity. Thus, the "aseptic meningitis syndrome" cannot be equated solely with aseptic meningitis of viral origin. It is useful to direct the work-up of the aseptic meningitis syndrome to two groups of diagnostic possibilities: (*1*) antimicrobial-requiring causes and (*2*) nonantimicrobial-requiring causes, in that order of priority. A systematic examination of these possible causes of meningitis should aid the physician in reaching an optimal therapeutic decision as rapidly as possible (Fig. 4).

The physician may decide to administer antimicrobial therapy for partially treated meningitis, but this decision should be ac-

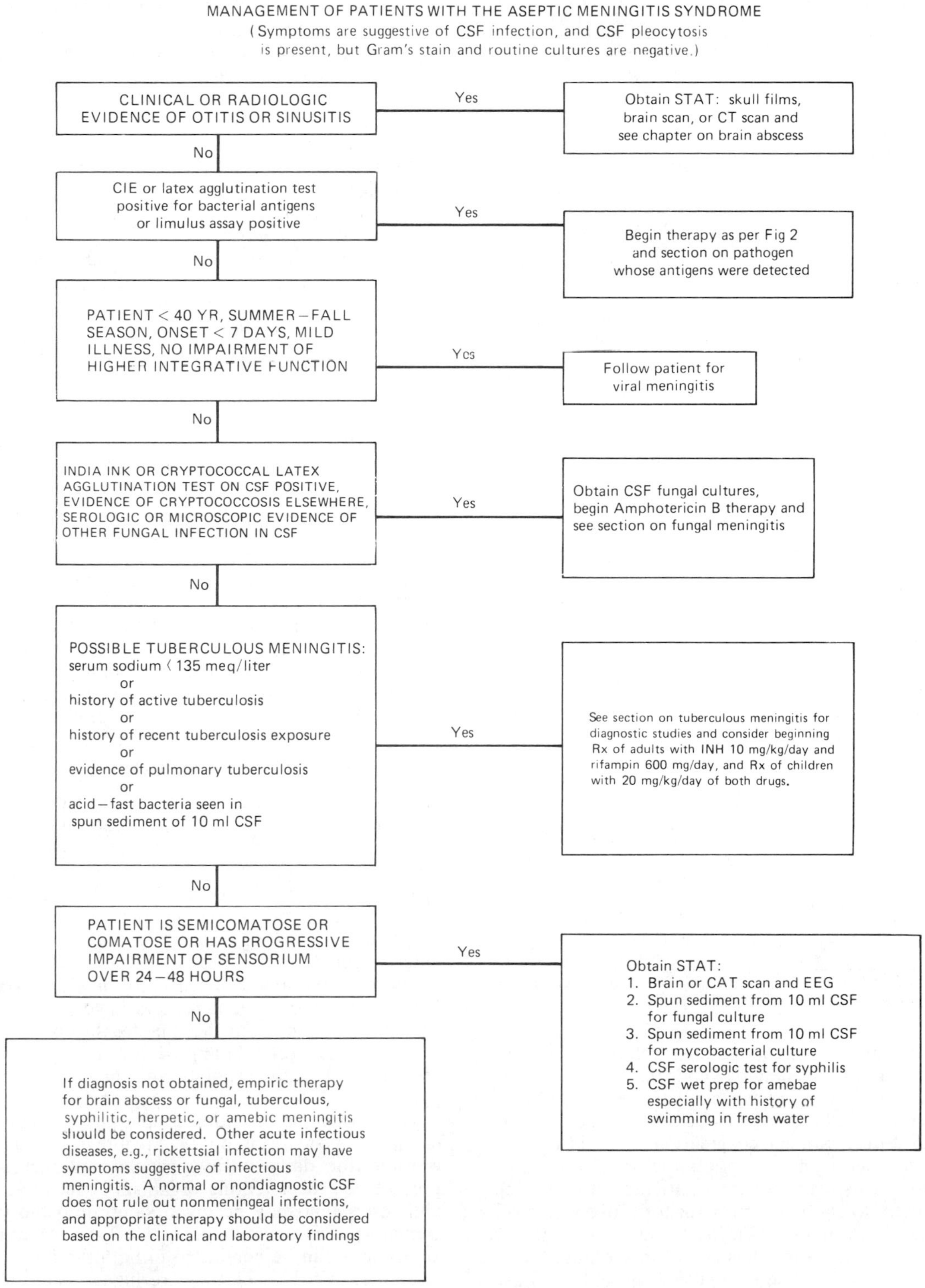

FIG. 4. Algorithm for management of patients with the aseptic meningitis syndrome.

TABLE 4. Laboratory Features in Patients with Suspected Infectious Meningitis

Laboratory Tests	*Interpretation*
Routine CSF evaluation	
Gram stain of centrifuged sediment	Usually positive in bacterial meningitis; more often negative in partially treated bacterial meningitis; always negative in nonbacterial meningitis; should be performed even with no increase in CSF white cells
Culture (include chocolate agar plates)	As above
White blood cell count	Greater than 1200[a] WBC/mm^3 suggests bacterial meningitis
Percent neutrophils	Less than 50%[a] suggests nonbacterial meningitis—but significant overlap
Glucose	Less than 30 mg/dl suggests bacterial, fungal, or tuberculous meningitis[a]
Protein	Greater than 150[a] mg/dl suggests bacterial meningitis
Special CSF evaluations (indicated when Gram stain is negative)	
Observations of supernatant	Orange color suggests subarachnoid hemorrhage
Counterimmunoelectrophoresis (CIE)	Specific for antigens of pneumococci, meningococci, or *H. influenzae*; test not very sensitive, false-negative results frequent
Lactic acid	>35 mg/dl suggests bacterial infection
Latex agglutination	Generally specific for antigens of pneumococci, meningococci, *H. influenzae*, group B streptococci and cryptococci; more sensitive and rapid than CIE
Limulus lysate assay	Positive indicates infection with gram-negative bacteria
Chloride	<110 mEq/liter suggests tuberculous infection if bacterial infection has been excluded
Acid-fast examination of sediment	Positive in >80% of tuberculous meningitis when >10 ml of CSF is spun and carefully evaluated
India ink	Cryptococci are diagnosed by this test; if ameboid movement is seen, *Naegleria* infection should be suspected
Tumor cytology	Tumor cells indicate CNS tumor—does not exclude infectious cause for meningitis
Wet mount	Ameboid movement of what look like monocytes may be amebas
Evaluation of peripheral blood	
Granulocyte count	>10,000 granulocytes/mm^3 suggest bacterial infection
Glucose	A baseline is helpful for comparison with CSF glucose
Serum sodium	<135 mEq/liter suggests inappropriate ADH
Culture	May yield agent causing meningitis when CSF cultures are sterile
Acute and convalescent sera	Important for diagnosis of viral and leptospiral meningitis
Other	
Sputum and bone marrow	Tuberculosis or fungal etiology often suspected by positive sputum or bone marrow examination

[a] Do not assume the converse of CSF parameters (For example, a WBC of <1200 does not imply viral infection since bacterial meningitis is also frequently associated with <1200 WBCs).

companied by an aggressive, continued search for other potential causes of the aseptic meningitis syndrome.

In any case of meningitis, but especially those caused by bacteria, the systemic effects of sepsis—acidosis, tissue hypoxia, and disseminated intravascular coagulation—should be monitored for and managed with appropriate therapy.

For those physicians who encounter patients with meningitis but who refer them to another facility (or for those who advise such physicians by telephone), the best course of action, regardless of whether the patient has acute presentation or not, is to follow those steps outline in Figure 2 through institution of empirical therapy. After intravenous therapy has been begun, the patient, accompanied by the physician's notes (history, physical findings, precise therapy), blood culture bottles, and at least one tube of CSF, should be sent by ambulance to the facility where definitive care can be given. Ideally CSF bacterial cultures, Gram stain, cell count, and protein and glucose level determinations should be performed at the referring facility after the patient has left, and the results of the tests phoned ahead. If this is not possible, the blood culture bottles and all tubes of CSF can be sent with the patient.

NEONATAL MENINGITIS

Neonatal meningitis differs from meningitis in older children and adults in at least two fundamental ways: (*1*) as described in the previous section, the signs and symptoms of meningitis are usually muted or lacking and (*2*) a different spectrum of bacterial pathogens predominates, the origin of these being the vaginal and perineal flora of the mother. The CSF laboratory values in newborns must be interpreted with caution. The CSF white cell count normally ranges from 0 to 30 with polymorphonuclear leukocytes accounting for over 50 percent of the cells. CSF protein concentration normally may be elevated to greater than 150 mg/dl.[13,20] The CSF cell count and protein or glucose concentration may be normal or only slightly altered despite the presence of serious meningitis. Although the CSF findings may thus suggest viral meningitis, when meningitis alone is present in neonates, viruses are seldom the cause; the physician should assume that the most likely pathogen is *E. coli*, group B streptococci, enterococci, or *L. monocytogenes*. Therefore initial therapy of suspected meningitis should include ampicillin (directed against group B streptococci, *Listeria*, and enterococci) and either an aminoglycoside or a third-generation cephalosporin (such as cefotaxime, directed against gram-negative bacilli). If the Gram stain or culture verifies group B streptococcal meningitis, penicillin G, 70,000 units/kg iv q8h, is optimal. Ampicillin, 100 mg/kg iv q8h, is usually adequate for *Listeria* and enterococci. Therapy for gram-negative bacillary meningitis with a third-generation cephalosporin (e.g., cefotaxime 50 mg/kg iv q6h) has been outlined above. Initial therapy of neonatal meningitis with ampicillin plus a third-generation cephalosporin has not yet been shown to be more effective than therapy with ampicillin plus an aminoglycoside. Details of this therapy are discussed in the section on gram-negative bacillary meningitis.

SHUNT-ASSOCIATED MENINGITIS

Approximately 10–30 percent of the patients who have emplacement of a ventriculoatrial or ventriculoperitoneal shunt develop meningitis.[93,94] Clinical illness ranges from low-grade fever to fulminant ventriculitis and sepsis. Coagulase-negative staphylococci (*S. epidermidis*) account for over half of the shunt infections, followed by coagulase-positive staphylococci, *Propionibacterium acnes*, gram-negative bacilli, and enterococci.[93,95]

Systemic therapy alone usually fails to eradicate shunt infection. Although recent reports have stressed that complete removal of the infected shunt under the cover of antimicrobials offers the most reliable approach to therapy, systemic plus intraventricular antimicrobials cure the meningitis in some of the patients without surgical manipulation of the shunt.[96]

Thus, a course of antibiotic therapy without removal of the shunt may be warranted if (*1*) the infection is not fulminant, (*2*) a route for daily intraventricular antimicrobial therapy is present, (*3*) the infecting organism is sensitive to bactericidal antibiotics that may be given safely into the ventricles (e.g., cephalosporins or aminoglycosides), or (*4*) antimicrobial concentrations can be generated in both the intracerebral and extracerebral CSF space that are higher than the mimimal bactericidal concentration for the infecting organisms during most of the interval between doses.

RECURRENT MENINGITIS

Recurrent bacterial meningitis most often signals the presence of a communication of the subarachnoid space with the paranasal sinuses, nasopharynx, middle ear, or skin. Communications with the skin are usually associated with congenital defects of the skull or dura such as cranial or lumbosacral midline dermal sinuses (Fig. 1), dermoid cysts, or myelomeningoceles. The meningitis that results from such lesions if often caused by gram-negative bacilli.[34] Communications with the paranasal sinuses, nasopharynx, and middle ear usually result from fractures of the paranasal sinuses, cribriform plate, or petrous bone, respectively. Some patients have experienced over 10 episodes of meningitis in association with such lesions.[29,34] The causative agent in over 80 percent of such instances is *S. pneumoniae*.[29] If the patient has received antimicrobial prophylaxis, especially with ampicillin, gram-negative bacilli are the more likely causative organisms. The value of such antimicrobial prophylaxis in skull fractures associated with CSF leak is not clear. The occurrence of meningitis in any patient with a history of head trauma—even years previously—should prompt a search for CSF rhinorrhea or otorrhea. This can be done by injecting metrizamide or radioactive tracer into the lumbar CSF and monitoring its appearance in the nose or ear. Testing for rhinorrhea can be done by measuring with glucose oxidase tape the glucose content of nasal secretions, which should be low relative to CSF. Note that this test may falsely indicate that rhinorrhea is only nasal secretions if the patient has a CSF leak with meningitis and hypoglycorrhachia. Any communications that are discovered should be repaired surgically after meningitis has resolved.

In patients with recurrent meningitis, a search should also be made for a parameningeal focus of infection such as those discussed in a previous section. In many cases surgical drainage or removal of such foci is a critical adjunct to antimicrobial therapy.

In diseases such as brucellosis, cryptococcosis, and leptospirosis there may be CNS manifestations; the fluctuation in intensity of clinical manifestations that characterize these diseases can be mistaken for recurrent meningitis.[79,90]

The defects of the immune system most frequently associated with recurrent meningitis include splenectomy, hypogammaglobulinemia, leukemia and lymphoma, sickle and other hemoglobinopathies, and selected defects of the complement system.[25,26,28,34] In some patients with recurrent meningitis no anatomic or functional defects can be found.[97]

A variety of other conditions, such as Mollaret's meningitis, that can cause recurrent meningitis are reviewed in an earlier section.

PREVENTION OF MENINGITIS

The two primary means of preventing meningitis are with antimicrobial prophylaxis (chemoprophylaxis) and with vaccination. They are applied in selected patients who are at increased risk of acquiring meningitis.

Chemoprophylaxis

In meningitis caused by meningococci, the risk to case contacts and the efficacy of chemoprophylaxis has been proved. The avoidance of panic in all the people casually exposed to a case of meningococcal meningitis requires a well-planned strategy on the part of the physician. As soon as the diagnosis is firm and therapy is under way, the physician should notify appropriate public health authorities about the case and work out a program for announcing promptly and aggressively *who should* and *who should not* receive antimicrobial prophylaxis. Prophylaxis should be administered only to intimate contacts of the patient (e.g., family, girlfriends or other intimates, and roommates). Unless there has been intimate contact, it generally is not necessary to provide prophylaxis for classmates, fellow office workers, or members of the bridge club. However, a recent report indicates that school-aged children may be at risk of secondary infection particularly when classrooms are crowded (average midchair distance ≤30 inches), when contact during lunch and recess is frequent, or both.[98] In the absence of prolonged intimate contact, such as might occur during mouth-to-mouth resuscitation, prophylaxis is not necessary for medical personnel caring for a case.[99]

The risk of *H. influenzae* spreading among case contacts in households and day care centers and resulting in serious secondary disease including meningitis approximates similar risks with meningococcal infection.[4,98,100] Rifampin should be given to adults and children in households and day care centers containing children 4 years old or younger, other than the index case, providing that exposure to *H. influenzae* type b was within the week before prophylaxis. The index case may still be a carrier despite successful therapy and should receive rifampin prophylaxis.

The drug of choice for chemoprophylaxis of contacts of patients with meningococcal or *H. influenzae* meningitis is rifampin; for *H. influenzae* prophylaxis of children and adults, one dose of 20 mg/kg (not to exceed 600 mg per dose) a day for each of 4 successive days is most effective.[4] For meningococcal case contacts, one dose of 10 mg/kg (not to exceed 600 mg per dose) twice a day for 2 days appears adequate.

Vaccination

Vaccines are available for protection against selected strains of three of the bacteria that most frequently cause meningitis—*S. pneumoniae* (pneumococcus), *N. meningitidis* (meningococcus), and *H. influenzae* (see Chapter 296).

The meningococcal polysaccharide vaccines licensed are monovalent serogroup A, monovalent serogroup C, bivalent A-C, and quadrivalent A/C/Y/W-135. Monovalent A or C vaccines are recommended for use in epidemics of serogroup A or C meningococcal disease. With the use of serogroup C vaccine in army recruits, the incidence of meningococcal meningitis decreased approximately 90 percent in immunized men as compared with those who received control injections.[101,102] Quadrivalent vaccine is recommended for military personnel and for persons traveling to countries where meningococcal disease is epidemic (e.g., Nigeria). Although there is no effective capsular vaccine for serogroup B, which causes a majority of serious meningococcal disease in the United States, a vaccine composed of type 2 outer membrane protein I, a porin protein, appears promising.[103] Note that meningococcal vaccine should not be used in place of chemoprophylaxis in persons exposed to a case; the protection from immunization is too group specific and too slowly generated in this situation. There is no firm evidence that vaccination is a useful adjunct to chemoprophylaxis. For help in determining whether an epidemic of meningococcal meningitis exists or in obtaining and planning administration of the vaccine, call the Centers for Disease Control ([404]639-3687).

Pneumococcal vaccine, originally released in 1978 composed of 14 capsular serotypes, has been reformulated to include 23 serotypes.[104] Although the spectrum of immunity elicited is broader, the new vaccine is still not expected to prevent all pneumococcal infections.[105] Pneumococcal vaccine is recommended for persons over 2 years of age who are at special risk because of (*1*) functional asplenia (e.g., sickle cell disease) or traumatic asplenia, (*2*) diabetes, and (*3*) cardiorespiratory, hepatic, or renal disease.[106] The vaccine is also recommended for persons over age 50—especially when entering chronic care institutions where pneumococcal infections are endemic or epidemic. For adults, polyvalent pneumococcal vaccine is given in a dose of 0.5 ml intramuscularly. No serious complications have been observed. The optimal interval for a booster is unknown, but booster injections should not be given at less than 3-year intervals.

Although children less than 1 year of age are at particular risk from meningitis caused by pneumococci, meningococci, *H. influenzae*, or *E. coli*, vaccines that protect against these microorganisms currently are not available or are ineffective in this age group. Two different vaccines are available for *H. influenzae* type b, both licensed for use in children 18 months of age or older.[107] One (HbPV) contains the polysaccharide polyribosephosphate (PRP) alone. In the other (HbCV), the PRP is conjugated to diphtheria toxoid. HbCV is currently the preferred vaccine because it elicits higher antibody titers than HbPV.

REFERENCES

1. Suhs RH, Feldman HA. Pneumococcal types detected in throat cultures from a population of "normal" families. Am J Med Sci. 1965;250:424.
2. Greenfield S, Sheehe PR, Feldman HA. Meningococcal carriage in a population of "normal" families. J Infect Dis. 1971;123:67.
3. Robbins JB, Schneerson R, Argaman M, et al. *Haemophilus influenzae* type b: Disease and immunity in humans. Ann Intern Med. 1973;78:259.
4. Glode MP, Daum RS, Halsey NA, et al. Rifampin alone and in combination with trimethoprim in chemoprophylaxis for infections due to *Haemophilus influenzae* type b. Rev Infect Dis. 1983;5:549S.
5. Kaiser AB, Hennekens CH, Saslaw MS, et al. Seroepidemiology and chemoprophylaxis of disease due to sulfonamide-resistant *Neisseria meningitidis* in a civilian population. J Infect Dis. 1974;130:217.
6. Beutler B, Cerami A. Cachectin: More than a tumor necrosis factor. N Engl J Med. 1987;316:379–85.
7. Waage A, Halstensen A, Espevik T. Association between tumour necrosis factor in serum and fatal outcome in patients with meningococcal disease. Lancet. 1987;1:355–7.
8. Guerina NG, Langermann S, Clegg HW, et al. Adherence of piliated *Haemophilus influenzae* type b to human oropharyngeal cells. J Infect Dis. 1982;146:564.
9. Stevens DS, McGee ZA. Attachment of *Neisseria meningitidis* to human mucosal surfaces: Influence of pili and type of receptor cell. J Infect Dis. 1981;143:525.
10. Stephens DS, Hoffman LH, McGee ZA. Interaction of *Neisseria meningitidis* with human nasopharyngeal mucosa: Attachment and entry into columnar epithelial cells. J Infect Dis. 1983;148:369.
11. McGee ZA, Stephens DS, Hoffman LH, et al. Mechanisms of mucosal invasion by pathogenic Neisseria. Rev Infect Dis. 1983;5:708S.
12. Robbins JB, McCracken GH Jr, Gotschlich EC, et al. *Escherichia coli* K1 capsular polysaccharide associated with neonatal meningitis. N Engl J Med. 1974;290:1216.
13. McCracken GH Jr. Neonatal septicemia and meningitis. Hosp Pract. 1976;2:89.
14. Stephens DS, McGee ZA. Association of virulence of *Neisseria meningitidis* with transparent colony type and low-molecular-weight outer membrane proteins. J Infect Dis. 1983;147:282.
15. Griffiss JM, Bertram MA. Immunoepidemiology of meningeal disease in military recuits. II. Blocking of serum bactericidal activity by circulating IgA in the course of invasive disease. J Infect Dis. 1977;136:733.
16. Hook EW, Kaye D. Prophylaxis of bacteria endocarditis. J Chronic Dis. 1962;15:635.
17. Feldman WE. Relation of concentrations of bacteria and bacterial antigen in cerebrospinal fluid to prognosis in patients with bacterial meningitis. N Engl J Med. 1977;296:433.
18. Moxon ER, Smith AL, Averill DR, et al. *Haemophilus influenzae* meningitis in infant rats after intranasal inoculation. J Infect Dis. 1974;129:154.
19. Gregorius FK, Johnson BL Jr, Stern WE, et al. Pathogenesis of hematogenous bacterial meningitis in rabbits. J Neurosurg. 1976;45:561.
20. Conly JM, Ronald AR: Cerebrospinal fluid as a diagnostic body fluid. Am J Med. 1983;75(1B):102.
21. Rahal JJ, Simberkoff MS. Host defense and antimicrobial therapy in adult gram-negative bacillary meningitis. Ann Intern Med. 1982;96:468.
22. Berman PH, Banker BQ: Neonatal meningitis: A clinical and pathological study of 29 cases. Pediatrics. 1966;38:6.
23. Rorke LB, Pitts FW: Purulent meningitis: The pathological basis of clinical manifestations. Clin Pediatr. 1963;2:64.
24. Young LS, LaForce FM, Head JJ, et al. A simultaneous outbreak of meningococcal and influenza infections. N Engl J Med. 1972;287:5.
25. Petersen BH, Lee TJ, Snyderman R, et al. *Neisseria meningitidis* and *Neisseria gonorrhoeae* bacteremia associated with C6, C7 or C8 deficiency. Ann Intern Med. 1979;90:917.
26. Griessmer DA, Winkelstein JA, Luddy R. Pneumococcal meningitis in patients with a major sickle hemoglobinopathy. J Pediatr. 1978;92:82.
27. Johnson RT, Mims CA. Pathogenesis of viral infections of the nervous system. N Engl J Med. 1968;278:23, 84.
28. Winston DJ, Schiffman G, Wang DC, et al. Pneumococcal infections after human bone-marrow transplantation. Ann Intern Med. 1979;91:835.
29. Hand WL, Sanford JP. Posttraumatic bacterial meningitis. Ann Intern Med. 1970;72:869.
30. Carpenter RR, Petersdorf RG: The clinical spectrum of bacterial meningitis. Am J Med. 1962;33:262.
31. Centers for Disease Control. Multiply resistant pneumococcus—Colorado. MMWR. 1981;30:197.
32. Bell WE, Silber DL. Meningococcal meningitis: Past and present concepts. Milit Med. 1971;136:601.
33. Koppes GM, Ellenbogen C, Gebhart RJ. Group Y meningococcal disease in United States Air Force recruits. Am J Med. 1977;62:661.
34. Swartz MN, Dodge PR. Bacterial meningitis: A review of selected aspects. N Engl J Med. 1965;272:725.
35. Gopal V, Bisno AL. Fulminant pneumococcal infections in "normal" asplenic hosts. Arch Intern Med. 1977;137:1526.
36. Dabernat HJ, Delmas C. Comparative activity of cefotaxime and selected β-lactam antibiotics against *Haemophilus influenzae* and aerobic gram-negative bacilli. Rev Infect Dis. 1983;4:401S.
37. Cherubin CE, Corrado ML, Nair SR, et al. Treatment of gram-negative bacillary meningitis: Role of the new cephalosporin antibiotics. Rev Infect Dis. 1983;4:453S.
38. Eigler JOC, Wellman WE, Rooke ED, et al. Bacterial meningitis. I. General review. Proc Mayo Clin. 1961;36:357.
39. Kaiser AB, McGee ZA. Unpublished results.
40. Bradley SL, Dines DE, Brewer NS. Disseminated *Strongyloides stercoralis* in an immunosuppressed host. Mayo Clin Proc. 1978;53:332.
41. Mangi RJ, Quintiliani R, Andriole VT: Gram-negative meningitis. Am J Med. 1975;59:829.
42. Ross S, Rodriguez W, Controni G, et al. Limulus lysate test for gram-negative bacterial meningitis: Bedside application. JAMA. 1975;233:1366.
43. Martin WJ. Rapid and reliable techniques for the laboratory detection of bacterial meningitis. Am J Med. 1983;75(1B):119.
44. Landesman SH, Shah PM, Armengaud M, et al. Past and current roles for cephalosporin antibiotics in treatment of meningitis. Am J Med. 1981;71:693.
45. Kaiser AB, McGee ZA: Aminoglycoside therapy of gram-negative bacillary meningitis. N Engl J Med. 1975;293:1215.
46. Wright PF, Kaiser AB, Bowman CM, et al. The pharmacokinetics and efficacy of an aminoglycoside administered into the cerebral ventricles in neonates: Implications for further evaluation of this route of therapy in meningitis. J Infect Dis. 1981;143:141.
47. Mangi RJ, Holstein LL, Andriole VT. Treatment of gram-negative bacillary meningitis with intrathecal gentamicin. Yale J Biol Med. 1977;50:31.
48. Lee EL, Robinson MJ, Thong ML, et al. Intraventricular chemotherapy in neonatal meningitis. J Pediatr. 1977;91:991.
49. Wirt TC, McGee ZA, Oldfield EH, et al. Intraventricular administration of amikacin for complicated gram-negative meningitis and ventriculitis. J Neurosurg. 1979;50:95.
50. Velvis H, Carrasco N, Hetherington S. Trimethoprim-sulfamethoxazole therapy of neonatal *Proteus mirabilis* meningitis unresponsive to cefotaxime. Pediatr Infect Dis. 1986;5:591–3.
51. McCracken GH Jr, Mize SG. A controlled study of intrathecal antibiotic therapy in gram-negative enteric meningitis of infancy. J Pediatr. 1976;89:66.
52. Lecour H, Sears A, Miranda AM, et al. Treatment of 160 cases of acute bacterial meningitis with cefotaxime. J Antimicrob Chemother. 1984;14(Suppl B):195–202.
53. Norrby SR. Role of cephalosporins in the treatment of bacterial meningitis in adults: Overview with special emphasis on ceftazidime. Am J Med. 1985;79(Suppl 2A):56–61.
54. Ralph ED, Behma RJ. Enterobacter meningitis—treatment complicated by emergence of mutants resistant to cefotaxime. Scand J Infect Dis. 1987;19:577–9.
55. Fong IW, Tompkins KB. Review of *Pseudomonas aeruginosa* meningitis with special emphasis on treatment with ceftazidime. Rev Infect Dis. 1985;7:604–12.
56. Barson WJ, Miller MA, Brady MT, et al. Prospective comparative trial of ceftriaxone vs conventional therapy for treatment of bacterial meningitis in children. Pediatr Infect Dis. 1986;4:362–8.
57. Jacobs RJ, Wells TG, Steele RM, et al. A prospective randomized comparison of cefotaxime vs ampicillin and chloramphenicol for bacterial meningitis in children. J Pediatr. 1985;107:1290–133.
58. Lebel MH, Freij BJ, Syrogiannopoulos GA, et al. Dexamethasone therapy for bacterial meningitis. Results of two double-blind, placebo-controlled trials. N Engl J Med. 1988;319:964–71.
59. Iwarson S, Lidin-Janson G, Svensson R. Listeric meningitis in the noncompromised host. Infection. 1977;5:204.
60. Schröter GPJ, Weil R III. *Listeria monocytogenes* infection after renal transplantation. Arch Intern Med. 1977;137:1395.
61. Schlech WF III. Listeriosis: New pieces to an old puzzle. Arch Intern Med. 1986;146:459–60.

62. Scheer MS, Hirschman SZ. Oral and ambulatory therapy of *Listeria* bacteremia and meningitis with trimethoprim-sulfamethoxazole. Mt Sinai J Med. 1982;49:411.
63. Converse GM, Gwaltney JM Jr, Strassburg DA, et al. Alteration of cerebrospinal fluid findings by partial treatment of bacterial meningitis. Pediatrics. 1973;83:220.
64. Dalton HP, Allison MJ. Modification of laboratory results by partial treatment of bacterial meningitis. Am J Clin Pathol. 1968;49:410.
65. Jarvis CW, Saxena KM. Does prior antibiotic treatment hamper the diagnosis of acute bacterial meningitis? Clin Pediatr. 1972;11:201.
66. Rytel MW: Counterimmunoelectrophoresis in diagnosis of infectious disease. Hosp Pract. 1975;10:75.
67. Baker AS, Ojemann RG, Swartz MN, et al. Spinal epidural abscess. N Engl J Med. 1975;293:463.
68. Schlossberg D, Shulman JA. Spinal epidural abscess. South Med J. 1977;70:669.
69. Nicoll AM. Fatal primary amoebic meningoencephalitis. NZ Med J. 1973;78:108.
70. Cerva L, Novak K. Amoebic meningoencephalitis: Sixteen fatalities. Science. 1968;160:92.
71. Goodman JS, Koenig MG. Amphotericin B: Specifics of administration. Mod Treat. 1970;7:581.
72. Anderson K, Jamieson A. Primary amoebic meningoencephalitis. Lancet. 1972:1:902.
73. Merritt HH, Moore M. Acute syphilitic meningitis. Medicine. 1935;14:119.
74. Tramont EC. Persistence of *Treponema pallidum* following penicillin G therapy. JAMA. 1976;236:2206.
75. Lukehart SA, Hook EW, Baker-Zander SA, et al. Invasion of the central nervous system by *Treponema pallidum*: Implications for diagnosis and treatment. Ann Intern Med. 1988;109:855–62.
76. Cooper DA, Gold J, Maclean P, et al. Acute AIDS retrovirus infection: Definition of a clinical illness associated with seroconversion. Lancet. 1985;1:537–40.
77. Meyer HM Jr, Johnson RT, Crawford IP, et al. Central nervous system syndromes of "viral" etiology: A study of 713 cases. Am J Med. 1960;29:334.
78. Pierce JF, Jabbari B, Shraberg D. Leptospirosis: A neglected cause of nonbacterial meningoencephalitis. South Med J. 1977;70:150.
79. Edwards GA, Domm BM. Human leptospirosis. Medicine. 1960;39:117.
80. Schwartz JF, Balentine JD. Recurrent meningitis due to an intracranial epidermoid. Neurology. 1978;28:124.
81. Gibbons RB. Chemical meningitis following spinal anesthesia. JAMA. 1969;210:900.
82. Kremer I, Ritz R. Aseptic meningitis as an adverse effect of co-trimoxazole. N Engl J Med. 1983;308:1481.
83. Derbes SJ. Trimethoprim-induced aseptic meningitis. JAMA. 1984; 252:2865–6.
84. Centers for Disease Control. Aseptic meningitis among kidney transplant recipients receiving a newly marketed murine monoclonal antibody preparation. MMWR. 1986;35:551–2.
85. Lockshin MD, Kagen LJ. Meningitic reactions after azathioprine. N Engl J Med. 1972;286:1321–2.
86. Jensen S, Torben KG, Bacher T, et al. Ibuprofen-induced meningitis in a male with systemic lupus erythematosus. Acta Med Scand. 1987;221:509–11.
87. Giansiracusa DF, Blumberg S, Kantrowitz FG. Aseptic meningitis associated with ibuprofen. Arch Intern Med. 1980;140:1553.
88. Ruppert GB, Barth WF. Tolmetin-induced aseptic meningitis. JAMA. 1981;245:67–8.
89. Sylvia LM, Forlenza SW, Brocavich JM. Aseptic meningitis associated with naproxen. Drug Intell Clin Pharm. 1988;22:399.
90. Hermans PE, Goldstein NP, Wellman WE. Mollaret's meningitis and differential diagnosis of recurrent meningitis. Am J Med. 1972;52:128.
91. Dillon HC, Gray BM. Bacterial meningitis in children. Guidelines Antibiot Ther. 1977;2:3.
92. Karandanis D, Shulman JA. Recent survey of infectious meningitis in adults: Review of laboratory findings in bacterial, tuberculous, and aseptic meningitis. South Med J. 1976;69:449.
93. Schoenbaum SC, Gardner P, Shillito J. Infections of cerebrospinal fluid shunts: Epidemiology, clinical manifestations and therapy. J Infect Dis. 1975;131:543.
94. Shurtleff DB, Christie D, Foltz EL. Ventriculoauriculostomy-associated infection: A 12-year study. J Neurosurg. 1971;35:686.
95. Simpson PB Jr, Warren GC, Smith RR. Intraventricular cephalothin in childhood ventriculitis. Surg Neurol. 1975;4:279.
96. McLaurin RL. Infected cerebrospinal fluid shunts. Surg Neurol. 1973;1:191.
97. Whitecar JP Jr, Reddin JL, Spink WW. Recurrent pneumococcal meningitis: A review of the literature and studies on a patient who recovered from eleven attacks caused by five serotypes of *Diplococcus pneumoniae*. N Engl J Med. 1966;274:1285.
98. Feigin RD, Baker CJ, Herwaldt LA, et al. Epidemic meningococcal disease in an elementary-school class room. N Engl J Med. 1982;307:1255.
99. Artenstein MS, Ellis RE. The risk of exposure to a patient with meningococcal meningitis. Milit Med. 1968;133:474.
100. Ward JI, Fraser DW, Baraff LJ, et al. *Hemophilus influenzae* meningitis: A national study of secondary spread in household contacts. N Engl J Med. 1979;301:122.
101. Gotschlich EC, Goldschneider I, Artenstein MS. Human immunity to the meningococcus. V. The effect of immunization with meningococcal group C polysaccharide on the carrier status. J Exp Med. 1969;129:1385.
102. Artenstein MS, Gold R, Zimmerly JG, et al. Prevention of meningococcal disease by group C polysaccharide vaccine. N Engl J Med. 1970;282:417.
103. Craven DE, Frasch CE. Protection against group B meningococcal disease: Evaluation of serotype II protein vaccines in a mouse bacteremia model. Infect Immun. 1979;26:110.
104. An expanded pneumococcal vaccine. Med Lett. 1983;25:91.
105. Kaiser AB, Schaffner W. Prospectus: The prevention of bacteremic pneumococcal pneumonia. JAMA. 1974;230:404.
106. Advisory Committee on Immunization Practices: Pneumococcal polysaccharide vaccine. MMWR. 1978;27:25.
107. Gilsdorf JR. *Haemophilus influenzae* type b vaccine efficacy in the United States. Pediatr Infect Dis. 1988;7:147–8.

67. CHRONIC MENINGITIS

MICHAEL KATZMAN
JERROLD J. ELLNER

A large number of infectious and noninfectious diseases can cause the clinical syndrome of chronic meningitis. The onset of symptoms in such cases typically is subacute to chronic with signs of meningoencephalitis such as fever, headache, lethargy, confusion, nausea, vomiting, and stiff neck. Cerebrospinal fluid (CSF) is abnormal with elevated protein concentrations, a pleocytosis that usually is predominantly lymphocytic, and sometimes a low glucose level. The major difficulty during initial evaluation is in distinguishing the rare patient with chronic meningitis from individuals with the more common syndromes of acute meningitis and encephalitis. If the neurologic symptoms and signs either persist or progress clinically and the CSF remains abnormal for a period of at least 4 weeks, the diagnosis of chronic meningitis is appropriate.[1–3] This duration of symptoms was derived empirically to optimize the distinction between patients with chronic progressive disease and those with self-limited processes. In practice, patients frequently are seen by a physician within 1–4 weeks of the onset of symptoms. Prompt diagnosis and institution of appropriate treatment, therefore, may abort the neurologic process before the criteria for chronic meningitis are fulfilled. The diagnosis of chronic meningitis has a number of implications; particularly important are those relating to etiology, management, and prognosis.

Central nervous system (CNS) involvement by most diseases causing chronic meningitis has a high morbidity and mortality. Successful intervention requires the early administration of specific, often potentially toxic forms of therapy. Furthermore, drugs appropriate for treating one cause of chronic meningitis may be contraindicated in others. Therefore, a precise etiologic diagnosis is critical in modifying the course of this syndrome, and broad empirical therapeutic regimens are a poor and sometimes hazardous substitute. While exact diagnosis may prove difficult, certain aspects of the presentation can be helpful in determining causality or at least in limiting the differential diagnosis.

HISTORY

The exposure history may be important in suggesting certain infectious diseases such as tuberculosis, coccidioidomycosis, histoplasmosis, brucellosis, cysticercosis, syphilis, Lyme disease, or the acquired immunodeficiency syndrome (AIDS) with its distinctive spectrum of pathogens. The exposure history should direct the evaluation to include specific serologic studies and other diagnostic tests.

The history also is of importance in distinguishing chronic meningitis from two superficially similar syndromes, acute men-

TABLE 1. Differential Diagnosis of Recurrent Meningitis

Parameningeal focus
Infection
Epidermoid cyst, craniopharyngioma
Post-traumatic (bacterial meningitis)
Aseptic meningitis
Mollaret's meningitis[5]
Systemic lupus erythematosus
Migrainous syndrome with pleocytosis[6]

ingitis or encephalitis with a protracted recovery and recurrent meningitis. In chronic meningitis, onset is insidious and symptoms chronic, although they may wax and wane. Episodes of acute neurologic deterioration sometimes punctuate the clinical course and may be caused by cerebral edema, hydrocephalus, cerebrovascular occlusions, and seizures. Even when symptoms temporarily regress, CSF abnormalities persist and reflect continued disease activity. One confusing syndrome that must be distinguished from chronic meningitis is that of a protracted recovery period that sometimes follows pyogenic or aseptic meningitis and viral encephalitis. In these patients, actual progression of disease is confined to the acute stages of the illness; clearing of the signs, symptoms, and CSF abnormalities, although gradual, may occur during observation. The second syndrome that must be differentiated from chronic meningitis is recurrent meningitis.[4] Patients with recurrent meningitis usually have repeated episodes of acute disease followed by symptom free periods during which signs and symptoms are absent and the CSF is normal (Table 1).

The history also is important in defining the cause of meningitis in those instances in which CNS extension typically occurs as a late manifestation of a previously diagnosed systemic disease. These conditions include acute leukemia, lymphoma, blastomycosis, and Behçet's disease. The history sometimes reveals an underlying disease associated with disordered cellular immunity. In such cases, the differential diagnosis shifts as considered below.

PHYSICAL EXAMINATION

Diagnostic physical findings are rare. However, physical examination may delineate signs of an associated systemic disease that provide a potential source of rapid diagnosis. Skin lesions, although infrequent, are particularly important for their diagnostic value. Even benign-appearing superficial lesions, subcutaneous nodules and abscesses, or draining sinuses should be cultured and biopsy specimens obtained. India ink preparations also should be prepared from expressed material. The eye examination may be helpful if such lesions as choroidal tubercles, sarcoid granulomas, or uveitis are demonstrable. The finding of papilledema also is of significance since it alters the course of the neurologic work-up and contraindicates lumbar puncture. Hepatomegaly may reflect systemic disease involving the liver and increases the potential diagnostic yield of a liver biopsy.

Neurologic examination is of obvious importance in delineating the extent of CNS involvement. However, it is of limited use in differentiating among specific etiologies since mental status changes, meningismus, oculomotor palsies, and less frequently, focal findings, evidence of increased intracranial pressure, and spinal cord signs may be caused by most processes associated with chronic meningitis. Focal signs, however, often reflect a parenchymal mass such as an abscess or granuloma that would dictate specific diagnostic and therapeutic maneuvers. Hydrocephalus may complicate chronic meningitis, and appropriate neuroradiographic evaluation should be initiated when the constellation of headache, nausea, vomiting, mental changes, ataxia, incontinence, and papilledema is present. The finding of hydrocephalus, particularly with associated cranial neuropathies, is suggestive of an infectious etiology with basilar leptomeningitis, although hydrocephalus also may complicate sarcoidosis and CNS tumor. Peripheral neuropathy is noted uncommonly in chronic meningitis and is suggestive of sarcoidosis or Lyme disease.

LABORATORY EVALUATION

The etiology of chronic meningitis ultimately must be established in the laboratory. Abnormalities on chest x-ray films may reflect systemic involvement by the underlying infectious process, carcinoma, or sarcoidosis. These findings should be pursued in an attempt to define the etiology of the meningitis. In more enigmatic cases, thoracotomy may be indicated and is associated with less morbidity and greater yield than a brain biopsy is.

The CSF formula is never itself diagnostic.[7] However, certain abnormalities and patterns are more characteristic of a restricted group of causes of chronic meningitis. A pleocytosis of fewer than 50 cells may occur in most diseases associated with chronic meningitis but is typical of sarcoidosis, carcinoma, and "chronic benign lymphocytic meningitis." Persistence of a neutrophilic pleocytosis suggests infection with *Nocardia, Actinomyces, Brucella*, or several fungi, especially *Candida, Aspergillus*, and the Zygomycetes,[8] although these agents all may present with a lymphocytic pattern. Hypoglycorrhachia limits the differential diagnosis of chronic meningitis somewhat to certain infectious diseases (tuberculosis, fungal infection, syphilis, toxoplasmosis, cysticercosis), sarcoidosis, and carcinoma. However, decreased CSF glucose levels may be found in lymphocytic choriomeningitis virus infection, in mumps meningoencephalitis, after subarachnoid bleeds, occasionally in "chronic benign lymphocytic meningitis," and in diseases associated with recurrent meningitis. Hypoglycorrhachia also may develop during the course of herpes simplex encephalitis, although it is uncommon (5 percent) during the first 3–5 days of hospitalization. Therefore, the finding of depressed CSF glucose early in the course of a patient with presumed herpes simplex virus encephalitis increases the likelihood of an alternative treatable infectious disease such as cryptococcosis or tuberculosis.[9]

Lumbar puncture needs to be repeated periodically both for culture and to follow the course of meningeal inflammation. India ink preparations should be prepared from the sediment of 3–5 ml of CSF. The entire slide must be examined since cryptococci may be present in small numbers. As opposed to artifacts that are seen commonly, encapsulated yeast has a regular, round, distinct capsule and a refractile central structure; budding yeast forms also may be found. The India ink preparation is more likely to be positive in patients with relatively acute presentations and/or immunosuppressed patients with lymphoma or AIDS. In the latter setting, yeast organisms often far outnumber leukocytes in the CSF. Cerebrospinal fluid cytologic studies are indicated in all patients with chronic meningitis. Multiple specimens may be necessary for the diagnosis of CNS involvement by tumor, and negative cytologic studies do not preclude this possibility. The demonstration of a clonal origin of CSF lymphocytes also is useful in the diagnosis of lymphomatous meningitis.[10]

Serologic studies of serum and CSF are extremely important in evaluating the patient for coccidioidomycosis, cryptococcosis, and syphilis and should be performed routinely. In the case of cryptococcal meningitis, relevant testing is for cryptococcal polysaccharide antigen. Serum antibodies to *Brucella* and *Toxoplasma* also may suggest these infections when they are present in high or increasing titers. Serum antibodies to *Histoplasma* are found in fewer than one-half of patients with *Histoplasma* meningitis. Complement-fixing antibodies to *Histoplasma* are found in most patients with CNS histoplasmosis, but there is an unacceptably high (25–50 percent) rate of false-positive test results in other fungal meningitides.[11,12] More promising is the detection of *H. capsulatum* antigen in serum, urine, or CSF by radioimmunoassay.[13] Recent studies indicate selective compartmentalization of lymphocytes and antibody-producing cells in the CNS. Cerebrospinal fluid lymphocytes may be more reactive to specific antigens than blood lymphocytes.[14] A relative or absolute increase in antibody levels in the CSF as compared with serum, indicative of local production rather than passive diffusion, may prove important in the diagnosis of tuberculosis[15] and other chronic infections as it has in herpes simplex encephalitis. Ultimately, the demonstration of constituents of the causative organism in CSF, so useful in the diagnosis of cryptococcal disease, may be extended to other infections; for example, tuberculostearic acid in CSF might be indicative of tuberculous meningitis.[16]

Skin testing should be limited to tuberculin purified protein derivative (PPD) and antigens to test for anergy. Repeated skin testing may be helpful when tuberculosis is a possibility. Fungal skin test antigens are of no use diagnostically and may cause confusion by altering the fungal serologies, particularly in the case of histoplasmosis.

Cultures are mandatory even when a specific diagnosis is suggested by serologies or other studies. Cerebrospinal fluid should be cultured at least three times for bacteria, acid-fast bacilli, and fungi and more numerous samples obtained and cultured in their entirety when the cause of the meningitis remains uncertain after the initial diagnostic evaluation is complete. The low density of fungi in the CSF and difficulty in culturing certain organisms may delay the diagnosis of some mycotic infections. In such cases, the yield can be improved by inoculating Sabouraud agar layered on the bottom of Erlenmeyer flasks with large volumes of CSF. The finding of even a single colony of an organism capable of causing chronic meningitis such as *Sporothrix schenckii* should never be disregarded as a contaminant.[17] In fact, it may be useful to continue to examine fungal cultures for at least 4–6 weeks because the growth of such organisms can be exceedingly slow. Ventricular CSF may have a higher cultural yield than lumbar CSF in certain infections.[18] Urine, sputum, gastric washings, stool, and blood cultures should be obtained and processed routinely and for mycobacteria and fungi even in the absence of clinical evidence of extraneural infection. These ancillary cultures frequently are positive in cases of cryptococcosis, tuberculosis, histoplasmosis, and blastomycosis. Special culture techniques such as anaerobiosis or increased carbon dioxide tension also are appropriate in the search for certain pathogens such as *Actinomyces* species and *Brucella abortus*, respectively.

Biopsy of specific tissues should be directed by abnormal findings on physical examination. Skin, lymph node, and liver biopsy specimens may demonstrate granulomas, sometimes with caseation and occasionally with an organism demonstrable on special staining. Caseation is suggestive of tuberculosis, histoplasmosis, and coccidioidomycosis. Focal necrosis may be found in brucellosis. All biopsy specimens should be cultured for bacteria, fungi, and mycobacteria. Bone marrow biopsy and culture are particularly useful in tuberculosis and histoplasmosis. Liver biopsy is indicated when miliary tuberculosis is suspected, even in the absence of hepatomegaly or abnormal liver function. Meningeal and brain biopsies should be performed and ventricular fluid sampled at the time of craniotomy for exploration of a mass or other focal lesion or indicated ventricular shunting procedures. In addition, despite the relatively low yield of nondirected meningeal and brain biopsies, these are indicated in patients with undiagnosed clinically progressive meningitis or in individuals with marked functional limitation.

Additional Radiographic Techniques

Computed axial tomography (CT) should be performed on all patients with chronic meningitis and allows a demonstration of inflammation at the base of the brain. The basal cisterns may be obscured, at least partly, by inflammatory tissue with attenuation similar to brain.[19] Areas of granulomatous inflammation show contrast enhancement. Similar findings occur with leptomeningeal infiltration by tumor. CT scanning also is useful to search for focal parenchymal lesions and hydrocephalus. The demonstration of hydrocephalus is not itself a sufficient indication for ventricular shunting since neurosurgical procedures have a high morbidity and failure rate in chronic meningitis. Furthermore, hydrocephalus may clear spontaneously with treatment of the underlying condition. Nonetheless, if clinical deterioration attributable to hydrocephalus occurs, a surgical approach must be considered. In enigmatic cases, magnetic resonance imaging has the potential to add further information, although the abnormalities often are not specific or diagnostic.

Ancillary procedures such as mammography and gastrointestinal radiographic series may be appropriate in the search for a primary carcinoma when meningeal carcinomatosis is suspected.

THERAPEUTIC TRIALS

Therapeutic trials are indicated when the specific etiology remains uncertain despite comprehensive evaluation. However, further attempts at establishing a diagnosis should be continued actively during such trials. The interpretation of the response to empirically administered drugs may be quite difficult since clinical improvement is often slow, even when the agent selected is appropriate. When the patient is stable, sequential trials are indicated, reserving amphotericin B for last and avoiding corticosteroids, which may have a disastrous effect on undiagnosed fungal infection.

An empirical trial of antituberculous drugs clearly is appropriate when the presentation and CSF formula are consistent with tuberculosis and there is evidence of active or prior tuberculous infection. Recent studies suggest that initial tuberculin skin test results are negative in up to 35 percent of patients with tuberculous meningitis.[20] Therefore, empirical antituberculous therapy in fact is indicated in most cases of undiagnosed chronic meningitis. Adequate cultures of CSF, urine, sputum, or gastric aspirates must be obtained before starting therapy and should include biopsy specimens of liver and bone marrow if miliary disease is suspected. Repeat intermediate-strength PPD skin testing after 2–4 weeks also may be of value if the initial studies are negative. The second-strength tuberculin skin test is less frequently negative than intermediate tests are and may be helpful. Positive cultures or a clinical response to antituberculous treatment despite negative cultures would be an indication to complete a full course of therapy.

An empirical trial of penicillin, 20 million units/day, or tetracycline, 2 g/day for 1 month, should be effective for meningitis due to actinomycosis and Lyme disease or brucellosis, respectively. Such treatment is indicated in the presence of a parameningeal focus suggesting actinomycosis when chronic meningitis occurs in late summer or early fall, particularly with confirmatory *Brucella* serologies and exposure history or in an area endemic for Lyme disease.

Empirical use of amphotericin B should be withheld as long as possible in view of its toxicity and the difficulty in determining the duration of administration even when the causative fungus is known. However, when chronic meningitis is caused by certain fungi (*Histoplasma, Blastomyces, Sporothrix*), cultures of lumbar CSF typically are negative. Generally empirical treatment with amphotericin B should be reserved for patients with progressive chronic meningitis who remain undiagnosed despite meningeal biopsy. Once initiated empirically, amphotericin B should be administered for 10–12 weeks intravenously. The development of nephrotoxicity should indicate a reduction in daily dose rather than discontinuation of the trial. Shorter-term trials of this drug are of little value. If patients respond to amphotericin B but relapse, a pattern suggestive of coccidioidal or cryptococcal meningitis, intrathecal therapy must be considered.

Empirical trials of corticosteroids are contraindicated because of potential catastrophic adverse effects on unrecognized fungal meningitis. In addition, the efficacy of this form of therapy has not been established in those forms of chronic meningitis generally considered to be corticosteroid responsive such as sarcoidosis.

DIFFERENTIAL DIAGNOSIS

A number of conditions may cause syndromes resembling chronic meningitis superficially but are usually distinguishable from it on clinical grounds at presentation or during evaluation and observation of the patient (Table 2). In addition, a careful history is important to differentiate between recurrent and chronic meningitis since the former syndrome connotes a different spectrum of diseases (Table 1).

Those infections causing the syndrome of chronic meningitis (Table 3) are discussed in detail in other chapters. Features that are important in establishing the cause of the chronic meningitis are reviewed here.

Tuberculous Meningitis

Tuberculous meningitis[20–29] results from rupture of a superficial infective focus into the subarachnoid space. In younger patients, this event typically is associated with active, progressive systemic disease. Stigmata of miliary tuberculosis may be present on physical examination and on chest x-ray films. Tuberculin skin test results frequently are negative initially, but "conversion" is noted on repeated skin testing. The diagnosis of tuberculosis usually is confirmed by smear, biopsy, and cultures obtained from extraneural specimens as well as CSF culture. In contrast, tuberculous meningitis in the adult more frequently results from the discharge of an old tuberculous focus into the subarachnoid space. As a result, physical examination, chest x-ray films, and extraneural cultures often are not helpful; despite presumably long-standing tuberculous infection, recent series indicate that the initial tuberculin skin test result is negative in up to 35 percent of patients. The diagnosis rests on the outcome of CSF cultures. As a result of the frequent early use of antituberculous therapy empirically, more cases now are "unproved" culturally, but the diagnosis of tuberculosis is suggested by an apparent response to treatment.[25] Overall there is nothing about the clinical syndrome of tuberculous meningitis that distinguishes it from other etiologies of chronic meningitis. About one-half of the patients have had symptoms for over 2 weeks. Ocular palsies, particularly due to involvement of nerve VI, are found in 30–70 percent of the cases. The typical CSF findings consist of a lymphocytic pleocytosis, usually of 100–500 cells, increased protein concentration and depressed glucose levels in two-thirds of the patients on the initial lumbar puncture. This formula also is not specific for tuberculous meningitis. However, in unclear cases, progressive decrease in CSF glucose in the absence of specific treatment may be useful in distinguishing tuberculosis from aseptic meningitis and viral encephalitis. Cytologic examination of CSF often shows activated monocytoid cells and rarely Langhans cells.[27] It should be noted that neutrophils may predominate, particularly during the first 10 days of symptoms. Cerebrospinal fluid smears contain acid-fast bacilli in 10–22 percent of the cases; a smear of the pellicle formed on standing may increase the diagnostic yield. Cerebrospinal fluid cultures are positive in 38–88 percent of the cases and sputum and gastric washings each in about 50 percent. Cerebrospinal fluid tests under evaluation for the presumptive diagnosis of tuberculous meningitis include adenosine deaminase levels (elevated due to release by T lymphocytes), bromide partitioning (abnormal due to alterations in the blood-brain barrier), and various antibody and antigen detection assays.[28] Conversion of the tuberculin skin test result from negative to positive is a supportive finding. In view of the 4- to 6-week delay often inherent in interpreting cultural results, empirical antituberculous therapy is appropriate in the patient with unexplained chronic meningitis. The duration of therapy needs to be individualized, with attention to the clinical course and results of repeat tuberculin skin testing if all cultures are negative after 6 weeks.

TABLE 2. Diseases That Sometimes Resemble Chronic Meningitis

Infectious etiologies
Aseptic meningitis
Viral and nonviral encephalitis
Partially treated bacterial meningitis
Parameningeal infections
Infective endocarditis
Noninfectious diseases
Metabolic and other encephalopathies
Brain tumor
Subarachnoid hemorrhage
Subdural hematoma
Multiple sclerosis
Systemic lupus erythematosus
Postinfectious encephalitis
Giant cell arteritis
Thrombotic thrombocytopenic purpura

TABLE 3. Infectious Diseases That May Be Manifest as Chronic Meningitis

Tuberculosis	Actinomycosis[a]
Cryptococcosis	Phaeohyphomycosis (chromomycosis)[a]
Coccidioidomycosis	Toxoplasmosis[a]
Histoplasmosis	Cysticercosis[a]
Candidiasis	Rarer infectious etiologies
Blastomycosis[a]	*Pseudallescheria boydii*
Syphilis	*Sporothrix schenckii*
Brucellosis	Agents of mucormycosis
Toxoplasmosis[a]	*Coenurus cerebralis*
Nocardiosis[a]	*Leptospira icterohaemorrhagiae*
Lyme disease	*Angiostrongylus cantonensis*

[a] More commonly occur as brain abscesses or focal lesions.

Cryptococcal Meningitis

Cryptococcal meningitis[20,29–34] presents in several different fashions, but the most characteristic, that of a subacute to chronic meningoencephalitis, is not at all distinctive among the etiologies of chronic meningitis. Exposure history is of little value clinically since this yeastlike fungus is a widespread saprophyte. Although one-half of patients in the pre-AIDS era lacked gross immunologic deficits, an underlying cellular immune dysfunction was known to predispose to this infection. The development of chronic meningitis in patients with Hodgkin's disease or lymphosarcoma, in persons receiving high-dose daily corticosteroid therapy, or in individuals at risk for AIDS, suggests this diagnosis. In the previously healthy person, cryptococcal meningitis may cause an extremely indolent illness with gradual progression of dementia. The India ink preparation frequently is negative in such cases. More commonly, the onset of disease is subacute, at times mimicking a brain tumor, particularly when signs of increased intracranial pressure are present. In patients with hematologic malignancies or AIDS, the initial manifestations of cryptococcosis may be unexplained fever. However, CNS involvement often evolves rapidly. Cerebrospinal fluid abnormalities include a lymphocytic pleocytosis, generally with 40–400 cells, and a depressed glucose level in 55 percent of the cases. In patients with AIDS, the CSF often shows little evidence of an inflammatory response.[33,34] Overall, the India ink preparation suggests the diagnosis of cryptococcal meningitis in over one-half of cases. The yield is highest in patients with an acute syndrome. More than 85 percent of patients have cryptococcal polysaccharide antigen in the CSF. However, serum also should be processed for this antigen; the overlap between significant antigen titers in the serum and CSF allows a presumptive diagnosis of cryptococcosis in 94 percent of the cases. Negative serologies do not exclude a diagnosis of cryptococcal meningitis. Cultural confirmation of the diagnosis is mandatory. The initial CSF culture is positive in three-quarters of patients; additional CSF cultures increase this yield and are indicated. Cultures of urine, sputum, stool, and blood also should be obtained. They have both diagnostic and prognostic value and frequently are positive in the absence of overt signs of extraneural infection. CSF cultures and serologies also are indicated in all patients with extraneural cryptococcal infection since they may have subclinical CNS disease.

Coccidioidal Meningitis

Exposure history is important in the diagnosis of coccidioidal meningitis since this infection is endemic in certain arid and semiarid areas of the Western Hemisphere.[35–40] Central nervous system infection may be a part of generalized coccidioidomycosis or may represent the sole extrapulmonary site of active clinical disease. Headache is the most prominent finding in patients with coccidioidal meningitis; the clinical syndrome is, however, in no way distinctive from the other causes of chronic meningitis. Skin tests with coccidioidin usually are negative in patients with meningitis. However, complement-fixing antibody to the causative organism is found in the CSF of 75–95 percent of such patients. A presumptive diagnosis is possible when chronic meningitis occurs in the presence of demonstrated systemic coccidioidomycosis or a serum complement fixation titer to *Coccidioides immitis* of at least 1:16. Cerebrospinal fluid findings resemble those of cryptococcal meningitis; CSF cultures are positive in one-third to one-half of the cases, and rarely, spherules of *C. immitis* may be present on a smear.

Histoplasma Meningitis

Although demonstrable spread to the CNS occurs in about one-quarter of the autopsied cases of disseminated histoplasmosis, neurologic symptoms usually are not prominent. *Histoplasma* meningitis[41–44] has been reported rarely and usually occurs without overt signs of extraneural infection. The clinical syndrome of *Histoplasma* meningitis is not differentiable from the other causes of chronic meningitis. A diagnosis of this entity may be extremely difficult in view of the absence of reliable serologic and skin tests and the paucity of viable fungi in the CSF. Nonetheless, serologies for antibody and *Histoplasma* antigen as discussed above and the repeated culture of large volumes of CSF sometimes have allowed a diagnosis to be made when initial cultures were negative.

Other Infectious Etiologies

Involvement of the CNS is common in disseminated candidiasis, but the clinical syndrome of chronic meningitis is less frequent. Most patients developing *Candida* meningitis[45,46] have significant underlying disease, although hematologic malignancy has not been prominent. Rather, *Candida* meningitis occurs in some of the other settings associated with disseminated candidiasis, i.e., prior antibiotic and corticosteroid therapy, indwelling bladder or venous catheters, and recent abdominal surgery. One-third of the patients are under 2 years of age. The expression of the meningitis is variable, but the average delay between the onset of symptoms and diagnosis has been 17 weeks. The mean CSF pleocytosis in one series was 600 cells; about one-half of the patients had lymphocytes predominating. Hypoglycorrhachia is present in 60 percent of the cases. Yeast cells have been noted on CSF smears in 43 percent of the cases, and results of CSF cultures usually are diagnostic. Overall, 71 percent of the patients with meningitis have active extraneural *Candida* infection, and an additional 14 percent have had antecedent invasive CNS procedures such as ventricular shunting or lumbar puncture, which are presumably responsible for introduction of the yeast into the subarachnoid space. Although spontaneous recovery has been recorded, antifungal therapy clearly seems indicated.

Syphilitic meningitis[47,48] is a rare but easily diagnosed and treated form of secondary syphilis. The disease is usually subacute, with the symptoms persisting for over 1 month in about one-quarter of the cases. Meningitis is the first overt sign of syphilis in 25 percent of meningitic patients. When extraneural manifestations have occurred, they generally preceded CNS involvement by less than 2 years. The clinical presentation and CSF abnormalities resemble those of the other causes of chronic meningitis. Hypoglycorrhachia is present in 55 percent of the cases. The diagnosis of syphilitic meningitis is suggested by positive CSF and serum serologies for syphilis. Transient dramatic deterioration of patients with meningitis after the initiation of penicillin therapy should suggest a Jarisch-Herxheimer reaction and the possibility of syphilis.

Borrelia burgdorferi, the cause of Lyme disease, is another spirochete associated with chronic meningitis. After the bite of an infected tick, the characteristic skin lesion of erythema chronicum migrans may or may not occur and is followed by neurologic symptoms in approximately one-third of cases. Cranial or peripheral neuropathies may be prominent.[49] The diagnosis is made by appropriate serologies in serum and CSF,[50] especially in the setting of tick exposure in an endemic area in late summer or early fall.

A meningoencephalomyelitis may follow the initial manifestations of brucellosis by 2 months to 2 years in fewer than 5 percent of cases.[51–55] Exposure to unpasteurized milk products or contact with cows, goats, sheep, swine, or their carcasses suggests the diagnosis. The patient also may have or have had symptoms and signs of systemic brucellosis such as night sweats, unexplained fever, orchitis, and hepatosplenomegaly. The clinical presentation of the meningitis and CSF abnormalities usually are nonspecific. However, transient episodes of hemianesthesia or paresthesia can be prominent in neurobrucellosis. Serologic studies often suggest the diagnosis of brucellosis. In chronic cases, calcified foci may be noted in the liver and spleen on abdominal x-ray films. Cultures should be maintained in an increased carbon dioxide atmosphere for 3 weeks. Cerebrospinal fluid cultures are positive for *Brucella* in fewer than one-half of the cases. Blood cultures are occasionally positive. *Sporothrix schenckii* has been described as a cause of chronic meningitis, and the CSF may demonstrate *Sporothrix* antibody before the fungus is recovered by culture.[56]

Central nervous system involvement by a large number of infections commonly is expressed as brain abscesses or other focal lesions occurring by hematogenous seeding or direct extension from clinically apparent extraneural sites. Rarely, the syndrome of chronic meningitis may be caused by these agents, sometimes without other stigmata of the infection. Infectious diseases belonging in this category include North American blastomycosis,[18,57,58] paracoccidioidomycosis,[59] cerebral dematiomycosis,[60] actinomycosis,[61–64] nocardiosis,[65,66] and toxoplasmosis.[67–69] One-half of patients with cerebral cysticercosis have the clinical syndrome of chronic meningitis; the frequent finding of hypoglycorrhachia is a somewhat confusing feature.[70–72]

Several infectious agents have been documented to cause chronic meningitis in unique epidemiologic circumstances (*Angiostrongylus cantonensis, Coenurus cerebralis*)[1] or in isolated case reports (*Leptospira icterohaemorrhagiae*, mucormycosis)[1,73] and will not be discussed. Other infections in which CNS involvement is a late manifestation with few related symptoms or leptomeningitis is noted pathologically but not clinically, also will not be reviewed.

Neoplastic Meningitis

The noninfectious diseases causing chronic meningitis may be difficult to diagnose and distinguish from occult infections (Table 4). Primary and metastatic, hematologic, and solid tumors all may involve the meninges diffusely to cause a similar clinical syndrome. In the case of acute leukemia and lymphoma,[74–76] CNS involvement usually occurs in the setting of known underlying malignancy. The major diagnostic problem involves distinguishing CNS involvement by the tumor from superimposed CNS infection and the uncommon paraneoplastic syndromes. Primary brain tumors including gliomas, pinealomas, ependymomas, and choroid plexus tumors may involve the meninges diffusely,[77] sometimes without gross parenchymal involvement. A diagnosis can be difficult in such cases. In metastatic "meningeal carcinomatosis,"[78–82] the nature of the meningeal process also may be difficult to ascertain. In one large series, the primary tumor had not been diagnosed at the onset of neurologic symptoms in 75 percent of the patients,[80] although the figure was 8 percent in patients selected by admission to an oncology center.[81] Typically, the onset of symptoms is subacute, with an intractable headache a prominent complaint along with mental changes. Cranial neuropathy occurs in 50 percent of the cases, and meningismus in about 20 percent. Fever usually is absent or when it occurs is associated with an intercurrent infection. Characteristically, neurologic signs far exceed symptoms and indicate widespread neurologic dysfunction; cerebral, cranial nerve, and spinal involvement are noted in one-half of the patients on initial physical examination. Cerebrospinal fluid is abnormal; 72 percent of the patients have a pleocytosis, often minimal, although occasional patients have a marked cellular response. The glucose content is depressed in 38 percent of the patients initially and in 72 percent during serial examinations. The finding of marked hypoglycorrhachia in the presence of minimal pleocytosis should suggest this diagnosis. In one series, CSF cytologies were diagnostic in 42 percent of patients on the first study and in 74 percent when multiple specimens were processed.[81] Of the ancillary neurodiagnostic tests, the myelogram was particularly helpful diagnostically and revealed multiple nodular deposits on nerve roots in 39 percent of the cases. The finding of markedly elevated CSF levels of β-glucuronidase is suggestive of meningeal carcinomatosis.[83] The most frequent primary sites of malignancy causing this syndrome are the breast, lung, stomach, pancreas, and skin (melanoma). Although neurologic signs may fluctuate and even partly regress, the course of meningeal carcinomatosis usually is rapidly progressive with involvement of all parts of the neuraxis. Since the primary tumor may be occult and extraneural metastatic sites lacking, cytologic examination of multiple CSF specimens is appropriate in all patients with undiagnosed chronic meningitis.

Sarcoid Meningitis

The neurologic manifestations of sarcoidosis are protean.[84–89] Chronic basilar granulomatous meningitis frequently occurs in the setting of characteristic systemic sarcoidosis. However, CNS involvement may be the presenting feature or the sole clinical manifestation of the disease. The clinical syndrome of sarcoid meningitis often includes cranial nerve palsies, long-tract and cerebellar abnormalities, and changes in mentation. The predilection for the basilar meninges with extension to the hypothalamus results in diabetes insipidus in 14–30 percent of the cases; this is of diagnostic significance because it rarely occurs in other forms of chronic meningitis. In addition, peripheral neuropathies accompany CNS sarcoidosis in 14 percent of patients but generally are unusual in chronic meningitis except for Lyme disease. Characteristic CSF abnormalities consist of a minimal lymphocytic pleocytosis in 60 percent of the patients and hypoglycorrhachia in 18 percent. The diagnosis of CNS sarcoidosis in patients with classic systemic manifestations of the disease is complicated by the necessity of excluding superimposed tuberculosis or cryptococcosis that occur with increased frequenty in sarcoidosis and in patients receiving corticosteroid therapy. The diagnosis is more difficult when disease is limited to the CNS. Even the demonstration of granulomas in meningeal biopsy specimens is not specific. Although corticosteroids are recommended for the treatment of CNS sarcoidosis, their efficacy has not been established rigorously. Low-dose irradiation of the CNS has been used with apparent advantage in one patient.[89]

TABLE 4. Noninfectious Causes of Chronic Meningitis

Neoplasm
Sarcoidosis
Granulomatous angiitis
Uveomeningoencephalitis
Behçet's disease
Chronic benign lymphocytic meningitis[a]
Chronic meningitis of unknown etiology[a]

[a] Some cases may be due to infecious agents.

Other Noninfectious Etiologies

Granulomatous angiitis is a necrotizing vasculitis of small leptomeningeal and perforating arteries and veins.[90–94] The process is usually manifested as a subacute meningoencephalitis in patients over 45 years of age. Cerebrospinal fluid findings include minimal lymphocytic pleocytosis and elevated protein levels. The major involvement by this syndrome has been limited to the CNS, although one patient developed a generalized granulomatous angiitis. The diagnosis can only be made from brain biopsy specimens or at autopsy. Corticosteroids may have had a saluatory effect in some cases, but the disease has been invariably fatal. On clinical and pathologic grounds, this syndrome is distinct from sarcoidosis, giant cell arteritis, and Wegener's granulomatosis. Central nervous system vasculitis also may accompany or follow ophthalmic zoster; in some instances, varicella-zoster virus has been cultured from involved cerebral blood vessels.

A subacute meningoencephalitis usually occurs early in the course of the Vogt-Koyanagi-Harada syndrome.[95–97] The diagnosis is established by the development of severe, protracted, granulomatous uveitis and depigmentary skin changes such as poliosis (whitening of the eyebrows and eyelashes) and vitiligo. The CNS disease gradually resolves spontaneously.

Of the patients with Behçet's disease (recurrent oral and genital ulcerations and iridocyclitis) 10–25 percent develop CNS involvement.[98] The neurologic manifestations are variable, severe, and progressive in most cases. Occasionally, they precede other features of the syndrome. All parts of the neuraxis may be involved. Cerebrospinal fluid abnormalities include a slight elevation of protein levels and minimal pleocytosis.

The syndrome of "chronic benign lymphocytic meningitis"[99] defines a small group of patients with unexplained headache and lymphocytic pleocytosis but no focal signs. In one series, clinical remission occurred in all patients within 7–25 weeks. The relationship of this syndrome to aseptic meningitis and benign intracranial hypertension is not clear. However, it seems likely that a small group of patients with unexplained chronic meningitis—chosen to exclude those with focal signs, progressive neurologic involvement, and marked CSF abnormalities—have a self-limited illness.

In contrast to the patients with unexplained minimal, self-limited disease, an additional group of patients have an enigmatic chronic meningitis with significant neurologic involvement, a high CSF protein concentration, and sometimes a depressed glucose level.[1] The prognosis in this group is poor. Therapeutic trials may alter the course of the disease, the cultures, and the pathologic findings. A specific diagnosis may be apparent at autopsy, but this is not always the case. A temporal response to antifungal therapy in some cases has implicated an infectious etiology, and mycotic meningitis too often is associated with negative CSF cultures (as discussed above) and only diagnosed postmortem. Therefore a thorough diagnostic evaluation followed ultimately by meningeal and brain biopsy and, if appropriate, an empirical trial of emphotericin B therapy is indicated in this type of patient.

THE IMMUNOCOMPROMISED PATIENT

Chronic meningitis in the immunosuppressed patient with impaired cellular immunity requires special consideration because of the distinctive differential diagnosis. Among renal transplant recipients and patients with lymphoma and leukemia, *Cryptococcus neoformans* is the most common etiology of chronic meningitis.[100] *Listeria monocytogenes, M. tuberculosis, Toxoplasma gondii, Nocardia, Histoplasma*, and *Coccidioides* also cause chronic meningitis more often in such patients.

In the severely immunocompromised patient, progressive multifocal leukoencephalopathy (caused by papovaviruses) may produce profound focal neurologic deficits with minimal or no abnormalities in the CSF. Computed tomographic scans in such cases demonstrate low-density, nonenhancing, progressive lesions in the white matter without mass effect. The list of opportunistic pathogens associated with chronic meningitis in patients with AIDS is long and continues to increase.[101,102] *Cryptococcus neoformans, Toxoplasma gondii, Mycobacterium avium-intracellulare*, and cytomegalovirus were noted early during the AIDS epidemic; they were followed later by papovavirus, *Mycobacterium tuberculosis, Treponema pallidum, Candida* sp., and others including the human immunodeficiency virus (HIV) itself. Aseptic meningitis may be associated with the initial seroconversion to HIV or may occur later in the course of HIV infection; occasionally it may be chronic or recurrent and involve cranial nerves V–VIII and XII.[103] The CSF usually shows a mononuclear pleocytosis, normal glucose, and mildly elevated protein levels. It is possible that infection of the meninges is a usual concomitant of HIV infection, even when asymptomatic.[104] Of greater concern is the AIDS dementia complex, a progressive decline in mentation and motor function that ultimately occurs in up to two-thirds of AIDS patients. Pathologic studies have demonstrated HIV in the brain, in particular in macrophages, microglia, and multinucleated cells derived from these, thus implicating the blood monocyte as a vehicle for entry of HIV into the CNS.

Patients with AIDS are also at risk for primary CNS lymphoma as well as metastatic neoplasms.[101,102] Recognition that a patient is at increased risk of AIDS, therefore, becomes crucial in considering the differential diagnosis of chronic meningitis.

REFERENCES

1. Ellner JJ, Bennett JE. Chronic meningitis. Medicine (Baltimore). 1976;55:341.
2. Wilhelm C, Ellner JJ. Chronic meningitis. Neurol Clin. 1986;4:115.
3. Salaki JS, Louria DB, Chmel H. Fungal and yeast infections of the central nervous system: A clinical review. Medicine (Baltimore). 1984;63:108.
4. Hermans PE, Goldstein NP, Wellman WE. Mollaret's meningitis and differential diagnosis of recurrent meningitis. Am J Med. 1972;52:128.
5. Haynes BF, Wright R, McCracken JP. Mollaret's meningitis: A report of three cases. JAMA. 1976;236:1967.
6. Bartleson JD, Swanson JW, Whisnant JP. A migrainous syndrome with cerebrospinal fluid pleocytosis. Neurology (NY). 1981;31:1257.
7. Swartz M. Chronic meningitis—many causes to consider. N Engl J Med. 1987;317:957.
8. Peacock JE Jr, McGinnis MR, Cohen MS. Persistent neutrophilic meningitis: Report of four cases and review of the literature. Medicine (Baltimore). 1984;63:379.
9. Sawyer J, Ellner J, Ransohoff DF. To biopsy or not to biopsy in suspected herpes simplex encephalitis: A quantitative analysis. Med Decis Making. 1988;8:95.
10. Goodson JD, Strauss GM. Diagnosis of lymphomatous leptomeningitis by cerebrospinal fluid lymphocyte cell surface markers. Am J Med. 1979;66:1057.
11. Plouffe JF, Fass RJ. *Histoplasma* meningitis. Diagnostic value of cerebrospinal fluid serology. Ann Intern Med. 1980;92:189.
12. Wheat J, French M, Batteiger B, et al. Cerebrospinal fluid *Histoplasma* antibodies in central nervous system histoplasmosis. Arch Intern Med. 1985;145:1237.
13. Wheat LJ, Kohler RB, Tewari RP. Diagnosis of disseminated histoplasmosis by detection of *Histoplasma capsulatum* antigen in serum and urine specimens. N Engl J Med. 1986;314:83.
14. Plouffe JF, Silva J, Fekety R, Baird I. Cerebrospinal fluid lymphocyte transformations in meningitis. Arch Intern Med. 1979;139:191.
15. Radin SB, Phair JP, Shaughnessy M, et al. Production of specific IgG antibody to purified protein derivative in the central nervous system in a patient with tuberculous meningitis (Abstract). Clin Res. 1982;30:738.
16. Mardh P-A, Larsson L. Hoiby N, et al. Tuberculostearic acid as a diagnostic marker in tuberculous meningitis. Lancet. 1983;1:367.
17. Ewing GE, Bose GJ, Petersen PK. *Sporothrix schenckii* meningitis in a farmer with Hodgkin's disease. Am J Med. 1980;68:455.
18. Kravitz GR, Davies SF, Eckman MR, et al. Chronic blastomycotic meningitis. Am J Med. 1981;71:501.
19. New FJ, Davis KR. The role of CT scanning in diagnosis of infections of the central nervous system. In: Remington JS, Swartz MN, eds. Current Clinical Topics in Infectious Diseases. v. 1. New York: McGraw-Hill; 1980:1.
20. Stocksill MT, Kauffman CA. Comparison of cryptococcal and tuberculous meningitis. Arch Neurol. 1983;40:81.
21. Rich AR, McCordock HA. The pathogenesis of tuberculous meningitis. Bull Johns Hopkins Hosp. 1933;52:5.
22. Merritt HH, Fremont-Smith F. Cerebrospinal fluid in tuberculous meningitis. Arch Neurol Psychol. 1935;33:516.
23. Lepper MH, Spies HW. The present status of the treatment of tuberculosis of the central nervous system. Ann NY Acad Sci. 1963;106:106.
24. Weiss W, Flippin HF. The changing incidence and prognosis of tuberculous meningitis. Am J Med Sci. 1965;50:46.
25. Barrett-Connor EB. Tuberculous meningitis in adults. South Med J. 1967;60:1061.
26. Kennedy DH, Fallon FJ. Tuberculous meningitis. JAMA. 1979;241:264.
27. Jeren T, Beus I. Characteristics of cerebrospinal fluid in tuberculous meningitis. Acta Cytol (Baltimore). 1982;26:678.
28. Daniel TM. New approaches to the rapid diagnosis of tuberculous meningitis. J Infect Dis. 1987;155:599.
29. Spickard A, Butler WT, Andriole V, et al. The improved prognosis of cryptococcal meningitis with amphotericin B therapy. Ann Intern Med. 1963;58:66.
30. Butler WT, Alling DW, Spickard A, et al. Diagnostic and prognostic value of clinical and laboratory findings in cryptococcal meningitis. A follow-up study of forty patients. N Engl J Med. 1964;270:59.
31. Littman ML, Walter JE. Cryptococcosis: Current status. Am J Med. 1968;45:922.
32. Diamond RD, Bennett JE. Prognostic factors in cryptococcal meningitis. A study of 111 cases. Ann Intern Med. 1974;80:176.
33. Kovacs JA, Kovacs AA, Polis M, et al. Cryptococcosis in the acquired immunodeficiency syndrome. Ann Intern Med. 1985;103:533.
34. Zuger A, Louie E, Holzman RS, et al. Cryptococcal disease in patients with the acquired immunodeficiency syndrome: Diagnostic features and outcome of treatment. Ann Intern Med. 1986;104:234.
35. Smith CE, Saito MT, Simons SA. Pattern of 39,500 serologic tests in coccidioidomycosis. JAMA. 1956;160:546.
36. Winn WA. The treatment of coccidioidal meningitis. The use of amphotericin B in a group of 25 patients. Calif Med. 1964;101:75.
37. Winn WA. Coccidioidal meningitis: A follow-up report. In: Ajello L, ed. Coccidiomycosis. Tucson: University of Arizona Press; 1967:55.
38. Candill RG, Smith CE, Reinarz JA. Coccidioidal meningitis. A diagnostic challenge. Am J Med. 1970;49:360.
39. Deresinski SC, Stevens DA. Coccidioidomycosis in compromised hosts. Medicine (Baltimore). 1974;54:377.
40. Bouza E, Dreyer JS, Hewitt WL, et al. Coccidioidal meningitis. An analysis of 31 cases and review of the literature. Medicine (Baltimore). 1981:60:139.
41. Tynes BS, Crutcher JC, Utz JP. Histoplasma meningitis. Ann Intern Med. 1963;59:615.
42. Smith JW, Utz JP. Progressive disseminated histoplasmosis. Ann Intern Med. 1972;76:557.
43. Gilden DH, Miller EM, Johnson WG. Central nervous system histoplasmosis after rhinoplasty. Neurology (Minn). 1974;24:874.
44. Gelfand JA, Bennett JE. Active *Histoplasma* meningitis of 22 years duration. JAMA. 1975;233:1294.
45. DeVita VT, Utz JP, Williams T, et al. *Candida* meningitis. Arch Intern Med. 1966;117:527.
46. Bayer AS, Edwards JE Jr, Seidel JS, et al. *Candida* meningitis. Medicine (Baltimore). 1976;55:477.
47. Merritt HH, Adams RD, Solomon HC. Neurosyphilis. New York: Oxford University Press; 1946:24.

48. Hooshmand H, Escobar MR, Kopf SW. Neurosyphilis, a study of 241 patients. JAMA. 1972;219:726.
49. Pachner AR, Steere AC. The triad of neurologic manifestations of Lyme disease: Meningitis, cranial neuritis, and radiculoneuritis. Neurology (NY). 1985;35:47.
50. Wilske B, Schierz G, Preac-Mursic V, et al. Intrathecal production of specific antibodies against *Borrelia burgdorferi* in patients with lymphocytic meningoradiculitis (Bannworth's syndrome). J Infect Dis. 1986;153:304.
51. Nelson-Jones A. Neurologic complications of undulant fever. Lancet. 1951;1:495.
52. Nichols E. Meningoencephalitis due to brucellosis. Ann Intern Med. 1951;35:673.
53. Fincham RW, Sahs AL, Joynt RJ. Protean manifestations of nervous system brucellosis. JAMA. 1963;184:97.
54. Reddin JL, Anderson RK, Jenness R, et al. Significance of 7S and macroglobulin brucella agglutinins in human brucellosis. N Engl J Med. 1965;272:1263.
55. Bouza E, Garcia de la Torre M, Parras F, et al. Brucellar meningitis. Rev Infect Dis. 1987;9:810.
56. Scott EN, Kauman L, Brown AC, et al. Serologic studies in the diagnosis and management of meningitis due to *Sporothrix schenckii*. N Engl J Med. 1987;317:935.
57. Wilhelmj CM. The primary meningeal form of systemic blastomycosis. Am J Med Sci. 1925;169:172.
58. Buechner HA, Clawson CM. Blastomycosis of the central nervous system. II. A report of nine cases from the Veterans Administration Cooperative Study. Am Rev Respir Dis. 1967;95:820.
59. Pereira WC, Raphael A, Tehuto RA, et al. Localizacao encefalica da blastomicose sul-Americana: Consideracoes a proposito de 9 casos. Arq Neuropsiquiat. 1965;23:113.
60. Bennett JE, Bonner H, Jennings AE, et al. Chronic meningitis caused by *Cladosporium trichoides*. Am J Clin Pathol. 1973;59:398.
61. Bolton CF, Ashenhurst EM. Actinomycosis of the brain. Case report and review of the literature. Can Med Assoc J. 1964;90:922.
62. Brown JR: Human actinomycosis. Hum Pathol. 1973;4:319.
63. Albright L, Toczek S, Brenner VJ, et al. Osteomyelitis and epidural abscess caused by *Arachnia proprionica*. J Neurosurg. 1974;40:115.
64. Smego RA Jr. Actinomycosis of the central nervous system. Rev Infect Dis. 1987;9:855.
65. King RB, Stoops WL, Fitzgibbons J, et al. *Nocardia asteroides* meningitis. A case successfully treated with large doses of sulfadiazine and urea. J Neurosurg. 1966;24:749.
66. Richter RW, Silva M, Neu HC, et al. The neurological aspects of *Nocardia asteroides* infection. Infect Nervous System. 1968;44:424.
67. Kramer W. Frontiers of neurological diagnosis in acquired toxoplasmosis. Psychiatr Neurol Neurochirg. 1966;69:43.
68. Townsend JJ, Wolinsky JS, Baringer JR, et al. Acquired toxoplasmosis. A neglected cause of treatable nervous system disease. Arch Neurol. 1975;32:335.
69. Grines C, Plouffe JF, Baird IM, et al. *Toxoplasma* meningoencephalitis with hypoglycorrhachia. Arch Intern Med. 1981;141:935.
70. Denti JH. Cysticercosis cerebri-cestode infestation of the human brain. JAMA. 1957;164:401.
71. Lombardo LL, Mateos JH. Cerebral cysticercosis in Mexico. Neurology (Minn). 1961;11:824.
72. Loo L, Braude A. Cerebral cysticercosis in San Diego. A report of 23 cases and a review of the literature. Medicine (Baltimore). 1982;61:341.
73. Jones PG, Gilman RM, Medeiros AA, et al. Focal intracranial mucormycosis presenting as chronic meningitis. JAMA. 1981;24:2063.
74. Moore EW, Thomas LB, Shaw RK, et al. The central nervous system in acute leukemia. Arch Intern Med. 1960;105:451.
75. Hyman CB, Boyle JM, Brubaker CA, et al. Central nervous system involvement by leukemia in children. Blood. 1965;25:1.
76. Griffin JW, Thompson RW, Mitchinson MJ, et al. Lymphomatous leptomeningitis. Am J Med. 1971;51:200.
77. Berg L. Hypoglycorrhachia of noninfectious origin: Diffuse meningeal neoplasia. Neurology (Minn). 1953;3:811.
78. Fischer-Williams M, Bosanquet FD, Daniel P. Carcinomatosis of the meninges. Brain. 1955;78:42.
79. Dinsdale HB, Taghavy A. Carcinomatosis of the meninges. Can Med Assoc J. 1964;90:505.
80. Vital C, Bruno-Martin F, Henry P, et al. La carcinomatose méningée. Bordeaux Med. 1970;12:2927.
81. Olson ME, Cherniak NL, Posner JB. Infiltration of the meninges by systemic cancer: A clinical and pathologic study. Arch Neurol. 1974;30:122.
82. Gonzalez-Vitale JC, Garcia-Bunvel R. Meningeal carcinomatosis. Cancer. 1976;37:2906.
83. Shuttleworth E, Allen N. CSF β-glucuronidase assay in the diagnosis of neoplastic meningitis. Arch Neurol. 1980;37:684.
84. Wiederholt WC, Siekert RB. Neurological manifestations of sarcoidosis. Neurology (Minn). 1965;15:1147.
85. Mathews WB. Sarcoidosis of the nervous system. J Neurol Neurosurg Psychiatry. 1965;28:23.
86. Gaines JD, Eckman PB, Remington JS. Low CSF glucose level in sarcoidosis involving the central nervous system. Arch Intern Med. 1970;125:333.
87. Douglas AC, Maloney AFJ. Sarcoidosis of the central nervous system. J Neurol Neurosurg Psychiatry. 1973;36:1024.
88. Delaney P. Neurological manifestations in sarcoidosis. Ann Intern Med. 1977;87:336.
89. Grizzanti JN, Knapp AB, Schecter AJ, et al. Treatment of sarcoid meningitis with radiotherapy. Am J Med. 1982;73:605.
90. Kolodny EM, Rebeiz JJ, Caviness VS, et al. Granulomatous angiitis of the central nervous system. Arch Neurol. 1968;19:510.
91. Nurick S, Blackwood W, Mair WGP. Giant cell granulomatous angiitis of the central nervous system. Brain. 1972;95:133.
92. Mohr JP, Powell HC. Clinicopathologic conference. Headache and progressive mental deterioration in a 45-year-old man. N Engl J Med. 1976;295:944.
93. Cupps TR, Moore PM, Fauci AS. Isolated angiitis of the central nervous system. Prospective diagnostic and therapeutic experience. Am J Med. 1983;74:97.
94. Reik L, Grunnet ML, Spencer RP, et al. Granulomatous angiitis presenting as chronic meningitis and ventriculitis. Neurology (NY). 1983;33:1609.
95. Cowper AR. Harada's disease and Vogt-Koyanagi syndrome. AMA Arch Ophthal. 1951;45:367.
96. Pattison EM. Uveomeningoencephalitis syndrome. Arch Neurol (Chicago). 1965;12:197.
97. Riehl J-L, Andrews JM. The uveomeningoencephalitis syndrome. Neurology (Minn). 1966;16:603.
98. Schotland DL, Wolf SM, White HH, et al. Neurologic aspects of Behçets disease. Am J Med. 1963;34:544.
99. Hopkins AP, Harvey PKP. Chronic benign lymphocytic meningitis. J Neurol Sci. 1973;18:443.
100. Hooper DC, Pruitt AA, Rubin RH. Central nervous system infection in the chronically immunosuppressed. Medicine (Baltimore). 1982;61:166.
101. Gopinathan G, Laubenstein LJ, Mondale B, et al. Central nervous system manifestations of the acquired immunodeficiency syndrome. (Abstract). Neurology (NY). 1983;33(Suppl):105.
102. Snider WD, Simpson DM, Nielsen S, et al. Neurological complications of the acquired immunodeficiency syndrome. Ann Neurol. 1983;14:403.
103. Bredesen DE, Lipkin WI, Messing R. Prolonged recurrent aseptic meningitis with prominent cranial nerve abnormalities: A new epidemic in gay men (Abstract). Neurology (NY). 33(Suppl):85.

68. ENCEPHALITIS, MYELITIS, AND NEURITIS

DIANE E. GRIFFIN
RICHARD T. JOHNSON

Encephalitis, myelitis, and *neuritis* mean inflammations of brain, spinal cord, and peripheral nerves, respectively. If sensory or motor spinal roots are specifically involved, the term *radiculitis* may be used. Since meningeal inflammation often accompanies these inflammatory processes, compounded terms such as *meningoencephalitis* and *meningoencephalomyelitis* are sometimes used. None of these terms, however, differentiates between the inflammatory diseases caused by direct invasion of agents and the post- or parainfectious demyelinating processes that may involve the brain, spinal cord, or peripheral nerve. Because of the diversity of clinical symptoms and signs that can occur with these inflammatory diseases, infectious or parainfectious causes must be entertained in the differential diagnosis of a great variety of neurologic diseases. As in the diagnosis of all neurologic disease, the differential diagnosis will be determined by the temporal evolution of signs and symptoms and by the localization of the disease process to one or more anatomic sites by physical findings. Systemic involvement of skin, lung, salivary glands, gastrointestinal tract, and so forth, or fever may suggest an infectious cause, but these may also be absent.

ENCEPHALITIS AND MYELITIS

This section will deal with infectious and postinfectious encephalitis and myelitis together since they are often considered in the same differential diagnosis and have considerable overlap in manifestation and causation. Peripheral neuropathies due to infectious agents are rare and will be considered, along with tetanus, in a separate section.

Pathogenesis and Pathologic Characteristics

Infectious agents can produce clinical symptoms and signs within the central nervous system (CNS) by either direct or indirect involvement of neural tissue. Infectious agents can invade the CNS by several pathways. The most common is via the blood. This is best documented for viral infections but probably is also important in rickettsial, bacterial, and fungal infections.[1–3] The initial site of entry of a pathogen and the primary site of replication may be the respiratory tract (measles, mumps, influenza, varicella-zoster, *Mycobacterium tuberculosis, Cryptococcus neoformans*), gastrointestinal tract (poliovirus, coxsackievirus, echovirus) or subcutaneous tissue (togaviruses, *Rickettsia rickettsia, R. typhi*, trypanosomes). Involvement of the CNS is, for the most part, an infrequent consequence of common infections.[1]

In certain viral infections, entry into the CNS occurs by way of the peripheral nerves. Transport systems within motor and sensory axons carry substances from the cell body to the periphery (anterograde transport) and from the periphery to the cell body (retrograde transport). The neural route of entry is important in viral infections such as rabies[4] and occasionally poliomyelitis.[5] Retrograde transport from the skin or mucous membranes moves herpes simplex and varicella-zoster viruses into sensory ganglia at the time of primary infection, and anterograde transport carries reactivated virus from the ganglia to the periphery during exacerbations.[6] On occasion reactivated virus may also be carried retrograde to the CNS. Retrograde transport of herpes simplex virus by nerves innervating the dura from the trigeminal ganglion may contribute to the unique temporal lobe localization of herpes simplex virus encephalitis.[7]

Entry of infectious agents into the CNS by way of the exposed olfactory nerves in the nasal mucosa has been demonstrated in experimental animals[8] but is of proven clinical importance only in the entry of free-living amebas into the olfactory and frontal lobes through the nasal mucosa and across the cribiform plate.[9]

Once within the CNS, only selected cells may be infected, giving rise to variations in clinical manifestations. Neuronal infection may cause seizure activity, which, depending on the areas involved, may be focal or generalized. Infection of oligodendroglia may cause demyelination alone. Cortical infection or reactive parenchymal swelling may give rise to changes in the state of consciousness,[10] and infection of specific brain stem neurons can cause coma or respiratory failure.[11]

In fatal viral encephalitis an inflammatory reaction is usually prominent in the meninges and in a perivascular distribution within the brain. Although the perivascular inflammatory reaction is composed predominantly of mononuclear cells, polymorphonuclear cells may be evident. Neural cells may show degenerative changes, and apparent phagocytosis of neurons by macrophages or microglial cells (neuronophagia) is often found. Myelin pallor, glial nodules, and giant cells containing viral antigen are found in the brain of patients with acquired immunodeficiency syndrome (AIDS)-related dementia.[12,13] Spinal cord lesions in human immunodeficiency virus infections may include vacuolar myelopathy[14] and gracile tract degeneration.[15] Whether these pathologic changes are direct or indirect consequences of virus infection is not yet clear. Intranuclear inclusion bodies are seen in herpesvirus,[6] adenovirus,[16] and subacute and chronic forms of measles virus infections.[17] Cytomegalovirus infections produce characteristic pathologic changes with the induction of cytomegalic cells containing inclusion bodies.[18] Negri bodies are found in rabies virus encephalitis.[19]

Rickettsiae tend to invade and to multiply in vascular endothelial cells, resulting in widespread vasculitis of capillaries, arterioles, and small arteries,[20] including the retina.

Infectious agents can give rise to signs or symptoms suggesting encephalitis or myelitis without actually invading CNS parenchyma. One mechanism is by the development of adhesive meningitis and vasculitis during the course of subacute or chronic leptomeningeal infections. In chronic tuberculosis, fungal or syphilitic meningitis, or in untreated or partially treated bacterial meningitis, the chronic meningeal reaction may cause obstruction of cerebrospinal fluid (CSF) flow, causing hydrocephalus, cranial nerve palsies, or gliosis in the underlying cerebral cortex. In addition, the vasculitis involving large vessels may lead to infarctions of brain and focal neurologic deficits. This sequence of events is frequently observed in tuberculosis,[21] aspergillosis,[22] and meningovascular neurosyphilis.[23] Syphilis of the meningovascular type appears relatively early in the course of this disease, and, in contrast to the parenchymatous manifestations (tabes dorsalis and paresis) that appear later, is inflammatory and often reversible. *Cryptococcus*, produces a chronic meningitis with little inflammatory reaction.[24] In chronic bacterial or fungal meningitis, organization of a subarachnoid exudate at the base of the brain may lead to communicating hydrocephalus and cranial nerve palsies.[25]

In the acute demyelinating diseases complicating viral exanthems or respiratory infections, it is not known whether invasion into the CNS is a prerequisite to disease. These diseases involve either central myelin (postinfectious myelitis or encephalomyelitis) or peripheral myelin (Guillain-Barré syndrome), and the pathogenesis of these syndromes is thought to be related to a sensitization of the infected person to central or peripheral myelin.[26] This mechanism is analogous to neurologic complications of neural tissue-derived rabies vaccines.[27,28]

The pathologic changes of postinfectious and postvaccinal encephalomyelitis are characterized by perivascular infiltration of mononuclear inflammatory cells and perivenous demyelination.[29,30] Acute hemorrhagic leukoencephalitis, characterized by fibrinoid necrosis of arterioles and hemorrhage as well as the perivenular demyelination, is thought to represent a more severe form of postinfectious encephalomyelitis.[30]

On the other hand, Reye syndrome is a distinct acute encephalopathy of unknown cause that usually follows a viral infection. This syndrome affects children and is characterized by acute fatty liver and a noninflammatory cerebral edema. Reye syndrome has been most commonly associated with influenza A and B virus infections, although cases have been reported after varicella and many other viral infections.[31] The pathogenesis of this disease and its relationship to the prior infection and/or medications taken during the prior illness are not completely understood.[32] Likewise, the role of the organism in the encephalopathy associated with cat-scratch disease is unknown.[33].

Clinical Findings

Infections limited to the leptomeninges manifest with signs and symptoms of meningeal irritation: headache, stiff neck, and pleocytosis. If the meningeal process is chronic, as in tuberculosis, manifesting symptoms and signs may be of a communicating hydrocephalus (headache, nausea and vomiting, mental deterioration, or spastic paraparesis) and/or of localized infarction secondary to vasculitis.[34] The chronic form of cryptococcal meningitis may manifest as progressive mental deterioration and headache, rather than with fever and meningismus, as seen in the more acute form.[25,35]

Patients with viral encephalitis usually have signs and symptoms of meningeal inflammation, but in addition to headache, fever, and nuchal rigidity, encephalitis is characterized by alterations of consciousness: Mild lethargy may progress to confusion, stupor, and coma. Focal neurologic signs usually develop, and seizures are common. Motor weakness, accentuated deep tendon reflexes, and extensor plantar responses may be observed. Abnormal movements are seen in some cases of encephalitis, and, rarely, a tremor characteristic of Parkinson's disease may develop. The hypothalamic pituitary area may be involved, causing severe hyperthermia or poikilothermia, diabetes insipidus, and inappropriate antidiuretic hormone secretion. Involvement of the spinal cord can lead to flaccid paralysis, depression of tendon reflexes, and paralysis of bowel and bladder. Increased intracranial pressure can cause papilledema and third and sixth cranial nerve palsies.

In herpes simplex encephalitis signs often include bizarre behavior, hallucinations, and aphasia, suggesting the temporal lobe localization typical of that infection.[36] Rabies may begin with local paresthesia at the site of the bite.[37] A parkinsonian syndrome is common in Japanese encephalitis.[38] Acute contralateral hemiparesis may occur after herpes zoster ophthalmicus related to a localized cerebral angiitis, causing frontal lobe infarction.[39] With Lyme disease, both peripheral and CNS complications occur, ranging from severe meningoencephalitis to isolated cranial nerve palsies.[40,41]

Myelitis can occur, with or without encephalitis. Transverse myelitis simulates acute transection of the cord with rostral limb weakness, sensory level, and the loss of control of bowel and bladder. Ascending myelitis leads to an ascending flaccid paralysis and rising sensory deficit and is characterized by early bowel and bladder involvement. Poliomyelitis, where anterior horn cells are involved primarily, typically causes flaccid paralysis and muscular pain without sensory loss or bladder dysfunction.

In postinfectious encephalomyelitis the time lapse between the primary viral infection, rash in measles, varicella, rubella, or parotid swelling in mumps, and the onset of symptoms referable to the nervous system ranges between 2 and 12 days. The onset is often abrupt, with depression of consciousness or seizure.[26,30,31]

Systemic findings of particular importance are the rashes of Lyme disease, Rocky Mountain spotted fever (palms and soles), typhus, varicella, and herpes zoster. An exanthem is also occasionally seen with *Mycoplasma*, coxsackievirus, and echovirus infections. A history of tick bite is usually obtained in Rocky Mountain spotted fever, Lyme disease, ehrlichiosis, and Colorado tick fever. A history of animal or bat bite may be obtained in rabies, although most patients in the United States never give such a history.[42]

Mycobacterial and fungal infections often present as chronic and, on occasion, fluctuating disease, but in certain cases (mucormycosis) they may progress very rapidly.

Bacterial infections usually manifest with an acute onset, but certain infections such as neurosyphilis, Lyme disease, relapsing fever, brain abscess, and Whipple's disease may have an insidious onset and an indolent, chronic, or even fluctuating course. The neurologic features of Whipple's disease may include dementia, supranuclear ophthalmoplegia, myoclonus, spastic paresis, ataxis, and papilledema. The patient may have neurologic signs and symptoms without significant manifestations of malabsorption.[43] The rickettsial diseases are usually acute in onset with fever, headache, and myalgias. Rocky Mountain spotted fever is associated with a rash before or after neurologic disease,[44] while there is no rash in ehrlichiosis.[45]

Viral infections also may be acute, subacute, or chronic. Encephalitis due to adenovirus and enteroviruses has occurred both as acute disease in immunologically healthy individuals[1,46] and as subacute disease in immunologically compromised individuals.[16,47] Certain of the "slow virus infections" such as Creutzfeldt-Jakob disease, subacute sclerosing panencephalitis, rubella panencephalitis, AIDS encephalopathy, tropical spastic paraparesis, and progressive multifocal leukoencephalopathy are slowly progressive disease with an insidious onset and absence of fever.[1,48–50]

Laboratory Findings

Peripheral blood counts are rarely helpful in this group of diseases since they may be normal or show a moderate leukocytosis or leukopenia. Peripheral blood smears may show atypical lymphocytes in Epstein-Barr virus infections, the diagnostic gametocytes of *Plasmodium falciparum* malaria, the morulae of *Ehrlichia*, the borreliae in relapsing fever, or the trypanosomes in trypanosomiasis. The serum amylase level may be elevated in mumps virus infection. Pulmonary infiltrates may accompany lymphocytic choriomeningitis virus, typhus, and *Mycoplasma* infections.

CSF examination is essential. The pleocytosis of viral encephalomyelitis is variable (10–2000 cells/mm^3), and mononuclear cells usually predominate, although early in any of these diseases, there may be no cells or polymorphonuclear cells may be present in considerable numbers. Repeat examination of the CSF in 24 hours is often useful.[51] Significant numbers of red blood cells may be found in herpesvirus,[52] acute necrotizing hemorrhagic leukoencephalitis,[53] and *Naegleria* encephalitis.[54] In the chronic fungal and bacterial meningitides a moderate mononuclear pleocytosis is usually found. Meningoencephalitis due to the free-living amebas, *Nocardia, Actinomyces, Candida,* and *Aspergillus* elicit a polymorphonuclear response.[54,55]

The CSF protein level is usually elevated, and in chronic infections an increased proportion of this protein is IgG (normal is <12 percent).[56] Under normal conditions CSF IgG is derived primarily from the serum, but antibodies are present at about $\frac{1}{200}$ the concentration.[57] During acute inflammatory reactions a transudate of protein occurs, including serum immunoglobulins. During convalescence plasma cells may produce a specific IgG within the CNS, as seen after mumps meningitis,[58] herpes simplex,[52] and zoster[59] encephalitis. In chronic infection examination of the CSF for specific antibody can be diagnostic in syphilis[60] Lyme disease,[61] tropical spastic paraparesis,[43] subacute sclerosing,[62] and rubella panencephalitis[63] and may be useful, when compared with serum levels, in the viral, rickettsial, and bacterial encephalitides for which antibody tests are available. If antibody to a particular pathogen is present at a comparable or higher amount in CSF compared with serum and the CSF protein is only moderately elevated, it is indicative of CNS infection with the agent.

For diagnosis by serum antibodies, it is important to obtain serum early in the course (acute phase) for comparison with serum taken after 1–3 weeks of illness to demonstrate a significant antibody increase.[64] This diagnosis is often of more than academic interest since presumptive therapy begun early may then be discontinued if a diagnosis is established. Tests for cold agglutinins and heterophile antibody may be suggestive but may yield false negatives in the diagnosis of *Mycoplasma* and Epstein-Barr virus infections, respectively; therefore, organism-specific antibody tests need to be done. Myelin basic protein may be present in diseases associated with central demyelination.[65]

The CSF glucose level is usually within the normal range during viral or rickettsial infections of CNS, although a mild depression may be seen. The glucose level is usually low in tuberculous,[66] fungal,[25] bacterial, or amoebic infections.[54]

Direct examination of the CSF by Gram stain for bacteria, by acid-fast stain for mycobacteria, and by India ink for *Cryptococcus* should be performed and may be diagnostic. Wet preparation of CSF may reveal *Naegleria*, and Giemsa stain will identify trypanosomes. Bacteria, mycobacteria, fungi, and viruses may also be recovered from the CSF by appropriate culture techniques, Microbial antigen detection methods are sometimes more sensitive than cultures and have proved particularly useful in cryptococcal meningitis.[35] Brain biopsy is necessary to diagnose herpes simplex virus encephalitis definitively.[36]

Etiology of Encephalomyelitis

Table 1 lists the viruses known to cause acute encephalitis or myelitis in the United States, as well as the viruses associated with postinfectious encephalomyelitis. Many of these infections have distinct seasonal variations that are helpful in narrowing the differential diagnosis (Fig. 1). The togavirus, flavivirus, and bunyavirus encephalitides (except rubella) are arthropod borne and therefore occur when their insect vectors are biting, generally in spring and summer. The mosquito-borne California and western equine encephalitides peak in August, and St. Louis encephalitis peaks somewhat later.[67,68] The tick-borne diseases occur most often in spring and early summer.[69–71] Enterovirus infections, and therefore their complications, are more common in late summer and fall, and mumps is most common in the winter and spring. In contrast, the herpesvirus encephalitides occur throughout the year. Lymphocytic choriomeningitis virus is most frequent in the winter when rodents come indoors, and leptospirosis is more common in the warm months when rodents and people are in contact with ponds and streams.[64]

In addition to the season, geographic occurrence and travel histories may be helpful in the diagnosis of vector-borne encephalitides. For instance, eastern equine encephalitis is confined to the Atlantic and Gulf Coast states, and California and St. Louis encephalitides are found primarily in the Midwestern United States. Colorado tick fever and western equine encephalitis are most common in the Western states.[1] Lyme disease is endemic in the Northeast and the upper Midwestern United States, Northern California, and Europe.[72] Japanese encephalitis is found in most of Asia,[73] and tick-borne encephalitis occurs over a wide area of Europe and the Soviet Union.[74]

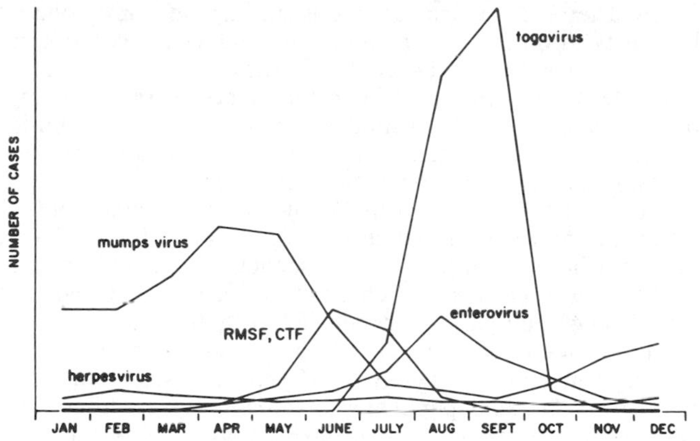

FIG. 1. Seasonal variation in the encephalitides caused by togaviruses, enteroviruses, mumps virus, herpesvirus, Rocky Mountain spotted fever (RMSF), and Colorado tick fever (CTF).

Infections with eastern equine encephalitis virus produce clinically evident encephalitis with high frequency in all age groups,[75] in contrast to the other alphaviruses, in which the majority of the infections are subclinical. Clinical disease with St. Louis encephalitis virus occurs in about 1 percent of infections, and infants and adults over age 50 are most likely to develop encephalitis.[76] California and western equine encephalitis viruses infect persons of all ages but produce encephalitis predominantly in children.[77,78] Venezuelan equine encephalitis virus primarily causes a flulike illness in humans but can produce encephalitis in any age group.[79]

Nonviral causes of encephalomyelitis are listed in Table 2. Some of these diseases are of known and others of unknown

TABLE 1. Viral Causes of Acute Encephalomyelitis

Direct Infection	Postinfection
TOGAVIRIDAE	TOGAVIRIDAE
Alphaviruses	Rubivirus
Eastern equine	Rubella
Western equine	MYXOVIRIDAE
Venezuelan equine	Influenzavirus
FLAVIVIRIDAE	Influenza A and B
St. Louis	PARAMYXOVIRIDAE
Murray Valley	Paramyxovirus
West Nile	Mumps
Japanese	Morbillivirus
Dengue	Measles
Tick-borne complex	POXVIRIDAE
BUNYAVIRIDAE	Orthopoxvirus
Bunyavirus	Vaccinia
California	HERPETOVIRIDAE
Rift Valley	Herpesvirus
PARAMYXOVIRIDAE	Varicella-zoster
Paramyxovirus	Epstein-Barr
Mumps	
Morbillivirus	
Measles	
ARENAVIRIDAE	
Arenavirus	
Lymphocytic choriomeningitis	
Machupo	
Lassa	
Junin	
PICORNAVIRIDAE	
Enterovirus	
Poliovirus	
Coxsackievirus	
Echovirus	
REOVIRIDAE	
Colorado tick fever	
RHABDOVIRIDAE	
Lyssavirus	
Rabies	
FILOVIRIDAE	
Ebola	
Marburg	
RETROVIRIDAE	
Lentivirus	
Human immunodeficiency	
HERPETOVIRIDAE	
Herpesvirus	
Herpes simplex types 1 and 2	
Varicella-zoster	
Epstein-Barr	
Cytomegalovirus	
ADENOVIRIDAE	
Adenovirus	

TABLE 2. Nonviral Causes of Encephalomyelitis

Rocky Mountain spotted fever
Typhus
Ehrlichia canis
Mycoplasma
Brucellosis
Subacute bacterial endocarditis
Listeria
Syphilis (meningovascular)
Relapsing fever
Lyme disease
Leptospirosis
Nocardia
Actinomycosis
Tuberculosis
Cryptococcus
Histoplasma
Naegleria
Acanthamoeba
Toxoplasma
Plasmodium falciparum
Trypanosomiasis
Whipple's disease
Behçet's disease
Cat-scratch disease
Vasculitis
Drug reactions

cause. They include drug reactions such as the neuroleptic malignant syndrome[80] and chemotherapy-induced leukoencephalopathy,[81] which may be confused with infection. Many are treatable. One of the most important concerns in evaluating a patient with encephalomyelitis is to rule out treatable entities.

The cause of encephalitis is different in immunodeficient patients. Patients with hypogammaglobulinemia may have chronic encephalitis with enterovirus.[47] Patients with defects in cell-mediated immunity have unusual forms of encephalitis or myelitis with herpesviruses,[18,82–84] a subacute inclusion body encephalitis with measles,[17] chronic encephalitis with adenovirus,[16] and granulomatous encephalitis with *Acanthamoeba*.[85] In acquired immunodeficiency disease a number of unusual agents, principally *Toxoplasma, Cryptococcus*, cytomegalovirus, *Nocardia*, and papovavirus (progressive multifocal leukoencephalopathy), may cause CNS disease, either singly or in combination.[42,86]

Transverse myelitis caused by a vasculitis of the anterior spinal artery has been seen in tuberculosis, syphilis, and schistosomiasis.[87] Postinfectious transverse myelitis has been associated with measles, rubella, mumps, and upper respiratory diseases, as well as with immunizations.[88,89] Direct involvement with varicella-zoster virus may also produce a transverse myelitis or an ascending necrotizing myelitis.[90] Infection with human T-lymphotropic virus type I causes disease primarily in the thoracic cord, leading to progressive spastic paraparesis.[49,50] Infection with human immunodeficiency virus causes myelopathy manifest by spastic paraparesis and sensory ataxia.[48] Dumb rabies after lower extremity bites by rabid vampire bats has also been described as producing an ascending myelitis.[91] The lower motor neuron variety of myelitis may be produced by poliovirus, coxsackievirus, or echovirus.

Presumptive Treatment

Specific therapy is available for most of the diseases listed in Table 2 and should be instituted as soon as possible if a presumptive diagnosis can be made. Tuberculous meningitis is, unfortunately, often a diagnosis of exclusion, and if the clinical picture is compatible and other diagnoses have been excluded, antituberculous therapy should be instituted.

For viral diseases vidarabine and acyclovir are of proven efficacy in herpes simplex virus encephalitis. They are equally efficacious in neonatal infection,[92] but acyclovir is superior in older individuals.[93] In immunocompromised patients acyclovir prevents visceral dissemination of varicella-zoster virus, including encephalitis.[94]

Patients in coma caused by encephalitis or postinfectious encephalomyelitis may make remarkable recoveries even after prolonged periods of unconsciousness. For this reason vigorous supportive treatment is indicated, and the complications of ventilator therapy, catheters, intravenous lines, and so forth, should be avoided if possible and should be treated vigorously if present. Blood glucose levels and electrolytes should be monitored closely, since the hypothalamic area may be involved in the encephalitic process. Seizures should be controlled, if they occur, with diphenylhydantoin. Some fever may be beneficial, but extreme hyperthermia, as well as hypoxia, may aggravate seizures. Cerebral edema can be damaging in itself and should be controlled with glycerol or mannitol, if possible, but steroids should be used if necessary for this purpose.

NEURITIS

Neuritis is an inflammatory disease involving the peripheral nerves. Only leprosy and trypanosomes are known to cause a direct infection leading to clinical signs of peripheral neuropathy, although human immunodeficiency virus and cytomegalovirus may cause disease directly as well.[95] Lyme disease is frequently associated with radiculoneuritis and cranial neuritis.[96] Herpes simplex virus and varicella-zoster virus infect sensory ganglia. Reactivation of herpes simplex virus type 2 has been associated with radiating radicular pain, which may mimic lumbar disk disease.[97] Radicular pain and segmental motor paralysis may accompany herpes zoster, and this may be followed by a postherpetic pain syndrome along the distribution of nerves supplied by the affected ganglia. Three bacterial toxins affect peripheral nerves either directly (diphtheria) or indirectly (tetanus, botulism), each causing distinct syndromes. The Guillain-Barré syndrome may represent a postinfectious inflammatory demyelinating process of peripheral nerves predominantly involving anterior roots.

Pathologic Characteristics and Pathogenesis

In lepromatous leprosy there is little if any immunologic response to the infection. There is a widespread distribution of *Mycobacterium leprae*. Nerves in the skin may exhibit only minor changes, but larger peripheral nerves contain many leprosy bacilli demonstrable in Schwann cells on acid-fast stains. These nerves show little inflammation. The organisms grow best in the cooler parts of the body, and nerves close to skin surface and distal nerves are affected preferentially. In late stages of the disease extensive axonal degeneration may occur.[98]

Tuberculoid leprosy is characterized by a marked granulomatous reaction to the infection and few demonstrable bacilli. Cutaneous nerves beneath the depigmented skin macules are destroyed, producing anesthesia. The peripheral nerves are nodular and thickened, with destruction of the normal architecture. Segmental demyelination and axonal degeneration result in nerve destruction and severe fibrosis.[98] *Trypanosoma cruzi, T. gambiense*, and *T. rhodesiense* all can invade and replicate in tissue of the peripheral as well as the central nervous system. *Trypanosoma cruzi* preferentially damages cells of the autonomic nervous system by replication in the supporting Schwann cells, satellite cells, and capsular fibroblasts rather than in the neurons. In African trypanosomiasis patients dying with encephalomyelitis often have evidence of neuritis.[99]

Tetanus toxin, produced by *Clostridium tetani* under anaerobic conditions, is transported up the axon and binds to the presynaptic endings on motor neurons in the anterior horns of the spinal cord blocking inhibitory input.[100,101] This results in uncontrolled motor input to skeletal muscle and the spasms typical of this disease. Because of this transport mechanism for entry into the CNS, patients may have only localized disease in the area of the *Clostridium*-containing wound.

Botulinum toxin is produced during anaerobic metabolism of *Clostridium botulinum* and may either be ingested as performed toxin or produced by organisms in the intestine (infant botulism) or introduced into a wound (wound botulism). Botulinum toxin binds to the presynaptic axon terminal of the neuromuscular junction, preventing release of acetylcholine and thus producing a flaccid paralysis.[101,102] Little, if any, histologic abnormality is seen in either tetanus or botulism.

Diphtheria toxin is produced by *Corynebacterium diphtheriae* lysogenized by a phage coding for this toxin. The toxin is a protein with two subunits; one (A) inhibits protein synthesis by blocking the adenosine diphosphate (ADP) ribosylation of elongation factor 2, whereas the second (B) binds to cell membranes and therefore enables the active subunit A to enter the cell.[103] The effect of this toxin on peripheral nerves is to cause a noninflammatory demyelination. Both cranial and peripheral nerves may be demyelinated, although cranial nerves are more frequently affected.

The Guillain-Barré syndrome often follows within 4 weeks of a respiratory or gastrointestinal infection, immunization, trauma, or metabolic insult. Infections with a wide spectrum of viruses as well as *Mycoplasma pneumoniae* have been associated with this syndrome. There is an increased incidence in individuals infected with human immunodeficiency virus.[95,104] A history of a nonspecific upper respiratory illness is, however, most common.[105] Nerves show segmental inflammation and demyelination. The inflammatory lesions are composed of mononuclear cells that are perivascular and focal. If nerve destruction has occurred, Wallerian degeneration may be present. Low-grade perivascular inflammation may persist for months to years after the episode.[106] Clinically and pathologically, the Guillain-Barré syndrome closely resembles experimental allergic neuritis, a disease induced in animals by immunization with peripheral nerve myelin.[107] The mechanism of the induction of this sensitization and whether the actual effector mechanism is humoral or cellular are unknown.

Clinical Findings

Leprosy has two distinctive manifestations, depending on whether the disease is of the tuberculoid or the lepromatous type. Tuberculoid leprosy produces a mononeuropathy beneath the sharply demarcated, hypopigmented skin patches. Peripheral nerves may be palpably and visibly enlarged, and the neurologic involvement is a prominent part of the disease. In lepromatous leprosy a distal hypesthesia with a selective loss of pain and temperature is most common, although a mononeuropathy may be present. Cooler areas of the body are more strikingly affected, and the loss of pain sensation results in mutilation and eventual loss of digits.[98]

Tetanus usually manifests with rigidity of muscles, which may be painful. The initial manifestation may be of ''local tetanus'' in which the rigidity affects only one limb or area of the body in which the *Clostridium*-containing wound is located. Stiffness of the jaw muscles causes trismus, and stiffness of the facial muscles may cause a change of expression. This mild picture may progress to generalized rigidity with reflex spasms and dysphagia. The history of a soil-contaminated puncture wound should be sought. The wound may have seemed insignificant at the time of the injury and may appear well healed at the time of the neurologic disease.[108]

Botulism characteristically manifests 12–36 hours after the ingestion of the toxin with weakness, dizziness, and dryness of the mouth. Neurologic symptoms follow within 12–72 hours with blurred vision, diplopia, dysphonia, dysphagia, and muscle weakness. On examination sensation is preserved, the tendon reflexes are depressed or absent, and the paralysis flaccid.[109] The same picture can develop more gradually in a patient with wound botulism. The original wound is usually of a rather severe traumatic nature and may appear to be healing well at the time of neurologic disease.[110]

The earliest sign of pharyngeal diphtheria (5–12 days) is paralysis of the palate, which produces a nasal quality of the voice and an increasing tendency to regurgitate fluids through the nose. Other cranial nerves (particularly the third, sixth, seventh, ninth and tenth) may become involved, with blurring of vision and inability to accommodate as early symptoms. Later in the course of the disease, when previous symptoms may have subsided (4–8 weeks), a predominantly motor polyneuropathy involving initial symmetrical weakness of distal extremities may appear similar to Guillain-Barré syndrome. There is a flaccid paralysis with loss of deep tendon reflexes that may be accompanied by the signs and symptoms of a diphtheritic myocarditis.[111]

Neuropathies associated with human immunodeficiency virus infection include acute and chronic inflammatory demyelinating polyneuropathies, sensory ganglioneuritis and polyradiculopathy early in infection, and a distal symmetrical polyneuropathy later when AIDS has developed.[95]

In approximately 60 percent of the cases, Guillain-Barré syndrome follows an infection or immunization. Clinically it manifests with subjective paresthesias and/or weakness, which may continue to progress for up to 4 weeks.[112] Examination typically reveals a flaccid paralysis with loss of deep tendon reflexes. Involvement of the autonomic nervous system resulting in lability of blood pressure, inappropriate antidiuretic hormone (ADH) secretion, and inability to compensate for volume changes occurs in approximately 20 percent of the cases.[113] These problems frequently necessitate the management of patients in an intensive care unit even though they may not require ventilatory assistance. The condition of an individual patient may change rapidly either during progression or during recovery. Improvement is often slow, however, and may continue for up to 12 months.[112]

Laboratory Findings

Routine blood chemistries are not helpful in this group of diseases. If botulinism is suspected serum for mouse inoculation should be procured. Cerebrospinal fluid should also be obtained. In Guillain-Barré syndrome or diphtheritic polyneuritis an increased protein level with few cells (albuminocytologic dissociation) in the CSF is the characteristic finding; some patients, however may have a normal protein level particularly early in the disease and others, particularly those with human immunodeficiency virus infection, will have a moderate pleocytosis.[104,114] The CSF findings are normal in tetanus, botulism, and leprosy. Neurometric tests that aid in localization of the pathologic changes and thus the diagnosis are (*1*) the measurement of nerve conduction times to look for the slowed conduction found in the peripheral nerve lesions of Guillain-Barré syndrome and diphtheria (F wave measurements may allow the identification of abnormalities if lesions are very proximal) and (*2*) the recording from muscle during repetitive nerve stimulation to look for the incremental response characteristic of botulism[109] and not found in Guillain-Barré syndrome. Nerve biopsies may be useful in identifying the granulomas and/or acid-fast bacilli of leprosy and the inflammatory demyelination of Guillain-Barré syndrome.[115]

Presumptive Treatment

In this group of clinically distinctive diseases it is important to recognize the disease and to treat it appropriately. Most patients with Guillain Barré syndrome benefit from plasmapheresis, especially when performed early in the disease.[104,116] Patients must be closely monitored for vital capacity, electrolytes, blood pressure, temperature, and heart rate and those with respiratory failure should be ventilated mechanically. Patients with autonomic nervous system dysfunction should be treated with short-acting drugs, since autonomic function in these patients may be very labile. A patient who is hypertensive in the morning may be distressingly hypotensive in the evening and vice versa. Patients may not adjust to abrupt changes in intravascular volume, so intravenous fluids should be carefully controlled.

REFERENCES

1. Johnson RT. Viral Infections of the Nervous System. New York: Raven Press; 1982.
2. Mims CA. The Pathogenesis of Infectious Diseases. 2d ed. London: Academic Pres; 1982.
3. Moxon ER, Murphy PA. *Hemophilus influenzae* bacteremia and meningitis resulting from survival of a single organism. Proc Natl Acad Sci USA. 1978;75:1534–6.
4. Murphy FA. Rabies pathogenesis: A brief review. Arch Virol. 1977;54:279.
5. Bodian D, Howe HA, Experimental studies on intraneural spread of poliomyelitis virus. Bull Johns Hopkins Hosp. 1941;68:248–67.

6. Baringer JR. Herpes simplex virus infection of nervous tissue in animals and man. Prog Med Virol. 1975;20:1–26.
7. Davis LE, Johnson RT. A possible explanation for the localization of herpes simplex encephalitis. Ann Neurol. 1979;5:2–5.
8. Monath TP, Cropp CP, Harrison AK. Mode of entry of a neurotropic arbovirus into the central nervous system. Reinvestigation of an old controversy. Lab Invest. 1983;48:399–410.
9. Martinez AJ, Duma RJ, Nelson EC, et al. Experimental *Naegleria* meningoencephalitis in mice. Penetration of the olfactory mucosal epithelium by *Naegleria* and pathologic changes produced: A light and electron microscopic study. Lab Invest. 1973;29:121.
10. Johnson RT. Selective vulnerability of neural cells to viral infection. Brain. 1980;103:447.
11. Johnson RT, Burke DS, Elwell M, et al. Japanese encephalitis: Immunocytochemical studies of viral antigen and inflammatory cells in fatal cases. Ann Neurol. 1985;18:567–73.
12. Navia BA, Cho ES, Petito CK, et al. The AIDS dementia complex II. Neuropathology. Ann Neurol. 1986;19:525–35.
13. Koenig S, Gendelman HE, Orenstein JM, et al. Detection of AIDS virus in macrophages in brain tissue from AIDS patients with encephalopathy. Science. 1986;233:1089–93.
14. Petito CK, Navia BA, Cho ES, et al. Vacuolar myelopathy pathologically resembling subacute combined degeneration in patients with the acquired immunodeficiency syndrome. N Engl J Med. 1985;312:874–9.
15. Rance NE, McArthur JC, Cornblath DR, et al. Gracile tract degeneration in patients with sensory neuropathy and AIDS. Neurology. 1988;38:265–71.
16. Chou SM, Roos R, Burrell R, et al. Subacute focal adenovirus encephalitis. J Neuropathol Exp Neurol. 1973;32:34.
17. Roos RP, Graves MC, Wollmann RL, et al. Immunologic and virologic studies of measles inclusion body encephalitis in an immunosuppressed host: The relationship to subacute sclerosing panencephalitis. Neurology. 1981;31:1263–70.
18. Dorfman LJ, Cytomegalovirus encephalitis in adults. Neurology. 1973;23:136.
19. Dupont JR, Earle KM. Human rabies encephalitis: A study of forty-nine fatal cases with a review of the literature. Neurology. 1965;15:1023.
20. Miller JQ, Price TR. The nervous system in Rocky Mountain spotted fever. Neurology. 1972;22:561.
21. Dastur DK, Lalitha VS, Udani PM, et al. The brain and meninges in tuberculous meningitis: Gross pathology in 100 cases and pathogenesis. Neurol India. 1970;18:86.
22. Young RC, Bennett JE, Vogel CL, et al. Aspergillosis: The spectrum of disease in 98 patients. Medicine. 1970;49:147–73.
23. Greenfield JG. Infectious diseases of the central nervous system: Neurosyphilis. In: Blackwood W, McMenemey WH, Meyer A, et al, eds. Greenfield's Neuropathology. Baltimore: Williams and Wilkins; 1963:164.
24. Baker RD, Haugen RK. Tissue changes and tissue diagnosis in cryptococcosis: A study of 26 cases. J Clin Pathol. 1955;25:14.
25. Ellner JJ, Bennett JE. Chronic meningitis. Medicine. 1976;55:341.
26. Johnson RT, Griffin DE, Hirsch RL, et al. Measles encephalomyelitis—Clinical and immunologic studies. N Engl J Med. 1984;310:137–41.
27. Hemachudha T, Griffin DE, Giffels JJ, et al. Myelin basic protein as an encephalitogen in encephalomyelitis and polyneuritis following rabies vaccination. N Engl J Med. 1987;316:369–74.
28. Hemachudha T, Phanuphak, Johnson RT, et al. Neurological complications of Semple type rabies vaccine: Clinical and immunologic studies. Neurology. 1987;37:550–6.
29. Miller HG, Stanton JB, Gibbons JL. Para-infectious encephalomyelitis and related syndromes: A critical review of the neurological complications of certain specific fevers. Q J Med. 1956;25:427–505.
30. Hart MN, Earle KM. Haemorrhagic and perivenous encephalitis: A clinical pathologic review of 38 cases. J Neurol Neurosurg Psychiatry. 1975;38:585–91.
31. Morens DM, Sullivan-Bolyai JZ, Slater JE, et al. Surveillance of Reye syndrome in the United States, 1977. Am J Epidemiol. 1981;114:406.
32. Hurwitz ES, Barrett MJ, Bregman D, et al. Public health service study on Reye's syndrome and medications: Report of the pilot phase. N Engl J Med. 1985;313:849–57.
33. Lewis DW, Tucker SH. Central nervous system involvement in cat scratch disease. Pediatrics. 1986;77:714–21.
34. Osuntokun BO, Adeuja AOG, Familusi JB. Tuberculous meningitis in Nigerians: A study of 194 patients. Trop Geogr Med. 1971;23:225.
35. Kovacs JA, Kovacs AA, Polis M, et al. Cryptococcosis in the acquired immunodeficiency syndrome. Ann Intern Med. 1985;103:533–8.
36. Whitley RJ, Soong S-J, Linneman C, et al. Herpes simplex encephalitis: Clinical assessment. JAMA. 1982;247:317.
37. Hattwick MAW. Human rabies. Public Health Rep. 1981;96:580–4.
38. Dickerson RB, Newton JR, Hansen JE. Diagnosis and immediate prognosis of Japanese B encephalitis. Am J Med. 1952;12:277–88.
39. Hilt DC, Buchholz D, Krumholz A, et al. Herpes zoster ophthalmicus and delayed contralateral hemiparesis due to cerebral angiitis: Diagnosis and management approaches. Ann Neurol. 1983;14:543.
40. Reik L, Steere AC, Bartenhagen NH, et al. Neurologic abnormalities of Lyme disease. Medicine. 1979;58:281.
41. Reik L, Burgdorfer W, Donaldson JO. Neurologic abnormalities in Lyme disease without erythema chronicum migrans. Am J Med. 1986;81:73–8.
42. Centers for Disease Control. Human rabies—California, 1987. MMWR. 1988;37:305–8.
43. Knox DL, Bayless TM, Pittman FE. Neurologic disease in patients with treated Whipple's disease. Medicine. 1976;55:467–76.
44. Helmick CG, Bernard KW, D'Angelo LJ. Rocky Mountain spotted fever: Clinical, laboratory, and epidemiological features of 262 cases. J Infect Dis. 1984;150:480–8.
45. Fishbein DB, Sawyer LA, Holland CJ, et al. Unexplained febrile illnesses after exposure to ticks. Infection with an *Ehrlichia*? JAMA. 1987;257:3100–4.
46. Kelsey DS. Adenovirus meningoencephalitis. Pediatrics. 1978;61:291.
47. McKinney RE Jr, Katz SL, Wilfert CM. Chronic enteroviral meningoencephalitis in agammaglobulinemic patients. Rev Infect Dis. 1987;9:334–56.
48. McArthur JC. Neurologic manifestations of human immunodeficiency virus infection. Medicine. 1987;66:407–37.
49. Osame M, Matsumoto M, Usuku K, et al. Chronic progressive myelopathy associated with elevated antibodies to human T-lymphotropic virus type 1 and adult T-cell leukemia-like cells. Ann Neurol. 1987;21:117–22.
50. Vernant JC, Maurs L, Gessain A, et al. Endemic tropical spastic paraparesis associated with human T-lymphotropic virus type I: A clinical and seroepidemiological study of 25 cases. Ann Neurol. 1987;21:123–30.
51. Feigin RD, Shackelford PG. Value of repeat lumbar puncture in the differential diagnosis of meningitis. N Engl J Med. 1973;289:571.
52. Koskiniemi M, Vaheri A, Taskinen E. Cerebrospinal fluid alterations in herpes simplex virus encephalitis. Rev Infect Dis. 1984;6:608–18.
53. Adams RD, Victor M. Multiple sclerosis and demyelinating disease: Acute hemorrhagic encephalomyelitis. In: Principles of Neurology. New York: McGraw-Hill; 1977:690.
54. Carter RF. Primary amoebic meningoencephalitis: An appraisal of present knowledge. Trans R Soc Trop Med Hyg. 1972;66:193–208.
55. Peacock JE Jr, McGinnis MR, Cohen MS. Persistent neutrophilic meningitis: Report of four cases and review of the literature. Medicine. 1984;63:379–95.
56. Link H, Muller R. Immunoglobulins in multiple sclerosis and infections of the nervous system. Arch Neurol. 1971;25:326–44.
57. Tourtellotte W. On cerebrospinal fluid immunoglobulin-G (IgG) quotients in multiple sclerosis and other diseases. J Neurol Sci. 1970;10:279.
58. Vandvik B, Nilsen RE, Vartdal F, et al. Mumps meningitis: Specific and nonspecific antibody responses in the central nervous system. Acta Neurol Scand. 1982;65:468–87.
59. Vartdal F, Vandvik B, Norrby E. Intrathecal synthesis of virus-specific oligoclonal IgG, IgA, and IgM antibodies in a case of varicella-zoster meningoencephalitis. J Neurol Sci. 1982;57:121–32.
60. Vartdal F, Vandvik B, Michaelson TE, et al. Neurosyphilis: Intrathecal synthesis of oligoclonal antibodies to *Treponema pallidum*. Ann Neurol. 1982;11:35.
61. Ackermann R, Rehese-Kupper B, Gollmer E, et al. Chronic neurologic manifestations of erythema migrans borreliosis. Ann NY Acad Sci. 1989;539:16–23.
62. Salmi AA, Norrby E, Panelius M. Identification of different measles virus-specific antibodies in the serum and cerebrospinal fluid from patients with subacute sclerosing panencephalitis and multiple sclerosis. Infect Immun. 1972;6:248.
63. Townsend JJ, Baringer JR, Wolinsky JS, et al. Progressive rubella panencephalitis: Late onset after congenital rubella. N Engl J Med. 1975;292:99.
64. Meyer HM, Johnson RT, Crawford IP, et al. Central nervous system syndromes of "viral" etiology: A study of 713 cases. Am J Med. 960;29:334–47.
65. Cohen SR, Herndon RM, McKhann GM. Radioimmunoassay of myelin basic protein in spinal fluid: An index of active demyelination. N Engl J Med. 1976;295:1455.
66. Ogawa SK, Smith MA, Brennessel DJ, et al. Tuberculous meningitis in an urban medical center. Medicine. 1987;66:317–26.
67. Lennette EH, Longshore WA. Western equine and St. Louis encephalitis in man. California 1945–1950. Calif Med. 1951;75:189.
68. Calisher CH, Thompson WE, eds. California Serogroup Viruses. New York: Alan R. Liss; 1983.
69. Spruance SL, Bailey A. Colorado tick fever: A review of 115 laboratory confirmed cases. Arch Intern Med. 1973;131:288.
70. Wilfert CM, MacCormack JN, Kleeman K, et al. Epidemiology of Rocky Mountain spotted fever as determined by active surveillance. J Infect Dis. 1984;150:469–79.
71. Ciesielski CA, Hightower AW, Horsley R, et al. The geographic distribution of Lyme disease in the United States. Ann NY Acad Sci. 1989;539:283–8.
72. Schmid GP. The global distribution of Lyme disease. Rev Infect Dis. 1985;7:41–50.
73. Rosen L. The natural history of Japanese encephalitis virus. Ann Rev Microbiol. 1986;40:395–414.
74. Monath TP. Flaviviruses. In: Fields BN, ed. Virology. New York: Raven Press; 1985:955–1004.
75. Goldfield M, Sussman O. The 1959 outbreak of Eastern encephalitis in New Jersey. I. Introduction and description of outbreak. Am J Epidemiol. 1968;87:1.
76. Southern PM, Smith JW, Luby JP, et al. Clinical and laboratory features of epidemic St. Louis encephalitis. Ann Intern Med. 1969;71:681.
77. Hilty HD, Haynes RE, Azimi PH, et al. California encephalitis in children. Am J Dis Child. 1972;124:530.

78. Earnest MP, Goolishian HA, Calverley JR, et al. Neurologic, intellectual and psychologic sequelae following western encephalitis. Neurology. 1971;21:969–74.
79. Ventura AK, Buff EE, Ehrenkranz NJ. Human Venezuelan equine encephalitis virus infection in Florida. Am J Trop Med Hyg. 1974;23:507.
80. Guze BH, Baxter LR Jr. Neuroleptic malignant syndrome. N Engl J Med. 1985;313:163–6.
81. Glass JP, Lee YY, Bruner J, et al. Treatment-related leukoencephalopathy: A study of three cases and literature review. Medicine. 1986;65:154–62.
82. Jemsek J, Greenberg SB, Taber L, et al. Herpes zoster-associated encephalitis: Clinicopathologic report of 12 cases and review of the literature. Medicine. 1983;62:81–96.
83. Linnemann CC, First MR, Alvira MM, et al. Herpes virus hominis type 2 meningoencephalitis following renal transplantation. Am J Med. 1976;61:703.
84. Morgello S, Cho ES, Nielson S, et al. Cytomegalovirus encephalitis in patients with acquired immunodeficiency syndrome: An autopsy study of 30 cases and a review of the literature. Human Pathol. 1987;18:289–97.
85. Martinez AJ. Is *Acanthamoeba* encephalitis an opportunistic infection? Neurology. 1980;30:567–74.
86. Elder GA, Sever JL. Neurologic disorders associated with AIDS retroviral infection. Rev Infect Dis. 1988;10:286–302.
87. Cohen J, Capildeo R, Rose FC, et al. Schistosomal myelopathy. Br Med J. 1977;1:1258.
88. Altrocchi PH. Acute transverse myelopathy. Arch Neurol. 1963;9:111.
89. Lipton HL, Teasdall RD. Acute transverse myelopathy in adults. Arch Neurol. 1973;28:252.
90. Hogan EL, Krigman MR. Herpes zoster myelitis: Evidence for viral invasion of spinal cord. Arch Neurol. 1973;29:309.
91. Hurst EW, Pawan JL. A further account of the Trinidad outbreak of acute rabic myelitis: Histology of the experimental disease. J Pathol Bacteriol. 1932;35:301.
92. Whitley R, Arvin A, Corey L, et al. Clinical factors which influence morbidity and mortality of herpes simplex virus. Pediatr Res. 1988;23:386A.
93. Whitley RJ, Alford CA, Hirsch MS, et al. Viradabine versus acyclovir therapy in herpes simplex encephalitis. N Engl J Med. 1986;314:144–9.
94. Balfour HH, Bean B, Laskin O, et al. Acyclovir halts progression of herpes zoster in immunocompromised patients. N Engl J Med. 1983;308:1448.
95. Parry GJ. Peripheral neuropathies associated with human immunodeficiency virus infection. Ann Neurol. 1988;23(Suppl):S49–S53.
96. Pachner AR, Steere AC. The triad of neurologic manifestations of Lyme disease: Meningitis, cranial neuritis, and radiculoneuritis. Neurology. 1985;35:47–53.
97. Hinthorn DR, Baker LH, Romig DA, et al. Recurrent conjugal neuralgia caused by herpes virus hominis type 2. JAMA. 1976;236:587.
98. Sabin TD, Swift TR. Leprosy. In: Dyck PJ, Thomas PK, Lambert EH, et al, eds. Peripheral Neuropathy. 1984;1955–87.
99. Palmieri JR, LaChance MA, Connon DH. Parasitic infection of the peripheral nervous system. In: Peripheral Neuropathy. Dyck PJ, Thomas PK, Lambert EH, et al, eds. 1984:1988–2009.
100. Prince DL, Griffin J, Young A, et al. Tetanus toxin: Direct evidence for retrograde intraaxonal transport. Science. 1975;188:945.
101. Simpson LL. Molecular pharmacology of botulinum toxin and tetanus toxin. Ann Rev Pharmacol Toxicol. 1986;26:427–53.
102. Black JD, Dolly JO. Interaction of ^{125}I-labelled botulinum neurotoxins with nerve terminals. II. Autoradiographic evidence for uptake into motor nerves by acceptor-mediated endocytosis. J Cell Biol. 1986;103:535–44.
103. Pappenheimer AM. Diphtheria toxin. Ann Rev Biochem. 1977;46:69–94.
104. Cornblath DR, McArthur JC, Kennedy PGE, et al. Inflammatory demyelinating peripheral neuropathies associated with human T-cell lymphotropic virus type III infection. Ann Neurol. 1987;21:32–40.
105. Server AC, Johnson RT. Guillain-Barré syndrome. In: Remington JS, Schwartz MN, eds. Current Clinical Topics in Infectious Diseases. vol. 3. New York: McGraw-Hill; 1982:74–96.
106. Asbury AK, Arnason BG, Adams RD. The inflammatory lesion in idiopathic polyneuritis: Its role in pathogenesis. Medicine. 1969;48:173–215.
107. Waksman BH, Adams RD. Allergic neuritis: An experimental disease of rabbits induced by the injection of peripheral nervous tissue and adjuvants. J Exp Med. 1955;102:213.
108. Weinstein L. Tetanus. N Engl J Med. 1973;289:1293.
109. Cherington M. Botulism: Ten-year experience. Arch Neurol. 1974;30:432.
110. Merson MH, Dowell VR Jr. Epidemiologic, clinical and laboratory aspects of wound botulism. N Engl J Med. 1973;289:1005.
111. McDonald WI, Kocen PS. Diphtheritic neuropathy. In: Dyck PJ, Thomas PK, Lambert EH, et al, eds. Peripheral Neuropathy. 1984:2010–7.
112. Masucci EF, Kurtzke JF. Diagnostic criteria for the Guillain-Barré syndrome: An analysis of 50 cases. J Neurol Sci. 1971;13:483.
113. Lichtenfeld P. Autoimmune dysfunction in the Guillain-Barré syndrome. Am J Med. 1971;50:772–80.
114. Wiederholt WC, Mulder DW, Lambert EH. The Landry-Guillain-Barré-Strohl syndrome or polyradiculoneuropathy: Historical review, report on 97 patients, and present concepts. Mayo Clin Proc. 1964;39:427.
115. McLeod JG, Walsh JC, Prineas JW, et al. Acute idiopathic polyneuritis: A clinical and electrophysiological follow-up study. J Neurol Sci. 1976;27:145–62.
116. The Guillain-Barré Syndrome Study Group: Plasmapheresis and acute Guillain-Barré syndrome. Neurology. 1985;35:1096–1104.

69. SLOW INFECTIONS OF THE CENTRAL NERVOUS SYSTEM

JAMES R. LEHRICH
KENNETH L. TYLER

The concept of "atypically slow infections" was introduced in 1954 by Sigurdsson,[1] an Icelandic pathologist who was particularly interested in visna, maedi, and scrapie, three diseases of sheep. By adapting his criteria, a slow infection may be defined as a progressive pathologic process caused by a transmissible agent that remains clinically silent during a prolonged incubation period of months to years, after which progressive clinical disease appears, usually ending months later in profound disability or death.[2]

Interest in slow infections of the human central nervous system (CNS) has been particularly keen since the experimental transmission of kuru from humans to chimpanzees. Several CNS diseases of humans can be classified as slow infections (Table 1), and there are diseases of other organ systems (e.g., infectious hepatitis) that might be considered slow infections as well. Two CNS diseases of known viral etiology (subacute sclerosing panencephalitis and progressive multifocal leukoencephalopathy) are described in Chapters 124 and 138. The transmissible spongiform encephalopathies (kuru and Creutzfeldt-Jakob disease), diseases caused by unnamed agents that may be viruses, and a common CNS disease for which a viral causation has been proposed (multiple sclerosis) are discussed in this chapter. The subject of prions, a putative agent of the transmissible spongiform encephalopathies, is discussed in Chapter 156.

The term *slow infection* is used rather than *slow virus* for two reasons: (*1*) for some of these diseases, the transmissible spongiform encephalopathies, the causative agent does not fit the conventional definition of virus, and (*2*) even in those slow infections that are caused by conventional viruses, it is the disease process and not the virus that is slow.

UNNAMED AGENTS OF CREUTZFELDT-JAKOB DISEASE AND KURU

Kuru, a neurologic disease found only among the primitive Fore tribes of the New Guinea highlands, was the first chronic, "degenerative" CNS disease of humans shown to be a transmissible slow infection. When intensive study began in 1956,[8] kuru was thought to be of genetic origin. In 1959, Hadlow[9] pointed out clinical and histopathologic similarities between kuru and scrapie, a disease of sheep that had been shown to be transmissible as long ago as 1936.[10] In both diseases, the CNS shows spongiform degeneration of gray matter, with severe loss of neurons, vacuolization of neuronal cytoplasm, marked proliferation of astrocytes, and little inflammation. Hadlow's suggestion led to intensified efforts to transmit kuru to experimental animals, and in 1965 Gajdusek and his colleagues reported that a kurulike disease developed in chimpanzees 20 months after intracerebral inoculation with suspensions of brain tissue from kuru patients.[11]

Creutzfeldt-Jakob disease (CJD),[12] a relatively uncommon dementing illness of humans that is found throughout the world, has spongiform neuropathologic changes that are similar to those seen in kuru. The successful transmission of kuru prompted similar attempts to transmit CJD to chimpanzees, and this was accomplished in 1968.[13] The most recent addition to the list of transmissible spongiform encephalopathies in humans is the Gerstmann-Straussler syndrome, an adult-onset chronic cerebellar ataxia in which dementia is a late feature.[14]

TABLE 1. Slow Infections of the Central Nervous System

Disease	Virus	Nucleic Acid
Subacute sclerosing panencephalitis (SSPE) (Chapter 138)	Measles	RNA
Progressive congenital rubella encephalomyelittis[3]	Rubella	RNA
Chronic progressive rubella panencephalitis[4,5]	Rubella	RNA
Rabies (Chapter 140)	Rabies	RNA
Acquired immune deficiency syndrome (AIDS) encephalopathy and vacuolar myelopathy (Chapter 108)[6,7]	HIV (HTLV-III)	RNA
Progressive multifocal leukoencephalopathy (PML) (Chapter 124)	JC and SV40-PML	DNA
Congenital cytomegalic inclusion disease (Chapter 120)	Cytomegalovirus	DNA
Transmissible spongiform encephalopathies Kuru (humans) Creutzfeldt-Jakob disease (humans) Scrapie (sheep) Transmissible mink encephalopathy (mink) Chronic wasting disease (mule, elk, deer)	Unnamed	?
Multiple sclerosis (possibly a slow infection)	?	?

The transmissible spongiform encephalopathies—kuru, Creutzfeldt-Jakob disease, scrapie, transmissible mink encephalopathy, and chronic wasting disease of mule, elk, and deer (Table 1)—are caused by transmissible agents that share the unusual properties of extremely small size, great resistance to chemical and physical agents, failure to induce either an inflammatory or an immune response, and a lack of demonstrable nucleic acid or non-host protein. Gajdusek[15] has called this group of unnamed agents "unconventional viruses," but it is still uncertain whether they are best considered viruses or some new group of microorganisms.

DESCRIPTION OF THE PATHOGEN

Much of the information about this group of agents comes from research on the more readily studied scrapie agent, which has been adapted to mice[16] and hamsters.[17] The agents of kuru and CJD had been transmissible only to primates until adaptation of the CJD agent to cats, mice, and guinea pigs and adaptation of the kuru agent to mink during the 1970s.

The infectivity of the agents of scrapie and transmissible mink encephalopathy are filterable to a 25 nm average pore diameter. The kuru and CJD agents are filterable to an average pore diameter of 100 nm. γ-Radiation inactivation studies of the scrapie agent indicate an equivalent target molecular mass of 150,000 daltons or less.[18] All replicate to 50 percent lethal dose (LD_{50}) titers of 10^5–10^{11}/g in infected brain tissue and can be assayed in either end point titration or incubation time interval bioassays. Infectivity is closely associated with cell membrane elements,[19] and complete destruction of the membrane is required to destroy infectivity. Thus, the agents are unusually resistant to inactivation by physical and chemical means, including formaldehyde, β-propiolactone, ethylenediamine tetraacetic acid (EDTA), proteases, nucleases, heat to 80°C, ultraviolet radiation (>20,000 J/m^2 at 254 nm), γ-radiation, and ultrasonic energy. They remain stable for many years at −70°C or after lyophilization. The agents can, however, be inactivated by autoclaving (121°C, 15 lb/in^2, 4.5 hours), or by three treatments with 1 N sodium hydroxide for 30 minutes at room temperature.[20]

The unusual properties of these agents, particularly their small size and resistance to inactivation, have raised questions as to whether they should be considered viruses. There are no detectable humoral or cellular immune responses to the agents,[21] and the scrapie agent does not influence interferon induction in mice.[22] No virions have been recognized in infected cells in tissue culture.[15] However, transmission experiments have shown that the agents of scrapie, kuru, and CJD persist in vitro in tissue culture explants from infected brain and that the scrapie agent replicates in cell culture.[23,24] Hunter[25] has postulated that the scrapie agent is an integral part of the cell membrane, possibly a replicable glycoprotein. Diener has suggested that these agents may be similar to viroids,[26] very small, naked, single-stranded RNA viruses of plants that are also extremely resistant to inactivation by ionizing and ultraviolet irradiation. Prusiner has introduced the term *prion* to denote small, proteinaceous infectious particles that resist inactivation by most procedures that modify nucleic acids.[27,28] (The subject is discussed in detail in Chapter 156).

It was not until recently that reliable and confirmed reports have appeared of characteristic fibrillar or rod-shaped particles specifically found in material prepared from the brains of humans infected with CJD or animals infected with scrapie. Previous reports[29–31] of virus-like or spiroplasma-like organisms have not been confirmed. In 1981, Merz and her colleagues described abnormal fibrils seen by electron microscopy in lysosomal fractions prepared from scrapie-infected brains.[32] They subsequently found similar fibrils in preparations of brain material from patients with CJD[33] and felt that these fibrils represented "infection specific particles" from the unconventional slow virus diseases.[34] Morphologically, the scrapie-associated fibrils (SAFs) resemble both the paired helical filaments of neurofibrillary tangles and the fibrils of amyloid. Rod-shaped particles can also be seen in purified preparations of prions made from the brains of scrapie-infected animals. These rods are typically 10–20 nm in diameter and 100–200 nm in length and appear to be composed almost exclusively of the prion protein PrP 27-30.[35,36] Extensive controversy continues about the relationship between SAFs and prion rods and whether or not they are in fact identical or closely related structures.[28,37]

EPIDEMIOLOGY

Kuru has been confined to a few primitive tribes in the mountainous highlands of eastern New Guinea. More than 80 percent of the cases have occurred among tribes of the Fore linguistic group. During the 1950s[8] there were more than 200 kuru deaths per year in that population, a prevalence rate that approached 1 percent per year. The disease affected all ages beyond infants, with an equal sex ratio among preadolescents but a striking excess in female adults. The number of deaths per year resulting from kuru has been declining gradually but steadily since 1957–8 when accurate statistics first became available. Since 1985 there have been fewer than 15 kuru-related deaths per year. This decline has been attributed to the cessation of ritual cannibalism, the consumption of dead kinsmen that had been practiced as a rite of mourning. No one born since cannibalism ceased in a given village has died of kuru. Gajdusek[38] has suggested that kuru was transmitted by autoinoculation of infected tissue through skin cuts, nasal mucosae, or ocular conjunctivae, thus infecting women and small children, the main participants in these ceremonies. The kuru agent has been shown to be transmissible to experimental animals orally as well as by peripheral routes of inoculation (see the section on "Pathogenesis"). The incubation period of kuru in humans can be more than 30 years.[39,40] The disease appears not to be contagious; there have been no secondary cases among contacts of kuru emigrants and no cases in immigrants to the endemic area.[41]

Creutzfeldt-Jakob disease has been found throughout the world, with a prevalence, annual incidence, and yearly mortality rate of about one per million reported from large population centers where the disease is more readily diagnosed.[15] A 30-fold higher incidence has been noted in Libyan Jews who had migrated to Israel, as compared with the incidence in Jews of European origin.[42] Other small geographic and temporal clusters of cases have been reported,[43,44] and there are two reports of a husband and wife dying of CJD within a few years of each other.[44,45] About 15 percent of the cases have been familial, and a pattern of occurrence that suggests autosomal dominant transmission has been described.[43,46] Most cases occur during the fifth to seventh decades of life, and men and women are affected equally. A study of cases in the United States[47] found no apparent relationship to occupation or exposure to other patients or animals. A possible association with the eating of animal brains or sheep eyeballs has been suggested but not confirmed to date.[47–49]

PATHOGENESIS

There is clear evidence that both kuru and CJD are caused by transmissible agents. In 1965, kuru was transmitted to chimpanzees, and they developed an ataxic illness quite similar to the human disease 18–30 months after the intracerebral inoculation of brain suspensions from kuru patients.[11] Subsequent studies have shown that kuru can be transmitted by peripheral or intracerebral inoculation to several species of new-world and old-world monkeys and to the mink and ferret; incubation periods vary from 8 months in the smaller animals to more than 8 years in the monkeys. CJD has been transmitted to new-world and old-world monkeys, goats, cats, guinea pigs, mice, and hamsters. Both agents can be passaged serially in experimental animals inoculated with infected tissues. Scrapie, kuru, and CJD have recently been orally transmitted by feeding infected tissues to squirrel monkeys.[50] Spongiform encephalopathy has been induced in monkeys inoculated with brain tissue suspensions from two patients with familial Alzheimer's disease, although subsequent attempts to confirm this result have not been successful.[51]

The agents are found in brain in 50 percent infective dose (ID_{50}) titers of over $10^8/g$[15] and also in lower titers in the liver, lymph nodes, and spleen; in addition, the CJD agent has been found in the lung, kidney, cornea, and cerebrospinal fluid (CSF) and also in leukocytes of infected guinea pigs.[52]

Creutzfeldt-Jakob disease has been transmitted from human to human through corneal transplants,[53] contaminated stereotactic brain electrodes,[57] dura mater grafts,[55,56] and the administration of human growth hormone derived from pools of pituitary glands obtained at autopsy and contaminated by tissue from patients who had CJD.[57–59] Thus CJD is transmissible from human to human, but probably only via direct inoculation. Of possible relevance are the increased incidence of recent brain or eye surgery that has been noted in CJD patients[44] and the experimental spongiform encephalopathy that has been produced in primates inoculated with brain tissue from a neurosurgeon who died after an atypical encephalopathy accompanied by vasculitis in skin and peripheral nerves and whose brain also showed pathologic changes of CJD.[62] No cases of CJD have been observed among virologists working with the disease or in pathologists, and there does not appear to be an excess of cases among medical personnel.[43] However, the unusual resistance of the agent to inactivation necessitates special precautions in dealing with patients and tissues, although special isolation procedures do not appear to be necessary.[63] Kuru is thought to be transmitted by autoinoculation during ritual cannibalism, as discussed previously.

The actual mechanisms by which the agents cause neurologic disease are unknown. There is no evidence of an inflammatory response in kuru- and CJD-infected brains and no significant humoral or cell-mediated immune response to any known infectious agent.[21] Autoantibodies that react with neurofilaments and with the paired helical filaments found in neurofibrillary tangles have been found not only in the sera of patients and animals afflicted with kuru, CJD, and scrapie[64,65] but also in some patients with other neurologic diseases and in some normal subjects. Reactivity is directed primarily against the 150 and 200 kD proteins of the neurofilament triplet and against the 62 kD neurofilament-associated protein.[66] Studies of the pathogenesis of mouse scrapie suggest that after inoculation at peripheral sites the scrapie agent replicates in spleen and lymphoid tissue before spreading via nerves to reach the CNS.[67] Neural spread may be mediated by slow axonal transport.[37] Neural spread of the scrapie agent within the CNS and from the CNS to the peripheral nervous system has also been reported.[68,69] Whether these pathways of spread also occur in human spongiform encephalopathies remains to be established.

PATHOLOGIC FINDINGS

Both kuru and CJD are spongiform encephalopathies; pathologic findings are limited to the CNS. Brains show diffuse losses of neurons, intense astrocytic proliferation with fibrous gliosis, and swelling and intracytoplasmic vacuolation of neuronal and astroglial processes that correspond to the spongy state.[70] The severity and distribution of the vacuolation has been variable in cases of kuru; in CJD it is most prominent in the early stage of the disease.[71] There are no inflammatory phenomena and no demyelination, although rare cases may show large areas of diffuse degeneration of white matter.[72] In 70 percent of kuru and 10 percent of CJD cases, argyrophilic, periodic acid–Schiff (PAS)-positive amyloid-like plaques are found, especially in the cerebellum. In kuru, the most severe changes are in the cerebellum and the areas to which it has afferent and efferent connections. In CJD, the frontal cortex is usually most severely affected, although there are some cases in which the occipitoparietal regions of the cerebral cortex are involved almost exclusively (Heidenhain type) and others in which there is severe granule cell atrophy of the cerebellum. The electron microscope has demonstrated the vacuoles within neurons and cytoplasmic processes of astrocytes as well as rupture of plasma membranes with accumulation of curled membrane fragments.[70,73] Golgi impregnations have shown a loss of dendritic spines of pyramidal neurons and unusual focal spherical distensions of dendritic and axonal processes.[73]

CLINICAL MANIFESTATIONS

Kuru

Almost all cases of this increasingly rare disease have occurred in individuals between the ages of 5 and 60 years.[8,20,38,40,51,74] The core syndrome is one of a rapidly progressive cerebellar degeneration to which features of cortical and brain stem dysfunction are conjoined. The disease is characterized by an insidious onset (without fever or evidence of systemic illness), cerebellar ataxia of gait and limbs, and a shivering tremor that involves the head, trunk, and legs more than the arms. Some patients experience a prodrome of headache or limb or joint pain that may last several months. *Kuru* is the Fore term for shivering. Dysarthria, signs of pyramidal and extrapyramidal involvement, strabismus, and mood changes are also found. These worsen progressively until the patient is unable to walk and cannot move without the ataxic tremors. During this stage, involuntary movements resembling chorea or athetosis and an exaggerated response to being startled (''startle myoclonus'') may be found. A dementia may supervene and can be associated with frontal release signs. Dysphagia develops, and patients usually die of inanition, pneumonia, or respiratory failure 3–12 months after onset.

The diagnosis is usually made based on the occurrence of the appropriate clinical findings in the correct epidemiologic setting. Laboratory tests have not been useful as aids to diagnosis. The electroencephalogram (EEG), electromyogram (EMG), CSF examination, blood count, and serum chemistries and electrolytes are typically normal. There are no reports to date of the use of computed tomography (CT) or magnetic resonance imaging (MRI).

Creutzfeldt-Jakob Disease

CJD is a relatively uncommon, rapidly evolving cerebral disease of late middle age, in which profound dementia is combined with ataxia and diffuse myoclonic jerking; rare cases in teenagers and octogenarians have been reported.[12,41,51,60,61,75–77] A presenile dementia with myoclonus is almost invariably CJD. The distribution is worldwide and the occurrence sporadic. In the early stages, there are changes in behavior, emotional responses, memory, and reasoning together with visual distortions or impaired visual acuity; patients often are delerious. Progression is rapid, and obvious deterioration can be detected from week to week. Most patients are profoundly demented within 6 months. Myoclonic contractions of various muscle groups appear eventually and can be triggered by sudden stimuli (noise, bright lights) or can occur spontaneously. Ataxia, dysarthria, and delerium progress to eventual stupor and coma. Death usually occurs in less than a year, often as a result of intercurrent infection. About 5–10 percent of patients have a clinical course of 2 years or more.

Certain laboratory tests may aid in the diagnosis. More than 50 percent of patients will have characteristic EEG findings at some point during their illness.[78] The most characteristic pattern is one of periodic-appearing (1 Hz), biphasic or triphasic, high-amplitude sharp waves, which may appear time locked to myoclonic jerks. This EEG appearance is quite different from what is seen in subacute sclerosing panencephalitis (SSPE) (see Chapter 138). A number of patients will never develop classic periodic sharp waves but instead show diffuse, polymorphic, high-amplitude, irregular slow (delta) waves. It is often helpful to obtain repeat EEGs at regular intervals because the characteristic periodic changes may become apparent only as the disease progresses. Even in patients without these changes, the EEG will often show progressive disorganization and deterioration with each successive recording.

The CSF is almost always normal. A mild elevation in protein levels is occasionally encountered. Significant pleocytosis, hypoglycorrachia, or an elevation in protein levels should prompt a search for other disorders or concomitant processes. A recent two-dimensional gel analysis report of the detection of abnormal proteins in the CSF of patients with CJD awaits confirmation.[79]

It has recently been reported that a 27 kD protein can be identified on Western blots of preparations of infected brain tissue from patients with CJD and kuru by using an antibody directed against a purified fraction of scrapie-infected hamster brain.[80] Whether this procedure will turn out to be sensitive and specific enough to aid in the diagnosis of CJD remains to be established.

Cerebral and cerebellar atrophy, sometimes rapidly progressive, may be shown by CT and MRI, although CT scans show normal anatomy in most cases.[81] The diagnosis may be confirmed by finding the characteristic neuropathologic features in a brain biopsy specimen or at autopsy. Cases with typical neuropathologic features ("spongiform encephalopathy") should be distinguished from similar cases that have been successfully transmitted to animals ("transmissible spongiform encephalopathy") and from cases of dementing diseases that lack the typical pathology but are transmissible to animals (which can be grouped under the more general label of "transmissible dementia").

PREVENTION AND TREATMENT

Kuru has been disappearing since the practice of cannibalism was eliminated among the Fore people between 1957 and 1962; cases are no longer seen among children or adolescents.[14] Our knowledge of the epidemiology of CJD is still incomplete, and little can be said about prevention of the disease as it occurs in nature. However, the evidence that CJD can be transmitted from person to person by corneal transplantation and accidental inoculation (see the section on pathogenesis) indicates that precautions are necessary in caring for patients and handling infected materials.[48,68] Certainly, demented patients should not be used as donors for tissue transplantation or blood or as sources of tissue for the preparation of biologic products to be used in humans (e.g., corneal transplants, dura mater, pituitary hormone, interferon). Needles, needle electrodes, scalpels, ophthalmic tonometers, autopsy instruments, and all other potentially contaminated materials should be sterilized, preferably by autoclaving at 121°C at 15 lb/in^2 for 4–5 hours or by three successive 30-minute immersions in 1 N sodium hydroxide at 25°C. Shorter treatment periods, lower dilutions of sodium hydroxide, or even the use of undiluted bleach are not consistently effective. Special isolation of CJD patients does not appear necessary, but clinical and pathologic laboratory specimens must be clearly marked, disposable gloves should be worn, and any skin contact with potentially infectious materials (especially blood, urine, or CSF), should be followed by washing with 1 N sodium hydroxide for several minutes.[20,63]

There is no treatment known to be effective for kuru or CJD, although there are unconfirmed reports of improvement in humans or experimental animals treated with amantidine, vidaribine, amphotericin B, high-molecular-weight dextran sulfate, and other agents.

AGENTS OF MULTIPLE SCLEROSIS

Multiple sclerosis (MS) is the most common and best known demyelinating disease of the human CNS. Demyelinating diseases are characterized by foci of destruction of the myelin sheaths of nerve fibers, with relative sparing of axons, nerve cell bodies, and the other elements of nervous tissue. It is important to use the term *demyelination* in this restricted sense since myelin is damaged in any disease in which there is necrosis or degeneration of white matter. Thus, progressive multifocal leukoencephalopathy (PML) (Chapter 124) is a demyelinating disease caused by papovavirus infection of oligodendrocytes. Subacute sclerosing panencephalitis (SSPE) (Chapter 138) and the acquired immunodeficiency syndrome (AIDS)-dementia complex (Chapter 108) are not considered demyelinating diseases, although there may be considerable damage to CNS myelin. A classification of the demyelinating diseases is given in Table 2.

The myelin sheath is formed from the cytoplasmic membrane of oligodendrocytes (central nervous system) or Schwann cells (peripheral nervous system) wrapped around the axon to form concentric layers of lipid and protein. Thus, demyelination could result from attacks on the oligodendrocyte or Schwann cell, attacks on the myelin itself, or disordered metabolism of myelin lipid or protein.

The pathogenesis of MS remains unknown, but a viral causation has often been proposed. The evidence in favor of the viral hypothesis remains indirect and incomplete but includes epidemiologic data, the inflammatory pathologic changes of MS, the oligoclonal immunoglobulins found in the CSF and synthesized within the neuraxis in MS, and the humoral and cell-mediated immunity to certain viral agents that have been detected in MS patients. The current evidence for and against a viral etiology of MS is summarized in this chapter. Several reviews of the subject are also available.[82–85]

TABLE 2. Central Nervous System Demyelinating Diseases of Humans

Multiple sclerosis
Acute disseminated encephalomyelitis (after viral infections or vaccination)
Acute necrotizing hemorrhage leukoencephalopathy
Schilder's disease (diffuse cerebral sclerosis)
Progressive multifocal leukoencephalopathy

EPIDEMIOLOGY

A relationship between the occurrence of MS and geographic latitude has been well established.[86] Rates of death, incidence, and prevalence increase with increasing latitudes, proceeding north or south from the equator, with especially high rates found above latitude 35 degrees in the northern hemisphere. For example, the prevalence in Rochester, Minnesota (latitude 45 degrees) is 60–70/100,000, while in New Orleans, Louisiana (latitude 30 degrees), it is 6/100,000. Similar gradients have been found in northern Europe and in the southern hemisphere, but there is a low prevalence of MS in Japan, latitudes at which North American and European cities have high prevalence.

It has also been shown that a person who migrates from a high-risk to a low-risk zone after early adolescence carries with him a high risk of developing MS, although the disease may not become apparent until 20 years after migration. Studies of immigrants from northern Europe to South Africa or Israel have indicated that there is a critical age of migration of 15 years.[86] If migration from the high-risk to the low-risk country takes place before the age of 15, the risk of MS equals that in the low-risk country; a person who migrates after the age of 15 carries with him the high risk of the native country. Patients with MS tend to have had measles and rubella later than the usual age.[87,88] A point-source epidemic of 24 cases of MS occurring between 1943 and 1960 in natives of the Faroe Islands and temporally related to the occupation of the Islands by British troops between 1940 and 1945 has also been described.[89] These data suggest that environmental factors, possibly related to an infectious agent, are significant in the genesis of MS. Studies of families have also been interpreted as consistent with exposure to an environmental factor before puberty.[86] MS is 15–20 times more common in first-degree relatives of MS patients than in unrelated persons, but there is increased prevalence in spouses of MS patients.

Clusters of extremely high prevalence have also been found. In the Shetland and Orkney islands off the north coast of Scotland (latitude 59 degrees) there are 128 cases of MS per 100,000 population.

Certain histocompatibility antigens are overrepresented in patients with MS as compared with controls.[90] These antigens are believed to provide markers for immune response genes and may affect susceptibility to an infectious agent or to an autoallergic mechanism in the causation of MS.

Reports of a possible association of MS with cats, dogs, and canine distemper have not been confirmed.[83,91–93]

These epidemiologic data do not establish which factors in the environment are significant in MS. Those lines of evidence that implicate viral infection are being considered here, but it should be recognized that the viral hypothesis may prove incorrect in the long run.

Humoral Antibodies to Viruses

In 1962, Adams and Imagawa[94] reported higher levels of serum antibodies to measles virus in patients with MS than in control subjects and the presence of measles antibodies in CSF from patients with MS but not controls. Since that time, there have been numerous investigations of measles antibodies in MS utilizing a variety of techniques. Although not all results have reached a level of statistical significance, most of these studies have shown elevations of mean antibody titer when larger numbers of MS and control sera were compared.[83] There has been particular interest in measles virus because a measleslike virus is the causative agent of subacute sclerosing panencephalitis (SSPE) (see Chapter 138). In MS, as in SSPE, the most impressive data have emerged from determinations of antibodies against the ribonucleoprotein components of measles virus, which are found elevated more consistently and to higher titers than are antibodies to the viral envelope.

The presence and probable local synthesis of measles antibodies in CSF in MS strongly imply a connection between the virus and the CNS disease. When antibody levels in CSF are compared with those in serum, there is a significantly lower serum:CSF ratio for measles antibodies than for several other viral antibodies tested.[95,96] This suggests the synthesis of measles antibodies within the CNS-CSF compartment; however, low serum:CSF ratios for other antibodies (for example, rubella, mumps, herpes simplex type 1, and vaccinia) have been reported in some patients with MS,[95,96] so the specificity of these findings is unclear.

Another observation consistent with local CNS production of viral antibodies is the presence in 35–100 percent of patients with MS (depending on the laboratory) of oligoclonal immunoglobulin G (IgG) appearing as multiple discrete γ-bands on agar gel electrophoresis of MS CSF.[97] These oligoclonal immunoglobulins suggest that a process of hyperimmunization goes on in MS. Their presence has been correlated with CSF lymphocytosis, CSF measles antibody titers, and reduced serum:CSF measles antibody ratios, and some investigators have been able to elute measles antibodies from the oligoclonal CSF IgG bands.[98,99] However, most of the immunoglobulins found in MS CSF have not been shown to be directed against specific viral antigens.[99] These observations should be compared with similar data from studies of SSPE (see Chapter 138), a disease in which levels of serum and CSF measles antibodies are much higher than in MS and in which dense oligoclonal IgG bands in serum, CSF, and brain tissue have been shown to contain antibodies to measles ribonucleoprotein antigens.[100]

Although most antibody studies of MS patients have concentrated on the measles virus, there have been data implicating herpes simplex type-2, varicella-zoster, vaccinia, rubella, and some other viruses.[82–84,99] By using highly sensitive radioimmunoassays, antibodies to more than one virus can be detected in the CSF in 67 percent of MS patients and 26 percent of controls.[101] It has been suggested that the antibodies to multiple viruses found in MS CSF are produced by preprogrammed B lymphocytes that enter the CNS and are then activated nonspecifically or released from normal immune regulation.[102]

The retrovirus human T-lymphotropic virus I (HTLV-I) has been implicated in patients with MS who were reported to have antiviral antibodies in serum and CSF; in four patients there were rare cells in the CSF that reacted with HTLV-I antigen by in situ hybridization under conditions of low stringency.[103] Using the polymerase chain reaction (PCR) technique, a recent study has identified DNA sequences related to HTLV-I in the peripheral blood mononuclear cells of 6 MS patients and in 1 of 20 healthy controls.[103a] Other neurologic syndromes have been associated with retroviruses: HTLV-I with tropical spastic paraparesis, HTLV-I–associated myelopathy in Japan,[104] the chronic leukoencephalitidies in sheep and goats caused by the visna and caprine arthritis-encephalitis viruses, as well as the encephalopathy (AIDS-dementia complex), myelopathy, and peripheral neuropathies that are common in patients infected with HIV (see Chapter 108). Several subsequent serologic and in situ hybridization studies have failed to confirm an association of retrovirus infection and MS, however,[104,105] and further studies in other laboratories are needed.[105a]

Some of the conflicting results reported in studies of humoral antibodies in MS may be accounted for by differences in control groups and in the viral antigens and antibody assay techniques used. Moreover, there is an increased prevalence in the MS population of the histocompatibility antigens HLA-A3, HLA-B7, HLA-BW18, and possibly others and of the mixed lymphocyte culture determinant HLA-Dw2 (present in up to 60 percent of MS patients in some studies); there is also evidence that persons carrying HLA-A3, HLA-B7, or HLA-BW18 have higher levels of serum antibodies to measles virus and to herpes simplex virus types 1 and 2, but not to parainfluenza virus type

1, than do persons lacking these HLA antigens, whether they suffer from MS or not.[82,90] It may be that the elevated levels of antibodies to measles and other viruses that are sometimes found in patients with MS reflect the overrepresentation in this disease of certain immune response (Ir) genes for which histocompatibility antigens and the HLA-Dw2 determinant provide a marker. Thus, persons carrying these antigens and an Ir gene linked to them may react to viral or to CNS antigens in a manner different from members of a control population. We do not know whether this difference is relevant to susceptibility to demyelinating disease.

Cell-Mediated Hypersensitivity to Viruses

Several studies of cell-mediated immunity to measles and other viruses in MS have been reported, but the results have been conflicting.[82–84,96] Some investigators have found impaired reactivity of lymphocytes to measles and other viral antigens, while others have found normal responses. Some of the apparent conflicts in these observations are, again, probably methodologic. Definite conclusions about cell-mediated hypersensitivity to viruses in MS have to await additional information.

Multiple sclerosis patients differ from controls in the distribution of T and B lymphocytes and their subpopulations. Suppressor T-cell activity as identified by suppression of lymphocyte mitogen responsiveness and numbers of suppressor-cytotoxic T cells labeled by monoclonal antibodies to phenotypic cell markers are in the low normal range in patients with stable disease. During acute attacks, suppressor activity and suppressor T-cell numbers are subnormal, rising to high normal levels as remission commences.[106,107] A relationship between suppressor activity and interferon production has also been described,[108] and decreased production of interferon by peripheral blood leukocytes in response to viruses and other interferon inducers have been found in some MS patients.[109]

Viral Isolation

Direct evidence of a viral causation of MS would require consistent and reproducible isolation of a viral agent from MS CNS tissue or body fluids and induction of demyelinating disease in experimental animals infected with that virus.

Early and unconfirmed reports[82] have included those of a rabies virus isolated in the Soviet Union and herpes simplex type 2 isolated in Iceland. Since then, there have been reports of isolation of virus or identification of virus antigen in brain and other tissues for a variety of agents, including parainfluenza type 1, measles, herpes simplex type 1, coronavirus and HTLV-I (see above). All these studies await confirmation.

There have also been many unsuccessful attempts to transmit disease to experimental animals by means of inoculation of affected CNS tissue. Reports of induction of a scrapielike disease in sheep and mice[110] and an MS-associated agent that caused a polymorphonuclear leukopenia in mice have not been reproducible.[111]

Electron Microscopic Studies

There have been numerous reports of "paramyxovirus-like" intranuclear and cytoplasmic filamentous rodlike profiles seen under the electron microscope within inflammatory cells near lesions in MS brains. Further study has led to general agreement that the profiles have the electron density of nuclear chromatin, are of homogeneous density, lack an inside tubular structure, and have an irregular diameter. This is in contrast to measles virus nucleocapsids (as observed in SSPE tissue, for example) and parainfluenza virus nucleocapsids, which are clearly tubular with a helical configuration, have a constant diameter (16 and 18 nm, respectively), and show clear-cut periodic striations. It is probable that the fuzzy rods seen in MS tissue are dispersed nuclear chromatin in damaged nuclei, similar to profiles seen in a wide variety of unrelated diseases and even in normal tissue.[112] A report of coronavirus-like particles seen within the cisterns of the rough endoplasmic reticulum of one patient has not been confirmed.[113]

PATHOGENESIS

The pathogenesis of MS is unknown. As noted earlier, demyelination could result from attacks on the oligodendrocyte, attacks on the myelin itself, or disordered metabolism of myelin lipid or protein. The ways in which viral infection or autoallergy may relate to MS remain to be elucidated. There is considerable indirect evidence indicating an autoallergic mechanism of cell-mediated destruction of myelin sheaths in MS. Multiple sclerosis has many histopathologic similarities to postinfectious or postvaccinal acute disseminated encephalomyelitis of humans and to experimental autoallergic encephalomyelitis (EAE), a disease induced in experimental animals by immunization with CNS myelin encephalitogenic basic protein in adjuvant. There have also been many studies of cell-mediated immunity to myelin encephalitogenic protein, cerebrosides, and oligodendrocytes in MS patients, but the results have been as confusing and conflicting as have the studies of delayed hypersensitivity to viral antigens. It is possible that an initial or persistent viral infection incites the disease and that the destruction of myelin is mediated by sensitized lymphocytes. Variations in the distribution of T and B lymphocytes, particularly suppressor-cytotoxic T cells, have been described (see above) and may be involved in the pathogenesis of the disease.

Several hypotheses concerning an infectious or immunologic pathogenesis of MS have been suggested: (*1*) suppressor cells may be damaged by viral infection or by some antigen or toxin released from CNS tissue during attacks; (*2*) a loss of suppressor cell function may permit autoallergic damage to tissue by effector lymphocytes or by antibodies; (*3*) the decreased numbers of suppressor-cytotoxic cells in peripheral blood during acute attacks may result from migration of cytotoxic effector lymphocytes into the CNS where they may damage myelin or oligodendrocytes directly; (*4*) suppressor cells may share an antigen, possibly viral-induced, with myelin or oligodendrocytes, and suppressor cells may thus be attacked as part of the disease; and (*5*) the inability of some MS patients to produce interferon in response to viral antigens may increase their susceptibility to persistent viral infection. It remains to be determined whether suppressor cell function or viral infection play any role in the pathogenesis of MS, however.

The reader should recall that, in contrast to MS, the viral etiology of progressive multifocal leukoencephalopathy (PML), another demyelinating disease, has been well substantiated (see Chapter 124). In PML, the mechanism of myelin destruction appears to be via direct infection and destruction of oligodendrocytes by a polyomavirus. That pathogenesis is unlikely in MS.

PATHOLOGIC FINDINGS

The characteristic lesion is the MS plaque, a zone of destruction of myelin that can be seen with the naked eye in the white matter of sectioned brain and spinal cord.[114] Plaques are especially common in the spinal cord, optic nerves, and paraventricular areas of the cerebrum, especially in proximity to veins. Under the microscope, recent lesions show a considerable degree of inflammation with perivenous infiltrates of mononuclear cells and lymphocytes. Later lesions contain microglial phagocytes and reactive astrocytes. Older "sclerotic" plaques contain relatively acellular fibroglial tissue (gliosis); at this stage, axis cylinders may no longer remain intact. As has been mentioned earlier, this sequence of pathologic changes has been interpreted as reflecting lymphocyte-mediated destruction of myelin, with late glial "scarring" in inactive lesions.

CLINICAL MANIFESTATION

The reader is referred to textbooks of neurology[86,115] for a detailed discussion of the clinical presentation of MS. The disease is characterized by episodes of focal disorder of the spinal cord, brain, and optic nerves that remit and recur, usually over a period of 20–30 years. Lesions are distributed in the CNS, although certain regions are affected preferentially. In the typical case, attacks and lesions are disseminated in time and space within the CNS. The more common sites of disease are the following:

1. *Optic nerve:* Optic neuritis is the initial episode in about 40 percent of patients with MS; probably about 40–60 percent of patients with acute optic neuritis eventually develop MS.
2. *Spinal cord:* Spinal cord lesions result in sensory symptoms and deficits (especially of posterior column function) and in pyramidal tract and bladder and bowel dysfunction.
3. *Brain stem and cerebellar connections:* Lesions may cause diplopia, nystagmus, internuclear ophthalmoplegia, gaze palsy, dysarthria, vertigo, facial anesthesia, facial weakness, trigeminal neuralgia, and cerebellar ataxia.
4. *Cerebrum:* Depression, euphoria, and dementia may appear as MS lesions accumulate.

Although the usual case is one of exacerbations and remissions, with gradually accumulating neurologic deficit and disability, MS may also be chronic and progressive, without remissions. Multiple sclerosis may also occur as an acute, fulminating disease, especially in childhood, as transverse myelitis or as neuromyelitis optica (myelitis plus optic neuritis), or it may be found incidentally at autopsy or by MRI, without a history of neurologic disease during life.

The CSF may contain increased numbers of mononuclear cells, especially in cases of acute onset or in exacerbation.[116] There are usually fewer than 10 cells/mm^3, rarely as many as 50/mm^3. The number of cells may correlate with the activity of the disease. Cerebrospinal fluid total protein levels are usually normal or slightly elevated; more than 100 mg/100 ml is highly unusual. Cerebrospinal fluid IgG levels are elevated (above 10–12 percent) in about 70 percent of the cases but do not correlate with the activity or severity of the disease; once elevated, the IgG level usually remains elevated. The CSF IgG/albumin ratio, the IgG/albumin index (derived from the CSF/serum ratio for both Ig and albumin), and the level of free κ-chains[117] are also abnormal in most patients with MS. In many patients (35–100 percent, depending on the laboratory), oligoclonal IgG bands can be demonstrated by agarose electrophoresis of CSF.[98] The IgG is probably synthesized within the CNS-CSF compartment. (The subject of CSF immunoglobulins in MS is reviewed by Desmond et al.[3] and Johnson and Nelson.[116]) Myelin basic protein components are often present in MS CSF, especially after acute exacerbations,[118,119] but also in other diseases in which there is active destruction of myelin. CSF glucose levels and pressure are normal.

Magnetic resonance imaging is quite sensitive in detecting the presence of plaques in the brain and less so in the spinal cord; the findings are not specific for MS, however.[120] Computed cranial tomography (CT scanning), especially delayed, contrast-enhanced scans, may reveal large MS plaques, although the test findings are normal in most cases.[121] Recordings of visual-, auditory-, and somatosensory-evoked responses have proved quite useful in documenting the presence of multiple CNS lesions that may be undetected by the neurologic examination.[122]

PREVENTION AND TREATMENT

Unfortunately, nothing is known about prevention. Moving from a higher latitude to a more tropical climate would have a theoretically protective effect, but only if the move were made in childhood (see the section on epidemiology).

Because of the usually unpredictable, exacerbating-remitting course of MS, the results of any therapeutic regimen are difficult to evaluate. Treatment with adrenocorticotrophic hormone (ACTH) or corticosteroids is used commonly, especially for acute exacerbations of the disease, and there are data indicating some benefit.[123,124] It has been presumed that these drugs act by suppressing lymphocyte-mediated myelin destruction in MS, although this is difficult to prove. Azathioprine, cyclophosphamide, cyclosporine A, anti-lymphocyte globulin, plasmapheresis, total lymphoid irradiation, and other immunosuppressive therapies have also been used in MS, but most studies have been uncontrolled or unconfirmed or are still in progress. Intensive immunosuppression with intravenous cyclophosphamide and ACTH has been reported in controlled studies to bring about 1 or 2 years of stabilization or improvement in most patients with severe, progressive MS.[125,126] Additional controlled studies are required for confirmation and extension of these findings.[127] Intrathecal interferon-β (IFN-β)[128] and subcutaneous IFN-α[129] have been reported to reduce exacerbation rates in relapsing-remitting MS. Interferon-γ administered intravenously has increased exacerbation rates, possibly as a result of its ability to augment the immune response.[130] The role of IFN in MS treatment remains unclear and subject to confirmation by further studies.[131]

At the present time, symptomatic and supportive measures such as drugs to treat spasticity, bladder dysfunction, and neuralgia continue to play a major role in the management of multiple sclerosis.

REFERENCES

1. Sigurdsson B. Observation on three slow infections of sheep. Br Vet J. 1954;110:255,307,341.
2. Johnson RT. Viral Infections of the Nervous System. New York: Raven Press; 1982.
3. Desmond MM, Wilson GS, Melnick JL, et al. Congenital rubella encephalitis: Course and early sequelae. J Pediatr. 1967;71:311.
4. Townsend JJ, Baringer JR, Wolinsky JS, et al. Progressive rubella panencephalitis: Late onset after congenital rubella. N Engl J Med. 1975;292:990.
5. Weil ML, Itabashi HH, Cremer NE, et al. Chronic progressive panencephalitis due to rubella virus simulating SSPE. N Engl J Med. 1975;292:994.
6. Price RW, Sidtis J, Rosenblum M. The AIDS dementia complex: Some current questions. Ann Neurol. 1988;23(Suppl):27–33.
7. Petito CK, Navia BA, Cho E-S, et al. Vacuolar myelopathy pathologically resembling subacute combined degeneration in patients with acquired immunodeficiency syndrome (AIDS). N Engl J Med. 1985;312:874–9.
8. Gajdusek DC, Zigas V. Degenerative disease of the central nervous system in New Guinea. The endemic occurrence of "kuru" in the native population. N Engl J Med 1957;257:974.
9. Hadlow WJ. Scrapie and kuru. Lancet 1959;2:289.
10. Cuille J, Chelle PL. La maladie dite tremblante du mouton est-elle inoculable? CR Acad Sci (Paris) 1936;203:1552.
11. Gajdusek DC, Gibbs CJ, Alpers M. Experimental transmission of a kuru-like syndrome to chimpanzees. Nature. 1966;209:794.
12. Kirschbaum WR. Jakob-Creutzfeldt Disease, New York: Elsevier Science Publishing; 1968.
13. Gibbs CJ, Gajdusek DC, Asher DM, et al. Creutzfeldt-Jakob disease (subacute spongiform encephalopathy): Transmission to the chimpanzee. Science. 1968;161:388.
14. Masters CL, Gajdusek DC, Gibbs DC Jr. Creutzfeldt-Jakob disease virus isolations from the Gerstmann-Straussler syndrome, with an analysis of the various forms of plaque deposition in the virus-induced spongiform encephalopathies. Brain. 1981;104:559–88.
15. Gajdusek DC. Unconventional viruses and the origin and disappearance of kuru. Science. 1977;197:943.
16. Chandler RL. Encephalopathy in mice produced with scrapie material. Lancet. 1961;2:1378.
17. Zlotnik I, Rennie JC. Experimental transmission of mouse passaged scrapie to goats, sheep, rats and hamsters. J Comp Pathol. 1965;75:147.
18. Gibbs CJ Jr, Gajdusek DC, Latarjet R. Unusual resistance to ionizing ra-

diation of the viruses of kuru, Creutzfeldt-Jakob disease and scrapie. Proc Natl Acad Sci USA. 1978;75:6268.
19. Millson GC, Hunter GD, Kimberlin RH. An experimental examination of the scrapie agent in cell membrane mixtures. II. The association of scrapie activity with membrane fractions. J Comp Pathol. 1971;81:255.
20. Prusiner SB. The biology of prion transmission and replication. In: Prusiner SB, McKinley M, eds. Prions. San Diego: Academic Press, 1987:83–112.
21. Brown P, Hooks J, Roos R, et al. Attempt to identify the agent of Creutzfeldt-Jakob disease by antibody relationship to known viruses. Nature. 1972;235:149.
22. Katz M, Koprowski H. Failure to demonstrate a relationship between scrapie and production of interferon in mice. Nature. 1968;219:639.
23. Gajdusek DC, Gibbs CJ, Rogers NG, et al. Persistence of viruses of kuru and Creutzfeldt-Jakob disease in tissue cultures of brain cells. Nature. 1972;235:104.
24. Clarke MC, Haig DA. Evidence for the multiplication of scrapie agent in cell culture. Nature. 1970;225:100.
25. Hunter GD. Scrapie. Prog Med Virol. 1974;18:289.
26. Diener TO. Viroids: The smallest known agents of infectious disease. Annu Rev Microbiol. 1974;28:23.
27. Prusiner SB. Prions and neurodegenerative diseases. N Engl J Med. 1987;317:1571–81.
28. Fields BN. Powerful prions? (Editorial). N Engl J Med. 1987;317:1597–8.
29. Baringer JR, Prusiner SB. Experimental scrapie in mice: Ultrastructural observations. Ann Neurol. 1970;4:205.
30. Cho HJ. Is the scrapie agent a virus? Nature. 1976;262:411.
31. Siakotos AN, Raveed D, Longa G. The discovery of a particle unique to brain and spleen subcellular fractions from scrapie-infected mice. J Gen Virol. 1979;43:417.
32. Merz PA, Somerville RA, Wisniewski HM, et al. Abnormal fibrils from scrapie infected brain. Acta Neuropathol (Berl). 1981;54:63–74.
33. Merz PA, Somerville RA, Wisniewski HM, et al. Scrapie associated fibrils in Creutzfeldt-Jakob disease. Nature. 1983;306:474–6.
34. Merz PA, Rohwer RG, Kascak R, et al. An infection specific particle from the unconventional slow virus diseases. Science. 1984;225:437–40.
35. Prusiner SB, Bolton DC, Groth DF, et al. Further purification and characterization of scrapie prions. Biochemistry. 1982;21:6942–50.
36. Prusiner SB, McKinley MP, Bowman KA, et al. Scrapie pions aggregate to form amyloid-like birefringent rods. Cell. 1983;35:349–58.
37. Gajdusek DC. Hypothesis: Interference with axonal transport of neurofilament as a common pathogenetic mechanism in certain disease of the central nervous system. N Engl J Med. 1985;312:714–9.
38. Gajdusek DC. Kuru in the New Guinea highlands. In: Spillane JD, ed. Tropical Neurology. V. 29. London: Oxford University Press; 1973:376.
39. Klitzman RL. Alpers MP, Gajdusek DC. The natural incubation period of kuru and the episodes of transmission in three clusters of patients. Neuroepidemiology. 1984;3:3–20.
40. Alpers M. Epidemiology and clinical aspects of Kuru. In: Prusiner SB, McKinley MP, eds. Prions. San Diego: Academic Press; 1987:451–65.
41. Brody JA, Gibbs CJ. Chronic neurological diseases: Subacute sclerosing panencephalitis, progressive multifocal leukoencephalopathy, kuru, Creutzfeldt-Jakob disease. In: Evans AS, ed. Viral Infections of Humans. New York: Plenum; 1976:519.
42. Kahana E, Alter M, Braham J, et al. Creutzfeldt-Jakob disease: A focus among Libyan Jews in Israel. Science. 1974;183:90.
43. Masters CL, Harris JO, Gajdusek DC, et al. Creutzfeldt-Jakob disease: Patterns of worldwide occurrence and the significance of familial and sporadic clustering. Ann Neurol. 1979;5:177.
44. Matthews WB. Epidemiology of Creutzfeldt-Jakob disease in England and Wales. J Neurol Neurosurg Psychiatry. 1975;38:210.
45. Jellinger VK, Seitelberger F, Heiss WD, et al. Konjugale Form der subakuten spongiosen Enzephalopathie (Jakob-Creutzfeldt-Erkrankung). Wein Klin Wochenschr. 1972;84:245.
46. Masters CL, Gajdusek DC, Gibbs CR Jr, et al. Familial Creutzfeldt-Jakob disease and other familial dementias: An inquiry into possible modes of transmission of virus-induced familial diseases. In: Prusiner SB, Hadlow WJ, eds. Slow Transmissible Diseases of the Nervous System. New York: Academic Press; 1979:143.
47. Bobowick AR, Brody JA, Matthews MR, et al. Creutzfeldt-Jakob disease: A case control study. Am J Epidemiol. 1971;98:381.
48. Herzberg L, Herzberg BW, Gibbs CJ, et al. Creutzfeldt-Jakob disease: Hypothesis for high incidence in Libyan Jews in Israel. Science. 1974;186:848.
49. Cavanipour Z, Alter M, Sobel E, et al. A case control study of Creutzfeldt-Jakob disease. Dietary risk factors. Am J Epidemiol. 1985;122:443–51.
50. Gibbs CJ Jr, Amyx HL, Bacote A, et al. Oral transmission of kuru. Creutzfeldt-Jakob disease and scrapie to nonhuman primates. J Infect Dis. 1980;142:205.
51. Brown P, Salazar AM, Gibbs CJ Jr, et al. Alzheimer disease and transmissible virus dementia (CJD). Ann NY Acad Sci. 1982;396:131–43.
52. Gajdusek DC, Gibbs CJ, Asher DM, et al. Precautions in medical care of, and in handling materials from, patients with transmissible virus dementia (Creutzfeldt-Jakob disease). N Engl J Med. 1977;297:1253.
53. Duffy P, Wolf J, Collins G, et al. Person-to-person transmission of Creutzfeldt-Jakob disease. N Engl J Med. 1974;299:692.
54. Bernoulli C, Siegfried J, Baumgartner G, et al. Danger of accidental person-to-person transmission of Creutzfeldt-Jakob disease by surgery. Lancet. 1977;1:478.
55. Rapidly progressive dementia in a patient who received a cadaveric dura mater graft. MMWR. 1987;36:49–55.
56. Update: Creutzfeldt-Jakob disease in a patient receiving a cadaveric dura mater graft. MMWR. 1987;36:324–5.
57. Brown P, Gajdusek DC, Gibbs CJ Jr, et al. Potential epidemic of Creutzfeldt-Jakob disease from human growth hormone therapy. N Engl J Med. 1985;313:728–31.
58. Bannister BA, McCormick A. Creutzfeldt-Jakob disease with reference to the safety of pituitary growth hormone. J Infect Dis. 1987;14:7–12.
59. Brown R. Human growth hormone therapy and Creutzfeldt-Jakob disease: A drama in three acts. Pediatrics. 1988;81:85–92.
60. Traub RD, Gajdusek DC, Gibbs CJ. Transmissible virus dementia: The relation of transmissible spongiform encephalopathy to Creutzfeldt-Jakob disease. In: Kinsbourne M, Smith L, eds. Aging, Dementia and Cerebral Function. New York: Spectrum Publications; 1977:91.
61. Nevin S, McMenemy WH, Behrman D, et al. Subacute spongiform encephalopathy: A subacute form of encephalopathy attributable to vascular dysfunction (spongiform cerebral atrophy). Brain. 1960;83:519.
62. Schoene WC, Masters CL, Gibbs CJ Jr, et al. Transmissible spongiform encephalopathy (Creutzfeldt-Jakob disease): Atypical clinical and pathological findings. Arch Neurol. 1981;38:473
63. Committee on Health Care Issues, American Neurological Association. Precautions in handling tissues, fluids, and other contaminated materials from patients with documented or suspected Creutzfeldt-Jakob disease. Ann Neurol. 1986;19:75–7.
64. Sotelo J, Gibbs CJ Jr, Gajdusek DC. Autoantibodies against axonal neurofilaments in patients with kuru and Creutzfeldt-Jakob disease. Science. 1981;210:190.
65. Aoki T, Gibbs CJ Jr, Sotelo J, et al. Heterogeneic autoantibody against neurofilament protein in the sera of animals with experimental kuru and Creutzfeldt-Jakob disease and natural scrapie infection. Infect Immun. 1982;38:316.
66. Toh BH, Gibbs CJ Jr, Gajdusek DC, et al. The 200- and 150-kDa neurofilament proteins react with IgG autoantibodies from chimpanzees with kuru or Creutzfeldt-Jakob disease; a 62-kDa neurofilament-associated protein reacts with sera from sheep with natural scrapie. Proc Natl Acad Sci USA. 1985;82:3894–6.
67. Kimberlin RH, Walker CA. Pathogenesis of mouse scrapie: Evidence for neural spread of infection to the CNS. J Gen Virol. 1980;51:183–87.
68. Kimberlin RH, Field HJ, Walker CA. Pathogenesis of mouse scrapie: Evidence for spread of infection from central to peripheral nervous system. J Gen Virol. 1983;64:713–6.
69. Fraser H. Neuronal spread of scrapie agent and targeting of lesions within the retino-tectal pathway. Nature. 1982;295:149–50.
70. Lampert PW, Gajdusek DC, Gibbs CJ. Subacute spongiform virus encephalopathies. Scrapie, kuru and Creutzfeldt-Jakob disease. Am J Pathol. 1972;68:626.
71. Masters CL, Richardson EP Jr. Subacute spongiform encephalopathy (Creutzfeldt-Jakob disease): The nature and progression of spongiform change. Brain. 1978;101:333.
72. Park TS, Kleinman GM, Richardson EP Jr. Creutzfeldt-Jakob disease with extensive degeneration of white matter. Acta Neuropathol (Berl). 1980;52:239–42.
73. Landis DMD, Williams RS, Masters CL. Golgi and electron-microscopic studies of spongiform encephalopathy. Neurology (NY). 1981;31:538.
74. Hornabrook RW. Slow virus infections of the central nervous system. In: Vinken PJ, Bruyn GW, Klawans HL, eds. Infections of the Nervous System. part II. Handbook of Clinical Neurology. V. 34. Amsterdam: Elsevier North Holland; 1978:275–90.
75. May WW. Creutzfeldt-Jakob disease. I. Survey of the literature and clinical diagnosis. Acta Neurol Scand. 1968;44:1.
76. Roos R, Gajdusek DC, Gibbs Jr. The clinical characteristics of transmissible Creutzfeldt-Jakob disease. Brain. 1973;96:1–20.
77. Brown P, Cathala F, Castaigne P, et al. Creutzfeldt-Jakob disease: Clinical analysis of a consecutive series of 230 neuropathologically verified cases. Ann Neurol. 1986;20:597–602.
78. Chiappa KH, Burke CJ, Young RR. Early evolution and incidence of electroencephalographic abnormalities in Creutzfeldt-Jakob disease. J Clin Neurophysiol. 1986;3:1–21.
79. Harrington MG, Merrill CR, Asher DM, et al. Abnormal proteins in the cerebrospinal fluid of patients with Creutzfeldt-Jakob disease. N Engl J Med. 1986;315:279–83.
80. Brown P, Coter-Vann M, Pomeroy K, et al. Diagnosis of Creutzfeldt-Jakob disease by Western blot identification of marker protein in human brain tissue. N Engl J Med. 1986;314:547–51.
81. Kovanen J, Erkinjuntti T, Iivanainen M, et al. Cerebral MRI and CT imaging in Creutzfeldt-Jakob disease. J Comput Assist Tomogr. 1985;9:125–128.
82. Lehrich JR, Arnason BGW. Virology of multiple sclerosis. In: Vinken PJ, Bruyn GW, eds. Handbook of Clinical Neurology. V. 34. New York: Elsevier Science Publishing; 1978:435.
83. Cook SD, Dowling PC. Multiple sclerosis and viruses: An overview. Neurology (NY). 1980;30:80.
84. McFarlin DE, McFarland HF. Multiple sclerosis. N Engl J Med. 1982;307:1183,1246.
85. Johnson RT. Viral Infections of the Nervous System. New York: Raven Press; 1982:263.

86. Matthews WB, Acheson ED, Batchelor JR, et al. McAlpine's Multiple Sclerosis. Edinburgh: Churchill Livingstone; 1985.
87. Sullivan CB, Visscher BR, Detels R. Multiple sclerosis and age at exposure to childhood diseases and animals: Cases and their friends. Neurology (NY). 1984;34:1144–8.
88. Compston DA, Vakarelis BN, Paul E, et al. Viral infection in patients with multiple sclerosis and HLA-DR matched controls. Brain. 1986;109:325–44.
89. Kurtzke JF, Hyllested K. Multiple sclerosis in the Faroe Islands: I. Clinical and epidemiological features. Ann Neurol. 1979;5:6.
90. Fog T. International symposium on the histocompatibility system in multiple sclerosis. Acta Neurol Scand. 1977;55(suppl 63):6.
91. Cook SD, Dowling PC. A possible association between house pets and multiple sclerosis. Lancet. 1977;1:980.
92. Alter M, Berman M, Kahana E. The year of the dog. Neurology (NY). 1979;29:1023.
93. Anderson LJ, Kibler RF, Kaslow RA, et al. Multiple sclerosis unrelated to dog exposure. Neurology (NY). 1984;34:1149–54.
94. Adams JM, Imagawa DT. Measles antibodies in multiple sclerosis. Proc Soc Exp Biol Med. 1962;111:562.
95. Salmi AA. Virus antibodies in patients with multiple sclerosis. Ann Clin Res. 1973;5:319.
96. Norrby E, Link H, Olsson JE, et al. Comparison of antibodies against different viruses in cerebrospinal fluid and serum samples from patients with multiple sclerosis. Infect Immun. 1974;10:688.
97. Link H, Müller R. Immunoglobulins in multiple sclerosis and infections of the nervous system. Arch Neurol. 1971;25:326.
98. Panelius M, Salmi A. Association of measles antibody activity with electrophoretic fractions of CSF in a patient with multiple sclerosis. Acta Neurol Scand. 1973;49:266.
99. Norrby E. Viral antibodies in multiple sclerosis. Prog Med Virol. 1978;24:1.
100. Salmi AA, Norrby E, Panelius M. Identification of different measles virus-specific antibodies in the serum and cerebrospinal fluid from patients with subacute sclerosing panencephalitis and multiple sclerosis. Infect Immun. 1972;6:248.
101. Forghani B, Cremer NE, Johnson KP, et al. Viral antibodies in cerebrospinal fluid of multiple sclerosis and control patients: Comparison between radio immunoassay conventional standards. J Clin Microbiol. 1978;7:63.
102. Cremer NE, Johnson KP, Fein G, et al. Comprehensive viral immunology of multiple sclerosis. II. Analysis of serum and CSF antibodies by standard serologic methods. Arch Neurol. 1980;37:610.
103. Koprowski H, DeFreitas E, Harper M, et al. Multiple sclerosis and human T cell lymphotropic retroviruses. Nature. 1985;318:154–60.
103a. Reddy EP, Sandberg-Wollheim M, Mettus RV, et al. Amplification and molecular cloning of HTLV-I sequences from DNA of multiple sclerosis patients. Science. 1989;243:529–533
104. Johnson RT. Myelopathies and retroviral infections. Ann Neurol. 1987;21:113–6.
105. Madden DL, Mundon FK, Tzan NR, et al. Antibody to human and simian retrovirus, HTLV-I, HTLV-II, HIV, STLV-III, and SRV-I not increased in patients with multiple sclerosis. Ann Neurol. 1988;23(Suppl):171–3.
105a. Waksman BH. Multiple sclerosis: Relationship to a retrovirus? Nature. 1989;337:599
106. Antel JP, Arnason BGW, Medof ME. Suppressor cell function in multiple sclerosis: Correlation with clinical disease activity. Ann Neurol. 1978;5:338.
107. Reinherz EL, Weiner HL, Hauser SL, et al. Loss of suppressor T cells in active multiple sclerosis. N Engl J Med. 1980;303:125.
108. Kadish AS, Tansey FA, Yu GSM, et al. Interferon as a mediator of human lymphocyte suppression. J Exp Med. 1980;151:637.
109. Neighbor PA, Miller AE, Bloom BR. Interferon responses of leukocytes in multiple sclerosis. Neurology (NY). 1981;31:561.
110. Palsson PA, Pattison IH, Field EJ. Transmission experiments with multiple sclerosis. In: Gajdusek DC, Gibbs CJ, Alpers M, eds. Slow, Latent and Temperate Virus Infections. NINDB Monograph No. 2. Washington, DC: US GPO; 1965:19.
111. Carp RI, Licursi PC, Merz PA, et al. Decreased percentage of polymorphonuclear neutrophils in mouse peripheral blood after inoculation with material from multiple sclerosis patients. J Exp Med. 1972;136:618.
112. Lampert F, Lampert P. Multiple sclerosis. Morphologic evidence of intranuclear paramyxovirus or altered chromatin fibers? Arch Neurol. 1975;32:425.
113. Tanaka R, Iwasaki Y, Koprowski H. Intracisternal virus-like particles in brain of a multiple sclerosis patient. J Neurol Sci. 1976;28:121.
114. Adams RD, Kubik CS. The morbid anatomy of the demyelinative diseases. Am J Med. 1977;12:510.
115. Adams RD, Victor M. Principles of Neurology. 3rd ed. New York: McGraw-Hill; 1985:699–717.
116. Johnson KP, Nelson BJ. Multiple sclerosis: Diagnostic usefulness of cerebrospinal fluid. Ann Neurol. 1977;2:425.
117. DeCarli C, Menegus MA, Rudick RA. Free light chains in multiple sclerosis and infections of the CNS. Neurology (NY). 1987;37:1334–8.
118. Cohen SR, Herndon RM, McKhann GM. Radioimmunoassay of myelin basic protein in spinal fluid: An index of active demyelination. N Engl J Med. 1976;295:1455.
119. Whitaker JN. Myelin encephalitogenic protein fragments in cerebrospinal fluid of persons with multiple sclerosis. Neurology (NY). 1977;27:911.
120. Uhlenbrock D, Seidel D, Gehlen W, et al. MR imaging in multiple sclerosis: Comparison with clinical, CSF, and visual evoked potential findings. AJNR. 1988;9:56–67.
121. Vinuela FV, Fox AJ, Debrun GM, et al. New perspectives in computed tomography of multiple sclerosis. AJNR. 1982;3:277.
122. Chiappa KH. Pattern shift visual, brainstem auditory, and short-latency somatosensory evoked potentials in multiple sclerosis. Neurology (NY). 1980;30:110.
123. Miller HG, Newell DJ, Ridley A. Multiple sclerosis. Treatment of acute exacerbations with corticotrophin (ACTH). Lancet 1961;2:1120.
124. Rose AA, Kuzma JW, Kurtzke JF, et al. Cooperative study in the evaluation of therapy in multiple sclerosis: ACTH vs. placebo: Final report. Neurology (NY). 1970;20:1.
125. Hauser SL, Dawson DM, Lehrich JR, et al. Intensive immunosuppression in progressive multiple sclerosis: A randomized, three-arm study of high-dose intravenous cyclophosphamide, plasma exchange, and ACTH. N Engl J Med. 1983;308:173.
126. Goodkin DE, Plencner S, Palmer-Saxerud J, et al. Cyclophosphamide in chronic progressive multiple sclerosis. Maintenance vs nonmaintenance therapy. Arch Neurol. 1987;44:823–7.
127. McFarlin DE. Treatment of multiple sclerosis (Editorial). N Engl J Med. 1983;308:215.
128. Jacobs L, Salazar AM, Herndon R, et al. Multicenter double-blind study of effect of intrathecally administered natural human fibroblast interferon on exacerbations of multiple sclerosis. Lancet. 1986;2:1411–3.
129. Knobler RL, Panitch HS, Braheny SL, et al. Systemic alpha interferon therapy of multiple sclerosis. Neurology (NY). 1984;34:1273–9.
130. Panitch HS, Hirsch RL, Schindler J, et al. Treatment of multiple sclerosis with gamma interferon. Exacerbations associated with activation of the immune system. Neurology (NY). 1987;37:1097–102.
131. McFarlin DE. Use of interferon in multiple sclerosis (Editorial). Ann Neurol. 1985;18:432–3.

70. BRAIN ABSCESS

BRIAN WISPELWEY
W. MICHAEL SCHELD

Brain abscess is a focal suppurative process within the brain parenchyma that continues to challenge the diagnostic acumen and therapeutic skill of the clinician. Despite the presence of potent and specific antimicrobial agents and improved neurosurgical technique, the mortality and morbidity from brain abscesses remained as high as in the preantibiotic era until relatively recently. A description of the disease together with a therapeutic proposal was found in an article dating back to the sixteenth century[1]; however, it was not until the late nineteenth century that the first encouraging results of surgical intervention were reported. MacEwen[2] reported the remarkable figure of a 80 percent (8 of 10) survival rate after neurosurgical drainage of temporal lobe abscesses.

Since that time, surgical techniques have continued to improve, and antibiotics have been introduced, but diagnostic delay has continued to be the major obstacle in the success of therapeutic intervention. Significant improvement in the mortality and moribidity of brain abscess has only occurred within the last 10–15 years. These improvements reflect advances in noninvasive diagnostic techniques allowing earlier diagnosis and more precise localization before mass effect leads to intracranial shifts, which result in irreversible brain damage or death. A combined medical–surgical approach is advisable; optimal management of a brain abscess requires cooperation between the medical physician and neurosurgeon.

EPIDEMIOLOGY

The incidence of brain abscess has remained relatively stable in the antibiotic era.[3–5] Although some series report a mild increase,[6] this may represent a bias of more sensitive diagnostic techniques.[7] It is estimated that brain abscess accounts for approximately 1 in 10,000 general hospital admissions and that 4–

10 cases are seen yearly on active neurosurgical services in hospitals of developed countries.[8,9] The etiology and incidence of brain abscesses varies among different geographic areas. In China, 65 percent of brain abscesses are thought to be secondary to otitis media but only 0.5 percent secondary to paranasal sinusitis.[10] This is contrasted to a 20–40 percent incidence secondary to otitis media and a 15–25 percent incidence secondary to paranasal sinusitis reported in series from Northern European countries.[11,12] Several authors[5,6,13] reported a male predominance (3:1) among patients with brain abscesses; more recently a series of 45 patients diagnosed between 1970 and 1983 revealed a male-to-female ratio of 2.7:1.[7] In another series of 257 patients (1973–1977), the ratio was only 1.2:1.[14,15] The median age of patients is 30–40 years[10,16,17]; however, the predominant age may vary somewhat by etiology. In some series, brain abscess due to otitis media displays a bimodal age distribution, with peaks in the pediatric age group and after 40 years of age,[18] whereas abscesses secondary to paranasal sinusitis more commonly occur between 10 and 30 years of age.[18,19] Approximately 25 percent of all brain abscesses occur in children less than 15 years of age,[6] with a peak incidence between ages 4 and 7.[20] A brain abscess before the age of 2 years is extremely rare.[21]

PATHOGENESIS

Brain abscesses develop in four clinical settings: (*1*) in association with a contiguous suppurative focus, (*2*) after hematogenous spread from a distant focus, (*3*) after trauma (e.g., open cranial fracture with a dural breach, postneurosurgery, pencil-tip injuries to the eye in children,[22] and more recently after lawn dart injuries to the head,[23] and (*4*) cryptogenic (no focus is recognized in approximately 20 percent of cases).[3,5,6,13,17] In approximate decreasing order of frequency a solitary abscess may involve various regions: frontal ≈ temporal > frontoparietal > parietal > cerebellar > occipital.[6] This distribution reflects the associated, often contiguous, focus of infection. Understanding the predisposing condition(s) in a given brain abscess case has important implications for its therapy (Table 1). Intrasellar, brain stem, basal ganglia, and thalamic abscesses are rare. Intrasellar abscesses are most common in the setting of pre-existing pituitary adenomas; however, cases have occurred in their absence.[25] Sinusitis, particularly sphenoid sinusitis, is a most important predisposing condition, with one series revealing pituitary abscesses in 16 of 126 patients with sphenoid sinusitis.[26] Brain stem abscesses arise most often from hematogenous spread from a distant focus; rare cases occur in association with a contiguous infection. In one-third of the 48 reported cases, no source was defined. These abscesses are often fusiform and extend over several levels of the brain stem; therefore, the clinical findings can be confusing. Before 1974, brain stem abscesses were uniformly fatal, but recent improvements in diagnosis and aggressive neurosurgical drainage have led to occasional survival.[27]

Most patients with brain abscesses demonstrate a contiguous focus of infection, usually sinusitis or otitis. Approximately 40 percent of brain abscesses were associated with otitis media and/or mastoiditis in earlier series; this is decreasing in most parts of the world. However, in areas where otitis media continues to be neglected or therapy is delayed, intracranial complications still present a serious threat.[28] As stated, a bimodal age distribution of brain abscess as a complication of otitis media is often seen, with cases in the youngest age groups often secondary to acute otitis media as opposed to the overwhelming preponderance of associated chronic otitis media in the older age group.[18] Overall, chronic otitis media and/or mastoiditis leads to intracranial extension four to eight times more frequently than does acute disease. Before the availability of antibiotic therapy it was estimated that about 3–6 percent of patients with otogenic suppuration developed an intracranial complication, with approximately 15 percent of those presenting as brain abscesses.[21,29] Current risk estimates are more difficult to assess; however, epidemiologic data from Scotland suggest that only 1 in 3500 cases of otitis media are complicated by intracranial spread.[30] Most otogenic brain abscesses are located in the temporal lobe, next is the cerebellum, but cases of frontal lobe and rare brain stem localizations have been reported. Most otogenic brain abscesses are solitary lesions.[3–6,9,13,17]

Brain abscess secondary to paranasal sinusitis also appears to be decreasing in incidence; however, sinusitis continues to be the major predisposing condition leading to subdural empyema. In a recent British review, sinusitis accounted for 15 percent of brain abscesses over a 30-year period.[19] The frontal lobe is almost exclusively involved as a complication of sinusitis; however, particularly with sphenoid sinusitis, the temporal lobe or sella turcica have been affected. Sphenoid sinusitis, despite its relative rarity when compared with frontoethmoidal or maxillary disease, has seemingly more frequent and severe complications. This stems from the difficulty in making this diagnosis and/or the lack of appropriately aggressive therapy for this condition.[31] Dental infection is a less frequent site of infection that can be complicated by brain abscess. Brain abscess appears more likely after infection of the molar teeth. A large majority of intracranial infections in this setting follow a recent tooth extraction. The site of the abscess is most com-

TABLE 1. Brain Abscess: Predisposing Condition, Site of Abscess, and Microbiology

Predisposing Conditions[a]	Site of Abscess	Usual Isolate(s) from Abscess
Contiguous site or primary infection		
Otitis media and mastoiditis	Temporal lobe or cerebellar hemisphere	Streptococci (anaerobic or aerobic), *Bacteroides fragilis*, Enterobacteriaceae
Frontoethmoidal sinusitis	Frontal lobe	Predominantly streptococci; *Bacteroides*, Enterobacteriaceae, *S. aureus*, and *Haemophilus* species
Sphenoidal sinusitis	Frontal or temporal lobe	Same as in frontoethmoidal sinusitis
Dental sepsis	Frontal lobe	Mixed *Fusobacterium*, *Bacteroides*, and *Streptococcus* species
Penetrating cranial trauma or postsurgical infection	Related to wound	*S. aureus*; streptococci, Enterobacteriaceae, *Clostridium*
Distant site of primary infection		
Congenital heart disease	Multiple abscess cavities; middle cerebral artery distribution common but may occur at any site	Viridans, anaerobic, and microaerophilic streptococci; *Haemophilus* species
Lung abscess, empyema, bronchiectasis	Same as in congenital heart disease	*Fusobacterium*, *Actinomyces*, *Bacteroides*, streptococci, *Nocardia asteroides*
Bacterial endocarditis	Same as in congenital heart disease	*S. aureus*, streptococci
Compromised host (immunosuppressive therapy or malignancy)	Same as in congenital heart disease	*Toxoplasma*, fungi, Enterobacteriaceae, *Nocardia*

[a] Predisposing conditions are identified in approximately 80 percent of cases.
(Data from Dacey et al.[24])

monly frontal, but temporal lobe localization can also occur by direct extension.[32] Many cases of cryptogenic brain abscess may be secondary to dental foci of infection. Facial or scalp infections are also important since they may lead to cavernous sinus thrombosis and attendant intracranial complications. Brain abscess rarely complicates meningitis; however, it should be strongly considered as an associated possibility in the neonate with meningitis, particularly meningitis due to gram-negative organisms. Abscess formation has been associated with >70 percent of cases of *Citrobacter diversus* meningitis in the infant.[33]

Brain abscesses from contiguous infection may occur by two major mechanisms: (*1*) direct extension through areas of associated osteitis or osteomyelitis and (*2*) retrograde thrombophlebitic spread via diploic or emissary veins into the intracranial compartment. Additional possibilities in the case of otogenic infection include spread through pre-existing channels (such as the internal auditory canal, cochlear and vestibular aqueducts, or between temporal suture lines). Hematogenous dissemination is occasionally implicated, particularly in cases of sinus or odontogenic origin.[8,9,32,34,35] None of these hypotheses explain the relative rarity of intracranial infection with sinusitis or otitis, how bacteria traverse an intact dura, the striking age and sex predominance of subdural empyema, or what determines the form of intracranial complication that eventually evolves (e.g., epidural abscess vs. brain abscess vs. subdural empyema) in the individual case with the same predisposing condition.

Hematogenous brain abscesses often share the following characteristics: (*1*) distant foci of infection, most often within the chest; (*2*) location in the distribution of the middle cerebral artery; (*3*) initial location at the gray-white matter junction where brain capillary flow is slowest; (*4*) poor encapsulation; and (*5*) high mortality. These abscesses are more commonly multiple and multiloculated as compared with those that have an origin in foci of contiguous infection.[3–6,8,9,13,17,35,36] Chronic pyogenic lung diseases (especially lung abscess, bronchiectasis, empyema, and cystic fibrosis) remain important diagnostic considerations.[6,8,9,37] Other distant foci of infection may be associated with brain abscesses and include wound and skin infections, osteomyelitis, pelvic infection, cholecystitis, and other forms of intra-abdominal sepsis. More recently, brain abscess has been described as a complication of esophageal dilation of caustic strictures and endoscopic sclerosis of varices, both of which can produce bacteremia.[38,39] Brain abscess rarely develops after bacteremia in the presence of a normal blood-brain barrier. Thus, brain abscess is rare in bacterial endocarditis, despite the presence of persistent bacteremia. In a series of 218 patients with infective endocarditis, only 9 cases of brain abscess were noted. In 8 of these cases, the brain abscesses were less than 1 cm^3, and in all cases multiple lesions were found.[40] In addition, only 4 of 148 brain abscesses in two large series were due to endocarditis.[5,17] Hereditary hemorrhagic telangiectasia is complicated by brain abscess with striking regularity, almost always presenting in those patients with pulmonary arteriovenous malformations. These abnormalities presumably allow septic microemboli to pass through the pulmonary circulation and avoid the normal pulmonary capillary filter, thereby affording direct access to the cerebral circulation. Cyanosis, clubbing, polycythemia, and hypoxemia were also found in those patients most likely to develop a brain abscess[41] and may be a necessary substrate. Cyanotic congenital heart disease (CCHD) is found in 5–10 percent of brain abscess cases, with some pediatric series revealing that it is the most common underlying condition in children. As many as 25 percent of all brain abscesses are attributable to this condition in this age group. Between 2 and 6 percent of children with CCHD develop a brain abscess, with tetralogy of Fallot and transposition of the great vessels being the most commonly cited.[1,6,21,42,43] The polycythemia associated with CCHD increases the viscosity, thus reducing brain capillary flow and perhaps leading to microinfarction and reduced tissue oxygenation. This may be the final common pathway of brain abscess from many etiologies. These insults can be caused by polycythemic thrombosis and hypoxia (as described), septic emboli, or a suppurative vasculitis from a contiguous infection. Experimental data suggest that infection is extremely difficult to establish in normal brain tissue.[44]

PATHOLOGY

Established infection recruits inflammatory cells and alters local vascular permeability. The evolution of an abscess includes four somewhat arbitrary histopathologic stages.[45] This staging process, described in animal models of brain abscess, correlates well with human brain abscess evolution.[46] An important feature of this description is its correlation with computed tomographic (CT) findings, which has direct implications for subsequent therapy. The four stages include early cerebritis (days 1–3), late cerebritis (days 4–9), early capsule formation (days 10–13), and late capsule formation (day 14 on). This sequence of events may be altered in the immunosuppressed host. Dogs immunosuppressed by azathioprine and prednisone therapy showed a decreased early inflammatory response and edema formation followed by a delayed increase in abscess size as compared with healthy controls.[47] Two repeated observations regarding encapsulation deserve special attention. First, capsule formation is frequently more complete on the cortical than on the ventricular side of the abscess.[35,45] Second, encapsulation is less extensive in abscesses from hematogenous spread as compared with those arising from a contiguous focus of infection.[48] These observations may be related to the requirement of oxygen for pro-α chains of collagen to form triple-helix strands.[49] Normal cortical gray matter is more vascular than is adjacent white matter, perhaps allowing greater fibroblast proliferation and collagen helix formation. This discrepancy probably explains the propensity for abscesses to rupture medially into the ventricles rather than into the subarachnoid space. Similarly, the infarct resulting from a septic embolus might impede optimal collagen formation by fibroblasts.[45] Two experimental models using organisms other than α-hemolytic streptococci, however, indicate that this view of abscess evolution may be overly stereotyped. In a model of *Bacteroides fragilis* brain abscess,[50] the same stages of evolution were observed, but the early and late capsule stages could not be differentiated due to a delay in encapsulation. *Staphylococcus aureus* inoculation in the same experimental model[51] resulted in larger lesions, earlier ependymitis, and delayed progress toward healing. Again, separation of the previously described stages was not as distinct. Additionally, the abscess reached maximum size in the late cerebritis stage, which suggests that the host was able to contain the infection before capsule formation and thereby contradicts the assumption that the capsule serves to contain infection.

Therefore, brain abscess formation is a continuum from cerebritis to a collagen-encapsulated necrotic focus; however, its maturity of development is dependent on many factors including local oxygen concentration, the offending organism, and the host immune response.

ETIOLOGIC AGENTS

In the preantibiotic era, analysis of intracranial pus revealed *Staphylococcus aureus* in 25–30 percent of cases, streptococci in 30 percent, coliforms in 12 percent, and no growth in about 50 percent.[14,15] With proper attention to techniques, the role of anaerobic agents in brain abscesses has become apparent. In one earlier study,[52] 14 of 18 abscesses grew anaerobes on culture, predominately streptococci in 66 percent with *Bacteroides* sp. in 60 percent. Recent series from the United Kingdom have stressed the role of anaerobic bacteria in brain abscesses, especially of otic origin.[14,15,53] In addition, some reports suggest that the proportion of abscesses due to staphylococci are decreasing in frequency, whereas those due to Enterobacteriaceae are now more prevalent.[3,6]

The current pattern of microbial isolates from brain abscesses is shown in Table 2.[14,15,53–57] *Staphylococcus aureus* causes 10–15 percent of brain abscesses, usually in pure culture, and is the most common pathogen in abscesses after trauma. The Enterobacteriaceae are found, usually in mixed culture, in 23–33 percent of cases.[14,15,60] *Proteus* sp., *Escherichia coli,* and *Pseudomonas* sp. appear in approximate order of decreasing frequency. Bacteria associated with pyogenic meningitis (*S. pneumoniae, H. influenzae*) cause fewer than 1 percent of brain abscesses. Various streptococci are implicated in 60–70 percent of cases. These streptococci are often microaerophilic but yield aerobic patterns by gas liquid chromotographic analysis.[14,15] The *S. milleri* group (*S. anginosus* and *S. intermedius*) has a predilection for causing focal suppurative disease, including brain abscesses.[61,62] These organisms were found in 13 of 16 (approximately 80 percent) cases in one recent analysis.[63] Most of the *S. milleri* group are placed within Lancefield group F and possess the group O III antigen,[14,15,62] a potential virulence factor for the suppuration characteristic of these organisms. *Bacteroides* sp., including *B. fragilis,* are isolated in 20–40 percent of cases of brain abscess, often in mixed culture.[14,15,53,57] Many other bacteria are occasionally found in brain abscess pus,[15,58] including *Clostridium* sp. (often trauma related), *Haemophilus* sp., *Fusobacterium* sp., other anaerobes,[9,14,15,59,64] *Actinomyces* sp., *Listeria monocytogenes,*[65,66] *Nocardia asteroides,*[67] and others. When *Citrobacter* sp.[68] and *Eikenella corrodens*[36] invade the central nervous system (CNS), abscess formation is very commonly present. *Citrobacter diversus* is the most common pathogen isolated from cerebral abscesses of neonates.[69] *Salmonella* brain abscess is rare, with the most common serotypes being typhi, typhimurium, and enteritidis.[70] It occurs more commonly in adults, with precipitating factors being meningitis, trauma, and intracranial hematoma. *Streptobacillus moniliformis,* the cause of the streptobacillary form of rat-bite fever, has also been reported as a rare cause of brain abscess.[71]

Yeasts and dimorphic fungi have assumed an increasing role, causing 9–17 percent of cases in a recent series from San Francisco.[72] Most cases occur in immunocompromised patients, and mortality remains extremely high.[73] A partial list of fungi causing intracerebral mass lesions includes *Aspergillus* sp.,[74] agents of mucormycosis, *Candida* sp.,[75] *Cryptococcus neoformans, Coccidioides immitis, Cladosporium trichoides, C. bantianum,*[76] *Pseudallescheria* (*Petriellidium*) *boydii, Bipolaris* sp., *Curvularia* sp., agents of chromoblastomycosis, *Blastomyces dermatitidis,* and rarely *Histoplasma capsulatum.* In addition to the rhinocerebral form found in diabetes with ketoacidosis or leukopenic hosts, cerebral mucormycosis with brain abscess formation also occurs in parenteral drug abusers.

Various protozoa and helminths may cause brain abscesses. In a well-documented case of multiple abscesses caused by *Strongyloides stercoralis,*[77] bacteria carried within the gut of the nematode were implicated in the abscesses found in the distribution of the middle cerebral artery. Brain abscesses caused by *Entamoeba histolytica, Schistosoma japonicum,* and *Paragonimus* species remain uncommon in the United States but are seen in other countries.[78,79] Cysticercosis is a major cause of brain lesions in the developing world. For example, cysticercosis accounted for 85 percent of all brain infections in Mexico City; tuberculomas were responsible in 11 percent, and only 3 percent were pyogenic abscesses.[9]

The patient's immune status is an important determinant of the microbiology of a brain abscess. The infecting organism can be predicted with some degree of certainty, or the differential diagnosis can be narrowed significantly by knowing which arm of the immune system is more severely altered.[80] Patient's with T-lymphocyte or mononuclear phagocytic defects are commonly encountered in most hospital settings. Common causes of brain abscess in this patient group are *Toxoplasma gondii* and *Nocardia asteroides.* Less common but still possible etiologies are *Cryptococcus neoformans, Mycobacterium* spp., and *Listeria monocytogenes. Nocardia asteroides* infection almost always has a pulmonary portal of entry, so patients with nocardial brain abscesses usually have a concomitant pulmonary lesion.[80,81] Central nervous system involvement with this organism has been reported in 18–44 percent of patients with nocardial infection elsewhere in the body. Nocardial abscesses are most often single, but multiple abscesses have been reported. *Toxoplasma gondii* is the most common cause of brain abscess in patients with the acquired immunodeficiency syndrome (AIDS)[81] (see below). *Cryptococcus neoformans* more commonly causes meningitis in the compromised host, but mass lesions have been described. *Listeria monocytogenes* is also more commonly associated with meningitis or meningoencephalitis, but single large abscesses as well as disseminated small abscesses with this organism have also been reported.[66,83] Neutrophil defects are most often due to chemotherapy-induced neutropenia. An increased incidence of brain abscess secondary to Enterobacteriaceae and *Pseudomonas aeruginosa* is seen to parallel their increased presence as a cause of meningitis in this group of patients.[80] Neutrophil abnormalities also lead to an increased occurrence of CNS fungal disease. Multiple agents have been described, as seen above, and prominent among these are infections with *Aspergillus* spp., Mucoraceae, or *Candida* spp. A fungal etiology of a brain abscess should be suspected in a patient with a protracted hospital course who has been neutropenic for more than 1 week and has been treated with broad-spectrum antibiotics.[81]

Focal CNS lesions of several etiologies can occur in patients with AIDS (Table 3), and multiple pathologic processes commonly coexist.[84] In one series, CNS toxoplasmosis occurred in 103 of 366 (28 percent) AIDS patients with CNS complications.[85] Single or multiple abscesses are characteristic and are difficult to distinguish from pyogenic lesions by CT. Unlike the situation in non-AIDS patients, serologic studies are rarely helpful; cases of CNS toxoplasmosis have been documented even in serology-negative patients.[84] In the same series, primary CNS lymphoma was the next most prevalent complication and occurred in 11 percent. Progressive multifocal leukoencephalopathy occurs in a significant minority, and abnormal focal CT findings are observed; however, the lack of mass effect, surrounding edema, or contrast enhancement and the confinement of the lesions to white matter helps differentiate this process

TABLE 2. Microbiologic Etiology of Brain Abscess

Organism	*Isolation Frequency (%)*
S. aureus	10–15
Enterobacteriaceae	23–33
S. pneumoniae	<1
H. influenzae	<1
Streptococci (*S. milleri* group, including *S. intermedius* and *S. anginosus*)	60–70
Bacteroides sp.	20–40
Fungi	10–15
Protozoa, helminths[a]	<1

[a] Heavily dependent on geographic locale (see the text).
(Data from Nielsen et al.,[6] Carey,[9] de Louvois et al.,[14,15,57,58] Ingham et al.,[53] and Brook.[59])

TABLE 3. Differential Diagnosis of Focal CNS Lesions in Patients with AIDS

Toxoplasmosis	*Candida* spp.
Primary CNS lymphoma	*Listeria monocytogenes*
Mycobacterium tuberculosis	*Nocardia asteroides*
Mycobacterium avium-intracellulare	*Salmonella* group B
Progressive multifocal leukoencephalopathy	*Aspergillus* spp.
Cryptococcus neoformans	

from toxoplasmosis or lymphoma. Additional less common infectious etiologies of mass lesions in this patient population include *Mycobacterium tuberculosis,*[86] *Mycobacterium avium-intracellulare, C. neoformans, Candida* spp., *Aspergillus* spp., *N. asteroides, L. monocytogenes,* and *Salmonella* group B.[84,87]

Location within the brain can predict the etiologic agent(s) (Table 1). For example, a frontal lobe abscess in association with sinusitis often yields one of the *S. milleri* group in pure culture.[14,15,57] Post-traumatic abscesses are usually caused by staphylococci, and abscesses from otitis media are virtually always polymicrobial in origin, with streptococci, *Bacteroides* sp., and gram-negative aerobic bacilli (particularly *Proteus* sp.) most often isolated in combination.[14,15,53,57] Thus, the location of the abscess may have important implications for antimicrobial therapy.

CLINICAL MANIFESTATIONS AND DIFFERENTIAL DIAGNOSIS

The course for a brain abscess patient may range from indolent to fulminant; in approximately 75 percent of patients, the duration of symptoms is 2 weeks or less.[13] Only a minority (≤50 percent) of patients display the classic triad of fever, headache, and focal neurologic deficit. The prominent clinical manifestations of brain abscesses are due to the space-occupying mass rather than to infection. A moderate to severe headache, often hemicranial but also generalized, is the most common symptom (approximately 70 percent of cases).[5,6,13,53] Fever occurs in only 45–50 percent of patients.[4,6,13] A change in mental status ranging from lethargy to frank coma occurs in most patients.[5,7,13] Focal neurologic findings are present in approximately 50 percent of cases and are dependent on the location and size of the lesion and concurrent surrounding edema; hemiparesis is the most common manifestation.[3–6,8,9,13] Nausea and vomiting afflict one-half of patients, presumably due to raised intracranial pressure. Seizures occur in 25–35 percent of patients; they most often appear generalized and are common with frontal lobe lesions.[6,8,9,13] Nuchal rigidity and papilledema each are present in about 25 percent of cases.[6,8,9,13,17] The clinical manifestations of a brain abscess, on rare occasions, may closely mimic pyogenic meningitis with a rapidly fulminant course. Other symptoms and signs are dependent on the intracranial location. Abscesses of the cerebellar hemispheres (10–18 percent of intracranial abscesses) often produce nystagmus, ataxia, vomiting, and dysmetria.[54,60] The clinical presentation of frontal lobe abscesses is often dominated by headache, drowsiness, inattention, and a generalized deterioration in mental function. Hemiparesis with unilateral motor signs and a motor speech disorder are the most common focal neurologic signs. A temporal lobe abscess may present with an early ipsilateral headache. If the abscess is in the dominant hemisphere, aphasia may be present. An upper homonymous quadrantanopia may also be demonstrated and may be the only sign of a right temporal lobe abscess.[88] Intrasellar abscesses often simulate a pituitary tumor and present with headache, visual field defects, and various endocrine disturbances.[25,89] Brain stem abscesses most frequently present with facial weakness, fever, headache, hemiparesis, dysphagia, and vomiting.[27] The symptoms and signs of the extracerebral focus of infection may be present and dominate the clinical picture. Neurologic findings, however subtle, in a patient with a predisposing condition outlined in Table 1, mandate investigation of the CNS to exclude a brain abscess and other intracranial complications of these disorders.[6,8,11,13]

The differential diagnosis of brain abscesses is broad and includes subdural empyema, epidural abscess, pyogenic meningitis, primary or metastatic cerebral neoplasms, viral (especially herpes simplex) encephalitis, hemorrhagic leukoencephalitis, echinococcosis, cysticercosis, cryptococcosis, cerebral infarction, CNS vasculitis, mycotic aneurysms, and chronic subdural hematoma. Computed tomography is often necessary but frequently not sufficient to accomplish this differentiation.

LABORATORY FINDINGS AND DIAGNOSIS

A moderate peripheral blood leukocytosis may be present in patients with abscesses but exceeds 20,000/mm^3 in only 10 percent of patients, while 40 percent display a completely normal leukocyte concentration.[5,6,64] The erythrocyte sedimentation rate is usually elevated with a mean of 45–50 mm/hr. Hyponatremia may be seen as a reflection of the syndrome of inappropriate antidiuretic hormone secretion.

Lumbar puncture is contraindicated in patients with a suspected or proven cerebral abscess since the diagnostic yield is poor and the procedure is dangerous. The cerebrospinal fluid (CSF) profile is nonspecific in patients with brain abscesses: hypoglycorrhachia in 25 percent; elevated protein in 67–81 percent; and a pleocytosis, usually <500/mm^3 and predominantly mononuclear, in 60–70 percent of cases.[5,6,9,13] Fewer than 10 percent of CSF cultures are positive, only increasing to 20 percent after ventricular rupture.[7] In addition, the removal of CSF may result in herniation. In one series,[3] 41 of 140 patients subjected to lumbar puncture deteriorated clinically in less than 48 hours; 25 of these 41 patients died (11 of these were fully alert or only mildly drowsy at the time of the procedure). Similarly, 7 of 44 patients deteriorated in less than 24 hours after lumbar puncture and 6 died.[65] In the analysis of Samson and Clark,[13] 22 of 44 patients with brain abscesses underwent lumbar puncture; 5 of the 22 developed signs of midbrain compression within 2 hours of the procedure. These sobering figures have been recently confirmed in a series of patients observed from 1970 to 1983. Sixty percent (27/45) of these patients were subjected to a lumbar puncture, and 4 of these 27 patients died within 24 hours of the procedure.[7] For these reasons, a lumbar puncture should be delayed in patients with a febrile CNS disorder with focal neurologic signs.[24,90] However, if pyogenic meningitis is also a strong consideration, blood cultures should be obtained and appropriate antibiotics started parenterally before obtaining the CT scan. In this case, if the CT scan findings are negative, a lumbar puncture is then performed.

The skull roentgenogram is usually normal in patients with brain abscesses but may show a pineal shift, signs of raised intracranial pressure, an effaced dorsum sellae (with intrasellar abscess), or pathognomonic collections of air within a cavity.[3–6,8,9,13,17] The electroencephalogram (EEG) is usually abnormal in patients with brain abscess and lateralizes to the side of the lesion.[5,6,13,17,64] In developing countries, the EEG is a useful (and often the only) screening procedure for the detection of brain abscesses.[9]

Arteriography and ventriculography are rarely necessary in the evaluation of patients with suspected brain abscesses since the advent of CT. Arteriograms are abnormal in about 80 percent of brain abscess patients and may show a "ring shadow" in 20–40 percent; the usual pattern is an avascular mass with surrounding hyperemia.[3–6,8,9,13,91] The absence of neovascularity may be helpful in excluding a necrotic tumor. Arteriography is essential if mycotic aneurysms due to endocarditis are suspected.

A technetium 99 brain scan is a very sensitive test for the detection of brain abscess and remains the procedure of choice in areas where CT scanning is unavailable. The results are abnormal in >95 percent of patients, and a "doughnut" lesion is detected in 25–35 percent.[92] Unfortunately, this radiographic appearance is also compatible with a necrotic tumor or infarction. The results of some series suggest that the brain scan is more sensitive than CT is in the early cerebritis stage of a brain abscess, but more information is necessary.[93] Compared with CT, localization is not as accurate; posterior fossa lesions are more difficult to visualize, and postoperative uptake can obscure the recognition of persistent or recurrent abscesses.[94] A

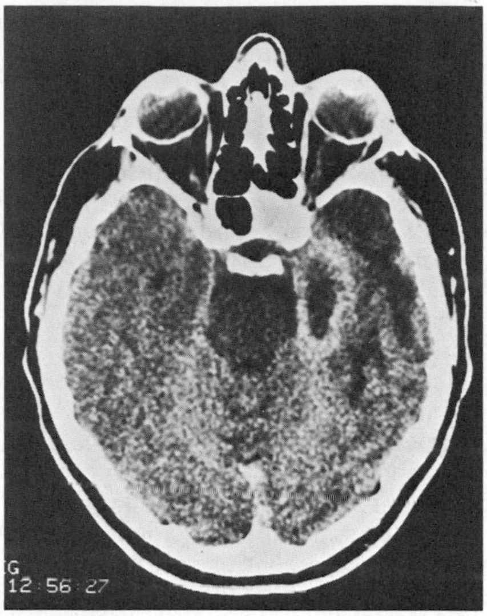

FIG. 1. CT scan after contrast administration in the axial projection of a 44-year-old woman with a history of chronic otitis media and documented sphenoid sinusitis. Note the ring enhancement around a hypodense lesion in the left medial temporal lobe with hypodense edema in the white matter. Aspiration revealed *S. anginosus* in pure culture.

brain scan or magnetic resonance imaging (MRI) (see below) should be performed when a brain abscess is suspected and CT findings are negative to exclude early cerebritis and alterations in the blood-brain barrier.

The introduction of CT revolutionized the diagnostic (and perhaps therapeutic) approach to brain abscess. CT has been shown to be superior to standard radiologic procedures for the evaluation of the paranasal sinuses, mastoids, and the middle ear; scans of these areas should be obtained, along with chest x-ray films, in all patients with suspected brain abscesses.[95] This technique is more sensitive (95–99 percent) than are traditional brain scans beyond the cerebritis stage and yields more information—the extent of surrounding edema, the presence of a midline shift, hydrocephalus, or imminent ventricular rupture.[96,97] The characteristic appearance (Figs. 1 and 2) is a hypodense center (leukocytes and necrotic debris) with an outlying uniform ring enhancement surrounded by a variable hypodense region of brain edema. Contrast enhancement is essential. The impressive sensitivity of CT is not paralleled by an equivalent specificity; a similar appearance is seen with neoplasms, granulomas, cerebral infarction, or resolving hematoma.[98,99] In addition, this characteristic appearance may be lost after ventricular rupture (Fig. 3). Features thought to discriminate abscesses from malignant tumors (thinner, more regular contrast-enhancing rim, and homogeneous enhancement of the capsule after infusion of contrast medium) do not always permit a precise diagnosis. Ependymal enhancement, when present, is indicative of ventriculitis and favors a diagnosis of brain abscess.[7] Holtas et al.[100] reported a series of 26 patients with brain abscesses wherein the CT and clinical findings in 8 were interpreted as representing a malignant tumor instead of abscess. In an effort to improve the diagnostic accuracy of CT, Coulam and associates[101] selected six parameters that could be used to differentiate between abscess and tumor, including patient age, ring thickness variability, outside ring diameter, lesion-to-ring ratio, maximum ring thickness, and CT mean value in the ring center. The overall classification accuracy in his study was still only 86 percent (84 percent for abscesses, 96 percent for tumors).

A diagnostic modality that may prove to be complimentary to CT is indium 111 labeled leukocyte scintigraphy, which has been useful in the diagnosis of occult abscesses elsewhere in the body and has been recently evaluated in the diagnosis of brain abscess. Radiolabeled leukocytes migrate to and accumulate in a focus of active inflammation, thus differentiating a brain abscess from other causes of mass lesions in the brain. In a study of 16 patients where CT was felt to be inconclusive in making a differentiation between tumor or abscess, leukocyte scintigraphy correctly predicted tumor in 10 of 11 patients and abscess in 4 of 5 patients for an overall diagnostic accuracy of 88 percent.[102] A second study of 20 patients yielded a sensitivity of 100 percent, specificity of 94 percent, and overall accuracy of 96 percent in making this differentiation.[103] Potential problems illustrated in these studies are that necrotic tumors can occasionally yield a false-positive result and that the concomitant use of steroids may be responsible for a false-negative scan finding.

Data regarding the utility of MRI (Fig. 4) in the diagnosis of a brain abscess is preliminary but encouraging. MRI appears to be more sensitive than CT is in the early detection of cerebritis as well as in detecting cerebral edema in healthy brain tissue adjacent to a cerebritic focus.[104–106] This increased sensitivity may be of limited clinical usefulness since there is already an obvious CT lesion when most brain abscess patients seek help. However, MRI may detect satellite lesions earlier. Contrast-enhanced MRI scans using the paramagnetic agent gadolinium diethylenetriamine penta-acetic acid (Gd-DTPA) increase the information obtained by MRI. This agent crosses a damaged blood-brain barrier and enhances proton relaxation, which in turn increases T1 signal intensity at the site of its accumulation. Gd-DTPA yields consistently increased enhancement of lesions relative to that seen with enhanced CT scans. Additionally, it differentiates three regions with greater accuracy: (*1*) the central abscess, (*2*) the surrounding enhancing rim, and (*3*) cerebral edema around the abscess.[105–107] Preliminary reports indicate that MRI may be superior to CT for the detection and characterization of a cerebral abscess, particularly in early stages of evolution. Its lack of ionizing radiation, greater tissue characterization, lack of bone artifact (which improves its sensitivity in posterior fossa lesions), and the decreased toxicity of Gd-

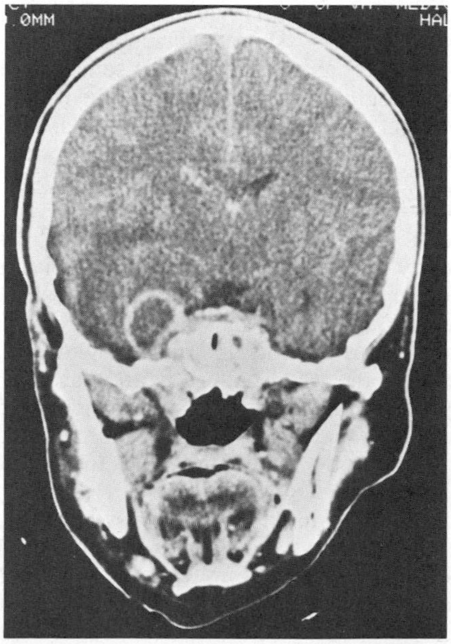

FIG. 2. CT scan after contrast administration, in the coronal projection, of the same patient shown in Fig. 1. Note the ring enhancement of the inferomedial left temporal lobe abscess, edema in the temporal lobe white matter, and effacement of the left lateral ventricle. Also note the proximity of the abscess to the petrous ridge and cavernous sinus. After abscess aspiration, drainage of sphenoid sinusitis, and 4 weeks of parenteral penicillin, the patient made a complete recovery without sequelae.

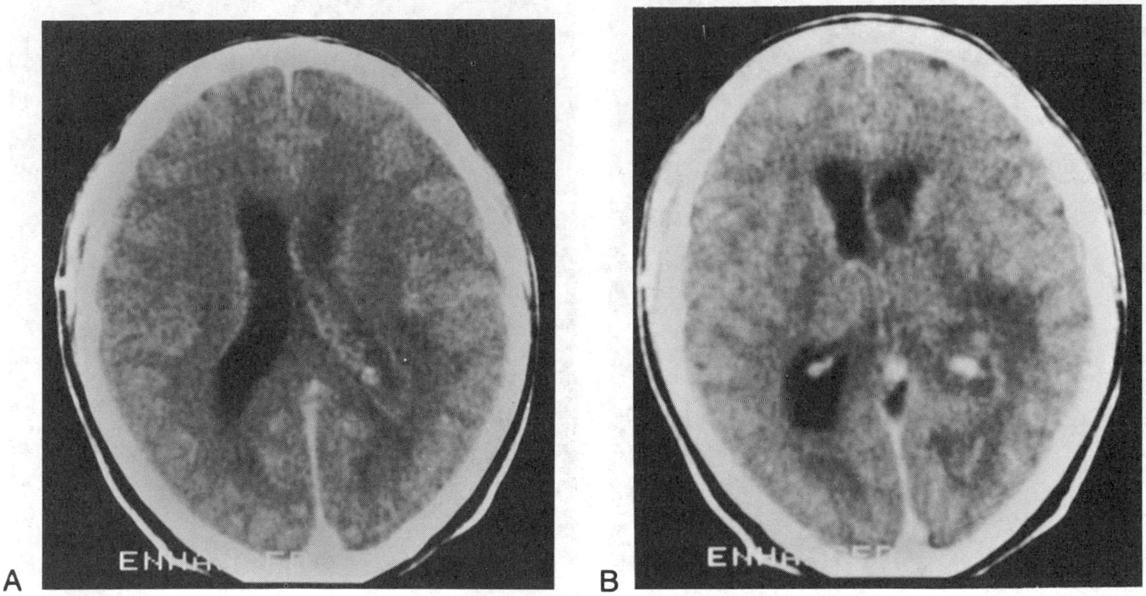

FIG. 3. CT scan after contrast administration in the axial projection. Note the loss of contrast enhancement in the original right hemispheric abscess after rupture into the right lateral ventricle. **(A)** Abscess enhancement is replaced by ependymal enhancement. **(B)** Abscess fluid/CSF interface in the right lateral ventricle.

DTPA as compared with CT contrast agents may make MRI the procedure of choice in the evaluation of brain abscesses.

ANTIBIOTIC THERAPY

Antibiotic Entry into Brain Abscess Pus

The various factors that determine the presentation of an antibiotic into the CSF[108] may not predict entry into brain tissue or abscess pus. The blood-brain barrier is altered in proximity to areas of cerebritis or an encapsulated abscess[109] and permits increased permeation of normally excluded antibiotics such as penicillin into the brain parenchyma. Few studies have addressed this issue in the treatment of brain abscesses.

An early study[110] examined brain tissue, CSF, and serum antibiotic concentrations in 27 patients subjected to a prefrontal lobotomy, presumably with an intact blood-brain barrier. After collection at various intervals after dosing, tetracycline entered both the CSF and the brain, streptomycin and erythromycin were found in the CSF but not in the brain, and penicillin was not present at either site, perhaps reflecting the low dose (600,000 units) and serum concentrations attained (0.06–2.0 μg/ml) 4 hours later when brain samples were analyzed. In patients undergoing excision of an intracranial neoplasm, a parenteral bolus of 2 g led to the following calculated brain-blood ratios: chloramphenicol, 9:1; cephalothin, 1:10; penicillin G, 1:23; and ampicillin, 1:56.[111] On the basis of this evidence and activity against anaerobic bacteria, chloramphenicol has often been included in recommended regimens for the treatment of brain abscesses.

Black et al.[112] analyzed antibiotic concentrations in brain abscess pus from 6 patients. Chloramphenicol, methicillin, and penicillin were detectable in the pus after standard dosages, whereas nafcillin was not. All six patients deteriorated clinically during medical treatment, and all cultures were still positive at surgery, thus indicating the need for surgical intervention. In the best analysis to date, de Louvois et al.[113] examined antibiotic concentrations in brain abscess pus obtained from 32 patients. Penicillin G was detectable consistently if the dose exceeded 24 million units daily (adults); however, the drug was ≥90 percent inactivated after incubation in pus for 1 hour in vitro[114] in 4 of 22 specimens. Fusidic acid entered the brain abscess pus readily, but concentrations of various cephalosporins and cloxacillin were low.[113] CSF and brain concentrations of clindamycin are low after conventional dosages[114]; however, potentially therapeutic concentrations in abscess fluid may be attainable.[115] Metronidazole attains high concentrations (approximately 35–45 μg/g) in brain abscess pus,[53] often exceeding serum concentrations after a dose of 400–600 mg every 8 hours. Due to these results and the bactericidal activity of metronidazole against strict anaerobes, this agent is often a component of antimicrobial regimens for brain abscesses.[116]

Trimethoprim-sulfamethoxazole, effective in cerebral nocardiosis[117,118] and gram-negative meningitis,[119] may have a role where susceptible organisms are present. In two studies, this drug combination was found to attain adequate brain abscess pus concentrations for the organisms being treated (*Proteus mirabilis* and *Nocardia asteroides*) and yielded successful results when combined with surgery.[118,120] In a recent report[121] vancomycin also attained acceptable concentrations in a single brain abscess.

Little information is currently available on the penetration of newer antimicrobial agents into brain abscesses or their clinical efficacy in this infection. Cefotaxime, ceftizoxime, ceftriaxone, ceftazidine and moxalactam have been shown to penetrate the CSF in therapeutic concentrations, but this does not necessarily predict activity in a brain abscess. A recent report demonstrated good penetration of moxalactam into brain abscess fluid,[122] and this agent has been used successfully in the treatment of neonatal brain abscess.[123] Aztreonam, a new monobactam derivative, has recently been shown to be effective in the treatment of experimental cerebritis,[124] but its penetration into brain tissue has not been evaluated, and it has not yet been evaluated in human brain abscesses.

Any study evaluating antibiotic penetration into the CNS must be interpreted cautiously. Considerable variation in tissue concentrations among different patients is often present as well as conflicting results between studies. A single tissue concentration may not represent the dynamics of antibiotic movement into the brain in the presence of inflammation.[125,126] The relevance of brain and abscess pus antibiotic concentrations or the necessity of bactericidal activity at the site of infection remains unknown.

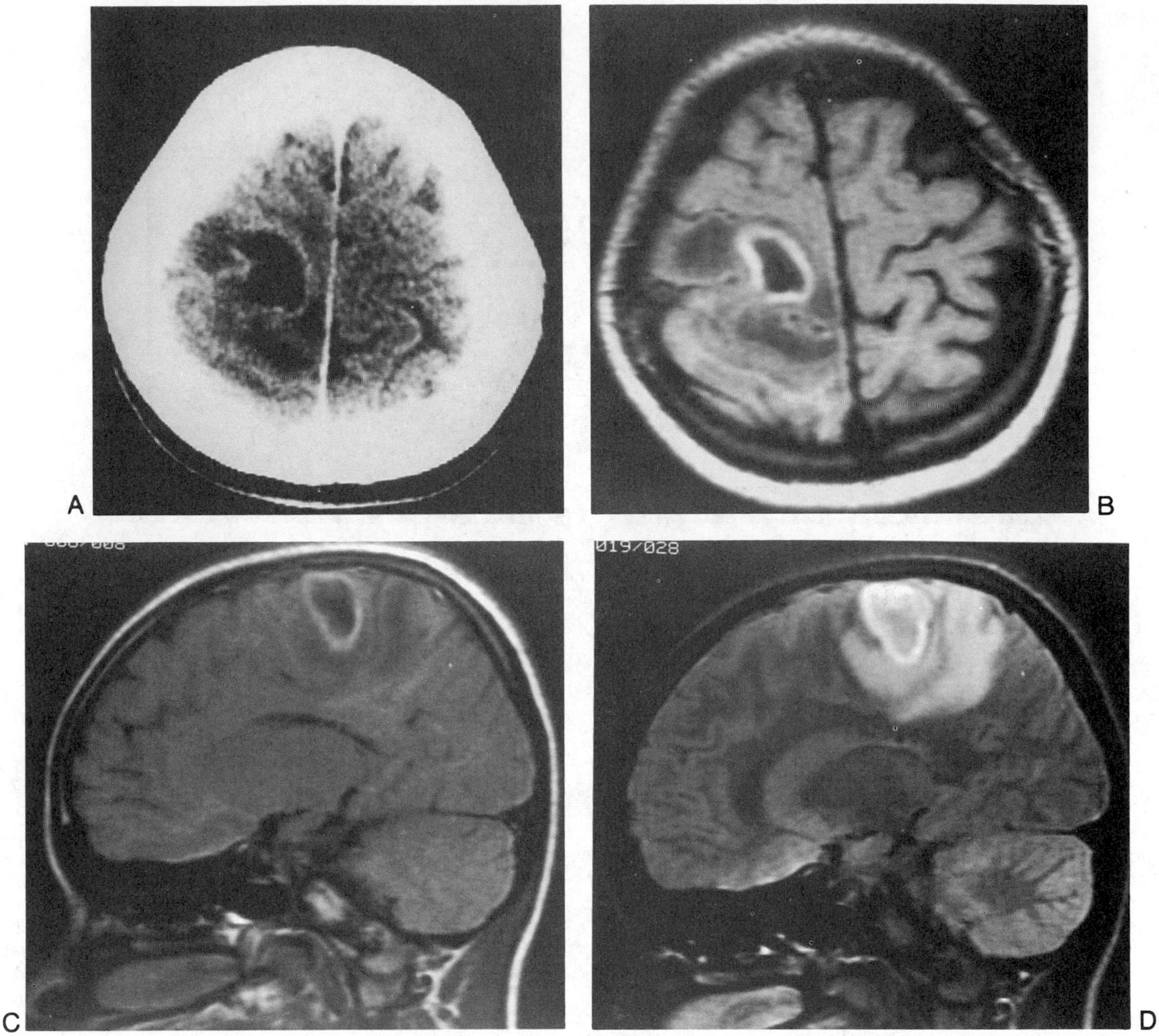

FIG. 4. MRI of a brain abscess in a teenage girl who developed seizures several days after esophageal dilation. **(A)** Contrast CT shows a thin-walled enhancing cystic lesion in the right parietal subcortical region. **(B)** T1-weighted MRI of a 5 mm thick axial section shows a thin-walled hyperintense rim abscess with surrounding hypointensity. Note, in comparison to the opposite side, the effacement of the sulci on the right. **(C)** Sagittal T1-weighted image of a 5 mm thick section shows the hyperintense thin-walled abscess. **(D)** Sagittal T2-weighted image of a 5 mm thick section shows a hyperintense abscess wall with high-signal contents (pus) and high-signal surrounding edema. (Courtesy of Dr. Robert Zimmerman, Department of Radiology, Hospital of the University of Pennsylvania, Philadelphia, PA.)

Choice of Antibiotic

The antimicrobial regimens commonly recommended for therapy for brain abscesses are empirical and reflect the considerations already noted as well as their in vitro activity against the usual pathogens. No controlled trials on the relative efficacy of various regimens have been performed. Since the early 1960s, a combination of penicillin G (20–24 million units/day) plus chloramphenicol (1.0–1.5 g intravenously q6h) has been advocated. Penicillin remains a mainstay of therapy[14,15,57] due to its excellent activity against streptococci in vitro and the favorable results obtained in experimental models of brain abscess.[127] The introduction of penicillin in the 1940s may have been instrumental in reducing brain abscess mortality from 50–80 percent to 20–30 percent by 1950.[128–131] Due to the important role of streptococci (especially the *S. milleri* group) in brain abscesses complicating contiguous foci of infection and pyogenic lung disease, penicillin should be employed in all such cases. Most anaerobes are also susceptible to penicillin with the notable exception of *Bacteroides fragilis*. Chloramphenicol is often administered concurrently with penicillin because its high lipid solubility results in concentrations in brain tissue often exceeding those in serum and its activity against anaerobic bacteria is significant. The use of metronidazole in brain abscesses has increased greatly in recent years because (*1*) metronidazole is bactericidal against *B. fragilis*, where chloramphenicol is frequently bacteriostatic; (*2*) metronidazole attains reproducibly excellent concentrations in brain abscess pus[53]; (*3*) metronidazole's entry into brain abscess pus is not affected by concomitant steroid treatment, unlike several other antibiotics[131];

(*4*) chloramphenicol may be degraded by deacetylation in pus (shown in experimental intra-abdominal abscesses); and (*5*) metronidazole may have a salutary effect on mortality as suggested by retrospective experience.[109] Metronidazole, when substituted for chloramphenicol, may lead to more rapid healing and lower mortality[40,116,132]; however, these two agents have never been compared in a prospective, randomized trial. Additionally, metronidazole may cause CNS side effects that are difficult to differentiate from clinical deterioration in brain abscess patients. An antianaerobic agent (e.g., chloramphenicol or metronidazole) is indicated in brain abscesses complicating otitis media, mastoiditis, or pyogenic lung disease since anaerobes (particularly *B. fragilis*) are often present. These agents may not be required in abscesses secondary to frontoethmoidal sinusitis because *B. fragilis* is an uncommon isolate.

When staphylococci are suspected (see Table 1) or grown, nafcillin (1.5 g q4h) is indicated.[133] Vancomycin should be substituted if the patient is either allergic to penicillin or a methicillin-resistant strain is isolated. European investigators favor fusidic acid for this indication,[14,15] but experience with this agent by physicians in the United States is limited.

The frequent isolation of Enterobacteriaceae in brain abscesses of otitic origin prompts many authorities to add a third-generation cephalosporin or trimethoprim-sulfamethoxazole to the regimen pending culture results. This approach appears to be reasonable, but the pathogenetic role of these organisms remains unsettled. Finally, the duration of therapy with any of the regimens as outlined remains unknown.

SURGICAL THERAPY

Although some patients with brain abscess respond to prolonged medical therapy alone, most require surgery for optimal management. The timing and type of surgical procedure remains controversial. Aspiration of the abscess after burr hole placement and complete excision after craniotomy have both been advocated, but no prospective randomized trial has ever been performed. By retrospective analysis, the two procedures appear to be equivalent as judged by outcome.[3–5,15] However, patients considered for excision are more often in a satisfactory neurologic condition, whereas aspiration is more often performed in the deteriorating neurologically compromised patient or for the drainage of inaccessible lesions (brain stem, thalamus, basal ganglia, etc.) where mortality is significant.[9] The procedure employed must be individualized in each patient and is dependent on the clinical course, size and location of the abscess, CT scan appearance, and other factors. Emergent surgery is mandatory when there is a progression of neurologic signs. Young and Frazee[134] advocate that abscesses exhibiting gas by CT or plain film should be considered for complete excision. In a review of five such patients, three of whom had unsuccessful aspiration procedures, a total excision was required, and a persistent extracranial communication was discovered. A brain abscess in a comatose patient carries a grave prognosis regardless of the form of treatment,[6,135] and surgery is indicated before this stage. Incomplete drainage of a multiloculated abscess is a major disadvantage of aspiration and is an important reason why reoperation is required more frequently after this procedure.[9] Excision is preferred for posterior fossa lesions and in fungal brain abscesses where antifungal therapy is limited. The incidence of postoperative seizures or other deficits is not clearly different after excision as compared with aspiration[9,136]; however, since the advent of CT, the data appear to favor more conservative surgical procedures, i.e., aspiration.[137] Instillation of antibiotics into the abscess cavity during aspiration (often bacitracin or penicillin) is frequently employed, although its efficacy has never been clearly established. Antibiotics given in this manner may potentially diffuse into surrounding brain tissue in high concentrations and cause seizures.[15,112,129,138] In cases where *Pseudomonas* spp. are implicated, direct instillation of specific antibiotics is probably warranted because adequate local antibiotic concentrations for this organism after systemic administration are difficult to obtain.[7]

Aspiration may be accomplished by stereotaxic CT guidance,[139] an extremely promising technique. This procedure affords the surgeon rapid, accurate (within 1 mm), and safe access to virtually any intracranial point. In a recent review of its use in 80 patients, recovery of tissue specific to establish a histologic diagnosis or the etiologic factors related to each disease process was realized in 94 percent of cases. There was no associated mortality and only 4 percent transient morbidity. The diagnosis of 20 cases of infection was made, 6 of which were pyogenic brain abscess, and in most instances the choice of antimicrobial therapy was significantly affected. In addition, this procedure allowed for successful drainage, even in two cases of multicompartment abscesses.[140] A second series of 102 patients[141] showed a diagnostic yield of 96 percent by this technique. There was no mortality and a 5.9 percent transient morbidity. The five abscesses that were encountered were definitively drained. Several recent evaluations confirm the efficacy and low morbidity of this procedure.[142–144] The risk of stereotaxic aspiration may be less than the risk of incorrect diagnosis and suboptimal choice of antibiotics, which makes it, in many cases, more difficult to support empirical therapy. Serial CT is useful in individual cases and may permit improved decisions regarding the need, timing, and type of surgery.

GENERAL MANAGEMENT

The CT scan, as noted earlier, has dramatically altered the diagnosis and treatment of brain abscesses. The results in animal models and humans suggest that focal bacterial infections of the brain parenchyma may be "staged" by sequential CT scans.[45,145] Cerebritis is characterized by an area of low density surrounded by ring enhancement (often thick and diffuse) that does not decay on delayed contrast scans obtained 60 minutes later (Table 4). In contrast, encapsulation is characterized by a faint ring on the unenhanced scan and ring enhancement that decays in the delayed CT scan. These parameters may prove useful in planning the combined medical–surgical approach.

Since 1971 it has been recognized that early antibiotic therapy alone could cure cerebritis without the later development of an encapsulated abscess.[146] Between 1975 and 1985, 67 cases of presumably established brain abscesses were reported to be cured by medical therapy alone.[147] These studies share the following features: (*1*) the initial diagnosis and resolution of brain abscess(s) were documented by sequential CT scans, (*2*) prolonged courses of high-dose antibiotic therapy (8 weeks or longer parenterally) were administered, and (*3*) there was a lack of surgical or histopathologic evidence of encapsulation.[9,137,148–153] Careful studies in animal models of brain abscess[45,154] and clinical observations[46,99,145,155] have clearly shown, however, that ring enhancement on the CT scan may be observed during the cerebritis stage. Thus, it is possible that these results with antimicrobial therapy represent successful resolution of bacterial cerebritis rather than a well-encapsulated abscess in some cases. This problem requires further study.

No general management guidelines can be formulated to en-

TABLE 4. "Staging" of Brain Abscesses with Computed Tomography

		Contrast Enhancement at	
Stage[a]	*Precontrast*	*10 min*	*60 min*
Cerebritis	Low density	Ring enhancement	No decay
Abscess	Capsule-faint ring around low density	Ring enhancement	Decay in contrast enhancement

[a] Both lesions may be surrounded by low-density areas of edema.
(Data from Britt et al.[46])

sure optimal results in the individual patient with a brain abscess. If the scanning suggests cerebritis and the patient is neurologically stable, antibiotic therapy (usually penicillin plus chloramphenicol or metronidazole) can be started and the patient observed. Criteria for nonoperative management also generally include (*1*) medical conditions that greatly increase the risk of surgery; (*2*) the presence of multiple abscesses, especially remotely distant from one another; (*3*) abscesses in a deep or dominant location; (*4*) concomitant meningitis or ependymitis; (*5*) early abscess reduction and clinical improvement attributable to antibiotic therapy; and (*6*) abscess size under 3 cm.[20,98,150,151] As noted, these criteria may be altered by the availability of stereotaxic CT guided aspiration. Neurologic deterioration mandates surgery, usually aspiration.[9] If the patient remains stable and the abscess is accessible, aspiration (CT guided, if possible) is desirable to make a specific bacteriologic diagnosis and narrow the antimicrobial regimen. Although this delay may render cultures negative, aspiration during the cerebritis stage may be dangerous with resultant hemorrhage.[155] Certain poor prognostic parameters, clinical or radiographic, may necessitate earlier aspiration.[135] If the lesion appears encapsulated by CT scan criteria, antibiotic treatment can be started and aspiration (for diagnosis and drainage) performed without delay.[46,145] Subsequent management is dependent on clinical and radiographic (CT) parameters. Later neurologic deterioration or failure of the abscess to decrease in size as detected by CT scan are indications for further surgery, often excision, if feasible. The duration of antimicrobial therapy remains unsettled. Many authorities treat parenterally for 4–6 weeks, often followed by prolonged oral therapy if a suitable agent is available against the isolated pathogens, for 2–6 months. It must be stressed that such regimens are empirical and may not be necessary; a cured brain abscess may continue to appear as nodular contrast enhancement on CT scans for 4–10 weeks to up to 6 months[46,98,99] after completion of successful therapy.

Steroids are often employed as adjunctives in the management of brain abscess, but their role remains controversial. These agents may be deleterious by reducing antibiotic entry into the CNS,[156,157] decreasing collagen formation and glial response,[158] or altering the CT scan appearance of ring enhancement as inflammation subsides,[159,160] which may obscure information from sequential studies or an assessment of cure. However, steroids may prove lifesaving in the patient with rapid neurologic deterioration and raised intracranial pressure. In this circumstance, intracranial pressure monitoring is advisable, and elevations in pressure should be controlled with steroids, forced hyperventilation, and mannitol if necessary. Anticonvulsants are appropriate in the patient having seizures.

PROGNOSIS

The mortality of brain abscesses was 40–60 percent in the preantibiotic era; some series report a decline after the introduction of penicillin.[3–6,8,9,13,17,64] An adverse prognosis is associated with (*1*) delayed or missed diagnosis; (*2*) poor localization, especially in the posterior fossa before the availability of CT scans; (*3*) multiple, deep, or multiloculated lesions; (*4*) ventricular rupture (80–100 percent mortality); (*5*) coma (Table 5) (80–100 percent mortality); (*6*) fungal etiology; and (*7*) inappropriate antibiotics.[6,9,135] Additional negative factors often cited include extremes of age, large abscesses, and metastatic abscesses.[7] More recently, a decreased mortality ranging between 0 and 24 percent has been reported in numerous series and is attributed to the introduction of CT scanning.[18,94,116,161] The incidence of neurologic sequelae ranges between 30 and 55 percent.[7] Most sequelae are mild, but up to 17 percent of patients may be incapacitated, with the severity of sequelae more often correlating with the patient's neurologic condition on admission than the form of treatment employed.[7,13,43,94] The likelihood of seizures is variable and ranges from 35 to >90 percent; these differences may relate to the length of follow-up. Anticonvulsant therapy appears to reduce this complication.[162] There is some recent suggestion that lesions treated conservatively (i.e., with antibiotics and/or aspiration vs. complete excision) have a lower incidence of post-treatment sequelae, correlating with less visible abnormalities on follow-up CT scans.[137] Earlier diagnosis, refinements in technology, and an aggressive medical–surgical approach may lead to a more consistent reduction in the morbidity and mortality of this still serious disease.

TABLE 5. Brain Abscess: Influence of Preoperative Mental Status on Mortality

Mental Status	*Patients (No.)*	*Mortality (%)*
Grade I (fully alert)	33	0
Grade II (drowsy)	55	4
Grade III (response to pain only)	61	59
Grade IV (coma, no pain response)	51	82

(Data from Nielsen et al.[6])

REFERENCES

1. Theophilo F, Markakis E, Theophilo L, et al. Brain abscess in childhood. Child Nerv Syst. 1985;1:324.
2. MacEwen W. Pyogenic Infective Diseases of the Brain and Spinal Cord. Glasgow: James MacLehose & Sons; 1893.
3. Garfield J. Management of supratentorial intracranial abscess: A review of 200 cases. Br Med J. 1969;2:7.
4. Beller AJ, Sahar A, Praiss I. Brain abscess. Review of 89 cases over 30 years. J Neurol Neurosurg Psychiatry. 1973;36:757.
5. Morgan H, Wood M, Murphy F. Experience with 88 consecutive cases of brain abscess. J Neurosurg. 1973;38:698.
6. Nielsen H, Glydensted C, Harmsen A. Cerebral abscess. Aetiology and pathogenesis, symptoms, diagnosis and treatment. Acta Neurol Scand. 1982;65:609.
7. Chun CH, Johnson JD, Hofstetter M, et al. Brain abscess. A study of 45 consecutive cases. Medicine (Baltimore). 1986;65:415.
8. Garvey G. Current concepts of bacterial infections of the central nervous system. Bacterial meningitis and bacterial brain abscess. J Neurosurg. 1983;59:735.
9. Carey ME. Brain abscesses. Contemp Neurosurg. 1982;3:1.
10. Yang SH. Brain abscess: A review of 400 cases. J Neurosurg. 1981;55:794.
11. Bradley PJ, Shaw MDM. Three decades of brain abscess in Merseyside. J R Coll Surg Edinb. 1983;28:223.
12. Van Alphen HAM, Driessen JJR. Brain abscess and subdural empyema. J Neurol Neurosurg Psychiatry. 1976;39:481.
13. Samson DS, Clark K. A current review of brain abscess. Am J Med. 1973;54:201.
14. de Louvois J, Gortvai P, Hurley R. Bacteriology of abscesses of the central nervous system. A multicentre prospective study. Br Med J. 1977;2:981.
15. de Louvois J. The bacteriology and chemotherapy of brain abscess. J Antimicrob Chemother. 1978;4:395.
16. Harrison MJG. The clinical presentation of intracranial abscesses. Q J Med. 1982;51:461.
17. Brewer NS, MacCarty CS, Wellman WE. Brain abscess: A review of recent experience. Ann Intern Med. 1975;82:571.
18. Small M, Dale BAB. Intracranial suppuration 1968–1982—a 15 year review. Clin Otolaryngol. 1984;9:315.
19. Bradley PJ, Manning KP, Shaw MDM. Brain abscess secondary to paranasal sinusitis. J Laryngol Otol. 1984;98:719.
20. Kaplan K: Brain abscess. Med Clin North Am. 1985;69:345.
21. Spires JR, Smith RJH, Catlin FI. Brain abscesses in the young. Otolaryngol Head Neck Surg. 1985;93:468.
22. Foy P, Skarr M. Cerebral abscesses in children after pencil-tip injuries. Lancet. 1980;2:662.
23. Tay JS, Garland JS. Serious head injuries from lawn darts. Pediatrics. 1987;79:261.
24. Dacey RG Jr, Winn HR. Brain abscess and perimeningeal infections. In: Stein JH, Cline MJ, Daly WJ, eds. Internal Medicine. Boston: Little, Brown; 1983:1213.
25. Berger SA, Edberg SC, David G. Infectious disease of the sella turcica. Rev Infect Dis. 1986;8:747.
26. Teed RW. Meningitis from the sphenoid sinus. Arch Otolaryngol. 1938;28:589.
27. Dake MD, McMurdo SK, Rosenblum ML, et al. Pyogenic abscess of the medulla oblongata. Neurosurgery. 1986;18:370.
28. Samuel J, Fernandes CMC, Steinberg JL. Intracranial otogenic complications: A persisting problem. Laryngoscope. 1986;96:272.

29. Gower D, McGuirt WF. Intracranial complications of acute and chronic infectious ear disease: A problem still with us. Laryngoscope. 1983;93:1028.
30. Browning GG. The unsafeness of safe ears. J Laryngol Otol. 1984;98:23.
31. Lew D, Southwick FS, Montgomery WW, et al. Sphenoid sinusitis. A review of 30 cases. N Engl J Med. 1983;309:1149.
32. Hollin SA, Hayashi H, Gross SW. Intracranial abscesses of odontogenic origin. Oral Surg. 1967;23:277.
33. Foreman SD, Smith EE, Ryan NJ, et al. Neonatal *Citrobacter* meningitis: Pathogenesis of cerebral abscess formation. Ann Neurol. 1984;16:655.
34. Brand B, Caparosa RJ, Lubic LG. Otorhinological brain abscess therapy—past and present. Laryngoscope. 1984;94:483.
35. Waggener JD. The pathophysiology of bacterial meningitis and cerebral abscesses: An anatomical interpretation. Adv Neurol. 1974;6:1.
36. Bronitsky R, Heim CR, McGee ZA. Multifocal brain abscesses: Combined medical and neurosurgical therapy. South Med J. 1982;75:1261.
37. Kline MW. Brain abscess in a patient with cystic fibrosis. Pediatr Infect Dis. 1985;4:72.
38. Schlitt M, Mitchem L, Zorn G, et al. Brain abscess after esophageal dilation for caustic stricture: Report of three cases. Neurosurgery. 1985;17:947.
39. Cohen FL, Koerner RS, Taub SJ. Solitary brain abscess following endoscopic injection sclerosis of esophageal varices. Gastrointest Endosc. 1985;31:331.
40. Pruit AA, Rubin RHJ, Karchmer AW, et al. Neurologic complications of bacterial endocarditis. Medicine (Baltimore). 1978;57:329.
41. Press OW, Ramsey PG. Central nervous system infections associated with hereditary hemorrhagic telangiectasia. Am J Med. 1984;77:86.
42. Fischbein CA, Rosenthal A, Fischer EG, et al. Risk factors for brain abscess in patients with congenital heart disease. Am J Cardiol. 1974;34:97.
43. Fischer EG, McLennan JE, Suzuki Y. Cerebral abscess in children. Am J Dis Child. 1981;135:746.
44. Molinari GF, Smith L, Goldstein MN, et al. Brain abscess from septic cerebral embolism: An experimental model. Neurology (NY). 1973;23:1205.
45. Britt RH, Enzmann DR, Yeager AS. Neuropathological and computerized tomographic findings in experimental brain abscess. J Neurosurg. 1981;55:590.
46. Britt RH, Enzmann DR. Clinical stages of human brain abscesses on serial CT scans after contrast infusion. Computerized tomographic, neuropathological, and clinical correlations. J Neurosurg. 1983;59:972.
47. Obana WG, Britt RH, Placone RC, et al. Experimental brain abscess development in the chronically immunosuppressed host. Computerized tomographic and neuropathological correlations. J Neurosurg. 1986;65:382.
48. Wood JH, Doppman JL, Lightfoote WE. Role of vascular proliferation on angiographic appearance and encapsulation of experimental traumatic and metastatic brain abscesses. J Neurosurg. 1978;48:264.
49. Prockop DJ, Kivirikko KI, Tuderman L, et al. The biosynthesis of collagen and its disorders. Part I. N Engl J Med. 1979;301:13.
50. Britt RH, Enzmann DH, Placone RC, et al. Experimental anaerobic brain abscess. J Neurosurg. 1984;60:1148.
51. Enzmann DR, Britt RH, Obana WG, et al. Experimental *Staphylococcus aureus* brain abscess. AJNR. 1986;7:395.
52. Heinnemann HS, Braude AI. Anaerobic infection of the brain. Observations on eighteen consecutive cases of brain abscess. Am J Med. 1963;35:682.
53. Ingham HR, Selkon JB, Roxby CM. Bacteriological study of otogenic cerebral abscesses: Chemotherapeutic role of metronidazole. Br Med J. 1977;2:991.
54. Arseni C, Ciurea AV. Cerebellar abscesses. A report on 119 cases. Zentralbl Neurochir. 1982;43:359.
55. Arseni C, Ciurea AV. Etiological data on cerebral abscesses. Zentralbl Neurochir. 1982;43:1.
56. Arseni C, Ciurea AV. Rhinogenic cerebral abscesses. Zentralbl Neurochir. 1982;43:12.
57. de Louvois J. Antimicrobial chemotherapy in the treatment of brain abscess. J Antimicrob Chemother. 1983;11:205.
58. de Louvois J. Bacteriological examinations of pus from abscesses of the central nervous system. J Clin Pathol. 1980;33:66.
59. Brook I. Bacteriology of intracranial abscess in children. J Neurosurg. 1981;54:484.
60. Shaw MDM, Russell JA. Cerebellar abscess—a review of 47 cases. J Neurol Neurosurg Psychiatry. 1975;38:429.
61. Murray HW, Gross KC, Masur H, et al. Serious infections caused by *Streptococcus milleri*. Am J Med. 1978;64:759.
62. Shlaes DM, Lerner PM, Wolinsky E, et al. Infections due to Lancefield group F and related streptococci (*S. milleri, S. anginosus*). Medicine (Baltimore). 1981;60:197.
63. Parker MT, Ball LC. Streptococci and aerococci associated with systemic infection in man. J Med Microbiol. 1976;9:275.
64. Carey ME, Chou SN, French LA. Experience with brain abscesses. J Neurosurg. 1972;36:1.
65. Lechtenberg R, Sierra MF, Pringle GF, et al. *Listeria monocytogenes:* Brain abscess or meningoencephalitis: Neurology (NY). 1979;29:86.
66. Nieman RE, Lorber B. Listeriosis in adults: A changing pattern. Report of eight cases and review of the literature. Rev Infect Dis. 1980;2:207.
67. Norden CW, Ruben FL, Selker R. Nonsurgical treatment of cerebral nocardiosis. Arch Neurol. 1983;40:594.
68. Levy RL, Saunders RL. *Citrobacter* meningitis and cerebral abscess in early infancy: Cure by moxalactam. Neurology (NY). 1981;31:1575.
69. Curless RG: Neonatal intracranial abscess: Two cases caused by *Citrobacter* and a literature review. Ann Neurol. 1980;8:269.
70. Rodriquez RE, Valero V, Watanakunakorn C. *Salmonella* focal intracranial infections: Review of the world literature (1884–1984) and report of an unusual case. Rev Infect Dis. 1986;8:31–41.
71. Dijkmans BAC, Thomeer RTWM, Vielvoye GJ, et al. Brain abscess due to *Streptobacillus moniliformis* and *Actinobacterium meyerii*. Infection. 1984;12:262.
72. Bell WE. Treatment of fungal infections of the central nervous system. Ann Neurol. 1981;9:417.
73. Chernik NL, Armstrong D, Posner JB. Central nervous system infections in patients with cancer. Medicine (Baltimore). 1973;52:563.
74. Beal MF, O'Carroll CP, Kleinman GM, et al. Aspergillosis of the nervous system. Neurology (NY). 1982;32:473.
75. Parker JC Jr, McCloskey JJ, Lee RS. The emergence of candidosis. The dominant postmortem cerebral mycosis. Am J Clin Pathol. 1978;70:31.
76. Sandhyamani S, Bhalia R, Mohapatra LN, et al. Cerebral cladosporiosis. Surg. Neurol. 1981;15:431.
77. Masdeu JC, Tantulavanich S, Gorelick PP, et al. Brain abscess caused by *Strongyloides stercoralis*. Arch Neurol. 1982;39:62.
78. Becker GL Jr, Knep S, Lance KP, et al. Amebic abscess of the brain. Neurosurgery. 1980;6:192.
79. Schmutzhard E, Mayr U, Rumpl E, et al. Secondary cerebral amebiasis due to infection with *Entamoeba histolytica*. Eur Neurol. 1986;25:161.
80. Armstrong D. Central nervous system infections in the immunocompromised host. Infection. 1984;12(Suppl 1):58.
81. Hooper DC, Pruitt AA, Rubin RH. Central nervous system infection in the chronically immunosuppressed. Medicine (Baltimore). 1982;61:166.
82. Horowitz SL, Bentson JR, Benson F, et al. CNS toxoplasmosis in acquired immunodeficiency syndrome. Arch Neurol. 1983;40:649–52.
83. Stamm SM, Dismukes WE, Simmons BP, et al. Listeriosis in renal transplant recipients: Report of an outbreak and review of 102 cases. Rev Infect Dis. 1982;4:589.
84. McArthur JC. Neurologic manifestations of AIDS. Medicine (Baltimore). 1987;66:407.
85. Levy RM, Bredesen DE, Rosenblum ML. Neurological manifestations of the acquired immunodeficiency syndrome (AIDS): Experience at UCSF and review of the literature. J Neurosurg. 1985;62:475.
86. Bishburg E, Sunderan EG, Reichman LB, et al. Central nervous system tuberculosis with the acquired immunodeficiency syndrome and its related complex. Ann Intern Med. 1986;105:210.
87. Helweg-Larsen S, Jakobsen J, Boesen F, et al. Neurological complications and concomitants of AIDS. Acta Neurol Scand. 1986;74:467.
88. Adams RD, Victor M. Nonviral infections of the nervous system. In: Adams RD, Victor M, eds. Principles of Neurology. New York: McGraw-Hill, 1985:552.
89. Domingue JN, Wilson CB: Pituitary abscesses. Report of seven cases and review of the literature. J Neurosurg. 1977;46:601.
90. Yoshikawa TT, Goodman SJ. Brain abscess. West J Med. 1974;121:207.
91. Nielsen H, Halaburt H. Cerebral abscess with special reference to the angiographic changes. Neuroradiology. 1976;12:73.
92. Crocker EF, McLaughlin AF, Morris JG, et al. Technetium brain scanning in the diagnosis and management of cerebral abscess. Am J Med. 1974;56:192.
93. Mascucci EF, Sauerbrunn BJL. The evolution of a brain abscess. The complementary roles of radionuclide and computed tomography scans. Clin Nucl Med. 1982;7:166.
94. Rosenblum ML, Hoff JT, Norman D, et al. Decreased mortality from brain abscesses since advent of computerized tomography. J Neurosurg. 1978;49:658.
95. Potter GD, ed. CT of the ear, nose and throat. Radiol Clin North Am. 1984;22:1.
96. New PFJ, Davis KR, Ballantine HT Jr. Computed tomography in cerebral abscess. Radiology. 1976;121:641.
97. Whelan MA, Hilal SK. Computed tomography as a guide in the diagnosis and follow-up of brain abscesses. Radiology. 1980;135:663.
98. Weisberg L. Clinical-CT correlations in intracranial suppurative (bacterial) disease. Neurology (NY). 1984;34:509.
99. Dobkin JF, Healton EB, Dickinson T, et al. Nonspecificity of ring enhancement in medically cured brain abscess. Neurology (NY). 1984;34:139.
100. Holtas S, Tornquist C, Cronqvist S. Diagnostic difficulties in computed tomography of brain abscesses. J Comput Assist Tomogr. 1982;6:683.
101. Coulam CM, Seshul M, Donaldson J. Intracranial ring lesions: Can we differentiate by computed tomography? Invest Radiol. 1980;15:103.
102. Rehncrona S, Brismar J, Holtas S. Diagnosis of brain abscesses with indium-111 labeled leukocytes. Neurosurgery. 1985;16:23.
103. Bellotti C, Aragno MG, Medina M, et al. Differential diagnosis of CT-hypodense cranial lesions with indium-111-oxine–labeled leukocytes. J Neurosurg. 1986;64:750.
104. Brant-Zawadzki M, Enzmann DR, Placone RC, et al. NMR imaging of experimental brain abscess: Comparison with CT. AJNR. 1983;4:250.
105. Runge VM, Clanton JA, Price AC, et al. Evaluation of contrast-enhanced MR imaging in a brain-abscess model. AJNR. 1985;6:139.
106. Grossman RI, Joseph PM, Wolf G, et al. Experimental intracranial septic infarction: Magnetic resonance enhancement. Radiology. 1985;155:649.

107. Davidson MD, Steiner RE. Magnetic resonance imaging in infections of the central nervous system. AJNR. 1985;6:499.
108. Scheld WM. Experimental animal models of bacterial meningitis. In: Zak O, Sande MA, eds. Experimental Models in Antimicrobial Chemotherapy. v. 1. Orlando, FL: Academic Press; 1986:139.
109. Oftedahl PR, Winn G, Rodeheaver G, et al. Changes in regional cerebral blood flow and blood brain barrier permeability in experimental brain abscess. J Cereb Blood Flow Metab. 1981;1(Suppl):38.
110. Wellman WE, Dodge HW, Heilmann FR, et al. Concentration of antibiotics in the brain. J Lab Clin Med. 1954;43:275.
111. Kramer PW, Griffith RS, Campbell RL. Antibiotic penetration of the brain. A comparative study. J Neurosurg. 1969;31:295.
112. Black P, Graybill JR, Charache P. Penetration of brain abscess by systemically administered antibiotics. J Neurosurg. 1973;38:705.
113. de Louvois J, Gortvai P, Hurley R. Antibiotic treatment of abscesses of the central nervous system. Br Med J. 1977;2:985.
114. Picardi JL, Lewis HP, Tan JS, et al. Clindamycin concentrations in the central nervous system of primates before and after head trauma. J Neurosurg. 1975;43:717.
115. de Louvois J, Hurley R. Inactivation of penicillin by purulent exudates. Br Med J. 1977;1:998.
116. Alderson D, Strong AJ, Ingham HR, et al. Fifteen year review of the mortality of brain abscess. Neurosurgery. 1981;8:1.
117. Smego R, Moeller MS, Gallis HA. Trimethoprim-sulfamethoxazole therapy for *Nocardia* infections. Arch Intern Med. 1983;143:711.
118. Maderazo EG, Quintiliani R. Treatment of nocardial infection with trimethoprim and sulfamethoxazole. Am J Med. 1974;57:671.
119. Levitz R, Quintiliani R. Trimethoprim-sulfamethoxazole for bacterial meningitis. Ann Intern Med. 1984;100:881.
120. Greene BM, Thomas FE Jr, Alford RH. Trimethoprim-sulfamethoxazole and brain abscess. Ann Intern Med. 1975;82:812.
121. Levy RM, Gutin PH, Baskin DS, et al. Vancomycin penetration of a brain abscess: Case report and review of the literature. Neurosurgery. 1986;18:633.
122. Preheim LC, McCracken GH, Jubeliver DP. Moxalactam penetration into brain abscess (abstract 738). In: Proceedings of the 21st Interscience Conference on Antimicrobial Agents and Chemotherapy. Chicago: American Society for Microbiology (ASM);1981.
123. Marcus MG, Atluru VL, Epstein N, et al. Conservative management of *Citrobacter diversus* meningitis with brain abscess. NY State J Med. 1984;84:252.
124. Scheld WM, Brodeur JP, Foresman PA, et al. Comparative evaluation of aztreonam in therapy for experimental bacterial meningitis and cerebritis. Rev Infect Dis. 1985;7(Suppl 4):635.
125. Neu HC. Uses of antimicrobial agents in brain abscesses. In: Nelson JD, Grassi C, eds. Current Chemotherapy and Infectious Disease. v. 1. Washington DC: American Society for Microbiology; 1980:41.
126. Norrby R. A review of the penetration of antibiotics into CSF and its clinical significance. Scand J Infect Dis. 1978;14(Suppl):296.
127. Haley EC Jr, Costello GT, Rodeheaver GT, et al. Treatment of experimental brain abscess with penicillin and chloramphenicol. J Infect Dis. 1983;148:737.
128. Ballantine HJ, White JC. Brain abscess. Influence of the antibiotic on therapy and morbidity. N Engl J Med. 1953;248:14.
129. Jooma OV, Pennybacker JB, Tutton GT. Brain abscess: Aspiration, drainage or excision? J Neurol Neurosurg Psychiatry. 1951;14:308.
130. Tutton GK: Cerebral abscess. The present position. Ann R Coll Surg Engl. 1953;13:281.
131. Holm S, Kourtopoulos H. Penetration of antibiotics into brain tissue and brain abscesses. An experimental study in steroid treated rats. Scand J Infect Dis. 1985;44(Suppl):68.
132. Warner J, Perkins RL, Cordero L. Metronidazole therapy of anaerobic bacteremia, meningitis, and brain abscess. Arch Intern Med. 1979;139:167.
133. Frame PT, Watanakunakorn C, McLaurin RL, et al. Penetration of nafcillin, methicillin, and cefazolin into human brain tissue. Neurosurgery. 1983;12:14.
134. Young RF, Frazee J. Gas within intracranial abscess cavities: An indication for surgical excision. Ann Neurol. 1984;16:35.
135. Karandanis D, Shulman JA. Factors associated with mortality in brain abscess. Arch Intern Med. 1975;135:1145.
136. Ohaegbulam SC, Saddeqi NU. Experience with brain abscesses treated by simple aspiration. Surg Neurol. 1980;13:289.
137. Rousseaux M, Lesoin F, Destee A, et al. Long term sequelae of hemispheric abscesses as a function of the treatment. Acta Neurochir. 1985;74:61.
138. LeBeau J, Creissard P, Harispe L, et al. Surgical treatment of brain abscess and subdural empyema. J Neurosurg. 1973;38:198.
139. Lunsford LD, Nelson PB. Stereotactic aspiration of a brain abscess using the therapeutic CT scanner. Acta Neurochir. 1982;62:25.
140. Apuzzo MLJ, Sabshin JK. Computed tomographic guidance stereotaxis in the management of intracranial mass lesions. Neurosurgery. 1983;12:277.
141. Lunsford D, Martinez AJ. Stereotactic exploration of the brain in the era of computed tomography. Surg Neurol. 1984;22:222.
142. Nauta HJW, Conteras FL, Weiner RL, et al. Brain stem abscess managed with computed tomography–guided stereotactic aspiration. Neurosurgery. 1987;20:476.
143. Itakura T, Yokote H, Ozaki F, et al. Stereotactic operation for brain abscess. Surg Neurology (NY). 1987;28:196.
144. Hall WA, Martinez AJ, Dummer JS, et al. Nocardial brain abscess; diagnostic and therapeutic use of stereotactic aspiration. Surg Neurol. 1987;28:114.
145. Enzmann DR, Britt RH, Placone R. Staging of human brain abscess by computed tomography. Radiology. 1983;146:703.
146. Heinnemann HS, Braude AI, Osterholm JL. Intracranial suppurative disease. Early presumptive diagnosis and successful treatment without surgery. JAMA. 1971;218:1542.
147. Rosenblum ML, Mampalam TJ, Pons VG. Controversies in the management of brain abscesses. Clin Neurosurg. 1986;33:603.
148. Berg B, Franklin G, Cuneo R, et al. Nonsurgical cure of brain abscess: Early diagnosis and follow-up with computerized tomography. Ann Neurol. 1978;3:474.
149. Rotheram EB Jr, Kessler LA. Use of computerized tomography in nonsurgical management of brain abscess. Arch Neurol. 1979;36:25.
150. Rosenblum ML, Hoff JT, Norman D, et al. Nonoperative treatment of brain abscesses in selected high-risk patients. J Neurosurg. 1980;52:217.
151. Boom WH, Tuazon CU. Successful treatment of multiple brain abscesses with antibiotics alone. Rev Infect Dis. 1985;7:189.
152. Daniels SR, Price JK, Towbin RB, et al. Nonsurgical cure of brain abscess in a neonate. Child Nerv Syst. 1985;1:346.
153. Keren G, Tyrrell DLJ. Nonsurgical treatment of brain abscesses: Report of two cases. Pediatr Infect Dis. 1984;3.331.
154. Enzmann DR, Britt RH, Yeager AS. Experimental brain abscess evolution: Computed tomographic and neuropathologic correlation. Radiology. 1979;133:113.
155. Epstein F, Whelan M. Cerebritis masquerading as brain abscess: Case report. Neurosurgery. 1982;10:757.
156. Scheld WM, Brodeur JP. Effect of methylprednisolone on entry of ampicillin and gentamicin into the cerebrospinal fluid in experimental pneumococcal and *E. coli* meningitis. Antimicrob Agents Chemother. 1983;23:108.
157. Kourtopoulos H, Holm SE, Norrby SR. The influence of steroids on the penetration of antibiotics into brain tissue and brain abscesses. An experimental study in rats. J Antimicrob Chemother. 1983;11:245.
158. Neuwelt EA, Lawrence MS, Blank NK. Effect of gentamicin and dexamethasone on the natural history of the rat *Escherichia coli* brain abscess model with histopathologic correlation. Neurosurgery. 1984;15:475.
159. Enzmann DR, Britt RH, Placone RC Jr, et al. The effect of short-term corticosteroid treatment on the CT appearance of experimental brain abscesses. Radiology. 1982;145:79.
160. Black KL, Farhat SM. Cerebral abscess: Loss of computed tomographic enhancement with steroids. Neurosurgery. 1984;14:215.
161. Gruszkiewicz J, Doron Y, Peyser E, et al. Brain abscess and its surgical management. Surg Neurol. 1982;18:7.
162. Calliauw WL, dePraetere P, Verbeke L. Postoperative epilepsy in subdural suppurations. Acta Neurochir. 1984;71:217.

71. SUBDURAL EMPYEMA

JOHN E. GREENLEE

The outer two layers of meninges, the dura and arachnoid, enclose a potential subdural space crossed by numerous small veins. Anatomic barriers to extension of infection within this space exist only at the falx cerebri, the tentorium cerebelli, the base of the brain, the foramen magnum, and the anterior spinal canal where arachnoid and dura are joined by penetrating nerves and vessels.[1] These structures divide the subdural space into several large compartments, within each of which subdural infection can spread but in which the infection will be confined to behave as a rapidly expanding mass lesion. Infection of the spinal subdural space is rare, but subdural empyema constitutes 13–23 percent of localized intracranial bacterial infections.[2,3] LeBeau has described subdural empyema as "the most imperative of all neurosurgical emergencies."[4]

ETIOLOGY AND PATHOGENESIS

In most cases, infection reaches the subdural space through emissary veins or by extension of an osteomyelitis of the skull, with accompanying epidural abscess.[5–9] In over half the cases, the source of infection is the paranasal sinuses, with the frontal and ethmoidal sinuses involved in 50–80 percent of the cases.[3,5–11] The middle ear and mastoid are the source in 10–

20 percent. In 5 percent of the cases, the infection is metastatic, principally from the lung.[2,8] Subdural empyema may also follow skull trauma, surgical procedures, or infection of a pre-existing subdural hematoma.[10–13]

BACTERIOLOGIC CHARACTERISTICS

Aerobic streptococci have been isolated in 35 percent of reported cases and staphylococci in 17 percent. A variety of other organisms including *Streptococcus pneumoniae, Haemophilus influenzae*, and gram-negative organisms have been recovered in 14 percent of cases.[2,7] Anaerobic organisms, particularly anaerobic and microaerophilic streptococci (including *Streptococcus anginosus*) and *Bacteroides fragilis*, have been reported in 12 percent of cases.[14] When careful anaerobic culturing is performed, however, these organisms are isolated in 33–100 percent of cases.[15] Polymicrobial infections are common.

PATHOLOGIC CHARACTERISTICS

The infection may involve one or both hemispheres and may occur at the base of the brain, over the convexity, or along the falx cerebri.[1,5–9] The posterior fossa is rarely involved. The subdural space contains an inflammatory exudate that is largest over the frontal lobes if the empyema follows sinusitis or over the temporal and occipital lobes if it follows otitis.[3] The empyema may be multiloculated and may be contralateral to the associated sinusitis. A focal, inflammatory reaction is frequently present within the subarachnoid space, but purulent meningitis occurs in only 14 percent of the cases. Focal osteomyelitis and/or epidural abscess is present in as many as 50 percent of the cases.[5–9] Septic thrombosis of veins within the empyema may extend into venous sinuses or cortical veins, causing hemorrhagic infarction and superficial abscess formation. Cerebral edema rapidly develops and may contribute greatly to mass effect early in the course of infection. Transtentorial herniation occurs unless there is prompt surgical intervention and may be precipitated by lumbar puncture.[2,5]

CLINICAL FEATURES

Subdural empyema may develop at any age but is most common in the second and third decades. Males are affected four times more frequently than are females.[2,3,5] In 60–90 percent of the cases there is an accompanying, frequently asymptomatic sinusitis or otitis. Extension of infection into the subdural space produces fever, focal headaches that later become generalized, vomiting, and signs of meningeal irritation.[2,6,9] Alteration in mental status may be insidious in onset and is present in 50 percent of the patients early in the infection.[3] Within 24–48 hours focal neurologic signs appear and progress rapidly to those of dysfunction of an entire cerebral hemisphere,[2] with hemiparesis, hemisensory deficit, and hemianopsia. Seizures, usually focal,[2] occur in 50 percent of the cases, and aphasia is common when the dominant hemisphere is involved.[3] Unless treatment is instituted, neurologic signs worsen, and signs of increased intracranial pressure appear, with transtentorial and tonsillar herniation. The course of the illness is sufficiently rapid that papilledema develops in less than 50 percent of the patients.[2,3]

Several exceptions exist to this clinical picture. Symptoms may be fulminant in onset or may develop over a period of several weeks. Development of symptoms in cases arising after craniotomy may be extremely insidious.[16] Prior antibiotic therapy may minimize systemic symptoms and may mask sinusitis or otitis, to make the clinical presentation that of brain abscess.[11] Infections metastatic to the subdural space or to a preexisting subdural hematoma may fail to produce sinus tenderness or systemic symptoms. In such cases, particularly in the alcoholic with an infected subdural hematoma, the patient often is seen late in the illness, and mortality is higher.

DIAGNOSIS

Subdural empyema should be suspected in any patient with meningeal signs and a focal neurologic deficit, particularly where the deficit indicates extensive dysfunction of one cerebral hemisphere. Sinusitis followed by meningeal signs should also suggest the diagnosis, for bacterial meningitis per se is rarely due to sinusitis.[17]

Sinusitis or otitis is present on skull x-rays or computed tomography (CT) in over two-thirds of patients.[18–20] Spinal fluid changes are nonspecific, and the danger of transtentorial herniation represents an absolute contraindication to lumbar puncture.[2,3] Magnetic resonance imaging (MRI) and CT with contrast enhancement are the diagnostic procedures of choice.[18–20] Both procedures are useful not only for identifying the empyema but also for detecting cerebral edema and concomitant brain abscess. MRI provides greater clarity of morphologic detail and may detect empyemas not clearly seen by CT scan.[20] The ability of MRI to view the brain in coronal and sagittal sections make it of particular value in identifying empyemas located at the base of the brain, along the falx cerebri, or in the posterior fossa. CT may show a poorly circumscribed extra-axial region of diminished density, often with a thin rim of contrast enhancement (Fig. 1; see also Chapter 72, Fig. 1).[18–20] CT, unlike currently available MRI, can be used to image bone and should be employed to supplement MRI when there are questions of penetrating injury or osteomyelitis. It must be kept in mind that CT early in the course of infection or with older equipment may show only loss of normal cortical markings or unilateral hemispheric swelling.[18–20] For this reason, failure of CT to demonstrate an empyema does not exclude the diagnosis. Angiography should be considered on an emergency basis when MRI is not available and subdural empyema is suspected despite a normal CT scan.[20] Because artifacts produced by patient movement may obscure positive findings on both MRI and CT, sedation should be used if required to achieve an optimal study. Occasionally, a subdural empyema may be diagnosed only by burr holes or craniotomy.

THERAPY

Aerobic and anerobic cultures of blood and other material should be obtained and antibiotics should be begun as described

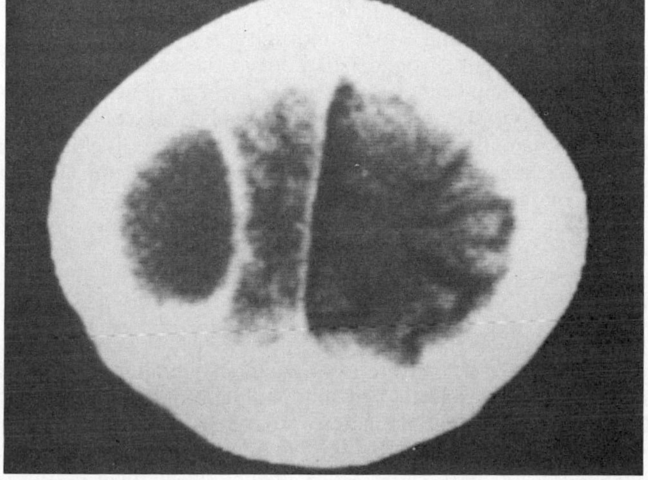

FIG. 1. Computed tomogram of subdural empyema overlying the left cerebral hemisphere. (Courtesy of Dr. Leon Morris, Charlottesville, VA.)

TABLE 1. Bacterial Etiology and Initial Antibiotic Therapy of Subdural Empyema, Epidural Abscess, and Septic Intracranial Thrombophlebitis

			Initial Therapy for Adults With Normal Renal Function	
Condition	*Site of Primary Infection*	*Probable Organisms*	*Suggested Initial Therapy (Intravenous)*	*Suggested Initial Therapy if Penicillin Allergy Present*
Subdural empyema, epidural abscess, or septic intracranial thrombophlebitis in adults[a]	Paranasal sinuses	Aerobic and anaerobic streptococci Other anaerobes *Staphylococcus aureus* (rarely facultative gram-negative bacilli)	Nafcillin 1.5 g q4h with either metronidazole or chloramphenicol[b]	Vancomycin 500 mg. IV q6h with either metronidazole or chloramphenicol[b]
	Otitis media or mastoiditis	*Staphylococcus aureus* Aerobic and anaerobic streptococci Other anaerobes Facultative gram-negative bacilli		
	Following cranial surgery	*Staphylococcus aureus* Facultative gram-negative bacilli	For suspected gram-negative bacilli infections see therapy for gram-negative meningitis (Chapter 66)	
	Hematogenous from distant and/or unknown site	Above organisms or organisms isolated from primary site		
Spinal or epidural abscess or subdural empyema	Extension of osteomyelitis or paravertebral infection Hematogenous spread	*Staphylococcus aureus* Aerobic and anaerobic streptococci Organisms isolated from distant source of sepsis	Nafcillin (1.5 g iv q4h) or antibiotic determined by organism isolated previously	Vancomycin (500 mg IV q6h)

[a] Subdural empyema in young children is almost always a complication of meningitis. See Chapter 66 for appropriate therapy.
[b] Metronidazole therapy is initiated with a loading dose of 1 g. The drug must be diluted and neutralized before intravenous use and is administered by slow intravenous infusion as 500 mg q6h. Chloramphenicol succinate is given intravenously as 1 g q6h.

in Table 1. Increased intracranial pressure may necessitate the preoperative use of mannitol, 1–1.5 g/kg infused over 10–15 minutes; hyperventilation to a P_{CO_2} of 30 torr; or dexamethasone, 10 mg iv, to be followed postoperatively by 4 mg every 6 hours (see Chapter 65). In rare cases, resolution of subdural empyemas has been reported with antibiotic therapy alone.[21] In most instances, however, the rapidly progressive nature of the infection and the fact that neuroradiologic studies may understate the actual size of the empyema necessitate emergency surgical as well as medical intervention. Craniotomy is believed by many workers to have a lower rate of complications than use of burr holes and may be essential in posterior fossa subdural empyema.[7,22–25] Use of burr holes and irrigation of the subdural space may be possible in early cases.[26] Empyema fluid should be submitted for culture, including culture for anaerobes. Otitis or sinusitis may require simultaneous surgery. The possibility of multiloculated or parafalcine infection must be kept in mind. Postoperative recurrence of the empyema may necessitate further surgery. Antibiotic therapy should be continued for at least 3 weeks.

PROGNOSIS

When treatment is prompt, there is good likelihood of neurologic recovery, but delay in therapy greatly increases the risk of permanent neurologic sequelae.[22] Overall mortality is 14–18 percent. If the patient is alert, mortality is 9 percent but if comatose, 75 percent. Prognosis is poor in the aged or when the infection is precipitous in onset. Late focal or generalized seizures develop in 42 percent of patients surviving subdural empyema and usually appear within 16 months. The likelihood of developing late seizures is not influenced by the presence or absence of seizures during the acute illness.[24]

SUBDURAL EMPYEMA IN INFANTS AND YOUNG CHILDREN

In children under 5 years of age,[27,28] intracranial subdural empyema almost invariably follows bacterial meningitis, and the causative organism is that of the meningitis itself, most often *H. influenzae*, or, in neonates, gram-negative bacilli. Early signs of irritability, poor feeding, or increase in head size are nonspecific and may cause delay in seeking medical help. By the time the child is seen by a physician, hemiparesis, convulsions, stupor, and coma are common, but fever may be absent. Examination may reveal increased head size and bulging fontanelle. Papilledema is unusual. The empyema fluid is often too turbid to allow transillumination. In infants, the diagnosis may be made by subdural taps, although this procedure will not detect a parafalcine empyema. Radiographic diagnosis and surgical therapy are as described for adults. Initial antibiotic therapy is that of the meningitis itself: a third-generation cephalosporin such as cefotaxime or alternatively ampicillin and gentamicin in neonates or ampicillin plus chloramphenicol in older infants and small children when *H. influenzae* is suspected (see Chapter 61).

SPINAL SUBDURAL EMPYEMA

Spinal subdural empyema is rare and virtually always metastatic.[29–32] Etiologic organisms are *Staphylococcus aureus* and less often, the streptococci. The empyema is usually posterior to the cord and involves the thoracic and lumbar cord more often than the cervical. Radicular pain and symptoms of cord compression may occur at multiple levels. Spinous process tenderness is often absent and vertebral osteomyelitis rare. High-resolution computed tomography may detect the lesion at one level but cannot, with equipment presently available, give accurate information as to the extent of the empyema. MRI is the diagnostic procedure of choice. Myelography should be employed when MRI is not available. Both MRI and myelography will reveal cord compression, block, or multiple extra-axial defects. Myelography, however, may not delineate the entire length of the empyema if complete obstruction of the subarachnoid space is present at multiple levels. If lower thoracic or lumbar empyema is suspected, myelography should be performed using a lateral cervical or cisternal route to avoid producing infection of the subarachnoid space. Therapy involves surgical drainage and antibiotics against penicillinase-producing staphylococci and streptococci (see Table 1). Unless therapy is begun early, cord necrosis is likely, and prognosis for recovery is poor.

REFERENCES

1. Courville CB. Subdural empyema secondary to purulent frontal sinusitis. Arch Otolaryngol. 1944;39:211–30.
2. Kaufman DM, Miller MH, Steigbigel NH. Subdural empyema: analysis of 17 recent cases and review of the literature. Medicine. 1975;54:485–98.
3. Hitchcock E, Andreadis A. Subdural empyema: a review of 29 cases. J Neurol Neurosurg Psychiatr. 1964;27:422–34.
4. LeBeau J, Creissard P, Harispe L, et al. Surgical treatment of brain abscess and subdural empyema. J Neurosurg. 1973;38:198–203.
5. Kaufman DM, Litman N, Miller MH. Sinusitis: induced empyema. Neurology. 1983;33:123–32.

6. Stephanov S, Joubert MJ, Welchman JM. Combined convexity and parafalx subdural empyema. Surg Neurol. 1979;11:147–51.
7. Mauser HW, Van Houwelingen HC, Tuleken CAF. Factors affecting the outcome in subdural empyema. J Neurol Neurosurg Psychiatr. 1987;50:1136–41.
8. Kubik CS, Adams RD. Subdural empyema. Brain. 1943;66:18–42.
9. Schiller F, Cairns H, Russell DS. The treatment of purulent pachymeningitis and subdural empyema with special reference to penicillin. J Neurol Neurosurg Psychiatr. 1948;11:143–82.
10. McLaurin RL. Subdural infection. In: Gurdjian ES, ed. Cranial and Intracranial Suppuration. Springfield, IL: Charles C Thomas; 1969:73–88.
11. Coonrod JD, Dans PE. Subdural empyema. Am J Med. 1972;53:85–91.
12. Balch RE. Wound infections complicating neurosurgical procedures. J Neurosurg. 1967;26:26:41–7.
13. Casson IR, Petel P, Blair D, et al. Subdural empyema caused by infection of a preexisting subdural hematoma. NY State Med J. 1981;81:389–91.
14. Blayney AW, Frootko NJ, Mitchell RG. Complications of sinusitis caused by *Streptococcus milleri*. J Laryngol Otol. 1984;98:895–9.
15. Yoshikawa TT, Chow AW, Guze LB. Role of anaerobic bacteria in subdural empyema. Am J Med. 1975;58:99–104.
16. Post EM, Modesti LM. "Subacute" postoperative subdural empyema. J Neurosurg. 1981;55:761–5.
17. Biehl JP. Subdural empyema secondary to acute frontal sinusitis: a neglected but curable emergency complication. JAMA. 1955;721–4.
18. Hodges J, Anslow P, Gillett G. Subdural empyema—continuing diagnostic problems in the CT scan era. Q J Med. 1986;228:387–93.
19. Weisberg L. Subdural empyema: clinical and computed tomographic correlations. Arch Neurol. 1986;43:497–500.
20. Moseley IF, Kendall BE. Radiology of intracranial empyemas, with special reference to computed tomography. Neuroradiology. 1984;333–45.
21. Mauser HW, Ravjist RAP, Elderson A, et al. Nonsurgical treatment of subdural empyema. J Neurosurg. 1985;63:128–30.
22. Bannister G, Williams B, Smith S. Treatment of subdural empyema. J Neurosurg. 1981;55:82–8.
23. Borzone M, Capuzzo T, Rivano C, et al. Subdural empyema: fourteen cases surgically treated. Surg Neurol. 1980;13:449–52.
42. Cowie R, Williams B. Late seizures and morbidity after subdural empyema. J Neurosurg. 1983;58:569–73.
25. Morgan DW, Williams B. Posterior fossa subdural empyema. Brain. 1985;108:983–92.
26. Miller ES, Dias PS, Uttley D. Management of subdural empyema: a series of 24 cases. J Neurol Neurosurg Psychiatr. 1987;50:1415–8.
27. Jacobsen PL, Farmer TW. Subdural empyema complicating meningitis in infants: improved prognosis. Neurology. 1981;31:190–6.
28. Farmer TW, Wise GR. Subdural empyema in infants, children and adults. Neurology. 1973;23:254–62.
29. Fraser RAR, Ratzan K, Wolpert SM, et al. Spinal subdural empyema. Arch Neurol. 1973;28:235–8.
30. Abbott KH. Acute pyogenic spinal epidural abscess. Bull Los Angeles Neurol Soc. 1952;17–18:91–103.
31. Dacey RG, Winn HR, Jane JA, et al. Spinal subdural empyema: report of two cases. Neurosurgery. 1978;3:400–3.
32. Heindel CC, Ferguson JP, Kumarasamy T. Spinal subdural empyema complicating pregnancy. J Neurosurg. 1974;40:654–6.

72. EPIDURAL ABSCESS

JOHN E. GREENLEE

An epidural abscess represents localized infection between the outermost layer of the meninges, the dura mater, and the overlying skull or vertebral column. Within the skull, the dura forms the inner layer of the cranial periosteum, and an intracranial epidural abscess must form by stripping periosteum from bone: such an abscess is almost always sharply confined and accompanied by focal osteomyelitis. Because of the ease with which infection can cross the cranial dura along emissary veins, subdural empyema is often present. Within the spinal canal, however, the dura mater is separated from the vertebrae by an epidural space filled with fat and vascular areolar tissue. Although the spinal dura itself is only rarely breached by bacteria, the spinal epidural space offers little resistance to the longitudinal spread of infection. For this reason, a spinal epidural abscess often occupies several vertebral segments and, within the narrow confines of the vertebral canal, may cause extensive cord compression and necrosis.

INTRACRANIAL EPIDURAL ABSCESS

The etiology, pathogenesis, and bacteriology of intracranial epidural abscess are identical to those described for intracranial subdural empyema (see Chapter 71).[1–4] Virtually all cases follow frontal sinusitis, craniotomy, or mastoiditis.[1,4] Epidural abscess may also develop during rhinocerebral mucormycosis.[5]

Pathologic Characteristics

Epidural abscess most often arises adjacent to the frontal sinuses. In almost all cases, osteomyelitis is present within overlying bones, and there is septic thrombosis of veins bridging skull and meninges. Subdural empyema is present in 81 percent of autopsied cases, with 38 percent of the cases also having meningitis and 17 percent brain abscess.[6] Rarely, infection of the bridging veins may produce venous necrosis and epidural hemorrhage rather than abscess.[7]

Clinical Features

The onset of symptoms may be insidious[4] and at first may be overshadowed by sinusitis or otitis. The abscess produces local pain followed by generalized headache, at times with alteration of mental state.[1,2,4] Focal neurologic signs and focal or generalized seizures then appear. An epidural abscess near the petrous bone may involve cranial nerves V and VI, with unilateral facial pain and lateral rectus weakness (Gradenigo syndrome).[8] As the abscess enlarges, papilledema and other signs of intracranial hypertension develop. Extension of the infection into the subdural space is accompanied by rapid neurologic deterioration.

Diagnosis

Persistent fever, leukocytosis, and focal or generalized neurologic signs in the setting of sinusitis or otitis suggest intracranial infection. Edema or cellulitis of face or scalp may be

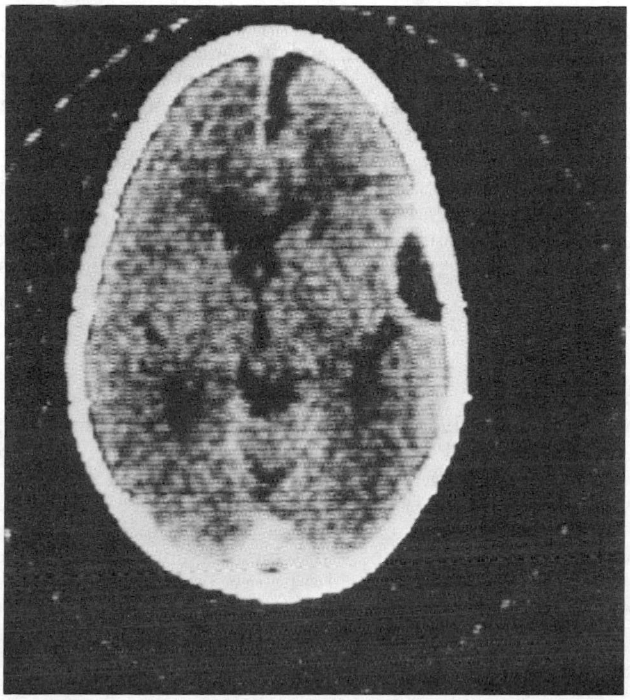

FIG. 1. Computed tomography of right-sided epidural abscess. A subdural empyema is also present between the falx cerebri and the medial aspect of the right frontal lobe. (Courtesy of Drs. D. M. Kaufman, N. E. Leeds and I. Kricheff; from Kaufman and Leeds,[9] with permission.)

present.[4] Skull x-ray films may demonstrate the sinusitis or otitis. Osteomyelitis may not be radiologically discernible if the infection is of recent onset. Magnetic resonance imaging (MRI) or computed tomography (CT)[8,9] (Fig. 1) will show a superficial, circumscribed area of diminished density; arteriography will outline an avascular mass, with inward displacement of cortical vessels and venous sinuses. Spinal fluid is usually sterile and CSF changes are nonspecific; the danger of tonsillar herniation contraindicates lumbar puncture. Successful medical therapy of intracranial epidural abscess without surgical intervention may be possible in lesions detected early in their course and followed closely by CT or MRI scans throughout treatment.[10] In general, however, intracranial epidural abscess should be drained as a neurosurgical emergency to avoid development of subdural empyema. Antibiotic therapy should be directed against aerobic and anaerobic streptococci and against *Staphylococcus aureus*, as outlined in Table 1 in Chapter 71. Concomitant surgery of infected sinuses or bone may be necessary.

SPINAL EPIDURAL ABSCESS

Etiology and Pathogenesis

Both acute and chronic spinal epidural abscess follow infection elsewhere in the body.[11–23] In most cases, infection reaches the epidural space by hematogenous spread, either by direct metastasis or by production of a vertebral osteomyelitis with extension into the spinal epidural space. Infection of the epidural space may also be caused by penetrating injuries or by extension of decubitus ulcers or paraspinal abscesses.[13] Epidural abscess has been reported following back surgery, lumbar puncture, and epidural anesthesia.[12,13,15] Rarely, infection may spread along a persistent dermal sinus. In 10–30 percent of the cases there is a history of back trauma and, less often, a history of diabetes mellitus, intravenous drug abuse, or pregnancy.[12,13,19,23]

Bacteriology

Staphylococcus aureus is the agent in 60–90 percent of both the acute and chronic cases and in some series is the only organism recovered.[11–14,16,17,19,23] Aerobic and anaerobic streptococci cause approximately 18 percent of the cases and gram-negative organisms, especially *Escherichia coli* and *Pseudomonas aeruginosa*, 13 percent.[13] Isolation of *Staphylococcus epidermidis*, pneumococcus, *Actinomyces israelii*, and gram-negative anaerobes has been reported.[13,18] Chronic epidural infection may occur during tuberculosis, frequently without other detectable evidence of infection, and may occasionally develop as a complication of echinococcosis.[19] In 10 percent of the cases, multiple organisms are present.[17]

Pathology

The abscess involves thoracic spine in 50–80 percent of the cases, lumbar in 17–38 percent, and cervical in 10–25 percent.[11–18] In children, cervical and lumbar spine are more often involved.[20] The abscess is posterior to the cord in 80–90 percent of the cases[13,21]; anterior abscesses usually occur at cervical levels, except in tuberculosis, in which the anterior thoracic or lumbar epidural spaces may also be involved. Vertebral osteomyelitis is present in 15 percent of acute and in over 50 percent of chronic epidural abscesses.[12,13,18] Acute abscesses consist of granulation tissue containing loculated pus; in chronic abscesses there may be a prominent fibroblastic component. The abscess usually occupies four or five vertebral segments but may extend the length of the cord. Enlargement of the abscess produces myelomalacia or cord necrosis both by compression and by invasion of the spinal venous plexus.[13,18] Extension of the infection into the subdural or subarachnoid spaces is unusual, except in anterior abscesses where meningitis may develop.[12,21]

Clinical Features

Epidural abscess is more common in males and may occur at any age. The abscess may develop acutely within hours to days or may pursue a chronic course over months. Most abscesses, however, pass through four clinical stages, differing only in time course: focal vertebral pain, root pain, deficits of motor, sensory, or sphincter function, and paralysis.[11] Acute metastatic infection of the epidural space produces rapid progression with prominent systemic symptoms and severe, focal pain. Patients usually seek medical help within the first few days of illness when radicular signs are already present. When epidural abscess arises following vertebral osteomyelitis, vertebral pain may develop over 2–3 weeks, but progression is rapid once radicular symptoms appear. Chronic epidural abscess may manifest with a course indistinguishable from that of an extrinsic neoplasm and without systemic signs. Where cervical cord is involved, respiratory function may be impaired.[22]

Diagnosis

Epidural abscess is a diagnostic consideration in any patient with localized back pain and radicular symptoms, especially when a source of infection is evident. Headache is a common additional complaint.[23] Nuchal rigidity and focal tenderness to percussion are almost universal.[11–13] In acute cases the white blood cell count and the erythrocyte sedimentation rate are elevated. X-ray films of the spine may show osteomyelitis but may also be normal. Magnetic resonance imaging is the diagnostic procedure of choice (Fig. 2), since it can visualize the cord and epidural space in both sagittal and transverse sections and can identify not only epidural abscess but also osteomyelitis, intra-

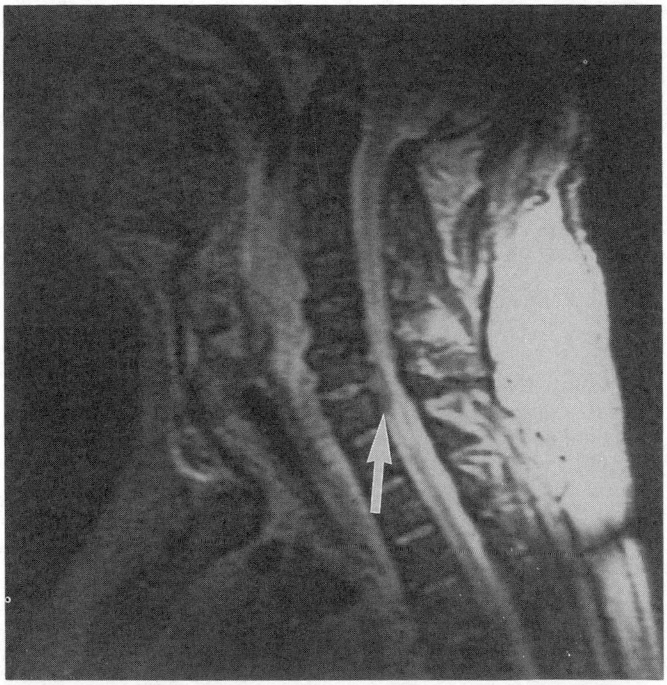

FIG. 2. Magnetic resonance scan of patient with anterior cervical epidural abscess. The abscess is seen as an area of diminished attenuation bulging into the spinal canal and compressing the spinal cord (arrow). The infection also involves the adjacent disc space. (Courtesy of Dr. J. Richard Baringer, Salt Lake City, UT.)

medullary spinal cord lesions, and joint space infection.[23,24] Myelography should be employed if MRI is not available or cannot be performed. Computed tomography with contrast enhancement may be helpful in differentiating subdural from epidural infections or in identifying osteomyelitis. CT is less sensitive than MRI, however, and may fail to define the longitudinal extent of the abscess. MRI should precede lumbar puncture when epidural abscess is suspected. In the absence of MRI, lumbar puncture should never be attempted without provision to introduce dye and carry out myelography before the needle is withdrawn. Spinal puncture, if indicated, should be performed well above or below the suspected area of involvement, and the needle should be advanced slowly with frequent aspiration to avoid contaminating the subdural or subarachnoid space. Artifacts produced by patient movement may obscure positive findings on MRI, CT, or myelography, and adequate sedation should be employed if required to achieve an optimal study. Spinal fluid is usually sterile, with nonspecific changes in cells, protein, and glucose. Blood and abscess material should be submitted for aerobic and anaerobic culture.

Therapy

The danger of spinal cord necrosis requires laminectomy and drainage as soon as the diagnosis is made. Antibiotic therapy should begin before surgery and, in the absence of a known causative organism, should be directed against penicillin-resistant *S. aureus*, with modification of antibiotic therapy based on Gram stain and culture. In certain carefully selected cases, the availability of highly sensitive, noninvasive methods of imaging the spine and epidural space has made it possible to treat spinal epidural abscess with antibiotics alone.[25,26] Such cases have included those who represent unacceptable surgical risks and also occasional patients without neurologic deficit in whom it is decided to defer surgery while monitoring the patient's neurologic status closely and following abscess size with serial MRI or CT scans. In such patients, surgery should be carried out immediately if neurologic findings appear despite antibiotic therapy. Antibiotic therapy should be continued for 3–4 weeks in spinal epidural abscess per se or for 8 weeks when there is an accompanying osteomyelitis. Prognosis for neurologic recovery is excellent if therapy is begun before or during the stage of radicular symptoms but worsens rapidly as evidence of cord injury appears. Mortality is 10–20 percent[13] but is higher, as is the likelihood of permanent neurologic deficit, if cervical cord is involved.[22,23]

HYPERTROPHIC SPINAL PACHYMENINGITIS

Rarely, chronic inflammation or infection within the spinal canal involves the dura mater alone, to produce a diffuse, fibrosing pachymeningitis. Cases have been attributed to syphilis and also to tuberculosis, but in many cases no etiologic organism can be identified.[27–29] The fibrosis compresses nerve roots and if extensive may injure the spinal cord. Early symptoms are pain, muscle weakness, and muscle atrophy occurring in a radicular pattern. Spinal fluid contains elevated protein but no cells. Electromyography may localize the process to nerve roots. In most cases, diagnosis has been made by myelography with lateral views. Newer techniques, however, such as myelography followed by CT or, in particular MRI with and without contrast enhancement with gadolinium may give much more precise information.[27,29] Treatment consists of surgical removal of the hypertrophied dura and antibiotic therapy of any diagnosed causative infection.

ACKNOWLEDGMENTS

Work on this chapter was supported in part by the Veterans Administration.

REFERENCES

1. Handel SF, Klein WC, Kim YW. Intracranial epidural abscess. Radiology. 1974;11:117–20.
2. Koenig RP, Craigmile TK. Epidural intracranial abscess. USAF Med J. 1957;8:120–4.
3. Norrell HA, Wilson CB. Primary intracranial extradural abscess diagnosed by carotid angiography. J Kentucky Med Assoc. 1967;65:1186–7.
4. French LA, Chou SN. Osteomyelitis of the skull and epidural abscess. In: Gurdjian ES, ed. Cranial and Intracranial Suppuration. Springfield, IL: Charles C Thomas; 1969:59–72.
5. Muresan A. A case of cerebral mucormycosis diagnosed in life, with eventual recovery. J Clin Pathol. 1960;13:34–6.
6. Slager UT. Infection and parainfectious inflammations. In: Basic Neuropathology. Baltimore: Williams & Wilkins; 1970:89–135.
7. Rajput AJ, Rozdilsky B. Extradural hematoma following frontal sinusitis. Arch Otolaryngol. 1971;94:83–5.
8. Lott T, El Gammal T, Dasilva R, et al. Evaluation of brain and epidural abscesses by computed tomography. Radiology. 1977;122:371–6.
9. Kaufman DMA, Leeds NE. Computed tomography (CT) in the diagnosis of intracranial abscesses. Neurology. 1977;27:1069–73.
10. Leys D, Destee A, Warot P. Empyeme extra-dural en fosse posterieure: traitement medical exclusif. Presse Med. 1983;12:1549.
11. Heusner AP. Nontuberculous spinal epidural infections. N Engl J Med. 1948;239:845–54.
12. Hulme A, Dott NM. Spinal epidural abscess. Br Med J. 1954;1:64–5.
13. Baker AS, Ojemann RG, Swartz MN, et al. Spinal epidural abscess. N Engl J Med. 1975;293:463–8.
14. Dandy WE. Abscesses and inflammatory tumors in the spinal epidural space (so-called pachymeningitis externa). Arch Surg. 1926;13:477–94.
15. Ferguson JF, Kirsch WM. Epidural empyema following thoracic extradural block. J Neurosurg. 1974;41:762–4.
16. Russell NA, Vaughan R, Morley TP. Spinal epidural infection. Can J Neurol Sci. 1979;6:325–8.
17. Dus V. Spinal peripachymeningitis (epidural abscess). J Neurosurg. 1960;17:972–83.
18. Browder J, Meyers R. Pyogenic infections of the spinal epidural space. Surgery. 1941;10:296–308.
19. Kaufman DM, Kaplan JG, Litman N. Infectious agents in spinal epidural abscess. Neurology. 1980;30:844–50.
20. Baker CJ. Primary spinal epidural abscess. Am J Dis Child. 1971;121:337–9.
21. Mixter WJ, Smithwick RH. Acute intraspinal epidural abscess. N Engl J Med. 1932;207:126–36.
22. Durity F, Thompson GB. Localized cervical extradural abscess. J Neurosurg. 1968;28:387–90.
23. Lasker BR, Harter DH. Cervical epidural abscess. Neurology. 1987;37:1747–53.
24. Modic MT, Feiglin DH, Piranio DW. Vertebral osteomyelitis: assessment using MRI. Radiology. 1985;157:157–66.
25. Leys D, Lesoin F, Viaud C, et al. Decreased morbidity from acute bacterial spinal epidural abscesses using computed tomography and nonsurgical treatment in selected patients. Ann Neurol. 1985;17:350–5.
26. Messer HD, Lenchner GS, Brust JCM, et al. Lumbar spinal abscess managed conservatively. J Neurosurg. 1977;46:825–9.
27. Bucy PC, Freeman W. Hypertrophic spinal pachymeningitis. J Neurosurg. 1952;9:564–78.
28. Guidetti B, LaTorre E. Hypertrophic spinal pachymeningitis. J Neurosurg. 1967;26:496–503.
29. Oonishi T, Ishiko T, Arai M, et al. Pachymeningitis cervicalis hypertrophica. Acta Pathol Jpn. 1982;32:163–71.

73. SUPPURATIVE INTRACRANIAL PHLEBITIS

JOHN E. GREENLEE

Septic intracranial thrombophlebitis most frequently follows infection of paranasal sinuses, middle ear, mastoid, face, or oropharynx. The infection spreads centrally along emissary veins.[1–5] Septic thrombophlebitis may also occur in association with epidural abscess, subdural empyema, or meningitis. Occasionally, the infection is metastatic from lungs or other distant sites.[3] The likelihood of thrombosis is increased by states altering blood viscosity or coagulability, including dehydration, polycythemia, pregnancy, oral contraceptive use, sickle cell disease, malignancy, or trauma.[4,6,7] *Staphylococcus aureus* is the most frequent isolate.[1] A minority of cases are due to *Staphylococcus epidermidis*, streptococci including *S. pneumoniae*, gram-negative bacilli,[1,2] and anaerobic organisms. Multiple infecting organisms may be present.[8]

PATHOLOGIC CHANGES

Septic intracranial thrombophlebitis may begin within veins or venous sinuses and may involve additional vessels by propagation or discontinuous spread.[1,9] The pathologic changes are those of both venous thrombosis and suppuration. Venous occlusion may produce no local injury, but if collateral veins are compromised, edema and hemorrhagic infarction result. The most common sites of infarction are the area of venous watershed immediately above the Sylvian fissue (see Chapter 65)[3] and the medial surfaces of the cerebral hemispheres.[3,4] Thrombosis of the anterior portion of the superior sagittal sinus or of the lateral sinuses may block reabsorption of cerebrospinal fluid with resultant communicating hydrocephalus. Local suppuration may produce venous necrosis and hemorrhage or may cause epidural abscess, subdural empyema, meningitis, or brain abscess.[1–4] Septic embolization may produce pulmonary infarction, abscesses in lungs or other organs, or mycotic aneurysm.[2–4,9]

CLINICAL FEATURES

Cortical Vein Thrombosis

If collateral venous drainage is adequate, septic venous thrombosis may produce only transient neurologic findings or may be silent except for its metastatic consequences. If the thrombus outstrips collateral flow, however, a progressive neurologic deficit will result and may mimic brain abscess, with impairment of consciousness, focal or generalized seizures, and increased intracranial pressure.[2,3] Focal neurologic findings include hemiparesis, which involves the face and hand if veins over the cerebral convexity are involved.[3] Thrombosis of veins along the falx cerebri may produce unilateral leg weakness, which becomes bilateral if propagation of the thrombus involves the veins of the contralateral hemisphere.[2,3] Aphasia is common when the dominant hemisphere is involved. Transient hemodynamic variation in venous collateral flow may cause considerable fluctation in neurologic signs.

Venous Sinus Thrombosis

The clinical findings vary with the sinus involved and are summarized in Table 1 (see Chapter 65, Fig. 5). Cavernous sinus, lateral sinus, and superior sagittal sinus are most often involved. Cavernous sinus thrombosis most commonly follows infections of the face or of the sphenoid and ethmoid sinuses.[1,9] Onset is abrupt, with diplopia, photophobia, orbital edema, and progressive exophthalmos.[9,10] Involvement of cranial nerves III, IV, V, and VI produces ophthalmoplegia, a midposition fixed pupil, loss of corneal reflex, and diminished sensation over the upper face. Obstruction of venous return from the retina results in papilledema, retinal hemorrhages, and visual loss. Similar findings appear in the opposite eye as the infection spreads to the contralateral cavernous sinus. Engorgement or thrombosis of facial veins may occur.

Thrombosis of the superior sagittal sinus produces bilateral leg weakness and may cause communicating hydrocephalus.[2,3,5] Occlusion of the lateral sinus produces pain over the ear and mastoid and may cause edema over the mastoid (Griesinger's sign).[4,11,12] Impairment of veins supplying cranial nerves V and VI produces ipsilateral facial pain and lateral rectus weakness (Gradenigo syndrome). Septic cortical vein or venous sinus occlusion may produce subdural empyema, meningitis, or brain abscess. The danger of septic pulmonary embolization is always present.

DIAGNOSIS

Septic intracranial thrombophlebitis may manifest as sepsis without neurologic signs or with stupor and focal neurologic signs in the presence of cranial infection. In the latter instance, septic thrombophlebitis may be indistinguishable from brain abscess or subdural empyema. Fever, leukocytosis, and elevated erythrocyte sedimentation rate are usually present. Skull x-rays should be evaluated for the presence of sinusitis or mastoiditis, with particular attention to frontal, ethmoidal, and sphenoidal sinuses. Lumbar puncture may reveal increased pressure, slight

TABLE 1. Symptoms of Intracranial Venous Sinus Occlusion

Venous Sinus Involved	*Associated Infection*	*Anatomic Structures Affected*	*Clinical Findings*
Cavernous sinus	Paranasal sinusitis, especially of frontal, ethmoidal or sphenoidal sinuses, infection of face or mouth	Venous drainage from orbit and eye. Cranial nerves III, IV, V, and VI within the cavernous sinus [venous supply of frontal lobe and pituitary]	Unilateral periorbital edema, exophthalmos, and chemosis; examination shows papilledema, ocular palsies, diminished pupillary reactivity, frequently diminished corneal reflex, and impaired sensation in the first and second divisions of V; extension to the contralateral sinus may duplicate these findings in the opposite eye [seizures, frontal lobe, deficits, hypopituitarism]
Lateral sinus	Otitis media or mastoiditis; rarely pharyngitis	Cranial nerves V and VI Venous route of CSF reabsorption [venous supply of temporal lobe, jugular bulb, cranial nerves IX, X, XI at jugular foramen]	Lateral rectus weakness; facial pain and altered facial sensation; increased intracranial pressure with papilledema if the other lateral sinus is also compromised [temporal lobe seizures; jugular foramen syndrome with ipsilateral palatal weakness, diminished gag reflex, and weakness of trapezius and sternomastoid]
Superior sagittal sinus	Infections of face, scalp, subdural or epidural spaces; meningitis	Venous drainage from medial portion of cerebral hemispheres; CSF reabsorption	Bilateral leg weakness; intracranial hypertension
Superior petrosal sinus	Otitis media or mastoiditis	Trigeminal ganglion [venous drainage from temporal lobe]	Ipsilateral pain or sensory deficit [temporal lobe seizures]
Inferior petrosal sinus	Otitis media or mastoiditis	Cranial nerves V and VI at tip of petrous bone	"Gradenigo syndrome"; ipsilateral facial pain and sensory deficit; ipsilateral lateral rectus palsy

Note: Brackets indicate structures affected or symptoms produced by extension of the sinus thrombus into cortical veins.

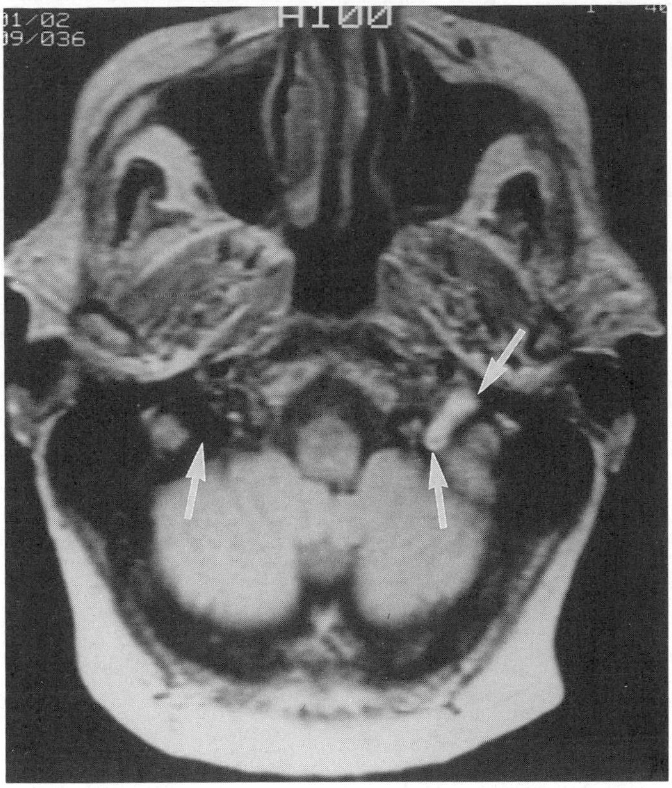

FIG. 1. Magnetic resonance scan in patient with left internal jugular vein thrombosis. There is bright signal, consistent with vessel occlusion, arising from the left internal jugular vein (double arrows). In contrast, the right internal jugular vein exhibits diminished signal (flow void) consistent with normal blood flow (single arrow). (Courtesy of Dr. Anne Osborn, Salt Lake City, UT.)

lymphocytic pleocytosis, and mild elevation of protein. Evidence of subarachnoid blood detectable by lumbar puncture is present in less than 15 percent of cases,[1,2] and cerebrospinal fluid is usually sterile. Magnetic resonance imaging (MRI), because of its ability to visualize vessels and to differentiate between normally flowing blood and thrombus, is the diagnostic procedure of choice (Fig. 1).[13–16] Computed tomography (CT) scanning, although considerably less sensitive and reliable than MRI, permits diagnosis of venous sinus thrombosis in many cases and should be employed as the initial diagnostic test when MRI is not available.[17–19] Magnetic resonance imaging and CT also provide information about concomitant subdural or epidural infections and allow visualization of brain infarction, hemorrhage, and edema. Angiography with close attention to the venous phase should be employed when venous sinus thrombosis is suspected despite negative MRI or CT.[20] Retrograde venography or digital subtraction angiography may prove useful in selected cases. Blood, spinal fluid, and all infected material should be cultured for both aerobic and anaerobic organisms.

TREATMENT

Appropriate antibiotic therapy, reversal of elevated intracranial pressure, and control of seizures are the goals of therapy. Initial antibiotics should be directed against *Staphylococcus aureus*, aerobic streptococci, and anaerobes (see Chapter 71, Table 1). Control of infection may require urgent surgery of infected cranial structures or drainage of intra- or extracranial abscess. Intracranial hypertension may require glucocorticoids, osmotic diuretics, or hyperventilation; an intracranial pressure monitor may be essential in assessing efficacy of therapy. Communicating hydrocephalus may require serial lumbar punctures or ventricular drainage. The use of anticoagulants is controversial[2,7,14] but may be necessary when there is progressive thrombosis or overt embolization in the face of antibiotic therapy. If anticoagulation is used, the danger of intracranial hemorrhage should always be kept in mind. Internal jugular vein ligation has been used with lateral sinus thrombosis,[11,12] and in a few instances thrombectomy has been successful.[21]

PROGNOSIS

Even when an apparently fixed neurologic deficit is present, intracranial venous infarction carries a better likelihood of functional recovery than does arterial infarction, but permanent deficits may occur. Overall mortality in suppurative intracranial thrombophlebitis is 34 percent. Mortality in complete occlusion of the superior sinus, however, is 78 percent.[1,22] Ominous prognostic signs are coma, progression of focal seizures to generalized ones, generalized seizures as an initial symptom, and bilateral signs, particularly bilateral flaccid hemiplegia.[1,2,21,23]

ACKNOWLEDGMENTS

Work on this chapter was supported in part by the Veterans Administration.

REFERENCES

1. Southwick FS, Richardson EP, Swartz MN. Septic thrombosis of the dural venous sinuses. Medicine. 1986;65:82–106.
2. Krayenbuhl HA. Cerebral venous and sinus thrombosis. Clin Neurosurg. 1967;14:1–24.
3. Stuart EA, O'Brien FH, McNally WJ. Cerebral venous thrombosis. Ann Otolaryngol. 1951;406–38.
4. Courville CB, Nielsen JM. Fatal complications of otitis media. Arch Otolaryngol. 1934;19:451–9.
5. Strauss SI, Stern NS, Mendelow H, et al. Septic superior sagittal sinus thrombosis after oral surgery. J Oral Surg. 1973;31:560–5.
6. Stehbens WE, ed. Pathology of the Cerebral Blood Vessels. St. Louis: CV Mosby; 1972:188–92.
7. Parsons M. Intracranial venous thrombosis. Postgrad Med J. 1967;43:409–14.
8. Pallares R, Santamaria J, Ariza X, et al. Polymicrobial anaerobic septicemia due to lateral sinus thrombophlebitis. J Laryngol Otolaryngol. 1984;98:895–9.
9. Shaw RE. Cavernous sinus thrombophlebitis: a review. Br J Surg. 1952;40:40–8.
10. Pascarelli E, Lemlich A. Diplopia and photophobia as premonitory symptoms in cavernous sinus thrombosis. Ann Rhinol Laryngol. 1964;73:210–7.
11. Jahrsdoerfer RA, Fitz-Hugh GS. Lateral sinus thrombosis. South Med J. 1968;61:1271–5.
12. Teichgraeber JF, Per-Lee JH, Turner JS. Lateral sinus thrombosis: a modern perspective. Laryngoscope. 1982;92:744–51.
13. Marchi PJ, Grossman RI, Gomori JM, et al. High field MR imaging of cerebral venous thrombosis. J Comput Assist Tomogr. 1986;10:10–5.
14. McArdle CB, Mirfakhraee M, Amparo EG, et al. MR imaging of transverse/sigmoid dural sinus and jugular vein thrombosis. J Comput Assist Tomogr. 1987;11:831–8.
15. Sze G, Simmons B, Krol G, et al. Dural sinus thrombosis: verification with spin-echo techniques. AJNR. 1988;9:679–86.
16. Snyder TC, Sachdev HS. MR imaging of dural sinus thrombosis. J Comput Assist Tomogr. 1986;10:889–92.
17. Goldberg AL, Rosenbaum AE, Wang H, et al. Computed tomography of dural sinus thrombosis. J Comput Assist Tomogr. 1986;10:16–20.
18. Virapongse C, Cazenave C, Quisling R, et al. The empty delta sign: frequency and significance in 76 cases of dural sinus thrombosis. Radiology. 1987;162:779–85.
19. Shinohara Y, Yoshitoshi M, Yoshii F. Appearance and disappearance of the empty delta sign in superior sagittal sinus thrombosis. Stroke. 1986;17:1282–4.
20. Askenasy HM, Kosary IZ, Braham J. Thrombosis of the longitudinal sinus. Neurology. 1962;12:288–92.
21. Kinal Me, Jaeger RM. Thrombophlebitis of dural sinuses following otitis media. J Neurosurg. 1960;17:81–9.
22. Kalbag RM, Woolf AL. Cerebral Venous Thrombosis. London: Oxford University Press; 1967:242–3.
23. Weber G. Treatment of cerebral venous and sinus thrombosis. Thromb Diath Haemorrh. 1966;21(Suppl):435–55.

SECTION I. SKIN AND SOFT TISSUE INFECTIONS

74. CELLULITIS AND SUPERFICIAL INFECTIONS

MORTON N. SWARTZ

Major attention should be directed to determination of the specific microbial cause of any infection involving the skin. In this chapter, bacterial and mycotic (exclusive of those due to the common dermatophytes) infections are considered. Classification of cutaneous infections on morphologic and clinical grounds can be most helpful in providing initial clues as to the most likely responsible infectious agents (Table 1).

PRIMARY PYODERMAS

Impetigo

Imeptigo is an initially vesicular, later crusted, superficial infection of the skin, usually due to group A streptococci. The majority of cases occur in children. *Staphylococcus aureus* is the etiologic agent in less than 10 percent of the cases, although it has been suggested recently that this figure may be increasing[1]; frequently, mixtures of streptococci and *S. aureus* are isolated from lesions, but in this situation the staphylococci are usually secondary invaders.

Pathologic Characteristics and Pathogenesis. Histopathologically, impetigo consists of a superficial, intraepidermal, unilocular vesicopustule. In epidemiologic studies, group A streptococcal acquisition on normal skin antedates the appearance of impetigo by about 10 days.[2] During that time, minor trauma (insect bites, abrasions) predisposes to the development of infected lesions. Impetigo is most common during hot, humid summer weather. Two to three weeks after skin acquisition of streptococci, pharyngeal colonization by the same organism occurs in about 30 percent of the children with skin lesions. (The sporadic cases of facial impetigo occurring in cooler climates probably result from contiguous spread from an initial nasopharyngeal infection, and the serotypes involved are those commonly causing pharyngeal disease.) In contrast, in the less common cases of staphylococcal impetigo (where *S. aureus* is the only pathogen), nasal colonization precedes that of the normal skin; skin lesions then follow such colonization.[3,4]

Impetigo is a highly communicable infection; spread in families (particularly among preschool children) is facilitated by crowding and poor hygiene.

Clinical Findings. Streptococcal impetigo begins as small vesicles, sometimes with narrow inflammatory halos, that rapidly pustulate and readily rupture. The purulent discharge dries, forming the characteristic thick, golden-yellow "stuck-on" crusts. Exposed areas are the most common sites of lesions. Pruritus is common, and scratching of lesions can spread infection. Occasionally, large crusts are produced by coalescence of smaller pustules. The lesions remain superficial and do not ulcerate or infiltrate the dermis. Mild regional lymphadenopathy is common. Healing occurs without scarring. The lesions are painless, and constitutional manifestations are minimal.

TABLE 1. Classification of Bacterial and Mycotic Infections of the Skin

Type of Lesion	*Etiologic Agents*
Primary pyodermas	
Impetigo	Group A streptococcus; *S. aureus*
Folliculitis	*S. aureus*; *Candida* ; *P. aeruginosa*; *Pityrosporum ovale*
Furuncles and carbuncles	*S. aureus*
Paronychia	*S. aureus*; Group A streptococcus; *Candida*; *P. aeruginosa*
Ecthyma	Group A streptococcus
Erysipelas	Group A streptococcus
Chancriform lesions	*T. pallidum*; *H. ducreyi*; *Sporothrix*; *B. anthracis*; *F. tularensis*; *M. ulcerans*; *M. marinum*
Membranous ulcers	*Corynebacterium diphtheriae*
Cellulitis	Group A streptococcus; *S. aureus*; rarely, various other organisms
Infectious gangrene and gangrenous cellulitis	
Streptococcal gangrene and necrotizing fasciitis	Group A streptococcus
Progressive bacterial synergistic gangrene	Anaerobic streptococci plus a second organism (*S. aureus*, *Proteus*)
Gangrenous balanitis and perineal phlegmon	Group A streptococcus; mixed infections with enteric bacteria (*E. coli*, *Klebsiella*, etc.) and anaerobes
Gas gangrene; crepitant cellulitis	*Clostridium perfringens* and other clostridial species; *Bacteroides*, peptostreptococci, *Klebsiella*, *E. coli*
Gangrenous cellulitis in immunosuppressed patients	*Pseudomonas*, *Aspergillus*, agents of mucormycosis
Erythrasma	*Corynebacterium minutissimum*
Nodular lesions	*Candida*; *Sporothrix*; *S. aureus* (botryomycosis); *M. marinum*
Hyperplastic (pseudoepitheliomatous) and proliferative lesions (mycetomas, etc.)	*Nocardia*; *Pseudoallescheria boydii*, *Blastomyces dermatitidis*; *Paracoccidioides brasiliensis*; *Phialophora*; *Cladosporium*
Annular erythema (erythema chronicum migrans)	*B. burgdorferi*
Secondary bacterial infections complicating pre-existing skin lesions such as the following:	
Burns	*P. aeruginosa*; *Enterobacter*; various other gram-negative bacilli; various streptococci; *S. aureus*; *Candida*; *Aspergillus*
Eczematous dermatitis and exfoliative erythrodermas	*S. aureus*; group A streptococcus
Chronic ulcers (varicose, decubitus)	Coliform bacteria; *P. aeruginosa*; peptostreptococci; enterococci, *Bacteroides*, *C. perfringens*
Dermatophytosis	*S. aureus*; group A streptococcus
Traumatic lesions (abrasions, animal bites, insect bites, etc.)	*P. multocida*; *C. diphtheriae*; *S. aureus*; group A streptococcus
Vesicular or bullous eruptions (varicella, pemphigus)	*S. aureus*; group A streptococcus
Acne conglabata	*Propionibacterium acnes*
Hidradenitis suppurativa	*S. aureus*, *Proteus* and other coliforms, streptococci, peptostreptococci, *Bacteroides*
Intertrigo	*S. aureus*, coliforms, *Candida*
Pilonidal and sebaceous cysts	Peptostreptococci; *Bacteroides*; coliforms
Pyoderma gangrenosa	*S. aureus*; peptostreptococci; *Proteus* and other coliforms; *P. aeruginosa*
Cutaneous involvement in systemic bacterial and mycotic infections	
Bacteremias	*S. aureus*; group A streptococcus (also other groups such as D); *N. meningitidis*; *N. gonorrhoeae*; *P. aeruginosa*; *S. typhi*; *H. influenzae*
Endocarditis	Viridans streptococci; *S. aureus*; group D streptococci, etc.
Fungemias	*Candida*; *Cryptococcus*; *B. dermatitidis*

(Continued)

TABLE 1. *(Continued)*

Type of Lesion	*Etiologic Agents*
Listeriosis	*Listeria monocytogenes*
Leptospirosis (Weil's disease and pretibial fever)	*L. interrogans* serotypes
Rat-bite fever	*Streptobacillus moniliformis; Spirillum minor*
Melioidosis	*P. pseudomallei*
Glanders	*P. mallei*
Carrion's disease (verruga peruana)	*Bartonella bacilliformis*
Scarlet fever syndromes	
Scarlet fever	Group A streptococcus; rarely *S. aureus*
Scalded skin syndrome	*S. aureus* (phage group II)
Toxic shock syndrome	*S. aureus* (pyrogenic toxin-producing strains)
Para- and postinfectious nonsuppurative complications	
Purpura fulminans	Group A streptococcus; *S. aureus*; pneumococcus
Erythema nodosum	Group A streptococcus; *M. tuberculosis; M. leprae; C. immitis; L. autumnalis; Y. Enterocolitica; L. pneumophila*
Erythema multiforme-like lesions (rarely)	Group A streptococcus

Laboratory Findings. Gram-stained smear of vesicles shows gram-positive cocci, usually streptococci. Culture of exudate beneath an unroofed crust reveals group A streptococci or a mixture of streptococci and *S. aureus*. The antistreptolysin O (ASLO) titer after streptococcal impetigo is scant, probably related to the inhibition of streptolysin O by skin lipids at the infection site. In contrast, the anti-DNase B response readily occurs (elevated titers in 90 percent of patients with nephritis complicating streptococcal skin infections).[5]

Etiologic Agents. Group A streptococci responsible for impetigo usually belong to different M serotypes (e.g., 2, 49, 52, 55, 57, 59–61) than the strains producing pharyngitis (e.g., 1, 2, 4, 6, 25). Group C and G streptococci rarely may cause impetigo; group B streptococci have been associated with impetigo in the newborn.

Differential Diagnosis. Although the initial vesicular lesions may resemble early varicella, the crusts of the latter are darker brown and harder. The central clearing of a confluent cluster of lesions of impetigo may suggest tinea circinata but can be distinguished by the thick crusts that are not formed in the fungus infection. When the vesicles of herpes simplex become turbid, they may look like impetigo.

Presumptive Therapy. Penicillin is the drug of choice in the treatment of ordinary impetigo because of the role of group A streptococci in the majority of cases and the possible occurrence of acute glomerulonephritis as a sequela. Whether penicillin therapy is effective (because of the delay in seeking medical attention for such a mild infection) in reducing the incidence of pyoderma-associated nephritis remains unclear. Penicillin is administered either as a single intramuscular injection of benzathine penicillin (300,000–600,000 units for children; 1,200,000 units for adults) or as oral penicillin (25,000–90,000 units/kg/day in divided doses every 6 hours for 10 days). Erythromycin (30–50 mg/kg/day in divided doses every 6 hours for 10 days for children; 250–500 mg orally every 6 hours for adults) is an alternative for the penicillin-allergic patient. Local care (removal of crusts by soaking with soap and water) is helpful.

Mixed streptococcal-staphylococcal impetigo has the same crusted lesions and clinical course as streptococcal impetigo and responds well to treatment with penicillin G.[6]

Topical antibiotic-containing (bacitracin-neomycin-polymyxin) ointments are inferior to systemic antibiotics in the treatment of impetigo, since they sterilize the lesions less rapidly and prevent transmission less promptly. However, among young children in close contact (e.g., in a day care center) during the peak impetigo season, application of such a topical antibiotic ointment several times daily to insect bites and minor abrasions can be effective in preventing the subsequent development of streptococcal pyoderma.[7]

A newer topical antibiotic, mupirocin, appears to be as effective in the topical treatment of impetigo as other more established topical agents. It has also been used topically to eradicate methicillin-resistent *S. aureus* from secondarily infected skin lesions and from colonized patients. However, since resistance in *S. aureus* strains has emerged sooner than anticipated after its introduction, particularly where long-term therapy has been employed, prolonged use should probably be avoided.

Bullous Impetigo

Clinical Findings. This form of impetigo is due to *S. aureus* of phage group II (usually type 71), occurs principally in the newborn and younger children, and comprises about 10 percent of all cases of impetigo. The lesions begin as vesicles that turn into flaccid bullae, initially containing clear yellow fluid. There is no erythematous areola, and the Nikolsky sign is absent. The bullae quickly rupture, leaving a moist red surface, and then form thin, "varnish-like" light brown crusts. Bullous impetigo, like the "staphylococcal scalded skin syndrome" (SSSS) and the staphylococcal scarlatiniform syndrome, represents a form of cutaneous response to the extracellular exfoliative toxins (ET) produced by *S. aureus* of phage group II. Staphylococci are regularly isolated from the skin lesions of bullous impetigo. Streptococcal superinfection rarely complicates bullous impetigo, probably because type 71 strains of *S. aureus* produce a bacteriocin that inhibits streptococci. Fever and constitutional symptoms are uncommon. Healing occurs without scarring.

Presumptive Therapy. Extensive bullous impetigo responds to treatment with a penicillinase-resistant penicillin (e.g., in the child, oxacillin, 50 mg/kg/day in divided doses orally every 6 hours) or erythromycin in the penicillin-allergic patient.

Staphylococcal Scalded Skin Syndrome

This is the most severe manifestation of infection with *S. aureus* strains producing an exfoliative exotoxin and is characterized by widespread bullae and exfoliation.[8–11] Pemphigus neonatorum (Ritter's disease) is the SSSS in the newborn. The more general term *toxic epidermal necrolysis* (*TEN*) is often used to encompass both SSSS and a morphologically identical syndrome due to various etiologies (drug reactions, viral illnesses). (See Chapter 173.)

Clinical Findings. SSSS usually occurs in younger children, but rarely it can develop in adults. Epidemics have occurred in neonatal nurseries.[12] It begins abruptly (sometimes a few days after a recognized staphylococcal infection) with fever, skin tenderness, and a scarlatiniform rash. The Nikolsky sign can be demonstrated. Large, flaccid, clear bullae form and promptly rupture, resulting in the separation of sheets of skin. New bullae appear over 2–3 days. Exfoliation exposes large areas of bright red skin surface (Fig. 1). With appropriate fluid replacement and antimicrobial therapy, the skin lesions heal within 2 weeks, in contrast to drug-induced TEN, where recovery is more prolonged, since the entire epidermis must be replaced, and where scarring is more frequent.

Presumptive Therapy. Intravenous use of a penicillinase-resistant penicillin (e.g., nafcillin, 50–100 mg/kg/day in the newborn, 100–200 mg/kg/day for older children) is indicated in the initial treatment of SSSS because of the presence of active staphylococcal infection and the rapid progression of the skin lesions. Topical treatment consists of cool saline compresses.

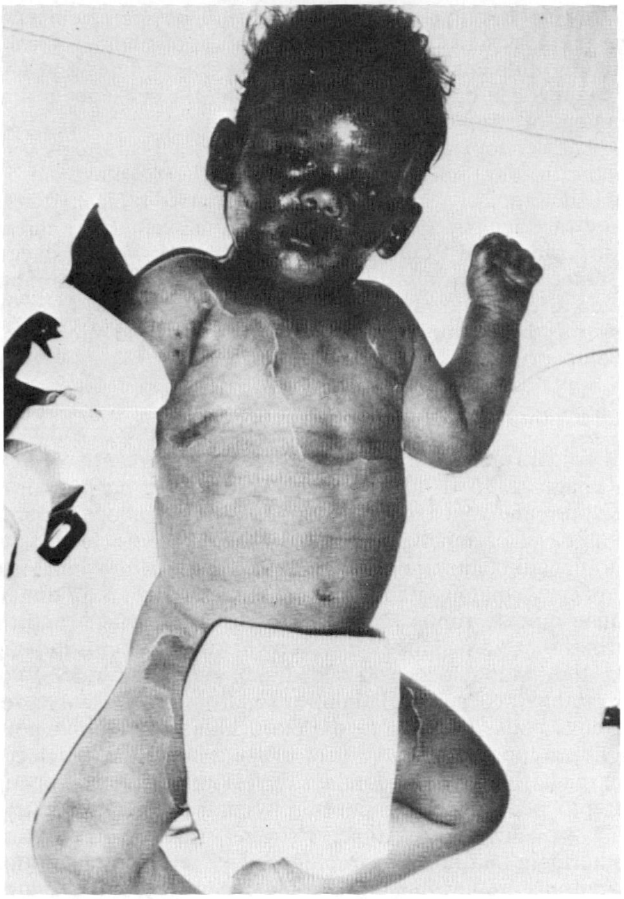

FIG. 1. Staphylococcal scalded skin syndrome in a young infant. Exfoliation has occurred on the face, chest, and groin, exposing areas of bright red skin surface.

Systemic corticosteroids alone should not be used in the treatment of SSSS, although they may be indicated in the therapy of drug-induced TEN.

Staphylococcal Scarlet Fever

This is fundamentally a forme fruste of SSSS (due to ET) that does not progress beyond the initial stage of a generalized erythematous eruption. At that stage the rash is indistinguishable from that of scarlet fever, and Pastia's lines can develop. However, pharyngitis is usually not present, and an enanthem does not develop. Desquamation, beginning on the face and involving most of the body, occurs 2–5 days after the onset of the scarlatiniform rash. Antibiotic treatment with penicillinase-resistant penicillins is indicated.

Toxic Shock Syndrome

The toxic shock syndrome (TSS) is another acute febrile illness with a generalized scarlatiniform eruption associated with *S. aureus* infection. Other elements of the syndrome include (*a*) hypotension (or shock), (*2*) functional abnormalities of three or more organ systems, and (*3*) desquamation in the evolution of the skin lesions[13–15] (see Chapter 173).

Folliculitis

Folliculitis is a pyoderma located within hair follicles and the apocrine regions. The lesions consist of small (2–5 mm) erythematous, sometimes pruritic, papules often topped by a central pustule. Sycosis barbae is a distinctive form of deep folliculitis, often chronic, occurring on the bearded areas. *Staphylococcus aureus* is the usual etiology of folliculitis. *Pseudomonas aeruginosa* (most often serotype 0–11) has been responsible for folliculitis acquired from swimming pools and whirlpools contaminated with large numbers of these organisms.[16] This type of skin infection produces pruritic papulourticarial lesions (appearing within 48 hours of exposure) that go on to pustule formation. Lesions in different stages of development are present simultaneously. Sites of predilection include the buttocks, hips, and axillae; the palms and soles are spared. Otitis externa is also a common manifestation. Healing occurs spontaneously, either by drainage or regression, within 5 days. Scarring develops rarely when an occasional pustule has progressed to furuncle formation. When acquired in a whirlpool, the lesions are sharply limited to the trunk below the upper chest or neck. Inadequate chlorine levels in whirlpools, hot tubs, and swimming pools have been responsible for many of the reported outbreaks. *Pseudomonas aeruginosa* can also cause superinfection in acne. In granulocytopenic or immunosuppressed hospitalized patients, *P. aeruginosa* 0–11 from tap water used for washing has been implicated in folliculitis that has rapidly progressed to ecthyma gangrenosum.[17]

Folliculitis due to Enterobacteriaceae can occur as a complication in patients with acne, usually during prolonged courses of oral antibiotic therapy.[18]

Candida is sometimes the etiology of folliculitis, producing pruritic satellite lesions surrounding areas of intertriginous candidiasis, particularly in patients on prolonged antibiotic or corticosteroid therapy. *Malassezia furfur*, common skin saprophytes, may also produce a folliculitis with pruritic erythematous papules and papulopustules on the trunk, upper extremities, and face, particularly in the setting of diabetes mellitus, corticosteroid administration, or granulocytopenia.[19,20] These lesions, particularly the early papular nodular ones, may suggest those of systemic candidiasis, a diagnosis that may seem to be supported by the presence of budding yeasts on Gram-stained material from unroofed lesions. Unlike *Candida, Malassezia furfur* requires lipid-supplemented media for primary isolation.

A rare pruritic dermatosis, eosinophilic pustular folliculitis, characterized by recurrent crops of follicular papules and pustules with eosinophilic infiltration of perifollicular dermis, resembles bacterial or mycotic folliculitis but is a sterile process.[21]

Local measures (saline compresses and topical antibacterials or antifungals such as clotrimazole) are usually sufficient to control the infection.

Furuncles and Carbuncles

Definition and Pathologic Characteristics. A furuncle is a deep inflammatory nodule, usually developing from a preceding folliculitis. A carbuncle is a more extensive process extending into the subcutaneous fat in areas covered by thick, inelastic skin. In the latter, multiple abscesses develop, separated by connective tissue septae, and drain to the surface along hair follicles. *Staphylococcus aureus* is almost invariably the etiologic agent (see also Chapter 173).

Clinical Findings. Furuncles occur in skin areas subject to friction and perspiration and containing hair follicles (neck, face, axillae, buttocks). Predisposing factors include obesity, blood dyscrasias, treatment with corticosteroids, defects in neutrophil function, and probably diabetes mellitus. A furuncle begins as a firm, tender, red nodule that soon becomes painful and fluctuant. Spontaneous drainage of pus commonly occurs and the lesion subsides. A carbuncle is a larger, deeper, indurated, more serious lesion, usually located at the nape of the neck, on the back, or on the thighs. Fever and malaise are frequent, and some patients are acutely ill. As the lesion progresses, drainage occurs externally along the course of multiple hair follicles. A leukocytosis occurs, particularly when the lesion contains a large amount of undrained pus or when there is a complicating cellulitis or bacteremia.

Blood stream invasion may occur unpredictably (but is sometimes precipitated by manipulation of the lesions), resulting in osteomyelitis, endocarditis, or other metastatic foci. Lesions about the upper lip and nose present the special problem of spread of infection via the facial and angular emissary veins to the cavernous sinus.

Presumptive Therapy. Most furuncles are satisfactorily treated by the application of moist heat, which promotes localization and drainage of the process. A carbuncle or a furuncle with surrounding cellulitis and/or fever, or if located about the midface, should be treated with an antistaphylococcal antibiotic (e.g., oxacillin, 0.5–0.75 g orally every 4–6 hours for an adult). In the penicillin-allergic adult, clindamycin (150–300 mg orally every 6 hours) or erythromycin (0.25–0.5 g orally every 6 hours) are alternatives. If the lesions are large and fluctuant, surgical drainage is indicated. Antibiotic treatment should be continued until evidences of acute inflammation have subsided.

Management of patients with recurrent furunculosis presents a troublesome problem. This disease does not appear to be due to specific staphylococcal strains with special biologic properties, and most patients do not have definable underlying defects in host defenses. Prophylaxis of recurrent episodes involves several measures:

1. *Antibiotic treatment.* Systemic antibiotic treatment, as described above, should be administered for the most recent episode. Prolonged treatment (2 months) is no more effective than a 10- to 14-day course in preventing recurrences.[22]
2. *General skin care.* Soap and water should be used to reduce the number of *S. aureus* organisms on the body surface, and careful handwashing should be performed after contact with lesions. A separate towel and washcloth (carefully washed in hot water before reuse) should be reserved for the patient. Some physicians prefer hexachlorophene or chlorhexidine to soap.
3. *Care of clothing.* Sheets and underclothing should be laundered at high temperatures and should be changed daily in problem patients.
4. *Care of dressings.* Draining lesions should be covered at all times with sterile dressings to prevent autoinoculation, and the dressings should be wrapped and promptly disposed of after removal.

Local (nasal) application of antibiotic ointments (bacitracin or neomycin) is sometimes used in refractory cases with the aim of reducing nasal carriage and subsequent shedding of *S. aureus* onto the skin. Occasionally, recurrent furunculosis occurs in a family, or sometimes other members of the family carry the same strain of *S. aureus* in their nares. Prophylaxis with antibiotic ointment in the nares twice daily for every fourth week for the patient and family members who are nasal carriers of the infecting strain has been employed.[22] Rifampin (600 mg orally daily for 10 days) is effective in eradicating coagulase-positive staphylococci from the majority of nasal carriers for periods of up to 12 weeks.[23] The use of rifampin for such a short period to eliminate nasal carriage of *S. aureus* and interrupt a continuing cycle of recurrent furunculosis might be considered in the patient in whom other measures have failed. However, selection of rifampin-resistant *S. aureus* strains can occur with such therapy. Thus we suggest cloxacillin, 500 mg po qid, along with the rifampin to reduce the emergence of rifampin-resistant organisms. Various staphylococcal vaccines have not proven effective in preventing recurrent furunculosis.

Ecthyma

Clinical Findings. The lesions of ecthyma begin in a fashion similar to those of impetigo but penetrate through the epidermis. Group A streptococci either produce the lesions de novo or secondarily infect pre-existing superficial lesions (insect bites, excoriations), resulting in the same clinical picture.[24] It is important to note that lesions with the same ultimate appearance can be produced in the course of *Pseudomonas* bacteremia (see below). The lesions most frequently occur on the lower extremities, particularly of children and the elderly. They consist of "punched-out" ulcers, covered by greenish yellow crusts, extending deeply into the dermis and surrounded by raised violaceous margins. Treatment is the same as for impetigo. Very extensive involvement with complicating bacteremia has occurred in a patient with the acquired immunodeficiency syndrome (AIDS).[25]

Chancriform Lesions

A variety of infections, often with systemic consequences, are characterized by an initial chancriform lesion (Table 1). Of the nonvenereal infections, anthrax has one of the most prominent chancriform lesions.

Anthrax. See Chapter 186 for a detailed discussion.

PATHOGENESIS. Anthrax is a very rare disease in the United States. Infections are limited to persons working with raw imported wool and other animal products contaminated with highly resistant spores of *Bacillus anthracis*. Routine safety measures for employees in wool plants and so forth virtually have eliminated anthrax from this group; sporadic cases still occur in transient workers in factories (e.g., ventilation repairmen) and in persons directly importing wool for their own weaving. Most infections occur on the face, neck, or arms in an area of a minor abrasion. Rarely, pulmonary infection follows inhalation of *B. anthracis*, or intestinal anthrax results from ingestion of the organism.

CLINICAL FINDINGS. After an incubation period of 1–3 days, a painless papule develops on an exposed area. The lesion enlarges, vesiculates ("malignant pustule"), and is surrounded by a wide zone of brawny, erythematous, gelatinous, nonpitting edema.[26] Malaise and low-grade fever are present. As the lesion evolves, the vesicle becomes hemorrhagic, necrotic, and covered by an eschar of variable dimensions (Fig. 2). At all stages the lesion remains painless. Bacteremic dissemination of infection from a skin site may occur, accompanied by high fever and

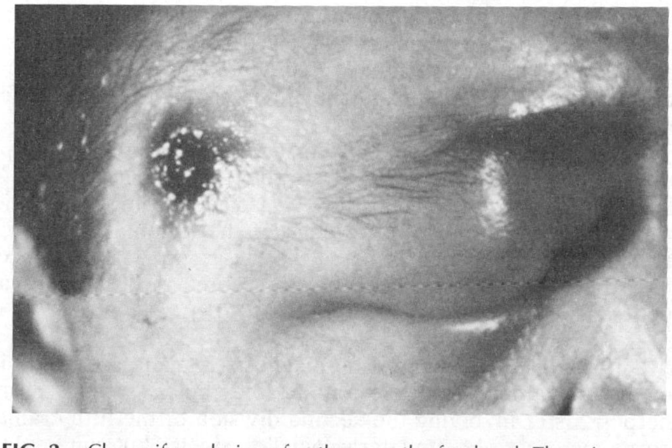

FIG. 2. Chancriform lesion of anthrax on the forehead. There is a prominent surrounding zone of gelatinous edema that is most evident on the eyelids. (Courtesy of Dr. Louis Weinstein, Boston, MA.)

hypotension. Meningitis may complicate either such a bacteremic infection or primary pulmonary anthrax.

The epidemiologic background and the striking appearance of extensive gelatinous edema serve to distinguish anthrax from other types of chancriform lesion. A staphylococcal pustule or carbuncle with a necrotic eschar may be mistaken for early anthrax. However, the former is very painful and tender, and the etiologic agent can usually be demonstrated on a Gram-stained smear of material from the lesion.

PRESUMPTIVE TREATMENT. Incision and débridement should be avoided, since they increase the likelihood of bacteremia. Parenteral penicillin G (1 million units every 4–6 hours) is used. In the penicillin-allergic patient, tetracycline (1.0–2.0 g/day intravenously in the adult) is an alternative.

Erysipelas

Erysipelas is a distinctive type of superficial cellulitis of the skin with prominent lymphatic involvement. It is almost always due to group A streptococci (uncommonly, group C or G). Group B streptococci have produced erysipelas in the newborn. Very rarely, a similar skin lesion is caused by *S. aureus*.

Clinical Findings. Erysipelas is more common in infants, young children, and older adults. Formerly, the face was most commonly involved, and an antecedent streptococcal respiratory tract infection preceded cutaneous involvement in about one-third of patients even though streptococci might not be found on culture at the time the skin lesion became evident. Now the localization of erysipelas has changed: 70–80 percent of the lesions are on the lower extremities and 5–20 percent are on the face.[27] Portals of entry are commonly skin ulcers, local trauma or abrasions, psoriatic or eczematous lesions, or fungal infections; in the neonate, erysipelas may develop from an infection of the umbilical stump. Predisposing factors include venous stasis, paraparesis, diabetes mellitus, and alcohol abuse. Patients with the nephrotic syndrome are particularly susceptible. Erysipelas tends to occur in areas of pre-existing lymphatic obstruction or edema (e.g., after a radical mastectomy). Also, because erysipelas itself produces lymphatic obstruction, it tends to recur in an area of earlier infection. Over a 3-year period, the recurrence rate is about 30 percent,[27] predominantly in individuals with venous insufficiency or lymphedema.

Streptococcal bacteremia occurs in about 5 percent of patients with erysipelas; group A, C, or G streptococci can be isolated on throat culture from about 20 percent of cases.[27]

Erysipelas is a painful lesion with a bright red, edematous, indurated (''peau d' orange'') appearance and an advancing, raised border that is sharply demarcated from the adjacent normal skin (Fig. 3). Fever is a feature. A common form of erysipelas involves the bridge of the nose and the cheeks. Uncomplicated erysipelas remains confined primarily to the lymphatics and the dermis. Occasionally, the infection extends more deeply, producing cellulitis, subcutaneous abscess, and necrotizing fasciitis.

A leukocytosis is common with erysipelas. Group A streptococci usually cannot be cultured from the surface of the skin lesion, and only rarely can they be isolated from tissue fluid aspirated from the advancing edge of the lesion. In cases of erysipelas complicating infected ulcers, group A streptococci have been isolated from the ulcerated area in 30 percent of patients.[27]

Differential Diagnosis. The diagnosis is made on the basis of the appearance of the lesion and the clinical setting. Early herpes zoster involving the second division of the fifth cranial nerve may resemble unilateral facial erysipelas but can be distinguished by the pain and hyperesthesia preceding the skin lesions. Occasionally contact dermatitis or giant urticaria may look like erysipelas but can be distinguished by the absence of fever and the presence of pruritus. Lesions closely resembling erysipelas, but apparently not due to streptococcal infection, may occur recurrently in patients with familial Mediterranean fever. Diffuse inflammatory carcinoma of the breast may mimic a low-grade erysipelas. Erythema chronicum migrans, the cutaneous lesion of Lyme disease, resembles erysipelas but is not painful and progresses much more slowly, and the associated fever is less marked.

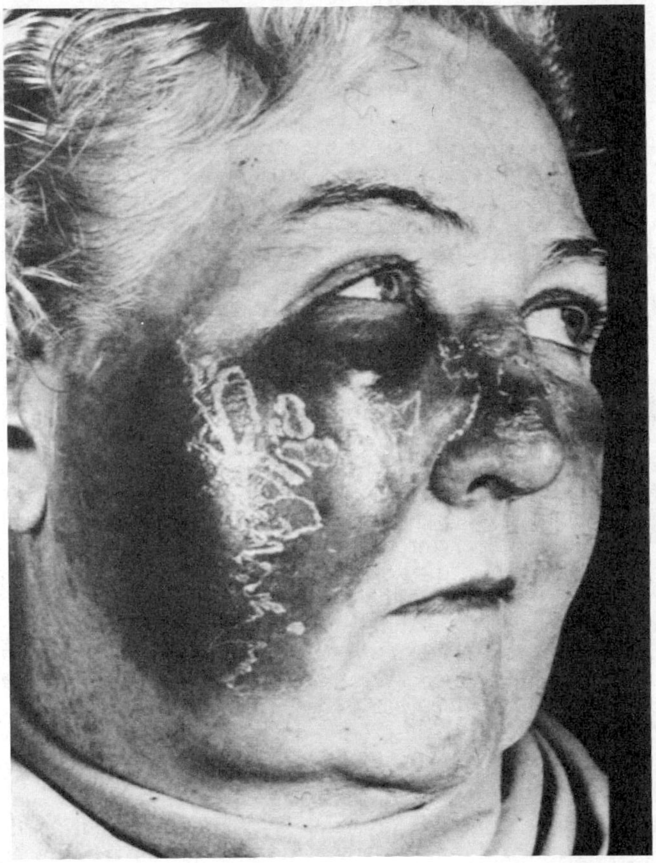

FIG. 3. Facial erysipelas involving both cheeks and the bridge of the nose. The sharp demarcation between the bright red area of erythema and the normal surrounding skin is evident. (From Fitzpatrick et al.,[28] with permission.)

Presumptive Therapy. Mild early cases of erysipelas in the adult may be treated with intramuscular procaine penicillin (600,000 units once or twice daily) or with oral penicillin V (250–500 mg every 6 hours). Erythromycin (250–500 mg orally every 6 hours) is a suitable alternative. For more extensive erysipelas, patients should be hospitalized and receive parenteral aqueous penicillin G (600,000–2,000,000 units every 6 hours).

Cellulitis

Cellulitis is an acute spreading infection of the skin extending deeper than erysipelas to involve the subcutaneous tissues. Group A streptococcus or *S. aureus* is most frequently the etiologic agent.

Clinical Findings. Previous trauma (laceration, puncture wound) or an underlying skin lesion (furuncle, ulcer) predisposes to the development of cellulitis; rarely, the latter may result from blood-borne spread of infection to the skin and subcutaneous tissues. Within several days of the inciting trauma, local tenderness, pain, and erythema develop and rapidly intensify. Malaise, fever, and chills develop. The involved area is often extensive and the lesion is very red, hot, and swollen. In contrast to erysipelas, the borders of an area of cellulitis are not elevated and sharply demarcated. Regional lymphadenopathy is common, and bacteremia can occur. Local abscesses may develop; small patches of overlying skin may subsequently undergo necrosis. Superinfection with gram-negative bacilli may supervene.

Cellulitis due to group A streptococci may occur as a postoperative wound infection. Although uncommon today, it is particularly noteworthy because of the rapidity with which it can spread and invade the blood stream. Such infection may manifest itself within 6–48 hours of surgery (comparable to the short incubation period of postoperative clostridial myonecrosis), earlier than the usual postoperative staphylococcal infection, which is not evident for at least several days after operation. Hypotension, often due to bacteremia, may be the initial sign of infection before significant erythema is evident about the incision. A thin serous discharge may be expressed on compression of the wound margins, and streptococci can be identified on a Gram-stained smear.

Cellulitis is a serious disease because of the propensity of infection to spread via the lymphatics and blood stream. Cellulitis of the lower extremities in older patients may be complicated by thrombophlebitis. In patients with chronic dependent edema, cellulitis may spread extremely rapidly.

A distinctive (by virtue of the clinical setting) form of cellulitis occurs in the lower extremities of patients whose saphenous veins have been removed for coronary artery bypass surgery.[29] Occasionally, an associated lymphangitis is present. In some patients, episodes of cellulitis are recurrent. Systemic manifestations such as chills, high fever, and toxicity are prominent. The area of cellulitis extends along the course of the saphenous venectomy. Edema, erythema, and tenderness are marked. Occasionally, the involved areas are somewhat similar to those of erysipelas (''pseudoerysipelas''). Although the bacterial etiology has not been defined in most cases, the available isolates from involved skin or blood implicate non-group A β-hemolytic streptococci (groups C, G, B) as major etiologies.[30] The portal of entry of the infection is often an associated area of tinea pedis. The combination of compromised lymphatic drainage and minor venous insufficiency secondary to saphenous venectomy may result in lower leg edema, a favorable setting for cellulitis. The inflammation from an initial episode of cellulitis, erysipelas, or lymphangitis obstructs lymphatic drainage, thus enhancing the predisposition to further episodes of infections.

Similar recurrent episodes of cellulitis or pseudoerysipelas due to group B and G streptococci have occurred in patients with lower extremity lymphedema secondary to radical pelvic surgery, radiation therapy, or neoplastic involvement of pelvic lymph nodes.[31] Typically, the cellulitis involves the vulva, inguinal areas, and both lower extremities. In this setting, recurrent episodes have occurred in association with recent coitus.[32]

An uncommon but distinctive form of cellulitis, perianal streptococcal (group A) cellulitis, occurs principally in children.[33] The clinical features consist of intense perianal erythema, pain on defecation, blood-streaked stools from anal fissures, and chronicity (months) if not treated with penicillin.

A rare but particularly troublesome, chronic, and progressive form of cellulitis, known as *dissecting cellulitis of the scalp* or *perifolliculitis capitis*, is probably similar to hydradenitis suppurativa and acne conglobata in pathogenesis. The clinical features consist of recurrent painful, fluctuant dermal and subcutaneous nodules, purulent drainage from burrowing interconnecting abscesses, scarring, and alopecia. The pathogenesis, as in hydradenitis suppurativa, is probably related to follicular plugging, secondary infection, and deep dissecting inflammation. *Staphylococcus aureus* is most commonly isolated. Effective treatment has involved wide excision and skin grafting.[34]

Lymphatic cutaneous metastases from neoplasms, particularly adenocarcinoma, may produce a localized, edematous, erythematous lesion resembling cellulitis. Inflammatory carcinoma of the breast, carcinoma erysipeloides, involves the skin overlying the site of the primary tumor.

A polymorphonuclear leukocytosis is usually present, regardless of the bacterial etiology.

Etiologic Agents. Group A streptococci and *S. aureus* are responsible for the overwhelming majority of cases of cellulitis, but other organisms may be involved occasionally. Streptococci belonging to other groups (group C, group G, and in neonates particularly, group B) are sometimes the etiologic agents.

Erysipelothrix rhusiopathiae is the etiologic agent of erysipeloid, a cellulitis occurring principally in persons handling saltwater fish, shellfish, poultry, meat, and hides (see Chapter 188). The infection, usually occurring in the summer, is introduced through an abrasion on the hands. A painful violaceous area appears within a week of the injury. As the process spreads peripherally with distinct raised borders, the central portion of the lesion clears. Ulceration is not a feature. Occasionally an adjacent joint is involved, and rarely, bacteremia and endocarditis may follow. The causative organism is generally not observed on Gram-stained drainage from the lesion but may be isolated on culture of a biopsy specimen taken from the advancing margin of the lesion. The development of a typical lesion in a person handling fish or meat products suggests the diagnosis. Other forms of bacterial cellulitis or erysipelas may resemble erysipeloid, particularly when the lesion is on the hand. A somewhat similar lesion of unknown etiology, ''seal finger,'' occurs in aquarium workers and veterinarians secondary to seal bites or trauma sustained in caring for these animals. While penicillin is the antibiotic of choice in the treatment of erysipeloid, it appears that seal finger responds to tetracycline.[35]

Rare cases of pneumococcal cellulitis acquired through the bacteremic route have been reported.[36] Soft tissue infections due to the pneumococcus can bear a striking resemblance to streptococcal erysipelas. A variety of bacteria (*Serratia, Proteus*, and other Enterobacteriaceae) and fungi (*Cryptococcus neoformans*) that are not the cause of cellulitis in normal individuals may produce cellulitis in the immunocompromised or granulocytopenic patient. Spontaneous *Escherichia coli* cellulitis occurs in children with the nephrotic syndrome in relapse.[37]

An environmental gram-negative bacillus, *Aeromonas hydrophila*, found particularly in lakes, rivers, and soil, may produce an acute cellulitis after introduction of the organism through a laceration acquired during swimming in fresh water.[38]

Cellulitis, bullous lesions, or necrotic ulcers may complicate infection of a traumatic wound sustained in salt water (or brackish inland waters) or exposed to drippings from raw seafood. Such infections, due to *Vibrio* spp. (e.g., *V. vulnificus, V. alginolyticus, V. parahaemolyticus*) can result in bacteremia and progress to necrosis, requiring extensive surgical débridement.[39] These vibrios are generally susceptible to chloramphenicol and tetracycline in vitro; most isolates are also susceptible to the aminoglycoside antibiotics.

Although needle aspiration of the lesion of erysipelas is commonly unsuccessful in providing a bacteriologic diagnosis (by Gram stain or culture), it is sometimes very helpful in defining the pathogen in cases of cellulitis. Using aspirates from the advancing edge of cellulitis, skin biopsy, and blood cultures, potential pathogens are isolated in only about 25 percent of patients.[40] When a site of origin (abrasion, ulcer) for the infection is present, isolates of potential pathogens (*S. aureus*, group A streptococci) can be obtained in about one-third of cases. The yield of potential pathogens may be higher if aspirates are obtained from the point of maximum inflammation (commonly the center) of areas of cellulitis rather than from the leading edge.[41]

The appearance and clinical features of a noninfectious process, eosinophilic cellulitis, may suggest the appearance of bacterial cellulitis on the extremities or trunk.[42] The involved area is moderately erythematous and edematous. The lesion develops rapidly, is often accompanied by fever, and enlarges over several days. It can be distinguished from the usual bacterial cellulitis by its minimal tenderness, lack of local heat, and its failure to respond to antibiotics. Biopsy of the early lesion shows marked infiltration of the dermis with eosinophils. The lesions resolve in several weeks but frequently recur.

Presumptive Therapy. If a mild early cellulitis is suspected to be of streptococcal etiology, it may be treated with an initial injection of aqueous penicillin G (600,000 units) followed by intramuscular procaine penicillin (600,000 units every 8–12 hours). When staphylococcal infection is suspected, or when there are no initial clues to the etiology, a penicillinase-resistant penicillin (e.g., oxacillin, 0.5–1.0 g orally every 6 hours) should be used. In adults allergic to penicillin, erythromycin (0.5 g orally every 6 hours) is an alternative. For more severe infections where both streptococcal and staphylococcal etiologies are considered, parenteral administration of a penicillinase-resistant penicillin (e.g., nafcillin, 1.0–1.5 g intravenously every 4 hours) should be used. Vancomycin (1.0–1.5 g/day intravenously) is an alternative for the highly penicillin-allergic patient. If the clinical setting suggests a gram-negative bacillus as a possible etiology of a serious cellulitis, an aminoglycoside such as gentamicin may be added to the semisynthetic penicillin initially while awaiting definitive bacteriologic results. Gentamicin, along with a penicillinase-resistant penicillin, is probably indicated in the initial treatment of a rapidly progressive cellulitis developing after a freshwater injury. *Aeromonas hydrophila* is usually susceptible to gentamicin and chloramphenicol (and to tetracycline to a slightly lesser degree).

Initial local care of cellulitis includes immobilization and elevation of the involved limb to reduce swelling and cool sterile saline dressing to decrease local pain. Subsequently, application of moist heat may aid in localization of the infection.

Patients with cellulitis at the saphenous site after coronary bypass surgery who have fungal infection in the intergidital spaces should be treated topically for the latter with miconazole or clotrimazole. The initial antibiotic (penicillin or nafcillin) should be given in high dosage by the intravenous route for 6–7 days to ensure prompt resolution before switching to other routes of therapy. Attention to the problem of tinea pedis before bypass surgery can prevent this form of cellulitis. Similar prompt attention to pedal epidermophytosis in patients who have had one such episode of cellulitis can obviate subsequent episodes.

Recurrent episodes of cellulitis usually occur in patients with peripheral edema. The use of support stockings and good skin hygiene can reduce its frequency or eliminate recurrences. In the occasional patient who continues to have frequent episodes of cellulitis or erysipelas despite such measures, prophylactic penicillin G (250–500 mg orally twice daily) may be indicated.

Membranous Ulcers

Infected ulcers of varied or mixed bacterial etiology may be covered at their base by a layer of necrotic debris resembling a membrane. The latter usually is not strongly adherent and can be removed without much difficulty. In addition, such a lesion has abundant purulent drainage attributable to infection with pyogenic bacteria. Membrane-covered lesions (both superficial and deep ulcers) also are produced by cutaneous infection with *Corynebacterium diphtheriae*.

Cutaneous Diphtheria. Cutaneous diphtheria (see Chapter 165) is uncommon in developed countries; most cases occur in unimmunized persons in overcrowded, underdeveloped parts of the world, particularly in tropical areas, and are associated with skin trauma and poor hygiene. Recent increases in cutaneous diphtheria have been noted in the Pacific Northwest and the South.

CLINICAL FINDINGS. Three types of cutaneous lesions have been described in cutaneous diphtheria: (*a*) *Wound diphtheria*—secondary infection with *C. diphtheriae* of a pre-existing wound, which becomes partially covered by a membrane and encircled by a zone of erythema; (*2*) *primary cutaneous diphtheria*—a disease of the tropics, which begins as a single or several pustules, usually on a lower extremity, and progresses to form a punched-out ulcer covered by a gray-brown membrane; and (*3*) *superinfection of eczematized skin lesions*—a superficial membranous infection; *C. diphtheriae* also have been isolated from lesions resembling impetigo, ecthyma, and infected insect bites, where they may represent true infections or merely a cutaneous carrier state.[43] Cutaneous diphtheria may be as contagious as the respiratory form of the disease among school children.

Occasionally, membranous pharyngitis may accompany cutaneous diphtheria. However, 20–40 percent of the patients with cutaneous diphtheria carry *C. diphtheriae* in their upper respiratory tract.[43,44] Myocarditis is extremely rare as a complication of cutaneous diphtheria, but cranial nerve palsies and Guillain-Barré syndrome occur in 3–5 percent of the patients with membranous diphtheritic skin ulcers.

LABORATORY FINDINGS. Characteristic beaded, metachromatically staining bacilli can be found in methylene blue-stained smears of the edge of the membrane. However, the diagnosis can be established only by isolation of *C. diphtheriae* from a suggestive skin lesion. Selective media (Loeffler's or tellurite agar) are necessary for isolation in order to inhibit other bacteria in skin ulcers. In addition to isolation of the organism, toxigenicity should be demonstrated by an Elek plate (agar diffusion precipitin reaction) or by guinea pig inoculation (dermonecrosis).

DIFFERENTIAL DIAGNOSIS. Pyogenic infection of ulcerated traumatic lesions is usually purulent, and the lesions are not covered by a membrane. Cutaneous fungal infections have more proliferative and irregular margins. The early stages of primary cutaneous diphtheria and of secondary infection of insect bites and abrasions with *C. diphtheriae* may closely resemble impetigo.

PRESUMPTIVE THERAPY. If a presumptive diagnosis of ulcerative cutaneous diphtheria is made on clinical grounds and on the basis of preliminary bacteriologic findings, antitoxin is administered (20,000–40,000 units intramuscularly or intravenously) after testing for sensitivity to horse serum. Antibiotic administration (erythromycin, 2.0 g/day orally, or procaine penicillin, 1.2–2.4 million units/day intramuscularly in the adult for 7–10 days) also assists elimination of the convalescent carrier state. Removal of necrotic debris aids in healing of the lesions.

Infectious Gangrene (Gangrenous Cellulitis)

Infectious gangrene is a cellulitis that has rapidly progressed, with extensive necrosis of subcutaneous tissues and overlying skin. Several different clinically distinguishable pictures may be produced, depending to varying extents on the specific causative organism, the anatomic location of the infection, and the predisposing conditions. Such clinical entities include (*1*) necrotizing fasciitis (streptococcal gangrene), (*2*) gas gangrene (clostridial myonecrosis and anaerobic cellulitis), (*3*) progressive bacterial synergistic gangrene, (*4*) synergistic necrotizing cellulitis (perineal phlegmon) and gangrenous balanitis, (*5*) gangrenous cellulitis in the immunosuppressed patient, and (*6*) very localized areas of skin necrosis complicating conventional cellulitis.

Pathologic Characteristics and Pathogenesis. The pathologic changes of gangrenous cellulitis are those of necrosis and some hemorrhage in skin and subcutaneous tissues. In most types of gangrenous cellulitis an abundant polymorphonuclear leukocytic exudate is present, but in clostridial gas gangrene the exudate is thin, consisting of fluid, fibrin, and gas, but with few leukocytes. In most types of gangrenous cellulitis (particularly streptococcal gangrene), fibrin thrombi are present in small arteries and veins of the dermis and subcutaneous fat.[45] In most instances, gangrenous cellulitis has developed secondary to introduction of the infecting organism at the infected site. It also may result from extension of infection from a deeper site to involve the subcutaneous tissues and skin (as in clostridial myonecrosis after intestinal surgery or in perineal phlegmon after dissection of infection from a perirectal abscess). Occasionally, gangrenous cellulitis may begin at a site of metastatic infection in the course of a bacteremia (gas gangrene due to *Clostridium septicum* at a peripheral site secondary to spread from an associated colonic neoplasm; *Pseudomonas* gangrenous cellulitis).

Clinical Findings. STREPTOCOCCAL GANGRENE. This is a rare form of gangrene, due to group A (or C or G) streptococci, which usually develops at a site of trauma on an extremity but may occur in the absence of an obvious portal of entry. The lesion begins as a local painful area of erythema and edema. Over the next 1–3 days the skin becomes dusky. Bullae containing yellowish to red-black fluid develop and rupture.[46] The lesion evolves into a sharply demarcated area covered by a necrotic eschar and surrounded by a border of erythema. The process at this point resembles a third-degree burn, for which it could be mistaken if a history were not available. Lymphangitis is rarely evident. Extensive necrotic sloughs can result because of deep penetration of the infection along fascial planes. Bacteremia, metastatic abscesses, and death may result from this life-threatening illness if appropriate antibiotic therapy is not initiated promptly. Secondary thrombophlebitis may be a complication when the lower extremities are involved. Streptococci can usually be cultured from the early bullous lesions and frequently from the blood.

PROGRESSIVE BACTERIAL SYNERGISTIC GANGRENE. This distinctive lesion usually follows infection at an abdominal operative wound site (frequently when wire sutures have been used), about an ileostomy or colostomy, at the exit of a fistulous tract, or in proximity to a chronic ulceration on an extremity.[47,48] It beings as a local tender area of swelling and erythema that subsequently ulcerates. The painful, shaggy ulcer gradually enlarges and is characteristically encircled by a margin of gangrenous skin (Fig. 4). Surrounding the latter is a violaceous zone that fades into an outer pink edematous border area. If untreated, the process extends slowly but relentlessly, ultimately producing an enormous ulceration. A related lesion, Meleney's ulcer, is essentially bacterial synergistic gangrene with the additional feature of burrowing necrotic tracts through tissue planes emerging at distant skin sites.

Microaerophilic or anaerobic streptococci can be recovered from aspirates of the advancing margin of the lesion, and *S. aureus* (or occasionally *Proteus* or other gram-negative bacilli) are present in the ulcerated area. Meleney has reproduced the same type of lesions by injecting both microaerophilic streptococci and *S. aureus* (but not either alone) into the skin of experimental animals.

GAS GANGRENE, ANAEROBIC CELLULITIS, AND OTHER FORMS OF CREPITANT CELLULITIS. See Chapters 75 and 76.

GANGRENOUS CELLULITIS IN THE PREDISPOSED HOST. The etiologic considerations in cellulitis occurring in the compromised host include agents that produce such infections in healthy persons, as well as a variety of other organisms not ordinarily regarded as causes of cellulitis, Mucormycotic gangrenous cellulitis may be engrafted on an extensive burn wound, or it may develop rarely in patients with diabetes mellitus or in those who are receiving immunosuppressive therapy. Local factors (open fracture sites, ileostomy stomas, fistulous tracts) also play a predisposing role in this type of infection. Spores of *Rhizopus* spp. (member of the Mucoraceae) contaminating Elastoplast tape used for occlusive dressings have resulted in progressive local and disseminated infection in immunosuppressed patients.[50] The infection may exhibit an indolent course with minimal fever and a slowly enlarging black ulcer, or it may follow a rapidly progressive febrile course. The characteristic lesion consists of a central anesthetic black necrotic area with a surrounding raised zone of violaceous cellulitis and edema.[51] Superficial vesicles may occur in the gangrenous area. Hematogenous dissemination is not ordinarily demonstrable, and the skin infection usually does not result from an initial pulmonary or rhinocerebral focus. Cultures of the necrotic skin or aspirates from the advancing margin usually do not reveal the fungus. Definition of the etiology is best obtained on biopsy specimens: fungal wet mount on a crushed tissue preparation, tissue sections stained with hematoxylin and eosin (showing tissue and vascular invasion by characteristic broad hyphae), and culture.

Pseudomonas bacteremia may also produce a gangrenous cellulitis (see the section on "Cutaneous Involvement in Systemic Bacterial and Mycotic Infections" later in this chapter) in immunocompromised hosts, patients with thermal burns, and so forth. In similar settings, gangrenous skin lesions may occur with disseminated aspergillosis.

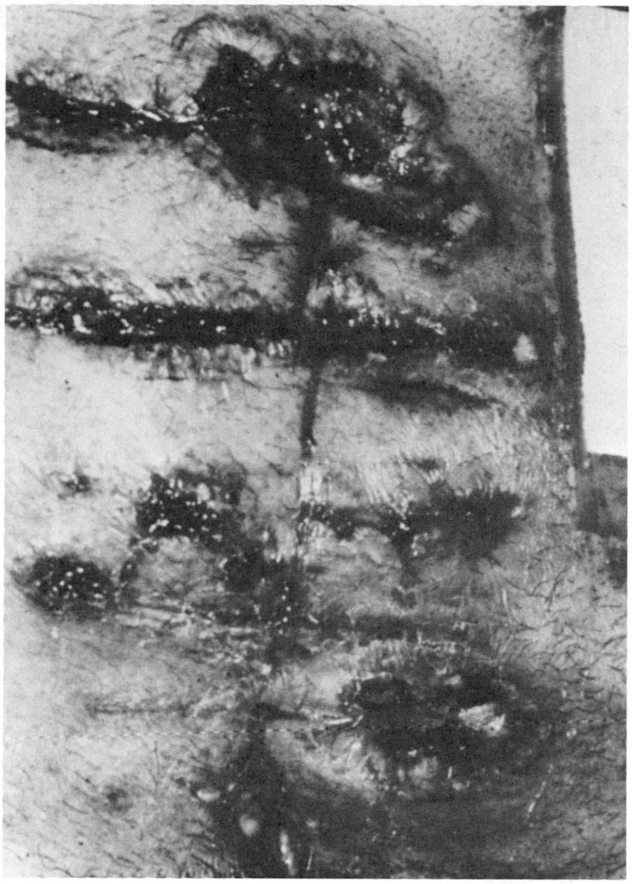

FIG. 4. Progressive bacterial synergistic gangrene of the abdominal wall. Ulcerated areas had developed about wire stay sutures that have since been removed. (From Bornstein et al.,[49] with permission.)

Differential Diagnosis. See Table 2. The bite of the brown recluse house spider can produce a necrotizing skin lesion that resembles infectious gangrenous cellulitis. The occurrence of fever and chills 24–48 hours after the bite enhances the mimicry.

TABLE 2. Differential Diagnosis of Infectious Gangrene and Gangrenous Cellulitis

	Progressive Bacterial Synergistic Gangrene	*Synergistic Necrotizing Cellulitis*	*Streptococcal Gangrene*	*Gas Gangrene*	*Necrotizing Cutaneous Mucormycosis*	*Bacteremic Pseudomonas Gangrenous Cellulitis*	*Pyoderma Gangrenosum*
Predisposing conditions	Surgery; draining sinus	Diabetes common	Occasionally diabetes or myxedema; after abdominal surgery	Local trauma	Diabetes; corticosteroid therapy	Burns, immunosuppression	Ulcerative colitis; rheumatoid arthritis
Pain	Prominent	Prominent	Prominent	Prominent	Minimal	Mild	Moderate
Systemic toxicity	Minimal	Marked	Marked	Very marked	Variable	Marked	Minimal
Course	Slow	Rapid	Very rapid	Extremely rapid	Rapid	Rapid	Slow
Fever	Minimal or absent	Moderate	High	Moderate or high	Low grade	High	Low grade
Anesthesia of lesion	–	–	±	–	+	±	–
Crepitus	–	Often present	–	+	–	–	–
Appearance of the involved area	Central shaggy, necrotic ulcer surrounded by dusky margin and erythematous periphery	Crepitant cellulitis; thick, copious, foul-smelling "dishwater" drainage from scattered areas of skin necrosis	Necrosis of subcutaneous tissue and fascia; black necrotic "burned" appearance of overlying skin	Marked swelling; yellow-bronzed discoloration of skin; brown bullae; green-black patches of necrosis; serosanguinous discharge	Usually a central black necrotic area with purple raised margin; also may present as just a black ulcer	A sharply demarcated necrotic area with black eschar and surrounding erythema, resembling a decubitus ulcer; may evolve from initial hemorrhagic bulla	Begin as bullae, pustules, or erythematous nodules that ulcerate deeply; often multiple, large and coalesce; usually on lower extremities or abdomen
Etiology	Microaerophilic streptococcus plus *S. aureus* (or *Proteus* sometimes)	Usually a mixture of organisms (e.g., *Bacteroides*, peptostreptococci, *E. coli*, etc.)	Primarily group A streptococci; when develops secondary to abdominal surgery, enteric bacteria also involved	*C. perfringens* (occasionally other clostridia)	*Rhizopus, Mucor, Absidia*	*P. aeruginosa*	Not an infection primarily; may be confused with such due to secondary colonization by Enterobacteriaceae, microaerophilic streptococci, *P. aeruginosa*, *S. aureus*

(Modified from Wilson et al.[51] with permission.)

Presumptive Therapy. Treatment of streptococcal gangrene consists of immediate surgical drainage with longitudinal incisions extending through the deep fascia and beyond the involved gangrenous and undermined areas.[46] Areas of cutaneous necrosis are excised. Antibiotic therapy consists of parenteral aqueous penicillin G (600,000–2,000,000 units every 4–6 hours). If there is any question as to the etiologic agent (e.g., possibly *S. aureus* rather than group A streptococcus), then nafcillin (1.5–2.0 g intravenously every 4–6 hours) should be used. The etiology of necrotizing fasciitis due to mixed anaerobes and facultative organisms (synergistic necrotizing cellulitis) can usually be suspected at the outset from the foul odor and the appearance of the exudate on a Gram-stained smear. After surgery the wound is treated with elevation and moist dressings. Skin grafting is usually required later.

Progressive bacterial synergistic gangrene is very difficult to treat. Local irrigations with bacitracin and systemic therapy with parenteral penicillin (4–6 million units/day intravenously) and a second drug (based on antibiotic susceptibility testing of bacteria other than microaerophilic streptococci isolated from the lesion) is sometimes helpful. However, wide excision of all necrotic tissue (extending well into normal tissue) combined with antibiotic treatment usually is required.

Erythrasma

Clinical Findings. Erythrasma is a common superficial bacterial infection of the skin characterized by slowly spreading, pruritic, reddish-brown macular patches, usually located in the genitocrural area.[52] The lesions are finely scaled and finely wrinkled, and they are more common in men and in obese individuals with diabetes mellitus. The disease may be asymptomatic or may undergo periodic exacerbations. The etiology appears to be bacterial: *Corynebacterium minutissimum*, a species that can be grown aerobically. Gram-stained imprints of the skin surface show large numbers of small gram-positive bacilli. Examination of the lesions under a Wood's lamp reveals a distinctive coral red fluorescence.

The principal superficial skin infections to be considered in the differential diagnosis are tinea versicolor lesions on the trunk and tinea cruris (a deeper, more inflammatory, and more rapidly progressive process).

Treatment with oral erythromycin (1.0 g/day orally for 5–7 days) is usually efficacious, clearing the lesions within several weeks. Topical treatment with an aqueous solution of 2% clindamycin hydrochloride can also be effective.[53]

SECONDARY BACTERIAL INFECTIONS COMPLICATING PRE-EXISTING SKIN LESIONS

A variety of skin lesions (burns, eczematous dermatitides, traumatic lesions, and so on) may become secondarily infected (Table 1). Such infected lesions usually do not exhibit distinctive morphologic characteristics based on the infecting organism; rather, the appearance of the lesions is determined to a large measure by the nature of the pre-existing injury or dermatosis. Several of these processes are considered in detail elsewhere (Chapters 75–77). Others are cared for primarily by dermatologists (dermatophytosis, acne conglabata). Several of the other secondarily infected dermatoses have some distinctive clinical and bacteriologic features and merit brief consideration here.

Chronic Superficial Skin Ulcers

A variety of aerobic and facultative organisms (*Pseudomonas*, *Proteus*, enterococci, and so on) colonize and secondarily infect decubitus ulcers. Only in recent years has the prominent role of anaerobic bacteria in such infections been recognized.[54] The character of the ulcers (extensive undermining and necrosis of tissue) and their location, frequently in proximity to the anus, provide the opportunity for invasion by anaerobes. *Bacteroides fragilis* and other Bacteroidaceae and *Clostridium perfringens* have commonly been isolated from infected decubitus ulcers. Such lesions have been the sources of symptomatic bacteremias.

Chronic foot infections in patients with diabetes mellitus are common and difficult problems. They usually begin after minor trauma in patients with peripheral neuropathy and arterial vascular insufficiency, and take the form of cellulitis, soft tissue necrosis, or osteomyelitis with a draining sinus. They are usually polymicrobial in etiology.[55,56] Deep tissue cultures provide the most reliable bacteriologic information. When these are not available, cultures and Gram-stained smears of material obtained from curettage of the base of the ulcer or from a purulent exudate may provide the needed information to guide antimicrobial therapy. Among the facultative bacteria involved in these infections, those most commonly isolated are *S. aureus*, enterococci, group B streptococci, and members of the Enterobacteriaceae (most commonly *Proteus* spp.).[56] Peptostreptococci, *B. fragilis*, and other *Bacteroides* spp. are the most frequently isolated anaerobes. When gas is present in surrounding tissues on radiologic examination, it may represent air introduced through the ulcer or gas generated in the soft tissues by the infecting anaerobic or coliform organisms.

Antibiotic treatment of infected diabetic foot ulcers is based on bacteriologic data. Initial treatment in a previously untreated patient with a mild infection might use a broad-spectrum cephalosporin such as cefoxitin. In patients with more severe infections, broader coverage with clindamycin and an aminoglycoside might be indicated, provided that renal function is not impaired. The oral route and broad spectrum of activity of the newer quinolones such as ciprofloxacin against the facultative bacteria involved in this process suggest that they will have an important role in the treatment of such chronic infections, either alone or in combination with another drug with activity against anaerobes.

Occupationally related contaminated traumatic wounds often involve loss of skin and subcutaneous tissues, with ensuing cellulitis and deeper infections. Comparison of the bacteriology of initial wounds sustained in factories with those on farms (associated with corn-harvesting machinery) indicates that gram-negative bacilli (particularly *Enterobacter* spp. and *Pseudomonas maltophilia*) are 10 times commoner in the latter.[57]

Post-Traumatic Opportunistic Skin Infections in Immunocompromised Patients

A variety of unusual pathogens may invade the skin of immunocompromised patients after some local, often minor laceration or abrasion. Such pathogens include fungi (*Paecilomyces, Penicillium, Trichosporon, Fusarium, Alternaria*), mycobacteria (*M. marinum*), and even algae (*Prototheca wickerhamii*).[50] The lesions are usually ulcerative but, in the case of *M. marinum*, may take the form of a nodular lymphangitis extending from the original focus. A typical dermatophyte, *Trichophyton rubrum*, which ordinarily produces only superficial skin infections, may invade the deeper subcutaneous tissues of immunosuppressed hosts and produce multiple nodular or fluctuant masses.[58]

Hydradenitis Suppurativa

This is an extremely troublesome, chronic, suppurative, cicatricial disease of apocrine glands in the axillary, genital, and perianal areas. The primary lesion appears to be an unexplained keratinous plugging of the ducts of the apocrine glands resulting in dilation and eventual rupture of the gland and surrounding tissue inflammation. The initial lesions are reddish-purple nodules that slowly become fluctuant and drain. Irregular sinus tracts are formed with repeated crops of lesions; reparative processes are only partially successful. Ultimately the involved areas show a mixture of burrowing, draining tracts, and cicatricial scarring. In some patients, hydradenitis suppurativa is associated with acne conglobata or dissecting cellulitis of the scalp. In such patients, a distinctive spondyloarthropathy may occur.[59]

Although not initially infected, the lesions frequently become so secondarily. Staphylococci, nonhemolytic streptococci, *E. coli, Proteus*, and *Pseudomonas* are often isolated from draining lesions. Anaerobic organisms (*Bacteroides*, anaerobic gram-positive cocci) also have been reported from such lesions.[54] The foul odor of the discharge from such lesions would suggest the presence of anaerobes.

Treatment of hidradenitis suppurativa is difficult, particularly when the process is chronic and extensive, because of the multiple deep-seated sites of secondary infection that are inaccessible to antibiotics. Antimicrobial therapy (based on Gram-stained smears and culture results) and local moist heat to establish drainage are helpful in the treatment of the initial phases of infection. Surgical drainage is required in the management of large abscesses. In very severe, resistant cases exhibiting chronicity and scarring, radical excision of most of the involved area followed by skin grafting may become necessary.

Self-Induced Skin Infections

Rarely, persisting unexplained skin ulcers are self-induced. Their colonization with a variety of gram-negative and gram-positive bacteria is inevitable. However, the continuing ulceration is the result of repeated, self-induced trauma rather than of bacterial infection per se. Very rarely, unexplained continuing or recurrent polymicrobial (oral or intestinal flora) cellulitis or a subcutaneous abscess is the result of injection of foreign material containing saliva or contaminated fluids into subcutaneous tissue. Examination of biopsy specimens from the involved area by polarizing microscopy may reveal the presence of birefringent foreign bodies, suggesting the true diagnosis.

CUTANEOUS INVOLVEMENT IN SYSTEMIC BACTERIAL AND MYCOTIC INFECTIONS

Cutaneous manifestations may be a feature of a variety of bacteremias, fungemias, and systemic bacterial infections[60] (Table 1). In leptospirosis, rat-bite fever, and listeriosis cutaneous manifestations are a small part of the total clinical picture and are considered elsewhere in chapters dealing with the responsible organisms. In some systemic infections cutaneous manifestations are noninfectious complications of the illness (erythema nodosum, purpura fulminans).

Bacteremias

Staphylococcus aureus. The occurrence of skin lesions (pustules, subcutaneous abscesses, purulent purpura) in the course of bacteremia or endocarditis due to *S. aureus* can provide a clue to the nature of the infecting organism. The most distinctive of these lesions is that of purulent purpura. This is a small area of purpura with a white, purulent center. Aspiration of the contents of the central portion reveals staphylococci and polymorphonuclear leukocytes. Rarely, scattered tender subcutaneous nodules may develop during *S. aureus* bacteremia.

Pseudomonas aeruginosa. Four types of skin lesion have been described in the course of *Pseudomonas* septicemia:

1. *Vesicles and bullae*. These occur as isolated bullae, or occasionally in small clusters, anywhere on the skin surface.

They rapidly become hemorrhagic and have a narrow encircling zone of dusky erythema. Occasionally, in infants, the lesions are surrounded by large, erythematous halos resembling insect bites or erythema multiforme.
2. *Ecthyma gangrenosum*. This is a round, indurated, ulcerated, painless area with a central gray-black eschar and a surrounding narrow zone of erythema. The lesions may develop de novo or may evolve from an initial bullous lesion.
3. *Gangrenous cellulitis*. This is either a superficial, sharply demarcated necrotic area that may resemble a decubitus ulcer or an area of cellulitis with edema and some necrosis of the overlying skin.
4. *Macular or maculopapular lesions*. These are small, oval, erythematous macules, located predominantly over the trunk, resembling the "rose spots" of typhoid fever. Such lesions have been reported, particularly in the tropics, in association with fever and diarrhea, the syndrome described as *Shanghai fever*.

The foregoing types of metastatic lesion contain numerous gram-negative bacilli but relatively few polymorphonuclear leukocytes. The development of such lesions in a febrile patient with leukemia undergoing induction chemotherapy or on uninvolved skin areas of a patient with extensive thermal burns should strongly suggest the presence of *Pseudomonas* bacteremia. Presumptive antibiotic management should be aimed at *P. aeruginosa* and includes a combination of ticarcillin with tobramycin or a similar aminoglycoside. Rarely, ecthyma gangrenosum occurs in the course of bacteremia due to other gram-negative bacilli or in disseminated candidiasis; or it may occur in the absence of bacteremia as progression of *Pseudomonas* folliculitis in an immunocompromised patient.[61]

Neisseria meningitidis. The skin lesions of acute meningococcemia consist of erythematous macules (initially), petechiae, purpura, and ecchymoses located on the extremities and trunk. Extensive gun-metal gray, hemorrhagic, necrotic patches can develop by confluence of petechial and purpuric lesions in fulminant meningococcemia. Symmetric peripheral gangrene and purpura fulminans occur with prominent disseminated intravascular coagulation. Occasionally, gram-negative diplococci can be observed on smears of serum obtained from the skin lesions of acute meningococcemia.

Skin lesions are an important feature of the unusual syndrome of chronic meningococcemia, characterized by recurrent cycles of fever, arthralgias, and rash over a period of 2–3 months.[62] The rash appears in crops, each consisting of a small number of individual lesions during febrile episodes. The lesions are generally located on the extremities, particularly about joints. They may consist of erythematous maculopapules, petechiae, petechiae with vesiculopustular centers, petechiae with small areolas of pale erythema, suggilations or tender erythema nodosum-like nodules. Biopsy specimens of the lesions reveal the histologic picture of leukocytoclastic angiitis, a finding that may erroneously direct attention toward a diagnosis of a small vessel hypersensitivity vasculitis and away from that of vasculitis secondary to systemic infection.

Neisseria gonorrhoeae. The skin lesions of gonococcemia consist of pustules surrounded by a thin zone of purpura, macules, papules, purpuric vesicles and bullae, and/or purpuric infarcts. The lesions are few, scattered over the distal extremities particularly, and frequently painful. They are part of the gonococcemic dermatitis-arthritis syndrome. In addition to arthralgias and frank arthritis, tenosynovitis may be a conspicuous feature.

Salmonella typhi. "Rose spots" frequently appear 7–10 days into the febrile course of untreated typhoid fever. The lesions are slightly raised, small (1–3 mm), pink papules that tend to occur in crops of 10–20 lesions. They are found most commonly on the upper abdomen, lower chest, and back. Rose spots are less frequently found in enteric fevers due to *Salmonella* spp. other than *S. typhi*. Early treatment with ampicillin or chloramphenicol will prevent the appearance of these skin lesions. *Salmonella typhi* can sometimes be found on Gram-stained preparations from the papules and isolated on culture.

Haemophilus influenzae. Cellulitis involving the face, neck, or upper extremities occasionally occurs with bacteremic *Haemophilus influenzae* type b infections in children, particularly under the age of 3 years. Although commonly described as having a peculiar purple-red or blue-red hue, the lesion most often is erythematous, indurated, and indistinguishable from cellulitis due to streptococci or staphylococci. The site of primary infection is in the pharynx, the middle ear, or elsewhere in the upper respiratory tract. Direct invasion across traumatized buccal mucous membranes by *H. influenzae* type b colonizing the respiratory tract has been suggested as the pathogenesis of most cases of buccal cellulitis in children.[63] Until very recently, this uncommon lesion had been described only in pediatric practice, but now cases have been reported in adults with epiglottitis and other forms of upper respiratory disease due to *H. influenzae*.[64] In view of the increasing incidence of ampicillin resistance in clinical strains of *H. influenzae* type b, provisional antibiotic therapy should use a third-generation cephalosporin (chloramphenicol, either alone or in combination with ampicillin), until the isolate can be tested for β-lactamase activity.

Infective Endocarditis

The cutaneous lesions of subacute bacterial endocarditis consist of petechiae, subungual "splinter" hemorrhages, Osler's nodes, and Janeway's lesions. Petechiae tend to occur in small crops, particularly in the conjunctivae, on the palate, and on the upper chest and extremities. These are the most common skin lesions of endocarditis. Rarely, petechiae are extremely numerous, particularly on the lower extremities, and suggest a primary vasculitis. Osler's nodes are split-pea sized, erythematous, tender nodules located principally on the pads of the fingers and toes. They are few at any given time and occur in about 15 percent of the patients with subacute bacterial endocarditis. The lesions are usually transient, clearing in 1–2 days. Similar lesions may also occur in acute endocarditis (e.g., due to *S. aureus*). Histologic examination of such lesions in several cases of acute endocarditis has suggested septic embolization in their pathogenesis.[65] The genesis of Osler's nodes in subacute bacterial endocarditis may have a different basis, perhaps an allergic vasculitis. Janeway's lesions are painless, small, erythematous macules or minimally nodular hemorrhages in the palms or soles occuring in either acute or subacute endocarditis (more commonly in the former, particularly when *S. aureus* is the etiology).

Fungemias

Candida albicans. Systemic candidiasis developing in the setting of leukemia, immunosuppression, extensive antibiotic therapy, hyperalimentation, heroin addiction, cardiac surgery, and so on may be difficult to diagnose clinically until the organism is isolated from routine blood cultures—often not until 5–7 days of incubation (more rapidly with lysis-centrifugation culture methods). The portal for disseminated candidiasis (or aspergillosis) may be an area of skin injured in the course of intravenous therapy (or trauma induced by adhesive tape or extravasation of intravenous fluid).[50] Examination of the optic fundi (for evidence of candidal ophthalmitis) and the search for *Candida* pseudohyphae and yeast forms on a smear of buffy coat of venous blood are sometimes helpful in making an early diagnosis of candidal fungemia while awaiting isolation of the organism from blood cultures. In occasional patients, the appearance of multiple discrete (2–5 mm) pink maculopapules (sometimes with pale centers) on the trunk or extremities can suggest the diagnosis.[66] In some of these patients severe diffuse muscle tenderness has been present, and muscle biopsy specimens have shown necrosis with yeast and pseudohyphal forms.[67] Occasionally, subcutaneous abscesses due to *Candida* may develop in the course of fungemia. Aspiration of such abscesses reveals the etiology on stained smear. Punch biopsy specimens of the maculopapular lesions provide a more accurate diagnosis than simple culture, since histologic sections can reveal *Candida* emboli in blood vessels and pseudohyphae in adjacent soft tissues. The isolation of *Candida* from an unroofed lesion may only represent surface colonization or may be consistent with *Candida* folliculitis rather than disseminated candidiasis.

REFERENCES

1. Schachner L, Taplin D, Scott GB, et al. A therapeutic update of superficial skin infections. Pediatr Clin North Am. 1983;30:397.
2. Ferrieri P, Dajani AS, Wannamaker LW, et al. Natural history of impetigo. I. Site sequence of acquisition and familial patterns of spread of cutaneous streptococci. J Clin Invest. 1972;51:2851.
3. Dajani AS, Ferrieri P, Wannamaker LW. Natural history of impetigo. II. Etiologic agents and bacterial interactions. J Clin Invest. 1972;51:2863.
4. Dillon HC. Impetigo contagiosa: Suppurative and non-suppurative complications. I. Clinical bacteriologic, and epidemiologic characteristics of impetigo. Am J Dis Child. 1968;115:530.
5. Dillon HC. Post-streptococcal glomerulonephritis following pyoderma. Rev Infect Dis. 1979;1:935.
6. Baltimore RS. Treatment of impetigo: A review. Pediatr Infect Dis. 1985;4:597.
7. Maddox JS, Ware JC, Dillon HC Jr. The natural history of streptococcal skin infection: Prevention with topical antibiotics. J Am Acad Dermatol. 1985;13:207.
8. Dajani AS. The scalded-skin syndrome: Relation to phage group II staphylococci. J Infect Dis. 1972;125:548.
9. Melish ME, Glascow LA, Turner MD, et al. The staphylococcal epidermolytic toxin: Its isolation, characterization, and site of action. Ann NY Acad Sci. 1974;236:317.
10. Elias PM, Fritsch P, Epstein EH Jr. Staphylococcal scalded skin syndrome: Clinical features, pathogenesis, and recent microbiological and biochemical developments. Arch Dermatol. 1977;113:207.
11. O'Reilly M, Dougan G, Foster TJ, et al. Plasmids in epidermolytic strains of *Staphylococcus aureus*. J Gen Microbiol. 1981;124:99.
12. Curran JP, Al-Salihi FL. Neonatal staphylococcal scalded skin syndrome: Massive outbreak due to an unusual phage type. Pediatrics. 1980;66:285.
13. Shands KN, Schmid GP, Dan BB, et al. Toxic-shock syndrome in menstruating women: Its association with tampon use and *Staphylococcus aureus* and the clinical features in 52 cases. N Engl J Med. 1980;303:1436.
14. Institute of Medicine, National Academy of Science: Conference on the Toxic Shock Syndrome. Ann Intern Med. 1978;96:835.
15. Todd JT, Fishaut M, Kapral F, et al. Toxic shock syndrome associated with phage-group-I staphylococci. Lancet. 1978;2:1116.
16. Gustafson LT, Band JD, Hutcheson RH, et al. *Pseudomonas* folliculitis: An outbreak and review. Rev Infect Dis. 1983;5:1.
17. El Baze P, Thyss A, Caldini C, et al. *Pseudomonas aeruginosa* 0-11 folliculitis: Development into ecthyma gangrenosum in immunosuppressed patients. Arch Dermatol. 1985;121:873.
18. Blankenship MI. Gram negative folliculitis. Arch Dermatol. 1984;120:1301.
19. Klotz SA, Drutz DJ, Huppert M, et al. *Pityrosporum* folliculitis. Its potential for confusion with skin lesions of systemic candidiasis. Arch Intern Med. 1982;142:2126.
20. Bufill JA, Lum LG, Caya JG, et al. Pityrosporum folliculitis after bone marrow transplantation. Ann Intern Med. 1988;108:560.
21. Buchness MR, Lim HW, Hatcher VA, et al. Eosinophilic pustular folliculitis in the acquired immunodeficiency syndrome. N Engl J Med. 1988;318:1183.
22. Hedstrom SA. Treatment and prevention of recurrent staphylococcal furunculosis: Clinical and bacteriologic follow-up. Scand J Infect Dis. 1985;17:55.
23. Wheat LJ, Kohler RB, Luft FC, et al. Long-term studies of the effect of rifampin on nasal carriage of coagulase-positive staphylococci. Rev Infect Dis. 1983;5:459S.
24. Allen AM, Taplin D, Twigg L. Cutaneous streptococcal infections in Vietnam. Arch Dermatol. 1971;104:271.
25. Hewitt WD, Farrar WE. Case report: Bacteremia and ecthyma caused by *Streptococcus pyogenes* in a patient with acquired immunodeficiency syndrome. Am J Med Sci. 1988;295:52.
26. Gold H. Anthrax: A report of 117 cases. Arch Intern Med. 1955;96:387.
27. Jorup-Ronstrom C. Epidemiological, bacteriological and complicating features of erysipelas. Scand J Infect Dis. 1986;18:519.
28. Fitzpatrick TB, Eisen AZ, Wolff K, et al, eds. Dermatology in General Medicine. New York: McGraw-Hill; 1971: PlateXXXVII.
29. Baddour LM, Bisno AL. Recurrent cellulitis after saphenous venectomy for coronary bypass surgery. Ann Intern Med. 1982;97:493.
30. Baddour LM, Bisno AL. Non-group A beta-hemolytic streptococcal cellulitis. Association with venous and lymphatic compromise. Am J Med. 1985;79:155.
31. Chmel H, Hamdy M. Recurrent streptococcal cellulitis complicating radical hysterectomy and radiation therapy. Obstet Gynecol. 1984;63:862.
32. Ellison RT III, McGregor JA. Recurrent postcoital lower extremity streptococcal erythroderma in women. Streptococcal-sex syndrome. JAMA. 1987;257:3260.
33. Spear RM, Rothbaum RJ, Keating JP, et al. Perianal streptococcal cellulitis. J Pediatr. 1985;107:557.
34. Williams CN, Cohen M, Ronan SG, et al. Dissecting cellulitis of the scalp. Plastic Reconstruct Surg. 1986;77:378.
35. Markham RB, Polk BF. Seal Finger. Rev Infect Dis. 1979;1:567.
36. Miyais S, Uwaydah M. Pneumococcal cellulitis. Infection. 1983;11:173.
37. Asmar BI, Bashour BN, Fleischmann LE. *Escherichia coli* cellulitis in children with idiopathic nephrotic syndrome. Clin Pediatr. 1987;26:592.
38. Hanson PG, Standridge J, Jarrett F, et al. Freshwater wound infection due to *Aeromonas hydrophila*. JAMA. 1977;238:1053.
39. Bonner JR, Coker AS, Berryman CR, et al. Spectrum of *Vibrio* infections in a gulf coast community. Ann Intern Med. 1983;99:464.
40. Hook EW III, Hooton TM, Horton CA, et al. Microbiologic evaluation of cutaneous cellulitis in adults. Arch Intern Med. 1986;146:295.
41. Howe PM, Fajardo JE, Orcutt MA. Etiologic diagnosis of cellulitis: Comparison of aspirates obtained from the leading edge and the point of maximal inflammation. Pediatr Infect Dis. 1987;6:685.
42. Saulsbury FT, Cooper PH, Bracikowski A, et al. Eosinophilic cellulitis in a child. J Pediatr. 1983;102:266.
43. Belsey MA, Sinclair M, Roder MR, et al. *Corynebacterium diphtheriae* skin infections in Alabama and Louisiana. A factor in the epidemiology of diphtheria. N Engl J Med. 1969;280:135.
44. Koopman JS, Campbell J. The role of cutaneous diphtheria infections in a diphtheria epidemic. J Infect Dis. 1975;131:239.
45. Barker FG, Leppard BJ, Seal DV. Streptococcal necrotizing fasciitis: Comparison between histological and clinical features. J Clin Pathol. 1987;40:335.
46. Strasberg SM, Silver MS. Hemolytic streptococcus gangrene. An uncommon but frequently fatal infection in the antibiotic era. Am J Surg. 1968;115:763.
47. Meleney FL. Bacterial synergism in disease processes with a confirmation of the synergistic bacterial etiology of a certain type of progressive gangrene of the abdominal wall. Ann Surg. 1931;94:961.
48. Husseinzadeh N, Nahas WA, Manders EK, et al. Spontaneous occurrence of synergistic bacterial gangrene following external pelvic irradiation. Obstet Gynecol. 1984;63:859.
49. Bornstein DL, Weinberg AN, Swartz MN, et al. Anaerobic infections. Review of current experience. Medicine. 1964;43:207.
50. Wolfson JS, Sober AJ, Rubin RH. Dermatologic manifestations in the compromised host. Ann Rev Med. 1983;14:205.
51. Wilson CB, Siber GR, O'Brien TF, et al. Phycomycotic gangrenous cellulitis. Arch Surg. 1976;111:532.
52. Sarkany I, Taplin D, Blank H. The etiology and treatment of erythrasma. J Invest Derm. 1961;37:283.
53. Sindhuphak W, MacDonald E, Smith EB. Erythrasma: Overlooked or misdiagnosed. Int J Dermatol. 1985;24:95.
54. Finegold SM. Infections of skin, soft tissue and muscle. In: Anaerobic Bacteria in Human Diseases. New York: Academic Press; 1977:386.
55. Sapico FL, Witte JL, Canawati HN, et al. The infected foot of the diabetic patient: Quantitative microbiology and analysis of clinical features. Rev Infect Dis. 1984;6(Suppl 1):S171.
56. Wheat LJ, Allen SD, Henry M, et al. Diabetic foot infections: Bacteriologic analysis. Arch Intern Med. 1986;146:1935.
57. Agger WA, Cogbill TH, Busch H Jr, et al. wounds caused by corn-harvesting machines: An unusual source of infection due to gram-negative bacilli. Rev Infect Dis. 1986;8:927.
58. Novick NL, Tapia L, Bottone EJ. Invasive *Trichophyton rubrum* infection in an immunocompromised host. Am J Med. 1987;82:321.
59. Rosner IA, Richter DE, Huettner TL, et al. Spondyloarthropathy associated with hydradenitis suppurativa and acne conglobata. Ann Intern Med. 1982;97:520.
60. Kingston ME, Mackey D. Skin clues in the diagnosis of life-threatening infections. Rev Infect Dis. 1986;8:1.
61. Huminer D, Siegman-Igra Y, Morduchowicz G, et al. Ecthyma gangrenosum without bacteremia: Report of six cases and review of the literature. Arch Intern Med. 1987;147:299.
62. Benoit FL. Chronic meningococcemia. Am J Med. 1963;35:103.
63. Chartrand SA, Harrison CJ. Buccal cellulitis reevaluated. Am J Dis Child. 1986;140:891.
64. Drapkin MS, Wilson ME, Shrager SM, et al. Bacteremic *Hemophilus influenzae* type B cellulitis in the adult. Am J Med. 1977;63:449.
65. Alpert JS, Krous HF, Dalen JE. Pathogenesis of Osler's nodes. Ann Intern Med. 1976;85:471.
66. Balandral L, Rothschild H, Pugh N, et al. A cutaneous manifestation of systemic candidiasis. Ann Intern Med. 1973;78:400.
67. Jarowski CI, Fialk MA, Murray HW, et al. Fever, rash, and muscle tenderness. A distinctive clinical presentation of disseminated candidiasis. Arch Intern Med. 1978;138:544.

75. SUBCUTANEOUS TISSUE INFECTIONS AND ABSCESSES

MORTON N. SWARTZ

Exact categorization of some bacterial infections of the soft tissues (skin, subcutaneous tissues, fascia, and skeletal muscle) may be difficult. While the differences between a superficial pyoderma and a necrotizing myositis like gas gangrene are readily apparent, distinctions between many other types of soft tissue infection are sometimes blurred. Classification is usually based on features such as the anatomic structure involved, the infecting organism(s), and the clinical picture. Unfortunately for convenience in categorization, some infections may involve several components of the soft tissues, and multiple bacterial species may produce infections with the same clinical appearance.

To compound the problem of classification further, a variety of designations have been given to closely related or virtually identical processes. For example, *streptococcal gangrene* has also been referred to as *necrotizing fasciitis*. Subsequent to the initial descriptions of this condition, it became apparent that it was sometimes caused by other bacteria than group A streptococci.[1] Thus, streptococcal gangrene can be considered the major subset of necrotizing fasciitis. For convenience, because a major feature of its manifestation is cutaneous gangrene, streptococcal gangrene has been considered in the preceding chapter with cellulitis and infectious cutaneous gangrene. Necrotizing fasciitis is reconsidered in this chapter on subcutaneous tissue infections, particularly in relation to its nonstreptococcal etiologies. Another example of the problems in nomenclature is that presented by infections that involve multiple soft tissue strata and that can be caused by a variety of bacterial species. Thus, the condition known as *synergistic necrotizing cellulitis* has also been described as *gram-negative anaerobic cutaneous gangrene* and *synergistic nonclostridial anaerobic myonecrosis*.[2,3] Because of the prominence of subcutaneous tissue involvement in this condition, it is considered primarily in this chapter, although it could be considered almost as readily in chapters on cellulitis or myositis.

CLOSTRIDIAL ANAEROBIC CELLULITIS

This is a necrotizing clostridial infection of devitalized subcutaneous tissues. Deep fascia is not appreciably involved, and ordinarily there is no associated myositis. Gas formation is common and often extensive. Anaerobic cellulitis is several times more common than gas gangrene in war wounds.

Pathogenesis and Pathologic Characteristics

Clostridial species, usually *Clostridium perfringens*, are introduced into subcutaneous tissues either through a dirty or inadequately debrided traumatic wound, through contamination at operation, or from a pre-existing localized infection. The last is frequently located in the perineum, abdominal wall, buttocks, and lower extremities, areas that are readily contaminated with fecal flora. The presence of foreign debris and necrotic tissue in the depths of a wound provides a suitable anaerobic milieu for clostridial proliferation.

Clinical Findings

The incubation period is several days, longer than the 1–2 days for clostridial myonecrosis. The onset is gradual but the process subsequently may spread rapidly.[4] Local pain, tissue swelling, and systemic toxicity are not prominent features, and the relative mildness of the process helps to distinguish it from true gas gangrene. The dark blebs and bronzing of the skin seen in gas gangrene are not usually features of clostridial cellulitis. A thin, dark, sometimes foul-smelling drainage (often containing fat globules) from the wound is characteristic, as is extensive tissue gas formation, more prominent than that observed in clostridial myonecrosis. Frank crepitus is present in the involved area and may extend very widely, even beyond the limits of the active infection.

Gram-stained smears of the drainage shows numerous blunt-ended, thick, gram-positive bacilli and variable numbers of polymorphonuclear leukocytes. Soft tissue x-ray films show abundant gas, but usually not in the feathery linear pattern in muscles observed in gas gangrene.

Etiologic Agents

Clostridium perfringens is the most common clostridial species responsible for this infection, but *C. septicum* and other species have been isolated. Sometimes, the clostridia are present in mixed culture with facultative organisms.

Differential Diagnosis

When crepitus is observed in a wound, a variety of possibilities must be considered in the differential diagnosis (Table 1). The first is gas gangrene because of the fulminant nature of the infection and the requirement for emergency surgery. At the same time, distinguishing between clostridial gas gangrene and anaerobic cellulitis is essential to avoid performing unnecessarily extensive surgery. Ultimately, the two processes are differentiated in the operating room when the wound is laid open and the viability and appearance of the muscle are observed. The muscle is normal (pink) in clostridial cellulitis but distinctly abnormal (discolored, fails to contract on stimulation, does not bleed from cut surface) in clostridial myonecrosis (see Chapter 76).

Presumptive Therapy

Surgical exploration is essential to determine the presence of any muscle involvement. If no myonecrosis is found, treatment should be limited to débridement of necrotic tissue and drainage of pus after the wound is opened widely. Penicillin in high dosage intravenously is indicated in management. Based on Gram-stained smears of exudate and tissue, an additional drug may be indicated for initial treatment of a potentially mixed infection.

NONCLOSTRIDIAL ANAEROBIC CELLULITIS

A clinical picture very similar to that of clostridial anaerobic cellulitis can be produced by infection with a variety of non-spore-forming anaerobic bacteria (various *Bacteroides* spp., peptostreptococci, peptococci—either alone or as mixed infections).[3] The anaerobic bacteria may be present along with facultative species (coliform bacilli, various streptococci, staphylococci) in a mixed infection. Gas-forming soft tissue infections have been produced by *Escherichia coli, Klebsiella, Aeromonas*, and perhaps other facultative bacteria.[5,6]

The surgical approach used is the same as in the treatment of clostridial anaerobic cellulitis. Antimicrobial therapy is initially based on the findings on Gram-stained smears of wound exudate. In view of the frequently mixed nature of the infections (and the spectrum of organisms involved), several antimicrobials (e.g., penicillin or ampicillin plus chloramphenicol) are probably indicated while awaiting the results of cultures.

TABLE 1. Differential Diagnosis of Crepitant Soft Tissue Wounds[a]

	Clostridial Cellulitis	*Nonclostridial Anaerobic Cellulitis*	*Gas Gangrene*	*Streptococcal Myositis*	*Necrotizing Fascitis*[b]	*Infected Vascular Gangrene*	*Synergistic Necrotizing Cellulitis*[c]	*Noninfectious Causes of Gas in Tissues*
Predisposing conditions	Local trauma or surgery	Diabetes mellitus; preexisting localized infection	Local trauma or surgery	Local trauma	Diabetes mellitus; abdominal surgery; perineal infection	Peripheral arterial insufficiency	Diabetes mellitus; cardiorenal disease; obesity; perirectal infection	Mechanical effects of penetrating trauma; injuries involving use of compressed air; entrapment of air under loosely sutured wounds or under ulcers; irrigation of wounds with hydrogen peroxide; intravenous catheter placement
Incubation period	Usually over 3 days	Several days	1–2 days	3–4 days	1–4 days	>5 days	3–14 days	Less than an hour
Onset	Gradual	Gradual or rapid	Acute	Not as rapid as gas gangrene	Acute	Gradual	Acute	Usually present immediately after trauma or manipulation; may not be recognized until examined several hours later
Pain	Mild	Mild	Marked	Occurs late; marked	Moderate or severe	Variable	Severe	Mild
Swelling	Moderate	Moderate	Marked	Moderate	Marked	Moderate or marked	Moderate or marked	Slight or absent
Skin appearance	Minimal discoloration	Minimal discoloration	Yellow-bronze; dark bullae; green-black patches of necrosis	Erythema	Erythematous cellulitis; areas of skin necrosis	Discolored or black	Scattered areas of skin necrosis	Only those due to initiating trauma
Exudate	Thin, dark	Dark pus	Serosanguinous	Abundant seropurulent	Seropurulent	0	"Dishwater" pus	0
Gas	+ + + +	+ + + +	+ +	±	+ +	+ + +	+ +	Variable but present; does not extend
Odor	Sometimes foul	Foul	Variable; slightly foul or peculiar sweet	Slight; "sour"	Foul	Foul	Foul	0
Systemic toxicity	Minimal	Moderate	Marked	Only late in course	Moderate or marked	Minimal	Marked	0
Muscle involvement	0	0	+ + + +	+ + +	0	Dead	+ +	0

Key: ±: rarely present; + +: present to mild extent; + + +: present to moderate extent; + + + +: extensive.

[a] In addition to the causes of crepitant infections listed in this table, *Aeromonas hydrophila* myostitis may be associated with gas in soft tissues.

[b] The term *necrotizing fascitis* is employed here to designate forms of this syndrome of streptococcal gangrene.

[c] Synergistic necrotizing cellulitis is essentially the same process as Type I necrotizing fasciitis. Since the former occasionally extends to involve muscle it is given a separate designation here; however, the two processes are clinically indistinguishable in most instances.

(Modified from Finegold,[3] with permission.)

NECROTIZING FASCIITIS

The term *necrotizing fasciitis* encompasses two bacteriologic entities[7,8]: *Type I* is the first entity, in which at least one anaerobic sp. (most commonly *Bacteroides* and *Peptostreptococcus* spp.) is isolated in combination with one or more facultative anaerobic sp. such as streptococci (other than group A) and members of the Enterobacteriaceae (e.g., *E. coli, Enterobacter, Klebsiella, Proteus*). An obligate aerobe such as *Pseudomonas aeruginosa* is only rarely a component of such a mixed infection. Cases in which only anaerobes are present appear to be rare.[8] *Type II* is the second entity (corresponding to the entity known also as *hemolytic streptococcal gangrene*) in which group A streptococci, either alone or in combination with other species, *Staphylococcus aureus* most commonly, are isolated. Streptococcal gangrene has been considered in Chapter 74 as a form of gangrenous cellulitis; the more general feature of necrotizing fasciitis will be considered here.

Clinical Findings

Necrotizing fasciitis is an uncommon severe infection involving the subcutaneous soft tissues, particularly the superficial (and often the deep) fascia. It usually is an acute process but rarely may follow a subacute progressive course. It can affect any part of the body but is most common on the extremities, particularly the legs. Other sites of predilection are the abdominal wall, perianal and groin areas, and postoperative wounds.[9] The portal of entry is usually a site of trauma (laceration, abrasion, burn, insect bite), a laparotomy performed in the presence of peritoneal soiling (penetrating abdominal trauma or perforated viscus) or other surgical procedure (e.g., hemorrhoidectomy or vasectomy), perirectal abscess, decubitus ulcer, or an intestinal perforation. The last may be secondary to occult diverticulitis,[10,11] rectosigmoid neoplasm, or a foreign body such as chicken bone or toothpick. Necrotizing fasciitis from such intestinal sources may occur in the lower extremity (extension along the psoas muscle), as well as in the groin or abdominal wall (via a colocutaneous fistula). Particular clinical settings in which necrotizing fasciitis may develop include diabetes mellitus, alcoholism, and parenteral drug abuse.[12]

In the newborn necrotizing fasciitis can be a serious complication of omphalitis. Initial swelling and erythema about the umbilicus can progress over several hours to several days, resulting in purplish discoloration and periumbilical necrosis.[13] Involvement of the anterior abdominal wall frequently extends to the flanks and even onto the chest wall.

The affected area initially is erythematous, swollen, without sharp margins, hot, shiny, exquisitely tender, and painful.[14] Lymphangitis and lymphadenitis are infrequent. The process progresses rapidly over several days, with sequential skin color changes from red-purple to patches of blue-gray. Within 3–5 days of onset, skin breakdown with bullae (containing thick pink or purple fluid) and frank cutaneous gangrene (resembling a thermal burn) occurs. By this time, the involved area is no longer tender but has become anesthetic secondary to thrombosis of small blood vessels and destruction of superficial nerves located in the necrotic undermined subcutaneous tissues. The development of anesthesia may antedate the appearance of skin necrosis, and this may provide a clue that the process is necrotizing fasciitis and not a simple cellulitis. Subcutaneous gas is often present in the polymicrobial form of necrotizing fasciitis, particularly in patients with diabetes mellitus. Systemic toxicity is prominent, and the temperature is elevated in the 102–105°F range. On probing of the lesion with a hemostat through a limited incision, easy passage of the instrument along a plane just superficial to the deep fascia occurs. This would not occur with ordinary cellulitis.

A leukocytosis is commonly present. Gram-stained smears of the exudate usually reveal a mixture of organisms or, in the case of streptococcal gangrene, chains of gram-positive cocci. In one instance, we observed numerous long gram-positive bacilli with subterminal spores (along with gram-negative bacilli) in the foul-smelling, purulent exudate of a patient with crepitant necrotizing fasciitis after a lower leg amputation for peripheral vascular disease. The presence of numerous spores in the wound exudate indicated that the gram-positive bacilli were unlikely to be *C. perfringens*. Before surgery the patient had had *Clostridium difficile* enterocolitis, and *C. difficile* was isolated, along with several members of the Enterobacteriaceae, from the wound drainage.

Blood cultures are frequently positive. Hypocalcemia (without tetany) may occur when necrosis of subcutaneous fat is extensive.

Fournier's Gangrene. A form of necrotizing fasciitis occurring about the male genitals is known as *Fournier's gangrene*[3] (*idiopathic gangrene of the scrotum, streptococcal scrotal gangrene, perineal phlegmon*). It may be confined to the scrotum or may extend to involve the perineum, penis, and abdominal wall. Predisposing factors include diabetes mellitus, local trauma, paraphimosis, periurethral extravasation of urine, perirectal or perianal infections, and surgery in the area (circumcision, herniorrhaphy). In cases originating in the genitalia, the infecting bacteria probably pass through Buck's fascia of the penis and spread along the dartos fascia of the scrotum and penis, Colles' fascia of the perineum, and Scarpa's fascia of the anterior abdominal wall. In view of the typical foul odor associated with this form of necrotizing fasciitis, a major role for anaerobic bacteria is likely. Mixed cultures containing facultative organisms (*E. coli, Klebsiella*, enterococci), along with anaerobes (*Bacteroides, Fusobacterium, Clostridium*, anaerobic or microaerophilic streptococci), have been obtained from the lesions in the limited number of cases studied. Group A streptococcal gangrene can, on rare occasions, also involve the male genital area.

The infection commonly starts as cellulitis adjacent to the portal of entry. Early on, the involved area is swollen, erythematous, and tender as the infection begins to involve the deep fascia. Pain is prominent; fever and systemic toxicity are marked.[15] The swelling and crepitus of the scrotum quickly increase, and dark purple areas develop and progress to extensive scrotal gangrene. If the abdominal wall becomes involved in an obese patient with diabetes, the process can spread like wildfire.

Differential Diagnosis

See Table 1.

Presumptive Therapy

Prompt diagnosis is of paramount importance because of the rapidity with which the process can progress. The mortality rate of necrotizing fasciitis ranges from 20 to 47 percent overall (13 and 22 percent for Fournier's gangrene).[14,15] Among patients (including those with either type I or type II necrotizing fasciitis) in whom the diagnosis is made within 4 days of appearance of the initial symptoms, the mortality rate is reduced to 12 percent.[16] Early clinical differentiation of necrotizing fasciitis from cellulitis may be difficult, since the initial signs, including pain, edema, and erythema, are not distinctive. However, the presence of marked systemic toxicity out of proportion to the local findings should alert the physician. Frozen section examination of biopsy specimens (including dermis, infected subcutaneous tissue, fascia, and underlying muscle) has been found to be helpful for early diagnosis.[16] Once the diagnosis is made, immediate surgical débridement is essential. In the patient in whom the diagnosis is clearly suspected on clinical grounds—deep pain with patchy areas of surface hypesthesia, or crepitation, or bullae and skin necrosis—direct operative intervention is indicated. Extensive incisions should be made through the skin and subcutaneous tissues, going beyond the area of involvement until normal fascia is found. Necrotic fat and fascia should be excised, and the wound should be left open. A second-look procedure may be necessary 24–48 hours later if there is any question as to the adequacy of the initial débridement. In the case of Fournier's gangrene, orchiectomy is almost never required, since the testes have their own blood supply independent of the compromised fascial and cutaneous circulation of the scrotum. Initial antimicrobial therapy is based on the evidence for prominent roles for anaerobic bacteria, Enterobacteriaceae, and various streptococci in this process and on the specific findings on Gram-stained smears. Antibiotics employed before obtaining bacteriologic data include combinations of ampicillin, gentamicin, and clindamycin; or ampicillin, gentamicin, and metronidazole.

SYNERGISTIC NECROTIZING CELLULITIS

Clinical Findings

Synergistic necrotizing cellulitis (gram-negative anaerobic cutaneous gangrene, necrotizing cutaneous myositis, synergistic nonclostridial anaerobic myonecrosis) is a variant of necrotizing fasciitis, one in which there is prominent involvement of skin and muscle as well as of subcutaneous tissue and fascia. Some cases of Fournier's gangrene extending onto the abdominal wall represent this condition. Predisposing factors include diabetes mellitus, obesity, advanced age, and cardiorenal disease. Most infections are located on the lower extremities or near the perineum (e.g., originating in a perirectal abscess).[2]

The lesion may first manifest with small skin ulcers draining foul-smelling reddish-brown ("dishwater") pus. Circumscribed areas of blue-gray gangrene surround these draining sites, but the intervening skin appears normal despite necrosis of underlying subcutaneous tissues, fascia, and muscle. Local pain and tenderness are marked. Tissue gas is noted in about a quarter of the patients. Systemic toxicity is a feature; about half the patients have bacteremia.

Etiologic Agents

Cultures consistently show mixtures of anaerobic (anaerobic streptococci and/or *Bacteroides*) and facultative bacteria (*Klebsiella-Enterobacter, E. coli, Proteus*).[2] *Bacteroides* has been reported as the major pathogen on occasion.[17]

Presumptive Therapy

Initial surgery involves incision and drainage, but radical débridement is often necessary because of extensive involvement of deep fascia and muscle.[2,17] Amputation may be required. Antibiotic management initially is based on the results of Gram-stained smears of wound exudates, but it should include an antimicrobial effective against *Bacteroides* (see "Presumptive Therapy" above for type I necrotizing fasciitis).

MISCELLANEOUS INFECTIONS SECONDARY TO TRAUMA

Bite Infections

See Chapter 80.

Burn Infections

See Chapter 79.

Injection Site Abscesses

Subcutaneous and intramuscular abscesses infrequently occur after therapeutic injections. *Staphylococcus aureus*, facultative gram-negative bacilli, and anaerobic bacteria are usually implicated. Hematomas may be the site of delayed infections. Gas gangrene has followed various injections, particularly epinephrine in oil.[5] Subcutaneous and intramuscular abscesses due to a variety of oral anaerobes and streptococci have occurred after "skin popping" or attempted intravenous injections by narcotic addicts.[3] In the case of subcutaneous abscesses secondary to intravenous drug abuse, appropriate débridement and drainage should include excision of involved veins, which often contain pus or an infected thrombus.[18]

Factitial Disease (Self-Induced Abscesses)

Occasionally, subcutaneous abscesses and cellulitis are produced when a patient deliberately injects or inserts into the skin contaminated substances.[19,20] Such abscesses often are recurrent and may be of mono- or polymicrobial etiology (often consisting of oral or fecal flora). Sterile abscesses may be induced by introduction of foreign material without bacterial contamination. Such foreign material may be identified by examination of biopsy specimens with polarizing microscopy.

SUBCUTANEOUS INFECTIONS ORIGINATING IN CONTIGUOUS FOCI

Osteomyelitis

In an occasional patient, most commonly a child, acute hematogenous osteomyelitis may manifest as a subcutaneous abscess. Under these circumstances, a subperiosteal abscess has ruptured through intervening tissues into the subcutaneous tissues. *Staphylococcus aureus* is the most common etiologic agent in such infections. It is important to recognize the nature of the process because of the different therapeutic programs required for osteomyelitis in contrast to a subcutaneous abscess of cutaneous origin. Involvement of subcutaneous tissues as a consequence of osteomyelitis may also occur in the form of a draining sinus associated with chronic osteomyelitis and sequestrum formation. Multiple draining sinuses may occur as a result of multiple foci of osteomyelitis in disseminated blastomycosis.

Actinomycosis

Subcutaneous abscesses frequently develop in the course of cervical, thoracic, or sometimes abdominal actinomycosis. Draining sinuses ultimately result (see Chapter 233).

Primary Pyodermas

On occasion, more superficial skin infections, beginning as folliculitis, furunculosis, or cellulitis, may progress into the deeper subcutaneous tissues and form a subcutaneous (sometimes "cold") abscess. *Staphylococcus aureus* is commonly the etiology. Such progression repeatedly might suggest certain underlying phagocytic cell defects such as chronic granulomatous disease of childhood or hyperimmunoglobulin E syndrome (Job syndrome).[21,22]

SUBCUTANEOUS ABSCESSES IN THE COURSE OF BACTEREMIC INFECTIONS

Metastatic pyogenic infections can occur during the course of bacteremias or endocarditis due to invasive organisms (e.g., *S. aureus*) in subcutaneous tissues as well as a variety of other organs and tissues. These abscesses are tender and fluctuant.

Rarely, multiple, firm, nodular subcutaneous lesions, clinically resembling those of Weber-Christian disease, occur in the course of a staphylococcal bacteremia. If promptly identified and treated, the process may be aborted before frank abscess formation occurs.

MYCETOMA

See Chapter 240.

REFERENCES

1. Wilson HD, Haltalin KC. Acute necrotizing fasciitis in childhood. Am J Dis Child. 1973;125:591.
2. Stone HH, Martin JJ Jr. Synergistic necrotizing cellulitis. Ann Surg. 1972;175:702.
3. Finegold SM. Anaerobic Bacteria in Human Disease. New York: Academic Press; 1977:Chap. 13.
4. MacLennan JD. The histotoxic clostridial infections of man. Bact Rev. 1962;26:177.
5. Bornstein DL, Weinberg AN, Swartz MN, et al. Anaerobic infections: A review of current experience. Medicine. 1964;43:207.
6. Bessman AN, Wagner W. Nonclostridial gas gangrene. JAMA. 1975;233:958.
7. Rea WJ, Wyrick WJ Jr. Necrotizing fasciitis. Ann Surg. 1970;172:957.
8. Giuliano A, Lewis F Jr, Hadley K, et al. Bacteriology of necrotizing fasciitis. Am J Surg. 1977;134:52.
9. Casali RE, Tucker WE, Petrino RA, et al. Postoperative necrotizing fasciitis of the abdominal wall. Am J Surg. 1980;140:787.
10. Galbut DL, Gerber DL, Belgraier AH. Spontaneous necrotizing fasciitis. Occurrence secondary to occult diverticulitis. JAMA. 1977;238:2302.
11. Barza MJ, Proppe KH. Case records of the Massachusetts General Hospital. N Engl J Med. 1979;301:370.
12. Schecter W, Meyer A, Schecter G, et al. Necrotizing fasciitis of the upper extremity. J Hand Surg. 1982;7:15.
13. Lally KP, Atkinson JB, Woolley MM, et al. Necrotizing fasciitis: A serious sequela of omphalitis in the newborn. Ann Surg. 1984;199:101.
14. Sudarsky LA, Laschinger JC, Coppa GF, et al. Improved results from a standardized approach in treating patients with necrotizing fasciitis. Ann Surg. 1987;206:661.
15. Nickel JC, Morales A. Necrotizing fasciitis of the male genitalia (Fournier's gangrene). Can Med Assoc J. 1983;129:445.
16. Stamenkovic I, Lew PD. Early recognition of potentially fatal necrotizing fasciitis: Use of frozen-section biopsy. N Engl J Med. 1984;310:1689.
17. Baxter CR. Surgical management of soft tissue infections. Surg Clin North Am. 1972;52:1483.
18. Biderman P, Hiatt JR. Management of soft-tissue infections of the upper extremity in parenteral drug abusers. Am J Surg. 1987;154:526.
19. Aduan RP, Fauci AS, Dale DC, et al. Factitious fever and self-induced infection: A report of 32 cases and review of the literature. Ann Intern Med. 1979;90:230.
20. Reich P, Gottfried LA. Factitious disorders in a teaching hospital. Ann Intern Med. 1983;99:240.
21. Dreskin SC, Gallin JI. Evolution of the hyperimmunoglobulin E and recurrent infection (HIE, JOB'S) syndrome in a young girl. J Allergy Clin Immunol. 1987;80:746.
22. Curnutte JT, Boxer LA. Clinically significant phagocytic cell defects. In: Remington JS, Swartz MN, eds. Current Clinical Topics in Infectious Diseases. v. 6. New York: McGraw-Hill; 1985:103–156.

76. MYOSITIS

MORTON N. SWARTZ

Infection of skeletal muscle (infectious myositis) is uncommon. When it occurs, a wide range of organisms may be responsible: bacteria, mycobacteria, fungi, viruses, and parasitic agents. Bacteria invade muscle either from contiguous sites of infection (skin and subcutaneous abscesses, penetrating wounds, decubitus ulcers, osteomyelitis) or by hematogenous spread from a distant focus. It is helpful to categorize infectious myositis on the basis of clinical manifestations. These may be very distinctive, as in clostridial gas gangrene, and suggest the specific etiologic agent; or they may be very nonspecific, as in the myalgias of viral infections and infective endocarditis (Table 1). In certain instances (e.g., psoas abscess), it is the anatomic location rather than the morphologic characteristics of the lesion or the nature of the infecting agent that distinguishes the particular type of muscle infection.

PYOMYOSITIS

Pyomyositis is an acute bacterial infection of skeletal muscle usually due to *Staphylococcus aureus*. The accumulation of pus is always intramuscular initially. Clinically, it is characterized by localized muscle pain, swelling, and tenderness.

Pathogenesis and Pathologic Characteristics

Bacterial infections of muscle usually occur after a penetrating wound, prolonged vascular insufficiency in an extremity, or a contiguous infection. Bacteremic spread of infection to skeletal muscle is extremely uncommon. Of fatal cases of staphylococcal septicemia, abscesses in skeletal muscle are found in less than 1 percent.[1] Pyomyositis (primary muscle abscess) is a bacterial infection of muscle occurring in the absence of a predisposing site of infection. *Staphylococcus aureus* is the most common etiology.[2] Blood cultures are positive in less than 5 percent of the cases at the time of clinical manifestation; metastatic infections in tissue other than muscle are rare.

Most cases of pyomyositis occur in the tropics, hence the term *tropical pyomyositis*. It accounts for 1–4 percent of hospital admissions in some tropical areas.[2,3] In the United States pyomyositis is very rare (only 31 cases reported up to 1984), occurring both in persons who have recently immigrated from the tropics and in those who have always resided in a temperate climate.[4–6] As yet, no convincing evidence to relate pyomyositis causally to predisposing circumstances peculiar to the tropics (malaria, filariasis, arbovirus infection) has been developed. Migration of the guinea worm, *Dracunculus medinensis*, in the deep connective tissues of the lower extremities may be complicated by staphylococcal abscesses. However, these are located between muscle groups and are not the intramuscular abscesses typical of pyomysitis. Staphylococcal myositis has been reported in immunosuppressed hosts in the temperate zone.[7,8]

Clinical Findings

Pyomyositis occurs at all ages. In 20–50 percent of cases, there has been recent trauma to the involved area. The onset is most often subacute, with localized muscle pain, then swelling, with induration and tenderness, developing over several days. Fever generally follows the onset of localizing symptoms by a few days. In an occasional patient the onset is acute, with malaise, chills, and high fever. In a rare patient, the clinical picture is combined with that of toxic shock syndrome.[9] The most frequent sites of involvement are the lower limb and trunk muscles.

Since the muscle abscesses are contained by the overlying fascia, local erythema and heat may be minimal until the process extends through to the subcutaneous tissues some days or weeks later. The initial local swelling is "woody" on palpation and pain may not be striking, directing attention away from an infectious etiology. Regional lymphadenitis is not prominent. Only a single muscle group is usually involved, but multiple muscle abscesses occur in up to 40 percent of the patients.

In addition to producing an occasional case of typical pyomyositis with abscess formation, on rare occasions group A streptococci cause a fulminant form of pyomyositis (peracute streptococcal pyomyositis, streptococcal necrotizing myositis, spontaneous streptococcal gangrenous myositis).[10,11] The entire clinical course may be telescoped to 2–3 days. Bacteremia and toxemia are prominent features and contribute to the very high mortality. Intramuscular pressure may lead to muscle necrosis,

TABLE 1. Classification of Infectious Myositis

Type of Process	*Clinical Pattern*	*Principal Specific Etiologies*
Pyogenic and predominantly localized (spreading by contiguity)	Pyomyositis	*S. aureus;* group A streptococcus (rarely)
	Gas gangrene	*C. perfringens;* occasionally other histotoxic clostridial species
	Nonclostridial (crepitant) myositis	
	Anaerobic streptococcal gangrene	*Peptostreptococcus* (plus group A streptococci or *S. aureus*)
	Synergistic nonclostridial anaerobic myonecrosis	Mixed infections: *Bacteroides* and other anaerobic non-spore-forming gram-negative bacilli; *Peptostreptococcus* and various streptococci; *E. coli; Klebsiella; Enterobacter*
	Infected vascular gangrene	Same as for synergistic nonclostridial anaerobic myonecrosis
	Aeromonas hydrophila myonecrosis	*Aeromonas hydrophila*
	Psoas abscess	Gram-negative bacilli; *S. aureus;* mixed infections; *M. tuberculosis*
Nonpyogenic and predominantly generalized	Myalgias	Viral infections (e.g., influenza, dengue); infective endocarditis; bacteremias (e.g., meningococcemia); rickettsioses (e.g., Rocky Mountain spotted fever); toxoplasmosis
	Pleurodynia	Coxsackievirus B
	Myalgias with eosinophilia	
	Trichinosis	*Trichinella spiralis*
	Cysticercosis (also subcutaneous nodules)	*Taenia solium*
	Muscle degeneration and destruction associated with infections elsewhere	
	Acute rhabdomyolysis	Viral influenza, echovirus, coxsackie and Epstein-Barr viruses, *Legionella*

much as in a compartment syndrome. This process differs from necrotizing fasciitis in that the skin and fascia are minimally if at all involved.[12,13]

A leukocytosis occurs. Eosinophilia is common in patients (even in the presence of a prominent leukocytosis) with tropical pyomyositis and appears to reflect the prevalence of parasitic infestation. Serum muscle enzyme levels may be elevated but frequently are normal despite gross muscle destruction. However, marked rhabdomyolysis with myoglobinuria and acute renal failure has developed in a patient with pyomyositis.[14]

Etiologic Agents

Staphylococcus aureus is responsible for 95 percent of the cases. Group A streptococci account for 1–5 percent of the cases. Other rare bacterial causes include *Streptococcus pneumoniae, Haemophilus influenzae, Escherichia coli, Klebsiella* spp., *Yersinia enterocolitica*, and other *Pseudomonas* spp. *Pseudomonas mallei* and *Pseudomonas pseudomallei* occasionally cause abscesses in muscle in the septicemic or chronic suppurative forms of the diseases they produce, glanders and meliodosis, respectively. *Aspergillus fumigatus* has caused localized myositis in a patient with myelodysplasia. Other causes of fungal myositis include disseminated cryptococcal and candidal infections.

Differential Diagnosis

Early in the course of pyomyositis, other diagnoses may be suspected, particularly in nontropical areas: osteomyelitis, septic arthritis, muscle hematoma, muscle rupture, and thrombophlebitis. Streptococcal necrotizing fasciitis, like gangrenous streptococal myositis, produces localized swelling, tenderness, and erythema, but it is less common and produces necrosis of fascia and skin. In the patient with multiple sites of muscle involvement and eosinophilia (from incidental parasitic infestation), the picture may suggest trichinosis. This resemblance ends when localized swellings become prominent and markedly tender. Rupture of the muscle abscess through the fascia into subcutaneous tissues may suggest the diagnosis of cellulitis. Radionuclide (^{67}Ga) scanning shows diffuse uptake in the involved area but does not distinguish an intramuscular abscess from necrotizing myositis or necrotizing fasciitis. Computed tomography can reveal low-density areas with loss of muscle planes characteristic of pyomyositis.

Presumptive Therapy

Surgical (open or ultrasound-guided percutaneous) drainage of all abscesses is essential. Initial antibiotic therapy should consist of intravenous administration of a β-lactamase-resistant penicillin because of the preponderance of penicillin-resistant *S. aureus* isolates from such abscesses. If a group A streptococcus is isolated, treatment should be changed to penicillin G. Continued fever after surgical drainage of a muscle abscess while the patient is receiving appropriate antimicrobial therapy should suggest the presence of other undrained suppurative foci. Streptococcal necrotizing myositis requires prompt radical débridement of all necrotic muscles.

GAS GANGRENE (CLOSTRIDIAL MYONECROSIS)

Gas gangrene is a rapidly progressive, life-threatening, toxemic infection of skeletal muscle due to clostridia (principally *Clostridium perfringens*). It usually follows muscle injury and contamination, as in a dirty traumatic wound, or sometimes surgery.

Pathogenesis and Pathologic Characteristics

Gas gangrene occurs in settings having in common muscle injury and contamination with soil or other foreign material containing spores of *C. perfringens* or other histotoxic clostridial species: (*1*) accidental traumatic civilian injuries such as compound fractures,[15] (*2*) penetrating war wounds,[16] (*3*) surgical wounds, particularly after bowel or biliary tract surgery,[17] and (*4*) arterial insufficiency in an extremity.[17] Rare cases of gas gangrene have occurred after parenteral injection of medication, particularly epinephrine in oil. A fulminant case has been described beginning at the site of a simple venipuncture in a granulocytopenic patient.[17] *Clostridium perfringens* are usually present in large numbers as normal flora in human feces and thus can endogenously contaminate skin surfaces. Despite a high frequency (up to 88 percent) of clostridial contamination of major traumatic, open wounds, the incidence of gas gangrene in this setting is only 1–2 percent,[18] emphasizing the importance of devitalized tissue and the presence of foreign bodies in the pathogenesis of gas gangrene. The minimal dose of *C. perfringens* needed to produce fatal gas gangrene in the experimental animal is reduced by a factor of 10^6 when injected into devitalized muscle contaminated with sterile dirt rather than into normal muscle. The policy of prompt, thorough débridement and of leaving wounds open has decreased the incidence of gas gangrene in wartime injuries; only 22 cases among 139,000 combat casualties in Vietnam have been reported.[19]

Gas gangrene may occasionally develop in the absence of an obvious external wound. It may manifest in the buttocks or flanks as the consequence of an intra-abdominal catastrophe, with extension of infection along the iliopsoas or other deep muscle groups. Such "idiopathic" gas gangrene may occur at a greater distance from the original intra-abdominal focus, spreading by the bacteremic route. *Clostridium septicum* has been involved, often with documented bacteremia, in clostridial infections occurring in the setting of neoplastic disease (particularly leukemia and carcinoma of the colon).[20,21] The primary source of the organism is probably mucosal ulceration or perforation of the intestinal tract.

The involved muscle undergoes rapid disintegration. Initially, it may exhibit only pallor, edema, and loss of elasticity. When examined in the operating room, it fails to contract on stimulation and does not bleed from a cut surface. Later it becomes discolored (reddish purple, then greenish purple and gangrenous) and friable. Histologically, the muscle fibers show coaglation necrosis, and the supporting connective tissue is destroyed; numerous gram-positive bacilli are present.

Clinical Findings

The usual incubation period between injury and the development of clostridial myonecrosis is 2–3 days, but it may be as short as 6 hours. The onset is acute. Pain is the earliest and most important symptom. It rapidly increases in intensity and is more severe than the pain that is generally associated with the preceding injury or surgical procedure. The patient soon appears severely ill, pale, and sweaty. The pulse is rapid, the blood pressure falls, and shock and renal failure follow. The patient may be apathetic or may be apprehensive and restless but mentally clear. Delirium, stupor, and unconsciousness may supervene. Fever is frequently present, but often with temperature elevations of less than 38.3°C (101°F). Hypothermia is a poor prognostic sign and is usually associated with shock. Jaundice may become evident. The process may rapidly progress over a period of hours, with a fatal outcome if not properly treated.

Appearance of the Local Lesion. Very early, tense edema and local tenderness may be the only findings. If an open wound is present, swollen muscle may herniate through. A serosanguineous, dirty-appearing discharge, containing numerous organisms but few leukocytes, escapes from the wound. The wound has a peculiar foul odor. Gas bubbles may be visible in the discharge. Crepitus is usually present but not prominent; sometimes it is completely obscured by very marked edema. The skin adjacent to the wound is initially swollen and white, but rapidly takes on a yellowish or bronze discoloration (Fig. 1). Tense blebs containing thin serosanguineous or dark fluid develop in the overlying skin, and areas of green-black cutaneous necrosis appear. In fulminant cases, progression of the

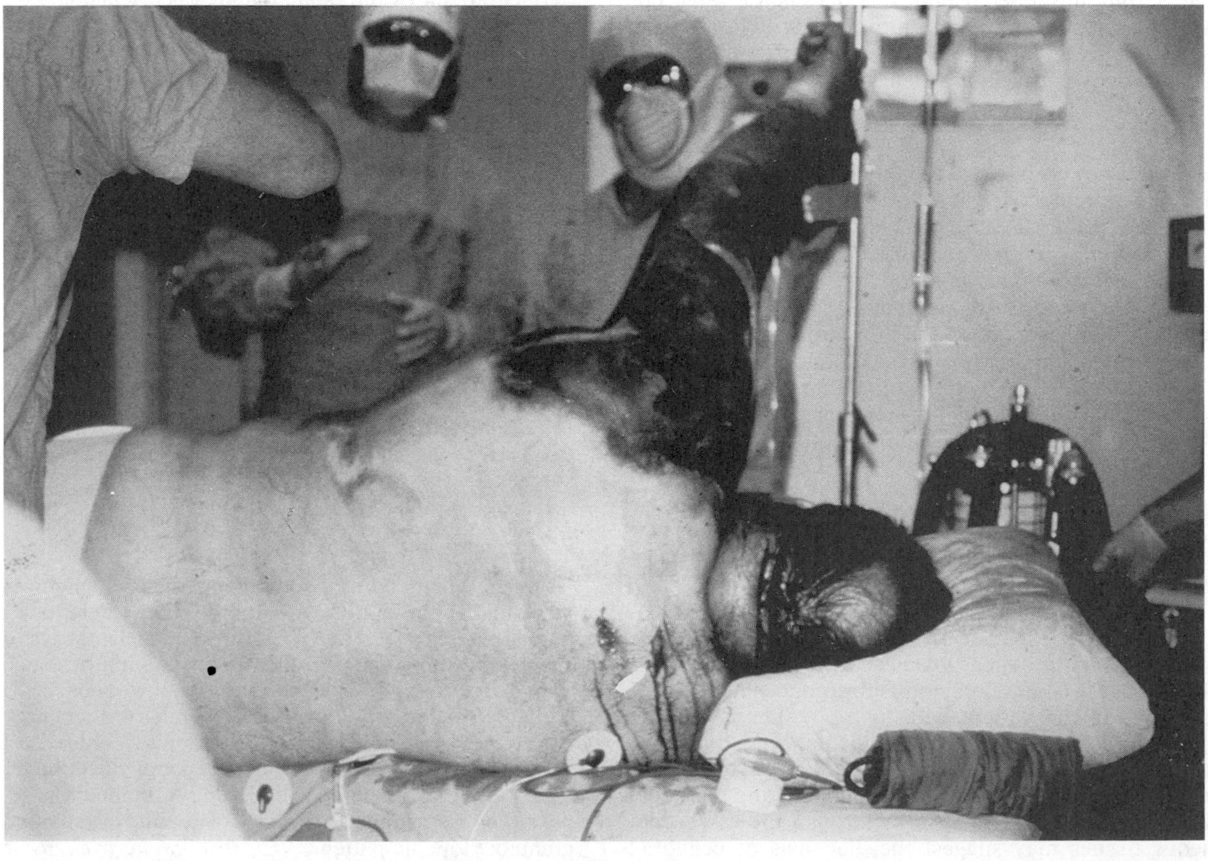

Fig. 1. Clostridial gas gangrene of the left upper extremity. There is prominent characteristic bronze discoloration of the skin extending over the shoulder. Crepitus could be palpated beyond the area of discoloration onto the back.

changes occurs over 2–4 hours, as indicated by the advance of the area of edema and crepitation.

Laboratory Findings

The hematocrit level is usually reduced. *Clostridium perfringens* bacteremia occurs in about 15 percent of the patients with gas gangrene.[22] Intense bacteremia (with associated intravascular hemolysis) is more likely to occur as a complication of uterine infection. A leukocytosis is common.

Gram-stained smear of the wound exudate or of an aspirate from one of the blebs reveals many large, gram-positive bacilli with blunt ends but few polymorphonuclear leukocytes (see Chapter 222, Fig. 1). In almost all cases, spores are not evident. Not infrequently, scattered gram-negative bacilli are also present, particularly in grossly contaminated wounds.

X-ray films of the involved areas show extensive and progressive gaseous dissection of muscle and fascial planes.

Etiologic Agents

Clostridium perfringens is most commonly isolated from the lesions of gas gangrene (80–95 percent of the cases).[15,19] *Clostridium novyi* is involved in 10–40 percent of the cases and *C. septicum* in 5–20 percent. Other clostridial species (*C. bifermentans, C. histolyticum, C. fallax*) have been implicated on rare occasions. In addition to clostridia, other organisms (*E. coli, Enterobacter*, enterococci, and so forth) are sometimes isolated from the lesions of gas gangrene, reflecting the contaminated character of the initiating trauma or lesion.[22]

Differential Diagnosis

The major considerations in differential diagnosis ae gas-forming infections of the soft tissues (clostridial anaerobic cellulitis, nonclostridial crepitant myositis, nonclostridial crepitant cellulitis). Clostridial anaerobic cellulitis (Chapter 74) is more gradual in onset and progression, and the systemic manifestations of illness are much milder than in gas gangrene. Local pain is relatively mild, and the skin lesions of gas gangrene (bronzing, dark blebs) do not develop. Gas formation is often much more extensive in clostridial cellulitis than in gas gangrene. Clinically, it is often difficult to distinguish between early clostridial cellulitis and myonecrosis. Definitive evaluation requires examination in the operating room for the characteristic changes of myonecrosis described earlier. The clinical picture of nonclostridial crepitant cellulitis is very similar to that of clostridial cellulitis. Although contamination of an operative or traumatic wound may be the source of infection in both types of cellulitis, nonclostridial crepitant cellulitis frequently develops in the setting of vascular insufficiency or perirectal infection. Bacteria isolated from nonclostridial crepitant cellulitis include facultative species (*E. coli, Klebsiella*, various streptococci) and anaerobic bacteria (*Bacteroides, Peptostreptococcus*, and so forth). Commonly, these are present in mixed culture and can be seen on Gram-stained smear of a wound aspirate.

Presumptive Therapy

Treatment includes emergency surgical exploration both to define the nature of the process (gas gangrene vs. crepitant cellulitis) by direct examination of muscles at the site of infection and to carry out appropriate débridement. Prompt and extensive surgery is the principle element in the treatment of gas gangrene. This includes excision of involved muscles (or amputation when necessary) and fasciotomies to decompress and to drain the swollen fascial compartments. Antibiotic therapy is an important adjunct to surgical management. Penicillin G is the antibiotic of choice and is administered intravenously in a dosage for the adult of 1–2 million units every 2–3 hours. A second antibiotic, such as chloramphenicol, is sometimes added initially when Gram-stained smears of the wound exudate show gram-negative bacilli as well as the predominant gram-positive bacilli. Chloramphenicol is also a good alernative drug in the highly penicillin-allergic patient; it is preferable to tetracycline or clindamycin in view of the resistance of some clostridia to these agents. Although the majority of *C. perfringens* isolates ae susceptible in vitro to first-, second-, and third-generation cephalosporins, the minimum inhibitory concentrations for at least 10 percent of isolates are above levels readily achievable in vivo.[23] The demonstration of plasmids mediating transferable drug resistance (tetracycline and chloramphenicol; perhaps erythromycin and clindamycin) in *C. perfringens*[24] suggests the need for periodic monitoring of antibiotic susceptibilities of clinical isolates. Recent evidence suggests that some strains of this organism may be showing somewhat less susceptibility in vitro to penicillin than was formerly the case.[23] *Clostridium perfringens* are susceptible in vitro to metronidazole, but experience with the use of this drug in clostridial myonecrosis is lacking.

The role of hyperbaric oxygen therapy is still under debate. Its most appropriate role at present would appear to be in the management of patients with extensive involvement of the trunk in whom surgical excision would be mutilating.[25] Initial hyperbaric oxygen therapy may reduce the extent of débridement necessary under these circumstances. The efficacy of intravenously administered polyvalent gas gangrene antitoxin has never been established clinically. It is no longer available. Ancillary therapy is essential in the management of gas gangrene. This includes attention to fluid and electrolyte replacement and maintenance of adequate hematocrit levels by transfusions.

NONCLOSTRIDIAL (CREPITANT) MYOSITIS

Nonclostridial (crepitant) myositis includes four relatively distinct entities, differing from gas gangrene in their clinical picture and bacteriologic characteristics: (*1*) anaerobic streptococcal myonecrosis, (*2*) synergistic nonclostridial anaerobic myonecrosis, (*3*) infected vascular gangrene and (*4*) *Aeromonas hydrophila* myonecrosis.

Anaerobic Streptococcal Myonecrosis

This is an acute interstitial myositis that clinically resembles subacute clostridial gas gangrene. The initial manifestations are swelling and a copious seropurulent exudate occurring 3–4 days after injury. Pain develops subsequently, unlike the early occurrence of pain in gas gangrene. Tissue gas is present in muscle and fascial planes but is not extensive. The wound has an unpleasant sour odor. The involved muscles are discolored but do react to stimulation. In contrast to gas gangrene, early cutaneous erythema is prominent. If not adequately treated, the infection progresses, with the development of toxemia, frank gangrene, and shock.

Numerous streptococci and polymorphonuclear leukocytes are present in the exudate. The infection is usually mixed (anaerobic streptococci with group A streptococci or *S. aureus*). A mixed infection of muscle with both peptostreptococci and *Bacillus subtilis* has been observed on several occasions in the setting of vascular injury. The clinical picture, along with the appearance of the Gram-stained smear, initially might suggest the diagnosis of clostridial myonecrosis.[26] Treatment involves the use of large doses of penicillin and surgical debridement.

Synergistic Nonclostridial Anaerobic Myonecrosis. This severe infection, also known as *synergistic necrotizing cellulitis* (Chapter 75), involves skin, subcutaneous tissue, fascia, and muscle. The most extensive involvement is in the subcutaneous tissues and fascia; changes in the overlying skin and underlying muscle are usually secondary.

Infected Vascular Gangrene[27]

This is a mixed infection developing in a group of muscles or in a limb devitalized as a result of arterial insufficiency, particularly in patients with diabetes mellitus. *Proteus, Bacteroides*, and anaerobic streptococci are among the bacteria found in such lesions. Gas formation and foul-smelling pus are prominent. The infection does not extend beyond the area of vascular gangrene to involve healthy muscle. *Bacillus cereus* infection has been associated with myonecrosis with slight crepitance after thrombosis of arterial grafts.[28]

Aeromonas Hydrophila Myonecrosis

Rapidly progressivve myonecosis due to *Aeromonas hydrophila*, a facultative, anaerobic, gram-negative bacillus, may follow penetrating trauma either in a freshwater environment or associated with fish or other aquatic animals.[29,30] In a few instances, myonecrosis has been accompanied by gas spreading extensively in soft tissue planes. The rapid onset (24–48 hours) and rapid progression after trauma resemble those of clostridial gas gangrene. The prominence of pain, marked edema, serosanguineous bullae, and toxicity, as well as the presence of gas in fascial planes, adds to the similarity of these conditions. Baceremia is frequently present. Treatment consists of extensive surgical débridement and prompt initiation of antimicrobial therapy. Most isolates of *Aeromonas* are susceptible in vitro to chloramphenicol, tetracyclines, gentamicin, tobramycin, and trimethoprim-sulfamethoxazole. Cefotaxime and moxalactam also appear to be active.[31]

PSOAS ABSCESS

Infection of the psoas muscle takes the form of either an abscess or a phlegmon. It is usually the consequence of spread of infection from an adjacent structure. Rarely, it develops by the hematogenous route; in children particularly, there may be no prior inciting event such as trauma or preceding infection, and *S. aureus* is the most common etiology in this setting. Psoas abscess usually is confined within the psoas fascia, but occasionally, due to anatomic relations, infection extends to the buttock, hip, or upper thigh. Psoas abscess may complicate pyogenic or tuberculous vertebral osteomyelitis. The latter was formerly the principle cause of a psoas abscess; now psoas abscesses most commonly result from direct extension of intra-abdominal infections (diverticulitis, appendicitis, Crohn's disease, and so on).[32] Occasionally, a psoas abscess results from extension of a perinephric abscess or from secondary infection of a retroperitoneal hematoma. The organisms involved in spread of infection from an intestinal site are usually members of the aerobic and anaerobic bowel flora. *Staphylococcus aureus* is the most common cause of psoas abscess secondary to vertebral osteomyelitis.

The iliacus muscle, applied to the ilium in the iliac fossa, forms a conjoined tendon with the lower portion of the psoas muscle. Osteomyelitis of the ilium or septic arthritis of the sacroiliac joint can penetrate the sheathes of either or both muscles in this location, producing an iliacus or psoas abscess.[33]

Clinical manifestations of a psoas abscess include fever, lower abdominal or back pain, or pain referred to the hip or knee. A limp may be evident and flexion deformity of the hip may develop from reflex spasm, suggesting septic arthritis of the hip. The psoas sign is evident. Often a tender mass can be palpated in the groin.

Roentgenograms may show a bulge produced by a psoas muscle abscess or the presence of gas within the psoas sheath. Calcification in a psoas abscess strongly suggests a tuberculous etiology.

Of the four noninvasive techniques currently available for visualization of the psoas (and iliacus) muscles, computed tomography (CT) scanning is the most rapid and sensitive. Ultrasound is less reliable for detecting small lesions or a phlegmon. Gallium scanning does not provide as sharp a localization and takes up to 72 hours; indium-labeled white blood cell scanning may be preferable to the latter. CT scanning may show diffuse enlargement of the psoas (phlegmon) or sharply circumscribed, low-density fluid collections (abscess) within the muscle, or may demonstrate the presence of gas within the muscle (indicative of abscess).[34]

Pyogenic psoas abscesses are treated by surgical drainage and provisional initial antibiotic therapy based on knowledge of the origin of the infection. CT scanning maybe of considerable value for guidance of direct needle aspiration of an abscess for culture or for drainage when the direct surgical approach is not preferable or warranted. When the process appears to be a phlegmon, repeated CT scanning during the course of antibiotic therapy can confirm resolution of the anatomic changes.

MYALGIAS

Myalgias are prominent features of a variety of infections such as dengue, influenza, and Rocky Mountain spotted fever. Little information is available on the presence of specific histologic findings indicative of myositis.

Influenza

Muscle aches are common early in the course of influenza. Occasionally, severe bilateral muscle pains in the lower limbs may develop in the recovery phase, particularly in young children.[35,36] Muscle tenderness, principally in the gastrocnemius and soleus muscles, is demonstrable and calf swelling may be present. Deep tendon reflexes and muscle strength are normal, but there is considerable difficulty in walking. The leg pains and muscle tenderness subside in less than a week. Mild elevations of serum levels of aldolase and creatine phosphokinase occur. The few biopsies performed have shown either nonspecific degenerative changes or muscle necrosis with polymorphonuclear leukocytic infiltration. Whether this "myositis" is due to direct viral invasion or to some immunologic or other response is unknown. However, influenza A virus has been isolated from the muscle biopsy specimen of an adult with generalized muscle weakness occurring during an influenza A outbreak.[37]

Infective Endocarditis

Prominent myalgias occur in about 15 percent of patients with infective endocarditis.[38] They may be either diffuse or localized. The pathogenesis is not known, but in one instance muscle biopsy specimens showed a small focus of muscle fiber destruction and leukocytic infiltration consistent with embolization to a small artery.[38]

Toxoplasmosis

The major features of acute acquired disseminated toxoplasmosis are those of meningoencephalitis, myocarditis, pneumonitis, skin rash, and occasionally hepatitis (Chapter 252). In rare instances, polymyositis may be a prominent clinical manifestation. Marked myalgias, muscle weakness and swelling, and fasciculations occur in such patients. Muscle biopsy specimens show interstitial myositis with destruction of muscle fibers, and pseudocysts of *Toxoplasma gondii* can be found in areas of muscle free of inflammatory reaction. In several cases *Toxoplasma* have been isolated by animal inoculation.[39,40]

Other Etiologies

Occasionally, the only clinical manifestations of initial infection with human immunodeficiency virus (HIV) retrovirus are those of polymyositis (myalgias, muscle weakness, and increased serum levels of muscle enzymes). HIV viral antigens can be found in OKT4 cells in areas of muscle fiber inflammation and necrosis.[41] Inflammatory myositis with a lymphoplasmacytic cellular response was the major feature in a case of Lyme disease.[42] Spirochetes morphologically similar to *Borrelia burgdorferi* were present on Dieterle silver stain of biopsied muscle. Rarely, *Sarcocystis* (an intracellular sporozoan parasite) infection has been observed in histologic sections of muscle of individuals, mainly from abroad, with muscle pain or weakness.[43] Microsporidia myositis has occurred in a patient with acquired immunodeficiency syndrome (AIDS).[44]

PLEURODYNIA SYNDROMES

Epidemic pleuodynia is an acute, febrile disease due to group B coxsackieviruses and is characterized by the sudden onset of sharp chest pain over the lower ribs or sternum (Chapter 150). Paroxysms of knife-like pain are precipitated by voluntary or respiratory movments. Muscle tenderness may be present. Abdominal pain may also be present in some patients; in others abdominal pain may be the sole manifestation, simulating intraperitoneal processes.

Group B coxsackieviruses produce visceral lesions and also some focal myositis in experimental animals. Myositis has not been demonstrated as a feature pathologically either in the fatal cases of severe neonatal coxsackievirus B infection or in the few biopsy specimens obtained from affected muscles of patients with epidemic pleurodynia.[45,46]

MYALGIAS WITH EOSINOPHILIA (PARASITIC MYOSITIS)

Trichinosis

The prominent clinical manifestations of trichinosis include fever, myositis, periorbital edema, and eosinophilia. An initial intestinal phase during the first week after infection is followed during the second week by larval invasion of skeletal muscle (Chapter 264). Serious complications in the form of myocarditis, meningoencephalitis, and pneumonitis can occur.[47] Myalgias, frequently accompanied by muscle swelling and weakness and occasionally associated with fasciculations, are present in most patients with the disease. Muscles commonly involved include the extraocular muscles, flexor muscles of the extremities, back muscles, and the muscles used in chewing and swallowing. Periorbital edema, chemosis, and conjunctival hemorrhages are related to larval invasion of extraocular muscles. The inflammatory response in muscle produces an elevation of serum levels of muscle enzymes.

Muscle biopsy specimens reveal encysted larval trichinae in necrotic muscle fibers surrounded by inflammatory cells (predominantly eosinophils and neutrophils, but also lymphocytes). Severe skeletal muscle involvement has been reported in a case of trichinosis in an immunosuppressed patient.[48] Although granulomatous reactions have been observed in the heart and lungs of fatal cases, larval encystment does not take place in organs other than skeletal muscle.

Cysticerosis (Cysticerus Cellulosal Myositis)

Human cysticerosis is rare in the United States but is common in Latin America and Asia. It results from the ingestion and subsequent hatching of viable eggs of *Taenia solium* into the larval form of the parasite *Cysticercus cellulosae* (Chapter 266). Eggs reach the upper intestinal tract from food contaminated by feces from a person parasitized by the adult worm. Autoinfection can occur through the fecal-oral route and possibly when reverse peristalsis introduces egg-laden proglottids back into the duodenum or stomach where they hatch. From there they are distributed widely (skeletal muscle, subcutaneous tissues, heart, eye).

Symptomatic involvement of muscle is uncommon. Occasionally, the stage of invasion is characterized by fever, muscle tenderness, and eosinophilia. More characteristically, asymptomatic calcified cysts (''puffed rice'' appearance) are detected in muscles on soft tissue x-ray films of patients with neurologic manifestations.

MUSCLE DEGENERATION ASSOCIATED WITH INFECTIONS AT OTHER SITES

Acute Rhabdomyolysis

Myoglobinuria occasionally follows an acute illness with symptoms suggesting an upper respiratory tract infection. Scattered cases in recent years have been shown to follow documented influenza A virus infections in children and adults,[49] legionnaires' disease, echovirus infections,[50] and infections due to coxsackie, Epstein-Barr, and adenovirus.[51] Diffuse muscle pains (especially in the extremities), weakness, swelling, and tenderness are prominent features, along with myoglobinuria. Rhabdomyolysis has occurred in patients who have had no previous episodes and no family history of this condition. Like the myositis after influenza occurring in children, it develops when respiratory symptoms are resolving.

Muscle Proteolysis and Mediators of Fever in Patients with Sepsis

Muscle involvement, in the form of myalgias and weakness, is common in the course of systemic infections. Accelerated catabolism of skeletal muscle contributes to the marked weakness and muscle wasting that can be observed in systemic infections. This appears to be part of a protective ''acute-phase'' host response to sepsis and trauma. The central role is played by interleukin-1 (IL-1), a polypeptide that appears identical to endogenous leukocytic pyrogen (EP). A polypeptide (possibly a breakdown product of IL-1) that produces a rapid increase in protein degradation in rat or human muscle preparations[52] has been observed in the plasma of patients with sepsis. Similar changes are produced by EP (IL-1) itself.[53] This accelerated proteolysis is effected through increased synthesis in muscle of prostaglandin E_2, which in turn activates proteases in muscle-cell lysosomes. This catabolic activity is accompanied by IL-1-stimulated hepatic protein synthesis (using the newly generated source of amino acids) and other elements of the acute-phase response, such as fever (also generated by IL-1 and mediated by prostaglandin E_2). The important role of prostaglandin E_2 in the generation of the muscle aches and fever of infection is consistent with the amelioration of these symptoms produced by prostaglandin synthesis inhibitors such as aspirin.

REFERENCES

1. Smith IM, Vickers AB. Natural history of 338 treated and untreated patients with staphylococcal septicaemia. Lancet. 1960;1:1318.
2. Levin MJ, Gardner P, Waldvogel FA. ''Tropical'' pyomyositis. An unusual infection due to *Staphylococcus aureus*. N Engl J Med. 1971;284:196.
3. Horn CV, Master S. Pyomyositis tropicans in Uganda. E Afr Med J. 1968;45:463.
4. Altrocchi PH. Spontaneous bacterial myositis. JAMA. 1971;217:819.
5. Echeverria P, Vaughn MC. ''Tropical pyomyositis.'' A diagnostic problem in temperate climates. Am J Dis Child. 1975;129:856.
6. Gibson RK, Rosenthal SJ, Lukert BP. Pyomyositis: Increasing recognition in temporate climates. Am J Med. 1984;77:768.
7. Jordan GW, Bauer R, Wong GA, et al. Staphylococcal myositis in a compromised host. West J Med. 1976;124:140.
8. Lachiewicz PF, Hadler NM. Spontaneous pyomyositis in a patient with Felty's syndrome: Diagnosis using computerized tomography. South Med J. 1986;79:1047.
9. Immerman RP, Greenman RL. Toxic shock syndrome associated with pyomyositis caused by a strain of *Staphylococcus aureus* that does not produce toxic-shock-syndrome toxin—1. J Infect Dis. 1987;156:505.

10. Svane S. Peracute spontaneous streptococcal myositis. Acta Chir Scand. 1971;137:155.
11. Moore DL, Delage G, Labelle H, et al. Peracute streptococcal pyomyositis: Report of two cases and review of the literature. J Pediatr Orthop. 1986;6:232.
12. Nather A, Wong FYH, Balasubramaniam P, et al: Streptococcal necrotizing myositis: A rare entity. Clin Orthop. 1987;215:206.
13. Yoder EL, Mendez J, Khatib R. Spontaneous gangrenous myositis induced by *Streptococcus pyogenes*: Case report and review of the literature. Rev Infect Dis. 1987;9:382.
14. Armstrong JH. Tropical pyomyositis and myoglobinuria. Arch Intern Med. 1978;138:1145.
15. Altemeier WA, Fullen WD. Prevention and treatment of gas gangrene. JAMA. 1971;217:806.
16. MacLennan JD. The histotoxic clostridial infections of man. Bact Rev. 1962;26:177.
17. Bornstein DL, Weinberg AN, Swartz MN, et al. Anaerobic infections: Review of current experience. Medicine. 1964;43:207.
18. Altemeier WA, Furste WL. Gas gangrene. Surg Gynecol Obstet. 1947;84:507.
19. Finegold SM. Anaerobic Bacteria in Human Disease. New York: Academic Press; 1977:424.
20. Alpern RJ, Dowell VR Jr. *Clostridium septicum* infections and malignancy. JAMA. 1969;209:385.
21. Jendrzejewski JW, Jones SR, Newcombe RL, et al. Nontraumatic clostridial myonecrosis. Am J Med. 1978;65:542.
22. Caplan ES, Kluge RM. Gas gangrene: Review of 34 cases. Arch Intern Med. 1976;136:788.
23. Marrie TJ, Haldane EV, Swantee CA, et al. Susceptibility of anaerobic bacteria to nine antimicrobial agents an demonstration of decreased susceptibility of *Clostridium perfringens* to penicillin. Antimicrob Agents Chemother. 1981;19:51.
24. Brefort G, Magot M, Ionesco H, et al. Characterization and transferability of *Clostridium perfringens* plasmids. Plasmid. 1977;1:52.
25. Shupak A, Halpern P, Ziser A, et al. Hyperbaric oxygen therapy for gas gangrene casualties in the Lebanon War, 1982. Isr J Med Sci. 1984;20:323.
26. Chambers CH, Bond GF, Morris JH. Synergistic necrotizing myositis complicating vascular injury. J Trauma. 1974;14:980.
27. Finegold SM. Anaerobic Bacteria in Human Disease. New York: Academic Press; 1977:425.
28. Johnson DA, Aulicino PL, Newby JG. *Bacillus cereus*-induced myonecrosis. J Trauma. 1984;24:267.
29. Davis WA, Kane JG, Garagusi VF. Human *Aeromonas* infections: A review of the literature and case report of endocarditis. Medicine. 1978;57:267.
30. Heckerling PS, Stine TM, Pottage JC, et al. *Aeromonas hydrophila* myonecrosis and gas gangrene in a nonimmunocompromised host. Arch Intern Med. 1983;143:2005.
31. Fass RJ, Barnishan J. In vitro susceptibilities of *Aeromonas hydrophila* to 32 antimicrobial agents. Antimicrob Agents Chemother. 1981;19:357.
32. Kyle J. Psoas abscess in Crohn's disease. Gastroenterology. 1971;61:149.
33. Simons GW, Sty JR, Starshak RJ, et al. Retroperitoneal and retrofascial abscesses. J Bone Joint Surg. 1983;65-A:1041.
34. Gordin F, Stamler C, Mills J. Pyogenic psoas abscesses: Noninvasive diagnostic techniques and review of the literature. Rev Infect Dis. 1983;5:1003.
35. Middleton PJ, Alexander RM, Szymanski MT. Severe myositis during recovery from influenza. Lancet. 1970;2:533.
36. Mejlszenkier JD, Safran AP, Healy JJ, et al. The myositis of influenza. Arch Neurol. 1973;29:441.
37. Kessler HA, Trenholme GM, Harris AA, et al. Acute myopathy associated with influenza A/Texas/1/77 infection. JAMA. 1980;243:461.
38. Churchill MA, Geraci JE, Hunder GG. Musculoskeletal manifestations of bacterial endocarditis. Ann Intern Med. 1977;87:754.
39. Greenlee JE, Johnson WD, Campa JF, et al. Adult toxoplasmosis presenting as polymyositis and cerebral ataxia. Ann Intern Med. 1975;82:367.
40. Kass EH, Andrus SB, Adams RD, et al. Toxoplasmosis in the human adult. Arch Intern Med. 1952;89:759.
41. Dalakas MC, Pezeshkpour GH, Gravell M, et al. Polymyositis associated with AIDS retrovirus. JAMA. 1986;256:2381.
42. Atlas E, Novak SN, Duray P, et al. Lyme myositis: Muscle invasion by *Borrelia burgdorferi*. Ann Intern Med. 1988;109:245.
43. Beaver PC, Gadgil RK, Morera P. Sarcocystis: A review and report of five cases. Am J Trop Med Hyg. 1979;28:819.
44. Ledford DK, Overman MD, Gonzalvo A, et al. Microsporidiosis myositis in a patient with the acquired immunodeficiency syndrome. Ann Intern Med. 1985;102:628.
45. Adams RD. Diseases of Muscle. A Study in Pathology, Hagerstown, Md.: Harper and Row; 1975:318.
46. Cherry JD. Enteroviruses. In: Remington JS, Klein JO, eds. Infectious Diseases of the Fetus and Newborn Infant. Philadelphia: WB Saunders; 1976:397.
47. Most H. Trichinosis: Preventable but still with us. N Engl J Med. 1978;298:1178.
48. Jacobson ES, Jacobson HG. Trichinosis in an immunosuppressed human host. Am J Clin Pathol. 1977;68:791.
49. Minow RA, Gorbach S, Johnson BL, et al. Myoglobinuria associated with influenza A infection. Ann Intern Med. 1974;80:359.
50. Josselson J, Pula T, Sadler JH. Acute rhabdomyolysis associated with an echovirus 9 infection. Arch Intern Med. 1980;140:1671.
51. Meshkinpour H, Vaziri ND. Acute rhabdomyolysis associated with adenovirus infection. J Infect Dis. 1981;143:133.
52. Clowes GHA Jr, George BC, Villee CA Jr, et al. Muscle proteolysis induced by a circulating peptide in patients with sepsis or trauma. N Engl J Med. 1983;308:545.
53. Baracos V, Rodemann HP, Dinarello CA, et al. Stimulation of muscle protein degradation and prostaglandin E_2 release by leukocytic pyrogen (Interleukin-1). A mechanism for the increased degradation of muscle proteins during fever. N Engl J Med. 1983;308:553.

77. LYMPHADENITIS AND LYMPHANGITIS

MORTON N. SWARTZ

LYMPHADENITIS

Lymphadenitis is an acute or chronic inflammation of lymph nodes. It may be restricted to a solitary node or to a localized group of nodes draining an anatomic area (regional lymphadenitis), or the involvement can be generalized during a systemic infection. The gross features may be those of nonsuppurative, suppurative, or caseous inflammation, depending on the nature of the infecting microorganism.

Pathogenesis and Pathologic Changes

Acute Lymphadenitis. Lymph nodes serve as filters, removing infectious agents from lymphatics draining areas of acute inflammation. The initial histologic response consists of swelling and hyperplasia of sinusoidal lining cells and the infiltration of leukocytes. Depending on the nature of the infecting organism, host defenses, and antimicrobial therapy, the process may or may not progress to abscess formation. With some microorganisms, more distinctive pathologic pictures may be seen—caseation necrosis with infections due to *Mycobacterium tuberculosis, Histoplasma capsulatum, Coccidioides immitis*, and various atypical mycobacteria; stellate abscesses surrounded by palisading epithelioid cells ("granulomatous abscess") with lymphogranuloma venereum and cat-scratch disease; reactive follicular hyperplasia with scattered clusters of epithelioid histiocytes, located in cortical and paracortical zones and characteristically blurring the margins of germinal centers, along with focal distension of subcapsular and trabecular sinuses by monocytoid cells (monocytoid B cells) in toxoplasmosis. The necrotizing granulomatous lymphadenitis that occurs in tularemia can resemble that occurring in cat-scratch disease but often exhibits more granulomatous inflammation. Yersinia (*Y. pseudotuberculosis* or *Y. enterocolitica*) infection in mesenteric lymph nodes can also cause a necrotizing lymphadenitis. Necrotizing nongranulomatous lymphadenitis may be a feature of processes to which an infectious etiology has not yet been ascribed: Kikuchi's necrotizing lymphadenitis, Kawasaki syndrome, and systemic lupus erythematosus.[2]

Chronic Lymphadenitis. Histologically, the response is proliferative with hyperplasia of reticuloendothelial cells, prominent germinal centers, and dilated lymph sinuses filled with mononuclear cells. This picture is nonspecific, can be seen with a variety of infections, and may be observed initially on biopsy in a patient subsequently proven to have a lymphoproliferative disorder.

Dermatopathic lymphadenitis is a distinctive form of chronic lymphadenitis involving lymph nodes draining sites of chronic pruritic dermatitides. Histologically, the enlarged nodes show hyperplasia of reticulum cells in the germinal follicles and of sinusoidal lining cells, as well as the accumulation of lipid and melanin in macrophages (released from the inflammatory process in the skin). The latter feature is the basis for the pathologic designation *lipomelanotic reticuloendotheliosis*. The hyperplastic appearance of such nodes may be so prominent as to suggest erroneously the diagnosis of a lymphoproliferative disorder.

Clinical Findings

Acute Regional Lymphadenitis Due to Pyogenic Bacteria. Palpable lymph nodes do not always indicate serious or ongoing disease. Some degree of inguinal lymphadenopathy is relatively common, reflecting prior episodes of infection on the lower extremities (e.g., interdigital web infections secondary to epidermophytosis); similarly, minor enlargement of cervical nodes may be the residual from previous pharyngeal or dental infections. Lymphadenopathy in certain anatomic areas (preauricular, posterior auricular, supraclavicular, deltoidopectoral, and pectoral) should be viewed with greater suspicion because they are not frequently enlarged as a result of local subclinical infections or minor trauma. Enlargement of superficial lymph nodes along the external jugular vein, as well as of nodes that drain the earlobe and the floor of the external acoustic meatus, is very infrequent but may be associated with superficial infection accompanying recent initial earring insertion. Rarely, a firm mass in the tail or lateral aspect of the breast, suggestive of carcinoma, proves to be an enlarged lymph node in an unusual location due to toxoplasmosis.[1]

Acute suppurative lymphadenitis is more common in children than in adults. In the past three decades, *Staphylococcus aureus* has superseded group A streptococci as the most frequent etiology. The most common sites of involvement are, in order, submandibular (submaxillary), anterior and posterior cervical, inguinal, and axillary lymph nodes. The portal of entry for infection is frequently difficult to determine in children when cervical lymph nodes are involved.

On examination the involved area is swollen and the node(s) is usually at least 3 cm in diameter and tender. Fever is commonly present. The node(s) may be very firm or frankly fluctuant. The overlying skin is warm and often erythematous and edematous.

Syndromes Due to Suppurative Lymphadenitis at Specific Anatomic Sites. CERVICAL LYMPHADENITIS. Acute unilateral adenitis of pyogenic origin occurs most often in pre-school-aged children. The temperature is usually elevated (100–101°F), and local swelling may have been present for some days before the patient is seen by a physician. In only a minority of the cases is there a history of sore throat. However, in the past, group A streptococci have been implicated in about 75 percent of the cases of untreated suppurative cervical lymphadenitis in children.[3,4] *Staphylococcus aureus*, or a combination of *S. aureus* and group A streptococci, is often the etiology of suppurative cervical lymphadenitis associated with pyodermas of the face and scalp.

On examination, there is prominent swelling of the neck or face due to the enlargement usually of a single node, which is often walnut sized. The node is exquisitely tender and firm but may be fluctuant. The swelling may be sufficiently marked to interfere with opening of the mouth. A leukocytosis of 12,000–25,000 white blood cells per cubic millimeter is commonly present.

Acute bilateral cervical adenitis usually involves multiple nodes that are enlarged and somewhat tender in association with viral pharyngitis, infectious mononucleosis, streptococcal pharyngitis, or periodontal infections. Such lymphadenopathy does not ordinarily go on to suppuration unless the symptomatic streptococcal pharyngitis or periodontal infections are ignored.

SUBPECTORAL LYMPHADENITIS. An unusual course may be taken occasionally by infection (usually streptococcal but sometimes staphylococcal) of the thumb or of the interdigital web between the thumb and index finger. Lymphatics from this area do not pass through the epitrochlear nodes but drain directly into the axillary nodes, which in turn communicate with the subpectoral nodes. If infection is not contained in the axillary nodes, subpectoral lymphadenitis develops.[5] Suppuration of these subpectoral nodes can follow. Infection in this area may dissect downward and manifest as cellulitis over the lower chest and upper abdomen or suggest an intra-abdominal infection. The suppurating nodes may drain onto the chest wall.

ACUTE SUPPURATIVE EPITROCHLEAR LYMPHADENITIS. The epitrochlear nodes receive lymphatic drainage from the middle, ring, and little fingers and from the medial portion of the hand and the ulnar aspect of the forearm. Acute suppurative epitrochlear lymphadenitis is uncommon. The predisposing infection in the majority of patients is a primary pyoderma or secondarily infected skin lesions. Unilateral tender swelling, erythema, and induration of the epitrochlear area develop and may subsequently spread along the medial aspect of the arm and forearm. Pain on movement of the elbow is evident. There is often a moderate fever and leukocytosis. The diagnosis is apparent when a discrete, tender nodular swelling can be palpated; but when the area is diffusely swollen and movement at the elbow is limited, the picture may suggest septic arthritis or osteomyelitis.[6] Group A streptococci and *S. aureus* are implicated most commonly.

SUPPURATIVE ILIAC LYMPHADENITIS. The iliac lymph nodes are located along the external and common iliac arteries in the anterior retroperitoneal space. They receive deep lymphatic drainage from the lower abdominal wall and afferents from the superficial and deep inguinal nodes. Iliac lymphadenitis may develop secondary to infection of the lower extremities, lower abdominal wall, perineum, and so forth, or rarely it may result from hematogenous infection. After infection develops, it appears to break through fascial compartments in the iliac fossa and abscess formation ensues. Formerly, most cases occurred in children and young adults, but more recently there appears to be no age predilection. The suppurative lymphadenitis progresses to abscess formation in the space between the posterior peritoneum and the psoas and iliacus fascia.[7] An unexplained limp may be the initial symptom; the acute onset with fever may not occur for some days or weeks. Back and hip pain becomes prominent; extension of the thigh is very painful, but abduction and adduction of the hip evoke minimal discomfort. The symptomatology and clinical findings direct attention to the diagnoses of septic arthritis and osteomyelitis. Only after some days or weeks does lower abdominal pain develop, and the patient becomes acutely ill with high fever and marked leukocytosis. Examination at this point reveals a tightly flexed hip, rectus muscle spasm on the affected side, possibly a tender posterolateral pelvic mass, or a tender inguinal mass suggesting an incarcerated inguinal hernia. By this stage, the abscess may be sizable and may produce elevation and medial displacement of the sigmoid colon and medial displacement of the lower one third of the ureter. When the symptoms are on the right side, the diagnosis of *retrocecal* appendicitis with abscess may be suggested, but the antecedent limp is an important clinical clue. Other diagnoses that may be suggested by the clinical manifestations include tuberculosis of the spine with psoas abscess formation, pelvic inflammatory disease, and tumor of the thigh.[8] Body computed tomography (CT) scanning can be very helpful in defining an inflammatory collection abutting the psoas and iliacus muscles. *Staphylococcus aureus* is the microorganism most commonly implicated, followed in frequency by streptococci.

Acute Regional Lymphadenitis Due to Infecting Agents Other Than Pyogenic Bacteria. A variety of organisms other than the common pyogens may produce localized lymphadenitis (in some cases, going on to abscess and sinus tract formation). These infections resemble pyogenic lymphadenitis but are distinguishable by a prolonged and indolent course, the atypical anatomic areas involved, the lack of prior pyogenic infection, and clues in the history (scratch by a cat, previous tuberculosis, recent sexual exposure, and so forth). Occasionally, the nature of the clinical setting broadens the spectrum of microorganisms to be considered in causing firm or fluctuant lymphadenitis. Mycotic (*Candida albicans, Aspergillus* spp.) cervical lymphadenitis has occurred after oral mucositis in neutropenic children with leukemia.[9] In patients with suppurative lymphadenitis complicating chronic granulomatous disease, the microbial etiology is usually a catalase-positive pathogen. In addition to the commonly involved *S. aureus*, these include Enterobacteriaceae (*Klebsiella, Serratia, Salmonella*), *Pseudomonas* (often *cepacia*), *Aspergillus, Nocardia*, Calmette-Guérin bacillus (BCG), and *Chromobacterium violaceum*.[10–12]

SPECIFIC TYPES OF NONPYOGENIC REGIONAL LYMPHADENITIS. *Scrofula* (Tuberculous Cervical Lymphadenitis). Tuberculous cervical adenitis, formerly a common disease in children and young adults, has become infrequent. It is still occasionally seen in older adults who many years earlier had immigrated to this country from endemic areas (British Isles, Europe, and the Far East) or who lived in rural areas in this country. In this setting it represents breakdown of prior cervical node tuberculosis, acquired either by ingestion of infected milk (bovine tuberculosis) or by lymphohematogenous spread of infection from an initial pulmonary focus to this group of lymph nodes. In this country mycobacterial cervical lymphadenitis (scrofula) is four to five times more frequently due to atypical mycobacteria, commonly *Mycobacterium scrofulaceum*,[13] than to *M. tuberculosis*. In certain areas of the United States, *M. avium-intracellulare* complex is the principal etiology.[14] In parts of the world where BCG vaccination of infants is commonly practiced, subcutaneous abscesses and regional lymphadenitis are not uncommon complications, occurring 2–8 weeks after vaccination, but usually heal spontaneously. Occasionally, the regional (axillary, supraclavicular, or cervical) lymphadenitis progressively enlarges and goes on to caseating suppuration.[15]

The onset of scrofula is insidious, and fever and other systemic manifestations are absent. Several nodes are enlarged and matted together; the mass so formed may develop a swollen fluctuant area, and this brings the patient to medical attention. The process is usually painless. In the majority of cases, clinical evidence of tuberculosis elsewhere is absent. Spontaneous drainage of caseous material onto the skin surface (scrofuloderma) may eventually occur.

Definition of the mycobacterial species involved is important. The atypical mycobacteria causing cervical lymphadenitis are frequently resistant to the usual antituberculous chemotherapy, and surgical excision of the involved fluctuant node(s) is indicated. Antituberculous therapy is usually not needed for BCG nonsuppurative lymphadenitis, but if suppurative lymphadenitis develops, complete excision and antituberculous chemotherapy are indicated.

Granulomatous Lymphadenitis Caused by Nondiphtheria Corynebacteria. Subacute or chronic relapsing lymphadenitis has been reported occasionally to be due to *Corynebacterium pseudotuberculosis* (*C. ovis*).[16] The majority of patients have had extensive contact with animals, particularly sheep. The histologic picture is that of a suppurative or necrotizing granulomatous process. Treatment consists of prolonged antibiotic (erythromycin or penicillin) therapy combined with surgical drainage or excision of the involved nodes.

Oculoglandular (Parinaud) Syndrome. Preauricular lymphadenopathy can occur secondary to granulomatous nodular conjunctival infection caused by the introduction of certain pathogens onto the external eye. Oculoglandular syndromes occur occasionally in tularemia, cat-scratch disease,[17] listeriosis, sporotrichosis, and lymphogranuloma venereum. Epidemic keratoconjunctivitis due to adenoviruses is often associated with an enlarged preauricular lymph node.

Cat-Scratch Disease.[17] This slowly progressive and sometimes chronic form of regional lymphadenitis is presumed to be infectious. Small, pleomorphic, gram-negative bacilli have been identified within the walls of capillaries, in macrophages lining sinuses near germinal centers, and in macrophages in necrotic areas of involved lymph nodes of patients with cat-scratch disease. The organisms have only rarely been noted within neutrophils or free in areas of necrosis. The organisms are most readily demonstrated with the Warthin-Starry silver impregnation stain.[18,19] Convalescent serum from a patient with clinical cat-scratch disease reacted (immunoperoxidase stain) with the bacilli in the lymph nodes of three patients with the same disease, suggesting both a similarity (or identity) of the organisms in these cases and the occurrence of an immune response in these patients. In a recent study, a pleomorphic, as yet unspeciated, gram-negative bacillus has been reported to have been isolated on culture, in biphasic brain-heart infusion medium, of material from lymph nodes of 10 of 19 patients with the clinical diagnosis of cat-scratch disease.[20] Three of seven patients with recent cat-scratch disease had fourfold or greater rises in indirect fluorescent antibody titer against the cultured bacilli. Although the process progresses to suppuration in 10–50 percent of cases, the course is slower than that of suppurative lymphadenitis due to pyogenic bacteria, and most patients are only mildly ill. The nodes are tender, acutely so when there is frank suppuration. Fever is present in only about one-third of patients and is low grade. Almost any peripheral lymph nodes may be involved, but the axillary nodes are most commonly affected. About 90 percent of patients give a history of contact with cats (most often kittens), and most have been scratched. A primary lesion (small papule or vesicle resembling an insect bite) develops at the site of a scratch 7–14 days after contact with the cat. The primary lesion lasts for 1–4 weeks and may be helpful in diagnosis. Lymphadenopathy develops within a week or two of the appearance of the skin papule.[21] There is no lymphangitis.

The diagnosis is made on the basis of a history of appropriate exposure, the clinical picture, the failure to isolate a known etiologic agent from aspirated pus, a bimorphic histologic picture (stellate abscesses with necrotic centers surrounded by epithelioid cells), and a positive intradermal skin test to a known preparation of cat-scratch skin test antigen. The latter (derived from pus from a suppurative node of cat-scratch disease) is not available commercially and must be prepared carefully to ensure complete inactivation of any hepatitis virus. In view of the recent acquired immunodeficiency syndrome (AIDS) epidemic, the use of this type of skin test reagent of human origin must be seriously questioned, particularly if the antigen has been prepared in the past 6 years. We have seen a male homosexual patient with typical cat-scratch disease who some months later developed the characteristic manifestations of AIDS. The preparation and use of cat-scratch skin antigen from such a source might serve as a vehicle for spread of human immunodeficiency virus (HIV) infection.

Inguinal Buboes of Venereal Origin. Inguinal lymphadenopathy due to pyogenic infections or cat-scratch disease is usually unilateral. Prominent bilateral (or unilateral) adenopathy, particularly in the adult man, is suggestive of several venereal diseases (see Chapter 93). The genital chancre of primary syphilis is usually accompanied by one or several discrete, firm, nonsuppurative, painless, enlarged nodes in one or both inguinal areas. Constitutional signs are lacking. The overlying skin is uninflamed. In secondary syphilis the lymphadenopathy is generalized.

In lymphogranuloma venereum (LGV), the primary genital lesion is usually transient and asymptomatic. The initial manifestation of the disease is usually the characteristic inguinal bubo, occurring 10–30 days after sexual exposure. The adenopathy is more commonly unilateral. Initially the node is tender, discrete, and movable, but subsequently the inflammatory process involves multiple nodes in the area. Chills, fever, and constitutional symptoms are common at this stage. As a result of periadenitis, the nodes become fixed and matted into an oval or lobulated mass. The latter is adherent to the overlying skin that is purplish in color. Foci of suppuration develop with multiple fistulous tracts. A central lengthwise linear depression (so-called groove sign of LGV) is produced by involvement of nodes above and below the inguinal ligament. Although characteristic of LGV, the groove sign may rarely be produced by suppurative bacterial lymphadenitis or by lymphomatous involvement of inguinal nodes.

Chancroid is usually accompanied by painful, tender inguinal adenopathy. The primary lesion is a papule or pustule that progresses to form an extremely painful and tender but nonindurated ulceration, quite in contrast to a syphilitic chancre. The adenopathy of chancroid develops about 1 week after the primary lesion appears and, unlike LGV, is present while the ulcer is still active. The chancroidal bubo is typically unilateral, made up of fused inguinal nodes, and is more painful than that of LGV. Unilocular suppuration may develop. However, in the majority of patients, the lymphadenitis subsides without suppuration.

Primary genital herpetic infection in men and women is often associated with tender inguinal adenopathy. Histologically, the nodes show paracortical hyperplasia (with a prominent admixture of immunoblasts, plasma cells, and macrophages), along with sinus histiocytosis, discrete foci of necrosis, and intranuclear inclusions within scattered mononuclear and giant cells. Similar, histologically proven, recurrent, localized herpetic lymphadenitis can occur in immunocompromised patients in the absence of overt mucocutaneous lesions.[22] The "pseudobuboes" of granuloma inguinale are produced by subcutaneous granulomatous infection rather than by suppurative lymphadenitis.

Suppurative inguinal lymphadenitis due to group A streptococci has been superimposed on chronic lymphadenopathy in homosexual males.[23]

Inguinal Buboes of Nonvenereal Origin. Inguinal or femoral buboes occur in bubonic plague, since the flea bite initiating the infection is commonly on a lower extremity.[24] However, involvement of most other peripheral nodes can occur. The disease begins with fever, malaise, headache, and tender regional adenopathy after an incubation period of 2–6 days. Only rarely is a lesion (papule, pustule) at the site of the insect bite evident at the onset of clinical illness. A large, matted collection of lymph nodes with surrounding edema quickly develops and may go on to suppuration and spontaneous drainage. If not treated promptly, the infection rapidly progresses to a septicemic phase. The diagnosis should be suspected in a febrile, acutely ill patient with a large cluster of extremely tender lymph nodes and a history of exposure to fleas, rodents, or rabbits in the western United States. (Tularemia may mimic the epidemiologic and clinical features of bubonic plague but is more likely to produce an *ulceroglandular syndrome* [Table 1], with a primary lesion at the site of inoculation.[25]) Diagnostic procedures include blood cultures (uniformly positive in the septicemic phase of plague), as well as cultures and stained smears (see Chapter 207) of carefully obtained bubo aspirates. Appropriate treatment (see below) should be instituted immediately while awaiting results of cultures if bubonic plague is suspected.

GENERALIZED LYMPHADENITIS ASSOCIATED WITH SYSTEMIC INFECTIONS. Widespread lymphadenitis is a feature of a variety of infections disseminated by the blood stream. In most instances, suppuration of the involved nodes does not occur. Generalized lymphadenopathy is a feature, for example, of secondary syphilis, infectious mononucleosis, leptospirosis, and miliary tuberculosis. Generalized lymphadenopathy associated with infections is commonly due to the presence of the invading microorganism in the nodes. Generalized lymph node enlargement is a feature of a variety of infectious diseases due to bacterial, rickettsial, chlamydial, spirochetal, viral, protozoal, and helminthic agents (Table 1).

Etiologic Agents and Differential Diagnosis

It is helpful for purposes of the differential diagnosis to consider infective lymphadenitis in several categories (Table 1): (*1*) regional lymphadenopathy, (*2*) regional lymphadenopathy with breakdown of nodes, (*3*) inguinal bubo formation, (*4*) ulceroglandular syndrome, (*5*) oculoglandular syndrome, and (*6*) generalized lymphadenopathy.

In distinguishing among the causes of fluctuant cervical lymphadenitis, the history may suggest a streptococcal (preceding tonsillitis), staphylococcal (recent facial or neck infection), tuberculous (prior exposure to tuberculosis), or cat-scratch disease (exposure to cat) etiology. In a study of suppurative cervical adenitis *S. aureus* was the etiology more frequently than group A streptococci (36 percent vs. 26 percent), and in another one-quarter of the cases a bacteriologic diagnosis could not be made.[26] A subacute clinical course with little fever and a normal leukocyte count would be more consistent with cat-scratch disease or tuberculous involvement. Sinus tract formation suggests infection due to *M. tuberculosis* or an atypical mycobacterium. Gram-stained and Ziehl-Neelsen smears and culture (including cultures for mycobacteria) of material aspirated or drained from suppurating nodes provides a diagnosis in about two-thirds of such cases of cervical lymphadenitis. Further information may be provided by skin tests (purified protein derivative; cat-scratch antigen [see earlier comment on the current risk in using this reagent]), serologic tests (antistreptolysin O antibody titer), and histologic examination (caseation necrosis suggesting mycobacterial infection; bimorphic appearance suggesting cat-scratch disease) of an excised node when culture of aspirated material is unrevealing. A variety of noninfectious processes may resemble unilateral cervical lymphadenitis. Lymphoma may be suggested by the indolent course of cat-scratch disease. Acute febrile mucocutaneous lymph node syndrome (Kawasaki syndrome), a disease of infants and young children of unknown etiology, is characterized by nonsuppurative cervical lymphadenopathy.[27] The age of the patient, febrile course, conjunctival injection, erythematous rash, and subsequent desquamation suggest the diagnosis. A recently described benign disorder of lymph nodes, histiocytic necrotizing lymphadenitis or Kikuchi's disease, was first recognized in Japan and now has been observed in the United States.[28] Clinically, its features consist of localized, sometimes tender, cervical lymphadenopathy, often with an upper respiratory prodrome and associated in some patients with fever. Most cases occur in women, commonly under 30 years of age. Mild leukopenia and lymphocytosis may suggest infectious mononucleosis. The illness does not respond to antibiotics, but it usually resolves spontaneously within 1 or 2 months. Histologically, biopsy specimens may be erroneously interpreted as lymphoma, but the principal findings are those of focal reticulum cell hyperplasia combined with patchy areas of necrosis. Although a viral etiology is suspected on the basis of the clinical features, serologic and ultrastructural studies have failed to identify a specific agent.

Bronchial cleft cysts and cystic hygromas may be mistaken for cervical lymphadenitis, particularly if infected; thyroglossal duct cysts may suggest infected submental nodes. Submaxillary sialadenitis or salivary gland tumors may mimic submandibular lymphadenitis. Bimanual (intraoral and submandibular) palpation can be helpful in distinguishing between these processes.

TABLE 1. Clinical Patterns and Microbial Etiologies of Infectious Lymphadenitis

		Form of Lymphadenitis					
Disease	*Infecting Organism*	*Regional*	*Regional with Suppuration (or Caseation)*	*Inguinal Bubo Formation*	*Ulceroglandular*	*Oculoglandular*	*Generalized*
Bacterial							
Pyogenic	Group A strep; S. aureus	+	+				
Scarlet fever	Group A strep.	+	+				+
Diphtheria	*C. diphtheriae*	+					
Fusospirochetal angina	*B. melaninogenicus;* peptostreptococci, etc.	+					
Scrofula	*M. tuberculosis*	+	+				
	M. scrofulaceum; M. avium-intracellulare	+	+				
Miliary tuberculosis	*M. tuberculosis*						+
Brucellosis	*Brucella*						+
Leptospirosis	*Leptospira*						+
Syphilis	*T. pallidum*	+					+
Chancroid	*H. ducreyi*			+			
Plague	*Y. pestis*	+	+	+			
Tularemia	*F. tularensis*		+		+	+	
Rat bite fever	*Streptobaccillus moniliformis;*	+					
	Spirillum minus	+			+		
Anthrax	*B. anthracis*	+			+		
Listeriosis	*L. monocytogenes*					+	
Melioidosis	*P. pseudomallei*	+	+				+
Glanders	*P. mallei*	+	+				+
Cat-scratch	? Unknown gram-negative bacillus	+	+		±	+	
Mycotic							
Histoplasmosis	*H. capsulatum*						+
	H. capsulatum var. duboisii	+					
Coccidioidomycosis	*Coccidioides immitis*	+					
Paracoccidioidomycosis	*P. brasiliensis*	+					
Rickettsial							
Boutonneuse fever, etc.	*R. conori*				+		
Scrub typhus	*R. tsutsugamushi*	+					+
Rickettsialpox	*R. akari*	+					
Chlamydial							
Lymphogranuloma venereum	*C. trachomatis*			+		+	+
Viral							
Measles	Measles virus						+
Rubella	Rubella virus						+
Infectious mononucleosis	EB virus						+
CMV mononucleosis	CMV virus						+
Dengue fever	Dengue virus						+
West Nile fever	West Nile virus						+
Epidemic (Far Eastern) hemorrhagic fevers	?						+
Lassa fever	Lassa virus						+
Genital herpes infection	HSV-type 2	+					
Pharyngoconjunctival fever	Adenovirus (types 3 and 7)	+				+	
Epidemic keratoconjunctivitis	Adenovirus (types 8 and 19)					+	
Cat-scratch	?	+	+		+	+	
Postvaccinial lymphadenitis	Vaccinia virus	+					
AIDS; AIDS-related complex	HIV						+
Protozoan							
Kala azar	*Leishmania donovani*						+
African trypanosomiasis	*Trypanosoma brucei*	+					+
Chagas disease	*T. cruzi*					+	+
Toxoplasmosis	*Toxoplasma gondii*						+
Helminthic							
Filariasis	*Wucheria bancrofti*						+
	Brugia malayi						+
Loiasis	*Loa loa*			+			
Oncocerciasis	*Oncocerca volvulus*			+			

Isolated inguinal lymphadenitis or bubo formation in the adult suggests venereal diseases (syphilis, LGV, chancroid). Distinctive associated primary lesions are usually features of syphilis and chancroid but not of LGV. The inguinal adenopathy of primary syphilis consists of painless, firm, discrete, movable nodes without erythema of the overlying skin. The nodes do not suppurate, whereas spontaneous rupture of the buboes of LGV and chancroid may occur. The groove sign is suggestive of LGV. The buboes of chancroid are characteristically painful. Axillary, cervical, and inguinal buboes may occur with plague and tularemia. In plague an inguinal location is common. The geographic locale and a history of animal exposure are important clues to the diagnosis. Inguinal and femoral nodes can be involved in cat-scratch disease, although much less frequently than axillary or cervical nodes.

Prominent painful lymphadenitis involving cervical, axillary, and particularly supraclavicular nodes (on the left side) occasionally follows smallpox immunization. This may become evident weeks after immunization, and thus this relevant event may be overlooked. The process is self-limited. However, if a node is biopsied because of a suspicion of lymphoma or tuberculosis, the histologic picture may superficially simulate that of a malignant lymphoma. The lymphadenopathy appears to represent a heightened immunoblastic response to the immunizing agent, similar to the changes observed in infectious mononucleosis.[29,30]

Generalized lymphadenopathy is frequently a manifestation of disseminated infection (Table 1). Clues may be provided by the age of the patient and the presence of a characteristic rash (childhood exanthems, secondary syphilis), geographic factors (dengue, filariasis, histoplasmosis), occupational and/or dietary history (brucellosis, toxoplasmosis), exposure to animals (leptospirosis), and the presence of atypical lymphocytes (infectious mononucleosis, cytomegalovirus infection). Diagnosis of toxoplasmic lymphadenitis in the immunocompetent patient is based primarily on serologic testing, although sometimes node biopsy is performed because of initial concern for lymphoma. A negative result in the Sabin-Feldman dye test or in a comparable test for toxoplasma IgG antibody (indirect fluorescent antibody [IFA] or agglutination test) practically excludes the diagnosis. Acute infection is likely if a high IgM antibody titer is present with a high IgG antibody titer (dye test or IFA test titers of >1:1000) in a single serum specimen.[1] Laboratory diagnosis of acute toxoplasmic lymphadenitis can also be made by seroconversion from a negative to a positive IgG antibody test or by demonstration of a fourfold titer rise over 3 weeks.

Widespread suppurative infections of lymph nodes occur as a result of the microbicidal defect characteristic of neutrophils and monocytes of patients with chronic granulomatous disease. Recurrent infections (skin, bones, lungs, and liver, as well as lymph nodes) beginning in childhood and due to *S. aureus* and certain gram-negative bacilli (*Escherichia coli*, salmonella, *Serratia marcescens*) suggest the diagnosis.

Widespread lymphadenopathy may be a feature of many noninfectious diseases, particularly infiltrative processes such as lymphoma and reticuloendothelioses. Prominent peripheral lymphadenopathy may be a feature of rheumatoid arthritis. Lymphadenopathy may occur as an adverse effect of prolonged use of phenytoin. Widespread lymphadenopathy is a feature of the syndrome of immunoblastic lymphadenopathy.

Generalized Lymphadenopathy with AIDS or with the AIDS-Related Complex. Patients with AIDS may have generalized lymphadenopathy in which involvement with opportunistic infection or neoplastic disease (particularly Kaposi sarcoma) is evident on histologic examination. The infections have included those due to cytomegalovirus and *M. avium-intracellulare*.[31] The latter usually show a few poorly formed or no granulomas and a prominent histiocytic reaction. Large clusters ("globi") of acid-fast bacilli are present within the cytoplasm of histiocytes. Kaposi sarcoma in patients with AIDS often follows the pattern of generalized lymph node involvement and a fulminant course with mucosal and visceral lesions.[32] In AIDS other neoplasms, primarily of the B-cell type (B-cell immunoblastic sarcoma; small noncleaved, Burkitt-like lymphoma; plasmacytoid lymphocytic lymphoma) have occurred in lymph nodes and extranodal sites.[33]

Lymphadenopathy occurs in almost 50 percent of patients at risk for AIDS who develop an acute illness after initial exposure to HIV.[34] It often is one feature of a mononucleosis-like syndrome consisting of fever, malaise, myalgias, headaches, sore throat, diarrhea, and a maculopapular rash. After the acute clinical illness subsides, lymphadenopathy may remain as persistant generalized lymphadenopathy (PGL), involving at least several extrainguinal sites, of at least 3 months' duration.[35] PGL may also occur in male homosexuals, intravenous drug abusers, and other individuals in high-risk groups without any history of prior clinically apparent initial HIV infection. The nodes are discrete and nontender; suppuration does not occur. HIV replication takes place in such lymph nodes,[36] which histologically show follicular hyperplasia or mixed follicular and interfollicular hyperplasia. With progression to AIDS, lymphocyte depletion supervenes. PGL is frequently one of the manifestations of what is termed the *AIDS-related complex*, a group of clinical manifestations (including fever, weight loss, diarrhea, fatigue, and night sweats) occurring in individuals at risk for developing AIDS but not as yet having any definable underlying infectious or neoplastic cause for the symptoms. Laboratory findings in this clinical syndrome include two or more of the following: (*1*) lymphopenia, (*2*) decreased numbers of helper T cells, (*3*) depressed helper/suppressor cell ratio, (*4*) increased levels of serum globulins, (*5*) decreased blastogenesis in response to mitogens, and (*6*) anergy to skin test antigens. A sizable number of patients with such chronic generalized lymphadenopathy go on eventually to develop AIDS, with its complicating opportunistic infections and Kaposi sarcoma.[31] Regression of the lymphadenopathy may occur after 8–19 months in some patients. However, opportunistic infections can develop in some patients following such regression.[37]

An abnormal distribution of T-helper and T-suppressor lymphocytes occurs in hyperplastic lymph nodes of homosexual men with lymhadenopathy[38]—a reduced helper/suppressor ratio and an increased number of suppressor cells in the germinal centers and mantle zones (locations in which ordinarily B cells and helper-inducer cells are found). In about 20 percent of cases of PGL in intravenous drug abusers, multinucleate giant cells of the Warthin-Finkeldey type ("mulberry cells") are found in the interfollicular areas.

Presumptive Treatment

Initial treatment of infective lymphadenitis requires some narrowing of the diagnostic possibilities (Table 1). Localized pyogenic lymphadenitis responds well to early antibiotic treatment. When cervical lymphadenitis has developed from a pharyngeal or peridontal portal, initial treatment with penicillin is appropriate (procaine penicillin G, 300,000–600,000 units intramuscularly every 12–24 hours initially to ensure receipt of therapy when the patient may be nauseated; subsequently 250–500 mg of penicillin V may be administered orally every 6 hours for at least 10 days for older children and adults). In patients who are more acutely ill, larger doses of aqueous penicillin G parenterally are indicated. Erythromycin (20–40 mg/kg/day orally in divided doses every 6 hours) is an alternative for patients allergic to penicillin.

Pyogenic lymphadenitis complicating skin infections may be staphylococcal or streptococcal in etiology, and a penicillinase-resistant penicillin is the drug of choice (e.g., oxacillin 0.5 g orally every 4–6 hours for the older child or an adult). In the more acutely ill patient, intravenous administration of the semisynthetic penicillin or a first generation cephalosporin should be employed. Failure to show improvement, or progression to suppuration, is an indication for percutaneous needle aspiration (for bacteriologic diagnosis and treatment) or surgical drainage.

If cat-scratch disease is suspected, the treatment is principally symptomatic; antibiotics are not effective. If the nodes become fluctuant, aspiration is the treatment of choice.

If the diagnosis of bubonic plague is suspected, antibiotic treatment should be instituted promptly. Streptomycin (1.0 g intramuscularly every 12 hours in adults) or tetracycline (0.5 g orally every 6 hours in adults) are the preferred drugs, and treatment is continued for 10 days.

LYMPHANGITIS

Lymphangitis is an inflammation of lymphatic channels, usually in the subcutaneous tissues. It occurs either as an acute process of bacterial origin or as a chronic process of mycotic, mycobacterial, or filarial etiology.

Pathologic Changes and Pathogenesis

The visible red streaking in acute lymphangitis stems from the inflammatory process in the walls (and surrounding tissue spaces) of dilated lymphatic channels. Lymphatic obstruction often occurs on healing, resulting sometimes in persistent lymphedema. Cutaneous lymphatic sporotrichosis, a form of chronic lymphangitis, produces a combined suppurative and granulomatous response.

Clinical Findings

Acute Lymphangitis. Acute lymphangitis develops when an infection, commonly on an extremity, is not contained locally but spreads along lymphatic channels. Such infections are most often due to group A streptococci. Systemic manifestations may develop rapidly before evidence of infection becomes apparent at the site of inoculation of organisms, and they may be more prominent than might be anticipated on the basis of local pain and erythema. Red linear streaks, a few millimeters to several centimeters in width, extend from the initial site of infection toward the regional lymph nodes, which are enlarged and tender. Peripheral edema of the involved extremity often occurs. The time course of this type of infection can be accelerated from initial lesion to lymphangitis to complicating bacteremia in 24–48 hours.

The peripheral white blood cell count is commonly elevated. The etiologic agent often can be identified on Gram-stained smears and cultures obtained from the initial lesion. Blood cultures also may reveal the causative organism.

Acute lymphangitis and/or lymphadenitis, usually involving the lower extremities, is a feature of filariasis due to *Wuchereria bancrofti* (and sometimes to *Brugia malayi*).[39] These mosquito-borne diseases are endemic to Africa, Southeast Asia and the Pacific, and tropical South America. The acute form of disease is characterized by recurrent episodes of headache, backache, lymphangitis, lymphadenitis, epididymitis, and orchitis. Fever is uncommon. The adult filariae reside in lymphatics and lymph nodes and discharge microfilariae into the blood stream. With prolonged exposure in an endemic area, chronic lymphatic obstruction can develop with elephantiasis of the skin and scrotum. In this setting, recurrent episodes of lymphangitis may be the result of both the parasitic infestation and superimposed streptococcal infections (to which the chronic lymphedema predisposes). Serologic tests for filariasis may be helpful in diagnosis if microfilariae are not found, but they are positive in many other filarial infections. Lymph node or lymphatic vessel biopsy may be necessary for diagnosis.

Chronic Granulomatous Lymphangitis. Unlike acute lymphangitis, this is an indolent process with little pain or systemic evidences of infection. Sporotrichosis is most commonly the underlying disease.[40] This infection frequently is introduced by minor trauma (e.g., from a thorn of a barberry or rose bush) into the skin of a gardener. An erythematous subcutaneous nodule (often becoming fluctuant) or a chancriform ulcer subsequently develops at the site of inoculation of *Sporothrix schenckii* (present on some plants and in sphagnum moss used in gardening) on the hand or finger.[41] The lesion does not respond to local treatment or to administration of the common antibacterial agents. Slowly, mutiple subcutaneous nodules appear and extend proximally along the course of regional lymphatics, which become thickened.

Cutaneous infection (''swimming pool granuloma'') with *Mycobacterium marinum*, an atypical mycobacterium that grows optimally at 25–32°C and is found in swimming pools and fish tanks, produces a chronic nodular, verrucous or ulcerative lesion at the site of an abrasion, usually about the knees or elbows. The lesion is usually solitary, but in an occasional patient new lesions develop proximally, as in sporotrichosis. Multiple sporotrichoid lesions have occurred in occasional infections due to *Nocardia brasiliensis*[42] and in rare infections due to *Mycobacterium kansasii* and *N. asteroides*.

Etiologic Agents

In the United States acute lymphangitis is most commonly due to group A streptococci, and chronic lymphangitis is usually caused by Sp. *schenckii*. Other infectious agents occasionally produce lymphangitis (Table 2).

Differential Diagnosis

The combination of a peripheral infection or traumatic lesion and the acute onset of fever with proximal red linear streaks directed toward regional lymph nodes is diagnostic of acute lymphangitis. In the legs, thrombophlebitis may produce linear areas of tender erythema, but the absence of an initiating lesion and of tender regional adenopathy is helpful in distinguishing it from lymphangitis. A history of rat bite and the subsequent development of lymphangitis suggest *Spirillum minus* infection. Filariasis is a consideration when an appropriate geographic history is obtained. Sporotrichosis is considered when chronic ulcerative lymphangitis develops in someone working with plants, soil, or timbers. *Mycobacterium marinum* is suggested as the etiology when sporotrichoid lesions develop in a person who has been around swimming pools and fish tanks.

Presumptive Therapy

Penicillin is the initial treatment of acute lymphangitis. In a mildly ill adult, 600,000 units of procaine penicillin G once or twice daily is administered initially, with supplementary oral penicillin V. More acutely ill patients in whom bacteremia may have developed should be hospitalized and treated with parenteral aqueous penicillin G (600,000–2,000,000 units every 4–6 hours). If a staphylococcal etiology is suspected, a penicillinase-resistant penicillin is used.

The initial treatment of presumptive lymphocutaneous sporotrichosis is potassium iodide. If sporotrichoid *M. marinum* infection is suspected, the diagnosis should be confirmed by demonstration of acid-fast bacilli and by isolation of the organism at 30°C on appropriate media. Localized swimming pool granulomas are often treated by surgical excision. Chemotherapy is reserved for more extensive and sporotrichoid forms of infection. On the basis of limited data, the combination of choice would appear to be rifampin and ethambutal.[43] Prolonged tetracycline or minocycline therapy has also been reported as successful in a small number of cases,[44] but in vitro resistance to and treatment failure with doxycycline have been reported.[45] Trimethoprim-sulfamethoxazole has been reported as effective in several studies. However, in vitro activity re-

TABLE 2. Causes of Lymphangitis

Clinical Form	*Etiologic Agent*	*Relative Frequency as Etiology of Lymphangitis*
Acute	Group A streptococcus	Common
	S. aureus	Occasional
	Pasteurella multocida	Occasional
	Spirillium minus (rat-bite fever)	Rare
	W. bancrofti; B. malayi (filariasis)	Rare (only in immigrants from endemic areas)
Chronic	*Sporothrix schenckii* (sporotrichosis)	Occasional
	M. marinum (swimming pool granuloma)	Occasional
	M. kansasii	Rare
	Nocardia brasiliensis	Rare
	W. bancrifti; B. malayi	Rare (only in immigrants from endemic areas)

quires drug concentrations greater than those usually achieved in serum and tissues.[46]

REFERENCES

1. McCabe RE, Brooks RG, Dorfman RF, et al. Clinical spectrum in 107 cases of toxoplasmic lymphadenopathy. Rev Infect Dis. 1987;9:754.
2. Strickler JG, Warnke RA, Weiss LM. Necrosis in lymph nodes. Pathol Annu. 1987;2:253.
3. Scobie WG. Acute suppurative adenitis in children. Scot Med J. 1969;14:352.
4. Dajani AS, Garcia RE, Wolinski E. Etiology of cervical lymphadenitis in children. N Engl J Med. 1963;268:1329.
5. Amren DP. Unusual forms of streptococcal disease. In: Wannamaker LW, Matsen JM, eds. Streptococci and Streptococcal Disease. New York: Academic Press; 1972:545.
6. Currarino G. Acute epitrochlear lymphadenitis. Pediatr Radiol. 1977;6:160.
7. Maull KI, Sachatello CII. Retroperitoneal iliac fossa abscess. A complication of suppurative iliac lymphadenitis. Am J Surg. 1974;127:270.
8. Oliff M, Chuang VP. Retroperitoneal iliac fossa pyogenic abscess. Radiology. 1978;126:647.
9. Shenep JL, Kalwinsky DK, Feldman S, et al. Mycotic cervical lymphadenitis following oral mucositis in children with leukemia. J Pediatr. 1985;106:243.
10. Curnutte JT, Boxer LA. Clinically significant phagocytic cell defects. In: Remington JS, Swartz MN, eds. Current Clinical Topics in Infectious Diseases. v. 4. New York: McGraw-Hill; 1985:103–55.
11. Sorensen RU, Jacobs MR, Shurin SB. *Chromobacterium violaceum* adenitis acquired in the northern United States as a complication of chronic granulomatous disease. Pediatr Infect Dis. 1985;4:701.
12. Kobayashi Y, Komazawa Y, Kobayashi M, et al. Presumed BCG infection in a boy with chronic granulomatous disease. A report of a case and review of the literature. Clin Pediatr. 1984;23:586.
13. Lincoln EM, Gilbert LA. Disease in children due to mycobacteria other than *Mycobacterium tuberculosis*. Am Rev Respir Dis. 1972;105:683.
14. Spark RP, Fried ML, Bean CK, et al. Nontuberculous mycobacterial adenitis of childhood. The ten-year experience at a community hospital. Am J Dis Child. 1988;142:106.
15. Victoria MS, Shah BR. Bacillus Calmette-Guérin lymphadenitis: A case report and review of the literature. Pediatr Infect Dis. 1985;4:295.
16. Lipsky BA, Goldberger AC, Tompkins LS, et al. Infections caused by nondiphtheria corynebacteria. Rev Infect Dis. 1982;4:1220.
17. Carithers HA, Carithers CM, Edwards RO Jr. Cat-scratch disease. Its natural history. JAMA. 1969;207:312.
18. Wear DJ, Margileth AM, Hadfield TL, et al. Cat-scratch disease: A bacterial infection. Science. 1983;221:1403.
19. Hadfield TL, Malaty RH, Van Dellen A, et al. Electron microscopy of the bacillus causing cat-scratch disease. J Infect Dis. 1985;152:643.
20. English CK, Wear DJ, Margileth AM, et al. Cat-scratch disease. Isolation and culture of the bacterial agent. JAMA. 1988;259:1347.
21. Carithers HA. Cat-scratch disease. An overview based on a study of 1,200 patients. Am J Dis Child. 1985;139:1124.
22. Epstein JI, Ambinder RF, Kuhajda, et al. Localized herpes simplex lymphadenitis. Am J Clin Pathol. 1986;86:444.
23. Ho DD, Murata GH. Streptococcal lymphadenitis in homosexual men with chronic lymphadenopathy. Am J Med. 1984;77:151.
24. Reed WB, Palmer DL, Williams RC, et al. Bubonic plague in southwestern United States. Medicine. 1970;49:465.
25. Young LS, Bicknell DS, Archer BG, et al. Tularemia epidemic: Vermont 1968. Forty-seven cases linked to contact with muskrats. N Engl J Med. 1969;280:1253.
26. Barton LL, Feigin RD. Childhood cervical lymphadenitis: A reappraisal. J Pediatr. 1974;84:846.
27. Feigin RD, Schleien CI. Kawasaki's disease. In: Remington J, Swartz MN, eds. Current Clinical Topics in Infectious Disease, v. 4. New York: McGraw-Hill; 1983:30.
28. Unger PD, Rappaport KM, Strauchen JA. Necrotizing lymphadenitis (Kikuchi's disease). Arch Pathol Lab Med. 1987;111:1031.
29. Hartsock RJ. Postvaccinial lymphadenitis. Hyperplasia of lymphoid tissue that simulates malignant lymphomas. Cancer 1968;21:632.
30. Childs CC, Parham DM, Berard CW. Infectious mononucleosis: The spectrum of morphologic changes simulating lymphoma in lymph nodes and tonsils. Am J Surg Pathol. 1987;11:122.
31. Fauci AS, Macher AM, Longo DL, et al. Acquired immunodeficiency syndrome: Epidemiologic, clinical, immunologic, and therapeutic considerations. Ann Intern Med. 1984;100:92.
32. Gottlieb MS, Groopman JE, Weinstein WM, et al. The acquired immunodeficiency syndrome. Ann Intern Med. 1983;99:208.
33. Levine AM, Meyer PR, Begandy MK, et al. Development of B-cell lymphoma in homosexual men: Clinical and immunological findings. Ann Intern Med. 1984;100:7.
34. Tindall B, Barker S, Donovan B, et al. Characterization of the acute clinical illness associated with human immunodeficiency virus infection. Arch Intern Med. 1988;148:945.
35. Biberfeld P, Porwit-Ksiazek A, Böttiger B, et al. Immunohistopathology of lymph nodes in HTLV-III infected homosexuals with persistent adenopathy or AIDS. Cancer Res. 1985;45(Suppl):4665S.
36. Biberfeld P, Chayt KJ, Marselle LM, et al. HTLV-III expression in infected lymph nodes and relevance to pathogenesis of lymphadenopathy. Am J Pathol. 1986;125:436.
37. Metroka CE, Cunningham-Rundles S, Pollack MS, et al. Generalized lymphadenopathy in homosexual men. Ann Intern Med. 1983;99:585.
38. Modlin RL, Meyer PR, Hofman FM, et al. T-lymphocyte subsets in lymph nodes from homosexual men. JAMA. 1983;250:1302.
39. Grove DI, Warren KS, Mahmoud AAF. Algorithms in the diagnosis and management of exotic diseases. VI. The filariases. J Infect Dis. 1975;132:340.
40. Orr ER, Riley HD Jr. Sporotrichosis in childhood: Report of ten cases. J Pediatr. 1971;78:951.
41. Duran RJ, Coventry MB, Weed LA, et al. Sporotrichosis: A report of twenty-three cases in the upper extremity. J Bone Joint Surg. 1957:39(A):1330.
42. Smego RA Jr, Gallis HA. The clinical spectrum of *Nocardia brasiliensis* infection in the United States. Rev Infect Dis. 1984;6:164.
43. Van Dyke JJ, Lake KB. Chemotherapy for aquarium granuloma. JAMA. 1975;233:1380.
44. Izumi AK, Hanke W, Higaki M. *Mycobacterium marinum* infections treated with tetracycline. Arch Dermatol. 1977;113:1067.
45. Ljungberg B, Christensson B, Grubb R. Failure of doxycycline treatment in aquarium-associated *Mycobacterium marinum* infections. Scand J Infect Dis. 1987;19:539.
46. Sanders WJ, Wolinsky E. In vitro susceptibility of *Mycobacterium marinum* to eight antimicrobial agents. Antimicrob Agents Chemother. 1980;18:529.

SECTION J. INFECTIONS RELATED TO TRAUMA

78. PROPHYLAXIS AND TREATMENT OF INFECTION IN TRAUMA

ROGER W. YURT
G. TOM SHIRES

Trauma is the leading cause of death in the first three decades of life in the United States and the fourth leading cause overall. Of the 50 million injuries that occur each year, 10 million of them are disabling.[1] The population at risk for infection associated with trauma is not only quantitatively large but is impressive from the standpoint of a large number of hospitalized patients who are prone to the development of nosocomial infections. The only real prophylaxis of infection in trauma is directed toward nosocomial infection. Initial regimens oriented toward the wound or injured tissue are in fact therapeutic since exogenous and endogenous contamination has already occurred. The magnitude of the infection problem after trauma is most dramatic in patients with severe burns in whom 50 percent of the mortality is related to infection.[2] The hypermetabolic state, depressed immune function, devitalized tissue, specific organ injury, foreign bodies, endogenous and exogenous contamination, and shock, individually or in combination, predispose the injured patient to and may potentiate infection.

THE INJURED PATIENT

The initial approach to the patient with major traumatic injury, that is, to maintain or achieve cardiovascular stability, is not only a lifesaving maneuver but is an attempt to reverse a loss of function on the cellular level. Although cellular dysfunction associated with trauma is reversible,[3] prolonged deficits in tissue perfusion can lead to organ dysfunction. Progressive devitalization of tissue enlarges the niche for infection. In addition, it is anticipated but not shown that the cellular components of the immune system are subject to the same dysfunction that has been documented in tissue and red blood cells.[4] The administration of a balanced salt solution and replacement of lost blood in the hypovolemic injured patient should be considered an integral part of the prophylaxis for infection.

Factors Associated with Infection

Several factors related to the type of injury are associated with the development of infection in the traumatized patient (Table 1). An appreciation for the contribution of devitalized tissue, visceral injury, and extent of contamination guides the therapeutic approach. Injury secondary to a high-velocity missile is anticipated to devitalize tissue, even in the absence of external signs, since cavitation within the wound may destroy large quantities of tissue. In addition, the kinetic energy of a projectile may be transmitted to viscera without obvious violation of body cavities, thereby leading to unsuspected injury. Significant infections related to retained single foreign bodies are rare but do occur. Contamination and infection in such cases are probably more related to the organs the missile passes through than to exogenous sources.[5] On the other hand, injuries caused by multiple fragments are often contaminated by exogenous sources since the wounds may contain pieces of clothing, wadding, and powder in addition to the multiple foreign bodies.

Stab wounds are rarely associated with large amounts of devitalized tissue but are of concern because of the potential for visceral injury and possible contamination with endogenous organisms. Likewise, blunt trauma causes organ injury, and with the rupture of a hollow viscus, endogenous contamination occurs. A high risk of infection is associated with multiple-organ injury and other major injuries, in particular, with an injury to viscera that contain bacteria (Table 2). That this is true is supported by reports that patients sustaining isolated colon injuries have a 12–71 percent chance of infection and a mortality rate of 3–15 percent.[6–9] In 43–100 percent of cases late mortality is due to infectious complications.[10,11] The National Research Council's classification[12] of operative and traumatic wounds, which emphasizes the extent of injury and contamination, includes the criteria outlined here.

TABLE 2. Organ-Specific Factors Associated with a High Risk of Infection

High-Risk Injury	*High Risk on Basis of Contamination*
Multiple organ	Perforated viscus
Pancreatic	Colon/rectum
Liver	Vagina
Esophageal	Biliary tract
	Urinary tract
	Small bowel
	Stomach
	Respiratory tract
	Other
	Mouth
	Anus

Effects of Trauma on Host Defense. In addition to the specific aspects of injury outlined, the trauma patient is at risk for infection due to suppression of the immune response at several levels. Balch studied patients after severe battle trauma and found a decreased ability of neutrophils to phagocytose bacteria in vitro for the first 24 hours after injury.[13] Several studies have shown impaired chemotactic activity, decreased neutrophil lysozomal enzymes, and lower serum immunoglobulin levels subsequent to thermal injury.[14–19] Davis et al.[20] have shown that chemotactic activity and random migration of neutrophils were depressed significantly during days 5–15 after injury. This study confirmed the inverse relationship between neutrophil chemotactic responsiveness and the extent of thermal injury, as well as a correlation between the severity of the neutrophil defect and the decrease in neutrophil lysozyme content. Such findings are consistent with neutrophil degranulation and subsequent depressed neutrophil responsiveness.

Studies from other laboratories[21,22] have demonstrated a cell-directed inhibitor of chemotaxis by serum from burn patients. All of these studies indicate that the burn patient develops a leukocyte chemotactic defect that is thought to predispose to infection. The difficulty in quantitating the extent of injury in other types of trauma contributes to the fact that few data are available in these patients with regard to neutrophil function after injury.

Current studies suggest that defects in human macrophages or function of the reticuloendothelial system (RES) may play a role in postinjury susceptibility to infection. Donovan[23] studied the clearance of iodine 125 microaggregated albumin immediately after surgery. He found a decreased clearance rate in eight out of nine patients, which correlated with the duration of the procedure and with decreased blood pressure. Scovill et al.[24] studied the effect of surgical trauma on the RES of animals. They observed a depressed RES function after surgery and decreased hepatic localization and increased pulmonary localization of labeled test particulate matter. Fibronectin, an α_2-opsonic glycoprotein, has been found to have depressed levels

TABLE 1. Factors Associated with Infection after Traumatic Injury

	Factors Associated with the Development of Infection				
			Contamination		
Type of Trauma	*Devitalized Tissue*	*Foreign Body*	*Exogenous*	*Endogenous*[a]	*Risk of Infection*
Penetrating					
Stab wound	±	–	±	+	+
Projectile					
Low velocity	+ +	+		+ + + +	+ + +
High velocity	+ + + +	+		+ + + +	+ + + +
Multiple fragments (shotgun, shrapnel)	+ + +	+ + +	+ + + +		+ +
Nonpenetrating					
Burn	+ + + +	–	–	–	+ + + +
Blunt	+ +	–	+	+ + +	+ +

[a] Location dependent.

24 hours after major operative procedures in patients who sustain severe trauma. This decrease in opsonic activity was transient and persisted over a 48- to 72-hour period postinjury. The trauma patient who ultimately died had lower levels of this circulating opsonic activity. Preliminary studies suggest that infusion of purified fibronectin may be of some benefit in patients who have depressed RES activity after major injury.

Depressed cellular immune function after major injury has been documented by reports of impaired delayed hypersensitivity reactions,[25,26] a prolongation of allograft and xenograft rejection times,[27–29] and altered mitogen and mixed lymphocyte responses.[30–32] Although these changes are incompletely characterized, there have been reports that T-cell function and numbers are affected such that increased suppressor activity[33] and decreased helper activity[34] may occur. Furthermore, immunologic suppression and fatal outcome have been associated with abnormal monocyte function.[35,36]

The only specific organ injury that has been associated with depressed host resistance is that of a loss of splenic tissue. In 1967, Eraklis and associates[37] reported that 5.4 percent of 467 patients died of postsplenectomy sepsis. Most of these deaths occurred within 4 years of splenectomy, and children seemed to have the greatest risk. Further reports of multicenter studies by Singer[38] suggested that the overall mortality due to sepsis in 2795 patients who underwent splenectomies was 2.52 percent. However, patients who underwent splenectomies for traumatic injury of the spleen had the lowest rate of septic mortality, which was nevertheless almost 60 times higher than that in the healthy population. Additional studies of adult populations suggest that the incidence of sepsis is increased in patients with (4.3 percent) and without (2.2 percent) chronic disease after splenectomy.[39] A more recent retrospective study[40] suggests that trauma patients have a higher rate of sepsis, both early and late after splenectomy, than do injured patients who have not undergone splenectomy. The primary cause of decreased host resistance to encapsulated bacteria after splenic loss is not fully delineated; however, the serum of these patients contains decreased amounts of opsonizing activity for pneumococci[41] and lower levels of IgM,[42] and tuftsin levels have been reported to be decreased.[43] The growing concern for the preservation of splenic tissue will be addressed under prophylaxis.

ACUTE PROPHYLAXIS AND TREATMENT

Coincident with the initiation of fluid resuscitation, systemic antibiotics are administered according to the extent, location, and type of injury. Data to support the use of preoperative antibiotics in the injured patient are based on the use of antibiotics before elective operative procedures (iatrogenic trauma). A recent review of 42 prospective studies of the use of antibiotics in the perioperative period in colon and rectal surgery reaffirms the value of short-term antibiotic administration.[44] These data confirm the necessity of achieving adequate tissue levels of antibiotics at the time of clean–contaminated operative procedures. Since traumatic injuries must be anticipated to equal or exceed this extent of contamination,[45] the standard approach has been to use perioperative antibiotics. However, in most cases contamination has occurred before medical care, and therefore, in a strict sense antibiotic administration must be viewed as therapy rather than as prophylaxis. The importance of the timing of antibiotic therapy is documented by animal studies in which antibiotics given 12 hours before were effective but those given 12 hours after infection were not.[46] Additional studies by Miles et al. and by Burke have indicated that antibiotics administered 4 hours after experimental infection were ineffective.[47,48] The value of preoperative administration of antibiotics after trauma has been shown by Fullen et al.[49] Stone et al.[50] have confirmed these clinical studies. When the interval from injury to the initiation of antibiotics was an average of 64 minutes, the wound infection rate from penetrating colon injuries was 11 percent, and no mortality was reported.[51]

Antibiotics, administered early after injury, are selected on the basis of the organisms that are anticipated to be present. Intra-abdominal contamination–infection is treated with antimicrobials active against aerobic and facultative organisms as well as anaerobes. The typical choice is combination antibiotic therapy; however, some have suggested that cefoxitin may be of equal value if administered soon after injury.[52] Penetrating injuries involving soft tissues are treated with agents that are penicillinase resistant and effective against gram-positive organisms. Injuries likely to be prone to clostridial infection are treated with penicillin. The treatment of soft tissue infections is specifically outlined in Chapters 74 and 75.

Any wound, including burn wounds, has the potential for harboring *Clostridium tetani*; therefore, patients who sustain penetrating injuries need adequate prophylaxis for tetanus. The following outline is a modification from the American College of Surgeons Committee on Trauma as presented by Sandusky[53]:

Immunization completed previously; last booster within 1 year: No additional toxoid required.

Immunization completed within the previous 10 years; no subsequent booster: Give 0.5 ml of Td.*

Immunization completed more than 10 years previously; last booster within the previous 10 years: Give 0.5 ml of Td* if wound is particularly tetanus prone. No booster necessary for minor wounds.

Immunization completed more than 10 years previously; no booster within the previous 10 years; wound minor and relatively clean, treated promptly and adequately: Give 0.5 ml of Td.*

Immunization completed more than 10 years previously; no booster within the previous 5 years; wound other than minor and relatively clean and/or not treated promptly: Give 0.5 ml of Td* and 250 units of TIG(H).† (If wound is considered prone to clostridial infection, give 500 units.)

No history or record of immunization; wound minor and very clean; wound surgery prompt and adequate: Begin immunization using 0.5 ml of Td*; give patient a written record of immunization, and schedule appointments for completion of immunization.

No history or record of immunization; wound other than minor and very clean, or not treated promptly or adequately: Give 250 units of TIG(H).† (If wound is considered prone to clostridial infection, give 500 units.) Begin immunization.

The Surgical Approach

A rapid and complete clinical and laboratory evaluation is essential to detect and anticipate injuries. Undiagnosed and therefore untreated injuries can lead to life-threatening infectious complications in the traumatized patient. For this reason x-ray films are taken to estimate the path of foreign bodies. Blunt trauma to the torso is evaluated clinically, but in the unresponsive patient or in those who are unable to be adequately examined, peritoneal lavage is used to detect intra-abdominal injury.[54] Hematuria demands a full work-up of the genitourinary tract,[55] and elevated serum amylase levels lead to a strong suspection of pancreatic, duodenal, and small bowel injury.[56] The value of computed tomography (CT) scanning in evaluating trauma to the head is well documented, and recent experience suggests that this is a valuable tool in detecting intra-abdominal injury. A comprehensive and quick preoperative evaluation minimizes the chance of infectious complications of missed injuries.

As with all surgical procedures, the goal is to minimize ad-

* Td: tetanus and diphtheria toxoid, adult type.

† TIG(H): tetanus immune globulin (human). When TD and TIG(H) are given concurrently, a separate syringe and needle and separate sites should be used.

ditional tissue injury. Necrotic and contaminated tissues are débrided, and dead space is minimized. Perforation of the gastrointestinal tract requires prompt identification and repair. Even if the secretions released into the abdominal cavity are not contaminated (i.e., bile), chemical peritonitis develops, which leads to ileus, edema of the bowel wall, and ultimately to a leakage of bacteria into the peritoneal cavity. On the other hand, gross contamination of the peritoneal cavity mitigates against primary repair of the violated gastrointestinal tract, particularly in relation to colon injury. The conservative approach in such injuries is to divert the colonic stream or to exteriorize all colonic injuries. Advocates of primary repair without colostomy have sited a significant complication rate related to the colostomy and its closure[57]; this has not been confirmed by additional studies.[58] Attempts to show that primary closure is acceptable in colon injury in highly selected patients have been difficult to interpret due to high baseline infection rates (57 percent wound and 29 percent abdominal) with the conservative approach[59] or the small number of patients studied.[60] The meticulous selection of patients with isolated right colon injuries suggests that primary closure of such injuries is safe without diversion. The study reported by Arango et al.[8] indicated that the mortality is only 3.2 percent and the morbidity 22 percent in 307 right colon cases treated in this manner.

The rationale behind external drainage of injured tissue stems from the high incidence of infection associated with dead space fluid collections, which are isolated from normal defense mechanisms. In addition, if leakage of corrosive material (e.g., pancreatic secretions) or bacteria-laden material is anticipated, drainage is carried out. Furthermore, drainage lessens the chance of the collection of blood from raw surfaces. Concern for draining such collections stems from the long-held belief that blood products potentiate infection in tissues. Current data implicate hemoglobin as a potentiating factor in experimental peritoneal infection and suggest that red blood cell stroma inhibits neutrophil function.[61] Residual blood and bacteria are diluted by irrigation of the peritoneal cavity, but localized contamination may be spread by such procedures, and hypothermia can ensue through the use of large volumes of room temperature fluids.

PROPHYLAXIS AND TREATMENT OF NOSOCOMIAL INFECTION

As already indicated, the early approach to infection in the trauma patient is therapeutic rather than prophylactic. Therefore, prophylaxis in the strict sense is only applicable to the development of hospital-acquired infection in these patients. That nosocomial infection is a substantial problem in severely traumatized patients cared for in critical care units is confirmed by the report of 639 such infections in 381 patients studied over a 2-year period.[62] Bacteremia without an apparent source occurred in 21 percent of these patients. The ability to ascertain whether infection is directly related to trauma or is a secondary occurrence is jaded by the fact that the patient with major injury is predisposed to infection. Cultures obtained initially from the wound or injured viscera assist in defining whether subsequent infection is primarily due to the injury.

If treatment of the injury and associated infection has been appropriate from a surgical standpoint, that is, necrotic tissue débrided, injured viscera repaired, and so on, then the primary concerns in preventing additional infection relate to appropriate antibiotic usage and the environment. The administration of antibiotics for presumed infection initially is limited to a short duration (three doses) unless overwhelming contamination, established infection in the tissue, or surgical débridement has been limited due to concern for removal of vital organs. Concern for the development of infection from resistant organisms selected by prophylactic antibiotics even in cases of major tissue injury such as burns has led to several studies that reveal that the use of such antibiotics in inpatients with major injury is of no benefit.[63] The judicious use of antibiotics for as short a term as possible is advocated to minimize nosocomial infections. Although multiple variables such as severity of the illness and frequency of the use of intravascular catheters contribute to the development of nosocomial infection, it appears that superinfection and especially fungal infection can be attributed to the prolonged use of antibiotics.[64]

There are now sufficient data to support the clinical observation that prolonged immobilization of patients leads to increased rates of infection. In a classic article[65] Seibel et al. have shown that early fixation of long-bone fractures and early mobilization can dramatically decrease the post-trauma complication rate. Not only is the infection rate decreased, but the development of adult respiratory distress syndrome (ARDS) is diminished. Such findings are also supported by studies of early mobilization of patients with disrupted pelvic rings.[66] A less clearly defined factor in these patients was the contribution of enteral feedings. Data are now accumulating to suggest that a decrease in gastrointestinal integrity may contribute to increased infection rates after injury. Enteral nutrition appears to maintain gastrointestinal integrity to a greater degree than does parenteral feeding.[67] Translocation of bacteria across the gastrointestinal barrier after injury has been shown,[68] but whether translocation of bacteria correlates with infection and sepsis is not yet known.

Indwelling Catheters

Infection at the site of intravenous catheters is more often the cause of sepsis than are contaminated intravenous solutions,[69] but contaminated infusion sets due to breaks in aseptic technique may also substantially contribute to sepsis in these immunodepressed patients.[70] The fibrin sheath that forms on the indwelling catheter may be infected from bacteria traveling along the catheter[71] or by hematogenous spread in the patient with prolonged venous cannulation. Most septic phlebitis has been attributed to peripheral intravenous cannulae in surgical patients,[72] especially from those placed in the emergency room.

Additional intravascular devices, including catheters connected to transducers used to measure intra-arterial and intravenous pressures, are sources for septicemia in these patients. Nosocomial outbreaks of bacteremia, candidemia, and hepatitis B have been associated with these devices.[73] Bacterial contamination has been associated with the use of stopcocks[74] and heparin-lock needles left in place for 4 days or longer.[75] Furthermore, ice baths used to cool arterial blood gas and cardiac output syringes have been implicated in outbreaks of infection.[76] Although purulent thrombophlebetis is overall an uncommon occurrence,[72] it carries a high mortality rate in traumatized patients even if appropriately treated.[77] In order to avoid these complications, all catheters are removed after 3 days.[78] A semiquantitative catheter culture technique has been reported that may assist in detecting these infections.[79]

Since the most common site for infection in patients in surgical intensive care units is the urinary tract, attempts should be made to minimize the duration of indwelling urinary catheters.

The Environment

The patient who sustains major trauma and requires intensive care in specialized units has a 50 percent risk of colonization by exogenous bacteria and a 23 percent chance of unit-acquired infection after only 3 days in the unit. This risk increases with time in the unit such that by 10 days colonization occurs in 90 percent of patients and the infection risk is 75 percent.[80] The primary vectors of these infections are personnel in the unit. Additional sources include respiratory equipment, endotracheal tubes, and the catheters listed above. Strict discipline with regard to handwashing, dress policy, cleaning policy, and aseptic technique is essential to minimize the development of nosocomial infection in these patients.[81]

Specific Organ Injury

With the accumulation of data indicating an increased susceptibility to infection in the postsplenectomy patient, emphasis has been placed on the preservation of splenic tissue. Although the risk of postsplenectomy sepsis has been reported to be less after splenectomy for trauma[38] than after splenectomy for other indications, there nevertheless is an increased risk of sepsis in patients after trauma-related splenectomy.[40] Recent studies have supported repair of the injured spleen as an alternative to splenectomy.[82,83] Such an approach is indicated when hemostasis can be obtained and when the abdominal cavity is not contaminated from additional injuries. A more radical approach, applied in children, has been that of nonoperative therapy for splenic injury.[84] This approach has yet to gain general acceptance due to the risks associated with missed additional intra-abdominal injury and the difficulty in applying this approach to the patient with multiple injuries. In general, consideration should be given to long-term prophylactic penicillin administration in patients who have undergone splenectomies as well as to immunization with pneumococcal and perhaps meningococcal vaccines.[85]

REFERENCES

1. Shires GT. Principles of Trauma Care. 3rd ed. New York: McGraw-Hill; 1985:xi.
2. Alexander JW, MacMillian BG. Hospital infections in burns. In: Bennett JV, Brachman P, eds. Nosocomial Infections. Boston: Little, Brown; 1979:335.
3. Shires GT, Cunningham JN, Baker CRF, et al. Alterations in cellular membrane function during hemorrhagic shock in primates. Ann Surg. 1972;176:288–95.
4. Yurt RW. Immunologic and molecular changes associated with trauma. New Dev Med. 1987;2:77–84.
5. Tzeng S, Swan KG, Rush BF. Bullets. A source of infection? Am Surg. 1982;48:239–40.
6. Haygood FD, Polk HC Jr. Gunshot wounds of the colon: A review of 100 consecutive patients with emphasis on complications and their causes. Am J Surg. 1976;131:213–8.
7. Kirkpatrick JR, Rajpal SG. The injured colon: Therapeutic considerations. Am J Surg. 1975;129:187–91.
8. Arango A, Baxter CR, Shires GT. Surgical management of traumatic injuries of the right colon: Twenty years of civilian experience. Arch Surg. 1979;114:703–6.
9. Chilimindris C, Boyd DR, Carlson LE, et al. A critical review of management of right colon injuries. J Trauma. 1971;11:651–60.
10. Mulherin JL, Sawyers JL. Evaluation of three methods for managing penetrating colon injures. J Trauma. 1975;15:580–7.
11. Schrock TR, Christensen W. Management of perforating injuries of the colon. Surg Gynecol Obstet. 1972;135:65–8.
12. Dudrick SJ, Baue AE, Eiseman B, et al. Manual of Preoperative and Postoperative Care: American College of Surgeons. Philadelphia: WB Saunders; 1983:110.
13. Balch HH. The effect of severe battle injury and of post-traumatic renal failure on resistance to infection. Ann Surg. 1955;142:145–63.
14. Warden JD, Mason AD Jr, Pruitt BA Jr. Evaluation of leukocyte chemotaxis in vitro in thermally injured patients. J Clin Invest. 1974;54:1001–4.
15. Grogan JB. Suppressed in vitro chemotaxis of burn neutrophils. J Trauma. 1976;16:985–8.
16. Fikrig SM, Karl SC, Suntharalingam L. Neutrophil chemotaxis in patients with burns. Ann Surg. 1977;136:746–8.
17. Alexander JW. Serum and leukocyte lysosomal enzymes. Arch Surg. 1967;95:482–91.
18. Munster AM, Hoagland HC, Pruitt BA Jr. The effect of thermal injury on serum immunoglobulins. Ann Surg. 1970;172:965–9.
19. Daniels JC, Larson DL, Abston S, et al. Serum protein profiles in thermal burns: I. Serum electrophoretic patterns, immunoglobulins and transport protein. J Trauma. 1974;14:137–52.
20. Davis JM, Dineen P, Gallin JI. Neutrophil degranulation and abnormal chemotaxis after thermal injury. J Immunol. 1980;127:1467–71.
21. Altman LC, Furukawa CT, Klebanoff SJ. Depressed mononuclear chemotaxis in thermally injured patients. J Immunol. 1977;119:199–205.
22. Warden GC, Mason AD, Pruitt BA Jr. Suppression of leukocyte chemotaxis in vitro by chemotherapeutic agents used in the management of thermal injuries. Ann Surg. 1975;181:363–9.
23. Donovan AJ. The effect of surgery on the reticuloendothelial cell function. Arch Surg. 1967;94:247–50.
24. Scovill WA, Saba TM, Blumenstock FA, et al. Opsonic alpha-2 surface binding glycoprotein therapy during sepsis. Ann Surg. 1979;188::521–9.
25. Rapaport FT, Milgrom F, Gesner B, et al. Immunologic sequelae of thermal injury. Ann NY Acad Sci. 1968;150:1004–8.
26. Munster AM, Eurenius K, Katz RM, et al. Cell mediated immunity after thermal injury. Ann Surg. 1973;177:139–43.
27. Polk HC. Prolongation of xenograft survival in patients with pseudomonas sepsis. Surg Forum. 1968;19:514–7.
28. Kay GD. Prolonged survival of a skin homograft in patients with extreme burns. Ann NY Acad Sci. 1957;64:767–74.
29. Ninneman JL, Fisher JC. Prolonged human allograft rejection to the spontaneous immunosuppression following thermal injury. Transplantation. 1978;25:69–72.
30. Miller CL, Baker CC. Changes in lymphocyte activity after thermal injury. J Clin Invest. 1979;63:202–10.
31. Mahler D, Batchelor JR. PHA transformation of lymphocytes in burned patients. Transplantation. 1971;12:409–11.
32. Daniels JC, Sakai H, Cobb ER. Evaluation of lymphocyte reactivity studies in patients with thermal burns. J Trauma. 1971;11:595–601.
33. Munster AM. Post-traumatic immunosuppression is due to activation of suppressor T-cells. Lancet. 1977;1:1319–21.
34. Antonacci AC, Good RA, Gupta S. T-cell subpopulations following thermal injury. Surg Gynecol Obstet. 1982;155:1–8.
35. Miller CL. Effect of surgery on quantity of lymphocyte subpopulations. J Surg Res. 1976;21:155–8.
36. Miller CL, Misholl RT. Differential regulatory effects of accessory cells on CMI. J Immunol. 1975;114:692–5.
37. Eraklis AJ, Kevy SJ, Diamond LK, et al. Hazard of overwhelming infection after splenectomy in childhood. N Engl J Med. 1967;276:1225–9.
38. Singer DB. Postsplenectomy sepsis. Perspect Pediatr Pathol. 1973;1:285–311.
39. O'Neal BJ, McDonald JC. The risk of sepsis in the asplenic adult. Ann Surg. 1981;194:775–8.
40. Sekikawa T, Shatney CH. Septic sequelae after splenectomy for trauma in adults. Am J Surg. 1983;145:667–73.
41. Winkelstein JA, Lambert GH, Swift A. Pneumococcal serum 81: Opsonizing activity in splenectomized children. J Pediatr. 1975;87:430–3.
42. Shumacher MJ. Serum immunoglobulin and transferrin levels after childhood splenectomy. Arch Dis Child. 1970;45:114–7.
43. Constantopoulos A, Najjar VA, Wish JB, et al. Defective phagocytosis due to tuftsin deficiency in splenectomized rats. Am Dis Child. 1973;124:663–5.
44. Bartlett SP, Burton RC. Effects of prophylactic antibiotics on wound infection after elective colon and rectal surgery: 1960 to 1980. Am J Surg. 1983;145:300–9.
45. Shires GT, Dineen P. Sepsis following burns, trauma, and intra-abdominal infections. Arch Intern Med. 1982;142:2012–22.
46. Alexander JW, McGloin JJ, Altemeier WA. Penicillin prophylaxis in experimental wound infections. Surg Forum. 1960;11:299–300.
47. Miles AA, Miles EM, Burke J. The value and duration of defense reactions of the skin to the primary lodgement of bacteria. Br J Exp Pathol. 1957;38:79–96.
48. Burke JF. The effective period of preventive antibiotic action in experimental incisions and dermal lesions. Surgery. 1961;50:161–8.
49. Fullen WD, Hunt J, Altemeier WA. Prophylactic antibiotics in penetrating wounds of the abdomen. J Trauma. 1972;12:282–9.
50. Stone HH, Haney BB, Kolb LD, et al. Prophylactic and preventive antibiotic therapy: Timing, duration and economics. Ann Surg. 1979;189:691–9.
51. Oreskovich MR, Dellinger EP, Lennard ES, et al. Duration of preventive antibiotic administration for penetrating abdominal trauma. Arch Surg. 1982;117:200–5.
52. Nichols RL, Smith JW, Trunkey DD, et al. Clindamycin-gentamicin versus cefoxitin for traumatic fecal soilage of the peritoneum (Abstract). In: Proceedings of the 21st Interscience Conference on Antimicrobial Agents and Chemotherapy. Chicago: 1981.
53. Sandusky WR. Prophylaxis of infection in trauma. In: Mandell GL, Douglas RG, Bennett JE, eds. Principles and Practice of Infectious Diseases. 2nd ed. New York: Churchill Livingstone; 1979:835.
54. Thal ER, Shires GT. Peritoneal lavage in blunt abdominal trauma. Am J Surg. 1973;125:64–71.
55. Shires GT. Trauma. In: Schwartz SI, Shires GT, Spenser FC, et al., eds. Principles of Surgery. New York: McGraw Hill; 1984:202.
56. Olsen WR. The serum amylase in blunt abdominal trauma. J Trauma. 1973;13:200–4.
57. Machiedo GW, Casey KF, Blackwood JM. Colostomy closure following trauma. Surg Gynecol Obstet. 1980;151:58–60.
58. Thal ER, Yeary EL. Morbidity of colostomy closure following colon trauma. J Trauma. 1980;20:287–91.
59. Stone HH, Fabian TL. Management of perforating colon trauma: Randomization between primary closure and exteriorization. Ann Surg. 1979;190:430–6.
60. Flint LM, Vitale GC, Richardson JD, et al. The injured colon: Relationship of management to complications. Ann Surg. 1981;193:619–23.
61. Dunn DL, Nelson RD, Condie RM, et al. Mechanisms of the adjuvant effect of hemoglobin in experimental peritonitis. VI. Effects of stroma-free hemoglobin and red blood cell stroma on mortality and neutrophil function. Surgery. 1983;93:653–9.

62. Caplan ES, Hoyt N. Infection surveillance and control in the severely traumatized patient. Am J Med. 1981;70:638–40.
63. Durtschi MB, Orgain C, Counts GW, et al. A prospective sutdy of prophylactic penicillin in acutely burned hospitalized patients. J Trauma. 1982;22:11–4.
64. Feingold DS. Hospital-acquired infections. N Engl J Med. 1970;283:1384–91.
65. Seibel R, LaDuca J, Hassett JM, et al. Blunt multiple trauma (ISS 36), femur traction, and the pulmonary failure-septic state. Ann Surg. 1985;202:283–93.
66. Goldstein A, Phillips T, Sclafani SJA, et al. Early open reduction and internal fixation of the disrupted pelvic ring. J Trauma. 1986;26:325–33.
67. Alexander JW. Nutrition and infection: New perspectives for an old problem. Arch Surg. 1986;121:966.
68. Deitch EA, Berg RD. Endotoxin but not malnutrition promotes bacterial translocation of the gut flora in burned mice. J Trauma. 1987;27:161–6.
69. Band JD, Maki DG. Safety of changing intravenous delivery systems at longer than 24 hours intervals. Ann Intern Med. 1979;91:173–8.
70. Duma RJ, Warner JF, Dalton HP. Septicemia from intravenous infusions. N Engl J Med. 1971;284:257–61.
71. Maki DG. The prevention and management of device-related infection in infusion therapy. J Med. 1980;11:239–53.
72. Baker CC, Petersen SR, Sheldon GF. Septic phelbitis: A neglected disease. Am J Surg. 1979;138:97–103.
73. Weinstein RA, Stamm WE, Kramer L, et al. Pressure monitoring devices overlooked source of nosocomial infection. JAMA. 1976;236:936–8.
74. Walrath JM, Abbott NK, Caplan E, et al. Stopcock bacterial contamination in invasive monitoring systems. Heart Lung. 1979;8:100–4.
75. Ferguson RL, Rosett W, Hodges GR, et al. Complications with heparin-lock needles. Ann Intern Med. 1976;85:583–6.
76. Stamm WE, Colella JJ, Anderson RL, et al. Indwelling arterial catheters as a source of nosocomial bacteremia: An outbreak caused by *Flavobacterium* species. N Engl J Med. 1975;292:1099–102.
77. Stein JM, Pruitt BA Jr. Suppurative thrombophlebitis: A lethal disease. N Engl J Med. 1976;282:1452–5.
78. Pruitt BA Jr, McManus WR, Kim SH, et al. Diagnosis and treatment of cannula-related intravenous sepsis in burn patients. Ann Surg. 1980;191:546–54.
79. Maki DG, Weise CE, Sarafin HW. A semiquantitative culture method for identifying intravenous catheter-related infections. N Engl J Med. 1977;296:1305–9.
80. Northey D, Adess ML, Hartsuck JM, et al. Microbial surveillance in a surgical intensive care unit. Surg Gynecol Obstet. 1974;139:321–5.
81. Centers for Disease Control. Isolation Techniques for Use in Hospitals. 2nd ed. Washington DC: Government Printing Office; DHEW Publication No. 76-8314. 1976.
82. Ratner M. Surgical repair of the injured spleen. J Pediatr Surg. 1977;12:1019–25.
83. Pachter HL, Hofstetter JR, Spencer FC. Evolving concepts in splenic surgery. Ann Surg. 1981;194:262–9.
84. Wesson DE, Filler RM, Ein SH, et al. Ruptured spleen: When to operate? J Pediatr Surg. 1981;16:324–6.
85. Dickerman JD. Traumatic asplenia in adults. A defined hazard? Arch Surg. 1981;116:361–3.

79. BURNS

ROGER W. YURT
G. TOM SHIRES

The disruption of homeostasis associated with severe burn injury exceeds that of any other injury or disease. With the advent of aggressive early resuscitation measures, mortality in the acute phase after injury is rare.[1] However, the mortality after burns of greater than 40 percent of the body surface area (BSA), which is primarily attributed to infection, continues to be high. Since the risk of developing infection relates directly to the extent of injury, the initial therapeutic approach is oriented toward limiting the progression of the injury by stabilization of the patient and maintenance of blood flow to the wound. The development and progression of the burn wound is well characterized as a dynamic process in which there are irreversible changes in the zone of coagulative necrosis and potentially reversible changes for as long as 3 days in the zones of stasis and hyperemia.[2,3] Since methods of manipulating the inflammatory response that may mediate the progression of the injury are not yet available, the primary goal of early burn therapy is to ensure adequate delivery of oxygen, nutrients, and circulating cells to the wound. Therefore, immediate burn care focuses on prevention of progression of injury and maintenance of a viable interface at which both specific and nonspecific defenses against infection can be mounted.

WOUND AND INFLAMMATORY PATHOPHYSIOLOGY

The evolution of the burn wound is dramatically seen in conversion of partial to full thickness wounds during difficult resuscitations, particularly in patients at the extremes of age in which cardiac output cannot meet the circulatory demand of large surface area injury. In such patients with progressive necrosis and limited defense at the viable tissue interface, early microbial invasion of wounds is to be anticipated. Similarly, decreases in body temperature due to heat loss to the environment or secondary to application of cool solutions or ice to the wound may lead to progressive deterioration of the wounds. Although circulating factors that depress myocardial function after burn injury have been postulated to exist,[4] the primary problem in maintenance of cardiovascular stability is ongoing intravascular volume depletion. Efforts are therefore directed at volume repletion, and α-adrenergic agents in particular are avoided in view of the deleterious result of further diminution of wound blood flow. Likewise, meticulous evaluation of blood flow in extremities with circumferential full thickness injury is necessary to avoid additional compromise of wound and muscular blood flow. When signs of compromised blood flow first appear, escharotomy is performed to diminish the developing pressure in the extremity.

In addition to the culture media provided by the necrotic tissue, the patient with large burns is predisposed to infection due to depression of nonspecific, humoral, and cellular immune function. Circulating levels of immunoglobulins are inversely proportional to the extent of injury,[5] and persistently decreased levels of IgG have been related to mortality.[6] Increased suppressor T-cell activity has been reported,[7,8] the number and function of helper T cells is decreased,[9] and monocyte defects have been reported,[10] leading to the hypothesis that depressed immune response in these patients is due to an imbalance in the cellular immune system. Based on prospective study of patients with large burns, however, it has been suggested that disorders of neutrophil function appear to be the major predisposing factors to the development of sepsis.[11]

That the response of the neutrophil to a site of injury and antigen challenge was depressed in patients with 40 percent or greater total body surface area burn was shown by McCabe et al.[12] using the skin window technique. Such findings of depressed neutrophil response in vivo have been confirmed by quantitating the response to heat-killed *Staphylococcus* in burn-injured patients.[13] The study of the mechanism of decreased neutrophil response to microbial invasion and injury has centered around in vitro study of neutrophil function. The chemotactic response of peripheral blood neutrophils after thermal injury is depressed early after injury in proportion to the extent of tissue damage[14] and correlates with mortality, presumably due to sepsis.[14,15] Although Grogan[15] did not find a factor in burn serum that depressed chemotaxis, others have suggested that such a factor exists and may be related to topical chemotherapy.[16] It has been postulated that consumption of complement components might account for depressed neutrophil response after burn injury[17]; however, even low levels of complement were sufficient to opsonize the invading bacteria.[18] More recent data from an animal model suggests that neutrophils do not respond to the burn wound as well after large burns. However, in vivo evaluation of neutrophil activity indicated that the cells were more responsive than after lesser injury.[19] These findings suggest that "indiscriminant" margination may be occurring after injury. Such a response would lead to depressed appropriate wound response and potentially cause distant tissue damage. Others have described similar events in infected patients and have correlated release of leukocyte enzymes with levels of chemotactic factors produced by complement activation.[20]

PREVENTION OF INFECTION

Although it is common practice to give prophylactic systemic antibiotics (penicillin) to outpatients with burns, current data do not support their general usage in the inpatient population.[21,22] Frequent evaluation of the wound and surrounding tissue allows early and appropriate therapy of cellulitis while sparing a majority of patients exposure to unnecessary antibiotics. However, it is well documented[23] that manipulation of the burn wound leads to bacteremia, and therefore antibiotics are administered immediately before and during burn wound excision. The choice of antibiotics is dictated by knowledge of the current flora in the burn center or more specifically by the burn wound flora of the individual patient. The cyclic nature of particular microorganisms causing burn wound invasion in this center is documented by the results of wound biopsies between January and June of 1982 (Table 1). *Enterobacter cloacae* was frequently isolated but was most prominent in March, April, and June. *Staphylococcus aureus*, which was methicillin-resistant, was most prominent in May, but no isolates were found in April. Based on such data, the current regimen for wound manipulation prophylaxis consists of intravenous vancomycin and amikacin.

The advent of effective topical antimicrobial therapy has decreased the incidence of conversion of partial thickness to full thickness wound by local infection. In addition, these agents may prolong the sterility of the full thickness burn wound; however, they have not eliminated the need for aggressive removal of the necrotic tissue and closure of the wound with autograft. Silver nitrate in a 0.5% solution is an effective topical agent when used before wound colonization. However, since this agent does not penetrate eschar, its broad spectrum gram-negative effectiveness is diminished once bacterial proliferation has occurred in the eschar. Additional disadvantages of this agent include the need for continuous occlusive dressings, which limit evaluation of wounds and range of motion. The black discoloration of the wound, as well as the environment, contributes to a decrease in use of silver nitrate.

The topical burn wound creams allow for open wound therapy and, except in an outpatient setting, are most commonly used without dressings. Mafenide acetate (Sulfamylon) cream has a broad spectrum of activity against gram-negative organisms but little activity against staphylococci. A significant advantage of this agent is that it penetrates the burn eschar and therefore is effective in the colonized wound. The disadvantages of Sulfamylon are transient burning sensation, an accentuation of postinjury hyperventilation, and inhibition of carbonic anhydrase activity. Silver sulfadiazine, on the other hand, is a soothing cream with good activity against gram-negative organisms. Since it does not penetrate the wound, it is best used as a prophylactic antimicrobial. Bacterial resistance to silver sulfadiazine has been reported.[24] Some centers have adopted an approach of alternating agents to take advantage of the attributes of both, such as at Brooke Army Medical Center, where silver sulfadiazine is applied at night and Sulfamylon during the day.[24] The current approach in our center is to initiate topical prophylaxis with silver sulfadiazine and to switch to Sulfamylon if wounds appear to deteriorate based on clinical and laboratory criteria.

TABLE 1. Distribution of Organisms in Burn Wound Biopsies

	Jan	*Feb*	*Mar*	*Apr*	*May*	*June*
Number of biopsies	189	141	244	201	162	69
Number of positive biopsies	84[a]	39	85	84	70	41
Enterobacter cloacae	29.8[b]	18.0	37.7	82.1	25.7	39.0
Staphylococcus aureus	27.4	28.2	22.4	0	42.9	17.1
Staphylococcus epidermidis	14.3	5.1	0	3.6	0	0
Enterococcus faecalis	10.7	12.8	4.7	2.4	11.4	17.1
Escherichia coli	7.1	7.6	11.8	6.0	4.3	12.2
Pseudomonas aeruginosa	2.4	5.1	20.0	6.0	8.6	12.2

[a] $\geq 10^5$ organisms/gram tissue.
[b] % of total positive biopsies.

The goal of burn therapy is to prevent burn wound infection by permanent closure of the wound as rapidly as possible. The recognition of the advantages of early removal of necrotic tissue and wound closure has led to an aggressive surgical approach in selected patients.[1] In such cases, full thickness wounds are excised as soon after injury as cardiovascular stability has been achieved. The advantages of this approach include removal of eschar before colonization, which typically is appreciated at 5–7 days after injury, and reduction of the overall extent of injury. The extent of excision of burn wound is usually limited to 20% of the body surface area at any one time, and blood loss is limited to one blood volume. Such an approach is most easily achieved by excision of full thickness injury to the level of the fascia, since blood loss is minimized under these conditions. The open wound is covered with autograft as donor sites are available or with allograft. This is repeated until the entire wound is closed. This aggressive surgical approach is modified by the age of the patient (ideal 15–35 years of age) and factors such as significant pre-existing disease and inhalation injury, which require a more conservative approach to the burn wound.

An additional difficulty with early excisional therapy is that one risks the possibility of excision of burned tissue that may heal if left alone over a 2–3-week period. If such a question arises, initial tangential excision of the eschar or biopsy may assist in evaluating the depth and the possibility of healing of the burn wound. Recent data suggests that a more conservative approach in which operative time is limited to 2 hours and blood loss to four units may contribute to improved survival from extensive burn injury.[25] In an effort to achieve burn wound closure more rapidly, Burke et al.[26] have advocated the use of immunosuppressive therapy to enhance allograft acceptance in children with extensive burns. These patients were kept in bacteria-controlled nursing units to minimize the possibility of infection during immunosuppresion. Attempts to follow a similar protocol in adults have been discouraging.[24]

Throughout the course of hospitalization, efforts are directed toward minimizing contamination of the patient's wounds. Cross-contamination is avoided by use of gowns, gloves, and masks by nursing, medical staff, and visitors. The patient is not touched except with a gloved hand, and each patient is restricted to his or her own monitoring and diagnostic equipment. Concern over the potential for cross-contamination in large burn centers has led to the diminished use of traditional Hubbard tanking of patients. A satisfactory alternative is showering and débridement on a covered or readily disinfected plinth. If adequate nursing care can be provided, it is preferable to isolate patients who have large open wounds in individual rooms. Burke's bacteria-controlled nursing unit[27] has been advocated as a means of protecting the patient and the environment. Such elaborate systems are not generally available.

DIAGNOSIS AND TREATMENT OF INFECTION

Wound Infection

Although surface cultures of burn wounds are helpful from the standpoint of evaluating the potential pathogens that exist on the patient and on a burn ward, they give no indication of the actual status of the wound itself. Biopsy of the wound, however, has been shown to give an accurate indication of the status of the wound.[28] Pruitt and Foley reported that quantitative cultures of 10^5 or more bacteria per gram of tissue or histologic evidence of bacterial invasion of viable tissue correlated with a high (75 percent) mortality rate.[28] In addition, serial biopsies that indicated advancing wound infection were associated with mortality rates of 85 percent, whereas stable or improving wounds were associated with an overall mortality rate of 55 percent. Direct correlation between biopsy and autopsy diagnosis was found in 26 of 32 patients. These data and that of others[29] support systematic evaluation of burn wounds with biopsy of all areas of wound change. Routine biopsy of full thickness burn wound on an every-other-day schedule has allowed detection of progressive wound infections.[30] The rapid fixation technique allows histologic diagnosis of invasive infection within 3 hours, whereas quantitative counts and identification of the organism is available within 24 hours. The combined use of histologic and culture techniques provides early diagnosis as well as identity and sensitivity of the organism to antimicrobials.

A change in wound appearance or character provokes the clinician to modify therapy and stimulates an aggressive diagnostic approach. Hemorrhage, rapid eschar separation, or greenish discoloration of eschar or subeschar fat suggest bacterial colonization or invasion of the wound. If clinical or biopsy data support a diagnosis of colonization, then a change in topical therapy and plans for excision would be entertained (Table 2). However, when the findings are consistent with invasive infection, then more aggressive therapy is instituted. In addition, if bacteremia is documented and other sources are eliminated, urgent surgical intervention is necessary. In the absence of documented bacteremia, signs of sepsis such as hypo- or hyperthermia, hypotension, decreased urinary output, hyperglycemia, thrombocytopenia, or neutropenia or neutrophilia support early intervention. When the wound is invaded with gram-negative organisms, surgical excision to the level of the fascia is the procedure of choice. In preparation for surgery or in those patients who require stabilization before general anesthesia is given, a penetrating topical agent is used (Sulfamylon), and subeschar clysis is initiated using an appropriate antibiotic. The choice of antibiotic is based on previous biopsy sensitivity data or data accumulated on sensitivities of the current flora in the patient population. Such a preoperative approach is based on recent data that indicated that Sulfamylon pulse therapy is effective in decreasing wound colony counts[31] and the previous data of Baxter et al.[30] supporting the efficacy of subeschar clysis. In general, systemic antimicrobials are not necessary, since the full daily dose of antibiotic administered by clysis is absorbed into the circulation. The direct administration of antibiotic into the viable—nonviable tissue interface is supported by concern that systemically administered antibiotics may not reach sufficient levels in the tissues with poor or absent vascularity. There are some data, however, that suggest that antibiotics administered at a distant site are effective[31] and that systemically administered antibiotics reach these tissues. Whether activity of the antimicrobial is maintained in these foci is not known.

In distinction to gram-negative invasion, gram-positive infection often presents as suppurative foci in the tissue or is associated with rapid eschar separation. In such cases, simple débridement with unroofing of involved areas, under the umbrella of appropriate systemic antibiotics, is sufficient acute therapy. Since surgical debridement should arrest this process, topical agents are of lesser importance; however, the wound should not be allowed to dessicate. Silver sulfadiazine, Dakin's solution, and triple antibiotic solutions have been used for this purpose.

Although gram-positive burn wound infection is anticipated to be primarily a suppurative type of infection, there appears to be a growing number of patients who present with primary nonsuppurative gram-positive infections. These infections are caused by methicillin-resistant *Staphylococcus aureus* (personal observation), and whether diminished neutrophil response or a change in the nature or virulence of such organisms[32] may explain this phenomenon is unknown. Burn wound invasion of this type seems to be best treated as are gram-negative invasive infections (Table 2).

Blackened discoloration of the burn wound should arouse suspicion of fungal infection. Such changes are more typical of the phycomycetes.[24] Confirmation of such organisms are best made on histologic sections of wound biopsies, where, in addition, a determination of invasion of viable tissue can be made. Reliance on culture data will prolong the time to diagnosis. Although silver sulfadiazine is active against *Candida* sp., a mixture of this agent or Sulfamylon with Mycostatin may be more effective in the topical therapy of superficial fungal infections. Since fungal infection is often preceded by bacterial infection and multiple antibiotic therapy, the use of Sulfamylon in such a mixture is preferred.[24] The treatment of fungal invasion is surgical excision to the level of noninvaded viable tissue. When invasion extends to the level of the investing fascia, the excision is carried deep to this level to viable muscle.[33] The cytotoxicity of currently available antifungal agents mitigates against their use for preoperative clysis. Recovery of the fungus from the blood mandates systemic therapy, which is often used even without positive blood cultures if invasion is documented and clinical signs are present.

Pulmonary Infection

With the advent of effective topical therapy for the burn wound, pulmonary complications have become a prominent problem in the burned patient.[34] In addition, the ability to salvage an increasing number of patients from the shock phase immediately after injury has led to a greater number of patients surviving to the time (2–3 days postinjury) when the effects of inhalation injury become clinically prominent.[35] In patients without inhalation injury but with large burns, postinjury hyperventilation

TABLE 2. Prophylaxis and Treatment of Burn Wound Infection

Diagnosis	Topical	Clysis	Systemic Therapy	Surgical
"Clean" burn	Silver sulfadiazine/ silver nitrate	No	No	Excision/debridement
Superficial/colonization	Silver sulfadiazine/ Sulfamylon	No	No	Excision/debridement
$Gram^-$ invasion	Sulfamylon	Yes	No	Excision to fascia
$Gram^+$ invasion				
Suppurative	Silver sulfadiazine	No	Yes	Unroof
Nonsuppurative		Yes	No	Excision to fascia
Fungus				
Superficial	Sulfamylon/Mycostatin	No	No	Excision
Invasive	Sulfamylon/Mycostatin	No	Yes	Exision to or deep to fascia

and subsequent decreases in tidal volume may lead to atelectasis and subsequent pneumonia. Furthermore, a recognized complication of circumferential full thickness chest burns is a decrease in compliance of the chest wall. Aggressive pulmonary toilet and escharotomy, respectively, are necessary to maintain pulmonary function. Since these patients frequently require large-volume feedings via nasogastric or nasojejunal tubes, aspiration must be guarded against. Diminished mucociliary functions and destruction of airways by inhalation of products of combustion lead to airway obstruction and infection.[36] Frequent diagnostic and therapeutic bronchoscopy are necessary in this group of patients.

Attempts at specific prophylaxis of the sequellae of inhalation injury, such as nebulization of antibiotics[37] and treatment with steroids,[38] have failed to show any benefit. Although hematogenous pneumonia is less frequent than in the past,[34] It remains a significant problem in the patient with burns. When it occurs, the source (most commonly wound or suppurative vein) must be defined and eradicated. Prophylactic antibiotics are not used for either bronchopneumonia or hematogenous pneumonia; specific therapy is based on knowledge of previous endobronchial culture, and sensitivity is substantial by repeat cultures at the time of diagnosis.

Miscellaneous Infections

Several additional types of infection are a significant problem in burned patients and should be mentioned here because of their frequency and peculiarities of clinical presentation. The diagnosis of suppurative thrombophlebitis in the presence of normal tissue (see Ch. 61) is often difficult to make. In the burned patient, the addition of injured and necrotic tissue compounds this difficulty. Less than 35 percent of suppurative veins in burned patients present with local findings.[39] The incidence of this disease in burned patients is at least as high as 5 percent, and the mortality, even in treated suppurative thrombophlebitis, reaches 60 percent.[39] In the absence of a septic venous source, persistent positive blood cultures in the burned patient should be attributed to endocarditis until proven otherwise.

In addition to superficial tissue damaged by direct heat, deeper tissue can be injured and present as a focus of infection. The vascular compromise associated with circumferential full thickness injury if not decompressed early leads to muscle necrosis and subsequent pyomyositis (see Ch. 76). A high index of suspicion is necessary to detect these changes in an already edematous extremity. Direct electrical contact can lead to deep muscular necrosis with delayed infection. Furthermore, significant visceral damage may occur after electrical injury, with subsequent abscess formation.[40]

CONCLUSIONS

The combination of injury-associated immunosuppression and the large area of nonviable tissue in the patient with greater than 30 percent surface area burns inevitably leads to infection. Success in treatment of these patients rests more with removal of necrotic tissue and achieving wound closure than through the use of antimicrobials. Current data support the judicious use of systemic antibiotics for therapy of documented infection and for prophylaxis during burn wound manipulation. The cyclic nature of the rise and fall of various bacteria and the rapid emergence of resistance to antibiotics in the burned patient population supplies ample evidence that there is always a niche that will be filled. Although contamination of the wound must be minimized and surveillance adequate to detect organisms before they invade the wound, closure of the wound is the primary prophylactic and therapeutic maneuver in the care of the burned patient.

REFERENCES

1. Curreri WP, Luterman A, Braun DW, et al. Burn injury analysis of survival and hospitalization time for 937 patients. Ann Surg. 1980;192:472–8.
2. Jackson DM. The diagnosis of the depth of burning. Br J Surg. 1953;40:588–96.
3. Noble HGS, Robson MC, Krizek TJ. Dermal ischemia in the burn wound. J Surg Res. 1977;23:117–25.
4. Baxter CR, Cook WA, Shires GT. Serum myocardial depressant factor of burn shock. Surg Forum. 1966;17:1–2.
5. Arturson G, Hogman CF, Johansson SGO, et al. Changes in immunoglobulin levels in severely burned patients. Lancet. 1969;1:546–8.
6. Munster AM, Hoagland HC, Pruitt BA Jr. The effect of thermal injury on serum immunoglobulins. Ann Surg. 1970;172:965–9.
7. Munster AM. Post-traumatic immunosuppression is due to activation of suppressor T-cells. Lancet. 1977;1:1319–21.
8. Ninnemann JL, Fisher JC. Prolonged human allograft rejection due to the spontaneous immunosuppression following thermal injury. Transplantation. 1978;25:69–72.
9. Antonacci AC, Good RA, Gupta S. T-cell subpopulation following thermal injury. Surg Gyn Obstet. 1982;155:1–8.
10. Shelby J, Merrell SW. In vivo monitoring of postburn immune response. J Trauma. 1987;27:213–6.
11. Alexander JW, Ogle CK, Stinnett JD, et al. A sequential prospective analysis of immunologic abnormalities and infection following severe thermal injury. Ann Surg. 1978;188:809–16.
12. McCabe WP, Rebuck JW, Kelly AP Jr, et al. Leukocyte response as a monitor of immunodepression in burn patients. Arch Surg. 1973;106:155–9.
13. Balch HH, Watters BS, Kelly D. Resistance to infection in burned patients. Ann Surg. 1963;157:1–19.
14. Warden GD, Mason AD Jr, Pruitt BA Jr. Evaluation of leukocyte chemotaxis *in vitro* in thermally injured patients. J Clin Invest. 1974;54:1001–14.
15. Grogan JB. Suppressed *in vitro* chemotaxis of burn neutrophils. J Trauma. 1976;16:985–8.
16. Warden GD, Mason AD Jr, Pruitt BA Jr. Suppression of leukocyte chemotaxis *in vitro* by chemotherapeutic agents used in the management of thermal injuries. Ann Surg. 1975;181:363–9.
17. Bjornson AB, Altemeier WA, Bjornson HS, et al. Host defense against opportunist microorganisms following trauma. I. Studies to determine the association between changes in humoral components of host defense and septicemia in burned patients. Ann Surg. 1978;188:93–101.
18. Bjornson AB, Altemeier WA, Bjornson HS. Complement, opsonins, and the immune response to bacterial infection in burned patients. Ann Surg. 1980;191:323–9.
19. Yurt RW, Pruitt BA. Decreased wound neutrophils and indiscriminate margination in the pathogenesis of wound infection. Surgery. 1985;95:191–8.
20. Solomkin JS, Jenkins MK, Nelson RD, et al. Neutrophil dysfunction in sepsis. II. Evidence for the role of complement activation products in cellular deactivation. Surgery. 1981;90:319–27.
21. Alexander JW: Prophylactic antibiotics in trauma. Am Surg. 1982;48:45–8.
22. Durtschi MB, Orgain C, Counts GW, et al. A prospective study of prophylactic penicillin in acutely burned hospitalized patients. J Trauma. 1982;22:11–4.
23. Sasaki TM, Welch GW, Herndon DN, et al. Burn wound manipulation-induced bacteremia. J Trauma. 1979;19:46–8.
24. Pruitt BA Jr. The burn patient: II. Later care and complications of thermal injury. Curr Probl Surg. 1979;XVI:1–95.
25. Demling RH. Improved survival after massive burns. J Trauma. 1983;23:179–84.
26. Burke JF, Quinby WC, Bondoc CC, et al. Immunosuppression and temporary skin transplantation in the treatment of massive third degree burns. Ann Surg. 1975;182:183–97.
27. Burke JF, Quinby WC, Bondoc CC, et al. The contribution of a bacterially isolated environment to the prevention of infection in seriously burned patients. Ann Surg. 1977;186:377–87.
28. McManus AT, Kim SH, Mason AD, et al. A comparison of quantitative microbiology and histopathology in divided burn wound biopsies. Arch Surg. 1987;122:74–6.
29. Loebl EC, Marvin JA, Heck EL, et al. The method of quantitative burn wound biopsy cultures and its routine use in the care of the burned patient. Am J Clin Pathol. 1974;61:20–4.
30. Baxter CR, Curreri PW, Marvin JA. The control of burn wound sepsis by the use of quantitative bacterial studies and subeschar clysis with antibiotics. Surg Clin North Am. 1973;53:1509–18.
31. McManus WF, Mason AD Jr, Pruitt BA Jr. Subeschar antibiotic infusion in the treatment of burn wound infection. J Trauma. 1980;20:1021–3.
32. Lacey RW, Chopra I. Effect of plasmid carriage on the virulence of *Staphylococcus aureus*. J Med Microbiol. 1975;8:137–47.
33. Levine BA, Sirinek KR, Pruitt BA Jr. Wound excision to fascia in burned patients. Arch Surg. 1978;113:403–7.

34. Pruitt BA Jr, Flemma RJ, DiVincenti FC, et al. Pulmonary complications in burn patients: a comparative study of 697 patients. J Thorac Cardiovasc Surg. 1970;59:7–20.
35. Bingham HG, Gallagher TJ, Powell MD. Early bronchoscopy as a predictor of ventilatory support for burned patients. J Trauma. 1987;27:1286–8.
36. Hunt JL, Agee RN, Pruitt BA Jr. Fiberoptic bronchoscopy in acute inhalation injury. J Trauma. 1975;15:641–9.
37. Levine BA, Petroff PA, Slade CL, et al. Prospective trials of dexamethasone and aerosolized gentamicin in the treatment of inhalation injury in the burned patient. J Trauma. 1978;18:188–93.
38. Welch GW, Lull RJ, Petroff PA, et al. The use of steroids in inhalation injury. Surg Gyn Obstet. 1977;145:539–44.
39. Pruitt BA Jr, McManus WF, Kim SH, et al. Diagnosis and treatment of cannula-related intravenous sepsis in burn patients. Ann Surg. 1980;191:546–54.
40. Newsome TW, Curreri PW, Eurenius K. Visceral injuries: an unusual complication of an electrical burn. Arch Surg 1972;105:494–7.

80. BITES

ELLIE J. C. GOLDSTEIN

Bite wounds are often mistakenly considered innocuous by both patients and physicians. Most data on the incidence of infection, the bacteriology, and the value of various medical and surgical methods of the treatment of bite wounds come from anecdotal case reports and noncomparable and retrospective studies that are further biased by the types of patients who elect to seek medical attention. Consequently, there are diverse approaches to the therapy for these common injuries. Bite wounds consist of lacerations, evulsions, punctures, and scratches. Although many patients never seek or need medical attention, there is a growing awareness of the magnitude of the infectious complications from bites. The bacteria associated with bite infections may come from the environment, from the victim's skin flora, or most frequently, from the "normal" oral flora of the biter.

ANIMAL BITES

It is estimated that 1–2 million people in the United States are bitten by dogs yearly.[1] Although the incidence of bites due to other animals remains undetermined, bite patients account for almost 1 percent of emergency room visits,[2] which results in over $30 million direct medical care costs.[3] Most dog bites are provoked attacks and involve the victim's own pet or a known animal.[4,5] Only 10 percent of attacks are caused by stray animals. Most injuries are caused by large dogs (more than 50 lb)[5] capable of jaw pressures of 200–450 lb/sq in. and result in extensive crush injury.[6] Most victims are men or boys under 20 years old; most incidents occur in the warm-weather months. Over 70 percent of bites are to the extremities, with the right upper extremity the most frequent site. Facial bites are more frequent in children under 10 years old and lead to 5–10 deaths per year, often due to exsanguination.[7]

There appear to be two distinct groups of patients who present for medical care[4]: those who present within 8 to 12 hours after injury and those who present more than 12 hours after injury. The patients in the first group are usually concerned with repair of disfiguring wounds or the need for rabies or tetanus therapy. Most of these patients will have attempted prior therapy, including washing their wounds with soap and water or hydrogen peroxide or applying topical salves. The effect of this first aid on the bacteriology of these wounds or their infection rate, is unknown. These early presenting wounds are almost always contaminated with multiple strains of aerobic and anaerobic bacteria similar to the spectrum found in documented bite infections. Patients who present after 12 hours of injury (often 24–48 hours) usually have established infection.[8–12] It was noted that the risk of infection was increased when the patient was over 50 years old, delayed seeking therapy, or had a puncture wound or a wound to the upper extremity.[8] It was also noted that 16 percent of wounds, including 4 percent of facial wounds, 12 percent of scalp wounds, and 28 percent of hand or arm wounds, later became infected despite various forms of therapy. Other studies note that between 1.6 and 29 percent of "treated" wounds will become infected.[3,4,6,8–14]

Infection is usually manifested by a localized cellulitis, pain at the site of injury, and a purulent discharge, often gray and malodorous. Temperature over 37.2°C, regional adenopathy, and lymphangitis occur in less than 20 percent of patients. Wounds close to bones or joints may penetrate these structures and cause septic arthritis, osteomyelitis, tenosynovitis, or local abscesses in any potential anatomic spaces. Puncture wounds more frequently result in abscess formation. Some patients may develop sepsis, endocarditis, meningitis, or brain abscess secondary to bites.

Several unusual clinical presentations of dog bite infection are recognized. Fiala et al.[15] reported a case of fatal sepsis associated with coagulopathy and renal thrombotic microangiopathy in a compromised host due to *Bacteroides* sp. Several reports have noted fatal infection due to the Centers for Disease Control (CDC)-designated bacteria DF-2 in association with splenectomy or severe hepatic disease.[16–19] This organism may be difficult to isolate and identify and may require up to 14 days of incubation to grow on blood culture. Brucellosis and blastomycosis have also been transmitted by dog bites.[20,21] Women who have undergone modified radical mastectomy may develop lymphangitis and sepsis. Lupus patients and those taking steroids may also have a greater tendency to develop sepsis after bite wounds.

Dog bite wound infections are considered to be predominantly related to the dog's oral flora.[22–25] Studies on the normal canine oral flora note the frequent isolation of *Pasteurella multocida* (12–60 percent), *Staphylococcus aureus* (18–42 percent), coagulase-negative staphylococci (32–40 percent), *Weeksiella zoohelcum* (38–90 percent), EF-4 (up to 74 percent), M5 (10–12 percent), and DF-2 (up to 8 percent). Other species isolated with varying frequency including *Streptococcus, Staphylococcus intermedius, Corynebacterium, Neisseria, Moraxella, Bacillus*, and various gram-negative rods.[26–28, 28a]

In England, Lee and Buhr[11] isolated *P. multocida* in 50 percent of infected dog bites. Other studies note much lower rates of isolation, usually about 20 percent.[4,8,24] Douglas[2] noted *S. aureus, Staphylococcus epidermidis*, and α-hemolytic streptococci to be the most frequently isolated pathogens.

When aerobic and anaerobic cultures are obtained, aerobic (including facultative) and anaerobic bacteria may be isolated from 74 and 41 percent of wounds, respectively.[4] Anaerobic bacteria, when present, were always isolated in mixed culture. Gram stains of the wounds were a specific but nonsensitive predictor of bacterial growth. Sixty-eight percent of noninfected early presenting wounds grew potential pathogens, and 88 percent of infected wounds grew bacterial pathogens. Streptococci were the most frequently isolated bacteria. Other bacteria frequently isolated included *P. multocida* (30 percent), *S. aureus* (30 percent), *Bacteroides* sp. (19 percent), and *Fusobacterium* sp. (19 percent). There was little difference in the types of bacteria isolated from noninfected early-presenting wounds and infected later-presenting wounds. All moderate to severe dog bite wounds, especially to the hands, except those that are not clinically infected and are more than 1 day old should be considered contaminated with potential pathogens.

Wounds inflicted by cats are frequently scratches or tiny punctures located on the lower extremities and are likely to become infected.[29,30] *Pasteurella multocida* has been isolated from the oropharynx of 50–70 percent of healthy cats and is a frequent pathogen in cat-associated wounds.[24,29–31] Tularemia has also been transmitted by cat bites.[32] People are also bitten by a wide variety of other animals, including unusual domestic pets, farm animals, wild animals, and laboratory animals.[2,10,33,34] Monkey bites cause more swelling and infection than do many other animal bites and may transmit B virus (herpesvirus simiae).

Management of Animal Bites

Tear wounds should be copiously irrigated. Puncture wounds may be irrigated by using a 20 ml syringe with a 19 gauge needle attached. Debris should be removed, and skin tags and devitalized tissue should be cautiously, surgically débrided.[35] Whether bite wounds that are clinically uninfected and are seen within 12 hours of injury should be surgically closed remains controversial.[3,4,8,11,35] Hand wounds may present a special situation due to their increased propensity to become infected and the disasterous consequences when infection does occur.

In conflict with most other studies,[4,13,35] one recent prospective study[3] noted the lack of value of early antimicrobial therapy. We feel that since these wounds are usually contaminated with potential pathogens it is advisable to treat hand bites and all bite wounds not trivial in nature with antibiotics. Penicillin (or ampicillin) is the most active agent against *P. multocida* and the other oral aerobic and anaerobic bacteria of dog oral flora. Some feel that amoxicillin/clavulanic acid should be used for empirical therapy since it covers *S. aureus, P. Multocida*, and the anaerobic bacteria likely to be found in bites. Tetracycline is a good alternative for penicillin-allergic patients but should not be used in pregnant women and young children. Erythromycin will be active against only 50 percent of *P multocida* isolates, and anaerobes may be or develop resistance.[36] Clindamycin and the penicillinase-resistant penicillins should be avoided because of their poorer activity against *P. multocida*.[37] Oral first-generation cephalosporins are not as active as penicillin against *P. multocida* and some anaerobes. Cefuroxime axetil, a second-generation oral cephalosporin, and the fluoroquinolones show good activity against *P. multocida* and many other bite isolates.[38] Patients who present early with uninfected wounds should receive antimicrobial therapy for 5 days. Despite the use of the above measures, between 8 and 16 percent of these wounds will become infected.

Patients who present with established infection should be managed similarly. They may need more extensive drainage and surgical débridement. Immobilization and elevation of the injured area is important and even required to achieve optimal healing. Infected wounds should not be closed primarily. Empirical antibiotic therapy should be changed according to specific cultural data and continued for 7–14 days depending on the severity of the infection and patient response.

Tetanus toxoid should be administered to patients requiring a booster. Rabies, cat scratch disease, tularemia, brucellosis, and other animal-associated diseases are discussed in the appropriate chapters.

VENOMOUS SNAKE BITES

Venomous snakes, usually vipers (rattlesnakes, copperheads, cottonmouths, or water moccasins), bite approximately 8000 people in the United States yearly.[39,40] Envenomization can cause extensive tissue destruction and devitalization that predisposes to infection from the snake's "normal" oral flora. Sparse data exist on the incidence and bacteriology of snake bite infections. In rattlesnakes, the oral flora appears to be fecal in nature since their live prey usually defecate in the snake's mouth coincident with ingestion. Common oral isolates include *Pseudomonas aeruginosa, Proteus* sp., coagulase-negative staphylococci, and *Clostridium* sp.[41,42] Other potential pathogens isolated from rattlesnakes mouths include *Bacteroides fragilis* and *Arizona hinshawii*. The role of empirical antimicrobial therapy for noninfected wounds is not well defined. Specific therapy based on cultural data of infected wounds should be instituted.

HUMAN BITES

Human bites have a higher complication and infection rate than do animal bites. Wounds of the lip and paronychia and infections of the structure surrounding the nail account for the majority of self-inflicted bite wounds that come to medical attention. Paronychia are more frequent in children who suck their fingers and result from the direct inoculation of the oral flora into the fingers. Brook[43] took cultures from 33 children with paronychia. Aerobes and anaerobes were each found in pure culture in 27 percent of the cases, whereas mixed infection were found in 46 percent of the cases. The most frequent aerobic organisms isolated were viridans streptococci, group A β-hemolytic streptococci, γ-hemolytic streptococci, *S. aureus, Haemophilus parainfluenzae, Klebsiella pneumoniae,* and *Eikenella corrodens*. The most frequently isolated anaerobic bacteria were *Bacteroides* sp., *Fusobacterium* sp., and anaerobic gram-positive cocci. Therapy should include drainage, appropriate antibiotics, and avoidance of further bacterial contamination.

Occlusional human bites may be to any part of the body but most often involve the distal phalynx of the long and/or index fingers of the dominant hand. Bites to the hand are more serious and more frequently become infected than do bites to other areas.[44–46]

Important prognostic factors for the development of infection include the extent of tissue damage, the depth of the wound and which compartments are entered, and the pathogenicity of the inoculated oral bactera.[45–52] Viridans streptococci were the most common wound isolates. *Staphylococcus aureus* occurred in 40 percent of wounds and was usually present in patients who had attempted self-débridement and presented 3–4 days postinjury. Although *Haemophilus influenzae* was occasionally isolated, no other penicillin-resistant gram-negative rods were isolated. *Bacteroides* sp., excluding *B. fragilis, Peptococcus* sp., *Peptostreptococcus* sp., and *Fusobacterium nucleatum* were also frequent isolates.[48] Up to 45 percent of the *Bacteroides* species isolated from human bite wounds may be penicillin resistant and β-lactamase–positive.[38,53]

Management of Human Bites

A Gram stain and aerobic and anaerobic cultures should be obtained on all infected wounds before any therapy. Wounds should be copiously irrigated, surgically débrided, and diagrammed and/or photographed. Immobilization of the affected area, including splinting if necessary, and elevation should be considered. Empirical antimicrobial therapy should be based on the Gram stain (specific but not sensitive) and/or knowledge of the susceptibility of the oral flora. Patients who present early with uninfected wounds should also be given antimicrobial therapy of shorter duration and may be considered for outpatient management. Penicillin is the drug of choice in bite patients unless *S. aureus* is suspected. In that case amoxicillin/clavulanic acid or penicillin plus a penicillinase-resistant penicillin should be used. First-generation cephalosporins are not as effective as the combination suggested due to resistance of some anaerobic bacteria and *E. corrodens*. Many patients will require hospitalization. Wounds in proximity to the bone should have baseline X-ray films taken to watch for osteomyelitis. Most physicians advise against primary closure even of uninfected human bite wounds, especially those of the hands. Facial wounds may present a special situation due to the possibility of scarring and disfigurement, and many authors recommend primary closure. Approximation of the wound margins or delayed primary closure (3–5 days) is often possible even in infected cases.

CLENCHED-FIST INJURIES

Clenched-fist injuries (CFIs) are traumatic lacerations that occur when one person strikes another in the mouth with a clenched fist. These are most common over the third and fourth metacarpophalangeal joints of the dominant hand, but they may also occur over the proximal interphalangeal joints. These lacerations are often only $\frac{1}{4}$–$\frac{1}{2}$ cm long but, despite their innocuous appearance, frequently lead to serious complications due to the proximity of the skin over the knuckles to the joint capsule and the potential spread of infection into subcutaneous, subfascial, subtendnous, subaponeurotic, and web spaces.

Typically, patients sustain a CFI and attempt to cleanse it or, more usually, ignore it until 3–24 hours postinjury when they awaken with a painful, throbbing, and swollen hand. The swelling usually spreads proximally but not distally and results in a decreased range of motion. A purulent discharge is often present. Lymphangitis, adenopathy, fever, or other signs of systemic infection are infrequent.

The bacteriology of CFIs is similar to that of human bites and usually consists of the normal oral flora. Viridans streptococci are the most frequent isolates, but *S. aureus* may be present in 20–40 percent of cases. Anaerobic bacteria can be recovered in over 55 percent of CFIs including *Bacteroides* sp., *Fusobacterium* sp. and peptostreptococci. *Eikenella corrodens* is an often overlooked but especially important pathogen in CFI infections.[54–59] It has a prevalence rate of 59 percent in human gingival plaque[60] and may be isolated in 25 percent of CFIs.[54] It can act synergistically with viridans streptococci and is a common cause of osteomyelitis. Although *E. corrodens* is susceptible to penicillin, it is resistant to penicillinase-resistant penicillins, clindamycin, and metronidazole and is variably resistant to cephalosporins.[61,62]

Management should include examination by an experienced hand surgeon to evaluate the nerve and muscular function and the extent of injury to tendons, bones, and joints. Débridement and copious irrigation is often required. Elevation and immobilization with a plaster splint from the fingers to the elbow are essential and should be continued until there is marked improvement. Aerobic and anaerobic cultures and x-ray films (to check for fracture and osteomyelitis) should be obtained. Many authors suggest the use of tetanus toxoid or both toxoid and antitoxin when indicated. Secondary débridement to remove necrotic bone and/or tissue or to drain abscesses may be advisable.

Antibimicrobial therapy is often intravenous and should include either cefoxitin or penicillin (or ampicillin) plus a penicillinase-resistant penicillin until cultures return. Failure of first-generation cephalosporins and penicillinase-resistant penicillins, when used alone, have been reported and are often due to *E. corrodens*.[54,55] If *S. aureus* is not present, treatment with the penicillinase-resistant penicillin may be discontinued. If resistant gram-negative rods are isolated, therapy should be altered according to cultural data. What role β-lactamase-positive *Bacteroides* species will have in the selection of antimicrobial therapy remains to be determined.

REFERENCES

1. Klien D. Friendly dog syndrome. NY State J Med. 1966;66.2306.
2. Douglas LG. Bite wounds. Am Fam Physician. 1975;11:93.
3. Elenbaas RM, McNabney WK, Robinson WA. Prophylactic oxacillin in dog bite wounds. Ann Emerg Med. 1982;11:248.
4. Goldstein EJC, Citron DM, Finegold SM. Dog bite wounds and infection: A prospective clinical study. Ann Emerg Med. 1980;9:508.
5. Harris D, Imperato PJ, Oken B. Dog bites—an unrecognized epidemic. Bull NY Acad Med. 1974;50:981.
6. Chambers GH, Payne JF. Treatment of dog-bite wounds. Minn Med. 1969;52:427.
7. Winkle WG. Human deaths induced by dog bites, United States, 1974–1975. Public Health Rep. 1977;92:425.
8. Callaham ML: Treatment of common dog bites: Infection risk factors. J Am Coll Emerg Med 1978;7:83.
9. Graham WP III, Calabretta AM, Miller SH. Dog bites. Am Fam Physician. 1977;15:132.
10. Hubbert WT, Rosen MN. *Pasteurella multocida* infection due to animal bites. Am J Public Health. 1970;60:1103.
11. Lee MLH, Buhr AJ. Dog-bites and local infection with *Pasteurella septica*. Br Med J. 1960;1:169.
12. Schultz RC, McMaster WC. The treatment of dog bite injuries, especially those of the face. *Plast Reconstr Surg*. 1972;49:494.
13. Callaham M. Prophylactic antibiotics in common dog bite wounds: A controlled study. Ann Emerg Med 1980;9:410.
14. Zook EG, Miller M, Van Beek AL, et al. Successful treatment protocol of canine fang injuries. J Trauma. 1980;20:243.
15. Fiala M, Bauer H., Khaleeli M, et al. Dog bite, *Bacteroides* infection, coagulopathy, renal microangiopathy. Ann Intern Med. 1977;87:248.
16. Butler T, Weaver RE, Ramani TKV, et al. Unidentified gram-negative rod infection: A new disease of man. Ann Intern Med. 1977;87:248.
17. Finding JW, Pohlmann GP, Rose H. Fulminant gram-negative bacillemia (DF-2) following dog bite in an asplenic woman. Am J Med. 1980;68:154.
18. Martone WJ, Zuehl RW, Minson GE, et al. Postsplenectomy sepsis with DF-2: Report of a case with isolation of the organism from the patient's dog. Ann Intern Med. 1980;93:457
19. Shankar PS, Scott JH, Anderson CL. Atypical endocarditis due to gram-negative bacillus transmitted by dog bite. South Med J. 1980;73:1640.
20. Swenson RM, Carmichael LE, Cundy KR. Human infection with *Brucella canis*. Ann Intern Med. 1972;76:435.
21. Gann JW Jr, Bressler GS, Bodet CA III, et al. Human blastomycosis after a dog bite. Ann Intern Med. 1983;98:48.
22. Goldstein EJC, Citron DM, Finegold SM. Role of anaerobic bacteria in bite wound infections. Rev Infect Dis. 1984;6(Suppl 1):5177.
23. Branson D, Bunkfeldt F Jr. *Pasteurella multocida* in animal bites of humans. Am J Clin Pathol. 1967;48:552.
24. Francis DP, Holmes MA, Brandon G. *Pasteurella multocida* infections after domestic animal bites and scratches. JAMA. 1975;233:42.
25. Hawkins LG. Local *Pasteurella multocida* infections. J Bone Joint Surg [Am] 1969;55A:363.
26. Baile WE, Stowe EC, Schmitt AM. Aerobic bacterial flora of oral and nasal fluids of canines with reference to bacteria associated with bites. J Clin Microbial. 1978;7:233.
27. Saphir DA, Carter GR. Gingival flora of the dog with special reference to bacteria associated with bites. J Clin Microbiol. 1976;3:344.
28. Nyby MD, Gregory DA, Kuhn DA, et al. Incidence of *Simonsiella* in the oral cavity of dogs. J Clin Microbiol. 1977;6:87.

28a. Talan DA, Goldstein EJC, Staatz D, et al. *Staphylococcus intermedius*: Clinical presentation of a new human dog bite pathogen. Annals Emerg Med. In press (1989).

29. Tindall JP, Harrison CM: *Pasteurella multocida* infections following animal injuries, especially cat bites. Arch Dermatol. 1972;105:412.
30. Lucas GL, Bartlett DH. *Pasteurella multocida* infection in the hand. Plast Reconstr Surg. 1981;67:49.
31. Torpy DE: *Pasteurella multocida* in dog and cat bite infections. Pediatrics. 1969;43:295.
32. Quenzer RW, Mostow SR, Emerson JK. Cat bite tularemia. JAMA. 1977;238:1845.
33. Dawson J, Cockel R. *Actinobacillus lingieresii* infection after a horse bite. Br Med J. 1981;283:583.
34. Marrie TJ, Bent JM, West AB, et al. Extensive gas in tissues of the forearm after horsebite. South Med J. 1979;72:1473.
35. Callaham M: Dog bite wounds. JAMA. 1980;244:2327.
36. Goldstein EJC, Citron DM, Richwald GA. Lack of in vitro efficacy of oral forms of certain cephalosporins, erythromycin and oxacillin against *Pasteurella multocida*. Antimicrob Agent Chemother. 1988;32:213.
37. Stevens DL, Higbee JW, Oberhofer TR, et al. Antibiotic susceptibility of human isolates of *Pasteurella multocida*. Antimicrob Agents Chemother. 1979;16:322.
38. Goldstein EJC, Citron DM. Comparative activity of cefuroxime, amoxicillin/clavulanic acid. ciprofloxacin, enoxacin and ofloxacin against aerobic and anaerobic bite wound bacteria. Antimicrob Agent Chemother. 1988;32:1143.
39. Parish HM. Incidence of treated snake bites in the United States. Public Health Rep. 1966;81:269.
40. Russell FE. Clinical aspects of snake venom poisoning in North America. Toxicon. 1969;7:33.
41. Goldstein EJC, Citron DM, Gonzalez H, et al. Bacteriology of rattlesnake venom and implications for therapy. J Infect Dis. 1979;140:818.
42. Williams FF, Freeman M, Kennedy E. The bacterial flora of the mouths of Australian venomous snakes in captivity. Med J Aust. 1934;2:190.
43. Brook I. Bacteriology study of paronychia in children. Am J Surg. 1981;141:703.
44. Mann RJ, Hoffeld TA, Farmer CB. Human bites of the hand: Twenty years of experience. J Hand Surg. 1977;2:97.
45. Welch CE: Human bite infections of the hand. New Engl J Med. 1936;215:901.
46. Boland FK: Morsus humanis. JAMA. 1941;116:127.
47. Barnes MN, Bibby BG. A summary of reports and a bacteriologic study of infections caused by human tooth wounds. J Am Dent Assoc. 1939;26:1163.
48. Goldstein EJC, Citron DM, Wield B, et al. Bacteriology of human and animal bite wounds. J Clin Microbiol. 1978;8:667.
49. Chuinard RG, D'Ambrosia RD. Human bite infections of the hand. J Bone Joint Surg [Am]. 1977;59:416.

50. Guba AM, Mulliken JB, Hoopes JE. The selection of antibiotics of human bites of the hand. Plast Reconstr Surg. 1975;56:538.
51. Peeples E, Boswick JA Jr, Scott FA. Wounds of the hand contaminated by human and animal saliva. J Trauma. 1980;20:383.
52. Shields C, Patzakis MJ, Meyers MJ, et al. Hand infections secondary to human bites. J Trauma. 1975;15:235.
53. Brook I. Microbiology of human and animal bite wounds in children. Pediatr Infect Dis. 1987;6:29.
54. Goldstein EJC, Miller TA, Citron DM, et al. Infections following clenched-fist injury: A new perspective. J Hand Surg. 1978;3:455.
55. Goldstein EJC, Barone M, Miller TA. *Eikenella corrodens* in hand infections. J Hand Surg. 1983;8:563.
56. Bilos ZJ, Kaucharchuk A, Metzger W. *Eikenella corrodens* in human bites. Clin Orthop. 1978;134:320.
57. Carruthers MM, Sommers HM. *Eikenella corrodens* osteomyelitis. Ann Intern Med. 1973;79:900.
58. Johnson SM, Pankey GA. *Eikenella corrodens* osteomyelitis, arthritis and cellulitis of the hand. South Med J. 1976;69:535.
59. McDonald I: *Eikenella corrodens* infections of the hand. Hand. 1979;11:224.
60. Goldstein EJC, Tarenzi LA, Agyare EO, et al. Prevalence of *Eikenella corrodens* in dental plaque. J Clin Microbiol. 1983;17:636.
61. Goldstein EJC, Sutter VL, Finegold SM. Susceptibility of *Eikenella corrodens* to ten cephalosporins. Antimicrob Agents Chemother. 1978;14:639.
62. Goldstein EJC, Gombert ME, Agyare EO: Susceptibility of *Eikenella ccrrodens* to newer beta-lactam antibiotics. Antimicrob Agents Chemother. 1980;18:832.

SECTION K. GASTROINTESTINAL INFECTIONS AND FOOD POISONING

81. PRINCIPLES AND SYNDROMES OF ENTERIC INFECTION

RICHARD L. GUERRANT

Gastrointestinal infections encompass a wide variety of symptom complexes and recognized infectious agents. With the exception of recently recognized *Campylobacter pylori* gastritis, the term *gastroenteritis* is applied to syndromes of diarrhea or vomiting that tend to involve noninflammatory infection in the upper small bowel or inflammatory infection in the colon. Other enteric infections and infestations cause predominantly systemic symptoms. Infections of the gastrointestinal tract, especially infectious diarrhea, are among the most common debilitating infectious diseases, afflicting people of all ages around the world. In many heavily populated areas, deaths from diarrheal illnesses exceed those from any other single cause.

In the absence of demonstrable causal forces, many descriptive terms have arisen through the years. Names such as "Montezuma's revenge," "Delhi belly," "Aden gut," "gyppi tummy," "Aztec two-step," "Greek gallop," "Rome runs," "Hong Kong dog," "Turkey trots," "La turista," "Basra belly," and "back door sprint" illustrate its widespread occurrence. Although an etiologic agent is not found in many cases, the infectious nature of most acute diarrheal diseases is suggested by their epidemiologic behavior showing case clustering, spread in families and other groups, and occurrence among travelers. In the last two decades, much has been learned about bacterial and viral agents capable of causing acute gastrointestinal illnesses. These include *Escherichia coli* that produce enterotoxins, which cause fluid secretion, other *E. coli* capable of causing tissue destruction and inflammation, newly appreciated and increasingly recognized pathogens such as *Yersinia*, *Campylobacter*, *Clostridium*, *Cryptosporidium*, rotaviruses, and Norwalk-like viruses. With the development of new tools for diagnosis, important information has been gained in our understanding of the etiologies, pathogenesis, epidemiology and control of acute gastrointestinal infections.

OCCURRENCE AND SCOPE OF GASTROINTESTINAL INFECTIONS

On a global scale, diarrheal diseases constitute the greatest single cause of morbidity and mortality,[1] far exceeding that from heart disease, cancer, or strokes in many populous areas.[2] The greatest mortality from diarrheal diseases and enteric infections occurs in infants and small children. Over 13 percent of the children born in certain parts of Latin America die before their fifth birthday. In more than half, diarrhea is the major or associated cause of death.[3] Although the global mortality is decreasing (especially with oral rehydration therapy),[4] some transitional areas have a worsening diarrhea mortality,[5] and prolonged diarrhea is emerging as the major cause of death.[6] In areas such as Bangladesh, Guatemala, and Brazil, the attack rates often exceed seven cases per person per year among children under 2 years of age.[7–10] The attack rate is highest at the time of weaning.[8–11] Studies from rural India reveal an annual death rate of 5.36 percent for children in their second 6 months of life.[11] Enteric infections doubtless account for a much larger submerged iceberg of morbidity, especially in association with malabsorption and malnutrition in the tropical developing world. Over 60 percent of the children dying with diarrhea in Latin America also had nutritional deficiencies as associated causes of death, suggesting that diarrhea may precipitate malnutrition.[3] Acute infectious diarrhea exacerbates nutritional deficiencies in several ways. As with any acute infection, caloric demands are increased and often catabolic steroids, glucagon, and adrenergic amines cause increased breakdown of structural proteins.[11] Through vicious cycles of transient malabsorption and anorexia, repeated bouts of acute diarrhea are major contributors to malnutrition.[12–16] The converse is also true; undernutrition appears to reduce resistance to acute infectious diarrhea. Increased attack rates and increased mortality from acute infectious diarrheal illnesses occur with progressive severity of malnutrition.[16–18] As a specific example, shigellae are shed longer and there is an increased relapse rate in children if they are malnourished.[17] In addition, malnutrition appears to predispose to more prolonged diarrheal illnesses.[19]

Military history indicates that acute diarrheal illnesses have played decisive roles in numerous campaigns. Diarrheal diseases and enteric infections comprised the major nontraumatic cause of hospitalization among U.S. troops in Vietnam and approached the number of hospitalizations resulting from injuries due to hostile action.[20] Although the mortality in the United States from diarrheal disease has been dramatically reduced with economic development and improved sanitation facilities in the last 50 years, diarrhea remains the third most frequent syndrome seen in general practice.[21] In studies of community illness among urban and suburban families in Cleveland, Dingle et al. identified "infectious gastroenteritis" as the second most common class of illnesses after common respiratory diseases.[22] In this community 1.5 bouts of gastroenteritis occurred per person each year and accounted for 16 percent of all illnesses. Although causative agents were not identified, the infectious nature of these diarrheal and febrile vomiting illnesses were confirmed by their passage to volunteers via stool filtrates. Data relevant to the epidemiology of diarrheal illnesses (even when the cause is unknown) can be applied to the prevention and control of the varied syndromes of gastrointestinal infections.[23]

EPIDEMIOLOGIC AND ENVIRONMENTAL FACTORS

The frequency, type, and severity of enteric infections are determined by *who* you are, *where* you are, and *when* you are there.

Who is at risk of acquiring a gastrointestinal infection varies greatly with age, living conditions, personal and cultural habits, and group exposures. Although the infant who is being breastfed is relatively protected from contaminated food and water and probably to some degree by maternal colostral antibodies and lactoferrin, at weaning there is a great increase in the risk of diarrheal illness. Adults, particularly if living for many years in the same environment, may become asymptomatic reservoirs of microorganisms that cause diarrhea in the immunologically untutored child or visitor. Living conditions often reflect socioeconomic conditions; type of housing, crowding, sanitation facilities, and water sources are major determinants of environmental exposure to enteric pathogens. The quantity of water available for hygienic and sanitation purposes is often as important as the quality of the water supply.[24] Personal hygienic habits determine how many organisms are ingested. Although the infectious dose varies with the organisms, relatively small inocula of certain organisms may result in disease. Shigellae are acquired with an unusually low infectious dose and are often spread by direct contact among children in day care centers. The majority of nonspecific diarrheal illnesses acquired in communities occur in family clusters, often with small children having the first illness. Of great importance whenever a patient has an enteric illness is a careful history of other illnesses in the family or community. Multiple illnesses and common exposure may be clues to a food-borne outbreak or to the causative agent.

The second epidemiologic determinant of risk for enteric infection is *where* one is. The pattern of illnesses and the etiologic agents vary greatly with climate. For example, *E. coli* that produce heat-labile or heat-stable (LT or ST) enterotoxins cause disease primarily in the tropics, where the heaviest burden of parasites also occurs. Viral causes of common enteric illlnesses have recently been found among young children in temperate and tropical climates. Despite their clustering, however, many community cases of diarrhea remain unexplained.

Finally, the third determinant of risk is *when* you are there. The majority of enteric illnesses in temperate climates occur during winter months. The opposite is true in tropical countries, where distinct summer peaks of illnesses are usual. The role of rainfall is uncertain, as some adjacent areas with similar monsoon climates have opposite seasons of major diarrheal illnesses, as illustrated by the peak seasons for cholera in different parts of Bengal. In Dhaka, endemic cholera consistently occurs during the winter dry months, whereas less than 200 miles away, the peak cholera season in Calcutta occurs during the summer monsoon.

HOST FACTORS

Considering the ubiquity of potential enteric pathogens, it is surprising that enteric infections are not even more common. After exposure to infectious agents, several host factors determine who becomes ill. Several enteric host defenses provide substantial protection against many intestinal pathogens (Table 1).

Host Species, Genotype and Age

Host species, genotype, and age are complex but major determinants of susceptibility to colonization and disease with enteric pathogens. While a broad spectrum of animal hosts are infected with pathogens such as *Salmonella enteritidis* and *Campylobacter jejuni*, only primates or humans are characteristically infected with *Salmonella typhi* or *Shigella* spp. In addition, the intestinal cell receptors for the K88, K99, and colonization factor (CF) attachment traits of enterotoxigenic *E. coli* are largely species specific.[25,26] Interspecies variation and host genotype are also important. Certain ABO blood groups in humans are associated with *Vibrio cholerae* infections.[27,28] Furthermore, Rutter et al. have bred a strain of piglets that do not have the single-locus dominant allele for the intestinal receptor for *E. coli* K88 adherence antigen and are consequently resistant to diarrhea caused by these organisms.[29] Such species or even genotype specificities play tremendously important roles in determining the host susceptibility as well as the epidemiology of these infections.

The role of age in determining host susceptibility is complex. In animals a narrow "age window" of susceptibility to specific enteric infections is well recognized. In humans, the tendency of rotaviral and enteropathogenic *E. coli* (EPEC) infections to affect young children is impressive. The explanations likely reside in age-related changes in gut mucus, cell surface factors, microbial flora, environmental exposure, and specific immune factors. In addition, specific receptors for microbial adhesins or toxins may be developmentally regulated, such as that recently described for *Shigella* toxin in rabbits.[30]

Specific receptor components or antagonists such as monosaccharides like *N*-acetyineuraminic acid (NANA) can be added exogenously and compete with intestinal binding sites for *E. coli*.[26,31] Conversely, lectin-like substances that bind to the intestinal cell receptors may compete with the bacterial attachment factors. Positive chemotaxis of *V. cholerae, E. coli* and *S. typhimurium* has been shown toward rabbit ileal mucosa and a role of negative chemotactic factors have been postulated as new types of host defense.[32]

Personal Hygiene

Whether or not we acquire an enteric infection depends first on the number of pathogens ingested. Nearly all agents of concern are acquired by the oral route. The majority of identified enteric pathogens have come from other mammalian intestinal tracts; often a human fecal–oral route can be traced. A plentiful, conveniently located supply of uncontaminated water, in conjunction with improved sanitary facilities, is critically important

TABLE 1. Enteric Host Defenses

Host species, genotype, and age
Personal hygiene
Gastric acidity and other physical barriers
Intestinal motility
Enteric microflora
Specific immunity
Phagocytic
Humoral
Cell mediated
Nonspecific protective factors and human milk
Intestinal receptors

in reducing this mode of spread.[24,33] Studies of presumptive viral agents that have not yet been defined (the "Marcy" and "Family Study" agents) strongly implicate the human fecal–oral route of infection.[34,35] In the cases of bacterial infections, a large number (100,000–100,000,000) of organisms must usually be ingested to overcome host defenses and to cause disease[36] (Table 2). Such numbers may require growth in food that is allowed to stand unrefrigerated for several hours after the initial contaminating inoculum. Exceptions to the large number of organisms usually required for an infecting dose are *Shigella* and cysts of certain parasites, which can be reproducibly transmitted with only 10–100 organisms. This small inoculum can be readily transmitted directly by person-to-person contact (as in day care centers). This is an unusual route of spread for other bacterial enteric pathogens in all but hosts with impaired defenses or newborn infants.

Gastric Acidity and Other Physical Barriers

The majority of bacterial pathogens ingested never reach the intestines because of the normal gastric acid barrier. When this barrier is neutralized with antacids, both the susceptibility and severity of several enteric bacterial and parasitic infections is increased. At the normal gastric pH (<4), over 99.9 percent of the ingested coliform bacteria are killed within 30 minutes. There is no reduction of an experimental bacterial inoculum in achlorhydric stomachs for 1 hour. Not surprisingly then, the gastric coliform flora in fasting subjects (normally fewer than 10/ml) exceed 10,000/ml in the majority of achlorhydric patients.[37] Excessive numbers of normal bacterial flora in the upper small bowel may contribute to malabsorption and diarrheal syndromes.[38,39]

The inoculum of *V. cholerae* required to cause disease can be reduced 10,000-fold (from 10^8 to 10^4 organisms) by neutralizing gastric acid with 2 g of sodium bicarbonate.[40] In an outbreak of cholera in Israel, 25 percent of the patients had had previous gastric resection, whereas none of a comparable control group had had gastric surgery.[41] The similar association of previous gastric surgery or achlorhydria with increased frequency and severity of *Salmonella* infections has also been noted in several studies.[42] Likewise, the frequency of enteric multiplication of a vaccine strain of *Shigella flexneri* increases threefold with sodium bicarbonate neutralization of gastric acid. With *Campylobacter jejuni*, a substantial range in infectious doses has been documented with different strains.[43] Although gastric acidity may enhance the process of excystation and infection by some parasites after ingestion of the ova, it may provide protection against other parasites. The fragile trophozoite of *Giardia lamblia* (requiring a pH of 6.4–7.1) causes more severe symptoms in association with hypochlorhydria or achlorhydria, perhaps by increased survival of trophozoites refluxed to the stomach and proximal duodenum. The association of achlorhydria and hypochlorhydria with symptomatic strongyloidiasis and other helminthic of the gastric mucosa has also been noted. Some have suggested that vitamin B_{12} deficiency occurs more often in association with fish tapeworm (*Diphyllobothrium latum*) in patients who are achlorhydric and who have high jeujunal infestations. Finally, certain parasitic, viral, or bacterial processes such as *Campylobacter pylori* infections may in themselves alter gastric acidity and thus increase host susceptibility to other enteric pathogens. The further importance of gastric acidity in preventing gastric, pharyngeal, and tracheal colonization by gram-negative bacilli and even nosocomial pneumonia has been shown by the increased risk of patients taking antacids or H2 blockers compared to sucralfate, which preserves gastric acidity.[44]

Other physical barriers such as mucus and mucosal tissue integrity are important resistance factors in healthy hosts and work in concert with gastric acidity and intestinal motility to clear many bacteria from the upper small bowel.[45] Continuous removal and renewal of gastrointestinal mucus may bind organisms and toxins and further aid in protecting the intact mucosa from enzymatic and microbial attack.[46]

TABLE 2. Infectious Doses of Enteric Pathogens

Shigella	10^{1-2}
Campylobacter jejuni	10^{2-6}
Salmonella	10^5
Escherichia coli	10^8
Vibrio cholerae	10^8
Giardia lamblia	10^{1-2} cysts
Entamoeba histolytica	10^{1-2} cysts

Intestinal Motility

Intestinal motility plays the following important roles in normal intestinal physiology: (*1*) in the fluid absorptive process, (*2*) in maintaining the appropriate distribution of indigenous enteric microflora, and (*3*) in ridding the host of pathogenic microorganisms. The role of motility in aiding fluid absorption has been demonstrated in a study done on human volunteers by Higgins et al.[47] Using methantheline bromide (Banthine), they showed that inhibition of normal intestinal motility resulted in impaired absorption of radiolabeled water and sodium. Whereas over 90 percent of a labeled saline bolus was normally absorbed in less than 10 minutes, less than 70 percent was absorbed over a half hour after methantheline bromide administration. Intraluminal distribution of a barium bolus in small bowel before and after methantheline bromide suggested that a reasonable explanation for this impaired absorption was a reduction in the absorptive surface area exposed to the intralumenal fluid. In contrast to the distribution within 2–3 minutes of the bolus of barium throughout the small bowel of healthy persons, methantheline bromide caused a puddling of barium near the injection site in the upper small bowel, which often persisted for over 60 minutes.

Motility also helps to maintain normal distribution and flow of microflora. The risk of bowel stasis is evident in the bacterial overgrowth syndromes in the small bowel and in the added risk of "toxic megacolon" in inflammatory bowel disease after antimotility drugs are administered.

In addition, intestinal motility appears to play a role in providing protection from enteric pathogens. Experimental animals are much more easily infected with enteric pathogens after the inhibition of gut motility with opiates.[48] *Salmonella* bacteremia may develop in patients after opiates are taken for relatively mild gastroenteritis.[49] A controlled study of adults with shigellosis treated with diphenoxylate hydrochloride with atropine (Lomotil) revealed that the antimotility drug abolished antibiotic effectiveness in reducing diarrhea and positive cultures and was associated with prolonged fever and shedding of the *Shigella* organisms.[50] Gut motility and diarrhea that help rid the host of offending pathogens may therefore be analogous to the cough in pulmonary infections as a mechanism to expel pathogens.

Normal Enteric Microflora

In recent years, there have been several developments in our understanding of the composition of intestinal microflora. With improved culture techniques[51] we now recognize that 99.9 percent of the normal enteric bacterial flora are anerobes (approximately 10^{11} organisms/g of normal feces). These organisms (*Bacteroides*, clostridia, peptostreptococci, peptococci, and others) far exceed the number of aerobes. The gram-negative aerobic coliform rods follow—*E. coli*: 10^8/g; *Klebsiella*, *Proteus*, enterococci, and other species: approximately 10^{5-7}/g. We are only beginning to appreciate the role of normal flora as an extremely important and often overlooked host defense. In several situations normal bacterial flora can be shown to be highly effective in resisting colonization by potentially pathogenic invaders. The loss of normal flora or a shift in their balance by antibiotics is often attended with their replacement by organisms such as *Pseudomonas*, *Klebsiella*, *Clostridium*, and *Candida*. When these organisms take up residence, there is a risk of their causing serious systemic infections, especially in a nosocomial setting. There are numerous examples of the increased susceptibility to infection of patients with reduced bacterial flora.[52,53] Several enteric infections, such as infant botulism, nosocomial salmonellosis, and enteropathogenic *E. coli*, occur with increased frequency in newborn infants who have not acquired a normal enteric flora. Diarrhea associated with the use of antibiotics is common and, in many cases, is likely related to an alteration in the balance of normal enteric microflora.

The basis for the resistance provided by normal bacterial flora in the intestinal tract has been elucidated in an elegant series of studies by Bohnhoff et al.[54] In experimental mice, the protective effect of normal flora is eradicated by a single injection of streptomycin. They showed that an infecting dose of *Salmonella typhimurium* was reduced over 100,000-fold by the administration of a single dose of streptomycin. This reduced resistance correlated with the reduction in the normal colonic flora and their toxic acidic products. Resistance was restored with the return of enteric flora (especially *Bacteroides*), either by inoculation or naturally. The importance of a reduced pH and volatile fatty acids from the anaerobic flora in colonization resistance has been further shown by Van der Waaj et al.[55] and by Que et al.[56] It has been shown that indigenous microbes such as *Lactobacillus*, *Bacteroides*, and *Clostridium* spp. attach to the intestinal epithelial surface and act synergistically with host immunity to interfere with experimental *S. typhimurium* challenge.[57] Enteric bacteria including *Proteus*, *Enterobacter*, and *E. coli* also act synergistically in mice with vibriocidal immunity from vaccination to antagonize *V. cholerae*.[58] The protective role of normal enteric bacterial flora in humans has been documented by the increased frequency of *Salmonella* infections among Swedish tourists who took a prophylactic antibiotic compared with those who took no antimicrobial agent.[53] In a huge outbreak of antimicrobial-resistant *S. typhimurium* enteritis involving nearly 200,000 people in Illinois in the spring of 1985, there was a significant association of illness with having taken antimicrobials the month before the illness. There was a fivefold increase (from 6 percent of well controls to 30 percent) of persons having taken antibiotics to which the outbreak strain was resistant.[59]

Intestinal Immunity

Enteric immunity is composed of phagocytic, humoral, and cell-mediated elements. Each component has specific contributions to host resistance to enteric infections. The normal intestinal mucosa demonstrates a state of "physiologic inflammation" in the lamina propria with numerous neutrophils, macrophages, plasma cells, and lymphocytes that suggest a constant battle of the host with luminal challenges to maintain the integrity of the mucosa. The importance of intact phagocytic immunity becomes evident when neutrophils are absent in hosts, who then become particularly susceptible to gram-negative rod infections that often originate in the gastrointestinal tract.[60] The importance of immunity is also demonstrated by the potentially severe adenoviral, rotaviral, coxsackieviral, and *Clostridium difficile* infections in bone marrow transplant patients.[61]

Diarrhea in patients with the acquired immunodeficiency syndrome (AIDS) is becoming increasingly common and raises a special set of diagnostic and therapeutic questions. The growing range of severe, recurring enteric infections in immunocompromised patients,[62] especially those with AIDS, demonstrates the critical role of immunity in resisting a broad range of viral, bacterial, parasitic, and fungal enteric infections. The majority of AIDS patients with diarrhea have a documentable infectious etiology such as cytomegalovirus, *Entamoeba histolytica*, *Cryptosporidium*, *Salmonella*, *Giardia*, *C. jejuni*, *Shigella*, *Mycobacterium* or Herpes simplex virus.[63,64] In Haiti and Africa, up to 95 percent of AIDS patients initially present with diarrhea; up to 50 percent may have *Crytosporidium* infections, followed by 15 percent with *Isospora belli*.[65–67] Still other patients may have the human immunodeficiency virus, which infects the bowel epithelium.[68]

Specific active humoral intestinal immunity (so-called coproantibody) arises either from a leakage of serum immunoglobulin (predominantly IgG or IgM) or from the formation of IgA by plasma cells located predominantly in the lamina propria. Secretory IgA (an 11S dimer [MW 390,000] with a secretory piece [MW 60,000] from the mucosal epithelial cells) is found in the lumen.[69] Both serum and secretory antibody responses have been demonstrated in response to parenteral and intraluminal challenge with cholera toxoid.[70] Secretory IgA is resistant to intraluminal degradation by enzymatic proteolysis and sulfhydryl reduction. The dynamics of local intestinal immunity have been elucidated in several experimental models. The most efficient method of eliciting a local antibody response is with a parenteral priming challenge followed by an intestinal booster antigen challenge. Studies of cholera toxoid immunity in rats suggest that the parenteral priming toxoid prepares a widespread distribution of precursor lymphocytes in areas like the Peyer's patches.[71] These cells are then capable of responding to a booster challenge to produce many large IgA-bearing lymphocytes that appear in the thoracic duct before "homing" back to the lamina propria as specific IgA-secreting plasma cells at or distal to this site of booster toxoid. Passively acquired IgA probably accounts for part of the protection against enteric infections in infants who are breast-fed. Colostral antibody against rotaviruses and the enterotoxins of *V. cholerae* and *E. coli* have been demonstrated in breast milk.[72,73]

Intestinal antibodies may be directed at any of a number of different bacterial antigens such as endotoxin, capsular material, or exotoxins and may have bactericidal, opsonic, or neutralizing effects. Although IgA can have hemagglutinating, precipitating, or virus-neutralizing properties, it does not appear capable of fixing complement in order to have the direct bactericidal effect that IgG and IgM may have. Selective IgA deficiency is often associated with a compensatory increase in IgM levels. Hereditary telangiectasia with IgA deficiency is associated with recurrent rhinopulmonary infection but is rarely associated with intestinal infection or dysfunction.[69] Although debated by others,[74] Zinneman and Kaplan[75] and Ament et al.[76] have suggested that patients with giardiasis have lower IgA levels and that hypogammaglobulinemic patients have more malabsorption and diarrhea with giardiasis. Patients with type 2 combined IgA and IgM deficiency and small intestinal lymphoid hyperplasia with a sparsity of plasma cells may have diarrhea, malabsorption, and giardiasis.[77] Crabbe and Heremans have described three patients with another type of selective IgA deficiency with spruelike intestinal symptoms and histopathologic changes.[78] The role of cell-mediated immune processes in the intestine is suggested by adjuvant enhancement of vaccine efficacy against intracellular infections such as *S. typhi*.[79]

Other Protective Factors in Human Milk and Serum

The protection afforded by breast-feeding likely relates to several passively transmitted factors, as well as to reduced exposure to a contaminated environment.[8–13,80,81] In addition to antibody, these include lactoferrin, lysozyme, phagocytes, high lactose, low protein, low phosphate, and low pH (in part from bifidobacteria).[80–85] The role of lactoferrin in human milk is suggested by the abolition of milk's bacteriostatic properties against *V. cholerae* and enteropathogenic *E. coli* by saturation with iron.[85] In addition, patients with chronic iron excess from hemolytic processes such as malaria, sickle cell anemia, and Oroya fever are at increased risk of infection with organisms such as *Salmonella*. Some of the bacteriostatic properties of normal serum were abolished when iron-binding proteins were saturated with iron.[85]

MICROBIAL FACTORS

A number of bacterial virulence traits determine the pathogenic mechanisms responsible for diarrhea. This entire range of traits is demonstrated by the various types of *E. coli*, as summarized in Table 3. This versatile species may represent the predominant normal colonic flora or may be a urinary or enteric pathogen. Depending largely on the transmissible virulence traits encoded on plasmids or phage, *E. coli* may produce one of three families of enterotoxins (LT, STa, or STb), may be invasive (EIEC), may cause hemorrhagic colitis (EHEC), or may exhibit three or four distinct types of adherence (class I and II EPC, with or without the plasmid-encoded focal HEp-2 cell enteroadherence factor, EAF; autoagglutinating enteroadherent *E. coli*, EAEC; and *E. coli* with one of the recognized or new colonization traits, CFAI, CFAII, E8775, 260-1, and 0159:H4). Study of *E. coli* with these varied pathogenic traits have greatly helped to unravel the way that enteric pathogens alter normal intestinal absorptive function to cause diarrheal diseases.[86–88]

Toxins

Toxic microbial components or products are implicated in the disease-producing capacity of several enteric pathogens. Culture filtrates of toxigenic microorganisms are capable of altering gastrointestinal structure or function in the absence of the organisms themselves. Toxins produced by enteric pathogens can be classified as *neurotoxins*, *enterotoxins*, or *cytotoxins* (Table 4). Neurotoxins are usually ingested as preformed toxins that often cause enteric symptoms. These include staphylococcal, *Bacillus cereus*, and botulinal toxins. Although staphylococcal food poisoning is an abrupt upper gastrointestinal syndrome attributed to staphylococcal enterotoxin, the effect appears to be due to the action of this toxin on the central autonomic nervous system rather than to destruction or fluid secretion in the intestine per se.[89] An exotoxin related to entertoxin A may cause fluid accumulation in rabbit ileal loops directly.[90,91] A different staphylococcal α-toxin elicits hyperperistalsis. Certain strains of *B. cereus* isolated from patients with acute food poisoning also produce a highly heat-stable emetic toxin (especially when cultured with rice) that is a small (Mr <5000), nonantigenic polypeptide capable of causing vomiting in monkeys, much like staphylococcal enterotoxin.[92,93] Botulinal toxin has a primary effect on the neuromuscular junction to prevent the release of acetylcholine from the presynaptic vesicle.[89]

True *enterotoxins* are defined as having a direct effect on the intestinal mucosa to elicit net fluid secretion. The classic enterotoxin, choleratoxin, has been extensively studied and causes fluid secretion through the activation of tissue adenylate cyclase to increase intestinal cyclic AMP (cAMP) concentrations.[94,95] Similar toxins both antigenically and mechanistically have been described for other closely related vibrios[96,97] and

TABLE 3. Different Pathogenic Mechanisms of *Escherichia coli* Diarrhea[a]

	Mechanism	*Model*	*Gene Code*	*Predominant Serogroups*
Enterotoxigenic E. coli (*ETEC*)				
LT *E. coli* (LTEC)	Adenylate cyclase-like choleratoxin	Rabbit loops (18h) CHO, Y1 cell immunoassay	Plasmid	LT: 06:K15, 08:K40 LT + St: 011:H27, 015, 020:K79, 025:K7, 027, 063, 080, 085, 0139
STa *E. coli* (STaEC)	Guanylate cyclase	Suckling mice	Plasmid	ST:O groups 12, 78, 115, 148, 149, 153, 159, 166, 167
STb *E. coli* (STbEC)	Noncyclic nucleotide-dependent bicarbonate secretion	Piglet loops	Plasmid	
Enterohemorrhagic E. coli (*EHEC*)	Shiga-like (Vero) toxin 1 or 2 inhibits protein synthesis	HeLa cell cytotoxicity	Phage	0157:H7, 026:H11/H⁻, 0128, 0139, 0111:K58:H8/H⁻, 0113:K75:H7/H21, 0121:H⁻, 0145:H⁻, rough
Enteroinvasive E. coli (*EIEC*)	Local mucosal invasion	Sereny test	Plasmid	O groups 11, 28ac, 29, 115, 124, 136, 144, 147, 152, 164
Enteropathogenic E. coli (*EPEC*)				
Attaching and effacing *E. coli* (AEEC or class I EPEC; EAF-positive EPEC)	Attach to and efface brush border epithelium	Focal HEp-2 cell adherence (EAF)	Plasmid (60 M DA, pMAR2)	055:K59(B5):H⁻/H6/H, 0111ab:K58(B4)H⁻/H5 H12, 0119:K69(B14), 0125ac:K70(B15)H21, 0126:K71, (B16)H⁻/H2, 0127a:K63(B8):H6,[b] 0128ab:K67(B12)H12, 0142, 0158
Class II EPEC (EAF-negative EPEC)	? Close enteroadherence (like class I EPEC)	Diffuse or no HEp-2 cell adherence	? Plasmid	044:K74, 086a:K61(B7), 0114:H2
Autoagglutinating enteroadherent *E. coli* (EAEC)	? Cytotoxic	Aggregative pattern of HEp-2 cell adherence	Plasmid	
Normal enteric flora	? Adherence traits	—	—	O groups 1, 2, 4, 6, 7, 25, 45, 75, 81
Genitourinary, blood stream or meningeal pathogens	? Capsular polysaccharide ± adherence pili	Several animals (mice, rabbits)	—	O groups 1, 2, 4, 6, 7, 11, 18, 22, 25, 62, 75 (K antigens 1, 2, 3, 5, 13)

[a] In addition, nontoxigenic *E. coli* with recognized or new colonization factor fimbriae can cause diarrhea, as documented in experimental animals and in human volunteers.
[b] 0127:H6 is the focally HEp-2 cell adherent strain (E2348) from which the plasmid pMAR-2 was isolated.
(Modified from Guerrant,[87] with permission.)

TABLE 4. Enteric Bacterial Toxins

Neurotoxin group
Clostridium botulinum
Staphylococcus aureus (enterotoxin B)
Bacillus cereus (emetic toxin)
True enterotoxin group
Vibrio cholerae (cAMP)
Noncholera vibrios
Escherichia coli—LT (cAMP)
E. coli—STa (cGMP)
E. coli—STb
Salmonella
Klebsiella
Clostridium perfringens (A)
Shigella dysenteriae
B. cereus
Cytotoxin group
Shigella
C. perfringens (A)
Vibrio parahemolyticus
S. aureus
Clostridium difficile
E. coli (certain O groups: 26, 39, 128, 157)

E. coli.[98,99] Because there are no reliable markers such as serotype or biotype for enterotoxigenicity, demonstration of the toxin itself is necessary to identify which *E. coli* are enterotoxigenic. The genetic codes for enterotoxigenicity reside on transmissible plasmids that can be lost or transferred to other *E. coli* by conjugation[100,101] or by phage transduction.[102] To recognize which *E. coli* are enterotoxigenic, we must identify enterotoxin activity in culture filtrates of the organisms in question. This has traditionally required inoculation into a ligated rabbit ileal segment[103] or into rabbit skin to test for toxin associated "permeability factor."[104] The ability of the heat-labile enterotoxin of *E. coli* to activate adenylate cyclase has been used in the development of tissue culture bioassays.[105,106] Its similar antigenicity to cholera toxin has provided immunoassay techniques as well.[107–109] Oligonucleotide gene probes for LT and STa are now available with nonradio-active enzyme markers and provide a simple, sensitive, and highly specific detection method for these enterotoxins.[110] The LT-producing *E. coli* are associated with watery diarrhea among adults in Asia,[111,112] travelers to Central America,[113–115] and children in a number of areas.[116–118]

Another plasmid-mediated but smaller, less antigenic, heat-stable toxin may be produced by *E. coli*. The ST-producing *E. coli*, first described as a cause of diarrhea in piglets and calves,[25,119] are capable of causing diarrhea in human volunteers as well.[120] It appears to be significantly associated with diarrhea among tourists to Central America,[121] occasional newborn nursery outbreaks in this country,[122] and among adults with noninflammatory diarrhea on a Navajo reservation[123] or in Brazil.[9,124] The mechanism of action of ST involves the specific activation of intestinal guanylate cyclase.[125–127] Like cyclic AMP, cyclic GMP analogues (such as 8 Br-cyclic GMP) can mimic the secretory effect of the enterotoxin.[125]

Other organisms capable of producing enterotoxic effects by causing fluid secretion in ligated small bowel segments of animal models such as rabbit ileum include *Clostridium perfringens* type A, *Shigella dysenteriae*, and *B. cereus*. A protein neuroenterotoxin isolated from *S. dysenteriae* I (that may be responsible for the headache, meningismus, and seizures) also causes fluid secretion in rabbit ileal loops.[128] Although experimental findings have been contradictory, the activation of adenylate cyclase by this *Shigella* enterotoxin has been demonstrated in rabbit ileal loops.[129] Noninflammatory secretion also occurs in the small bowel of experimental monkeys infected with *S. flexneri* 2A,[130] and 80 percent of the patients infected with *S. flexneri* or *Shigella sonnei* develop neutralizing antibodies to the toxin.[131] However, the toxin alone does not appear to be sufficient to cause *Shigella* diarrhea, because toxigenic, noninvasive opaque colonial mutants of virulent *Shigella* are totally avirulent.[132,133] Certain strains of *B. cereus* have also been reported to produce a heat-labile, adenylate-cyclase-activating rabbit ileal loop-positive, dermonecrotic, and intestinonecrotic enterotoxin.[92,93,134,135]

Certain strains of *S. typhimurium* may cause severe watery cholera-like diarrhea[136,137] that can be prevented in experimental models by indomethacin. As noted in Chapter 83, the products of an inflammatory response could act to cause mucosal secretion.[138] Sandefur and Peterson have described a heat-labile enterotoxinlike effect in rabbit skin and Chinese hamster ovary cell models after separation from an inhibitor.[139] Others have described a heat-stable enterotoxin from *Salmonella*.[140] Other enteric organisms with which enterotoxin-like activity has been reported include *Klebsiella*, *Citrobacter*, *Aeromonas*, and *Enterobacter* spp.[141–145] Both heat-labile and heat-stable toxins have been reported. Although these enterotoxigenic organisms appear to be infrequent at the present time, much needs to be learned about the occurrence and the mechanism of action of enterotoxins from these organisms other than *E. coli*.

Cytotoxic products of several enteric pathogens are responsible for the mucosal destruction that often results in inflammatory colitis. Bacillary dysentery is a colonic mucosal destructive process in which a cytotoxin isolated from *S. dysenteriae* type 1 may play a role.[146,147] Whether this cytotoxin is a component or a digestive product of the larger neuroenterotoxin mentioned above is unknown. *Clostridium perfringens* enterotoxin also produces cytotoxicity similar to that of *S. dysenteriae* toxin in HeLa cell and in animal models.[148] More recent studies have used Vero cells to detect cytotoxicity in fecal filtrates that is neutralized by specific antiserum or toxin fragments.[149–151] These methods have enabled studies to be done that implicate enterocytotoxigenic *C. perfringens* in geriatric institutions and with antibiotic-associated diarrhea.[152–154] Another enteric pathogen for which a cytotoxin has been described is *Vibrio parahemolyticus*. Although some have reported the presence of a true enterotoxin with this organism,[155] others have described a cytotoxin[156]; still others note the tendency of *V. parahemolyticus* to penetrate and cause bacteremia in animal models[157] or an invasive colitis in patients.[158] *Vibrio parahemolyticus* typically causes explosive watery diarrhea in food-borne outbreaks in coastal areas of the United States.[159] *Staphylococcus aureus* produce a nonantigenic Δ-toxin that impairs water absorption and causes cytotoxic disruption of intestinal mucosa or cells in tissue culture.[160] The clindamycin-resistant *C. difficile* isolated from patients with antibiotic-associated pseudomembranous enterocolitis produces a potent cytotoxin capable of causing cytotoxicity in tissue culture and lethality in a hamster model,[161–163] as well as an enterotoxic product that causes hemorrhagic fluid secretion in rabbit ileal loops.[163,164] Data have emerged that associate the capacity to produce one or two *Shiga*-like Vero cell cytotoxins with certain serotypes of *E. coli* that cause hemorrhagic colitis or the hemolytic uremic syndrome (0 groups 26, 39, 111, 113, 121, 128, and 157).[165–169] Two groups have reported the transfer of Vero toxin production to recipient *E. coli* or its association with a large plasmid,[167,169] whereas others have associated the production of Shiga-like toxins I and II with bacteriophages in *E. coli* 0157:H7.[170] The heat-labile Vero cytotoxin, initially found in *E. coli* 026:H11, 0128, and 039, has a slight secretory effect in 18-hour ligated rabbit ileal loops.[166] The multistate outbreak of hemorrhagic colitis with *E. coli* 0157:H7 in 1982[168] was followed by studies showing the near identity (one amino acid difference) of verocytotoxin to Shiga toxin (hence the term *Shiga-like toxin, SLT*) and the association of these enterohemorrhagic *E. coli* (EHEC) with numerous outbreaks and sporadic cases of hemorrhagic colitis or childhood hemolytic uremic syndrome in schools, day care centers, nursing homes, and communities.[168,171–173] Like Shiga toxin, *E. coli* SLT has binding and active subunits, is neutralized by anti-Shiga toxin antibody, and inhibits protein synthesis by cleaving an *N*-glycoside bond at nucleotide position 4324 in the target cell 60S ribosomal RNA, much like the plant lectin ricin. SLT-II acts similarly to SLT but is not neutralized by anti-SLT-I and is about 60 percent homologous by deduced amino acid sequence. The receptor for SLT-I and -II appears to be a globotriosyl ceramide.[174]

Attachment

The ability of many enteric pathogens to cause disease depends not only on the organisms's ability to penetrate the mucosa or to produce enterotoxin or cytotoxin but also on their ability to adhere to and colonize the mucosa. This adherence capacity has been well described with enterotoxigenic *E. coli*, which, in order to cause disease, must not only produce an enterotoxin but also must first adhere to and colonize in the upper small bowel of humans or animals. This adherence capacity for *E. coli* is variously called *K88*, *K99*, or *colonization factor antigen* (*CFA*) for piglet, calf, and human strains, respectively. As with enterotoxigenicity, the production of these adherence antigens also appears to be genetically encoded by transmissible plasmids. These fimbriate bacterial surface adhesins are distinct from type 1 pili and from recognized urinary tract adhesins[175–177] and usually cause hemagglutination that is mannose resistant.[178,179] Although these adhesins hold great promise for immunization against colonization, there are now at least five different types of CFAs among human enterotoxigenic *E. coli* CFAI, CFAII, E8775, 260-1, and O159:H4.[178–183]

In addition, attachment of EPEC to intestinal mucosa appears to be important, and attachment by certain strains has been associated with transferrable plasmids as well.[184–189] Adherence to HEp-2 cells in tissue culture has been helpful as a model of different types of adherence among EPEC strains.[190–196] Focal HEp-2 cell adherence (EAF) is associated with pathogenicity and an approximately 60 MDa plasmid among many EPEC serotypes now being referred to as *class I EPEC*[86,191,192] (see Table 3). These *E. coli* attach and efface the brush border epithelium of human and piglet enterocytes[186,189,197,198] in a manner similar to that seen with HEp-2 cells in culture.[199] Other EPEC serotypes may also attach closely to brush border epithelium but do not exhibit focal HEp-2 adherence ("EAF-negative EPEC"). These *E. coli* exhibit diffuse or no HEp-2 cell adherence and have been called *class II EPEC*.[86,192] Still other *E. coli* (usually not of classically recognized EPEC serotypes) exhibit autoagglutination and a distinct aggregative pattern of adherence to HEp-2 cells that some have referred to as *enteroadherent E. coli* (*EAEC*) and that may be independently associated with diarrhea[86,192,193] (see Table 3). Finally, *E. coli* with the colonization traits mentioned above, but without enterotoxin production, are capable of causing diarrhea in animals[25,200] and in human volunteers fed *E. coli* with the colonization trait as a potential vaccine.[201] Whether such colonizing *E. coli* are responsible, alone or in part, for naturally occurring acute or prolong diarrhea remains to be determined.

The enterohemorrhagic, Shiga toxin-producing *E. coli* (EHEC) 026 has been shown to adhere to the mucosa of human fetal small intestinal tissue in vitro in a mannose-resistant fashion, a trait that is transmissible by a colicinogenic conjugative plasmid.[183] In addition, EHEC strain 0157:H7 has been shown to have a 60 MDa plasmid that encodes a new type of fimbriea that appear to mediate attachment to Henle 407 cells in tissue culture.[195]

Invasiveness

The capacity of organisms such as *Shigella* and certain invasive strains of *E. coli* to invade and destroy epithelial cells is responsible for the inflammatory or dysenteric diarrhea they cause. This capacity is demonstrated in the laboratory by the guinea pig conjunctivitis (Sereny) test.[202] There is cell destruction and superficial inflammatory invasion of the cornea similar to that noted in colonic mucosa. Modifications in the specific components of the O side chain of the cell wall lipopolysaccharide alter this invasive property in *Shigella*.[203,204] There is also evidence that the invasiveness of certain *E. coli* may be reflected in their O antigens or serotype.[205,206] Recent evidence has associated invasiveness with large 120–140-Mdal plasmids in *S. sonnei*,[129] *S. flexneri*,[207] and invasive *E. coli*.[208] HeLa cell, rabbit loop, and Sereny test invasiveness can be genetically constructed by the sequential transfer of defined chromosomal and plasmid genes for *Shigella flexneri* to *E. coli* K12.[209] As discussed above, cytotoxic exotoxins may well play roles in the invasive and destructive properties of certain shigellae, *V. parahemolyticus*, staphylococci, and clostridia.

Other Virulence Factors

In addition to enterotoxin production and adherence, an orchestrated set of additional virulence traits appear to be critical to the ability of pathogen such as *V. cholerae* to succeed in colonizing the intestinal mucosa. These include motility,[210,211] chemotaxis,[32,211] and mucinase production,[212,213] any one of which can be missing and lead to reduced virulence. The virulence of certain enteric pathogens such as *S. typhi* appears to be related to the Vi antigen[214] and to the polysaccharide composition of the O side chain of its lipopolysaccharide cell wall content,[215,216] both of which have been used in vaccine production.[201,217,218] The virulence factors that enable enteric pathogens such as *Yersinia enterocolitica* to cause an enteric fever-like illness or mesenteric adenitis are less clear.

Another potential enteric pathogen that is increasingly recognized with improved culture techniques is *Campylobacter*. *Campylobacter jejuni* tends to cause more diarrhea than *C. fetus*; some *C. jejuni* have been reported to produce an LT-like enterotoxin,[219] or a cytotoxin,[220] and *C. fetus* causes more febrile systemic illness with bacteremia. The mechanisms by which *Campylobacter* cause disease still remain unclear.[221]

Still another way that organisms may cause diarrhea involves the selective destruction of absorptive cells (villus tip cells) in the mucosa, leaving secretory cells (crypt cells) intact.[2,222] Thus it is not surprising that both the rotaviruses and the Norwalk-like viruses, which selectively infect and disrupt the villus tip cells, alter the normal absorptive fluid balance as well as reduce the brush border digestive enzymes present during active infection.[2,223–225] Such an imbalanced disruption of the specialized absorptive surface may also be involved in other small bowel infections that are often associated with villus tip flatening or microvillus destruction, including bacterial overgrowth syndromes, EPEC infections, giardiasis, strongyloidiasis, and cryptosporidiosis.

MAJOR SYNDROMES OF DERANGED GASTROINTESTINAL PHYSIOLOGY

The elements of net fluid balance in the healthy adult intestinal tract are shown diagrammatically in Figure 1. With a daily oral intake of 1.5 liters, salivary, gastric, biliary, and pancreatic secretions contribute a total of approximately 8.5 liters of fluid that enters the upper gastrointestinal tract each day. However, daily fecal fluid excretion is normally less than 150 ml, indicating a net absorption in excess of 8 liters each day by the intestinal tract. Over 90 percent of this net absorption occurs in the small bowel, where there is a massive bidirectional flux that probably exceeds 50 liters a day. We can readily see how a relatively slight shift in the bidirectional flux can result in substantial overload of the colonic absorptive capacity that rarely exceeds 2–3 liters a day. As in the kidney, there are analogous hormonal, physical, and osmotic factors active in the intestinal tract. Aldosterone, for example, enhances intestinal sodium absorption at the expense of potassium.[226,227] Excessive

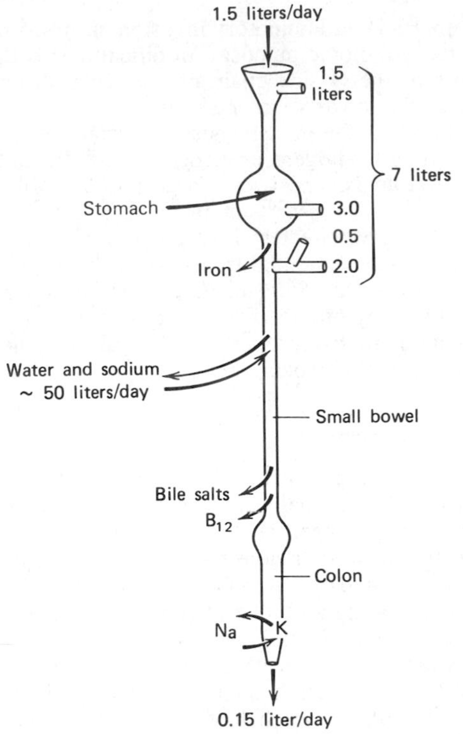

FIG. 1. Diagram of fluid balance in the healthy adult gastrointestinal tract.

fluid volume results in a ''third factor'' effect that may elicit or prolong diarrhea,[228] and osmotic laxatives are as familiar as osmotic diuretics.

Enteric disease can be produced by the microbe–host interaction that alters normal gastrointestinal physiology in one or more of these three ways: (*1*) a shift in the delicate balance of bidirectional water and electrolyte fluxes in the upper small bowel by intraluminal processes such as enterotoxin action, (*2*) inflammatory destruction of the ileal or colonic mucosa, or (*3*) penetration through an intact mucosa to the reticuloendothelial system. These three types of enteric infections are outlined in Table 5.

They can often be distinguished by a quick, simple examination. Mucus from a fresh stool specimen is mixed with a drop of methylene blue on a slide and examined for the presence of fecal leukocytes.[229,230] In the majority of cases, no leukocytes will be noted. This suggests a noninflammatory process in which diarrhea usually arises from the upper small bowel by the action of a true enterotoxin or by agents such as *Giardia* or viruses. The secretory effects of certain enterotoxins share similar mechanisms with noninfectious endocrine causes of diarrhea such as non-β-cell islet tumors, medullary carcinoma of the thyroid, carcinoid tumors, and other benign or malignant neoplasms that are associated with increased serum prostaglandins, vasoactive intestinal polypeptide, or changes in cyclic nucleotide concentrations.[231] Impaired small bowel absorption is important in tropical sprue, enzyme deficiencies, and solute loads. Enhanced colonic secretion without an inflammatory response characteristic of microbial or ulcerative colitis may result from excessive bile salts or fatty acids or from malignancies such as villous adenomas.

The presence of numerous polymorphonuclear leukocytes documents an inflammatory or invasive process that usually arises from the colon or distal small bowel. Amebic colitis can often be distinguished from bacterial dysenteries by microscopic fecal examination. In addition to the amebic trophozoites or cysts, fecal neutrophils are usually pyknotic or absent with amebiasis, probably because of the cytopathic effect of virulent amebae on mammalian cells, including neutrophils.[232,233] Impaired colonic absorption may contribute to the diarrhea in inflammatory colitis due to shigellosis, pseudomembranous enterocolitis, amebic colitis, or idiopathic ulcerative colitis. In addition, recent evidence suggests that the products of the lipoxygenase pathways in neutrophils may also contribute to a secretory process.[138] Agents that cause an inflammatory colitis may require specific antimicrobial intervention, as well as supportive fluid therapy.[230]

The third type of enteric infection is caused by organisms that penetrate the intact intestinal mucosa, often in the distal small bowel, to multiply in the lymphatic or reticuloendothelial cells. This usually results in a febrile systemic illness with or without diarrhea. If diarrhea is present, mononuclear leukocytes may be found in the stools of these patients.[229] Cultural documentation of the pathogen is important, since a bacteremia that necessitates specific antimicrobial therapy may result in this setting.

DIAGNOSTIC APPROACH TO ENTERIC INFECTIONS

The appropriate diagnostic approach to diarrheal illness is determined by the patient's age, severity of illness, duration of illness, type of illness, and the available facilities. Of greatest importance in patients with diarrhea are a careful history, physical examination, and examination of a fresh stool specimen for fecal leukocytes. A *history* of recent antibiotic use, weight loss, underlying diseases, other illnesses in the family or in other contacts, or of travel outside the United States, to the seacoast, or to rural mountainous areas should elicit a more careful investigation of specific etiologic agents. A prompt evaluation of

TABLE 5. Three Types oe Enteric Infection

	I	II	III
Mechanism:	Noninflammatory (enterotoxin)	Inflammatory (invasion ?cytotoxin)	Penetrating
Location	Proximal small bowel	Colon	Distal small bowel
Illness:	Watery diarrhea	Dysentery	Enteric fever
Stool exam:	No fecal leukocytes	Fecal polymorphonuclear leukocytes	Fecal mononuclear leukocytes
Examples	*Vibrio cholerae* *Escherichia coli* (LT) *E. coli* (ST) *Clostridium perfringens* *Bacillus cereus* *Staphylococcus aureus* ?*Salmonella* ?*Vibrio parahemolyticus* *Giardia lamblia* Rotavirus Norwalk-like viruses *Cryptosporidium*	*Shigella* Invasive *E. coli* *Salmonella enteritidis* *V. parahemolyticus* ?*Clostridium difficile* ?*Campylobacter jejuni* *Entamoeba histolytica*[a]	*Salmonella typhi* *Yersinia enterocolitica* ?*Campylobacter fetus*

[a] Although amebic dysentery involves tissue inflammation, the leukocytes are characteristically pyknotic or absent, having been destroyed by the virulent amebae.[232]

physical signs of fever, toxicity, or severe dehydration may result in lifesaving supportive fluid therapy. Particularly worrisome signs of severe dehydration, especially in children, include lethargy, postural hypotension and tachycardia, sunken fontanelles, and dry skin (with decreased turgor), dry eyes, or dry mucous membranes. As noted in Figure 2, if the history of physical findings indicate anything more than a mild, isolated, afebrile illness, examination of a fresh *stool* specimen, preferably collected in a cup, is particularly valuable. First, it provides the physician with an objective determination of the patient's subjective complaints. Second, a gross description of the stool as either watery, mucoid, or bloody will provide important clues about its cause and appropriate management. Third, a microscopic examination for fecal leukocytes, as described above, may reveal heavy parasitic intestinal infestations or maldigested fat or meat fibers, suggesting pancreatic insufficiency, or lipid droplets suggesting malabsorption with steatorrhea. If fever or fecal neutrophils are present, the physician should selectively take a culture for the most commonly recognized invasive pathogens—*C. jejuni*, *Salmonella*, and *Shigella*.[230] Cup specimens, when promptly examined for leukocytes, provide a highly sensitive screen for invasive processes such as shigellosis or *C. jejuni* enteritis.[234,235] Swab or diaper specimens appear to be less sensitive.[235] The history of recent antibiotic use, weight loss, and chronic diarrhea (>10 days), seacoast or other exposures, or immunocompromised states should prompt the physician to consider other agents as noted.

Other diagnostic studies that can be made on fecal specimens include special stains for fat or muscle and determinations of pH and reducing substances. A Sudan stain may reveal many large (10–75 μm) orange-stained globules of fat suggesting malabsorption or smaller (1–4 μm) globules or needle-like crystals

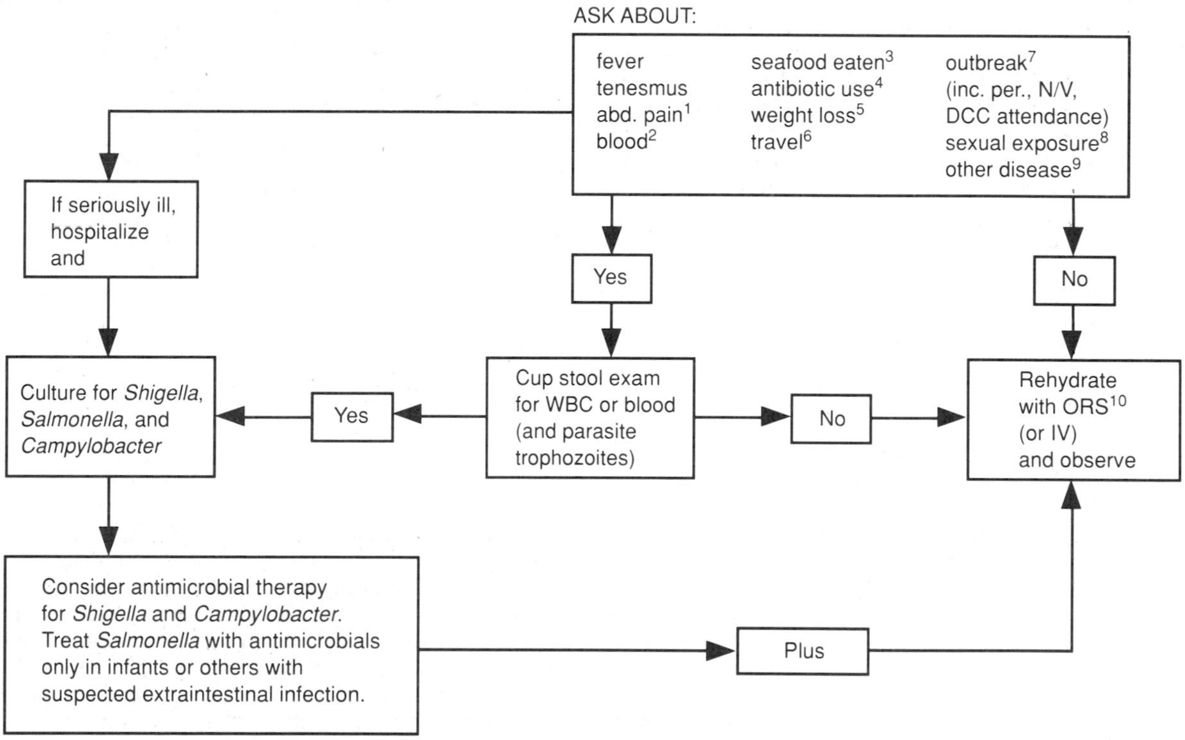

FIG. 2. Initial evaluation and management of diarrhea. Special considerations include the following:

1. If unexpained abdominal pain and fever persist or suggest and appendicitis-like syndrome, culture for *Y. enterocolitica* with cold enrichment.
2. Bloody diarrhea, especially if without fecal leukocytes, suggests enterohemorrhagic (Shiga toxin-producing) *E. coli* 0157 or amebiasis (in which leukocytes are destroyed by the parasite).
3. Ingestion of inadequately cooked seafood should prompt consideration of *Vibrio* infections or Norwalk-like viruses.
4. Associated antibiotics should be stopped if possible and cytotoxigenic *C. difficile* considered.
5. Persistence (>10 days) with weight loss should prompt consideration of giardiasis or cryptosporidiosis.
6. Travel to tropical areas increases the chance of developing enterotoxigenic *E. coli* as well as viral (Norwalk-like or rotaviral), parasite (*Giardia, Entamoeba, Strongyloides, Crytosporidium*), and, if fecal leukocytes are present, invasive bacterial pathogens, as noted in the algorithm.
7. Outbreaks should prompt consideration of *S. aureus, B. cereus,* anisakiasis (incubation period <6 hours), *C. perfringens,* ETEC, *Vibrio, Salmonella, Campylobacter, Shigella,* or EIEC infection. Consider saving *E. coli* for LT, ST, invasiveness, adherence testing, serotyping, and stool for rotavirus, and stool plus paired sera for Norwalk-like virus testing.
8. Sigmoidoscopy in symptomatic homosexual men should distinguish proctitis in the distal 15 cm only (caused by herpesvirus, gonococcal,chlamydial, or syphilitic infection) from colitis (*Campylobacter, Shigella, C. difficile,* or chlamydial [LGV serotypes] infections) or noninflammatory diarrhea (due to giardiasis).
9. In immunocompromised hosts, a wide range of viral (cylomegalovirus, herpes simplex virus, coxsackievirus, rotavirus), bacterial (*Salmonella, M. avium-intracellulare*), and parasitic (*Cryptosporidium, Isospora, Strongyloides, Entamoeba,* and *Giardia*) agents should be considered.
10. ORS can be prepared by adding 3.5 g NaCl (or ¾ teaspoon table salt), 2.5 g $NaHCO_3$ (or 2.9 g Na citrate or 1 teaspoon baking soda), 1.5 g KCl (or one cup orange juice or two bananas) and 20 g glucose (or 40 g sucrose or 4 tablespoons sugar) per liter (1.05 qt) of clean water. This makes approximately Na 90, K 20, HCO_3 30, glucose 110 mM/liter.

(Data from Guerrant et al.[230,234])

of fatty acid that may be normal. Numerous undigested muscle fibers may be seen with an aqueous 2% eosin stain that suggest pancreatic insufficiency and maldigestion.

An acidic stool pH may be helpful in the identification of lactose intolerance, especially in children with diarrhea. Although breast-fed infants have a fecal pH ranging from 4.7 to 5.1, stool pH usually exceeds 7.0 if the infant is on a regular milk-containing diet. On a regular diet, a fecal pH less than 5.0 suggests the presence of lactic acid from the action of colonic bacterial flora on unabsorbed lactose. Stool-reducing substances may also be helpful in the detection of carbohydrate malabsorption. A simple test uses copper sulfate (Clinitest) tablets. Mix 1 ml stool with 2 ml water, add 15 drops of this mixture to a test tube, and then add one copper sulfate tablet. A reduction positive for "sugar" indicates reducing substances. Positive tests for blood may suggest an invasive process such as amebiasis or shigellosis. Although this is usually evident from a gross examination of the stool, tests for occult blood are much more sensitive but less specific. Tests for hemoglobin peroxidase use orthotolidine, benzidine, or guaiac reagents in descending order of sensitivity. Some are so sensitive that they may be positive with ingested meat myoglobin. Twenty-four-hour determinations for fecal fat (normal <7.2 g/day fecal fat or <150–200 g/day total stool weight) may also be of value.

For culture of enteric pathogens, the specimen should be inoculated onto culture plates as promptly as possible.[236] The media used are selective and often contain indicator substances that aid in initial identification. Routine techniques must now include selective culture for *C. jejuni*, one of the most common causes of inflammatory diarrhea throughout the world.[237] For optimal results, this requires a highly selective atmosphere of reduced oxygen (4–6 percent) and increased carbon dioxide (6–10 percent) and an increased incubator temperature (42°C). Selective media and means to obtain the proper atmosphere are now available.[237–240] When culturing stool from homosexual men with diarrhea, it should be kept in mind that *Campylobacter cinaedi* and *C. ferinelliae* will not grow at 42°C. Routine stool culture also includes a medium, such as MacConkey's or eosin methylene blue (EMB) agar, that inhibits gram-positive organisms and selects predominantly for aerobic gram-negative rods. In addition more selective media (such as xylose-lysine-deoxycholate [XLD] or *Salmonella–Shigella* [SS] agar) and enrichment broth (such as gram-negative GN, selenite, or tetrathionate) that inhibit most organisms except *Salmonella* and *Shigella* should be used. However, since highly selective media are also more inhibitory, we should also examine the less selective MacConkey's and EMB agar for non-lactose-fermenting (colorless) colonies that may be salmonellae or shigellae. Even the best techniques with fresh specimens may miss fragile organisms such as shigella.[236,239] Fecal cultures failed to yield shigellae in 40 percent of volunteers with inflammatory diarrhea from experimental *Shigella* infection.[229] When immediate culture of specimen is impossible, specimens may be transported to a laboratory in a non-nutrient-holding medium, such as Cary-Blair soft agar, which prevents drying and overgrowth of normal flora.

Culture of vibrios (*V. cholerae*, *V. parahemolyticus*, and others), which should be suspected after any exposure to coastal areas or seafood, requires the highly selective thiosulfate citrate bile salt sucrose (TCBS) agar.[240] Selective culture for *C. difficile* and examination for fecal cytotoxin[158,159,241] may be indicated in patients with refractory antibiotic-associated diarrhea or colitis. Culture of *Y. enterocolitica* may require the selective process of "cold enrichment" on sheep blood agar or phosphate buffered saline for 2–3 weeks.[242]

Escherichia coli that grow readily as dry lactose-fermenting (purple) colonies on EMB or MacConkey's agar are major aerobic constituents of normal fecal flora but should also be considered as potential pathogens. Certain serotypes have been associated with inflammatory diarrhea,[203] recently with bloody diarrhea,[165–170] with outbreaks of diarrhea in newborn nurseries, and even with some enterotoxigenic *E. coli*.[243] However, detection of enterotoxigenicity depends not on serotypes but on detection of the toxin itself. Therefore, routine serotyping of *E. coli* in sporadic cases is of limited value at present and should be considered a special tool for investigating epidemic diarrhea in settings such as nurseries for newborns or unexplained dysentery. Special tests for the cholera-like, heat-labile, adenylate-cyclase-activating enterotoxin may use rabbit ileal loop,[103] rabbit skin permeability,[104] Chinese hamster ovary cell,[105] Y-1 adrenal cell,[106] immunoassay,[107–109] or direct assay for the enterotoxin genome.[110,244] The heat-stable enterotoxin acts through a different mechanism and currently requires the suckling mouse assay for its detection.[245,246] Invasive *E. coli* may be identified by inoculation into the conjunctival sac of guinea pigs (Sereny test).[202]

When diarrhea persists unexplained, especially with blood or weight loss, examinations for *Entamoeba*, *Giardia*, or *Strongyloides* parasites are indicated, using concentration or special staining techniques.[247,248] In immunosuppressed patients with persisting unexplained diarrhea, sugar flotation or modified Kinyoun's acid-fast stains should be done for cryptosporidiosis.[249]

Proctoscopic examination may be very helpful in the differential diagnosis, especially when inflammatory colitis is present. Although necrotic ulcers may be seen in acute shigellosis, discrete ulcers are more suggestive of amebiasis or Crohn's disease. Mucosal friability is more suggestive of inflammatory bowel disease such as ulcerative colitis. The appearance of raised, plaque-like pseudomembranes is diagnostic of pseudomembranous colitis that may be associated with staphylococci or antibiotics such as clindamycin. Large amounts of mucus may be present in "mucous colitis" or with a villous adenoma; melanosis coli may suggest laxative abuse.

Rectal mucosal biopsy specimens, especially when ulcers are present, may be of great help in the identification of the parasite *Entameba histolytica*, granulomata, amyloidosis (with Congo red stain), or Whipple's disease (with periodic acid-Schiff [PAS] stain). Small bowel biopsy specimens may also be diagnostic in Whipple's disease, giardiasis, amyloidosis, a β-lipoproteinemia, lymphoma, coccidiosis, or mast cell disease. Characteristic but not necessarily diagnostic histopathologic changes may be seen in celiac disease, tropical sprue, eosinophilic gastroenteritis, dermatitis herpetiformis, and dysgammaglobulinemia. However, several conditions, including Crohn's disease, bacterial overgrowth syndrome, and pancreatic or bile salt insufficiency, may be associated with normal small bowel histologic findings or with nonspecific changes.

Radiologic studies of the intestinal tract may reveal toxic megacolon, pancreatic calcifications, or nodular adrenal calcifications suggestive of tuberculosis or histoplasmosis. Colonic mucosal edema with a "thumbprint" appearance has been reported on barium enema studies of patients with bloody diarrhea and *E. coli* 0157 infection.[168] Although barium studies may reveal nonspecific changes in the small bowel (giardiasis) or colon (inflammatory colitis), they are less useful in diagnosing microbial diarrheas. Indeed, the barium contrast material renders a microscopic examination of stool virtually useless.

Bacterial overgrowth syndrome may result in deconjugation of bile salts that can be tested with a ^{14}C-glycocholic acid breath test. Carbon-14 labeled carbon dioxide in the breath represents the degradation product of bacterial deconjugation of bile salts.

APPROACH TO PREVENTION, CONTROL, AND THERAPY

The public health measures of improved water supply and sanitation facilities are most important for the control of the majority of enteric infections. Another important area for intervention in the spread of enteric infection lies in the quality control of commercial products such as bottled water and beverages. These may be responsible for outbreaks of significant enteric infections such as those of cholera in Portugal[250] or typhoid fever in Mexico.[251]

Nonspecific host factors should be appreciated to minimize their violation. Examples include careful personal hygiene and limited judicious use of antacids, antimotility drugs, or antimicrobial agents.

Vaccines may be used to boost specific immune processes that may be directed against bacteria themselves, adherence appendages, cytotoxins, or enterotoxins (Chapter 75). Perhaps the most promising are the newly developed live gal-epimerase mutant typhoid vaccine,[214] and the new Vi polysaccharide capsule vaccine against typhoid fever.[217,218] Several additional live and killed bacterial vaccines are currently under study,[201] and new rotavirus vaccines are being studied.[224] To date, there are no effective vaccines against a parasitic enteric infection, and much new work is required to improve the understanding of host defenses against enteric parasitic processes.

New possibilities for pharmacologic antagonists to microbial adherence or to toxin action are now on the horizon. New types of "antibiotics" may work by blocking the formation of bacterial adherence factors, binding bacterial adherence appendages, or lectin-like competitors for the host cell receptors that enable microorganisms to colonize the gastrointestinal tract.[252] Finally, specific competitors for either the binding or the action of enterotoxins hold promise. For example, monosialoganglioside (G_{m1}) successfully binds cholera toxin or the heat-labile enterotoxin of *E. coli* in vitro and in animal experiments. Pharmacologic reversal of the cyclic nucleotide-associated secretory process may also be possible. Such a mechanism has been suggested for bismuth subsalicylate (Pepto-Bismol).[253]

Specific antimicrobial chemotherapy may be indicated, especially in inflammatory processes such as shigellosis or in parasitic diseases such as giardiasis or amebiasis.

Of greatest importance in the treatment of microbial diarrhea, regardless of the cause or category, is fluid replacement. The degree of volume depletion must be first assessed by examining the turgor of the skin and mucous membranes, by noting the amount of lacrimation, and by obtaining a history of urinary output. Postural light-headedness with changes in pulse and blood pressure are helpful objective parameters in volume depletion. Recent observations have documented that, despite the severest form of secretory derangement in cholera, glucose absorption and its coupled sodium and water absorption remain intact in the upper small bowel. Thus, many patients can be completely rehydrated and maintained by a simple oral-glucose-containing electrolyte solution. A controlled study of patients with cholera and other noninflammatory watery diarrhea in Dacca, Bangladesh, documents the efficacy of sucrose (table sugar) as well as glucose in the oral therapy solution.[254] Electrolyte losses in severe watery diarrhea are similar to the electrolyte composition of serum, and fluid replacement should contain approximately these concentrations of electrolytes. A standard oral fluid regimen contains 3.5 g NaCl, 2.5 g $NaHCO_3$, 1.5 g KCl, and 20 g glucose per liter of boiled water. This corresponds to sodium 90, potassium 20, bicarbonate 30, chloride 80, and glucose 110 mM/liter.[255] A similar solution may be prepared with 4 level tablespoons of sugar, $\frac{3}{4}$ teaspoon salt, 1 teaspoon sodium bicarbonate in 1 cup of orange juice to make up 1 liter (1.05 qt) in water. If there is concern about hypertonicity, particularly in children, the salt can be reduced in cases of milder diarrhea or the solution can be given with ad lib water. The electrolyte contents of commonly available soft drinks are quite variable, although solutions of similar electrolyte composition to the ideal as described above can be made in dilute solutions of bouillon or gelatin water. New developments in oral rehydration therapy under study include the use of rice powder or other glucose polymers and the use of amino acids such as glycine, alanine, and glutamine, which enhance sodium absorption independently of glucose.

REFERENCES

1. Walsh JA, Warren KW. Selective primary health care: An interim strategy for disease control in developing countries. N Engl J Med. 1979;301:967.
2. Guerrant RL. Pathophysiology of the enterotoxic and viral diarrheas. In: Chen LC, Scrimshaw NS, eds. Diarrhea and Malnutrition. New York: Plenum Press; 1983:chap 2.
3. Puffer RR, Serrano CV. Patterns of Mortality in Childhood. Washington, DC: Pan American Sanitary Bureau, Regional Office, World Health Organization; 1975.
4. Impact of oral rehydration therapy on hospital admission and case-fatality rates for diarrhoeal disease: Results from 11 countries. WHO Wkly Epidemiol Rec No. 8. 1988;49–52.
5. Yunes J. Evaluation of infant mortality and proportional infant mortality in Brazil. World Health Stats Q. 1981;34:200–19.
6. McAuliffe JF, Shields DS, de Souza MA, et al. Prolonged and recurring diarrhea in the northeast of Brazil: Examination of cases from a community-based study. J Pediatr Gastroenterol Nutr. 1986;5:902–6.
7. Black RE, Brown KH, Becker S, et al. Longitudinal studies of infectious diseases and physical growth of children in rural Bangladesh. Am J Epidemiol. 1982;115:315–24.
8. Mata LJ. The Children of Santa Maria Cauque: A Prospective Field Study of Health and Growth. Cambridge, Mass.: MIT Press; 1978.
9. Guerrant RL, Kirchhoff LV, Shields DS, et al. Prospective study of diarrheal illness in northeastern Brazil: Patterns of disease, nutritional impact, etiologies and risk factors. J Infect Dis. 1983;148:986.
10. Guerrant RL, Hughes JM, Lima NL, et al. Microbiology of diarrhea in developed and developing countries. Rev Infect Dis. In press.
11. Gordon JE, Chitkara ID, Wyon JB. Weanling diarrhea. Am J Med Sci. 1963;245:345.
12. Gordon JE, Scrimshaw NS. Infectious disease in the malnourished. Med Clin North Am. 1970;54:1495.
13. Lindenbaum J. Malabsorption during and after recovery from acute intestinal infection. Br Med J. 1965;2:326.
14. Hirschhorn N, Molla A. Reversible jejunal disaccharidase deficiency in cholera and other acute diarrheal diseases. J Hopkins Med J. 1969;125:291.
15. Lindenbaum J, Kent TH, Sprinz H. Malabsorption and jejunitis in American Peace Corps volunteers in Pakistan. Ann Intern Med. 1966;65:1201.
16. Chen LC, Scrimshaw NS, eds. Diarrhea and Malnutrition: Interactions, Mechanisms and Interventions. New York: Plenum Press; 1983.
17. Gordon JE, Guzman MA, Ascoli W, et al. Acute diarrhoeal disease in less developed countries. 2. Patterns of epidemiological behaviour in rural Guatemalan villages. Bull WHO. 1964;31:9.
18. Bowie MD. Malnutrition and diarrhea. S Afr Med J. 1960;34:344.
19. Black RE, Brown RH, Becker S. Malnutrition is determining factor in diarrheal duration, but not incidence, among young children in a longitudinal study in rural Bangladesh. Am J Clin Nutr. 1984;37:87–94.
20. Sheehy TW. Digestive diseases as a national problem. VI. Enteric disease among United States troops in Vietnam. Gastroenterology. 1968;55:105.
21. Hodgkin K. Towards Earlier Diagnosis. A Family Doctor's Approach. Baltimore: Williams & Wilkins; 1963.
22. Dingle JH, Badger GF, Jordan WS Jr. Illnesses in the Home, A Study of 25,000 Illnesses in a Group of Cleveland Families. Cleveland: The press of Western Reserve University; 1964.
23. Gordon JE, Behar M, Scrimshaw NS. Acute diarrhoeal disease in less developed countries. 1. An epidemiological basis for control. Bull WHO. 1964;31:1.
24. Hollister AC, Beck MD, Gittelsohn AM, et al. Influence of water availability on shigella prevalence in children of farm labor families. Am J Public Health. 1955;45:354.
25. Smith HW, Linggood MA. Observations of the pathogenic properties of the K88, Hly and Ent plasmids of *Escherichia coli* with particular reference to porcine diarrhea. J Med Microbiol. 1971;4:467.
26. Evans DG, Silver RP, Evans DJ, et al. Plasmid-controlled colonization factor associated with virulence in *Escherichia coli* enterotoxigenic for humans. Infect Immun. 1975;12:656.
27. Levine MM, Nalin DR, Rennels MB, et al. Genetic susceptibility to cholera. Ann Hum Biol. 1979;6:369–374.
28. Zisman M. Blood group A and giardiasis. Lancet. 1977;2:1285.
29. Rutter JM, Burrows MR, Sellwood R, et al. A genetic basis for resistance to enteric disease caused by *E. coli*. Nature. 1975;257:135.
30. Mobaselleh M, Donohue-Rolfe A, Jacewicz M, et al. Pathogenesis of *Shigella* diarrhea: Evidence for a developmentally regulated glycolipid receptor for Shiga toxin involved in the fluid secretory response of rabbit small intestine. J Infect Dis. 1988;157:1023–31.
31. Bergman MJ, Evans DG, Sullivan JA, et al. Attachment of *E. coli* to human intestinal epithelial cells: A functional in vitro test for intestinal colonization factor. Trans Assoc Am Physicians. 1978;91:80.
32. Allweiss B, Dostal J, Carey KE, et al. The role of chemotaxis in the ecology of bacterial pathogens of mucosal surfaces. Nature. 1977;266:448.
33. Briscoe J. A role for water supply and sanitation in the child survival revolution. PAHO Bull. 1987;21(2):93–105.

34. Gordon I, Ingraham HS, Korns RF. Transmission of epidemic gastroenteritis to human volunteers by oral administration of fecal filtrate. J Exp Med. 1947;86:409.
35. Jordan WS, Gordon I, Dorrance WR. A Study of Illness in a group of Cleveland families. VII. Transmission of acute nonbacterial gastroenteritis to volunteers: Evidence for two different etiologic agents. J Exp Med. 1953;98:461.
36. Blacklow NR, Dolin R, Fedson DS, et al. Acute infectious nonbacterial gastroenteritis: Etiology and pathogenesis. Ann Intern Med. 1972;76:993.
37. Giannella RA, Broitman SA, Zamcheck N. Gastric acid barrier to ingested microorganisms in man: Studies in vivo and in vitro. Gut. 1972;13:251.
38. Gorbach SL. Progress in gastroenterology: Intestinal microflora. Gastroenterology. 1971;60:1110.
39. Roberts SH, James O, Jarvis EH. Bacterial overgrowth syndrome without "blind loop": A cause for malnutrition in the elderly. Lancet. 1977;2:1193.
40. Hornick RB, Musik SI, Wenzel R, et al. The Broad Street pump revisited: Response to volunteers to ingested cholera vibrios. Bull NY Acad Med. 1971;47:1181.
41. Gitelson S. Gastrectomy, achlorhydria and cholera. Isr J Med Sci. 1971;7:663.
42. Giannella RA, Broitman SA, Zamcheck N. Influence of gastric acidity on bacterial and parasitic enteric infections: A perspective. Ann Intern Med. 1973;78:271.
43. Black RE, Levine MM, Clements ML, et al. Experimental *Campylobacter jejuni* infection in humans. J Infect Dis. 1988;157:472–9.
44. Driks MR, Craven DE, Celli BR, et al. Nosocomial pneumonia in intubated patients given sucralfate as compared with antacids or histamine type 2 blockers. The role of gastric colonization. N Engl J Med. 1987;317:1376.
45. Dixon JMS. The fate of bacteria in the small intestine. J Pathol Bacteriol. 1960;79:131.
46. Schrager J. The chemical composition and function of gastrointestinal mucus. Gut. 1970;11:450.
47. Higgens JA, Code CF, Orvis AL. The influence of motility on the rate of absorption of sodium and water from the small intestine of healthy persons. Gastroenterology. 1956;31:708.
48. Formal SB, Abrams GD, Schneider H, et al. Experimental *Shigella* infections. VI. Role of the small intestine in an experimental infection in guinea pigs. J Bacteriol. 1963;85:119.
49. Sprinz H. Pathogenesis of intestinal infections. Arch Pathol. 1969;87:556.
50. DuPont HL, Hornick RB. Adverse effect of Lomotil therapy in shigellosis. JAMA. 1973;226:1525.
51. Holdeman LV, Cato EP, Moore WEC, eds. Anaerobe Laboratory Manual. Blacksburg, Va.: Virginia Polytechnic and State University Anaerobe Laboratory; 1977.
52. Price DJE, Sleigh JD. Control of infection due to *Klebsiella* aerogenes in a neurosurgical unit by withdrawal of all antibiotics. Lancet. 1970;2:1213.
53. Mentzing LO, Ringertz O. *Salmonella* infection in tourists. 2. Prophylaxis against salmonellosis. Acta Pathol Microbiol Scand. 1968;74:405.
54. Bohnhoff M, Miller CP, Martin WR. Resistance of the mouse's intestinal track to experimental *Salmonella* infections. J Exp Med. 1964;120:805.
55. Van der Waaj D, Berguis JM, Lekkerkerk JEC. Colonization resistance of the digestive tract of mice during systemic antibiotic treatment. J Hyg. 1972;70:605–10.
56. Que JU, Casey SW, Hentges DJ. Factors responsible for increased susceptibility of mice to intestinal colonization after treatment with streptomycin. Infect Immun. 1986;53:116–23.
57. Tannock GW, Savage DC. Indigenous microorganisms prevent reduction in fecal size induced by *Salmonella typhimurium* in vaccinated gnotobiotic mice. Infect Immun. 1976;13:172.
58. Schrank GD, Verwey WF. Distribution of cholera organisms in experimental *Vibrio cholerae* infections: Proposed mechanisms of pathogenesis and antibacterial immunity. Infect Immun. 1976;13:195.
59. Ryan CA, Nickels MK, Hargrett-Bean NT, et al. Massive outbreak of antimicrobial-resistant salmonellosis traced to pasteurized milk. JAMA. 1987;258:3269–74.
60. Bodey GP, Buckley M, Sathe YS, et al. Quantitative relationships between circulating leukocytes and infection in patients with acute leukemia. Ann Intern Med. 1966;64:328.
61. Yolken RH, Bishop CA, Townsend TR, et al. Infectious gastroenteritis in bone-marrow-transplant recipients. N Engl J Med. 1982;306:1009.
62. Bodey GD, Fainstein V, Guerrant RL. Infections of the gastrointestinal tract in the immunocompromised patient. Ann Rev Med. 1986;37:271–81.
63. Smith PD, Lane C, Gill VJ, et al. Intestinal infections in patients with the acquired immunodeficiency syndrome (AIDS). Ann Intern Med. 1988;108:328–33.
64. Sperber SJ, Schlenpner CJ. Salmonellosis during infection with human immunodeficiency virus. Rev Infect Dis. 1987;9:925–34.
65. Soave R, Johnson WD. *Cryptosporidium* and *Isospora belli* infections. J Infect Dis. 1988;157:225–9.
66. Colebunders R, Franastt, Mann J, et al. Persistent diarrhea, strongly associated with HIV infection in Kinshasa, Zaire. Am J Gastroenterol. 1987;82:859–64.
67. Sewankambo N, Mugerwa RD, Goodgame R, et al. Enteropathic AIDS in Uganda. An endoscopic, histological and microbiological study. AIDS. 1987;1:9–13.
68. Nelson JA, Reynolds-Kohler C, Margaretten W, et al. Human immunodeficiency virus detected in bowel epithelium from patients with gastrointestinal symptoms. Lancet. 1988;1:259–62.
69. Bull DM, Tomasi TB: Deficiency of immunoglobulin A in intestinal disease. Gastroenterology. 1968;54:313.
70. Pierce NF, Reynolds HY: Immunity to experimental cholera. II. Secretory and humoral antitoxin response to local and systemic toxoid administration. J Infect Dis. 1975;131:383.
71. Pierce NF, Gowans JL. Cellular kinetics of the intestinal immune responses to cholera toxoid in rats. J Exp Med. 1975;142:1550.
72. Stoliar OA, Pelley RP, Kaniecki-Green E, et al. Secretory IgA against enterotoxins in breast-milk. Lancet. 1976;1:1258.
73. Brown SE III, Sauer KT, Nations-Shields M, et al. Comparison of paired whole milk and dried filter paper samples for antienterotoxin and anti-rotavirus activities. J Clin Microbiol. 1982;16:103.
74. Jones EG, Brown WR. Serum and intestinal fluid immunoglobulins in patients with giardiasis. Am J Dig Dis. 1974;19:791.
75. Zinneman HH, Kaplan AP. The associate of giardiasis with reduced intestinal secretory immunoglobulin A. Am J Dig Dis. 1972;17:793.
76. Ament ME, Ochs HD, Davis SD. Structure and function of the gastrointestinal tract in primary immunodeficiency syndromes: A study of 39 patients. Medicine. 1973;52:227.
77. Hermans PE, Huizenga KA, Hoffman HN, et al. Dysgammaglobulinemia associated with nodular lymphoid hyperplasia of the small intestine. Am J Med. 1966;40:78.
78. Crabbe PA, Heremans JF. Lack of gamma A-immunoglobulin in serum of patients with steatorrhea. Gut. 1966;7:119.
79. Collins FM, Carter PB. Cellular immunity in enteric disease. Am J Clin Nutr. 1974;27:1424.
80. Welsh JK, May JT. Anti-infective properties of breast milk. J Pediatr. 1979;94:1.
81. McClelland DBL, McGrath J, Samson RR. Antimicrobial factors in human milk: Studies of concentration and transfer to the infant during the early stages of lactation. Acta Paediatr Scand. 1978;271(Suppl):1.
82. Arnold RR, Cole MF, McGhee JR. A bactericidal effect for human lactoferrin. Science. 1977;197:263.
83. Griffiths E, Humphreys J. Bacteriostatic effect of human milk and bovine colostrum on *Escherichia coli*: Importance of bicarbonate. Infect Immun. 1977;15:396.
84. Bullen JJ, Rogers HJ, Leight L. Iron-binding proteins in milk and resistance to *Escherichia coli* infection in infants. Br Med J. 1975;1:69.
85. Hanson LA, Winberg J. Breast milk and defence against infection in the newborn. Arch Dis Child. 1972;47:845.
86. Levine MM. *Escherichia coli* that cause diarrhea: Enterotoxigenic enteropathogenic, enteroinvasive, enterohemorrhagic, and enteroadherent. J Infect Dis. 1987;155:377–88.
87. Guerrant RL. *Escherichia coli* and related enteric pathogens. In: Warren KS, Malmoud AAF, eds. *Tropical and Geographical Medicine*. New York: McGraw-Hill; 1989: in press.
88. Schlager TA, Guerrant RL. Seven possible pathogenic mechanisms for *Escherichia coli* diarrhea. Infect Dis Clin North Am. 1988;2:1–18.
89. Lamanna C, Carr CJ. The botulinal, tetanal, and enterostaphylococcal toxins: A review. Clin Pharmacol Ther. 1967;8:286.
90. Koupal A, Deibel RH. Rabbit intestinal fluid accumulation by an enterotoxigenic factor of *Staphylococcus aureus*. Infect Immun. 1977;18:298–303.
91. Freer JH, Arbuthnott JP. Toxins of *Staphylococcus aureus*. In: Dorner F, Drews J, eds. Pharmacology of Bacterial Toxins. Oxford: Pergamon Press; 1986;581–633.
92. Terranova W, Blake PA. *Bacillus cereus* food poisoning. N Engl J Med. 1978;298:143.
93. Turnbull PCB. *Bacillus cereus* toxins. In: Dorner F, Drews J, eds. Pharmacology of Bacterial Toxins. Oxford: Pergamon Press; 1986;397–448.
94. Chen LC, Rohde JE, Sharp GWG. Intestinal adenyl-cyclase activity in human cholera. Lancet. 1971;1:939.
95. Guerrant RL, Chen LC, Sharp GWG. Intestinal adenyl-cyclase activity in canine cholera: Correlation with fluid accumulation. J Infect Dis. 1972;125:377.
96. Honda T, Shimizu M, Takeda Y, et al. Isolation of a factor causing morphological changes of Chinese hamster ovary cells from the culture filtrates of *Vibrio parahemolyticus*. Infect Immun. 1976;14:1028.
97. Blake PA, Weaver RE, Hollis DG. Diseases of humans (other than cholera) caused by vibrios. Ann Rev Microbiol. 1980;34:341.
98. Evans DJ Jr., Chen LC, Curlin GT. Stimulation of adenyl cyclase by *Escherichia coli* enterotoxin. Nature (New Biol). 1972;236:137.
99. Guerrant RL, Ganguly U, Casper AGT, et al. Effect of *Escherichia coli* on fluid transport across canine small bowel: Mechanism and time-course with enterotoxin and whole bacterial cell. J Clin Invest. 1973;52:1707.
100. Skerman FJ, Formal SB, Falkow S. Plasmid-associated enterotoxin production in a strain of *Escherichia coli* isolated from humans. Infect Immun. 1972;5:622.
101. Lathe R, Hirth P. Cell-free synthesis of enterotoxin of *E. coli* from a cloned gene. Nature. 1980;284:473.
102. Takeda Y, Murphy J. Bacteriophage conversion of heat-labile enterotoxin in *Escherichia coli*. J Bacteriol. 1978;133:172.
103. Evans DG, Evans DJ Jr, Pierce NF. Differences in the response of rabbit small intestine to heat-labile and heat-stable enterotoxins of *Escherichia coli*. Infect Immun. 1973;7:873.
104. Craig JP. A permeability factor (toxin) found in cholera stools and culture filtrates and its neutralization by convalescent cholera sera. Nature. 1965;207:614.

105. Guerrant RL, Brunton LL, Schnaitman TC, et al. Cyclic adenosine monophosphate and alteration of Chinese hamster ovary cell morphology: A rapid, sensitive in vitro assay for the enterotoxins of *Vibrio cholerae* and *Escherichia coli*. Infect Immun. 1974;10:320.
106. Donta ST, Moon HW, Whipp SC. Detection of heat-labile *Escherichia coli* enterotoxin with the use of adrenal cells in tissue culture. Science. 1974;183:334.
107. Greenberg HB, Sack DA, Rodriguez W, et al. A microtiter solid-phase radioimmunoassay for detection of *Escherichia coli* heat-labile enterotoxin. Infect Immun. 1977;17:541.
108. Yolken RH, Greenberg HB, Merson MH, et al. Enzyme-linked immunosorbent assay for detection of *Escherichia coli* heat-labile enterotoxin. J Clin Microbiol. 1977;6:439.
109. Honda T, Tage S, Takeda Y, et al. Modified Elek test for detection of heat-labile enterotoxin of enterotoxigenic *E. coli*. J Clin Microbiol. 1981;13:1.
110. Sommerfelt H, Svennerholm AM, Kalland KH, et al. Comparative study of colony hybridizations with synthetic oligonucleotide probes and enzyme-linked immunosorbent assay for identification of *Escherichia coli*. J Clin Microbial. 1988;26:530–4.
111. Gorbach SL, Banwell JG, Chatterjee BD, et al. Acute undifferentiated human diarrhea in the tropics. I. Alterations in intestinal microflora. J Clin Invest. 1971;50:881.
112. Ryder RW, Sack DA, Kapikian AZ, et al. Enterotoxigenic *Escherichia coli* and reovirus-like agent in rural Bangladesh. Lancet. 1976;1:659.
113. Gorbach SL, Kean BH, Evans DG: Traveler's diarrhea and toxigenic *Escherichia coli*. N Engl J Med. 1975;292:933.
114. Merson MH, Morris GK, Sack DA, et al. Travelers' diarrhea in Mexico: A prospective study. Abstract 149 presented at the 15th Interscience Conference on Antimicrobial Agents and Chemotherapy: September 1975.
115. Guerrant RL, Rouse JD, Hughes JM. Turista among members of the Yale Glee Club in Latin America. Am J Trop Med Hyg. 1980;29:895.
116. Gorbach SL, Khurana CM. Toxigenic *Escherichia coli*: A cause of infantile diarrhea in Chicago. N Engl J Med. 1972;287:791.
117. Sack RB, Hirschhorn N, Brownlee I, et al. Enterotoxigenic *Escherichia coli*-associated diarrheal disease in Apache children. N Engl J Med. 1975;292:1041.
118. Guerrant RL, Moore RA, Kirschenfeld PM, et al. Role of toxigenic and invasive bacteria in acute diarrhea of childhood. N Engl J Med. 1975;293:567.
119. Gyles CL. Heat-labile and heat-stable forms of the enterotoxin from *E. coli* strains enteropathogenic for pigs. Ann NY Acad Sci. 1971;176:315.
120. Levine MM, Caplan ES, Waterman D, et al. Diarrhea caused by *Escherichia coli* that produce only heat-stable enterotoxins. Infect Immun. 1977;17:78.
121. Sack DA, Wells JG, Merson MH. Diarrhoea associated with heat-stable enterotoxin-producing strains of *Escherichia coli*. Lancet. 1975;2:239.
122. Ryder RW, Wachsmuth IK, Buxton AE, et al. Infantile diarrhea produced by heat-stable enterotoxin *Escherichia coli*. N Engl J Med. 1976;295:849.
123. Hughes JM, Rouse JD, Barada FA, et al. Etiology of summer diarrhea among the Navajo. Am J Trop Med Hyg. 1980;29:613.
124. Korzeniowski OM, Dantas W, Trabulsi LR, et al. A controlled study of endemic sporadic diarrhoea among adult residents of southern Brazil. Trans R Soc Trop Med Hyg. 1984;78:363–9.
125. Hughes JM, Murad F, Chang B, et al. Role of cyclic GMP in the action of heat-stable enterotoxin of *Escherichia coli*. Nature. 1978;271:755.
126. Field M, Graf LH, Jr, Laird WJ, et al. Heat stable enterotoxin of *E. coli*. In vitro effects on guanylate cyclase activity, cyclic GMP concentration, and ion transportin small small intestine. Proc Natl Acad Sci USA. 1978;75:2800.
127. Guerrant RL, Hughes JM, Chang B, et al. Activation of intestinal guanylate cyclase by heat-stable enterotoxin of *E. coli*: Studies of tissue specificity, potential receptors and intermediates. J Infect Dis. 1980;142:220.
128. Keusch GT, Grady GF, Mata LJ, et al. The pathogenesis of *Shigella* diarrhea. I. Enterotoxin production by *Shigella dysenteriae* 1. J Clin Invest. 1972;51:1212.
129. Charney AN, Gots RE, Formal SB, et al. Activation of intestinal mucosal adenylate cyclase by *Shigella dysenteriae* I enterotoxin. Gastroenterology. 1976;70:1085.
130. Rout WR, Formal SB, Giannella RA, et al. Pathophysiology of *Shigella* diarrhea in the rhesus monkey: Intestinal transport, morphological and bacteriological studies. Gastroenterology. 1975;68:270.
131. Keusch FT, Jacewicz M. Serum enterotoxin neutralizing antibody in human shigellosis. Nature (New Biol). 1973;241:31.
132. Kopecko DJ, Washington O, Formal SB. Genetic and physical evidence for plasmid control of *Shigella sonnei* form I cell surface antigen. Infect Immun. 1980;29:207.
133. Keusch GT. Invasive bacterial diarrhea. In: LC Chen, NS Scrimshaw, eds. Diarrhea and Malnutrition. New York: Plenum Press; 1983: Chap 3, p 45.
134. Turnbull PCB: Studies on the production of enterotoxins by *Bacillus cereus*. J Clin Pathol. 1976;29:941–949.
135. Gilbert RJ, Kramer JM. *Bacillus ceseus* enterotoxins: Present status. Biochem Soc Trans. 1984;12:198–200.
136. Giannella RA, Formal SB, Dammin GJ, et al. Pathogenesis of salmonellosis. Studies of fluid secretion, mucosal invasion, and morphologic reaction in the rabbit ileum. J Clin Invest. 1973;52:441.
137. Giannella RA, Gots RE, Charney AN, et al. Pathogenesis of *Salmonella*-mediated intestinal fluid secretion: Activation of adenylate cyclase and inhibition by indomethacin. Gastroenterology. 1975;69:1238.
138. Musch MW, Miller RJ, Field M, et al. Stimulation of colonic secretion by lipoxygenase metabolites of arachidonic acid. Science. 1982;217:1255.
139. Sandefur PD, Peterson JW. Neutralization of *Salmonella* toxininduced elongation of Chinese hamster ovary cells by cholera antitoxin. Infect Immun. 1977;15:988.
140. Koupal LR, Deibel RH. Assay, characterization and localization of an enterotoxin produced by *Salmonella*. Infect Immun. 1975;11:14.
141. Klipstein FA, Holdeman LV, Corcino JJ. Enterotoxigenic intestinal bacteria in tropical sprue. Ann Intern Med. 1973;79:632.
142. Guerrant RL, Dickens MD, Wenzel RP, et al. Toxigenic bacterial diarrhea: Nursery outbreak involving multiple bacterial strains. J Pediatr. 1976;89:885.
143. Wasdtrom T, Aust-Kettis A, Habte D, et al. Enterotoxin-producing bacteria and parasites in stools of Ethiopian children with diarrhoeal disease. Arch Dis Child. 1976;51:865.
144. Wachsmuth K, Wells J, Shipley P, et al. Heat-labile enterotoxin production in isolates from a shipboard outbreak of human diarrheal illness. Infect Immun. 1979;24:793–7.
145. Ljungh A, Popoff M, Wadstrom T. *Aeromonas hydrophila* in acute diarrhea disease: Detection of enterotoxin and biotyping of strains. J Clin Microbiol. 1977;6:96.
146. Kcusch GT, Jacewicz M. The pathogenesis of *Shigella* diarrhea. V. Relationship of Shiga enterotoxin, neurotoxin and cytotoxin. J Infect Dis. 1975:131S:S33.
147. Keusch GT. Invasive bacterial diarrheas. In: Chen LC, Scrimshaw NS, eds. Diarrhea and Malnutrition. New York: Plenum Press; 1983:45–72.
148. McDonel JL, Duncan CL. Histopathological effect of *Clostridium perfringens* enterotoxin in the rabbit ileum. Infect Immun. 1975;12:1214.
149. Bartholomew BA, Stringer MF. Observations on the purification of *Clostridium perfringens* type A enterotoxin and the production of a specific antiserum. Fems Microbiol Lett. 1983;18:43–8.
150. Bartholomew BA, Stringer MF. *Clostridium perfringens* enterotoxin: A brief review. Biochem Soc Trans. 1984;12:195–7.
151. Horiguchi Y, Akai T, Sakaguchi G. Isolation and function of a *Clostridium perfringens* enterotoxin fragment. Infect Immun. 1987;55:2912–5.
152. Borriello SP, Barclay F, Welch AR, et al. Epidemiology of diarrhea caused by enterotoxigenic *Clostridium perfringens*. J Med Microbiol. 1985;20:363–72.
153. Borriello SP, Welch AR, Larson HE, et al. Enterotoxigenic *Clostridium perfringens*: A possible cause of antibiotic associated diarrhea. Lancet. 1984;1:305–7.
154. Larson HE, Borriello SP. Infectious diarrhea due to *Clostridium perfringens*. J Infect Dis. 1988;157:390–2.
155. Bhattacharya S, Bose AK, Ghosh AK: Permeability and enterotoxic factors of nonagglutinable vibrios *V. alcaligenes* and *V. parahaemolyticus*. Appl Microbiol. 1971;22:1159.
156. Carruthers MM. Cytotoxicity of *Vibrio parahemolyticus* in HeLa cell culture. J Infect Dis. 1975;132:555.
157. Calia FM, Johnson DE. Bacteremia in suckling rabbits after oral challenge with *Vibrio parahemolyticus*. Infect Immun. 1975;11:1222.
158. Bolen JL, Zamiska SA, Grennough WB III. Clinical features in enteritis due to *Vibrio parahemolyticus*. Am J Med. 1974;57:638.
159. Barker WH, MacKowiak PA, Fishbein M, et al. *Vibrio parahaemolyticus* gastroenteritis outbreak in Covington, Louisiana in August 1972. Am J Epidemiol. 1974;100:316.
160. Kapral FA, O'Brien AD, Ruff PD, et al. Inhibition of water absorption in the intestine by *Staphylococcal aureus* delta toxin. Infect Immun. 1976;13:140.
161. Bartlett JG, Chang TW, Gurwith M, et al. Antibiotic-associated pseudomembranous colitis due to toxin-producing clostridia. N Engl J Med. 1978;298:531.
162. Rifkin GD, Fekety FR, Silva J Jr, et al. Antibiotic-induced colitis: Implication of a toxin neutralized by *Clostridium sordelli* antitoxin. Lancet. 1977;2:1103.
163. Taylor NS, Thorne GM, Bartlett JG. Comparison of two toxins produced by *Clostridium difficile*. Infect Immun. 1981;34:1036.
164. Lima AAM, Lyerly DM, Wilkins TD, et al. Effects of *Clostridium difficile* toxins A and B in rabbit small and large intestine in vivo and on culltured cells in vitro. Infect Immun. 1988;56:582–8.
165. Konowalchuk J, Speirs JI, Stavric S. Vero response to a cytotoxin of *Escherichia coli*. Infect Immun. 1977;18:775.
166. Konowalchuk J, Dickie N, Stavric S, et al. Properties of an *Escherichia coli* cytotoxin. Infect Immun. 1978;10:575.
167. Scotland SM, Day NP, Willshaw GA, et al. Cytotoxic enteropathogenic *Escherichia coli*. Lancet. 1980;1:90.
168. Riley LW, Remia RS, Helgerson SD, et al. Outbreaks of hemorrhagic colitis associated with a rare *Escherichia coli* serotype. N Engl J Med. 1983;308:681.
169. Johnson WM, Lior H, Bezanson GS. Cytotoxic *Escherichia coli* 0157:H7 associated with hemorrhagic colitis in Canada. Lancet. 1983;1:76.
170. Strockbine NA, Marques LRM, Newland JW, et al. Two toxin-converting phages from *E. coli* 0157:H7 strains 933 encode antigenically distinct toxins with similar biologic activities. Infect Immun. 1986;53:135–40.
171. Karmali MA, Petric M, Lim C, et al. The association between idiopathic hemolytic uremic syndrome and infection by verotoxin producing *E. coli*. J Infect Dis. 1985;151:775–82.
172. Pai CH, Gordon R, Sims HU, et al. Sporadic cases of hemorrhagic colitis associated with *E. coli* 0157:H7. Ann Intern Med. 1984;101:738–42.
173. Carter AO, Borczyk AA, Carlson AK, et al. A severe outbreak of *E. coli* 0157:H7 associated hemorrhagic colitis in a nursing home. N Engl J Med. 1987;317:1496–1500.

174. Edelman R, Karmali, MA, et al. Summary of the International Symposium and Workshop on Infections due to Verocytotoxin (Shiga-like Toxin)-Producing *E. coli*. J Infect Dis. 1988;157:1102–4.
175. Salit IE, Gostchlich EC. Type I *Escherichia coli* pili: Characterization of binding to monkey kidney cells. J Exp Med. 1977;146:1182.
176. Silverblatt FJ. Host parasitic in the rat renal pelvis: A possible role for pili in the pathogenesis of pyelonephritis. J Exp Med. 1974;140:1696.
177. Eden CS, Hausson S, Jodal U, et al. Host–parasite interaction in the urinary tract. J Infect Dis. 1988;157:421–6.
178. Evans DG, Satterwhite TK, Evans DJ Jr, et al. Differences in serological responses and excretion patterns of volunteers challenged with enterotoxigenic *Escherichia coli* with and without the colonization factor antigen. Infect Immun. 1978;19:883.
179. Bergman MJ, Updike WS, Wood SJ, et al. Attachment factors among enterotoxigenic *Escherichia coli* from patients with acute diarrhea from diverse geographic areas. Infect Immun. 1981;32:881.
180. Thomas LV, Cravioto A, Scotland SM, et al. New fimbrial antigenic type E8775 that may represent a colonization factor in enterotoxigenic *E. coli* in humans. Infect Immun. 1982;35:1119–24.
181. Honda T, Arita M, Miwatani T: Characterization of new hydrophobic pili of human enterotoxigenic *Escherichia coli*: A possible new colonization. Infect Immun. 1984;43:959–65.
182. Tacket CO, Maneval DR, Levine MM. Purification, morphology, and genetics of a new fimbrial putative colonization factor of enterotoxigenic *Escherichia coli* 0159:H4. Infect Immun. 1987;55:1063–9.
183. Williams PH, Sedgwick MI, Evans N, et al. Adherence of an enteropathogenic strain of *Escherichia coli* is mediated by a colicinogenic conjugative plasmid. Infect Immun. 1978;22:393.
184. Edelman R, Levine MM. Summary of NIAID workshop on enteropathogenic *E. coli* (EPEC). J Infect Dis. 1983;147:1108.
185. Levine MM, Nalin DR, Hornick RB, et al. *Escherichia coli* strains that cause diarrhea but do not produce heat-labile or heat-stable enterotoxins and are noninvasive. Lancet. 1978;1:1119.
186. Ulshen MH, Rollo JL. Pathogenesis of *Escherichia coli* gastroenteritis in man: Another mechanism. N Engl J Med. 1980;302:99.
187. Polotsky YE, Dragunskaya EM, Seliverstova VG, et al. Pathogenic effect of enterotoxigenic *Escherichia coli* and *Escherichia coli* causing infantile diarrhoea. Acta Microbiol Acad Sci Hung. 1977;24:221.
188. Guerrant RL. Yet another pathogenic mechanism for *Escherichia coli* diarrhea? N Engl J Med. 1980;302:113.
189. Rothbaum R, McAdams AJ, Giannella R, et al. A clinicopathologic study of enterocyte-adherent *Escherichia coli*: A cause of protracted diarrhea in infants. Gastroenterology. 1982;83:441.
190. Cravioto A, Gross RJ, Scotland S, et al. An adhesive factor found in strains of *Escherichia coli* belonging to the traditional infantile enteropathogenic serotypes. Curr Microbiol. 1979;3:95–9.
191. Baldini MM, Kaper JB, Levine MM, et al. Plasmid mediated adhesion of enteropathogenetic *Escherichia coli*. J Pediatr Gastroenterol Nutr. 1983;2:534–8.
192. Nataro JP, Kaper JB, Robins-Browne R, et al. Patterns of adherence of diarrheagenic *Escherichia coli* to HEp-2 cells. Pediatr Infect Dis J. 1987;6:829–31.
193. Mathewson JJ, Johnson PC, Dupont HL, et al. Pathogenicity of enteroadherent *Escherichia coli* in adult volunteers. J Infect Dis. 1986;154:524–7.
194. Bray J, Beavan TED. Slide agglutination of *Bacterium coli* var. *neapolitanum* in summer diarrhoea. J Pathol. 1948;60:395–401.
195. Karch H, Heesemann J, Laufs R, et al. A plasmid of enterohemorrhagic *Escherichia coli* 0157:H7 is required for expression of a new fimbrial antigen and for adhesion to epithelial cells. Infect Immun. 1987;55:455–61.
196. Scaletsky ICA, Silva MLM, Toledo MRF, et al. Correlation between adherence to HeLa cells and serogroups, serotypes, and bioserotypes of *Escherichia coli*. Infect Immun. 1985;49:528–32.
197. Moon HW, Whipp SC, Argenzio RA, et al. Attaching and effacing activities of rabbit and human enteropathogenic *Escherichia coli* in pig and rabbit intestines. Infect Immun. 1983;41:1340–51.
198. Tzipori S, Robins-Browne RM, Gonis G, et al. Enteropathogenic *Escherichia coli* enteritis: Evaluation of the gnotobiotic piglet as a model of human infection. Gut. 1985;26:570–8.
199. Knutton S, Lloyd D, McNeish A. Adhesion of enteropathogenic *Escherichia coli* to human intestinal enterocytes and cultured human intestinal mucosa. Infect Immun. 1987;55:69–77.
200. Wanke C, Guerrant RL. Small-bowel colonization alone is a cause of diarrhea. Infect Immun. 1987;55:1924–6.
201. Levine MM, Kaper JB, Black RE, et al. New knowledge on pathogenesis of bacterial enteric infections as applied to vaccine development. Microbiol Rev. 1983;47:510–50.
202. Sereny B. Experimental *Shigella* keratoconjunctivitis: A preliminary report. Acta Microbiol Acad Sci Hung. 1955;2:293.
203. Gemski P Jr, Sheahan DG, Washington O, et al. Virulence of *Shigella flexneri* hybrids expressing *Escherichia coli* somatic antigens. Infect Immun. 1972;6:104.
204. Keusch GT. *Shigella* infections. Clin Gastroenterol. 1979;8:645.
205. Trabulsi LR, Fernandes MFR. *Escherichia coli* serogroup 0115 isolated from patients with enteritis: Biochemical characteristics and experimental pathogenicity. Rev Inst Med Trop Sao Paulo. 1969;11:358.
206. DuPont HL, Formal SB, Hornick RB, et al. Pathogenesis of *Escherichia coli* diarrhea. N Engl J Med. 1971;285:1.
207. Sansonetti PJ, Kopecko DJ, Formal SB. Involvement of an plasmid in the invasive ability of *Shigella flexneri*. Infect Immun. 1982;35:852.
208. Harris JR, Wachsmuth IK, Davis BR, et al. High-molecular-weight plasmid correlates with *Escherichia coli* invasiveness. Infect Immun. 1982;37:1295.
209. Sansonetti PJ, Hale TL, Oaks EV. Genetics of virulence in enteroinvasive *Escherichia coli*. Microbiology. 1985;74–7.
210. Guentzel MN, Berry LJ. Mortality as a virulence factor for *Vibrio cholerae*. Infect Immun. 1975;2:890–7.
211. Freter R, Allweiss B, O'Brien PCM, et al. Role of chemotaxis in the association of motile bacteria with intestinal mucosa: In vitro studies. Infect Immun. 1981;34:241–9.
212. Schneider DR, Parker CD. Isolation and characterization of protease-deficient mutants of *Vibrio cholerae*. J Infect Dis. 1978;138:143–51.
213. Schneider DR, Parker CD. Purification and characterization of the mucinase of *Vibrio cholerae*. J Infect Dis. 1982;145:474–82.
214. Hornick RB, Greisman SE, Woodward TE, et al. Typhoid fever: Pathogenesis and immunologic control. N Engl J Med. 1970;283:686.
215. Robbins PW, Uchida T. Determinants of specificity in *Salmonella*: Changes in antigenic structure mediated by bacteriophage. Immunochemistry. 1962;21:702.
216. Germanier R, Furer E. Isolation and characterization of Gal E Mutant Ty 21a of *Salmonella typhi*: A candidate strain for a live, oral typhoid vaccine. J Infect Dis. 1975;131:553.
217. Acharva IL, Lowe CU, Thapa R, et al. Prevention of typhoid fever in nepal with the Vi capsular polysaccharide of *Salmonella typhi*. N Engl J Med. 1987;317(18);1102–4.
218. Klugman KP, Koornhof H, Schneerson R, et al. Protective activity of Vi capsular polysaccharide vaccine against typhoid fever. Lancet. 1987;2:1165–7.
219. Ruiz-Palacios GM, Torres J, Torres NI, et al. Cholera-like enterotoxin produced by *Campylobacter jejuni*. Characterization and clinical significance. Lancet. 1983;2:250.
220. Guerrant RL, Wanke CA, Pennie RA, et al. Production of a unique cytotoxin by *Campylobacter jejuni*. Infect Immun. 1987;55:2526–30.
221. Guerrant RL, Lahita RG, Winn WC, Jr, et al. Campylobacteriosis in man: Pathogenic mechanisms and review of 91 bloodstream infections. Am J Med. 1878;65:584.
222. Field M. Cholera toxin, adenylate cyclase, and the process of active secretion in the small intestine. The pathogenesis of diarrhea in cholera. In: Andreoli TE, Hoffman JF, Fauestil DD, eds. Physiology of Membrane Disorder. New York: Plenum Press; 1978.
223. Davidson GP, Barnes GL. Structural and functional abnormalities of the small intestine in infants and young children with rotavirus enteritis. Acta Paediatr Scand. 1979;68:181.
224. Hamilton JR. Viral enteritis. Pediatr Clin North Am. 1988;35:89–102.
225. Agus SG, Dolin R, Wyatt RG, et al. Acute infectious nonbacterial gastroenteritis: Intestinal histopathology, histologic and enzymatic alterations during illness produced by Norwalk agent in man. Ann Intern Med. 1973;79:18.
226. Levitan R, Ingelfinger FJ. Effect of *d*-aldosterone on salt and water absorption from the intact human colon. J Clin Invest. 1965;44:801.
227. Guerrant RL, Chen LC, Rohde JE. Effect of spironolactone on stool electrolyte losses during human cholera. Gut. 1972;13:197.
228. Guerrant RL, Carpenter CCJ. Diarrheagenic effect of volume expansion: Intestinal fluid secretion without mucosal adenyl cyclase stimulation. Johns Hopkins Med J. 1975;136:209.
229. Harris JC, DuPont HL, Hornick RB. Fecal leukocytes in diarrheal illness. Ann Intern Med. 1972;76:697.
230. Guerrant RL, Shields DS, Thorson SM, et al. Evaluation and diagnosis of acute infectious diarrhea. Am J Med. 1985;78:91–8.
231. Said SI, Faloona GR. Elevated plasma and tissue levels of vasoactive intestinal polypeptide in the watery-diarrhea syndrome due to pancreatic, bronchogenic and other tumors. N Engl J Med. 1975;293:155.
232. Guerrant RL, Brush JE, Ravdin JI, et al. The interaction between *Entamoeba histolytica* and human polymorphonuclear leukocytes. J Infect Dis. 1981;143:83.
233. Ravdin JI, Guerrant RL. A review of the parasite cellular mechanisms involved in the pathogenesis of amebiasis. Rev Infect Dis. 1982;4:1185.
234. Guerrant RL. *Campylobacter* enteritis. In: Wyngaarden JB, Smith LH Jr, eds. Cecil Textbook of Medicine. Philadelphia: Saunders; 1988:1648–51.
235. Korzeniowski OM, Basada FA, Rouse JD, et al. Value of examination for fecal leukocytes in the early diagnosis of shigellosis. Am J Trop Med Hyg. 1979;28:1031–5.
236. Rahaman MM, Huq I, Dey CR: Superiority of MacConkey's agar over *Salmonella-Shigella* agar for isolation of *Shigella dysenteria* type 1. J Infect Dis. 1975;131:700.
237. Blaser MJ, Reller LB. Campylobacter enteritis. N Engl J Med. 1981;305:1444.
238. Kaplan RL, Barrett JE: Monograph: Campylobacter. Marion Scientific, Kansas City, Mo.; 1981.
239. Rahaman MM, Khan MM, Azi KMS, et al. An outbreak of dysentery caused by Shigella dysenteriae type I on a coral island in the Bay of Bengal. J Infect Dis. 1975;132:15.
240. Feeley JC, Balows A. Vibrio. In Lennette EH, Spaulding EH, Truant JP eds. Manual of Clinical Microbiology. Washington, DC, American Society for Microbiology; 1974:238.
241. Ryan RW, Kwasnik I, Tilton RC. Rapid detection of *Clostridium difficile* in human feces. J Clin Microbiol. 1980;12:776.

242. Morris GK, Feeley JC, Martin WT, et al. Isolation and identification of *Yersinia enterocolitica*. Public Health Lab. 1977;35:217.
243. Merson MH, Black RE, Gross RJ, et al. Use of antisera for identification of enterotoxigenic *E. coli*. Lancet. 1980;2:222.
244. Moseley SL, Escheverria P, Seriwatana J, et al. Identification of enterotoxigenic *E. coli* by colony hybridization using three enterotoxin fene probes. J Infect Dis. 1982;145:863.
245. Dean AG, Ching Y-C, Williams RG, et al. Test for *Escherichia coli* using infant mice: Application in a study of diarrhea in children in Honolulu. J Infect Dis. 1972;125:407.
246. Giannella RA. Suckling mouse model for detection of heat-stable *Escherichia coli* enterotoxin: Characteristic of the model. Infect Immun. 1976;14:95.
247. Brown HW, Neva FA. Basic Clinical Parasitology. Norwalk, Conn. Appleton-Century-Crofts, 1983.
248. Lima JP, Delgado PG. Diagnosis of stronygloidiasis: Importance of Baermann's method. Am J Dig Dis. 1961;6:899.
249. Current WL, Reese NC, Ernst JV, et al. Human cryptosporidiosis in immunocompetent and immunodeficient persons: Studies of an outbreak and experimental transmission. N Engl J Med. 1983;21:1252.
250. Blake PA, Rosenberg ML, Florencia J, et al. Cholera in Portugal, 1974. Am J Epidemiol. 1977;105:344.
251. Lee JA, Kean BH. International Conference on the Diarrhea of Travelers. New Directions in Research: A summary. J Infect Dis. 1978;137:360.
252. Costerton JW, Geesey GG, Cheng K-J. How bacteria stick. Sci Am. 1977;1:86.
253. Ericsson CD, Evans DG, DuPont HL, et al. Bismuth subsalicylate inhibits activity of crude toxins of *Escherichia coli* and *Vibrio cholerae*. J Infect Dis. 1977;136:693.
254. Palmer DL, Koster FT, Islam AFRM, et al. A comparison of sucrose and glucose in oral electrolyte treatment of cholera and other severe diarrheas. N Engl J Med. 1977;297:1107.
255. Oral glucose/electrolyte therapy for acute diarrhea, editorial. Lancet. 1975;1:79.

82. NAUSEA, VOMITING, AND NONINFLAMMATORY DIARRHEA

RICHARD L. GUERRANT

The vast majority of acute gastrointestinal illnesses do not involve a recognizable inflammatory process.[1–3] Although there is considerable inflammatory enteritis during summer months in warm areas with poor sanitation, most cases of diarrhea in these areas are noninflammatory, which suggests an enterotoxic bacterial, viral, or noninvasive parasitic process.[4–9]

EPIDEMIC DIARRHEA IN NEWBORN NURSERIES

Epidemic infantile diarrhea has long been recognized as a potentially serious problem that occurs in newborn nurseries. Its mortality has been as high as 24–50 percent.[10,11] Epidemic diarrhea among hospitalized newborns has been associated with certain "enteropathogenic" serotypes of *Escherichia coli* (EPEC). Enteropathogenic *E. coli* serotypes have been associated with diarrhea in hospitalized infants under 4 months of age.

The unusual susceptibility of newborns may be explained by their unique host status; they have not yet acquired a normal intestinal flora or specific immunity. Infants in special care nurseries have this situation compounded by severe underlying diseases such as prematurity or congenital cardiac or pulmonary disease. The consequences of diarrhea in the newborn are unusually severe because of poorly developed homeostatic mechanisms and limited water and electrolyte reserves. Nosocomial transmission may occur since the newborn nurseries may be crowded with susceptible infants.[12] A nursery outbreak can go unrecognized since infants may develop diarrhea after being discharged.

The onset is insidious, with the development of listlessness, irritability, and poor feeding over a period of 3–6 days.[11,13,14] Vomiting and fever are infrequent, and the stools tend to be watery, yellow-green, and usually without mucus, pus, or blood. Early signs such as failure to gain weight or a slight weight loss and abdominal distension may be subtle. The disease may progress to more severe signs of dehydration and shock with depressed sensorium, drowsiness, coma, sunken eyes, circumoral cyanosis, and grayish discoloration of the skin. Shock without hyperpnea often occurs in this setting despite the development of severe acidosis. Poorly nourished infants with decreased protein and potassium reserves may have severe hypokalemia, hyponatremic dehydration, and paradoxical edema. The illness usually lasts 5–15 days but may persist or relapse over the course of several weeks. Complications may include intercurrent otitis media, pneumonia, bacteremia, peritonitis, and renal vein or cerebral sinus thrombosis. Dissemination of EPEC to the lungs has been demonstrated by immunofluorescent staining of tissue at autopsy.[15] While the mortality may be quite high as noted above, South and Kaslow et al. have reported a milder illness with lower morbidity and mortality in recent years.[16,17] However, in many areas such as South Africa and southern Brazil, EPEC remain among the most common causes of diarrhea in infants and young children, especially during the summer months.[18–20] Endemic childhood diarrheal illness in areas like England and Canada also remain associated with EPEC in 6–18 percent of cases.[18,19]

Several potentially life-threatening processes may mimic this infantile diarrhea syndrome. So-called parenteral diarrhea is the well-recognized, but poorly understood tendency for systemic or localized infections elsewhere (such as otitis or meningitis) to be manifested clinically with diarrhea. Likewise, a strangulated hernia, intussusception, or torsion of an ovary or testis may be manifested by abdominal pain or diarrhea.

Appropriate antibiotic therapy must be tailored to the specific sensitivity pattern of the organism isolated. While neomycin or colistin have been used successfully, EPEC may develop resistance to these agents as well as to chloramphenicol and gentamicin.[16] Because the illness is often mild, oral nonabsorbable antibiotics such as neomycin or gentamicin are usually adequate. However, if systemic infection is suspected, parenteral therapy should be started and should be tailored to the antibiotic sensitivity pattern of the organism isolated. Appropriate preventive measures include cohorting of nursery admissions, avoidance of overcrowding in nurseries, utilization of individual units and equipment, careful formula preparation, isolation of infants with diarrhea, and careful hand washing by hospital personnel.

The association of a certain strain of *E. coli* with infantile diarrhea was first demonstrated by slide agglutination by Bray and Beavan in 1945 and reported in further detail in 1948.[21] They identified serologically homogeneous *E. coli* in most infants with summer diarrhea (87.5 percent vs. 4 percent of the controls), half of which was hospital acquired. Varela et al.[22] and Olarte and Varela[23] subsequently found this strain (called *E. coli*-"gomez" by Varela) in cases of infantile diarrhea in Mexico. A second serotype, initially designated as "beta" to distinguish it from the earlier serotype called "alpha," was described by Giles and Sangster as the cause of an outbreak of infantile gastroenteritis in Aberdeen.[24]

Escherichia coli strains are classified into a large number of serotypes on the basis of three major types of antigens: the "O" or heat-stable somatic antigen (lipopolysaccharide endotoxin), which forms the basis for 169 serogroups; an outer, heat-labile "capsular" antigen called "K" that may inhibit O agglutination; and for motile organisms, the "H" or flagellar antigen, which is also heat labile. Three different kinds of "K" antigen have been identified; L, A, and B, the latter being of importance in the identification of EPEC serotypes. The original alpha- and beta-serotypes of *E. coli* were subsequently associated with several outbreaks of infantile epidemic gastroenteritis and were classified as serotypes of O111:B4 and O55:B5, respectively, by Kaufmann and Dupont.[25] As shown in Table 1, exclusive of certain invasive serotypes (see Table 2 in Chapter 84), there are some 14 classically recognized EPEC *E. coli* serotypes, beginning with O111:K58 (alpha), O55:K59 (beta), O127:K63, O128:K67, O26:B6, O86:K61, O119:K69, O125:K70, O126:K71, O20:B7, and O44:K74. Additional serotypes recently recognized as causes of epidemic infantile diarrhea include O114,[10,29,30] O142,[12,27] and O158.[28] With the recent association of *E. coli* O157:H7 with hemorrhagic diarrhea in several outbreaks as well as sporadic cases, yet another EPEC serotype (if not another mechanism of pathogenesis) has been introduced.[31–33]

The evidence that EPEC serotypes are responsible for infantile diarrhea has been outlined.[11,18] There is a strong association for these organisms with cases of epidemic infantile diarrhea, and these organisms are infrequently encountered in healthy infants, children, or adults not exposed to cases of diarrhea. However, the mechanism by which most EPEC organisms cause disease is poorly understood. Although most are not invasive and do not produce conventionally recognized heat-labile or heat-stable enterotoxins, these organisms are capable of causing diarrheal disease in human volunteers, from whom the organism can be reisolated and in whom an antibody response can be documented.[13,34] As noted in Table 3 in Chapter 75, these EPEC serotypes differ from those *E. coli* isolated from patients with nonenteric infections.[35]

Epidemic infantile diarrhea may also be caused by enterotoxigenic organisms that are not limited to certain serotypes of *E. coli*. An outbreak has been described in which multiple serotypes of different organisms (*E. coli, Klebsiella,* and *Citrobacter*) that were demonstrated to be transiently enterotoxigenic were isolated,[36] which suggests the transmission of enterotoxigenicity among etiologic strains by plasmids[37] or by bacteriophages.[38] A subsequent outbreak of diarrhea on a cruise ship also documented the association of enterotoxigenic *Klebsiella* and *Citrobacter* as well as *E. coli* with watery diarrhea.[39] Another report of sporadic diarrhea among infants and children in Africa has shown that enteric organisms other than *E. coli* may produce an enterotoxin.[6] Enterotoxigenicity is by no means limited to specific serotypes, and most EPEC serotypes do not produce recognizable enterotoxins.[5–7,40] There do, however, tend to be a number of serotypes of *E. coli* that are more often enterotoxigenic, as shown in Table 2.[26,41] Whether these organisms are better recipients for enterotoxin plasmids or whether they are simply better adapated to maintaining these plasmids is not known.

TABLE 1. Enteropathogenic *E. coli* Serotypes Classically Recognized in Infantile Diarrhea Outbreaks[a]

Serotype	*Difco Serogroup and References*
Class I (EAF-positive) EPEC	
O55:K59(B5):H$^-$/6/7	A (24–26)
O111ab:K58(B4):H$^-$/5/12	A (21–23,25,26)
O127a:K63(B8):H6	A (26)
O119:K69(B14)	B (26)
O125ac:K70(B15):H21	B (26)
O126:K71(B10):H$^-$/H2	B (26)
O128ab:K67(B12)	B (26)
O142	(12,26,27)
O158	(26,28)
Class II (EAF-negative) EPEC	
O44:K74	C (26)
O114	(10,26,29,30)
O86a:K61(B7)	B (26)
Enterohemorrhagic *E. coli* (EHEC)	
O157:H7	(31–33)
O26:B6	A (26)

Abbreviation: EAF: enteroadherence factor probe for focal HEp-2 cell adherence plasmid pMAR2.[a]
[a] See also Table 3, Chapter 81.

TABLE 2. Serotypes of *E. coli* That Appear with Increased Frequency among Enterotoxigenic Isolates

LT *E. coli*
O6:K15:H16
O8:K40:H9, O8:K25:H9
LT + ST *E. coli*
O11:H27
O15:H22
O20:H—, O20:H11
O25:K7:H42, O25:K98:H—
O27:H7
O63:H12
O80, O85, O139
ST *E. coli*
O78:H11, O78:H12
O115:H40
O128:H7
O148:H28
O149:H10
O153
O159:H20
O166, O167

A 9-month-long outbreak of diarrhea in the special care nurseries of a pediatric hospital has been reported in association with a multiple drug-resistant *E. coli* O78 that produced only the heat-stable type of enterotoxin.[42] Another outbreak of diarrhea lasting 3 months in a newborn nursery in Scotland was related to ST-producing *E. coli* O159.[43]

Shigellosis[44] and epidemic salmonellosis[45,46] may readily spread in the newborn nursery setting. Echoviruses,[47] coxsackieviruses,[48] adenoviruses,[49] and rotaviruses[50–52] are potential viral causes of epidemic infantile diarrhea. Echovirus 18 was isolated from 10 of 12 infants who had watery noninflammatory diarrhea in a 21-patient premature nursery. The virus was also isolated from two nurses, one of whom was implicated in the spread of the agent to five other babies in another ward.[47] While there are conflicting interpretations of the significance of isolation of enteroviruses and adenoviruses among controls as well as patients, some have suspected that they may cause summer or winter gastroenteritis, respectively. Hospital acquisition of rotaviruses may be common among newborns; some suggest that mild diarrhea develops relatively infrequently.[53] However, rotaviruses have been clearly implicated in epidemic neonatal diarrhea[50–52] as well as in sporadic infantile diarrhea after the neonatal period.

WEANLING DIARRHEA

Weanling diarrhea usually occurs in the second year of life in areas where sanitation is poor. In contrast to cases of diarrhea where EPEC are still found in many areas,[18–21] EPEC were not found in the relatively infrequent cases of diarrhea among breast-fed neonates studied in rural Guatemala.[54] The greatest attack rate of diarrhea in the community occurs at the time of weaning, usually between 6 and 24 months of age.[9,11,12,55] As noted in the previous chapter, weanling diarrhea is a major cause of mortality around the world. The increased susceptibility of a recently weaned infant relates to several factors.[56] In areas with poor sanitation the infant ingests large numbers of many new organisms at the time of weaning. A second contributing factor is the deteriorating nutritional status that may occur with weaning in many parts of the world.[57,58] Finally there are cellular and humoral factors passively transferred in human breast milk that convey resistance to agents that commonly cause diarrhea in this age group.[59–63] Weanling diarrhea is manifested clinically as an acute, sporadic, watery diarrheal illness that occurs with increased frequency, especially in the summer months, in areas with poor sanitation. In the well-nourished infant, the disease is usually short-lived and resolves within 2–3 days with adequate hydration. A low-grade fever may be present, and vomiting is common.[5,55] Diarrhea in the malnourished child tends to persist or to recur and is often much more severe.

Weanling diarrhea is usually an acute, noninflammatory process. Acute diarrhea in children 6–24 months of age has been commonly associated with rotaviruses[2–4] and with enterotoxigenic *E. coli*.[5–7] Shigellosis may also occur in this setting. From 16 to 83 percent of acute diarrheal illnesses among infants and young children have been associated with enterotoxigenic *E. coli*.[5–7,64] Most of these reports involve studies of the summer peak of diarrhea in areas with poor sanitation. The presence of antibody to the heat-labile enterotoxin (LT) of *E. coli* in colostrum[59,60] may provide some protection against LT-producing *E. coli* diarrhea among breast-fed infants exposed to unsanitary conditions. The recent demonstration of passive protection against experimental enterotoxigenic *E. coli* infections in human volunteers with immune bovine colostrum further documents the potential protective role of passive antibody in colostrum or milk.[65] The role of enterotoxigenic *E. coli* in causing infantile diarrhea in temperate climates is less clear. Enterotoxigenic *E. coli* serotypes are uncommon among children with diarrhea in Massachusetts and Virginia.[66–68]

The ability of enteric organisms other than *E. coli* to produce enterotoxins has been suggested, but these organisms appear to be considerably less common than enterotoxigenic *E. coli*. Studies from Ethiopia suggested that young children with sporadic diarrhea may have *Klebsiella, Citrobacter, Aeromonas,* or *E. coli* that produce an LT-like toxin.[6] However, in Brazil enterotoxigenic *Klebsiella* organisms were found in only 2 of 40 patients, both of whom also had enterotoxigenic *E. coli*.[5] Diarrhea produced by the heat-labile enterotoxin shares the adenylate cyclase–activating mechanism with cholera toxin,[69–73] while the heat-stable toxin (STa) activates intestinal guanylate cyclase.[74–76]

The major nonbacterial causes of weanling diarrhea are rotaviruses. While most adults have demonstrable antibody to rotaviruses that may protect against symptomatic disease, children less than 2 years of age throughout temperate and tropical climates appear to be highly susceptible to rotavirus diarrhea, which occurs most frequently in the winter or cooler, dry months[2,4,66,77–84] and occasionally in the summer months.[85] Rotavirus diarrhea appears to be associated with low humidity and possibly indoor crowding to a greater extent than with temperature or inadequate sanitation.[86–88] The illness tends to have a more insidious onset and to last slightly longer than bacterial diarrheas do, is slightly more common in males than in females, is usually mild and without fever, and is often associated with vomiting.[2,4,89] Rotaviruses probably account for most cases of "pseudocholera infantum" or hakuri ("white stool diarrhea") in Japan.[80] They have been associated with initial bouts of weanling diarrhea in Aboriginal communities,[90] and anti-rotavirus antibody has been demonstrated in human colostrum among patients in Costa Rica and Brazil.[60,63] There is a high frequency of rotavirus shedding or seroconversion among parents and other household contacts of cases of rotavirus-associated diarrhea.[2,91,92] Up to 40 percent of these infected adult contacts may develop mild abdominal cramps or diarrhea.[93]

The human rotaviruses demonstrate antigenic cross reaction with several animal strains including the Nebraska calf diarrhea virus (NCDV), the agent of epizootic diarrhea of infant mice (EDIM), simian rotavirus (SA-11), and the "O" agent of monkeys.[2,94] However, there are three to five different antigenic types of rotaviruses,[95–98] so multiple attacks may occur.[99]

The laboratory diagnosis of rotavirus diarrhea may be made by examining the stool directly for viruses or the rotaviral RNA genome or by testing for an antibody titer increase in serum. Rotaviruses can be detected in fecal material by direct electron microscopy or by using immunologic techniques such as the enzyme-linked immunosorbent assay (ELISA),[100] radioimmunoassay,[101] counterimmunoelectrophoresis,[102] or fluorescent antibody staining of stool or biopsy specimens.[103,104] Immunoassays for rotaviral antigen are available, with ELISA being the most sensitive. Simple rapid latex agglutination assays with 86 percent sensitivity and 95 percent specificity have been developed.[105] Detection of rotaviral genomic RNA in stools by using "dot" hybridation with labeled RNA probes appears to be sensitive, specific, and convenient.[106] Methods for detecting serum antibody titers to rotaviruses use their cross-reactivity with NCDV, SA-11, or O agents of animals that can be cultivated in bovine embryonic kidney or in African green monkey kidney cells in tissue culture. Serum antibody has been measured by using immune electron microscopy,[79,107] complement fixation,[2,79] and immunofluorescence[66] with one of the substitute antigens.

In vitro studies were initially difficult because rotaviruses do not grow in most widely used tissue culture systems. Human rotaviruses incorporate into human embryonic gut monolayers,[108] guinea pig intestinal monolayers,[109] and human embryonic kidney cells in tissue culture.[110] Gnotobiotic piglets[111] and colostrum-deprived newborn rhesus monkeys[112] also acquire diarrhea after experimental infection with human rotaviruses. After the initial adaptation of human rotavirus type 2 in African green monkey kidney cell cultures after 11 passages through gnotobiotic newborn piglets,[113] several reports demonstrate the primary isolation of two human rotaviral types in MA104 cells in tissue culture with demonstrable cytopathic effects and without requiring animal passage.[114–116]

Much has been learned about the pathogenesis and the pathologic characteristics of intestinal rotavirus infections. Biopsy specimens from confirmed cases have shown transient, patchy, irregular inflammatory responses in the lamina propria and immature, cuboidal epithelium with 70–90 nm rotavirus particles in the distended cisternae of the endoplasmic reticulum.[77] Normal columnar epithelium at the villus tips was replaced by irregular cuboidal cryptlike cells. As would be expected from the destruction of villous tip epithelial cells, a transient brush border disaccharidase deficiency in the duodenal and upper jejunal mucosa and, despite the efficacy of oral therapy with glucose–electrolyte solutions, increased fecal reducing substances have been noted in children with rotavirus diarrhea.[117–120] The degree of microvillus damage parallels the severity of diarrhea and dehydration.[121] As with transmissible gastroenteritis in piglets, experimental rotaviral infections in animals confirm the shortened villi, reduced sucrase activity, increased thymidine kinase activity, no change in cyclic AMP concentrations, and blunted glucose-induced sodium absorption.[122,123] As noted in Chapter 81, this loss of absorptive villus tip cells may be responsible for the fluid imbalance and nutritional impact of rotaviral infections.

The availability, convenience, and cost-effectiveness of enzyme immunoassays or latex agglutination tests for rotavirus infections may enable improved diagnosis and epidemiologic control.[105] Therapy should be directed first at the immediate restoration of fluid balance by intravenous or oral glucose–electrolyte therapy and then at restoring the nutritional state to normal. Although several candidate live oral rotavirus vaccines (including bovine, rhesus monkey, and reassortant rotaviruses) show promise, questions remain about their efficacy in infants (<1 year old), especially in developing countries, and about the optimal means of delivery, age, and serotype to provide protection with minimal side effects.[124,125] Reasonable preventive measures include the provision of improved sanitation facilities and safe water supplies as well as efforts to develop protective antibacterial, antitoxic, or antiviral immunity.

ACUTE NAUSEA AND VOMITING (WINTER VOMITING DISEASE)

The syndrome of acute nausea and vomiting, "intestinal flu," or "viral gastroenteritis" commonly occurs in winter months in temperate climates. While there is some overlap of this syndrome with rotavirus-associated infantile gastroenteritis, rotaviruses appear to be relatively uncommon causes of winter vomiting disease in older children and adults. The Cleveland family studies of Dingle et al.[1] showed that enteritis was second only to upper respiratory infection as a cause of illness in homes. Gastrointestinal illnesses were most common between the ages of 1 and 10 years, when approximately two illnesses occurred per person per year. The peak season of these gastrointestinal illnesses was November through February, with June being the lowest point of the year over this continuous study period. Most illnesses were of less than 1–3 days' duration; 20 percent occurred with respiratory symptoms, and 20 percent involved only diarrhea.

Illnesses tended to occur in one of two patterns: (*1*) mild afebrile illness with watery diarrhea or (*2*) a more severe febrile illness with vomiting, headache, and constitutional symptoms. Although etiologic agents were rarely identified, these two patterns of illness subsequently developed among volunteers who ingested filtrates prepared from the feces of ill patients.[126–128] Studies done in 1975–1977 in Charlottesville, Virginia, confirmed this pattern of winter illnesses with clustering in families, highest attack rates in children, and the absence of identifiable etiologic agents in most cases despite the application of techniques for virologic and enterotoxin studies.[67,68]

Although there has been little consistent documentation of enteroviruses in association with febrile winter vomiting disease, echovirus type 11 has been demonstrated in association with a small laboratory outbreak of febrile vomiting disease.[129] Abdominal pain and vomiting have been described with influenza B infections in children between the ages of 4 and 10 years.[130]

Careful evaluation of specimens from an outbreak of winter vomiting disease in an elementary school revealed a 27 nm parvovirus-like agent.[131–133] Typical winter vomiting disease, first described in 1929 by Zahorsky,[134] occurred over a 2-day period in late October 1968 in Norwalk, Ohio. Fifty percent of 232 students and teachers in an elementary school developed a mild illness characterized by nausea, vomiting, and abdominal cramps that usually lasted only 12–24 hours. Diarrhea occurred in fewer than half, and a low-grade fever occurred in approximately one-third. A remarkable 32 percent secondary attack rate in family contacts occurred approximately 48 hours later. A bacteria-free fecal suspension from a secondary case from the Norwalk outbreak caused an illness with low-grade fever and diarrhea in two of three volunteers. A second passage in volunteers produced either a febrile vomiting disease or an afebrile diarrheal disease, and illness was also produced in one of four volunteers who ingested an inoculum after three passages in human fetal intestinal organ culture.[132] From the stool of a second human passage in these volunteers, Kapikian and his colleagues used convalescent serum to identify a 27 nm agent by immune electron microscopy.[133] Antibody in the convalescent serum of other volunteers and three of five patients with naturally acquired illness was shown to coat and to aggregate these particles. Biopsy specimens revealed an intact small intestinal mucosa but blunted villi, shortened microvilli, and dilatation of the endoplasmic reticulum with intracellular multivesiculate bodies. Dilated mitochondria and intercellular spaces were also observed.[135] There was also a transient decrease in the activities of the brush border enzymes, alkaline phosphatase, sucrase, and trehalase. All changes had returned to normal by 2 weeks after the illness. The colon is relatively spared, and fecal leukocytes are absent in this noninflammatory type of diarrhea.

The pathophysiologic features of winter vomiting disease caused by Norwalk-like agents may be parallel in some respects to that mentioned in the previous section for rotaviruses. Both cause mucosal villus destruction and transient brush border enzyme deficiencies in the upper portion of the small bowel without any alteration in adenylate cyclase activity.[97,136,137] The roles of transient enzyme deficiency, malabsorption of xylose and lactose, and the slight increase in the number of bacteria present during the Norwalk illness remain unclear.[136,138]

Similar outbreaks of vomiting disease have occurred elsewhere with either documented or suspected Norwalk-like agents. In March 1971, all four members of a household in Honolulu, Hawaii, developed a vomiting illness over a 4-day period with an apparent 44- to 48-hour incubation period, and in June 1971, another family of four in Montgomery County, Maryland, developed illnesses at 24- to 48-hour intervals that were characterized by vomiting, diarrhea, and occasional myalgias.[139] Fecal specimens from these patients revealed 27 nm Norwalk-like particles, and subsequent cross-challenge volunteer studies suggested that the Norwalk and Montgomery County agents were antigenically similar and conferred cross-immunity while the Hawaii agent appeared to be antigenically different and failed to confer cross-immunity to the other agents.[139] Other Norwalk-like agents include the Snow Mountain and Taunton agents.[140] Clarke and associates reported an outbreak from a boys' boarding school in Britain. The illness was transmitted to volunteers with filtered extracts of feces from one ill boy (W agent).[141] Another outbreak in a primary school in Ditchling, England, in October 1975 revealed 26 nm particles that aggregated in convalescent serum and appeared to be antigenically similar to the W agent but different from the Hawaii and Norwalk agents.[142] Another 27 nm Norwalk-like agent was associated with an outbreak of gastroenteritis in a winter resort camp in Colorado.[143] From a convalescent hospital in Marin County, California, and a social gathering nearby, outbreaks of acute gastroenteritis have been associated with yet another viral agent capable of causing gastroenteritis, the Marin County agent.[144]

Several small (ranging from 20 to 35 nm in diameter), round (variably structured) viral agents of gastroenteritis have been grouped into four categories.[140,145] The first three categories have a better-defined surface morphology: (*1*) Norwalk-like viruses (including Norwalk or Montgomery County agent, Hawaii, Snow Mountain and Taunton agents); (*2*) caliciviruses, with characteristic "chalicelike" surface hollows (including agents described in the United Kingdom, UK1-4, and Japan); (*3*) astroviruses, with five- or six-pointed starlike surface structure (including Marin County, UK1-5, and Japan agents; and (*4*) Other less well defined, small round viruses (including Wollan, Wor Ditchling agent, Cockle, Paramatta, and other agents). Except for certain astrovirus and calicivirus strains, these have not yet been cultivated in vitro, and the lack of a convenient animal model has restricted their study. The roles of other viral agents, including enteroviruses (especially echovirus types 11, 14, and 18), enteric adenoviruses (said to cause up to 9 percent of pediatric inpatient diarrhea[146]), human coronaviruses (reported from infants with gastroenteritis[147,148], and the recently reported pestiviruses[149] are beyond the scope of this chapter. Over one-third of outbreaks of nonbacterial gastroenteritis in the United States have been associated with the Norwalk virus.[150,151]

Identification of Norwalk-like agents capable of causing winter vomiting disease requires immune electron microscopy[133] or radioimmunoassay for demonstration of a serologic response.[152] It is clear that there are multiple antigenic types of these agents that are capable of causing similar disease and that resistance may relate to individual (genetic) differences rather than to lasting protective immunity after symptomatic infection.[140,153] The detection of other viral causes of gastroenteritis includes monoclonal antibody-based enzyme immunoassay,[149,154] tissue culture,[155] or gene probes.[156]

ACUTE NONINFLAMMATORY DIARRHEA IN ADULTS

In temperate climates, acute noninflammatory diarrhea in adults may be caused by rotaviruses[157,158] or by Norwalk-like viruses.[93,97,132,157] The association of rotaviruses as well as adenoviruses, coxsackieviruses and toxigenic *Clostridium difficile* with diarrhea, abdominal cramps, and a higher mortality among adult bone marrow transplant recipients has also been noted.[159] Additionally, several agents of food poisoning such as *Clostridium perfringens, Bacillus cereus,* or *Staphylococcus aureus* commonly cause noninflammatory diarrheal syndromes in adults (see Chapter 86).

In adults living in areas with poor sanitation, several other agents commonly cause sporadic noninflammatory diarrhea. In certain areas in South Asia, cholera is an endemic cause of severe watery diarrhea. With the increased infection-to-case ratio of El Tor cholera, the seventh pandemic has swept most of the continents of the Eastern Hemisphere including Asia, Africa, and the Mediterranean portions of Europe.[160] Isolated cases have also occurred in the United States.[161,162] Outbreaks have been related to contaminated mineral water[163] or to undercooked shellfish.[164,165] One should suspect cholera in any patient who has severe dehydration and watery diarrhea, especially if the patient has a history of recent travel to a cholera-endemic area. The disease can be so fulminant as to cause hypovolemic shock and death from the outpouring of fluid into the upper portion of the small bowel before the first diarrheal stool occurs.[166] As discussed in detail in Chapter 192, the entire dehydrating syndrome of cholera appears to be related to the activation of intestinal adenylate cyclase by the potent cholera enterotoxin.[69,70] To make the diagnosis of cholera bacteriologically, one should culture stool specimens onto thiosulfate citrate bile salts sucrose agar. Of prime importance in therapy is fluid replacement either intravenously with isotonic fluids or orally with glucose electrolyte solutions.

Patients from whom *Vibrio cholerae* cannot be isolated may also have a cholera-like syndrome. In 1956, De et al. demonstrated that *E. coli* isolated from adults and children with this syndrome caused fluid accumulation similar to that seen with *V. cholerae* in ligated rabbit ileal loops.[167] In the early 1960s Trabulsi, working in São Paulo, reported a similar finding with "toxigenic" *E. coli*.[168] Subsequent studies by Taylor et al.[169,170] demonstrated that enterotoxigenicity correlated poorly with classic serotypes and that viable organisms were not required. Smith and Halls identified several enterotoxigenic strains in association with animal diarrhea.[171] Other workers showed that several adult cases of "acute undifferentiated diarrhea" in tropical Bengal were due to enterotoxigenic *E. coli* strains that were usually not of the classically recognized pathogenic serotypes.[172–175] These strains were transiently present during acute illness and elicited a net jejunal fluid secretion. The toxic material present in the culture filtrate of these *E. coli* strains was demonstrated to be heat labile and nondialyzable and was precipitated in 40% ammonium sulfate. Subsequent studies have demonstrated that two types of enterotoxin are produced by *E. coli,* a heat-labile enterotoxin (LT) and a heat-stable enterotoxin (ST).[176] Like cholera toxin, the *E. coli* heat-labile enterotoxin activates mucosal adenylate cyclase.[58–60] Heat-labile enterotoxin is larger, inactivated by heating at 60°C for 30 minutes, and antigenically and mechanistically similar to cholera toxin with a lag period before the activation of adenylate cyclase. Heat-labile enterotoxin is detected by several bioassay systems that use the adenylate cyclase activating property of this toxin[177–179] or by immunoassay methods.[180] In contrast, ST activates guanylate cyclase,[74–76] has an earlier onset of action,[176] has greater tissue specificity,[76] and has a much lower molecular weight than LT does.[181] It is assayed in suckling mice.[182] The role of yet a different type of enterotoxin, STb, that causes secretion in piglets without altering intestinal cyclic AMP or cyclic GMP remains unclear in humans at present.[183–185]

Methods for demonstrating enterotoxigenic *E. coli* are limited by the lack of a selective culture process (as routinely used, for example, to identify salmonellae or shigellae) and the necessity to pick a few random colonies of *E. coli* for enterotoxin testing. Data from a common-source outbreak of enterotoxigenic *E. coli* diarrhea in Crater Lake National Park in Oregon demonstrate the insensitivity of nonselective culture methods.[186] Fourteen patients in this outbreak had enterotoxigenic *E. coli* diarrhea by epidemiologic and clinical criteria, and each had multiple, random *E. coli* stool isolates tested for enterotoxin as well as paired sera examined for antitoxic immunity. Only 43 percent had enterotoxigenic *E. coli* identified, 36 percent had significant serum antitoxic antibody titer increases, and only 64 percent had either one or the other. Thirty-six percent of the cases could not be confirmed by current, nonselective methods. The lack of a serum antibody response in many patients with this intralumenal toxinosis is not surprising.

Other studies have shown that, in addition to the association with diarrhea in children, LT-only, ST-only, and LT-plus-ST–producing strains are associated with adult diarrhea.[3] Adults living in areas of poor sanitation may often carry LT-producing *E. coli* asymptomatically.[187,188] In contrast, ST-producing *E. coli* strains are significantly associated with diarrheal disease and are less frequently present in asymptomatic control patients living in areas with poor sanitation. However, studies suggest that enterotoxigenic *E. coli* serotypes are uncommonly associated with diarrhea in the United States.[66,67]

A newly recognized cause of acute, noninflammatory, self-limited diarrhea among those exposed to infected animals and patients is cryptosporidiosis.[189–191] This tiny coccidian protozoan parasite causes more severe, watery, prolonged diarrhea in immunocompromised hosts.

Treatment of diarrhea in adults consists primarily of rehydration. If glucose or sucrose accompany the isotonic fluid taken orally, the coupled absorption of sodium and water are often sufficient to replace fluid loss.[192] Pepto-Bismol may reduce enterotoxin action,[193] and if there is no significant febrile or inflammatory process, low doses of antimotility agents may offer some relief with minimum risk if cramping is severe.

DIARRHEA IN AIDS PATIENTS

Patients with the acquired immunodeficiency syndrome (AIDS) often develop or present with diarrhea. Among AIDS patients in the United States, 50–60 percent present with diarrhea,[194,195] a number that reaches 95 percent in tropical developing areas such as Africa or Haiti.[195] In many of these patients, diarrhea becomes prolonged and life-threatening and may present major difficulties in management. Although some have reported an enteropathy without identifiable pathogens[196,197] or with primary human immunodeficiency virus (HIV) infection of enterochromaffin cells in the bowel mucosal crypts and lamina propria,[198] others report one or more enteric pathogens in 55–85 percent of patients with AIDS and diarrhea.[199,200] Sexually promiscuous homosexual males often become infected with *Giardia lamblia, Entamoeba histolytica, Campylobacter jejuni, Shigella, Chlamydia trachomatis, C. difficile,* or (with proctitis) *N. gonorrheae,* herpes simplex virus, or *Treponema pallidum*.[201] As shown in Table 3, the leading agents found in AIDS patients with diarrhea are cytomegalovirus, *Cryptosporidium, E. histolytica, G. lamblia, Salmonella, Campylobacter, Shigella, C. difficile, Vibrio parahaemolyticus, Mycobacterium,* sp.,[199,200] and microsporidia. Even *Pneumocystis carinii* can occasionally involve the intestinal tract in this setting.[202] Although eradicative treatment may be difficult, most of these patients respond to specific antimicrobial or antiparasitic therapy, thus

TABLE 3. Possible Enteric Pathogens in AIDS Patients

Pathogen	Diarrhea (%) (n = 69)	No Diarrhea (%) (n = 48)
Cytomegalovirus	27–45	0–15
Cryptosporidium	15–16	0
Entamoeba histolytica	0–25	0
Giardia lamblia	4–15	0–5
Salmonella sp.	0–15	0
Campylobacter sp.	10–11	5–8
Shigella sp.	5–10	0
Clostridium difficile toxin	7	0
Vibrio parahaemolyticus	4	0
Mycobacterium sp.	2–5	0
Isospora belli	2	0
Blastocystis hominis	15	0–16
Candida albicans	53	0–24
Herpes simplex	5–18	0–40
Chlamydia trachomatis	11	0–13
Intestinal spirochetes	11	0–11
One or more pathogens	55–85	5–39

(Data from Smith et al.[199] and Laughon et al.[200])

emphasizing the need to specifically diagnose the etiologies of these infections whenever possible. The antiviral agent ganciclovir (DHPG) can transiently reverse intestinal cytomegalovirus infection,[203] and most bacterial and parasitic agents can be treated with some improvement. *Cryptosporidium,* which infects 3–21 percent of AIDS patients in the United States, can be found in as many as 50 percent of patients in Africa and Haiti with AIDS and diarrhea.[195] *Cryptosporidium* may also extend into the biliary tract as well in this setting. The same acid-fast stain that detects *Cryptosporidium* or *Mycobacterium* in fecal specimens may also reveal *Isosora belli* in 2–15 percent of AIDS patients with diarrhea in the United States and Africa, respectively.[195] Nontyphoidal *Salmonella* infections occur with an estimated 20-fold increase in frequency as well as increased severity in AIDS patients.[204–207] Nevertheless, these infections, as those with *Campylobacter jejuni* and other species, are treatable. Other common enteric infections include esophagitis or stomatitis with *Candida* or herpes simplex virus.

DIARRHEA IN INSTITUTIONS

Institutions provide special host and environmental settings for the acquisition of certain enteric pathogens. As with diarrhea in AIDS patients and travelers' diarrhea, most cases are still noninflammatory; however, an increased frequency of certain causes of inflammatory diarrhea should prompt a careful search for fecal leukocytes in sporadic or clustered cases in hospitals, chronic care facilities, or day care centers.[208]

Hospitals

Nosocomial diarrhea is among the most common of reported nosocomial outbreaks to the Centers for Disease Control and accounts for 21 percent of all 223 nosocomial outbreaks reported from 1956 to 1979.[209] However, its frequency is often overlooked, and it has been suggested to be the most common nosocomial infection in some areas.[210] Furthermore, nosocomial diarrhea appears to be a significant predisposing factor to other nosocomial infections such as urinary tract infections.[211] Overall rates range from 2.3 to 4.1 illnesses per 100 admissions on pediatric wards[210,212] and from 7.7 per 100 admissions to 41 percent of adults hospitalized in intensive care units.[210,213] From limited available data, *C. difficile* appears to be associated with most cases with a recognized etiology (45 percent), followed by *Salmonella* (12 percent).[214] *Salmonella* is the commonest cause among reported outbreaks of nosocomial gastroenteritis.[209] In young children and in immunocompromised hosts, viral agents (rotaviruses, adenoviruses, coxsackieviruses, and others) are often found as well.[212,215]

Chronic Care Facilities

Diarrheal illnesses are also significant problems in extended care facilities for the elderly. Conservative estimates based on passively reported illness rates are that one-third of patients in chronic care facilities experience diarrhea each year.[216,217] About one-quarter of these patients have *C. difficile* cytotoxin, one-third of whom are symptomatic with diarrhea.[218] Over 20 percent have fecal cytotoxin on admission, and a comparable number acquire cytotoxigenic *C. difficile* in the institution.[218] When those with diarrhea are studied, 18–53 percent have cytotoxin or *C. difficile,* respectively.[219] The frequency of potentially transmissible enteric pathogens emphasizes the importance of careful hand washing in situations where hygiene is often difficult. Similar problems have been long recognized in mental institutions where hepatitis, *Strongyloides,* and amebiasis are readily acquired.

Day Care Centers

Another special institutional setting where hygiene is difficult and enteric infections are increasingly appreciated is in day care centers. Numerous outbreaks have been reported in association with viruses, bacteria, or parastites. Most common in infants and children <2 years old are rotaviruses, while older toddlers are more likely to acquire *Giardia lamblia.*[220] An identical clinical syndrome of prolonged noninflammatory diarrhea may be seen with *Cryptosporidium* in day care centers.[221–223] Outbreaks of inflammatory diarrhea in the day care center setting include those due to *Shigella, Campylobacter jejuni,* and *Clostridium difficile.*[224,225]

THE DIARRHEA OF TRAVELERS (TURISTA)

Whether it "arouses one from bed with a start at 4 A.M. for a record-breaking race to the bathroom to begin a stacatto ballet"[226] or it produces the poetry of the Psalmist, "I am poured out like water . . . my heart like wax is melted in the midst of my bowels,"[227] travelers' diarrhea has a major impact each year on the 300 million international travelers and probably on the distribution of $100 billion in international tourism receipts.[228] Sixteen million people (8 million from the United States) travel from industrialized to developing countries. It is by far the most common and among the most feared illnesses that threaten the traveler. Many studies have focused on North Americans and northern Europeans who appear to be the groups at greatest risk when they travel to Latin America, Southern Europe, Africa, or Asia.[229–232] Travelers' diarrhea, which may be severe and incapacitating (albeit rarely if ever fatal), is by far the most common health problem encountered with travel to developing countries.[233] The global nature of the problem and some suggested causal forces are illustrated by its more euphemistic names: "Delhi belly," "Gyppi tummy," "GIs," "Rome runs," "Greek gallop," "Turkey trots," "Montezuma's revenge," "Aztec two-step," "Aden gut," "San Franciscitis," "Basra belly," "La turista," "backdoor sprint," "summer complaint," "coeliac flux," "Canary disease," "passion," "Hong Kong dog," "Poona poohs," "Casablanca crud," "tourist trots," "Malta dog," and many more.

The onset of the vast majority of travelers' diarrhea is usually between 5 and 15 days after arrival, with a range from 3 to 31 days in several reported series.[226,234–240] The illness is typically manifested by malaise, anorexia, and abdominal cramps, followed by the sudden onset of watery diarrhea. Nausea and vomiting may accompany 10–25 percent of the illnesses. The diarrhea is usually noninflammatory, without blood or pus. A low-grade fever may be present in approximately one-third of the cases. The duration is usually 1–5 days, but a significant number of people (19–50 percent) have an illness that continues beyond 5–10 days.

TABLE 4. Etiologies of Travelers' Diarrhea

Characteristics	Latin America (15 Studies)	Africa (3 Studies)	Asia (8 Studies)
Duration of stay (days)	21 (2–42)[a]	28 (28–35)	(28–42)
Attack rate (%)	52 (21–100)	54 (36–62)	(39–57)
Percentage with			
Enterotoxigenic *E. coli*	46 (28–72)	36 (31–75)	(20–34)
Shigella	0 (0–30)	0 (0–15)	(4–7)
Salmonella	0 (0–16)	0 (0–0)	(11–15)
C. jejuni	—	—	(2–15)
V. parahaemolyticus	—	—	(1–13)
Rotavirus	23 (0–36)	0 (0–0)	—

[a] Median (range) from 26 studies.[241,242]

The attack rate ranges from 7 percent after 2 weeks in Aden[235] to 54 percent after 8 days in Mexico,[229] and was 4–51 percent over a 14-day period among 17,280 Swiss tourists, depending on where they went.[232] One report of British tourists notes an attack rate ranging from 26 percent in Africa to 7.7 percent in North America. In descending order of risk after Africa in this study were the Middle East, Southern Europe, Central Europe, Asia (including India and Pakistan), South America, Australia, and North America.[240] In general, it appears that one approaches a 50 percent risk of acquiring turista during travel to a tropical country from a temperate climate for 2 weeks or more. The attack rate also appears to decrease with age after 25 years, an observation that may reflect different habits and exposure rather than inherent susceptibility.[226,232]

For many years, the etiology of turista was an enigma; only infrequently have parasites or bacteria such as amebas, *Giardia, Salmonella,* or *Shigella* been identified. Likewise viral studies have failed to elucidate significant viral etiologies of travelers' diarrhea. The first suggestion that an infectious bacterial process was likely came from the effective reduction in the attack rate by the use of prophylactic antimicrobial agents.[185,191,234,240] Studies by Kean suggested that *E. coli* of certain enteropathogenic serotypes might be involved in up to one-third of the cases.[226] The involvement of *E. coli* was further confirmed in an outbreak of travelers' diarrhea among the British troops in Aden, where *E. coli* 0148 was identified among 54 percent of British troops with diarrhea.[235]

Subsequent studies have demonstrated enterotoxigenic *E. coli* (ETEC) in approximately 50 percent (range, 20–75 percent) of cases of travelers' diarrhea in Latin America, Africa, and Asia (Table 4).[241,242] The attack rate ranged from 20 to 100 percent (median, 52–54 percent) in 26 studies reviewed (Table 4).[241,242] Enterotoxigenic *E. coli* organisms were almost never present before the travel; they were acquired by only 14 of 111 (12.6 percent) fellow travelers who did not become ill.[237–239] The type of enterotoxin produced by *E. coli* associated with travelers' diarrhea may be the heat-labile type (LT), the heat-stable type (ST), or both LT and ST (Table 5). In contrast to adults who live in tropical areas and may often carry enterotoxigenic *E. coli* asymptomatically, the traveler appears to be susceptible to illness caused by enterotoxin-producing *E. coli.* Salmonellae, shigellae, or vibrios are present in only 1–16 percent of the patients with travelers' diarrhea. Rotavirus infections have been described in 0–36 percent of cases of travelers' diarrhea, often in association with bacterial or parasitic pathogens.[243] In a study of Panamanian tourists to Mexico, rotavirus or Norwalk viruses were found in 41 percent, *Campylobacter* in 11 percent, and ETEC in only one case of diarrhea.[244] Cholera is rarely a problem for U.S. travelers.[232,245]

In contrast to the frequent identification of potential etiologic agents among travelers to tropical areas who develop diarrhea, careful studies of a group of marines who developed diarrhea upon arrival in temperate South Korea (21 percent in 3 weeks) failed to reveal any evidence of bacterial, parasitic, or rotaviral pathogens.[246] Travelers to certain areas such as Russia and national parks in the United States may be especially prone to the more insidious watery diarrhea seen with giardiasis or cryptosporidiosis.[247–250] Strongyloidiasis may also be acquired in tropical areas and may cause noninflammatory diarrhea, abdominal pain, and eosinophilia.[251]

Several other potentially serious infections may be acquired by travelers whose major complaint is diarrhea or abdominal pain. Malaria may be manifested initially as "gastroenteritis" with nausea, vomiting, diarrhea, or abdominal pain in 30–50 percent of the cases.[252] The physician caring for world travelers should also remember to consider typhoid fever and other infections that may be manifested with a "typhoidal pattern" including plague, meloidosis, typhus, and arboviral hemorrhagic fevers.[252,253]

The desire to control the bothersome problem of diarrhea in travelers has led to extreme and sometimes irrational attempts at its control.[226] Some travelers persist in using iodochlorhydroxquin (Entero-Vioform, clioquinol), which has been shown not only to be ineffective for travelers' diarrhea[229,254] but also to carry a risk of severe subacute myelo-optic atrophy.[255] Other commonly used remedies such as diphenoxylate-atropine (Lomotil) and kaolin-pectin suspension were of no value in treating children with acute diarrhea in Guatemala.[256] The former and other antimotility agents may actually worsen the illness with inflammatory processes such as shigellosis.[257] Bismuth subsalicylate (Pepto-Bismol) has been shown to inhibit enterotoxin activity in experimental animal models[193] and has been recommended for symptomic therapy and, in doses as low as 1.05 g/day (2 tablets bid), for prophylaxis.[258,259]

The mainstay of therapy, as with any diarrheal illness, is adequate hydration with an oral glucose– or sucrose–electrolyte solution.

Prevention of travelers' diarrhea should be directed toward reducing the consumption of infectious agents in food and water. Salads, raw vegetables, and untreated water (or ice) are high-risk foods.[260] Bottled, noncarbonated water cannot be considered safe since outbreaks of cholera[163] and typhoid fever[261,262] have been traced to bottled water and beverages, respectively. It has been suggested that even brief, 10-minute heating to 50–55°C (the temperature of some hot tap water, "too hot for the hand to tolerate") may kill many enteric bacterial

TABLE 5. Frequency of Enterotoxigenic *E. coli* in Association with Travelers' Diarrhea in Latin America, Africa, and Asia

	Study				
Feature	Gastroenterologists in Mexico[146]	Peace Corps Volunteers in Kenya[147]	Yale Glee Club in Latin America[148]	Japanese Travelers Returning to Tokyo from India, Southeast Asia, Orient[242]	Total
Illness attack rate (%)	49% in 16 days	69% in 5 wk	74% in 1 mon	—	
Type of enterotoxin					
LT only	16%	33%	25%	4.8%	21%
LT and ST	16%	15%	12.5%	11.8%	38%
ST only	9.8%	2%	19%	13.6%	41%
Total	21/51 cases	14/27 cases	9/16 cases	226/749 cases	270/843 cases
(Percentage of illness with ETEC)	(41%)	(52%)	(56%)	(30.2%)	(32%)

Abbreviations: LT: heat-labile; ST: heat-stable.

and parasitic pathogens.[263] Care in eating and drinking may reduce one's risk even in highly endemic areas to <15 percent.[260,264]

The efficacy of prophylactic antimicrobial agents has been documented in several studies.[234,240,265] However, multiple drug-resistant enterotoxigenic *E. coli* occur and have demonstrated cotransfer of enterotoxigenicity and drug resistance.[266,267] The increased risk of acquiring a more severe infection such as salmonellosis,[268] the risk of drug side effects (such as photosensitivity in the tropics), and the emergence of drug-resistant organisms should preclude the widespread use of antibiotic prophylaxis at this time. Until more widespread resistance develops,[269,270] treatment of travelers' diarrhea with trimethoprim, sulfamethoxazole-trimethoprim, bicozamycin, or ciprofloxacin may reduce a 3- to 4- day illness to 1–1½ days.[271–273]

DIFFERENTIAL DIAGNOSIS OF ACUTE NONINFLAMMATORY DIARRHEA

Acute noninflammatory diarrhea may also be the consequence of several noninfectious processes. As with agents that effect an osmotic diuresis, nonabsorbable agents such as sorbitol may cause diarrhea if consumed in excess. Ipecac fluid extract used by mistake instead of ipecac syrup may cause watery diarrhea instead of vomiting. Heavy metal poisoning (As, Sn, Fe, Cd, Hg, Pb) is often associated with diarrhea, probably as a result of toxic effects on the rapidly growing mucosal epithelium. Endocrine causes of diarrhea that may share the adenylate cyclase–activating mechanism with enterotoxins include non-β islet cell tumors, medullary carcinoma of the thyroid, carcinoid tumors, and others that are associated with increased serum prostaglandins or vasoactive intestinal polypeptide (VIP).[274] Patients with thyrotoxicosis and adrenal or parathyroid insufficiency may also have diarrhea. Congenital and acquired enzyme deficiencies include lactase deficiency and pancreatic or biliary insufficiency in which inadequately degraded or absorbed nutrients may promote an osmotic diarrhea. A child with diarrhea as well as with edema, hypertension, or petechiae should be suspected of having hemolytic-uremic syndrome with or without enterohemorrhagic *E. coli* O157:H7. Patients with dermatitis herpetiformis may also have diarrhea that may respond to sulfone or sulfapyridine therapy or to a gluten-free diet.

CHRONIC NONINFLAMMATORY DIARRHEA

Syndromes of chronic noninflammatory diarrhea of infectious etiology include giardiasis, tropical spruelike syndromes, syndromes of bacterial "overgrowth," and *Cryptosporidium* or *Isospora belli* infection (especially in immunocompromised hosts).[189,190,195,249,275]

The patient with weight loss, malaise, and watery or fatty stools should be suspected of having giardiasis or some other cause of a malabsorption syndrome. This syndrome may also be associated with hypocalcemia, with iron or folate deficiency anemia, or with vitamin D, vitamin K, or protein deficiency.

Giardiasis may go undiagnosed for weeks. While it is endemic throughout most of the United States and much of the world, giardiasis received attention when acquired in Rocky Mountain ski resorts and in Leningrad.[247,248] Effective management requires a high index of suspicion followed by a careful search by a competent experienced person for the trophozoite or cyst of *G. lamblia* in multiple stool specimens or in a small bowel aspirate or "string" (Enterotest; Hedeco, Palo Alto, CA) sample. Recommended therapy is quinacrine (Atabrine), 100 mg tid for 5–7 days, with a reported 95 percent cure rate, or metronidazole (Flagyl), 250 mg tid for 7–10 days, with a reported 70 percent cure rate.[275] Higher doses of metronidazole may be more effective. Furazolidone, which is available in liquid form for pediatric use, divided into three daily doses with meals (total, 8 mg/kg/day) for 10 days is often used in children.[276]

The diagnosis of *Cryptosporidium* or *Isospora belli* infection is best made by phase microscopic or modified Kinyoun acid-fast stain examination of fecal specimens with or without sugar floatation.[189,195,277]

BACTERIAL OVERGROWTH SYNDROMES

Many syndromes have been described in which impaired absorption was attributed to abnormal bacterial colonization in the upper segment of the small bowel.[278] Whether these organisms are virulent pathogens or simply normal colonic flora abnormally distributed is currently unclear.

Normally, the upper portion of the small bowel is relatively sparsely populated with fewer than 10^5 organisms/ml that are predominantly facultative gram-positive organisms (diptheroids, streptococci, and lactobacilli).[279] The organisms most often incriminated in bacterial overgrowth syndromes in the small bowel are aerobic enteric coliforms (Enterobacteriaceae) and anerobic gram-negative fecal flora (*Bacteroides* and other genera). Other organisms such as *Plesiomonas shigelloides* may occasionally be responsible.[280] Bacterial colonization in the upper part of the small bowel may be associated with malabsorption or chronic diarrhea in the absence of significant histopathologic changes. Small bowel overgrowth is usually associated with a predisposing bowel abnormality such as achlorhydria, (from gastritis, pernicious anemia, or gastric surgery), blind-loop syndromes, cholangitis, impaired motility (scleroderma, diabetic neuropathy, vagotomy), surgery, strictures, diverticula, or radiation damage.[281,282] Malnutrition, especially with protein, folate, or B_{12} deficiency, may also render the bowel more susceptible to microbial colonization and injury.[279,283] An episode of acute infectious diarrhea may also provide the initiating event in the establishment of small bowel colonization and chronic diarrhea.[279,284,285] Lindenbaum et al. described spruelike morphologic changes in the upper portion of the small bowel in association with increased numbers of bacteria and malabsorption among Peace Corps volunteers living in Pakistan.[286]

The mechanism by which fecal flora in the small bowel cause malabsorption may involve bacterial binding or utilization of nutrients (such as vitamin B_{12} or carbohydrates, respectively), deconjugation of bile salts by bacteria such as enterococci and anerobes,[287] or the toxic effects of bacterial products such as fatty acids or amines.[279] Indeed, colonizing *E. coli* without other recognized virulence traits have been shown to cause prolonged diarrhea in a rabbit model,[288] with an associated impairment in water and electrolyte absorption as well as disaccharidase activity.[289]

The approach to the patient suspected of having bacterial "overgrowth" as a cause of malabsorption or chronic diarrhea should include quantitative aerobic and anerobic cultures of the upper small bowel contents obtained by intubation or "string" passage. Since the critical number of organisms appears to be approximately 10^5 organisms/ml, semiquantitative estimates from a Gram stain analogous to the urine Gram stain may also prove to be of value. Roberts et al. have suggested that unexplained malnutrition in the elderly may be due to clinically inapparent bacterial overgrowth that can be detected by the ^{14}C-glycocholic acid breath test for bacterial deconjugation of bile salts.[284] Tests for urinary indican (from bacterial conversion of tryptophan) have proved to be insensitive and nonspecific for bacterial overgrowth syndromes.[290]

Patients with diarrhea or malabsorption and bacterial overgrowth should be considered for antibiotic therapy, especially if predisposing conditions like achlorhydria, scleroderma, or diabetes are present. Depending on results of quantitative cultures of upper small bowel aspirates, therapy may need to be directed against anerobes as well as aerobic coliform organisms.[279,284] While small amounts of antibiotics have been used to improve the nutritional status of animals and poultry and even of malnourished children,[291] the potential risks of widespread antibiotic use[292] must be weighed against potential benefits.

Noninfectious causes of chronic noninflammatory diarrhea should also be considered in the differential diagnosis. These include congenital deficiency syndromes and food allergies, certain neoplastic and endocrine processes, and less well understood functional disorders. In the first categories one may consider milk allergies, disaccharidase deficiencies, gluten enteropathy, acrodermatitis enteropathica, β-lipoprotein deficiency, familial hyperchloremic alkalosis (congenital "chloridorrhea") Leiner's disease, and Wiskott-Aldrich syndrome. Neoplastic and endocrine causes of diarrhea include carcinoid, Werner syndrome (multiple endocrine adenomatosis), Zollinger-Ellison syndrome (gastrinoma), "pancreatic cholera" syndromes, medullary carcinoma of the thyroid, and thyrotoxicosis. Patients with partial mechanical bowel obstruction or pellagra may also have chronic diarrhea. Finally, frequent small stools may suggest an irritable bowel syndrome of presumed functional etiology. However, a search for treatable infectious agents reviewed in this chapter should always precede this latter diagnosis.

REFERENCES

1. Dingle JH, Badger GF, Jordan WS Jr. Illnesses in the Home: A Study of 25,000 Illnesses in a Group of Cleveland Families. Cleveland: Press of Western Reserve University; 1964.
2. Kapikian AZ, Kim H-W, Wyatt RG, et al. Human reovirus-like agent as the major pathogen associated with "winter" gastroenteritis in hospitalized infants and young children. N Engl J Med. 1976;294:965.
3. Black RE, Merson MH, Huq I, et al. Incidence and severity of rotavirus and *E. coli* diarrhea in rural Bangladesh. Lancet. 1981;1:141.
4. Ryder TW, Sack DA, Kapikian AZ, et al. Enterotoxigenic *Escherichia coli* and reovirus-like agent in rural Bangladesh. Lancet. 1976;1:659.
5. Guerrant RL, Moore RA, Kirschenfeld PM, et al. Role of toxigenic and invasive bacteria in acute diarrhea of childhood. N Engl J Med. 1975;293:567.
6. Wadstrom T, Aust-Kettis A, Habte D, et al. Enterotoxin-producing bacteria and parasites in stools of Ethiopian children with diarrhoeal disease. Arch Dis Child. 1976;51:865.
7. Sack RB, Hirschhorn N, Brownlee I, et al. Enterotoxigenic *Escherichia coli*-associated diarrheal disease in Apache children. N Engl J Med. 1975;292:1041.
8. Black RE, Brown KH, Becker S, et al. Longitudinal studies of infectious diseases and physical growth of children in rural Bangladesh. I. Patterns of morbidity. Am J Epidemiol. 1982;115:305.
9. Guerrant RL, Kirchoff LV, Shields DS, et al. Prospective study of diarrheal illnesses in Northeastern Brazil: Patterns of disease, nutritional impact and risk factors. J Infect Dis. 1983;148:986.
10. Jacobs SI, Holzel A, Wolman B, et al. Outbreak of infantile gastroenteritis caused by *Escherichia coli* 0114. Arch Dis Child. 1970;45:656.
11. Neter E. Enteritis due to enteropathogenic *Escherichia coli:* Present-day status and unsolved problems. J Pediatr. 1959;55:223.
12. Hone R, Fitzpatrick S, Keane C, et al. Infantile enteritis in Dublin caused by *Escherichia coli* 0142. Med Microbiol. 1973;6:505.
13. Levine MM, Nalin DR, Hornick RB, et al. *Escherichia coli* strains that cause diarrhea but do not produce heat-labile or heat-stable enterotoxins and are noninvasive. Lancet. 1978;1:1119.
14. Nelson JD, Haltalin KC. Accuracy of diagnosis of bacterial diarrheal disease by clinical features. J Pediatr. 1971;78:519.
15. Drucker MM, Polliack A, Yeivin R, et al. Immunofluorescent demonstration of enteropathogenic *Escherichia coli* in tissues of infants dying with enteritis. Pediatrics. 1970;46:855.
16. South MA: Enteropathogenic *Escherichia coli* disease: New developments and perspectives. J Pediatr. 1971;79:1.
17. Kaslow RA, Taylor A, Dweck HS, et al. Enteropathogenic *Escherichia coli* infection in a newborn nursery. Am J Dis Child. 1974;128:797.
18. Levine MM, Edelman R. Enteropathogenic *Escherichia coli* of classic serotypes associated with infant diarrhea: Epidemiology and pathogenesis. Epidemiol Rev. 1984;6:31–51.
19. Gurwith M, Hinde D, Gross R, et al. A prospective study of enteropathogenic *E. coli* in endemic diarrheal disease. J Infect Dis. 1978;137:292.
20. Toledo MRF, Alvariza MCB, Murahovschi J, et al. Enteropathogenic *Escherichia coli* serotypes and endemic diarrhea in infants. Infect Immun. 1983;39:586–589.
21. Bray J, Beavan TED. Slide agglutination of *Bacterium coli* var. *Neapolitanum* in summer diarrhea. J Pathol Bacteriol. 1948;60:395.
22. Varela G, Aguirre A, Grillo J. *Escherichia coli*-gomez, nueva especie aislada de un caso mortal de diarrea. Bol Medico del Hospital Infantil Mexico. 1946;3:3.
23. Olarte J, Varela G. A complete somatic antigen common to *Salmonella adelaide, Escherichia coli-gomez* and *Escherichia coli* 0111:B4. J Lab Clin Med. 1952;40:252.
24. Giles C, Sangster G. An outbreak of infantile gastro-enteritis in Aberdeen. J Hyg (Camb) 1948;46:1.
25. Kaufmann F, Dupont A. *Escherichia* strains from infantile epidemic gastroenteritis. Acta Pathol Microbiol Scand. 1950;27:552.
26. Ørskov I, Ørskov F, Jann B, et al. Serology, chemistry and genetics of O and K antigens of *Escherichia coli*. Bacteriol Rev. 1977;41:667.
27. Rowe B, Gion RJ. *Escherichia coli* 0142 and infantile enteritis in Scotland. Lancet. 1971;1:649.
28. Rowe B, Gross J, Lindop R, et al. A new *E. coli* O group 0158 associated with an outbreak of infantile enteritis. J Clin Pathol. 1974;27:832.
29. Rogers KB, Cracknell VM. Epidemic infantile gastro-enteritis due to *Escherichia coli* type 0114. J Pathol Bacteriol. 1956;72:27.
30. Charter RE. *Escherichia coli* type 0114 isolated from infantile diarrhea and calf scours. J Pathol Bacteriol. 1956;72:33.
31. Riley LW, Remis RS, Helgerson SD, et al. Outbreaks of hemorrhagic colitis associated with a rare *Escherichia coli* serotype. N Engl J Med. 1983;308:681.
32. Johnson WM, Lior H, Bezanson GS. Cytotoxic *Escherichia coli* 0157:H7 associated with hemorrhagic colitis in Canada. Lancet. 1983;1:76.
33. Outbreak of hemorrhagic colitis—Ottawa, Canada. MMWR. 1983;32:133.
34. Neter E, Shumway CN: *E coli* serotype D433: Occurrence in intestinal and respiratory tracts, cultural characteristics, pathogenicity, sensitivity to antibiotics. Proc Soc Exp Biol Med. 1950;74:504.
35. Ørskov F. Virulence factors of the bacterial cell surface. J Infect Dis. 1978;137:630.
36. Guerrant RL, Dickens MD, Wenzel RP, et al. Toxigenic bacterial diarrhea: Nursery outbreak involving multiple bacterial strains. J Pediatr. 1976;89:885.
37. Skerman FJ, Formal SB, Falkow S. Plasmid-associated enterotoxin production in a strain of *Escherichia coli* isolated from humans. Infect Immun. 1972;5:622.
38. Takeda Y, Murphy J. Bacteriophage conversion of heat labile enterotoxin in *Escherichia coli*. J Bacteriol. 1978;133:172.
39. Wachsmith K, Wells J, Shipley P, et al. Heat-labile enterotoxin production in isolates from a shipboard outbreak of human diarrheal illness. Infect Immun. 1979;24:793–7.
40. Sack RB. Human diarrheal disease caused by enterotoxigenic *Escherichia coli*. Annu Rev Microbiol. 1975;29:333.
41. Merson MH, Black RE, Gross RJ, et al. Use of antisera for identification of enterotoxigenic *E. coli*. Lancet.. 1980;2:222.
42. Ryder RW, Wachsmuth IK, Buxton AE, et al. Infantile diarrhea produced by heat-stable enterotoxigenic *Escherichia coli*. N Engl J Med. 1976;295:849.
43. Gross RJ, Rowe B, Henderson A, et al. A new *Escherichia coli* O-group, 0159, associated with outbreaks of enteritis in infants. Scand J Infect Dis. 1976;8:195.
44. Haltalin KC. Neonatal shigellosis. Am J Dis Child. 1967;114:603.
45. Schroeder SA, Aserkoff B, Brachman PS. Epidemic salmonellosis in hospitals and institutions. N Engl J Med. 1968;279:674.
46. Rice PA, Craven PC, Wells JG: *Salmonella heidelberg* enteritis and bacteremia. An epidemic on two pediatric wards. Am J Med. 1976;60:509.
47. Eichenwald HF, Ababio A, Arky AM, et al. Epidemic diarrhea in premature and older infants caused by echo virus type 18. JAMA. 1958;166:1563.
48. Yow MD, Melnick JL, Blattner RJ, et al. The association of viruses and bacteria with infantile diarrhea. Am J Epidemiol. 1970;92:33.
49. Moffet HL, Shulenberger HK, Burkholder ER. Epidemiology and etiology of severe infantile diarrhea. J Pediatr. 1968;72:1.
50. Murphy AM, Albrey MB, Crew EB. Rotavirus infections of neonates. Lancet. 1977;2:1149.
51. Cameron DJS, Bishop RF, Davidson GP, et al. New virus associated with diarrhea in neonates. Med J Aust. 1976;1:85.
52. Bishop RF, Hewstone AS, Davidson GP, et al. An epidemic of diarrhea in human neonates involving a reoviruslike agent and "enteropathogenic" serotypes of *Escherichia coli*. J Clin Pathol. 1976;29:46.
53. Chrystie IL, Totterdell BM, Banatvala JE. Asymptomatic endemic rotavirus infections in the newborn. Lancet. 1978;1:1176.
54. Mata LJ, Urrutia JJ. Intestinal colonization of breast-fed children in a rural area of low socioeconomic level. Ann NY Acad Sci. 1971;176:93.
55. Gordon JE, Chitkara ID, Wyon JB. Weanling diarrhea. Am J Med Sci. 1963;245:345.
56. Welsh JK, May JT. Anti-infective properties of breast-milk. J Pediatr. 1979;94:1.
57. Gordon JE, Guzman MA, Ascoli W, et al. Acute diarrhoeal disease in less developed countries. Bull WHO. 1964;31:9.
58. Reddy V, Rashuramulu N, Bhaskaram C. Secretory IgA in protein-calorie malnutrition. Arch Dis Child. 1976;51:871.
59. Stoliar OA, Kaniecki-Green E, Pelley RP, et al. Secretory IgA against enterotoxins in breast milk. Lancet. 1976;1:1258.
60. Brown SE III, Sauer KT, Nations MK, et al. Comparison of paired whole milk and dried filter paper samples for anti-enterotoxin and antirotavirus activities. J Clin Microbiol. 1982;16:103.
61. Bullen CL, Willis AT. Resistance of the breast-fed infant to gastroenteritis. Br Med J. 1971;3:338.
62. Bullen JJ, Rogers HJ, Leigh L. Iron-binding proteins in milk and resistance of *Escherichia coli* infection in infants. Br Med J. 1972;1:69.
63. Simhon A, Mata L. Anti-rotavirus antibody in human colostrum. Lancet. 1978;1:39.

64. Gorbach SL, Khurana CM. Toxigenic *Escherichia coli:* A cause of infantile diarrhea in Chicago. N Engl J Med. 1972;287:791.
65. Tacket CO, Losonsky G, Link H, et al. Protection by milk immunoglobulin concentrate against oral challenge with enterotoxigenic *Escherichia coli.* N Engl J Med. 1988;318:1240–3.
66. Echeverria P, Blacklow NR, Smith DH. Role of heat-labile toxigenic *Escherichia coli* and reovirus-like agent in diarrhea in Boston children. Lancet. 1975;2:1113.
67. Hughes JM, Gwaltney JM, Hughes DH, et al. Acute gastrointestinal illness in Charlottesville: A prospective family study (Abstract). Clin Res. 1978;26:24.
68. Guerrant RL, Hughes JM, Lima NL, et al. Microbiology of diarrhea in developed and developing countries. Rev Inf Dis. 1989. In press.
69. Chen LC, Rohde JE, Sharp GWG. Intestinal adenyl-cyclase activity in human cholera. Lancet. 1971;1:939.
70. Guerrant RL, Chen LC, Sharp GWG. Intestinal adenyl-cyclase activity in canine cholera: Correlation with fluid accumulation. J Infect Dis. 1972;125:377.
71. Evans DJ Jr, Chen LC, Curlin GT, et al. Stimulation of adenyl cyclase by *Escherichia coli* enterotoxin. Nature. 1972;236:137.
72. Guerrant RL, Ganguly U, Casper AGT, et al. Effect of *Escherichia coli* on fluid transport across canine small bowel: Mechanism and time course—with enterotoxin and whole bacterial cells. J Clin Invest. 1973;52:1707.
73. Kantor HS, Tao P, Gorbach SL. Stimulation of intestinal adenyl cyclase by *Escherichia coli* enterotoxin: Comparison of strains from an infant and an adult with diarrhea. J Infect Dis. 1974;129:1.
74. Hughes JM, Murad F, Chang B, et al. Role of cyclic GMP in the action of heat stable enterotoxin of *Escherichia coli.* Nature. 1978;271:755.
75. Field M, Graf LH Jr, Laird WJ, et al. Heat-stable enterotoxin of *Escherichia coli:* In vitro effects on guanylate cyclase activity, cyclic GMP concentration, and ion transport in small intestine. Proc Natl Acad Sci USA. 1978;75:2800.
76. Guerrant RL, Hughes JM, Chang B, et al. Activation of intestinal guanylate cyclase by heat stable enterotoxin of *E. coli:* Studies of tissue specificity, potential receptors, and intermediates. J Infect Dis. 1980;142:220.
77. Bishop RF, Davidson GP, Holmes IH, et al. Virus particles in epithelial cells of duodenal mucosa from children with acute non-bacterial gastroenteritis. Lancet. 1973;2:1281.
78. Flewett TH, Bryden AS, Davies H. Virus particles in gastroenteritis. Lancet. 1973;2:1497.
79. Kapikian AZ, Kim HW, Wyatt RG, et al. Reoviruslike agent in stools: Association with infantile diarrhea and development of serologic tests. Science. 1974;185:1049.
80. Kanno T, Suzuki H, Ishida N. Reovirus-like agent in Japanese infants with gastroenteritis. Lancet. 1975;1:918.
81. Virus of infantile gastroenteritis, editorial. Br Med J. 1975;3:555.
82. Rotaviruses of man and animals, (editorial). Lancet. 1975;1:257.
83. Mata L, Simhon A, Padilla R, et al. Diarrhea associated with rotaviruses, enterotoxigenic *E. coli, Campylobacter,* and other agents in Costa Rican children, 1976–1981. Am J Trop Med Hyg. 1983;32:146.
84. Black RE, Merson MH, Rahman ASMM, et al. A two-year study of bacterial, viral, and parasitic agents associated with diarrhea in rural Bangladesh. J Infect Dis. 1980;142:660.
85. Echeverria P, Ho MT, Blacklow NR, et al. Relative importance of viruses and bacteria in the etiology of pediatric diarrhea in Taiwan. J Infect Dis. 1977;136:383.
86. Paul MO, Erinle EA. Influence of humidity on rotavirus prevalence among Nigerian infants and young children with gastroenteritis. J Clin Microbiol. 1982;15:212.
87. Brandt CD, Kim HW, Rodriguez WJ. Rotavirus gastroenteritis and weather. J Clin Microbiol. 1982;16:478.
88. Gurwith M, Wenman W, Gurwith D, et al. Diarrhea among infants and young children in Canada: A longitudinal study in three Northern communities. J Infect Dis. 1983;147:685.
89. Shepherd RW, Truslow S, Walker-Smith JA. Infantile gastroenteritis: A clinical study of reovirus-like agent infection. Lancet. 1975;2:1082.
90. Sexton M, Davidson GP, Bishop RF, et al. Viruses in gastroenteritis. Lancet. 1974;2:355.
91. Tallett S, MacKenzie C, Middleton P, et al. Clinical, laboratory, and epidemiologic features of a viral gastroenteritis in infants and children. Pediatrics. 1977;60:217.
92. Kim HW, Brandt CD, Kapikian AZ, et al. Human reoviruslike agent infection. Occurrence in adult contacts of pediatric patients with gastroenteritis. JAMA. 1977;238:404.
93. Wenman WM, Hinde D, Feltham S, et al. Rotavirus infection in adults: Results of a prospective family study. N Engl J Med. 1979;301:303.
94. Kapikian AZ, Dienstag JL, Purcell RH. Immune electron microscopy as a method for the detection, identification, and characterization of agents not cultivable in an in vitro system. In: Rose NR, Friedman H, eds.: Manual of Clinical Immunology. Washington, DC: American Society for Microbiology; 1976.
95. Zissis G, Lambert JP. Different serotypes of human rotaviruses. Lancet. 1978;1:38.
96. Beards GM, Pilford JN, Thouless ME, et al. Rotavirus serotypes by serum neutralization. J Med Virol. 1980;5:231.
97. Blacklow NR, Cukor G. Viral gastroenteritis. N Engl J Med. 1981;304:397.
98. Urasawa S, Urasawa T, Taniguchi K. Three human rotavirus serotypes demonstrated by plaque neutralization of isolated strains. Infect Immun. 1982;38:781.
99. Fonteyne J, Zissis G, Lambert JP. Recurrent rotavirus gastroenteritis. Lancet. 1978;1:983.
100. Yolken R, Kim HW, Clem T, et al. Enzyme immunoassay (ELISA) for the detection of human reovirus-like agent in human stools. Lancet. 1977;2:263.
101. Kalica AR, Purcell RH, Sereno NM, et al. Microtiter solid phase radioimmunoassay for detection of the human reovirus-like agent in stools. J Immunol. 1977;118:1275.
102. Middleton PJ, Petrie M, Hewitt CM, et al. Counter-immunoelectroosmophoresis for the detection of infantile gastroenteritis virus (orbi group) antigen and antibody. J Clin Pathol. 1976;29:191.
103. Middleton PJ, Szymanski MT, Abbott GD, et al. Orbivirus acute gastroenteritis of infancy. Lancet. 1974;1:1241.
104. Davidson GP, Goller I, Bishop RF, et al. Immunofluorescence in duodenal mucosa of children with acute enteritis due to a new virus. J Clin Pathol. 1975;28:263.
105. Thomas EE, Puterman ML, Kawano E, et al. Evaluation of seven immunoassays for detection of rotavirus in pediatric stool samples. J Clin Microbiol. 1988;26:1189–93.
106. Flores J, Purcell RH, Perez I, et al. A dot hybridization assay for detection of rotavirus. Lancet. 1983;1:555.
107. Flewett TH, Bryden AS, Davies H, et al. Relation between viruses from acute gastroenteritis of children and newborn calves. Lancet. 1974;2:61.
108. Purdham DR, Purdham PA, Evans N, et al. Isolation of human rotavirus using human embryonic gut monolayers. Lancet. 1975;2:977.
109. Banatvala JE, Totterdell B, Chrystie IL, et al. In vitro detection of human rotaviruses. Lancet. 1975;2:821.
110. Wyatt RG, Gill VW, Sereno MM, et al. Probable in vitro cultivation of human reovirus-like agent of infantile diarrhea. Lancet. 1976;1:98.
111. Middleton PJ, Petric M, Szymanski MT. Propagation of infantile gastroenteritis virus (orbi-group) in conventional and germfree piglets. Infect Immun. 1975;12:1276.
112. Wyatt RG, Sly DL, London WT, et al. Induction of diarrhea in colostrum deprived newborn rhesus monkeys with human reovirus-like agent of infantile gastroenteritis. Arch Virol. 1976;50:17.
113. Wyatt RG, James SD, Bohl EH, et al. Human rotavirus type 2: Cultivation in vitro. Science. 1980;207:189.
114. Sato K, Inaba Y, Shinozuka T, et al. Isolation of human rotavirus in cell cultures. Arch Virol. 1981;69:155.
115. Urasawa T, Urasawa S, Taniguchi K. Sequential passages of human rotavirus in MA-104 cells. Microbiol Immunol. 1981;25:1025.
116. Kutsuzawa T, Konno T, Suzuki H, et al. Isolation of human rotavirus subgroups 1 and 2 in cell culture. J Clin Microbiol. 1982;16:727.
117. Guerrant RL. Pathophysiology of the enterotoxic and viral diarrheas. In Chen LC, Scrimshaw NS, eds. Diarrhea and Malnutrition: Interactions, Mechanisms and Interventions. New York: Plenum; 1983.
118. Middleton PJ, Szymanski MT, Abbott GD, et al. Orbivirus acute gastroenteritis of infancy. Lancet. 1974;1:1241.
119. Davidson GP, Goller I, Bishop RF, et al. Immunofluorescence in duodenal mucosa of children with acute enteritis due to a new virus. J Clin Pathol. 1975;28:263.
120. Sack DA, Chowdhury AMAK, Eusof A, et al. Oral hydration in rotavirus diarrhea: A double blind comparison of sucrose with glucose electrolyte solution. Lancet. 1978;2:280.
121. Davidson GP, Barnes GL. Structural and functional abnormalities of the small intestine in infants and young children with rotavirus enteritis. Acta Paediatr Scand. 1979;68:181.
122. Shepherd RW, Butler DG, Cutz E, et al. The mucosal lesion in viral enteritis: Extent and dynamics of the epithelial response to virus invasion in transmissible gastroenteritis of piglets. Gastroenterology. 1979;76:770.
123. Davidson GP, Gall DG, Petric M, et al. Human rotavirus enteritis induced in conventional piglets: Intestinal structure and transport. J Clin Invest. 1977;60:1402.
124. Vesikari T, Isolauri E, D'Hondt E, et al. Protection of infants against rotavirus diarrhea: R1T 4237 attenuated bovine rotavirus vaccine. Lancet. 1984;1:977–980.
125. Edelman R. Perspective on the development and deployment of rotavirus vaccines. Pediatr Infect Dis. 1987;6:704.
126. Gordon I, Ingraham HS, Korns RF. Transmission of epidemic gastroenteritis to human volunteers by oral administration of fecal filtrates. J Exp Med. 1947;86:409.
127. Jordan WS, Gordon I, Dorrance WR. A study of illness in a group of Cleveland families. VII. Transmission of acute nonbacterial gastroenteritis to volunteers: Evidence for two different etiologic agents. J Exp Med. 1953;98:461.
128. Kojima S, Fukumi H, Kusama H, et al. Studies on the causative agent of the infectious diarrhea; records of the experiments on human volunteers. Jpn Med J. 1948;1:467.
129. Klein JO, Lerner AM, Finland M. Acute gastroenteritis associated with echo virus, type II. Am J Med Sci. 1960;240:749.
130. Kerr AA, McQuillin J, Downham MAPS, et al. Gastric "flu" influenza B causing abdominal symptoms in children. Lancet. 1975;1:291.
131. Adler JL, Zickl R. Winter vomiting disease. J Infect Dis. 1969;119:668.
132. Dolin R, Blacklow NR, DuPont H, et al. Transmission of acute infectious nonbacterial gastroenteritis to volunteers by oral administration of stool filtrates. J Infect Dis. 1971;123:307.

133. Kapikian AZ, Wyatt RG, Dolin R, et al. Visualization by immune electron microscopy of a 27-nm particle associated with acute infectious nonbacterial gastroenteritis. J Virol. 1972;10:1075.
134. Zahorsky J. Hyperemesis hiemis or the winter vomiting disease. Arch Pediatr. 1929;46:391.
135. Agus SG, Dolin R, Wyatt RG, et al. Acute infectious nonbacterial gastroenteritis. Intestinal histopathology. Ann Intern Med. 1973;79:18.
136. Schreiber DS, Trier JS, Blacklow NR. Recent advances in viral gastroenteritis. Gastroenterology. 1977;73:174.
137. Levy AG, Widerlite L, Schwartz CJ, et al. Jejunal adenylate cyclase activity in human subjects during viral gastroenteritis. Gastroenterology. 1976;70:321.
138. Blacklow NR, Dolin R, Fedson DS, et al. Acute infectious nonbacterial gastroenteritis: Etiology and pathogenesis. Ann Intern Med. 1972;76:993.
139. Wyatt RG, Dolin R, Blacklow NR, et al. Comparison of three agents of acute infectious nonbacterial gastroenteritis by cross-challenge in volunteers. J Infect Dis. 1974;129:709.
140. Dolin R, Treanor JJ, Madore HP. Novel agents of viral enteritis in humans. J Infect Dis. 1987;155:365–76.
141. Clarke SKR, Cook GT, Egglestone SI, et al. A virus from epidemic vomiting disease. Br Med J. 1972;3:86.
142. Appleton H, Buckley M, Thom BT, et al. Virus-like particles in winter vomiting disease. Lancet. 1977;1:409.
143. Morens DM, Zweighaft RM, Vernon TM. A waterborne outbreak of gastroenteritis with secondary person-to-person spread. Lancet. 1979;1:964.
144. Oshiro LS, Haley CE, Roberto RR, et al. A 27-nm virus isolated during an outbreak of acute infectious nonbacterial gastroenteritis in a convalescent hospital: A possible new serotype. J Infect Dis. 1981;143:791.
145. Caul EO, Appleton H. The electron microscopical and physical characteristics of small round human fecal viruses: An interim scheme for classification. J Med Virol. 1982;9:257–65.
146. Brandt CD, Kim HW, Rodriguez WJ, et al. Adenoviruses and pediatric gastroenteritis. J Infect Dis. 1985;151:437–43.
147. Gerna G, Passarani N, Battaglia M, et al. Human enteric coronaviruses: Antigenic relatedness to human coronavirus OC43 and possible etiologic role in viral gastroenteritis. J Infect Dis. 1985;151:796–802.
148. Battaglia M, Passarani N, DiMatteo A, et al. Human enteric coronaviruses: Further characterization and immunoblotting of viral proteins. J Infect Dis. 1987;155:140–3.
149. Yolken R, Santosham M, Reid R, et al. Pestiviruses: Major etiological agents of gastroenteritis in human infants and children (Abstract) Clin Res. 1988;36:780.
150. Greenberg HB, Valdesuso J, Yolken RH, et al. Role of Norwalk virus in outbreaks of nonbacterial gastroenteritis. J Infect Dis. 1979;139:564.
151. Kaplan JE, Gary GW Jr, Baron RC, et al. Epidemiology of Norwalk gastroenteritis and the role of the Norwalk virus in outbreaks of nonbacterial gastroenteritis. Ann Intern Med. 1982;96:756.
152. Greenberg HB, Wyatt RG, Valdesuso J, et al. Solid-phase microtiter radioimmunoassay for detection of the Norwalk strain of acute nonbacterial, epidemic gastroenteritis virus and its antibodies. J Med Virol. 1978;2:97.
153. Parrino TA, Schreiber DS, Trier JS, et al. Clinical immunity in acute gastroenteritis caused by Norwalk agent. N Engl J Med. 297:86–89, 1977;297:86–9.
154. Herrmann JE, Perron-Henry DM, Blacklow NR. Antigen detection with monoclonal antibodies for the diagnosis of adenovirus gastroenteritis. J Infect Dis. 1987;155:1167–71.
155. Shinozaki T, Araki K, Ushijima H, et al. Use of Graham 293 cells in suspension for isolating enteric adenoviruses from the stools of patients with acute gastroenteritis. J Infect Dis. 1987;156:246.
156. Neil C, Gomes SA, Leite JPG, et al. Direct detection and differentiation of fastidious and nonfastidious adenoviruses in stools by using a specific nonradioactive probe. J Clin Microbiol. 1986;24:785–9.
157. von Bonsdorff CH, Hovi T, Makela P, et al. Rotavirus associated with acute gastroenteritis in adults. Lancet. 1976;2:423.
158. Wenman WM, Hinde D, Feltham S, et al. Rotavirus infection in adults. Results of a prospective study. N Engl J Med. 1979;301:306.
159. Yolken RH, Bishop CA, Townsend TR, et al. Infectious gastroenteritis in bone-marrow transplant recipients. N Engl J Med. 1982;306:1099.
160. Goodgame RW, Greenough WBIII. Cholera in Africa: A message for the west. Ann Intern Med. 1975;82:101.
161. Weissman JB, DeWitt WE, Thompson J, et al. A case of cholera in Texas, 1973. Am J Epidemiol. 1975;100:487.
162. Blake PA, Allegra DT, Snyder JD, et al. Cholera: A possible endemic focus in the United States. N Engl J Med. 1980;302:305.
163. Blake PA, Rosenberg ML, Florencia J, et al. Cholera in Portugal, 1974. II. Transmission by bottled mineral water. Am J Epidemiol. 1977;105:344.
164. Baine WB, Mazzotti M, Greco D, et al. Epidemiology of cholera in Italy in 1973. Lancet. 1974;2:1370.
165. Gitelson S. Gastrectomy, achlorhydria and cholera. Isr J Med Sci. 1971;7:663.
166. Snow J. On the Mode of Communication of Cholera. 2nd ed. London: Churchill; 1855.
167. De SN, Bhattacharya K, Sarkar JK. A study of the pathogenicity of strains of *Bacterium coli* from acute and chronic enteritis. J Pathol Bacteriol. 1956;71:201.
168. Trabulsi LR. Revelação de colibacilos associados as diarreias infantis pelo metodo da infeccão experimental da alca ligade do intestino do coelho. Rev Inst Med Trop Sao Paulo. 1964;6:197.
169. Taylor J, Wilkins MP, Payne JM. Relation of rabbit gut reaction to enteropathogenic *Escherichia coli*. Br J Exp Pathol. 1961;42:43.
170. Taylor J, Bettlelheim KA. The action of chloroform-killed suspensions of enteropathegenic *Escherichia coli* on ligated rabbit-gut segments. J Gen Microbiol. 1966;42:309.
171. Smith HW, Halls S. Studies on *Escherichia coli* enterotoxin. J Pathol Bacteriol. 1967;93:531.
172. Gorbach SL, Banwell JG, Chatterjee BD, et al. Acute undifferentiated human diarrhea in the tropics. I. Alterations in intestinal microflora. J Clin Invest. 1971;50:881.
173. Banwell JG, Gorbach SL, Pierce NF, et al. Acute undifferentiated human diarrhea in the tropics. II. Alterations in intestinal fluid and electrolyte movements. J Clin Invest. 1971;50:890.
174. Sack RB, Gorbach SL, Banwell JG, et al. Enterotoxigenic *Escherichia coli* isolated from patients with severe cholera-like disease. J Infect Dis. 1971;123:378.
175. DuPont HL, Formal SB, Hornick RB, et al. Pathogenesis of *Escherichia coli* diarrhea. N Engl J Med. 1971;285:1.
176. Evans DG, Evans DJ Jr, Pierce NF. Differences in the response of rabbit small intestine to heat-labile and heat-stable enterotoxins of *Escherichia coli*. Infect Immun. 1973;7:873.
177. Guerrant RL, Brunton LL, Schnaitman TC, et al. Cyclic adenosine monophosphate and alteration of Chinese hamster ovary cell morphology: A rapid, sensitive in vitro assay for the enterotoxins of *Vibrio cholerae* and *Escherichia coli*. Infect Immun. 1974;10:320.
178. Donta ST, Moon HW, Whipp SC. Detection of heat-labile *Escherichia coli* enterotoxin with the use of adrenal cells in tissue culture. Science. 1974;183:334.
179. Guerrant RL, Brunton LL. Characterization of the Chinese hamster ovary cell assay for the enterotoxins of *Vibrio cholerae* and *Escherichia coli* and for antitoxin: Differential inhibition by gangliosides, specific antisera, and toxoid. J Infect Dis. 1977;135:720.
180. Honda T, Arita M, Takeda Y, et al. Further evaluation of the Biken test (modified Elek test) for detection of enterotoxigenic *E. coli* producing heat-labile enterotoxin and application of the test to sampling of heat-stable enterotoxin. J Clin Microbiol. 1982;16:60.
181. Alderete JF, Robertson DC. Purification and chemical characterization of the heat-stable enterotoxin produced by porcine strains of enterotoxigenic *Escherichia coli*. Infect Immun. 1978;19:1021.
182. Dean AG, Ching YC, Williams RG, et al. Test for *Escherichia coli* enterotoxin using infant mice: Application in a study of diarrhea in children in Honolulu. J Infect Dis. 1972;125:407.
183. Gyles CL. Limitations of the infant mouse test for *E. coli* heat-stable enterotoxin. Can J Comp Med. 1979;43:371–9.
184. Kennedy, DJ, Greenberg RN, Dunn JA, et al. Effects of *Escherichia coli* heat stable enterotoxin STb on intestines of mice, rats, rabbits and piglets. Infect Immun 1984;46:639–43.
185. Weikel CS, Mellans HN, Guerrant RL. In vivo and in vitro effects of a novel enterotoxin, STb, produced by *Escherichia coli*. J Infect Dis. 1986;153:893–901.
186. Rosenberg ML, Koplan JP, Wachsmuth IK, et al. Epidemic diarrhea at Crater Lake from enterotoxigenic *Escherchia coli*. A large, waterborne outbreak. Ann Intern Med. 1977;86:714.
187. Korzeniowski OM, Dantas W, Trabulsi LR, et al. A controlled study of endemic sporadic diarrhea among adult residents of southern Brazil. Trans R Soc Trop Med Hyg. 1984;78:363–9.
188. Hughes JM, Rouse JD, Barada FA, et al. Etiology of summer diarrhea among the Navajo. Am J Trop Med Hyg. 1980;29:613.
189. Current WL, Reese NC, Ernst JV, et al. Human cryptosporidiosis in immunocompetent and immunodeficient persons. N Engl J Med. 1983;308:1252.
190. Tzipori S. Cryptosporidiosis in animals and humans. Microbiol Rev. 1983;47:84.
191. Wolfson JS, Richter JM, Waldron MA, et al. Cryptosporidiosis in immunocompetent patients. N Engl J Med. 1985;312:1278–82.
192. Palmer DL, Koster FT, Islam AFMR, et al. A comparison of sucrose and glucose in oral electrolyte therapy of cholera and other severe diarrheas. N Engl J Med. 1977;297:1107.
193. Ericsson CD, Evans DG, DuPont HL, et al. Bismuth subsalicylate inhibits activity of crude toxins of *Escherichia coli* and *Vibrio cholerae*. J Infect Dis. 1977;136:693.
194. Gelb A, Miller S. AIDS and gastroenterology. Am J Gastroenterol. 1986;81:619–22.
195. Soave R, Johnson WD. *Cryptosporidium* and *Isospora belli* infections. J Infect Dis. 1988;157:225–29.
196. Kotler DP, Goetz HP, Lange M, et al. Enteropathy associated with the acquired immunodeficiency syndrome. Ann Intern Med. 1984;101:421–28.
197. Gillin JS, Shike M, Alcock N, et al. Malabsorption and mucosal abnormalities of the small intestine in the acquired immunodeficiency syndrome. Ann Intern Med. 1985;102:619–22.
198. Nelson JA, Reynolds-Kohler G, Margaretten W, et al. Human immunodeficiency virus detected in bowel epithelium from patients with gastro-intestinal symptoms. Lancet 1988;1:259–62.
199. Smith PD, Lance C, Gill VJ, et al. Intestinal infections in patients with the

acquired immunodeficiency syndrome (AIDS). Ann Intern Med. 1988;108:328–33.
200. Laughon BE, Druckman DA, Vernon A, et al. Prevalence of enteric pathogens in homosexual men with and without Acquired Immunodeficiency Syndrome. Gastroenterology. 1988;94:984.
201. Quinn TC, Stamm WE, Goodell SE, et al. The polymicrobial origin of intestinal infections in homosexual men. N Engl J Med. 1983;309:576–82.
202. Carter TR, Cooper PH, Petri WA Jr, et al. *Pneumocystis carinii* infection of the small intestine in a patient with aquired immune deficiency syndrome. Am J Clin Pathol. 1988;89:679–83.
203. Chachoua A, Dieterich D, Krasinski K, et al. 9-(1,3-dihydroxy-2-propoxymethyl) guanine (ganciclovir) in the treatment of cytomegalovirus gastrointestinal disease with the acquired immunodeficiency syndrome. Ann Intern Med. 1987;107:133–7.
204. Celum CL, Chaisson RE, Rutherford GW, et al. Incidence of salmonellosis in patients with AIDS. J Infect Dis. 1987;156:998–1002.
205. Jacobs JL, Gold JWM, Murray HW, et al. *Salmonella* infections in patients with the acquired immunodeficiency syndrome. Ann Intern Med. 1985;102:186–88.
206. Glaser JB, Morton-Kute L, Berger SR, et al. Recurrent *Salmonella typhimurium* bacteremia associated with the acquired immunodeficiency syndrome. Ann Intern Med. 1985;102:189–93.
207. Sperber SJ, Schleupner CJ: Salmonellosis during infection with human immunodeficiency virus. Rev Infect Dis. 1987;9:925–34.
208. Guerrant RL, Hughes JM, Lima NL, et al. Microbiology of diarrhea in developed and developing countries. Rev Infect Dis. 1989. In press.
209. Stamm WE, Weinstein RA, Dixon RE. Comparison of endemic and epidemic nosocomial infections. Am J Med. 1981;70:393–97.
210. Lima N, Searcy M, Guerrant R. Nosocomial diarrhea rates exceed those of other nosocomial infections on ICU and pediatric wards (Abstract 1050). In: Proceedings of the 26th Interscience Conference on Antimicrobial Agents and Chemotherapy, New Orleans, 1986.
211. Lima NL, Guerrant RL, Kaiser DL, et al. Nosocomial diarrhea: A possible risk factor for nosocomial infections (Abstract). Clin Res. 1988;36:580.
212. Welliver RC, McLaughlin S. Unique epidemiology of nosocomial infection in a children's hospital. Am J Dis Child. 1984;138:131–35.
213. Kelly WJ, Patrick MR, Hillman KM. Study of diarrhea in critically ill patients. Crit Care Med. 1983;1:7–9.
214. Hughes JM, Jarvis WR. Nosocomial gastrointestinal infections. In: Wenzel RP, ed. Prevention and Control of Nosocomial Infections. Philadelphia: Williams & Wilkins; 1987.
215. Yolken RH, Bishop CA, Townsend R, et al. Infectious gastroenteritis in bone marrow transplant recipients. N Engl J Med. 1982;306:1009–12.
216. Farber BF, Brennen JC, Puntereri AJ, et al. A prospective study of nosocomial infections in a chronic care facility. J Am Geriatr Soc. 1984;32:499.
217. Nicolle LE, McIntyre M, Zacharias H, et al. Twelve-month surveillance of infections in institutionalized elderly men. J Am Geriatr Soc. 1984;32:513.
218. Bender BS, Laughon BE, Gaydos C, et al. Is *Clostridium difficile* endemic in chronic-care facilities? Lancet. 1986;2:1279.
219. Treolar AJ, Kalra L. Mortality and *Clostridium difficile* diarrhoea in the elderly. Lancet. 1987;2:1279.
220. Pickering LK, Evans DG, Dupont HL, et al. Diarrhea caused by *Shigella,* rotavirus and *Giardia* in day care centers: Prospective study. J Pediatr. 1981;99:51–56.
221. Centers for Disease Control. Cryptosporidiosis among children attending day-care centers: Georgia, Pennsylvania, Michigan, California, New Mexico. MMWR. 1984;33:599.
222. Alpert G, Bell LM, Kirkpatrick CE, et al. Cryptosporidiosis in a day-care center. N Engl J Med. 1984;311:860–1.
223. Taylor JP, Perdue JN, Dingley D, et al. Cryptosporidiosis outbreak in a day-care center. Am J Dis Child. 1985;139:1023–5.
224. Bartlett AV, Moore M, Gary GW, et al. Diarrheal illness among infants and toddlers in daycare centers. I Epidemiology and pathogens. J Pediatr. 1985;107:495–502.
225. Guerrant RL, Lohr JA, Williams EK. Acute infectious diarrhea. I. Epidemiology, etiology, and pathogenesis. Pediatr Infect Dis. 1986;5:353–59.
226. Kean BH. The diarrhea of travelers to Mexico. Summary of five-year study. Ann Intern Med. 1963;59:605.
227. Psalms 22:14.
228. Consensus development conference statement on travelers' diarrhea. Rev Inf Dis. 1986;8(Suppl):227–33.
229. Lowenstein MS, Balows A, Gangarosa EJ. Turista at an international congress in Mexico. Lancet. 1973;1:529.
230. Editorial. The diarrhea of travelers. Turista. JAMA. 1962;180:402.
231. Higgens AR. Observations on the health of United States personnel living in Cairo, Egypt. Am J Trop Med Hyg. 1955;4:970.
232. Steffen R. Epidemiologic studies of travelers' diarrhea, severe gastrointestinal infections, and cholera. Rev Infect Dis. 1986;8(Suppl 2):122–30.
233. Steffen R, Rickernbach M, Wilhelm U, et al. Health problems after travel to developing countries. J Infect Dis. 1987;156:84–91.
234. Kean BH, Schaffner W, Brennan RW. The diarrhea of travelers. V. Prophylaxis with phthalysulfathiazole and neomycin sulphate. JAMA. 1962;180:367–71.
235. Rowe B, Taylor J, Bettelheim KA. An investigation of travelers' diarrhea. Lancet. 1970;1:1.
236. Gorbach SL, Kean BH, Evans DG, et al. Travelers' diarrhea and toxigenic *Escherichia coli.* N Engl J Med. 1975;292:933.
237. Merson MH, Morris GK, Sack DA, et al. Travelers' diarrhea in Mexico, a prospective study of physicians and family members attending a congress. N Engl J Med. 1976;294:1299.
238. Sack DA, Kaminsky DC, Sack RB, et al. Enterotoxigenic *Escherichia coli* diarrhea of travelers: A prospective study of American Peace Corps volunteers. Johns Hopkins Med J. 1977;141:63.
239. Guerrant RL, Rouse JD, Hughes JM. Turista among members of the Yale Glee Club in Latin America. Am J Trop Med Hyg. 1980;29:895.
240. Turner AC. Travelers' diarrhoea: A survey of symptoms, occurrence, and possible prophylaxis. Br Med J. 1967;4:453–4.
241. Black RE. Pathogens that cause travelers' diarrhea in Latin America and Africa. Rev Infect Dis. 1986;8(Suppl 2):131–5.
242. Taylor DN, Echeverria P. Etiology and epidemiology of travelers' diarrhea in Asia. Rev Infect Dis. 1986;8(Suppl 2):136–41.
243. Bolivar R, Conklin RH, Vollet JJ, et al. Rotavirus in travelers' diarrhea: Study of an adult student population in Mexico. J Infect Dis. 1978;137:324.
244. Ryder RW, Oquist CA, Greenberg H, et al. Travelers' diarrhea in Panamanian tourists in Mexico. J Infect Dis. 1981;144:442.
245. Snyder JD, Blake PA. Is cholera a problem for US travelers? JAMA. 1982;247:2268.
246. Echeverria P, Hodge FA, Blacklow NR, et al. Travelers' diarrhea among United States marines in South Korea. Am J Epidemiol. 1978;108:68.
247. Wolfe MS. Current concepts in parasitology. Giardiasis. N Engl J Med. 1978;298:319.
248. Brodsky RE, Spencer HC Jr, Schultz MG. Giardiasis in American travelers to the Soviet Union. J Infect Dis. 1974;130:319.
249. Soave R, Armstrong D. *Cryptosporidium* and cryptosporidiosis. Rev Infect Dis. 1986;8:1012–23.
250. Jokipii L, Pohjola S, Jokipii AMM. *Cryptosporidium:* A frequent finding in patients with gastrointestinal symptoms. Lancet. 1983;2:358–360.
251. Kean BH, Reilly PC. Malaria–the mime. Recent lessons from a group of civilian travelers. Am J Med. 1976;61:159.
252. Pearson RD, Hewlett EL, Guerrant RL. Tropical diseases in North America. DM. 1984;30:1–68.
253. Hill DR, Pearson RD. Health advice for international travel. Ann Intern Med. 1988;108:839–52.
254. Kean BH, Waters SR. Diarrhea of travelers. III. Drug prophylaxis in Mexico. N Engl J Med. 1959;261:71.
255. Oakley GP. The neurotoxicity of the halogenated hydroxyguinolines. JAMA. 1973;225:395.
256. Portnoy BL, DuPont HL, Pruitt D, et al. Antidiarrheal agents in the treatment of acute diarrhea in children. JAMA. 1976;236:844.
257. DuPont HL, Hornick RB. Adverse effect of Lomotil therapy in shigellosis. JAMA. 1973;226:1525.
258. DuPont HL, Sullivan P, Pickering LK, et al. Symptomatic treatment of diarrhea with bismuth subsalicylate among students attending a Mexican university. Gastroenterology. 1977;73:715.
259. Steffen R, Heusser R, DuPont HL. Prevention of travelers' diarrhea by nonantibiotic drugs. Rev Infect Dis. 1986;8(Suppl 2):151–9.
260. Blaser MJ. Environmental interventions for the prevention of travelers' diarrhea. Rev Inf Dis. 1986;8(Suppl 2):142–50.
261. Gonzales-Cortez A, Gangarosa EJ, Parrilla C, et al. Bottled beverages and typhoid fever: The Mexican epidemic of 1972–3. Am J Public Health. 1982;72:844.
262. Harris JR. Are bottled beverages safe for travelers? Am J Public Health. 1982;72:787.
263. Neumann HH. Travellers' diarrhea. Lancet. 1970;1:420.
264. Tjoa W, DuPont HL, Sullivan P, et al. Location of food consumption and travelers' diarrhea. Am J Epidemiol. 1977;106:61.
265. Sack DA, Kaminsky DC, Sack RB, et al. Prophylactic doxycycline for travelers' diarrhea, results of a prospective double-blind study of Peace Corps volunteers in Kenya. N Engl J Med. 1978;298:758.
266. Echeverria P, Verhaert L, Ulyangco CV, et al. Antimicrobial resistance and enterotoxin production among isolates of *Escherichia coli* in the Far East. Lancet. 1978;2:589.
267. Murray BE. Resistance of *Shigella Salmonella* and other selected enteric pathogens. Rev Infect Dis. 1986;8(Suppl 2):172–81.
268. Mentzing LO, Ringertz O. *Salmonella* infection in tourists. 2. Prophylaxis against salmonellosis. Acta Pathol Microbiol Scand. 1968;74:405.
269. Murray BE, Rensimer ER, DuPont HL. Emergence of high level trimethoprim resistance in fecal *E. coli* during oral administration of trimethoprim or trimethoprim/sulfamethoxazole. N Engl J Med. 1982;306:130.
270. Tiemens KM, Shipley PL, Correia RA, et al. Sulfamethoxazole-trimethoprim resistant *Shigella flexneri* in northeastern Brazil. Antimic Ag Chemother. 1984;25:653–54.
271. DuPont HL, Reves RR, Galindo E, et al. Treatment of travelers' diarrhea with trimethoprim/sulfamethoxazole and with trimethoprim alone. N Engl J Med. 1982;307:841–4.
272. Ericsson CD, DuPont HL, Sullivan P, et al. Bicozamycin, a poorly absorbable antibiotic, effectively treats travelers' diarrhea. Ann Intern Med. 1983;98:20.
273. Ericsson CD, Johnson PC, DuPont HL, et al. Ciprofloxacin or trimethoprim-sulfamethoxazole as initial therapy for travelers' diarrhea. Ann Intern Med. 1987;106:216–20.
274. Said SI, Faloona GR. Elevated plasma and tissue levels of vasoactive intestinal polypeptide in the watery diarrhea syndrome due to pancreatic, bronchogenic, and other tumors. N Engl J Med. 1975;293:155.

275. Wolff MS. Giardiasis. JAMA. 1975;233:1362.
276. Murphy TV, Nelson JD. Five vs ten days' therapy with furazolidone for giardiasis. Am J Dis Child. 1983;137:267.
277. Ma P, Soave R. Three-step stool examination for cryptosporidiosis in 10 homosexual men with protracted watery diarrhea. J Infect Dis. 1983;147:824.
278. Donaldson RM Jr. Small bowel bacterial overgrowth. Adv Intern Med. 1970;16:191.
279. Gorbach SL. Intestinal microflora. Gastroenterology. 1971;60:1110.
280. Penn RG, Giger DK, Knoop FC, et al. *Plesiomonas shigelloides* overgrowth in the small intestine. J Clin Microbiol. 1982;15:869.
281. Scott AJ, Khan GA. Partial biliary obstruction with cholangitis producing a blind loop syndrome. Gut. 1968;9:187.
282. Vantrappen G, Janssens J, Hellemans J, et al. Interdigestive motor complex of normal subjects and patients with bacterial overgrowth of the small intestine. J Clin Invest. 1977;59:1158.
283. Heyworth B, Brown J. Jejunal microflora in malnourished Gambian children. Arch Dis Child. 1975;50:27.
284. Roberts SH, James O, Jarvis EH. Bacterial overgrowth syndrome without "blind loop": A cause for malnutrition in the elderly. Lancet. 1977;2:1193.
285. Ruiz-Palacios GM, DuPont HL. Bacterial overgrowth syndrome after acute nonspecific diarrhoea. Lancet. 1978;1:337.
286. Lindenbaum J, Kent TH, Sprinz H. Malabsorption and jejunitis in American Peace Corps Volunteers in Pakistan. Ann Intern Med. 1966;65:1201.
287. Shimada K, Brickenll KS, Finegold SM. Deconjugation of bile acids by intestinal bacteria: Review of literature and additional studies. J Infect Dis. 1969;119:273.
288. Wanke CA, Guerrant RL. Small bowel colonization alone is a cause of diarrhea. Infect Immun. 1987;55:1924–6.
289. Schlager TA, Guerrant RL. Net fluid secretion and impaired villous function induced by small intestinal colonization by non-toxigenic, colonizing *E. coli*. Abst. No. 1133, 28th Intersc Conf Antimic Ag Chemother. 1988;310.
290. Hamilton JD, Dyer NH, Dawson AM, et al. Assessment and significance of bacterial overgrowth in the small bowel. Q J Med. 1970;39:265.
291. MacDougall LG. The effect of aureomycin on undernourished African children. J Trop Pediatr. 1957;3:74.
292. Levy SB, FitzGerald GB, Macone AB. Changes in intestinal flora of farm personnel after introduction of a tetracycline-supplemented feed on a farm. N Engl J Med. 1976;295:583.

83. ANTIBIOTIC-ASSOCIATED COLITIS

ROBERT FEKETY

HISTORICAL PERSPECTIVE

Although antibiotics are the most important precipitating cause of pseudomembranous colitis (PMC), it is noteworthy that this disease was recognized in the preantibiotic era[1]; thus, other factors are important in pathogenesis. Many cases diagnosed soon after antibiotics were introduced were attributed to *Staphylococcus aureus,* but in retrospect many investigators believe that this association may have been coincidental. PMC was rarely recognized from 1960 to 1970, but it was often diagnosed thereafter in patients treated with lincomycin, clindamycin, or broad-spectrum β-lactam antibiotics. In these patients, staphylococci could not be implicated, and many patients died because no effective therapy was known. Furthermore, we now realize that a type of diarrhea unassociated with PMC is common in patients treated with antibiotics. At the University of Michigan Hospitals in 1976, 19 (8 percent) of 242 patients receiving ampicillin or clindamycin developed diarrhea.[2] Only 3 of these 19 patients had PMC, while the rest had a benign diarrhea of unknown cause that was believed to be related to change in the bowel flora.

In order to better understand PMC, investigators administered antibiotics to various species of animals in the hope of producing a model of the human disease. They found that golden Syrian hamsters were highly susceptible to diarrhea and fatal enterocolitis after being given any of many antibiotics either orally or parenterally.[3] After a cytotoxin neutralizable by *Clostridium sordellii* antitoxin was detected in the feces of these hamsters,[4] cultural studies revealed large numbers of *Clostridium difficile* in their feces and showed that this organism produced a cytotoxin neutralizable by *C. sordellii* antitoxin.[1] Hamsters inoculated with cell-free filtrates of broth cultures of *C. difficile* developed enterocolitis,[1] and hamsters passively immunized with *C. sordellii* antitoxin did not develop colitis after being given antibiotics.[5] After *C. difficile* was shown to be susceptible to vancomycin, antibiotic-treated hamsters were given vancomycin prophylactically, and it was found that they did not develop colitis.[6]

When humans with PMC were studied, it was found that *C. difficile* and/or its cytotoxin were almost always present in their stools.[7,8] It was also learned that many patients with antibiotic-associated colitis (AAC) did not have pseudomembranes and that both PMC and AAC could be treated successfully by the oral administration of vancomycin. However, most patients with antibiotic-associated diarrhea had neither colitis nor *C. difficile* or its toxin in their stools. This more common and benign type of diarrhea was found to be treatable by discontinuing antibiotic therapy and replacing fluid and electrolyte losses.

As a result of these studies, *C. difficile* has become recognized as the most frequent cause of AAC. Recently, a comprehensive review and a state-of-the-art book on *C. difficile* and its role in intestinal disease have been published.[9,10]

PATHOLOGY

The important characteristic of the disease is acute colitis. Pseudomembranes may be absent or extensive or consist of small and discrete yellow-white plaques or nodules that are easily dislodged (Fig. 1). The pseudomembrane consists of fibrin, mucus, necrotic epithelial cells, and leukocytes adherent to the underlying inflamed tissues. Colitis usually affects only the epithelium and superficial lamina propria, but in severe cases deeper tissues are involved. In many cases, pseudomembranes are not visible to the naked eye but are detectable microscopically if a biopsy specimen is obtained. These patients are usually categorized as having nonspecific colitis until *C. difficile* and its toxins are detected in their stools. Pseudomembranes occur throughout the colon but are usually most prominent in the rectosigmoid area; the ileum is rarely involved. AAC is uncommon in infants, but cases have been recognized.[12] Some

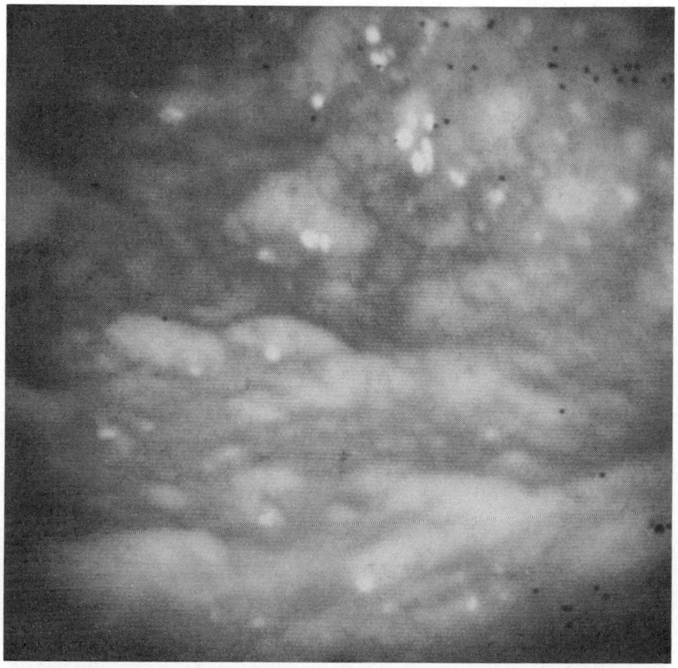

FIG. 1. Proctoscopic view of pseudomembranous colitis in a patient who received clindamycin. Note the 4 to 8 mm raised, white plaques overlying an erythematous mucosa. (From Tedesco et al.,[11] with permission.)

infants with chronic diarrhea and positive stools for *C. difficile* and its toxin have undergone rectal biopsies that revealed cryptitis, and some of them became well after treatment with oral vancomycin.[13]

MICROBIOLOGY, EPIDEMIOLOGY, AND PATHOGENESIS

Clostridium difficile is a spore-forming, gram-positive, obligate anaerobic bacillus. It is part of the normal intestinal flora of about 3 percent of healthy adults. Colonization rates may be much higher in hospitalized persons. We found small numbers of *C. difficile* in the stools of 15 percent of medical patients without diarrhea in our hospital, and 71 percent of asymptomatic infants were positive on a pediatric ward where there was a case of AAC.[14] The organism has been isolated from healthy dogs and cats, waterfowl, horses, camels, donkeys, seals, hamsters, and guinea pigs,[15] but animals are not considered important in transmission to humans. Because the organism was not easily distinguished from *Clostridium sporogenes* and other organisms commonly found in stools, it was difficult to detect with ordinary cultural techniques and was overlooked as a cause of colitis until 1977.[1] In 1979, George and his associates reported that a selective medium that contained cycloserine, cefoxitin, and fructose in agar (CCFA) was helpful in isolating *C. difficile* from stools.[16] The addition of 0.2% highly purified sodium taurocholate to CCFA increased its ability to detect small numbers of spores in stools or on surfaces.[17] *Clostridium difficle* can also be detected on agar because of its production of *p*-cresol from *p*-hydroxyphenylacetic acid.[18] Alcohol shock also facilitates isolation of the organism from stools.[19]

Staphylococcus aureus is now a very rare cause of AAC, and many doubt that it can cause the disease, although our experiences indicate that it can.[20] As observed in earlier times, staphylococcal enterocolitis involved the ileum and cecum more often than it did the colon and rectum, and it usually followed the use of tetracyclines or chloramphenicol, antibiotics that are now rarely associated with colitis. *Clostridium perfringens* type C and salmonellae have been implicated in solitary cases of PMC.[21,22]

Clostridium difficile colitis occurs at all ages but is most frequent in elderly and debilitated patients. Other groups at high risk include women, patients with cancer or burns, and patients undergoing surgery (especially abdominal surgery) or who are in intensive care units.[14] Even short courses of antibiotics given for prophylaxis or treatment of minor infections may permit the organism to overgrow, produce toxin, and cause colitis. AAC may follow oral, intramuscular, intravenous, or topical administration of antibiotics. The list of inciting agents includes penicillin G, ampicillin, amoxicillin, carbenicillin, ticarcillin, cephalothin, cefazolin, cephalexin, cefamandole, cefoxitin, cefotaxime, moxalactam, cefoperazone, ceftizoxime, ceftazidime, ceftriaxone, imipenem-cilastatin, ciprofloxacin, clindamycin, lincomycin, metronidazole, vancomycin, tetracycline, erythromycin, trimethoprim-sulfamethoxazole, chloramphenicol, and rifampin. A few cases have been related to the oral administration of aminoglycosides.[1,14] The relative risk of various antimicrobials in inducing AAC is not known with precision because antibiotic-specific attack rates in well-controlled studies of well-matched patient groups have not been reported. The incidence of AAC in adults treated with clindamycin has ranged from 1 in 10,000 to 1 in 10 in various reports.[2] The high rates reported from some hospitals suggest that the disease can be transmitted nosocomially, either via the hands of personnel or by direct contact with patients or infected surfaces or objects.[14] Most cases reported within the past decade have been related to clindamycin or lincomycin (to which *C. difficile* is often resistant), to ampicillin (to which it is usually susceptible), or to cephalosporins (to which susceptibility varies).[6] This paradox is not completely understood, but β-lactamase production by intestinal bacteria seems important in the pathogenesis of cases associated with ampicillin or cephalosporins.

Since alteration of the intestinal flora is so important in the pathogenesis of AAC, it is not surprising that almost every antibiotic used in treating humans has been implicated at least once. The components of the normal intestinal flora that suppress colonization, overgrowth, or toxin production by *C. difficile* are not known, but the suspects include *Escherichia coli*, enterococci, lactobacilli, *Bacteroides*, and *Clostridium*. Factors predisposing to colitis presumably inhibit or eliminate these competing organisms, but antibiotics may also operate by stimulating toxin production by *C. difficile*. Normal hamsters inoculated orally with large numbers of *C. difficile* remained well, while antibiotic-treated hamseters given only 2 colony-forming units (cfu) of *C. difficile* developed lethal enterocolitis.[8] The effects of antibiotics on stool flora may persist for long periods, and acquisition and overgrowth of *C. difficile* with production of colitis may occur up to 6 weeks after discontinuation of treatment with an antibiotic. Many reported patients with pseudomembranous colitis had received no antibiotics; these cases suggest that dietary changes, anesthesia, uremia, and various nonantibiotic medications (such as methotrexate or gold salts) may precipitate the disease.[23]

Clostridium difficile has been isolated from the hands of hospital personnel caring for colonized patients. The spores of *C. difficile* persist on fomites and surfaces for long periods. They have been found in abundance in the environment of patients with AAC.[14] Instruments inserted into the gastrointestinal tract should be cleaned and disinfected after use on patients with AAC. While vegetative forms of the organism are oxygen-sensitive and easily killed, spores are very resistant to adverse conditions, including most of the disinfectants used in hospitals. Alkaline glutaraldehyde, sodium hypochlorite, and chlorine dioxide are most effective against spores. Enteric isolation precautions and careful handwashing after contact with patients with AAC are recommended.

Colitis results from toxin production by the organism within the intestinal lumen. *Clostridium difficile* is rarely invasive. Isolates from patients with colitis usually produce at least two and possibly more toxins.[24,25] Some isolates are nontoxigenic, but these are never associated with colitis. The two best-characterized toxins are toxins A and B. Because it is difficult to purify these toxins, their characteristics and mechanisms of action are not completely understood. The toxins may attack the membranes or microfilaments of cells and produce contraction, hemorrhage, necrosis, inflammation, and loss of protein into the lumen.[26,27] They also increase intestinal myoelectric responses and peristalsis.[28] They may induce secretion of fluid and electrolytes by purely biochemical mechanisms. The reported molecular weights of toxins A and B have ranged widely (50,000–600,000). Toxin A is lethal for certain rodents and causes intestinal hemorrhage and fluid secretion. Toxin B is detectable by its cytotoxic or actinomorphic effects on cell culture monolayers. Diarrhea associated with *C. difficile* toxins in well-studied humans has almost always been associated with inflammatory mucosal lesions.[1,29]

Newborn infants may be colonized with toxigenic *C. difficile* organisms and yet remain well despite the presence of large amounts of toxins in their stools. Colonization rates as high as 50–60 percent have been reported in newborns.[13,30] In one study, the environment appeared to be the main source of the organism[31]; in another, hand transmissions by nursery personnel from infant to infant seemed responsible (Bacon A, Fekety R: unpublished observations). A glycoprotein found in milk (fetulin) or a subunit of it may interfere with the action of these toxins on the cecum.[32] In addition, the toxins may not bind to the intestinal mucosa.[33] As newborn infants acquire their normal intestinal flora, the rate of isolation of *C. difficile* and its toxins from their stools declines toward the rates in adults.

Hamsters immunized with toxoids prepared from both toxin

A and B (but not those immunized with either one alone) were protected against AAC.[34] Toxin B is a poor immunogen. Neutralizing or other serum antibodies to toxins of *C. difficile* have been detected in adults,[35–37] but their function is unknown. In one report, antibodies against *C. difficile* antigens were found much less often in sera from elderly than young adults[34]; this is of interest because AAC is more common in elderly patients.

CLINICAL MANIFESTATIONS

The range of severity of the symptoms associated with *C. difficile* colitis is wide.[1,29,38–40] Early reports consisted mostly of severe cases documented at the time of surgery or autopsy. Now that there is a high index of suspicion of AAC and noninvasive tests are available to aid in diagnosis, mild cases not only have been documented but also have been shown to be commonplace.

In the typical patient, profuse watery or mucoid green, foul-smelling diarrhea begins along with cramping abdominal pain 4–9 days after starting antibiotics. In some patients, diarrhea does not begin until after antibiotic treatment has been discontinued. Sometimes the diarrhea is guaiac-positive or bloody. *Clostridium difficile* is not reliably identifiable on Gram-stained smears of stools, but leukocytes are found in smears from about 50 percent of patients. High fever (temperatures of 103–105°F), marked abdominal tenderness, a leukocyte count as high as 35,000/mm^3, and hypoalbuminemia are common and point to the diagnosis of colitis rather than benign diarrhea. Sometimes patients with AAC have little or no diarrhea but have an acute abdominal syndrome with toxic megacolon, colonic perforation, or peritonitis. Acute arthritis resembling Reiter syndrome may complicate the illness.[41]

The pseudomembranous nodules or plaques of *C. difficile* colitis are usually most numerous in the distal colon, sigmoid, and rectum and are easily detected by sigmoidoscopy (Fig. 1). In about 10 percent of cases, lesions are present only in the cecum or transverse colon; this form of the illness is difficult to detect without performing colonoscopy but should be suspected when patients with diarrhea and toxin-positive stools have no visible lesions during proctosigmoidoscopy. Diarrhea caused by *C. difficile* without colitis has been postulated but has not been proved to be caused by *C. difficile*.[42] This putative mechanism includes a purely secretory diarrhea or a diarrhea caused by a motility-altering factor.[27,43] Some patients with leukemia or granulocytopenia or who are receiving antineoplastic chemotherapy have ileocecitis (typhlitis) similar to the disease seen in hamsters.[44,45] If *C. difficile* colitis goes unrecognized and untreated, the outcome may be fatal. Death rates of 10–20 percent were reported in untreated elderly or chronically debilitated patients. Hypovolemic shock, cecal perforation, secondary sepsis, and hemorrhage are the most serious complications that can result in death.

Clostridium difficile colitis can cause symptoms that may be eroneously interpreted as an exacerbation of an underlying chronic inflammatory bowel disease. This presentation usually occurs during or within a month of treatment with antibiotics.[46] Some of the diarrhea attributed to the effects of cancer chemotherapeutic agents on the intestinal mucosa may actually be due to *C. difficile* colitis.[47,48]

LABORATORY DIAGNOSIS

The laboratory tests most useful in confirmation of the diagnosis of AAC include CCFA stool cultures for *C. difficile* and tests for the presence of *C. difficile* toxins in stools.

Clostridium difficile has a characteristic chartreuse fluorescence and gross appearance on CCFA. CCFA can detect as few as 100 cfu of *C. difficile* per gram of stool.[16] Patients with AAC usually have many more organisms than that (10^4–10^5/g), but asymptomatic carriers may have only a few organisms per gram. Almost all patients with AAC are culture-positive if the stool is processed properly. Vegetative forms are easily killed by exposure to air or other adverse conditions; spores are hardy but less numerous and harder to detect. Anaerobe jars incubated at 35–37°C provide adequate cultural conditions. When using CCFA, it is possible to isolate *C. difficile* (presumptively) in just a few days. Confirmation is not difficult when using either biochemical reactions, gas–liquid chromatography to detect the production of fatty acids, or tests of toxin production.[49,50] Few fecal organisms that resemble *C. difficile* can grow on CCFA. *Clostridium sporogenes* is similar but does not produce a cytotoxin.[49] While not all isolates of *C. difficile* are toxigenic, those that are not have not caused colitis or diarrhea.[51]

The isolation of *C. difficile* from stools does not in itself prove that the patient has colitis. As mentioned previously, 60–70 percent of healthy newborns can carry it in their stools for a few weeks, and 3 percent or more of healthy adults may be asymptomatic carriers. In some hospitals where AAC is frequent, 20–30 percent of asymptomatic patients carry the organism.[14] Nevertheless, a positive culture may be useful in making therapeutic decisions. In our hospital, about 85 percent of adults with antibiotic-associated diarrhea and positive stool cultures have had colitis. Since the cytotoxin is heat and acid labile, stools from patients with AAC may be toxin-negative but culture-positive. Cultures also are useful in detecting post-treatment carriers who appear to be at an increased risk of relapse, but there is no effective treatment for eradication of the carrier state.

Tests to detect *C. difficile* toxin B usually employ monolayer cultures of fibroblasts or other cell lines.[4,49,50] These are difficult to maintain and are not available in many hospitals. However, demonstration of cytotoxin in stools is very helpful to the clinician. In our hospital, 95 percent of adults with antibiotic-associated diarrhea and *C. difficile* cytotoxin-positive stools have had documentable colitis. When proctosigmoidoscopy performed on patients with toxin titers greater than 1:10 shows normal mucosa, it is likely that they have colitis at a more proximal site. Isolated cecitis (typhlitis) is more common in patients treated with ampicillin or penicillin G or who have leukemia or granulocytopenia.[45] Colonoscopy or radionuclide scans using gallium or indium may be helpful in detecting and localizing colitis in these patients.

With tests for cytotoxin, a cytopathic effects may be seen within 4–6 hours but usually is not definite until 18–24 hours. Nonspecific (false-positive) toxicity can occur with concentrated specimens but is not neutralizable by antitoxin. Thus, it is necessary to confirm all positive results by demonstrating neutralization of cytotoxicity by incubation with *C. difficile* or *C. sordellii* antitoxin (these reagents are equivalent). Patients with AAC usually have large amounts of toxin in their stool filtrates and have positive titers at dilutions of 10^{-3}–10^{-5} or more. However, the value of the toxin B titer in individual patients does not correlate well with the severity of the illness[39,52]; the discrepancy may be either artifactual or indicative of the greater importance of toxin A in determining disease severity.

More than one toxin (or more than one aggregate of toxin subunits) produced by *C. difficile* can be found in stools of patients with AAC.[24,25,53] Enzyme-linked immunosorbent assays (ELISA) for toxin A have been developed and used for research purposes but are not yet available for routine clinical use. Usually both toxins A and B are present when either one is present in stools of patients with colitis.

Clostridium difficile produces other antigenic substances in addition to toxins A and B. One of these is immunologically similar to proteins produced by other microbial species. Counterimmunoelectrophoresis (CIE) has been used as a rapid method for detecting toxin B in fecal extracts. Since this test uses nonspecific antisera, it may detect these other antigens and is therefore subject to frequent false-positive results. False-negative results also occur.[54–56] A rapid and inexpensive latex agglutination test to aid in the diagnosis of diarrhea caused by *C. difficile* has become available recently.[57] The test was originally thought to detect toxin A; it is now known that it actually detects a nontoxic protein that is distinct from toxin A and of unknown function.[58] Nontoxigenic isolates of *C. difficile* produce the antigen, as do several other species of organisms that are found in the intestinal tract.[58] Both false-negative and false-positive latex results occur; the latter are more common. The clinical significance of a positive latex test result is roughly equivalent to that of a positive culture for *C. difficile*.

Staphylococcal toxins can produce cytopathic effects in Walker rat carcinoma cells (as do *C. difficile* toxins) but not in the fibroblast monolayers used to detect *C. difficile* toxins.[20] This difference may be useful in the diagnosis of staphylococcal enterocolitis.

CLINICAL DIAGNOSIS

When patients with antibiotic-associated diarrhea have high fevers, severe abdominal pain and tenderness, bloody stools, or large numbers of leukocytes in their stools, benign diarrhea is ruled out, and colitis is probably present. The diagnosis of AAC is most rapidly and certainly established by endoscopy, which detects evidence of inflammation (colitis) or pseudomembranous lesions. Colonoscopy may be required to detect isolated proximal colonic lesions. Colonic biopsy is not needed when typical gross findings are seen but may aid in the diagnosis of clostridial colitis when so-called nonspecific colitis is visualized because it may reveal pseudomembranes too small to be seen grossly.

Air-contrast barium enema studies may show signs of PMC, but these signs are not specific and are often absent early in the illness. In severe colitis, barium studies may precipitate toxic megacolon, perforation, or other complications, and they are not recommended.

In patients with nonspecific colitis associated with antibiotic usage, it is important also to consider Crohn's disease, idiopathic ulcerative colitis, and ischemic colitis. Infection with other intestinal pathogens such as *Salmonella, Edwardsiella, Shigella,* invasive *E. coli* (especially the 0157:H7 serotype if the colitis is hemorrhagic), *Entamoeba histolytica, Campylobacter, Yersinia,* and *Strongyloides* should be considered. Enterotoxin-producing organisms that can cause diarrhea without colitis include *E. coli, Bacillus cereus, Aeromonas, Vibrio,* and possibly other Enterobacteriaceae and pseudomonads.

TREATMENT

Antibiotics

Clostridium difficile is very susceptible to vancomycin, metronidazole and rifampin, and most isolates are susceptible to bacitracin. The minimal inhibitory concentrations for these are about 1μg/ml or less. Since resistance to rifampin can develop rapidly, this drug is not used alone in the treatment of AAC. Isolates resistant to metronidazole have been reported. Vancomycin-resistant isolates have never been detected. *Clostridium difficile* is often susceptible to tetracycline, erythromycin, ampicillin, cefamandole, cefazolin, and other antibiotics[6,52]; however, all of these except bacitracin have induced AAC and have not been very useful for treating the disease.

Not all patients with AAC need to be treated with antimicrobials. When patients have mild or moderate symptoms, it is sufficient to discontinue treatment with the precipitating antibiotic and give supportive therapy with fluids and electrolytes. If the patient improves within 48 hours, supportive therapy can be continued, and diarrhea usually subsides within 7–10 days. If treatment with the inducing antibiotic must be continued, specific antimicrobial treatment should be started promptly, even if symptoms are mild. Patients with high fever, leukocytosis, marked abdominal pain, and signs of peritoneal inflammation should be treated promptly with specific antibiotics, as should patients who are elderly, toxic, debilitated, or unresponsive to supportive therapy or cholestyramine.

Discontinuation of treatment with the inducing antibiotic, although desirable, is probably not essential if specific therapy for AAC is given. For example, the antibacterial effects of vancomycin on *C. difficile* in vitro are not antagonized by clindamycin, and the continuation of clindamycin therapy in patients treated with oral vancomycin has not been harmful. Furthermore, many of the antibiotics chosen as alternative therapy are capable of inducing AAC.

Vancomycin. Vancomycin given orally is expensive therapy but still the treatment of choice for severe AAC.[38,52,55] Metronidazole[56] and bacitracin[59] are less expensive alternatives for treating mild or moderately severely ill patients or when vancomycin is unavailable. The efficacy of vancomycin has been so well documented in different parts of the world that it must be considered the most reliable treatment. *Clostridium difficile* is usually susceptible to vancomycin at concentrations of less than 5 μg/ml, and no isolate has been identified that required more than 16 μg/ml. Since vancomycin is poorly absorbed from the gastrointestinal tract, it is nontoxic, and concentrations far exceeding 16 μg/ml are easily achieved in stools. When 500 mg is given orally four times daily, stool concentrations average 2000 μg/ml or more. When 125 mg is given four times daily, concentrations reach 300–1000 μg/ml. Even patients with profuse diarrhea achieve adequate concentrations with these regimens. Vancomycin has been detected in the urine of patients treated orally, but only in low concentrations after oral administration. Vancomycin is usually undetectable in serum, but concentrations were 5–30 μg/ml when it was detectable. Systemic toxic reactions have been very rare with oral vancomycin, even in patients with an inflamed colonic mucosa.[38,52,55]

Oral vancomycin was evaluated in a controlled study and was found to be significantly better than placebo in the treatment of *C. difficile* toxin-positive postoperative diarrheal syndromes.[55] The dose was 125 mg every 6 hours for 5 days. Vancomycin-treated patients who had *C. difficile*-negative antibiotic-associated diarrhea fared no better than did placebo-treated patients. Many patients with *C. difficile* colitis have been treated with oral vancomycin in uncontrolled studies. The clinical response almost invariably has been excellent unless the disease was far advanced when treatment was begun or oral therapy was not possible. Antibacterial activity within colonic tissues does not appear necessary; cessation of toxin production within the lumen or at the mucosal surface seems sufficient and indeed essential.

Patients treated with oral vancomycin usually show improvement in fever, diarrhea, abdominal cramps, and malaise within 48 hours. Toxin titers in stools decline shortly after treatment is begun. Treatment should continue until stools no longer contain toxin. Diarrhea and fever may require a week or more to resolve. Treatment should continue for at least 5–7 days but is rarely needed for more than 10 days. Some investigators believe that therapy should not be discontinued until toxin is no longer detected in stools.

The major disadvantages to the use of vancomycin are its expense ($16–$25 or more per day), its short supply in some parts of the world, and its bitter taste. A less expensive tablet form of vancomycin for oral use has recently been made available in the United States.

In about 50 patients entered into a randomized study, there were no significant differences in the overall clinical or bacteriologic responses of those treated with oral vancomycin every 6 hours in dosages of either 500 or 2000 mg/day.[59b] Although diarrhea in very ill patients ceased slightly sooner with the higher dose. The 500 mg/day regimen is less expensive and is therefore preferable except for extremely ill patients. For the treatment of infants and children with AAC, a dose of 500 mg/ 1.73 m^2 every 6 hours orally has been recommended.[12]

Vancomycin is also the drug of choice for the treatment of staphylococcal PMC, which may be suspected when Gram-stained smears of stools show very little except gram-positive cocci.

Patients who are unable to take vancomycin orally should be given it via a nasogastric tube, but patients with adynamic ileus may still not achieve adequate concentrations within the colonic lumen where it is needed to stop toxic production. These patients pose a formidable therapeutic problem since there is no parenteral regimen that is of proven benefit. When healthy adults were given intravenous vancomycin, their stool concentrations ranged from 0 to 100 μg/ml.[60] Thus, some patients with colitis treated intravenously might not achieve adequate concentrations within the bowel lumen. A few patients with colitis appear to have responded to intravenous vancomycin,[61] but other seriously ill patients have failed to respond. Recent evidence suggests that metronidazole given intravenously may also reach therapeutic concentrations in the colonic lumen in some patients. Reliance upon either intravenous metronidazole or vancomycin for the treatment of AAC, to the exclusion of oral therapy, is *not* recommended.

When parenteral therapy is essential (as in patients with paralytic ileus), we recommend treatment with both intravenous vancomycin and metronidazole (see below) supplemented by vancomycin given via nasogastric tube (500 mg four times per day for adults), into ileostomies and colostomies, or by enema. Oral metronidazole plays no role in this setting since, if small amounts of the drug pass down the gastrointestinal tract, they will be absorbed in the small intestine and none will reach the colon.

Metronidazole. Metronidazole is very active against *C. difficile* and has been effective in the treatment of patients with AAC.[56,62,63] It is inactive against staphylococci and has no value in treatment of staphylococcal enterocolitis. In a randomized comparative study, oral metronidazole was associated with a cure rate within 7 days of 92 percent; the rate was 100 percent with vancomycin, but the difference was not statistically significant.[64] Metronidazole was well tolerated, significantly less expensive than vancomycin, and associated with about the same rate of post-treatment carriage and relapse as was vancomycin. The usual oral dose is 500–750 mg three times daily or 250 mg four times daily. The drug is so well absorbed from the small intestine that concerns have been raised about whether the concentrations achieved within the colonic lumen are adequate in all patients, especially seriously ill patients. Some seriously ill patients have failed to respond to metronidazole.[45] We reserve metronidazole for mildly or moderately ill patients with AAC. Metronidazole has a number of side effects, some serious, and is not recommended for use in pregnant women or children. Furthermore, one case of colitis with a metronidazole-resistant organism has been reported.[65] Recent reports have encouraged the use of intravenous metronidazole to treat patients with AAC who are too sick to be treated via the oral route.[66,67] The usual intravenous dose was 500 mg every 6–8 hours. Metronidazole was detected in stools of patients and in rat intestinal tissues when using a chemical assay.[68] However, adequate bioactivity within the colonic lumen of patients has not been documented. Further, it is possible the biliary excretion of metronidazole was responsible for the clinical improvement noted in these patients, most of whom apparently did not have decreased intestinal motility. Since no form of parenteral therapy has been proved to be reliably effective in AAC, it should be used only when oral therapy is not possible. In such patients, both metronidazole and vancomycin should probably be given intravenously. Vancomycin (500 mg four times per day for adults) should also be given via nasogastric tube with intermittent clamping, and the administration of vancomycin by enema or by direct instillation through an ileostomy or colostomy should be considered. A high proportion of these patients ultimately require an emergent colectomy as a lifesaving measure.

Bacitracin. Chang et al. and Tedesco and associates[59,62] reported several patients whose PMC improved with treatment with oral bacitracin. The dosage was 25,000 units (about 500 mg) four times per day for 7–19 days. One patient relapsed after this therapy and then was treated successfully with vancomycin. Bacitracin has a bitter taste and is very nauseating if not given in capsule form (which requires special preparation). Although bacitracin is a useful alternative to vancomycin and metronidazole, the response to bacitracin is slower and less certain than with vancomycin; furthermore, carrier rates and stool toxin titers decline less rapidly, and it is not as reliable.[69,70] More experience with it is needed. Most isolates of *C. difficile* are susceptible to bacitracin, but some require more than 20 units/ml (about 1000 μg/ml) for inhibition, which may indicate resistance since these concentrations may not be achieved in the stools of some patients with diarrhea. Some absorption of the drug occurs when it is given orally. The systemic absorption and safety of bacitracin in patients with an inflamed intestinal mucosa as well as the frequency of relapse after treatment with this drug need better documentation. Bacitracin is often unavailable and is slightly less expensive than vancomycin is. It is also active against staphylococci. It may become available soon in a more palatable oral preparation.

Other Antibiotics. Fusidic acid is highly active against *C. difficile* and has been used successfully for the oral treatment of 15 patients with AAC.[71] It is also active against staphylococci. Tetracycline and erythromycin have been used occasionally in treatment of AAC of unknown cause, but many isolates of *C. difficile* are resistant to these antibiotics, and their use is not recommended.

Cholestyramine

This anion-exchange resin (as well as others) was used in treatment of PMC before the cause of the disease was known and was based on speculation that secretory bile acids might be responsible for antibiotic-associated diarrhea or colitis.[72] Studies in hamsters suggested that secretory bile acids were unlikely to cause antibiotic-associated diarrhea.[73] Cholestyramine binds *C. difficile* toxin B (and probably also toxin A), which is its presumed mechanism of action in this condition. It may also bind vancomycin, so their simultaneous use should be avoided.[74] Since many patients with AAC respond slowly or not at all to cholestyramine and require a change to treatment with antibiotics, it is usually reserved for mild illness. The usual oral dose of cholestyramine for adults is 4 g three or four times per day. Obstipation is the most serious side effect.

Antidiarrheal Agents

Opiates and other antiperistaltic agents should be avoided in patients with AAC. They are especially dangerous in infants. While they often provide symptomatic relief, they may promote more severe damage to the colon because of toxin retention; some patients have become worse when given these drugs.[75]

Adrenal Steroids

These are not of proven value in this disease. Reported mortality is higher in patients who received steroids, but such patients have tended to be sicker on the average before treatment.

Relapse or Recurrence of Colitis

More than one episode of colitis has been observed in 10–20 percent or more of patients treated with vancomycin, metronidazole, or bacitracin.[38,76–79] Recurrences respond to retreatment with vancomycin or, if the organism is susceptible, to metronidazole or bacitracin. Recurrences may be caused by germination of persistent spores or by reinfection from environmental or human contacts; persistence appears more common on the basis of typing studies. Treatment of carriers with oral vancomycin until discharge or transfer in a hospital unit where there is a high rate of the disease may have been useful in terminating outbreaks. The use of sodium hypochlorite diluted 1:500 to disinfect contaminated surfaces has also been recommended for control of nosocomial outbreaks. Careful hand washing by staff after contact with cases or carriers is urged. Not all patients who remain fecal carriers of the organism after treatment relapse. Unfortunately, the carrier state cannot be reliably eradicated with antimicrobials or any other regimen. Most relapses are spontaneous and occur within a few weeks of the first episode. Little is known about local, humoral, or cellular immunity to either the toxins, the organism, or the disease. Serum antibodies to the toxins have been detected in most healthy adults and in a minority of patients who recovered from the disease.[35,37,80] One patient developed neutralizing antibodies to toxin B in serum after eight episodes of colitis. He suffered no further recurrences despite the presence of large amounts of toxin in his stools (Buggy B, Fekety R: Unpublished observations).

Patients who relapse may be treated with oral vancomycin, metronidazole, or bacitracin for 7–10 days or until their diarrhea ceases. Longer courses do not appear more efficacious in preventing recurrences. Indeed, short courses may permit more rapid restoration of the normal fecal flora, which seems inhibitory for *C. difficile*.

Although most patients have only one relapse, some unfortunate persons relapse repeatedly. No reliable way to manage them is known, but anecdotal experiences suggest they may respond to long courses (4–6 weeks) of oral vancomycin or metronidazole, followed by a gradual tapering of the dose[81]; to intermittent short periods (5–7 days) of treatment alternating with periods of nontreatment; to postantibiotic therapy with cholestyramine to suppress symptoms by binding toxin while a normal flora is being reestablished; to recolonization by supplementation of antibiotics with oral lactobacillus preparations; or even to enemas with feces from healthy persons.[82,83] Oral vancomycin plus rifampin has been useful in a few cases[84] in an uncontrolled study. Since recent evidence suggests lactobacilli, enterococci, *Saccharomyces,* and nontoxigenic *C. difficile* isolates are important inhibitors of *C. difficile* within the gut, interest in their use for treatment of patients who relapse is growing.[85–89] A nontoxigenic strain of *C. difficile* has been useful in two patients with relapsing disease in an uncontrolled study.[88]

Surgical Measures

Before specific antibiotic therapy was available for AAC, diversion of the fecal stream or resection of the diseased bowel was often necessary. These drastic measures are now rarely performed except in life-threatening situations such as with toxic megacolon or cecal perforation. Sometimes a colostomy or ileostomy is needed to facilitate instillation of vancomycin or metronidazole into the colonic lumen of patients with ileus.[78]

Prevention

Eventually it may be possible to immunize patients against the toxins or other virulence factors of *C. difficile*, but this is not yet possible. Passive immunization of hamsters with *C. sordellii* antitoxin, which cross reacts with toxin B of *C. difficile*, protected them against clindamycin-induced colitis.[5] However, it has been difficult to purify the toxins and to prepare potent toxoids from them. Ordinary immune serum globulin does not appear useful. Prophylaxis with antibiotics such as vancomycin or metronidazole in patients at high risk of AAC is not of proven value; it is expensive and theoretically undesirable and should not be given.[4] Bacteriophage and bacteriocin typing systems as well as immunologic and antibiogram systems for typing *C. difficile* have recently become available, and their use in epidemiologic studies may lead to new or better preventive measures.[90–94]

REFERENCES

1. Bartlett JG. Antibiotic-associated pseudomembranous colitis. Rev Infect Dis. 1979;1:530.
2. Lusk RH, Fekety FR, Silva J, et al. Gastrointestinal side effects of clindamycin and ampicillin therapy. J Infect Dis. 1977;135(Suppl):111.
3. Lusk RH, Fekety FR, Silva J, et al. Clindamycin-induced enterocolitis in hamsters. J Infect Dis. 1978;137:464.
4. Rifkin GD, Fekety FR, Silva J, et al. Antibiotic-induced colitis: Implication of a toxin neutralized by *Clostridium sordellii* antitoxin. Lancet. 1977;2:1103.
5. Allo M, Silva J, Fekety FR, et al. Prevention of clindamycin-induced colitis in hamsters by *Clostridium sordellii* antitoxin. Gastroenterology. 1979;76:351.
6. Fekety R, Silva J, Toshniwal R, et al. Antibiotic-associated colitis: Effects of antibiotics upon *Clostridium defficile* and the disease in hamsters. Rev Infect Dis. 1979;1:386.
7. Borriello SP, Barclay FE. An in vitro model of colonization resistance to *Clostridium difficile* infection. Med Microbiol. 1986;21:299–309.
8. Larson HE, Price AB, Honour P, et al. *Clostridium difficile* and the aetiology of pseudomembranous colitis. Lancet. 1978;1:1063.
9. Lyerly DM, Krwan HC, Wilkins TD. *Clostridium difficile*: Its disease and toxins. Clin Microbiol Rev. 1988;1:1–18.
10. Rolfe RD, Finegold SM, eds. *Clostridium difficile*: Its role in intestinal disease. San Diego: Academic Press; 1988:408.
11. Tedesco FJ et al. Clindamycin-associated colitis: A prospective study. Ann Intern Med. 1974;81:432.
12. Scapa E. Pseudomembranous colitis in a 5 week old infant. Br Med J. 1982;284:824.
13. Batts DH, Martin D, Holmes R, et al. Treatment of antibiotic-associated *Clostridium difficile* diarrhea with oral vancomycin. J Pediatr. 1980;97:151.
14. Fekety R, Kim K-H, Brown D, et al. Epidemiology of antibiotic-associated colitis. Isolation of *Clostridium difficile* from the hospital environment. Am J Med. 1981;70:906.
15. Borriello SP, Honour P, Turner T, et al. Household pets as a potential reservoir for *Clostridium difficile* infection. J Clin Pathol. 1983;36:84.
16. George WL, Sutter VL, Citron D, et al. Selective and differential medium for isolation of *Clostridium difficile*. J Clin Microbiol. 1979;9:214.
17. Wilson KH, Kennedy MJ, Fekety FR. Use of sodium taurocholate to enhance spore recovery on a medium selective for *Clostridium difficile*. J Clin Microbiol. 1982;15:443.
18. Phillips KD, Rogers PA. Rapid detection and presumptive identification of *Clostridium difficile* by *p*-cresol production on a selective medium. J Clin Pathol. 1981;36:642.
19. Borriello SP, Honour P. Simplified procedure for the routine isolation of *Clostridium difficile* from faeces. J Clin Pathol. 1981;34:1124.
20. Batts DH, Silva J, Fekety R. Staphylococcal enterocolitis, in Nelson JD, Grassi C, eds. Current Chemotherapy and Infectious Disease. v. 2. Washington, DC: American Society for Microbiology; 1980:944.
21. Schwartz JN, Hamilton JP, Fekety R, et al. Ampicillin-induced enterocolitis: Implication of toxigenic *Clostridium perfringens* type C. J Pediatr. 1980;97:661.
22. Hovius SER, Rietra PJ. *Salmonella* colitis clinically presenting as a pseudomembranous colitis. Neth J Surg. 1982;34:81.
23. Peikin SR, Galdibini J, Bartlett JG. Role of *Clostridium difficile* in a case of nonantibiotic-associated pseudomembranous colitis. Gastroenterology. 1980;79:948.
24. Banno Y, Kobayashi T, Watanabe K, et al. Two toxins (D-1 and D-2) of *Clostridium difficile* causing antibiotic-associated colitis: Purification and some characterization. Biochem Int. 1981;2:629.
25. Taylor NS, Thorne GM, Bartlett JG. Comparison of two toxins produced by *Clostridium difficile* Infect Immun. 1981;34:1036.
26. Thelestam M, Bronnegard M. Interaction of cytopathogenic toxin from *Clostridium difficile* with cells in tissue culture. Scand J Infect Dis. 1980;22(Suppl):16.
27. Lima AA, Lyerly DM, Wilkins TD, et al. Effects of *Clostridium difficile* toxins A and B in rabbit small and large intestines in vivo and on cultured cells in vitro. Infect Immun. 1988;56:582–8.

28. Justus TG, Martin JL, Goldberg DA, et al. Myoelectric effects of *Clostridium difficile*: Motility-altering factors distinct from its cytotoxin and enterotoxin in rabbits. Gastroenterology. 1982;83:836.
29. Fekety R, Silva J, Armstrong J, et al. Treatment of antibiotic-associated enterocolitis with vancomycin. Rev Infect Dis. 1981;3(Suppl):273.
30. Welch DF, Marks MI. Is *Clostridium difficile* pathogenic in infants? J Pediatr. 1982;100:393.
31. Delmee M, Verellen G, Avesani V, et al. *Clostridium difficile* in neonates: Serogrouping and epidemiology. Eur J Pediatr. 1988;147:36–40.
32. Griffin GE, Heath J, Knox P. The action of *Clostridium difficile* cytotoxin is inhibited by specific glycoproteins (Abstract 596). Proceedings of the 22nd Interscience Conference on Antimicrobial Agents and Chemotherapy. Washington, DC: American Society for Microbiology; 1982.
33. Chang TW, Sullivan NM, Wilkins TD. Insusceptibility of fetal intestinal mucosa and fetal cells to *Clostridium difficile* toxins. Acta Pharmacol Sin. 1986;7:448–53.
34. Libby JM, Wilkins TD. Production of antitoxins to two toxins of *Clostridium difficile* and immunological comparison of the toxins by cross-neutralization studies. Infect Immun. 1982;35:374.
35. Nakamura S, Mikawa M, Nakashio S, et al. Identification of *Clostridium difficile* from the feces and the antibody in sera of young and elderly adults. Microbiol Immunol. 1981;25:345.
36. Viscidi R, Yolken R, Laughon B, et al. Serum antibody response to toxins A and B of *Clostridium difficile* (Abstract 595). Proceedings of the 22nd Interscience Conference on Antimicrobial Agents and Chemotherapy. Washington, DC: American Society for Microbiology; 1982.
37. Lishman AH, Al-Jumaili IJ, Record CO: Antitoxin production in antibiotic-associated colitis? J Clin Pathol. 1981;34:414.
38. Silva J, Batts DH, Fekety R. Treatment of *Clostridium difficile* colitis and diarrhea with vancomycin. Am J Med. 1981;71:815.
39. Burdon DW, George RH, Mogg G, et al. Faecal toxin and severity of antibiotic-associated pseudomembranous colitis. J Clin Pathol. 1981;34:548.
40. Thompson Jr CM, Gilligan PH, Fisher MC, et al. *Clostridium difficile* cytotoxin in a pediatric population. Am J Dis Child. 1983;137:271.
41. Puddey IB. Reiter's syndrome following antibiotic-associated colitis. Aust NZ J Med. 1982;12:292.
42. Gerding DN, Olson MM, Peterson LR et al. *Clostridium difficile*-associated diarrhea and colitis in adults. A prospective case-controlled epidemiologic study. Arch Intern Med. 1986;146:95–100.
43. Lashner BA, Todorczvk J, Sahm DF, et al. *Clostridium difficile* culture-positive toxin-negative diarrhea. Am J Gastroenterol. 1986;81:940–3.
44. Ikard RW: Neutropenic typhlitis in adults. Arch Surg. 1981;116:943.
45. Rampling A, Warren RE, Berry PJ, et al. Atypical *Clostridium difficile* colitis in neutropenic patients. Lancet. 1982;2:162.
46. Trnka YM, LaMont JT. Associations of *Clostridium difficile* toxin with symptomatic relapse of chronic inflammatory bowel disease. Gastroenterology. 1981;80:693.
47. Cudmore MA, Silva J, Fekety R, et al. *Clostridium difficile* colitis associated with cancer chemotherapy. Arch Intern Med. 1982;142:333.
48. Fainstein V, Bodey GP, Fekety R. *Clostridium difficile* colonization in cancer patients admitted to laminar air-flow units (Abstract). Clin Res. 1982;30:365.
49. Larson L, Holst E, Gemmell CG, et al. Characterization of *Clostridium difficile* and its differentiation from *Clostridium sporogenes* by automatic headspace gas chromatography. Scand J Infect Dis. 1980;22(Suppl):37.
50. Chang TW, Lauermann M, Bartlett JG. Cytotoxicity assay in antibiotic-associated colitis. J Infect Dis. 1979;140:765.
51. Chang TW. *Clostridium difficile* toxin and antimicrobial agent-induced diarrhea. J Infect Dis. 1978;137:854.
52. Tedesco F, Markham R, Gurwith M, et al. Oral vancomycin for antibiotic-associated pseudomembranous colitis. Lancet. 1978;2:226.
53. Aronsson B, Granstrom M, Molby R, et al. Toxin A (enterotoxin) from *Clostridium difficile* in antibiotic-associated colitis. Lancet. 1982;2:1279.
54. Levine HG, Kennedy M, LaMont JT. Counterimmunoelectrophoresis vs. cytotoxicity assay for the detection of *Clostridium difficile* toxin. J Infect Dis. 1982;145:398.
55. Keighley MRB, Burdon DW, Arabi Y, et al. Randomized controlled trial of vancomycin for pseudomembranous colitis and postoperative diarrhea. Br Med J. 1978;2:1667.
56. Pashby NL, Bolton RP, Sherriff RJ. Oral metronidazole in *Clostridium difficile* colitis. Br Med J. 1979;1:1605.
57. Sherman ME, Degirolami PC, Thorne G, et al. Evaluation of a latex agglutination test for diagnosis of *Clostridium difficile* associated colitis. Am J Clin Pathol. 1988;89:228–33.
58. Lyerly DA, Ball DW, Toth J, et al. Characterization of cross-reactive proteins detected by culturette brand rapid latex test for *Clostridium difficile*. J Clin Microbiol. 1988;26:397–400.
59a. Chang T-W, Gorbach SL, Bartlett JG, et al. Bacitracin treatment of antibiotic-associated colitis and diarrhea caused by *Clostridium difficile* toxin. Gastroenterology. 1980;78:1584.
59b. Fekety R, Silva J, Kauffman C, et al. Treatment of *Clostridium difficile* antibiotic-associated colitis with oral vancomycin: Comparison of two dosage regimens. Am J Med. 1989;86:15.
60. Geraci JE, Heilman FR, Nichols DR, et al. Some laboratory and clinical experiences with a new antibiotic, vancomycin. Proc Staff Meet Mayo Clin. 1956;31:564.
61. Donta ST, Lamps GM, Summers KW, et al. Cephalosporin-associated colitis and *Clostridium difficile* Arch Intern Med. 1980;140:574–7.
62. Tedesco FJ. Bacitracin therapy in antibiotic-associated pseudomembranous colitis. Dig Dis Sci. 1980;25:783.
63. Cherry RD, Portnoy D, Jabbari M, et al. Metronidazole: An alternate therapy for antibiotic-associated colitis. Gastroenterology. 1982;82:849.
64. Teasley DG, Gerding DN, Olson MN, et al. Prospective randomized trial of Metronidazole versus vancomycin for the treatment of *Clostridium difficile* associated diarrhea and colitis. Lancet. 1983;2:1043–6.
65. Saginur R, Hawley CR, Bartlett JG. Colitis associated with metronidazole therapy. J Infect Dis. 1980;141:772.
66. Bolton RF, Culshaw MA. Faecal metronidazole concentrations during oral and intravenous therapy for antibiotic-associated colitis due to *Clostridium difficile* Gut. 1986;27:1169–72.
67. Kleinfeld DI, Sharpe RJ, Donta ST. Parenteral therapy for antibiotic associated pseudomembranous colitis. J Infect Dis. 1988;157:389.
68. Bergan T, Solhaug JH, Soreide O, et al. Comparative pharmacokinetics of metronidazole and tinidazole and their tissue penetration. Scand J Gastroenterol. 1985;20:945–50.
69. Young GP, Ward PB, Bayley N, et al. Antibiotic-associated colitis due to *Clostridium difficile*: Double-blind comparison of vancomycin with bacitracin. Gastroenterology. 1985;89:1038–45.
70. Dudley MN, McLauglin JC, Carrington G, et al. Oral bacitracin vs vancomycin therapy for *Clostridium difficile*-induced diarrhea. A randomized double-blind trial. Arch Intern Med. 1986;146:1101–4.
71. Cronberg S, Castor B, Thoren A. Fusidic acid for the treatment of antibiotic-associated colitis induced by *Clostridium difficile*. Infection. 1984;12:276–79.
72. Kreutzer EW, Milligan FD. Treatment of antibiotic-associated pseudomembranous colitis with cholestyramine resin. Johns Hopkins Med J. 1978;143:67.
73. Fekety R, Browne RA, Silva J, et al. Fecal bile acids and cholestyramine in hamsters with clindamycin-associated colitis (Abstract 129). Proceedings of the 18th Interscience Conference on Antimicrobial Agents and Chemotherapy. Atlanta: American Society for Microbiology; 1978.
74. King CY, Barriere SL. Analysis of the in vitro interaction between vancomycin and cholestyramine. Antimicrob Agents Chemother. 1981;19:326.
75. Novak E, Lee JG, Seckman E, et al. Unfavorable effect of atropine-diphenoxylate (Lomotil) therapy in lincomycin-caused diarrhea. JAMA. 1976;235:1451–4.
76. George WL, Volpicelli NA, Stiner DB, et al. Relapse of pseudomembranous colitis after vancomycin therapy. N Engl J Med. 1979;301:414.
77. Bartlett JG, Tedesdo FJ, Shull S, et al. Symptomatic relapse after oral vancomycin therapy of antibiotic-associated pseudomembranous colitis. Gastroenterology. 1980;78:431.
78. George WL, Rolfe RD, Finegold SM. Treatment and prevention of antimicrobial agent-induced colitis and diarrhea. Gastroenterology. 1980;79:366.
79. Walters BAJ, Roberts R, Stafford R, et al. Relapse of antibiotic-associated colitis: Endogenous persistence of *Clostridium difficile* during vancomycin therapy. Gut. 1983;24:206.
80. Silva J, Lusk R, Kekety R, et al. Immune responses of hamsters and humans with antibiotic associated colitis. In: Lambe DW Jr, Genco RJ, Mayberry-Carson KJ, eds. Anaerobic Bacteria: Selected Topics. New York: Plenum; 1980:295.
81. Tedesco FJ. Treatment of recurrent antibiotic-associated pseudomembranous colitis. Am J Gastroenterol. 1982;77:220.
82. Schwan A, Sjolin S, Trottestan U. Relapsing *Clostridium difficile* enterocolitis cured by rectal infusion of homologous faeces. Lancet. 1983;2:845.
83. Schwan A, Sjolin S, Trottesam U, et al. Relapsing *Clostridium difficile* enterocolitis cured by rectal infusion of normal faeces. Scand J Infect Dis 1984;16:211–5.
84. Buggy BP, Fekety R, Silva J. Therapy of relapsing *Clostridium difficile*-associated diarrhea and colitis with the combination of vancomycin and rifampin. J Clin Gastroenterol. 1987;9:155–9.
85. Wilson KH, Sheagren JH, Freter R, et al. Gnotobiotic models for study of the microbial ecology of *Clostridium difficile* and *Eschericia coli*. J Infect Dis. 1986;153:547–51.
86. Borriello SP, Barclay FP. An in vitro model of colonisation resistance to *Clostridium difficile* infection. J Med Microbiol. 1986;21:299–309.
87. Elmer G, McFarland LV. Suppression by *Saccharomyces boulardii* of toxigenic *Clostridium difficile* overgrowth after vancomycin treatment of hamsters. Antimicrob Agents Chemother. 1987;31:129–31.
88. Seal D, Borriello SP, Barclay FE, et al. Treatment of relapsing *Clostridium difficile* diarrhoeae by administration of a non-toxigenic strain. Eur J Clin Microbiol. 1987;6:51–3.
89. Wilson KH, Silva J, Fekety FR. Suppression of *Clostridium difficile* by normal hamster cecal flora and prevention of antibiotic-associated cecitis. Infect Immun. 1981;34:626.
90. Wilson KH, Sheagren JN. Antagonism of toxigenic *Clostridium difficile* by non-toxigenic *C. difficile*. J Infect Dis. 1983;147:733.
91. Rolfe RD, Helebian S, Finegold SM. Bacterial interference between *Clostridium difficile* and normal fecal flora. J Infect Dis. 1981;143:470.
92. Malamoa-Lodas H, Tabaqchali S. Inhibition of *Clostridium difficile* by fecal streptococci. J Med Microbiol. 1982;15:569.
93. Wust J, Sullivan NM, Hardegger U, et al. Investigation of an outbreak of antibiotic-associated colitis by various typing methods. J Clin Microbiol. 1982;16:1096.
94. Sell TL, Schaberg DR, Fekety FR. Bacteriophage and bacteriocin typing scheme for *Clostridium difficile*. J Clin Microbiol. 17:1148,1983.

84. INFLAMMATORY ENTERITIDES

RICHARD L. GUERRANT

The acute inflammatory enteritides include several specific distal small bowel and colonic infections such as campylobacteriosis salmonellosis, shigellosis, and amebiasis as well as the syndromes of necrotizing enteritis and antibiotic-associated pseudomembranous enterocolitis. Several other infectious agents cause chronic enteric inflammatory processes that may result in syndromes of abdominal pain, weight loss, diarrhea, or malabsorption. These include such processes as gastrointestinal mycoses, mycobacterioses, bacterial infections, and certain parasitic infections such as coccidiosis.

ACUTE DYSENTERY

Syndromes of acute dysentery with fecal blood and pus have been well recognized since the days of Hippocrates. Dysentery implies frequent, small bowel movements accompanied by blood and mucus with tenesmus or pain on defecation. This syndrome implies an inflammatory invasion of the colonic mucosa resulting from bacterial, cytotoxic, or parasitic destruction.

The pathologic changes of inflammatory colitis range from a superficial intense exudative inflammatory process involving the colonic mucosa by shigellae or invasive *Escherichia coli* to deeper, penetrating, "flask-shaped" ulcers with undermined edges as seen in amebic dysentery. The pathogenesis of the inflammatory colitides may involve cytotoxic products of shigellae,[1] certain *E. coli*,[2] clostridia, or other organisms.

The epidemiologic patterns of acute dysenteric syndromes are influenced by the unusually low inoculum required by organisms such as shigellae or amebae for infection. As few as 10^2 shigellae or as few as 10 cysts of enteric parasites such as *Entamoeba coli* or *Giardia lamblia* may cause infection in adult volunteers.[3,4] Consequently, there is a substantial risk of person-to-person spread in day care centers,[5] institutions, or other areas where nonhygienic conditions may allow direct fecal–oral spread. The cysts of parasites such as *Entamoeba histolytica* or *Balantidium coli* often resist chlorination and therefore may cause water-borne outbreaks of dysenteric illnesses. Saltwater or seafood exposure should lead one to consider *Vibrio parahaemolyticus* as a cause of inflammatory colitis, and farm or domestic animal exposure might lead one to consider nontyphoid *Salmonella* sp., *Campylobacter jejuni*, or *Yersinia enterocolitica*. In addition, when typhoid fever is present with diarrhea in an endemic area, the diarrhea is often inflammatory with many fecal polymorphonuclear leukocytes seen on microscopic examination.[6] Travel to areas of poor sanitation might implicate any of the aforementioned pathogens. Finally, venereal exposure, particularly among male homosexuals, might implicate the gonococcus, herpes simplex virus, *Chlamydia trachomatis*, or *Treponema pallidum* as causes of proctitis or *Campylobacter, Shigella, Chlamydia trachomatis* (lymphogranuloma venereum serotypes), *E. histolytica*, or *Clostridium difficile* as causes of colitis.[7]

Examination for fecal leukocytes often reveals sheets of polymorphonuclear leukocytes in clumps of mucus even in the absence of gross blood in the stool specimen[8,9] (Fig. 1). Fewer, pyknotic leukocytes are reported in amebic dysentery[10–12]; this may be attributable to the deeper, undermining ulcers characteristic of intestinal amebiasis or to a toxic effect of the ameba on leukocytes. A prompt culture of fresh specimens onto appropriate enteric culture media is very important in the isolation of shigellae.[13] Specialized techniques are required to isolate *Vibrio* (thiosulfate citrate bile salt agar),[14] *Yersinia* (cold enrichment),[15] or *Campylobacter jejuni*.[16] Leukocytosis or even a leukemoid reaction has been described. Sigmoidoscopic examination may be useful in the diagnosis of a pseudomembranous enterocolitis or in the identification of parasites such as *E. histolytica* or *B. coli*. Amebic colitis is associated with discrete small ulcerations with undermined edges amid relatively normal mucosa. Acute shigellosis causes more widespread, shallow, 3 to 7 mm ulcers with a more intense inflammatory exudate. Barium studies are unnecessary and are relatively contradicted in toxic patients with acute colitis. Therapy consists of careful supportive fluid management with specific antimicrobial therapy directed at a specific pathogen if suspected by the epidemiologic setting or culture results.

The potential etiologies of acute dysentery are listed in Table 1.

Bacillary Dysentery (Shigellosis and Enteroinvasive E. coli)

Shigella sp. (types A–D: *dysenteriae*, *flexneri*, *sonnei*, and *boydii*) may cause acute bloody dysentery with high fever and systemic manifestations of malaise, headache, and abdominal pain. The incubation period ranges from 6 hours to 9 days but is usually <72 hours. This syndrome may be particularly severe in poorly nourished children. As noted previously, this organism may be spread with relatively small inocula by direct contact as well as in food or water.

Despite the intense superficial destructive process in the colonic epithelium that typifies acute shigellosis, bacteremia and disseminated infection are relatively rare. A complication of severe shigellosis in childhood is a hemolytic-uremic syndrome that may be associated with a leukemoid reaction, pseudomembranous colitis, circulating immune complexes, and circulating endotoxin, usually in the absence of demonstrable bacteremia.[17] Other more common extraintestinal manifestations of shigellosis include headache, meningismus, and even seizures, especially in children.[18] These findings may be attributable to a neurotoxin that has been demonstrated with *Shigella dysenteriae* type I.[1,19] A serous arthritis similar to that seen in Reiter syndrome has been described in up to 10 percent of the patients 2–5 weeks after the dysenteric illness that characteristically occurs in patients with histocompatibility antigen HLA-B27.[20,21] Culture-positive conjunctivitis during acute shigellosis has also been described and may represent autoinoculation of the conjunctiva analogous to that induced in the guinea pigs in the Sereny test.[22] Arthritis syndromes have also been described after inflammatory colitis with *Yersinia enterocolitica* or *Salmonella enteritidis*, again in association with HLA-B27.

Certain *E. coli* strains may produce an identical syndrome to that seen with acute shigellosis. The incubation period is usually 2–3 days after ingestion. Although invasive *E. coli* organisms appear to be limited to certain serotypes[22,23] (Table 2), to identify invasive *E. coli* one should demonstrate that their invasive potential in the guinea pig conjunctivitis (Sereny) test,[26] in Hela cells,[27] or identify the 120–140 megadalton plasmid that is associated with invasiveness in *Shigella* and invasive *E. coli*.[28–30] Invasive *E. coli* organisms were responsible for a single widespread outbreak of dysentery associated with imported French Camembert cheese.[25,31] While they have been identified as occasional causes of diarrhea in Brazil,[22] invasive *E. coli* do not appear to be frequent causes of sporadic diarrhea in the United States. Because they are often slow to ferment lactose in the laboratory, invasive *E. coli* may be initially mistaken for shigellae,[22,25,32] to which it is closely related. Invasive *E. coli* are also usually lysine-negative and often nonmotile.[33] There is also antigenic relatedness among invasive *E. coli* and *Shigella*.[34]

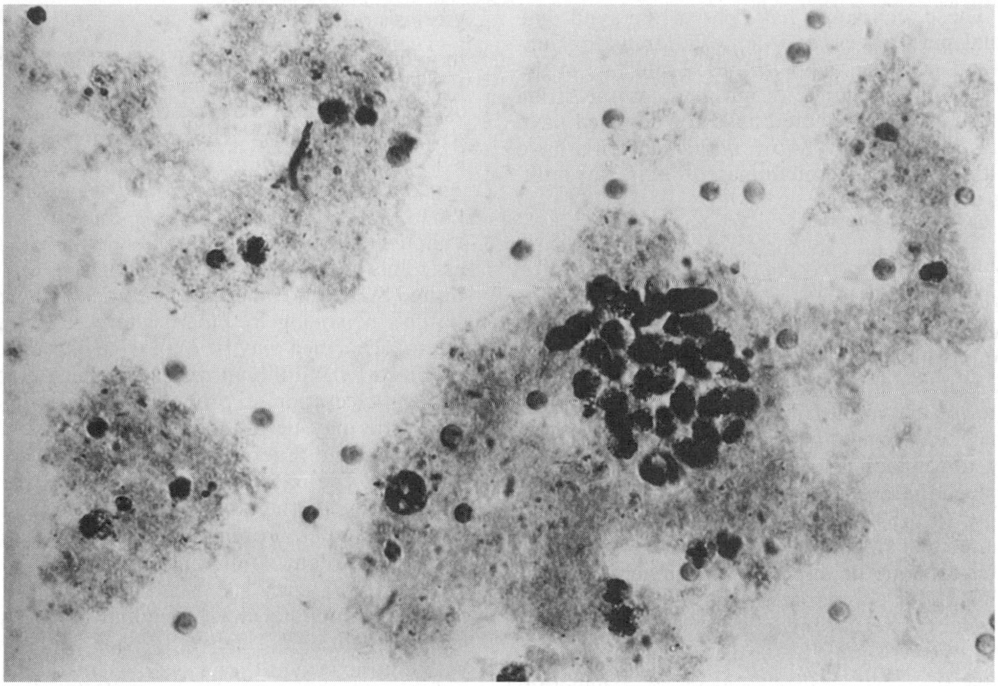

FIG. 1. Methylene blue stain of fecal leukocytes found in colitis. This exudative response may be seen in shigellosis, salmonellosis, *Campylobacter* infection, and colitis due to invasive *E. coli*.

Enterohemorrhagic E. coli Diarrhea

Although the frequency with which it causes inflammatory diarrhea is not clear, a significant cause of bloody diarrhea is now recognized to be enterhemorrhagic *E. coli* (EHEC) that produce relatively large amounts of Shiga-like (Vero) cytotoxin.[2,35] While they account for only 0.8–3.0 percent of all diarrhea in the United States and Canada, EHEC (of serotype 0157) are estimated to account for 15–36 percent of cases of bloody diarrhea.[2,36] The majority of recognized EHEC are of serotype O157; others include O26:K60:H11; O103:H2; O91:H2; O145:H–; O111:K58:H–; O38:H21; O6:H–; O5:H– O128; O139; O113:K75; and O121.[2,24,36] EHEC were the most commonly recognized cause of diarrhea (3 percent) among 5415 patients studied in Calgary in Canada where they showed a summer seasonal peak.[36] In addition to causing 15–36 percent of all cases of bloody diarrhea, including outbreaks of hemorrhagic colitis, EHEC are associated with 75–90 percent of cases of hemolytic-uremic syndrome in North America, a complication that develops in 8 percent of EHEC infections.[2] After binding to a globotriosylceramide receptor, the Shiga-like toxin cleaves adenosine from an *N*-glycoside bond at nucleotide residue 4324 on the 60 S ribosomal RNA to block protein synthesis by inhibiting EF1-dependent aminoacyl t-RNA binding.[2,37,38] The diagnosis is suspected on clinical grounds and confirmed by serotyping sorbitol-negative *E. coli* insolates or by using tissue culture or gene probes to detect the cytotoxin.

TABLE 1. Differential Diagnoses of Acute Dysentery and Inflammatory Enterocolitis

Specific infectious processes
Bacillary dysentery (*Shigella dysenteriae, flexneri, sonnei, boydii; invasive E. coli*)
Campylobacteriosis (*Campylobacter jejuni*)
Amebic dysentery (*Entamoeba histolytica*)
Ciliar dysentery (*Balantidium coli*)
Bilharzial dysentery (*Schistosma japonicum, mansoni*)
Other parasites (*Trichinella spiralis*)
Vibriosis (*Vibrio parahaemolyticus*)
Salmonellosis (*Salmonella typhimurium*)
Typhoid fever (*Salmonella typhi*)
Enteric fever (*Salmonella choleraesuis, paratyphi*)
Yersiniosis (*Yersinia enterocolitica*)
Spirillar dysentery (*Spirillum* sp.)
Proctitis
Gonococcal (*Neisseria gonorrhoeae*)
Herpetic (herpes simplex virus)
Chlamydial (*Chlamydia trachomatis*)
Syphilitic (*Treponema pallidum*)
Other syndromes
Necrotizing enterocolitis of the newborn
Enteritis necroticans
Pseudomembraneous enterocolitis (*Chlamydia difficile*)
Syndromes without known infectious etiology
Idiopathic ulcerative colitis
Crohn's disease

Campylobacter Enteritis

Campylobacter jejuni (formerly *C. fetus* or "*Vibrio fetus*") systemic infections have been recognized for many years. While the majority of *Campylobacter* blood stream infections in humans are with *C. fetus* (old subspecies, *intestinalis*),[39] *Campylobacter jejuni* commonly causes an enteric infection in all ages. This organism was recognized many years ago as a cause of swine dysentery.[40] Commercially available techniques of fecal culture have enabled the culture of *C. jejuni* on highly selective media at 42°C from fecal specimens of patients

TABLE 2. Enteroinvasive *E. coli* Serotypes

Serotype	*Difco Serogroup*	*References*
O28 ac	C	22, 23
O29		24
O112 a, c	C	23
O124	B	22, 23, 25
O136	C (Trabulsi's 193-T-64)	23, 25
O143		23
O144		23, 25
O152	(Trabulsi's 185-T-64)	23, 25
O164		23
O167		24

with diarrhea.[16,41] These techniques have revealed a syndrome of severe abdominal pain, fever, and acute inflammatory enteritis that may result in dysentery with blood and pus in the stools.[41–43] Reports from Belgium, England, and central Africa reveal that 5–14 percent of unselected cases of diarrhea have *C. jejuni*,[42–44] and outbreaks of *Campylobacter* enteritis have been associated with ingestion of contaminated water, raw milk, or uncooked meat or poultry.

Amebic Dysentery

Entamoeba histolytica cysts are ingested, pass through the gastric acidity, and have the capsule digested in the small bowel. Trophozoites then invade the colonic mucosa and produce shallow, flasklike undermining ulcers. The capacity of this parasite to invade tissue may be attributed to histolytic enzymes or products that may be delivered on contact of the ameba with cells[45–48] and may depend on associated viable bacteria.[49,50] Amebae may then seed the liver via the portal vein, from which extension may occur to the skin, diaphragm, lung, or pericardium. While extraintestinal amebiasis occurs with less than one-tenth the frequency of symptomatic intestinal amebic dysentery, dissemination is reportedly more common in states of undernutrition, cytotoxic or steroid medication, late pregnancy, carcinoma, or other overwhelming systemic diseases. Asymptomatic cyst carriage occurs in 1–5 percent of the population in the southern United States. The frequency of amebiasis is greater in rural and lower socioeconomic groups and in institutions where fecal–oral spread of this human parasite may occur.[51] The role of amebic infections that are highly prevalent among promiscuous male homosexuals in producing symptoms or invasive disease remain unclear.[52,53]

Ciliar Dysentery

Balantidium coli is the only ciliate parasite that is pathogenic for humans. The most common reservoir is swine. Like *E. histolytica*, this parasite excysts in the small bowel, invades the terminal ileum and colon, and may cause appendicitis or a dysenteric syndrome with rectosigmoid ulceration (with heaped-up 1.5 to 3 cm ulcers) and secondary bacteremia. However, there is no extraintestinal extension of *B. coli* as one may see with amebiasis. The diagnosis is made by scraping the margin of the ulcer and examining microscopically for the ciliate trophozoite. Mucosal invasion is usually limited to the rectal vault. Symptoms may last for 1–4 weeks and may recur several times a year if the diagnosis is not suspected. Treatment is usually successful with tetracycline.

Bilharzial Dysentery

Schistosomiasis may cause acute bloody diarrhea, abdominal pain, and weight loss when the adult schistosomes (usually *S. japonicum* or *S. mansoni*) migrate to the intestinal tract where they begin egg deposition. This occurs 3–8 weeks after initial skin exposure to the cercariae and may last for several weeks. Fecal examination reveals blood, pus, and numerous ova. Fever, leukocytosis, and increasing eosinophilia may be associated with this illness, and hepatosplenic disease may follow. *S. mansoni* may also cause chronic blood or protein loss via inflammatory "polyps."

Other Parasites

Another potential parasitic cause of inflammatory enteritis is acute trichinosis. Approximately 24 hours after the ingestion of infested pork, the larvae excyst and invade the intestinal mucosa, often resulting in nausea, vomiting, diarrhea, and abdominal pain. This precedes the systemic manifestations of periorbital edema, fever, myositis, and eosinophilia by 1–2 weeks.

Vibriosis

In addition to classic and El Tor *Vibrio cholerae* O1, non-O1 *V. cholerae* and several halophilic *Vibrio* species are now recognized to cause diarrhea and occasional wound or blood stream infections.[54,55] The most common and best characterized is *V. parahaemolyticus*. *Vibrio parahaemolyticus* has been recognized since 1950 in Japan and was identified as a *Vibrio* in 1963. *V. parahaemolyticus* is a cause of seafood poisoning 9–25 hours after the ingestion of inadequately cooked fish or shellfish. This has been reported throughout the coastal areas of the United States and on cruise ships and is the most common cause of food poisoning in Japan where raw seafood is commonly eaten.[56] Diarrhea may be explosive and watery or may be characterized by full-blown dysentery with blood and pus and superficial ulceration on proctoscopic examination.[57,58] The latter syndrome may be associated with cramps, nausea, vomiting, headache, and fever. The illness usually is self-limited within 3–4 days. The pathogenic Kanagawa-positive strains from patients produce β-hemolysis on special (Wagatsuma) medium—in contrast to environmental isolates—and are best isolated as blue-green colonies (alkaline) on thiosulfate citrate bile salt sucrose (TCBS) agar.[14]

Other halophilic vibrios include *V. alginolyticus, fluvialis, hollisase, damsella*, and *vulnificus*, which have been associated with enteric, wound, or systemic infections in humans.[54,55] *V. vulnificus* has been associated with life-threatening septicemia within 24 hours of ingesting raw oysters.[55,59]

Salmonellosis

Salmonella enterocolitis is characterized by fever, cramping, abdominal pain, and diarrhea that begins 8–48 hours after ingestion of an infectious dose, usually with food, and usually lasts 3–5 days. The diarrheal stools of patients with salmonellosis often contain a moderate number of polymorphonuclear leukocytes, usually fewer than is typical of shigellosis.

While salmonella enteritis predominantly involves the lamina propria in the small bowel, several reports have noted colitis due to *S. typhimurium*, with crypt abscesses and erosion and ulcerations of the colonic mucosa that resulting in blood and pus in the stool.[60–64] Certain other strains of salmonella (*S. choleraesuis* and *S. paratyphi*), like *S. typhi*, tend to elicit a mononuclear response and cause a bacteremia characteristic of enteric fever.

Typhoid Fever

Typhoid fever may lead to an erosion of the blood vessels in Peyer's patches that, if untreated, may result in gross blood in the feces in 10–20 percent of the patients. Severe intestinal hemorrhage may compliate approximately 2 percent of the cases late in the course of untreated typhoid fever. Such intestinal bleeding may precede perforation, another complication of typhoid fever.[65]

Yersiniosis

Yersinia enterocolitica is another increasingly recognized enteric pathogen that may be responsible for an enteric feverlike illness, mesenteric adenitis, or an inflammatory ileitis or ulcerative colitis syndrome with fecal neutrophils and mononuclear cells.[66–68] *Yersinia* may also be associated with migratory polyarthritis, Reiter syndrome, or erythema nodosum. A syndrome with acute diarrhea and vomiting is especially common in young children.[69] The organism may cause disseminated abscesses in the liver and spleen[70] or an inflammatory colitis.[71] The causative agent, a gram-negative member of the family Enterobacteriaceae, is in the same genus as the plague bacillus *Y.*

pestis and is sometimes mistaken for *Proteus* on initial culture plates. Cultivation may require "cold enrichment."[15]

Gonococcal Proctitis

Neisseria gonorrhoeae may be the cause of ulcerative proctitis, particularly in male homosexuals who may have acquired this infection by venereal exposure.[7] The resultant purulent proctitis appears with an erythematous friable mucous membrane in the rectal vault and occasional abscess or fistula formation. While copious purulent discharge, tenesmus, and burning rectal pain may be noted, two-thirds of the culture-positive patients with anorectal gonococcal infection are asymptomatic.[72,73]

Spirillar Dysentery

"Spirillar" or "spirochetal" dysentery has been reported to occur in southern France and has been attributed to *Spirillum* species.[74] While severe mucoid diarrhea or dysentery has been associated with intestinal spirochetes, their frequency and role in causing enteric disease is unclear.[75]

Approach to Diagnosis and Treatment of Acute Dysentery

Any of the aforementioned microorganisms may cause an acute dysentery syndrome with blood and pus in the stool; examination for leukocytes may suggest one of the above etiologies even if blood is not present in the stool on gross examination. Other diagnoses to be considered in the differential diagnosis of inflammatory colitis are pseudomembranous enterocolitis, which may be associated with antibiotic use, and the potentially rapidly progressive necrotizing enterocolitis syndromes, which are discussed in the subsequent sections. These diagnoses are suspected by clinical course, history, and radiologic and proctoscopic examination. Noninfectious syndromes that may be manifested with acute inflammatory enterocolitis include idiopathic ulcerative colitis and Crohn's disease.

Presumptive therapy for the inflammatory colitides varies greatly with the suspected etiology (see "Algorithm" in Chapter 81). For example, an acute febrile dysenteric illness in a young child with day care exposure or in an area where shigellosis is common should be treated with an appropriate absorbable antimicrobial agent such as ampicillin or sulfamethoxazole-trimethoprim. If the *Shigella* organism is sensitive, prompt therapy can successfully reduce the diarrhea, systemic symptoms, and shedding of the organisms in the feces.[76–78] Nonabsorbable antibiotics such as colistin or aminoglycosides are ineffective, possibly because they do not prevent the spread of shigellae to adjacent epithelial cells.[79] Because shigellae are increasingly antibiotic resistant,[80,81] one must be familiar with the local resistance pattern of shigellae to appropriately treat acute shigellosis early when it is first suspected. The quinolone antibiotics may offer a considerable advance in treating inflammatory diarrhea. Not only are they effective in treating otherwise resistant shigellosis, but they appear to reduce fecal shedding and the duration of illness with *Campylobacter jejuni* and, in preliminary studies, even *Salmonella* infections.[82,83]

Amebic dysentery is usually diagnosed by direct examination of wet mounts of fresh fecal or proctoscopic specimens, which reveal *E. histolytica* trophozoites or cysts in 60–80 percent of the cases. The cysts and trophozoites are characterized by four or fewer delicate nuclei with central karyosomes. Additional patients may be diagnosed by biopsy, where trophozoites or cysts may be found in the undermining ulcer in the lamina propria, or by a serum indirect hemagglutinating antibody (IHA) test, which is positive in approximately 90 percent of the patients with intestinal amebiasis.[84] While the systemic amebacide metronidazole is effective in eradicating hepatic amebiasis and may eradicate intestinal disease, some would use the lumenocide diiodohydroxyquin to eradicate intestinal infection. The therapy for balantidiasis is tetracycline or diiodohydroxyquin. Praziquantel is used for significant schistosomal infections. The optimal therapies for *V. parahaemolyticus*, *Y. enterocolitica*, and *C. jejuni* infections are not well established and should be tailored to the specific sensitivity pattern of the organism isolated. Gonococcal proctitis may be difficult to eradicate but should first be treated with penicillin or, in areas with significant penicillin resistance (>3 percent), ceftriaxone (250 mg im).

As with all diarrheas, the therapy for *Salmonella* gastroenteritis is supportive fluid management. With the exception of the preliminary experience with ciprofloxacin,[82] oral antibiotics are of no benefit and may actually prolong shedding of the organism and even be associated with increased risk of relapse in children.[85,86]

NECROTIZING ENTEROCOLITIS IN THE NEWBORN

The syndrome of diffuse fulminating necrotizing colitis has been increasingly recognized among infants since reports by Waldhausen et al. in 1963[87] and Mizrahi and colleagues in 1965.[88] This syndrome probably represents the same entity described as "spontaneous" intestinal perforation and peritonitis as early as 1838.[89–91] While milder forms of the syndrome doubtless exist, the syndrome of necrotizing enterocolitis (NEC) is defined by air in the wall of the intestine, portal venous system, or peritoneal cavity or by necrosis of the bowel wall with mucosal sloughing. This fulminant syndrome often leads to intestinal perforation, peritonitis, and bacteremia. It is a major cause of mortality in low-birth-weight infants (<1500 g) after the first week of life.[92] The diffuse necrotic changes that characterize this syndrome most often occur in the terminal ileum but may be seen in the colon or in the proximal portion of the gastrointestinal tract.

The pathogenesis of NEC appears to involve mucosal injury that is most often ischemic from hypoxemic or hypotensive episodes that may occur in premature infants or infants with complicating features such as an umbilical vein exchange transfusion. Ischemia may also result from the effects of endotoxemia followed by the effects of epinephrine, to which the vessels supplying the terminal ileum may be especially sensitive. Other predisposing factors to mucosal ischemia include asphyxia in association with hyaline membrane disease in premature infants or cyanotic heart disease. Increased intraluminal pressures may contribute to ischemia and pneumatosis, a process that may also play a role in previously normal infants who develop necrotizing colitis after protracted periods of diarrhea.[93] Others have suggested a localized Schwarzman reaction to endotoxemia or gram-negative bacteria.[94] The absence of lysozyme (normally present in human breast milk) may allow overgrowth of gram-negative bacilli. McKay and Wahle have reported the association of "enteropathogenic" *E. coli* serotype 0111:B4 with necrotizing enterocolitis.[95] Because of the association with umbilical vein polyvinylchloride catheters and feeding tubes, the toxic effect of plasticizers leached from the polyvinylchloride materials has been suggested.[96] Reports of outbreaks of necrotizing enterocolitis in newborn intensive care units[97–100] have led to a careful search for infectious agents including viral, fungal, or bacterial pathogens.[101–103] Among bacteria, *Pseudomonas*,[88] *Klebsiella*,[101,102] certain *E. coli*,[95,104,105] *Salmonella*,[106] and most recently, *Clostridium butyricum*[99] have been implicated in NEC. The roles of both ischemia and bacteria have been suggested by Barlow et al. with work in an experimental rat model of NEC in which breast milk was also shown to be protective.[107]

Clinical features of this serious condition in newborn infants include apneic spells, vomiting, abdominal distension, and occasionally bloody diarrhea. Most infants are less than 1 week of age, and there is an association with prematurity, maternal infections during delivery (such as anmionitis with prolonged ruptured membranes), and exchange transfusion via the umbilical vein. There is no sexual or seasonal predilection. The disease often progresses rapidly to intestinal perforation, shock, septicemia, and pneumatosis intestinalis. Air may also be evident in the portal venous system or biliary tract on plain roentgenograms. This syndrome is associated with mortality rate that is often in excess of 70 percent.

The diagnosis of NEC should be considered in any premature infant with altered gastrointestinal function, abdominal distension, or apneic spells. It may be further suspected by examination of the stool for occult blood and for the presence of reducing substances.[108] Plain abdominal roentgenograms may reveal air in the bowel wall, peritoneal cavity, or portal venous system, and there may be bloody diarrhea late in the course of the disease. Management must be initiated early and aggressively for any infant suspected of having NEC. Umbilical catheters should be removed, oral feeding should be stopped, and nasogastric aspiration should be initiated. Intravenous fluid therapy is of paramount importance. Laparotomy and excision of the necrotic bowel is often necessary and should be done aggressively if there is any evidence of peritonitis or obstruction.[109]

Prevention of NEC includes avoidance of risk factors and careful infection control measures in newborn intensive care units. Hypertonic elemental formulas have been implicated and should be avoided in high-risk patients.[110] Necrotizing enterocolitis rarely occurs in breast-fed infants. Explanations of the advantage of human breast milk include the presence of lysozyme, antibodies, and cellular elements that may play a protective role against potential infectious agents. While oral prophylactic nonabsorbable antibiotics have been suggested,[111] serious questions remain about the use of prophylactic antibiotics, even in high-risk newborn infants weighing less than 1500 g.[112]

DARMBRAND, PIG-BEL, NECROTIZING ENTERITIS IN ADULTS (ENTERITIS NECROTICANS)

First described as "Darmbrand" (meaning "fire bowels") in epidemics of enteritis necroticans in northern Germany in the immediate postwar period in the mid-1940s,[113] a severe necrotizing jejunitis has also been recognized in both epidemic and sporadic forms after pork feasting in the highlands of New Guinea.[114] "Pig-bel" was the name given to the syndrome of abdominal discomfort that followed a large pork meal, commonly eaten after a large "pig kill," which takes place every 3–10 years among the highland Melanesians of New Guinea. Sporadic cases have been reported from other parts of the world including the United States.[115,116]

The pathologic findings involved are acute patchy, necrotizing disease of the small bowel in previously healthy people that may proceed rapidly to segmental gangrene with small amounts of gas in the mucosa, mesentery, or nodes.

Several theories of pathogenesis have been suggested, most of which involve the toxic products of *C. perfringens* type C, including α- and β-toxins. Sporadic cases of necrotizing enterocolitis have been noted in association with nutritional disorders, alcoholism, and malabsorption and after pancreatic or gastric resection.[117,118] After gastric surgery, increased numbers of *C. perfringens* and α-toxin have been noted in the upper small bowel and stomach.[119] Whether α- or β-toxins are capable of causing the necrotizing enteritis alone or whether they initiate the invasion of the mucosa by other organisms such as gram-negative rods is currently unclear. An attractive hypothesis has been suggested by Lawrence and Walker that could explain the association of necrotizing enteritis with poor nutrition and episodic dietetic overindulgence.[118] The low-protein diet of New Guinea highlanders is associated with low levels of digestive proteases in the intestinal lumen that can be shown to inactivate the β-toxin. The proteases can be further blocked by the oral intake of trypsin inhibitors, which are found in such dietary staples as sweet potatoes. Proteases return with improved diet,[120] as occurred in postwar Germany. This hypothesis has been confirmed in an animal model that required protease inhibitors for symptomatic infection.[121]

The clinical syndromes of necrotizing enteritis range from anorexia, vomiting, severe abdominal pain, and bloody diarrhea to fulminant toxemia and shock. Acute complications that require emergency surgery include paralytic ileus, strangulation, and bowel perforation with peritonitis. These complications are common in the first 2 weeks of illness. Later complications that may also require surgery include scarring that may lead to stenosis, obstruction, malabsorption, or fistulas. Necrotizing enteritis occurs with greater frequency and greater severity in children under 10 years of age. In contrast to European controls, 70 percent of the healthy adults in New Guinea have demonstrable antibody to clostridial β-toxin.[114,118]

The syndrome is defined pathologically but must be suspected in patients who develop severe abdominal pain, bloody diarrhea, ileus, and toxemia. The course is often too fulminant for detection of air in the bowel wall radiologically to be of any diagnostic value.

Etiologic agents held responsible for necrotizing enteritis include *C. perfringens* type C, once designated as type F in the older classification of *Clostridium welchii*. The majority of surgically resected bowel samples with necrotizing enteritis contain *C. perfringens*, over half of which are type C. Furthermore, 12 of 21 cases described had a significant change in serum β-antitoxin titer after illness with "pig-bel" in New Guinea.[114] While polyvalent gas gangrene antiserum was ineffective, administration of type C antiserum resulted in a 30 percent decrease in the need for surgery and a reduced mortality from 43 to 19 percent.[114] Furthermore, active immuization against the β-toxin has also proved effective in preventing "pig-bel."[122]

Others have suggested that type A *C. perfringens*, staphylococci, or even hepatitis virus may be responsible for necrotizing enteritis.[123] The syndrome of "enteritis gravis" has been described in association with infectious hepatitis, although no viral etiology has been documented.

The differential diagnosis of necrotizing enteritis include acute shigellosis, acute food poisoning syndromes, antibiotic-associated pseudomembranous colitis, and acute ulcerative colitis. The absence of colonic involvement, the epidemiologic setting, especially in poorly nourished patients, and the rapid progression to toxemia and shock are strongly suggestive of necrotizing enteritis.

Therapy for necrotizing enteritis includes careful supportive care and bowel decompression. Fluid requirements may be substantially greater than what is indicated by fecal output. Resection of the involved bowel must be considered if there is a persistence of paralytic ileus, a rapid increase in signs of toxemia, localized or diffuse signs of peritonitis, persistent pain, or a palpable mass lesion. If subacute obstruction or malabsorption is suspected on the basis of weight loss, elective surgery may be required up to 6 months after the acute illness. Raw peanut or soybean diets should be avoided since they contain trypsin inhibitors. *C. perfringens* type C antiserum containing β-antitoxin or the active β-toxin vaccine should be available and should be used in areas where necrotizing enteritis may be expected to occur.

PSEUDOMEMBRANOUS ENTEROCOLITIS (C. DIFFICILE COLITIS)

First reported by Coats in 1883[124] and described by Finney as postoperative diphtheritic enteritis in 1893,[125] the syndrome of pseudomembranous enterocolitis has received increasing attention in recent years as different host and etiologic factors have been unraveled. Pettit and colleagues characterized pseudomembranous entercolitis as occurring typically 4–5 days after abdominal surgery, often for colonic obstruction due to a carcinoma.[126] The association of pseudomembranous enterocolitis with antibiotics was first noted by Reiner et al. in 1952.[127] While this disease occurred in the pre-antibiotic era in association with intestinal obstruction, surgery, uremia, pneumonia, myocardial infarction, and sepsis,[128,129] most reports in the last decade have identified an association with the administration of antimicrobial agents, especially those with a broad antianaerobic spectrum. Diarrhea constitutes a major side effect of many antibiotics. From 4 to 50 percent of the patients taking tetracycline, chloramphenicol, penicillin, ampicillin, lincomycin, and clindamycin will develop diarrhea. Furthermore, each of these antibiotics has also been associated with the potentially life-threatening pseudomembranous enterocolitis.

Pseudomembranous enterocolitis is defined by the protoscopic appearance of small 1 to 5 mm raised whitish yellow plaques of "pseudomembrane" that may become confluent and overlie an erythmatous, minimally friable, colonic mucosa (Fig. 2).[130] It is often necessary to remove a thick layer of mucus to identify the characteristic "pseudomembrane." Ulcers and erosions as seen in amebic, bacillary, or ulcerative colitis are usually absent in pseudomembranous enterocolitis. The "pseudomembrane" is composed microscopically of epithelial debris, fibrin, and polymorphonuclear leukocytes and may be found on biopsy if the whole plaque is obtained (Fig. 2).[131] The appearance of filling defects or "thumb printing" on plain and barium roentgenograms is inconstant and not reliable for diagnosis.

The pathogenesis of pseudomembranous enterocolitis associated with surgery, intestinal obstruction, debilitating diseases, or antibiotics undoubtedly involves multiple factors. Theories have ranged from circulatory failure with intravascular coagulation[132] and localized Schwartzman reaction or lumenal obstruction to toxic substances that are ingested or produced in the intestinal tract by microorganisms locally on the bowel mucosa. However, the pathologic changes are quite distinct from the hemorrhagic lesions of ischemic colitis or vasculitic processes. Some antibiotics such as neomycin have direct effects on binding bowel salts that may result in diarrhea.[133] Other antibiotics that inhibit protein synthesis may have direct effects

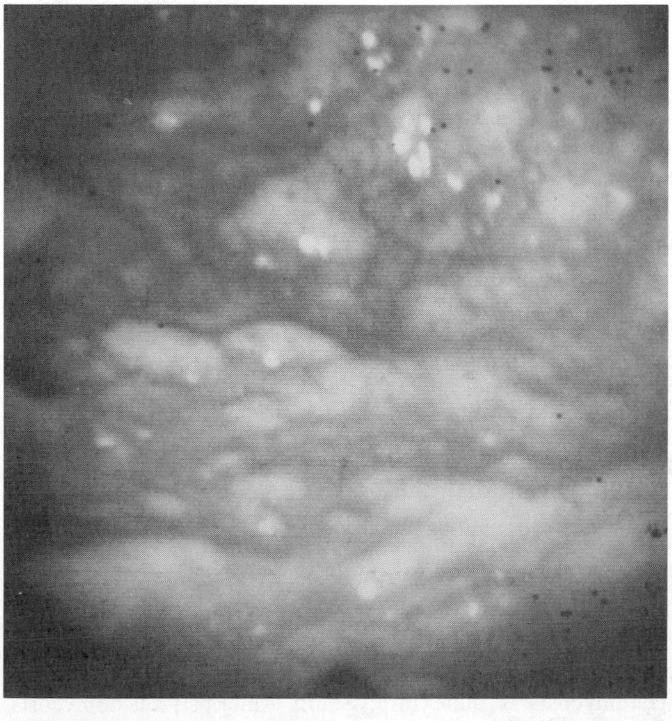

FIG. 2. Proctoscopic view of pseudomembranous colitis in a patient who received clindamycin. Note the 4 to 8 mm raised, white plaques overlying an erythematous mucosa. (From Tedesco et al,[130] with permission.)

on mammalian cells as well. Antibiotics may also induce toxin production by bacteria. Lincomycin enhances enterotoxin productin by *V. cholerae* and enterotoxigenic *E. coli*.[134] Still others have described the appearance of viral particles in the intestinal mucosa of patients with antibiotic-associated colitis.[135] However, the majority of cases involve the alteration of normal bowel flora, especially of anaerobes, which allows the emergence of resistant organisms such as *Clostridium difficile* that are capable of producing cytotoxic substances that alter mucosal function and integrity. While *Candida* often appears in the stools of patients taking broad-spectrum antibiotics and may be associated with diarrhea,[136] a double-blind, controlled trial of antifungal therapy failed to reduce the high frequency of gastrointestinal symptoms with oral tetracycline.[137] Pseudomembranous colitis in humans and animals has been associated with overgrowth of staphylococci in the stool.[138,139] While there is debate about their role in causing colitis,[140] staphylococci are capable of producing a cytotoxic Δ-toxin that causes tissue destruction and cell damage and elicits a net secretory response in animal models.[141]

Most cases of antibiotic-associated pseudomembranous colitis are now associated with cytotoxigenic *C. difficile*[142] (see Chapter 83). Larson et al. reported a nondialyzable heat-labile cytotoxin in the stools of five of six patients with antibiotic-associated pseudomembranous colitis that produced a cytopathic effect.[143] Using a hamster model described by Small in 1968,[144] investigators obtained a heat-labile cytotoxic material from patients with clindamycin-associated pseudomembranous colitis that caused cecal damage and death in hamsters similar to that resulting from administering clindamycin to the animals.[140,141] This effect is neutralized by pentavalent clostridial antiserum, by human immune serum globulin, and by *Clostridium difficile* or *C. sordellii* antiserum but not by specific antisera against *Clostridium perfringens* (*welchii*), *septicum*, *novyi*, or *histolyticum*. Bartlett and colleagues[145] and George et al.[146] have further demonstrated such cytotoxic activity in the broth culture filtrates of strains of *Clostridium difficile* isolated from patients with antibiotic-associated colitis.[147] This organism was described and noted to be pathogenic for guinea pigs and rabbits by Hall and O'Toole in 1935,[148] who found the organism in 4 of 10 newborn infants. Snyder had noted in 1937 that certain strains of this organism produced a thermolabile toxin that was lethal for guinea pigs and that the guinea pigs could be protected with specific antiserum.[149]

The association of pseudomembranous enterocolitis with several antibiotics is well documented.[150,151] Pseudomembranous colitis is said to occur in 0.1–10 percent of the patients given clindamycin irrespective of dose.[152,153] While it occurs more frequently with oral than with parenteral antibiotic, there are several cases in which it has followed intravenous or intramuscular drug administration. There is a slight predominance of females over males and of adults over children in most series. However, children have been reported with the syndrome as well.[154] In one series, clindamycin-associated diarrhea was reported to occur in 46 percent of the patients 60 years old or older.[155] The discrepant incidence figures for pseudomembranous colitis with clindamycin may have their explanation in the apparent clustering of cases in several reports.[156,157] Case clusters suggest that the agent responsible for pseudomembranous colitis may be transmitted in the nosocomial setting.

The onset of clinical illness is usually abrupt, often with fever and abdominal pain. While most patients develop symptoms after receiving antibiotics for 4–9 days, several cases have been reported to begin 2–4 weeks after the discontinuation of clindamycin therapy. Early diagnosis and discontinuation of treatment usually result in resolution of symptoms within 1 week. However, the continuation of the drug or the occurrence of colitis after a full course of antibiotic may lead to diarrhea of 6–10 weeks' duration that may cause severe electrolyte abnormalities and protein loss with significant mortality.

The etiologies of antibiotic-associated diarrhea and of the syndrome pseudomembranous colitis may involve direct effects of antimicrobial agents on gastrointestinal function, effects of antimicrobial agents on microorganisms, or indirect effects of surgery, debilitating disease, or antimicrobial agents on intestinal flora that allow an overgrowth of abnormal, sometimes cytotoxigenic organisms such as staphylococci or clostridia. *Clostridium difficile* colitis is increasingly recognized in immunocompromized patients (those receiving chemotherapy, after marrow transplants, or with human immunodeficiency virus [HIV] infection) and in day care centers or institutions for the elderly.[158]

Any patient who develops diarrhea while taking antibiotics should stop taking the antibiotic immediately if at all possible. If symptoms are severe or persistent or if an inflammatory process is noted by fecal leukocyte examination, one should perform a proctoscopic examination to make the diagnosis of pseudomembranous colitis.

Therapy, after discontinuing treatment with the antibiotic, is mainly supportive. Most patients will improve within a week. The potential risk of *increased* diarrheal symptoms when antimotility drugs are used has been documented with lincomycin-associated colitis.[159] Oral vancomycin or the less expensive metronidazole are used for treating pseudomembranous enterocolitis.[146,160,161] Although vancomycin protects Syrian hamsters against lethal clindamycin-associated enterocolitis,[162] symptoms may recur after vancomycin therapy, and vancomycin itself can cause colitis in experimental animals[163] and should be used only when symptoms persist or worsen. (See Chapter 83 for a complete discussion of diagnosis and therapy.)

CHRONIC INFLAMMATORY PROCESSES

Chronic inflammatory enteritides are often indolent, slowly progressive infections. Often there is a history of weeks or months of fever, abdominal pain, weight loss, or other systemic manifestations. Recurring or relapsing symptoms may be seen with *Campylobacter jejuni* or *Salmonella* gastroenteritis. In addition, 16 percent of cases of shigellosis may become prolonged for 3 weeks or longer.[164] Any diarrheal illness that extends beyond 2 weeks identifies a high-risk child for severe diarrhea and nutritional morbidity in tropical, developing areas.[165]

Chronic E. coli Diarrhea

"Enteropathogenic" *E. coli* organisms that cause acute diarrhea in infants by largely unknown mechanisms may rarely be associated with an insidious persistent or relapsing diarrheal illness.[166] *E. coli* in O groups 1, 2, 4, 7, and 75 that produce hemolysin and necrotoxin have been isolated from patients with ulcerative colitis. These toxic organisms were not present in healthy people or in patients with acute diarrheal syndromes.[167]

Gastrointestinal Tuberculosis

Intestinal tuberculosis, once considered common, has become a relatively rare disease. Intestinal involvement with tuberculosis may be either *primary*, from ingestion of the organism or from spread of miliary tuberculosis, or *secondary*, usually from a pulmonary source.

Primary intestinal tuberculosis without pulmonary disease often results in hypertrophic mucosal changes. Sixty-four percent of the cases of acute miliary tuberculosis may also have gastrointestinal involvement.[168] Primary intestinal tuberculosis may present with abdominal pain, fever, and a tender, fixed palpable mass in the ileocecal area.[169] Primary hypertrophic intestinal tuberculosis continues to occur in the Near East[170] and in India[171] where infection is most often due to the human strain *M tuberculosis*.[172]

Intestinal involvement secondary to pulmonary tuberculosis may result from swallowing infected sputum or from biliary excretion of the organism from an infected liver. The frequency of secondary intestinal tuberculosis increases to 25–80 percent with far-advanced pulmonary disease.[173] Hippocrates stated: "diarrhea attacking a person with phthisis is a mortal symptom."[174]

Tuberculosis may involve any part of the gastrointestinal tract, but most ulcerative and hypertrophic types occur in the ileocecal region where there is a predominance of submucosal lymphatic tissue.[175] The most common features are fever and abdominal pain that is often relieved by defecation or vomiting. Weight loss is more common in secondary intestinal tuberculosis. Only one-third of the patients with gastrointestinal tuberculosis have diarrhea. Diarrhea may be related to exacerbations of abdominal pain and occasionally occurs with extensive involvement of the small intestine that may cause steatorrhea and a malabsorption syndrome. While ulceration and mucous diarrhea are relatively common with secondary intestinal tuberculosis, hemorrhage and the presence of gross blood in the stool are distinctly uncommon, perhaps because of the obliterative endarteritis.

The diagnosis of gastrointestinal tuberculosis may be very difficult radiologically and even histologically. It must be distinguished from regional enteritis, sarcoidosis, actinomycosis, ameboma, carcinoma, and periappendiceal abscess. In contrast to Crohn's disease, gastrointestinal tuberculosis rarely causes anal lesions, fistulas, or perforation; is often associated with miliary nodules on the serosa, rarely causes strictures longer than 3 cm, and may cause circumferential transverse ulcers. Tuberculosis may also cause fibrosis of the muscularis mucosa, pyloric metaplasia, and epithelial regeneration.[176] There may be minimal or no radiologic changes in the bowel mucosa. Small mucosal ulcerations may result in tiny calcified nodules in the mucosa in association with calcified mesenteric lymph nodes analogous to the pulmonary Ghon complex. The ileocecal region often reveals radiologic evidence of irritability and hypermotility, with hypersegmentation of the mucosal folds or poor filling of the ileocecal region detected by barium enema. Occasionally, frank ulcerations can be noted on contrast studies, and late in the course there is scarring. The diagnosis requires a careful examination of involved tissue for acid-fast bacilli by special stain and culture. Caseous necrosis is more frequently found in the mesenteric nodes than in intestinal tissue itself. Complications of intestinal tuberculosis include perforation, peritonitis, and obstruction from either hypertrophy, scarring, or tuberculoma.

Candidiasis

Chronic inflammatory enteritis may be caused by local or disseminated systemic fungal infections, often in association with antibiotic alteration of normal flora or with other host impairment. Candidal involvement of the gastrointestinal tract includes gastric bezoarlike masses after partial gastrectomy.[177] Secondary candidal infection of tumors or ulcerative disease (peptic, amebic, or idiopathic) in the stomach or colon may also occur,[178,179] and *C. albicans* can be seen in over half of patients with diarrhea and the acquired immunodeficiency syndrome (AIDS).[180] Retrosternal pain, dysphagia, or gastrointestinal bleeding in patients with predisposing illnesses should alert one to suspect candidal esophagitis and to proceed with a barium esophagogram and endoscopy for diagnosis.[173]

South American Blastomycosis

While gastrointestinal involvement with the North American blastomycosis is quite rare, South American blastomycosis (*Paracoccidioides brasiliensis*) often presents as lesions of the skin, oral mucosa, or intestinal tract where it causes granulomatous or ulcerative disease.[181] The most common intestinal sites of involvement are the appendix, cecum, and anorectal areas. There is often abscess formation and lymphatic spread to regional nodes and to the spleen, liver, or even the lungs. The major symptoms are abdominal pain and ulcerative, granulomatous lesions, especially in the oropharynx. Palpable, tender abdominal masses in the ileocecal region may be noted on physical examination. Peritoneal signs are often absent. Diagnosis is made by biopsy, stain, and culture of the ulcerative lesion.

Phycomycosis

Other fungi usually involve the intestinal tract only as one feature of disseminated granulomatous disease, some of which may be acquired through a gastrointestinal portal of entry. Phycomycosis (*Absidia, Rhizopus*, and *Mucor* spp.) may invade the predisposed host via the gastrointestinal tract[182] or may involve the gastrointestinal tract by hematogenous spread and cause abdominal pain, diarrhea, gastrointestinal bleeding, and peritonitis.[183]

Histoplasmosis

Histoplasmosis may also involve the intestinal tract as a part of disseminated infection. In the gastrointestinal tract, histoplasmosis presents as ulceration, bleeding, obstruction, or rarely, protein-losing enteropathy.[184–186] Lesions tend to be single and may be considered initially to be neoplastic.

Syphilis

Syphilis can also involve the gastrointestinal tract, usually in the upper part of the small bowel or stomach. An acute erosive and infiltrative gastritis with motile spirochetes and positive specific treponemal immunofluorescence test response has been reported in late secondary syphilis.[187] The initial complaints are upper abdominal pain, vomiting, and weight loss. More classic are the late gastrointestinal manifestations of lues with pyloric obstruction, "hourglass" constriction, or linitis plastica of the stomach. Less commonly, gumma may be seen in the small bowel or colon.

Parasites

Parasitic enteritides that should be considered among causes of chronic inflammatory bowel processes include coccidiosis, chronic or recurrent amebiasis, and the rare invasive, inflammatory form of giardiasis.

Human coccidiosis is an upper small bowel inflammatory process caused by *Isospora belli* that should be considered in patients with obscure chronic diarrhea and eosinophilia,[188,189] especially in AIDS patients.[180,190] Weight loss, fever, headache, and colicky abdominal pain may also be present with steatorrhea and malabsorption. This infection is common in Chile and has occurred in nontraveling United States residents. It is likely that it often is unrecognized. This unicellular sporozoan parasite undergoes asexual schizogony in the intestinal epithelial cells from which merozoites are released. Like malarial plasmodia, the merozoite may then invade other cells and repeat the asexual schizogony cycle or may mature into sexual gametocytes and form a zygote and then a sporulated oocyst that ruptures to yield sporozoites that restart the enterocyte cycle. Sporulated oocysts are the infective form and have caused laboratory-acquired infections. The diagnosis is made by careful examination of multiple serial sections of intestinal biopsy specimens for any stage of the parasite or by examining small bowel contents for oocysts. Stool oocysts may be seen with a modified acid-fast stain as for *Cryptosporidium*[190] or may rarely be demonstrated with some difficulty by incubating a specimen at room temperature for 1–2 days to permit their maturation before examining using a concentration technique such as zinc sulfate flotation. While many therapeutic agents have been used unsuccessfully (including quinacrine, nitrofurantoin, tetracycline, metronadizole), pyramethamine and sulfadiazine in combination have been effective.[189,190]

The related protozoan parasite, *Cryptosporidium*, is a cause of severe chronic diarrhea in immunosuppressed hosts.[190–192] It may also cause diarrhea that is self-limited in normal hosts.[192] Unlike *Isospora*, cryptosporidia usually infect only the surface of the mucosal epithelium, and the process is usually noninflammatory. The organism may be identified by sugar floatation or modified acid-fast stains of fecal specimens.[190,193]

Invasive syndromes may occur over a long period of time or in a recurring pattern with intestinal amebiasis. This syndrome may even extend into an entity called "ulcerative postdysenteric colitis" that may no longer respond to antiamebic therapy.[194]

Inflammatory small bowel disease may occur with unusually severe *Giardia lamblia* infection. This may result in severe villus atrophy, with dense plasma cell infiltration and acute inflammation in the lamina propria.[195]

The differential diagnosis of chronic inflammatory diarrhea includes several syndromes of noninfectious or unknown etiology. Idiopathic inflammatory bowel disease including regional enteritis, granulomatous colitis, and ulcerative colitis may be difficult to distinguish from infectious enteritides. Other processes that often require biopsy and culture to exclude infectious processes are intestinal involvement with sarcoidosis, lymphoma, or carcinoma. Radiation enterocolitis, ischemic colitis, and diverticulitis may also be manifested with chronic inflammatory diarrhea.

Few generalizations can be made about the management of infectious chronic inflammatory enteritides. The causes are so varied that the diagnosis often requires a careful search outside the gastrointestinal tract or surgical biopsy of the involved bowel. Only after the diagnosis is made can specific, effective therapy be instituted.

REFERENCES

1. Keusch GT, Jacewicz M. The pathogenesis of *Shigella* diarrhea. V. Relationship of Shiga enterotoxin, neurotoxin and cytotoxin. J Infect Dis. 1975;131(Suppl):33.
2. Edelman R, Karmali MA, Fleming PA. Summary of the International Symposium and Workshop on Infections due to Verocytotoxin (Shiga-like toxin)-Producing *Escherichia coli*. J Infect Dis. 1988;157:1102–4.
3. Blacklow NR, Dolin R, Fedson DS, et al. Acute infectious nonbacterial gastroenteritis: Etiology and pathogenesis. Ann Intern Med 1972;76:993.
4. Rendtorff RC. The experimental transmission of human intestinal protozoan parasites. Am J Hyg 1954;59:196.
5. Weissman JB, Schmerler A, Gangarosa EJ, et al. Shigellosis in day-care centres. Lancet. 1975;1:88.
6. Roy SK, Speelman P, Butler T, et al. Diarrhea associated with typhoid fever. J Infect Dis. 1985;151:1138–43.
7. Quinn TC, Stamm WE, Goodell SE, et al. The polymicrobial origin of intestinal infections in homosexual men. N Engl J Med. 1983;309:576.
8. Korzeniowski OM, Barada FA, Rouse JD, et al. Value of examination for fecal leukocytes in the early diagnosis of shigellosis. Am J Trop Med Hyg. 1979;28:1031.
9. Pickering LK, DuPont HL, Olarte J, et al. Fecal leukocytes in enteric infections. Am J Clin Pathol. 1977;68:562–5.
10. Haugwout FG. The microscopic diagnosis of the dysenteries at their onset. JAMA. 1924;83:1156.
11. Guerrant RL, Brush JE, Ravdin JI, et al. Interaction between *Entamoeba histolytica* and human polymorphonuclear neutrophils. J Infect Dis. 1981;143:83–93.
12. Speelman P, McGlaughlin R, Kabir I, et al. Differential clinical features and stool findings in shigellosis and amebic dysentery. Trans R Soc Trop Med Hyg. 1987;81:549–51.
13. Rahaman MM, Khan MM, Azi KMS, et al. An outbreak fo dysentery caused by *Shigella dysenteriae* type I on a coral island in the Bay of Bengal. J Infect Dis. 1975;132:15.
14. Feeley JC, Balows A. *Vibrio*. In: Lennette EH, Spaulding EH, Truant JP, eds. Manual of Clinical Microbiology. Washington, DC: American Society for Microbiology; 1974:238–45.
15. Morris GK, Feeley JC, Martin WT, et al. Isolation and identification of *Yersinia enterocolitica*. Public Health Lab. 1977;35:217.

16. Skirrow MB. *Campylobacter enteritis*: A "new" disease. Br Med J 1977;2:9.
17. Koster F, Levin J, Walker L, et al. Hemolytic uremic syndrome after shigellosis. Relation to endotoxemia and circulating immune complexes. N Engl J Med. 1978;298:927.
18. Barrett-Connor E, Connor JD. Extraintestinal manifestations of shigellosis. Am J Gastroenterol. 1970;53:234.
19. Keusch GT, Grady GF, Mata LJ, et al. The pathogenesis of *Shigella* diarrhea. I. Enterotoxin production by *Shigella dysenteriae* 1. J Clin Invest. 1972;51:1212.
20. Calin A, Fries JF. An "experimental" epidemic of Reiter's syndrome revisted. Follow-up evidence on genetic and environmental factors. Ann Intern Med. 1976;84:564.
21. Aho K, Ahvonen P, Alkio P, et al. HLA-27 in reactive arthritis following infection. Ann Rheum Dis. 1975;34(Suppl):29.
22. Trabulsi LR, Fernandes MFR, Zuliani ME. Noval bacterias pathogenicas para o intestino do homen. Rev Inst Med Trop Sao Paulo. 1967;9:31.
23. Ørskov F. Virulence factors of the bacterial cell surface. J Infect Dis. 1978;137:630.
24. Levine MM. *Escherichia coli* that cause diarrhea: Enterotoxigenic, enteropathogenic, enteroinvasive, enterohemorrhagic, and enteroadherent. J Infect Dis. 1987;155:377–89.
25. Tulloch EF Jr, Ryan KJ, Formal SB, et al. Invasive enteropathic *Escherichia coli* dysentery. An outbreak in 28 adults. Ann Intern Med. 1973;79:13.
26. Sereny B. Experimental shigella keratoconjunctivitis: A preliminary report. Acta Microbiol Acad Sci Hung. 1955;2:293.
27. DuPont HL, Formal SB, Hornick R. Pathogenesis of *E. coli* diarrhea. N Engl J Med. 1971;285:1–9.
28. Harris JR, Wachsmuth IK, Davis BF, et al. High molecular weight plasmid correlates with *E. coli* enteroinvasiveness. Infect Immun. 1982;37:1295–8.
29. Sansonetti PS, d'Hauteville H, Ecobiochon C. Moleculare comparison of virulence in *Shigella* and enteroinvasive *E. coli* (Abstract). Ann Microbiol (Paris). 1983;134:295–318.
30. Silva RM, Toledo MRF, Trabulsi LR. Correlation of invasiveness with plasmids in enteroinvasive strains of *E. coli*. J Infect Dis. 1982;146:706.
31. Marier R, Wells JG, Swanson RC, et al. An outbreak of enteropathogenic *Escherichia coli* foodborne disease traced to imported French cheese. Lancet. 1973;2:1376.
32. DuPont HL, Formal SB, Hornick RB, et al. Pathogenesis of Escherichia coli diarrhea. N Engl J Med 1971;285:1.
33. Silva RM, Toledo MRF, Trabulsi LF. Biochemical and cultural characteristics of invasive Escherichia coli. J Clin Microbiol 1980;11:441.
34. Pal T, Pasca S, Emody L, et al. Antigenic relationship among virulent enteroinvasive E. coli, Shigella flexneri and Shigella sonnei detected by ELISA. Lancet. 1983;2:102.
35. O'Brien AD, Newland JW, Miller SF, et al. Shiga-like toxin-converting phages from *Escherichia coli* strains that cause hemorrhagic colitis or infantile diarrhea. Science. 1984;226:694–6.
36. Pai CH, Ahmed N, Lior H, Johnson WM, Sims HV, Woods DE. Epidemiology of sporadic diarrhea due to Verocytotoxin-producing *Escherichia coli*: A two-year prospective study. J Infect Dis. 1988;157:1054–7.
37. Obrig TG, Moran TP, Brown JE. The mode of action of shigatoxin on peptide elongation of eukaryotic protein synthesis. Biochem J. 1987;244:287–94.
38. Takeda Y, Yutsudo T, Igarashi K, Endo Y. Mode of action of Vero toxins (VT1 and VT2) from *Escherichia coli* and of Shiga toxin. p104. Twenty-third US-Japan Joint Conference on Cholera. Williamsberg, Va., 1987.
39. Guerrant RL, Lahita RG, Winn WC, et al. Campylobacteriosis in man: Pathogenic mechanisms and review of 91 bloodstream infections. Am J Med 1978;65:584.
40. Doyle LP. A vibrio associated with swine dysentery. Am J Vet Res. 1944;5:3.
41. Dekeyser P, Gossuin-Detrain M, Butzler JP, et al. Acute enteritis due to related Vibrio: First positive stool cultures. J Infect Dis 1972;125:390.
42. Butzler JP, Dekeyser P, Detrain M, et al. Related vibrio in stools. J Pediatr. 1973;82:493.
43. Blaser MJ, Reller LB. Campylobacter enteritis. N Engl J Med. 1981;305:1444.
44. DeMol P, Bosmans E. Campylobacter enteritis in Central Africa. Lancet. 1978;1:604.
45. Ravdin JI, Croft BY, Guerrant RL. Cytopathogenic mechanisms of Entamoeba histolytica. J Exp Med. 1980;152:377.
46. Lynch EC, Rosenberg IM, Gitler C. An ion-channel forming protein produced by Entamoeba histolytica. EMBO. 1982;1:801.
47. Young JDE, Young TM, Lu LP, et al. Characterization of a membrane poreforming protein from Entamoeba histolytica. J Exp Med. 1982;156:1677.
48. Ravdin JI, Guerrant RL. A review of the parasite cellular mechanisms involved in the pathogenesis of amebiasis. Rev Infect Dis. 1982;4:1185–207.
49. Wittner M, Rosenbaum RM. Role of bacteria in modifying virulence of Entamoeba histolytica: Studies of amebae from axenic cultures. Am J Trop Med Hyg. 1970;19:755.
50. Bracha R, Mirelman D. Virulence of *Entamoeba histolytica* trophozoites. Effects of bacteria, microaerobic conditions and metronidazole. J Exp Med. 1984;160:353.
51. Krogstad DJ, Spencer HC Jr, Healy GR, et al. Amebiasis: Epidemiologic studies in the United States, 1971–1974. Ann Intern Med. 1978;88:89.
52. Kean BH. Venereal amoebiasis. NY State J Med. 1967;76:930.
53. Keystone JS, Keystone DL, Proctor LM. Intestinal parasitic infections in homosexual men: Prevalence, symptoms, and factors in transmission. Can Med Assoc J. 1980;123:512.
54. Blake PA. Disease of humans (other than cholera) caused by vibrios. Annu Rev Microbiol. 1980;34:341.
55. Morris JG, Black RE. Colera and other vibrioses in the United States. N Engl J Med. 1985;312:343.
56. Hughes JM, Boyce JM, Aleen ARMA, et al. *Vibrio parahemoliticus* enterocolitis in Bangladesh: Report of an outbreak. Am J Trop Med Hyg. 1978;27:106.
57. Bolen JL, Zamiska SA, Greenough WB III. Clinical features in enteritis due to *Vibrio parahemolyticus*. Am J Med. 1974;57:638.
58. Barker WH. *Vibrio parahemolyticus* outbreaks in the United States. Lancet. 1974;1:551.
59. Blake PA, Merson MH, Weaver RE, et al. Disease caused by a marine vibrio: Clinical characteristics and epidemiology. N Engl J Med. 1979;300:1.
60. Mandal BK, Mani V. Colonic involvement in salmonellosis. Lancet. 1976;1:887.
61. Thomas M, Tillett H. Colonic involvement in salmonellosis. Lancet. 1976;1:1129.
62. Boyd JF. Colonic involvement in salmonellosis. Lancet. 1976;1:1415.
63. Appelbaum PC, Scragg J, Schonland MM. Colonic involvement in salmonellois. Lancet. 1976;2:102.
64. Radsel-Medvescek A, Zargi R, Acko M, et al. Colonic involvement in salmonellosis. Lancet. 1977;1:601.
65. Rowland HAK. The complications of typhoid fever. J Trop Med Hyg. 1961;64:143.
66. Sonnenwirth AC, Weaver RE. *Yersinia enterocolitica*. N Engl J Med. 1970;283:1468.
67. Black RE, Jackson RJ, Tsai T, et al. Epidemic *Yersinia enterocolitica* infection due to contaminated chocolate milk. N Engl J Med. 1978;298:76.
68. Leino R, Kalliomaki JL. Yersiniosis as an internal disease. Ann Intern Med. 1974;81:458.
69. Ahvonen P. Human yersiniosis in Finland. II. Clinical features. Ann Clin Res. 1972;4:39.
70. Rabson AR, Hallett AF, Koornhof HJ. Generalized *Yersinia enterocolitica* infection. J Infect Dis. 1975;131:447.
71. Bradford WD, Noce PS, Gutman LT. Pathologic features of enteric infection with *Yersinia enterocolitica*. Arch Pathol. 1974;98:7.
72. Kilpatrick AM. Medical intelligence—current concepts: Gonorrheal proctitis. N Engl J Med. 1972;287:967.
73. Klein EJ, Fisher LS, Chow AW. Anorectal gonococcal infection. Ann Intern Med. 1977;86:340.
74. Dantec LE. Dysenterie spirillaire. CR Soc Biol. 1903;55:617.
75. Lee FD, Kraszewski A, Gordon J, et al. Intestinal spirochaetosis. Gut. 1971;12:126.
76. Haltalin KC, Nelson JD, Ring R III, et al. Double-blind treatment study of shigellosis comparing ampicillin, sulfadiazine, and placebo. J Pediatr. 1967;70:970.
77. Tong MJ, Martin DG, Cunningham JJ, et al. Clinical and bacteriological elevation of antibiotic treatment in shigellosis. JAMA. 1970;214:1841.
78. Barada FA, Guerrant RL. Sulfamethoxazole-trimethoprim versus ampicillin in treatment of acute invasive diarrhea in adults. Antimicrob Agents Chemother. 1980;17:961.
79. Osada Y, Une T, Ogawa H. Inhibition of cell to cell transfer of *Shigella* by treatment with some antibiotics. Jpn Microbiol. 1973;17:233.
80. Farrar WE Jr, Eidson M: Antibiotic resistance to *Shigella* mediated by R factors. J Infect Dis. 1971;123:477.
81. Ross S, Controni G, Khan W. Resistance of shigellae to ampicillin and other antibiotics. Its clinical and epidemiological implications. JAMA. 1972;221:45.
82. Pichler HET, Diridl G, Sticklerk, et al. Clinical efficacy of ciprofloxacin compared with placebo in bacterial diarrhea. Am J Med. 1987;82(Suppl 4A):329–32.
83. DuPont HL, Ericsson CD, Robinson A, et al. Current problems in antimicrobial therapy for bacterial enteric infection. Am J Med. 1987;82(Suppl 4A):324–8.
84. Healy GR. Laboratory diagnosis of amebiasis. Bull NY Acad Med. 1971;47:478.
85. Aserkoff B, Bennett JV. Effect of antibiotic therapy in acute salmonellosis on the fecal excretion of salmonellae. N Engl J Med. 1969;281:636.
86. Nelson JD, Jusmiesz H, Jackson LH, et al. Treatment of *Salmonella* gastroenteritis with ampicillin, amoxicillin or placebo. Pediatrics. 1980;65:1125.
87. Waldhausen JA, Herendeen T, King H. Necrotizing colitis of the newborn: Common cause of perforation of the colon. Surgery. 1963;54:365.
88. Mizrahi A, Barlow O, Berdon W, et al. Necrotizing enterocolitis in premature infants. J Pediatr. 1965;66:697
89. Simpson JY. Peritonitis in the fetus in uterus. Edinburgh Med Surg J. 1838;15:390.
90. Genersich A. Bauchfellentzondung beim Neugeboreneh in Folg von Perforation des Ileums. Arch Pathol Anat. 1891;126:485.
91. Thelander HE. Perforation of the gastrointestinal tract of the newborn infant. Am Dis J Child. 1939;58:371.
92. Wilson R, Kanto WP, McCarthy BJ, et al. Epidemiologic characteristics of necrotizing enterocolitis: A population-based study. Am J Epidemiol. 1981;114:880.
93. Fairborn RA. Etiology of necrotising enterocolitis. Lancet. 1977;1:956.
94. Hermann RE. Perforation of the colon from necrotizing colitis in the newborn: Report of a survival and new etiologic concept. Surgery. 1965;58: 436.

95. McKay DG, Wahle GH. Epidemic gastroenteritis due to *Escherichia coli* 0111B4. Arch Pathol. 1955;60:679.
96. Rogers AF, Dunn PM. Intestinal perforation, exchange transfusion and P.V.C. Lancet. 1969;2:1246.
97. Virnig NL, Reynolds JW. Epidemiological aspects of neonatal necrotizing enterocolitis. Am J Dis Child. 1974;128:186.
98. Book LS, Overall JC, Herbst JJ, et al. Clustering of necrotizing enterocolitis. Interruption by infection-control measures. N Engl J Med. 1977;297:984.
99. Howard FM, Flynn DM, Bradley JM, et al. Outbreak of necrotising enterocolitis caused by *Clostridium butyricum*. Lancet. 1977;2:1099.
100. Ryder RW, Buxton AE, Wachsmuth IK. Heat-stable enterotoxigenic *Escherichia coli* and necrotizing enterocolitis: Lack of an association. J Pediatr. 1977;91:302.
101. Olarte J, Ferguson WW, Henderson NI, et al. *Klebsiella* strains isolated from diarrheal infants. Am J Dis Child. 1961;101:763.
102. Frantz ID, L'Heureux P, Engel RR, et al. Necrotizing enterocolitis. J Pediatr. 1975;86:259.
103. Levin SE, Isaacson C. Spontaneous perforation of the colon in the newborn infant. Arch Dis Child. 1960;35:378.
104. Speer ME, Taber LH, Yow MD, et al. Fulminant neonatal sepsis and necrotizing enterocolitis associated with a "nonenteropathogenic" strain of *Escherichia coli*. J Pediatr. 1976;89:91.
105. Drucker MM, Polliack A, Yeivin R, et al. Immunofluorescent demonstration of enteropathogenic *Escherichia coli* in tissue of infants dying with enteritis. Pediatrics. 1970;46:855.
106. Stein H, Beck J, Solomon A, et al. Gastroenteritis with necrotizing enterocolitis in premature babies. Br Med J. 1972;2:616.
107. Barlow B, Santulli TV, Heird WC, et al. An experimental study of acute neonatal enterocolitis—the importance of breast milk. J Pediatr Surg. 1974;9:587.
108. Book LS, Herbst JJ, Jung AL. Carbohydrate malabsorption in necrotizing enterocolitis. Pediatrics. 1975;57:201.
109. Stevenson JK, Oliver TK, Graham CB, et al. Aggressive treatment of neonatal necrotizing enterocolitis: Thirty-eight patients with 25 survivors. J Pediatr Surg. 1971;6:28.
110. Book LS, Herbst JJ, Atherton SO, et al. Necrotizing enterocolitis in low-birth-weight infants fed on elemental formula. J Pediatr. 1975;87:602.
111. Egan EA, Mantilla G, Nelson RM, et al. A prospective controlled trial of oral kanamycin in the prevention of neonatal necrotizing enterocolitis. J Pediatr. 1976;89:467.
112. Nelson JD. Commentary. J Pediatr. 1976;89:471.
113. Hansen K, Jeckeln E, Jochims J, et al. Darmbrand-Enteritis Necroticanss. Stuttgart: Georg Thiem Verlag, 1949.
114. Murrell TGC, Roth L, Egerton J, et al. Pig-bel: Enteritis necroticans. Lancet. 1966;1:217.
115. Patterson M, Rosenbaum HD. Enteritis necroticans. Gastroenterology. 1952;21:110.
116. Fick KA, Wolken AP. Necrotic jejunitis. Lancet. 1949;1:519.
117. Williams MR, Pullan JM. Necrotising enteritis following gastric surgery. Lancet. 1953;2:1013.
118. Lawrence G, Walker PD. Pathogenesis of enteritis necroticans in Papua, New Guinea. Lancet. 1976;1:125.
119. Howie JW, Duncan IBR, Mackie LM. Growth of *Clostridium welchii* in the stomach after partial gastrectomy. Lancet. 1953;2:1018.
120. Kumar R, Banks PA, George PK, et al. Early recovery of exocrine pancreatic function in adult protein-calorie malnutrition. Gastroenterology. 1975;68:1593.
121. Lawrence G, Coake R. Experimental pigbel: The production and pathology of necrotizing enteritis due to *Clostridium welchii* type C in the guinea pig. Br J Exp Pathol. 1980;61:261–71.
122. Lawrence G, Shann F, Frestone DS, et al. Prevention of necrotising enteritis in Papua New Guinea by active immunization. Lancet. 1979;1:227–30.
123. Kravetz RE, Brazenas NV. Viral hepatitis associated with enteritis gravis. Arch Intern Med. 1963;112:179.
124. Coats J. A Manual of Pathology. Philadelphia: Henry C Lea's Sons; 1883:567.
125. Finney JMT. Gastroenterostomy for cicatrizing ulcer of the pylorus. Bull John Hopkins Hosp. 1893;4:53.
126. Pettet JD, Baggenstoss AH, Dearing WH, et al. Postoperative pseudomembranous enterocolitis. Surg Gynecol Obstet. 1954;98:546.
127. Reiner L, Schlesinger MJ, Miller GM. Pseudomembranous colitis following aureomycin and chloramphenicol. Arch Pathol. 1952;54:39.
128. Hardaway RM, McKay DG. Pseudomembranous enterocolitis. Are antibiotics wholly responsible? Arch Surg. 1959;78:446.
129. Goulston SJM, McGovern VJ. Pseudo-membranous colitis. Gut. 1965;6:207.
130. Tedesco FJ, Barton RW, Alpers DH. Clindamycin-associated colitis. Ann Intern Med. 1974;81:429.
131. Sumner HW, Tedesco FJ. Rectal biopsy in clindamycin-associated colitis. Arch Pathol. 1975;99:237.
132. McKay DG, Hardaway RM, Whale GH, et al. Experimental pseudomembranous enterocolitis. Arch Intern Med. 1955;95:779.
133. Antibiotic diarrhea (Editorial). Br Med J. 1975;4:243.
134. Levner M, Wiener FP, Rubin BA. Introduction of *Escherichia coli* and *Vibrio cholerae* enterotoxins by an inhibition of protein synthesis. Infect Immun. 1977;15:132.
135. Steer HW. The pseudomembranous colitis associated with clindamycin therapy—a viral colitis. Gut. 1975;16:695.
136. Kane JG, Chretien JH, Garagusi VF. Diarrhoea caused by *Candida*. Lancet. 1976;1:335.
137. Comparison of side-effects of tetracycline and tetracycline plus nystatin. Report to the Research Committee of the British Tuberculosis Association by the Clinical Trials Subcommittee. Br Med J. 1968;4:411.
138. Dearing WH, Baggenstoss AH, Weed LA. Studies on the relationship of *Staphylococcus aureus* to pseudomembranous enteritis and to postantibiotic enteritis. Gastroenterology. 1960;38:441.
139. Bennett IL, Wood JS Jr, Yardley JH. Staphylococcal pseudomembraneous enterocolitis in chinchillas: A clinico-pathologic study. Trans Assoc Am Physicians. 1956;69:116.
140. Bartlett JG, Gorbach SL. Pseudomembranous enterocolitis (antibiotic-related colitis). Adv Intern Med. 1977;22;455.
141. Kapral FA, O'Brien AD, Ruff PD, et al. Inhibition of water absorption in the intestine by *Staphylococcus aureus* delta toxin. Infect Immun. 1976;13:140.
142. Bartlett JG, Chang TW, Taylor NS, et al. Colitis induced by *Clostridium difficile*. Rev Infect Dis. 1979;1:370.
143. Larson HE, Parry JV, Price AB, et al. Undescribed toxin in pseudomembranous colitis. Br Med J. 1977;1:1246.
144. Small JD. Fatal enterocolitis in hamsters given lincomycin hydrochloride. Lab Anim Care. 1968;18:411.
145. Bartlett JG, Chang TW, Gurwith M, et al. Antibiotic-associated pseudomembranous colitis due to toxin-producing clostridia. N Engl J Med. 1978;298:531.
146. George RH, Symonds JM, Dimock F, et al. Identification of *Clostridium difficile* as a cause of pseusomembranous colitis. Br Med J. 1978;1:695.
147. Rifkin GD, Fekety FR, Silva J, et al. Antibiotic-induced colitis: Implications of a toxin neutralized by *Clostridium sordellii* antitoxin. Lancet. 1977;2:1103.
148. Hall IC, O'Toole E. Intestinal flora in new-born infants with a description of a new pathogenic anaerobe, *Bacillus difficilis*. Am J Dis Child. 1935;49:390.
149. Snyder ML: Further studies on *Bacillus difficilis*. J Infect Dis. 1937;60:223.
150. Silva J, Fekety R, Werk C, et al. Inciting and etiologic agents of colitis. Rev Infect Dis. 1984;6(Suppl):214–21.
151. Aronsson B, Mollby R, Nord CE. Antimicrobial agents and *Clostridium difficile* in acute enteric disease: Epidemiological data from Sweden, 1980–1982. J Infect Dis. 1985;151:476–81.
152. Colitis associated with clindamycin. Med Lett. 1974;16:73.
153. Tedesco FJ, Stanley RJ, Alpers DH. Diagnostic features of clindamycin-associated pseudomembranous colitis. N Engl J Med. 1974;290:841.
154. Buts J-P, Weber AM, Roy CC, et al. Pseudomembranous enterocolitis in childhood. Gastroenterology. 1977;73:823.
155. Tedesco FJ. Clindamycin-associated colitis—review of the clinical spectrum of 47 cases. Am J Digest Dis. 1976;21:26.
156. Kabins SA. Outbreak of clindamycin-associated colitis. Ann Intern Med. 1975;83:830.
157. Keefe EB, Katon RM, Chan TT, et al. Pseudomembranous enterocolitis. Resurgence related to newer antibiotic therapy. West J Med. 1974;121:462.
158. Guerrant RL, Hughes JM, Lima NL, et al. Microbiology of diarrhea in developed and developing countries. Rev Infect Dis. 1989, in press.
159. Novak E, Lee JG, Seckman CE, et al. Unfavorable effect of atropine-diphenoxylate (Lomotil) therapy in lincomycin caused diarrhea. JAMA. 1976;235:1451.
160. Khan MY, Hall WH. Staphylococcal enterocolitis—treatment with oral vancomycin. Ann Intern Med. 1966;65:1.
161. Keighley MRB, Burdon DW, Arabi Y, et al. Randomised controlled trial of vancomycin for pseudomembranous colitis and postoperative diarrhoea. Br Med J. 1978;2:1667.
162. Bartlett JG, Onderdonk AB, Cisneros RL. Clindamycin-associated colitis in hamsters: Protection with vancomycin. Gastroenterology. 1977;73:772.
163. Browne RA, Fekety Jr, Silva J Jr, et al. The protective effect of vancomycin on clindamycin-induced colitis in hamsters. John Hopkins Med J. 1977;141:183.
164. Black RE, Merson MH, Rahaman SMM, et al. Prospective study of bacterial, viral, and parasitic agents associated with diarrhea in rural Bangladesh. J Infect Dis. 1980;142:660.
165. McAuliffe JF, Shields DS, de Souza MA, et al. Prolonged and recurring diarrhea in the northeast of Brazil: Examination of cases from a community-based study. J Pediatr Gastroenterol Nutr. 1986;5:902–6.
166. Nelson JD, Haltalin KC. Accuracy of diagnosis of bacterial diarrheal disease by clinical features. J Pediatr. 1971;78:519.
167. Cooke EM. Properties of strains of *Escherichia coli* isolated from the feces of patients with ulcerative colitis, patients with acute diarrhea and normal persons. J Pathol Bacteriol. 1968;95:101.
168. Cullen JH. Intestinal tuberculosis—a clinic pathologic study. Q Bull Sea View Hosp. 1940;5:143.
169. Davis AA. Hypertrophic intestinal tuberculosis. Surg Gynecol Obstet. 1933;56:907.
170. Hamandi WJ, Thamer MA. Tuberculosis of the bowel in Iraq: A study of 86 cases. Dis Colon Rectum. 1965;8:158.
171. Anand SS. Hypertrophic ileo-cecal tuberculosis in India with a record of fifty hemicolectomies. Ann R Coll Surg Engl. 1956;19:205.
172. Blacklock JWS. Tuberculous diseases in children. Medical Research Council, Spec Rep Ser 1972. London: His Majesty's Stationery Office; 1932.
173. Blumberg A. Pathology of intestinal tuberculosis. J Lab Clin Med. 1928;13:405.

174. Walsh J. Diagnosis of intestinal tuberculosis. Trans Natl Assoc Prev Tuberc London. 1909;5:217.
175. Paustian FF, Monto GL. Tuberculosis of the intestines. In: Bockus HL, ed. Gastroenterology. v. 2. Philadelphia: WB Saunders; 1976:750–77.
176. Tandon HD, Prakach A. Pathology of intestinal tuberculosis and its distinction from Crohn's disease. Gut. 1972;13:260.
177. Borg I, Hejjkenskjold F, Nilehn B, et al. Massive growth of yeasts in resected stomach. Gut. 1966;1:244.
178. Eras P, Goldstein MJ, Sherlock P. *Candida* infection of the gastrointestinal tract. Medicine (*Baltimore*). 1972;51:367.
179. Bensaude A, Breging E. Examen anorecto-sigmoidien au cours des colopathies a *Candida albicans*. Ann Gastroent Hepat. 1972;8:199.
180. Smith PD, Lane C, Gill VJ, et al. Intestinal infections in patients with the acquired immunodeficiency syndrome (AIDS): Etiology and response to therapy. Ann Intern Med. 1988;108:328–33.
181. Restrepo A, Robledo M, Gutierrey F, et al. Paracoccidioidomycosis (South American blastomycosis). Am J Trop Med Hyg. 1970;19:68.
182. Satir AA, Alla MD, Mahgoub S, et al. Systemic phycomycosis. Br Med J. 1971;1:440.
183. Smith JMB. Mycoses of the alimentary tract. Gut. 1969;10:1035.
184. Bank S, Trey C, Gans I, et al. Histoplasmosis of the small bowel with "giant" intestinal villi and secondary protein-losing enteropathy. Am J Med. 1965;39:492.
185. Shull HJ. Human histoplasmosis. Disease with protean manifestations, often with digestive system involvement. Gastroenterology. 1953;25:582.
186. Kirk ME, Lough J, Warner HA. Histoplasma colitis: An electron microscopic study. Gastroenterology. 1971;61:46.
187. Sachar DB, Klein RS, Swerdlow F. Erosive syphilitic gastritis: Dark-field and immunofluorescent diagnosis from biopsy specimen. Ann Intern Med. 1974;80:512.
188. Brandborg LL, Goldberg SB, Breidenbach WC. Human coccidiosis—a possible cause of malabsorption. The life cycle in small-bowel mucosal biopsies as a diagnostic feature. N Engl J Med. 1970;24:1306.
189. Trier JS, Moxey PC, Schimmel EM, et al. Chronic intestinal coccidiosis in man: Intestinal morphology and response to treatment. Gastroenterology. 1974;66:923.
190. Soave R, Johnson WD Jr. *Cryptosporidium* and *Isospora belli* infections. J Infect Dis. 1988;157:225.
191. Tzipori S. Cryptosporidiosis in animals and humans. Microbiol Rev. 1983;47:84.
192. Current WL, Reese NC, Ernst JV, et al. Human cryptosporidiosis in immunocompetent and immunodeficient persons. N Engl J Med. 1983;308:1252.
193. Ma P, Soave R. Three-step stool examination for cryptosporidiosis in homosexual men with protracted watery diarrhea. J Infect Dis. 1983;147:824.
194. Powell SJ, Wilmot AJ. Ulcerative post-dysenteric colitis. Gut. 1966;7:438.
195. Blenkinsopp WK, Gibson JA, Haffenden GP. Giardiasis and severe jejunal abnormality. Lancet. 1978;1:994.

85. ENTERIC FEVER AND OTHER CAUSES OF ABDOMINAL SYMPTOMS WITH FEVER

RICHARD D. PEARSON
RICHARD L. GUERRANT

Several enteric infections are characterized by clinical syndromes of abdominal pain and fever distinct from acute gastroenteritis. The portal of entry of the responsible infectious agents is usually the gastrointestinal tract, but several other infections and some noninfectious conditons may mimic enteric fever. After a systemic phase, these infections may subsequently involve intestinal tissue and are then manifest as one of three clinical syndromes: (*1*) Enteric fever, characterized by sustained fever, headache, abdominal pain, bacteremia, and often skin rash and splenomegaly, is the most serious of these syndromes and may result from infection by several bacteria. A range of systemic bacterial, rickettsial, viral, fungal, and parasitic infections may mimic enteric fever, and these are discussed later in the chapter. (*2*) Mesenteric adenitis, a syndrome that may mimic acute appendicitis, may be caused by several bacteria. (*3*) Eosinophilia, associated with abdominal cramps or diarrhea often accompanied by fever, may be caused by a number of parasites, usually helminths, and several diseases of unknown cause.

This chapter will focus on the differential diagnosis of these syndromes. Important clinical and epidemiologic features, appropriate diagnostic approaches, and antimicrobial therapeutic considerations will be discussed.

ENTERIC FEVER

The classic syndrome of enteric fever is an acute illness, the first typical manifestations of which are fever, headache, abdominal pain, relative bradycardia, splenomegaly, and leukopenia.[1] The prototype of the syndrome is typhoid fever caused by *Salmonella typhi* (see chapter 86), in which fever is present in 75–100 percent of cases[2,3] and is often initially of the remittent type, rising in a stepwise fashion during the first week of illness, after which it becomes sustained.[4,5] Annually, 300–500 cases of typhoid fever are reported in the United States, over half of which are imported, often from Mexico or India.[6,7]

Pathogenesis

Organisms that cause the enteric fever syndrome must be ingested and must survive exposure to gastric acid before gaining access to the small bowel, where they penetrate the intestinal epithelium possibly via microfold (M) cells over Peyer's patches and then multiply in intestinal lymphoid tissue before systemic dissemination via the lymphatic or hematogenous route. Organisms causing enteric fever grow intracellularly, primarily in reticuloendothelial cells in lymph nodes, liver, and spleen. An animal model for this syndrome in which mice are infected orally with *Salmonella enteritidis* has been developed.[8] After multiplication in ileal and distal mesenteric lymphoid tissue, organisms disseminate with the production of microabscesses in the liver and spleen.

Clinical Features

The organisms classically responsible for the enteric fever syndrome is *S. typhi*. Other salmonellae (especially *Salmonella paratyphi* A and B, *S. choleraesuis,* and other salmonella serotypes) may cause a similar clinical illness (Table 1). Other diseases that may mimic enteric fever early in their course and that must be included in the differential diagnosis of enteric fever are also summarized in Table 1; important clinical and epidemiologic clues to these specific diagnoses are indicated.

Symptoms. Classic "typhoidal" fever begins with a remittent fever pattern that becomes sustained over the first few days of illness. The frequencies of reported symptoms from several series of patients infected by *S. typhi* and *S. paratyphi* A and B are summarized in Table 2. Most patients report fever and headache. Although reports from the preantibiotic era suggest that constipation occurs more frequently than diarrhea (79 vs. 43 percent),[5] more recent reports suggest that these symptoms occur with approximately equal frequency[2,9] or that diarrhea may be more common.[10–13] Extraintestinal symptoms reported by patients include cough and conjunctivitis. Although enteric fever caused by salmonellae other than *S. typhi* is usually less severe and of shorter duration than typhoid fever,[14] the syndromes are not sufficiently different to permit clinical separation of the individual case.[9–13]

Physical Findings. In evaluating patients with possible enteric fever syndrome, physical examination should focus on characteristics of the fever curve and accompanying pulse, skin, eyes, oral cavity and oropharynx, chest, abdomen, and lymph

TABLE 1. Clinical, Epidemiologic, and Laboratory Clues to the Causes of Enteric Fever and Conditions That May Mimic Enteric Fever

Etiologic Agent or Disease	*Clinical Clues*	*Epidemiologic Clues*	*Laboratory Clues*
Causes of Enteric Fever			
Salmonella typhi, *Salmonella paratyphi A, B*, *Salmonella choleraesuis*	Relative bradycardia, splenomegaly, rose spots, conjunctivitis	Young adults, travel,[a] exposure to known carrier	Cultures (B, BM, U, F), leukopenia
Yersinia enterocolitica, *Yersinia pseudotuberculosis*	Stigmata of chronic liver disease, arthritis, erythema nodosum	Older adults ± pet exposure	Cultures (B, F. J), serology
Campylobacter fetus	Stigmata or chronic liver disease	Older adults, ± farm or small animal contact	Cultures (B, F), serology
Acute brucellosis	Paucity of physical findings	Occupation (abattoir employee, butcher), animal contact (goats, sheep, cattle), diet (unpasteurized cheese)	Cultures (B, BM), serology, leukopenia
Typhoidal tularemia	Severe prostration, splenomegaly	Animal contact (especially rabbits), vector exposure (ticks)	Serology
Conditions that mimic enteric fever			
Bacterial Infections			
Septicemic plague	Severe prostration	Rodent contact, vector exposure (fleas), travel	Cultures (B), serology
Intestinal anthrax	Severe prostration	Travel,[a] diet (undercooked meat)	Cultures (B, F)
Septicemia melioidosis	Severe prostration, pustular skin lesions	Travel[a]	Cultures (B), serology, chest x-ray
Acute bartonellosis	Severe prostration, renal failure	Travel,[a] vector exposure (sandfly)	Cultures (B), blood smear, acute hemolysis
Leptospirosis	Relative bradycardia, conjunctival suffusion	Occupation (farmers, abattoir and sewer workers, veterinarians), animal contact (especially cattle, dogs) swimming[b]	Cultures (B, CSF, U), serology, hepatorenal dysfunction
Relapsing fever	Fever pattern, conjunctival suffusion, splenomegaly, skin rash	Travel,[a] vector exposure (louse, tick)	Blood smear
Legionellosis	Pneumonia, CNS symptoms	Normal or compromised host	Chest radiogram, purulent sputum, DFA of sputum
Intestinal tuberculosis	Stigmata of tuberculosis	Exposure to known case, ± travel[a] ± diet (unpasteurized milk and milk products), malnourished children	Cultures (S, G, BM, L), x-ray (UGI, SBFT)
Abdominal actinomycosis	Abdominal mass, fistula	Adult males	Culture (FD, A), radiograph (UGI, SBFT)
Intra-abdominal abscess	Spiking daily fever, reduced diaphragmatic excursion, intraabdominal or diaphragmatic pain	Previous surgery, bowel or biliary tract disease	Leukocytosis, computed tomography, gallium scan, sonography, fluoroscopy
Viral Infections			
Hepatitis	Jaundice, arthritis (with hepatitis B)	Exposure to known case, drug abuse, travel[a]	Liver dysfunction, antigen detection
Dengue	Relative bradycardia, conjunctival suffusion, rash, lymphadenopathy	Travel,[a] vector exposure (mosquito)	Culture (B), serology, leukopenia
Infectious mononucleosis	Pharyngitis, lymphadenopathy, splenomegaly, rash	Young adults	Serology, lymphocyte morphology
Rickettsial Infection			
Epidemic typhus	Conjunctival suffusion, rash, severe prostration	Travel,[a] vector exposure (louse)	Serology
Brill-Zinsser disease	Rash	Older adults, remote travel[a] history	Serology
Endemic typhus	Conjunctival suffusion, rash, splenomegaly	Rat contact, vector exposure (flea)	Serology
Scrub typhus	Conjuntival suffusion, rash, lymphadenopathy	Travel,[a] vector exposure (mites)	Serology
Q fever	Pneumonia, hepatitis	Animal contact (especially livestock), ± travel, ± diet (especially unpasteurized milk)	Serology, chest radiograph, liver dysfunction
Mycotic Infections			
Disseminated histoplasmosis	Mucocutaneous lesions, adrenal insufficiency	Travel,[a] animal contact (chicken, birds, bats), hobby (cave exploration)	Culture (B, BM, L, MM), biopsy (BM, L, MM), chest radiograph
Parasitic Infections			
Malaria	Fever pattern, splenomegaly	Travel,[a] vector exposure (mosquito)	Blood smear
Amebiasis	Colitis, liver abscess	Travel[a]	Stool examination, serology, liver scan, sonography, computed tomography, colon biopsy
Babesiosis	Paucity of physical findings	Travel,[a] vector exposure (tick)	Blood smear, serology
Toxoplasmosis	Lymphadenopathy	Animal contact (cat); diet (undercooked pork)	Serology, biopsy (lymph node), lymphocyte morphology
Trichinosis	Periorbital edema, muscle tenderness	Diet (undercooked pork or bear meat)	Serology, eosinophilia, biopsy (muscle)

(*Continued*)

TABLE 1. *(Continued)*

Etiologic Agent or Disease	*Clinical Clues*	*Epidemiologic Clues*	*Laboratory Clues*
Katayama fever (Acute schistosomiasis)	Urticaria, lymphadenopathy	Travel,[a] swimming	Eosinophilia
Visceral larva migrans	Hepatosplenomegaly, rash, bronchospasm, ocular lesions	Young children with history of pica, animal contact (dog, cat)	Serology, biopsy (L), eosinophilia
Noninfectious causes			
Malignancy Hematologic, Intra-abdominal	Adenopathy, anergy, weight loss	Family history or prior malignancy	Sonography, computed tomography, gallium scan, lymphangiography
Vasculitic or granulomatous disease (e.g., sarcoidosis, granulomatous hepatitis, Crohn's disease, Still's disease)	Skin lesions, arthritis, serositis	Family history	Biopsy of involved tissue, serology (ANA, C'), exclusion of other causes

Abbreviations for cultures: B: blood; BM: bone marrow; U: urine; F: feces; J: joint fluid; S: sputum; CSF: cerebrospinal fluid; G: gastric aspirate; L: liver; FD: fistula drainage; A: abscess; T: throat; N: nasal; MM: mucous membrane.
Abbreviations for x-rays: UGI, SBFT: upper gastrointestinal tract with small bowel follow-through.
Abbreviations for serology: ANA: antinuclear antibody; C': complement; DFA: direct fluorescent antibody test.
[a] Travel to endemic areas, either domestic or foreign.
[b] Swimming in contaminated surface water.

nodes. The frequencies of commonly reported physical findings are summarized in Table 2. Fever is present in most series in over 90 percent of the cases. However, bacteriologic confirmation of typhoid fever has been obtained in patients who were afebrile when the culture was obtained.[10,11] Classically, the fever is remittent during the first week, rising in a stepwise fashion in both naturally acquired infection[5] and volunteer studies[4,15]; after the first week, the fever is usually sustained. Deviations from this classic pattern frequently occur, however, particularly in endemic areas. In two studies from India, fever was remittent in 30 and 60 percent of the case, sustained in 22–25 percent, and intermittent in 15–46 percent.[3,12] Relative bradycardia suggests the diagnosis of enteric fever. The presence of rose spots, although not pathognomonic, is extremely helpful in confirming the impression of enteric fever[16]; however, they are observed in less than half of the patients and are even less frequently in dark-skinned people.[5] Rose spots may be observed more frequently in infection caused by *S. typhi* than in other forms of enteric fever.[9,13,17] Conjunctivitis is reported in up to 44 percent of the patients with enteric fever[9] but is usually less common.[5] Pharyngitis is infrequent and is usually not a prominent feature of the illness. Rales or other auscultatory abnormalities in the chest may be present. Abdominal tenderness may be diffuse or localized, most often in the right lower quadrant. Splenomegaly is noted more frequently than heptomegaly. Two physical findings that may be useful in suggesting alternative diagnoses because they are rarely reported in patients with enteric fever are lymphadenopathy and herpes simplex labialis.

TABLE 2. Frequency of Symptoms and Physical Findings in Patients with Enteric Fever

	Typhoid Fever[a] *(%)*	*Paratyphoid A and B*[b] *(%)*
Symptoms		
Fever	39–100	92–100
Headache	43–90	60–100
Nausea	23–36	33–58
Vomiting	24–35	22–45
Abdominal cramps	8–52	29–92
Diarrhea	30–57	17–68
Constipation	10–79	2–29
Cough	11–86	10–68
Physical findings		
Fever	98–100	100
Abdominal tenderness	33–84	6–29
Splenomegaly	23–65	0–74
Hepatomegaly	15–52	16–32
Relative bradycardia	17–50	11–100
Rose spots	2–46	0–3
Rales or rhonchi	4–84	2–87
Epistaxis	1–21	2–13
Meningismus	1–12	0–3

[a] Data from Refs. 2, 3, 5, 9–12.
[b] Data from Refs. 9, 13, 17.

Laboratory Findings. The definitive diagnosis of enteric fever is made by isolating *S. typhi* or another *Salmonella* from blood, bone marrow, stool, or urine. Several cultures of blood, stool, and urine should be obtained from every patient with a syndrome compatible with enteric fever before the initiation of antimicrobial therapy. If multiple blood cultures are obtained, 73–97 percent[5,9] of the cases can be confirmed. Culture of the blood clot after the serum is removed may yield more positive results.[2,9,18] Bone marrow cultures may be positive when blood cultures are negative.[13,19,20] Stool cultures are positive in less than half the patients,[5,19] and urine cultures are even less frequently positive.[5,19] Detection of *S. typhi* antigens in urine by slide coagglutination is a promising rapid diagnostic technique,[21] although lack of specificity may be a problem.[22] When patients have already received antimicrobial therapy, blood cultures may be positive in only 40 percent of the cases. In these cases, cultures of biopsy specimens of rose spots may be useful; these cultures may be positive in nearly two-thirds of the patients, including some who have received previous antimicrobial therapy.[19] Counterimmunoelectrophoresis of serum may reveal circulating *S. typhi* antigen in patients who have received prior antimicrobial therapy.[23,24]

The role of serologic testing (Widal's reaction) in the diagnosis of typhoid fever is controversial. The minimum positive titer must be determined in individual geographic areas and is higher in endemic regions.[10] Cross-reactions occur with both non-*S. typhi* group D salmonellae[25] and salmonellae from other groups .[26] Antibody titers to the O antigen, especially if paired sera demonstrate a fourfold or greater increase, are generally more useful than antibodies to the H antigen that are often elevated after vaccination.[25,27] However, on at least one occasion, antibody titers to the H antigen have been more helpful.[28] Widal's reactions have been reported positive in 46–94 percent of the case of typhoid fever.[3,27,29] The test is most reliable in areas in which data on Widal's titer results in control groups of patients without enteric fever are available; the sensitivity of the test can be improved when diseases such as rheumatoid arthritis associated with false-positive reactions are identified.[27] Although single elevated titers ($O \geq 1{:}40$ and $H \geq 1{:}80$) may suggest the diagnosis of typhoid fever in unvaccinated people in nonendemic areas or in children under 10 years of age in endemic areas,[30] the consensus is that the diagnostic role of Widal's rection is limited.[31] Widal's reaction is not helpful in the diagnosis of enteric fever caused by organisms other than *S. typhi*. The roles of the enzyme-linked immunoabsorbent assay (ELISA) using a cell envelope antigen or lipopolysaccharide (LPS) of *S. typhi*[31–33] or a purified Vi antigen[34,35] and radial counterimmunoelectrophoresis[36] in the serodiagnosis of acute typhoid fever need to be defined.

Additional laboratory tests that may be of value include the white blood cell count and differential, liver function tests, urinalysis, and chest radiograph. Leukopenia is reported in 16–46 percent of the cases.[10,11] In two series, two-thirds of patients had no eosinophils on peripheral smear,[3,9] a finding that may be especially helpful in areas in which parasitic diseases are prevalent and eosinophilia is common. Liver function tests may reveal a mildly elevated bilirubin[9] and a slight to threefold elevation in alkaline phosphatase and transaminase levels in from one-third to two-thirds of the patients[9,11]; on occasion, hepatic manifestations may be prominent.[37] Urinalysis frequently reveals proteinura, pyuria, and casts[5,9]; immune complex glomerulonephritis with red blood cell casts occasionally occurs.[38] Coagulation abnormalities compatible with mild disseminated intravascular coagulation are common, but the syndrome is rarely clinically apparent.[39] Chest radiographic films may reveal pneumonia in 2–11 percent of the cases.[2,5] In patients with diarrhea, a methylene blue stain of a fresh stool specimen for fecal leukocytes may reveal mononuclear cells.[40]

Epidemiology

Certain epidemiologic data may be of value in the diagnosis of enteric fever. Typhoid fever is most common in children and young adults both in the United States[6] and abroad.[9,10] In the United States, cases occur throughout the year. Since humans are the only reservoir for *S. typhi,* history of contact with a known typhoid case or carrier may be extremely useful but is obtained in the minority of cases.[6,7] Over the past 10 years, the proportion of the cases in the United States that were acquired abroad has increased dramatically; during 1977–1979, 62 percent of the cases were acquired abroad, most frequently in Mexico and India.[7] The attack rate was highest for travelers to Pakistan and India.[7] Patients who acquired infection abroad were older than those who acquired disease in the United States.[6] The importance of the microbiology laboratory as a source of domestic *S. typhi* infection has also been recognized.[41,42] In most cases, *S. typhi* had been used for proficiency testing or research.[41] Most patients with enteric fever caused by *S. paratyphi* A or B acquire their infection abroad; *S. paratyphi* B is only occasionally and *S. paratyphi* A is rarely isolated in the United States.

Differential Diagnosis

Enteric Fever-like Syndromes. *Yersinia enterocolitica, Yersinia pseudotuberculosis,* and *Campylobacter fetus* may each produce an enteric fever-like illness characterized by fever, headache, and abdominal pain, which may be clinically indistinguishable from enteric fever caused by *S. typhi* or other salmonellae (see Table 1). However, certain features of these infections may serve to differentiate them from true enteric fever. Acute diarrhea is often a prominent feature of enteric fever-like illnesses caused by *Y. enterocolitica*[43,44] and occasionally *Y. pseudotuberculosis*.[45] Diarrhea is less frequent in enteric fever-like illness caused by *C. fetus*; the acute gastrointestinal symptoms of nausea, vomiting, abdominal cramps, and diarrhea were present in only 27 percent of bacteremic illnesses caused by *C. fetus*.[46] A clue to the diagnosis of *Campylobacter* infection is associated phlebitis.[46,47,48]

The enteric fever-like syndromes caused by *Y. enterocolitica, Y. pseudotuberculosis,* and *C. fetus* more frequently occur in patients with significant underlying disease. Of 31 patients with *Y. enterocolitica* bacteremia for whom information was available 12 had cirrhosis of the liver; 4 others had thalassemia and 1 had kwashiorkor.[44] Only 5 were known to be free of underlying disease. In another series, 5 out of 7 patients with the acute septicemic or typhoidal form of *Y. enterocolitica* infection had evidence of liver disease; in addition all 6 patients with the subacute, localized form of the disease characterized by hepatic and splenic abscesses had cirrhosis of the liver.[43] Of 20 patients with the enteric fever-like syndrome caused by *Y. psuedotuberculosis* 11 had evidence of significant underlying disease; the liver was involved in 10 of these patients.[45] This syndrome has also been reported in a patient with amyloidosis and *Y. pseudotuberculosis* bacteremia.[49] In a series of patients with bacteremic *C. fetus* illness, 73 percent had a significant underlying disease, frequently involving the liver.[46]

Epidemiologic clues in differentiating true enteric fever from these enteric fever-like syndromes include the patient's age, residence, and recent travel history. Patients with *Salmonella*-induced enteric fever are most often less than 30 years of age,[6] whereas the vast majority of patients with non-*Salmonella* enteric fever-like syndromes are over 40.[43–46,50] As in typhoid fever, men are more frequently affected than women. Patients with *Salmonella*-induced enteric fever frequently have a history of recent foreign travel, most often to developing countries. Disease caused by *Y. enterocolitica* and *Y. pseudotuberculosis* appears to be common in Europe, particularly in Scandinavia,[51,52] and in South Africa[41] and is not frequently reported from developing countries. Infections due to both *Y. enterocolitica* and *Y. pseudotuberculosis* may be acquired in the United States as well.[45,53–55] Although bacteremic *C. fetus* infection is relatively rarely documented, the majority of cases have been reported from the United States, and foreign travel has not appeared to be a significant predisposing factor.[46,50]

A pulse–temperature deficit similar to that observed in typhoid fever has been reported in enteric fever-like illness caused by *Y. enterocolitica*[44,55–57] and *Y. pseudotuberculosis*[45,51] but not with *C. fetus*.[46] An additional clue may be provided by the fever pattern. In contrast to *Salmonella*-induced enteric fevers in which sustained fever is common, intermittent fever throughout the illness caused by *Y. enterocolitica* has been reported.[58] Because of the increased frequency of chronic liver disease in patients with these enteric fever-like syndromes, physical examination is more likely to reveal stigmata of chronic liver disease such as spider angiomata, gynecomastia, ascites, and testicular atrophy. In addition, hepatomegaly is frequent and may be more pronounced than in patients with typhoid fever.[44] Both erythema nodosum and polyarthritis occur in patients with illness caused by *Y. enterocolitica* and *Y. pseudotuberculosis*; in one series 55 percent of the patients with yersiniosis had arthritis, and 88 percent of these had multiple joint involvement.[51] Nonsuppurative arthritis is more common in infections caused by *Y. enterocolitica* (43 percent) than in those caused by *Y. pseudotuberculosis* (10 percent).[59] Patients with bacteremic infection caused by *Y. enterocolitica* and *C. fetus* may also have acute septic arthritis,[44,50,55,57] a condition that is infrequently found in patients with classic enteric fever. Erythema nodosum has been reported in 15–24 percent of patients with *Yersinia* and may be slightly more common with *Y. pseudotuberculosis* infection than with *Y. enterocolitica* infection.[51,59] Thrombophlebitis has been reported in patients with *C. fetus* bacteremia and may be an additional diagnostic clue.[60]

As in the *Salmonella* induced enteric fevers, blood cultures are the key to the diagnosis. Each of the three organisms is more frequently isolated from blood than from other specimens.[43–46,50]; the isolation rate from stool cultures may be improved if cold-enrichment techniques are used for *Yersinia*[61] and if special selective media are used for *Campylobacter*.[62,63] However, because of its sensitivity to cephalosporins, *C. fetus* cannot be cultured on commonly used *C. jejuni* selective agars if they contain cephalosporins. In addition, serologic tests are available for documenting infection with *Y. enterocolitica* and *Y. pseudotuberculosis* and appear to be more sensitive and more specific than those for *Salmonella* infection.[52,64] Leukopenia is infrequent in patients with enteric fever-like syndromes; its presence may suggest that *Salmonella* are responsible. Findings on liver, abdominal CT scan, or ultrasound suggestive of hepatic or splenic abscesses may favor the diagnosis of yersioniosis.[43,65] Glomerulitis complicating both typhoid fever and *Y. enterocolitica* has been reported; therefore, the presence of protein, red blood cells, and red blood cell casts in the urine is compatible with either of these syndromes.[38,66]

Patients with typhoidal tularemia may be clinically indistinguishable from those with enteric fever. The epidemiologic history may be of value; a history of rabbit or tick exposure within 7 days before the onset of illness supports the diagnosis of tularemia.[67] Although potentially dangerous, *Francisella tularensis* may be isolated from blood if the appropriate medium is used; serologic tests may confirm the diagnosis of tularemia.

Acute brucellosis may manifest with fever, myalgias, and splenomegaly.[68] As in typhoid fever, white blood cell counts are frequently normal or low. Skin lesions are uncommon in brucellosis. Blood and bone marrow cultures and serologic testing should permit separation of these entities.

Systemic Infections That May Mimic Enteric Fever. A number of other potentially fatal infections such as malaria in travelers or plague in endemic areas such as the southwestern United States may present with fever and abdominal pain or diarrhea and may be initially confused with enteric fever. Similarly, other common extraintestinal infections such as otitis or pneumococcal pneumonia may present with enteric symptoms. These infections are treatable and must be properly considered and diagnosed.

Septicemic plague may mimic enteric fever. The diagnosis of plague may be suggested by the sudden onset and rapid progression of the illness. Epidemiologic history may again provide a clue to the differentiation of these entities; plague is endemic in wild rodents in the southwestern United States, and a history of travel to this area with rodent exposure during the previous 2 weeks would support the diagnosis of plague.[69] In addition, a history of recent foreign travel to countries in which plague is endemic may suggest the diagnosis. Blood cultures, methylene blue stains of peripheral blood,[70] and serologic testing may aid in the separation of these entities.

Intestinal anthrax may be characterized by fever and severe abdominal pain. However, intestinal anthrax is acute in onset and rapid in progression, and patients usually die during the first few days of their illness. A history of ingestion of raw or undercooked meat in an area in which anthrax is endemic should suggest the diagnosis.[71]

Acute septicemic melioidosis may be confused clinically with enteric fever; this disease is endemic in Southeast Asia. Physical findings that may support the diagnosis of septicemic melioidosis are pustular skin lesions.[72] In melioidosis, the chest radiographic film may reveal nodular pulmonary densities. Blood cultures and serologic studies may again permit differentiation of these syndromes.

Acute bartonellosis (Oroya fever) may manifest with fever, headache, and abdominal pain. Since this disease occurs only in certain valleys in the Andes in Peru, Ecuador, and Columbia, a travel history for the preceding month may be helpful in excluding this possibility.[73] Evidence of acute hemolysis may suggest the diagnosis. Since the causative organisms are frequently seen on the stained peripheral blood smear, this procedure may be helpful in ruling out this diagnosis. Since Oroya fever predisposes to *Salmonella* induced bacteremia, both infections may be encountered simultaneously.[74]

Rat-bite fever caused by *Streptobacillus moniliformis* may mimic enteric fever when the rat puncture site is not clinically evident or when the infection is food borne.[75] This illness may also mimic enteric fever-like syndromes since polyarthritis is frequent. History of a recent rat bite may suggest the diagnosis.[75] Cultures of blood and joint fluid may confirm this diagnosis; serologic tests may also be helpful. The other cause of rat-bite fever, *Spirillum minor,* causes subacute fever, headache, nausea, and vomiting, often with an urticarial rash (soduku) 1–4 weeks after an initial rat bite injury that heals with residual regional adenopathy.[76,77] Spirillary fever causes a false-positive serologic test for syphilis in the majority of cases; *Spirillum minor* requires mouse inoculation for its isolation or demonstration of the 2- to 5-μm twisted gram-negative rod in tissue or blood for diagnosis. Like relapsing fever, spirillary fever is often associated with a Herxheimer's reaction when treatment is started with penicillin G.

Leptospirosis frequently manifests with fever and headache and is most frequent in young adults; abdominal pain occurs in approximately 30 percent of cases.[78] Diarrhea and constipation are less frequent. Muscle pain and tenderness occur in nearly 70 percent of the cases, more frequently than in enteric fever. Additional differentiating features are the fever curve and clinical course; leptospirosis is characteristically a biphasic illness.[79] Evidence of liver dysfunction is present in approximately 50 percent of the patients with leptospirosis.[78] Although conjunctival suffusion is characteristic of leptospirosis and is reported in one-third of patients, conjunctivitis occurs in enteric fever as well. Two findings that would favor the diagnosis of leptospirosis are azotemia (26 percent of cases) and cerebrospinal fluid pleocytosis (47 percent of cases).[78] Serologic tests are of value in confirming the diagnosis of leptospirosis.

Relapsing fever due to *Borrelia recurrentis* may simulate enteric fever. The lack of a history of travel during the previous 3 weeks to an area where louse-borne relapsing fever is endemic (Ethiopia, South America, Far East) permits exclusion of this diagnosis. However, tick-borne relapsing fever may be acquired in the western United States.[80] Conjunctivitis, rash, and hepatosplenomegaly are common. However, in contrast to patients with enteric fever, those with tick-borne relapsing fever resolve their fever in a crisis during the first week of their illness.[81] Giemsa or Wright stain of the spirochetes in peripheral blood during a febrile episode may confirm the diagnosis of relapsing fever.

Patients with intestinal tuberculosis may present with fever and findings referable to the gastrointestinal tract. In addition radiologic studies of the terminal ileum may show evidence of a terminal ileitis that can be confused with the terminal ileitis sometimes associated with typhoid fever or *Y. enterocolitica* infection.[82] This disease is currently extremely rare in the United States in the absence of active pulmonary tuberculosis. Abdominal tuberculosis remains an important, treatable disease in developing areas, especially in malnourished children.[83] Evidence of clinical tuberculosis elsewhere or of delayed hypersensitivity to tuberculin would support the diagnosis.

Abdominal actinomycosis may also mimic enteric fever. Physical examination may reveal an abdominal mass; the presence of a draining sinus tract strongly favors this diagnosis.[84]

Intra-abdominal pyogenic abscesses pose difficult diagnostic challenges and remain high on the list of fatal undiagnosed causes of fever of unknown origin.[85] They should be suspected when fever persists or recurs and may be detected by sonography, fluoroscopy of the diaphragms, computed tomography, or gallium scans.

Patients with *Mycoplasma pneumoniae* infection may rarely be confused clinically with those with enteric fever. Fever and headache may be prominent in infection caused by this organism. The presence of pneumonia determined by physical examination or on the chest radiographic film may suggest this diagnosis, although pneumonia may also occur in patients with enteric fever. The presence of bullous myringitis also suggests *M. pneumoniae* infection but is uncommon in naturally acquired infection.[86] The appearance of upper or lower respiratory illness in other members of the patient's family also favors this diagnosis. Serologic studies may be helpful in confirmation of *M. pneumoniae* infection.

Patients with psittacosis frequently have an illness characterized by fever, headache, myalgia, abdominal pain, vomiting, and diarrhea. On physical examination a faint macular rash may be noted; splenomegaly occurs in some patients.[87] A history of exposure to birds may suggest the diagnosis, and serologic testing is helpful in confirmation.

Several rickettsial infections, especially epidemic typhus, Brill-Zinsser disease, endemic typhus, Rocky Mountain spotted fever, scrub typhus, and Q fever are characterized by fever, headache, myalgia, and, except in Q fever, skin rash. Of these, Rocky Mountain spotted fever and endemic typhus are most likely to be encountered in the United States.[88,89] The gastrointestinal manifestations of Rocky Mountain spotted fever include abdominal pain, diarrhea, vomiting and upper gastrointestinal tract bleeding, and an initial diagnosis of appendicitis, cholecystitis, or gastroenteritis is often considered.[90–92] History of recent tick or louse exposure may suggest the diagnosis. Although failure of the characteristic rash to develop may lead to fatal delay in diagnosis and treatment,[93] once the characteristic rashes associated with these illnesses appear, the diagnostic confusion is lessened. Serologic testing may provide documentation of rickettsial infection. In addition, fluorescent antibody techniques may be used to demonstrate the etiologic agent of Rocky Mountain spotted fever in biopsy specimens of involved skin.[94] Q fever may be associated with cat or wild rabbit exposure.[95] Sporadic cases of epidemic typhus associated with flying squirrels have been reported in the United States since 1976.[96,97] The majority of cases have occurred in the southeastern states during the winter months.

Legionella infections in normal or compromised hosts often present with gastrointestinal symptoms of abdominal pain, nausea, vomiting, or diarrhea (usually watery, noninflammatory) in up to 47 percent of patients.[98–100] Patients with disseminated histoplasmosis may have fever, abdominal pain, nausea, vomiting, and diarrhea.[101] The diagnosis may be suggested by the presence of mucous membrane lesions or adrenal insufficiency. Biopsy specimens and cultures of liver, blood, urine, and bone marrow may be useful in confirming the diagnosis.

Several acute viral infections have gastrointestinal manifestations. Abdominal pain, nausea, and vomiting are frequent symptoms in patients with hepatitis. However, the severity of jaundice and extent of transaminase increases are much greater than those observed in enteric fever. Influenza (particularly type B) may manifest with fever, headache, and abdominal pain. Throat cultures and serologic studies may distinguish these illnesses. In dengue, headache, severe myalgias, and leukopenia are common. The maculopapular skin rash that characteristically appears on the trunk on the third to fifth day of illness and subsequently spreads peripherally, the biphasic clinical course, and a history of recent travel to areas in which dengue is endemic may suggest the diagnosis. Infectious mononucleosis may mimic enteric fever, particularly when acute pharyngitis is not a prominent part of the syndrome. Examination of a peripheral blood smear and a heterophil antibody determination are helpful in differentiating this illness from enteric fever.

A number of protozoan and helmintic infections may mimic the enteric fever syndrome. Malaria is endemic in many areas of the world in which enteric fever also occurs. Both may present with fever, headache, abdominal pain, and other gastrointestinal symptoms. Two-thirds of 25 cases of malaria recently reviewed presented with prominent gastrointestinal symptoms (nausea, vomiting, abdominal pain, or diarrhea) that may initially mislead one away from an early diagnosis of malaria.[102] The intermittent fever in malaria is a useful diagnostic clue but may not always be present. Peripheral blood smear may confirm the diagnosis of malaria. Fever chills and hemolytic anemia in an area with the soft tick (nymphal stage of *Ixodes dammini,* the same vector as for Lyme disease) and white-foot mice (*Peromyscus*) or white-tailed deer (*Odocoileus virginianus*) may represent infection with the malaria-like sporozoan *Babesia microti,* especially in an asplenic patient.[103,104] Either intestinal or hepatic amebiasis may mimic acute enteric fever. In patients with hepatic abscesses, documentation of a single abscess cavity somewhat favors the diagnosis of amebiasis.[105] The diagnosis may be confirmed either by demonstration of *Entamoeba histolytica* in stool or colonic mucosal biopsy or by means of the indirect hemagglutination serologic test.

Patients with trichinosis may have fever, headache, myalgias, abdominal pain, and diarrhea; however, the presence of eosinophilia rather than the eosinopenia frequently noted in enteric fever should suggest the diagnosis, which can be confirmed serologically or by muscle biopsy. The history of recent ingestion of raw or undercooked pork may suggest the diagnosis. Patients with acute schistosomiasis (Katayama fever) may be thought to have an enteric fever syndrome. Eosinophilia may again be useful in separating these possibilities; the history of swimming in fresh water during the previous month in areas in which schistosomiasis is endemic also favors this diagnosis. Patients with visceral larva migrans may be confused with those with enteric fever. Patients with visceral larva migrans frequently have fever and hepatomegaly; in more severe infections, splenomegaly, rashes, and pneumonitis may also occur. In contrast to enteric fever, visceral larva migrans is most common in children less than 5 years of age; the diagnosis may be suggested by a history of pica. Serologic tests may confirm the diagnosis of visceral larva migrans.

Noninfectious causes of fever and abdominal pain, such as eosinophilic gastroenteritis, hematologic and other malignancies involving abdominal lymph nodes or organs, and vasculitic and granulomatous diseases, must also be considered. Diagnosis often requires biopsy of involved tissues, scans, serologic tests, or exclusion of other processes.[85] See Chapter 36 for a discussion of the differential diagnosis of fever of unknown origin.

Therapy for Enteric Fever

In some patients with the enteric fever syndrome, antimicrobial therapy may have to be initiated before the diagnosis is documented. Chloramphenicol has been the drug of choice for the treatment of *Salmonella* induced enteric fevers.[106] Alternative drugs are amoxicillin, ampicillin, trimethoprim–sulfamethoxazole, third-generation cephalosporins, and the quinolones.[107–109] Chloramphenicol resistance among *S. typhi* has been reported from Mexico[110] and Southeast Asia[111,112] as well as from the United States, India, and Taiwan. Ampicillin resistance has also been reported, most often from Mexico.[7,113] A patient's recent travel history should be considered before initial empiric antimicrobial therapy is selected. For chloramphenicol-sensitive strains of *S. typhi,* chloramphenicol remains the drug of choice for patients who are seriously ill.[114,115] Strains may occasionally acquire resistance during therapy.[116]

MESENTERIC ADENITIS

Patients with mesenteric adenitis typically have a history of fever and abdominal pain, frequently with localization in the right lower quadrant. The illness closely mimics acute appendicitis. Few data on the incidence of this syndrome are available. In the preantibiotic era, mesenteric adenitis was present in 43 of 2140 patients (2 percent) undergoing appendectomy.[117] In a report from the antibiotic era, 20 of 93 (22 percent) of patients undergoing appendectomy for suspected appendicitis had mesenteric adenitis.[118]

Etiologic Agents and Pathogenesis

In the preantibiotic era, hemolytic streptococci were frequently reported as etiologic agents in this syndrome; in one study, 19 of 36 patients (53 percent) with mesenteric adenitis in whom cultures were obtained grew hemolytic streptococci; 4 (11 percent) grew *Escherichia coli*. Of interest is the fact that 37 of 39 patients (97 percent) had throat cultures positive for hemolytic streptococci, and 35 of these had a history of a recent sore throat.[117] In another report from the preantibiotic era, of 2 patients with mesenteric abscess secondary to suppurative mesenteric adenitis, 1 had enterococci and an unidentified hemolytic bacillus isolated from the abscess, whereas the other had both *Bacteroides* and *Clostridium* species isolated; in both cases the appendix was normal.[119] Hemolytic streptococci appear to be responsible for a few cases of mesenteric adenitis in the antibiotic era as well. Asch et al. reported on one patient from whom β-hemolytic streptococci were isolated from an inflamed mesenteric node and in whom subsequent studies revealed an elevated ASO titer.[120] In another case, both a β-hemolytic streptococcus and a coagulase-positive staphylococcus were isolated from an inflamed mesenteric node in an infant.[120] Of two 9-year-old children, β-hemolytic streptococci were isolated from one and *Staphylococcus aureus* from the other.[121] *Giardia lamblia* has also been reported as a cause of mesenteric adenitis in an adult in Spain.[122] A viral cause has also been suspected for this syndrome; however, 17 well-studied patients in one series had no evidence of viral infection.[118]

At present, the most frequently reported etiologic agents in the syndrome of mesenteric adenitis are *Y. enterocolitica* and *Y. pseudotuberculosis*. Again, few valid data on incidence are available. Of the 20 patients with mesenteric adenitis reported by Mair et al., 17 were adequately studied; 3 (18 percent) had evidence of infection with *Y. pseudotuberculosis*.[118] In another report, 5 of 8 patients (63 percent) who had mesenteric adenitis confirmed at surgery also had serologic evidence of recent *Y. enterocolitica* infection.[123]

In a mouse model after intragastric administration of *Y. enterocolitica*, polymorphonuclear leukocytes appear in Peyer's patches within 24 hours. The infection then spreads to the mesenteric lymph nodes, where abscesses develop.[124] The invasive potential of pathogenic strains of *Y. enterocolitica* has also been demonstrated in HeLa cells in tissue culture[125,126] and in the guinea pig conjunctival (Sereny) test.[126,127] Invasiveness is plasmid-mediated,[128,129] but the correlation of this and other plasmid-mediated traits with the production of human disease is unclear at present.

Clinical Features

Symptoms. *Yersinia enterocolitica* produces a spectrum of disease including acute enterocolitis, terminal ileitis, and mesenteric adenitis. *Yersinia pseudotuberculosis,* which commonly infects animals, is a less frequent cause of human disease. When it infects humans, it usually produces mesenteric adenitis, especially in older children and adults. Patients with mesenteric adenitis have an illness clinically indistinguishable from acute appendicitis.[130] Symptoms reported by ill people in four common-source outbreaks are summarized in Table 3.[131–133] Fever, abdominal pain, vomiting, and diarrhea are frequent. In a series of 37 sporadic cases of *Yersinia*-induced enteritis reported from Belgium, 84 percent of the patients had abdominal pain, 78 percent had diarrhea, 43 percent had fever, and 22 percent reported anorexia; only 13 percent had nausea and 8 percent vomited.[134] Patients with sporadic cases of mesenteric adenitis caused by *Yersinia* may have a history of biphasic illness[135] or experience of similar illnesses in the remote past.[118] Consumption of raw pork in the two weeks before illness has been strikingly associated with *Y. enterocolitica* infection in the most highly endemic country, Belgium.[136]

Physical Examination. Regardless of cause, the clinical syndrome of mesenteric adenitis typically includes fever, right-lower-quadrant tenderness, and rebound tenderness.[59,133] In the setting of a common-source outbreak, rectal tenderness was present in nearly one-third of people examined.[133] In contrast to the enteric fever syndromes, a pulse–temperature deficit is not reported.

Laboratory Findings. Leukocytosis is usually present in patients with mesenteric adenitis[135–140]; white blood cell counts typically are between 10,000 and 15,000/mm^3. A methylene blue examination of fresh feces may reveal polymorphonuclear leukocytes.[141] Blood cultures are rarely positive in this syndrome; however, both *Y. enterocolitica* and *Y. pseudotuberculosis* have been isolated from stool cultures. Frequency of isolation is improved by use of cold enrichment techniques.[61,142] Stool cultures were positive in 56 percent of the hospitalized patients with the syndrome in a recent common-source outbreak[133]; isolation of *Y. pseudotuberculosis* from feces may be less frequent but has been reported.[143] Serologic testing may help in the diagnosis, although agglutinins are rarely present during the first week of illness,[52,134] and cross-reactions can occur with *Brucella* species, *Vibrio* species, and some Enterobacteriaceae. Serologic confirmation was made in 84 percent of the hospitalized patients in one outbreak.[133] The isolation of *Y. enterocolitica* from a stool culture should be considered significant; the organism was isolated from only 1 out of 974 controls in one study and from none of 545 controls in another.[144,145]

Sonographic or radiologic contrast studies of the small bowel may provide a clue to the diagnosis, particularly if ileitis is associated with the mesenteric adenitis. Sonography, using graded compression, may help distinguish appendicitis from mesenteric adenitis. Of 170 patients presenting with a clinical syndrome suggesting acute appendicitis 14 had only enlarged mesenteric nodes with mural thickening of the terminal ileum (without visualization of the appendix); none of the 14 had appendicitis; and 8 (of 9 cultured) had *Y. enterocolitica* in the stool.[146] In a series of 37 adult patients with documented *Y. enterocolitica* infection, 40 percent of whom had symptoms compatible with appendicitis, 21 of the 24 patients studied had a radiologic abnormality of the terminal ileum consisting of coarse mucosal folds in 67 percent, nodularity in 45 percent, and ulceration in 45 percent.[134] Although radiologic studies of the colon were normal in these patients, sigmoidoscopic or colonoscopic examination in 13 revealed evidence of colitis in 6 and aphthoid ulceration in 2, indicating that colonic involvement may occur.[134] In another series of 25 patients with *Yersinia* infection with the clinical diagnosis of acute appendicitis who underwent appendectomy, acute terminal ileitis was confirmed

TABLE 3. Symptoms in Four Outbreaks of Mesenteric Adenitis Caused by *Y. enterocolitica*

Location	Japan (114)	Japan (115)	Japan (115)	United States (116)
Serotype	03	03	03	08
Number ill	198	188	544	38
Percentage with				
Abdominal pain	76	86	64	97
Fever	61	76	50	100
Diarrhea	36	60	32	47
Vomiting	12	4	11	
Percentage undergoing appendectomy	2			42

at surgery. When these patients were examined within 1 week of surgery by a barium contrast study of the small bowel, abnormalities were confined to the distal 20 cm of the ileum. The lesions evolved from an initial nodular pattern to an edematous pattern before resolution within 10 weeks in all cases.[147]

At surgery, patients with mesenteric adenitis may also have evidence of acute appendicitis, but the organ is rarely severely inflamed or ruptured. Patients may also have evidence of acute terminal ileitis.[123,130,137,138,140,147] Culture of the terminal ileum at surgery may yield the organism.[139]

Histopathologic examination of resected mesenteric lymph nodes in cases of *Y. enterocolitica* infection frequently reveals histiocytic infiltration and presence of large pyroninophilic cells; abscesses are typically absent.[148,149] In contrast, although reticulum cell hyperplasia is frequently seen in nodes infected with *Y. pseudotuberculosis*,[118,138,139,150] granulomas, polymorphonuclear leukocyte infiltration, and abscess formation are more frequent.[118,139,148,150] In both infections, tissue Gram's stain may reveal the responsible organisms. Two fatal cases occurred in a *Y. enterocolitica* outbreak among four families in North Carolina.[151] Postmortem examination revealed extensive ulceration and necrosis extending from the stomach or small bowel to the colon. Mesenteric lymph nodes were necrotic in one case, and the sinusoids were filled with leukocytes and mononuclear cells. In the second case, the lymph nodes were large, firm, and edematous. There was reticuloendothelial hyperplasia with abundant histiocytes and plasma cells within the sinusoids.[141]

Epidemiology

Mesenteric adenitis caused by *Y. enterocolitica* or *Y. pseudotuberculosis* is a syndrome of children and young adults,[118] is most frequent in people between 5 and 14 years of age,[59] is more common in boys.[118,144] and is most often encountered during the winter and spring. This seasonal pattern is reported from both the preantibiotic[117] and antibiotic eras.[137,152]

The mode of transmission of *Y. enterocolitica* and *Y. pseudotuberculosis* has not been well defined; outbreaks involving several members of several families[151] have been reported. In these and other episodes of *Yersinia* infection, simultaneous documentation of infection in family pets has been obtained[153]; whether these animals were the source of the human infection or merely acquired the infection simultaneously is unknown. Person-to-person spread to family members does occur.[145] Large common-source outbreaks of mesenteric adenitis have also been reported[131–133,154–155]; in one of these, chocolate milk was the vehicle of transmission.[133] *Yersinia enterocolitica* has been isolated from drinking water,[156,157] but water-borne transmission of these organisms has not been well documented. Results of one study in Wisconsin suggested that *Y. enterocolitica* infection was more common in rural areas.[158]

Differential Diagnosis

The major consideration in the differential diagnosis of mesenteric adenitis is acute appendicitis. Other inflammatory diseases characteristically involving the terminal ileum, such as tuberculosis and actinomycosis, should also be considered. *Angiostrongylus costaricensis* can also produce an appendicitis-like syndrome, but usually is associated with eosinophilia as described below.[159]

Therapy

Mesenteric adenitis is a self-limited illness in the vast majority of cases. Specific antimicrobial therapy is often not required. In patients with the syndrome who are severely ill, the selection of an antimicrobial agent should be based, if possible, on the results of antimicrobial sensitivity tests. When these data are not available, therapeutic agents to be considered include tetracycline, chloramphenicol, trimethoprim–sulfamethoxazole, and third-generation cephalosporins, to which *Y. enterocolitica* is sensitive in vitro.[160,161] The trimethoprim–sulfamethoxazole combination has been shown to be synergistic against 100 percent of 23 human *Y. enterocolitica* isolates.[160] Although *Y. enterocolitica* isolates may also be sensitive in vitro to aminoglycosides[162] these drugs should probably not be the initial choice for treatment of this syndrome because of their toxicity and their reported failure to eradicate effectively systemic infection caused by these organisms.[43] *Y. pseudotuberculosis* is usually sensitive to ampicillin, tetracycline, chloramphenicol, cephalosporins, and aminoglycosides. Persons with septicemic disease should receive antibiotic therapy because of the high mortality.

THE SYNDROME OF ABDOMINAL PAIN AND/OR DIARRHEA WITH EOSINOPHILIA

The differential diagnosis and etiologic considerations for the syndrome of abdominal pain, diarrhea, and eosinophilia as well as useful diagnostic tests are summarized in Table 4. Most cases are caused by helminths. Additional diagnostic considerations include five diseases of unknown cause: eosinophilic gastroenteritis, dermatitis herpetiformis, periarteritis nodosa, regional enteritis, and ulcerative colitis. In addition, lymphomas and some solid tumors may manifest with abdominal pain and eosinophilia. Epidemiologic data, particularly dietary and travel histories, may provide important clues to the diagnosis in patients with this syndrome. Valuable laboratory tests in these patients include examination of stool and small bowel contents for ova and parasites, specific serologic tests, and, in some cases, tissue biopsy and radiologic studies.

Differential Diagnosis

Strongyloides stercoralis is unique among intestinal nematodes in its ability to persist for many years through autoinfection and to produce life-threatening hyperinfection in immunocompromised hosts.[163] It infects people in areas where sanitation is poor. Patients with strongyloidiasis frequently have abdominal pain, diarrhea, or bloating with eosinophilia. In a study of 100 hospitalized adult men, abdominal pain was reported by 79 percent and diarrhea by 36 percent.[164] Pain was most often epigastric, although some patients reported pain in the right-upper and right-lower quadrants and in the periumbilical region. Ninety percent of these patients had eosinophilia. More than 30 cases of severe strongyloidiasis hyperinfection after renal transplantation or in association with Hodgkin's disease or cimetidine use have been reported.[165–167] Hyperinfection is often associated with secondary bacteremia, meningitis, urinary tract infection, or pneumonia due to enteric bacteria.

In the United States, strongyloidiasis is most often found in residents of the southeast, immigrants, or veterans who served in endemic areas. Prolonged infections have been demonstrated in troops and former prisoners of World War II who served in Southeast Asia.[168–171] A prospective study in rural Tennessee documented *S. stercoralis* in 6.1 percent of patients at a Veterans Administration hospital and 2.6 percent of their household contacts.[172] Diagnosis is made by demonstration of larvae in fresh concentrated stool specimens or in duodenal contents obtained either by intestinal intubation or by use of the Enterotest capsule.[173] Serologic tests currently play no role. Eosinophilia is often not present in immunocompromised patients, particularly those taking corticosteroids.[165,166]

Most patients infected with *Ascaris lumbricoides* are asymptomatic. Although ascariasis is not usually associated with diarrhea, severe abdominal pain may occur when patients with heavy worm burdens develop intestinal obstruction, or adult worms occlude the biliary or pancreatic ducts. These compli-

TABLE 4. Etiologic Agents and Useful Laboratory Studies in the Differential Diagnosis of Infectious Causes of the Syndrome of Abdominal Pain and/or Diarrhea with Eosinophilia

Etiologic Agents or Disease	*Stool Examination*	*Small Bowel Fluid Examination or Biopsy*	*Tissue Biopsy*	*Serology*	*Radiologic and Other Studies*
Nematodes					
Strongyloides stercoralis	+	+	−	−	−
Trichinella spiralis	−	−	+(Muscle)	+	−
Ascaris lumbricoides	+	+	−	−	±(Small bowel)
Visceral larva migrans	−	−	+(Liver)	+	−
Anisakiasis	−	+	−	−	+(endoscopy)
Capillaria philippinensis	+	+	−	−	−
Angiostrongylus costaricensis	−	−	+(Ileum, colon)	−	+(UGI series; small bowel)
Trematodes					
Schistosomiasis	+	−	+(Rectum)	+	−
Fasciola hepatica	+	−	−	−	−
Fasciolopsis buski	+	−	−	−	−
Clonorchis sinensis	+	−	−	−	±(Biliary tract abnormalities)
Opisthorchis species	+	−	−		±(Biliary tract abnormalities)
Cestodes					
Echinococcosis	−	−	−	±	+(Chest radiograph, abdominal ultrasound or CT scan)
Protozoa					
Isospora belli	+	+	−	−	−
Dientamoeba fragilis	+	−	−	−	−
Diseases of unknown etiology					
Eosinophilic gastroenteritis	−	+	−	−	+(UGI series; small bowel)
Periarteritis nodosa	−	−	+(Skin, muscle, kidney)	−	+(Angiography)
Inflammatory bowel disease	−	−	+(Colon)	−	+(Small bowel, colonoscopy)
Malignancies	−	±	+(Lymph nodes, liver, bone marrow)	−	+(UGI Series, barium enema, CT scan)

Key: +: feature present; −: feature absent.

cations are most frequent in young children.[174–175] Ascariasis is most common in areas in which sanitation is poor; the eggs may be ingested in contaminated food or water or, by children, in dirt. In the United States, this infection is most common in the southeastern states,[174] but symptomatic infections are rare. The diagnosis is made by demonstration of the typical eggs in stool specimens. Eosinophilia may or may not be present. Since a single worm produces large numbers of eggs, concentration of feces is not necessary. In patients with intestinal or biliary tract obstruction, radiologic studies and liver or pancreatic enzyme elevations may provide a clue to the diagnosis.

Patients with toxocariasis (visceral larva migrans) caused by animal nematodes such as *Toxocara canis* or *Toxocara cati* may have abdominal pain and eosinophilia. In temperate climates, *T. canis* is the more important etiologic agent.[176] The abdominal pain may be associated with the presence of tender hepatomegaly. Clinical clues to the diagnosis include the simultaneous occurrence of splenomegaly or pneumonitis with bronchospasm.[177–179] Patients may have pruritic rashes on the trunk or lower extremities. The presence of a granuloma in the ocular fundus or other evidence of ocular inflammation, high titers of isoagglutinins, and hypergammaglobulinemia provide additional diagnostic clues. The total white count is often elevated, and eosinophils may exceed 50 percent. Patients are usually young children; additional epidemiologic clues are a history of pica or close contact with dogs or cats. Between 10 and 30 percent of the soil samples in public playgrounds and parks in the United States have been found to be contaminated with *Toxocara* eggs.[176] Serologic tests are available; an ELISA seems to be the most sensitive and specific.[177–179] On occasion, larvae are identified in biopsies of hepatic granulomas.

Infection with *Trichinella spiralis* may be characterized initially by diarrhea, which occurs in approximately 40 percent of the cases; abdominal pain, which occurs in approximately 20 percent; or even by constipation.[180,181] The intestinal symptoms are attributed to the presence of adult worms or invading larvae in the intestinal tract, occur during the first week of illness, and may precede the appearance of eosinophilia. Approximately 100 cases are reported annually in the United States.[182] Infection occurs by the ingestion of raw or undercooked pork or pork products such as sausage, bear meat, and horse meat, and occasionally by other vehicles such as ground beef contaminated during processing with pork.[181–185] Prolonged diarrhea has been the dominant symptom among Inuit inhabitants of northern Canada who acquired *Trichinella nativa* from contaminated, uncooked walrus meat. Myalgia and muscle weakness were less prominent complaints.[186] The presence of myalgias, periorbital edema, muscle tenderness, splinter hemorrhages, and evidence of myocarditis or central nervous system involvement may suggest the diagnosis. The diagnosis may be confirmed serologically with either the bentonite flocculation or immunofluorescence test, which typically do not become positive until several weeks into infection.[187] Definitive diagnosis may be made by demonstration of larvae in specimens from a muscle biopsy, but biopsy is seldom necessary.

Patients with anisakiasis caused by nematodes of the family Anisakidae, ascarid parasites of marine animals, may have an acute illness characterized by epigastric pain, nausea, and vomiting or more commonly a chronic illness characterized by abdominal pain and fever. The disease is caused by larvae that penetrate the gastrointestinal tract. The stomach, small bowel, and colon may be involved. Necrotizing eosinophilic granulomatous inflammation with peripheral eosinophilia may occur.[188] The pathologic and radiologic manifestations may resemble regional enteritis[189]; mass lesions resembling malignancies may also occur.[190] The disease is rarely reported in the United States and is most common in the Netherlands and Japan. The infection is acquired by the ingestion of raw or undercooked marine fish such as cod, salmon, and herring. In Japan, raw or pickled marine fish are common vehicles; in the Netherlands, raw or slightly salted herring is the most common source of infection.[188] Therefore, a travel or a dietary history may suggest the diagnosis. Confirmation is obtained by identification of the larvae by endoscopy or in tissue specimens.

Patients with capillariasis typically give a history of several weeks of vague abdominal pain followed by voluminous watery diarrhea. The illness is characterized by a protein-losing enteropathy and malabsorption. Electrolyte abnormalities and hypoproteinemia are common. Weight loss, muscle wasting, weakness, hyporeflexia, and edema occur.[191,192] The worms are found in the small bowel, especially in the jejunum, and the adults are partially embedded in the mucosa.[193] The intestinal villi are flattened in focal areas.[193] The disease is most common in the Philippines; a few cases have also been reported from Thailand. Although the epidemiology of the disease has not been completely characterized, freshwater fish eaten raw or poorly cooked appear to be the vehicle of transmission.[194] The diagnosis is made by demonstration of the typical eggs of *Capillaria philippinensis* in fecal specimens. The finding of eggs, adult worms, and larvae in the small bowel contents suggest that autoinfection may occur.[193,194] Travel and dietary histories may provide a clue to the diagnosis.

Angiostrongylus costaricensis lives in the lumen of mesenteric arteries of the ileocecal region of rodents and occasionally involves the same site in humans. Eggs form emboli to terminal branches of the mesenteric arteries, where they hatch and invade the intestinal wall. Disease, usually encountered in children, may present as an acute abdominal infection with fever, nausea, vomiting, pain, and sometimes a right lower quadrant mass. Leukocytosis and eosinophilia (11–82 percent) are usually present. It may be impossible to distinguish infection with *A. costaricensis* from acute appendicitis.[159] Other patients experience a visceral larva migrans-like syndrome.[195] Humans are thought to become infected by ingesting material contaminated by infected slugs or snails, which are intermediate hosts. *Angiostrongylus costaricensis* is found in areas of Central and South America.

Patients with trematode infection may occasionally have a syndrome characterized by abdominal pain and/or diarrhea and eosinophilia. Katayama fever, a clinical syndrome characterized by fever, headache, diarrhea, hepatosplenomegaly, generalized lymphadenopathy, urticaria, and eosinophilia, may occur within 4–8 weeks after primary exposure to schistosomes. This syndrome is most common in the presence of heavy infections and occurs most frequently with *Schistosoma japonicum* infection, less frequently with *Schistosoma mansoni* infection, and very rarely with *Schistosoma haematobium* infection.[196] This acute manifestation of schistosomiasis is usually self-limited, although deaths may occur. The diagnosis may be suspected in patients with a serum sickness-like illness accompanied by eosinophilia who have had exposure during the previous 4–8 weeks, through swimming or bathing, to fresh water in an area in which schistosomiasis is endemic.[197,198] As *S. japonicum* is found mainly in China, Japan, and Southeast Asia,[197] a history of recent travel to these areas would suggest the diagnosis. Diagnosis is made by demonstration of the characteristic eggs in either a Kato thick smear of feces[196] or a rectal biopsy specimen. Serologic tests provide suggestive evidence of infection.

Acute infection with the liver fluke *Fasciola hepatica*, which is found in many sheep raising areas of the world, is often characterized by fever and pain in the right upper quadrant, hepatomegaly, and often marked eosinophilia.[199–201] Human infections are acquired by ingestion of encysted metacercariae on aquatic plants such as wild watercress. Infections have been reported from South America, Africa, Europe, China, and Australia. The laboratory diagnosis is based on identification of characteristic ova in the feces or bile. Concentration techniques increase the likelihood of finding eggs.

Another trematode that may be associated with abdominal pain or diarrhea and eosinophilia is the intestinal fluke *Fasciolopsis buski*. Although infection with *F. buski* is usually asymptomatic, patients with heavy infections may have both abdominal pain and diarrhea.[202,203] The diagnosis may be suggested by a history of travel to the Far East and Southeast Asia, where the disease is endemic.[203] Infection is acquired through the ingestion of water chestnuts or the peeling of other freshwater plants with the teeth before ingestion. Diagnosis is made by demonstration of *F. buski* eggs in feces and usually requires a concentration technique.[203]

Acute infections with the liver flukes, *Clonorchis sinensis* and *Opisthorchis* species, may be associated with fever, abdominal pain, diarrhea, hepatomegaly, and eosinophilia. Although at increased risk of ascending cholangitis and cholangiocarcinoma, persons with established infection are usually free of specific symptoms and eosinophilia.[204,205]

Abdominal pain and/or diarrhea and eosinophilia are very uncommon in cestode (tapeworm) infections.[206] Eosinophilia may occur in conjunction with abdominal pain in a few patients with echinococcosis when cysts rupture. Laboratory studies may reveal a cystic lesion(s), in the liver, or other organs. The diagnosis should be suspected in patients who have lived in or traveled to areas in which the disease is endemic. In the United States, endemic areas include California, Utah, and Alaska. Other endemic areas include sheep and cattle raising areas of Australia, South America, South Africa, the Soviet Union, and Mediterranean countries.[207] The diagnosis is usually made on the basis of radiologic or ultrasound findings and serologic tests.[208]

Patients with protozoal infections (e.g., *Entamoeba histolytica*) typically do not have eosinophilia. *Isospora belli* is an important exception.[209,210] It can cause abdominal pain, watery diarrhea, and malabsorption in association with eosinophilia. The disease occurs throughout the world, but it is most prevalent in the tropics where sanitation is poor. In healthy adults, *Isospora belli* produces a self-limited disease. The diagnosis may be suggested by an appropriate history of travel. *Isospora belli* is an important cause of severe, chronic diarrhea and weight loss in Haitians with acquired immunodeficiency syndrome (AIDS).[211] Infection has been documented in a few patients with AIDS in the United States.

The diagnosis of *Isospora belli* is established by the demonstration of oocysts in feces[211]; concentration techniques may be necessary. Examination of duodenal contents or small bowel biopsy specimens are more sensitive diagnostic techniques. Mucosal abnormalities are frequently seen on small bowel biopsy specimens and include blunted villus tips, shortened villi, hypertrophied crypts, and eosinophilic infiltration of the lamina propria.[209] *Dientamoeba fragilis* is another protozoan that can cause diarrhea and abdominal discomfort and has been associated with eosinophilia.[212,213]

Eosinophilic gastroenteritis is a disease of adults with protean clinical manifestations that may include abdominal pain, diarrhea, gastrointestinal bleeding, protein-losing enteropathy, a malabsorption syndrome, and gastric outlet obstruction.[214] Manifestations depend both on the part of bowel involved (stomach, duodenum, jejunum, or ileum) and on the layer of bowel involved (mucosa, muscular layer, or submucosa). The stomach and small intestine are the most common sites of involvement, but eosinophilic ileocolitis has also been reported.[215] Patients frequently have a history compatible with an allergic diathesis.[216] The sedimentation rate is usually normal or mildly elevated. Additional clues to the diagnosis include peripheral blood eosinophilia and presence of Charcot-Leyden crystals in stools.[216–217] Radiologic studies may reveal polypoid gastric or duodenal mucosal folds and rigid dilated loops of jejunum with a sawtooth mucosal pattern.[218] Diagnosis may be made by peroral or endoscopic biopsy. Histologic examination of involved tissue reveals eosinophilia in the absence of both granulomas and vasculitis.[216] Since the involvement may be patchy, multiple biopsies are usually required. All biopsies may be negative if the disease involves only the muscular or subserosal layers. In the latter case, the presence of eosinophils in ascitic fluid may suggest the diagnosis.[216] The disease is chronic and occasionally fatal,[219] but most patients respond to corticosteroid therapy.[214,216]

Gastrointestinal involvement with eosinophilia may occur as manifestations of vasculitis.[220–224] Gastrointestinal involvement appears in up to 25 percent of the patients with periarteritis nodosa and may be the initial manifestation of the disease in 15 percent of the patients.[215,221,222] Abdominal pain is a prominent symptom, and eosinophilia is frequent. The clue to the diagnosis, which may be confirmed by biopsy or angiography, is provided by the systemic nature of the disease with frequent involvement of the kidneys, heart, musculoskeletal, and nervous systems. In allergic angiitis and granulomatosis of the Churg-Strauss syndrome type, lung involvement is pronounced, patients manifest prominent eosinophilia, and there is a strong allergic diathesis, often with asthma.[220] Some of the patients with this syndrome also have abdominal involvement and have been classified as having a polyangiitis overlap syndrome.[223,224]

Abdominal pain and diarrhea accompanied by eosinophilia may occur in patients with regional enteritis, Whipple's disease, and ulcerative colitis.[225] In one series, 32 percent of the patients with radiologically or surgically proven regional enteritis had eosinophilia on more than one occasion.[226] The average elevated eosinophil count was 6.2 percent; the range was from 4 to 22 percent.[226] The characteristic extraintestinal manifestations in patients with these inflammatory bowel diseases may provide clues to their diagnosis.[227]

Patients with solid tumors and lymphomas may also have abdominal pain and eosinopilia.[225] Eosinophilia is most commonly associated with solid tumors after metastasis has occurred.[228,229] Among these solid tumors, frequently implicated malignancies are gastric, colonic, lung, pancreatic, and uterine carcinomas.[228,230] A history of weight loss and the presence of melena or guaiac positive stools and anemia may suggest the diagnosis, which may be confirmed by appropriate radiographic, endoscopic, or cytologic studies. Both Hodgkin's disease and non-Hodgkin's lymphomas may also be associated with eosinophilia and abdominal pain when abdominal or retroperitoneal nodes are involved.

REFERENCES

1. Christie AB. Typhoid and paratyphoid fevers. In: Infectious Diseases: Epidemiology and Clinical Practice, 2nd ed. Churchill Livingstone; New York: 1974:55–130.
2. Walker W, ed. The Aberdeen typhoid outbreak of 1964. Scott Med J 1965;10:466–79.
3. Gulati PD, Saxena SN, Gupta PS, et al. Changing pattern of typhoid fever. Am J Med. 1968;45:544–8.
4. Hornick RB, Greisman SE, Woodward TE, et al. Typhoid fever: Pathogenesis and immunologic control. N Engl J Med. 1970;283:686–91.
5. Stuart BM, Pullen RL: Typhoid, Clinical analysis of three hundred and sixty cases. Arch Intern Med. 1946;78:629–61.
6. Rice PA, Baine WB, Gangarosa EJ. *Salmonella typhi* infections in the United States, 1967–1972: Increasing importance of international travelers. Am J Epidemiol. 1977;106:160–6.
7. Taylor DN, Pollard RA, Blake PA. Typhoid fever in the United States and the risk to international travelers. J Infect Dis. 1983;148:599–602.
8. Carter PB, Collins FM. The route of enteric infection in normal mice. J Exp Med. 1974;139:1189–1203.
9. Kamat SA, Herzog C. Typhoid: Clinical picture and response to chloramphenicol: Prospective study in Bombay (1972). Infection. 1977;5:85–91.
10. Wicks ACB, Holmes GS, Davidson L. Endemic typhoid fever: A diagnostic pitfall. Q J Med. 1971;40:341–54.
11. Hoffman TA, Ruiz CJ, Counts GW, et al. Waterborne typhoid fever in Dade County, Florida: Clinical and therapeutic evaluation of 105 bacteremic patients. Am J Med. 1975;59:481–7.
12. Samantray SK, Johnson SC, Chakrabarti AK. Enteric fever: An analysis of 500 cases. Practitioner. 1977;218:400–8.
13. Wahab MFA, Robertson RP, Raasch FO. Paratyphoid A fever, Cairo, Egypt. Ann Intern Med. 1969;70:913–7.
14. Black PH, Kunz LJ, Swartz MN. Salmonellosis: A review of some unusual aspects. N Engl J Med. 1960;262:811–7.
15. Sprinz H, Gangarosa EJ, Williams M, et al. Histopathology of the upper small intestines in typhoid fever: Biopsy study of experimental disease in man. Am J Dig Dis. 1966;11:615–24.
16. Litwack, KD, Hoke AW, Borchardt KA. Rose spots in typhoid fever. Arch Dermatol. 1972;105:252–5.
17. Meals RA. Paratyphoid fever: A report of 62 cases with several unusual findings and a review of the literature. Arch Intern Med. 1976;136:1422–8.
18. Watson KC. Laboratory and clinical investigation of recovery of *Salmonella typhi* from blood. J Clin Microbiol. 1978;7:122–6.
19. Gilman RH, Terminel M, Levine MM, et al. Relative efficacy of blood, urine, rectal swab, bone-marrow, and rose-spot cultures for recovery of *Salmonella typhi* in typhoid fever. Lancet. 1975;1:1211–3.
20. Guerra-Caceres JG, Gotuzzo-Herencia E, Crosby-Dagnino E, et al. Diagnostic value of bone marrow culture in typhoid fever. Trans R Soc Trop Med Hyg. 1979;73:680–3.
21. Rockhill RC, Rumans LW, Lesmana M, et al. Detection of *Salmonella typhi* D, Vi, and d antigens, by slide coagglutination, in urine from patients with typhoid fever. J Clin Microbiol. 1980;11:213–6.
22. Taylor DN, Harris JR, Barrett TJ, et al. Detection of urinary Vi antigen as a diagnostic test for typhoid fever. J Clin Microbiol. 1983;18:872–6.
23. Tsang RSW, Chau PY. Serological diagnosis of typhoid fever by counter-immunoelectrophoresis. Br Med J. 1981;282:1505–7.
24. Sundararaj T, Ilango B, Subramanian S. A study on the usefulness of counter immuno-electrophoresis for the detection of *Salmonella typhi* antigen in the sera of suspected cases of enteric fever. Trans R Soc Trop Med Hyg. 1983;77:194–7.
25. Schroeder SA. Interpretation of serologic tests for typhoid fever. JAMA. 1968;206:839–40.
26. Reynolds DW, Carpenter RL, Simon WH. Diagnostic specificity of Widal's reaction for typhoid fever. JAMA. 1970;214:2192–3.
27. Senewiratne B, Chir B, Senewiratne K. Reassessment of the Widal test in the diagnosis of typhoid. Gastroenterology. 1977;73:233–6.
28. Brodie J: Antibodies and the Aberdeen typhoid outbreak of 1964:I. The Widal reaction. J Hyg. 1977;79:161–80.
29. Buck RL, Escamilla J, Sangalang RP, et al. Diagnostic value of a single, pre-treatment Widal test in suspected enteric fever cases in the Philippines. Trans R Soc Trop Med Hyg. 1987;81:871–3.
30. Levine MM, Grados O, Gilman RH, et al. Diagnostic value of the Widal test in areas endemic for typhoid fever. Am J Trop Med Hyg. 1978;27:795–800.
31. Editorial: Typhoid and its serology. Br Med J. 1978;1:389.
32. Beasley WJ, Joseph SW, Weiss E: Improved serodiagnosis of *Salmonella* enteric fevers by an enzyme-linked immunosorbent assay. J Clin Microbiol 1981;13:106–114.
33. Petchclai B, Ausavarungnirun R, Manatsathit S. Passive hemagglutination test for enteric fever. J Clin Microbiol. 1987;25:138–41.
34. Nolan CM, Feeley JC, White PC Jr, et al. Evaluation of a new assay for Vi antibody in chronic carriers of *Salmonella typhi*. J Clin Microbiol. 1980;12:22–6.
35. Barrett TJ, Blake PA, Brown SL, et al. Enzyme-linked immunosorbent assay for detection of human antibodies to *Salmonella typhi* Vi antigen. J Clin Microbiol. 1983;17:625–7.
36. Gupta AK, Rao KM. Radial counter-immunoelectrophoresis for rapid serodiagnosis of typhoid fever. J Immunol Methods. 1981;40:373–6.
37. Ramachandran S, Godfrey JJ, Perera MVF. Typhoid hepatitis. JAMA. 1974;230:236–242.
38. Sitprija V, Pipatanagul V, Boonpucknavig V, et al. Glomerulitis in typhoid fever. Ann Intern Med. 1974;81:210–3.
39. Butler W, Bell WR, Levin J, et al. Typhoid fever: Studies of blood coagulation, bacteremia, and endotoxemia. Arch Intern Med. 1978;138:407–10.
40. Harris JC, DuPont HL, Hornick RB. Fecal leukocytes in diarrheal illness. Ann Intern Med. 1972;76:697–703.
41. Blaser MJ, Hickman FW, Farmer JJ III, et al. *Salmonella typhi:* The laboratory as a reservoir of infection. J Infect Dis. 1980;142:934–8.
42. Blaser MJ, Lofgren JP. Fatal salmonellosis originating in a clinical microbiology laboratory. J Clin Microbiol. 1981;13:855–8.
43. Rabson AR, Hallett AF, Koornhof HJ, Generalized *Yersinia enterocolitica* infection. J Infect Dis. 1975;131:447–51.
44. Spira TJ, Kabins SA. *Yersinia enterocolitica* septicemia with septic arthritis. Arch Intern Med. 1976;136:1305–8.
45. Marlon A, Gentry L, Merigan TC. Septicemia with *Pasteurella pseudotuberculosis* and liver disease. Arch Intern Med. 1971;127:947–9.
46. Guerrant RL, Lahita RG, Winn WC Jr, et al. Campylobacteriosis in man: Pathogenic mechanisms and review of 91 bloodstream infections. Am J Med. 1978;65:584–92.
47. Schmidt U, Chmel H, Kaminski Z, et al. The clinical spectrum of *Campylobacter fetus* infection: Report of 5 cases and review of the literature. Q J Med. 1980;49:431–42.
48. Carbone KM, Heinrich MC, Quinn TC. Thrombophlelitis and cellulitis due to *Campylobacter fetus ssp fetus*. Medicine. 1984;64:244–50.
49. Bevanger L. *Yersinia pseudotuberculosis* as the cause of septicemia in a patient with amyloidosis. Acta Pathol Microbiol Scand [B]. 1976;84:461–2.
50. Bokkenheuser, V. *Vibrio fetus* infection in man: I. Ten new cases and some epidemiologic observations. Am J Epidemiol. 1970;91:400–9.
51. Leino R, Kalliomäki JL. Yersiniosis as an internal disease. Ann Intern Med. 1974;81:458–61.
52. Ahvonen P. Human yersiniosis in Finland: I. Bacteriology and serology. Ann Clin Res. 1972;4:30–8.
53. Hubbert WT, Petenyi CW, Glasgow LA, et al. *Yersinia pseudotuberculosis* infection in the United States: Septicemia, appendicitis, and mesenteric lymphadenitis. Am J Trop Med Hyg. 1971;20:679–84.
54. Yamashiro KM, Goldman RH, Harris D, et al. *Pasteurella pseudotuberculosis:* Acute sepsis with survival. Arch Intern Med. 1971;128:605–8.
55. Keet EE. *Yersinia enterocolitica* septicemia: Source of infection and incu-

bation period identified. NY State J Med. 1974;74:2226–30.
56. Sonnenwirth AC. Bacteremia with and without meningitis due to *Yersinia enterocolitica, Edwardsiella tarda, Comamonas terrigena*, and *Pseudomonas maltophilia*. Ann NY Acad Sci. 1970;174:488–502.
57. Taylor BG, Zafarzai MZ, Humphreys DW, et al. Nodular pulmonary infiltrates and septic arthritis associated with *Yersinia enterocolitica* bacteremia. Am Rev Respir Dis. 1977;116:525–9.
58. Bliddal J, Kaliszan S. Prolonged monosymptomatic fever due to *Yersinia enterocolitica*. Acta Med Scand. 1977;201:387–9.
59. Ahvonen P. Human yersiniosis in Finland: II. Clinical features. Ann Clin Res. 1972;4:39–48.
60. Franklin B, Ulmer DD. Human infection with *Vibrio fetus*. West J Med. 1974;120:200–4.
61. Greenwood JR, Flanigan SW, Pickett MJ, et al. Clinical isolation of *Yersinia enterocolitica:* Cold temperature enrichment. J Clin Microbiol. 1975;2:559–60.
62. Skirrow MB. Campylobacter enteritis: A "new" disease. Br Med J. 1977;2:9–11.
63. Lauwers S, DeBoeck M, Butzler JP. Campylobacter enteritis in Brussels. Lancet. 1978;1:604–5.
64. Bokkenheuser V. *Vibrio fetus* infection in man: A serological test. Infect Immun. 1972;5:222–226.
65. Reinicke V, Korner B. Case report: Fulminant septicemia caused by *Yersinia enterocolitica* Scand J Infect Dis. 1977;9:249–51.
66. Forrström J, Viander M, Lehtonen A, et al. Case report: *Yersinia enterocolitica* infection complicated by glomerulonephritis. Scand J Infect Dis. 1977;9:253–6.
67. Guerrant RL, Humphries MK Jr, Butler JE, et al. Tickborne oculoglandular tularemia. Arch Intern Med. 1976;136:811–3.
68. Buchanan TM, Faber LC, Feldman RA. Brucellosis in the United States, 1960–1972: An abattoir-associated disease: I. Clinical features and therapy. Medicine. 1974;53:403–13.
69. Reed WP, Palmer DL, Williams RC Jr, et al. Bubonic plague in the southwestern United States: A review of recent experience. Medicine. 1970;49:465–86.
70. Cantey JR. Plague in Vietnam: Clinical observations and treatment with kanamycin. Arch Intern Med. 1974;133:280–3.
71. Nalin DR, Sultana B, Sahunja R, et al. Survival of a patient with intestinal anthrax. Am J Med. 1977;62:130–2.
72. Brundage WG, Thuss CJ Jr, Walden DG. Four fatal cases of melioidosis in U.S. soldiers in Vietnam: Bacteriologic and pathologic characteristics. Am J Trop Med Hyg. 1968;17:183–91.
73. Schultz MG. A history of bartonellosis (Carrión's disease). Am J Trop Med Hyg. 1968;17:503–15.
74. Cuadra M. Salmonellosis complication in human bartonellosis. Tex Rep Biol Med. 1956;14:97–113.
75. Cole JS, Stoll RW, Bulger RJ. Rat-bite fever: Report of three cases. Ann Intern Med. 1969;71:979–81.
76. Kowal J. Spirillum fever: Report of a case and review of the literature. N Engl J Med. 1961;264:123–8.
77. Anderson LC, Leary SL, Manning PJ. Rat bite fever in animal research laboratory personnel. Lab Anim Sci. 1983;33:292–4.
78. Heath CW Jr, Alexander AD, Galton MM. Leptospirosis in the United States: Analysis of 483 cases in man, 1949–1961. N Engl J Med. 1965;273:857–64.
79. Edwards GA, Domm BM. Human leptospirosis. Medicine. 1960;39:117–56.
80. Boyer KM, Munford RS, Maupin GO, et al. Tick-borne relapsing fever: An interstate outbreak originating at Grand Canyon National Park. Am J Epidemiol. 1977;105:469–79.
81. Southern PM Jr, Sanford JP. Relapsing fever: A clinical and microbiological review. Medicine. 1969;48:129–49.
82. Lewis EA, Kolawole RM. Tuberculous ileo-colitis in Ibadan: A clinico-radiological review. Gut. 1972;13:646–53.
83. Johnson CAC, Hill ID, Bowie MD. Abdominal tuberculosis in children: A survey of cases at the Red Cross War Memorial Children's Hospital. 1976–1985. S Afr Med J. 1987;72:20–2.
84. Weese WC, Smith IM. A study of 57 cases of actinomycosis over a 36-year period: A diagnositc "failure" with good prognosis after treatment. Arch Intern Med. 1975;135:1562–8.
85. Larson EB, Featherstone HJ, Petersdorf RG. Fever of undetermined origin: Diagnosis and follow-up of 105 cases, 1970–1980. Medicine. 1982;61:269–92.
86. Murray HW, Masur H, Senterfit LB, et al. The protean manifestations of *Mycoplasma pneumoniae* infection in adults. Am J Med. 1975;58:229–42.
87. Schaffner W, Drutz DJ, Duncan GW, et al. The clinical spectrum of endemic psittacosis. Arch Intern Med. 1967;119:433–43.
88. Hattwick MAW, O'Brien RJ, Hanson BF. Rocky Mountain spotted fever: Epidemiology of an increasing problem. Ann Intern Med. 1976;84:732–9.
89. Woodward TE. A historical account of the rickettsial diseases with a discussion of unsolved problems. J Infect Dis. 1973;127:583–94.
90. Walker DH. Gastroenterology of Rocky Mountain spotted fever. Practical Gastroenterol. 1986;10:25–39.
91. Jiminez J, Byrne WJ, Seibert JJ, et al. Gastrointestinal symptoms in Rocky Mountain spotted fever: Histopathologic finding of ulcerative enteritis with vasculitis. Clin Pediatr. 1982;21:581–4.
92. Middleton DB. Rocky Mountain spotted fever: Gastrointestinal and laboratory manifestations. South Med J. 1978;71:629–32.
93. Westerman EL. Rocky Mountain spotless fever: A dilemma for the clinician. Arch Intern Med. 1982;142:1106–7.
94. Woodward TE, Pedersen CE Jr, Oster CN, et al. Prompt confirmation of Rocky Mountain spotted fever: Identification of rickettsiae in skin tissues. J Infect Dis. 1976;134:297–301.
95. Marrie TJ, Schlech WF III, Williams JC, et al. Q fever pneumonia associated with exposure to wild rabbits. Lancet 1986;1:427–9.
96. Duma RJ, Sonenshine DE, Bozeman FM, et al. Epidemic typhus in the United States associated with flying squirrels. JAMA. 1981;245:2318–23.
97. Centers for Disease Control. Epidemic typhus associated with flying squirrels: United States. MMWR. 1982;31:555–61.
98. Yu VL, Kroboth FJ, Shonnard J, et al. Legionnaires' disease: New clinical perspective from a prospective pneumonia study. Am J Med. 1982;73:357–61.
99. Kirby BD, Snyder KM, Meyer RD, et al. Legionnaires' disease: Report of 65 nosocomially acquired cases and a review of the literature. Medicine. 1980;59:188–205.
100. Chow JW, Lu VL. New perspectives on *Legionella* pneumonia: Diagnosis, management and prevention. J Crit Illness. 1988;3:17–27.
101. Sturim HS, Kouchonkos NT, Ahlvin RC. Gastrointestinal manifestations of disseminated histoplasmosis. Am J Surg. 1965;110:435–40.
102. Gordon S, Brennessel DJ, Goldstein JA, et al. Malaria: A city hospital experience. Arch Intern Med. 1988;148:1569–71.
103. Steketee RW, Eckman MR, Burgess EC, et al. Babesiosis in Wisconsin: A new focus of disease transmission. JAMA. 1985;253:2675–8.
104. Ruebush TK II, Cassaday PB, Marsh HJ, et al. Human babesiosis on Nantucket Island: Clinical features. Ann Intern Med. 1977;86:6–9.
105. May RP, Lehmann JD, Sanford JP. Difficulties in differentiating amebic from pyogenic liver abscess. Arch Intern Med. 1967;119:69–74.
106. Robertson RP, Wahab MFA, Raasch FO. Evaluation of chloramphenicol and ampicillin in salmonella enteric fever. N Engl J Med. 1968;278:171–6.
107. Butler T, Rumans L, Arnold K. Response of typhoid fever caused by chloramphenicol-susceptible and chloramphenicol-resistant strains of *Salmonella typhi* to treatment with trimethoprim–sulfamethoxazole. Rev Infect Dis. 1982;4:551–61.
108. Bryan JP, Rocha H, Scheld WM. Problems in salmonellosis: Rationale for clinical trials with newer Beta-lactam agents and quinolones. Rev Infect Dis. 1986;8:189–207.
109. Soe GB, Overturf GD. Treatment of typhoid fever and other systemic salmonellosis with cefotaxime, ceftriaxone, cefoperazone and other newer cephalosporins. Rev Infect Dis. 1987;9:719–36.
110. Baine WB, Farmer JJ III, Gangarosa EJ. Typhoid fever in the United States associated with the 1972–1973 epidemic in Mexico. J Infect Dis. 1977;135:649–53.
111. Butler T, Arnold K, Linh NN, et al. Chloramphenicol-resistant typhoid fever in Vietnam associated with R factor. Lancet. 1973;2:983–91.
112. Brown JD, Mo DH, Rhoades ER. Chloramphenicol-resistant *Salmonella typhi* in Saigon. JAMA. 1975;231:162–6.
113. Olarte J, Galindo E. *Salmonella typhi* resistant to chloramphenicol, ampicillin and other antimicrobial agents: Strains isolated during an extensive typhoid fever epidemic in Mexico. Antimicrob Agents Chemother. 1973;4:597–603.
114. Snyder MJ, Gonzalez O, Palomino C, et al. Comparative efficacy of chloramphenicol, ampicillin, and co-trimoaxazole in the treatment of typhoid fever. Lancet. 1976;2:1155–7.
115. Butler T, Linh NN, Arnold K, et al. Therapy of antimicrobial-resistant typhoid fever. Antimicrob Agents Chemother. 1977;11:645–50.
116. Datta N, Richards H, Datta C. *Salmonella typhi* in vivo acquires resistance to both chloramphenicol and co-trimoxazole. Lancet. 1981;1:1181–3.
117. Collins DC. Mesenteric lymphadenitis in adolescents simulating appendicitis. Can Med Assoc J. 1936;34:402–5.
118. Mair NS, Mair HJ, Stirk EM, et al. Three cases of acute mesenteric lymphadenitis due to *Pasteurella pseudotuberculosis*. J Clin Pathol. 1960;13:432–9.
119. Dudley HAF, MacLaren IF. Primary mesenteric abscess. Lancet. 1956;2:1182–4.
120. Asch MJ, Amoury RA, Touloukian RJ, et al. Suppurative mesenteric lymphadenitis: A report of two cases and review of the literature. Am J Surg. 1968;115:570–3.
121. Constantinides CG, Davies MRQ, Cywes S. Suppurative mesenteric lymphadenitis in children: Case reports. S Afr Med J. 1981;60:629–31.
122. Rey C, Escribano JC, Foz M, et al. Mesenteric adenitis secondary to *Giardia lamblia*. Dig Dis Sci. 1980;25:968–71.
123. Winblad S, Nilehn B, Sternby NJ. *Yersinia enterocolitica* (Pasteurella X) in human enteric infections. Br Med J. 1966;2:1363–6.
124. Carter PB. Pathogenicity of *Yersinia enterocolitica* for mice. Infect Immun. 1975;11:164–70.
125. Une T. Studies on the pathogenicity of *Yersinia enterocolitica:* II. Interaction with cultured cells in vitro. Microbiol Immunol. 1977;21:365–77.
126. Kay BA, Wachsmuth K, Gemski P, et al. Virulence and phenotypic characterization of *Yersinia enterocolitica* isolated from humans in the United States. J Clin Microbiol. 1983;17:128–38.
127. Feeley JC, Wells JG, Tsai TF, et al. Detection of enterotoxigenic and invasive strains of *Yersinia enterocolitica*. Contrib Microbiol Immunol. 1979;5:329–34.
128. Zink DL, Feeley JC, Wells JG, et al. Plasmid-mediated tissue invasiveness in *Yersinia enterocolitica*. Nature. 1980;283:224–6.

129. Kay BA, Wachsmuth K, Gemski P. New virulence-associated plasmid in *Yersinia enterocolitica*. J Clin Microbiol. 1982;15:1161–3.
130. Jepsen OB, Korner B, Lauritsen KB, et al. *Yersinia enterocolitica* infection in patients with acute surgical abdominal disease: A prospective study. Scand J Infect Dis. 1976;8:189–94.
131. Zen-Yoji H, Maruyama T, Sakai S, et al. An outbreak of enteritis due to *Yersinia enterocolitica* occurring at a junior high school. Jpn J Microbiol. 1973;17:220.
132. Asakawa Y, Akahane S, Kagata N, et al. Two community outbreaks of human infection with *Yersinia enterocolitica*. J Hyg (Camb). 1973;71:715–23.
133. Black RE, Jackson RJ, Tsai T, et al. Epidemic *Yersinia enterocolitica* infection due to contaminated chocolate milk. N Engl J Med. 1978;298:76–9.
134. Vantrappen G, Agg HO, Ponette E, et al. *Yersinia* enteritis and enterocolitis: Gastroenterological aspects. Gastroenterology. 1977;72:220–7.
135. Jansson E, Wallgren GR, Ahvonen P. *Yersinia enterocolitica* as a cause of acute mesenteric lymphadenitis. Acta Paediatr Scand. 1968;57:448–50.
136. Tauxe RV, Vandepitte J, Wauters G, et al. *Yersinia enterocolitica* infections and pork: The missing link. Lancet. 1987;1:1129–32.
137. Knapp W. Mesenteric adenitis due to *Pasteurella pseudotuberculosis* in young people. N Engl J Med. 1958;259:776–8.
138. Randall KJ, Mair NS. Family outbreak of *Pasteurella pseudotuberculosis* infection. Lancet. 162;1:1042–3.
139. Weber J, Finlayson NB, Mark JBD. Mesenteric lymphadenitis and terminal ileitis due to *Yersinia pseudotuberculosis*. N Engl J Med. 1970;283:172–4.
140. Saari TN, Triplett DA. *Yersinia pseudotuberculosis* mesenteric adenitis. J Pediatr. 1974;85:656–9.
141. Bradford WD, Noce PS, Gutman LT. Pathologic features of enteric infection with *Yersinia enterocolitica*. Arch Pathol. 1974;98:17–22.
142. Weissfeld AS, Sonnenwirth AC. *Yersinia enterocolitica* in adults with gastrointestinal disturbances: Need for cold enrichment. J Clin Microbiol. 1980;11:196–7.
143. Daniëls JJHM. Enteral infection with *Pasteurella pseudotuberculosis:* Isolation of the organism from human feces. Br Med J. 1961;2:997.
144. Niléhn B, Sjöström B. Studies on *Yersinia enterocolitica*. Acta Pathol Microbiol Scand. 1967;71:612–28.
145. Marks MI, Pai CH, Lafleur L, et al. *Yersinia enterocolitica* gastroenteritis: A prospective study of clinical, bacteriologic, and epidemiologic features. J Pediatr. 1980;96:26–31.
146. Puylaert JB. Mesenteric adenitis and acute terminal ileitis: Ultrasound evaluation using graded compression. Radiol. 1986;161:691–5.
147. Ekberg O, Sjöström B, Brahme F. Radiological findings in *Yersinia* ileitis. Radiology. 1977;123:15–9.
148. Ahlqvist J, Ahvonen P, Räsänen JA, et al. Enteric infection with *Yersinia enterocolitica:* Large pyroninophilic cell reproduction in mesenteric lymph nodes associated with early production of specific antibodies. Acta Pathol Microbiol Scand [A]. 1971;79:109–22.
149. Braunstein H, Tucker EB, Gibson BC. Mesenteric lymphadenitis due to *Yersinia enterocolitica:* Report of a case. Am J Clin Pathol. 1971;55:506–10.
150. El-Maraghi NRH, Mair NS. The histopathology of enteric infection with *Yersinia pseudotuberculosis*. Am J Clin Pathol. 1979;71:631–9.
151. Gutman LT, Ottesen EA, Quan TJ, et al. An inter-familial outbreak of *Yersinia enterocolitica* enteritis. N Engl J Med. 1973;288:1372–7.
152. Arvastson B, Damgaard K, Winblad S. Clinical symptoms of infection with *Yersinia enterocolitica*. Scand J Infect Dis. 1971;3:37–40.
153. Wilson HD, McCormick JB, Feeley JC. *Yersinia enterocolitica* infection in a 4-month-old infant associated with infection in household dogs. J Pediatr. 1976;89:767–8.
154. Tacket CO, Narain JP, Sattin R, et al. A multistate outbreak of infections caused by *Yersinia enterocolitica* transmitted by pasteurized milk. JAMA. 1984;251:483–6.
155. Nolan C, Harris N, Ballard J, et al. Outbreak of *Yersinia enterocolitica:* Washington State. MMWR. 1982;31:562.
156. Laasen J. *Yersinia enterocolitica* in drinking-water. Scand J Infect Dis. 1972;4:125–7.
157. Highsmith AK, Feeley JC, Skaliy P, et al. Isolation of *Yersinia enterocolitica* from well water and growth in distilled water. Appl Environ Microbiol. 1977;34:745–50.
158. Snyder JD, Christenson E, Feldman RA. Human *Yersinia enterocolitica* infections in Wisconsin. Am J Med. 1982;72:768–74.
159. Loría-Cortés R, Lobo-Sanahuja JF. Clinical abdominal angiostrongylosis: A study of 116 children with intestinal eosinophilic granuloma caused by *Angiostrongylus costaricensis*. Am J Trop Med Hyg. 1980;29:538–44.
160. Gutman LT, Wilfert CM, Quan T. Susceptibility of *Yersinia enterocolitica* to trimethoprim–sulfamethoxazole. J Infect Dis. 1973;128(Suppl):S538.
161. Hornstein MJ, Jupeau AM, Scavizzi MR, et al. *In vitro* susceptibilities of 126 clinical isolates of *Yersinia enterocolitica* to 21 β-lactam antibiotics. Antimicrob Agents Chemother. 1985;27:806–11.
162. Hammerberg S, Sorger S, Marks MI. Antimicrobial susceptibilities of *Yersinia enterocolitica* biotype 4, serotype 0:3. Antimicrob Agents Chemother. 1977;11:566–8.
163. Grove DI, Warren KS, Mahmoud AAF. Algorithms in the diagnosis and management of exotic diseases: III. Strongyloidiasis. J Infect Dis. 1975;131:755–8.
164. Jones CA. Clinical studies in human strongyloidiasis: I. Semeiology. Gastroenterology. 1950;16:743–56.
165. Purtilo DT, Meyers WM, Connor DH. Fatal strongyloidiasis in immunosuppressed patients. Am J Med. 1974;56:488–93.
166. Morgan JS, Schaffner W, Stone WJ. Opportunistic strongyloidiasis in renal transplant recipients. Transplantation. 1986;42:518–24.
167. Cadranel JF, Eugene C. Another example of *Strongyloides stercoralis* infection associated with cimetidine in an immunosuppressed patient. Gut. 1986;27:1229.
168. Pelletier LL Jr, Baker CB, Gam AA, et al. Diagnosis and evaluation of treatment of chronic strongyloidiasis in ex-prisoners of war. J Infect Dis. 1988;157:573–6.
169. Gill GV, Bell DR. *Strongyloides stercoralis* infection in former Far East prisoners of war. Br Med J [Clin Res]. 1979;2:572–4.
170. Grove DI. Strongyloidiasis in Allied ex-prisoners of war in south-east Asia. Br Med J [Clin Res]. 1980;280:598–601.
171. Pelletier LL Jr. Chronic strongyloidiasis in World War II Far East ex-prisoners of war. Am J Trop Med Hyg. 1984;33:55–61.
172. Berk SL, Verghese A, Alvarez S, et al. Clinical and epidemiologic features of strongyloidiasis: A prospective study in rural Tennessee. Arch Intern Med. 1987;147:1257–61.
173. Beal CB, Viens P, Grant RGL, et al. A new technique for sampling duodenal contents: Demonstration of upper small bowel pathogens. Am J Trop Med Hyg. 1970;19:399–52.
174. Blumenthal DS, Schultz MG. Incidence of intestinal obstruction in children infected with *Ascaris lumbricoides*. Am J Trop Med Hyg. 1975;24:801–5.
175. Krige JEJ, Lewis G, Bornman PC. Recurrent pancreatitis caused by a calcified ascaris in the duct of Wirsung. Am J Gastroenterol. 1987;82:256–7.
176. Schantz PM, Glickman LT. Toxocaral visceral larva migrans. N Engl J Med. 1978;298:436–9.
177. Taylor MRH, Keane CT, O'Connor P, et al. The expanded spectrum of toxocaral disease. Lancet. 1988;1:692–5.
178. Thompson DE, Bundy DAP, Cooper ES, et al. Epidemiological characteristics of *Toxocara canis* zoonotic infection of children in a Caribbean community. *Bull WHO*. 1986;64:283–90.
179. Glickman LT, Magnaval J-F, Domanski LM, et al. Visceral larva migrans in French adults: A new disease syndrome. Am J Epidemiol. 1987;125:1019–34.
180. Grove DI, Warren KS, Mahmoud AAF. Algorithms in the diagnosis and management of exotic diseases: VII. Trichinosis. J Infect Dis. 1975;132:485–8.
181. Campbell WC. Trichinella and Trichinosis. New York: Plenum Press; 1983.
182. Stehr-Green JK, Schantz PM, Chisolm EM. Trichinosis surveillance, 1984. MMWR. 1985;35:11–15SS.
183. Singal M, Schantz PM, Werner SB. Trichinosis acquired at sea: Report of an outbreak. Am J Trop Med Hyg. 1976;25:675–81.
184. Petri WA Jr, Holsinger JR, Pearson RD. Common-source outbreak of trichinosis associated with eating raw home-butchered pork. South Med J. 1988;81:1056–8.
185. Trichinosis outbreaks associated with horsemeat. Parasitol Today. 1986;2:295.
186. Viallet J, MacLean JD, Goresky CA, et al. Arctic trichinosis presenting as prolonged diarrhea. Gastroenterology. 1986;91:938–46.
187. Kagan IG. Serodiagnosis of trichinosis. In: Cohen S, Sadun EH, eds. Immunology of Parasitic Infections. Oxford: Blackwell Scientific; 1976:143–51.
188. Pinkus GS, Coolidge C. Intestinal anisakiasis: First case report from North America. Am J Med. 1975;59:114–20.
189. Richman RH, Lewicki AM. Right ileocolitis secondary to anisakiasis. Am J Roentgen Rad Ther Nucl Med. 1973;119:329–31.
190. Yokogawa M, Yoshimura H. Clinicopathologic studies on larval anisakiasis in Japan. Am J Trop Med Hyg. 1967;16:723–34.
191. Whalen GE, Strickland GT, Cross JH, et al. Intestinal capillariasis: A new disease in man. Lancet. 1969;1:13–6.
192. Watten RH, Beckner WM, Cross JH, et al. Clinical studies of capillariasis philippinensis. Trans R Soc Trop Med Hyg. 1972;66:828–34.
193. Fresh JW, Cross JH, Reyes V, et al. Necropsy findings in intestinal capillariasis. Am J Trop Med Hyg. 1972;21:169–73.
194. Cross JH, Banzon T, Clarke MD, et al. Studies on the experimental transmission of *Capillaria philippinensis* in monkeys. Trans R Soc Trop Med Hyg. 1972;66:819–27.
195. Morera P, Perez F, Mora F, et al. Visceral larva migrans-like syndrome caused by *Angiostrongylus costaricensis*. Am J Trop Med Hyg. 1982;31:67–70.
196. Mahmoud AA. Schistosomiasis. N Engl J Med. 1977;297:1329–31.
197. Warren KS. Schistosomiasis japonicum. In Marsden PD, ed. Clinics in Gastroenterology. v. 17. no. 1: Intestinal Parasites. London: WB Saunders; 1978:77–85.
198. Farid Z, Trabolsi B, Hafez A. Acute schistosomiasis mansoni (Katayama syndrome). Ann Trop Med Parasitol. 1986;80:563–4.
199. Hardman EW, Jones RLH, Davies AH. Fascioliasis—a large outbreak. Br Med J. 1970;3:502–5.
200. Stork MG, Venables GS, Jennings SMF, et al. An investigation of endemic fascioliasis in Peruvian village children. J Trop Med Hyg. 1973;76:231–5.
201. Jones EA, Kay JM, Milligan HP, et al. Massive infection with *Fasciola hepatica* in man. Am J Med. 1977;63:836–42.
202. Plaut AG, Kampanart-Sanyakorn C, Manning GS. A clinical study of *Fasciolopsis buski* infection in Thailand. Trans R Soc Trop Med Hyg. 1969;63:470–8.

203. Warren KS, Mahmoud AAF. Algorithms in the diagnosis and management of exotic diseases. XXI. Liver, intestinal and lung flukes. J Infect Dis. 1977;135:692–6.
204. Lin AC, Chapman SW, Turner HR, et al. Clonorchiasis: An update. South Med J. 1987;80:919–22.
205. Brockelman WY, Upatham ES, Viyanant V, et al. Measurement of incidence of the human liver fluke, *Opisthorchis viverrini*, in northeast Thailand. Trans R Soc Trop Med Hyg. 1987;81:327–35.
206. Warren KS, Mahmoud AAF. Algorithms in the diagnosis and management of exotic diseases: XIV. Tapeworms. J Infect Dis. 1976;134:108–12.
207. Grove DI, Warren KS, Mahmoud AAF. Algorithms in the diagnosis and management of exotic diseases. X. Echinococcosis. J Infect Dis. 1976;133:354–8.
208. Kagan IG. Current status of serologic testing for parasitic diseases. Hosp Pract. 1974;9:157–63.
209. Trier JS, Moxey PC, Schimmel EM, et al. Chronic intestinal coccidiosis in man: Intestinal morphology and response to treatment. Gastroenterology. 1974;66:923–35.
210. Liebman WM, Thaler MM, DeLorimier A, et al. Intractable diarrhea of infancy due to intestinal coccidiosis. Gastroenterology. 1980;78:579–84.
211. DeHovitz JA, Pape JW, Boncy M, et al. Clinical manifestations and therapy of *Isospora belli* infection in patients with the acquired immunodeficiency syndrome. N Engl J Med. 1986;315:87–90.
212. Spencer MJ, Garcia LS, Chapin MR. *Dientamoeba fragilis:* An intestinal pathogen in children? Am J Dis Child. 1979;133:390–3.
213. Yang J, Scholten TH. *Dientamoeba fragilis:* A review with notes on its epidemiology, pathogenicity, mode of transmission, and diagnosis. Am J Trop Med Hyg. 1977;26:16–22.
214. Blackshaw AJ, Levison DA. Eosinophilic infiltrates of the gastrointestinal tract. J Clin Pathol. 1986;39:1–7.
215. Tedesco FJ, Huckaby CB, Hamby-Allen M, et al. Eosinophilic ileocolitis: Expanding spectrum of eosinophilic gastroenteritis. Dig Dis Sci. 1981;26:943–8.
216. Klein NC, Hargrove L, Sleisenger MH, et al. Eosinophilic gastroenteritis. Medicine. 1970;49:299–319.
217. Leinbach GE, Rubin CE. Eosinophilic gastroenteritis: A simple reaction to food allergens? Gastroenterology. 1970;59:874–89.
218. Goldberg HI, O'Kieffe D, Jenis EH, et al. Diffuse eosinophilic gastroenteritis. Am J Roentgen Rad Therapy Nucl Med. 1973;119:342–51.
219. Tytgat GN, Grijm, R, Dekker W, et al. Fatal eosinophilic enteritis. Gastroenterology. 1976;71:479–83.
220. Cupps TR, Fauci AS. The Vasculitides. Philadelphia: WB Saunders; 1981.
221. Mowrey FH, Lundberg EA. The clinical manifestations of essential polyangiitis (periarteritis nodosa), with emphasis on the hepatic manifestations. Ann Intern Med. 1954;40:1145–64.
222. Nightingale EJ. The gastroenterological aspects of periarteritis nodosa. Am J Gastroenterol. 1959;31:152–65.
223. Leavitt RY, Fauci AS. Polyangiitis overlap syndrome. Am J Med. 1986;81:79–85.
224. Churg J, Strauss L. Allergic granulomatosis, allergic angiitis and periarteritis nodosa. Am J Pathol. 1951;27:277–301.
225. Finch SC. Granulocytosis. In: Williams WJ, Beutler E, Erslev AJ, et al. eds. Hematology. New York: McGraw-Hill; 1977:746–755.
226. Haeberle MG, Griffen WO Jr. Eosinophilia and regional enteritis: A possible diagnostic aid. Am J Dig Dis. 1972;17:200–4.
227. Glotzer DJ, Gardner RC, Goldman H, et al. Comparative features and course of ulcerative and granulomatous colitis. N Engl J Med. 1970;282:582–7.
228. Isaacson NJ, Rapoport P. Eosinophilia in malignant tumors: Its significance. Ann Intern Med. 1946;25:893–902.
229. Banerjee RN, Narang RM. Haematological changes in malignancy. Br J Haematol. 1967;13:829–43.
230. Beeson P. Cancer and eosinophilia. N Engl J Med. 1983;309:792–3.

86. FOOD-BORNE DISEASE

JAMES M. HUGHES
ROBERT V. TAUXE

Food-borne disease syndromes result from ingestion of a wide variety of foods contaminated with pathogenic microorganisms, microbial toxins, or chemicals. From 1972 to 1982, between 300 and 600 outbreaks of food-borne disease affecting 10,000–18,000 people in the United States were reported annually to the Centers for Disease Control (CDC).[1–5] These figures certainly underestimate the magnitude of the problem. The actual incidence of food-borne disease is unknown but has been estimated to be 9,000,000 illnesses annually.[6]

Although a wide variety of microorganisms and toxins can

TABLE 1. Etiology of Food-borne Disease Outbreaks of Known Etiology Reported to the CDC, 1972–1986

Etiology	*Number of Outbreaks*	*Percentage of Total*
Bacterial		
Salmonella	753	27.4
S. aureus	395	14.4
C. botulinum	220[a]	8.0
C. perfringens	187	6.8
Shigella	99	3.6
B. cereus	52	1.9
C. jejuni	49	1.8
V. parahaemolyticus	25	0.9
Y. enterocolitica	5	0.2
V. cholerae 01	5[b]	0.2
Verotoxigenic *E. coli*	4	0.1
L. monocytogenes	3	0.1
Other	30	1.1
Chemical		
Ciguatera	206	7.5
Histamine fish poisoning (scombroid)	182	6.6
Mushrooms	64	2.3
Heavy metals	53	1.9
Paralytic shellfish poisoning (PSP)	20	0.7
Chinese restaurant syndrome	19	0.7
Neurotoxic shellfish poisoning (NSP)	2	0.1
Other	111	4.0
Parasitic[c]	147	5.4
Viral	114	4.1
Total	2745	99.8

[a] Excludes cases of infant botulism.
[b] Includes outbreaks on Guam[7] and in Louisiana.[8]
[c] Includes first two reported food-borne outbreaks caused by *Giardia lamblia*.[9,10]

cause food-borne disease, this discussion will focus on food-borne disease syndromes that are acute (onset of symptoms usually within 72 hours of ingestion) and whose clinical features include gastrointestinal manifestations. The diseases to be discussed and the frequency with which outbreaks were reported to the CDC from 1972 to 1986 are indicated in Table 1.

PATHOGENESIS AND CLINICAL FEATURES

The diagnosis of food-borne disease should be considered when an acute illness with gastrointestinal or neurologic manifestations affects two or more persons who have shared a meal during the previous 72 hours. Important clues to the etiologic agent are provided by both the symptoms and incubation period.

Food-borne Disease Due to Microbial Agents or Their Toxins (Table 2)

Nausea and Vomiting within 1–6 Hours. The major etiologic considerations are *Staphylococcus aureus* and *Bacillus cereus*. The relatively short incubation period reflects the fact that these diseases are caused by a preformed enterotoxin. Staphylococcal food poisoning is characterized by vomiting (76 percent of the cases) and diarrhea (77 percent); fever is relatively uncommon (23 percent).[11] Staphylococci responsible for episodes of food poisoning produce one or more enterotoxins; five immunologically distinct heat-stable proteins (A, B, C, D, E) with molecular weights ranging from 28,000 to 35,000 daltons have been identified.[12] Another staphylococcal protein, enterotoxin F, is produced by the majority of *S. aureus* strains causing toxic shock syndrome[13] but has not been reported to cause food-borne disease. Although the mechanism of action of these enterotoxins in humans has not been clarified, studies in monkeys and cats suggest that the enterotoxin produces its emetic action after interaction with abdominal viscera.[14,15] The sensory stimulus is carried to the vomiting center in the brain by the vagus and sympathetic nerves.[14] Other studies suggest that diarrhea may result from inhibition of water and sodium absorption in the small intestine by enterotoxin.[16]

TABLE 2. Pathogenic Mechanisms in Bacterial Food-borne Disease

Preformed Toxin	*Toxin Production in Vivo*	*Tissue Invasion*	*Toxin Production and/or Tissue Invasion*
S. aureus	*C. perfringens*	*C. jejuni*	*V. parahaemolyticus*
B. cereus (short incubation)	*B. cereus* (long incubation)	*Salmonella*	*Y. enterocolitica*
C. botulinum	*C. botulinum* (infant botulism)	*Shigella*	
	Enterotoxigenic *E. coli*	Invasive *E. coli*	
	V. cholerae 01		
	V. cholerae non-01		
	Verotoxigenic *E. coli*		

Enterotoxigenic staphylococci isolated from implicated foods in outbreaks are most often lysed by group III phages; less commonly, they are lysed by both group I and group III phages or by group I phages alone.[17] Over 99 percent of enterotoxigenic staphylococci associated with food poisoning are coagulase positive; occasionally, an outbreak caused by enterotoxigenic *Staphylococcus epidermidis* is reported.[18] In the past, strains producing type A enterotoxin alone accounted for 44–69 percent of the reported outbreaks of staphylococcal food poisoning in the United States and England.[19,20] Strains producing type D enterotoxin, either alone or in combination with type A, were the next most frequently implicated. Strains producing enterotoxins B, C, or E alone accounted for fewer than 10 percent of the outbreaks. During 1979–1981, all reported staphylococcal food-borne outbreaks in the United States of known toxin type were caused by strains producing type A enterotoxin alone.[21]

Bacillus cereus strains can cause two types of food poisoning syndromes: one characterized primarily by nausea and vomiting with an incubation period of 1–6 hours (short-incubation "emetic" syndrome) and a second manifested primarily by abdominal cramps and diarrhea with an incubation period of 8–16 hours (long-incubation "diarrhea" syndrome).[22,23] Recent evidence suggests that the short-incubation syndrome, which is characterized by vomiting (100 percent of the cases), abdominal cramps (100 percent), and, less frequently, diarrhea (33 percent)[24] may be caused by a heat-stable toxin produced by some *B. cereus* strains and capable of causing vomiting when fed to monkeys.[25] The mechanism and site of action of this toxin, which has a molecular weight of less than 5000, are unknown.[26]

Another clue to the cause of both staphylococcal and short-incubation *B. cereus* outbreaks is provided by the fact that the illnesses are of short duration, usually lasting less than 12 hours.[11,24]

Abdominal Cramps and Diarrhea within 8–16 Hours. The major etiologic considerations for this syndrome, which is also enterotoxin mediated, are *Clostridium perfringens* and *B. cereus*. In contrast to staphylococcal food poisoning and the short-incubation *B. cereus* disease, which are caused by ingestion of preformed enterotoxins in food, *C. perfringens* and long-incubation *B. cereus* food poisoning are caused by toxins produced in vivo, accounting for the longer incubation period. In *C. perfringens* food poisoning, the most common symptoms are diarrhea and abdominal cramps. Although nausea may occur, vomiting and fever are uncommon, occurring in less than 10 percent of the patients.[27,28] Only *C. perfringens* type A strains have been associated with this food poisoning syndrome.[28,29] *Clostridium perfringens* enterotoxin is a heat-labile protein with a molecular weight of approximately 35,000 daltons[30] synthesized during sporulation of the vegetative cells of *C. perfringens* in the gastrointestinal tract; the enterotoxin is released during lysis of the sporangium.[31] Studies in rabbits and rats indicate that the enterotoxin is active throughout the small intestine, with greatest activity in the ileum, in which net secretion of sodium and fluid and inhibition of chloride and glucose absorption occur.[32,33] The enterotoxin damages brush borders of epithelial cells at villus tips.[33]

Bacillus cereus strains, which cause a similar syndrome characterized by diarrhea (96 percent) and abdominal cramps (75 percent), sometimes vomiting (33 percent), and rarely fever,[24] elaborate a heat-labile enterotoxin with a molecular weight of approximately 50,000[26] that activates intestinal adenylate cyclase and results in intestinal fluid secretion.[34] This enterotoxin appears to also have cytotoxic properties in rabbit small intestine and guinea pig skin.[26,34]

Although nausea occurs in many patients with *C. perfringens* and long-incubation *B. cereus* food poisoning, vomiting occurs infrequently. In fact, occurrence of vomiting in greater than one-third of affected people suggests that these organisms are not involved. Although these illnesses last longer than staphylococcal and short-incubation *B. cereus* food poisoning, symptoms usually resolve within 24 hours.[24,35] However, in one large long-incubation *B. cereus* outbreak involving elderly patients in a chronic disease hospital, the mean duration of illness was 2.3 days, and one patient was ill for 10 days.[36]

Fever, Abdominal Cramps, and Diarrhea within 16–48 Hours. The major etiologic considerations for this syndrome are salmonellae, shigellae, *Campylobacter jejuni, Vibrio parahaemolyticus*, and invasive *Escherichia coli*. These organisms cause this syndrome after tissue invasion.[37–42] Vomiting occurs in 35–80 percent of the patients.[43–46] These illnesses usually resolve within 2–7 days.

Campylobacter jejuni is the most common food-borne bacterial pathogen.[47,48] The frequency of fecal blood and polymorphonuclear leukocytes[49] and colitis[50] suggests that this organism also causes this syndrome after tissue invasion. In contrast to the illnesses caused by other organisms in this group, *C. jejuni* food poisoning is characterized by vomiting in only 15–25 percent of cases[49,51,52] and a longer incubation period of 1–7 days.[47] The duration of illness is usually less than 1 week, but relapses may occur in untreated patients.[53]

The diarrhea experienced by patients with *Vibrio cholerae* non-01 infection is sometimes bloody, and fever may be present.[54–56]

Abdominal Cramps and Watery Diarrhea within 16–72 Hours. The major etiologic considerations in this syndrome are enterotoxigenic strains of *E. coli, V. parahaemolyticus, V. cholerae* non-01, and in endemic areas, *V. cholerae* 01; *C. jejuni*, salmonellae, and shigellae may also cause this syndrome. Enterotoxins synthesized in vivo are responsible for the syndrome caused by *V. cholerae* 01.[57] *Vibrio cholerae* non-01,[58,59] and enterotoxigenic strains of *E. coli*[60]; enterotoxigenic and/or cytotoxic substances may also play a role in the pathogenesis of this syndrome when caused by salmonellae,[61,62] shigellae,[63–65] and *V. parahaemolyticus*.[66,67]

Fever and vomiting occur in a minority of cases.[68–71] With the exception of cholera, which may last for 5 days, and disease due to *V. cholerae* non-01, which may last for 2–12 days, these illnesses usually resolve within 72–96 hours. However, in one documented enterotoxigenic *E. coli* outbreak, the median duration of illness was 7 days.[72]

Food-borne transmission of the Norwalk agent, a 27-nm virus, may be common.[73–76] In contrast to the illness produced by bacterial agents causing this syndrome, vomiting is a prominent feature of Norwalk agent gastroenteritis and occurs in the majority of cases.[73] The duration of illness is usually 24–48 hours. The occurrence of secondary cases in close contacts not exposed to the suspected food is an important clue to the possibility of a Norwalk agent etiology. A Norwalk-like virus (Snow Mountain agent) has recently been reported to be transmitted by food.[77] The importance of food in transmission of other similar viral agents (e.g., Hawaii, Ditchling, Colorado, and Marin County agents) remains to be determined.[78]

Fever and Abdominal Cramps within 16–48 Hours. *Yersinia enterocolitica* has been incriminated as a cause of food-borne outbreaks in the United States and is a more common cause of food-borne disease in Northern Europe and Canada.[79–82] Although some strains of this organism have been reported to produce a heat-stable enterotoxin,[83,84] the frequent occurrence of fever and mesenteric adenitis suggests that this organism causes disease as a result of tissue invasion. In older children and adults, the clinical illness may closely resemble acute appendicitis; nausea and vomiting are relatively uncommon, occurring in less than 25–40 percent of the cases.[81,85] Diarrhea is the most common symptom in infants.[86] Duration of the illness may range from 24 hours to 4 weeks.[81,85]

Bloody Diarrhea without Fever within 72–120 Hours. The distinctive syndrome of hemorrhagic colitis has been linked to verotoxigenic strains of *E. coli*, most often serotype 0157:H7.[87–89] These strains, which cause diarrhea in infant rabbits,[87,90] produce a cytotoxin for Vero cells, which has been neutralized by antiserum to shiga toxin.[91,92] The illness is characterized by abdominal cramps and diarrhea, which is initially watery but subsequently grossly bloody. Patients with uncomplicated infection usually remain afebrile. The mean incubation period in two outbreaks was 4 days. The duration of uncomplicated illness ranges from 1 to 12 days. The development of fever and leukocytosis may herald complications, which include hemolytic-uremic syndrome, thrombotic thrombocytopenic purpura, and death.[88,93–95] Case fatality rates in two nursing home outbreaks were 16 and 35 percent.[88,93]

Nausea, Vomiting, Diarrhea, and Paralysis within 18–36 Hours. The occurrence of acute gastrointestinal symptoms simultaneously with or just before the onset of descending weakness or paralysis strongly suggests the diagnosis of food-borne botulism. Constipation is common once the neurologic syndrome is well established, but nausea and vomiting occur at onset in 50 percent of the patients, and diarrhea occurs in approximately 20–25 percent.[96–98] The pathogenesis of the acute gastrointestinal symptoms is not understood; the botulinal toxins, which inhibit acetylcholine release from nerve endings,[99,100] do not appear to be responsible. The disease in humans is usually caused by one of three immunologically distinct heat-labile protein neurotoxins designated A, B, and E,[101] which are produced after germination of *Clostridium botulinum* spores in inadequately processed foods. The disease in older children and adults results from ingestion of preformed toxin. The syndrome of infant botulism appears to result from ingestion of spores with subsequent toxin production in vivo.[102–104] Both illnesses last from several weeks to several months. Clinical suspicion is critical if the disease is to be correctly diagnosed.[105]

Food-borne Disease due to Chemicals of Nonmicrobial Origin

Nausea, Vomiting, and Abdominal Cramps within 1 Hour. The major etiologic considerations for this syndrome are heavy metals; copper, zinc, tin, and cadmium have caused food-borne outbreaks.[106–110] Incubation periods most often range from 5 to 15 minutes. Nausea, vomiting, and abdominal cramps result from irritation of the gastric mucosa and usually resolve within 2–3 hours after removal of the offending agent during emesis.

Paresthesias within 1 Hour. When patients have this symptom, fish poisoning, shellfish poisoning (Table 3), and the "Chinese restaurant syndrome," and niacin poisoning are the major possibilities.

Histamine fish poisoning (scombroid) is characterized by symptoms resembling those of a histamine reaction. Burning of the mouth and throat, flushing, headache, and dizziness are common; abdominal cramps, nausea, vomiting, and diarrhea also occur in a majority of the cases.[111] In severe cases, urticaria and bronchospasm may also occur. Symptoms are thought to result from histamine and inhibitors of histamine degradation produced in fish flesh by the enzymatic decarboxylation of histidine by certain marine bacteria.[112–115] In an outbreak traced to tuna sashimi,[116] a strain of *Klebsiella pneumoniae* capable of producing large quantities of histamine was implicated.[117] Symptoms usually resolve in a few hours.

Two types of shellfish poisoning should be considered: paralytic (PSP) and neurotoxic (NSP).[118] PSP is characterized by paresthesias of the mouth, lips, face, and extremities.[119–123] In severe cases, dyspnea, dysphagia, muscle weakness or frank paralysis, ataxia, and respiratory insufficiency may occur.[119,122] Respiratory failure may occur during the first 12 hours of the illness.[122] Some patients also have nausea, vomiting, and diarrhea.[118] The disease is caused by neurotoxic substances in dinoflagellates, one of which is known as *saxitoxin*. Bivalve mollusks feed on these dinoflagellates; the toxins are concentrated in their flesh but do not affect the mollusks.[119] Saxitoxin appears to be the only neurotoxin produced by *Gonyaulax catenella*, whereas *Gonyaulax tamarensis* produces saxitoxin and several additional neurotoxic substances.[124–126] The structure of saxitoxin has been determined[127]; it is heat stable and blocks the propagation of nerve and muscle action potentials by interfering with the increase in sodium permeability by acting at a metal cation binding site in the sodium channels of nerve membranes.[128–130] The mechanism of action of the other neurotoxins is unknown. Duration of the illness ranges from a few hours to a few days.[118]

Although many patients with PSP experience the onset of symptoms within 1 hour of ingestion, the incubation period is often inversely related to the amount of toxin ingested. A European outbreak involved 120 cases after the ingestion of contaminated mussels; the median incubation period in this outbreak was 3.5 hours, with a range of 1–10 hours.[121]

The clinical features of NSP are similar to those of PSP, but

TABLE 3. Fish and Shellfish Poisoning Syndromes

Syndrome	Incubation Period	Duration	Geographic Location[a]	Season
Histamine fish poisoning (scombroid)	5 min–1 hr	Few hours	Primarily coastal areas (Hawaii, California)	Year round
Ciguatera	1–6 hr	Few days–few months	35°–35°S latitude (Hawaii, Florida)	Feb.–Sept.
Paralytic shellfish poisoning	5 min–4 hr	Few hours–few days	Above 30°N and below 30°S latitude (New England, West Coast)	May–Nov.
Neurotoxic shellfish poisoning	5 min–4 hr	Few hours–few days	Gulf and Atlantic coasts of Florida (Florida)	Spring, fall

[a] Location of U.S. outbreaks in parentheses.

paralysis does not occur.[118,119] Several poorly characterized neurotoxins responsible for this illness are found in *Gymnodinium breve*, the responsible dinoflagellate.[131–133] One of these neurotoxins stimulates postganglionic cholinergic nerve fibers.[134] Duration of the illness ranges from a few hours to a few days.[118]

The Chinese restaurant syndrome is characterized by a burning sensation in the neck, chest, abdomen, or arms and by a sensation of tightness over the face and chest.[135] Headache, flushing, diaphoresis, lacrimation, weakness, nausea, abdominal cramps, and thirst frequently occur.[135,136] Symptoms appear to be caused by excessive amounts of monosodium L-glutamate in foods, although other undefined substances may also play a role.[135,136] The illness usually resolves within several hours.

Niacin poisoning produces a burning facial erythema within 20 minutes of ingestion, which rapidly resolves.[137]

Paresthesias within 1–6 Hours. The major diagnostic considerations for this syndrome are PSP and ciguatera fish poisoning (Table 3), which is often characterized by the onset of abdominal cramps, nausea, vomiting, and diarrhea preceded or followed by numbness and paresthesias of the lips, tongue, and throat.[138–140] Malaise, headache, pruritus, dry mouth, metallic taste, myalgias, arthralgias, blurred vision, photophobia, and transient blindness have also been reported.[141–143] Sharp shooting pains in the legs and a sensation of looseness and pain in the teeth are characteristic.[139] In severe cases, reversal of hot and cold temperature sensations, sinus bradycardia, hypotension, cranial nerve palsies, and respiratory paralysis may occur.[140,141,144]

The illness is caused by ciguatoxin, a poorly characterized lipid-soluble, relatively heat-stable compound,[145] which is acquired by fish through the food chain.[146] The dinoflagellate, *Gambierdiscus toxicus*, has been identified as the source of the toxin in the food chain.[147] Ciguatoxin inhibits red blood cell cholinesterase activity,[148] increases membrane sodium permeability,[149] and changes the electrical potential of cells through its action on sodium channels.[150,151] Duration of the acute illness ranges from a few days to a few months; pain in the extremities has been reported to occur intermittently for years after an episode of ciguatera.

Miscellaneous Mushroom Poisoning Syndromes within 2 Hours. At least five clinical syndromes may occur within 2 hours of ingestion of toxic mushrooms[152–155] (Table 4). Species containing ibotenic acid and muscimol cause an illness mimicking acute alcoholic intoxication characterized by confusion, restlessness, and visual disturbances followed by lethargy; symptoms resolve within 24 hours. Species containing muscarine cause an illness characterized by evidence of parasympathetic hyperactivity, for example, salivation, lacrimation, diaphoresis, blurred vision, abdominal cramps, and diarrhea. Some patients experience miosis, bradycardia, and bronchospasm. Symptoms usually resolve within 24 hours. Species containing the toxic substances psilocybin and psilocin cause an acute psychotic reaction manifested by hallucinations and inappropriate behavior, which usually resolves within 12 hours. The mushroom *Coprinus atramentarius* contains a disulfiram-like substance that can result in headache, flushing, paresthesias, nausea, vomiting, and tachycardia if alcohol is consumed during the 48-hour period after ingestion. The fifth clinical syndrome is characterized by nausea, vomiting, abdominal cramps, and diarrhea after the ingestion of mushrooms containing gastrointestinal irritants that are not well characterized.

Abdominal Cramps and Diarrhea within 6–24 Hours Followed by Hepatorenal Failure. Species of poisonous mushrooms containing amatoxins and phallotoxins are responsible for this syndrome[152,153,155] (Table 4). The most common implicated species are *Amanita phalloides, A. virosa*, and *A. verna*.[156,157] The illness is typically biphasic; the abdominal cramps and diarrhea, which may be quite severe, usually resolve within 24 hours. The patient then remains well for 1–2 days before evidence of hepatic and renal failure supervenes. A mortality of 30–50 percent has been reported.[158,159]

A similar clinical syndrome follows the ingestion of mushrooms of the *Gyromitra* genus, which contain the toxic substance gyromitrin. However, this toxin does not cause acute renal failure.[160]

Chronic Diarrhea within 1–3 Weeks. A new food-borne disease, chronic watery diarrhea, has recently been described among persons drinking raw milk.[161] After a mean incubation period of 15 days, affected persons developed acute watery diarrhea with marked urgency and abdominal cramps. Diarrhea persisted for a mean period of 2 years. No etiologic agent was identified. A second restaurant-associated outbreak of a similar illness suggests that vehicles other than raw milk may also be involved.[162]

Water-borne Disease. The evaluation of a suspected food-borne outbreak may reveal that water was the vehicle. Pathogens incriminated in water-borne outbreaks are different from those most often responsible for food-borne disease; the responsible etiologic agents for water-borne outbreaks reported to the CDC from 1972 through 1985 are shown in Table 5.[163–176] *Giardia lamblia* is the single most frequently recognized pathogen in the United States and has been responsible for several large outbreaks traced to a municipal water supply.[177–179] This illness is characterized by abdominal pain, bloating, flatulence, and occasionally malabsorption. The incubation period is typi-

TABLE 4. Mushroom Poisoning Syndromes

Syndrome	*Mushroom Species*	*Toxins*
Short incubation		
Delirium	*Amanita muscaria* *A. pantherina*	Ibotenic acid, muscimol
Parasympathetic hyperactivity	*Inocybe* spp. *Clitocybe* spp.	Muscarine
Hallucinations	*Psilocybe* spp. *Panaeolus* spp.	Psilocybin, psilocin
Disulfiram reaction	*Coprinus atramentarius*	Disulfiram-like substance
Gastroenteritis	Many	?
Long incubation		
Gastroenteritis, hepatorenal failure	*Amanita phalloides* *A. virosa* *A. verna* *Galerina autumnalis* *G. marginata* *G. venenata*	Amatoxins, phallotoxins
Gastroenteritis, hepatic failure	*Gyromitra* spp.	Gyromitrin

TABLE 5. Etiology of Water-borne Disease Outbreaks of Known Etiology Reported to the CDC, 1972–1985

Etiology	*Number of Outbreaks*	*Percentage of Total*
G. lamblia	85	38.6
Shigella	26	11.8
Hepatitis A	17	7.7
Norwalk-like agents	15	6.8
C. jejuni	10	4.5
Nontyphoid salmonella	10	4.5
S. typhi	5	2.3
Enterotoxigenic *E. coli*	1	0.5
V. cholerae 01	1	0.5
Y. enterocolitica	1	0.5
Rotavirus	1	0.5
Cryptosporidium	1	0.5
E. histolytica	1	0.5
Miscellaneous chemicals	46	20.9
	Total 220	100.1

TABLE 6. Etiology of Food-borne Disease Outbreaks by Food, Season, and Geographic Predilection

Etiology	Foods	Season	Geographic Predilection
Bacterial			
Salmonella	Beef, poultry, eggs, dairy products	Summer	None
S. aureus	Ham, poultry, egg salads, pastries	Summer	None
C. jejuni	Poultry, raw milk	Spring, summer	None
C. botulinum	Vegetables, fruits, fish, honey (infants)	Summer, fall	West, Northeast
C. perfringens	Beef, poultry, gravy, Mexican food	Fall, winter, spring	None
Shigella	Egg salads, lettuce	Summer	None
V. parahaemolyticus	Crabs	Spring, summer, fall	Coastal states
B. cereus	Fried rice, meats, vegetables	Year round	None
Y. enterocolitica	Milk, tofu, pork	Winter	Unknown
V. cholerae 01	Shellfish	Variable	Tropical, Gulf Coast
V. cholerae non-01	Shellfish	Unknown	Tropical, Gulf Coast
Verotoxigenic *E. coli*	Beef, raw milk	Summer, fall	Unknown
Viral			
Norwalk agent	Shellfish, salads	Year round	Northeast
Chemical			
Ciguatera	Barracuda, snapper, amberjack, grouper	Spring, summer (in Florida)	Tropical
Histamine fish poisoning (scombroid)	Tuna, mackerel, bonito, skipjack, mahi-mahi	Year round	Coastal
Mushroom poisoning	Mushrooms	Spring, fall	Temperate
Heavy metals	Acidic beverages	Year round	None
Monosodium-L-glutamate	Chinese food	Year round	None
Paralytic shellfish poisoning	Shellfish	Summer, fall	Temperate
Neurotoxic shellfish poisoning	Shellfish	Spring, fall	Subtropical

cally 1–4 weeks, and duration of the illness may be several weeks. Large water-borne outbreaks caused by shigellae,[180] hepatitis A,[181] *Salmonella typhi*,[182] nontyphoid salmonellae,[183] enterotoxigenic *E. coli*[184] *C. jejuni*,[185–187] the Norwalk agent,[188,189] and a Norwalk-like virus, the Colorado agent,[190] have been reported. The majority of water-borne outbreaks are of unknown etiology.

Miscellaneous Food-borne Diseases. This discussion has focused on diseases often transmitted by foods and manifested primarily by gastrointestinal or neurologic symptoms and signs. Other infectious diseases with primary symptoms outside the gastrointestinal and neurologic systems, which are occasionally or usually transmitted by foods and their most common vehicles of transmission, include group A β-hemolytic streptococci (potato and egg salds), brucellosis (goat's milk cheese), anthrax (meat), tularemia (water), listeriosis (cole slaw, milk, cheese), *Vibrio vulnificus* (raw oysters), tuberculosis (milk), Q fever (milk), hepatitis A (shellfish, salads), trichinoisis (pork), toxoplasmosis (beef), anisakiasis (fish), and tapeworms (beef, pork, fish).

EPIDEMIOLOGY

In addition to the clinical syndrome and incubation period, additional clues to the cause of an outbreak of food-borne disease may be provided by the type of food responsible and the setting in which it is eaten[191] (Table 6).

Foods

Outbreaks of staphylococcal food poisoning are associated with foods of high protein content, such as ham, poultry, potato and egg salads, and cream-filled pastries, that are thought to be contaminated during preparation by a food handler. The nasal carrier rate for *S. aureus* has been reported to range from 30 to 50 percent, whereas 14–40 percent of healthy people harbor staphylococci on their hands or wrists.[192] Other studies suggest that as many as 38 percent of *S. aureus* isolates from humans are capable of producing an enterotoxin.[193] Although in the classic staphylococcal food-borne outbreak a food handler has a purulent skin lesion on his or her hand, in actuality this is true in only a minority of outbreaks. In contrast, outbreaks of *B. cereus* food poisoning of the short-incubation type are most often associated with fried rice that has been cooked and held warm for extended periods. The growth of *B. cereus* under similar experimental conditions in rice has been well documented.[194] The vehicle in a recently reported outbreak was macaroni and cheese that was mishandled after preparation; investigation revealed that powdered milk was the source of the organism.[195] The short-incubation syndrome is most often caused by serotype 1 strains,[196] possibly because these strains are more heat resistant than strains of other serotypes.[197]

Clostridium perfringens outbreaks usually follow the ingestion of meat (especially beef and poultry) and gravies; organisms have been isolated from 16–85 percent of raw meat, poultry, and fish specimens.[198–200] Outbreaks are more likely to occur when these items are prepared in large quantities for banquets or in institutional settings when food is prepared well in advance without adequate final reheating.[201] Long-incubation *B. cereus* food poisoning is also frequently associated with meat or vegetable dishes. In addition to the frequent contamination of raw meats, vegetables, and milk products with *B. cereus*, the organism has been isolated from 25 percent of dried foods such as seasoning mixes, spices, and dried potatoes[202] and from over 50 percent of dried beans and cereals.[203] A long-incubation *B. cereus* outbreak has also been traced to a "meals-on-wheels" operation in which food was held at and above room temperature for an extended period.[204]

Salmonella food-borne outbreaks most frequently follow the ingestion of poultry, beef, egg, or dairy products. The role of raw milk in the transmission of *Salmonella* infections has recently been re-emphasized.[205–207] Two large international outbreaks have been caused by contaminated chocolate candy.[208,209] A recently recognized contamination of shell eggs is associated with a large number of outbreaks due to *Salmonella enteriditis*.[210] *Shigella* outbreaks are most often associated with cool, moist foods such as potato and egg salads. In a recent outbreak caused by *Shigella dysenteriae* type 2, the vehicle was raw vegetables served at a salad bar.[211] *Campylobacter jejuni* outbreaks most often follow the ingestion of raw milk and poultry.[48,212] *Vibrio parahaemolyticus* outbreaks in the United States are associated with the ingestion of bivalve mollusks and crustaceans[213,214]; in Japan, these outbreaks are more often associated with the ingestion of a variety of saltwater fish.[215] *Vibrio cholerae* 01 and non-01 outbreaks have been traced to contaminated shellfish eaten raw or inadequately cooked.[56,216,217] Crabs, shrimp, and raw oysters have been implicated as the vehicles of transmission of a unique epidemic strain of *V. cholerae* in Louisiana.[8,218–221] Sporadic cases of diarrhea associated with *V. cholerae* non-01 strains in the United States have also been linked to shellfish ingestion.[54,55] Food-borne outbreaks in the United States due to *Y. enterocolitica* were caused by contaminated milk[79,80] and tofu.[81] In Europe, this illness is associated with eating raw pork.[82] The single food-borne outbreak caused by invasive *E. coli* followed the ingestion of cheese.[46] Travelers' diarrhea caused by enterotoxigenic *E. coli* has been associated with consumption of salads in Mexico,[222] a recent food-borne outbreak of enterotoxigenic *E. coli* followed the ingestion of imported cheese,[223]and enterotoxigenic isolates have been obtained from a variety of foods including hamburger, sausage, seafood, and cheese in the United States.[224] Botulism outbreaks are most often associated with the ingestion of low-acid (pH ≥ 4.4) home-canned vegetables, fruits, and fish. Recent outbreaks of botulism followed ingestion of unusual vehicles including baked potatoes, sauteed onions, and chopped garlic.[105,225] Honey may have been the source of *C. botulinum* in some cases of infant botulism.[226] In Norwalk agent outbreaks, oysters[74,227,228] and salads[229] have been implicated. In a recent large outbreak, cake and frosting were implicated.[230] Contamination of food by an ill food handler has been documented.[231] Food-borne transmission of the Snow Mountain agent has been associated with clams.[77]

Outbreaks of heavy metal poisoning are most often associated with acidic beverages such as lemonade, fruit punch, and carbonated drinks that have been stored in corroded metallic containers such as punch bowls[108] or that have been in contact with metallic tubing (e.g., in vending machines)[232] for periods of time sufficient to leach the metallic ions from the container. Histamine fish poisoning outbreaks are associated with scombroid fish, the most common of which are tuna, mackerel, bonito, and skipjack. In addition, the nonscombroid fish mahi-mahi has caused outbreaks of scombroid-like fish poisoning. Ciguatera fish poisoning has been associated with over 400 species of fish. Barracuda, red snapper, amberjack, and grouper are most commonly implicated. The disease is more often associated with large fish; in one study, 69 percent of red snapper weighing 2.8 kg or more was toxic, compared to only 18 percent of smaller fish.[233] PSP and NSP follow the ingestion of bivalve mollusks, most often oysters, clams, and mussels. The most common Chinese food item associated with the Chinese restaurant syndrome is soup, which is frequently the first item ingested at a meal; the absorption of monosodium L-glutamate is most rapid when the stomach is empty.[135]

Seasonality

The time of year may also provide a clue to the cause of a food-borne outbreak. Outbreaks caused by the bacterial pathogens *S. aureus, Salmonella*, and *Shigella*, are most common during the summer months. *C. jejuni* outbreaks are more common during the spring and fall, *C. perfringens* outbreaks occur throughout the year but least often during the summer months, and botulism outbreaks are more common during the summer and fall.

In general, chemical food poisoning occurs throughout the year. Exceptions are PSP, which often occurs in association with a red tide[234] and is most common in the summer and fall; ciguatera, which is most common in the spring and summer in Florida;[235] and mushroom poisoning, which is most common in the spring, late summer, and fall.

Geographic Location

The geographic setting may provide a clue to the cause of food-borne disease. *Vibrio parahaemolyticus* outbreaks are most frequently reported from coastal states. The initial 13 outbreaks reported in the United States all occurred in coastal states.[213] An outbreak of cholera and sporadic cases of *V. cholerae* 01 and non-01 infection have been reported from the Gulf Coast of the United States.[8] Type A botulism outbreaks are most common west of the Mississippi River, whereas type B outbreaks are most common in the East, and type E outbreaks are most common in the Great Lakes Region.[101]

Ciguatera outbreaks occur in tropical and subtropical regions between 35°N and 35°S latitudes. Over 90 percent of outbreaks in the United States have been reported from Florida and Hawaii.[118] Ciguatera is common in the West Indies,[237] and travelers who return with the characteristic syndrome should be questioned regarding fish consumption. PSP and NSP outbreaks occur in coastal areas. *Gonyaulax tamarensis* is the dinoflagellate responsible for shellfish contamination along the New England Coast, whereas *G. catenella* is the responsible organism along the Pacific Coast. *Gymnodinium breve* is the dinoflagellate responsible for outbreaks of neurotoxic shellfish poisoning on the Gulf Coast of Florida.

Epidemiologic Assessment

For a food to provide a clue to the cause of a food-borne outbreak, it must be identified. Once a common meal is identified through interviews with ill people, food-specific attack rates should be determined for all foods and beverages served at the meal (see example in Table 7). People who ate the same meal but did not become ill must also be interviewed to serve as controls. Food-specific attack rates may identify the responsible vehicle of transmission. To be adequately incriminated, a food must have a significantly higher attack rate for those who ate it than for those who did not, and most of those who became ill must have eaten the food. On occasion, more than one food

TABLE 7. Example of Use of Food-Specific Attack Rates and Cross-Table Analysis to Identify Food Vehicle in a Food-borne Outbreak

	Food-Specific Attack Rates					
	No. of People Eating Food			*No. of People Not Eating Food*		
Food	*Total*	*Ill*	*Percent Ill*	*Total*	*Ill*	*Percent Ill*
Meat loaf	100	88	88[a]	10	2	20[a]
Gravy	80	80	100[b]	30	10	33[b]
Potatoes	95	78	82	15	12	80
Salad	90	74	82	20	16	80
Water	70	58	82	40	32	80
	Cross-Table Analysis					
	No. of People Eating Meat Loaf			*No. of People Not Eating Meat Loaf*		
	Total	*Ill*	*Percent Ill*	*Total*	*Ill*	*Percent Ill*
No. eating gravy	75	67	89[c]	5	1	20[d]
No. not eating gravy	25	21	84[c]	5	1	20[d]

[a] $p < .05$ (Fisher's exact test).
[b] $p < .05$ (Chi-square analysis).
[c] $p > .05$ (Chi-square analysis).
[d] $p > .05$ (Fisher's exact test).

item may be incriminated. On these occasions, simple cross-table analysis may indicate whether both items were contaminated by the etiologic agent or whether both were eaten by most people at the meal (e.g., meat and gravy) (Table 7). For example, if meat loaf and gravy were both incriminated, subsequent analysis may indicate that attack rates were equally high for those who ate meat loaf, regardless of whether or not they ate gravy, and were similarly low for those who did not eat meat loaf, regardless of whether or not they ate gravy, indicating that the meat loaf alone was responsible for the outbreak.

LABORATORY DIAGNOSIS

Appropriate specimens for laboratory confirmation vary with the etiologic agents but include feces, vomitus, serum, and blood (Table 8). In addition, cultures of the food preparation environment and food handlers may be indicated. The laboratory should be alerted to suspected causes so that special techniques can be used for isolation of *C. perfringens*, vibrios, *C. jejuni, E. coli* 0157:H7 and *Y. enterocolitica* and so that organisms considered part of the normal flora (other *E. coli, B. cereus*) are not overlooked.

Outbreaks of staphylococcal food poisoning may be confirmed by the isolation of *S. aureus* of the same phage type from vomitus or feces of ill people and from the incriminated food or skin lesion or hand of a food handler, by the isolation of more than 10^5 *S. aureus* organisms per gram of incriminated food, or by the demonstration of staphylococcal enterotoxin in the food by gel diffusion, radioimmunoassay (RIA), or the enzyme-linked immunosorbent assay (ELISA), which have sensitivities of 0.1–3 ng/g of food.[238–242] *Bacillus cereus* outbreaks may be documented by the isolation of organisms from the feces of ill people who shared the same meal or by the isolation of 10^5 or more *B. cereus* per gram of incriminated food. Serotyping, if available, may be of value in confirming that isolates were derived from a common source, since 14 percent of healthy adults have been reported to have transient gastrointestinal colonization with *B. cereus*.[243] Plasmid analysis may also be useful.[244]

The laboratory confirmation of *C. perfringens* outbreaks is more difficult. Since both heat-sensitive and heat-resistant strains of *C. perfringens* type A have been implicated as causes of food poisoning, selective isolation procedures involving heat treatment of food and fecal specimens should not be used. Because *C. perfringens* organisms are variably reported as normal flora in 42–100 percent of healthy people,[245,246] organisms of the same serotype[247–249] or bacteriocin type[250] should be demonstrated in stools of ill people and the incriminated food or in stools of ill people and not in those of people who ate the same meal but did not become ill, or median counts of 10^6 or more *C. perfringens* spores per gram of feces obtained within 48 hours after onset of illness should be demonstrated.[247,251] Alternatively, counts of 10^5 or more organisms per gram of food provide etiologic confirmation. For serotyping, approximately 90 *C. perfringens* antisera, including the original 13 Hobbs serotypes, are available, but many isolates cannot be typed. In the United Kingdom, serotyping implicates a specific serotype in nearly two-thirds of outbreaks,[248] whereas in the United States serotyping is helpful in only approximately 20 percent of outbreaks.[252] Alternative confirmatory tests, which remain experimental, are the demonstration of enterotoxin in the stools of ill people and not in control subjects or a fourfold rise in antitoxin titers in serum by counterimmunoelectrophoresis or reverse passive hemagglutination techniques.[253–255] Because 65–100 percent of healthy people have antibody to *C. perfringens* enterotoxin,[253,256] a single elevated titer is inadequate confirmation. Reverse passive hemagglutination (sensitivity 1 ng/ml) is the most sensitive method of enterotoxin detection.[257]

Salmonella, Shigella, C. jejuni, V. cholerae 01 and non-01, *V. parahaemolyticus*, and *Y. enterocolitica* outbreaks may be confirmed by the isolation and serotyping of the organisms from the feces of ill people. In *Salmonella* outbreaks in which it is uncertain whether a common vehicle is responsible, plasmid profiling may be necessary.[258,259] Strains of *V. parahaemolyticus* isolated from patients are hemolytic on special blood agar medium (Kanagawa-positive strains). Isolation and serotying of salmonellae, shigellae, *C. jejuni*, vibrios, and *Y. enterocolitica* from the incriminated food may also be confirmatory. Because *V. parahaemolyticus* in low numbers are a frequent contaminant of shellfish, counts of 10^5 or more organisms per gram are required for confirmation; food isolates are usually Kanagawa negative. Serologic testing of acute and convalescent sera may be helpful in confirming the diagnosis in patients in *Y. enterocolitica*, cholera, and typhoid fever outbreaks but currently plays no important role in the investigation of nontyphoid *Salmonella, Shigella, C. jejuni*, and *V. parahaemolyticus* outbreaks.

Verotoxigenic *E. coli* may be implicated by isolating sorbitol-negative *E. coli* from stools of ill persons and confirming them

TABLE 8. Appropriate Laboratory Specimens for Documentation of Etiology of a Food-borne Outbreak

	Patient			*Food Handler*				
	Stools	*Vomitus*	*Blood*	*Stools*	*Nose*	*Hands*	*Food*	*Food-Preparation Environment*
Bacterial								
Salmonella	C		C	C			C	C
S. aureus	C	C			C	C	C, T	
C. jejuni	C			C			C	C
C. botulinum	C, T	C, T	T				C, T	
C. perfringens	C, T						C	
Shigella	C			C			C	
V. parahaemolyticus	C						C	C
B. cereus	C	C					C	
Y. enterocolitica	C		S	C			C	C
V. cholerae 01 and non-01	C		S	C			C	C
Verotoxigenic *E. coli*	C, T						C, T	
Viral								
Norwalk agent	I		S					
Chemical								
Ciguatera							T	
Histamine fish poisoning (scombroid)							T	
Mushroom	T	T	T				T	
Heavy metals							T	
Monosodium-L-glutamate							T	
Paralytic shellfish poisoning							T	
Neurotoxic shellfish poisoning							T	

Abbreviations: C: culture; T: toxin testing; S: serology; I: immune electron microscopy.

as serotype 0157:H7,[260] by demonstrating free verotoxin in stools, or by isolating other verotoxigenic strains from stools from ill individuals.[95] Enterotoxigenic *E. coli* may be implicated by demonstrating the presence of isolates producing the heat-labile enterotoxin (LT) in tissue culture assays,[261,262] ELISA,[263] or the Biken test[264] or isolates producing the heat-stable enterotoxin (ST) in the suckling mouse assay[265] in ill people and not in control subjects. Invasive strains may be identified using the Sereny test.[266] Since *E. coli* serotypes have been shown to cause diarrhea in volunteers in the absence of detectable enterotoxin production or invasiveness,[267] serotyping of *E. coli* isolates from both patients and controls may also be useful in outbreak settings if cases are found to have a serotype absent from controls.

Botulism outbreaks may be confirmed by the demonstration of botulinal toxin in the serum or stool of ill people or in incriminated food by the mouse neutralization test or by the isolation of *C. botulinum* from the feces of ill people or from the incriminated food.[268,269] Laboratory confirmation by testing of clinical specimens can be obtained in approximately 70–75 percent of the cases of botulism.[268,269] Norwalk agent outbreaks may be confirmed by the demonstration of viral particles in stools of ill people by immune electron microscopy[270] or of a serologic response by a biotin-avidin immunoassay procedure.[271]

Outbreaks caused by heavy metals may be documented by the demonstration of the metallic ion in the incriminated food. Histamine fish poisoning may be confirmed by the demonstration of histamine in the fish; concentrations of 100 mg in 100 g of fish flesh correlate with toxicity. The diagnosis of ciguatera is based on the clinical picture.[272] However, ciguatera outbreaks may be documented by the demonstration of ciguatoxin in the incriminated fish using a bioassay in the mongoose, rat, or cat; RIA and ELISA techniques have been developed but are not generally available.[273,274] Shellfish poisoning may be confirmed either by demonstrating the toxin in mollusks by the mouse bioassay technique or by finding elevated numbers of the responsible dinoflagellate in the water from which the mollusks were obtained. Outbreaks of Chinese restaurant syndrome may be confirmed by the demonstration of elevated monosodium L-glutamate levels in the food. Mushroom poisoning may be confirmed either by the identification of the responsible toxin in gastric contents, blood, urine, or fecal specimens by thin-layer chromatography or RIA or by the identification of the mushroom by a mycologist.

An additional diagnostic tool that may be of value in food-borne disease outbreaks characterized by diarrhea is the fecal leukocyte examination.[275] The presence of leukocytes implies that the responsible organism has invaded the intestinal tract, suggesting that salmonellae, shigellae, *C. jejuni*, invasive *E. coli, V. parahaemolyticus*, or *Y. enterocolitica* are responsible for the illness.

Over 50 percent of the reported food-borne disease outbreaks in the United States are of unknown cause. In some cases, appropriate diagnostic procedures are not conducted. In others, no agent is identified, raising the possibility that other etiologic agents are responsible. Possibilities include *Aeromonas hydrophila, Plesiomonas shigelloides*, rotaviruses, and Norwalk-like agents. In several outbreaks in England traced to cockles, 25–26 nm viral particles similar to Norwalk-like agents have been seen in stool specimens.[276] Although enterococci and gram-negative rods (*Klebsiella, Enterobacter, Proteus, Citrobacter*, and *Pseudomonas* spp.) have been reported as causes of food-borne outbreaks on rare occasions, their role in the cause of food-borne outbreaks has not been well documented. Because these latter organisms may be part of the normal fecal flora, documentation of their presence in ill people and their absence from well people will be required to confirm their role in food-borne outbreaks. That the gram-negative organisms might be responsible for some outbreaks is suggested by reports of the production of LT[277,278] and ST enterotoxins[279,280] by some of these organisms.

THERAPY

Supportive measures are the mainstay of therapy in most cases of food poisoning. The majority of these illnesses are self-limited; exceptions are botulism, long-incubation mushroom poisoning, and PSP, which may be fatal in previously healthy people, and listeriosis, which is often fatal in neonates and immunocompromised persons. In addition, fatalities occasionally occur due to staphylococcal and *C. perfringens* food poisoning, salmonellosis, verotoxigenic *E. coli* infections, and shigellosis in infants, the elderly, and debilitated people (Table 9).

Gastrointestinal fluid losses should be replaced either orally or parenterally. Antimicrobial agents may be used in the therapy for shigellosis, cholera, and typhoid fever but should be avoided in uncomplicated gastrointestinal infection caused by nontyphoid salmonellae. Tetracycline shortens both the duration of clinical cholera and the excretion of *V. cholerae* 01. Erythromycin eradicates carriage of *C. jejuni* and can shorten the duration of illness if given early in the disease.[281] The role of antimicrobial agents in the management of food poisoning due to *V. parahaemolyticus*, enterotoxigenic, verotoxigenic, and invasive *E. coli*, and *Y. enterocolitica* is unsettled but probably minimal. Antimicrobial agents are of no value in the management of staphylococcal, *C. perfringens*, or *B. cereus* food poisoning. Antiperistaltic agents appear to be of little if any benefit in controlling diarrhea and are contraindicated in patients with fever or fecal leukocytes, which suggest a syndrome associated with an invasive pathogen. Patients with botulism present several additional therapeutic problems, which are discussed in Chapter 221.

Patients with PSP and occasional patients with ciguatera may require ventilatory support; in these illnesses, this support is usually required for only a few days. A recent report suggests that intravenous mannitol may ameliorate the acute symptoms of ciguatera rapidly.[282] Therapy is otherwise supportive; no antitoxins are available. If not contraindicated by the presence of ileus, enemas or cathartics may be administered to these patients in an effort to remove unabsorbed toxin from the intestinal tract. Because of the severe dysesthesias associated with ciguatera, analgesics may also be required. Symptoms of histamine fish poisoning may be relieved by antihistamines. In severe cases with bronchospasm, epinephrine or aminophylline may be required.

Therapy for short-incubation-period types of mushroom poisoning is primarily supportive.[283] Patients who have ingested species containing pharmacologically active amounts of muscarine and who manifest evidence of parasympathetic hyperactivity may be treated with atropine. Patients who are severely ill after ingestion of species containing ibotenic acid and mus-

TABLE 9. Etiology of Food-borne Disease Deaths Reported to the CDC, 1972–1986

Etiology	*Number of Deaths*	*Percentage of Total*
Salmonella	88	28.9
L. monocytogenes	56	18.4
C. botulinum	49	16.1
Unknown	36	11.8
Miscellaneous	18	5.9
C. perfringens	13	4.3
V. cholerae 01	12	3.9
Mushrooms	11	3.6
Trichinella	6	2.0
Verotoxigenic *E. coli*	4	1.3
Shigella	4	1.3
Ciguatera	3	1.0
S. aureus	2	0.7
C. jejuni	2	0.7
Paralytic shellfish poisoning	1	0.3
	Total 305	100.2

cimol may be treated with physostigmine. Therapy for the long-incubation illness includes cathartics and enemas in an effort to remove unabsorbed toxin, as well as a number of specific and supportive measures.[283] Since hypoglycemia often occurs, intravenous glucose may be required. Thioctic acid is an experimental drug that appears to be an effective antidote in these patients[153]; the drug may be obtained from Burton M. Berkson, M.D., Ph.D., in Las Cruces, New Mexico (505-523-3284 or 523-3276). Pyridoxine is indicated in the management of patients poisoned with *Gyromitra* species.

Therapy for acute heavy metal poisoning is supportive. Emesis should be induced if it does not occur spontaneously. Antiemetics are contraindicated, since retention of the toxic ions in the gut with subsequent systemic absorption may result. In severe cases with systemic manifestations of heavy metal toxicity, use of specific antidotes may be considered but is rarely necessary in these outbreaks.

PREVENTION

Food-borne disease can be prevented if food is selected, prepared, and stored properly. In outbreaks reported to the CDC, the most common error is storage of food at inappropriate temperatures; this error is most often identified in staphylococcal, short- and long-incubation *B. cereus, C. perfringens*, and *Salmonella* outbreaks. Bacterial pathogens grow in food at temperatures ranging from 40 to 140°F; growth may be prevented if cold food is adequately refrigerated and if hot food is held at temperatures above 140°F before serving.

Another food-handling deficiency that frequently contributes to staphylococcal, *Shigella*, and typhoid fever outbreaks and appears to be important in some Norwalk agent outbreaks is poor personal hygiene by food handlers. Although thorough cooking of food just before consumption will eliminate the risk of many illnesses, protection against staphylococcal food poisoning is not provided, since the staphylococcal enterotoxins are heat stable. Inadequate heat processing may lead to botulism, and the use of contaminated equipment such as knives and meat slicers may result in nontyphoid salmonellosis.[284] Particular care in handling and cooking raw poultry, raw beef, raw pork, raw shellfish, and raw eggs is important in preventing many food-borne diseases. Avoiding consumption of raw milk is important in preventing *Salmonella* and *C. jejuni* outbreaks.[285]

Food-handling errors resulting in chemical intoxication are different from those leading to bacterial outbreaks. Heavy metal poisoning occurs when acidic beverages are stored in defective metallic containers or when valves in vending machines malfunction. Ciguatera and shellfish poisoning occur when fish or shellfish are obtained from unsafe sources. Items contaminated with these toxins appear and taste normal; in addition, cooking of these items does not provide protection, since the toxins are heat stable.

Food-borne disease outbreaks should be reported to public health authorities. Reporting is essential if investigations are to be conducted to identify the food-handling error so that these deficiencies can be corrected. Prompt reporting may also lead to the prevention of additional cases; there are well-documented episodes of botulism[105,286] and salmonellosis[287] in which recognition and reporting of the initial illness could have prevented subsequent cases. Reporting may lead to recognition of illnesses with the potential for intrafamilial spread (e.g., shigellosis), so secondary transmission can be prevented. Finally, reporting is vital if the 1–2 percent of all reported outbreaks that are caused by commercially distributed foods are to be identified before large numbers of people become ill.

REFERENCES

1. Sours HE, Smith DG. Outbreaks of foodborne disease in the United States, 1972–1978. J Infect Dis. 1980;142:122.
2. Centers for Disease Control. Foodborne Disease Surveillance Annual Summary 1979. April 1981.
3. Centers for Disease Control. Foodborne Disease Surveillance Annual Summary 1980. February 1983.
4. Centers for Disease Control. Foodborne Disease Surveillance Annual Summary 1981. June 1983.
5. MacDonald KL, Griffin PM. Foodborne disease outbreaks, annual summary, 1982. CDC surveillance summaries. Morb Mort Weekly Rep. 1986;35(No 1SS):7–16SS.
6. Bennett JV, Holmberg SD, Rogers MF, et al. Infectious and parasitic diseases. In: Amler RW, Dull HB, eds. Closing the Gap: The Burden of Unnecessary Illness. New York: Oxford University Press; 1987;102–14.
7. Merson MH, Martin WT, Craig JP, et al. Cholera on Guam, 1974: Epidemiologic findings and isolation of non-toxinogenic strains. Am J Epidemiol. 1977;105:349.
8. Blake PA, Allegra DT, Snyder JD, et al. Cholera: A possible endemic focus in the United States. N Engl J Med. 1980;302:305.
9. Osterholm MT, Forfang JC, Ristinen TL, et al. An outbreak of foodborne giardiasis. N Engl J Med. 1981;304:24.
10. Petersen LR, Cartter ML, Hadler JL. A food-borne outbreak of *Giardia lamblia*. J Infect Dis. 1988;157:846–8.
11. Feig M. Staphylococcal food poisoning. A report of two related outbreaks, and a discussion of the data presented. Am J Public Health. 1950;40:279.
12. Bergdoll MS. The enterotoxins. In: Cohen JO, ed. The Staphylococci. New York: Wiley; 1972:301.
13. Bergdoll MS, Crass BA, Reiser RF, et al. A new staphylococcal enterotoxin, enterotoxin F, associated with toxic-shock-syndrome *Staphylococcus aureus* isolates. Lancet. 1981;1:1017.
14. Sugiyama H, Hayama T. Abdominal viscera as site of emetic action for staphylococcal enterotoxin in the monkey. J Infect Dis. 1965;115:330.
15. Clark WG, Vanderhooft GF, Borison HL. Emetic effect of purified staphylococcal enterotoxin in cats. Proc Soc Exp Biol Med. 1962;111:205.
16. Elias J, Shields R. Influence of staphylococcal enterotoxin on water and electrolyte transport in the small intestine. Gut. 1976;17:527.
17. Gilbert RJ. Staphylococcal food poisoning and botulism. Postgrad Med J. 1974;50:603.
18. Breckinridge JC, Bergdoll MS. Outbreak of foodborne gastroenteritis due to a coagulase-negative enterotoxin-producing staphylococcus. N Engl J Med. 1971;284:541.
19. Merson MH. The epidemiology of staphylococcal foodborne disease. Proc Staph in Foods Conf. University Park, PA: Pennsylvania State University; 1973:20.
20. Šimkovičova M, Gilbert RJ. Serological detection of enterotoxin from food-poisoning strains of *Staphylococcus aureus*. J Med Microbiol. 1971;4:19.
21. Holmberg SD, Blake PA. Staphylococcal food poisoning in the United States: New facts and old misconceptions. JAMA. 1984;251:487.
22. Mortimer PR, McCann G. Food-poisoning episodes associated with *Bacillus cereus* in fried rice. Lancet. 1974;1:1043.
23. Midura T, Gerber M, Wood R, et al. Outbreak of food poisoning caused by *Bacillus cereus*. Public Health Rep. 1970;85:45.
24. Terranova W, Blake PA. *Bacillus cereus* food poisoning. N Engl J Med. 1978;298:143.
25. Melling J, Capel BJ, Turnbull PCB, et al. Identification of a novel enterotoxigenic activity associated with *Bacillus cereus*. J Clin Pathol. 1976;29:938.
26. Turnbull PCB, Kramer JM, Jorgensen K. Properties and production characteristics of vomiting, diarrheal, and necrotizing toxins of *Bacillus cereus*. Am J Clin Nutr. 1979;32:219.
27. Hobbs BC, Smith ME, Oakley CL, et al. *Clostridium welchii* food poisoning. J Hyg. 1953;51:75.
28. Shandera WX, Tacket CO, Blake PA. Food poisoning due to *Clostridium perfringens* in the United States. J Infect Dis. 1983;147:167.
29. Smith LDS. *Clostridium perfringens*. The Pathogenic Anaerobic Bacteria. Springfield, Ill: Charles C Thomas; 1975:115.
30. Stark RL, Duncan CL. Purification and biochemical properties of *Clostridium perfringens* type A enterotoxin. Infect Immun. 1972;6:662.
31. Duncan CL. Time of enterotoxin formation and release during sporulation of *Clostridium perfringens* type A. J Bacteriol. 1973;113:932.
32. McDonel JL, Duncan CL. Regional localization of activity of *Clostridium perfringens* type A enterotoxin in the rabbit ileum, jejunum, and duodenum. J Infect Dis. 1977;136:661.
33. McDonel JL. The molecular mode of action of *Clostridium perfringens* enterotoxin. Am J Clin Nutr. 1979;32:210.
34. Turnbull PCB. Studies on the production of enterotoxins by *Bacillus cereus*. J Clin Pathol. 1976;29:941.
35. Loewenstein MS.Epidemiology of *Clostridium perfringens* food poisoning. N Engl J Med. 1972;286:1026.
36. Giannella RA, Brasile L: A hospital food-borne outbreak of diarrhea caused by *Bacillus cereus*. Clinical, epidemiologic, and microbiologic studies. J Infect Dis. 1979;139:366.
37. Giannella RA, Formal SB, Dammin GJ, et al. Pathogenesis of salmonellosis: Studies of fluid secretion, mucosal invasion, and morphologic reaction in the rabbit ileum. J Clin Invest. 1973;52:441.
38. Rout WR, Formal SB, Giannella RA, et al. Pathophysiology of shigella diarrhea in the rhesus monkey: Intestinal transport, morphological, and bacteriological studies. Gastroenterology. 1975;68:270.
39. Bolen JL, Zamiska SA, Greenough WB III. Clinical features in enteritis due to *Vibrio parahaemolyticus*. Am J Med. 1974;57:638.

40. Hughes JM, Boyce JM, Aloem ARMA, et al. *Vibrio parahaemolyticus* enterocolitis in Bangladesh: Report of an outbreak. Am J Trop Med Hyg. 1978;27:106.
41. Boutin BK, Townsend SF, Scarpino PV, et al: Demonstration of invasiveness of *Vibrio parahaemolyticus* in adult rabbits by immunofluorescence. Appl Environ Microbiol. 1979;37:647.
42. Tulloch EF, Ryan KJ, Formal SB, et al. Invasive enteropathic *Escherichia coli* dysentery: An outbreak in 28 adults. Ann Intern Med. 1973;79:13.
43. Horwitz MA, Pollard RA, Merson MH, et al. A large outbreak of foodborne salmonellosis on the Navaho Nation Indian Reservation: Epidemiology and secondary transmission. Am J Public Health. 1977;67:1071.
44. Weissman JB, Williams SV, Hinman AR, et al. Foodborne shigellosis at a country fair. Am J Epidemiol. 1974;100:178.
45. Chatterjee BD, Neogy KN, Gorbach SL. Studies of *Vibrio parahaemolyticus* from cases of diarrhea in Calcutta. Indian J Med Res. 1970;58:234.
46. Marier R, Wells JG, Swanson RC, et al. An outbreak of enteropathogenic *Escherichia coli* foodborne disease traced to imported French cheese. Lancet. 1973;2:1376.
47. Blaser MJ, Reller LB. *Campylobacter* enteritis. N Engl J Med. 1981; 305:1444.
48. Tauxe RV, Bean NH, Patton CH. *Campylobacter* isolates in the United States, 1982–1986. CDC surveillance summaries. MMWR. 1988;37(No SS-2):1–13.
49. Blaser MJ, Wells JG, Feldman RA. *Campylobacter* enteritis in the United States: A multicenter study. Ann Intern Med. 1983;98:360.
50. Lambert ME, Schofield PF, Ironside AG, et al. *Campylobacter* colitis. Br Med J. 1979;1:857.
51. Taylor DN, Porter BW, Williams CA, et al. *Campylobacter* enteritis: A large outbreak traced to commercial raw milk. West J Med. 1982;137:365.
52. Blaser MJ, Checko P, Bopp C, et al. *Campylobacter* enteritis associated with foodborne transmission. Am J Epidemiol. 1982;116:886.
53. Blaser MJ, Berkowitz ID, LaForce FM, et al. *Campylobacter* enteritis: Clinical and epidemiologic features. Ann Intern Med. 1979;91:179.
54. Hughes JM, Hollis DG, Gangarosa FJ, et al. Non-*cholera vibrio* infections in the United States: Clinical, epidemiologic, and laboratory features. Ann Intern Med. 1978;88:602–6.
55. Morris JG Jr, Wilson R, Davis BR, et al. Non-0 group 1 *Vibrio cholerae* gastroenteritis in the United States: Clinical, epidemiologic, and laboratory characteristics of sporadic cases. Ann Intern Med. 1981;94:656.
56. Wilson R, Lieb S, Roberts A, et al. Non-0 group 1 *Vibrio cholerae* gastroenteritis associated with eating raw oysters. Am J Epidemiol. 1981;114:293.
57. Carpenter CCJ Jr. Cholera enterotoxin: Recent investigations yield insights into transport processes. Am J Med. 1971;50:1.
58. Zinnaka Y, Carpenter CCJ Jr. An enterotoxin produced by noncholera vibrios. Johns Hopkins Med J. 1972;131:403.
59. Craig JP, Yamamoto K, Takeda Y, et al. Production of cholera-like enterotoxin by a *Vibrio cholerae* non-01 strain isolated from the environment. Infect Immun. 1981;34:90.
60. Sack RB. Human diarrheal disease caused by enterotoxigenic *Escherichia coli*. Ann Rev Microbiol. 1975;29:333.
61. Sandefur PD, Peterson JW. Neutralization of *Salmonella* toxin-induced elongation of Chinese hamster ovary cells by cholera antitoxin. Infect Immun. 1977;15:988.
62. Sedlock DM, Deibel RH. Detection of *Salmonella* enterotoxin using rabbit ileal loops. Can J Microbiol. 1978;24:268.
63. Keusch GT, Donta ST. Classification of enterotoxins on the basis of activity in cell culture. J Infect Dis. 1975;131:58.
64. Keusch GT, Jacewicz M. The pathogenesis of *Shigella* diarrhea. IV. Toxin and antitoxin in *Shigella flexneri* and *Shigella sonnei* infections in humans. J Infect Dis. 1977;135:552.
65. O'Brien AD, Gentry MK, Thompson MR, et al. Shigellosis and *Escherichia coli* diarrhea: Relative importance of invasive and toxigenic mechanisms. Am J Clin Nutr. 1979;32:229.
66. Honda T, Shimizu M, Takeda Y, et al. Isolation of a factor causing morphological changes of Chinese hamster ovary cells from the culture filtrate of *Vibrio parahaemolyticus*. Infect Immun. 1976;14:1028.
67. Carruthers MM. Cytotoxicity of *Vibrio parahaemolyticus* in HeLa cell culture. J Infect Dis. 1975;132:555.
68. Banwell JG, Gorbach SL, Pierce NF, et al. Acute undifferentiated human diarrhea in the tropics. II. Alterations in intestinal fluid and electrolyte movements. J Clin Invest. 1971;50:890.
69. Barker WH Jr, Mackowiak PA, Fishbein M, et al. *Vibrio parahaemolyticus* gastroenteritis outbreak in Covington, Louisiana, in August 1972. Am J Epidemiol. 1974;100:316.
70. Aldova E, Lázničková K, Stěpánková E, et al. Isolation of nonagglutinable vibrios from an enteritis outbreak in Czechoslovakia. J Infect Dis. 1968;118:25.
71. Carpenter CCJ Jr, Mitra PP, Sack RB. Clinical studies in Asiatic cholera. I. Preliminary observations, November, 1962–March, 1963. Bull Johns Hopkins Hosp. 1966;118:165.
72. Taylor WR, Schell WL, Wells JG, et al. A foodborne outbreak of enterotoxigenic *Escherichia coli* diarrhea. N Engl J Med. 1982;306:1093.
73. Kaplan JE, Gary GW, Baron RC, et al. Epidemiology of Norwalk gastroenteritis and the role of Norwalk virus in outbreaks of acute nonbacterial gastroenteritis. Ann Intern Med. 1982;96:756.
74. Murphy AM, Grohmann GS, Christopher PJ, et al. An Australia-wide outbreak of gastroenteritis from oysters caused by Norwalk virus. Med J Aust. 1979;2:329.
75. Morse DL, Guzewich JJ, Hanrahan JP, et al. Widespread outbreaks of clam- and oyster-associated gastroenteritis: Role of Norwalk virus. N Engl J Med. 1986;314:678–81.
76. Kaplan JE, Feldman R, Campbell DS, et al. The frequency of a Norwalk-like pattern of illness in outbreaks of acute gastroenteritis. Am J Public Health. 1982;72:1329–32.
77. Truman BI, Madore HP, Menegus MA, et al. Snow Mountain Agent gastroenteritis from clams. Am J Epidemiol. 1987;126:516–25.
78. Dolin R, Treanor JJ, Madore HP. Novel agents of viral enteritis in humans. J Infect Dis. 1987;155:365–76.
79. Black RE, Jackson RJ, Tsai T, et al. Epidemic *Yersinia enterocolitica* infection due to contaminated chocolate milk. N Engl J Med. 1978;298:76.
80. Tacket CO, Narain JP, Sattin R, et al. A multistate outbreak of infections caused by *Yersinia enterocolitica* transmitted by pasteurized milk. JAMA. 1984;251:483.
81. Centers for Disease Control. Outbreak of *Yersinia enterocolitica*: Washington State. Morb Mort Wkly Rep. 1982;31:652.
82. Tauxe RV, Vandepitte J, Wauters G, et al. *Yersinia enterocolitica* infections and pork: The missing link. Lancet. 1987;1:1129–32.
83. Pai CH, Mors V. Production of enterotoxin by *Yersinia enterocolitica*. Infect Immun. 1978;19:908.
84. Boyce JM, Doyle DJ Jr, Evans DG, et al. Production off heat-stable, methanol-soluble enterotoxin by *Yersinia enterocolitica*. Infect Immun. 1979;25:532.
85. Asakawa Y, Akahane S, Kagata N, et al. Two community outbreaks of human infection with *Yersinia enterocolitica*. J Hyg (Camb). 1973;71:715.
86. Arvastson B, Damgaard K, Winblad S. Clinical symptoms of infection witih *Yersinia enterocolitica*. Scand J Infect Dis. 1971;3:37.
87. Riley LW, Remis RS, Helgerson SD, et al. Hemorrhagic colitis associated with a rare *Escherichia coli* serotype. N Engl J Med. 1983;308:681.
88. Ryan CA, Tauxe RV, Hosek GW, et al. *Escherichia coli* 0157:H7 diarrhea in a nursing home: Clinical, epidemiological, and pathological findings. J Infect Dis. 1986;154:631–8.
89. Riley L. The epidemiological, clinical, and microbiologic features of hemorrhagic colitis. Ann Rev Microbiol. 1987;41:383–407.
90. Farmer JJ III, Potter ME, Riley LW, et al. Animal models to study *Escherichia coli* 0157:H7 isolated from patients with haemorrhagic colitis. Lancet. 1983;1:702.
91. Johnson WM, Lior H, Bezanson GS. Cytotoxic *Escherichia coli* 0157:H7 associated with haemorrhagic colitis in Canada. Lancet. 1983;1:76.
92. O'Brien AD, Lively TA, Chen ME, et al. *Escherichia coli* 0157:H7 strains associated with haemorrhagic colitis in the United States produce a *Shigella dysenteriae* 1 (shiga) like cytotoxin. Lancet. 1983;1:702.
93. Carter AO, Borczyk AA, Carlson JAK, et al. A severe outbreak of *Escherichia coli* 0157:H7-associated hemorrhagic colitis in a nursing home. N Engl J Med. 1987;317:1496–1500.
94. Centers for Disease Control. Thrombotic thrombocytopenic purpura associated with *Escherichia coli* 0157:H7-Washington. Morb Mort Weekly Rep. 1986;35:549–51.
95. Karmali MA, Petric M, Lim C, et al. The association between idiopathic hemolytic uremic syndrome and infection by verotoxin-producing *Escherichia coli*. J Infect Dis. 1985;151:775–82.
96. Koenig MG, Spickard A, Cardella MA, et al. Clinical and laboratory observations of type E botulism in man. Medicine. 1964;43:517.
97. Barker WH Jr, Weissman JB, Dowell VR Jr, et al. Type B botulism outbreak caused by a commercial food product. JAMA. 1977;237:456.
98. Hughes JM, Blumenthal JR, Merson MH, et al. Clinical features of types A and B food-borne botulism. Ann Intern Med. 1981;95:442.
99. Kao I, Drachman DB, Price DL. Botulinum toxin: Mechanism of presynaptic blockade. Science. 1976;193:1256.
100. Simpson LL. The origin, structure, and pharmacological activity of botulinum toxin. Pharmacol Rev. 1981;33:155.
101. Horwitz MA, Hughes JM, Merson MH, et al. Food-borne botulism in the United States, 1970–1975. J Infect Dis. 1977;136:153.
102. Midura TF, Arnon SS. Infant botulism: Identification of *Clostridium botulinum* and its toxins in feces. Lancet. 1976;2:934.
103. Arnon SS, Midura TF, Clay SA, et al. Infant botulism: Epidemiological, clinical, and laboratory aspects. JAMA. 1977;237:1946.
104. Sugiyama H, Mills DC. Intraintestinal toxin in infant mice challenged intragastrically with *Clostridium botulinum* spores. Infect Immun. 1978;21:59.
105. St Louis ME, Shaun HS, Peck MB, et al. Botulism from chopped garlic: Delayed recognition of a major outbreak. Ann Intern Med. 1988;108:363–8.
106. Semple AB, Parry WH, Phillips DE. Acute copper poisoning: An outbreak traced to contaminated water from a corroded geyser. Lancet 1960;2:700.
107. Brown MA, Thom JV, Orth GL, et al. Food poisoning involving zinc contamination. Arch Environ Health. 1964;8:657.
108. Centers for Disease Control. Illness associated with elevated levels of zinc in fruit punch: New Mexico. Morb Mort Weekly Rep. 1983;32:257.
109. Barker WH Jr, Runte V. Tomato juice-associated gastroenteritis, Washington and Oregon, 1969. Am J Epidemiol. 1972;96:219.
110. Baker TD, Hafner WG. Cadmium poisoning from a refrigerator shelf used as an improvised barbecue grill. Public Health Rep. 1961;76:543.
111. Merson MH, Baine WB, Gangarosa EJ, et al. Scombroid fish poisoning: Outbreak traced to commercially canned tuna fish. JAMA. 1974;228:1268.
112. Kawabata T, Ishizaka K, Miura T. Studies on the allergy-like food poisoning

associated with putrefaction of marine products. III. Physiological and pharmacological action of "saurine," a vagusstimulant of unknown structure recently isolated by the authors, and its characteristics in developing allergy-like symptoms. Jpn J Med Sci Biol. 1955;8:521.
113. Foo, LY. Scombroid poisoning: Recapitulation on the role of histamine. NZ Med J. 1977;85:425.
114. Geiger E, Courtney G, Schnakenberg G. The content and formation of histamine in fish muscle. Arch Biochem. 1944;3:311.
115. Taylor SL. Histamine food poisoning: Toxicology and clinical aspects. CRC Crit Rev Toxicol. 1986;17:91–128.
116. Lerke PA, Werner SB, Taylor SL, et al. Scombroid poisoning: Report of an outbreak. West J Med. 1978;129:381.
117. Taylor SL, Guthertz LS, Leatherwood M, et al. Histamine production by *Klebsiella pneumoniae* and an incident of scombroid fish poisoning. Appl Environ Microbiol. 1979;37:274.
118. Hughes JM, Merson MH. Fish and shellfish poisoning. N Engl J Med. 1976;295:1117.
119. Halstead BW, Courville DA. Poisonous and Venomous Marine Animals of the World. v. 1. Invertebrates. Washington, Government Printing Office; 1965:157.
120. McCollum JPK, Pearson RCM, Ingham HR, et al. An epidemic of mussel poisoning in North-East England. Lancet 1968;2:767.
121. Zwahlen A, Blanc MH, Robert M. Epidémie d'intoxication par les moules ("Paralytic Shellfish Poisoning"). Schweiz Med Wochenschr. 1977;107:226.
122. Acres J, Gray J. Paralytic shellfish poisoning. Can Med Assoc J. 1978; 119:1195.
123. Porkiss MEE, Horstman DA, Harpur D. Paralytic shellfish poisoning: A report of 17 cases in Cape Town. S Afr Med J. 1979;55:1017.
124. Proctor NH, Chan SL, Trevor AJ: Production of saxitoxin by cultures of *Gonyaulax catenella*. Toxicon 1975;13:1.
125. Ghazarossian VE, Schantz EJ, Schnoes HK, et al. Identification of a poison in toxic scallops from a *Gonyaulax tamarensis* red tide. Biochem Biophys Res Comm. 1974;59:1219.
126. Shimizu Y, Buckley LJ, Alam M, et al. Structures of gonyautoxin II and III from the East Coast toxic dinoflagellate *Gonyaulax tamarensis*. J Am Chem Soc. 1976;98:5414.
127. Schantz EJ, Ghazarossian VE, Schnoes HK, et al. The structure of saxitoxin. J Am Chem Soc. 1975;97:1238.
128. Henderson R, Ritchie JM, Strichartz GR. The binding of labelled saxitoxin to the sodium channels in nerve membranes. J Physiol. 1973;235:783.
129. Henderson R, Ritchie JM, Strichartz GR. Evidence that tetrodotoxin and saxitoxin act at a metal cation binding site in the sodium channels of nerve membrane. Proc Natl Acad Sci USA. 1974;71:3936.
130. Catterall WA. Neurotoxins that act on voltage-sensitive sodium channels in excitable membranes. Ann Rev Pharmacol Toxicol. 1980;20:15.
131. McFarren EF, Tanabe H, Silva FJ, et al. The occurrence of a ciguatera-like poison in oysters, clams, and *Gymnodinium breve* cultures. Toxicon. 1965;3:111.
132. Spiegelstein MY, Paster Z, Abbott BC. Purification and biological activity of *Gymnodinium breve* toxins. Toxicon. 1973;11:85.
133. Kim YS, Padilla GM. Purification of the ichthyotoxic component of *Gymnodinium breve* (red tide dinoflagellate) toxin by high pressure liquid chromatography. Toxicon. 1976;14:379.
134. Grunfeld Y, Spiegelstein MY. Effects of *Gymnodinium breve* toxin on the smooth muscle preparation of guinea-pig ileum. Br J Pharmacol. 1974;51:67.
135. Schaumburg HH, Byck R, Gerstl R, et al. Monosodium L-glutamate: Its pharmacology and role in the Chinese restaurant syndrome. Science. 1969;163:826.
136. Reif-Lehrer L. A questionnaire study of the prevalence of Chinese restaurant syndrome. Fed Proc. 1977;36:1617.
137. Hudson PJ, Vogt RL. A foodborne outbreak traced to niacin overenrichment. J Food Protection. 1985;48:249–51.
138. Barkin RM. Ciguatera poisoning: A common source outbreak. South Med J. 1974;67:13.
139. Halstead BW. Fish poisoning: The diagnosis, pharmacology and treatment. Clin Pharmacol Ther. 1964;5:615.
140. Russell FE. Ciguatera poisoning: A report of 35 cases. Toxicon. 1975;13:383.
141. Halstead BW, Courville DA. Poisonous and Venomous Marine Animals of the World, V. 2. Vertebrates. Washington, DC: Government Printing Office; 1967:63.
142. Engleberg NC, Morris JG Jr, Lewis J, et al. Ciguatera fish poisoning: A major common-source outbreak in the U.S. Virgin Islands. Ann Intern Med. 1983;98:336.
143. Bagnis R, Kuberski T, Laugier S. Clinical observations on 3,009 cases of ciguatera (fish poisoning) in the South Pacific. Am J Trop Med Hyg. 1979;28:1067.
144. Morris JG Jr, Lewin P, Hargrett NT, et al. Clinical features of ciguatera fish poisoning: A study of the disease in the U.S. Virgin Islands. Arch Intern Med. 1982;142:1090.
145. Scheuer PJ, Takahashi W, Tsutsumi J, et al. Ciguatoxin: Isolation and chemical nature. Science. 1967;155:1267.
146. Helfrich P, Banner AH. Experimental induction of ciguatera: Toxicity in fish through diet. Nature. 1963;197:1025.
147. Bagnis R, Chanteau S, Chungue E, et al. Origins of ciguatera fish poisoning: A new dinoflagellate, *Gambierdiscus toxicus* Adachi and Fukuyo, definitively involved as a causal agent. Toxicon. 1980;18:199.
148. Li K-M. Ciguatera fish poison: A cholinesterase inhibitor. Science. 1965;147:1580.
149. Halstead BW. Current status of marine biotoxicology: An overview. Clin Toxicol. 1981;18:1.
150. Le Grand AM, Galonnier M, Bagnis R. Studies on the mode of action of ciguateric toxins. Toxicon. 1982;20:311–5.
151. Bidard JN, Vijverberg HPM, Frelin C, et al. Ciguatoxin is a novel type of Na^+ channel toxin. J Biol Chem. 1984;259:8353–7.
152. Lampe KF. Current concepts of therapy in mushroom intoxication. Clin Toxicol. 1974;7:115.
153. Becker CE, Tong TG, Boerner U, et al. Diagnosis and treatment of *Amanita phalloides*-type mushroom poisoning: Use of thioctic acid. West J Med. 1976;125:100.
154. McCormick DJ, Avbel AJ, Gibbons RB. Nonlethal mushroom poisoning. Ann Intern Med. 1979;90:332.
155. Lampe KF. Toxic fungi. Ann Rev Pharmacol Toxicol. 1979;19:85.
156. Paaso B, Harrison DC. A new look at an old problem: Mushroom poisoning. Am J Med. 1975;58:505.
157. Hughes JM, Horwitz MA, Merson MH, et al. Foodborne disease outbreaks of chemical etiology in the United States, 1970–1974. Am J Epidemiol. 1977;105:233.
158. Editorial: Death-cap poisoning. Lancet. 1972;1:1320.
159. Centers for Disease Control: Mushroom poisoning among Laotian refugees: 1981. Morb Mort Weekly Rep. 1982;31:287.
160. Wieland T, Wieland O. The toxic peptides of *Amanita* species. In: Kadis S, Ciegler A, Aji SJ, eds. Microbiol Toxins. v. 8. Fungal Toxins. New York: Academic Press; 1972:249.
161. Osterholm MT, Macdonald KL, White KE, et al. An outbreak of a newly recognized chronic diarrhea syndrome associated with raw milk consumption. JAMA. 1986;256:484–90.
162. Martin DL, Hoberman LJ. A point source outbreak of chronic diarrhea in Texas: No known exposure to raw milk. JAMA. 1986;256:469.
163. Merson MH, Barker WH Jr, Craun GF, et al. Outbreaks of waterborne disease in the United States, 1971–1972. J Infect Dis. 1974;129:614.
164. Hughes JM, Merson MH, Craun GF, et al. Outbreaks of waterborne disease in the United States, 1973. J Infect Dis. 1975;132:336.
165. Horwitz MA, Hughes JM, Craun GF. Outbreaks of waterborne disease in the United States, 1974. J Infect Dis. 1976;133:588.
166. Black RE, Horwitz MA, Craun GF. Outbreaks of waterborne disease in the United States, 1975. J Infect Dis. 1978;137:370.
167. Centers for Disease Control: Foodborne and Waterborne Disease Outbreaks Annual Summary 19876. October 1977.
168. Centers for Disease Control: Foodborne and Waterborne Disease Surveillance Annual Summary 1977. August 1979.
169. Centers for Disease Control: Water-Related Disease Outbreaks Surveillance Annual Summary 1978. May 1980.
170. Centers for Disease Control: Water-Related Disease Outbreaks Surveillance Annual Summary 1979. September 1981.
171. Centers for Disease Control: Water-Related Disease Outbreaks Surveillance Annual Summary 1980. February 1982.
172. Centers for Disease Control: Water-Related Disease Outbreaks Surveillance Annual Summary 1981. September 1982.
173. Centers for Disease Control. Water-Related Disease Outbreaks Surveillance Annual Summary 1982. Centers for Disease Control. 1983;1–15.
174. Centers for Disease Control. Water-Related Disease Outbreaks Surveillance Annual Summary 1983. Centers for Disease Control. 1984;1–15.
175. Centers for Disease Control. Water-Related Disease Outbreaks Surveillance Annual Summary 1984. Centers for Disease Control. 1985;1–15.
176. St Louis ME. Centers for Disease Control. Water-Related Disease Outbreaks, 1985. CDC surveillance summaries. Morb Mort Weekly Rep. 1986;37(No SS-2):15–24.
177. Shaw PK, Brodsky RE, Lyman DO, et al. A community wide outbreak of giardiasis with evidence of transmission by a municipal water supply. Ann Intern Med. 1977;87:426.
178. Lopez CE, Dykes AC, Juranek DD, et al. Waterborne giardiasis: A community-wide outbreak of disease and a high rate of asymptomatic infection. Am J Epidemiol. 1980;112:495.
179. Dykes AC, Juranek DD, Lorenz RA, et al. Municipal waterborne giardiasis: An epidemiologic investigation. Ann Intern Med. 1980;92:165.
180. Weissman JB, Craun GF, Lawrence DN, et al. An epidemic of gastroenteritis traced to a contaminated public water supply. Am J Epidemiol. 1976;103:391.
181. Mosley JW. Water-borne infectious hepatitis. N Engl J Med. 1959;261:703.
182. Feldman RE, Baine WB, Nitzkin JL, et al. Epidemiology of *Salmonella typhi* infection in a migrant labor camp in Dade County, Florida. J Infect Dis. 1974;130:334.
183. A collaborative report. A waterborne epidemic of salmonellosis in Riverside, California, 1965: Epidemiologic aspects. Am J Epidemiol. 1971;93:33.
184. Rosenberg ML, Koplan JP, Wachsmuth IK, et al. Epidemic diarrhea at Crater Lake from enterotoxigenic *Escherichia coli*. A large waterborne outbreak. Ann Intern Med. 1977;86:714.
185. Mentzing LO. Waterborne outbreaks of *Campylobacter* enteritis in central Sweden. Lancet. 1981;2:352.
186. Vogt RL, Sours HE, Barrett T, et al. *Campylobacter* enteritis associated with contaminated water. Ann Intern Med. 1982;96:292.
187. Palmer SR, Gully PR, White JM, et al. Water-borne outbreak of *Campylobacter* gastroenteritis. Lancet. 1983;1:287.
188. Wilson R, Anderson LJ, Holman RC, et al. Waterborne gastroenteritis due to the Norwalk agent: Clinical and epidemiologic investigation. Am J Public Health. 1982;72:72.

189. Kaplan JE, Goodman RA, Schonberger LB, et al. Gastroenteritis due to Norwalk virus: An outbreak associated with a municipal water system. J Infect Dis. 1982;146:190.
190. Morens DM, Zweighaft RM, Vernon TM, et al. A waterborne outbreak of gastroenteritis with secondary person-to-person spread. Lancet. 1979;1:964.
191. Horwitz MA. Specific diagnosis of foodborne disease. Gastroenterology. 1977;73:375.
192. Williams REO. Healthy carriage of *Staphylococcus aureus*: Its prevalence and importance. Bacteriol Rev. 1963;27:56.
193. Wieneke AA. Enterotoxin production by strains of *Staphylococcus aureus* isolated from foods and human beings. J Hyg (Camb). 1974;73:255.
194. Gilbert RJ, Stringer MF, Peace TC. The survival and growth of *Bacillus cereus* in boiled and fried rice in relation to outbreaks of food poisoning. J Hyg (Camb). 1974;73:433.
195. Holmes JR, Plunkett T, Pate P, et al. Emetic food poisoning caused by *Bacillus cereus*. Arch Intern Med. 1981;141:766.
196. Gilbert RJ, Parry JM. Serotypes of *Bacillus cereus* from outbreaks of food poisoning and from routine foods. J Hyg (Lond). 1977;78:69.
197. Parry JM, Gilbert RJ. Studies on the heat resistance of *Bacillus cereus* spores and growth of the organisms in boiled rice. J Hyg (Lond). 1980;84:77.
198. Strong DH, Canada JC, Griffiths BB. Incidence of *Clostridium perfringens* in American foods. Appl Microbiol. 1963;11:42.
199. Hall HE, Angelotti R. *Clostridium perfringens* in meat and meat products. Appl Microbiol. 1965;13:352.
200. Smart JL, Roberts TA, Stringer MF, et al. The incidence and serotypes of *Clostridium perfringens* on beef, pork and lamb carcasses. J Appl Bacteriol. 1979;46:377.
201. Petersen LR, Mshar R, Cooper GH Jr, et al. A large *Clostridium perfringens* foodborne outbreak with an unusual attack rate pattern. Am J Epidemiol. 1988;127:605–11.
202. Kim HU, Goepfert JM. Enumeration and identification of *Bacillus cereus* in foods. I. 24-hour presumptive test medium. Appl Microbiol. 1971;22:581.
203. Blakey LJ, Priest FG. The occurrence of *Bacillus cereus* in some dried foods including pulses and cereals. J Appl Bacteriol. 1980;48:297.
204. Jephcott AE, Barton BW, Gilbert RJ, et al. An unusual outbreak of food-poisoning associated with meals-on-wheels. Lancet. 1977;2:129.
205. Werner SB, Humphrey GL, Kamei I. Association between raw milk and human *Salmonella dublin* infection. Br Med J. 1979;2:238.
206. Small RG, Sharp JCM. A milk-borne outbreak due to *Salmonella dublin*. J Hyg (Lond). 1979;82:95.
207. Galbraith NS, Forbes P, Clifford C. Communicable disease associated with milk and dairy products in England and Wales 1951–80. Br Med J. 1982;284:1761.
208. Gill ON, Bartlett CLR, Sockett PN, et al. Outbreak of *Salmonella napoli* infection caused by contaminated chocolate bars. Lancet. 1983;1:574.
209. Craven PC, Baine WB, Mackel DC, et al. International outbreak of *Salmonella eastbourne* infection traced to contaminated chocolate. Lancet. 1975;1:788.
210. St Louis ME, Morse DL, Potter ME, et al. The emergence of grade A eggs as a major source of *Salmonella enteritidis* infections. JAMA. 1988; 259:2103–7.
211. Centers for Disease Control. Hospital-associated outbreak of *Shigella dysenteriae* type 2: Maryland. Morb Mort Weekly Rep. 1983;32:250.
212. Robinson DA, Jones DM. Milk-borne *Campylobacter* infection. Br Med J. 1981;282:1374.
213. Barker WH Jr. *Vibrio parahaemolyticus* outbreaks in the United States. Lancet. 1974;1:551.
214. Lawrence DN, Blake PA, Yashuk JC, et al. *Vibrio parahaemolyticus* gastroenteritis outbreaks aboard two cruise ships. Am J Epidemiol. 1979;109:71.
215. Kudoh Y, Sakai S, Zen-Yoji H, et al. Epidemiology of food poisoning due to *Vibrio parahaemolyticus* occurring in Tokyo during the last decade. In: Fujino T, Sakaguchi G, Sakazaki R, et al, eds. International Symposium on Vibrio parahaemolyticus. Tokyo: Saikon; 1974:9.
216. Baine WB, Zampieri A, Mazzotti M, et al. Epidemiology of cholera in Italy in 1973. Lancet. 1974;2:1370.
217. Dutt AK, Alwi S, Velauthan T. A shellfish-borne cholera outbreak in Malaysia. Trans R Soc Trop Med Hyg. 1971;65:815.
218. Barrett TJ, Blake PA. Epidemiological usefulness of changes in hemolytic activity of *Vibrio cholerae* biotype El Tor during the seventh pandemic. J Clin Microbiol. 1981;13:126.
219. Kaper JB, Bradford HB, Roberts NC, et al. Molecular epidemiology of *Vibrio cholerae* in the U.S. Gulf Coast. J Clin Microbiol. 1982;16:129.
220. Pavia AT, Campbell JF, Blake PA, et al. Cholera from raw oysters shipped interstate. JAMA. 1987;258:2374.
221. Klontz KC, Tauxe RV, Cook WL, et al. Cholera after the consumption of raw oysters: A case report. Ann Intern Med. 1987;107:846–8.
222. Merson MH, Morris GH, Sack DA, et al. Travelers' diarrhea in Mexico. N Engl J Med. 1976;294:1299.
223. MacDonald KL, Eidson M, Strohmeyer C, et al. A multistate outbreak of gastrointestinal illness caused by enterotoxigenic *Escherichia coli* in imported semisoft cheese. J Infect Dis. 1985;151:716–20.
224. Sack RB, Sack DA, Mehlman IF, et al. Enterotoxigenic *Escherichia coli* isolated from food. J Infect Dis. 1977;135:313.
225. MacDonald KL, Cohen ML, Blake PA. The changing epidemiology of adult botulism in the United States. Am J Epidemiol. 1986;124:794–9.
226. Arnon SS. Infant botulism. Ann Rev Med. 1980;31:541.
227. Linco SJ, Grohmann GS. The Darwin outbreak of oyster-associated viral gastroenteritis. Med J Aust. 1980;1:211.
228. Gunn RA, Janowski HT, Lieb S, et al. Norwalk virus gastroenteritis following raw oyster consumption. Am J Epidemiol. 1982;115:348.
229. Griffin MR, Surowiec JJ, McCloskey DI, et al. Foodborne Norwalk virus. Am J Epidemiol. 1982;115:178.
230. Kuritsky JN, Osterholm MT, Greenberg HB, et al. Norwalk gastroenteritis: A community outbreak associated with bakery product consumption. Ann Intern Med. 1984;100:519.
231. Reid JA, Caul EO, White OG, et al. Role of infected food handler in hotel outbreak of Norwalk-like viral gastroenteritis: Implications for control. Lancet. 1988;2:321–3.
232. Hopper SH, Adams HS. Copper poisoning from vending machines. Public Health Rep. 1958;73:910.
233. Hesse IDW, Halstead BW, Peckham NH. Marine biotoxins. I. Ciguatera poison: Some biological and chemical aspects. Ann NY Acad Sci. 1960;90:788–97.
234. Collins JC, Bicknell WJ. The red tide: A public-health emergency. N Engl J Med. 1974;288:1126.
235. Lawrence DN, Enriquez MB, Lumish RM, et al. Ciguatera fish poisoning in Miami. JAMA. 1980;244:254.
236. Kelly MT, Peterson JW, Sarles HE Jr, et al. Cholera on the Texas Gulf Coast. JAMA. 1982;247:1598.
237. Morris JG Jr, Lewin P, Smith CW, et al. Ciguatera fish poisoning: Epidemiology of the disease on St. Thomas, U.S. Virgin Islands. Am J Trop Med Hyg. 1982;31:574.
238. Casman EP, Bennett RW. Detection of staphylococcal enterotoxin in food. Appl Microbiol. 1965;13:181.
239. Pober Z, Silverman GJ. Modified radioimmunoassay determination for staphylococcal enterotoxin B in foods. Appl Environ Microbiol. 1977;33:620.
240. Saunders GC, Bartlett ML. Double-antibody solid-phase enzyme immunoassay for the detection of staphylococcal enterotoxin. A. Appl Environ Microbiol. 1977;34:518.
241. Stiffler-Rosenberg G, Fey H. Simple assay for staphylococcal enterotoxins A, B, and C: Modification of enzyme-linked immunosorbent assay. J Clin Microbiol. 1978;8:473.
242. Freed RC, Evenson ML, Reiser RF, et al. Enzyme-linked immunosorbent assay for detection of staphylococcal enterotoxins in foods. Appl Environ Microbiol. 1982;44:1349.
243. Ghosh AC. Prevalence of *Bacillus cereus* in the faeces of healthy adults. J Hyg (Lond). 1978;80:233.
244. De Buono BA, Brondum J, Kramer JM, et al. Plasmid, serotypic, and enterotoxin analysis of *Bacillus cereus* in an outbreak setting. J Clin Microbiol. 1988;26:1571–4.
245. Mansson I, Colldahl H. The intestinal flora in patients with bronchial asthma and rheumatoid arthritis: With special reference to *Clostridium perfringens*. Acta Allergy. 1965;20:94.
246. Akama K, Otani S. *Clostridium perfringens* as the flora in the intestine of healthy persons. Jpn J Med Sci Biol. 1970;23:161.
247. Hauschild AHW. Criteria and procedures for implicating *Clostridium perfringens* in food-borne outbreaks. Can J Public Health. 1975;66:388.
248. Stringer MF, Turnbull PCB, Gilbert RJ. Application of serological typing to the investigation of outbreaks of *Clostridium perfringens* food poisoning, 1970–1978. J Hyg (Lond). 1980;84:443.
249. Harmon SM, Kautter DA, Hatheway CL. Enumeration and characterization of *Clostridium perfringens* spores in the feces of food poisoning patients and normal controls. J Food Protection. 1986;49:23–8.
250. Watson GN, Stringer MF, Gilbert RJ, et al. The potential of bacteriocin typing in the study of *Clostridium perfringens* food poisoning. J Clin Pathol. 1982;35:1361.
251. Schiemann DA. Laboratory confirmation of an outbreak of *Clostridium perfringens* food poisoning. Health Lab Sci. 1977;14:35–8.
252. Hatheway CL, Whaley DN, Dowell VR Jr. Epidemiological aspects of *Clostridium perfringens* foodborne illness. Food Technol. 1980;34:77.
253. Naik HS, Duncan CL. Detection of *Clostridium perfringens* enterotoxin in human fecal samples and anti-enterotoxin in sera. J Clin Microbiol. 1978;7:337.
254. Skjelkvåle R, Uemura T. Detection of enterotoxin in faeces and anti-enterotoxin in serum after *Clostridium perfringens* food poisoning. J Appl Bacteriol. 1977;42:355.
255. Birkhead G, Vogt RL, Heun EM, et al. Characterization of an outbreak of *Clostridium perfringens* food poisoning by quantitative fecal culture and fecal enterotoxin measurement. J Clin Microbiol. 1988;26:471–4.
256. Niilo L, Bainborough AR. A survey of *Clostridium perfringens* enterotoxin antibody in human and animal sera in western Canada. Can J Microbiol. 1980;26:1162.
257. Genigeorgis C, Sakaguchi G, Riemann H. Assay methods for *Clostridium perfringens* type A enterotoxin. Appl. Microbiol. 1973;26:111.
258. Taylor DN, Wachsmuth IK, Shangkuan YH. Salmonellosis associated with marijuana: A multistate outbreak traced by plasmid fingerprinting. N Engl J Med. 1982;306:1249.
259. Riley LW, Cohen ML. Plasmid profiles and *Salmonella* epidemiology. Lancet. 1982;1:573.
260. Farmer JJ III, Davis BR. H7 antiserum-sorbitol fermentation medium: A single tube screening medium for detecting *Escherichia coli* 0157:H7 associated with hemorrhagic colitis. J Clin Microbiol. 1985;22:620–5.

261. Guerrant RL, Brunton LL, Schnaitman TC, et al. Cyclic adenosine monophosphate and alteration of Chinese hamster ovary cell morphology: A rapid, sensitive in vitro assay for the enterotoxins of *Vibrio cholerae* and *Escherichia coli*. Infect Immun. 1974;10:320.
262. Donta ST, Moon HW, Whipp SC. Detection of heat-labue *Escherichia coli* enterotoxin with the use of adrenal cells in tissue culture. Science. 1974;183:334.
263. Svennerholm AM, Wiklund G. Rapid GMl-enzyme-linked immunosorbent assay with visual reading for identification of *Escherichia coli* heat-labile enterotoxin. J Clin Microbiol. 1983;17:596.
264. Honda T, Arita M, Takeda Y, et al. Further evaluation of the Biken test (modified Elek test) for detection of enterotoxigenic *Escherichia coli* producing heat-labile entertoxin and application of the test to sampling of heat-stable enterotoxin., J Clin Microbiol. 1982;16:60.
265. Giannella RA. Suckling mouse model for detection of heat-stable *Escherichia coli* enterotoxin: Characteristics of the model. Infect Immun. 1976;14:95.
266. Sereny B. Experimental *Shigella* keratoconjunctivitis: A preliminary report. Acta Microbiol Acad Sci Hung. 1955;2:293.
267. Levine MM, Berquist EJ, Nalin DR, et al. *Escherichia coli* strains that cause diarrhoea but do not produce heat-labile or heat-stable enterotoxins and are non-invasive. Lancet. 1978;1:1119.
268. Dowell VR Jr, McCroskey LM, Hatheway CL, et al. Coproexamination for botulinal toxin and *Clostridium botulinum*. JAMA. 1977;238:1829.
269. Mann JM, Hatheway CL, Gardiner TM. Laboratory diagnosis in a large outbreak of type A botulism. Am J Epidemiol. 1982;115:598.
270. Kapikian AZ, Wyatt RG, Dolin R et al. Visualization by immune electron microscopy of a 27-nm particle associated with acute infectious nonbacterial gastroenteritis. J Virol. 1972;10:1075.
271. Gary GW Jr, Kaplan JE, Stine SE, et al. Detection of Norwalk virus antibodies and antigen with a biotin-avidin immunoassay. J Clin Microbiol. 1985;22:274–8.
272. Morris JG Jr. Ciguatera fish poisoning. JAMA. 1980;244:273.
273. Withers NW. Ciguatera fish poisoning. Annu Rev Med. 1982;33:97.
274. Hokama Y, Abad MA, Kimura LH. A rapid enzyme-immunoassay for the detection of ciguatoxin in contaminated fish tissues. Toxicon. 1983;21:817–24.
275. Harris JC, DuPont HL. Hornick RB. Fecal leukocytes in diarrheal illness. Ann Intern Med. 1972;76:697.
276. Appleton H, Pereira MS. A possible virus etiology in outbreaks of food-poisoning from cockles. Lancet. 1977;1:780.
277. Guerrant RL, Dickens MD, Wenzel RP, et al. Toxigenic bacterial diarrhea: Nursery outbreak involving multiple bacterial strains. J Pediatr. 1976;89:885.
278. Wadström T, Aust-Kettis A, Habte D, et al. Enterotoxin-producing bacteria and parasites in stools of Ethiopian children with diarrhoeal disease. Arch Dis Child. 1976;51:865.
279. Klipstein FA, Engert RF. Purification and properties of *Klebsiella pneumoniae* heat-stable enterotoxin. Infect Immun. 1976;13:373.
280. Klipstein FA, Engert RF. Partial purification and properties of *Enterobacter cloacae* heat-stable enterotoxin. Infect Immun. 1976;13:1307.
281. Salazar-Lindo E, Sack RB, Chea-Woo E, et al. Early treatment with erythromycin of *Campylobacter jejuni*-associated dysentery in children. J Pediatr. 1986;109:355–60.
282. Palafox NA, Jain LG, Pinano AZ, et al. Successful treatment of ciguatera fish poisoning with intravenous mannitol. JAMA. 1988;259:2740–2.
283. Mitchel DH. *Amanita* mushroom poisoning. Annu Rev Med. 1980;31:51.
284. Jordan MC, Powell KE, Corothers TE, et al. Salmonellosis among restaurant patrons: The incisive role of a meat slicer. Am J Public Health. 1973;63:982.
285. Chin J. Raw milk: A continuing vehicle for the transmission of infectious disease agents in the United States. J Infect Dis. 1982;146:440.
286. Horwitz MA, Marr JS, Merson MH, et al. A continuing common-source outbreak of botulism in a family. Lancet. 1975;2:861.
287. Payne DJH, Scudamore JM. Outbreaks of salmonella food poisoning over a period of eight years from a common source. Lancet. 1977;1:1249.

87. TROPICAL SPRUE

FREDERICK A. KLIPSTEIN

Although apparently familiar to medical practitioners in India for centuries, it was not until the colonization of Asia by the European maritime powers early in the eighteenth century that Western physicians first became aware of tropical sprue. The disease was recognized among the British in India, the French in Indochina, the Dutch in Java, and somewhat later, the Americans in the Philippines and West Indies.

EPIDEMIOLOGY

Sprue can afflict visitors to the tropics within weeks, months, or years after arrival, the most common time interval being between 1 and 2 years.[1] It can occur as an isolated case or in epidemic proportions, as happened among British and Indian troops serving in the India–Burma theater of operations during the Second World War.[2] The disorder occurs among both sexes and all age groups, although it is less common in children than in adults. Symptoms of tropical sprue may persist after a return to a temperate climate and, in some instances, first become manifested there.[3]

The geographic regions in which sprue occurs are known (Fig. 1), but the exact prevalence of the disorder among people in these areas is uncertain, due largely to the relatively complex diagnostic procedures required to make the diagnosis. A disorder thought to be sprue was recognized in the southern part of the United States early in this century,[3] and more recently, "temperate sprue" has been described among some people who acquired transient intestinal malabsorption syndrome in temperate climates.[4] Long considered incorrectly to occur principally or even exclusively among European expatriates in the tropics, it is now recognized that sprue occurs more often among native populations of endemic areas. Although the disorder can occur among affluent, well-nourished people, its prevalence among indigenous populations appears to be more common among those living in substandard economic and sanitary conditions.

Abnormalities of small bowel structure and function develop in sprue as sequelae to an episode of acute enteritis; these abnormalities become progressively more severe, cause persistent gastrointestinal symptoms, and eventually result in nutritional deficiencies. In addition to overt sprue, many asymptomatic native residents of the tropics as well as expatriates who have lived in the tropics for more than 6 months are found to have mild-to-moderate small bowel abnormalities that are qualitatively indistinguishable from those present in sprue.[5,6] This condition is referred to as tropical enteropathy; it differs from sprue in a number of aspects: (*1*) the intestinal abnormalities in sprue relentlessly become more severe, whereas those in tropical enteropathy vary over time, either improving or worsening spontaneously. Further, unlike in sprue, the intestinal abnormalities in tropical enteropathy disappear within about a year after either active residents or expatriates move to a temperate climate.[7] (*2*) The intestinal abnormalities in sprue consistently result in nutritional deficiencies, but those in tropical enteropathy contribute to the development of nutritional deficiencies only in people subsiding on marginal or suboptimal diets. (*3*) Treatment with folic acid[8,9] and/or antimicrobials[10,11] either improves or completely heals the intestinal lesion in sprue, but the effect of this form of therapy is variable and usually limited in tropical enteropathy.[12]

ETIOLOGY

The clinical and epidemiologic aspects of sprue strongly suggest that it has an infectious cause: (*1*) It is acquired only by visitors to or residents of endemic areas; (*2*) it can occur in epidemic form among both visitors to and native residents of endemic areas; (*3*) both the epidemics among visitors to India and the occurrence of the disease among the indigenous population of Puerto Rico have a peak seasonal incidence[13]; (*4*) "sprue houses"—dwellings in which there is a high prevalence of the disease among the occupants—have long been recognized in India and Ceylon[14]; and (*5*) treatment with broad-spectrum antibiotics or sulfa preparations is curative.[10,11] Other observations indicate that sprue often occurs as a sequela to epidemics of acute enteritis. During an annual seasonal epidemic of enteritis of unknown cause among Americans in the Philippines,

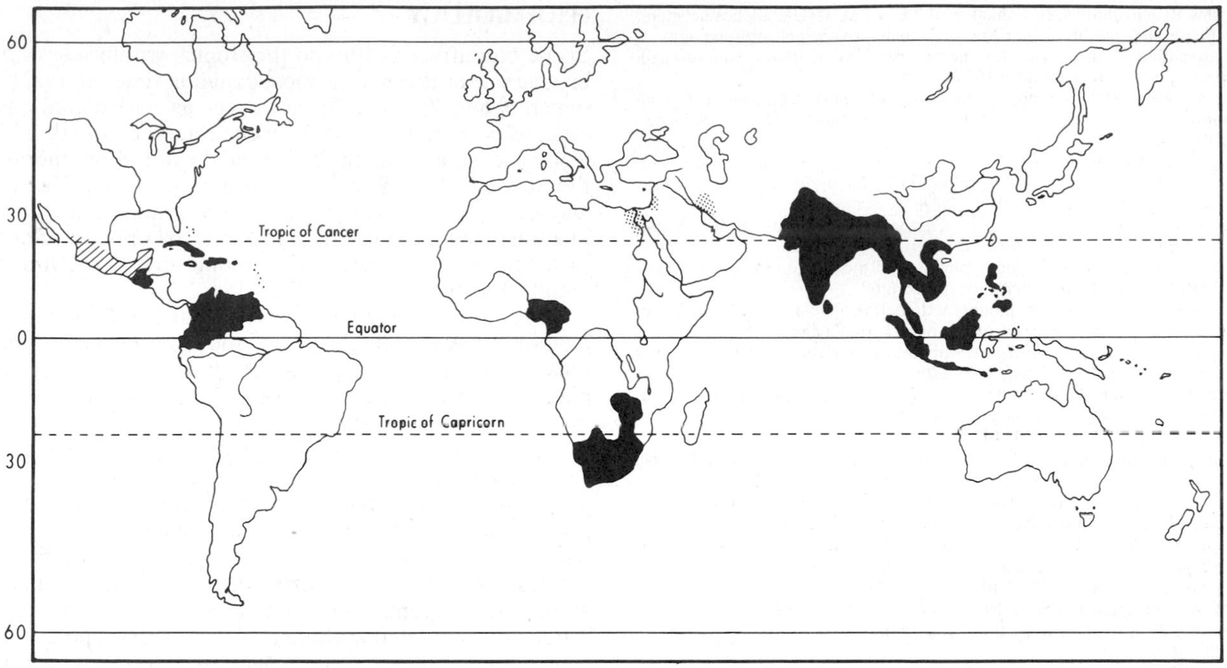

FIG. 1. Geographic distribution of tropical malabsorption. Black indicates those areas where overt tropical sprue occurs; cross-hatching, areas where a disorder resembling sprue occurs; and stippling, areas where only subclinical abnormalities of small intestinal structure or function have been observed.

one-fifth of affected people subsequently developed chronic symptoms and abnormalities of intestinal structure and function characteristic of sprue that were cured by treatment with folic acid or tetracycline.[15] Similar observations have been made after epidemics of acute enteritis that occurred in South Indian villages.[16]

Despite this circumstantial evidence, no single specific infectious agent has been isolated by culture techniques or visualized within the intestinal mucosa by light or electron microscopy. Examinations for fungus or algae with known pathogenic properties have been negative[17,18]; enterovirus- and parovirus-like agents such as the Norwalk and Hawaii agents have not been found, but no studies have been reported in which rotaviruses were searched for; strict anaerobic cultures of jejunal aspirates have not grown any obligate anaerobes,[19] and cultures of *Mycoplasma* have been negative. On the other hand, most patients with sprue who were studied in Calcutta,[20] Puerto Rico,[19] and Haiti[21] as well as expatriates who acquired sprue in Asia[22] have been found to have small intestinal contamination by coliform bacteria, most commonly with *Klebsiella pneumoniae* and less often with *Escherichia coli* and *Enterobacter cloacae*. The evidence suggests that patients with sprue have chronic contamination by a specific coliform strain and that this is not a transient colonization due to constant exposure from an unsanitary environment: (*1*) sprue patients are usually contaminated by a single biotype (as determined by API profile) of a single species; (*2*) the coliforms persist within the small intestine for months in those expatriates who return to a temperate climate,[22] and (*3*) coliforms are rarely isolated from the jejunum of healthy residents of the tropics.[19–21]

The coliform bacteria that are isolated do not have invasive properties; they yield a negative Sereny test response and are not found by immunofluorescent techniques to penetrate the mucosa after instillation with rabbit ileal ligated loops. They do produce two metabolic products that are potentially injurious to the mucosa. The first, ethanol, which is one of the principal fermentation products of coliforms, is found in the jejunal aspirate of most patients with sprue who have coliform overgrowth.[19] The second, enterotoxins, are produced by all three coliform species; these toxins are not produced by similar species of coliform bacteria isolated from the jejunum of people with the blind loop syndrome.[23] These toxins have been identified by the ability of cell-free filtrates to cause fluid secretion in rabbit ligated ileal loops[19] and the ability of semipurified ultrafiltration fractions to cause water secretion when perfused in vivo through the rat jejunum.[23,24] The toxins also impair the absorption of solutes such as xylose and are capable of producing abnormalities of intestinal structure in various experimental animal models.[24] Two toxin forms have been identified: a large-molecular-weight heat-labile form and a low-molecular-weight heat-stable form. Their precise nature remains to be determined; in most cases, they are negative in standard assays for the classic *E. coli* heat-labile (LT) and heat-stable (ST) toxins such as the Y1 adrenal cell tissue culture assay for LT and the suckling mouse assay for ST.[25]

Transient contamination of the small intestine by toxigenic forms of coliform bacteria is a common cause of acute diarrheal episodes among persons in the tropics (see Chapter 81). The finding that toxigenic strains of the same species also chronically colonize the small intestine in tropical sprue has led to the suggestion that sprue is a sequela to acute diarrhea in which failure to eliminate the toxigenic coliform bacteria results in chronic colonization by these organisms during which persistent exposure of the intestinal mucosa to the bacterial toxins results in the development of abnormalities of intestinal structure and function.[26] The milder abnormalities present in those with tropical enteropathy are viewed as sequelae of repeated episodes of transient bowel contamination. In accordance with this concept are the observations that (*1*) intestinal structure is usually normal and transport abnormalities limited to those of water and xylose during the initial phase of sprue,[27] (*2*) postinfective malabsorption is well documented in some cases,[4] and (*3*) eradication of the coliform bacteria by antibiotic treatment in sprue results in cure.[20,22]

The factors responsible for persistent contamination of the small intestine by coliform bacteria are unknown. There is suggestive evidence that the coliforms may be unusually adherent to the intestinal mucosa,[28] but no information is available concerning whether this is due to the presence of plasmid-induced specific fimbrial antigens, as is the case with strains of classic enterotoxigenic *E. coli*. Intestinal motility can be delayed in sprue, and this may contribute to persistent colonization.[29] Immunoglobulins, including mucosal IgA, are normal in people with sprue.[30] Several lines of evidence have suggested that dietary lipids may be of relevance[13]: (*1*) Sprue is endemic in areas in which and among people whose dietary lipid consists principally of long-chain unsaturated fatty acids, but it does not occur in those areas (such as Jamaica) or among those groups (such as Ghurkas) whose dietary lipid is mainly short-chain, saturated fatty acids; (*2*) epidemiologic studies have pointed toward a correlation between the occurrence of outbreaks of sprue and periods of high intake of a diet rich in linoleic acid among the population of Puerto Rico. These observations have led to the suggestion that dietary linoleic acid creates an intestinal milieu favorable for colonization by coliforms by means of its well-recognized capacity to inhibit the growth of the normally resident gram-positive organisms.[13] This sequence of events has been shown to occur in a continuous culture chemostat system,[31] but its relevance to humans remains to be established.

The failure to culture coliform bacteria from the small intestine of some persons with sprue, particularly those in South India[32] and South Africa,[33] raises the possibility that other, unrecognized enteric pathogens such as a virus may be the pathogenic factor in these cases.

The improvement in intestinal structure, particularly of crypt cell morphology, and transport that attends treatment with folic acid indicates that the eventual development of folate deficiency of the intestinal mucosa plays a perpetuating role once the intestinal abnormalities are established in sprue.

CLINICAL MANIFESTATIONS

Diarrhea is usually the first manifestation of tropical sprue and is present in 90 percent of patients; it is usually accompanied by borborygmi, abdominal distension, and cramps. Visitors to the tropics can often date exactly the onset of the disease; in these people, this usually consists of an explosive episode of diarrhea, sometimes accompanied by a flulike illness with malaise, fever, weakness, and nausea, that within a week resolves into chronic gastrointestinal symptoms. Native residents of the tropics who are accustomed to intermittent bouts of gastrointestinal upsets often find it difficult to precisely date the onset of symptoms. Many patients develop milk intolerance due to lactase deficiency, and some develop alcohol intolerance. Within 1–3 months, folate stores become depleted, and this leads to the development of anorexia, decreased dietary intake, and progressive weight loss. After 4–6 months, most develop glossitis and, eventually, symptoms of anemia. Tetany or neurologic manifestations of vitamin B_{12} deficiency are rare.

In those who were well nourished before the onset of the disease, abnormal findings on physical examination are usually confined to pallor, glossitis, increased bowel sounds, evidence of recent weight loss, and in some elderly people with severe anemia, evidence of cardiac decompensation. Among persons who were marginally or poorly nourished before the onset of sprue, signs and symptoms related to the development of nutritional deficiencies develop more rapidly and are often more prominent. These individuals can develop night blindness, stomatitis, hyperpigmentation or a pellagralike rash, koilonychia, edema, and severe emaciation.

INTESTINAL ABNORMALITIES

Function

The function of the stomach and both segments of the small intestine can be impaired in people with chronic sprue. Gastric secretion of both intrinsic factor and hydrochloric acid may be reduced. In the jejunum, there is a net secretion of water and electrolytes; glucose-facilitated water transport remains intact, however, and the administration of glucose reverses water transport to absorption. The absorption of xylose, glucose, minerals such as calcium and magnesium, and both folic acid and its dietary form polyglutamate folate are impaired. Fat absorption is reduced, due in part to a reduced bile salt pool and in part to impaired reesterification within the enterocyte; the absorption of the fat-soluble vitamins A, D, E, and K is commonly reduced. Amino acid absorption is impaired, and there may be an excess loss of albumin into the intestinal lumen. Disaccharidase concentrations of the brush border are reduced with resultant impaired hydrolysis and malabsorption of disaccharides such as lactose. There is malabsorption of vitamin B_{12} and bile salts from the ileum. Vitamin B_{12} absorption returns to normal in most patients only after antibiotic therapy has been given for several months, thus indicating that the basic defect was malabsorption due to ileal disease. In a few, it returns to normal within 1–2 weeks after the institution of antibiotic treatment, which suggests that uptake of this vitamin by the coliform bacteria was the basic abnormality. In vitro studies have shown that the coliform bacteria isolated from sprue patients incorporate vitamin B_{12} but synthesize folate.

Morphology

When observed under the dissecting microscope, the villi are usually thickened and coalesced to form leaves that, in many cases, fuse together to give the more abnormal appearance of ridges and convolutions; the flat pavementlike appearance that is characteristic of biopsy specimens from patients with gluten enteropathy is unusual. Histologic sections of the jejunum (Fig. 2) show changes of variable severity consisting of lengthening of the crypt area, broadening and shortening of the villi, and infiltration by chronic inflammatory cells; fewer than 10 percent have a flat appearance. Abnormalities of the surface epithelial cells and enzymatic activity within these cells, as detected by histochemical stains, are usually directly related to the severity of villus structural abnormality. Crypt cell nuclei often show megalocytic changes. The basement membrane beneath the surface epithelium appears to be thickened on light microscopy; electron microscopy has shown that the basal lamella itself is normal but that directly subjacent to it is a dense collagenous material. The precise identity of this material is unknown, but it has been suggested that it represents an antigen–antibody complex.

DIAGNOSIS

The diagnosis of sprue is based to a degree on the exclusion of other pathologic entities. To be considered are all of those conditions present in a temperate climate that are associated with gastrointestinal symptoms, malabsorption, and the development of nutritional deficiencies. In addition to the usual tests of intestinal function, radiologic examination of the small intestine is helpful in excluding disorders such as blind loops, strictures, and regional enteritis. A jejunal biopsy must be performed to exclude the diagnosis of gluten enteropathy, which is associated with complete villus atrophy (a rare finding in sprue), or infiltrative disease of the submucosa such as lymphoma or Whipple's disease. Conditions that are particularly common in the tropics must also be considered. These include intestinal infestation by parasites including *Giardia lamblia, Strongyloides stercoralis, Capillaria philippensis*, and *Coccidia*. These conditions can be excluded by examination of the stool.

The differential diagnosis among expatriates returning from the tropics who have chronic diarrhea, weight loss, and malabsorption usually rests between sprue and giardiasis.[1] The

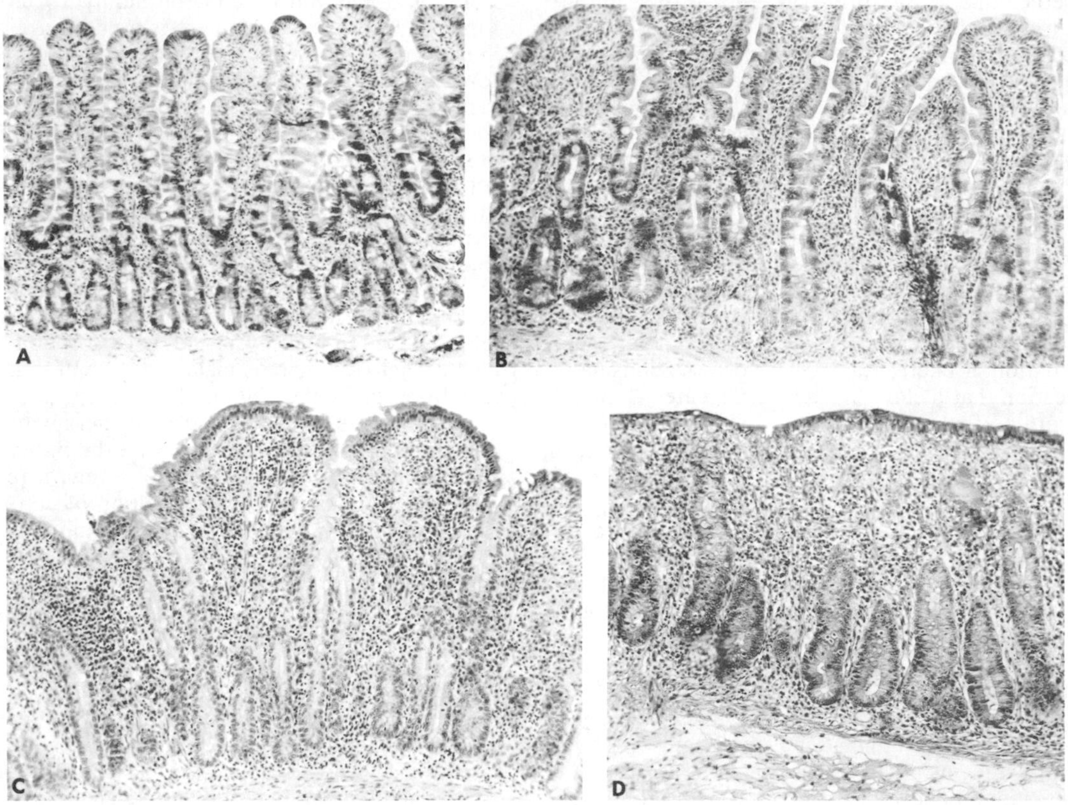

FIG. 2. Jejunal structure in tropical sprue: microscopic changes. (H&E, ×100). (**A**) Mild (1+) abnormality; (**B**) moderate (2+) abnormality; (**C**) severe (3+) abnormality; (**D**) very severe (4+) abnormality, a flat mucosa. (From Gerson,[7] with permission.)

presence of *Giardia* can be confirmed by microscopic examination of stool specimens or jejunal aspirates and biopsy specimens. Some expatriates infected with giardiasis also have small bowel contamination with coliform bacteria.[34]

In our experience with 60 consecutively studied Puerto Ricans with sprue, all had malabsorption of a 25 g oral dose of xylose, 96 percent had reduced absorption of vitamin B_{12} as tested by the Schilling test, and 69 percent had steatorrhea as assessed by fecal fat determination on a 72-hour collection; all had abnormalities of varying degrees of severity of the jejunal mucosa. Patients examined early in the course of the disorder will have none or few nutritional deficiencies. Most of those with chronic sprue have a megaloblastic anemia due to a combined deficiency of folate and vitamin B_{12}; about one-half have reduced serum albumin and cholesterol levels, and one-third mild hypocalcemia. The final confirmatory evidence to the diagnosis of sprue is improvement with the appropriate therapy.

TREATMENT

Supportive measures such as fluid or blood replacement are occasionally required in severely ill patients, but in most cases the institution of specific therapy is all that is required. Before the introduction of liver extract in 1931 and folic acid in 1946, no such therapy was available, and the therapeutic programs used then, such as dietary manipulations, often met with a variable and sometimes fatal result. Treatment with either folic acid or vitamin B_{12} is associated with prompt clinical improvement including a hematologic remission, the disappearance of glossitis, the return of appetite and weight gain, and in some, a progressive decrease in gastrointestinal symptoms. Earlier workers felt that folic acid cures sprue; however, when techniques to examine intestinal function and morphology in detail became available in the early 1960s, it became apparent that such is rarely the case in patients with chronic sprue, most of whom continue to have chronic intestinal abnormalities.[9] An exception to this is that treatment with folic acid alone can be curative in some visitors to the tropics who have been symptomatic for relatively short periods of time.[8,27]

During the Second World War, sulfaguanidine was found to alleviate or halt intestinal symptoms in British military personnel with sprue in India and Burma.[2] Subsequently, workers in England and Puerto Rico showed that combined therapy with a sulfa preparation and tetracycline for 2–3 weeks improved the intestinal abnormalities in most cases. Prolonged antibiotic therapy for 6 months was then shown to result in a complete cure in nearly all Puerto Ricans with sprue.[10] Tetracycline or poorly absorbed sulfonamides are equally effective,[11] erythromycin is said to be ineffective, and the effect of other antimicrobials has not been tested. Since most patients have only been evaluated after 6 months of treatment, it remains uncertain as to whether a shorter course of therapy might be equally effective. Recent studies in Puerto Rico have shown that there is a high rate of recurrence of intestinal abnormalities within several years after the cessation of antibiotic therapy among persons living in the tropics[35]; experience among similarly treated people living in New York City[3] suggests that such is not the case in a temperate zone.

Optimum therapy for chronic sprue consists of folic acid, 5 mg/day by mouth for 6 months, plus tetracycline, 250 mg qid for 1 month followed by the same dose bid for 5 months, and 1000 μg of vitamin B_{12} given intramuscularly several times initially and then at monthly intervals during this period. This therapeutic regimen results in prompt clinical improvement and in eventual healing of the mucosal lesion in nearly all cases.

REFERENCES

1. Klipstein FA. Tropical sprue in travelers and expatriates living abroad. Gastroenterology. 1981;80:590.
2. Keele KD, Bound JP. Sprue in India: Clinical survey of 600 cases. Br Med J. 1946;1:77.
3. Klipstein FA, Falaiye JM. Tropical sprue in expatriates from the tropics living in the continental United States. Medicine (Baltimore). 1969;48:475.
4. Montgomery RD, Beale DJ, Sammons HG, et al. Postinfective malabsorption: A sprue syndrome. Br Med J. 1973;2:265.
5. Lindenbaum J, Kent TH, Sprinz H. Malabsorption and jejunitis in American Peace Corps volunteers in Pakistan. Ann Intern Med. 1966;65:1201.
6. Thomas G, Clain DJ, Wicks ACB. Tropical enteropathy in Rhodesia. Gut. 1976;17:888.
7. Gerson CD, Kent TH, Saha JR, et al. Recovery of small-intestinal structure and function after residence in the tropics. II. Studies in Indians and Pakistanis living in New York City. Ann Intern Med. 1971;75:41.
8. Sheehy TW, Cohen WC, Wallace DK, et al. Tropical sprue in North Americans. JAMA. 1965;194:1069.
9. Sheehy TW, Baggs B, Perez-Santiago E, et al. Prognosis of tropical sprue. A study of the effect of folic acid on the intestinal aspects of acute and chronic sprue. Ann Intern Med. 1962;57:892.
10. Guerra R, Wheby MS, Bayless TM. Long-term antibiotic therapy in tropical sprue. Ann Intern Med. 1965;63:619.
11. Maldonado N, Horta E, Guerra R, et al. Poorly absorbed sulfonamides in the treatment of tropical sprue. Gastroenterology. 1969;57:559.
12. Klipstein FA, Samloff IM, Smarth G, et al. Treatment of overt and subclinical malabsorption in Haiti. Gut. 1969;10:315.
13. Klipstein FA, Corcino JJ. Seasonal occurrence of overt and subclinical tropical malabsorption in Puerto Rico. Am J Trop Med Hyg. 1974;23:1189.
14. Mathan VI, Ignatius M, Baker SJ. A household epidemic of tropical sprue. Gut. 1966;7:490.
15. Jones TC, Dean AG, Parker GW. Seasonal gastroenteritis and malabsorption at an American military base in the Philippines. II. Malabsorption following the acute illness. Am J Epidemiol. 1972;95:128.
16. Mathan VI, Baker SJ. Epidemic tropical sprue and other epidemics of diarrhea in South Indian villages. A comparative study. Am J Clin Nutr. 1968;21:1077.
17. Swanson VL, Haley LD, Wheby MS. Mycological study of jejunal biopsy specimens from patients with tropical sprue. Am J Trop Med Hyg. 1965; 14:1066.
18. Klipstein FA, Schenk EA. Prototheca and sprue. Gastroenterology. 1975;69:1372.
19. Klipstein FA, Holdeman LV, Corcino JJ, et al. Enterotoxigenic intestinal bacteria in tropical sprue. Ann Intern Med. 1973;79:632.
20. Gorbach SL, Banwell JG, Jacobs B, et al. Tropical sprue and malnutrition in West Bengal. I. Intestinal microflora and absorption. Am J Clin Nutr. 1970;23:1545.
21. Klipstein FA, Short HB, Engert RF, et al. Contamination of the small intestine by enterotoxigenic coliform bacteria among the rural population of Haiti. Gastroenterology. 1976;70:1035.
22. Tomkins AM, Drasar BS, James WPT. Bacterial colonisation of jejunal mucosa in acute tropical sprue. Lancet. 1975;1:59.
23. Klipstein FA, Engert RF, Short HB. Enterotoxigenicity of colonising coliform bacteria in tropical sprue and blind-loop syndrome. *Lancet*. 1978;2:342.
24. Klipstein FA, Horowitz IR, Engert RF, et al. Effect of *Klebsiella pneumoniae* enterotoxin on intestinal transport in the rat. J Clin Invest. 1975;56:799.
25. Klipstein FA, Guerrant RL, Wells JG, et al. Comparison of assay of coliform enterotoxins by conventional techniques versus in vivo intestinal perfusion. Infect Immun. 1979;25:146.
26. Klipstein FA. Sprue and subclinical malabsorption in the tropics. Lancet. 1979;1:277.
27. O'Brien W, England NWJ. Tropical sprue amongst British servicemen and their families in South-East Asia. In: Tropical Sprue and Megaloblastic Anaemia. London: Churchill Livingstone; 1971:25.
28. Drasar, BS, Agostini C, Clarke D, et al. Adhesion of enteropathogenic bacteria to cells in tissue culture. Dev Biol Stand. 1980;46:83.
29. Cook GC. Delayed small-intestinal transit in tropical malabsorption. Lancet. 1978;2:238.
30. Ross IN, Mathan VI. Immunological changes in tropical sprue. Q J Med. 1981;50:435.
31. Mickelson MJ, Klipstein FA. Enterotoxigenic intestinal bacteria in tropical sprue. IV. Effect of linoleic acid on growth interrelationships of *Lactobacillus acidophilus* and *Klebsiella pneumoniae*. Infect Immun. 1975;12:1121.
32. Bhat P, Shantakumari S, Rajan D, et al. Bacterial flora of the gastrointestinal tract in southern Indian control subjects and patients with tropical sprue. Gastroenterology. 1972;62:11.
33. Appelbaum PC, Moshal MG, Hift W, et al. Intestinal bacteria in patients with tropical sprue. S Afr Med J. 1980;57:1081.
34. Tomkins AM, Wright SG, Drasar BS, et al. Bacterial colonization of jejunal mucosa in giardiasis. Trans R Soc Trop Med Hyg. 1978;72:33.
35. Rickles FR, Klipstein FA, Tomasini J, et al. Long-term follow-up of antibiotic-treated tropical sprue. Ann Intern Med. 1972;76:203.

88. WHIPPLE'S DISEASE

WILLIAM O. DOBBINS III

Whipple's disease, first described in 1907,[1] is a systemic bacterial illness affecting primarily middle-aged, white men. It is characterized morphologically by the presence of macrophages in virtually all organ systems, and these macrophages are intensely stained by the periodic acid–Schiff (PAS) stain. There may be a subtle cell-mediated immune deficit that predisposes to the infection. Whipple organisms have all the structural characteristics of bacteria.[2–4] Their uniform light and electron microscopic appearance and the antigenic structure of the bacilli as determined by immunofluorescence staining[5,6] strongly suggest that a single microorganism is etiologic. However, this putative microorganism has not been cultured in vitro, and the disease has not been reproduced in animals. Most patients respond to treatment with antibiotics.

PATHOGENESIS AND PATHOLOGIC CHARACTERISTICS

Sieracki and Fine first emphasized the presence of systemic involvement when they found characteristic PAS-positive macrophages in body tissues.[7] The PAS-positive material usually occurred in the form of discrete sickle-shaped masses scattered throughout the cytoplasm of macrophages, described by Sieracki as "characteristic cells containing sickle-form particles" (SPC cells). The PAS reaction has a strong affinity for glycoproteins, and electron microscopic studies have shown that the rod-shaped masses found within macrophages are actually masses of intact and degenerating bacteria, the walls of which are apparently in part composed of glycoproteins.[3,4] Greatest involvement occurs in the lamina propria of the small intestine and its lymphatic drainage, in the heart (with valvular lesions being particularly prominent), and in the central nervous system (CNS).

Electron microscopic studies from many laboratories have documented the presence of bacilli in involved tissues,[3] both intracellularly and extracellularly. The bacilli are usually reported to be gram-positive, but sometimes they have been found to be gram-negative. These bacilli have been remarkably uniform in appearance and are approximately 0.2 μm wide by 1.5–2.5 μm long (Fig. 1). The organism possesses a trilaminar plasma membrane that is surrounded by a homogeneous cell wall approximately 20 nm thick. The cell wall itself is enclosed within an outer trilaminar "membrane."[3] This latter feature is more characteristic of gram-negative bacilli. Tubules and vesicles are located centrally within the bacilli and resemble the mesosomes that are characteristic of gram-positive bacteria. Nucleoids can often be identified within the core of the bacilli. Binary fission is often present. The Whipple bacillus is present within a variety of cells, including macrophages, intestinal epithelial cells, lymphatic and capillary endothelial cells, smooth muscle cells, polymorphonuclear leukocytes, plasma cells, mast cells, and even intraepithelial lymphocytes.[8] The intracellular bacilli are often intact in structure, which suggests that these organisms may be intracellular pathogens.[4] Immunofluorescence studies have shown that the material found within macrophages has a strong antigenic similarity to material found within streptococci groups B and G.[5,6]

Because the disease has not been reproduced in laboratory animals and because the organism has not been convincingly cultured in vitro, the only sure assay for Whipple's disease is the structural characteristic of the organism as seen by electron microscopy and possibly its antigenic structure as defined by immunofluorescence staining. Thus, the remarkable similarity

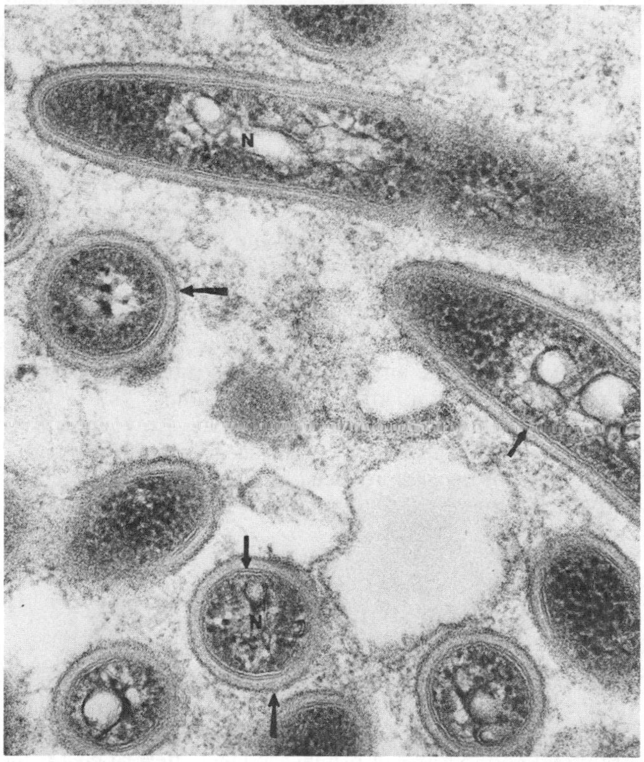

FIG. 1. Electron micrograph showing the characteristic appearance of the Whipple bacilli, many of which have been cut obliquely. These bacilli are up to 0.25 μm wide and, when sectioned lengthwise, up to 2.5 μm long. The nucleoid (N) is enclosed within a typical trilaminar plasma membrane (small arrows). A homogeneous cell wall about 20 nm thick surrounds the plasma membrane, and the cell wall itself is surrounded by a less well characterized "membrane," which has a trilaminar appearance (large arrows). The bacilli have electron microscopic characteristics, therefore, of both gram-positive and of gram-negative bacilli. (×100,000)

of the Whipple bacillus to the "unidentified erythrocyte-associated bacterium" described by Archer et al. as a cause of human infection suggests that the latter disease may be an unusual presentation of Whipple's disease.[9]

Microscopic pathology in the proximal small intestine shows the presence of typical club-shaped villi containing PAS-positive macrophages. The macrophages are found chiefly in the gastrointestinal tract, the mesenteric and retroperitoneal nodes, the heart, and the CNS. Occasional involvement has been found in the lungs, spleen, pancreas, and peripheral lymph nodes. Minimal changes have been noted in the genitourinary tract, adrenals, joints, skin, bone marrow, and skeletal muscle.

There is evidence supporting the presence of cell-mediated immune deficiency. Even after successful treatment, the cutaneous response to antigens and the responsiveness of lymphocytes to nonspecific mitogens, although improved, are subnormal. There may be an increased association with HLA-B27 (28 percent of Whipple's patients and 10 percent of healthy people).[10]

CLINICAL AND LABORATORY FINDINGS

The patient is usually a middle-aged white man with a history of intermittent arthralgia involving multiple joints over a period of years.[11] The actual illness develops gradually, with diarrhea followed by the development of steatorrhea, weight loss, and finally a progressive downhill course. Rarely, there is no diarrhea, and the illness is characterized by nondescript abdominal pain and low-grade fever. The arthralgias may appear 10–30 years before the development of gastrointestinal symptoms and are usually migratory. Usually the large joints are most prominently involved.

Evidence of weight loss is usual. The abdomen is often distended and tender to palpation, and abdominal nodes may be palpable. Hypotension is often present, and hyperpigmentation of the skin is found in 50 percent of patients. Fever is usually low grade, but on occasion spiking temperatures to 103°F are present. Peripheral lymphadenopathy is often present. Cardiac murmurs (often with marantic endocarditis) have been noted in 25 percent of patients. Ascites is uncommon, and splenomegaly and hepatomegaly occur in less than 5 percent of patients. All of the manifestations of advanced malabsorption may be present in those patients diagnosed late in their clinical course. Neurologic abnormalities are often present and include ophthalmoplegia, dementia, ataxia, myoclonus, hyperreflexia, paresis, and sensory changes such as hearing loss and visual disturbances. The patient may present with neurologic and personality changes as the initial manifestation in the absence of significant gastrointestinal signs or symptoms.[12–14] Exceedingly rarely, Whipple's disease of the CNS has been reported in the absence of involvement of the gastrointestinal tract.

Laboratory findings include a normocytic, normochromic anemia in 90 percent of the patients. Occasional patients have iron deficiency. Megaloblastic anemia is rare. The white blood cell count is usually not elevated, and the differential count is usually normal. Hypoalbuminenia, hypocholesterolemia, hypokalemia, and prolonged prothrombin times are usually present. Steatorrhea is present in 93 percent and decreased D-xylose absorption in 78 percent of patients, whereas decreased vitamin B_{12} absorption is found in only 15 percent of patients.[11]

DIAGNOSIS

Whipple's disease should be suspected in people with the four most prominent symptoms—weight loss, diarrhea, arthralgia, and abdominal pain.[11] If the arthralgias precede the other symptoms, the diagnosis deserves very serious consideration. Histologically, the most severe and consistent changes are seen in the proximal small intestine. Thus, small bowel biopsy is the diagnostic procedure of choice. Rarely, the intestinal mucosa will contain numerous macrophages in patients with diffuse histoplasmosis and in patients with acquired immune deficiency syndrome (AIDS). Macrophages found in these diseases are not intensely PAS-positive and can be easily distinguished from those found in Whipple's disease by using special stains (for *Histoplasma capsulatum* in histoplasmosis and for intracellular *Mycobacterium avium* in AIDS).

PAS-positive macrophages can also be found in most tissues from healthy subjects. This is particularly true in the rectal and colonic mucosa. PAS-positive macrophages in the small intestinal mucosa but not in other tissues are unique and may be considered diagnostic. It is helpful to have electron microscopic confirmation of the presence of the characteristic Whipple bacilli, although these bacilli can be seen by light microscopy in properly prepared specimens.[15]

Occasionally, biopsy specimens of a lymph node or other tissue may permit the diagnosis, but they require electron microscopic confirmation.[16] Even brain biopsy specimens have been used to establish the diagnosis in the rare person with CNS Whipple's disease in the absence of intestinal involvement.[13]

Antibiotics are the treatment of choice, and good responses have been reported to a variety of antibiotics.[17–19] The appropriate duration of the therapy is unclear, but because occasional patients have had a relapse after several weeks to a few months of treatment, antibiotics should be given for 1 year.[11,17–19]

Initial treatment should consist of parenteral penicillin G (1.2 million units) plus streptomycin (1.0 g) daily for 10–14 days followed by one double-strength tablet of trimethoprim–sulfamethoxazole (TMP/SMX) given twice daily for 1 year. TMP/SMX penetrates the blood-brain barrier well. Indeed, two patients who presented with CNS Whipple's disease have responded to treatment with TMP/SMX.[17,18] If the patient is severely ill, the double-strength tablet may be given three times per day for 2 weeks and then given twice daily for 1 year. Folic acid deficiency is a potential complication of such therapy, especially in a malnourished individual. Folinic acid in a dose of 3 mg twice weekly should prevent this complication and should be administered routinely during the 2-week period that patients are given three double-strength tablets on a daily basis.

CNS relapses have not developed in patients treated with the earlier recommended regimen of parenteral penicillin and streptomycin, with or without subsequent administration of oral tetracycline.[17] Thus one could argue that treatment with parenteral penicillin and streptomycin for 10 to 14 days followed by oral tetracycline is appropriate. However, patients so treated do not receive antibiotics that cross the blood-brain barrier. In the patient allergic to or unable to tolerate sulfonamides, treatment with parenteral penicillin and streptomycin for 10–14 days followed by oral penicillin (penicillin V, 250 mg four times per day) for 1 year is recommended. Reed et al.[19] elected to treat their patient with high doses (20 million units per 24 hours) of penicillin initially for 30 days because of the *suspicion* of subclinical cerebral involvement. Because patients with Whipple's disease may be severely malnourished, folate, vitamin B_{12}, vitamin K, iron, and other dietary supplements may be beneficial.

The duration of therapy should not be determined by the presence or absence of PAS-positive macrophages within the intestinal lamina propria. The macrophages may persist within the lamina propria for many years after successful treatment, whereas free bacilli clear very rapidly and have never been reported to last longer than 9 weeks after the initiation of treatment. Routine follow-up intestinal biopsies are thus not necessary. However, it is becoming apparent that many successfully treated patients will develop a clinical relapse years after treatment, with or without intestinal symptoms. Thus, all treated patients should be followed up by careful clinical evaluation on a yearly basis. If a relapse is suspected, then intestinal biopsy specimens should be obtained and the presence or absence of free bacilli determined. An empirical trial of antibiotics may still be appropriate.

Treatment of relapse is the same as that outlined for initial therapy. If a patient with CNS relapse fails to respond to parenteral penicillin and streptomycin followed by oral TMP/SMX, treatment with oral chloramphenicol, 1 g/day (250 mg qid) for 6 to 12 months is indicated. Chloramphenicol, like TMP/SMX, results in a relatively high CNS concentration of the drug. Failure of the patient with non-CNS relapse to respond to TMP/SMX may require trials of oral penicillin (penicillin V, 250 mg four times per day) or oral tetracycline (250 mg four times per day).

REFERENCES

1. Whipple GH. A hitherto undescribed disease characterized anatomically by deposits of fat and fatty acids in the intestinal and mesenteric lymphatic tissues. Johns Hopkins Hosp Bull. 1907;18:382.
2. Dobbins WO III. Whipple's Disease. Springfield, IL: Charles C Thomas; 1987:242.
3. Silva MT, Macedo PM, Moura Nunes JF. Ultrastructure of bacilli and the bacillary origin of the macrophage inclusions in Whipple's disease. J Gen Microbiol. 1985;131:1001.
4. Dobbins WO III, Kawanishi H. Bacillary characteristics in Whipple's disease: An electron microscopic study. Gastroenterology. 1981;80:1468.
5. Keren DF, Weisburger WR, Yardley J, et al. Whipple's disease: Demonstration by immunofluorescence of similar bacterial antigens in macrophages from three cases. Johns Hopkins Med J. 1976;139:51.
6. Kent SP, Kirkpatrick PM. Whipple's disease: Immunological and histochemical studies of eight cases. Arch Pathol Lab Med. 1980;104:544.
7. Sieracki JC, Fine G. Whipple's disease: Observation on systemic involvement. I. Gross and histologic observation. *Arch Pathol.* 1959;67:81.
8. Austin LL, Dobbins WO III. Intraepithelial leucocytes of the intestinal mucosa in normal man and in Whipple's disease: A light and electron microscopic study. Dig Dis Sci. 1982;27:311.
9. Archer GL, Coleman PH, Cole RM, et al. Human infection from an unidentified erythrocyte-associated bacterium. N Engl J Med. 1979;301:897.
10. Dobbins WO III. HLA antigens in Whipple's disease. Arthritis Rheum. 1987;30:102–5.
11. Maizel H, Ruffin JM, Dobbins WO III. Whipple's disease. A review of 19 patients from one hospital and a review of the literature since 1950. Medicine (Baltimore) 1970;49:175.
12. Finelli PF, McEntee WJ, Lessel S, et al. Whipple's disease with predominantly neuroophthalmic manifestations. Ann Neurol. 1977;1:247.
13. Johnson L, Diamond I. Cerebral Whipple's disease: Diagnosis by brain biopsy. Am J Clin Pathol. 1979;74:486.
14. Schmitt BP, Richardson H, Smith E, et al. Encephalopathy complicating Whipple's disease. Ann Intern Med. 1981;94:51.
15. Trier JS, Phelps PC, Eidelman S, et al. Whipple's disease: Light and electron microscope correlation of jejunal mucosal histology with antibiotic treatment and clinical status. Gastroenterology. 1965;48:684.
16. Mansbach CM II, Shelburne FA, Stevens RD, et al. Lymph node bacilliform bodies resembling those of Whipple's disease in a patient without intestinal involvement. Ann Intern Med. 1978;89:64.
17. Keinath RD, Merrell DE, Vlietstra R, et al. Antibiotic treatment and relapse in Whipple's disease: Long-term followup of 88 patients. Gastroenterology. 1985;88:1867–73.
18. Ryser RJ, Locksley RM, Eng SC, et al. Reversal of dementia associated with Whipple's disease by trimethoprim-sulfamethoxazole, drugs that cross the blood-brain barrier. Gastroenterology. 1984;86:745.
19. Reed JI, Sipe JD, Wohlgethan JR, et al. Response of the acute phase reactants to antibiotic treatment of Whipple's disease. Arthritis Rheum. 1985;28:352–5.

SECTION L. BONE AND JOINT INFECTIONS

89. INFECTIOUS ARTHRITIS

JAMES W. SMITH

An inflammatory reaction in the joint space (arthritis) follows infection with many different microorganisms. Bacterial invasion of the joint generally leads to a suppurative arthritis, principally of one joint (monarticular). Certain bacteria, however, may produce symptoms in multiple joints, particularly during the bacteremic stage of their infection, as well as induce inflammation in the neighboring tendon sheaths, for example, *Neisseria gonorrhoeae*. Infections of the joint due to viruses frequently involve multiple joints and demonstrate inflammation without suppuration. A chronic granulomatous monarticular arthritis may be seen with mycobacteria or fungi that must be differentiated from other causes of chronic monarticular arthritis. In addition, a sterile arthritis may be associated with an infection either preceding the typical clinical syndrome, as with hepatitis B, or following the infection as postinfectious arthritis with *Shigella* or *Salmonella*. Infectious arthritis is associated with a low case fatality rate and few residual symptoms if recognized and treated properly. Since a number of other clinical entities may be confused with infectious arthritis, the approach to any person with an inflamed joint must include infection among the differential possibilities.

PATHOGENESIS AND PREDISPOSING FACTORS

Infectious arthritis follows hematogenous inoculation of the pathogenic organism in a great majority of instances since only a few have a history of recent intra-articular injection before infection.[1,2] The infection may develop as a direct infection of the synovial space or may represent extension from infected bone. Infectious arthritis in infants below the age of 1 year may occur secondary to extension from a primary osteomyelitis focus since capillaries still perforate the epiphyseal growth plate.[3] However, children over the age of 1 are more likely to develop infection of the joint alone since the growth plate contains the infection. Many patients with bacterial arthritis give a history of trauma (Table 1) that may enable bacteria, mycobacteria, or fungi to penetrate the synovial space more easily. Extra-articular infections are found in approximately one-quarter of both adults and children with bacterial arthritis (Table 1). In contrast to children, adults frequently have one or more significant systemic conditions predisposing to bacterial arthritis.[1,4] These factors vary from the administration of corticosteroids, either orally or after intra-articular injection, to the presence of a systemic disease as diabetes mellitus or hematologic malignancies. Patients with rheumatoid arthritis and osteoarthritis appear to be predisposed to infectious arthritis more than would be expected by chance alone.[5] Joint infections in rheumatoid patients tend to occur in older people with debilitating arthritis of longer than 10 years' duration.[6]

Endocrine factors appear to be important in the genesis of the disseminated gonococcal syndrome since this syndrome tends to occur in women during a particularly susceptible period in pregnancy (the second or third trimester) and during menstruation.[7,8] Not only is endocervical shedding of the *N. gonorrhoeae* maximal during menstruation, but also access to the blood stream would be greatest at this time. In contrast, infection is rarely seen in the third week of the menstrual cycle when the shedding of *N. gonorrhoeae* is minimal and the pH is not optimal for growth of the bacteria.[8] Arthritis due to particular viral infections also relates to certain endocrine factors since rubella arthritis principally occurs in postpubertal women whereas mumps arthritis is seen exclusively in postpubertal men.[9]

Arthritis that occurs in the convalescent period of infection has been postulated in a number of instances to relate to the immune response to the microorganism. Arthritis has been noted late in the course of infections with meningococci and lymphocytic choriomeningitis virus.[10,11] However, it cannot be clearly established whether these infections represent active infection or are more likely postinfectious arthritis due to the immune response of the organism. Arthritis in patients with hepatitis B infection has been shown to relate to antigen–antibody complexes.[12] Circulating complexes in patients with arthritis have high quantities of IgG, IgM, and IgA, especially IgG1 and IgG3, the complement-fixing globulins. In addition, C3, C4, and C5 have been demonstrated in the immune complexes. As the arthritis disappears with the onset of jaundice, the complement components can no longer be demonstrated in the immune complexes.

The postinfectious arthritis that develops in persons after *Shigella, Salmonella, Campylobacter,* and *Yersinia* infections of the gastrointestinal tract frequently have the specific histocompatibility antigen HLA-B27 (Table 2).[13–16] Persons with arthritis after one outbreak of shigellosis had Reiter syndrome with active disease for up to 10 years.[13] It has been calculated that the likelihood of a B27-positive patient developing Reiter syndrome varies from 16 to 37 percent and that a B27-positive patient has a 50 times greater risk of developing arthritis after *Yersinia* infection than a person who is not B27-positive.[13,14]

TABLE 1. Predisposing Factors in Bacterial Arthritis

Factor	In Adults[a] %	In Children %
Corticosteroid administration	33	
Pre-existing arthritis	24	
Intra-articular injection	23	
Other infection	22	26
Diabetes mellitus	13	
Trauma	12	28
Other diseases	19	3
None	8	43

[a] More than one predisposing factor existed in some patients.
(Data from Kelly et al.,[1] and Nelson et al.[2])

TABLE 2. Frequency of HLA-B27 in Patients with Arthritis After Infectious Diarrhea

Group	*Infecting Pathogens* *Shigella*	*Yersinia*	*Salmonella*
Control	7[a]	14	10
No arthritis		15	8
Arthritis	80	88	69

[a] Values are percentages of the groups expressing HLA-B27.
(Data from Calin et al.,[13] Aho et al.,[14] and Hakansson et al.[15])

CLINICAL FEATURES

Site of Infection

The site of infection in cases with bacterial or suppurative arthritis is monarticular in 90 percent of children and adults.[1,2,4,17,18] The knee is the most commonly affected joint in both children and adults with bacterial arthritis as well as in infections with *Mycobacterium tuberculosis*[19] (Table 3). The hip is the next most commonly involved joint, with variation in the frequency of involvement of other joints. Adults tend to have more involvement of the shoulder, sternoclavicular, and sacroiliac joints, especially in parenteral drug abusers,[20,22] whereas children tend to have infection more commonly of the ankle and elbow.[2] The wrist and interphalangeal joints of the hand are infrequently involved with suppurative arthritis due to bacteria, although these joints are commonly involved in patients with infections with *N. gonorrhoeae*[8] and with *M. tuberculosis*.[19] Infectious arthritis of viral etiology (e.g., rubella) tends to involve multiple joints, with most having symptoms in the interphalangeal joints of the hands, the wrist, as well as the knees, ankles, and elbows[9,21] (Table 3).

TABLE 3. Frequency (Percentages) of Joint Involvement in Infectious Arthritis[a]

Joint	*Bacterial (Suppurative)* *Children*	*Adults*	*Mycobacterial*	*Viral*
Knee	41	48	24	60
Hip	23	24	20	4
Ankle	14	7	12	30
Elbow	12	11	8	20
Wrist	4	7	20	55
Shoulder	4	15	4	5
Interphalangeal and metacarpal	1.4	1	12	75
Sternoclavicular	0.4	8	0	0
Sacroiliac	0.4	2	0	0

[a] More than one joint may be involved, so the percentages exceed 100 percent.
(Data from refs. 1, 2, 4, 9, 17, 19, 20, 21.)

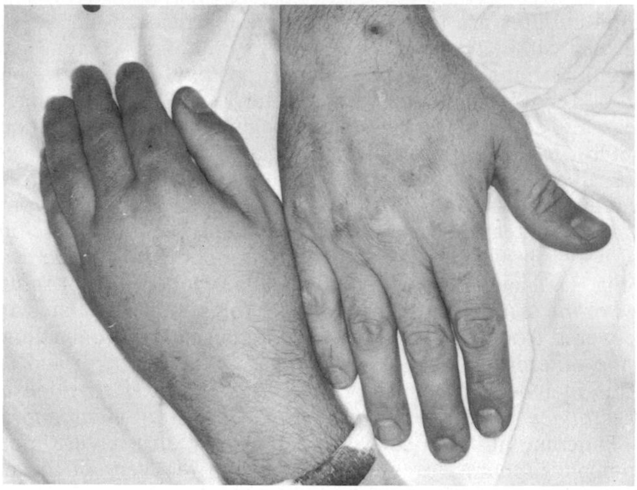

FIG. 1. Patient with chromic gonococcemia with swollen hand and skin lesions over dorsal surface of wrist. (Courtesy of *Current Prescribing*, April, 1979.)

Persons with bacterial (suppurative) arthritis generally have fever and symptoms in a single joint with pain on motion, limitation of motion, and swelling. The joints may vary from minimal tenderness to severe tenderness. Joint effusion can be demonstrated in 90 percent of the joints that can be examined easily. In 10 percent of persons, multiple joints may be involved with bacterial infection. Infections with mycobacteria or certain fungi such as *Sporothrix schenckii* may be so insidious and slow to evolve that an infection may not be considered.[19,23] A diagnosis of bacterial infection of hip joints is difficult since the symptoms may be minimal and effusions may be difficult to demonstrate.[5]

Inflammation of the tendon sheaths (tenosynovitis) occurs commonly with the disseminated gonococcal syndrome[8] (Fig. 1). Tenosynovitis also may be seen with other infections such as *Moraxella*, rubella, atypical mycobacteria, and sporotrichosis. Carpal tunnel syndrome (paresthesias of the hands), with or without joint symptoms, occurs with rubella, atypical mycobacteria, sporotrichosis, and histoplasmosis.

Septic bursitis is usually due to *Staphylococcus aureus* and more commonly follows local trauma.[24] The olecranon and prepatellar bursae are the usual sites. Occasionally, organisms of low pathogenicity cause chronic olecranon bursitis, such as nontuberculous *Mycobacterium, Prototheca,* and *Phialophora*.

LABORATORY FINDINGS

Patients with infectious arthritis, whether bacterial, viral, or mycobacterial, have an elevated erythrocyte sedimentation rate (ESR). The ESR is higher in those with bacterial infection and in those with an infection of long duration. Anemia may be noted, particularly in those with chronic infections or in those who develop infectious arthritis secondary to underlying joint disease such as rheumatoid arthritis. Children tend to have elevated white blood cell counts with a predominance of polymorphonuclear leukocytes, whereas many adults do not have an elevated peripheral blood leukocyte count.[1,2]

Joint fluid from monarticular bacterial arthritis generally appears turbid or purulent, although 10–20 percent have serosanguineous fluid. The joint leukocyte count is greater than $100,000/mm^3$ in one-third to one-half, and most have a differential count of more than 90 percent polymorphonuclear leukocytes.[18] However, this finding is not specific for bacterial arthritis since many other joint conditions such as rheumatoid arthritis, rheumatic fever, and crystalline joint disease may be associated with a preponderance of polymorphonuclear leukocytes and, conversely, not all cases of bacterial infection have an elevated leukocyte count. Protein levels are generally elevated, but this has little specificity for joint infection. Although a low synovial fluid glucose content or a synovial fluid glucose content less than 40 mg/dl of the blood glucose is suggestive of suppurative arthritis,[5,17] this difference is valid only if the blood and synovial fluid specimens have been obtained simultaneously. Low joint fluid glucose concentrations have been found in only one-half of adult patients[25] and in an even smaller proportion of children with bacterial arthritis.[17] Other conditions are associated with a low joint fluid glucose value including rheumatoid arthritis; hence this test does not have the specificity of predictive value as a low cerebrospinal fluid glucose value does for bacterial meningitis. Viral arthritis may be associated with a modest elevation of the synovial fluid leukocyte count. In most instances the preponderant cell is mononuclear, although some cases with proven rubella arthritis have had a majority of polymorphonuclear leukocytes. In tuberculous arthritis, most patients had an elevated leukocyte count and a predominance of polymorphonuclear leukocytes.[26] A significantly decreased joint fluid glucose level was found in 61 percent. Leukocyte counts exceeding $1000/mm^3$ are characteristic of staphylococcal bursitis.[24]

Smears of joint fluid stained for bacteria from persons with bacterial arthritis show the organisms in slightly over one-half of the cases.[5] The Gram stain can give false-positive results (positive test results not confirmed by a positive culture). The methylene blue stain is probably a more reliable stain. Both blood and joint fluid should be cultured aerobically and anaerobically. In addition, other appropriate cultures such as on spinal fluid should be done if there are central nervous system manifestations. Pharyngeal, rectal, and cervical or urethral cultures should be done if the disseminated gonococcal syndrome is considered. Blood cultures have been positive in 10–60 percent of the cases in adults and in 29 percent of children with bacterial arthritis.[1,4,17] Joint cultures are positive in up to 90 percent of those in whom a diagnosis of bacterial arthritis has been established and in 79 percent of those with tuberculosis.[26]

The most frequent roentgenographic abnormality in bacterial arthritis is distension of the joint capsule and soft tissue swelling in the adjacent space. However, these findings are not pathognomonic for infection. Destructive changes are rarely noted in bacterial infections save in those who are seen late (more than 2 weeks) in the course of infection, as with hip infection.[1] If the infection complicates rheumatoid arthritis, then cortical destruction and erosion is a more constant feature; however, these changes cannot be distinguished from rheumatoid arthritis without infection. Mycobacterial infection of the joint leads to joint space narrowing, metaphyseal and subchondral erosions, and cyst formation.[19] Viral infections rarely produce roentgenographic changes unless significant quantities of fluid are present and result in distension of the joint capsule.

PATHOLOGIC CHANGES

In experimental arthritis produced by the intra-articular injection of *Staphylococcus aureus* into rabbits, early pathologic changes were noted in the surface and in the matrix of the superficial zone of the articular surface by electron microscopy within 24 hours.[27] At this time, the joint cavity showed polymorphonuclear leukocytes, and lysosomal bodies were present in the synovial cells. By 3 days, the destruction of articular cartilage was more extensive and was even visible with light microscopy. The matrix appeared loose in the superficial zones, and degeneration of chondrocytes was noted in deeper zones. In chronic arthritis due to mycobacteria or fungi, histologic evidence of a granulomatous inflammation occurs with dense mononuclear inflammatory infiltrates consisting of lymphocytes.[26] Palisading of histiocytes may be detected around a foci of coagulation necrosis.[23,26] Organisms were demonstrated with special stain in only 19 percent with *M. tuberculosis* and rarely in fungal infections, but culture of the biopsy tissue was positive for the particular infecting organism.[23,26]

ETIOLOGIC AGENTS

Bacterial (Suppurative) Arthritis

The frequency of the etiologic agents that induce bacterial arthritis varies with age (Table 4). *Haemophilus influenzae* type b is the preponderant causative organism in children under 2 years of age. Although it is rarely seen after 5 years of age,[2,5] adults can develop septic arthritis with *H. influenzae* if they have immune defects.[28] In infants under 1 month of age, group B streptococci, gram-negative bacilli, and *S. aureus* are causative organisms. *Staphylococcus aureus* is the most frequent organism causing bacterial arthritis in children over 2 years of age[2,17] and is the causative organism in the vast majority of cases of suppurative arthritis in adults.[1,4,18] *Neisseria gonorrhoeae* is the preponderant cause of bacterial arthritis in adults under 30 years.[25] The frequency of streptococcal infections as a cause of bacterial arthritis is relatively constant from childhood through the adult years (13–17 percent). The most frequently isolated type in both children and adults is group A β-hemolytic streptococci; however, group B (in the neonate and adult diabetic), viridans streptococci, and microaerophilic and anaerobic streptococci have been isolated. *Streptococcus pneumoniae* is rarely encountered now as a cause of suppurative arthritis. It has been noted to be the causative organism of septic arthritis in children with sickle disease.[29] The course of suppurative arthritis, the frequency of multiple joint involvement, the sites of infection, and the laboratory abnormalities do not differ significantly with any of these major causative agents of bacterial arthritis.[25]

Infectious arthritis due to gram-negative bacilli (other than *H. influenzae*) as causative organisms is seen in 9–17 percent of the cases of infectious arthritis.[1,4,18,25] Most had either a chronic debilitating disease or a chronic arthritis in the infected joint along with an intercurrent urinary tract infection or had the clinical picture of gram-negative bacteremia.[30] Infection with these organisms was associated with a poor outcome since a large proportion of the patients died and most survivors developed significant flexion contractions, an ankylosing joint, or chronic effusions. Heroin addicts who develop septic arthritis are more likely to have *Pseudomonas* as the causative organism than any other group, with more frequent sternoclavicular and sacroiliac joint infections.[20] Septic arthritis due to *Salmonella* species occurs preponderantly in children but bears no association with sickle cell disease, unlike *Salmonella* osteomyelitis.

Gonococcal arthritis, one of the more commonly recognized features of disseminated gonococcal infections,[7,8] exists in either of two forms. (*1*) Patients have systemic symptoms with fever, shaking chills, skin lesion, and a polyarticular syndrome. Blood cultures are frequently positive, particularly if patients are seen within 2 days of the onset of symptoms, whereas synovial fluid cultures are rarely, if ever, positive. *N. gonorrhoeae* can be recovered if cultures of genital, rectal, and pharyngeal areas are done. The skin lesions begin as tiny erythematous papules, frequently petechiae, and may evolve to become vesicles or even be pustular (Fig. 1). These lesions are fairly transient and last 3–4 days. An occasional patient who fails to come to medical attention may have recurrent episodes of skin lesions and polyarthralgias for periods up to 3 months[8] (as in the case in Fig. 1). The organism is occasionally recovered from scrapings of the skin lesion, although more frequently organisms are recovered from blood. Other microorganisms to be considered in the differential diagnosis of patients with skin rash and arthritis include *Haemophilus influenzae, Moraxella osloensis, Streptobacillus moniliformis,* and *Neisseria meningitidis*. (*2*) Patients with gonococcal infection may also have a monarticular, suppurative joint infection with recovery of the organism from joint fluid. These patients may give a history of having had transient polyarthralgias before the monarticular arthritis developed and may even have a history of skin lesions; however, skin lesions are rarely present in those with a monarticular arthritis. Infection with *N. meningitidis* may mimic the disseminated gonococcemia syndrome with a high probability of greater than 100 skin lesions.[31] In addition, patients with meningococcemia may develop joint effusions 5–10 days after the onset of the infection. Sterile effusions are found in multiple joints and resolve rather rapidly regardless of antimicrobial therapy. An uncommon variety of meningococcal infection is chronic meningococcemia in which symptoms are present for more than a week without meningeal involvement.[10] These patients have low-grade fever; a rash that may be macular, papular, or petechial; joint involvement; and headache. Two-thirds of the patients have polyarthralgias, and one-third have arthritis with joint effusions. Infections with *Streptobacillus moniliformis* occur 2–3 days after rat bites with the onset of chills, a macular rash of the palms and soles, and arthralgias in large joints.[32] The organism, a pleomorphic gram-negative bacillus, can be grown in blood cultures but not from joint fluid. Intermittent attacks of a migratory polyarticular arthritis lasting weeks to months, usually in large joints, occur late in the disease course of many patients with Lyme disease.[33] This spirochetal infection transmitted by tick bite (Chapter 217) also rarely can result in a long-standing chronic arthritis of the knee joint.[33]

Obligate anaerobic bacteria rarely are the causative agents in bacterial arthritis, even when anaerobic cultures are performed routinely on joint fluid, but can result in a long-standing chronic arthritis of the knee joint.[34] The predominant obligate anaerobic bacteria causing septic arthritis in adults have been gram-negative cocci, especially after surgery.[34] *Bacteroides* species are less often encountered. The most frequent anaerobic arthritis in children is due to *Clostridium* species.[2]

TABLE 4. Etiologic Agents as Causes of Bacterial (Suppurative) Arthritis (Percentages)

	Children		
Agent	*<5 Yr*	*>5 Yr*	*Adults*
Staphylococcus aureus	12	33	70
Haemophilus influenzae, type b	29	1	<1
Streptococcus sp[a]	12	13	17
Gram-negative bacilli	5	6	8
Anaerobic	0	1	<1
Neisseria	5	8	[b]
Other	2	5	0
Unknown	35	34	3

[a] Includes *Streptococcus pneumoniae*, groups A and B streptococci, viridans group streptococci, and microaerophilic and anaerobic streptococci.
[b] Excluded from most series of adult suppurative arthritis.
(Data from refs. 1, 4, 17, 18.)

Mycobacterial Infections

Chronic monarticular arthritis with a granulomatous reaction on pathologic examination may be caused by variety of organisms (Table 5). Mycobacterial infections of the joint are chronic, slowly progressive monarticular infections that may also involve the tendon sheaths, particularly the carpal tunnel area of the wrist. A granulomatous reactions of the synovium is seen pathologically, but organisms are rarely demonstrated save by appropriate culture of synovial tissue. Small particulate matter representing fibrinous deposits, called *rice bodies*, may be seen in synovial fluid or tissue with mycobacterial infections, brucellosis, and sporotrichosis.[19,23,35] Infections with *M. tuberculosis* principally involve the knee, followed by the hip, ankle, and wrist.[19] A number of nontuberculous mycobacteria produce infections of the joints (Table 5). *Mycobacterium kansasii* was the most common cause of monarticular synovitis seen in Dal-

TABLE 5. Infectious Causes of Chronic Monarticular Arthritis

Bacterial	
	Brucella sp.
Eubacteria	
	Mycobacterium tuberculosis
	M. kansasii
	M. marinum
	M. intracellulare
	M. fortuitum
	Nocardia asteroides
Fungi	
	Sporothrix schenckii
	Coccidioides immitis
	Blastomyces dermatitidis
	Candida albicans
	Pseudallescheria boydii

las, Texas.[36] This organism has a propensity to involve the wrist and hands and cause a flexor tenosynovitis, a carpal tunnel syndrome, and rarely olecranon bursitis.[36] *M. kansasii* may localize to a joint after trauma from a pulmonary focus. These patients do not usually have extra-articular infection. *Mycobacterium marinum* would be suspected in a patient with arthritis who develops the infection after exposure to tropical fish aquariums or marine life.[37] Synovial tissue from a patient with a chronic monarticular arthritis should be cultured for mycobacteria, observed at a few days (to recognize *M. fortuitum*, a rapid grower), and incubated at 30°C (*M. marinum* grows better at this temperature than at 37°C).

Fungal Arthritis

Sporothrix schenckii can cause infections of the joints.[23,38] The organism commonly infects the knee, the wrist, and the elbow. The ankle or small joints of the hand may be infected, but shoulders and hips are spared (Figs. 2 and 3). Sporotrichotic arthritis or tenosynovitis is not usually a sequel of cutaneous inoculation but may result from occult pulmonary infection. The course is progressive over months and years, usually without fever. With time, infection appears in contiguous bursae or bones as well as in distant joints. Diagnosis is by culture of fluid or tissue.

A chronic monarticular arthritis is seen with *Coccidioides immitis* with or without other evidence of disseminated infection.[39] The knee is the most frequently involved joint. The joint fluid may show either a polymorphonuclear or a lymphocytic cellular response, but smears and cultures are often negative. X-ray films show little evidence of bony destruction even after many months of clinical evidence. Diagnosis is made by culture of synovium. Patients' sera also have positive complement fixation responses with *Coccidioides* antigen.

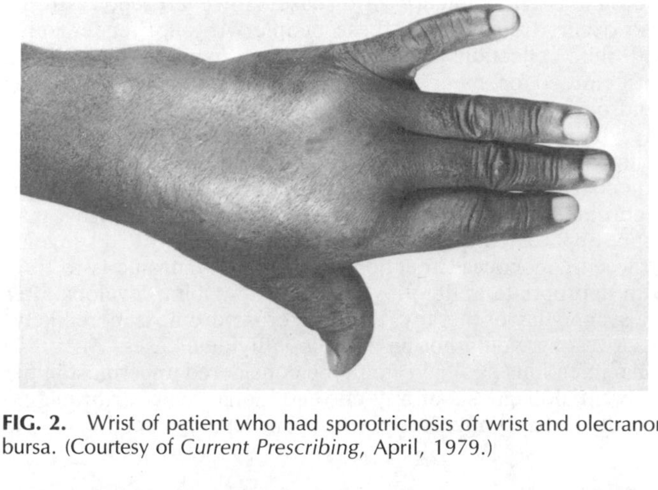

FIG. 2. Wrist of patient who had sporotrichosis of wrist and olecranon bursa. (Courtesy of *Current Prescribing*, April, 1979.)

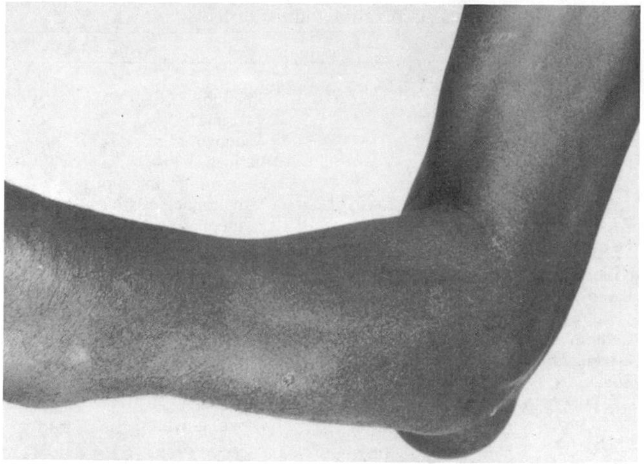

FIG. 3. Elbow of patient who had sporotrichosis of wrist and olecranon bursa. (Courtesy of *Current Prescribing*, April, 1979.)

Joint infection in patients with blastomycosis primarily spreads from osteomyelitis.[40] The diagnosis can be made by examination of synovial tissue and by appropriate culture of surgical material. Complement fixation tests are usually not helpful.

Infections of the joint with *Candida* species generally follows hematogenous spread of the organism, most frequently *Candida albicans*. Or the fungus may be introduced accidentally during intra-articular corticosteroid injection.[41] Synovial fluid shows a polymorphonuclear leukocytic response, and acute and chronic inflammatory cells are noted on microscopic examination. The knee is the most commonly involved joint, with hip, elbow, and other joints also noted. More than one joint may demonstrate infection. Migratory polyarthritis, usually in association with skin lesions or erythema nodosum and erythema multiforme, has been seen with acute histoplasmosis.[42] Carpal tunnel syndrome has also been noted in patients with disseminated histoplasmosis. *Pseudallescheria (Petriellidium) boydii* arthritis has occurred in several patients with penetrating trauma of the knee.

Viral Arthritis

Viral agents associated with symptoms and signs of arthritis are listed in Table 6. Arthritis is a reasonably frequent event and thus can be considered a common manifestation of infection with some agents such as rubella or mumps. Single or only a few cases have been reported with a number of other viruses, so arthritis occurs as an atypical manifestation of infection with these agents, for example, varicella, adenovirus, echovirus. Epidemic smallpox was associated with arthritis (with a frequency of 0.2–0.5 percent) exclusively in infants or children under 7 years of age.[43]

Patients with sporadic or epidemic hepatitis B have been noted to develop arthritis, frequently in association with urticaria.[44] The frequency of arthritis and urticaria is highly variable but was seen in 25 percent of the persons in one epidemic, with skin rash (urticaria, angioneurotic edema, and other erythematous reactions) in 42 percent of those who subsequently developed jaundice.[44] The joint and skin manifestations appear a few days to a few weeks before the onset of the jaundice, and in the great majority, the symptoms disappear with the onset of the jaundice.[45] The hands are most frequently involved. Joint effusions are scanty when present and reveal predominantly mononuclear cells. Hepatitis B antigen is frequently found in the serum at the time of the onset of the arthritis and has been detected in joint fluid in a few cases.[21] Circulating immune com-

TABLE 6. Viral Agents Associated with Arthritis

Group	Virus
Deoxyribonucleic acid viruses	
Poxvirus	Smallpox
	Vaccinia[a]
Adenovirus	Adenovirus[a]
Herpesvirus	Varicella[a]
	Epstein-Barr (infectious mononucleosis)[a]
Parvovirus	Erythema infectiosum
Hepadnavirus	Hepatitis B
Ribonucleic acid viruses	
Paramyxoviruses	Mumps
	Rubeola[a]
Orthomyxoviruses	Influenza[a]
Picornavirus	Echovirus[a]
Togavirus	
Alphavirus	Chikungunya
	O'nyong-nyong
	Sindbis
	Ockelbo disease
	Ross River virus
Rubivirus	Rubella
Arenavirus	Lymphocytic choriomeningitis virus

[a] Unusual manifestation of infection.

plexes containing immunoglobulin and complement components are detected in serum.[12] Joint symptoms may rarely persist up to 6 months, but no residual deformity or sequelae have been noted.

Arthritis occurs in association with mumps with a frequency of 0.44 percent and is seen more commonly in men.[9] The arthritis begins from 1 day before to 15 days after the onset of parotitis, with multiple large and small joints affected. Effusions are infrequent. Symptoms subside within 2 weeks, although arthritis may persist for up to 3 months.[46]

A number of alphaviruses of the togavirus family have arthritis as a frequent manifestation of the illness they cause. Chikungunya derives its name from its characteristic clinical finding (that which bends up). This disease is characterized by an abrupt onset of fever, chills, and severe incapacitating pain in the large joints, although hot, swollen joints are infrequently seen.[47] Maculopapular eruption occurred over the trunk and extensor surface of the extremities in 80 percent of those with the disease. A similar illness in Uganda in 1959 was given the name O'nyong-nyong fever (weakening of the joints).[48] The onset of O'nyong-nyong fever was also abrupt, with symmetric involvement of most of the large joints with excruciating pain. All eventually made a full recovery. Sindbis virus and Sindbis-related diseases such as Ockelbo disease in Sweden have been noted to have arthritis as a prominent manifestation of the illness.[49] In Australia, epidemics of polyarthritis with rash have been observed since 1928 that are due to the recently identified alphavirus, the Ross River agent.[50]

Arthritis due to rubella occurs principally in women.[9,21] The onset of the joint symptoms occurs either with the rash or within 3 days after the eruption. The small joints of the hand are most frequently involved, with knees, wrists, and ankles less commonly affected. Synovial fluid shows a predominance of mononuclear cells, and virus is rarely isolated from the joint fluid. The course is self-limited in most people, although symptoms will rarely last for longer than a month. Rubella vaccine induces joint symptoms with a frequency of 3 percent in children of both sexes but in 39 percent of susceptible postpubertal women.[51] The vaccine virus has rarely been recovered from synovial fluid, but persons with arthralgias or arthritis developed a significantly higher antibody titer than did those without joint reaction. Thus, the use of rubella vaccine in susceptible postpubertal women entails a risk of significant joint symptoms.

Lymphocytic choriomeningitis, caused by an arenavirus, was associated with arthritis in one outbreak among laboratory personnel.[11] Hence, the development of a severe influenza-like disease with headache and arthritis may be due to lymphocytic choriomeningitis virus rather than influenza, a disease in which arthritis is an uncommon complication. In outbreaks of epidemic erythema infectiosum, an infection caused by a parvovirus, a symmetric arthritis was noted in adults, particularly in women.[52]

Parasites

Joint manifestations are not a feature of any of the commonly recognized parasitic infections. However, in the Sepik district of Papua, New Guinea, arthritis in association with filarial infections was the most frequent cause of arthritis.[53] The knee was the most frequently involved joint and showed warmth, tenderness, and limitation of motion. Joint effusions were present in slightly less than one-half of the cases, and the fluid aspirated was creamy yellow. X-ray films showed no articular destruction, only soft tissue swelling. Microfilariae were present in the blood. The patients responded promptly to treatment with diethylcarbamazine, with improvement in the joint symptoms and loss of microfilariae in the blood.

APPROACH TO THE PATIENT

Differential Considerations

Any person with an acute monarticular arthritis should be suspected of having septic arthritis of bacterial etiology. However, a number of conditions may show a single joint involvement with effusions, including acute rheumatoid arthritis, gout, and chondrocalcinosis (pseudogout). In each of these conditions up to 90 percent of the synovial fluid cell count can demonstrate polymorphonuclear leukocytes. The synovial fluid glucose content may be diminished in rheumatoid arthritis and is not reliably diminished in bacterial arthritis. Hence, the ultimate diagnosis must be based on multiple studies including cultures of joint fluid and blood. Synovial fluid from any adult with monarticular arthritis should be examined for crystals, both for negatively birefringent (uric acid) and positively birefringent (calcium pyrophosphate) crystals. Simultaneous bacterial infection and crystalline joint disease has been reported.[54] Serologic studies including rheumatoid factor, LE cell and anti-nuclear antibody tests, and acute and convalescent studies for anti-streptolysin O (ASO) should be performed if more than one joint is affected. A small proportion of cases of suppurative arthritis (10 percent) do involve more than one joint. This may be particularly perplexing in the patient with rheumatoid arthritis since the involvement of a number of joints may herald an exacerbation of their underlying disease. However, septic arthritis also occurs frequently in these people. Any hot tender joints with fluid collections should be aspirated, and the fluid should be submitted for smear and culture. Gonococcal arthritis, Reiter syndrome, and acute rheumatic fever should be suspected in any young adult having fever and multiple joint involvement, although skin lesions are the clinical clue to the disseminated gonococcal syndrome. The other features of the triad of Reiter syndrome, the conjunctival manifestations and urethritis, may not be apparent initially. Frequently, the only way to distinguish between gonococcal infection and Reiter syndrome is to treat with appropriate antibiotics, and if a new joint develops after the second day of therapy, then Reiter syndrome is more likely. HLA testing would not be done in individual cases.

An infectious etiology should be considered uppermost in the differential diagnosis of any chronic monarticular arthritis, especially if tenosynovitis is present. The leading infectious cause is infection with nontuberculous mycobacteria, followed closely by *Sporothrix schenckii*. Infection with *M. tuberculosis* is less often seen today. In addition, Lyme arthritis should be considered if patient is from an endemic area.[33] A synovial biopsy should be done in any person with a chronic monarticular involvement whose synovial fluid cultures are negative, and the tissue should be cultured for fungus and acid-fast organisms. In Lyme arthritis, the infectious agent can be demonstrated by Dieterle silver stain in 25 percent, but all should have a diagnostic titer in a serum indirect immunofluorescent assay of 1:256 or greater.[33] Pathologic examination of the tissue and the culture results provide a clue to whether an infection or other rheumatic disease is the cause of chronic arthritis in most cases.

In any patient with an acute arthritis in whom a diagnosis of bacterial infection cannot be established and in whom other systemic manifestations consistent with a viral infection are present, a diagnosis of viral arthritis should be considered. Unfortunately, it is not usually possible to isolate virus from the joint fluid, so serologic confirmation of the infection is necessary using acute and convalescent sera. In general, the course is the major determinant in distinguishing between viral arthritis and rheumatic disorders such as adult Still's disease since the former has a self-limited course with no residual joint abnormalities.

Specific Antimicrobial Therapy

Most antimicrobial agents achieve therapeutic levels in the infected joint equal to or higher than serum levels.[55,56] Not only does intravenous administration lead to adequate levels of penicillin G, ampicillin, nafcillin, and cephalothin, but also adequate levels have been achieved after the oral administration of cloxacillin and penicillin V. However, borderline adequate levels of synovial fluid have been achieved with oral penicillin G, erythromycin,[56,57] and gentamicin. Thus, therapy with these latter antimicrobial agents must be followed carefully, and organisms must be subjected to in vivo testing. Intra-articular injection of antibiotics is not required, and in fact penicillin has induced a sterile synovitis after intra-articular injection.[4]

The appropriate antimicrobial therapy for bacterial arthritis varies with the age group. In very young infants (infants less than 1 month of age) organisms with widely varying antimicrobial susceptibilities may be the causative agent; empirical therapy must be directed at potential pathogens such as *S. aureus*, gram-negative organisms, and group B streptococci.[17] Initial therapy then would include a penicillinase-resistant synthetic penicillin such as nafcillin, 150 mg/kg/day, combined with gentamicin, 6 mg/kg/day.[17] Therapy would then be altered depending on the antimicrobial susceptibility of the infecting organism. Initial therapy for children under 5 years of age could also include a cephalosporin such as cefuroxime administered at a dose of 75 mg/kg/day.[58] The drug is useful because of the possibility of ampicillin-resistant *Haemophilus influenzae*. If *Haemophilus* is isolated and is β-lactamase-negative, then ampicillin can be substituted. For children over 5 years of age and for adults, initial therapy would be either nafcillin or cefuroxime unless the smear shows another organism. Since there are individual cases of streptococcal infections that do not appear to respond to the antistaphylococcal agents, if the Gram stain shows gram-positive cocci in chains or if the culture is positive for streptococci, then the patient's regimen should be switched to penicillin G intravenously. Initial therapy in all these cases should be with parenteral antibiotics. Oral antibiotics can be used later in the course with success, but adequacy of serum levels must be ensured.[58] If a person is allergic to penicillin, then alternative agents as vancomycin or clindamycin can be chosen.[17] Therapy for a renal dialysis patient with staphylococcal infection would be vancomycin, which can be given once a week to maintain adequate circulating levels. Therapy for gram-negative arthritis could include any third-generation cephalosporin, aztreonam, or imipenem-cilastatin, depending on susceptibility testing. The usual duration of therapy for suppurative arthritis is 2 weeks for *H. influenzae*, streptococci, or gram-negative cocci and 3 weeks for staphylocci or gram-negative bacilli.[59] In most cases, joint fluid cultures are negative within 7 days of therapy, but exceptions do occur.[60]

Recommended therapy for gonococcal arthritis is ceftriaxone 1.0 g i.v. or i.m. daily for 7–10 days. If the infecting organism is fully susceptible to penicillin or tetracycline, many patients who are improving after 3 days can be switched to amoxicillin 500 mg 4 times a day, doxycycline or tetracycline to complete a 7–10 day course.[(61,62)] Initiating therapy with a 3-day course of high dose intravenous penicillin is appropriate if the isolate is already known to be fully susceptible to penicillin. Arthritis due to Lyme disease agent can be treated successfully with penicillin, 20 million units daily for 10 days.[33]

Appropriate therapy for mycobacterial infection consists of isoniazid and rifampin for 9 months for *M. tuberculosis* and *M. kansasii* and rifampin and ethambutol for 6–12 weeks for *M. marinum*.[63,64] Treatment of other mycobacteria must be tailored to the results of in vitro susceptibility testing with a large number of agents since these organisms are relatively resistant to usually administered antituberculous drugs. Amphotericin B is the treatment of choice for arthritis due to fungi.[38–42] Intra-articular amphotericin B may benefit arthritis due to *S. schenckii*.[38] The proper duration and dose of amphotericin is not clearly established, although treatment periods of 6–10 weeks and a total dosage of 2 g or more have been used with some success.[23,38,41] Oral ketaconazole has proved useful in the chronic suppression of coccidioidal arthritis.[65]

Other Therapeutic Modalities

Most people with suppurative arthritis respond adequately to appropriate antimicrobial agents after an initial joint aspiration for diagnosis. Repeated needle aspiration for recurrent joint effusions has been used with success during the first 5–7 days of treatment.[66,67] If the volume of synovial fluid, the cell count, and the percentage of polymorphonuclear leukocytes decreases with each aspiration, then the combination of antimicrobial therapy and aspiration as needed should be adequate. Persistence of effusion beyond 7 days is evidence that surgical drainage is required.[66] Suppurative arthritis of the hip frequently requires surgical drainage since this joint is difficult to evacuate via needle aspiration.[1] There is no evidence that surgical drainage is required for persons with a suppurative arthritis in a joint with underlying joint disease since these patients do well with aspiration alone.[67] If open surgical drainage is performed, there is no evidence that continued irrigation of the joint after the drainage is of any value. Treatment with systemic antimicrobial agents should be continued for up to a week after open drainage, and the wound should be allowed to close by secondary closure.

In the usual case of septic arthritis, immobilization of the infected joint is not necessary, although weight bearing should be avoided until signs of inflammation and pain have disappeared. The joint should be maintained in the functional position, and passive motion may be instituted early, once the symptoms of pain have subsided. As the inflammation diminishes, active exercises may be instituted, and weight bearing may be permitted when all signs of inflammation have disappeared and no evidence of effusion is present.

Course of the Illness

Many persons with bacterial arthritis now recover with no long-term residual abnormalities.[5,67] The major determinants of a poor long-term response include (*1*) failure to recognize and to treat the infection within 7 days of onset,[5] (*2*) infection of the hip joint,[1] (3) infections with gram-negative bacilli, and age over 60 years.[18,30,59] The frequency of sequelae in children was shown to be 27 percent,[68] including slight limitation of movement, impairment of ambulation, and shortening of the extremity. These residua were more common with hip and ankle infection. In adults, up to 50 percent had limitation of motion or persistence of pain.[25] Infectious causes of chronic monarticular arthritis are occasionally associated with substantial residua even after maximal therapy.[23,36] Synovectomy has been combined with chemotherapy to achieve an inactive joint infection.[23,39]

REFERENCES

1. Kelly PJ, Martin WJ, Coventry MB. Bacterial (suppurative) arthritis in the adult. J Bone Joint Surg [Am]. 1970;52:1595–602.
2. Nelson JD, Koontz WC. Septic arthritis in infants and children: A review of 117 cases. Pediatrics. 1966;38:966–71.
3. Trueta J. The three types of acute haematogenous osteomyelitis. J Bone Joint Surg [Br]. 1959;41:671–80.
4. Argen RJ, Wilson CH Jr, Wood P. Suppurative arthritis. Arch Intern Med. 1966;117:661–6.
5. Ward JR, Atcheson SG. Infectious arthritis. Med Clin North Am. 1977;61:313–29.
6. Rimoin DLK, Wennberg JE. Acute septic arthritis complicating chronic rheumatoid arthritis. JAMA. 1966;196:617–21.
7. Keiser H, Ruben FL, Wolinsky E, et al. Clinical forms of gonococcal arthritis. N Engl J Med. 1968;279:234–40.
8. Holmes KK, Counts GW, Beaty HN. Disseminated gonococcal infection. Ann Intern Med. 1968;74:979–93.
9. Smith JW, Sanford JP. Viral arthritis. Ann Intern Med. 1967;67:651–9.
10. Kidd BL, Hart HH, Grigor RR. Clinical features of meningococcal arthritis: A report of four cases. Ann Rheum Dis. 1985;44:790–2.
11. Baum SG, Lewis AM Jr, Rowe WP, et al. Epidemic nonmeningitic lymphocytic-choriomeningitis-virus infection. N Engl J Med. 1966;274:934–6.
12. Wands JR, Mann E, Alpert E, et al. The pathogenesis of arthritis associated with acute hepatitis-B surface antigen–positive hepatitis: Complement activation and characterization of circulating immune complexes. J Clin Invest. 1975;55:930–6.
13. Calin A, Fries JF. An "experimental" epidemic of Reiter's syndrome revisited. Ann Intern Med. 1976;84:564–6.
14. Aho K, Ahvonen P, Lassus A, et al. HLA-27 in reactive arthritis. Arthritis Rheum. 1974;17:521–6.
15. Hakansson V, Low B, Eitren B, et al. HLA-27 and reactive arthritis in an outbreak of salmonellosis. Tissue Antigens. 1975;6:366–7.
16. Keat A. Reiter's syndrome and reactive arthritis in perspective. N Engl J Med. 1983;309:1606–15.
17. Jackson MA, Nelson JD. Etiology and medical management of acute suppurative bone and joint infections in pediatric patients. J Pediatr Orthop. 1982;2:313–23.
18. Cooper C, Cawley MID. Bacterial arthritis in an English health district: A 10 year review. Ann Rheum Dis. 1986;45:458–63.
19. Berney S, Goldstein M, Bishko F. Clinical and diagnostic features of tuberculous arthritis. Am J Med. 1972;53:36–42.
20. Gifford DB, Patzakis M, Ivler D, et al. Septic arthritis due to *Pseudomonas* in heroin addicts. J Bone Joint Surg [Am]. 1975;57:631–5.
21. Medical Staff Conference: Arthritis caused by viruses. Calif Med. 1973;119:38–44.
22. Gordon G, Kabins SA. Pyogenic sacroilitis. Am J Med. 1980;69:50–6.
23. Wilson DE, Mann JJ, Bennett JE, et al. Clinical features of extracutaneous sporotrichosis. Medicine (Baltimore). 1967;46:265–79.
24. Ho G Jr, Tice AD, Kaplan SR. Septic bursitis in the prepatellar and olecranon bursae. An analysis of 25 cases. Ann Intern Med. 1978;89:21–7.
25. Sharp JT, Lidsky MD, Duffy J, et al. Infectious arthritis. Arch Intern Med. 1979;139:1125–30.
26. Wallace R, Cohen AS. Tuberculous arthritis. A report of two cases with review of biopsy and synovial fluid findings. Am J Med. 1976;61:277–82.
27. Roy S, Bhawan J. Ultrastructure of articular cartilage in pyogenic arthritis. Arch Pathol. 1975;99:44–47.
28. Borenstein DG, Simon GL. *Haemophilus influenzae* septic arthritis in adults. A report of four cases and a review of the literature. Medicine (Baltimore). 1986;65:191–201.
29. Syrogiannopoulos GA, McCracken GH Jr, Nelson JD. Osteoarticular infections in children with sickle cell disease. Pediatrics. 1986;78:1090–6.
30. Goldenberg DL, Brandt KD, Cathcart ES, et al. Acute arthritis caused by gram-negative bacilli: A clinical characterization. Medicine (Baltimore). 1974;53:197–208.
31. Rompalo AM, Hook EW, Roberts PL, et al. The acute arthritis–dermatitis syndrome. The changing importance of *Neisseria gonorrhoeae* and *Neisseria meningitidis*. Arch Intern Med. 1987;147:281–3.
32. Roughgarden JW. Antimicrobial therapy of rat-bite fever. Arch Intern Med. 1965;116:39–54.
33. Goldings EA, Jericho J. Lyme disease. Clin Rheum Dis. 1986;12:343–67.
34. Fitzgerald RH Jr, Rosenblatt JE, Tenney JH. Anaerobic septic arthritis. Clin Orthop. 1982;164:141–8.
35. Kelly PJ, Martin WJ, Schirger MD, et al. Brucellosis of the bones and joints. JAMA. 1960;174:347–53.
36. Sutker WL, Lankford LL, Tompsett R. Granulomatous synovitis: The role of atypical mycobacteria. Rev Infect Dis. 1979;1:729–35.
37. Jolly HW Jr, Seabury JH. Infections with *Mycobacterium marinum*. Arch Dermatol. 1972;106:32–6.
38. Bayer AS, Scott VJ, Guze LB. Fungal arthritis. III. Sporotrichal arthritis. Semin Arthritis Rheum. 1979;9:66–74.
39. Bayer AS, Guze LB. Fungal arthritis. II. Coccidioidal synovitis: Clinical diagnostic, therapeutic, and prognostic considerations. Semin Arthritis Rheum. 1979;8:200–11.
40. Witorsch P, Utz JP. North American blastomycosis: A study of 40 patients. Medicine (Baltimore). 1968;47:169–200.
41. Bayer AS, Guze LB. Fungal arthritis. I. *Candida* arthritis: Diagnostic and prognostic implications and therapeutic considerations. Semin Arthritis Rheum. 1978;8:142–50.
42. Bayer AS, Choi C, Tilman DB, et al. Fungal arthritis. V. Cryptococcal and histoplasmal arthritis. Semin Arthritis Rheum. 1980;9:218–27.
43. Cockshott P, MacGregor M. Osteomyelitis variolosa. Q J Med. 1958;37:369–87.
44. Steigman AJ. Rashes and arthropathy in viral hepatitis. Mt. Sinai J Med. 1973;40:752–7.
45. Fernandez R, McCarty DJ. The arthritis of viral hepatitis. Ann Intern Med. 1971;74:207–11.
46. Gordon SC, Lauter CB. Mumps arthritis: A review of the literature. Rev Infect Dis. 1984;6:338–44.
47. Robinson MC. An epidemic of virus disease in Southern Province, Tanganyika Territory, in 1952–53. Trans R Soc Trop Med Hyg. 1955;49:28–32.
48. Shore H. O'nyong-nyong fever: An epidemic virus disease in East Africa. III. Some clinical and epidemiological observations in the North Province of Uganda. Trans R Soc Trop Med Hyg. 1961;55:361–73.
49. Niklasson B, Espmark A, Lundstrom J. Occurrence of arthralgia and specific IgM antibodies three to four years after Ockelbo disease. J Infect Dis. 1988;157:832–5.
50. Fraser JRE. Epidemic polyarthritis and Ross River virus disease. Clin Rheum Dis. 1986;12:369–88.
51. Lerman SJ, Nankervis GA, Heggie AD, et al. Immunologic response, virus excretion, and joint reactions with rubella vaccine. Ann Intern Med. 1971;74:67–73.
52. Reid DM, Brown T, Reid TMS, et al. Human parvovirus-associated arthritis: A clinical and laboratory description. Lancet 1985;1:422–5.
53. Salfield S. Filarial arthritis in the Sepik District of Papua New Guinea. Med J Aust. 1975;1:264–7.
54. Baer PA, Tenenbaum J, Fam AG, et al. Coexistent septic and crystal arthritis. Report of four cases and literature review. J Rheumatol. 1986;13:604–7.
55. Nelson JD. Antibiotic concentrations in septic joint effusions. N Engl J Med. 1971;284:349–53.
56. Parker RH, Schmid R. Antibacterial activity of synovial fluid during therapy of septic arthritis. Arthritis Rheum. 1971;14:96–104.
57. Chow A, Hecht R, Winters R. Gentamicin and carbenicillin penetration into the septic joint. N Engl J Med. 1971;285:178–9.
58. Nelson JD, Bucholz RW, Kusmiesz H, et al. Benefits and risks of sequential parenteral–oral cephalosporin therapy for suppurative bone and joint infections. J Pediatr Orthop. 1982;2:255–62.
59. Syrogiannopoulos GA, Nelson JD. Duration of antimicrobial therapy for acute suppurative osteoarticular infections. Lancet 1988;1:37–40.
60. Ho G Jr, Su EY. Therapy for septic arthritis. JAMA. 1982;247:797–800.
61. Treatment of sexually transmitted diseaese. Medical letter. 1988;30:5–10.
62. Bush LM, Boscia JA. Disseminated multiple antibiotic-resistant gonococcal infection: Needed changes in antimicrobial therapy. Ann Intern Med. 1987;107:692–3.
63. Dutt AK, Moers D, Stead WW. Short-course chemotherapy for extrapulmonary tuberculosis. Nine year's experience. Ann Intern Med. 1986;104:7–12.
64. Donta ST, Smith PW, Levitz RE, et al. Therapy of *Mycobacterium marinum* infections: Use of tetracyclines vs. rifampin. Arch Intern Med. 1986;146:902–4.
65. Catanzaro A, Einstein H, Levin B, et al. Ketoconazole for treatment of disseminated coccidioidomycosis. Ann Intern Med. 1982;96:436–40.
66. Schmid FR, Parker RH. Ongoing assessment of therapy in septic arthritis. Arthritis Rheum. 1969;12:529–34.
67. Goldenberg DL, Brandt KD, Cohen AS, et al. Treatment of septic arthritis. Arthritis Rheum. 1975;18:83–90.
68. Howard JG, Highgenboten CL, Nelson JD. Residual effects of septic arthritis in infancy and childhood. JAMA. 1976;236:932–5.

90. INFECTIONS WITH PROSTHESES IN BONES AND JOINTS

BARRY D. BRAUSE

Over the past 2 decades joint replacement surgery has become commonplace due to the magnificent success of these procedures in restoring function to disabled arthritic individuals. Initially, total prosthetic hip implantation techniques were devised. Subsequently, total knee replacement, total shoulder replacement, and total elbow replacement procedures using many of the same orthopedic principles became available. Patients receiving total joint replacements number in the hundreds of thousands each year worldwide, and virtually millions of people have indwelling prosthetic articulations. One to five percent of indwelling prostheses becomes infected; this is a calamity for the patient and is associated with significant morbidity and occasionally death. Prosthesis removal, which usually is necessary to treat these infections, produces large skeletal defects, shortening of the extremity, and severe functional impairment. The health care cost of treating septic prosthetic articulations has been estimated conservatively at 40–80 million dollars per year in the United States alone.[1] The patient faces protracted hospitalization, sizable financial expense, and potentially renewed disability.

PATHOGENESIS

Certain patient populations have been identified as predisposed toward infection of their prosthetic joints including those with prior surgery at the site of the prosthesis, rheumatoid arthritis, corticosteroid therapy, diabetes mellitus, poor nutritional status, obesity, and extremely advanced age.[2,3] Infection usually occurs in osseous tissue adjacent to the foreign body. Since most prostheses are cemented in place with polymethylmethacrylate, infection develops at the bone–cement interface. Sepsis involving cementless prostheses develops in the bone contiguous with the metallic alloy.

Prosthetic joints become infected by two different pathogenetic routes: locally introduced and hematogenous types of osteomyelitis. The locally introduced form of infection is the result of wound sepsis contiguous to the prosthesis or operative contamination. Any factor or event that delays wound healing increases the risk of infection. Ischemic necrosis, infected wound hematomas, wound infection (with or without identifiable cellulitis), and suture abscesses are common preceding events for joint replacement sepsis. During the early postimplantation period when these superficial infections develop, the fascial layers have not yet healed, and the deep, periprosthesis tissue is not protected by the usual physical barriers. Generally these infections are caused by a single pathogen, but polymicrobial sepsis with as many as five different organisms is also observed. *Staphylococcus epidermidis* is the most common etiologic agent in this clinical setting. Infrequently, latent foci of chronic, quiescent osteomyelitis are reactivated by the disruption of tissue associated with implantation surgery. Although bone cultures at the time of the joint replacement operation are sterile, old *Staphylococcus aureus* and *Mycobacterium tuberculosis* infections can recrudesce postoperatively.

Any bacteremia can induce infection of a total joint replacement by the hematogenous route.[4–6] Dentogingival infections and manipulations are known causes of viridans streptococcal and anaerobic (*Peptococcus, Peptostreptococcus*) infections in prostheses. Pyogenic skin processes can cause staphylococcal (*S. aureus, S. epidermidis*) and streptococcal (groups A, B, C, and G streptococci) infections of joint replacements. Genitourinary and gastrointestinal tract procedures or infections are associated with gram-negative bacillary, enterococcal, and anaerobic infections of prostheses. Twenty to forty percent of prosthetic joint infections arise by the hematogenous route, the remainder being of the locally introduced type.

TABLE 1. Bacteriology of Prosthetic Joint Infection

Pathogens	*Frequency (%)*
Staphylococci	53
S. epidermidis	28
S. aureus	25
Streptococci	20
β-Hemolytic streptococci	12
Viridans streptococci	8
Gram-negative aerobic bacilli	20
Anaerobes	7

The frequency of specific microorganisms etiologic in prosthetic joint sepsis varies among the published studies, but a general view of the spectrum of this bacteriology as well as the prominence of certain microbial groups is seen in Table 1. Staphylococci (*S. epidermidis* and *S. aureus*) are the principal causative agents, aerobic streptococci and gram-negative bacilli are each responsible for approximately 20 percent, and anaerobes represent 5–10 percent of these infections. The spectrum of microbial agents capable of causing prosthetic joint infection is unlimited and includes organisms ordinarily considered "contaminants" of cultures such as corynebacteria (aerobic diphtheroides), propionibacteria (anaerobic diphtheroids), and members of the *Bacillus* genus. Rarely have infections with fungi (particularly *Candida*) and mycobacteria been described.

As foreign bodies, the indwelling metallic prosthesis and the polymethylmethacrylate cement, which binds the metal alloy to adjacent bone, predispose both joint space and osseous tissue to septic processes. Foreign substances contribute to local sepsis experimentally by decreasing the quantity of bacteria necessary to establish infection and by permitting pathogens to persist on their avascular surface, sequestered from circulating immunologic defenses (leukocytes, antibodies and complement) as well as systemic antibiotics.[3,7] Polymethylmethacrylate cement appears to predispose toward infection to an extent beyond that of other inert foreign substances. The cement in unpolymerized form has been shown to inhibit phagocytic, lymphocytic, and complement function in vitro.[8,9] The polymerization process itself appears to enhance the risk of infection, possibly due to the substantial heat generated by this in vivo reaction.[8] In an effort to provide total joint replacement without polymethylmethacrylate, cementless prostheses have been designed. These devices have textured surfaces to provide fixation by the growth of adjacent bone into the "porous" interface of the prosthesis. The performance and durability of this new form of arthroplasty is uncertain.

Host responses to methylmethacrylate also may play a role in the pathogenesis of infection. Fibronectin, a connective tissue and plasma glycoprotein, appears to enhance *S. aureus* adherence to polymethylmethacrylate in vivo and thus may contribute to the occurrence of sepsis.[10] Microbial products may assist the development and persistence of infection in association with foreign substances. In the presence of prosthetic devices, many bacteria elaborate a fibrous exopolysaccharide material called *glycocalyx*. Organisms can grow within this matrix and form thick biofilms that are protected at least in part from host defense mechanisms[2,11] (see Chapter 2).

CLINICAL PRESENTATION

Prosthetic joint sepsis produces the cardinal symptoms of inflammation with a wide spectrum of severity. Most patients

TABLE 2. Presenting Symptoms of Prosthetic Joint Infection

Symptom	*Frequency (%)*
Joint pain	95
Fever	43
Periarticular swelling	38
Wound or cutaneous sinus drainage	32

present with a long indolent course characterized by a progressive increase in joint pain and occasionally the formation of cutaneous draining sinuses but no fever, soft tissue swelling, or systemic toxicity. Others present with an acute, fulminant illness with high fever, severe joint pain, local swelling, and erythema. The frequencies of these presenting symptoms are listed in Table 2.[12]

The pattern of clinical presentation is determined largely by three factors: (*1*) the virulence of the infecting pathogen, (*2*) the nature of the host tissue in which the microorganism grows, and (*3*) the route of infection. *Staphylococcus aureus* is a particularly virulent pathogen in this setting and usually produces a fulminant infection (occasionally with septic shock). β-Hemolytic streptococci and aerobic gram-negative bacilli are also capable of causing this clinical picture. Alternatively, the relatively avirulent but tenacious *S. epidermidis* is consistently associated with an indolent course. Characteristics of the involved tissue can influence the type of presentation on the basis of their support of microbial growth. Wound hematomas (as well as seromas and hemarthroses), fresh operative wounds, ischemic wounds, and tissues in diabetic and steroid-treated patients all enhance the ability of bacteria to multiply rapidly in expansive tissue planes. These factors promote the development of a more fulminant infection when a large inoculum of bacteria is allowed access to deep tissue compartments during surgery or in a slowly healing wound postoperatively. The hematogenous route of infection theoretically seeds the bone–cement interface with a relatively small number of organisms. When a blood-borne infection arises in a prosthetic joint several months or years after implantation surgery, the fully healed connective tissue often is capable of restricting the septic process to a relatively small but critical focus at the bone–cement interface. Joint pain is the principal symptom of deep tissue infection irrespective of the mode of presentation and suggests either acute inflammation of periarticular tissue or loosening of the prosthesis due to subacute erosion of bone at the bone–cement interface.

DIAGNOSIS

The clinical manifestations previously described (i.e., joint pain, swelling, erythema, and warmth) all reflect an underlying inflammatory process in the surrounding tissues but are not specific for infection. When a painful prosthesis is accompanied by a fever or purulent drainage from overlying cutaneous sinuses, infection may be presumed, pending further confirmatory tests. However, in the vast preponderance of cases, infection must be differentiated from aseptic and mechanical problems (e.g., hemarthrosis, gout, bland loosening, and dislocation), which are more common causes of pain and inflammatory symptoms in these patients.

Constant joint pain is suggestive of infection, whereas mechanical loosening commonly causes pain only with motion and weight bearing.[2] Plain x-ray films can reveal (*1*) abnormal lucencies greater than 2 mm in width at the bone–cement interface, (*2*) changes in the position of prosthetic components, (*3*) cement fractures, (*4*) periosteal reaction, or (*5*) motion of components on stress views. In addition, the intra-articular injection of dye (arthrography) may reveal abnormal communications between the joint space and multiple defects in the bone–cement interface. These radiologic abnormalities (Fig. 1) are found in 50 percent of septic prostheses. They are generally related to the duration of infection since it may require 3–6 months to manifest such changes. When both distal and proximal components of a prosthetic joint demonstrate radiographic pathology, sepsis is a more likely than is simple mechanical loosening. However, these changes seen on x-ray films are not specific for infection because they are also seen frequently with aseptic processes.

Radioisotopic scans with technetium diphosphonate demonstrate increased uptake in areas of bone with enhanced blood supply or increased metabolic activity. Increased technetium uptake is seen routinely around normal prostheses for 6 months after arthroplasty. Positive scan findings after this period are abnormal and reflect inflammation and possible loosening but not specifically infection of the implant. Sequential technetium-gallium bone scanning is also nondiagnostic due to unacceptable sensitivity (66 percent) and specificity (81 percent).[13] Indium-labeled leukocyte scanning, although very sensitive, also provides only nonspecific results.[14] Therefore normal or negative technetium or indium leukocyte scan findings can be considered strong evidence against the presence of infection, but they are not definitive in establishing the diagnosis. Elevated peripheral white blood cell counts and erythrocyte sedimentation rates, although suggestive, also are inadequate in diagnosing sepsis in this clinical setting.

The specific diagnosis of joint replacement infection is de-

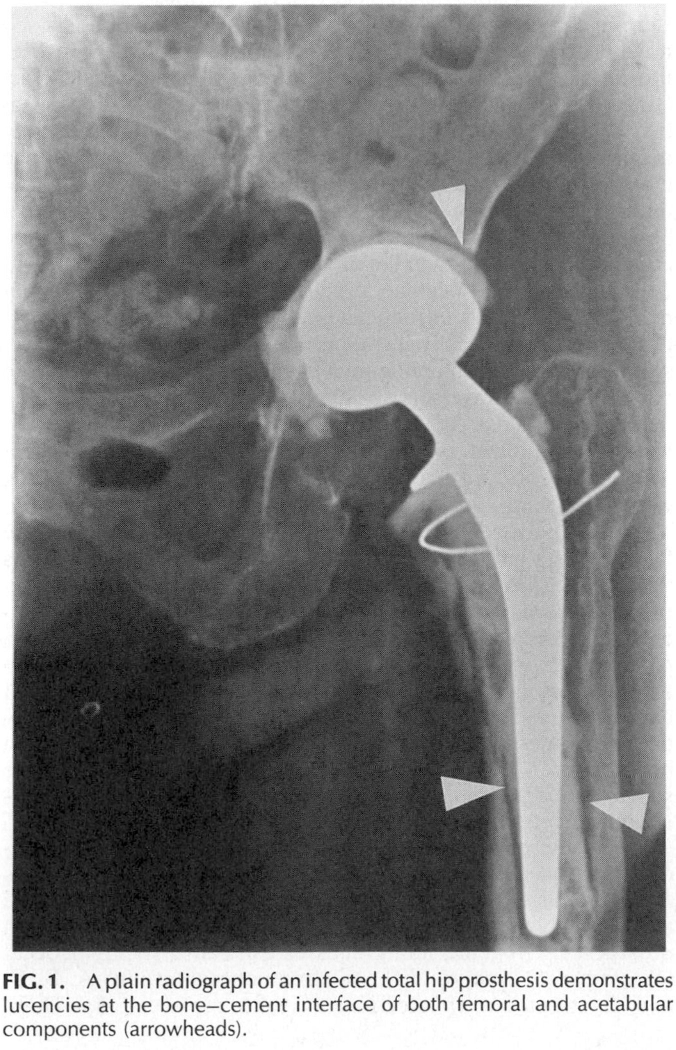

FIG. 1. A plain radiograph of an infected total hip prosthesis demonstrates lucencies at the bone–cement interface of both femoral and acetabular components (arrowheads).

pendent, in large part, upon isolation of the pathogen by aspiration of joint fluid or by culture of tissue obtained at arthrotomy.[15] Analysis of joint fluid often reveals a high leukocyte count (mainly polymorphonuclear cells), a high protein content, and a low glucose concentration. However the changes are only variably present and are neither prerequisites for making the diagnosis of joint replacement infection nor specific for this entity. Histopathologic examination of periprosthetic tissue frequently reveals an infiltration of polymorphonuclear leukocytes indicative of an acute inflammatory reaction, but this parameter is positive in only 55 percent of infected patients and also may not be sufficiently specific. Therefore the single observation that delineates the presence of implant infection is isolation of the pathogen by arthrocentesis or surgical débridement.

Since fastidious microorganisms, including anaerobes, may be etiologic agents in prosthetic arthroplasty infections, multiple specimens should be obtained and rapidly cultured in appropriate media. Arthrocentesis demonstrates the pathogen in 85–98 percent of cases.[15,16] Gram stain is positive in 32 percent. Fluoroscopic guidance and arthrography are useful in documenting accurate needle placement. When difficulty is encountered in obtaining intra-articular fluid, irrigation with sterile normal saline (without antiseptic preservative additives) can be used to provide the necessary fluid for culture. When initial cultures reveal a relatively avirulent organism (*S. epidermidis*, corynebacteria, propionibacteria, *Bacillus* sp.), a second aspirate should be considered to reconfirm the bacteriologic diagnosis and to eliminate the possibility that the isolate is artifactual. Operative cultures are definitively diagnostic; therefore the patient should not receive antimicrobial therapy for several weeks before the procedure. Multiple specimens of tissue and fluid should be submitted for culture. The results of these microbiologic techniques should confirm the presence and nature of the infection as well as allow for optimal treatment. In the uncommon circumstance when the clinical suggestion of sepsis is strong but the cultures are sterile, fastidious organisms (particularly anaerobes) should be suspected. In order to design efficacious and the least toxic antimicrobial therapy the patient's infecting strain of bacteria must be available for in vitro evaluation as described later in this chapter.

THERAPY

Successful treatment of a total joint arthroplasty infection depends upon extensive and meticulous surgical débridement and effective antimicrobial therapy. Simple surgical drainage (with retention of the prosthesis in situ) followed by a nonstandardized, finite course of antibiotic therapy has been only 20 percent successful.[17] In response to this 80 percent failure rate, two different approaches to more effective treatment of prosthetic joint infection have evolved over the past decade. Complete removal of all foreign materials (metallic prosthesis and cement) is an essential component of both regimens.

The most successful protocol incorporates standardized antimicrobial therapy with a two-stage surgical procedure. Removal of the prosthesis and cement is followed by a 6-week course of bactericidal antibiotic therapy chosen on the basis of in vitro susceptibility studies. Reimplantation is performed at the conclusion of the 6-week antibiotic course. With this protocol a 90 percent success rate has been achieved in total hip replacement infections, and a 97 percent success rate has been obtained in total knee replacement infections.[18–20] The success of this regimen relies on thorough débridement techniques and effective antimicrobial therapy. In this manner, both gram-positive bacteria (including multidrug-resistant staphylococci and enterococci) as well as gram-negative bacteria (including *Pseudomonas aeruginosa*) can be eliminated if the specific sensitivities of each isolate allow eradication. The empirical selection of a 6-week duration of antibiotic therapy may be critical for efficacy. Others have employed a similar approach to therapy but only a 2-week course of antibiotic treatment before reinsertion of the prosthesis.[21] With this protocol the pathogen was eradicated in only 79 percent of the cases, and only 35 percent of the patients obtained good function in the new prosthesis.

The alternative method of treatment involves metallic joint and cement extraction with immediate reimplantation of a new prosthesis in a one-stage surgical procedure (exchange operation) accompanied by nonstandardized antimicrobial therapy. Methylmethacrylate cement impregnated with an antibiotic (usually gentamicin or tobramycin) is employed during reimplantation. The antimicrobial agent leaches out from the hardened plastic to produce variable but high initial release as well as protracted diffusion of antibiotic into surrounding tissues at the bone–cement interface.[22] The protocol is effective in 70–80 percent of cases.[23–25] When using repeated exchange operations (in the 20–30 percent failure group) incorporating antibiotic-laden cement, the success rate is increased to 90 percent.[24] It has been suggested that this mode of therapy is applicable only to infections with the less virulent microorganisms since high failure rates are observed when *S. aureus* or gram-negative bacilli are the pathogens.[26] Systemic antibiotics are administered rarely and without standardization in this regimen. Moreover, the selection of an aminoglycoside as a component in the recementing phase of these operations may not have reflected the susceptibility of the pathogen being treated.

Future therapeutic approaches will likely include the most efficacious parts of these two protocols: combining the specific, standardized 6-week antibiotic regimen and two-stage prosthesis removal-reimplantation surgery with the incorporation of antibiotic-impregnated cement during arthroplasty reinsertion. In those clinical situations in which adequate antimicrobial potency cannot be achieved, arthrodesis or resection arthroplasty is recommended rather than attempting prosthesis reimplantation. However, with the advent of antibiotic-impregnated cement even these difficult cases may be candidates for another total joint arthroplasty.

SUPPRESSIVE ANTIBIOTIC THERAPY

Although removal of the implanted prosthesis is necessary to eradicate deep infection associated with these devices, this therapeutic approach is not always available. Occasionally surgical excision is contraindicated due to medical and surgical conditions or patient refusal. Since it is likely that the pathogen will be able to persist at the undébrided bone–cement interface despite high-dose, finite systemic antimicrobial therapy, lifelong oral antibiotic treatment can be considered to suppress the infection and retain the usefulness of the total joint replacement. In selected cases in which (*1*) prosthesis removal is not possible, (*2*) the pathogen is relatively avirulent, (*3*) the pathogen is exquisitely sensitive to an orally absorbed antibiotic, (*4*) the patient can tolerate an appropriate oral antibiotic, and (*5*) the prosthesis is not loose, suppressive oral antimicrobial therapy may be of value. Preliminary observations suggest that this form of therapy is effective only when all of these five criteria are fulfilled. Successful retention of the functioning arthroplasty has been seen in 63 percent of patients in this unusual clinical setting. The suppressive approach is not without risk. Serial radiographs are needed over the course of treatment to monitor for progressive bone resorption at the bone–cement interface that could reduce the success of any future revision surgery. Despite continual antibiotic therapy the localized septic process could extend into adjacent tissue compartments or become a systemic infection. Moreover, the patient would be subjected to the potential side effects of chronic antibiotic administration.

PREVENTION OF JOINT PROSTHESIS INFECTION

In view of the catastrophic effects of prosthetic arthroplasty infection, prevention of these septic processes is of prime importance. In anticipation of elective total joint replacement surgery, the patient should be evaluated for the presence of pyogenic dentogingival pathology, obstructive uropathy, and dermatologic conditions that might predispose to infection and bacteremia. Strong consideration should be given to reducing the risks represented by these factors (i.e., dental extraction, prostatic resection, control of dermatitis) before insertion of the prosthesis. Perioperative antibiotic prophylaxis has been shown to effectively reduce deep wound infection in total joint replacement surgery.[27] Oxacillin or cefazolin are commonly administered as antistaphylococcal agents immediately before the operation and for 1–2 days thereafter. Filtered laminar airflow systems in the operating room further reduce infection rates, especially when whole-body, exhaust-ventilated suits are worn by the operating team.[28,29]

For patients with indwelling joint prostheses, early recognition and prompt therapy for infection in any location is critical to reduce the risk of seeding the joint implant hematogenously. Situations likely to cause bacteremia should be avoided. The use of prophylactic antibiotics in anticipation of bacteremic events (i.e., dental surgery, cystoscopy, colonoscopic biopsy, surgical procedures on infected or contaminated tissues) has been suggested on the same empirical basis upon which endocarditis prophylaxis is recommended.[3,5] This approach to prevention is controversial at the present time, and no data are available to determine the adequacy or the cost-effectiveness of such measures. Clinical decisions regarding prophylactic antibiotics for expected bacteremias in patients with prosthetic joints should be made on an individual basis.

REFERENCES

1. Salvati EA, Small RD, Brause BD, et al. Infections associated with orthopedic devices. In: Sugarman B, Young EJ, eds. Infections Associated with Prosthetic Devices. Boca Raton, FL: CRC Press; 1984:181–218.
2. Gristina AG, Kolkin J. Total joint replacement and sepsis. J Bone Joint Surg [Am] 1983;65:128–34.
3. Brause BD. Infections associated with prosthetic joints. Clin Rheum Dis. 1986;12:523–36.
4. Ahlberg A, Carlsson AS, Lindberg L. Hematogenous infection in total joint replacement. Clin Orthop. 1978;137:69–75.
5. Lattimer GL, Keblish PA, Dickson TB, et al. Hematogenous infection in total joint replacement. JAMA. 1979;242:2213–4.
6. Lindqvist C, Slatis P. Dental bacteremia—a neglected cause of arthroplasty infections? Acta Orthop Scand. 1985;56:506–8.
7. Petty W, Spanier S, Shuster JJ, et al. The influence of skeletal implants on incidence of infection. J Bone Joint Surg [Am]. 1985;67:1236–44.
8. Petty W. The effect of methylmethacrylate on bacterial inhibiting properties of normal human serum. Clin Orthop. 1978;132:266–77.
9. Petty W. The effect of methylmethacrylate on bacterial phagocytosis and killing by human polymorphonuclear leukocytes. J Bone Joint Surg [Am]. 1978;60:752–7.
10. Vaudaux P, Suzuki R, Waldvogel FA, et al. Foreign-body infection: Role of fibronectin as a ligand for the adherence of *Staphylococcus aureus*. J Infect Dis. 1984;150:546–53.
11. Costerton JW, Irvin RT, Cheng K-J. The bacterial glycocalyx in nature and disease. Annu Rev Microbiol 1981;35:299–324.
12. Inman JN, Gallegos KV, Brause BD, et al. Clinical and microbial features of prosthetic joint infection. Am J Med. 1984;77:47–53.
13. Merkel KD, Brown ML, Fitzgerald RH. Sequential technetium-99m HMDP-gallium-67 citrate imaging for the evaluation of infection in the painful prosthesis. J Nucl Med. 1986;27:1413–7.
14. Pring DJ, Henderson RG, Rivett AG, et al. Autologous granulocyte scanning of painful prosthetic joints. J Bone Joint Surg [Br]. 1986;68:647–52.
15. O'Neill DA, Harris WH. Failed total hip replacement: Assessment by plain radiographs, arthrograms and aspiration of the hip joint. J Bone Joint Surg [Am]. 1984;66:540–6.
16. Eftehar NS. Wound infection complicating total hip joint arthroplasty. Orthop Rev. 1979;8:49–64.
17. Fitzgerald RH, Nolan DR, Ilstrup DM, et al. Deep wound sepsis following total hip arthroplasty. J Bone Joint Surg [Am]. 1977;59:847–55.
18. Callaghan JJ, Salvati EA, Brause BD, et al. Reimplantation for salvage of the infected hip. In: The Hip: Proceedings of the 14th Open Scientific Meeting of The Hip Society. St Louis: CV Mosby; 1986:65–94.
19. Insall JN, Thompson FM, Brause BD. Two-stage reimplantation for the salvage of infected total knee arthroplasty. J Bone Joint Surg [Am] 1983;65:1087–98.
20. Salvati EA, Chekofsky KM, Brause BD, et al. Reimplantation in infection. Clin Orthop. 1982;170:62–75.
21. Rand JA, Bryan RS. Reimplantation for the salvage of an infected total knee arthroplasty. J Bone Joint Surg [Am]. 1983;65:1081–6.
22. Trippel SB. Antibiotic-impregnated cement in total joint arthroplasty. J Bone Joint Surg [Am]. 1986;68:1297–302.
23. Buchholz HW, Elson RA, Lodenkamper H. The infected joint implant. In: McKibbin B, ed. Recent Advances in Orthopedics. Edinburgh: Churchill Livingstone; 1979:139–61.
24. Buchholz HW, Elson R, Engelbrecht E. Management of deep infection of total hip replacement. J Bone Joint Surg [Br]. 1981;63:342–53.
25. Carlsson AS, Josefsson G, Lindberg L. Revision with gentamicin-impregnated cement for deep infection in total hip arthroplasties. J Bone Joint Surg [Am]. 1978;60:1059–64.
26. Fitzgerald RH, Jones DR. Hip implant infection. Am J Med. 1986;78(Suppl 6B):225–8.
27. Norden C. A critical review of antibiotic prophylaxis in orthopedic surgery. Rev Infect Dis. 1983;5:928–32.
28. Lidwell O, Lowbury E, Whyte E. Effect of ultraclean air in operating rooms on deep sepsis in the joint after total hip or total knee replacement. Br Med J. 1982;285:10–4.
29. Salvati EA, Robinson RP, Zeno SM, et al. Infection rates after 3175 total hip and total knee replacements performed with and without a horizontal unidirectional filtered air-flow system. J Bone Joint Surg [Am]. 1982;64:525–35.

91. OSTEOMYELITIS

CARL W. NORDEN

Osteomyelitis continues to pose difficulties both in diagnosis and management and causes serious morbidity and, less frequently, mortality. Antibiotics have significantly altered the mortality and outcome of osteomyelitis, but chronic disease still occurs as a sequela. There are differences of opinion about the choice of antibiotic, the duration of treatment, the type of surgical intervention needed, and the effect of these factors on prognosis.

PATHOPHYSIOLOGY AND PATHOLOGY

Osteomyelitis may develop in any bone of the body. However, the predisposition of the disease for certain bones can be better understood after reviewing its structure. Bone is a metabolically active tissue with high rates of synthesis and resorption, processes that depend on an adequate vascular supply. Acute hematogenous osteomyelitis usually involves rapidly growing bone and characteristically affects the metaphysis of long bones. The anatomy of the vasculature in this area provides some explanation for this specific localization of bacteria. The capillary ramifications of the nutrient arteries supplying bone make sharp loops in the area of the epiphyseal growth plates and enter a system of sinusoidal veins connected with the venous network of the medullary cavity. The afferent loops of these metaphyseal capillaries lack phagocytic lining cells, and the efferent loops contain functionally inactive phagocytic cells. In the loops of the capillaries, flow becomes considerably slower and more turbulent. The capillary loops adjacent to the epiphyseal growth plates are essentially end-artery branches of the nutrient artery, and obstruction of these vessels results in areas of avascular necrosis.

In the prepubescent person, infection presumably starts in the metaphyseal sinusoidal veins, is contained by the growth plate, and spreads laterally where it breaks through the cortex and lifts the loose periosteum to result in a subperiosteal collection. In adults, the periosteum is firmly attached to the underlying bone, and because of this, subperiosteal abscess formation and intense periosteal proliferation are less frequently seen. Once infection has started, it provokes an acute suppurative response that contributes to necrosis of tissue, breakdown of bone, and removal of calcium. Infection may extend to neighboring bony structures through the Haversian and Volkmann canals, thereby shutting off the vascular supply and causing the death of more bone. At this point, the chronic phase of osteomyelitis may be established as large segments of avascular bone separate and form sequestra. There is also frequently deposition of new bone, an involucrum, under the elevated periosteum.

MANIFESTATIONS OF OSTEOMYELITIS

In any consideration of bone infections, it is logical to divide them into three main types: osteomyelitis resulting from hematogenous spread of infection, osteomyelitis that is secondary to a contiguous focus of infection, and osteomyelitis associated with vascular insufficiency (see Table 1 for a summary of the features of each). Other specific clinical situations and problems can then be considered.

Hematogenous Osteomyelitis

Age Distribution. Although classically described as a disease of children, hematogenous osteomyelitis is being reported with increased frequency in older age groups. One form, involving the vertebrae, is commonly a disease of individuals over the age of 50.

Bones Involved. Most frequently involved are the long bones of the lower extremities and the humerus (Fig. 1). The vertebrae are often the sites of infection in adults. Multiple bone involvement may occur in up to 15 percent of the patients.

Bacteriology. In most cases of acute hematogenous osteomyelitis, a determined diagnostic effort results in the identification of an etiologic agent. The most useful procedures for recovery of the etiologic agent are bone biopsies, blood cultures, and cultures of draining pus. *Staphylococcus aureus* has been the most common agent, but gram-negative bacilli (*Escherichia coli, Klebsiella, Salmonella, Proteus,* and *Pseudomonas*) are being found with increasing frequency.

Clinical Features. The classic presentation of acute hematogenous osteomyelitis in children is that of an abrupt onset of high fever, systemic toxicity, and physical findings of local suppuration about the involved bone. In adults, such a classic picture is less frequently seen. About one-half of the patients may have symptoms of pain, swelling, chills, and fever for less than 3 weeks before admission. Other patients may have had vague symptoms for 1 or 2 months with few constitutional complaints; the major complaint is pain in the involved limb. Drainage is an infrequent occurrence.

If chronic osteomyelitis supervenes, systemic signs such as toxicity and high fever are relatively uncommon. Local tenderness, swelling, and erythema are less frequent than in acute osteomyelitis. Drainage from a sinus tract is often the herald of an exacerbation of chronic osteomyelitis.

Laboratory Data. Sedimentation rates and white blood cell counts are frequently elevated, although the latter rarely exceed 15,000/mm^3. The magnitude of these values is of little help in predicting the outcome of disease.

Osteomyelitis Secondary to a Contiguous Focus of Infection

This form of osteomyelitis represents a direct infection of bone from an exogenous source or the spread of infection from a nearby infected focus. The most common precipitating factor is postoperative infection such as that after open reduction of fractures. Nonsurgically induced infections develop from soft tissue infections, infected teeth, or infected sinuses (Fig. 2). After animal bites, spread of locally inoculated organisms may occur with consequent development of osteomyelitis (most commonly due to *Pasteurella multocida*).

Age Distribution. Most cases of this type of osteomyelitis are seen in patients over the age of 50, presumably because the precipitating factors such as hip fractures or neurosurgery occur more frequently in older persons.

Bones Involved. Although any bone in the body may be involved, the long bones of the lower extremity (femur and tibia) are most frequently involved since these are often the site of fracture and open reduction. Pressure sores (decubitus ulcers) may overlie a focus of osteomyelitis. The diagnosis is not always easy and frequently requires a combination of x-ray films, bone scans, and bone biopsy for histologic examination. Culture of bone biopsy samples usually discloses anaerobic bacteria, gram-negative bacilli, or both. The diagnosis of osteomyelitis must be strongly considered if a pressure sore does not respond to local therapy.[1]

The skull and mandible are also frequent sites of osteomyelitis after neurosurgery, oral surgery, or dental infections. Sternal osteomyelitis is an uncommon but highly morbid complication of median sternotomy incisions for cardiac surgery. Mediastin-

TABLE 1. Major Types of Osteomyelitis

Feature	*Hematogenous*	*Secondary to Contiguous Focus of Infection*	*Due to Vascular Insufficiency*
Age distribution (yr)	Peaks at 1–20 and ≥50	≥50	≥50
Bones involved	Long bones Vertebrae	Femur, tibia, skull, mandible	Feet
Precipitating factors	Trauma (?) Bacteremia	Surgery Soft-tissue infections	Diabetes mellitus Peripheral vascular disease
Bacteriology	Usually only one organism *S. aureus* Gram-negative organisms	Often mixed infection *S. aureus* Gram-negative organisms Anaerobic organisms	Usually mixed infections *S. aureus or epidermidis* Streptococci Gram-negative organisms Anaerobic organisms
Episode Major clinical findings	Initial Fever Local tenderness Local swelling Limitation of motion Recurrent Drainage	Initial Fever Erythema Swelling Heat Recurrent Drainage Sinus	Initial and Recurrent Pain Swelling Erythema Drainage Ulceration

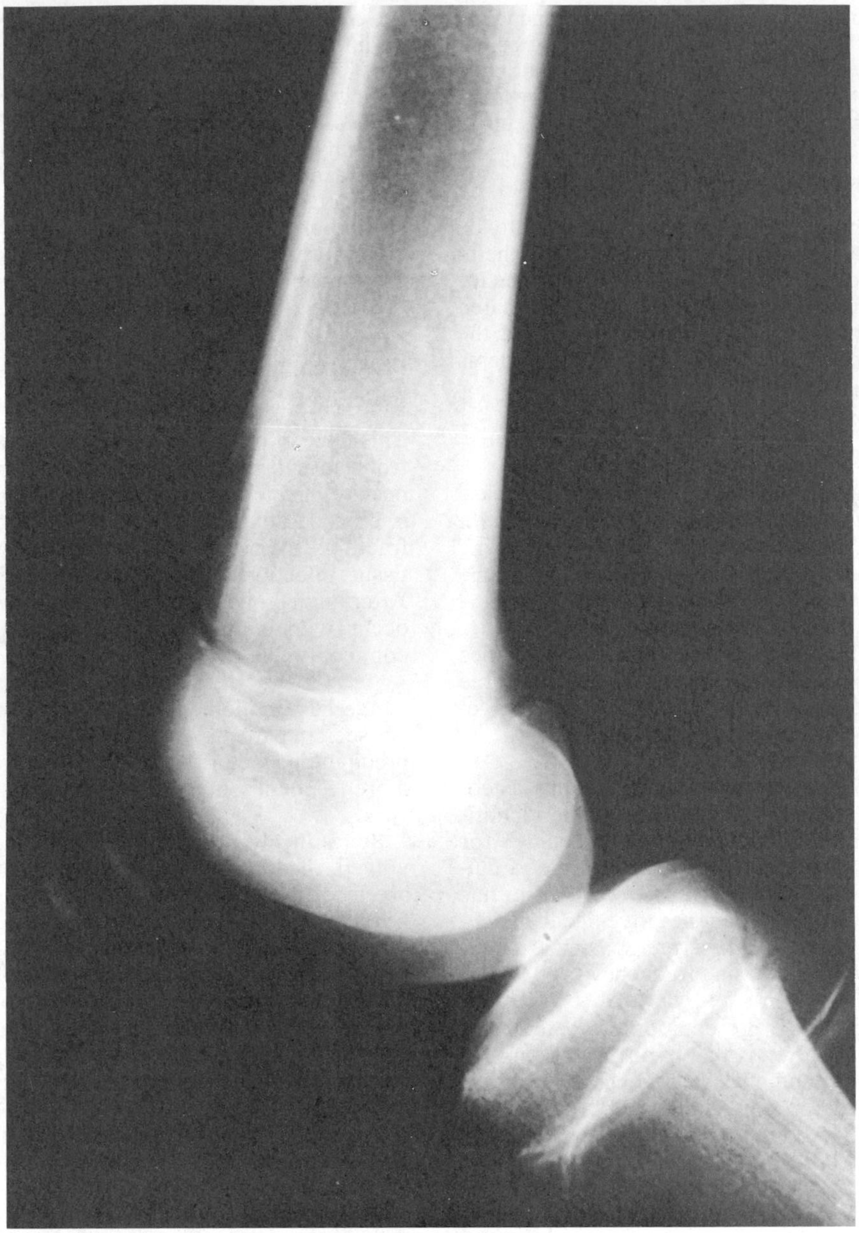

FIG. 1. Chronic hematogenous osteomyelitis. The patient is a 15-year-old boy with a 1 month history of pain in his leg, fever, and a swollen knee. Arthrocentesis revealed purulent but sterile fluid. At surgery, pus, which grew *S. aureus* when cultured, was curetted from the bone cavity. Full recovery followed intensive antibiotic therapy, with total disappearance of the lytic lesion.

itis regularly accompanies sternal infection. Initial manifestations include fever, leukocytosis, and erythema of the wound. With time, bone dissolution at the sternal edges leads to sternal instability despite the presence of sutures. Gram-positive and gram-negative bacteria as well as atypical mycobacteria are etiologic agents in this disease. Cure almost always requires reoperation for irrigation of the mediastinum and débridement of necrotic sternum.[2] When most of the sternum must be resected, closure is delayed until bilateral pectoralis muscle flaps can be placed over the wound.

Bacteriology. Unlike hematogenous osteomyelitis where a single organism is usually responsible, osteomyelitis secondary to a contiguous focus of infection is often associated with more than one species of bacteria. *Staphylococcus aureus* is still the most common infecting organism, but it is frequently found as part of a mixed infection. The value of culturing sinus tract drainage, even if it is purulent, is open to question.

A study comparing cultures of sinus tracts with cultures of operative specimens from patients with chronic osteomyelitis revealed that less than half the sinus tract cultures contained the operative pathogen. Isolation of *S. aureus* from sinus tracts correlated to some degree with the finding of this organism in bone; in contrast, isolation of bacteria other than *S. aureus* from sinus tracts had a low likelihood of predicting the pathogen isolated from bone.[3]

Clinical Signs. In the initial episodes, fever, swelling, and erythema are seen in approximately one-half of the cases. During recurrences, sinus formation and drainage are the two major presenting signs, and patients generally show fewer systemic signs in recurrences than in initial episodes.

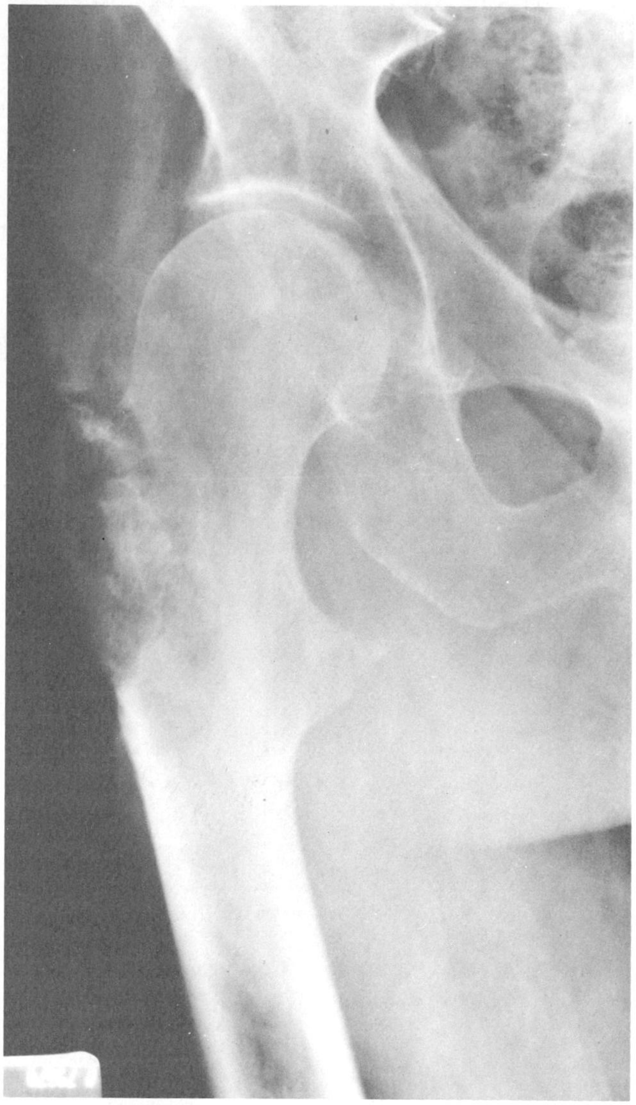

FIG. 2. Osteomyelitis secondary to a contiguous focus of infection. The patient is a debilitated 76-year-old man with a large decubitus ulcer overlying the right greater trochanter. Cultures of pus revealed mixed anaerobic–aerobic infection. An x-ray film reveals a soft-tissue defect as well as irregular loss of bone around the region of the greater trochanter.

Osteomyelitis Associated with Vascular Insufficiency

Patients with osteomyelitis associated with vascular insufficiency present difficult problems of management. Such patients nearly always have diabetes or severe atherosclerosis.

Age Distribution. Most patients are between 50 and 70 years old and have had diabetes mellitus from 2 to more than 10 years before infection occurs.

Bones Involved. The toes or other small bones of the feet are usually affected.

Bacteriology. Most cultures obtained from either surgical specimens or from the wound will show several different species of organisms. Staphylococci are most commonly isolated, but gram-negative aerobic organisms and gram-positive and gram-negative anaerobic bacteria are also recovered frequently.[4]

Clinical Signs. Local symptoms dominate the picture, and few patients manifest systemic signs. Patients may have long-standing chronic draining ulcers on their toes or feet or may be admitted because of cellulitis manifested by pain, swelling, and redness of the lower extremity. Fever and septicemia are uncommon. Such patients usually have evidence of long-standing diabetes with neuropathy and retinopathy. Peripheral pulses may be palpable in the face of vascular insufficiency since this is a disease of small vessels.

SPECIFIC CLINICAL SITUATIONS

Vertebral Osteomyelitis

Vertebral osteomyelitis is a diagnostic pitfall for practicing physicians since it is often protean and subtle in its presenting manifestations.[5,6] The infection generally occurs in drug addicts, after trauma (often surgical), or after hematogenous spread from another focus of infection (usually the urinary tract). It is postulated that infection disseminates from the urinary tract to the vertebral column via the posterior venous plexus and the vertebral venous system (Batson's veins).

The infecting bacteria may be isolated from blood cultures or from material aspirated from the vertebral body, disk space, or adjacent areas. Although *S. aureus* continues to be the predominant organism, Enterobacteriaceae (presumably from the urinary tract) have been responsible with increasing frequency.

The clinical diagnosis is based on the finding of localized pain and tenderness over one or more vertebrae in patients with fever. Symptoms may be minimal, and the initial presentation may be only that of malaise and low back pain. Fever can be low grade or absent. However, about 10 percent of patients are bacteremic and acutely ill on admission. Perhaps the most useful laboratory test is the sedimentation rate; the finding of an elevated sedimentation rate in association with low back pain, with or without fever, should make one think of vertebral osteomyelitis. Conventional roentgenograms as well as bone scans can suggest the appropriate diagnosis (Fig. 3).

Complications of vertebral osteomyelitis include subluxation of the atlantoaxial joint (in cervical spine disease), abscesses and local extension of infection, and significant neurologic lesions. A spinal epidural abscess, most often caused by *S. aureus,* may occur secondary to osteomyelitis; the major neurologic manifestations include spinal ache, foot weakness, paraparesis, and paraplegia. Diagnosis by myelography, magnetic resonance imaging (MRI), or computed tomography (CT) scan with subsequent evacuation of pus from the epidural space is critical for full recovery of neurologic function.

Until recently, it was common practice to immobilize patients with vertebral osteomyelitis, usually in a body cast. Several reports now strongly suggest that antibiotic therapy with simple bed rest suffices to cure pyogenic vertebral osteomyelitis, that external stabilization is not needed, and that we should avoid the inconvenience and hazards of body casts.

Osteomyelitis Due to Gram-Negative Organisms

Because the clinical patterns of osteomyelitis due to gram-negative organisms are somewhat different from those described in previous sections, it is appropriate to discuss them separately. *Pseudomonas aeruginosa* was the most frequent pathogen in one series, although *Proteus, E. coli, Salmonella,* and *Klebsiella* spp. were also encountered.[7] *Brucella* spondylitis will not be discussed here. The femur was the most frequently involved bone, followed by infection of the metatarsals. Draining wounds were seen in over half the patients when first examined. About one-third of the patients had underlying diseases such as malignancy, alcoholism, or collagen-vascular disease, which may have contributed to their susceptibility to infection. Surgery or a breach of the skin as from a puncture wound was an antecedent factor in many patients with osteomyelitis due

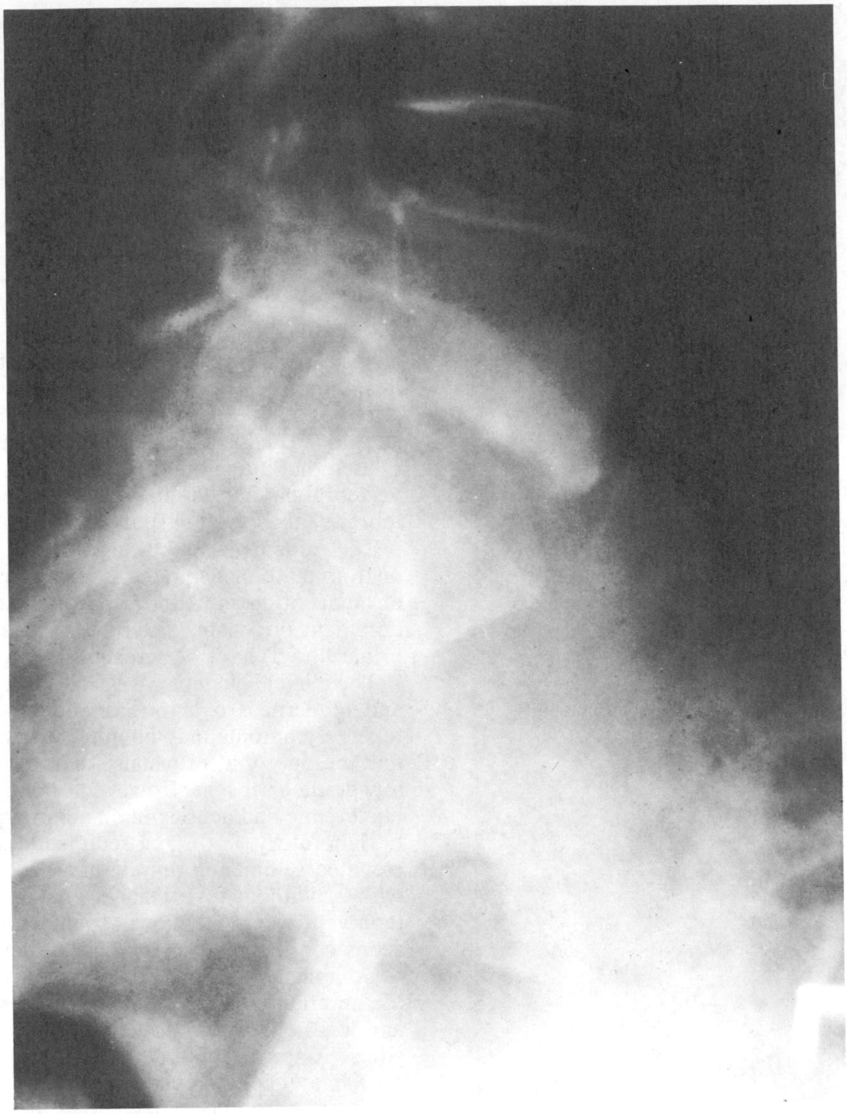

FIG. 3. Osteomyelitis involving vertebrae, in a 42-year-old man with postoperative infection of the fifth lumbar vertebral body. *Staphylococcus aureus* was recovered on biopsy. The tomogram reveals an irregular destructive process at the inferior surface of the L5 vertebral body as well as narrowing of the L5-S1 intervertebral space. With appropriate antibiotic therapy, the patient made an excellent recovery.

to *Pseudomonas*. Heroin addicts may also have osteomyelitis due to gram-negative organisms. Therapy for osteomyelitis caused by gram-negative organisms consists of appropriate antibiotic management as well as necessary surgical intervention. One of the difficulties with the treatment of gram-negative osteomyelitis has been that the minimal inhibitory concentrations (MICs) of gram-negative organisms are generally sufficiently high to make oral therapy, with its attendant lower levels of antibiotic in serum, less effective than similar oral therapy would be for osteomyelitis due to gram-positive organisms. Further, for organisms such as *P. aeruginosa*, there were no effective oral agents available. In one series, only half of the patients with osteomyelitis were successfully treated; this is a higher incidence of therapeutic failures than is generally reported for gram-positive organisms. It is possible that the use of quinolones may improve the prognosis for patients with osteomyelitis due to these organisms, but clinical trials will be required to verify this.[8,9]

Osteomyelitis Due to Anaerobic Organisms

Anaerobic organisms are found in osteomyelitis with some frequency and would probably be recovered more often if optimal techniques for isolation were used. In one series spanning 28 months, anaerobic bacteria were isolated from tissue obtained during débridement for osteomyelitis in 40 of 182 patients.[10] In 9, only anaerobic bacteria were recovered; in the rest, mixed aerobic–anaerobic infections were present. As a group, the patients in whom only anaerobes were isolated were older and had a short duration of symptoms (1 month or less in 7 of the 9), and in 7 the infection was associated with a metallic foreign body.

In a review of the literature, anaerobic osteomyelitis was found most frequently in long bones (40 percent) and skull and facial bones (27 percent).[11] The most common predisposing factors were previous fractures, diabetes, and human bites. *Bacteroides fragilis* and *Bacteroides melaninogenicus* were the anaerobes most frequently isolated. Suggested settings in which anaerobic osteomyelitis should be suspected include (*1*) hand infections after human bites, (*2*) infection of the pelvis after abdominal sepsis, (*3*) sacral osteomyelitis after decubitus ulcers, (*4*) osteomyelitis of the skull or facial bones, (*5*) chronic nonhealing indolent ulcers of the feet, (*6*) the presence of foul-smelling exudate, and (*7*) when there is a failure to grow bacteria from clinical specimens, particularly when the Gram stain has shown organisms. The role of anaerobes in cases of osteomyelitis that also yield aerobic organisms is unclear; whether they are primary pathogens or act synergistically with other bacteria remains to be determined. However, it seems wise to treat both the anaerobes and aerobes in mixed infections. Actinomycosis can cause osteomyelitis by the hematogenous route or by contiguous spread from lesions in the chest or abdomen. The diagnosis is made by a culture of deep tissue or by the demonstration of sulfur granules. Further details are given in Chapter 233.

Osteomyelitis Caused by Fungi

Hematogenous osteomyelitis is a frequent complication of blastomycosis and disseminated coccidioidomycosis. Both tend to present as indolent osteolytic lesions with pus in the contiguous soft tissue. Whereas osteomyelitis often accompanies sporotrichosis arthritis, the appearance on x-ray films is only a subtle decrease in trabeculation. *Candida* osteomyelitis is a rare, late complication of candidemia that usually presents as a single osteolytic lesion.[12]

Osteomyelitis in Hemodialysis Patients

Bacterial infections, usually staphylococcal, are common in hemodialysis patients in whom indwelling cannulae allow portals of bacterial entry. Osteomyelitis is a complication of chronic hemodialysis. Ribs and the thoracic vertebral column are the most common sites of involvement. Infection is probably hematogenous since most patients have prior bacteremias and the organisms infecting bone are the same as those found by blood culture. The diagnosis of osteomyelitis is usually made 12–72 months after the initiation of hemodialysis.

The patient may have a fever of unknown origin, the clinical and x-ray film signs may mimic those of renal osteodystrophy, and infection may not be recognized. Surgical intervention and antibiotic treatment can result in cure of the infection.

Osteomyelitis in Patients with Sickle Cell Disease

In a large series reviewing sickle cell disease and osteomyelitis, it was reported that 20 of 70 patients with complete hemoglobin defects had at least one hospitalization for the treatment of osteomyelitis during a 10-year study period.[13] In essentially all cases, the infecting organisms in patients with sickle cell disease were gram-negative rods. *Salmonella* sp. accounted for approximately 80 percent. In contrast, from the same hospital, records of 117 patients with osteomyelitis but with normal hemoglobin included only a single patient with *Salmonella* infection of the bone.

It is difficult to differentiate thrombotic marrow crisis from osteomyelitis in patients with sickle cell disease. In some children, there is a history of bone pain and fever that, after an interval of 5 days to 2 weeks, is followed by the onset of spiking fever, chills, and leukocytosis. Such a sequence is suggestive of osteomyelitis after a crisis. Children with sickle cell disease may have multiple sites of bone infection simultaneously. Frequently, because the symptoms may be insidious and mimic those of marrow crisis, early cultures of blood and stool offer the only clue to the correct diagnosis. Presumptive antibiotic therapy in children with sickle cell disease who are suspected of having osteomyelitis should include agents effective against *Salmonella* (generally ampicillin, a cephalosporin, or trimethoprim-sulfamethoxazole). X-ray films of patients appropriately treated will usually show complete healing of the changes of osteomyelitis.

Osteomyelitis in Heroin Addicts

One of the complications associated with drug addiction is osteomyelitis.[14] Generally, the clinical course is indolent, and fever is infrequent; sites of infection may be any bone including the vertebrae, pubis, and clavicles. The organisms causing infection generally reflect the spectrum of pathogens infecting addicts: staphylococci, gram-negative rods, and yeast. Primary infection of bone should be considered in narcotic addicts having localized pain. Roentgenographic changes may be initially absent, only to appear after several weeks, thus necessitating serial x-ray films. Surgical exploration is often required to make a bacteriologic diagnosis, particularly in view of the fact that the spectrum of organisms seen is much broader than that commonly associated with osteomyelitis.

Brodie's Abscess

Brodie's abscess is the name given to a chronic, localized bone abscess. While the more subacute cases may have fever, pain, and periosteal elevation, truly chronic cases are often afebrile and present with dull pain of weeks' to months' duration. The lesion is typically single and located near the metaphysis. About 75 percent of the patients reported were less than 25 years of age. The distal part of the tibia is the most common site. Surgical débridement is often curative, but antimicrobial therapy is also recommended.[15]

Gaucher's Disease

Patients with Gaucher's disease, particularly children, may develop all the signs and symptoms of acute bacterial osteomyelitis.[16] These bone crises have an acute onset of bone pain, usually over the tibia, that is often accompanied by high fever, leukocytosis, and an elevated sedimentation rate. The overlying skin may be warm and the area tender to palpation. Even the bone scan findings may be compatible with osteomyelitis. Although biopsy shows bone necrosis, the etiology is noninfectious. This entity of "pseudo-osteomyelitis" is important to recognize because bone biopsy is associated with a high incidence of chronic infection and persistent drainage from the operative site.[17]

Tuberculosis

Skeletal tuberculosis is presumably caused by dissemination of bacilli via the blood stream early in the course of the initial infection. In some cases, spread to bone appears to result from lymphatic drainage from another infected area such as the pleura or kidney. In both children and adults, skeletal involvement may be the only manifestation of systemic disease and, like the pulmonary form, may smolder for years before being discovered.

The basic lesion almost always is a combination of osteomyelitis and arthritis. An inflammatory reaction is followed by formation of granulation tissue that begins to erode and destroy cartilage and eventually cancellous bone, ultimately leading to demineralization and necrosis. The healing process involves deposition of fibrous tissue.

In adults, skeletal tuberculosis usually occurs in weight-bearing joints.[18] The spine is the most frequent site (Pott's disease) followed by the hip and the knee. Tuberculosis is the most common inflammatory process involving the ribs. More than one bone may be affected, and a patient presenting with multiple osteolytic lesions should have the diagnosis of widespread dissemination of bone tuberculosis considered.

Pain is generally the most common complaint. X-ray film evaluations should be followed by specimen collection and culture. Biopsy may be necessary to obtain tissue: a pathology report of granulomatous tissue compatible with tuberculosis is sufficient evidence to begin therapy since organisms may not be grown.

One of the most important radiologic distinctions is between tuberculous spondylitis and pyogenic infection of the spine. In tuberculosis, the first change noted in the spine is a slight narrowing of the intervertebral space. Later, adjacent vertebral bodies are destroyed with eventual collapse and formation of kyphosis and scoliosis (gibbus formation). Generally, pyogenic osteomyelitis involves the disk early and produces rapid sclerosis by 3 or 4 months, whereas tuberculous spondylitis moves more slowly, and the course can be measured over years.

Valuable clinical trials, carried out by the British Medical Research Council, have established that properly prescribed and adequately controlled chemotherapy is sufficient for the routine treatment of tuberculosis of the spine. Cases in which there are complications may need further measures, but for the uncomplicated case, immobilization, plaster jackets, and surgery are unnecessary. Chemotherapy with appropriate antituberculous drugs should provide adequate therapy.

Nontuberculous Mycobacterial Infections

Osteoarticular infections with nontuberculous mycobacteria fall into three distinct types: tenosynovitis, synovitis, and osteomyelitis. Multiple diverse species including *M. marinum, M. avium-intracellulare, M. fortuitum,* and *M. gordonae* have all been associated with infection. Many of these infections seem to respond well to surgery alone; the role of antituberculous therapy, particularly with organisms like *M. avium-intracellulare,* is not clear.[19]

DIAGNOSIS

Roentgenologic Observations

In most patients with hematogenous osteomyelitis, no changes on x-ray film are visible until 10 days after the onset of illness. Although roentgenographic bone changes are rather late events, deep soft tissue swelling and obliteration of the planes between muscles occur early and may provide the first diagnostic clue to the presence of osteomyelitis. The delay in roentgenographic bone changes is probably due to the time needed for more than 50 percent of the bone matrix to be removed before a lytic process can be visualized. Generally, changes of destruction precede new bone formation. In addition, periosteal reaction, cortical irregularity, demineralization, and sequestrum formation may be seen. Computed tomography may be of value for the study of the articular surface of bone and periarticular soft tissues, delineation of the extent of involvement, and demonstration of sequestra.[20] However, its use has not been compared systematically with that of either routine roentgenographic studies or radionuclide studies, and its role in the diagnosis and management of osteomyelitis is still unclear.

MRI with T1- and T2-weighted images is a technique that is currently under active investigation for the detection of inflammatory disease involving the musculoskeletal system. In vertebral osteomyelitis, MRI was as accurate and sensitive as radionuclide scanning in the detection of osteomyelitis. Although MRI can also be helpful in infection of the appendicular skeleton, it is unclear under what circumstances MRI can add significantly to other techniques in diagnosing bone infection.[21] It is probably better than radionuclide studies for differentiating soft tissue infection with periostitis from osteomyelitis. Its role in the immediate postoperative period in the presence of metallic implants is probably very limited. The current data base regarding MRI is small, and further studies of its role in the evaluation of inflammatory processes will be needed.[22]

Radionuclide Studies

The use of radionuclide scanning techniques has enhanced our ability to make an early diagnosis in cases of osteomyelitis.[23] Scanning agents are laid down in newly formed collagen; bone scan results are positive when there is either accelerated bone turnover or increased blood supply to the involved bone. Inflammatory processes, tumor, acute trauma with repair, synovitis, and arthritis may all give positive scan findings. The interpretation of a positive bone scan must depend on the clinical picture to distinguish between these different processes.

The most widely studied technique is technetium scanning, which is extremely sensitive and misses only a small percentage of infections in the musculoskeletal system. The major drawback to technetium scanning is specificity. Some workers feel that this can be improved by the three-phase bone scan, which allows some differentiation of osteomyelitis from soft tissue infection. The addition of gallium scans or indium-labeled white blood cell scintigraphy may be useful in patients with infection superimposed on previous surgery or trauma. In summary, it is fair to say that, although the more recent scanning techniques show promise for the identification of early osteomyelitis in patients with negative findings on x-ray films and technetium bone scanning, they remain expensive procedures whose precise sensitivity, specificity, and predictive value have not yet been firmly established.[23,24]

Microbiologic Studies

The importance of making a precise bacteriologic diagnosis of the infecting organism cannot be overemphasized. Since we are committing patients to prolonged courses of therapy and since there is no distinctive clinical or roentgenographic pattern by which we can make a precise diagnosis of the etiologic agents, it behooves the physician to do whatever tests are necessary to recover the responsible agent. In a comprehensive review of acute osteomyelitis in infants and children, bacteria were recovered in 85 percent of the episodes of osteomyelitis.[25] The frequency of positive cultures in relation to the sources of specimens in that same series was 57 percent for blood, 69 percent for needle aspirate of bone, 65 percent for bone pus obtained at surgery, 83 percent for joint fluid, and 100 percent for wound drainage. Comparable figures are not available for osteomyelitis cases in adults, but we would expect a similarly high percentage of recovery of bacteria for appropriate diagnostic procedures. Cultures for fungi and mycobacteria should be done when clinical suspicion of such infection exists.

Since osteomyelitis, in its chronic form, may persist for years despite antibiotic therapy, the question of the role of protoplasts (L-forms or cell wall-deficient forms) has been raised. Despite a careful search, no protoplasts were found in patients with osteomyelitis in one large series. There are well-documented reports of a few cases in which these forms were recovered. It would seem reasonable in a case of persistent osteomyelitis (particularly one previously treated with antibiotics) from which no bacteria have been recovered that cultures in appropriate hypertonic medium be performed to recover these fastidious forms.

TREATMENT

Antibiotics

Vital questions such as the optimal antibiotics to use, duration over which the agents should be administered, and importance of penetration of antibiotics into bone remain unanswered. Further, it is unlikely that answers will be forthcoming from clinical studies because of the tremendous number of variables involved in assessing the treatment of chronic osteomyelitis. Animal models that mimic the human disease offer some hope for providing rational guidelines.

"Levels" of different antibiotics in bone have been measured after antibiotic administration to patients undergoing surgery. It is difficult to compare the results of these studies since different assay techniques were used. Furthermore, many variables affect the uptake of antibiotics in bone tissue such as the vascularity, the presence of concomitant disease, and the anatomy of the bone chosen for study. Among the agents tested, clindamycin was found in a higher bone-to-serum ratio than were drugs such as methicillin, oxacillin, or cephalothin. Similar observation has been made in experimental animals. The clinical significance of "bone levels" is unknown; studies in experimental animals suggest that it is not necessarily a significant factor in predicting the success of therapy.[26]

When using a well-standardized technique, concentrations of methicillin, dicloxacillin, cephaloridine, or cefazolin were measured in pus and bone from children with osteomyelitis.[27] The penetration of the antibiotics into pus and bone was similar for the two penicillins and for the two cephalosporins despite the disparate protein-binding affinities of these drugs; both penicillins achieved higher bone-to-serum ratios than did the cephalosporins. These four agents attained tissue concentrations that were at least severalfold greater than the MIC values for the infecting *S. aureus* strains.

A model of chronic staphylococcal osteomyelitis in rabbits has been used to test various antimicrobial regimens.[28] Oxacillin, cephalothin, cephaloridine, lincomycin, and rifampin were all found to be associated with a significant number of failures to sterilize diseased bone when administered for 4 weeks. In contrast, it was found that the combinations of rifampin with an aminoglycoside or cephalothin or the combination of oxacillin with an aminoglycoside sterilized the bones of significantly more animals than these agents administered alone did. Because of the need to extrapolate these experimental data to the clinical situation, a controlled, multicenter trial was carried out in chronic staphylococcal osteomyelitis that compared nafcillin and rifampin to nafcillin alone. Although statistical significance was not reached, 80 percent of the patients receiving the two drugs had favorable responses with a minimum of a 2-year follow-up as compared with 50 percent of those receiving nafcillin alone.[29] These results suggest that the combination of nafcillin and rifampin is extremely effective in chronic staphylococcal osteomyelitis involving long bones and should be considered for refractory or difficult cases in particular.

A multicenter collaborative study was carried out to determine whether a standardized serum bactericidal test could be a predictor of therapeutic efficacy in acute and chronic osteomyelitis.[30] The authors evaluated 48 episodes of osteomyelitis (30 acute and 18 chronic) and concluded that patients with acute osteomyelitis should have serum bactericidal titers of 1:2 or greater at all times and that patients with chronic osteomyelitis should have serum bactericidal titers of 1:4 or greater at all times. In general, trough titers appeared to have better predictive value than do peak titers. The study was well done and carefully controlled, but certain caveats are in order. The number of treatment failures was small (four and six, respectively, in the acute and chronic patients), thus making interpretation of the predictive values of titers more difficult. It is my conclusion, based on the results of this study, that it is desirable to aim for a trough serum bactericidal titer of 1:2 or greater but that one must balance the potential toxicity of too high doses of drugs in attempting to obtain such level. I would recommend using these levels as a guide to therapy but not adhering to them rigidly.

Acute Osteomyelitis

The best measure of success of antibiotic therapy in acute osteomyelitis is the incidence of recurrent or chronic disease. In an excellent review of osteomyelitis in infants and children, Dich et al.[25] found a failure rate (defined as recurrent or chronic disease developing) of 19 percent in the patients who received antibiotic therapy for fewer than 21 days after the onset of illness. In contrast they found only 1 failure in 50 patients receiving antibiotics for more than 3 weeks. Their recommendations for the management of acute osteomyelitis should probably be followed until controlled studies indicate that other approaches would be as effective; similar recommendations seem appropriate for adults. They recommend immediate needle aspiration whenever osteomyelitis is suspected. If subperiosteal pus is not obtained, the needle is inserted into the bone, and if any amount of pus is obtained, the patient is taken to surgery for drainage. Antibiotic therapy is based on Gram stain and culture of aspirated material. Therapy is carried out with parenteral antibiotics in high dosage for 4 weeks; oral antibiotics are not subsequently administered. Other investigators have demonstrated that oral antimicrobial therapy after a brief course of parenterally administered drug has been successful in treating acute osteomyelitis.

Chronic Osteomyelitis

In contrast to these clear recommendations for the treatment of acute osteomyelitis, appropriate therapy for chronic osteomyelitis remains a conundrum. Since chronic osteomyelitis is associated with necrotic bone that may serve to sequester bacteria and because it is believed that the organisms are not rapidly multiplying but are relatively dormant, most feel that it is necessary to attain high levels of antibiotics over a prolonged period of time in the infected tissue. This logic has been translated into a recommendation for giving parenteral antibiotics for 1–2 months followed by oral antibiotics for another period of months.

The above recommendation has little hard data to support it. Furthermore, it may not be applicable to cases of chronic osteomyelitis caused by certain gram-negative organisms whose MIC is sufficiently high that orally administered antibiotics could not attain levels in serum or bone that would be adequate to inhibit the organism. Thus, the recommendation generally applies to staphylococcal osteomyelitis. Our present recommendation for chronic staphylococcal osteomyelitis is to establish the precise bacteriologic diagnosis by the culture of bone or pus and then to treat it with a penicillinase-resistant penicillin given intravenously for 4–6 weeks to be followed by an orally administered penicillinase-resistant penicillin for another 2 months. The addition of rifampin to a β-lactam antibiotic may be useful in recurrent or refractory staphylococcal osteomyelitis. Surgical intervention with removal of dead tissue and adequate débridement is an essential part of this therapy.

Because the administration of parenteral antibiotics for 4–6 weeks is expensive and time-consuming, there has been some effort to examine the outcome of treatment with orally administered antibiotics only. The most impressive data come from studies by Bell[31] who has used oral cloxacillin in doses of 5 g plus probenecid in doses of 2 g each day. Patients were treated for a minimum of 6 months and some as long as 1 year. Follow-up study has now continued in approximately 19 patients for 7–9 years with good results, that is, closure of sinuses and absence of clinical recurrences. These results, although highly encouraging, need confirmation before we can confidently recommend this approach. In an era of diagnosis-related groups (DRGs) and shortened hospitalizations, effort have been made to find ways to reduce the period of in-hospital treatment in patients with osteomyelitis. One approach has been to administer long-acting parenteral antimicrobial agents to outpatients; these have resulted in cost savings but paradoxically may increase the expense to patients unless third-party payers show an increased willingness and interest in paying for such programs.[32] Oral antimicrobial therapy with newer agents that may attain effective concentrations is also a promising approach; there needs to be further study with larger numbers of patients to be sure that such approaches are effective.[33]

Perfusion or Irrigation. Because of the difficulty of attaining adequate antibiotic concentrations in avascular necrotic bone, efforts have been made to deliver higher concentrations of antimicrobial agents to the infected area by special means. One such technique is regional perfusion of an extremity, similar to that used in the treatment of neoplasms. There are no controlled data to evaluate the efficacy of this form of treatment, and at present we cannot recommend it.

Another attempt to improve the results of treatment of chronic osteomyelitis involves postoperative irrigation with antibacterial solutions of the surgical wound. Once again, there are no controlled data to support the efficacy of this technique, and there is the potential hazard (often real based on personal experience) that irrigation itself may introduce superinfection with organisms resistant to the antimicrobial agents being used. Antibiotic-impregnated polymethylmethacrylate beads are being used with increased frequency for both the prevention and treatment of bone infections.[34] To date, most of the studies have been with aminoglycoside-impregnated bone cement or beads. There appears to be a paucity of controlled data comparing this approach with standard therapy; further studies are needed before this becomes an accepted method of treatment.

Other Therapeutic Measures. The role of surgery in the treatment of chronic osteomyelitis is an important one. The necessity for removing sequestra and necrotic tissue cannot be overemphasized. There are recent reports that microvascular techniques allowing transplantation of a muscle flap to distant areas have been used successfully in the management of chronic osteomyelitis in infected exposed bone.[35] Optimal management of chronic osteomyelitis is probably best achieved by a combined medical and surgical approach.

COMPLICATIONS

Secondary amyloidosis was once a frequent complication of osteomyelitis of long duration (and other chronic suppurative diseases) but appears to occur infrequently since the advent of antibiotics. The nephrotic syndrome, without secondary amyloidosis, has been reported in association with chronic osteomyelitis; renal biopsy specimens revealed membranoproliferative glomerulonephritis. Neither antibiotic treatment nor therapy with adrenal steroids proved beneficial.

Epidermoid carcinoma may arise in a draining sinus of chronic osteomyelitis with a latent period up to 30 years but frequently a much shorter period. Many of the signs such as pain, increased drainage, and increased bone destruction can occur with either carcinoma or infection alone, and the distinction may be difficult.

PROGNOSIS

The prognosis in acute osteomyelitis is good. The two major variables that affect the outcome are the duration of symptoms before antibiotic therapy is begun (patients generally do well if treated within 3–5 days after the onset of symptoms) and the duration of antibiotic therapy (in adequate dosages) of over 3 weeks. If these two conditions are met, the incidence of recurrent or chronic disease should be extremely low.

Once chronic osteomyelitis supervenes, the prognosis is significantly poorer. In one series, from the Mayo Clinic, of chronic osteomyelitis of hematogenous origin, 55 of 81 patients were treated successfully, 7 were improved, and 19 showed no improvement.[36] In the Massachusetts General Hospital series[37] treatment failure was reported in 13 of 18 cases with "recurrences of hematogenous osteomyelitis." It was also noted that the largest number of failures occurred in patients treated with "limited" antibiotic therapy (less than 4 weeks of parenterally administered antibiotics). Answers to the question "What is optimal therapy for chronic osteomyelitis?" should be forthcoming with further study and may help to improve the prognosis of this disease.

REFERENCES

1. Sugarman B, Hawes S, Musher D, et al. Osteomyelitis beneath pressure sores. Arch Intern Med. 1983;143:683–8.
2. Johnson P, Frederikson J, Sanders J, et al. Management of chronic sternal osteomyelitis. Ann Thorac Surg. 1985;40:69–73.
3. Mackowiak P, Jones S, Smith JW. Diagnostic value of sinus tract cultures in chronic osteomyelitis. JAMA. 1978;239:2772–5.
4. Wheat LJ, Allen SD, Henry M, et al. Diabetic foot infections. Bacteriologic analysis. Arch Intern Med. 1986;146:1935–40.
5. Sapico F, Montgomerie J. Pyogenic vertebral osteomyelitis: Report of nine cases and review of the literature. Rev Infect Dis. 1979;1:754–76.
6. Silverthorn KG, Gillespie WJ. Pyogenic spinal osteomyelitis: A review of 61 cases. NZ Med J. 1986;99:62–5.
7. Meyers B, Berson B, Gilbert M, et al. Clinical patterns of osteomyelitis due to gram-negative bacteria. Arch Intern Med. 1973;131:228–33.
8. Lesse A, Freer C, Salata R, et al. Oral ciprofloxacin therapy for gram-negative bacillary osteomyelitis. Am J Med. 1987;82(Suppl 4A):247–53.
9. Greenberg R, Tice A, Marsh P, et al. Randomized trial of ciprofloxacin compared with other antimicrobial therapy in the treatment of osteomyelitis. Am J Med. 1987;82(Suppl 4A):266–9.
10. Hall B, Fitzgerald R, Rosenblatt J. Anaerobic osteomyelitis. J Bone Joint Surg [Am]. 1983;65:30–5.
11. Raff M, Melo J. Anaerobic osteomyelitis. Medicine (Baltimore). 1978;57:83–103.
12. Gathe J Jr, Harris R, Garland B, et al. *Candida* osteomyelitis. Report of 5 cases and review of the literature. Am J Med. 1987;82:927–37.
13. Engh C, Hughes J, Abrams R, et al: Osteomyelitis in the patient with sickle cell disease. J Bone Joint Surg [Am]. 1971;53:1–15.
14. Chandresekar P, Narula A. Bone and joint infections in intravenous drug abusers. Rev Infect Dis. 1986;8:904–11.
15. Miller W, Murphy W, Gilula L. Brodie abscess: Reappraisal. Radiology 1979;132:15–23.
16. Beighton P, Goldblatt J, Sacks S. Bone involvement in Gaucher disease. In: Desnick RJ, Gatt S, Grabowski GA, eds. Gaucher Disease: A Century of Delineation and Research. New York: Alan R Liss; 1982:107–109.
17. Noyes FR, Smith WS. Bone crises and chronic osteomyelitis in Gaucher's disease. Clin Orthop. 1971;79:132–40.
18. Davidson P, Horowitz I. Skeletal tuberculosis. Am J Med. 1970;48:77–4.
19. Marchevsky A, Damsker B, Green S, et al. The clinicopathological spectrum of non-tuberculous mycobacterial osteoarticular infection. J Bone Joint Surg [Am]. 1985;67:925–9.
20. Azouz E. Computed tomography in bone and joint infections. J Can Assoc Radiol. 1981;32:102–6.
21. Tang J, Gold R, Bassett L, et al. Musculoskeletal infection of the extremities: Evaluation with MR imaging. Radiology 1988;166:205–9.
22. Modic M, Pflanze W, Feiglin D, et al. Magnetic resonance imaging of musculoskeletal infections. Radiol Clin North Am. 1986;24:247–58.
23. Wheat J. Diagnostic strategies in osteomyelitis. Am J Med. 1985;78(Suppl 6B):218–24.
24. Merkel K, Fitzgerald RH Jr, Brown M. Scintigraphic evaluation in musculoskeletal sepsis. Orthop Clin North Am. 1984;15:401–16.
25. Dich V, Nelson J, Haltalin K. Osteomyelitis in infants in children. Am J Dis Child. 1975;129:1273–8.
26. Norden C. Experimental osteomyelitis II. Therapeutic trials and measurement of antibiotic levels in bone. J Infect Dis. 1971;124:565–71.
27. Tetzlaff T, Howard J, McCracken G, et al. Antibiotic concentrations in pus and bone of children with osteomyelitis. J Pediatr. 1978;92:135–40.
28. Norden C. Experimental osteomyelitis IV. Therapeutic trials with rifampin alone and in combination with gentamicin, sisomicin, and cephalothin. J Infect Dis. 1975;132:493–9.
29. Norden C, Bryant R, Palmer D, et al. Chronic osteomyelitis caused by *Staphylococcus aureus*: Controlled clinicial trial of nafcillin therapy and nafcillin-rifampin therapy. South Med J. 1986;79:947–51.
30. Weinstein M, Stratton C, Hawley HB, et al. Multicenter collaborative evaluation of a standardized serum bactericidal test as a predictor of therapeutic efficacy in acute and chronic osteomyelitis. Am J Med. 1987;83:218–22.
31. Bell S. Further observations on the value of oral penicillins in chronic staphylococcal osteomyelitis. Med J Aust. 1976;2:591–3.
32. Eisenberg J, Kitz D. Savings from outpatient antibiotic therapy for osteomyelitis. Economic analysis of a therapeutic strategy. JAMA. 1986;255:1584–8.
33. Black J, Hunt TL, Godley PJ, et al. Oral antimicrobial therapy for adults with osteomyelitis or septic arthritis. J Infect Dis. 1987;155:968–72.
34. Seligson D. Antibiotic-impregnated beads in orthopedic infectious problems. J Ky Med Assoc. 1984;82:25–9.
35. Fitzgerald RH Jr, Ruttle P, Arnold P, et al. Local muscle flaps in the treatment of chronic osteomyelitis. J Bone Joint Surg [Am]. 1985;67:175–85.
36. Kelly P, Wikowski C, Washington J. Comparison of gram-negative bacillary and staphylococcal osteomyelitis of the femur and tibia. Clin Orthop 1973;96:70–5.
37. Waldvogel R, Medoff G, Swartz M. Osteomyelitis: A review of clinical features, therapeutic considerations, and unusual aspects. N Engl J Med. 1970;282:198–206.

SECTION M. DISEASES OF THE REPRODUCTIVE ORGANS AND SEXUALLY TRANSMITTED DISEASES

92. SKIN AND MUCOUS MEMBRANE LESIONS

MICHAEL F. REIN

The skin of the genital area is subject to many of the same diseases that affect other areas of the body. Wilson[1] provides an extensive list of nonvenereal and noninfectious conditions that can involve the genital epithelium alone or as part of the more generalized disease process. Among adults, sexually transmitted diseases are a frequent cause of genital lesions, and a sympathetically obtained sexual history and diligent search for extragenital manifestations of sexually transmitted diseases should be a part of the initial work-up.

HISTORY

Age

Candida albicans and herpes simplex can infect the neonatal genitalia, and herpetic vulvitis occurs occasionally in young children as the initial manifestation of exposure to the virus. Molluscum contagiosum is a common pediatric infection that only occasionally involves the genitalia, probably by autoinfection. Among adults, the sexually transmitted infections are considerably more common, but the presence of sexually transmitted lesions such as herpes genitalis,[2] condylomata accuminata,[3–5] and *exclusively* genital molluscum contagiosum[6] in a child should prompt an evaluation for sexual abuse.

Sexual History

Exposure to multiple partners increases the risk of sexually acquired infection. Orogenital contact can inoculate sexually transmitted pathogens into the oral or pharyngeal mucosa.[7–9] Receptive anal intercourse predisposes to perianal, anal, and rectal infection.[8–11] A history of genital symptoms or recent treatment of a sexual partner may be helpful diagnostically. Specific sexual practices such as particularly vigorous coitus or masturbation[12] or a history of being bitten by a sexual partner should be sought.

Incubation Period

We can occasionally estimate the incubation period for sexually transmitted infection by obtaining a history of a single sexual contact or specific exposure to a new partner. Genital lesions developing within hours of sexual exposure suggest trauma or allergy.[1,12–14] Localized penile edema occurring within hours of vigorous coitus has been reported.[12] The swelling decreased spontaneously, and no specific therapy was required. Incubation periods of less than 24 hours are occasionally noted in chancroid.[15,16] Some patients experience reactivation of herpes genitalis within 12 hours after coitus.[10,17] Somewhat longer incubation periods of 2–5 days are usually seen with chancroid[15,16] and most cases of herpes genitalis.[10,17] Although the mean incubation period for primary genital herpes is about 6 days,[10,17] clinical manifestations may follow infection by as much as 2–3 weeks for both these diseases. An incubation period of 1–3 weeks is usually seen with syphilis,[9] 4–12 weeks with venereal warts,[11] and about 4 weeks for pubic lice[18] and scabies (Chapters 269 and 270). The incubation period for molluscum contagiosum is not well documented and may range from 2 to 26 weeks.[19,20] The incubation periods for donovanosis is poorly defined[15] but in recent series averages around 2 weeks.[21,22] The incubation period for syphilis[9] ranges from 1 to 12 weeks, and for genital warts, it is about 2–3 months.[11]

Residence and Travel

Chancroid and lymphogranuloma venereum are considerably more common in Africa and the Far East than in the United States.[15] Outbreaks of chancroid have occurred recently in the United States,[23] but in general the disease accounts for only about 1 percent of genital ulcers in North America and Europe.[24–27] On the other hand, chancroid was diagnosed in from 40 percent to 90 percent of patients with genital ulcerations in some African and Indian series,[25,28–32] and the relative prevalence of genital herpes infection was correspondingly reduced. Donovanosis is endemic in India, New Guinea, the West Indies, and some parts of Africa and South America, but it is now rare in the United States.[15,21,22,33]

Use of Antibiotics

Antibiotics and other drugs have been reported to cause fixed drug eruptions that occasionally involve the genitalia.[1,34,35] The tetracyclines, commonly used in the treatment of genital infections, are incriminated with particular frequency.[35] Antibiotics may predispose to the development of candidiasis and may alter or completely eliminate the lesions of syphilis.[36]

Underlying Diseases

Immunodeficiency states predispose to a variety of genital lesions. Balanitis due to *Candida* occurs in neutropenic patients,[37] and balanitis caused by gram-negative bacteria[38] is seen in patients wearing condom catheters. The acquired immunodeficiency syndrome (AIDS) is associated with chronic necrotizing and recurrent genital[39] and perianal[40] herpes simplex virus (HSV) infections.

Mode of Onset and Course

Because lesions often change over time, a history of the initial manifestation may be crucial to making the diagnosis. Thus, the patient with genital ulcerations who can state with surety that the lesions began as vesicles has helped to make a diagnosis of herpes genitalis. Vesicles often rupture quickly so that this stage of the lesions goes unnoticed by women.[17] A prodrome of local paresthesia preceding the appearance of lesions is reported by 50–90 percent of patients with recurrent genital herpes.[8,17,41] Venereal warts and molluscum contagiosum may remain relatively static for long periods of time after their initial appearance. The lesions of syphilis often last for many weeks and then heal without antibiotic intervention.[9] Pearly penile papules are a completely benign condition appearing in single or multiple rows around the penile corona at puberty.[42]

A recurrence of the lesions at intervals strongly suggests genital herpes. The rate of recurrence varies strikingly among individuals, but the average rate of recurrence among patients genitally infected with HSV type 2 is 0.33 per month, whereas genital infections with HSV type 1 recur at an average rate of but 0.02 per month.[43] Indeed, whereas 90 percent of patients with type 2 genital infections report a recurrence within a year, recurrences are experienced by only 25 percent of the patients genitally infected with HSV type 1.

Pain

Although the syphilitic chancre is usually described as nontender, up to 30 percent of the patients with primary syphilis describe either pain or tenderness of the lesions.[36] The relative indolence of the lesions of donovanosis[15,33,44] sometimes results in long delays before the patient seeks medical attention. Pain usually accompanies the lesions of chancroid,[15,45] herpes genitalis,[8,17] tularemia,[46,47] and amebiasis.[48–50]

Pruritis

Itching is associated with herpes genitalis and is described by 50–90 percent of patients with recurrent disease,[8,17,41] particularly in the prodromal period. Pruritus accompanies 90 percent of infestations with pubic lice,[18] and severe itching increased by warming the skin, either in bed or when taking a bath, suggests scabies. Although *severe* pruritis is uncommon in secondary syphilis,[9] 42 percent of patients describe at least mild itching.[51] Itching also characterizes candidal balanitis, which is observed occasionally in male sexual partners of women with vulvovaginal candidiasis.[52,53]

Vaginal Discharge

Many infectious vaginitides are associated with vulvar lesions. The vulvovaginitis syndrome is discussed in Chapter 95.

Fever

Fever is described in 5–8 percent of the patients with secondary syphilis[9,51] and in many patients with disseminated gonococcal infection.[54,55] Fever accompanies primary herpes genitalis in 70 percent of women and 40 percent of men but is uncommon in recurrent disease.[8,17,41]

Other

Sacral root neurologic symptoms suggest herpes,[8,17] and a urethral discharge suggests gonorrhea or, rarely, Reiter syndrome (Chapter 95).

MORPHOLOGIC CHARACTERISTICS OF GENITAL LESIONS

Careful examination of the entire genital area is essential and will be facilitated by a good light source and a hand lens. A differential diagnosis can often be made on the basis of the morphologic characteristics of genital lesions, but variations from the typical morphologic features and clinical overlap among the various diseases are unfortunately common.[36,56,57] A clinical differential diagnosis of genital ulcers is perhaps the most difficult[30,56,58] with the most common error involving the overdiagnosis of chancroid.[26] Nonetheless, the morphologic characteristics of genital lesions often supply the first and most important clue to their cause. Table 1 provides a morphologic classification of genital lesions but can serve only as a rough guide.

TABLE 1. Morphologic Classification of Genital Lesions

Ulcers	Vesicles
Herpes genitalis	Herpes genitalis
Syphilis	Crusts
Trauma	Scabies
Chancroid	Herpes genitalis
Lymphogranuloma venereum	Miscellaneous lesions
Tularemia	Nits: crabs
Behçet's syndrome	Hypertrophic: donovanosis
Malignancy	Diffuse inflammation: drug reaction, candidiasis, trauma
Histoplasmosis	Linear tracks: scabies
Donovanosis (granuloma inguinale)	Reddish flecks: crab excreta
Candidiasis	Maculae caeruleae (sky blue spots): crabs
Mycobacterioses	Crepitus: anaerobes[62]
Amebiasis	
Fixed drug eruption	
Gonorrhea[29]	
Trichomoniasis[27]	
Papules	
Venereal warts	
Scabies	
Molluscum contagiosum	
Syphilis	
Pearly penile papules	
Candidiasis	

Genital Ulcers

As noted earlier, the causes of genital ulcers vary markedly in different parts of the world.[24,25,28–32] Because of the relative rarity of chancroid in the United States and its similarities to herpes simplex genital infection, we should regard a clinical diagnosis of chancroid with some suspicion.[56] Rare causes of destructive penile ulcerations include tuberculosis[59–62] and amebiasis.[48–50]

Number. The classic chancre of primary syphilis is a single lesion[9] (Figs. 1 and 2); however, in some series, almost half of the patients with proven primary syphilis had more than one

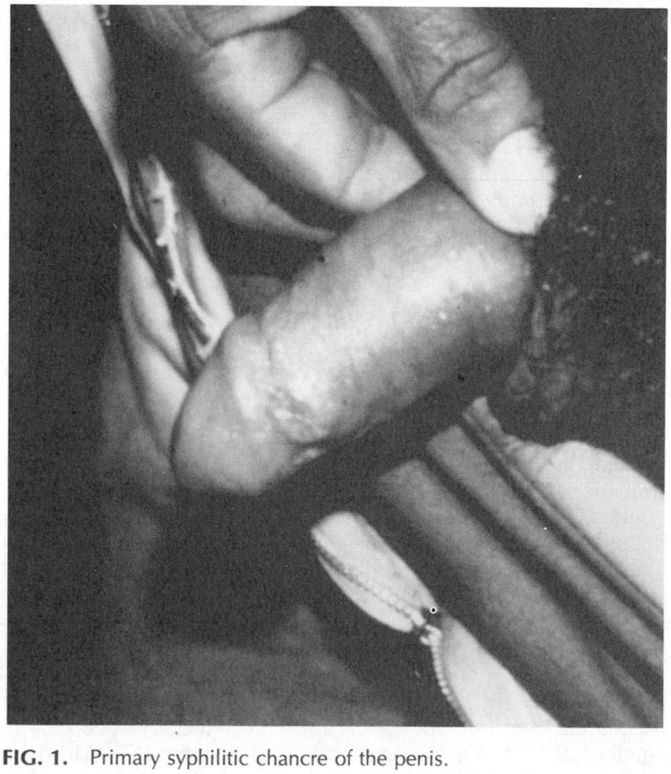

FIG. 1. Primary syphilitic chancre of the penis.

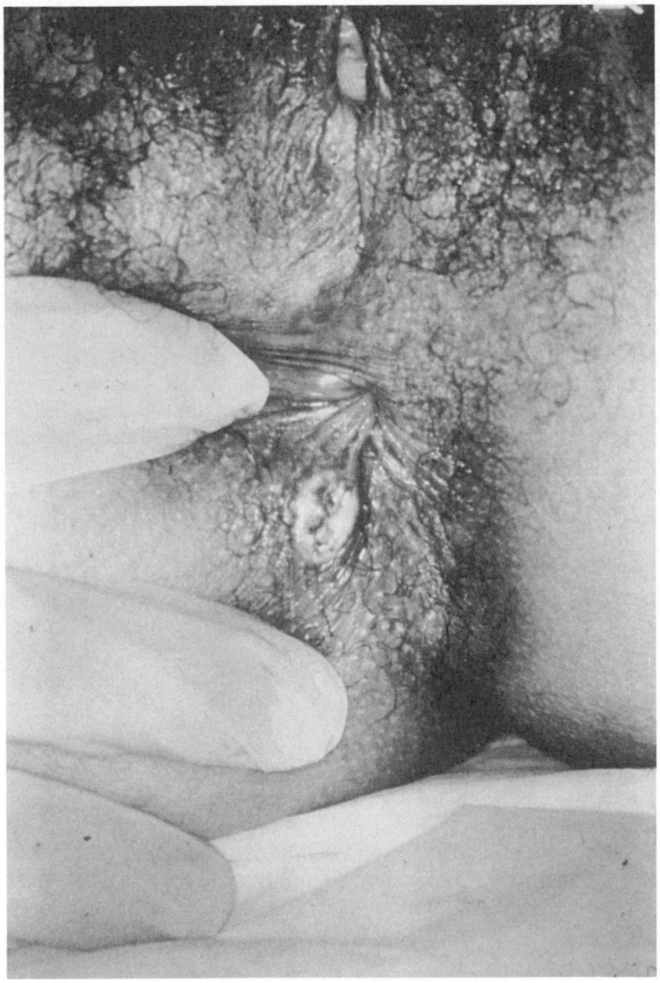

FIG. 2. Primary syphilitic chancre of the perineum.

penile ulcer.[27,36] Chancroid is usually said to be present as multiple ulcerations, yet in some series 40–70 percent of the affected men had but a single lesion.[45,63] The genital lesion of tick-borne tularemia is single.[46] Herpes genitalis characteristically produces multiple ulcerations in groups surrounded by an erythematous border (Fig. 3).[8,17,41] The vagina per se is involved in only 4 percent of cases.[8,17,36] Although the multiple lesions of syphilis and herpes are generally of uniform size, the lesions of chancroid may vary in an individual patient.[15] A rare cause of recurrent, multiple, genital ulcerations in the United States is Behçet syndrome,[64] an inflammatory disease of unknown cause that usually also involves the oral, conjunctival, and synovial membranes. Behçet's ulcers involve the scrotum and vulva more frequently than they do the penis, anus, and vagina, and scars from previous episodes may be present.[64] Ulcers are rarely observed in vulvovaginal or penile[24] candidiasis. Intravaginal ulcers may follow tampon use,[65] but infectious and neoplastic causes must be ruled out in these cases.

Tenderness. Tenderness on palpation may be extreme with herpes genitalis,[8,17] and chancroid[15,45] is present in 30 percent of syphilitic chancres[36] and characterizes tularemia.[46] Even massive ulcerated lesions of donovanosis are nontender.[15,33]

Ulcer Base. The lesions of chancroid are usually ragged and have a necrotic base.[15,30,45] On the other hand, syphilitic and herpetic ulcers are relatively clean (Figs. 1–3). The ulcers of Behçet syndrome often have a yellow, necrotic base.[64] Donovanosis produces ulcers with granulation tissue at the base yielding a beefy red lesion that often becomes exuberantly hypertrophic and produces large, friable, ulcerated masses projecting above the skin.[15,33]

Ulcer Edge. The ulcers of chancroid are characteristically undermined, but the edge is not indurated.[15,16,45,30,66] An indurated lesion is highly suggestive of syphilis[9,27] (and some rare conditions[60]), and occurs in 92 percent of the infected patients.[36] An erythematous border is seen both with herpes[8,17] and with chancroid.[15,45] The border of the lesion in donovanosis is often a stark white, which is characteristic of no other genital infection.[44] Lesions of donovanosis also often manifest a thickening of the edge that yields a rolled appearance.[33]

Serpiginous lesions, progressing in one area as they heal in another, are characteristic of donovanosis[15,33] and less so of chancroid.[15]

Genital Papules

Careful examination of the papules with the aid of a hand lens often yields an immediate etiologic diagnosis. Papules may be the transient, initial state of a variety of genital infections including syphilis.[36] scabies,[67] lymphogranuloma venereum,[68] chancroid,[15] and herpes.[8,17] Early condylomata accuminata usually appear as simple papules and can be identified when the hand lens reveals the beginning of a verrucous cap or tiny blood vessels at the base.

Pearly penile papules are normal and occur in 8–25 percent of men.[42] They are found more commonly in uncircumcised men

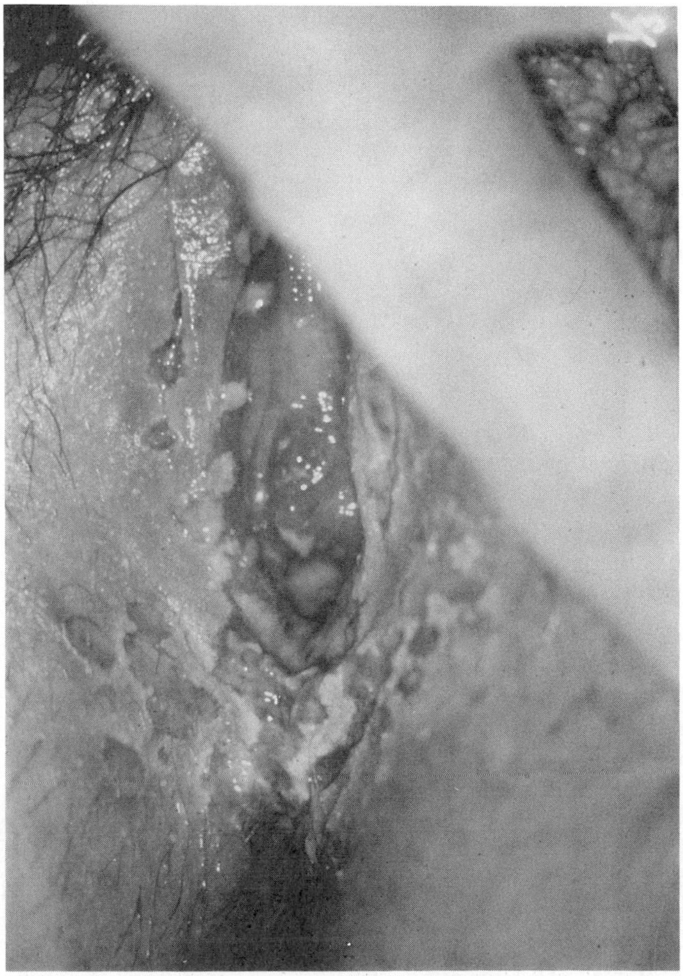

FIG. 3. Herpes (HSV-II) of the vulva.

and present as one or more rows of grayish white or pink papules along the corona or in the coronal sulcus. They usually appear at puberty and are of no pathologic significance. Patients concerned about venereal disease will occasionally notice the lesions and will seek medical attention. Although the histologic appearance is characteristic, biopsy is rarely warranted because the diagnosis can be made clinically.

Umbilication. The hand lens will reveal tiny umbilications at the vertex of the lesions of molluscum contagiosum[19,20] (Fig. 4, Chapter 116). The umbilications often appear to contain keratin plugs. These 1 to 5 mm papules occur singly or in small clusters on the penile shaft, glans, labia majora, thighs, and buttocks. In children, the disease is nonvenereally acquired and usually affects the trunk and extremities. The lesions are nonpruritic and may coalesce to form larger masses.[19,20] Squeezing expresses caseous material from the umbilication. Curettage easily removes the entire lesion and leaves a shallow, slightly hemorrhagic ulceration that heals without scarring. If the diagnosis is in doubt, a papule may be removed by curetting and crushed between two microscope slides. Wright or Giemsa stains reveal cells distended by intracytoplasmic inclusions (Chapter 116).

Verrucous papules suggest a diagnosis of condylomata accuminata (venereal warts). The lesions are usually multiple and may show a satelliting phenomenon wherein a larger wart is surrounded by smaller lesions. Stalked or sessile, the warts can be found anywhere on the external genitalia and in the vagina or on the cervix. Perianal warts in women may occur as a result of the spread from a genital focus. Perianal condylomas in men are associated with receptive anal intercourse,[10,11,69] and such men should be evaluated for intra-anal warts[19] and other anorectal infections as well.[70] In moist areas warts may become relatively elongated. The major source of diagnostic difficulty is differentiating these from the moist lesions of secondary syphilis, condylomata lata. The syphilitic lesions tend to be flatter and often have a more grayish appearance.[9] A differential diagnosis is best made by carefully abrading the lesions and performing a darkfield examination, for condylomata lata are teeming with spirochetes. Unfortunately, anaerobic spirochetes occasionally superinfect condylomata accuminata and may give an initial appearance of darkfield positivity. Venereal warts, particularly flat warts of the cervix, are strongly associated with cervical intraepithelial neoplasia and cancer[71] (Chapter 123), and culposcopy or biopsy may be indicated for suspicious lesions.

Although acetic acid applications have long been used to identify subclinical papillomavirus infections of the cervix and vagina, the technique has recently been employed to detect otherwise invisible lesions in men.[72–76] Acetic acid, 3–5%, is applied to the penis for 3–5 minutes, and the skin is examined with the colposcope. Flat, white lesions are revealed in 40–80 percent of the male partners of women with warts, and 60–80 percent of such lesions are identified as human papillomavirus infection by biopsy.[72–76] The accuracy of histologic diagnosis and the significance of "acetowhite" lesions are, at the present time, somewhat controversial.

Candidal balanitis occurs in up to 10 percent of the men who are the sexual partners of women with candidal vulvovaginitis[52,53] and is usually manifestated as an intensely pruritic papular lesion of the glans, foreskin, or shaft of the penis. The raised erythematous area may be surrounded by small, discrete papules, or satellite lesions, which are helpful diagnostically. Similar papular or papulopustular lesions accompany candidal infection of the groin, scrotum, and vulva.

Crusted Lesions. Herpetic ulcers heal by crusting over. Crusts are also characteristic of scabies (see Chapter 270, Fig. 2) and may be accompanied by moist papules[37] and burrows. These threadlike lesions, often stippled, may be 1–10 mm long and are specific for scabies. They may be dramatically demonstrated by covering a papule with ink (as from a fountain pen) and then wiping it off, with an alcohol swab. In about two-thirds of cases, the burrow, now filled with ink, is readily visualized.[77]

Diffuse Erythematous Lesions

Superficial infection with tinea or *Candida* may cause diffusely erythematous, intensely pruritic lesions of the genitalia and

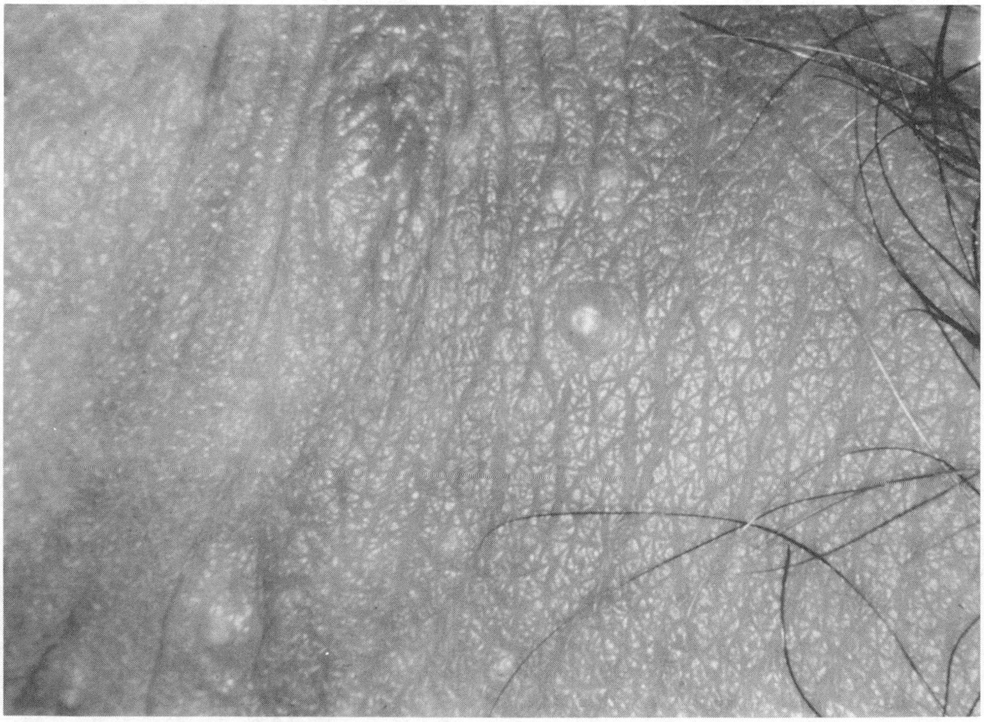

Fig. 4. Molluscum contagiosum: penile lesions displaying characteristic keratin-plugged umbilications.

groin area. Candidal lesions are often more intensely erythematous, whereas lesions caused by tinea are usually somewhat brown and may show central clearing. Involvement of the scrotum or the appearance of small papules or pustules beyond the main border of the lesion suggests candidal infection.

Group B streptococci have caused balanitis.[78] *Gardnerella vaginalis* is also felt to cause some cases of balanitis in uncircumcized men[79] in whom it is associated with the same fishy odor that characterizes bacterial vaginosis. Likewise, the condition responds to metronidazole.

Pubic Hair

Crab lice are usually manifested in very small numbers, an average infestation consisting of fewer than 10.[80] The lice are, however, observed in 97 percent of infested patients who have not treated themselves before seeking medical attention.[18] Examination of the pubic hair with a hand lens reveals them as gray-brown creatures climbing along the shafts or partially buried at the bases. They are found in perianal hair in about 50 percent of patients and in abdominal hair in about 17 percent of patients.[18] If the organisms themselves are not observed, the diagnosis can be made in 80 percent of patients by recognizing the eggs or nits, 0.5 mm ovoids adherent to the hair shafts, and a careful examination may reveal tiny reddish spots of louse excreta at the base of the hair in about 15 percent of patients.[18] Crab bites sometimes result in round to oval, 0.5–1.5 mm, bluish red macules called maculae caeruleae or sky blue spots.[18,81]

EXTRAGENITAL DERMATOLOGIC MANIFESTATIONS OF SEXUALLY TRANSMITTED DISEASES

Patients should be questioned about orogenital and receptive anal practices since these may result in direct inoculation of sexually transmitted pathogens into extragenital sites. Additionally, sexually transmitted infections may disseminate and result in secondary extragenital manifestations.

Mouth

Direct inoculation of sexually transmitted viruses can result in oral lesions. Intraoral condylomata accuminata are reported,[7] and lesions resemble those of the genital mucous membranes. Herpes simplex has been transmitted from the genital tract to the mouth and vice versa.[8,17,43] Genital lesions produced by HSV type 1 are indistinguishable from those produced by type 2. Likewise, oral inoculation can result in fever blisters, a primary gingivostomatitis, or a herpangina-like picture,[8,17,82] with clusters of vesicles and ulcers on the hard palate.

Although the oral mucosa is generally resistant to gonococcal infection, occasional cases of gonococcal stomatitis, presumably resulting from the direct inoculation, have been reported.[83] Chancres of the lip, buccal mucous membranes, gingiva, and tonsils are becoming relatively more common. They are usually painless and may be difficult to diagnose because normal oral spirochetes confound the darkfield examination.[9] Disseminated infections may also affect the mouth. Mucous patches occur in about 20 percent of patients with secondary syphilis[9,51] and appear on the oral mucous membranes and the tongue as painless, relatively clean, shallow ulcerations, often with a yellow or gray base and a small amount of surrounding erythema.[9] Palatal petechiae may accompany gonococcal bacteremia. Recurrent oral and genital ulcers suggest Behçet syndrome.[64]

Anorectum

A similar spectrum of diseases affects the rectal mucosa.[70] Perianal warts[10,11,69] and herpetic lesions[40,84] are seen in homosexual men who practice receptive anal intercourse. Both types of lesions can involve women in the same manner, but in women they may also have extended to the anus from a primary genital focus. Among patients with AIDS, herpetic proctitis may be chronic and relentlessly destructive.[40] Destructive perianal lesions occasionally result from amebiasis in endemic areas.[85]

Other Skin

The generalized rash of secondary syphilis frequently involves the genitalia. In fact, a generalized eruption sparing the genital area and the oral mucous membranes is unlikely to be syphilis.[9] The rash is highly variable, and the differential diagnosis is challenging.[51,57] One should consider secondary syphilis in the differential diagnosis of any generalized, relatively indolent eruption, particularly if the palms and soles are involved, if there is accompanying generalized lymphadenopathy (70–86 percent), or if there is a patchy hair loss.[9,51] The lesions are usually macular, maculopapular (70 percent), or papulosquamous[9,51] and symmetrically distributed. Markedly pruritic or vesicular lesions in an adult are unlikely to be syphilis.

About 33–50 percent of the patients with disseminated gonococcal infections will have small numbers of skin lesions, usually found on the distal portions of the extremities and occasionally involving the palms and the soles. The lesions are relatively pleomorphic and may be macular, maculopapular, petechial, vesicular, pustular, or necrotic.[55] The typical lesion is an erythematous or hemorrhagic spot 2–5 mm in diameter that is surmounted by a gray pustule, sometimes displaying a small eschar in its center.[54] The lesions of subacute meningococcemia may be similar and represent an important differential diagnosis.

The interdigital webs, wrists, and ankles are often involved with scabies.[86] Secondary papular lesions, thought to occur as a hypersensitivity phenomenon, may occur on the abdomen or the pelvic girdle area. Burrows, described above, are pathognomonic of scabies.[77] Maculae caerulae (see above) often occur on the anterior and lateral portions of the abdomen and thorax.[81]

Patients with AIDS may demonstrate a variety of skin lesions, including Kaposi sarcoma, at some distance from sexual orifices (Chapter 108).

Herpes genitalis involves the thigh or buttock in some 15 percent of infected women.[87,88]

LABORATORY EXAMINATIONS

Sufficiently accurate etiologic diagnoses can often be made on the basis of clinical examination when the lesions are typical. In many situations, particularly in the etiologic diagnosis of genital ulcers, laboratory examination is required.

Direct Microscopic Examinations

Any ulcerated genital lesion or hypertrophic lesion in a moist area may be examined by darkfield microscopy. Gloves must be worn. The lesion is cleaned with a dry gauze pad and is then abraded with gauze until some blood is seen. The blood is blotted until bleeding ceases, and a small amount of serous fluid is expressed by squeezing the edges of the lesion. A drop of this material may be picked up directly on a glass coverslip, which is then inverted on a microscope slide and is examined for characteristic motile spirochetes with darkfield illumination.

The diagnosis of chancroid is sometimes confirmed by cleaning the lesion with gauze and swabbing material from the undermined edge. Gram staining of this material sometimes reveals chains of streptobacilli suggestive of *Haemophilus ducreyi*,[45] but the smear technique has a low sensitivity and specificity, and is not useful in a clinical setting.[29,32,63,89]

A smear of material from the base of a freshly ruptured vesicle may be stained with Wright or Giemsa stains and examined for multinucleated giant cells that are diagnostic of herpes infection.[8,17] This Tzanck test is not generally helpful, however, because the presence of vesicles is essentially diagnostic of herpetic infection and the test is insensitive on genital ulcers, being positive in fewer than 40 percent of culture-proven cases.[90] Several recent developments appear likely to improve rapid diagnostic capabilities. Monoclonal antibodies will detect herpes viral antigens in material from 75 percent of herpetic lesions by direct examination with fluorescence microscopy,[91,92] and the technique also differentiates type 1 virus from type 2. DNA hybridization with radiolabeled probes has identified HSV in 80 percent of lesions.[93,94]

Bits of tissue from a hypertrophic lesion may be crushed between microscope slides, treated with Wright or Giemsa stains and examined for the characteristic intracytoplasmic bacterial inclusions of donovanosis.[15,21,22,33]

Papular lesions may be scraped, crushed, stained with a variety of agents, and examined for the balloonlike cells of molluscum contagiosum.[20] Heating such scrapings with 10% potassium hydroxide will destroy the squamous elements and may reveal tinea, *Candida*, or the mite or larvae of scabies.[67] Mixing scrapings with mineral oil rather than potassium hydroxide may have an advantage in the diagnosis of scabies, for unlike potassium hydroxide, mineral oil preserves mite fecal pellets and motility.[94a]

Scrapings or aspirations of the peripheral lesions of disseminated gonococcal infection reveal the organisms only infrequently by Gram stain but may be subjected to immunofluorescent microscopy, which will be diagnostic in about half the cases.[55,95]

Serologic Tests

Serologic tests are occasionally misleading in the diagnosis of syphilis. From 20 to 30 percent of the patients with a chancre, particularly if the lesion has just appeared, will have nonreactive nontreponemal tests for syphilis.[96–98] About 10–17 percent of the patients may have a reactive fluorescent treponemal antibody absorption (FTA-ABS) test even if the nontreponemal tests (e.g., Venereal Disease Research Laboratory [VDRL], rapid plasma reagin [RPR], automated reagin test [ART]) (see Chapter 213) are nonreactive.[96–98] The clinician may therefore wish to obtain an FTA-ABS test on patients with suspicious genital lesions, even if the nontreponemal test result is negative. In many areas, the microhemagglutination test for *Treponema pallidum* antibodies (MHA-TP) has replaced the more demanding FTA-ABS as the confirmatory treponemal test. The tests are not entirely equivalent since the MHA-TP is only about 89 percent sensitive in primary syphilis and will therefore miss about 10 percent of cases that would be detected by the FTA-ABS.[98] The vast majority of patients will have positive nontreponemal test findings within the week after the appearance of the chancre, and repeated serologic testing and darkfield examination may be necessary to make the diagnosis.

The sensitivity of nontreponemal and treponemal tests is almost 100 percent in secondary syphilis. Thus, a negative serologic examination essentially rules out this diagnosis.[96,98]

Serologic testing has almost no current role in the routine clinical diagnosis of genital HSV infection[17,94,99] because of cross-reactions resulting from highly prevalent herpes simplex type 1 infections. Serologic tests for chancroid and donovanosis are not available.

Culture

Tissue culture for herpes simplex is the most sensitive way to diagnose this infection. It is 70 percent sensitive in lesions that have ruptured and formed ulcers even in initial infections when cytologic findings are negative. Once the lesions have crusted over, however, sensitivity of the culture is reduced to about 30 percent.[100] The sensitivity is lower in recurrent disease, dropping to 30 percent in ulcers and to less than 20 percent in crusted lesions.[92]

The edge of a clean lesion may be cultured for *H. ducreyi*.[103] The medium employed dramatically affects sensitivity,[103] which is, even under the best circumstances, probably no higher than 80 percent.[30,31,63,103] Material from the lesion suspected of being molluscum contagiosum may be inoculated into tissue culture, and a cytopathic effect may be observed (Chapter 115). Culture for the agent of donovanosis is unreliable and not generally available.[33]

INITIAL APPROACH TO THERAPY

So diverse are the causes of the lesions in the genital area that initial therapy must be based on highly presumptive or definitive etiologic diagnosis. In most cases, it is possible to delay therapy until such a diagnosis has been reached. When dealing with multiple infections, it is important to avoid the situation in which treatment for one infection interferes with the diagnosis of another. Thus, if one is treating gonorrhea in the presence of a suspicious genital lesion, spectinomycin may be the treatment of choice because it does not interfere with the subsequent darkfield or serologic diagnosis of syphilis.

REFERENCES

1. Wilson JF. The nonvenereal diseases of the genitals: Their differentiation from venereal lesions. Med Clin North Am. 1964;48:787.
2. Hibbard RA. Herpetic vulvovaginitis and child abuse. Am J Dis Child. 1985;139:542–5.
3. Schachner L, Hankin DE. Assessing child abuse in childhood condyloma accuminatum. J Am Acad Dermatol. 1985;12:157–60.
4. Shelton TB, Jerkins GR, Noe HN. Condylomata accuminata in the pediatric patient. J Urol. 1986;135:548–9.
5. Bender ME. New concepts of condyloma accuminata in children. Arch Dermatol. 1986;122:1121–4.
6. Bargman H, Schachner L, Hankin D. Is genital molluscum contagiosum a cutaneous manifestation of sexual abuse in children? J Am Acad Dermatol. 1986;14:847–9.
7. Choukass NC, Toto PD. Condyloma accuminatum of the oral cavity. Oral Surg. 1982;54:480.
8. Corey L, Adams HG, Brown ZA, et al. Genital herpes simplex infection: Clinical manifestations, course, and complications. Ann Intern Med. 1983;98:958.
9. Stokes JH, Beerman H, Ingraham NR. Modern Clinical Syphilology. 3rd ed. Philadelphia: WB Saunders; 1944.
10. Carr G, William DC. Anal warts in a population of gay men in New York City. Sex Transm Dis. 1977;4:56.
11. Oriel JD. Genital warts. Sex Transm Dis. 1981;8:326.
12. Wilde H, Canby JP. Penile venereal edema. Arch Dermatol. 1973;108:263.
13. Fried FA. Glans penis dermatitis after treatment of wife's vaginitis. JAMA. 1981;245:2532.
14. Gochfeld M, Burger J. Sexual transmission of nickel and poison oak contact dermatitis. Lancet. 1983;1:589.
15. Hart G. Chancroid, Donovanosis, Lymphogranuloma Venereum. DHEW publication (CDC) 75-8302. 1975.
16. Fiumara NJ. A guide to lesions of the penis. Hosp Med. March: 1970.
17. Pazin GJ. Management of oral and genital herpes simplex virus infections: Diagnosis and treatment. DM 1986;32:725–824.
18. Chapel TA, Katta T, Kuszmar T, et al. Pediculosis pubis in a clinic for sexually transmitted diseases. Sex Transm Dis. 1979;6:257.
19. Margolis S. Genital warts and molluscum contagiosum. Urol Clin North Am. 1984;11:163–70.
20. Brown ST, Nalley JF, Kraus SJ. Molluscum contagiosum. Sex Transm Dis. 1981;8:227.
21. Sehgal VN, Shyam Prasad AL. Donovanosis: Current concepts. Int J Dermatol. 1986;25:8–16.
22. Rosen T, Tschen JA, Ramsdell W, et al. Granuloma inguinale. J Am Acad Dermatol. 1984;433–7.
23. Blackmore CA, Limpakarnjanarat K, Rigau-Perez JG, et al. An outbreak of chancroid in Orange County, California: Descriptive epidemiology and disease control measures. J Infect Dis. 1985;151:840–4.
24. Chapel T, Brown WJ, Jeffries C, et al. The microbiological flora of penile ulcerations. J Infect Dis. 1978;137:50.
25. Meheus A, Van Dyck E, Ursi JP, et al. Etiology of genital ulcerations in Swaziland. Sex Transm Dis. 1983;10:33.
26. Sturm AW, Stolting GJ, Cormane RH, et al. Clinical and microbiological evaluation of 46 episodes of genital ulceration. Genitourin Med. 1987;63:98–101.
27. Diaz-Mitoma F, Benningen G, Slutchuk M, et al. Etiology of nonvesicular genital ulcers in Winnipeg. Sex Transm Dis. 1987;14:33–6.

28. Nsanze H, Fast MV, D'Costa LJ. Genital ulcers in Kenya: Clinical and laboratory study. Br J Vener Dis. 1981;57:378.
29. Cooradia YM, Kharsany A, Hoosen A. The microbial aetiology of genital ulcers in black men in Durban, South Africa. Genitourin Med. 1985;61:266–9.
30. Plummer FA, D'Costa LJ, Nsanze H, et al. Clinical and microbiologic studies of genital ulcers in Kenyan women. Sex Transm Dis. 1985;12:193–7.
31. Fast MV, D'Costa LJ, Nsanze H, et al. The clinical diagnosis of genital ulcer disease in men in the tropics. Sex Transm Dis. 1984;11:72–6.
32. Sehgal VN, Prasad ALS. Chancroid or chancroidal ulcers. Dermatologica. 1985;170:136–41.
33. Kuberski T. Granuloma inguinale (donovanosis). Sex Transm Dis. 1980;7:29.
34. Talbot MD. Fixed genital drug eruption. Practitioner. 1980;224:823.
35. Dodds PR, Chi T-N. Balanitis as a fixed drug eruption to tetracycline. J Urol. 1981;133:1044–5.
36. Chapel TA. The variability of syphilitic chancres. Sex Transm Dis. 1978; 5:68.
37. Morrissey R, Xavier A, Nguyen N, et al. Invasive candidal balanitis due to a condom catheter in a neutropenic patient. South Med J. 1985;78:1247–9.
38. Manian FA, Alford RH. Nosocomial infectious balanoposthitis in neutropenic patients. South Med J. 1987;80:909–11.
39. Maier JA, Bergman A, Ross MG. Acquired immunodeficiency syndrome manifested by chronic primary genital herpes. Am J Obstet Gynecol. 1986;155:756–8.
40. Siegal FP, Lopez C, Hammer GS, et al. Severe acquired immunodeficiency in male homosexuals manifested by chronic perianal herpes simplex lesions. N Engl J Med. 1981;305:1439–44.
41. Guinan ME, MacCalman J, Kern ER, et al. The course of untreated recurrent genital herpes simplex infection in 27 women. N Engl J Med. 1981;304:759.
42. Rehbein HM. Pearly penile papules: Incidence. Cutis. 1977;19:54.
43. Lafferty WE, Coombs RW, Benedetti J, et al. Recurrences after oral and genital herpes simplex virus infection. Influence of site of infection and viral type. N Engl J Med. 1987;316:1444–9.
44. D'Aunoy R, Von Hamm E. Granuloma inguinale. Am J Trop Med. 1937;17:747.
45. Asin J. Chancroid: A report of 1402 cases. Am J Syph Gonorr Vener Dis. 1952;36:483.
46. Dienst FT. Tularemia: A perusal of 339 cases. J La State Med Soc. 1963;115:114.
47. Evans ME, Gregory DW, Schaffner W, et al. Tularemia: A 30 year experience with 88 cases. Medicine (Baltimore). 1985;64:251–69.
48. Parkash S, Ramakrishnan K, Ananthakrishnan N, et al. Amoebic ulcer of the penis. Postgrad Med J. 1982;58:375.
49. Veliath AJ, Bansal R, Sankaran V, et al. Genital amebiasis. Int J Gynaecol Obstet. 1987;25:249–56.
50. O'Leary RK, Posen J. Amoebiasis of the penis. S Afr Med J. 1984;65:113–6.
51. Chapel TA. The signs and symptoms of secondary syphilis. Sex Transm Dis. 1980;7:161.
52. Oriel JD, Partridge BM, Denny MJ, et al. Genital yeast infections. Br Med J. 1972;4:761.
53. Diddle AW. Oral contraceptive medication and vulvovaginal candidiasis. Obstet Gynecol. 1969;34:373.
54. Holmes KK, Counts GW, Beaty HN. Disseminated gonococcal infection. Ann Intern Med. 1971;74:979.
55. Masi AT, Eisenstein BI. Disseminated gonococcal infection (DGI) and gonococcal arthritis (GCA): II. Clinical manifestations, diagnosis, complications, treatment, and prevention. Semin Arthritis Rheum. 1981;10:173.
56. Chapel TA, Brown WJ, Jeffries C, et al. How reliable is the morphologic diagnosis of penile ulcerations? Sex Transm Dis. 1977;4:150.
57. Chapel TA. Physician recognition of the signs and symptoms of secondary syphilis. JAMA. 1981;246:250.
58. Verdich J. *Hemophilus ducreyi* infection resembling granuloma inguinale. Acta Derm Venereol (Stokh). 1984;64:452–5.
59. Vekataramaiah NR, van Raalte JA, Dutta SN. Tuberculous ulcer of the penis. Postgrad Med J. 1982;58:59.
60. Nishigori C, Taniguchi S, Hayakawa M, et al. Penis tuberculosis: Papulonecrotic tuberculosis on the glans penis. Dermatologica. 1986;172:93–7.
61. Kumar B, Skarma VK. Papulonecrotic tuberculids on glans penis. Dermatologica. 1987;174:151–3.
62. Carroll PR, Cattolica EV, Turzan CW, et al. Necrotizing soft-tissue infections of the perineum and genitalia. Etiology and early reconstruction. West J Med. 1986;144:174–8.
63. D'Costa LJ, Bowmer I, Nsanze H, et al. Advances in the diagnosis and management of chancroid. Sex Transm Dis. 1986;13:189–91.
64. Shimizu T, Ehrlich GE, Inaba G, et al. Behçet disease (Behçet syndrome). Semin Arthritis Rheum. 1979;8:223.
65. Weissberg SM, Dodson MG. Recurrent vaginal and cervical ulcers associated with tampon use. JAMA. 1983;250:1430.
66. Kraus SJ. Evaluation and management of acute genital ulcers in sexually active patients. Urol Clin North Am. 1984;11:155–62.
67. Shelley WB, Wood MG. Larval papule as a sign of scabies. JAMA. 1976;236:1144.
68. Schachter J, Dawson CR, Human Chlamydial Infection. Littleton, MA: PSG Publishing; 1978:45.
69. Oriel JD. Genital warts. Sex Transm Dis. 1977;4:153.
70. Quinn TC, Stamm WE, Goodell SE, et al. The polymicrobial origin of intestinal infections in homosexual men. N Engl J Med. 1983;309:576.
71. Campion MJ, Singer A, Clarkson PK, et al. Increased risk of cervical neoplasia in consorts of men with penile condylomata accuminata. Lancet. 1985;1:943–6.
72. Rosemberg SK. Subclinical papilloma viral infection of male genitalia. Urology. 1985;26:554–7.
73. Sand PK, Baven LW, Blischke PA, et al. Evaluation of male consorts of women with genital human papilloma virus infection. Obstet Gynecol. 1986;68:679–81.
74. Schultz RE, Skelton HG. Value of acetic acid screening for flat genital condylomata in men. J Urol. 1988;139:777–9.
75. Sedlack TV, Cunnane M, Carpiniello V. Colposcopy in the diagnosis of penile condyloma. Am J Obstet Gynecol. 1986;154:494–6.
76. Krebs H-B, Schneider V. Human papillomavirus-associated lesions of the penis: Colposcopy, cytology, and histology. Obstet Gynecol. 1987;70:299–304.
77. Woodley D, Saurat JH. The burrow ink test and the scabies mite. J Am Acad Dermatol. 1981;4:715.
78. Lucks DA, Venezio FR, Lakin CM. Balanitis caused by group B streptococcus. J Urol. 1986;135:1015.
79. Burdge DR, Bowie WR, Chow A. *Gardnerella vaginalis*-associated balanoposthitis. Sex Transm Dis. 1986;13:159–62.
80. Ackerman A. Crabs: The resurgence of *Phthirus pubis*. N Engl J Med. 1968;278:950.
81. Miller RA. Maculae ceruleae. Int J Dermatol. 1986;25:383–4.
82. Chang TW. Herpetic angina following orogenital exposure. J Am Vener Dis Assoc. 1975;1:163.
83. Jamsky RJ, Christen AG. Oral gonococcal infections. Oral Surg. 1982;53:358.
84. Goodell SE, Quinn TC, Mkrtichian PA-C, et al. Herpes simplex virus proctitis in homosexual men. Clinical, sigmoidoscopic and histopathological features. N Engl J Med. 1983;308:868.
85. deLeon JC. Cutaneous amebiasis. In: Padilla y Padilla CA, Padilla GM eds. Amebiasis in Man. Springfield, IL: Charles C Thomas; 1974:110.
86. Burkhart CG. Scabies: An epidemiologic reassessment. Ann Intern Med. 1983;98:498.
87. Weisman K, Secher L, Hjorth N. Recurrent genital herpes on the buttocks: "Herpes disciformis". Cutis. 1987;40:166–8.
88. Wickett WH, Miller RD. Sites of multiple lesions in recurrent genital herpes. Am Fam Physician. 1985;32:145–52.
89. Nsanze H, Fast MV, D'Costa LJ, et al. Genital ulcers in Kenya: Clinical and laboratory study. Br J Vener Dis. 1981;57:378.
90. Brown ST, Jaffe HW, Zaidi A, et al. Sensitivity and specificity of diagnostic tests for genital infection with *Herpesvirus hominis*. Sex Transm Dis. 1979;6:10.
91. Goldstein LC, Corey L, McDougall JK, et al. Monoclonal antibodies to herpes simplex viruses: Use in antigenic typing and rapid diagnosis. J Infect Dis. 1983;47:829.
92. Lafferty WE, Krofft S, Remington M, et al. Diagnosis of herpes simplex virus by direct immunofluorescence and viral isolation from samples of external genital lesions in a high prevalence population. J Clin Microbiol. 1987;25:323–6.
93. Redfield DC, Richman DD, Albanil S, et al. Detection of herpes simplex virus in clinical specimens by DNA hybridization. Diagn Microbiol Infect Dis. 1983;1:117.
94. Corey L. Laboratory diagnosis of herpes simplex virus infections. Principles guiding the development of rapid diagnostic tests. Diagn Microbiol Infect Dis. 1986;4(Suppl):111–9.
94a. Austin VH, Topham EB. Mineral oil versus KOH for *Sarcoptes*. J Am Acad Dermatol. 1982;7:555.
95. Tronca E, Handsfield HH, Wiesner PJ, et al. Demonstration of *Neisseria gonorrhoeae* with fluorescent antibody in patients with disseminated gonococcal infection. J Infect Dis. 1974;129:583.
96. Deacon WE, Lucas JB, Price EV. Fluorescent treponemal antibody absorption (FTA-ABS) test for syphilis. JAMA. 1966;198:624.
97. Duncan W, Knox J, Wende R. The FTA-ABS test in darkfield positive primary syphilis. JAMA. 1974;228:859.
98. Larsen SA, Hambie EA, Pettit DE, et al. Specificity, sensitivity, and reproducibility among the fluorescent treponemal antibody absorption test, the microhemagglutination assay for *Treponema pallidum* antibodies, and the hemagglutination treponemal test for syphilis. J Clin Microbiol. 1981;14:441.
99. Corey L, Holmes KK. Genital herpes simplex virus infections: Current concepts in diagnosis, therapy, and prevention. Ann Intern Med. 1983;98:973.
100. Moseley RC, Corey L, Benjamin D, et al. Comparison of viral isolation, direct immunofluorescence, and indirect immunoperoxidase techniques for detection of genital herpes simplex virus infection. J Clin Microbiol. 1981;13:913.
101. Hammond GW, Lian CJ, Witt JC, et al. Comparison of specimen collection and laboratory techniques for isolation of *Hemophilus ducreyi*. J Clin Microbiol. 1978;7:39.
102. Nobre GN. Identification of *Hemophilus ducreyi* in the clinical laboratory. J Med Microbiol. 1982;15:243.
103. Nsanze H, Plummer FA, Maggwa AB, et al. Comparison of media for the primary isolation of *Haemophilus ducreyi*. Sex Transm Dis. 1984;11:6–9.

93. INGUINAL ADENOPATHY

MICHAEL F. REIN

Inguinal and femoral adenopathies may be asymptomatic but more commonly produce noticeable pain, stiffness, or swelling in the groin. These symptoms may be the initial manifestation of an inflammatory or neoplastic process that will eventually involve many other groups of lymph nodes. Isolated inguinofemoral adenopathy usually results from infection or neoplasm of the external genitalia or lower extremities, but processes arising in the lower portion of the abdomen or internal genitalia occasionally involve these nodes, and conditions other than adenopathy may be manifested as swellings around the inguinal ligament.

CONDITIONS PRODUCING A MASS IN THE GROIN

The etiologic spectrum varies markedly with the age, general life-style (e.g., urban or rural), sexual practices, and geographic location of the patient population.

Sexually Transmitted Diseases

Among sexually active people, genital infections are common causes of inguinofemoral adenopathy. The inguinal nodes drain the distal part of the urethra in both sexes. It must be remembered that the proximal portion of the vagina and cervix are drained by deep inguinal and iliac nodes, and women with primary infections of the proximal aspect of the vagina and cervix do not manifest superficial inguinal or femoral adenopathy. Tender inguinal adenopathy has been reported in up to 40 percent of the patients with acute gonococcal urethritis,[1] but it is felt by most observers to occur less often and followed only 5 percent of experimentally induced infections.[2] The mechanism is unclear, but in two cases gonococci were isolated from aspirates of an inguinal node.[2,3] It is interesting that in both of these cases the precipitating urethral infection was asymptomatic. Similar adenopathy appears to accompany only about 1 percent of the cases of nongonococcal urethritis.[1] With either infection, the nodes are usually discrete and not fixed to the overlying skin.

Relatively painless and usually bilateral,[4] inguinal adenopathy (satellite bubo) appears in 50–70 percent of the cases of primary syphilis.[5] Nodes usually become enlarged about 7 days after the appearance of the chancre. The examiner usually palpates a chain of nodes rather than a single node, and these are discrete, firm, and freely movable. Suppuration is extremly rare.

Relatively tender adenopathy affects 80 percent of the patients with primary herpes genitalis and is seen in 20 percent of men and 30 percent of the women who have recurrent herpes.[4] The adenopathy is described as lasting about 9–14 days in patients with primary infection and 7–9 days in patients with recurrent infection.[6] The diagnosis is generally made on the basis of the characteristic skin lesions (Chapter 118). Occasionally, the adenopathy actually precedes the appearence of skin lesions.[7] Herpetic inguinal lymphadenopathy has been described in elderly patients with immunologic impairments.[8]

Tender buboes are observed in 25–60 percent of the patients with chancroid. Adenopathy is noted by only about one-third of patients at the time of initial presentation[9] with the ulcer but appears in most 7–10 days later. It is frequently unilateral and is often accompanied by reddening of the overlying skin. Outbreaks of chancroid have occurred in California.[10] The disease is edemic in Southeast Asia, Africa, and other tropical and subtropical regions. Its painful ulcers may be confused with herpes genitalis, but they are usually larger and have a more ragged appearance.[11]

The initial genital lesion of lymphogranuloma venereum (LGV) is unnoticed by 70–95 percent of the patients,[11–13] and inguinal adenopathy is the most common initial complaint. Unilateral in 70 percent of the cases, it is initially noted as a stiffness or aching in the groin 2–6 weeks after the infecting sexual contact.[11–13] The nodes become matted and attached to the overlying skin, which is said to develop a purplish color.[11] If untreated, the nodes frequently suppurate in 7–10 days[13] and rupture, and chronic lymphadenopathy develops in about 5 percent of the patients.[11–12] Lymphogranuloma venereum is uncommon in the United States, with fewer than 1000 civilian cases reported each year,[14–15] but it must be considered in the differential diagnosis of inguinal adenopathy without an obvious primary source.

Generalized lymphadenopathy is a frequent manifestation of infection with human immunodeficiency virus (HIV). The involved nodes are usually nontender and chronically enlarged (see Chapter 108).

Nonvenereal Infections

Streptococci and staphylococci are frequent causes of inguinal lymphadenitis in children and not uncommon causes in adults.[16–18] Although extension from the lower extremity is the most likely route of infection of the glands, the primary site often escapes detection. If the infection does not respond to antibiotics, the nodes are likely to suppurate and require surgical intervention. Pneumococcal[19] and even yersinial[20] inguinal adenopathies have been described in adults. In all cases, the nodes were fluctuant. Sexual transmission of these pathogens has been considered in some cases.

Cat-scratch disease (Chapter 228), the specific agent of which appears to be a bacillus, results in tender and poorly defined lymph nodes draining an area scratched by a domestic cat. A history of the cat scratch is obtained in somewhat more than half of the infected patients,[21] and the adenopathy appears 1–9 weeks after the initial injury. Inguinal or femoral nodes are involved in 10–25 percent of the patients,[22,23] and the adenopathy is bilateral in about 2 percent of the cases.[21–23] The adenopathy characteristically lasts for 2–4 months, and 12–33 percent of the nodes will suppurate. The skin test antigen is not generally available, and the diagnosis is often assumed on the basis of a consistent history, characteristic histopathology of excised lymph nodes,[24] and the absence of alternative diagnoses.

Isolated, painful, inguinal or femoral adenopathy is the most common manifestation of bubonic plague. About 25 percent of the patients exhibit inguinal and about 40 percent femoral adenopathy.[25] One-fourth of the patients complain of obvious pain in the groin preceding the swelling, and the adenopathy may be accompanied by erythema and edema of the overlying skin (Chapter 207). Patients are often systemically ill and have a leukocytosis with increased numbers of immature leukocytes.

Although rabbit-associated tularemia usually involves the nodes of the upper extremity, tick-borne infections frequently produce inguinal adenopathy, which is observed in 20–50 percent of the cases overall[26,27] and is more common in adults than in children.[26] The tick prefers warm moist areas, and the initial lesion, which may be pustular, crusted, or ulcerated, is often found on the scrotum or penis or in the groin itself.[28] The lesion may be very subtle and is absent in the so-called glandular form of the disease. Affected nodes are enlarged and tender and are usually firm, discrete, and not attached to the overlying skin. Along the lymphatic channels proximal to the site of inoculation, one may observe occasional nodules that mimic sporotrichosis. The peripheral white blood cell count is low, normal, or elevated, and the differential count is usually normal. Tick-borne disease occurs most frequently in the warm months.[27]

Enlargement of inguinal or femoral nodes occurs in 8 percent of the patients with brucellosis,[29] but other groups of nodes are always involved simultaneously. The nodes are often tender.

Typical and atypical mycobacteria rarely produce isolated inguinal adenopathy in children and adults.[30] Cervical nodes are involved far more frequently.[31,32] Early on, the affected nodes are discrete, firm, and movable, but later they become matted together and may undergo caseous necrosis and drain through the overlying skin to form chronic sinuses.

Infectious mononucleosis is rarely manifested as isolated inguinofemoral adenopathy.[33] Other groups of nodes are likely to be involved later in the course of the disease. Likewise, toxoplasmosis, which characteristically results in generalized lymphadenopathy, involves the inguinal nodes in 10–20 percent of cases[34,35] and presents as isolated inguinal adenopathy in perhaps 1 percent of the infections.[34]

Onchocerciasis produces inguinal lymphadenopathy and a loss of local elastic fibers that may be so pronounced as to create sacs that droop over the thigh yielding so-called hanging groin.[36] In African onchocerciasis the nodes themselves are usually atrophic and contain microfilariae, whereas the Arabian form (sowda) has hyperplastic nodes in which microfilariae have only recently been described.[37] Usually only single groups of nodes are involved.

Intravenous drug use may be associated with regional lymphadenopathy.[38] Addicts making use of veins on the foot or leg may have isolated inguinal or femoral lymphadenopathy that is usually relatively indolent. The observation of needle tracks is helpful diagnostically. Repeated minor infections of the feet can lead to the development of chronic indolent lymphadenopathy, which is more common in people who habitually go barefoot.[39] Malignancy arising in the genital tract[40,41] or lower extremities[42] or of an unknown primary[43] may metastasize to inguinal nodes and produce nontender adenopathy, and lymphoma is manifested as inguinal adenopathy in about 10 percent of patients.[44]

Conditions Mimicking Inguinal Adenopathy

Abscesses of the skin or soft tissue overlying the groin may produce a tender mass inviting confusion with inguinal adenopathy. Such infection may arise in a hair follicle. The mass cannot be moved independently of the overlying skin, and the examiner may be able to press his fingers behind the mass to establish its separation from the inguinal or femoral lymphatic chains. Such local infection may, however, elicit true local lymphadenopathy to confuse the picture. An intra-abdominal abscess such as a psoas abscess from tuberculous spondylitis occasionally points through the groin area or dissects into the inguinal canal. An inguinal or femoral hernia may also be manifested as a mass in the groin, but its softness and variation with respiration usually suggest its identity. A hematoma or pseudoaneurysm sometimes presents as a groin mass. Ultrasonography or computed tomography (CT) helps to distinguish these conditions from true adenopathy.

Donovanosis (granuloma inguinale), a sexually transmitted infection extremely rare in the United States, produces granulomatous lesions in the groin that may be confused with true adenopathy (Chapter 227). Genital lesions are common, but 3 percent of the cases have only inguinal involvement.[45] The initial inguinal mass or pseudobubo is indolent and doughy. It is clearly superficial and fixed to the overlying intact skin.[46] Genital and groin lesions break down into ulcerations and exuberant growths of beefy granulation tissue.[11,47] The diagnosis is based on biopsy specimens of the lesions (Chapter 227). Although not primrily a disease of the lymphatics, inguinal and femoral nodes may become secondarily involved.[48]

APPROACH TO THE PATIENT WITH INGUINAL ADENOPATHY

The initial work-up is aimed at detecting infection of the external and internal genitalia, infection of the lower extremities, and involvement of other groups of lymph nodes.

History

Age. Among children under the age of 10 years, staphylococci and streptococci are numerically significant causes of inguinal adenopathy.[16] Once the patient enters the age of sexual activity, sexually transmitted infections are more likely. Malignancy is somewht more likely in elderly patients.

Occupation. Brucellosis should be considered in patients having dairy- or farm animal-related occupations. Patients with outdoor occupations are at greater risk for tick-borne tularemia.

Residence. Plague is extremely rare in patients who have not lived in or passed through endemic areas in the southwestern United States or in Southeast Asia. Chancroid is prevalent in many areas of African and Asia. Tropical causes of inguinal adenopthy must be considered if residence in appropriate areas is documented.

Duration. Because painless adenopathy may go unnoticed, the patient's history is a minimum estimate of the duration of an indolent process. Most infections produce a relatively acute enlargement of the affected nodes, but fungal and mycobacterial infections, cat-scratch disease, and neoplastic processes are more often relatively chronic. Persistent swelling may result from diverse acute processes, and gradually increasing indolent adenopathy may accompany repeated minor injuries to the lower extremities.

Pain. Pain or tenderness accompanies many acute infections and is characteristic of brucellosis,[29] tularemia,[28,49] yersinial inguinal lymphadenitis,[20] chancroid,[11] herpes genitalis,[6] gonorrhea,[1–3] cat-scratch disease,[21,22] and infection with pyogenic cocci.[16,19] Tenderness is often less pronounced with LGV[11–13] and is unusual in nodes involved by syphilis,[50,51] lymphoma,[44] or other malignancies.[40–43]

Trauma. A history of nonspecific trauma to the lower extremity may be useful. A definite history of a cat scratch suggests cat-scratch disease, but such a history is obtained in only 50 percent of the affected patients.[21–23] Bites by domestic animals frequently result in regional adenopathy and may suggest infection with *Pasturella multocida* (Chapter 206).

Genital Lesions. The history of a painless papule or ulcer of the external genitalia that has disappeared is consistent with LGV but is reported by fewer than 25 percent of the infected patients.[11–15] An indurated, indolent, genital ulcer that heals spontaneously is also suggestive of syphilis.[5] For most other genital infections, lesions and adenopathy are concurrent and will be discussed as part of the physical examination.

Genital Discharge. This history directs attention toward infectious urethritis or cervicitis including gonococcal, nonspecific, and herpetic. Urethritis and cervicitis may be asymptomatic. Adenopathy rarely accompanies trichomoniasis or vulvovaginal candidiasis.

Sexual History. A history of prior sexually transmitted disease increases the probability that the patient currently suffers from a genital infection. A history of new or multiple sexual partners or of genital symptoms among sexual partners also points toward sexually transmitted infection as the cause of the patient's adenopathy. A history of male homosexual contacts increases concern regarding the acquired immunodeficiency syndrome (AIDS) (Chapter 106).

Drug Abuse. The intravenous or subcutaneous administration of drugs into the lower extremity can result in progressive inguinal adenopathy even in the absence of acute infectious episodes.[38] Intravenous drug abusers are at increased risk for infection with HIV. Recently, syphilis has recrudesced in heterosexual populations in association with the use of cocaine.[52]

Examination of the Nodes

Bilaterality. The satellite bubo of syphilis is usually bilateral,[5] as is the adenopathy associated with chancroid[11] and herpes genitalis.[6] Bilaterality is observed in one-third of the patients with LGV[11–14] and in some patients with gonorrhea.[1] Bilateral adenopathy directs attention away from disease processes of the lower extremities but has been reported rarely in cat-scratch disease.[21–23]

Tenderness has essentially the same diagnostic significance as pain.

Firmness. Firm nodes accompany most acute inflammatory processes and are of little differential diagnostic value. Hard nodes are characteristic of lymphoma and other malignancies.

If unchecked, many acute inflammatory adenopathies will result in fluctuance, which is particularly characteristic of plague[25] and other yersinial infections,[20] pyogenic cocci,[16–19] cat-scratch disease[21,23] and LGV.[11–14] It occurs in from 25[28] to 50 percent[49] of the patients with tularemia. It is rare in infectious mononucleosis,[33] syphilis,[5] and herpes genitalis.[6–8]

Matting together of nodes may accompany any intense inflammatory process but is rare in syphilis.[5]

Sign of the Groove. Inguinal adenopathy above and below Poupart's ligament gives the appearance of a single lymphoid mass bisected by a groove. This phenomenon is observed in 15–20 percent of the patients with LGV[12,13] and is highly suggestive but not diagnostic of this infection.[11–13] It has been reported with lymphoma[44] and can probably be seen with adenopathy of other causes.

Color. Redness of the skin overlying the nodes is frequently observed in chancroid[11] and tularemia[49] and less frequently with plague.[25] It has been described in mycobacterial infection[30] but is distinctly unusual with syphilis[5] and viral infections. A purple tinge in the skin overlying the affected nodes has been described in some cases of LGV[11] but is also seen in metastatic melanoma[42] and rarely in other conditions.[53]

Associated Findings

Urethral Discharge. Urethritis is almost invaribly sexually transmitted. Gonorrhea is more frequently associated with inguinal adenopathy than is nongonococcal urethritis.[1–3] Urethral discharge accompanies a few cases of LGV, presumably on the basis of an intraurethral primary lesion.[12]

Genital Lesions (Chapter 92). Groups of vesicles in the genital area are diagnostic of herpes genitalis. Early in the disease, the vesicles are sometimes observed to be umbilicated, and they quickly rupture to form groups of painful shallow ulcers,[6] which in dry skin sites heal by crusting. In primary herpetic infection, the lesions usually precede the adenopathy by 1–2 weeks,[6] although the reverse is occasionally true.[7] A history of recurrent vesicles in the same area or a prodrome of local paresthesia 6–12 hours before the eruption supports the diagnosis of recurrent disease. Observing one or two larger, ragged ulcers is more suggestive of chancroid.[11] A single painless ulcer with an indurated border suggests syphilis.[5] A single pustular or crusted lesion or a tender, shallow ulcer may be seen in tularemia.[28] A papule, sometimes slightly eroded, often initiates LGV but is observed in fewer than 50 percent of men and only very rarely in women.[11–13]

Lesions of the Lower Extremity. The lesions of herpes genitalis and syphilis may appear in the inguinal area. Chancroid may also involve the thigh and characteristically produces a "kissing lesion" immediately opposed to a similar lesion on the shaft of the penis.[11] Trauma to the lower extremity, including animal bites and splinters, are helpful diagnostically, particularly if there is local inflammation or if lymphatic streaking can be observed proximal to the lesion. Animal bites (Chapter 80) raise the possibility of infection with *P. multocida* (Chapter 206). A peripheral lesion of tularemia can be very small and may be missed by all but the most careful examination. It may be crusted or pustular or be manifested as the shallow ulcer giving the name to the ulceroglandular form of the disease that makes up 50–80 percent of the cases.[28] Careful examination of the interdigital spaces is important. Needle tracks should not be overlooked.[38]

Lymphangitis. Erythema and tenderness over lymphatic channels may accompany any acute infection. A series of nodules appearing along the course of the lymphatic channels suggests sporotrichosis but has also been reported in tularemia.[28] In either case the nodules may break down. Nontender, firm inflammation of the lymphatic channels, particularly in the penis, may be associated with syphilis and is referred to as *pipestem lymphangitis*.[5]

Coincident adenopathy at distant sites should be assiduously sought. Its presence changes the etiologic spectrum.

Laboratory Investigations

Peripheral leukocytosis is a regular feature of plague and is usually accompanied by an increased number of immature neutrophils.[25] Peripheral leukocytosis is also common with staphylococcal and streptococcal infections but is found only variably with other conditions. A high percentage of atypical lymphocytes supports a diagnosis of infectious mononucleosis, and bizzare forms may suggest lymphoma.

The diagnosis of herpes genitalis can usually be made clinically but may be confirmed with the Tzanck test. An intact vesicle is unroofed, and material from the base is smeared on a microscope slide and stained with Giemsa or Wright stain or with methylene blue. The preparation is observed under low (100×) and high (400×) power for the presence of multinucleated giant cells diagnostic of infection with a herpes group virus. The Tzanck test is insensitive on lesions that have spontaneously ruptured to become shallow ulcers,[54] and the diagnosis is best made in these cases by isolating the virus from a swab of the lesion.[55–57] Monoclonal antibodies can be used to identify herpesvirus in direct smears from lesions and, although less sensitive than culture is, may enable a rapid, specific diagnosis.[55–57] Once the lesions have crusted over, the virus can be recovered only with difficulty,[56] but by this time, the adenopathy should be resolving. Other techniques such as enzyme-linked immunosorbent assay (ELISA) and DNA hybridization offer promise.[55]

Ulcerated lesions for which an alternative diagnosis is not obvious should be subjected to darkfield examination for *Treponema pallidum* (Chapter 213).

A Gram-stained smear of an ulcerated lesion will occasionally reveal short gram-negative rods, sometimes in a parallel array resembling a school of fish. This finding is highly suggestive of chancroid but is seen in relatively few cases.[9] The edge of the lesion is the best site for obtaining this material. Fluid from the edge of the lesion can be cultured for *Haemophilus ducreyi*; however, the organism is quite fastidious.[9]

Urethral discharge (Chapter 94) should be stained with Gram stain and examined for the presence of gram-negative, cell-associated diplococci, which diagnose gonorrhea. The presence of neutrophils alone indicates nongonococcal urethritis. A urethral swab should be taken from asymptomatic men, and Gram staining will reveal gonococci in about two-thirds of the infected patients (Chapter 190). A urethral swab should be cultured for *Neisseria gonorrhoeae* before initiating therapy.

Before the development of effective antimicrobial chemotherapy, aspiration of enlarged nodes often resulted in sinus formation. The risk is now very small, and needle aspiration may reveal the cause if other diagnostic maneuvers have failed. This procedure is contraindicated if the inguinal mass may be an incarcerated hernia or aneurysm. Ultrasonography may help to resolve such questions. Fluctuant areas, if present, are appropriate targets. The overlying skin should be prepared with an iodophore that is allowed to dry and is washed off with alcohol. The skin may be infiltrated with a small amount of a local anesthetic agent, or it may be numbed with an ethyl chloride spray. Frequently, the approach producing the least total discomfort is to perform the aspiration without prior anesthesia. The femoral artery should be located by palpation and studiously avoided. A 21 gauge needle on a 6 ml syringe is introduced briskly through the skin and into the node. The plunger should be drawn back in an attempt to aspirate pus. If syphilis is suspected, the needle is plunged in various directions within the node while suction is applied to the syringe.[5] Material recovered from nonfluctuant nodes should be examined by darkfield microscopy. A good specimen contains about 10 lymphocytes per oil-immersion field and reveals spirochetes in about 95 percent of the cases of syphilis.[5] Pus from fluctuant nodes should be stained with Gram stain and examined for pyogenic cocci. Wayson stain will diagnose plague with a sensitivity of 60–85 percent.[25] The aspirate should be cultured for gonococci, pyogenic cocci, and *H. ducreyi*.[9]

If no material is obtained from a fluctuant node, the syringe may be disconnected from the needle and replaced with another containing a small amount of saline free of bacteriostatic agents. This saline is introduced into the node, reaspirated into the syringe, and processed as above. In general, surgical incision and drainage of the nodes should be avoided.

Serologic tests for plague, tularemia, and brucellosis are available but generally confirm a diagnosis only in retrospect. Serologic tests for syphilis are almost always positive in patients with inguinal adenopathy,[5,50,58] and a nonreactive fluorescent treponemal antibody absorption (FTA-ABS) test essentially rules out syphilis. The microhemagglutination test for *T. pallidum* (MHA-TP) is somewhat less sensitive in primary syphilis. The complement fixation test with chlamydial antigen will show a high ($\geq$1:32) or rising titer in 95 percent of the patients with LGV.[11–13] The test is sometimes positive in the presence of other chlamydial infections such as psittacosis, nongonococcal urethritis, or trachoma, but a negative examination with acute and convalescent sera rules out LGV. The older Frei test, an intradermal test with chlamydial antigen, is much less sensitive, and the antigen is no longer available. Serologic tests are useful in the diagnosis of toxoplasmosis.[59]

Eventually, biopsy may be necessary to establish a diagnosis. Few pathologic features are differentially diagnostic in acute infection. Noncaseating granulomas are frequently observed and may be seen with gonorrhea,[2] LGV,[11–13,58] and syphilis.[51] Langhans-type giant cells may be seen with LGV and syphilis and are not specific for mycobacterial infection. Stellate microabscesses are described in LGV[11–13] but can also be seen in other conditions including syphilis.[51] Highly suggestive of syphilis is the finding of fibrosis of the capsule and pericapsular tissues and phlebitis or endarteritis.[51] The combination of follicular hyperplasia, granulomas with giant cells, and microabscesses in the same specimen is highly suggestive of cat-scratch disease.[24] Follicular and sinusoidal hyperplasia and packing of the sinusoids with monomorphologic round cells are seen in nodes from patients with AIDS.[60]

In an unselected series of node biopsy specimens in general hospital admissions, 71 percent of inguinal nodes showed inflammatory disease, 21 percent showed carcinoma, and 8 percent showed lymphoma.[61]

Initial Therapeutic Approach

If a specific diagnosis can be made initially, the patient should, of course, be treated with the agent having the narrowest spectrum and the least toxicity. Systemically ill patients should be hospitalized. If there is a suspicion of plague or tularemia, initial therapy should include coverage for these diseases, probably with streptomycin. Treatment of indolent, slowly progressive, inguinal adenopathy may await the results of laboratory investigations. If plague and tularemia are not considerations and the patient is sexually active, initial therapy with ceftriaxone, 250 mg im, followed by erythromycin, 500 mg orally four times a day, will adequately cover gonorrhea, most cases of syphilis, nongonococcal urethritis, chancroid, LGV, and staphylococcal and streptococcal infections. Close follow-up study is required while the definitive diagnosis is awaited. Substantiation of an accurate diagnosis may lead to more appropriate therapy.

REFERENCES

1. Akers WA. Tender inguinal lymph nodes and gonococcal urethritis. Milit Med. 1972;137:107.
2. Dahl R, Dans PE. Gonococcal lymphadenitis. Arch Intern Med. 1974;134:1116.
3. DeHertogh DA, Murcia ES. Gonococcal inguinal lymphadenitis. Arch Intern Med. 1984;144:391.
4. Drusin LM. Syphilis: Clinical manifestations, diagnosis, and treatment. Urol Clin North Am. 1984;11:121–30.
5. Stokes JH, Beerman H, Ingraham NR. Modern Clinical Syphilology. 3rd ed. Philadelphia: WB Saunders; 1944.
6. Corey L, Adams HG, Brown ZA, et al. Genital herpes simplex virus infections: Clinical manifestations, course, and complications. Ann Intern Med. 1983;98:958.
7. Taxy JB. Herpes simplex lymphadenitis. An unusual presentation with necrosis and viral particles. Arch Pathol Lab Med. 1985;109:1043–4.
8. Epstein JL, Ambinder R, Kuhajada FP, et al. Localized herpes simplex lymphadenitis. Am J Clin Pathol. 1986;86:444–8.
9. D'Costa LJ, Bowmer I, Nsanze H, et al. Advances in the diagnosis and management of chancroid. Sex Transm Dis. 1986;3:189–91.
10. Blackmore CA, Limpokarnjanaratk, Rigau-Perez JG, et al. An outbreak of chancroid in Orange County, California: Descriptive epidemiology and disease control measures. J Infect Dis. 1985;151:840–4.
11. Hart G. Chancroid, Donovanosis, Lymphogranuloma Venereum. Atlanta: US DHEW; 1974.
12. Schachter J, Dawson CR: Human Chlamydial Infection. Littleton, MA: PSG Publishing; 1978:45.
13. Thorsteinsson SB. Lymphogranuloma venereum: Review of clinical manifestations, epidemiology, diagnosis, and treatment. Scand J Infect Dis. 1982;32(suppl):127.
14. McLelland BA, Anderson PC Lymphogranuloma venereum: Outbreak in a university community. JAMA. 1976;235:56.
15. Schachter J, Dawson CR. Lymphogranuloma venereum (Letter). JAMA. 1976;236:915.
16. Scobie WG. Acute suppurative adenitis in children: A review of 964 cases. Scott Med J. 1969;14:352.
17. Pattman RS. Two unusual manifestations of infection with *Staphylococcus aureus* presenting to a clinic for sexually transmitted diseases. Br J Clin Pract. 1983;37:228–9.
18. Ho DD, Murata GH. Streptococcal lymphadenitis in homosexual men with chronic lymphadenopathy. Am J Med. 1984;77:151–3.
19. Lebowitz AS, Tierno PM. Suppurative pneumococcal inguinal adenitis. NY State J Med. 1985;85:509–10.
20. Zimmerman RS, Hamilton JD. *Yersinia enterocolitica* inguinal lymphdenitis. Diagn Microbiol Infect Dis. 1986;5:265–8.
21. Spaulding WB, Hennessy JN. Cat scratch disease: A study of 83 cases. Am J Med. 1960;28:504.
22. Margileth AM. Cat scratch disease: Nonbacterial regional lymphadenitis. Pediatrics. 1968;42:803.

23. Carithers HA. Cat-scratch disease. An overview based on a study of 1200 patients. Am J Dis Child. 1985;139:1124–33.
24. Campbell JAH. Cat scratch disease Pathol Annu. 1977;12:277.
25. Butler T, Bell WR, Linh NN, et al. *Yersinia pestis* infection in Vietnam: 1. Clinical and hematologic aspects. J Infect Dis. 1974;129:578.
26. Jacobs RF, Condrey YM, Yamauchi T. Tularemia in adults and children: A changing presentation. Pediatrics. 1985;76:818–22.
27. Evans ME, Gregory DW, Schoffner W, et al. Tularemia: A 30 year experience with 88 cases. Medicine (Baltimore). 1985;64:251–69.
28. Dienst FT. Tularemia: A perusal of 339 cases. J La State Med Soc. 1963;115:114.
29. Bloomfield AL. Enlargement of superficial lymph nodes in brucella infection. Am Rev Tuberc. 1942;45:741.
30. Andringa CL, Cherry JD. Bilateral inguinal adenitis due to a nonphotochromogenic atypical mycobacterium: Report of a case. JAMA. 1966;198:785.
31. Spark RP, Fried MC, Bean CK, et al. Nontuberculous mycobacterial adenitis of childhood. The ten-year experience at a community hospital. Am J Dis Child. 1988;142a;106–8.
32. Martin T, Hoeppner VH, Ring ED. Superficial mycobacterial lymphadenitis in Saskatchewan. Can Med Assoc J. 1988;138:431–4.
33. Wechsler HF, Rosenblum AH, Sills CT. Infectious mononucleosis: Report of an epidemic in an army post. Ann Intern Med. 1946;25:113.
34. McCabe RE, Brooks RG, Dorfman RF, et al. Clinical spectrum in 107 cases of toxoplasmic lymphdenopathy. Rev Infect Dis. 1987;9:754–74.
35. Rafaty FM. Cervial adenopathy secondary to toxoplasmosis. Arch Otolaryngol. 1977;103:547–9.
36. Gibson DW, Connor DH. Onchocercal lymphadenitis: Clinicopathological study of 34 patients. Trans Soc Trop Med Hyg. 1978;72:137–54.
37. Abdel-Hameed AA, Voah MS, Schacher JF, et al. Lymphadenitis in sowda. Trop Geogr Med. 1987;39:73–6.
38. Geller SA, Stimmel B. Diagnostic confusion from lymphatic lesions in heroin addicts. Ann Intern Med. 1973;78:703.
39. Wapinick S, MacKintosh M, Mauchaza B. Shoelessness, enlarged femoral lymph nodes and femoral hernia: A possible association. Am J Surg. 1973;126:108.
40. Stein M, Steiner M, Suprun H, et al. Inguinal lymph node metasteses from testicular tumor. J Urol. 1985;134:144–5.
41. Sedlis A, Homasley H, Bundy BN, et al. Positive groin lymph nodes in superficial squamous cell vulvar cancer. A Gynecologic Oncology Group Study. Am J Obstet Gynecol. 1987;156:1159–64.
42. Singletary SE, Shallenbergen R, Guinee VF, et al. Melonoma with metasteses to regional axillary or inguinal lymph nodes: Prognostic factors and results of surgical treatment in 714 patients. South Med J. 1988;81:5–9.
43. Guarischi A, Keane TJ, Elhakim T. Metastatic inguinal nodes from an unknown primary neoplasm. A review of 56 cases. Cancer. 1987;59:572–7.
44. Murphy JF, Fred HL. Infectious lymphadenitis or lymphoma? Seven lessons. JAMA. 1976;235:742.
45. Lal S, Nicholas C. Epidemiological and clinical features in 165 cases of granuloma inguinale. Br J Vener Dis. 1970;47:461.
46. Davis CM. Granuloma inguinale: A clinical, histological and ultrastructural study. JAMA. 1970;211:632.
47. Sehgal VN, Shyam Prasad AL. Donovanosis: Current concepts. Int J Dermatol. 1986;25:8–16.
48. Greenblatt RB, Dienst RB, Pund ER, et al. Experimental and clinical granuloma inguinale. JAMA. 1939;113:1109.
49. Simpson SM. Tularemia: Histology, Pathology, Diagnosis, and Treatment. New York: Paul B Hoeber; 1929:67.
50. Bergstrom JF, Navin JJ. Luetic lymphadenitis: Lymphographic manifestations simulating lymphoma. Radiology. 1973;106:287.
51. Hartsock RJ, Halling LW, King FM. Luetic lymphadenitis: A clinical and histologic study of 20 cases. Am J Clin Pathol 1970;53:304.
52. Centers for Disease Control. Recommendations for diagnosing and treating syphilis in HIV-infected patients. MMWR. 1988;37:600–8.
53. Rheaume T, Robertson DI, Urbanski SJ, et al. Inguinal intranodal blue nevus: A case report. Can J Surg. 1986;29:282–3.
54. Brown ST, Jaffe HW, Zaidi A, et al. Sensitivity and specificity of diagnostic tests for genital infection with Herpesvirus hominis. Sex Transm Dis. 1979;6:10.
55. Corey L. Laboratory diagnosis of herpes simplex virus infections. Principles guiding the development of rapid diagnostic tests. Diagn Microbiol Infect Dis. 1986;4(Suppl):115.
56. Lafferty WE, Kroft S, Remington M, et al. Diagnosis of herpes simplex virus by direct immunofluorescence and viral isolation from samples of external genital lesions. J Clin Microbiol. 1987;25:323–6.
57. Goldstein LC, Corey L, McDougall JK, et al. Monoclonal antibodies to herpes simplex viruses: Use in antigenic typing and rapid diagnosis. J Infect Dis. 1983;47:829.
58. King FM. Case for diagnosis: Syphilitic lymphadenitis. Milit Med. 1972;137:155.
59. Brooks RG, McCabe RE, Remington JS. Role of serology in the diagnosis of toxoplasmic lymphadenopathy. Rev Infect Dis. 1987;9:1055–62.
60. Guarda LA, Buttler JJ, Mansell P, et al. Lymphdenopathy in homosexual men: Morbid anatomy with clinical and immunologic correlations. Am J Clin Pathol. 1983;79:559.
61. Lee Y-TN, Terry R, Lukes RJ: Biopsy of peripheral lymph nodes. Am Surg. 1982;48:536.

94. URETHRITIS

MICHAEL F. REIN

Urethritis affects an estimated 4 million American men each year.[1] The symptoms range from the trivial and often overlooked to the disabling. Urethral discharge is more frequently recognized by men than by women. It may be apparent at all times during the day and may be present in sufficient quantity to stain undergarments, or it may be so scanty that it is noted only on arising as a small bead of moisture or crust at the meatus. It may be completely clear, mucopurulent, or frankly purulent, and it may be white, yellow, green, or brown. Some patients complain only of a deviation of the first morning urine stream. Occasionally, urethral discharge comes to the attention of the patient through the observation of mucous strands in the urine specimen.

The urine stream transiently eliminates most inflammatory discharges; thus, scanty discharges are best observed on arising before the passage of any urine. Micturation immediately preceding urethral examination may completely eliminate signs of infection.

The discomfort of urethritis can take several forms. Dysuria is common, and men variously localize it to the meatus, the distal portion of the penis, or anywhere along the shaft. Discomfort is sometimes increased by the acidity or solute content of the urine and, therefore, may be most marked during the passage of a concentrated first morning urine. Dysuria may be increased in the presence of irritants such as alcohol, which is an observation that sometimes leads the patient to attribute his disease to the ingestion of specific foods or fluids. Discomfort may persist between micturations and is perceived as pain, itching, frequency, urgency, or a feeling of heaviness in the genitals. Women may complain of dysuria, but urethral pain between micturations is uncommon.

Discomfort only during ejaculation, deep pelvic pain, or pain radiating to the back is infrequent in uncomplicated urethritis and suggests prostatitis or inflammation involving other portions of the urogenital tract such as the epididymis. Hematuria, particularly if painless, or blood in the ejaculate are uncommon in urethritis.[2] The persistence of symptoms after cure of urethritis demands a thorough urologic evaluation.[2]

EXAMINATION OF THE URETHRA

Men should stand before the seated examiner so that the external genitalia are approximately eye level. A good light source is essential. The patient should lower his pants and underwear so the entire genital area may be observed. The underwear may reveal stains of dried discharge, which suggest that it is being produced in large amounts. This observation is particularly useful if the patient has recently urinated.

The patient is preferably examined at least 2 hours after his last micturation. If advised to restrict his fluids during the day preceding the examination, he may be able to present for evaluation before passing his first urine of the day, which sometimes permits the recovery of very small amounts of discharge.[3]

The entire genital area should be carefully examined since other sexually transmitted infections are relatively common in patients with urethritis. Inguinal adenopathy should be sought, and tenderness should be noted. The skin of the entire pubic area, scrotum, groin, and penis should be examined for lesions, and the hair should be examined for nits. The testes and the spermatic cords should be palpated for masses or tenderness. The foreskin should be completely retracted and the glans examined. The urethral meatus is examined for dried crusts, redness, and spontaneous discharge. If no discharge is present, the urethra should be gently stripped by placing the gloved thumb along the ventral surface of the base of the penis and the forefinger on the dorsum and then applying gentle pressure. The examiner's hand is moved slowly toward the meatus. This will frequently expell a discharge that may be collected on a swab for examination as described below.

If no discharge is delivered by this maneuver, the third and fourth fingers should be used to grip the penis lightly, just behind the glans. The thumb and forefinger can then spread open the meatus to examine for urethral redness or the presence of small amounts of discharge. Unless the patient has recently urinated or has been in a state of sexual arousal, virtually no fluid should be expressible from the urethra or observed by spreading the meatus.

If expressed material cannot be collected at the meatus, a specimen must be recovered from inside the urethra. This is best accomplished with a calcium alginate urethral or nasopharyngeal swab.[4] The swab should be inserted gently at least 2 cm into the urethra while taking care not to attempt to force the tip past an obstruction. The patient should be warned that the examination is uncomfortable; also, the insertion and removal of the swab should be accomplished as quickly as possible. Occasional patients will tolerate the examination better if they are supine. If additional specimens are required for multiple examinations or cultures, separate swabs should be used while taking care to insert each at least 1 cm deeper than that preceding it.

Regular cotton swabs should not be used for urethral examination, because their larger diameter makes insertion extremely uncomfortable and because of the possibility that the cotton or the wooden shaft may be toxic to some fastidious pathogens. A small platinum loop is effective, but it must be sterilized in a flame and carefully cooled between uses.

A woman's urethra is best examined when she is in the lithotomy position. The entire genital area should be examined for lesions, and the vagina should be examined as described in Chapter 95. The urethral meatus may be directly visualized, and the urethra may be gently stripped by placing the gloved finger inside the vagina and gently moving it along the urethra. A calcium alginate swab may be inserted a short distance within the meatus to obtain a urethral specimen.

EXAMINATION OF THE URETHRAL SPECIMEN

A swab that contains material from the urethra should be rolled across a clean microscope slide. Rolling rather than streaking the swab brings all its surfaces into contact with the slide and better preserves cellular morphologic characteristics. The material may be air-dried and fixed by gentle heating or by rinsing with methanol. Gram staining of urethral material is particularly useful in the work-up of urethritis and the specimen should be examined by using the oil-immersion objective. Specimens obtained from within the urethra generally reveal urethral epithelial cells. When recovered from near the meatus, these are typical squamous cells with a very large cytoplasmic/nuclear ratio, or when obtained from further within the urethra, they are cuboidal epithelial cells, which are smaller and have relatively larger, less dense nuclei.

Urethral material from patients with acute urethritis will contain polymorphonuclear neutrophils (PMNs). The area of the smear that contains most PMNs should be sought. More than four PMNs per oil-immersion microscopic field is always abnormal and is seen in 60–90 percent of all patients with acute symptomatic urethritis.[4–6] However, 16–50 percent of all men with documented urethral infection will not show four PMNs in maximally dense oil-immersion fields.[7–12] The number of PMNs in the smear is reduced by recent micturation[13]; also, there often is considerable observer variation in the number of PMNs detected in a single specimen.[14] Thus, although purulent discharges may reveal sheets of PMNs, the minimal number of these cells that indicate disease is not known. In general, the presence of even rare PMNs suggests infection, particularly in the patient who has urethral symptoms or who is found to have a small amount of discharge on examination.

The distal centimeter of the urethra is colonized by normal skin or introital flora. One usually will observe a variety of gram-positive and gram-negative organisms that have no particular significance. Of great diagnostic value, however, is the presence of typical gram-negative, "intracellular" diplococci (Fig. 1). These organisms are not randomly distributed among the cells but are seen in large numbers in a few PMNs. They will be observed in more than 95 percent of all symptomatic patients with gonococcal urethritis and in fewer than 2 percent of all symptomatic men who cannot be shown to have gonorrhea by culture.[15–17] Some strains of *Neisseria gonorrhoeae* are inhibited by the concentrations of vancomycin that usually are employed in selective isolation media; these organisms will not be recovered by standard culture techniques. Extracellular diplococci indicate gonorrhea in only 10–29 percent of all cases, and this predictive value is even further reduced in populations with a low prevalence of gonorrhea.[17,18] A shortcoming of the Gram-stained smear is that it cannot diagnose coincidental nongonococcal urethritis (NGU) in the presence of gonorrhea. Although a smear that does not reveal gram-negative intracellular diplococci strongly suggests NGU, a smear revealing these organisms does not rule out NGU.

In men with adequate amounts of urethral discharge, one can use commercially available kits to test for the presence of gonococcal oxidase. Experience with the technique is limited; however, preliminary data suggest a sensitivity of 96 percent but a specificity of only 85 percent.[19] Furthermore, the Gram stain provides information on the degree of inflammation present. Limulus lysate assays for gonococcal endotoxin, although greater than 95 percent sensitive and specific,[20] are of limited clinical utility because many patients have inadequate amounts of discharge.[21]

Candida may be recognized as gram-positive or beaded, oval bodies about 3×6 μm. Observing small numbers of yeast cells does not prove a candidial etiology for the urethritis since *Candida* may be recovered from normal patients, particularly if they are uncircumcised.

Trichomonads are very difficult to identify on Gram-stained smears.

Urethral material may be mixed with a small amount of saline and observed as a wet mount with the substage condenser racked down or the substage diaphragm partially closed. Motile trichomonads occasionally are observed but are rarely seen unless the examination is carried out before the first voiding. A positive wet mount diagnoses trichomoniasis, but the wet mount will be negative (even under ideal circumstances) in 10–50 percent of infected men.[22,23]

After the patient's urethra has been carefully examined, he may be asked to provide a divided urine specimen. The patient delivers the first 10 ml of urine into one container and the remainder of the urine specimen into a second. Mucous strands in the first fraction that clear in the second portion suggest urethritis. Equal aliquots of the fractions may be centrifuged and the sediments examined as wet mounts. Observing more white blood cells in the initial than in the second fraction suggests urethritis, while observing equal numbers of white cells in both fractions suggests cystitis or infection higher in the urinary tract.[2,3] A total of more than 15 white blood cells in five $400\times$ microscopic fields of the sediment from the initial fraction strongly suggests urethritis,[4,7,10] but the minimum significant number of white blood cells is unknown. More than 10 PMNs per high-power field have been observed in 90 percent of all men with chlamydial urethritis,[7] and *N. gonorrhoeae* or *Chlamydia trachomatis* can be recovered from 90 percent of men

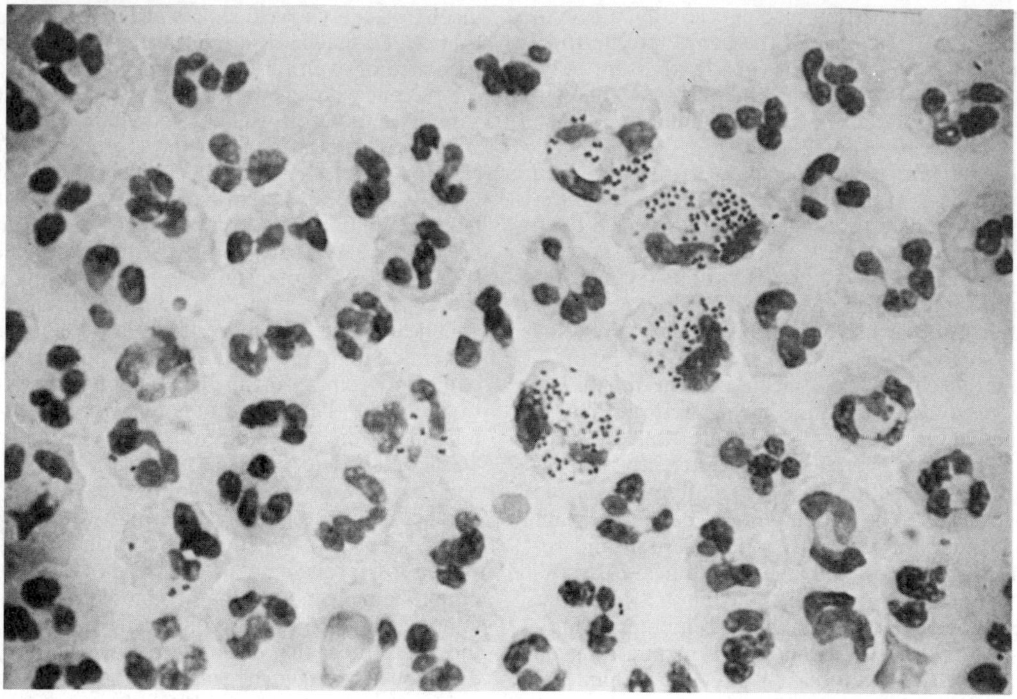

FIG. 1. Gram stain of urethral exudate from a man with gonorrhea. Several neutrophils contain many gram-negative cell-associated diplococci.

demonstrating this level of pyuria.[24] White blood cells or mucous strands in the initial urine fraction provide no clue to the etiology of the urethritis. If the urine specimen is a first morning micturation, motile trichomonads may be observed in the sediment from almost 80 percent of infected men, and they are recovered by culture in 95 percent of the cases.[13] Trichomonads are infrequently recovered from patients who have already voided during the day.

Material recovered from the urethra can be cultured with appropriate media for *N. gonorrhoeae* and *Trichomonas vaginalis*. Culture systems for *C. trachomatis* are becoming more generally available and less costly. Enzyme-linked immunosorbent assay (ELISA) and immunofluorescence techniques for identifying *C. trachomatis* in genital specimens have been developed (see Chapter 158) and are changing our approach to these infections. Their sensitivity in urethritis, however, may be as low as 70 percent.[25] Cultures for *Ureaplasma urealyticum* are less frequently performed; also, their interpretation is complicated by the high prevalence of colonization in asymptomatic, sexually active people. Although present in the distal urethra, normal skin flora (such as *Staphylococcus epidermidis*, α-hemolytic streptococci, and propionibacteria), normal vaginal flora (such as *Candida albicans*, lactobacilli, and *Escherichia coli*), and other organisms (such as *Gardnerella vaginalis*) are of no diagnostic significance.[26,27]

NONINFECTIOUS URETHRITIS

So psychically important is the genital tract that trivial symptoms often receive patients' frightened attention. The "worried well" make up a significant fraction of men who are seen in venereal disease clinics and in private practices. Sympathetic questioning as to why the patient thinks he has contracted a genital infection may reveal guilt over an act such as masturbation, which does not put the patient at significant risk of infection. The urethral specimen in these cases usually reveals normal epithelial cells and no white blood cells. Some patients confuse dried remnants of semen with inflammatory discharge. Microscopic examination again fails to reveal inflammatory cells, but spermatozoa may be recognized on the Gram stain as gram-positive ovoids whose coloration fades gradually toward the achrosomal cap or may be recognized on the wet mount. However, the physician must remember that symptoms and signs of true urethritis can be trivial and that microscopic examination may miss minimal inflammation, particularly if the patient has recently voided. Symptomatic patients with negative examinations should be asked to return in several days, by which time the symptoms may have resolved or examination may provide a diagnosis. An occasional patient who complains of a discharge is really suffering from urinary incontinence.

Chronic irritation of the urethra can elicit a clear, mucoid discharge. Occasional patients, concerned that they may have contracted a venereal disease, vigorously strip the urethra looking for a discharge. After several days of this, a clear discharge obligingly appears that may contain a few white blood cells. A history of vigorous urethral stripping is helpful diagnostically. Patients treated for other forms of urethritis should be cautioned not to examine themselves too vigorously for fear that such a traumatic discharge may confuse the clinical picture. Very rarely, patients will insert foreign bodies into the urethra and produce a discharge that may be blood-tinged.[28] This sort of self-abuse should be considered in retarded or psychotic individuals.

A heavy precipitation of crystals in the urine can suggest a discharge, and the presence of large amounts of crystalline material or calculous gravel may produce urinary discomfort. The intermittent nature of pain associated with the passage of gravel or the obvious presence of crystals on microscopic examination of the urine sediment usually confirms this diagnosis. White blood cells may be present.

Urethritis may accompany noninfectious systemic diseases such as Stevens-Johnson syndrome or Wegener's granulomatosis.

Chemicals may irritate the urethra, and alcohol has long been known to produce mild dysuria. The ingestion of alcohol during the treatment for gonorrhea was at one time thought to be responsible for the syndrome of postgonococcal urethritis discussed later, although it is now known to have an infectious etiology. An occasional patient may develop urethral symptoms on contact with vaginal chemicals used by a sexual partner. The history of discomfort immediately after sexual contact may be suggestive. This uncommon condition should be diagnosed only after other etiologies have been excluded. Shampoos and other bath products have produced urethritis in children.[29]

INFECTIOUS URETHRITIS

Gonococcal and Nongonococcal Urethritis

The major single specific etiology of acute urethritis is *Neisseria gonorrhoeae*. Urethral inflammation of all other etiologies is referred to collectively as NGU. As with gonorrhea, most cases of NGU are sexually acquired; also, over the past 15 years, the incidence of both infections has increased. NGU is twice as common as gonorrhea in the United States and in much of the developed world as well.[30–32] In some underdeveloped areas, however, gonorrhea accounts for 80 percent of the cases of acute urethritis. As with many other sexually transmitted diseases (STDs) gonococcal and nongonococcal urethritis have an increased incidence during the summer months,[31,32] presumably because of a seasonal increase in sexual activity. Although a number of reports have suggested that the incidence of NGU is increasing more rapidly than is that of gonorrhea, such conclusions must be viewed with caution. Public interest has focused on NGU, and patients may now be more likely to seek medical attention for mild genital symptoms than they had been in the past.[30] Indeed, except in Great Britain, the ratio of NGU to gonorrhea has remained relatively stable over the past decade.[30]

The ratio of nongonococcal to gonococcal urethritis has been thought to be greater among groups with higher socioeconomic status.[33] This differential distribution is most likely related to differences in health care behavior, with wealthier and better educated individuals more likely to seek medical care for milder symptoms. There are, however, some studies suggesting that blacks are more susceptible than are whites to gonococcal infection.[30]

Compared with gonorrhea, NGU is relatively less prevalent among homosexual than among heterosexual men with urethritis. Examining consecutive men attending an STD clinic, Stamm and colleagues recovered gonococci from 12 percent of heterosexual and 25 percent of homosexual men, whereas they recovered chlamydia from 14 percent of heterosexual but only 5 percent of homosexual men.[9]

Historically, there has been considerable interest in the possible contribution of circumcision in the epidemiology of STD. Such studies are difficult to interpret because certain behavioral factors are associated with circumcision.[34] The presence of a foreskin may mask a urethral discharge and delay patients from presenting for evaluation, but other roles remain speculative.[34]

The spectrum of gonorrhea differs from that of NGU, but there is sufficient clinical overlap so that an accurate differential diagnosis must be based on microscopic examination of the urethral specimen. Seventy-five percent of men acquiring urethral gonorrhea develop symptoms within 4 days[3] and 80–90 percent within 2 weeks.[30,35,36] The incubation period for NGU is much more variable and is often longer, usually between 7 and 14 days, but incubation periods ranging from 2 to 35 days have been described,[30,33,35] and almost 50 percent of the men with NGU developed urethral symptoms within 4 days.[3,30,35] Thus, an incubation period of less than 1 week is not a reliable factor in the differential diagnosis.[3,30,35,37] The incubation period of either infection can be prolonged by the ingestion of subcurative doses of antibiotics.[38]

The urethral discharge is described as frankly purulent in three-quarters of the patients with gonorrhea but in only 11–33 percent of the patients with NGU.[15,33,39] A purulent discharge issuing from the meatus without stripping the urethra correlates strongly with the diagnosis of gonorrhea but is also seen in 4 percent of patients with NGU.[15,39] Mucopurulent discharge, consisting of thin cloudy fluid or mucoid fluid with purulent flecks, is seen in about 50 percent of the patients with NGU but in only 25 percent of the patients with symptomatic gonorrhea.[15,39] The discharge is completely clear and moderately viscid in 10–50 percent of the patients with NGU, principally those who are minimally symptomatic, but in only 4 percent of symptomatic patients with gonorrhea.[15,39,40] A differential diagnosis on the basis of the clinical characteristics of the urethral discharge is unreliablc and yields a correct diagnosis in only 73 percent of all cases, even under optimal circumstances.[39] Microscopic examination always should be part of the initial evaluation.

Dysuria has been described in 53–75 percent of the patients with NGU and in 73–88 percent of the patients wiht symptomatic gonorrhea.[15,41] Only about 10 percent of the patients complaining of dysuria without discharge have gonorrhea; the remainder suffer from NGU.[15] A combination of dysuria and discharge is seen in 71 percent of the patients with gonococcal urethritis but in only 38 percent of the patients with NGU. Thus, the combination of discharge and dysuria is associated with gonorrhea, while the appearance of one without the other is more frequently seen with NGU. The association is insufficiently specific for a differential diagnosis. Urethral discomfort may mimic cystitis in men and women and result in urinary frequency and urgency.

Symptoms of gonorrhea often begin abruptly, and the patient may remember the specific time of day when they were first noted. Nongonococcal urethritis usually has a less acute onset, with symptoms increasing over several days. A urethral discharge may appear days in advance of dysuria; the symptoms may wax and wane, even to the point of transiently disappearing before the patient seeks therapy. The mildness and variability of the symptoms may erroneously convince the patient with NGU that he does not have a significant disease; such patients often delay seeking medical attention.[15,41]

The symptoms of infectious urethritis will, in most cases, resolve even if the patient remains untreated. Ninety-five percent of untreated patients with acute gonogoccal urethritis will be free of symptoms 6 months after contracting the disease,[36] and the symptoms of NGU gradually subside over a period of 1–3 months in 30–70 percent of the patients.[42] How many of these asymptomatic patients remain infected and potentially infectious is unknown. Untreated gonococcal urethrits may subside to a chronic state characterized by little or no urethral discomfort and a small amount of mucoid discharge called "gleet." This discharge contains small numbers of gonococci and PMNs.

So great are the clinical overlaps between nongonococcal and gonococcal urethritis that a differential diagnosis should not be made on clinical grounds alone. A Gram-stained smear of urethral discharge material will reveal typical, gram-negative, "intracellular" diplococci in about 95 percent of the cases of gonococcal urethritis and will be negative in about 97 percent of the patients with NGU.[15–17] Thus, in a population in which about 50 percent of the acute urethritis is gonococcal, a positive Gram stain suggests gonorrhea, and a negative Gram stain suggests NGU with 98 percent accuracy.[15,17] The observation of typically shaped *extracellular* diplococci diagnoses gonorrhea with an accuracy of 10–30 percent.[17,18] The Gram stain is equivocal in about 15 percent of cases.[15] Other techniques for diagnosing gonococcal urethritis are described above.[19–21]

The sensitivity of the culture for *N. gonorrhoeae* is less than 100 percent, partly because some gonococci are inhibited by the vancomycin concentrations used in selective media. The chances of isolating the organism are further reduced if the patient has recently taken antibiotics or if there is a delay in processing the culture. Thus, it seems likely that most of the few patients with positive Gram stains and negative cultures actually have gonorrhea. In most cases of acute symptomatic urethritis it is unnecessary to culturally confirm a Gram stain diagnostic of gonorrhea. It must be remembered that the Gram stain will be negative in as many as 5 percent of such patients who have gonorrhea, so a Gram stain suggestive of NGU should be confirmed with a culture, although therapy need not be delayed until the results are known. The Gram stain cannot be used to make a diagnosis of simultaneous NGU in the presence of gonorrhea. Because of the frequency with which trichomonads may be missed with direct microscopic techniques, patients in whom trichomonal urethritis is suspected should be evaluated by culture as well as by wet mount.

There is no doubt that urethritis is sexually transmitted. It occurs most frequently during the ages of peak sexual activity and in groups with a high prevalence of other STDs. It is found with increased frequency in persons with a history of other sexually transmitted genital infections.[30,33] It frequently follows sexual exposure to a new partner and is (except as a part of some systemic conditions) almost never seen in virgins. As the etiologic agents of urethritis have been defined, they have been isolated with high frequency from the female and homosexual male sexual partners of infected men where, however, they usually are carried asymptomatically.

Recognizing urethritis as an STD is important for several practical reasons. It allows one to define a population at very high risk for carrying the agents, namely, the sexual partners of infected patients. The prevalence of colonization with these agents is sufficiently high among sexual partners to justify their treatment on epidemiologic grounds, even if they are asymptomatic. Many episodes of recurrent NGU are terminated only by the treatment of an asymptomatic sexual partner of the infected patient. Since persons with one STD are at increased risk for others, it is important to screen patients with urethritis for other STDs.

Etiology of NGU

The organism most clearly associated with nongonococcal urethritis, *Chlamydia trachomatis*, is discussed in detail in Chapter 158. This obligate intracellular parasite causes 30–50 percent of the cases of NGU.[7,26,31,43,44] *Chlamydia trachomatis* is sensitive to several drugs, including the tetracyclines, sulfonamides, and erythromycin. Significantly, it is not reliably eradicated by penicillins, cephalosporins, or spectinomycin in doses used in the treatment of uncomplicated gonorrhea.

Chlamydiae are not recovered from at least 50 percent of the men with NGU. Although the clinical features of *Chlamydia*-negative NGU are very similar to those of *Chlamydia*-positive NGU,[30,45] some workers have suggested that less discharge is produced in patients who are positive for *Chlamydia* than in those who are not, and the mean incubation period may be slightly shorter.[30,45]

The agents responsible for *Chlamydia*-negative NGU remain to some extent unidentified. *Ureaplasma urealyticum*, formerly known as the T-strain mycoplasma, has been recovered from 81 percent of the men with *Chlamydia*-negative NGU, which is significantly higher than the 60 percent isolation rate from asymptomatic controls.[26,46] Furthermore, *U. urealyticum* can be recovered in larger numbers from men with *Chlamydia*-negative NGU than from control subjects.[46–48] Supporting the hypothesis that these free-living agents (see Chapter 163) cause some cases of NGU is the observation that sulfa drugs or rifampin, to which the organisms are insensitive, fail to cure most patients with *Chlamydia*-negative NGU.[49,50] Conversely, spectinomycin, which is active against ureaplasmas but inactive against *Chlamydia*, cures patients with NGU from whom only *U. urealyticum* has been isolated.[49] Additional support comes from experiments in which two investigators inoculated themselves with ureaplasmas; both developed NGU.[51] Further, some patients with NGU show rises in IgM and IgG antibody titers against *U. urealyticum*.[52] *Mycoplasma hominis* is not a cause of NGU,[53,54] but a new mycoplasma, christened *M. genitalum*, has been recovered from a few patients with NGU[55] and shown to cause inflammation in the urethras of experimental animals.[56,57]

As with *Chlamydia*, the ureaplasmas are susceptible to erythromycin and, usually, tetracyclines—the agents that have been most successful in treating NGU. Some patients, however, are infected with tetracycline-resistant *U. urealyticum*[5,58–61]; about 20 percent of such patients are not cured by tetracycline therapy. Sixteen percent of men with NGU do not carry either *C. trachomatis* or *U. urealyticum*,[49,50,62,63] and it would not be surprising if other agents were in the future identified as causes of NGU. Patients with nonchlamydial, nonureaplasmal NGU have a higher recurrence rate after therapy than do men with chlamydial urethritis.[50,62,63]

Uncommon Causes of Nongonococcal Urethritis

Dysuria is described by 83 percent of women and 44 percent of men with primary herpes simplex genital infection. Some men notice a clear, mucoid discharge that seems disproportionately mild when compared with the amount of dysuria that they experience. Herpes simplex virus (HSV) is recovered from the urethras of about 80 percent of women and 30 percent of men with primary infection, and HSV must be regarded as a cause of some cases of NGU. Urethral involvement is less common in recurrent disease, and dysuria is described by only 27 percent of women and 9 percent of men.[64]

Trichomonas vaginalis has been isolated from 3–15 percent of the patients with NGU,[22,23,27] and it causes a small percentage of the cases. The syndrome is not clinically distinguishable from NGU of other etiologies, although the discharge often is so scant that it may be noticed only as a small bead at the meatus on arising in the morning.

Pre-existing urethral stricture, particularly in the presence of other infectious agents, may (it is said) produce a urethritis-like syndrome. Urethral infection with gram-negative rods can occur in patients with phimosis or with urethral trauma after instrumentation or indwelling catheterization.[65] Periurethral abscesses may occur in this setting. Somewhat fewer than 3 percent of the cases are due to infection higher up in the urinary tract. Syphilis, with an endourethral chancre, occasionally may be manifested as a urethral discharge. Intraurethral condylomata acuminata occasionally cause a urethral discharge.

A few investigators have attributed some cases of NGU to *Clostridium difficile, Branhamella catarrhalis, Haemophilus influenzae, Neisseria meningitidis*, corynebacteria, *Gardnerella vaginalis*, various anaerobes including bacteroides[66,67] and fusobacteria,[66,67] adenoviruses,[68] and shistosomes. These observations, however, are uncontrolled for the presence of such important pathogens as *C. trachomatis* and *U. urealyticum* and must be considered unproven. Indeed, other studies have recovered corynebacteria and *G. vaginalis* less frequently from patients with NGU than from asymptomatic controls.[26,46] Rhinosporidial infection produces a nonvenereal urethritis that is manifested as a friable, meatal mass and is seen primarily on the Indian subcontinent.[69]

POSTGONOCOCCAL URETHRITIS

Some patients who are correctly treated for acute gonococcal urethritis experience prompt resolution followed in a few days by a recurrence of symptoms—usually a mucoid or mucopurulent discharge and sometimes mild dysuria. Other patients may note that their symptoms never entirely disappeared and, after initial rapid improvement, stabilized at a low level. This syndrome is referred to as postgonococcal urethritis (PGU) and should be suspected if signs, symptoms, or laboratory evidence of urethritis is found 4–7 days after completing therapy for gonorrhea.[70,71] It is a manifestation of double urethral infection. The gonococcus and the agents of NGU are extremely prevalent in sexually active populations, and they are carried simultaneously and asymptomatically by many women. Male sexual partners of these women acquire both agents during the same sexual exposure. In the presence of gonorrhea, coincident NGU cannot be diagnosed by Gram stain. β-Lactam therapy eradicates the gonococci (eliminating the symptoms of gonorrhea), but it usually leaves the agents of NGU. When the incubation period of NGU is exceeded, the patient experiences a recurrence or persistance of milder symptoms that is consistent with the latter infection.

Although originally thought to result from the consumption of alcohol or other irritants during therapy for gonorrhea, PGU is now well established as a dual infection. *Chlamydia trachomatis* has been recovered from 11–50 percent of men with gonorrhea[43]; 75–100 percent of patients with gonorrhea who are also culture-positive for *Chlamydia* will develop PGU if their gonorrhea is treated with an agent that does not eradicate *Chlamydia*.[70–74] *Chlamydia trachomatis* can be recovered from almost 50 percent of the patients with PGU, which is similar to the recovery rate in NGU. Postgonococcal urethritis, however, also develops in 20–50 percent of the patients with gonorrhea, even if *Chlamydia* is also not recovered[70,71,73]; some of these cases appear to be associated with ureaplasmal infection.[71] As one might expect, if gonorrhea is treated with a regimen active against the agents of NGU, the incidence of PGU is lower.[74–76]

Patients suffering persistence or recurrence of urethral symptoms after therapy for acute gonococcal urethritis may indeed have PGU, but the physician also should remember the possibilities of gonococcal reinfection or frank treatment failure. The patient who is having recurrent urethritis must be treated like a new patient to differentiate gonococcal from nongonococcal infections.

ASYMPTOMATIC URETHRAL INFECTION

Many patients without specific complaints that are referable to the urethra will be found to have signs of urethritis on physical examination; sexually transmitted pathogens can be recovered from some patients who have neither symptoms nor signs of urethritis. Infected adolescents are less likely to complain of urethral symptoms than are adults.[77]

The importance of asymptomatic urethral gonococcal infection in men is well recognized.[78] Prolonged asymptomatic urethral carriage of gonococci occurs in about 2–3 percent of newly infected men[78]; however, since these men do not seek treatment, the prevalence of asymptomatic urethral infections in many populations is distinctly higher than 3 percent and may have considerable epidemiologic significance. Random screening of asymptomatic populations is unrewarding[78] except in high-risk populations.[79] Most cases of asymptomatic urethral infection are detected when gonorrhea is diagnosed in female sexual partners or if complications subsequently develop in the infected man. Asymptomatic urethral infection, therefore, is particularly prevalent among the male sexual partners of women who develop symptomatic complications of gonorrhea or where gonorrhea is detected by screening.[78] Up to 40 percent of the asymptomatic sexual partners of women with disseminated gonococcal infection or pelvic inflammatory disease are found to be infected[78]; 60 percent of the infected men may be asymptomatic. Asymptomatic urethral infection also is prevalent among men with the gonococcal dermatitis–arthritis syndrome.[78] Asymptomatic gonorrhea may be diagnosed by a Gram stain of urethral material collected on a swab with a sensitivity of about 70 percent.[78]

Part of the controversy over the etiologic role of *Ureaplasma urealyticum* is its recovery from 59 percent of sexually active, asymptomatic men attending venereal disease clinics.[26,46] *Chlamydia trachomatis* is recovered from about 3 percent of such men.[26,46] Most men harboring trichomonads are asymptomatic[22] and represent an important vector of infection.

Asymptomatic urethritis in many cases can be rapidly detected by observing PMNs in material recovered from the urethra with a swab or loop. About 25 percent of asymptomatic men with four or more PMNs per oil-immersion microscopic field were found to carry *C. trachomatis* in their urethras.[80]

Because of the frequency of asymptomatic, sexually transmitted urethral infections in men, asymptomatic sexual partners of infected women or homosexual men should always be evaluated. Since immediate diagnostic techniques are of relatively low sensitivity, such men should probably be treated at the time of their initial presentation (epidemiologic treatment).

URETHRAL SYMDROME AND RELATED DISEASES OF WOMEN

Dysuria, frequency, urgency, and nocturia are frequent symptoms of bacterial cystitis in women. A similar syndrome occurs in women who do not have classic bacterial infection of the lower urinary tract. Such women are said to have the acute urethral syndrome.[81] The usual work-up for bacterial urinary tract infection is unrewarding because fewer than 10^5 organisms are recovered from each milliliter of urine. The urine sediment contains PMNs, and the symptoms frequently respond to antimicrobial therapy. Some of these patients appear to suffer from bacterial cystitis, although bacteria are recovered from the urine in smaller than traditional numbers.[81,82] Other patients' symptoms, however, appear to be related to urethritis rather than to cystitis. *Escherichia coli* sometimes apparently causes urethritis in the absence of cystitis.[83] When ordinary bacterial pathogens associated with urinary tract infections are not isolated (even in small numbers), the condition appears to be due to sexually transmitted agents.[81,82]

Neisseria gonorrhoeae can affect the urethra in women as it does in men, and it occasionally causes the urethral syndrome.[84] Gently stripping the urethra may deliver a purulent discharge that with a Gram stain will reveal typical gram-negative, cell-associated diplococci. The Gram-stained smear from the female urethra has a sensitivity of about 50 percent for gonorrhea.[85] About three-quarters of these women also will have gonococci recoverable from the endocervix.[84] The syndrome responds to standard therapy for uncomplicated anogenital gonorrhea (see Chapter 190).

Chlamydia trachomatis is frequently recovered from women with dysuria, frequency, and pyuria.[81,82] Indeed, urinary tract symptoms are described by 53 percent of women from whom *C. trachomatis* is isolated from the urethra.[86,87] This association suggests that, in some cases, the urethral syndrome is the clinical manifestation of NGU in women. If such patients are initially treated with antimicrobial agents that are active against chlamydiae (e.g. tetracyclines, sulfonamides, sulfamethoxazole-trimethoprim [SMX-TMP]), their symptoms are likely to respond. Relapses, however, are frequent and may reflect reinfection from an asymptomatic male sexual partner. *Ureaplasma urealyticum* has not been statistically associated with the urethral syndrome[81,82,86–88] except among women with $>10^3$ organisms/ml and pyuria.[89] The acute urethral syndrome, which is associated with pyuria, must be differentiated from the chronic urethral syndrome. The latter is not associated with pyuria and responds poorly to antimicrobial therapy.[90–93] It may require traditional treatments such as dilation.[82]

Dysuria is a common complaint of women with trichomoniasis. The parasite is recovered from the urethra and periurethral glands of over 90 percent of women with the infestation (Chapter 258) and is associated with pyuria.[94] Dysuria also may result from vulvar irritation such as that accompanying vaginal candidiasis. It is far less common in patients with *G. vaginalis*-associated vaginitis.

The urethral syndrome has been treated with steroids[82] or

with surgery, particularly when it is seen in postmenopausal women. Among sexually active women, however, gonococcal infection should be ruled out; NGU or trichomoniasis should be considered before other therapies are tried.

Chlamydia trachomatis can be recovered from the endocervix of 45–90 percent of the sexual partners of infected men[31,42,78,95–97] and from the urethra alone in about 15–25 percent of these women.[86,94,98,99] Although infected women usually are asymptomatic, the organism is far from benign (see Chapter 158). Chlamydial infection can be documented in almost 50 percent of the women with hypertrophic or ulcerative cervicitis who are attending a VD clinic. Indeed, cervical abnormalities, often mild, may be seen in 80 percent of the women from whom *C. trachomatis* is recovered. *Chlamydia trachomatis* may be a cause of acute salpingitis and bartholinitis. In addition, babies born to infected women may develop chlamydial ophthalmia neonatorum or pneumonia, and asymptomatic women undoubtedly are a reservoir for recurrent NGU. The carriage of ureaplasmas has been linked to infertility, although the causal nature of the relationship is controversial.[53,54,100] These considerations support the routine treatment of female sexual partners of men with NGU.

COMPLICATIONS OF URETHRITIS

Both *Neisseria gonorrhoeae* and *Chlamydia trachomatis* have been identified as causes of acute epididymitis among sexually active men.[101,102] In 20–30 percent of the men with NGU prostatic involvement is documented; however, it is usually asymptomatic[5,103] and responds to standard treatments. The role of chlamydia in the development of clinical prostatitis remains controversial. The organism has been recovered from 2 to 56 percent of men with subacute or chronic prostatitis,[104–106] and the condition appears to respond to treatment with tetracyclines. The role of *Ureaplasma urealyticum* is even more controversial. The organism has been associated with prostatitis in some series[53,107] but not in others.[54] An association with male infertility and abnormal semen specimens has been described, but it also is regarded as controversial.[54,100,107] Stricture may follow gonococcal or nongonococcal urethritis. *Chlamydia trachomatis* can infect the conjunctiva (Chapter 158). Also, an oculogenital syndrome consisting of NGU and conjunctivitis may be seen in about 4 percent of the patients with NGU[108,109]; it responds to standard therapy with tetracyclines and must be differentiated from Reiter syndrome.

THERAPY

Specific forms of urethritis including chlamydial and ureaplasmal infections, gonorrhea, trichomoniasis, and syphilis should be treated as discussed in the appropriate chapters in Part III. As a syndrome, NGU has been treated with a variety of regimens, but a tetracycline (to which *C. trachomatis* and most *U. urealyticum* strains are both sensitive) probably is the drug of choice. Treatment for 7 days will cure 65–94 percent of the patients.[8,9,44,49,50,62,70,110–113] Although longer treatment for 14–21 days has been tried, there is little convincing evidence that full-dose regimens exceeding 7 days have any additional benefits.[42,63,111] Although in the interval immediately after therapy there may be some difference in relapse rate, after 6 weeks from the initiation of therapy, relapse rates appear to be about the same with therapy of either duration. Tetracycline hydrochloride may be administered in doses of 500 mg four times a day,[8,9,44,49,50,62,70,110–113] which appears superior to 250 mg four times a day.[111,113] The patient should be instructed to take the drug on an empty stomach and not accompanied by milk or antacids. Alternatively, doxycycline can be administered in a dose of 100 mg orally twice daily for 7 days.[114,115] This drug is highly effective and well tolerated by patients; however, its use is limited by cost and by an increased tendency to produce photosensitivity reactions. Minocycline has no apparent advantages over doxycycline, and it produces dizziness in many patients.[63,116]

Erythromycin is as effective as tetracycline,[8,117] and it may be of particular use in the pregnant patient for whom tetracycline is relatively contraindicated. It is active against tetracycline-resistent ureaplasmas.[5,61] Erythromycin has the additional theoretic advantage of producing higher prostatic levels than tetracycline hydrochloride does, and it may be of use in the retreatment of patients whose symptoms are relieved by tetracycline but return after therapy is completed. Such patients may have a prostatic focus of infection that is not cured by tetracycline.[8,118] A few anecdotal cases support this use of erythromycin. Gastrointestinal discomfort is an unfortunately common adverse effect of erythromycin therapy. Instead, patients who are not tolerating a dose of 500 mg four times daily for 7 days might be treated with 250 mg four times daily, a regimen that is almost as effective in NGU.[8,117]

Sulfa drugs (e.g., sulfisoxazole, 500 mg orally four times daily for 10 days) can be used to treat chlamydial NGU,[117] but they are ineffective in *Chlamydia*-negative infection.[49,115] Although SMX-TMP (two tablets twice daily) is more effective, it is not as good as tetracycline.[115,119]

Even if untreated, the symptoms of nongonococcal urethritis will resolve within 2 weeks in 14–30 percent of the patients[110,120]; up to 70 percent of the patients will have a complete resolution of symptoms within 6 months.[42] Resolution of symptoms does not, of course, mean that the infection is cured. Such asymptomatic patients may remain infected and infectious. Conversely, the inflammatory response accompanying NGU may take some time to resolve, even after the pathogens have been eliminated.[51]

During treatment, the symptoms of NGU frequently resolve before the patient has completed his therapy. Patients should be cautioned to complete the entire course of antibiotics since a relapse is considerably more common if therapy is aborted. To differentiate reliably a relapse from reinfection and to protect sexual partners, patients undergoing treatment for urethritis should refrain from coitus until post-treatment reexamination documents cure.

The treatment of women carrying the agents of NGU is the same as for men. Erythromycin may fail to eradicate ureaplasmas from the vagina, possibly in part because vaginal acidity interferes with the action of the drug.[59]

Because coincident chlamydial infection is very common in men with gonorrhea, the Centers for Disease Control have suggested that uncomplicated gonococcal urethritis should be treated with a combined regimen consisting of a single dose of a suitable β-lactam antibiotic followed by 7 days of tetracycline hydrochloride (500 mg orally four times daily), doxycycline hyclate (100 mg orally twice daily), or erythromycin (500 mg orally four times daily). This regimen has the advantage of providing effective single-dose therapy for gonorrhea and effective therapy for coincident, undiagnosed NGU.[121] Its disadvantages include increased cost, potential for adverse reactions, and the need to delay post-treatment tests of cure cultures for gonorrhea until after the completion of tetracycline therapy. The combination, however, may be of increasing importance because an increase in gonococcal resistance to tetracycline has been accompanied by a decreased effectiveness of tetracycline regimens for this disease. In the past, tetracycline regimens for NGU were at least 95 percent effective in uncomplicated gonococcal infections as well. At present, however, it probably is more prudent to use the combined regimen for urethritis of undetermined etiology. The failure of patients to complete a multidose tetracycline regimen has been a major concern, and it also influences the choice of therapy.[1,122]

Patients who are being treated for urethritis should be examined for other STDs and should be tested serologically for syphilis at the initial visit.

An initial work-up for trichomoniasis probably is not indicated in most routine settings since the infection accounts for only about 3–5 percent of the cases.[22] Additionally, direct microscopic examination of a urethral specimen usually is unrewarding unless the patient can be seen before first morning micturation. If the patient's urethritis has not been cured by previous antibacterial therapy or if symptoms or signs in the sexual partner suggest trichomonal infection, the patient's urine sediment can be examined as a wet mount or can be cultured on suitable media. Observation of motile trichomonads in the urine is an indication for therapy.

Patients treated for gonorrhea should return at least 3 days after completing therapy and should have a urethral specimen recultured to document cure because insufficient therapy may eliminate the symptoms without eradicating the pathogen in up to 50 percent of patients.[123] Men treated for nongonococcal urethritis should be reexamined to document the disappearance of urethral inflammation. One should probably wait for several weeks after completion of therapy before performing a test of cure for chlamydial infection. The sensitivity of the immunofluorescence or ELISA technique in this setting is undefined.

Patients initially treated for NGU whose symptoms are not eliminated by tetracycline should be suspected of having infection with *Trichomonas* or tetracycline-resistant *Ureaplasma*.[5,58,59,61] Because these infections may be impossible to differentiate clinically, such patients may be empirically treated with a single 2 g dose of metronidazole followed by erythromycin, 500 mg orally four times daily for 7 days. It is, of course, important that their sexual partners be treated with the same regimen.

Some men report that their urethral symptoms disappeared while they were taking tetracycline but reappeared days to weeks after completing therapy. Such recurrences are seen in about 20 percent of patients with chlamydial NGU and in about 40 percent of patients with nonchlamydial infection. Among NGU patients from whom neither chlamydiae nor ureaplasmas are isolated, the recurrence rate is greater than 50 percent.[50,62,63] Eighty percent of recurrent NGU occurs in patients in whom neither organism is initially recovered,[63] and 70–80 percent of men with recurrent NGU are culture-negative for both organisms at the time of recurrence.[85]

Men with recurrent disease should be questioned closely about the possibility of reexposure, and attention should be given to ensuring simultaneous treatment of all sexual partners. If reexposure is likely, the patient may be retreated with the initial tetracycline regimen. If the patient has not been reexposed, a recurrence of urethritis suggests the possibility that some pathogens remained in a relatively antibiotic protected site. Such men are sometimes cured by retreating them with a 3- to 6-week course of tetracycline.[85,124,125] Prostatic involvement is common in NGU. It is possible that some men may have a prostatic focus of infection that is not eradicated by treatment with tetracycline because it penetrates rather poorly into the prostate gland.[62] Men with repeated relapses occasionally are successfully treated with a 3- to 6-week course of doxycycline or erythromycin, which are active against *Chlamydia* and *Ureaplasma* and achieve better prostatic levels than does tetracycline hydrochloride. Patients whose relapses are not eliminated by these maneuvers should be referred for urologic evaluation to rule out anatomic abnormalities.[118,124] Such men most likely are not infected with *Chlamydia* or *Ureaplasma*. About one-quarter will be found to have a partial obstruction to urine flow, and about half of these will have urethral strictures.[118] They and their sexual partners do not appear to be at significant risk for complications.[125] Long-term antimicrobial suppression is useful in this setting.[125]

Sexual partners of patients with sexually transmitted urethritis should be treated simultaneously. Asymptomatic male sexual partners of women known to have gonorrhea or trichomoniasis should be treated even if direct microscopic examinations are negative. Sexual partners of men with gonococcal, nongonococcal, or trichomonal urethritis should be treated at the initial visit. A woman who has been the sexual partner of a man with urethritis of undetermined etiology should be treated with a regimen that is effective against gonococci, chlamydiae, and ureaplasmas. The combined β-lactam/tetracycline regimen described above is suitable in nonpregnant women. Erythromycin may be substituted for tetracycline in pregnancy.

REITER SYNDROME

Some cases of nongonococcal urethritis appear as one element of Reiter syndrome, which also includes arthritis, uveitis, and often, lesions of the skin and mucous membranes. The syndrome complicates 1–2 percent of the cases of NGU[124,126–128] and is felt to be the most common peripheral inflammatory arthritis in young men.[129] Its pathogenesis is unclear, but it probably represents an abnormal host response to any of a number of infections.[130] The idiosyncratic nature of the host's response is supported by a strong correlation between the development of Reiter syndrome and the presence of the HLA-B27 histocompatibility antigen. This antigen has been found in 60–96 percent of the patients with Reiter syndrome,[128,129,131,132] and it also has been related to uveitis and sacroileitis.[128] Although possibly providing a clue to pathogenesis, its diagnostic value has been questioned.[133]

The inciting infection is of two types. Reiter syndrome may follow sexually transmitted urethritis, and most cases in North American and Europe seem to occur in sexually active young people.[134,135] Many cases occur after contact with a new partner, and some cases have been epidemiologically linked.[128,136] In one series, 9 percent of cases followed gonococcal urethritis, although 50 percent of these patients subsequently developed PGU.[137] *Chlamydia trachomatis* has been impicated in the pathogenesis of Reiter syndrome[138] since it has been recovered from the urethras of 16–44 percent of the patients with Reiter syndrome and from 69 percent of those men who had signs of urogenital inflammation at the time of examination.[135,139,140] In addition, antibodies to *Chlamydia* have been detected in 46–67 percent and cell-mediated immunity in 72 percent of patients with Reiter syndrome.[130,140,141] Chlamydial antigens have been identified in synovial membranes,[142] and chlamydial elementary bodies have been observed in joint fluid[143] in a few patients. The significance of these recent observations is not yet defined, but the failure of antichlamydial therapy to influence the course of disease argues against it.

Reiter syndrome also follows bacterial gastroenteritis and has been described after infection with *Salmonella, Shigella, Yersinia,* and *Campylobacter*[127–129,131,137,144–148] and after antibiotic-associated colitis.[149] Postdysenteric Reiter syndrome has occurred in 0.24–1.50 percent of the patients after epidemics of gastrointestinal infection[145,147]; it is considerably more common among patients who are HLA-B27–positive. Antibodies reacting with *Yersinia* proteins occur in the sera of many patients with Reiter syndrome.[150]

Clinically, Reiter syndrome after genital infection is indistinguishable from that following bacterial gastroenteritis; indeed, 12–80 percent of the patients with postdysenteric Reiter syndrome have genital symptoms.[128,151] The age- and sex-specific attack rates, however, are different; 94–99 percent of the cases of Reiter syndrome after sexually transmitted infections occur in men. However, a much larger fraction—up to 10 percent—of the cases of postdysenteric Reiter syndrome occur in women.[134,147,152,153] It also is reported in sexually inactive children.[134,146]

Clinical Features

Nongonococcal urethritis is the initial manifestation in 80 percent of the patients.[128,129] As with other forms of nongonococcal urethritis, it usually occurs 7–14 days after sexual exposure.[128] The urethritis may be mild and may be unnoticed by the patient,[127] and it may be detectable only by physical examination performed before the first micturation. Gonococcal urethritis sometimes sets the stage for Reiter syndrome.[137] The discharge may be purulent or mucopurulent, and patients may or may not complain of dysuria. Accompanying prostatitis has been described by some authors.[127,129,151,153] If present, it usually is asymptomatic. Cystitis without urethritis is also reported and may be a common manifestation, particularly in women.[151] Cervicitis is associated with Reiter syndrome[154] and may represent female genital infection with the inciting microorganism.

The other features of Reiter syndrome develop 1–5 weeks after the onset of urethritis.[151] Arthritis begins within 4 weeks of the onset of urethritis in four-fifths of patients,[127,128] but it precedes urethritis in about 15 percent.[134] The knees are the most frequently involved, followed by the ankles and small joints of the feet. Sacroileitis, either symmetric[151] or more frequently asymmetric,[134,146,153] may develop later in up to two-thirds of patients.[151] It is more frequent in patients with the HLA-B27 antigen.[146] Ankylosing spondylitis, which occurs in only about 1 percent of the general population, complicates one-quarter to one-third of the cases of Reiter syndrome[128,132,146,155]; also, back pain is reported by 60 percent of all patients.[129] Ninety percent of patients with the HLA-B27 antigen who develop Reiter syndrome develop ankylosing spondylitis,[155,156] which is rare in patients without the antigen.[156] Spurring of the calcaneus may be seen in up to one-quarter of the patients with Reiter syndrome[134,153] and may produce heel pain. A dactylitis resulting in sausage-shaped swelling of the digits is also characteristic.[134] Arthritis is the most persistent feature of the syndrome and may last for 2–6 months after other manifestations have disappeared.[134,151]

Mild bilateral conjunctivitis, iritis, or uveitis is sometimes present but often lasts for only a few days.[127,151,153,157] It is occasionally accompanied by a purulent discharge or frank keratitis.[151,157] Unlike the conjunctivitis caused by direct infection with *Chlamydia trachomatis*, the inflamed conjunctivae in Reiter syndrome do not manifest follicular hypertrophy.

Dermatologic manifestations affect 50 percent of the patients.[127–129] The initial lesions are waxy papules, which often display a central yellow spot and occur most frequently on the soles and palms[151] and with decreasing frequency on the nails, scrotum, scalp, and trunk.[127] The papules epithelialize and thicken to produce keratoderma blenorrhagicum in about 10–25 percent of the patients.[129,154] Circinate balanitis is usually painless and occurs in about 25–40 percnet of all patients.[128,129,151] Circinate and ulcerative vulvitis also are described.[158] Painless erosions on the dorsum of the tongue and fauces occur most commonly with the initial episode and less frequently with recurrences.[153,154]

Incomplete Reiter syndrome consisting of urethritis and arthritis or arthritis alone has been reported.[129,144,159]

The initial episode of Reiter syndrome usually lasts for 2–6 months, but episodes lasting for 1 year have been described.[129,151,153] Most patients feel completely well after the attack subsides, but the disease recurs in 35–70 percent of the patients[128,129,134,153,155] at a rate of about 15 percent in each 5-year period after the initial attack.[160] During recurrences, the genital symptoms are usually less marked and may be entirely absent.[161,162] About 60–80 percent of the patients will have active disease 15–20 years after the initial episode,[125,129,132,155,160] with the risk of residuals being somewhat higher among patients with the HLA-B27 antigen.[163] Almost 50 percent of the affected patients develop some degree of permanent disability.[132,155]

Rare complications of Reiter syndrome include pericarditis,[154] myocarditis,[151] first-degree atrioventricular block,[153,164] and aortic insufficiency.[132,153] Thrombophlebitis, radiculitis,[154] and myelopathy[165] are occasionally described.

Laboratory Features

Anemia is common,[129] and the erythrocyte sedimentation rate is elevated in about 50 percent of the patients.[134,154] Fluid recovered at the same time from different joints is often different.[151] Synovial fluid may contain 1000–200,000 white blood cells, more than two-thirds of which are PMNs.[151] Complement levels in the fluid are generally elevated, which allows differentiation from rheumatoid arthritis,[146] and the glucose is low in about 50 percent of the joints.[151] Synovial biopsy specimens reveal infiltration by PMNs.[154]

Therapy

Treatment of Reiter syndrome is quite controversial. Because of the possibility that the inciting infection may be sexually transmitted NGU, treatment with tetracycline for 7 days is recommended[127,154] and has been said by some to reduce or eliminate the urethritis.[166] Others, however, have seen no effect on the arthritis or on the overall course of the disease.[154–161] The relative safety of oral tetracycline and the frequency with which chalmydiae are isolated from patients with Reiter syndrome makes a course of tetracycline reasonable.

Nonsteroidal anti-inflammatory drugs, particularly phenylbutazone given as 400–600 mg/day in divided doses, probably is the most effective treatment.[129] Indomethacin or tolmetin are favored by some workers,[167] and all of these are superior to salicylates or corticosteroids. Cytotoxic agents may be of value in recalcitrant cases.[167]

REFERENCES

1. Braun P, Sherman H, Komaroff AL. Urethritis in men: Benefits, risks, and costs of alternative strategies of management. Sex Transm Dis. 1982;9:188.
2. Amarasuriya KL. Haematuria presenting in outpatients attending a department of genitourinary medicine. Br J Vener Dis. 1979;55:214.
3. Swartz SL. Diagnosis of nongonococcal urethritis. In: Hobson D, Holmes KK, eds. Nongonococcal Urethritis and Related Infections. Lake Placid, NY: American Society for Microbiology; 1976:15.
4. Bowie WR. Comparison of the Gram stain and first-voided urine sediment in the diagnosis of urethritis. Sex Transm Dis. 1978;5:39.
5. Root TE, Edwards LD, Spengler PJ. Nongonococcal urethritis: A survey of clinical and laboratory features. Sex Trasnm Dis. 1980;7:59.
6. Swartz SL, Kraus SJ, Herrmann KL, et al. Diagnosis and etiology of nongonococcal urethritis. J Infect Dis. 1978;138:445.
7. Desai K, Robson HG. Comparison of the Gram-stained urethral smear and first-voided urine sediment in the diagnosis of nongonococcal urethritis. Sex Transm Dis. 1982;9:21.
8. Scheibel JH, Kristensen JK, Hentzler B, et al. Treatment of chlamydial urethritis in men and *Chlamydia trachomatis* positive female partners: Comparison of erythromycin and tetracycline in treatment courses of one week. Sex Transm Dis. 1982;9:128.
9. Stamm WE, Koutsky LA, Benedetti JK, et al. *Chlamydia trachomatis* urethral infections in men: Prevalence, risk factors, and clinical manifestations. Ann Intern Med. 1984;100:47.
10. Perera SA. Use of the Kova-Slide II with grid and uncentrifuged segmented urine specimens in the diagnosis of nongonococcal urethritis: A quantitative technique. Sex Transm Dis. 1985;12:14.
11. Veeravahu M, Smyth RW, Clay JC. Detection of leukocyte esterase in urine: A new screening test for nongonococcal urethritis compared with two microscopic methods. Sex Transm Dis. 1987;14:180.
12. Perera SAB, Jones C, Srikantha V, et al. Leukocyte esterase test as rapid screen for non-gonococcal urethritis. Genitourin Med. 1987;63:380–3.
13. Simmons PD. Evaluation of the early morning smear investigation. Br J Vener Dis. 1978;54:128.
14. Willcox JR, Adler MW, Belsey EM. Observer variation in the interpretation of Gram stained urethral smears. Br J Vener Dis. 1981;57:134.
15. Jacobs NF, Kraus SJ. Gonococcal and nongonococcal urethritis in men: Clinical and laboratory differentiation. Ann Intern Med. 1975;82:7.
16. Kraus SJ. Semiquantitation of urethral polymorphonuclear leukocytes as objective evidence of nongonococcal urethritis. Sex Transm Dis. 1982;9:52.
17. Goodhart ME, Ogden J, Zaidi AA, et al. Factors affecting the performance of smear and culture tests for the detection of *Neisseria gonorrhoeae*. Sex Transm Dis. 1982;9:63.
18. Kleris GS, Arnold AJ. Differential diagnosis of urethritis: Predictive value and therapeutic implications of the urethral smear. Sex Transm Dis. 1981;8:110.

19. Janda WH, Jackson T. Evaluation of Gonodecton for the presumptive diagnosis of gonococcal urethritis in men. J Clin Microbiol. 1985;21:143.
20. Prior RB, Spagna VA. Improved utility of Gonoscreen, a limulus amoebocyte lysate assay, in the evaluation of urethral discharges in men. J Clin Microbiol. 1985;22:141.
21. Judson FN, Werness BA, Shahan MR. Lack of utility of a limulus amoebocyte lysate assay in the diagnosis of urethral discharges in men. J Clin Microbiol. 1985;21:152.
22. Krieger JN. Urologic aspects of trichomoniasis. Invest Urol. 1981;18:412.
23. Kuberski T. *Trichomonas vaginalis* associated with nongonococcal urethritis and prostatitis. Sex Transm Dis. 1981;7:135.
24. Adger H, Shafer MA, Sweet RL, et al. Screening for *Chlamydia trachomatis* and *Neisseria gonorrhoeae* in adolescent males: Value of first catch urine examination. Lancet. 1984;2:944.
25. Chernsky MA, Mahony JB, Castriciano S, et al. Detection of *Chlamydia trachomatis* antigens by enzyme immunoassay and immunofluorescence in genital specimens from symptomatic and asymptomatic men and women. J Infect Dis. 1986;154:41.
26. Bowie WR, Pollock HM, Forsyth PS, et al. Bacteriology of the urethra in normal men and men with nongonococcal urethritis. J Clin Microbiol. 1977;6:482.
27. Wong JL, Hines PA, Brasher MD. The etiology of nongonococcal urethritis in men attending a venereal disease clinic. Sex Transm Dis. 1977;4:4.
28. Bacci M. Masturbation injury resulting from intraurethral introduction of spaghetti. Am J Forensic Med Pathol. 1986;7:254.
29. Rogers WB. Shampoo urethritis. Am J Dis Child. 1985;139:748.
30. McCutchen JA. Epidemiology of venereal urethritis: Comparison of gonorrhea and nongonococcal urethritis. Rev Infect Dis. 1984;6:669.
31. Judson FN. Epidemiology and control of nongonococcal urethritis and genital chlamydial infections: A revoew. Sex Transm Dis. 1981;8:117.
32. Wright RA, Judson FN. Relative and seasonal incidences of the sexually transmitted diseases: A two-year statistical review. Br J Vener Dis. 1978;54:433.
33. McChesney JA, Zedd A, King H, et al. Acute urethritis in male college students. JAMA. 1973;226:37.
34. Smith GL, Greenup R, Takafuji ET. Circumcision as a risk factor for urethritis in racial groups. Am J Public Health. 1987;77:452.
35. Boyd JT, Csonka GW, Oates JK. Epidemiology of nonspecific urethritis. Br J Vener Dis. 1958;34:40.
36. Holmes KK. Gonococcal infection: Clinical, epidemiologic and laboratory perspectives. Adv Intern Med. 1974;19:259.
37. Schofield CBS. Some factors affecting the incubation period and duration of symptoms of urethritis in men. Br J Vener Dis. 1982;58:184.
38. Harrison WO, Hooper R, Wiesner PJ, et al. Minocycline given after exposure to prevent gonorrhea. N Engl J Med. 1979;300:1074.
39. Rothenberg R, Judson FN. The clinical diagnosis of urethral discharge. Sex Transm Dis. 1983;10:24.
40. Lee Y-H, Rosner B, Alpert S, et al. Clinical and microbiological investigation of men with urethritis. J Infect Dis. 1978;158:798.
41. Volk J, Kraus SJ. Nongonococcal urethritis: A venereal disease as prevalent as epidemic gonorrhea. Arch Intern Med. 1974;134:511.
42. Oriel JD. Treatment of nongonococcal urethritis. In: Hobson D, Holmes KK, eds. Nongonococcal Urethritis and Related Infections. Lake Placid, NY: American Society for Microbiology; 1976:38.
43. Johannisson G, Lowhagin GB, Nilsson S. *Chlamydia trachomatis* and urethritis in men. Scand J Infect Dis. [Suppl] 1982;32:87.
44. Handsfield HH, Alexander ER, Wang S-P, et al. Differences in the therapeutic response of chlamydia-positive and chlamydia-negative forms of nongonococcal urethritis. J Am Vener Dis Assoc. 1976;2:5.
45. Jacobs NF, Arum ES, Kraus SJ. Nongonococcal urethritis: The role of *Chlamydia trachomatis*. Ann Intern Med. 1977;86:313.
46. Bowie WR, Wang SP, Alexander ER, et al. Etiology of non-gonococcal urethritis: Evidence for *Chlamydia trachomatis* and *Ureaplasma urealyticum*. J Clin Invest. 1977;59:735.
47. Viarengo J, Hebrant F, Piot P. *Ureaplasma urealyticum* in urethra of healthy men. Br J Vener Dis. 1980;56:169.
48. Hunter JM, Smith IW, Peutherer JF, et al. *Chlamydia trachomatis* and *Ureaplasma urealyticum* in men attending a sexually transmitted diseases clinic. Br J Vener Dis. 1981;57:130.
49. Bowie WR, Floyd JF, Miller Y, et al. Differential response of chlamydial and ureaplasma-associated urethritis to sulfafurazole (sulfisoxazole) and aminocyclitols. Lancet. 1976;2:1276.
50. Coufalike ED, Taylor-Robinson D, Csonka GW. Treatment of nongonococcal urethritis or the rifampicin as a means of defining the role of *Ureaplasma urealyticum*. Br J Vener Dis. 1979;55:36.
51. Taylor-Robinson D, Csonka GW, Prentice MJ. Human intraurethral inoculation of ureaplasmas. Q J Med. 1977;46:309.
52. Brown MB, Cassel GH, Taylor-Robinson D. Measurement of antibody to *Ureaplasma urealyticum* by an enzyme-linked immunoassay and detection of antibody responses in patients with nongonococcal urethritis. J Clin Microbiol. 1983;17:288.
53. Cassell GH, Cole BC. Mycoplasmas as agents of human disease. N Engl J Med. 1981;304:80.
54. Taylor-Robinson D, McCormack WM. The genital mycoplasmas. N Engl J Med. 1980;302:1003,1063.
55. Tully JG, Cole RM, Taylor-Robinson D, et al. A newly discovered mycoplasma in the human urogenital tract. Lancet. 1981;1:1288.
56. Taylor-Robinson D, Furr PM, Hetherington CM. The pathogenicity of a newly discovered human mycoplasma (Strain G37) for the genital tract of marmosets. J Hug (Lond). 1982;89:449.
57. Taylor-Robinson D, Tully JG, Barile MF. Urethral infection in male chimpanzees produced experimentally by *Mycoplasma genitalium*. Br J Exp Pathol. 1985;66:95.
58. Magalhaes M. Persistent nongonococcal urethritis associated with a minocycline-resistant strain of *Ureaplasma urealyticum*. Sex Transm Dis. 1983;10:151.
59. Arya OP, Pratt BC. Persistent urethritis due to *Ureaplasma urealyticum* in conjugal or stable partnerships. Genitourin Med. 1986;62:329.
60. Magalhaes M, Veras A. Minocycline resistance among clinical isolates of *Ureaplasma urealyticum*. J Infect Dis. 1984;149:117.
61. Stimson JB, Hale J, Bowie WK, et al. Tetracycline-resistant *Ureaplasma urealyticum*: A cause of persistent nongonococcal urethritis. Ann Intern Med. 1981;94:192.
62. Bowie WR. Urethritis and infections of the lower urogenital tract. Urol Clin North Am. 1980;7:17.
63. Bowie WR, Alexander ER, Stimson JB, et al. Therapy for non-gonococcal urethritis: double blind, randomized-comparison of two doses and two durations of minocycline. Ann Intern Med. 1981;95:306.
64. Corey L, Adams HG, Brown ZA, et al. Genital herpes simplex virus infection: Clinical manifestations, course, and complications. Ann Intern Med. 1983;98:958.
65. Nacey JN, Tulloch AGS, Ferguson AF. Catheter-induced urethritis: A comparison between latex and silicone catheters in a prospective clinical trial. Br J Urol. 1985;57:325.
66. Fontaine EAR, Bryant TN, Taylor-Robinson D, et al. A numerical toxonomic study of anaerobic gram-negative bacilli classified as *Bacteroides ureolyticus* isolated from patients with nongonococcal urethritis. J Gen Microbiol. 1986;132:3137.
67. Fontaine EA, Borriello SP, Taylor-Robinson D, et al. Characteristics of a gram negative anaerobe isolated from men with nongonococcal urethritis. J Med Microbiol. 1984;17:129.
68. Harnett GB, Phillips PA, Gollors MM. Association of genital adenovirus infection with urethritis in men. Med J Aust. 1984;141:337.
69. Sasidharan K, Subramonian P, Moni VN, et al. Urethral rhinosporidiosis. Analysis of 27 cases. Br J Urol. 1987;59:66.
70. Arya OP, Mallinson H, Pareek SS, et al. Postgonococcal cervicitis and postgonococcal urethritis: A study of their epidemiologic correlation and the role of *chlamydia trachomatis* in their etiology. Br J Vener Dis. 1981;57:395.
71. Bowie WR, Alexander ER, Holmes KK. Etiologies of post-gonococcal urethritis in homosexual and heterosexual men: Roles of *Chlamydia trachomatis* and *Ureaplasma urealyticum*. Sex Transm Dis. 1978;5:151.
72. Terho P. *Chlamydia trachomatis* in gonococcal and non-gonococcal urethritis. Br J Vener Dis. 1978;54:326.
73. Oriel JD, Ridgway GL, Reeve P, et al. The lack of effect of ampicillin plus probenecid given for genital infections with *Neusseria gonorrhoeae* on associated infections with *Chlamydia trachomatis*. J Infect Dis. 1976;133:568.
74. Stamm WE, Guinan ME, Johnson C, et al. Effect of treatment regimens for *Neisseria gonorrhoeae* on simultaneous infection with *Chlamydia trachomatis*. N Engl J Med. 1984;310:545.
75. Patrone P, Negosanti M, Ghetti P, et al. A combined treatment in prevention of postgonococcal urethritis. Dermatologica. 1984;168:300.
76. Holmes KK, Johnson DW, Floyd TM, et al. Studies of venereal disease: II observations on the incidence, etiology, and treatment of the postgonococcal urethritis syndrome. JAMA. 1967;202:467.
77. Chambers CV, Shafer M-A, Adger H, et al. Microflora of the urethra in adolescent boys: Relationships to sexual activity and nongonococcal urethritis. J Pediatr. 1987;110:314.
78. Handsfield HH, Lipman TO, Harnisch JP, et al. Asymptomatic gonorrhea in men: Diagnosis, natural course, prevalence, and significance. N Engl J Med. 1974;290:117.
79. Smith JA, Linder CW, Jay MS, et al. Isolation of *Neisseria gonorrhoeae* from the urethra of asymptomatic adolescent males. Clin Pediatr (Phila). 1986;25:566.
80. Swartz SL, Kraus SJ. Persistent urethral leukocytosis and asymptomatic chlamydial urethritis. J Infect Dis. 1979;140:614.
81. Stamm WE. Etiology and management of the acute urethral syndrome. Sex Transm Dis. 1981;8:235.
82. Stamm WE, Wagner KF, Amsel R, et al. Causes of the acute urethral syndrome in women. N Engl J Med. 1980;303:409.
83. Fihn SD, Johnson C, Stamm WE. *Escherichia coli* urethritis in women with symptoms of acute urinary tract infection. J Infect Dis. 1988;1:196.
84. Curran JW. Gonorrhea and the urethral syndrome. Sex Transm Dis. 1977;4:119.
85. Goh BT, Varia KB, Aylifte PF, et al. Diagnosis of gonorrhea by gram stained smears and cultures in men and women: Role of the urethral smear. Sex Transm Dis. 1985;12:135.
86. Paavonen J. *Chlamydia trachomatis*-induced urethritis in female partners of men with nongonococcal urethritis. Sex Transm Dis. 1979;6:69.
87. Paavonen J, Vesterinen E. *Chlamydia trachomatis* in cervicitis and urethritis in women. Scand J Infect Dis [Suppl]. 1982;32:45.
88. Hunter JM, Young H, Harris AB. Genitourinary infection with *Ureaplasma*

urealyticum in women attending a sexually transmitted disease clinic. Br J Vener Dis. 1981;57:338.
89. Stamm WE, Running K, Hale J, et al. Etiologic role of *Mycoplasma hominis* and *Ureaplasma urealyticum* in women with the acute urethral syndrome. Sex Transm. Dis. 1983;10:318.
90. Fihn SD, Stamm WE. The urethral syndrome. Semin Urol. 1983;1:121.
91. Latham RH, Stamm WE. Urethral syndrome in women. Urol Clin North Am. 1984;11:95.
92. Scotti RJ, Ostergard DR. The urethral syndrome. Clin Obstet Gynecol. 1984;27:515.
93. Bump RC, Copeland WE Jr. Urethral isolation of the genital mycoplasmas and *Chlamydia trachomatis* in women with chronic urologic complaints. Am J Obstet Gynecol. 1985;152:38.
94. Feldman RG, Johnson AL, Schober PC, et al. Aetiology of urinary symptoms in sexually active women. Genitourin Med. 1986;62:333.
95. Ghadirian FD, Robson HG. *Chlamydia trachomatis* genital infections. Br J Vener Dis. 1979;55:415.
96. Paavonen J, Karsa M, Sackku P, et al. Examination of men with nongonococcal urethritis and their sexual partners for *Chlamydia trachomatis* and *Ureaplasma urealyticum*. Sex Transm Dis. 1978;5:93.
97. Thelin I, Mardh P-A. Contact tracing in genital chlamydial infection. Scand J Infect Dis. [Suppl]. 1982;32:163.
98. Johannisson G, Lowhagen G-B, Lycke E. Genital *Chlamydia trachomatis* infection in women. Obstet Gynecol. 1980;56:671.
99. Wallin JE, Thompson SE, Zaidi A, et al. Urethritis in women attending an STD clinic. Br J Vener Dis. 1981;57:50.
100. Toth A, Lesser ML, Brooks C, et al. Subsequent pregnancies among 161 couples treated for T-mycoplasma genital-tract infection. N Engl J Med. 1983;308:505.
101. Berger RE. Acute epididymitis. Sex Transm Dis. 1981;8:286.
102. Berger RE, Alexander ER, Harnish JP, et al. Etiology and therapy of acute epididymitis: Prospective study of 50 cases. J Urol. 1979; 121:750.
103. Holmes KK, Handsfield HH, Wang S-P, et al. Etiology of nongonococcal urethritis. N Engl J Med. 1975;292:1199.
104. Bruce AW, Chadwick P, Willett WS, et al. The role of chlamydiae in genitourinary disease. J Urol. 1982;126:625.
105. Mardh PA, Ripa KT, Colleen S, et al. Role of *Chlamydia trachomatis* in nonacute prostatitis. Br J Vener Dis. 1978;54:330.
106. Nilsson S, Johannisson G, Lycke E. Isolation of *Chlamydia trachomatis* from the urethra and from prostatic fluid in men with signs and symptoms of acute urethritis. Acta Derm Venereol (Stockh). 1981;61:456.
107. Cassell GH, Younger JB, Brown MB, et al. Microbiologic study of infertile women at the time of diagnostic laparoscopy: Association of *Ureaplasma urealyticum* with a defined subpopulation. N Engl J Med. 1983;308:502.
108. Mordhorst CH. Clinical epidemiology of oculogenital chlamydial infections. In: Hobson D, Holmes KK, eds. Nongonococcal Urethritis and Related Infections. Lake Placid, NY: American Society for Microbiology; 1976:126.
109. Ronnerstam R, Persson K. Chlamydial eye infections in adults. Scand J Infect Dis [Suppl]. 1982;32:111.
110. Holmes KK, Johnson DW, Floyd TM. Studies of venereal disease: III. Double-blind comparison of tetracycline hydrochloride and placebo in treatment of nongonococcal urethritis. JAMA. 1967;201:474.
111. Arya OP, Alergant CD, Annels EH, et al. Management of nonspecific urethritis in men: Evaluation of six treatment regimens and effect of other factors including alcohol and sexual intercourse. Br J Vener Dis. 1978;54:414.
112. Thambar IV, Simmons PD, Thin RN, et al. Double-blind comparison of two regimens in the treatment of nongonococcal urethritis: Seven-day vs 21-day courses of triple tetracycline (Deteclo). Br J Vener Dis. 1979;55:284.
113. Bowie WR, Yu JS, Fawcett A, et al. Tetracycline in nongonococcal urethritis. Comparison of 2 g and 1 g daily for seven days. Br J Vener Dis. 1980;56:332.
114. Juvakowski T, Lauharanta J, Kanerva L, et al. One-week treatment of chlamydia-positive urethritis with doxycycline and tetracycline chloride in males. Acta Derm Venereol (Stockh). 1981;61:273.
115. Lassus A, Juvakoski T. Treatment of uncomplicated genital *Chlamydia trachomatis* infections in males. Scand J Infect Dis [Suppl]. 1982;32:169.
116. Oriel JD, Ridgway GL. Comparison of tetracycline and minocycline in the treatment of nongonococcal urethritis. Br J Vener Dis. 1983;59:245.
117. Bowie WR, Manzon LM, Borrie-Hume CJ. Efficacy of treatment regimens for lower urogenital *Chlamydia trachomatis* infection of women. Am J Obstet Gynecol. 1982;142:125.
118. Krieger JN, Hooton TM, Brust PJ, et al. Evaluation of chronic urethritis: Defining the role for endoscopic procedures. Arch Intern Med. 1988;148:703.
119. Willcox RR, Sparrow RW. Cotrimoxazole in the treatment of nongonococcal urethritis. Acta Derm Venereol (Stockh). 1974;54:317.
120. Willcox RR. "Triple tetracycline" in the treatment of nongonococcal urethritis in males. Br J Vener Dis. 1972;48:137.
121. Centers for Disease Control. Sexually transmitted diseases treatment guidelines, 1985. MMWR. 1985;34(Suppl 4):1.
122. Jordan WC. Doxycycline vs tetracycline in the treatment of men with gonorrhea: The compliance factor. Sex Transm Dis. 1981;8:105.
123. Schmid GP, Johnson RE, Brenner ER, et al. Symptomatic response to therapy of men with gonococcal urethritis: Do all need posttreatment cultures? Sex Transm Dis. 1987;14:37.
124. Kaufman RE, Wiesner PJ. Current concepts: Nonspecific urethritis. N Engl J Med. 1974;291:1175.
125. Berger RE. Recurrent nongonococcal urethritis. JAMA. 1983;249:409.
126. Csonka GW. Course of Reiter's disease. Br Med J. 1958;1:1088.
127. Morton RS. Reiter's disease. Practitioner. 1972;209:631.
128. Keat A. Reiter's syndrome and reactive arthritis in perspective. N Engl J Med. 1983;309:1606.
129. Arnett FC Jr. Reiter's syndrome. Johns Hopkins Med J. 1982;150:39.
130. Ford DK, daRoza DM, Schulzer M. The specificity of synovial mononuclear cell-responses to microbiological antigens in Reiter's syndrome. J Rheumatol. 1982;9:561.
131. Lehman DH. Postdysenteric Reiter's syndrome. West J Med. 1977;126:405.
132. Sairanen E, Paronen I, Mahonen H. Reiter's syndrome: A followup study. Acta Med Scand. 1969;185:57.
132. Kahn M, Kahn M. Diagnostic value of HLA-B27 testing in ankylosing spondylitis and Reiter's syndrome. Ann Intern Med. 1982;96:70.
134. Hawkes JG. Clinical and diagnostic features of Reiter's disease: A followup study of 39 patients. NZ Med J. 1973;78:347.
135. Kousa M, Saikku P, Richmond S, et al. Frequent association of chlamydial infection with Reiter's syndrome. Sex Transm Dis. 1978;5:57.
136. Rustin MHA, Wedzicha JA, Keat AC, et al. Sexually transmitted arthritis? Two informative cases. J Rheumatol. 1982;9:646.
137. Leirisalo M, Skylv G, Kousa M, et al. Followup study on patients with Reiter's disease and reactive arthritis with special reference to HLA-B27. Arthritis Rheum. 1982;25:249.
138. Editorial. Is Reiter's syndrome caused by chlamydia? Lancet. 1985;1:317.
139. Keat AC, Thomas BJ, Taylor-Robinson D, et al. Evidence of *Chlamydia trachomatis* infection in sexually acquired reactive arthritis. Ann Rheum Dis. 1980;39:431.
140. Kousa M. Evidence of chlamydial involvement in the development of arthritis. Scand J Infect Dis [Suppl]. 1982;32:116.
141. Inman RD, Johnston MEA, Chici B, et al. Immunochemical analysis of immune response to *Chlamydia trachomatis* in Reiter's syndrome and nonspecific urethritis. Clin Exp Immunol. 1987;69:246.
142. Schumacher HR Jr, Cherian PV, Sieck M, et al. Ultrastructural identification of chlamydial antigens in synovial membrane in acute Reiter's syndrome (Abstract 115). Arthritis Rheum. 1986;29(Suppl 4):531.
143. Keat A, Thomas B, Dixey J, et al. *Chlamydia trachomatis* and reactive arthritis: The missing link. Lancet. 1987;1:72.
144. Jones RAK. Reiter's disease after *Salmonella typhimurium* enteritis. Br Med J. 1977;1:1391.
145. Noer HR. An "experimental" epidemic of Reiter's syndrome. JAMA. 1966;197:693.
146. Calin A. Reiter's syndrome. Med Clin North Am. 1977;61:365.
147. Paronon E. Reiter's disease: A study of 244 cases observed in Finland. Acta Med Scand. 1948;131(Suppl 212):1.
148. Urman JD, Zurier RB, Rothfield NF. Reiter's syndrome associated with *Campylobacter fetus* infection. Ann Intern Med. 1977;86:444.
149. Puddey I. Reiter's syndrome following antibiotic associated colitis. Aust NZ J Med. 1982;12:292.
150. Kobayashi S, Ogasawara M, Maeda K, et al. Antibodies against *Yersinia enterocolitica* in patients with Reiter's syndrome. J Lab Clin Med. 1985;105:380.
151. Weinberger HW, Ropes MW, Kulka JP, et al. Reiter's syndrome, clinical and pathologic observations. Medicine (Baltimore). 1962;41:35–91.
152. Smith DL, Bennett RM, Regan MG. Reiter's disease in women. Arthritis Rheum. 1980;23:335.
153. Good AE. Reiter's disease. Postgrad Med. 1977;61:153.
154. Catterall RD. Reiter's disease. In: Danielsson D, Juhlin L, Mardh P-A, eds. Genitall Infections and Their Complications. Stockholm: Almquist & Widsell; 1975:205.
155. Marks JS, Holt PJL. The natural history of Reiter's disease—21 years of observations. Q J Med. 1986;60:685.
156. Morris R, Metzger AL, Bluestone R, et al. HL-A W27—a clue to the diagnosis and pathogenesis of Reiter's syndrome. N Engl J Med. 1974;290:554.
157. Mark DB, McCulley JB. Reiter's keratitis. Arch Ophthalmol. 1982;100:781.
158. Daunt SO, Kotowski KE, O'Reilly AP, et al. Ulcerative vulvitis in Reiter's syndrome. Br J Vener Dis. 1982;58:405.
159. Arnett FC, McClusley OE, Schacter BZ, et al. Incomplete Reiter's disease: Discriminating features and HL-A W27 in diagnosis. Ann Intern Med. 1976;84:8.
160. Csonka GW. Recurrent attacks in Reiter's disease. Arthritis Rheum. 1960;3:164.
161. Catterall RD. The role of microbiol infection in Reiter's syndrome. In: Dumonde DC, ed. Infection and Immunology in the Rheumatic Diseases. Oxford: Blackwell Scientific Publications; 1976:147.
162. Butler J, Russell AS, Percy JS, et al. A followup study of 48 patients with Reiter's syndrome. Am J Med. 1979;67:808.
163. Calin A, Fried JF. An "experimental" epidemic of Reiter's syndrome revisited. Ann Intern Med. 1976;84:564.
164. Ruppert GB, Lindsay J, Barth WF. Cardiac conduction abnormalities in Reiter's syndrome. Am J Med. 1982;73:335.
165. Montanaro A, Bennett RM. Myelopathy in Reiter's disease. J Rheumatol. 1984;11:540.
166. Ford DK. Reiter's syndrome: Current concepts of etiology and pathogenesis. In: Hobson D, Holmes KK, eds. Nongonococcal Urethritis and Related Infection. Lake Placid, NY: American Society for Microbiology; 1976:64.
167. Editorial. Treating Reiter's syndrome. Lancet. 1987;2:1125.

95. VULVOVAGINITIS AND CERVICITIS

MICHAEL F. REIN

THE NORMAL VAGINA

Under the influence of estrogens, the vaginal epithelium becomes cornified and supports a prodigious microbial flora. This adult microenvironment may develop transiently in neonates because of transplacentally acquired maternal estrogens[1] but resolves within several weeks as they are metabolized. The prepubescent vagina supports a flora rich in anaerobic bacteria, in particular, more *Bacteroides* species than are commonly found in the adult.[2] *Staphylococcus epidermidis* is frequently recovered,[2] and yeasts and *Gardnerella vaginalis* are isolated from 10 percent.[2,3] The vagina again matures in the immediate premenarchal period. In its mature state the vagina is colonized by a variety of bacteria,[4–8] primarily obligate and facultative anaerobes. More than 10^5 lactobacilli/ml of vaginal material are recovered from three-quarters and viridans streptococci and *Staphylococcus epidermidis* from almost half of asymptomatic women of childbearing age. Surprisingly, 10^5 *Bacteroides* were recovered from only one-sixth of these women[4,5,7,8] and *Gardnerella vaginalis* from 30–90 percent.[9,10] *Staphylococcus aureus* is recovered from the vaginas of only about 5 percent of healthy women.[11] Pregnancy has little effect on the distribution of most of the bacteria,[6,7] although the flora varies slightly during the menstrual cycle. Yeasts are carried by about 15–20 percent of healthy women.[12] With the onset of sexual activity, statistically significant increases are observed in the prevalence of *G. vaginalis*, lactobacilli, mycoplasmas, and ureaplasmas, but the prevalences of group B streptococci, *S. aureus*, and yeasts are not significantly altered.[13] It is of interest that ureaplasmas and *G. vaginalis* are recovered from 20–25 percent of young women who have not commenced sexual activity.[13]

Although our descriptive knowledge of vaginal microbiology has increased, our understanding of the factors controlling the flora remains primitive.[14] Specific and nonspecific vaginal host defenses have been catalogued, but again, their precise significance is unclear.[15]

Mucoid endocervical secretions combine with sloughed vaginal epithelial cells and normal bacteria to form a physiologic vaginal discharge. This material is usually unnoticed but may produce symptomatic "leukorrhea." It is often increased during pregnancy or with the use of oral contraceptives.

VULVOVAGINITIS

Vulvovaginitis is a common clinical syndrome and is diagnosed in more than one-quarter of women attending sexually transmitted disease clinics.[16] Treatment should be based on a specific etiologic diagnosis that can usually be made at the time of the initial evaluation.[17]

Candidiasis

The archaic term *moniliasis* should be discarded.[18] *Candida albicans* is isolated from about 80 percent of cases of vulvovaginal candidiasis, and other species of *Candida* account for about 15 percent.[19] *Candida tropicalis* infections may be associated with a higher rate of recurrence after standard treatments.[20] *Torulopsis glabrata* accounts for 3–16 percent of vaginal yeast isolates.[9,19] Symptomatic vaginitis caused by this organism is not distinguished from that caused by other *Candida* species in terms of clinical features or response to therapy,[21,22] and it is not dealt with separately.

Vulvovaginal candidiasis (VC) accounts for about one-third of vaginitis cases seen in private practice.[23] Some workers have estimated that 75 percent of adult women suffer at least one episode of VC during their lifetimes.[12] Yeast carried vaginally in small numbers and producing no symptoms may be considered part of the normal vaginal flora. If conditions in the vagina change so as to give the yeast an advantage over competing normal vaginal bacteria, VC may result. Inhibition of normal bacterial flora by broad-spectrum antibiotics favors the growth of yeasts. Thus yeasts were isolated from about 10 percent of women before but from 30 percent of women after 2- to 3-week courses of various tetracyclines.[9] Vulvovaginal candidiasis is said to follow 6–8 percent of single doses and 26 percent of 1-week courses of metronidazole.[24]

Overgrowth of yeasts is apparently favored by high estrogen levels. Vulvovaginal candidiasis is more common in pregnancy; it occurs in 10 percent of first-trimester women and 36–55 percent of women in their third trimesters.[9] Symptomatic disease has eventually developed in 60–90 percent of pregnant carriers, and old inoculation studies confirm the increased susceptibility of pregnant women.[9] Some nonpregnant women note recurrent or increasing symptoms preceding each menstrual period. The association with oral contraceptives surprisingly remains somewhat controversial.[9] The prevalence of vaginal carriage of *Candida* is higher among users of oral contraceptives than among women using other methods of birth control, and the percentage of these women developing symptoms is about the same in both groups.[25] Sequential regimens seem to predispose less than does a combination tablet.[9,26] Small series and anecdotal reports suggest that some patients with recurrent VC can be cured only when oral contraceptives are discontinued.[9] The mechanism of estrogenic predisposition is unclear, although some investigators have suggested that increased vaginal glycogen stores may play a role[9] or that estrogens influence vaginal pH in a way that makes the milieu more hospitable to the fungi.[12] An estrogen receptor in the cytosol of *C. albicans* suggests a possible direct effect of gestational hormones on the organism.[27] This mechanism has also been adduced to explain the association of VC with poorly controlled diabetes melitus.

It has been suggested that tight, insulating clothing predisposes to VC by increasing vulvar warmth and moisture. In a prospective study, a higher prevalence of candidal carriage and higher concentrations of organisms were found among women wearing tight rather than loose clothing.[28–30] Impaired immunity also predisposes to VC, and severe, refractory disease plagues women with the acquired immunodeficiency syndrome (AIDS).[31]

The mechanism by which *Candida* produces disease is not well defined. Strains isolated from symptomatic women are not demonstrably different in the laboratory than are isolates from asymptomatic carriers.[32] Filamentous forms (hyphae and pseudohyphae) are associated with active disease.[18] Pseudohyphae have been observed to penetrate vaginal epithelial cells[33] and are more adherent to cells than are blastospores.[34] Adherence appears to be an important pathogenic feature of *Candida* species,[35] and sublethal concentrations of antifungals may ameliorate disease by reducing adherence.[36]

The severity of symptoms in VC is not directly related to the number of yeasts present.[9] Indeed, very small numbers of yeasts may be present in vaginal material recovered from highly symptomatic women.[9,25]

Patients with candidal vulvovaginitis generally complain of perivaginal pruritus, often with little or no discharge. Dysuria is occasionally noted and is likely to be perceived as vulvar rather than urethral. The labia may be pale or erythematous, and excoriations may be noted. Tiny satellite papules or papulopustules just beyond the main area of erythema are helpful diagnostically. The vaginal walls may be erythematous. Candidal discharge is classically thick and adherent and contains curds. It may, however, be thin and loose and thus resemble the discharges of other vaginitides.

The vaginal pH is generally normal (approximately 4.5) in women with VC[37–39] in contrast to trichomoniasis or bacterial vaginosis. Thus, demonstrating a normal pH (see below) in a woman with signs and symptoms of vaginitis suggests that she has candidiasis rather than one of the other infections. The addition of 10% KOH to vaginal discharge on a slide or in the speculum (see below) fails to elicit a fishy odor in most women with VC. Such an odor (a positive "whiff test") suggests other infections.

An attempt should be made to demonstrate the organism on a wet mount of vaginal discharge. Although classic descriptions and most textbook pictures suggest that extensive tangles of filamentous forms can be seen, many patients in fact carry only small numbers of yeasts. Indeed, direct microscopic examination fails to reval fungi in 30–50 percent of infected women,[12,40,41] and a presumptive diagnosis must occasionally be made on other grounds with confirmation by culture or by antigen detection tests.[42] The discharge usually contains relatively few polymorphonuclear neutrophils.

Because many women carry yeasts in their vaginas, the examining physician faces a problem in interpretation: can a patient's vaginitis be attributed to the small number of yeasts present in her vagina, or has the vaginitis another etiology with the *Candida* present only by coincidence? Candidal vulvovaginitis should be diagnosed only after careful consideration of the total clinical picture of the history, physical examination, and laboratory data. Simultaneous infection with other organisms is not rare.

Vulvovaginal candidiasis is usually treated with the topical application of an antifungal agent. The striking variety of available drugs and regimens attests to the difficulty often encountered in satisfactorily managing this infection.[43]

Commercially available preparations are characterized by high patient acceptability and safety in pregnancy. Most of the commercially available drugs are polyenes (e.g., candicidin, which is no longer available in the United States, and nystatin) or imidazoles (e.g., clotrimazole, miconazole, butoconozole, terconazole, and econazole). They are available in a variety of forms including creams, tablets, and coated tampons.[39] It is difficult to compare therapies directly because of the variety of protocols used in various studies. Odds reviewed studies published through 1975 and concluded that in general imidazoles cured about 90 percent of patients and were superior to polyenes, which cured about 80 percent.[44] He could find no significant difference between delivery systems consisting of creams or vaginal tablets. More recent reviews generally support Odds' observations.[9,43]

Current interest centers on shorter courses of therapy. Seven days of treatment with miconazole cream yields cure rates ranging from 80 to 94 percent, results that are not significantly different from those obtained by the older 14-day regimen,[9] and a currently recommended therapy consists of a 100 mg intravaginal dose nightly for 7 nights. Tampons coated with 100 mg of miconazole are available in Europe.[39] Intravaginal treatment with 100 mg of clotrimazole for 6 or 7 days has produced cure rates of 88–94 percent.[9] Recent studies support the use of 200 mg of clotrimazole or miconazole or 100 mg of butoconazole inserted daily for 3 days, which produces approximately equivalent cure rates,[45–51] although some reviews suggest marginally better results with 7 days of therapy.[45] Because patients' compliance is likely to be better, it seems reasonable to recommend the 3-day regimen. Econazole is not currently marketed in the United States but produces effects roughly equivalent to those seen with clotrimazole. Mild systemic symptoms have followed its topical use.[43]

A few studies have examined the efficacy of single-dose treatments with larger amounts of imidazoles such as 500 mg of clotrimazole.[46,47,52,53] Such regimens may be preferred for the sake of convenience in the treatment of mild infections. Cure rates obtained in some studies have not quite matched those obtained with longer courses. Treatment in pregnancy is more often unsuccessful, and the longer-course regimens may be preferred in this setting.

Nystatin is a polyene that has been used in the United States for many years in a regimen consisting of one 100,000 unit tablet inserted intravaginally daily for 14 days. Although older series suggested a cure rate of about 80 percent,[44] recent studies have yielded cure rates in excess of 90 percent, approximately equivalent to those obtained with the imidazoles.[9] It must be remembered, however, that treatment with nystatin requires 2 weeks as compared with shorter-course regimens now recommended for the imidazoles.

Ketoconazole is an orally administered and well-absorbed imidazole of great value in treatment of systemic mycoses. A number of different regimens have been found effective in the treatment of VC.[9,54–56] Results do not appear to be substantially superior to those obtained with topical regimens, and the clinician must carefully consider the need for systemic therapy for VC in view of the potential toxicities of ketoconazole (see Chapter 33). Other orally absorbed imidazoles such as itraconazole and fluconazole may also have a future therapeutic role.[57]

Gentian violet, a classic treatment, has a low patient acceptability because it stains clothing. Povidone-iodine cures about 65 percent of patients.[58] It should probably be avoided in pregnancy because absorption of iodine might suppress fetal thyroid development.[59] In a single study, treatment with 600 mg of boric acid powder in gelatin capsules inserted intravaginally each evening for 14 days cured 92 percent of women.[60] Treatment of VC with various lactobacillus preparations has long been recommended in published anecdotes and in the lay press. Theoretically acting by restoring a normal bacterial flora that can successfully compete with yeasts, these regimens have not be evaluated in well-controlled trials.

Recurrent Infection. When patients treated for VC are recultured 3–6 weeks after the completion of therapy, a sizable proportion are found once again to harbor the yeasts. Results from a large number of studies[9,52,57,61] suggest a late recolonization rate of 21 ± 12 percent (mean ± SD), which is largely independent of the regimen used and often precedes symptomatic recurrence by 1–2 months.[54]

Recurrent symptomatic infection is a major problem. The mechanisms of recurrence remain obscure, but what is known has recently been analyzed by Sobel and colleagues.[12] Techniques for subspeciation of *Candida* are useful tools that will increase our understanding.[62,63] Such analyses suggest that about 40 percent of women with recurrent disease are demonstrably infected with new strains of *Candida*.[19] Obviously, women whose recurrence is associated with reappearance of the same strain might have suffered either recurrence or reinfection. The source of reinfection is poorly defined. Sexual transmission may be implicated in some cases. About 15 percent of women associate recurrences with sexual contact.[12] Yeasts are carried by 5 to 26 percent of male partners,[12,19] and 80 percent of the female partners of infected men are vaginally colonized.[17] Conjugal partners always carry the same strain.[12] Simultaneous treatment of male partners can delay symptomatic recurrence,[54] although the effect on vaginal recolonization is minimal.[54,57] Reinfection from contaminated douche equipment has also been proposed.[12]

Vaginal reinfection from a persistent rectal focus has been alleged, but support for this contention is weak. Admittedly, 40–70 percent of women with VC have positive rectal cultures, and 80 percent of doubly colonized women carry the same strain in rectal and vaginal sites,[12,19,64] but simultaneous treatment of a rectal focus with oral nystatin[65,66] or systemic ketoconazole[54–56] does not significantly lower recolonization or recurrence rates over vaginal therapy alone. One large recent study, however, suggests a benefit of oral nystatin,[67] with decreased colonization and symptomatic relapse rates during a relatively short 3–7 week follow-up period. The study population is not well defined but does not appear to have been specifically composed of women with frequently recurring disease. Care must be taken in interpreting these results. Whether certain individual women might benefit from coincident gastrointestinal therapy is unclear.

Endogenous vaginal relapse from small numbers of yeasts that survive chemotherapy has also been suggested. Intracellular residence may protect some fungal cells from antimycotic agents.[12,19] Small numbers of yeasts would certainly be invisible on wet mount and even by culture,[12] so early post-treatment evauation might erroneously suggest a cure.

As Lossick has remarked, the frequency with which *Candida* is carried asymptomatically suggests that mere reinoculation of yeasts is not an adequate cause of symptomatic recurrence.[68] Host susceptibility must also play a role. In addition to the risk factors described above, some women with recurrent VC appear to be mildly zinc deficient[69] or have defective cell-mediated immunity to yeasts.[70] The significance of these findings is unclear. Tolerance may be induced by chronic infection rather than acting as its cause.[12]

If our lack of understanding is dispiriting, our lack of effective therapy for recurrent VC is dramatically frustrating to patients and clinicians. One should attempt to reduce or eliminate the aforementioned risk factors. Short courses of antifungal therapy administered on the 5th–11th days of the menstrual cycle may reduce the rate of recurrence,[71] but such treatment rapidly becomes oppressively expensive. Simultaneous treatment of a rectal focus with oral nystatin or systemic treatment with ketoconazole does not significantly reduce the relapse rate.[56,65,66] Continuous treatment with ketoconazole, 100 mg orally per day, prevents recurrences but only for the duration of treatment.[55] Intermittent treatment at the time of menses permitted breakthrough recurrences in about one-quarter of the women.[54,55] In some cases of frequently recurrent VC, a switch to lower doses or to sequential oral contraceptives or even a discontinuance of oral contraceptives may be indicated. Oral glucose tolerance tests in such women have very low yield and are not routinely recommended.[12] Rarely, examination of sexual partners may reveal candidal balanitis, which could conceivably be a source of exogeneous reinfection.

The contribution of sexual transmission to vaginal candidiasis is apparently considerably smaller than for other forms of vaginitis. Balanitis, however, has been reported in 3–10 percent of the male sexual partners of women with candidal vulvovaginitis, and this condition is clearly sexually transmitted.[12,25,37,72] It responds to antifungal creams or ointments and treatment of the involved women. Some men develop pruritus within minutes of sexual contact. Symptoms usually resolve by the following day, and the syndrome may result from hypersensitivity to a partner's vaginal yeast.[12]

Trichomoniasis

Estimates based on the amount of metronidazole sold in this country suggest that 3 million Americans are infected with *Trichomonas vaginalis* each year. The disease is almost always sexually acquired and usually produces a combination of vaginal discharge and vulvovaginal irritation. About 25 percent of the women carrying trichomonads are asymptomatic, and the parasite has been recovered from up to 5 percent of sexually active asymptomatic women in Great Britain. The infection is discussed in detail in Chapter 258, to which the reader is referred.

Bacterial Vaginosis

Many young women with vulvovaginal signs or symptoms are not infected with *T. vaginalis* or *C. albicans*. Such women have been said to have "nonspecific vaginitis." This is an unfortunate term because it suggests an unknown etiology or a collection of undifferentiated diseases. Indeed, most of these women appear to have a specific condition first described by Gardner and Dukes in 1955, [73] and the condition is now usually referred to (perhaps unfortunately from the linguistic standpoint) as bacterial vaginosis (BV).[74] Inflammation and perivaginal irritation are often considerably milder than in trichomoniasis or candidiasis. Dysuria and dyspareunia are correspondingly rare. Affected women are sexually active and often complain predominantly of vaginal odor. This odor is described as "fishy" in the textbooks more frequently than by the patients. About 90 percent of patients also notice a mild to moderate discharge. Abdominal discomfort is occasionally present, but it is usually mild and should prompt evaluation for coincident infections including salpingitis.

Discharge is often present at the introitus and visible on the labia minora. The labia and vulva are generally not erythematous or edematous. On speculum examination the vaginal walls usually appear uninflamed. The vagina often contains a grayish, thin, homogeneous discharge manifesting small bubbles. This discharge differs from normal, physiologic discharge in that the latter has a floccular appearance and bubbles are absent. Although the discharge may be heavy enough to pool in the posterior fornix, it is usually present in smaller amounts. In some patients, the discharge may be so slight that it does not conspicuously pool. Because it is relatively thin but adherent to the vaginal walls, it is often apparent only as an increased light reflex. A distinct, pungent odor may be noted by the examiner.

The endocervix is unaffected by the process, and cervical discharge should be physiologic and therefore mucoid. The presence of a purulent cervical discharge or frank cervicitis is not rare but results from coincident gonococcal, chlamydial, or herpetic infection.[75] Abnormalities on bimanual examination are distinctly unusual and should prompt a search for other pathologic processes.

Other vaginal infections may closely resemble BV; an accurate differential diagnosis depends on laboratory examination of the genital specimen. The pH of vaginal discharge is elevated above the normal of 4.5 in about 90 percent of women with BV.[73,76,77] Although the pH may also be elevated in trichomoniasis, it is usually normal in vulvovaginal candidiasis. A vaginal pH ≥ 6 strongly suggests infection.[78] If 10% KOH is added to vaginal discharge samples either in the speculum blade or on a microscope slide, a distinctively pungent, fishy odor is generated.[8,9,76,79–81] This positive "whiff test" has been used as part of the case definition of BV by some workers and has been found to be positive in about 70 percent of cases in other series.[76,80] The accuracy of this test appears to improve with experience,[81] but the test is also positive in some patients with trichomoniasis, and its predictive value is therefore limited in populations with a high prevalence of the protozoal infection.

Bacterial vaginosis is perhaps most easily differentiated from trichomoniasis on the basis of direct microscopic examination of vaginal discharge. A wet mount of the discharge from patients with BV reveals clue cells, which are vaginal epithelial cells studded with tiny coccobacilli. These organisms are best appreciated at the edges of the cell (Fig. 1) but may be dense enough partially to obscure the nucleus. Not all cells in the specimen are clue cells, but some clue cells are seen in over 90 percent of patients with BV.[81,82] Predominant bacterial flora can also be assessed on a wet mount slide. In healthy women, the predominant morphotype is a large rod (presumably *Lactobacillus* species). In the discharge from a patient with BV, these rods have been completely supplanted by clumps of coccoba-

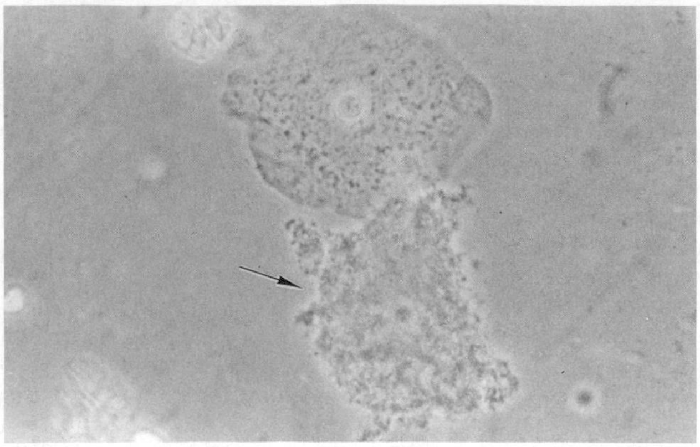

FIG. 1. A wet mount of vaginal discharge from a patient with bacterial vaginosis shows a normal epithelial cell (above) and a clue cell (below, arrow). (Phase microscopy, ×400)

cilli. Similar discrimination can be made on the basis of a Gram stain of the vaginal discharge.[9] Discharge in BV contrains few polymorphonuclear neutrophils (PMNs). This may in part explain the absence of the green or yellow color that frequently characterizes the discharge in trichomoniasis. About one PMN per epithelial cell is considered normal in a vaginal wet mount. Finding increased numbers of PMNs in a patient with BV suggests the presence of a second inflammatory process, often coincidental cervicitis.[75]

Culture for *Gardnerella vaginalis* is easily accomplished on a variety of media (Chapter 202). The organism is isolated from 98 percent of women with BV,[81] but also is recovered in smaller numbers[82] from up to 70 percent of some populations of asymptomatic women,[2,3,9,10,13,83,84] and its presence does not therefore prove that the patient has BV.[84] Thin-layer chromatography, gas–liquid chromatography, and enzyme assays can be used to diagnose BV by identifying specific bacterial products.[9,77,85,86] These techniques are not routinely available, but provide insight into the pathophysiology of BV.

Amsel et al.[81] suggest that the clinician look for a pH greater than 4.5; homogeneous, white, adherent vaginal discharge; a positive whiff test; and clue cells. Finding any three of these four signs strongly supports the diagnosis of BV, although an abnormal discharge, an elevated pH, and a positive whiff test often accompany trichomoniasis as well. The final diagnosis and decision to treat depends, however, on a complete evaluation of the patient. An isolated finding of clue cells in asymptomatic women does not demand treatment.

Pathophysiology. Microscopic examination of vaginal discharge in BV characteristically reveals a predominant flora of coccobacilli. On the basis of morphology this organism was originally called *Haemophilus vaginalis*[73] It has been transferred to its own genus and is now called *Gardnerella* in honor of Dr. Gardner's initial observations (Chapter 203).[87]

Several observations suggest a less than straightforward relationship between *G. vaginalis* and BV. Although Gardner and Dukes regularly produced BV by inoculating fresh vaginal discharge from patients into the vaginas of healthy recipients, inoculation of pure cultures of *G. vaginalis* was far less likely to produce disease.[73] In addition, *G. vaginalis* is isolated from 30–70 percent of asymptomatic women,[2,3,9,10,13,81,83,84] and only 50 percent of women with heavy vaginal colonization by *G. vaginalis* actually have BV.[84] Finally, the in vitro sensitivity of *G. vaginalis* to antimicrobial agents does not match the effectiveness of these agents in clinical disease. Metronidazole is highly effective therapy for BV[76,79,88–92] despite the fact that *G. vaginalis* is relatively resistant to the drug in vitro.[76,90,93]

An explanation for all these observations is that *G. vaginalis* is not the single cause of BV. There is considerable experimental support for the hypotheseis that BV is actually a synergistic infection involving not only *G. vaginalis* but certain anaerobic bacteria as well.[8,9,76,77,80,86,92,94] Various *Bacteroides* species other than *B. fragilis* and various peptococci are principally involved. Asymptomatic carriers of *G. vaginalis* might lack the anaerobic synergants. Pure cultures of *G. vaginalis* would not be able to produce clinical disease in patients lacking the other necessary bacteria, but the vaginal discharge from symptomatic women would be expected to contain all the necessary bacterial components. Drugs relatively inactive against *G. vaginalis* might still cure the disease if they acted against the other bacteria, and metronidazole is highly active against most strict anaerobes. The characteristic odor of BV is due to various aromatic amines such as putrescine and cadaverine, which are produced by anaerobes but not by *G. vaginalis*.[77] These aromatic diamines are volatilized at basic pH, which explains the positive whiff test associated with this infection.

Mycoplasmas are isolated from the vaginas of many women with BV.[13,14,95,96] A role in the production of BV has not been established.

Treatment. Many studies[76,79,88–92,97–100] have now shown that BV is most successfully treated with metronidazole, 500 mg orally twice daily or 250 mg orally three times daily for 7 days. Cure rates of over 90 pecent are reported. Most studies suggest that single doses of metronidazole are inadequate,[9,89–91,97–101] but tinidazole, a nitroimidazole with a longer half life that is available in Europe, cured 80 percent of patients after a single 2 g administration.[102] Ampicillin is highly active in vitro against *G. vaginalis*, with minimum inhibitory concentrations (MICs) of less than 2 μg/ml for most strains.[9,92,98] BV has been treated with 500 mg of ampicillin administered four times daily for 7 days. Although some studies have yielded a cure rate of about 90 percent,[82,92] others have yielded cure rates of only 40–70 percent.[76,88] Amoxicillin in the same doses is minimally if at all superior.[91,92] The inferiority of ampicillin to metronidazole probably derives in part from its inactivation by penicillinase elaborated by *Bacteroides* species in the vagina[76,92]; however, the combination of amoxicillin with clavulanic acid is still inferior to metronidazole.[91] Ampicillin or amoxicillin treatment blocks recolonization of the vagina by normal lactobacilli, whereas metronidazole does not.[92] Recolonization with lactobacilli may be part of the recovery process from BV. A recent study suggests that clindamycin, 300 mg orally, twice daily for 7 days, is effective therapy for BV.[102a]

The value of oral cephalosporins for BV remains controversial. Gardner and Dukes praise them anecdotally,[73,103] as do other workers. Indeed, cephalexin, 500 mg taken four times daily for 1 week, has cured some women whose disease relapsed after repeated treatments with metronidazole. Oral therapy with tetracyclines or erythromycin has been disappointing.[9]

Topical therapy with clindamycin cream is under investigation and appears promising. Sulfanilamide-aminacrine-allantoin and providone-iodine have unacceptably low cure rates.[9] Triple sulfa preparations have been used topically for some decades, but small series suggest that the compounds are ineffective.[76,104] Topical therapy with yogurt does not work.[105]

Although BV behaves epidemiologically as if it were a sexually transmitted disease, there are no data supporting the need to treat asymptomatic male sexual partners initially.[9] *Gardnerella vaginalis* is recovered from the urethras of 80 percent of the male sexual partners of women with BV,[76] and recolonization with the organism is far more common in women reexposed to untreated male partners than to those who are not.[76] Some women suffer from frequently relapsing disease that can be controlled only by the simultaneous treatment of male sexual partners. These men carry *G. vaginalis*, and it is unclear whether they should be treated with metronidazole or ampicillin.

Asymptomatic carriage of *G. vaginalis* is common and need not be treated.

Other Infections with G. vaginalis. *Gardnerella vaginalis* has been identified in urine obtained by suprapubic aspiration from pregnant women, but the organisms are usually present in very small numbers, and pyuria is distinctly unusual.[106] Urinary tract infection in a man, a possible perinephric abscess in a transplanted kidney, and balanoposthitis have all been reported.[9] *Gardnerella vaginalis* has been carried asymptomatically in the urethras of sexually active men, but it is not associated with nongonoccal urethritis.

Gardnerella vaginalis and the associated anaerobic bacteria and mycoplasmas are frequently isolated from the endometrium and blood of patients with postpartum fever and endometritis.[95,107–111] Premature labor has been associated with BV.[109]

Curved Anaerobic Rods. Considerable recent interest concerns vaginitis associated with motile, curved anaerobic rods that are gram-negative or gram-variable.[112–118] These organisms, classified in the new genus *Mobiluncus,*[119] are sensitive to ampicillin, but some species are relatively resistant to metronidazole.[114,117] The precise pathogenic role of these organisms remains to be elucidated.

Staphylococci. *Staphylococcus aureus* is recovered from the vaginas of only about 5 percent of healthy women.[11] The organism is isolated, however, from most women with menstruation-associated toxic shock syndrome.[120,121] (Chapter 173). Frank vaginitis with a vaginal discharge has been observed in about one-third to three-quarters of these women, and a history of vaginitis is associated with an increased incidence of toxic shock syndrome.[122] The disease is usually characterized by vulvar edema and vulvar and vaginal erythema.[121] A vaginal discharge, purulent but often scanty, is observed in about one-quarter to one-third of these patients.[120,121] Vaginal ulceration was noted in about 7 percent of these women.[121] The pathogenesis of the vaginitis is not entirely understood. Toxic shock syndrome is manifested as a polymucositis, and vaginitis is also reported in about one-third of women who have nonmenstrual toxic shock syndrome, sometimes with the staphylococcal source at sites other than the vagina. Thus, the vaginitis may reflect direct infection or may be a secondary effect of staphylococcal toxin. The ulcerations sometimes observed may result from tampon use, with which toxic shock syndrome is associated (see below).

Foreign Body Vaginitis. Secondary anaerobic infections may be associated with foreign bodies in the vagina. In adults, the most common of these are the forgotten vaginal tampon and various contraceptive devices such as the diaphragm, cervical cap, or a condom that has slipped off during coitus. Objects apparently used in masturbation are occasionally implicated.[123] In children and the mentally incompetent, a variety of objects may be found.[1] These infections often produce an intensely foul odor, and the discharge is usually scanty and contains small amounts of blood. Therapy often requires only the removal of the offending object, but oral metronidazole may speed recovery.

Tampon use has been observed to affect the vaginal mucosa.[124–127] Extended tampon use, particularly of superabsorbent tampons, may produce local drying and peeling of the vaginal mucosa and result in frank ulceration of the vaginal wall and exocervix. Tampon fibers have been observed within ulcerations.[126] Microscopic ulcers have been noted in up to one-fifth of women using tampons,[123] and larger lesions are occasionally observed.[125,127] Ulceration may be associated with vaginal bleeding and pain on insertion of the tampons. Because of possible confusion with other ulcerating vaginal diseases including malignancy, a thorough work-up is essential.[127]

Herpes Simplex Virus. The adult vaginal epithelium is relatively resistant to herpetic infection. Vaginal lesions have been observed in only about 4 percent of infected women.[128,129] Fourteen percent of women with primary genital herpes developed vulvovaginal candidiasis during the second week of infection.[128,129] Treatment of these secondary infections, however, must be done carefully because the topical antifungal miconazole cream appears to be associated with delayed healing of genital herpetic lesions.[130] Indeed, the application of any occulsive preparation to herpetic lesions should probably be avoided,[128,129] and oral ketoconazole might be useful in this setting.

Other Specific Infections

True vaginal infections with other specific agents such as *Mycobacterium tuberculosis*, salmonellae, Enterobacteriaceae, actinomycetes, and schistosomes are rare and usually occur in patients with underlying diseases or who are systemically ill. Group A streptococcal vaginitis has been described in children aged 3–5 years old. It is manifested as a blood-tinged discharge, "firey red" vaginal mucosae, and dysuria. A Gram stain is usually negative, and the disease responds promptly to penicillin G.[131]

Pre-existing lesions due to other diseases may become secondarily infected with a mixed anaerobic flora of fusobacteria and spirochetes. Such "fusospirochetal" infections can progress rapidly. Metronidazole, 250 mg orally three times daily, is recommended therapy.

Pinworms are an occasional cause of perivaginal itching, especially in children.[1] Perianal pruritus that becomes worse at night may suggest this diagnosis. True vaginal infestation has been described.[132]

Neisseria gonorrhoeae and *C. trachomatis* can cause frank vaginitis in prepubescent girls.[133]

"Doderlein cytolysis", a condition characterized by irritative symptoms exacerbating in the premenstrual interval and theoretically caused by microbially induced hyperacidity, is poorly substantiated. It is said to result from an overgrowth of lactobacilli and to respond to alkalinizing douches.[134]

Noninfectious Vulvovaginitis

Genital neoplasm may produce an abnormal vaginal discharge. Such conditions are more common in older women and are usually manifested by the gradual onset of a thin, often foul-smelling discharge that may be blood tinged.

In postmenopausal women, the absence of estrogen stimulation results in atrophy of the vaginal epithelium, which may lead to an atrophic vaginitis. The vaginal walls become secondarily infected with a number of different organisms, but treatment of the primery disease often requires estrogenic supplementation.

Occasional cases of vulvovaginal inflammation from chemicals including deodorant sprays[135] and allergic reactions to semen[136] and nickel[137] have been reported.

Desquamative or purulent vaginitis is characterized by a vaginal discharge containing large numbers of polymorphonuclear neutrophils. The etiology and therapy of the condition are unknown, but lichen planus should be considered in the differential diagnosis.[138,139]

Conditions Imitating Vulvovaginitis

Physiologic or normal vaginal discharge is sometimes referred to as leukorrhea and generally consists of cervical mucus combined with desquamated vaginal epithelial cells. This material passes through the vaginal introitus where it is noted by the patient as a vaginal discharge. Neonates may have a transient physiologic discharge until transplacentally acquired maternal estrogens are metabolized. In the adult, the output of the endocervical glands is highly responsive to hormonal levels and sometimes increases at the time of ovulation or in the immediate premenstrual period. Oral contraceptives may increase the cervical component, and women sometimes note a new discharge when they start to use these agents. This leukorrhea may cause considerable concern since it often begins coincidentally with first sexual exposures, thus raising the specter of venereal disease. Physiologic discharge accounted for 10 percent of women attending a private practice with vaginal complaints.[23] It may be heavy enough to stain underwear and may dry to a brown residue, which patients sometimes associate with infectious vaginitis. Unlike most infections, it is usually not associated with perineal burning or pruritus, dyspareunia, or dysuria, but odor is sometimes described.[140] Abdominal pain does not occur unless another process is present. Microscopic examination reveals normal vaginal flora and few polymorphonuclear neutrophils (PMNs). More than one PMN per epithelial cell is unusual in physiologic vaginal discharge.

Infectious cervicitis due to any of several different organisms may result in an inflammatory cervical discharge that passes through the vagina. This condition is discussed in a later section of this chapter.

A variety of inflammatory diseases confined to the perineum may produce symptoms suggesting vaginitis to the patient. The lesions of herpes genitalis or chancroid produce considerable perineal discomfort. Intertrigo may result in burning, an unpleasant odor, and staining of underwear. Infection of Bartholin's glands and Skene's glands sometimes produce perineal discomfort and a discharge and is dealt with in a later section of this chapter. Inflammatory diseases of the rectum occasionally result in a discharge that suggests vaginitis to the patient. Dysuria may be a symptom of urinary tract infection.

Of particular interest is a condition referred to as focal vulvitis or vestibular adenitis.[141,142] Affected women suffer vulvar pain and significant dyspareunia. They frequently undergo repeated treatments for vulvovaginal candidiasis, and they are often thought to be neurotic. Physical examination reveals rather subtle but exquisitely tender, erythematous patches, usually along the posterior portion of the introital ring. Biopsy demonstrates nonspecific inflammation of vestibular glands. Current therapy is surgical excision of the affected areas. An infectious etiology has not been demonstrated.

Vaginitis emphasematosa is an uncommon condition in which the vaginal walls contain submucosal, gas-filled cysts.[143] The exocervix too may be involved.[144] This benign condition is frequently associated with trichomoniasis.

Obstruction of the pelvic nodes is a rare cause of lymphatic weeping of the vagina. Massive lymphedema of the lower extremities usually accompanies this finding, and the diagnosis is not difficult.

There are small numbers of women who complain of vaginal discharge, discomfort, or odor without any objective findings.[145] Such women may be motivated by a neurotic fear of uncleanliness, guilt concerning sexual activities (or a desire to avoid them), or anxiety about venereal disease whether or not sexual exposure has actually taken place. These patients have often sought advice from numerous physicians and have symptoms that have failed to respond to a variety of standard therapies. They require careful and complete medical evaluation. The diagnosis of "worried well" must not be made without a thorough examination for physical disease. Women with psychosomatic complaints may respond to a careful and sympathetic explanation of the results of the examination and psychotherpay.[145]

Scabies, pediculosis, or enterobiasis may produce intense perivaginal itching and soreness.

APPROACH TO THE PATIENT WITH VAGINAL COMPLAINTS

History

The etiologic diagnosis of vaginitis depends on a careful evaluation of the history, physical examination, and immediate laboratory tests. Historical features are relatively nonspecific,[9] but they may direct clinical suspicion toward certain causes.

Age. Neonates can acquire trichomonal or candidal vulvovaginitis during passage through an infected birth canal, an argument for treating these infections in pregnant women before term. Neonatal vaginal thrush responds promptly to topical antifungal medications such as nystatin.[1] Neonatal trichomoniasis often does not require specific therapy and disappears when the estrogens are metabolized.[146] Thereafter, any vaginal discharge is abnormal and should prompt a vigorous search for disease. Immediately before menarche, physiologic discharge may reappear. Prepubescent vaginal epithelium is not cornified, and the entire vagina is susceptible to infection with *Neisseria gonorrhoeae* or *Chlamydia trachomatis*. Gonococcal vulvovaginitis often causes profuse vaginal discharge, and the rectum is almost always involved. Vaginal candidiasis is extremely rare in prepubescent girls.[147] A diagnosis of sexually transmitted disease in a young girl should raise the suspicion of child abuse, although some agents have been transmitted to children in the absence of frank sexual contact.

Patients in the sexually active years are more likely to have a sexually transmitted disease. Genital neoplasia is more common among older women, and postmenopausal women are more likely to have atrophic vaginitis.

Mode of Onset. An abrupt and identifiable time of onset of symptoms suggests infection. Vaginal discharge associated with neoplasia, estrogen depletion, or a foreign body often has a subacute onset with symptoms progressing over a period of weeks. Symptoms beginning during or immediately after the menstrual period are somewhat suggestive of trichomoniasis, and a premenstrual onset more frequently accompanies candidiasis.

Quantity of Discharge. The amount of discharge is highly variable in all conditions. Patients with candidiasis often have scanty discharge or note no discharge at all. Atrophic or neoplastic discharges are commonly scanty unless infection has supervened.

Perineal Irritation. Physiologic discharge is rarely associated with perineal discomfort. Pruritus with a scanty or absent discharge is frequently seen in candidiasis and less commonly with trichomoniasis. Perineal discomfort is an infrequent complaint in BV. Severe episodic perineal pain sometimes preventing urination is strongly suggestive of herpes genitalis, which affects the labia but usually spares the vagina per se.[128,129] Chronic discomfort, often interfering with sexual activity, should prompt consideration of focal vulvitis.[141,142]

Odor. An unpleasant odor accompanies many vaginal infections and sometimes physiologic discharge as well.[140] Vaginal odor in the absence of other symptoms is the initial complaint in many cases of BV. A feculent odor may accompany anaerobic superinfection of genital lesions or may be noted in the presence of a foreign body.

Abdominal Pain. Abdominal discomfort is rare in uncomplicated vulvovaginitis except for occasional cases of trichomoniasis. Women complaining of abdominal pain should be examined carefully for evidence of coincidental infections including cystitis and pelvic inflammatory disease.

Sexual History. Exposure to a new sexual partner increases the likelihood of sexually transmitted disease. A history of genital symptoms in a sexual partner is helpful diagnostically. The commencement of oral contraceptive use may be associated with increased physiologic discharge. The use of tampons, particularly the prolonged use of superabsorbent tampons, may be associated with ulcerative vaginitis.[124–127]

Other Diseases. Diabetes, AIDS,[31] malignancy and treatment thereof, and possibly hypoparathyroidism increase the risk of candidal vaginitis. Diseases known to impair host defenses may predispose to otherwise rare infections. Other diseases may be treated with drugs that predispose to vaginal infection.

Medication. Systemic or local medication may influence the spectrum of vaginal infection. Antibiotics, particularly tetracyclines and ampicillin, are active against much of the normal bacterial flora of the vagina, and their use predisposes to candidal vaginitis. Metronidazole is active against vaginal anaerobes and also predisposes to candidal infection, but less frequently than with many other antimicrobials. Low doses of many antibiotics can interfere with the isolation of *N. gonorrhoeae* and possibly *G. vaginalis*. Low-dose antibiotics may result in the development of atypical syphilitic chancres or may eliminate the primary stage of syphilis entirely.

Patients taking corticosteroids or oral contraceptives are at increased risk for developing candidal vaginitis. Oral contraceptive use may also be associated with the development of a physiologic vaginal discharge.

Local medication including vaginal douches may produce a chemical vaginitis, but douching immediately before examination may make etiologic diagnosis difficult.

Examination of the Female Genitalia

With the patient supine on the examining table, the pubic hair should be examined for the presence of crab lice or nits. The inguinofemoral areas are palpated for adenopathy. Superpubic and lower abdominal tenderness or masses are sought by palpation.

With the patient in the lithotomy position, the labia and the perineum should be examined for erythema, lichenification, excoriation, and discrete lesions. Diffuse perineal erythema may accompany trichomoniasis or candidiasis. Diffuse reddening with small satellite lesions, usually papular or papulopustular, suggests candiadiasis. The degree of perineal irritation is quite variable with all infectioins, but severe perivaginal irritation is uncommon with BV. Labial edema may accompany severe irritation.

Careful examination of all the extravaginal surfaces may reveal lesions of herpes genitalis, syphilis, condyloma accuminatum, molluscum contagiosum, scabies (which are discussed in Chapter 92) or focal vulvitis. Even though the patient's chief complaint may strongly suggest a true vaginitis, examination of the external genitalia for coincident infections is very important because multiple, coexistent sexually transmitted diseases are common.

By spreading the labia with the gloved hand, the urethral meatus is examined. The urethra may be gently stripped with the finger placed inside the introitus. Urethral discharge is not a common finding, but if delivered, such material should be examined microscopically and cultured. The introitus and the internal surfaces of the labia minora should be examined for lesions.

Vaginal discharge is sometimes observed on the labia or actually running out onto the perineum. Such copius discharge is usually associated with trichomoniasis but may accompany other infections.

If the patient has had a hysterectomy, a calcium alginate urethral swab should be inserted gently into the urethra and recovered material inoculated for gonococcal culture. This is unnecessary if the cervix is present since gonococci are more often recovered from the cervix than from the urethra. The urethra is frequently the only site from which *C. trachomatis* can be recovered.

A vaginal speculum moistened with warm water is gently inserted. In the presence of severe herpes genitalis or, occasionally, trichomoniasis, insertion of the speculum may be impossible because of the patient's discomfort. In such a case, a preliminary diagnosis is sometimes made from material recovered on a cotton swab gently inserted into the vagina.

After the speculum has been inserted, the vaginal walls are examined. Candidal or trichomonal vaginitis is often accompanied by erythema of the vaginal walls. The degree of erythema, however, is often very difficult to assess in an individual patient. Punctate hemorrhages of the vaginal walls strongly suggest trichomoniasis. A diffuse sheen, manifested by an increased light reflex, may be caused by thin discharge adhering to the walls. This is seen most frequently with BV but may accompany other infections. Fingerlike projections within the vagina may be condylomata accuminata, but these must be differentiated from hymenal tags. The latter are normal but are usually found only near the introitus.

The surface of the cervix may be inflamed. Punctate hemorrhages are rarely observed in patients with severe trichomoniasis (strawberry cervix), and ulcerations may be present with herpetic cervicitis. Mucoid material is normally observed at the cervical os and is present in increased amounts in women taking oral contraceptives. A normal cervical discharge may be clear or white. A purulent or mucopurulent discharge is associated with infectious cervicitis, primarily chlamydial, gonococcal, or herpetic.

Bimanual examination for adnexal tenderness and masses should be a part of the examination. Adnexal tenderness is uncommon with local vaginal infections and suggests salpingitis; palpation of abnormal adnexal mass may indicate a tuboovarian abscess or ectopic pregnancy and requires prompt gynecologic or surgical consultation.

The anus should be examined for the presence of discharge, chancres, or condylomata. A glove used in vaginal examination should never be introduced into the rectum since this may inoculate the rectum with gonococci, chlamydia, or herpes simplex virus.

Other Bedside Evaluation. After the speculum is withdrawn, the pH of vaginal secretions can be determined by inserting a strip of indicator paper in the material collected in the lower lip of the speculum. We have found nitrazine paper with a pH range of 4.5–7.0 to be useful. A normal pH of 4.5 is seen in most patients with vulvovaginal candidiasis, whereas a pH elevated to 5.0 or above is associated with BV and trichomoniasis.

If several drops of 10% KOH then added to the material on the speculum elicit a pungent, fishy, aminelike odor, this would constitute a positive "whiff test." The whiff test is positive in more than 90 percent of patients with BV and in many patients with trichomoniasis. It is negative in women with vulvovaginal candidiasis. The whiff test may also be performed on a slide that has been prepared for KOH microscopic examination.

Laboratory Examination

A wet mount is of greatest value in the differential diagnosis of a vaginal discharge, and the specimen may be prepared in several ways. A swab of vaginal discharge may be agitated in a tube containing about 1 ml of normal saline. One drop of the resulting suspension is put on a microscope slide, and a coverslip is applied. Alternatively, the examiner may place a drop of saline on the slide and mix in a loopful of vaginal material, after which a coverslip is applied. The slide is examined initially under low power on a brightfield microscope with the substage condenser racked down or with the substage diaphragm closed down to increase the contrast. Phase-contrast microscopy is becoming more widely available in clinical settings and provides an excellent means of examining vaginal wet mounts.

The relative numbers of epithelial cells and polymorphonuclear neutrophils (PMNs) should be noted. PMNs are present in physiologic endocervical discharge[148] that collects in the vagina, so small numbers of PMNs may be observed in the vaginal material recovered from healthy women. A finding of more than one PMN per epithelial cell should raise the examiner's suspicion of cervical or vaginal inflammation. Observing relatively few PMNs, however, does not rule out vaginal infection. Vaginal candidiasis often produces a discharge containing small numbers of PMNs.[38] The relative absence of PMNs is characteristic of the discharge of BV.[9] In fact, finding many PMN in the vaginal discharge of a patient with BV should prompt the examiner to search for simultaneous infection such as trichomoniasis, gonorrhea, or chlamydial cervicitis.

Large clumps of pseudohyphae suggest vaginal candidiasis, but the examiner often sees only moderate or even very small numbers of yeasts in this condition. Indeed, some patients with vulvovaginal candidiasis have organisms identified only by culture. The wet preparation should be scanned for motile trichomonads.

The wet mount should then be observed under high power (×400). Normal squamous epithelial cells have transparent cytoplasm and small nuclei. Epithelial cells covered with tiny coccobacillary forms (Fig. 1) are called "clue cells" and are associated with BV. Clue cells are best recognized by observing the edges of epithelial cells, which may be obscured by the adherent coccobacilli. Some cells are so heavily encrusted that the nuclei are obscured. Trichomonads are best be recognized by their characteristic twitching motility (Fig. 2). The flagella and undulating membrane may be observed by carefully focusing the microscope and adjusting the light source. Trichomonad motility is improved by gently warming the preparation. Unfortunately, the wet mount is negative in about 30 percent of the women with trichomoniasis (Chapter 258), and a negative wet mount does not rule out this infection, particularly in relatively asymptomatic women. A negative wet mount should be confirmed with a culture. Small numbers of *Candida* are frequently observed and do not necessarily indicate that the patient's vaginitis is of candidal etiology. Large numbers of *Candida*, frequent budding, and the presence of pseudohyphae add strength to the contention that *Candida* is the etiologic agent.

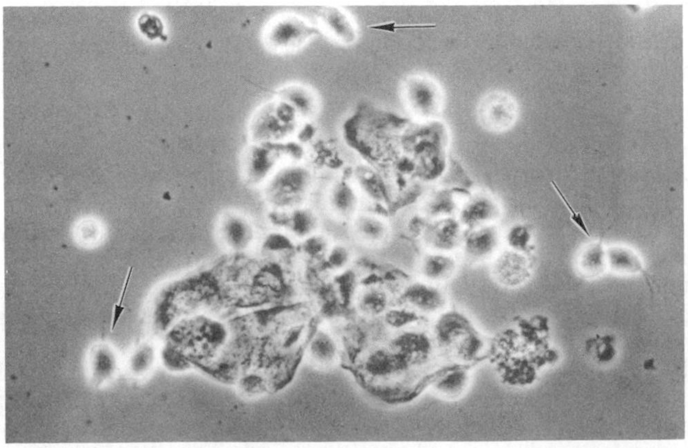

FIG. 2. A wet mount of vaginal discharge from a patient with trichomonal vaginitis shows epithelial cells, neutrophils, and trichomonads (arrows). (Phase microscopy, ×400)

The bacterial flora can often be assessed on the wet mount. Normal vaginal flora consist primarily of rods. In BV, the predominant flora is tiny coccobacilli.

Spermatozoa may be observed as long as 10 days after the last coitus. Motile sperm suggests sexual contact within the preceding 24 hours.[149]

Combining a drop of 10% or 20% KOH with the vaginal material on a microscope slide, applying a coverslip, and gently heating destroy epithelial cells and most microbial flora, leaving fungal elements behind. The potassium hydroxide preparation cannot be used for a microscopic diagnosis of trichomoniasis or BV, but elaboration of a fishy odor from the slide suggests these infections.

A Gram stain of vaginal material is generally less useful for the differential diagnosis than the wet mount. Normal vaginal flora consists primarily of gram-positive rods, which are presumably lactobacilli. In BV the normal flora is replaced by sheets of gram-variable coccobacilli, which may often be seen overlying the surface of epithelial cells. Small numbers of *Candida* are occasionally observed as dense, gram-positive ovoids, but the Gram stain is positive in fewer than one-third of the women from whom *Candida* can be cultured.[40] Women with active vaginal candidiasis often have large numbers of budding yeasts and pseudohyphae recognizable as thick gram-positive or beaded tubes. The Gram stain of vaginal material should not be used for the diagnosis of gonorrhea or trichomoniasis. Trichomonads are recognized only with difficulty on a Gram stain, and gonorrhea is a cervicitis rather than vaginitis in the adult.

Material recovered from the endocervix can be Gram stained. Cervical discharge always contains moderate numbers of PMNs, and their presence is not necessarily an indication of specific inflammation.[148] Large numbers of PMNs indicate cervicitis. Gram-negative, intracellular diplococci accurately diagnose gonorrhea (see Chapter 190), but extracellular diplococci are of no significance since nonpathogenic *Neisseria* is part of the normal flora of the female genital tract. Unfortunately, the cervical Gram stain is positive in only about one-half of the women with cervical gonorrhea, and a negative Gram stain does not rule out the infection.[40] Trichomonads are only infrequently found in the endocervix, and cervical material should not be used to examine for trichomoniasis. Cervical material recovered from women at risk should be cultured for *N. gonorrhoeae* and evaluated for *C. trachomatis*. The Papanicolaou smear may reveal *T. vaginalis* or clue cells, but neither of these findings is sufficiently sensitive for a negative result to rule out infection. Direct staining of cervical specimens using the Giemsa or Papanicolaou methods is insufficiently sensitive for the diagnosis of chlamydial cervicitis (Chapter 158).

CERVICITIS

Under the influence of estrogens, the normal vaginal epithelium cornifies and becomes relatively resistant to infection with a number of pathogens. The endocervix, however, is lined with columnar epithelium, which remains susceptible to many of these infections. Therefore, the examiner frequently finds infectious cervicitis in the absence of vaginitis and vice versa. Studies of the etiology of cervicitis have been hampered by the lack of a reliable definition of the syndrome.[74,150,151] Erythema around the cervical os may indicate infection or may merely represent cervical *erosion* or *eversion*, terms applied to the migration of endocervical epithelium over the surface of the cervix. Such lesions are usually symmetric about the os and are not particularly friable. They are more common in women taking oral contraceptives, and it may be impossible on clinical grounds alone to differentiate these from true infection. *Hypertrophic cervicitis*, on the other hand, is manifested as an intensely erythematous, raised, irregular lesion that bleeds easily.[75,150–152] Normal cervical discharge is clear and mucoid. Purulent or mucopurulent discharge is associated with gonococcal or chlamydial infection.[75,153–155] The color and quality of the cervical discharge can be assessed by obtaining endocervical material on a swab and comparing its consistency and color against a well-illuminated sheet of white paper or cloth. Polymorphonuclear neutrophils are normally present in the endocervix,[148] but abnormally increased numbers can be detected crudely on a Gram stain of endocervical material. After the exocervix has been cleaned off, a swab is inserted into the cervix and gently rotated, and the recovered material is applied to a microscope slide by rolling the swab over an area about 1 × 2 cm. The specimen is then Gram stained. Observing more than 10 polymorphonuclear neutrophils per oil-immersion field in the densest portion of the slide correlates statistically with the presence of gonococci or chlamydiae,[75,154,156] but the sensitivity and positive predictive value of the observation are far too low for a definitive diagnosis.

Specific Etiologies of Acute Cervicitis

The clinical features of specific cervical infections overlap too much to permit an accurate etiologic diagnosis without laboratory assistance.[75,150,157] Multiple infections are common[157] and may be missed if the diagnosis is attempted on clinical grounds alone.

Acute gonococcal cervicitis has been known for hundreds of years. The endocervix is the site from which gonococci are most frequently isolated in women with uncomplicated gonococcal infections. In typical cases the cervical os is reddened and productive of a purulent discharge.[158] A Gram stain of this material reveals typical gram-negative cell-associated diplococci in only about one-half of the infected women[40] (Fig. 3), and a negative Gram stain must never be used as an argument against treating women for uncomplicated gonorrhea. Examination for gonococcal cervicitis must include an appropriate culture. The sensitivity of the endocervical culture is disputed but is generally held to be on the order of 90 percent. Most women with uncomplicated gonococcal cervicitis are asymptomatic, but about one-third note vaginal discharge.[148,158]

Chlamydia trachomatis can be recovered from the endocervix of 60–90 percent of the sexual partners of men with chlamydial urethritis.[148,150–152,159,160] Cervical abnormalities, often subtle, have been observed in 80–90 percent of chlamydiae-positive women.[148,150–152,159,160] Most of these women are asymptomatic, but about one-third note a discharge from the vagina[148] that actually originates in the inflamed cervix. Chlamydiae have been isolated from 50–90 percent of sexually active patients with hypertrophic cervicitis.[148] Only 19–32 percent of women with chlamydial cervical infection manifest hypertrophic cervicitis, and only about 30 percent have a mucopurulent or purulent cervical discharge.[148,150,151,153,161] On examination 20–70 percent[153,161] of women have a completely normal cervix. Therefore, physical examination is never adequate to exclude chlamydial infection, similar to the situation with gonococcal cervicitis. Because chlamydiae are isolated from over 40–50 percent of the female partners of men with chlamydial nongonoccal urethritis, female partners should be epidemiologically treated even before the diagnosis of chlamydial infection is confirmed by laboratory techniques.

Chlamydiae can be identified in cervical specimens from 75 to 95 percent of infected women by using immunofluoresence microscopy.[153,161–163] An enzyme immunoassay is also about

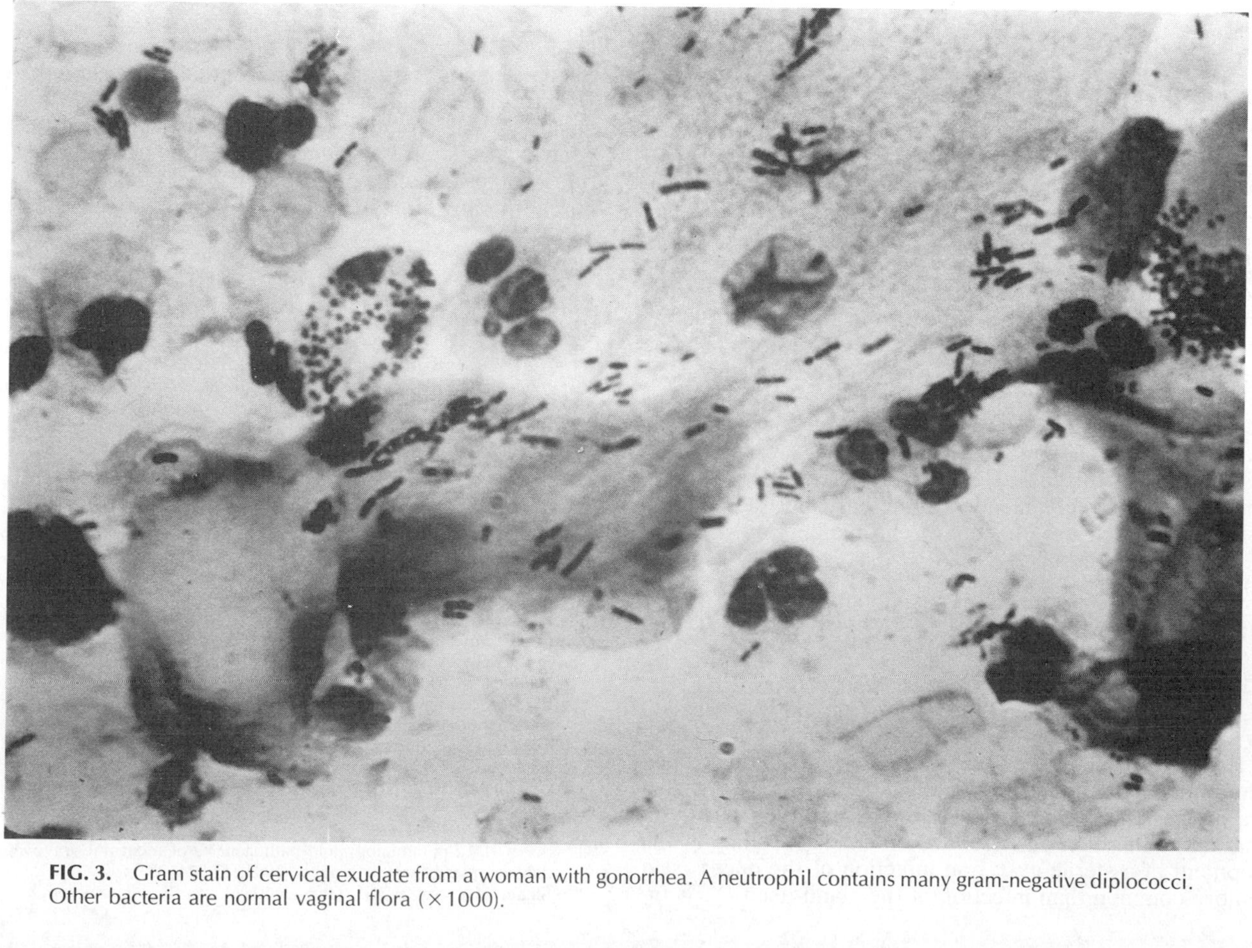

FIG. 3. Gram stain of cervical exudate from a woman with gonorrhea. A neutrophil contains many gram-negative diplococci. Other bacteria are normal vaginal flora (×1000).

80–90 percent sensitive in women.[136] The lower cost of these culture-independent tests has made selective screening for chlamydiae advisable in certain populations.[164] Routine cervical cytology is not useful because of its low sensitivity.[153,161,165] Colposcopy has revealed a typical follicular appearance in most cases and may be useful diagnostically.[166,167]

Herpes simplex virus is isolated from the cervix in 88 percent of women with primary infection but only from 12 percent of women with recurrent herpetic infection.[128,129] Cervicitis may be present without external lesions. Cervicitis is seen on physical examination in about 90 percent of culture-positive women.[128,129] The cervix usually displays diffuse friability and less frequently, frank ulcers or necrosis.[108] Cervical discharge is usually mucoid, but it is occasionally mucopurulent, and in one series, herpetic cervical infection caused 8 percent of cases of mucopurulent cervicitis.[75] Affected patients may have lower abdominal pain, but inguinal adenopathy is rare unless the disease is accompanied by lesions of the external genitalia.[168] The diagnosis may be made cytologically by observing multinucleated giant cells, often with intranuclear inclusions.[169] In the presence of severe necrosis, however, cellular architecture is so distorted that cytologic examination becomes insensitive, and the diagnosis is best made by recovering the virus in tissue culture or by immunofluorescent staining.[170]

Cancer of the cervix behaves epidemiologically as if it is a sexually transmitted disease.[171] A variety of sexually transmitted agents causing cervical infection have been more or less strongly associated with cervical malignancy. These include herpes simplex virus[128,129,171] and *Chlamydia trachomatis*,[166,167] but the strongest association has been established for some types of human papillomavirus[172] (see Chapter 123).

Other organisms occasionally considered causes of cervicitis include adenovirus,[173] type C viruses,[174] cytomegalovirus,[175] *Enterobius vermicularis*,[176] *Mycobacterium tuberculosis*,[177] group B streptococci,[178] and actinomycetes,[179] the last usually in association with the use of intrauterine contraceptive devices.

Therapeutic Approach to Cervicitis

Specifically diagnosed gonococcal cervicitis should be treated as recommended in Chapter 190. Because 30–60 percent of women with gonococcal cervicitis also have chlamydial infection, simultaneous treatment for both infections is advised when gonorrhea is diagnosed.[180] Cervicitis in patients who are the sexual partners of men with nongonococcal urethritis should be treated with tetracycline, 500 mg orally four times daily; doxycycline, 100 mg orally twice daily; or erythromycin, 500 mg orally four times daily, each for 7 days. Because none of these regimens can still be assumed to cure gonorrhea reliably, cervicitis of unknown etiology should probably be treated with one of the aforementioned regimens plus antigonococcal therapy such as ceftriaxone, 250 mg im. Therapy for cervicitis due to herpes simplex is discussed in Chapter 118. A variety of douches have been recommended in the past, but there are no data supporting their use in acute or chronic cervicitis.

INFECTIONS OF BARTHOLIN'S AND SKENE'S GLANDS

Bartholinitis

In the adult, Bartholin's gland is a 1 cm structure on each side of the vagina near the base of the labia minora. The healthy gland is not palpable and nontender. A 2 cm long duct lined with columnar epithelium opens on the inner surface of the labia minora at the junction of the posterior and middle thirds. Inflammation of the duct can produce blockage resulting in the development of a sterile cyst, and infection of the duct is said to be more common than infection of the gland itself.[181,182] Infection of the gland behind a blocked duct can result in the development of a Bartholin's gland abscess.

The frequency with which specific organisms infect Bartholin's glands is unclear. Early writers felt that clinically significant bartholinitis accompanied 2–50 percent of gonococcal infections.[181–183] Rees recovered gonococci from the glands of 28 percent of the women with gonorrhea, most of whom were asymptomatic,[182] but Lee et al. recovered gonococci from only 12 percent of a series of patients with Bartholin's gland abscess.[184] Gonococcal bartholinitis is usually asymptomatic, but about 1 in 5 women has a palpable enlargement or tenderness of the glands, and 1 in 20 has edema.[182] The examiner should attempt to palpate the glands during the pelvic examination. If material can be expressed from the duct opening, it should be examined with the Gram stain, and it should be cultured.

Chlamydia trachomatis is an apparent cause of bartholinitis,[185] although its incidence is undefined. Infection with normal genital flora is also significant. Single or mixed species of anaerobes have been recovered from up to 90 percent of the infected glands.[184,186–188] *Escherichia coli* and *Proteus mirabilis* are also frequently recovered.[184,186,188,189] *Staphylococcus aureus* is apparently a rare cause of abscess, but streptococci are frequently isolated.[184,186,190]

Lee et al. recovered *Ureaplasma urealyticum* from two-thirds of Bartholin's gland abscesses.[184] Occasionally, herpes genitalis involves the duct and produces a recurrent but transient swelling of the gland.

Bartholinitis accompanying gonococcal infection can be treated like acute gonorrhea,[182] although some workers have recommended repeating the treatment daily for 3 days.[181] The optimal initial therapy for bartholinitis of uncertain etiology is not known. A tetracycline, in doses adequate for chlamydial infection, and metronidazole might be considered. A failure of bartholinitis to respond to antibiotic therapy may require surgical drainage of the abscess.[191]

Skenitis

Skene's glands are small structures that empty into the urethra. Dysuria is the usual complaint of patients with infection of these glands,[181] and sometimes a bead of pus can be expressed. The gonococcus is felt to produce some cases of skenitis,[181] but the role of other potential pathogens has not been determined. Empirical therapy similar to that for bartholinitis may be tried.

REFERENCES

1. Lang WR. Pediatric vaginitis. N Engl J Med. 1955;253:1153.
2. Hammerschlag MR, Alpert S, Onderdonk AB, et al. Anaerobic microflora of the vagina in children. Am J Obstet Gynecol. 1978;131:853–60.
3. Hammerschlag MR, Alpert S, Rosner I, et al. Microbiology of the vagina in children: Normal and potentially pathogenic organisms. Pediatrics. 1978;62:57–62.
4. Levison ME, Corman LC, Carrington ER, et al. Quantitative microflora o the vagina. Am J Obstet Gynecol. 1977;127:80.
5. Tashjian JH, Coulam CB, Washington JA. Vaginal flora in asymptomatic women. Mayo Clin Proc. 1976;51:557.
6. Brown WJ. Variations in the bacterial flora: A preliminary report. Ann Intern Med. 1982;96:131.
7. Larsen B, Galask RP. Vaginal microbial flora: Composition and influences of host physiology. Ann Intern Med. 1982;96(Suppl 6):926.
8. Spiegel CA, Amsel R, Eschenbach D, et al. Anaerobic bacteria in nonspecific vaginitis. N Engl J Med. 1980;303:601.
9. Rein MF, Holmes KK. "Nonspecific vaginitis," vulvovaginal candidiasis, and trichomoniasis. In: Remington JS, Swartz MN, eds. Current Clinical Topics in Infectious Diseases. v. 4. New York: McGraw-Hill; 1983:281.
10. Easmon CSF, Ison CA. *Gardnerella vaginalis*. Lancet. 1983;2:343.
11. Guinan ME, Dan BB, Guidotti RJ, et al. Vaginal colonization with *Staphylococcus aureus* in healthy women: A review of four studies. Ann Intern Med. 1982;94:944.
12. Sobel JD. Epidemiology and pathogenesis of recurrent vulvovaginial candidiasis. Am J Obstet Gynecol. 1985;152:924–35.
13. Shafer MA, Sweet RL, Ohm-Smith MJ, et al. Microbiology of the lower

gential tract in postmenarchal adolescent girls: Differences in sexual activity, contraception, and presence of nonspecific vaginitis. J Pediatr. 1985;107:974–81.

14. Hill GB, Eschenbach DA, Holmes KK. Bacteriology of the vaginia. Scand J Urol Nephrol. 1984;18(Suppl 86):23–80.
15. Cohen MS, Black JR, Proctor RA, et al. Host defenses and the vaginal mucosa: A reevaluation. Scand J Urol Nephrol. 1984;8(Suppl 86):13–22.
16. Centers for Disease Control. Nonreported sexually transmitted diseases. MMWR. 1979;28:61.
17. Sweet RL. Importance of differential diagnosis in acute vaginitis. Am J Obstet Gynecol. 1985;152:921–3.
18. Odds FC. *Candida* and Candidiosis. Baltimore: University Park Press; 1979:4.
19. O'Connor MI, Sobel JD. Epidemiology of recurrent vulvovaginal candidiasis: Identification and strain differentiation of *Candida albicans*. J Infect Dis. 1986;154:358–63.
20. Horowitz BJ, Edelstein SW, Lippman L. *Candida tropicalis* vulvovaginitis. Obstet Gynecol. 1985;66:229–32.
21. Clark JFJ, Faggett T, Peters B, et al. Ulcerative vaginitis due to *Torulopsis glabrata*: A case report. J Natl Med Assoc. 1978;70:913.
22. Boquet-Jimenez E, San Cristobal AA. Cytologic and microbiologic aspects of vaginal torulopsis. Acta Cytol (Baltimore). 1978;22:331.
23. Fleury FJ. Adult vaginitis. Clin Obstet Gynecol. 1981;24:407.
24. Heary FJ. Recurrent *Candida* vulvovaginitis. Chemotherapy. 1982;28(Suppl 1):48–50.
25. Oriel JD, Partridge BM, Denny MJ, et al. Genital yeast infections. Br Med J. 1972;4:761.
26. Jackson JL III, Spain WT. Comparative study of combined and sequential anti-ovulatory therapy on vaginal moniliasis. Am J Obstet Gynecol. 1968;101:1134.
27. Powell BL, Frey CL, Drutz DJ. Estrogen receptor in *Candida albicans*. A possible explanation for hormonal influences in vaginal candidiasis (Abstract 751). In: Proceedings of the 23rd 23 ICAAC. Las Vegas, 1983.
28. Elegbe IA, Botu M. A preliminary study on dressing patterns and incidence of candidiasis. Am J Public Health. 1982;72:176.
29. Elgebe IA, Elgebe I. Quantitative relationships of *Candida albicans* infections and dressing patterns in Nigerian women. Am J Public Health. 1983;73:450–2.
30. Heidrich FE, Berg AO, Bergman JJ. Clothing factors and vaginitis. J Family Pract. 1984;19:491–4.
31. Rhoads JL, Wright DC, Redfield RR, et al. Chronic vaginal candidiasis in women with human immunodeficiency virus infection. JAMA. 1987;257:3105–9.
32. Odds FC. Genital candidosis. Clin Exp Dermatol. 1982;7:345–54.
33. Garcia-Tamayo J, Castillo G, Martinez AJ. Human genital candidiasis: Histochemistry, scanning and transmission electron microscopy. Acta Cytol (Baltimore). 1982;26:7.
34. Kimura LH, Pearsall NH. Relationship between germination of *Candida albicans* and increased adherence to human buccal epithelial cells. Infect Immun. 1980;28:464.
35. King RD, Lee JC, Morris AL. Adherence of *Candida albicans* and other *Candida* species to mucosal epithelial cells. Infect Immun. 1980;27:667.
36. Sobel JD, Muller G. Ketoconazole in the prevention of experimental candidal vaginitis. Antimicrob Agents Chemother. 1984;25:281–2.
37. Drake SM, Evans BA, Gerken A. Vaginal pH and microflora related to yeast infections and treatment. Br J Vener Dis. 1980;56:107.
38. Peeters F, Snauwaert R, Segers J, et al. Observation on candidal vaginitis: Vaginal pH, microbiology. Am J Obstet Gynecol. 1972;112:80.
39. Baldson MJ. Comparison of miconazole-coated tampons with clotrimazole vaginal tablets in the treatment of vaginal candidosis. Br J Vener Dis. 1981;57:275.
40. Rothenberg RB, Simm R, Chipperfield E, et al. Efficacy of selected diagnostic tests for sexually transmitted diseases. JAMA. 1976;235:49.
41. Pattman RS. Evaluation of a culture in the diagnosis of vaginal candidosis. Br J Vener Dis. 1981;57:67.
42. Rajakumar R, Lacey CJN, Evans EGV, et al. Use of a slide latex agglutination test for rapid diagnosis of vaginal candidosis. Genitourin Med. 1987;63:192–5.
43. Anonymous. Terconazole for candida vaginitis. Med Lett Drugs Ther. 1988;30:118–9.
44. Odds FC. Cure and relapse with antifungal therapy. Proc R Soc Med. 1977;70(Suppl 4):24.
45. Weisberg M. Treatment of vaginal candidiasis in pregnant women. Clin Ther. 1986;8:563–7.
46. Lebherz T, Guess E, Wolfson N. Efficacy of single- venous multiple-dose clotrimazole therapy in the management of vulvovaginal candidiasis. Am J Obstet Gynecol. 1985;152:965–7.
47. Heary F, Hughes D, Floyd R. Therapeutic results obtained in vaginal mycoses after single-dose treatment with 500 mg clotrimazole vaginal tablets. Am J Obstet Gynecol. 1985;152:968–70.
48. Anonymous. Butoconazole for vulvovaginal candidiasis. Med Lett Drugs Ther. 1986;28:68.
49. Loendersloot EW, Goormans E, Wiesenhann E, et al. Efficacy and tolerability of single-dose versus six-day treatment of candidal vulvovaginitis with vaginal tablets of clotrimazole. Am J Obstet Gynecol. 1985;152:953–5.
50. Bradbeer CS, Mayhew SR, Barlow D. Butoconazole and miconazole in treating vaginal candidiasis. Genitourin Med. 1985;61:270–2.
51. Droegemueller W, Adamson DG, Brown D, et al. Three-day treatment with butoconazole nitrate for vulvovaginal candidiasis. Obstet Gynecol. 1984;64:530–4.
52. Cohen L. Single dose treatment of vaginal candidosis: Comparison of clotrimazole and isoconazole. Br J Vener Dis. 1984;60:42–4.
53. Milson I, Forssman L. Treatment of vaginal candidosis with a single 500 mg clotrimazole pessary. Br J Vener Dis. 1982;58:124.
54. Sobel JD. Management of recurrent vulvovaginal candidiasis with intermittent ketoconazole prophylaxis. Obstet Gynecol. 1985;65:435–40.
55. Sobel JD. Recurrent vulvovaginal candidiasis. A prospective study of the efficacy of maintenance ketoconazole therapy. N Engl J Med. 1986;315:1455–8.
56. Eschenbach DA, Hummel D, Gravett MG. Recurrent and persistant vulvovaginal candidiasis: Treatment with ketoconazole. Obstet Gynecol. 1985;66:248–54.
57. Calderón-Márquez JJ. Itraconzole in the treatment of vaginal candidosis and the effect of treatment of the sexual partner. Rev Infect Dis. 1987;9(Suppl 1):143–5.
58. Clayton YM. Antifungal drugs in current use: A review. Proc R Soc Med. 1977;70(Suppl 4):15.
59. Vorherr H, Vorherr UF, Mehta P, et al. Vaginal absorption of povidone-iodine. JAMA. 1980;244:2628.
60. van Slyke KK, Michel VP, Rein MF. Treatment of vulvovaginal candidiasis with boric acid powder. Am J Obstet Gynecol. 1981;141:145.
61. Cohen L. Is more than one application of an antifungal necessary in the treatment of acute vaginal candidiasis. Am J Obstet Gynecol. 1985;152:961–4.
62. Odds FC, Abbott AB. A simple system for the presumptive identification of *Candida albicans* and differentiation of strains within the species. Sabouraudia. 1980;18:301–17.
63. Odds FC, Abbott AB. Modification and extension of tests for differentiation of *Candida* species and strains. Sabouraudia. 1983;21:79–81.
64. Hill LVH, Embil JA. Vaginits: Current microbiological and clinical concepts. Can Med Assoc J. 1986;134:3221–31.
65. Milne JD, Warnock DW. Effect of simultaneous oral and vaginal treatment on the rate of cure and relapse in vaginal candidosis. Br J Vener Dis. 1979;55:362.
66. Velupillai S, Thin RN. Treatment of vulvovaginal yeast infection with nystatin. Practitioner. 1977;219:897.
67. Nystatin Multicenter Study Group. Therapy of candidal vaginitis: The effect of eliminating intestinal *Candida*. Am J Obstet Gynecol. 1986;155:651–5.
68. Lossick JG. Sexually transmitted vaginitis. Semin Adolesc Med. 1985;2:131–42.
69. Edman J, Sobel JD, Taylor ML. Zinc status in women with recurrent vulvovaginal candidiasis. Am J Obstet Gynecol. 1986;155:1082–5.
70. Witkin SS, Yu IR, Ledger WJ. Inhibition of *Candida albicans*-induced lymphocyte proliferation by lymphocytes and sera from women with recurrent vaginitis. Am J Obstet Gynecol. 1983;147:809–11.
71. Davidson F, Mould RF. Recurrent genital candidosis in women and the effect of intermittent prophylactic treatment. Br J Vener Dis. 1978;54:176.
72. Waugh MA. Clinical presentation of candidal balanitis—its differential diagnosis and treatment. Chemotherapy. 1982;28(Suppl 1):56–60.
73. Gardner HL, Dukes CD. *Haemophilus vaginalis* vaginitis: A newly defined specific infection previously classified "non-specific" vaginitis. Am J Obstet Gynecol. 1955;69:962.
74. Mårdh PA, Taylor-Robinson D, eds. Bacterial vaginosis. Scand J Urol Nephrol. 1984;18(Suppl 86):1–270.
75. Brunham RC, Paavonen J, Stevens CE, et al. Mucopurulent cervicitis—the ignored counterpart in women of urethritis in men. N Engl J Med. 1984;311:1–6.
76. Phiefer TA, Forsyth PS, Durfee MA, et al. Nonspecific vaginitis: Role of *Haemophilus vaginalis* and treatment with metronidazole. N Engl J Med. 1978;298:1429.
77. Chen KCS, Forsyth PS, Buchanan TM, et al. Amine content of vaginal fluid from untreated and treated patients with nonspecific vaginitis. J Clin Invest. 1979;63:828.
78. Hanna NF, Taylor-Robinson D, Kalodiki-Karamanoli M, et al. The relation between vaginal pH and the microbiological status in vaginitis. Br J Obstet Gynaecol. 1985;92:1267–71.
79. Baldson MJ, Taylor GE, Pead L, et al. *Corynebacterium vaginale* and vaginitis: A controlled trial of treatment. Lancet. 1980;1:501.
80. Vontver LA, Eschenbach DA. The role of *Gardnerella vaginalis* in nonspecific vaginitis. Clin Obstet Gynecol. 1981;24:439.
81. Amsel R, Totten PA, Spiegel CA, et al. Nonspecific vaginitis: Diagnostic criteria and microbial and epidemiological associations. Am J Med. 1983;74:14.
82. Bhattycharyya MN, Jones BM. *Haemophilus vaginalis* infection: Diagnosis and treatment. J Reprod Med. 1980;24:71.
83. Ratnam S, Fitzgerald BL. Semiquantitative culture of *Gardnerella vaginalis* in laboratory determination of nonspecific vaginitis. J Clin Microbiol. 1983;18:344.
84. Totten PA, Amsel R, Hale J, et al. Selective differential human blood bilayer media for isolation of *Gardnerella* (*Haemophilus*) *vaginalis*. J Clin Microbiol. 1982;15:141–7.
85. Thomason JL, Gelbart SM, Wilcoski LM. Proline aminopeptidase activity as a rapid diagnostic test to confirm bacterial vaginosis. Obstet Gynecol. 1988;71:607–71.

86. Chen KCS, Amsel R, Eschenbach DA, et al. Biochemical diagnosis of vaginitis: Determination of diamines in vaginal fluid. J Infect Dis. 1982;145:337.
87. Greenwood JR, Picket MJ. Transfer of *Haemophilus vaginalis* to a new genus, *Gardnerella: G. vaginalis* (Gardner and Dukes) comb. nov. Int J Syst Bacteriol. 1980;30:170.
88. Malouf M, Fortier M, Morin G, et al. Treatment of *Hemophilus vaginalis* vaginitis. Obstet Gynecol. 1980;57:711.
89. Monhanty KC, Deighton R. Comparison of 2 g single dose of metronidazole, nimorazole and tinidazole in the treatment of vaginitis associated with *Gardnerella vaginalis*. J Antimicrob Chemother. 1987;19:393–9.
90. Mohanty KC, Deighton R. Comparison of two different metronidazole regimens in the treatment of *Gardnerella vaginalis* infection with or without trichomoniasis. J Antimicrob Chemother. 1985;16:799–803.
91. van der Meijden WI, Piot P, Loriaux SM, et al. Amoxycillin, amoxycillin-clavulanic acid and metronidazole in the treatment of clue cell positive discharge. A comparative clinical and laboratory study. J Antimicrob Chemother. 1987;20:735–42.
92. Amsel R, Critchlow CW, Spiegel CA, et al. Comparison of metronidazole, ampicillin, and amoxicillin for treatment of bacterial vaginosis (nonspecific vaginitis): Possible explanation for the greater efficacy of metronidazole. In: Finegold S, ed. United States Metronidazole Conference. Proceedings from a Symposium, Tarpon Springs, Florida, February 18–20, 1982. New York: Biomedical Information Corp; 1982:225.
93. Shanker S, Munro R. Sensitivity of *Gardnerella vaginalis* to metabolites of metronidazole and tinidazole. Lancet. 1982;1:167.
94. Taylor E, Blackwell AL, Barlow D, et al. *Gardnerella vaginalis*, anaerobes, and vaginal discharge. Lancet. 1982;1:1376.
95. Eschenbach DA, Gravett MG, Chen KCS, et al. Bacterial vaginosis during pregnancy: An association with prematurity and postpartum complications. Scand J Urol Nephrol. 1984;18(Suppl 86):213–22.
96. Paavonen J, Miettinen A, Stevens CE, et al. *Mycoplasma hominis* in nonspecific vaginitis. Sex Transm Dis. 1983;10:271–5.
97. Swedberg J, Steiner JF, Deiss F, et al. Comparison of single-dose vs. one-week course of metronidazole for symptomatic bacterial vaginosis. JAMA. 1985;254:1046–9.
98. Alawattegama AB, Jones BM, Kinghorn GR, et al. Single-dose versus seven-day metronidazole in *Gardnerella vaginalis* associated non-specific vaginitis. Lancet. 1984;1:1355–7.
99. Eschenbach DA, Critchlow CW, Watkins H, et al. A dose-duration study of metronidazole for the treatment of nonspecific vaginosis. Scand J Infect Dis. 1983;40(Suppl):73–6.
100. Jones BM, Geary I, Alawattegama AB, et al. *In vitro* and *in vivo* activity of metronidazole against *Gardnerella vaginalis*, *Bacteroides* spp. and *Mobiluncus* spp. in bacterial vaginosis. J Antimicrob Chemother. 1985;16:189–97.
101. Ison CA, Taylor RFH, Link C, et al. Local treatment for bacterial vaginosis. Br Med J. [Clin Res] 1987;295:886.
102. Bardi M, Maneti G, Mattioni D, et al. Metronidazole for nonspecific vaginitis. Lancet. 1980;1:1029.
102a. Greaves WL, Chungafung J, Morris B, et al. Clindamycin versus metronidazole in the treatment of bacterial vaginosis. Obstet Gynecol. 1988;72:799–802.
103. Garnder HL. *Hemophilus vaginalis* vaginitis after twenty-five years. Am J Obstet Gynecol. 1980;137:385–92.
104. Piot P, Van Dyck E, Godts P, et al. A placebo-controlled, double blind comparison of tinidazole and triple sulfonamide cream for the treatment of nonspecific vaginitis. Am J Obstet Gynecol. 1983;147:85–9.
105. Fredicsson B, Englund K, Weintraub L, et al. Ecological treatment of bacterial vaginosis. Lancet. 1987;1:276.
106. McDowall DRM, Buchanan JD, Fairley KF, et al. Anaerobic and other fastidious microorganisms in asymptomatic bacteriuria in pregnant women. J Infect Dis. 1981;144:114.
107. Rosene K, Eschenbach DA, Tompkins LS, et al. Polymicrobial early postpartum endometritis with facultative and anaerobic bacteria, genital mycoplasmas, and *Chlamydia trachomatis*: Treatment with piperacillin or cefoxitin. J Infect Dis. 1986;153:1028–37.
108. Lamey JR, Eschenbach DA, Mitchell SH, et al. Isolation of mycoplasmas and bacteria from the blood of postpartum women. Am J Obstet Gynecol. 1982;143:104–12.
109. Gravett MG, Hummel DH, Eschenbach DA, et al. Preterm labor associated with subclinical amniotic fluid infection and with bacterial vaginosis. Obstet Gynecol. 1986;67:229–37.
110. Venkataramani TK, Rathbun HK. *Corynebacterium vaginale* (*Hemophilus vaginalis*) bacteremia: Clinical study of 29 cases. Johns Hopkins Med J. 1976;139:93.
111. Reimer LG, Reller LB. *Gardnerella vaginalis* bacteremia: A review of 30 cases. Obstet Gynecol. 1984;65:170–2.
112. Darieux R, Dublanchet A. Les "vibrions" anaerobics des leucorrhees. I: Technique d'isolement et sensibilite aux antibiotiques. Med Mal Infect. 1980;10:109.
113. Sprott MS, Pattman RS, Ingham HR, et al. Anaerobic curved rods in vaginitis. Lancet. 1982;1:54.
114. Hjelm E, Hallen A, Forsum U, et al. Motile anaerobic curved rods in nonspecific vaginitis. Eur J Sex Transm Dis. 1982;1:9.
115. Spiegel CA, Eschenbach DA, Amsel R, et al. Curved anaerobic bacteria in bacterial vaginosis and their response to antimicrobial therapy. J Infect Dis. 1983;148:817.
116. Thomason JL, Schreckenberger PC, Spellacy WN, et al. Clinical and microbiological characterization of patients with nonspecific vaginosis associated with motile, curved anaerobic rods. J Infect Dis. 1984;149:801–9.
117. Spiegel CA. New developments in the etiology and pathogenesis of bacterial vaginosis. Adv Exp Med Biol. 1987;224:127–34.
118. Thomason JL and the Working Group. Diagnosis of infection with anaerobic cervical rods. Scan J Urol Neophrol. 1984;18(Suppl 86):261–2.
119. Spiegel CA, Roberts, M. *Mobiluncus* gen nov, *Mobiluncus curtisii* subspecies *curtisii* sp. nov., *Mobiluncus curtisii* subspecies *holmesii* subsp. nov., and *Mobiluncus mulieris* sp. nov; curved rods from the human vagina. Int J Syst Bacteriol. 1984;34:177–184.
120. Shands KN, Schmid GP, Dan BB, et al. Toxic shock syndrome in menstruating women: Association with tampon use and *Staphylococcus aureus* and clinical features in 52 cases. N Engl J Med. 1980;303:1436.
121. Tofte RW, Williams DN. Clinical and laboratory manifestations of toxic shock syndrome. Ann Intern Med. 1982;96:843.
122. Lanes SF, Poole C, Dreyer NA. Toxic shock syndrome, contraceptive methods, and vaginitis. Am J Obstet Gynecol. 1986;154:989–91.
123. Zaaijman JD, deBeer J. An unusual vaginal foreign body. S. Afr Med J. 1982;61:33.
124. Friedrich EG, Siegesmund KA. Tampon associated vaginal ulcerations. Obstet Gynecol. 1980;55:149.
125. Friedrich EG. Tampon effects on vaginal health. Clin Obstet Gynecol. 1981;24:295.
126. Jimerson SD, Becker JD. Vaginal ulcers associated with tampon usage. Obstet Gynecol. 1980;56:97.
127. Weissberg SM, Dodson MG. Recurrent vaginal and cervical ulcers associated with tampon use. JAMA. 1983;250:1430.
128. Corey L, Adams HG, Brown AZ, et al. Genital herpes simplex virus infections: Clinical manifestations, course, and complications. Ann Intern Med. 1983;98:958.
129. Pazin GH. Management of oral and genital herpes simplex viral infections: Diagnosis and treatment. DM. 1986;32:725–824.
130. Corey L, Holmes KK. The use of 2-deoxy-D-glucose for genital herpes. JAMA. 1980;243:29.
131. Ginsburg CM. Group A streptococcal vaginitis in children. Pediatr Infect Dis. 1982;1:36.
132. Symmers WStC. Pathology of oxyuriasis. Arch Pathol. 1950;50:475.
133. Dump RC. *Chlamydia trachomatis* as a cause of prepubertal vaginitis. Obstet Gynecol. 1985;65:384–8.
134. Cibley LF, Cibley LJ. Diagnostic considerations in vulvovaginal candidiasis. J Reprod Med. 1986;31(Suppl 7):648–9.
135. Fisher AA. Allergic reactions to feminine hygiene sprays. Arch Dermatol. 1973;108:801.
136. Chang T. Familial allergic seminal vulvovaginitis. Am J Obstet Gynecol. 1976;126:442.
137. Gochfeld M, Burger J. Sexual transmission of nickel and poison oak contact dermatitis. Lancet. 1983;1:589.
138. Gardner HL. Desquamative inflammatory vaginitis: A newly defined entity. Am J Obstet Gynecol. 1968;102:1102–5.
139. Edwards L, Friedrich EG. Desquamative vaginitis: Lichen planus in disguise. Obstet Gynecol. 1988;71:832–6.
140. Huggins GR, Preti G. Vaginal odors and secretions. Clin Obstet Gynecol. 1981;24:355.
141. Friedrich EG. The vulvar vestibule. J Reprod Med. 1983;28:773–7.
142. Peckham BM, Maki DG, Patterson JJ, et al. Focal vulvitis: A characteristic syndrome and cause of dyspareunia. Features, natural history, and management. Am J Obstet Gynecol. 1986;154:855–64.
143. Kramer K, Jobón H. Vaginitis emphasematosa. Arch Pathol Lab Med. 1987;111:746–9.
144. McCallion JS, Parkin DE. Emphasematous vaginitis masquerading as carcinoma of the cervix. Case report. Br J Obstet Gynecol. 1988;95:309–11.
145. Dodson MG, Friedrich EG. Psychosomatic vulvovaginitis. Obstet Gynecol. 1978;51(Suppl):23.
146. Al-Saliki FL, Curran JP, Wong J-S. Neonatal *Trichomonas vaginalis*: Report of three cases and review of the literature. Pediatrics. 1974;53:196.
147. Paradise JE, Campos JM, Friedman HM, et al. Vulvovaginitis in premenarchal girls: Clinical features and diagnostic evaluation. Pediatrics. 1982;70:193.
148. Rees E, Tait IA, Hobson D, et al. Chlamydia in relation to cervical infection and pelvic inflammatory disease. In: Hobson D, Holmes KK, eds. Nongonococcal Urethritis and Related Infections. Lake Placid, NY: American Society for Microbiology; 1976.
149. Silverman EM, Silverman AG. Persistence of spermatozoa in the lower genital tracts of women. JAMA. 1978;240:1875.
150. Tait IA, Rees E, Hobson D, et al. Chlamydial infection of the cervix in contacts of men with non-gonococcal urethritis. Br J Vener Dis. 1980;56:37.
151. Mardh P-A, Moller BR, Paavonen J. Chlamydial infection of the female genital tract with emphasis on pelvic inflammatory disease. A review of Scandinavian studies. Sex Transm Dis. 1981;8:140.
152. Paavonen J, Vesterinen E. *Chlamydia trachomatis* in cervicitis and urethritis in women. Scand J Infect Dis. 1982;32(Suppl):45.
153. Spence MR, Barbacci M, Kappus E, et al. A correlative study of Papanicolaou smear, fluorescent antibody, and culture for the diagnosis of *Chlamydia trachomatis*. Obstet Gynecol. 1986:68:691–5.
154. Paavonen J, Critchlow CW, DeRouen T, et al. Etiology of cervical inflammation. Am J Obstet Gynecol. 1986;154:556–64.

155. Harrison HR, Costin M, Meder JB, et al. Cervical *Chlamydia trachomatis* infection in university women: Relationship to history, contraception, ectopy, and cervicitis. Am J Obstet Gynecol. 1985;153:224–51.
156. Moscicki B, Shafer MA, Millstein SG, et al. The use and limitations of endocervical Gram stains and mucopurulent cervicitis as predictors for *Chlamydia trachomatis* in female adolescents. Am J Obstet Gynecol. 1987;157:65–71.
157. Wentworth BB, Bonin P, Holmes KK, et al. Isolation of viruses, bacteria and other organisms from venereal disease clinic patients: Methodology and problems associated with multiple isolations. Health Lab Sci. 1973;10:75.
158. Curran JW, Rendtorff RC, Chandler RW, et al. Female gonorrhea: Its relationship to abnormal uterine bleeding, urinary tract symptoms and cervicitis. Obstet Gynecol. 1975;45:195.
159. Hilton AL, Richmond SJ, Milne JD, et al. Chlamydia A in the female genital tract. Br J Vener Dis. 1974;50:1.
160. Oriel JD, Powis PA, Reeve P, et al. Chlamydial infection of the cervix. Br J Vener Dis. 1974;50:11.
161. Quinn TC, Gupta PK, Burkman RT. Detection of *Chlamydia trachomatis* cervical infections: A comparison of Papanicolaou and immunofluorescent staining with cell cultures. Am J Obstet Gynecol. 1987;157:394–9.
162. Stamm WE, Harrison HR, Alexander ER, et al. Diagnosis of *Chlamydia trachomatis* infections by direct immunofluorescence staining of genital secretions: A multicenter trial. Ann Intern Med. 1984;101:638–42.
163. Hipp SS, Han V, Murphy D. Assessment of enzyme immunoassay and immunofluorescence tests for detection of *Chlamydia trachomatis*. J Clin Microbiol. 1987;25:1983–92.
164. Phillps RS, Aronson MD, Taylor WC, et al. Should tests for *Chlamydia trachomatis* cervical infection be done during routine gynecological visits? An analysis of the costs of alternative strategies. Ann Intern Med. 1987;107:188–94.
165. Purola E, Paavonen J. Routine cytology as a diagnostic aid in chlamydial cervicitis. Scand J Infect Dis. 1982;32(Suppl):55.
166. Hare MJ, Toone E, Taylor-Robinson D, et al. Follicular cervicitis: Colposcopic appearances and association with *Chlamydia trachomatis*. Br J Obstet Gynecol. 1981;88:174.
167. Paavonen J, Vesterinen E, Meyer B, et al. Colposcopic and histological findings in cervical chlamydial infection. Obstet Gynecol. 1982;59:712.
168. Willcox RR. Necrotic cervicitis due to primary infection with the virus of herpes simplex. Br Med J. 1968;1:610.
169. Morse AR, Coleman DV, Gardner SD. An evaluation of cytology in the diagnosis of herpes simplex virus infection and cytomegalovirus infection of the cervix uteri. J Obstet Gynecol Br Commonwealth. 1974;81:393.
170. Corey L. Laboratory diagnosis of herpes simplex virus infections. Principles guiding the development of rapid diagnostic tests. Diagn Microbiol Infect Dis. 1986;4(Suppl):1115–95.
171. Aurelian L. The "viruses of love" and cancer. Am J Med Tech. 1974;40:496.
172. Pfister H. Relationship of papillomaviruses to anogenital cancer. Obstet Gynecol. Clin North Am. 1987;14:349–62.
173. Laverty CR, Russell P, Black J, et al. Adenovirus infection of the cervix. Acta Cytol (Baltimore). 1977;21:114.
174. Marquart K-H, Cunderlik VN. Oncornavirus-like particles in biopsy material from a glandular erosion of the human uterine cervix. Acta Cytol (Baltimore). 1976;29:335.
175. Deppisch LM. Cytomegalovirus inclusion body endocervicitis: Significance of CMV inclusions in endocervical biopsies. Mt. Sinai J Med. 1981;48:418.
176. Wong JV, Becker SN. *Enterobius vermicularis* ova in routine cervicovaginal smears. Light a scanning electron microscopic observations. Acta Cytol (Baltimore). 1982;26:484.
177. Tang LCH. Postmenopausal tuberculous cervicitis. Acta Obstet Gynecol Scand. 1986;65:279–81.
178. Buttigieg G. Cervicitis and urethritis caused by group B streptococcus: Case report. Genitourin Med. 1985;61:343–4.
179. Mao K, Guillebaud J. Influence of removal of intrauterine contraceptive devices on colonization of the cervix by *Actinomyces*-like organisms. Contraception. 1984;30:535–44.
180. Washington AE, Browner WS, Korenbrot CC. Cost-effectiveness of combined treatment for endocervical gonorrhea. Considering coinfection with *Chlamydia trachomatis*. JAMA. 1987;257:2056–60.
181. Morton RS. Gonorrhea. London: WB Saunders; 1977:108.
182. Rees E: Gonococcal bartholinitis. Br J Vener Dis. 1967;43:150.
183. Norris CC: Gonorrhea in Women. Philadelphia; WB Saunders; 1913:202.
184. Lee Y-H, Rankin JS, Alpert S, et al. Microbiological Investigation of Bartholin's gland abscesses and cysts. Am J Obstet Gynecol. 1977;129:150.
185. Davies JA, Rees E, Hobson D, et al. Isolation of *Chlamydia trachomatis* from Bartholin's duct. Br J Vener Dis. 1978;54:409.
186. Swensen RM. Anaerobic bacteria in infections of the female genital tract. In: Balows A, DeHaan RM, Dowell VR, et al., eds. Anaerobic Bacteria Role in Disease. Springfield, IL: Charles C Thomas, 1974.
187. Swenson RM, Michaelson TC, Dayl MJ, et al. Anaerobic bacterial infections of the female genital tract. Obstet Gynecol. 1973;42:538.
188. Kubitz R, Hoffman K. Bartholin's gland abscess in an infant. A case report. J Reprod Med. 1986;31:67–9.
189. Carson GD, Smith LP. *Escherichia coli* endotoxic shock complicating Bartholin's gland abscess. Can Med Assoc J. 1980;122:1397.
190. Morton BD, McCarthy LR. Bartholinitis: An unusual etiologic agent. Obstet Gynecol. 1980;55(Suppl):97.
191. Azzan BB. Bartholin's cyst and abscess: A review of treatment of 53 cases. Br J Clin Pract. 1978;32:101.

96. INFECTIONS OF THE FEMALE PELVIS

WILLIAM J. LEDGER

In most soft tissue infections of the female, multiple bacterial species are recovered, and frequently some or all of these organisms are anaerobes. In recent years, there has been increasing awareness of the importance of *Chlamydia trachomatis* in many of these pelvic infections.

PATHOGENESIS

Animal model studies of peritoneal infection have suggested a biphasic response to massive bacterial contamination of bowel flora,[1] with early-onset peritonitis and septicemia with gram-negative aerobic organisms, followed later by intra-abdominal abscess formation with anaerobic bacteria.[2] The significance of any animal model evaluation is only as great as the parallel with human experience, and it is clear that early-onset septicemia and late-onset abscess formation are recognizable clinical syndromes. The only variation from the animal model seen in female patients with infections of the pelvis is the frequency (25 percent or more) of anaerobic bacteria and gram-positive aerobic blood stream isolates in early-onset bacteremia.[3–5]

Microbiology

The diagnostic microbiology laboratory can be very helpful in the management of these women. However, the laboratory report will only be as good as the specimen submitted by the physician. Since there is an abundant normal anaerobic flora on the surface of the mucous membranes of the lower genital tract, a surface swab of the vagina or endocervix is not acceptable for the evaluation of cases of deep pelvic infections such as postabortion infection, postpartum endomyometritis, or salpingo-oophoritis. Sheathed containers can be used to obtain specimens from the endometrial cavity.[6] Needle sampling of the peritoneal cavity or direct aspiration of an abscess yields good material for the laboratory to isolate anaerobic bacteria (Fig. 1). This sample can be transported to the laboratory for processing in an air-free container, such as the syringe in which it is collected. Since serious infections usually occur late at night, either the laboratory should provide 24-hour coverage or the physician should be taught to plate the specimens directly and to incubate the plates in an anaerobic environment.[7] Agar dilution testing of gram-negative anaerobes is required for antibiotic sensitivity testing. This is important because it has been

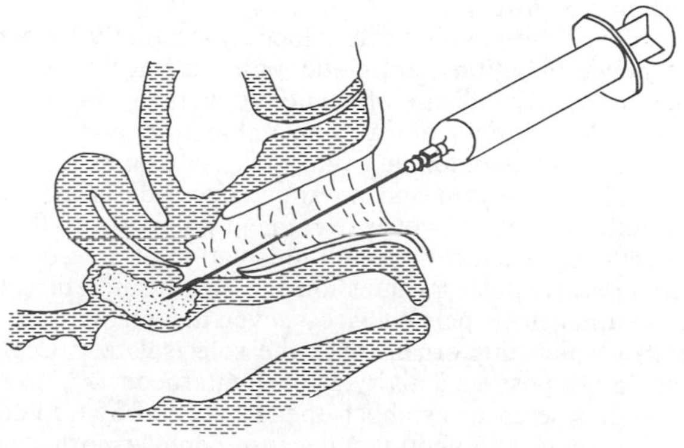

FIG. 1. Appropriate microbiologic sampling technique for the patient with acute salpingitis.

reported that the antibiotic susceptibility of *Bacteroides fragilis* varies considerably from institution to institution.[8] There has been increasing concern about the role of chlamydia in salpingitis in the United States. The inability to grow this organism from peritoneal fluid samples[9] has led to a new use of the endometrial biopsy to obtain the culture for this organism.[10] Tissue culture isolation systems are not available in all hospitals, but monoclonal antibody testing for *Chlamydia* is a feasible technique for all laboratories. Although not as specific as tissue culture (i.e., some positive tests are not culture positive), the test has good sensitivity.

The selection of antibiotics for the patient with a soft tissue pelvic infection should be guided by an awareness of the organisms frequently involved. Most patients are young, with intact hose defense mechanisms. Few have serious underlying diseases that require multiple hospital admissions or stays in nursing homes. As a result, resistant organisms are seldom a problem. Instead, more common gram-negative aerobic organisms, such as *Escherichia coli*, are usually isolated, in addition to anaerobes, *Chlamydia* strains, and enterococci.

Antibiotics

The aminoglycosides, cephalosporins, and penicillins, are used to treat the most common infections seen by obstetrician-gynecologists. The choice of antibiotic should be based upon the recent antibiotic susceptibility patterns of such organisms in the hospital, because the patterns of gram-negative aerobic antibiotic susceptibility vary from hospital to hospital. Aminoglycoside dosage should be based upon an accurate assessment of the patient's age and weight, on frequent studies of renal function, and on peak and trough antibiotic levels to assess the individual patient's response. Since most obstetric-gynecologic patients are young with good renal function, the major problem with aminoglycosides is underdosing. Despite this, aminoglycoside failures are few.[11]

For treatment of anaerobic organisms, additional antibiotics should be considered. In addition to gram-positive anaerobes, including peptostreptococci and clostridia, the major concern is gram-negative anaerobic rods. These include *B. fragilis, B. melaninogenicus, B. bivius, B. disiens*, and *Fusobacterium* strains. Clindamycin and metronidazole, have been approved by the Food and Drug Administration (FDA) for use in these situations. Newer penicillins given in high doses intravenously are effective against a high percentage of anaerobes. These include carbenicillin, ticarcillin, piperacillin, mezlocillin, and azlocillin. In addition, penicillins such as ticarcillin or ampicillin, with an added β-lactamase inhibitor, clavulanate, or sulbactam, are also effective. Cefoxitin, a cephamycin, and cefotetan have significant activity against anaerobes, including *B. fragilis*, and are useful agents in the treatment of pelvic infections. Metronidazole is the most bactericidal agent in laboratory tests against *B. fragilis*.

Since coagulase-positive staphylococci are rarely isolated in female pelvic infections, antibiotics, targeted against such organisms are rarely indicated for initial coverage.

None of these agents, alone or incombination, provides complete coverage of all potential pathogens. For example, the combination of clindamycin and an aminoglycoside is ineffective against enterococci. However, treatment failures with this regimen occur less frequently than the isolation of enterococci.[12] Thus, some investigators question the significance of enterococci as pathogens in pelvic abscess, even though there are case reports in which this organism is the sole isolate.[13] Cephalosporins do not possess activity against enterococci.[14] More detailed studies seem to establish the role of these streptococci in hospital-acquired infections, because cephalosporins are so frequently prescribed in the United States.[15]

An important consideration in the treatment of female pelvic infections is the development of abscesses. Patients with a pelvic abscess often require operative intervention for cure. However, some patients with a pelvic abscess will respond to medical treatment alone. Treatment with antibiotics is the important first step toward cure. The problem for the clinician is the patient who fails to respond to systemic antibiotics. In the past, physicians assumed that patients who failed medical treatment had antibiotic-resistant organisms at the site of infection; in such patients, other antibiotics were tried before resorting to operative intervention. In women with a suspected pelvic abscess, the physician should use antibiotics that are effective against gram-negative anaerobes from the beginning of therapy. If this is done and there is no clinical response, operative drainage or removal is necessary. One study of multiple-antibiotic therapy for the treatment of serious pelvic infections documented 40 patients who failed to respond and who required some form of operative intervention. In only 2 of these 40 women were the bacteria recovered from the abscess resistant in vitro to the antibiotics used.[16] In these cases, continued spiking fevers were not due to antibiotic resistance but to the unique environment of the abscess, which inhibited antibiotic effectiveness. Imaging techniques have been helpful in the management of the patient with a persistent fever. Ultrasound can demonstrate the presence of a fluid-filled mass, but in some cases, it will not differentiate an inflammatory cyst from an abscess. Computed tomography scanning and magnetic resonance imaging usually give better resolution of the pelvic findings and can guide directed needle aspiration of abscesses.[17] Clinical observation is important. Patient deterioration in the form of tachycardia, hypotension, or tachypnea may indicate loss of integrity of the abscess capsule with intra-abdominal leaking. In the face of these signs of clinical deterioration, continued physician dependence upon medical therapy is not in the patient's best interests. If the decision is made to operate, the least extensive operation compatible with cure should be used. If the abscess is amenable to extraperitoneal drainage, this alone should suffice. If not, operative extirpation will be necessary.

HOSPITAL-ACQUIRED INFECTIONS

Postpartum Endomyometritis

It is surprising that infection of the uterus is an infrequent postpartum event, since so many factors that can contribute to infection are present in abundance. The lower genital tract (i.e., the vagina and endocervix) has a heavy flora of bacteria, many of which can be pathogenic. During the course of every observed labor, many internal examinations are performed, each of which forces some bacteria above the endocervical canal into the uterus. In many women, invasive indwelling monitoring equipment consisting of a fetal scalp electrode and an intra-amniotic catheter will be used for many hours. Delivery, either vaginally or by cesarean section, is nearly always accompanied by tissue trauma, operative repair with the use of suture, a foreign material, and blood loss of 1–2 units even in uncomplicated cases. The combination of bacterial contamination and compromise of local host defense mechanisms by these operative procedures yields a high probability of a postpartum uterine infection. The observation that such infections occur in only a minority of women is evidence of the usual adequacy of host defense mechanisms in normal young patients with healthy tissues.

There are a number of recognized events that lower the risk of maternal postpartum infection. There is a remarkable change in the bacterial flora of the lower genital tract during the course of pregnancy; anaerobic organisms, particularly gram-negative ones, decrease late in pregnancy.[18] Amniotic fluid studies demonstrate increasing antibacterial activity as term approaches, which may be due in part to the activity of lysozymes,[19] β-lysin,[20] transferrin,[21] immunoglobulins,[22] peroxidase,[23] and another antibacterial substance,[24] which rises progressively until the 40th week of gestation, when a secondary fall is again seen.[24–27] The useful efficiency of these local host defense mechanisms in clearing the uterus of bacteria has been demonstrated by Spore et al.,[28] who found no bacteria in the uterine cavity at the time of elective tubal ligation postpartum. Normal women with no clinical evidence of infection have elevated white blood cell counts during pregnancy, labor, and the puerperium.[29] In addition, there is evidence of increased white blood cell activity, manifested by a higher percentage of women free of infection who have an elevated number of nitroblue tetrazolium dye-positive leukocytes.[29]

There are a number of factors that probably increase the risk of a postpartum uterine infection. In recent years, invasive monitoring techniques have been widely used in obstetrics. These techniques undoubtedly increase the risk of infection, but the degree of risk seems to be small. An increased risk can be demonstrated in middle-class private patients[30] but not in patients of the lower socioeconomic classes.[31] The percentage of women in the latter category who develop an infection after vaginal delivery is less than 4 percent. This is not the case among women undergoing cesarean section, which is more commonly performed for fetal indications than in the past. The infection rate is higher and the infections are more serious than those in women who have delivered vaginally.[32] Any analysis of infection in postpartum women is difficult because of the multiplicity of factors involved. The length of labor, invasive monitoring, ruptured membranes, number of vaginal examinations, and so on may be less important than the socioeconomic status of the patient. Major differences have been noted in an institution whose patients have different socioeconomic backgrounds.[31]

The organsms involved in postpartum uterine, pelvic, and abdominal wound infections are often found in the lower genital tract of asymptomatic patients. The most frequent isolates include aerobes such as *E. coli, Klebsiella* spp., group B β-hemolytic streptococci, enterococci, and anaerobes such as peptostreptococci, *B. fragilis, B. bivius*, and *B. disiens*. In most situations, the clinical diagnosis of an infection will be made before culture reports are available, and the initial antibiotic prescription must be made empirically. The selection of antibiotic agents before the receipt of culture reports should focus on the most commonly isolated bacteria. *Chlamydia trachomatis* should not be considered normal flora. It is involved in many cases of late postpartum endomyometritis.[33] A number of other pathogenic organsms are also occasionally associated with serious illness in this setting. These include group A β-hemolytic streptococci and the coagulase-positive staphylococci. Since these are uncommon isolates, they should not be a primary consideration when ordering the initial antibiotic postpartum.

Antibiotic therapy for the postpartum patient with a soft tisue infection is empiric and is not based on a prospective study documenting the best therapeutic approach. Data obtained from hospital surveillance are helpful.[34] Following vaginal delivery, I recommend a single antibiotic, either cefoxitin or a newer penicillin, in patients with no evidence of a urinary tract infection.

Two categories of patients who have undergone vaginal delivery have a more serious prognosis. First, women with extensive extrauterine soft tissue infection after pudendal or paracervical block anesthesia have complicated and protracted courses.[35] The most important early clinical sign is the patient's refusal to walk because of severe pain with any leg movement and the discovery on physical examination of a partially flexed lower extremity that is painful with any passive movement. Although these infections have been associated with the isolation of multiple organisms, anaerobes seem particularly important because of the clinical success seen when metronidazole was used.[36] Another rare but life-threatening infection is synergistic necrotizing fascitis that follows vaginal delivery and episiotomy repair.[37] Because of the rapid progression of gangrene and the risk of death, early operative débridement is critical.

The most serious postpartum infections occur in women who have undergone a cesarean section. Current clinical strategy employs antibiotics effective against gram-negative aerobes and anaerobes. This strategy is based upon the results of a comparison of a penicillin-gentamicin combination to clindamycin-gentamicin in postpartum cesarean section patients who developed clinical evidence of an endomyometritis.[12] The results demonstrate the clear superiority of the clindamycin-gentamicin regimen, with less protracted clinical courses and fewer maternal complications. These results indicate that early coverage of anaerobes, particularly *B. fragilis*, yields excellent results in postpartum cesarean section patients. Good results have also been achieved with cephalosporins, including cefoxitin, cefotetan, and the penicillins, including carbenicillin, ticarcillin, piperacillin, mezlocillin, and ampicillin with sulbactam added. Metronidazole has not been widely used in the United States because of theoretical concerns about the exposure of the breast-feeding baby to this agent.

Another approach to the problem of serious postpartum infection after cesarean section is the use of preventive antibiotics. Many of the factors that increase the infection rate in cesarean section seem amenable to systemic antibiotic prophylaxis. The surgical field at the time of cesarean section is usually contaminated with bacteria.[38] A number of prospective studies of antibiotic prophylaxis in cesarean section have been performed. In general, the reports have been enthusiastic. Such prophylaxis is a standard form of treatment for the patient in labor who requires this operation.

Operative strategies play an important role in both the prevention and treatment of pelvic infection after cesarean section. Techniques in the operating room on the patient in labor may alter the postoperative course of morbidity. One form of preventive operative therapy is the extraperitoneal approach at the time of the initial operation.[39] This does not eliminate postpartum infection, but it does eliminate intraperitoneal infection. The major drawbacks are the relative lack of experience with this operative technique in most medical centers and the awareness that the majority of patients can be safely managed without it.

Operative therapy for serious postpartum infections is uncommon, but it can be important for cure. In women who have developed a pelvic abscess, operative drainage or removal is imperative if antibiotic treatment fails. The decision concerning the approach is based on the location of the abscess. If extraperitoneal drainage can be easily accomplished, drainage will usually suffice. If the abscess is high in the pelvis, laparotomy with removal of the infected tissue is indicated. Laparotomy is the most frequently used therapeutic approach at present.

POSTOPERATIVE SOFT TISSUE GYNECOLOGIC INFECTIONS

A number of factors are involved in postoperative soft tissue gynecologic infections. Bacterial contamination occurs if the vagina is part of the operative field. This is the case with both vaginal and abdominal hysterectomy despite thorough preoperative cleansing of the vagina to remove the abundant normal flora. At least part of this subsequent bacterial contamination comes from the resident bacterial flora of the endocervix, which will not be eliminated by the usual surface preparation techniques. Some patients undergoing hysterectomy are more at risk than others for postoperative infections. In a nationwide evaluation of over 12,000 women undergoing hysterectomy, it was noted that blacks had a higher incidence of postoperative fever and received antibiotics more frequently than whites.[40] Whether these differences were related to the socioeconmic status of the population or to the presence of a population risk factor such as sickle cell trait is not known. In addition, many different evaluations have documented populations at risk for a postoperative pelvic abscess. These include premenopausal women who undergo vaginal hysterectomy,[41] particularly when the operation is performed on the clinic service.[42] It is not known whether the increased number of abscesses seen in these young women in the era before antibiotic prophylaxis was due to differences in the bacterial flora present in the lower genital tract; difficulty in obtaining hemostasis when performing vaginal hysterectomy in the more vascular pelvis of premenopausal women; or recurrent postoperative ovulation, which breaks the protective surface and exposes the interior of the ovary to the risk of infection. Whatever the mechanism, the premenopausal woman undergoing vaginal hysterectomy is at increased risk for a postoperative adnexal abscess. Although this has occurred much less frequently since the introduction of prophylactic antibiotics, these abscesses are still seen in premenopausal women.[43] The microorganisms involved in these infections are similar to those previously noted in the discussion of postpartum infections.

Antibiotic therapy for postoperative pelvic infections is empiric, since no prospective studies have been done. In view of the results of an experimental study[2] and clinical observations, early antibiotic coverage of gram-negative aerobes and of all anaerobes seems important. The use of prophylactic preoperative antibiotics have become routine in many situations, a subject that is discussed in Chapter 285.

The operative management of an established postoperative pelvic infection is very important for cure in the occasional patient who does not respond to antibiotic treatment. The basic management is drainage or removal of an infected, purulent collection. One diagnostic ritual in the evaluation of the febrile postoperative patient is the search by physical examination for an infected collection that can be drained. After hysterectomy, an uncommon infection is a vaginal cuff collection. If present, adequate drainage is easily accomplished and usually yields a cure. Other febrile patients seen a week or more postoperatively may have a pelvic abscess. The decision about the appropriate approach to these abscesses is based upon their location. If they are bulging into the vagina, vaginal drainage can easily be accomplished, with good therapeutic results.[44] If the abscess is high in the pelvic cavity and is not amenable to extraperitoneal drainage, laparotomy with removal of the abscess is necessary for cure.[41–43] These active therapeutic measures are important, for such pelvic abscesses can rupture into the peritoneal cavity, resulting in life-threatening illness and death.[41]

COMMUNITY-ACQUIRED INFECTIONS

The Infected Abortion

There have been dramatic changes in the past two decades in the clinical presentation of infected abortion in the United States. There has been a remarkable drop in the frequency of this syndrome. Of even greater significance is the decrease in the severity of the infections seen in this clinical population.[32] Before these changes occurred, septic abortion with endotoxic shock, as well as life-threatening myometritis due to *Clostridium perfringens*, were commonplace. The reasons for this dramatic change in clinical presentation were not due solely to better methods of therapy for the symptomatic patient. Instead, vast changes in health care delivery have had a major impact on this problem. More widespread availability of better methods of contraception to women from all social classes has decreased the number of women with unwanted pregnancies. The greatest impact occurred when restrictions on pregnancy termination in the hospital were lifted nationwide in the early 1970s. A poor woman with an unwanted pregnancy was no longer forced to seek the services of unskilled nonmedical personnel to terminate the pregnancy. The results were immediately apparent in urban hospitals, as both infected abortions and serious infection decreased.

The cornerstone of therapy for the patient with an infected abortion is the surgical removal of retained products of conception. Chow et al.[45] demonstrated that curettage was more beneficial than systemic antibiotics in the control of abortion-related infections. These products of conception are a nidus of continuing infection, and treatment with systemic antibiotics alone can be ineffective. There are also other situations in which operative intervention can be lifesaving. A syndrome of life-threatening sepsis in spontaneous mid-first trimester abortion has been reported in women wearing a large Dalkon Shield,[46] and at least part of the problem is continual bacterial seeding caused by the the heavily contaminated multifilamented tail.[47] Operative removal of this source of contamination may prove to be crucial for a clinical cure. Other situations include more extensive uterine damage in which the pelvic infection cannot be controlled by systemic antibiotics and curettage. This was not uncommon when necrosis-producing substances were used to induce abortion and an infection with potentially lethal agents like *Cl. perfringens* was established. In these women, surgical removal of the pelvic organs may be necessary for cure.

Antibiotic therapy for the patient with an infected abortion is usually empiric. Few prospective studies have been done, and those reported contain small numbers of patients. The best microbiologic study of women with an infected abortion was reported by Rotheram and Schick.[48] They found a high incidence of anaerobic organism bacteremia and suggested that an appropriate antibiotic strategy should include coverage of anaerobes, particularly *B. fragilis*. This is probably not necessary for all patients. In another study of a small number of patients, good results were noted when antibiotic coverage specifically for *B. fragilis* was not used as primary therapy.[49] This has been our clinical impression and probably reflects the overriding importance of curettage in therapy. In the infected abortion patient with septic shock, we recommend treatment for anaerobic organisms, as well as for the gram-negative aerobes usually associated with shock, since the septic shock syndrome can occur in women with anaerobic bacteremia.[50]

Salpingo-Oophoritis

A rational approach to patients with this infection is presented in Figure 2. The major grouping on the right focuses on the small percentage of the total population who are potential candidates for surgery. This is the smallest group in numbers, but these women with acute abdominal findings suggestive of an intraperitoneal abscess rupture have the most serious prognosis. Warning signs include upper abdominal rigidity and rebound, tenderness, tachycardia, and free pus on peritoneal aspiration. Although antibiotic coverage of aerobic and anaerobic organisms is important, immediate operative intervention with extirpation of the infected tissue and thorough peritoneal toilet is necessary for survival and cure.[51] Fortunately, this is a rare clinical picture. A more common event, although it is still found in a minority of the patients with salpingitis, is the presence of a pelvic mass. This may be a pelvic abscess that will eventually require operative intervention, either drainage or removal for cure. Since *B. fragilis* is frequently involved in pelvic abscesses, it is important to provide antibiotic coverage for this anaerobe from the onset of therapy.[52] Clinically, less than half of the

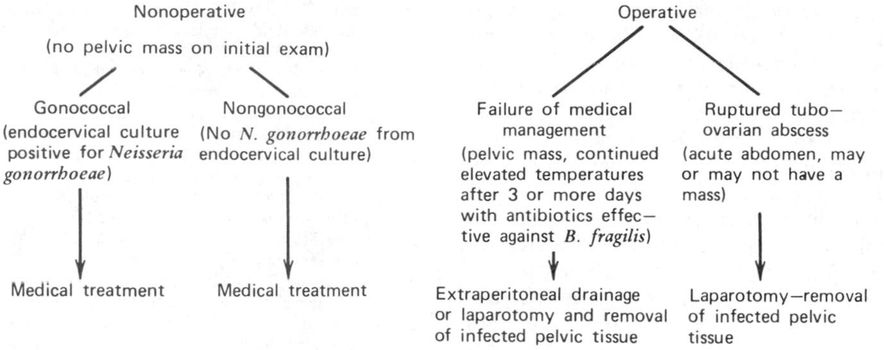

FIG. 2. Clinical classification of salpingo-oophoritis.

patients with a pelvic mass will require an operation.[53] Some abscesses are cured medically, and often the palpated mass is an inflammatory response to the infection rather than an abscess.

The majority of patients with salpingitis have neither a pelvic mass nor evidence suggesting an intraperitoneal accident. These women can be classified as having gonococcal or nongonococcal salpingitis. The physician should suspect gonococcal salpingitis in a woman with the first clinical episode of salpingitis, particularly when the symptoms occur with or just after menses and when the temperature is above 38°C. The key to this classification is the recovery of *Neisseria gonorrhoeae* from the endocervical culture. Obviously, this information will not be available at the onset of therapy, so the clinician should make a judgment based upon the Gram stain findings of an endocervical smear. Eschenbach et al.[54] found a good correlation between positive Gram stains and cultures positive for *N. gonorrhoeae*. In their study, approximately one-third of the women who had positive cultures did not have a positive smear, but all the women with a positive smear had positive cultures. The designation of gonococcal salpingitis has clinical significance. These women have a more favorable response to antibiotics than those with nongonococcal salpingitis.[55] They become afebrile more rapidly than women with nongonococcal salpingitis, seem less likely to develop a pelvic abscess during antibiotic therapy, and are more likely to be free of tubal damage after treatment. Since many men have positive cultures and are symptom free, it is important to culture and to treat the sexual partners of women with positive cultures.

Risk factors have been associated with either an increased frequency or an increased severity of infection. These risks have been assigned on the basis of clinical observations or by a case control method, but not by prospective study. An increased frequency of salpingo-oophoritis among women who use in intrauterine device for contraception has been reported in a number of studies.[56,57] The highest rate of pelvic infection has been noted in young nulliparous women.[58] In addition to the increased frequency of infection with an intrauterine device, there is evidence that the presentation of infection varies among intrauterine device users. Serious pelvic infections due to *Actinomyces bovis* have been reported among intrauterine device wearers.[59] These organisms can be detected on the cytology smear of women using this form of contraception, and these changes disappear when the intrauterine device is removed.[60] Another new phenomenon is the observation of unilateral tuboovarian abscesses among patients who use intrauterine devices. Although one study indicated that this finding only occurred in women who have used this method,[61] unilateral abscess in women who had never used this contraceptive has been reported.[62] Nevertheless, there was a greater than expected number of patients with unilateral pelvic abscess among intrauterine device wearers, and this was particularly true for those women with a Dalkon Shield in place. A strong clinical impression has been that infections are more severe among patients using an intrauterine device, but one prospective evaluation did not show this correlation.[16] The patient who has had salpingitis is more likely to have other episodes in the future. The mechanism is not known. It may reflect either changes in host defense mechanisms or simply exposure of these patients to sexual partners who reinfect them.

The antibiotic therapy of salpingo-oophoritis should have a number of goals. There should be a rapid clinical response without pelvic abscess formation, and the patient should have a pelvis free of adhesions or tubal abnormalities in which fertility is possible, since each episode of salpingitis increases the risk of infertility.[58,63] Unfortunately, few data are available on the long-term follow-up and subsequent fertility of women with salpingitis.

A number of treatment regimens can be used in the patient with salpingitis. The recommendations of the Centers for Disease Control are noted in Table 1.[64]

A few patients with salpingo-oophoritis require operative intervention for cure. In some instances, the decision to operate is relatively easy. The woman with a ruptured tuboovarian abscess has an operative emergency and requires immediate pel-

TABLE 1. Combination Regimens with Broad Activity Against Major Pathogens in Pelvic Inflammatory Disease

Regimen A (preferred when *Neisseria gonorrhoeae* or *Chlamydia trachomatis* is suspected as the primary pathogen):

Doxycycline: 100 mg IV twice a day
Plus
Cefoxitin: 2 g IV four times a day

Continue drugs IV for at least 4 days and for at least 48 hours after the patient improves (defervescence, decreased symptoms and signs). Then continue doxycycline, 100 mg by mouth twice a day, to complete 10–14 days of total therapy.

Regimen B (preferred when facultative gram-negative bacilli or anaerobes are suspected as the primary pathogens):

Clindamycin: 900 mg IV three times a day
Mixed in same infusion with
Gentamicin: 2 mg/kg IV

followed by 1.5 mg/kg, three times a day, for patients with normal renal function. Serum gentamicin levels should be monitored and dose or dose interval adjusted to maintain a gentamicin serum level of 5–10 μg/ml 30 minutes postadministration. Continue drugs IV for at least 4 days and at least 48 hours after the patient improves. Then continue clindamycin, 450 mg, by mouth four times a day, to complete 10–14 days of therapy.

Ambulatory Regimen

When the patient is not hospitalized, the following regimen is recommended:

Ceftriaxone: 250 mg IM in one dose
plus
Doxycycline: 100 mg by mouth twice a day for 10–14 days

(Data from Centers for Disease Control.[64])

vic tissue extirpation, plus thorough peritoneal cavity lavage for cure. Such patients are seen rarely today. The patient with a large pelvic abscess pointing into the posterior cul de sac is an excellent candidate for surgical drainage and usually has a rapid defervescence of temperature.[44] Alternatively, transabdominal needle aspiration of the pelvic abscess with imaging guidance[17] or needle aspiration at the time of laparoscopy can be done.[65] Both procedures are well tolerated by the patient and involve less morbidity than exploratory laparotomy. A patient who has had an exploratory laparotomy for suspected intraperitoneal rupture and is found to have acute salpingitis with no abscess formation is an easy therapeutic decision. The abdomen should be closed, antibiotics continued, and a cure can be expected. Antibiotics reduce the number of anaerobic bacteria in a model that simulates an abscess.[52] Since one therapeutic goal of antibiotic therapy is to eliminate anaerobic organisms at the site of infection, the use of antibiotics effective against anaerobes is indicated. A decision to operate should be made only when there is no response to this therapy.

REFERENCES

1. Weinstein WM, Onderdonk AB, Bartlett JG, et al. Experimental intra-abdominal abscesses in rats: Development of an experimental model. Infect Immun. 1974;10:1250.
2. Weinstein WM, Onderdonk AB, Bartlett JG, et al: Antimicrobial therapy of experimental intra-abdominal sepsis. J Infect Dis. 1975;132:282.
3. Ledger WJ, Norman M, Gee C, et al. Bacteremia on an obstetric-gynecologic service. Am J Obstet Gynecol. 1975;121:205.
4. Blanco JD, Gibbs RS, Castaneda YS. Bacteremia in obstetrics: Clinical course. Obstet Gynecol. 1981;58:621.
5. Bryan CS, Reynolds KL, Moore, EE. Bacteremia in obstetrics and gynecology. Obstet Gynecol. 1984;64:2.
6. Kauppel RA, Scerbo JC, Dzink J, et al. Quantitative transcervical uterine cultures with a new device. Obstet Gynecol. 1981;57:243.
7. Ledger WJ, Gee CL, Pollin P, et al. The use of pre-reduced media and portable jars for the collection of anaerobic organisms from clinical sites. Am J Obstet Gynecol. 1966;125:677.
8. Cuchoral GJ Jr, Tally FP, Jacobus NV, et al. Susceptibility of the *Bacteroides fragilis* group in the United States: Analysis by site of isolation. Antimicrob Agents Chemother. 1988;32:717.
9. Sweet RL, Mill J, Hadley KW, et al. Use of laparoscopy to determine the microbiologic etiology of acute salpingitis. Am J Obstet Gynecol. 1979;134:68.
10. Sweet RL, Schachter J, Robbie MO. Failure of beta-lactam antibiotics to eradicate *Chlamydia trachomatis* from the endometrium of patients with acute salpingitis despite apparent clinical cure. JAMA. 1983;250:2641.
11. Wood CA, Norton DR, Kohlhepp SJ, et al. The influence of tobramycin dosage regimens on nephrotoxicity-ototoxicity and antibacterial efficacy in a rat model of subcutaneous abscess. J Infect Dis. 1988;158:13.
12. Di Zerega G, Yonekura L, Roy S, et al. A comparison of clindamycin, gentamicin, and penicillin-gentamicin in the treatment of postcesarean endomyometritis. Am J Obstet Gynecol. 1979;134:238.
13. Gibbs RS, Listwa HM, Dreskin RB. A pure enterococcal abscess after cesarean section. J Reprod Med. 1977;19:17.
14. Moellering RC Jr, Enteroccal infections in patients treated with moxalactam. Rev Infect Dis. 1982;4:S708.
15. Terpenning MS, Zervos MJ, Schaberg DR, et al. Enterococcal infections: An increasing problem in hospitalized patients. Infect Cont Hosp Epidemiol 1988;9:457.
16. Ledger WJ, Moore DE, Lowensohn RI, et al. A fever index evaluation of chloramphenicol or clindamycin in patients with serious pelvic infections. Obstet Gynecol. 1977;50:523.
17. Gerzol SG, Robbins AH, Johnson WC, et al. Percutaneous catheter drainage of abdominal abscesses. N Engl J Med. 1981;305:653.
18. Goplerud CP, Ohm MJ, Galask RP. Aerobic and anaerobic flora of the cervix during pregnancy and the puerperium. Am J Obstet Gynecol. 1976;126:858.
19. Cherry SH, Filler M, Harvey H. Lysozyme content of amniotic fluid. Am J Obstet Gynecol. 1973;116:639.
20. Ford LC, Delange RJ, Lebherz TB. Identification of a bactericidal factor (B-lysin) in amniotic fluid at 40 weeks gestation. Am J Obstet Gynecol. 1977;127:788.
21. Larsen B, Synder IS, Galask RP. Transferrin concentration in human amniotic fluid. Am J Obstet Gynecol. 1973;117:952.
22. Cederqvist LL, Ewol LC, Bonsnas RW, et al. Detectability and pattern of immunoglobulins in normal amniotic fluid throughout gestation. Am J Obstet Gynecol. 1978;130:220.
23. Larsen B, Galask RP, Synder IS. Muramidase and peroxidase activity of human amniotic fluid. Obstet Gynecol. 1974;44:219.
24. Larson JW, Goldkrand JW, Hanson TM, et al. Intrauterine infection on an obstetric service. Obstet Gynecol. 1974;43:838.
25. Florman AL, Teubner D. Enhancement of bacterial growth in amniotic fluid by meconium. J Pediatr. 1969;74:111.
26. Blanco JD, Gibbs RS, Krebs, LF, et al. The association between the absence of amniotic fluid bacterial inhibitory activity and intra-amniotic infection. Am J Gynecol. 1982;143:749.
27. Tafari N, Ross SM, Naeye RL, et al. Failure of bacterial growth inhibition by amniotic fluid. Am J Obstet Gynecol. 1977;128:187.
28. Spore WW, Moskal PA, Nakamura RM, et al. The bacteriology of the postpartum oviducts and endometrium. Am J Obstet Gynecol. 1970;107:572.
29. Ledger WJ, Nakamura RM. Measurement of infectious disease morbidity in obstetrics and gynecology. Clin Obstet Gynecol. 1976;19:195.
30. Perloe M, Curet LB. The effect of internal fetal monitoring on cesarian section morbidity. Obstet Gynecol. 1979;53:354.
31. Anstey JT, Sheldon GW, Blythe JG. Infectious morbidity after primary cesarean section in a private institution. Am J Obstet Gynecol. 1980;136:205.
32. Ledger WJ, Kriewall TJ, Gee C. The fever index. A technic for evaluating the clinical response to bacteremia. Obstet Gynecol. 1975;45:603.
33. Wager GP, Martin DH, Koutsky L, et al. Puerperal infectious morbidity: Relationship to route of delivery and to antepartum *Chlamydia trachomatis* infection. Am J Obstet Gynecol. 1980;138:1028.
34. Ledger WJ, Reite AM, Headington JT. A system for infectious disease surveillance on an obstetric service. Obstet Gynecol. 1971;37:769.
35. Hibbard LT, Snyder EN, McVann RE. Subgluteal and retropsoal infection in obstetric practice Obstet Gynecol. 1972;39:172.
36. Ledger WJ, Lewis W, Golde S, et al. The use of metronidazole in obstetric and gynecologic infections. In: Finegold SM, McFadzean JA, Roe FJC, eds. Metronidazole. Princeton, N.J.: Excerpta Medica; 1977:353.
37. Golde S, Ledger WJ. Necrotizing fasciitis in postpartum patients. A report of four cases. Obstet Gynecol. 1977;50:670.
38. Wong R, Gee C, Ledger WJ. Prophylactic use of cefazolin in monitored patients undergoing cesarean section. Obstet Gynecol. 1978;51:407.
39. Imig JR, Perkins RP. Extraperitoneal cesarean section: A new need for old skills. Am J Obstet Gynecol. 1976;125:51.
40. Ledger WJ, Child M. The hospital care of patients undergoing hysterectomy. An analysis of 12,026 women from the Professional Activity Study. Am J Obstet Gynecol. 1973;117:423.
41. Ledger WJ, Campbell C, Willson JR. Postoperative adnexal infection. Obstet Gynecol. 1968;31:83.
42. Willson JR, Black JR. Ovarian abscess. Am J Obstet Gynecol. 1964;90:34.
43. Livengood CH III, Addison WA. Adnexal abscess as a delayed complication of vaginal hysterectomy. Am J Obstet Gynecol. 1982;143:596.
44. Rubenstein PR, Mishell DR, Ledger WJ. Colpotomy drainage of pelvic abscess. Obstet Gynecol. 1976;48:142.
45. Chow AW, Marshall JR, Guze LB. A double-blind study comparison of clindamycin with penicillin plus chloramphenicol in treatment of septic abortions. J Infect Dis. 1977;135:S35.
46. Christian CD. Maternal deaths associated with an intrauterine device. Am J Obstet Gynecol. 1974;119:441.
47. Tatum HJ, Schmidt FH, Phillips D, et al. The Dalkon Shield controversy. Structural and bacteriological studies of IUD tails. JAMA. 1975;231:711.
48. Rotheram EB, Schick SF. Nonclostridial anaerobic bacteria in septic shock. Am J Med. 1969;46:80.
49. Ostergard DR. Comparison of two antibiotic regimens in the treatment of septic abortion. Obstet Gynecol. 1970;36:473.
50. Ledger WJ, Gee CL, Lewis WP, et al. Comparison of clindamycin and chloramphenicol in treatment of serious infections of the female genital tract. J Infect Dis. 1977;135:S30.
51. Collins CG, Nix FG, Cerha HT. Ruptured tubo-ovarian abscess. Am J Obstet Gynecol 1956;72:820.
52. Bartlett JG, Recent developments in the management of anaerobic infections. Rev Infect Dis. 1983;5:235.
53. Ledger WJ. Selection of antimicrobial agents for the treatment of infections of the female genital tract. Rev Infect Dis. 1983;5:S98.
54. Eschenbach DA, Buchanan TM, Pollock HM, et al. Polymicrobial etiology of acute pelvic inflammatory disease. N Engl J Med. 1975;293:166.
55. Cunningham FG, Hauth JC, Strong JD, et al. Tetracyclines or penicillin-ampicillin for pelvic inflammatory disease. N Engl J Med. 1977;296:1380.
56. Westrom L, Bangtsson L, Mardh P. The risk of developing pelvic inflammatory disease in women using intrauterine devices as compared to non-users. Lancet. 1976;2:221.
57. Osser S, Liedholm P, Sjobert NO. Risk of PID among users of intrauterine devices, irrespective of previous pregnancy. Am J Obstet Gynecol. 1980;138:864.
58. Westrom L. Incidence, prevalence and trends of PID and its consequences in industrialized countries. Am J Obstet Gynecol. 1980;138:880.
59. Schiffer MA, Elquezobal A, Sultana M, et al. Actinomycosis infections associated with IUCD's Obstet Gynecol. 1975;45:67.
60. Gupta PK, Hollander SH, Frost JK. Actinomycetes in cervicovaginal smears. An associated with IUD usage. Acta Cytol. 1976;20:295.
61. Taylor ES, McMille JH, Greer BF, et al. The IUD and tubo-ovarian abscess. Am J Obstet Gynecol. 1975;123:338.
62. Golde SH, Israel R, Ledger WJ. Unilateral tubo-ovarian abscess. A distinct entity. Am J Obstet Gynecol. 1977;127:802.
63. Westrom L. Effects of acute PID on fertility. Am J Obstet Gynecol. 1975;121:707.
64. Centers for Disease Control. STO Treatment Guidelines 1987. MMWR. 1987;36(Suppl 55).
65. Henry-Sacket J, Soler A, Wilfredo V. Laparoscopic treatment of tubo-ovarian abscess. J Reprod Med. 1984;29:579.

97. PROSTATITIS, EPIDIDYMITIS, AND ORCHITIS

JOHN N. KRIEGER

ANATOMY AND PHYSIOLOGY OF THE TESTES AND MALE ACCESSORY SEX ORGANS

The testicle has two functional components, seminiferous tubules and interstitial cells. Sperm production is the primary function of the seminiferous tubules. Interstitial cells, located between the seminiferous tubules, are primarily responsible for hormone production. After spermatogenesis spermatozoa are transported from the testis into the epididymis (Fig. 1). Sperm then move into the vas deferens, a muscular tube approximately 12 inches long that is easily palpable in the scrotum. Fructose from the seminal vesicles is the major energy source for ejaculated sperm. In addition, the seminal vesicles provide a number of proteins that cause coagulation of the ejaculate. Liquification of the semen occurs within 5–30 minutes after ejaculation as a result of proteolytic enzymes from the prostate.[1]

HOST DEFENSES OF THE MALE LOWER UROGENITAL TRACT

Organisms ascend via the urethra to cause most infections of the urogenital ducts and accessory sex organs.[2] Thus, mechanical factors such as the flushing action of micturition and ejaculation should provide some protection against infection, although the relative significance of such defenses is unclear.

A zinc-containing polypeptide known as the prostatic antibacterial factor is the most important antimicrobial substance secreted by the prostate.[2,3] Men with well-documented chronic bacterial prostatitis have significantly lower levels of zinc in their prostatic fluid than do healthy men, but their serum zinc levels are within normal limits.[3] It is unclear whether reduced zinc concentrations precede the development of prostatic infection or represent a secretory dysfunction resulting from such infections. Prostatic secretions of patients with bacterial prostatitis contain high concentrations of immunoglobulins.[4,5] Several studies have demonstrated antigen-specific antibody coating of bacteria isolated from the lower urinary tracts of patients with prostatitis syndromes. The antigen-specific antibody response in prostatic secretions (predominately secretory IgA) is significantly greater than is the serologic response.[5]

The presence of leukocytes is characteristic of many conditions of the male lower urinary tract, including prostatitis.[6] Phagocytosis of abnormal sperm by leukocytes in some infertile men with pyosemina has been observed.

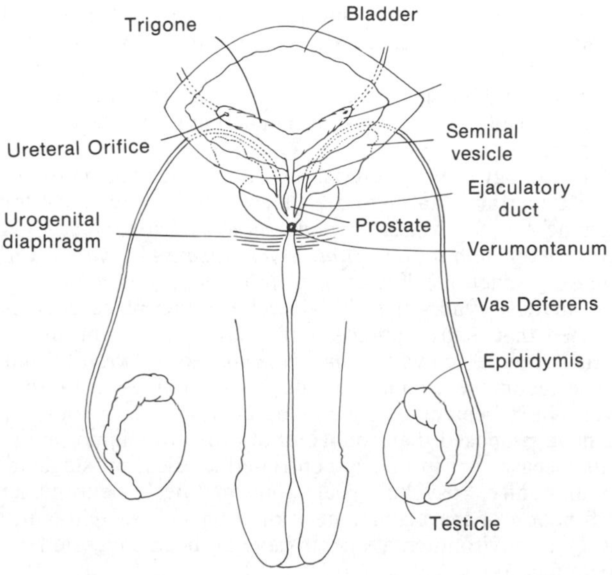

FIG. 1. Anatomy of the male sex organs and lower urinary tract.

PROSTATITIS

Classification of Prostatitis

The term *prostatitis* is employed clinically to describe a large group of adult men with a variety of complaints referable to the lower urogenital tract and perineum.[2,7] It has been estimated that 50 percent of men will experience symptoms of prostatitis at some time in their lives.[2] It is of critical importance to distinguish patients with lower urinary tract complaints associated with bacteriuria, such as patients who may have bacterial prostatitis, from the larger number of patients without bacteriuria. Further classification of patients with prostatitis depends on careful bacteriologic assessment of the lower urinary tract that is based on sequential urine cultures obtained during micturition[7,8] (Table 1). On the basis of results of lower urinary tract localization, men with prostatitis syndromes may be classified into four major groups: acute bacterial prostatitis, chronic bacterial prostatitis, nonbacterial prostatitis, and prostatodynia[7] (Table 2). In addition, rare patients develop granulomatous prostatitis.

Bacterial prostatitis is a frequent diagnosis in general clinical practice, but well-documented bacterial infections of the prostate, whether acute or chronic, are uncommon.[2,5] The great majority of patients with a diagnosis of prostatitis are adult men with perineal, lower back, or lower abdominal pain; urinary discomfort; or ejaculatory complaints. Most of these patients have no history of bacteriuria, and there is little objective evidence of bacterial infection of the prostate. Thus, most patients with prostatitis may be classified in the groups of nonbacterial prostatitis or prostatodynia, conditions about which there are few firm data to base therapeutic decisions.

Acute Bacterial Prostatitis. Acute bacterial prostatitis is usually not a subtle or difficult diagnosis. Patients complain of symptoms associated with lower urinary tract infection such as urinary frequency and dysuria. Patients may also experience lower urinary tract obstruction due to acute edema of the prostate. Signs of systemic toxicity are common. On physical examination patients may have a high temperature and lower abdominal or suprapubic discomfort due to bladder infection. The rectal examination is frequently impressive, with an exquisitely

TABLE 1. Lower Urinary Tract Localization Using Segmented Urine Cultures[a]

Specimen	*Symbol*	*Description*
Voided bladder 1	VB_1	Initial 5–10 ml of urinary stream
Voided bladder 2	VB_2	Midstream specimen
Expressed prostatic secretions	EPS	Secretions expressed from prostate by digital massage after midstream specimen
Voided bladder 3	VB_3	First 5–10 ml of urinary stream immediately after prostatic massage

[a] Unequivocal diagnosis of bacterial prostatitis requires that the colony count in the VB_3 specimen greatly exceed the count in the VB_1 specimen, preferably by at least 10-fold.[2,8] Many patients who have chronic bacterial prostatitis, however, harbor only small numbers of bacteria in their prostates. In such patients, direct culture of the prostatic secretions is particularly useful. Microscopic examination of the EPS is useful for identifying white blood cells and "oval fat bodies," large lipid-laden macrophages characteristic of the prostatic inflammatory response.[2,7]

TABLE 2. Classification of Prostatitis Syndromes on the Basis of Lower Urinary Tract Localization Studies

Condition	*Bacteriuria*[a]	*Infection Localized to Prostate*[b]	*Inflammatory Response in EPS*[c]	*Abnormal Rectal Examination of Prostate*[d]	*Systemic Illness*[e]
Acute bacterial prostatitis	+	+	+	+	+
Chronic bacterial prostatitis	+	+	+	−	−
"Nonbacterial" prostatitis	−	−	+	−	−
Prostatodynia	−	−	−	−	−

[a] Documented with an identical organism that is shown to localize to a prostatic focus when the midstream urine culture is negative.
[b] Refer to the text for diagnostic criteria.
[c] Prostatic secretions containing ≥ 12 WBC/HPF in a patient with no objective evidence of urethritis.
[d] Abnormal findings include exquisite tenderness and swelling that may be associated with signs of lower urinary tract obstruction.
[e] Systemic findings frequently include fever and rigors and may include signs of bacteremia.

tender, tense prostate on palpation. Urinalysis is abnormal, with evidence of pyuria, and cultures are positive. Bacteremia may be present spontaneously or may result from overly vigorous rectal examinations.

Results of antimicrobial therapy for acute bacterial prostatitis are often dramatic. Many drugs that do not penetrate into the prostate under normal conditions are effective in acute bacterial prostatitis.[2] Thus, drugs that would be appropriate in patients with bacteremia caused by Enterobacteriaceae, pseudomonads, and enterococci should be administered once specimens have been obtained for urine and blood cultures. General measures are also indicated including hydration, analgesics, and bed rest. The most important complications of acute bacterial prostatitis include prostatic abscess, prostatic infarction, chronic bacterial prostatitis, and granulomatous prostatitis.

Chronic Bacterial Prostatitis. Chronic bacterial prostatitis is an important cause of bacterial persistence in the male lower urinary tract. Patients characteristically experience recurrent bacterial urinary tract infections caused by the same organism.[2] Patients are generally asymptomatic between episodes of bladder bacteriuria. The prostate gland is usually normal on either rectal or endoscopic evaluation. Thus, careful lower urinary tract localization studies are the cornerstone on which to base a diagnosis of chronic bacterial prostatitis.[8] Diagnosis of chronic bacterial prostatitis based solely on symptoms, the number of leuckoytes in expressed prostatic secretions, or the use of prostate biopsy specimens is inadequate.

Gram-negative rods (Enterobacteriaceae or pseudomonads) are by far the most important pathogens in chronic bacterial prostatitis. Gram-positive cocci such as *Enterococcus faecalis* or, perhaps, *Staphylococcus saprophyticus,* may be the etiologic organisms in a few cases. Reports implicating many other organisms are generally difficult to evaluate due to methodologic problems with case definition or a lack of documentation of bacteriuria by the alleged pathogen.

Medical management is effective in curing or suppressing bacterial infections of the prostate. Trimethoprim has two useful characteristics: it achieves good levels in the prostatic parenchyma and is effective against most of the common bacterial pathogens.[2] Available studies have most commonly employed the combination of trimethoprim and sulfamethoxazole for the treatment of patients with well-documented chronic bacterial prostatitis. Long treatment courses result in symptomatic and bacteriologic cure in approximately one-third of patients, symptomatic improvement while receiving therapy in approximately one-third of patients who relapse after the drug therapy is stopped, and no improvement in the remaining patients.[9] Many other orally administered antimicrobial agents have been used for the treatment of patients with chronic bacterial prostatitis. Most of these studies are hampered by imprecise case definitions, a lack of sufficient microbiologic documentation or follow-up, or an abundance of patients infected with organisms generally considered urethral contaminants. In early studies, several of the new quinolones have shown promise as agents for the treatment of chronic bacterial prostatitis.[10–11]

Bacteria isolated from patients with chronic bacterial prostatitis, even after multiple episodes of symptomatic bacteriuria and prolonged courses of antibiotics, are generally antibiotic-sensitive strains.[2,9] Several findings may explain the disappointing results of antibiotic therapy including poor diffusion of most drugs into the prostatic parenchyma, changes in prostatic fluid pH level that are associated with infection, and infected calculi that may serve as persistent foci for bacteria.[9,13]

Patients with chronic bacterial prostatitis who are not cured may be rendered asymptomatic by long-term, suppressive treatment. Since patients are usually asymptomatic between episodes of bacteriuria, the goal of suppressive therapy is to prevent symptomatic episodes despite the persistence of bacteria in the prostate. Very low doses of agents such as penicillin, tetracycline, nitrofurantoin, nalidixic acid, or trimethoprim-sulfamethoxazole are remarkably effective in preventing episodes of symptomatic bladder infection in patients with chronic bacterial prostatitis.[2]

Nonbacterial Prostatitis and Prostatodynia. Patients with nonbacterial prostatitis and prostatodynia have no history of bacteriuria and lack objective evidence of bacterial infection of their prostatic secretions on careful lower urinary tract localization studies (Table 2).[7] Such patients may complain of a variety of perineal and pelvic symptoms. Pain or vague discomfort is common and may be suprapubic, infrapubic, scrotal, or inguinal in location. The discomfort may be described as either continuous or spasmodic and is commonly described as a "dull ache." Occasional patients complain of increased urinary frequency or dysuria, and ejaculatory complaints are not infrequent. Systemic symptoms or signs are absent. Physical examination is generally unremarkable.

Nonbacterial prostatitis and prostatodynia are distinguished by microscopic examination of the expressed prostatic secretions. Patients with nonbacterial prostatitis have objective evidence of an inflammatory response in their prostatic secretions, while patients with prostatodynia have no evidence of inflammation.

The etiology of nonbacterial prostatitis and prostatodynia remains uncertain. Mardh and Colleen found no evidence for an etiologic role for *Neisseria gonorrhoeae, Trichomonas vaginalis, Ureaplasma urealyticum, Mycoplasma hominis, Candida albicans,* anaerobic bacteria, *Chlamydia trachomatis,* or viruses in these syndromes.[14,15] However, other researchers have reported that many patients with "subacute or chronic prostatitis" are infected with *C. trachomatis*[16] or *U. urealyticum.*[17–19] The techniques, control groups, and findings in these later studies have been questioned by other workers.[2,20] Some workers have proposed that nonbacterial prostatitis is not an infectious disease.[21,22] In poorly controlled studies, prostaglandins, autoimmunity, psychological abnormalities, neuromuscular dysfunction of the bladder neck or urogenital diaphragm, and allergy to environmental agents have all been suggested as etiologic factors.

Current therapy for symptomatic patients with nonbacterial prostatitis is unsatisfactory. There is little objective evidence that patients with nonbacterial prostatitis or prostatodynia benefit from empirical antimicrobial therapy.

Granulomatous Prostatitis. Granulomatous prostatitis is a characteristic histologic reaction of the prostate to a variety of insults, with granulomas containing lipid-laden histiocytes, plasma cells, and scattered giant cells. In most cases granulomatous prostatitis follows an episode of acute bacterial prostatitis.[23,24] There are also a number of specific infectious causes of granulomatous reaction by the prostate. Tuberculous prostatitis is usually secondary to tuberculosis elsewhere in the genital tract.[25,26] Most patients have no symptoms referable to prostatic infection. On biopsy the granulomas may contain typical Langhans giant cells and may be associated with caseous necrosis. Such infections are most often caused by *Mycobacterium tuberculosis* but have also been reported to be caused by atypical mycobacteria.[27] Prostatitis may be secondary to systemic involvement with many of the deep mycoses.[28] Most cases of mycotic prostatitis reported have been associated with blastomycosis,[28] coccidioidomycosis,[29] and cryptococcosis.[30] However, paracoccidioidomycosis occasionally involves the prostate.[28] Other reported causes of granulomatous prostatitis include actinomycosis, candidiasis, syphilis, brucellosis, and sacral herpes zoster.[23]

Granulomatous prostatitis is most important in the differential diagnosis of an indurated, firm, or nodular prostate. The rectal examination of such patients raises the suspicion of prostatic carcinoma. Biopsy is usually necessary for diagnosis, and it is important that appropriate stains be used for the detection of specific etiologic agents.

Prostatic Abscess

Prostatic abscess is a rare complication in patients who receive appropriate treatment for acute bacterial prostatitis.[31] Most prostatic abscesses occur in patients with diabetes, in immunocompromised patients, and in patients who have not received appropriate therapy for acute prostatitis. The presence of a foreign body or urinary tract obstruction are other predisposing factors. In the past, *N. gonorrhoeae* was a common pathogen, but most cases are now caused by the common uropathogens. Infection generally occurs by the ascending route. On occasion, *Staphylococcus aureus* is the pathogen, which suggests the possibility of hematogenous infection. Patients are usually febrile with irritative voiding symptoms, and they may have signs of urosepsis. Thus, the clinical presentation closely resembles that of acute bacterial prostatitis. Classically, the abscess presents as a fluctuant area in the prostate that can be palpated during rectal examination. However, the presentation may be more subtle. The use of ultrasonography[32] or computed tomography[33] of the pelvis is helpful for confirming the diagnosis or in patients with equivocal clinical findings. Treatment includes draining the abscess, via either a perineal or transurethral route in addition to appropriate antimicrobial therapy.

EPIDIDYMITIS

Epididymitis is an inflammatory reaction of the epididymis to a variety of infectious agents or to local trauma. Epididymitis is common, accounting for over 600,000 visits to physicians per year in the United States. Acute epididymitis is responsible for more days lost from military service than any other disease and is responsible for 20 percent of urologic admissions in military populations.[35]

Patients with epididymitis usually complain of painful swelling of the scrotum. The onset may be acute over 1 or 2 days or more gradual and is often associated with dysuria or irritative lower urinary tract symptoms. Many patients have a urethral discharge.[34] Specific attention should be directed to eliciting a past history of genitourinary tract disease or sexual exposure. Some patients may have only a nonspecific finding of fever or other signs of infection. This is particularly frequent in hospitalized patients who have recent urinary tract manipulation and may be obtunded by medication.

Tender swelling, frequently accompanied by erythema, generally unilateral, may be noted primarily in the posterior aspect of the scrotum. If the patient is examined early in the course of the disease, the swelling may be localized to one portion of the epididymitis. Later, involvement of the ipsilateral testis is frequent, producing an epididymo-orchitis, and it may be difficult to distinguish the testicle from the epididymis within the inflammatory mass. Scrotal examination commonly reveals the presence of a hydrocele caused by the secretion of inflammatory fluid between the layers of the tunica vaginalis. Urethral discharge may be apparent on inspection or stripping of the urethra.

There are two common types of epididymitis, nonspecific bacterial epididymitis and sexually transmitted epididymitis. In addition, epididymitis may occur rarely after genital trauma or with disseminated infections.

Classification of Epididymitis

Nonspecific Bacterial Epididymitis. The most common cause of epididymitis in men over 35 years old is infection with coliform or *Pseudomonas* species.[34,36] In most series, gram-negative aerobic-rods caused over two-thirds of cases of bacterial epididymitis.[34,36,37] However, gram-positive cocci are also important pathogens and were the most common organisms in some reports.[39]

Many patients who develop bacterial epididymitis have underlying urologic pathology or have a history of recent genitourinary tract manipulation.[34,36] The development of epididymitis after surgery or urethral catheterization may occur weeks or rarely months after the manipulation. Epididymitis is particularly likely in patients who undergo urinary tract surgery or instrumentation while they are bacteriuric. Acute and chronic bacterial prostatitis are other important predisposing conditions for the development of bacterial epididymitis.

Bacterial epididymitis may be an important focus of organisms causing bacteremia and local morbidity in patients with indwelling transurethral catheters. Genitourinary tract complications of acute bacterial epididymitis include testicular infarction, scrotal abscess, pyozele, a chronic draining scrotal sinus, chronic epididymitis, and infertility.[39,40]

Tuberculous epididymitis generally occurs after involvement of the prostate and seminal vesicles.[25] There is characteristic scrotal swelling with ''beadlike'' enlargement of the vas deferens. Chronic draining scrotal sinuses may be present. The systemic mycoses may rarely cause epididymitis; blastomycosis is the most common pathogen.

Medical management is appropriate for most patients with bacterial epididymitis. Initial empirical treatment with agents appropriate for both gram-negative rods and gram-positive cocci should be initiated pending urine culture and sensitivity results. Nonspecific measures such as bed rest, scrotal elevation analgesics, and local ice packs are helpful. Surgery may be necessary for complications of acute epididymal infections.

Sexually Transmitted Epididymitis. Sexually transmitted epididymitis is the most common type of epididymitis in young men. *C. trachomatis* and *N. gonorrhoeae* are the major pathogens in this population. Chlamydiae have recently been identified as the most common cause of epididymitis in younger, sexually active populations.[41,42] Such patients were formerly considered to have ''idiopathic,'' nonspecific epididymitis. Berger et al. documented infections with *C. trachomatis* in 17 of 34 cases of epididymitis in patients less than 35 years old and only 1 of 16 cases of epididymitis in patients older than 35. Patients with chlamydial epididymitis frequently did not complain of urethral discharge. However, 11 of 17 patients with epididymitis caused by chlamydiae had demonstrable discharge, usually the scant, watery discharge characteristic of nonspecific urethritis. The median interval from the last sexual exposure was 10 days and ranged from 1 to 45 days. Thus, patients may carry chlamydiae for long periods before the development of overt epididymitis.

Before the availability of penicillin, it was estimated that epididymitis occurred in 10–30 percent of men with gonococcal urethritis.[40] In more recent studies, *N. gonorrhoeae* was identified as the cause of acute epididymitis in 16 percent of cases in military populations[43] and in 21 percent of cases of epididymitis in civilians less than 35 years old.[34] Many patients with gonococcal epididymitis do not have a history of urethral discharge, and a discharge may be demonstrable in only 50 percent of such patients.

Underlying genitourinary tract abnormalities are uncommon in this population. Diagnosis depends on a high index of clinical suspicion, evaluation for presence of urethritis (which may be asymptomatic), and appropriate cultures. Specific antibiotic therapy, generally employing drugs appropriate for both chlamydiae and gonococci (i.e., tetracycline, 500 mg po four times daily for at least 10 days), is the most important aspect of treatment.[44] Patients should be evaluated for other sexually transmitted pathogens, and treatment of sexual partners is important. In general, a complete urologic work-up is not indicated for patients with uncomplicated sexually transmitted epididymitis. Complications of sexually transmitted epididymitis include abscess formation, testicular infarction, chronic epididymitis, and infertility.

ORCHITIS

Orchitis is significantly less common than is either prostatitis or epididymitis. Orchitis differs from infections of the male accessory sex glands in two important respects: blood-borne dissemination is the major route of infection, and viruses are clearly implicated as important pathogens.

Classification of Orchitis

Viral Orchitis. Viral infections, particularly mumps, are associated with most cases of orchitis. Although mumps rarely causes orchitis in prepubertal boys, orchitis occurs in approximately 20 percent of postpubertal patients with mumps.[45] Testicular pain and swelling usually begin 4 to 6 days after the onset of parotitis but may occur without parotid involvement. Orchitis is unilateral in approximately 70 percent of cases. Contralateral testicular swelling may occur 1 to 9 days after involvement of the first side. The clinical course is variable and ranges from mild testicular discomfort and swelling to severe testicular pain and marked swelling accompanied by nausea, vomiting, prostration, high fever, and constitutional symptoms. Epididymitis and inflammation of the spermatic cord may be noted on physical examination. Resolution of mild cases may occur in 4 or 5 days. More severe cases usually resolve in 3 to 4 weeks. Approximately one-half of the involved testes undergo some degree of atrophy. In older series, sterility was reported in 25 percent of patients with bilateral disease. However, more recent studies have found that mumps orchitis seldom results in infertility.[45] Coxsackie B virus produces a disease that clinically and histologically resembles mumps orchitis.

Bacterial Orchitis. With the exception of viral diseases, acute genitourinary tract infections involving only the testis are distinctly unusual. Pyogenic bacterial orchitis usually occurs as a consequence of the contiguous spread from an inflammatory process in the epididymis to cause an epididymo-orchitis. Thus, most cases of pyogenic orchitis are caused by *Escherichia coli, Klebsiella pneumoniae, Pseudomonas aeruginosa,* staphylococci, or streptococci. Occasionally, acute orchitis may be caused by other organisms as a result of metastatic seeding.

The patient with pyogenic orchitis appears acutely ill with a high fever and marked discomfort and swelling of the involved testicle. Generally the pain is described as radiating to the inguinal canal and is frequently accompanied by nausea and vomiting. On examination, there is usually an acute hydrocele, and the testis is swollen and exquisitely tender. The overlying scrotal skin is generally erythematous and edematous. Complications of pyogenic bacterial orchitis include testicular infarction, abscess formation, and pyocele of the scrotum. Surgery is usually required for treatment of these conditions. Orchitis can be caused by tuberculosis and blastomycosis, but by extension from the epididymis. Involvement of the testicle without palpable abnormality in the adjacent epididymis has rarely been observed with these agents.

REFERENCES

1. Jenkins AD, Turner TT, Howards SS. Physiology of the male reproductive system. Urol Clin North Am. 1978;5:437.
2. Stamey TA: Pathogenesis and Treatment of Urinary Tract Infections. Baltimore: Williams & Wilkins; 1980:1, 342.
3. Fair WR, Couch J, Wehner N. Prostatic antibacterial factor: Identity and significance. Urology. 1976;7:169.
4. Shortliffe LMD, Wehner N, Stamey TA. Use of solid-phase radioimmunoassay and formalin-fixed whole bacterial antigen in the detection of antigen-specific immunoglobulin in prostatic fluid. J Clin Invest. 1981;67:780.
5. Fowler JE Jr, Mariano M. Immunologic response of the prostate to bacteriuria and bacterial prostatitis: II. Antigen specific immumoglobulin in prostatic flud. J Urol. 1982;128:165.
6. Schaeffer AJ, Wendel EF, Dunn JK, et al. Prevalence and significance of prostatic inflammation. J Urol. 1981;125:215.
7. Drach GW, Meares EM, Fair WR, et al. Classification of benign diseases associated with prostatic pain: Prostatitis or prostatodynia? J Urol. 1978;120:266.
8. Meares EM, Stamey TA. Bacteriologic localization patterns in bacterial prostatitis and urethritis. Invest Urol. 1968;5:492.
9. Fair WR, Crane DB, Schiller N, et al. Re-appraisal of treatment in chronic bacterial prostatitis. J Urol. 1979;121:437.
10. Weidner W, Schiefer HG. Treatment of bacterial prostatitis with ciprofloxacin: Results of a one-year follow-up study. Am J Med. 1987;82(Suppl 4A):280.
11. Comhaire FH. Concentration of pefloxacine in split ejaculates of patients with chronic male accessory gland infection. J Urol. 1987;138:828.
12. Malinverni R, Glausser MP. Comparative studies of fluoroquinolones in the treatment of urinary tract infections. Rev Infect Dis. 1988;10(Suppl 1):153.
13. Eykyn S, Bultitude MI, Mayo ME, et al. Prostatitic calculi as a source of recurrent bacteriuria in the male. Br J Urol. 1974;46:527.
14. Mardh PA, Colleen S. Search for uro-genital tract infections in patients with symptoms of prostatitis. Scand J Urol Nephrol. 1975;9:8.
15. Mardh PA, Ripa KT, Colleen S et al. Role of *Chlamydia trachomatis* in nonacute prostatitis. Br J Vener Dis. 1978;54:330.
16. Weidner W, Arens M, Krauss H, et al. *Chlamydia trachomatis* in "abacterial" prostatitis: Microbiological cytological, and serological studies. Urol Int. 1983;38:146.
17. Weidner W, Brunner H, Krause W. Quantitative culture of *Ureaplasma urealyticum* in patients with chronic prostatitis or prostatosis. J Urol. 1980;124:622.
18. Poletti F, Medici MC, Alinovi A, et al. Isolation of *Chlamydia trachomatis* from the prostatic cells in patients affected by nonacute abacterial prostatitis. J Urol. 1985;134:691.
19. Schacter J. Is *Chlamydia trachomatis* a cause of prostatitis? J Urol 1985;134:711.
20. Taylor-Robinson D. The role of chlamydiae in genitourinary disease (Letter). J Urol. 1982;128:156.
21. Segura JW, Opitz JL, Green LF. Prostatosis prostatitis or pelvic floor tension myalgia? J Urol. 1979;122:168.
22. Nilsson JK, Colleen S, Mardh PA. Relationship between psychological and laboratory findings in patients with symptoms of non-acute prostatitis. In: Danielsson D, Juhlin L, Mardh PA, eds. Genital Infections and Their Complications. Stockholm: Almquist and Wiksell; 1975:133.
23. Kreiger JN. Prostatitis syndromes: Pathophysiology, differential diagnosis and treatment. Sex Transm Dis. 1984;11:100.
24. O'Dea MJ, Hunting DB, Greene LF. Nonspecific granulomatous prostatitis. J Urol 1977;118:58.
25. Venema RJ, Lattimer JK. Genital tuberculosis in the male. J Urol. 1957;78:65.
26. Simon HB. Genitourinary tuberculosis: Clinical features in a general hospital population. Am J Med. 1977;63:410.
27. Brooker WJ, Aufderheide AC. Genitourinary tract infections due to atypical mycobacteria. J Urol. 1980;124:242.
28. Schwarz J: Mycotic prostatitis. Urology. 1982;19:1.

29. Price MJ, Lewis EL, Carmalt JE. Coccidioidomycosis of prostate gland. Urology. 1982;19:653.
30. Hinchley WW, Someren A. Cryptococcal prostatitis. Am J Clin Pathol. 1981;75:257.
31. Meares EM Jr. Postatic Abscess. J Urol. 1986;136:1281.
32. Suago H, Takiuchi H, Sakurai T. Transrectal longitudinal ultrasonography of prostatic abscess. J Urol. 1986;136:1316.
33. Vaccaro JA, Belville WD, Kiesling VJ Jr, et al. Prostatic abscesses: Computerized tomography scanning as an aid to diagnosis and treatment. J Urol 1986;136:1318.
34. Berger RE, Alexander ER, Harnisch JP, et al. Etiology, manifestations and therapy of acute epididymitis: Prospective study of 50 cases. J Urol. 1979;121:750.
35. Bormel P: Current concepts on the etiology and treatment of epididymitis. Med Bull US Army, Europe. 1963;20:332.
36. Berger RE, Alexander ER, Monda GD, et al. *Chlamydia trachomatis* as a cause of acute "idiopathic" epididymitis. N Engl J Med. 1978;298:301.
37. Mittemeyer BT, Lennox KW, Borski AA. Epididymitis—a review of 610 cases. J Urol. 1966;95:390.
38. Witherington R, Harper WM IV. The surgical management of acute bacterial epididymitis with emphasis on epididymotomy. J Urol. 1982;128:722.
39. Nilsson S, Obrant KD, Persson PS: Changes in the testes parenchyma caused by acute nonspecific epididymitis. Fertil Steril. 1968;19:748.
40. Nickel WR, Plumb RT. Other infections and inflammations of the external genitalis. In: Harrison JH, Gittes RF, Perlmutter AD, et al, eds. Campbell's Urology. v. 1. ed 4. Philadelphia: WB Saunders; 1978:640.
41. Shapiro FR, Breschi LC: Acute epididymitis in Viet Nam. Review of 52 cases. Milit Med. 1973;138:643.
42. Harnisch JP, Berger RE, Alexander ER, et al. Aetiology of acute epididymitis. Lancet. 1977;1:819.
43. Watson RA. Gonorrhea and acute epididymitis. Milit Med. 1979;144:785.
44. Drotman PD. Epidemiology and treatment of epididymitis. Rev Infect Dis. 1982;4(Suppl):788.
45. Beard CM, Benson RC, Kelalis PP, et al. The incidence and outcome of mumps orchitis in Rochester, Minn. Mayo, 1935–1974. Mayo Clin Proc. 1977;52:3.

SECTION N. EYE INFECTIONS

98. CONJUNCTIVITIS

PETER J. McDONNELL
W. RICHARD GREEN

The most common eye disease in the Western Hemisphere is conjunctivitis. The normal flora of the conjunctiva, various sources of infection in conjunctivitis, and factors important in the resistance of the conjunctiva to infections have been well described.[1–15]

ETIOLOGIC AGENTS

The numerous agents that may cause conjunctivitis are listed in Table 1.

CLINICAL MANIFESTATIONS

The most obvious clinical manifestation of conjunctivitis is hyperemia of the conjunctiva. The dilatation and congestion of the vessels are greater near the periphery of the bulbar conjunctiva and become less marked as the limbus is approached.

The presence of secretion is almost always a feature of conjunctivitis. This is due to an exudation of inflammatory cells and a fibrin-rich edematous fluid from the blood, and the exudate is combined with denuded epithelial cells and mucus. The secretion may be purulent, mucopurulent, fibrinous, or serosanguineous, depending on the cause and severity of the disease. When the exudate dries, the eyelids may stick together.

Conjunctival edema (chemosis) may be present in parts of the conjunctiva that are freely movable over the globe and lids. The normal transparency of the conjunctiva may be lost, and it may appear thickened due to the infiltration of the tissues with leukocytes. If there is diffuse leukocytic infiltration of the conjunctival stroma, with hyperplasia of the overlying epithelium, papillae form. A papilla contains a central blood vessel in its core. This vessel branches on the surface of the papilla. Papillae usually occur in the tarsal conjunctiva. The conjunctiva may have a velvety appearance from numerous small papillae. When large, the papillae have the appearance of cobblestone excrescences. This is unusual in acute infectious conjunctivitis but more common in allergic and chronic conjunctivitis.

Normal conjunctiva has an occasional follicle in its substantia propria, especially in the fornices. In some forms of conjunctivitis, a follicular reaction may predominate. Follicles and papillae may be differentiated clinically because follicles resemble white grains whereas papillae are red with a central vascular tuft.

Membrane formation is also seen in some cases of conjunctivitis. This membrane consists of a superficial fibrinous layer connected to subconjunctival granulation tissue. When this membrane is excised, a raw bleeding surface is exposed.

The cornea is sometimes involved in viral conjunctivitis, and this may lead to photophobia, grittiness, and pain.

The various forms of conjunctivitis have many of the aforementioned signs and symptoms in common, with none having pathognomonic features. A morphologic diagnosis is rarely possible unless there are associated corneal changes (e.g., in epidemic keratoconjunctivitis or herpes simplex keratoconjunctivitis).

BACTERIAL CONJUNCTIVITIS

Bacterial conjunctivitis is the most common type of infectious conjunctivitis.

In adults, the most common bacterial isolates from an acute conjunctivitis are *Streptococcus pneumoniae, Staphylococcus aureus*, and *Staphylococcus epidermidis*. The role of the latter two organisms in causation is, however, disputed.[16–18]

In children, the chief organisms causing acute conjunctivitis are *Haemophilus influenzae, Streptococcus pneumoniae*, and perhaps *Staphylococcus aureus*.[19–21]

The bacterial etiology of chronic bacterial conjunctivitis is less well defined.

Anaerobic bacteria have been isolated from conjunctivitis patients in association with aerobic organisms thought to be the cause of the conjunctivitis.[19] The same organisms have been isolated in immunodeficient patients, in whom acute and chronic conjunctivitis are more common than in normal patients.[22] Table 1 identifies bacteria that probably have been responsible for conjunctivitides.

TABLE 1. Etiologic Agents of Conjunctivitis

Bacteria
Streptococcus
Staphylococcus aureus
Haemophilus influenzae
Neisseria gonorrhoeae
Haemophilus aegyptius (Koch-Weeks)
Haemophilus ducreyi
Neisseria meningitidis
Streptococci of the viridans group
Proteus vulgaris
Morax-Axenfeld (*Moraxella lacunata*)
Corynebacterium diphtheriae
Mycobacterium tuberculosis
Francisella tularensis
Treponema pallidum
Branhamella catarrhalis
Shigella flexneri
Yersinia enterocolitica
Staphylococcus epidermidis
Acinetobacter calcoaceticus var. *anitratus*
Aeromonas hydrophila
Peptostreptococcus
Propionibacterium
Cat scratch bacillus
Viruses
Adenoviridae
Poxviruses (variola, vaccinia, molluscum contagiosum)
Herpesviruses (herpes simplex, varicella-zoster, Epstein-Barr virus)
Papillomaviruses (papilloma virus)
Influenza
Paramyxoviruses (measles, mumps, Newcastle disease virus)
Picornaviruses (echovirus, enterovirus, coxsackievirus, and poliovirus)
Chlamydia trachomatis
Fungi
Candida sp.
Sporothrix schenckii
Rhinosporidium seeberi
Parasites
Onchocerca volvulus
Loa loa
Wuchereria bancrofti
Oestrus ovis (myiasis)

The significance of most studies of bacterial cultures during conjunctivitis remains to be explored. However, there seems little argument that bacterial and viral conjunctivitis may be mistakenly identified clinically one for the other, and that few bacterial conjunctivitides have pathognomonic features that identify their cause.[16]

The cause of epidemics of bacterial conjunctivitis has been better established, for example, *Streptococcus pneumoniae*.[23]

Of special interest is gonococcal conjunctivitis, in which the conjunctiva is markedly injected and chemotic, with a profuse purulent discharge.[24] The eyelids become swollen and difficult to open. Serious complications of untreated gonococcal conjunctivitis may include corneal ulceration and subsequent perforation. Sometimes gonococcal conjunctivitis has a prolonged asymptomatic course, in a manner similar to some of the genital infections.[25]

Membrane formation may be seen in any severe infection of the conjunctiva, but it is typically present in infections with streptococci and *Corynebacterium diphtheriae*. These membranes may lead to a spectrum of changes from fine corneal scarring to obliteration of the fornices. In contrast to most other types of conjunctivitis, pain is a common symptom with *C. diphtheriae* infection. Diphtheritic conjunctivitis does not occur as the sole manifestation of diphtheria, and so other manifestations of the disease should be sought.

Moraxella lacunata produces a localized ''angular'' conjunctivitis associated with fissuring and dermatitis of the external canthi and a scanty conjunctival discharge.

Certain nonpyogenic organisms (*Mycobacterium tuberculosis, Francisella tularensis, Treponema pallidum*) produce an atypical clinical picture characterized by unilateral conjunctival nodules that tend to ulcerate. Moderate localized conjunctival injection, minimal discharge, and a palpable preauricular lymph node on the affected side are present.

The pleomorphic gram-negative cat-scratch disease bacillus, first identified in lymph nodes,[26] produces a unilateral follicular conjunctivitis associated with prominent enlargement of the ipsilateral preauricular lymph node.[27] *Yersinia* infection has been implicated[28] in a syndrome similar to Reiter syndrome and consisting of a self-limited conjunctivitis, acute myalgia, fever, gastrointestinal symptoms, and a prolonged anterior uveitis, polyarthritis, sacroiliitis, and HLA-B27 association. Similar syndrome complexes were seen within family groups. *Yersinia entercolitica* has also been associated with an isolated conjunctivitis.[29]

Haemophilus ducreyi,[30] *Pasteurella multocida*,[31] *Francisella tularensis*,[32] *Neisseria meningitidis*,[33] streptococci,[34] *Acinetobacter calcoaceticus* (*Herellea vaginicola*),[35] and *Aeromonas hydrophila*[36] have caused isolated cases of acute conjunctivitis.

VIRAL CONJUNCTIVITIS

Viral conjunctivitis is fairly common, causing 20 percent of nonepidemic cases of conjunctivitis in one study in children[20] and 14 percent of adult patients in another study.[16] The morphology of associated corneal changes, the time course, systemic involvement, and epidemic characteristics will usually permit identification that the conjunctivitis is of viral origin. The actual causative virus usually cannot be implicated by ocular morphologic characteristics alone but requires cultures and serologic studies. Most viral conjunctivitides are self-limited and highly contagious, with low morbidity. The discharge is usually watery rather than purulent. A generalized conjunctival injection, moderate tearing, and mild itching are present. Follicle formation may be prominent. Preauricular lymphadenopathy is common, and occasionally the conjunctivitis is associated with an upper respiratory tract infection.

Adenoviruses are responsible for the most frequent epidemics of viral conjunctivitis in the United States.

Serotypes of adenoviruses typically associated with pharyngoconjunctival fever (PCF) are 3 and 7, with occasional involvement by types 1, 2, 4, 5, 6, 8, and 14. The clinical complex of pharyngitis, fever, and conjunctivitis, inferior forniceal follicles, and rarely, keratitis may help identify this conjunctivitis. Spontaneous resolution within 1 to 2 weeks is the rule.[37]

Epidemic keratoconjunctivitis (EKC) has most commonly resulted from infection with serotype 8, but types 2, 3, 4, 7, 9, 10, 11, 14, 16, 19, and 29 have been reported.[38–45] The clinical picture includes pharyngitis, preauricular lymphadenopathy, and follicular conjunctivitis, and there is a 7- to 10-day incubation period with a 5- to 12-day interval before characteristic (but inconsistent) corneal subepithelial infiltrates develop. These epidemics are sometimes propagated by eye health care personnel. Despite a wide spectrum of symptoms ranging from severe photophobia to mild irritation only, this disease is usually self-limited and is rarely associated with visual loss from corneal changes.[46,47] Occasional reports have described raised intraocular pressure[48] and chronic keratitis and a Stevens-Johnson syndrome[49] as a result of epidemic keratoconjunctivitis. Chronic adenovirus conjunctivitis has been reported.[50,51]

Reports of recent epidemics in Florida have emphasized the emergence of a picornavirus as a factor in epidemic hemorrhagic conjunctivitis (EHC) in the United States. Previous reports have been mainly from Africa.[52,53] Enterovirus, type 70, coxsackievirus A24, and adenovirus 11 have all resulted in a similar clinical picture[54–60] (Fig. 1). This consists of bilateral follicular conjunctivitis of sudden onset, with (rarely) corneal changes and systemic symptoms, a short (4–5 day) symptomatic course, and bulbar conjunctival hemorrhages.[62] Spontaneous resolution with low morbidity is the usual course, although occasional reports have described Bell's palsy, radiculomyelitis,

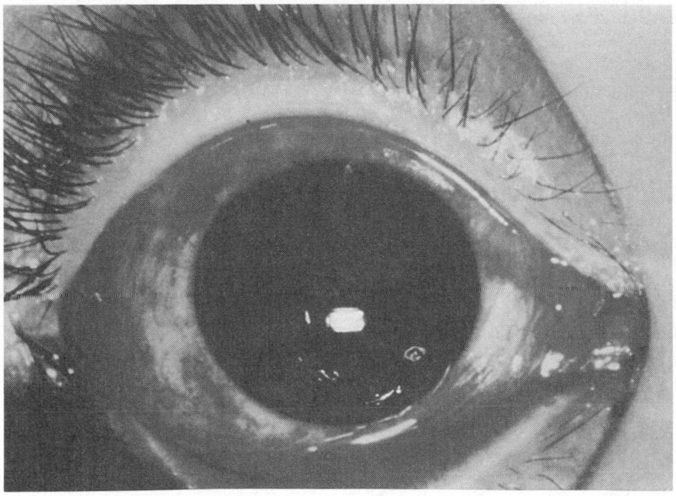

FIG. 1. Acute hemorrhagic conjunctivitis due to enterovirus 70. (From Kono et al,[61] with permission.)

cranial nerve palsies, and other types of central nervous system involvement.[63–66]

Ocular infection with vaccinia virus occurs when the virus is accidentally transferred from the site of medical inoculation to the eye. Vesicles appear on the lid margin,[67] and a conjunctivitis may follow. Conjunctivitis without lid lesions has also been reported.[68]

Molluscum contagiosum virus produces small, waxy, elevated lid-margin tumors with umbilicated centers that are associated with a chronic follicular conjunctivitis caused by the toxic effect of shed incomplete virions.[69]

Herpes simplex virus, types 1 and 2, varicella-zoster virus, and the Epstein-Barr virus can cause conjunctivitis.[70,71] Herpes simplex is responsible for the majority of cases of nonepidemic follicular conjunctivitis in young children.[72] Vesicular lid lesions and preauricular adenopathy may be present, and transient keratitis may be noted. The conjunctivitis is self-limited and is rarely associated with significant morbidity.

In patients with chickenpox, papules may develop on the lids and conjunctiva and at the limbus during the infection. These papules may become pustules and ulcerate. Vesicles may be found on the conjunctiva, particularly on the semilunar fold. Four percent of patients with chickenpox have conjunctival and corneal manifestations.[73] In herpes zoster ophthalmicus, a follicular conjunctivitis with regional adenopathy rarely occurs. In less than 5 percent of patients with infectious mononucleosis, a mild conjunctivitis is present.[74,75]

Human papillomavirus may produce lesions on the tarsal and bulbar conjunctivae and on the lid margin. A catarrhal conjunctivitis may result, and the cornea may show multiple punctate erosions. The presence of viral antigen and DNA sequences in some dysplastic epithelial lesions of the conjunctiva has raised concern that the virus may have a role in the development of conjunctival epithelial malignancies, similar to its suspected role in the female genital tract.[76]

Congenital rubella is associated with numerous ocular abnormalities.[77,78] Epidemic rubella in young children has produced a follicular conjunctivitis associated with occasional corneal epithelial changes.

The influenza viruses often cause catarrhal conjunctivitis and occasionally an acute follicular conjunctivitis. This ocular manifestation of influenza has been reported in both 48 percent[79] and 60 percent[80] of patients.

Infections due to the measles (rubeola) virus may be associated with mild paralimbal conjunctival epithelial erosion; the epithelia contain measles antigens that develop during the prodrome before the skin rash.[81] An epithelial keratitis with photophobia may occur after the skin rash occurs. Koplik's spots may be found on the semilunar fold.[82]

Conjunctivitis occurs rarely with mumps.[83] Newcastle disease virus (which causes a fatal pneumoencephalitis in fowl) may produce a self-limited, unilateral follicular conjunctivitis in humans.[84] Echo 11[85] and polio virus[86] have occasionally been described as a cause of follicular conjunctivitis.

Parinaud oculoglandular syndrome is a clinical complex of conjunctivitis, prominent preauricular lymphadenopathy, and a febrile illness with various possible causes, including infectious mononucleosis[87] and cat-scratch fever,[88] syphilis, tuberculosis, and sarcoidosis.

CHLAMYDIAL CONJUNCTIVITIS

Trachoma, one of the leading causes of blindness in the world,[89,90] is caused by a chlamydial organism that has a low infectivity. In the United States, the disease is largely confined to certain Native American populations that are characterized by poverty and poor communal hygiene. Repeated infections appear necessary to establish clinical trachoma. The conjunctivitis is characterized by a follicular reaction in the superior tarsal conjunctiva that is often associated with a concurrent papillary response. As follicles resolve, they appear to be replaced with fine subconjunctival scars. The degree of scarring seems to be related to the intensity of the follicular response and also to the presence of secondary bacterial infection. The subconjunctival scarring may in time lead to distortion of the tarsal plate and result in trichiasis.

Also associated with trachoma is the development of a superior limbic pannus with opacification of the corneal stroma and neovascularization. Follicles may occur in the limbus, and when these resolve, a clear depression persists (Herbert's pit).

Inclusion conjunctivitis is a fairly common infection caused by *Chlamydia trachomatis* that is venereally transmitted.[91,92] Since an infant may acquire the organism during his passage through the birth canal, it is one of the causes of ophthalmia neonatorum. Because the conjunctiva in the newborn does not form follicles, the injected appearance of this conjunctivitis in newborns is nonspecific. In adults, numerous papillae and follicles form on the tarsal conjunctiva and are more pronounced on the lower. The disease is usually bilateral, and the discharge is often profuse. Inclusion conjunctivitis is differentiated from trachoma by two important features: (*1*) corneal scarring rarely occurs in inclusion conjunctivitis; and (*2*) in trachoma the upper tarsal conjunctiva is more involved than the lower, although occasionally inclusion conjunctivitis may take on the characteristics of trachoma and various corneal changes have been described in inclusion conjunctivitis. Associated urethritis and cervicitis is common.[93]

Conjunctivitis is a rare manifestation of systemic lymphogranuloma venereum that is caused by certain immunotypes (L-1, L-2, L-3) of *C. trachomatis*. Moderate unilateral conjunctival injection, slight conjunctival discharge, and extreme edema of the upper and lower lids are present. In addition, ipsilateral preauricular, parotid, and submaxillary lymphadenopathy is present.[94] Types A, B, Ba, and C have been most commonly found in hyperendemic areas of trachoma.

OPHTHALMIA NEONATORUM

The incidence of acute conjunctivitis of the newborn (ophthalmia neonatorum) is reported to be as high as 12 percent of all newborns.[95] It has been most commonly the result of mild chemical irritation after ocular silver nitrate prophylaxis. This self-limited conjunctivitis appears within the first 24 hours, and it lasts 1–2 days. However, chlamydial conjunctivitis is becoming much more common, with an incidence of approximately 2.8 percent of all births at one clinic and occurring in more than

35 percent of the infants who are born to mothers with proven chlamydial cervicitis.[96] This has been substantiated by other studies.[97,98] The onset generally occurs within 5 to 19 days, with no pathologic features except for an association with other systemic chlamydial infections such as pneumonia and otitis media.[99,100] It has been suggested that the organism in these cases gains entry to the neonate through the conjunctival mucosa. There have been reports of occasional cases of chlamydial conjunctivitis in infants delivered by cesarean section.[101]

Bacterial conjunctivitis is most often the result of *Staphylococcus aureus* infection, with *Streptococcus pneumoniae* and *Haemophilus influenzae* the next most common.[102,103] There are no pathognomonic features of these infections, and they may occur as early as 24 hours after birth. Streptococcal infections may be associated with acute dacryocystitis of the newborn, and *Pseudomonas* sp. have been reported as an occasional cause.[104] Cases of staphylococcal "scalded skin" syndrome have been attributed to primary staphylococcal conjunctivitis.[105] *H. influenzae* conjunctivitis has been implicated in neonatal meningitis. *Shigella flexneri* has caused ethmoiditis and conjunctivitis.[106] *Branhamella catarhalis* is being more frequently diagnosed[107–109] and has been confused with true gonococcal ophthalmia neonatorum.

The prevailing incidence of gonococcal ophthalmia neonatorum is not known, but it is usually seen 1–2 days after birth and is characterized by a florid course and the threat of corneal ulceration and perforation. Recent cases of penicillin-resistant strains[110,111] and occasional cases with a deceptively mild course have made diagnosis and management more difficult.[112]

Infants born to mothers with herpes simplex virus cervicitis may develop a conjunctivitis within a few days of birth. The conjunctivitis is usually self-limited but may be associated with corneal epithelial changes and, rarely, stromal keratitis.

OTHER INFECTIVE AND NONINFECTIVE CONJUNCTIVITIDES

Ophthalmomyiasis,[113] nematode,[114] and trematode[115] infections have been described. Conjunctival inflammation (chemosis and injection and discharge) is seen as a result of many noninfectious conditions, but particularly as an allergic mucosal response. The agents responsible include drugs and devices such as hard and soft contact lenses,[116,117] contact lens sterilizing solutions (usually the preservative thiomerasol)[118,119] that cause giant papillary conjunctivitis, prostheses,[120,121] topical timolol,[122] atropine, antiviral agents, and other drugs,[123–127] cosmetics,[128] and external allergens that cause vernal keratoconjunctivitis.[129] Conjunctivitis may occur as a response to toxic agents such as gentian violet,[130] latex,[131] and ultraviolet irradiation.[132–134] Phlyctenular keratoconjunctivitis has occurred in patients with increased tuberculin sensitivity[135] and staphylococcal hypersensitivity.[136]

The exact causes of numerous other conditions with fairly specific clinical features have not been identified. These include keratoconjunctivitis sicca, superior limbic keratoconjunctivitis, ligneous conjunctivitis, mucocutaneous lymph node syndrome, and Reiter syndrome. Immune-mediated conjunctivitis has been implicated in mucous membrane pemphigoid[137] and in the conjunctivitis associated with graft-vs.-host disease in bone marrow transplant patients.[138]

DIFFERENTIAL DIAGNOSIS

Other serious, sight-threatening conditions that present as "red eye" may superficially resemble a conjunctivitis. The points of difference are highlighted in Table 2. Chronic, unilateral conjunctivitis in which a specific diagnosis is not made should alert the physician to the possibility of a meibomian gland carcinoma.[139]

TABLE 2. Comparison of Conjunctivitis and Other Conditions

Characteristic	*Conjunctivitis*	*Uveitis*	*Acute Angle-Closure Glaucoma*
Prominent symptoms	Discharge, irritation	Photophobia, visual loss	Pain, visual loss
Vision	Usually normal	Normal and occasionally decreased	Markedly reduced
Ocular injection	Conjunctival injection generalized	Paralimbal injection (ciliary flush)	Paralimbal injection
Cornea	Usually clear	Usually clear	Edematous and cloudy
Pupil	Normal	May be normal or small	Usually middilated, irregular, and immobile
Intraocular pressure	Normal	Normal or slightly elevated	Markedly elevated

LABORATORY INVESTIGATIONS

Mild conjunctivitis is rarely investigated, and it usually is treated empirically. Reports differ on the value of culturing suspected bacterial conjunctivitis.[140,141] Scrapings of the superior and inferior tarsal conjunctiva may be taken (after the administration of proparacaine HCl, 0.5%) for smears and cultures in a manner similar to that described in Chapter 99. Cultures are usually taken from both conjunctival sacs and separately from both lids in suspected conjunctivitis.[142] Chlamydial cultures are taken with a dry calcium alginate swab, which is then placed in chlamydial culture medium.

All cases of suspected ophthalmia neonatorum should have cultures and smears performed for bacteria, chlamydia, and herpes simplex virus. Acute and convalescent serologic tests for adenovirus and picornavirus may help in diagnosing epidemic conjunctivitis, but these are generally not required because of the self-limited nature of the infection, the nonspecific treatment available, and the diagnostic characteristics of the epidemic features. Serodiagnostic testing of tears in serum by using microimmunofluorescent tests has been described for patients with *C. trachomatis* inclusion conjunctivitis.[143] Serologic testing for SS-A and SS-B autoantibodies has assisted in the early diagnosis of keratoconjunctivitis sicca that is a prodrome of Sjögren syndrome.[144]

In a conjunctival scraping from a normal healthy eye, epithelial cells and occasional goblet cells are present. In acute bacterial infection, the scraping shows large numbers of neutrophils. Bacteria may be present within or outside leukocytes. In chronic bacterial infections, there is a decrease in neutrophils and an increase in lymphocytes and large mononuclear cells. In viral conjunctivitis, lymphocytes and monocytes are predominant. In herpes simplex infections, multinucleated epithelial cells may be seen. In chlamydial infections, a mixed inflammatory cell population (polymorphonuclear leukocytes and lymphocytes) is present, and basophilic intracytoplasmic inclusion bodies may be seen in epithelial cells; the latter finding is common in children and less common in adults. Immunofluorescent techniques promise to provide more sensitivity in identification. In allergic conjunctivitis, scrapings characteristically reveal eosinophils.[145] They are found in greatest abundance in vernal conjunctivitis. Between attacks of vernal conjunctivitis, mast cells and no eosinophils are seen.

Scrapings from patients with keratoconjunctivitis sicca and superior limbic keratoconjunctivitis reveal keratinized epithelial cells or condensed chromatin patterns when using the Papanicolaou staining technique.[146]

Impression cytology may offer an alternative to the conjunctival scraping method.[147] Immunoelectron microscopy and immunofluorescent techniques may aid in diagnosing viral conjunctivitis.[148,149]

TREATMENT

Most types of mild bacterial conjunctivitis and most types of viral conjunctivitis are self-limited, benign conditions that require no treatment. Topical gentamicin or tobramycin[150] for gram-negative rod infections; and erythromycin, bacitracin, chloramphenicol, or neomycin/polymixin for gram-positive infections, given every 2–4 hours for 7–10 days, are usually effective.[18,141] Often an organism reported to be resistant to a specific antibiotic in the laboratory will respond to that antibiotic clinically because of the high concentrations achievable in the tear film by topical application.

Gonococcal conjunctivitis requires urgent therapy with parenteral penicillin, topical penicillin, and frequent instillations of normal saline. Penicillinase-producing *Neisseria gonorrhoeae* (PPNG) require systemic ceftriaxone or another third generation cephalosporin. A single intramuscular dose of 125 mg of ceftriaxone resulted in a 100 percent cure rate for gonococcal ophthalmia neonatorum without the need for concomitant topical therapy.[151]

Herpes simplex virus conjunctivitis may be treated with topical trifluridine every 2 hours for 7 days, although this condition is usually benign and self-limited.

Adult inclusion conjunctivitis requires a 3-week course of either erythromycin or sulfamethoxazole and trimethoprim orally, supplemented with topical tetracycline ointment or erythromycin drops. A similar therapy is effective in treating trachoma, but prevention of reinfection and bacterial superinfection are equally important.

The place of interferon and interferon inducers in treating viral conjunctivitis remains conjectural.

Allergic and immune-mediated conjunctivitis responds best to topical corticosteroids, of which prednisolone acetate, 1%, is the most potent. The long-term use of topical steroids may be associated with glaucoma and cataracts, whereas short-term use may accelerate herpes simplex epithelial keratitis. Nonsteroidal anti-inflammatory agents such as aspirin[152] and cromolyn sodium[153,154] are becoming increasingly useful.

PROPHYLAXIS OF OPHTHALMIA NEONATORUM

There is considerable debate over the relative efficacy of 1% silver nitrate vs. topical antibiotics such as 0.5% erythromycin or 1% tetracyclines. Silver nitrate is still extremely effective, particularly against gonococcal infection, but it has little impact on the increasing incidence of chlamydial infections. Topical erythromycin seems the most effective agent in preventing this infection.[155] In infants born to mothers with known genital chlamydial infection, the routine use of erythromycin ointment will eliminate chlamydial conjunctivitis, but systemic erythromycin estolate is preferred to prevent nasopharyngeal colonization.[156,157]

Children born to mothers with known gonococcal genital infections should be treated with parenteral penicillin or ceftriaxone, depending on susceptibility.

REFERENCES

1. Allansmith MR, Ostler HB, Butterworth M. Concomitance of bacteria in various areas of the eye. Arch Ophthalmol. 1969;82:37.
2. Lucic H. Bacteriology of the normal conjunctival sac. Am J Ophthalmol. 1927;10:829.
3. Khorazo D, Thompson R. The bacterial flora of the normal conjunctiva. Am J Ophthalmol. 1935;18:1114.
4. Gowen GH. Source of staphylococci on normal conjunctiva of human eye. Am J Ophthalmol. 1934;17:36.
5. Locatcher-Khorazo D, Benham RW, Silva-Hunter M. Incidence of fungi from clinically healthy eyes of 508 young people 10–18 years of age and in 1347 adults 19–80 years of age. In: Locatcher-Khorazo D, Seegal BC, eds. Microbiology of the Eye. St Louis: CV Mosby; 1972;213.
6. Hammeke JC, Ellis PP. Mycotic flora of the conjunctiva. Am J Ophthalmol. 1960;49:1174.
7. Williamson J, Gordon AM, Wood R, et al. Fungal flora of the conjunctival sac in health and disease: Influence of topical and systemic steroids. Br J Ophthalmol. 1968;52:127.
8. Nema HV, Ahuja OP, Bal A, et al. Mycotic flora of the conjunctiva. Am J Ophthalmol. 1966;62:968.
9. Locatcher-Khorazo D, Guiterrez E. Eye infections following cataract extraction, with special reference to the role of *Staphylococcus aureus*. Am J Ophthalmol. 1956;41:981.
10. Allen HF, Mangiaracine AB. Bacterial endophthalmitis after cataract extraction. II. Incidence in 36,000 consecutive operations, with special reference to preoperative topical antibiotics. Trans Am Acad Ophthalmol Otolaryngol. 1973;77:581.
11. McMeel JW, Wapner JM. Infections and retina surgery. I. Bacteriologic contamination during scleral buckling surgery. Arch Ophthalmol. 1965;74:42.
12. Howard HJ. Role of the epithelial cell in conjunctival and corneal infections. Am J Ophthalmol. 1924;7:909.
13. Halbert SP, Locatcher-Khorazo D, Sonn-Kazar C, et al. Further studies on the incidence of antibiotic-producing microorganisms of the ocular flora. Arch Ophthalmol. 1957;58:66.
14. Halbert SP, Swick LS. Antibiotic-producing bacteria of the ocular flora. Am J Ophthalmol. 1952;35(5 Pt 2):73.
15. Halbert SP, Swick LS, Sonn C, et al. Ocular antibiotic-producing bacteria in normal eyes and in conjunctivitis. Arch Ophthalmol. 1954;51:7.
16. Leibowitz HM, Pratt MV, Flagstad IJ, et al. Human conjunctivitis. A diagnostic evaluation. Arch Ophthalmol. 1976;94:1747.
17. Brook I, Pettit TH, Martin WJ, et al. Anaerobic and aerobic bacteriology of acute conjunctivitis. Ann Ophthalmol. 1979;11:389.
18. Seal DV, Barrett SP, McGill JI. Aetiology and treatment of acute bacterial infection of the external eye. Br J Ophthalmol. 1982;66:357.
19. Brook I. Anaerobic and aerobic bacterial flora of acute conjunctivitis in children. Arch Ophthalmol. 1980;98:833.
20. Gigliotti F, Williams WT, Hayden FG, et al. Etiology of acute conjunctivitis in children. J Pediatr. 1981;98:531.
21. Levin RM, Ticknor W, Jordan C, et al. Etiology of conjunctiviits. J Pediatr. 1981;99:831.
22. Friedlaender MH, Masi RJ, Osumoto M, et al. Ocular microbial flora in immunodeficient patients. Arch Ophthalmol. 1980;98:1211.
23. Shayegani M, Parsons LM, Gibbons WE Jr, et al. Characterization of nontypable *Streptococcus pneumoniae*-like organisms isolated from outbreaks of conjunctivitis. J Clin Microbiol. 1982;16:8.
24. Valenton MJ, Abendanio R. Gonorrhea conjunctivitis. Can J Ophthalmol. 1973;8:421.
25. Tight RR. Gonococcal conjunctivitis. JAMA. 1982;247:2499.
26. English CK, Wear DJ, Margileth AM, et al. Cat-scratch disease, isolation and culture of the bacterial agent. JAMA. 1988;259:1347–52.
27. Wear DJ, Malaty RH, Zimmerman LE, et al. Cat scratch disease bacilli in the conjunctiva of patients with Parinaud's oculoglandular syndrome. Ophthalmology. 1985;92:1282–7.
28. Saari KM, Laitinen O, Leirisalo M, et al. Ocular inflammation associated with Yersinia infection. Am J Ophthalmol. 1980;89:84.
29. Crichton EP. Suppurative conjunctivitis caused by *Yersinia enterocolitica*. Can Med J. 1978;118:22.
30. Gregory JE, Henderson RW, Smith R. Conjunctivitis due to *Haemophilus ducreyi* infection. Br J Vener Dis. 1980;56:414.
31. Eschete ML, Rambin ED, West BC. *Clostridium pseudotetanicum* bacteremia in a patient with *Pasteurella multocida* conjunctivitis. J Clin Microbiol. 1978;8:509.
32. Guerrant RL, Humphries MK, Butler JE, et al. Tickborne oculoglandular tularemia. Case report and review of seasonal and vectorial associations in 106 cases. Arch Intern Med. 1976;136:811.
33. Brook I, Bateman JB, Pettit TH. Meningococcal conjunctivitis. Arch Ophthalmol. 1979;97:890.
34. Cohn H, Mondino BJ, Brown SI, et al. Marginal corneal ulcers with acute beta streptococcal conjunctivitis and chronic dacryocystitis. Am J Ophthalmol. 1979;87:541.
35. Abel R, Shulman J, Boyle GL, et al. Herellea vaginicola and ocular infections. Ann Ophthalmol. 1975;7:1485.
36. Smith JA. Ocular *Aeromonas hydrophila*. Am J Ophthalmol. 1980;89:449.
37. Bell JA, Rowe WP, Engler JI, et al. Pharyngoconjunctival fever: Epidemiological studies of a recently recognized disease entity. JAMA. 1955;175:1083.
38. O'Day DM, Guyer B, Hierholzer JC, et al. Clinical and laboratory evaluation of epidemic keratoconjunctivitis due to adenovirus types 8 and 19. Am J Ophthalmol. 1976;81:207.
39. Aoki K, Kato M, Ohtsuka H, et al. Clinical and aetiological study of adenoviral conjunctivitis, with special reference to adenovirus types 4 and 19 infections. Br J Ophthalmol. 1982;66:776.
40. Tullo AB, Higgins PG. An outbreak of adenovirus type 14 conjunctivitis. Br J Ophthalmol. 1980;64:489.
41. D'Angelo LJ, Hierholzer JC, Holman RC, et al. Epidemic keratoconjunctivitis caused by adenovirus type 8: Epidemiologic and laboratory aspects of a large outbreak. Am J Epidemiol. 1981;113:44.
42. Darougar S, Pearce R, Gibson JA, et al. Adenovirus type 21 keratoconjunctivitis. Br J Ophthalmol. 1978;62:836.
43. Taylor JW, Chandler JW, Cooney MK. Conjunctivitis due to adenovirus type 19. J Clin Microbiol. 1978;8:209.

44. Schaap GJP, deJong JC, van Bijsterveld OP, et al. A new intermediate adenovirus type causing conjunctivitis. Arch Ophthalmol. 1979;97:2336.
45. Newland JC, Cooney MK. Characteristics of an adenovirus type 19 conjunctivitis isolate and evidence for a subgroup associated with epidemic conjunctivitis. Infect Immun. 1978;21:303.
46. Beale AJ, Doane F, Ornsby HL. Studies on adenovirus infections of the eye in Toronto. Am J Ophthalmol. 1957;43:26.
47. Boniuk M, Phillips CA, Hines MJ, et al. Adenovirus infections of the conjunctiva and cornea. Trans Am Acad Ophthalmol Ortolaryngol. 1966;70:1016.
48. Hara J, Ishibashi T, Fujimoto F, et al. Adenovirus type 10 keratoconjunctivitis with increased intraocular pressure. Am J Ophthalmol. 1980;90:481.
49. Kiernan JP, Schanzlin DJ, Leveille AS. Stevens-Johnson syndrome associated with adenovirus conjunctivitis. Am J Ophthalmol. 1981;92:543.
50. Pettit TH, Holland GN. Chronic keratoconjunctivitis associated with ocular adenovirus infection. Am J Ophthalmol. 1979;88:748.
51. Darougar S, Quinlan MP, Gibson JA, et al. Epidemic keratoconjunctivitis and chronic papillary conjunctivitis in London due to adenovirus type 19. Br J Ophthalmol. 1977;61:76.
52. Epidemiology: Acute haemorrhagic conjunctivitis. Br Med J. 1982;284:833.
53. Hoffman M. Acute haemorrhagic conjunctivitis. S Afr Med J. 1982;62:311.
54. Christopher S, Theogaraj S, Godbole S, et al. An epidemic of acute hemorrhagic conjunctivitis due to coxsackievirus A24. J Infect Dis. 1982;146:16.
55. Langford MP, Stanton GJ, Barber JC, et al. Early-appearing antiviral activity in human tears during a case of picornavirus epidemic conjunctivitis. J Infect Dis. 1979;139:653.
56. Goh KT, Doraisingham S, Yin-Murphy M. An epidemic of acute conjunctivitis caused by enterovirus-70 in Singapore in 1980. Southeast Asian J Trop Med Public Health. 1981;12:473.
57. Hatch MH, Malison MD, Palmer EL. Isolation of enterovirus 70 from patients with acute hemorrhagic conjunctivitis in Key West, Florida. N Engl J Med. 1981;305:1648.
58. Kono R, Miyamura K, Yamazaki S, et al. Seroepidemiologic studies of acute hemorrhagic conjunctivitis virus (enterovirus type 70) in West Africa. II. Studies with human sera collected in West African countries other than Ghana. Am J Epidemol. 1981;114:274.
59. Bernard KW, Hierholzer JC, Dugan JB, et al. Acute hemorrhagic conjunctivitis in Southeast Asian refugees arriving in the United States: Isolation of enterovirus 70. Am J Trop Med Hyg. 1982;31:541.
60. Minami K, Otatsume S, Mingle JAA, et al. Seroepidemiologic studies of acute hemorrhagic conjunctivitis virus (enterovirus type 70) in West Africa. I. Studies with human sera from Ghana collected eight years after the first outbreak. Am J Epidemiol. 1981;114:267.
61. Kono R, Uchida Y. Acute hemorrhagic conjunctivitis. Ophthalmol Dig. 1977;39(April):14.
62. Wolken SH. Acute hemorrhagic conjunctivitis. Surv Ophthalmol. 1974;19:71.
63. Wadia NH, Wadia PN, Katrak SM, et al. Neurological manifestations of acute haemorrhagic conjunctivitis. Lancet. 1981;2:528.
64. Thakur LC. Cranial nerve paralyses associated with acute haemorrhagic conjunctivitis. Lancet. 1981;2:584.
65. Katiyar BC, Surendra M, Singh RB, et al. Neurological syndromes after acute epidemic conjunctivitis. Lancet. 1981;2:866.
66. John TJ, Christopher S, Abraham J. Neurological manifestation of acute haemorrhagic conjunctivitis due to enterovirus 70. Lancet. 1981;2:1283.
67. Bybee JD, Phillips CA, Ory EM, et al. Vaccinia of the eyelid. JAMA. 1967;199:126.
68. Croffead GW, Harrison SW. Vaccinia conjunctivitis. Am J Ophthalmol. 1962;53:531.
69. Denis J, Chauvaud D, Savoldelli M, et al. Fine structure of palpebral molluscum contagiosum and its secondary conjunctival lesions. Graefe Arch Ophthalmol. 1978;208:207.
70. North RD. Presumptive viral keratoconjunctivitis, mononucleosis, and the oncogenic viruses. Int Ophthalmol Clin. 1975;15:211.
71. Darougar S, Hunter PA, Viswalingam M, et al. Acute follicular conjunctivitis and keratoconjunctivitis due to herpes simplex virus in London. Br J Ophthalmol. 1978;62:843.
72. Jones BR. The management of ocular herpes. Trans Ophthalmol Soc UK. 1959;79:425.
73. Stucchi CA, Bianchi G. Complications oculaires graves post-varicelleuses chez l'adulte. Ophthalmologica. 1970;161:108.
74. Carter RL, Penman HG. Infectious Mononucleosis. Oxford: Blackwell Scientific Publications; 1969.
75. Wilhelmus KR. Ocular involvement in infectious mononucleosis. Am J Ophthalmol. 1981;91:117.
76. McDonnell JM, McDonnell PJ, Green WR, et al. Demonstration of papillomavirus capsid antigen in human conjunctival neoplasia. Arch Ophthalmol. 1986;104:1801.
77. Roy FH, Hiatt RL, Korones SB, et al. Ocular manifestations of congenital rubella syndrome. Arch Ophthalmol. 1966;75:601.
78. Hara J, Fujimoto F, Ishibashi T, et al. Ocular manifestations of the 1976 rubella epidemic in Japan. Am J Ophthalmol. 1979;87:642.
79. Holland WW. A clinical study of influenza in the Royal Air Force. Lancet. 1957;2:840.
80. Jordan WS Jr, Denny FW Jr, Badger GF, et al. A study of illness in a group of Cleveland families. Am J Hyg. 1958;68:190.
81. Nommensen FE, Dekkers NWHM. Detection of measles antigen in conjunctival epithelial lesions staining by lissamine green during measles virus infection. J Med Virol. 1981;7:157.
82. Deckard PS, Bergstrom TJ. Rubeola keratitis. Ophthalmology. 1981;88:810.
83. Riffenburgh RS. Ocular manifestations of mumps. Arch Ophthalmol. 1961;66:739.
84. Lippman O. Human conjunctivitis due to the Newcastle-disease virus of fowls. Am J Ophthalmol. 1952;35:1021.
85. Spalton DJ, Palmer S, Logan LC. Echo 11 conjunctivitis. Br J Ophthalmol. 1980;64:487.
86. Kasova V, John J, Koza J, et al. Poliovirus type 3 keratoconjunctivitis. J Infect Dis. 1980;42:292.
87. Meisler DM, Bosworth DE, Krachmer JH. Ocular infectious mononucleosis manifested as Parinaud's oculoglandular syndrome. Am J Ophthalmol. 1981;92:722.
88. Loftus MJ, Sweeney G, Goldberg MH. Parinaud oculoglandular syndrome and cat-scratch fever. J Oral Surg. 1980;38:218.
89. Schachter J, Dawson CR. Human Chlamydial Infections. Littleton, MA: PSG Publishing; 1978.
90. Darougar S. Chlamydial ocular infection. J Antimicrob Chemother. 1981;8:350.
91. Schacter J. Chlamydial infections. N Engl J Med. 1978;298:428.
92. Holmes KK. The Chlamydia epidemic. JAMA. 1981;245:1718.
93. Stenson S. Adult inclusion conjunctivitis. Clinical characteristics and corneal changes. Arch Ophthalmol. 1981;99:605.
94. Macnie JP. Ocular lymphogranuloma venereum. Arch Ophthalmol. 1941;25:255.
95. Pierce JM, Ward ME, Seal DV. Ophthalmia neonatorum in the 1980s: Incidence, aetiology and treatment. Br J Ophthalmol. 1982;66:728.
96. Schachter J, Holt J, Goodner E, et al. Prospective study of chlamydial infection in neonates. Lancet. 1979;2:377.
97. Heggie AD, Lumicao GG, Stuart LA, et al. *Chlamydia trachomatis* infection in mothers and infants. A prospective study. Am J Dis Child. 1981;135:507.
98. Persson K, Ronnerstam R, Svanberg L, et al. Maternal and infantile infection with *Chlamydia* in a Swedish population. Acta Paediatr Scand. 1981;70:101.
99. Schachter J, Lum L, Goodnig CA, et al. Pneumonitis following inclusion blennorrhea. J Pediatr. 1975;87:779.
100. Beem MO, Saxon EM. Respiratory-tract colonization and a distinctive pneumonia syndrome in infants infected with *Chlamydia trachomatis*. N Engl J Med. 1977;296:306.
101. Givner LB, Rennels MB, Woodward CL, et al. *Chlamydia trachomatis* infection in infant delivered by cesarean section. Pediatrics. 1981;68:420.
102. Stenson S, Newman R, Fedukowicz H. Conjunctivitis in the newborn: Observations on incidence, cause, and prophylaxis. Ann Ophthalmol. 1981;13:329.
103. Cohen KL, McCarthy LR. *Haemophilus influenzae* ophthalmia neonatorum. Arch Ophthalmol. 1980;98:1214.
104. Cole GF, Davies DP, Austin DJ. *Pseudomonas* ophthalmia neonatorum: A cause of blindness. Br Med J. 1980;281:440.
105. Fox KR, Golomb HS. Staphylococcal ophthalmia neonatorum and the staphylococcal scalded skin syndrome. Am J Ophthalmol. 1979;88:1052.
106. Overton ME, Heath JD, Stapleton FB. Conjunctivitis and ethmoiditis due to *Shigella flexneri* in an infant. Clin Pediatr (Phila). 1981;20:231.
107. Garvey RJP, Reed TAG. Ophthalmia neonatorum due to *Branhamella* (*Neisseria*) *catarrhalis*. Case reports. Br J Vener Dis. 1981;57:346.
108. Spark RP, Dahlberg PW, LaBelle JW. Pseudogonococcal ophthalmia neonatorum. *Branhamella* (*Neisseria*) *catarrhalis* conjunctivitis. Am J Clin Pathol. 1979;72:471.
109. Lue YA, Simms DH, Ubriani R, et al. Ophthalmia neonatorum caused by penicillin-resistant *Branhamella catarrhalis*. NY State J Med. 1981;81:1775.
110. Pang R, Teh LB, Rajan VS. Gonococcal ophthalmia neonatorum caused by beta-lactamase–producing *Neisseria gonorrhoeae*. Br Med J. 1979;280:380.
111. Dunlop EMC, Rodin P, Seth AD, et al. Ophthalmia neonatorum due to beta-lactamase–producing gonococci. Br Med J. 1980;281:483.
112. Podgore JK, Holmes KK. Ocular gonococcal infection with minimal or no inflammatory response. JAMA. 1981;246:242.
113. Wong D. External ophthalmomyiasis caused by the sheep bot *Oestrus ovis*. Br J Ophthalmol. 1982;66:786.
114. Ashton N, Cook C. Allergic granulomatous nodules of the eyelid and conjunctiva. The XXXV Edward Jackson Memorial Lecture. Am J Ophthalmol. 1979;87:1.
115. Mimori T, Hirai H, Kifune T, et al. *Philophthalmus* sp. (Trematoda) in a human eye. Am J Trop Med Hyg. 1982;31:859.
116. Stenson S. Superior limbic keratoconjunctivitis associated with soft contact lens wear. Arch Ophthalmol. 1983;101:402.
117. Allansmith MR, Baird RS, Greiner JV. Vernal conjunctivitis and contact lens–associated giant papillary conjunctivitis compared and contrasted. Am J Ophthalmol. 1979;87:544.
118. Binder PS, Rasmussen RM, Gordon M. Keratoconjunctivitis and soft contact lens solutions. Arch Ophthalmol. 1981;99:87.
119. Wright P, Mackie I. Preservative-related problems in soft contact lens wearers. Trans Ophthalmol Soc UK. 1982;102:3.
120. Srinivasan RB, Jakobiet FA, Iwamoto T, et al. Giant papillary conjunctivitis with ocular prostheses. Arch Ophthalmol. 1979;97:892.
121. Meisler DM, Krachmer JH, Goeken JA. An immunopathologic study of giant papillary conjunctivitis associated with an ocular prosthesis. Am J Ophthalmol. 1981;92:368.

122. Baldone JA, Hankin JS, Zimmerman TJ. Allergic conjunctivitis associated with timolol therapy in an adult. Ann Ophthalmol. 1982;14:364.
123. Vizel M, Oster MW. Ocular side effects of cancer chemotherapy. Cancer. 1982;49:1999.
124. Ostler HB. Acute chemotic reaction to cromolyn. Arch Ophthalmol. 1982;100:412.
125. Umez-Eronini EM. Conjunctivitis due to ketoprofen. Lancet. 1978;2:737.
126. Flach AJ, Peterson JS, Mathias CGT. Photosensitivity to topically applied sulfisoxazole ointment. Evidence for a phototoxic reaction. Arch Ophthalmol. 1982;100:1286.
127. Wilson FM II. Adverse external ocular effects of topical ophthalmic medications. Surv Ophthalmol. 1979;24:57.
128. Jacobson JH. Blepharitis and secondary conjunctivitis. Am J Ophthalmol. 1980;89:609.
129. Neumann E, Gutman MJ, Blumenkrantz N, et a. A review of 400 cases of vernal conjunctivitis. Am J Ophthalmol. 1959;47:166.
130. Parker WT, Binder PS. Gentian violet keratoconjunctivitis. Am J Ophthalmol. 1979;87:340.
131. Biedner BZ, Sachs U, Witztum A. *Euphorbia peplus* latex keratoconjunctivitis. Ann Ophthalmol. 1981;13:739.
132. Backman HA. The effects of PUVA on the eye. Am J Optom Physiol Opt. 1982;59:86.
133. Halperin W, Altman R, Black K, et al. Conjunctivitis and skin erythema. Outbreak caused by a damaged high-intensity lamp. JAMA. 1978;240:1980.
134. Rose RC, Parker RL. Erythema and conjunctivitis. Outbreak caused by inadvertent exposure to ultraviolet light. JAMA. 1979;242:1155.
135. Philip RN, Comstock GW, Shelton JH. Phlyctenular keratoconjunctivitis among Eskimos in southern Alaska: I. Epidemiologic characteristics. Am Rev Respir Dis. 1965;91:171.
136. Ostler HB, Lanier JD. Phlyctenular keratoconjunctivitis with special reference to the staphylococcal type. Trans Pac Coast Otoophthalmol Soc Annu Meet. 1974;55:237.
137. Mondino BJ, Brown SI, Lempert S, et al. The acute manifestations of ocular cicatricial pemphigoid: Diagnosis and treatment. Ophthalmology. 1979;86:543.
138. Hirst LW, Jabs DA, Tutschka PJ, et al. The eye in bone marrow transplantation. I. Clinical Study. Arch Ophthalmol. 1983;101:580.
139. Perlman E, McMahon RT. Sebaceous gland carcinoma of the eyelid. Am J Ophthalmol. 1978;86:699.
140. Stenson S, Newman R, Fedukowicz H. Laboratory studies in acute conjunctivitis. Arch Ophthalmol. 1982;100:1275.
141. Leibowitz HM, Pratt MV, Flagstad IJ, et al. Human conjunctivitis. II. Treatment. Arch Ophthalmol. 1976;94:1752.
142. Jones DB, Liesegang TJ, Robinson NM. Laboratory diagnosis of ocular infections. Cumitech. 1980;13:1.
143. Darougar S, Treharne JD, Minassian D, et al. Rapid serological test for diagnosis of chlamydial ocular infections. Br J Ophthalmol. 1978;62:503.
144. Forstot SL, Forstot JZ, Peebles CL, et al. Serologic studies in patients with keratoconjunctivitis sicca. Arch Ophthalmol. 1981;99:888.
145. Abelson MB, Madiwale N, Weston JH. Conjunctival eosinophils in allergic ocular disease. Arch Ophthalmol. 1983;101:555.
146. Wander AH, Masukawa T. Unusual appearance of condensed chromatin in conjunctival cells in superior limbic keratoconjunctivitis. Lancet. 1981;2:42.
147. Hershenfeld S, Kazdan JJ, Mancer K, et al. Impression cytology in conjunctivitis. Can J Ophthalmol. 1981;16:76.
148. Rodrigues MR, Leennette DA, Arentsen JJ, et al. Methods for rapid detection of human ocular viral infections. Ophthalmology. 1979;86:452.
149. Van Rij G, Klepper L, Peperkamp E, et al. Immune electron microscopy and a cultural test in the diagnosis of adenovirus ocular infection. Br J Ophthalmol. 1982;66:317.
150. Liebowitz HM, Hyndiuk RA, Smolin GR, et al. Tobramycin in external eye disease. A double-masked study vs gentamicin. Curr Eye Res. 1981;1:259.
151. Laga M, Naamara W, Brunham RC, et al. Single-dose therapy of gonococcal ophthalmia neonatorum with ceftriaxone. N Engl J Med. 1986;315:1382.
152. Abelson MB, Butrus SI, Weston JH. Aspirin therapy in vernal conjunctivitis. Am J Ophthalmol. 1983;95:502.
153. Foster CS, Duncan J. Randomized clinical trial of topically administered cromolyn sodium for vernal keratoconjunctivits. Am J Ophthalmol. 1980;90:175.
154. Friday GA, Biglan AW, Hiles DA, et al. Treatment of ragweed allergic conjunctivitis with cromolyn sodium 4% ophthalmic solution. Am J Ophthalmol. 1983;95:169.
155. Hammerschlag MR, Chandler JW, Alexander ER, et al. Erythromycin ointment for ocular prophylaxis of neonatal chlamydial infection. JAMA. 1980;244:2291.
156. Patamasucon P, Rettig PJ, Faust KL, et al. Oral versus topical erythromycin therapies for chlamydial conjunctivitis. Am J Dis Child. 1982;136:817.
157. Rees E, Tait A, Hobson D, et al. Persistence of chlamydial infection after treatment for neonatal conjunctivitis. Arch Dis Child. 1981;56:193.

99. KERATITIS

PETER J. McDONNELL
W. RICHARD GREEN

Keratitis or inflammation of the cornea may be produced by infectious organisms or by noninfectious stimuli such as trauma, hypersensitivity, and other immune-mediated reactions. Since the corneal epithelium and conjunctival epithelium are continuous, forming the ocular surface, agents causing conjunctival disease may also affect the cornea. Before most infectious agents and some mediators of the immune reaction can invade the corneal stroma, a defect in the ocular surface must be present. This defect may be caused by various kinds of external trauma, including trauma from contact lenses, trichiasis, entropion, or abnormal lid margins, or chronic surface problems such as dry eyes, exposure, or neurogenic corneal anesthesia. Systemic diseases such as diabetes mellitus or immunodeficiency states decrease the corneal host resistance when the ocular surface has been broached by one of the above mechanisms.

Any corneal inflammation should be considered potentially sight threatening, and it requires prompt management. Corneal perforation and loss of the eye can occur within 24 hours after a severe inflammatory episode or infection by organisms such as *Pseudomonas aeruginosa* or *Staphylococcus aureus*. Even minor corneal ulcers in the visual axis can cause severe visual loss.

ETIOLOGIC AGENTS

The various etiologic agents known to cause keratitis are listed in Table 1.

Clinical Manifestations

The most common symptom of inflammatory lesions of the cornea is pain. The movement of the eyelids over the cornea increases the pain. The examination of such patients is greatly facilitated by first instilling a drop of topical anesthetic on the eye (preferably proparacaine hydrochloride, 0.5%).

Unlike conjunctival infections, a keratitis is usually accompanied by a variable decrease in vision. Discharge, which is a distinctive feature of conjunctivitis, is generally absent in patients with keratitis unless a purulent bacterial corneal ulcer is present. Reflex tearing, photophobia, and blepharospasm are common.

Since the cornea is normally avascular, the clinical appearance of an inflammatory reaction in the cornea is different from that in other tissues. After a noxious agent enters the cornea, inflammatory cells enter the cornea from dilated limbal vessels (ciliary flush) and from the tear film. The first sign of keratitis is therefore a subtle loss of corneal transparency, localized or generalized, and frequently a localized epithelial defect that is observed best with a cobalt light after instillation of fluorescein. The most important result of the inflammatory reaction with invasion by any of the agents in Table 1 is a loss of corneal substance (ulcer formation), which may rapidly lead to perforation if untreated or to a corneal scar (leukoma) even if successful therapy is initiated promptly.

In severe keratitis there is frequently an invasion of the cornea by blood vessels. After the inflammation subsides, residual empty blood channels (ghost vessels) that are not visible to the naked eye may be the only evidence of a previous inflammatory condition.

Some degree of corneal edema accompanies almost all inflammatory conditions of the cornea, leading to a loss of corneal transparency and a decrease in vision. Edema fluid may also

TABLE 1. Some Infectious Agents That Cause Keratitis

- Bacteria
  - Gram-positive cocci
    - *Staphylococcus aureus*
    - *Staphylococcus epidermidis*
    - *Streptococcus pneumoniae*
    - Streptococci of the viridans group
    - *Streptococcus pyogenes* (group A)
    - *Enterococcus* (*Streptococcus*) *faecalis*
    - *Peptostreptococcus*
  - Gram-negative bacilli
    - *Pseudomonas aeruginosa, P. mallei, P. fluorescens, P. pseudomallei, P. acidovorans, P. stutzeri*
    - *Proteus mirabilis*
    - *Morganella moragnii*
    - *Klebsiella pneumoniae*
    - *Serratia marcescens*
    - *Escherichia coli*
    - *Aeromonas hydrophila*
    - Cat-scratch bacillus
  - Gram-negative coccobacilli
    - *Moraxella lacunata, M. nonliquefaciens*
    - *Acinetobacter calcoaceticus*
    - *Pasteurella multocida*
    - *Neisseria gonorrhoeae*
    - *Branhamella catarrhalis*
  - Gram-positive bacilli
    - *Bacillus coagulans, B. laterosporus, B. cereus, B. licheniformis, B. brevis*
    - *Corynebacterium diphtheriae*
    - *Clostridium perfringens, C tetani*
  - Spirochetes
    - *Treponema pallidum*
  - Mycobacteria
    - *Mycobacterium tuberculosis, M. fortuitum, M. chelonae*
  - Actinomycetes
    - *Nocardia* sp.
- Chlamydia
  - *Chlamydia trachomatis*
- Viruses
  - Herpes simplex
  - Adenovirus
  - Varicella-zoster virus
  - Epstein-Barr virus
  - Poxviruses (variola, vaccinia, molluscum contagiosum)
  - Rubeola (measles)
- Fungi
  - *Acremonium* sp.
  - Fusarium
  - *Bipolaris* sp.
  - *Candida* sp.
  - *Aspergillus* sp.
  - *Pseudallescheria boydii*
  - *Penicillium*
  - *Paecilomyces*
  - *Neurospora*
  - *Phialophora*
  - *Curvularia*
- Parasites
  - *Onchocerca volvulus*
  - *Acanthamoeba polyphaga, A. castellanii*
  - *Leishmania brasiliensis*
  - *Trypanosoma* spp.

accumulate under the corneal epithelium and form bullae that cause severe "foreign body" pain when they rupture.

An associated intraocular inflammation is common. Early changes may be seen only by slit-lamp examination (flare and cells). Severe inflammation may lead to a layering of fibrin and white blood cells in the inferior portion of the anterior chamber (hypopyon) by gravity. The aqueous and vitreous remain sterile in most microbial corneal ulcers until a late stage, when infective endophthalmitis may occur.

BACTERIAL KERATITIS

Bacterial keratitis accounts for approximately 65–90 percent of all microbial corneal infections.[1–3] In the United States the most common infecting organisms are *Staphylococcus aureus, Streptococcus pneumoniae, Pseudomonas aeruginosa,* and *Moraxella. Staphylococcus aureus, S. pneumoniae,* and *P. aeruginosa* by themselves account for more than 80 percent of all bacterial corneal ulcers. The clinical appearance of various bacterial ulcers does *not* usually provide a basis for specific diagnosis. The prevalence of organisms incriminated in corneal ulcers has changed little during the last 10 years. Any apparent changes that have occurred result from improved isolation techniques from the cornea, an increase in the population of patients who are systemically immunosuppressed, an increase in topical steroid administration, and an increase in the use of soft contact lenses,[4–6] especially for extended wear. There have been occasional cases as a result or organ-cultured and M-K medium–stored corneal buttons used for corneal transplantation.[7] A geographic variation in causes of microbial keratitis has also been noted. The inoculation of the organisms into the corneal stroma may occur via obvious exogenous penetrating trauma (cat-scratch bacillus[8]), through intact corneal epithelium (*Neisseria gonorrhoeae, Listeria, Corynebacterium diphtheriae,* and *Haemophilis aegypticus*), or more often via inapparent minor corneal epithelial abrasions such as from contaminated mascara.[9,10]

Strains of staphylococci causing extensive corneal ulcers are the same ones that are found as inhabitants in other noninfected parts of the body.[11,12] Paralimbal corneal ulcers found in association with conjunctival cultures that are positive for staphylococci have been thought to be due to toxins or hypersensitivity reactions to these bacteria. *Staphylococcus epidermidis* and streptococci can cause corneal ulceration, usually in an immunocompromised host and occasionally in association with chronic dacryocystitis,[13] in which a peripheral ulcer may occur that is similar in appearance to the staphylococcal hypersensitivity ulcer described above.[14] A toxic factor (exopeptidase) has been implicated in the pathogenesis of corneal ulceration caused by *S. pneumoniae.*[15]

Pseudomonas aeruginosa is recognized for its particularly swift course to perforation because of its proteolytic enzyme production,[16] which degrades the corneal stroma. In comatose patients with corneal exposure and tracheostomies colonized by *P. aeruginosa,* the danger of corneal infection is greatly increased.[17] Unusual extension of the corneal ulcer into the sclera has been reported.[18,19] Other *Pseudomonas* species such as *P. acidovorans* and *P. stutzeri,* have caused corneal ulcers with a less malignant course.[20] Corneal ulcers due to *Morganella morganii* may be clinically indistinguishable from those *Pseudomonas* ulcers. *Serratia marcescens* corneal ulcers have been associated with contact lens wear[21] and contaminated eyedrops.[22] *Moraxella* ulcers have been described in debilitated alcoholic patients in whom the organism is also frequently a nasopharyngeal commensual[23] and in otherwise well patients when chronic ocular surface disease is present.[24] The infrequency of isolation of this bacterium may perhaps be explained by its fastidious nature in culture and the inhibitory topical anesthetic agents used to obtain the corneal cultures.

Neisseria gonorrhoeae may cause a keratitis during an episode of untreated or inadequately treated conjunctivitis. It is one of the few organisms that can penetrate an intact corneal epithelium. It is essential that the presence of the gonococcus be verified by culture because *Acinetobacter,* which is morphologically identical to the gonococcus and is penicillin resistant, can cause corneal perforation.

Gram-positive aerobic bacilli are widespread in nature and are of low virulence. They produce infections of the cornea when host resistance is lowered.[25] *Corynebacterium diphtheriae* may penetrate an intact corneal epithelium to produce a keratitis.[26]

Primary tuberculous keratitis is now extremely rare.

Atypical mycobacteria (*Mycobacterium fortuitum* and *M. chelonae*) are known to cause a keratitis.[27,28] These corneal ulcers usually follow removal of a foreign body and have a slow, progressive course without much anterior chamber reaction.

The incidence of ocular lesions of leprosy varies from about 15 percent of the patients with tuberculoid leprosy to about 100 percent of the patients with long-standing lepromatous leprosy.[29–31] Many other bacteria have been involved in corneal ulcers, including *Azobacter,*[32] *Branhamella catarrhalis,*[33] *Aeromonas hydrophila,*[34] *Pasteurella multocida,*[35] *Clostridium perfringens,*[36] *Bacillus licheniformis,*[37] *B. thuringiensis,*[38] and anaerobic streptococci.[39] Polymicrobial keratitis was seen in about 8 percent of one series of bacterial and fungal ulcers and is associated with the use of therapeutic soft "bandage" contact lenses in diseased corneas.

VIRAL KERATITIS

About 20 percent of infants born with herpes simplex virus types I or II infections have ocular changes.[40] Seven percent will have keratitis with either punctate keratopathy, dendritic ulcers, or disciform keratitis. Of these, 30 percent are infected by herpes simplex, type I. Keratouveitis may occasionally be present at the time of birth. Prophylactic silver nitrate use is not uniformly successful in preventing ocular disease in neonates born to infected mothers. Atypically, the primary keratitis may present as subepithelial dendritic opacities.[41] Morphologically the lesions of herpes simplex, types I and II, are identical.

Ocular herpes simplex acquired during childhood usually presents as a follicular conjunctivitis and is frequently undiagnosed. Transient epithelial lesions are common. However, very similar changes to those described below in adults may also be encountered.[42]

In adults with documented previous corneal herpetic infection, the recurrence rates are approximately 25 percent within 12 months of the last attack and 33 percent within 24 months.[43] Another study suggested a 40 percent recurrence rate for all cases of corneal epithelial herpes and a 25 percent recurrence rate in the form of stromal disease or keratouveitis.[44] Six percent developed visual loss secondary to stromal scarring.

The pattern of epithelial disease is either *dendritic* or *geographic,* with active viral replication in the ulcer margin in the epithelium. The geographic type is notable for a prolonged course. Both diseases are known to heal spontaneously within 10 to 14 days in 80 percent of cases. Stromal involvement is usually seen in recurrent attacks, and the cornea has not been conclusively shown to harbor active viral particles. This form of the disease (*disciform keratitis*) is thought to be an immune-mediated reaction. This process frequently leads to some stromal scarring, commonly with thinning and occasionally with perforation. An associated *uveitis* is common. Recurrent ocular herpes simplex is thought to result from reactivation of latent herpes in the trigeminal ganglion and centripetal spread to the eye.[45,46] Active virus has not been isolated from the lacrimal gland, tears, cornea, or iris between episodes. Corneal hypoesthesia,[47] which worsens with repeated attacks, is present.

The pattern of disease is different in immunosuppressed patients.[48,49] They may have bilateral corneal involvement, which is seen in only 5 percent of other patients, and may also have extensive and multiple lesions on the cornea and conjunctiva. These lesions tend to persist or recur with topical antiviral therapy until immunosuppressive therapy is reduced.

Some of the factors that may precipitate recurrent episodes are exposure to sunlight, menstruation, psychiatric disturbances, and fever.[50] Acute illnesses may temporarily suppress the immune mechanisms, and the most common cause of a unilateral red eye in a hospitalized patient is herpes simplex keratitis. The exact mechanisms involved are unknown. Topical and systemic steroids and immunosuppressive agents may provoke recurrences in corneal epithelium, and they enhance replication in established lesions.[51]

The subepithelial corneal opacities occurring in epidemic keratoconjunctivitis caused by an adenovirus probably represent an immune phenomenon. These opacities tend to appear 10–14 days after symptoms commence. The natural course of the corneal lesions is resolution over 2–3 weeks, although patients may be very photophobic during this period. The lesions tend to clear dramatically with the use of topical steroids, with occasional reappearance when the steroid therapy is discontinued.[52]

In about 10 percent of the patients with herpes zoster infections the ophthalmic division of the trigeminal nerve is involved. The various ocular manifestations include vesicles on the lid and conjunctiva, iridocyclitis, secondary glaucoma, ophthalmoplegia, neuroretinitis, optic neuritis, and retinal vascular occlusion.[53,54] Corneal findings include decreased corneal sensation, epithelial and subepithelial punctate keratitis, dendritic figures, disciform keratitis, segmental keratitis, and corneal vascularization. The corneal disease may occur after the skin eruption is healed, and it can be prolonged.[55] Visual loss may result from peripheral and central stromal involvement.[56]

In varicella infections (chickenpox), ocular involvement is usually limited to the appearance of vesicles on the lids, conjunctiva, and limbus. Superficial punctate keratitis, interstitial and disciform keratitis, and uveitis have also been reported.[57] Epithelial dendritic figures that are identical to those seen in herpes zoster keratitis may occur immediately or up to several months after the skin eruption.[58]

Vaccinia infections of the eye occur from accidental autoinoculation.[59] Corneal complications occur in one-third of the patients with ocular vaccinia, and they consist of superficial punctate keratitis, epithelial ulcers, and (rarely) disciform keratitis. The epithelial ulcers may superficially resemble herpetic keratitis.[60,61]

The keratitis that is occasionally associated with measles (rubeola) infections causes punctate or dendritic epithelial defects in the cornea.[62] In one adult population study, all rubeola patients had epithelial keratitis that followed a benign course.[63] The changing immune status of the population after vaccination programs is changing the pattern of the clinical disease—from a childhood illness to an adult disease and perhaps a different ocular expression of measles infection. In developing countries, vitamin A deficiency and malnutrition sometimes makes measles keratitis a blinding disease with secondary bacterial infection and perforation of the globe.

Infectious mononucleosis has been associated with a peripheral nummular interstitial keratitis with a benign course.[64] More recently, ring-shaped granular anterior stromal opacities have been associated with Epstein-Barr viral infection.[65]

There have been occasional reported cases of Jacob-Kreutzfeldt disease[66] and rabies transmission[67] by the use of infected donor tissue in corneal transplantation. Human immunodeficiency virus (HIV) has been demonstrated to be present within corneal epithelium.[68] Donor corneas from such patients should never be used.

OTHER CAUSES OF KERATITIS

In one series of culture-positive corneal ulcers,[3] approximately 35 percent were of fungal origin, whereas another study found 20 percent to have a fungal origin.[1] While the incidence appeared to be related to geographic location, with higher rates in Florida and decreased incidence in northern states, seasonal fluctuations were not remarkable. Although 35 genera have been associated with corneal ulcers, *Fusarium solani* is the most common offending agent and has been isolated in up to 65 percent of cases.[69–71] *Aspergillus*[72] and *Candida* are also commonly isolated.[73] More rarely, *Acremonium* and *Curvularia* may be found. An antecedent vegetable injury may have occurred, and the use of broad-spectrum topical antibiotics and steroids has been implicated in the development of fungal ulcers. In patients with local ocular surface abnormalities—such as with dry eyes, extended-wear contact lens use, exposure keratitis, and previous herpes simplex keratitis or with systemic immunosuppression—infection with *Candida* is more common. The morphology of a fungal ulcer is not pathognomonic, but a torpid course, prominent hypopyon, and stromal infiltrates surrounded by satellite lesions are signs suggestive of fungal etiology.

Nocardia[74] and *Bacterionema matruchotii*[75] are rare causes of corneal ulcers, and the lesions are indistinguishable from those of a fungal origin. Cases have been reported of corneal ulcers from infection with *Pullularia,*[76] *Helminthosporium,*[77] *Rhodotorula,*[75] *Scedosporium,*[79] *Phialophora bubakii,*[80] and *Tritirachium roseum.*[81]

Parasitic infestations in certain parts of the world are major causes of blindness. Sclerosing keratitis and stromal opacification occur from invasion of the corneal stroma by microfilariae of *Onchocerca volvulus*.[82–85] Leishmania may produce a similar keratitis.[85]

Corneal changes secondary to trachoma conjunctivitis are a major cause of worldwide blindness.[86] In developed countries, sexually transmitted *Chlamydia trachomatis* infection may mimic the morphology of true trachoma.

Acanthamoeba is being recognized more often as a cause of recalcitrant keratitis, frequently leading to a loss of vision or the eye.[87] Patients who develop infection with this organism often have a history of contact lens wear (using a homemade saline solution) or exposure to soil or standing water.[88] Extreme pain and a ring infiltrate in the cornea should suggest the diagnosis.

Perhaps the most common cause of keratitis is thought to be from a hypersensitivity reaction to the exotoxin of *Staphylococcus*. Typically, inferior punctate epithelial defects that stain with fluorescein dye, marginal corneal infiltrates, and ulcers are manifestations of this allergy. Histologically, lymphocytes and plasma cells are present in peripheral cornea, but the cornea is free of organisms.

Ring ulcers of the cornea may give the appearance of coalesced marginal ulcers. They are more dangerous to the eye than are the usual marginal ulcers because they may lead to total corneal destruction. Their cause is uncertain, but they are sometimes associated with acute systemic diseases such as influenza, bacillary dysentery, brucellosis, gonococcal arthritis, dengue fever, herpes zoster ophthalmicus, diabetes mellitus, and hookworm infestation. They may also be associated with a number of autoimmune diseases such as periarteritis nodosa, rheumatoid arthritis,[89] Wegener's granulomatosis,[90] systemic lupus erythematosus, and giant cell arteritis.[91]

The two major types of interstitial keratitis encountered clinically are due to syphilis and tuberculosis. About 90 percent of all the cases of interstitial keratitis are caused by congenital syphilis. Mycobacteria other than *M. tuberculosis* rarely cause a similar keratitis. The best explanation for the occurrence of interstitial keratitis in these two main conditions is as a host-immune response rather than an active microbial infection.

Ocular involvement with syphilis may be acquired or congenital. The chancre of acquired primary syphilis has been reported to have occurred in the conjunctiva.[92] Among patients with acquired secondary syphilis the incidence of ocular complications is 4.5 percent.[93] These include papulosquamous lesions of the skin of the lids, temporary loss of the eyebrows, diffuse papillary conjunctivitis, scleroconjunctivitis,[92] interstitial keratitis, iritis, chorioretinitis,[94,95] and optic[96] and retrobulbar neuritis.[97] The most common eye lesion in secondary syphilis is iridocyclitis, which accounts for about 75 percent of all the eye lesions of the early acquired disease.[98] The diagnosis here is not difficult because in almost all cases there are other manifestations of early syphilis. Iritis may also develop as a complication of antisyphilitic therapy in the Jarisch-Herxheimer reaction.

Interstitial keratitis is a rare complication of acquired primary or secondary syphilis. Fewer than 3 percent of all cases of interstitial keratitis occur in acquired syphilis. In acquired late syphilis, gummas of the conjunctiva, lids, sclera, cornea, iris, ciliary body, and orbit are rare occurrences. The most common ocular inflammatory lesion of late acquired syphilis is iridocyclitis.[99]

There are two clinical forms of congenital syphilis: infantile, or early, and tardive, or late. Interstitial keratitis occurs rarely in early congenital syphilis.[92] However, it is the most common lesion of late congenital syphilis and occurs in about 52 percent of untreated patients. It typically occurs in the early teens, with most of the cases occurring in patients between the ages of 5 and 20 years. In the acute stage the patients have decreased visual acuity, photophobia, pain, blepharospasm, and lacrimation. The corneal stroma becomes hazy within a few days and has a ground-glass appearance, with marked reduction in vision. A severe iridocyclitis is present in the early stages. Over a period of months, new vessels grow into the corneal stroma from the limbus at all levels. When the vessels meet in the center of the cornea, there is a dramatic regression of the disease; the corneal infiltrates are resorbed, and the vessels are partially obliterated. The final visual prognosis in these patients is surprisingly good. Seventy percent have 20/20 to 20/100 acuity, and only ten percent have poorer than 20/200 acuity.[92]

The most common mechanical cause of keratitis is a foreign body embedded in the cornea. Corneal exposure from improper lid closure may also result in keratitis. This occurs in patients with Bell's palsy and proptosis due to Graves disease and in comatose patients. Trichiasis secondary to abnormal lid structure (e.g., entropion) may cause a keratitis.

A severe liquefactive keratitis may develop secondarily to decreased tear production, which may be idiopathic[100,101] or due to decreased corneal sensation after local corneal disease (e.g., herpes zoster infection), to neurologic lesions of the ophthalmic division of the trigeminal nerve, or to medullary infarction. This problem is greatly compounded when associated with inadequate lid closure. Rarely, superficial or deep keratitis may be associated with dermatoses and/or systemic conditions, including ichthyosis, epidermal nevus syndrome, anhydrotic ectodermal dysplasia, pulmonary and plantar hyperkeratosis, and tyrosinemia.[102] Isolated epithelial keratitis of unknown etiology such as Thygeson's migratory keratitis occurs infrequently.[103]

The association of Reiter syndrome and a keratitis with stromal infiltrates needs to be further investigated.[104] Finally, one of the major causes of blindness in the third-world countries is xerophthalmia, in which vitamin A deficiency results in corneal opacification and stromal liquefaction and leads to perforation.[105]

LABORATORY FEATURES

Because the morphologic features of corneal ulcers and keratitis are rarely pathognomonic, great emphasis must be placed on adequate laboratory work-up of suspected cases. The possibility of rapid progression to perforation requires early scrapings of the ulcer for smears and cultures. Methods for culture taking vary considerably but may be summarized by the following: (*1*) scrapings with a heat-sterilized Kimura platinum spatula (with or without the use of topical proparacaine hydrochloride, 0.5%), transferred to glass slides for Gram, Giemsa, periodic acid–Schiff (PAS), and methenamine silver stains; (*2*) multiple inoculations with the Kimura spatula on blood agar held at room temperature and at 37°C, chocolate agar, thioglycolate or Schaedler broth or brain–heart infusion, Sabouraud agar, and a reduced blood agar in an anaerobic environment. Special cultures may require non-nutrient agar or media for culturing mycobacteria. In most cases, concomitant cultures of the conjunctiva and lid, on the involved and uninvolved eye, are frequently taken to ascertain the person's flora and to assist in assessing the significance of positive corneal cultures taken from the ulcer. The type and number of positive cultures needed to support a microbial diagnosis are still unsettled.[106–108] Negative cultures obtained from scrapings as described above, in the face of a suspicious corneal ulcer, should lead to a superficial keratectomy or corneal biopsy specimens taken in the operating room under microscopic control. These may prove positive when superficial scrapings were previously negative since fungi and acanthamoebae are characteristically deep in corneal parenchyma and conspicuously absent on the surface.[109]

Viral keratitis does not often require culture, and the diagnosis is sustained by the morphology of the lesions. Careful débridement of the corneal epithelium and transfer to viral transport media will usually suffice to grow herpes simplex virus, types I and II, and adenovirus. Herpes zoster virus is rarely isolated from corneal lesions. In doubtful cases, transmission electron microscopy may occasionally be helpful in establishing the viral etiology.[110]

The limulus lysate assay has been used in the diagnosis of corneal ulcers when gram-negative organisms are suspected.[111] Sensitivity testing should proceed according to the usual laboratory techniques, although laboratory sensitivity testing of fungi remains unsatisfactory.

TREATMENT

Early specific therapy is the prime requisite for successful management of corneal ulcers. Because of the rapid evolution to perforation of some ulcers and the visual loss by central corneal scarring, most patients with bacterial keratitis with significant ulceration should be hospitalized. There are several methods of antibiotic therapy. These include topical antibiotic drops and ointment, subconjunctival injection, continuous lavage, and parenteral administration.

Topical antibiotics in solution are preferred over ointments because hospital pharmacies can readily prepare highly concentrated solutions by using commercially available ocular lubricants and parenteral antibiotic preparations.[112]

Subconjunctival administration of antibiotics, although painful, provides a higher transient peak concentration of drug within the corneal stroma than is usually obtainable with topical therapy.[113]

Continuous lavage of the cornea with antibiotic solutions has been described.[114] The advantages of this method are the increased drug levels obtained within the aqueous humor[115] and the lack of dependence on nursing personnel for frequent drop instillations.

Parenteral (intramuscular or intravenous) administration of antibiotics is reserved for deep corneal ulcers with impending perforation. The choice of antibiotics is dictated by the Gram-stained smears and then is modified according to culture results. Initial broad-spectrum antibiotic cover with a cephalosporin and gentamicin is commonly advocated.[116]

Supportive therapy in the treatment of infectious keratitis consists of cycloplegics, enzyme inhibitors, therapeutic soft contact lenses, and topical steroids. Since a severe anterior chamber reaction may occur with a bacterial keratitis, cycloplegics should be used to prevent the formation of synechiae and to relieve the discomfort of ciliary spasm.

If corneal ulceration is marked, the temporary use of a therapeutic soft contact lens or "bandage" lens may facilitate stromal repair and promote reepithelialization by protecting the corneal surface from the mechanical trauma of lid movement. Topical medication may be continued after the contact lens insertion.

The use of topical corticosteroids in the management of bacterial keratitis is a controversial issue. It has been suggested that steroids in conjunction with specific antibacterial therapy minimize the inflammatory sequelae of bacterial keratitis.[114,115]

The treatment of the epithelial keratitis in herpes simplex infections consists of simple débridement of the epithelium[117] and use of an antiviral agent; this is effective in most cases of corneal dendritic ulcers. Extensive involvement, central lesions, geographic lesions, or resistant lesions are usually treated with a 10-day course of antiviral agents. Trifluridine and acyclovir are the preferred agents because of their lower corneal toxicity.[118] The use of corticosteroids is contraindicated in isolated epithelial herpes. Herpetic uveitis may resolve spontaneously, but most ophthalmologists would use cycloplegia and topical corticosteroids to reduce the damaging effect of prolonged stromal and anterior chamber inflammation. The use of an antiviral "umbrella" while the patient is being administered corticosteroids to prevent the recurrence of epithelial herpes is still widely debated.[119,120] Other methods of therapy such as topical interferon[121] and cryotherapy have been used. Uncontrolled herpetic stromal keratitis and secondary stromal scarring may require corneal transplantation.[122,123]

Epidemic keratocon junctivitis rarely requires more therapy than mild cycloplegics and antibiotic cover. Severe photophobia, incapacitating irritation, and decreased vision during the acute episodes may be relieved with use of topical corticosteroids. It is unclear whether their use prolongs the course of the disease.

Stromal keratitis caused by herpes zoster will frequently require corticosteroids to reduce the inflammatory response and resultant corneal destruction, although some authors have suggested that the use of the steroids alone has a deleterious effect on this keratitis.[120,124]

Fungal ulcers require the prolonged use of topical antifungal therapy and occasionally parenteral therapy. Topical natamycin, 5%, is a valuable addition to ocular therapy.[71] Topical miconazole (10 mg/ml) and fluocytosine, 1%, and amphotericin B drops (1 mg/ml) may occasionally be used, although the latter has definite epithelial toxicity.[107,108]

Resistant fungal ulcers may require the use of parenteral amphotericin B, flucytosine, or ketoconazole.[125] Corneal transplantation or conjunctival flaps may be needed to stabilize the eye. The addition of corticosteroids to therapy when a response to the antifungal agent has been observed remains controversial, but it may help to reduce corneal destruction caused by host response.

Nocardia asteroides has been reported to respond to topical and parenteral sulfadiazine administration.[74]

Currently recommended medical therapy for *Acanthamoeba* keratitis includes topical propamadine isethionate, dibromopropamadine isethionate, and neomycin. Although one patient has been successfully treated medically,[126] most cases require corneal transplantation and medical therapy to eradicate the infection.

The drug management of onchocerciasis is changing, with the recent addition of ivermectin as the therapeutic agent of choice.[127]

Since syphilitic interstitial keratitis is a manifestation of an immune phenomenon, specific antiluetic therapy does not greatly affect the course of the acute inflammation. However, therapy reduces the chances of recurrence from 27 percent in untreated cases to 3.6 percent in treated cases. Treatment also reduces the likelihood of bilateral ocular involvement. Topical steroids are used during the acute stages of the keratitis to avoid severe postinflammatory sequelae.[92]

Noninfected corneal ulcers with associated destruction of the stroma may require systemic immunosuppressive[128] or other supportive therapy, including corneal transplantation or tissue adhesive application.[129] Corneal changes in xerophthalmia can be reversed by topical or systemic vitamin A administration[130] if given early enough.

Foreign bodies embedded in the cornea are removed with a metal spud. This is usually followed by the use of a topical antibiotic, a cycloplegic, and patching of the eye. In exposure keratitis the lids may be taped. Artificial tears, topical ointments at night, and hydrophilic lenses are useful. In neuroparalytic keratitis, short-term taping of the eyelids usually is followed by partial tarsorraphy or a conjunctival flap.

REFERENCES

1. Jones DB. Polymicrobial keratitis. Trans Am Ophthalmol Soc. 1981;79:153.
2. Asbell P, Stenson S. Ulcerative keratitis. Survey of 30 years' laboratory experience. Arch Ophthalmol. 1982;100:77.
3. Liesegang TJ, Forster RK. Spectrum of microbial keratitis in south Florida. Am J Ophthalmol. 1980;90:38.
4. Eichenbaum JW, Feldstein M, Podos SM. Extended-wear aphakic soft contact lenses and corneal ulcers. Br J Ophthalmol. 1982;66:663.
5. Wilson LA, Schlitzer RL, Ahearn DG. *Pseudomonas* corneal ulcers associated with soft contact-lens wear. Am J Ophthalmol. 1981;92:546.
6. Krachmer JH, Purcell JJ. Bacterial corneal ulcers in cosmetic soft contact lens wearers. Arch Ophthalmol. 1978;96:57.
7. Escapini H Jr, Olson RJ, Kaufman HE. Donor cornea contamination with McCarey-Kaufman medium preservation. Am J Ophthalmol. 1979;88:59.
8. Udell IJ, Kelly CG, Wolf TC, et al. Cat scratch keratitis. Ophthalmology. 1987;94(Suppl):124.
9. Wilson LA, Ahearn DG. *Pseudomonas* induced corneal ulcers associated with contaminated eye mascaras. Am J Ophthalmol. 1977;84:112.
10. Reid FR, Wood TO. *Pseudomonas* corneal ulcer. The causative role of contaminated eye cosmetics. Arch Ophthalmol. 1979;97:1640.
11. Locatcher-Khorazo D, Butierrez E. Bacteriophage typing of *Staphylococcus aureus:* A study of normal, infected eyes and environment. Arch Ophthalmol. 1960;63:774.
12. Locatcher-Khorazo D, Sullivan N, Gutierrez E. *Staphylococcus aureus* isolated from normal and infected eyes: Phage types and sensitivity to antibacterial agents. Arch Ophthalmol. 1967;77:370.
13. Kim HB, Ostler HB. Marginal corneal ulcer due to β-*Streptococcus*. Arch Ophthalmol. 1977;95:454.
14. Cohn H, Mondino BJ, Brown SI, et al. Marginal corneal ulcers with acute beta streptococcal conjunctivitis and chronic dacryocystitis. Am J Ophthalmol. 1979;87:541.
15. Johnson MK, Allen JH. Ocular toxin of the pneumococcus. Am J Ophthalmol. 1971;72:175.
16. Brown SI, Bloomfield SE, Wai-Fong IT. The cornea-destroying enzyme of *Pseudomonas aeruginosa*. Invest Ophthalmol. 1974;13:174.
17. Hutton WL, Sexton RR. Atypical *Pseudomonas* corneal ulcers in semicomatose patients. Am J Ophthalmol. 1972;73:37.
18. Codere F, Brownstein S, Jackson WB. *Pseudomonas aeruginosa* scleritis. Am J Ophthalmol. 1981;91:706.
19. Raber IM, Laibson PR, Kurz GH, et al. *Pseudomonas* corneoscleral ulcers. Am J Ophthalmol. 1981;92:353.
20. Brinser JH, Torczynski E. Unusual *Pseudomonas* corneal ulcers. Am J Ophthalmol. 1977;84:462.
21. Lass JH, Haaf J, Foster CS, et al. Visual outcome in eight cases of *Serratia marcescens* keratitis. Am J Ophthalmol. 1981;92:384.
22. Templeton WC, Eiferman RA, Snyder JW, et al. *Serratia keratitis* transmitted by contaminated eyedroppers. Am J Ophthalmol. 1982;93:723.
23. Baum J, Fedukowicz HB, Jordan A. A survey of *Moraxella* corneal ulcers in a derelict population. Am J Ophthalmol. 1980;90:476.
24. Cobo LM, Coster DJ, Peacock J. *Moraxella* keratitis in a nonalcoholic population. Br J Ophthalmol. 1981;65:683.
25. van Bijsterveld OP, Richards RD. *Bacillus* infections of the cornea. Arch Ophthalmol. 1965;74:91.
26. Chandler JW, Milam DF. Diphtheria corneal ulcers. Arch Ophthalmol. 1978;96:53.
27. Turner L, Stinson I. *Mycobacterium fortuitum* as a cause of corneal ulcer. Am J Ophthalmol. 1965;60:329.
28. Meisler DM, Friedlaender MH, Okumoto M. *Mycobacterium chelonei* keratitis. Am J Ophthalmol. 1982;94:398.
29. Allen JH, Byers JL. The pathology of ocular leprosy. I. Cornea. Arch Ophthalmol. 1960;64:216.
30. Elliott DC. An interpetation of the ocular manifestations of leprosy. Ann NY Acad Sci. 1951;54:84.
31. Pillat A. Leprosy bacilli in the scraping from the diseased cornea in a leper, and comments on keratitis punctata superficialis leprosa. Arch Ophthalmol. 1930;3:306.
32. Liesegang TJ, Jones DB, Robinson NM. *Azotobacter* keratitis. Arch Ophthalmol. 1981;99:1587.
33. Wilhelmus KR, Peacock J, Coster DJ. *Branhamella* keratitis. Br J Ophthalmol. 1980;64:892.
34. Feaster FT, Nisbet RM, Barber JC. *Aeromonas hydrophilia* corneal ulcer. Am J Ophthalmol. 1978;85:114.
35. Purcell JJ, Krachmer JH. Corneal ulcer caused by *Pasteurella multocida*. Am J Ophthalmol. 1977;83:540.
36. Stern GA, Hodes BL, Stock EL. *Clostridium perfringens* corneal ulcer. Arch Ophthalmol. 1979;97:661.
37. Tabbara KF, Tarabay N. *Bacillus licheniformis* corneal ulcer. Am J Ophthalmol. 1979;87:717.
38. Samples JR, Buettner H. Corneal ulcer caused by a biologic insecticide (*Bacillus thuringiensis*). Am J Ophthalmol. 1983;95:258.
39. Ostler HB, Okumoto M. Anaerobic streptococcal corneal ulcer. Am J Ophthalmol. 1976;81:518.
40. Nahmias AJ, Visintine AM, Caldwell DR, et al. Eye infections with herpes simplex viruses in neonates. Surv Ophthalmol. 1976;21:100.
41. Stern GA, Zam ZS, Gutgesell VJ. Primary herpes simplex subepithelial dendritic keratitis. Am J Ophthalmol. 1981;91:496.
42. Poirier RH. Herpetic ocular infections of childhood. Arch Ophthalmol. 1980;98:704.
43. Shuster JJ, Kaufman HE, Nesburn AB. Statistical analysis of the rate of recurrence of herpesvirus ocular epithelial disease. Am J Ophthalmol. 1981;91:328.
44. Wilhelmus KR, Coster DJ, Donovan HC, et al. Prognostic indicators of herpetic keratitis. Analysis of a five-year observation period after corneal ulceration. Arch Ophthalmol. 1981;99:1578.
45. Stevens JG, Nesburn AB, Cook M. Latent herpes simplex virus recovered from trigeminal ganglia of rabbits with recurrent eye infection. Nature. 1972;235:216.
46. Baringer J, Swoveland P. Recovery of herpes simplex virus from human trigeminal ganglions. N Engl J Med. 1973;288:648.
47. Norn MS. Dendritic (herpetic) keratitis. IV. Follow-up examination of corneal sensitivity. Acta Ophthalmol. 1970;48:383.
48. Bloomfield SE, Lopez C. Herpes infections in the immunosuppressed host. Ophthalmology. 1980;87:1226.
49. Howcroft MJ, Breslin CW. Herpes simplex keratitis in renal transplant recipients. Can Med Assoc J. 1981;124:292.
50. Cleobury JF, Skinner GRB, Thouless ME, et al. Association between psychopathic disorder and serum antibody to herpes simplex virus (type 1). Br Med J. 1971;261:438.
51. Patterson A, Jones BR. Management of ocular herpes. Trans Ophthalmol Soc UK. 1967;87:59.
52. Theodore FH. Allergic keratitis. In: King JH, McTigue JW, eds: The Cornea World Congress. Washington, DC: Butterworths; 1965;197.
53. Womack LW, Liesegang TJ. Complications of herpes zoster ophthalmicus. Arch Ophthalmol. 1983;101:42.
54. Hedges TR III, Albert DM. The progression of the ocular abnormalities of herpes zoster. Histopathologic observations of nine cases. Ophthalmology. 1982;89:165.
55. Edgerton AE. Herpes zoster ophthalmicus: Report of cases and review of literature. Arch Ophthalmol. 1945;34:40.
56. Mondino BJ, Brown SI, Mondzelewski JP. Peripheral corneal ulcers with herpes zoster ophthalmicus. Am J Ophthalmol. 1978;86:611.
57. Strachman J. Uveitis associated with chickenpox. J Pediatr. 1955;46:327.
58. Uchida Y, Kaneko M, Hayashi K. Varicella dendritic keratitis. Am J Ophthalmol. 1980;89:259.
59. Frampton G, Smith C. Primary vaccinia of the eyelid. Br J Ophthalmol. 1952;36:214.
60. Bedell AJ. Multiple vaccination of the eyelids. Trans Am Ophthalmol Soc. 1919:17, 273.
61. Darrell RW, Vrabec F. Vaccinia virus infection of the rabbit cornea. Arch Ophthalmol. 1971;86:568.
62. Sachs U, Marcus M. Bilateral herpetic keratitis during measles. Am J Ophthalmol. 1981;91:796.
63. Deckard PS, Bergstrom TJ. Rubeola keratitis. Ophthalmology. 1981;88:810.
64. Pinnolis M, McCulley JP, Urman JD. Nummular keratitis associated with infectious mononucleosis. Am J Ophthalmol. 1980;89:791.
65. Matoba AY, Wilhemus KR, Jones DB. Epstein-Barr viral stromal keratitis. Ophthalmology. 1986;93:746–51.
66. Manuelidis EE, Angelo JN, Gorgacz EJ, et al. Experimental Creutzfeldt-Jakob disease transmitted via the eye with infected cornea. N Engl J Med. 1977;296:1334.
67. Houff SA, Burton RC, Wilson RW, et al. Human-to-human transmission of rabies virus by corneal transplant. N Engl J Med. 1979;300:603.
68. Salahuddin SZ, Palestine AG, Heck E, et al. Isolation of the human T-cell leukemia/lymphotrophic virus type III from the cornea. Am J Ophthalmol. 1986;101:149–52.
69. Jones BR, Richards AB, Morgan G. Direct fungal infection of the eye in Britain. Trans Ophthalmol Soc UK. 1969;89:727.
70. DeVoe AG, Silva-Hutner M. Fungal infections of the eye. In: Locatcher-Khorazo D, Seegal BC, eds. Microbiology of the Eye. St Louis; CV Mosby; 1972;208.
71. Jones DB, Forster RK, Rebell G. *Fusarium solani* keratitis treated with natamycin (pimaricin): 18 consecutive cases. Arch Ophthalmol. 1972;88:147.
72. Searl SS, Udel IJ, Sadun A, et al. *Aspergillus* keratitis with intraocular invasion. Ophthalmology. 1981;88:1244.
73. Polack FM, Kaufman HE, Newmark E. Keratomycosis: Medical and surgical treatment. Arch Ophthalmol. 1971;85:410.
74. Hirst LW, Harrison GK, Merz WG, et al. *Nocardia asteroides* keratitis. Br J Ophthalmol. 1979;63:449.
75. Wilhelmus KR, Robinson NM, Jones DB. *Bacterionema matruchotii* ocular infections. Am J Ophthalmol. 1979;87:143.
76. Jones FR, Christensen GR. *Pullularia* corneal ulcer. Arch Ophthalmol. 1974;92:529.
77. Krachmer JH, Anderson RL, Binder PS, et al. Helminthosporium corneal ulcers. Am J Ophthalmol. 1978;85:66.
78. Francois J, Rijsselaere. Corneal infections by rhodotorula. Ophthalmologica. 1979;178:241.
79. Zapater RC, Albesi EJ. Corneal monosporiosis. A review and report of 1 case. Ophthalmologica. 1979;178:142.
80. Eiferman RA, Snyder JW, Barbee JV Jr. Corneal chromomycosis. Am J Ophthalmol. 1982;95:255.
81. Rodrigues MM, Laibson P, Kaplan W. Exogenous corneal ulcer caused by *Tritirachium roseum*. Am J Ophthalmol. 1979;80:804.

82. Taylor HR. Treatment of onchocerciasis in the 1980s Postgrad Doctor Afr. 1983;5:74.
83. Buck AA, ed. Onchocerciasis: Symptomatology, pathology, diagnosis. Geneva: World Health Organization; 1974.
84. Gibson DW, Heggie C, Connor DH. Clinical and pathologic aspects of onchocerciasis. Pathol Ann. 1980;15:195.
85. Roizenblatt J. Interstitial keratitis caused by American (mucocutaneous) leishmaniasis. Am J Ophthalmol. 1979;87:175.
86. Dawson CR, Jones BR, Tarizzo ML. Guide to trachoma control in programmes for the prevention of blindness. Geneva: World Health Organization; 1981.
87. Ma P, Willaert E, Juechter KB, et al. A case of keratitis due to *Acanthamoeba* in New York, New York, and features of 10 cases. J Infect Dis. 1981;143:662.
88. Mannis MJ, Tamaro R, Roth AM, et al. *Acanthamoeba* sclerokeratitis. Determining diagnostic criteria. Arch Ophthalmol. 1986;104:1313–17.
89. Eiferman RA, Carothers DJ, Yankeelow JA. Peripheral rheumatoid ulceration and evidence for conjunctival collagenase production. Am J Ophthalmol. 1979;87:703.
90. Austin P, Green WR, Sallyer DC, et al. Peripheral corneal degeneration and occlusive vasculitis in Wegener's granulomatosis. Am J Ophthalmol. 1978;85:311.
91. Gerstle CC, Friedman AH. Marginal corneal ulceration (limbal guttering) as a presenting sign of temporal arteritis. Ophthalmology. 1980;87:1173.
92. Duke-Elder S. System of Ophthalmology. v. 8. Diseases of the Outer Eye. St Louis: CV Mosby; 1965;237, 239, 539, 828, 829, 1032.
93. Woods AC. Syphilis of the eye. Am J Syph Gonor Vener Dis. 1943;27:133.
94. Ballantyne AJ, Michaelson IC: Textbook of the Fundus of the Eye. Baltimore: Williams & Wilkins; 1962;564.
95. Knapp A. Bilateral circumpapillary chorioretinitis with detachment of the retina in syphilis. Trans Am Acad Ophthalmol Otolaryngol. 1920;25:132.
96. Stokes JH, Beerman H, Ingraham NR. Modern Clinical Syphilology. Philadelphia: WB Saunders; 1949:59.
97. Carrol FD. Retrobulbar neuritis. Arch Ophthalmol. 1940;24:44.
98. Hogan MJ, Zimmerman LE, eds. Ophthalmic Pathology. 3rd ed. Philadelphia: WB Saunders; 1968;397.
99. Moore JE. Syphilitic iritis. Am J Ophthalmol. 1931;14:110.
100. Krachmer JH, Laibson PR. Corneal thinning and perforation in Sjögren's syndrome. Am J Ophthalmol. 1974;78:917.
101. Pfister RR, Murphy GE. Corneal ulceration and perforation associated with Sjögren's syndrome. Arch Ophthalmol. 1980;98:89.
102. Charlton KH, Binder PS, Wozniak L, et al. Pseudodendritic keratitis and systemic tyrosinemia. Ophthalmology. 1981;88:355.
103. Tabbara KF, Ostler HB, Dawson C, et al. Thygeson's superficial punctate keratitis. Ophthalmology. 1981;88:75.
104. Mark DB, McCulley JB. Reiter's keratitis. Arch Ophthalmol. 1982;100:781.
105. Sommer A, Tarwotjo I, Hussaini G, et al. Incidence, prevalence, and scale of blinding malnutrition. Lancet. 1981;1:1407.
106. Jones DB, Liesgang TJ, Robinson NM. Laboratory diagnosis of ocular infections. Cumitech 13. 1981.
107. Forster RK, Rebell G. The diagnosis and management of keratomycoses. II. Medical and surgical management. Arch Ophthalmol. 1975;93:1134.
108. Jones DB. Decision-making in the management of microbial keratitis. Ophthalmology. 1981;88:814.
109. Naumann G, Green WR, Zimmerman LE. Mycotic keratitis. A histopathologic study of 73 cases. Am J Ophthalmol. 1967;64:668–82.
110. Boerner CF, Lee FK, Wichliffe CL, et al. Electron microscopy for the diagnosis of ocular viral infections. Ophthalmology. 1981;88:1377.
111. Wolters RW, Jorgensen JH, Calzada E, et al. Limulus lysate assay for early detection of certain gram-negative corneal infections. Arch Ophthalmol. 1979;97:875.
112. Chaudhuri PR, Godfrey B. Treatment of bacterial corneal ulcers with concentrated antibiotic eye drops. Trans Ophthalmol Soc UK. 1982;102:11.
113. Baum J, Barza M. Topical vs subconjunctival treatment of bacterial corneal ulcers. Ophthalmology. 1983;90:162.
114. Aronson SB, Moore TE Jr, O'Day DM. The effects of structural alteration on anterior ocular inflammation. Am J Ophthalmol. 1970;70:886.
115. Golden B, Fingerman LH, Allen HF. *Pseudomonas* corneal ulcers in contact lens wearers. Arch Ophthalmol. 1971;85:543.
116. Baum JL. Initial therapy of suspected microbial corneal ulcers: I. Broad antibiotic therapy based on prevalence of organisms. Surv Ophthalmol. 1979;24:97.
117. Wilhelmus KR, Coster DJ, Jones Br. Acyclovir and debridement in the treatment of ulcerative herpetic keratitis. Am J Ophthalmol. 1981;91:323.
118. LaLau C, Oosterhuis A, Versteeg J, et al. Acyclovir and trifluorothymidine in herpetic keratitis: A multicentre trial. Br J Ophthalmol. 1982;66:506.
119. Jones BR, Falcon MG, Williams HP, et al. Symposium on herpes simplex eye disease. Objectives in therapy of herpetic eye disease. Trans Ophthalmol Soc UK. 1977;97:305.
120. Ostler HB. The management of ocular herpesvirus infections. Surv Ophthalmol. 1976;21:136.
121. Jones BR, Coster DJ, Falcon MG, et al. Topical therapy of ulcerative herpetic keratitis with human inteferon. Lancet. 1976;2:128.
122. Cobo LM, Coster DJ, Rice NSC, et al. Prognosis and management of corneal transplantation for herpetic keratitis. Arch Ophthalmol. 1980;98:1755.
123. Foster CS, Duncan J. Penetrating keratoplasty for herpes simplex keratitis. Am J Ophthalmol. 1981;92:336.
124. Bergaust B, Westby RK. Zoster ophthalmicus: Local treatment with cortisone. Acta Ophthalmol. 1967;45:787.
125. Ishibashi Y. Oral ketoconazole therapy for keratomycosis. Am J Ophthalmol. 1983;95:342.
126. Wright P, Worhurst D, Jones BR. *Acanthamoeba* keratitis successfully treated medically. Br J Ophthalmol. 1985;69:778–82.
127. White AT, Newland HS, Taylor HR, et al. Controlled trial and dose-finding study of ivermectin for treatment of onchocerciasis. J Infect Dis. 1987;156:463–70.
128. Foster CS. Immunosuppressive therapy for external ocular inflammatory disease. Ophthalmology. 1980;87:140.
129. Kenyon KR. Decision-making in the therapy of external eye disease. Noninfected corneal ulcers. Ophthalmology. 1982;89:44.
130. Sommer A. Nutritional Blindness: Xerophthalmia and Keratomalacia. New York: Oxford University Press; 1982

100. ENDOPHTHALMITIS

PETER J. McDONNELL
W. RICHARD GREEN

Endophthalmitis is defined as an inflammatory process that involves an ocular cavity and adjacent structures and may be classified according to the type of etiologic agent, the mode of entry, and the location within the eye. Infectious etiologic agents include bacteria, fungi, viruses, protozoa, and parasites (Table 1). The infectious agent may be introduced directly into the eye as in cases of surgical and nonsurgical trauma or may reach the eye by hematogenous spread from a distant site of infection. Noninfectious stimuli causing endophthalmitis in-

TABLE 1. Infectious Agents That Cause Endophthalmitis

- Bacteria
  - Aerobic
    - Gram-positive cocci
      - *Staphylococcus aureus, S. epidermidis*
      - *Streptococcus pneumoniae,* other species of *Streptococcus*
    - Gram-positive bacilli
      - *Bacillus cereus, B. subtilis,* other *Bacillus* species
      - *Corynebacterium pseudodiphtheriticum* (*C. hofmannii*), *C. xerosis,* other *Corynebacterium* species
      - *Listeria monocytogenes*
    - Gram-negative cocci
      - *Neisseria meningitidis*
    - Gram-negative bacilli
      - *Acinetobacter* species
      - *Alcaligenes faecalis*
      - *Enterobacter* species
      - *Escherichia coli*
      - *Flavobacterium meningosepticum*
      - *Haemophilis influenzae*
      - *Klebsiella* species
      - *Moraxella* species
      - *Proteus* species
      - *Pseudomonas aeruginosa*
      - *Salmonella typhimurium*
      - *Serratia marcescens*
  - Anaerobic
    - *Clostridium* species
    - *Propionibacterium acnes*
  - Spirochetes
    - *Treponema pallidum*
  - Higher bacteria
    - *Actinomyces israelii*
    - *Mycobacterium tuberculosis, M. leprae, M. avium-intracellulare*
    - *Nocardia* species
- Fungi
  - *Acremonium* (*Cephalosporium*) species
  - *Aspergillus* species
  - *Blastomyces dermatitidis*
  - *Candida* species
  - *Cladosporium* species
  - *Coccidioides immitis*
  - *Cryptococcus neoformans*
  - *Exophiala jeanselmei*
  - *Fusarium* species
  - *Graphium* species
  - *Histoplasma capsulatum*
  - *Mucor* species
  - *Neurospora sitophila*
  - *Rhizopus* species
  - *Paecilomyces* species
  - *Penicillium* species
  - *Pseudallescheria* (*Petriellidium*) *boydii* (*Scedosporium apiospermum*)
  - *Sporothrix schenckii*
  - *Torulopsis glabrata*
  - *Trichosporon* species
  - *Volutella* species
- Viruses
  - Herpes simplex virus
  - Herpes zoster virus
  - Cytomegalovirus
  - Rubella
  - Rubeola
- Parasites
  - *Onchocerca volvulus*
  - *Taenia solium* (cysticercosis)
  - *Toxocara canis* and *cati*
  - *Toxoplasma gondii*

clude retained lens material, foreign materials introduced at the time of surgery, blood, and intraocular neoplasms. The inflammatory process may be localized to specific tissues within the eye or may involve the intraocular contents in a generalized fashion. When the episclera participates significantly in the inflammatory process, a panophthalmitis is said to be present. Pain, especially on movement of the eye, is a prominent feature of panophthalmitis.

BACTERIAL ENDOPHTHALMITIS

Bacteria are the most common infectious agents that cause endophthalmitis. Typically, a bacterial endophthalmitis develops suddenly and progresses rapidly.[1,2] The symptoms and signs become manifested in the first 24 to 48 hours after surgical or nonsurgical trauma. If, in the early postoperative period, the patient complains of increasing pain with progressive blurred vision and exhibits any unexpected degree of hyperemia, chemosis, lid edema, corneal edema, and anterior-chamber and vitreous reaction, bacterial endophthalmitis should be strongly suspected. Careful slit-lamp examination and direct or indirect ophthalmoscopy are necessary if the earliest signs of endophthalmitis are to be detected.

Bacterial endophthalmitis usually occurs as a complication of ocular surgery. The usefulness of prophylactic antibiotics topically or subconjunctivally, before, during, or after surgery, remains unproven, although preoperative topical antibiotics are widely used.[3–6] It should be emphasized that the ocular surface microflora are responsible for the majority of infections and probably gain access to the eye during surgery. *Staphylococcus aureus* is responsible for 50 percent of the cases of endophthalmitis after cataract extraction.[5] Infections due to *S. aureus* and *Pseudomonas* are usually manifested in a fulminating fashion in the early postoperative period. Virtually any bacterial microorganism, including those previously considered saprophytic, may cause endophthalmitis[7–25] (Table 1).

The incidence of endophthalmitis after cataract extraction varies from 0.078 percent[5,26] to 0.496 percent[6] and 0.533 percent,[27] and it occurs in 0.2 percent of cases after penetrating keratoplasties.[28] Contamination of intraocular lenses has produced isolated endophthalmitis.[29–31] Short-term storage of corneal buttons in McCarey-Kaufman media[32] has resulted in endophthalmitis.

Bacterial endophthalmitis may follow surgical procedures for glaucoma,[33–35] retinal detachment,[36] strabismus,[37] pterygia,[38] myopia,[39] and corneal transplantation.[32,40] Postoperative complications such as wound leaks,[41] unplanned filtering blebs,[42,43] vitreous wick syndromes,[44] deep sutures, epithelial ingrowth, and retained lens material[45] may predispose to bacterial endophthalmitis. An incidence of 1.2–9 percent has been reported for late endophthalmitis in patients who have had glaucoma procedures.[46,34] The use of contact lenses in patients with inadvertent postoperative blebs may lead to endophthalmitis.[42] Recently, persistent low-grade infections with organisms of low virulence such as *Propionibacterium acnes* have been recognized to cause chronic inflammation after cataract extraction.[47]

Bacterial endophthalmitis is surprisingly rare after penetrating nonsurgical trauma.[48–50] *Bacillus* species are most commonly isolated in this setting.[51] The development of systemic tetanus has been reported after penetrating ocular trauma.[52,53]

If there is a sudden onset of endophthalmitis in an unoperated nontraumatized eye, hematogenous spread from a distant focus of infection should be suspected.[54–60] The clinical picture is similar to that seen in postoperative bacterial endophthalmitis except that the posterior segment of the eye is usually involved and the patients are usually extremely ill and often immunologically compromised.[57,61–63] Dental procedures have occasionally preceded the developement of bacterial endophthalmitis.[64,65] Neonates and women in the puerperal period may also occasionally develop endogenous endophthalmitis.[66–68] The most common features are decreased visual acuity, pain, hypopyon or severe anterior uveitis, and conjunctival hyperemia. Within hours, a focal chorioretinitis occurs. Vitreous infection and finally an acute panophthalmitis may follow. Endophthalmitis may also occur as a result of progressive severe bacterial corneal ulceration.

In hematogenous bacterial endophthalmitis, a septic focus is usually apparent before intraocular inflammation occurs. In a review[60] of 20 such cases, meningitis, abdominal infection, endocarditis, pneumonia, otitis media, breast abscess, paronychia, pharyngitis, and lymphangitis were implicated as septic foci. The etiologic agent was the pneumococcus in 30 percent of the cases. Meningococci and staphylococci were each responsible for 15 percent of the cases. Since the etiologic agents are usually of low virulence in subacute bacterial endocarditis, ocular findings may be minimal. Conjunctival and retinal hemorrhages are the most frequent findings. Retinal hemorrhages that have white centers called *Roth spots* may represent septic retinitis. These lesions are characteristic but not pathognomonic of subacute bacterial endocarditis. Hemorrhages with white centers due to the accumulation of platelets and fibrin may be seen in other diseases. Bacterial endophthalmitis due to *Bacillus cereus* has been reported after transfusion with contaminated blood and in heroin addicts. Various agents including *Haemophilus influenzae, Streptococcus,* and *Neisseria meningitidis* have been implicated in unilateral and bilateral endophthalmitis associated with meningitis.[58,59,70]

In miliary tuberculosis, small elevated yellow-white choroidal nodules with indistinct borders may be seen.[71] Tuberculous retinitis and endophthalmitis have been observed.[72]

In congenital syphilis the severe chorioretinitis leads to extensive chorioretinal scarring with a variety of patterns.[72]

In secondary and late-acquired syphilis, iridocyclitis is the most frequent ocular finding.[73] Other inflammatory features include retinal vasculitis, phlebitis, periarteritis, panuveitis, "posterior uveitis," multifocal choroiditis, chorioretinitis, papillitis, and neuroretinitis.[72]

Nocardia asteroides is a higher bacteria. Disseminated nocardiosis occurs via hematogenous spread from a pulmonary lesion. There have been 11 reported cases of intraocular involvement. With ocular involvement, the patients complain of blurred vision and pain. On fundus examination, central or paracentral foci of necrotizing chorioretinitis are seen.[74,75] A vitreous abscess may occasionally occur. Of the 14 reported cases with intraocular involvement, 3 occurred after surgery or trauma, 1 occurred after carotid endarterectomy, and 10 were associated with systemic diseases and reduced immune competence.[72]

In Whipple's disease, macrophages with phagocytosed bacilli in varying stages of breakdown may be present in the vitreous cavity and retina.[76]

MYCOTIC ENDOPHTHALMITIS

The incidence of systemic mycotic infections has increased markedly in the past 3 decades. This increase is thought to be related in part to the widespread use of antibiotics, corticosteroids, chemotherapy, and immunosuppressive therapy; to an increased addictive drug usage[77–82]; and to hyperalimentation.[83–85]

Fungi generally considered to be saprophytes can cause endophthalmitis. Over 20 different fungal agents have been isolated from cases of intraocular mycoses.[86]

Fungal endophthalmitis may occur from exogenous and endogenous sources. Exogenous sources include extension of a fungal corneal ulcer and surgical or nonsurgical trauma,[87] including outbreaks of fungal endophthalmitis due to contaminated ophthalmic irrigation solutions.[88]

The main difference between bacterial and fungal endophthalmitis after trauma or surgery is the time of onset of symptoms and signs. Typically in a fungal endophthalmitis, there is a greater delay in the onset of symptoms and signs than in a bacterial endophthalmitis. After intraocular surgery, there may be a lapse of several weeks before the onset of ocular pain, ciliary injection, and signs of a nonspecific uveitis. On slit-lamp examination, a localized gray-white area may be seen in the anterior vitreous adjacent to the pupillary border. A transient hypopyon may occur, and additional satellite lesions occur in the anterior vitreous. In rare instances, the site of infection and abscess formation may occur in the anterior chamber, usually near the chamber angle.

The incidence of fungal endophthalmitis after cataract surgery is very low. In one series of 36,000 cataract extractions, only two cases of infection were reported.[89] However, epidemic fungal endophthalmitis has occurred after intraocular lens implantation[90,91] and in isolated cases after retinal reattachment surgery[92] and penetrating keratoplasty using cryopreserved or organ-icultured tissue.[93,94] Fungi isolated postoperatively have included *Volutella* species,[95] *Neurospora sitophila,*[96] *Scedosporium apiospermum,*[97] *Candida parapsilosis,*[98] *Trichosporon cutaneum,*[99] *Paecilomyces lilacinus,*[90,100] *Acremonium* (*Cephalosporium*),[94] and *Torulopsis glabrata*[93] (Table 1).

After penetrating nonsurgical trauma, signs of fungal endophthalmitis may develop in an indolent fashion many weeks later.[101–103] Extension of fungal corneal ulcer may also lead to endophthalmitis.[104,105]

In hematogenous fungal endophthalmitis, the ocular involvement may be the first or only manifestation. Evidence of non-ocular foci of metastatic fungal disease may not be present. Of 133 patients who died after fungemia, 14 (10.5 percent) were found to have ocular involvement (11 with *Candida,* 2 with *Aspergillus,* and 1 with *Cryptococcus*).[106] Reduction of vision is the usual initial symptom. At first, only a slight preretinal vitreous haze may be seen. Within a few days, fluffy white balls of exudate occur in the vitreous just anterior to the retina. The degree of inflammation may vary from a localized abscess to a total endophthalmitis. Chorioretinal or vitreoretinal scarring may result in a severe reduction of vision or even loss of the eye.

Candida albicans is the most frequently reported cause of endogenous fungal endophthalmitis[107–113] (Chapter 234). There has been an impressive increase in *Candida* endophthalmitis over the last 3 or 4 decades, which is only partly accounted for by increased clinical suspicion and improved culture techniques.[114] Although intravenous drug addiction clearly has contributed to the problem, the major causal factor appears to be the extensive use of intravascular catheters.[80,83–85]

In a review of 100 reported cases of *Candida* endophthalmitis, it was determined that 85 patients had received broad-spectrum antibiotic therapy, 17 patients had received corticosteroids, and 8 patients had received both concurrently.[114] Fifty-three patients had undergone abdominal, thoracic, or cardiac surgery within a short time preceding the development of candidiasis. One-quarter of the abdominal procedures were performed for malignancy. Nine patients had diabetes mellitus, and six were alcoholics with cirrhosis of the liver. Blood cultures were positive in 41 patients, and urine cultures were positive in 25 patients. In 14 cases, culture of material from intravenous catheter tips yielded *Candida*.

There is an average delay of 18 days between the time a positive culture for *Candida* is obtained and the onset of ocular symptoms.[114] Blurred vision, pain, and ciliary injection may occur. A casual diagnosis of conjunctivitis or, in comatose patients, of exposure keratitis may be made. All too often, symptoms are reported late because the patient is comatose, on a respirator, or gravely ill. Periodic funduscopic examinations are indicated in patients with known or suspected candidemia. The earliest lesion is a small, yellow-white retinal exudate that may be mistaken for a lesion of diabetes mellitus, acute leukemia, or systemic lupus erythematosus. This early lesion, which may be unilateral or bilateral, may resolve spontaneously or progress slowly to a vitreous abscess. As extension to the vitreous occurs, margins of the lesion become hazy, the vitreous becomes progressively clouded, and one or more balls of yellowish white exudate protrude into the vitreous. Although the ciliary body or iris may on occasion be the site of an initial lesion, extension to the anterior chamber is usually a late finding.[115] Prognosis for the return of normal visual acuity in an eye with a *Candida* vitreous abscess is guarded despite appropriate therapy.[107–109] Recognition of an early funduscopic lesion may not only preserve vision but may provide useful evidence of disseminated candidiasis. In one autopsy series of 15 cases with *Candida* endophthalmitis, 13 had *Candida* in other organs.[108]

Twenty-two cases of endophthalmitis due to *Aspergillus* have been reported or presented.[72,114] Of these, 14 patients had underlying systemic debilitating conditions. Antibiotics, corticosteroids, and immunosuppressive therapy, alone or in combination, were used in about one-half the patients before the onset of infection. Intravenous injection of illicit drugs is another cause.[77,82] The most common sign is an iridocyclitis or a vitritis with associated yellow-white retinal lesions. Retinal hemorrhages, hypopyon, scleritis, and panophthalmitis are also seen. Endophthalmitis due to *Aspergillus* has also been observed after accidental and surgical trauma.[116]

Cryptococcal infection usually involves the central nervous system. Ocular manifestations include papilledema, nystagmus, extraocular muscle paresis, and optic atrophy.[117] Intraocular involvement may occur as a complication of disseminated cryptococcosis or as the sole manifestation. The most common ocular symptom is blurred vision. Intraocular signs include uveitis, papilledema, retinal hemorrhages, exudates, and detachment. Discrete yellow choroidal or chorioretinal lesions may be seen. As with other fungal infections, cryptococcosis tends to occur in patients with lymphomas or other disorders of the reticuloendothelial system and in patients receiving long-term corticosteroid therapy (Chapter 240).

Pulmonary infection is the most common systemic manifestation of coccidioidomycosis (Chapter 243). Hematogenous spread usually leads to bone or skin lesions. Coccidioidomycosis tends to occur in otherwise healthy persons. Ocular symptoms include blurred vision, pain, and photophobia. Multiple yellow-white chorioretinal lesions that are 0.1 to 0.5 optic disk diameter in size are present, often with pigmented borders. Juxtapapillary chorioretinal lesions, retinal exudates,[118] recurrent uveitis,[119,120] secondary glaucoma, perivascular sheathing, and serous retinal detachment overlying a lesion in the macular area have been reported.[121,122] In a 1980 study, 4 of 10 consecutive patients with chronic pulmonary and disseminated disease had chorioretinal involvement.[118]

The usual form of ocular involvement with *Sporothrix schenckii* is a lid or conjunctival nodule. With intraocular sporotrichosis, the most common presenting sign is anterior uveitis.[114,123] Of 22 reported cases of sporotrichosis,[72] 18 were endogenous. A lid or conjunctival lesion was present in 4 patients. In eight patients there was no evidence of systemic sporotrichosis or other ocular lesions.

Lid lesions are the most common ocular manifestations of North American blastomycosis. In the rare patient with intraocular involvement, blurred vision and pain may occur. An anterior uveitis and secondary glaucoma can be present.[124] Yellow nodules on the iris and yellow-white posterior fundus lesions may also be seen. Of the six cases of intraocular blastomycosis reported, endophthalmitis was observed in three, an iritis or iridocyclitis in two, and bilateral choroiditis in one.

In mucormycosis, the orbit is involved by direct extension from infection of the sinuses. No cases of hematogenous *Mucor* endophthalmitis have been reported.[114] In craniofacial mucormycosis, however, eyes examined histopathologically have shown changes varying from normal to panophthalmitis with ophthalmic artery and central retinal artery occlusion or thrombosis.[125]

Presumably during the course of unrecognized systemic histoplasmosis, multifocal choroiditis may occur scattered throughout the fundus, in the peripapillary area, and sometimes in the macular area.[72] The lesions heal with variable chorioretinal scarring. This pattern of chorioretinal scars is the principal basis on which the diagnosis of the ocular histoplasmosis syndrome is made. Clinical diagnosis is enhanced by corroborative evidence of a previous infection such a pulmonary calcification and a positive histoplasmin skin test response. Years later, macular and, sometimes, lesions at other sites may become "active." Such activity is due to leakage and hemorrhage from choroidal neovascularization tissue that extends to the scar. This sequence of change may threaten vision. The mechanism by which the macular lesion develops neovascularization and its sequelae are unknown. Recurrent low-grade inflammation, presumably related to residual organisms or *Histoplasma* antigen, may play a role. It has been shown that argon laser photocoagulation of vision-threatening macular lesions can significantly reduce the risk of visual loss.[126] *Histoplasma* organisms have been identified in eyes in 13 cases.[127] In an additional case, positive indirect immunofluorescence to *Histoplasma* antigen was observed. Of the 14 eyes with organisms present, 6 were said to have had the features of the ocular histoplasmosis syndrome. In the other eight cases, ocular involvement was associated with systemic histoplasmosis.

VIRAL INFECTIONS

Herpes Simplex

In herpes simplex keratitis, generally from herpes simplex virus, type 1, intraocular inflammation in the form of a persistent nongranulomatous iridocyclitis is often present. Occasionally, an iridocyclitis is seen in the absence of keratitis. In a few cases, herpes simplex virus has been isolated from the aqueous humor.[128]

The intraocular inflammation from herpes simplex is usually located in the anterior segment of the eye. However, posterior involvement has been documented,[129–132] especially in the newborn,[128,133–135] usually as a result of herpes simplex virus type 2 infection. Large patches of yellowish white retinal exudates accompanying perivascular and vitreous inflammatory infiltrates are present. The posterior pole of the fundus is usually more extensively involved than is the periphery. When the lesions heal, sharply circumscribed punched-out chorioretinal scars that may be confused with toxoplasmic scars are seen.

Histopathologically, areas of retinal necrosis are present.[76] Inflammatory cells are noted in the vitreous and choroid adjacent to these areas of necrosis. By electron microscopy, viral particles consistent with herpes simplex virus are present in the retinal pigment epithelium,[136] retinal ganglion cell, and inner nuclear layers.[137]

Varicella-Zoster Virus

Herpes zoster keratitis is commonly followed by iridocyclitis. A diffuse choroiditis may occur. The characteristic histopathologic feature of ocular herpes zoster infection is a chronic nongranulomatous infiltration around posterior ciliary nerves and vessels.[72] Occlusive vasculitis may lead to iris and ciliary body necrosis and anterior chamber hemorrhage. A perivasculitis and vasculitis of retinal vessels may lead to hemorrhagic retinopathy. Viral inclusions have been described in the necrotizing retinopathy of herpes zoster ophthalmicus.[138] An optic neuritis may occur secondary to a periarteritis.[139] Varicella-zoster virus is at least one cause of the acute retinal necrosis syndrome.[76,140]

In varicella infections, uveitis may develop either during the acutely infectious stage or during convalescence.

Cytomegalovirus

Congenital cytomegalovirus infection is a well-recognized cause of chorioretinitis[141] and occurs in 23–29 percent of the neonates with the disease.[142] Iritis, cataracts, and optic atrophy may also accompany congenital infection.

Symptomatic acquired cytomegalovirus infection in adults is uncommon.[143–145] It may occur in patients receiving chemotherapy for acute leukemia and malignant lymphomas.[146] However, most frequently it occurs in patients with the acquired immunodeficiency syndrome (AIDS) and in patients receiving immunosuppressive therapy after renal transplantation.[143,147–152] Patients usually complain of blurred vision and scotomas. Initially, this visual impairment is mild; but with progression of the disease, severe and permanent visual loss occurs. Ocular pain is usually not present. Fundus examination reveals retinal edema, scattered intraretinal hemorrhages, yellow-white exudates, vessel attenuation, and sheathing.[76] The picture of a branch vein occlusion or a necrotizing vasculitis may be simulated.[152] As the initial lesions heal, retinal and pigment epithelial atrophy occurs. Adjacent areas of active infection may be seen to progress through the same exudative, hemorrhagic, and atrophic stages.[147] The appearance of the fundus is quite distinctive and is the first clinical manifestation of systemic viral infection in the majority of cases.[144] Therefore, it is recommended that regular ophthalmoscopic examinations be performed in all organ transplant recipients.[144,153]

Rubeola and Rubella

Measles (rubeola) retinopathy (maculopathy) occurs 6–12 days after the skin rash and is clinically manifested by acute blindness. It may or may not accompany measles encephalitis. In the early stages, retinal edema, attenuated vessels, and a stellate macular figure are seen in the fundus.[76] In the later stages of the disease, there is frequently a return of useful vision and the occurrence of a secondary pigmentary retinopathy that may have a salt-and-pepper appearance.[154]

Subacute sclerosing panencephalitis (SSPE) is a progressive, invariably fatal disease caused by the measles virus, and it appears years after an attack of clinical measles. Chorioretinitis is a common ocular complication occurring in about 30 percent of the cases.[155] Optic atrophy, papilledema, and cortical blindness may also occur.[156]

The ocular complications of rubella virus infection include congenital cataracts, glaucoma, and a pigmentary retinopathy.[157]

PARASITIC ENDOPHTHALMITIS

Toxoplasma gondii is a protozoan that causes retinochoroiditis.[76] Since the *Toxoplasma* are found primarily in an area of coagulative necrosis of the retina, with a secondary granulomatous choroiditis, the term *retinochoroiditis* is applied to the ocular lesion.

Ocular involvement is present in both the congenital and acquired forms of the disease. A retinochoroiditis usually affecting the macula is present in 80 percent of the patients with congenital toxoplasmosis. The eye is rarely affected in the acquired form of the disease, but it has been suggested that almost all cases of ocular toxoplasmosis are congenital.[158]

In the active stage, the fundus lesion is whitish yellow, with indistinct borders and an overlying hazy vitreous. In recurrent disease, an active focus of inflammation is present at the border of an area of an inactive healed scar of retinochoroiditis. An iridocyclitis is usually present, and posterior vitreous detachment with vitreous precipitates on its detached surface is common. As the activity of the retinochoroiditis subsides, its color changes from yellowish white to gray, and the vitreous haze recedes. Glaucoma, cataract, vitreous hemorrhage, and retinal detachment are possible complications.

The nematode *Toxocara* is the most common parasitic cause of endophthalmitis.[159,160] The second-stage larva of this nematode is responsible for both endophthalmitis and visceral larva migrans. The average age of patients affected is 7.5 years, with a range of 2 to 31 years. Children become infected by the ingestion of ova present is soil contaminated with the excrement of dogs or cats. Nematode endophthalmitis has been diagnosed in 2 percent of 1000 eyes enucleated in children under 15 years of age[161] and is thought to be responsible for 10 percent of the cases of uveitis in children.[162]

The infestation may present as a diffuse chronic endophthalmitis, as a posterior-pole granuloma, or as a peripheral granuloma in a quiet eye[163]; a cloudy vitreous, cyclitic membrane, and posterior synechiae may be present. A *Toxocara* granuloma is typically white and hemispheric, with a diameter roughly equal to or bigger than the disk. It is primarily located in the retina. It may be present at the macula or at the periphery of the fundus. Other ocular manifestations of *Toxocara* infestation include a localized vitreous abscess, papillitis,[164] pars planitis, iridocyclitis, hypopyon,[165] preretinal and vitreous hemorrhages, and very rarely, central retinal artery occlusion.[166] In the presence of systemic disease (visceral larva migrans), ocular involvement is rare. Nematode granulomas in the eye have often been confused with retinoblastoma, and the differential diagnosis is important.

Diffuse unilateral neuroretinitis (DUSN) is a syndrome characterized by a loss of vision, vitritis, papillitis, and recurrent crops of gray-white retina lesions; the syndrome progresses to optic atrophy, retinal vessel narrowing, and diffuse pigmentary changes. DUSN may be caused by at least two different nematodes.[167]

Ocular infestation with *Cysticercus cellulosae* may occur in 13 percent[168] of patients with cysticercosis (Chapter 264). The parasite may be found in the vitreous cavity or in the subchoroidal space.[169] Ocular inflammation and charactistic retinal tracks may be seen with fly larvae (myiasis).[170] Onchocerciasis (river blindness) is usually manifested in the eye as keratitis, but iridocyclitis, glaucoma, and choroiditis also may occur (Chapter 262).

NONINFECTIOUS ENDOPHTHALMITIS

Other intraocular inflammatory syndromes such as sympathetic ophthalmia, idiopathic uveitis, and pars planitis may be confused with the previously described infectious diseases. Sterile endophthalmitis has resulted from surgical chemical contamination of the intraocular contents by starch particles[171] and from probable ethylene oxide/polymer by-products of the intraocular lens sterilization process.[172]

LABORATORY FINDINGS

Rapid and accurate diagnosis of the etiologic agent is essential if useful vision is to be salvaged in bacterial endophthalmitis. The site from which material is obtained for smears and cultures is important. Conjunctival cultures are inadequate and misleading in bacterial endophthalmitis. The anterior chamber, vitreous cavity, wound abscesses, and wound dehiscenses are the sites from which material should be cultured.[173–175]

All cases of traumatic and postsurgical endophthalmitis should have aqueous and vitreous aspiration for cultures and smears. In a study of 140 cases of endophthalmitis, an agent was isolated by vitreous and aqueous tap in 78 cases. In 27 of these, the organism was isolated from the vitreous alone, with a negative aqueous culture.[173] The vitreous specimen should be specially prepared for cytology,[176] and centrifugal cytology may be helpful.[177]

Material from each site should be separately stained with Gram, Giemsa, periodic acid–Schiff (PAS), and methenamine silver stains and should be cultured on blood and chocolate agar, thioglycollate media, or Schaedler broth or brain–heart infusion, Sabouraud agar, and on reduced blood agar kept in an anaerobic environment.[178] Vitreous irrigate material from vitrectomy can be centrifuged and smeared or can be passed through a Millipore filter, which can be stained and cultured. The limulus lysate test on aqueous and vitreous material may help in the rapid detection of gram-negative endophthalmitis.[179] Vitreous glucose estimations have been used to differentiate sterile from bacterial endophthalmitis. In patients with leukokoria and suspected nematode endophthalmitis, aqueous cytology revealing eosinophils and normal lactate dehydrogenase levels[180] may prevent enucleation as a result of a misdiagnosis of retinoblastoma. Enzyme-linked immunosorbent assay (ELISA) testing of aqueous humor material may aid in the diagnosis.[181,182]

TREATMENT

Effective therapy for endophthalmitis requires a low threshold of suspicion for diagnosing endophthalmitis of infective origin, early diagnostic aspirates, and immediate broad-spectrum antibiotic cover, followed by appropriate therapy to reduce the host immune and anti-inflammatory response and modification of the antibiotic therapy in view of culture results.[173,174,183,184] Animal and human studies demonstrate that the visual outcome is greatly influenced by the virulence of the etiologic agent. *Staphylococcus epidermidis* endophthalmitis, which appears to be increasing in frequency, responds well to relatively conservative therapy with topical, subconjunctival, and intravenous antibiotics together with corticosteroids.[174,185]

Unfortunately, reliable and rapid diagnosis of the organism involved remains difficult. Destruction of the eye by virulent organisms such as *Pseudomonas aeruginosa* and *Staphylococcus aureus* may occur within 24 hours, so aggressive therapy appears warranted if the type of organism is in doubt. There is no consensus, however, on what constitutes aggressive therapy. It may include early vitrectomy[186–189]; intravitreal antibiotics (gentamicin, cefazolin)[190]; early systemic, topical, and perhaps intravitreal corticosteroids[174]; and intravenous broad-spectrum antibiotics such as a third-generation cephalosporin. In cases of post-traumatic endophthalmitis, intravitreal and systemic clindamycin therapy should be added because of the risk of *Bacillus cereus* endophthalmitis.[191] Successful eradication of *Propionibacterium acnes* infection may require removal of all residual lens material by using vitrectomy instrumentation combined with intravitreal antibiotic therapy.[47]

The rationale for the use of early corticosteroids as an addition to therapy is based on the recognition of the visually destructive secondary processes that can occur after the successful inflammatory and immune response mounted by the host in response to the causative organism. Unlike various infections elsewhere, successful elimination of the organism is not the only criterion of successful treatment of endophthalmitis. If vision is to be retained, control of the inflammatory and immune response is crucial.

Data on the choice of antibiotics, route of administration and the degree of intraocular penetration of the antibiotics has been obtained from animal studies only. The results of these studies are not necessarily to be extrapolated to human endophthalmitis.

Therapy for suspected fungal endophthalmitis is more difficult still, with commonly a delay in diagnosis, and less information is available on the pharmacokinetics and sensitivity testing with the preferred antifungal agents. Currently, the combined use of topical natamycin, oral flucytosine, intravenous amphotericin B, and possibly intraocular amphotericin B is recommended.[192] This should be combined with a vitrectomy of any intravitreal abscess formation. The use of corticosteroids, either orally or intravitreally, together with antifungal agents remains extremely controversial.

Candida endophthalmitis appears to be best treated with intravenous amphotericin B.[114,193] As the retinal lesions resolve, scarring is a common occurrence. Once vitreous invasion is present, significant intraocular morbidity occurs despite treatment. Vitreous organization and vitreous traction leading to retinal detachment may occur.[109]

Candida endophthalmitis not involving the vitreous has been noted to rarely resolve spontaneously without antifungal treatment.[83] Presumably, these patients have relatively intact immunologic systems.

Combined therapy with amphotericin B and flucytosine appears to provide a syngergistic effect in vitro. This combination has been reported to be successful in the treatment of endogenous and postsurgical *Candida* endophthalmitis.[194] Pars plana vitrectomy is both a diagnostic and therapeutic modality that may be used in the management of *Candida* endophthalmitis. It facilitates diagnosis by making tissue available for culture and microscopic evaluation.[176] It plays a therapeutic role by removing replicating fungi in the vitreous body, by improving the diffusion of systematically administered antifungal agents into the vitreous cavity, and by preventing future vitreoretinal traction.[195] Because of toxicity, the place of intravitreal amphotericin B is unclear,[196–198] but 5–10 μg of amphotericin B have been injected into the vitreous with some success.

Intravenous amphotericin B successfully eradicates sytemic aspergillosis, but organisms usually remain in the eye[199] in endogenous *Aspergillus* endophthalmitis. Successful treatment of endogenous *Aspergillus* endophthalmitis has been accomplished in only two instances that combined surgical removal of infected vitreous and antifungal agents.[76,77]

Of five patients who received amphotericin B for cryptococcal endophthalmitis, two were successfully treated.[200,201]

Of 12 patients with endophthalmitis secondary to *Coccidioides immitis*[114] were treated with amphotericin B. There was dramatic improvement in both systemic and ocular disease manifestations in two patients.

In the ocular histoplasmosis syndrome, systemic steroids have been repoted to be of some value in treating the early stage of serous and/or hemorrhagic detachment of the retina and/or retinal pigment epithelium that occurs in an old macular scar.[202] Corticosteroids do not activate any latent histoplasmosis in such patients, nor is antifungal therapy of benefit in patients with this syndrome. In almost all instances, there is no evidence of actively replicating fungal organisms in these lesions, and the photocoagulation of macular lesions not involving the fovea has been proved to reduce the risk of visual loss.[126]

Topical corticosteroids and atropine are the mainstay of therapy for herpetic keratouveitis. The usefulness of an antiviral "umbrella" to prevent the recurrence of epithelial herpetic disease remains unproven. Acyclovir has been shown to be effective in the treatment of retinitis associated with varicella-zoster virus.[140,203] Herpetic retinitis may also may also be treated with short courses of systemic corticosteroids.[128]

Herpes zoster iridocyclitis is best treated with topical corticosteroids and cycloplegia. The role of acyclovir in the management of this condition is unclear.

In the treatment of cytomegalovirus infection in adults, early reduction or discontinuation of immunosuppressive therapy, if possible, should help in limiting the progression of the ocular and systemic infection.[204] Ganciclovir is an effective means of therapy for cytomegalovirus retinitis, but it must be given chronically to prevent reactivation.[205]

In the treatment of ocular toxoplasmosis, mydriatics, topical corticosteroids, systemic and/or periocular depot administration of corticosteroids, pyrimethamine, and triple sulfonamides have been recommended.[206] Some authorities only treat cases with extensive involvement or those in which the macula is threatened. Experimental studies in mice have shown that clindamycin may destroy encysted forms of the parasite in chronically infected tissues, and it has been combined with sulfadiazine to treat human ocular toxoplasmosis.[207]

To prevent ocular toxocariasis, prophylaxis should include avoidance of eating dirt and handling of puppies that have not been dewormed. Thiabendazole is effective in the treatment of visceral larva migrans. However, intraocular inflammation develops when the *Toxocara* larvae die within the eye. Therefore, systemic or periocular injection of corticosteroids is the usual therapy of choice.[160,208] Removal of the encysted larvae by vitrectomy may offer a solution.[209,210] Diethylcarbamazine treatment of onchocerciasis may cause intense ocular inflammation due to the death of microfilariae. Ocular corticosteroids are often administered to ameliorate this complication. Less inflammation may result if ivermectin is used to treat onchocerciasis.[211]

Intensive topical and systemic steroids most effectively treat the sterile endophthalmitis induced by intraocular lens sterilizing methods and other chemical agents.

REFERENCES

1. Forster RK. Etiology and diagnosis of bacterial postoperative endophthalmitis. Ophthalmology. 1978;85:320.
2. Theodore FH. Etiology and diagnosis of fungal postoperative endophthalmitis. Ophthalmology. 1978;85:327.
3. Allen HF. Prevention of postoperative endophthalmitis. Ophthalmology. 1978;85:386.
4. Binder PS, Abel R Jr, Bellows R. Postoperative bacterial endophthalmitis. Section II. Ann Ophthalmol. 1976;6:1129.
5. Allen HF, Mangiaracine AB. Bacterial endophthalmitis after cataract extraction. II. Incidence in 36,000 consecutive operations with special reference to preoperative topical antibiotics. Arch Ophthalmol. 1974;91:3.
6. Christy NE, Lall P. Postoperative endophthalmitis following cataract surgery. Effects of subconjunctival antibiotics and other factors. Arch Ophthalmol. 1973;90:361.
7. Brinser JH, Hess JB. Meningococcal endophthalmitis without meningitis. Can J Ophthalmol. 1981;16:100.
8. Wassermann HE. Avian tuberculosis endophthalmitis. Arch Ophthalmol. 1973;89:321.
9. Ebright JR, Lentino JR, Juni E. Endophthalmitis caused by *Moraxella nonliquefaciens*. Am J Clin Pathol. 1982;77:362.
10. Salceda SR, Lapuz J, Vizconde R. *Serratia marcescens* endophthalmitis. Arch Ophthalmol. 1973;89:163.
11. Bigger JF, Miltzer G, Mandell A, et al. *Serratia marcescens* endophthalmitis. Am J Ophthalmol. 1971;72:1102.
12. Oesterle CS, Kronenberg HA, Peyman GA. Endophthalmitis caused by an *Erwinia* species. Arch Ophthalmol. 1977;95:824.
13. Peyman GA, Vastine DW, Diamond JG. Vitrectomy and intraocular gentamicin management of *Herellea* endophthalmitis after incomplete phacoemulsification. Am J Ophthalmol. 1975;80:764.
14. Wahl JW. *Vibrio* endophthalmitis. Arch Ophthalmol. 1974;91:423.
15. Smolin G. *Proteus* endophthalmitis. Arch Ophthalmol. 1974;91:419.
16. Tabbara KF, Juffali F, Matossian RM. *Bacillus laterosporus* endophthalmitis. Arch Ophthalmol. 1977;95:2187.
17. Snead JW, Stern WH, Whitcher JP, et al. *Listeria monocytogenes* endophthalmitis. Am J Ophthalmol. 1977;84:337.
18. Friedman E, Peyman GA, May DR. Endophthalmitis caused by *Propionibacterium acnes*. Can J Ophthalmol. 1978;13:50.
19. Hanscom T, Maxwell WA. *Corynebacterium* endophthalmitis. Laboratory studies and report of a case treated by vitrectomy. Arch Ophthalmol. 1979;97:500.
20. Ballen PH, Loffredo FR, Painter B. *Listeria* endophthalmitis. Arch Ophthalmol. 1979;97:101.
21. Abbott, RL, Forster RK, Rebell G. *Listeria monocytogenes* endophthalmitis with a black hypopyon. Am J Ophthalmol. 1978;86:715.
22. Cooperman EW, Friedman AH. Exogenous *Moraxella liquefaciens* endophthalmitis. Ophthalmologica. 1975;171:177.
23. O'Day DM, Smith RS, Gregg CR, et al. The problem of *Bacillus* species infection, with special emphasis on the virulence of *Bacillus cereus*. Ophthalmology. 1981;88:833.
24. Bagnarello AG, Berlin AJ, Weinstein AJ, et al. *Listeria monocytogenes* endophthalmitis. Arch Ophthalmol. 1977;95:1004.
25. Werner EB, Herschorn BR. Exogenous endophthalmitis. Am J Ophthalmol. 1983;95:123.
26. Allen HF. Symposium: Postoperative endophthalmitis. Introduction: Incidence and etiology. Ophthalmology. 1978;85:317.
27. Fahmy JA. Endophthalmitis following cataract extraction. A study of 24 cases in 4,498 operations. Acta Ophthalmol. 1975;53:522.
28. Leveille AS, McMullan D, Cavanagh HD. Endophthalmitis following penetrating keratoplasty. Ophthalmology. 1983;90:38.

29. Zaidman GW, Mondino BJ. Postoperative pseudophakic bacterial endophthalmitis. Am J Ophthalmol. 1982;93:218.
30. Schanzlin DJ, Goldberg DB, Brown SI. *Staphylococcus epidermidis* endophthalmitis following intraocular lens implantation. Br J Ophthalmol. 1980;64:684.
31. Gerding DN, Poley BJ, Hal WH, et al. Treatment of *Pseudomonas* endophthalmitis associated with prosthetic intraocular lens implantation. Am J Ophthalmol. 1979;88:902.
32. Shaw EL, Aquavella JV. Pneumococcal endophthalmitis following grafting of corneal tissue from a (cadaver) kidney donor. Ann Ophthalmol. 1977;9:435.
33. Hattenhauer JM, Lipsich MP. Late endophthalmitis after filtering surgery. Am J Ophthalmol. 1971;72:1097.
34. Kanski JJ: Treatment of late endophthalmitis associated with filtering blebs. Arch Ophthalmol. 1974;91:339.
35. Freedman J, Gupta M, Bunke A. Endophthalmitis after trabeculectomy. Arch Ophthalmol. 1978;96:1017.
36. Pusin SM, Green WR, Tasman W, et al. Simultaneous bacterial endophthalmitis and sympathetic uveitis after retinal detachment surgery. Am J Ophthalmol. 1976;81:57.
37. Salamon SM, Friberg TR, Luxenberg MN. Endophthalmitis after strabismus surgery. Am J Ophthalmol. 1982;93:39.
38. Tarr KH, Constable IJ. *Pseudomonas* endophthalmitis associated with scleral necrosis. Br J Ophthalmol. 1980;64:676.
39. Gelender H, Flynn HW, Mandelbaum SH. Bacterial endophthalmitis resulting from radial keratotomy. Am J Ophthalmol. 1982;93:323.
40. LeFrancois M, Baum JL. *Flavobacterium* endophthalmitis following keratoplasty. Use of a tissue culture medium-stored cornea. Arch Ophthalmol. 1976;94:1907.
41. Gelender H. Bacterial endophthalmitis following cutting of sutures after cataract surgery. Am J Ophthalmol. 1982;94:528.
42. Bellows AR, McCulley JP. Endophthalmitis in aphakic patients with unplanned filtering blebs wearing contact lenses. Ophthalmology. 1981;88:839.
43. Swan KC, Campbell L. Unintentional filtration following cataract surgery. Arch Ophthalmol. 1964;71:43.
44. Ruiz, RS, Teeters VW. The vitreous wick syndrome. A late complication following cataract extraction. Am J Ophthalmol. 1970;70:483.
45. Allen HF. Recent advances in aseptic surgical technique. Trans Am Acad Ophthalmol Otolaryngol. 1960;64:493.
46. Sugar HS, Zekman T. Late infection of filtering conjunctival scar. Am J Ophthalmol. 1971;72:1097.
47. Meisler DM, Palestine AG, Vastine DW, et al. Chronic *Propionibacterium* endophthalmitis after extracapsular cataract extraction and intraocular lens implantation. Am J Ophthalmol. 1986;102:733.
48. Mason GI, Peyman GA, Jampol LM, et al. Peptostreptococcal endophthalmitis with a relapsing course. Arch Ophthalmol. 1978;96:1813.
49. Mason GI, Bottone EJ, Podos SM. Traumatic endophthalmitis caused by an *Erwinia* species. Am J Ophthalmol. 1976;82:709.
50. Lass JH, Thoft RA, Bellows AR, et al. Exogenous *Nocardia asteroides* endophthalmitis associated with malignant glaucoma. Ann Ophthalmol. 1981;13:317.
51. Affeldt JC, Flynn HW, Forster RK, et al. Microbial endophthalmitis resulting from ocular trauma. Ophthalmol. 1987;94:407.
52. Wetzel JO. Tetanus following eye injury. Report of a case: Review of literature. Am J Ophthalmol. 1942;25:933.
53. Muddappa TM, Rao RNS. Ocular tetanus. Indian J Ophthalmol. 1982;30:163.
54. Burns CL. Bilateral endophthalmitis in acute bacterial endocarditis. Am J Ophthalmol. 1979;88:809.
55. Jensen AD, Naidoff MA. Bilateral meningococcal endophthalmitis. Arch Ophthalmol. 1973;90:396.
56. Shammas HF. Endogenous *E. coli* endophthalmitis. Surv Ophthalmol. 1977;21:429.
57. Weinstein JM, Elliott J, Tilford RH. Metastatic endophthalmitis due to *Salmonella typhimurium*. Arch Ophthalmol. 1982;100:293.
58. Taylor JRW, Cibis GW, Hamtil LW. Endophthalmitis complicating *Haemophilus influenzae* type B meningitis. Arch Ophthalmol. 1980;98:324.
59. Hull DS, Patipa M, Cox F. Metastatic endophthalmitis: A complication of meningococcal meningitis. Ann Ophthalmol. 1982;14:29.
60. Gamel JW, Allansmith MR. Metastatic staphylococcal endophthalmitis presenting as chronic iridocyclitis. Am J Ophthalmol. 1974;77:454.
61. Rogers SJ, Johnson BL. Endogenous *Nocardia* endophthalmitis: Report of a case in a patient treated for lymphocytic lymphoma. Ann Ophthalmol. 1977;9:1123.
62. Nigrin J, Tyrrell DIJ, Jackson FL, et al. *Listeria monocytogenes* endophthalmitis in an immune-suppressed host. Can Med Assoc J. 1977;116:1378.
63. Bloomfield SE, David DS, Cheigh JS, et al. Endophthalmitis following staphylococcal sepsis in renal failure patients. Arch Intern Med. 1978;138:706.
64. Folk JC, Lobes LA Jr. Bacterial endophthalmitis and traumatic hyphema resulting from ocular injuries during dental procedures. Can J Ophthalmol. 1981;16:151.
65. May DR, Peyman GA, Raichand M, et al. Metastatic *Peptostreptococcus intermedius* endophthalmitis after a dental procedure. Am J Ophthalmol. 1978;85:662.
66. Weintraub MI, Otto RN. Pneumococcal meningitis and endophthalmitis in a newborn. JAMA. 1972;219:1763.
67. Berger BB. Endophthalmitis complicating neonatal group B streptococcal septicemia. Am J Ophthalmol. 1981;92:681.
68. Jain MR, Sharma HR. Puerperal sepsis leading to bilateral fulminating purulent endophthalmitis with tenonitis. Br J Ophthalmol. 1973;57:698.
69. Kerkenezov N. Panophthalmitis after a blood transfusion. Responsible organism *Bacillus cereus*. Br J Ophthalmol. 1953;37:632.
70. McLendon BF, Bron AJ, Mitchell CJ. *Streptococcus suis* type II (group R) as a cause of endophthalmitis. Br J Ophthalmol. 1978;62:729.
71. Massaro D, Katz S, Sachs M. Choroidal tubercles: A clue to hematogenous tubercles. *Ann Intern Med*. 1964;60:231.
72. Green WR. Uvea. In Spencer WH, ed. Ophthalmic Pathology. An Atlas and Textbook. v. 5. Philadelphia: WB Saunders; 1985:1352–2071.
73. Moore JE. Syphilitic iritis: A study of 249 patients. Am J Ophthalmol. 1931,14:110.
74. Jampol LM, Strauch BS, Albert DM. Intraocular nocardiosis. Am J Ophthalmol. 1973;76:568.
75. Meyer SL, Front RL, Shaver RP. Intraocular nocardiosis. Report of three cases. Arch Ophthalmol. 1970;83:536.
76. Green WR. Retina. In: Spencer WH, ed. Ophthalmic Pathology. An Atlas and Textbook. v. 2. Philadelphia: WB Saunders; 1985:589–1291.
77. Doft BH, Clarkson JG, Febell G, et al. Endogenous *Aspergillus* endophthalmitis in drug abusers. Arch Ophthalmol. 1980;98:859.
78. Elliott JH, O'Day DM, Gutow GS, et al. Mycotic endophthalmitis in drug abusers. Am J Ophthalmol. 1979;98:66.
79. Getnick RA, Rodrigues MM. Endogenous fungal endophthalmitis in a drug addict. Am J Ophthalmol. 1974;77:680.
80. Aguilar GL, Blumenkrantz MS, Egbert PR, et al. *Candida* endophthalmitis after intravenous drug abuse. Arch Ophthalmol. 1979;97:96.
81. Sugar HS, Mandell GH, Shalev J. Metastatic endophthalmitis associated with injection of addictive drugs. Am J Ophthalmol. 1971;71:1055.
82. Michelson JB, Freedman SD, Boyden DG. *Aspergillus* endophthalmitis in a drug abuser. Ann Ophthalmol. 1982;14:1051.
83. Dellon AL, Stark WJ, Chretien PB. Spontaneous resolution of endogenous *Candida* endophthalmitis complicating intravenous hyperalimentation. Am J Ophthalmol. 1978;79:648.
84. Henderson DK, Edwards JE, Montgomerie JZ. Hematogenous *Candida* endophthalmitis in patients receiving parenteral hyperalimentation fluids. J Infect Dis. 1981;143:655.
85. Freeman JB, Davis PL, MacLean LD. *Candida* endophthalmitis associated with intravenous hyperalimentation. Arch Surg. 1974;108:237.
86. François J, Rysselaere M. Oculomycoses. Springfield, MA: Charles C Thomas; 1972.
87. Fine BS, Zimmerman LE. Exogenous intraocular fungus infections: With particular reference to complications of intraocular surgery. Am J Ophthalmol. 1959;48:151.
88. McCray E, Rampell N, Solomon SL, et al. Outbreak of *Candida parapsilosis* endophthalmitis after cataract extraction and intraocular lens implantation. J Clin Microbiol. 1986;24:625.
89. Allen HF. Amphotericin B and exogenous mycotic endophthalmitis after cataract extraction. Arch Ophthalmol. 1972;88:640.
90. Pettit TH, Olson RJ, Foos RY, et al. Fungal endophthalmitis following intraocular lens implantation. Arch Ophthalmol. 1980;98:1025.
91. O'Day DM. Fungal endophthalmitis caused by *Paecilomyces lilacinus* after intraocular lens implantation. Am J Ophthalmol. 1977;83:130.
92. Landott E, Zuccoli A. Mycotic endophthalmitis after retinal surgery. Ophthalmologica. 1970;161:237.
93. Larsen PA, Lindstrom RL, Doughman DJ. *Torulopsis glabrata* endophthalmitis after keratoplasty with an organ-cultured cornea. Arch Ophthalmol. 1978;96:1019.
94. Rao GN, Aquavella JV. *Cephalosporium* endophthalmitis following penetrating keratoplasty. Ophthalmic Surg. 1979;10:34.
95. Foster JBJ, Almeda E, Liltman ML, et al. Some intraocular and conjunctival effects of amphotericin B in man and the rabbit. Arch Ophthalmol. 1958;60:555.
96. Theodore FH, Littman ML, Almeda E. Endophthalmitis following cataract extraction: Due to *Neurospora sitophila,* a so-called nonpathogenic fungus. Am J Ophthalmol. 1962;53:35.
97. Glassman MI, Henkind P, Alture-Werker E. *Monosporium apiospermum* endophthalmitis. Am J Ophthalmol. 1973;76:821.
98. Rosen R, Friedman AH. Successfully treated postoperative. *Candida parakrusei* endophthalmitis. Am J Ophthalmol. 1973;76:574.
99. Sheikh HA, Mahgoub S, Badi K. Postoperative endophthalmitis due to *Trichosporon cutaneum*. Br J Ophthalmol. 1974;58:591.
100. Miller GR, Rebell G, Magoon RC, et al. Intravitreal antimycotic therapy and the cure of mycotic endophthalmitis caused by a *Paecilomyces lilacinus* contaminated pseudophakos. Ophthalmic Surg. 1978;9:54.
101. Searl SS, Udell IJ, Sadun A, et al. *Aspergillus keratitis* with intraocular invasion. Ophthalmology. 1981;88:1244.
102. Rodrigues MM, MacLeod D. Exogenous fungal endophthalmitis caused by *Paecilomyces*. Am J Ophthalmol. 1975;79:687.
103. Elliott ID, Halde C, Shapiro J. Keratitis and endophthalmitis caused by *Petriellidium boydii*. Am J Ophthalmol. 1977;83:16.
104. Rowsey JJ, Acers TE, Smith DL, et al. *Fusarium oxysporum* endophthalmitis. Arch Ophthalmol. 1979;97:103.
105. Apostol JG, Meyer SL. *Graphium* endophthalmitis. Am J Ophthalmol. 1972;73:566.

106. McDonnell PJ, McDonnell JM, Brown RH, et al. Ocular involvement in patients with fungal infections. Ophthalmology. 1985;92:706.
107. Fishman LS, Griffin JR, Sapico FL, et al. Hematogenous *Candida* endophthalmitis: A complication of candidemia. N Engl J Med. 1972;286:675.
108. Griffin JR, Pettit TH, Fishman LS, et al. Bloodborne *Candida* endophthalmitis: A clinical and pathological study of 21 cases. Arch Ophthalmol. 1973;88:450.
109. Michelson PE, Stark WJ, Reeser F, et al. Endogenous *Candida* endophthalmitis: Report of 13 cases of 16 from the literature. In: Smith ME, ed. International Ophthalmology Clinics: Ocular Pathology. v. 2. Boston: Little, Brown; 1971:125.
110. Edwards JE Jr, Foos RY, Montgomerie JF, et al. Ocular manifestations of *Candida* septicemia: Review of seventy-six cases of hematogenous *Candida* endopthalmitis. Medicine (Baltimore). 1974;53:47.
111. Michelson PE, Rupp R, Efthimiadis B. Endogenous *Candida* endophthalmitis leading to bilateral corneal perforation. Am J Ophthalmol. 1975;80:800.
112. Cantrill HL, Rodman WP, Ramsay RC, et al. Postpartum *Candida* endophthalmitis JAMA. 1980;243:1163.
113. Baley JE, Annabele WL, Kliegman RM: *Candida* endophthalmitis in the premature infant. J Pediatr. 1981;98:458.
114. Clarkson JG, Green WR. Endogenous fungal endophthalmitis. In: Duane TD, ed. Clinical Ophthalmology. v. 4. Hagerstown, MD: Harper & Row, 1976.
115. Meyers BR, Lieberman TW, Ferry AP. *Candida* endophthalmitis complicating candidemia. Ann Intern Med. 1973;79:647.
116. Roney P, Barr CC, Chun CH, et al. Exogenous *Aspergillus* endophthalmitis. Rev Infect Dis. 1986;8:955.
117. Okun E, Butler WT. Ophthalmologic complications of cryptococcal meningitis. Arch Ophthalmol. 1964;71:52.
118. Blumenkranz MS, Stevens DS. Endogenous coccidioidal endophthalmitis. Ophthalmology 1980;87:974.
119. Bell R, Font RL. Granulomatous anterior uveitis caused by *Coccidioides immitis*. Am J Ophthalmol. 1972;74:93.
120. Cutler JE, Binder PS, Paul TO, et al. Metastatic coccidioidal endophthalmitis. Arch Ophthalmol. 1978;96:689.
121. Rainin EA, Little HL. Ocular coccidioidomycosis: A clinico-pathological case report. Trans Am Acad Ophthalmol Otolaryngol. 1972;76:645.
122. Glasgow BJ, Brown HH, Foos RV. Miliary retinitis in coccidioidomycosis. Am J Ophthalmol. 1987;104:24.
123. Cassady JR, Foerster HC. *Sporotrichum schenckii* endophthalmitis. Arch Ophthalmol. 1977;85:71.
124. Font RL, Spaulding AB, Green WR. Endogenous mycotic panophthalmitis caused by *Blastomyces dermatitidis*. Arch Ophthalmol. 1967;77:217.
125. Straatsma BR, Zimmerman LE, Gass JDM. Phycomycosis: A clinicopathologic study of fifty-one cases. Lab Invest. 1962;2:963.
126. Macular Photocoagulation Study Group. Argon laser photocoagulation for ocular histoplasmosis: Results of a randomized clinical trial. Arch Ophthalmol. 1983;101:1347.
127. Scholz R, Green WR, Kutys R, et al. *Histoplasma capsulatum* in the eye. Ophthalmology. 1984;91:1100.
128. Pavan-Langston D, Brockhurst RJ. Herpes simplex panuveitis. Arch Ophthalmol. 1969;81:783.
129. Bloom JN, Katz JI, Kaufman HE. Herpes simplex retinitis and encephalitis in an adult. Arch Ophthalmol. 1964;95:1798.
130. Cibis GW, Flynn JT, David EB. Herpes simplex retinitis. Arch Ophthalmol. 1978;96:299.
131. Partamian LG, Morse PH, Klein HZ. Herpes simplex type 1 retinitis in an adult with systemic herpes zoster. Am J Ophthalmol. 1981;92:215.
132. Uninsky E, Jampol LM, Kaufman S, et al. Disseminated herpes simplex infection with retinitis in a renal allograft recipient. Ophthalmology 1983;90:175.
133. Nahmias AJ, Hagler WS. Ocular manifestations of herpes simplex in the newborn (neonatal ocular herpes). In: Boniuk M, ed. Rubella and Other Intraocular Viral Diseases in Infancy. International Ophthalmology Clinics. v. 12. 1972:191.
134. Cibis A, Burde RM. Herpes simplex virus–induced congenital cataracts. Arch Ophthalmol. 1971;85:220.
135. Yanoff M, Allman FI, Fine BS. Congenital herpes simplex virus, type 2, bacterial endophthalmitis. Trans Am Ophthalmol Soc. 1977;75:325.
136. Minckler DS, McLean EB, Shaw CM, et al. *Herpesvirus hominis* encephalitis and retinitis. Arch Ophthalmol. 1976;94:89.
137. Cibis GW, Flynn JT, Davis EB. Herpes simplex retinitis. Arch Ophthalmol. 1978;94:299.
138. Schwartz JN, Cashwell F, Hawkins HK, et al. Necrotizing retinopathy with herpes zoster ophthalmicus: A light and electron microscopic study. Arch Pathol Lab Med. 1976;100:386.
139. Bartlett RE, Mumma CS, Irvine AR. Herpes zoster ophthalmicus with bilateral hemorrhagic retinopathy. Am J Ophthalmol. 1951;34:45.
140. Culbertson WW, Blumenkranz MS, Pepose JS, et al. Varicella zoster virus is a cause of the acute retinal necrosis syndrome. Ophthalmology. 1986;93:559.
141. Boniuk I. The cytomegaloviruses and the eye. Int Ophthalmol Clin. 1979;12:169.
142. Lonn LI. Neonatal cytomegalic inclusion disease chorioretinitis. Arch Ophthalmol. 1972;88:434.
143. deVenecia G, Zu Rhein GM, Pratt MV, et al. Cytomegalovirus retinitis in adults: A clinical, histopathologic, and ultrastructural study. Arch Ophthalmol. 1971;86:44.
144. Murray HW, Knox DL, Green WR, et al. Cytomegalovirus retinitis in adults: A manifestation of disseminated viral infection. Am J Ophthalmol. 1977;63:574.
145. Egbert PR, Pollard RB, Gallagher JG, et al. Cytomegalovirus retinitis in immunosuppressed hosts. II. Ocular manifestations. Ann Intern Med. 1980;93:664.
146. Smith ME. Retinal involvement in adult cytomegalic inclusion disease. Arch Ophthalmol. 1964;72:44.
147. Aaberg TM, Cesarz TJ, Rytel MW. Correlation of virology and clinical course of cytomegalovirus retinitis. Am J Ophthalmol. 1972;74:407.
148. Porter R. Acute necrotizing retinitis in a patient receiving immunosupressive therapy. Br J Ophthalmol. 1972;36:555.
149. Wyhinny GJ, Apple DJ, Guastella FR, et al. Adult cytomegalic inclusion retinitis. Am J Ophthalmol. 1973;76:773.
150. Newman NM, Mandel MR, Gullett J, et al. Clinical and histologic findings in opportunistic ocular infections. Arch Ophthalmol. 1983;101:396.
151. Holland GN, Gottlieb MS, Yee RD, et al. Ocular disorders associated with a new severe acquired cellular immunodeficiency syndrome. Am J Ophthalmol. 1982;93:393.
152. Astle JN, Ellis PP. Ocular complications in renal transplant patients. Ann Ophthalmol. 1974;6:1269.
153. Porter R, Crombie Al, Gardner PS, et al. Incidence of ocular complications in patients undergoing renal transplantation. Br Med J. 1972;3:133.
154. Scheie HG, Morse PH. Rubeola retinopathy. Arch Ophthalmol. 1972;88:341.
155. Robb RM, Walters GV. Ophthalmic manifestations of subacute sclerosing panencephalitis. Arch Ophthalmol. 1970;83:426.
156. La Piana FG, Tso MOM, Jenis EH. The retinal lesions of subacute sclerosing panencephalitis. Ann Ophthalmol. 1974;6:603.
157. Krill AE. Retinal disease of rubella. Arch Ophthalmol. 1967;77:445.
158. Perkins ES. Ocular toxoplasmosis. Br J Ophthalmol. 1973;57:1.
159. Molk R. Ocular toxocariasis: A review of the literature. Ann Ophthalmol. 1983;15:216.
160. Shields JA. Ocular toxocariasis. A review. Surv Ophthalmol. 1984;28:361.
161. Leopold IH. Is the dog really man's best friend? Am J Ophthalmol. 1965;59:717.
162. Perkins ES. Pattern of uveitis in children. Br J Opthalmol. 1966;50:169.
163. Wilkinson CP, Welch RB: Intraocular *Toxocara*. Am J Ophthalmol. 1971;71:921.
164. Bird AC, Smith JL, Curtin VT. Nematode optic neuritis. Am J Ophthalmol. 1970;69:72.
165. Smith PH, Greer CH. Unusual presentation of ocular *Toxocara* infestation. Br J Ophthalmol. 1971;55:317.
166. Schlaegel TF Jr, Knox DL. Uveitis and parasitoses. In: Duane TD, ed. Clinical Ophthalmology. v. 4. Hagerstown, MD: Harper & Row; 1976.
167. Gass JDM, Braunstein RA. Further observations concerning the diffuse unilateral subacute neuroretinitis syndrome. Arch Ophthalmol. 1983;101:1689.
168. Malik SRK, Gupta AK, Chounhry S. Ocular cysticercosis. Am J Ophthalmol. 1968;66:1168.
169. Topilow HW, Yimoyines DJ, Freeman HM, et al. Bilateral multifocal intraocular cysticercosis. Ophthalmology. 1981;88:1166.
170. Rapoza PA, Michels RG, Semeraro RJ, et al. Vitrectomy for excision of intraocular larva (*Hypoderma* species). Retina. 1986;6:99–104.
171. Aronson SB. Starch endophthalmitis. Am J Ophthalmol. 1972;73:570.
172. Stark WJ, Rosenblum P, Maumenee AE, et al. Postoperative inflammatory reactions to intraocular lenses sterilized with ethylene-oxide. Ophthalmology. 1980;87:385.
173. Forster RK, Zachary IG, Cottingham AJ Jr, et al. Further observations on the diagnosis, cause, and treatment of endophthalmitis. Am J Ophthalmol. 1976;81:52.
174. Forster RK, Abbott RL, Gelender H. Management of infectious endophthalmitis. Ophthalmology. 1980;87:313.
175. Engel HM, Green WR, Michels RG, et al. Diagnostic vitrectomy. Retina. 1981;1:121.
176. Engel H, de la Cruz ZC, Jimenes-Abalahin LD, et al. Cytopreparatory techniques for eye fluid specimens obtained by vitrectomy. Acta Cytol (Baltimore). 1982;26:551.
177. Stulting RD, Leif RC, Clarkson JG, et al. Centrifugal cytology of ocular fluids. Arch Ophthalmol. 1982;100:822.
178. Jones DB, Liesegang TJ, Robinson NM. Laboratory diagnosis of ocular infections. Cumitech. 1981;13:16.
179. Ellison AC. The limulus lysate test. A rapid test for diagnosis of *Pseudomonas* keratitis or endophthalmitis. Arch Ophthalmol. 1978;96:1268.
180. Shields JA, Lerner HA, Felberg NT. Aqueous cytology and enzymes in nematode endophthalmitis. Am J Ophthalmol. 1977;84:319.
181. Felberg NT, Shields JA, Federman JL. Antibody to *Toxocara canis* in the aqueous humor. Arch Ophthalmol. 1981;99:1563.
182. Searl SS, Moazed K, Albert DM, et al. Ocular toxocariasis presenting as leukocoria in a patient with low ELISA titer to *Toxocara canis*. Ophthalmology. 1981;88:1302.
183. Forster RK. Endophthalmitis. Diagnostic cultures and visual results. Arch Ophthalmol. 1974;92:387.
184. Baum JL. The treatment of bacterial endophthalmitis. Ophthalmology. 1978;83:350.
185. O'Day DM, Jones DB, Patrinely J, et al. *Staphylococcus epidermidis* en-

dophthalmitis. Visual outcome following noninvasive therapy. Ophthalmology. 1982;89:354.
186. Eichenbaum DM, Jaffe NS, Clayman HM, et al. Pars plana vitrectomy as a primary treatment for acute bacterial endophthalmitis. Am J Ophthalmol. 1978;86:167.
187. Diamond JG. Intraocular management of endophthalmitis. A systematic approach. Arch Ophthalmol. 1981;99:96.
188. Algvere P, Alanko H, Dickhoff K, et al. Pars plana vitrectomy in the management of intraocular inflammation. Acta Ophthalmol. 1981;59:727.
189. Peyman GA, Raichand M, Bennett TO. Management of endophthalmitis with pars plana vitrectomy. Br J Ophthalmol. 1980;64:474.
190. Baum J, Peyman GA, Barza M. Intravitreal administration of antibiotic in the treatment of bacterial endophthalmitis. III. Consensus. Surv Ophthalmol. 1982;26:204.
191. Schemmer GB, Dricke WJ. Post Traumatic *Bacillus cereus* endophthalmitis. Arch Ophthalmol. 1987;105:342.
192. Jones DB. Therapy of postsurgical fungal endophthalmitis. Ophthalmology. 1978;85:357.
193. Blumenkranz MS, Stevens DA. Therapy of endogenous fungal endophthalmitis. Miconazole or amphotericin B for coccidioidal and candidal infection. Arch Ophthalmol. 1980;98:1216.
194. Jones DB. Therapy of postsurgical fungal endophthalmitis. Ophthalmology. 1978;85:357.
195. Snip RC, Michels RG. Pars plana vitrectomy in the management of endogenous *Candida* endophthalmitis. Am J Ophthalmol. 1976;82:699.
196. Perraut LE Jr, Perraut LE, Bleiman B, et al. Successful treatment of *Candida albicans* endophthalmitis with intravitreal amphotericin B. Arch Ophthalmol. 1981;99:1565.
197. Axelrod AJ, Peyman GA, Apple DJ. Toxicity of intravitreal injection of amphotericin B. Am J Ophthalmol. 1973;76:578.
198. Souri EN, Green WR. Intravitreal amphotericin B toxicity. Am J Ophthalmol. 1974;78:77.
199. Naidoff MA, Green WR. Endogenous *Aspergillus* endophthalmitis occurring after kidney transplant. Am J Ophthalmol. 1975;79:502.
200. Grieco MH, Freilich DB, Louria DB. Diagnosis of cryptococcal uveitis with hypertonic media. Am J Ophthalmol. 1971;72:171.
201. Cameron ME, Harrison A. Ocular cryptococcosis in Australia: With a report of two further cases. Med J Austr. 1970;1:935.
202. Schlaegel TF Jr. Recent advances in uveitis. Ann Ophthalmol. 1972;4:525.
203. Jabs DA, Schachat AP, Liss R, et al. Presumed varicella zoster retinitis in immunocompromised patients. Retina. 1987;7:9.
204. Dorfman LJ. Cytomegalovirus encephalitis in adults. Neurology (Minn). 1973;23:136.
205. Henderly DE, Freeman WR, Causey DM, et al. Cytomegalovirus retinitis and response to therapy with ganciclovir. Ophthalmology. 1987;94:425.
206. Schlaegel TF Jr. Toxoplasmosis. In: Duane TD, ed. Clinical Ophthalmology. v. 4. Hagerstown, MD: Harper & Row; 1976:12.
207. Tabbara KF, O'Connor GR. Treatment of ocular toxoplasmosis with clindamycin and sulfadiazine. Ophthalmology. 1980;87:129.
208. Byers B, Kimura SJ. Uveitis after death of a larva in the vitreous cavity. Am J Ophthalmol. 1974;77:63.
209. Belmont JB, Irvine A, Benson W, et al. Vitrectomy in ocular toxocariasis. Arch Ophthalmol. 1982;100:1912.
210. Grand MG, Roper-Hall G. Pars Plana vitrectomy for ocular toxocariasis. Retina. 1981;1:258.
211. White AT, Newland HS, Taylor HR, et al. Controlled trial and dose-finding study of ivermectin for treatment of onchocerciasis. J Infect Dis. 1987;156:463.

101. PERIOCULAR INFECTIONS

L. NEAL FREEMAN
W. RICHARD GREEN

When considering infections involving periocular structures, the anatomic areas of concern are the eyelids, the components of the lacrimal apparatus, the orbit, and the paranasal and cavernous sinuses.

EYELIDS

Inflammations affecting the eyelids are commonly seen in an ophthalmologic practice. They include marginal blepharitis, hordeola (or sties), and chalazia. The eyelids show signs of inflammation very readily because the overlying skin is thin and the subcutaneous layer is composed of loose strands of connective tissue without fat. Bacteria are responsible for most infections of the eyelids, with *Staphylococcus* being the most common cause.[1]

The term *blepharitis* refers to inflammation of the lid margins and is usually chronic and bilateral. There are two main types: staphylococcal and seborrheic. The chief symptoms in both types are irritation of the eyes, a burning sensation, and itching of the lid margins.

Staphylococcal blepharitis is usually chronic and is manifested by hyperemia and small ulcerations of the lid margins, crusted exudate in the form of dry scales around the base of the lashes, and loss of the lashes. Although *Staphylococcus aureus* is the organism most commonly responsible, *Staphylococcus epidermidis* is increasingly being recognized as a cause of marginal blepharitis. Exotoxins elaborated by these bacteria may cause nonspecific conjunctivitis, inferior punctuate epithelial keratitis, and peripheral corneal infiltrates.[2] Associated seborrhea of the scalp and brows may be found. Acne rosacea is associated with a chronic blepharitis and occasional keratitis. Mascara use has been implicated in some cases of blepharitis.[3]

A *hordeolum* is a common acute purulent infection of the glands of the eyelids that is usually caused by *Staphylococcus*. Depending on the glands affected, a hordeolum can be classified into two types—internal and external.

An internal hordeolum is an infection of the meibomian glands, which are modified sebaceous glands located within the connective tissue tarsal plate of the lid. Hordeola may be associated with diffuse lid swelling, erythema, and tenderness. They may point toward the skin or the conjunctival surface of the lid.

An external hordeolum (or sty) is an infection of the glands of Zeis, which are small sebaceous glands connected with the follicles of the eyelashes, and the glands of Moll, which are apocrine sweat glands in the skin of the lid. External hordeola are smaller and more superficial than internal hordeola. They are discrete, elevated, erythematous tender pustules and point toward the skin surface of the lid, usually near the margin.

A *chalazion* is a nontender, sterile, chronic granulomatous inflammation of a meibomian gland and has a tendency to recur. It presents as a lid nodule and may begin with inflammation and tenderness similar to a hordeolum. However, a fully developed chalazion is differentiated from a hordeolum by the absence of acute inflammatory signs. If a chalazion becomes secondarily infected, signs of acute inflammation are evident. The majority of these lesions point toward the conjunctival surface of the lid, and they may be large enough to press on the globe and distort vision or be a cosmetic blemish. Since sebaceous gland carcinoma of the lid may be confused clinically with a chalazion, any recurrent chalazion should be examined histopathologically. The main histopathologic feature of a chalazion is a chronic granulomatous inflammatory reaction centered around clear spaces. These spaces represent areas of lipid material that are dissolved out during processing of the tissue.

If a chalazion ruptures through the tarsal conjunctiva, there may be an outgrowth of granulation tissue that results in a rapidly enlarging, painless, polypoid mass called a granuloma pyogenicum. Histopathologically it is composed of capillaries in a radiating pattern and is separated by a loose connective tissue with an acute and chronic inflammatory cell infiltrate.

Blepharitis and dermatitis may also be caused by molluscum contagiosum, herpes simplex virus,[4] *Pseudomonas*,[5] *Proteus mirabilis*,[6] and *Moraxella*[7] and may be secondary to contact allergies caused by agents such as cosmetics[8] and eye drops. The role of the hair follicle mites *Demodex folliculorum* and *D. brevis* in disease of the lids is unclear.[9–11] *Phthirus pubis* (pubic lice) may cause an irritating bloody blepharitis and is commonly transmitted as a venereal disease.[12]

LACRIMAL APPARATUS

The lacrimal apparatus has two major functions. The main lacrimal gland (located anteriorly in the superotemporal quadrant of the orbit) and the accessory lacrimal glands of Krause and Wolfring (located in the conjunctiva) produce the aqueous component of the tear film. The lacrimal puncta, the superior and inferior canaliculi, the common canaliculus, the lacrimal sac, and the nasolacrimal duct are concerned with the drainage of tears from the conjunctival cul-de-sac and tear lake to the nasal cavity. Pathologic processes affecting the main and the accessory lacrimal glands result in diminished tear production, whereas those affecting the lacrimal drainage apparatus cause obstruction resulting in epiphora (or "tearing").

Canaliculitis is a low-grade chronic inflammation in the canaliculi, that is usually due to infection from the anaerobic, gram-positive filamentous organisms *Actinomyces* or *Arachnia propionica*.[13] Other organisms that may be responsible include *Pityrosporum pachydermatis*,[14] *Fusobacterium*,[15] *Enterobacter cloacae*,[16] *Nocardia asteroides, Candida albicans*, and *Aspergillus niger*.[17] Viruses implicated in canaliculitis include herpes simplex,[18–20] herpes zoster,[18,19] and vaccinia.[19] Inflammation leads to obstruction of the lumen of the canaliculus,[21] which results in epiphora, chronic conjunctivitis, and a tender swollen nasal lid margin that may go undiagnosed for years. Typically, the punctum has a slightly distended appearance. In cases due to *Arachnia*, a gritty sensation is felt when the canaliculus is probed.

Dacryocystitis is inflammation of the lacrimal sac. It is clinically useful to divide dacryocystitis into chronic and acute forms. Chronic dacryocystitis is usually caused by a single site of partial or complete obstruction within the lacrimal sac or within the nasolacrimal duct. The infection is usually the result and not the cause of obstruction.

There are many causes of obstruction. In about 5 percent of all newborns the distal end of the nasolacrimal duct is not patent at birth, but in most cases there is spontaneous opening of the duct during the first few days or weeks of life.[22,23]

True congenital lacrimal sac mucoceles are uncommon and may require early probing.[24] Trauma causing fractures in the nasoethmoid region may obstruct the drainage system at the junction of the lacrimal sac and the nasolacrimal duct. Infection of the lacrimal sac by *Aspergillus, Candida albicans*, or *Actinomyces* may occur. With partial or complete obstruction of the nasolacrimal duct, a laminated concretion (dacryolith) may develop in the lacrimal sac and often is associated with bacterial and fungal infections.[25] Benign and malignant tumors of the lacrimal sac may cause obstruction of the outflow system. Obstruction in the area of the sac–duct junction from a silicone implant used for an orbital floor fracture repair has been reported; a chronic dacryocystitis developed.[26] Foreign bodies such as wood or cilia are rare causes of obstruction of the drainage apparatus.

Streptococcus pneumoniae is most commonly isolated from cases of chronic dacryocystitis. However, a mixed infection with *Staphylococcus, Streptococcus*, and *Pseudomonas aeruginosa* can occur, Sarcoidosis[27,28] and *Chlamydia trachomatis*[29] may cause a chronic recurrent dacryocystitis.

Epiphora is usually the only clinical finding in patients with chronic dacryocystitis. On palpation of the tear sac area, a mucoid discharge may be expressed through the lacrimal puncta.

Acute dacryocystitis occurs when both the proximal and distal ends of the drainage system become partially or totally obstructed. The obstruction may be due to trauma, dacryoliths acting as ball valves, or the flare-up of a chronic dacryocystitis or lacrimal sac sarcoidosis. The major symptom in patients with acute dacryocystitis is pain in the tear sac area. Erythema and swelling of the lacrimal sac area, a purulent discharge, and epiphora are signs of acute dacryocystitis. On palpation, tenderness in the tear sac area is present, and purulent material can be expressed in a retrograde fashion through the lacrimal puncta. A serious complication of acute dacryocystitis is orbital cellulitis (see below).[30,31] This occurs if the inflammatory process involving the lacrimal sac spreads posterior to the orbital septum; this is more likely in older patients with attenuated septa.[30] Marginal corneal ulcers have been described in β-streptococcal dacryocystitis.[32]

The common pathogens in acute dacryocystitis are *Staphylococcus aureus* and *Haemophilus influenzae* in children.[30]

Histopathologic study of bone from the area adjacent to the lacrimal sac showed normal bone in approximately one-half of patients undergoing dacryocystorhinostomy for acute or chronic dacryocystitis in a recent study. The other half of the bone samples revealed evidence of bone remodeling or woven bone, but no inflammation was present. The periosteum of the lacrimal fossa may help prevent bony changes in dacryocystitis.[33]

Dacryoadenitis refers to inflammation of the main lacrimal gland. Acute bacterial infections of the gland are uncommon. Infection may occur from an exogenous site on the skin, or the gland may be seeded during a bacteremia. Local trauma is a predisposing factor. The palpebral lobe of the gland is more frequently involved than is the orbital lobe.[34] Pyogenic bacteria such as *Staphylococcus aureus* and streptococci are often implicated as causes. Rarely, gonococcal bacteremia may result in an acute dacryoadenitis. *Cysticercus cellulosae* dacryoadenitis has been reported.[35] Viral infections of the lacrimal gland cause acute inflammation and usually occur in children. The two viral diseases that most often involve the gland are mumps[36] and infectious mononucleosis.[37] Clinically inapparent infection of the lacrimal gland may occur with cytomegalovirus, coxsackievirus A, echoviruses, or herpes zoster virus infections.[38] Patients with acute dacryoadenitis complain of severe pain in the lacrimal gland region, and signs of inflammation including erythema of overlying skin, swelling, and tenderness on palpation of this region are noted. Ocular motility defects such as combined abduction and elevation deficiency or isolated abduction deficiency may be seen.[34,39] In some cases (particularly in children), fever and leukocytosis occur.[38]

Chronic infections of the lacrimal gland may occur in tuberculosis,[40] syphilis, leprosy, and schistosomiasis.[41] Clinically, painless enlargement of one or both lacrimal glands may occur, and signs of acute inflammation are not present. Similar clinical features may be present in sarcoidosis.[42]

Fungal infections that may involve the lacrimal gland include blastomycosis, histoplasmosis, nocardiosis, and sporotrichosis.[38]

ORBIT AND CAVERNOUS SINUS

Orbital cellulitis is an acute infection of the orbital contents. It is most commonly caused by bacteria, although it may be caused by fungi in debilitated patients. It is a serious infection because of the risk of visual loss and the possibility of posterior spread to involve the cavernous sinus, which may lead to thrombosis and death.

There are many causes of orbital cellulitis. Most cases occur by spread from contiguous structures such as the paranasal sinuses. The potentially serious nature of this condition is frequently underestimated.[43] Any of the sinuses may be involved. The lamina papyracea separating the ethmoid air cells from the orbit is thin and may permit the spread of infection. Congenital or traumatic breaks may further compromise this barrier. Additionally, the anterior and posterior ethmoidal foramina allow communication between the sinus and orbit. The bones separating the frontal and maxillary sinuses from the orbit are also thin. In children, since the ethmoid sinuses are the first to pneumatize, ethmoiditis is the most common source.[45–48] In one large series, 84 percent of the children with orbital cellulitis had roentgenographic evidence of sinusitis. This sinusitis was bilateral in almost half the cases.[49] In adults, a frontal sinusitis is a common cause.

Direct inoculation of organisms may occur after puncture wounds to the orbit when they perforate the orbital septum. Retained orbital foreign bodies are another source of infection.[50] Orbital cellulitis may occur as a complication of orbital fractures, even in the absence of adjacent sinusitis.[51] Certain surgical procedures can rarely cause orbital infections. These include exploration for orbital tumors, retinal reattachment procedures, and strabismus operations.[52,53] Foreign materials such as sutures, encircling ocular bands, and sponges may serve as the nidus in postoperative orbital infections, and such materials must be removed to eliminate the infection. Acute dacryocystitis[30,51,54] or posterior perforation of the lacrimal sac during therapeutic probing may result in orbital cellulitis. Rare cases from bites by house pets and rats have been reported.[55] Dental and intracranial infections may extend into the orbit and produce an orbital cellulitis.

In adults, infection of the orbit by blood-borne bacterial metastases from a distant site is extremely rare. In children, however, orbital cellulitis may develop secondarily to a bacteremia caused by *Haemophilus influenzae*.[47] *Enterococcus (Streptococcus) faecalis* causing a bacteremia with the subsequent development of orbital cellulitis has also been reported.[56] Systemic diseases that may result in orbital infection include influenza, subacute bacterial endocarditis, scarlet fever, vaccinia, herpes simplex, and herpes zoster.[44] In newborns, intrauterine infections have been implicated in the causation of orbital cellulitis.[57] Anaerobes are frequently present in cases of chronic sinusitis and should be suspected in orbital cellulitis associated with long-standing sinus disease. Multiple anaerobic strains may be found.[58,59] Trauma with resultant inoculation of earthen material is a cause of orbital cellulitis due to *Clostridium perfringens*.[60]

The bacteria most commonly causing orbital cellulitis are *Staphylococcus aureus, Streptococcus pyogenes,* and *Streptococcus pneumoniae*.[47,48] Of these, *Staphylococcus* is the most common etiologic agent. However, given the variability of organisms found on the skin and conjunctiva and from foreign bodies, a mixed infection is usual. In children under 5 years of age, *H. influenzae* is the most common cause.[61] Anaerobic organisms found in infected paranasal sinuses can also cause orbital cellulitis.[58] If crepitation is present, the possibility of cellulitis secondary to clostridial organisms should be considered.[62,63] In patients receiving immunosuppressive drugs, atypical mycobacteria may rarely cause orbital cellulitis.[64]

Regardless of the source of the infection, many of the symptoms and signs of orbital cellulitis are distinctive. However, in some cases it may be difficult to establish an early diagnosis. For example, after severe injuries, hemorrhage and edema in the lids and orbit may prevent early recognition of the signs of infection. Likewise, nonseptic inflammation after intraorbital surgical procedures often mimics bacterial cellulitis by the presence of lid edema, chemosis, orbital edema, and restricted ocular motion. These factors may cause a delay in diagnosis. Therefore, it is imperative that the clinician maintain a high index of suspicion of the possibility of infection in such cases. After trauma, symptoms and signs of orbital cellulitis usually begin within 48 to 72 hours. However, occasionally a retained intraorbital foreign body may reveal signs of infection only several months later.

Fever, lid edema, and rhinorrhea are the most frequent early signs. They are followed by orbital pain, tenderness on palpation of the lids, and headache. Vision is usually normal during the early stages. As the infection progresses, the lids acquire a dark red discoloration and increased warmth. Conjunctival hyperemia, chemosis, and proptosis follow. The direction of proptosis may help to indicate the primary site of involvement in the orbit. There is limitation of ocular motility, with pain on attempted motion and increased resistance to retropulsion of the globe. Increased intraocular pressure, reduced corneal sensation, congestion of retinal veins, and chorioretinal striae may be present later in the course of the infection. In severe cases of orbital cellulitis, gangrene and sloughing of the lids have been reported.[65] Acute infarction of the choroid and retina from involvement of the posterior ciliary vessels and ophthalmic artery may rarely occur.[66] A leukocytosis with a WBC count greater than 15,000/mm^3 is usually present.

A different clinical course is seen in "posterior" orbital cellulitis.[67] These patients manifest an orbital apex syndrome in which profound visual loss and ophthalmoplegia develop with minimal external inflammatory signs.[67–69] This condition occurs as a result of contiguous spread into the orbit from an adjacent sphenoidal and/or ethmoidal sinusitis. The cause of visual loss in posterior orbital cellulitis is probably vascular compromise, but vasculitis of the optic nerve vasculature may also be of etiologic importance.[67,68] In the few cases reported, the visual loss has been almost uniformly irreversible. Posterior orbital cellulitis is less common than is orbital cellulitis; this is probably because of the thicker bony barrier and the more firmly attached periosteum of the posterior orbit.[67]

Preseptal and postseptal (orbital) cellulitis secondary to paranasal sinusitis may be classified into five clinical stages.[70] In the first stage (preseptal cellulitis), bacteria are not present within the orbit, but inflammatory orbital edema produced by the proximity of a suppurative sinusitis is present. During the second stage there is direct extension through bone, with infiltration of the orbital contents by bacteria and inflammatory cells. The third stage occurs after the infection has extended beneath bone, thereby leading to formation of a subperiosteal abscess. The fourth stage is reached when the infection within the orbit consolidates as an abscess. This may be clinically verifiable by the subcutaneous induration of the lids, as mentioned above, and by fluctuance in the orbit that is detectable on retropulsion of the globe. This is quite unlike the usual loss of resiliency and the difficulty in retropulsion that accompanies orbital cellulitis without abscess formation. Occasionally, the abscess may rupture through the orbital septum and present beneath the skin of the lid.[71] The fifth, or final, stage is that of cavernous sinus thrombosis.

Before antibiotics became available, about 19 percent of the patients with orbital cellulitis died of intracranial complications. About 20 percent of the patients were blinded in the involved eye, and an additional 13 percent suffered some visual loss from the infection.[72] Additional complications include osteomyelitis, strabismus, an afferent pupillary defect, a chronic draining sinus, and a scarred upper eyelid.[73] With antibiotic therapy, the prognosis in cases of orbital cellulitis has markedly improved.

Tuberculous involvement of the orbit is very rare, occurs by a hematogenous route, and is unassociated with miliary tuberculosis.[74] The patients are apparently healthy, without pulmonary disease or other signs of systemic tuberculosis.

Syphilitic gummas in the orbit are rare. They may occur in the extraocular muscles, the orbital nerves, and the optic nerve.[75]

The two most common fungal infections causing orbital infection are mucormycosis (Chapter 237) and aspergillosis (Chapter 236). Conditions predisposing to orbital mucormycosis and the clinical and pathologic features of the infection have been well described.[76–81]

The *Aspergillus* organism is an opportunistic fungus that is common in the air of many localities. The infection develops in a sinus and rarely spreads to the orbit.[82,83] Chronic sinus aspergillosis usually occurs in persons who are 40–60 years of age and who have a chronically obstructed sinus due to allergic diathesis, a deviated nasal septum, or nasal polyps. There appears to be a geographic factor related to humidity.[84] A similar syndrome produced by *Bipolaris, Curvularia,* and *Drechslera* species appears to be geographically disperse. Orbital infection with these fungi in the normal host is a slowly progressive, granulomatous, fibrosing disease. Thus, patients may be asymptomatic for extended periods of time, and the duration of symptoms may range from several months to 16 years. The chief symptoms and signs are ocular pain, decreased vision, and unilateral proptosis. The fibrosing nature of the granulomatous inflammation in the orbit may cause optic nerve damage with optic disk swelling, venous engorgement, and central retinal artery occlusion. Other signs of inflammation—such as lid edema, chemosis, fever, and leukocytosis—are usually absent.

Aspergillosis in the sinus of an immunosuppressed patient is typically an acute infection resembling mucormycosis.[83] As a third clinical form, *Aspergillus* may form a fungus ball in a chronically obstructed maxillary sinus without invading the sinus lining.

Orbital infections caused by other fungi[85–88] and parasites[76,89–96] are rare.

The nematode *Trichinella spiralis* may invade the extraocular muscles and result in periorbital edema and pain on movement of the eyes.[92]

Orbital inflammation may be due to a wide variety of noninfectious causes. The differential diagnosis of orbital inflammation has been well reviewed.[97]

Cavernous sinus thrombosis may be difficult to distinguish from mucormycosis and orbital cellulitis. Most often, cavernous sinus thrombosis results from blood-borne infection from the face, nasal cavity, paranasal sinuses, and ear.[98,99] It may also occur as a rare complication of orbital cellulitis.[100,101] Evidence of orbital infection was found in all of six cases of cavernous sinus thrombosis that came to autopsy in one series.[102] This suggests that although orbital cellulitis often occurs without involvement of the cavernous sinus most cases of cavernous sinus thrombosis will have coinvolvement of the orbit.[103] Aseptic thrombosis of the sinus is uncommon, and it usually follows surgical and/or nonsurgical trauma.[104]

The symptoms and signs of cavernous sinus thrombosis are graver than those of orbital cellulitis. The early onset of internal and external ophthalmoplegia is a suggestive feature. Decreased sensation about the eye, indicating involvement of the trigeminal nerve, and signs of bilaterality with paretic muscles in the contralateral eye are strong evidence of cavernous sinus thrombosis. Altered consciousness and other signs of meningitis indicate the seriousness of this clinical entity.

LABORATORY FEATURES

Patients with blepharitis may often be more symptomatic than the clinical findings seem to warrant. In such cases, bacteriologic culture of the lid margins may reveal a dense population of *Staphylococcus*.

In canaliculitis from *Arachnia* the recovery of concretions is diagnostic. Gram stain will demonstrate gram-positive filamentous organisms. Fluorescein-labeled antisera may aid in diagnosis.[13] Cultures should be obtained for confirmation, but the organisms may be difficult to isolate.[13]

When obstruction of the lacrimal drainage system is suspected, several procedures are available to evaluate its patency. When the drainage apparatus is fully patent, 2% fluorescein dye instilled in the conjunctival sac may usually be collected on a nasal applicator passed beneath the inferior turbinate (Jones I test). If no dye is recovered, the fornices are irrigated to remove residual fluorescein. The nasolacrimal sac is then cannulated and irrigated with saline (Jones II test). If dye is recovered with the Jones II test when none could be recovered with the Jones I test, a partial nasolacrimal duct obstruction is probably present. Probing of the lacrimal passages may provide information regarding the site of the obstruction.

Several other techniques have been devised to assess the patency and status of the lacrimal drainage system. Thermography, a process by which body surface temperatures are recorded in the form of thermal images, has been used to study lacrimal system obstructions and inflammations.[105,106] Inflammation induces hyperthermia, and canaliculitis and acute dacryocystitis may be demonstrated by comparisons to a normal contralateral side. Radiographic studies that have been used to evaluate the patency of the drainage system include plain film dacryocystography with contrast injection (distension dacryocystography), macrodacryocystography, scintillography, and tomography (including computed tomography).[107–109] Computed tomography of the outflow system after topical instillation of a contrast agent is useful as a physiologic test with good anatomic resolution.[109]

In cases of orbital cellulitis, the isolation of the causative agent is often difficult because external drainage is often absent, aspiration of fluid from the orbit is contraindicated (unless an abscess is present), and results of efforts to isolate organisms in periorbital and orbital cellulitis are variable. The assistance of an otolaryngologist is essential in the management of this infection because infectious sinusitis is the most common cause of orbital cellulitis. Careful clinical examination of the sinuses with microbiologic investigation of purulent material obtained from the nasopharynx, nasal mucosa, and conjunctiva is important. Blood cultures are essential and are most likely to be positive in children under 5 years of age with periorbital cellulitis associated with an upper respiratory tract infection.[48] Microbiologic investigation should consist of Gram and PAS stains and inoculation of blood agar, chocolate agar, Sabouraud agar and thioglycollate broth, and reduced blood agar in an anaerobic environment.

Ultrasonography is useful in the diagnosis of orbital cellulitis and orbital abscess. B-scan ultrasound may indicate fingerlike clear areas in the retrobulbar space in cases of cellulitis, and an abscess may be manifested as an area of low or medium reflectivity.[44] Plain orbital and sinus films are helpful in these cases and may show sinus opacification, air–fluid levels, bony abnormalities, or foreign bodies.

Computed tomography (CT) is the technique providing the most important information in patients with suspected orbital cellulitis with or without abcess formation.[44,110] Studies with and without contrast agent with multiple sections and views should be obtained when feasible. A correlation of CT findings with the clinical stages of orbital cellulitis mentioned previously has been recently proposed.[110] In stage II disease (orbital cellulitis without abcess), a low-density fluid collection is present between the periosteum and the adjacent rectus muscle. In stage III (subperiosteal abcess), the periosteum is elevated and the rectus muscle displaced by an abscess defined by an enhancing periosteal border. An orbital abscess (stage IV) is manifested by a homogeneous, heterogeneous, or ringlike mass within the orbital space.[111] CT will also delineate sinus and bony abnormalities and most orbital foreign bodies. Orbital venography may show attenuation of the superior ophthalmic vein from increased orbital pressure, which is compatible with cellulitis.

In cases of suspected cavernous sinus thrombosis, any of a number of diagnostic studies may be helpful. Carotid arteriography is of diagnostic usefulness, but is potentially dangerous. Orbital venography is effective in the region of the cavernous sinus, and modification of this technique by digital subtraction has also been used to diagnose thrombosis.[112] Contrast-enhanced computed tomography has been beneficial in some cases of cavernous sinus thrombosis.[103,113,114] It has recently been suggested that high-field magnetic resonance imaging may be the neuroimaging modality of choice in cases of suspected cavernous sinus thrombosis.[115] The cerebrospinal fluid will often show pleocytosis with an abundance of polymorphonuclear cells and an increased protein level.[103] Cultures of the cerebrospinal fluid, although, are often negative in cases of cavernous sinus thrombosis. Blood cultures are usually positive.[116]

In cases of mucormycosis, positive cultures are often difficult to obtain, and the diagnosis is usually made by histologic examination of excised tissue. Otolaryngologic consultation is necessary, and a biopsy and scraping samples from any necrotic area of the nasal mucosa or palate are essential. On tissue sections, nonseptate branching hyphae that are large (6–20 μm wide) and irregularly thick are found. A mainly acute suppurative inflammatory response is usually seen, although sometimes a granulomatous response is present at the sites of thrombosis and in surrounding necrotic tissues.

TREATMENT

In staphylococcal blepharitis, the use of a topical antibiotic (bacitracin, sulfacetamide, or erythromycin) or antibiotics/steroid combination ointment and lid scrubs with or without diluted shampoo applied to the lid margins may decrease lid inflammation.[117] Resistant cases or those associated with acne rosacea may benefit from the long-term, low-dose use of oral tetracyclines. Topical steroid drops are occasionally used to decrease ocular surface inflammation.

Any internal or external hordeolum should be treated with topical antibiotics and warm compresses until the inflammation subsides. The use of systemic antibiotics is rarely indicated, and surgical drainage is rarely required.

Because most chalazia seldom subside spontaneously and they show chronic or subacute inflammation, surgical curettage and excision may be done on chalazia. However, simple observation is reasonable because they tend to decrease in size with time. The use of intralesional corticosteroids has been suggested. *Phthirus pubis* may be treated by manual epilation of involved lashes together with the use of gamma benzene hexachloride shampoo on the body hair of the patient and that of other family members and sexual contacts.[12] In more widely involved cases, the application of a pediculocide—such as yellow mercuric oxide twice a day for a week, 0.25% physostigmine ointment twice a day for 10 days, or 20% fluorescein topically—may be used.[118]

The value of topical antiviral ointment to treat ulcerative herpes simplex blepharitis is unclear, although a short course of trifluridine or vidarabine ointment is reasonable in an effort to prevent inoculation of the ocular surface with herpes simplex virus.

Antibiotic irrigation of the canaliculi combined with topical antibiotic eyedrops is useful in the treatment of canaliculitis. Penicillin G (160,000 units/ml as an irrigant, 60,000 units/ml as drops) is used for *Arachnia* and *Actinomyces;* amphotericin B (1–5 mg/ml) is used against *Candida* and *Aspergillus*.[17] Systemic penicillin, erythromycin, or cephalosporins should be part of the treatment regimen in cases due to *Arachnia*.[17,119] When concretions are present, they should be removed by canaliculotomy and curettage. The canaliculus should then be reconstructed; silicone intubation may be needed.[120] Cases of canalicular obstruction associated with herpes simplex virus infection may require surgical intervention more frequently than in cases caused by bacteria. A possible explanation is that, in the situation with herpes, the epithelial lining of the canaliculi is damaged with resultant adherence of the subepithelial layers with scar formation. In the cases of bacterial infection, however, the epithelium remains intact, and the obstruction is due to edema, which is more reversible.[20]

Parents of infants with nasolacrimal duct obstruction should be taught to firmly massage the lacrimal sac area several times daily. Topical antibiotic eyedrops may be used for lid mattering. If symptoms persist for 6–8 months, the lacrimal drainage apparatus should be irrigated and probed. Probing is more successful in cases of lacrimal duct obstruction due to membranous obstruction than in cases due to narrowing of the duct. If probing is unsuccessful, repeat probing is done a few months later. Silicone intubation of the drainage apparatus is performed if the repeat probing also fails to succeed.[23]

In adults with acute dacryocystitis, treatment with warm compresses and systemic antibiotics should be given. If β-hemolytic streptococci are isolated or suspected, oral penicillin is used.[17] Staphylococci are best treated with a penicillinase-resistant penicillin.[17,30] After the acute infection is controlled, the patient should be taught to perform digital massage of the lacrimal sac, and topical antibiotic drops should be used. If epiphora persists, a dacryocystorhinostomy is performed in most cases to obtain adequate tear drainage.

Bacterial dacryoadenitis is treated with systemic antibiotics. If an orbital abscess forms, surgical drainage is necessary.

In treating orbital cellulitis, intravenous antibiotics and decongestion of the paranasal sinuses are vital. The bacterial agents most commonly responsible for this infection were mentioned above. In adults, nafcillin or oxacillin (1.5 g) every 4 hours should be the initial therapy. In cases of penicillin allergy, cefotaxime (if the allergic response was nonanaphylactic), clindamycin, chloramphenicol, or vancomycin may be substituted.[73,121] Because *H. influenzae* is the most common cause of orbital cellulitis in young children, ampicillin (200 mg/kg/day in divided doses) should be given intravenously along with nafcillin or oxacillin (100 mg/kg/day). If *H. influenzae* is isolated, it should be tested for sensitivity to ampicillin. A third-generation cephalosporin, such as cefotaxime or ceftriaxone, or chloramphenicol (100 mg/kg/day) is used in cases of suspected or confirmed resistance to ampicillin.[70,121,122] Methods of sinus decongestion include nasal sprays, oral decongestants, and oral antihistamines. If the sinusitis persists, surgical drainage of the sinuses should be performed. If the infection progresses and the clinical situation deteriorates despite adequate intravenous antibiotic therapy, it is probably due to the development of a subperiosteal or orbital abscess, and surgical drainage is imperative.[46–48] Material obtained from such drainage should have the complete microbiologic evaluation mentioned previously. In cases of radiographically suspected subperiosteal abscess that seem to be responding to conservative measures, surgery may be deferred, but inflammatory signs may persist much longer than in those patients treated by drainage.[110,123,124]

If the management of patients with orbital mucormycosis is to be successful, the combined efforts of internists, mycologists, otolaryngologists, and ophthalmologists are essential. The underlying disease, for example, diabetic ketoacidosis, should be treated. Intravenous amphotericin B is of value if begun early in the disease.[125,126] The drug may also be injected directly into the involved orbital, paranasal, or pharyngeal tissues, although the value of this type of regional therapy has not been proved.[127] Surgical débridement of devitalized tissue is extremely important. Frequently the involved eye may need to be sacrificed to obtain adequate orbital débridement.

In the treatment of chronic orbital aspergillosis, surgical excision appears to be the best method. Amphotericin B is only of ancillary help.

Cavernous sinus thrombosis is treated with high-dose intravenous antibiotics. Corticosteroids have been used successfully in this entity.[103,128] The role of anticoagulants is still unclear.[98,129,130]

REFERENCES

1. Smolin G, Okumoto M. Staphylococcal blepharitis. Arch Ophthalmol. 1977;95:812.
2. Valenton MJ, Okumoto M. Toxin-producing strains of *Staphylococcus epidermidis* (*albus*). Isolates from patients with staphylococcic blepharoconjunctivitis. Arch Ophthalmol. 1973;89:186.
3. Wilson LA, Julian AJ, Ahearn DG. The survival and growth of microorganisms in mascara during use. Am J Ophthalmol. 1975;79:596.
4. Egerer I, Stary A. Erosive-ulcerative herpes simplex blepharitis. Arch Ophthalmol. 1980;98:1760.
5. Rosenoff SH, Wolfe ML, Chabner BA. *Pseudomonas* blepharoconjunctivitis. A complication of combination chemotherapy. Arch Ophthalmol. 1974;90:490.
6. Parunovic A. *Proteus mirabilis* causing necrotic inflammation of the eyelid. Am J Ophthalmol. 1973;76:543.

7. van Bijsterveld OP. The incidence of *Moraxella* on mucous membranes and the skin. Am J Ophthalmol. 1972;74:72.
8. van Ketel WG, Liem DH. Eyelid dermatitis from nickel contaminated cosmetics. Contact Dermatitis. 1981;4:217.
9. Rufli T, Mumcuoglu Y. The hair follicle mites *Demodex folliculorum* and *Demodex brevis:* Biology and medical importance. A review. Dermatologica. 1981;162:1.
10. Roth AM. *Demodex folliculorum* in hair follicles of eyelid skin. Ann Ophthalmol. 1979;11:37.
11. Gutgesell VJ, Stern GA, Hood CI. Histopathology of meibomian gland dysfunction. Am J Ophthalmol. 1982;94:383.
12. Couth JM, Green WR, Hirst LW, et al. Diagnosing and treating *Phthirus pubis palpebrarum.* Surv Ophthalmol. 1982;26:219.
13. Hirst LW, Merz WB, Kaufmann CS, et al. *Actinomyces/Arachnia* lacrimal canaliculitis. Cornea. 1982;1:259.
14. Romano A, Segal E, Blumenthal M. Canaliculitis with isolation of *Pityrosporum pachydermatis*. Br. J Ophthalmol. 1978;62:732
15. Weinberg RJ, Sartoris MJ, Buerger GF Jr, et al. *Fusobacterium* in presumed *Actinomyces* canaliculitis. Am J Ophthalmol. 1977;84:371
16. Chumbley LC. Canaliculitis caused by *Enterobacter cloacae:* Report of a case. Br J Ophthalmol. 1984;68:364–6.
17. Starr MB. Lacrimal drainage system infections. In: Smith BC, Della Rocca RC, Nesi FA, et al, eds. Ophthalmic Plastic and Reconstructive Surgery. St Louis: CV Mosby; 1987:947–5.
18. Bouzas A. Canalicular inflammation in ophthalmic cases of herpes zoster and herpes simplex. Am J Ophthalmol. 1965;60:713–6.
19. Bouzas AG. Virus aetiology of certain cases of lacrimal obstruction. Br J Ophthalmol. 1973;57:849–51.
20. Harris GJ, Hyndiuk RA, Fox MJ, et al. Herpetic canalicular obstruction. Arch Ophthalmol. 1981;99:282–3.
21. Wolter JR. *Pityrosporum* species associated with dacryoliths in obstructive dacryocystitis. Am J Ophthalmol. 1977;84:806.
22. Korchmaros I, Szalay E. Cannula-probing combined with nasal procedure for dacryocystitis neonatorum. Acta Ophthalmol. 1978;56:357.
23. Kushner BJ. Congenital nasolacrimal system obstruction. Arch Ophthalmol. 1982;100:597.
24. Weinstein GS, Biglan AW, Patterson JH. Congenital lacrimal sac mucoceles. Am J Ophthalmol. 1982;94:106.
25. Berlin AJ, Rath R, Rich L. Lacrimal system dacryoliths. Ophthalmic Surg. 1980;11:435.
26. Mauriello JA, Fiore PM, Kotch M. Dacryocystitis—late complication of orbital floor fracture repair with implant. Ophthalmology. 1987;94:248–50.
27. Harris GJ, Williams GA, Clarke GP. Sarcoidosis of the lacrimal sac. Arch Ophthalmol. 1981;99:1198.
28. Coleman SL, Brull S, Green WR. Sarcoid of the lacrimal sac and surrounding area. Arch Ophthalmol. 1972;88:645.
29. Bahnasawi SA, Abdalla MI, Ghaly AF, et al. Trachoma of the lacrimal sac. Bull Ophthalmol Soc Egypt. 1976;69:619.
30. Hurwitz JJ, Rodgers KJA. Management of acquired dacryocystitis. Can J Ophthalmol. 1983;18:213–6.
31. Ahrens-Palumbo MJ, Ballen PH. Primary dacryocystitis causing orbital cellulitis. Ann Ophthalmol. 1982;14:600.
32. Cohn H, Mondino BJ, Brown SI, et al. Marginal corneal ulcers with acute beta streptococcal conjunctivitis and chronic dacryocystitis. Am J Ophthalmol. 1979;87:541.
33. Hinton P, Hurwitz JJ, Cruickshank B. Nasolacrimal bone changes in diseases of the lacrimal drainage system. Ophthalmic Surg. 1984;15:516–21.
34. Ulman S, Sergott R. Abduction deficit secondary to presumed bacterial dacryoadenitis. Arch Ophthalmol. 1986;104:1127–8.
35. Sen DK. Acute suppurative dacryoadenitis caused by a *Cysticercus cellulosa*. J Pediatr Ophthalmol Strabismus. 1982;19:100.
36. Riffenburgh RS. Ocular manifestations of mumps. Arch Ophthalmol. 1961;56:739.
37. Jones BR. Lacrimal disease associated with infectious mononucleosis. Trans Ophthalmol Soc UK. 1955;75:101.
38. Jakobiec FA, Jones IS. Orbital inflammations. In: Duane TD, ed. Clinical Ophthalmology. v. 2. Philadelphia: Harper & Row; 1987:65.
39. Duke-Elder S. The ocular adnexa. In: Duke-Elder S, ed. System of Ophthalmology. v. 13. St. Louis: CV Mosby; 1974:601.
40. Baghdassarian SA, Zakharia H, Asdourian KK. Report of a case of bilateral caseous tuberculous dacryoadenitis. Am J Ophthalmol. 1972;74:744.
41. Jakobiec FA, Gess L, Zimmerman LE. Granulomatous dacryoadenitis caused by *Schistosoma haematobium*. Arch Ophthalmol. 1977;95:278.
42. Obernauf CD, Shaw HE, Sydnor CJ, et al. Sarcoidosis and its ophthalmic manifestations. Am J Ophthalmol. 1978;86:648.
43. Check WA. Many misjudge severity of orbital cellulitis. JAMA. 1982;247:1236.
44. Hornblass A, Herschorn BJ, Stern K, et al. Orbital abcess. Surv Ophthalmol. 1984;29:169–78.
45. Macy JI, Mandelbaum SH, Minckler DS. Orbital cellulitis. Ophthalmology. 1980;87:1309.
46. Brook I, Friedman EM, Rodriguez WJ, et al. Complications of sinusitis in children. Pediatrics. 1980;66:568.
47. Noel LP, Clark WN, Peacocke TA. Periorbital and orbital cellulitis in childhood. Can J Ophthalmol. 1981;16:178.
48. Weiss A, Friendly D, Eglin K, et al. Bacterial periorbital and orbital cellulitis in childhood. Ophthalmology. 1983;90:195.
49. Watters EC, Wallar PH, Hiles DA, et al. Acute orbital cellulitis. Arch Ophthalmol. 1976;94:785–8.
50. Ferguson EC III. Deep wooden foreign bodies of the orbit: A report of two cases. Trans Am Acad Ophthalmol Otolaryngol. 1970;74:778.
51. Goldfarb MS, Hoffman DS, Rosenberg S. Orbital cellulitis and orbital fractures. Ann Ophthalmol. 1987;19:97–9.
52. Von Noorden GK. Orbital cellulitis following extraocular muscle surgery. Am J Ophthalmol. 1972;74:627.
53. Wilson ME, Paul TO. Orbital cellulitis following strabismus surgery. Ophthalmic Surg. 1987;18:92–4.
54. Allen MV, Cohen KL, Grimson BS. Orbital cellulitis secondary to dacryocystitis following blepharoplasty. Ann Ophthalmol. 1985;17:498–9.
55. Diwan R, Sen DK, Sood GC. Rat bite orbital cellulitis. Br J Ophthalmol. 1970;54:211.
56. Biedner BZ, Marmur U, Yassur Y. *Streptococcus faecalis* orbital cellulitis. Ann Ophthalmol. 1986;18:194–5.
57. Appalanarasayya K, Murthy ASR, Viswanath CK, et al. Proptosis in a newborn due to orbital infection: Case report. Int Surg. 1971;55:149.
58. Frederick J, Braude AL. Anaerobic infection of the paranasal sinuses. N Engl J Med. 1974;290:135.
59. Partamian LG, Jay WM, Fritz KJ. Anaerobic orbital cellulitis. Ann Ophthalmol. 1983;15:123–6.
60. Crock GW, Heriot WJ, Janakiraman P, et al. Gas gangrene infection of the eyes and orbits. Br J Ophthalmol. 1985;69:143–8.
61. Londer L, Nelson DL. Orbital cellulitis due to *Haemophilus influenzae*. Arch Ophthalmol. 1974;91:89.
62. Gorbach SL, Bartlett JG. Anaerobic infections. Part I. N Engl J Med. 1974;290:1177.
63. Sevel D, Tobias B, Sellars SL, et al. Gas in the orbit associated with orbital cellulitis and paranasal sinusitis. Br J Ophthalmol. 1973;57:133.
64. Levine RA. Infection of the orbit by an atypical mycobacterium. Arch Ophthalmol. 1969;82:608.
65. Ross J, Kohlhepp PA. Gangrene of the eyelids. Ann Ophthalmol. 1973;5:84.
66. El-Shewy TM. Acute infarction of the choroid and retina: A complication of orbital cellulitis. Br J Ophthalmol. 1973;57:204.
67. Slavin ML, Glaser JS. Acute severe irreversible visual loss with sphenoethmoiditis—"posterior" orbital cellulitis. Arch Ophthalmol. 1987;105:345–8.
68. Kjoer I. A case of orbital apex syndrome in collateral pansinusitis. Acta Ophthalmol. 1945;23:357–66.
69. Jarrett WH, Gutman FA. Ocular complications of infection in the paranasal sinuses. Arch Ophthalmol. 1969;81:683–8.
70. Chandler JR, Langenbrunner DJ, Stevens ER. The pathogenesis of orbital complications in acute sinusitis. Laryngoscope. 1970;80:1414–28.
71. Sen DK. Surgical treatment of "collar-stud" orbital abscess. Int Surg. 1970;54:379.
72. Birch-Hirshfield, cited by Duke-Elder S. The ocular adnexa. In: Textbook of Ophthalmology. v. 5. St Louis: CV Mosby; 1952:5420–44.
73. Bergin DJ, Wright JE. Orbital cellulitis. Br J Ophthalmol. 1986;70:174–8.
74. Mortada A. Tuberculoma of the orbit and lacrimal gland. Br J Ophthalmol. 1971;55:565.
75. Whitfield R, Wirotsko E. Ocular syphilis. In: Locatcher-Khorazo D, Seegal BC, eds. Microbiology of the Eye. St Louis: CV Mosby; 1972:322.
76. Jakobiec FA. Orbital infections. In: Spencer WH, ed. Ophthalmic Pathology: An Atlas and Textbook. 3rd ed. Philadelphia: WB Saunders; 1986:2812–31.
77. Gass JDM. Ocular manifestations of acute mucormycosis. Arch Ophthalmol. 1961;65:226.
78. Baum JL. Rhino-orbital mucormycosis occurring in an otherwise apparently healthy individual. Am J Ophthalmol. 1967;63:335.
79. Hale LM. Orbital-cerebral phycomycosis: Report of a case and a review of the disease in infants. Arch Ophthalmol. 1971;86:39.
80. Blodi FC, Hannah FT, Wadsworth JAC. Lethal orbitocerebral phycomycosis in otherwise healthy children. Am J Ophthalmol. 1969;67:698.
81. Straatsma BR, Zimmerman LE, Gass JDM. Phycomycosis: A clinico-pathologic study of fifty-one cases. Lab Invest. 1962;11:963.
82. Green WR, Font RL, Zimmerman LE. Aspergillosis of the orbit: Report of ten cases and review of the literature. Arch Ophthalmol. 1969;82:302.
83. Houle TV, Ellis PP. Aspergillosis of the orbit with immunosuppressive therapy. Surv Ophthalmol. 1975;20:35.
84. Miloshev B, Davidson CM, Gentles JC, et al. Aspergilloma of the paranasal sinuses and orbit in northern Sudanese. Lancet. 1966;1:746.
85. Morris FH Jr, Spock A: Intracranial aneurysm secondary to mycotic orbital and sinus infection: Report of a case implicating *Penicillium* as an opportunistic fungus. Am J Ophthalmol. 1969;68:14.
86. Olurin O, Lucas AO, Oyediran ABO. Orbital histoplasmosis due to *Histoplasma duboisii*. Am J Ophthalmol. 1969;68:14.
87. Vida L, Moel SA. Systemic North American blastomycosis with orbital involvement. Am J Ophthalmol. 1974;77:240.
88. Streeten BW, Rabuzzi DD, Jones DB. Sporotrichosis of the orbital margin. Am J Ophthalmol. 1974;77:750.
89. Baghdassarian SA, Zakheria H. Report of three cases of hydatid cyst of the orbit. Am J Ophthalmol. 1971;71:1081.
90. Mehra KS, Banerjee C, Somani PN, et al. Hydatid cyst in orbit. Acta Ophthalmol. 1965;43:761.
91. Talib H. Orbital hydatid cyst in Iraq. Br J Surg. 1972;59:391.

92. Kagan IG. Trichinosis: A review of biologic, serologic and immunologic aspects. J Infect Dis. 1960;107:65.
93. Hamed HH. Orbital affection with *Cysticercus cellulosae*. Bull Ophthalmol Soc Egypt. 1968;61:253.
94. Jones BR. Inflammatory pseudotumors of the orbit: A probable case of microfilarial granuloma of the orbit. Trans Ophthalmol Soc UK. 1970;90:299.
95. Mathur SP, Makhija JM. Invasion of the orbit by maggots. Br J Ophthalmol. 1967;51:406.
96. Wood TR, Slight JR. Bilateral orbital myiasis. Arch Ophthalmol. 1970;84:692.
97. Blodi FC. Orbital inflammations. Symposium on diseases and surgery of the lids, lacrimal apparatus, and orbit. Trans New Orleans Acad Ophthalmol. 1982:1–17.
98. Clune JP. Septic thrombosis within the cavernous chamber: Review of the literature with recent advances in diagnosis and treatment. Am J Ophthalmol. 1963;56:33.
99. Yarington CR Jr. The prognosis and treatment of cavernous sinus thrombosis: A review of 878 cases in the literature. Ann Otol Rhinol Layngol. 1961;70:263.
100. Price CD, Hameroff SB, Richards RD. Cavernous sinus thrombosis and orbital cellulitis. South Med J. 1971;64:1243.
101. Bell RW. Orbital cellulitis and cavernous sinus thrombosis caused by rhabdomyosarcoma of the middle ear. Ann Ophthalmol. 1972;4:1090.
102. Walsh FB. Ocular signs of thrombosis of the intracranial sinuses. Arch Ophthalmol. 1937;17:46.
103. Clifford-Jones RE, Ellis CJK, Stevens JM, et al. Cavernous sinus thrombosis. J Neurol Neurosurg Psychiatry. 1982;45:1092.
104. Geggel HS, Isenberg SJ. Cavernous sinus thrombosis as a cause of unilateral blindness. Ann Ophthalmol. 1982;14:569.
105. Raflo GT, Chart P, Hurwitz JJ. Thermographic evaluation of the human lacrimal drainage system. Ophthalmic Surg. 1982;13:119–24.
106. Rosenstock T, Chart P, Hurwitz JJ. Inflammation of the lacrimal drainage system—assessment by thermography. Ophthalmic Surg. 1983;14:229–37.
107. Galloway JE, Kavic TA, Raflo GT. Digital subtraction macrodacryocystography: A new method of lacrimal system imaging. Ophthalmology 1984;91:956.
108. Rossomondo RM, Carlton WH, Trueblood JH, et al. A new method of evaluating lacrimal drainage. Arch Ophthalmol. 1972;88:523.
109. Freeman LN, Zinreich SJ, Iliff NT. Radiography of the lacrimal system using topical CT dacryocystography (Abstract). Ophthalmology 1987;94:142.
110. Eustis HS, Amstrong DC, Buncic JR, et al. Staging of orbital cellulitis in children: Computed tomography characteristics and treatment guidelines. J Pediatr Ophthalmol. Strabismus 1986;23:246–51.
111. Harr DL, Quencer RM, Abrams GW. Computed tomography and ultrasound in the evaluation of orbital infection and pseudotumor. Radiology. 1982;152:395.
112. Fiandaca MS, Spector RH, Hartmann TM, et al. Unilateral septic cavernous sinus thrombosis—a case report with digital orbital venographic documentation. J Clin Neuro-ophthalmol. 1986;6:35–8.
113. Kline LB, Acker JD, Post MJD, et al. The cavernous sinus: A computed tomographic study. Am J Neurol Radiol. 2:299, 1981.
114. Lew D, Southwick FS, Montgomery WW, et al. Sphenoid sinusitis: A review of 30 cases. N Engl J Med. 1983;309:1149.
115. Savino PJ, Grossman RI, Schatz NJ, et al. High-field magnetic resonance imaging in the diagnosis of cavernous sinus thrombosis. Arch Neurol. 1986;43:1081–2.
116. Taylor PJ. Cavernous sinus thrombophlebitis. Br J Ophthalmol. 1957;41:228–37.
117. Aragones JV. The treatment of blepharitis: A controlled double blind study of combination therapy. Ann Ophthalmol. 1973;5:49.
118. Mathew M, D'Souza P, Mehta DK. A new treatment of pthiriasis palpebrarum. Ann Ophthalmol. 1982;14:439.
119. Seal DV, McGill J, Flanagan D. Lacrimal canaliculitis due to *Arachnia (Actinomyces) propionica*. Br J Ophthalmol. 1981;65:10–13.
120. Campbell CB, Flanagan JC, Schaefer AJ. Acquired lacrimal disorders. In: Smith BC, Della Rocca RC, Nesi FA, eds. Ophthalmic Plastic and Reconstructive Surgery. St Louis: CV Mosby; 1987:956.
121. Krohel G. Orbital cellulitis and abscess. In: Fraunfelder F, Roy H, eds. Current Ocular Therapy. 2nd ed. Philadelphia: WB Saunders; 1985:451.
122. Gutman L. Appropriate antibiotics in orbital cellulitis. Arch Ophthalmol. 1977;95:170.
123. Tannenbaum M, Tenzel J, Byrne SF, et al. Medical management of orbital abscess. Surv Ophthalmol. 1985;30:211–2.
124. Gold SC, Arrigg PG, Hedges TR. Computed tomography in the management of acute orbital cellulitis. Ophthalmic Surg. 1987;18:753–6.
125. Best M, Obstbaum SA, Friedman B, et al. Survival in orbital phycomycosis. Am J Ophthalmol. 1971;71:1078.
126. Bullock JD, Jampol LM, Fezza AJ. Two cases of orbital phycomycosis with recovery. Am J Ophthalmol. 1974;78:811.
127. Jones DB. Microbial preseptal and orbital cellulitis. In: Duane TD, ed. Clinical Ophthalmology. v. 4. Hagerstown, MD: Harper & Row; 1976:17.
128. Solomon OD, Moses L, Volk M. Steroid therapy in cavernous sinus thrombosis. Am J Ophthalmol. 1962;54:1122–5.
129. Parsons M. Intracranial venous thrombosis. Postgrad Med J. 1967; 43:409–14.
130. Lyons C. Treatment of staphylococcal cavernous sinus thrombophlebitis with heparin and chemotherapy. Ann Surg. 1941;113:113–7.

SECTION O. HEPATITIS

102. ACUTE VIRAL HEPATITIS

JAY H. HOOFNAGLE

Acute viral hepatitis is a common and serious infectious disease caused by several viral agents and marked by necrosis and inflammation of the liver. This disease was traditionally separated into two types: type A, or infectious hepatitis caused by the hepatitis A virus (HAV), and type B, or serum hepatitis caused by the hepatitis B virus (HBV).[1] In the last 25 years it has become clear that there are many agents that cause acute viral hepatitis. At present, five hepatitis virus agents have been identified: HAV[2]; HBV[3,4]; the hepatitis delta virus[5,6]; a parenterally transmitted, classic non-A, non-B hepatitis agent[7,8]; and an enterically transmitted, epidemic non-A, non-B hepatitis agent.[9,10] The five forms of acute viral hepatitis are similar clinically, but the agents that cause them are quite distinct.

Hepatitis A, B, delta, and the two forms of non-A, non-B hepatitis are primary infectious diseases of the liver; their main manifestations are those of hepatocellular necrosis and hepatic inflammation, and there is little evidence to suggest that they infect other organs to a major extent. Several other viral agents can secondarily affect the liver and induce a viral hepatitis-like syndrome. The most important of these agents are the Epstein-Barr virus (EBV) and cytomegalovirus (CMV); however, liver disease also can occur with infections with herpes simplex viruses; varicella-zoster virus; measles, rubella, rubeola, and coxsackie B viruses; and adenoviruses. While these agents can cause diagnostic confusion by producing some degree of liver inflammation and dysfunction, they are not considered to be primary causes of acute or chronic viral hepatitis.

Acute viral hepatitis is a common disease. Yearly estimates from the U.S. Centers for Disease Control suggest that the incidence of acute viral hepatitis has been rising slowly over the last 20 years.[11] During 1985, there were approximately 60,000 cases of viral hepatitis reported, among which an estimated 29 percent were due to hepatitis A, 44 percent to hepatitis B, and 27 percent to non-A, non-B hepatitis. These reports suggest that the annual incidence of acute viral hepatitis in the United States is 0.25 per 1000 population. This is clearly an underestimate.

Attempts at quantifying the degree of underreporting of viral hepatitis[12] have suggested that the true incidence is five to eight times that reported each year (thus 1–2 per 1000 population). Indeed, the use of serologic markers for evidence of previous HAV and HBV infections reveals that by the age of 50 years, 70 percent of middle-class white Americans have had HAV infection and 7 percent have had HBV infection.[13] These prevalences of antibody markers are higher among lower socioeconomic groups and among foreign-born U.S. citizens.

Acute viral hepatitis is a serious disease. The mortality rate for icteric viral hepatitis overall is approximately 1 percent. The mortality rate of acute hepatitis is higher in older persons, and some of the variation in the reported mortality rates of this disease relates to the age of the affected patients. In addition, fulminant cases occur more commonly in delta hepatitis than in the other forms of acute viral hepatitis. In various outbreaks of delta hepatitis, the mortality rate has been reported to be between 2 and 20 percent.[6,14] Finally, the epidemic form of non-A, non-B hepatitis has a striking characteristic of a high mortality rate (~10 percent) in pregnant women.[10]

In addition to mortality from the acute disease, viral hepatitis also has serious sequelae including chronic liver disease and cirrhosis, polyarteritis nodosa, cryoglobulinemia, glomerulonephritis, aplastic anemia, and hepatocellular carcinoma.[15–17] In the United States and Western Europe, chronic viral hepatitis is probably the second most frequent cause of cirrhosis, second only to alcohol abuse. The chronic forms of hepatitis B, delta hepatitis, and non-A, non-B hepatitis are frequent causes of terminal liver disease for which hepatic transplantation is performed. On a worldwide scale, chronic hepatitis B infection is the most important cause of cirrhosis and is a major cause of cancer mortality. It is estimated that 5 percent of the world's population has chronic HBV infection (the chronic carrier state) and up to 40 percent of these persons may ultimately develop hepatocellular carcinoma.[18]

The many advances that have been made in understanding viral hepatitis during the past 25 years are just now being translated into means of preventing and treating this disease. Serologic markers have been developed for all five forms of viral hepatitis and promise to have a major effect in preventing post-transfusion hepatitis and defining the epidemiology, natural history, and means of controlling sporadic viral hepatitis. A highly effective hepatitis B vaccine made from plasma has been available since 1982 and a "second-generation," recombinant hepatitis B vaccine since 1986.[19] Recently, experimental vaccines against hepatitis A have been developed and are being evaluated in selected human populations. Therapies for chronic viral hepatitis have been developed and are now under investigation as treatment for acute hepatitis. Such advances hold promise for the ultimate goal of controlling this common and serious infection.

CLINICAL MANIFESTATIONS

Symptoms

Acute viral hepatitis is such a sufficiently distinct clinical syndrome that it usually poses no difficult in diagnosis. It is conveniently separated into four stages: incubation period, preicteric phase, icteric phase, and convalescence. The timing and major symptoms of each of these stages are shown diagrammatically in Figure 1.

The incubation period of acute viral hepatitis varies from as short as a few weeks to as long as 6 months. The incubation period of type A hepatitis averages 30 days (range, 15–45 days), that of type B hepatitis averages 70 days (range, 30–180 days), that of classic non-A, non-B hepatitis averages 50 days (range, 15–150 days), and that of epidemic non-A, non-B hepatitis averages 40 days (range, 15–60 days). The incubation period of delta hepatitis has not been well documented. Because delta hepatitis invariably occurs in conjunction with type B hepatitis, its incubation period probably is similar.

The initial symptoms of acute hepatitis are nonspecific; in the typical case, the patient develops malaise and weakness, followed shortly by anorexia, intermittent nausea, vomiting, and a vague, dull, right upper quadrant pain. These symptoms of the preicteric phase usually last 3–10 days. The onset of jaundice and/or dark urine then ushers in the icteric phase. It is these symptoms that usually bring the patient to the doctor—the iatrogenic stimulus. The duration of icterus is, of course, quite variable; but, it usually lasts 1–3 weeks. In the average case, the patient often will begin to feel better quite soon after jaundice appears; the appetitie returns, nausea abates, and a sense of well-being returns, even while jaundice persists. Ma-

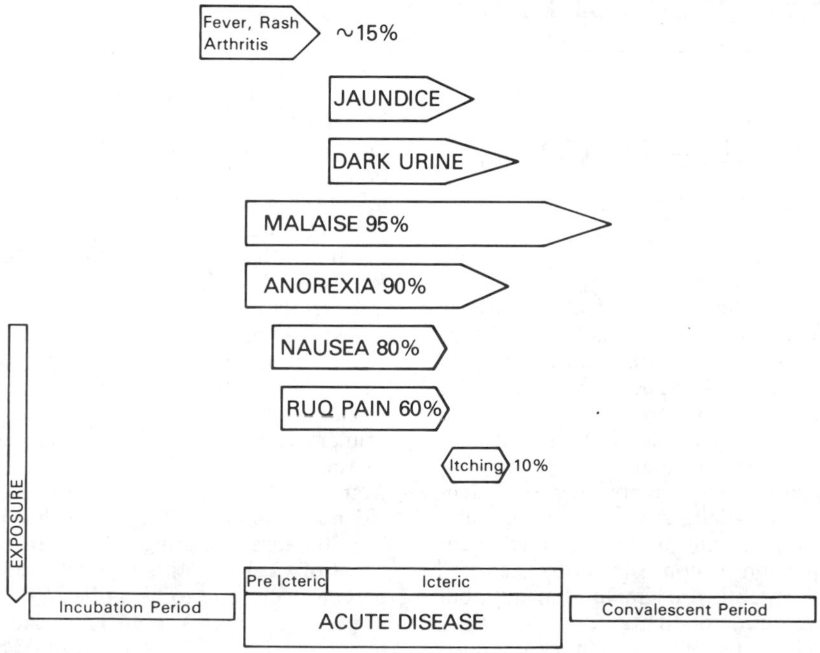

FIG. 1. The course of acute viral hepatitis. The timing and frequency of the major symptoms of viral hepatitis are shown.

laise usually is the last symptom to disappear, often concurrent with or shortly before jaundice clears.

While this may represent the "typical" case, one must stress that such cases probably represent a minority of hepatitis virus infections. The most characteristic feature of viral hepatitis is the variability of clinical expression. Icteric cases (which, for convenience, can be defined as those with a bilirubin level of ≥2.5 mg/dl, the approximate level at which jaundice can be visually detected) account for only 20–50 percent of hepatitis virus infections. The remainder pass unnoticed, without symptoms or with such mild and few symptoms that they are dismissed as inconsequential ("indigestion" or "the flu"). The spectrum of hepatitis virus infections ranges from inapparent to anicteric (but symptomatic) to icteric to fulminant. Any discussion of the clinical manifestations of viral hepatitis must take into account that only a part of this spectrum is being described.

The *onset* of viral hepatitis either can be sudden (most typical of type A hepatitis) or insidious (more typical of type B or non-A, non-B hepatitis), but it usually can be dated quite well. *Malaise* is no doubt the earliest, most common (~95 percent) and reliable symptom of this disease. It is variously reported as weakness, lethargy, easy fatigability, drowsiness, or just feeling low or ill. It usually is the first symptom to appear and the last to leave. *Anorexia* is almost as frequent (~90 percent) as malaise in symptomatic viral hepatitis, but it typically is one of the first symptoms to abate. It also assumes several forms—lack of desire for food, change in food preferences, easy satiety, or the provocation of nausea, indigestion, or abdominal pain by smell, taste, or ingestion of food. The end result is decreased food intake; weight loss of 5–20 lb (2–10 kg) is common during viral hepatitis. A loss of the taste for cigarettes is another form of the anorexia or dysgeusia of acute hepatitis. While it is said to be typical of acute viral hepatitis, this symptom actually is characteristic of any acute liver disease. *Nausea* and vomiting occur in about 80 percent of the patients with symptomatic viral hepatitis. The nausea is typically intermittent and rarely intractable. Nausea, as with malaise, may be absent early in the day and then appear and worsen as the day progresses. Abdominal *pain* can accompany acute viral hepatitis (~60 percent), and it usually consists of a dull, right upper quadrant, aching discomfort. It usually is not severe and is unaffected by meals, antacids, stool patterns, or position.

At least 25 percent of the patients with viral hepatitis describe the onset of their disease as an "influenza-like" illness with weakness, headaches, myalgias, chilliness, and fever. This onset is most common with type A hepatitis. The *headaches* are generalized, dull, and mild to moderate. *Fever*, if present, is low grade. In some instances, symptoms of an upper respiratory infection such as a sore throat and cough may be present. These symptoms are short-lived (1–3 days) and are replaced by the more typical symptoms of anorexia, nausea, and then jaundice. Fever, in particular, rarely persists into the icteric phase. Jaundice with high fever is *not* characteristic of viral hepatitis.

A smaller percentage of patients with acute hepatitis (5–10 percent) experience a "serum sickness-like syndrome" at the onset of their illness.[20] This consist of a triad of symptoms—fever, rash, and arthritis. This syndrome occurs during the preicteric phase and almost invariably will resolve dramatically with the onset of jaundice. *Fever* is usual but not invariable. The *rash* is typically urticarial, with pruritic hives appearing and disappearing in a largely peripheral distribution. More exanthem-like macular-papular lesions can also occur as well as fleeting irregular patches of erythema. The *arthritis* is mild to moderate, nondeforming, polyarticular, migratory. Major joints involved are the elbows, wrists, knees, and small joints of the hands. Arthralgias probably are more common than frank arthritis. This syndrome is most common with type B hepatitis, but it also has been reported in type A and in non-A, non-B hepatitis. It probably is a manifestation of immune complex (virus/antibody) deposition. In children with type B hepatitis, a condition perhaps related to this syndrome has been described—papular acrodermatitis (Gianotti's disease).[21] Isolated reports of other manifestations such as Raynaud's phenomenon, bullous formation, and erythema nodosum also have been described in acute hepatitis (but are rare).

Jaundice and dark urine are the most distinctive symptoms of this disease, but they can be unreliable. Many patients (and some physicians) may not recognize scleral icterus, even with a serum bilirubin level as high as 10 mg/dl. *Dark urine* often is more noticeable than scleral icterus, because the urine can turn dark before the icterus is visible. Dark urine also is helpful in indicating that the jaundice is accompanied by conjugated (direct) hyperbilirubinemia (not found with jaundice due to hemolysis or Gilbert syndrome). While jaundice and dark urine usually occur after a 4- to 10-day preicteric phase, some patients have jaundice only and deny any prodrome of malaise, anorexia, or nausea. Light stools also can occur with the jaundice of viral hepatitis, reflecting the absence of bile pigments being added to the intestinal contents. The lightening of stool color in viral hepatitis, however, usually is not as great as in obstructive jaundice, and white or chalky stools are uncommon. Persons with prominent jaundice will also often complain of *pruritus*. Approximately 40 percent of jaundiced patients will complain of itching at the peak of icterus or sometime into convalescence.

Diarrhea or *constipation* can occur during acute viral hepatitis, but they usually are not prominent. These changes in bowel habits may reflect changes in activity or diet rather than an effect of the viral infection.

Fulminant viral hepatitis is defined by the appearance of symptoms and signs of hepatic failure or encephalopathy during the course of viral hepatitis. Fulminant hepatic failure can occur at any time—early or late—during the course of the disease. The first symptoms usually are *lethargy*, *somnolence*, and a *change in personality*. There may be abnormal behavior with an unexpected display of sexual or aggressive activity or a subtle change in personality with untidiness, mild confusion, or a loss of the usual inhibitions. Patients may be excited, euphoric, and unruly. These symptoms are followed in more severe cases by *stupor* and then *coma*.

Physical Findings

The physical findings in acute viral hepatitis are few. In general, the patient may appear acutely but not chronically ill. Acute hepatitis, by and large, is a disease of the healthy; wasting or undernutrition are not part of this disease. The patient usually is afebrile. Vital signs are normal, although bradycardia can occur when significant hyperbilirubinemia is present. Icterus can be detected if the billirubin level exceeds 2.5–3.0 mg/dl. It is seen most easily in the sclera or under the tongue. In light-skinned people, the skin may have a yellowish hue. Natural light is mandatory in assessing mild degrees of jaundice. Also, a deliberate search for icterus should be included in the physician's evaluation of every ill patient.

The abdomen appears grossly normal. Bowel sounds are present. Palpation often demonstrates an enlarged and slightly tender liver. However, in acute viral hepatitis, the liver usually is only modestly enlarged (9–13 cm in breadth by percussion), and its edge is smooth, regular, and firm (not flabby or hard). Tenderness can be elicited by direct palpation of the edge or by gentle percussion of the lower ribs with the fist (comparing the right with the left side). A spleen tip is felt in 5–25 percent of the patients. Signs of portal hypertension (ascites, edema, prominent splenomegaly, abdominal venous patterns) are not seen in acute hepatitis except in late, severe disease (as with subacute hepatic necrosis). The rest of the examination is rarely helpful. Adenopathy, if present, is not prominent.

There are several skin findings in acute viral hepatitis. Vascular spiders often are found in light-skinned persons, but they are few and small. Excoriations will occur with severe pruritus. Multiple forearm venipuncture marks can suggest drug addiction, a common source of hepatitis virus infection. Patients with the serum sickness-like syndrome will have urticaria or a mild, fleeting erythematous rash and (occasionally) red, warm, and tender joints. Finally, acne-prone persons may exhibit an exacerbation of this condition with acute hepatitis, especially during recovery.

When fulminant hepatitis supervenes, signs of hepatic encephalopathy appear. These consist of lethargy, somnolence, untidiness, confusion, forgetfulness, and then stupor and full coma. Typical of hepatic encephalopathy is asterixis—the asynchronous irregular flapping of the forcibly dorsiflexed, outstretched hands. In stage I coma, mild mental changes are present, but asterixis is minimal or absent. Stage II coma is marked by worsening of mental changes and definite asterixis. In stage III coma, the patient develops stupor and semicoma but can still be roused. With stage IV coma, the patient no longer is arousable, and there may or may not be a response to deep pain stimuli. Patients with hepatic failure may demonstrate other neurologic signs—flapping of the tongue, involuntary movements, long-tract signs, and decerebrate posturing. They also may demonstrate the sweetish smell of fetor hepaticus.

Laboratory Findings

While the symptoms and signs of acute viral hepatitis are frequently nonspecific or vague, laboratory findings are quite characteristic. The typical ranges of key serum enzyme and bilirubin levels in acute viral hepatitis and other common liver diseases are shown in Figure 2. Most distinctive of viral hepatitis are the dramatic elevations in the *aminotransferases*—asparate aminotransferase (AST, SGOT) and alanine aminotransferase (ALT, SGPT). In acute viral hepatitis, concentrations of the two aminotransferases are both elevated (usually greater than eight times normal when jaundice appears) and to the same degree.[22] The ALT level is the most important because this serum enzyme is quite specific for liver injury (it also may be slightly elevated in muscle disease). In acute hepatitis, the ALT level usually is as high or higher than the AST (although above 20–40 times normal this distinction is less reliable). The *alkaline phosphatase* and other serum enzyme levels that denote biliary obstruction or cholestasis (leucine aminopeptidase, 5′-nucleotidase) are only mildly elevated (one to three times normal). The *lactic dehydrogenase* (LDH) concentration usually is mildly elevated in acute viral hepatitis (one to three times normal). The *creatine phosphokinase* (CPK) level, which is elevated in muscle and heart injury, is normal in viral hepatitis. Indeed, the dramatic elevation of both AST and ALT levels, with only mild elevation in alkaline phosphatase and LDH levels, is virtually diagnostic of ''acute hepatitis'' or ''acute necroinflammatory disease of the liver.'' Given this enzyme pattern, one need then only to resolve whether this acute hepatitis is due to a hepatitis virus, a hepatotoxic drug, a toxin, or a nonspecific liver injury (anoxia, shock, or severe heart failure).

The AST and ALT levels become abnormal during the late incubation period of this disease. They are invariably abnormal once symptoms occur, usually rise during the preicteric phase, and peak early in the icteric phase. With recovery, the aminotransferase levels quickly fall but almost always remain slightly abnormal for several weeks after the jaundice and symptoms have abated.

The *bilirubin* level is variably elevated in icteric viral hepatitis. This elevation involves both the direct and indirect fractions, with the ratio being approximately 1:1. Disproportionate elevations in direct bilirubin concentration suggest cholestasis, whereas the preponderance of indirect bilirubin (≥80 percent)

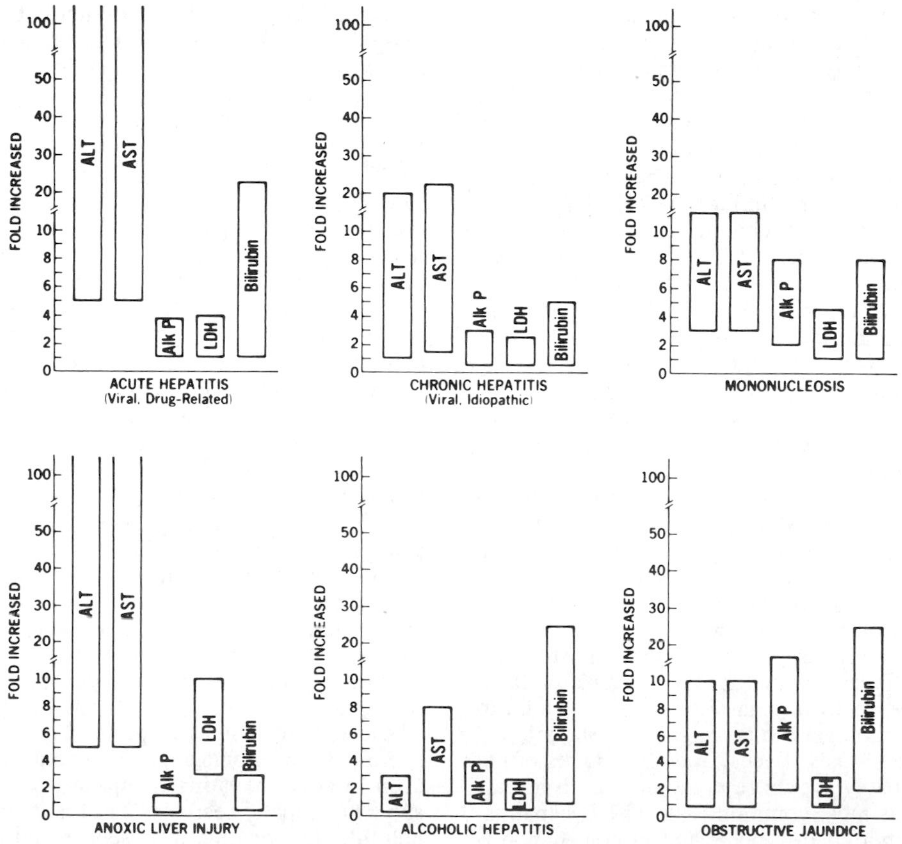

FIG. 2. The range of elevation of key serum enzyme levels in acute viral hepatitis, and other common liver diseases. ALT: alanine aminotransferase; AST: asparate aminotransferase; Alk P: alkaline phosphate; LDH: lactic dehydrogenase.

suggests hemolysis. Persons with underlying hemolytic states (glucose-6-phosphate dehydrogenase [G6PD] deficiency or thalassemia minor) may suffer accelerated hemolysis with many viral infections and especially viral hepatitis.[23] These persons may become markedly jaundiced and yet have relatively mild symptoms and aminotransferase level elevations.

The *prothrombin time* generally is normal in typical acute viral hepatitis, but it is invariably elevated in fulminant hepatitis. Abnormalities in the prothrombin time are the most reliable indicators of prognosis in acute hepatitis. Any elevation should be regarded as a serious sign. The *partial thromboplastin time* is not as sensitive or reliable a measure as the prothrombin time. Assays for the separate liver-synthesized coagulation factors (e.g., factors V, VII, and X) may be more sensitive and reliable measures of liver dysfunction than the prothrombin time. However, they are technically demanding and expensive, and their relative advantages have yet to be proved.

The *serum albumin* and *globulin* levels usually are normal in acute viral hepatitis. While the serum albumin level may fall and the serum globulin level may rise slightly during the course of the disease, this pattern of low albumin and high globulin levels should point once more toward a diagnosis of chronic liver disease.

Other laboratory test results rarely are abnormal. *Hemoglobin* and hematocrit values remain normal (decreased values should suggest hemolysis, chronic liver disease, or unrelated anemia). A *white blood cell count* is either normal or slightly low. A mild lymphocytosis can occur. The *platelet count* remains normal except with fulminant hepatitis, in which case disseminated intravascular coagulation can supervene.

Patients with acute viral hepatitis often develop low levels of anti-DNA and smooth muscle antibodies (SMA). Biologic false-positive VDRL test reactions are rare. Tests for other "autoantibodies" (rheumatoid factor, antinuclear antibody, lupus erythematosus phenomenon, and so on) usually are negative or normal. The sedimentation rate is normal or minimally elevated. Serum *complement* levels can be depressed in the preicteric phase of illness, especially in those patients with the serum sickness-like syndrome of polyarthritis, fever, and rash.[20] Serum *immunoglobulin* levels usually are normal except in type A hepatitis, in which case the serum IgM level may double during the course of the disease.

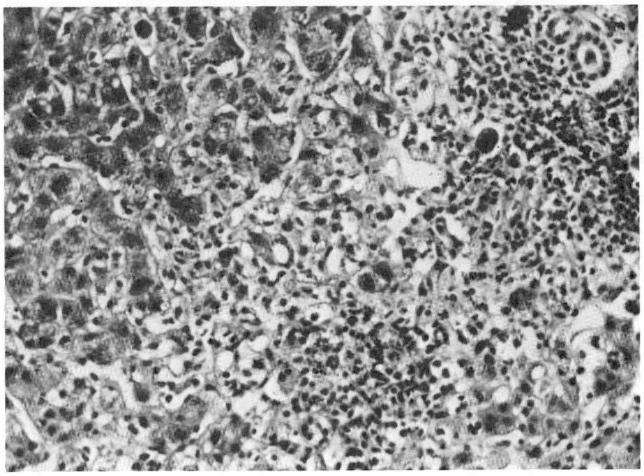

FIG. 3. Liver biopsy specimen from a patient with acute viral hepatitis. Note the lobular disarray, the occurrence of eosinophilic degeneration, free hyaline bodies, and spotty hepatocellular necrosis and the prominent mononuclear cell infiltrates in the portal zone and areas of parenchyma. (H&E, ×240) (Photomicrograph courtesy of Dr. Kamal Ishak, Washington, DC:AFIP negative No. 65-12490.)

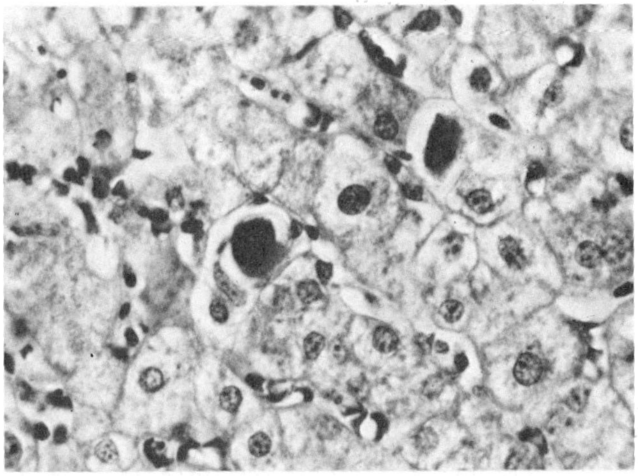

FIG. 4. The free hyaline body and eosinophilic generation typical of acute viral hepatitis. (H&E, ×660) (Photomicrograph courtesy of Dr. Kamal Ishak, Washington, DC:AFIP negative No. 68-8127.)

Pathologic Findings

The clinical history and pattern of serum enzyme levels in acute viral hepatitis are sufficiently characteristic that a percutaneous liver biopsy specimen is rarely necessary for diagnosis. However, when several possible causes of acute liver disease are present or when therapy is a consideration, a liver biopsy specimen can be helpful. The typical liver biopsy findings of acute viral hepatitis are the following: (*1*) lobular disarray, (*2*) ballooning and eosinophilic degeneration, (*3*) liver cell necrosis, (*4*) mononuclear cell infiltration of the parenchyma and portal tracts, and (*5*) variable degrees of cholestasis.[24] These changes are diffuse and generalized; therefore, sampling error from needle biopsy usually is not a problem. Lobular disarray refers to a loss of the orderly pattern of hepatic sinusoidal cords, the result of widespread anisocytosis, liver cell degeneration, regeneration, or death (Fig. 3). Liver cells demonstrate two forms of degeneration: ballooning degeneration (in which there is swelling of the liver cell and rarefaction of the cytoplasm) and eosinophilic degeneration (in which the cell shrinks and becomes a deeper red and more angular). The end result of eosinophilic degeneration is the free hyaline body (Fig. 4). There also may be "smudging" of hepatocytes with indistinctness of cell outline as well as cell "dropout"—with or without associated inflammatory cell reaction. Küpffer cells appear to be more numerous and enlarged. Areas of lymphocytic infiltration are common both in the parenchyma and in portal tracts. Polymorphonuclear leukocytes are not numerous. A few plasma cells and eosinophils may be found, but a prominence of portal tract plasma cells suggests chronic hepatitis; also, unusual numbers of eosinophils suggest drug addiction or a drug-related hepatitis. Cholestasis (bile staining of liver cells and bile "plugs") may be seen on liver biopsy specimens and generally correspond in degree to the height of the serum bilirubin level. The portal bile ducts, however, usually appear to be normal.

In typical viral hepatitis, cell necrosis is spotty and focal. More severe hepatitis may be accompanied by coalescent or bridging necrosis (between portal zones or from portal zones to central veins), multilobular necrosis, or massive necrosis.[24,25] Bridging necrosis found during acute viral hepatitis indicates a serious lesion that can progress to postnecrotic cirrhosis. Multilobular or massive necrosis is seen in severe and fulminant disease.

Fluorescence and electron microscopy of liver biopsy specimens in acute viral hepatitis rarely is helpful. Viral antigens and particles can be found in liver tissue during type A, type

B, and delta hepatitides. However, the techniques to detect these antigens in tissue are less sensitive and far more difficult than are the available serologic tests for viral antigens and antibodies in serum.[26]

DIFFERENTIAL DIAGNOSIS

Diseases that need to be excluded in the differential diagnosis of acute viral hepatitis are not so much other infectious diseases as other forms of liver disease (e.g., alcoholic hepatitis, cholecystitis, and Gilbert syndrome). The first step in the differential diagnosis should be the demonstration that acute necroinflammatory disease (acute hepatitis) is present. This distinction is based largely on the pattern of serum enzyme concentrations—dramatic elevations in aminotransferase levels with mild elevations in the alkaline phosphatase level. The second step in the differential diagnosis should be the exclusion of the nonviral causes of acute hepatitis. These include bacterial infections (pneumococcal pneumonia, leptospirosis), various drugs (acetaminophen, isoniazid), toxins (carbon tetrachloride), and nonspecific injury (shock, heart failure). These types of acute hepatitis usually can be excluded by a careful history with some support from laboratory data. Finally, with viral hepatitis diagnosed, the third step should be the identification of the responsible viral agent and the source of infection. Most cases of acute viral hepatitis are caused by one of five agents: HAV, HBV, delta, and the agents of non-A, non-B hepatitis. The diseases that these agents cause are quite similar. They overlap so much in symptoms and severity that they cannot be distinguished on clinical grounds, by biochemical tests, or even by liver biopsy findings. Fortunately, specific serologic assays and (in certain circumstances) typical epidemiologic features can separate and identify these five types of viral hepatitis.

Type A Hepatitis

Hepatitis A has certain clinical features that may help to distinguish it from other forms of acute viral hepatitis. In general, it is an acute self-limited disease. Type A hepatitis characteristically has an acute, sudden, influenza-like onset with a prominence of myalgia, headache, fever, and malaise.[1,27,28] This type of onset is less common with type B, delta, and non-A, non-B hepatitides, which tend to have a more gradual, insidious onset. Type A hepatitis usually is not as severe or as long lasting as type B hepatitis. However, a relapsing course occurs more commonly in hepatitis A than in other forms.[29] Furthermore, a prolonged cholestasis appearing late in the acute phase and lasting for several months is most typical of hepatitis A.[30] Both of these unusual forms of hepatitis A are often benign; the mortality rate of hepatitis A is low (~2/1000),[28] and the disease ultimately resolves. Hepatitis A does not lead to a chronic hepatitis or a carrier state.[31]

Epidemiologic features can be helpful in distinguishing hepatitis A from other forms of viral hepatitis.[11,32] Type A hepatitis is spread predominantly by the fecal–oral route. It is highly contagious and spreads rapidly. Type A hepatitis can occur in outbreaks that may have an identifiable point source (often a person in the incubation period of acute disease). Type A hepatitis has been shown to be spread (*1*) by contaminated water, milk, or food[33]; (*2*) after a breakdrown in the usual sanitary conditions or after floods or natural disasters[34]; (*3*) by the ingestion of raw or undercooked shellfish (oysters, clams, and mussels) from contaminated waters[34]; (*4*) during travel to areas of the world with poor hygienic conditions where hepatitis A is endemic[35]; (*5*) in institutionalized children and adults[1]; and (*6*) after exposure to recently imported chimpanzees or apes.[36]

Three other epidemiologic sources have recently been shown to be important in the spread of hepatitis A: exposure to children in day care centers,[32,37] male homosexuality,[38] and intravenous drug addiction.[11,32] Day care centers can serve as sources of outbreaks of hepatitis A—especially when there are children who are still not toilet trained in the centers. Male homosexuals have a high incidence of hepatitis A that probably is related to high degrees of promiscuity and practices of oral–anal and genital–anal intercourse. Drug addicts have recently been found to have a high incidence of hepatitis A, which may relate more to socioeconomic and hygienic standards than to the repeated parenteral exposures that occur with drug abuse. Yet, despite all these epidemiologic features, hepatitis A may be difficult to distinguish from other forms of viral hepatitis, and some cases occur without any known point source of infection. Blood transfusion is a very rare mode of transmission of hepatitis A.[11]

Unless hepatitis occurs as a part of a clear-cut epidemic with a definable incubation period, it usually is not possible to reliably diagnose hepatitis A without specific serologic assays. The serologic course of a typical case of hepatitis A is shown in Figure 5. Hepatitis A virus (HAV) and hepatitis A antigen can be detected in the stool during both the incubation period and early symptomatic phase of illness. Levels of virus in stool usually are decreasing and no longer may be detectable at the time of the onset of jaundice. Antibody to HAV (anti-HAV) is detectable in serum by the time of the onset of disease. Initially, the anti-HAV consists of both IgG and IgM class antibodies. After 3–12 months, IgM anti-HAV disappears, whereas IgG anti-HAV persists in high titer. Indeed, IgG anti-HAV seems to be long lasting and is associated with lifelong immunity. The diagnosis of acute hepatitis A can be made by the finding of IgM anti-HAV in a patient with either clinical symptoms or biochemical evidence of acute hepatitis.[39] Immunoassays are now available for IgM anti-HAV and for total anti-HAV. These assays allow for both diagnosis (IgM anti-HAV) as well as assessment of immunity (total anti-HAV) to hepatitis A.

Several research assays such as radioimmunoassay for hepatitis A antigen in serum and stool,[2] identification of virion HAV RNA in serum and stool,[29] direct culture of HAV in susceptible cell lines, and assay for neutralizing anti-HAV[28] have proved to be invaluable in study of the biology, natural history, and pathogenesis of hepatitis A but are not generally available for use in routine clinical settings.

Type B Hepatitis

Type B hepatitis appears to be a more serious disease than type A hepatitis, and it has a definite propensity to chronicity. It usually has a more insidious onset and a more prolonged course than type A hepatitis. In the individual case, however, type B

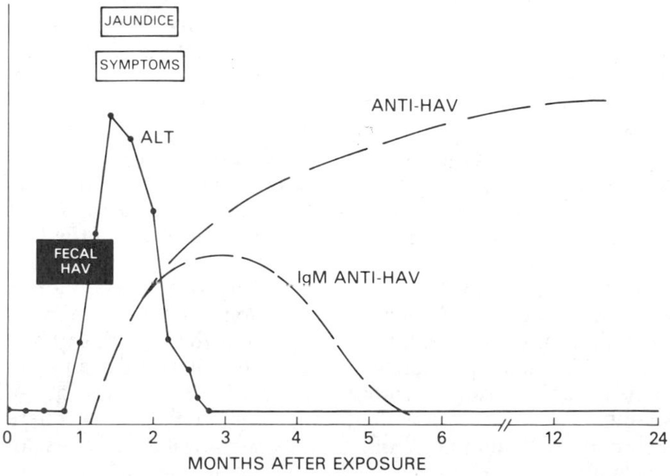

FIG. 5. The clinical and serologic course of a typical case of type A hepatitis. HAV: hepatitis A virus; ANTI-HAV: antibody to hepatitis A virus; ALT: alanine aminotransferase.

hepatitis cannot be distinguished from type A hepatitis or from non-A, non-B hepatitis on clinical grounds alone. The occurrence of the serum sickness-like syndrome of fever, rash, and polyarthritis during the preicteric phase favors the diagnosis of type B hepatitis (but also occurs in non-A, non-B hepatitis).

Epidemiologic features can strongly suggest hepatitis B virus (HBV) infection. This disease has a long incubation period (40–180 days) and is more likely to occur as sporadic rather than epidemic hepatitis.[1] It is spread predominantly by the parenteral route. Thus, type B hepatitis often occurs in persons with exposure to blood or blood products (multiply transfused patients, hemophiliacs, renal dialysis, and oncology ward patients), with exposure to contaminated needles and syringes (medical personnel with accidental needlesticks, drug addicts), with multiple sexual contacts (homosexuals, prostitutes, the sexually active),[40] and with exposure to saliva or other potentially infectious excreta (children in institutions for the mentally retarded).[1]

However, these same epidemiologic features also can be found in cases of non-A, non-B hepatitis and (occasionally) also in type A hepatitis. In at least 50 percent of acute type B hepatitis cases, no history of parenteral exposure is uncovered. Whether these cases were acquired by "nonparenteral" routes or by inapparent parenteral routes is not known.

The diagnosis of type B hepatitis should rest on specific serologic testing, with the finding of hepatitis B surface antigen (HBsAg) in the serum during the acute disease (Fig. 6). HBsAg appears in the serum during the incubation period 2–7 weeks before the onset of symptoms. It usually persists in the blood throughout the illness and disappears with convalescence.[41,42] Almost all patients (95 percent) will be HBsAg-positive at the onset of symptoms and jaundice. In some patients, however, HBsAg is cleared rapidly and may be absent by the time the patient is tested. In this situation, tests for antibody must be used to make this diagnosis. Antibody to HBsAg (anti-HBs) usually arises during convalescence from type B hepatitis and, indeed, may not be detectable for some time into the recovery phase. Antibody to hepatitis B core antigen (anti-HBc) is a more reliable marker of HBV infection and usually appears at or about the time of onset of symptoms. Sensitive and specific immunoassays are now available for assaying both anti-HBs and anti-HBc. However, neither of these assays are particulary helpful in the serodiagnosis of acute type B hepatitis. Both anti-HBs and anti-HBc are long-lived. The finding of either of these antibodies in the serum of a patient with acute hepatitis does not prove that the disease is due to HBV infection. Recently, immunoassays for IgM anti-HBc have been developed that promise to be of some help in the diagnosis of type B hepatitis. IgM anti-HBc arises early in the illness of patients with acute type B hepatitis, but it rapidly decreases in titer and no longer may be detectable 6–24 months after the illness.[43] Both false-positive and false-negative results can occur with the IgM anti-HBc test, but they are rare.

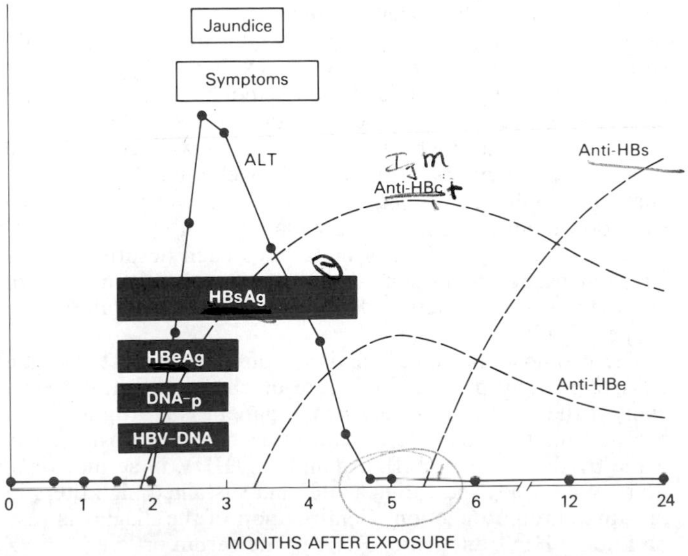

FIG. 6. The clinical and serologic course of a typical case of acute type B hepatitis. HBsAg: hepatitis B surface antigen; HBeAg: hepatitis B e antigen; DNA-p: DNA polymerase; HBV-DNA: hepatitis B virus DNA; ALT: alanine aminotransferase; Anti-HBc: antibody to hepatitis B core antigen; anti-HBe: antibody to HBeAg; anti-HBs: antibody to HBsAg.

Patients with acute type B hepatitis also develop hepatitis B e–antigen (HBeAg) as well as direct markers for the presence of HBV in serum such as HBV-DNA (as detected by molecular hybridization) and DNA polymerase (the endogenous polymerase of this virus). These are markers of active viral replication and are detected early in the course of acute hepatitis. By the peak of clinical illness and jaundice, levels of HBV in serum usually are decreasing or absent. Indeed, the seroconversion from HBeAg to antibody to HBeAg (anti-HBe) can be considered a favorable serologic sign indicating that the height of the viral replication has passed and that the infection is on the wane.

From 5 to 10 percent of patients with HBV infection do not clear HBsAg but become HBsAg carriers.[1,42] These people typically have mild, often anicteric and asymptomatic disease, which may explain why most chronic HBsAg carriers do not give a history of acute hepatitis. As many as 0.2–1.0 percent of adults in the United States are chronic HBsAg carriers. The prevalence of the carrier state is even higher in "high-risk" populations such as male homosexuals (6 percent), iv drug abusers (7 percent), hemophiliacs (7 percent), and renal dialysis patients (2–15 percent).[42] Most chronic HBsAg carriers are asymptomatic of their infection and have minimal or no accompanying liver injury.

The development of the chronic HBsAg carrier state as a result of symptomatic acute viral hepatitis is not common, but it does occur. Progression to a chronic carrier state should be suspected if the patient remains HBeAg-positive or if HBsAg titers do not decrease for more than 8 weeks after the onset of illness.[41]

The presence of the chronic HBsAg carrier state also can create diagnostic confusion in the serodiagnosis of acute viral hepatitis. A patient with acute viral hepatitis who is HBsAg-positive does not necessarily have acute type B hepatitis; the patient may be a chronic HBsAg carrier and have a superimposed and unrelated form of acute liver injury. This possibility is not as unlikely as it may seem. People who are at high risk for developing type B hepatitis and, therefore, the chronic HBsAg carrier state often are at high risk for developing other forms of acute viral hepatitis. Indeed, delta hepatitis represents just this phenomenon of an acute viral hepatitis being superimposed on the chronic HBsAg carrier state.[6] In this situation, testing for IgM anti-HBc can be helpful. This marker of acute type B hepatitis should be absent if the patient is a chronic HBsAg carrier with another form of acute hepatocellular injury.[43]

Delta Hepatitis

The delta agent was discovered in 1977 by Rizzetto and coworkers from Turin, Italy.[5] Subsequently, delta hepatitis has been shown to be caused by the delta hepatitis virus (HDV), an incomplete RNA virus that requires HBsAg for replication.[6,44] Delta infection occurs only in patients who have HBsAg in their serum and thus have either acute or chronic HBV infection. In the United States and Western Europe, delta hepatitis occurs most commonly in persons who have multiple parenteral exposures such as iv drug addicts, hemophiliacs, and persons who have multiple transfusions.[44] Delta infection is uncommon in medical care workers and male homosexuals. There are several areas of the world with a high prevalence of delta infection among carriers in the general population, including the Amazon Basin in South America, Central Africa, southern Italy, and Middle Eastern countries. Why delta infection became established among HBsAg carriers in those areas of the world and not in others such as China and Southeast Asia (where hepatitis B is very common) is not known.

Acute delta infection occurs in two forms depending upon the state of the underlying HBV infection: (*1*) as a coinfection in which acute delta hepatitis occurs simultaneously with acute hepatitis B (Fig. 7) and (*2*) as a superinfection in which acute delta hepatitis is superimposed upon chronic hepatitis B (Fig. 8).[45] Delta antigen can sometimes be detected in the serum during the early phase of acute delta hepatitis; with the disappearance of antigen, anti-HDV arises.[46] However, the appearance of anti-HDV may be delayed, short-lived, and low in titer. Thus, many patients with acute delta hepatitis will test negative for anti-HDV during the acute illness and will only become positive in convalescence and then only in low titer. A radioimmunoassay for anti-HDV is commercially available,[47] but anti-HDV tests are not always reliable for the diagnosis of acute HDV infection.

Most patients with acute delta coinfection recover; as the hepatitis B resolves and HBsAg is cleared from the serum, the HDV infection also resolves. Thus, fewer than 5 percent of cases of acute delta coinfection result in chronic delta hepatitis. In contrast, most patients with acute delta superinfection are left with chronic delta hepatitis; because HBsAg persists, the HDV infection can persist. More than 70 percent of cases of delta superinfection result in chronic hepatitis (Fig. 8).[46] The diagnosis of chronic is easier than that of acute delta hepatitis; high titers of anti-HDV (>1:100 by commerical radioimmunoassay) indicate ongoing delta infection. Furthermore, patients with chronic delta hepatitis will have HDV antigen in the liver and persistence of IgM anti-HDV in serum.[46] HDV antigen is readily detectable in liver when using immunoperoxidase techniques.

Recently, two new research assays have provided new information regarding the natural history and biology of HDV infection: tests of HDV antigen in serum and liver by using Western blotting (immunoblotting)[48] and tests for HDV RNA in serum and liver by using molecular hybridization with a cloned cDNA or RNA ("riboprobe").[49] The finding of HDV

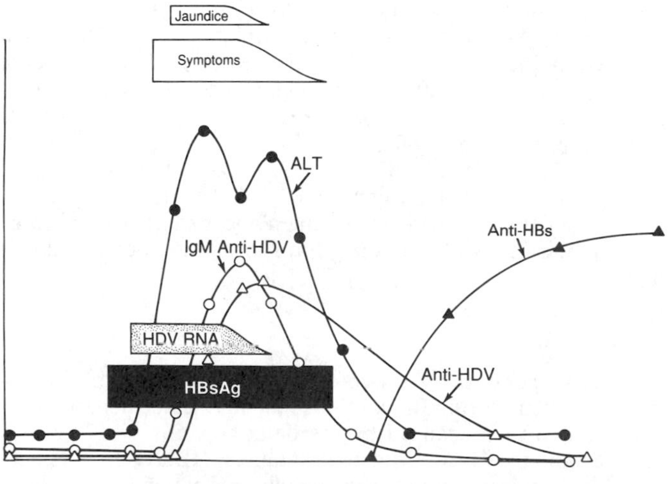

FIG. 7. The clinical and serologic course of a typical case of acute delta coinfection. ALT: alanine aminotransferase; HDV: hepatitis delta virus; HBsAg: hepatitis B surface antigen; anti-HBs: antibody to HBsAg; anti-HDV: antibody to HDV.

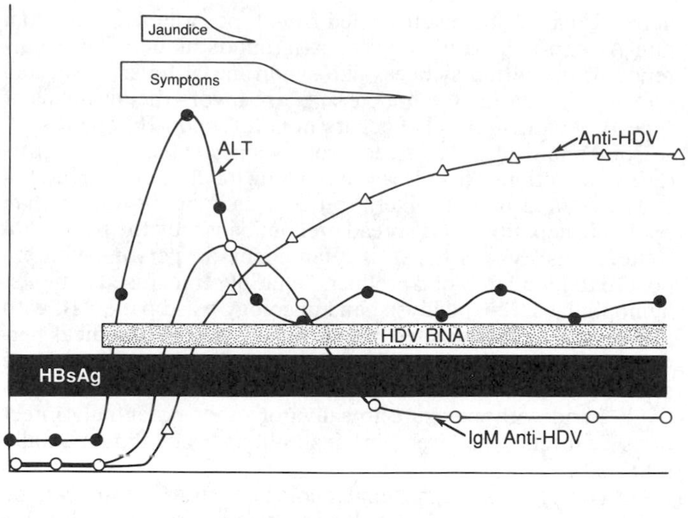

FIG. 8. The clinical and serologic course of a typical case of acute delta superinfection that leads to chronic delta hepatitis. ALT: alanine aminotransferase; HDV: hepatitis delta virus; HBsAg: hepatitis B surface antigen; Anti-HDV: antibody to HDV.

antigen or RNA in serum is a direct demonstration of the presence of virus and documents active viral replication. Hepatitis D virus antigen and RNA are typically present transiently during the early phases of acute delta hepatitis and for prolonged periods in chronic delta hepatitis. The sensitivity of these assays is still not well documented; only 50–80 percent of patients with chronic delta hepatitis (as shown by the presence of delta antigen in liver by immunoperoxidase) have detectable HDV antigen or RNA in their serum.

Clinically, delta hepatitis tends to be a severe illness. Acute delta hepatitis has a mortality of 2–20 percent.[44] The illness also often has a biphasic and protracted course. Chronic delta hepatitis is also a severe illness and is more likely to result in serious morbidity or mortality than is chronic hepatitis B alone or non-A, non-B hepatitis. In large series, 60–70 percent of patients with chronic delta hepatitis eventually developed cirrhosis, and most of these patients died of liver disease.[50] The progression to cirrhosis usually takes 10–15 years, but it can be quite rapid, within 2 years of the onset of infection.[44]

The epidemiology of delta hepatitis indicates that it is usually spread by parenteral exposure, which explains why this disease is common among drug addicts and hemophiliacs. Other modes of spread are less well defined. In some areas of the world intrafamilial spread has been documented as well as spread between sexual partners.[51] Interestingly, delta hepatitis often occurs in indolent, prolonged, severe epidemics that strike susceptible populations (i.e., populations with a high HBsAg carrier rate).[14] Epidemics of delta have been described in the Amazon basin and in central Africa, as well as among communities of drug addicts and institutionalized, mentally handicapped children.[44]

The diagnosis of delta hepatitis should be suspected in any HBsAg-positive patient with acute or chronic hepatitis, especially if the disease is severe or the patient is a drug addict or has had multiple parenteral exposures. The diagnosis can be made by the finding of HBsAg and anti-HDV in serum: rising titers of antibody indicating acute, and sustained high titers indicating chronic infection. Confirmation of the diagnosis rests on finding HDV antigen or RNA in the serum or liver.

Classic Non-A, Non-B Hepatitis

Non-A, non-B hepatitis is defined as an acute or chronic viral hepatitis-like syndrome in which serologic evidence of HAV or

HBV infection does not appear and no other cause of liver injury is apparent.[52,53] Despite attempts to identify the non-A, non-B hepatitis agent by many investigators during the last 15 years, the etiologic agent of non-A, non-B hepatitis has remained elusive, and the diagnosis is still made by the exclusion of other causes. Fortunately, this situation may soon change. In 1988, Houghton and coworkers from the Chiron Corporation in California announced the identification and cloning of a viral genome that appeared to be related to the agent of classic, parenterally transmitted non-A, non-B hepatitis.[8] By using molecular biologic techniques they developed a radioimmunoassay for antibody to this agent, which they have called the hepatitis C virus (HCV). Preliminary and as yet unpublished data indicated that this assay for anti-HCV successfully identified 50–90 percent of cases of acute and chronic non-A, non-B hepatitis.

Non-A, non-B hepatitis is a form of serum hepatitis. It is the most common cause of post-transfusion hepatitis and is commonly spread by the parenteral route,[52] the disease being frequent among dialysis patients, hemophiliacs, drug addicts, and medical care workers. This disease also occurs sporadically and without obvious parenteral exposure. In recent U.S. surveys, non-A, non-B hepatitis was considered to be the cause of 20–40 percent of cases of sporadic acute viral hepatitis.[32,53,54] Furthermore, analysis of the incidence of non-A, non-B hepatitis resulting from blood transfusion has indicated that as many as 1 percent of American blood donors harbor the agent of non-A, non-B hepatitis.[52] Thus, non-A, non-B hepatitis must be spread by intrafamilial, intimate, or sexual exposure, although proof of such transmission had yet to be demonstrated.

Clinically, non-A, non-B hepatitis is similar to hepatitis B. Approximately 25 percent of cases of acute disease are icteric, and the death rate is less than 1 percent.[52] Non-A, non-B hepatitis has several distinctive clinical and biochemical characteristics. On the average, non-A, non-B hepatitis has a more indolent and prolonged course than hepatitis B does. Serum aminotransferases often fluctuate widely and peak at levels (10–20 times normal) somewhat lower than those in hepatitis B (20–50 times normal) (Fig. 9). Non-A, non-B hepatitis also tends to have an insidious onset and a protracted, relapsing course.

Perhaps the most distinctive feature of non-A, non-B hepatitis is its propensity to progress to chronic hepatitis. In prospective studies, 50–70 percent of persons with acute non-A, non-B hepatitis have been left with biochemical evidence of chronic hepatitis.[52,55] Furthermore, the chronicity rate tends to be just as high after sporadic as after transfusion-related non-A, non-B hepatitis.[54] Chronic non-A, non-B hepatitis tends to be indolent and often silent. However, long-term follow-up studies of patients with this disease have shown that 20–25 percent ultimately develop cirrhosis of the liver.[55] It is often with the development of end-stage liver disease that symptoms first appear. Chronic non-A, non-B hepatitis is one of the major causes of cirrhosis in the United States and ranks as one of the most common indications for liver transplantation in adults.

Advances in knowledge about non-A, non-B hepatitis have been stymied by the lack of a sensitive and specific serologic assay for this infection. The recent development of an assay for anti-HCV promises to correct this lack. Preliminary data indicate that the classic non-A, non-B hepatitis agent (HCV) is a medium-sized (30–60 nm) RNA virus that is present in the blood in acute and chronic infections in low titer. This virus particle has not been visualized, but the genome has been cloned and characterized as a 10.5 kilobase [kb], single-stranded (+) RNA that produces a single polyprotein. Antibody to HCV (anti-HCV) can be detected with immunoassays using an expressed protein from the cDNA clone of this viral genome. Anti-HCV was detected in most cases of non-A, non-B hepatitis. However, the antibody arose rather late in the course of acute disease, often during convalescence. This feature made anti-HCV testing an unreliable diagnostic marker for non-A, non-B hepatitis during the acute illness. Anti-HCV testing was, however, quite reliable in identifying cases of chronic non-A, non-B hepatitis. Preliminary results showed that anti-HCV was detected in 80–90 percent of pedigreed cases of chronic non-A, non-B hepatitis. It follows from these results that screening of donor blood for anti-HCV may identify most infectious donors and make post-transfusion non-A, non-B hepatitis as rare as post-transfusion hepatitis B. Further information regarding these assays for anti-HCV is eagerly awaited, as is the commercial availability of this antibody test.

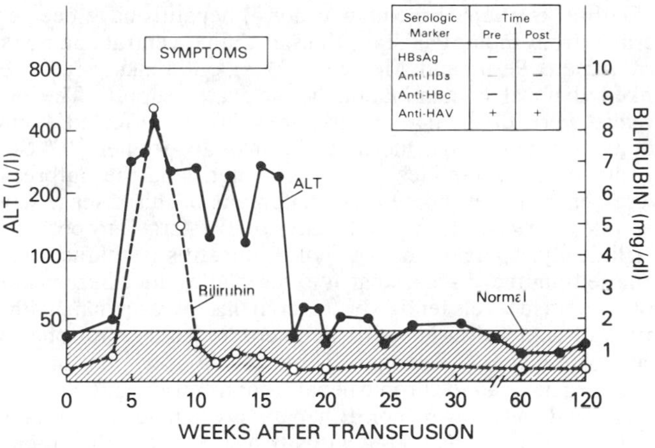

FIG. 9. The clinical and serologic course of a typical case of post-transfusion non-A, non-B hepatitis. ALT: alanine aminotransferase; HBsAg: hepatitis B surface antigen; Anti-HBs: antibody to HBsAg; Anti-HBc: antibody to hepatitis B core antigen; Anti-HAV: antibody to hepatitis A virus.

Epidemic Non-A, Non-B Hepatitis

Not all cases of non-A, non-B hepatitis are associated with parenteral exposure. In recent years, several large outbreaks of viral hepatitis linked to water contamination have been shown to be unrelated to either HBV or HAV infection.[10,56,57] These outbreaks have been studied extensively and shown to be caused by a non-A, non-B hepatitis agent that is distinct from the classic, parenterally transmitted form of disease (Table 1). This disease has been referred to as "epidemic" or "enterally transmitted" non-A, non-B hepatitis. The identification of the virus by immune electron microscopy,[9] the development of serologic assays for antibody to this agent,[58,59] and the announcement that the genome of the virus has been cloned indicate that this agent is distinct from HCV and warrants being referred to as hepatitis E virus (HEV).

TABLE 1. Comparison of Classic and Epidemic Non-A, Non-B Hepatitis

Feature	*Classic*	*Epidemic*
Mode of spread	Parenteral	Enteral
Pattern of spread	Endemic Exposure to blood	Epidemics Water contamination
Viral agent	Unknown	Unknown
Genome	RNA	RNA
Size	30–60 nm	27–34 nm
Location	Serum	Stool
Similarity	HBV-like	HAV-like
Incubation period		
Mean (range)	50 (20–90) days	40 (15–60) days
Mortality	<1%	<1%, but higher in pregnant women
Chronicity	50–70%	None

(Data from Refs. 3, 7, 54–57.)

Outbreaks of epidemic non-A, non-B hepatitis have been described from India, Pakistan, Russia, China, central and northern Africa, Peru, and Mexico.[10] Most outbreaks have been linked to fecal contamination of the water supply. The outbreaks were distinctive in that they largely affected young adults and had a high mortality in pregnant women.[57,58] Secondary cases in families were uncommon, and the outbreaks were generally self-limited. No outbreaks of this disease have been described in the United States or Western Europe.

Clinically, epidemic non-A, non-B hepatitis is characterized as a self-limited disease that is often cholestatic. Serum aminotransferase levels tend to be lower in this disease than in other forms of acute viral hepatitis and serum alkaline phosphatase somewhat higher.[57] Prolonged jaundice can occur, but this disease does not lead to chronic hepatitis or a carrier state. In many ways, epidemic non-A, non-B hepatitis resembles hepatitis A.

The HEV is a small RNA virus that is found in the stool of patients during the incubation period and early acute phase of illness.[9,58] Evidently, the amount of HEV shedding in stool is not as great as the amount of HAV shedding that occurs in hepatitis A. These features may explain why secondary spread of epidemic non-A, non-B hepatitis is uncommon.

Antibody to HEV (anti-HEV) can be detected by immune electron microscopy or by the inhibition of immunofluorescence detection of HEV antigen in hepatocyte cytoplasm.[58,59] Both techniques are cumbersome but have shown that this antibody develops early during the course of illness. Cases of hepatitis associated with large-scale epidemics of non-A, non-B hepatitis have invariably demonstrated the development of anti-HEV. In contrast, none of a large number of cases of sporadic non-A, non-B hepatitis from the United States have demonstrated anti-HEV reactivity. These preliminary results suggest that epidemic non-A, non-B hepatitis, which may be the most common cause of jaundice and acute hepatitis in the underdeveloped world, is a very rare cause of hepatitis in the United States.

Serodiagnosis of Acute Viral Hepatitis

A guide to the serodiagnosis of acute viral hepatitis is given in Table 2. Patients with acute hepatitis should be tested for IgM anti-HAV and HBsAg. The presence of IgM anti-HAV establishes the diagnosis of hepatitis A. The presence of HBsAg suggests the diagnosis of hepatitis B, but two further tests may be helpful to confirm the diagnosis: IgM anti-HBc and anti-HDV. The presence of IgM anti-HBc confirms the diagnosis of *acute* hepatitis B; its absence suggests that the patient is actually a chronic carrier of HBsAg and that the hepatitis is either due to an exacerbation of the underlying chronic hepatitis B or due to superinfection with another hepatitis agent. The presence of anti-HDV suggests the diagnosis of delta hepatitis, although it is not conclusive and does not indicate whether the delta infection is resolved or ongoing, acute or chronic. The titer of anti-HDV can help to separate acute (rising titers) or chronic delta hepatitis (sustained high titers).

Non-A, non-B hepatitis is marked by the absence of IgM anti-HAV, HBsAg, and IgM anti-HBc, but other causes should also be excluded before the diagnosis is made (see below). Tests for anti-HCV and anti-HEV are not currently available. Anti-HCV testing is likely to become a valuable adjunct to serologic diagnosis, but it may not be particularly reliable during the acute illness and may require retesting in convalescence. Anti-HEV testing is rarely necessary because epidemic non-A, non-B hepatitis is uncommon in the United States and can usually be suggested by epidemiologic features such as occurrence in an epidemic or travel to an endemic area.

A careful history and physical examination are of prime importance in diagnosis of the form of viral hepatitis. Often, epidemiologic features or a history of exposure to hepatitis will provide the necessary confirmation of the diagnosis, especially if tests for IgM anti-HAV and HBsAg are negative. Research tests may also be helpful in special situations by providing definitive evidence of the type of hepatitis. These confirmatory research tests include molecular hybridization assays for HAV RNA, HBV DNA and HDV RNA in serum or liver tissue as well as more conventional immunoassays for HAV, HBV, or HDV antigens in liver biopsy samples. Nevertheless, use of the standard, commercially available serologic tests and a careful clinical history should indicate the accurate diagnosis in more than 90 percent of cases of acute hepatitis.

TABLE 2. Serodiagnosis of Acute Viral Hepatitis

IgM Anti-HAV	*HBsAg*	*IgM Anti-HBc*	*Interpretation*
+	−	−	Acute hepatitis A
−	+ (or −)	+	Acute hepatitis B
−	+	−	Chronic hepatitis B[a]
−	−	−	Non-A, non-B hepatitis

[a] In this situation, delta hepatitis should be considered.

Chronic Hepatitis

Chronic hepatitis with an acute exacerbation can mimic acute viral hepatitis and can represent a significant problem in the differential diagnosis. This is best demonstrated for HBsAg-positive chronic hepatitis. These patients occasionally can be asymptomatic, except for recurrent bouts of jaundice and symptoms of hepatitis that can occur with almost seasonal regularity. Several features should suggest the presence of chronic hepatitis. These include previous bouts of hepatitis or jaundice, a prolonged and indolent preicteric phase of disease, protracted and only mild-to-moderate elevations in aminotransferase and serum bilirubin levels (Fig. 2), and increased globulin and decreased serum albumin levels. In most instances the presence of HBsAg with absence of IgM anti-HBc confirms the diagnosis of chronic infection. In the final analysis, however, differentiation requires the test of time. The persistence of symptoms or abnormal serum enzyme levels for more than 6 months indicates chronic hepatitis. A liver biopsy specimen usually can be helpful if it demonstrates chronic hepatitis with fibrosis or with ground-glass cells. However, it may not clearly differentiate acute from chronic hepatitis at the height of an acute exacerbation. Other features of chronic hepatitis will be discussed in the next chapter.

Acute Hepatitis Due to Other Viruses

Several other common viral infections can secondarily affect the liver and can cause an acute hepatitis-like picture. The liver disease associated with these infections usually is mild, self-limited, subclinical, and overshadowed by the other symptoms in these diseases.

Of prime importance as a secondary cause of viral hepatitis is the Epstein-Barr virus (EBV), the agent of heterophile-positive infectious mononucleosis. When sought, mild elevations in serum aminotransferase levels (two to five times normal) are very common in acute mononucleosis. This syndrome should offer no diagnostic confusion with acute viral hepatitis; the liver disease is mild and subclinical. However, on rare occasions, EBV infection can be manifested as acute icteric hepatitis without the usual symptoms of mononucleosis.[22] Physical examination may reveal little or no evidence of pharyngitis or lymphadenopathy. Several features of the hepatitis should suggest that it is due to EBV infection. First, fever (which usually is not prominent in acute viral hepatitis) is prominent and persistent in mononucleosis. High fever lasting into the icteric phase should suggest infectious mononucleosis. Second, the serum enzyme levels in mononucleosis are not entirely typical of those in acute viral hepatitis. The alkaline phosphatase and LDH levels usually are higher than expected from the degree of jaundice and aminotransferase elevation (Fig. 2). Most suggestive, however, is the presence of a significant lymphocytosis (>50 percent) with atypical lymphocytes (>20 percent). Without this, hepatitis cannot be readily ascribed to EBV infection. Finally, the mononucleosis slide test or heterophile antibody is usually but not invariably reactive. Absolute confirmation of infectious mononucleosis rests on the appearance of anti-EBV or on a fourfold rise in titer when tested on paired sera. Because most adults have anti-EBV, a single positive specimen is not meaningful. Liver biopsy findings in acute mononucleosis hepatitis are quite characteristic but add little. A diagnosis of acute hepatitis as being due to infectious mononucleosis requires only a typical pattern of serum enzyme levels, atypical lymphocytosis, and a positive heterophile test.

Much of what is said about EBV-related hepatitis can be repeated for the cytomegalovirus (CMV). However, the role of CMV infection in causing a hepatitis in adults still is subject to debate, especially as it relates to post-transfusion hepatitis.[55,60,61] The problem centers on relating changes in anti-CMV titers and/or excretion of the virus to an episode of hepatitis. Such changes can occur in totally asymptomatic patients and are frequent after blood transfusions (regardless of the occurrence of hepatitis).[60] There is no doubt that primary CMV infection can cause a heterophile-negative mononucleosis syndrome that frequently is accompanied by hepatosplenomegaly and minor elevations of serum aminotransferase levels.[61] Whether CMV can induce a purely hepatitis-like syndrome is unclear. If it can, it probably is rare in adults. The diagnosis rests either on the finding of atypical lymphocytosis with acute liver injury, the absence of heterophile antibody, and the appearance or titer rise of anti-CMV (without anti-EBV rise) or on the excretion of the virus in urine or oropharyngeal secretions.

Several other common human viruses (including rubella rubeola, and mumps viruses; and coxsackie B virus) can induce mild abnormalities in liver enzymes.[62] These changes are not common and rarely are accompanied by jaundice. In the immunosuppressed host, however, several usually benign viruses can cause a disseminated infection, part of which may be hepatic involvement. Chief among these are the herpes simplex virus, CMV, and the varicella-zoster virus.[60–63] These are all herpesviruses that are ubiquitous and common benign infections in humans. In the patient with poor host defenses, dissemination with these viruses can occur. Hepatic necrosis, marked elevations in the serum aminotransferase levels, icterus, and even death from hepatic failure have been described. In the immunosuppressed or the immunoincompetent host with fulminant hepatic failure, a search for these viruses should be made. Liver biopsy specimens may demonstrate inclusion bodies and/or intranuclear herpesvirus particles. These viruses, however, are not common causes of sporadic acute hepatitis in the otherwise healthy host.

One more virus that is responsible for severe hepatic failure should be mentioned as a rare cause of acute viral hepatitis—yellow fever virus. Yellow fever has not been reported in the United States for over 40 years. It is, however, still enzootic in Central America, South America, and central Africa. Clinically, it is marked by a short incubation period (3–7 days), severe hepatitis with high aminotransferase level elevations, and a high mortality (approximately 20 percent).[64] It need be considered only in the recent traveler to enzootic areas who has not received adequate immunization. The diagnosis is made by isolating the virus from the blood, by finding a significant rise in antibody titers on paired sera, or by characteristic pathologic findings in the liver.

Hepatitis Due to Nonviral Infectious Diseases

Elevations in serum enzyme levels and liver dysfunction can occur with many nonviral infectious diseases due to bacteria, mycobacteria, rickettsia, and fungi. Thus jaundice with mild elevations in aminotransferase and alkaline phosphatase levels (two to five times normal) can be seen with several types of sepsis as well as with pneumococcal pneumonia.[22,65] Furthermore, minor elevations of liver enzyme levels without jaundice often are seen with many severe infections that usually do not primarily involve the liver—pulmonary and miliary tuberculosis,[66] brucellosis, tularemia, plague, gram-negative sepsis, legionnaires' disease, and so on. Liver biopsy specimens usually show nonspecific changes and focal areas of necrosis. However, at times (as in miliary tuberculosis), a liver biopsy specimen can be very helpful in establishing the primary diagnosis.

Three nonviral infectious agents that can produce an acute hepatitis-like syndrome deserve special note: syphilis, leptospirosis, and Q fever. Early syphilis, either primary or early secondary, can be accompanied by significant serum aminotransferase level elevations (three to eight times normal).[67] Jaundice, however, is rare, and the chancre of primary syphilis or the rash of secondary syphilis should be present. The liver enzyme tests, as in mononucleosis hepatitis, show atypically high elevations of alkaline phosphatase levels (four to eight times normal) when compared with the extent of aminotransferase abnormalities. Diagnosis is established by the finding of a reactive VDRL and fluorescent treponemal antibody (FTA) as well as by the typical clinical setting and response to treatment.

Leptospirosis is a well-known but rare cause of jaundice and hepatitis in the United States. The disease is caused by at least 15 serotypes of *Leptospira interrogans*.[59] The serotypes that are responsible for most of the infections in this country are *(1) icterohemorrhagiae* (30–40 percent), which is enzootic in rats; *(2) canicola* (30 percent), enzootic in dogs; and *(3) pomona* (10–20 percent), enzootic in cattle and swine. The history usually points to exposure to these animals or their urine (lake water, swimming holes). The clinical manifestations include malaise, fever, chills, severe myalgias, and headache.[68] Later symptoms of cough, sputum production, prostration, and hepatic and renal involvement appear. Hepatic involvement is most common with the serotype *icterohemorrhagiae*. Evaluation may demonstrate fever, prostration, severe muscle tenderness, hepatosplenomegaly, and pneumonitis. Laboratory abnormalities include leukocytosis and a left shift in the differential count. The urinalysis may show albuminuria, casts, and white and red blood cells. In severe cases, the urine output falls, and the blood urea nitrogen level rises; central nervous system manifestations and pneumonitis also may appear. Liver function tests reveal jaundice that is often out of proportion to the degree of serum enzyme level elevations. As with the jaundice of pneumococcal pneumonia,[65] the jaundice in leptospirosis appears to be a result of a defect in bilirubin excretion, rather than the result of hepatic necrosis.[68] The diagnosis is made by finding a high titer or a significant rise in leptospiral agglutinins. It is unclear whether early antibiotic treatment ameliorates this disease. A differential diagnosis from typical acute viral hepatitis usually is not difficult.

Q fever is the third nonviral infectious disease that may be mistaken for acute viral hepatitis. This rare disease is caused by the rickettsial agent *Coxiella brunetti*. In this disease, as in leptospirosis, constitutional symptoms are prominent with fever, chills, and pneumonitis. Overt jaundice occurs in only about 5 percent of the cases, although subclinical hepatic involvement is quite common. In rare cases, hepatitis without pneumonitis occurs, and a differentiation from acute viral hepatitis may be difficult.[69] Epidemiologic features should reveal exposure to farm or wild animals (cows, goats, sheep). Clinically, persistent fever, pneumonitis, and prostration are more prominent than in viral hepatitis. Liver function tests reveal jaundice with only mild elevations in aminotransferase levels (two to five times normal) and sometimes marked elevations in the alkaline phosphatase concentration. The diagnosis is made by demonstration of a rise in agglutination titers against *C. burnetii* in paired sera. As in leptospirosis, early antibiotic treatment has not been found to be helpful in this rickettsial disease.

Drug-Related Acute Hepatitis

The major differential diagnosis in acute hepatitis is between viral and drug-related hepatitis. Every patient with hepatitis should be questioned carefully about all medications that he uses and should be specifically asked about "over-the-counter" products. Drug-related acute liver injury is not nearly as common as acute viral hepatitis, but it often is much more serious and is a prominent cause of fulminant hepatic failure.[70] Many drugs and toxins have been shown to induce hepatic injury, but few have actually been repeatedly implicated as causing an acute hepatitis-like syndrome. The major common medications available in the United States that are associated with significant hepatotoxicity are listed in Table 3 by the type of injury usually seen and with an approximate incidence. This is not an exhaustive list. Any patient who develops hepatitis while taking a drug that is a known or potential hepatotoxin should have treatment with the medication stopped until the full clinical picture can be evaluated. The most serious mistake that can be made in caring for patients with acute hepatitis injury is to underestimate the role of drugs and to continue administering them in the face of acute hepatitis. The suspicion of drug-induced liver injury should be the greatest when epidemiologic features are not absolutely typical of acute viral hepatitis (e.g., in the elderly, in patients with underlying diseases, and in patients who develop fulminant hepatitis). However, even when epidemiologic features are appropriate for acute viral hepatitis, the role of drugs should not be dismissed: the renal dialysis patient taking methyldopa or the drug addict receiving isoniazid who develop acute hepatitis should have treatment with these medications stopped until adequate evaluation dismisses their role.

Some of the most commonly encountered causes of drug-related acute hepatitis are aspirin, acetaminophen, isoniazid, rifampin, phenytoin, and the anesthetic halothane. *Aspirin* (acetylsalicylic acid) can cause dramatic elevations in serum enzyme levels (two to five times normal), but it rarely causes jaundice. Aspirin hepatotoxicity seems to occur only with a high maintenance dosage, usually with serum salicylate levels of 20 mg/dl or greater. Characteristically, the biochemical abnormalities subside rapidly on withdrawing the drug. *Acetaminophen* (paracetamol) regularly causes severe hepatic necrosis similar to acute viral hepatitis when taken in large amounts (especially >15 g), as with a suicide attempt. Acetaminophen overdose seems to be becoming a more popular method of suicide and has become a major cause of fulminant hepatic failure both in the United States and England. The liver disease appears 2–5 days after the overdose. Interestingly, the liver injury can be averted if the patient is treated within 10 hours of the overdose with large doses of glutathione precursors (cysteamine, methionine, *N*-acetyl cysteine). Liver injury from the chronic use of acetaminophen in high doses also has been described.[71] Unexplained fulminant hepatitis should lead the physician to consider an acetaminophen overdose, the history of which the patient

TABLE 3. Common Causes of Drug-Related Liver Injury

Agent Class	*Agent*	*Frequency of Occurrence*[a]	*Type of Injury*
Analgesic	Acetaminophen	Dose-related	Hepatitis
	Aspirin	Dose-related	Hepatitis
Anesthetic	Halothane	Rare (0.01–0.1%)	Hepatitis
	Methoxyflurane	Rare	Hepatitis
Antiarthritic	Allopurinol	Rare	Granuloma/hepatitis
	Indomethacin	Very rare	Hepatitis
	Phenylbutazone	Rare	Granuloma/mixed
Antibacterial	Carbenicillin	Low[b]	Hepatitis
	Erythromycin estolate	Low	Cholestasis
	Nitrofurantoin	Rare	Mixed
	Oxacillin	Rare	Hepatitis
	Sulfonamides/sulfones	Rare	Hepatitis
	Tetracycline	Dose-related	Steatosis/necrosis
Antifungal	Ketoconazole	Rare	Hepatitis
Antineoplastic	Azathioprine	Rare[b]	Cholestasis
	6-Mercaptopurine	Common[b] (10–35%)	Hepatitis
	Methotrexate	Dose-related	Fibrosis
	Mithromycin	Rare[b]	Necrosis
Antituberculosis	Isoniazid	Low (1%)	Hepatitis
	Para-aminosalicylic acid	Low (0.1–1%)	Hepatitis
	Rifampin	Low	Hepatitis
Cardiovascular	Methyldopa	Low	Hepatitis
	Quinidine	Rare	Granuloma/hepatitis
	Thiazides	Very rare	Mixed
	Amiodarone	Low (1–3%)	Steatosis/necrosis
Endocrinologic	17-Alkylated androgens	Dose-related	Cholestasis
	Chlorprompamide	Rare	Cholestasis
	Oral contraceptives	Rare	Cholestasis
	Propylthiouracil	Rare	Hepatitis
	Tolbutamide	Very rare	Cholestasis
Neuro- and psychopharmacologic	Dantrolene	Low (1–2%)	Hepatitis
	Monoamine oxidase inhibitors	Low	Hepatitis
	Phenothiazines	Low (1–2%)	Cholestasis
	Phenytoin	Rare	Hepatitis
	Valproic acid	Low (1–2%)	Steatosis/necrosis

[a] The frequency of occurrence is an estimate from the literature[70]: common ≃ >2 percent, low ≃ 0.1–2 percent, rare <0.1 percent, very rare = isolated case reports only.
[b] Dose-related to some degree.

may have denied. Both *isoniazid* and *rifampin* have been implicated in causing an acute hepatitis-like syndrome; both have been associated with fulminant hepatic failure. Rifampin hepatic injury usually has its onset within the first weeks of therapy, whereas isoniazid hepatotoxicity is most common after 1–2 months of therapy. The incidence of isoniazid hepatotoxicity is approximately 1 percent, but it is definitely higher in older age groups and approaches 10 percent in patients over the age of 40. Treatment with these drugs should be discontinued if symptoms of hepatitis or jaundice appear or if aminotransferase levels are persistently elevated more than five times normal. Phenytoin can cause an acute hepatitis, usually within 1–6 weeks of starting the medication and associated with other manifestations of hypersensitivity such as fever, rash, lymphadenopathy, and eosinophilia. It has a mortality of approximately 10 percent. Therapy with this drug should be stopped in any patient showing evidence of acute hepatitis. The anesthetic agents *halothane* and *methoxyflurane* perhaps are the most controversial drugs incriminated in causing acute hepatic necrosis. A recent cooperative study on halothane-induced hepatitis suggested that approximately 1/10,000 patients given this anesthetic for the first time and 1/1000 given it more than once develop fulminant hepatic necrosis.[72] While halothane-induced hepatitis is rare, it nevertheless is a significant cause of death from hepatic failure. Clinically, halothane-related jaundice appears within 3–14 days of its use and resembles an acute, severe viral hepatitis. Fever is very characteristic early in the course; many patients have an accompanying leukocytosis and eosinophilia. Halothane-induced hepatitis usually is not confused with post-transfusion hepatitis because of its early onset after surgery and anesthesia.

Many other medications have been implicated or cited as causes of acute hepatic injury. Every agent that a person with acute hepatitis is taking should be held in suspicion. The suspicion of drug-induced liver injury should weigh heavily in the performance of a liver biopsy procedure. In many situations, liver biopsy findings can help to identify the cause of hepatic injury and can aid in the future use of the implicated drugs.

Anoxic Liver Injury

A syndrome resembling acute viral hepatitis can occur after anoxic injury to the liver due to a period of hypotension, severe left- or right-sided heart failure, or cardiopulmonary arrest.[73] The clinical and historical features usually can distinguish this nonspecific type of liver injury from acute viral hepatitis. However, in some cases, no clear history of an anoxic episode is obtained, or the patient is brought to the hospital comatose and unable to give an adequate history. In these situations, a diagnosis usually can be made on the basis of serum enzymes. Within hours of an anoxic episode, there are marked elevations of aminotransferase levels into the range seen with acute viral hepatitis (Fig. 2). The alkaline phosphatase level remains only minimally elevated or is normal. The LDH level, conversely, is dramatically elevated (as is the CPK level), and it may be most helpful in suggesting this diagnosis. Most typical of anoxic liver injury, however, is the rapid resolution of these enzyme abnormalities. The aminotransferase levels often decrease by half each day and can fall from 50–100 times elevated to normal within a week. Jaundice is uncommon and mild; it generally occurs several days after injury. In some cases, aminotransferase levels remain elevated to two to five times normal for 5–14 days after the injury, in which case differentiation from acute viral hepatitis may be difficult and may require a liver biopsy procedure (which will show a bland centrozonal necrosis). While a liver biopsy specimen is diagnostic, it generally is not needed for the diagnosis when the clinical history and pattern of enzyme levels are typical.

Alcoholic Liver Disease

Alcohol abuse is the most common cause of serious liver disease in the United States. Alcoholic liver disease (i.e., fatty liver, alcoholic hepatitis, and Laennec cirrhosis) usually can be readily differentiated from acute viral hepatitis by history and biochemical tests. Acute alcoholic hepatitis is the syndrome that, perhaps, is most easily confused with viral hepatitis. These patients have the gradual and imprecisely dated onset of malaise, anorexia, weight loss, nausea and vomiting, fever, chills, abdominal swelling, and jaundice or dark urine. The history of alcohol intake should suggest the diagnosis, but many patients conceal or underestimate the amount of alcohol they consume. The lower limit of alcohol intake said to lead to alcoholic liver disease is 80 g/day—the equivalent to a half-pint of 86 proof whiskey, four conventional "cocktails," five to six cans (12 oz) of beer, or 1 quart of wine each day.[70,74] Alcoholic liver disease is rarely manifested until after 10 or more years of excessive drinking.

Clinically, the patient usually appears chronically ill and typically is older than the average patient with viral hepatitis. Fever and tachycardia are common. Examination may reveal evidence of *chronic* liver disease and alcohol abuse that is not seen with acute viral hepatitis—wasting, parotid enlargement, palmar erythema, vascular spiders, gynecomastia, testicular atrophy, significant hepatomegaly, and signs of portal hypertension (ascites, edema, splenomegaly, and prominent abdominal veins). The laboratory data are most helpful.[22] The white blood cell count is usually elevated with a left shift. The hematocrit may be slightly decreased, and the red blood cell indices reveal macrocytosis (with or without folate deficiency). Liver function tests reveal hyperbilirubinemia and typically a low albumin level and a prolonged prothrombin time. The aminotransferase values are most characteristic (Fig. 2) in that the AST levels almost always are elevated, but rarely more than eight times normal. Furthermore, the AST level is elevated out of proportion to the ALT level (which can be slightly elevated, normal, or even low). Thus, the aminotransferase levels in alcoholic hepatitis differ greatly from those in viral hepatitis—not only in the degree of elevation but also by the relative elevation of the AST to the ALT level. The alkaline phosphatase level can be quite variable in alcoholic liver disease and sometimes is quite high. The LDH values are variable. If the clinical and biochemical pictures are unclear, acute alcoholic hepatitis can be readily diagnosed by a liver biopsy procedure, which is also helpful in judging the severity of liver injury and in gauging the prognosis.

Cholestatic Liver Disease

Cholestatic liver disease refers to a host of diseases marked by bile retention. Cholestasis can be due either to extrahepatic biliary obstruction (from gallstones, stricture, pancreatitis, or cancer) or to intrahepatic causes (from primary biliary cirrhosis, several childhood cholestatic syndromes, and drug-induced cholestasis from phenothiazines or methyltestosterone). These patients have the nonspecific symptoms of acute liver disease with jaundice, but the differentiation from acute viral hepatitis rarely is difficult. In general, signs and symptoms of cholestasis are prominent; the degree of jaundice, lightening of stools, and itching overshadow the amount of anorexia or malaise. Laboratory data are confirmatory and show modest abnormalities in aminotransferase levels but marked elevations in alkaline phosphatase levels (Fig. 2). Gallstone obstruction perhaps most closely mimics acute viral hepatitis, with its typical manifestation being fever, chills, malaise, right upper quadrant pain, nausea, vomiting, jaundice, and dark urine. Fever is prominent and often hectic, thus pointing away from viral hepatitis. Furthermore, the liver usually is quite tender, and there may be signs of localized peritonitis. Leukocytosis and a left shift usually are present; although aminotransferase levels can be quite high (up to 10–15 times normal), the alkaline phosphatase level usually is also markedly elevated.

Other Liver Diseases

Few other causes of jaundice pose a problem in the differential diagnosis of acute hepatitis. Rare causes of an acute hepatitis-like syndrome include Wilson's disease,[75] sickle cell crisis,[76] acute Budd-Chiari syndrome or veno-occlusive disease,[77] and massive replacement of the liver by tumor.[78] These causes usually are associated with a fulminant or severe hepatitis. Patients with hemolytic anemia may have vague nonspecific symptoms and jaundice, but the urine will have no bilirubin, and the aminotransferase levels will be normal. Patients with congenital disorders of bilirubin metabolism (Gilbert and Dubin-Johnson syndromes) may become notably jaundiced, especially during intercurrent viral illnesses, but serum enzyme levels should be normal.

Patients who are found, on routine blood tests (either during a screening test or during evaluation for other problems), to have abnormal aminotransferase levels sometimes are suspected of having anicteric or preicteric acute viral hepatitis. Actually, such patients with asymptomatic elevations in aminotransferase levels are far more likely to have chronic liver disease, and their evaluation should proceed with that in mind.

MANAGEMENT

Supportive Care

There is no specific therapy for acute viral hepatitis. Good management consists of supportive measures, relief of symptoms, and avoidance of further injury.

Hospitalization. Most patients with acute viral hepatitis do not require hospitalization. Little can be done for most patients in the hospital that is not available at home; also, for many, hospitalization is a heavy emotional and financial burden. However, several factors should be weighed when deciding not to hospitalize the patient with acute hepatitis. Home care should be reserved for patients who have only mild to moderate symptoms, who have someone at home to care for and feed them, and who can return for regular medical evaluation without difficulty. Hospitalization is advisable in any patient whose prothrombin time shows any prolongation or who has any clinical evidence of hepatic failure. The duration of hospitalization, of course, will vary with the severity of illness. Once symptoms have abated, the patient usually can be discharged to continue convalescence at home. There is no need to continue hospitalization until laboratory test values return to normal.

Rest. Bed rest should be prescribed for patients with acute viral hepatitis during the period of symptoms. However, the bed rest should not be absolute; use of the bathroom and periods of being up each day should be encouraged. Traditionally, it has been recommended that bed rest be continued until recovery is complete and liver function test values have returned to normal. While most patients are willing to remain at bed rest for the duration of the symptoms, most—and especially the young—will be anxious to return to normal activity once the symptoms abate. Indeed, controlled studies have shown that after the symptoms have cleared normal activity and even strenuous exercise does not slow recovery, induce relapses, or predispose to chronic liver disease.[79] It is unnecessarily restrictive to insist on bed rest until the aminotransferase levels return to normal or until HBsAg is negative. A gradual return to activity with monitoring of liver function test values is warranted once the symptoms have abated. Relapses of symptoms should be treated with a return to bed rest.

Alcohol. Alcohol traditionally has been prohibited not only during the acute illness but also for an extended period into convalescence. However, there are no data to suggest that moderate alcohol intake leads to a worsening of acute hepatitis or predisposes to chronic hepatitis. While it is prudent to advise abstinence during the acute symptomatic phase of viral hepatitis, the recommendation of total abstinence for 6–12 months after viral hepatitis is unnecessarily strict.

Diet. There is little evidence that any dietary regimen has any effect on the course of acute hepatitis. A generally nutritious diet should be encouraged. During the symptomatic phase, patients frequently are anorexic and may have distinct likes and dislikes. The person with anorexia cannot be forced to eat; however, some encouragement can come from the use of frequent small feedings and a diet low in fat but high in carbohydrates. Forced or nasogastric tube feedings should be avoided.

Drugs. Most medications are best avoided during acute hepatitis. Antibiotics are not indicated. Immune serum globulin has no effect. No single drug has yet been shown to significantly shorten or to ameliorate the course of the disease. Symptomatic therapy for nausea, pain, or sleeplessness may be needed at times. Antiemetics can be helpful, but chlorpromazine (because of its potential to cause intrahepatic cholestasis) should be avoided. Among analgesics, acetaminophen is preferable to aspirin (because of its effects on platelet function and the gastric mucosa) and codeine or morphine derivatives (because of their sedative effects). Sedatives should not be used at all, if possible. Mild sleeping medications such as triazolam or flurazepam often have been prescribed without incident, but they should not be considered routine. Previous data have suggested that estrogens might worsen the course of typical acute viral hepatitis; however, prospective studies of women with acute viral hepatitis who were taking oral contraceptives have failed to support this.[80] Nevertheless, it is advisable that treatment with all but the most necessary medications be discontinued during the acute phase of viral hepatitis. Vitamins often are given but have not been shown to be beneficial in patients with acute hepatitis. If the prothrombin time is prolonged, a trial of vitamin K (1–5 mg im) can be given. The administration of vitamin K, however, will have little or no effect on the prothrombin time in typical viral hepatitis unless there has been prolonged cholestasis.

Treatment

There are no specific therapies for acute viral hepatitis. Corticosteroids have not been shown to shorten the course or to aid in the healing of acute viral hepatitis.[81,82] Indeed, some studies have indicated that corticosteroids may predispose to more prolonged illness, more relapses, and more chronic liver disease.[82] Corticosteroids are definitely not indicated for the typical case of acute viral hepatitis.

Corticosteroids have sometimes been recommended for two situations in acute viral hepatitis: fulminant hepatic failure and cholestatic hepatitis. In prolonged cholestasis after acute viral hepatitis, corticosteroids can decrease serum bilirubin levels and ameliorate symptoms of fatigue and itching. The use of corticosteroids in this situation, however, should be limited to cases of hepatitis A in which the possibility of transition to chronic hepatitis is not present. In fulminant hepatitis, corticosteroids are often used, frequently because no other options are available. However, controlled clinical trials have failed to demonstrate any benefit of corticosteroids in acute viral hepatitis, and some have indicated that the adverse side effects of high doses of corticosteroids outweigh their potential benefit.[82]

Antiviral medications that have shown promise as therapy in chronic viral hepatitis[83,84] also hold promise as therapy for acute disease. So far, the only studies of antiviral treatment in severe acute viral hepatitis have been nonrandomized trials in small numbers of patients. In a study from Israel,[85] five patients with fulminant hepatitis were treated with interferon-α, and three survived, which led the authors to suggest that antiviral therapy might be helpful in a subset of patients with severe or fulminant hepatitis. However, in a later study from Spain,[86] only 2 of 12 patients with fulminant hepatitis B or delta who were treated with high doses of parenteral interferon-α survived, thus indicating that this medication is unlikely to be of benefit in reversing fulminant viral hepatitis.[86] Nevertheless, the possible role of interferon-α or other antiviral agents in typical acute or in severe hepatitis deserves further evaluation. The absence of a beneficial effect of therapy in fulminant hepatitis does not necessarily indicate that the therapy will have no effect in patients with less advanced or severe hepatic injury.

Monitoring

Monitoring during acute viral hepatitis should be regular and specific. While the patient is hospitalized, a daily check on major symptoms is important. The patient should be examined for the degree of icterus, liver size, and the presence of asterixis or other evidence of hepatic encephalopathy. The ALT, AST, alkaline phosphatase, and bilirubin levels and the prothrombin time should be monitored once or twice a week during hospitalization and every 1–2 weeks thereafter until they return to normal. Initially, the patient should be tested for HBsAg. If positive, the test is best repeated every 1–2 months until HBsAg disappears. The continued presence of HBsAg 4–6 months after acute viral hepatitis indicates the establishment of the chronic HBsAg carrier state. Other specialized testing of liver function or structure such as bromosulfophthalein retention, indocyanine green excretion, ultrasonography, computed tomography (CT), and liver–spleen radionuclide scanning are not helpful, nor are they needed in acute viral hepatitis.

A percutaneous liver biopsy specimen in acute viral hepatitis may well establish the diagnosis, but generally it is not necessary. However, in two situations, liver biopsy is indicated: (*1*) when the diagnosis is in doubt; if diagnostic confusion remains despite clinical, biochemical, and serologic data; if more than one explanation of acute liver injury exists; or if drug-related acute hepatitis is a possibility; and (*2*) when therapy is being considered.

Fulminant Viral Hepatitis

The management of fulminant viral hepatitis should begin with its early recognition. The initial signs and symptoms of hepatic encephalopathy may be subtle (nightmares, slight changes in personality, restlessness) or dramatic (unexpected aggressive physical or sexual activity). It is important to recognize these signs for what they are and not respond to them by using sedative or physical restraints.

At the first sign of encephalopathy, vigorous management should be started.[85] This should include bed rest, a low-protein diet (20–30 g/day), the administration of enemas to cleanse the bowel, and the use of oral neomycin (1.0–1.5 g every 6 hours) or lactulose (30–60 cc in sorbitol every 2–6 hours until loose stools are achieved). Treatment with all sedatives should be stopped. With deepening coma, the patient may require iv fluids, a central venous pressure line, a nasogastric tube, and a urinary bladder catheter. Coagulation defects may require correction with the use of freshly frozen plasma (the coagulation factor concentrates such as fibrinogen and prothrombin complex should not be used). The patient should be carefully monitored for gastrointestinal bleeding. Cimetidine (300–500 mg iv every 6 hours) or vigorous antacid therapy may be begun to help prevent upper gastrointestinal bleeding. Most important is careful attention to all the details of "routine" medical management (fluid and electrolyte balance, acid-base balance, pulmonary toilet, iv and bladder catheter care, skin care, and monitoring for signs of blood loss or superinfection). Corticosteroids may be used as outlined above. More aggressive approaches such as exchange transfusions, "total body washout," charcoal hemoperfusion, cross-circulation with a human or baboon liver, and immunotherapy with antibody to HBsAg each have had their advocates, but none has been repeatedly shown to be more effective than "conventional" medical management is.

The most promising new therapy for fulminant hepatic failure is emergency hepatic transplantation.[87,88] Since the early 1980s and the introduction of cyclosporine A as an immunosuppressive agent, liver transplantation has become a successful and well-accepted approach to severe liver disease. At present, 1200–1500 liver transplants are done yearly in the United States in 40–50 different medical centers. Approximately 7 percent of patients undergo liver transplantation for fulminant or subacute hepatic failure. The 1- to 2-year survival rates have ranged between 60 and 90 percent.[87]

The major reason to avoid liver transplantation in fulminant hepatic failure is the possibility of spontaneous recovery. The survival rate of patients with fulminant hepatitis in stage III–IV coma averages 20–30 percent. Features that predict a poor outcome include age (either less than 10 or greater than 40 years), non-A, non-B hepatitis or medications as a cause of the liver injury, and a prothrombin time greater than 50 seconds.[89] The decision for transplantation needs to be made before severe complications supervene, in particular decerebration, after which recovery is unlikely even with liver transplantation. Interestingly, the cause of liver injury usually does not recur in the transplanted liver[90]: hepatitis B causing fulminant hepatitis rarely infects the new liver. Thus, at the first sign of hepatic failure, the physician should refer the patient with acute viral hepatitis to a liver transplant center. The criteria for transplantation in fulminant hepatitis are currently changing, and the decision for organ transplantation should be made by a team of physicians with experience in treating fulminant hepatic failure.

Prevention

Specifics of prevention in viral hepatitis will be presented in later chapters. Management of needlestick injuries in hospital employees is discussed in Chapters 282 and 283. Certain nonspecific measures regarding the patient with acute hepatitis should be stressed here.

If the patient is hospitalized, he should be placed in a private room with separate toilet facilities. The major reason for such isolation is to prevent the spread of type A hepatitis. Even with lax precautions, such spread is very rare; most patients with type A hepatitis are no longer excreting virus once they have become symptomatic. Nevertheless, there are exceptions, and isolation is prudent. Secretions and blood products should be handled with care. Gowns, masks, and gloves are not necessary, but a prominent sign reading "needle and blood precautions" is appropriate. Labeling of blood specimens, as from a patient with hepatitis, is a common practice. It should be stressed, however, that all blood from any patient should be handled as if potentially infectious.

If at home, the patient should be advised about care in personal hygiene—use of a private bathroom, if possible, and careful hand washing. Attention also should be paid to blood and blood products and the handling of cuts and lacerations.

Recommendations regarding the prevention of acute hepatitis are governed by the type of viral hepatitis that is being considered. In the case of acute type A hepatitis, all family members and close personal contacts should receive immune serum globulin (ISG) at a dosage of 2–5 ml im as soon as possible after exposure. Office, factory, and school contacts do not need to be treated. Immune serum globulin can be given for up to 4 weeks after exposure, but it probably is only effective if given within 7–14 days. In the case of acute type B hepatitis, prophylaxis only needs to be provided for "regular" sexual contacts. The best form of protection is argued. Hepatitis B immune globulin (HBIG) at a dosage of 5 ml im as soon as possible and again 1 month later has been the conventional recommendation in this situation. However, the efficacy of HBIG in preventing the sexual spread of acute type B hepatitis has not been well proved.[91] In addition, there is now evidence that postexposure immunization with HBV vaccine can attentuate or prevent acute type B hepatitis.[92,93] In view of this, a practical approach is the administration of one injection of HBIG and the simultaneous initiation of vaccination. Vaccine should be given in 20 μg amounts (0.5–1.0 cc) im as soon as possible and then 1 month and 6 months later. In the case of acute delta hepatitis, the recommendations are the same as for type B hepatitis. Prevention of type B hepatitis also will prevent delta hepatitis. In the case of non-A, non-B hepatitis, there is little or no information concerning the efficacy of any mode of prevention. Prophylaxis probably is unnecessary, except for household contacts. Sexual partners may be at highest risk. Because ISG is inexpensive and safe and may have some effect in preventing icteric disease, it often is recommended for the regular sexual contacts of patients with acute non-A, non-B hepatitis.

There often is a delay between the diagnosis of acute viral hepatitis and the identification of whether the disease is due to type A, type B, delta, or non-A, non-B hepatitis. Indeed, serologic testing sometimes is not available. The recommendations given above require that the prophylaxis of family and intimate contacts of patients be postponed until the results of serologic testing are known. A simplified approach to prophylaxis is to administer ISG immediately to all family, household, and intimate contacts and to begin HBV vaccination of the sexual contact(s) if the disease is subsequently shown to be type B (or delta) hepatitis. This schema could be modified if the hepatitis is obviously not due to HAV (e.g., post-transfusion hepatitis). This approach is appealing because of its simplicity and also because the titers of anti-HBs (the protective antibody in type B hepatitis) in standard preparations of ISG have been increasing over the past 10–15 years.[91] Thus, ISG that is currently being produced may be partially effective in preventing type B hepatitis.

Finally, it should be stressed that viral hepatitis is a reportable disease. Once the diagnosis is verified and serologic testing data are available, they should be reported to the local or state department of health.

REFERENCES

1. Krugman S, Giles JP, Viral hepatitis. New light on an old disease. JAMA. 1970;212:1019.
2. Feinstone SM, Kapikian AZ, Purcell RH. Hepatitis A: Detection by immune electron microscopy of a virus-like antigen associated with acute illness. Science. 1973;182:1026.
3. Blumberg BS, Alter HJ, Visnich S. A "new" antigen in leukemia sera. JAMA. 1965;191:541.
4. Tiollais P, Pourcel C, Dejean A. The hepatitis B virus. Nature. 1985;317:489.
5. Rizzetto M, Canese MG, Arico S, et al. Immunofluorescence detection of a new antigen–antibody system (δ/anti-δ) associated with hepatitis B virus in liver and serum of HBsAg carriers. Gut. 1977;18:997.
6. Rizzetto M. The delta agent. Hepatology. 1983;3:729.
7. Feinstone SM, Kapikian AZ, Purcell RH, et al. Transfusion-associated hepatitis not due to viral hepatitis type A or B. N Engl J Med. 1975;292:767.
8. Houghton M, Wiener J, Rutter WJ, et al. Non-A, non-B agent. News conference. 1988.
9. Balayan MS, Andjaparidze AG, Savinskaya SS, et al. Evidence for a virus in non-A/non-B hepatitis transmitted via the fecal oral route. Intervirology. 1983;20:23.
10. Gust ID, Purcell RH. Waterbourne non-A, non-B hepatitis. J Infect Dis. 1987;156:630.
11. Centers for Disease Control. Hepatitis surveillance report. No. 51:13, 1987.
12. Koff RS, Chalmers TC, Culhane PO, et al. Underreporting of viral hepatitis. Gastroenterology. 1973;64:1194.
13. Szmuness W, Dienstag JL, Purcell RH, et al. Distribution of antibody to hepatitis A antigen in urban adult populations. N Engl J Med. 1976;295:755.
14. Hadler SC, de Monzon M, Ponzetto A, et al. An epidemic of severe hepatitis due to delta virus infection in Yucpa Indians of Venezuela. Ann Intern Med. 1984;100:339.
15. Hoofnagle JH, Shafritz DA, Popper H. Chronic type B hepatitis and the "healthy" HBsAg carrier state. Hepatology. 1987;7:758.
16. Zeldis JB, Dienstag JL, Gale RP. Aplastic anemia and non-A, non-B hepatitis. Am J Med. 1983;74:64.
17. Beasley RP, Hwang LY, Lin CC, et al. Hepatocellular carcinoma and hepatitis B virus. A prospective study of 22,707 men in Taiwan. Lancet. 1981;2:1129.
18. Beasley RP. Hepatitis B virus as the etiologic agent in hepatocellular carcinoma—epidemiologic considerations. Hepatology. 1982;2(Suppl):21.
19. Stevens CE, Taylor PE. Hepatitis B vaccine: Issues, recommendations, and new developments. Semin Liver Dis. 1986;6:23.
20. Alpert E, Isselbacher KJ, Schur PH. The pathogenesis of arthritis associated with viral hepatitis. N Engl J Med. 1971;285:185.
21. Gianotti F. Hepatitis B antigen in papular acrodermatitis of children. Br Med J. 1974;3:169.
22. Zimmerman HG. The differential diagnosis of jaundice. Med Clin North Am. 1968;52:1417.
23. Salen G, Goldstein F, Haurani F, et al. Acute hemolytic anemia complicating viral hepatitis in patients with glucose-6-phosphate dehydrogenase deficiency. Ann Intern Med. 1966;65:1210.
24. Ishak KG. Light microscopic morphology of viral hepatitis. Am J Clin Pathol. 1976;65:787.
25. Boyer JL, Klatskin G. Pattern of necrosis in acute viral hepatitis. Prognostic value of bridging (subacute hepatic necrosis). N Engl J Med. 1970;283:1063.
26. Mathiesen LR, Fauerholt L, Moller Am, et al. Immunofluorescence studies for hepatitis A virus and hepatitis B surface and core antigen in liver biopsies from patients with acute viral hepatitis. Gastroenterology. 1979;77:623.
27. Boggs JD, Melnick JL, Conrad ME, et al. Viral hepatitis, clinical and tissue culture studies. JAMA. 1970;214:1041.
28. Lemon S. Type A viral hepatitis. New developments in an old disease. N Engl J Med. 1985;313:1059.
29. Sjogren MH, Tanno H, Fay O, et al. Hepatitis A virus in stool during clinical relapse. Ann Intern Med. 1987;106:221.
30. Gordon SC, Reddy KR, Schiff L, et al. Prolonged intrahepatic cholestasis secondary to acute hepatitis A. Ann Intern Med. 1984;101:635.
31. Rakela A, Redeker AF, Edwards VM, et al. Hepatitis A virus infection in fulminant hepatitis and chronic active hepatitis. Gastroenterology. 1978;74:879.
32. Francis DP, Hadler SC, Prendergast TJ, et al. Occurrence of hepatitis A, B, and non-A, non-B hepatitis in the United States—CDC Sentinel County hepatitis study I. Am J Med. 1984;76:69.
33. Dienstag JL, Routenberg JA, Purcell Rh, et al. Foodhandler-associated outbreak of hepatitis type A. An immune electron microscopic study. Ann Intern Med. 1975;83:647.
34. Mackowiak PA, Caraway CT, Portnoy EL. Oyster-associated hepatitis. Lessons from the Louisiana experience. Am J Epidemiol. 1976;103:181.
35. Woodson RD, Clinton JJ. Hepatitis prophylaxis abroad. Effectiveness of immune serum globulin in protecting Peace Corps volunteers. JAMA. 1968;109:1053.
36. Pattison CP, Maynard JE, Bryan JS. Subhuman primate-associated hepatitis. J Infect Dis. 1975;132:478.
37. Hadler SC, Erben JJ, Francis DP, et al. Risk factors for hepatitis A in daycare centers. J Infect Dis. 1982;145:255.
38. Corey L, Holmes KK. Sexual transmission of hepatitis A in homosexual men. Incidence and mechanism. N Engl J Med. 1980;302:435.
39. Decker RH, Kosakowski SM, Vanderbilt AS, et al. Diagnosis of acute hepatitis A by Havab-M, a direct radioimmunoassay for IgM anti-HAV. Am J Clin Pathol. 1981;76:140.
40. Szmuness W, Much MI, Prince AM, et al. On the role of sexual behavior in the spread of hepatitis B infection. Ann Intern Med. 1975;83:489.
41. Krugman S, Overby LR, Mushahwar IK, et al. Viral hepatitis type B. Studies on the natural history and prevention reexamined. N Engl J Med. 1979;300:101.
42. Hoofnagle JH, Seeff LB, Bales ZB, et al. Serologic responses in type B hepatitis. In: Vyas GN, Cohen SN, Schmid R, eds. Viral Hepatitis. Philadelphia: Franklin Institute Press; 1978:219–44.
43. Chau KH, Hargie MP, Decker RH, et al. Serodiagnosis of recent hepatitis B infection by IgM class anti-HBc. Hepatology. 1983;3:142.
44. Rizzetto M, Gerin JL, Purcell RH, eds. Hepatitis Delta Virus and Its Infection. New York: Alan R Liss; 1987.
45. Hoofnagle JH. Type D hepatitis. JAMA. 1989;261:1321.
46. Farci P, Gerin JL, Aragona M, et al. Diagnostic and prognostic significance of the IgM antibody to the hepatitis delta virus. JAMA. 1986;255:1443.
47. Mushawar IK, Decker RH. Prevalence of delta antigen and antidelta detected by immunoassays in various HBsAg positive populations. In: Vyas GN, Dienstag JL, Hoofnagle JH, eds. Viral Hepatitis and Liver Disease. Orlando, FL: Grune & Stratton; 1984:617.
48. Bergmann KF, Gerin JL. Antigens of hepatitis delta virus in the liver and serum of humans and animals. J Infect Dis. 1986;514:702.

49. Smedile A, Baroudy BM, Bergmann KF, et al. Clinical significance of HDV RNA in HDV disease. In: Rizzetto M, Gerin JL, Purcell RH, eds. Hepatitis Delta Virus and Its Infection. New York: Alan R. Liss; 1987:231–4.
50. Rizzetto M, Verme G, Recchia S, et al. Chronic HBsAg hepatitis with intrahepatic expression of delta antigen. An active and progressive disease unresponsive to immunosuppressive treatment. Ann Intern Med. 1983;98:437.
51. Rocca G, Poli G, Gerardo P, et al. Familial clustering of delta infection. In: Verme G, Bonino F, Rizzetto M, eds. Viral Hepatitis and Delta Infection. New York: Alan R Liss; 1984:133–7.
52. Dienstag JL. Non-A, non-B hepatitis. I. Recognition, epidemiology, and clinical features. Gastroenterology. 1983;85:439.
53. Dienstag JL. Non-A, non-B hepatitis. II. Experimental transmission, putative virus agents and markers, and prevention. Gastroenterology. 1983;85:743.
54. Alter MJ, Gerety RJ, Smallwood LA, et al. Sporadic non-A, non-B hepatitis: Frequency and epidemiology in an urban U.S. population. J Infect Dis. 1982;145:886.
55. Alter HJ, Hoofnagle JH. Non-A, non-B. Observations on the first decade. In: Vyas GN, Dienstag JL, Hoofnagle JH, eds. Viral Hepatitis and Liver Disease. Orlando, FL: Grunc & Stratton; 1984:345–55.
56. Wong DC, Purcell RH, Sreenivasan MA, et al. Epidemic and endemic hepatitis in India: Evidence for non-A/non-B hepatitis virus etiology. Lancet. 1980;2:876.
57. Khuroo SM. Study of an epidemic of non-A, non-B hepatitis. Possibility of another human hepatitis virus distinct from post-transfusion non-A, non-B type. Am J Med. 1980;68:818.
58. Kane MA, Bradley DW, Shrestha SM, et al. Epidemic non-A, non-B hepatitis in Nepal: Recovery of a possible etiologic agent and transmission studies in marmoset. JAMA. 1984;252:3140.
59. Kraczynski K, Bradley DW, Kane MA. Virus associated antigen of epidemic non-A, non-B hepatitis and specific antibodies in outbreaks and in sporadic cases of NANB hepatitis. Hepatology. 1988;8:1223.
60. Purcell RH, Walsh JH, Holland PV, et al. Seroepidemiological studies of transfusion-associated hepatitis. J Infect Dis. 1981;123:406.
61. Lamb SG, Stern H. Cytomegaolovirus hepatitis. Lancet. 1966;2:1003.
62. Gavish D, Kleinman Y, Morag A, et al. Hepatitis and jaundice associated with measles in young adults. Arch Intern Med. 1983;143:674.
63. Shalev-Zimels H, Weizman Z, Lotan C, et al. Extent of measles hepatitis in various ages. Hepatology. 1988;8:1138.
64. Francis TI, Moore DL, Edington GM, et al. A clinicopathological study of human yellow fever. Bull WHO. 1972;46:659.
65. Zimmerman HG, Fang M, Utili R, et al. Jaundice due to bacterial infection. Gastroenterology. 1979;77:362.
66. Bowry S, Chan CH, Weiss H, et al. Hepatic involvement in pulmonary tuberculosis. Histologic and functional characteristics. Am Rev Respir Dis. 1970;101:941.
67. Lee RV, Thornton GF, Conn HO. Liver disease associated with secondary syphilis. N Engl J Med. 1971;284:1423.
68. Heath CW Jr, Alexander AD, Galton MM. Leptospirosis in the United States. Analysis of 483 cases in man, 1949–1961. N Engl J Med. 1965;273:857.
69. Bernstein M, Edmondson HA, Barhour BH. The liver lesion in Q fever. Clinical and pathologic features. Arch Intern Med. 1965;116:491.
70. Zimmerman HJ. Hepatotoxicity. The Adverse Effects of Drugs and Other Chemicals on the Liver. New York: Appleton-Century-Crofts; 1978.
71. Johnson GK, Tolman KG. Chronic liver disease and acetaminophen. Ann Intern Med. 1977;87:302.
72. Subcommittee on the National Halothane Study of the Committee on Anesthesia. Possible association between halothane anesthesia and postoperative hepatic necrosis. JAMA. 1966;197:775.
73. Bynum TE, Boinoit JK, Maddrey WC. Ischemic hepatitis. Am J Dig Dis. 1979;24:129.
74. Lieber CS. Biochemical and molecular basis of alcohol-induced injury to the liver and other tissues. N Engl J Med. 1988;319:1639.
75. Roche-Sicot J, Benhamou JP. Acute intravascular hemolysis and acute liver failure associated as a first manifestation of Wilson's disease. Ann Intern Med. 1977;86:301.
76. Rosenblate HJ, Eisenstein R, Halmes AW. The liver in sickle cell anemia. Arch Pathol Lab Med. 1970;90:235.
77. Parker RGF. Occlusion of the hepatic veins in man. Medicine (Baltimore). 1959;38:369.
78. Harrison HB, Middleton HM III, Crosby JH, et al. Fulminant hepatic failure. An unusual presentation of metastatic liver disease. Gastroenterology. 1981;80:820.
79. Repsher LH, Freebern RK. Effects of early and vigorous exercise on recovery from infectious hepatitis. N Engl J Med. 1969;281:1393.
80. Schweitzer IL, Weiner JM, McPeak CM, et al. Oral contraceptives in acute viral hepatitis. JAMA. 1975;233:979.
81. Blum AI, Stutz R, Haemmerli UP, et al. A fortuitously controlled study of steroid therapy in acute viral hepatitis. I. Acute disease. Am J Med. 1969;47:82.
82. Gregory PB, Knauer CM, Miller R, et al. Steroid therapy in severe viral hepatitis. N Engl J Med. 1976;294:681.
83. Sherlock S, Thomas HC. Treatment of chronic hepatitis due to hepatitis B virus. Lancet. 1985;2:1343.
84. Hoofnagle JH, Mullen KD, Jones DB, et al. Treatment of chronic non-A, non-B hepatitis with recombinant human alpha interferon. N Engl J Med. 1986;315:1575.
85. Levin S, Hahn T. Interferon system in acute viral hepatitis. Lancet. 1982;1:592.
86. Sanchez-Tapias JM, Mas A, Costa J, et al. Recombinant alpha 2c interferon therapy in fulminant viral hepatitis. J Hepatol. 1987;5:205.
87. Peleman RR, Gavaler JS, Van Thiel DH, et al. Liver transplantation for acute and subacute hepatic failure. Hepatology. 1985;5:1045.
88. Vickers C, Neuberger J, Buckels J, et al. Transplantation of the liver in adults and children with fulminant hepatic failure. J Hepatol. 1988;7:143.
89. Bernuau J, Gordeau A, Poynard T, et al. Multivariate analysis of prognostic factors in fulminant hepatitis. Hepatology. 1986;6:648.
90. Auslander MO, Gitnick GL. Vigorous medical management of acute fulminant hepatitis. Arch Intern Med. 1977;137:599.
91. Seeff LB, Hoofnagle JH. Immunoprophylaxis of viral hepatitis. Gastroenterology. 1979;77:161.
92. Center for Disease Control. Post-exposure prophylaxis of hepatitis B. Ann Intern Med. 1984;101:351.
93. Beasley RP, Hwang LY, Lee GC, et al. Prevention of perinatally transmitted hepatitis B virus infections with hepatitis B immune globulin and hepatitis B vaccine. Lancet. 1983;2:1099.

103. CHRONIC HEPATITIS

SHALOM Z. HIRSCHMAN

Chronic hepatitis is defined as an abnormality in liver function that persists for 6 or more months.[1] Two broad classes of chronic hepatitis have been established through the study of liver histology, i.e., chronic persistent hepatitis and chronic active hepatitis (Table 1).[2] The former is most often a benign entity requiring no therapy, while the latter frequently leads to hepatic cirrhosis. The histologic separation of the two is by no means always clear, and the total clinical status of the patient must be considered in arriving at a diagnosis.[3]

CHRONIC PERSISTENT HEPATITIS

The overall architecture of the liver is usually normal in patients with chronic persistent hepatitis. The portal triads may be normal or moderately increased in size and contain an inflammatory cell infiltrate consisting mainly of lymphocytes and mononuclear cells (Fig. 1). Most important, the limiting plate of liver cells between portal zones and the lobule is intact (Fig. 1). Even if necrosis of these cells is present, it is not extensive. Minimal collections of inflammatory cells or foci of parenchymal cell necrosis may be present in the lobule. Piecemeal necrosis, that is, the destruction of liver cells at an interface between par-

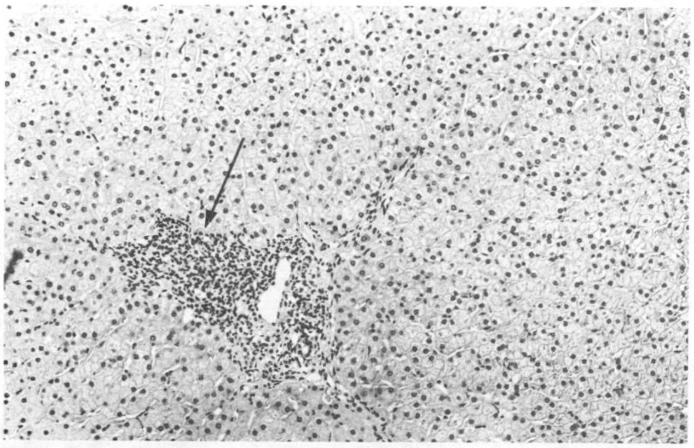

FIG. 1. Chronic persistent hepatitis with inflammatory infiltrate confined to the enlarged portal tract. The limiting plate of the liver cells (arrow) between the portal zone and liver lobule is intact. (H&E, ×40) (Courtesy of Dr. Fenton Schaffner, New York, NY.)

TABLE 1. Chronic Hepatitis

Type	*Etiology*	*Histology*	*Prognosis*	*Therapy*
Chronic persistent hepatitis	Hepatitis B virus; non-A, non-B virus(es) Drugs Unknown cause	Unresolved hepatitis with minimal periportal inflammation and no necrosis of the liver plate	Benign	Periodic reassessment
Chronic active hepatitis	Hepatitis B virus Non-A, non-B hepatitis virus(es) Autoimmune Drugs	With no cirrhosis Portal piecemeal necrosis and inflammation Bridging hepatic necrosis Periportal piecemeal necrosis with bridging hepatic necrosis With cirrhosis	Results in liver failure	Corticosteroid and/or azathioprine for autoimmune hepatitis

enchyma and connective tissue, together with a predominantly lymphocytic plasma cell infiltrate is not seen. Although the abnormalities of chronic persistent hepatisis may remain for many years, the prognosis for eventual complete recovery is excellent.

CHRONIC ACTIVE HEPATITIS

Chronic active hepatitis, formerly called chronic aggressive hepatitis as defined by an international group of hepatologists,[4] is a chronic inflammatory and fibrosing liver lesion of varied etiology and variable histologic features. The features common to all untreated cases are piecemeal necrosis together with new fiber formation and lymphocytic infiltration of portal tracts and lobules (Fig. 2). Other infiltrating cells, including neutrophils, may also be found, and features of acute hepatitis such as spotty necrosis (hepatocytolysis) may be superimposed. Passive septa formed by collapse after bridging (Fig. 3) or multilobular liver cell necrosis may be present. Cirrhosis is not a necessary defining criterion but can develop (Fig. 4). Liver cell regeneration is seen in chronic active hepatitis, and the borderline between chronic active hepatitis and cirrhosis in the more severe cases is not sharp. The severity of chronic active hepatitis varies with the degree of piecemeal and confluent necrosis and the density of the inflammatory infiltrate.

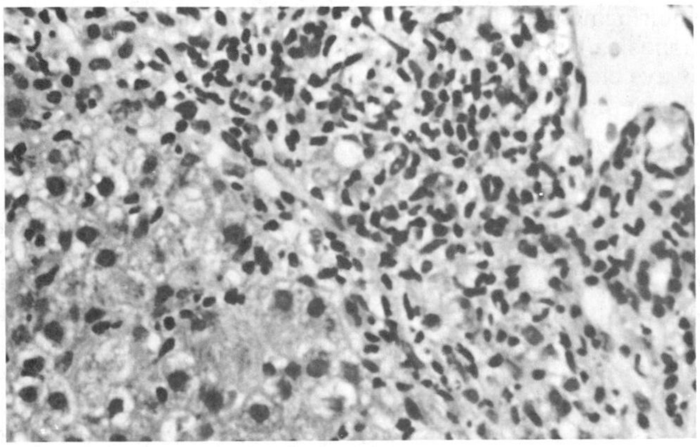

FIG. 2. Piecemeal necrosis in chronic active hepatitis. The border zone between the portal tract on the upper right and parenchymal liver cells on the lower left is obscured by necrosis of liver cells and inflammatory infiltrate. (H&E, ×250) (Courtesy of Dr. Fenton Schaffner, New York, NY.)

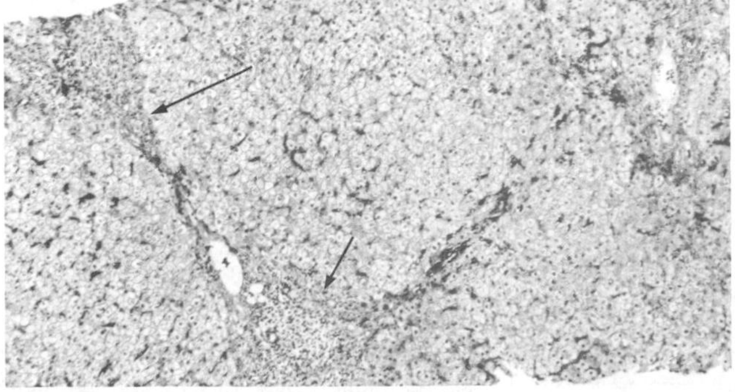

FIG. 3. Chronic active hepatitis with bridging necrosis (arrows) dissecting lobular parenchyma. (H&E, ×40) (Courtesy of Dr. Fenton Schaffner, New York, NY.)

Piecemeal necrosis is a major characteristic of chronic active hepatitis (Fig. 2). The process may be seen either at the edges of portal tracts or the septa of cirrhotic liver or at the margins of septa resulting from collapse after confluent necrosis. Therefore, it is not necessarily confined to the periportal areas of hepatic lobules. The inflammatory infiltrate contains lymphocytes and plasma cells; polymorphonuclear leukocytes may also be present. The lymphocytes are closely associated with hepatocytes, and within the lymphoid infiltrate, hepatocytes may be seen singly or in groups. At the advancing edge of piecemeal necrosis, the liver cells show hydropic swelling and are at times arranged in abnormal configuration such as liver cell rosettes.

Several histologic subgroups of chronic active hepatitis have been defined. These have been conveniently divided into those with or without morphologic evidence of cirrhosis.

Chronic Active Hepatitis without Evidence of Cirrhosis

This subgroup of chronic active hepatitis is characterized by either a portal inflammatory infiltrate with substantial necrosis of the limiting plate of lvier cells (Fig. 2), bridging necrosis (Fig. 3) that interconnects between the two portal triads or with a central vein, or both. The portal triads are swollen with inflammatory infiltrate consisting mainly of lymphocytes and plasmacytes. The limiting plate of liver cells is destroyed to a variable degree by cell necrosis occurring in irregular fashion (piecemeal necrosis). Inflammatory infiltrates extend from the portal triads into the lobules and form septa that are often associated with increases in collagen. With more extensive necrosis, cell collapse extends between portal triads or between portal triads and central veins to create recognizable necrotic and inflammatory bridges known as bridging hepatic necrosis (Fig. 3). This portal–central or portal–portal bridging type of parenchymal cell necrosis was originally termed *subacute hepatic necrosis*[5] or *subacute hepatitis*.[6]

Chronic Active Hepatitis with Evidence of Cirrhosis

In this type of histologic pattern of chronic active hepatitis, the cirrhosis is usually quite active, and regenerating nodules and fibrosis coexist with areas of more recent parenchymal cell necrosis and collapse (Fig. 4). The cell necrosis may be piecemeal, bridging, or multilobular in pattern. Bridging fibrosis, repre-

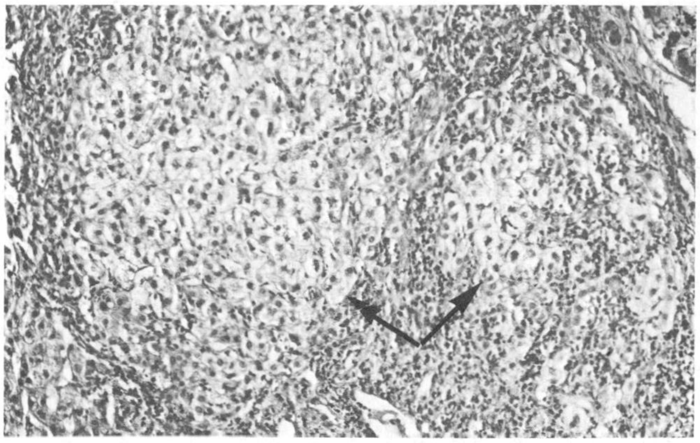

FIG. 4. Chronic active hepatitis with a transition to cirrhosis and the formation of two adjacent nodules (arrows) of liver cells. (H&E, ×100) (Coutesy of Dr. Fenton Schaffner, New York, NY.)

senting the final stage int he progression of necrotic lesions with condensation of reticulin fibers and an increase in fibrosis, may also be present.

Most workers believe that piecemeal necrosis is the most important pathologic process in the development of chronic active hepatitis.[4] However, attention also has been drawn to the nonhomogeneous nature of liver cell damage, to focal hepatocytolysis with inflammatory cell infiltration, and to unevenly distributed regeneration as important features. Bridging hepatic necrosis was considered by some to be the most important lesion in the development of chronic active hepatitis.[5,7] Undoubtedly, all these processes, including piecemeal necrosis, bridging hepatic necrosis, and focal hepatocytolysis and regeneration, are involved in the pathogenesis of chronic active hepatitis and cirrhosis. Confluent necrosis alone is usually followed by healing, leaving either a scarred or a substantially normal liver. This is well documented in the complete recovery of some patients from severe necrotizing acute hepatitis and from nonfatal hepatic necrosis due to shock, carbon tetrachloride, or acetaminophen. In these situations, inflammatory infiltration is usually slight, and piecemeal necrosis is absent. Chronic hepatitis due to hepatitis B virus (HBV) and the non-A, non-B type cannot be distinguished histopathologically unless hepatocytes containing hepatitis B surface antigen (HBsAg) are demonstrated.[8]

CLINICAL PRESENTATIONS OF CHRONIC PERSISTENT HEPATITIS

The clinical presentation usually does not differentiate the patient with chronic persistent hepatitis from the patient with chronic active hepatitis. The patient with chronic persistent hepatitis may complain of fatigue, and jaundice may be present. As a general rule symptoms in patients with chronic persistent hepatitis tend to be mild, and features of cirrhosis do not develop.

CLINICAL PRESENTATIONS OF CHRONIC ACTIVE HEPATITIS

Symptoms and Signs

The patient usually complains of a slow onset of increasing fatigue and fluctuating jaundice. Fatigue is a very important symptom and usually increases in the afternoon and evening. Amenorrhea is common. Examination of the patient shows malnutrition, and arachnoid nevi (spiders) may be found on the upper part of the body. Hepatosplenomegaly may be present. Features of cirrhosis such as hepatic encephalopathy, edema, ascites, and bleeding esophageal varices develop late in the advanced stage of the disease. However, the process may be quite insidious, and cirrhosis may develop in patients without significant symptoms or an antecedent history of jaundice. Therefore, liver biopsy is necessary in asymptomatic patients with chronic abnormalities in liver function.

Biochemical Abnormalities

The biochemical abnormalities are quite variable. The serum bilirubin level may or may not be elevated. The serum glutamic oxaloacetic transaminase (SGOT) and serum glutamic pyruvic transaminase (SGPT) levels are usually increased to at least five times the normal values. The serum alkaline phosphatase and γ-glutamyl transpeptidase values are also increased to at least twice normal. The serum γ-globulin concentration is usually elevated and is of polyclonal type. Serum albumin levels remain within normal limits until the late stage of the disease.

The biochemical abnormalities cannot be used to differentiate chronic persistent from chronic active hepatitis, although elevation of the γ-globulin level is much more common in the latter. In addition, serum bile acid concentrations are more likely to be elevated in patients with chronic active hepatitis than in patients with chronic persistent hepatitis.[9,10]

Immunologic Abnormalities

Patients with chronic active hepatitis due to HBV infection show a selective sensitization of peripheral blood T lymphocytes to hepatitis B core antigen (HBcAg). The specific proliferation was limited to the CD4+ cells.[11] The percentage of resting T cells expressing HLA class II antigens is higher in patients with chronic hepatitis than in controls.[12] Chronic HBsAg carriers have increased proportions of suppressor/cytotoxic T cells in their peripheral blood.[13] Liver damage in hepatitis B appears to be due to a loss of hepatocytes replicating virus rather than a cytotoxic effect of the virus itself.[14]

There is a reduction in γ-interferon production by peripheral blood mononuclear cells of patients with chronic liver disease.[15] Some hepatitis B carriers have a reduced capacity to produce both α- and γ-interferon.[16] No serum interferon was detected in patients with acute or chronic hepatitis when compared with controls.[17]

ETIOLOGY OF CHRONIC HEPATITIS

Chronic Active Hepatitis Associated with Hepatitis B Virus

Chronic active hepatitis is an important complication of HBV infection. Positive serologic tests for HBsAg have been observed in a substantial percentage of patients with chronic active hepatitis, ranging from 10 to 67 percent of the cases. After acute hepatitis B infection, approximately 80 percent of the patients recover completely, and 20 percent develop chronic hepatitis. Of the latter, about 15 percent have chronic persistent hepatitis, and 5 percent have chronic active hepatitis. Only about 2.5 percent of patients progress to cirrhosis. Non-A, non-B acute hepatitis also seems to carry a definite risk for the development of chronic active hepatitis.[18] On the other hand, epidemiologic studies have not demonstrated a risk for the development of chronic active hepatitis after hepatitis A virus (HAV) infection.[19]

Factors Indicating Risk for Chronic Active Hepatitis B

Several factors are useful in pointing to a greater risk of chronicity (Table 2). Clinically, the type of acute attack of HBV infection is helpful in indicating possible progression to chronicity.[20] The patient with an explosive onset of acute hepatitis and deep jaundice usually recovers completely. Survivors of fulminant viral hepatitis rarely progress to chronic disease de-

TABLE 2. Factors Indicating Increased Risk of Chronic Hepatitis B

Age: infants and elderly	
Sex: males	
Insidious and mild acute hepatitis B	
Immunosuppression	
Increased exposure to hepatitis B virus (drug addicts, homosexuals, health workers and renal dialysis units, multiple blood transfusions)	
Geographic location: Mediterranean area, China, Africa	
Persistence of serum	HBsAg
	HBcAg
	DNA polymerase
	HBeAg
Chronic delta virus infection	
Absence of serum	Anti-HBe
	Anti-Hbs
Genetic: ?HLA-B8	

spite the extreme hepatic necrosis during the acute illness. These patients appear to have normal immunologic mechanisms that can clear the virus. Similarly, cholestatic acute viral hepatitis, despite deep jaundice, rarely progresses to chronic hepatitis. In contrast, the patient with an insidious onset with mild prodromal symptoms, slight or even absent jaundice, and continued fatigue seems more likely to slip into chronic disease. Patients receiving immunosuppressive therapy or corticosteroids during the acute attack may also have an increased risk of developing chronic hepatitis.

The very young and very old are at greater risk of developing chronic hepatitis. This may be related to impaired cellular immunity that may be present both in the elderly and in the very young. Men are more often affected than are women during epidemics of hepatitis B infection. Thus, chronic hepatitis B is a disease that predominantly affects men, usually in the 30- to 50-year age range.

Serologic markers for delta hepatitis virus in patients with chronic hepatitis B infection are associated with symptomatic chronic disease and chronic hepatitis.[21,22] Moreover, patients with serologic markers for delta hepatitis more often progress from chronic hepatitis B to cirrhosis.[23] Persistent IgM antibodies to delta antigen indicate chronic delta virus infection.[24]

Patients with acute hepatitis B infection who suffer from chronic diseases that depress immunologic competence such as patients with renal failure, neoplastic disease, or renal transplantation are at particular risk of chronic hepatitis. Persons continually exposed to HBV are also at risk. Health workers such as physicians and laboratory personnel, drug addicts, and homosexuals are at risk. Both patients and personnel in dialysis units are at great risk of exposure. HBV infection is more prevalent in certain geographic areas such as the Mediterranean area, China, and Africa. Patients receiving multiple blood transfusions are also at greater risk of hepatitis developing.

The presence of HBsAg in liver cells of biopsy specimens can be suspected by the ground glass appearance of the cytoplasm. The presence of HBsAg can be confirmed by the orcein stain of Shikata and colleagues[25] or preferably by the presence of cytoplasmic immunofluorescence using anti-HBs. Hepatitis B core antigen (HBcAg) can be identified in the nucleus of the liver cell by immunofluorescent staining. Core particles of HBV with diameters of 27 nm can also be visualized in the nuclei of hepatocytes by electron microscopy.

Patients with persistent HBsAg, HBcAg, and DNA polymerase activity in serum after an acute attack of HBV infection are at greater risk of developing chronic hepatitis. Circulating immune complexes containing HBsAg and IgM usually disappear within 4 weeks of the onset of hepatitis B. Persistence of such complexes after the early phase of acute viral hepatitis B is a predictor of progression to chronic disease.[26] Patients with persistent e antigen (HBeAg) and without anti-HBe appear to be at greater risk of progressing to chronic active hepatitis.[27–29] Patients who develop chronic active hepatitis tend to have persistent anti-HBc in their serum and often have no detectable anti-HBs. HBeAg is present particularly in chronic active and chronic persistent hepatitis. Anti-HBe is found in healthy carriers and in patients with cirrhosis and hepatocellular carcinoma.[30] Most patients who recover without sequelae from acute HBV infection develop anti-HBc before anti-HBs, and the anti-HBc disappears more quickly. Anti-HBs titers fall slowly over the subsequent years. HBeAg, HBcAg, and DNA polymerase appear early in acute disease and disappear rather quickly in those who recover completely.

Many patients with chronic-type B hepatitis eventually undergo a spontaneous remission in clinical and biochemical evidence of active disease, which is usually indicated by the disappearance of HBeAg, HBcAg, and DNA polymerase. Patients who remain HBeAg-positive continue to have elevated aminotransferase levels.[31]

There is some evidence that chronic active hepatitis is more apt to develop in patients who have had acute HBV infection and who are of HLA type B8.[32] Thus, there appears to be a genetic predisposition to development of chronic active hepatitis after acute HBV infection.

By using a radiolabeled 50-base oligonucleotide complementary with the measles virus gene encoding the nucleocapsid as a probe, Robertson and coworkers[33] identified a persistent measles virus genome in the lymphocytes of 12 of 18 patients with autoimmune chronic active hepatitis. These findings raise the possibility that persistent measles virus infection may be a cause of autoimmune chronic active hepatitis. Indeed, the persistence of the measles genome in these patients was correlated with high levels of antibodies to measles.

Clinical Presentation of Chronic Hepatitis B

Chronic hepatitis B may be recognized as unresolved acute viral hepatitis, with persistent abnormalities in lvier function, particularly when HBsAg positivity continues for more than 3 months. About one-half of the patients have established liver disease or a positive test for serum HBsAg. The serum bilirubin, transaminase, and γ-globulin levels are moderately increased, but jaundice is rarely severe. Smooth muscle antibody is most often absent and if present is of low titer. Antimitochondrial antibody is usually absent. Histologic liver sections show the classic features of chronic active hepatitis.

Autoimmune Chronic Hepatitis

Despite documented virus- and drug-related chronic hepatitis, the cause of most chronic cases remains obscure. Chronic active hepatitis of unknown etiology is more commonly associated with autoimmune phenomena including hypergammaglobulinemia, antinuclear factor, a positive lupus erythematosus (LE) cell test, and other serologic tests that suggest an underlying abnormality of the immune response. Chronic active hepatitis has often been described in young women who have arthralgia, amenorrhea, signs of hypercortisolism, and high levels of immunoglobulins.[34] The disease has variously been termed *lupoid hepatitis, plasma cell hepatitis, Waldenström's chronic active hepatitis*, and *active juvenile cirrhosis*. The disease is strongly associated with other clinical manifestations believed to be related to autoimmunity including ulcerative colitis, diabetes mellitus, Coombs-positive hemolytic anemia, pericarditis and myocarditis, pleurisy, pulmonary infiltrations, glomerulitis, renal tubular acidosis, thyroiditis, thrombocytopenic purpura, nondeforming migratory arthritis, leg ulcers, acne and other skin lesions, fibrosing alveolitis, and neurologic lesions.[1] This multisystem involvement indicates that there is a more generalized disorder of immune function. Suppressor T-cell activity is decreased especially in hepatitis B-negative chronic active hepatitis.[35–37] However, increased prostaglandin-producing suppressor cell activity was found in both hepatitis B-positive and

B-negative chronic active hepatitis.[38] Patients with "autoimmune" or hepatitis B-negative chronic hepatitis more often have autoantibodies to liver-specific protein (LSP).[39,40] There is also evidence that genetic factors may determine the type of immune response in patients with chronic hepatitis. The incidence of HLA-A1 and -8 is as high as 70 percent in some of these patients,[41] and there is an increased incidence of antimitochondrial antibodies and other serologic abnormalities in first-degree relatives including an association with familial hypergammaglobulinemia.[1] The clinical characteristics of chronic "autoimmune" hepatitis are compared with those of chronic hepatitis B in Table 3.

Autoimmune hepatitis commonly affects women between the ages of 15 and 25 years and recurs about the time of menopause. Illness often begins insidiously but may resemble acute viral hepatitis in onset. Fever is present in those who are acutely ill. Arachnoid nevi are often present, as is hepatosplenomegaly. Skin striae, acne, and moon face are common. Serologic tests show a positive antinuclear factor in more than 50 percent of cases and smooth muscle antibody in about 67 percent. The serum γ-globulin is quite high, and LE cells are present in about 15 percent of cases. Thrombocytopenia and leukopenia are frequent even before the onset of portal hypertension. The prothrombin time may be prolonged even in the early stages of the disease. Liver biopsy specimen shows histologic evidence of chronic active hepatitis. This type of chronic active hepatitis is most amenable to therapy, and the prognosis currently is very good.

Drug-Related Chronic Hepatitis

Drugs are increasingly implicated in both acute and chronic hepatitis. Chronic hepatitis may result from a direct hepatotoxic effect of the drug or drug metabolite or from an idiosyncratic drug allergy directed toward hepatic tissue. Drugs that are most commonly associated with chronic hepatitis include methotrexate, acetylsalicylic acid, isoniazid, α-methyldopa, and oxyphenacetin. Prolonged administration of nitrofurantoin also has been associated with hepatic necrosis and chronic active hepatitis.[42,43] Abnormalities in liver function often improve after withdrawal of the drug. The clinical and histologic characteristics of drug-related chronic hepatitis are frequently indistinguishable from other forms of chronic hepatitis when eosinophilia or extrahepatic manifestations of drug allergy are absent. In such instances, it is often difficult to establish a relationship between chronic liver disease and the drug.

Oxyphenacetin, found in some laxatives, is no longer used in the United States and was the first drug to be associated with chronic active hepatitis. Isoniazid, used in the treatment of tuberculosis, has been associated with the picture of chronic active hepatitis and may result in fatal disease. α-Methyldopa is used in the treatment of hypertension, and severe, even fatal hepatitis has been reported with this drug; the acute hepatitis may progress to chronic active hepatitis. Thus, it is important to take an accurate history of drug usage in all patients with chronic active hepatitis.

Isoniazid can lead to serious hepatotoxic disease resulting in death.[44] About one-half of the cases are recognized during the first 2 months of therapy and the other half up to a period of 1 year. Hepatic injury presenting after 2 months of therapy is more likely to prove fatal. Approximately 50 percent of the patients have gastrointestinal complaints including anorexia, nausea, vomiting, and abdominal distress. About 40 percent of the patients complain of symptoms suggestive of "viral" illness either with or without gastrointestinal complaints, and the remaining 10 percent have jaundice. Fever is rarely observed, and hepatomegaly is seen in about a third of the patients. Serum transaminase and alkaline phosphatase levels are usually elevated. Marked hyperbilirubinemia is generally associated with more severe disease and a poorer prognosis. Histologic examination of the liver shows hepatocellular damage. Most often the liver cellular structure resembles that of acute viral hepatitis with ballooning degeneration, sinusoidal acidophilic bodies, and focal necrosis. Some patients show bridging hepatic necrosis. A histologic picture resembling chronic active hepatitis is seen in about 10 percent of the patients. Most patients respond to discontinuing isoniazid therapy.

Methyldopa can also lead to liver cellular patterns resembling that of chronic active hepatitis.[45] Nausea, vomiting, and fatigue begin within 1 to 2 weeks after drug administration. Jaundice supervenes if the therapy is continued. The serum transaminase levels are elevated. Liver biopsy specimens show a predominantly mononuclear infiltrate in the portal triads. The LE cell preparation and the anti–smooth muscle antibody test may be positive. The hepatitis resolves when the drug is removed, although residual fibrosis due to extensive cell necrosis may be present.

TABLE 3. Clinical Characteristics of Chronic Active Hepatitis

Characteristic	Autoimmune	Hepatitis B
Predominant sex	Female	Male
Age	15–25; menopause	Older adults; neonates
Serum HBsAg	Negative	Usually positive
Serum HBcAg	Negative	May be positive
Serum hepatitis B DNA polymerase	Negative	May be positive
Serum HBeAg	Negative	May be positive
Serum γ-globulin	Markedly increased	Normal or moderately increased
Smooth muscle antibody	High	Absent or low
Associated autoimmune disease	Common	Uncommon
Frequent HLA type	A1, A8	B8
Response to immunosuppressive therapy	Good	Poor

DIFFERENTIAL DIAGNOSIS OF CHRONIC ACTIVE HEPATITIS

The differential diagnosis of chronic hepatitis includes prolonged viral hepatitis, primary biliary cirrhosis, alcoholic liver disease, pericholangitis with inflammatory bowel disease, Wilson's disease (hepatolenticular degeneration), granulomatous hepatitis, and α_1-antitrypsin deficiency.

Prolonged Viral Hepatitis

It is often difficult to distinguish relapsing or unresolved acute hepatitis from which recovery will be complete from chronic hepatitis. Needle liver biopsy is mandatory, but at times the interpretation can be difficult. In instances where the diagnosis is doubtful, several needle biopsies may be required to elucidate the nature of the disease.

Primary Biliary Cirrhosis

Primary biliary cirrhosis, a chronic obstructive, granulomatous cholangitis, usually is seen in middle-aged women with a predominant cholestasis and marked pruritus.[46] Antimitochondrial antibody is usually present in high titer, and the serum IgM level is raised in 80 percent of patients. Histologic sections of the liver show inflammation of the bile ductules with lymphocytes and plasma cells. Granulomas are found next to damaged intrahepatic bile ductules and in lymph nodes outside the liver, hepatic hilum, omentum, and lungs, especially in early stages of the disease.

Alcoholic Liver Disease

Patients with alcoholic liver disease tend to be older. There is a history of the chronic use of large amounts of alcohol, and the patient shows many arachnoid nevi. Histologic sections of the liver show fatty infiltration, Mallory's hyaline bodies, and a central zonal type of liver damage.

Pericholangitis with Inflammatory Bowel Disease

Inflammatory bowel disease including ulcerative colitis, granulomatous colitis, and regional enteritis may be complicated by pericholangitis. The serum globulin levels are usually normal, and the alkaline phosphatase level is very elevated. Liver biopsy specimens show a portal zone of inflammation, especially around the bile ducts. Anti-smooth muscle and anti-mitochondrial antibodies are usually absent.

Wilson's Disease

Patients with this disease may have all the typical features of chronic active hepatitis, often with ascites or with acute hemolysis.[47] There may be a history of parental consanguinity or a familial history of liver disease. Examination of the cornea by slit lamp may show Kaiser-Fleischer rings indicating copper deposition. The serum ceruloplasmin levels are low, and the serum copper level is high. Urinary copper and the copper content of the liver are also high. The disease can be treated with D-penicillamine and a low-copper diet.

Granulomatous Hepatitis

The presentation of granulomatous hepatitis often may be confused with chronic active hepatitis (see Chapter 104).

α_1-Antitrypsin Deficiency

α_1-Antitrypsin is a glycoprotein with a molecular weight of 50,000 that occupies the α_1-globulin position on standard serum protein electrophoresis.[48] The electrophoretic phenotype, called the protease inhibitor (Pi) type, is determined by codominant genes. In most populations 85 percent are PiM, containing about 2.2 mg/ml of serum α_1-antitrypsin. Serum protease inhibitor concentrations of 1.8 mg/ml or less are found in Pi types ZZ, SZ, (−) null, S (−), and Z (−), the first two being more common. These patients develop familial emphysema beginning early in life. There is an increased prevalence of the MZ phenotype in patients with α_1-antitrypsin deficiency and chronic active hepatitis or cryptogenic cirrhosis.[49] Neonatal hepatitis and cirrhosis also are associated with α_1-antitrypsin deficiency. Although these patients usually have neonatal jaundice progressing to cholestasis during childhood, chronic active hepatitis has been reported.[50] The diagnosis can be made by measuring the concentration of α_1-antitrypsin in the serum.

TREATMENT OF CHRONIC PERSISTENT HEPATITIS

It is generally agreed that chronic persistent hepatitis is a benign disease that does not evolve into cirrhosis, although hepatic inflammation may be present for many years. Therefore, steroid and immunosuppressive therapy is not used in this condition. Unfortunately, most cases of chronic persistent hepatitis have been observed only for short periods of time, so the ultimate prognosis of such patients cannot be certain. Therefore, these patients must be reexamined periodically. Repeat liver biopsy may be necessary to establish a definitive diagnosis.

TREATMENT OF CHRONIC ACTIVE HEPATITIS

Chronic active hepatitis is a progressive disease that often responds to corticosteroid therapy with improvement in liver function and reduction in mortality. However, there is evidence that the prognosis of patients with chronic active hepatitis depends on the specific etiology of the liver disease and the type of liver lesion.[51–53] Patients with periportal piecemeal necrosis without bridging necrosis or fibrosis respond well to corticosteroid therapy and do not progress to cirrhosis. On the other hand, patients with bridging necrosis or multilobular necrosis have a high incidence of progression to cirrhosis even with corticosteroid therapy. Moreover, patients with an active stage of cirrhosis on liver biopsy are more likely to be refractory to steroid therapy and relapse more frequently when steroid treatment is withdrawn. There is also increasing evidence that patients with chronic active hepatitis after HBV infection with chronic carriage of HBsAg are more refractory to corticosteroid therapy, and indeed, the lesions may worsen with such therapy. Prednisolone was found to have a deleterious effect in patients with HBsAg-positive chronic active hepatitis.[54,55] Immunosuppressive therapy appears to favor the replication of HBV in patients with HBsAg-positive chronic active hepatitis.[56–58]

There is general agreement that patients with autoimmune chronic active hepatitis respond well to corticosteroid therapy and that the prognosis is quite good. These patients lose their feelings of fatigue, the menses return, and liver function test findings become normal. The hepatic lesions are arrested. Prednisolone therapy significantly improves survival by reducing mortality in the early active phase of hepatitis B-negative chronic active hepatitis.[59] However, clinical deterioration can occur unpredictably after cessation of corticosteroid therapy.[60]

Most treatment regimens use prednisone or prednisolone. The choice of whom to treat or not to treat is often quite difficulte. Moreover, the type of therapy must be individualized with each patient. Generally, the initial dose of prednisone or prednisolone is 30–50 mg/day for 1 week with reduction over the following weeks to a maintenance dose of 10–20 mg/day. The maintenance dose is adjusted so that the patient is asymptomatic and liver function test results are relatively normal. Alternate-day prednisone therapy has also been used in an attempt to minimize side effects. However, such therapy cannot be used in every patient because the liver cells may not respond.

Liver biopsy and liver function tests should be performed before beginning corticosteroid therapy. Clinical examination and follow-up liver function tests should then be done at approximately monthly intervals. Liver biopsy should be repeated by 6 months to determine the effect of therapy on liver histology.

Azathioprine has been added to prednisone in those patients who do not respond or in those patients who have side effects with larger doses of prednisone and the dose must be reduced.[53] In such cases, azathioprine has often been effective. White blood cell counts should be checked at regular intervals in patients receiving azathioprine. The drug may be teratogenic and should not be given to pregnant patients. Moreover, when used as long-term therapy, the drug has been associated with the development of neoplasms in patients with renal transplants. Azathioprine is used usually at a dose of 50–100 mg/day.

A satisfactory remission is characterized by the absence of symptoms, normal serum globulin levels, and normal or minimally elevated transaminase levels. Histologic liver sections show no evidence of piecemeal necrosis or other signs of active hepatitis. Almost 90 percent of the patients who respond should achieve a clinical and biochemical remission after about a year and a half of therapy, whereas only 60 percent show a histologic remission. Relapse is uncommon after a full clinical and biochemical remission of 6 months' duration. In most patients the total duration of therapy is at least 2 years, and in many it is much longer.

In addition to immunosuppressive therapy patients should be urged to eat a balanced diet and to obtain adequate amounts of rest and sleep, and they should be given an individualized exercise program to promote a general sense of well-being. Failure of immunosuppressive therapy occurs in about 20 percent of the patients, and these may develop liver failure. In such patients, the dose of prednisone and azathioprine is increased in the hope of inducing a remission.

Several experimental modalities of therapy have been applied to patients with chronic active hepatitis B. Early studies indicated that the combination of human leukocyte interferon with vidarabine showed some promise in eliminating viral replication in chronic hepatitis B infection[61]; the use of vidarabine monophosphate (ara-AMP) administered intramuscularly allowed outpatient therapy.[62,63] Recombinant α-interferon administered to patients with chronic hepatitis B mediated a decrease in serum viral DNA polymerase activity.[64] It appears that a major effect of α-interferon on immunoregulation in patients with chronic type B hepatitis is the inhibition of late stages of B-cell differentiation into immunoglobuline-producing and -secreting plasma cells.[65] However, the results of a more recent large randomized study did not support the use of ara-AMP and human leukocyte interferon in chronic persistent or chronic active hepatitis B.[66]

Acyclovir does not appear to inhibit the replication of HBV.[67,68] However, patients with chronic HBV infection had greater decreases in serum viral DNA polymerase and HBeAg when treated with interferon and acyclovir in combination than when treated with either agent alone.[69] Suramin, an inhibitor of retroviral DNA polymerases, is not useful in treating chronic hepatitis B.[70] There have been reports, as yet unconfirmed, that cianidanol may be useful in treating HBeAg-positive chronic active hepatitis.[71] Long-term therapy with the immune modulator levamisole showed a trend toward normalization of serum aminotransferase activities and suppression of viral replication in patients with chronic hepatitis B.[72] Recombinant interleukin-2 (r-IL2) decreased serum viral DNA polymerase activity and resulted in a loss of serum HBeAg in two of five patients.[73]

Prolonged treatment of chronic non-A, non-B hepatitis with recombinant α-interferon resulted in a sustained improvement in serum aminotransferase levels.[74] Three patients with hypogammaglobulinemia given α-interferon for chronic non-A, non-B hepatitis showed striking decreases in serum aminotransferase levels after the start of each course of therapy.[75] Further studies are needed to define the role, if any, of α-intereferon in therapy for non-A, non-B hepatitis.

REFERENCES

1. Sherlock S. Chronic hepatitis. Gut. 1974;15:581.
2. DeGroote J, Desmet VJ, Gedigk P, et al. A classification of chronic hepatitis. Lancet. 1968;2:626.
3. Boyer JL. Chronic hepatitis: A perspective on classification and determinants of prognosis. Gastroenterology. 1976;70:1161.
4. Bianchi CC, Mulligan R, Sherlock S. Controlled prospective trial of corticosteroid therapy in active chronic hepatitis. Q J med. 1971;40:159.
5. Boyer JL, Klatskin G. Pattern of necrosis in acute viral hepatitis: Prognostic value of bridging (subacute hepatic necrosis). N Engl J Med. 1970;283:1063.
6. Tisdale WA. Subacute hepatitis. N Engl J Med. 1963;268:85.
7. Ware AJ, Eigenbrodt EH, Combes B. Prognostic significance of subacute hepatic necrosis in acute hepatitis. Gastroenterology. 1975;68:519.
8. Thorne CH, Higgins GR, Ulrich TR, et al. A histologic comparison of hepatitis B with non-A, non-B chronic active hepatitis. Arch Pathol Lab Med. 1982;106:433.
9. Jones MB, Weinstock S, Koretz RL, et al. Clinical value of serum bile acid levels in chronic hepatitis. Dig Dis Sci. 1981;26:978.
10. Monroe PS, Baker AL, Schneider JF, et al. The aminopyrine breath test and serum bile acids reflect histologic severity in chronic hepatitis. Hepatology. 1982;2:317.
11. Ferrari C, Penna A, Sansoni P, et al. Selective sensitization of peripheral blood T lymphocytes to hepatitis B core antigen in patients with chronic active hepatitis type B. Clin Exp Immunol. 1986;66:497.
12. Scudeletti M, Indiveri F, Pierri I, et al. T cells from patients with chronic liver diseases: Abnormalities on PHA-induced expression of HLA class II antigens and in autologous mixed-lymphocyte reactions. Cell Immunol. 1986;102:227.
13. Alexander GJ, Mondelli M, Naumor NV, et al. Functional characterization of peripheral blood lymphocytes in chronic HBsAg carriers. Clin Exp Immunol. 1986;63:498.
14. Chu CM, Karayiannis P, Fowler MJ, et al. Natural history of chronic hepatitis B virus infection in Taiwan: Studies of hepatitis B virus DNA in serum. Hepatology. 1985;5:431.
15. Fuji A, Kakumu S, Ohtani Y, et al. Interferon-gamma production by peripheral blood mononuclear cells of patients with chronic liver disease. Hepatology. 1987;7:577.
16. Ikeda T, Lever AM, Thomas HC. Evidence for a deficiency of interferon production in patients with chronic hepatitis B virus infection acquired in adult life. Hepatology. 1986;6:962.
17. Pieovino M, Aguet M, Huber M, et al. Absence of detectable serum interferon in acute and chronic viral hepatitis. Hepatology. 1986;6:645.
18. Hoofnagle JH, Garety RJ, Tabor E, et al. Transmission of non-A, non-B hepatitis. Ann Intern Med. 1977;87:14.
19. Dienstag JL, Ezmuness W, Stevens CE, et al. Hepatitis A virus infection: New insights from seroepidemiologic studies. J Infect Dis. 1978;137:328.
20. Sherlock S. Predicting progression of acute type B hepatitis to chronicity. Lancet. 1976;2:354.
21. Shields MT, Czaja AJ, Taswell HF, et al. Frequency and significance of delta antibody in acute and chronic hepatitis B. A United States experience. Gastroenterology. 1985;89:1230.
22. Hadziyannis SJ, Sherman M, Lieberman HM, et al. Liver disease activity and hepatitis B virus replication in chronic delta antigen–positive hepatitis B virus carriers. Hepatology. 1985;5:544.
23. Fattovich G, Boscaro S, Noventa F, et al. Influence of hepatitis delta virus infection on progression to cirrhosis in chronic hepatitis type B. J Infect Dis. 1987;155:931.
24. Aragona M, Macagno S, Caredda F, et al. Serological response to the hepatitis delta virus in hepatitis D. Lancet 1987;1:478.
25. Shikata T, Uzawa T, Yoshiwara N, et al. Staining methods of Australia antigen in paraffin sections: Detection of cytoplasmic inclusion bodies. Jpn J Exp Med. 1974;44:25.
26. Careoda F, de Fravebis R, D'Arminio Monforte A, et al. Persistence of circulating HBsAg/IgM complexes in acute viral hepatitis, type B: An early marker of chronic evolution. Lancet. 1982;2:358.
27. Nielsen JO, Dietrichson O, Juhl E. Incidence and meaning of the "e" determinant among hepatitis B antigen positive patients with acute and chronic liver disease. Lancet. 1974;2:913.
28. Vogten AJM, Schalm SW, Sumemrskill WHJ, et al. Behavior of e antigen and antibody during chronic active liver disease: Relation to HB antigen-antibody system and prognosis. Lancet. 1976;2:126.
29. Trepo CG, Magnius LO, Schaefer RA, et al. Detection of e antigen and antibody: Correlations with hepatitis B surface and hepatitis B core antigens, live disease, and outcome in hepatitis B infections. Gastroenterology. 1976;71:804.
30. Viola LA, Barrison IG, Coleman JC, et al. The HBe antigen-antibody system and its relationship to clinical and laboratory findings in 100 chronic HBsAg carriers in Great Britain. J Med Virol. 1981;8:169.
31. Hoofnagle JH, Dusheiko GM, Seeff LB, et al. Seroconversion from hepatitis B e antigen to antibody in chronic type B hepatitis. Ann Intern Med. 1981;94:744.
32. Page AR, Sharp HL, Greenberg LJ, et al. Genetic analysis of patients with chronic active hepatitis. J Clin Invest. 1975;56:530..
33. Robertson DAG, Guy EC, Zhang SL, et al. Persistent measles virus genome in autoimmune chronic active hepatitis. Lancet. 1987;2:9–11.
34. Sherlock S. Waldenstrom's chronic active hepatitis. Acta Med Scand. 1966;445(suppl):426.
35. Tremolada F, Fattovich G, Panebianco G, et al. Suppressor cell activity in viral and non-viral chronic active hepatitis. Clin Exp Immunol. 1980;40:89.
36. Nonomura A, Tanino M, Kurumaya H, et al. Disordered immunoregulatory functions in patients with chronic active hepatitis. Clin Exp Immunol. 1982;47:595.
37. Carella G, Chatenoud L, Degos F, et al. Regulatory T cell-subset imbalance in chronic active hepatitis. J Clin Immunol. 1982;2:93.
38. Krawitt EL, Albertini RJ, Webb DD, et al. Immune regulation and HLA types in chronic hepatitis. Hepatology. 1981;1:300.
39. Manns M, Meyer zum Buschenfelde KH, Hutteroth TH, et al. Detection and characterization of liver membrane autoantibodies in chronic active hepatitis by solid-phase radioimmunoassay. Clin Exp Immunol. 1980;42:263.
40. Meliconi R, Baraldini M, Stefanini GF, et al. Antibodies against human liver-specific protein (LSP) in acute and chronic viral hepatitis types A, and B and non-A, non-B. Clin Exp Immunol. 1981;46:382.
41. MacKay IR, Morris PJ. Association of autoimmune chronic active hepatitis with HL-A1,8. Lancet. 1972;2:793.
42. Sharp JR, Ishak KG, Zimmerman JH. Chronic active hepatitis and severe hepatic necrosis associated with nitrofurantoin. Ann Intern Med. 1980;92:14.
43. Black M, Rabin L, Schatz N. Nitrofurantoin-induced chronic active hepatitis. Ann Intern Med. 1980;92:62.
44. Black M, Mitchell JR, Zimmerman HJ, et al. Isoniazid-associated hepatitis in 114 patients. Gastroenterology. 1975;69:289.
45. Maddrey WC, Boitnott JK. Severe hepatitis from methyldopa. Gastroenterology. 1975;68:351.
46. Sherlock S. Primary biliary cirrhosis. Mt Sinai J Med. 1977;44:790.
47. Sternleib I, Scheinberg IH. Chronic hepatitis as a first manifestation of Wilson's disease. Ann Intern Med. 1972;76:59.
48. Norum RA, Kearn AG, Briscoe WA, et al. Alpha-1-antitrypsin and disease. Mt Sinai J Med. 1977;44:827.
49. Hodges JR, Millward-Sadler GH, Barbatis C, et al. Heterozygous MZ alpha-1-antitrypsin deficiency in adults with chronic active hepatitis and cryptogenic cirrhosis. N Engl J Med. 1981;304:557.
50. Fisher RL, Taylor L, Sherlock S. Alpha-1-antitrypsin deficiency in liver disease: The extent of the problem. Gastroenterology. 1976;71:651.
51. Cook GC, Mulligan R, Sherlock S. Controlled prospective trial of corticosteroid therapy in active chronic hepatitis. Q J Med. 1971;40:159.

52. Soloway RD, Summerskill WHJ, Baggenstoss AH, et al. Clinical, biochemical and histological remission of severe chronic active liver disease: A controlled trial of treatments and an early prognosis. Gastroenterology. 1972;63:820.
53. Summerskill WHJ, Korman MG, Ammon HV, et al. Prednisone for chronic active liver disease: Dose titration, standard and combination with azothioprine compared. Gut. 1975;16:876.
54. Lam KC, Lai CL, Trepo C, et al. Deleterious effect of prednisolone in HBsAg-positive chronic active hepatitis. N Engl J Med. 1981;304:380.
55. Hoofnagle JH, Davis GL, Pappas SC, et al. A short course of prednisolone in chronic type B hepatitis. Report of a randomized, double-blind, placebo controlled trial. Ann Intern Med. 1986;104:12.
56. Weller IV, Bassendine MF, Murray AK, et al. Effects of prednisolone/azathioprine in chronic hepatitis B viral infection. Gut. 1980;23:650.
57. Sagnelli E, Manzillo G, Maio G, et al. Serum levels of hepatitis B surface and core antigens during immunosuppressive treatment of HBsAg-positive chronic active hepatitis. Lancet. 1980;2:395.
58. Sherlock S, Thomas HC. Treatment of chronic hepatitis due to hepatitis B virus. Lancet. 1985;2:1343.
59. Kirk AP, Jain S, Pocock S, et al. Late results of the Royal Free Hospital prospective controlled trial of prednisolone therapy in hepatitis B surface antigen negative chronic active hepatitis. Gut. 1980;21:78.
60. Czaja AJ, Ludwig J, Baggenstoss AA, et al. Corticosteroid-treated chronic active hepatitis in remission: Uncertain prognosis of chronic persistent hepatitis. N Engl J Med. 1981;304:5.
61. Scullard GH, Pollard RB, Smith JL, et al. Antiviral treatment of chronic hepatitis B virus infection. I. Changes in viral markers with interferon combined with adenine arabinoside. J Infect Dis. 1981;143:772.
62. Smith CI, Kitchen LW, Scullard GH, et al. Vidarabine monophosphate and human leukocyte interferon in chronic hepatitis B infection. JAMA. 1982;247:2261.
63. Weller IV, Bassendine MF, Craxi A, et al. Successful treatment of HBs and HBeAg positive chronic liver disease: Prolonged inhibition of viral replication by highly soluble adenine arabinoside 5′-monomphosphate(ARA-AMP). Gut. 1982;23:717.
64. Eisenberg M, Rosno S, Garcia G, et al. Preliminary trial of recombinant fibroblast interferon in chronic hepatitis B virus infection. Antimicrob Agents Chemother. 1986;29:122.
65. Peters H, Walling DM, Kelly K, et al. Immunologic effects of interferon-alpha in man: Treatment with human recombinant interferon-alpha suppresses in vitro immunoglobulin production in patients with chronic type B hepatitis. J Immunol. 1986;137:3147.
66. Garcia G, Smith CI, Weisberg JI, et al. Adenine arabinoside monophosphate (vidarabine phosphate) in combination with human leukocyte interferon in the treatment of chronic hepatitis B. A randomized, double-blind, placebo controlled trial. Ann Intern Med. 1987;107:278.
67. Smith CI, Scullard GH, Gregory PB, et al. Preliminary studies of acyclovir in chronic hepatitis B. Am J Med. 1982;73:267.
68. Alexander GJ, Fagan EA, Hegarty JE, et al. Controlled trial of acyclovir in chronic hepatitis B virus infection. J Med Virol. 1987;21:81.
69. Schalm SW, Heytink RA, van Buuren HR, et al. Acyclovir enhances the antiviral effect of interferon in chronic hepatitis B. Lancet. 1985;2:358.
70. Loke RH, Anderson MG, Coleman JC, et al. Suramin treatment for chronic active hepatitis B—toxic and ineffective. J Med Virol. 1987;21:97.
71. Suzuki H, Yamamoto S, Hirayama C, et al. Cianidanol therpay for HBe-antigen–positive chronic hepatitis: A multicenter, double blind study. Liver. 1986;6:35.
72. Fattovich G, Brollo L, Pontisso P, et al. Levamisole therapy in chronic type B hepatitis. Results of a double-blind randomized trial. Gastroenterology. 1986;91:692.
73. Nishioka M, Kagawa H, Shirai M, et al. Effects of human recombinant interleukin 2 in patients with chronic hepatitis B: A preliminary report. Am J Gastroenterol. 1987;82:438.
74. Hoofnagle JH, Muller KD, Jones DB, et al. Treatment of chronic non-A, non-B hepatitis with recombinant human alpha interferon. A preliminary report. N Engl J Med. 1986;315:1575.
75. Thomson BJ, Doran M, Lever AM, et al. Alpha-interferon therapy for non-A, non-B hepatitis transmitted by gammoglobulin replacement therapy. Lancet. 1987;1:539.

104. GRANULOMATOUS HEPATITIS

ANTHONY S. FAUCI
GARY S. HOFFMAN

Granulomas in the liver are histopathologic manifestations of a broad range of disease processes that may be of diverse etiologies, both infectious and noninfectious. They do not represent a distinct disease; also, in and of themselves, they rarely are diagnostic of a particular disease entity since their etiology is seldom determined purely on histologic criteria.[1] Most often (74 percent), they reflect a systemic granulomatous disease. Less frequently (21 percent), they represent a process that primarily is neither a systemic granulomatous nor a hepatic disease; only rarely (4 percent) do they represent an isolated hepatic disease.[1] In this regard, the demonstration of hepatic granulomas may serve to confirm documented underlying disease, or it may present a diagnostic challenge requiring an organized and directed approach in determining its underlying etiology. Since the histopathologic features of granulomas resulting from infectious and noninfectious etiologies may be identical and since the treatment regimens (particularly corticosteroids) used in diseases with hepatic granulomata of noninfectious etiologies are directly contraindicated in most disorders of infectious etiologies, it is imperative to appreciate the intricacies of this clinicopathologic process.

PATHOPHYSIOLOGIC MECHANISMS OF GRANULOMA FORMATION

It is now fairly well established that granulomas form by a stepwise series of events that include the migration of monocyte–macrophages into an area of inflammatory or immunologic reactivity and the transformation of these cells into epithelioid cells, which may remain as such or may fuse to form the characteristic multinucleated giant cells.[2–5] The morphologic changes that impart an epithelial-like appearance to the macrophage are accompanied by functional changes. The macrophage–phagocyte becomes a nonphagocytic epithelioid cell having increased organelles for enzyme and other protein synthesis and secretion.[6,7] The persistence of incompletely degraded foreign matter in tissues represents one type of stimulus for such cellular transformation. An example is found in tuberculosis, the clinically most common microbial cause of granulomata. It has been demonstrated that mycobacterial lipids persist within the macrophage and trigger its transformation.[8] Although this is an excellent example of persistence of microbial intracellular antigen-enhancing granuloma formation, persistent extracellular stimuli such as schistosome eggs lead to similar responses.[7] In addition, nonmicrobial particles may also stimulate granuloma formation (e.g., silica, metal salts), although in these examples nonimmunologic mechanisms appear to activate macrophages.

It is quite clear that undegraded materials are not the only stimuli of epithelioid cell transformation and granuloma formation since antigen persistence cannot adequately explain many of the granulomatous responses of hypersensitivity etiology.[3] Pure foreign body granulomas in which antigen persistence triggers the reaction fall on one end of the spectrum, and pure hypersensitivity responses in which it is highly unlikely that antigen persistence is operable forms the other end of the spectrum.[9] In the latter circumstance, sensitized lymphocytes on exposure to antigen (which, in many cases, is soluble) amplify the immune response by release of mediators. Monocyte–macrophages accumulate, most likely in response to mediators, and subsequently undergo transformation as described above. In experimental animals, cyclosporine A has been demonstrated to markedly reduce the granulomatous response induced with a variety of mycobacterial agents.[6] This observation suggests that, at least in this setting, granuloma formation is highly dependent upon T-lymphocyte mediators that may inhibit migration and cause activation of macrophages (e.g., γ-interferon).[10,11]

Most infectious diseases in which granulomas occur constitute an overlap of mechanisms since microbes can serve both as a foreign body and as an antigen for an immunologic response. In addition, immune complexes made up of host antibody and microbial or nonmicrobial antigen may, under certain circumstances, stimulate granuloma formation. Finally,

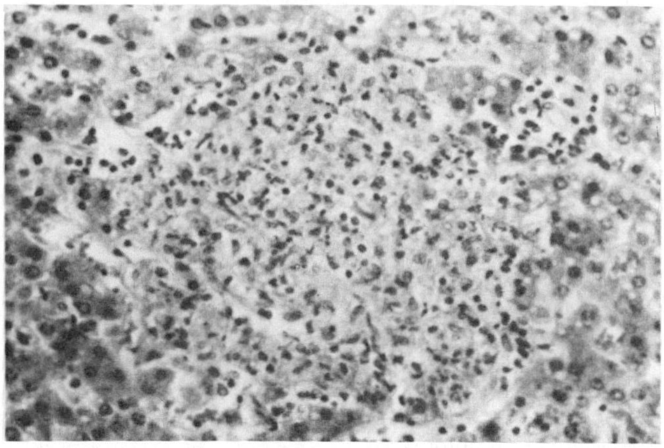

FIG. 1. Liver biopsy specimen from a patient with disseminated histoplasmosis. A typical granuloma is shown with epithelioid cells and mononuclear cell infiltration. (H&E, ×220)

certain T-lymphocyte neoplasms may secrete soluble factors that activate macrophages,[12] an alternative mechanism for granuloma formation in diseases such as lymphomatoid granulomatosis.[13]

The liver serves as a particularly susceptible target organ for granuloma formation. It is an extremely large organ rich in reticuloendothelial cells. In addition to their phagocytic ability, certain of these cells possess receptors such as those for the Fc portion of immunoglobulin,[14] thus allowing for nonspecific (as well as a degree of immunologically specific) clearance of circulting antigens, unopsonized and opsonized microorganisms, and immune complexes. It is clear then why hepatic granulomas are found in such a high proportion of diseases with systemic granulomatous responses and why a liver biopsy specimen provides such a high-yield source of diagnostic tissue in such diseases (Fig. 1).

Histopathologically, hepatic granulomas are characterized by the presence of generally discrete nodular infiltrates of epithelioid cells interspersed with greater or lesser degrees of mononuclear cells. The epithelioid cells usually are compactly arranged and may merge to form typical multinucleated giant cells. However, the presence of these giant cells is not necessary to make the diagnosis of a granulomatous reaction. This histopathologic picture of hepatic granulomas is clearly distinguishable from portal triaditis, which is more commonly seen in a number of inflammatory conditions and which is characterized by the infiltration of mononuclear cells as well as granulocytes around the portal tract areas. Thus, it is not strictly correct to term granulomatous hepatitis a true "hepatitis" since classic inflammatory responses are rarely seen and, as will be discussed below, significant hepatocellular dysfunction is rare.[15,16]

DISEASES CHARACTERIZED BY HEPATIC GRANULOMAS

Infectious Diseases

Infectious diseases clearly are the most common underlying causes of granulomas in general and of hepatic granulomas in particular.[17–19] Table 1 lists some of the various types of infectious diseases that may be associated with granulomas in the liver. Tuberculosis continues to lead the list as the most common infectious disease cause of hepatic granulomas.[17–19] Even when one considers all causes of hepatic granulomas (infectious and noninfectious), tuberculosis still ranks very high in incidence. In Klatskin's series[1] of 433 patients with documented granulomatous diseases in other organs, tuberculosis ranked

TABLE 1. Infectious Disease Causes of Granulomatous Hepatitis

Bacterial
Mycobacteriosis
Tuberculous
Nontuberculous
Lepromatous leprosy
Brucellosis (*Brucella abortus*)
Tularemia
Granuloma inguinale
Melioidosis
Listeriosis
Fungal
Histoplasmosis
Coccidioidomycosis
Candidiasis
Viral
Cytomegalovirus
Infectious mononucleosis
Viral hepatitis
Parasitic
Schistosomiasis (*Schistosoma mansoni*)
Visceral larva migrans (*Toxocara canis* or *catis*)
Fascioliasis (*Fasciola hepatica*)
Capillaria hepatica
Rickettsial
Q fever (*Coxiella burnetii*)
Spirochetal
Syphilis

second to sarcoidosis in the incidence of demonstrable hepatic granulomas. Of 164 tuberculous patients 70 had granulomas on liver biopsy specimens. Caseating granulomas are the classic findings in tuberculosis. However, noncaseating granulomas also are quite common in tuberculous hepatic involvement. In one series reporting noncaseating granulomas of infectious and noninfectious etiology in 50 liver biopsy specimens, tuberculosis again ranked second to sarcoidosis and accounted for 10 percent of the total.[20] In other studies of hepatic granulomas unrestricted in regard to the presence or absence of caseous changes, fewer than 15 percent of patients found to have tuberculosis had caseous necrosis in the liver.[21,22] Certain consistent findings emerge from various series on the diagnostic import of liver biopsy specimens in patients who ultimately are proved to have tuberculosis. Thirty-one percent of the patients with "isolated" active pulmonary tuberculosis were shown to have hepatic granulomas.[1] In series of patients with documented pulmonary and extrapulmonary tuberculosis (exclusive of miliary involvement), 70–80 percent had hepatic granulomas.[1,23] In cases of miliary tuberculosis, greater than 90 percent of the patients will have hepatic granulomas.[1,24] There is no question that the tubercule bacillus can be demonstrated by appropriate staining techniques as well as by culture from liver biopsy specimens.[23–26] Yet, when one looks at all cases of hepatic granulomas associated with tuberculosis of any extent, this demonstration is rather uncommon.[27,28] However, in a series of 23 liver biopsies in documented miliary tuberculosis, 43 percent either had a positive culture or smear.[24]

Other mycobacterial infections that may cause hepatic granulomas are disseminated atypical mycobacterial disease,[29] lepromatous leprosy,[39] and BCG-osis after Calmette-Guérin bacillus (BCG) vaccination, immunotherapy for neoplasms, or intravesical therapy in the treatment of bladder cancer.[31–33] It is noteworthy that, in the hepatic granulomas associated with lepromatous leprosy, organisms are plentiful and can be easily demonstrated within Küpffer cells.[30] It is of interest that granulomatous tissue reactions rarely are found; if present, they are poorly formed in the *Mycobacterium avium-intracellulare* infections that are commonly seen in patients with acquired immunodeficiency syndrome (AIDS).[34] This is likely due to the fact that these patients have markedly suppressed inducer–helper T-lymphocyte numbers and function,[35] which is required for the immunologic component of the granulomatous response to mycobacteria.

Brucellosis is quite commonly associated with hepatic granulomas.[35] In infections with *Brucella abortus*, the granulomas are well formed and discrete. Infection with *Brucella suis* and *Brucella melitensis* results in less distinct changes in the liver, which may be manifested merely as isolated areas of necrosis.[28,36]

Although tularemia often is cited as one of the bacterial diseases that can lead to hepatic granulomas, in reality this is not the case. Classic well-formed granulomas with multinucleated giant cells are seldom seen in this disease. The most common finding is scattered necrotic nodules with neutrophil infiltration.[37]

Other uncommon bacterial causes of hepatic granulomas are granuloma inguinale,[39] melioidosis,[39] and disseminated infection with *Listeria monocytogenes*, particularly in a rare syndrome in neonates called miliary granulomatosis or granulomatosis infantisepticum.[40]

Fungi are another common cause of hepatic granulomas. Depending on the reported series and geographic location, they may be the most common infectious disease cause, surpassing even tuberculosis in some individual reports.[20] In the United States, disseminated histoplasmosis is the most common of the fungal etiologies of hepatic granulomas. A hepatic biopsy specimen is a more fruitful source of diagnostic tissue in histoplasmosis as compared with tuberculosis.[41] In a prospective study of 26 patients with disseminated histoplasmosis at the National Institutes of Health, 21 of 26 patients had liver function abnormalities; in the 8 in whom liver biopsy specimens were obtained, 5 had granulomas.[42] Furthermore, *Histoplasma* was cultured from four of the eight biopsy specimens and was demonstrated by staining techniques in three of the four cultured specimens.

Other disseminated mycotic infections such as coccidioidomycosis, candidiasis, and aspergillosis rarely may cause hepatic granulomas. However, the other organ system manifestations of these diseases in their disseminated form far overshadow the hepatic granulomas when present. For the most part, the finding of hepatic granulomas in this setting adds little to an already obvious clinicopathologic setting.

It is now well established that viral infections may cause hepatic granulomas. Cytomegalovirus and infectious mononucleosis,[1] in particular, have been associated with granulomatous hepatitis. In addition, in a large biopsy series of hepatitis of various causes, granulomas were demonstrated in the liver biopsy specimens of 2 percent of the patients with acute viral hepatitis and 12 percent of the patients with chronic active hepatitis.[1]

It is uncertain whether influenza virus may cause granulomatous hepatitis. There has been an association of influenza B infection and granulomatous hepatitis,[43] but the two may have been unrelated.[17]

Several parasites encountered throughout the world may cause hepatic granulomas.[17,44] Of particular importance are schistosomiasis (resulting from *Schistosoma mansoni*) and visceral larva migrans (caused by *Toxocara canis* or *Toxocara cati*). Granuloma formation in these disorders most likely results from a deposition of eggs in the liver, with a subsequent combination foreign body reaction to the eggs themselves and a cell-mediated or delayed hypersensitivity reaction to antigenic determinants of the parasite. Another potential cause of parasite-related granulomatous reaction in the liver is fascioliasis caused by the liver fluke *Fasciola hepatica*.

Of the rickettsioses, *Coxiella burnettii*, which is the agent causing Q fever, most often is associated with granulomatous hepatitis.[45,46] Q fever is not associated with an exanthem (characteristic of the other rickettsioses); in some cases, it may present with a clinical syndrome identical to viral hepatitis. Thus, the finding of granulomas on a liver biopsy specimen in such a clinical setting should suggest Q fever as part of the differential diagnosis.

The liver may be involved in secondary and tertiary syphilis. During the era when late syphilis was much more common than it is at present, variable degrees of hepatic involvement were frequently seen. Hepatic gummas and hepar lobatum are the typical changes of late syphilitic liver involvement, and interstitial hepatitis is the typical finding in congenital syphilis.[28] Well-formed granulomas, however, are not characteristic but may be found in certain cases.

Noninfectious Diseases

Among diseases in which a diagnosis is ultimately made, sarcoidosis is the most common noninfectious disease cause of hepatic granulomas[1,17]; in addition, it is the most common cause—infectious and noninfectious—of noncaseating hepatic granulomas.[20] It is the histopathologic prototype of the classic noncaseating granuloma.

Other noninfectious disease causes of granulomatous hepatitis are listed in Table 2 and have been reviewed in detail elsewhere.[46–48] Of particular interest in this group, with regard to infectious diseases, are erythema nodosum and chronic granulomatous disease (CGD) of childhood.

Erythema nodosum is a hypersensitivity manifestation of several different clinical entities that is characterized predominantly by tender subcutaneous nodules over the anterior surface of the lower extremities beneath the knees and (occasionally) elsewhere.[49] It can be associated with granulomatous hepatitis as part of the syndrome complex itself. In addition, some of the infectious disease entities with which it is associated (e.g., tuberculosis, coccidioidomycosis, histoplasmosis, and lepromatous leprosy), in and of themselves, can cause hepatic granulomas; this makes the diagnostic approach even more complex when hepatic granulomas are found in erythema nodosum.

In up to 29 percent of patients with hepatic granulomas, medications have been suspected causes. Granulomas are said to always be noncaseating and often contain large numbers of eosinophils (>5–10 per granuloma), a finding that would be very unusual in tuberculosis or sarcoidosis. In a minority of cases, drug-induced granulomas may be found in extrahepatic sites such as lymph nodes and bone marrow. Eosinophilic granulomas may also occur in schistosomiasis, visceral larva migrans, Hodgkin's disease, and histoplasmosis. In the absence of these disorders, the question of drug-induced disease should be considered.[50] The terms "probable" and "possible" have been applied to drug-suspected cases when the withdrawal of a drug has been associated with resolution of symptoms, normalization of liver function test results (if these had been abnormal), and diminution or absence of granulomas in a repeat liver biopsy specimen. A "definite" diagnosis of drug-induced disease would require the demonstration of recurrent abnormalities

TABLE 2. Noninfectious Disease Causes of Granulomatous Hepatitis

Sarcoidosis
Hypersensitivity diseases
Erythema nodosum
Berylliosis
Hypersensitivity drug reactions
Primary liver disease
Primary biliary cirrhosis
Rarely, others such as Laennec's cirrhosis, postnecrotic cirrhosis, alcoholic hepatitis, or chronic active hepatitis
Neoplasms
Hodgkin's disease and, rarely, other lymphomas and solid tumors
Host defense defects
Chronic granulomatous disease of childhood
Immune deficiencies (hypogammaglobulinemia)
Others
Temporal arteritis—polymyalgia rheumatica syndrome
Allergic granulomatosis
Idiopathic granulomatous hepatitis
Ulcerative colitis
Crohn's disease

after reinstitution of the suspected agent. Both moral and legal considerations should discourage intentional manipulations to establish such definite relationships unless the medication in question was considered essential and another with similar properties, but chemically unrelated, was not available. Since it is conceivable that many different medications may play a role in granuloma formation, it would be judicious to discontinue treatment with any nonessential drugs and follow the patient's clinical course and, when indicated, hepatic histopathology up to 8 weeks later before a diagnosis of either sarcoidosis or idiopathic granulomatous hepatitis is considered.

Patients with the host defense defect of CGD frequently have disseminated granulomas with a predominance of liver involvement.[51] It is felt that the mechanism of granuloma formation in this disease is an intracellular persistence of microorganisms or their products that is related to the well-established microbial killing defect. This triggers the epithelioid cell transformation with subsequent granuloma formation as described above. Granulomas persist in these patients, and it is difficult to recover microorganisms from the liver tissue. Hence, although the syndrome of CGD is not an infectious disease per se, the granulomatous reaction results from an inability to normally handle a variety of microorganisms.

Hodgkin's disease and other lymphomas are recognized as the most common malignancies associated with hepatic granulomas. Although other tumors (renal cell, rectal, nasopharyngeal, and primary hepatocellular carcinoma) have also been noted to share this association, those examples are not as well documented.[22,48,50] Further confusion is added by the observation that malignancies related to hepatic granulomas may not become apparent until months or even several years after the initial evaluation. Preliminary data have suggested that individuals who later (4–40 months) demonstrate lymphomas are more likely to have at initial presentation (*1*) prolonged (>4 weeks) unexplained fevers, (*2*) liver or (*3*) spleen size extending more than 4 cm below the costal margins, and (*4*) eosinophilia of greater than 4 percent of the peripheral white blood cell count. The presence of any two of these features had an 80 percent specificity in distinguishing hepatic granulomas and lymphoma from other causes of such hepatic abnormalities. The sensitivity of having at least two of four features for lymphoma was 100 percent.[52]

Another interesting and perplexing category of granulomatous hepatitis is that group of patients in whom the etiology of the granulomatous reaction remains unknown despite extensive diagnostic investigation.[53] In various series, this group of idiopathic granulomatous hepatitis ranged to as high as 36 percent of the cases with documented hepatic granulomas.[17,19,27,30] In addition, in a group of 72 patients with hepatic granulomas whose underlying disease did not appear to be hepatic or granulomatous in nature, 37 of these remained undiagnosed.[1] These patients do not have extra-abdominal granulomas, and other criteria for sarcoidosis are absent.[44] This group probably represents hypersensitivity states that are clinically and histopathologically reflected primarily in the liver, with the responsible antigen remaining unidentified.

GRANULOMATOUS HEPATITIS AND FEVER

Fever is a major manifestation in most cases of granulomatous hepatitis. In fact, in one large series, over 40 percent of the patients with hepatic granulomas had fevers of unknown origin.[17] This is not difficult to understand when one considers the current theories on the pathogenesis of fever. It has been demonstrated that the final common mediators of fever are proteins called endogenous pyrogens, which are synthesized by phagocytic cells of the host. On release from these cells, these pyrogens act on specific neurons of the anterior hypothalamus–preoptic region of the brain, with resulting elevation of body temperature.[54] The liver is rich in phagocytic Küpffer cells, which are highly efficient producers of endogenous pyrogen.[54] Triggering of these cells by antigens, immune complexes, or microorganisms in the pathogenesis of granuloma formation can potentially lead to the release of pyrogen. This is of particular relevance in the diagnostic challenge of granulomatous hepatitis with regard to infectious disease etiologies. On the one hand, an infectious agent that may be the underlying cause of the hepatic granulomas can cause fever; conversely, the hepatic granulomas, whether resulting from infectious or noninfectious causes, can of themselves be the sources of fever. Finally, it has been recently demonstrated that the pyrogen molecule is, in fact, identical to interleukin-1, which is secreted by monocyte–macrophages and which is critically involved in the activation of T lymphocytes.[55] This observation lends further support to the complex relationship among immunologic reactions, granuloma formation, and the presence of a febrile response.

DIAGNOSTIC APPROACH TO HEPATIC GRANULOMAS

Hepatic granulomas really are quite common and may be found in up to 10 percent of specimens from liver biopsy procedures performed in general hospitals.[17] Although laparotomy with a biopsy specimen of a substantial amount of tissue is the obvious highest-yield approach, it is now clear that percutaneous needle biopsy is a safe and efficient procedure for obtaining tissue for diagnostic and extent-of-disease work-up as well as for follow-up of the clinical course and therapeutic response. In particular, its value in certain circumstances in the diagnostic approach to fevers of unknown origin is well established.[56] Once hepatic granulomas have been histologically demonstrated and the underlying diagnosis is still not established, a stepwise diagnostic approach should be undertaken. Bearing in mind that infectious diseases are the leading causes of all types of hepatic granulomas, bacterial, fungal, and mycobacterial cultures should be performed. In addition, special staining techniques should be applied to histologic sections, and appropriate skin tests and diagnostic serologic tests should be used. Also, viral infections such as cytomegalovirus and infectious mononucleosis infrequently may cause granulomatous hepatitis (Table 1). The diagnostic culture yield of tissue for the recovery of virus is so low that the diagnosis, when suspected, can be best made on clinical and serologic grounds.

If infectious disease causes have been ruled out and the diagnosis is still unknown, an orderly diagnostic approach that includes clinical, histopathologic, serologic, and radiologic parameters should be used to rule out other noninfectious disease causes (Table 2). Recently provided (within 6 months) medications should be suspected and treatment with all nonessential medications discontinued. If after this diagnostic approach one is still left with a diagnosis of granulomatous hepatitis of unknown etiology, then careful follow-up, subsequent reevaluation, and (in some cases) empirical therapy (discussed below) are indicated.

There may be specific laboratory abnormalities associated with various diseases in which granulomatous hepatitis may be a manifestation.[13,20,53] However, the laboratory abnormalities usually associated with hepatic granulomas as such are generally nonspecific. The erythrocyte sedimentation rate is almost invariably elevated. Liver function test findings may be completely normal or, in most cases, mildly abnormal. Increased serum levels of alkaline phosphatase and transaminase are frequent abnormalities. Hyperbilirubinemia is most unusual except in cases of primary biliary cirrhosis. Mild hyperglobulinemia may be found, and prothrombin elevations are unusual.

TREATMENT OF GRANULOMATOUS HEPATITIS

When the underlying cause of the granulomatous hepatitis is known, treatment obviously should be directed toward that etiology, whether infectious or noninfectious. The disappearance of granulomas usually parallels the therapeutic response of the underlying disease. After successful therapy for the underlying disease, there usually is little if any histopathologic residue of the granulomas.[47,53]

In the clincal setting where one has ruled out as far as possible infectious and other causes of granulomatous hepatitis and where the diagnosis of idiopathic granulomatous hepatitis remains, corticosteroids often lead to clinical and histopathologic improvement.[53] Since the obvious danger in this situation is to administer corticosteroids to a patient with an underlying, but undetectable infection (particularly tuberculosis), there is a place for empirical antituberculous therapy. Several cases of what appeared to be granulomatous hepatitis in which tuberculosis could not be demonstrated responded to antituberculous drugs. Conversely, occasional patients who have lacked evidence for tuberculosis and were treated with steroids for idiopathic granulomatous hepatitis have died of disseminated tuberculosis.[22] Due to these observations, it is recommended that all patients with granulomatous hepatitis in whom an etiology cannot be established should be given an empirical trial of two-drug antituberculous therapy. If a clinical response is seen, the drugs are continued for the usual recommended course. If no clinical response is seen after 2 months, corticosteroids are added. If the patient is tuberculin skin test–positive, a single drug (isoniazid) should be continued with the corticosteroid. Therapeutic responses should be monitored by clinical and laboratory parameters as well as by repeat liver biopsy procedures every 6–12 months. Once improvement occurs, it is highly recommended to attempt to convert the therapeutic regimen to alternate-day corticosteroids since granulomatous hepatitis can be controlled quite adequately in many patients with alternate-day corticosteroid regimens.[53]

REFERENCES

1. Klatskin G. Hepatic granulomata: Problems in interpretation. Ann NY Acad Sci. 1976;278:427.
2. Silverman L, Shorter RG. Histogenesis of the multinucleated giant cell. Lab Invest. 1963;12:985.
3. Epstein WL. Granulomatous hypersensitivity. Prog Allergy. 1967;11:36.
4. Epstein WL, Krasnobrod H. The origin of epithelioid cells in experimental granulomas of man. Lab Invest. 1968;18:190.
5. Gillman T, Wright LJ. Probable in vivo origin of multinucleated giant cells from circulating mononuclears. Nature. 1963;209:263.
6. Muller-Hermelink HK, Kaiserling E, Sonntag HG. Modulation of epitheloid cell granuloma formation to apathogenic mycobacteria by cyclosporin A. Pathol Res Pract. 1982;175:80.
7. Williams GT, Williams WJ. Granulomatous inflammation—a review. J Clin Pathol. 1983;36:723.
8. Rich AR. The Pathogenesis of Tuberculosis. Springfield, IL: Charles C Thomas; 1951:13.
9. Warren KS. Granulomatous inflammation. In: Lepow IH, Ward PW, eds. Inflammation: Mechanisms and Control. New York: Academic Press; 1972:203.
10. Weinberg JB, Hobbs MM, Misukonis MA. Recombinant human γ-interferon induces human monocyte polykaryon formation. Proc Natl Acad Sci USA 1984;81:4554.
11. Block CM, Catterall JR, Remington JS. In vivo and in vitro activation of alveolar macrophges by recombinant interferon-γ. J Immunol. 1987;138:491.
12. Simrell CR, Crabtree GR, Cossman J, et al. Stimulation of phagocytosis by a T cell lymphoma derived lymphokine. In: Vitetta E, Fox CF, eds. B and T Cell Tumors: Biological and Clinical Aspects. UCLA Symposia on Molecular and Cellular Biology. v. 24. New York: Academic Press; 1982:247.
13. Fauci AS, Haynes BF, Costa J, et al. Lymphomatoid granulomatosis. Prospective clinical and therapeutic experience over 10 years. N Engl J Med. 1982;306:68.
14. Atkinson JP, Frank MM. Studies on the in vivo antibody and complement in the immune clearance and destruction of erythrocytes in man. J Clin Invest. 1974;54:339.
15. Sherlock S. Hepatic granulomas. In: Sherlock S, ed. Diseases of the Liver and Biliary System, ed 5. Oxford, Blackwell Scientific Publications; 1975:598.
16. Harrington PT, Gutierrez JJ, Ramirez-Ronda CH, et al. Granulomatous hepatitis. Rev Infect Dis. 1982;4:638.
17. Guckian JC, Perry JE. Granulomatous hepatitis. An analysis of 63 cases and review of the literature. Ann Intern Med. 1969;65:1081.
18. Gold J, Wigderson A, Leiman E, et al. Report of a case with review of the literature. Gastroenterology. 1957;33:113.
19. Bowry S, Chan CH, Weiss H, et al. Hepatic involvement in pulmonary tuberculosis. Histologic and functional characteristics. Am Rev Respir Dis. 1970;101:941.
20. Mir-Madjlessi SH, Farmer RG, Hawk WA. Granulomatous hepatitis. A review of 50 cases. Am J Gastroenterol. 1973;60:122.
21. Irani SK, Dobbins WO III. Hepatic granulomas: A review of 73 patients from one hospital and survey of the literature. J Clin Gastroenterol. 1979;1:131.
22. Cunningham D, Mills PR, Quigley EMM, et al. Hepatic granulomas: Experience over a 10-year period in West of Scotland. Q J Med. 1982;51:162.
23. Korn RJ, Kellow WF, Heller P, et al. Hepatic involvement in extrapulmonary tuberculosis. Histologic and functional characteristics. Am J Med. 1959;27:60.
24. Cucin RL, Coleman M, Eckardt JJ, et al. The diagnosis of miliary tuberculosis: Utility of peripheral blood abnormalities, bone marrow and liver needle biopsy. J Chronic Dis. 1973;26:355.
25. Healey RJ, Leff AH, Rosenak BD. Needle biopsy in tuberculosis of the liver, with culture of acid-fast bacilli. Am J Dig Dis. 1959;4:638.
26. Rumball JM, Baum GL. Liver biopsy culture in the diagnosis of miliary tuberculosis: A case report. Gastroenterology. 1952;22:124.
27. Wagoner GP, Anton AT, Gall EA, et al. Needle biopsy of the liver. VII. Experiences with hepatic granulomas. Gastroenterology. 1953;25:487.
28. Rubin E. Interpretation of the liver biopsy. Diagnostic criteria. Gastroenterology. 1963;45:400.
29. Koenig MG, Collins RD, Heyssel RM. Disseminated mycobacteriosis caused by Battey type mycobacteria. Ann Intern Med. 1966;64:145.
30. Browne SG. The liver in leprosy: A review. W Afr Med J. 1964;13:35.
31. Marans HY, Bekirov HM. Granulomatous hepatitis following intravesical bacillus Calmette-Guerin therapy for bladder carcinoma. J Urol. 1987;137:111.
32. Hunt JS, Silverstein MJ, Spark FC, et al. Granulomatous hepatitis: A complication of BCG immunotherapy. Lancet. 1973;2:820.
33. Bodurtha A, Kim YH, Laucius JF, et al. Hepatic granulomas and other hepatic lesions associated with BCG immunotherapy for cancer. Am J Clin Pathol. 1974;61:714.
34. Greene JB, Sidhu GS, Lewin S, et al. *Mycobacterium avium-intracellulare*: A cause of disseminated life-threatening infection in homosexuals and drug abusers. Ann Intern Med. 1982;97:539.
35. Fauci AS. The syndrome of Kaposi's sarcoma-opportunisitc infections: An epidemiolologically restricted disorder of immunoregulation. Ann Intern Med. 1982;96:777.
36. Spink WW, Hoffbauer FW, Walher WW, et al. Histopathology of the liver in human brucellosis. J Lab Clin Med. 1949;34:40.
37. Foshay L. Tularemia: A summary of certain aspects of the disease including methods for early diagnosis and the results of serum treatment in 600 patients. Medicine (Baltimore). 1940;19:1.
38. Lyford J III, Johnson RW Jr, Blackman S, et al. Pathologic findings in a fatal case of disseminated granuloma inguinale with miliary bone and joint involvement. Bull Johns Hopkins Hosp. 1946;79:349.
39. Borchardt KA, Stansifer P, Albano PM. Osteomyelitis due to *Pseudomonas pseudomallei*. JAMA. 1966;196:660.
40. Ray CJ, Wedgewood RJ. Neonatal listeriosis; six case reports and a review of the literature. Pediatrics. 1964;34:378.
41. Schiff L. The clinical value of needle biopsy of the liver. Ann Intern Med. 1951;34:948.
42. Smith JW, Utz JP. Progressive disseminated histoplasmosis. A prospective study of 26 patients. Ann Intern Med. 1972;76:557.
43. Klatskin G, Yesner R. Hepatic manifestations of sarcoidosis and other granulomatous diseases. Yale J Biol Med. 1950;23:207.
44. Marcial Rojas RA. Helminthic diseases. In: Schiff L, ed. Diseases of the Liver. ed 2. Philadelphia: JB Lippincott; 1963:800.
45. Dupont HL, Hornick RB, Levin HS, et al. Q fever hepatitis. Ann Intern Med. 1971;74:198.
46. Travis LB, Travis WD, Li C-Y, et al. Q fever: A clinicopathologic study of five cases. Arch Pathol Lab Med 1986;110:1017.
47. Fauci AS, Wolff SM. Granulomatous hepatitis. In: Popper H, Schaffner F, eds. Progress in Liver Diseases. v. 5. New York: Grune & Stratton; 1976:609.
48. Anderson CS, Nicholls J, Rowland R, et al. Hepatic granulomas: A 15-year experience in the Royal Adelaide Hospital. Med J Aust. 1988;148:71.
49. Epstein WL. Erythema nodosum. In: Samter M, ed. Immunological Diseases. v. 2. Boston: Little, Brown; 1971:944.
50. McMaster KR III, Hennigar GR. Drug-induced granulomatous hepatitis. Lab Invest. 1981;44:61.
51. Good RA, Quie PG, Windhorst DB, et al. Fatal (chronic) granulomatous disease of childhood: A hereditary defect of leukocyte function. Semin Hematol. 1968;5:215.
52. Aderka D, Kraus M, Weinberger A, et al. Parameters which can differentiate patients with "idiopathic" from patients with lymphoma-induced liver granulomas. Am J Gastroenterol. 1985;80:1004.
53. Simon HB, Wolff SM. Granulomatous hepatitis and prolonged fever of unknown origin: A study of 13 patients. Medicine (Baltimore). 1973;52:1.
54. Dinarello CA, Wolff SM. Exogenous and endogenous pyrogen. In: Brazier MAB, Coceani F, eds. Brain Dysfunction in Infantile Febrile Convulsions. v. 2. New York: Raven Press; 1976:117.
55. Oppenheim JJ, Gery I. Interleukin 1 is more than an interleukin. Immunol Today. 1982;3:113.
56. Wolff SM, Simon HB. Granulomatous hepatitis and prolonged fever of unknown origin. Trans Am Clin Climatol Assoc. 1973;84:149.

SECTION P. ACQUIRED IMMUNODEFICIENCY SYNDROME

105. INTRODUCTION

R. GORDON DOUGLAS, JR.

Acquired immunodeficiency syndrome (AIDS) was first recognized in 1981. Since then, modern science has discovered its cause as a novel retrovirus known as human immunodeficiency virus (HIV), defined the nature of the immune defect, developed tests to detect antibodies to determine the presence of infection and to screen blood and blood products for HIV, and developed a specific antiviral treatment that, although not a cure, significantly prolongs life. Research progress continues at a great rate. More is being learned about the basic properties and behavior of the virus as well as the immune defects. Such research is yielding new ideas for chemotherapeutic agents, immunologic stimulators and modifiers, and potential vaccines, and clinical trials to test these agents are under way.

Despite these remarkable accomplishments, the epidemic progresses unchecked, resulting in enormous demands on health care facilities and health care providers. Clinicians have had to learn to cope with new, difficult, and confusing opportunistic infections. Yet advances in the treatment and prevention of these illnesses have benefited many AIDS victims.

What appears to have happened with AIDS is the rapid introduction of an infectious agent into an immunologically naive population. In this case, the virus probably originated from primates in central Africa and has rapidly adapted to humans.[1] History of such introductions of new infectious agents to naive populations indicates the prospect for a devastating outcome: for example, influenza in 1918, bubonic plague in the 14th century, measles in island populations.[2,3] This bleak outlook for mankind is further supported by the failure of antibody that is neutralizing in vitro to be protective in vivo in humans or chimpanzees. Despite these dismal predictions, in the developed world, the disease is difficult to transmit from person to person and thus is restricted primarily to certain population groups, namely, male homosexuals or bisexuals and intravenous drug abusers (IVDA). It is this epidemiologic restriction that limits the magnitude of the epidemic. With time, the primary epidemic population has shifted from homosexuals and bisexuals to the IVDA population, mostly due to modification of behavior on the part of the former groups. Further, antibody testing has virtually eliminated transfusion of blood and blood products as a source of HIV infection.

The concentration of AIDS in these groups and the very skewed geographic distribution of cases in the United States has led to a mixed public reaction to recognition of the importance of the disease and, consequently, to public support for health care and research.

Increasing the controversies surrounding the disease are concerns related to the Federal Drug Administration's lengthy approval process for new drugs and the issue of confidentiality of HIV antibody testing—who should and should not be tested and who has a right to know the results. Vaccine development produces several concerns of its own. For example, candidate vaccines will convert an individual from seronegative to seropositive for HIV with all the attendant risks, such as uninsurability and possible loss of job, housing, and schooling.

Infectious disease specialists have felt the brunt of the epidemic.[4,5] They are often asked to be the role models and standard-bearers for professional behavior. They have shouldered much of the responsibility for the health care of AIDS victims and for performance of the clinical investigations related to specific antiviral agents and immunomodulators versus HIV, treatment for opportunistic infections, and vaccine development.[6,7]

Thus, major textbooks of infectious diseases must present comprehensive, up-to-date material related to all aspects of AIDS and HIV infection. AIDS was not mentioned in the first edition of this text published in 1979. In the second edition, published in 1985, only one short chapter was devoted to AIDS. For the present edition, the section on AIDS was completely reorganized and rewritten. AIDS is treated as a syndrome, as is proper, and thus most of the material related to AIDS appears in Part II, "Syndromes," with separate chapters on Epidemiology (Chapter 106), Immunology (Chapter 107), Clinical Manifestations (Chapter 108), Detection of HIV Infections (Chapter 109), Therapy (Chapter 110), and Vaccines (Chapter 111). The chapter concerning Human Immunodeficiency Virus (HIV) (Chapter 147) appears in Part III, in the section on Retroviridae. Also in keeping with the organization of the book, the chapter on HIV in the health care setting (Chapter 283) appears in the section in Part IV dealing with nosocomial infections. Other sections of the book contain important information on AIDS. For example, the section on anti-infective therapy in Part I discusses antiviral agents versus HIV and drugs used to treat opportunistic infections. Specific organisms that opportunistically infect patients with AIDS are discussed in the relevant chapters of Part III.

REFERENCES

1. Gallo RC. HIV—the cause of AIDS: An overview on its biology, mechanisms of disease induction, and our attempts to control it. J Acquired Immune Deficiency Syn. 1988;1:521–35.
2. Ludmerer KM. Patients Beyond the Pale: Historical View. Fifth Conference on Health Policy, Cornell University Medical College. 1989;1:1–20.
3. Sigerist HE. Civilization and Disease. New York: Cornell University Press; 1943:112–7.
4. Loewy EH. Duties, fears and physicians. Social Sci Med. 1986;22:1364.
5. Zuger A, Miles SH. Physicians, AIDS, and occupational risk. JAMA. 1987;258:1924–5.
6. Ada GL. Prospects for HIV vaccines. J Acquired Immune Deficiency Syn. 1988;1:295–303.
7. Oberg B. Antiviral therapy. J Acquired Immune Deficiency Syn. 1988;1:257–66.

106. EPIDEMIOLOGY AND PREVENTION OF AIDS AND HIV INFECTION

MARY E. CHAMBERLAND
JAMES W. CURRAN

Acquired immunodeficiency syndrome (AIDS) is the most severe manifestation of a clinical spectrum of illness after infection with a retrovirus, human immunodeficiency virus (HIV).

The syndrome is defined by the development of serious opportunistic infections, neoplasms, or other life-threatening manifestations resulting from progressive HIV-induced immunosuppression. AIDS was first recognized in mid-1981 when unusual clusters of *Pneumocystis carinii* pneumonia and Kaposi sarcoma were reported in young, previously healthy homosexual men in New York City, Los Angeles, and San Francisco.[1,2] The subsequent documentation of cases among persons with hemophilia, blood transfusion recipients, and heterosexual iv drug abusers and their sex partners suggested that a transmissible agent was the primary cause of the immunologic defects characteristic of AIDS.[3] In 1983, more than 2 years after the first reports of AIDS, a cytopathic retrovirus was isolated from persons with AIDS and associated conditions such as chronic lymphadenopathy.[4–6]

SURVEILLANCE AND REPORTING OF AIDS

All 50 states require AIDS cases to be reported. Surveillance of AIDS cases has been ongoing in the United States since 1981. In 1981, before the etiology of AIDS was known and a specific diagnostic test was available, the Centers for Disease Control (CDC) developed a surveillance case definition.[7] The initial case definition included a limited number of specific opportunistic diseases diagnosed by reliable methods in patients with no other known causes of immunodeficiency. Although the surveillance definition excluded other less severe manifestations of illness, it was highly specific, uniformly interpreted, and permitted a consistent evaluation of trends of severe underlying immunodeficiency caused by what was then an unknown agent. The definition was adopted worldwide for surveillance of AIDS in all industrialized nations.

The discovery of HIV as the cause of AIDS and the subsequent development of serologic tests to detect HIV resulted in an increased appreciation of the spectrum of HIV-associated clinical and immunologic manifestations. In addition, a review of death certificates in 1985 in four cities showed that reported AIDS cases underestimated the actual incidence of AIDS-related deaths: 13 percent of deaths were attributed to *P. carinii* pneumonia, Kaposi sarcoma, and other opportunistic diseases that had been diagnosed without the recommended rigorous histologic or cultural techniques required to meet the surveillance definition.[8] To more completely and effectively monitor serious HIV-associated morbidity, the original case definition was modified in 1985 and again in September 1987.[9,10] The 1987 revision incorporated a broader range of AIDS-indicative diseases, most notably HIV encephalopathy and wasting syndrome; included patients whose indicator diseases were diagnosed presumptively, without confirmatory laboratory evidence of the opportunistic disease; and took advantage of the increasing use of HIV diagnostic tests to further improve the sensitivity and specificity of the definition (Table 1).

The impact of the 1987 revision on the reported number of AIDS cases will depend on the use and reporting of HIV antibody tests and employment of presumptive methods to diagnose the indicator diseases.[11] These factors are likely to vary with geographic location, hospital size, patients' socioeconomic status and/or method of payment, physicians' clinical experience, and availability of HIV testing. In the first 8 months after implementation of the September 1987 revised case definition, 17,969 AIDS cases were reported to the CDC, of which 2279 (13 percent) were diagnosed presumptively and 2944 (16 percent) involved indicator diseases (such as wasting syndrome or HIV encephalopathy) that met the revised criteria only. During this period, New York and California accounted for 45 percent of reported AIDS cases that met the pre-1987 case definition but only 24 percent of cases that met the 1987 revision. Cases reported in heterosexual iv drug abusers were more likely than those in exclusively homosexual or bisexual men to fulfill only 1987 criteria (44 vs 22 percent). A higher proportion of blacks (36 percent) and Hispanics (35 percent) than whites (24 percent) met the new definition categories of presumptive diagnoses, HIV encephalopathy, and HIV wasting syndrome.

TABLE 1. Revised Surveillance Case Definition for AIDS, Centers for Disease Control, September 1987

I. Indicator diseases diagnosed definitively in the absence of other causes of immunodeficiency and laboratory tests for HIV
   - Candidiasis of the esophagus, trachea, bronchi, or lungs
   - *Cryptococcus*, extrapulmonary
   - Cryptosporidiosis with diarrhea >1 mon
   - Cytomegalovirus disease exclusive of liver, spleen, or lymph nodes in patients >1 mon of age.
   - Herpes simplex virus infection causing a mucocutaneous ulcer >1 mon or bronchitis, pneumonitis, or esophagitis in patients >1 mon of age
   - Kaposi sarcoma in patients <60 yr of age
   - Lymphoma of the brain (primary) in patients <60 yr of age
   - Lymphoid interstitial pneumonia and/or pulmonary lymphoid hyperplasia in patients <13 yr of age
   - *Mycobacterium avium* complex or *M. kansasii* disease, disseminated
   - *Pneumocystis carinii* pneumonia
   - Progressive multifocal leukoencephalopathy
   - Toxoplasmosis of the brain in patients >1 mon of age

II. Indicator diseases diagnosed definitively regardless of other causes of immunodeficiency and laboratory evidence of HIV present
   - All indicator diseases listed in Section I
   - Bacterial infections, recurrent or multiple, in patients <13 yr of age that are caused by *Haemophilus*, *Streptococcus*, or other pyogenic bacteria
   - Coccidioidomycosis, disseminated
   - HIV encephalopathy
   - Histoplasmosis, disseminated
   - Isosporiasis with diarrhea >1 mon
   - Kaposi sarcoma at any age
   - Primary lymphoma of the brain at any age
   - Non-Hodgkin's lymphoma of B cell or unknown immunologic phenotype including small noncleaved lymphoma or immunoblastic sarcoma
   - Mycobacterial disease exclusive of *M. tuberculosis*, disseminated
   - *M. tuberculosis*, extrapulmonary
   - *Salmonella* septicemia, recurrent
   - HIV wasting syndrome

III. Indicator diseases diagnosed presumptively with laboratory evidence of HIV infection
   - Candidiasis, esophageal
   - Cytomegalovirus retinitis with loss of vision
   - Kaposi sarcoma
   - Lymphoid interstitial pneumonia and/or pulmonary lymphoid hyperplasia in patients <13 yr of age
   - Mycobacterial disease, disseminated
   - *Pneumocystis carinii* pneumonia
   - Toxoplasmosis, brain, in patients >1 mo of age

IV. Indicator diseases diagnosed definitively in the absence of other causes of immunodeficiency and negative laboratory tests results for HIV
   - *Pneumocystis carinii* pneumonia
   - Other indicator diseases listed in Section I and a T-helper/inducer (CD4) lymphocyte count <400/mm^3

Several studies have documented high levels of case reporting,[8,12,13] but the timeliness of reporting to state and local health departments and to the CDC has diminished somewhat, given the increasing number of case reports.[14] In 1987, the median and mean intervals between diagnosis and report were 2.9 and 4.8 months respectively, with 80 percent of cases reported within 6 months of diagnosis.

AIDS IN ADULTS

Incidence of AIDS in the United States

As of May 1988, 60,000 cases of AIDS in adults were reported in the United States. The number of cases has increased rapidly over time. The first 15,000 cases were reported over a 54-month period between June 1981 and November 1985. In contrast, the fourth quartile of 15,000 cases was reported over a 6-month period between November 1987 and May 1988. Based on an empirical mathematic model, 80,000 AIDS cases are projected to be diagnosed in 1992 alone, and the cumulative number of diagnosed cases is estimated to total 365,000 by the end of 1992

(Fig. 1).[15] These projections do not take into account AIDS cases that are never diagnosed or reported to the CDC and other HIV-related illnesses and deaths that do not meet the 1987 surveillance case definition. Factors that may alter the projected course of the epidemic include the development of effective therapeutic modalities and intervention and prevention efforts to reduce HIV transmission.

Transmission Groups

For surveillance purposes, AIDS cases are classified into a hierarchy of mutually exclusive risk or transmission groups (Table 2). Patients with more than one risk factor are ordered in the highest ranking transmission group. Of the first 60,000 reported cases, 13 percent of patients with AIDS had two or more reported risk factors for infection. The largest overlaps occurred in homosexual/bisexual men and iv drug abusers (4445 patients) and among heterosexual iv drug abusers and persons with heterosexual sex partners in risk groups (971 patients).

Since 1981, cases in homosexual and bisexual men have consistently represented the largest proportion (63 percent). However, the proportion of homosexual and bisexual men decreased from 66 percent of the third quartile of 15,000 cases (reported between February 1987 and October 1987) to 56 percent of the fourth quartile of cases (reported between November 1987 and May 1988). This declining trend was similar for homosexual and bisexual men who abused iv drugs as well. There has been a corresponding increase in the proportion of AIDS cases attributable to iv drug abuse by heterosexuals. When analyses are restricted to patients meeting only the pre-1987 case definition, there are no significant changes in the proportion of cases in homosexual men and iv drug abusers, which suggests that diagnostic and reporting practices involving the use of HIV antibody tests and presumptive diagnostic methods vary by transmission group and need to be considered when evaluating trend data.

The proportion of cases in persons with hemophilia or other coagulation disorders requiring iv administration of clotting factors has remained stable at 1 percent. Recipients of transfused blood or blood components account for 3 percent of all AIDS cases. While there has been a small but steady increase in the proportion of transfusion-associated cases, from 2 percent of the first quartile of 15,000 cases to 3 percent of the fourth quartile of cases, all but a few of these cases reflect transmission from blood products received before screening for HIV antibody was available.[16] Because of the long period from the date of transfusion to the development of AIDS, additional transfusion-associated cases will be diagnosed and reported.[17,18]

Heterosexual transmission cases comprise persons who report either specific heterosexual contact with a person with or at increased risk for HIV infection or persons who were born in areas such as Haiti or central Africa where heterosexual transmission is a major route of HIV infection. Of the 2468 persons in the heterosexual transmission category, 1464 (59 percent) reported contact with a specific at-risk partner, and 1004 (41 percent) were born in Haiti or central Africa. While the overall proportion of heterosexually acquired AIDS cases has remained constant at 4 percent, there has been a striking change in the composition of this group over time. Of the 594 heterosexual transmission cases reported between June 1981 and November 1985 in the first quartile of 15,000 cases, 378 (64 percent) were in persons of Haitian or central African origin. In contrast, only 208 (31 percent) of the 668 heterosexual transmission cases in the fourth quartile were in persons from Haiti or central-Africa. The decline in cases among Haitians may reflect a concomitant decline in immigration to the United States.[19] The vast majority of Haitians in the United States immigrated before 1978. However, 75,000–150,000 additional Haitians entered the United States between 1978 and 1981. Since 1981, immigration has declined to the pre-1978 rate of 6,000–9,000 persons per year. Most AIDS cases in Haitians in the United States have occurred in relatively recent immigrants, thus suggesting that

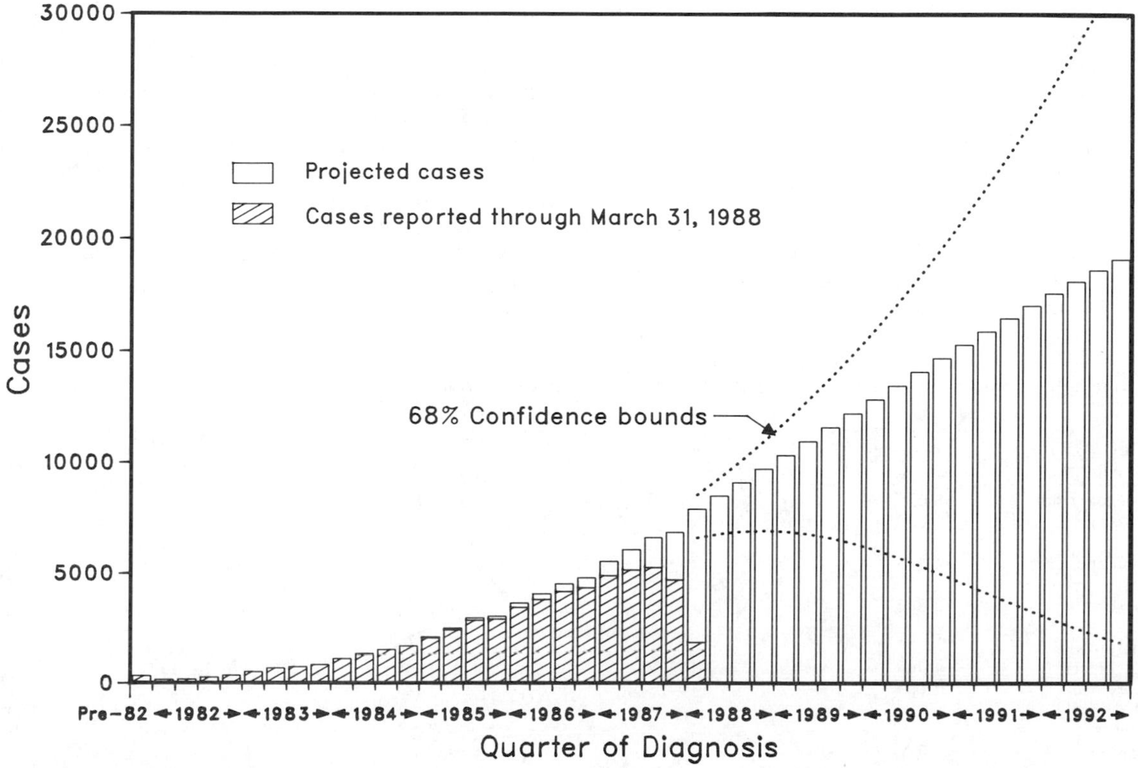

FIG. 1. Reported and projected incidence of AIDS in the United States by quarter year of diagnosis through 1992. The projections are based on a statistical extrapolation from cases reported to the CDC through March 1988 and diagnosed through June 1987.

TABLE 2. Distribution of Adults with AIDS by Transmission Group for Each Quartile of 15,000 Reported Cases[a]

	Reported Cases (%)				
Transmission Group	*First 15,000*	*Second 15,000*	*Third 15,000*	*Fourth 15,000*	*Total*
Homosexual/bisexual man	65	66	66	56	63
Heterosexual iv drug abuser	18	17	15	24	19
Homosexual man and iv drug abuser	8	8	8	7	7
Hemophilia/coagulation disorder	1	1	1	1	1
Heterosexual transmission					
Heterosexual contact	1	2	3	3	2
Born in country with high incidence of heterosexual transmission	3	2	1	1	2
Transfusion recipient	2	2	3	3	3
Undetermined	2	2	3	5	3

[a] The first quartile of 15,000 cases was reported between June 1981 and November 1985, the second 15,000 between December 1985 and January 1987, the third 15,000 between February 1987 and October 1987, and the fourth 15,000 between November 1987 and May 1988.

HIV infection was acquired before leaving Haiti and that AIDS was relatively uncommon in Haiti until the late 1970s.[19,20] Studies of Haitians with AIDS have shown that most are heterosexual men and women often with a history of sexually transmitted diseases (STDs), sexual contact with female prostitutes, or multiple heterosexual partners—findings that suggest acquisition of HIV through heterosexual contact.[20,21]

The index partners for 70 percent of patients with heterosexually acquired AIDS (exclusive of persons born in Haiti or central Africa) are iv drug abusers. In addition, 12 percent of the partners are bisexual men (female patients only), 3 percent were born in Haiti or central Africa, and 3 percent have received blood or blood components; for 12 percent the risk of the partner is unreported or under investigation.

Overall, 3 percent of all AIDS cases have no risk factor reported and are classified as undetermined. When follow-up information is available, risk factors can be identified for over 70 percent of these patients, and they are reclassified into the appropriate transmission categories.[22] As of May 1988, 1880 patients were classified in the undetermined category: 16 percent could not be reclassified after follow-up investigation; 20 percent had died, refused to be interviewed, or were lost to follow-up; and 64 percent were still under investigation. The proportion of AIDS patients with undertermined risk has increased from 2 percent of the first 15,000 cases to 5 percent of the most recently reported 15,000 cases. However, 92 percent of the cases reported in the last quartile are still under investigation; other risk factors for HIV infection will be identified for most of these persons when investigations have been completed, thus lowering this proportion.[22] The race/ethnicity and gender of AIDS patients with an undetermined risk are demographically distinctive within the U.S. population (Table 3), which suggests that they probably represent a mixture of persons who either have risk factors that they are unwilling to report or are sex partners of persons in risk groups.[22–25] The possibility of infection through heterosexual contact can be inferred from follow-up investigations of patients with undetermined risk: nearly 40 percent report a history of STDs, and one-third of interviewed men give a history of heterosexual contact with a prostitute.[22]

Demographic Characteristics

Eighty-nine percent of adults with AIDS are 20–49 years of age; only 10 percent are older than 49 years. Transfusion recipients have the highest mean and median ages (53.9 and 58.0 years, respectively), similar to that of all recipients of blood transfusions in the United States (Table 3).

Overall, 59 percent of reported AIDS cases are in white persons, 26 percent in blacks, and 14 percent in Hispanics (Table 3). The racial/ethnic group distribution of AIDS patients has been affected by the 1987 revision of the case definition: the proportion of cases in whites decreased from 63 percent of the third quartile of 15,000 cases to 54 percent of the fourth quartile of cases. The proportion of cases among blacks and Hispanics increased commensurately during this period from 36 to 45 percent. This is consistent with the observed change in the proportion of cases among homosexual and bisexual men and iv drug abusers. Blacks and Hispanics have higher relative risks of AIDS than do whites (defined as the ratio of the number of cases per million population of blacks or Hispanics to the number of cases per million population of whites) in all transmission categories except hemophilia and associated coagulation disorders in which the relative risk for black men is 0.5[26,27] Black

TABLE 3. Demographic Characteristics of the First 60,000 Adults with AIDS Reported in the United States, by Transmission Group

		Age at Diagnosis (yrs)		Sex (%)		Race/Ethnicity (%)			
Transmission Group	*No. Cases*	*Mean*	*Range*	*Male*	*Female*	*White*	*Black*	*Hispanic*	*Other*
Homosexual/bisexual man	38,055	37.1	13–80	100	0	74	15	10	1
Heterosexual iv drug abuser	11,086	35.3	15–72	78	22	19	51	29	1
Homosexual man and iv drug abuser	4,445	34.0	15–75	100	0	62	24	13	1
Hemophilia/coagulation disorder	588	35.7	13–86	96	4	85	6	7	2
Heterosexual transmission									
Heterosexual contact	1,464	34.9	15–78	22	78	29	48	22	1
Born in country with high incidence of heterosexual transmission	1,004	33.2	16–73	78	22	<1	99	1	0
Transfusion recipient	1,478	53.9	13–90	65	35	74	15	8	3
Undetermined	1,880	39.9	17–85	79	21	37	40	21	2
Total	60,000	36.9	13–90	92	8	59	26	14	1
U.S. population				49	52	80	12	6	2

women are 13.4 times and Hispanic women 9.5 times more likely than are white women to have AIDS. The disproportionate incidence rates of AIDS among black and Hispanic women as compared with white women are most striking for those who report iv drug abuse (18.9 and 10.0 times greater than whites, respectively) or heterosexual contact with a male iv drug abuser (20.2 and 20.5 times greater). The risk of AIDS in exclusively homosexual men without a history of iv drug abuse is 1.4 and 1.8 times greater in black and Hispanic men, respectively, than in white men. For bisexual men with AIDS, the relative risks are higher (3.9 and 2.9 in blacks and Hispanics, respectively). In contrast, heterosexual black and Hispanic men who report iv drug abuse are each 20 times more likely than white heterosexual men are to have AIDS.

Men account for 92 percent of all AIDS cases, which reflects the large number of cases in homosexual and bisexual men and male iv drug abusers (Table 3). However, there has been a small but significant increase from 1981 to 1988 in the proportion of women with AIDS, from 7 percent of the first 15,000 reported cases to 10 percent of the most recent 15,000 cases reported. Heterosexual contact is the only transmission group with a predominance of women. The smaller number of men with heterosexually acquired AIDS is undoubtedly partly due to the much smaller reservoir of infection in women and the possible lower efficiency of female-to-male transmission.[28,29]

Geographic Distribution of Cases

The first reports of AIDS were clustered among homosexual men and iv drug abusers residing in major metropolitan areas on the east and west coasts.[30] Since then, cases of AIDS have been reported from all 50 states, the District of Columbia, Puerto Rico, the Virgin Islands, and Guam. Although five states—New York, California, Florida, Texas, and New Jersey—have reported most cases (68 percent), there has been a steady decrease in the proportion of cases from these states from 75 percent of the first quartile of 15,000 cases to 63 percent of the fourth quartile. This trend is primarily due to the more rapid increase in the number of cases reported from the remaining 45 states. In general, the cumulative reported incidence of AIDS by state roughly parallels the prevalence of HIV infection in military recruits, with the sex-adjusted prevalence of HIV in recruit applicants through March 1988 3–10 times higher than the cumulative incidence of reported AIDS (Fig. 2).

The distribution of cases by state of residence varies among the transmission groups. Nearly half the AIDS cases in homosexual or bisexual men have been reported from California and New York. Sixty-seven percent of cases in heterosexual iv drug abusers have been reported from New Jersey and New York; in contrast these two states account for 32 percent of AIDS cases overall. Most patients who acquired AIDS through heterosexual contact with an iv drug abuser also have been from New York and New Jersey. Florida and New York account for three-fourths of heterosexually acquired AIDS cases in persons born outside the United States, primarily in Haiti. AIDS patients with hemophilia or who received transfusions are distributed throughout the United States. These geographic patterns reflect the rapidity and magnitude of the introduction of HIV into various susceptible populations.

Opportunistic Diseases

The most frequently reported opportunistic disease among adults with AIDS is *P. carinii* pneumonia (62 percent) followed by Kaposi sarcoma (17 percent), esophageal or bronchial candidiasis (15 percent), extrapulmonary cryptococcosis (7 percent), disseminated *Mycobacterium avium* complex (5 percent), cytomegalovirus disease (5 percent), HIV wasting syndrome (4 percent), herpes simplex (4 percent), toxoplasmosis of the brain (4 percent), chronic cryptosporidiosis (3 percent), HIV encephalopathy (2 percent), non-Hodgkin's lymphoma (2 percent), extrapulmonary tuberculosis (1 percent), and other disseminated mycobacterial diseases (1 percent). Other opportunistic infections or cancers that have been reported in fewer than 1 percent of all AIDS patient are disseminated histoplasmosis, cytomegalovirus retinitis, progressive multifocal leukoencephalopathy, primary lymphoma of the brain, recurrent *Salmonella* septicemia, chronic isosporiasis, and disseminated coccidioidomycosis. The reported frequency of each of these opportunistic diseases represents a minimum estimate of the actual incidence among AIDS patients since there is substantial underreporting of opportunistic diseases diagnosed after the initial case report to the CDC. For example, only 5 percent of AIDS patients reported to the CDC have a diagnosis of disseminated *M. avium* complex; in contrast, in one series of 71 AIDS patients, 24 (34 percent) developed infection secondary to *M. avium* complex at some point in the course of their illness.[31]

P. carinii pneumonia is the most commonly reported opportunistic infection overall and for every transmission group (Table 4). When analyzed by year of diagnosis, the percentage of AIDS patients initially presenting with *P. carinii* pneumonia has increased from 31 percent in 1981 to 72 percent in 1988. The reason for this increase is unknown but does not appear to be related to changes in the distribution of cases by transmission group, race/ethnicity, geographic location, or the use of presumptive diagnostic measures.[32]

One of the strongest associations between a particular disease and the various transmission categories is the high frequency of Kaposi sarcoma in homosexual and bisexual men. Kaposi sarcoma accounts for nearly eight times the proportion of cases reported in homosexual and bisexual men when compared with heterosexual iv drug abusers. In heterosexuals, Kaposi sarcoma is most frequently reported for persons born in other countries (predominantly Haitians) and persons classified in the undetermined group. The reason for the relatively higher frequency of Kaposi sarcoma in homosexual men is unknown. The use of nitrite inhalants by homosexual men has been proposed as a possible cofactor in the development of Kaposi sarcoma. While nitrites may have some immunosuppressive effects that theoretically could result in increased susceptibility to infection or malignancy,[33,34] nitrite use has been inconsistently associated with Kaposi sarcoma and HIV infection in homosexual men.[35–40] Similarly, cytomegalovirus has also been suggested as a cofactor in the etiology of Kaposi sarcoma.[41–43] While many homosexual men have serologic evidence of cytomegalovirus infection, not all develop Kaposi sarcoma. In addition, a cohort study of HIV-infected homosexual men demonstrated no association between Kaposi sarcoma and elevated cytomegalovirus antibody titer.[44] When analyzed by year of diagnosis, the percentage of AIDS patients initially presenting with Kaposi sarcoma has decreased from 28 percent in 1981 to 9 percent in 1988. This decline was observed in every transmission group with the exception of heterosexual contact cases (exclusive of persons born in Haiti or Central Africa) and transfusion-associated cases. Studies in San Francisco suggest that the decline in Kaposi sarcoma is not secondary to diagnostic bias or selective underreporting of Kaposi sarcoma.[45] The proportional decrease in new cases of AIDS with Kaposi sarcoma suggests the possibility of a concomitant decrease in exposure to a cofactor necessary for the development of Kaposi sarcoma. However, none of several cofactors evaluated in a cohort of homosexual men in San Francisco were associated with the diagnosis of Kaposi sarcoma, including a history of STDs, enteric infections, iv drug use, and specific sexual practices.[45]

Since many HIV-associated infections result from the endogenous reactivation of previously acquired pathogens,[46,47] geographic residence and the associated higher prevalence of asymptomatic infection with certain pathogens influences the frequency of reported opportunistic infections. For example,

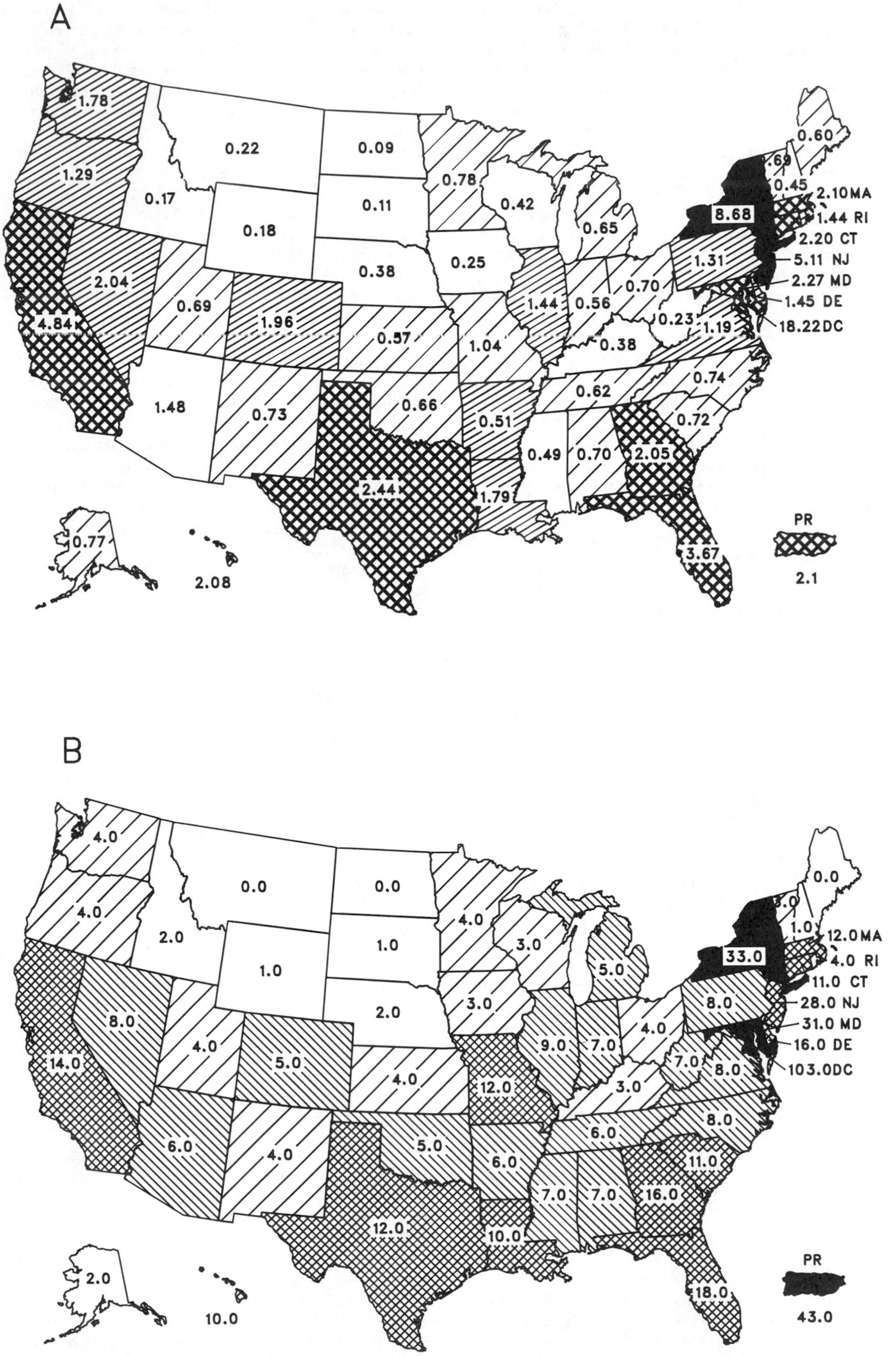

Source: Department of Defense

FIG. 2. **(A)** Reported cumulative incidence rates of AIDS as of May 1988, and **(B)** HIV seroprevalence rates in U.S. military recruit applicants, by state, from November 1985 through March 1988. Rates are per 10,000 population; military recruit applicant data are sex adjusted.

TABLE 4. Distribution of Selected Opportunistic Diseases by Transmission Group for the First 60,000 Adults with AIDS, United States

		Opportunistic Disease (%)[a]									
Transmission Group	*No. Cases*	Pneumocystis carinii *Pneumonia*	*Kaposi Sarcoma*	*Esophageal or Bronchial Candidiasis*	*Extrapulmonary Cryptococcosis*	*Disseminated* Mycobacterium avium	*Cytomegalovirus disease*	*Herpes Simplex*	*Cryptosporidiosis*	*Toxoplasmosis*	*Extrapulmonary Tuberculosis*
Homosexual/bisexual man	38,055	63	23	12	6	5	5	4	3	3	1
Heterosexual iv drug abuser	11,086	60	3	19	9	4	2	3	1	5	2
Homosexual man and iv drug abuser	4,445	59	20	16	8	6	5	5	3	4	2
Hemophilia/ coagulation disorder	588	62	1	23	9	5	4	2	3	3	1
Heterosexual transmission											
Heterosexual contact	1,464	69	2	19	6	4	4	5	3	4	2
Born in country with high incidence of heterosexual transmission	1,004	44	7	19	11	3	4	5	4	15	8
Transfusion recipient	1,478	63	3	24	7	4	6	3	2	4	1
Undetermined	1,880	64	7	17	8	4	5	4	3	5	2

[a] Row percentages may total more than 100 percent because some patients had more than one disease.

the proportion of Haitian-born adults with AIDS and toxoplasmosis and disseminated tuberculosis is five and six times higher, respectively, than in non-Haitian-born adults. Similarly, disseminated histoplasmosis is diagnosed and reported more frequently in AIDS patients residing in the Mississippi valley states, while disseminated coccidioidomycosis is more common among AIDS patients residing in Arizona than in all other states.[32]

Several reports have noted a significant increase in tuberculosis associated with HIV infection.[48–50] In New York City, AIDS patients with and without tuberculosis were similiar in median age at AIDS diagnosis (34 compared with 36 years) and in sex (predominantly male).[50] However, AIDS patients with tuberculosis were more likely to be non-Haitian black, Haitian, Hispanic, and iv drug abusers than AIDS patients without tuberculosis.

Mortality of Patients with AIDS

Fifty-nine percent of the first 60,000 patients with AIDS are reported to have died. Reported fatalities increase as time from diagnosis of AIDS increases, with 31 percent of patients reported to have died within 1 year of diagnosis and 56 and 76 percent reported to have died 2 and 3 years, respectively, after diagnosis. However, reporting of deaths is known to be incomplete. In one study, when intensive follow-up was undertaken of 147 persons with AIDS who were not reported to have died after 3 years, 31 percent had died, 30 percent were lost to follow-up, and 39 percent were alive.[51] Factors that may influence survival include type of opportunistic disease at diagnosis, age, race/ethnicity, sex, mode of HIV transmission, and specific antiviral therapy (e.g., zidovudine [AZT]). Longer survival has been consistently associated with the diagnosis of Kaposi sarcoma.[51–55] Reported median survival times for patients with only Kaposi sarcoma range from 11 to 25 months as compared with 7–13 months for patients with Kaposi sarcoma and other opportunistic infections and 7–13 months for persons with opportunistic infections but not Kaposi sarcoma.[52–55] In patients with Kaposi sarcoma, younger age at diagnosis, no other opportunistic diseases, and earlier stages of clinical illness, as manifested by immunologic parameters, have been correlated with a more favorable prognosis.[51–56]

One measure of the impact of premature mortality is the years of potential life lost before the age of 65 (YPLL). This measure emphasizes deaths of children and young adults, whereas crude mortality statistics represent all deaths, which largely occur among the elderly. The leading causes of YPLL have changed only minimally from 1979 to 1986, except for AIDS. Fewer than five AIDS deaths were retrospectively identified in 1979, but by 1986 AIDS had become the eighth leading cause of YPLL in the United States.[57] The impact of AIDS on patterns of premature death is particularly important in areas such as New York City and San Francisco where AIDS has been the leading cause of YPLL for single men aged 25–44 since 1984.[58] AIDS is the leading cause of death for men aged 30–39 years and for women aged 25–29 years in New York City.[59,60] In New York City, mortality rates secondary to AIDS differ significantly by race/ethnicity: for black and Hispanic men, mortality rates as compared with white males are 1.6 and 1.5 times higher, respectively.[59] Black and Hispanic women have mortality rates 6.0 and 5.2 times higher than white women do.

AIDS IN CHILDREN

Less than 1½ years after AIDS was first recognized in adults the first cases of unexplained immunodeficiency were reported in children.[61–64] For national reporting, pediatric cases of AIDS include children less than 13 years of age who have an illness characterized by essentially the same range of "indicator" diseases as adults with AIDS (Table 1). Two important exceptions are the inclusion of recurrent bacterial infections and lymphoid interstitial pneumonia and/or pulmonary lymphoid hyperplasia (LIP/PLH complex) affecting a child less than 13 years of age. Toxoplasmosis, herpes simplex virus infection, and cytomegalovirus disease must be diagnosed after 1 month of age.

As of May 1988, the first 1000 cases of AIDS in children were reported in the United States. The date of initial infection with HIV can be estimated for most children as either the year of birth for those with perinatally acquired infection or the year of transfusion for those who acquired HIV through blood transfusions. For perinatally acquired cases, the earliest year of birth is 1977; the first reported transfusion of blood that transmitted HIV to a child was administered in 1977 (Fig. 3).

Children born to mothers known to be infected with HIV or at increased risk for infection account for approximately three-quarters of reported cases. Of these mothers 72 percent were iv drug abusers or had sexual contact with an iv drug abuser, 19 percent acquired their infection through heterosexual contact with infected men other than iv drug abusers, 3 percent had a history of a blood transfusion, and 6 percent had AIDS or infection with HIV, but the specific route of transmission was unreported. Risk factors for the remaining children include receipt of transfusion (14 percent) and hemophilia (6 percent); 4 percent had an undetermined risk. When follow-up information is available, most children who are initially reported with an undetermined risk are reclassified; in one study, half of those reclassified had mothers who used iv drugs or were partners of men who used iv drugs.[65]

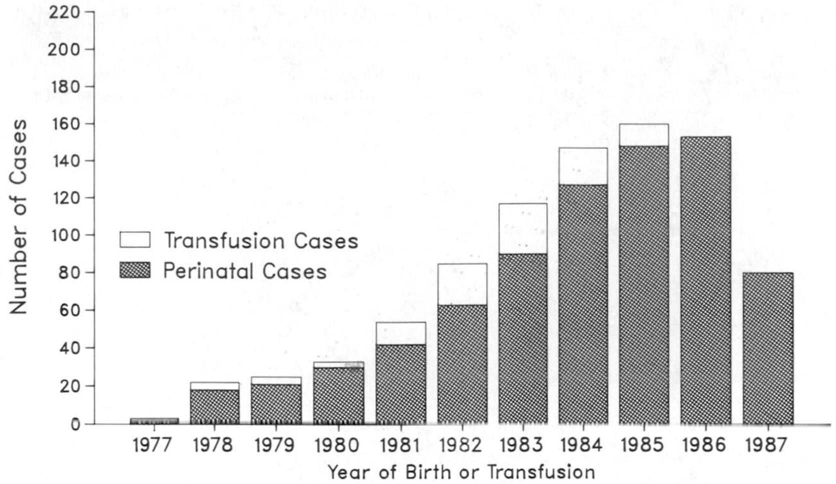

FIG. 3. Children in the United States with AIDS reported through May 1988 by year of birth for perinatally acquired cases and by year of transfusion for transfusion-acquired cases.

Most reported cases of AIDS in children are initially diagnosed at less than 2 years of age (64 percent), with 24 percent less than 6 months of age; only 11 percent are older than 5 years. Children with hemophilia have the highest mean and median ages (8.7 and 9.1 years, respectively).

The demographic characteristics of children with AIDS are very similar to those of heterosexual adult patients with AIDS: 53 percent are black, 22 percent are Hispanic and 23 percent are white. The cumulative incidence rates in black and Hispanic children are 11.2 and 7.4 times the rate for white children, with the highest rates of AIDS reported for transmission categories associated with iv drug abuse. For children whose mothers are iv drug abusers, the rates for blacks and Hispanics are 24.3 and 17.0 times greater than that for whites, respectively, and for children whose mothers have sex partners who are iv drug abusers, 17.2 and 17.9 times greater, respectively. The racial/ethnic distribution of children with AIDS varies by transmission group: of the 771 children who acquired AIDS perinatally, 84 percent were black or Hispanic as compared with 43 percent of 135 children with transfusion-associated AIDS and 23 percent of children with hemophilia. The racial/ethnic distribution of children with an undetermined risk is nearly identical to that of children with perinatally acquired infection.

There is an equal distribution by sex for perinatal cases and cases with an undetermined risk. Males are overrepresented in hemophilic children (95 percent) and transfusion recipients (62 percent). The sex distribution of transfusion-acquired cases is similar to that of all transfused infants in the United States in that more male than female infants receive transfusions.[66]

AIDS in children has been reported from 40 states, the District of Columbia, and Puerto Rico. Four states—New York, California, Florida, and New Jersey—have reported most of the cases (64 percent). However, there has been an increase in the proportion of children with AIDS residing in states other than these four, from 27 percent of the first 250 cases (which were reported over a 3-year period) to 41 percent of the most recent 250 cases (reported over a 6-month period). The geographic distribution of perinatally acquired cases is similar to that for women with AIDS in that 69 percent were reported from New York, New Jersey, Florida, and California as compared with 44 percent of the transfusion-acquired cases and 33 percent of hemophilia-associated cases in children.

Overall, 59 percent of children with AIDS are reported to have died. However, reported death rates vary significantly by age: 71 percent of infants younger than 1 year at diagnosis are reported to have died as compared with 51 percent of children older than 1 year. Similar to adult AIDS cases, mortality data are underreported in children with AIDS; actual fatality rates for reported cases are undoubtedly much higher. The length of survival is likely influenced by age at diagnosis and by type of opportunistic disease at initial presentation. The reported median survival time for infants (4.0 months) is significantly less than for children older than 1 year (11.2 months). Children with *P. carinii* pneumonia have been reported to have shorter survival times, while children with lymphocytic interstitial pneumonitis have been reported to live longer.[67]

MODES OF TRANSMISSION

HIV is transmitted almost exclusively through sexual contact, parenteral exposure to blood or blood products, and perinatally from infected mothers to their infants.

Sexual Transmission

Sexual transmission is the predominant mode of HIV transmission throughout the world. In general, the risk of acquiring HIV infection through a single sexual contact depends on several factors including specific sex practices, the infectivity of the source partner, the susceptibility of the recipient partner, and possibly the viral strain.[68] As the prevalence of infection in the population increases, the likelihood of encountering an infected partner also increases.

Homosexual and bisexual men, the population in the United States in whom AIDS was first recognized, have continued to account for most U.S. AIDS cases. Multiple epidemiologic studies have identified specific risk factors associated with HIV infection in homosexual men, including increased number of sex partners, receptive anal intercourse, and other practices associated with rectal trauma such as "fisting" and douching.[35–39,69–72] While no sexual activities involving exposure to semen or blood have been shown to be without risk, the precise risk of specific sexual activities, such as fellatio, is difficult to ascertain because most homosexual men report engaging in multiple sex practices. Nonetheless, several reports suggest that the risks of HIV transmission that are associated with insertive anal intercourse and oral intercourse are less than that associated with receptive anal intercourse.[38,39,71–74]

Two instances of female-to-female transmission of HIV have been reported after traumatic sex practices.[75,76]

Bidirectional heterosexual transmission of HIV infection is well documented, but the relative efficiency of male-to-female as compared with female-to-male transmission is not clearly established.[77–85] The approximate 1:1 sex ratio of cases in Africa has been cited as evidence of equal bidirectional efficiency. Actually, the male-to-female ratio of AIDS and HIV infection in many African areas varies by age, e.g., in Kinshasa, Zaire, for persons 20–29 years, the male-to-female ratio of AIDS case rates is 1:2.7; for those 30–39 years, 1.3:1; and for those 40–49 years, 4.2:1.[86,87] These sex and age distributions are similar to other STDs both in industrialized and developing countries where disease incidence and associated morbidity are higher among younger women. Other factors related to HIV infection and transmission among heterosexuals of African or Haitian descent include high rates of concurrent STDs, particularly those causing genital ulceration, large numbers of different heterosexual partners, and to a lesser extent, the possibility of parenteral exposures to contaminated needles.[20,21,85–90]

The highest reported rates of heterosexual transmission of HIV have been reported for the partners of infected iv drug abusers and persons born in Haiti or central Africa, although the duration of unprotected sexual contact has not been adequately controlled for in all studies.[14] The difference in these rates may reflect biologic factors such as concurrent infections in either the index patient or the partner, behavioral factors such as unreported drug abuse by the partner, or varying levels of infectivity in the source patient over the course of infection. Epidemiologic and laboratory data suggest that infectivity may be related to the source partner's clinical stage of infection. In a prospective study of infected hemophilic men and their female sex partners, transmission of HIV was associated with the development of severe immunodeficiency in the men, as manifested by very low numbers of T4 cells.[91] This is consistent with the observation that the ability to isolate HIV in vitro significantly increases as the number of T-helper cells declines and the clinical course advances.[92]

Most heterosexual transmission of HIV occurs through penile–vaginal contact, but in two studies receptive anal intercourse was associated with an increased risk of transmission between heterosexual partners.[82,93] Transmission of HIV has been reported after a single heterosexual contact,[84] but other studies have reported no evidence of heterosexual transmission even after hundreds of contacts.[77,80–84]

Case–control studies of homosexual men have documented an association between HIV infection and STDs such as syphilis, gonorrhea, and genital herpes.[35,36,38,39,70,72] STDs reflect, in part, a sexually active life-style that usually includes large numbers of sex partners. In addition, STDs may play a direct role in facilitating HIV transmission by disrupting genital epithelium. Additional studies of homosexual men show an association between syphilis and herpes simplex virus type 2 and HIV infection that is independent of the number of partners and specific sex practices.[94,95] Similarly, genital ulcer disease, particularly chancroid, has been associated with HIV infection in both heterosexual men and female prostitutes in Kenya.[88,90,96–98] Given these data, the recent increases in primary and secondary syphilis and chancroid in heterosexual men and women in the United States are of concern.[99]

Parenteral Exposure to Blood or Blood Products

Among iv drug abusers, HIV is transmitted by parenteral exposure to HIV-contaminated needles and other equipment used for injection. Specific risk factors that have been associated with HIV seropositivity include duration of iv drug use since 1978, needle sharing, number of persons with whom needles are shared, number of injections, median number of injections in "shooting galleries," and residence in an area with a high prevalence of HIV infection.[100–102]

AIDS in persons with hemophilia and recipients of transfusions has clearly implicated blood as a major vehicle of HIV transmission. Whole blood, blood cellular components, plasma, and clotting factors have transmitted HIV.[103,104] Several epidemiologic and laboratory studies have shown that recipients of other products prepared from blood or plasma including hepatitis B immune globulin, immune serum globulin, $Rh_o(D)$ immune globulin, and hepatitis B vaccine have not developed serologic evidence of HIV infection.[105–107] These products are prepared by using one of several fractionation processes that are effective in removing and inactivating HIV.[108]

The likelihood of becoming infected with HIV after receiving a single-donor blood product documented to be HIV-seropositive approaches 100 percent.[109] Investigation of donors of blood given to patients who later developed AIDS has often identified a donor infected with HIV and/or at high risk for AIDS.[103,110] Because many donors are asymptomatic at donation, effective screening of blood for transfusion depends on the use of serologic tests to detect HIV antibody. It has been estimated that between 1978 and 1984, before the implementation of HIV antibody testing of donated blood, as many as 29,000 transfusion recipients in the United States received a unit of blood infected with HIV and that approximately 12,000 are still alive.[18] Serologic screening of blood for HIV and donor deferral procedures have vastly reduced transmission of HIV by transfusion. The rare exception is recently infected donors who have not yet developed detectable HIV antibody. The rate of such transmission by HIV-seronegative blood has been estimated to be 26 per 1 million transfusions in the United States.[16]

The risk of HIV infection for patients with hemophilia who receive concentrated clotting factors composed of blood components from potentially thousands of donors was substantial before 1984–1985.[111] This risk has been reduced to a very low level with the implementation of heat treatment of clotting factor concentrates, HIV antibody testing of donated blood, and donor deferral procedures.[112]

Transmission of HIV has also been linked to recipients of organs, tissues, and semen from donors at increased risk for or documented to have HIV infection.[113–115] The U.S. Public Health Service has recommended that potential donors of organs, tissues, or semen be screened for HIV antibody and that organs from HIV-seropositive donors not be used for transplantation except under extremely unusual circumstances and with informed consent.[114,116]

Parenteral, nonintact skin, and mucous membrane exposures to blood have infrequently resulted in occupationally acquired HIV infections in health care workers.[117] Data from several prospective surveillance projects of health care workers indicate that the risk of seroconversion after needlestick exposures to blood from HIV-infected patients is less than 1 percent and that the level of risk associated with the exposure of nonintact skin or mucous membranes is far less.[117–120] In one study, 179 health care workers reported 2703 cutaneous exposures to HIV-infected blood; none of these workers became infected with HIV.[121] The increasing number of persons being treated for HIV-associated illnesses makes it likely that more health care workers will encounter patients and laboratory specimens infected with HIV. The risk of transmission can be minimized if health care workers adhere to published recommendations and use universal precautions when caring for all patients.[122–124]

Perinatal Transmission

HIV can be transmitted from an infected woman to her fetus or newborn in the following ways: antepartum through the maternal circulation, during delivery through exposure to blood or other infected fluids, and postpartum through breast-feeding. The occurrence of intrauterine infection is supported by the detection of HIV in fetal tissues[125,126] and the isolation of HIV from cord blood.[127] The isolation of HIV from breast milk[128] as well as several case reports of breast-feeding mothers who became infected after delivery and subsequently transmitted HIV to their infants indicate that breast-feeding can transmit HIV.[129–131]

Precise estimates of the frequency of perinatal transmission are lacking because of the unavailability of a reliable method to detect HIV infection in newborn infants. Prospective studies indicate perinatal transmission rates ranging from 23 to 45 percent.[132–136] Preliminary data suggest that the risk of perinatal transmission increases with the progression of HIV-associated immunosuppression and disease in the mother.[127,137]

Other Modes of Transmission

Sexual contact, exposure to blood, and perinatal transmission are the major modes of HIV infection, but there is concern that alternate, albeit rare, modes of transmission exist.[138,139] HIV has been isolated from blood,[4–6] semen,[140] vaginal secretions,[141,142] the uterine cervix,[143] saliva,[144–146] breast milk,[128] tears,[147] urine,[146] cerebrospinal fluid,[146,148] alveolar fluid,[149] and amniotic fluid.[150] However, isolation of virus from a body fluid does not necessarily implicate that body fluid as an important source of infection. For example, although virus has been isolated from saliva, it is recovered much less frequently from saliva than from blood.[145,146] Additionally, in vitro laboratory data indicate that both whole saliva and saliva filtrates contain components that inactivate HIV.[151] Contact with HIV-contaminated saliva has occurred through human bites and in the health care setting. A case report of two siblings infected with HIV suggested a bite as the route of transmission for the previously uninfected sibling.[152] Because the bite did not break the skin or result in bleeding, the precise mode of transmission remains unclear. Fifteen other persons have been reported who did not become infected with HIV after a human bite from a person known to be infected with HIV.[153,154] More than 100 health care workers have been followed prospectively after parenteral, mucous membrane, or nonintact skin exposure to the saliva of HIV-infected persons, and none have become infected with HIV.[117–121] Over 1800 dental professionals have been evaluated in other studies, and only one dentist without a history of behavioral risk factors for AIDS was HIV-seropositive.[155–157] The infected dentist reported several needlestick injuries and trauma to his hands and did not routinely wear gloves when providing dental care; whether saliva or blood was the mode of transmission cannot be determined.[155] Thus, epidemiologic evidence has not conclusively documented transmission of HIV by saliva and suggests that the risk of HIV infection after such extensive exposure to saliva, if present at all, is extremely low.[139]

To examine the risk of HIV transmission through casual contact, more than 700 nonsexual household contacts of both adults and children with HIV infection have been evaluated.[78,80,81,84,138,139,158–160] Many of these household members shared bathroom and kitchen facilities including toilets, baths, and eating utensils with the AIDS patient. In addition, close personal interaction frequently occurred, including hugging and kissing on the cheek and lips. No transmission of HIV has been documented exclusive of sex partners, children both to infected mothers, and persons who themselves had risk factors for AIDS.

Laboratory and epidemiologic studies have failed to demonstrate either replication of HIV within insects or transmission of HIV through biting or bloodsucking insects.[161,162] The role of insect-mediated HIV infection was evaluated in a case–control study of residents in Belle Glade, Florida; HIV infection was not associated with either epidemiologic or laboratory evidence of exposure to mosquitoes, as measured by the presence of antibodies to five arboviruses.[163] Furthermore, HIV infection was not detected in any adults older than 60 years or in children aged 2–10 years. The high rate of HIV infection in this community appears to be the result of transmission through sexual contact and iv drug abuse and not insect vectors. Additional studies in Haiti and Africa have failed to establish an association between the presence of dengue or malaria antibodies and HIV.[164,165]

HIV INFECTION OTHER THAN AIDS

Spectrum and Progression of HIV Infection

Patients infected with HIV may present with a spectrum of clinical manifestations ranging from asymptomatic infection to severe immunodeficiency associated with serious secondary infections, neoplasms, and other conditions.[165a]

Various systems have been proposed to classify the manifestations of HIV infection in both children and adults (Tables 5 and 6).[166–169] Staging criteria generally include serologic evidence of HIV infection; the presence or absence of clinical signs and symptoms of disease; and various immunologic parameters such as T-helper (T4) lymphopenia, decreased T-helper/T-suppressor (T4/T8) ratio, and evidence of cutaneous anergy. These systems have both clinical and public health applications including disease surveillance and reporting, design and analysis of epidemiologic studies, development and implementation of prevention and control strategies, formulation of health policy and strategy, and facilitation of scientific communication regarding HIV infection.[170]

An acute, mononucleosis-like illness has been described in association with initial infection with the virus.[171–172a] Features of this illness include fever, lymphadenopathy, sweats, myalgia, arthralgia, rash, malaise, lethargy, sore throat, anorexia, nausea, vomiting, headaches, photophobia, and diarrhea. *Candida* esophagitis during the acute retroviral illness has also been reported.[173] The rate of symptomatic primary HIV infection is difficult to determine because symptoms tend to be nonspecific, may cause little discomfort, pass largely unnoticed by the patient, and are often assessed retrospectively. For example, of 54 HIV-infected transfusion recipients, only 13 (24 percent) recalled an illness compatible with the acute retroviral syndrome.[174] Among patients with well characterized exposures to HIV and compatible symptoms, the interval between exposure

TABLE 5. Centers for Disease Control Classification Systems for Human Immunodeficiency Virus

I.	Classification system for HIV infection in adults
Group I.	Acute infection
Group II.	Asymptomatic infection
Group III.	Persistent generalized lymphadenopathy
Group IV.	Other diseases
Subgroup A.	Constitutional disease including HIV wasting syndrome in the CDC surveillance definition for AIDS
Subgroup B.	Neurologic disease including HIV encephalopathy in the CDC surveillance definition for AIDS
Subgroup C.	Secondary infectious diseases
Category C-1.	Specified secondary infectious diseases in the CDC surveillance definition for AIDS
Category C-2.	Other specified secondary infectious diseases
Subgroup D.	Secondary cancers in the CDC surveillance definition for AIDS
Subgroup E.	Other conditions
II.	Classification system for HIV infection in children under 13 years of age
Class P-0.	Indeterminate infection
Class P-1.	Asymptomatic infection
Subclass A.	Normal immune function
Subclass B.	Abnormal immune function
Subclass C.	Immune function not tested
Class P-2.	Symptomatic infection
Subclass A.	Nonspecific findings
Subclass B.	Progressive neurologic disease including HIV encephalopathy in the CDC surveillance definition for AIDS
Subclass C.	Lymphoid interstitial pneumonitis in the CDC surveillance definition for AIDS
Subclass D.	Secondary infectious diseases
Category D-1.	Specified secondary infectious diseases in the CDC surveillance definition for AIDS
Category D-2.	Recurrent serious bacterial infections in the CDC surveillance definition for AIDS
Category D-3.	Other specified secondary infectious diseases
Subclass E.	Secondary cancers
Category E-1.	Specified secondary cancers in the CDC surveillance definition for AIDS
Category E-2.	Other cancers possibly secondary to HIV infection
Subclass F.	Other diseases possibly due to HIV infection

(Modified from refs. 168 and 169.)

TABLE 6. The Walter Reed Staging Classification for HIV Infection in Adults

Stage	HIV Antibody and/or Virus Isolation	Clinic Lymphadenopathy	T-Helper Cells/mm^3	Cutaneous Anergy	Thrush	Opportunistic Infection
0	−	−	>400	Normal	−	−
1	+[a]	−	>400	Normal	−	−
2	+[a]	+[a]	>400	Normal	−	−
3	+[a]	+/−	<400[a]	Normal	−	−
4	+[a]	+/−	<400[a]	Partial[a]	−	−
5	+[a]	+/−	<400	Complete and/or	+[a]	−
6	+[a]	+/−	<400	Partail or complete	+/−	+[a]

[a] Essential criteria for assignment to each stage.
(Modified from Redfield et al.,[167] with permission.)

and symptomatic illness ranges from 6 to 58 days (Horsburgh CR Jr: Unpublished data, 1988).

Observations in persons with primary HIV infection indicate that HIV antigen can be detected within 1–4 weeks, followed by the development of HIV anti-core (p24) and anti-envelope antibodies (gp41).[171,172,175–176b] HIV antibodies usually develop within 3–12 weeks of the infection and evidence suggests that infection with HIV is persistent and lifelong. In one study, the virus was isolated from 22 (96 percent) of 25 blood donors who had been infected for 1–4 years.[110] Virus has been recovered from some homosexual men as long as 6 years after the initial detection of HIV antibody.[177] Loss of serologically detectable antibodies to HIV is rare in asymptomatic, latently infected persons. In a longitudinal study of 1000 HIV-seropositive homosexual men without AIDS, serologic tests for HIV antibody for 4 men (0.4 percent) apparently reverted from positive to negative, although polymerase chain reaction (gene amplification) assays demonstrated HIV provirus in all 4.[178] Long-term follow-up will be required to determine whether serologic reexpression of HIV occurs and whether clinical evidence of infection develops.

The period of time between the initial infection with HIV and the development of AIDS is usually long. While the risk for disease progression increases with the duration of infection, the risk is not uniform over time. Typically, a low rate of disease progression is observed in the first few years after infection. Of 6700 homosexual and bisexual men enrolled from 1978 to 1980 for studies of hepatitis B in San Francisco, 70 percent are estimated to be infected with HIV.[179] For a sample of 184 men from this study who had known dates of seroconversion, the cumulative proportion who have developed AIDS after 10 years is 48 percent.[180] Fewer than 5 percent were diagnosed with AIDS in the first 2 years after infection, however. In studies of persons with hemophilia, the rate of disease progression to AIDS is similar to that reported for homosexual men. For hemophilic persons followed 7 years after HIV seroconversion, the actuarial AIDS incidence is 22 percent.[180–181a] Transfusion recipients may have a more rapid rate of progression to AIDS. In one study, 23 percent of 71 transfusion recipients followed for a median of 4 years developed AIDS.[182]

The average period of time between infection with HIV and the development of AIDS is underestimated from such follow-up studies because persons with longer incubation periods who have not yet become ill are selectively excluded from analysis. To adjust for this limitation, various mathematic models have been developed. When using a model-based approach, the mean incubation period for both homosexual men and for adults with transfusion-associated AIDS is estimated to be approximately 8 years[183,183a] In contast, the calculated mean incubation period for infants with transfusion-mediate infection is 2 years.[183,184]

Prevalence and Incidence of HIV Infection

Because of the long incubation period, surveillance data for AIDS cannot be used to accurately monitor the incidence of HIV infection. The Public Health Service estimated in 1988 that approximately 1–1.5 million persons were infected with HIV in the United States.[185] The highest rates of infection are concentrated among persons known to be at an increased risk.

Reported HIV seroprevalence rates in homosexual and bisexual men range from 10 percent to as high as 70 percent, with most between 20 and 50 percent.[185] While the prevalence of HIV infection among iv drug abusers varies more widely, consistently high rates (usually > 50 percent) have been reported from New York, New Jersey, and Puerto Rico.[185] In contrast, the prevalence of HIV infection in hemophilic persons varies according to the severity of disease and tends to be uniformly distributed throughout the country. Overall, approximately 70 percent of persons with hemophilia A (factor VIII deficiency) and 35 percent of persons with hemophilia B (factor IX deficiency) are seropositive.[185]

Female prostitutes are at risk of HIV infection because of iv drug abuse and multiple sex partners. In a multicenter study of prostitutes in various settings in selected cities, 65 (10 percent) of 670 women had antibody to HIV.[186] Seroprevalence rates for HIV ranged from 0 percent of prescreened prostitutes in southern Nevada who were seen at STD clinics to 69 percent of prostitutes being treated for drug addition in northern New Jersey. Among prostitutes who were studied, the major risk factor for HIV infection was iv drug abuse. In a study of prostitutes in southern Florida in 1987, 37 (41 percent) of 90 inner-city prostitutes were HIV antibody-positive, including 29 (46 percent) of 63 women who abused iv drugs and 8 (30 percent) of 27 women who denied abusing iv drugs.[187] These data indicate that female prostitutes are at high risk for HIV infection and represent a potential source for heterosexual transmission.

Few specific data are available on the transmission of HIV among heterosexuals in the United States who are not the direct sex partners of iv drug abusers or other persons at high risk. The level of HIV infection in persons attending STD clinics who do not acknowledge homosexual contact, iv drug abuse, or sexual contact with persons at high risk varies, depending on the method used to ascertain risk history (i.e., self-administered questionnaire vs. in-person interview), the population being tested, and geographic location. In surveys conducted in three cities, seroprevalence rates in persons who did not report any high-risk behavior ranged from 2.7 percent of men and 1.8 percent of women in Baltimore[188] to 1.4 percent of men and 0.4 percent of women in New York City[189] and 0.2 percent of men and 0 percent women in Denver.[190] A survey of 602 parturient women in New York City identified 12 (2 percent) who were infected with HIV; 5 of the 12 women had no identified risk factors.[191] These studies suggest that patients at perinatal or STD clinics, particularly those located in areas where HIV seroprevalence is high among iv drug abusers, represent a group at increased risk for HIV infection. Beginning in 1988, a comprehensive family of HIV surveys and a national household-based seroprevalence survey will be undertaken by the U.S. Public Health Service in collaboration with local and state health departments and other agencies.[192] This surveillance approach will help monitor the levels and trends of HIV infection in the United States.

HIV seroprevalence data are more extensive from blood donors and military recruit applicants. Because these two populations are screened to select out homosexual men, iv drug abusers, and persons with hemophilia, the observed prevalence of HIV infection in these groups is much lower than the actual prevalence in the general population. For these same reasons, the relative proportion of unrecognized heterosexual and unexplained transmission will probably be higher in those who are seropositive for HIV. Among blood donors, 0.020 percent of 12.6 million American Red Cross blood donations collected between April 1985 and May 1987 were seropositive for HIV.[185] The overall level decreased from 0.035 percent in mid-1985 to 0.012 percent in mid-1987, primarily as a result of eliminating previously identified seropositive persons from the donor pool. Among first-time donors, who provide a measure of the prevalence of infection in the geographic area from which they are drawn, the level of HIV seropositivity averaged 0.043 percent during 1985–1987.[185] The overall prevalence of HIV infection among military recruits remained relatively stable at 0.15 percent between October 1985 and September 1987 and decreased slightly between October 1987 and March 1988.[185a] Among active-duty U.S. Army personnel who were tested more than once for HIV, 7.7 per 10,000 per year became infected since their initial test.[185]

HIV antibody prevalence for childbearing women has been ascertained by blinded surveys of blood samples collected on filter paper from newborns for routine metabolic assays such as phenylketonuria. These surveys provide unbiased population-based estimates of HIV infection in women bearing children. In Massachusetts, of over 30,000 specimens tested, 81 (0.3 percent) were confirmed as HIV-positive.[193] The prevalence of HIV infection varied by type and location of the hospital and ranged from 8.0 per 1000 in inner-city hospitals to 0.9 per 1000 in suburban and rural hospitals. In New York, HIV seroprevalence rates ascertained by this method were 1.6 percent in New York City and 0.2 percent for the remainder of the state.[194]

AIDS AND HIV INFECTION OUTSIDE THE UNITED STATES

Soon after the initial reports of AIDS in the United States, similar cases were identified in Europe.[195] Most of the initial European patients were homosexual and bisexual males. By early 1983, cases were recognized in Caribbean and central African expatriates residing in Europe.[195,196] Studies in Haiti and central Africa confirmed that homosexuality and iv drug abuse did not appear to be common risk factors in these patients.[21,88,89,197] These studies and the approximately equal proportion of cases among men and women suggested the occurrence of heterosexual transmission.[86–89]

The origin and global dissemination of HIV infection is of considerable interest. Antibodies to HIV have been detected in stored serum specimens obtained as early as 1959 in Zaire[198] and 1963 in Burkina Faso.[199] These observations suggest that sporadic cases of AIDS and HIV infection antedated the recognized epidemic in Africa as well as in the United States and other areas.[200] In retrospect, clinical evidence of the syndrome was not recognized with any regularity in Africa until the late 1970s and early 1980s when increases in several opportunistic infections and cancers were documented, including esophageal candidiasis,[197] unusually severe Kaposi sarcoma,[201] as well as wasting syndrome or "slim disease."[202]

Through May 1988, 96,433 cases of AIDS were reported to the World Health Organization (WHO).[203] However, WHO estimates that as many as 150,000 cases of AIDS may have occurred worldwide through 1987.[204] Precise enumeration of the number of AIDS cases is not possible, particularly in developing countries, because of the inability to obtain definitive diagnostic studies including HIV antibody tests and the absence of formalized disease surveillance and reporting systems. A systematic, hospital-based program of surveillance was initiated in Kinshasa, Zaire, in 1984 that used a modified version of the CDC surveillance case definition.[86] Even though the ability to diagnose many opportunistic diseases in this setting (most notably *P. carinii* pneumonia) was limited, an incidence rate of 55–100 per 100,000 Kinshasa residents was calculated. This was similar to the incidence rate of 82–100 per 100,000 calculated for recent Haitian entrants into the United States that same year.[19,58]

While similar modes of transmission exist worldwide, their geographic distribution and relative importance vary considerably. In western Europe, North America, Australia, New Zealand, and parts of South America, homosexual and bisexual men and iv drug abusers initially exposed to the virus in the mid-1970s or early 1980s remain the predominantly affected population group.[204,205] In Africa, the Caribbean, and some areas of South America, heterosexual sexual transmission, perinatal transmission, and receipt of HIV-infected blood are the primary modes of infection. Significant rates of HIV infection have been documented among women of childbearing age: between 3 and 11 percent of pregnant women in some urban areas of central and East Africa are seropositive.[127,132,206–208] Prostitutes studied in central and East Africa have also had high rates of HIV seroprevalence reported.[90,96,197] A retrospective, longitudinal seroepidemiologic study of prostitutes in Nairobi documented a steady increase in HIV seroprevalence from 4 percent in 1981 to 61 percent in 1985.[90] A concomitant rise in seroprevalence occurred in men treated for chancroid at a Nairobi STD clinic: 0 percent in 1981 to 15 percent in 1985. High rates of HIV infection in heterosexuals in these areas have resulted in a substantial and growing burden of perinatally acquired HIV infection in infants.[127,132,206–208]

In Kinshasa, Zaire, treatment of malaria-associated anemia with blood transfusions is an important factor in the exposure of children to HIV infection. In one hospital alone, an estimated 561 transfusions of HIV-seropositive blood were given to children with malaria over a 1-year period.[165] Receipt of injections and scarifications have been inconsistently associated with HIV infection,[206,209] the role of these and other nonsexual cultural practices in the transmission of HIV is not clear.[210]

HIV-2

A second retrovirus, HIV-2, has been isolated and associated with the development of serious opportunistic diseases that are clinically indistinguishable from AIDS caused by HIV-1. HIV-1 and HIV-2 are genetically and immunologically distinct. HIV-2 has only 40 percent DNA homology with HIV-1.[211] Serologic screening tests for HIV-1 antibodies have been estimated to detect 42–96 percent of HIV-2 infections.[212] While serum samples reactive to antigens of both viruses have been reported, this dual seropositivity is most often secondary to cross-reactivity of HIV-1-positive serum with HIV-2 antigens.[213,214]

Most cases of HIV-2 infection have been reported from countries in West Africa, but several well-documented cases have also been reported in Europeans and in West Africans residing in Europe and the United States.[213,215,216] Although the reported spectrum of disease is as broad as that for HIV-1-associated infection, the relative pathogenicity of the two viruses is unknown. Most persons infected with HIV-2 in West Africa have not progressed to develop AIDS.[217] Preliminary epidemiologic studies indicate that the modes of HIV-2 transmission are the same as those of HIV-1.[213,217]

PREVENTION OF AIDS AND HIV INFECTION IN THE COMMUNITY

In the absence of vaccines and only a limited number of effective antiviral agents or other therapeutic modalities, prevention of HIV infection must be based on strategies that interrupt sexual, blood-borne, and perinatal transmission of the virus.[218] Such strategies must be grounded in an understanding of the epidemiology of HIV infection. Application of such epidemiologic information is therefore critical in the design, implementation, and evaluation of prevention efforts.[219]

Prevention of Transmission

The risk of sexual transmission of HIV can be completely eliminated by either abstention from sexual activity or participation in a mutually monogamous relationship with an uninfected person. Other approaches that will reduce (but not completely eliminate) the risk of transmission include reduction of number of sex partners and efforts to minimize the likelihood of genital or oral mucous membrane exposure to blood, semen, saliva, cervical secretions, and vaginal secretions during intercourse.[220] The correct and consistent use of condoms and possibly condoms in conjunction with spermicides can reduce transmission of HIV by preventing exposure to infectious secretions and lesions. Laboratory testing has demonstrated latex condoms to be effective mechanical barriers to HIV as well as a number of other sexually transmitted pathogens.[221] Epidemiologic studies suggest that the usage of condoms may be associated with a reduction in acquisition of HIV from sexual partners either known to have AIDS or at increased risk of infection.[81,222] Most condom failures result from incorrect use, but breakage does occur.[221]

Examination of trends in self-reported sexual behaviors among homosexual and bisexual men point to significant reductions in certain high-risk behaviors such as the number of nonsteady partners and insertive anal intercourse.[223,224] Declining rates of rectal and pharyngeal gonorrhea among males in New York City and, more importantly, reductions in incident HIV infections among men in San Francisco provide additional evidence that the sexual transmission of HIV can be reduced.[225–266a] Comparable data to suggest significant changes in sexual behavior by heterosexual men and women in response to AIDS are not available. There is ample evidence that, while both homosexual and heterosexual persons are generally aware of the risk of sexually acquired HIV infection, many continue not to take precautions to protect themselves against AIDS and other STDs.[70,81,99,223,224,226–228]

Prevention of HIV infection through transmission by blood and blood products depends on deferral of blood and plasma donation by persons at increased risk for HIV infection, serologic screening of donated blood and plasma for HIV antibody, and heat treatment of clotting factor concentrates.[112,229–232] These measures have vastly reduced transmission of HIV by blood and blood products in the United States and other industrialized nations.[16,233] Although there is evidence that high-risk donors are voluntarily refraining from donation,[234] follow-up of seropositive donors has shown that most have a risk factor for HIV infection.[16,232,235,236] Therefore, additional strategies to reduce the already very low incidence of HIV transmission by blood or plasma transfusion need to focus on learning why some persons at risk for HIV infection continue to donate blood, improving educational programs to dissuade such persons from donating, and implementing more sensitive serologic assays to detect HIV as they become available.[16,233]

Strategies to prevent the transmission of HIV through iv drug abuse need to be tailored specifically to three target groups: (*1*) persons who have not yet begun iv drug abuse; (*2*) persons who are willing to enter treatment programs to eliminate iv drug use; and (*3*) persons who are unwilling to enter treatment.[237] A creative blend of educational, therapeutic, and law enforcement approaches and a substantial amount of resources will be required for each target group. The Presidential Commission on the HIV Epidemic has recommended that prevention and treatment of iv drug abuse must be a national priority and that treatment capacity must be greatly expanded in the United States.[238] Data are limited but indicate that many current abusers are aware of the risk associated with injection, and that some have decreased their risk by reduced needle sharing, increased procurement of sterile needles, and increased needle cleaning practices.[237,239]

Primary prevention of perinatally acquired HIV infection should center on routine, voluntary counseling and HIV antibody testing of childbearing age women in settings where HIV prevalence is moderate to high (e.g., 0.5 percent or higher) and in women with identified risks for HIV infection.[240] Women at increased risk for HIV infection include those who have used iv drugs; engaged in prostitution; had sex partners who were infected or at risk for HIV infection because they were bisexual, iv drug abusers, or hemophilic; lived in communities or were born in countries where there is a known or suspected high prevalence of infection in women; or received a blood transfusion before blood was being screened for HIV antibody but after HIV infection occurred (e.g., in the United States from 1978 to 1985). Because a substantial proportion of women may not initially acknowledge high-risk behavior or not have complete knowledge of the infection status of their partners, routine HIV counseling and testing must be considered a standard of care in areas of high prevalence (e.g., 0.5 percent or higher) and not be reserved for those women with self-reported risk histories.[191]

HIV-infected women should be advised to avoid pregnancy in view of the significant probability that they will transmit HIV to their unborn children[132–136] and the possibility that pregnancy may accelerate the progression of their HIV disease.[241,242] To avoid postnatal transmission to a child who may not be infected, breast-feeding is not recommended for HIV-infected women living in countries where alternative and effective infant nutrition is widely available.[243] In developing countries where the risk of infant mortality is significantly higher for bottle-fed than for breast-fed infants, the documented benefits of breast-feeding need to be weighed against the risk of transmission of HIV through breast-feeding.[244,245] In such settings, the WHO recommended in 1987 that breast-feeding should remain the feeding method of choice, even for HIV-infected mothers.[244]

In many developed countries, the effective treatment of iv drug abuse remains an essential adjunct to preventing perinatal transmission of HIV because mothers of most children with perinatally acquired AIDS either abuse iv drugs themselves or are the sex partners of men who do.

Counseling and HIV Antibody Testing

Counseling and HIV antibody testing programs are important to facilitate behavioral changes needed to prevent HIV transmission. The U.S. Public Health Service, in consultation with other public health agencies, has formulated guidelines for counseling and testing for HIV antibody.[240] Specific population groups or settings in which testing is recommended include the following:

Persons who seek treatment for an STD
IV-drug abusers
Persons who consider themselves at risk
Women of childbearing age with identifiable risks for HIV infection
Persons planning marriage
Persons undergoing medical evaluation or treatment for selected clinical conditions that may indicate underlying HIV infection such as generalized lymphadenopathy; unexplained dementia; unexplained fever, diarrhea, weight loss; diseases such as tuberculosis, generalized herpes, and chronic candidiasis
Persons admitted to hospitals to determine HIV seroprevalence in age groups at highest risk for infection

Persons in correctional systems
Prostitutes
Other health care settings where the prevalence of unsuspected HIV infection is moderate to high.

The U.S. Public Health Service, the Presidential Commission, and the American Medical Association have recommended that partner notification and/or contact tracing of HIV-infected persons should be incorporated in HIV prevention, counseling, and testing programs.[238,240,246] In addition, these guidelines stress the need for ensuring quality performance of laboratory tests for HIV through employment of trained personnel, establishment of quality controls, and participation in performance evaluation systems. Confidentiality and avoidance of discrimination toward persons who test seropositive must be ensured.

Preliminary studies indicate that antibody testing and counseling may have useful public health outcomes in terms of reductions in high-risk behavior in persons tested. However, such testing is often accompanied by adverse psychological consequences such as anxiety and depression.[247–249]

CONCLUSION

HIV infection and AIDS are now major causes of morbidity and mortality in the United States and other areas of the world. Although the basic epidemiology of the disease and its modes of transmission have been established, important questions remain regarding the incidence and prevalence of HIV infection, the efficiency of transmission and the role of cofactors in facilitating transmission of HIV, the natural history of infection in various population groups, and the effectiveness of various prevention strategies. In addition to the clinical and epidemiologic aspects of the epidemic, its economic impact is substantial—in terms of both the cost of providing medical and psychosocial services and losses incurred from disability and premature death. The control and prevention of HIV infection will require a coordinated, sustained, and costly global commitment that will extend into the next century.

REFERENCES

1. *Pneumocystis* pneumonia—Los Angeles. MMWR. 1981;30:250–2.
2. Kaposi's sarcoma and *Pneumocystis* pneumonia among homosexual men—New York City and California. MMWR. 1981;30:305–8.
3. Curran JW. AIDS—two years later (Editorial). N Engl J Med. 1983;309:609–11.
4. Barre-Sinoussi F, Chermann JC, Rey F, et al. Isolation of a T-lymphotropic retrovirus from a patient at risk for acquired immune deficiency syndrome (AIDS). Science. 1983;220:868–71.
5. Gallo RC, Salahuddin SZ, Popovic M, et al. Frequent detection and isolation of cytopathic retroviruses (HTLV-III) from patients with AIDS and at risk for AIDS. Science. 1984;224:500–3.
6. Levy JA, Hoffman AD, Kramer SM, et al. Isolation of lymphocytopathic retroviruses from San Francisco patients with AIDS. Science. 1984;225:840–2.
7. Update on acquire immune deficiency syndrome (AIDS)—United States. MMWR. 1982;31:507–14.
8. Hardy AM, Starcher ET II, Morgan WM, et al. Review of death certificates to assess completeness of AIDS case reporting. Public Health Rep. 1987;102:386–91.
9. Revision of the case definition of acquired immunodeficiency syndrome for national reporting—United States. MMWR. 1985;34:373–5.
10. Revision of the CDC surveillance case definition for acquired immunodeficiency syndrome. MMWR. 1987;36(Suppl 1):1–15.
11. Starcher ET II, Biel JK, Castano RR, et al. The impact of presumptively diagnosed opportunistic infections and cancers on national reporting of AIDS (Abstract) In: Proceedings of the Third International Conference on AIDS, June 1–5, 1987. Washington, DC: The U.S. Department of Health and Human Services and the WHO; 1987:125.
12. Chamberland ME, Allen JR, Monroe JM, et al. Acquired immunodeficiency syndrome in New York City. Evaluation of an active surveillance system. JAMA. 1985;254:383–7.
13. Rauch, KJ, Rutherford GW, Badran C, et al. Surveillance of acquired immunodeficiency syndrome in San Francisco: Evaluation of the completeness of reporting (Abstract). In: Proceedings of the International Conference on AIDS, June 23–25, 1986. Paris: The U.S. Department of Health and Human Services and the WHO; 1986:152.
14. Curran JW, Jaffe HW, Hardy AM, et al. Epidemiology of HIV infection and AIDS in the United States. Science. 1988;239:610–6.
15. Report of the Second Public Health Service AIDS Prevention and Control Meeting. Public Health Rep. 1989;103:10–8.
16. Ward JW, Holmberg SD, Allen JR, et al. Transmission of human immunodeficiency virus (HIV) by blood transfusions screened as negative for HIV antibody. N Engl J Med. 1988;318:473–8.
17. Peterman TA, Jaffe HW, Feorino PM, et al. Transfusion-associated acquired immunodeficiency syndrome in the United States. JAMA 1985;254:2913–17.
18. Peterman TA, Lui K-J, Lawrence DN, et al. Estimating the risks of transfusion-associated acquired immune deficiency syndrome and human immunodeficiency virus infection. Transfusion. 1987;27:371–4.
19. Hardy AM, Allen JR, Morgan WM, et al. The incidence rate of acquired immunodeficiency syndrome in selected populations. JAMA. 1985;253:215–20.
20. The Collaborative Study Group of AIDS in Haitian-Americans. Risk factors for AIDS among Haitians residing in the United States. Evidence of heterosexual transmission. JAMA. 1987;257:635–9.
21. Pape JW, Liautaud B, Thomas F, et al. The acquired immunodeficiency syndrome in Haiti. Ann Intern Med. 1985;103:674–8.
22. Castro KG, Lifson AR, White CR, et al. Investigations of AIDS patients with no previously identified risk factors. JAMA. 1988;259:1338–42.
23. Chamberland ME, Castro KG, Haverkos HW, et al. Acquired immunodeficiency syndrome in the United States: An analysis of cases outside high-incidence groups. Ann Intern Med. 1984;101:617–23.
24. Lekatsas AM, Walker J, O'Donnell R, et al. Identification of risk in persons with AIDS in New York City: When is "no risk" without risk? (Abstract). In: Proceedings of the Internationl Conference on AIDS, June 23–25, 1986. Paris: L'Association pour la Recherche sur les Déficits Immunitaire Viro-Induits (ARDIVI); 1986:151.
25. Potterat JJ, Phillips L, Muth JB. Lying to military physicians about risk factors for HIV infections (Letter). JAMA. 1987;257:1727.
26. Acquired immunodeficiency syndrome (AIDS) among blacks and Hispanics—United States. MMWR. 1986;35:655–8, 663–6.
27. Selik RM, Castro KG, Pappaioanou M. Racial/ethnic differences in the risk of AIDS in the United States. Am J Public Health. 1988;78:1539–45.
28. Guinan ME, Hardy A. Epidemiology of AIDS in women in the United States. 1981 through 1986. JAMA. 1987;257:2039–42.
29. Chamberland ME, Dondero TJ Jr. Heterosexually acquired infection with human immunodeficiency virus (HIV). A view from the III International Conference on AIDS (Editorial). Ann Intern Med. 1987;107:763–6.
30. Jaffe HW, Bregman DJ, Selik RM. Acquired immune deficiency syndrome in the United States: The first 1,000 cases. J Infect Dis. 1983;148:339–45.
31. Agins B, Spicehandler D, Della-Latta P, et al. *M. avium-intracellulare* infection in AIDS (Abstract). In: Proceedings and abstracts of the 24th Interscience Conference on Antimicrobial Agents and Chemotherapy, October 8–10, 1984. Washington, DC: The American Society for Microbiology; 1984:229.
32. Selik RM, Starcher ET, Curran JW. Opportunistic diseases reported in AIDS patients: Frequencies, associations, and trends. AIDS. 1987;1:175–82.
33. Newell GR, Adams SC, Mansell PWA, et al. Toxicity, immunosuppressive effects and carcinogenic potential of volatile nitrites: Possible relationship to Kaposi's sarcoma. Pharmacotherapy. 1984;4:284–91.
34. Goedert JJ, Neuland CY, Wallen WC, et al. Amyl nitrite may alter T lymphocytes in homosexual men. Lancet. 1982;1:412–6.
35. Marmor M, Friedman-Kien AE, Laubenstein L, et al. Risk factors for Kaposi's sarcoma in homosexual men. Lancet. 1982;1:1083–7.
36. Jaffe HW, Choi K, Thomas PA, et al. National case–control study of Kaposi's sarcoma and *Pneumocystis carinii* pneumonia in homosexual men: Part 1, epidemiologic results. Ann Intern Med. 1983;99:145–51.
37. Melbye M, Biggar RJ, Ebbeson P, et al. Seroepidemiology of HTLV-III antibody in Danish homosexual men: Prevalence, transmission, and disease outcome. Br Med J. 1984;289:573–5.
38. Darrow WW, Echenberg DF, Jaffe HW, et al. Risk factors for human immunodeficiency virus (HIV) infections in homosexual men. Am J Public Health. 1987;77:479–83.
39. Moss AR, Osmond D, Bacchetti P, et al. Risk factors for AIDS and HIV seropositivity in homosexual men. Am J Epidemiol. 1987;125:1035–47.
40. Haverkos HW, Pinsky PF, Drotman DP, et al. Disease manifestion among homosexual men with acquired immunodeficiency syndrome: A possible role of nitrites in Kaposi's sarcoma. Sex Transm Dis. 1985;12:203–8.
41. Giraldo G, Beth E, Huang E-S. Kaposi's sarcoma and its relationship to cytomegalovirus (CMV). III. CMV DNA and CMV early antigens in Kaposi's sarcoma. Int J Cancer. 1980;26:23–9.
42. Drew WL, Mintz L, Miner RC, et al. Prevalence of cytomegalovirus infection in homoosexual men. J Infect Dis. 1981;143:188–92.
43. Drew WL, Conant MA, Miner RC, et al. Cytomegalovirus and Kaposi's sarcoma in young homosexual men. Lancet. 1982;2:125–7.
44. Polk BF, Fox R, Brookmeyer R, et al. Predictors of the acquired immunodeficiency syndrome developing in a cohort of seropositive homosexual men. N Engl J Med. 1987;316:61–6.
45. Lifson AR, Darrow WW, O'Malley PM, et al. Decline in Kaposi's sarcoma among homosexual and bisexual men and analysis for cofactors (Abstract). In: Proceedings of the Fourth International Conference on AIDS, Book 1,

June 12–16, 1988. Stockholm: The Swedish Ministry of Health and Social Affairs; 1988:290.
46. Blaser MJ, Cohn DL. Opportunistic infections in patients with AIDS: Clues to the epidemiology of AIDS and the relative virulence of pathogens. Rev Infect Dis. 1986;8:21–30.
47. Glatt AE, Chirgwin K, Landesman SH. Treatment of infections associated with human immunodeficiency virus. N Engl J Med. 1988:318:1439–48.
48. Tuberculosis and acquired immunodeficiency syndrome—Florida. MMWR. 1986;35:587–90.
49. Tuberculosis and AIDS—Connecticut. MMWR. 1987;36:133–5.
50. Tuberculosis and acquired immunodeficiency syndrome—New York City. MMWR. 1987;36:785–90, 795.
51. The Long-Term Survivor Collaborative Study Group, Hardy AM. Characterization of long-term survivors (LTS) of AIDS (Abstract). In: Proceedings and abstracts of the 27th Interscience Conference on Antimicrobial Agents and Chemotherapy, October 4–7, 1987. New York: The American Society for Microbiology; 1987:98.
52. Bacchetti P, Osmond D, Chaisson RE, et al. Survival patterns in San Francisco AIDS patients (Abstract). In: Proceedings and abstracts of the 27th Interscience Conference on Antimicrobial Agents and Chemotherapy, October 4–7, 1987. New York: The American Society for Microbiology; 1987:98.
53. Moss AR, McCallum G, Volberding PA, et al. Mortality associated with mode of presentation in the acquired immune deficiency syndrome. JNCI. 1984;73:1281–4.
54. Marasca G, McEvoy M. Length of survival of patients with acquired immune deficiency syndrome in the United Kingdom. Br Med J. 1986;292:1727–9.
55. Rothenberg R, Woelfel M, Stoneburner R, et al. Survival with the acquired immunodeficiency syndrome. Experience with 5833 cases in New York City. N Engl J Med. 1987;317:1297–302.
56. Vadhan-Raj S, Wong G, Gnecco C, et al. Immunological variables as predictors of prognosis in patients with Kaposi's sarcoma and the acquired immunodeficiency syndrome. Cancer Res. 1986;46:417–25.
57. Changes in premature mortality—United States, 1979–1986. MMWR. 1986,37.47–8.
58. Curran JW, Morgan WM, Hardy AM, et al. The epidemiology of AIDS: Current status and future prospects. Science. 1985;229:1352–7.
59. Kristal AR. The impact of the acquired immunodeficiency syndrome on patterns of premature death in New York City. JAMA. 1986;255:2306–10.
60. Chiasson MA, Fleisher E, Petrus D, et al. Epidemiologic characteristics of women with AIDS in New York City (Abstract). In: Proceedings of the Third International Conference on AIDS, June 1–5, 1987. Washington DC: The U.S. Department of Health and Human Services and the WHO; 1987:174.
61. Unexplained immunodeficiency and opportunistic infections in infants—New York, New Jersey, California. MMWR. 1982:31:665–7.
62. Oleske J, Minnefor A, Cooper R, et al. Immune deficiency syndrome in children. JAMA. 1983;249:2345–9.
63. Rubinstein A, Sicklick M, Gupta A, et al. Acquired immunodeficiency with reversed T4/T8 ratios in infants born to promiscuous and drug-addicted mothers. JAMA. 1983;249:2350–6.
64. Thomas PA, Jaffe HW, Spira TJ, et al. Unexplained immunodeficiency in children. A surveillance report. JAMA. 1984;252:639–44.
65. Lifson AR, Rogers MF, White C, et al. Unrecognized modes of transmission of HIV: Acquired immunodeficiency syndrome in children reported without risk factors. Pediatr Infect Dis. 1987;6:292–3.
66. Friedman BA, Burns TL, Schork MA. A study of national trends in transfusion practice. Ann Arbor: The University of Michigan Medical School and School of Public Health; 1980:1–283.
67. Thomas PA, O'Donnell RE, Lessner L. Survival analysis of children reported with AIDS in New York City, 1982–1986 (Abstract). In: Proceedings of the Third International Conference on AIDS, June 1–5, 1987. Washington, DC: The U.S. Department of Health and Human Services and the WHO; 1987:75.
68. Peterman TA, Curran JW. Sexual transmission of human immunodeficiency virus. JAMA. 1986;256:2222–6.
69. Goedert JJ, Sarngadharan MG, Biggar RJ, et al. Determinants of retrovirus (HTLV-III) antibody and immunodeficiency conditions in homosexual men. Lancet. 1984;2:711–6.
70. Stevens CE, Taylor PE, Zang EA, et al. Human T-cell lymphotropic virus type III infection in a cohort of homosexual men in New York City. JAMA. 1986;255:2167–72.
71. Winkelstein W, Lyman DM, Padian N, et al. Sexual practices and risk of infection by the human immunodeficiiency virus. The San Francisco Men's Health Study. JAMA. 1987;257:321–5.
72. Kingsley LA, Detels R, Kaslow R, et al. Risk factors for seroconversion to human immunodeficiency virus among male homosexuals. Results from the Multicenter AIDS Cohort Study. Lancet 1987;1:345–9.
73. Mayer KH, DeGruttola V. Human immunodeficiency virus and oral intercourse (Letter). Ann Intern Med. 1987;107:428–9.
74. Lyman D, Winkelstein W, Ascher M, et al. Minimal risk of transmission of AIDS-associated retrovirus infection by oral-genital contact (Letter). JAMA. 1986;255:1703.
75. Marmor M, Weiss LR, Lyden M, et al. Possible female-to-female transmission of human immunodeficiency virus (Letter). Ann Intern Med. 1986;105:969.
76. Monzon OT, Capellan JMB. Female-to-female transmission of HIV (Letter). Lancet. 1987;2:40–1.
77. Kreiss JK, Kitchen LW, Prince HE, et al. Antibody to human T-lymphotropic virus type III in wives of hemophiliacs. Evidence for heterosexual transmission. Ann Intern Med. 1985;102:623–6.
78. Redfield RR, Markham PD, Salahuddin SZ, et al. Frequent transmission of HTLV-III among spouses of patients with AIDS-related complex and AIDS. JAMA. 1985;253:1571–3.
79. Allain J-P. Prevalence of HTLV-III/LAV antibodies in patients with hemophilia and in their sexual partners in France (Letter). N Engl J Med. 1986;315:517–8.
80. Jason JM, McDougal JS, Dixon G, et al. HTLV-III/LAV antibody and immune status of household contacts and sexual partners of persons with hemophilia. JAMA. 1986;255:212–5.
81. Fischl MA, Dickinson GM, Scott GB, et al. Evaluation of heterosexual partners, children, and household contacts of adults with AIDS. JAMA. 1987;257:640–4.
82. Padian N, Wiley J, Winkelstein W. Male-to-female transmission of human immunodeficiency virus (HIV): Current results, infectivity rates, and San Francisco population seroprevalence estimates (Abstract). In: Proceedings of the Third International Conference on AIDS, June 1–5, 1987. Washington, DC: The U.S. Department of Health and Human Services and the WHO; 1987:171.
83. Smiley L, White GC II, Macik G, et al. Transmission of human immunodeficiency virus from hemophiliacs to their sexual partners: Role of parenteral exposures (Abstract). In: Proceedings of the Third International Conference on AIDS, June 1–5, 1987. Washington, DC: 1987:23.
84. Peterman TA, Stoneburner RL, Allen JR, et al. Risk of human immunodeficiency virus transmission from heterosexual adults with transfusion-associated infections. JAMA. 1988;259:55–8.
85. Padian NS. Heterosexual transmission of acquired immunodeficiency syndrome: International perspectives and national projections. Rev Infect Dis. 1987;9:947–60.
86. Mann JM, Francis H, Quinn T, et al. Surveillance for AIDS in a central African city. Kinshasa, Zaire. JAMA. 1986;255:3255–9.
87. Quinn TC, Mann JM, Curran JW, et al. AIDS in Africa: An epidemiologic paradigm. Science. 1986,234.955–63.
88. Piot P, Quinn TC, Taelman H, et al. Acquired immunodeficiency syndrome in a heterosexual population in Zaire. Lancet. 1984;2:65–9.
89. Clumeck N, Van de Perre P, Carael M, et al. Heterosexual promiscuity among African patients with AIDS (Letter). N Engl J Med. 1985;313:182.
90. Piot P, Plummer FA, Rey M-A, et al. Retrospective seroepidemiology of AIDS virus infection in Nairobi populations. J Infect Dis. 1987;155:1108–12.
91. Goedert JJ, Eyster ME, Biggar RJ. Heterosexual transmission of human immunodeficiency virus (HIV): Association with severe T4-cell depletion in male hemophiliacs (Abstract). In: Proceedings of the Third International Conference on AIDS, June 1–5, 1987. Washington, DC: The U.S. Department of Health and Human Services and the WHO; 1987:106.
92. Redfield RR, Wright DC, Khan NC, et al. Correlation of HIV isolation rate and stage of infection (Abstract). In: Proceedings of the Third International Conference on AIDS, June 1–5, 1987. Washington, DC: The U.S. Department of Health and Human Services and the WHO; 1987:180.
93. Steigbigel NH, Maude DW, Feiner CJ, et al. Heterosexual transmission of infection and disease by the human immunodeficiency virus (HIV) (Abstract). In: Proceedings of the Third International Conference on AIDS, June 1–5, 1987. Washington, DC: The U.S. Department of Health and Human Services and the WHO; 1987:106.
94. Handsfield HH, Ashley RL, Rompalo AM, et al. Association of anogenital ulcer disease with human immunodeficiency virus infection in homosexual men (Abstract). In: Proceedings of the Third International Conference on AIDS, June 1–5, 1987. Washington, DC: The U.S. Department of Health and Human Services and the WHO; 1987:206.
95. Holmberg SD, Stewart JA, Gerber AR, et al. Prior herpes simplex virus type 2 infection as a risk factor for HIV infection. JAMA. 1988;259:1048–50.
96. Kreiss JK, Koech D, Plummer FA, et al. AIDS virus infection in Nairobi prostitutes. Spread of the epidemic to East Africa. N Engl J Med. 1986;314:414–8.
97. Greenblatt RM, Lukehart SL, Plummer FA, et al. Genital ulceration as a risk factor for human immunodeficiency virus infection in Kenya (Abstract). In: Proceediings of the Third International Conference on AIDS, June 1–5, 1987. Washington, DC: The U.S. Department of Health and Human Services and the WHO; 1987:174.
98. Cameron DW, Plummer FA, Simonsen JN, et al. Female to male heterosexual transmission of HIV infection in Nairobi (Abstract). In: Proceedings of the Third International Conference on AIDS, June 1–5, 1987. Washington, DC: The U.S. Department of Health and Human Services and the WHO; 1987:25.
99. Increases in primary and secondary syphilis—United States. MMWR. 1987:36:393–7.
100. Schoenbaum EE, Selwyn PA, Klein RS, et al. Prevalence of and risk factors associated with HTLV-III/LAV antibodies among intravenous drug abusers in methadone program in New York City (Abstract). In: Proceedings of the International Conference on AIDS, June 23–35, 1986. Paris: L'Association pour la Recherche sur les Déficits Immunitaire Viro-Induits (ARDIVI); 1986:111.
101. Weiss SH, Ginzberg HM, Altman R, et al. Risk factors of HTLV-III/LAV infection and the development of AIDS among drug abusers (DA) (Abstract). In: Proceedings of the International Conference on AIDS, June 23–25, 1986.

Paris: L'Association pour la Recherche sur les Déficits Immunitaire Viro-Induits (ARDIVI); 1986:124.

102. Chaisson RE, Moss AR, Onishi R, et al. Human immunodeficiency virus infection in heterosexual intravenous drug users in San Francisco. Am J Public Health. 1987;77:169–72.
103. Curran JW, Lawrence DN, Jaffe H, et al. Acquired immunodeficiency syndrome (AIDS) associated with transfusions. N Engl J Med. 1984;310:69–75.
104. Evatt BL, Ramsey RB, Lawrence DN, et al. The acquired immunodeficiency syndrome in patients with hemophilia. Ann Intern Med. 1984;100:499–504.
105. Safety of therapeutic immune globulin preparations with respect to transmission of human T-lymphotropic virus type III/lymphadenopathy-associated virus infection. MMWR. 1986;35:231–3.
106. Lack of transmission of human immunodeficiency virus through Rh_0(D) immune globulin (human). MMWR. 1987;36:728–9.
107. Hepatitis B vaccine: Evidence confirming lack of AIDS transmission. MMWR. 1984;33:685–7.
108. Wells MA, Wittek AE, Epstein JS, et al. Inactivation and partition of human T-cell lymphotrophic virus, type III, during ethanol fractionation of plasma. Transfusion. 1986;26:210–3.
109. Ward JW, Deppe DA, Samson S, et al. Risk of human immunodeficiency virus infection from blood donors who later developed the acquired immunodeficiency syndrome. Ann Intern Med. 1987;106:61–2.
110. Feorino PM, Jaffe HW, Palmer E, et al. Transfusion-associated acquired immunodeficiency syndrome. Evidence for persistent infection in blood donors. N Engl J Med. 1985;312:1293–6.
111. Stehr-Green JK, Holman RC, Jason JM, et al. Hemophilia-associated AIDS in the United States, 1981 to September 1987. Am J Public Health. 1988;78:439–42.
112. Survey of non-U.S. hemophilia treatment centers for HIV seroconversions following therapy with heat-treated factor concentrates. MMWR. 1987;36:121–4.
113. L'age-Stehr J, Schwarz A, Offermann G, et al. HTLV-III infection in kidney transplant recipients (Letter). Lancet. 1985;2:1361–2.
114. Human immunodeficiency virus infection transmitted from an organ donor screened for HIV antibody—North Carolina. MMWR. 1987;36:306–8.
115. Stewart GJ, Tyler JPP, Cunningham AL, et al. Transmission of human T-cell lymphotropic virus type III (HTLV-III) by artificial insemination by donor. Lancet. 1985;2:581–5.
116. Testing donors of organs, tissues, and semen for antibody to human T-lymphotropic virus type III/lymphadenopathy-associated virus. MMWR. 1985;34:294.
117. Update: Acquired immunodeficiency syndrome and human immunodeficiency virus infection among health-care workers. MMWR. 1988;37:229–34,239.
118. Marcus R and The CDC Cooperative Needlestick Surveillance Group. Surveillance of health care workers exposed to blood from patients infected with the human immunodeficiency virus. N Engl J Med. 1988;319:118–23.
119. Henderson DK, Saah AJ, Zak BJ, et al. Risk of nosocomial infection with human T-cell lymphotropic virus type III/lymphadenopathy-associated virus in a large cohort of intensively exposed health care workers. Ann Intern Med. 1986;104:644–7.
120. Gerberding JL, Bryant-LeBlanc CE, Nelson K, et al. Risk of transmitting the human immunodeficiency virus, cytomegalovirus, and hepatitis B virus to health care workers exposed to patients with AIDS and AIDS-related conditions. J Infect Dis. 1987;156:1–8.
121. Henderson DK, Fahey BJ, Willy ME. Frequency and intensity of cutaneous exposures to blood and body fluids among health care providers in a referral hospital (Abstract). In: Proceedings of the Fourth International Conference on AIDS, Book 1, June 12–16, 1988. Stockholm: The Swedish Ministry of Health and Social Affairs; 1988:480.
122. 1988 agent summary statement for human immunodeficiency virus and report on laboratory-acquired infection with human immunodeficiency virus. MMWR. 1988;37(Suppl 4):1–22.
123. Recommendations for prevention of HIV transmission in health-care settings. MMWR. 1987:36(Suppl 2):1–18.
124. Update: Universal precautions for prevention of transmission of human immunodeficiency virus, hepatitis B virus, and other bloodborne pathogens in health-care settings. MMWR. 1988;37:377–82, 387–8.
125. Jovaisas E, Koch MA, Shafer A, et al. LAV/HTLV-III in 20-week fetus (Letter). Lancet. 1985;2:1129.
126. Lapointe N, Michaud J, Pekovic D, et al. Transplacental transmission of HTLV-III virus (Letter). N Engl J Med. 1985;312:1325–6.
127. Nzilambi N, Ryder RW, Behets F, et al. Perinatal HIV transmission in two African hospitals (Abstract). In: Proceedings of the Third International Conference on AIDS, June 1–5, 1987. Washington, DC: The U.S. Department of Health and Human Services and the WHO; 1987:158.
128. Thiry L, Sprecher-Goldberger S, Jonckheer T, et al. Isolation of AIDS virus from cell-free breast milk of three healthy virus carriers (Letter). Lancet. 1985;2:891–2.
129. Ziegler JB, Stewart GJ, Penny R, et al. Breast feeding and transmission of HIV from mother to infant (Abstract). In: Proceedings of the Fourth International Conference on AIDS, Book 1, June 12–16, 1988. Stockholm: The Swedish Ministry of Health and Social Affairs; 1988:339.
130. Colebunders R, Kapita B, Nekwei W, et al. Breastfeeding and transmission of HIV (Letter). Lancet. 1988;2:1487.
131. Weinbreck F, Loustaud V, Denis F, et al. Postnatal transmission of HIV infection. Lancet. 1988;1:482.
132. Ryder RW, Rayfield M, Quinn T, et al. Transplacental HIV transmission in African newborns (Abstract). In: Proceedings of the Fourth International Conference on AIDS, Book 1, June 12–16, 1988. Stockholm: The Swedish Ministry of Health and Social Affairs; 1988:345.
133. The European Collaborative Study. Mother-to-child transmission of HIV infection. Lancet. 1988;2:1039–43.
134. Blanche S, Rouzioux C, Tricoire J, et al. Prospective study on newborns of HIV seropositive women (Abstract). In: Proceedings of the Fourth International Conference on AIDS, Book 1, June 12–16, 1988. Stockholm: The Swedish Ministry of Health and Social Affairs; 1988:434.
135. Scott G, Hutto C, Mastrucci T, et al. Probability of perinatal infections in infants of HIV-1 positive mothers (Abstract). In: Proceedings of the Fourth International Conference on AIDS, Book 2, June 12–16, 1988. Stockholm: The Swedish Ministry of Health and Social Affairs; 1988:292.
136. Mendez H, Willoughby A, Hittelman J, et al. Infants of HIV seropositive (SP) women and their seronegative (SN) controls (Abstract). In: Proceedings of the Fourth International Conference on AIDS, Book 2, June 12–16, 1988. Stockholm: The Swedish Ministry of Health and Social Affairs; 1988:295.
137. Mok JQ, Giaquinto C, De Rossi A, et al. Infants born to mothers seropositive for human immunodeficiency virus. Preliminary findings from a multicentre European study. Lancet. 1987;1:1164–8.
138. Friedland GH, Klein RS. Transmission of the human immunodeficiency virus. N Engl J Med. 1987;317:1125–35.
139. Lifson AR. Do alternate modes for transmission of human immunodeficiency virus exist? A review. JAMA. 1988;259:1353–6.
140. Zagury D, Bernard J, Leibowitch J, et al. HTLV-III in cells cultured from semen of two patients with AIDS. Science. 1984;226:449–51.
141. Vogt MW, Witt DJ, Craven DE, et al. Isolation of HTLV-III/LAV from cervical secretions of women at risk for AIDS. Lancet. 1986;1:525–7.
142. Wofsy CB, Cohen JB, Hauer LB, et al. Isolation of AIDS-associated retrovirus from genital secretions of women with antibodies to the virus. Lancet. 1986;1:527–9.
143. Pomerantz RJ, de la Monte SM, Donegan SP, et al. Human immunodeficiency virus (HIV) infection of the uterine cervix. Ann Intern Med. 1988;108:321–7.
144. Groopman JE, Salahuddin SZ, Sarngadharan MG, et al. HTLV-III in saliva of people with AIDS-related complex and healthy homosexual men at risk for AIDS. Science. 1984;226:447–9.
145. Ho DD, Byington RE, Schooley RT, et al. Infrequency of isolation of HTLV-III virus from saliva in AIDS (Letter). N Engl J Med. 1985;313:1606.
146. Levy JA, Kaminsky LS, Morrow WJW, et al. Infection by the retrovirus associated with the acquired immunodeficiency syndrome. Clinical, biological, and molecular features. Ann Intern Med. 1985;103:694–9.
147. Fujikawa LS, Salahuddin SZ, Palestine AG, et al. Isolation of human T-lymphotropic virus type III from the tears of a patient with the acquired immunodeficiency syndrome. Lancet. 1985;2:529–30.
148. Ho DD, Rota TR, Schooley RT, et al. Isolation of HTLV-III from cerebrospinal fluid and neural tissues of patients with neurologic syndromes related to the acquired immunodeficiency syndrome. N Engl J Med. 1985;313:1493–7.
149. Ziza J-M, Brun-Vezinet F, Venet A, et al. Lymphadenopathy-associated virus isolated from bronchoalveolar lavage fluid in AIDS-related complex with lymphoid interstitial pneumonitis (Letter). N Engl J Med. 1985; 313:183.
150. Mundy DC, Schinazi RF, Gerber AR, et al. Human immunodeficiency virus isolated from amniotic fluid (Letter). Lancet. 1987;2:459–60.
151. Fultz PN. Components of saliva inactivate human immunodeficiency virus (Letter). Lancet. 1986;2:1215.
152. Wahn V, Kramer HH, Voit T, et al. Horizontal transmission of HIV infection between two siblings (Letter). Lancet. 1986;2:694.
153. Rogers MF, White CR, Sanders R. Can children transmit HTLV-III/LAV infection? (Abstract). In: Proceedings and abstracts of the 26th Interscience Conference on Antimicrobial Agents and Chemotherapy, September 28–October 1, 1986. New Orleans: The American Society for Microbiology; 1986:284.
154. Tsoukas C, Hadjis T, Theberge L, et al. Risk of transmission fo HTLV-III/LAV from human bites (Abstract). In: Proceedings of the International Conference on AIDS, June 23–25, 1986, Paris: L'Association pour la Recherche sur les Déficits Immunitaire Viro-Induits (ARDIVI); 1986:125.
155. Klein RS, Phelan JA, Freeman K, et al. Low occupational risk of human immunodeficiency virus infection among dental professionals. N Engl J Med. 1988;318:86–90.
156. Flynn NM, Pollet SM, Van Horne JR, et al. Absence of HIV antibody among dental professionals exposed to infected patients. West J Med. 1987;146:439–42.
157. Gerberding JL, Nelson K, Greenspan D, et al. Risk to dental professionals (DP) from occupational exposure to human immunodeficiency virus (HIV): Followup (Abstract). In: Proceedings and abstracts of the 27th Interscience Conference on Antimicrobial Agents and Chemotherapy, October 4–7, 1987. New York: The American Society for Microbiology; 1987:219.
158. Berthier A, Chamaret S, Fauchet R, et al. Transmissibility of human immunodeficiency virus in haemophilic and non-haemophilic children living in a private school in France. Lancet. 1986;2:598–601.
159. Mann JM, Quinn TC, Francis H, et al. Prevalence of HTLV-III/LAV in household contacts of patients with confirmed AIDS and controls in Kinshasa, Zaire. JAMA. 1986;256:721–4.
160. Friedland GH, Kahl P, Feiner C, et al. The effect of AIDS diagnosis upon

close personal interaction among family members of AIDS patients (Abstract). In: Proceedings of the Third International Conference on AIDS, June 1–5, 1987. Washington, DC: The U.S. Department of Health and Human Services and the WHO; 1987;196.

161. Srinivasan A, York D, Bohan C. Lack of HIV replication in arthropod cells (Letter). Lancet. 1987;1:1094–5.
162. Miike L. Do insects transmit AIDS? Washington, DC: Health Program, Office of Technology Assessment, U.S. Congress; 1987:1–43.
163. Castro KG, Lieb S, Jaffe HW, et al. Transmission of HIV in Belle Glade, Florida: Lessons for other communities in the United States. Science. 1988;239:193–7.
164. Pape JW, Stanback ME, Pamphile M, et al. Pattern of HIV infection in Haiti: 1977–1986 (Abstract). In: Proceedings of the Third International Conference on AIDS, June 1–5, 1987. Washington, DC: The U.S. Department of Health and Human Services and the WHO; 1987:6.
165. Greenberg AE, Nguyen-Dinh P, Mann JM, et al. The association between malaria, blood transfusions, and HIV seropositivity in a pediatric population in Kinshasa, Zaire. JAMA. 1988;259:545–9.
165a. Stoneburner RL, Des Jarlais DC, Benezra D, et al. A larger spectrum of severe HIV-I related disease in intravenous drug users in New York City. Science. 1988;242:916–9.
166. Haverkos HW, Gotlieb MS, Killen JY, et al. Classification of HTLV-III/LAV-related diseases (Letter). J Infect Dis. 1985;152:1095.
167. Redfield RR, Wright DC, Tramont EA. The Walter Reed staging classification for HTLV-III/LAV infection. N Engl J Med. 1986;314:131–2.
168. Classification system for human T-lymphotropic virus type III/lymphadenopathy-associated virus infections. MMWR. 1986;35:334–9.
169. Classification system for human immunodeficiency virus (HIV) infection in children under 13 years of age. MMWR. 1987;36:225–36.
170. Solomon SL, Curran JW. Public health applications of a classification system for human immunodeficiency virus infection (Editorial). Ann Intern Med. 1987;106:319–21.
171. Ho DD, Sarngadharan MG, Resnick L, et al. Primary human T-lymphotropic virus type III infection. Ann Intern Med. 1985;103:880–3.
172. Cooper DA, Gold J, Maclean P, et al. Acute AIDS retrovirus infection. Definition of a clinical illness associated with seroconversion. Lancet. 1985;1:537–40.
172a. Tindall B, Barker S, Donovan B, et al. Characterization of the acute clinical illness associated with human immunodeficiency virus infection. Arch Intern Med. 1988;148:945–9.
173. Pedersen C, Gerstoft J, Lindhardt BO, et al. *Candida* esophagitis associated with acute human immunodeficiency virus infection (Letter). J Infect Dis. 1987;156:529–30.
174. Ward JW, Deppe D, Perkins H, et al. Risk of disease in recipients of blood from donors later found infected with human immunodeficiency virus (HIV) (Abstract). In: Proceedings of the Third International Conference on AIDS, June 1–5, 1987. Washington, DC: The U.S. Department of Health and Human Services and the WHO; 1987:2.
175. Allain J-P, Laurian Y, Paul DA, et al. Serological markers in early stages of human immunodeficiency virus infection in haemophiliacs. Lancet. 1986;2:1233–6.
176. Gaines H, von Sydow M, Sonnerborg A, et al. Antibody response in primary human immunodeficiency virus infection. Lancet. 1987;1:1249–53.
176a. Simmonds P, Lainson FAL, Cuthbert R, et al. HIV antigen and antibody detection: Variable responses to infection in the Edinburgh haemophiliac cohort. Br Med J. 1988;296:593–8.
176b. Ward JW, Schable C, Dickinson GM, et al. Acute human immunodeficiency virus (HIV) infection: Antigen detection and seroconversion in immunosuppressed patients. Transplantation. In press.
177. Jaffe HW, Feorino PM, Darrow WW, et al. Persistent infection with human T-lymphotropic virus type III/lymphadenopathy-associated virus in apparently healthy homosexual men. Ann Intern Med. 1985;102:627–8.
178. Farzadegan H, Polis MA, Wolinsky SM, et al. Loss of human immunodeficiency virus type 1 (HIV-1) antibodies with evidence of viral infection in asymptomatic homosexual men. A report from the Multicenter AIDS Cohort Study. Ann Intern Med. 1988;108:785–90.
179. Hessol NA, Rutherford GW, Lifson AR, et al. The natural history of HIV infection in a cohort of homosexual and bisexual men: A decade of follow-up (Abstract). In: Proceedings of the Fourth International Conference on AIDS, Book 1, June 12–16, 1988. Stockholm: The Swedish Ministry of Health and Social Affairs; 1988:283.
180. Lifson AR, Rutherford GW, Jaffe HW. The natural history of human immunodeficiency virus infection. J Infect Dis. 1988;158:1360–7.
181. Eyster ME, Goedert JJ. Predictive value of T4 cell count and HIV antigen in antibody positive hemophiliacs (Abstract). In: Proceedings of the Fourth International Conference on AIDS, Book 2, June 12–16, 1988. Stockholm: The Swedish Ministry of Health and Social Affairs; 1988:365.
181a. Jason J, Lui K-J, Ragni MV, et al. Risk of developing AIDS in HIV-infected cohorts of hemophilic and homosexual men. JAMA. In press.
182. Ward J, Perkins H, Pepkowitz S, et al. Dose response or strain variation may influence disease progression in HIV-infected blood recipients (Abstract). In: Proceedings of the Fourth International Conference on AIDS, Book 2, June 12–16, 1988. Stockholm: The Swedish Ministry of Health and Social Affairs; 1988:352.
183. Medley GF, Anderson RM, Cox DR, et al. Incubation period of AIDS in patients infected via blood transfusion. Nature. 1987;328:719–21.
183a. Lui K-J, Darrow WW, Rutherford GW III. A model-based estimate of the mean incubation period for AIDS in homosexual men. Science. 1988; 240:1333–5.
184. Lui K-J, Peterman TA, Lawrence DN, et al. A model-based approach to characterize the incubation period of paediatric transfusion-associated acquired immunodeficiency syndrome. Stat Med. 1988;7:395–401.
185. Human immunodeficiency virus infection in the United States: A review of current knowledge. MMWR. 1987;36(Suppl 6):1–48.
185a. Trends in human immunodeficiency virus infection among civilian applicants for military service—United States, October 1985–March 1988. MMWR. 1988;37:677–9.
186. Darrow WW, Cohen JB, French J, et al. Multicenter study of HIV antibody in U.S. prostitutes (Abstract). In: Proceedings of the Third International Conference on AIDS, June 1–5, 1987. Washington, DC: The U.S. Department of Health and Human Services and the WHO; 1987:105.
187. Fischl MA, Dickinson GM, Flanagan S, et al. Human immunodeficiency virus (HIV) among female prostitutes in south Florida (Abstract). In: Proceedings of the Third International Conference on AIDS, June 1–5, 1987. Washington, DC: The U.S. Department of Health and Human Services and the WHO; 1987:105.
188. Quinn TC, Glasser D, Cannon RO, et al. Human immunodeficiency virus infection among patients attending clinics for sexually transmitted diseases. N Engl J Med. 1988;318:197–203.
189. Stoneburner RL, Chiasson MA, Lifson AR, et al. HIV-1 infection in persons attending a sexually transmitted disease clinic in New York City (Abstract). In: Proceedings of the Fourth International Conference on AIDS, Book 1, June 12–16, 1988. Stockholm: The Swedish Ministry of Health and Social Affairs; 1988:377.
190. Judson FN, Douglas J, Cohn D. HIV seroprevalence in heterosexual men and women, Denver Metro STD Clinic, 1985–1987 (Abstract). In: Proceedings of the Fourth International Conference on AIDS, Book 1, June 12–16, 1988. Stockholm: The Swedish Ministry of Health and Social Affairs; 1988:263.
191. Landesman S, Minkoff H, Holman S, et al. Serosurvey of human immunodeficiency virus infection in parturients. Implications for human immunodeficiency virus testing programs of pregnant women. JAMA. 1987;258:2701–3.
192. Dondero TJ Jr, Pappaioanou M, Curran JW. Monitoring the levels and trends of HIV infection: The Public Health Service's HIV surveillance program. Public Health Rep. 1988;103:213–20.
193. Hoff R, Berardi VP, Weiblen BJ, et al. Seroprevalence of human immunodeficiency virus among childbearing women. Estimation by testing samples of blood from newborns. N Engl J Med. 1988;318:525–30.
194. Quarterly report to the Domestic Policy Council on the prevalence and rate of spread of HIV and AIDS in the United States. MMWR. 1988;37:223–6.
195. Update: Acquired immunodeficiency syndrome—Europe. MMWR. 1984;33:607–9.
196. Clumeck N, Sonnet, J, Taelman H, et al. Acquired immunodeficiency syndrome in African patients. N Engl J Med 1984;310:492–7.
197. Van de Perre P, Rouvroy D, Lepage P, et al. Acquired immunodeficiency syndrome in Rwanda. Lancet. 1984;2:62–5.
198. Nahmias AJ, Weiss J, Yao X, et al. Evidence for human infection with an HTLV III/LAV-like virus in central Africa, 1959 (Letter). Lancet. 1986;1:1279–80.
199. Epstein JS, Moffitt AL, Mayner RE, et al. Antibodies reactive with HTLV-III found in freezer-banked sera from children in West Africa (Abstract). In Proceedings and abstracts of the 25th Interscience Conference on Antimicrobial Agents and Chemotherapy, September 29–October 1, 1985. Minneapolis: The American Society for Microbiology; 1985:130.
200. Huminer D, Rosenfeld JB, Pitlik SD. AIDS in the pre-AIDS era. Rev Infect Dis. 1987;9:1102–8.
201. Bayley AC. Aggressive Kaposi's sarcoma in Zambia, 1983. Lancet. 1984;1:1318–20.
202. Serwadda D, Mugerwa RD, Sewankambo NK, et al. Slim disease: A new disease in Uganda and its association with HTLV-III infection. Lancet. 1985;2:849–52.
203. World Health Organization. Acquired immunodeficiency syndrome (AIDS)—data as at 31 May 1988. Weekly Epidemiol Rec. 1988;63:173–4.
204. Piot P, Plummer FA, Mhalu FS, et al. AIDS: An international perspective. Science. 1988;239:573–9.
205. Holmberg SD, Curran JW. The epidemiology of HIV infection in industrialized nations. In: Holmes KK, Mardh P-A, Sparling PF, et al., eds. Sexually Transmitted Diseases. 2nd ed. New York: McGraw-Hill; In press.
206. Mann JM, Francis H, Davachi F, et al. Risk factors for human immunodeficiency virus seropositivity among children 1–24 months old in Kinshasa, Zaire. Lancet. 1986;2:654–7.
207. Francis H, Lubaki N, Duma MP, et al. Immunologic profiles of mothers in perinatal transmission of HIV infection (Abstract). In: Proceedings of the Third International Conference on AIDS, June 1–5, 1987. Washington, DC: The U.S. Department of Health and Human Services and the WHO; 1987:214.
208. Braddick M, Kreiss J, Embree J, et al. Vertical transmission of HIV in Nairobi (Abstract). In Proceedings of the Fourth International Conference on AIDS, Book 1, June 12–16, 1988. Stockholm: The Swedish Ministry of Health and Social Affairs; 1988:346.
209. N'Galy B, Ryder R, Bila K, et al. Human immunodeficiency virus infection among employees in an African hospital. N Engl J Med. 1988;319: 1123–7.

210. Hrdy DB. Cultural practices contributing to the transmission of human immunodeficiency virus in Africa. Rev Infect Dis. 1987;9:1109–19.
211. Guyader M, Emerman M, Sonigo P, et al. Genome organization and transactivation of the human immunodeficiency virus type 2. Nature. 1987;326:662–9.
212. Denis F, Leonard G, Mounier M, et al. Efficacy of five enzyme immunoassays for antibody to HIV in detecting to HTLV-IV (Letter). Lancet. 1987;1:324–5.
213. AIDS due to HIV-2 infection—New Jersey. MMWR. 1988;37:33–5.
214. Foucault C, Lopez O, Jourdan G, et al. Double HIV-1 and HIV-2 seropositivity among blood donors (Letter). Lancet. 1987;2:165–6.
215. Brun-Vezinet F, Rey MA, Katlama C, et al. Lymphadenopathy-associated virus type 2 in AIDS and AIDS-related complex. Clinical and virological features in four patients. Lancet. 1987;1:128–32.
216. Clavel F, Mansinho K, Chamaret S, et al. Human immunodeficiency virus type 2 infection associated with AIDS in West Africa. N Engl J Med. 1987;316:1180–5.
217. Horsburgh CR Jr, Holmberg SD. The global distribution of human immunodeficiency virus type 2 (HIV-2) infection. Transfusion. 1988;28:192–5.
218. Francis DP, Chin J. The prevention of acquired immunodeficiency syndrome in the United States. An objective strategy for medicine, public health, business, and the community. JAMA. 1987;257:1357–66.
219. Allen JR, Curran JW. Prevention of AIDS and HIV infection: Needs and priorities for epidemiologic research. Am J Public Health. 1988;78:381–6.
220. Additional recommendations to reduce sexual and drug abuse-related transmission of human T-lymphotropic virus type III/lymphadenopathy-associated virus. MMWR. 1986;35:152–5.
221. Condoms for prevention of sexually transmitted diseases. MMWR. 1988;37:133–7.
222. Mann J, Quinn TC, Piot P, et al. Condom use and HIV infection among prostitutes in Zaire (Letter). N Engl J Med. 1987;316:345.
223. Self-reported changes in sexual behaviors among homosexual and bisexual men from the San Francisco City Clinic Cohort. MMWR. 1987;36:187–9.
224. Martin JL. The impact of AIDS on gay male sexual behavior patterns in New York City. Am J Public Health. 1987;77:578–81.
225. Declining rates of rectal and pharyngeal gonorrhea among males—New York City. MMWR. 1984;33:295–7.
226. Winkelstein W Jr, Samuel M, Padian NS, et al. The San Francisco Men's Health Study: III. Reduction in human immunodeficiency virus transmission among homosexual/bisexual men, 1982–86. Am J Public Health. 1987; 77:685–9.
226a. Winkelstein W Jr, Wiley JA, Padian NS, et al. The San Francisco Men's Health Study: Continued decline in HIV seroconversion rates among homosexual/bisexual men. Am J Public Health. 1988;78:1472–4.
227. Positive HTLV-III/LAV antibody results from sexually active female members of social/sexual clubs—Minnesota. MMWR. 1986;35;697–9.
228. HIV infection and pregnancies in sexual partners of HIV-seropositive hemophilic men—United States. MMWR. 1987;36:593–5.
229. Prevention of acquired immune deficiency syndrome (AIDS): Report of inter-agency recommendations. MMWR. 1983;32:101–3.
230. Provisional Public Health Service inter-agency recommendations for screening donated blood and plasma for antibody to the virus causing acquired immunodeficiency syndrome. MMWR. 1985;34:1–5.
231. Update: Revised Public Health Service definition of persons who should refrain from donating blood and plasma—United States. MMWR. 1985;34:547–8.
232. Ward JW, Grindon AJ, Feorino PM, et al. Laboratory and epidemiologic evaluation of an enzyme immunoassay for antibodies to HTLV-III. JAMA. 1986;256:357–61.
233. Zuck TF. Greetings—a final look back with comments about a policy of a zero-risk blood supply (Editorial). Transfusion. 1987;27:447–8.
234. Grindon A. Efficacy of voluntary self-deferral of donors at high risk of AIDS (Abstract). Transfusion. 1984;24:434.
235. Rabkin CS, Van Devanter N, Ewing WE, et al. Risk factors for antibody to HIV in New York blood donors: Validation of AIDS risk classification and of confidential donor self-exclusion at the time of donation (Abstract). In: Proceedings of the Third International Conference on AIDS, June 1–5, 1987. Washington, DC: The U.S. Department of Health and Human Services and the WHO; 1987:103.
236. Ward JW, Kleinman JH, Douglas DK, et al. Epidemiologic characteristics of blood donors with antibody to human immunodeficiency virus. Transfusion. 1988;28:298–301.
237. Des Jarlais DC, Friedman SR. Editorial review. HIV infection among intravenous drug users: Epidemiology and risk reduction. AIDS. 1987;1:67–76.
238. Report of the Presidential Commission on the Human Immunodeficiency Virus Epidemic. Submitted to the President of the United States, June 24, 1988. Washington, DC: U.S. Government Printing Office; 1988:1–201.
239. Des Jarlais DC, Friedman SR, Hopkins W. Risk reduction for the acquired immunodeficiency syndrome among intravenous drug users. Ann Intern Med. 1985;103:755–9.
240. Public Health Service guidelines for counseling and antibody testing to prevent HIV infection and AIDS. MMWR. 1987;36:509–15.
241. Scott GB, Fischl MA, Klimas N, et al. Mothers of infants with the acquired immunodeficiency syndrome. Evidence for both symptomatic and asymptomatic carriers. JAMA. 1985;253:363–6.
242. Minkoff HL. Care of pregnant women infected with human immunodeficiency virus. JAMA. 1987;258:2714–7.
243. Recommendations for assisting in the prevention of perinatal transmission of human T-lymphotropic virus type III/lymphadenopathy-associated virus and acquired immunodeficiency syndrome. MMWR. 1985;34:721–6,731–2.
244. World Health Organization. Breast-feeding/breast milk and human immunodeficiency virus (HIV). Weekly Epidemiol Rec. 1987;62:245–6.
245. Oxtoby MJ. Breast milk and human immunodeficiency virus: placing the issues in broader perspective. Pediatr Infect Dis J. 1988;7:825–35.
246. Abraham L. AIDS contact tracing, prison testing stir debate. American Medical News 1988 July 8/15:4.
247. Coates TJ, Morin SF, McKusick L. Behavioral consequences of AIDS antibody testing among gay men (Letter). JAMA. 1987;258:1889.
248. McCusker J, Stoddard AM, Mayer KH, et al. Effects of HIV antibody test knowledge on subsequent sexual behaviors in a cohort of homosexually active men. Am J Public Health. 1988;78:462–7.
249. Casadonte PP, Des Jarlais D, Smith T, et al. Psychological and behavioral impact of learning HTLV-III/LAV antibody test results (Abstract). In: Proceedings of the International Conference on AIDS, June 23–25, 1986. Paris: L'Association pour la Recherche sur les Déficits Immunitaire Viro-Induits (ARDIVI); 1986.163.

107. IMMUNOLOGY OF AIDS AND HIV INFECTION

MARGARET A. HAMBURG
SCOTT KOENIG
ANTHONY S. FAUCI

A remarkable recent development in the field of infectious diseases has been the relatively sudden appearance and rapid spread of the acquired immune deficiency syndrome (AIDS). Infection with the human immunodeficiency virus (HIV), the etiologic agent of AIDS, results in a wide range of immunologic abnormalities involving a variety of immunopathogenic mechanisms. While patients with AIDS may share certain laboratory and clinical features in common with other disorders caused by defects in the immune system—particularly those with primary immunodeficiencies such as the severe combined immunodeficiencies (SCID)—the pathophysiology and spectrum of clinical manifestations associated with HIV infection and AIDS is quite unique.[1–6]

HIV infection can occur through sexual contact, infected blood, or blood products, and from mother to infant. The clinical syndrome of AIDS follows infection with HIV after a variable, often prolonged, period of time. Although multiple components of the immune system are at least indirectly affected in individuals with HIV infection, it is the impairment of T-cell mediated responses that appears to produce the most significant clinical consequences. Because the T4 cell is pivotally involved in virtually all immune responses, a major host defense defect results from T4 cell depletion and renders the body highly susceptible to "opportunistic" infections and unusual neoplasms.[1–9] Moreover, the pathogens for these opportunistic infections may alter immune function independent of HIV.[10] The long and variable latent period from initial infection to symptomatic disease is a demonstration of the fact that despite rapid cytopathicity of HIV for T lymphocytes in vitro,[11,12] the virus can persist in cells in a state of low-level or latent infection for prolonged periods in vivo. In addition, it has been demonstrated that cells of the monocyte/macrophage lineage, including bone marrow precursor cells, can be infected without cyytopathic effects and may serve as a reservoir for HIV in the body.[13] HIV also has a tropism for the brain leading to neuropsychiatric abnormalities. While components of the host immune system respond to infection with HIV, these responses appear to be minimally protective against HIV infection or disease progression.

This chapter will examine these characteristics of HIV infection and the range of mechanisms—many of which remain to be fully elucidated—whereby HIV relentlessly compromises and ultimately destroys the immune system and produces central nervous system disease.

THE ETIOLOGIC AGENT

In order to understand the pathogenic mechanisms and immune response to HIV infection, it is important to examine the infectious agent (see also Chapter 147). HIV is an RNA retrovirus belonging to the lentivirus family.[14–16] Two major forms of HIV have been described in humans, HIV-1[17–20] and HIV-2.[21–25] HIV-1 is the more common form and has been studied fairly extensively. Most current knowledge regarding immunologic changes associated with AIDS has derived from studies of individuals infected with HIV-1, which is widely disseminated throughout the world. HIV-2 shares serologic reactivity and polynucleotide sequence homology with simian immunodeficiency virus (SIV),[22,26] which produces disease in a limited number of simian species.

The HIV Genome

As visualized by electron microscopy, the mature virion has a dense cylindrical core that encases two molecules of the viral RNA (see also Chapter 147). A spherical lipid envelope, acquired as the virion buds from the surface of an infected cell, surrounds the central core. The HIV proviral genome measures approximately 10 kilobases in length.[27] It consists of three structural genes, *gag, pol*, and *env*, located between shorter segments called long terminal repeat (LTR) sequences. The *gag* gene codes for components of the viral core, *pol* codes for the viral enzymes involved in replication (reverse transcriptase, a protease, and integrase), and *env* codes for the internal and external envelope proteins. Adjacent to or within the LTR segments are the genes coding for the regulatory proteins required for HIV replication. Other genes identified in the HIV-1 genome include *tat* (transactivator), *rev* (regulator of expression of virion proteins), *vif* (virion infectivity factor), *nef* (negative factor), *vpr* (viral protein R), and *vpu* (viral protein U).[28] The expression of these genes has significant impact on the immunopathogenic mechanisms of the virus.

IMMUNOPATHOGENIC MECHANISMS OF HIV INFECTION

It has been clearly established that infection with HIV results in selective defects in immune function. The most prominent feature of the immunopathogenesis of HIV infection–AIDS is depletion of the T4 (helper–inducer) subset of T lymphocytes. Multiple other arms of the immune system are at least indirectly affected, and a wide spectrum of immunologic abnormalities has been observed to accompany HIV infection.

HIV and CD4 as Receptor

From an immunopathogenic perspective, a critical structural feature of HIV appears to be the outer envelope. It has been well documented that the glycoprotein portion, gp120, interacts avidly and specifically with the CD4 molecule, which is expressed predominantly on the T4 cells and acts as a high-affinity receptor for HIV.[12,29,30] In fact, the gp120 portion of HIV has the capability of specifically binding to the CD4 molecule with an affinity that is greater than that for the CD4 molecule's natural ligand, the class II major histocompatibility complex (MHC) molecule.[12,29,30] In vitro studies have demonstrated that monoclonal antibodies to the CD4 molecule could prevent infection.[12,29] Furthermore, certain epitopes of the CD4 molecule appear more essential to viral binding.[31] In one study, various antibodies to CD4 manifested differential capacities for blocking infection.[31] In a more recent report, synthetic CD4 peptide fragments were used as competitive blockers and demonstrated markedly different abilities to inhibit HIV infection and cytopathicity.[32]

A number of other experiments have also shown convincingly that the initial step in HIV infection is the binding of the virus to a cellular receptor such as the CD4 molecule. One such demonstration comes from studies in which cells from the human HELA line were transfected with the cloned CD4 gene, resulting in the expression of the CD4 protein and consequent susceptibility to infection by HIV.[33] By contrast, murine cells made to express the human CD4 molecule could not be infected with HIV. Nonetheless, those cells could support HIV replication following transfection with the HIV genome, suggesting that other mechanisms may facilitate HIV entry. Some researchers have proposed that the HLA-DR molecule may provide another receptor mechanism for HIV entry into cells. In this regard, it has been shown that HLA-DR expression decreases transiently after viral exposure. This occurs in association with a more persistent decline in CD4 expression from those same cells.[34] Further study is currently being directed at the characterization of the role of HLA-DR in the infective process.

Since the binding of the virus to a cellular receptor is a crucial step in HIV infection, virtually any cell expressing the CD4 surface molecule may be a target for infection. In addition to the T4 cell, which represents a major target cell for HIV infection, cells of the monocyte–macrophage lineage and others are capable of binding and becoming infected with HIV.[35–40] After binding to the CD4 molecule, the virus is internalized, uncoated, and, through the action of viral reverse transcriptase, the virion RNA is transcribed into DNA. This can then exist either in an unintegrated form or as a provirus integrated into the cellular DNA. Following integration of provirus, the infection may enter a latent phase within the host cell until cellular activation occurs. Once the infected cell is activated, the proviral DNA transcribes viral genomic RNA and messenger RNA. Subsequent protein synthesis, processing, and viral assembly leads ultimately to the budding of the mature virion from the surface of the cell[41] (Fig. 1).

T-Cell Abnormalities

One of the earliest laboratory abnormalities recognized in AIDS patients was a striking depletion of T4 lymphocytes, characterized not only by an overall reduction in lymphocyte numbers, but also a marked alteration in the ratio of T4 to T8 cells in the circulating T-lymphocyte pool.[1] This depression of the T4/T8 ratio and depletion of the T4 population correlates to some degree with severity of disease, particularly at the extremes of the spectrum. HIV-infected but asymptomatic individuals tend to have higher T4 counts than patients with frank disease.[42] Although not absolute, low T4 cell counts (less than 200/mm^3) in HIV-seropositive individuals often portends imminent development of full-blown AIDS with an opportunistic infection.[43–45] However, there is marked variation in the rate of depletion of T4 cells among HIV-infected individuals. Following an initial drop in number, many individuals maintain relatively normal or slightly lower than normal levels of T4 cells for prolonged periods of time, often followed by a precipitous decline. The rapid fall in T4 cells may coincide with notable increases in circulating p24 antigen (Lane HC, unpublished data.) Other patients may experience a continual, progressive decline in CD4+ cells, with a rapid and unfavorable clinical course.[46,47] A recent study indicates that virulence of HIV may increase in the later stages of disease progression.[48]

Alterations in the numbers of CD8+, or suppressor T cells,

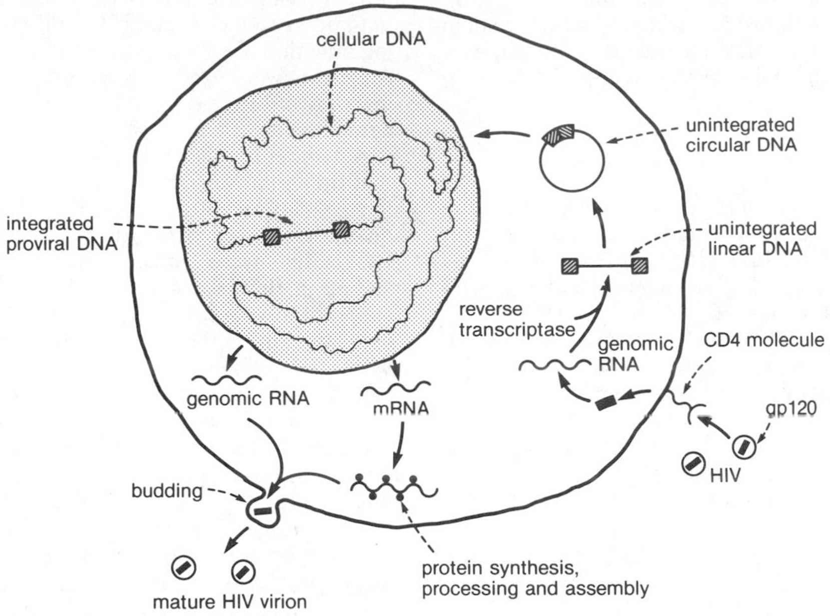

FIG. 1. Schematic diagram of the life cycle of HIV. (From Fauci,[41] with permission.)

have also been noted with HIV infection. Early in the course of HIV infection, many healthy HIV-seropositive individuals, as well as those with lymphadenopathy syndromes, were found to have measurable increases in CD8+ cells. Expansion of the CD8+ cell population may reflect the instigation of cytotoxic responses against HIV or other pathogens. An alternative explanation is that CD8+ suppressor cells may be stimulated to down-modulate other immune responses, such as the polyclonal activation of B cells found in seropositive patients. Interestingly, it has been observed that HIV can be more easily isolated from peripheral blood cultures of seropositive individuals if the CD8+ cells were removed; addition of the CD8+ cells back into the culture suppressed HIV propagation.[49] Although conclusive evidence is lacking, it would seem likely that the CD8+ population may act, at least in part, to suppress HIV replication in vivo, even in symptomatic patients.

Later in the course of disease, AIDS patients with opportunistic infection are often depleted of virtually all lymphoid cells, including the CD8+ population.[42] The mechanism for this depletion remains to be clarified.

Cytopathic Mechanisms of T4 Cell Depletion. The mechanisms by which HIV actually destroys the cells it infects remain unknown. Compared with most other retroviruses, an unusual feature of HIV infection is the accumulation of large amounts of unintegrated viral DNA in the infected cells.[50] When such a phenomenon does occur in other retroviral systems, it is generally associated with a significant cytopathic effect.[50] Such a process has been proposed to be responsible for the cytopathic effects of HIV, although no experimental evidence has yet to directly implicate the finding of unintegrated viral DNA in HIV cytotoxicity.

Another proposed mechanism for the cytopathic effect of HIV on CD4+ cells is the production and budding off from the cell surface of large amounts of virus with a resulting massive increase in cell membrane permeability and eventual cell lysis.[50a] Others have suggested that the cytopathic effects of HIV are a function of the density of the CD4 molecule on the surface of cells. This was proposed in conjunction with the observation that the cell lines with the highest CD4 density appeared to be the most susceptible to cell death. It was speculated that complexing of CD4 with the envelope protein of HIV in the cytoplasm might be cytopathic for cells.[51,52] Such a hypothesis, however, is not supported by recent evidence that there are marked cytopathic effects of HIV even in cell lines that express only modest amounts of CD4 on their surface membrane (Rabson AB, unpublished data). A potentially important mode of T-cell destruction studied in vitro involves syncytia formation. Following HIV infection of CD4+ cells and integration of the viral genome, the HIV envelope glycoprotein is expressed on the surface of the cell. Uninfected T4 cells, with CD4 molecules on their surface that can serve as potential receptors for the virus or for envelope proteins, may bind to those infected cells and lead to the formation of multinucleated giant cells (syncytia)[53–56] (Fig. 2). Multinucleated giant cells have been observed in lymph nodes[57] and brain specimens[58] from HIV-infected patients, but it is uncertain whether they form as result of cell fusion. While syncytia formation has been proposed as a mechanism of HIV cytopathicity in vivo, there is considerable debate as to whether or not it plays a major role.

In addition to the possible direct cytopathic effects of HIV discussed above, other indirect mechanisms almost certainly contribute to the depletion of T4 lymphocytes in vivo. Immune-mediated responses may play an important role.[59,60] For example, HIV-infected cells expressing viral antigens on their surface may be eliminated by HLA-restricted and -unrestricted cytotoxic cells as part of routine immune surveillance. Arguing somewhat against this explanation, the use of fluoresceinated antibodies against viral encoded proteins and in situ hybridization techniques to detect cells expressing viral proteins or mRNA has demonstrated that only an extremely small percentage (perhaps 1 in 100,000) of T4 cells in the peripheral blood of HIV-infected individuals expresses viral proteins at any given time.[61] Given the normal turnover of T lymphocytes in the body, it would seem possible for the T-cell pool to compensate for such a seemingly low rate of destruction.[41] However, impaired maturation of stem cells coupled with progressive depletion may make this proposal feasible (see below). Also, if a large proportion of cells is latently infected, significant cell losses could occur due to viral persistence, reactivation of latent virus, and progressive dissemination to uninfected cells over time. The development of the polymerase chain reaction

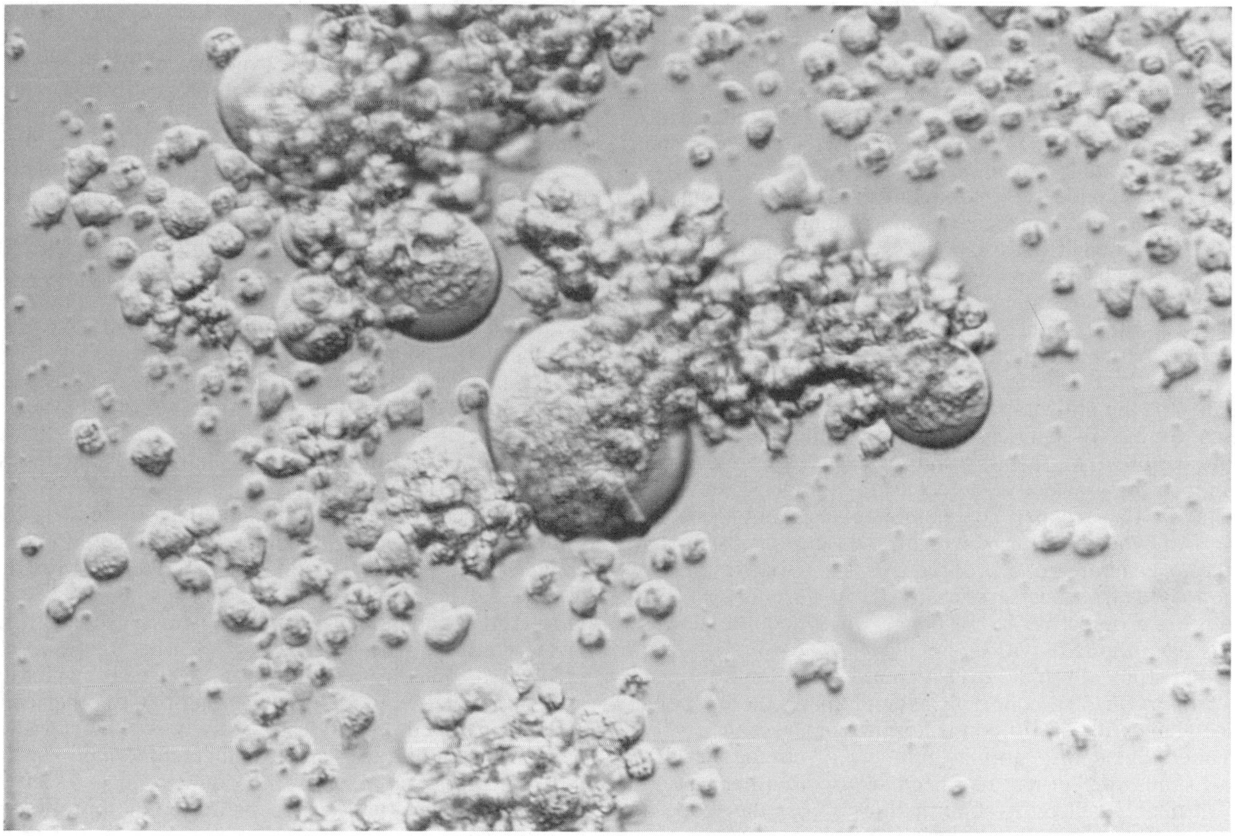

FIG. 2. Light micrograph of syncytia formation between HIV-infected cells and uninfected CD4+ cells. (Courtesy of Dr. Cecil Fox, Bethesda, MD.)

(PCR) technique—a selective DNA amplification approach that enables direct detection of exceedingly small amounts of proviral DNA—may help shed new light on this area.[62]

Additional mechanisms underlying lymphodepletion may involve concomitant failure of hematopoietic organs to produce mature cells. For example, HIV might infect a T4 cell precursor or stem cell, leading to an inability to regenerate depleted lymphocytes. In this regard, it has been demonstrated that AIDS patients have a decreased capacity to generate T-cell colonies.[63] Furthermore, colony formation of granulocytes–macrophages (CFU-GM) and erythrocytes (BFU-E) from bone marrow of AIDS patients is inhibited when cultured in the presence of their sera. It is possible to isolate HIV from some of those cultures.[64]

Recent studies indicate that HIV can infect certain bone marrow cells. These infectible cells belong to the myelomonocytic cell lineage that develops into monocytes–macrophages. These studies found that HIV can propagate and remain within those bone marrow cells. Thus these cells may represent important reservoirs of HIV in the body.[13]

Emerging evidence suggests that autoimmune phenomena may be partially responsible for the cytopathic effects and T4 cell depletion associated with HIV infection. An autoimmune process may be induced through the interaction of the CD4 molecule with HIV envelope proteins; the binding of free HIV envelope proteins to the CD4 molecule on uninfected cells may result in the immune system responding to these cells as nonself,[65] with consequent elimination by immune clearance or by antibody-dependent cellular toxicity (ADCC).[66] Another autoimmune theory involves immune system clearance of cells bearing the class II MHC molecule.[60] This theory derives from the fact that the CD4 molecule on the T4 cell recognizes and binds a portion of the class II MHC molecule. Because the HIV envelope binds to the CD4 molecule as well, it may mimic the configuration of a portion of the class II MHC antigen. It is conceivable that an immune response—either antibodies or cytotoxic lymphocytes—directed against the envelope proteins may result in a cross-reactive response against class II MHC-bearing cells as well as an anti-idiotypic response against cells expressing CD4.[60] Recent data indicate that T4 cells can process and present antigens, such as gp120, in conjunction with class II MHC molecules in a CD4-mediated process. Thus CD4+ T cells may be targeted for destruction by gp120-specific cytotoxic cells via a CD4-dependent autocytolytic mechanism.[67,68] To what degree, if any, such phenomena play a role in the cytopathicity of HIV infection is unclear at present.

Functional Impairment of CD4+ Lymphocytes. Although quantitative depletion of CD4+ lymphocytes is the most prominent immunologic abnormality in HIV-infected individuals, there is growing evidence that HIV can cause a qualitative or functional impairment of immune cells in the absence of a cytopathic effect. Unfractionated peripheral blood mononuclear cells (PBMC) from AIDS patients manifest profound decreases in responses to mitogens, alloantigens, and soluble antigens.[69–71] The degree of these functional changes is variable, but depression of T-cell function appears more pronounced in AIDS patients with opportunistic infections than in individuals with other HIV-related conditions.[42]

When unfractionated PBMC from uninfected individuals and from AIDS patients were stimulated with common mitogens such as pokeweed, concanavalin A (con A), and phytohemagglutinin (PHA), the cells from AIDS patients consistently demonstrated a diminution of response. Depresssed mitogenic responses by PBMC of AIDS patients could be restored by increasing the absolute number of CD4+ lymphocytes so that cultures from both control and AIDS patients contained equivalent numbers of such cells.[70,72] This indicates that this functional T-cell defect is intimately related to the depletion of CD4 cells. By contrast, reconstituting PBMC from AIDS patients to normal proportions of CD4 cells did not result in the restoration of an absent response to tetanus toxoid (TT) antigen, suggesting that antigen-responsive CD4 cells are either selectively depleted or, in fact, functionally impaired.

Evidence for a selective impairment in antigen responsiveness during HIV infection comes from a number of sources. Cutaneous hypersensitivity responses, which depend on the subset of CD4 cells that recognizes and responds to soluble antigen, are selectively deficient in AIDS patients.[69] Correspondingly, purified populations of these CD4 lymphocytes from AIDS patients also do not proliferate normally to soluble antigen in vitro.[69] This defect does not appear to be due to an abnormality of the antigen-presenting cells necessary for such responses. Studies of identical twins, in which one sibling had AIDS and the other was healthy and seronegative, provide further evidence for a selective defect in the antigen-responsive CD4 cells. In these experiments, monocytes from the seronegative twin, when cocultured with his own autologous T cells, were able to generate good proliferative TT responses. However, monocytes from the seronegative twin were incapable of reconstituting a defective TT response when cocultured with CD4 cells from the twin with AIDS.[73]

In another study of proliferative responses to soluble antigen, a large proportion of a cohort of asymptomatic, seropositive homosexual men demonstrated the absence of a response to TT even in individuals with normal numbers of circulating CD4 cells.[73] A similar defect has also been seen with other test antigens,[74] probably reflecting abnormalities across the scope of the antigen-specific T-cell repertoire. If this loss of responsiveness simply reflected the depletion of antigen-responsive cells, one would expect a cumulative quantitative loss of most of the CD4 cells, which was not the case. This finding strongly supports the contribution of a functional impairment of CD4 lymphocytes in the abnormal antigen responses. Because the decreased response to soluble antigen appears early in the course of HIV infection, even in those individuals with total lymphocyte numbers above 1000 cells/mm^3,[69] a functional impairment of T4 cells may represent a critical initial step in the progressive immune defects seen with HIV infection.

There is evidence of functional abnormalities of T4 cells caused by exposure to HIV without the development of a productive or cytopathic infection. In one series of experiments, exposure of PBMC stimulated in vitro with a soluble antigen to noncytopathic concentrations of HIV resulted in a marked inhibition of response to soluble antigen and a lesser inhibition of mitogen response.[75] Other studies have shown that certain purified subunits of HIV, particularly gp120 envelope protein, could inhibit antigen-specific responses when exposed to lymphocytes, even though they would be incapable of producing infection.[76]

Several potential mechanisms could explain this impairment of T4 cell function by exposure to HIV, but not actual infection of the cell. Antigen-specific responses of T4 cells require the interaction of the CD4 molecule expressed on the surface of the T4 cell with the class II MHC molecule of the antigen-presenting cell as part of the presentation of processed antigen to the CD3-Ti antigen receptor complex on the T4 cell.[77] It is conceivable that since the HIV envelope binds avidly to the CD4 molecule on the T4 cell,[12,29,30] this could interfere with the normal interaction of the CD4 molecule with the class II MHC molecule on the antigen-presenting cell.[77,78] Responses of T4 cells to mitogens are not critically dependent on the CD4–class II MHC molecule interaction.[73] The cellular activation pathway of mitogen stimulation could bypass this step, inducing an essentially normal proliferative response in cells rendered refractory to antigenic stimulation. This would be consistent with the observations noted earlier of normal mitogen responses under certain circumstances in which a selective defect in antigen responses is seen.[69]

Another hypothesis is that exposure of T cells to HIV or its products might cause a postreceptor signal transduction defect that mitogen, but not antigen, can at least partially override. Since the triggering of cells by soluble antigens and mitogens occurs through different pathways,[79] it is possible that the virus-induced block in T-cell function occurs following ligand binding to the CD4 molecule and may offer an explanation of the discrepancy between suppression of antigen responses as opposed to mitogen responses.[69] It has recently been observed that HIV-infected T cells have a defect in the calcium mobilization necessary for activation when stimulated through the CD3-Ti complex but not through the CD2 pathway.[80]

IL-2 has an important role in the generation of T-cell activation and response. A functional defect in IL-2 gene expression may contribute to the antigen-specific defect that requires IL-2 for amplification of response in cells displaying a noncytopathic infection with HIV.[41]

In addition to the deficiencies noted in proliferative responses to antigen, AIDS patients demonstrate impaired cytotoxic responses. For instance, depressed HLA class I-restricted cytotoxic T-lymphocyte (CTL) responses against cytomegalovirus (CMV) and influenza have been observed in patients early in the course of their disease.[74,81–83] This depressed function involves responses mediated by CD8+ cells, which typically are not infected with HIV, suggesting that another component must be involved. Class I CTL activity is characteristically dependent on the intact T4-cell inducer function. The observed impairment of this response no doubt reflects T-cell dysfunction. This implies that the reconstitution of appropriate T4 cell function should ameliorate this cytotoxic defect if the effector function of CD8+ cells is intact. Supporting this notion, in vitro T-cell-mediated cytotoxicity to CMV was restored with the addition of IL-2, possibly by bypassing the usual CD4+ inductive signals.[84] Correspondingly, CD8+ cytotoxic responses against alloantigens appear to be relatively preserved in AIDS patients. CD4+ cells are not considered necessary for induction of those alloreactive responses.[85]

Role of Monocytes–Macrophages

Infection. It is now well established that monocytes and macrophages can be infected with HIV and thus play an important role in the pathogenesis of HIV infection.[35–40] The virus can infect cells of the monocyte–macrophage lineage through attachment to the CD4 molecule expressed on the surface of certain subsets of the cells, or via phagocytic engulfment.[35–40] Virus can be isolated from these cells in the blood and various organs of HIV-infected individuals.[39,40] An important difference in HIV infection of monocytes–macrophages and T lymphocytes is that the monocyte is relatively refractory to the cytopathic effects of the virus. Not only can the virus survive within cells of the monocyte–macrophage lineage, but it can replicate within the cell. Electron micrographs demonstrate that the replicating virions bud inward into intracytoplasmic vesicles and thus can remain sequestered from immune surveillance by the host.[86] A critical implication of this phenomenon is that the monocyte–macrophage has the potential to harbor the virus and serve as a reservoir of infection in the host. Persistence of HIV infection in monocytes may help to partially explain the inability of an HIV-specific immune response to clear the body of virus. Furthermore, because monocytes–macrophages circulate, these cells may be responsible for disseminating the virus to various parts of the body, including the brain, the lung, and perhaps the bone marrow.

Functional Abnormalities. There is a growing appreciation of the major role played by monocytes–macrophages in the propagation and pathogenesis of HIV infection. The ability of

HIV to infect and persist within cells of the monocyte–macrophage lineage has been well documented, and was discussed above. Although many monocyte activities appear to be preserved in AIDS patients, a number of functional abnormalities of these cells have also been reported, including defective chemotaxis and killing of certain organisms.[87–89] Certain of these abnormalities may reflect direct infection of monocytes by HIV. However, given the relatively low number of infected circulating monocytes, it is more likely that multiple influences are at work. Many of the functional defects observed in monocyte function may reflect deficient inductive signals from CD4 cells. For example, γ-interferon produced by normal CD4 cells is capable of reconstituting certain defective functions of monocytes,[90] although following prolonged courses of intravenous γ-interferon, impaired monocyte respiratory burst activity persists in these AIDS patients.[91]

Chemotaxis is the monocyte function most frequently observed to be impaired in HIV-infected patients,[87,89] but this defect is not necessarily specific for HIV infection, since many patients chronically ill from other viral and malignant disorders also have depressed chemotactic responses. Reports from many studies indicate that a range of functions appears to remain intact in monocytes derived from HIV-infected patients. These include phagocytic activity,[92] ADDC,[89] tumoricidal activity, cytotoxicity against *Toxoplasma gondii* and *Chlamydia psittaci* in response to γ-interferon,[90] and fungicidal activity against *Aspergillus fumigatus, Cryptococcus neoformans*, and *Thermoascus crustaceus*,[92] as well as *Candida*.[93]

Macrophages from AIDS patients also appear to function reasonably well in soluble antigen presentation, in both syngeneic and class II MHC-compatible systems. Minimal abnormalities have been observed in soluble antigen presentation by circulating monocytes in a syngeneic system using highly enriched cell populations derived from healthy identical twins.[73] Similar results have been found by others using class II MHC-compatible presenting cells,[94] although one report indicates decreased expression of class II antigens on monocytes of patients with AIDS.[95] Compared with normal individuals, a higher proportion of HIV-infected lymphadenopathy patients demonstrated a low proliferative response to anti-T3 antibody. This could be augmented by the addition of normal allogeneic macrophages, suggesting a defect of accessory cell function in this T-cell dependent response.[89]

HIV infection may directly and/or indirectly influence secretion of monokines such as IL-1 and tumor necrosis factor (TNF, formerly called cachectin).[41] Although it has generally been felt that IL-1 production and secretion by monocytes was relatively preserved,[96,97] some findings suggest that inhibitors of IL-1 may be present in the circulation of AIDS patients.[97] These issues, and their clinical significance, require further clarification.

Related Pathogenic Effects. HIV INFECTION OF THE BRAIN. It is well established that HIV can cause brain disease, ranging from asymptomatic infection to meningoencephalitis and dementia.[98] Neuropsychiatric manifestations occur to a greater or lesser degree in about 60 percent of HIV-infected patients.[98] Circulating infected monocytes may be responsible for the initiation of infection in the brain. Brain tissue studies demonstrate that the predominant cell type infected with HIV is the monocyte–macrophage.[40]

Pathologic findings from patients with AIDS-related dementia complex suggest several potential indirect mechanisms of brain tissue damage in which infected monocytes–macrophages may play a role. Infected monocytes–macrophages may release chemotactic factors that lead to the infiltration of the brain with inflammatory cells.[98] Alternatively, activated and infected macrophages may release factors toxic for the growth of neurons and may stimulate reactive glial cell growth. Reactive glial cells have been found in intimate contact with macrophages in the brains of AIDS patients.[99] Glial cells, which sometimes express CD4 molecules and under certain circumstances bind virus, may be permissive for HIV replication.[100,101] Infected macrophages may be the primary source of HIV for these cells. However, there is little evidence of infection in neurons, oligodendrocytes, or astrocytes.[40,99]

It has been observed in vitro that the HIV envelope protein can inhibit neuronal growth. A putative nerve growth factor, neuroleukin, has been implicated in this process.[102] One proposed pathogenic mechanism involves a partial sequence homology between HIV gp120 and neuroleukin and suggests that the HIV envelope could compete for binding to the growth factor receptor on neurons[103] and inhibit neuroleukin-induced neuronal growth. Whether infected macrophages in the central nervous system release high concentrations of viral envelope that is inhibitory to neuron growth in vivo is unclear at present.

HIV INFECTION OF BONE MARROW CELLS. HIV-infected individuals manifest a wide range of hematologic abnormalities, including leukopenia, anemia, and thrombocytopenia, as well as myelodysplasia.[104,105] The presence of these hematologic disorders led researchers to examine the possible role of HIV infection of bone marrow progenitor cells; a major obstacle to the study of HIV infection of human bone marrow, however, has been the inability to obtain purified bone marrow precursor cells devoid of mature T lymphocytes. Using a newly developed cell fractionation technique, researchers have been able to show infection in vitro of monocytic progenitor cells with HIV.[13] Virus production in these cells occurs predominantly intracellularly, producing minimal cytopathic effect and displaying intracellular budding of virus particles into cytoplasmic vesicles rather than from the surface of the cell membrane. Electron microscopic analysis reveals that the virus load in these cells can be of such magnitude that, in many instances, entire regions of cytoplasm are replaced with mature virions. The extent to which HIV-infected bone marrow cells contribute to the hematologic abnormalities observed in AIDS patients is uncertain at present.

HIV INFECTION OF OTHER CELL TYPES. Other cell types capable of infection with HIV include Langerhans cells of the skin,[106] endothelial cells,[107] colorectal cells,[108] cervical cells,[109] retinal cells,[110] pulmonary macrophages,[38] and transformed B cells.[111] Some but not all of these cell types have been shown to express CD4 mRNA or protein. The physiologic significance and contribution of HIV infection in these cells to the pathogenesis and clinical manifestations of AIDS remains to be determined.

Other Immunologic Abnormalities

B-Cell Involvement. B-cell function and humoral immunity is markedly abnormal in patients with AIDS. Beyond the consequences of deficient CD4+ T-helper cells in initiating specific antibody production, intrinsic B-cell physiology and activity is abnormal in HIV-infected individuals. AIDS patients characteristically develop polyclonal B-cell activation, manifested by hypergammaglobulinemia, spontaneous B-cell proliferation, and increased spontaneous secretion of immunoglobulin in vitro.[1,2,112–117] In symptomatic individuals, serum levels of IgG, IgA, and IgD are elevated,[112–114,118] with more variable changes noted in IgM. Generally IgM levels appear to be relatively normal in adults with AIDS,[116] although IgM hypergammaglobulinemia is frequently noted in pediatric AIDS.[116]

In contrast to the increased spontaneous activity noted in B cells from AIDS patients, antigen-specific and -nonspecific B-cell responses are impaired.[112] In vitro proliferative responses to antigens and mitogens are decreased, as are pokeweed mitogen (PWM)-induced immunoglobulin synthesis.[115] In vivo responses to primary and secondary immunizations of AIDS patients are poor, with reduced specific antibody production shown to both protein and polysaccharide antigens.[112,116] An inability to mount an adequate IgM response to antigenic challenge is an obvious and clinically significant humoral defect.

Consequences of this are most severe in HIV-infected infants and children who have not previously been exposed to a variety of pathogenic bacterial organisms and must rely on an initial IgM response for immune protection.[119] Certain adult AIDS patients also appear to have an increased susceptibility to certain pyogenic bacteria, which probably reflects defective humoral responses.[120]

The polyclonal hyperactivity of the B-cell limb of the immune response in AIDS patients no doubt reflects multiple factors. Several well-established polyclonal B-cell activators such as Epstein-Barr virus (EBV) and cytomegalovirus are frequently found to coinfect this patient population and may contribute to such hyperactivity.[117,124]

Increased spontaneous transformation of B cells of AIDS patients by EBV in vitro has been reported and is thought to reflect impaired T-cell and natural killer (NK)-cell surveillance,[121] not necessarily related to intrinsic B-cell dysfunction. This phenomenon may be associated with the increased incidence of B-cell lymphomas observed in AIDS patients. It is important to note, however, that despite the ability of HIV to infect EBV-transformed cells in vitro, there is no evidence of HIV integration in the B-cell lymphomas of AIDS patients.[122] The high incidence of these lymphomas in AIDS patients may be associated with increased transformation by EBV and may simply reflect the high incidence of coinfection with EBV in these individuals.

The mechanisms of B-cell dysfunction in HIV infection remain somewhat poorly understood. There is no current indication that nontransformed B cells can be infected with HIV, nor have HIV-infected B cells been identified in HIV-seropositive individuals. Despite the apparent inability of HIV to infect these cells directly, the effects of viral proteins on B-cell activity may account for some of the observed in vivo changes. Both intact infectious HIV and disrupted viral particles induce polyclonal activation of normal B cells with proliferative responses and immunoglobulin synthesis comparable to that of other B-cell mitogens.[117,121,123] Whether these responses reflect direct effects solely on B cells, or whether they require T cells to secrete soluble factors or to "present" concentrated virions, remains to be resolved.

In addition to the stimulatory effects of viral particles on B cells, HIV has been found to suppress EBV-induced immunoglobulin production by purified B cells.[124] The mechanism of this process is unclear, but because EBV is mitogenic for B cells in the absence of T cells or accessory cells, it raises the possibility of a direct effect of HIV on B cells.

Natural Killer Cell Impairment. A group of phenotypically distinct cell types associated with the functional properties of NK cells are included in this classification. The majority of these cells composes a relatively small circulating population of large granular lymphocytes (LGL) and bear CD16 on their surface. A smaller circulating population of CD16 cells expressing the product of the γ-δ-T-cell receptor gene have also been shown to have NK cell activity.[125] These NK cells are capable of killing virally infected cells, tumor cells, and allogeneic cells. They are thought to have a central role in immunosurveillance against viral infections and spontaneously developing tumors.

The number of circulating NK cells does not appear to be significantly decreased with HIV infection, even in those patients who have developed AIDS. These cells bind normally to their target cells[126]; however, compared with uninfected individuals, their cytotoxic capability is diminished.[126,127] Using lysis of tumor cell lines as a standard of NK activity, NK cell function measured in unfractionated populations of mononuclear cells from AIDS patients has been found to be depressed as compared with healthy seronegative controls.[84,126–130] NK function can be enhanced or restored to normal levels when activated by IL-2, concanavalin A, or phorbol ester and calcium ionophore.[126,131] Thus, NK cells from AIDS patients appear to be intrinsically able to perform their cytolytic function once activated, but manifest a postbinding or "triggering" defect that interferes with the normal pathway for delivery of a transmembrane signal for activation when in contact with an appropriate target.[132]

Other Immune Factors

A number of other factors have been proposed to account for some of the immune defects seen in AIDS patients. In addition to hypergammaglobulinemia,[111] circulating autoantibodies[133–137] and circulating immune complexes have been detected in AIDS patients.[138,139] The clinical consequences of an elevation in circulating immune complexes are unclear but may have relevance to certain symptoms such as arthritis, nephritis, and thrombocytopenia, which are sometimes seen in HIV-infected individuals.

Elevated levels of acid-labile α-interferon,[140,141] α-1-thymosin,[142] and β-2-microglobulin[143] have been reported in patients with AIDS but are of unknown clinical significance. Antibodies to α-1-thymosin appear to cross react with p17 and may be effective in viral neutralization.[144]

HIV Variation and Possible Selective Cell Tropism

An important topic for current debate in the virology of AIDS concerns whether or not individuals can harbor several forms of HIV, manifesting different selective tropisms for particular cell types in vivo. In the laboratory it has been documented that some HIV isolates obtained from brain and lung of AIDS patients exhibit selective tropism for monocytes and are capable of only feeble infection of T cells.[39] Conversely, peripheral blood HIV isolates that were passaged in vitro through T cells were unable to infect monocytes. Recent studies from another group support these observations of differential cell tropisms using a culture system that enhances the growth of macrophages in vitro. Of particular interest is that CD4 could not be detected on the surface of these monocytes, suggesting that another receptor or mechanism may allow viral entry into monocytes.[86]

Another group reported dual infection of the central nervous system by HIV isolates with distinct cellular tropisms.[145] These two structurally dissimilar viruses were obtained from frontal cortex tissue and cerebrospinal fluid (CSF) of a patient with encephalopathy. In contrast to the other studies, both of these viral isolates were passaged in lectin-stimulated lymphocytes. Following this, the viral isolate from the cortex infected macrophages as well, whereas the CSF-derived isolate infected glioma cells but not macrophages.

The nature, control, and ultimate significance of HIV variation and selective cell tropism are not yet fully understood. The selective cell tropisms observed in viral isolates may be coded by genes for viral-specific envelope sequences or by acquisition of a receptor from the host cell membrane during the process of budding. Molecular cloning of these biologically different isolates should provide future insight into this issue.

ACTIVATION OF LATENT HIV INFECTION

Significant gaps exist in the present understanding of the events that surround the progression of illness in HIV-infected individuals from asymptomatic infection to immunosuppression and full-blown AIDS. Recent clinical observations suggest that early in the course of infection with HIV, rising levels of the HIV structural protein, p24, can be detected in patients. With the onset of antibody production against the virus, these levels generally decline. This p24 antigenemia is felt to reflect active viral replication, and it is interesting to note that during the period of asymptomatic infection, small intermittent bursts of p24 antigenemia that usually return to baseline may be detected. However, late in the course of infection, the HIV-infected individual may manifest sustained p24 antigenemia (Lane HC, unpublished data). These rising levels of p24 antigen have important prognostic implications for the development of AIDS, although the mechanisms and triggers underlying this phenomenon are not understood.

It has been observed in vitro that while inactivated cells can be infected with HIV, productive infection requires an activation signal. Virus isolation from HIV-infected patients requires the stimulation of PBMC cultures. Early experiments demonstrated that HIV replication could be induced in latently infected cells following exposure of the cells to PHA.[11,14] However, for the HIV-infected individual, exposure to antigenic stimuli is much more likely to have physiologic relevance than exposure to mitogens. When similar experiments were undertaken using specific antigenic stimuli, it was demonstrated that PBMC that had been activated by antigen (such as the soluble antigens TT and keyhole impact hemocyanin [KLH]) prior to exposure to HIV were 10 to 100 times more susceptible to viral replication than PBMC that had been preincubated without antigen.[75]

Heterologous viruses represent one possible source of antigenic stimulation to which HIV-infected individuals may be exposed during the course of their infection. There is reason to suspect that concurrent infections with viral pathogens such as cytomegalovirus, Epstein-Barr virus, hepatitis B, and herpes simplex virus could activate latent HIV and induce viral expression in those individuals infected with HIV.[146] It has been shown in vitro that HIV expression can be up-regulated in cells following transfection with heterologous viruses.[147,148] More recently, it has been shown that HIV reverse transcriptase activity increases when a full-length infectious HIV clone is cotransfected with heterologous viral DNAs.[149]

In addition to mitogens, antigens, and coinfecting viruses, normal physiologic stimuli such as cytokines appear to play a role in the induction of productive HIV infection from a latent or low-level chronic infection. Studies using chronically infected cell lines indicate that exposure to a variety of cytokines, including granulocyte–macrophage-colony stimulating factor (GM-CSF) and particularly TNF-α, can produce physiologic cellular inductive signals with consequent upregulation of HIV infection. Further investigation of this phenomenon suggests that enhanced HIV expression by cytokines reflects induction of the promotor region of HIV by the transactivating effect of a DNA binding protein (Rubson A, personal communication). Full understanding of the mechanisms of activation of latent HIV infection will be essential in attempting to develop strategies to limit progression of HIV-induced disease.

IMMUNE RESPONSES TO HIV

Once diagnosed with AIDS, the life expectancy of an individual is approximately 2 years or less, depending on the initial clinical manifestations and response to treatment. The availability of the antiretroviral agent azidothymidine (AZT)—the only drug presently approved for the treatment of AIDS—has led to modest but significant increases in life span for those who can tolerate its potentially toxic side effects.[150] New agents under development may improve prospects for the future. Investigations into the nature and course of the immune response to HIV infection offer some insight into approaches to prevention and control of the relentless progression of HIV infection.

Multiple conditions can influence the outcome of an individual's exposure to HIV and the clinical sequelae of HIV infection. Factors such as the route of viral entry, the integrity of skin and other protective barriers to entry, the size of the viral inoculum, the virulence of the viral isolate, the presence of coinfecting pathogens, the number of contacts, the nutritional state, and the response of the immune system of the exposed individual may all determine whether or not that individual will become infected with HIV or manifest symptoms. Interestingly, there are reports of individuals with documented exposure to HIV, such as the wives of HIV-infected hemophiliacs, who remain uninfected, even after multiple contacts, while others with similar exposure seroconvert rapidly.[151] A resistance to infection based on HLA association has been looked for but not found. One study reported a relationship between an individual's group-specific component (Gc) type and resistance or susceptibility to infection and ultimate progression of disease.[152] However, subsequent studies did not corroborate this initial observation.[153,154]

The best available evidence indicates that infection with HIV leads to viral DNA integration and lifelong chronic infection of lymphocytes, monocytes, and other cells expressing the CD4 surface molecule. Seropositivity, reflecting the production of antibodies to HIV, develops approximately 3 to 12 weeks following infection and persists thereafter. Characteristically, there is a variable but relatively long period of time from initial infection to the development of AIDS. What proportion of infected individuals will develop AIDS over an extended time period remains undetermined. Current estimates indicate that approximately 37 percent of HIV-seropositive individuals will develop an AIDS-associated condition within 7 years of infection.[155] Unless an effective therapy is developed, it may well be the case that virtually all of those infected with HIV will ultimately die from AIDS. Despite a few isolated reports of asymptomatic seropositive individuals reverting to a seronegative state, reexamination of those cases using the newly developed gene amplification technique of polymerase chain reaction (PCR) suggests that those individuals remain latently infected with HIV.[156]

The conditions influencing disease course and clinical sequelae following HIV infection are unclear. Many factors similar to those bearing on initial susceptibility to infection may also influence the postinfectious course; such factors include the virulence of a particular viral isolate, the size of the initial inoculum, or the type and nature of other pathogens coinfecting individuals. Undoubtedly, a major determinant of clinical outcome in an individual is the capacity of their immune system to contain or eliminate the virus. The conditions necessary for development of effective immunity in an exposed or infected individual have not been established.

Many different responses, involving multiple limbs of the immune system, may participate in the body's attempt to mount a protective immune response to HIV. Humoral responses would include the production of neutralizing and cytolytic antibodies. Activation of the complement cascade may occur, with resultant killing of free and cell-bound virions. The development of cell-mediated responses, such as cytotoxic T cells, antibody-dependent cytotoxicity, and NK cell activity, may play an even more critical role in providing immune protection against HIV.

Neutralizing Antibodies

For virtually all individuals, HIV infection is associated with humoral immune response that produces antibodies to multiple viral proteins[157,158] but appears inadequate in preventing HIV propagation and clinical progression. Low titers of antibodies with neutralizing capacity have been detected in seropositive individuals at all stages of clinical disease. However, the finding of neutralizing antibodies in roughly equivalent levels in both AIDS patients and healthy seropositive individuals suggests that their presence may have little clinical significance. In several studies, no clear correlation of the in vitro effects of such neutralizing antibodies with clinical course or ability to prevent disease could be determined.[159–162]

The specificity of neutralizing antibody—determined by the ability of sera to inhibit viral isolates—may be type-specific (responding only to a restricted range of closely related strains) or group-specific (responding to a broad, heterogenous group of viral isolates). The potential specificity differences for neutralizing antibodies results from the diversity found within the HIV envelope, where variable regions demonstrating less than 50 percent homology among HIV strains are interposed with sequences that are more highly conserved.

Attempts to stimulate neutralizing antibody production experimentally with a variety of recombinant and purified proteins have been successful in both uninfected animals and humans.[163,164] Glycosylation of these proteins does not appear to be necessary to induce antibodies with neutralizing capability, although theoretically it may yield some qualitative advantages.[165,166] However, not all of the experimentally induced antibodies are neutralizing. For example, antibodies generated against the amino-terminal half of gp120 and gp41 envelope protein components could bind but not neutralize HIV.[165]

The specificity of neutralizing antibody has been examined in animal models as well as in individuals infected with HIV. This area of research has important implications for the feasibility of and approach to developing a successful vaccine against HIV. Most neutralizing antibody responses that have been generated in animal models by immunization with envelope protein appear to be type-specific. For example, in one recent study, antibody produced in response to immunization with envelope from the HIV-1 III-B strain could not neutralize the HIV-1 RF strain, and vice versa.[167] However, using other immunogenic epitopes of HIV, it may be possible to generate group-specific responses. Support for this comes from recent work in a rabbit model, which demonstrated that a peptide within a conserved portion of the envelope region could generate a group-specific neutralizing response against both HIV-1 III-B and HIV-1 RF isolates.[168] Studies in humans indicate the appearance of both patterns of neutralizing activity, but neither seems to confer a particular protective advantage to the individual.

In addition, there may be an important dichotomy in the regions that can induce antibody formation and T-cell proliferation. Virally induced antibodies found in sera from HIV-exposed patients reacted strongly with recombinant proteins from the carboxy terminus of gp120, but only bound weakly to proteins from the amino terminus. Conversely, T cells from those same patients demonstrated marked proliferative responses to the gp120 amino-terminus proteins, but poor response to the carboxy-terminus gp120.[169] Found within a conserved region of gp120, a specific sequence has been demonstrated to stimulate T-helper cell responses in mice immunized with HIV envelope proteins.[167] This sequence portion of the HIV envelope was predicted to be immunogenic based on the location within amphipathic α-helical regions. Cells from mice that were immunized with purified envelope proteins showed proliferative responses to a 16-residue synthetic peptide derived from that epitope.[167] However, the study did not determine whether neutralizing antibodies were produced to this peptide.

There is a concern that even if high-titered neutralizing antibodies could be stimulated in uninfected individuals, the very nature of HIV may hinder full and persistent protection against infection. It has been well demonstrated that a biologic property of HIV is easy and rapid mutation, resulting in the frequent creation of new strains.[19] There appears to be strong selective pressures for inducing changes within the envelope regions in particular. Neutralizing antibodies may in fact hasten this selection process, a phenomenon noted in vitro for HIV[170] and seen in vivo in other lentiviral diseases.[171] In a study of chimpanzees immunized with purified gp120, neutralizing antibodies were formed in response to immunization, but despite this, the animals became infected after challenge with HIV.[172] Ethical considerations clearly preclude direct investigation into the ability of neutralizing antibody to confer protection in human subjects against challenge with HIV, but accumulated evidence suggests that neutralizing antibodies have only a limited role in inhibiting HIV propagation and clinical progression of disease. There is no evidence to support the notion that the presence of neutralizing antibody to HIV could be protective for the uninfected individual exposed to HIV.

Cell-Mediated Cytotoxicity

The development of cellular cytotoxic immune responses may play a more critical role than neutralizing antibody formation in providing protection against HIV and other retroviruses. In a murine system using the Friend leukemia virus, it has been demonstrated that animals that developed cell-mediated cytotoxic responses to HIV along with neutralizing antibodies were protected against the development of leukemia following viral challenge, whereas animals that developed only neutralizing antibodies succumbed to leukemia.[173] The nature and scope of cellular immune responses in HIV infection is the subject of considerable current investigation. Protective cell-mediated responses against HIV may include ADCC, CTL, and NK cell responses.

Antibody-Dependent Cellular Cytotoxicity

ADCC may prove to be a key feature of the immune response to HIV. It has been shown that sera from HIV-seropositive individuals can mediate ADCC activity in vitro.[174–176] Some studies suggest that the level of this activity may correlate roughly with the clinical condition of the individual; sera derived from individuals with AIDS demonstrate less activity as compared with those of healthy seropositives.[174] However, this decrease in ADCC activity may simply reflect a more global defect in immune function in clinically advanced disease. One study attempted to compare ADCC specific antibody titer and anti-HIV antibody titer as measured by the ELISA assay, but no correlation was evident.[176] Presence or absence of antibody to a particular viral protein may be more critical than total anti-HIV antibody titers. ADCC activity appears to correlate best with the presence of antibodies to HIV envelope protein, although antibodies directed against other viral proteins may be involved as well. In one fairly recent report, ADCC activity was undetectable when anti-envelope activity was absent[176] but was present in sera without anti-p24 activity. The relationship of ADCC activity to anti-p24 activity is somewhat unclear, however, given an earlier study indicating that ADCC activity correlated best with anti-p24 activity.[174] In another study, although ADCC activity was not specifically examined, it was shown in a cohort of healthy seropositive homosexual men followed over a 3-year period that those individuals who remained healthy also demonstrated substantially greater anti-p24 activity.[177] No significant difference in neutralizing activity was observed between those who became symptomatic and those who remained healthy. Large-scale, careful examination of sera from HIV-infected individuals, looking at both neutralizing antibodies and ADCC activity, should be done—either prospectively or retrospectively—and correlated with clinical progression. In this manner, important insights may be gained into the potential components of effective immune response to HIV.

Natural Killer Cells

As mentioned earlier, natural killer cells appear to participate in the host elimination of HIV-infected cells. Several different cell phenotypes may be involved in this response, including those that express CD16 and Leu19. In addition, certain T cells, those with the γ-δ-T-cell receptor rearrangement in particular, may be involved in the lysis of HIV-infected cells in an MHC-unrestricted manner.[178] Large granular lymphocytes (LGLs) are the predominant cells containing NK activity. Purified populations of LGLs from seronegative individuals have been shown to mediate a small cytolytic response against HIV-infected targets. This response could be markedly augmented by culture in the presence of IL-2.[179] A similar enhancement of HLA-unrestricted cytotoxic activity was found when unfractionated cells from both seronegative and seropositive individuals were cultured in the presence of IL-2.[83] It has been demonstrated that the majority of HIV envelope-specific cytoxicity in the peripheral blood of HIV-seropositive individuals is HLA-unrestricted and mediated by cells expressing CD16.[180] The activity of these cells appeared to correlate with the patient's clinical status in that the healthier individuals demonstrated greater activity. Since cells that bear CD16 can participate in either NK-mediated lysis or ADCC activity, a portion of these cells may effect lysis through an ADCC-dependent mechanism.

Cytotoxic T Cells

T cells with cytotoxic activities have been detected in the circulation and lungs of HIV-infected individuals, and, with a variety of different assay systems, have been demonstrated to lyse target cells expressing HIV or HIV-associated proteins. An important area of current research concerns the delineation of the antigens recognized by cytotoxic T lymphocytes in infected individuals, as well as attempts to further characterize the cytotoxic effector cell population and the nature of the cytotoxic response to HIV proteins.

One group has reported the presence of CTL to HIV envelope and *gag* proteins in PBMC from HIV-infected individuals, using target cells infected with a recombinant vaccinia virus expressing HIV proteins.[181] These peripheral blood cells could lyse envelope- and *gag*-expressing targets that were either MHC class I- or class II-matched to the effector cells. It was later reported that PBMC from HIV-seropositive individuals could lyse target cells expressing the *pol* gene product and reverse transcriptase. In most patients this cytotoxic response could be blocked with antibody to CD8 or CD3.[182] CTL activity was present in all seropositive patients studied, including those with ARC and AIDS, and some features of HLA restriction were noted.[183] Other investigators have reported similar activity in a large proportion of healthy HIV-seropositive individuals studied, some patients with ARC, and rare AIDS patients with Kaposi sarcoma, but not in those AIDS patients with opportunistic infections.[184] This activity did not appear to be HLA class I-restricted. Another group studying anti-envelope responses following in vitro priming, reported finding low but statistically significant HLA class I-restricted CTL in some seropositive individuals.[185] In another study using a somewhat different approach, cytotoxic cell lines were generated from the bronchiolar lavage fluids from HIV-infected patients with interstitial pneumonitis. These cells were able to lyse macrophages infected with HIV, as well as target cells expressing envelope HLA class I-matched proteins. Further study demonstrated that these cytotoxic cells expressed CD8, and the response appeared to be HLA-A2-restricted in the individuals tested.[186]

In an animal model of HIV immune response, peripheral blood cells obtained from chimpanzees immunized with recombinant vaccinia viruses expressing HIV envelope proteins demonstrated proliferative responses to purified whole and envelope proteins.[185] Cells cloned from these immunized chimpanzees were cytotoxic for target cells infected with vaccinia virus expressing the recombinant envelope protein. However, these cytotoxic cells proved to be CD4+.

Efforts to characterize further the cell types involved in the cytolytic response to HIV clearly indicate that several cell types may be involved in the process. Using envelope-expressing targets derived from HIV isolates with envelope regions differing by at least 21 percent, it has been demonstrated that a group-specific cytotoxic response against envelope proteins is present in the majority of seropositive individuals. Recent evidence indicates that such a group-specific response against envelope-expressing target cells can be MHC-restricted.[178]

It remains to be determined whether both class I and class II HIV-specific CTL activity is generated in the course of natural infection and with immunization with recombinant proteins, and whether the CTL process confers any protection to the uninfected and immunized host.

CONCLUSIONS

In the relatively short period of time since this new disease entity was established and the causal virus discovered, an extraordinary amount of information has been gained about HIV, the pathogenesis of infection, and the immune response to the virus. Laboratory studies of HIV and the cells it infects are providing important insights into how the virus produces disease. Virtually the entire HIV genome has now been deciphered and the function of the major viral proteins determined. Infection with HIV can result in a complex array of immunopathogenic effects (Fig. 3). While the precise mechanisms whereby HIV infection leads to the immunosuppression and clinical manifestations characteristic of the disorder are complex and incompletely understood, it is evident that the depletion and functional impairment of T4 lymphocytes plays a central role. Defects in these cells—which occupy a prominent position in all the body's major defense mechanisms—produce consequential abnormalities in other immune effector cells, including B cells, T cells, and monocytes.

Many critically important but as yet poorly understood functional changes occur early in the course of HIV infection, often preceding significant losses of T4 lymphocytes. The mechanisms of T4 lymphocyte loss in vivo remain to be clarified, although virally induced cytotoxic and fusogenic processes along with autoimmune phenomena all appear to be contributors. In addition, cells of the monocyte–macrophage lineage may play an important role in the initiation and propagation of HIV infection and may serve as a reservoir of infection in the host. Experimentally, activation of HIV from latent or low-level chronic infection to productive infection may occur through mitogens, antigens, other infections, or through cytokines involved in the normal immune response. These represent potential mechanisms by which HIV infection in individuals can progress from an asymptomatic state to clinical AIDS. It is also evident that HIV infection of a given cell can result in modulation of expression of certain cellular genes and thereby has the potential to compound immunoregulatory abnormalities. Clearly, a greater understanding of these complex issues will be essential in developing effective treatment strategies for HIV infection and AIDS.

Further knowledge of protective immune responses to HIV will be critical to efforts to prevent infection or limit the clinical progression of disease. Major gaps persist in understanding the nature of protective immunity against HIV, including the relationship between the quantity and type of antibody produced and an individual's clinical status, as well as the role of cell-mediated immunity. Development of an effective vaccine against HIV will depend upon such information. Major efforts are currently under way, and the first candidate vaccines are being tested in humans in the United States and Africa.[187] However, given the long latency for development of AIDS in seropositive individuals, as well as the myriad ethical complexities of large-scale trials of an AIDS vaccine in humans, determining the efficacy of a vaccine may prove difficult.

Although devastating in its consequences, the discovery of HIV and its role in the development of AIDS and AIDS-related conditions has opened up exciting new avenues of research. Concerted efforts to elucidate the immunopathogenesis and immune response to HIV should ultimately lead to successful strategies to combat HIV-induced disease and will have important, broader implications for understanding the mechanisms of normal and aberrant regulation of the human immune system.

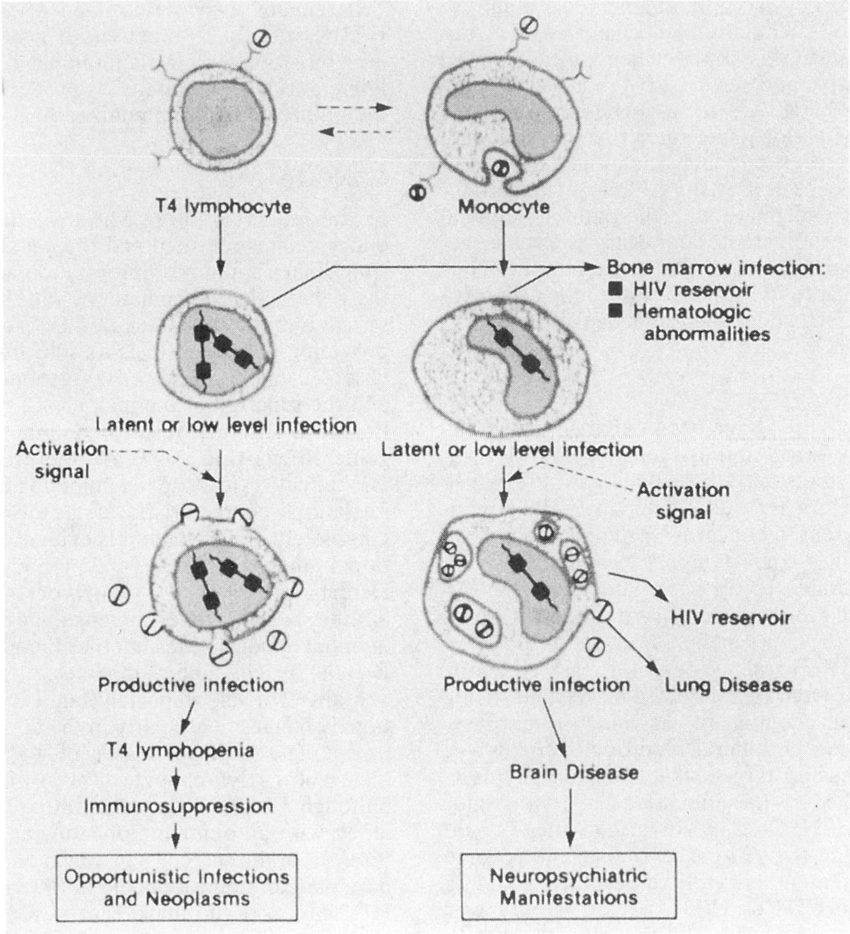

FIG. 3. Schematic diagram of the pathogenic mechanisms of HIV infection.

REFERENCES

1. Gottlieb MS, Schroff R, Schanker HM, et al. *Pneumocystis carinii* pneumonia and mucosal candidiasis in previously healthy homosexual men: evidence of a new acquired cellular immunodeficiency. N Engl J Med. 1981;305:1425–1.
2. Masur H, Michelis MA, Greene JB, et al. An outbreak of community-acquired *Pneumocystis carinii* pneumonia: initial manifestation of cellular immune dysfunction. N Engl J Med. 1981;305:1431–8.
3. Siegel FP, Lopez C, Hammer GS, et al. Severe acquired immunodeficiency in male homosexuals, manifested by chronic perianal ulcerative herpes simplex lesions. N Engl J Med. 1981;305:1439–4.
4. Centers for Disease Control. Acquired immunodeficiency syndrome weekly surveillance report, September 19, 1988. Centers for Disease Control, Atlanta, GA.
5. Public Health Service, DHHS. Quarterly report to the domestic policy council on the prevalence and rate of spread of HIV in the United States, July, 1988. Centers for Disease Control, Atlanta, GA.
6. Piot P, Plummer FA, Mhalu FS, et al. AIDS: an international perspective. Science. 1988;239:573–9.
7. Fauci AS, Masur H, Gelmann EP, et al. The acquired immunodeficiency syndrome: an update. Ann Intern Med. 1985;102:800–3.
8. Poon MC, Landay A, Prasthofer EF, et al. Acquired immunodeficiency syndrome with *Pneumocystis carinii* pneumonia and *Mycobacterium avium-intracellulare* infection in a previously healthy patient with classic hemophilia. Ann Intern Med. 1983;98:287–90.
9. Hymesk, Cheung T, Greene JB, et al. Kaposi's sarcoma in homosexual men: a report of eight cases. Lancet. 1981;2:598–600.
10. Reinherz E, O'Brien C, Rosenthal P, et al. The cellular basis for viral-induced immunodeficiency: analysis by monoclonal antibodies. J Immunol. 1980;125:1264–4.
11. Klatzmann D, Barré-Sinoussi F, Nugeyre MT, et al. Selective tropism of lymphadenopathy associated virus (LAV) for helper-inducer T lymphocytes. Science. 1984;225:59–63.
12. Dalgleish AG, Beverly CL, Clapham PR, et al. The CD4 (T4) antigen is an essential component of the receptor for the AIDS retrovirus. Nature. 1984;312:763–7.
13. Folks, TM, Kessler, SW, Orenstein, JM, et al. Infection and replication of human immunodeficiency virus-1 (HIV-1) in highly purified progenitor cells from normal human bone marrow. Science. 1988;242:919–22.
14. Gallo RC, Salahuddin SZ, Popovic M, et al. Frequent detection and isolation of cytopathic retrovirus (HTLV-III) from patients with AIDS and at risk for AIDS. Science. 1984;224:500–3.
15. Levy JA, Hoffman AD, Kramer SM, et al. Isolation of lymphocytopathic retroviruses from San Francisco patients with AIDS. Science. 1984;225:840–2.
16. Coffin J, Haase A, Levy JA, et al. Human immunodeficiency viruses. Science. 1986;232:697.
17. Barré-Sinoussi F, Chermann JC, Rey F, et al. Isolation of a T lymphotropic retrovirus from a patient at risk for acquired immune deficiency syndrome (AIDS). Science. 1983;220:868–71.
18. Popovic M, Sarngadharan MG, Read E, et al. Detection, isolation, and continuous production of cytopathic retroviruses (HTLV-III) from patients with AIDS and pre-AIDS. Science. 1984;224:497–500.
19. Fisher AG, Ensoli B, Looney D, et al. Biologically diverse molecular variants within a single HIV-1 isolate. Nature. 1988;334:444–7.
20. Benn S, Rutledge R, Folks T, et al. Genomic heterogeneity of AIDS retroviral isolates from North American and Zaire. Science. 1985;230:949.
21. Brun-Vezinet F, Rey MA, Katlama C, et al. Lymphadenopathy-associated virus type 2 in AIDS and AIDS-related complex. Lancet. 1987;1:128–32.
22. Clavel F, Guyader M, Guetard D, et al. Molecular cloning and polymorphism of the human immune deficiency virus type 2. Nature. 1986;324:691–5.
23. Horsburgh CR, Holmberg SD. The global distribution of human immunodeficiency virus type 2 (HIV-2). Infection. 1988;28:192–5.
24. Clavel F, Mansinho K, Chamaret S, et al. Human immunodeficiency virus type 2 infection associated with AIDS in West Africa. N Engl J Med. 1987;316:1180–5.
25. Public Health Service, DHHS. AIDS due to HIV-2 infection—New Jersey. MMWR. 1988;37:33–5.
26. Letvin N, Daniel MD, Sengal PK, et al. Induction of AIDS-like disease in

macaque monkeys with T-cell tropic retrovirus STLV-III. Science. 1985;230:71–3.
27. Rabson AB, Martin MA. Molecular organization of the AIDS retrovirus. Cell. 1985;40:477–80.
28. Gallo R, Wong-Staal F, Montagnier L, et al. HIV/HTLV gene nomenclature. Nature. 1988;333:504.
29. Klatzmann D, Champagne E, Charmaret S, et al. T-lymphocyte T4 molecule behaves as the receptor for human retrovirus LAV. Nature. 1984;312:767–8.
30. McDougal JS, Kennedy MS, Sligh JM, et al. Binding of HTLV-III/LAV to T4+ T cells by a complex of the 110 K viral protein and the T4 molecule. Science. 1985;231:382–5.
31. Sattentau QJ, Dalgleish AG, Weiss RA, et al. Epitopes of the CD4 antigen and HIV infection. Science. 1986;234:1120.
32. Lifson JD, Hwang KM, Nara PL, et al. Synthetic CD4 peptide derivatives that inhibit HIV infection and cytopathicity. Science. 1988;241:712–6.
33. Maddon PJ, Dagleish AG, McDougal JS, et al. The T4 gene encodes the AIDS virus receptor and is expressed in the immune system and the brain. Cell. 1986;47:333–8.
34. Mann DL, Lesane F, Blattner WA, et al. HLA-DR is involved in the HIV receptor (Abstract). In: III International Conference on Acquired Immunodeficiency Syndrome (AIDS). Washington, DC: U.S. Department of Health and Human Services. 1987;209.
35. Levy JA, Shimabukuro J, McHugh T, et al. AIDS-associated retrovirus (ARV) can productively infect other cells besides human T helper cells. Virology. 1985;147:441–8.
36. Ho DD, Rota TR, Hirsch MS. Infection of monocyte/macrophages by human T lymphotropic virus type III. J Clin Invest. 1986;77:1712–5.
37. Nicholson JKA, Cross GD, Callaway CS, et al. In vitro infection of human monocytes with human T-lymphotropic virus type III/lymphadenopathy-associated virus (HTLV-III/LAV). J Immunol. 1986;137:323–9.
38. Salahuddin SZ, Rose RM, Groopman JE, et al. Human T lymphotropic virus type II infection by human alveolar macrophages. Blood. 1986;68:281–4.
39. Gartner S, Markovits P, Markovits DM, et al. The role of mononuclear phagocytes in HTLV-III/ALV infection. Science. 1986;233:215–24.
40. Koenig S, Gendelman HE, Orenstein JM, et al. Detection of AIDS virus in macrophages in brain tissue from AIDS patients with encephalopathy. Science. 1986;233:1089–193.
41. Fauci AS. The human immunodeficiency virus: infectivity and mechanisms of pathogenesis. Science. 1988;239:617–22.
42. Lane HC, Masur H, Gelmann EP, et al. Correlation between immunologic function and clinical subpopulations of patients with the acquired immune deficiency syndrome. Am J Med. 1985;78:417–22.
43. Mittelman, Wong G, Safai B, et al. Analysis of T cell subsets in different clinical subgroups of patients with the acquired immune deficiency syndrome. Am J Med. 1985;78:951–6.
44. Polk BF, Fox R, Bookmeyer R, et al. Predictors of the acquired immunodeficiency syndrome developing in a cohort of seropositive homosexual men. N Engl J Med. 1987;316:61–6.
45. Goedert JJ, Bigga RJ, Melbye M, et al. Effect of T4 count and cofactors on the incidence of AIDS in homosexual men infected with human immunodeficiency virus. JAMA. 1987;257:331–4.
46. Kaplan JA, Spira TJ, Fishbein DB, et al. Lymphadenopathy syndrome in homosexual men: evidence for continuing risk of developing the acquired immunodeficiency syndrome. JAMA. 1987;257:335–7.
47. Fahey JL, Giorgi J, Martinez-Maza O, et al. Immune pathogenesis of AIDS and related syndromes. Ann Inst Pasteur Immunol. 1987;138:245–52.
48. Cheng-Mayer C, Seto D, Tateno M, et al. Biologic features of HIV-1 that correlate with virulence in the host. Science. 1988;240:80–2.
49. Walker CM, Moody DJ, Stites DP, et al. $CD8^+$ lymphocytes can control HIV infection in vitro by suppressing virus replication. Virology. 1986;234:1563.
50. Rabson, AB. The molecular biology of HIV infection: clues for possible therapy. In: Levy JA, ed. AIDS Pathogenesis and Treatment. New York: Marcel Dekker; 1988.
50a. Leonard R, Zagury D, Desportes I, et al. Cytopathic effect of human immunodeficiency virus in T4 cells is linked to the last stage of virus infection. Proc Natl Acad Sci USA. 1988;85:3570–4.
51. Hoxie JA, Alpers JD, Rackowski JL, et al. Alterations in T4 (CD4) protein and mRNA synthesis in cells infected with HIV. Science. 1986;234: 1123–7.
52. Asjö B, Ivhed I, Gidlund M, et al. Susceptibility to infection by the human immunodeficiency virus (HIV) correlates with T4 expression in a parental monocytoid cell line and its subclones. Virology. 1987;157:359–65.
53. Sodrowski J, Goh WC, Rosen C, et al. Role of the HTLV-III/LAV envelope in syncytium formation and cytopathicity. Nature. 1986;322:470–4.
54. Lifson JD, Reyes, McGrath MS, et al. AIDS retrovirus induced cytopathology: giant cell formation and involvement of CD4 antigen. Science. 1986;232:1123–7.
55. Lifson JD, Feinberg MB, Reyes GR, et al. Induction of CD4-dependent cell fusion by the HTLV-III/LAV envelope glycoprotein. Nature. 1986;323:725–8.
56. Yoffe B, Lewis DE, Petrie BL, et al. Fusion as a mediator of cytolysis in mixtures of uninfected CD4+ lymphocytes and cells infected by human immunodeficiency virus. Proc Natl Acad Sci USA. 1987;84:1429–33.
57. Ewing EP, Chandler FW, Spira TJ, et al. Primary lymph node pathology in AIDS and AIDS-related lymphadenopathy. Arch Pathol Lab Med. 1985; 109:977.
58. Epstein LG, Sharer LR, Joshi VV, et al. Progressive encephalopathy in children with acquired immune deficiency syndrome. Annal Neurol. 1985;17:488–96.
59. Klatzmann D, Montagnier L. Approaches to AIDS therapy. Nature. 1986;319:10–1.
60. Ziegler JL, Stites DP. Hypothesis: AIDS is an autoimmune disease directed at the immune system and triggered by a lymphotropic retrovirus. Clin Immunol Immunopathol. 1986;41:305–13.
61. Harper ME, Marselle LM, Gallo RC, et al. Detection of lymphocytes expressing human T-lymphotropic virus type III in lymph nodes and peripheral blood from infected individual by *in situ* hybridization. Pro Natl Acad Sci USA. 1986;83:772–6.
62. Ou CY, Kwok S, Mitchell SW, et al. DNA amplification for direct detection of HIV-1 in DNA of peripheral blood mononuclear cells. Science. 1988;239:295–7.
63. Winkelstein A, Klein RS, Evans TL, et al. Defective in vitro T cell colony formation in the acquired immunodeficiency syndrome. J Immunol. 1985;134:151–6.
64. Donahue RE, Johnson MM, Zon LI, et al. Suppression of in vitro haematopoiesis following human immunodeficiency virus infection. Nature. 1987;326:200–5.
65. Klatzmann D, Gluckman JC. HIV infection: facts and hypotheses. Immunol Today. 1986;7:291–6.
66. Katz JD, Nishanian P, Mitsuyasu R, et al. Antibody-dependent cellular cytotoxicity (ADCC)-mediated destruction of human immunodeficiency virus (HIV)-coated CD4+ T lymphocytes by acquired immunodeficiency syndrome (AIDS) effector cells. Clin Immunol. 1988;8:453–8.
67. Siliciano RF, Lawton T, Knall C, et al. Analysis of host-virus interactions in AIDS with anti-gp120 T cell clones: effect of HIV sequence variation and a mechanism for CD4+ cell depletion. Cell. 1988;54:561–6.
68. Lanzavecchia A, Roosnek E, Gregory T, et al. T cells can represent antigens such as HIV gp120 targeted to their own surface molecules. Nature. 1988;334:530.
69. Lane HC, Depper JM, Greene WC, et al. Qualitative analysis of immune function in patients with the acquired immunodeficiency syndrome. N Engl J Med. 1985;313:79–84.
70. Smolen JS, Bettelheim P, Köller U, et al. Deficiency of the autologous mixed lymphocyte reaction in patients with classic hemophilia treated with commercial factor VIII concentrate. J Clin Invest. 1985;75:1828–34.
71. Gupta S, Gillis S, Thornton M, et al. Autologous mixed lymphocyte reaction in man. XIV. Deficiency of the autologous mixed lymphocyte reaction in acquired immune deficiency syndrome (AIDS) and AIDS related complex (ARC). In vitro effect of purified interleukin-1 and interleukin-2. Clin Exp Immunol. 1984;58:395–401.
72. Lane HC, Fauci AS. Immunologic reconstitution in the acquired immunodeficiency syndrome. Ann Intern Med. 1985;103:714–8.
73. Fauci AS. AIDS: immunopathogenic mechanisms and research strategies. Clin Res. 1987;35:503–10.
74. Shearer GM, Salahuddin SZ, Markham PD, et al. Prospective study of cytotoxic T lymphocyte responses to influenza and antibodies to human T lymphotropic virus-III in homosexual men. J Clin Invest. 1985;76:1699–704.
75. Margolick JB, Volkman DJ, Folks TM, et al. Amplification of HTLV-III/LAV infection by antigen-induced activation of T cells and direct suppression by virus of lymphocyte blastogenic responses. J Immunol. 1987;138:1719–23.
76. Shalaby MR, Krowka JF, Gregory TJ, et al. The effects of human immunodeficiency virus recombinant envelope glycoprotein on immune cell functions in vitro. Cell Immunol. 1987;110:140–8.
77. Gay D, Maddon P, Sekaly R, et al. Functional interaction between human T-cell protein CD4 and the major histocompatibility complex HLA-DR antigen. Nature. 1987;626–9.
78. Doyle C, Strominger JL. Interaction between CD4 and class II MHC molecules mediates cell adhesion. Nature. 1987;330:256–9.
79. Alcover A, Ramarli D, Richardson NE, et al. Functional and molecular aspects of human T lymphocyte activation via T3-T1 and T11 pathways. Immunol Rev. 1987;95:5–6.
80. Linette GP, Hartzmann RJ, et al. HIV-1-infected T cells show a selective signaling defect after perturbation of CD3/antigen receptor. Science. 1988;241:573–576.
81. Shearer GM, Payne SM, Joseph LJ, et al. Functional T lymphocyte immune deficiency in a population of homosexual men who do not exhibit symptoms of acquired immune deficiency syndrome. J Clin Invest. 1984;74:496.
82. Sheridan JF, Aurelian L, Donnenberg AD, et al. Cell-mediated immunity of cytomegalovirus (CMV) and herpes simplex virus (HSV) antigens in the acquired immune deficiency syndrome: interleukin-1 and interleukin-2 modify in vitro responses. J Clin Immunol. 1984;4:304.
83. Rook AH, Manischewitz JD, Frederick WR, et al. Deficient, HLA-restricted, cytomegalovirus-specific cytotoxic T cells and natural killer cells in patients with the acquired immunodeficiency syndrome. J Infect Dis. 1985;152:627–8.
84. Rook AH, Masur H, Lane HC, et al. Interleukin-2 enhances the depressed natural killer and cytomegalovirus-specific cytotoxic activities of lymphocytes from patients with the acquired immune deficiency syndrome. J Clin Invest. 1983;72:398–403.

85. Mizuochi T, Goldberg H, Rosenberg AS, et al. Both L3T4$^+$ and Lyt-2$^+$ helper cells initiate cytotoxic T lymphocyte responses against allogeneic major histocompatibility antigens but not against trinitrophenyl-modified self. J Exp Med. 1985;162:427–33.
86. Gendelman HE, Orenstein JM, Martin MA, et al. Efficient isolation and propagation of human immunodeficiency virus on recombinant colony- stimulating factor 1-treated monocytes. J Exp Med. 1988;167:1428–31.
87. Smith PD, Ohura K, Masur H, et al. Monocyte function in the acquired immune deficiency syndrome. J Clin Invest. 1984;74:2121–8.
88. Prince HE, Moody DJ, Shubin BI, et al. Defective monocyte function in acquired immune deficiency syndrome (AIDS): evidence from a monocyte-dependent T-cell proliferative system. J Clin Immunol. 1985;5:21–5.
89. Poli G, Bottazzi B, Acero R, et al. Monocyte function in intravenous drug abusers with lymphadenopathy syndrome and in patients with acquired immunodeficiency syndrome: selective impairment of chemotaxis. Clin Exp Immunol. 1985;62:136–42.
90. Murray HW, Rubin BY, Masur H, et al. Impaired production of lymphokines and immune (gamma) interferon in the acquired immunodeficiency syndrome. N Engl J Med. 1984;310:883–9.
91. Pennington JE, Groopman JE, Small GJ, et al. Effect of intravenous recombinant gamma interferon in the respiratory burst of blood monocytes from patients with AIDS. J Infect Dis. 1986;153:609–12.
92. Washburn RG, Tuazon CU, Bennett JE. Phagocytic and fungicidal activity of monocytes from patients with acquired immunodeficiency syndrome. J Infect Dis. 1985;151:565.
93. Estevez ME, Ballart IJ, Diez RA, et al. Early defect of phagocytic cell function in subjects at risk for acquired immunodeficiency syndrome. Scand J Immunol. 1986;24:215–21.
94. Hofmann B, Odum N, Jakobsen BK. Immunological studies in the acquired immunodeficiency syndrome. Scand J Immunol. 1986;23:669–78.
95. Heagy W, Kelley VE, Strom TB, et al. Decreased expression of human class II antigens on monocytes from patients with acquired immune deficiency syndrome. J Clin Invest. 1984;74:2089–96.
96. Kleinerman ES, Ceccorulli LM, Zwelling LA, et al. Activation of monocyte-mediated tumoricidal activity in patients with acquired immunodeficiency syndrome. J Clin Oncol. 1985;3:1005–12.
97. Enk C, Gerstoft J, Moller S, et al. Interleukin 1 activity in the acquired immunodeficiency syndrome. Scand J Immunol. 1986;23:491–7.
98. Price RW, Brew B, Sidtis J, et al. The brain in AIDS: central nervous system HIV-1 infection and AIDS dementia complex. Science. 1988;239:586–92.
99. Gyorkey JF, Melnick JL, Gyorkey P. Human immunodeficiency virus in brain biopsies of patients with AIDS and progressive encephalopathy. J Infect Dis. 1987;155:870–6.
100. Dewhurst S, Bresser J, Stevenson M, et al. Susceptibility of human glial cells to infection with human immunodeficiency virus (HIV). FEBS Lett. 1987;213:138–43.
101. Chiodi F, Fuerstenberg S, Gidlund M, et al. Infection of brain-derived cells with the human immunodeficiency virus. J Virol. 1987;93:1244–7.
102. Gurney ME, Apatof BR, Spear GT, et al. Neuroleukin: a lymphokine product of lectin-stimulated T cells. Science. 1986;234:574–81.
103. Lee MR, Ho DD, Gurney ME. Functional interaction and partial homology between human immunodeficiency virus and neuroleukin. Science. 1987;237:1047–51.
104. Spivak JL, Bender BS, Quinn TC. Hematologic abnormalities in the acquired immune deficiency syndrome. Am J Med. 1984;77:224–8.
105. Delacretaz F, Perey L, Schmidt PM, et al. Histopathology of bone marrow in human immunodeficiency virus infection. Virchows Arch [A]. 1987; 411:543–51.
106. Belsito DV, Sanchez MR, Baer RL, et al. Reduced Langerhan's cell 1a antigen and ATPase activity in patients with the acquired immunodeficiency syndrome. N Engl J Med. 1984;310:1279–82.
107. Tschler E, Groh V, Popvic M, et al. Epidermal Langerhans cells—a target for HTLV-III/LAV infection. J Invest Dermatol. 1987;88:233–7.
108. Adachi A, Koenig S, Gendelman HE, et al. Productive, persistent infection of human colorectal cell lines with human immunodeficiency virus. J Virol. 1987;61:209–13.
109. Pomerantz RJ, de la Monte SM, Donegan SP, et al. Human immunodeficiency virus (HIV) infection of the uterine cervix. Ann Intern Med. 1988;108:321–7.
110. Pomerantz RJ, Kuritzkes DR, De La Monte SM, et al. Infection of the retina by human immunodeficiency virus type 1. N Engl J Med. 1987;317:1643–7.
111. Montagnier L, Gruest J, Chamaret S, et al. Adaption of lymphadenopathy associated virus (LAV) to replication in EBV-transformed B lymphoblastoid cell lines. Science. 1984;225:63–6.
112. Lane HC, Masur H, Edgar LC, et al. Abnormalities of B-cell activation and immunoregulation in patients with the acquired immunodeficiency syndrome. N Engl J Med. 1983;309:453–8.
113. Chess Q, Daniels J, North E, et al. Serum immunoglobulin elevations in the acquired immunodeficiency syndrome (AIDS): IgG, IgA, IgM, and IgD. Diagn Immunol. 1984;148–53.
114. Papadopoulos NM, Frieri M. The presence of immunoglobulin D in endocrine disorders and diseases of immunoregulation, including the acquired immunodeficiency syndrome. Clin Immunol Immunopathol. 1984;132:248–52.
115. Anderson KC, Boyd AW, Fisher DC, et al. Isolation and functional analysis of human B cell populations. J Immunol. 1985;134:820–7.
116. Pahwa SG, Quilop MTJ, Lange M, et al. Defective B-lymphocyte function in homosexual men in relation to the acquired immunodeficiency syndrome. Ann Intern Med. 1984;101:757–63.
117. Pahwa S, Pahwa R, Saxinger C, et al. Influence of the human T-lymphotropic virus/lymphadenopathy-associated virus on functions of human lymphocytes: evidence of immunosuppressive effects and polyclonal B cell activation by banded viral preparation. Proc Natl Acad Sci USA. 1985;82:8198–202.
118. Ammann AJ, Abrams D, Conant M, et al. Acquired immune dysfunction in homosexual men: immunologic profiles. Clin Immunol Immunopathol. 1983;27:315–52.
119. Ammann AJ, Schiffman G, Abrams D, et al. B-cell immunodeficiency in acquired immune deficiency syndrome. JAMA. 1984;251:1447–9.
120. Polsky B, Gold JWM, Whimbey E, et al. Bacterial pneumonia in patients with the acquired immunodeficiency syndrome. Ann Intern Med. 1986; 104:38–41.
121. Yarchoan R, Redfield RR, Broder S. Mechanisms of B cell activation in patients with acquired immunodeficiency syndrome and related disorders. J Clin Invest. 1985;78:439–47.
122. Pelicci PG, Knowles DM, Arlin ZA, et al. Multiple monoclonal B-cell expansions and c-myc oncogene rearrangements in AIDS-related lymphoproliferative disorders: implications for lymphomagenesis. J Exp Med. 1986;164:2049–60.
123. Schnittman SM, Lane HC, Higgins SE, et al. Direct polyclonal activation of human B lymphocytes by the acquired immune deficiency syndrome virus. Science. 1986;233:1084–6.
124. Pahwa S, Pahwa R, Good RA, et al. Stimulatory and inhibitory influences of human immunodeficiency virus on normal B lymphocytes. Proc Natl Acad Sci USA. 1986;83:9124–8.
125. Borst J, van de Griend RJ, van Oostveen JW, et al. A T-cell receptor γ/CD3 complex found on cloned functional lymphocytes. Nature. 1987;325:683–8.
126. Rook AH, Hooks JJ, Quinnan GV, et al. Interleukin 2 enhances the natural killer cell activity of acquired immunodeficiency syndrome patients through a γ-interferon-independent mechanism. J Immunol. 1985;134:1503–7.
127. Reddy MM, Chinoy P, Grieco MH. Differential effects of interferon-α_2 and interleukin-2 on natural killer cell activity in patients with acquired immune deficiency syndrome. J Biol Response Mod. 1984;3:379–86.
128. Lew F, Tsang P, Solomon S, et al. Natural killer cell function and modulation of α-IFN and IL-2 in AIDS patients and prodromal subjects. Clin Lab Immunol. 1984;14:115–21.
129. Creemers PC, Stark DF, Boyko WJ. Evaluation of natural killer cell activity in patients with persistent generalized lymphadenopathy and acquired immunodeficiency syndrome. Clin Immunol Immunopathol. 1985;36:141–50.
130. Hersh EM, Gutterman JU, Spector S, et al. Impaired in vitro interferon, blastogenic, and natural killer cell responses to viral stimulation in acquired immune deficiency syndrome. Cancer Res. 1985;45:406–10.
131. Bonavida B, Katz J, Gottlieb M. Mechanism of defective NK cell activity in patients with acquired immunodeficiency syndrome (AIDS) and AIDS-related complex. J Immunol. 1986;137:1157–63.
132. Katzman M, Lederman MM. Defective postbinding lysis underlies the impaired natural killer activity in factor VIII-treated, human T lymphotropic virus type III seropositive hemophiliacs. J Clin Invest. 1986;77:1057–62.
133. Pollack MS, Callaway C, LeBlanc D, et al. Lymphocytotoxic antibodies to non-HLA antigens in the sera of patients with acquired immunodeficiency syndrome (AIDS). In: Cohen E, Singal DP, eds. Non-HLA antigens in Health, Aging, and Malignancy. New York: Alan R. Liss; 1983: 209–13.
134. Kloster BE, Tomar RH, Spira TJ. Lymphocytotoxic antibodies in the acquired immune deficiency syndrome (AIDS). Clin Immunol Immunopathol. 1984;30:330–5.
135. Williams RC Jr, Masur H, Spira TJ. Lymphocyte-reactive antibodies in acquired immune deficiency syndrome. J Clin Immunol. 1984;4:118–23.
136. Dorsett B, Cronin W, Chuma V, et al. Anti-lymphocyte antibodies in patients with the acquired immune deficiency syndrome. Am J Med. 1985;78:621–6.
137. Tomar RH, John PA, Hennig AK, et al. Cellular targets of antilymphocyte antibodies in AIDS and LAS. Clin Immunol Immunopathol. 1985;37:37–47.
138. McDougal JS, Hubbard M, Nicholson JKA. Immune complexes in the acquired immunodeficiency syndrome (AIDS). J Clin Immunol. 1985;5:130–8.
139. Gupta S, Licorish K. Circulating immune complexes in AIDS. N Engl J Med. 1984;310:1530–1.
140. DeStefano E, Friedman RM, Friedman-Kien AE, et al. Acid-labile human leukocyte interferon in homosexual men with Kaposi's sarcoma and lymphadenopathy. J Infect Dis. 1982;146:451–5.
141. Buimovici-Klein E, Lange M, Klein RJ, et al. Long-term follow-up of serum-interferon and its acid-stability in a group of homosexual men. *AIDS Research*. 1986:99–108.
142. Hersh EM, Reuben JM, Rios A, et al. Elevated serum thymosin alpha$_1$ levels associated with evidence of immune dysregulation in male homosexuals with a history of infectious diseases or Kaposi's sarcoma. N Engl J Med. 1983;308:45.
143. Bhalla RB. Abnormally high concentrations of beta 2 microglobulin in acquired immunodeficiency syndrome (AIDS) patients. Clin Chem. 1983;29:1560.
144. Sarin PS, Sun DK, Thornton AH, et al. Neutralization of HTLV-III/LAV replication by anti-serum to thymosin α_1. Science. 1986;232:1135–7.
145. Koyanagi Y, Miles S, Mitsuyasu RT, et al. Dual infection of the central

nervous system by AIDS viruses with distinct cellular tropisms. Science. 1987;236:819–22.
146. Gendelman HE, Phelps W, Feigenbaum L, et al. Transactivation of the human immunodeficiency virus terminal repeat sequence by DNA viruses. Proc Natl Acad Sci USA. 1986;83:9759–63.
147. Mosca JD, Bednarik DP, Raj NBK, et al. Herpes simplex virus type-1 can reactivate transcription of latent human immunodeficiency virus. Nature. 1987;325:67–70.
148. Davis MG, Kenney SC, Kamine J, et al. Immediate-early gene region of human cytomegalovirus transactivates the promotor of human immunodeficiency virus. Proc Natl Acad Sci USA. 1987;84:8642–6.
149. Ostrove JM, Leonard J, Weck KE, et al. Activation of the human immunodeficiency virus by herpes simplex virus by type 1. J Virol. 1987;61:3726–32.
150. Broder S, Fauci AS. Progress in the development of drug therapies for AIDS. Public Health Rep. May-June 1988;103:224–8.
151. Smiley ML, White II GC, Becherer P, et al. Transmission of human immunodeficiency virus to sexual partners of hemophiliacs. Am J Hematol. 1988;28:27–32.
152. Eales LJ, Ke N, Parkin JM, et al. Genetic factors in susceptibility to HIV infection and to HIV related diseases: variation in Gc subtypes. Lancet. 1987;1:999–1002.
153. Gilles K, Louie L, Newman B, et al. Genetic susceptibility to AIDS: absence of an association with group-specific component. N Engl J Med. 1987; 317:630–41.
154. Daiger SP, Brewton GW, Rios AA, et al. Letter. N Engl J Med. 1987;17:631–2.
155. Curran JW, Jaffe HW, Hardy AM, et al. Epidemiology of HIV infection and AIDS in the United States. Science. 1988;239:610–6.
156. Farzadegan H, Polis MA, Wolinsky SM, et al. Loss of HIV-1 antibodies with evidence of viral infection in asymptomatic homosexual men. Ann Intern Med. 1988;108:785–90.
157. Sarngadharan MF, Veronese FM, Lee S, et al. Immunological properties recognized by sera of patients with AIDS and AIDS-related complex and of asymptomatic carriers of HTLV-III infection. Cancer Res. 1985;45:4574–7.
158. Montagnier L, Clavel F, Kurst B, et al. Identification and antigenicity of the major envelope glycoprotein of lymphadenopathy-associated virus. Virology. 1985;141:283–9.
159. Robert-Guroff M, Brown M, Gallo RC. HTLV-III-neutralizing antibodies in patients with AIDS and AIDS-related complex. Nature. 1985;316:72–4.
160. Weiss RA, Clapham PR, Cheingsong-Popov R, et al. Neutralization of human T-lymphotropic virus type III by sera of AIDS and AIDS-risk patients. Nature. 1985;316:69–72.
161. Weiss RA, Clapham PR, Weber JN, et al. Variable and conserved neutralization antigens of human immunodeficiency virus. Nature. 1986;324:572.
162. Matthews TJ, Langlois AJ, Robey WG, et al. Restricted neutralization of divergent human T-lympnotropic virus type III isolates by antibodies to the major envelope glycoprotein. Proc Natl Acad Sci USA. 1986;83:9709–13.
163. Lasky LA, Groopman JE, Fennie CW, et al. Neutralization of the AIDS retrovirus by antibodies to a recombinant envelope glycoprotein. Science. 1986;233:209–12.
164. Zagury D, Bernard J, Cheynier R, et al. A group specific anamnestic immune reaction against HIV-1 induced by a candidate vaccine against AIDS. Nature. 1988;332:728–31.
165. Putney SD, Matthews TJ, Robey WG, et al. HTLV-III/LAV-neutralizing antibodies to an *E. coli*-produced fragment of the virus envelope. Science. 1986;234:1392–5.
166. Krohn K, Robey WG, Putney S, et al. Specific cellular immune response and neutralizing antibodies in goats immunized with native or recombinant envelope proteins derived from human T-lymphotropic virus type III_B and in human immunodeficiency virus-infected men. Proc Natl Acad Sci USA. 1987;84:4994–8.
167. Cease KB, Margalit H, Cornette JL, et al. Helper T-cell antigenic site identification in the acquired immunodeficiency syndrome virus gp120 envelope protein and induction of immunity in mice to the native protein using a 16-residue synthetic peptide. Proc Natl Acad Sci USA. 1987;84:249–53.
168. Ho DD, Kaplan JC, Rackauskas IE, et al. Second conserved domain of gp120 is important for HIV infectivity and antibody neutralization. Science. 1988;239(4843):1021–3.
169. Ahearne PM, Matthews TJ, Lyerly HK, et al. Cellular immune response to viral peptides in patients exposed to HIV. AIDS Res Hum Retroviruses. 1988;4:259–67.
170. Robert-Guroff M, Reitz MS, Robey WG, et al. In vitro generation of an HTLV-III variant by neutralizing antibody. J Immunol. 1986;137:3306–9.
171. Montelaro RC, Parakh B, Orrego A, et al. Antigenic variation during persistent infection by equine infectious anemia virus, a retrovirus. J Biol Chem. 1984;259:10539–44.
172. Prince AM, Horowitz B, Baker L, et al. Failure of an HIV immune globulin to protect chimpanzees against experimental challenge with HIV. Proc Natl Acad Sci US. 1988;85:6944–8.
173. Earl P, Moss B, Morrison RP, et al. T-lymphocyte priming and protection against Friend leukemia by vaccinia-retrovirus env gene recombinant. Science. 1986;234:728–31.
174. Rook AH, Lane HC, Folks T, et al. Sera from HTLV-III/LAV antibody-positive individuals mediate antibody-dependent cellular cytotoxicity against HTLV-III/LAV-infected T cells. J Immunol. 1987;138:1064–7.
175. Ojo-Amaize EA, Nishanian P, Keith DE, et al. Antibodies to human immunodeficiency virus in human sera induce cell-mediated lysis of human immunodeficiency virus-infected cells. J Immunol. 1987;139:2458.
176. Ljunggren K, Böttiger B, Biberfeld G, et al. Antibody-dependent cellular cytotoxicity-inducing antibodies against human immunodeficiency virus. J Immunol. 1987;139:2263.
177. Weber JN, Clapham, Weiss RA, et al. Human immunodeficiency virus infection in two cohorts of homosexual men: neutralizing sera and association of anti-gag antibody with prognosis. Lancet. 1987;1:119.
178. Koenig S, Earl P, Powell D, et al. Group specific, major histocompatibility complex class I restricted cytotoxic responses to human immunodeficiency virus-1 envelope proteins by cloned peripheral blood T cells from an HIV infected individual. Proc Natl Acad Sci USA. 1988;85:8638–42.
179. Ruscetti FW, Mikovits JA, Kalyanaraman VS, et al. Analysis of effector mechanism against HTLV-1 and HTLV-III/LAV infected lymphoid cells. J Immunol. 1986;136:3619–24.
180. Weinhold KJ, Lyerly HK, Matthews TJ, et al. Cellular anti-GP120 cytolytic reactivities in HIV-1 seropositive individuals. Lancet. 1988;1:902–905.
181. Walker BD, Chakrabarti S, Moss B, et al. HIV-specific cytotoxic T lymphocytes in seropositive individuals. Nature. 1987;328:345–8.
182. Walker BD, Flexner C, Paradis TJ, et al. HIV-1 reverse transcriptase is a target for cytotoxic T lymphocytes in infected individuals. Science. 1988;240:64–66.
183. Quinnan GV. Detection of HLA restricted human immunodeficiency virus (HIV) envelope antigen-specific cytotoxic lymphocytes (CTL) [Abstract]. In: III International Conference on Acquired Immunodeficiency Syndrome (AIDS). Washington, DC: U.S. Department of Health and Human Services; 1987:59.
184. Koenig S, Earl P, Powell D, et al. Cytotoxic T cells directed against target cells expressing HIV-1 proteins [Abstract]. In: III International Conference on Acquired Immunodeficiency Syndrome (AIDS). Washington, DC: U.S. Department of Health and Human Services; 1987:59.
185. Zarling JM, Eichberg JW, Moran PA, et al. Proliferative and cytotoxic T cells to AIDS virus glycoproteins in chimpanzees immunized with a recombinant vaccinia virus expressing AIDS virus envelope glycoproteins. J Immunol. 1987;139:988–90.
186. Plata F, Autran B, Pedroza Martins L, et al. AIDS virus-specific cytotoxic T lymphocytes in lung disorders. Nature. 1987;328:348.
187. Koff WC, Hoth DF. Development and testing of AIDS vaccines. Science. 1988;241:426–32.

108. CLINICAL MANIFESTATIONS OF HIV INFECTION

RICHARD E. CHAISSON
PAUL A. VOLBERDING

Infection with the human immunodeficiency virus (HIV) results in a wide range of clinical consequences from asymptomatic carriage to life-threatening opportunistic infections and malignancies. The disease state called acquired immunodeficiency syndrome (AIDS) is at the terminal stage of this axis when the infected host can no longer control opportunistic organisms or malignancies that rarely cause illness in immunocompetent individuals. In persons infected with HIV, the sequential decline and ablation of cell-mediated immunity result in diverse manifestations of opportunistic disease. Those manifestations may vary according to the individual's age, race, geographic location, and behavioral history. This chapter will review the clinical features of HIV infection from the acquisition of the virus to death with AIDS and discuss the classification and evaluation of HIV-related syndromes.

HISTORY

Disease caused by HIV-induced immunosuppression was first described in late 1980 and early 1981 when physicians in Los

Angeles, New York, and San Francisco observed opportunistic infections in homosexual men.[1–4] Simultaneously, an outbreak of Kaposi sarcoma, a previously rare malignancy, was reported in young homosexual men from the same three cities.[5,6] These patients also had a selective defect in cell-mediated immunity that was manifested by low numbers of CD4+ T lymphocytes and the development of opportunistic infections.

That opportunistic diseases occurred in homosexual men who had been healthy previously suggested that immunodeficiency developed because of an acquired rather than a congenital trait. In 1982, the Centers for Disease Control (CDC) developed a case definition, based on the clinical, immunologic, and epidemiologic features of the first clusters of cases, for what was called the acquired immunodeficiency syndrome[7] (AIDS). AIDS was defined as the occurrence of a reliably diagnosed disease at least moderately indicative of underlying cellular immunodeficiency in a person without a condition known to be associated with an increased incidence of diseases related to cellular immunodeficiency.[6,8] AIDs became a reportable condition in 1983. Soon after the initial case reports of AIDS, additional cases were observed in persons other than homosexual men. In 1981 and 1982, heterosexual intravenous drug users and immigrants from Haiti were reported to have AIDS.[2,9–12] AIDS cases in hemophiliacs, recipients of blood transfusions, and Africans were also soon reported.[13,14]

While the groups of persons at risk for AIDS expanded, clinicans noted an increasing spectrum of clinical manifestations of AIDS-associated immunodeficiency. Unexplained generalized lymphadenopathy, idiopathic thrombocytopenia, oral candidiasis, herpes zoster, and a constitutional wasting syndrome were observed in persons from AIDS risk groups who had deficits in cellular immunity.[15–19] The term *AIDS-related complex* (ARC) was coined in 1984 to describe the symptoms of immunodeficiency recognized with increasing frequency in persons at risk for AIDS.[20] In 1982–1983, several investigators postulated an asymptomatic carrier state of the AIDS agent in healthy homosexual men, heterosexual partners of iv drug users, and Haitians who were noted to have laboratory evidence of impaired cellular immunity.[21] As discussed elsewhere, HIV was first described in 1983 by Barre-Sinoussi et al.[22] Gallo and coworkers and Levy and associates[23,24] confirmed the pathogenic nature and continuous culture of HIV in 1983–1984. Serologic tests to identify persons infected with HIV were developed shortly thereafter, and this allowed large serologic surveys of risk group members to estimate the number of individuals infected with the virus and to delineate the spectrum of HIV-associated diseases. The CDC expanded its case definition of AIDS in 1985 and again in 1987 (Table 1) to accommodate the increased number of manifestations of impaired cellular immunity that had become associated with chronic HIV infection.[7,25,26] The World Health Organization also promulgated a case definition for AIDS for use in developing countries that lacked sophisticated diagnostic resources (Table 2).[27] As the epidemic continues to grow and additional cases are observed, the list of diseases recognized as complications of HIV infection will undoubtedly be modified.

TABLE 1. CDC Surveillance Case Definition for AIDS

Diseases diagnosed definitively without confirmation of HIV infection in patients without other causes of immunodeficiency
Candidiasis of the esophagus, trachea, bronchi, or lungs
Cryptococcosis, extrapulmonary
Cryptosporidiosis >1 mon duration
Cytomegalovirus (CMV) infection of any organ except the liver, spleen, or lymph nodes in patients >1 mon old
Herpes simplex infection, mucocutaneous (>1 mon duration) or of the bronchi, lungs, or esophagus in patients? 1 mon duration
Kaposi sarcoma in patients <60 yr old
Primary CNS lymphoma in patients <60 yr old
Lymphoid interstitial pneumonitis (LIP) and/or pulmonary lymphoid hyperplasia (PLH) in patients <13 yr old
Mycobacterium avium complex or *M. kansasii* disseminated
Pneumocystis carinii pneumonia
Progressive multifocal leukoencephalopathy
Toxoplasmosis of the brain in patients >1 mon old
Diseases diagnosed definitively with confirmation of HIV infection
Multiple or recurrent pyogenic bacterial infections in patients <13 yr old
Coccidioidomycosis, disseminated
Histoplasmosis, disseminated
Isosporiasis >1 mon duration
Kaposi sarcoma, any age
Primary CNS lymphoma, any age
Non-Hodgkin's lymphoma (small, noncleaved lymphoma; Burkitt or non-Burkitt type; or immunoblastic sarcoma)
Mycobacterial disease other than *M. tuberculosis*, disseminated
M. tuberculosis, extrapulmonary
Salmonella septicemia, recurrent
Diseases diagnosed presumptively with confirmation of HIV infection
Candidiasis of the esophagus
CMV retinitis
Kaposi sarcoma
LIP/PLH in patients <13 yr old
Disseminated mycobacterial disease (not cultured)
Pneumocystis carinii pneumonia
Toxoplasmosis of the brain in patients >1 mon old
HIV encephalopathy
HIV wasting syndrome

(From Centers for Disease Control.[25])

TABLE 2. World Health Organization Adult Case Definition for AIDS

Major signs[a]
>10% weight loss
Diarrhea >1 mon duration
Fever >1 mon duration
Minor signs[a]
Cough >1 mon duration
General pruritic dermatitis
Recurrent herpes zoster
Oropharyngeal candidiasis
Progressive, disseminated herpes simplex
Generalized lymphadenopathy
Diagnostic of AIDS
Cryptococcal meningitis
Disseminated Kaposi sarcoma

[a] The presence of at least two major signs and one minor sign is diagnostic of AIDS.
(From World Health Organization,[27] with permission.)

CLASSIFICATION OF HIV INFECTION AND RELATED DISEASES

HIV is a pathogen that causes a variety of specific and nonspecific defects in immune function that result in diverse clinical consequences. AIDS, the end stage of HIV infection, currently affects only a small proportion of persons infected with HIV. HIV infection therefore represents the underlying disease process and will probably result in serious immunologic and clinical consequences (discussed below). While individuals who are HIV infected but asymptomatic should not be classified as being ill, they do have a chronic and progressive disease that may result ultimately in significant impairment and/or death.

Several systems to classify HIV infection and disease have been proposed.[26,29] The CDC bases its classification system for HIV infection on clinical manifestations. HIV-infected persons are placed into four categories: group I, acute infection; group II, asymptomatic seropositive; group III, persistent generalized lymphadenopathy; and group IV, symptomatic HIV disease (Table 3). Although clinically based, the CDC system has several drawbacks. The system is hierarchic (persons in a higher category are presumed to have more advanced disease); however, the categories do not reflect disease progression. A number of prospective studies have shown, for instance, that persistent, generalized lymphadenopathy (group III) is not associated with a greater degree of immunopathology or an increased risk of developing AIDS or other opportunistic processes than is asymptomatic infection without lymphadenopathy (group II).[30] Moreover, some manifestations of group IV (e.g., aseptic meningitis, subgroup IVB), may be early mani-

TABLE 3. CDC Classification System of HIV Infection

Group I. Acute infection
Group II. Asymtomatic infection
Group III. Persistent generalized lymphadenopathy
Group IV. Other diseases
Subgroup A. Constitutional disease
Subgroup B. Neurologic disease
Subgroup C. Secondary infections diseases
Category C-1. Specified secondary infections diseases listed in the CDC surveillance definition for AIDS[a]
Category C-2. Other specified secondary infections diseases
Subgroup D. Secondary cancers
Subgroup E. Other conditions

[a] Includes those patients whose clinical presentation fulfills the definition of AIDS used by the CDC for national reporting.

festations of HIV infection and unrelated to its subsequent course.[31] Most importantly, the CDC system contains no prognostic variables and cannot be used to predict future immunologic deterioration and progression of the disease. The system has proved useful for surveillance and administrative purposes and has fostered the concept that an individual with HIV infection can be considered to have AIDS-related illness without manifesting life-threatening opportunistic diseases.

The Walter Reed (WR) staging system for HIV infection (Table 4) classifies patients on the basis of CD4 lymphocyte counts, skin test responsiveness, and the presence of lymphadenopathy, oral candidiasis, and opportunistic infections. The stages of the WR system are hierarchic, and they roughly parallel the natural history of HIV in infected individuals. This system is limited by several factors. While the predictive value of both CD4 lymphocyte counts and oral candidiasis have been established, cutaneous anergy and lymphadenopathy have not attained similar prognostic importance. The strata of CD4 cell counts used in the WR system may not be sensitive enough to give precise prognostic information. The system requires that skin tests be performed routinely—a practice that is often clinically cumbersome and impractical in managing large numbers of patients. As many as 30–70 percent of HIV-seropositives cannot be placed into WR stages because they have >400 CD4+ cells but are anergic.[32,33] The Walter Reed system must be prospectively evaluated before it is recommended for widespread application. Adding other laboratory markers of immunosuppression, discussed below, may strengthen the Walter Reed system.

We prefer to classify HIV-infected patients according to clinical and prognostic parameters (Table 5). Clinical outcomes can be categorized relative to acquiring the infection as early, middle, or late complications. Prognostic variables are laboratory measures that assess the degree of immunopathology caused by HIV and predict subsequent clinical deterioration and disease progression. Those laboratory markers are discussed below.

DIAGNOSIS OF HIV INFECTION

The diagnosis of HIV infection (see also Chapter 109) is best accomplished by detecting specific antibodies against viral antigens serologically. Directly detecting viral antigens and cocultivating the virus in cell culture are also possible; however, the former is relatively insensitive, and the latter is very expensive. Other diagnostic tests are being developed, including the use of polymerase chain reaction assays and other methods for detecting the viral genome. Use of the enzyme-linked immunosorbant assay (ELISA) for HIV antibodies, however, is the most sensitive, efficient, and practical way to diagnose HIV infection.

Detecting anti-HIV antibodies by ELISA is highly sensitive (>99 percent) and specific (95–99 percent). As with any diagnostic test, the predictive value of a positive test result depends on the prevalence of infected persons in the population being tested. A number of conditions including collagen-vascular diseases, chronic hepatitis, malaria, and certain HLA phenotypes have been associated with false-positive results on ELISA. The use of assays with recombinant antigens, which do not require culture in human cell lines, may significantly reduce the proportion of false-positive results. The cost-effectiveness of recombinant ELISA testing has not been demonstrated. Serum samples that are reactive by ELISA should be retested; repeatedly positive specimens should then be confirmed with a

TABLE 4. Walter Reed Staging System for HIV Disease

Stage	*HIV (Antibody/Antigen)*	*Lymphadenopathy*	*CD4+ Lymphocytes/mm³*	*Skin Tests*	*Thrush*	*Opportunistic Infection*
WR 0	−	−	>400	NL	−	−
WR 1	+	−	>400	NL	−	−
WR 2	+	+	>400	NL	−	−
WR 3	+	±	<400	NL	−	−
WR 4	+	±	<400	Partial anergy	−	−
WR 5	+	±	<400	Complete anergy	+	−
WR 6	+	±	<400	Complete anergy	+	+

Abbreviations: NL: normal.
(From Redfield et al.,[29] with permission.)

TABLE 5. Staging of HIV Disease

Stage	*Clinical*	*T4*	*p24Ag*	*β_2-Microglobulin*	*Hct*
Acute	Mononucleosis-like illness	Normal	+	Normal	Normal
Early	Asymptomatic or Persistent generalized lymphadenopathy Aseptic meningitis Dermatologic manifestations	>400	−	Normal	Normal
Middle	Asymptomatic or Persistent generalized lymphadenopathy Thrush Hairy leukoplakia Idiopathic thrombocytopenic purpura, etc.	200–400	±	Moderately high	Normal or low
Late	Opportunistic infections Malignancy Wasting Dementia	<200	±	High	Low

highly specific test such as an immunofluorescence assay (IFA) or a Western blot (WB). Other specific methods such as radioimmunoprecipitation assay are not practical for routine use in clinical laboratories. When confirmed reactive by IFA or WB, specimens should be considered true positives. Individuals positive by these tests should be informed that they are infected with HIV, counseled about the implications of HIV infection, and advised to eliminate behaviors that might result in transmitting the virus to others. Medical screening and follow-up should be offered to all HIV-seropositives.

The serologic response to HIV infection is shown in Figure 1. Shortly after exposure to the virus, a period of viremia and p24 antigenemia occurs. Antigenemia generally occurs within 2 weeks of exposure and lasts for several weeks. Both IgM and IgG antibodies to core (p24) and envelope (gp41, gp120) antigens develop 1–3 months after exposure, although longer periods of seroconversion have been documented. As a rule, infection with HIV and seropositivity for antibodies are lifelong. Rare cases of seroreversion (loss of specific antibodies after a period of antibody positivity) have been reported.[34] However, all four persons who seroreverted had HIV genome detected by polymerase chain reaction (in peripheral blood mononuclear cells).

Months to years after seroconversion, a significant proportion of HIV-infected individuals begin to lose antibodies to core antigens, although antibodies to envelope antigens, reverse transcriptase, and regulatory proteins remain. Most such individuals then develop core antigenemia; a minority may have antigen detected in the cerebrospinal fluid (CSF). Developing antigenemia presumably reflects an antigen-excess state, with anti-core antibodies consumed in immune complexes. This excess of antigen may signal increasing replication of the virus and carries a poor prognosis.

HIV antibody testing should be performed only for a valid medical or public health purpose. Patients being tested for HIV antibody should be told why they are being tested and should give consent for the procedure. Some states require written, informed consent before testing. Like all medical data, HIV antibody test results should be kept confidential; unauthorized disclosure should be vigorously avoided.

NATURAL HISTORY OF HIV INFECTION

The number of asymptomatic carriers of HIV far exceeds the number of persons with late complications or with AIDS. A number of studies have focused on the rate at which infected individuals progress to clinical disease and death. Initial reports indicated that fewer than 5 percent of seropositive individuals developed AIDS during several years of follow-up. Goedert and coworkers evaluated five small cohorts of HIV-seropositives and found 3-year progression rates of 5–36 percent.[35] Larger prospective studies now show that the rate of progression is high and grows as the length of time from infection increases.[36–38]

The rate at which AIDS develops in seropositive persons has been estimated by several studies to be approximately 4–10 percent per year of infection, with a low incidence in the first several years and an inflection upwards in the incidence curve thereafter. Eyster and colleagues studied a group of 85 hemophiliacs for whom seroconversion dates were known for a median of 4.5 years.[39] They found an actuarial rate of progression to AIDS at 18 percent 6 years after infection. Adults had a significantly higher progression rate (34 percent at 6 years) than did hemophiliacs less than 22 years old (10 percent at 6 years). The San Francisco Department of Public Health and the CDC have studied a cohort of 132 homosexual men in whom serconversion dates are known for a median of 8 years.[36,40] In this group, the actuarial progression rate to AIDS at 9 years was 42 percent; an additional 32 percent developed symptomatic conditions (ARC) that are not AIDS defining by surveillance criteria. Both of these studies, although small, show an increasing incidence of AIDS as the infection persists.

Studies of prevalent HIV infections have shown similar rates of progression to AIDS. Moss and associates followed 288 HIV-seropositive homosexual men for 3 years; they estimated that the median duration of infection was 6 years.[38] The 3-year actuarial rate of progression to AIDS was 22 percent; an additional 19 percent developed ARC (oral candidiasis, hairy leukoplakia, chronic diarrhea, or persistent constitutional symptoms). Moreover, the projected rate of progression to AIDS is 50 percent and to ARC is 25 percent at 6 years (or 9 years from infection) by extrapolating from predictors of progression at 3 years. Long-term projections of disease progression show that most seropositive subjects will develop illness in the 10–15 years after infection.[41]

Clinical and laboratory findings may help predict how the disease develops in seropositive subjects. Oral candidiasis (thrush), itself an opportunistic infection, is an early clinical marker of immunosuppression and heralds the development of AIDS in many patients.[42] Carne and colleagues studied 100 homosexual men with generalized lymphadenopathy and found that the risk of developing AIDS over an 18-month period increased 12-fold for subjects with thrush when compared with subjects without this finding.[43] Hairy leukoplakia, an opportunistic infection associated with Epstein-Barr virus (EBV), also predicts the development of AIDS. Greenspan et al. found that a referred population of homosexual men with hairy leukoplakia had an actuarial progression rate to opportunistic infection of 48 percent at 16 months and 83 percent at 31 months.[44] Dermatomal or disseminated outbreaks of herpes zoster appear

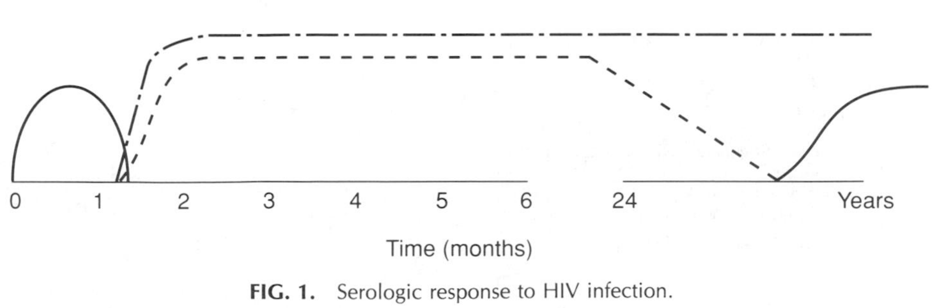

FIG. 1. Serologic response to HIV infection.

to be associated with the HIV infection, per se, but not with the progressive development of AIDS. One study of 112 homosexual men in New York City who had had an episode of shingles between 1980 and 1986 found that 73 percent had developed AIDS 6 years after the outbreak.[45] This finding, however, probably reflects an incubation period of HIV before full-blown AIDS symptoms developed. Prospective studies of seropositive homosexual men have failed to confirm zoster as a risk factor for progression to immunodeficiency. Generalized lymphadenopathy has also been proposed as a predictor of progression to AIDS, but prospective studies have failed to confirm this. One study found that average CD4+ lymphocyte counts were higher in homosexual men with lymphadenopathy than in seropositives without enlarged nodes.[30]

A number of laboratory tests have correlated progressive immunodeficiency and the development of AIDS.[46] CD4+ lymphocyte counts, a specific test for HIV-induced immunopathology, have sensitively predicted the development of AIDS and ARC. Goedert et al. found that CD4 cell counts <300/mm^3 were associated with a progression rate of 18.5 cases/100 person-years in seropositive homosexual men as compared with 1.5 cases/100 person-years for men with >550 CD4 cells/mm^3.[47] Polk and associates also showed that the development of AIDS was associated with a CD4 cell count of less than 300/mm^3 during a 15-month period of follow-up.[48] Moss and coworkers associated a baseline CD4 cell count of 200/mm^3 or less with a 3-year progression rate to AIDS of 89 percent; the rate for those with baseline CD4 counts of 200–400/mm^3 was 46 percent, and those with more than 400 cells/mm^3 had a 15 percent progression rate (Table 6).[38] Other studies have shown similar findings. Several studies have focused on the ratio of CD4 to CD8 cells and have shown higher rates of progression in individuals with ratios of less than 0.6.[48] Most studies find no independent association with the CD4:CD8 ratio when it is controlled for CD4 count. Likewise, the absolute number of CD8 cells falls in advanced infection with HIV and does not independently predict outcome. Other cell determinations that predict the development of AIDS in a seropositive individual include a total lymphocyte count of less than 1000, a total white blood cell count of less than 4000, a hematocrit of less than 40, and a low proportion of lymphocytes with the CD4 phenotype, regardless of the total CD4 count.[38,43]

As discussed earlier, the presence of HIV core antigen in the serum reflects either recent infection or an antigen-excess state from unchecked viral replication. In chronically infected subjects, HIV antigenemia is associated with a high rate of disease progression. Moss et al. compared initially antigenemic subjects with antigen-negative subjects. Of the antigenemic subjects 59 percent developed AIDS, and 30 percent developed ARC in 3 years as compared with 16 and 17 percent, respectively, for antigen-negative subjects.[38] Approximately 7 percent of antigen-negative subjects became antigenemic annually. Allain and coworkers showed that in hemophiliacs HIV antigenemia was a better predictor of progression to disease than was the CD4 cell count.[49] DeWolf and associates also found a higher rate of disease progression in antigenemic homosexual men in Amsterdam.[50] Conversely, Polk et al. reported that the rate of disease progression was higher in subjects who had lower titers of HIV antibody by ELISA,[48] a finding that probably reflects the loss of anti-core antibodies in persons with advanced disease. Weber and colleagues associated the loss of anti-p24 with the development of AIDS in a cohort of infected homosexual men.[51] Moss et al. found, however, that the absence of p24 antibodies did not predict disease progression independently of p24 antigen.

Levels of serum β_2-microglobulin, a low-molecular-weight immunoglobulin that forms the light chain of the class I major histocompatibility center (MHC) receptor, are elevated in HIV infection, particularly in subjects with advanced disease. A β_2-microglobulin level greater than 5 μg/ml was associated with a 3-year actuarial rate of AIDS of 69 percent in one study.[38] Subjects with a β_2-microglobulin level greater than 5 μg/ml had a seventeenfold greater hazard for developing AIDS than did seropositive subjects with normal levels. Both cytomegalovirus (CMV) infection and acid-labile interferon-α (INF-α) induce the synthesis of β_2-microglobulin. High titers of anti-CMV antibodies and acid-labile, INF-α have also been shown to predict disease activity in seropositive subjects.[48,52]

A number of researchers have extensively studied behavioral factors as predictors of disease progression; however, no convincing evidence has been found that individuals decrease the risk of becoming ill by modifying their behavior. In vitro, HIV replication can be induced by coinfection with herpesviruses. It has been theorized that in vivo exposure to potentially activating pathogens such as herpes simplex virus (HSV) or syphilis may lead to a greater degree of viral replication. Large prospective studies have not associated sexual activities, a history of sexually transmitted diseases, or exposure to specific infectious agent(s) with disease progression.[53] Epidemiologic cohort studies detect such influences poorly, however, and as a result, it is prudent to advise seropositive individuals to avoid other sexually transmitted diseases. Similarly, inactivated-virus vaccines stimulate and activate CD4 cells and, theoretically, may increase viral replication.[54] The use of influenza and pneumococcal vaccines in adults with HIV infection carries the same theoretic risk, but no in vivo evidence of harm exists.[55]

Antigenic stimulation by foreign proteins contaminating unsterile hypodermic needles (such as those used by iv drug users to inject drugs) may also increase the rate of progression of disease in seropositive drug users. DesJarlais et al. studied declines in CD4 cell counts in 163 HIV-infected drug users and found that subjects who continued to inject drugs had a greater loss of cells than did those who were abstinent.[56] While it is again prudent to advise seropositive addicts to avoid drug injection or needle sharing, the decline in CD4 cell counts during a very short period of follow-up cannot be assumed to reflect differential rates of developing AIDS. Continued drug injection, particularly cocaine injection, increases the risk of non-AIDS-associated infections such as absesses and endocarditis.[57]

Striking racial differences in the prevalence of AIDS and HIV infection, particularly among iv drug users, has led some investigators to speculate that genetic factors may lead to higher rates in acquiring the disease. Studies of HIV infection in drug users, however, suggest that racial differences are largely behavioral.[58] A widely reported study by Eales and associates in London stated that allelic differences in the group-specific pro-

TABLE 6. Predictors of Progression to AIDS in HIV Seropositive Homosexual Men

Variable	*Category*	*3-Year Rate of Progression*[a] *(%)*	*Relative Hazard*
CD4+ lymphocyte count	<200/mm^3	87	13.4
	200–400/mm^3	46	3.6
	>400/mm^3	16	1.0
CD4+ lymphocyte proportion (of total lymphocytes)	<25%	48	5.1
	≥25%	12	1.0
HIV p24 antigen	Positive	59	4.6
	Negative	15	1.0
Anti-p24 antibody	Negative	43	3.2
	Positive	16	1.0
β-2 microglobulin	>5 μg/ml	69	16.9
	3.1–5 μg/ml	33	4.5
	≤3 μg/ml	12	1.0
Hemoglobin	<13.5 g/dl	50	4.5
	≥13.5 g/dl	21	1.0

[a] Actuarial progression rate by product-limit method
(From Moss et al.,[38] with permission.)

tein (GC) predicted both HIV infection and the development of AIDS in infected subjects.[59] These investigators later retracted their findings and blamed malfunctioning laboratory equipment for generating erroneous data.[59a] The predilection of Kaposi sarcoma (KS) for certain racial and ethnic groups suggests a genetic predisposition that may explain the occurrence of KS in some persons with HIV infection. An early study found that KS was associated with the HLA-DR5 phenotype, but this finding has not been confirmed for other groups. Nevertheless, genetic differences in susceptibility to HIV infection or disease may exist.

Biologic differences in disease progression do exist. Age is an important factor in the rate at which AIDS develops in seropositive subjects. Eyster et al. reported that disease progression was three- to fivefold higher in adult hemophiliacs with HIV infection when compared with subjects under 21 years old.[39] Moss and associates observed a relative hazard of 2.2 for developing AIDS, independent of the CD4 cell count, in seropositive homosexual men over 35 years old.[38] Bacchetti et al. studied the first 500 AIDS cases in San Francisco and found that patients over the age of 40 had significantly shorter survival than did patients 20–39 years old.[60] This difference was most pronounced for patients with an initial diagnosis of Kaposi sarcoma. While immunocompetence is known to decline with senescence, the striking differences in disease progression and mortality by age are poorly understood.

Acute Retroviral Syndrome

In 1985 Cooper and colleagues in Australia identified an acute mononucleosis-like syndrome in 11 of 12 homosexual men who became antibody-positive for HIV antibodies.[61] Similar reports of a characteristic syndrome occurring in all AIDS risk groups, including health care workers exposed to accidental parenteral inoculation of HIV, were soon published.[62] The CDC classification system lists the acute retroviral syndrome as category I of HIV disease.

The incidence of the acute retroviral syndrome is not precisely known. Retrospective studies of homosexual men infected with HIV find a low prevalence of seroconversion illness.[63,64] A prospective study of homosexual men showed a 55 percent incidence of a mononucleosis-like illness in 22 subjects who become antibody-positive as compared with 21 percent in 44 nonconverting controls.[65] Other studies show a higher incidence of the syndrome. In a follow-up study to the report of Cooper et al., Tindall and associates evaluated 39 homosexual men known to have become antibody-positive and found that 36 (92 percent) recalled an illness consistent with the acute retroviral syndrome during the time when their tests showed seroconversion.[66] Forty percent of a seronegative control group also reported a mononucleosis-like illness, however. Most health care workers with occupational acquisition of HIV had the acute retroviral syndrome after exposure.[62,68] Overall, this syndrome is probably underreported and underdiagnosed; its true incidence may be between one-third and two-thirds of all persons who acquire HIV infection.

The clinical features of the acute retroviral syndrome are nonspecific and variable. The onset of the illness ranges from 1 to 6 weeks after exposure to the virus. Fever, sweats, malaise, myalgias, anorexia, nausea, diarrhea, and a nonexudative pharyngitis are prominent symptoms.[69,70] Many patients report headaches, photophobia, and meningismus. One-quarter to one-half of patients may have a truncal exanthem that may be maculopapular, roseola-like, or urticarial.[71] In addition to aseptic meningitis, neurologic symptoms occur in a minority of patients and may include encephalitis, peripheral neuropathy, and an acute, ascending polyneuropathy (Guillain-Barré syndrome).[72–77] Physical examination frequently reveals cervical, occipital, or axillary lymphadenopathy; rash; and less commonly, hepatosplenomegaly. Oral aphthous ulcerations have been reported in several cases; these may involve the esophagus. Oral and esophageal candidiasis during the seroconversion illness has been reported.[78] The remainder of the physical examination is usually unremarkable.

Laboratory evaluation of patients with the syndrome reveals a reduced total lymphocyte count, elevated sedimentation rate, negative heterophil-antibody test, and elevated transaminase and alkaline phosphatase levels.[66,79,80] When lymphocyte phenotyping is performed, a characteristic pattern is observed.[81] Initially, the total lymphocyte count decreases with a normal ratio of CD4 to CD8 T lymphocytes. Within several weeks, both the CD4 and CD8 cell populations begin to increase. The rise in CD8 cell numbers is relatively greater than is that in CD4 cells, and the CD4:CD8 ratio is inverted. In the weeks that follow, the CD8 cell population increases rather markedly. The total lymphocyte count also increases, and atypical lymphocytes may be seen on the peripheral smear. The ratio of CD4:CD8 cells usually remains inverted as the acute illness resolves (primarily due to excess numbers of CD8 cells). In patients with neurologic symptoms, cerebrospinal fluid may show a lymphocytic pleocytosis with normal levels of protein and glucose.[76,82]

Serologic studies of patients with the acute illness may be useful in making an early diagnosis. HIV core (p24) antigen may be detected in the serum and cerebrospinal fluid of patients with primary infection within 2 weeks of exposure, often coincidently with the onset of symptoms.[69,83] Antigenemia can persist for several weeks or months and generally resolves when antibodies to p24 are produced in sufficient quantity to form complexes with free antigen. The ELISA for HIV antibodies remains negative for an average of 2–3 months despite the appearance of specific antibodies on a Western blot of the patient's serum. Anti-p24 appears on the Western blot shortly before seroconversion is detected by ELISA and the appearance of antibodies to other antigens.[84] Prolonged seronegative, antigen-positive states have been reported, although the frequency of these states is not known.[85] Most investigators have observed seroconversion within several months of acute illness and the appearance of antigenemia.

The differential diagnosis of the acute retroviral syndrome includes a number of other illnesses: infectious mononucleosis; other viral infections such as influenza, measles, rubella, and herpes simplex; and secondary syphilis. Evaluation of patients presenting with an illness consistent with acute retroviral infection should include a careful history to elicit risks for HIV infection, laboratory tests to rule out mononucleosis and syphilis, HIV antibody and antigen tests, and complete blood counts and differential. Sera should be saved so that acute and convalescent titers of HIV and other viral antibodies can be performed.

Therapy for primary HIV infection is symptomatic and supportive. Fever, myalgias, and headaches may be treated with acetaminophen or nonsteroidal anti-inflammatory drugs. Bed rest and hydration may be necessary. Specific antiviral therapy has been proposed as postexposure prophylaxis for persons with known HIV exposures; however, the therapy is likely to be less effective after clinical symptoms appear than as an immediate intervention.

Persistent Generalized Lymphadenopathy

Infection with HIV is associated with a high prevalence of generalized lymphadenopathy, often beginning with the acute retroviral syndrome. In the early 1980s, clinicians in New York and San Francisco recognized persistent generalized lymphadenopathy (PGL) and suggested a prodromal state to the development of AIDS in homosexual men who were otherwise healthy.[15,16,86] The syndrome of PGL was defined as the presence of two or more extrainguinal sites of lymphadenopathy for a minimum of 3–6 months for which no other explanation could be found. Biopsy specimens of lymph nodes from such patients usually revealed a follicular hyperplasia without specific pathogens. An increasing proportion of these patients developed AIDS over time, thus linking PGL and AIDS before HIV was discovered.[87]

After becoming antibody-positive, approximately 50–70 percent of infected individuals develop PGL. The most frequently involved node groups are the posterior and anterior cervical, submandibular, occipital, and axillary chains; epitrochlear and femoral nodes may also be enlarged. Mediastinal and hilar adenopathy are not characteristic of the syndrome; however, abdominal computed tomography (CT) often reveals enlarged mesenteric and retroperitoneal adenopathy in HIV-infected persons. Although first described in homosexual men, PGL appears to occur with equal frequency in all infected groups. The natural history of PGL does not differ significantly from that of the HIV infection itself, although the CDC defines PGL as a separate category in its classification system for HIV disease (category III). Persistent generalized lymphadenopathy is a very sensitive marker of HIV infection: this finding in an individual who has no other reason for lymphadenopathy should prompt an evaluation for HIV, including HIV serologic testing.

Physical examination usually reveals symmetric, mobile, rubbery, lymph nodes ranging from 0.5 to 2 cm and distributed as previously described. Pain and tenderness are uncommon. Localized (i.e., asymmetric) adenopathy and rapid nodal enlargement are not characteristic and suggest an infectious or malignant process. The remainder of the physical examination is often unremarkable, although other complications of HIV infection may be found such as thrush or hairy leukoplakia. Laboratory evaluation is generally unrewarding, with the exception of HIV serology and T-cell subset phenotyping.

The differential diagnosis of PGL includes HIV infection and a wide variety of other processes that are associated with generalized lymphadenopathy: sarcoid, secondary syphilis, and Hodgkin's disease, for example. In patients with HIV infection, lymphadenopathy may also be caused by mycobacterial infections, Kaposi sarcoma, and lymphoma.[88] If not already known, the HIV serostatus should be determined with the patient's consent. Many patients who assume that they are infected with HIV decline to undergo serologic testing, although this preference is changing as both the knowledge of the natural history and the treatment of HIV advance. Aspiration of lymph nodes usually reveals benign cells.[89] Biopsy specimens show follicular hyperplasia, with the normal architecture distorted by greatly expanded germinal centers composed of B lymphocytes. The peripheral blood may also show a B-cell lymphocytosis and a polyclonal gammopathy.

Management of lymphadenopathy in a patient with known or suspected HIV infection should include node aspiration or biopsy in certain circumstances. Patients who may have been previously infected with *Mycobacterium tuberculosis* (e.g., iv drug users and persons from developing countries) have an increased risk of tuberculous adenitis and should be evaluated by aspiration or biopsy. A purified protein derivative (PPD) test should be administered to all patients. In addition, the presence of constitutional symptoms such as fever and weight loss with PGL merits a work-up to rule out lymphoma or opportunistic infection.[90,91] Likewise, localized or rapidly enlarging lymphadenopathy suggests an underlying infection or malignancy and should be evaluated by needle aspiration or biopsy. Fine-needle aspiration by an experienced pathologist is an acceptable alternative to biopsy and identifies infections and lymphomas very sensitively.[89,90] Follow-up biopsies for immunocytologic studies may need to be performed when a lymphoma is diagnosed by needle aspiration.

Most patients with PGL require no invasive evaluation and can be managed expectantly for the occurrence of other AIDS-related manifestations.

Immune Thrombocytopenia and Hematologic Manifestations

Thrombocytopenia was identified early in the AIDS epidemic in persons with high-risk groups. In homosexual men, thrombocytopenia was often diagnosed simultaneously with lymphadenopathy, while isolated thrombocytopenia was reported in iv drug users from the New York area. Prospective studies of persons with HIV infection now indicate that 5–15 percent of HIV-seropositives may have persistent thrombocytopenia (platelet count, $<100,000/mm^3$; a smaller proportion have platelet counts $<50,000/mm^3$). The natural history of HIV infection does not appear to differ in persons with immune thrombocytopenia and in nonthrombocytopenic persons, and specific risk factors for developing immune thrombocytopenia have not been identified.

HIV-related immune thrombocytopenia may be manifested by easy bruising, petechiae, bleeding gums, and prolonged bleeding from minor cuts and abrasions. Most patients are asymptomatic and are found to have low platelet counts incidently during routine clinical evaluation. More severe bleeding complications such as gastrointestinal (GI) hemorrhage or cerebrovascular bleeding are very rare. Platelet counts typically remain low for months to years, although platelet counts increase in some patients as HIV disease advances.

The pathophysiology of immune thrombocytopenia has been studied in both homosexual men and drug users, and the primary mechanism of disease has been identified as the peripheral destruction of platelets. Examination of the bone marrow usually shows normal or increased production of megakaryocytes and erythroid hyperplasia. Deposition of immune complexes on platelets has been postulated as one mechanism of destruction. Investigation of homosexual men with HIV-related immune thrombocytopenia showed the presence of a specific platelet membrane antigen against which antibodies were directed.[92] The same antigen and antibodies were also found, however, in HIV-infected controls without immune thrombocytopenia. Splenomegaly is often found on physical examination and is frequently present when abdominal CT scans are performed.[93]

A limited differential diagnosis of isolated thrombocytopenia in an HIV-infected person includes drug-induced thrombocytopenia, particularly in heroin addicts and alcoholics, consumptive thrombocytopenia, or splenic sequestration. Some patients with thrombocytopenia may also present with leukopenia or anemia. The presence of constitutional symptoms and pancytopenia suggests an opportunistic infection, particularly disseminated mycobacterial or fungal infection, or a lymphoma. Patients with these clinical findings should undergo bone marrow aspiration and biopsy, with appropriate stains and cultures. Isolated immune thrombocytopenia in an HIV-infected person can be managed expectantly by advising the patient to avoid aspirin and drugs that may exacerbate thrombocytopenia. Managing drugs associated with thrombocytopenia (e.g., rifampin) depends on the need for the drug and the degree of thrombocytopenia. If the patient does not have significant bleeding and maintains a platelet count above $20,000/mm^3$, the medication can be continued with close observation. If an alternative agent can be reasonably substituted, this should be done. Some patients with advanced HIV disease who are taking azidothymidine (AZT) may present with pancytopenia. While AZT is clearly associated with anemia and leukopenia, it does not cause thrombocytopenia; in fact, it significantly increases platelet counts in most patients.[94] This finding should be evaluated with appropriate diagnostic studies.

Other Hematologic Manifestations

HIV infection is associated with other abnormalities of the blood. Thrombotic thrombocytopenic purpura (TTP) has been reported in a small number of persons with HIV disease, and its clinical features appear to be similar to other populations. Intravascular hemolysis and thrombocytopenia are pronounced. The prevalence of TTP appears to be extremely low, and it is unclear whether HIV itself or another infectious agent is responsible for TTP in HIV-infected patients.

Anemia is a prominent feature of HIV disease. Most patients with advanced disease, particularly those with opportunistic infections, have a normochromic, normocytic anemia. The anemia is generally mild (hemoglobin content, 11–14 g/dl) and nonprogressive, although patients with a history of multiple opportunistic infections may have a hemoglobin level as low as 8–9 g/dl. Anemia is caused by a number of factors. HIV may infect erythroid precursors in the bone marrow[95] and inhibit the production of red cells; however, AIDS patients with anemia usually show normal myeloid and erythroid precursors and adequate iron stores upon aspiration and biopsy of the bone marrow. Sequestration of red cells in the spleen and, to a lesser extent, the liver may contribute to the anemia. Concurrent opportunistic infections or malignancies frequently depress the hematocrit value. Suppression of erythropoietin production may also affect red cell production.

The differential diagnosis of anemia in a person with HIV disease should include blood loss, infiltration of the bone marrow by opportunistic pathogens (e.g., *Mycobacterium avium* complex, *Histoplasma capsulatum*), malignancy, and drug toxicity. Depression of all cell lines suggests opportunistic disease, whereas isolated, mild anemia is most often associated with HIV. Bone marrow biopsy is not usually indicated in the latter situation. Although HIV-induced anemia generally does not require specific therapy, a low hematocrit predicts disease progression in asymptomatic HIV-seropositives.[38]

Constitutional Disease

Prolonged infection with HIV is often completely asymptomatic; however, a minority of patients complain of nonspecific constitutional symptoms in the months or years after primary infection. Patients commonly complain of being easily fatigued and report the need to reduce their normal activities somewhat. Debilitating fatigue is uncommon in the early years of infection. Low-grade fevers (temperature, <38°C), occasional night sweats, and intermittent diarrhea are also reported. The exact incidence of these findings is not known, and attributing them solely to HIV infection may be mistaken. The differential diagnosis of these findings includes intercurrent minor illnesses and psychological disorders. Anxiety and depression are common responses to knowledge or suspicion of HIV infection.[96] Many patients infected with HIV may have underlying psychiatric conditions. Intravenous drug users, in particular, have a high prevalence of affective disorders that may result in somatic complaints. Moreover, the physical effects of opiates and withdrawal from stimulants such as cocaine and amphetamines cause fatigue and other constitutional symptoms.

In patients with more advanced HIV disease and severe depletion of CD4+ cells, constitutional disease may primarily reflect immunosuppression or may herald the onset of opportunistic infections or malignancies. For example, the prodrome of *P. carinii* pneumonia (PCP) often consists of a month or more of fevers, weight loss, and fatigue before respiratory complaints develop. Disseminated mycobacterial infections typically cause fatigue, fever, night sweats, and diarrhea. In African patients with HIV infection, a wasting illness termed "slim disease" has been described.[97] These patients have debilitating fatigue, fevers, sweats, protracted diarrhea, and severe weight loss. Opportunistic or conventional pathogens are not revealed upon evaluation, but the patients waste away and die of severe malnutrition and terminal secondary infections. This illness has been encountered in developed countries as well, but far less commonly than in Africa—a pattern that suggests underdiagnosis of opportunistic diseases in Africa. One study of African patients with enteropathic slim disease found that most (16/22) had enteric pathogens or microsporidia found when a thorough evaluation was performed.[97a] In the United States, the CDC considers that an individual has AIDS when he has an unexplained constitutional disease for more than 1 month with a temperature greater than 38.3°C, diarrhea, and a loss of more than 10 percent of baseline body weight in the presence of HIV infection.[25]

Patients with progressive constitutional symptoms should be evaluated carefully for opportunistic pathogens. A history of respiratory, neurologic, gastrointestinal, and dermatologic symptoms should be elicited and a thorough physical examination completed. The skin may reveal characteristic lesions of Kaposi sarcoma or localized viral or bacterial infections. The oral cavity may show thrush (a finding extremely common in *P. carinii* pneumonia), hairy leukoplakia, oral Kaposi sarcoma, or other opportunistic processes. Asymmetric adenopathy should prompt an evaluation as outlined above. The chest findings are often normal, although rales or rhonchi indicating pulmonary infection may be heard. Abdominal examination may reveal hepatosplenomegaly or tenderness, particularly in the presence of retroperitoneal adenopathy. A rectal examination may show perirectal ulceration, vesicles, or erythema. A careful neurologic examination may identify evidence of global or focal neurologic impairment.

Laboratory evaluation should include a complete blood count, chemistry panel, and determination of T-cell subsets (if recent values are not available). An elevated erythrocyte sedimentation rate (ESR) is a sensitive, although nonspecific finding. A chest radiograph may reveal infiltrates, even though respiratory complaints are absent. When diarrhea is present, the stool should be evaluated as discussed below. Some clinicians find whole-body gallium scanning useful to evaluate systemic symptoms in HIV-infected patients because a focal uptake of gallium can identify clinically occult sites of opportunistic infection. Often, however, gallium may be taken up in the spleen and the transverse colon although a specific diagnosis is never reached. A physician should ascribe severe constitutional symptoms to HIV-induced wasting syndrome and diagnose AIDS *only* after a thorough evaluation.

Oral Disease

Abnormalities of the oral cavity occur throughout the course of HIV infection. Primary HIV infection has been associated with severe aphthous stomatitis and with oropharyngeal and esophageal candidiasis.[78] As the infection progresses and immunologic impairment proceeds, numerous oral complications arise. In the late stages of disease, oral manifestations are universal and frequently severe.[98,100]

Oral Candidiasis. *Candida* infections of the hard and soft palates, buccal mucosa, tongue, pharynx, and hypopharynx are observed frequently. Contrary to systemic *Candida* infections, which appear to result from defects in phagocyte function and number, mucosal candidal infections result from impaired cellular immunity. The incidence of candidiasis increases with progressive cellular immunodeficiency, particularly as CD4+ lymphocyte counts fall below 200–300/mm^3. Since oral candidiasis itself is an opportunistic infection, it predicts the disease progression and development of other AIDS-related infections.

A variety of manifestations of candidiasis have been described in HIV-infected patients. The most common form is thrush (pseudomembranous candidiasis). Characteristic cottage cheese plaques that can be removed with a tongue blade are seen on the soft palate, tonsils, and buccal mucosa. Less often, thrush involves the lateral and posterior aspects of the tongue, the hard palate, and the hypopharynx. *Candida* infection can produce flat, erythematous plaques distributed in the same way as the pseudomembranous form of the disease, but without the characteristic white exudate. This atrophic form of candidiasis is underdiagnosed because many clinicians are unfamiliar with its appearance. *Candida* can also cause a nonscrapable white plaque similar to hairy leukoplakia (see below). This hypertrophic form of disease may involve the lateral border of the tongue, the palate, and the buccal mucosa.

The diagnosis of candidiasis is frequently made on the basis of physical examination alone. A KOH preparation of scraped material from a plaque is diagnostic and can be performed easily in most clinical settings. Cultures for *Candida* are rarely necessary. Biopsy specimen of oral lesions can distinguish various forms of leukoplakia. A therapeutic trial of antifungal agents can also help to establish a diagnosis. *Candida* infection of the corners of the mouth (angular cheilitis) can cause pain, fissures, and difficulty opening the mouth. Physical examination, KOH preparation, and the response to antifungal therapy establish the diagnosis.

Hairy Leukoplakia. Originally described in 1984 by Greenspan et al., hairy leukoplakia (HL) is a raised, white lesion of the oral mucosa that is unique to HIV infection.[101] The lesion was initially described in homosexual men; it has subsequently been observed in all other groups of persons at risk for HIV infection.[102] Hairy leukoplakia appears asymptomatically when immunodeficiency has progressed to an advanced stage. In one prospective study of patients referred for evaluation of HL, the actuarial rate of progression to an AIDS-defining opportunistic infection was 85 percent at 2 years.[44] Other studies have shown a less dramatic (although substantial) rate of progression to AIDS after the diagnosis of HL.

The cause of HL is not completely understood, but it appears to be related to the replication of Epstein-Barr virus (EBV) in the epithelium of keratinized cells on the surface of the tongue and buccal mucosa.[104] Other herpesviruses have also been isolated from cultures of biopsied lesions; however, their role in the pathogenesis of HL is unclear. HIV is not routinely cultured from specimens and is not found with DNA probes. The diagnosis of HL is established by visual inspection, failure of the lesion to scrape off with a tongue blade, failure to respond to antifungal therapy, and by biopsy material or scrapings in which EBV can be identified.[104] Hairy leukoplakia is usually asymptomatic, although large lesions may impair taste, hinder eating, and cause discomfort.

Severe gingivitis and periodontitis have been observed in patients with HIV disease.[98] The onset of symptoms is often insidious but may be abrupt. Pain is often severe; patients may note foul breath, bleeding gums, and loosening of teeth. Physical examination may reveal a bright red marginal line on the gingiva, necrosis and ulceration of interdental papillae, gingival erosion, exfoliation of enamel, and loose teeth. The etiology of gingivitis and periodontitis is unclear. Mixed cultures of aerobic and anaerobic flora have been obtained from gingival biopsy samples. More severe, ulcerating gingivitis can be caused by infections with gram-negative bacilli, particularly *Klebsiella pneumoniae* and *Enterobacter cloacae*. Infections tend to be chronic, but topical antiseptic agents or metronidazole therapy may control some cases.

Peripheral Neuropathy

In most patients with AIDS, the peripheral nervous system is involved, and 20–40 percent of patients may have symptomatic peripheral nerve disease.[105,106] Symptoms may occur at any time during the course of HIV infection. Each stage of the infection is associated with specific neuropathies, as outlined in Table 7. The most common peripheral neuropathy, a distal, predominantly sensory polyneuropathy, accounts for at least 50 percent of cases.[107] Patients with this neuropathy usually complain of chronic, symmetric, painful dysesthesias in a stocking distribution, particularly in the soles; numbness; and (less often) weakness. Some patients feel pain when lightly touched. Sensory deficits, decreased or absent ankle jerks, and weakness may also be observed on examination, and patellar reflexes may be brisk. Electromyography shows a combined sensory and motor neuropathy consistent with demyelination in the lower extremities. Nerve biopsy may reveal axonal degeneration. Distal, sensory neuropathy is most often found in patients with advanced symptomatic HIV disease.

TABLE 7. Peripheral Neuropathies in HIV Disease by Stage

Disorder	*Seropositive*	*ARC*	*AIDS*
Guillain-Barre Syndrome	———	——→	
Chronic inflammatory demyelinating polyneuropathy	———	———	——→
Multiple mononeuropathy		———	——→
Sensory neuropathy		———	——→

Abbreviation: ARC: AIDS-related complex.
(Adapted from McArthur,[106] with permission.)

Chronic inflammatory demyelinating polyneuropathy (CIDP), the second most common peripheral neuropathy, tends to occur before other clinical manifestations of HIV develop.[108,109] Acute, inflammatory, demyelinating polyneuropathy (Guillain-Barré syndrome) is also reported early in the course of HIV disease. Patients report motor weakness that occurs acutely or gradually and have minimal sensory complaints. Weakness and areflexia are often noted on examination; a CSF pleocytosis is often present and the CSF protein level elevated. Nerve biopsy shows mononuclear cell infiltration and demyelination. The clinical course may wax and wane, and some patients recover spontaneously. Inflammatory demyelinating polyneuropathies may be associated with CMV infection, although the etiology may be autoimmune.[110]

Other rarer neuropathies include multiple mononeuropathy, possibly associated with vasculitis, herpesvirus and CMV radiculitis, and neuropathies of vitamin deficiency.

Musculoskeletal Complications

Polymyositis complicates HIV infection in a small number of patients.[111,112] Clinical features include myalgias, weakness of the proximal muscles, muscle tenderness, wasting, and fatigue. Creatinine kinase and other muscles enzyme concentrations are usually elevated, and electrophysiologic studies are consistent with a myopathy. Biopsies reveal muscle fiber necrosis and inflammatory infiltrates. Recent reports suggest that patients taking zidovudine (AZT) may be at increased risk for myopathy, although this not not been proved in prospective studies.[113]

Several reports have postulated the existence of an HIV-associated arthropathy.[114,115] Defining a specific arthropathy caused by HIV is difficult because many patients with HIV infection are already at increased risk for inflammatory joint disease. Intravenous drug users, for example, may develop septic arthritis caused by pyogenic bacteria, particularly *Staphylacoccus aureus*. Homosexual men may have increased risk of gonococcal arthritis or reactive arthritis associated with genital or gastrointestinal tract infections (Reiter syndrome). In patients with HIV infection, immune complex deposition or hepatitis B infection may also contribute to arthritis. HIV-associated arthropathy probably does exist since retrovirally induced arthritis is seen in other species.

Rheumatologic complications of HIV are highly prevalent. One prospective study of patients with HIV infection found that 71 percent had rheumatic manifestations (Table 8).[116] Arthralgias, arthritis, Reiter syndrome, and an oligoarticular painful syndrome were the most common findings. Arthralgias were intermittent and involved primarily the knees, shoulders, ankles, and elbows. Arthritis in HIV-seropositive patients may be due to a variety of conventional causes, or it may be unexplained and associated temporally with AIDS-related opportunistic infections. In the latter case, a painful mono- or oli-

TABLE 8. Frequency of Rheumatologic Manifestations in 101 Patients with HIV Disease

Manifestation	*Patients (%)*
Arthralgias	35
Arthritis	12
Reiter syndrome	10
Painful articular syndrome	10
Psoriatic arthritis	2
Polymyositis	2
Vasculitis	1
Total	71

(From Berman et al.,[116] with permission.)

goarticular inflammatory arthritis is present, often affecting the large joints.[114–116] The arthritis is nondeforming and nonerosive.

Aspirating the synovial fluid is generally unremarkable, and synovial biopsy specimens show mononuclear cell infiltrates. HIV has been cultured from the synovial fluid of one patient, although the meaning of this finding is not clear. The erythrocyte sedimentation rate may be elevated; other studies are nonspecific. Some patients may be HLA-B27–positive. In one series, a precipitating infection was detected in only 3 of 13 patients, although 7 additional patients had diarrhea and/or urethritis of undetermined etiology.[114]

The clinical course is often progressive. Some patients show little response to anti-inflammatory drugs, and most clinicians are reluctant to use cytotoxic or immunosuppresive drugs in such patients.

Reiter syndrome in HIV-infected persons can be particularly severe. Patients with this syndrome are usually HLA-B27–positive and present with an asymmetric oligoarticular arthritis and sacroiliitis with a variety of extra-articular signs and symptoms.[117] Reiter syndrome may occur in advanced HIV infection because of yet-unexplained immunologic mechanisms or the susceptibility of this population to infections with arthritogenic agents. Managing these patients clinically is difficult because the symptoms may not respond to nonsteroidal anti-inflammatory agents.

Berman et al. have described a painful articular syndrome in patients with advanced HIV infection.[116] This syndrome is characterized by excrutiating, oligo- or monoarticular pain that starts abruptly and resolves in several hours to 1 day. Physical examination of the joints is negative. The cause of this syndrome is not known, and it has not been widely reported.

Other rheumatic manifestations of HIV that have been reported include psoriatic arthritis, sicca syndrome, and vasculitis.[118] Prospective studies of populations of HIV-infected persons are necessary to further delineate the spectrum of HIV-associated musculoskeletal conditions.

Cutaneous Manifestations

Dermatologic consequences of HIV infection include primary cutaneous opportunistic infections and malignancies (that may also disseminate to the viscera) and systemic, opportunistic diseases with skin involvement. Examples of the former include Kaposi sarcoma (discussed subsequently) and dermatophytoses; the latter are exemplified by herpesvirus infections, syphilis, and fungal infections such as cryptococcosis.

Viral Infections of the Skin and Mucus Membranes. A wide range of viruses involve the skin in HIV-immunosuppressed patients. Herpesviruses in particular cause frequent morbidity in patients with advanced HIV disease. Serology documents previous infection with HSV-2 in more than 90 percent of homosexual men with HIV infection; it is less prevalent in other AIDS risk group members.[229] While HSV-2 recurs frequently even in nonimmunosuppressed hosts, it occurs frequently and for prolonged periods in patients with HIV infection. The CDC considers chronic mucocutaneous HSV-2 disease (<1 month) diagnostic of AIDS by its surveillance criteria. HSV-2, a common pathogen of the sacral root dermatomes, often causes outbreaks in the buttocks, perineum, scrotum or vulva, and the shaft and glans of the penis. Characteristic lesions of herpes appear first as painful erythematous papules; later they vesiculate and ulcerate, and in superinfection, pustules may form. Chronic ulcers may become granulated and bloody. Herpes proctitis is associated with severe rectal pain, fever, tenesmus, and obstipation. External lesions may be absent, and the diagnosis is established by anoscopic or sigmoidoscopic examination and cultures. Giant perirectal ulcers that yield thymidine kinase–resistant strains of HSV-2 have been reported in patients who were previously treated with acyclovir. Herpes simplex virus infections are diagnosed by the typical appearance and distribution of the lesions and culture. Tzanck preparations may show giant cells, which suggests HSV infection. Some physicians base their diagnoses on how patients respond to an empirical trial of acyclovir. Orolabial HSV infections in HIV-infected persons may be caused by either HSV-1 or HSV-2. While primary infections may occur after patients acquire HIV, recurrences are more common. Often, a prodrome of tingling and pain precedes the appearance of painful vesicles and ulcers. Lesions may be found on the lips, buccal mucosa, gingiva, soft palate, uvula, and tongue. Herpes simplex virus disease may recur chronically in patients with advanced immunosuppression.

In persons with HIV infection, varicella-zoster virus (shingles) often reactivates. As a result, the virus has been proposed as a marker of disease progression.[230] Prospective clinical trials have failed, however, to associate shingles and the subsequent development of AIDS. Dermatomal outbreaks are most common, and a substantial proportion of patients may have several dermatomes involved. Shingles is often characterized by radicular pain and itching several days before erythematous papules appear, and vesiculation occurs within several days. Lesions are often extremely pruritic, and excoriation with secondary bacterial infection commonly occurs. Over a period of 4–7 days lesions form bullae and crust and begin to heal, although some patients have zoster chronically. Cranial and thoracic dermatomes, followed by lumbar and sacral roots, are most often involved. Outbreaks along the ophthalmic branch of the trigeminal nerve may result in corneal involvement and lead to scarring and opacification that impair vision. Varicella-zoster virus appears to disseminate less often in patients with HIV infection than in other immunosuppressed patients. A substantial proportion of patients may experience post-herpetic scarring and pain. Although considered extremely rare before AIDS, recurrences of zoster have been reported from a number of patients with HIV infection. Chronic or nonremitting zoster has also been observed.

Molluscum contagiosum, a cutaneous poxvirus infection, is seen more often in HIV-infected persons than in other populations. The agent is transmitted by sexual or other close contact; reactivation of remote infection may cause outbreaks in immunosuppressed hosts. Molluscum lesions are small, firm papules with a pearly white surface distributed on the face, trunk, or genital areas. The lesions are usually painless and can be differentiated from herpetic lesions by the absence of erythema and the smaller size and resolution of lesions without ulcerating or crusting. Molluscum lesions can become superinfected with bacteria if they become excoriated, but otherwise they do not cause complications. Liquid nitrogen is used effectively to treat this condition.

LATE SYNDROMES

Gastrointestinal Syndromes

As HIV infection progresses, diseases of the gastrointestinal tract occur with greater frequency. Virtually every component of the gut represents a potential site of pathologic involvement.[119] Functional alimentation and nutrition are deranged, and this poses an additional burden on patients. Besides opportunistic disease resulting from HIV-induced immunodeficiency, persons with AIDS may have more common gastrointestinal problems exacerbated by advanced systemic illness. Therefore, clinicians evaluating gastrointestinal complaints in HIV-infected patients must consider conventional gut pathology.

Esophageal Disease. Several specific agents cause esophageal pathology in HIV infection. Esophagitis secondary to infections by *Candida*, cytomegalovirus, and herpes simplex viruses are the most common opportunistic manifestations of HIV disease in the upper GI tract.[120–123] In approximately 3 percent of AIDS cases in the United States, esophageal candidiasis is the presenting AIDS diagnosis. Other esophageal infections are less common. The subsequent development of esophageal disease after another index AIDS diagnosis is not unusual.

These processes most commonly present with odynophagia, often associated with persistent or intermittent retrosternal pain, nausea, anorexia, and weight loss. Dysphagia without pain is also encountered and may be associated with opportunistic infection, particularly esophageal candidiasis. The duration of symptoms may be brief or prolonged, and other manifestations of immunodeficiency often coincide. In particular, the finding of oral candidiasis in a patient with odynophagia strongly suggests esophageal involvement. While one site of another pathogen (e.g., CMV retinitis) may suggest a secondary esophageal process with the same organism, multiple etiologies of diverse organ system disease in AIDS is remarkably common.

Evaluation of patients with symptoms of esophagitis begins with a careful physical examination. The finding of oropharyngeal candidiasis strongly suggests esophageal candidiasis, and physicians may elect a trial of antifungal therapy. If symptoms resolve, the diagnosis can be established empirically. In patients who do not have oral thrush or who fail to respond to empirical antifungal therapy, upper gastrointestinal contrast radiography may show characteristic abnormalities that suggest a specific diagnosis. *Candida* esophagitis is associated with a classic pattern of diffuse ulcerations and plaques that creates a cobblestone appearance. Cytomegalovirus esophagitis frequently causes numerous, large, shallow ulcerations, although single ulcers are also reported. Herpes simplex infection of the esophagus usually produces multiple, deep ulcers. Esophageal endoscopy is a highly sensitive procedure to establish a diagnosis in patients with odynophagia or dysphagia. Friable cheesy plaques that may be easily removed with biopsy forceps are characteristic in candidal esophagitis, while diffuse erythematous ulcers are more common in viral esophagitis.[119] Lesions should be biopsied and tissue sections prepared for histopathologic stains to identify viral inclusion bodies or invasive yeast forms. Cultures for fungi and viruses should also be obtained from biopsy specimens. The yield of contrast radiography and of endoscopy with biopsy and culture are extremely high; additional diagnostic manuevers are not usually required. Additional pathology that may be found in evaluating esophageal symptoms in HIV-infected patients includes reflux esophagitis, esophageal Kaposi sarcoma, lymphoma, carcinoma, or peptic ulcer disease.

Disorders of the Stomach, Small Bowel, and Hepatobiliary System. As with esophageal diseases in HIV-infected patients, gastric disease may be opportunistic or may be unrelated to immunodeficiency. Common complaints include nausea, early satiety, anorexia, vomiting, hematemesis, and abdominal pain. Esophageal pathology may also involve the stomach. Cytomegalovirus gastritis has been described alone or associated with esophageal CMV ulcers. Cytomegalovirus gastritis causes an intense inflammatory response, ulceration, enlargement of ruggal folds, and edema. Cytomegalovirus gastritis may appear on a radiograph to be a mass lesion engulfing the entire stomach. Gastric Kaposi sarcoma is a common complication of cutaneous KS and is often asymptomatic.[124] The GI tract is the organ system most involved in visceral KS, and gastric lesions may occur in 25 percent of patients who undergo endoscopy. Occasionally, gastrointestinal KS may be associated with nausea, early satiety, severe pain, and gastrointestinal hemorrhage.

Barium contrast radiographs aid in evaluating an HIV-seropositive patient with gastric symptoms. They may show typical abnormalities such as duodenal ulcers, gastroesophageal reflux, or gastritis. Patients with a history of alcohol abuse may develop any of the upper GI complications of chronic alcoholism. When radiographic studies suggest non–AIDS-related pathology, standard therapy should be offered. If no response is observed, further diagnostic procedures are warranted. Upper GI contrast radiographs may reveal specific lesions consistent with an opportunistic process. Gastric KS appears in radiographs as an ulcerated, target lesion with underlying submucosal masses.

Definitive diagnoses of upper GI pathology may be made by endoscopic observation, biopsy, and culture. Kaposi sarcoma typically appears as a violet-blue submucosal mass without mucosal ulceration or bleeding. Biopsy of these lesions results in a histologic diagnosis in only about one-third of the cases—presumably because of the nonmucosal location of the tumor.[119] When other KS lesions are histologically confirmed, observing characteristic lesions on endoscopy is sufficient to make a diagnosis. Gastric lymphomas are diagnosed by endoscopic biopsy with histologic and immunohistochemical stains. Like KS, AIDS-related lymphomas are almost always multifocal, so a biopsy of the most accessible lesion can establish a diagnosis. Gastric ulcers and mass lesions should be sent for viral culture, and standard histologic stains should be performed to identify viral inclusion bodies.

Acalculous cholecystitis has been associated with both *Cryptosporidium* and CMV infections.[125,126] The usual presentation is postprandial pain, fever, right upper quadrant pain and tenderness, and an elevated alkaline phosphatase level. Ultrasonography or computed tomography may reveal typical findings of cholecystitis as well as a thickened gallbladder wall and obliteration of the bladder lumen. On histologic study, Cryptosporidia have been seen in the gallbladder mucosa, as have CMV inclusions.

Papillary stenosis and sclerosing cholangitis have been documented in a growing proportion of AIDS patients who present with right upper quadrant pain and tenderness, fever, and an elevated alkaline phosphatase level.[127,128] Dilatation of intrahepatic and extrahepatic ducts is noted on ultrasonography, and papillary stricture is frequently observed. In 75 percent of the patients studied, Cello and coworkers reported that endoscopic retrograde cholangiopancreatography identified cholangitis, ductal sclerosis, isolated papillary stenosis, or a combination of these findings.[119] Papillary stenosis was associated with *Cryptosporidium* or CMV in almost one-half of the cases. Jacobson et al. found that 12 of 36 patients with CMV end-organ disease had cholestatic liver enzyme abnormalities, and one-third of those undergoing ultrasound had biliary dilatation.[129] A significantly higher proportion of AIDS patients with CMV cultured from the blood have elevated liver enzymes than patients with negative blood cultures. Endoscopic sphincterotomy may significantly relieve pain and normalize the alkaline phosphatase level in patients with sclerosing cholangitis.

Liver disease in AIDS patients is extremely common.[130–132] It may result from previous injury (e.g., hepatitis B infection, non-A, non-B hepatitis, or alcoholic liver disease) or HIV disease. Right upper quadrant pain, hepatomegaly, and elevated liver function test values are the common presenting features. Both *M. avium* complex (MAC) and Kaposi sarcoma are frequently found in the liver. In one series, KS was the most common postmortem diagnosis, and MAC was the most frequently identified pathogen when a percutaneous liver biopsy was performed.[132] Forty percent of biopsies and autopsies demonstrated HIV-related pathologies. In addition to MAC and KS, other diagnoses included lymphoma, tuberculosis (TB), CMV infection, and viral hepatitis. Alcohol-related pathology was also commonly identified. Frequently, patients whose clinical findings suggest liver disease may be diagnosed on the basis of noninvasive tests or biopsies of other organs. When a primary hepatic process appears likely or when other diagnostic procedures fail to reveal a cause of the symptoms, percutaneous liver biopsy is indicated. Specimens should undergo standard histologic and microbiologic staining and should be cultured for viruses, fungi, and mycobacteria. Hepatotoxicity of drugs used to treat HIV-related disorders should also be considered when evaluating patients with liver dysfunction. Rarer causes of infiltrative liver disease in patients with HIV disease include hepatic pneumocystosis, leishmaniasis, histoplasmosis, and other fungal infections.

Enterocolitis. Small and large bowel infections and disease processes may cause symptoms in association with HIV infection. Table 9 lists the principal causes of lower gastrointestinal tract disease in patients with AIDS. A variety of infectious agents may produce diarrhea, abdominal cramping, and pain, and they may be managed less readily by a host with HIV-induced immunosuppression. Before the AIDS epidemic, both symptomatic and asymptomatic gastrointestinal infections were found to be prevalent in homosexual men. Asymptomatic carriage of some pathogens has also been observed in patients with HIV infection and AIDS.[133] The incidence of gastroenteritis in patients with HIV infection is high, and some specific infections (e.g., *Salmonella*, *Cryptosporidium*, *Isospora*, CMV, *Microsporidia*) have been found to occur more frequently in AIDS patients.

Small bowel infections generally produce bloating, nausea, cramping, and profuse diarrhea and may be associated with significant weight loss. Colitis and proctitis more often cause lower quadrant cramping and pain, urgency, tenesmus, and smaller, more frequent stools. Distinguishing small bowel infections and colitis clinically may be difficult, however, and some infections may cause a panenteritis. The differential diagnosis of enterocolitis includes bacteria (such as *Salmonella*, *Shigella*, *Campylobacter*, mycobacteria) protozoa (such as *Entamoeba histolytica*, *Giardia lamblia*, *Cryptosporidium*, *Isospora*), and cytomegalovirus. In addition, *Clostridium difficile*-associated colitis may be more common in patients with HIV disease, particularly in those who have previously received antimicrobial therapy.

TABLE 9. Lower Gastrointestinal Tract Disease in Patients with HIV Infection

Causes of enterocolitis
Bacteria
Campylovacter jejuni and other spp.
Salmonella spp.
Shigella flexneri
Mycobacterium avium-complex
Clostridium difficile (toxin)
Parasites
Cryptosporidium spp.
Entamoeba histolytica
Giardia lamblia
Isospora spp.
Viral
Cytomegalovirus
HIV (?)
Causes of proctocolitis
Bacteria
Chlamydia trachomatis
Neisseria gonorrhoeae
Treponema pallidum
Viral
Herpes simplex

Patients with AIDS and diarrhea frequently have an enteric pathogen that is identified when stool studies are performed. Infectious agents have been found in 55–85 percent of AIDS patients who present with diarrhea[134]; from 10 to 40 percent of AIDS patients without diarrhea are infected with an enteric pathogen.[133] Asymptomatic HIV-seropositive patients also carry intestinal pathogens at a high rate. Treatable pathogens are found in about one-half of patients studied. Cytomegalovirus and *Cryptosporidium* are the most often identified enteric pathogens in symptomatic patients; next are *Giardia*, *Salmonella*, *Campylobacter* and *C. difficile*. More extensive, invasive diagnostic evaluations probably yield a higher number of pathogens.

Renal Disease

Renal abnormalities have been described in a variety of patients with AIDS, but it is still debated whether a specific AIDS-associated nephropathy (AAN) exists. Ascribing renal dysfunction to HIV infection or AIDS is problematic because some AIDS patients have a high risk for renal disease. Intravenous drug use, hepatitis B infection, fluid and electrolyte disorders, therapy with nephrotoxic drugs, and concomitant opportunistic infections and malignancies are all associated with renal dysfunction. In 1984, Rao and colleagues reported on 11 AIDS patients who had renal disease.[135] The patients were characterized clinically by proteinuria and mildly elevated serum creatinine levels and pathologically by focal and segmental glomerulosclerosis. While this entity is similar to heroin-associated nephropathy, only one-half of the patients studied gave a history of iv drug use. In a review of 75 consecutive AIDS patients in Miami, 43 percent of the patients had proteinuria >0.5 g/24 hr; 9 percent had >3 g/24 hr.[136] In 36 autopsied patients, 17 (47 percent) had renal pathology, 5 had focal glomerulosclerosis, and 12 had mesangial proliferation. A subsequent review of the same patient population found that patients with a history of iv drug use had the highest incidence of renal disease; however, Haitians, homosexual men, and children with perinatally acquired HIV infection also developed proteinuria and glomerulosclerosis.[137] In another series of patients, renal disease was observed in 13 of 32 patients and included focal glomerulosclerosis, mesangial proliferation, and glomerulonephritis.[138] Renal disorders developed in association with fungal infections, disseminated *Mycobacterium avium-intracellulare* infection, hypotension, and the use of nephrotoxic drugs (such as aminoglycosides or amphotericin B). AIDS-associated nephropathy appears more frequently in the eastern United States where large numbers of iv drug users with AIDS are found. Large numbers of patients followed in San Francisco and other cities have not had as much kidney involvement as those seen in New York and Miami. Moreover, AAN is more commonly reported in blacks than in other racial groups, which suggests a biologic susceptibility to this disorder. Further prospective studies of how HIV-seropositives develop renal disease are needed.

Renal dysfunction in AIDS patients is usually diagnosed incidently when patients present with opportunistic infections. Asymptomatic proteinuria, up to 5 g/day, is often the initial finding, and the serum creatinine level is often normal or only mildly elevated. The albumin concentration is almost always low (as is true for most AIDS patients with opportunistic infections), and the blood pressure is usually normal. Renal biopsy most often shows focal and segmental glomerulosclerosis with tubular dilatation and atrophy, fibrosis, and a mononuclear cell infiltrate. Immunofluorescence studies often reveal deposits of IgM and C3, and electron micropsy shows electron-dense mesangial deposits and mesangial hypocellularity. One report of intranuclear and intracytoplasmic inclusion bodies, which suggest a viral etiology of renal pathology, has been published.

The clinical course of AAN progresses quickly, usually because many other opportunistic processes occur simultaneously. Rao et al.[135] originally reported death with renal failure in 8 of 11 patients with AAN in less than 4 months. Since AAN is diagnosed late in the course of HIV disease, it is difficult to determine the effect of renal dysfunction on survival. Rao and associates have also reported on 18 patients who developed AIDS while receiving hemodialysis for end-stage renal disease. They survived a median of 1 month beyond their AIDS diagnosis.[139] Other centers have also reported that patients with AIDS responded poorly to maintenance by hemodialysis.[140] Activating the cellular immune system through chronic dialysis may accelerate HIV pathology. On the other hand, AIDS patients who have acute renal failure from a reversible insult (such as hypotension or nephrotoxic drugs) respond to conservative measures and the brief use of hemodialysis.

Pulmonary Disease

Opportunistic pulmonary diseases are the most common cause of acute illness and death in patients with HIV infection.[141] In the United States, approximately 65 percent of AIDS-defining illnesses are pulmonary opportunistic infections; most of these are *P. carinii* pneumonia (PCP). Moreover, pulmonary diseases (such as PCP) are assuming a greater role in the clinical spectrum of AIDS as the relative prevalence of Kaposi sarcoma as an AIDS-defining diagnosis decreases.[142] Before the AIDS epidemic, PCP was a rare opportunistic pathogen encountered in patients with severe malnutrition, hematologic malignancies, and iatrogenic immunosuppression. As of June 1989, approximately 55,000 AIDS patients in the United States had had an index AIDS diagnosis of PCP. It has been estimated that an additional 16,000–18,000 patients had PCP as a secondary AIDS diagnosis not reported to public health authorities. Reports of the prevalence of PCP in AIDS patients are substantially lower in developing countries than in industrial nations; however, significant underdiagnosis and underreporting of PCP may be caused by the lack of sophisticated diagnostic facilities.

The multiple etiologies of pulmonary disease in patients with HIV infection are listed in Table 10. In addition to *P. carinii*, other common infectious agents that cause pneumonitis in AIDS are mycobacteria (particularly *M. tuberculosis*), fungi (such as *Cryptococcus*), encapsulated bacteria, cytomegalovirus, and possibly HIV itself.[143,144] Kaposi sarcoma is found frequently in the lungs of patients with mucocutaneous lesions and is associated with an accelerated clinical course.[145] The differential diagnosis of respiratory complaints in an HIV-seropositive patient is quite extensive. Patients with known or suspected HIV infection who present with pulmonary symptoms should be expeditiously evaluated with reliable diagnostic procedures to achieve a specific diagnosis so that therapy can be initiated

TABLE 10. Pulmonary Complications of AIDS

Protozoa
Pneumocystis carinii
Bacteria
Mycobacterium tuberculosis
Mycobacterium avium-intracellulare
Streptococcus pneumoniae
Haemophilus influenzae
Legionella pneumophila
Nocardia asteroides
Fungi
Cryptococcus neoformans
Histoplasma capsulatum
Coccidioides immitis
Candida albicans
Viruses
Cytomegalovirus
? Human immunodeficiency virus
Tumors
Kaposi sarcoma
Non-Hodgkin's lymphoma
Nonspecific pneumonitis
? Human immunodeficiency virus

as soon as possible. Empirical antimicrobial therapy is often appropriate while the diagnostic evaluation proceeds.

A clinical history is useful in evaluating patients who may have AIDS-related pulmonary disease. In AIDS patients (as opposed to other immunocompromised hosts), PCP often has an insidious onset.[146] Patients have a constitutional prodrome of fevers, night sweats, weight loss, and oral candidiasis for weeks followed by increasing respiratory distress—with shortness of breath at first on exertion and finally dyspnea at rest. Approximately 80 percent of patients with PCP note a dry cough, and many report retrosternal irritation on deep breathing. About 5–10 percent of patients with PCP may initially deny respiratory symptoms. These same symptoms may occur in patients with other pulmonary pathogens. Bacterial pneumonias in HIV-seropositive individuals tend to have a more abrupt and severe onset.[147,148,149] In one study, the median duration of symptoms for AIDS patients with pneumonia caused by *H. influenzae* and *S. pneumoniae* was 5 days vs. 21 days in patients with PCP.[150] Seventy percent of patients with bacterial pneumonia may report pleuritic chest pain (uncommon in PCP), and most have a fever, a productive cough, and progressive dyspnea. Patients with cryptococcal pneumonitis generally have disseminated disease and may have a paucity of pulmonary complaints.

Tuberculosis in HIV-seropositive patients most often presents as pulmonary disease and often has an accelerated clinical course.[151,152] In patients already diagnosed as having AIDS, tuberculosis may be a multiorgan, disseminated disease and may present as a systemic illness. Pulmonary Kaposi sarcoma may be a primary lesion but most commonly occurs in patients with extensive tumor(s) elsewhere.[145] Respiratory symptoms tend to progress slowly at first, and constitutional symptoms may be minimal. Upper respiratory tract infections are common in AIDS patients and are most often remarkable for pronounced cough without dyspnea.

A variety of upper respiratory tract symptoms and signs may be elicited. Rales are often detected in patients with PCP and other opportunistic infections. Bacterial pneumonias tend to be focal and may result in localized findings of consolidation on auscultation. Pulmonary Kaposi sarcoma is frequently associated with pleural effusions that are detected by dullness to percussion and diminished breath sounds at the lung bases. Many patients will have normal chest examination findings despite the presence of active pulmonary infection or malignancy. Physical examination may be of limited value to establish a specific diagnosis, and all patients with respiratory symptoms should undergo further diagnostic work-up as outlined below.

Figure 2 shows the diagnostic algorithm employed in the authors' institutions to evaluate patients with suspected AIDS-related pulmonary disease. The protocol has proved to be efficient, cost-effective, and reliable in expeditiously diagnosing both hospitalized and ambulatory patients. A chest radiograph is performed initially. It may be read as normal or have one or more of the following abnormalities: interstitial infiltrates, focal infiltrate with or without cavitation, pleural effusion, intrathoracic adenopathy, or nodules (Table 11). Although 5–10 percent of patients with proven PCP may present with normal chest film findings, PCP is most often associated with interstitial infiltrates.[153] Since a patient with diffuse infiltrates probably has PCP, immediate specific tests for *P. carinii* are indicated. In most institutions, initial pulmonary specimens are obtained by induction of sputum with an ultrasonic nebulizer.[154–156] Patients whose respiratory symptoms are due to PCP, tuberculosis, fungal disease, nonspecific pneumonitis, upper respiratory disease, severe anemia, and other conditions may, however, have normal chest films. Since PCP is less likely in patients with normal chest films, a nonspecific but noninvasive evaluation is useful. Arterial oxygen tension is useful to screen for PCP, although the arterial PaO_2 is both insensitive and nonspecific. Determining the PaO_2 does assess a patient's need for supplemental

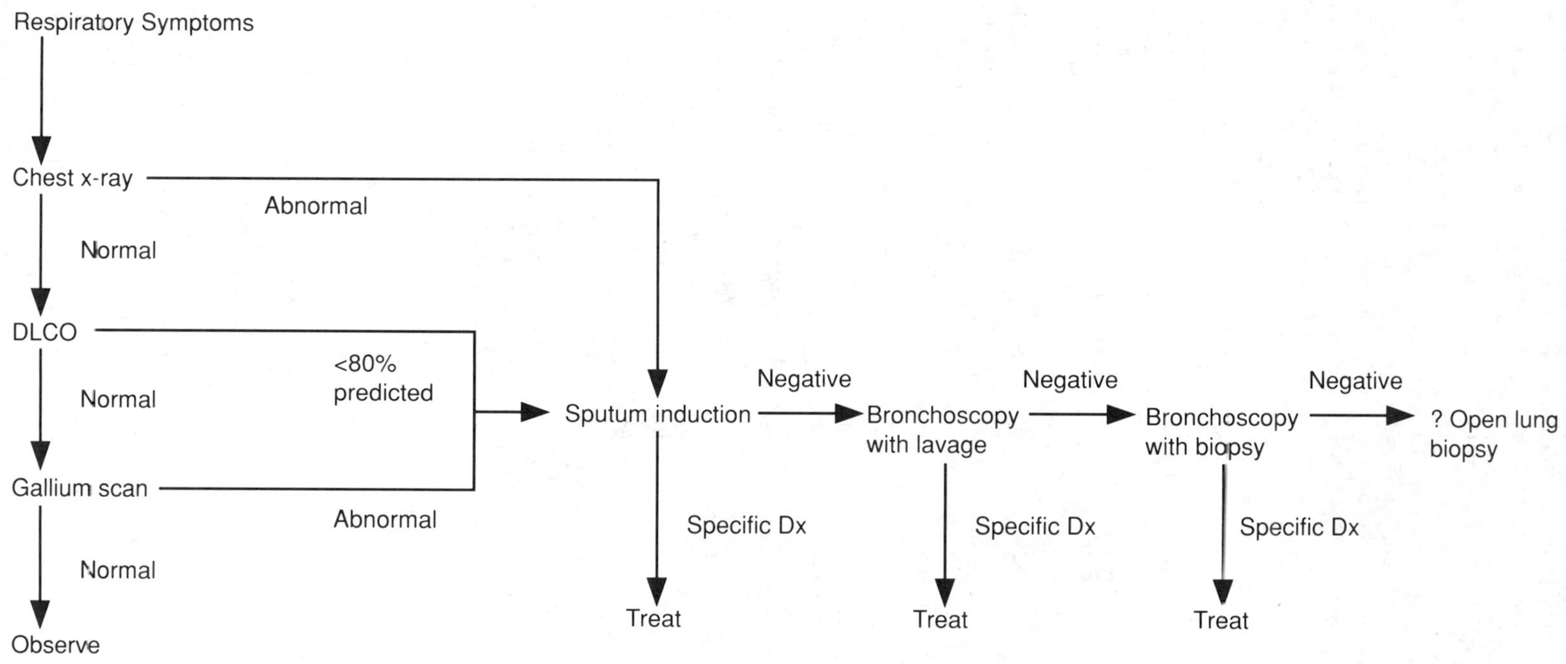

FIG. 2. Algorithm for evaluating pulmonary disease in patients with HIV.

TABLE 11. Chest Radiographic Findings in AIDS Patients with Respiratory Disease

CXR Pattern	Illnesses
Normal	No disease *Pneumocystis carinii* pneumonia Disseminated fungal infection
Focal infiltrate	Pyogenic pneumonia Tuberculosis Cryptococcal pneumonia *Pneumocystis carinii* pneumonia
Pleural effusion	Kaposi sarcoma Pyogenic pnumonia Tuberculosis
Mediastinal adenopathy	Tuberculosis/Mycobacterium avium complex Lymphoma
Interstitial infiltrate	*Pneumocystis carinii* pneumonitis Tuberculosis Lymphocytic interstitial pneumonia Nonspecific pneumonitis Pyogenic pneumonia

oxygen. Arterial blood gases have been evaluated in patients after exercise to screen patients with normal chest radiographs for PCP. The baseline A-aO_2 gradient is compared with the gradient after 3 minutes of exercise.[131] Recruitment of underventilated areas of the lungs during exercise normally decreases the A-aO_2 gradient; however, the A-aO_2 gradient often increases in patients with PCP. This procedure is about 80 percent sensitive, but it is not widely used, primarily because of its inconvenience. Determining the diffusing capacity of carbon monoxide (DLCO) provides a very sensitive test for PCP. Of patients with PCP, 95 percent have a DLCO of less than 80 percent of the predicted value (corrected for hemoglobin). In one study, the mean DLCO for patients with PCP was 62 percent of the predicted value.[156a] This test is nonspecific, however; in the same study, patients without PCP had an average DLCO that was 72 percent of the predicted value. Other abnormalities of pulmonary function are frequently encountered in patients with PCP, including a decreased total lung capacity and vital capacity. These maneuvers are less sensitive than is the DLCO. Patients who present with an abnormal DLCO should be evaluated specifically for *P. carinii*.

Gallium lung scanning is also used to evaluate pulmonary disease in patients with HIV infection.[157] Patients receive an injection of 5–8 mCu of ^{67}Ga and undergo scintigraphic scanning 48 and/or 72 hours later. Scans may be interpreted by qualitative or semiquantitative methods. Typically, PCP results in a diffuse uptake of gallium in the lungs. Any pulmonary uptake is abnormal and should prompt additional specific studies to diagnose pulmonary infection. Gallium scanning, like pulmonary function testing, is nonspecific, and PCP should never be diagnosed on the basis of a positive gallium scan alone.

Examination of induced sputum is now widely used initially to identify *P. carinii*. Specimens should be collected and processed properly, and only well-trained laboratory personnel should review stained specimens to identify organisms. Table 12 describes how to obtain and prepare samples of induced sputum. An ultrasonic nebulizer and 3% to 5% saline solution are essential, as is processing of the sputum specimen with a mucolytic agent. A number of reagents may be used to stain *P. carinii*. A modified Giemsa stain (Dif-Quik), silver methenamine, and toluidine blue O have all produced good results. Silver methenamine, which stains *P. carinii* cysts, may be less sensitive than trophozoite stains are (such as Giemsa). In institutions with staff experienced in the procedure, the overall sensitivity of sputum induction is about 80 percent. Obtaining a second sample of induced sputum may increase the yield and reduce the need for subsequent bronchoscopy from patients with initially negative results. Both direct and indirect immunofluorescence assays (IFA) have recently been developed; they may increase the sensitivity of sputum induction to nearly 90 percent.[155] False-positive results may be obtained with IFA however. Additional studies are required to determine the specificity of these assays. A sample of sputum that is obviously purulent should have a Gram stain and bacterial culture, and antibacterial therapy is appropriate. Laboratories should also perform acid-fast smears and mycobacterial cultures on induced sputum, especially where tuberculosis is more prevalent. Fungal and viral cultures of induced sputum may also be performed, particularly if *P. carinii* is found and subsequent bronchoscopy will not be performed. The yield for these tests, however, is low.

TABLE 12. Method for Sputum Induction

Patient preparation	
	Overnight fast
	Thorough mouth cleansing with saline
	Inhalation of 3% saline from ultrasonic nebulizer
Specimen preparation	
	Digestion (dithiothreitol)
	Centrifugation
	Smear, air-dry, and heat fix
	Giemsa, silver methanamine, or fluorescent antibody stain

Since the negative predictive value of sputum induction is no more than 60 percent, patients who do not have a pathogen identified by this method should undergo a bronchoscopic procedure to establish a diagnosis. Fiber-optic bronchoscopy is an effective, low-morbidity procedure that has a high yield for diagnosing pulmonary pathogens in patients with HIV infection.[158–161] The combination of bronchoalveolar lavage (BAL) and transbronchial biopsy has a diagnostic yield of >95 percent for all pathogens in AIDS patients, and its yield is 100 percent for *P. carinii*. Bronchoalveolar lavage alone has a sensitivity of 85–95 percent and can be performed safely in most patients with suspected PCP. Brush biopsies are not sensitive and are not taken in many institutions. In the our institutions, BAL alone is performed initially. Centrifuged specimens are stained with Giemsa, silver methenamine, and an AFB stain and are also cultured for mycobacteria and fungi. When this procedure does not establish a diagnosis, a repeat bronchoscopic examination is performed, and BAL and transbronchial biopsies are done. Six biopsies of the right lower lobe are generally taken—again without fluoroscopic guidance—unless a focal abnormality is present on the chest radiograph. Fresh biopsy material is examined by touch imprints. Formalin-fixed specimens are stained with hematoxylin and eosin (H&E), Giemsa, acid-fast stains, and silver methenamine. Performance of transbronchial biopsy is not recommended for patients who require mechanical ventilation or have an uncorrectable coagulopathy, although BAL may be performed in such instances. Bronchoalveolar lavage can result in hypoxemia transiently after the procedure. A transbronchial biopsy results in pneumothorax in about 10 percent of patients, at least 50 percent of whom require tube thoracostomy for reexpansion.

Although open lung biopsy (OLB) was previously considered the gold standard for diagnosing PCP, its use is now restricted to several unusual circumstances in patients with HIV-related pulmonary disease. Rarely, a patient with progressive respiratory impairment will have a nondiagnostic sputum induction and bronchoscopy or will have a coagulopathy that contraindicates transbronchial biopsy. Such patients may benefit from OLB.

The serologic diagnosis of PCP has been evaluated in patients who have undergone bone marrow transplant. Neither anti-*P. carinii* antibodies nor *P. carinii* antigen were sensitive or specific in diagnosing PCP. Serologic studies of this population have proved unhelpful: the prevalence of *P. carinii* antibodies is relatively high, and the antibody titers may not increase significantly after the disease is reactivated.

Specific Pathogens. PNEUMOCYSTIS CARINII. *Pneumocystis carinii* (see Chapter 256) is generally considered to be a protozoon, although recent studies suggest that it may be more closely related to fungi.[163] Infection with *P. carinii* is common early in life and does not generally result in symptomatic disease in immunocompetent hosts. Patients with chronic HIV infection develop disease caused by *P. carinii* very frequently—principally an intra-alveolar pneumonitis. *Pneumocystis carinii* pneumonia often presents as a slowly progressive pneumonitis associated with fever, sweats, weight loss, increasing cough, and dyspnea. Kovacs and colleagues compared patients with AIDS-related PCP with patients with PCP and other types of immunodeficiency.[146] The median duration of symptoms was prolonged in the AIDS group (28 vs. 5 days in non-AIDS patients), and AIDS patients with PCP tended to have less fever, a lower respiratory rate, and a higher arterial PO_2. Similar studies by other authors have confirmed the difference between AIDS and non-AIDS PCP. The longer prodrome of PCP in AIDS patients may reflect a better host response to *P. carinii* or may be secondary to other infectious processes (e.g., CMV, mycobacteria, or HIV itself).

Pathologically, PCP causes air space consolidation because a protein-rich exudate consisting of numerous *P. carinii* trophozoites fills the alevoli and causes intrapulmonary right-to-left shunting and arterial hypoxemia. Alveolar membranes become thickened, and parenchymal inflammation, edema, and fibrosis occur. Patients with advanced PCP may have what physiologically appears to be the adult respiratory distress syndrome. Alveolar capillaries leak solutes into the air spaces, pulmonary fluids increase and worsen the shunting of pulmonary capillary blood flow, and arterial hypoxemia increases. Hughes has proposed a histopathologic staging system for PCP in adults that reflects the natural progression of pneumonitis caused by the organism.[164] In stage 1 (early infection), scattered *P. carinii* cysts can be seen in the alveolar wall, but no inflammatory response is evident. Neither autopsy nor biopsy materials for asymptomatic HIV-infected patients have demonstrated that this stage of the disease is common before patients develop symptomatic PCP. Stage 2 is marked by an increase in the number of *P. carinii* cysts in the alveolar wall, alveolar septal inflammation, and desquamation of alveolar cells into the lumen. In addition, *P. carinii* trophozoites can be seen by electron microscopy. In stage 3, alveolar hypertrophy occurs along with a mononuclear cell infiltration and extensive alveolar desquamation; numerous *P. carinii* cysts and trophozoites are found in pulmonary macrophages. After acute PCP is resolved, *P. carinii* cysts or trophozoites may be found in up to 60 percent of patients, although it is not known whether the organisms are viable. Over time the recovery of *P. carinii* declines. Alveolar hypertrophy, interstitial fibrosis, and nonspecific inflammation may be found on biopsy or at autopsy. Approximately 20–25 percent of patients with an initial episode of PCP die acutely—a proportion that has not changed significantly over the course of the epidemic. A study conducted at the National Institutes of Health suggests that early mortality can be predicted by histopathologic findings when the lungs are biopsied.[165] Patients with more extensive edema, fibrosis, and inflammation (stage 3 disease) have a significantly higher mortality rate than do those with less severe disease. Consequently, earlier diagnosis and treatment may improve survival of the first episode of PCP. Patients dying of respiratory failure due to PCP are frequently found to have additional pathogens in the lungs at autopsy (most commonly CMV), but how other infections contribute to the morbidity of PCP is not yet known.

Although most patients with disease caused by *P. carinii* appear to have pneumonitis alone, several reports of extrapulmonary pneumocystosis have been published.[166–169] *Pneumocystis carinii* has been identified in specimens obtained from the middle ear, mastoid, retina, liver, lymph nodes, spleen, and bone marrow. More extensive extrapulmonary dissemination has been reported in patients without HIV infection. How *P. carinii* disseminates and how prevalent extrapulmonary disease is in patients with PCP are both unknown (although the prevalence is felt to be low). Autopsies of patients dying of AIDS only occasionally have identified *P. carinii* outside the lungs.[170]

MYCOBACTERIA. Both tuberculosis and atypical mycobacterial disease (see Chapters 229 and 231) are common manifestations of chronic HIV infection. Disease caused by *M. tuberculosis* may occur early in the course of HIV-induced immunosuppression.[171] Infections with the generally avirulent, atypical organisms (e.g., *M. avium* complex) probably manifest later severe immunodeficiency. Other mycobacteria that cause disease in AIDS patients are *M. kansasii*, *M. xenopi*, *M. cheloni*, *M. gordonae*, and *M. bovis*.[172–174]

In HIV disease, tuberculosis may be the initial manifestation of immunodeficiency in patients who were previously infected with *M. tuberculosis*.[175] Tuberculosis appears more frequently in populations that have an increased risk of the disease, particularly iv drug users, blacks, and Hispanics in the United States and residents of developing countries where tuberculosis may emerge as the predominant AIDS-related opportunistic infection.[176] In Miami, approximately 60 percent of Haitian AIDS patients have tuberculosis.[151] At a tuberculosis sanitorium in Zaire, 33 percent of those with pulmonary tuberculosis were infected with HIV.[177]

In the United States, tuberculosis has recently become more prevalent, primarily because of the HIV epidemic.[178] The number of cases of tuberculosis rose from 1985 to 1986 by 2.6 percent, with New York City reporting the largest increase. Demographically, tuberculosis increased in both sexes, in people aged 25–44, and in blacks and Hispanics. AIDS and tuberculosis registries in New York, San Francisco, and Florida have been matched and reveal that between 2 and 10 percent of AIDS patients have tuberculosis.[179,180] Studies in Miami and San Francisco show that approximately 30 percent of individuals newly diagnosed with tuberculosis have HIV infection[171,181]; most patients had no other clinical evidence of AIDS.

Clinical features of tuberculosis in AIDS patients vary with the degree of immunosuppression. Most patients appear to have been infected previously with *M. tuberculosis*, and the infection is reactivated by progressive immunodeficiency. These patients may have tuberculosis months to years before the diagnosis of AIDS. The pattern of tuberculosis in these individuals is typical of the reactivation seen in other populations; characteristic pulmonary symptoms and clinical findings are the rule. Most patients (60–80 percent), despite moderately severe CD4 lymphopenia, respond to intradermal tuberculin. Chest radiographs show localized or diffuse lung abnormalities in half of the patients. Tuberculosis most commonly affects the pulmonary system, although 20–40 percent of patients may have extrapulmonary disease concomitantly. Tuberculosis is diagnosed by examinating pulmonary specimens with stains for acid-fast organisms and by culture for mycobacteria. Clinicians should employ the diagnostic algorithm for pulmonary disease described above. In some patients with AIDS, tuberculosis may appear as a late opportunistic complication coinciding with or following other opportunistic diseases.[182–184] Clinically, this type of tuberculosis often differs from early reactivation. Constitutional symptoms are more pronounced; chest radiographic findings are usually atypical, with diffuse infiltrates and intrathoracic adenopathy predominant; a response to tuberculin testing occurs at a rate of only 30–40 percent; and extrapulmonary dissemination is found in 50–70 percent of the cases.[175] The lungs remain the site where the organism is most frequently isolated and an important source to spread the infection to other susceptible individuals.

The pathology of tuberculosis in HIV-infected persons reflects the stage of immunosuppression at which disease occurs. In patients whose earlier TB is reactivated, well-formed granulomas may be found on biopsy or autopsy. A brisk inflammatory response is reflected in localized pulmonary symptoms, radiographic infiltrates, and tuberculin reactivity. As immunosuppression advances, pathologic findings become more atypical, and poorly formed granulomas without caseation may be found. Although tuberculosis responds excellently to chemotherapy, the overall prognosis for patients infected with TB and AIDS is very poor. In one study, the median survival rate was 6 months.[179] Most patients, however, die of other opportunistic diseases.

Early in the AIDS epidemic, clinicians recognized infections caused by nontuberculous mycobacteria as complications of HIV-induced immunosuppression. In 1981–1982 investigators found high-grade, disseminated infections with *M. avium* complex in patients with AIDS.[185,186] Approximately 4 percent of AIDS cases have nontuberculous mycobacterial infections as an index AIDS diagnosis[187]; 97 percent are caused by *M. avium* complex, and 3 percent are due to *M. kansasii*, *M. xenopi*, *M. gordonae*, and others.[187] As many as 25–50 percent of AIDS patients may subsequently develop nontuberculous mycobacterial disease. It may be difficult to diagnose *M. avium* complex (MAC) while patients are alive; autopsy series show that over 50 percent of these infections may be clinically undetected.[170,188] Nontuberculous mycobacterial disease appears to be equally prevalent in males and females, in all age groups, and in different geographic regions. *Mycobacterium avium* complex, a common environmental saprophyte, may be acquired orally or inhaled. In several studies, researchers have isolated MAC in the respiratory system before its dissemination in 50–75 percent of the cases.[189–191] Others have reported little association between colonization in the respiratory tract and subsequent systemic spread. One study found numerous mycobacteria in macrophages of the lamina propria in the small bowel—a finding consistent with acquiring the gastrointestinal infection.[192] Since nontuberculous mycobacteria are distributed uniformly among different risk groups, the disease caused by MAC is probably a new infection rather than a previous infection reactivated.

In AIDS patients, nontuberculous mycobacterial disease is characterized pathologically by continuous bacteremia, with as many as 10^4 to 10^5 colony-forming-units per milliliter of blood.[193,194] *Mycobacterium avium* complex can infect numerous organs: bone marrow, liver, spleen, gut, lymph nodes, lungs, skin, brain, adrenals, and kidneys. There is little histologic response despite relatively large numbers of organisms. Granulomas, when present, are usually poorly formed. Some studies suggest that MAC disease may be associated with abnormal levels of lymphokines and the dysfunction of macrophages rather than the intrinsic loss of helper-inducer T lymphocytes.[195] In infected patients, macrophages may be packed with organisms that have not been killed in the cells themselves with antimicrobial therapy. Mycobacteremia may fail to clear because of impaired host defenses or because of intrinsic resistance to these agents.[198] How MAC infection contributes to AIDS mortality is not known. One study suggested that survival improved when MAC disease was treated.[199] The study was, however, prone to significant lead-time bias because cases were diagnosed earlier in their clinical course than historical controls. One study followed 161 patients from the date PCP was diagnosed; they found that those who had or subsequently developed MAC infection had a marginally longer median survival rate than did patients without MAC.[191] This finding probably reflects an increased incidence of MAC over time, with longer survivors most likely to acquire the organism. Several autopsy series have found MAC postmortem in a large proportion of subjects; however, in one series (where cause of death was listed), only 1 of 36 (3 percent) AIDS deaths was attributed to MAC.[170] It appears that nontuberculous mycobacterial infections mark severe, cellular immunodeficiency associated with an extremely poor prognosis, but they may not directly affect survival.

In patients with PCP, recovery of MAC from pulmonary specimens is often an incidental finding, and most patients recover with anti-*Pneumocystis* therapy alone. Abundant clinical data, however, show significant morbidity from MAC. A minority of patients, may have respiratory tract disease caused by MAC alone, an infection that results in diffuse pulmonary infiltrates, arterial hypoxemia, and progressive pulmonary deterioration.[200] Clinicians should evaluate patients carefully for other pulmonary pathogens before ascribing respiratory findings to MAC.

Mycobacterium avium complex disease most commonly presents as a systemic illness with fevers, night sweats, fatigue, and weight loss. Gastrointestinal symptoms such as abdominal pain and persistent diarrhea are also often reported. Patients usually appear emaciated and have generalized lymphadenopathy and other findings associated with immunodeficiency (e.g., oral candidiasis). Abdominal examination may show diffuse tenderness and hepatosplenomegaly. Laboratory evaulation is usually nonspecific, although anemia and leukopenia are usually pronounced. Computed tomography scans of the abdomen may show marked hepatosplenomegaly and diffuse lymphadenopathy (often with central attenuation). The bowel wall is often thickened—consistent with an inflammatory colitis. Gallium scans may show intense colonic uptake. Biopsy or autopsy specimens of the colon show acute and chronic inflammation and numerous acid-fast bacilli in the mucosa and submucosa. Concurrent infections with *Cryptosporidium*, CMV, and other pathogens may be found. The small bowel may also be involved and result in a histologic appearance similar to Whipple's disease and the chronic diarrhea syndrome. *Mycobacterium avium* complex has been found in enlarged periportal lymph nodes in patients whose extrahepatic bile ducts were extrinsically obstructed. *Mycobacterium avium* complex has also been found in the adrenals of patients with acute adrenal insufficiency (although CMV is most often associated with this clinical entity), in brain abscesses and in the bone biopsy of patients with osteomyelitis.

PYOGENIC BACTERIA. Infections with pyogenic bacteria occur more frequently in patients with HIV disease, particularly in children and iv drug users. The incidence of bacterial pneumonia, for example, is increased greatly in HIV-seropositive iv drug users when compared with seronegative controls.[201] Encapsulated bacteria (particularly *Streptococcus pneumoniae* and *Haemophilus influenzae*) are the most common pathogens.[202] Table 13 lists bacteria that cause serious infections in HIV-infected persons.

In HIV-infected patients, bacterial infections involve primarily the skin, lungs, sinuses, and middle ear. Children appear to have a high prevalence of otitis media and pneumonia caused by *S. pneumoniae* and *H. influenzae*. In adults, pyogenic infections are manifested most commonly as skin and soft tissue infections, sinusitis, and pneumonia. Persistent impetigo, furunculosis, folliculitis, and skin abscesses in adults with HIV infection; streptococci and *Staphylococcus aureus* are usually responsible. In patients with HIV infection, sinusitis may be

TABLE 13. Bacteria Causing Serious Infections in Patients with HIV Infection

	Organism	Site(s) of Disease
Gram-positive	*Streptococcus pneumoniae*	Lung, sinuses, blood
	Streptococcus spp.	Lung
	Staphylococcus aureus	Skin, blood, lung, perineum
	Listeria monocytogenes	Meninges, blood
	Nocardia asteroides	Lung, brain
Gram-negative	*Haemophilus influenzae*	Lung, blood
	Haemophilus spp.	Lung
	Branhamella catarrhalis	Lung
	Salmonella spp.	Gut, blood, brain
	Shigella spp.	Gut
	Campylobacter spp.	Gut
	Legionella pneumophila	Lung
Spirochetes	*Treponema pallidum*	Skin, meninges, brain

caused by *S. pneumoniae*, *H. influenzae* other or *Haemophilus* species, *Branhamella catarrhalis*, or other organisms. The clinical presentation is often subacute; congestion, cough, and headache are the most prominent symptoms. Sinus tenderness is uncommon, but sinus x-ray films frequently reveal sinus thickening and air–fluid levels within the paranasal sinuses. Aspirating the sinus fluids may be both diagnostic and therapeutic.

Bacterial pneumonias (discussed earlier) present as clinically distinct from PCP. Bacterial pneumonia may occur more frequently in iv drug users, cigarette smokers, and children with HIV infection and bacterial bronchitis, more commonly in the HIV-infected population. Patients usually complain of a chronic cough with scant sputum production and minimal dyspnea. Evaluation reveals rhonchi or wheezes, and chest films are normal. Sputum Gram staining may show polymorphonucleocytes (PMNs) and gram-positive diplococci or gram-negative coccobacillary organisms. Although bronchitis is rarely associated with bacteremia, bacterial pneumonias in AIDS patients are often bacteremic. Up to 80 percent of patients with *S. pneumoniae* pneumonia and 25 percent of patients with *H. influenzae* pneumonia have bacteremia.[148,202,203] Infection may be more difficult to eradicate in these patients, and relapses after appropriate therapy are common.

Reports suggest that bacteremia occurs more frequently in patients with advanced HIV disease. One report found 22 cases of *Staphylococcus aureus* bacteremia in patients with AIDS or advanced HIV disease.[204] Six of those patients had intravenous catheters in place. Many physicians have reported a high rate of catheter-related sepsis in AIDS patients, particularly those with central venous lines who are receiving intravenous therapy at home. The organisms responsible for catheter-related sepsis are predominantly *S. aureus* or *epidermidis*; gram-negative bacilli are encountered less frequently. Why the risk of infection increases is not known: AIDS patients may be more likely to employ inadequate hygienic techniques than are other patient groups with indwelling venous catheters, and host mechanisms that control integumental defense may be impaired. Patients with HIV infection who have a central venous catheter should receive careful instructions on how to control infection, adequate nursing supervision, and medical follow-up.

Neurologic Complications

HIV is a neurotrophic virus with a variety of clinical manifestations in the central and peripheral nervous systems.[206] Numerous neurologic opportunistic infections occur in AIDS patients in addition to the direct, immunologic sequelae of HIV infection, so the neurologic complications of HIV infection can best be considered primary and secondary consequences.

Aseptic Meningitis. When HIV directly infects the central nervous system, several distinct clinical syndromes result. In approximately 25 percent of the cases, an aseptic meningitis characterizes the acute retroviral syndrome (described previously). Although cranial neuropathies have been reported, meningeal signs may be minimal and laboratory evaluation remarkable for only a slight CSF pleocytosis and elevation of the CSF protein.[207,208] Culture of CSF may reveal HIV, and free viral core antigen may be detected.[209–211] Seroconversion can result in the intrathecal production of anti-HIV antibodies. Patients with this presentation may wax and wane clinically for months. HIV-related meningitis was reported in one series of 14 patients who presented no evidence of recently acquiring HIV.[207] The symptoms that prompted evaluation lasted from 10 days to more than 10 months. Signs of immunodeficiency were found in eight cases (57 percent). A mild CSF pleocytosis was noted in all patients, and both CSF protein levels and opening pressure were elevated in five patients. Eighty percent of patients tested had positive HIV cultures. A CSF pleocytosis, detection of HIV antigen, and viral cocultivation can also be found in asymptomatic HIV-seropositive patients, however, so attributing meningitis in HIV-infected persons to HIV itself is speculative.

HIV Encephalopathy. A progressive neurologic syndrome (now termed HIV encephalopathy) can be caused when HIV infects the central nervous system (CNS) white matter. Ninety percent of patients with AIDS have cognitive, affective, and psychomotor abnormalities[213]; patients with less advanced opportunistic disease have a lower frequency of these abnormalities. A study of asymptomatic, seropositive subjects found no encephalopathic abnormalities before overt clinical opportunistic disease developed elsewhere. HIV-encephalopathy can be divided into two phases, early and late, and each has a distinct clinical presentation. In early HIV encephalopathy, the major symptoms are memory loss, impaired concentration, and mental slowness. Patients also demonstrate affective symptoms, apathy, behavior change, and motor complaints. Patients with early HIV encephalopathy may have hyperreflexia, hypertonia, frontal-release signs, tremor, psychomotor slowing, ataxia, and abnormal results of mental status examination. Laboratory evaluation is essential to rule out opportunistic infection, tumor, or other causes of mental status changes. In 70–90 percent of patients, CT scans of the head show generalized atrophy that is usually inconsistent with the patient's age.[214] Magnetic resonance imaging (MRI) also shows cerebral atrophy, often with marked abnormalities of the subcortical white matter and an increased signal intensity that is distributed multifocally. Magnetic resonance image scanning is more specific but less sensitive than CT scanning.[214] A slight CSF pleocytosis is found in a minority of individuals and normal glucose and elevated CSF protein levels (primarily CSF IgG) in more than half of the patients. Oligoclonal bands may be present in a small proportion of subjects tested. HIV isolation and antigen detection assays may be positive, although these tests are both nonspecific and insensitive for predicting and diagnosing HIV encephalopathy. Other diagnostic test findings, e.g., electroencephalography (EEG), may be abnormal but have not been adequately evaluated to be helpful.

Late HIV encephalopathy is a more fulminant process. Patients present with marked cognitive abnormalities, memory loss, behavioral change, and significant, psychomotor impairment. Profound weakness, neglect, tremor, seizures, and psychosis may also be noted. Computed tomography and MRI scanning findings are often more severely abnormal; extreme cerebral atrophy and white matter changes are common. Other diagnostic studies are used to rule out opportunistic infections. A clinical diagnosis of HIV encephalopathy is made by excluding other causes of encephalopathy and documenting HIV infection. Characteristic findings on history and examination, suggestive radiographic or imaging findings, and the absence of space-occupying lesions, opportunistic pathogens, or intoxicating drugs all support the diagnosis. Brain biopsy has been performed in some patients with results consistent with autopsy findings; however, the yield of brain biopsy in reaching a treatable diagnosis is very low in the absence of localizing lesions by noninvasive imaging studies. Consequently, routine biopsy cannot be recommended. In children infected with HIV, CNS involvement appears very frequently. It can be manifested by a failure to thrive, cognitive deficits, abnormalities of muscle tone, and paraparesis. Seizures have been reported occasionally as a late complication in both children and adults.

In the brains of patients with HIV encephalopathy, pathologic findings are varied. Seventy-five percent of patients had cerebral atrophy that was most pronounced in the frontal and temporal lobes. Almost all patients have gliosis and focal necrosis. Microglial nodules of macrophages, lymphocytes, and microglia are reported in up to 70 percent of patients. Demyelination and myelin pallor are common; focal perivascular myelin rarefaction or demyelination and vacuolation are also frequently noted. The basal ganglia are commonly involved. Multinucleated giant cells, produced by direct HIV infection in the brain, can be found scattered throughout the cerebral cortex and white matter. Perivascular and leptomeningeal inflammation may also be found.

Intracranial Mass Lesions. Central nervous system dysfunction from intracranial mass lesions is a late complication of HIV disease. Processes associated with mass lesions of the brain are listed in Table 14. Cerebral toxoplasmosis is the most common cause of intracranial masses in patients with AIDS, followed by CNS lymphoma, progressive multifocal leukoencephalopathy (PML), and other infectious agents (e.g., *M. tuberculosis*, *Cryptococcus*, *Candida*). As many as 10 percent of biopsied or autopsied intracranial masses have nondiagnostic histopathology.[214] In many cases, neither the clinical presentation nor the neuroradiologic appearance of CNS lesions permits a definitive diagnosis. Patients with opportunistic CNS disease may present with a variety of signs and symptoms. Headache may occur in one-third to three-quarters of patients and altered sensorium in 50–90 percent. Incoordination, ataxia, hemiparesis, and cranial neuropathies are present in fewer than 25 percent of patients with intracranial mass lesions.[215] The radiographic appearance of various CNS lesions may be distinct but not pathognomonic. A diagnosis of CNS disease is challenging without examining tissue. However, because brain biopsy is not always feasible, empiric therapy for toxoplasmosis is warranted in selected patients. A clinical response establishes the diagnosis reliably (see below). Figure 3 presents a diagnostic algorithm for evaluating patients with HIV infection and suspected intracranial mass lesions.

Patients who present with clinical findings suggestive of intracranial pathology should be evaluated with a brain imaging study. Both CT and MRI have been shown to be sensitive for assessing CNS disease in HIV infection. Double-dose, delayed-contrast CT scanning identifies ring-enhancing abscesses and other mass lesions more sensitively than do single-dose studies. Lesions are typically hypodense with surrounding edema and may have a mass effect. Characteristically, abscesses are enhanced by contrast in tuberculoma, cryptococcoma, nocardiosis, and pyogenic brain abscesses. A lack of enhancement is more often associated with PML and lymphomas. Multiple ring-enhancing lesions are the sine qua non of toxoplasmosis; however, many toxoplasmic abscesses are not detected by CT scanning. Therefore, the appearance of a single ring-enhancing lesion by CT does not rule out toxoplasmosis. Toxoplasmosis is frequently associated with bilateral lesions, and most patients have basal ganglia involvement.[214] Lesions are often small (1–3 cm) and hemorrhage rare. Progressive multifocal leukoencephalopathy is a demyelinating disease that results in diffuse, nonenhancing, hemispheric, white matter lesions without edema or mass effect. Primary CNS lymphoma usually produces single, hyperdense lesions that enhance unevenly. Multiple lesions may be found in some patients, particularly in serial studies of untreated individuals. CT scanning may have normal findings, or it may reveal cerebral atrophy. Up to one-half of patients with HIV encephalopathy and a substantial proportion of patients with other CNS pathology may have atrophy. In patients with HIV infection, normal CT scan results do not rule out CNS disease. If clinical findings suggest intracranial mass lesions, a negative CT scan should be followed by an MRI scan. High-field strength, T 2-weighted MRI scans are more sensitive than CT scans are in detecting cerebral abscesses and other CNS pathology.[216] Magnetic resonance imaging often reveals multiple high-intensity target lesions (which suggest toxoplas-

TABLE 14. Causes of Intracranial Mass Lesions in AIDS

Infections	
	Toxoplasma gondii
	Progressive multifocal leukoencephaly (JC virus)
	M. tuberculosis
	Cryptococcus neoformans
	Nocardia asteroides
	Histoplasma capsulatum
	Cytomegalovirus
	Herpes simplex virus
	Human immunodeficiency virus
	Candida albicans
Neoplasms	
	Primary CNS lymphoma
	Metastatic lymphoma
	Kaposi sarcoma
Unidentified	
	Nonspecific gliosis

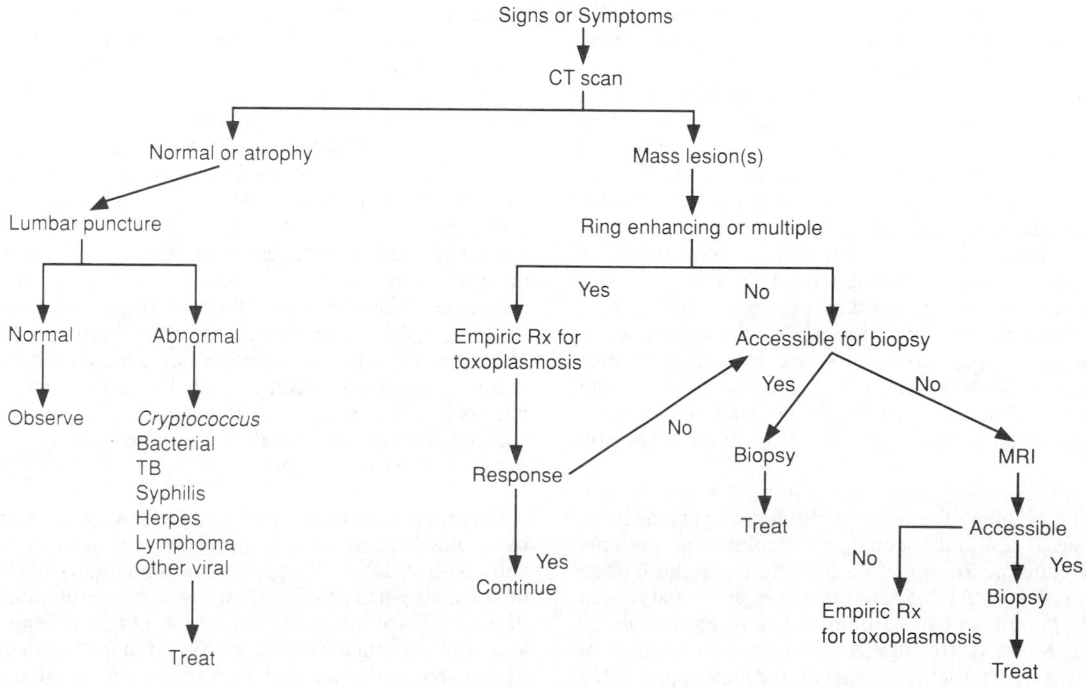

FIG. 3. Algorithm for evaluating neurologic abnormalities in patients with HIV.

mosis) when the CT scan shows only a single ring-enhancing lesion. Magnetic resonance image scanning also reveals lesions in the basal ganglia in virtually all patients with toxoplasmosis. When multiple lesions and basal ganglia lesions are absent in MRI scanning, this finding strongly suggests a diagnosis other than toxoplasmosis. Progressive multifocal leukoencephalopathy characteristically causes hemispheric, white matter lesions; on MRI scans, multiple, high-signal, nonenhancing white matter lesions are found. Solitary lesions on MRI scans may be CNS lymphomas, cryptococcomas, tuberculomas, or viral encephalitides.

Patients with suspected CNS mass lesions can first be evaluated with a CT scan. If the scan reveals no mass effect, a lumbar puncture can be performed. Cerebrospinal fluid should be sent for a cell count and differential; protein and glucose determination; cryptococcal antigen assay; bacterial, mycobacterial, viral, and fungal culture; cytology; and VDRL testing. *Toxoplasma* serology may be peformed; however, it is nonspecific and insensitive and should not be relied on to determine treatment options.[217] If the CT scan findings are normal or show only atrophy and no alternative diagnosis is established by clinical examination or laboratory studies, an MRI scan should be performed. Similarly, if the CT scan finds only a single focal lesion and biopsy of the lesion is not feasible (e.g., a basal ganglion lesion), MRI scanning should be performed. Previously, focal lesions on the CT or MRI scan of an immunocompromised patient required a brain biopsy to make a specific diagnosis. In recent years, empirical anti-*Toxoplasma* therapy has been accepted as an alternative to biopsy in selected patients because a growing number of AIDS patients have intracranial masses and among such patients toxoplasmosis is prevalent. Patients who may be empirically treated include the following:

1. Patients who have typical CT or MRI scan findings (multiple ring-enhancing lesions) and consistent clinical presentation
2. Patients with no lesion accessible for biopsy
3. Patients who refuse biopsy.

Empirical therapy is not indicated for patients with a single lesion detected by MRI scan; patients with tuberculosis, cryptococcosis, other fungal infection, or malignancy at an anatomic site outside the CNS; or patients allergic to anti-*Toxoplasma* drugs. Empirical treatment should be avoided in patients with mass effect who require steroid therapy because the response to steroids alone may confuse the clinical picture and render later biopsy results uninterpretable. These patients and those who have not had a clinical and radiographic response after 10 to 14 days of empirical therapy should undergo brain biopsy. Stereotactic needle biopsy is a safe and relatively nonmorbid way to obtain brain tissue for histologic study. In patients with impending herniation, open biopsies should be performed.

Biopsy material obtained from the periphery of an abscess has the highest diagnostic yield, particularly for toxoplasmosis. Fresh tissue may be used for touch preparations and should be cultured for viruses, bacteria, mycobacteria, and fungi. Specimens should be stained with standard cytochemical stains (e.g., hematoxylin and eosin); however, the sensitivity of hematoxylin-eosin staining for *toxoplasma* may be less than 50 percent.[218] Staining with immunoperoxidase greatly increases the diagnostic yield and should be used routinely to evaluate brain biopsy specimens when standard stains fail to make a specific diagnosis.

Serologic tests for toxoplasmosis have limited value. Serum IgG antibodies (detected by the Sabin-Feldman dye test or hemagglutination assay) are nonspecific, particularly in patients from areas with endemic *Toxoplasma* infections. In the United States 30–50 percent of AIDS patients have previously been infected with *T. gondii* and have demonstrable antibodies.[219] At the Memorial Sloan Kettering Cancer Center, one-third of the IgG-positive AIDS patients studied later developed CNS toxoplasmosis.[219] Conversely, IgG-negative patients with biopsy-confirmed CNS toxoplasmosis have been reported.[213,220] In patients with AIDS, increases in baseline IgG titers indicate active toxoplasmosis unreliably.[222] IgM antibody levels against *Toxoplasma* are frequently increased in nonimmunosuppressed patients with acute toxoplasmosis but are rarely elevated in AIDS-related, reactivated disease.[223–225] The intrathecal production of anti-*Toxoplasma* IgG has been proposed as a relatively sensitive and specific test that suggests CNS toxoplasmosis when positive (ratio >1). This method is limited clinically because treatment often must be given long before test results are available. Moreover, this technique has not been sufficiently assessed to determine its sensitivity and specificity. Consequently, treatment decisions should not be based on serologic test results alone.

Specific Etiologies of Opportunistic CNS Disease. TOXOPLASMOSIS. Toxoplasmosis (see Chapter 255) causes most intracranial mass lesions in AIDS patients. CNS toxoplasmosis is the index diagnosis of AIDS in approximately 2 percent of patients in the United States, and it occurs as a secondary diagnosis in an additional 2–5 percent.[226] In geographic areas where the underlying prevalence of remote infection with *T. gondii* is high (e.g., France, Haiti), cerebral toxoplasmosis among AIDS patients is very prevalent. Of those AIDS patients who have mass lesions revealed by CT head scans, 50–70 percent have toxoplasmosis.[214]

Central nervous system toxoplasmosis presents as a global encephalitis with altered mental status in up to 75 percent of patients. Fifty percent of patients report headaches, although those headaches are not typically severe. About 50 percent may have focal neurologic signs (i.e., seizure, hemiparesis, or ataxia); fewer than 50 percent may have fever. Symptoms often have a subscute onset—over a period of days to several weeks—with a median of 22 days in one series.[206] Pathologically, toxoplasmosis results in a diffuse encephalitis with focal areas of intense inflammation and necrosis. Abscesses show acute and chronic inflammation and infiltration by PMNs, lymphocytes, and histiocytes. The abscess centers are necrotic, with scant organisms. On the periphery of an abscess, numerous *T. gondii* tachyzoites may be found, while cyst forms can be seen in non-necrotic tissue. In small vessels surrounding abscesses, vasculitis may be present; reactive astrocytosis is seen adjacently.

PROGRESSIVE MULTIFOCAL LEUKOENCEPHALOPATHY. PML (see Chapter 124), a demyelinating disease of cerebral white matter, is characterized by multiple, discrete foci of disease. A papovavirus, JC virus, is consistently identified in oligodendrocytes in affected areas of the syndrome. In the United States, fewer than 1 percent of patients with AIDS have PML reported to the CDC.[226] The symptoms of PML include headache, ataxia, hemiparesis, confusion, and other mental status changes. Computed tomography scans most often reveal nonenhancing, low-density lesions of the periventricular white matter. Magnetic resonance imaging scans show high-signal intensity lesions without enhancement. Cerebrospinal fluid studies are usually unrevealing; the diagnosis is established by brain biopsy. JC virus can be identified by typical electron microscopy morphology, by immunofluorescence staining, or by gene amplification techniques. Clinically, patients deteriorate progressively. Death occurs on average in less than 3 months, although spontaneous remission has been reported.[228]

Cryptococcus neoformans. The CDC reports disease caused by *C. neoformans* (see Chapter 241) in up to 10 percent of persons with AIDS.[231] Cryptococcal meningitis occurs in approximately 80 percent of patients with symptomatic cryptococcal disease. Cryptococcosis is more common among iv drug users and ethnic minorities with AIDS and in the south-central United States. No seasonal variation in the occurrence of cryptococcosis has been reported. A number of other clinical syndromes including pneumonitis, multiple skin lesions resembling molluscum contagiosum, fungemia, and prostatitis may also be seen. Cryptococcal meningitis often presents clinically with nonspecific symptoms. Eighty percent of patients complain only of fever, night sweats, malaise, and a dull headache.[232] Severe headache, photophobia, meningismus, and an altered sensorium occur in 2–20 percent of patients. Focal neurologic complaints such as seizures, cranial nerve abnormalities, or hemiparesis are rare. Many patients may have only low-grade fever. Other symptoms may be elicited retrospectively after cryptococcosis is diagnosed. Clinicians need to be vigilant to detect cryptococcal disease early in its course before it disseminates and fulminant disease develops.

The diagnosis of cryptococcal meningitis is made by detecting cryptococcal antigen and growth of *Cryptococcus* in the cerebrospinal fluid. Patients with suspected cryptococcal meningitis should be carefully examed neurologically and ophthalmologically. If no focal neurologic abnormalities are noted and papilledema is absent, a lumbar puncture may be performed with small risk of complication. If neurologic abnormalities or altered sensorium are noted, a CT scan of the head should be obtained before performing a lumbar puncture. In many institutions, clinicians perform CT scanning on all patients before a lumbar puncture. The CSF findings of cryptococcal meningitis in AIDS is usually benign, with a pleocytosis of 5–50 mononuclear cells/mm^3, slightly elevated protein levels, and a normal glucose concentration. India ink examination reveals organisms in 50–90 percent of cases, and the cryptococcal antigen is positive in more than 95 percent of patients. Cultures of the CSF are invariably positive in primary disease but may be negative in patients who are relapsing from previously treated cryptococcosis. A rising antigen titer in the CSF strongly suggests relapse in this setting, particularly if the lysis-centrifugation technique is used.

Cryptococcal infections are acquired by inhaling the organism into the lungs. The primary pulmonary infection is often asymptomatic, even in immunodeficient hosts; however, cryptococcal pneumonia does occur in patients with advanced HIV infection. The clinical features of cryptococcal pneumonia include the insidious onset of fever, night sweats, malaise, cough, and dyspnea. The radiograph may show focal lobar infiltrates, sometimes with cavitation. Examination of induced sputum (using silver methenamine stain) may show yeast. Bronchoalveolar lavage fluid and transbronchial biopsy specimens may also show yeast, and cultures may yield *C. neoformans*. Cryptococcal antigenemia is present variably, and fungal blood cultures may grow *Cryptococcus*.

Other extraneural sites of disease are less common in AIDS patients with cryptococcosis. Fungemia is present in >80 percent of patients with cryptococcal meningitis, but other organs are not usually involved. The organism has been found in the bone marrow, liver, spleen, kidneys, skin, and other organs, and it may compromise organ function in some cases.

Cytomegalovirus. Cytomegalovirus (see Chapter 120) is ubiquitous in patients with HIV infection and causes serious morbidity in AIDS. Cytomegalovirus is transmitted by the same routes as HIV, and almost all patients with sexually acquired HIV infection are also infected with CMV. Like other herpesviruses, CMV may infect cells latently and reactivate when host defenses are impaired. Asymptomatic CMV viruria and viremia may be found in more than 50 percent of patients with AIDS,[233] but whether this predicts the subsequent development of CMV disease is uncertain. Ultimately, between 2 and 10 percent of AIDS patients have organs involved with CMV, and most AIDS patients autopsied have evidence of CMV infection.[170]

CMV RETINITIS. The eye is the end organ most often involved in CMV disease.[234] Cytomegalovirus retinitis is the index diagnosis of AIDS in 1–2 percent of patients and occurs subsequently in 4–6 percent. The onset of CMV retinitis may be insidious or rapid. Patients complain of painless, progressive visual loss, blurring, and "floaters." Cytomegalovirus retinitis usually presents unilaterally, although it may subsequently progress to the contralateral retina. Funduscopic examination of the involved eye typically reveals coalescing white exudates in a vascular pattern with surrounding hemorrhage and edema.

Often, lesions are peripheral initially, involve the fovea later, and result in visual loss. Retinal detachment may occur as a late complication.

Patients complaining of ocular symptoms should undergo a thorough ophthalmologic examination. The differential diagnosis of retinal lesions includes cotton wool spots, ischemic retinopathy, Roth spots, and toxoplasmic retinitis. Cotton wool spots are very prevalent in patients with AIDS but do not appear to predict the development of other retinal disease. The cotton-wool spots are distributed in a vascular pattern similar to CMV, but do not have the irregular pattern of exudate and hemorrhage that is characteristic of CMV retinitis. Similarly, *Toxoplasma* retinitis shows discrete, rounded, pale exudates. Autopsy studies of persons dying with CMV retinitis have shown retinal necrosis, hemorrhage, and mononuclear cell infiltration. Cytomegalovirus (but not HIV) DNA and RNA can be detected in affected cells. An ophthalmologist or other highly trained observer can make a premortem diagnosis by visually inspecting the lesions. Cultures of the blood and urine yield CMV in 80–100 percent of cases, respectively. At autopsy, one quarter of patients with CMV retinitis may also have CMV encephalitis.[234a]

MALIGNANCIES IN THE HIV-INFECTED PATIENT

Along with opportunistic infections and clinical problems directly attributed to HIV itself, malignant neoplasms are frequent causes of severe morbidity and mortality. The recognition and management of these cancers are key components of comprehensive AIDS care, and research into their etiology and pathogenesis is expected to shed additional light on oncogenesis in non–HIV-infected patients.

Early Reports of AIDS-Related Cancers

Cases of Kaposi sarcoma (KS) in young homosexual men in the early 1980s helped alert the medical community to the AIDS epidemic. Before this, KS had been a rare and relatively indolent cutaneous neoplasm of elderly men in the United States and elsewhere[235] and also an endemic malignancy in parts of central Africa.[236–238] Additionally, KS had been reported as a complication of exogenous corticosteroids taken to prevent organ transplant rejection.[239–245] Although an interesting disease because of these unusual geographic patterns and postulated associations with CMV infection[246,247] and iatrogenic immune suppression, KS was not a clinically significant problem in the United States.

In 1980 several cases of KS were diagnosed in homosexual men in New York, and these and similar cases from California were described in a series of reports in 1981 and 1982.[248–250] Several aspects of these cases were distinctly unusual (Table 15). First, they affected a much younger population than prior ("classic") KS in the United States, Second, the tumor was much more aggressive, with early and wide dissemination the rule. Finally, the patients often had the same spectrum of unusual infections being diagnosed simultaneously in other homosexual men but had no known reason for immune deficiency. The combination of these striking findings in similar "risk" populations soon led to the recognition of a common underlying disorder, AIDS.

The second malignancy recognized as part of the AIDS epidemic was non-Hodgkins lymphoma (NHL). Sporadic cases of NHL of CNS origin in individuals with other manifestations of AIDS resulted in the early inclusion of this cancer in AIDS surveillance definitions.[251–253] Subsequently, NHL of peripheral origin was also reported in association with AIDS.[254–264] Since 1984, NHL in both sites has become increasingly common, and its clinical appearance, biology, and management have been the subject of several reviews and ongoing clinical trials. The severe clinical problems caused by NHL make it, like KS, an important disease for the clinician to understand.

In addition to KS and NHL, an increasing variety of other cancers have been diagnosed in HIV-infected individuals. Although less common than KS and NHL and less clearly linked causally to HIV infection, these tumors may also offer insight into the relationship between HIV, immune deficiency, and oncogenesis. While the wide variety of these cancers and their relative rarity precludes extensive discussion in this chapter, their diagnosis should be considered when clinically appropriate.

Epidemiology of AIDS-Related Malignancies—Kaposi Sarcoma

Kaposi sarcoma (KS) is, by far, the most common neoplasm in HIV-infected patients.[265–267] Overall, 9 percent of all AIDS cases reported to the CDC have been initially diagnosed with KS as compared with <1 percent with NHL, the next most common cancer. Many more patients develop KS or lymphoma later in their disease course. Kaposi sarcoma is, in fact, one of the most common clinical manifestations of HIV-disease, and as mentioned, its increased incidence was an early indicator of the AIDS epidemic.

Kaposi sarcoma, for reasons still unclear, disproportionately affects HIV-infected male homosexuals.[265–268] In the first several years of the epidemic, for example, 47 percent of newly diagnosed AIDS cases in homosexual and bisexual men had KS as compared with 3.9 percent in intravenous drug users.[269] Kaposi sarcoma is rare in all heterosexuals with HIV disease except black Africans.[270,271] In Africa, KS is more common and clinically more aggressive in the HIV-infected population when compared with reports before the HIV epidemic.[272–276] While precise incidence figures are not available, KS does seem more common in African AIDS patients than in other groups of heterosexuals.[277,278] Kaposi sarcoma in children with AIDS has been reported but is rare.[279] Recent work suggests that even when adjusted for risk-group category KS may be more common in whites than blacks.[280]

Adding even more to the interest in KS are studies showing that it is an epidemiologic "moving target." For example, its incidence in homosexual men is clearly decreasing in the United States.[281,282] Compared with initial rates of 36 percent of AIDS cases at diagnosis, more recent work now shows a 6 percent incidence of KS.[269]

Not only is the incidence of KS declining, but its mortality rate also appears to be worsening. In a preliminary study from San Francisco the median duration of survival for a group of KS patients diagnosed in 1982–1983 was 24 months, while a cohort diagnosed from 1984 to 1986 had a 14-month median survival.[283] In this study, HIV p24 antigen was more frequently detectable in the more recent group (76 vs. 43 percent, p = .03), which suggests that KS had been diagnosed at a later point in the course of the HIV infection.

Explanations for the unusual epidemiologic profile of KS in the AIDS epidemic are yet being developed.[284] The relative restriction to homosexuals has been speculated secondary to recreational drug use[285,286] or to a second, as yet unidentified sexually transmitted virus. Either theory could at least partially explain the change in KS incidence (decreasing exposure to a second "cofactor"), but neither clarifies the more rapid disease course now being seen.

Ideally, information from epidemiology studies could contribute to our knowledge of the pathogenesis of KS, but this is not yet the case. No recreational drug used primarily by homosexual men, including the inhaled nitrites once popular, have been clearly shown to be carcinogenic or particularly immunosuppressive. Similarly, despite some early speculation, no coincident "KS virus" has been found. Recent work points to HIV-induced endothelial growth factors as potentially involved in KS formation, but to date this theory is not reconciled with the complex and variable epidemiology of KS in different HIV-infected populations.

Clinical Appearance and Pathophysiology of Kaposi Sarcoma in HIV Infection. Kaposi sarcoma (Table 15) is considered by most an endothelial neoplasm of either capillary or lymphatic origin.[287–289] Histologically, the tumor is typified by a proliferation of vascular structures, often with large malignant-appearing endothelial cells, set against a background of a bland proliferation of spindle-shaped cells and extravasated erythrocytes.[236,290–294] Efforts to establish KS cell lines in culture have made little headway,[295,296] and direct tumor transplants to immunodeficient animals have been unsuccessful. This and the not uncommonly indolent clinical behavior have led to speculation that KS is not in the truest sense a malignancy at all but rather a striking benign cellular proliferation[297] in response to some circulating "growth factor."

Laboratory support for a KS growth factor comes from the preliminary work of Dr. Robert Gallo. Here, inoculation of immunodeficient mice with cells cultured from human KS tumors led to the appearance of vascular tumors in the mouse. Interestingly, however, these tumors were of murine rather than human genetic origin.[295,296]

The clinical pattern of KS is usually not difficult to recognize and can be somewhat predicted from the histologic appearance. Kaposi sarcoma lesions are typically nodular, pigmented, and initially asymptomatic. Size varies from several millimeters to confluent tumor plaques 5–10 cm in diameter. Violaceous to red pigmentation is common, but KS in dark-skinned persons may be nearly black, and occasionally patients irrespective of race have subcutaneous lesions that are nonpigmented. Nodularity of KS lesions is typical, and even small lesions are usually palpable. Many areas of the body can be affected by KS, although some are rarely involved. For example, KS is frequently seen on the skin and in the oral cavity, and while the soles are one of the most common KS sites, the tumor rarely affects the palms.[249,298–308]

Kaposi sarcoma is a multicentric tumor, and numerous lesions can appear simultaneously in widely scattered areas of the body. Kaposi sarcoma in the HIV-infected patient, unlike most other KS populations, often involves visceral structures.[309] Kaposi sarcoma in the gastrointestinal tract is seen in almost 50 percent of cases, most commonly in the stomach, duodenum, and rectum. Another important visceral site of KS is the lung. Both sites will be discussed below.

The lymphatic endothelial origin postulated for KS is often reflected in the gross clinical appearance of the disease. Linearity of lesions following cutaneous lymphatic drainage patterns is particularly common across the chest and back. Lymphedema, often out of proportion to the visible extent of tumor,

TABLE 15. Kaposi Sarcoma in AIDS—Distinguishing Characteristics

Extent of disease	Unlike "traditional" KS, AIDS/KS is *rarely* limited to a single anatomic region
Site of involvement	The head and neck are common primary sites (including the face, oral cavity)
Visceral involvement	Common, rarely symptomatic except for pulmonary KS, which is *rapidly* fatal
Opportunistic infections	Almost uniform during the course of disease; usual cause of death
Social problems	The stigma of AIDS is exacerbated by visible lesions

is seen in some patients and usually affects either the lower extremities or face. In extreme cases, lymphedema of the lower portion of the body to the level of the diagphragm is observed.

Gastrointestinal Kaposi Sarcoma. The GI tract is the most common visceral site of KS.[310–313] As many as 50 percent of patients with KS have lesions in the GI tract even early in the course of their disease. Gastrointestinal KS is seldom symptomatic and is rarely if ever fatal. In some cases, however, GI KS can cause intestinal obstruction, bleeding, or enteropathy. Essentially, any segment of the GI tract may be involved with KS, although the stomach and duodenum are most commonly affected.[314]

The diagnosis of GI KS is most often made by the endoscopic visualization of typical lesions.[311,315] Endoscopy is not routinely recommended in all KS patients and should be reserved for those with GI symptoms. Radiographic visualization of KS is possible, with contrast studies showing raised, smooth, rounded intraluminal masses. The diagnostic accuracy of these studies, however, is not as high as with endoscopy.[316,317]

On endoscopy, KS lesions are nodular and raised and appear highly vascular. As with cutaneous lesions, they vary in size from several millimeters to several centimeters in diameter. Any number may be present, but confluent tumor masses are unusual. Despite their ready visualization, GI KS lesions are not easily diagnosed by biopsy because the tumor is subcutaneous, beyond the depth of the biopsy forceps in 77 percent of cases.[315] If biopsy confirmation is considered essential for patient management, a higher yield may be achieved with loop biopsy technique (Cello J, personal communication, 1988).

Pulmonary KS. Pulmonary parenchymal involvement by KS is less commonly recognized than gastrointestinal spread is but, when present, is more often symptomatic.[318–321] In fact, the general principle that KS, even in the HIV-infected patient, is not directly fatal is not true with symptomatic pulmonary disease where the median duration of survival is approximately 3 months.[319]

The symptoms of pulmonary KS, described in several reviews,[318–320,322] usually consist of dyspnea, a severe but minimally productive cough, chest tightness, and less commonly, fever. These symptoms clearly overlap with those of *Pneumocystis carinii* and CMV and mycobacterial pneumonias, which are the main diseases to be considered in a differential diagnosis.

The diagnosis of pulmonary KS is to some degree one of exclusion, particularly of PCP. The chest x-ray findings in pulmonary KS tend to show a more nodular pattern with less even infiltration than is typical of PCP. Pleural effusions are also more suggestive of pulmonary KS. These effusions are frequently bloody, but cytologic examination is usually nondiagnostic. Pulmonary gallium scan can provide useful information in some cases, generally showing no uptake in patients with pulmonary KS in contrast to those with infectious pneumonias.[322,323]

Bronchoscopy provides the strongest evidence of pulmonary KS. Although the pulmonary parenchyma is the principle site of disease, in most cases endobronchial lesions are easily visualized by an experienced bronchoscopist. Lesions are several millimeters or more in diameter and appear redder and more vascular than cutaneous KS lesions are. Biopsy is relatively contraindicated because of possible hemorrhage, but transbronchial biopsy has been used to diagnose KS in some cases. Patients with pulmonary KS almost always have extensive cutaneous KS as well, although primary pulmonary KS has been reported.[318,324] At any rate, the presence of typical pulmonary symptoms and diagnostic tests in the absence of an infectious pneumonia should be considered adequate to warrant management for pulmonary KS.

Diagnosis of Cutaneous Kaposi Sarcoma. A clinician should, with some experience, have no difficulty in recognizing typical cutaneous KS lesions, but biopsy confirmation should be obtained, particularly if this information will be used to make an initial AIDS diagnosis. A punch biopsy (ideally ≥4 mm in diameter) is usually sufficient. The biopsy can be safely performed in an outpatient setting with local anesthesia. Despite the vascular nature of KS, hemorrhage is rarely encountered. While KS has been diagnosed from fine-needle aspiration cytology specimens, this technique is almost certainly less sensitive and specific, and its use should be limited.

Oral Kaposi Sarcoma. The oral cavity is an extremely common site of KS.[302,325,326] In as many as one-third of patients this represents the first site of disease, while it appears later in the course of KS in many others. Intraoral lesions are most common on the hard palate but are not uncommon on the posterior pharyngeal wall or the gingiva.[327] The tongue is an uncommon site of KS, and the buccal mucosa is almost always spared.

The appearance of oral KS is typical and similar to cutaneous disease. Lesions on the hard palate, however, are often not palpable and are blue to violet in color. Biopsy (usually by an oral surgeon) can be performed, and this should be done if other, more easily sampled cutaneous lesions are not present.[307,328]

Intraoral KS is generally asymptomatic until late in the disease course. Then, the lesions can become bulky, with superficial necrosis leading to pain, bleeding, and occasionally difficulty in swallowing. Gingival KS can additionally contribute to the periodontal disease seen in many AIDS patients.

Staging, Clinical Course, and Management of Kaposi Sarcoma. PROGNOSTIC FACTORS/STAGING Staging of KS (Table 16) by estimates of tumor burden have been proposed by several groups.[306,329] Usually, KS in these systems is categorized by the number, size, appearance, site of involvement, and the rate of growth. Although most experienced clinicians are convinced that KS patients can be divided into those with "minimal" tumor burden and those with "advanced" KS, no common definitions have been accepted. This is problematic for the individual patient and practitioner who would like more precise information available to better discuss the prognosis and plan therapy, but it is of even more concern for the design and comparison of clinical investigations.

Admitting limitations, some broad staging guidelines of KS extent can be proposed. Patients with "few" lesions (for example, <25), those without known visceral or intraoral disease, and those with an established history of "slow" tumor growth are judged more stable than are those patients with many lesions or with any extracutaneous involvement. Similarly, patients with a history of minimal increase in lesion size or number over a several month period (not an uncommon observation at the time of actual biopsy) have a better prognosis than do patients in whom new lesions are rapidly appearing. Some feel that the prognosis is improved when the lesions are geographically con-

TABLE 16. Prognostic Variables in Kaposi Sarcoma

Predicts Indolent Course	*Predicts Aggressive Course*
Few lesions (<25)	Many KS lesions
Low rate of growth	Rapid appearance of new lesions
No visceral KS identified	Intraoral or visceral lesions
No fevers, drenching night sweats, or weight loss	One or more constitutional symptoms
No prior opportunistic infection	One prior or concurrent opportunistic infection
Absolute CD4+ count, >400/mm^3	CD4+ cell count, <200/mm^3
Normal ESR	ESR, >40 mm/hr
HIV p24 antigen not detectible	HIV p24 detectable
Normal β_2-microglobulin	β_2-microglobulin, >5
Normal blood counts	Leukopenia or anemia present

fined to one body area, for example, the skin of one extremity, No firm data exist to support this, however. Certainly, the prognosis is worsened if visceral KS is diagnosed. The median duration of survival is less than 4 months, for example, in patients with pulmonary KS. While the effect of gastrointestinal and intraoral KS on survival duration is less clear, disease in these sites is also felt to imply a worsened prognosis.

Along with estimates of KS tumor burden, it is known that the symptomatic status of the patient is important in the prognosis. Similar to Hodgkin's and non-Hodgkin's lymphoma, KS patients with chronic systemic symptoms such as unexplained fevers, night sweats, and weight loss have a decrease in median survival duration.[330] Also, this effect is cumulative, and the prognosis is additionally limited in patients with multiple constitutional symptoms. Whether one or more specific symptoms have a greater impact is now being investigated.

A final means of staging KS involves laboratory tests grouped into those of general value an those specifically estimating HIV burden and/or immunologic impairment.[298,300,331,332] Survival duration is decreased in patients with severe anemia or neutropenia or with erythrocyte sedimentation rates above 40 mm/hr. Abnormalities in serum chemistry test results have not been shown to be of independent value, although elevated serum globulin levels are common in KS as in other HIV-infected patients.

Probably the strongest laboratory predictors of outcome in KS are likely to be those that are more directly involved in HIV and its immune effects. HIV p24 antigen, for example, if present in AIDS patients in detectable concentrations, implies a poor prognosis,[333] which is also correlated with severe depression in the number of circulating CD4+ cells. This general observation is likely to hold true in patients with KS. Similar speculations can be made for other markers such as β_2-microglobulin.

As with other methods of staging KS, laboratory abnormalities are often closely correlated with other poor prognostic markers. Rather than enabling the clinician or clinical investigator to precisely define the stage of disease or prognosis, all staging information must be taken into account. It is, from a clinical practice standpoint, probably adequate to group KS patients into those with a reasonably high likelihood of a 1-year survival without secondary opportunistic infections or rampant KS growth and into others where these clinical events are much more probable. Using this information, the clinician can better advise the patient concerning opportunistic infection prophylaxis and the need for specific antineoplastic therapy. A summary of the prognostic and staging variables discussed is shown in Table 16.

INITIAL EVALUATION OF THE PATIENT WITH KAPOSI SARCOMA. The goals of an initial evaluation of a patient with suspected KS vary depending on the patients' prior health status. If KS represents the initial AIDS-defining process, biopsy is essential. If, on the other hand, the patient has had prior opportunistic infections and if the KS is not likely to require treatment either because of poor baseline prognosis or because the extent of KS is still minimal, biopsy may not be required, especially if the lesion sites are on visible skin or are intraoral.

The initial evaluation can, overall, be divided into those tests that would be performed in any new AIDS patient to estimate viral burden and immune damage and to rule out opportunistic infections. The specific application of these tests to the new KS patient is to estimate the prognosis and plan treatment. To this end, a careful examination of the entire body surface is essential, with recording of the number, size, site, and general appearance of visible KS lesions. Photography of selected areas can be useful for later establishing progression or response to treatment. The examination should include a digital rectal exam to palpate possible KS lesions and a careful examination of the pharynx to identify intraoral KS lesions on the palate, posterior oral pharynx, or gingiva. Routine gastrointestinal endoscopy is not recommended unless indicated for specific symptomatology.

The initial (and each subsequent) medical history should inquire about the constitutional symptoms discussed previously and about any symptoms potentially related to opportunistic infections. Because these are often the cause of death in patients with KS,[334] their diagnosis, prophylaxis, and treatment must be considered at *all* times by treating physicians.

Laboratory studies in the KS patient should include a complete blood count, determination of the ESR, and a routine chemistry panel. As with all parts of the spectrum of HIV disease, HIV infection must be established with HIV antibody tests, and all patients should be tested for serologic evidence of syphilis and active hepatitis B infection. HIV status can be additionally evaluated with an HIV p24 antigen and indirectly with β_2-microglobulin determination. Immunologic testing should include T-lymphocyte subset testing with enumeration of CD4+ and CD8+ populations. Given recent evidence, these can probably be expressed most accurately as their percentages of the total T-lymphocyte population, although following their absolute number (a further calculated estimate) is more commonly used.[298,300] The use of skin testing for delayed hypersensitivity reactivity is advocated by some groups but is probably of limited additional value when compared with the other tests discussed.

As soon as the results of the initial examination are available, the patient should be informed of the results. This discussion should attempt to give the patient a better sense of the disease prognosis to help further decision making. Specific counseling should address the need for considering antiretroviral therapy and the importance of recognizing, treating, and if possible, preventing opportunistic infections. The options for treating the KS directly should also be frankly reviewed. This discussion should, of course, include the possibility of not treating the KS per se if that seems an option and should also address the common concerns about the visible nature of KS and the fear that antineoplastic treatment—particularly chemotherapy and radiation therapy—may cause further immune impairment or may further compromise the ability to tolerate zidovudine administration.

Therapy for Kaposi Sarcoma. Although perhaps less dramatic than progress in antiretroviral drug development, research in the treatment of KS has improved overall patient care. Kaposi sarcoma therapy (Table 17) currently reflects the growing realization that the tumor, which while not a true malignancy according to some definitions,[297] has a heterogeneous natural history ranging from indolent to rapidly fatal that takes place against a backdrop of progressive HIV-induced immune depletion. Thus, recent reports include both local treatments and increasingly aggressive chemotherapy regimens as well as attempts to combine antineoplastic drugs with agents of antiviral potential such as zidovudine. These approaches are summarized in Table 17, which stresses the individualization of treatment based on the patient's estimated prognosis.

LOCAL THERAPY. Many patients experience more problems from individual lesions than from their overall disease. This is especially common in patients with bulky intraoral KS, those with scattered facial lesions, and those with lesions in areas subjected to recurrent minor trauma (e.g., the ankle). Surgical excision or local radiation therapy remain good options for some of these situations, and increasingly, topical or intralesional treatments are also being evaluated. Radiation therapy rapidly shrinks individual KS lesions and is also frequently administered to somewhat broader areas of the body to control plaques of coalesced lesions or to reduce KS-associated lymphedema.[335–344] Although tumor responses to relatively low doses of radiation therapy (2000–3000 rads) are gratifying, local toxicity remains a problem for some patients. Particularly common

TABLE 17. Guidelines for Kaposi Sarcoma Treatment

Patient Status	*Options*
Favorable prognostic indicators[a]	Expectant observation Alternating single-agent chemotherapy such as vinblastine/vincristine Interferon-α with or without zidovudine Experimental treatment trials
Unfavorable prognostic indicators[a]	Early initiation of therapy Alternating vincristine/vinblastine chemotherapy Other single-agent chemotherapy (e.g., Adriamycin) Combination chemotherapy (e.g., Adriamycin, bleomycin, vincristine)
Local tumor problems	Radiation therapy Topical liquid nitrogen Intralesional dilute vinblastine Surgical excision

[a] See Table 15.

are moderate to severe mucositis from radiating large intraoral KS lesions and cutaneous erythema from radiating larger lesions on the feet. These local toxicities are temporary and, in the case of intraoral mucositis, can be reduced by scrupulous attention to oral hygiene and control of minor infections such as with *Candida albicans*.

Intralesional or topical treatments being investigated for KS include some that are not directly antineoplastic in the usual sense such as cryotherapy with liquid nitrogen or topical applications of dinitrochlorobenzene (DNCB). Other local treatments include injections of intralesional tumor necrosis factor or dilute vinblastine, agents that are presumably directly active on the tumor cells.

One observation only now being actively studied is that agents that cause a local inflammatory reaction can lead to KS regression. The most straightforward of these is the topical application of liquid nitrogen. This therapy (personal communication, Alvin Friedman-Kien, 1988) consists of applying liquid nitrogen by a cotton applicator to the lesion until a "halo" of surrounding erythema is observed. A mild inflammation results, and the lesion flattens as this resolves. Larger lesions may require repeated applications at approximately 2-week intervals. Small lesions may completely disappear with this therapy; larger ones may leave a residual hemosiderin "tattoo."

A similar result has been reported with injections of small volumes of dilute vinblastine directly into the KS lesion.[345] Here, a 0.2 mg/cc solution of sterile vinblastine is prepared and injected through a fine-gauge needle placed perpendicular to the skin surface in the center of small KS lesions. Larger lesions (>1 cm) may require two or more such injections at separate sites. Sufficient volume is injected into the lesion (usually less than 0.5 cc). Because of the low dose, multiple lesions can be treated simultaneously. As with liquid nitrogen application, a mild inflammatory reaction ensues, but cutaneous ulcerations are not common, and small lesions typically heal without scarring. Therapy can be repeated every 2 weeks if required. This therapy has also been applied to intraoral lesions, but these, if extensive, are probably best treated with radiation therapy even considering the frequent mucositis seen in HIV-infected patients with this therapy.

Other local therapies under investigation include intralesional injections of recombinant tumor necrosis factor.[346] This is supposedly directly cytotoxic to the KS lesion. Because even local injections of tumor necrosis factor have led to systemic side effects, this therapy is currently considered appropriate for experimental uses only. Similarly, groups are investigating intralesional injections of interferon-α, an agent recently approved for systemic use in KS.

SYSTEMIC CHEMOTHERAPY. Even early in the AIDS epidemic, recognition of the variable natural history of KS and the many uncertainties of staging led to concern that overly aggressive chemotherapy—particularly the use of combinations of agents—might be inappropriate in some patients. Awareness of the underlying immune deficiency caused fears of the immunologic toxicity resulting from the aggressive use of cytotoxic drugs. Thus, most subsequent efforts were directed at single-agent chemotherapy—giving this more frequently but in lower doses or in alternating regimens with other single-agent therapy. This direction has been of value; single-agent chemotherapy with vinblastine alone[347] at a dose of 4–8 mg weekly or alternated with vincristine[348] at 1–2 mg/dose is considered by many as a standard for HIV-related KS, especially if the disease is relatively indolent. Recently, equal or increased activity has been shown for single-agent Adriamycin given in attenuated doses (10–30 mg total dose) intravenously every 1–2 weeks.[349] In a study of the National Institute of Allergy and Infectious Diseases (NIAID)-supported AIDS Clinical Trials Group, for example, Adriamycin therapy administered weekly at a dose of 15 mg/m^2 resulted in a 16 percent partial remission in a group of 32 previously untreated patients. Also, vincristine as a single-drug treatment regimen is used for KS patients who are thrombocytopenic. This regimen has a high response rate—over 50 percent—with acceptable neurotoxicity.[350]

Although concern about immune toxicity is still appropriate, more information suggests that some combination chemotherapy can be used safely.[351,352] The group of KS patients with rapidly progressing and often fatal disease may, in fact, benefit from these more aggressive chemotherapeutic approaches. Gill et al. have reported recently that a combination of Adriamycin, bleomycin, and vincristine results in rapid and often complete KS responses with no apparent increase in expected rates of opportunistic infections. Doses of each agent are as follows: Adriamycin, 20 mg/m^2; bleomycin, 10 mg/m^2; vincristine, 1.4 mg/m^2, all given intravenously every other week.[353] Because of the cardiac, pulmonary, and neurologic toxicities of these agents, this regimen should probably be reserved for patients with poor overall prognoses. Its use should be accompanied by careful monitoring of toxicities.

INTERFERON-α. Systemic recombinant interferon-α has an established level of activity in treating HIV-related KS and recently earned Food and Drug Administration (FDA) approval for this indication. Objective response rates of approximately 40 percent can be expected and are even higher in selected patients with a more favorable overall prognosis.[354–358] The doses used have varied widely in reported trials, but daily doses of greater than 10 million units may be required for the optimum antineoplastic effect. The major predictor of poor response in several studies is the presence of chronic constitutional symptoms or a prior AIDS diagnosis when therapy with interferon is initiated. The drawbacks to single-agent interferon-α therapy are the side effects seen with the high doses required and the need for parenteral injection. Toxicities are primarily subjective—fever, malaise, nausea—but neutropenia is not uncommon, and central nervous system effects including confusion are also seen.

Recent studies in New York and Miami (again, supported by the NIAID AIDS Clinical Trials Group) show antineoplastic activity with low doses (9–18 million units) of recombinant or lymphoblastoid interferon-α along with low doses (100 mg every 4 hours) of zidovudine.[359–361] Hematologic toxicity was seen in these studies but was considered moderate and usually manageable by the investigators. Although this combination employs drugs readily available by prescription in the United States, physicians might be advised to await publication of final study results to permit a more detailed assessment of the attendant risks and benefits.

CHEMOTHERAPY WITH ZIDOVUDINE. Although carefully designed clinical trials of cytotoxic chemotherapy combined with zidovudine are not yet reported, considerable clinical experience has been collected that suggests that this will be difficult to administer. This is unfortunate because the rationale of this combination is attractive considering the dual problems of KS and the underlying HIV infection. Both zidovudine and many cytotoxic regimens used in KS induce some degree of myelosuppression, which is expected to be at least additive when these drugs are combined. Because of a lack of published investigation, no firm guidelines can be provided; however, in general, it seems prudent to maintain patients on a regimen of zidovudine as long as possible to achieve the expected survival benefit. Kaposi sarcoma can then be managed either by increasing the use of local therapies or by the use of non–marrow-toxic agents such as bleomycin and/or vincristine.

Antibiotic Prophylaxis of Opportunistic Infections. It is clear that most KS patients die not of their tumor but of opportunistic infections.[334] In the United States the most common of these is *Pneumocystis carinii* pneumonia. Recent studies show that this infection can be largely prevented by the use of appropriate antibiotics. In a Miami study by Fischl et al.[362] oral trimethoprim-sulfamethoxazole, when tolerated, completely prevented PCP in KS patients, whereas a concurrent group had an incidence of 53 percent without prophylaxis. The toxicity of this prophylaxis was reduced in the investigators' opinion by the inclusion of 5 mg/day of oral leucovorin. Still, 17 percent of subjects experienced toxicity including rash and myelosuppression, which required discontinuation of treatment.

Another attractive option for PCP prophylaxis is pentamidine isethionate given as an inhaled aerosol.[362–364] Although careful prospective results of clinical trials have not been published, this form of prophylaxis may avoid the problems of side effects common with trimethoprim-sulfamethoxazole.

Non-Hodgkin's Lymphoma

The second most common HIV-associated malignancy, non-Hodgkin's lymphoma (NHL), bears little epidemiologic resemblance to KS. Non-Hodgkin's lymphoma is less frequent than KS is; it is seen in <1 percent of reported cases of AIDS in the United States, but is not seemingly restricted to any specific risk group. Nor does the relative frequency of diagnosed NHL seem to be changing, although the absolute number of cases is increasing with the epidemic.[255,261,365]

The pathogenesis of HIV-associated NHL is unknown but is the subject of active laboratory investigation, although some of the tumor's biologic characteristics are understood.[366] Non-Hodgkin's lymphoma in AIDS is a B-lymphocyte neoplasm of unfavorable histologic grade.[260] Most are either large cell, undifferentiated, or immunoblastic types with a clinical presentation and natural history that matches their highly malignant pathologic appearance. No single cytogenetic abnormality has been found, but several different gene rearrangements have been reported.[367–369] A relationship to EBV has been proposed, but again, laboratory studies have been inconclusive, with EBV-related DNA sequences found in some, but not all specimens from several tumor sites in a single affected individual.[370]

Non-Hodgkin's lymphoma in HIV can be present in single or multiple sites, and the clinical problems are determined, in part, by areas of involvement, by the rate of tumor growth, and by the presence or absence of underlying or pre-existing HIV-related opportunistic infections. Malignant lymphocytes are often found in the peripheral blood of NHL patients with HIV, but it is uncommon for the lymphoma to present without easily identifiable solid tumor masses.

Central Nervous System Non-Hodgkin's Lymphoma. Non-Hodgkin's lymphoma occurring in the CNS in AIDS patients was recognized early in the epidemic, well before the peripheral lymphomas were reported, and thus the early CDC surveillance definitions of AIDS included NHL only of CNS origin.[253,371–373]

Central nervous system lymphomas cause the array of clinical problems expected from space-occupying intracranial masses, but these tumors have been surprisingly difficult to diagnose.[252,374] In part, diagnosis is difficult because of the other CNS processes that are more common in HIV infection, especially *Toxoplasma* encephalitis. In several autopsy series, CNS lymphomas have been surprisingly frequent, further attesting to the need to consider them in differential diagnoses and obtain a brain biopsy to establish the diagnosis.

Patients with NHL in the CNS may complain of motor deficits, but others present with cranial neuropathies, headache, or seizures, and frequently some combination of these are present. The onset of symptoms is usually rapid, and death can occur quickly in the absence of therapy.

The diagnosis of CNS NHL relies on a combination of suggestive imaging studies and brain biopsy. Either CT or MRI head scanning are commonly employed, but MRI is probaby a more sensitive test. In contrast to toxoplasmosis, NHL usually presents with a single mass lesion, but tumors occurring along the base of the skull can be missed by imaging. A brain biopsy must be used to finally establish the NHL diagnosis, especially if an empirical course of therapy for toxoplasmosis fails to rapidly (1–2 weeks) lead to a decrease in mass size. Examination of the CSF is not of significant value and should be deferred until large intracranial mass lesions are excluded by imaging studies.

Peripheral Non-Hodgkin's Lymphoma. The clinical presentation of NHL outside the CNS is highly varied because essentially any organ can be affected. In contrast to NHL in non–HIV-infected patients, extralymphatic disease is extremely common, with 63 percent of patients having stage IV disease.[253,254,260,263,375] Also, NHL in the HIV-infected group presents with disease in sites otherwise rarely seen. These have included primary lymphoma in the liver, common bile duct, rectum, soft tissue, duodenum, and lung.[254,376,377]

The clinical course and prognosis of NHL in the HIV infected is not surprising considering the tumor's aggressive histology. Patients often have fulminant disease progression, even developing the tumor lysis syndrome before initiation of therapy due to rapid tumor cell turnover. The prognosis of NHL in HIV infection is extremely grave. In several reports from Los Angeles, New York, and San Francisco, the median survival from diagnosis was <12 months.[254,255,364] Markers of prognosis include histologic type and stage as with the non–HIV-infected patient, but the most important factor is whether or nor the lymphoma represents the patient's first HIV-induced opportunistic disease. Patients with a prior history of AIDS have a median survival of 3 months as compared with 12 months for those initially diagnosed with AIDS on the basis of the lymphoma.[254] In fact, some would generally discourage treatment for patients with a prior AIDS diagnosis because of the poor prognosis and limited ability to tolerate the aggressive chemotherapy otherwise essential to control the lymphoma.

The relationship between persistent generalized lymphadenopathy (PGL) and NHL has been widely discussed but is still quite unclear. It is obvious that in some HIV-infected individuals B-cell proliferation results in diffuse and persisting lymph node enlargment. Occasionally, NHL arises in patients with PGL, but it is not certain that the factors responsible for PGL are the same as those causing the malignant proliferation. What is clear is that the usual caveats against biopsying nodes in patients with PGL need revision if one nodal group is rapidly enlarging. Because this is often due to NHL, immediate biopsy is essential.[378,379]

The diagnosis of NHL should ideally be made by histologic examination of tissue obtained by incisional or excisional biopsy. This permits a more accurate assessment of histologic type for special stains and immunologic subtyping. It may be possible, however, to make an adequate diagnosis from needle aspiration cytology, and this may be required if the patient's clinical condition is critical or deteriorating rapidly.[378] Because the disease is so often widespread, the initial clinical evaluation of the NHL patient should include imaging of the head, chest, and abdomen[380,381]; bone marrow aspiration and biopsy; and lumbar puncture. Once staging is completed, therapy, if it is to be recommended, should be initiated promptly and should be coordinated by an oncologist experienced with these extremely complex patients.

Therapy for HIV-Related Non-Hodgkin's Lymphoma. Therapy for HIV-related NHL is still under active investigation. If therapy is to be employed (potentially excluding those with extremely poor prognoses), an aggressive regimen must be used to achieve acceptable complete response rates. However, because patients with HIV infection have a limited bone marrow reserve, the clinician is frequently faced with the dilemma of selecting a regimen and dose of chemotherapy that controls the tumor without precipitating death from secondary infections. For NHL confined to the CNS, these questions are less urgent since primary therapy usually consists of whole brain radiation with intrathecal chemotherapy.[373]

CHEMOTHERAPY FOR NON-HODGKIN'S LYMPHOMA IN HIV-INFECTED PATIENTS. Few definite guidelines are possible for the treatment of HIV-related NHL. As with all aggressive lymphomas, the use of combinations of drugs is essential. In most reports, cyclophosphamide has been the primary agent,[254,260,263,382] however, because of the compromised marrow reserve at least one investigator favors an attenuated dose at the beginning and subsequent dose escalation. Older combinations such as Cytoxan, Adriamycin, vincristine, and prednisone (CHOP) are often avoided because their relatively prolonged dosing intervals may allow rapid tumor growth between cycles. Most clinicians favor attenuated doses of aggressive regimens such as M-BACOD (methotrexate, leucovorin rescue, bleomycin, doxorubicin, cyclophosphamide, vincristine, and dexamethasone (M-BACOD); methotrexate with leucovorin rescue, doxorubin, cyclophosphamide, vincristine, prednisone, and bleomycin (MACOP-B); cyclophosphamide, vincristine, prednisone, bleomycin, doxorubicin, and procarbazine (COP-BLAM); or cyclophosphamide, vincristine, methotrexate with leucovorin rescue, and cytarabine (COMLA). Even these general guidelines, however, should not be accepted as established because further clinical trials are clearly needed.

Drug regimens for peripheral NHL must include intrathecal therapy, which can be relatively brief in the absence of identified CNS involvement. Specific guidelines are available in recent clinical reviews from Los Angeles[262,382] and San Francisco.[254]

The newer areas of therapy such as the use of zidovudine to treat the concomitant HIV infection and hematopoietic hormones such as granulocyte colony-stimulating factor (G-CSF) and granulocyte-macrophage colony-stimulating factor (GM-CSF) to permit more aggressive lymphoma chemotherapy are especially relevant to the treatment of HIV-related NHL. Zidovudine, because of its associated myelotoxicity, should, in general, be avoided in the early chemotherapy of HIV-related NHL. Most clinicians would consider it more critical to attain a complete tumor response but would then try to combine zidovudine in standard doses with any ongoing maintenance chemotherapy.

One group of studies just being initiated are designed to use the hematopoietic hormone GM-CSF to ameliorate the myelotoxicity of aggressive chemotherapy in HIV-associated NHL. This drug has already shown a remarkable activity in elevating peripheral leukocyte counts in chemotherapy for other cancers, and it is hoped that positive results will be forthcoming in HIV-related NHL.

A final area of NHL therapy deserving attention is the prophylaxis of opportunistic infections. Even more than in KS, these are a frequent cause of mortality for patients with NHL.[254] Although no controlled series have been published, it would seem advisable to use prophylactic aerosolized pentamidine, thus avoiding the additional myelotoxicity of trimethoprim-sulfamethoxazole. Clinicians should follow the results of ongoing clinical trials in this area closely, but 300 mg of pentamidine delivered monthly by a Respigard II nebulizer is recommended.

TABLE 18. Cancers in the HIV Epidemic

Incidence increased:
Kaposi sarcoma
CNS non-Hodgkin's lymphoma
Peripheral non-Hodgkin's lymphoma
Cases reported
Hodgkin's lymphoma
Squamous carcinoma
Small cell carcinoma
Testicular cancer
Basal cell cancer
Melanoma
Anticipated relationship:
Hepatocellular carcinoma

Other Cancers in HIV Infection

In addition to those cancers described with a presumed etiologic relationship to HIV, many other neoplasms have been reported in HIV-infected subjects (Table 18). In some, the number of reports begin to suggest an etiologic relationship while in others the connection is uncertain. Irrespective of the causal role of HIV, there is a suspicion that the natural history of tumors and their response to therapy may be affected by the HIV infection.

One tumor relatively commonly seen in HIV is Hodgkin's lymphoma.[383–393] Although Hodgkin's disease has been commonly reported in HIV-infected patients, several studies have not shown it to occur at a higher than expected frequency. When seen with HIV infection, however, Hodgkin's disease tends to be more advanced and responds less completely to therapy. Most centers still attempt "curative" chemotherapy; however, the meaning of "cure" is uncertain given the HIV infection status. Thus some have suggested using less aggressive chemotherapy designed primarily to control rather than cure the malignancy. No recent findings have changed this recommendation, and large-scale clinical trials are not yet underway. Until more is known, these patients should be treated with conventional regimens such as melphalan, vincristine, procarbazine, and prednisone (MOPP) or this alternating with Adriamycin, bleomycin, vincristine, and dacarbazine (ABVD). As with NHL, PCP prophylaxis should be considered due to a high risk of opportunistic infections.

Other cancers reported in HIV-infected individuals include malignant melanoma,[393] squamous cell carcinomas,[394–396] testicular cancers of all histologies,[397–399] small cell carcinomas,[394–396] basal cell cancers,[400,401] carcinoid tumors,[402] liposarcoma,[403] and colonic adenocarcinoma.[404] Each of these has been seen in insufficient numbers to draw any strong inference as to etiology, but a growing clinical impression is that their natural history is also more aggressive.

REFERENCES

1. Gottlieb MS, Schroff R, Schanker HM, et al. *Pneumocystis carinii* pneumonia and mucosal candidiasis in previously healthy homosexual men: Evidence of a new acquired cellular immunodeficiency. N Engl J Med. 1981;305:1425–31.
2. Masur H, Michelis MA, Greene JB, et al. An outbreak of community-acquired *Pneumocystis carinii* pneumonia: Initial manifestation of cellular immune dysfunction. N Engl J Med. 198;305:1431–8.
3. Siegal FP, Lopez C, Hammer GS, et al. Severe acquired immunodeficiency in male homosexuals manifested by chronic perianal ulcerative herpes simplex lesions. N Engl J Med. 1981;305:1431–8.
4. Follansbee SE, Busch DF, Wofsy CB, et al. An outbreak of *Pneumocystis carinii* pneumonia in homosexual men. Ann Intern Med. 1982;96:705–13.

5. Centers for Disease Control. Kaposi's sarcoma and *Pneumocystis pneumonia* among homosexual men—New York City and California. MMWR. 1982;30:305–8.
6. Centers for Disease Control. Opportunistic infections and Kaposi's sarcoma among Haitians in the United States. MMWR. 1982;31:353–61.
7. Centers for Disease Control. Update on acquired immunodeficiency syndrome (AIDS)—United States. MMWR. 1982;31:507–14.
8. Centers for Disease Control. Update: Acquired immunodeficiency syndrome—United States. MMWR. 1985;34:245–8.
9. Pape JW, Liautaud B, Thomas F, et al. Characteristics of the acquired immunodeficiency syndrome (AIDS) in Haiti. N Engl J Med. 1983;309:945–50.
10. Pape JW, Liautaud B, Thomas F, et al. The acquired immunodeficiency syndrome in Haiti. Ann Intern Med. 1985;103:674–8.
11. Malebranche R, Annoux E, Guerin JM, et al. AIDS with severe gastrointestinal manifestations in Haiti. Lancet. 1983;2:873–8.
12. Centers for Disease Control. *Pneumocystis carinii* pneumonia among persons with hemophilia A. MMWR. 1982;31:365–7.
13. Centers for Disease Control. Update on acquired immune deficiency syndrome (AIDS) among patients with hemophilia A. MMWR. 1982;31:644–6,52.
14. Centers for Disease Control. Possible transfusion-associated acquired immune deficiency syndrome AIDS—California. MMWR. 1982;31:652–4.
15. Abrams DI, Lewis BJ, Beckstead JP, et al. Persistent diffuse lymphadenopathy in homosexual men: Endpoint or prodrome? Ann Intern Med. 1984;100:801–8.
16. Abrams DI. Lymphadenopathy syndrome in male homosexuals. In: Gallin JI, Fauci AS, eds. Acquired Immunodeficiency Syndrome. Advances in Host Defense Mechanisms. v. 5. New York: Raven Press, 1985:75–97.
17. Morris L, Distenfeld A, Amorosi E, et al. Autoimmune thrombocytopenic purpura in homosexual men. Ann Intern Med. 1982;96:714–7.
18. Walsh CM, Nardi MA, Karpatkin S. On the mechanism of thrombocytopenic purpora in sexually active homosexual men. N Engl J Med. 1984;311:635–9.
19. Abrams DI, Volberding PA, Linker CA, et al. Immune thrombocytopenic purpura in homosexual men: Clinical manifestations and treatment results (Abstract). Blood. 1983;62:1082.
20. Abrams DI. AIDS-related conditions. Clin Immunol Allergy. 1986;6:581.
21. Harris C, Small CB, Klein RS, et al. Immunodeficiency in female sexual partners of men with the acquired immunodeficiency syndrome. N Engl J Med. 1984;308:1181–4.
22. Barre-Sinoussi F, Chermann JC, Rey F, et al. Isolation of a T-lymphotropic retrovirus from a patient at risk for acquired immunodeficiency syndrome (AIDS). Science. 1983;220:868–71.
23. Gallo RC, Salahudin SZ, Popovic M, et al. Frequent detection and isolation of cytopathic retroviruses (HTLV-III) from patients with AIDS and at risk for AIDS. Science. 1984;224:500–3.
24. Levy JA, Hoffman AD, Kramer SD, et al. Isolation of lymphocytopathic retrovirus from San Francisco patients with AIDS. Science. 1984;225:840–2.
25. Centers for Disease Control. Revision of the CDC surveillance case definition for acquired immunodeficiency syndrome. MMWR. 1987;36(Suppl):1.
26. Centers for Disease Control. Current trends: Classification system for human T lymphotropic virus type III/lymphadenopathy associated virus infections. MMWR. 1986;35:334–39.
27. World Health Organization. Acquired immunodeficiency syndrome (AIDS). Weekly Epidemiol Rec 1986;61:69–73.
28. Centers for Disease Control. Current trends: Classification system for human T lymphotropic virus type III/lymphadenopathy associated virus infections. MMWR. 1986;35:334–39.
29. Redfield RR, Wright DC, Tramont EC: The Walter Reed staging classification for HTLV-III/LAV infection. N Engl J Med. 1986;314:131–2.
30. Osmond D, Chaisson RE, Moss AR, et al. Lymphadenopathy in asymptomatic patients seropositive for HIV. New Engl J Med. 1987;317:246.
31. McArthur JC, Johnson RT. Primary infection with human immunodeficiency virus. In: Rosenblum ML, Levy RM, Bredesen DE, et al., eds. AIDS and the Nervous System. New York: Raven Press; 1988.
32. MacDonnell KB, Chmiel JS, Goldsmith J, et al. Prognostic usefulness of the Walter Reed staging classification for HIV infection. J AIDS. 1988;1:367–74.
33. Terragna A, Dodi F, Anselmo M, et al. The Walter Reed staging classification in the follow-up of HIV infection. N Engl J Med. 1986;315:1355–6.
34. Farzadagen H, Polis MA, Wolinsky SM, et al. Loss of human immunodeficiency virus type 1 (HIV-1) antibodies with evidence of viral infection in asymptomatic homosexual men: A report from the multicenter AIDS cohort study. Ann Intern Med. 1988;108:785–790.
35. Goedert JJ, Biggar RJ, Weiss SH, et al. Three-year incidence of AIDS in five cohorts of HTLV-III-infected risk group members. Science. 1986;231:992–5.
36. Jaffe HW, Darrow WW, Echenberg DF, et al. The acquired immunodeficiency syndrome in a cohort of homosexual men: A six year follow-up study. Ann Intern Med. 1985;103:210–4.
37. Melbye M, Biggar RJ, Ebbesen P, et al. Long-term HTLV-III seropositive homosexual men without AIDS develop measurable immunologic and clinical abnormalities: A longitudinal study. Ann Intern Med. 1986;104:496–500.
38. Moss AR, Bacchetti P, Osmond D, et al. Seropositivity for HIV and the development of AIDS or ARC: Three year follow-up of the San Francisco General Hospital cohort. Br Med J. 1988;296:745–50.
39. Eyster ME, Gail MH, Ballard JO, et al. Natural history of human immunodeficiency virus infections in hemophiliacs: Effects of T-cell subsets, platelet counts and age. Ann Intern Med. 1987;107:1–6.
40. Hessol NA, Rutherford GW, Lifson AR, et al. The natural history of HIV infection in homosexual and bisexual men: a decade of followup. (Abstract 4096) Proceedings of the 4th International Conference on AIDS. Stockholm, Sweden, June 12–16, 1988.
41. Bacchetti P, Moss AR. The incubation period of AIDS in San Francisco. Nature. In press.
42. Klein RS, Harris CA, Small CB, et al. Oral candidiasis in high-risk patients as the initial manifestation of the acquired immunodeficiency syndrome. N Engl J Med. 1984;311:354–8.
43. Carne CA, Weller IVD, Loveday C, et al. From persistent generalized lymphadenopathy to AIDS: Who will progress? Br Med J. 1987;294:868–9.
44. Greenspan D, Greenspan JS, Hearst NG, et al. Relation of oral hairy leukoplakia to infection with the human immunodeficiency virus and the risk of developing AIDS. J Infect Dis. 1987;155:475.
45. Melbye M, Grossman RJ, Goedert JJ, et al. Risk of AIDS after herpes zoster. Lancet. 1987;1:728–30.
46. Moss AR. Predicting progression to AIDS. Br Med J. 1988;297:1067–8.
47. Goedert JJ, Bigga RJ, Melbye M, et al. Effect of T4 count and cofactors on the incidence of AIDS in homosexual men infected with human immunodeficiency virus. JAMA. 1987;257:331–4.
48. Polk BF, Fox R, Brookmeyer R, et al. Predictors of the acquired immunodeficiency syndrome developing in a cohort of seropositive homosexual men. N Engl J Med. 1987;316:61–6.
49. Allain J-P. Laurian Y, Paul DA, et al. Long-term evaluation of HIV antigen and antibodies to p24 and gp41 in patients with hemophilia. N Engl J Med. 1987;317:1114–21.
50. De Wolf F, Goudsmit J, Paul DA, et al. Risk of AIDS related complex and AIDS in homosexual men with persistent antigenemia. Br Med J. 1987;295:569–72.
51. Weber JN, Clapham PR, Weiss RA, et al. Human immunodeficiency virus infection in two cohorts of homosexual men: Neutralising sera and association of anti-*gag* antibody with prognosis. Lancet. 1987;1:119–21.
52. Eyster ME, Goedert JJ, Poon MC, et al. Acid-labile interferon: A possible preclinical marker for the acquired immunodeficiency syndrome in hemophilia. N Engl J Med. 1983;309:583–6.
53. Holmberg SD, Gerber AR, Stewart JA, et al. Herpesviruses as co-factors in AIDS (Letter). Lancet. 1988;2:746–7.
54. Oxtoby MS, Mvula M, Ryder R, et al. Measles and measles immunization in African children with human immunodeficiency virus (Abstract 1353). In Proceedings of the 28th Inter Science Conference on Antimicrobial Agents and Chemotherapy. Am Soc Microbiol, Washington, DC: American Society for Microbiology; 1988.
55. Nelson KE, Clements ML, Miotti P, et al. The influence of human immunodeficiency virus (HIV) infection on antibody responses to influenza vaccines. Ann Intern Med. 1988;109:383–8.
56. DesJarlais DC, Friedman SR, Marmor M, et al. HTLV-III/LAV-associated disease progression and co-factors in a cohort of IV drug users. AIDS. 1987;1:105–11.
57. Chambers HF, Morris DL, Tauber MG, et al. Cocaine use and the risk of endocarditis in intravenous drug users. Ann Intern Med. 1987;106:833–6.
58. Chaisson RE, Bacchetti P, Osmond D, et al. Cocaine use and HIV infection in intravenous drug users in San Francisco. JAMA. 1989;261:561–65.
59. Eales LS, Nye KE, Parkin SM, et al. Association of different allelic forms of group specific component with susceptibility to and clinical manifestation of human immunodeficiency virus infection. Lancet. 1987;1:999–1002.
59a. Eales LJ, Nye KE, Pinching AJ. Group-specific component and AIDS: erroneous data. Lancet. 1988;1:936.
60. Bacchetti P, Osmond D, Chaisson RE, et al. Patterns of survival in the acquired immunodeficiency syndrome. J Infect Dis. 1988;157:1044–7.
61. Cooper DA, Gold J, MacLean P, et al. Acute AIDS retrovirus infection. Definition of a clinical illness associated with seroconversion. Lancet. 1985;1:537–40.
62. Anonymous. Needlestick transmission of HTLV-III from a patient infected in Africa. Lancet. 1984;2:1376–7.
63. Moss AR, Osmond D, Bacchetti P, et al. Risk factors for AIDS and HIV seropositivity in homosexual men. Am J Epidemiol 1987;125:1035–47.
64. Jaffe HW, Hardy AM, Morgan WM, et al. The acquired immunodeficiency syndrome in gay men. Ann Intern Med. 1985;103:662–4.
65. Fox R, Eldred LJ, Fuchs EJ, et al. Clinical manifestations of acute infection with human immunodeficiency virus in a cohort of gay men. AIDS. 1987;1:35–8.
66. Tindall B, Barker S, Donovan B, et al. Characteristics of the acute clinical illness associated with human immunodeficiency virus infection. Arch Intern Med. 1988:148(4):945–49.
67. Pyun KH, Ochs HD, Dufford MTW, et al. Perinatal infection with human immunodeficiency virus. Specific antibody responses by the neonate. N Engl J Med. 1987;317:611–4.
68. Stricof RL, Morse DL. HTLV-III/LAV seroconversion following a deep intramuscular needlestick injury. N Engl J Med. 1986;314:1115.
69. Kessler HA, Blaauw B, Spear J, et al. Diagnosis of human immunodeficiency virus infection in seronegative homosexuals presenting with an acute viral syndrome. JAMA. 1987;258:1196–9.

70. Valle S-L. Febrile pharyngitis as the primary sign of HIV infection in a cluster of cases linked by sexual contact. Scand J Infect Dis. 1987;19:13–7.
71. Rustin MHA, Ridely CM, Smith MD, et al. The acute exanthem associated with seroconversion to human T-cell lymphotropic virus III in a homosexual man. J Infect Dis. 1986;12:161–3.
72. Carne CA, Tedder RS, Smith A, et al. Acute encephalopathy coincident with seroconversion for anti-HTLV-III. Lancet. 1985;2:1206–8.
73. Denning DW, Anderson J, Rudge P, et al. Acute myelopathy associated with primary infection with human immunodeficiency virus. Br Med J. 1987;294:143–4.
74. Elder G, Dalakas M, Pezeshkpour G, et al. Ataxic neuropathy due to ganglioneuritis after probable acute human immunodeficiency virus infection. Lancet. 1986;2:1275–6.
75. Farthing C, Gazzard B: Acute illnesses associated with HTLV-III seroconversion. Lancet. 1985;1:935–6.
76. Ho DD, Sarngadharan MG, Resnick L, et al. Primary human T-lymphotropic virus type III infection. Ann Intern Med. 1985;103:880–3.
77. Piette AM, Tusseau F, Vignon D, et al. Acute neuropathy coincident with seroconversion for anti-LAV/HTLV-III. Lancet. 1986;1:852.
78. Podzamczer D, Casanova A, Santa-Maria P, et al. Esophageal candidiasis in the diagnosis of HIV-infected patients. JAMA. 1988;259:1328–9.
79. Cooper DA, Imrie AA, Penny R. Antibody response to human immunodeficiency virus after primary infection. J Infect Dis. 1987;155:1113–8.
80. Cooper DA, Tindall B, Wilson E, et al. Characterization of T lymphocyte responses during primary HIV infection. J Infect Dis. 1988;157(5):889–96.
81. Cooper DA, Tindall B, Wilson EJ, et al. Characterization of T lymphocyte responses during primary infection with human immunodeficiency virus. J Infect Dis. 1988;157:889–96.
82. Goudsmit J, De Wolf F, Paul DA, et al. Expression of human immunodeficiency virus antigen (HIV-Ag) in serum and cerebrospinal fluid during acute and chronic infection. Lancet. 1986;2:177–80.
83. Allain J-P, Laurian Y, Paul DA, et al. Serological markers in early stages of human immunodeficiency virus infection in hemophiliacs. Lancet. 1986;2:1233–6.
84. Gaines H, Sonnerborg A, Czajkowski J, et al. Antibody response in primary human immunodeficiency virus infection. Lancet. 1987;1:1249–53.
85. Ranki A, Valle S-L, Krohn M, et al. Long latency period precedes overt seroconversion in sexually transmitted human-immunodeficiency-virus infection. Lancet. 1987;2:589–93.
86. Metroka CE, Cunningham-Rundles S, Pollack MS, et al. Persistent generalized lymphadenopathy in homosexual men. Ann Intern Med. 1983;99:585.
87. Abrams DI, Kirn DH, Feigal DW, et al. Lymphadenopathy: Update of a 60 month prospective study (Abstract). In: Proceedings of the III International Conference on AIDS. Washington, DC:USDH and WHO; 1987:118.
88. Hewlett D, Duncanson FP, Jagadha V, et al. Lymphadenopathy in an inner-city population consisting principally of intravenous drug abusers with suspected acquired immunodeficiency syndrome. Am Respir Rev Dis. 1988;137:1275–9.
89. Bottles K, McPhaul LW, Volberding P. Fine-needle aspiration biopsy of patients with the acquired immunodeficiency syndrome (AIDS): Experience in an outpatient clinic. Ann Intern Med. 1988;108:42–5.
90. Hales M, Bottles K, Miller T. Diagnosis of Kaposi's sarcoma by fine-needle aspiration biopsy. Am J Clin Pathol. 1987;88:20–5.
91. Abrams DI. AIDS-related lymphadenopathy: The role of biopsy. J Clin Oncol. 1986;4:126–7.
92. Stricker RB, Abrams DI, Corash L, et al. Target platelet antigen in homosexual men with immune thrombocytopenia. N Engl J Med. 1985;313:1375–80.
93. Federle MP, Megibow AJ, Naidich DP, eds. Radiology of AIDS. New York: Raven Press; 1988.
94. The Swiss Group for Clinical Studies on AIDS, Luthy R, Chairman. Zidovudine for the treatment of thrombocytopenia associated with human immunodeficiency virus (HIV): A prospective study. Ann Intern Med. 1988;109:718–21.
95. Folks TM, Kessler SW, Orenstein JM, et al. Infection and replication of HIV-1 in purified progenitor cells of normal human bone marrow. Science. 1988;242:919–22.
96. Ochitill HN, Dilley JW. Neuropsychiatric aspects of acquired immunodeficiency syndrome. In: Rosenblum ML, Levy RM, Bredesen DE, eds. AIDS and the Nervous System. New York: Raven Press; 1988.
97. Serwadda D, Mugerwa RD, Sewankambo NK, et al. Slim disease: A new disease in Uganda and its association with HTLV-III infection. Lancet. 1985;2:1849.
97a. Sewankambo N, Mugerwa R, Goodgame R, et al. Enteropathic AIDS in Uganda: An endoscopic, histologic and microbiologic study. AIDS. 1987;1:9–14.
98. Greenspan D, et al., eds. AIDS and the Dental Team. Copenhagen; 1986.
99. Greenspan JS, Greenspan D, Winkler JR. Diagnosis and management of the oral manifestations of HIV infection and AIDS. Infect Dis Clin N Am. 1988;2:373–85.
100. Greenspan JS, Greenspan D, Winkler JR. Diagnosis and management of the oral manifestations of HIV infection and AIDS. In: Sande ME, Volberding PA, eds. The Medical Management of AIDS. Philadelphia: WB Saunders Co; 1988:127–40.
101. Greenspan D, Greenspan JS, Conant M, et al. Oral "hairy" leukoplakia in male homosexuals: Evidence of association with both papillomavirus and a herpes-group virus. Lancet. 1984;2:831–4.
102. Greenspan D, Hollander H, Freidman-Kein A, et al. Oral hairy leukoplakia in two women, a haemophiliac, and a transfusion recipient. Lancet. 1986;2:978–9.
103. Jaffe HW, Darrow WW, Echenberg DF, et al. The acquired immunodeficiency syndrome in a cohort of homosexual men: A six year follow-up study. Ann Intern Med. 1985;103:210.
104. Greenspan JS, Greenspan D, Lennette ET, et al. Replication of Epstein-Barr virus within the epithelial cells of oral "hairy" leukoplakia and AIDS-associated lesion. N Engl J Med. 1985;313:1564–71.
105. Levy RM, Bredesen DE, Rosenblum ML. Neurological manifestations of the acquired immunodeficiency syndrome (AIDS): Experience at UCSF and review of the literature. J Neurosurg. 1985;62:475.
106. McArthur JC. Neurologic manifestations of AIDS. Medicine (Baltimore). 1987;66:407–37.
107. Cornblath DR, McArthur JC. Predominantly sensory neuropathy in patients with AIDS and AIDS-related complex. Neurology (NY). 1988;38:794–6.
108. Cornblath DR, McArthur JC, Kennedy PG, et al. Inflammatory demylinating peripheral neuropathies associated with human T-cell lymphotrophic virus type III infection. Ann Neurol. 1987;21:32–40.
109. Lipkin WI, Parry G, Kiprov D, et al. Inflammatory neuropathy in homosexual men with lymphadenopathy. Neurology (NY). 1985;35:1479–83.
110. Bredesen DE, et al. Inflammatory polyradiculoneuropathy with culture of cytomegalovirus from nerve. Neurology (NY). In press.
111. Dalakas MC, Pezeshkpour GH, Gnavall M, et al. Polymyositis associated with AIDS retrovirus. JAMA. 1986;256:2381–3.
112. Simpson DM, Beuder AN. HTLV-II-associated myopathy. Neurology (NY). 1987;37(Suppl):319.
113. Helbert M, Fletcher T, Peddle B, et al. Zidovudine-associated myopathy. Lancet. 1988;2:689–90.
114. Forster SM, Seeifert MH, Keat AC, et al. Inflammatory joint disease and human immunodeficiency virus infection. Br Med J. 1988;296:1625–7.
115. Rynes RI, Goldenberg DL, DiGiacomo R, et al. Acquired immunodeficiency syndrome-associated arthritis. Am J Med. 1988;84:810–6.
116. Berman A, Espinoza LR, Diaz JD, et al. Rheumatic manifestations of human immunodeficiency virus infection. Am J Med. 1988;85:59–64.
117. Winchester R, Bernstein DH, Fischer HD, et al. The co-occurrence of Rieter's syndrome and acquired immunodeficiency. Ann Intern Med. 1987;106:19–26.
118. Couderc LJ, D'Agay MF, Danon F, et al. Sicca complex and infection with human immunodeficiency virus. Arch Intern Med. 1987;147:898–901.
119. Cello JP. Gastrointestinal manifestations of HIV infection. Infect Dis Clin North Am. 1988;2:387–96.
120. Freedman PG, Weiner BC, Balthazan ES. Cytomegalovirus esophagogastritis in a patient with acquired immunodeficiency syndrome. Am J Gastroenterol. 1985;80:434–7.
121. Rabeneck L, Boyko WJ, McLean DM, et al. Unusual esophageal ulcers containing enveloped virus-like particles in homosexual men. Gastroenterology. 1986;90:1882.
122. St Onge G, Bezahler GH. Giant esophageal ulcer associated with cytomegalovirus. Gastroenterology. 1983;83:127.
123. Tavitian A, Raufman JP, Rosenthal LE. Oral candidiasis as a marker for esophageal candidiasis in the acquired immunodeficiency syndrome. Ann Intern Med. 1986;104:54.
124. Friedman SL, Wright TL, Altman DF. Gastrointestinal KS in patients with acquired immunodeficiency syndrome: Endoscopic and autopsy findings. Gastroenterology. 1985;89:102–8.
125. Blumberg RS, Kelsey P, Perrone T, et al. Cytomegalovirus- and *Cryptosporidium*-associated acalculous gangrenous cholecystitis. Am J Med. 1984;76:1118.
126. Kavin H, Jonas RB, Chowdhury L, et al. Acalculous cholecystitis and cytomegalovirus infection in the acquired immunodeficiency syndrome. Ann Intern Med. 1986;104:53.
127. Margulis SJ, Honig CL, Soave R, et al. Biliary tract obstruction in the acquired immunodeficiency syndrome. Ann Intern Med. 1986;105:207.
128. Schneiderman DJ, Cello JP, Laing FC. Papillary stenosis and sclerosing cholangitis in the acquired immunodeficiency syndrome. Ann Intern Med. 1987;106:546.
129. Jacobson MA, Cello JP, Sande MA. Cholestasis and disseminated cytogalovirus disease in patients with acquired immunodeficiency syndrome. Am J Med. 1987;84:218–24.
130. Glasgow BJ, Anders K, Layfield LJ, et al. Clinical and pathologic finding of the liver in the acquired immune deficiency syndrome. Am J Clin Pathol. 1985;83:582.
131. Lebovics E, Thung SN, Schaffner F, et al. The liver in the acquired immunodeficiency syndrome: A clinical and histologic study. Hepatology. 1985;5:293.
132. Schneiderman DJ, Arenson DM, Cello JP, et al. Hepatic disease in patients with acquired immune deficiency syndrome (AIDS). Hepatology. 1987;7:925.
133. Laughon BE, Druckman DA, Vernon A, et al. Prevalence of enteric pathogens in homosexual men with and without AIDS. Gastroenterology. 1988;94:984–93.
134. Smith PD, Lane HC, Gill VJ, et al. Intestinal infections in patients with the acquired immunodeficiency syndrome (AIDS). Etiology and response to therapy. Ann Intern Med. 1988;108:328–33.
135. Rao TKS, Filippone EJ, Nicastri AD, et al. Associated focal and segmental

glomerulosclerosis in the acquired immunodeficiency syndrome. N Engl J Med. 1984;310:669–73.
136. Pardo V, Aldana M, Colton RM, et al. Glomerular lesions in the acquired immunodeficiency syndrome. Ann Intern Med. 1984;101:429–34.
137. Pardo V, Meneses R, Ossa L, et al. AIDS-related glomerulopathy: Occurrence in specific risk groups. Kidney Int. 1987;31:1167–73.
138. Gardenswartz MH, Lerner CW, Seligson GR, et al. Renal disease in patients with AIDS: A clinicopathologic study. Clin Nephrol. 1984;21:197–204.
139. Rao TKS, Friedman EA, Nicastri AD. The types of renal disease in the acquired immunodeficiency syndrome. N Engl J Med. 1987;316:1062–8.
140. Ortiz C, Meneses R, Jaffe D, et al. Outcome of patients with human immunodeficiency virus on maintenance hemodialysis. Kidney Int. 1988;34:248–53.
141. Hopewell PC, Luce JM. Pulmonary involvement in the acquired immunodeficiency syndrome. Chest. 1984;87:104–12.
142. Selik R, Curran JW. Frequency of opportunistic infections in AIDS. AIDS. 1987;1:175–82.
143. Murray JF, Felton CP, Garay SM et al. Pulmonary complications of the acquired immunodeficiency syndrome: Report of a National Heart, Lung and Blood Institute Workshop. N Engl J Med. 1984;310:1682–8.
144. Stover DE, White DA, Romano PA, et al. Spectrum of pulmonary diseases associated with the acquired immunodeficiency syndrome. Am J Med. 1985;78:429–37.
145. Ognibene FP, Steis RG, Macher AM, et al. Kaposi's sarcoma causing pulmonary infiltrates and respiratory failure in the acquired immunodeficiency syndrome. Ann Intern Med. 1985;102:471–5.
146. Kovacs JA, Hiemenz JW, Macher AM, et al. *Pneumocystis carinii* pneumonia: A comparison between patients with the acquired immunodeficiency syndrome and patients with other immunodeficiencies. Ann Intern Med. 1984;100:663–71.
147. Simberkoff MS, El-Sadr W, Schiffman G. *Streptococcus pneumoniae* infections and bacteremia in patients with acquired immune deficiency syndrome, with report of a pneumococcal vaccine failure. Am Rev Respir Dis. 1984;145:837–40.
148. Polsky B, Gold JWM, Whimbey E, et al. Bacterial pneumonia in patients with the acquired immunodeficiency syndrome. Ann Intern Med. 1986;104:38–41.
149. Chaisson RE. Infections due to encapsulated bacteria, *Salmonella, Shigella* and *Campylobacter* (medical management of AIDS). Infect Dis Clin North Am. 1988;2:475–84.
150. Gerberding JL, Krieger J, Sande MA. Recurrent bactermic infection with *S. pneumoniae* in patients with AIDS virus (AV) infection (Abstract 443). In: Proceedings of the 26th ICAAC. Washington, DC: American Society for Microbiology; 1986.
151. Pitchenik AE, Cole C, Russell BW, et al. Tuberculosis, atypical mycobacteriosis and the acquired immunodeficiency syndrome among Haitian and non-Haitian patients in South Florida. Ann Intern Med. 1984;101:641–5.
152. Chaisson RE, Schecter GF, Theuer CP, et al. Tuberculosis in patients with the acquired immunodeficiency syndrome: Clinical features, response to therapy and outcome. Am Rev Respir Dis. 1987;136:570–4.
153. Goodman PC, Broaddus VC, Hopewell PC. Chest radiographic patterns in the acquired immunodeficiency syndrome. Am Rev Respir Dis. 1984;129:36.
154. Bigby TD, Margolskee D, Curtis JL, et al. The usefulness of induced sputum in the diagnosis of *Pneumocystis carinii* pneumonia in patients with the acquired immunodeficiency syndrome. Am Rev Respir Dis. 1986;133:515–8.
155. Kovacs JA, Ng VL, Masur H, et al. Diagnosis of *Pneumocystis carinii* pneumonia: Improved detection in sputum with use of monoclonal antibodies. N Engl J Med. 1988;318:589–93.
156. Pitchenik AE, Ganjei P, Torres A, et al. Sputum examination for the diagnosis of Pneumocystis carinii pneumonia in the acquired immunodeficiency syndrome. Am Rev Resp Dis. 1986;133:226–9.
156a. Curtis J, Goodman P, Hopewell PC. Noninvasive tests in the diagnostic evaluation for P. carinii pneumonia in patients with or suspected of having AIDS. Am Rev Resp Dis. 1986;132:A182.
157. Coleman DL, Hattner RS, Luce JM, et al. Correlation between gallium lung scans and fiberoptic bronchoscopy in patients with suspected *Pneumocystis carinii* pneumonia and the acquired immunodeficiency syndrome. Am Rev Respir Dis. 1984;130:1155–9.
158. Coleman DL, Dodek PM, Luce JM, et al. Diagnostic utility of fiberoptic bronchoscopy in patients with *Pneumocystis carinii* pneumonia and the acquired immunodeficiency syndrome. Am Rev Respir Dis. 1983;128:795–9.
159. Ognibene FP, Shelhamer S, Gill V, et al. The diagnosis of *Pneumocystis carinii* pneumonia in patients with the acquired immunodeficiency syndrome using subsegmental bronchoalveolar lavage. Am Rev Respir Dis. 1984;130:659–62.
160. Stover DE, White DA, Romano PA, et al. Diagnosis of pulmonary disease in acquired immunodeficiency syndrome (AIDS): Role of bronchoscopy and bronchoalveolar lavage. Am Rev Respir Dis. 1984;102:747–52.
161. Broaddus C, Dake MD, Stulbarg MS, et al. Bronchoalveolar lavage and transbronchial biopsy for the diagnosis of pulmonary infections in the acquired immunodeficiency syndrome. Ann Intern Med. 1985;102:747–52.
162. Milligan SA, Luce JM, Golden J, et al. Transbronchial biopsy without fluoroscopy in patients with diffuse roentgenographic infiltrates and the acquired immunodeficiency syndrome. Am Rev Respir Dis. 1988;137:486–8.
163. Edman JC, Kovacs JA, Masur H, et al. Ribosomal RNA sequence shows *Pneumocystis carinii* to be a member of the fungi. Nature. 1988;334:519–22.
164. Hughes WT. *Pneumocystis carinii*. Boca Raton, FL: CRC Press; 1987.
165. Brenner M, Ognibene FP, Lack EE, et al. Prognostic factors and life expectancy of acquired immunodeficiency syndrome patients with *Pneumocystis carinii* pneumoniae. Am Rev Respir Dis. 1987;136:1199–206.
166. Gherman CR, Ward RR, Basis ML: *Pneumocystis carinii* otitis media and mastoiditis as the initial manifestation of the acquired immunodeficiency syndrome. Am J Med. 1988;85:250–2.
167. Pilon A, Echols RM, Celo JS, et al. Disseminated *Pneumocystis carinii* infection in AIDS. N Engl J Med. 1987;316:1410–1.
168. Grimes MM, LaPook JD, Bar MH, et al. Disseminated *Pneumocystis carinii* infection in a patient with acquired immunodeficiency syndrome. Hum Pathol. 1987;18:307–8.
169. Schinella RA, Breda SD, Hammerschlag PE. Otic infection due to *Pneumocystis carinii* in an apparently healthy man with antibody to the human immunodeficiency virus. Ann Intern Med. 1987;106:399–400.
170. Welch K, Finkbeiner W, Alpers CE, et al. Autopsy findings in the acquired immune deficiency syndrome. JAMA. 1984;252:1152–9.
171. Theuer CP, Chaisson RE, Schecter GF, et al. Human immunodeficiency virus infection in tuberculosis patients in San Francisco (Abstract). Am Rev Respir Dis. 1988;137:121.
172. Horsburgh CR, Selik RA. Mycobacterial infections in patients with AIDS. Am Rev Respir Dis. 1989. In press.
173. Sherer R, Sable R, Sonnenburg M, et al. Disseminated infection with *Mycobacterium kansasii* in the acquired immunodeficiency syndrome. Ann Intern Med. 1986;105:710–2.
174. Chan J, McKitrick JC, Klein RS. *Mycobacterium gordonae* in the acquired immunodeficiency syndrome. Ann Intern Med. 1984;101:400.
175. Chaisson RE, Slutkin G. Tuberculosis in patients with human immunodeficiency virus infection. J Infect Dis. 1989;159:96–100.
176. Selwyn PA, Hartel D, Lewis VA, et al. A prospective study of the risk of tuberculosis among intravenous drug users with human immunodeficiency virus infection. New Engl J Med. 1989;320:545–50.
177. Mann J, Snider DE Jr, Francis H, et al. Association between HTLV-III/LAV infection and tuberculosis in Zaire (Letter). JAMA. 1986;256:346.
178. Centers for Disease Control. Tuberculosis, final data—United States, 1986. MMWR. 1988;36:817–20.
179. Chaisson RE, Schecter GF, Theuer CP, et al. Tuberculosis in patients with the acquired immunodeficiency syndrome: Clinical features, response to therapy, and survival. Am Rev Respir Dis. 1987;136:570–4.
180. Tuberculosis and acquired immunodeficiency syndrome—New York City. MMWR. 1987;36:785–95.
181. Pitchenik AE, Burr J, Suarez M, et al. Human T-cell lymphotrophic virus III (HTLV-III) seropositivity and related disease among 71 consecutive patients in whom tuberculosis was diagnosed. Am Rev Respir Dis. 1987;135:875–90.
182. Sunderam G, McDonald RJ, Maniatis T, et al. Tuberculosis as a manifestation of the acquired immunodeficiency syndrome. JAMA. 1986;256:362–6.
183. Louie E, Rice LB, Holzman RS. Tuberculosis in non-Haitian patients with acquired immunodeficiency syndrome. Chest. 1986;90:542–5.
184. Handwerger S, Mildvan D, Senie R, et al. Tuberculosis and the acquired immunodeficiency syndrome at a New York City Hospital: 1978–1985. Chest. 1987;91:176–80.
185. Greene JB, Sidhu GS, Lewis S, et al. *Mycobacterium avium-intracellulare:* A cause of disseminated life-threatening infection in homosexuals and drug abusers. Ann Intern Med. 1982;97:539–46.
186. Macher AM, Kovacs JA, Gill V, et al. Bacteremia due to *Mycobacterium avium-intracellulare* in the acquired immunodeficiency syndrome. Ann Intern Med. 1983;99:782–5.
187. Horsburgh CR, Selik RM. The epidemiology of disseminated nontuberculous mycobacterial infection in AIDS. Am Rev Respir Dis. 1989;139:4–7.
188. Wilkes MS, Fortin AH, Felix JC, et al. Value of necropsy in acquired immunodeficiency syndrome. Lancet. 1988;2:85–8.
189. Mess TP. *Mycobacterium avium* complex isolated from the lung only, does it disseminate? (Abstract WP217). In: Proceedings of the III International Conference on AIDS. Washington, DC, June 1–5, 1987.
190. Tenholder MF, Moser RJ, Tellis CJ. Mycobacteria other than tuberculosis: Pulmonary involvement in patients with acquired immunodeficiency syndrome. Arch Intern Med. 1988;148:953–5.
191. Demopulos P, Sande MA, Bryant C, et al. Influence of *Mycobacterium avium-intracellulare* infection on morbidity and survival in patients with *Pneumocystis carinii* pneumonia and the acquired immunodeficiency syndrome (Abstract 745). In: Proceedings of the 25th Interscience Conference on Antimicrobial Agents and Chemotherapy. Washington, DC: American Society for Microbiology; 1985.
192. Hawkins CC, Gold JWM, Whimbey E, et al. *Mycobacterium avium* complex infections in patients with the acquired immunodeficiency syndrome. Ann Intern Med. 1986;105:184–8.
193. Jacobson MA. Mycobacterial diseases: Tuberculosis and *Mycobacterium avium* complex. Infect Dis Clin North Am 1988;2:465–74.
194. Young LS. *Mycobacterium avium* complex infection. J Infect Dis. 1988;157:863–7.
195. Bermudez LE, Young LS. Interaction between macrophages and *M. avium complex* (MAC) from AIDS patients (Abstract D129). In: Proceedings of the Annual Meeting of the American Society for Microbiology. Washington, DC: American Society for Microbiology; 1986.
196. Beutler B. The presence of cachectin/tumor necrosis factor in human disease states. Am J Med. 1988;85:287–8.

197. Lahdevirta J, Maury CPJ, Teppo AM, et al. Elevated levels of circulating cachetin/tumor necrosis factor in patients with acquired immunodeficiency syndrome. Am J Med. 1988;85:289–91.
198. Yajko DM, Nassos PS, Hadley WK. Therapeutic implications of inhibition versus killing of *Mycobacterium avium* complex by antimicrobial agents. Antimicrob Agents Chemother. 1987;31:117–20.
199. Agins B, Spicehandler D, Zuger A, et al. *M. avium*-complex (MAC) infections in AIDS: Significance of respiratory isolates and therapy (Abstract 746). In: Proceedings of the 25th Interscience Conference on Antimicrobial Agents and Chemotherapy. Washington, DC: American Society for Microbiology; 1985.
200. Packer SJ, Cesario T, Williams JH Jr. *Mycobacterium avium* complex infection presenting an endobronchial lesions on immunosuppressed patients. Ann Intern Med. 1988;109:389–93.
201. Selwyn PA, Feingold AR, Hartel D, et al. Increased of bacterial pneumonia in HIV-infected intravenous drug abusers without AIDS. AIDS. 1988;2:267–72.
202. Schlamm HT, Yancovitz SR. *Haemophilus influenzae* pneumonia in young adults with AIDS, ARC or risk of AIDS. Am J Med. 1989;86:11–14.
203. Gerberding JL, Kreiger J, Sande MA. Recurrent bacteremic infection with *S. pneumoniae* in patients with AIDS virus (AV) infection (Abstract 443). In: Proceedings of the 26th Interscience Conference on Antimicrobial Agents and Chemotherapy. Washington, DC: American Society for Microbiology; 1986:177.
204. Jacobson MA, Gellermann H, Chambers H. *Staphylococcus aureus* bacteria and recurrent staphylococcal infection in patients with acquired immunodeficiency syndrome and AIDS-related complex. Am J Med. 1988;85:172–6.
205. Jacobson MA, Gellermann H, Chambers H. *Staphylococcus aureus* bacteremia amd recurrent staphylococcal infection in patients with acquired immunodeficiency syndrome and AIDS-related complex. Am J Med. 1988;85:172–6.
206. Levy RM, Bredesen DE, Rosenblum ML. Neurological manifestations of the acquired immunodeficiency syndrome (AIDS): Experience of UCSF and review of the literature. J Neurosurg. 1985;62:75–95.
207. Hollander H, Stringari S. Human immunodeficiency virus-associated meningitis. Clinical course and correlations. Am J Med. 1987;83:813–16.
208. Hollander H, Levy JA. Neurologic abnormalities and recovery of human immunodeficiency virus from cerebrospinal fluid. Ann Intern Med. 1987;106:692.
209. Levy JA, Shimabukuro J, Hollander H, et al. Isolation of AIDS-associated retroviruses from cerebrospinal fluid and brain of patients with neurological symptoms. Lancet. 1985;2:586–8.
210. Goudsmit J, deWolf F, Paul DA, et al. Expression of human immunodeficiency virus antigen (HIV-Ag) in serum and cerebrospinal fluid during acute and chronic infection. Lancet. 1986;2:177.
211. Goudsmit J, Wolters EC, Bakker M, et al. Intrathecal synthesis of antibodies to HTLV-III in patients without AIDS or AIDS related complex. Br Med J. 1986;292:1231.
212. Hollander H, Stringari. Human immunodeficiency virus-associated meningitis. Clinical course and correlations. Am J Med. 1987;83:813–6.
213. McArthur JC. Neurologic manifestations of AIDS. Medicine (Baltimore). 1987;66:407–37.
214. De la Paz R, Enzmann D. Neuroradiology of the acquired immunodeficiency syndrome. In: Rosenblum ML, Levy RM, Bredesen DE, eds. AIDS and the Nervous System. New York: Raven Press; 1988.
215. Levy RM, Bredesen DE. Central nervous system dysfunction in acquired immunodeficiency syndrome. In: Rosenblum ML, Levy RM, Bredesen DE, eds. AIDS and the Nervous System. New York: Raven Press, 1988.
216. Levy RM, Mills CM, Posin JP, et al. The superiority of cranial magnetic resonance imaging to computed tomographic (CT) brain scans for the diagnosis of cerebral lesions in patients with AIDS (Abstract 146). In: Proceedings of the Second International Conference on AIDS. Paris, June 23–25, 1986.
217. Potasman I, Resnick L, Luft BJ, et al. Intrathecal production of antibodies against *T. gondii* in patients with toxoplasmic encephalitis and AIDS. Ann Intern Med. 1988;108:49–51.
218. Luft BJ, Brooks RG, Conley FK. Toxoplasmic encephalitis in patients with acquired immune deficiency syndrome. JAMA. 1984;252:913–7.
219. Grant IH, Gold JWM, Armstrong D. Risk of CNS toxoplasmosis in patients with acquired immune deficiency syndrome (Abstract 441). Proc 26th ICAAC Washington, DC: American Society for Microbiology; 1986.
220. Leoung GS, Mills J, Hadley WK, et al. Cerebral toxoplasmosis (CNS-T) in AIDS patients: Clinical presentation with laboratory, radiographic and histologic correlations (Abstract). In: Proceedings of the First International Conference on AIDS. Atlanta, Georgia, April 14–17, 1985.
221. McArthur JC. Neurologic manifestations of AIDS. Medicine (Baltimore). 1987;66:407–37.
222. Snider WD, Simpson DM, Nielson S, et al. Neurologic complications of the acquired immunodeficiency syndrome: Analysis of 50 patients. Ann Neurol. 1983;14:403–14.
223. Anonymous: Toxoplasmosis diagnosis and immunodeficiency. Lancet. 1984;1:605.
224. McCabe RE, Gibbons D, Brookes RG, et al. Agglutination test for diagnosis of toxoplasmosis in AIDS. Lancet. 1983;2:680.
225. Wong B, Gold JWM, Brown AE, et al. Central-nervous-system toxoplasmosis in homosexual men and parenteral drug abusers. Ann Intern Med. 1984;100:36–42.
226. Levy RM, Janssen RS, Bush TJ, et al. Neuroepidemiology of acquired immunodeficiency syndrome. In: Rosenblum ML, Levy RM, Bredesen DE, eds. AIDS and the Nervous System. New York: Raven Press; 1988:13–27.
227. Levy RM, Bredesen DE, Rosenblum ML. Neurological manifestations of the acquired immunodeficiency syndrome (AIDS): Experience at UCSF and review of the literature. J Neurosurg. 1985;62:475–95.
228. Berger JR, Mucke L. Neurologic recovery and prolonged survival in progressive multifocal leukoencephalopathy with HIV infection. In: Proceedings of the Third International Conference on AIDS. Washington, DC, June 1–5, 1987.
229. Rogers MF, Morens DM, Stewart JA, et al. National case control study of Kaposi's sarcoma and *Pneumocystis carinii* pneumonia in homosexual men. Part 2. Laboratory results. Ann Intern Med. 1983;99:151–8.
230. Friedman-Kien AE, Lafleur FL, Gendler E, et al. Herpes zoster: A possible early clinical sign for development of acquired immunodeficiency syndrome in high-risk individuals. J Am Acad Dermatol. 1986;14:1023–8.
231. Horsburgh CR, Selik R. Extrapulmonary cryptococcosis (CC) in AIDS patients: Risk factors and association with decreased survival (Abstract 564). In: Proceedings of the 28th Interscience Conference on Antimicrobial Agents and Chemotherapy. Microbiology, Washington, DC: American Society for Microbiology; 1988:207.
232. Kovacs JA, Kovacs AA, Polis M, et al. Cryptococcosis in the acquired immunodeficiency syndrome. Ann Intern Med. 1985;103:533–8.
233. Quinnan GV, Masur H, Rook AH, et al. Herpesvirus infections in the acquired immune deficiency syndrome. JAMA. 1984;252:72–7.
234. Jacobson MA, Mills J. Serious cytomegalovirus disease in acquired immunodeficiency syndrome (AIDS). Clinical findings, diagnoses, and treatment. Ann Intern Med. 1988;108:585–94.
234a. Pepose JS, Holland GN, Nestor MSA, et al. Acquired immune deficiency syndrome: pathogenic mechanisms of ocular disease. Ophthalmology. 1985;92:472–84.
235. Safai B, Good RA. Kaposi's sarcoma: A review and recent developments. Clin Bull. 1980;10:62–8.
236. Templeton AC. Kaposi's sarcoma. Pathol Annu. 1981;16:315–36.
237. Hutt MSR. The epidemiology of Kaposi's sarcoma. Antibiot Chemother. 1981;29:3–8.
238. Taylor JF, Templeton AC, Vogel CL, et al. Kaposi's sarcoma in Uganda: A clinico-pathological study. Int J Cancer. 1971;8:122–35.
239. Zisbrod Z, Haimov M, Schanzer H, et al. Kaposi's sarcoma after kidney transplantation. Transplantation. 1980;30:383–4.
240. Myers BD, Kessler E, Levi J, et al. Kaposi's sarcoma in kidney transplant recipients. Arch Intern Med. 1974;133:307–11.
241. Penn I. Kaposi's sarcoma in immunosuppressed patients. J Clin Lab Immunol. 1983;12:1–10.
242. Little PJ, Al Khader A, Farthing CF, et al. Kaposi's sarcoma in a patient after renal transplantation. Postgrad Med J. 1983;59:325–6.
243. Meyers AM, Rice GC, Kaye S, et al. Kaposi's sarcoma in an immunosuppressed renal allograft recipient. S Afr Med J. 1976;50:1299–300.
244. Stribling J, Weitzner S, Smith GV. Kaposi's sarcoma in renal allograft recipients. Cancer. 1978;42:442–6.
245. Klepp O, Dahi O, Stenwig JT. Association of Kaposi's sarcoma and prior immunosuppressive therapy. Cancer. 1978;42:2626–30.
246. Giraldo G, Beth E, Huang E-S. Kaposi's sarcoma and its relationship to cytomegalovirus (CMV) III. CMV DNA and CMV early antigens in Kaposi's sarcoma. Int J Cancer. 1980;26:23–9.
247. Giraldo G, Beth E, Coeur P, et al. Kaposi's sarcoma: A new model in the search for viruses associated with human malignancies. JNCI. 1972;49:1495–507.
248. Urmacher C, Myskowski P, Ochoa M, et al. Outbreak of Kaposi's sarcoma with cytomegalovirus infection in young homosexual men. Am J Med. 1982;72:569–75.
249. Friedman-Kien AE, Laubenstein LJ, Rubinstein P, et al. Disseminated Kaposi's sarcoma in homosexual men. Ann Intern Med. 1982;96:693–700.
250. Friedman-Kien AE. Kaposi's sarcoma and *Pneumocystis* pneumonia among homosexual men—New York City and California. MMWR. 1981;30:305–8.
251. Editor. Revision of the case definition of acquired immunodeficiency syndrome for national reporting—United States. N Engl J Med. 1987;34:373–5.
252. Levy RM, Pons VG, Rosenblum ML. Central nervous system mass lesions in the acquired immunodeficiency syndrome (AIDS). J Neurosurg. 1984;61:9–16.
253. Rosenblum ML, Levy RM, Bredesen DE, et al. Primary central nervous system lymphomas in patients with AIDS. Ann Neurol. 1988;23(Suppl):13–6.
254. Kaplan LD. AIDS-associated lymphomas. Infect Dis Clin North Am. 1988;2:525–32.
255. Ioachim HL, Cooper MC, Hellman GC. Lymphomas in men at high risk for acquired immune deficiency syndrome (AIDS). Cancer. 1985;56:2831–42.
256. Hoffken G, Kramer A, Dienemann B, et al. Malignant tumors other than Kaposi's sarcoma in persons at high risk for AIDS (Abstract). Tumor Biol. 1987;286.
258. Monfardini S, Italian Cooperative Group for AIDS-Related tumors. Malignant lymphomas in patients with or at risk for AIDS in Italy. JNCI. 1988;80:855–60.
259. Nasr SA, Brynes RK, Garrison CP, et al. Peripheral T-cell lymphoma in a

patient with acquired immune deficiency syndrome. Cancer. 1988;61:947–51.
260. Di Carlo EF, Amberson JB, Metroka CE, et al. Malignant lymphomas and the acquired immunodeficiency syndrome (Abstract). Arch Pathol Lab Med. 1986;110:1012–6.
261. Ziegler JL, Beckstead JA, Volberding PA, et al. Non-Hodgkin's lymphoma in 90 homosexual men. N Engl J Med. 1984;311:565–70.
262. Kreiss JK, Kitchen LW, Prince HE, et al. Antibody to human T-lymphotropic virus type III in wives of hemophiliacs. Ann Intern Med. 1985;102:623–6.
263. Levine AM, Gill PS, Meyer PR, et al. Retrovirus and malignant lymphoma in homosexual men. JAMA. 1985;254:1921–5.
264. Ahmed T, Wormser GP, Stahl RE, et al. Malignant lymphomas in a population at risk for acquired immune deficiency syndrome. Cancer. 1987;60:719–23.
265. Levine AM. Non-Hodgkin's lymphomas and other malignancies in the acquired immune deficiency syndrome. Semin Oncol. 1987;14:34–9.
266. Haverkos HW, Drotman DP. Prevalence of Kaposi's sarcoma among patients with AIDS. N Engl J Med. 1985;312:1518.
267. Rogers MF, Morens DM, Stewart JA, et al. National case-control study of Kaposi's sarcoma and *Pneumocystis carinii* pneumonia in homosexual men: Part 2, laboratory results. Ann Intern Med. 1983;99:151–8.
268. Jaffe HW, Keewhan C, Thomas P, et al. National case-control study of Kaposi's sarcoma and *Pneumocystis carinii* pneumonia in homosexual men: Part 1, epidemiologic results. Ann Intern Med. 1983;99:145–51.
269. DeJarlais DC, Marmor M, Thomas P, et al. Kaposi's sarcoma among four different AIDS risk groups. Lancet. 1988;1:1119.
270. Jaffe HW, Bregman D, Selik RM. Acquired immune deficiency syndrome in the United States: The first 1,000 cases. J Infect Dis. 1983;148:339–45.
271. Cohn DL, Judson FN. Absence of Kaposi's sarcoma in hemophiliacs with the acquired immunodeficiency syndrome. Ann Intern Med. 1984;101:401.
272. Garrett TJ, Lange M, Ashford A, et al. Kaposi's sarcoma in heterosexual intravenous drug users. Cancer. 1985;55:1146–8.
273. Van de Perre P, Lepage P, Kestelyn P, et al. Acquired immunodeficiency syndrome in Rwanda. Lancet. 1984;2:62–5.
274. Kestens L, Melbye M, Biggar RJ, et al. Endemic African Kaposi's sarcoma is not associated with immunodeficiency. Int J Cancer. 1985;36:49–54.
275. Bayley AC, Cheingsong-Popov R, Dalgleish AG, et al. HTLV-III serology distinguishes atypical and endemic Kaposi's sarcoma in Africa. Lancet. 1985;359–61.
276. Downing RG, Eglin RP, Bayley AC. African Kaposi's sarcoma and AIDS. Lancet. 1984;478–80.
277. Bayley AC. Aggressive Kaposi's sarcoma in Zambia, 1983. Lancet. 1988;1318–22.
278. Montgomery AB, Luce JM, Turner J, et al. Aerosolised pentamidine as sole therapy for *Pneumocystis carinii* pneumonia in patients with acquired immunodeficiency syndrome. Lancet. 1987;480–3.
279. Safai B. Pathophysiology and epidemiology of epidemic Kaposi's sarcoma. Semin Oncol. 1987;14:7–12.
280. Buck BE, Scott GB, Valdes-Dapena M, et al. Kaposi's sarcoma in two infants with acquired immune deficiency syndrome. J Pediatr. 1983;103:911–3.
281. Haverkos HW, Amsel Z, Drotman DP, et al. Kaposi's sarcoma in homosexual men with AIDS, by race. Lancet. 1988;1075.
282. Drew WL, Mills J, Hauer LB, et al. Declining prevalence of Kaposi's sarcoma in homosexual AIDS patients paralleled by fall in cytomegalovirus transmission. Lancet. 1988;66.
283. Declines in proportion of Kaposi's sarcoma among cases of AIDS in multiple risk groups in New York City. Lancet. 1987;1024.
284. Volberding PA, Kusick P, Feigal DW. HIV antigenemia at diagnosis with Kaposi's sarcoma: Predictors of shortened survival (Abstract). In: Proceedings of the Fourth International Conference on AIDS. 1988:136.
285. Marmor M, Laubenstein LJ, William DC, et al. Risk factors for Kaposi's sarcoma in homosexual men. Lancet. 1982;1083–6.
286. Haverkos HW. Factors associated with the pathogenesis of AIDS. J Infect Dis. 1987;156:251–7.
287. Newell GR, Mansell PWA, Spitz MR, et al. Volatile nitrites use and adverse effects related to the current epidemic of the acquired immune deficiency syndrome. Am J Med. 1985;78:811–6.
288. Hashimoto H, Muller H, Falk S, et al. Histogenesis of Kaposi's sarcoma associated with AIDS: A histologic, immunohistochemical and enzyme histochemical study. Pathol Res Pract. 1987;182:658–68.
289. Nadji M, Morales AR, Ziegles-Weissman J, et al. Kaposi's sarcoma: Immunohistologic evidence for an endothelial origin. Arch Pathol Lab Med. 1981;105:274–5.
290. Beckstead JH, Wood GS, Fletcher V. Evidence for the origin of Kaposi's sarcoma from lymphatic endothelium. Am J Pathol. 1985;119:294–300.
291. Dorfman RF. Kaposi's sarcoma revisited. Hum Pathol. 1984;15:1013–7.
292. McNutt NS, Fletcher V, Conant MA. Early lesions of Kaposi's sarcoma in homosexual men. Am J Pathol. 1983;111:62–77.
293. Jones RR, Spaull J, Spry C, et al. Histogenesis of Kaposi's sarcoma in patients with and without acquired immune deficiency syndrome (AIDS). J Clin Pathol. 1986;39:742–9.
294. Green TL, Beckstead JH, Lozada-Nur F, et al. Histopathologic spectrum of oral Kaposi's sarcoma. Oral Surg. 1984;58:306–14.
295. Lesbordes JL, Martin PMV, Ravisse P, et al. Clinical and histopathological aspects of Kaposi's sarcoma in Africa: Relationship with HIV serology. 1988;139:197–203.
296. Nakamura S, Salahuddin SZ, Biberfeld P, et al. Kaposi's sarcoma cells: Long-term culture with growth factor from retrovirus-infected CD4 T cells. Science. 1988;242:426–30.
297. Salahuddin SZ, Nakamura S, Biberfeld P, et al. Angiogenic properties of Kaposi's sarcoma-derived cells after long-term culture in vitro. Science. 1988;242:430–3.
298. Costa J, Rabson AS. Generalised Kaposi's sarcoma is not a neoplasm. Lancet. 1983;58.
299. Mitsuyasu RT. Clinical variants and staging of Kaposi's sarcoma. Semin Oncol. 1987;14:13–8.
300. Safai B, Sarngadharan MG, Koziner B, et al. Spectrum of Kaposi's sarcoma in the epidemic of AIDS. Cancer Res. 1985;45(Suppl):4646–8.
301. Vadhan-Raj S, Wong G, Gnecco C, et al. Immunological variables as predictors of prognosis in patients with Kaposi's sarcoma and the acquired immunodeficiency syndrome. Cancer Res. 1986;46:417–25.
302. Rawlinson KF, Zubrow AB, Harris MA, et al. Disseminated Kaposi's sarcoma in pregnancy: A manifestation of acquired immune deficiency syndrome. Obstet Gynecol 1984;63(Suppl):2–6.
303. Patow CA, Steis R, Longo DL, et al. Kaposi's sarcoma of the head and neck in the acquired immune deficiency syndrome. Otolaryngology. 1984;92:255–60.
304. Real FX, Oettgen HF, Krown SE. Kaposi's sarcoma and the acquired immunodeficiency syndrome: Treatment with high and low doses of recombinant leukocyte A interferon. J Clin Oncol. 1986;4:544–51.
305. Hymes KB, Greene JB, Marcus A, et al. Kaposi's sarcoma in homosexual men—a report of eight cases. Lancet. 1981;598–600.
306. Seftel AD, Sadick NS, Waldbaum RS. Kaposi's sarcoma of the penis in a patient with the acquired immune deficiency syndrome. J Urol. 1986;136:673–5.
307. Mitsuyasu RT, Taylor J, Glaspy J, et al. Heterogeneity of epidemic Kaposi's sarcoma. Cancer. 1986;57:1657–61.
308. Lumerman H, Freedman PD, Kerpel SM, et al. Oral Kaposi's sarcoma: A clinicopathologic study of 23 homosexual and bisexual men from the New York metropolitan area. Oral Surg. 1988;65:711–6.
309. Gnepp DR, Chandler W, Hyams V. Primary Kaposi's sarcoma of the head and neck. Ann Intern Med. 1984;100:107–14.
310. Moskowitz LB, Hensley GT, Gould EW, et al. Frequency and anatomic distribution of lymphadenopathic Kaposi's sarcoma in the acquired immunodeficiency syndrome: An autopsy series. Hum Pathol. 1985;16:447–56.
311. Lustbader I, Sherman A. Primary gastrointestinal Kaposi's sarcoma in a patient with acquired immune deficiency syndrome. Am J Gastroenterol. 1987;82:894–5.
312. Rose HS, Balthazar EJ, Megibow AJ, et al. Alimentary tract involvement in Kaposi sarcoma: Radiographic and endoscopic findings in 25 homosexual men. AJR. 1982;139:661–6.
313. Scott LF, Wright TL, Altman DF. Gastrointestinal Kaposi's sarcoma in patients with acquired immunodeficiency syndrome. Gastroenterology. 1988;89:102–8.
314. Dworkin B, Wormser GP, Rosenthal WS, et al. Gastrointestinal manifestations of the acquired immunodeficiency syndrome: A review of 22 cases. Am J Gastroenterol. 1985;80:774–8.
315. Barrison IG, Foster S, Harris JW, et al. Upper gastrointestinal Kaposi's sarcoma in patients positive for HIV antibody without cutaneous disease. Br Med J. 1988;296:92–3.
316. Friedman SL, Wright TL, Altman DF. Gastrointestinal Kaposi's sarcoma in patients with acquired immunodeficiency syndrome. Gastroenterology. 1985;89:102–8.
317. Federle MP. A radiologist looks at AIDS: Imaging evaluation based on symptom complexes. Radiology. 1988;166:553–62.
318. Frager DH, Frager JD, Brandt LJ, et al. Gastrointestinal complications of AIDS: Radiologic features. Radiology. 1986;158:597–603.
319. Rucker L, Meador J. Kaposi's sarcoma presenting as homogeneous pulmonary infiltrates in a patient with acquired immunodeficiency syndrome. West J Med. 1985;142:831–3.
320. Ognibene FP, Steis RG, Macher AM, et al. Kaposi's sarcoma causing pulmonary infiltrates and respiratory failure in the acquired immunodeficiency syndrome. Ann Intern Med. 1985;102:471–5.
321. Caray SM, Belenko M, Fazzini E, et al. Pulmonary manifestations of Kaposi's sarcoma. Chest. 1987;91:39–43.
322. Meduri GU, Stover D, Lee M, et al. Pulmonary Kaposi's sarcoma in the acquired immune deficiency syndrome. Am J Med. 1986;81:11–8.
323. Kaplan LD, Hopewell PC, Jaffe HW, et al. Kaposi's sarcoma involving the lung in patients with the acquired immunodeficiency syndrome. J AIDS. 1988;1:23–30.
324. Nash G, Fligiel S. Kaposi's sarcoma presenting as pulmonary disease in the acquired immunodeficiency syndrome: Diagnosis by lung biopsy. Hum Pathol. 1984;15:999–1001.
325. Kornfeld H, Axelrod JL. Pulmonary presentation of Kaposi's sarcoma in a homosexual patient. Am Rev Respir Dis. 1983;127:248–9.
326. Keeney K, Abaza NA, Tidwel O, et al. Oral Kaposi's sarcoma in acquired immune deficiency syndrome. J Oral Maxillofac Surg. 1987;45:815–21.
327. Lozada F, Silverman S, Migliorati CA, et al. Oral manifestations of tumor and opportunistic infections in the acquired immunodeficiency syndrome (AIDS): Findings in 53 homosexual men with Kaposi's sarcoma. Oral Surg. 1983;56:491–4.
328. Emery CD, Wall SD, Federle MP, et al. Pharyngeal Kaposi's sarcoma in patients with AIDS.; AJR. 1986;147:919–22.

329. Green TL, Beckstead JH, Lozada-Nur F, et al. Histopathologic spectrum of oral Kaposi's sarcoma. Oral Surg. 1984;58:306–14.
330. Krigel RL, Laubenstein LJ, Muggia FM. Kaposi's sarcoma: A new staging classification. Cancer Treat Rep. 1983;67:531–4.
331. Volberding PA. The role of chemotherapy for epidemic Kaposi's sarcoma. Semin Oncol. 1987;16(Suppl 3):23–6.
332. Taylor J, Afrasiabi R, Fahey JL, et al. Prognostically significant classification of immune changes in AIDS with Kaposi's sarcoma. Blood. 1986;67:666–71.
333. Lane HC, Masur H, Gelmann EP, et al. Correlation between immunologic function and clinical subpopulations of patients with the acquired immune deficiency syndrome. Am J Med. 1985;78:417–22.
334. Moss AR. Predicting who will progress to AIDS. Br Med J. 1988;297:1067–8.
335. Moss AR, McCallum G, Volberding PA, et al. Mortality associated with mode of presentation in the acquired immune deficiency syndrome. JNCI. 1984;73:1281–4.
336. El-Akkad S, Bull CA, El-Senoussi MA, et al. Kaposi's sarcoma and its management by radiotherapy. Arch Dermatol. 1986;122:1396–9.
337. Holecek MJ, Harwood AR. Radiotherapy of Kaposi's sarcoma. Cancer. 1978;41:1733–8.
338. Hill DR. The role of radiotherapy for epidemic Kaposi's sarcoma. Semin Oncol. 1987;14:19–22.
339. Groopman JE. AIDS-related Kaposi's sarcoma: Therapeutic modalities. Semin Hematol. 1987;24:5–8.
340. Cooper JS, Fried PR. Treatment of aggressive epidemic Kaposi's sarcoma of the conjunctiva by radiotherapy. Arch Ophthalmol. 1988;106:20–1.
341. Cooper JS, Fried PR, Laubenstein LJ. Initial observations of the effect of radiotherapy on epidemic Kaposi's sarcoma. JAMA. 1984;252:934–5.
342. Volberding PA. Therapy of Kaposi's sarcoma in AIDS. Semin Oncol. 1984;11:60–7.
343. Harris JW, Reed TA. Kaposi's sarcoma in AIDS: The role of radiation therapy. Front Radiat Ther Oncol. 1985;19:126–32.
344. Nisce LZ, Safai B, Poussin-Rosillo H. Once weekly total and subtotal skin electron beam therapy for Kaposi's sarcoma. Cancer. 1981;47:640–4.
345. Nobler MP, Leddy ME, Huh SH. The impact of palliative irradiation on the management of patients with acquired immune deficiency syndrome. J Clin Oncol. 1987;5:107–12.
346. Brambilla L, Boneschi V, Beretta G, et al. Intralesional chemotherapy for Kaposi's sarcoma. Dermatology. 1984;169:149–55.
347. Kahn J, Kaplan LD, Jaffe HW, et al. Intralesional recombinant tumor necrosis factor for AIDS related Kaposi's sarcoma (Abstract). In: Proceedings of the Fourth International Conference on AIDS. Washington, DC: Bio-Data Publishers; 1988:324.
348. Volberding PA, Abrams DI, Conant MA, et al. Vinblastine therapy for Kaposi's sarcoma in the acquired immunodeficiency syndrome. Ann Intern Med. 1985;103:335–8.
349. Kaplan LD, Abrams DI, Volberding PA. Treatment of Kaposi's sarcoma in acquired immunodeficiency syndrome with an alternating vincristine vinblastine regimen. Cancer Treat Rep. 1986;70:1121–2.
350. Fischl MA, Krown S, O'Boyle K, et al. Weekly doxorubicin in the treatment of patients with AIDS-related Kaposi's sarcoma (Abstract). In: Proceedings of the Fourth International Conference on AIDS. Washington, DC: Bio-Data Publishers; 1988:202.
351. Mintzer DM, Real FX, Jovino L, et al. Treatment of Kaposi's sarcoma and thrombocytopenia with vincristine in patients with the acquired immunodeficiency syndrome. Ann Intern Med. 1985;102:200–2.
352. Laubenstein LJ, Krigel RL, Odajnyk CM, et al. Treatment of epidemic Kaposi's sarcoma with etoposide or a combination of doxorubicin, bleomycin, and vinblastine. J Clin Oncol. 1984;2:1115–20.
353. Gill PS, Krailo MD, Slater L, et al. Results of a randomized trial of ABV (Adriamycin, bleomycin, vincristine) vs an advanced epidemic Kaposi's sarcoma. (Abstract). In: Proceedings of the Fourth International Conference on AIDS. Washington, DC: Bio-Data Publishers; 1988:323.
354. Flepp, M, Tauber MG, Luthy R, et al. Kaposi's sarcoma in AIDS patients: Long-term treatment with recombinant interferon alpha-2A and chemotherapy. Klin Wochenschr. 1988;66:437–42.
355. Gelmann EP, Preble OT, Steis R, et al. Human lymphoblastoid interferon treatment of Kaposi's sarcoma in the acquired immune deficiency syndrome. Am J Med. 1985;78:737–41.
356. Krown SE, Real FX, Cunningham-Rundles S, et al. Preliminary observations on the effect of recombinant leukocyte A interferon in homosexual men with Kaposi's sarcoma. N Engl J Med. 1983;308:1071–6.
357. Redfield RR, Markham PD, Salshuddin SZ, et al. Frequent transmission of HTLV-III among spouses of patients with AIDS-related complex and AIDS. JAMA. 1985;253:1571–3.
358. Rios A, Mansell PWA, Newell GR, et al. Treatment of acquired immunodeficiency syndrome-related Kaposi's sarcoma with lymphoblastoid interferon. J Clin Oncol. 1985;3:506–12.
359. Krigel RL, Slywotzky CM, Lonberg M, et al. Treatment of epidemic Kaposi's sarcoma with a combination of interferon-alpha 2b and etoposide. J Biol Response Mod. 1988;7:359–64.
360. Krown SE, Bundow D, Tong WP, et al. Interferon-alpha plus azidothymidine (AZT) in AIDS-associated Kaposi's sarcoma (KS). J Interferon Res. 1987;7:688–9.
361. Krown S, Bundow D, Gansbacher B, et al. Interferon-alpha plus zidovudine: A phase I trial in AIDS-associated Kaposi's sarcoma (KS) (Abstract). In: Proceedings of the Fourth International Conference on AIDS. Washington, DC: Bio-Data Publishers; 1988:173.
362. Fischl MA, Dickinson GM, LaVoie L. Safety and efficacy of sulfamethoxazole and trimethoprim chemoprophylaxis for *Pneumocystis carinii* pneumonia in AIDS. JAMA. 1988;259:1185–9.
363. Girard PM, Brun-Pascaud M, Farinotti, R, et al. Pentamidine aerosol in prophylaxis and treatment of murine *Pneumocystis carinii* pneumonia (Abstract). Antimicrob Agents Chemother. 1987;31:978–81.
364. Lowery S, Fallat R, Feigal DW, et al. Changing patterns of *Pneumocystis carinii* pneumonia (PCP) on pentamidine aerosol prophylaxis (Abstract). In: Proceedings of the Fourth International Conference on AIDS. Washington, DC: Bio-Data Publishers; 1988:419.
365. Levine AM. Non-Hodgkin's lymphomas and other malignancies in the acquired immune deficiency syndrome. Semin Oncol. 1987;14:34–9.
366. Biggar RJ, Horm J, Lubin JH, et al. Cancer trends in a population at risk of acquired immunodeficiency syndrome. JNCI. 1985;74:793–7.
367. Rechavi B, Ben-Bassat B, Berkowicy M, et al. Molecular analysis of Burkitt's leukemia in two hemophilic brothers with AIDS. Blood. 1987;70:1713–7.
368. Groopman JE, Sullivan JL, Mulder C, et al. Pathogenesis of B cell lymphoma in a patient with AIDS. Blood. 1986;67:612–5.
369. Lippman SM, Volk JR, Spier CM, et al. Clonal ambiguity of human immunodeficiency virus-associated lymphomas. Arch Pathol Lab Med. 1988;112:128–32.
370. Subar M, Neri A, Inghirami G, et al. Frequent c-*myc* oncogene activation and infrequent presence of Epstein-Barr virus genome in AIDS-associated lymphoma. Blood. 1988;72:667–71.
371. Loeffler JS, Ervin TJ, Mauch P, et al. Primary lymphomas of the central nervous system: Patterns of failure and factors that influence survival. J Clin Oncol. 1985;3:490–4.
372. Elkin CM, Leon E, Grenell SL, et al. Intracranial lesions in the acquired immunodeficiency syndrome. JAMA. 1985;253:393–6.
373. So YT, Beckstead JH, Davis RL. Primary central nervous system lymphoma in acquired immune deficiency syndrome: A clinical and pathological study (Abstract). Ann Neurol. 1986;20:566–72.
374. Levy RM, Bredesen DE, Rosenblum ML. Neurologic manifestations of the acquired immunodeficiency syndrome (AIDS): Experience at UCSF and review of the literature. J Neurosurg. 1985;62:475–95.
375. Knowles DM, Chamulak GA, Subar M, et al. Lymphoid neoplasia associated with the acquired immunodeficiency syndrome (AIDS). Ann Intern Med. 1988;108:744–53.
376. Ioachim HL, Weinstein MA, Robbins RD, et al. Primary anorectal lymphoma: A new manifestation of the acquired immune deficiency syndrome (AIDS). Cancer. 1987;60:1449–53.
377. Caccamo D, Pervez NK, Marchevsky A. Primary lymphoma of the liver in the acquired immunodeficiency syndrome. Arch Pathol Lab Med. 1986;110:553–5.
378. Bottles K, McPhaul LW, Volberding PA. Fine needle aspiration biopsy of patients with acquired immunodeficiency syndrome (AIDS): Experience in an outpatient clinic. Ann Intern Med. 1988;108:42–5.
379. Abrams DI, Kaplan LD, McGrath MS, et al. AIDS-related benign lymphadenopathy and malignant lymphoma: Clinical aspects and virology interactions. AIDS Res. 1986;2:131–40.
380. Jeffrey RB, Nyberg DA, Bottles K, et al. Abdominal CT in acquired immunodeficiency syndrome. AJR. 1986;146:7–13.
381. Nyberg DA, Jeffrey RB, Federle MP, et al. AIDS-related lymphomas: Evaluation by abdominal CT. Radiology. 1986;159:59–63.
382. Gill PS, Levine AM, Krailo MD, et al. AIDS-related malignant lymphoma: Results of prospective treatment trials. J Clin Oncol. 1987;5:1322–8.
383. Schoeppel SL, Hoppe RT, Dorfman RF, et al. Hodgkin's disease in homosexual men with generalized lymphadenopathy. Ann Intern Med. 1985;102:68–70.
384. Robert NJ, Schneiderman H. Hodgkin's disease and the acquired immunodeficiency syndrome. Ann Intern Med. 1984;100:142–3.
385. Ioachim HL, Cooper MC, Hellman GC. Hodgkin's disease and the acquired immunodeficiency syndrome. Ann Intern Med. 1984;101:876–7.
386. Unger PD, Strauchen JA. Hodgkin's disease in AIDS complex patients. Cancer. 1986;4:821–5.
387. Baer DM, Anderson ET, Wilkinson LS. Acquired immune deficiency syndrome in homosexual men with Hodgkin's disease. Am J Med. 1986;80:738–40.
388. Gongora-Biachi RA, Gonzalez-Martinez P, Bastarrachea-Ortiz J. Hodgkin's disease as the initial manifestation of acquired immunodeficiency syndrome. Ann Intern Med. 1987;107:112.
389. Mitsuyasu RT, Coman MF, Sun NCJ. Simultaneous occurrence of Hodgkin's disease and Kaposi's sarcoma in a patient with the acquired immune deficiency syndrome. Ann J Med. 1986;80:954–8.
390. Picard O, De Gramont A, Krulik M, et al. Rectal Hodgkin disease and the acquired immunodeficiency syndrome. Ann Intern Med. 1987;106:775.
391. Unger PD, Strauchen JA. Hodgkin's disease in AIDS complex patients. Cancer. 1986;58:821–5.
392. Robert NJ, Scheiderman H. Hodgkin's disease and the acquired immunodeficiency syndrome. Ann Intern Med. 1988;101:142–43.
393. Krause W, Mittag H, Gieler U, et al. A case of malignant melanoma in AIDS-related complex. Arch Dermatol. 1987;123:867–8.
394. Frager DH, Wolf EL, Competiello LS, et al. Squamous cell carcinoma of the esophagus in patients with acquired immunodeficiency syndrome. Gastrointest Radiol. 1988;13:358–60.

395. Kaplan MJ, Sabio H, Waneba HJ, et al. Squamous cell carcinoma in the immunosuppressed patient: Fanconi's anemia. Laryngoscope. 1985;95:771–5.
396. Enck RE. Squamous cell cancers and the acquired immunodeficiency syndrome. Ann Intern Med. 1987;106:773.
397. Tessler AN, Catanese A. AIDS and germ cell tumors of testis. Urology. 1987;203–4.
398. Logothetis CJ, Newell GR, Samuels ML. Testicular cancer in homosexual men with cellular immune deficiency: Report of 2 cases. J Urol. 1985;133:484–6.
399. Quang TN, Beuzeboc P, Lurie A, et al. Cancer du testicule chez deux homosexuels avec anticorps anti HIV. Ann Med Interne (Paris). 1987;138:233–40.
400. Slazinski L, Stall JR, Mathews CR. Basal cell carcinoma in a man with acquired immunodeficiency syndrome. J Am Acad Derm. 1984;11:140–1.
401. Sitz KV, Keppen M, Fohnson DF. Metastatic basal cell carcinoma in acquired immunodeficiency syndrome-related complex (Abstract). JAMA. 1987;257:340–3.
402. Weitberg AB, Mayer KH, Miller ME, et al. Dysplastic carcinoid tumor and AIDS-related complex. N Engl J Med. 1986;314:1455.
403. Grieger T, Carl M, Liebert H, et al. Mediastinal liposarcoma in a patient infected with the human immunodeficiency virus. Am J Med. 1988;84:366.
404. Cappell MSI, Yao F, Cho KC. Colonic adenocarcinoma associated with the acquired immune deficiency syndrome. Cancer. 1988;62:617–9.

109. DETECTION OF HIV-1 INFECTION

CHARLES J. SCHLEUPNER

In 1983–1984 as the isolation of human immunodeficiency virus (HIV-1) was first reported, serologic tests were described that recognized antibodies to HIV-1 in the sera of patients with the acquired immunodeficiency syndrome (AIDS).[1–7] The first assay for screening blood donors became licensed for commercial use on March 2, 1985, when blood centers initiated screening of all donated blood for antibody to HIV-1.[8] The "first generation" of these enzyme immunoassays (EIAs) were adaptations of assays using antigens derived from lysed HIV-1-infected cell cultures.[6] They were designed for sensitivity of detection of HIV infection; the EIA gained specificity only upon repeated testing with positive results and "confirmatory" evaluation with Western blot (WB). The test was clearly successful at its primary purpose, making the blood supply safer.[8,9]

To prevent individuals in high-risk groups from using blood banks for diagnostic testing (thereby increasing the risk of contamination of the blood supply), alternate test sites were also established where patients in high-risk groups could have EIA evaluations (and WB if indicated) performed anonymously or confidentially and without charge after appropriate counseling. Therefore, continued self-deferral of high-risk donors was facilitated.[10]

Through counseling, another goal of EIA testing for antibody to HIV-1 evolved, i.e., prevention of infection or spread thereof to others. In December 1985, the Centers for Disease Control (CDC) extended its recommendation for EIA testing to pregnant women and women who might become pregnant while being at high risk for HIV-1 infection.[11] In the spring of 1986, serologic testing was additionally recommended for persons attending sexually transmissible disease (STD) clinics and clinics for prostitutes and intravenous drug abusers.[12] Testing was further advised for recipients of transfusions between 1978 and 1985 and all patients with tuberculosis.[13]

At the same time that the target high-risk populations for diagnostic testing were being extended, the limitations of the "first-generation" EIAs were acknowledged; the rate of false positivity was high in low-risk populations (80–90 percent), which resulted in an unnecessary reduction in the sources of the nation's blood supply and unwarranted emotional stress for individuals receiving such erroneous information.[14–16] With the purpose of increasing the specificity of both screening and confirmatory tests, EIAs using specific HIV-1 proteins produced by recombinant technology were developed.[17] With the application of these assays together with the development of an EIA for HIV core antigen,[18–20] the use of serologic assays has been extended to include a better understanding of the pathogenesis of HIV-1 infection, evaluation of the success of therapy, and definition of the strategies for earlier initiation of therapy.[21,22]

SEROLOGIC RESPONSE TO HIV INFECTION

The serologic response to HIV is best understood by an appreciation of the major protein products of the viral genome (see Chapter 147). The temporal course of the appearance of serum HIV antigen and antibodies to several viral proteins is shown in Figure 1. After infection, p24 antigen is the first serologic marker to be detected.[23,24] The appearance of antibody to p24 is temporally associated with falling p24 antigen levels and with immune complexes of these reactants.[18,23,25–27] Antibodies to the carboxy terminal envelope cleavage product (gp41) of gp160 are often detectable before anti-p24 (Fig. 1) by WB, competitive EIA using recombinant antigens (CIA-RA), or radioimmunoprecipitation (RIPA).[23,28] Months or years after the development of antibodies to both the core and envelope proteins, the core antigen may reappear (Fig. 1); this is usually coincident with the loss of anti-p24 and correlates with the development of AIDS.[19,22,29–35]

HIV-1 ANTIBODY ASSAYS

Enzyme Immunoassays

All seven licensed "first-generation" EIAs for the detection of antibody to HIV-1 use virus derived from lysed cell cultures.[36–38] All kits use the human T-cell leukemia/lymphoma virus (HTLV-III) strain of HIV-1, except for the Genetic Systems assay, which uses the lymphadenopathy-associated virus (LAV) strain. The cell source of HIV-1 varies according to each manufacturer. The Abbott, Dupont, Electronucleonics (ENI), Organon-Teknika, Cellular Products, and Ortho kits use the H-9 cell line. Genetic Systems uses the CEM-F line.[38,39] (The Organon-Teknika kit is an improved version of what was formerly the Litton EIA.) The partially purified virus is bound to a microtiter well or to a latex or a polystyrene-coated metal bead (the solid phase; Table 1). Most EIAs are indirect; viral antigen is exposed to a patient specimen (serum, cerebrospinal fluid [CSF], other body fluid) and incubated to allow antigen–antibody binding. The solid phase is then washed to remove unbound immunoglobulin and is exposed to an enzyme-labeled anti-human globulin (e.g., horseradish peroxidase or alkaline phosphatase). After binding has occurred, these complexes are exposed to a substrate for the attached enzyme to allow a colorimetric reaction to occur, which is proportional to the amount of bound anti-HIV-1 globulin in the patient specimen. Both strongly and weakly reactive controls as well as negative con-

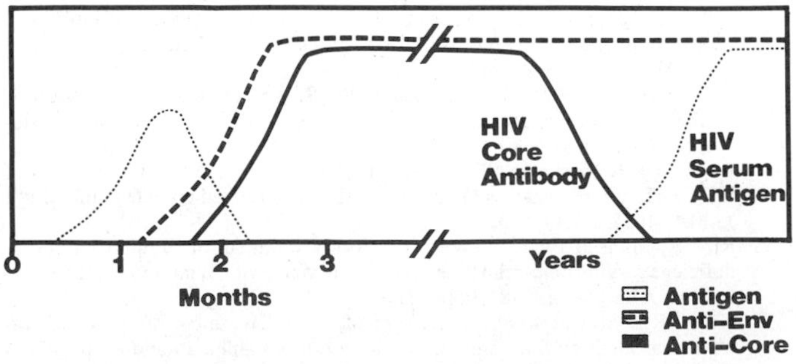

FIG. 1. Chronology of HIV-1 infection defined by the presence of core (p24) antigen and antibodies to core protein and envelope (gp41) glycoprotein. (Courtesy of Abbott Diagnostics Division, Abbott Laboratories, North Chicago, IL.)

TABLE 1. Summary of Methodology for Six Commonly Used Screening EIAs for HIV-1 Antibody

Features	*ABB*	*DU*	*ENI*	*GS*	*OT*	*OR*
Viral antigen source						
HTLV-III	X	X	X		X	X
LAV				X		
H-9 cell line	X	X	X		X	X
CEM-F cell line				X		
Antigen-coated beads	X				X	
Latex	X					
Plastic-coated ferrous metal					X	
Antigen-coated wells		X	X	X		X
Assay performed in						
Microtiter plate		X	X	X	X	X
Test tube	X					
Anti-human IgG						
Peroxidase conjugated	X		X	X	X	X
Alkaline phosphatase conjugated		X				
Substrate						
O-phenylenediamine	X		X			X
Para-nitrophenyl-phosphate		X				
2,2′-Azino-di-[3-ethylbenzthiazoline sulfonate]					X	
Tetramethylbenzidine				X		
Total test time (hr)	4.4	2.5	2.0	3.0	3.0	3.0

Abbreviations: ABB: Abbott; DU: Dupont; ENI: Electronucleonics; GS: Genetic Systems; OT: Oganon/Teknika; OR: Ortho Diagnostics.

trols are run in parallel on each occasion that unknown sera are assayed. Some more recent kits use a competitive inhibition enzyme immunoassay. In the latter assay, the color reaction is inversely proportional to the amount of bound anti-HIV-1 globulin in the patient specimen. An EIA assay takes up to 4 hours to perform (Table 1).

With either indirect or competitive EIA, the optical density (OD) of each unknown (individual or paired) and each control is measured at the optimal wavelength for substrate absorption after undergoing the colorimetric reaction. A cutoff OD is then calculated by using negative and/or positive control values (the equation varies with each kit), and a ratio of sample to cutoff OD is calculated. For the indirect or "sandwich" EIA, values ≥ 1.0 are considered positive; for the competitive EIA, values <1.0 are positive. These EIAs are usually performed with serum, but an EIA has been reported to detect HIV-1 antibodies in saliva with a sensitivity equal to that in serum.[40]

Burke et al. have shown that OD readings vary with the intensity of various WB banding patterns.[41] While the Abbott EIA has greatest sensitivity for antibodies to gp41 and the polymerase gene products, the Dupont, ENI, and Litton EIAs are more sensitive for antibodies to the gag (core) proteins.[41] This has relevance to the sensitivity of each EIA for HIV-1 antibody during various stages of infection; for example, during AIDS when anti-p24 has usually disappeared, the latter EIAs may be less sensitive for detecting infection due to their greater sensitivity for p24 antibody. Cooper et al. have compared four EIAs for their ability to identify infection during acute HIV-1 illness[42]; the ENI assay was the most sensitive for early diagnosis, while the Abbott EIA was the least.

If a blood or plasma collection center or a referral laboratory detects HIV-1 antibody by EIA in a plasma or serum sample, a repeat EIA is performed on a second specimen (Fig. 2). If the repeated assay is positive, a confirmatory test is ordered (usually a WB), and the donor or patient is notified. If the repeated test is negative, a different EIA should be performed.[8] In either case, the unit of blood or plasma is discarded, and the donor is referred to a private physician, a health department, or an alternate testing site for evaluation and counseling. For specimens indeterminate by WB analysis, a repeat specimen obtained in 2–3 months should be evaluated, and/or the specimen can be examined by another confirmatory test method (e.g., RIPA).

Because the EIA for anti-HIV-1 has been used for serologic evaluation of high-risk populations in addition to volunteer blood donors,[15,16,38] any discussion of the validity of test results must take into account the population tested and its overall seropositivity rate. In blood donor populations, initial reports of the performance of the screening "first-generation" EIA (usually the Abbott test) showed positive predictive values of 3.8–27.3 percent.[9,43] These predictive values varied depending on the EIA OD reactivity, with low positive OD values being associated with greater degrees of false positivity.[43–45] Other early studies compared various EIA tests against the same sera, usually from a group of patients with a spectrum of risk for HIV-1 infection.[46–49] While the Abbott and the Wellcome Diagnostics EIAs were usually among the most sensitive, the Abbott assay had the highest false-positive rate among low-risk groups (i.e., blood donors), followed by the Organon, Dupont, and Litton assays. The sensitivity and specificity for most man-

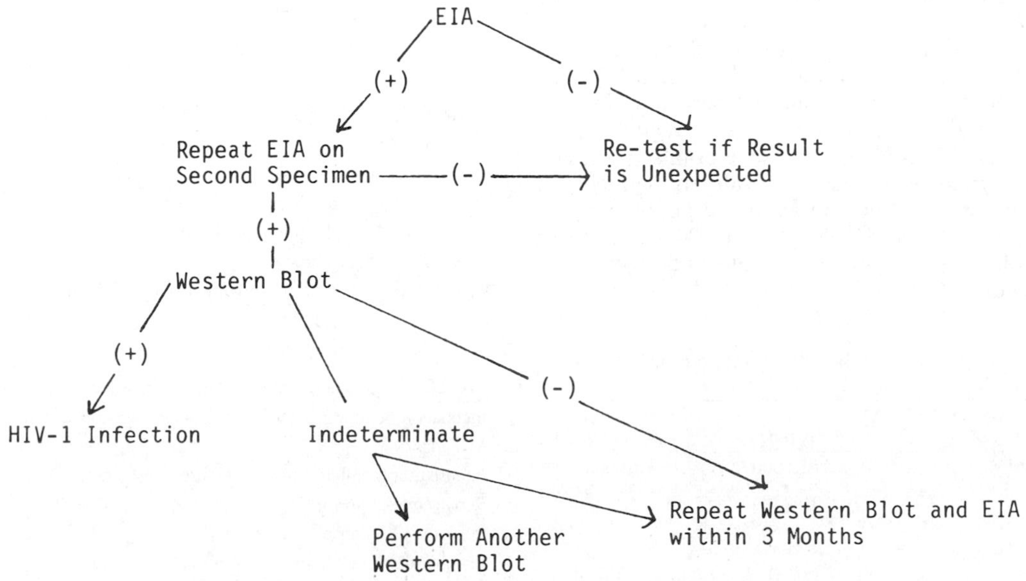

FIG. 2. An algorithm for the management of HIV-1 serologic results.

ufacturers' assays were 97.2–100 percent and 99.6–100 percent, respectively, when using sera from patients in high-risk groups,[47] except for one report of low specificity for the Abbott test in this risk group.[50]

Subsequent reports have evaluated the Genetic Systems EIA, along with the others mentioned previously, by using sera from a similar spectrum of patients.[28,44,45,51] The Genetic Systems EIA repeatedly ranked best in these studies in terms of sensitivity, specificity, and reproducibility. The most recent studies, some using EIA assays with more purified disrupted viral antigens, further confirm the excellence of the Genetic Systems and the new, improved Organon-Teknika EIAs.[34,52–54] A number of recent studies have also pointed out the relevance of the distribution of positive and negative OD values above and below the cutoff to differentiate true positive from negative results.[44,53,54] It is evident that an EIA with many OD determinations clustered around the OD cutoff will be subject to more false-positive and/or negative results (e.g., Litton, ENI, and Ortho).[44,53,54] A recent CDC survey of health department and American Red Cross laboratories identified similar problems with specimens having OD results around cutoff values.[55] It was noteworthy that, despite a confirmation of higher false-positive rates with the Abbott EIA, 80–85 percent of laboratories reported using this assay; another 3–8 percent of laboratories reported using the ENI or Organon-Teknika kits. Schwartz et al. recently discussed arguments for varying the OD cutoff values defining positive and negative specimens.[56] Since a rise of the OD cutoff of the noncompetitive EIA increases the specificity at the cost of sensitivity, these authors argued for raising cutoff values when these tests are being used for diagnostic rather than screening purposes. Future experience will determine whether such variations of definition of reactive specimens are warranted.

Variations of specificity and positive predictive value are codependent upon the prevalence of HIV-1 infection in the population tested, as shown in Table 2. For any laboratory test, methodologic error, regardless of source, occurs with a relatively fixed frequency; therefore, for each population tested, regardless of risk for HIV-1 infection, the number of false-positives per 1000 tests will be approximately the same. However, in a low-risk population (with few true positives), the number of false-positives will be a much greater percentage of those called positive than for the high-risk population. Therefore, the positive predictive value of such a screening test in a low-risk population may only be 10%, while it would be as high as 97.3% in a high-risk population.[15,16] This is anticipated since these screening EIAs were designed for optimum sensitivity at the expense of specificity.[15]

The relevance of false positivity in a low-risk population is apparent from American Red Cross data[9,39] (Table 3). Among 2.58 million volunteer blood donors, only 3.5 percent of initially positive EIAs and only 13 percent of repeatedly reactive EIAs were reactive by WB.[39] This high prevalence of false positivity in low-risk groups brings into focus the relatively high cost of identifying one truly infected person in such a population, estimated conservatively to be $35,000 to $40,000 per infected person (for example, if all hospital admissions underwent mandatory screening annually).

TABLE 2. Example of Problems with the HIV-1 Antibody EIA When Applied to High- and Low-Risk Populations

Assay Result	*High-Risk Population*	*Low-Risk Population*
No. tested	10,000	10,000
Percentage positive	10%	0.3%
Total no. positive	1000	30
No. false-positives[a]	27	27
No. true positives	973	3
Positive predictive value	973/1000 (97.3%)	3/30 (10%)

[a] False-positives due to intrinsic methodologic inaccuracies, regardless of the population tested.

TABLE 3. Correlation between EIA and Western Blot Positivity for 2.58 Million American Red Cross Blood Donors

	Blood Donor Results	
Assay Result	*Number*	*Percent*
EIA, initially positive	25,800	1
Repeat EIA positive	6966	0.27
WB positive	903	0.035
Positive predictive values		
Initial EIA	—	3.5
Repeat EIA	—	13

The false-positive and false-negative results obtained with EIAs are due to a variety of clinical and technical variables.[57] It has been noted that heat-inactivated sera (treated to enhance laboratory safety) cause false-positive reactions with the Abbott EIA.[48,58,59] Sera with rapid plasma reagin (RPR) reactivity have also been reported to cause false-positive EIAs for HIV-1 antibody only with the Abbott kit; the false-positive rate with RPR-positive sera when using the most recent viral lysate Abbott EIA has been reduced to approximately 3 percent.[60] Other factors are also associated with erroneous results, as noted in Tables 4 and 5.[38,43,49,61–71] By far the most important cause of false positivity is cross-reacting antibodies in serum to HLA class II antigens present in HIV-1 preparations harvested from H-9 cells.[43,61–65] The Genetic Systems and Wellcome assays avoid this problem by use of CEM-F cells for virus propogation; this cell line lacks such HLA reactivity[53,56] (Table 1). While too insensitive to assay for HIV-2 antibodies, anti-HIV-1 EIAs, especially competitive EIAs, can be falsely positive due to cross-reacting core antibodies with HIV-2.[72]

Using WB and the Dupont EIA, Tribe et al. have also recognized some sera that are repeatedly reactive by EIA but nonreactive by WB blot criteria due to their EIA reactivity with gag proteins of HIV-1.[73] These sera react predominantly with p15/p17 and less frequently with p24, but they lack anti-env reactivity. Such individuals must be excluded from blood donation until the reasons for this continued reactivity are clarified (e.g., cross-reactivity with other [retro] viruses or tissue proteins).

Despite the foregoing comments, the probability of a false-positive result after the complete testing sequence (Fig. 2) has been estimated to be 1–5 per 100,000 persons screened.[13] Per-

TABLE 4. Causes of False-Positive EIA Reactions to HIV-1

Antibody against smooth muscle, parietal cell, mitochondrial, nuclear, leukocyte, and T-cell antigens; anti-HAV-IgM and anti-HBc-IgM
Antibodies against class II leukocyte antigens (HLA-DR4, -DQw3) present on H-9 cells (more frequently observed in multiparous women, multiply transfused patients)
Severe alcoholic liver disease, primary biliary cirrhosis, sclerosing cholangitis
Heat inactivation or RPR positivity of serum tested (Abott EIA only)
Hematologic malignancies, lymphoma
Acute DNA viral infections, HIV-2 infection
Renal transplants, chronic renal failure
Stevens-Johnson syndrome
Passively acquired HIV-1 antibody (hepatitis B immunoglobulin)

TABLE 5. Causes of False-Negative EIA Reactions to HIV-1

Incubation period or acute disease before seroconversion ("window-period")
Malignancy
Intensive or long-term immunosuppressive therapy
Replacement transfusion
Bone marrow transplantation
Kits that detect antibody to p24 primarily
B-cell dysfunction

haps more important from a clinical perspective, estimates of the false-negative rate of EIAs for HIV-1 antibody range from 1 in 40,000 to 1 in 1 million.[74] The causes of such false negativity are presented in Table 5. This problem has been recently reviewed with regard to the transfusion-related transmission of HIV-1.[75]

The most recently developed "second-generation" EIAs for antibody to HIV-1 use polypeptide antigens of the HIV-1 core and envelope that are produced by recombinant DNA technology. None is yet licensed, apparently due to the lack of acceptance by regulatory agencies of recombinant proteins for the detection of antibody. While Dupont, Cambridge Bioscience, and Smith Kline Bioscience Laboratories are developing similar assays, Abbott has produced a competitive enzyme immunoassay (CIA-RA) using recombinant HIV-1 antigens (p24 and gp41) individually and an indirect EIA combining these two proteins (Envacore); each has been evaluated for screening and confirmatory purposes. The inital report with CIA-RAs demonstrated sensitivity superior to both "first-generation" (viral lysate antigen) EIAs and WB.[23] Subsequent studies confirmed this initial impression and demonstrated greater specificity for CIA-RA.[34,35,50,76]

Other authors reported similarly enhanced sensitivity and specificity for the Cambridge Bioscience assay (recombinant envelope protein only) and another recombinant EIA for HIV-1 antibody.[17,77,78] These studies noted that the enhanced sensitivity of such recombinant protein assays for antibody were dependent to a significant extent upon the presence of envelope-patterned peptides, including both gp160 and gp41,[17,35,38,77,78] since antibodies to gp160/120 and gp41 develop before anti-p24 and remain after anti-p24 disappears.[23,35,38]

Some theoretic limitations of these recombinant protein assays include (*1*) the lack of glycosylation of env proteins, which may limit interactions with serum antibodies, and (*2*) limited cross-reactions with HIV-1 variants (e.g., HIV-2).[17,38] These assays retain the limitations of all antibody assays in that they fail to detect p24 antigen before antibody seroconversion.[17] Their advantages are significant, however, including safety, reproducibility of antigen content, and lack of contaminating cellular proteins that cause false positivity.[38] Due to their technical ease, assays for antibody to individual recombinant antigens may be useful as (or replace) confirmatory tests such as WB.[38]

Western Blot

The WB was developed as a method for separating proteins obtained from HIV-1 harvested from cell lysates and thereby analyzing sera for antibody content to these specific proteins. HIV-1 is allowed to replicate in continuous lymphoid cell lines, usually HUT-78 (H-9) cells. Cells are lysed to release viral and precursor proteins; virus is then partially purified by centrifugation[29,79,80] (Fig. 3). The viral protein is then electrophoresed in polyacrylamide gel. The lower-molecular-weight proteins (p17, p24) migrate farther in the gel, with the higher-molecular-weight proteins (gp160/120) remaining near the origin. The proteins are then blotted (or transferred) to nitrocellulose paper electrophoretically, and the paper is dried and cut into strips (or lanes) of approximately 5 mm width. The strips are subsequently exposed to a dilution of patient serum, washed, and incubated with anti-human IgG labeled with an enzyme that produces a colored band upon exposure to its substrate. Molecular weight standards as well as positive and negative control sera are incorporated into each assay. This reference WB technique is performed according to the Towbin method[80]; Figure 4 depicts test strips developed by using the Dupont licensed WB kit, which provides nitrocellulose paper strips with pre-electrophoresed disrupted viral proteins blotted onto the strips.

The WB has the advantage over nonrecombinant EIAs that antibodies to individual viral proteins can be assayed. The WB is more sensitive for the assay of anti-p24 than anti-gp41 since the latter glycosolated proteins do not transfer as well to nitrocellulose paper.[23,37,45,51] Western blot is also less sensitive for the detection of antibody to gp160/120 than are other confirmatory assays (e.g., RIPA) because of less resolving power. This is due to clumping of higher-molecular-weight antigens at the origin.[28,45] During the spectrum of HIV-1 infection, WB is insensitive during early HIV-1 infection (similar to EIA due to lack of anti-p24 and/or anti-gp41) and in patients with AIDS (due to a loss of anti-p24 late in disease).[28,29,51]

The definition of a positive WB result has been in a state of flux for some time. In addition to the cumbersome nature of the assay, which allows for the possibility of multiple technical errors, the test is also subjective in interpretation (reading the presence or absence of faint bands). The CDC has variably

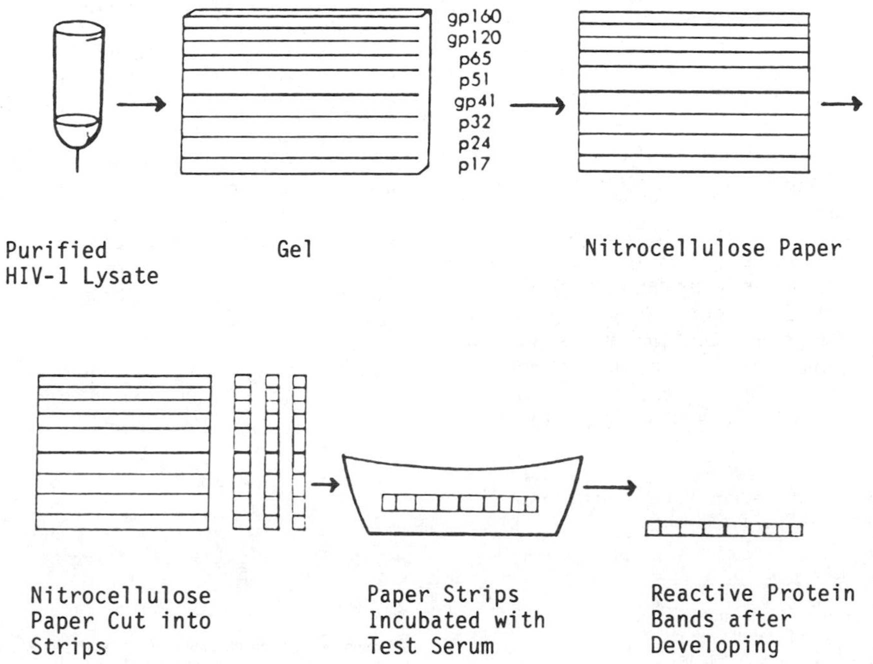

FIG. 3. Western blot procedure in diagramatic format. (Modified from Griffith et al.,[79] with permission.)

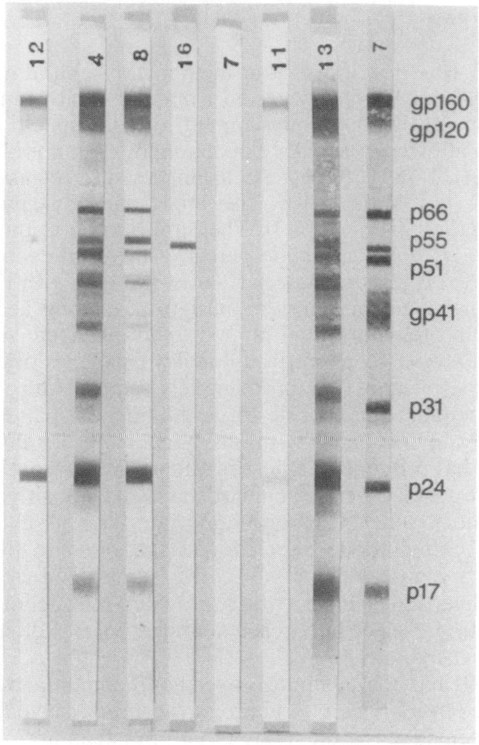

FIG. 4. Typical Western blot result using the Dupont immunoblot kit. Number 12 is indeterminate serum; numbers 4, 8, and 13 are positive sera; numbers 7 (middle), 11, and 16 are negative sera; and number 7 (right) is a positive control.

called WB with anti-p24 or anti-gp41 bands positive.[36,37] The licensed Dupont kit defines the presence of anti-p24, either anti-gp41 or gp160, and anti-p31 as a positive test[36,37,56,57]; the American Red Cross uses a similar definition,[56] while the U.S. Army accepts the presence of either anti-gp41 or both anti-p24 and anti-p55 bands.[57,81] Most recently, the Association of State and Territorial Public Health Laboratory Directors published recommended guidelines.[82] A *reactive* WB must contain two of three major bands of diagnostic significance (anti-gp160/120, anti-gp41, anti-p24); a *nonreactive* WB is defined as one without any HIV-1-specific bands, and an *indeterminate* WB contains one or more viral specific bands but insufficient bands to meet the definition of reactive (above). Such an indeterminate WB should be repeated and, if still indeterminate, followed with a repeat blot in 2–3 months (Fig 2).

A recent report has compared three different WB techniques, one similar to the Towbin method and two commercially available kits, Bio-Rad and Dupont.[83] The Dupont kit had the best sensitivity (dilutional reactivity) and specificity (lack of reaction with cellular and subcellular antisera). It was noted that antibodies to HLA class I cellular antigens tend to cause false-positive anti-gp41 bands, while antibodies to HLA class II antigens primarily caused false-positive anti-p31 bands; a parallel WB of uninfected H-9 cellular proteins was recommended to detect these false-positive reactions. Unexplained occasional anti-HIV-1 gag protein bands (falsely positive) were also noted by these authors[83] and others,[34,81,84,85] as has been noted for EIAs.[73] Overall, false-positive WB results are estimated to occur no more frequently than 1 in 20,000[37]; the potential cross-reacting antibodies are noted in Table 6.[81,84,85] Their false positivity is determined by a negative RIPA or immunofluorescence assay.

False-negative reactions by WB occur usually very early after HIV-1 infection or late after the development of AIDS.[28,29,36,37,51] HIV-1 culture positivity has been noted in WB-negative patients.[37,43,71,86,87] In conjunction with serial EIA determinations, the false-negative rate of WB for blood donors is estimated to be 1 in 250,000.[37] Should the prevalence of HIV-2 infection increase in the United States, it may become necessary to incorporate both HIV-1 and HIV-2 antigens in both EIA and WB assays because these viruses only cross react with antibodies to p24.[37]

TABLE 6. Causes of False-Positive Western Blot Reactions to HIV-1 Antigens (gag, env, and pol Proteins)

Cross reactions with
Normal human ribonucleoproteins
Other human retroviruses
Antibody to mitochondrial, nuclear, T-cell, and leukocyte antigens
Antibodies to HLA antigens (classes I and II)
Globulins produced during polyclonal gammopathy

Indirect Immunofluorescence Assay

The indirect immunofluorescence assay (IFA) is a rapid and reliable supplemental test using uninfected and HIV-1-infected H-9 (or HUT-78) cells in the logarithmic growth phase. The cells are air-dried and fixed to a fluorescent glass microscope slide.[37] A small quantity of a 1:10–1:20 test serum dilution is applied to each well, incubated to allow antibody to react with antigen, washed, and air-dried. Subsequently, anti-human IgG labeled with fluorescein isothiocyanate is applied to each well, followed again by incubation, washing, drying, and mounting. The use of known positive and negative control sera with both infected and uninfected cells in each assay allow for correction due to nonspecific fluorescence. Specimens are evaluated for fluorescence intensity, the percentage of fluorescent cells, and the fluorescent pattern; each test serum is determined to be qualitatively positive or negative but may be quantitatively assayed by the use of serial dilutions. Through the use of anti-human globulin specific for IgM, this immunoglobulin response can be also differentiated.

The IgM and IgG antibody responses to acute HIV-1 infection can be detected by IFA earlier than other currently available antibody assays[42] (Table 7). Sandstrom et al. found excellent overall agreement of IFA results with those of WB for both low- and high-risk populations; IFA was also shown to be more sensitive than EIA.[88] Others have suggested similar sensitivity and specificity for high-risk patients.[29,89–91] However, for a low-risk population, Lennette et al. noted nonspecific staining patterns that could be absorbed by noninfected HUT-78 cell antigens,[91] perhaps accounting for the false-positives reported by Carlson et al. when a similar population was screened by IFA in their study.[92] Most authors concur that IFA requires less technical expertise, is quicker to perform (<2 hours), and is less costly than WB, while being equally sensitive and specific.[89–91] Infrequently, however, false-negative assays have been identified.[87,88] The sensitivity of IFA may vary according to the cell line in which the virus is grown.[28] Generally, IFA interpretation is subjective and requires an experienced observer.[37]

TABLE 7. Comparison of IFA and Western Blot: Day of Acute Illness When Initially Positive for Indicated Antibody

	Day of Illness According to Test	
Antibody	*IFA*	*WB (8)[a]*
IgM	5 (5)	—
IgG	11 (6)[a]	—
p24/gp41	—	24
p55	—	40
p68	—	57
p34	—	71

[a] The number of patients evaluated are in parentheses.
(From Cooper et al.,[42] with permission.)

Radioimmunoprecipitation Assay

The radioimmunoprecipitation assay is a research technique confined to laboratories capable of propagation of HIV-1 in cell culture. The virus is grown in H-9 cells to logarithmic growth and then exposed to a radiolabeled amino acid or other substance that allows isotopic incorporation in or transfer to viral proteins.[37,93] Cells are subsequently lysed, thereby releasing labeled viral proteins. Cell lysates are exposed to test serum, the IgG content of which has been previously bound to the "Fc" receptors of protein A coated Sepharose beads. The immunoprecipitates are then eluted from the beads and separated electrophoretically on polyacrylamide gels, as for WB. The HIV-1 antigen–antibody complexes are detected in the gel by autoradiography (due to isotopic labeling); the bands are similar to those of WB except that the gp160 and gp120 bands are better separated and defined.[28,37,45,51,93]

RIPA is more sensitive than WB for the detection of antibodies to the higher-molecular-weight proteins of HIV-1; due to this sensitivity, gp 160/120 antibodies may be detected with RIPA before anti-p24 or anti-gp41, thereby potentially allowing for earlier detection of seroconversion.[28,51,93] In contrast, RIPA has been found to be less sensitive than WB at detecting antibodies to p24 in most studies,[28,51] while one group reported greater sensitivity for anti-p24 by RIPA as compared with WB.[93] Generally, RIPA is more sensitive late during HIV-1 infection when WB may revert to negativity.[51] Few false-positives have been detected,[28,34] and RIPA is usually negative among blood donors when WB may be falsely reactive with anti-p24 bands.[28,93] There are rare false-negatives by RIPA.[51,87] RIPA has also been applied to the detection of salivary antibodies.[94]

Overall, RIPA is slightly more sensitive and specific than WB and, therefore, can be used to supplement WB assays when the results are indeterminate.[28,37] Theoretic reasons for the advantages of this assay include (*1*) retention of three-dimensional structure by soluble proteins, which allows for more specific antibody binding; (*2*) greater multivalent binding by antibody in a liquid medium, thereby increasing sensitivity; and (*3*) the formation of more stable antigen–antibody complexes in a soluble phase, thereby detecting low-avidity antibodies.[93] Despite these advantages, whether real or theoretic, RIPA will remain a supplemental test confined to research laboratories due to its being labor intensive, expensive, and requiring the use of HIV-1-infected cell lines and radioisotopes.

Latex Agglutination

For developing countries many of the screening tests described above are not practical due to lack of needed equipment, biohazard containment facilities, sufficient skilled technicians and/or sufficient financial resources. Furthermore, current EIAs are recognized to give a high rate of false positivity with African sera,[95] possibly due to cross-reactivity with other retroviruses.[39,72] Riggin et al. have reported the development of a rapid latex agglutination (LA) assay using recombinant envelope antigen (CBre3) to detect HIV-1 antibodies.[96] This antigen incorporates the immunodominant regions of gp120 and gp41 and has been used by others for a recombinant EIA.[17,77] Riggin et al. showed complete agreement of LA with WB and only one discordant result with EIA among 211 serum specimens (95 positive by WB and EIA)[96]; most positive specimens were strongly reactive by LA and easy to interpret. Similar results have been reported by others with this Cambridge Bioscience kit when using sera from 300 African patients[52] and 2820 sera from many areas of the globe (the Carribean, Africa, North and South America, and Europe).[97] Van de Perre et al. did note a need to dilute sera for the LA test to avoid a prozone phenomenon causing false-negative results[52]; these authors believed that LA results did not require confirmation. Quinn et al. cautioned about the need for positive and negative LA controls and a trained observer due to the subjective determination of reactivity with LA.[97] The need for such training, its limited shelf life, and need for refrigeration of reagents may unfortunately limit the use of LA in developing countries.[98] The LA does appear to be an excellent screening (and possibly confirmatory) assay for future use. However, its applicability to low-risk population screening (e.g., blood donors) requires evaluation due to anticipated increases in rates of false positivity.

Other Antibody Tests

Van de Perre et al. have described a dipstick screening test for HIV-1 antibodies.[52] An HIV-1-infected H-9 cell lysate is coated onto a polystyrene stick, which is then reacted with test serum and immunoenzymatic reagents modified from an EIA. The color reaction is observer visible after three 15-minute incubations. This assay was 98 percent sensitive but suffered from false positivity (90 percent specific). Confirmation of results was needed when using the dipstick as a screen. Its low cost and lack of equipment requirements may make this assay applicable as a screening test in developing countries.

A rapid dot immunobinding assay for HIV-1 antibodies has been described recently for screening purposes.[99,100] The lysate of HIV-1-infected cells[100] or a recombinant HIV-1 envelope polypeptide is spotted onto nitrocellulose paper and reacted with test sera; this is followed by typical EIA immunoenzymatic reactions resulting in the development of color. The color intensity is judged as positive or negative by the observer when compared with both positive and negative controls.[101] The test has the advantage of being simple, rapid (30 minutes), stable, and requiring no equipment, but it is subject to observer variability. It also does not detect HIV-1 antibodies to defined viral antigens. The assay was sensitive and specific when compared with the Genetic Systems EIA and WB. It may have applicability in developing countries.

The most recent development regarding screening for HIV-1 infection uses the patient's own blood, with autologous red cell agglutination being a positive test.[102] A nonagglutinating murine monoclonal antibody was made to human red blood cells; to this monoclonal antibody was bound a synthetic peptide containing the immunoreactive portion of gp41. The addition to this monoclonal antibody–peptide complex results in binding of the antibody to red blood cells and agglutination if HIV-1 envelope antibodies are present in the patient's blood. This assay can be performed with 0.01 ml of the patient's blood and takes 2 minutes. The sensitivity reported was 98 percent for patients with AIDS; a false-positive rate of 0.1 percent with sera from healthy blood donors was noted, as compared with a 0.2 percent rate when using the Genetic Systems EIA on the same samples. This assay, pending the results of further tests, may have major applications as a screening test in the future, especially considering its simplicity and speed.

A confirmatory technique has been recently described and marketed, although not licensed for clinical use, that incorporates recombinant HIV-1 antigens with a protein electrophoretic immunoblot technique.[103] In this Chiron immunoblot, recombinant p24, p31, gp41, and gp120 are electrophoresed and blotted onto nitrocellulose sheets, which are cut into strips. These strips are sold in kits similar to the Dupont WB kit. Controls include an antibody-negative serum and two sera with high and low levels of antibody. With this kit, the bands are sharp, well separated, and defined; this assay also requires less reaction time with the patient's serum than the WB.[103] Data on the sensitivity and specificity of this assay are lacking. Calarco et al. reported on the sequence in which antibodies appear during acute HIV-1 infection when using this recombinant technology, i.e., antibodies to gp41 and/or p24, followed by anti-p31, and finally anti-gp120.[103]

Hofbauer et al. have reported on a similar recombinant envelope (gp41) immunoblot.[104] This recombinant blot was easier to read than was the WB when using viral lysate. This assay detected anti-gp41 before anti-p24 was detected by the conventional WB, lacked any false-positives, and was more sensitive than either the conventional WB or IFA. Further studies are needed to define the use of these recombinant antigen immunoblots in the diagnosis of HIV-1 infection.

Some virologists consider the ability of serum to neutralize the infectivity of a virus to be a reference serologic test. With HIV-1, this is a tedious assay requiring its culture in H-9 cells and is confined to laboratories with stringent biohazard capabilities. There are few reports of the assay of neutralizing antibody. Several authors have reported the association of neutralizing antibody with a lack of symptoms and the progression to symptomatic HIV-1 infection with a loss of such antibodies.[105,106] Weber et al. did show a similar trend but were unable to associate neutralizing antibody with anti-p24 activity.[32] The complexity of the assay will limit its application and availability in the future.

HIV-1 ANTIGEN DETECTION

The detection of the p24 antigen in serum and CSF has become important for experimental protocols in the diagnosis and treatment of HIV-1 infection since the Abbott EIA became available in 1986 (for research use only). A Genetic Systems antigen EIA is also currently available for research use, while Dupont and Coulter have similar assays in development or pending licensure.

The detection of the p24 antigen viral marker differs from antibody detection in two ways: (*1*) only low antigen concentrations are present, and (*2*) p24 forms immune complexes with its antibody that are not detected by the antigen assay. The EIA for p24 antigen only detects free antigen in excess of antibody, and this implies the presence of active viral replication.

With this indirect EIA for p24 antigen, the test specimen is incubated overnight with polystyrene beads or in a microtiter well coated with polyclonal HIV-1 antibody. After rinsing, the bead or well is allowed to react with rabbit or goat anti-HIV-1. After rinsing, the bead or well is then exposed to an enzyme-linked anti-rabbit or anti-goat immunoglobulin. The substrate is added to allow the color to develop, after which absorbance is measured. The OD is proportional to the amount of antigen present, with the limit of detection for the assay being between 50 and 100 pg/ml.[18,30] The entire assay consumes 24–30 hours.[37]

For a specimen that is repeatedly reactive, the specificity of the assay must be confirmed by the use of a blocking ("neutralizing") antibody.[37,82] The specimen as well as positive and negative controls are incubated with reference human sera with or without antibody to HIV-1 and then reassayed for the presence of detectable p24 antigen. Specificity is confirmed by a concomitant reduction (50 percent or greater) in OD with the specimen exposed to human anti-HIV-1 or by an OD of the nonneutralized specimen equal to or greater than the cutoff value.[37] Including repetition and the blocking assay, confirmation of a positive p24 antigen assay may take 3–4 days.

The major advantages of this assay over viral culture include working with noninfectious HIV-1 antigen and the lack of HLA determinants contaminating the antigen preparation used in the former assay. A major disadvantage is the complexity and duration of the assay itself, especially when coupled with confirmatory tests. Additionally, this assay is not a screening test and must be used in conjunction with an antibody assay.

Suggested uses for the antigen assay are (*1*) detection of HIV-1 in cell culture, (*2*) prediction of disease progression (by the reappearance of p24), (*3*) monitoring antiviral therapy, and (*4*) assessing the HIV-1 infection status of neonates born to seropositive mothers.[82,107] Cerebrospinal fluid can also be assayed for p24 to provide evidence for HIV-1 central nervous system involvement.[19]

TABLE 8. Correlation of the Clinical Status of HIV-1 Infection with p24 Antigen Detection

Clinical Status	*Percentage with p24 Antigenemia*
Asymptomatic	4
AIDS-related complex	56
AIDS	70

(From Kenny et al.,[113] with permission.)

During acute infection, p24 antigenemia precedes seroconversion, usually resolves within 2–3 weeks as antibodies to p24 appear,[18,25,27,108–110] but may persist for 6–14 months before seroconversion.[24,25] However, during early infection, antigen detection is not as sensitive as viral culture.[111] Additionally, while detection of p24 antigen has been shown to correlate with virus culture positivity, the antigen assay is an insensitive test for infection due to its usual negativity during asymptomatic illness when patients remain culture-positive.[37,112] Its sensitivity improves as HIV-1-related disease develops[113] (Table 8). As the infection progresses clinically with the development of AIDS, p24 antibodies decline, and p24 antigen reappears.[19,22,27,30,31,110,112–114]

The specificity of p24 antigen positivity by EIA is very good since Stute found only a 0.43 percent false positivity rate among volunteer blood donors.[115] Such specificity provides a rationale for including p24 antigen testing with antibody screening of all blood donors in the future.

The p24 antigen assay has been useful for following HIV-1-infected patients receiving azidothymidine (AZT).[20,116] During therapy, falling p24 levels have correlated with diminished symptoms, rising CD4 cell counts, and a better prognosis. Before therapy, a high serum antigen concentration has correlated with a poor prognosis.[116]

In addition to the detection of soluble antigen in serum, HIV-1 antigens have also been detected on the surface of peripheral blood lymphocytes from HIV-1-infected patients by direct and indirect immunofluorescence.[117]

HIV-1 DETECTION

Viral Culture

The in vitro propagation of HIV-1 was initially reported in 1983 and was followed by improvements in culture techniques by other researchers.[3–5] While the virus was initially identified in cell culture by electron microscopy,[2] most laboratories today detect HIV-1 indirectly by assaying for reverse transcriptase (RT) activity in cell culture supernatants. This enzyme is produced by HIV-1-infected cells in large quantities. Interestingly, the lack of universal culture positivity among patients with HIV-1 seropositivity may be at least partially attributable to the presence of an inhibitor of RT.[118] Reverse transcriptase activity is not specific for HIV-1 since it is also produced by other retroviruses.[119] More specific indirect assays for the presence of HIV-1 in cell culture have been described, including HIV-1 antigen (p24) detection in culture supernatants by EIA,[21,37,120–122] antigen detection by a dot immunoenzymatic binding assay,[123] and a radioimmunoassay (RIA) designed for antigen detection in cell culture.[121]

Each of these indirect methods of viral detection requires HIV-1 culture, which is cumbersome, costly, and time-consuming (weeks) and exposes personnel to an infectious risk.[37] A typical HIV-1 culture requires (*1*) separation of peripheral blood mononuclear cells (PBMC) from other blood components, (*2*) incubation of patient PBMC with PBMC from a HIV-1-seronegative donor for several weeks in the presence of interleukin-2 and phytohemagglutinin, and (*3*) once- or twice-weekly assay of supernatants from these cultures for RT activity or p24 antigen.[3–5,37] In culture supernatants, antigen detection is more sensitive and positive earlier than the RT assay for HIV-1[21,37,120,122,124]; 60–94 percent of supernatants are positive by the p24 detection assay at day 10 of culture as compared with 20–25 percent by the RT assay. The RIA and EIA are equally sensitive.[121] Technically, however, antigen detection has numerous advantages over RIA and the RT assay.[37,120–122]

The clinical indications for HIV-1 culture are similar to those for p24 antigen detection, but culture is the more sensitive technique. Cultures may be used to assess strain virulence (proportional to the rate of replication), viral inoculum (inversely proportional to the time of culture positivity), and efficacy of therapy.[37] However, due to the many technical difficulties with HIV-1 culture, it will remain confined to a limited number of laboratories.[37,82]

DNA Probes

A recently used alternative method for the detection of HIV-1 in culture-negative patients is molecular hybridization using DNA-probes and peripheral blood nonlymphoid mononuclear cells.[24,37] Previous attempts at direct detection of the HIV-1 circular proviral genome in the host cell nucleus with hybridization were quite insensitive.[37] To enhance sensitivity, subsequent attempts have relied upon amplification of the virus in host cells before hybridization by cocultivation in vitro[125] or by oligonucleotide probes of DNA extracted from mononuclear cells and blotted on nitrocellulose.[37,124] These probes of subgenomic size are made by inserting fragments of the HIV-1 genome into plasmids, by allowing the plasmids to replicate, and then by extracting the subgenomic fragments from the plasmids.[124] These fragments are then isotopically labeled. DNA is extracted from a patient's mononuclear cells and blotted onto nitrocellulose paper. Hybridization is then attempted with the blotted cellular DNA extract and the labeled subgenomic HIV-1 DNA fragments. Blots are subsequently washed, dried, and exposed to film for the detection of hybridized, labeled DNA. Such hybridization assays have been shown to be at least as sensitive and specific as HIV-1 culture.[24,124] The method is time-consuming and technically difficult but faster and easier than culture.[124] As few as 1 in 10,000 PBMC may express HIV-1 RNA by hybridization.[125]

Much excitement has been generated by the development of far more sensitive amplification techniques for the detection of as little as one genome of nonreplicating HIV-1 in mononuclear cells; these techniques may totally circumvent the need for HIV-1 culture in the future.[125] Molecular hybridization without amplification requires an actively replicating HIV-1 infection. The polymerase chain reaction (PCR) involves annealing two short DNA chains to the viral genome after DNA denaturation, one onto each strand of the HIV-1 proviral DNA. This template-directed replication of the HIV-1 genome is initiated by the addition of DNA polymerase; the products of this replication serve as templates for repeated cycles (up to 25) of denaturation, annealing, and replication until there are sufficient numbers of oligonucleotides to be detected by a complementary, labeled oligonucleotide DNA probe. This technique has the capability of detecting latent HIV-1 infection in the nonreplicative state in patients who are seronegative.[126–128] This assay takes about 1 day to complete.

Potential applications for the PCR include (*1*) identification of all HIV-1-infected blood donors; (*2*) confirmation of the diagnosis of HIV-1 infection, especially when false-positive screening and/or confirmatory tests are suspected; (*3*) identification of seronegative infected patients; (*4*) early diagnosis of infection before seroconversion; and (*5*) confirmation of infection in newborns. Until further simplifications of the PCR assay are developed and cost reduced, broad applicability will not be feasible, however. While hybridization and PCR technologies hold great promise, they are not currently recommended for general use.[82]

TABLE 9. Population Groups Currently Screened for HIV-1 Antibody

Mandatory
Blood donors
Federal prisoners
Military recruits and active duty personnel
Foreign service officers
Aliens seeking immigration
With consent
Patients in STD clinics, prostitutes
Intravenous drug users
Women of childbearing age with a recognized risk for HIV-1 infection
Persons planning marriage (in a few states)
Hospital admissions in high-risk groups

TABLE 10. Considerations for Determining Justification for Mandatory Screening Programs for Antibody to HIV

The population selected should have a reservoir of infected persons so that disproportionate numbers of uninfected persons do not have to submit to intrusive testing
The population must pose a significant risk of communication of infection
Knowledge of results should allow for the reduction of transmission
Benefits must outweigh the ill effects of testing
No less intrusive/restrictive alternatives are available

(From Gostin et al.,[133] with permission.)

APPLICATION OF HIV-1 ANTIBODY SCREENING

Since the screening EIA became available in March 1985, much discussion and debate have ensued among the public and among legal and health care professionals as to the appropriateness of broad-based screening programs for HIV-1 antibody. Arguments have been presented for and against premarital and preoperative mandatory screening as well as screening employees in the workplace.[129–131] Issues of ethics, confidentiality, and informed consent have been raised.[132–135] Appropriate hospital policies have been debated.[136,137] At present, in the United States, the population groups undergoing mandatory and voluntary screening are defined in Table 9. Proposed justifications for mandatory screening are enumerated in Table 10. As the sensitivity and especially the specificity of the current means for diagnosing HIV-1 infection improve,[56] screening tests for HIV-1 infection will gain broader applicability.

REFERENCES

1. Centers for Disease Control. Prevention of acquired immunodeficiency syndrome (AIDS): Report of inter-agency recommendations. MMWR. 1984;32:101–3.
2. Barre-Sinoussi F, Chermann JC, Rey F, et al. Isolation of a T-lymphotropic retrovirus from a patient at risk for acquired immune deficiency syndrome (AIDS). Science. 1983;220:868–71.
3. Popovic M, Sarngadharan MG, Read E, et al. Detection, isolation, and continuous production of cytopathic retroviruses (HTLV-III) from patients with AIDS and pre-AIDS. Science. 1984;224:497–500.
4. Gallo RC, Salahuddin SZ, Popovic M, et al. Frequent detection and isolation of cytopathic retroviruses (HTLV-III) from patients with AIDS and at risk for AIDS. Science. 1984;224:500–2.
5. Levy JA, Hoffman AD, Kramer SM, et al. Isolation of lymphocytopathic retroviruses from San Francisco patients with AIDS. Science. 1984;225:840–2.
6. Sarngadharan MG, Popovic M, Bruch L, et al. Antibodies reactive with human T-lymphotropic retroviruses (HTLV-III) in serum of patients with AIDS. Science. 1984;224:506–8.
7. Brun-Vezinet F, Barre-Sinoussi F, et al. Detection of IgG antibodies to lymphadenopathy-associated virus in patients with AIDS or lymphadenopathy syndrome. Lancet. 1984;1:1253–6.
8. Centers for Disease Control. Provisional Public Health Service inter-agency recommendations for screening donated blood and plasma for antibody to the virus causing acquired immunodeficiency syndrome. MMWR. 1985;34:1–5.
9. Schorr JB, Berkowitz A, et al. Prevalence of HTLV-III antibody in American blood donors. N Engl J Med. 1985;313:384–5.

10. Centers for Disease Control. Human T-lymphotropic virus type III/lymphadenopathy-associated virus antibody testing at alternate sites. MMWR. 1986;35:284–7.
11. Centers for Disease Control. Recommendations for assisting in the prevention of perinatal transmission of human T-lymphotropic virus type III/lymphadenopathy-associated virus and acquired immunodeficiency syndrome. MMWR. 1985;34:721–6,731–3.
12. Centers for Disease Control. Additional recommendations to reduce sexual and drug abuse-related transmission of human T-lymphotropic virus type III/lymphadenopathy-associated virus. MMWR. 1986;35:152–5.
13. Centers for Disease Control. Perspectives in disease prevention and health promotion: Public Health Service guidelines for counseling and antibody testing to prevent HIV infection and AIDS. MMWR. 1987;36:509–15.
14. Weiss SH, Goedert JJ, et al. Screening test for HTLV-III (AIDS agent) antibodies; specificity, sensitivity, and applications. JAMA. 1985;253:221–5.
15. Carlson JR, Bryant ML, et al. AIDS serology testing in low and high risk groups. JAMA. 1985;253:3405–8.
16. Sivak SL, Wormser GP. Predictive value of a screening test for antibodies to HTLV-III. Am J Clin Pathol. 1986;85:700–3.
17. Burke DS, Brandt BL, et al. Diagnosis of human immunodeficiency virus infection by immunoassay using a molecularly cloned and expressed virus envelope polypeptide; comparison to Western blot on 2707 consecutive serum samples. Ann Intern Med. 1987;671–6.
18. Goudsmit J, Paul DA, et al. Expression of human immunodeficiency virus antigen (HIV-Ag) in serum and cerebrospinal fluid during acute and chronic infection. Lancet. 1986;2:177–80.
19. Lange JMA, Paul DA, et al. Persistent HIV antigenaemia and decline of HIV core antibodies associated with transition to AIDS. Br Med J. 1986;293:1459–62.
20. Chaisson RE, Allain JP, et al. Significant changes in HIV antigen level in the serum of patients treated with azidothymidine. N Engl J Med. 1986;315:1610–11.
21. Diggs JL. Testing for HIV antigen. Infect Control Hosp Epidemiol. 1988;9:353–4.
22. Allain JP, Laurian Y, et al. Long-term evaluation of HIV antigen and antibodies to p24 and gp41 in patients with hemophilia. N Engl J Med. 1987;317:1114–21.
23. Allain JP, Laurian Y, et al. Serological markers in early stages of human immunodeficiency virus infection in haemophiliacs. Lancet. 1986;2:1233–6.
24. Ranki A, Krohn M, et al. Long latency precedes overt seroconversion in sexually transmitted human-immunodeficiency-virus infection. Lancet. 1987;1:589–93.
25. Simmonds P, Lainson FAL, et al. HIV antigen and antibody detection: Variable responses to infection in the Edinburgh haemophiliac cohort. Br Med J. 1988;296:593–8.
26. Cooper DA, Tindall B, et al. Characterization of T lymphocyte responses during primary infection with human immunodeficiency virus. J Infect Dis. 1988;157:889–96.
27. Von Sydow M, Gaines H, et al. Antigen detection in primary HIV infection. Br Med J. 1988;296:238–40.
28. Gaines H, Sonnerborg A, et al. Antibody response in primary human immunodeficiency virus infection. Lancet. 1987;1:1249–53.
29. Pan LZ, Cheng-Mayer C, Levy JA. Patterns of antibody response in individuals infected with the human immunodeficiency virus. J Infect Dis. 1987;155:626–32.
30. Goudsmit J, Lange JMA, et al. Antigenemia and antibody titers to core and envelope antigens in AIDS, AIDS-related complex, and subclinical human immunodeficiency virus infection. J Infect Dis. 1987;155:558–60.
31. Mayer KH, Falk LA, et al. Correlation of enzyme-linked immunosorbent assays for serum human immunodeficiency virus antigen and antibodies to recombinant viral proteins with subsequent clinical outcomes in a cohort of asymptomatic homosexual men. Am J Med. 1987;83:208–12.
32. Weber JN, Weiss RA, et al. Human immunodeficiency virus infection in two cohorts of homosexual men: Neutralising sera and association of anti-gag antibody with prognosis. Lancet. 1987;1:119–21.
33. Schupbach J, Haller O, et al. Antibodies to HTLV-III in Swiss patients with AIDS and pre-AIDS and in groups at risk for AIDS. N Engl J Med. 1985;312:265–70.
34. Lelie PN, Reesink HW, Huisman H. Evaluation of three second-generation and three confirmatory assays for antibodies to human immunodeficiency virus. Vox Sang. 1988;54:84–91.
35. Dawson GJ, Heller JS, et al. Reliable detection of individuals seropositive for the human immunodeficiency virus (HIV) by competitive immunoassays using *Escherichia coli*-expressed HIV structural proteins. J Infect Dis. 1988;157:149–55.
36. Steckelberg JM, Cockerill FR. Serologic testing for human immunodeficiency virus antibodies. Mayo Clin Proc. 1988;63:373–80.
37. Jackson JB, Balfour HH Jr. Practical diagnostic testing for human immunodeficiency virus. Clin Microbiol Rev. 1988;1:124–38.
38. Allain JP, Hojvat S. Development in HIV serology. In: de la Maza LM, Peterson EM, eds. Proceedings of the 1987 International Symposium on Medical Virology. Anaheim, CA. Amsterdam: Elsevier Science Publishing; 1987:315–30.
39. Houn HY, Pappas AA, Walker EM Jr. Status of current clinical tests for human immunodeficiency virus (HIV): Applications and limitations. Ann Clin Lab Sci. 1987;17:279–85.
40. Parry JV, Perry KR, Mortimer PP. Sensitive assays for viral antibodies in saliva: An alternative to tests on serum. Lancet. 1987;2:72–5.
41. Burke DS, Redfield RR, et al. Variations in Western blot banding patterns of human T-cell lymphotropic virus type III/lymphadenopathy-associated virus. J Clin Microbiol. 1987;25:81–4.
42. Cooper DA, Imrie AA, et al. Antibody response to human immunodeficiency virus after primary infection. J Infect Dis. 1987;155:1113–8.
43. Ward JW, Grindon AJ, et al. Laboratory and epidemiologic evaluation of an enzyme immunoassay for antibodies to HTLV-III. JAMA. 1986;256:357–61.
44. Nishanian P, Taylor JMG, et al. Significance of quantitative enzyme-linked immunosorbent assay (ELISA) results in evaluation of three ELISAs and Western blot tests for detection of antibodies to human immunodeficiency virus in a high risk population. J Clin Microbiol. 1987;25:395–400.
45. Handsfield HH, Wandell M, et al. Screening and diagnostic performance of enzyme immunoassay for antibody to lymphadenopathy-associated virus. J Clin Microbiol. 1987;25:879–84.
46. Voeller B. Evaluation of eight ELISA kits for the detection of anti-LAV/HTLV-III antibodies. Lancet. 1986;1:1152–3.
47. Reesink HW, Huisman JG, et al. Evaluation of six enzyme immunoassays for antibody against human immunodeficiency virus. Lancet. 1986;2:483–6.
48. Evans RP, Shanson DC, Mortimer PP. Clinical evaluation of Abbott and Wellcome enzyme linked immunosorbent assays for detection of serum antibodies to human immunodeficiency virus (HIV). J Clin Pathol. 1987;40:552–5.
49. Burkhardt U, Mertens Th, Eggers HJ. Comparison of two commercially available anti-HIV ELISAs: Abbott HTLV III EIA and Du Pont HTLV III-ELISA. J Med Virol. 1987;23:217–24.
50. Deinhardt F, Eberle J, Gurtler L. Sensitivity and specificity of eight commercial and one recombinant anti-HIV ELISA tests. Lancet. 1987;1:40.
51. Saah AJ, Farzadegan H, et al. Detection of early antibodies in human immunodeficiency virus infection by enzyme-linked immunosorbent assay, Western blot, and radioimmunoprecipitation. J Clin Microbiol. 1987;25:1605–10.
52. Van De Perre P, Nzaramba D, et al. Comparison of six serological assays for human immunodeficiency virus antibody detection in developing countries. J Clin Microbiol. 1988;26:552–6.
53. Ozanne G, Fauvel M. Performance and reliability of five commercial enzyme-linked immunosorbent assay kits in screening for anti-human immunodeficiency virus antibody in high-risk subjects. J Clin Microbiol. 1988;26:1496–500.
54. Engle JC, Schleupner CJ. Performance evaluation of six commercially available enzyme linked immunosorbent assays kits for antibody to human immunodeficiency virus (Abstract). In: de la Maza LM, Peterson EM, eds. Proceedings of the 1987 International Symposium on Medical Virology. Anaheim, CA. Amsterdam: Elsevier Science Publishing; 1987:357.
55. Taylor RN, Przybyszewski VA. Summary of the Centers for Disease Control human immunodeficiency virus (HIV) performance evaluation surveys for 1985 and 1986. Am J Clin Pathol. 1988;89:1–13.
56. Schwartz JS, Dans PE, Kinosian BP. Human immunodeficiency virus test evaluation, performance, and use. JAMA. 1988;259:2574–9.
57. Centers for Disease Control. Update: Serologic testing for antibody to human immunodeficiency virus. MMWR. 1988;36:833–45.
58. Van Den Akker R, Hekker AC, Osterhaus ADME. Heat inactivation of serum may interfere with HTLV-III/LAV serology. Lancet. 1985;2:672.
59. Jungkind DL, DiRenzo SA, Young SJ. Effect of using heat-inactivated serum with the Abbott human T-cell lymphotropic virus type III antibody test. J Clin Microbiol. 1986;23:381–2.
60. Kvinesdal B, Pedersen NS. False-positive HIV antibody tests in RPR-reactive patients. JAMA. 1988;260:923–4.
61. Kuhnl P, Seidl S, Holzberger G. HLA DR4 antibodies cause positive HTLV-III antibody ELISA results. Lancet. 1985;1:1222–3.
62. Ameglio F, Dolei A, et al. Antibodies reactive with nonpolymorphic epitopes on HLA molecules interfere in screening tests for the human immunodeficiency virus. J Infect Dis. 1987;156:1034–5.
63. Wartick MG, McCarroll DR, Wiltbank TB. A second discriminator for biological false positive results in enzyme-linked immunosorbent assays for antibodies to human immunodeficiency virus (HTLV-III/LAV). Transfusion. 1987;27:109–11.
64. Blanton M, Balakrishnan K, et al. HLA antibodies in blood donors with reactive screening tests for antibody to the immunodeficiency virus. Transfusion. 1987;27:118–9.
65. Smith DM, Dewhurst S, et al. False-positive enzyme-linked immunosorbent assay reactions for antibody to human immunodeficiency virus in a population of midwestern patients with congenital bleeding disorders. Transfusion. 1987;127:112.
66. Mendenhall CL, Roselle GA, et al. False positive tests for HTLV-III antibodies in alcoholic patients with hepatitis. N Engl J Med. 1986;314:921–2.
67. Marlink RG, Allain JS, et al. Low sensitivity of ELISA testing in early HIV infection. N Engl J Med. 1986;315:1549.
68. Biberfeld G, Bredberg-Raden U, et al. Blood donor sera with false-positive Western blot reactions to human immunodeficiency virus. Lancet. 1986;2:289–91.
69. Albersheim SG, Smyth JA, et al. Passively acquired human immunodeficiency virus seropositivity in a neonate after hepatitis B immunoglobulin. J Pediatr. 1988;112:915–6.

70. Saag MS, Britz J. Asymptomatic blood donor with a false-positive HTLV-III western blot. N Engl J Med. 1986;314:118.
71. Goetz DW, Hall SE, et al. Pediatric acquired immunodeficiency syndrome with negative human immunodeficiency virus antibody response by enzyme-linked immunosorbent assay and Western blot. Pediatrics. 1988;81:356–9.
72. Denis F, Leonard G, et al. Comparison of 10 enzyme immunoassays for detection of antibody to human immunodeficiency virus type 2 in West African sera. J Clin Microbiol. 1988;26:1000–4.
73. Tribe DE, Reed DL, et al. Antibodies reactive with human immunodeficiency virus gag-coded antigens (gag reactive only) are a major cause of enzyme-linked immunosorbent assay reactivity in a blood donor population. J Clin Microbiol. 1988;26:641–7.
74. Hickman M, Mortimer JY, Rawlinson VI. Donor screening for HIV: How many false negatives? Lancet. 1988;1:1221.
75. Ward JW, Holmberg SD, et al. Transmission of human immunodeficiency virus (HIV) by blood transfusions screened as negative for HIV antibody. N Engl J Med. 1988;318:473–8.
76. Navarro MDR, Pineda JA, et al. Recombinant EIA for anti-HIV testing is more specific than conventional EIA. Vox Sang. 1988;54:62–3.
77. Thorn RM, Beltz GA, et al. Enzyme immunoassay using a novel recombinant polypeptide to detect human immunodeficiency virus env antibody. J Clin Microbiol. 1987;25:1207–12.
78. Gnann JW Jr, Schwimmbeck PL, et al. Diagnosis of AIDS by using a 12-amino acid peptide representing an immunodominant epitope of the human immunodeficiency virus. J Infect Dis. 1987;156:261–7.
79. Griffith BP, Ferguson D, Landry ML. Detection of antibodies to human immunodeficiency virus: Principles, use and interpretation. VA Practitioner. 1988;5:50–61.
80. Towbin H, Staehelin T, et al. Electrophoretic transfer of proteins from polacrylamide gels to nitrocellulose sheets: Procedure and some applications. Proc Natl Acad Sci USA. 1979;76:4350–4.
81. Burke DS, Redfield RR. False-positive Western blot tests for antibodies to HTLV-III. JAMA. 1986;256:347.
82. Hausler WJ Jr. Report of the Third Consensus Conference on HIV Testing sponsored by the Association of State and Territorial Public Health Laboratory Directors. Infect Control Hosp Epidemiol. 1988;9:345–9.
83. Blomberg J, Klasse PJ. Specificities and sensitivities of three systems for determination of antibodies to human immunodeficiency virus by electrophoretic immunoblotting. J Clin Microbiol. 1988;26:106–10.
84. Mathex D, Leibovitch J, et al. LAV/HTLV-III seroconversion and disease in hemophiliacs treated in France. N Engl J Med. 1986;314:118–9.
85. Courouce AM, Muller JY, Richard D. False-positive Western blot reactions to human immunodeficiency virus in blood donors. Lancet. 1986;2:921–2.
86. Salahuddin SZ, Groopman JE, Markham PD, et al. HTLV-III in symptom-free seronegative persons. Lancet. 1984;2:1418–20.
87. Groopman JE, Hartzband PI, et al. Antibody seronegative human T-lymphotropic virus type III (HTLV-III)-infected patients with acquired immunodeficiency syndrome or related disorders. Blood. 1985;66:742–4.
88. Sandstrom EG, Schooley RT, et al. Detection of human anti-HTLV-III antibodies by indirect immunofluorescence using fixed cells. Transfusion. 1985;25:308–12.
89. Gallo D, Diggs JL, et al. Comparison of detection of antibody to the acquired immune deficiency syndrome virus by enzyme immunoassay, immunofluorescence, and Western blot methods. J Clin Microbiol. 1986;23:1049–51.
90. Hedenskog M, Dewhurst S, et al. Testing for antibodies to AIDS-associated retrovirus (HTLV-III/LAV) by indirect fixed cell immunofluorescence: Specificity, sensitivity, and applications. J Med Virol. 1986;19:325–34.
91. Lennette ET, Karpatkin S, Levy JA. Indirect immunofluorescence assay for antibodies to human immunodeficiency virus. J Clin Microbiol. 1987;25:199–202.
92. Carlson JR, Yee J, et al. Comparison of indirect immunofluorescence and Western blot for detection of anti-human immunodeficiency virus antibodies. J Clin Microbiol. 1987;25:494–7.
93. Tersmette M, Lelie PN, et al. Confirmation of HIV seropositivity: Comparison of a novel radioimmunoprecipitation assay to immunoblotting and virus culture. J Med Virol. 1988;24:109–16.
94. Archibald DW, Zon LI, et al. Salivary antibodies as a means of detecting human T cell lymphotropic virus type III/lymphadenopathy-associated virus infection. J Clin Microbiol. 1986;24:873–5.
95. Biggar RJ, Gigase PL, et al. ELISA HTLV retrovirus antibody reactivity associated with malaria and immune complexes in healthy Africans. Lancet. 1985;2:520–3.
96. Riggin CH, Beltz GA, et al. Detection of antibodies to human immunodeficiency virus by latex agglutination with recombinant antigen. J Clin Microbiol. 1987;25:1772–3.
97. Quinn TC, Riggin CH, et al. Rapid latex agglutination assay using recombinant envelope polypeptide for the detection of antibody to the HIV. JAMA. 1988;260:510–3.
98. Heyward WL, Curran JW. Rapid screening tests for HIV infection. JAMA. 1988;260:542.
99. Carlson JR, Yee JL, et al. Rapid, easy, and economical screening test for antibodies to human immunodeficiency virus. Lancet. 1987;1:361–2.
100. Heberling RL, Kalter SS, et al. Dot immunobinding assay compared with enzyme-linked immunosorbent assay for rapid and specific detection of retrovirus antibody induced by human or simian acquired immunodeficiency syndrome. J Clin Microbiol. 1988;26:765–7.
101. Heberling RL, Kalter SS. Rapid dot-immunobinding assay on nitrocellulose for viral antibodies. J Clin Microbiol. 1986;23:109–13.
102. Kemp BE, Rylatt DB, et al. Autologous red cell agglutination assay for HIV-1 antibodies: Simplified test with whole blood. Science. 1988;241:1352–4.
103. Calarco TL, Polito AJ, et al. Nitrocellulose cellulose strip ELISA for antibodies to human immunodeficiency virus employing recombinant antigens. In: de la Maza LM, Peterson EM, eds. Proceedings of the 1987 International Symposium on Medical Virology. Anaheim, CA. Amsterdam: Elsevier Science Publishing; 1987:293–314.
104. Hofbauer JM, Schulz TF, et al. Comparison of Western blot (immunoblot) based on recombinant-derived p41 with conventional tests for serodiagnosis of human immunodeficiency virus infections. J Clin Microbiol. 1988;26:116–20.
105. Anderson KC, Gorgone BC, et al. Transfusion-acquired human immunodeficiency virus infection among immunocompromised persons. Ann Intern Med. 1986;105:519–27.
106. Robert-Guroff M, Brown M, Gallo RC. HTLV-III-neutralizing antibodies in patients with AIDS and AIDS-related complex. Nature. 1985;316:72–4.
107. Borkowsky W, Paul D, et al. Human-immunodeficiency-virus infections in infants negative for anti-HIV by enzyme-linked immunoassay. Lancet. 1987;1:1168–71.
108. Kessler HA, Blaauw B, et al. Diagnosis of human immunodeficiency virus infection in seronegative homosexuals presenting with an acute viral syndrome. JAMA. 1987;258:1196–9.
109. Wall RA, Denning DW, Amos A. HIV antigenaemia in acute HIV infection. Lancet. 1987;1:566.
110. Goudsmit J, Paul DA. Circulation of HIV antigen in blood according to stage of infection, risk group, age and geographic origin. Epidemiol Infect. 1987;99:701–10.
111. Gaines H, Albert J, et al. HIV antigenaemia and virus isolation from plasma during primary HIV infection. Lancet. 1987;1:1317–8.
112. Wittek AE, Phelan MA, et al. Detection of human immunodeficiency virus core protein in plasma by enzyme immunoassay. Ann Intern Med. 1987;107:286–92.
113. Kenny C, Parkin J, et al. HIV antigen testing. Lancet. 1987;1:565–6.
114. Lange J, Goudsmit J. Decline of antibody reactivity to HIV core protein secondary to increased production of HIV antigen. Lancet. 1987;1:488.
115. Stute R. HIV antigen detection in routine blood donor screening. Lancet. 1987;1:566.
116. Jackson GG, Paul DA, et al. Human immunodeficiency virus (HIV) antigenemia (p24) in the acquired immunodeficiency syndrome (AIDS) and the effect of treatment with Zidovudine (AZT). Ann Intern Med. 1988;108:175–80.
117. Pekovic DD, Chausseau JP, et al. Detection of HTLV-III/LAV antigens in peripheral blood lymphocytes from patients with AIDS. Arch Virol. 1986;91:11–9.
118. Sano K, Lee MH, et al. Antibody that inhibits human immunodeficiency virus reverse transcriptase and association with inability to isolate virus. J Clin Microbiol. 1987;25:2415–7.
119. Poiesz BJ, Ruscetti FW, et al. Detection and isolation of type C retrovirus particles from fresh and cultured lymphocytes of a patient with cutaneous T-cell lymphoma. Proc Natl Acad Sci USA. 1980;77:7415–9.
120. Viscidi R, Farzadegan H, et al. Enzyme immunoassay for detection of human immunodeficiency virus antigens in cell cultures. J Clin Microbiol. 1988;26:453–8.
121. Gupta P, Balachandran R, et al. Detection of human immunodeficiency virus by reverse transcriptase assay, antigen capture assay, and radioimmunoassay. J Clin Microbiol. 1987;25:1122–5.
122. Feorino P, Forrester B, et al. Comparison of antigen assay and reverse transcriptase assay for detecting human immunodeficiency virus in culture. J Clin Microbiol. 1987;25:2344–6.
123. Blumberg RS, Hartshorn KL, et al. Dot immunobinding assay for detection of human immunodeficiency virus-associated antigens. J Clin Microbiol. 1987;25:1989–92.
124. Richman DD, McCutchan JA, Spector SA. Detecting human immunodeficiency virus RNA in peripheral blood mononuclear cells by nucleic acid hybridization. J Infect Dis. 1987;156:823–7.
125. Ou CY, Kwok S, et al. DNA amplification for direct detection of HIV-1 in DNA of peripheral blood mononuclear cells. Science. 1988;239:295–7.
126. Farzadegan H, Polis MA, et al. Loss of human immunodeficiency virus type 1 (HIV-1) antibodies with evidence of viral infection in asymptomatic homosexual men. Ann Intern Med. 1988;108:785–90.
127. DeRossi A, Amadori A, et al. Polymerase chain reaction and in-vitro antibody production for early diagnosis of paediatric HIV infection. Lancet. 1988;2:278.
128. Loche M, Mach B. Identification of HIV-infected seronegative individuals by a direct diagnostic test based on hybridization to amplified viral DNA. Lancet. 1988;2:418–21.
129. Cleary PD, Barry MJ, et al. Compulsory premarital screening for the human immunodeficiency virus; technical and public health considerations. JAMA. 1987;258:1757–62.
130. Hagan MD, Meyer KB, Pauker SG. Routine preoperative screening for HIV; does the risk to the surgeon outweigh the risk to the patient? JAMA. 1988;259:1357–9.
131. HIV testing in the workplace (Editorial). Lancet. 1988;2:199–200.
132. Bayer R, Levine C, Wolf SM. HIV antibody screening: An ethical framework for evaluating proposed programs. JAMA. 1986;256:1768–74.

133. Gostin L, Curran WC. AIDS screening, confidentiality, and the duty to warn. Am J Public Health. 1987;77:361–5.
134. Dixon RE. Sacred secrets: Confidentiality, informed consent, and diagnostic testing in the AIDS era. Infect Control Hosp Epidemiol. 1988;9:187–8.
135. Sherer R. Physician use of the HIV antibody test; the need for consent, counseling, confidentiality, and caution. JAMA. 1988;259:264–5.
136. Eickhoff TC. Hospital policies on HIV antibody testing. JAMA. 1988;259:1861–2.
137. Henry K, Willenbring K, Crossley K. Human immunodeficiency virus antibody testing: A description of practices and policies at US infectious disease-teaching hospitals and Minnesota hospitals. JAMA. 1988;259:1819–22.

110. THERAPY FOR AIDS

HENRY MASUR

Experience in the United States with the first 80,000 cases of the acquired immunodeficiency syndrome (AIDS) from 1979 to 1988 has clearly demonstrated that the quality and duration of patient survival are dismal. The 1-year survival rate for AIDS patients in New York City (1981–1985) was less than 45 percent for patients initially presenting with *Pneumocystis* pneumonia, less than 72 percent for patients initially presenting with Kaposi sarcoma, and less than 39 percent for patients presenting with other AIDS-defining illnesses.[1] One-year survival probabilities for the first 500 patients in San Francisco, calculated by different techniques, were no better.[2] In addition to the duration of patient survival being distressingly short, the quality of patient survival has usually been poor as manifested by decreasing performance scores and repeated needs for inpatient or outpatient medical interventions. The development of an effective antiretroviral drug, zidovudine (also known as azidothymidine or AZT), has been a major advance in the management of AIDS patients since its chronic administration clearly decreases the number (and probably the severity) of life-threatening illnesses and prolongs survival. Zidovudine is not a cure for AIDS, however, since patients chronically treated with this drug continue to develop serious tumors and infections and die prematurely.

Until more effective antiretroviral and immunomodulating agents can be developed, the management of AIDS patients will have to rely on zidovudine and on strategies that either prevent or more effectively treat the severe and life-threatening processes that are caused by the human immunodeficiency virus (HIV) itself, by immunologically mediated processes, or by opportunistic infections and tumors.[3] Autopsy studies suggest that almost 90 percent of life-threatening illnesses and deaths have been due to opportunistic infections.[4–6] Thus, a major focus in the management of HIV-infected patients must be placed on infectious processes. An increasing amount of data indicate that aggressive efforts to prevent opportunistic infections and aggressive efforts to diagnose complications expeditiously and intervene with therapy early can improve the prognosis for patients with this epidemic disease.

Some clinicians and patients question the utility of expending resources and subjecting patients to uncomfortable procedures and therapies when the underlying retroviral process is inevitably fatal.[7] The goals for the management of AIDS patients should be no different, however, from goals for the management of other incurable diseases such as cancer or atherosclerosis: to improve the quality and duration of survival in a manner that is reasonable in terms of the individual patient's wishes, a realistic assessment of the immediate prognosis, and the medical resources that are available. Experience is accumulating that shows that some patients with AIDS clearly benefit from surgical procedures, ventilatory support, and prolonged intensive care and survive for many months outside the hospital after such events.[7–9] Clinicians need considerable knowledge about the natural history of HIV infection, its complications, and the patient's wishes in order to make such decisions rationally.

THERAPY FOR UNDERLYING RETROVIRAL DISEASE

Since the clinical manifestations of AIDS are a direct consequence of HIV or the consequences of the effect of this virus on immune response, the most logical therapeutic strategy against AIDS would be to eradicate the HIV and to restore immune function to normal levels. During the 1980s, there has been an explosion in knowledge about the immunopathogenesis of AIDS. A variety of logical therapeutic strategies have been proposed, and many antiretroviral and immunomodulating agents with promising in vitro properties have been identified (Table 1). It is important to recognize that in vitro activity is not synonymous with clinical efficacy and safety. Before any therapeutic agent is introduced into standard clinical practice, there must be convincing demonstration that the new agent has therapeutic activity and is safe. In addition, advantage over existing therapy in terms of enhanced efficacy, decreased toxicity, decreased cost, or increased convenience of administration are desirable. Although many new agents are highly promising, as of May 1989 zidovudine was the only drug among the antiretroviral agents that had unequivocally been demonstrated to provide objective clinical benefit to HIV-infected patients (interferon-α has antiretroviral activity, but the only proven clinical benefit to date is its activity against Kaposi sarcoma, hairy cell leukemia, and papillomavirus infections). It is important for clinicians to avoid being influenced to use a drug solely because of aggressive advocacy by the drug's sponsor or enthusiastic interest on the part of patient groups.

In assessing antiretroviral and immunomodulating agents, a variety of laboratory assays are currently being used such as HIV cultures of circulating mononuclear cells, serum p24 antigen levels, drug levels, and the peripheral CD4-positive lymphocyte number.[10–12] The utility of any of these markers for predicting efficacy or avoiding toxicity is currently being assessed. The optimal laboratory parameters to follow are likely to change rapidly as technology becomes increasingly sophisticated. The ultimate criteria for the efficacy of any agent are not laboratory parameters, however, but are objective clinical markers showing improved quality or duration of survival.

Zidovudine (AZT) inhibits HIV replication in vitro at concentrations greater than 0.1 μmol (greater than 0.37 μg/ml), while uninfected lymphocytes or bone marrow progenitor cells are inhibited by concentrations of about 0.9 μmol[13–15] (see also Chapter 34). Zidovudine has little or no known direct activity against the common opportunistic pathogens associated with

TABLE 1. Examples of Antiretroviral and Immunomodulating Agents Undergoing Clinical Trials as Therapy for AIDS

Antiretroviral Agents	*Immunomodulating Agents*
Zidovudine (AZT)	Interferon-α
Dideoxycytidine (DDC)	Interferon-γ
Dideoxyinosine (DDI)	Interleukin-2 (IL-2)
Dideoxyadenosine (DDA)	Interferon-β
3′-deoxy-2′,3′-didehydrothymidine (D4T)	Isoprinosine
AL721	Ampligen
Interferon-α	Granulocyte-macrophage colony–stimulating factor
Dextran sulfate	Tumor necrosis factor
Intravenous immunoglobulin	Methionine enkephalin
Soluble CD4	Imreg
Antisense oligonucleosides	AS101
Ribavirin	

AIDS. Zidovudine is converted by a cellular thymidine kinase to a monophosphate form and ultimately into a triphosphate form that inhibits HIV reverse transcriptase about 100 times more effectively than mammalian polymerases. Zidovudine is available as an oral drug and as an investigational intravenous preparation. The oral drug is rapidly absorbed. Chronic administration of 250 mg every 4 hours results in peak and trough levels of 0.62 and 0.16 μg/ml, respectively.[15–17] The mean half-life is about 1 hour, and metabolism occurs primarily by hepatic glucuronidation, with total urinary recovery of about 90 percent. The drug penetrates the blood-brain barrier. Antiviral concentrations can be obtained in cerebrospinal fluid (CSF) when oral doses of 200–250 mg q4h are given.[15]

A multicenter, placebo-controlled trial of zidovudine (250 mg orally every 4 hours) was completed in 1986 with 282 patients who had either AIDS (first episode of *Pneumocystis* pneumonia within the preceding 120 days) or symptomatic AIDS-related complex (ARC).[16,17] Significant differences between the zidovudine- and placebo-treated patients were found in terms of the occurrences of opportunistic infections and deaths in both the AIDS and ARC patients. In the placebo-treated group, 19 patients died as compared with only 1 who was treated with zidovudine, and 45 opportunistic infections occurred in the placebo-treated group as compared with 24 opportunistic infections in the zidovudine-treated group.

Indicators of improved general clinical status such as increased body weight and higher Karnofsky performance status were also noted in zidovudine recipients. Psychometric testing demonstrated that zidovudine-treated patients showed significant cognitive improvement when compared with placebo-treated patients.[18,19] This improvement was often noted during the first 1–3 weeks of therapy. On the basis of this trial, zidovudine was licensed by the Food and Drug Administration for the management of patients with HIV infection who have a history of confirmed *Pneumocystis* pneumonia or who are symptomatic and have an absolute peripheral CD4 lymphocyte count of less than 200/mm^3 before therapy is initiated. The dose recommended was 200 mg orally six times per day.

The beneficial effects of zidovudine appear to persist beyond the 6-month period of observation reported in the initial trial, but opportunistic infections and deaths do continue to occur.[20,21] The magnitude of the benefit after the initial 6 months of therapy needs to be more clearly defined. A review of compassionate plea data suggests that sustained benefit is less likely in patients who did not start their zidovudine within 120 days of their episode of *Pneumocystis* pneumonia or in patients with very low peripheral CD4 lymphocyte counts.[20] Preliminary results of one large study of zidovudine for patients who have had a recent episode of *Pneumocystis* pneumonia suggest that, if specific anti-*Pneumocystis* therapy is not administered, a second episode of *Pneumocystis* pneumonia will occur in about 30 percent of patients still taking zidovudine after 6 months and 60 percent of patients still taking zidovudine after 12 months.

Zidovudine also has been shown to have benefit for HIV-infected patients with thrombocytopenia. All 10 patients in one study demonstrated elevations in platelet counts that averaged 54,000/mm^3.[22] Zidovudine may thus be preferable to other treatment modalities for severe HIV-related thrombocytopenia.[22,23] Zidovudine also appears to decrease the size of enlarged lymph nodes, liver, and spleen. Whether such decreases in organomegaly correlate with increased survival remains to be determined. Preliminary studies suggest that zidovudine does not have a major effect on Kaposi sarcoma lesions.

Whether zidovudine produces clinical benefit for other HIV-infected patient populations is not yet certain. It is logical to consider the possibility that zidovudine could improve the quality or duration of survival for asymptomatic patients with high peripheral CD4 lymphocyte counts, patients with Kaposi sarcoma and high or low peripheral CD4-positive lymphocyte counts, or patients with recent sexual or percutaneous or mucosal exposure to HIV. Such studies have not yet been completed and analyzed, however, and thus there are currently no data on which to base treatment recommendations for these patient groups.

The clinical benefit that zidovudine provides for patients with symptomatic AIDS or ARC does not clearly correlate with objective immunologic improvement. Peripheral CD4-positive lymphocyte counts may peak after a month of zidovudine therapy; they rise an average of 90/mm^3 in AIDS patients and 98/mm^3 in ARC patients.[16] The increase persists for only 16–20 weeks in AIDS patients. These modest increases may be more sustained in ARC patients. Other studies assessing patients with better initial immune function have been unable to demonstrate any benefit of zidovudine in terms of CD4-positive lymphocyte counts. Serum IgG and IgM levels diminish during zidovudine therapy, however, which suggests that zidovudine may influence polyclonal B-cell activation.

Zidovudine does have a measurable effect on HIV activity. Serum p24 antigen levels, a marker of the *gag* gene product, decrease during the initial 2–4 weeks of therapy in most antigen-positive patients.[10–12] Most HIV-infected patients remain culture-positive for HIV during zidovudine therapy even if they convert their serum p24 antigen from positive to negative (many HIV-infected patients have no measurable p24 antigen in their serum, however, during long periods of serial study). This suggests that zidovudine induces a decrease in active viral replication as manifested by a decrease in p24 antigen but that the drug has no effect on latent or slowly replicating virus. It may also be that zidovudine has only incomplete or intermittent antiviral activity. It is important to note that some patients who show an initial antiviral response may manifest rising serum p24 levels after many months of zidovudine therapy. Whether this represents the development of drug resistance or an alteration in zidovudine pharmacokinetics over time remains to be determined.

Zidovudine therapy has been associated with considerable toxicity.[17] Nausea, myalgias, insomnia, and severe headaches were reported substantially more often in zidovudine-treated patients as compared with the placebo-treated group in the initial controlled trial.[17] Occasionally these symptoms can be so severe that dose reduction or discontinuation of zidovudine therapy is necessary. Confusion, anxiety, and tremulousness can also occur, especially when high doses of zidovudine are used.[17,19,20] Zidovudine can also produce a bluish pigmentation in the nail beds of black patients.

The major toxicity of zidovudine is hematologic suppression.[17,20,21] A dose-dependent anemia is the most common effect recognized. During the second week of therapy, a macrocytosis is initially seen. In the initial placebo-controlled zidovudine trial, a 50 percent decrease in the hemoglobin level was seen in 8.4 percent of zidovudine-treated patients as compared with 0.7 percent of control patients.[17] Transfusions were administered to 31 percent of zidovudine recipients but only 11 percent of placebo recipients. Transfusions are usually necessary 6–15 weeks after the initiation of zidovudine therapy. Zidovudine appears to cause anemia by a direct effect on the bone marrow: erythroid hypoplasia or pure red cell aplasia are usually seen without peripheral evidence of hemolysis.[24] Serum erythropoietin levels are usually elevated.[24] A fall in reticulocyte count is usually the earliest predictor of toxicity. Interestingly, those patients who develop a markedly increased mean corpuscular volume are usually those patients who are less likely to develop substantial anemia and require transfusions. Many clinicians provide patients receiving zidovudine with enough transfusions to maintain their hemoglobin levels above 100 g/liter.

Leukopenia and granulocytopenia are also common occurrences in patients treated with zidovudine. A 50 percent decrease in neutrophil counts was seen in 52 percent of zidovudine-treated patients as compared with 10 percent of controls.[17] Complications of granulocytopenia are rarely seen. Thrombocytopenia is not a frequent occurrence due to zidovudine. Platelet counts usually rise even when initial values are above 100,000/mm^3. Toxicity required 45 percent of patients in the placebo-controlled trial to have their dose of zidovudine reduced or suspended.[17] There is little information about the efficacy of doses lower than 200–250 mg orally five times per day, although some European experience suggests that 250 mg orally four times per day has an antiviral effect.[22] It seems logical to use reduced doses of zidovudine rather than no drug at all if full doses cannot be tolerated while further studies are in progress. When the dose of zidovudine is reduced or terminated, an acute meningoencephalitis characterized by fever, headache, and confusion has been reported.[25] This syndrome appears to occur more commonly in patients who had neurologic dysfunction before the institution of zidovudine. This syndrome may remit spontaneously after 5–7 days, although one patient with this syndrome died. How often this syndrome occurs in the setting of a dose reduction is unknown. It has been suggested that the concurrent use of zidovudine and acetaminophen may predispose to toxicity. Patients who have low hemoglobin levels, low CD4 counts, low serum B_{12} levels, and constitutional symptoms are the subpopulation most likely to develop toxicity. Whether acetaminophen really predisposes to toxicity or whether patients who take acetaminophen are those who have symptoms attributable to severe HIV disease for which they coincidentally take acetaminophen has not been delineated. The recommendation to avoid acetaminophen while taking zidovudine is thus based on suggestive but inconclusive evidence.

There are very few data to date concerning how various drugs interact with zidovudine in terms of altering efficacy, toxicity, or pharmacokinetics. Many drugs used to treat opportunistic infections or tumors such as ganciclovir, trimethoprim-sulfamethoxazole, pentamidine, flucytosine, or cyclophosphamide have hematologic toxicities that may be difficult to distinguish from the toxicities of zidovudine or that may produce toxicities that are additive to those of zidovudine. Moreover, drugs such as amphotericin that may alter renal function or drugs such as flucytosine or phenytoin (Dilantin) that may alter hepatic function could alter zidovudine pharmacokinetics. Clinicians need to be aware of these potential interactions when managing HIV-infected patients who are receiving multiple drugs.

An expanding spectrum of agents with antiretroviral properties are being introduced into clinical trials (Table 1). None of these agents other than zidovudine has been proved to produce improved patient longevity. Certain nucleoside analogues such as dideoxycytidine appear to produce decreases in serum p24 antigen levels, although the toxicities of dideoxycytidine require that modifications from the doses used in initial trials be made. Recombinant interferon-α has been shown to reduce serum p24 antigen levels as well as the size of Kaposi sarcoma lesions in two small trials, especially in patients with relatively high CD4 counts.[26,27] Improved immunologic status was not observed to occur. Larger studies with longer follow-up are needed to determine whether recombinant interferon-α can prolong survival. Fatigue, myalgia, weight loss, hepatitis, thrombocytopenia, and leukopenia can occur with the interferon regimens employed in these studies. A reversible cardiomyopathy has also been reported.

OPPORTUNISTIC INFECTIONS

As indicated in Table 2, most opportunistic pathogens that cause disease in HIV-infected patients can be successfully treated with available anti-infective agents.[3,28] The opportunistic pathogens commonly seen in HIV-infected patients can be categorized into two groups: those that may respond to conventional or experimental drugs but have a high likelihood of recurring or relapsing when therapy is discontinued and those for which no therapy currently appears to be effective. The successful management of those opportunistic infections that are treatable depends on (*1*) prompt diagnosis and initiation of therapy before the clinical syndrome is severe, (*2*) recognition that a poor response to therapy may indicate that a pathogen other than the one initially identified may have been present or may have developed subsequently and requires additional therapy, and (*3*) recognition that some therapies must be lifelong to prevent relapses or recurrences.

TABLE 2. Therapy for Common Opportunistic Pathogens in HIV-Infected Patients

Pathogens that may respond to therapy but frequently recur or relapse
Pneumocystis carinii
Toxoplasma gondii
Isospora belli
Leishmania donovani
Herpes simplex virus
Varicella-zoster virus
Cytomegalovirus
Candida species
Cryptococcus neoformans
Histoplasma capsulatum
Coccidioides immitis
Salmonella species
Campylobacter species
Shigella species
Mycobacterium tuberculosis
Streptococcus pneumoniae
Pathogens for which no therapy currently appears to be effective
Cryptosproridia
Epstein-Barr virus
Microsporidia
Mycobacterium avium-intracellulare

The management of opportunistic infections in HIV-infected patients differs from management in other patient populations because the natural history of specific processes like *Pneumocystis* pneumonia or cryptococcal meningitis is different from non-AIDS patients, because the tolerance of HIV-infected patients for therapeutic agents such as trimethoprim-sulfamethoxazole or flucytosine may be less than for other patient populations, and because consideration must be given to interactions between the drugs directed against opportunistic pathogens and drugs directed against HIV itself or the immune defect or associated tumors such as the potential interaction between ganciclovir and zidovudine or the potential interaction between interferon-α and zidovudine. When feasible, specific therapy (Table 3) for an identified pathogen is preferable to empirical therapy due to the predilection of AIDS patients to have adverse drug reactions and the prospect that drug interactions may present management problems for a population that is often taking many drugs chronically.

PNEUMOCYSTIS PNEUMONIA

The likelihood that an AIDS patient will survive an episode of *Pneumocystis* pneumonia (see also Chapter 256) depends on the severity of pulmonary dysfunction at the time therapy is initiated, the patient's ability to tolerate available regimens, and the severity of the patient's immunologic dysfunction. A poor prognosis correlates with an alveolar–arterial gradient greater than 30 mmHg, a severely abnormal chest radiograph, a high number of organisms detected on lavage or biopsy, and an episode that is the second or greater episode rather than a first episode of *Pneumocystis* pneumonia.[29] Thus any drug therapy is more likely to be successful if the patient is having a first episode of *Pneumocystis* pneumonia, if therapy is started at a time when pulmonary dysfunction is mild, and if other severe opportunistic infections are absent. Patients who have been receiving the full recommended dose of zidovudine for at least 6 weeks also appear to have a better prognosis.

TABLE 3. Therapy for Frequent Infectious Diseases in AIDS Patients

Clinical Disease	*Drug*	*Usual Daily Adult Dose*	*Interval between Divided Doses*	*Route*	*Minimum Duration*[a]
Protozoa					
Pneumocystis pneumonia	Trimethoprim-sulfamethoxazole	15–20 mg/kg trimethoprim with 75–100 mg/kg sulfamethoxazole	q6–8h	iv, po	14–21 days
	or				
	Pentamidine isethionate	3–4 mg/kg	qd	iv	14–21 days
	or				
	Trimethoprim-dapsone	1200 mg trimethoprim with 100 mg dapsone	trimethoprim q6h, dapsone qd	po	14–21 days
Toxoplasmosis	Pyrimethamine	75 mg once, then 25 mg	qd	po	28 days
	and				
	Sulfadiazine	4 g	q6h	po	28 days
Cryptosporidiosis	None	—	—	—	—
Fungi					
Oral thrush (*Candida*)	Nystatin or	3×10^6 units	q4h	po	7–10 days
	Ketoconazole	400 mg	q12h	po	7–10 days
Candida esophagitis	Amphotericin B	0.6 mg/kg	qd	iv	7–10 days
	or				
	Ketoconazole	400 mg	q12h	po	7–10 days
Cryptococcosis	Amphotericin B with or without	0.4 mg/kg	qd	iv	42 days
	Flucytosine	150 mg/kg	q6h	po, iv	42 days
Isosporiasis	Trimethoprim	640 mg	q6h	po	7–10 days
	and				
	Sulfamethoxazole	3200 mg	q6h	po	7–10 days
Viruses					
Mucocutaneous herpes simplex	Acyclovir	15 mg/kg	q8h	iv, po	7 days
Disseminated herpes zoster	Acyclovir	30 mg/kg	q8h	iv	7 days
CMV	Ganciclovir or	10 mg/kg	q12h	iv	21 days
	Foscarnet	180 mg/kg	q8h	iv	21 days
Bacteria					
Mycobacterium avium-intracellulare	None	—	—	—	—
Mycobacterium tuberculosis	INH and	300 mg	q24h	po, im	9 mon
	Rifampin and	600 mg	q24h	po, iv	9 mon
	Ethambutol	15 mg/kg	q24h	po	9 mon

[a] Before the maintenance regimen.

Trimethoprim-sulfamethoxazole and parenteral pentamidine isethionate are effective agents for the treatment of *Pneumocystis* pneumonia in AIDS patients.[30,31] The survival rate for all patients treated with these two regimens is about 75 percent. The survival rate for certain AIDS populations such as patients with first episodes of *Pneumocystis* pneumonia, no serious concomitant opportunistic infections, and an alveolar–arterial gradient less than 30 mmHg is probably better than 90 percent.[29–31] Intravenous trimethoprim-sulfamethoxazole, oral trimethoprim-sulfamethoxazole, oral trimethoprim-dapsone, and parenteral pentamidine are all probably equally effective. Oral trimethoprim-sulfamethoxazole is the regimen of choice for most clinicians because of the convenience of administration, the high degree of efficacy, and the manageability of associated toxicities. There is no clear reason to prefer intravenous over oral trimethoprim-sulfamethoxazole in compliant patients with no obvious gastrointestinal dysfunction. Monitoring serum drug concentrations is probably more useful for managing toxicity than for maximizing efficacy. Peak serum sulfamethoxazole levels should probably be maintained at 100–150 μg/ml. The major disadvantages of trimethoprim-sulfamethoxazole and parenteral pentamidine are that they are less than 100 percent effective and adverse reactions are frequent.[30–32] Adverse reactions can occur in 50–100 percent of AIDS patients treated with trimethoprim-sulfamethoxazole or parenteral pentamidine. Because adverse reactions are so common and because *Pneumocystis* is responsible for only about 40–60 percent of the pulmonary syndromes that present in this population, empirical therapy is less desirable than is the establishment of a specific diagnosis followed by the institution of specific therapy.

For trimethoprim-sulfamethoxazole, common adverse reactions include skin rash, granulocytopenia, transaminase elevations, nephritis, nausea, and vomiting (see Chapter 29). These adverse reactions do not invariably require discontinuation of trimethoprim-sulfamethoxazole therapy.[33] The skin rashes, which commonly occur between the 8th and 12th days of therapy, may be limited in extent and associated with a degree of pruritus that the patient can tolerate for 21 days. Life-threatening mucocutaneous sloughing such as the Stevens-Johnson syndrome are extraordinarily rare in AIDS patients, although a few fatal cases have been reported. Thus, the development of a rash associated with trimethoprim-sulfamethoxazole therapy is not necessarily an indication to discontinue this drug regimen. Granulocytopenia appears to be a dose-related phenomenon that may resolve partially or completely if the dose of trimethoprim-sulfamethoxazole is reduced by 25 percent.[33] Granulocytopenia only rarely responds to leucovorin administration. Nausea and vomiting can be troublesome complications of trimethoprim-sulfamethoxazole therapy: severe nausea may be due to very high sulfonamide levels and may improve if the dose is reduced. Clinical hepatitis is less often a clinically important complication of trimethoprim-sulfamethoxazole therapy. Transaminase levels may fluctuate until therapy is stopped; however, at which time they usually return promptly to baseline values. Overall, adverse reactions have in the past required discontinuation of trimethoprim-sulfamethoxazole therapy in about 25 percent of cases. Although it has not been proved by a prospective study, adverse reactions can probably be reduced without sacrificing efficacy by lowering the recommended dose of trimethoprim-sulfamethoxazole from trimethoprim, 20 mg/kg/day, with sulfamethoxazole, 100 mg/kg/day, to trimethoprim, 15 mg/kg/day, with sulfamethoxazole, 75 mg/kg/day.[33]

Parenteral pentamidine is effective therapy for *Pneumocystis* pneumonia (see Chapter 36). This regimen is inconvenient to administer, however, and the adverse reactions associated with it can be life-threatening. Renal dysfunction, hypoglycemia, hyperglycemia, granulocytopenia, and hypotension are reported in 10–50 percent of patients.[30,31,33] For many years pentamidine was administered intramuscularly because early reports had described fatal hypotension when the drug was given intravenously. Intramuscular administration of pentamidine is no longer recommended except in unusual circumstances, however, because the intramuscular injections are often associated with painful sterile abscesses that can also become superinfected. Moreover, the hypotension originally associated with intravenous pentamidine was probably related to the rate of infusion. When pentamidine is administered over a 60-minute period in 100–150 ml of dextrose in water, clinically important hypotension is unusual. The renal dysfunction associated with pentamidine can be severe. If the serum creatinine level rises by more than 1.0–2.0 mg/dl, strong consideration should be given to withholding therapy for a few days or switching to an alternative agent. Hypoglycemia can be a life-threatening complication of pentamidine therapy and occurs at any juncture during therapy or after therapy has been completed.[34] Hypoglycemia occurs more frequently in patients who also develop renal dysfunction due to pentamidine. The unpredictability of the hypoglycemia adds an element of danger to the inpatient or outpatient use of this drug. Life-threatening hypoglycemia is sufficiently uncommon, however, that this effective agent is still recommended for trimethoprim-sulfamethoxazole–intolerant or trimethoprim-dapsone intolerant patients. Toxicity may be reduced without sacrificing efficacy by lowering the dose of parenteral pentamidine from 4 to 3 mg/kg/day.[33,35]

The relapse rate after conventional therapy with trimethoprim-sulfamethoxazole or parenteral pentamidine is about 60 percent per 12 months for AIDS patients receiving zidovudine but no specific anti-*Pneumocystis* prophylaxis. The likelihood of a relapse cannot be predicted from clinical features of an episode or the rate of response to acute therapy. Every patient who completes a course of therapy for *Pneumocystis* pneumonia and every patient whose CD4 count is less than 200/mm^3, especially those with oral candidiasis or fever, should receive anti-*Pneumocystis* prophylaxis.

There are several investigational therapies that show promise for the treatment of *Pneumocystis* pneumonia in AIDS patients. Aerosolized pentamidine isethionate has been used successfully to treat some patients with mild to moderately severe disease.[35,36] Since *Pneumocystis* is almost always confined to the lungs, this therapy has the virtue of delivering high concentrations of drug to the target organ with little systemic absorption and little serious toxicity when compared with intravenous administrations. The delivery of pentamidine to the lungs depends on the particle size generated by the specific nebulizer used as well as the tubing length, the baffles, and the patient's ventilatory pattern. Aerosol delivery may not provide optimal drug concentrations in the upper lobes. Since this delivery system was designed to avoid substantial serum concentrations of pentamidine, it will also be important to determine whether extrapulmonary *Pneumocystis* becomes a substantially more common occurrence in patients treated only by the aerosol route. Cases of disseminated *Pneumocystis* infection with involvement of multiple visceral organs, skin, and lymph nodes have been reported in patients who were receiving aerosol pentamidine prophylaxis and in patients who had been receiving no prophylaxis at all. Toxicity of aerosolized pentamidine has been uncommon and consists primarily of reversible bronchospasm, especially in smokers. Hypoglycemia has also been reported. Where aerosolized pentamidine will fit into the anti-*Pneumocystis* armamentarium remains to be determined by controlled trials comparing this promising therapy with conventional approaches.

Dapsone (100 mg po qd) plus trimethoprim (5 mg/kg po q6h or 300 mg po q6h) appears to be as effective as trimethoprim-sulfamethoxazole but less toxic in limited experience.[37] Skin rashes are very common among AIDS patients treated with dapsone, but a 21-day course of therapy can usually be completed without interruption. This regimen may therefore be preferable to trimethoprim-sulfamethoxazole because of the reduced toxicity. Dapsone alone has some efficacy when 100 mg po qd is used for 21 days, but higher doses may be necessary to achieve a satisfactory response rate. Whether higher doses would be well tolerated remains to be determined.

Trimetrexate is a potent inhibitor of dihydrofolate reductase that is effective therapy against *Pneumocystis* pneumonia when used either alone (30–45 mg/m^2 iv qd) or in combination with a sulfonamide.[38] Since trimetrexate inhibits the dihydrofolate reductase of human cells as well as the enzyme of *Pneumocystis*, it must be given in conjunction with high-dose leucovorin (20 mg/kg iv or po q6h), which rescues mammalian cells without diminishing the anti-*Pneumocystis* effect. Trimetrexate appears to be well tolerated. Reversible leukopenia is its major adverse effect. The efficacy of trimetrexate as compared with trimethoprim-sulfamethoxazole is being assessed by controlled trials. It remains to be documented whether or not any very potent dihydrofolate reductase inhibitor such as trimetrexate (or piritrexim, a structurally similar compound) can be as effective as a combination regimen that includes a dihydrofolate reductase inhibitor plus a sulfonamide or sulfone. At this juncture it is uncertain to what extent the sulfonamide contributes to efficacy when dihydrofolate reductase inhibitors are used in conjunction with sulfonamides in regimens such as trimethoprim-sulfamethoxazole, pyrimethamine-sulfadiazine, or trimetrexate-sulfadiazine. The relapse rate after trimetrexate therapy is high: 40–60 percent of patients relapse within the first 60 days if no prophylactic regimen is employed.

Difluoromethylornithine (DFMO), an inhibitor of polyamine synthesis, and primaquine-clindamycin have been used to treat AIDS patients with *Pneumocystis* pneumonia, but there are currently inadequate data to assess their potential roles. Corticosteroids have been advocated as an adjunct to conventional anti-*Pneumocystis* agents for patients who present with substantial pulmonary dysfunction, but the results of trials comparing such a regimen to conventional therapies are not yet available.[39]

When an AIDS patient with *Pneumocystis* pneumonia fails to improve when receiving conventional therapy, there are no controlled data to indicate what modifications in therapy are optimal. The mean time to improvement for AIDS patients treated with conventional therapy is 5–6 days, so patients should probably not be considered therapeutic failures until they have received 7–10 days of therapy.[30,31] Clinicians often feel compelled to alter therapy earlier, however, especially if the patient is deteriorating rapidly. If a patient has not improved after 7–10 days of therapy, a repeat diagnostic procedure should be considered to determine whether another treatable pathogen is present. Bronchoscopy with transbronchial biopsies is the procedure of choice since lung tissue is usually necessary to assess the presence of cytomegalovirus (CMV) or perhaps fungal diseases, which are the major diagnostic considerations. *Pneumocystis* will usually be present in lavage or tissue for at least 3–4 weeks after initiating therapy even in patients who respond promptly, so their presence after 7–10 days of therapy does not necessarily imply ineffective therapy. The presence of extensive intra-alveolar exudate after 7–10 days of therapy is probably a more ominous sign. Open lung biopsy should rarely be necessary to supplement bronchoalveolar lavage and transbronchial biopsy given the very high yield of bronchoscopy for most treatable infections. Kaposi sarcoma of the lung is one treatable process that is difficult or impossible to reliably diagnose from transbronchial biopsy specimens. Nodular lesions on chest computed axial tomography (CAT) scan, progressing skin lesions, and the presence of a bloody pleural effusion may be helpful clues.[40]

If *Pneumocystis* is the only identifiable cause of the pulmonary dysfunction after 7–10 days of therapy and the patient has failed to improve, there are several therapeutic alternatives: (*1*) switch from trimethoprim-sulfamethoxazole to parenteral pentamidine or vice versa, (*2*) add corticosteroids to conventional therapy, (*3*) switch to trimetrexate, (*4*) switch to difluoromethylornithine, or (*5*) switch to clindamycin-primaquine. Each of these approaches has been demonstrated to be successful in some cases. A controlled trial is needed to determine the best approach. Whether AIDS patients with *Pneumocystis* pneumonia should be aggressively supported with intensive care, mechanical ventilation, or other interventions is a controversial issue.[7–9] The most reasonable approach would appear to be to individualize each patient in terms of how many days of therapy have been received, what therapeutic alternatives are available, what concomitant processes are present, what the patient's wishes are, and what resources are available. There is published literature indicating that AIDS patients with *Pneumocystis* pneumonia can survive intubation and mechanical ventilation and lead independent lives for several months after hospital discharge.[7–9] The best candidates for intensive care and mechanical ventilation would be those patients presenting with an initial episode of *Pneumocystis* pneumonia and no other serious opportunistic processes, those who have received less than 7 days of therapy, and those who have clearly articulated a desire for aggressive support.

The prevention of *Pneumocystis* pneumonia is a major priority given the high frequency of this life-threatening infection among AIDS patients (at least 65 percent will have one or more episodes) and the high likelihood for a second episode if no prophylaxis is administered after the first episode (about 60 percent over a period of 12 months even if chronic zidovudine therapy is given). Candidate patients especially well-suited for prophylaxis include those who have had an episode of *Pneumocystis* pneumonia (secondary prophylaxis) and those HIV-positive patients who have fewer than 200 circulating CD4-positive cells/mm^3 (primary prophylaxis), especially those with oral candidiasis or fever. The only placebo-controlled trial of prophylaxis for AIDS patients has demonstrated that trimethoprim, 160 mg, with sulfamethoxazole, 800 mg po q12h, plus leucovorin, 5 mg po qd, is highly effective as primary prophylaxis.[41] Adverse reactions occurred in 27 percent of treated patients, but prophylaxis had to be discontinued because of toxicity in only 17 percent. Whether other trimethoprim-sulfamethoxazole regimens employing fewer doses per week would be equally effective (in pediatric cancer patients 3 consecutive days per week are as effective as 7 days per week) remains to be determined. Aerosolized pentamidine is used widely for prophylaxis. Preliminary assessment of ongoing trials suggests a high degree of efficacy and low toxicity when pentamidine is administered according to protocol. How often the *Pneumocystis* disease that does occur during aerosolized pentamidine prophylaxis will be atypical, extrapulmonary, or difficult to treat remains to be determined. Other drugs with potential as prophylactic agents include dapsone, dapsone plus trimethoprim, or pyrimethamine plus sulfadoxine.

TOXOPLASMA GONDII

When an HIV-infected patient with substantial immunodeficiency presents with a space-occupying cerebral lesion that involves gray matter, the differential diagnosis primarily includes toxoplasmosis (see Chapters 36 and 255) and lymphoma.[42–46] Fungal, mycobacterial, and viral processes present as space-occupying lesions only rarely, and progressive multifocal leukoencephalopathy should primarily involve white matter. The definitive diagnostic study (i.e., brain biopsy) has some morbidity associated with it, and the diagnostic yield is often only 50 percent if toxoplasmosis is the etiology. The cysts and tachyzoites of *T. gondii* can be very difficult to recognize in fragments of necrotic brain tissue, and even several small needle biopsy samples may miss the area that has abundant organisms. Since toxoplasmosis is the only common etiology for gray matter lesions that clearly benefits from therapy and because brain needle biopsy has diagnostic limitations, empirical therapy with pyrimethamine (75 mg po the first day followed by 25 mg po qd) and sulfadiazine (1–2 g po q6h) is reasonable. Some clinicians use higher doses of both drugs, but there is no clear evidence that higher doses are more effective, and they almost certainly produce more toxicity. If there is not unequivocal improvement by clinical and radiologic criteria within 14–21 days, a biopsy should be performed to establish whether the etiology is an infectious or neoplastic process other than toxoplasmosis.[42–44] Corticosteroids to reduce inflammation may be necessary in patients with substantial or progressive neurologic dysfunction or signs of increased intracranial pressure. The administration of corticosteroids may make evaluation of the clinical and radiologic response to specific therapy difficult since the observed improvement may be solely due to corticosteroid therapy and may be unrelated to the anti-*Toxoplasma* regimen employed. Chronic antiseizure medication should routinely be instituted. For patients who do respond, anti-*Toxoplasma* therapy should be continued for life since relapses do occur in the same sites as those presenting initially if therapy is discontinued, even after 8–12 months.[44] Whether the chronic suppressive regimen will be as effective if both pyrimethamine and sulfadiazine are not included at full doses remains to be demonstrated.

Treatment failures are very unusual for patients with toxoplasmosis who are able to tolerate both pyrimethamine and sulfadiazine.[45] Radiologically proven failures in patients who are unequivocally taking their drugs should raise the possibility that toxoplasmosis is not the correct diagnosis. Adverse reactions to sulfadiazine (leukopenia, rash, elevated transaminase level, nausea, nephritis) and to pyrimethamine (leukopenia, thrombocytopenia) are common. The leukopenia often will not respond to leucovorin therapy, although a short course of leucovorin (10–20 mg po or iv q6h) should be attempted. There are no alternative regimens that are clearly effective for patients who cannot tolerate both pyrimethamine and sulfadiazine. Alternatives that are currently being assessed include higher doses of pyrimethamine alone (50–150 mg po qd with or without leucovorin), clindamycin, clindamycin plus pyrimethamine, dapsone plus pyrimethamine, trimetrexate, and spiramycin. Clindamycin (intravenous three times daily) plus pyrimethamine has been effective in some patients and is currently the most promising alternative to pyrimethamine and sulfadiazine. Oral clindamycin plus pyrimethamine may not be as effective as intravenous clindamycin plus pyrimethamine.

HERPES SIMPLEX AND VARICELLA-ZOSTER VIRUS INFECTIONS

Acyclovir (200 mg po q4h) is very effective therapy for herpes simplex viral perirectal lesions, proctitis, oral lesions, digital lesions, and esophagitis (see Chapters 34, 118, and 119).[47] Disseminated herpes simplex viral infections almost never occur in HIV-infected patients. Intravenous therapy is rarely necessary unless the patient has a major gastrointestinal disorder that prevents oral absorption. Topical acyclovir has not been demonstrated to be effective in AIDS patients. Acyclovir-resistant disease or acyclovir-resistant isolates have been very uncommon. The response of herpes simplex lesions is usually prompt and occurs within 3–10 days. Therapy should continue until the lesions are crusted over or epithelialized. Relapses occur with high frequency. If relapses occur quickly or often, therapy may have to be continuous for life. Whether daily doses lower than those used for therapy would be adequate prophylaxis has not been determined. Some therapeutic benefits of the combination of zidovudine plus acyclovir have been suggested but need to be confirmed in larger trials.

Dermatomal herpes zoster does not usually need to be treated in HIV-infected patients because dissemination of the virus has rarely followed.[48] Local involvement in more than one dermatome is seen. Even when extensive disseminated cutaneous lesions have been observed, however, clinically apparent visceral disease has rarely been documented. Whether acyclovir therapy has any role in hastening the crusting of lesions or in preventing recurrences in HIV-infected patients is not known. Patients with persistent or recurrent lesions or zoster ophthalmicus might be logical candidates for high-dose oral acyclovir (400–800 mg po q4h). Whether acyclovir is beneficial in decreasing the severity or duration of post-herpetic neuralgia has not been determined. Corticosteroid therapy to prevent post-herpetic neuralgia is not recommended in AIDS patients because of the potentially adverse effect of corticosteroids on immune function and on Kaposi sarcoma activity.

CYTOMEGALOVIRUS

Cytomegalovirus infection (see Chapters 34 and 120) is almost universal among HIV-infected patients as assessed by serology. HIV-infected patients with fewer than 100–200 circulating CD4 cells are often viremic and viruric with CMV, but only a few of these patients develop specific organ damage that needs to be treated. Retinitis is the most commonly recognized disorder caused by CMV.[49] Cytomegalovirus retinitis has the potential to rapidly involve the macula and optic disk and result in visual impairment and ultimately in blindness. When lesions are recognized close to the macula or disk or when extensive lesions are present, therapy is warranted. Whether patients benefit from prompt treatment of peripheral lesions rather than close observation until the lesions progress remains to be determined. Cytomegalovirus retinitis responds to either ganciclovir (DHPG) administered at a dose of 5 mg/kg iv q12h or foscarnet (phosphonoformate) at 60 mg/kg iv q8h.[49–56] Empirical therapy without a specific histologic or virologic diagnosis is reasonable since obtaining retinal or vitreous material for examination is risky (detached retinas or secondary infection may result), the ophthalmologic appearance of CMV retinitis is quite characteristic to an experienced ophthalmologist, and CMV causes almost all the retinitis that occurs in HIV-infected patients.[57] The response to ganciclovir is quite prompt. New lesions or progressive disease may be identified during the first 7 days of therapy and do not necessarily imply a poor response. Considerable improvement in inflammation, edema, and hemorrhage will be recognized in responders before the end of 21 days of therapy. Without maintenance suppressive therapy, relapse at the same site as the initial lesions and at new sites almost invariably occurs within a few weeks or months. Maintenance regimens using ganciclovir, 5–6 mg/kg iv qd 5–7 days per week, are often administered, but these regimens seem only to prolong the interval until relapse. They do not prevent relapses from occurring. At the time of relapse, patients will usually respond to reinstitution of ganciclovir, 5 mg/kg iv q12h. Ganciclovir's major toxicity is bone marrow suppression with neutropenia and thrombocytopenia. Confusion, nausea, vomiting, transaminase elevation, and inhibition of spermatogenesis also occur. Some AIDS patients will be unable to tolerate parenteral ganciclovir therapy. Intravitreal injections of ganciclovir have been assessed in a few hundred patients. This therapy appears to be effective and relatively safe, although retinal detachment resulting from repeated injections is a concern.[54] When patients with sight threatening CMV lesions become neutropenic due to ganciclovir, the clinician and patient must often make a choice between saving vision and accepting neutropenia. When neutropenia occurs during ganciclovir therapy, other infectious, neoplastic, immunologic, and drug-related causes of the neutropenia should be sought. Alternatively, another therapy such as intravitreal ganciclovir or parenteral foscarnet may be tried. Foscarnet has in vitro and clinical antiviral activity against CMV.[55,56] It also has activity against HIV. This drug is nephrotoxic but not bone marrow toxic. Its efficacy, as determined in much more limited trials, appears to be generally similar to that of ganciclovir. Acyclovir, even in high doses, has not convincingly been shown to have anti-CMV activity.

Esophagitis, enteritis, colitis, and pneumonitis are life-threatening syndromes caused by CMV that have been documented to respond to ganciclovir therapy.[50,51,53,58,59] For these syndromes, a specific diagnosis should be established by histology since the syndromes are indistinguishable from those caused by other pathogens if clinical criteria alone are used. Culture of CMV from tissue or secretions or excretions is probably too nonspecific to be used as a basis for therapy.

For patients with esophagitis, colitis, or rectal ulcers, improvement in clinical symptoms is usually noted during the first week of therapy. Improved performance status and increased weight is often noted, especially if therapy results in less dysphagia or less diarrhea. There is considerably less experience with ganciclovir therapy for CMV pneumonia. There are reports of successful therapy for CMV pneumonia in a patient with AIDS.[50] There is no consensus about the specific criteria for establishing the diagnosis, however, and some patients who failed ganciclovir therapy had very severe lung damage before ganciclovir treatment was started. Ganciclovir therapy alone has not been reported to be effective in bone marrow transplant recipients unless immune serum globulin or hyperimmune globulin is given concurrently.[60,61] How often ganciclovir will be effective in AIDS patients either alone or in conjunction with immunoglobulin remains to be determined.

EPSTEIN BARR VIRUS

Epstein Barr virus (EBV) (see Chapter 121) can be cultivated from the oropharynx and peripheral mononuclear cells of a substantial proportion of AIDS patients. This virus has been implicated in the pathogenesis of hairy leukoplakia and may have a role in the pathogenesis of nonspecific pneumonitis, lymphadenopathy, lymphoma, fever, or wasting. There is insufficient evidence to warrant specific therapy for EBV at this point, nor is there a drug that would clearly be effective.

PROGRESSIVE MULTIFOCAL LEUKOENCEPHALOPATHY

Progressive multifocal leukoencephalopathy (see Chapter 124) is caused by JC and SV-40 viruses. No therapy is known to be effective. Management should consist of early diagnosis so that arrangements for appropriate supportive care can be made.

CANDIDA SPECIES

Stomatitis, esophagitis, vaginitis, and proctitis due to *Candida* species (see Chapters 33 and 235) will respond to topical therapy (nystatin or clotrimazole), oral therapy (ketoconazole or fluconazole), or intravenous therapy (amphotericin B).[62,63] Ketoconazole (200 mg po q12h) is often the most convenient regimen, although the longer half-life for the investigational agent fluconazole may make this agent more convenient. There is usually no urgency to institute amphotericin B for any of these disorders: esophagitis is rarely associated with bleeding, perforation, fungemia, or disseminated fungal disease. Stomatitis, esophagitis, and proctitis often recur when therapy is discontinued. Ketoconazole administration may thus have to be continued for life. Occasional patients who do not respond to topical or oral therapy, especially those who are extremely debilitated or immunosuppressed, may respond to amphotericin B.

Disseminated candidiasis is not a common occurrence in AIDS patients unless they are receiving drug therapy that makes them neutropenic (especially cytotoxic antineoplastic therapy) or they have an infected intravenous catheter. Treatment is similar to that in other patient populations, with particular attention directed at removing infected intravenous lines or discontinuing therapies that may be producing neutropenia.

CRYPTOCOCCUS NEOFORMANS, HISTOPLASMA CAPSULATUM, COCCIDIOIDES IMMITIS

Cryptococcosis (see Chapters 241, 242, 244, and 33) is very difficult to cure in patients with AIDS. Even among those responding to therapy, relapse is usual.[64–66] Isolation of *Cryptococcus neoformans* from any body fluid is diagnostic and should prompt a careful assessment to determine the extent of dissemination. Culture of CSF, blood, and urine as well as a determination of the serum and CSF antigen titers are useful. The lysis–centrifugation technique is superior to other methods for isolating *C. neoformans* from blood.

The therapy of choice for cryptococcosis in AIDS is amphotericin B, 0.4–0.6 mg/kg daily or double that dose on alternate days. It is not known in this group of patients whether flucytosine can be used to permit a reduced dose of amphotericin B. The common occurrence of worsening hepatic or bone marrow function during flucytosine therapy makes this drug difficult to use in AIDS patients.

Almost all patients with cryptococcosis are switched from intensive to long-term, intermittent amphotericin B at some point in therapy, but that point remains to be defined, as does the optimum maintenance regimen.[64–66] One strategy is to continue daily or alternate-day therapy until at least 2.0–2.5 g of amphotericin B have been received and until cultures have become negative. At that juncture, treatment with amphotericin B, 1.0 mg/kg one to three times per week, is often chosen. It is probably unrealistic to continue intensive therapy until the CSF smears and antigen titers are negative because that goal is rarely attainable.

Oral fluconazole is being evaluated in a multicenter trial for maintenance suppressive therapy in cryptococcal meningitis. There is early evidence that this drug may be useful not only in the maintenance but also in acute treatment of some patients with cryptococcosis.[67–69]

Disseminated histoplasmosis in AIDS patients has not responded to ketoconazole and has often relapsed after treatment with amphotericin B.[70,71] Maintenance daily ketoconazole or weekly intravenous amphotericin B has been used to prevent relapse. Disseminated coccidioidomycoses in AIDS patients have proved difficult to control even with amphotericin B.[72]

MYCOBACTERIUM SPECIES

Mycobacterium avium-intracellulare (see Chapters 32, 229, and 231) is a common pathogen among HIV-infected patients, but what role this organism plays in contributing to morbidity or mortality is uncertain. A variety of antimicrobial agents have some activity against *Mycobacterium avium-intracellulare*, including ansamycin (rifabutin), clofazimine, imipenem, various quinolones, amikacin, cycloserine, pyrazinamide, and ethambutol.[73–75] Isoniazid and rifampin rarely have in vitro activity. There has been no convincing in vivo evidence that any antimicrobial regimen has clinical or microbiologic effect.[75–77] All therapeutic regimens must therefore be considered to be experimental.

Mycobacterium tuberculosis isolates from AIDS patients appear to be identical to isolates from other patients in terms of susceptibility to antimicrobacterial drugs. A regimen of isoniazid (300 mg po qd), rifampin (600 mg po qd), and ethambutol (15 mg/kg/day po) for 9 months (and a minimum of 6 months after cultures become negative) is recommended, although lifelong therapy may be more prudent.[78]

ENTERIC PATHOGENS: SALMONELLA SPECIES, SHIGELLA SPECIES, CAMPYLOBACTER SPECIES, ENTAMEBA HISTOLYTICA, GIARDIA LAMBLIA, CRYPTOSPORIDIA, ISOSPORA BELLI, MICROSPORIDIA

When *Salmonella* species, *Shigella* species, and *Campylobacter* species cause persistent diarrhea, severe diarrhea, or bacteremic disease, therapy is indicated. The antimicrobial susceptibility of these pathogens does not appear to differ from that in other patients.[79–82] Appropriate antibiotic therapy will usually control the bacteremia or diarrhea, but eradication of the organism can often not be accomplished. Chronic suppressive regimens with quinolones, trimethoprim-sulfamethoxazole, erythromycin, or ampicillin may be necessary (depending on the specific isolate), often in conjunction with antimotility drugs.

Amebiasis and giardiasis in AIDS patients do not appear to be associated with any more severe disease than that seen in HIV-negative homosexual men. Therapy can thus follow routine guidelines.

Cryptosporidia can cause severe gastrointestinal or biliary disease, but there is no specific therapy for it (see Chapter 261). Spiramycin does not appear to be effective. Antimotility drugs are often useful. Total parenteral nutrition may benefit patients who are becoming debilitated due to severe diarrhea if the patient and health care team deem this type of intervention to be appropriate.

Isospora belli (see Chapter 260) responds to trimethoprim-sulfamethoxazole (trimethoprim, 160 mg, plus sulfamethoxazole, 800 mg po q6h for 7–10 days), but the relapse rate is high and necessitates chronic suppression with trimethoprim-sulfamethoxazole.[83,84] Metronidazole, quinacrine, or pyrimethamine may be alternatives for patients with severe intolerance to trimethoprim-sulfamethoxazole.

TREPONEMA PALLIDUM

Syphilis is often recognized in HIV-infected patients either because of characteristic lesions of primary or secondary disease or because a screening serology for *T. pallidum* (see also Chapter 213) is positive. It is becoming increasingly apparent that, in patients with primary and secondary syphilis, central nervous system involvement is more common than was previously thought.[85,86] As many as 40 percent of patients with primary or secondary syphilis will have serologic or microbiologic evidence of *T. pallidum* in their cerebrospinal fluid regardless of their HIV status if careful diagnostic studies are employed.[83] It is also becoming increasingly apparent that, in HIV-infected patients with primary, secondary, or latent syphilis, a single dose of 2.4 mIU benzathine penicillin may be inadequate to cure the central nervous system or to prevent systemic relapses as measured by subsequent rises in serum VDRL titers. The optimal treatment for HIV-infected patients with early or latent syphilis is not established: procaine penicillin (1.2 mIU daily for 10–14 days) may be preferred over serial doses of benzathine penicillin (2.4 mIU every week for 3 or 4 weeks).[87]

KAPOSI SARCOMA

Although Kaposi sarcoma can often involve extensive areas of skin and mucous membranes on physical examination and although postmortem examination may reveal many visceral lesions, Kaposi sarcoma does not directly cause death in most patients with this tumor.[4–6] Kaposi sarcoma can cause cosmetically unpleasant lesions such as those on the face or hands, and Kaposi sarcoma can cause painful lesions such as those overlying joints or on the sole of the feet. Kaposi sarcoma lesions can also become impressively extensive. Most patients with Kaposi sarcoma ultimately die of opportunistic infections. Thus a major principal of therapy for this tumor is to avoid potentially toxic therapeutic modalities until the bulk of the tumor is extensive or until a vital organ is compromised.

When patients have individual lesions that are unattractive or painful or when lymphatic obstruction causes extensive lower extremity edema, radiation therapy may be beneficial.[88,89] Kaposi sarcoma lesions tend to recur despite intensive radiation therapy. When the oropharynx is radiated, mucositis seems to be especially common.

When cutaneous Kaposi sarcoma is extensive, recombinant interferon-α therapy (10–30 million units/m^2 im, iv, or sc qd) can be useful, especially for patients with circulating CD4 counts greater than 100–200/mm^3.[90–92] Objective tumor responses can be seen in 4–8 weeks, with maximal responses in 12–24 weeks. Late initial responses after many months of therapy occasionally occur. Tumor response may persist for over 1 year, especially when maintenance therapy is given. Because the tumor response is not rapid, interferon-α therapy is not desirable for urgent, life-threatening situations. Adverse effects of interferon-α include confusion, fatigue, myalgias, leukopenia, thrombocytopenia, hepatitis, and cardiomyopathy.

Kaposi sarcoma can cause life-threatening disease by obstructing a vital structure such as the larynx, bronchus, biliary tract, or bowel. Kaposi sarcoma can occasionally infiltrate a vital organ such as the lung and cause fatal hypoxemia. In these life-threatening situations, either radiation therapy or cytotoxic chemotherapy is necessary to produce a rapid and substantial response. The optimal mode of therapy depends on the location and extent of tumor. In appropriate clinical settings, short-term palliation of life-threatening symptoms rather than long-term survival is the therapeutic goal, and thus the immunosuppressive nature of some therapies is not the overriding concern. A variety of chemotherapeutic regimens have been used with some success including vinblastine; etoposide; vincristine; vincristine and vinblastine; vinblastine and bleomycin; doxorubicin, bleomycin, and vincristine.[93,94] The optimal drug regimen for specific situations has not been determined.

Lymphomas of the Hodgkin, non-Hodgkin, and Burkitt types generally are associated with short patient survival regardless of the therapeutic modality chosen. A variety of cytotoxic regimens and irradiation have been used in order to reduce tumor size or palliate specific syndromes such as neurologic dysfunction caused by central nervous system lesions. The response rate has been lower in AIDS patients than in non-AIDS patients, and relapses have been prompt and frequent.[46,95] Whether any regimen prolongs survival and which regimen is optimal have not yet been determined. Patients die as a direct result of lymphoma, as a result of AIDS-related infections, and as a result of chemotherapy-associated infections.

REFERENCES

1. Rothenberg R, Woelfel M, Stoneburner R, et al. Survival with the acquired immunodeficiency syndrome: Experience with 5833 cases in New York City. N Engl J Med. 1987;317:1297–302.
2. Bacchetti P, Osmond D, Chaisson RE, et al. Survival patterns of the first 500 patients with AIDS in San Francisco. J Infect Dis. 1988;157:1044–7.
3. Sande MA, Volberding PA, eds. The Medical Management of AIDS. Philadelphia: WB Saunders; 1988.
4. Moskowitz L, Hensley GT, Chen JC, et al. Immediate causes of death in acquired immunodeficiency syndrome. Arch Pathol Lab Med. 1985;109:735–8.
5. Niedt GW, Schinella RA. Acquired immunodeficiency syndrome. Clinicopathologic study of 56 autopsies. Arch Pathol Lab Med. 1985;109:727–34.
6. Welch K, Finkbeiner W, Alpers C, et al. Autopsy findings in the acquired immune deficiency syndrome. JAMA. 1984;252:1152–9.
7. Lo B, Raffin TA, Cohen NH, et al. Ethical dilemmas about intensive care for patients with AIDS. Rev Infect Dis. 1987;9:1163–7.
8. El Sadr W, Simberkoff M. Survival and prognostic factors in severe *Pneumocystis carinii* pneumonia requiring mechanical ventilation. Am Rev Respir Dis. 1988;137:1264–7.
9. Rogers PL, Lane HC, Henderson DK, et al. Admissions of AIDS patients to a medical intensive care unit: Cause and outcome. Crit Care Med. 1989;17:113–7.
10. Jackson GG, Paul DA, Falk LA, et al. Human immunodeficiency virus (HIV) antigenemia (p24) in the acquired immunodeficiency syndrome and the effect of treatment with zidovudine (AZT). Ann Intern Med. 1988;108:175–80.
11. De Wolf F, Gaudsmit J, DeGans J, et al. Effect of zidovudine on serum human immunodeficiency virus antigen levels in symptom free subjects. Lancet. 1988;1:373–6.
12. Chaisson RE, Leuther MD, Allain JP, et al. Effect of zidovudine on serum human immunodeficiency virus core antigen levels. Arch Intern Med. 1988;148:2151–3.
13. Mitsuya H, Weinhold KJ, Furman PA, et al. 3′-Azido-3′-deoxythymidine (BW A509U): An antiviral agent that inhibits the infectivity and cytopathic effect of human T lymphotropic virus type III 1 (lymphadenopathy associated virus) in vitro. Proc Natl Acad Sci USA. 1985;82:7096–100.
14. Sommadossi JP, Carlisle R. Toxicity of 3′-azido-3′-deoxythymidine and 9-(1,3-dihydroxy-2-propoxymethyl) guanine for normal human hematopoietic progenitor cells in vitro. Antimicrob Agents Chemother. 1987;31:452–4.
15. Hirsch MS. Azidothymidine. AIDS commentary. J Infect Dis. 1988;157:427–30.
16. Fischl MA, Richman DD, Grieco MH, et al. The efficacy of azidothymidine (AZT) in the treatment of patients with AIDS and AIDS-related complex. N Engl J Med. 1987;317:185–202.
17. Richman DD, Fischl MA, Grieco MH, et al. The toxicity of azidothymidine (AZT) in the treatment of patients with AIDS and AIDS related complex. A double blind, placebo controlled trial. N Engl J Med. 1987;317:192–7.
18. Schmitt FA, Bigley JW, McKinnis R, et al. Neuropsychologic outcome of zidovudine (AZT) treatment of patients with AIDS and AIDS related complex. N Engl J Med. 1988;319:1573–8.
19. Pizzo PE, Eddy J, Falloon J, et al. Effect of continuous intravenous infusion of zidovudine (AZT) in children with symptomatic HIV infection. N Engl J Med. 1988;319:889–96.
20. Creagh-Kirk T, Doi P, Andrews E, et al. Survival experience among patients with AIDS receiving zidovudine: Follow-up of patients in a compassionate plea program. JAMA. 1988;260:3009–15.
21. Dournon E, Matheron S, Rozenbaum W, et al. Effects of zidovudine in 365 consecutive patients with AIDS or AIDS related complex. Lancet. 1988;2:1297–302.
22. The Swiss Group for Clinical Studies on the Acquired Immunodeficiency Syndrome (AIDS). Zidovudine for the treatment of thrombocytopenia associated with human immunodeficiency virus. Ann Intern Med. 1988;109:718–21.
23. Pottage JC, Benson CA, Spear JB, et al. Treatment of human immunodeficiency virus related thrombocytopenia with zidovudine. JAMA. 1988;260:3045–8.
24. Walker RE, Parker RI, Kovacs JA, et al. Anemia and erythropoiesis in patients with acquired immunodeficiency syndrome (AIDS) and Kaposi sarcoma treated with zidovudine. Ann Intern Med. 1988;108:372–6.
25. Helbert M, Peddle B, Kocsis A, et al. Acute meningoencephalitis on dose reduction of zidovudine. Lancet. 1988;1:1249–52.
26. Lane HC, Kovacs JA, Feinberg J, et al. Antiretroviral effects of interferon-alpha in AIDS associated Kaposi's sarcoma. Lancet. 1988;2:1218–22.
27. De Wit R, Schattenkerk JKME, Boucher CAB, et al. Clinical and virologic effects of high dose recombinant interferon alpha in disseminated AIDS related Kaposi's sarcoma. Lancet. 1988;2:1214–7.
28. Glatt AE, Chirgwin K, Landesman SH. Treatment of infections associated with human immunodeficiency virus. Current concepts. N Engl J Med. 1988;3189:1439–48.
29. Brenner M, Ognibene FP, Lack EE, et al. Prognostic factors and life expectancy of acquired immunodeficiency syndrome patients with *Pneumocystis carinii* pneumonia. Am Rev Respir Dis. 1987;136:1199–206.
30. Kovacs JA, Hiemenz JW, Macher AM, et al. *Pneumocystis carinii* pneumonia: A comparison between patients with the acquired immunodeficiency syndrome and patients with other immunodeficiencies. Ann Intern Med. 1984;100:663–71.
31. Wharton JM, Coleman DL, Wofsy CB, et al. Trimethoprim-sulfamethoxazole or pentamidine for *Pneumocystis carinii* pneumonia in the acquired immunodeficiency syndrome. A prospective randomized trial. Ann Intern Med. 1986;195:37–44.
32. Gordin FM, Simon GL, Wofsy CB, et al. Adverse reactions to trimethoprim-sulfamethoxazole in patients with the acquired immunodeficiency syndrome. Ann Intern Med. 1984;100:495–9.
33. Sattler FR, Cowan R, Nielsen DM, et al. Trimethoprim-sulfamethoxazole versus pentamidine for therapy of *Pneumocystis* pneumonia: A prospective non crossover study in patients with AIDS. Ann Intern Med. 1988;109:280–7.
34. Waskin H, Stehr-Green JK, Helmick CG, et al. Risk factors for hypoglycemia associated with pentamidine therapy for *Pneumocystis* pneumonia. JAMA. 1988;260:345–7.
35. Conte JE Jr, Hollander H, Golden JA. Inhaled or reduced dose intravenous pentamidine for *Pneumocystis carinii* pneumonia. A pilot study. Ann Intern Med. 1987;107:495–8.

36. Montgomery AB, Debs RJ, Luce JM, et al. Aerosolised pentamidine as sole therapy for *Pneumocystis carinii* pneumonia in patients with acquired immunodeficiency syndrome. Lancet. 1987;2:480–3.
37. Leoung GS, Mills J, Hopewell PC, et al. Dapsone-trimethoprim for *Pneumocystis carinii* pneumonia in the acquired immunodeficiency syndrome. Ann Intern Med. 1986;105:45–8.
38. Allegra CJ, Chabner BA, Tuazon CU, et al. Trimetrexate for the treatment of *Pneumocystis carinii* pneumonia in patients with acquired immunodeficiency syndrome. N Engl J Med. 1987;317:978–85.
39. MacFadden DK, Edelson JD, Hyland RH, et al. Corticosteroids as adjunctive therapy in treatment of *Pneumocystis carinii* pneumonia in patients with acquired immunodeficiency syndrome. Lancet. 1987;1:1477–9.
40. Ognibene FP, Steis RG, Macher AM, et al. Kaposi's sarcoma causing pulmonary infiltrates and respiratory failure in the acquired immunodeficiency syndrome. Ann Intern Med. 1985;102:471–5.
41. Fischl M, Dickinson GM, LaVoie L. Safety and efficacy of sulfamethoxazole and trimethoprim chemoprophylaxis for *Pneumocystis carinii* pneumonia in AIDS. JAMA. 1988;259:1185–9.
42. Navia BA, Petito CK, Gold JWM, et al. Cerebral toxoplasmosis complicating the acquired immune deficiency syndrome: Clinical and neuropathological findings in 27 patients. Ann Neurol. 1986;19:224–38.
43. Luft BJ, Remington JS. Toxoplasmic encephalitis. AIDS commentary. J Infect Dis. 1988;157:1–6.
44. Wanke C, Tuazon CU, Kovacs JA, et al. *Toxoplasma* encephalitis in patients with acquired immune deficiency syndrome: Diagnosis and response to therapy. Am J Trop Med Hyg. 1987;36:509–16.
45. Leport C, Raffi F, Matheron S, et al. Treatment of central nervous system toxoplasmosis with pyrimethamine/sulfadiazine combination in 35 patients with acquired immunodeficiency syndrome. Efficacy of long term continuous therapy. Am J Med. 1988;84:94–100.
46. So YT, Beckstead JH, Davis RL. Primary central nervous system lymphoma in acquired immunodeficiency syndrome: A clinical and pathological study. Ann Neurol. 1986;20:566–72.
47. Kalb RE, Grossman ME. Chronic perianal herpes simplex in immunocompromised hosts. Am J Med. 1986;80:486–90.
48. Melbye M, Grossman RJ, Goedert JS, et al. Risk of AIDS after herpes zoster. Lancet. 1987;1:728–31.
49. Jacobson MA, Mills J. Serious cytomegalovirus disease in the acquired immunodeficiency syndrome (AIDS): Clinical findings, diagnosis, and treatment. Ann Intern Med. 1988;108:585–94.
50. Masur H, Lane HC, Palestine A, et al. Effect of 9-(1,3-dihydroxy-2-propoxymethyl) guanine on serious cytomegalovirus disease in eight immunosuppressed homosexual men. Ann Intern Med. 1986;104:41–4.
51. Laskin OL, Stahl-Bayliss CM, Kalman CM, et al. Use of ganciclovir to treat serious cytomegalovirus infections in patients with AIDS. J Infect Dis. 1987;155:323–7.
52. Felsenstein D, D'Amico DJ, Hirsch MS, et al. Treatment of cytomegalovirus retinitis with 9-[(2-hydroxy-2-(hydroxymethyl)ethoxymethyl)] guanine. Ann Intern Med. 1985;103:377–80.
53. Collaborative DHPG Treatment Study Group. Treatment of serious cytomegalovirus infections with 9-(1,3-dihydroxy-2-propoxymethyl) guanine in patients with AIDS and other immunodeficiencies. N Engl J Med 1986;314:801–5.
54. Henry K, Cantrill H, Fletcher C, et al. Use of intravitreal ganciclovir (dihydroxy propoxy methyl guanine) for cytomegalovirus retinitis in a patient with AIDS. Am J Ophthalmol. 1987;103:17–23.
55. Jacobson MA, O'Donnell JJ, Mills J. Tolerance and efficacy of intermittent intravenous foscarnet therapy for cytomegalovirus retinitis in AIDS patients (Abstract 7179). In: Proceedings of the Fourth International Conference on AIDS. Stockholm: 1988.
56. Walmsley SL, Chew E, Read SE, et al. Treatment of cytomegalovirus retinitis with trisodium phosphonoformate hexahydrate (foscarnet). J Infect Dis. 1988;157:569–72.
57. Bloom JN, Palestine AG. The diagnosis of cytomegalovirus retinitis. Ann Intern Med. 1988;109:963–9.
58. Chachoua A, Dieterich D, Krasinski K, et al. 9-(1,3-2-Propoxymethyl) guanine (ganciclovir) in the treatment of cytomegalovirus gastrointestinal disease with the acquired immunodeficiency syndrome. Ann Intern Med. 1987;107:133–7.
59. Mansell P, Roston K, Hoy J, et al. Treatment of CMV infections in patients with AIDS or following bone marrow transplantation with DHPG (Abstract). In: Proceedings of the International Conference on AIDS. Paris: 1986:62.
60. Reed EC, Bowden RA, Dandliker PS, et al. Treatment of cytomegalovirus pneumonia with gancyclovir and intravenous cytomegalovirus immunoglobulin in patients with bone marrow transplants. Ann Intern Med. 1988;109:783–8.
61. Emanuel D, Cunningham I, Jules-Elysee K, et al. Cytomegalovirus pneumonia after bone marrow transplantation successfully treated with the combination of gancyclovir and high dose intravenous immune globulin. Ann Intern Med. 1988;109:777–82.
62. Klein RS, Harris CA, Small CB, et al. Oral candidiasis in high-risk patients as the initial manifestation of the acquired immunodeficiency syndrome. N Engl J Med. 1984;311:354–8.
63. Rhoads JL, Wright DC, Redfield RR, et al. Chronic vaginal candidiasis in women with human immunodeficiency virus infection. JAMA. 1987;257:3105–7.
64. Dismukes WE. Cryptococcal meningitis in patients with AIDS. J Infect Dis. 1988;157:624–8.
65. Zuger A, Louie E, Holzman RS, et al. Cryptococcal disease in patients with the acquired immunodeficiency syndrome: Diagnostic features and outcome of treatment. Ann Intern Med. 1986;104:234–40.
66. Kovacs JA, Kovacs AA, Polis M. Cryptococcosis in the acquired immunodeficiency syndrome. Ann Intern Med. 1985;103:533–8.
67. Byrne WR, Wajszczuk CP. Cryptococcal meningitis in the acquired immunodeficiency syndrome (AIDS); Successful treatment with fluconazole after failure of amphotericin B. Ann Intern Med. 1988;108:384–5.
68. Stern JJ, Hartman BJ, Sharkey P, et al. Oral fluconazole therapy for patients with acquired immunodeficiency syndrome and cryptococcosis: Experience with 22 patients. Am J Med. 1988;85:477–80.
69. Sugar AM, Saunders C. Oral fluconazole as suppressive therapy of disseminated *Cryptococcus* in patients with acquired immunodeficiency syndrome. Am J Med. 1988;85:481–9.
70. Wheat IJ, Slama TG, Zeckel ML. Histoplasmosis in the acquired immune deficiency syndrome. Am J Med. 1985;78:203–10.
71. Johnson PC, Khardori N, Najjor AF, et al. Progressive disseminated histoplasmosis in patients with acquired immunodeficiency syndrome. Am J Med. 1988;85:152–8.
72. Bronnimann DA, Adam RD, Galgiani JN. Coccidioidomycosis in the acquired immunodeficiency syndrome. Ann Intern Med. 1987;106:372–9.
73. Young LS. *Mycobacterium avium* complex infection. AIDS commentary. J Infect Dis. 1988;157:863–7.
74. Inderlied CB, Young LS, Yamada JK. Determination of in vitro susceptibility of *Mycobacterium avium* complex isolates to antimycobacterial agents by various methods. Antimicrob Agents Chemother. 1987;31:1697–702.
75. Agins BD, Berman DS, Spicehandler D, et al. Effect of combined therapy with ansamycin, clofazimine, ethambutol, and isoniazid for *Mycobacterium avium* infection in patients with AIDS. J Infect Dis. 1989;159:784–7.
76. Masur H, Tuazon CU, Gill V, et al. Effect of combined clofazimine and ansamycin therapy of *Mycobacterium avium-Mycobacterium intracellulare* bacteremia in patients with AIDS. J Infect Dis. 1985;151:523–7.
77. Hawkins CC, Gold JWM, Whimbey E. *Mycobacterium avium* complex infections in patients with the acquired immunodeficiency syndrome. Ann Intern Med. 1986;105:184–8.
78. American Thoracic Society, Centers for Disease Control. Mycobacterioses and the acquired immunodeficiency syndrome. Am Rev Resp Dis. 1987;136:492–6.
79. Schroeder S, Sande MA, Root RK, et al. Incidence of salmonellosis in patients with AIDS. J Infect Dis. 1987;156:998–1002.
80. Perlman DM, Ampel NM, Schifman RB, et al. Persistent *Campylobacter jejuni* infections in patients infected with human immunodeficiency virus (HIV). Ann Intern Med. 1988;108:540–6.
81. Sperber SJ, Schleupner CJ. Salmonellosis during infection with human immunodeficiency virus. Rev Infect Dis. 1987;9:925–34.
82. Smith PD, Lane HC, Gill VJ, et al. Intestinal infections in patients with acquired immunodeficiency syndrome: Etiology and response to therapy. Ann Intern Med. 1988;108:328–33.
83. DeHovitz JA, Pape JW, Boncy M, Johnson WD Jr. Clinical manifestations and therapy of isospora belli infection in patients with the acquired immunodeficiency syndrome. N Engl J Med. 1986;315:87–90.
84. Pape JW, Verdier R, Johnson WD. Treatment and prophylaxis of *Isospora belli* infection in patients with the acquired immunodeficiency syndrome. N Engl J Med. 1989;320:1044–7.
85. Johns DR, Tierney M, Felsenstein D. Alteration in the natural history of neurosyphilis by concurrent infection with human immunodeficiency virus. N Engl J Med. 1987;315:1569–72.
86. Lukehart SA, Hook EW, Baker-Zander SA, et al. Invasion of the central nervous system by *Treponema pallidum*: Implications for diagnosis and treatment. Ann Intern Med. 1988;109:855–62.
87. Musher D. How much penicillin cures early syphilis? Ann Intern Med. 1988;109:849–51.
88. Chak LY, Gill PS, Levine A, et al. Radiation therapy for acquired immunodeficiency syndrome-related Kaposi's sarcoma. J Clin Oncol. 1988;6:863–7.
89. Cooper JS, Eried PR. Defining the role of radiation therapy in the management of epidemic Kaposi's sarcoma. Int J Radiat Oncol Biol Phys. 1987;13:35–9.
90. Volberding PA, Mitsuyasu RT, Golando JP, Spiegel RJ. Treatment of Kaposi's sarcoma with interferon alfa-2b (Intron A). Cancer. 1987;59:620–5.
91. Groopman JE, Gottlieb MS, Goodman J. Recombinant alpha-2 interferon therapy for Kaposi's sarcoma associated with the acquired immunodeficiency syndrome. Ann Intern Med. 1984;100:671–6.
92. Oettgen HF, Safai B. Preliminary observations on the effect of recombinant leukocyte A interferon in homosexual men with Kaposi's sarcoma. N Engl J Med. 1983;308:1071.
93. Volberding PA, Abrams DI, Conant M. Vinblastine therapy for Kaposi's sarcoma in the acquired immunodeficiency syndrome. Ann Intern Med. 1985;103:335–8.
94. Kaplan L, Abrams D, Volberding P. Treatment of Kaposi's sarcoma in acquired immunodeficiency syndrome with an alternating vincristine-vinblastine regimen. Cancer Treat Rep. 1986;70:1121–2.
95. Gill PS, Levine PM, Krailo M, et al. AIDS related malignant lymphoma: Results of prospective treatment trials. J Clin Oncol. 1987;5:1322–8.

111. AIDS VACCINES

MARY LOU CLEMENTS

Since human immunodeficiency virus type 1 (HIV-1) can be incorporated into the human genome and persist there in a dormant state for an indefinite period, it is unlikely that antiviral treatment will ever eradicate the virus in an infected person. For this reason, an effective vaccine is the only foreseeable intervention to prevent HIV-1 transmission, infection, and disease. Recent advances in molecular biology, immunology, and biochemistry have made it possible to develop and produce new vaccines and approaches for immunization against HIV-1 infection. The fact that most or all HIV-infected individuals will eventually develop the acquired immunodeficiency syndrome (AIDS) makes it necessary to design a vaccine that will not only protect against disease but will prevent HIV-1 infection. Such a goal will undoubtedly be difficult to achieve since none of the current, highly effective vaccines have been able to provide complete protection against virus infection. Moreover, the paucity of knowledge of the immune correlates of protection against HIV-1 infection, the high mutation rate of HIV-1 strains, and the potential for immunopathogenicity of HIV-1 viral products and immune enhancement all pose special challenges to the goal to develop and evaluate an effective HIV-1 vaccine. Several obstacles and strategies for HIV-1 vaccine development that have been reviewed elsewhere are discussed in this chapter.[1–11]

ISSUES RELATED TO VACCINE DEVELOPMENT

Genetic Variation

One potential obstacle in the development of an effective HIV-1 vaccine is the high mutation rate of HIV-1 strains that results in considerable genetic diversity of HIV-1 isolates and immunologically different subtypes.[12–18] Several constant and variable domains that contain antigenic sites that evoke neutralizing antibodies to HIV-1 have been identified in the envelope glycoprotein 120 (gp120).[19–24] The most substantial variation among HIV-1 isolates is located in the NH_2 terminal region (referred to as the hypervariable region) of gp120.[25] Differences in amino acid content in this region range from 3 to 30 percent in U.S. isolates[13,14,21] and up to 50 percent in African isolates.[13,16,26] Such sequence variations in the envelope gene of HIV-1 may be an important feature that enables the virus to escape host immune surveillance mechanisms.[14,25,27] For lentiviruses related to HIV-1 such as visna virus, there is evidence that progressive changes in the envelope gene lead to changes in envelope antigenicity and the inability for antibodies to effectively neutralize subsequent virus variants.[28] This could pose a particular problem for vaccine development since an effective vaccine to prevent HIV-1 infection would need to elicit an immune response against a number of HIV-1 strains or subtypes.[18]

Mode of HIV-1 Transmission

An effective vaccine strategy must take into account whether HIV-1 infection is transmitted by virus-infected cells, free virus particles, or both.[7] Since HIV-1 infection is likely to be transmitted by virus-infected cells as well as by free virus particles, it is unlikely that humoral antibody alone will be able to protect a person against dormant or proviral forms of HIV-1 that are hidden in lymphocytes or macrophages. In this case, other forms of immunity, such as cell-mediated cytotoxic reactions, will be required for killing virus-infected cells before or after they express viral proteins.

Correlates of Immunity

Much of the current understanding of the immune responses to HIV-1 is derived from responses of individuals who have already been infected with HIV-1 and who are at various stages of the clinical spectrum.[29–31] Other factors are likely to influence the outcome of an HIV-1 infection including the route of virus entry, the size of the virus inoculation, the virulence of the infecting virus and of subsequent progeny viruses,[17] the presence of coinfecting pathogens, the duration of infection, the underlying nutritional and immunologic status of the individual, the age and sex of the person, and possibly genetic factors.

Most individuals infected with HIV-1 develop a variety of humoral and cell-mediated immune responses to HIV-1 in the face of persistent viral replication or latency.

Neutralizing Antibody. Neutralizing antibody that blocks or restricts viral replication is an important correlate of protective immunity for many viral diseases.[31a] Vaccines that stimulate the production of neutralizing antibodies have been shown to be highly effective in preventing such diseases as hepatitis B, polio, and influenza.[31a] Neutralizing antibodies to HIV-1 appear to be directed primarily against the viral envelope of gp120,[18,20–22,29] but they may also be directed to some extent against the core (gag) protein.[32]

Low levels of antibodies with neutralizing activity have been detected in serum of HIV-1-seropositive individuals at all stages of clinical infection.[29–31,33] Some studies have reported a correlation between the ability of a patient's serum to neutralize HIV-1 in vitro and disease status,[22,29–31] but others have not.[21,33] This suggests that the presence of neutralizing antibody per se does not fully protect HIV-1-infected individuals against the development of disease. The levels of neutralizing activity detected may have been influenced in part by the sensitivity of the assay employed and a general decline in immune competence of infected individuals with progressive disease.

The relevance of titers of neutralizing antibody to protective immunity is not known. Cats with weak neutralizing antibody titers of only 1:2 to 1:8 to the retrovirus feline leukemia virus were able to resist virus challenge.[34] However, a recent study conducted in chimpanzees by Prince and coworkers failed to demonstrate any protective effect of high-titered neutralizing antibody against intravenous challenge with a 400 ($TCID_{50}$) tissue culture infectious dose of HIV-1.[35] It is possible that the high challenge dose may have overwhelmed any protective effect of neutralizing antibody.

The high rate of mutation among HIV-1 strains resulting in genomic heterogeneity within the *env* gene that encodes for gp120 poses a significant problem since neutralizing antibodies induced in animals against gp120 derived from HIV-1-infected cells appear to be type specific.[18,20,21,36] A key question is whether an antigen representing conserved epitopes from a single virus type will induce antibodies that will neutralize less related variants. If so, the design of effective polyvalent synthetic HIV-1 vaccines may depend on the selection of conserved regions of gp120 that contain neutralizing epitopes.[18,36]

Cell-Mediated Immune Responses. Relatively little is known about which cell-mediated immune responses might provide protection against HIV-1 infection or disease. In a murine retrovirus system, mice that developed cell-mediated cytotoxic responses to Friend murine leukemia virus were protected against leukemia, whereas those that developed only neutralizing antibody died.[37] This observation and studies in other viral systems suggest that cellular anti-HIV-1 immune responses may be required to destroy HIV-1-infected cells and restrict virus replication.[38,39]

ANTIBODY-DEPENDENT CELLULAR CYTOTOXICITY. One of the immune responses against murine or feline retroviruses is antibody-dependent, cell-mediated cytotoxicity (ADCC) directed against virus-infected cells.[40–43] ADCC killing depends on effector cells with Fc receptors for immunoglobulin (Ig) that bind and kill Ig-coated target cells that express viral gene products. Antibodies active in ADCC are present in serum from patients infected with HIV-1.[44–48] Also, there is evidence that sera from healthy HIV-1-seropositive individuals mediate higher levels of ADCC activity as compared with sera obtained from subjects with AIDS.[44,48] This suggests that ADCC may represent a protective immune response, or as with cytomegalovirus,[38] it may be important for recovery from viral infection.

Protective immunity in animals against disease with passively administered antibodies has been induced 1 month after virus inoculation with Friend murine leukemia virus or feline leukemia virus.[43,49–51] This suggests that serum antibody with potent ADCC activity might help control cell-to-cell spread of the virus by killing HIV-1-infected cells early in the infection. ADCC might also contribute to host surveillance against residual virus-infected cells that remain dormant but could emerge and express viral protein on their cell surface at a later time.[47,48]

Different studies suggest that the location of the determinant for ADCC activity is within the transmembrane gp41,[45] the gp120,[41,47] or the p24[44] protein.

NATURAL KILLER CYTOLYTIC ACTIVITY. One study demonstrated that HIV-1-infected peripheral blood mononuclear cells that mediated HLA-unrestricted natural killer (NK) cytolytic activity appeared to be higher in healthy HIV-1-infected individuals than in those with AIDS.[46] This suggests that NK cells may also be important in early infection.

CYTOTOXIC T-CELL ACTIVITY. Cytotoxic T lymphocytes specific for HIV-1 proteins, including the envelope and gag proteins and those with reverse transcriptase activity, have been detected in HIV-1-seropositive persons.[52–54] Weinhold and colleagues[54] detected cell-mediated cytotoxicity (CMC) against autologous target cells bearing the HIV-1 gp120 envelope protein in HIV-1-seropositive patients but not in HIV-1-seronegative individuals. Healthy HIV-1-infected persons had the highest CMC, whereas those with the AIDS-related compex (ARC) or AIDS showed progressively less reactivity. The gp120-specific cytolysis appeared to be mediated by non-T-cell effectors that resembled NK cells phenotypically. CMC was not restricted by the major histocompatibility complex and was highly augmented by interleukin-2 (IL-2). Whether all or part of CMC might be antibody dependent is not known. A totally antibody-independent lytic mechanism would require induction of a specific receptor, whereas antibody-dependent lysis would make use of existing antibodies that are capable of interacting with resident cells bearing Fc receptors.[54]

Cytotoxic cells, with their inherent ability to recognize and lyse virally infected cells, could limit cell-to-cell spread. On the other hand, they could cause a deleterious immune response if the HIV-1 vaccine is not fully protective. For example, when gp120 is liberated from cells during viral replication, it could bind to normal CD4-bearing cells and make them targets for lympholysis mediated by HIV-1 gp120 effector cells. Studies by Plata and coworkers[55] suggest that CD8-positive T lymphocytes with cytotoxic activities induce local inflammation in the lungs by their interaction with HIV-1-infected macrophages.

COMPLEMENT-MEDIATED CYTOTOXIC ANTIBODY. It is important to determine which components of the immunologic responses protect chimpanzees that have been infected with HIV-1 against the development of disease. One immunologic difference between HIV-1-infected humans and inoculated chimpanzees that has been noted is the development of complement-mediated cytotoxic antibody (ACC) for HIV-1 cells in chimpanzees but not in humans, despite the presence of a high titer of broadly reactive neutralizing antibodies in both species.[56] The pre-existence of broadly reactive ACC and neutralizing antibody ready to kill a cell that has just begun to express virus might be important in preventing or eliminating disease.

Secretory Mucosal Immunity. Secretory antibodies in the mucosal secretions are important mediators of protection in other viral diseases,[57] but their role in protective immunity against HIV-1 replication and infection is not known. Several investigators have found secretory IgA in blood, saliva, and other mucosal fluids of HIV-1 patients with AIDS and ARC.[58] To protect against sexually transmitted HIV-1 infection, an effective AIDS vaccine may need to stimulate secretory immunity to prevent viral entry and replication through mucosal sites.

Risks of Immunopathology

No experiments to date have indicated that HIV-1 vaccine candidates using HIV envelope or core proteins as antigens cause toxic effects in animals[59] or in humans. However, some experts have expressed concern that immunization with vaccine preparations that contain certain viral proteins of HIV-1 might cause immunosuppression and immunopathology.[59–63]

Several regions within the envelope protein of HIV-1 bind with high affinity to CD4 lymphocytes.[64,65] The binding of the gp120 vaccine component could mask epitopes of CD4 that would otherwise function in immunologic recognition.[66] In addition, it has been suggested that HIV-1 envelope proteins such as gp41 are partly responsible for T-cell loss and the decline in function that occurs with AIDS.[67–69] Similar immunodeficiencies that occur after infection with murine and feline leukemia virus are ascribed to the transmembrane protein.[70] Viral gp41 or a factor related to this protein may also be partially responsible for in vivo impairment of monocyte chemotaxis or the ability of monocytes to migrate to the foci of inflammation.[70]

Anti-CD4 antibodies and HIV-1 gp120 share binding sites on the CD4 molecule,[71] and anti-CD4 antibodies may mimic gp120.[63] Since CD4 serves as a receptor for both HIV-1 and class II histocompatibility molecules, an immune response to HIV-1 might result in a cross-reactive response against class II bearing cells and an idiotypic response against cells expressing CD4.[41,63] Such autoimmune mechanisms may be involved in CD4 depletion with AIDS. This suggests that HIV-1-seronegative persons vaccinated against HIV-1 might be subject to more severe disease if the vaccine is not protective and they become infected with HIV-1.[63]

Structural homologies have been identified between HIV-1 proteins and the following endogenously produced regulatory proteins: HIV-1 gag (core) protein and thymosin α_1,[32] gp120 and neuroleukin,[72] and gp41 and IL-2.[73] These relationships raise the question about whether an antibody response to HIV-1 proteins will cross react with lymphoid and thymic epithelial cells involved in the production of these peptides.[59] Clearly, evidence of these toxic effects should be sought in extensive animal testing of vaccine candidates before they are evaluated in humans.

Immune Enhancement

The phenomenon of immune enhancement has been associated with vaccination against dengue[74] and is of theoretic concern with HIV-1 vaccines.[62,62a] Robinson and coworkers have identified heat-stable and heat-labile factors in the serum of HIV-infected patients that in combination appear to enhance HIV-1 infection in vitro. The enhancing activity appears to be related to antibody (possibly to viral protein) and activation of the alternate pathway of complement.[75] Data in vitro and in vivo suggest that the alternate pathway of complement is chronically activated in patients with ARC more than in those with lymphadenopathy syndrome.[76] Thus, high HIV-1-enhancing activity mediated by antibodies may result in a depletion of complement and worsening of disease. HIV-1 vaccine candidates should be evaluated for their ability to stimulate antibody formation that enhances infection.

PRECLINICAL TESTS

Before a candidate AIDS vaccine is evaluated in humans, a number of tests to assess the safety, toxicity, and immunogenicity of the vaccine are usually conducted in vitro, in small animals, and subsequently in primates.[1,7]

In Vitro Tests

A major constraint in the development and evaluation of AIDS vaccines is the lack of uniform reference reagents and standardized methods to assess neutralization titers, cell-mediated immune responses, and immunopathogenicity of vaccine candidates.[7] Several methods have been used to measure neutralizing antibodies to HIV-1, and all are subject to technical limitations.[3,77] One approach involves inoculating cell cultures with HIV 1 and subsequently quantitating the virus production by detecting reverse transcriptase activity or core antigen.[29,78] Another, more sensitive and convenient method involves the use of vesicular stomatitis virus to form pseudotype viruses with envelopes bearing HIV-1 antigens and then monitoring their cytopathic effect.[33] Other methods measure cytolytic effects of HIV-1 in human T-cell leukemia/lymphoma virus-1 (HTLV-1)-infected cell lines.[21,79] The relevance of antibodies for the neutralization of HIV-1 as measured by each of these tests is not clear. More recently, a plaque reduction microassay to measure neutralizing antibodies was developed.[80] This assay, which measures the percent reduction of giant cells (syncytia formation) in the presence of test serum, may be more sensitive than are the other assays.

Tests in Animals

Another major problem in the development of a safe, effective AIDS vaccine is the lack of relevant animal models to evaluate whether immunization with a candidate AIDS vaccine will prevent HIV-1 infection and development of disease.[7] Candidate HIV-1 vaccines are generally administered to small animals (e.g., mice, guinea pigs, and rabbits) initially to determine whether they stimulate the production of neutralizing antibodies in serum and other immune responses to the HIV-1.[7]

The chimpanzee is the only animal model that can be readily infected with HIV-1.[81–84] After intravenous inoculation with HIV-1, virus can be recovered from peripheral mononuclear cells, and HIV-1-specific immune responses can be detected in the blood.[81,82] However, with few exceptions, infected chimpanzees, some of whom have been followed for as long as 5 years, remain clinically and immunologically well in contrast to HIV-1-infected humans, who develop AIDS.[81,82] These issues together with their endangered status, limited availability, and cost make the use of chimpanzees for screening of AIDS vaccines problematic.[3,77,85,86] For these reasons, many experts question the validity of the chimpanzee model for human AIDS vaccine.[77,85,86] Yet others believe that a candidate HIV-1 vaccine should demonstrate an ability to induce protective immunity in chimpanzees before the vaccine is tested in humans.[7,77,87] Since many of the chimpanzees designated for AIDS vaccine testing have already been infected with hepatitis B or non-A, non-B viruses, it is possible that those chimpanzees that are infected with another infectious agent may have an altered immune response to an HIV-1 vaccination, challenge, or both.

To date, there has been no standardization of the protocols for vaccination (i.e., number of doses, spacing of doses) or for virus challenge (i.e., dose and route of virus inoculation, cell-free vs. cell-associated virus inoculum, or homologous versus heterologous challenge) in chimpanzees or other animals. As yet, chimpanzees previously immunized with various prototype AIDS vaccines and subsequently challenged with HIV-1 have not been protected against virus infection.[2,85,87] However, the challenge doses used have been as high as 300,000 HIV-1 tissue culture infectious doses ($TCID_{50}$) and all challenges to date have been given intravenously. Experimental HIV-1 infection resulting from virus challenge that employs such high doses and the intravenous route of transmission probably does not mimic human HIV-1 infection transmitted by sexual activity.

An alternate animal model is the rhesus macaque monkey, which can be persistently infected with simian immunodeficiency virus (SIV).[7,85,88–90] SIV rapidly induces an immune deficiency syndrome remarkably similar to AIDS, with wasting, opportunistic infections, and a high fatality rate.[89] Studies in the SIV system may provide insights about the role of cell-mediated immune responses and neutralizing antibody in protection against virus infection and the development of simian AIDS. Prototype vaccine candidates can also be developed in the SIV system and tested for safety and efficacy in macaques. Whether genetic and biologic differences between the two viruses and their hosts will limit the usefulness of this model for vaccine screening is not known.

Lentiviruses, which are genetically and biologically similar to HIV-1, have been isolated from household cats, domestic cattle, and several other ungulate (hoofed) mammals.[91–93] The availability of cats and cattle in contrast to primates and the ability of these lentiviruses to induce disease after infection make them potential animal models for the evaluation of vaccines applicable to HIV-1. Animal studies with ungulate and feline retroviruses may also provide insights about host-specific immunologic responses and vaccine-induced immune enhancement to retrovirus infections. One study in which goats were immunized with inactivated caprine arthritis-encephalitis virus suggested that a vaccine-enhanced immune response to CAEV virus caused severe destructive arthritis.[94]

VACCINE APPROACHES

An ideal vaccine should possess all of the antigens capable of protecting against infection with HIV-1 and its antigenic variants but not cause the harmful immunologic effects that occur with natural infection. In addition, the vaccine should be easily administered, inexpensive, stable, and readily available. Several vaccine approaches are listed in Table 1.

The most common approach used to develop an HIV-1 vaccine is to employ protein subunits of the virus that are produced by genetic engineering and recombinant DNA methods. This approach offers several advantages[65]: (*1*) recombinant proteins are safe to prepare, and no genetic material is used for vaccination; (*2*) purified recombinant proteins can be more efficiently produced than can purified native viral proteins obtained from virus-infected cells; and (*3*) synthetic peptides can be prepared that bear neutralizing epitopes representing a spectrum of envelope sequences.

There are also several concerns with the subunit approach for an HIV-1 vaccine. First, a single viral protein such as the envelope might not be immunogenic enough because the antigen may not be presented or structurally configured to be recog-

TABLE 1. Potential HIV-1 Vaccine Approaches

Immunization of HIV-1–seronegative persons
Subunit preparations:
Recombinant envelope glycoproteins (gp120, gp160)
Native envelope glycoproteins
Synthetic envelope peptides
Synthetic core proteins
Live non-HIV virus recombinants (vaccinia or adenovirus)
Inactivated (killed) HIV-1 vaccine
Live attenuated (nonpathogenic) HIV-1 strains
Anti-idiotypes
Passive immunization
Immunization of HIV-1–seropositive persons
Inactivated HIV-1 virus vaccine
Hyperimmunization with non–HIV-1 vaccines

nized by the host immune system. Second, a subunit vaccine may protect against only one strain rather than against multiple variants. Thus, a combination of antigens rather than a single peptide or protein may be required to stimulate protective immunity.[7]

Subunit Vaccines: Recombinant Envelope Proteins

The HIV-1 envelope protein is a 160 kD glycosylated protein (gp160) that is composed of a gp120 external glycoprotein and a gp41 transmembrane protein.[95–97] The envelope glycoprotein is an accessible target for antibody-directed neutralization and cytotoxic immunity because of its location on the outer surface of the virus.[20,65,95–101] On the basis of animal retroviral models[102–104] it may be possible to prevent primary virus infection with a vaccine incorporating all or part of the envelope gp120 and, to a lesser extent, the transmembrane gp41. One approach to constructing such a vaccine is to clone the appropriate gene sequences of envelope glycoproteins and to express these proteins through genetic engineering techniques in eukaryotic (mammalian, insect, or yeast) or prokaryotic (*Escherichia coli*) cell cultures.[5,7,41,65,100,105–108] Such recombinant glycoproteins have induced neutralizing antibodies in animals and in vitro against the homologous virus but not against less related HIV-1 variants.[7,20,21,97,98,100] This suggested that an effective gp120 vaccine might need to incorporate envelope proteins or peptides containing selected sequences from the variable regions of different isolates to provide group-specific neutralizing antibodies.

Native gp120 is heavily glycosylated.[101] However, recombinant envelope proteins lacking natural sugar residues appear to be effective immunogens since these sugars are not required for the induction of neutralizing antibodies.[7,65] Krohn and colleagues[109] have shown that gp120 also contains an immunogenic T-cell epitope that will evoke a group-specific cellular immune response.

A recombinant gp120 envelope vaccine preparation expressed in Chinese hamster ovary cells stimulated neutralizing antibodies in rabbits and guinea pigs,[99,108] but it failed to protect chimpanzees against experimental challenge with HIV-1[109a] and has not been tested in humans. The first vaccine preparation that has been evaluated in humans in the United States is a recombinant envelope gp160 gene product.[105,106,108] The HIV-1 gp160 gene was inserted into the baculovirus genome, and the recombinant baculovirus was cultured in an insect cell line from which the gp160 was extracted and purified.[105,108] The vaccine stimulated neutralizing antibodies but no toxic reactions in animals.[2] This subunit envelope protein vaccine prototype does appear to elicit immunologic responses in humans,[2] but the functional significance of these antibodies is not yet known.

Subunit Vaccines: Native Proteins

Another subunit approach is to isolate and purify natural gp120 envelope glycoprotein from cells infected with HIV-1.[7,9] Goats, horses, rhesus monkeys, and chimpanzees immunized with native gp120 developed low to moderate titers of neutralizing antibodies but no toxic reactions.[7,109,110] However, the production of native HIV-1 products is hazardous for laboratory workers.

Subunit Vaccines: Synthetic Envelope Peptides

Another subunit approach involves the chemical synthesis of peptide segments of HIV-1 protein, and it has the advantage that large quantities of peptide antigens without other contaminating material can be produced.[111–113] To be effective immunogens, synthetic peptides or polypeptides must incorporate the amino acid sequences that are important for binding or cellular attachment and for inducing neutralizing antibody, cellular reactivity, or both.[111] Synthetic peptides must also be presented in the appropriate steric configuration so that they will be accessible to antibodies and B cells and T cells will recognize the different antigenic determinants on the molecules.[113–115] Several methods can be used to predict the amino acid sequences that contain epitopes from conserved regions of different isolates that are recognized by both B and T cells.[114,115] Since synthetic peptides are weak immunogens, they will require appropriate adjuvants and delivery systems and possibly need a carrier molecule before they can be used as a potent vaccine.[116]

Non-neutralizing domains should be excluded since they could sterically hinder critical epitopes or elicit blocking antibodies and interfere with the action of neutralizing antibodies.[74] In addition, coating of HIV-1 by non-neutralizing antibodies could lead to enhancement of virus uptake by Fc receptor–bearing cells such as monocytes and macrophages,[62a] as has been reported for dengue virus.[74] This may be important since human monocytes and macrophages are capable of supporting HIV-1 replication.[117]

Immunogenic peptide products include C21E, peptide sequences 732–735, and PB1. Antibodies against a conserved part of the central region of gp120, referred to as C21E, have been shown to block virus replication and mediate ADCC.[24] Peptide sequences 735–752 mimic epitopes found in native HIV-1 transmembrane gp41.[109] PB1, a 180 amino acid peptide of gp120 expressed in *E. coli*, elicited high titers of cross-neutralizing antibody in goats.[109]

Subunit Vaccine: Synthetic Core Proteins

Yet another approach is to use a synthetic protein (p17) that is part of the core proteins of HIV-1.[32] There is evidence in humans that HIV-1-infected persons who remain asymptomatic have higher titers of antibodies to p24 (the core protein) than do those who manifested AIDS or ARC.[118,119] An antiserum prepared against a naturally occurring peptide from the thymus gland, thymosin α_1, which is similar in amino acid composition to the (core) protein of HIV-1, weakly neutralized HIV-1 and blocked its replication in H9 cells in vitro.[32] In addition, a synthetic p17 protein induced neutralizing antibodies in rabbits.[32] Since the core region is highly conserved among HIV-1 isolates, a vaccine directed against this protein might overcome the problem of genetic drift of HIV-1 strains.

Live Virus Recombinants

In another approach, genes encoding for the HIV-1 envelope protein can be inserted in a non-HIV-1, which then serves as a vehicle for producing the HIV-1 protein. Vectors used for this purpose include vaccinia virus, the virus used for smallpox vaccine,[120–123] and an attenuated adenovirus that is used to immunize army recruits against respiratory disease caused by adenovirus.[124]

Buller and colleagues[125] constructed thymidine kinase–negative (tk−) vaccinia virus recombinants by inserting a variety of DNA coding sequences into the thymidine kinase gene of vaccinia virus and demonstrated that the tk− recombinants were less pathogenic for mice than was wild-type virus. This genetic modification attenuated the vaccinia virus, as evidenced by a reduction in its ability to initiate and maintain a viremia.[125] Moreover, with the insertion of foreign genes into the thymidine kinase gene, reversion of tk− to tk+ virus is unlikely to occur.

Several investigators have inserted cloned genes encoding HIV-1 envelope gp120 or gp160 from the HIV-1 into the DNA of vaccinia.[121,122] Chakrabarti and coworkers demonstrated that the envelope protein expressed by a gp160-recombinant vaccinia virus reacted by immunoprecipitation with sera from unrelated AIDS patients and that a single inoculation with purified recombinant HIV-1 vaccinia induced antibodies to gp120 in mice.[122]

Several studies have demonstrated that primates immunized

with a recombinant vaccinia virus expressing the complete HIV gp160 envelope gene developed cell-mediated immune responses to HIV-1 envelope glycoproteins.[121,126,127] In one study, the chimpanzees were subsequently challenged with a 100 tissue culture infectious dose ($TCID_{50}$) of HIV-1.[2] The results indicated that prior immunization with the HIV-1 gp160–vaccinia recombinant had primed the immune system of the chimpanzees for developing neutralizing antibodies to HIV-1 envelope proteins but did not prevent HIV-1 infection.[2]

Zagury and others conducted a small trial in Zaire to determine the safety and immunogenicity of an HIV-1 gp160–vaccinia recombinant virus in healthy HIV-1-seronegative adult volunteers.[128,129] Twelve volunteers were inoculated intradermally with recombinant vaccinia virus that expressed the complete gp160 envelope protein of the $HTLV\text{-}III_B$ strain of HIV-1. No adverse effects or immune defects were detected after immunization. The vaccine induced antibodies to vaccinia and a low level of neutralizing antibodies to $HTLV\text{-}III_B$ antigens. About 3 months after the primary vaccination, one vaccinated individual was boosted with intravenously administered, paraldehyde-fixed autologous cells that had been infected in vitro with the $HTLV\text{-}III_B$ gp160–vaccinia virus recombinant. He was boosted again 10 and 12 months after primary vaccination with a gp160 preparation derived from an $HTLV\text{-}III_B$ clone by using a hybrid vaccinia virus/bacteriophage T7 expression system.[129] This complicated immunization induced neutralizing antibodies against two divergent HIV-1 strains that persisted for over a year after the original vaccination and elicited group-specific, cell-mediated immune responses and cell-mediated cytotoxicity against infected T4 cells. Since these results were observed in only one individual, they should be viewed with caution. Nevertheless, this trial demonstrated for the first time that group-specific cell-mediated and humoral immune responses to vaccination against HIV-1 can be induced in humans. This vaccination approach is not feasible for use on a larger scale unless another method for boosting can be used to replace the autologous vaccinia virus recombinant–infected cells.[129] Another trial with a vaccinia recombinant expressing the genes for HIV gp160 has been initiated in the United States.[2,130]

The low cost, ease of administration, and high degree of stability under field conditions make this type of vaccine approach attractive for use in developing countries.[120] However, there are several possible disadvantages to this approach. Infrequent (but severe) complications that have been associated with smallpox vaccination include generalized vaccinia, encephalitis, vaccinia necrosum, and accidental self-inoculation.[131] The ability of the vaccinia virus to produce a progressive infection in immunodeficient individuals is a serious risk,[131] and a reaction of this type in an asymptomatic man infected with HIV-1 was recently reported.[132] Of special concern is the use of vaccinia–HIV-1 recombinants in persons who may have contact with immunosuppressed, HIV-1-infected persons since transmission of vaccinia virus infection from a vaccinated individual to an unvaccinated person can occur.

It may be possible to further attenuate the vaccinia virus by incorporating the gene for a lymphokine such as IL-2 into its genome.[133] IL-2 is secreted by CD4 lymphocytes in response to antigenic stimulation and is important for the activation of specific and nonspecific immune responses.[133] Ramshaw and colleagues showed that thymic nude mice infected with the vaccinia–IL-2 recombinant cleared their virus infection rapidly whereas mice infected with the unaltered vaccinia strain developed progressive vaccinia disease.[134] This suggests that live virus vaccines that express IL-2 might minimize or eliminate the complications associated with inadvertent transmission of vaccine virus to immunodeficient persons. Concomitant expression of IL-2 or other lymphokines with HIV-1 antigens in live recombinant vaccines may be particularly important for the wide-scale use of an HIV-1–vaccinia recombinant vaccine in populations where HIV-1 is endemic and prior screening is not practical.[134]

Killed Virus Vaccine

To prepare a safe whole HIV-1 vaccine, it will be necessary to destroy (inactivate) the infectivity of the virus by disrupting the function of the viral nucleic acid but preserving the functional activity of the relevant protective antigens.[135] Inactivation of the virus can be accomplished by the use of formalin, psoralen, B propriolactone, irradiation, or heat.

Protection against retroviral disease has been induced by inactivated virus vaccines in animal studies.[136] Immunization of rhesus monkeys with formalin-inactivated whole SIV, type C, retrovirus containing the adjuvant threonyl muramyl dipeptide provided full protection against intravenous challenge with a heterologous (type D) retrovirus.[136] However, in other trials, inactivated type C SIV vaccine given with immune stimulatory complexes (ISCOMS) or threonyl muranyl dipeptides failed to protect rhesus monkeys or macaques against intravenous challenge with a homologous rhesus SIV.[86] In another study an inactivated whole SIV (type C) vaccine with an adjuvant appeared to partially protect macaques against experimental challenge with homologous SIV administered intramuscularly 1 week after the fifth immunization (R. Derrosier et al., manuscript in preparation). After challenge, two of six vaccinated macaques remained clinically and immunologically well, with no evidence of viremia or anamnestic antibody response, whereas all seven unvaccinated challenged macaques became infected and most died. Additional studies are needed to further investigate the protective capability of inactivated SIV and HIV-1 vaccines.

Immunization of HIV-1-Seropositive Individuals

Another approach has been taken by Salk and others[135,139] in an attempt to protect persons already infected with HIV-1 and to prevent infants born to HIV-1-infected mothers from developing AIDS. The rationale for this strategy is based on the long incubation period between HIV-1 infection and the development of disease.[137,138] This suggests that a postinfection intervention, like that for hepatitis B virus infection,[140] might be feasible to prevent the progression of immunologic disease in healthy HIV-1 carriers and, possibly, to halt deterioration in symptomatic carriers whose disease is not far advanced. This would be accomplished by inducing cytotoxic mechanisms to destroy HIV-1 and HIV-1 antigen-producing cells.[135] If successful, HIV-1 would remain as a latent infection in a proviral form within infected cells. Also, immunized HIV-1 carriers might have a reduced ability to transmit the infection. The availability of an effective intervention for HIV-1-seropositive individuals could increase voluntary HIV-1 testing, identification of cases, and the opportunity to initiate early treatment of infected persons.[135]

A postexposure vaccine trial with killed SIV is being conducted in rhesus monkeys.[139] Also, a small trial with an HIV-1 preparation inactivated by γ-irradiation has been initiated in HIV-1-seropositive persons in California.[135,139] Yet another postinfection trial in which 10 patients with AIDS are receiving their own infected cells and inactivated HIV-1 is being conducted in Zaire.[139]

Nonpathogenic Variants

It is possible to produce genetically engineered nonpathogenic variants by rendering them unable to replicate but able to express all other antigens.[141] A mutant of HIV-1 (designated X10-1) that has a deletion of a 200 base pair segment spanning the last 14 base pairs of the envelope gene and the 3′ *orf* genes was able to replicate in and infect cells but did not kill normal human

T cells in vitro.[141] Such a noncytopathic mutant might be used to make an inactivated virus vaccine that would be less likely to cause disease than would a vaccine prepared from a pathogenic virus.

Anti-idiotype

HIV-1 isolates appear to use CD4 as a receptor.[142] Thus, one approach to vaccines to prevent HIV-1 infection is to generate an antibody-based vaccine, such as an anti-CD4 idiotype vaccine that would mimic the CD4 antigen and bind to HIV-1 envelope glycoprotein.[143,144] Koprowski and colleagues immunized mice with a protein from the HIV-1.[7,144] They then immunized mice with the first antibody (Ab1) and induced the animals to make a second antibody (Ab2) whose binding site resembled the original antigen from the HIV-1. Subsequently, Ab2 was used as an antigen to induce mice to make a third generation of antibodies (Ab3) that should bind to the HIV-1. Thus, Ab3 would mimic the CD4 receptor for the HIV-1.[143] Such anti-idiotype vaccines might induce a broadly reactive response, and no infectious material or antigens from HIV-1 would be used.[144]

One monoclonal anti-idiotype raised against a monoclonal antibody (Leu3a) to CD4 in mice reacted with gp120 in Western blot analysis and partly neutralized one HIV-1 isolate.[145] Dalgleish and colleagues[143] showed that a repeated-dose regimen in mice stimulated polyclonal anti-idiotypic antibodies that neutralized three different isolates of HIV-1 and one isolate of HIV-2. This suggests that this approach might overcome the diversity in HIV-1 isolates.

Immunizing with an anti-CD4 preparation could be harmful since anti-idiotype antibodies to CD4 could block CD4 epitopes on T cells that are responsible for helper activity.[146] Immunosuppression in mice has been observed when large quantities of anti-CD4 were given,[147] but it is hoped that the low quantities of anti-CD4 needed to induce an anti-idiotype response against HIV-1 would not be immunosuppressive.[143,146]

PASSIVE IMMUNOTHERAPY

Passive immunotherapy has been suggested as a way to prevent HIV-1 infection in infants born to HIV-1-infected mothers and to prevent the development of ARC and AIDS in HIV-1-infected persons. Preliminary studies were conducted by Prince and colleagues with anti-HIV-1 globulin extracted from HIV-1-infected individuals.[35] The serum was fractionated and purified to inactivate HIV-1. One unimmunized chimpanzee and four chimpanzees immunized with serum (1 or 10 ml/kg of body weight) containing high titers of neutralizing antibody were challenged with 400 tissue culture infectious doses of HIV-1. All of the chimpanzees became infected; the high-titered anti-HIV-1 globulin preparation did not alter the incubation period between the virus challenge and manifestation of viremia or seroconversion. However, it is possible that the dose employed for challenge may have overwhelmed any protective effect of neutralizing antibody. Studies using a lower dose of virus for challenge should answer the question about what role if any neutralizing antibody plays in the prevention of HIV-1 infection or progression of disease.

HYPERIMMUNIZATION

One brief report suggested that chronic nonspecific hyperimmunization may ameliorate symptoms of HIV-1 infection.[148] In this study, four HIV-1-infected patients who received inactivated polio vaccine subcutaneously three times a week for 3–12 months experienced improvement or resolution of their symptoms of fatigue, lymphadenopathy, or thrush. A potential risk associated with this approach is that antigenic stimulation by non-HIV-1 immunogens might accelerate virus expression in CD4+ lymphocytes and result in their destruction.[149]

ADJUVANTS

A suitable adjuvant is needed to augment and prolong the immune response of HIV-1 vaccine antigens without causing side effects.[116,150,151] Adjuvants appear to work by at least two mechanisms[116]: (*1*) by slowing the excretion of antigen and thereby extending the time of interaction between antigen and antigen-presenting cells and (*2*) by attracting immunocompetent cells to the site of injection and possibly by directing antigen to T-cell-containing areas in regional lymph nodes. Aluminum salt compounds are the only adjuvants licensed by the Federal Drug Administration. While aluminum salts are generally safe and induce humoral immunity,[116,150] more potent adjuvants that elicit cell-mediated immunity are needed for HIV-1 vaccine preparations. Other new potential adjuvants include muramyl dipeptides, which can be used with viral antigens (administered by the parenteral or oral routes), synthetic peptides, and nonpyrogenic subunits of lipopolysaccharides.[116,151,152] When muramyl dipeptide is administered in liposomes or is made lipophilic by the addition of glycerol mycolate,[153] it markedly increases cell-mediated immunity.[154]

Liposomes, concentric spheres consisting of phospholipid bilayers separated by aqueous compartments, have been used effectively as carriers of diphtheria toxoid proteins and other antigens.[152] Liposomes are a potentially promising vehicle for HIV-1 vaccine antigens since liposome–antigen complexes appear to elicit both humoral and cell-mediated immunity.[116,155] The potency of these complexes can be increased by the inclusion of bacterial lipopolysaccharides[156] or muramyl dipeptides[154,157] within the liposomes.

Another promising adjuvant system consists of immune-stimulating complexes (ISCOMS), which are matrices composed of quil A, an extract from the bark of the *Quillaja sonponaria molina* tree.[158–160] ISCOMS are composed of subunits of about 12 nm each that are held together by hydrophobic interactions between the matrix, lipids, and amphipathic antigens.[158,159] ISCOM-bound antigens stimulate an immune response that is generally 10-fold higher when compared with the same antigen packaged in a micelle or in a virus particle.[158,160] Potent cell-mediated immune responses have been elicited after parenteral immunization of monkeys with ISCOMS containing cytomegalovirus antigens and after inoculation with ISCOMS containing hepatitis B surface antigen.[160–162] Furthermore, ISCOMS containing gp120 from feline leukemia virus induced both neutralizing antibody and protective immunity in cats when compared with vaccines consisting of whole killed virus, which failed to induce neutralizing antibody or protective immunity.[34] Vaccine candidates incorporating HIV-1 envelope proteins or synthetic peptides in ISCOMS appear to be safe and immunogenic in gibbons and apes.[163] After repeated immunizations with HIV-1 protein products p17, p41, and gp120 incorporated into ISCOMS, antibodies to all of the proteins were induced in several animal species.[163] However, this ISCOM preparation only stimulated a low level of neutralizing activity against the homologous HIV-1, possibly because it did not contain enough gp120.[163]

CLINICAL TRIALS IN HUMANS

Human trials of four candidate AIDS vaccines have already been initiated in the United States, England, and Africa, with the expectation that they will provide useful information about the safety of and immune response to HIV-1 immunogens in humans.[2] In general, the clinical trials will be carried out in three phases to assess the safety and immunogenicity of candidate vaccines.[1,3,10,85] In phase I trials, different doses of vaccine are generally evaluated in about 10–30 healthy adults per dose group in a double-blinded, placebo-controlled, dose-escalating manner. If the vaccine is found to be safe and sufficiently immunogenic, phase II trials would then be conducted to evaluate the safety and immunogenicity of the vaccine candidate in larger numbers of persons, approximately 40–80 persons per dose. Information regarding the optimal dose and interval between booster doses will be sought from phase I and II trials, each of which will take 1 to 2 years to complete. Only after a vaccine has been shown to be safe and highly immunogenic will it be considered for phase III efficacy testing in humans.

To assess the tolerability and reactogenicity of the vaccine, local and systemic reactions and a variety of laboratory and immunologic parameters of recipients of HIV-1 vaccine will be compared with those of placebo recipients. In one phase I HIV-1 gp160 vaccine trial, yeast-derived recombinant hepatitis B vaccine was used as a control in addition to a placebo so that variations in certain test results (e.g., numbers of CD4+ cells) that might occur after immunization with a recombinant protein could be differentiated from those that might be due specifically to vaccination with the HIV-1 recombinant protein.[75,108] The determination of which group of adults should be selected for vaccine trials will depend to some extent on the phase of the trial and type of vaccine to be evaluated.[1,3,10,85] In general, there are two reasons for selecting persons at low risk for acquiring HIV-1 infection for phase I trials (and possibly for phase II trials) instead of persons at high risk. First, persons at high risk may already be infected with HIV-1 before vaccination or may become infected during the vaccine trial. If this happens, it would be difficult to distinguish their immune responses to the vaccine from those resulting from intercurrent HIV-1 infection. Second, since persons at high risk for acquiring HIV-1 infection are often infected with other agents, they may respond differently to the HIV-1 vaccine than do persons not infected with other agents.[164]

Populations at high risk for HIV-1 infection should be targeted for phase III vaccine efficacy trials.[1,3,10] The sample size required to assess vaccine efficacy will depend on the current incidence of infection and the confidence levels sought to signify significant protection from infection. Finding an adequate volunteer population for phase III vaccine efficacy studies will be difficult.[10,85] It is possible that by the time of the phase III trials the homosexual risk group will have an incidence of infection too low for participation in a vaccine trial. The number of sexual partners of hemophiliacs constitute too small a group to study. Other high-risk populations such as intravenous drug users and prostitutes may not be compliant with the long-term follow-up (7–10 years) required to assess protection against disease. It is possible that trials to determine vaccine efficacy may have to be targeted for populations in Africa where the incidence of HIV-1 infection remains high.[3,10]

ETHICAL ISSUES

Special ethical considerations must be taken into account in the design and conduct of HIV-1 vaccine trials.[1,3,10,165] The consent form not only must clearly state all of the risks associated with the vaccine candidate, but it must educate the volunteer about how to reduce the risk of acquiring HIV-1 infection. In addition, all volunteers who participate in AIDS vaccine trials must be counseled about how to avoid becoming infected with HIV-1. The counseling itself may lower the overall rate of infection in both the unvaccinated control group and the vaccinees and thus increase the amount of time required to determine the efficacy of a vaccine.

Maintenance of strict confidentiality of the study participants throughout these trials is of utmost importance since the volunteers who might be identified as members of high-risk groups could be subjected to discrimination or abuse.[1,165] Of paramount concern is the fact that persons immunized with HIV-1 vaccine candidates who mount an immune response may test positive for HIV-1 antibody by the enzyme-linked immunosorbent assay (ELISA) used for screening.[1,3,10,165] It is possible that persons who seroconvert after receiving an HIV-1 vaccine preparation may not be able to travel to foreign countries where HIV-1 testing is required by immigration, donate blood, enter the military or foreign service, or obtain a marriage license or health and life insurance.[1,3,10,165] Clearly, the risks of social and economic hazards associated with HIV-1 seroconversion have already had a negative impact on recruitment efforts for AIDS vaccine trials.

The urgent need to control the transmission of HIV-1 has fueled efforts to develop HIV-1 vaccines. The application of modern molecular biotechnology and the identification of the specific function of amino acid sequences and peptides of HIV-1 proteins has made the task of vaccine development somewhat less formidable.[9] The need to expedite the development of an effective HIV-1 vaccine warrants the evaluation of different vaccine strategies simultaneously.[5] Finally, the issue of potential liability for producers of HIV-1 vaccines and those who conduct the clinical trials is a problem that could block the eventual availability of an HIV-1 vaccine and, therefore, needs to be resolved.[7,166]

REFERENCES

1. Koff WC, Hoth DF. Development and testing of AIDS vaccines. Science. 1988;241:426–32.
2. Barnes DM. Obstacles to an AIDS vaccine. Science. 1988;240:719–21.
3. Homsy J, Steimer K, Kaslow R. Towards an AIDS vaccine: Challenges and prospects. Immunol Today. 1987;8:193–7.
4. Purdy BD, Plaisance KI. Current concepts in clinical therapeutics: Immunologic treatment of human immunodeficiency virus infections. Clin Pharmacol. 1987;6:851–65.
5. Dreesman GR, Eichberg JW, Chanh TC, et al. Use of vaccination in prevention of HIV infection. In: AIDS. Acquired Immunodeficiency Syndrome and Other Manifestations of HIV Infections. Park Ridge, NJ: Noyes Publications; 1987:1037–52.
6. Fischinger PJ, Gallo RC, Bolognesi DP. Toward a vaccine against AIDS: Rationale and current progress. Mt Sinai J Med. 1986;53:639–47.
7. Barnes DM. Strategies for an AIDS vaccine. Science. 1986;233:1149–53.
8. Vogt M, Hirsch MS. Prospects for the prevention and therapy of infections with the human immunodeficiency virus. Rev Infect Dis. 1986;8:991–1000.
9. Fischinger PJ, Robey WG, Koprowski H, et al. Current status and strategies for vaccines against diseases induced by human T-cell lymphotropic retroviruses (HTLV-1, -II, -III). Cancer Res. 1985;45(Suppl):4694–9.
10. Francis DP, Petricciani JC. The prospects for and pathways toward a vaccine for AIDS. N Engl J Med. 1985;313:1586–90.
11. Hunsmann G. Subunit vaccines against exogenous retroviruses: Overview and perspectives. Cancer Res. 1985;45(Suppl):4691–3.
12. Wong-Staal F, Shaw GM, Hahn BH, et al. Genomic diversity of human T-lymphotropic virus type III (HTLV-III). Science. 1985;229:759–62.
13. Benn S, Rutledge R, Folks T, et al. Genomic heterogeneity of AIDS retroviral isolates from North America and Zaire. Science. 1985;230:949–51.
14. Starcich BR, Hahn BH, Shaw GM, et al. Identification and characterization of conserved and variable regions in the envelope gene of HTLV-III/LAV, the retrovirus of AIDS. Cell. 1986;45:637–48.
15. Hahn BH, Shaw GM, Taylor ME, et al. Genetic variation in HTLV-III/LAV over time in patients with AIDS or at risk for AIDS. Science. 1986;232:1548–53.
16. Willey RL, Rutledge RA, Dias S, et al. Identification of conserved and divergent domains within the envelope gene of the acquired immunodeficiency syndrome retrovirus. Proc Natl Acad Sci USA. 1986;83:5038–42.
17. Cheng-Mayer C, Seto D, Tateno M, et al. Biologic features of HIV-1 that correlate with virulence in the host. Science. 1988;240:80–2.
18. Cheng-Mayer C, Homsy J, Evans LA, et al. Identification of human immunodeficiency virus subtypes with distinct patterns of sensitivity to serum neutralization. Proc Natl Acad Sci USA. 1988;85:2815–9.
19. Barin F, McLane MF, Allan JS, et al. Virus envelope protein of HTLV-III represents major target antigen for antibodies in AIDS patients. Science. 1985;228:1094–6.
20. Matthews TJ, Langlois AJ, Robey WG, et al. Restricted neutralization of divergent human T-lymphotropic virus type III isolates by antibodies to the major envelope glycoprotein. Proc Natl Acad Sci USA. 1986;83:9709–13.
21. Weiss RA, Clapham PR, Weber JN, et al. Variable and conserved neutralization antigens of human immunodeficiency virus. Nature. 1986;324:572–5.
22. Ho DD, Sarngadharan MG, Hirsch MS, et al. Human immunodeficiency virus neutralizing antibodies recognize several conserved domains on the envelope glycoproteins. J Virol. 1987;61:2024–8.

23. Modrow S, Hahn BH, Shaw GM, et al. Computer-assisted analysis of envelope protein sequences of seven human immunodeficiency virus isolates: Prediction of antigenic epitopes in conserved and variable regions. J Virol. 1987;61:570–8.
24. Ho DD, Kaplan JC, Rackauskas IE, et al. Second conserved domain of gp120 is important for HIV infectivity and antibody neutralization. Science. 1988;239:1021–3.
25. Hahn BH, Gonda MA, Shaw GM, et al. Genomic diversity of the acquired immune deficiency syndrome virus HTLV-III: Different viruses exhibit greatest divergence in their envelope genes. Proc Natl Acad Sci USA. 1985;82:4813–7.
26. Alizon M, Wain-Hobson S, Montagnier L, et al. Genetic variability of the AIDS virus: Nucleotide sequence analysis of two isolates from African patients. Cell. 1986;45:63–74.
27. Sanchez-Pescador R, Power MD, Barr PJ, et al. Nucleotide sequence and expression of an AIDS-associated retrovirus (ARV-2). Science. 1985;227:484–92.
28. Clements JE, Pedersen FS, Narayan O, et al. Genomic changes associated with antigenic variation of visna virus during persistent infection. Proc Natl Acad Sci USA. 1980;77:4454–8.
29. Robert-Guroff M, Brown M, Gallo RC. HTLV-III–neutralizing antibodies in patients with AIDS and AIDS-related complex. Nature. 1985;316:72–4.
30. Robert-Guroff M, Oleske JM, Connor EM, et al. Relationship between HTLV-III neutralizing antibody and clinical status of pediatric acquired immunodeficiency syndrome (AIDS) and AIDS-related complex cases. Pediatr Res. 1987;21:547–50.
31. Ranki A, Weiss SH, Sirkka-Liisa V, et al. Neutralizing antibodies in HIV (HTLV-III) infection: Correlation with clinical outcome and antibody response against different viral proteins. Clin Exp Immunol. 1987;69:231–9.
31a. Murphy BR, Chanock RM. Immunization against viruses. In: Fields BN, Knipe DN, Chanock RM, et al., eds. Virology. New York: Raven Press; 1985:349–70.
32. Sarin PS, Sun DK, Thornton AH, et al. Neutralization of HTLV-III/LAV replication by antiserum to thymosin α1. Science. 1986;232:1135–7.
33. Weiss RA, Clapham PR, Cheingson-Popov R, et al. Neutralization of human T-lymphotropic virus type III by sera of AIDS and AIDS-risk patients. Nature. 1985;316:69–72.
34. Osterhaus A, Weijer K, Uytdehagg F, et al. Induction of protective immune response in cats by vaccination with feline leukemia virus ISCOM. J Immunol. 1985;135:591–6.
35. Prince AM, Horowitz B, Baker L, et al. Failure of a human immunodeficiency virus (HIV) immune globulin to protect chimpanzees against experimental challenge with HIV. Proc Natl Acad Sci USA. 1988;85:6944–8.
36. Palker TJ, Clark ME, Langlois AJ, et al. Type-specific neutralization of the human immunodeficiency virus with antibodies to *env*-encoded synthetic peptides. Proc Natl Acad Sci USA. 1988;85:1932–6.
37. Earl PL, Moss B, Morrison RP, et al. T-lymphocyte priming and protection against Friend leukemia by vaccinia-retrovirus env gene recombinant. Science. 1986;234:728–31.
38. Quinnan GV, Kirmani N, Rook AH, et al. HLA-restricted T-lymphocyte and non T-lymphocyte cytotoxic responses correlate with recovery from cytomegalovirus infection in bone-marrow-transplant recipients. N Engl J Med. 1982;307:7–13.
39. Yap KL, Braciale TJ, Ada GL. Role of T-cell function in recovery from murine influenza infection. Cell. 1979;43:341–51.
40. Tam MR, Green WR, Nowinski RC. Cytotoxic activities of monoclonal antibodies against the envelope proteins of murine leukemia virus. Cancer Res. 1980;40:3850–3.
41. Lyerly HK, Matthews TJ, Langlois AJ, et al. Human T-cell lymphotropic virus IIIB glycoprotein [gp120] bound to CD4 determinants on normal lymphocytes and expressed by infected cells serves as target for immune attack. Proc Natl Acad Sci USA. 1987;84:4601–5.
42. Grant CK, Essex M, Pedersen NC, et al. Lysis of feline lymphoma cells by complement-dependent antibodies in feline leukemia virus contact cats. Correlation of lysis and antibodies to feline oncornavirus-associated cell membrane antigen. JNCI. 1978;60:161–6.
43. Matthews TJ, Weinhold KJ, Langlois AJ, et al. Immunologic control of a retrovirus-associated murine adenocarcinoma. VI. Augmentation of antibody-dependent killing following quantitative and qualitative changes in host peritoneal cells. JNCI. 1985;75:703–8.
44. Rook AH, Lane HC, Folks T, et al. Sera from HTLV-III/LAV antibody–positive individuals mediate antibody-dependent cellular cytotoxicity against HTLV-III/LAV–infected T cells. J Immunol. 1987;138:1064–7.
45. Blumberg RS, Paradis T, Hartshorn KL, et al. Antibody-dependent cell-mediated cytotoxicity against cells infected with the human immunodeficiency virus. J Infect Dis. 1987;156:878–84.
46. Ojo-amaize EA, Nishanian P, Keith DE Jr, et al. Antibodies to human immunodeficiency virus in human sera induce cell-mediated lysis of human immunodeficiency virus–infected cells. J Immunol. 1987;139:2458–63.
47. Spickett GP, Dalgleish AG. Cellular immunology of HIV-infection. Clin Exp Immunol. 1988;71:1–7.
48. Ljunggren K, Bottiger B, Biberfeld G, et al. Antibody-dependent cellular cytotoxicity-inducing antibodies against human immunodeficiency virus. J Immunol. 1987;139:2263–7.
49. DeNoronha F, Schafer W, Essex M, et al. Influence of antisera to oncornavirus glycoprotein (gp 71) on infections of cats with feline leukemia virus. Virology. 1978;85:617–21.
50. Schwarz H, Ihle JN, Wecker E, et al. Properties of mouse leukemia viruses. XVII. Factors required for successful treatment of spontaneous AKR leukemia by antibodies against gp71. Virology. 1981;111:568–78.
51. Ward EC, Iglehart JD, Weinhold KJ, et al. Immunotherapy of a murine leukemia virus–infected, chemically induced murine sarcoma with antiviral antibodies. JNCI. 1982;69:509–14.
52. Walker BD, Chakrabarti S, Moss B, et al. HIV-specific cytotoxic T lymphocytes in seropositive individuals. Nature. 1987;328:345–7.
53. Walker BD, Flexner C, Paradis TJ, et al. HIV-1 reverse transcriptase is a target for cytotoxic T lymphocytes in infected individuals. Science. 1988;240:64–6.
54. Weinhold KJ, Lyerly HK, Matthews TJ, et al. Cellular anti-gp120 cytolytic reactivities in HIV-1 seropositive individuals. Lancet. 1988;1:902–5.
55. Plata F, Autran B, Martins LP, et al. AIDS virus–specific cytotoxic T lymphocytes in lung disorders. Nature. 1987;328:348–51.
56. Nara PL, Robey WG, Gonda MA, et al. Absence of cytotoxic antibody to human immunodeficiency virus–infected cells in humans and its induction in animals after infection or immunization with purified envelope glycoprotein gp120. Proc Natl Acad Sci USA. 1987;84:3797–801.
57. Ogra PL, Karzon DT. Distribution of poliovirus antibody in serum, nasopharynx and alimentary tract following segmental immunization of lower alimentary tract with poliovaccine. J Immunol. 1968;102:1423–30.
58. Archibald DW, Barr CE, Torosian JP, et al. Secretory IgA antibodies to human immunodeficiency virus in the parotid saliva of patients with AIDS and AIDS-related complex. J Infect Dis. 1987;155:793–6.
59. Barnes DM. Solo actions of AIDS virus coat. Science. 1987;237:971–3.
60. del Guercio P, Zanetti M. The CD4 molecule, the human immunodeficiency virus and anti-idiotypic antibodies. Immunol Today. 1987;8:204–5.
61. Ellrodt A, Le Bras P. The hidden dangers of AIDS vaccination. Nature. 1987;325:765.
62. Robinson WE Jr, Montefiori DC, Mitchell WM. Antibody-dependent enhancement of human immunodeficiency virus type 1 infection. Lancet. 1988;1:790–4.
62a. Takeda A, Tuazon CU, Ennis FA. Antibody-enhanced infection by HIV-1 via Fc receptor-mediated entry. Science. 1988;242:580–3.
63. Martinez AC, Marcos MAR, de la Hera A, et al. Immunological consequences of HIV infection: Advantage of being low responder casts doubts on vaccine development. Lancet. 1988;1:454–7.
64. Dalgleish AG, Beverley PCL, Clapham PR, et al. The CD4 (T4) antigen is an essential component of the receptor for the AIDS retrovirus. Nature. 1984;312:763–7.
65. Putney SD, Matthews TJ, Robey WG, et al. HTLV-III/LAV–neutralizing antibodies to an *E. coli*–produced fragment of the virus envelope. Science. 1986;234:1392–5.
66. Lasky LA, Nakamura G, Smith JH, et al. Delineation of a region of the human immunodeficiency virus type 1 (HIV-1) gp120 glycoprotein critical for interaction with the CD4 receptor. Cell. 1987;50:975–85.
67. Lifson JD, Feinberg MB, Reyes GR, et al. Induction of CD4-dependent cell fusion by the HTLV-III/LAV envelope glycoprotein. Nature. 1986;323:725–8.
68. Sodroski J, Goh WC, Rosen C, et al. Role of the HTLV-III/LAV envelope in syncytium formation and cytopathicity. Nature. 1986;322:470–4.
69. Tas M, Drexhage HA, Goudsmit J. A monocyte chemotaxis inhibiting factor in serum of HIV infected men shares epitopes with the HIV transmembrane protein gp41. Clin Exp Immunol. 1988;71:13–8.
70. Mathes LE, Olsen RG, Hedebrand LC. Immunosuppressive properties of a virion polypeptide, a 15,000-dalton protein, from feline leukemia virus. Cancer Res. 1979;39:950–5.
71. McDougal JS, Mawle A, Cort SP, et al. Cellular tropism of the human retrovirus HTLV-III/LAV. I. Role of the T cell activation and expression of the T4 antigen. J Immunol. 1985;135:3151–62.
72. Gurney ME, Apatoff BR, Spear GT, et al. Neuroleukin: A lymphokine product of lectin-stimulated T cells. Science. 1986;234:574–81.
73. Reiher WE, Blalock JE, Brunck TK. Sequence homology between acquired immunodeficiency syndrome virus envelope protein and interleukin 2. Proc Natl Acad Sci USA. 1988;83:9188–92.
74. Halsted SB, O'Rourke EJ. Dengue viruses and mononuclear phagocytes. I. Infection enhancement by non-neutralizing antibody. J Exp Med. 1977;146:201–17.
75. Anonymous. First AIDS vaccine to enter clinical trials. Innovations. 1987;2:1,7.
76. Perricone R, Fontana L, DeCarolis C, et al. Evidence for activation of complement in patients with AIDS related complex (ARC) and/or lymphadenopathy syndrome (LAS). Clin Exp Immunol. 1987;70:500–7.
77. Barnes DM. The challenge of testing potential AIDS vaccines. Science. 1986;233:1151.
78. Wittek AE, Phelan MA, Wells MA, et al. Detection of human immunodeficiency virus core protein in plasma by enzyme immunoassay. Association of antigenemia with symptomatic disease and T-helper cell depletion. Ann Intern Med. 1987;107:286–92.
79. Harada S, Koyanagi Y, Yamamoto N. Infection of HTLV-III/LAV in HTLV-1-carrying cells MT-2 and MT-4 and application in a plaque assay. Science. 1985;229:563–6.
80. Vujcic LK, Shepp DH, Klutch M, et al. Use of sensitive neutralization assay to measure the prevalence of antibodies to the human immunodeficiency virus. J Infect Dis. 1988;157:1047–50.
81. Fultz PN, McClure HM, Swenson RB, et al. Persistent infection of chim-

panzees with human T-lymphotropic virus type III/lymphadenopathy-associated virus: A potential model for acquired immunodeficiency syndrome. J Virol. 1986;58:116–24.
82. Nara PL, Robey WG, Arthur LO, et al. Persistent infection of chimpanzees with human immunodeficiency virus: Serological responses and properties of reisolated viruses. J Virol. 1987;61:3173–80.
83. Alter JH, Eichberg JW, Masur H, et al. Transmission of HTLV-III infection from human plasma to chimpanzees: An animal model for AIDS. Science. 1984;226:549–52.
84. Gajdusek DC, Gibbs CJ, Rodgers-Johnson P, et al. Infection of chimpanzees by human T-lymphotropic retroviruses in brain and other tissues from AIDS patients. Lancet. 1985;1:55–6.
85. Barnes DM. Broad issues debated at AIDS vaccine workshop. Science. 1987;236:255.
86. Newmark P. Problems with AIDS vaccines. Nature. 1986;324:304–5.
87. Barnes D. AIDS vaccine trial OKed. Science. 1987;237:973.
88. Daniel MD, Letvin NL, King NW, et al. Isolation of T-cell tropic HTLV-III-like retrovirus from macaques. Science. 1985;228:1201–4.
89. Letvin NL, Daniel MD, Sehgal PK, et al. Induction of AIDS-like disease in macaque monkeys with T-cell tropic retrovirus STLV-III. Science. 1985;230:71–3.
90. Bryant ML, Yamamoto J, Luciw P, et al. Molecular comparison of retroviruses associated with human and simian AIDS. Hematol Oncol. 1985;3:187–97.
91. Gonda MA, Wong-Staal F, Gallo RC. Sequence homology and morphologic similarity of HTLV-III and visna virus, a pathogenic lentivirus. Science. 1985;227:173–7.
92. Pedersen NC, Ho EW, Brown ML, et al. Isolation of a T-lymphotropic virus from domestic cats with an immunodeficiency-like syndrome. Science. 1987;235:790–3.
93. Gonda MA, Braun MJ, Carter SG, et al. Characterization and molecular cloning of a bovine lentivirus related to human immunodeficiency virus. Nature. 1987;330:388–91.
94. McGuire TC, Adams DS, Johnson GC, et al. Challenge exposure of vaccinated or persistently infected goats. Am J Vet Res. 1986;47:537–40.
95. Allan JS, Coltigan JE, Barin F, et al. Major glycoprotein antigens that induce antibodies in AIDS patients are encoded by HTLV-III. Science. 1985;228:1091–4.
96. Veronese FD, DeVico AL, Copeland TD, et al. Characterization of gp41 as the transmembrane protein coded by the HTLV-III/LAV envelope gene. Science. 1985;229:1402–5.
97. Robey WG, Safai B, Oroszlan S, et al. Characterization of envelope and core structural gene products of HTLV-III with sera from AIDS patients. Science. 1985;228:593–5.
98. Robey WG, Arthur LO, Matthews TJ, et al. Prospect for prevention of human immunodeficiency virus infection: Purified 120-kDa envelope glycoprotein induces neutralizing antibody. Proc Natl Acad Sci USA. 1986;83:7023–7.
99. Lasky LA, Groopman JE, Fennie CW, et al. Neutralization of the AIDS retrovirus by antibodies to a recombinant envelope glycoprotein. Science. 1986;233:209–12.
100. Crowl R, Ganguly K, Gordon M, et al. HTLV-III env gene products synthesized in *E. coli* are recognized by antibodies present in the sera of AIDS patients. Cell. 1985;41:979–86.
101. Ratner L, Gallo RC, Wong-Staal F. HTLV-III, LAV, ARV are variants of the same AIDS virus. Nature. 1985;313:636–7.
102. Lewis MG, Mathes LE, Olson RG. Protection against feline leukemia by vaccination with a subunit vaccine. Infect Immun. 1981;34:888–94.
103. Onuma M, Hodatsu T, Yamamoto S, et al. Protection by vaccination against bovine leukemia virus infection in sheep. Am J Vet Res. 1984;45:1212–5.
104. Hunsmann G, Schneider J, Schulz A. Immunoprevention of Friend virus–induced erythroleukemia by vaccination with viral envelope glycoprotein complexes. Virology. 1981;113:602–12.
105. Jasny BR. Insect viruses invade biotechnology. Science. 1987;238:1653.
106. Rusche JR, Lynn DL, Robert-Guroff M, et al. Humoral immune response to the entire human immunodeficiency virus envelope glycoprotein made in insect cells. Proc Natl Acad Sci USA. 1987;84:6924–8.
107. Chang NT, Chanda PK, Barone AD, et al. Expression in *Escherichia coli* of open reading frame gene segments of HTLV-III. Science. 1985;228:93–6.
108. Wright K. AIDS protein made. Nature. 1986;319:525.
109. Krohn K, Robey WG, Putney S, et al. Specific cellular immune response and neutralizing antibodies in goats immunized with native or recombinant envelope proteins derived from human T-lymphotropic virus type III_B and in human immunodeficiency virus–infected men. Proc Natl Acad Sci USA. 1987;84:4994–8.
109a. Berman PW, Groopman JE, Gregory T, et al. Human immunodeficiency virus type 1 challenge of chimpanzees immunized with recombinant envelope glycoprotein gp120. Proc Natl Acad Sci USA. 1988;85:5200–4.
110. Arthur LO, Pyle SW, Nara PL, et al. Serological responses in chimpanzees inoculated with human immunodeficiency virus glycoprotein (gp120) subunit vaccine. Proc Natl Acad Sci USA. 1987;84:8583–7.
111. Cease KB, Margalit H, Cornette JL, et al. Helper T-cell antigenic site identification in the acquired immunodeficiency syndrome virus gp120 envelope protein and induction of immunity in mice to the native protein using a 16-residue synthetic peptide. Proc Natl Acad Sci USA. 1987;84:4249–53.
112. Kennedy RC, Henkel RD, Pauletti D, et al. Antiserum to a synthetic peptide recognizes the HTLV-III envelope glycoprotein. Science. 1986;231:1556–1559.
113. Steward MW, Howard CR. Synthetic peptides: A next generation of vaccines? Immunol Today. 1987;8:51–7.
114. Hopp TP, Woods KR. Prediction of protein antigenic determinants from amino acid sequences. Proc Natl Acad Sci USA. 1981;78:3824–8.
115. DeLisi C, Berzofsky JA. T-cell antigenic sites tend to be amphipathic structures. Proc Natl Acad Sci USA. 1985;82:7048–52.
116. Warren HS, Vogel FR, Chedid LA. Current status of immunological adjuvants. Annu Rev Immunol. 1986;4:369–88.
117. Gartner S, Markovits P, Markovitz DM, et al. The role of mononuclear phagocytes in HTLV-III/LAV infection. Science. 1986;233:215–9.
118. Weber JN, Clapham PR, Weiss RA, et al. Human immunodeficiency virus infection in two cohorts of homosexual men: Neutralising sera and association of anti-gag antibody with prognosis. Lancet. 1987;1:119–22.
119. Groopman JE, Chen FW, Hope JA, et al. Serological characterization of HTLV-III infection in AIDS and related disorders. J Infect Dis. 1986;153:736–42.
120. Brown F, Schild GC, Ada GL. Recombinant vaccinia viruses as vaccines. Nature. 1986;319:549–50.
121. Hu S-L, Kosowski SG, Dalrymple JM. Expression of AIDS virus envelope gene in recombinant vaccinia viruses. Nature. 1986;320:537–40.
122. Chakrabarti S, Robert-Guroff M, Wong-Staal F, et al. Expression of the HTLV-III envelope gene by a recombinant vaccinia virus. Nature. 1986;320:535–7.
123. Moss B, Flexner C. Vaccinia virus expression vectors. Annu Rev Immunol. 1987;5:305–24.
124. Davis AR, Kostek B, Mason BB, et al. Expression of hepatitis B surface antigen with a recombinant adenovirus. Proc Natl Acad Sci USA. 1985;82:7560–4.
125. Buller RML, Smith GL, Cremer K, et al. Decreased virulence of recombinant vaccinia virus expression vectors is associated with a thymidine kinase-negative phenotype. Nature. 1985;317:813–5.
126. Hu S-L, Fultz PN, McClure HM, et al. Effect of immunization with a vaccinia-HIV *env* recombinant on HIV infection of chimpanzees. Nature. 1987;328:721–3.
127. Zarling JM, Morton W, Moran PA, et al. T-cell responses to human AIDS virus in macaques immunized with recombinant vaccinia viruses. Nature. 1986;323:344–6.
128. Zagury D, Leonard R, Fouchard M, et al. Immunization against AIDS in humans. Nature. 1987;326:249–50.
129. Zagury D, Bernard J, Cheynier R, et al. A group specific anamnestic immune reaction against HIV-1 induced by a candidate vaccine against AIDS. Nature. 1988;332:728–31.
130. Ezzell C. Another AIDS vaccine. Nature. 1987;328:509.
131. Chapter 7. Developments in vaccination and control between 1900 and 1966. In: Fenner F, Henderson DA, Arita I, et al, eds. Smallpox and Its Eradication. Geneva: World Health Organization; 1988:277–314.
132. Redfield RR, Wright DC, James WD, et al. Disseminated vaccinia in a military recruit with human immunodeficiency virus (HIV) disease. N Engl J Med. 1987;316:673–6.
133. Flexner C, Hugin A, Moss B. Prevention of vaccinia virus infection in immunodeficient mice by vector-directed IL-2 expression. Nature. 1987;330:259–62.
134. Ramshaw IA, Andrew ME, Phillips SM, et al. Recovery of immunodeficient mice from a vaccinia virus/IL-2 recombinant infection. Nature. 1987;329:545–6.
135. Salk J. Prospects for the control of AIDS by immunizing seropositive individuals. Nature. 1987;327:473–6.
136. Marx PA, Pedersen NC, Lerche NW, et al. Prevention of simian acquired immune deficiency syndrome with a formalin-inactivated type D retrovirus vaccine. J Virol. 1986;60:431–5.
137. Ranki A, Krohn M, Allain JP, et al. Long latency precedes overt seroconversion in sexually transmitted human-immunodeficiency-virus infection. Lancet. 1987;2:589–93.
138. Francis DP, Jaffe HW, Fultz PN, et al. The natural history of infection with the lymphadenopathy-associated virus human T-lymphotropic virus type III. Ann Intern Med. 1985;103:719–22.
139. Ezzell C. Killed HIV treatment in clinical trials. Nature. 1988;332:668.
140. Szmuness W, Stevens CE, Harley EJ, et al. Hepatitis B vaccine. Demonstration of efficacy in a controlled clinical trial in a high risk population in the United States. N Engl J Med. 1980;303:833–41.
141. Fisher AG, Ratner L, Mitsuya H, et al. Infectious mutants of HTLV-III with changes in the 3′ region and markedly reduced cytopathic effects. Science. 1986;233:655–9.
142. Klatzmann D, Champagne E, Chamaret S, et al. T-lymphocyte T4 molecule behaves as the receptor for human retrovirus. Nature. 1984;312:767–8.
143. Dalgleish AG, Thomson BJ, Chanh TC, et al. Neutralisation of HIV isolates by anti-idiotypic antibodies which mimic the T4(CD4) epitope: A potential AIDS vaccine. Lancet. 1987;2:1047–50.
144. Koprowski H. Unconventional vaccines: Immunization with anti-idiotype antibody against viral disease. Cancer Res. 1985;45(Suppl):4689–90.
145. Chanh TC, Dreesman GR, Kennedy RC. Monoclonal antiidiotypic antibody mimics the CD4 receptor and binds human immunodeficiency virus. Proc Natl Acad Sci USA. 1987;84:3891–5.
146. Dalgleish AG. The T4 molecule. Immunol Today. 1986;7:142–4.

147. Benjamin RJ, Waldmann H. Introduction of tolerance by monoclonal antibody therapy. Nature. 1986;320:449–51.
148. Pitts FN Jr, Allen RE, Haraszti JS, et al. Improvement of four patients with HIV-1 related symptoms after hyperimmunization with killed poliomyelitis (Salk) vaccine. Clin Immunol Immunopathol. 1988;46:167–8.
149. Kehrl JH, Fauci AS. Activation of human B lymphocytes after immunization with pneumococcal polysaccharides. J Clin Invest. 1983;71:1032–40.
150. Edelman R. Vaccine adjuvants. Rev Infect Dis. 1980;2:370–83.
151. Chedid L, Audibert F, Lefrancier P, et al. Modulation of the immune response by a synthetic adjuvant and analogs. Proc Natl Acad Sci USA. 1976;73:2472–5.
152. Allison AC, Gregoriadis G. Liposomes as immunological adjuvants. Nature. 1974;252:252.
153. Parant M, Audibert F, Chedid L, et al. Immunostimulant activities of a lipophilic muramyl dipeptide derivative and of desmuramyl peptidolipid analogs. Infect Immun. 1980;27:826–31.
154. Masek K, Zaoral M, Jezek J, et al. Immunoadjuvant activity of synthetic *N*-acetylmuramyl dipeptide. Experimentia. 1978;34:1363–4.
155. Sanchez Y, Ionescu-Matiu I, Dreesman GR, et al. Humoral and cellular immunity to hepatitis B virus–derived antigens: Comparative activity of Freund complete adjuvant, alum and liposomes. Infect Immun. 1980;30:728.
156. Desiderio JV, Campbell SG. Immunization against experimental murine salmonellosis with liposome-associated O-antigen. Infect Immun. 1985; 48:658–63.
157. Jolivet M, Sache E, Audibert F. Biological studies of lipophilic MDP derivatives incorporated into liposomes. Immunol Commun. 1981;10:511–22.
158. Morein B. The iscom antigen–presenting system. Nature. 1988;332:287–88.
159. Morein B, Sundquist B, Hoglund S, et al. Iscom, a novel structure for antigenic presentation of membrane proteins from enveloped viruses. Nature. 1984;308:457–60.
160. Morein B, Lovgren K, Hoglund S, et al. Iscom: An immune stimulating complex. Immunol Today. 1987;8:333–8.
161. Wahren B, Nordlund S, Akesson A, et al. Monocyte and ISCOM enhancement of cell-mediated response to cytomegalovirus. Med Microbiol Immunol. 1987;176:13–9.
162. Howard CR, Sundquist B, Allen J, et al. Preparation and properties of immune-stimulating complexes containing hepatitis B virus surface antigen. J Virol. 1987;68:2281–9.
163. Newmark P. Human and monkey virus puzzles. Nature. 1987;327:458.
164. Nabel GJ, Rice SA, Knipe DM, et al. Alternative mechanisms for activation of human immunodeficiency virus enhancer in T cells. Science. 1988;239:1299–302.
165. Walters L. Ethical issues in the prevention and treatment of HIV infection and AIDS. Science. 1988;239:597–603.
166. Barnes DM. Will an AIDS vaccine bankrupt the company that makes it? Science. 1986;223:1035.

INFECTIOUS DISEASES AND THEIR ETIOLOGIC AGENTS

PART III

SECTION A. VIRAL DISEASES

112. INTRODUCTION TO VIRUSES AND VIRAL DISEASES

KENNETH L. TYLER
BERNARD N. FIELDS

HISTORY

The history of virology encompasses virtually the entire time span of recorded history.[1] Viral diseases have the distinction of being among both the oldest recorded human diseases (e.g., rabies, polio) as well as some of the most recently described (acquired immunodeficiency syndrome [AIDS]). The tempo of advances in the history of virology began to accelerate during the nineteenth century. First, careful clinical observations led to the identification and differentiation of a number of viral illnesses (e.g., smallpox from chickenpox and measles from rubella). Second, this improved clinical definition of illnesses combined with improvements in pathologic techniques and methods, exemplified by Virchow, allowed the pathologic substrate of many viral diseases to be identified. Finally, the work of Pasteur ushered in the systematic use of laboratory animals to study the pathogenesis of disease.

As the nineteenth century ended and the twentieth century began, the first viruses were identified. Beijerinck identified tobacco mosaic virus and Loeffler and Frosch discovered foot and mouth disease virus. This was quickly followed by the discovery of the first human disease-causing virus, yellow fever virus, and the seminal work on the pathogenesis of yellow fever by Walter Reed and the Army Yellow Fever Commission.[2] By the end of the 1930s tumor viruses, bacteriophages, influenza viruses, mumps, and many arboviruses had been identified. This process of discovery has continued unabated through the present, with the human immunodeficiency (HIV) and human T-cell lymphotropic viruses being the most recent additions to the catalog of human disease-causing viruses.

In the 1940s, using bacteriophages as a model, Delbruck, Luria, and others established many of the basic principles of microbial genetics and molecular biology and identified the major events in the viral growth cycle.[3,4] The pioneering experiments of Avery and associates on the transformation of pneumococcal types, which established that DNA was the genetic material,[5] set the stage for the experiments by Hershey and Chase[6] showing that the genetic material of bacteriophages was also DNA. In the late 1940s, Enders and colleagues grew poliovirus in tissue culture.[7] This work led to the subsequent development of both formalin-inactivated (Salk) and live attenuated (Sabin) vaccines for polio[8,9] and ushered in the modern era of virology.

Technical advances such as the development of electron microscopy, ultracentrifugation, and techniques for the electrophoresis of nucleic acids and proteins set the stage for improved understanding of viral structure and for a detailed biochemical analysis of purified virion components and their biologic properties.

In the modern era the use of x-ray crystallography has allowed structural definition of viruses and their components at a near-atomic level. By using the techniques of molecular biology, the entire genomes of many viruses have been sequenced. Monoclonal antibodies have enabled specific domains on viral proteins to be defined with a precision previously impossible. These techniques and others are already being applied to the development of new strategies for the diagnosis of viral illness and the design of effective antiviral therapy. For example, the polymerase chain reaction (PCR) technique allows small amounts of nucleic acid, for example, the integrated DNA of a retrovirus such as HIV that is present in some circulating host cells, to be dramatically amplified, which greatly facilitates its subsequent detection. Techniques such as this may prove to be greatly superior to conventional serologic approaches to diagnosis of viral diseases. Among the challenges for the future will be the application of these powerful new techniques to expand our understanding at the molecular level of how viruses interact with target cells to alter function, how the interaction of viruses and cells within a living host produce disease, and how events in the infected host result in the transmission of disease and the maintenance of infectious viruses in the environment. Improved understanding of these aspects of viral infection should lead to new approaches to the diagnosis, prevention, and cure of viral diseases.

VIRUS STRUCTURE AND CLASSIFICATION

The first classification of viruses as a group distinct from other microorganisms was based almost exclusively on their ability to pass through filters of a small pore size (''filterable agents''). Initial subdivisions were based primarily on pathologic properties such as specific organ tropism (e.g., enteroviruses) or on common epidemiologic features such as tranmission by arthropod vectors (e.g., arboviruses). Since the 1950s classification has depended predominantly on morphologic and physicochemical criteria.[10] More recently, the availability of an increasing body of knowledge concerning the nucleic acid properties of many viral genomes has led to attempts to reorganize classification along lines of genetic relatedness. The key constituents of current classification systems are (*1*) the type and structure of the viral nucleic acid and the strategy used in its replication, (*2*) the type of symmetry of the virus capsid (helical vs. icosahedral), and (*3*) the presence or absence of an envelope (see Table 1). Each of these features will be discussed in more detail in subsequent sections.

Much of our current knowledge about viral structure has been gained from the examination of electron micrographs of negatively stained viral particles (virions). The use of high-resolution x-ray crystallographic techniques has recently provided views of viral structure at the atomic level. Identification of key structural motifs such as receptor binding sites or immunodominant domains can provide the framework for beginning to understand structural features involved in virus–cell interactions.

The genetic information of viruses is encoded in nucleic acids, which occurs in individual viral families in a wide variety of forms and sizes (Table 1 and Fig. 1). The nucleic acid may be composed of either RNA or DNA. Its size can range from 10^6 daltons in small viruses such as the Parvoviridae to $>200 \times 10^6$ daltons in complex viruses such as the Poxviridae. The genomes of the smallest viruses probably encode only three or four unique proteins, whereas those of the largest viruses may encode several hundred proteins. The DNA and RNA can occur in either single- or double-stranded forms and can be either circular (i.e., closed) or linear (i.e., open ended) in shape. Viruses with linear RNA may have either a single piece of nucleic acid

TABLE 1. Classification of Viruses

Family	*Example*	*Type of Nucleis Acid*	*Genome Size (Kilobases or Kilobase Pairs)*	*Envelope*	*Capsid Symmetry*
Picornaviridae	Poliovirus	SS (+) RNA	7.2–8.4	No	I
Caliciviridae	Norwalk virus	SS (+) RNA	8	No	I
Togaviridae	Rubella virus	SS (+) RNA	12	Yes	I
Flaviviridae	Yellow fever virus	SS (+) RNA	10	Yes	Unk
Coronaviridae	Coronaviruses	SS (+) RNA	16–21	Yes	H
Rhabdoviridae	Rabies virus	SS (−) RNA	13–16	Yes	H
Filoviridae	Marburg virus	SS (−) RNA	13	Yes	H
Paramyxoviridae	Measles virus	SS (−) RNA	16–20	Yes	H
Orthomyxoviridae	Influenza viruses	8 SS (−) RNA segments[a]	14	Yes	H
Bunyaviridae	California encephalitis virus	3 circular SS (−) RNA segments	13–21	Yes	H
Arenaviridae	Lymphocytic choriomeningitis virus	2 circular SS (−) RNA segments	10–14	Yes	H
Reoviridae	Rotaviruses	10–12 DS RNA[2] segments	16–27	No	I
Retroviridae	HIV-1	2 identical SS (+) RNA segments	3–9	Yes	I—capsid H—nucleocapsid (probable)
Hepadnaviridae	Hepatitis B	DS DNA with SS portions	3	Yes	Unk
Parvoviridae	Human parvovirus B-19	SS (+) or (−) DNA	5	No	I
Papoviridae	JC virus	Circular DS DNA	8	No	I
Adenoviridae	Human adenoviruses	DS DNA	36–38	No	I
Herpesviridae	Herpes simplex virus	DS DNA	120–220	Yes	I
Poxviridae	Vaccinia	DS DNA with covalently closed ends	130–280	No	Complex

Abbreviations: DS: double stranded; SS: single stranded; (+): message sense; (−): anti-message sense; I: icosahedral; H: helical; Unk: unknown.
(From Murphy,[10] with permission.)
[a] Influenza C: seven segments.
[b] Reovirus, orbivurus: 10 segments; rotavirus: 11 segments; Colorado tick fever: 12 segments.

or a variable number of segments. The number of RNA segments can vary in number from as few as 2 (Arenaviridae) to as many as 12 (some Reoviridae).

The viral nucleic acid is packaged in a protein coat (capsid) that is composed of multiple, nearly identical repeating protein subunits (capsomeres). The combination of the viral nucleic acid and the surrounding protein capsid is often referred to as the nucleocapsid (Fig. 2). A number of general principles have emerged from studies of virus structure.[13,14] First, in almost all cases the capsid is composed of a repeating series of structurally similar subunits, each of which is in turn composed of at most only a few different proteins. The parsimonious use of structural proteins in a repetitive motif minimizes the amount of the viral genome that must be committed to encode the capsid components. The use of only a few different types of proteins and the repetition of subunits also leads to structural arrangements of virus capsids with symmetric features. All but the most complex viruses exhibit one of two types of capsid symmetry (Table 1). In helically symmetric viruses the repeating protein subunits of the capsid are bound periodically along the helical spiral formed by the viral nucleic acid. Interestingly, all animal viruses that show this type of symmetry have RNA genomes.

The second major type of capsid symmetry is icosahedral. Viruses with this type of symmetry typically have a nearly spherical shape, with twofold, threefold, and fivefold axes of rotational symmetry. The nucleic acid, which can be either DNA or RNA, is tightly packed inside the spherical core and is also intimately associated with specific viral capsid proteins, although the details of this interaction are not as well understood as they are for helically symmetric viruses.

The use of repeating subunits with symmetric protein–protein interactions undoubtedly facilitates the assembly of the viral capsid. In most cases this appears to be an autocatalytic process that occurs spontaneously under the appropriate physiologic conditions. In some viruses such as the bacteriophages, assembly of the capsid may proceed through a series of intermediates or subassemblies, each of which seems to nucleate the addition of subsequent components in the sequence.

One of the most poorly understood aspects of viral assembly is the process that ensures that the viral nucleic acid is correctly packaged into the capsid. In the case of helically symmetric viruses there may be an initiation site on the nucleic acid to which the initial capsomere subunit binds, triggering the addition of subsequent subunits. In preparations of many icosahedral viruses, it is not uncommon to find empty capsids (i.e., capsids lacking nucleic acid), which indicates that assembly may proceed to completion without a requirement for the presence of the viral genome.

In some viruses the nucleocapsid is surrounded by a lipid envelope acquired as the virus particle buds from host cell cytoplasmic or nuclear membranes or the endoplasmic reticulum. Into this lipid bilayer are inserted virally encoded proteins (e.g., the hemagglutinin [HA] and neuraminidase [NM] of influenza), which are exposed on the outside of the virus particle. These viral proteins typically contain a glycosylated hydrophilic external portion and internally positioned hydrophobic domains that span the lipid membrane and serve to anchor the proteins. In some cases another viral protein may associate with the internal (cytoplasmic) surface of the lipid envelope where it can interact with the cytoplasmic domains of the envelope glycoproteins. These matrix (M) proteins may play a role in directing the insertion of viral glycoproteins into host cell membranes, in stabilizing the interaction between these proteins and the lipid envelope, or in facilitating viral budding.

Viruses belonging to the family Reoviridae, which includes the human rotaviruses, have an outer protein shell that surrounds the nucleocapsid. The mechanisms by which the two capsids are assembled in proper relationship to each other remains to be identified.

VIRUS–CELL INTERACTIONS

The interaction between a virus and a target cell begins with attachment of the virus particle to the cell surface.[15] This process is initiated by a random collision between a virus particle and the cell surface. Tighter binding is facilitated by appropriate ionic and pH conditions in the extracellular milieu. Attachment may involve the interaction between specific proteins on the

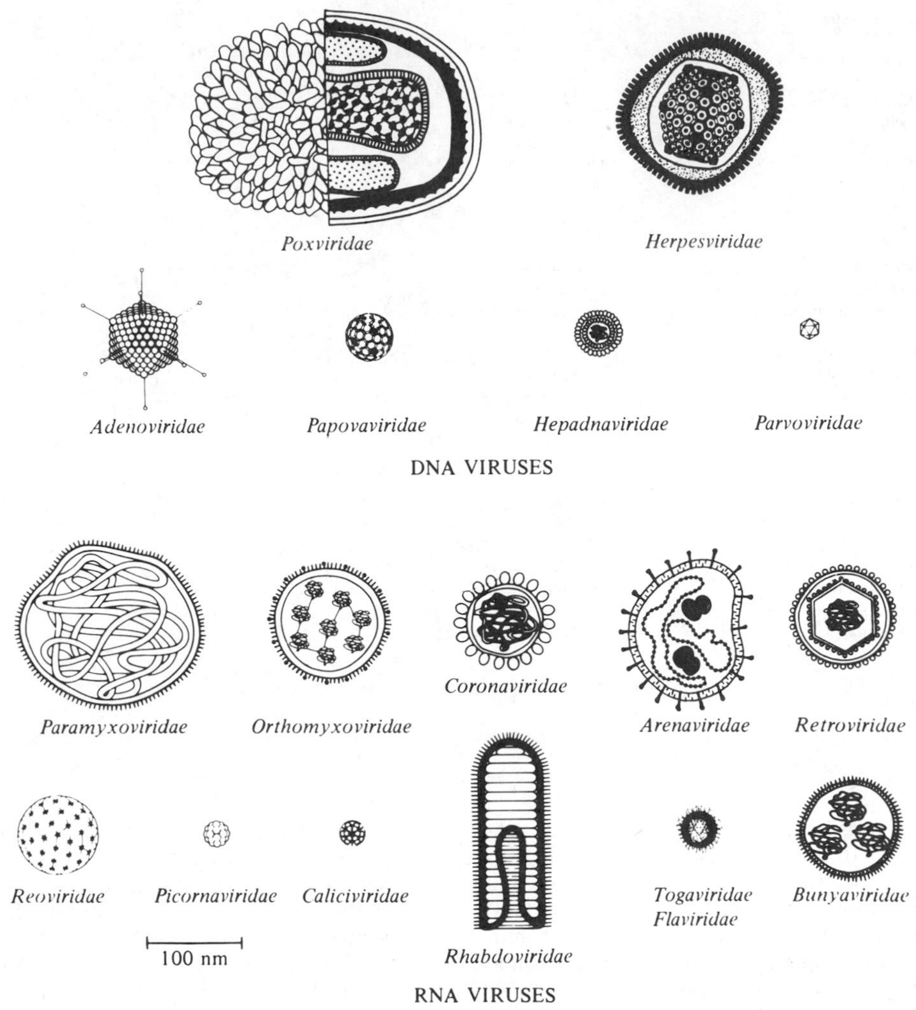

FIG. 1. Diagrams illustrating the general sizes and shapes of animal viruses belonging to families known to be pathogenic to humans. (From White et al.,[11] with permission.)

viral surface (virion attachment protein [VAP]) and specific receptors in the target cell membrane. The nature of the VAP has been identified for a number of viruses. In the case of enveloped viruses the VAP is typically one of the envelope glycoproteins such as the HA glycoprotein of influenza. Outer capsid proteins typically serve as the VAPs for nonenveloped viruses. For some viruses more then one surface protein may be involved in receptor binding.

Using high resolution x-ray crystallography it has been possible to obtain detailed views of the three-dimensional structure of the VAPs of a number of viruses including influenza and several of the picornaviruses (polio, rhino, mengo, encephalomyocarditis [EMC], Theiler).[16–20] The receptor binding domain of the flu HA is located at the distal end of its globular head (Fig. 3). The receptor-binding sites of the picornaviruses appear to take the form of depressions or indentations in the surface topology of the virion. These depressions can take the form of "pits" (mengovirus), "canyons" (rhinovirus), or "valleys" (poliovirus) and are clearly visible on electron density maps of the virus particles.

One of the most dynamic areas of current research in virology deals with the identification of viral receptors on host cells. A number of putative viral receptors have now been identified (Table 2); however, in many cases considerable controversy concerning these identifications still exists.

A number of important principles have emerged from studies of VAPs and host cell receptors. First, cells presumably did not evolve with viral receptors on their surfaces. Instead, viruses have adapted to "parasitize" host-cell surface molecules designed to subserve a variety of normal cellular functions. These may either be highly specialized proteins with somewhat limited distribution such as neurotransmitters, hormones, and complement receptors or may be more ubiquitous components of cellular membranes such as sialoglycoproteins or phospholipids. Second, it appears that some viruses may use more then one type of host cell receptor or possibly both specific receptor-mediated and other nonspecific pathways to enter cells. Finally, it has been frequently demonstrated that not all cells carrying the receptor for a particular virus can be productively infected by that virus. Therefore, although receptor binding may be a first step in the interaction between viruses and cells, subsequent events in the viral life cycle must also be successfully completed for productive infection to occur.

Once attachment has occurred, the virus must penetrate the plasma membrane of the cell, and then the capsid must undergo a series of conformational changes (uncoating) that prepares the virus for subsequent replication. Many enveloped and nonenveloped viruses penetrate cells through a process analogous to the receptor-mediated endocytosis of nonviral ligands such as hormones, growth factors, and toxins[23–25] (Fig. 4). In this schema viral–receptor complexes aggregate at distinct sites on the plasma membrane where specialized pits lined with the protein clathrin ("clathrin-coated pits") occur. These pits then invaginate to form coated vesicles, which are subsequently uncoated and form endosomes. The acidic pH of the interior of endosomes may trigger pH-dependent conformational changes

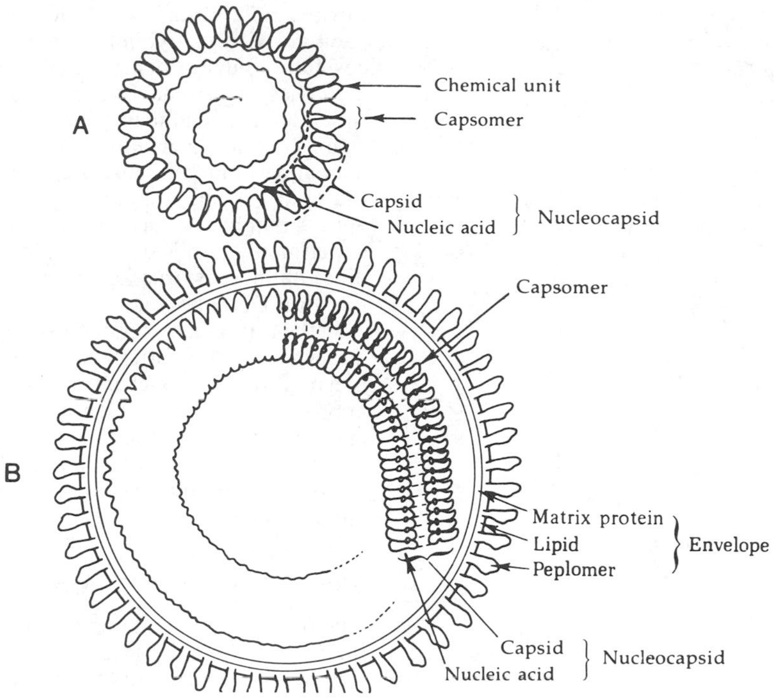

FIG. 2. Schematic diagrams of the structure of a nonenveloped icosahedral virus (**A**) and an enveloped helical virus (**B**). (Modified from Caspar et al.,[12] with permission.)

TABLE 2. Putative Viral Receptors

Virus	*Receptor*
Cytomegalovirus	β_2-Microglobulin/MHC
Encephalomyocarditis virus	Glycophorin A (RBCS)
Epstein-Barr virus	C3d receptor (CR2)
Human immunodeficiency virus	CD4 (T4 antigen)
Influenza virus	Glycophorin A (RBCS)
	Sialic acid
Lactate dehydrogenase–elevating virus	Ia
Rabies virus	Acetylcholine receptor
Reovirus type 3 (Dearing)	β-adrenergic–related receptor
	Glycophorin A (RBCS)
Semliki Forest virus	HLA, H-2 antigens
Sendai virus	Sialic acid
Vaccinia virus	Epidermal growth factor receptor
Vesicular stomatitis virus	Phospho- or glycolipids

(Data from Crowell et al.[21] and Marsh et al.[22])

in specific viral proteins. These conformational changes may uncover protein domains capable of mediating fusion between the viral envelope or capsid and the endosomal membrane, thereby allowing escape of the viral nucleocapsid into the cytoplasm. Endosomal vesicles may subsequently fuse with lysosomes. Proteolytic enzymes present in lysosomes may also trigger partial digestion of viral capsid proteins, which leads to activation of viral transcription.

Viruses may also enter cells through nonendocytic pathways such as direct translocation across the plasma membrane. For some enveloped viruses this may be mediated by direct fusion of the viral envelope with the outer membrane of target cells with subsequent entry of the nucleocapsid into the cytoplasm.[26]

Once a virus has successfully entered a target cell, it must replicate both its genome and the associated structural and nonstructural proteins. A discussion of the many strategies of replication used by different families of viruses is beyond the scope of this chapter (see Fields and Knipe[27]). However, certain basic principles are worth noting. First, there is no enzymatic mechanism in host cells to replicate RNA from an RNA template (i.e., no RNA-dependent RNA polymerases). Second, the host cell enzymes for making mRNA from DNA are all located in the nucleus and are therefore not accessible to DNA viruses whose replication is exclusively cytoplasmic.

There are two basic replication strategies used by single-stranded RNA viruses. If the genomic RNA is (+)sense it can serve directly as messenger RNA. For example, after infection of target cells with picornaviruses such as poliovirus, the viral genomic RNA serves directly as messenger RNA and is translated on target cell ribosomes into a large polyprotein. This protein is subsequently cleaved into several smaller proteins. One of these proteins is a RNA-dependent RNA polymerase, which serves to replicate the viral RNA. A different strategy is required for viruses with (−)sense genomic RNA since this RNA cannot serve directly as mRNA. These viruses all contain an RNA-dependent RNA polymerase that transcribes a (+)sense RNA segment from the original (−)sense genomic RNAs. These (+)sense RNAs can serve both as mRNAs and as templates for the replication of more genomic (−)sense RNAs.

RNA viruses belonging to the family Reoviridae have a segmented double-stranded RNA genome. These viruses contain a double-stranded RNA–single-stranded RNA polymerase that allows the production of (+)sense single-stranded RNA from the double-stranded RNA segments by using the (−)sense strand as a template. The reovirus (+)sense RNAs are capped at their 5′-terminal end by virally encoded enzymes and then extruded from the viral core through a channel formed by the core spike protein and serve as mRNAs. The (+)sense RNAs also serve as the templates for the viral polymerase to make (−)sense RNA segments that can then anneal with the complementary (+)sense strands to form new genomic double-standed RNAs.

Perhaps the most intriguing RNA replicative strategy is that used by the retroviruses. The viral genomic RNA is (+)sense and single stranded. However, unlike the case with the picornaviruses, it does not serve directly as mRNA. It is transcribed into DNA through the operation of a virally encoded RNA-dependent DNA polymerase ("reverse transcriptase"). The virally encoded DNA is then translocated into the host cell nu-

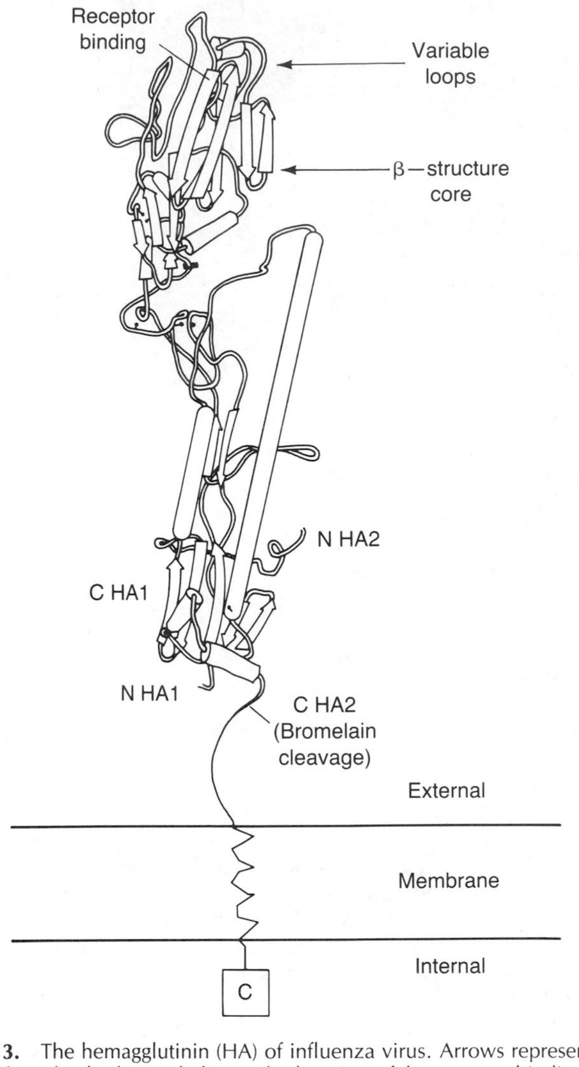

FIG. 3. The hemagglutinin (HA) of influenza virus. Arrows represent β-strands and cylinders, α-helices. The location of the receptor binding site is indicated. (Modified from Wilson,[17] with permission.)

cleus where it becomes integrated into the chromosomal DNA of the host ("provirus"). Transcription of this integrated DNA then falls under the control of the same transcriptase enzymes used by the host to replicate its own DNA. This transcription produces both mRNAs that encode viral proteins and genomic-length RNAs for packaging into progeny virions. The factors that govern whether this integrated viral DNA remains latent and untranscribed or is actively transcribed to produce progeny virions remains one of the unsolved mysteries of viral replication.

Viruses whose genomes are in the form of DNA did not have to develop as complex replicative strategies as those outlined above for RNA viruses. These viruses, which typically replicate in the nucleus of target cells, can use host cell enzymes for the production of mRNA from their DNA. In most cases, as exemplified by the herpesviruses, the viral mRNA encodes a DNA polymerase that serves to replicate the viral genomic DNA. A further degree of complexity is added by the fact that some DNA viruses can remain latent in the host. Unlike the case with retroviruses, the viral DNA does not typically integrate into host cell chromosomes but instead exists in episomal form. The factors that govern the reactivation from latency to active infection are currently the subject of active investigation.[28,29]

Knowledge of the replicative strategies of viruses has provided insights into critical steps in the viral life cycle that can serve as potential targets for antiviral therapy (see Shannon[30]). For example, drugs can be designed that interfere with the capacity of viruses to bind to their target cell receptors or to successfully undergo penetration-uncoating once receptor attachment has occurred. Two currently available antiviral agents, rimantadine and amantadine, which are effective in prophylaxis against influenza A infections, probably act by inhibiting viral uncoating in target cells. Steps involved in the transcription of the viral genome are another obvious target for antiviral therapy. A number of currently available (acylovir, vidarabine) and experimental (phosphonoformic acid, bromovinyldeoxyuridine) antiherpesvirus agents act, at least in part, by inhibiting the viral DNA polymerase.

In the future, a better understanding of viral replicative strategies will undoubtedly pave the way for the design and testing of a multitude of novel antiviral agents. One of the most exciting approaches to this problem will be to use high resolution x-ray crystallography to study the interaction between antiviral drugs and virions at the molecular level.[31] As more viral structures are solved, this approach may allow the design of highly specific antiviral agents.

VIRUS–HOST INTERACTION

One of the most fundamental challenges in virology is trying to integrate lessons learned from the study of virus–cell interaction in tissue culture into a conception of how viruses interact with an intact living host in order to produce the signs and symptoms of disease. The process by which a virus produces disease in an animal host is referred to as *pathogenesis*. The capacity of a virus to produce illness or death in susceptible animals is referred to as *virulence*, and it is often measured in terms of the amount of virus required to kill or cause infection in 50 percent of a cohort of mice infected under defined conditions. Pathogenesis and virulence were initially defined in largely descriptive terms. Specific stages in the pathogenesis of particular viral infections were identified and their associated pathologic substrates defined. More recently it has been possible, in some cases, to begin to identify the role played by specific viral genes and the proteins they encode at specific stages in viral pathogenesis and the importance of specific viral genes in determining viral virulence. The goal for future studies of pathogenesis will be to continue to define at a genetic and molecular level viral components involved at discrete steps in disease production.

The first step in the process of virus–host interaction is exposure of a susceptible host to infectious virus under conditions that are propitious for transmission.[32] The infecting virus may be present in respiratory droplets or aerosols, in fecally contaminated food or water, or in a body fluid or tissue (e.g., blood, saliva, urine, semen, or a transplanted organ) to which the susceptible host is exposed. In some cases the virus is inoculated directly into the host through the bite of an insect or animal vector or through the use of a sullied needle.

Infection can also be transmitted vertically, from a mother to her fetus or newborn child, through virus carried in the germ cell line, virus that has infected the placenta or maternal birth canal, or virus in maternal milk. In some cases acute viral infection results from the reactivation of endogenous latent virus that had previously lain dormant in the host (e.g., shingles, recurrent herpes labialis or genitalis), rather than from de novo exposure to exogenous virus.

One of the most important routes of transmission of infection to a susceptible host is through infected respiratory droplets or aerosols. A simple cough can generate up to 10,000 small potentially infectious aerosol particles and a sneeze, nearly 2 million! The distribution of these particles depends on a variety of ambient environmental factors, the most important of which are probably temperature, humidity, and air currents. Amother critical factor is particle size. In general, smaller particles remain airborne longer than do larger ones. Airborne particles are inspired through the nasopharynx, after which their ultimate fate

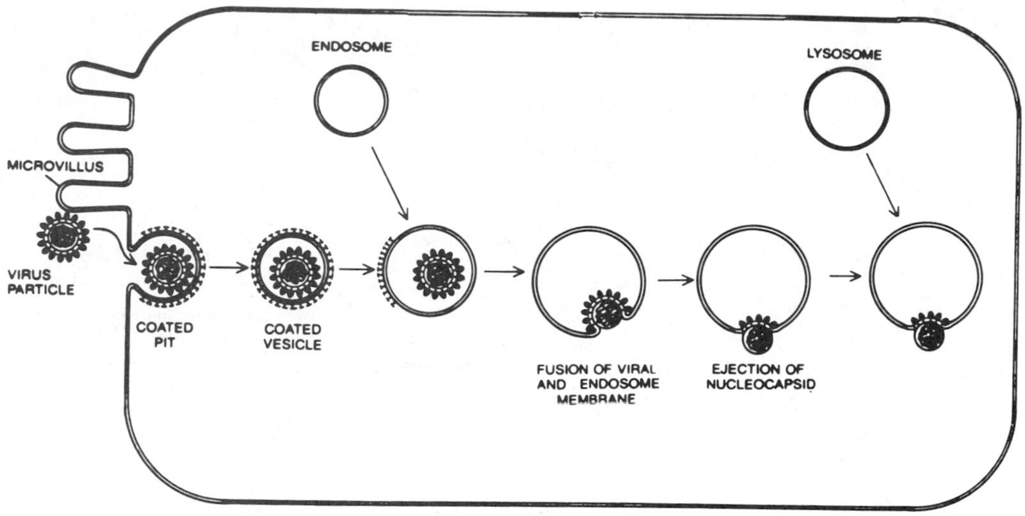

FIG. 4. Pathway of viral entry into cells. (Modified from Simons et al.,[25] with permission.)

depends largely on their size. Larger particles (>6 μm) are generally trapped in the nasal turbinates, whereas smaller particles may find their way into the tracheae and the bronchi of the upper respiratory tract or the alveolar spaces of the lower respiratory tract.

A second common route of viral transmission is through "fecal–oral" spread. Food, water, or hands contaminated by infected fecal material can allow the entry of virus via the mouth into the upper gastrointestinal (GI) tract. Once a virus has reached the upper GI tract, it faces a formidable physicochemical environment. Gastric juice is extremely acidic, at times approaching pH 2.0. Bile and proteolytic enzymes secreted from the gallbladder and pancreas enter the duodenum. The intestinal epithelial cells are covered by a carpet of mucous secreted by adjacent goblet cells. Secretory immunoglobulin (IgA) as well as non-immunoglobulin-inhibitory substances are also present.

The physicochemical environment of the GI tract essentially mandates that viruses infecting via this route have certain prescribed physical properties. They must be acid stable to survive transit through the stomach. Since bile salts are extremely destructive of the lipids present in viral envelopes, most enteric viruses are also nonenveloped. Finally, many viruses infecting via the GI tract have become adapted so that partial proteolytic digestion, rather than inhibiting viral infectivity, may actually be a necessary first step in the viral replicative cycle. This appears to be the case during rotavirus infection in which partial proteolytic digestion of the viral outer capsid actually enhances viral infectivity.

The lumens of the GI, respiratory, and genitourinary tracts can be considered extensions of the external environment. In order to produce systemic disease, a virus must cross the mucosal barrier that separates these luminal compartments from the host's parenchymal tissues. Studies with reovirus have illustrated a strategy by which, after entry into the GI tract, viruses can invade the host, by crossing mucosal barriers, thereby initiating systemic infection.[33,34] After oral inoculation of mice, reovirions adhere to the surface of intestinal microfold cells (M cells) that overlie collections of intestinal lymphoid tissue (Peyer's patches). In electron micrographs, virions can be followed sequentially as they are transported within vesicles from the luminal to the abluminal surface of M cells. Virions subsequently appear within Peyer's patches and, in the case of reovirus type 1, can subsequently spread to regional lymph nodes and to extraintestinal lymphoid organs such as the spleen. Although the use of M cells to transport virus has only been specifically described for reoviruses, it would appear likely that this represents a more ubiquitous pathway for invasion of the host from the GI tract by enteric viruses.

Once a virus has entered the host via respiratory, GI, or genitourinary routes or through direct inoculation, it may either produce a local infection or spread from its site of entry to distant target organs to produce systemic disease (Fig. 5). Examples of localized infections in which viral entry, primary replication, and tissue tropism all occur at the same anatomic site include the upper and lower respiratory infections caused by the rhinoviruses and the myxoviruses, the enteric illness produced by rotaviruses, and the dermatologic diseases produced by papillomavirus (warts) and paravaccinia virus (milker's nodules). Conversely, enteroviruses (e.g., poliovirus) must spread from the GI tract to the central nervous system (CNS) to produce meningitis, encephalitis, or poliomyelitis. Measles and varicella enter the host through the respiratory tract but then spread to the skin to produce exanthemal lesions and often to visceral organs as well.

The primary pathways of spread used by viruses to reach target organs are through the lymphatic system, through the blood stream, or through nerves. Rabies virus, herpes simplex and simiae, varicella-zoster virus, bornavirus, and the scrapie agent all spread via nerves.[35] A number of viruses including rabies have been shown to accumulate at the neuromuscular junctions after inoculation and subsequent multiplication in skeletal muscle. In the case of rabies it has been suggested that the acetylcholine receptor (AChR) may serve as a viral receptor that enables virus to enter the distal axon terminals of motor neurons.[36,37] Interestingly, the major envelope glycoprotein of rabies (G protein) has areas of amino acid sequence similarity with certain snake neurotoxins that are known to also bind to the AChR.[38] Herpes simplex virus also appears to enter nerve cells via receptors that are located primarily at synaptic endings rather than on the nerve cell body.[39] Spread of both of these viruses to the CNS can be inhibited by interruption of the appropriate nerves or by chemical agents that inhibit axonal transport.[40–42]

Certain strains of poliovirus can also be shown to spread through nerves to reach the CNS in infected animals, although the importance of neural spread in human infection has never been conclusively established.[42–45] Studies of the kinetics of the neural spread of herpes, rabies, and polio suggest that the neural spread of these viruses is probably due to fast axonal transport. Recent studies of the neural spread of reovirus type 3 (Dearing) also indicate that this virus spreads to the CNS via nerves.[48] By using selective pharmacologic inhibitors of either fast or

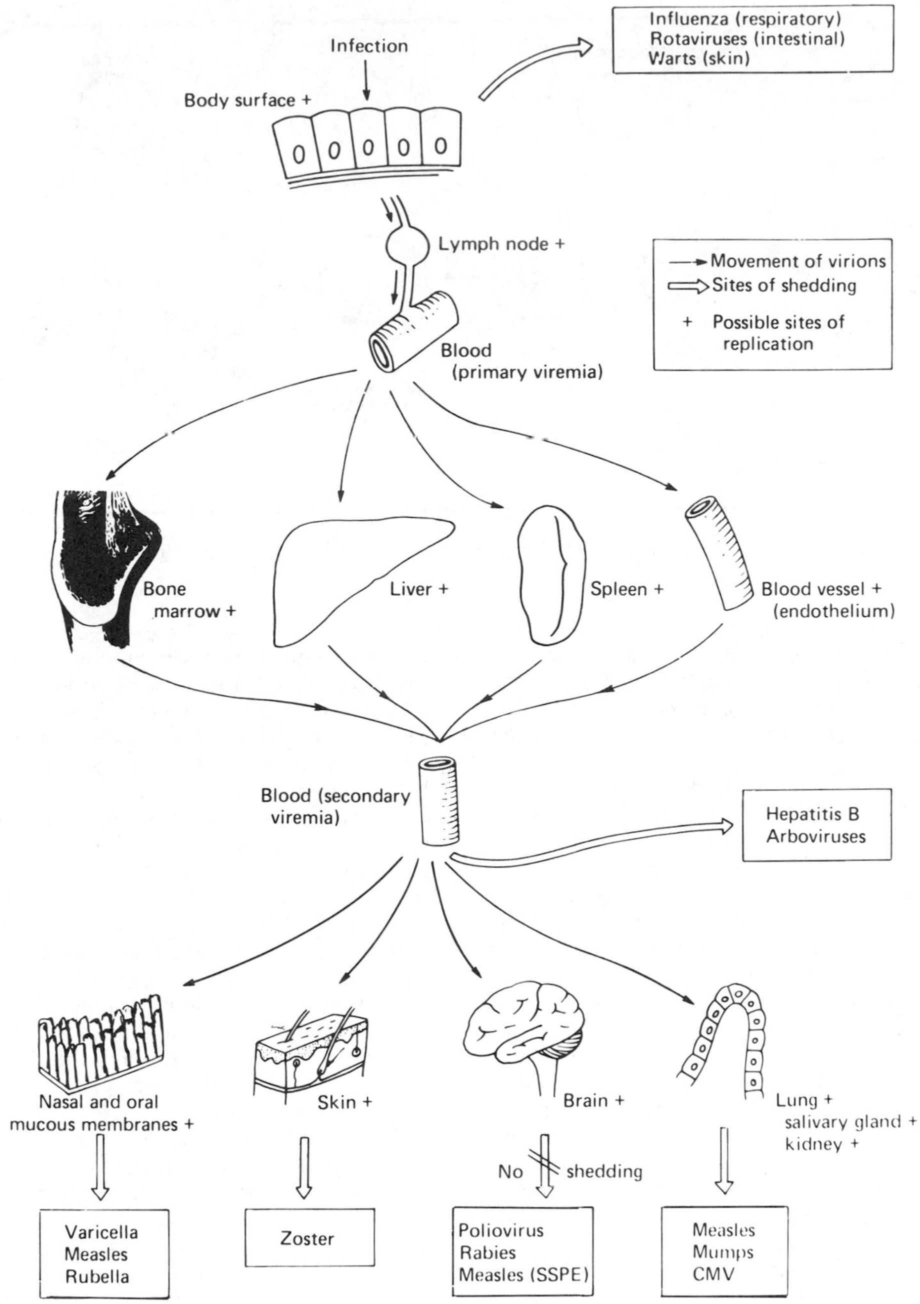

FIG. 5. The spread of virus through the body in human viral infections. Also shown are potential sites for shedding of virus, with examples of diseases in which that route of excretion is important. (Modified from Mims et al.,[32] with permission.)

slow axonal transport it was shown that the spread of reovirus type 3 is also mediated by the microtubule-associated system of fast axonal transport. Kinetic studies of the spread of the scrapie agent to the CNS after peripheral inoculation, or within the CNS after intracerebral or intraocular inoculation, suggest that this agent also travels via nerves.[47,48] The rate of spread was extremely slow which suggests that this agent may actually use the intermediate filament-associated system of slow axonal transport rather then the microtubule-based system of fast axonal transport.

A second major pathway for the spread of viruses from their site of primary replication to distant target tissues is through the blood stream.[32] In some cases virus may enter the blood stream directly, as when a patient is transfused with contaminated blood or blood products or when an addict uses a dirty needle for injecting drugs. More commonly, virus enters the blood stream after replication at some primary site. Important sites of primary replication include Peyer's patches and mesenteric lymph nodes for enteric viruses, epithelial and alveolar cells for respiratory viruses, and skeletal muscle, subcutaneous tissues, and brown fat for togaviruses and some enteroviruses.

Classic studies by Fenner with mousepox suggested that an initial low-titer viremia ("primary viremia") served to seed virus to a variety of organs where a period of further replication led to a much larger high-titer viremia ("secondary viremia") that served to disseminate virus to target organs.[49] It is often exceedingly difficult to identify "primary" and "secondary" viremias in naturally occurring viral infections; however, multiplication of many viruses in reticuloendothelial organs (liver, spleen, lymph nodes, bone marrow), muscle, fat, and even vascular endothelial cells often plays an important role in maintaining viremia.

A virus that reaches the blood stream may travel either free in the plasma (e.g., picornaviruses, togaviruses) or in association with specific cellular elements.[32] A number of viruses are known to travel in association with macrophages (e.g., lentiviruses including HIV) and lymphocytes (e.g., Epstein-Barr virus, HIV). Although many viruses have the capacity to agglutinate red cells in vitro (hemagglutination), only in exceptional cases (e.g., Colorado tick fever virus) have red cells been shown to be important in transporting virus.

The maintenance of viremia appears to depend on the interplay between factors contributing to the maintenance of viremia (e.g., continued virus replication) and host mechanisms designed to remove virus from the circulation ("clearance") or inactivate circulating virus (e.g., neutralizing antibody). A number of factors have been identified that can alter the outcome of these events.[32] In general, the larger the viral particle, the more efficiently it is cleared. Studies of the clearance of reoviruses from the circulation indicate that the outer capsid protein sigma-1 plays a role in determining the pattern of clearance of these viruses and that this pattern can be altered by the presence of antibody bound to the virion.[50] This type of study suggests that the nature of specific components of the virion, especially those present on the outer surface, may be important in determining patterns of clearance in the infected host. Inhibition of the capacity of cells in the host reticuloendothelial system (RES) to phagocytose circulating viruses can also lead to prolongation and magnification of the viremic state. This can be accomplished experimentally by giving animals compounds such as silica or thorotrast, which are avidly phagocytosed by RES cells and seem to "block" their capacity to subsequently clear circulating virus.

Little is known about how specific viral genes and the proteins they encode determine the pathways used by viruses to spread from their site of entry in the host to the ultimate target tissues. Recent experiments with reoviruses have provided some insights into how viruses "choose" between blood-borne and neural routes of spread.[46] Reovirus type 1 (Lang) spreads via the blood stream, and reovirus type 3 (Dearing) spreads via nerves to reach the spinal cord after intramuscular inoculation. By using reovirus reassortants containing different combinations of genes derived from these two parents it was shown that a single viral gene encoding a surface (outer capsid) protein determines the pattern of spread used by these viruses. Studies using intertypic recombinants between herpes simplex virus types 1 and 2 have also identified specific regions in the genome of herpes simplex virus that are important in determining the neural spread of these viruses.[51,52] The region of the genome initially identified as important in determining the capacity of herpes simplex type 1 to spread via nerves from the eye to the brain (0.31–0.44 m.u.) was rather large and encoded a number of proteins (including the DNA polymerase, the major nucleocapsid protein, an immediate early DNA binding protein [ICP8], and a major envelope glycoprotein, gB). Subsequent studies strongly suggest that it is the gene encoding the DNA polymerase that is important,[52] although the mechanism of action remains obscure. Interestingly, studies comparing the neuroinvasiveness of two strains of herpes simplex type 1 identified an overlapping region of the genome (0.25–0.53 m.u.) as critical for neuroinvasiveness.[53] Thus, as illustrated by both reoviruses and herpesviruses, there is evidence that the nature of the pathways used by viruses to spread in the infected host is genetically determined.

It is important to recognize that viruses are not limited to using only a single route of spread. Varicella-zoster virus, for example, is believed to spread from its site of initial entry in the host through the respiratory tract to the skin via the blood stream. Infection of the skin produces the characteristic exanthem of chickenpox. The virus subsequently travels retrogradely up the distal terminals of sensory neurons to reach the dorsal root ganglia where it remains latent. Reactivation of virus from the latent state results in transport of virus down the sensory nerve axon to produce zoster (shingles).[54] Polioviruses represent another example of viruses that appear capable of spreading via both neural and hematogenous routes. Polioviruses are generally believed to travel from the GI tract to the CNS via the blood stream, although the alternative suggestion that they may travel via autonomic nerves in the gut to reach the brain stem and spinal cord has never been conclusively excluded.[55,56] Once the virus reaches the CNS, axonal transport appears to be its major route of dissemination.[45]

In a series of papers nearly 30 years ago, Holland and McLaren suggested that the capacity of poliovirus to injure specific tissues while sparing others during acute poliomyelitis paralleled the capacity of homogenates of these tissues to bind poliovirus in vitro.[57] They also suggested that several types of cells that were not naturally susceptible to infection with poliovirus would support a single cycle of viral replication if transfected with poliovirus RNA. These studies helped establish the principle that the presence or absence of receptors on specific cells was a major determinant of the capacity of viruses to selectively infect and injure these cells ("tropism").

It is important to recognize that the interaction between virion attachment proteins and host cell receptors is not the only determinant of tropism. Obviously, in order for a virus to infect a specific population of cells it must first reach these cells. The route of entry and pathway of spread used by a virus to infect the host can therefore profoundly influence tropism.[58] It is commonly recognized that a wide variety of host factors can dramatically affect the ultimate tropism of a virus. These can include the age, immune status, genetic composition, and nutritional state of the host. Examples of age-related susceptibility and/or resistance to viral infection abound. Similarly, the pathogenesis of viral infection differs markedly in an immune as compared with a nonimmune host. The basis for genetic determinants of viral susceptibility are extremely complex.[59] Studies with inbred strains of mice suggest that a variety of different mechanisms for genetic-related variations in susceptibility exist. These may involve differences in immune responses, the induction of antiviral mediators such as interferon, the presence or absence of genes encoding viral receptors, and in the case of certain retroviruses, the existence of defective endogenous proviruses in the genome. In many cases, although the existence of genetic factors that determine susceptibility is clear, their mechanism of action remains unknown. Nutritional factors such as starvation or malnutrition may act by altering the host's immune responsiveness or through yet unidentified modes of action.

It is important to recognize that the events, including receptor binding, that bring a virus into contact with susceptible cells in target tissues are merely the first steps along a pathway that may lead to replication of viral genomes and production of progeny virions. As discussed in the section dealing with virus–cell interactions, a complex series of events are initiated by virus attachment to host cell receptors. It is necessary for all of these events to proceed successfully for infectious progeny virions to be produced.

An important recent development in understanding viral tropism has been the recognition that some viruses contain elements in their genome that act to stimulate the transcription of specific sets of viral genes in a tissue-specific fashion.[60] Enhancers are one of the most important tissue-specific genetic elements. Enhancers are short strings of nucleotides, often repeated in tandem, that act in a position- and orientation-independent fashion to stimulate the transcription of specific sets of viral genes. In some cases these enhancers are "promiscuous," that is, they seem to be active in virtually all types of cells. Other enhancers show exquisite tissue specificity. For example, the JC virus promoter–enhancer region seems to be specifically active in human cultured fetal glial cells but not in HeLa or CV-1 cells.[61] This correlates well with the capacity of this virus, under certain circumstances, to produce a disease known as progressive multifocal leukoencephalopathy (PML) in which permissive infection is limited to oligodendroglia in the CNS.

One of the most exciting technological advances in molecular biology has been the development of transgenic mice. Transgenic mice are produced when a fertilized mouse egg is microinjected with foreign DNA and this DNA becomes incorporated into the somatic cell line as the embryo matures. Transgenic mice have been produced that contain the enhancer regions of SV40, JC virus, and more recently portions of the genome of the human immunodeficiency virus (HIV-1).[62,63] Studying the tissue-specific pattern of viral gene expression in these mice has provided a valuable method to investigate and identify tissue-specific elements in the genomes of these viruses.

In a simplified sense, viral virulence reflects the capacity of a virus to successfully complete these stages and subsequently injure or kill the host. One of the most important areas of recent research in viral pathogenesis has been to try to identify the role played by specific viral genes and the proteins they encode in determining viral virulence. It has been possible to identify specific "virulence determinants" in the genomes of a number of types of viruses including the togaviruses, bunyaviruses, reoviruses, herpesviruses, rhabdoviruses, myxoviruses, and picornaviruses. Although the nature of these virulence determinants varies for each viral group, a common theme is for the involved protein(s) to be viral surface proteins and frequently to include the virion cell attachment protein (e.g., the G glycoprotein of rabies, the sigma-1 protein of reovirus, the HA of influenza).

One of the important continuing themes in the study of viral–host interactions will be the further definition at a molecular and genetic level of the role played by individual viral genes and the proteins they encode at specific stages in the pathogenesis of an increasing number of viral infections. These studies will be complemented by studies designed to identify precise cellular targets, such as receptors, that are involved in viral–host interactions. One can predict that, as viral–host interactions are understood at an increasingly basic level, this will pave the way toward new strategies for preventing or treating viral diseases.

VIRUS–ENVIRONMENT INTERACTIONS

For a virus to propagate itself in nature, the outcome of virus–host interaction must be the shedding of infectious virus into the environment in a manner that optimizes the possibility for infection of subsequent susceptible hosts (Fig. 6). As discussed earlier, infectious virus may be shed from an infected host through a variety of mediums. Virus may be expelled from the respiratory tract in the form of aerosols generated by coughing or sneezing. Virus may be contained in saliva and transmitted through biting or intimate personal contact. Virus contained in feces may contaminate food or water that is subsequently ingested. Virus in semen or genital secretions may be transmitted during sexual intercourse. Each of these modes of transmission requires that virus be stable (i.e., remain infectious) under specific defined environmental conditions. Largely because of the obvious implications of this information for the inactivation and sterilization of viruses or virally infected material, the effects of temperature, pH, and of a variety of chemical and physical agents on the infectivity of a number of viruses has been extensively investigated. For example, polioviruses are resistant to inactivation by ether, chloroform, bile, detergents, and acidic pH but are quite susceptible to heat, dessication, ultraviolet (UV) irradiation, formalin, and chlorine. However, it was not until recently that it became possible to begin to correlate the susceptibility of viruses to specific agents of this type with specific aspects of their structural composition. In the case of poliovirus, many of the conditions that inactivate the virus (e.g., heating, UV irradiation, high pH) seem to result in a loss or alteration of the outer capsid protein VP4.[65] This in turn may create a "hole" in the viral capsid that allows the viral RNA to leak out. Obviously particles lacking RNA ("empty capsids") will not be infectious. Extensive studies of the effects of a variety of chemical and physical inactivating agents on the inactivation of reoviruses of different serotypes indicate that the surface proteins of the virus appear to play a critical role in determining the relative susceptibility of these viruses to inactivation.[66] The outer capsid protein sigma-1 was important in determining susceptibility to alkaline pH and guanidine, the outer capsid protein sigma-3 in determining susceptibility to sodium dodecyl sulfate (SDS) and high temperature, and the outer capsid protein mu-lc in determining sensitivity to phenol and ethanol. It is easy to appreciate how some

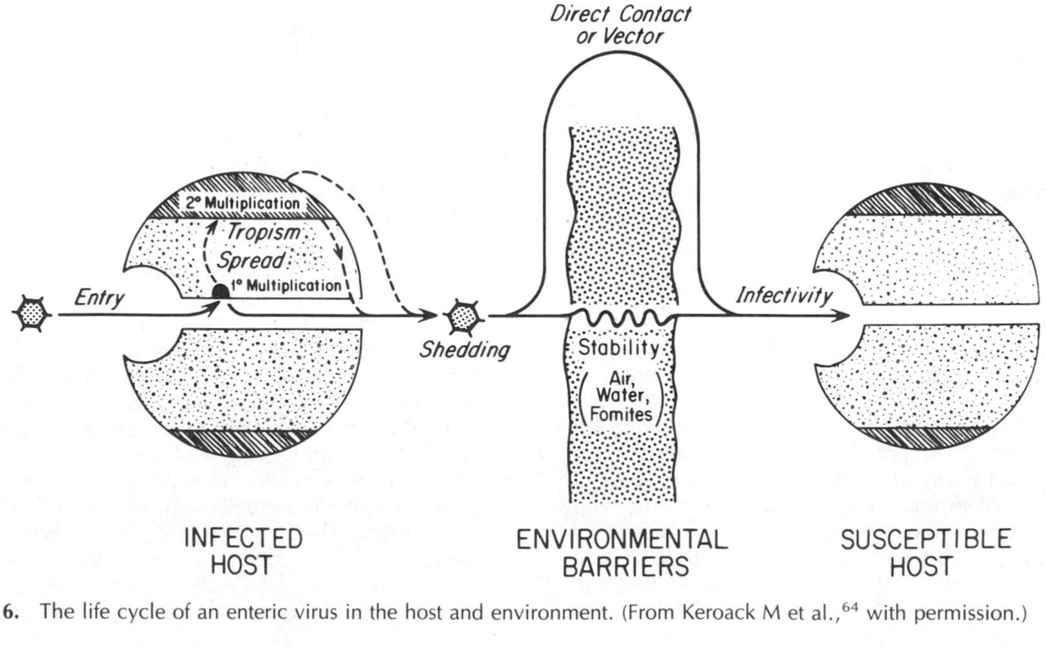

FIG. 6. The life cycle of an enteric virus in the host and environment. (From Keroack M et al.,[64] with permission.)

of the physical and chemical manipulations correlated with viral structure (e.g., temperature and pH sensitivity) may have direct relevance to understanding how viruses survive in the environment.

The future direction of research on how viruses interact with the environment will focus in part on defining in better detail, for a variety of viral systems, how specific structural components of virions determine the stability of these particles in defined physicochemical settings. This type of knowledge should be directly applicable to improving understanding of key factors in virion structure and chemistry that allow viruses to survive in the environment. This in turn may allow for better methods of decontamination of virally infected materials and for the design of public health strategies that will serve to interrupt the cycle of virus transmission through the environment.

REFERENCES

1. Waterson AP, Wilkinson L. An Introduction to the History of Virology. London: Cambridge University Press; 1978.
2. Reed W. Recent researches concerning the etiology, propagation and prevention of yellow fever by the United States Army Commission. J Hyg 1902;2:101–19.
3. Delbruck M. The growth of bacteriophage and lysis of the host. J Gen Physiol. 1940;23:643.
4. Luria SE. Bacteriophage: An essay on virus reproduction. Science. 1950; 111:507–11.
5. Avery OT, MacLeod CM, McCarty M. Studies on the chemical nature of the substance inducing transformation of pneumococcal types. Induction of transformation by a desoxyribonucleic acid fraction isolated from pneumococcus type III. J Exp Med. 1944;79:137–58.
6. Hershey AD, Chase M. Independent functions of viral protein and nucleic acid in the growth of bacteriophage. J Gen Physiol. 1952;36:39–56.
7. Enders JF, Weller TH, Robbins FC. Cultivation of the Lansing strain of poliomyelitis virus in cultures of various human embryonic tissues. Science. 1949;109:85–7.
8. Salk JE, Bennett BL, Lewis LJ, et al. Studies in human subjects on active immunization against poliomyelitis. I. A preliminary report of experiments in progress. JAMA. 1953;151:1081–98.
9. Sabin AB, Boulger LR. History of Sabin attenuated poliovirus oral live vaccine strains. J Biol Stand. 1973;1:115–8.
10. Murphy FA. Virus taxonomy. In: Fields BN, Knipe DM, eds. Fundamental Virology. New York: Raven Press; 1986:7–25.
11. White DO, Fenner FJ. Medical Virology. 3rd ed. San Diego: Academic Press, 1986.
12. Caspar D, Dulbecco R, Klug A, et al. Proposals. Cold Spring Harbor Symp Quant Biol. 1962;27:49.
13. Harrison S. Principles of virus structure. In: Fields BN, Knipe DM, eds. Fundamental Virology. New York: Raven Press; 1986:27–44.
14. Wiley DC. Viral membranes. In: Fields BN, Knipe DM, eds. Fundamental Virology. New York: Raven Press; 1986:45–67.
15. Lonberg-Holm K. Attachment of animal viruses to cells: An introduction. In: Lonberg-Holm K, Philipson L, eds.: Virus Receptors. part 2. London: Chapman & Hall; 1981:3–20.
16. Wilson IA, Skehel JJ, Wiley DC. Structure of the haemagglutinin membrane glycoprotein of influenza virus at 3 angstrom resolution. Nature. 1981; 289:366–73.
17. Wilson IA. The three-dimensional structures of surface antigens from animal viruses. In: Notkins AL, Oldstone MBA, eds. Concepts in Viral Pathogenesis II. New York: Springer Publishing; 1986:15–24.
18. Hogle JM, Chow M, Filman DJ. Three dimensional structure of poliovirus at 2.9 angstrom resolution. Science. 1985;229:1358–65.
19. Rossmann MG, Arnold E, Erickson JW, et al. Structure of a human common cold virus and functional relationship to other picornaviruses. Nature. 1985;317:145–53.
20. Luo M, Vriend G, Kamer G, et al. The atomic structure of Mengo virus at 3 angstrom resolution. Science. 1987;235:182–91.
21. Crowell RL, Hsu K-HL. Isolation of cellular receptors for viruses. In: Notkins AL, Oldstone MBA, eds. Concepts in Viral Pathogenesis II. New York, Springer Publishing; 1986:117–25.
22. Marsh M, Helenius A. Virus entry into animal cells. Adv Virus Res. 1988. In press.
23. Goldstein JL, Anderson RW, Brown MS. Coated pits, coated vesicles, and receptor mediated endocytosis. Nature. 1979;21:679–85.
24. Helenius A, Kartenbeck J, Simons K, et al. On the entry of Semliki Forest virus into BHK-21 cells. J Cell Biol. 1980;84:404–20.
25. Simons K, Garoff H, Helenius A. How an animal virus gets into and out of its host cell. Sci Am. 1982;246:58–66.
26. White J, Killian M, Helenius A. Membrane fusion proteins of enveloped animal viruses. Q Rev Biophys. 1981;16:151–95.
27. Fields BN, Knipe DM, eds. Fundamental Virology. New York: Raven Press; 1986.
28. Deatly AM, Spivack JG, Lavi E, et al. RNA from an immediate early region of the type 1 herpes simplex virus genome is present in the trigeminal ganglia of latently infected mice. Proc Natl Acad Sci USA. 1987;84:3204–8.
29. Stevens JG, Wagner EK, Devi-Rao GB, et al. RNA complementary to a herpesvirus alpha gene mRNA is prominent in latently infected neurons. Science. 1987;235:1056–9.
30. Shannon WM. Mechanisms of action and pharmacology: Chemical Agents. In: Galasso GJ, Merigan TC, Buchanan RA, eds. Antiviral Agents and Viral Diseases of Man. 3rd ed. New York: Raven Press; 1984:55–121.
31. Smith TJ, Kremer MJ, Luo M, et al. The site of attachment in human rhinovirus 14 for antiviral agents that inhibit uncoating. Science. 1986;233:1286–93.
32. Mims CA, White DO. Viral Pathogenesis and Immunology. Oxford: Blackwell Scientific Publications; 1984.
33. Wolf JL, Rubin DH, Finberg R, et al. Intestinal M cells: A pathway for entry of reovirus into the host. Science. 1981;212:471–2.
34. Wolf JL, Kauffman RS, Finberg R, et al. Determinants of reovirus interaction with the intestinal M cells and absorptive cells of murine intestine. Gastroenterology. 1983;85:291–300.
35. Johnson RT: Viral Infections of the Nervous System. New York: Raven Press; 1982:37–60.
36. Lentz TL, Burrage TG, Smith AL, et al. Is the acetylcholine receptor a rabies virus receptor? Science. 1982;215:182–4.
37. Burrage TG, Tignor GH, Smith AL. Rabies virus binding at neuromuscular junctions. Virus Res. 1985;2:273–89.
38. Lentz TL, Wilson PT, Hawrot E, et al. Amino acid sequence similarity between rabies virus glycoprotein and snake venom curaremimetic neurotoxins. Science. 1984;226:847–8.
39. Ziegler RJ, Herman RE. Peripheral infection in culture of rat sensory neurons by herpes simplex virus. Infect Immun. 1980;28:620.
40. Tsiang H. Evidence for intraaxonal transport of fixed and street rabies virus. J Neuropathol Exp Neurol. 1979;38:286–97.
41. Lycke E, Tsiang H. Rabies virus infection of cultured rat sensory neurons. J Viol. 1987;61:2733–41.
42. Kristensson K, Lycke E, Sjostrand J. Spread of herpes simplex virus in peripheral nerves. Acta Neuropathol (Berl). 1971;17:44–53.
43. Howe HA, Bodian DB. Neural Mechanisms of Poliomyelitis. New York: Commonwealth Fund; 1942.
44. Nathanson N, Bodian D. Experimental poliomyelitis following intramuscular virus injection. I. The effect of neural block on a neurotropic and a pantropic strain. Bull J Hopkins Hosp. 1961;108:308–33.
45. Jubelt B, Narayan O, Johnson RT. Pathogenesis of human poliovirus infection in mice. II. Age-dependency of paralysis. J Neuropathol Exp Neurol. 1980;39:149–59.
46. Tyler KL, McPhee DA, Fields BN. Distinct pathways of viral spread in the host determined by the reovirus S1 gene segment. Science. 1986;233:770–4.
47. Fraser H. Neuronal spread of scrapie agent and targeting of lesions within the retino-tectal pathway. Nature. 1982;295:149–50.
48. Kimberlin RH, Walker CA. Pathogenesis of mouse scrapie: Evidence for neural spread of infection to the CNS. J Gen Virol. 1980;51:183–7.
49. Fenner F. The pathogenesis of acute exanthems. Lancet. 1948;2:915.
50. Verdin EM, Lynn SP, Fields BN, et al. Uptake of reovirus serotype 1 by the lungs from the bloodstream is mediated by the viral hemagglutinin. J Virol. 1988;62:545–51.
51. Oakes JE, Gray WL, Lausch RN. Herpes simplex virus type 1 DNA sequences which direct spread of virus from the cornea to central nervous system. Virology. 1986;150:513–7.
52. Day SP, Lausch RN, Oakes JE. Evidence that the gene for herpes virus type 1 DNA polymerase accounts for the capacity of an intertypic recombinant to spread from eye to central nervous system. Virology. 1988;163:166–73.
53. Thompson RL, Cook ML, Devi-Rao GB, et al. Functional and molecular analysis of the avirulent wild-type herpes simplex virus type 1 strain KOS. J Virol. 1986;58:203–11.
54. Gelb LD. Varicella-zoster virus. In: Fields BN, ed. Virology. New York: Raven Press; 1985:591–627.
55. Bodian D. Poliomyelitis: Pathogenesis and histopathology. In: Rivers TM, Horsfall FL, eds. Viral and Rickettsial Infections of Man. 3rd ed. Philadelphia: JB Lippincott; 1959:479–518.
56. Sabin AB. Paralytic poliomyelitis: Old dogmas and new perspectives. Rev Infect Dis. 1981;3:543–64.
57. Holland JJ. Receptor affinities as major determinants of enterovirus tissue tropisms in humans. Virology. 1961;15:312–26.
58. Tyler KL. Host and viral factors that influence viral neurotropism. Trends Neurosci. 1987;10:455–60,492–7.
59. Rosenstreich DL, Weinblatt AC, O'Brien AD. Genetic control of resistance to infection in mice. CRC Crit Rev Immunol. 1982;3:263–300.
60. Khoury G, Gruss P. Enhancer elements. Cell. 1983;33:313–4.
61. Kenney S, Natarajan V, Strike D, et al. JC virus enhancer–promoter active in human brain cells. Science. 1984;226:1337–9.
62. Palmiter R, Chen H, Messing A, et al. SV40 enhancer and large-T-antigen are instrumental in development of choroid plexus tumors in transgenic mice. Nature. 1985;316:457–60.
63. Small J, Scangos G, Cork L, et al. The early region of human papovavirus JC induces dysmyelination in transgenic mice. Cell. 1986;46:13–8.
64. Keroack M, Bassel-Duby R, Fields B, et al. Genetic alterations in reovirus and their impact on host and environment. In: Fields BN, Martin MA, Kamely D, eds. Genetically Altered Virus and the Environment. Cold Spring Harbor, NY: Cold Spring Harbor Laboratory; 1985.

65. Rueckert R. Picornaviruses and their replication. In: Fields BN, ed. Virology. New York: Raven Press; 1985:705–38.
66. Drayna D, Fields BN. Biochemical studies on the mechanism of chemical and physical inactivation of reovirus. J Gen Virol. 1982;63:161–70.

DNA VIRUSES

Poxviridae

113. INTRODUCTION

JOHN M. NEFF

The pox viruses are a complex group of viruses whose classification is based primarily on the morphology of the virion and the viral nucleic acid.[1] This group of viruses represents the largest of all viruses. These viruses replicate in cytoplasm, rather than in the nucleus of cells, and by this characteristic differ from most other DNA viruses. The genomes of these agents are virtually homologous along 25–62 percent of the length of the internal segment.[2] The virus particles are asymmetric and brick-shaped, with round corners, and are very resistant to chemical and physical inactivation. They contain double-stranded DNA and have specific enzymes not found in other DNA viruses that allow them to replicate in the cytoplasm. Within the cytoplasm, they produce eosinophilic inclusions called *Guanieri bodies*. Originally, the pox viruses were classified according to their capability to produce vesicular skin lesions or cytoplasmic inclusion bodies. Since 1966, with the establishment of the International Committee on the Nomenclature of Viruses, the classification of these viruses has depended on the large shape of the virion and the presence of a large single linear molecule of double-stranded DNA.[3] The accepted classification of poxviruses of vertebrates is as follows: family: Poxviridae; subfamily: Chordopoxvirinae; genera: *Orthopoxvirus, Avipoxvirus* (fowlpox), *Capripoxvirus* (sheep pox), *Leporipoxvirus* (myxoma), *Parapoxvirus* (milker's nodule), *Suipoxvirus* (swinepox), unclassified (molluscum contagiosum, tanapox).

The genus *Orthopoxvirus* includes at least nine different species that are generally very homogeneous. They are the causative agents for vaccinia, variola, cowpox, monkeypox, ectromelia, camelpox, taterapox, raccoonpox, and Uasin Gishu disease.

The two major viruses of the *Orthopoxvirus* genus, vaccinia and variola, are closely related and have similar chemical and physical characteristics. Morphologically, they cannot be distinguished. The viral surface is composed of tubular structures surrounding a central nucleoid with a dense dumbbell-shaped core. On either side of the nucleoid core, inside the viral coat, is an elliptical body that gives the virion an appearance of central swelling.[2]

The virions are generally resistant to drying agents and many disinfectants. They may maintain infectivity for months at room temperature and for years below −20°C. They can be inactivated by autoclaving, by heating at 60°C for 10 minutes, and by the chlorine preparations, formaldehyde, iodophores, and quaternary ammonium compounds.[4]

The vaccinia and variola viruses share common antigens. Infection produces hemagglutination-inhibition (HAI) and neutralizing (N) antibodies. Because of the close antigenic similarity of these viruses, routine serologic testing is, in general, not useful in distinguishing variola infection from vaccinia infection or the different strains of variola from each other.[5] The enzyme-linked immunosorbent assay (ELISA) technique and radioimmunoassay have provided more sensitive differentiation between the antibodies produced by infection with these agents, as well as among the other viruses that make up the *Orthopoxvirus* genus group.[6,7] The monoclonal antibody technique may provide an even more specific differentiation.[8]

REFERENCES

1. Fenner F, Henderson DA, Arita L, et al. Smallpox and Its Eradication. Geneva: World Health Organization; 1988:69–103.
2. Dales S, Pogo BGT. Biology of poxviruses. Virol Monogr 1981;18:1.
3. Matthews REF. A Critical Appraisal of Viral Taxonomy, Boca Raton, Fla: CRC Press; 1983.
4. WHO Technical Report Series, No 283, WHO Expert Committee on Smallpox, First Report. Geneva: World Health Organization; 1964.
5. Bedson HS, Dumbell KR. Smallpox and vaccinia. Br Med Bull 1967;23:119.
6. Marennikova SS, Malceva NN, Habahpaseva NA. ELISA: A simple test for detecting and differentiating antibodies to closely related orthopoxviruses. Bull WHO 1981;59(3):365.
7. Walls HH, Ziegler DW, Nakano JH. Characterization of antibodies to orthopoxviruses in human sera by radioimmunoassay. Bull WHO 1981;59(2):253.
8. Kitamoto N, Tanimoto S, Hiroi K, et al. Monoclonal antibodies to cowpox virus: Polypeptide analyses of several major antigens. J Gen Virol 1987;68:239–46.

114. VACCINIA VIRUS (COWPOX)

JOHN M. NEFF

Little is known about the origins of vaccinia virus.[1] The virus was used for vaccination before there was any ability to characterize it or standardize its use. Vaccinia itself now has no natural host. One plausible theory of origin is that it derived from the cowpox virus, but in the early nineteenth century it was gradually transformed into the current virus as a result of person-to-person vaccination.

Edward Jenner, in his "Inquiry into the Causes and Effects of the Variolae Vaccinae" in 1798, was the first to observe that pustular material from the lesions of cowpox, when inoculated into humans, protected them from infection with smallpox.[2] Following Jenner's work, Woodville and Pearson of the Smallpox Hospital in London experimented extensively with this technique and distributed vaccination material to many physicians throughout England. The practice of vaccination then spread throughout the world and has been directly responsible for eradication of smallpox.[3]

VACCINES AND VACCINATION TECHNIQUES

Several years ago, many vaccine strains were in use, and there was much uncertainty about the protective value or risk of a given vaccine. Under the leadership of the World Health Organization (WHO), the use of strains was reduced generally to the derivatives of one of three strains: Elstree strain (Lister Institute), the EM63 strain (Moscow Research Institute of Virus Preparation), and the New York Board of Health strain.[4] WHO also established standards for production and use.[5] In general, smallpox vaccines are produced from a seed virus propagated on the skin of calves and then processed to eliminate bacterial contamination. The final vaccine is stored in liquid form or as a freeze-dried preparation. The latter preparations may maintain their titer even after incubation at 37°C for 4 weeks.[4] With the development of freeze-dried vaccines, it has been possible to distribute standard vaccines to remote and temperate countries throughout the world without loss of titer.

To pass WHO standards, a vaccine should be able to produce major reactions in 95 percent of the primary vaccinees and in 90 percent of those who were vaccinated more than 10 years previously. To obtain such results, most vaccines should have a titer of at least 10^8 pock-forming units per milliliter.

Vaccinations should be made over the deltoid region of the upper arm. The preferred method of vaccination is to use a bifurcated needle that has been dipped into the vaccine. The needle is then held perpendicular to the skin and pressed in and out 5 times for primary vaccinees and 15 times for revaccinees. Pressure should be sufficient to produce a trace of blood on the skin. Successful vaccination produces a major response in both primary vaccinees and revaccinees. A *major* response is defined by WHO as a "pustular lesion or an area of definite induration or congestion surrounding a central lesion (scab or ulcer) 6–8 days after vaccination." Any other response is called *equivocal*.[4]

Primary vaccinees in general demonstrate a vesicle within 3–5 days after vaccination. This becomes pustular and reaches its maximum size approximately 9 days after vaccination. The lesion forms a scab and ultimately leaves a small circular scar approximately 1 cm in diameter. Revaccinations yield variable results, ranging from an accelerated reaction, which become vesicular within 1–2 days after vaccination, to lesions that are very similar to primary reactions. Usually revaccinations do not result in scar formation even in remote revaccinees.

IMMUNITY RESULTING FROM VACCINATION

After vaccination there is local replication of virus. There also may be some replication of virus in the regional lymph nodes. Viremia, however, has not been demonstrated in uncomplicated vaccinations using modern, standardized vaccines.[6] Protection against smallpox that results from vaccination is probably due to both T and B cell-mediated antibodies. The dermal reaction that results from revaccination is a rough measurement of T-cell function and the circulating antibodies of B-cell function. The dermal evidence of immunity and circulating antibodies can be demonstrated within 4–5 days and increases up to 4 weeks after vaccination.[7,8] Circulating antibodies may persist for years after vaccination, and the dermal response after vaccination may demonstrate evidence of modification for up to 20 years. Although a primary vaccinee may rarely demonstrate seroconversion without a dermal response, the absence of a primary take and a following scar is considered to be an inadequate response to immunization.[4,9]

Successful vaccination is highly protective against smallpox even though the exact factors responsible for this protection have not been accurately defined. In general, protection against smallpox is nearly 100 percent for the first 1–3 years after vaccination. Persons who have not been vaccinated within 3 years may acquire smallpox on exposure, but this is a modified and nonfatal form of the disease. This modification can occur for up to 20 years after vaccination. After 20 years, there is very little remaining protection from vaccination.[4]

PASSIVE IMMUNITY

Hyperimmune vaccinial gamma globulin obtained from recent revaccinees is probably effective in reducing the incidence and severity of smallpox in intimate family contacts of an index case. If administered shortly after exposure and simultaneously with vaccination, there is limited evidence indicating that the resulting morbidity and mortality from smallpox will be less than would be expected in those who receive only a vaccination.[10]

COMPLICATIONS RESULTING FROM VACCINATION

In the majority of situations, primary vaccination results in modified swelling and tenderness at the site of vaccination, some regional lymphadenopathy, and occasionally a low-grade fever at the peak of the dermal response. At times, the pustular lesion itself may be as large as 4 cm but usually does not exceed 2 cm in diameter. Occasionally, abnormal reactions occur that may be mild or may be severe enough to result in fatality. Complications that result from vaccination have been broadly classified into (*1*) central nervous system, (*2*) dermal, and (*3*) other.[11,12]

Central Nervous System Complications

The principal central nervous system complication that results from vaccination is a postinfectious encephalitis,[13–24] which is similar to the encephalitis that occurs after measles and a few other acute viral illnesses. The vaccinia virus cannot be isolated from the central nervous system lesions. Most cases occur 1–2 weeks after vaccination, and the signs and symptoms are those of a generalized encephalitis. There also may be spinal cord signs when there is transverse myelitis or, rarely, focal neurologic signs. Routine diagnostic tests are of little help, except to rule out other possible causes of the illness. Treatment is supportive and symptomatic. The extent and severity of residual neurologic problems depend on the severity and location of the original lesions. Mortality is generally in the range of 10–30 percent. There is no known predilection for this disorder.[18]

The reported incidence of this disease has varied considerably from country to country, and the explanation for this variance has not been absolutely clear.[19] The incidence of this complication in the United States, where the New York Board of Health strain was used, was a little more than 1 in 100,000 primary vaccinees. This incidence was slightly higher when vaccination occurred before the first birthday. Similar rates have been observed in Great Britain, where the Elstree strain was used.[13] Although some countries have reported a higher incidence of this complication in adult primary vaccinees, as compared with children, this has not been observed either in the United States or in Great Britain.

Dermal Complications

The most frequent complications reported after smallpox vaccination are dermal. These can be roughly classified as those that are associated with an underlying illness and those that are not.[11,25,26] The former include vaccinia necrosum, or progressive vaccinia, and eczema vaccinatum; the latter, accidental infection, generalized vaccinia, and erythematous urticarial eruptions.

Vaccinia Necrosum. Vaccinia necrosum is the most severe complication occurring after smallpox vaccination.[27–31] It invariably results when a person with an immunologic deficiency is inadvertently vaccinated. The disease is insidious. The lesion begins as a normal vaccination but continues to progress, and in fatal cases shows no evidence of resolution. Paradoxically, the patient initially may have no systemic signs, no regional lymphadenopathy or erythema, but only progressive necrosis at the site of vaccination. As the disease continues, the patient develops metastatic lesions throughout the body. Vaccinia virus can easily be isolated from any of the lesions.

Eczema Vaccinatum. Patients with atropic dermatitis are unusually susceptible to two viral infections—herpes simplex and vaccinia. In both infections the clinical picture, Kaposi's varicellaform eruption, is similar, and the syndrome can be distinguished only by the history and viral isolation. Eczema vaccinatum is the clinical result of local spread and/or dissemination of vaccinia virus infections in such persons[32–34] (Dr. J. M. Neff, unpublished data). The complication may be a result of inadvertent vaccination or of intimate contact with a recently vaccinated person.

The treatment of eczema vaccinatum is to administer vaccinia immune globulin (VIG) in the therapeutic dose of 0.6 cc/kg/24 hr, repeated daily until no new lesions appear.

Accidental Infection. Not uncommonly, a healthy person may acquire vaccinial lesions accidentally as a result of either autoinoculation at the time of vaccination or intimate body contact with a person who had been recently vaccinated.[14,15] These lesions almost always occur in primary vaccinees. They are identical to a primary vaccination and are self-limited. When autoinoculation occurs, it is generally a coprimary reaction on a mucous membrane, the palpebral margins of the eyelid (ocular vaccinia), the nose, mouth, or anus.[35,36]

Generalized Vaccinia. *Generalized vaccinia* is a nonspecific term that is used to describe a vesicular rash that develops after vaccination. If cases of eczema vaccination and vaccinia necrosum (illnesses that truly represent a generalized vaccinia) are excluded, it is extremely rare to document a generalized, systemic viral dissemination resulting from vaccination. On the other hand, it is not uncommon to see, at about 7–12 days after vaccination, a patient who develops a rash characterized by multiple small vesicular lesions, each with an erythematous base.[14,15,25,26,32] The patient is nontoxic and often afebrile. Vaccinia virus cannot be isolated from the blood or the peripheral lesions. These cases have often been reported as generalized vaccinia. They occur in primary vaccinees and are seen most frequently in children vaccinated before their first birthday. The etiology is not known, and there is no specific treatment.

Erythematous Urticarial Eruptions. There are several erythematous rashes similar to enterovirus- or roseola-like rashes that are frequently observed 7–12 days after vaccination.[37] These are self-limited reactions lasting no more than a few days. The patients are not acutely ill and require no specific treatment. The pathogenesis is unknown.

Other Complications

Many other complications of vaccinations have been reported. These include myocarditis, thrombocytopenia, arthritis, and pericarditis. There also have been cases of malignant melanoma occurring in vaccination scars, as well as reports of acute erythema nodosum leprosum or lepra reactions after vaccination of patients with lepromatous leprosy.[11,38]

Three more frequent but still rare reactions should be noted: (*1*) bullous erythema multiforma, (*2*) overwhelming viremia resulting in sudden death in infancy, and (*3*) fetal vaccinia.

Further Attenuated Vaccines

Two strains that have been tested most widely have been those that were derived from the CV-1 and CV-2 strains of Rivers. In the United States the CV-1 strain has been studied most thoroughly.[39] It was found to be safe when administered to over 1000 eczematous children as a preimmunizing agent.[40] In healthy children, it has also been demonstrated to be more attenuated than standard calf lymph vaccine, and it may not provide full protection against smallpox. Since the successful eradication of smallpox, vaccination has not been performed frequently on a worldwide basis. Fortunately, the resulting complications have become rare.

There may, however, be new situations that could result in more frequent use of vaccinia and in a reappearance of complications. The first is the continuation of vaccination of military personnel because of the concern of biologic warfare.[41] This potential risk has been demonstrated in a report of disseminated vaccinia occurring in a military recruit who was immunologically impaired because of a concurrent infection with human immunodeficiency virus (HIV).[42] The second potential risk is from the use of new, experimental recombinant live virus vaccines.[43] In these vaccines, vaccinia is used as the biologic carrier for immunizing genes. Extensive work has already been done in this field, recombining vaccinia with genes for several other immunizing agents, including respiratory syncytial virus (RSV), HIV, parainfluenza, rotavirus, malaria, hepatitis B, and herpes simplex viruses.[44–49] Vaccinia is an ideal agent for such recombinant research because of its large size and extraordinary stability. This may be an important advance allowing the simultaneous delivery of several immunizing antigens through one vehicle. This agent, because of its stability, ease of storage, and mode of delivery, can be used in areas of the world where the use of other vaccines may not be practical. Vaccinia is also being used experimentally in a melanoma oncolysate to stimulate the production of antimelanoma antibodies in high-risk melanoma patients.[50] On a very preliminary basis, it has also been used as treatment for a patient with IgA multiple myeloma.[51]

This ongoing experimental use of vaccinia virus will require knowledge and evaluation of its immunogenic characteristics and its complications as an immunizing agent and as a recombinant.

REFERENCES

1. Baxby D. The origins of vaccinia virus. J Infect Dis. 1977;136:453.
2. Downie AW. Jenner's cowpox inoculation. Br Med J. 1951;2:251.
3. Dixon CW. Smallpox. London: Churchill Livingstone; 1962:249.
4. WHO Technical Report, Series No 493, WHO Expert Committee on Smallpox Eradication, Second Report. Geneva: World Health Organization; 1972.
5. WHO Technical Report, Series No 323, WHO Expert Group on Requirements for Biological Substances. Geneva: World Health Organization; 1965.
6. Glattner RJ, Norman JO, Hays FM, et al. Antibody response to cutaneous inoculation with vaccinia virus: Viremia and viruria in vacc children. J Pediatr. 1964;64:839.
7. Pincus WB, Flick JA. The role of hypersensitivity in the pathogenesis of vaccinia virus infection in humans. J Pediatr. 1963;62:57.
8. Wulff H, Chin TDY, Wenner HA. Serological responses of children after primary vaccination and revaccination against smallpox. Am J Epidemiol. 1969;90:312.
9. Pincus WB, Flick JA. Successful vaccinia infection without a local lesion. Am J Public Health. 1963;53:898.
10. Kempe CH, Bowles C, Meiklejohn G, et al. The use of vaccinia hyperimmune gamma globulin in the prophylaxis of smallpox. Bull WHO. 1961;25:41.
11. Lane JM, Millar JD, Neff JM. Smallpox and smallpox vaccination policy. Ann Rev Med. 1971;22:251.
12. Kempe CH. Studies on smallpox and complications of smallpox vaccination. Pediatrics. 1960;26:176.
13. Conybeare ET. Illness attributed to smallpox vaccination during 1951–60. Part II. Illness reported as affecting the central nervous system. Monthly Bull Ministry Health Public Health Lab Serv. 1964;23:150.
14. Neff JM, Lane JM, Pert JH, et al. Complications of smallpox vaccination, I National Survey in the United States, 1963. N Engl J Med. 1967;276:125.
15. Lane JM, Ruben FL, Neff JM, et al. Complications of smallpox vaccination 1968. National Surveillance in the United States. N Engl J Med. 1969;281:1201.
16. de Vries E. Postvaccinial Perivenous Encephalitis. Amsterdam: Elsevier; 1960.
17. Scott TFM. Postinfectious and vaccinial encephalitis. Med Clin North Am. 1967;51:701.
18. Keuter EJW. Predisposition of Post Vaccinial Encephalitis. Amsterdam: Elsevier; 1969.
19. Stuart G. Memorandum on post-vaccinial encephalitis. Bull WHO. 1947;1:36.
20. Nanning W. Prophylactic effect of antivaccinia gamma-globulin against post-vaccinial encephalitis. Bull WHO. 1962;27:317.
21. Noordaan J van der, Dekking F, Posthuma J, et al. Primary vaccination with an attenuated strain of vaccinia virus. Arch Gesamte Virusforsch. 1967;22:210.
22. Ehrengut W, Ehrengut-Lang J. Non-infectious smallpox vaccine in the prophylaxis of postvaccinial encephalitis. Int Symp Smallpox Vaccine, Bilthoven. 1972;19:319.
23. Polak MF. Complication of smallpox vaccination in the Netherlands 1959–1970. Int Symp Smallpox Vaccine, Bilthoven. 1972;19:235.
24. Berger K, Heinrich W. Decrease of postvaccinial deaths in Austria and in-

troduction of less pathogenic virus strain. Int Symp Smallpox Vaccine, Bilthoven. 1972;19:119.
25. Sarkany I, Caron GA. Cutaneous complications of smallpox vaccination. Trans St John Hosp Dermatol Soc. 1963;48:163.
26. Conybeare ET. Illness attributed to smallpox vaccination during 1951–60. Part I. Illnesses reported as "generalized vaccinia." Monthly Bull Ministry Health Public Health Lab Serv. 1964;23:126.
27. Fulginiti VA, Kempe CH, Hathaway WE, et al. Progressive vaccinia in immunologically deficient individuals. In: Bergsma D, ed. Birth Defects: Immune Deficiency Diseases of Man. v. 4. New York: The National Foundation—The March of Dimes; 1968:129.
28. Rosen FS, Janeway CA. The gamma globulins. III. The antibody deficiency syndrome. N Engl J Med. 1966;275:709.
29. O'Connell CJ, Karzon DT, Barron AL. Progressive vaccinia with normal antibodies. Ann Intern Med. 1964;60:282.
30. Lane JM, Ruben FL, Abrutyn E, et al. Deaths attributed to smallpox vaccination 1959 to 1966, 1968. JAMA. 1970;212:441.
31. Neff JM, Lane JM. Vaccinia necrosum following smallpox vaccination for chronic herpetic ulcers. JAMA. 1970;213:123.
32. Lane JM, Ruben FL, Neff JM, et al. Complications of smallpox vaccination, 1968 II. Results of ten statewide surveys. J Infect Dis. 1970;122:303.
33. Copeman PWM, Wallace HJ. Eczema vaccinatum. Br Med J. 1964;2:5415, 902.
34. Rachelefsky GS, Opelz G, Mickey R. Defective T cell function in atopic dermatitis. J Allergy Clin Immunol. 1976;57:569.
35. Ruben FL, Lane JM. Ocular vaccinia, an epidemiologic analysis of 348 cases. Arch Ophthalmol. 1970;84:45.
36. Fulginiti VA, Winograd LA, Jackson M, et al. Therapy of experimental vaccinial keratitis: Effect of idoxuridine and VIG. Arch Ophthalmol (Chicago). 1965;74:539.
37. Neff JM, Drachman RH. Complications of smallpox vaccination 1968. Surveillance in a comprehensive care clinic. Pediatrics. 1972;50:481.
38. Conybeare ET. Illness attributed to smallpox vaccination during 1951–60. Part III. Fatal illnesses reported as associated with vaccination (but not as generalized vaccinia or as post-vaccinial encephalomyelitis). Monthly Bull Ministry Health Public Health Lab Serv. 1964;23:182.
39. Galasso GJ, Karzon DT, Katz SL, et al, eds. Clinical and serological study of four smallpox vaccines comparing variations of dose and routes of administration. J Infect Dis. 1977;135:131.
40. Kempe CH, Fulginiti V, Minamitani M, et al. Smallpox vaccination of eczematous patients with a strain of attenuated live vaccinia (CVI-78). Pediatrics. 1968;42:980.
41. Halsey NA, Henderson DA. HIV infection and immunization against other agents. N Engl J Med. 1987;316:683–5.
42. Redfield RR, Wright DC, James WD, et al. Disseminated vaccinia in a military recruit with human immunodeficiency virus disease. N Engl J Med. 1987;316:673–6.
43. Quinnan GV. Vaccinia vectors for vaccine antigens. Proceedings of the Workshop on Vaccinia Viruses as Vectors for Vaccine Antigens, Held November 13–14, 1984, in Chevy Chase, Maryland. New York: Elsevier; 1985.
44. Stott EJ, Taylor G, Ball LA, et al. Immune and histopathological responses in animals vaccinated with recombinant vaccinia viruses that express individual genes of human respiratory syncytial virus. J Virol. 1987;61:3855–61.
45. Spriggs MK, Murphy BR, Prince GA, et al. Expression of the F and HN glycoproteins of human parainfluenza virus type B by recombinant vaccinia virus: Contribution of the individual proteins to host immunity. J Virol. 1987;61:3416–23.
46. Mackett M. Vaccinia virus recombinants: Potential vaccines. Acta Trop (Basel). 1987;445(Suppl 12):94–7.
47. Andrew ME, Boyle DB, Coupar BE, et al. Vaccinia virus recombinants expressing the SA 11 rotavirus VP7 glycoprotein gene induce serotype-specific neutralizing antibodies. J Virol. 1987;61:1054–60.
48. Langford CJ. Live viruses for the delivery of malaria vaccines. Papua New Guinea Med J. 1986;29:103–8.
49. Hu SL, Kosowski SG, Dalrymple JM. Expression of AIDS virus envelope gene for recombinant vaccinia virus. Nature. 1986;320:537–40.
50. Hersey P, Edwards A, Coates A, et al. Evidence that treatment with vaccinia melanoma cell lysates may improve survival of patients with Stage II melanoma. Cancer Immunol Immunother. 1987;25:257–65.
51. Kawa A, Arakawa S. The effect of attenuated vaccinia virus as strain on multiple myeloma; a case report. Jpn J Exp Med. 1987;57:79–81.

115. VARIOLA (SMALLPOX) AND MONKEYPOX VIRUSES

JOHN M. NEFF

Although a great deal is known about the chemical and biologic properties of vaccinia virus, the study of variola virus has been limited because of the obvious laboratory hazards involved. Where comparative studies have been possible, very similar characteristics between the two viruses have been found. Therefore, what has been noted about the morphology and biochemistry of vaccinia also applies to variola. The differences between variola and vaccinia lie in their predilection for certain hosts and their different growth characteristics in the laboratory.[1] Whereas vaccinia virus infects a wide range of hosts, variola infection is limited to humans and, under certain circumstances, to monkeys. In the laboratory, the two viruses can be distinguished by the appearance of the pock lesions formed on the chorioallantoic membrane of the chick embryo.[2] The pocks caused by variola are small and gray-white, while those caused by vaccinia are large and sometimes hemorrhagic. The two viruses can also be distinguished by their different growth characteristics in tissue culture.

There are at least two different strains of variola virus. The most virulent strain causes variola major, with a mortality of 20–50 percent. Variola minor, or alastrim, has a mortality of less than 1 percent. These two strains can easily be distinguished by their temperature-sensitive growth characteristics on the chorioallantoic membrane.

LABORATORY DIAGNOSIS OF SMALLPOX

One of the most important factors in the control of smallpox was the availability of rapid diagnostic techniques that differentiated smallpox from other vesicular illnesses.[7] The two techniques that are most commonly used are electron microscopy and gel diffusion. In both tests, vesicular scrapings are used. By using the electron microscope the pox virus particles can be distinguished from herpes or chickenpox. In situations where this technique is not available, variola viral particles, Guarnieri bodies, may be seen under light microscopy after staining by the Gispens method. Gel diffusion tests the vesicular fluid antigen against known hyperimmune vaccinia antiserum. It is not as sensitive as the electron microscope or as direct virus isolation on the chorioallantoic membrane. It is, however, a good, rapid diagnostic tool in a laboratory where an electron microscope is not available.[3,4] None of these tests help to distinguish vaccinia from variola. For this differentiation, the growth characteristics on the chorioallantoic membrane, mentioned above, are used.

CLINICAL ILLNESS

Variola no longer exists in an indigenous state in nature since the implementation of the successful worldwide eradication program. The last reported case was in Somalia in October 1977.[5] In 1980 the World Health Organization (WHO) Global Commission for the Certification of Smallpox Eradication officially declared that smallpox eradication had been achieved throughout the world.[6] Since 1977, there have been no indigenous cases of variola despite extensive surveillance.

The history, epidemiology, and clinical manifestations of smallpox have been well documented. The best of the most recent summaries can be found in the 1988 WHO publication *Smallpox and Its Eradication*.[7] Clinically, smallpox is a homogeneous illness that begins after an incubation period of 12 days, with a prodromal period of 2–4 days during which the virus can easily be isolated from the blood. The ensuing rash progresses in a uniform pattern as follows: maculopapules to vesicles to pustules and scabs over 1–2 weeks. The rash follows a centrifugal pattern. The progress of the disease may vary anywhere from death, occurring before the appearance of any rash in its most fulminant form, to a discrete form following a full course to recovery. Except when the disease appears in its toxic or vaccinio-modified form, it is easily diagnosed.

Smallpox is a relatively noncontagious disease requiring close contact for spread. It can easily be contained by careful identification and vaccination of contacts.

MONKEYPOX

Monkeypox is the only other member of the *Orthopoxvirus* species that has any significant clinical application to humans (Ref. 7, pp. 1287–1311). This virus creates a vesicular illness in monkeys that is very similar to variola. It occurs mostly in monkeys from the tropical rain forests of western and central Africa, and has infected humans sporadically in this same area. When the illness occurs in humans, it produces a vesicular rash very much like variola and generally does not pass on to other generations. This occurs occasionally, however, and there is one report of its spread through four generations.[8] WHO is carefully investigating all sporadic cases of monkeypox and has an active surveillance program in the geographic area where monkeypox is likely to occur. Most of the cases by far have occurred in Zaire, where 331 cases in a population of 5 million were identified in 3 years. It is considered to be a rare disease in humans (Ref. 7, pp. 1310–11).

It is unlikely that any of the other orthopoxviruses will cause any significant pathologic disease in humans. There is no natural reservoir of variola, and it is extremely unlikely that the genomes of any of the other orthopoxviruses will alter in nature to a form that infects and persists in humans. The only credible source of variola is from infection in a laboratory where the virus is stored.[9] At present, only two such laboratories in the world contain the virus (Ref. 1, pp. 1338–41). If for any reason this virus were once again introduced to humans, the resulting disease could be easily contained by vaccination of identified contacts. Control depends on the early recognition of a case and knowledge of its clinical and epidemiologic characteristics.

REFERENCES

1. Bedson HS, Dumbell KR. Smallpox and vaccinia. Br Med Bull. 1967;23:119.
2. World Health Organization: Guide to the Laboratory Diagnosis of Smallpox for Smallpox Eradication Programs. Geneva: World Health Organization; 1969.
3. Mitra AC, Sarkar SK, Mukherjee MK, et al. Evaluation of the precipitation-in-gel reaction in the diagnosis of smallpox. Bull WHO. 1973;49:555.
4. Nakano JH. Evaluation of virological laboratory methods in smallpox diagnosis. Bull WHO. 1973;48:529.
5. Deria A, Jezek Z, Markvart K, et al. The world's last endemic case of smallpox. Bull WHO. 1980;58:279–83.
6. WHO Declaration of global eradication of smallpox. Weekly Epidemiol Rec. 1980;55:145–52.
7. Fenner F, Henderson DA, Arita I, et al. Smallpox and Its Eradication. Geneva: World Health Organization; 1988.
8. Jezek Z, Arita I, Mutombo M, et al. Four generations of probably person to person transmission of human monkeypox. Am J Epidemiol. 1986;123:1004–12.
9. Dumbell K. What should be done about smallpox virus? Lancet. 1987;2:957–8.

116. PARAPOXVIRUSES AND MOLLUSCUM CONTAGIOSUM AND TANAPOX VIRUSES

JOHN M. NEFF

Within the Poxviridae family there are a few other viruses, other than the orthopoxvirus genus, that produce diseases in humans. They are the unclassified molluscum contagiosum and tanapox viruses, and the milker's node virus and bovine pustular stomatitis virus (orf) of the parapoxvirus genus.[1]

MOLLUSCUM CONTAGIOSUM

Molluscum contagiosum is a benign human disease that occurs worldwide and may be spread by close human contact including sexual intercourse. The disease is characterized by small firm umbilicated papules that are present on exposed epithelial surface areas of children or the genital areas of adults. The lesions resolve spontaneously without significant associated systemic symptoms. The virus has not been cultivated. Electron microscopy studies, however, have revealed a virus indistinguishable from other poxviruses.[2,3]

Recently, molluscum contagiosum has occurred as an opportunistic infection in patients with the acquired immune deficieny synrome (AIDS). Clinically the presentation is the same as described in healthy people except that the lesions may not resolve spontaneously but instead may continue to increase in size, number, and severity. Diagnosis is confirmed by histologic and electron microscopic examination.[4]

TANAPOX VIRUS

The tanapox virus is the source of a recently identified disease occurring in humans along the Tana river in Kenya and in Zaire. This disease is similar to monkeypox.[5]

MILKER'S NODE VIRUS

Milker's node virus produces a cutaneous disease in cattle that may be transmitted to humans through intimate contact. The disease in cattle is manifested by vesicular lesions of the udder or teets and in humans by watery, painless small nodules on exposed surfaces. The lesions in humans are self-limited, with complete recovery in 4–8 weeks. The immunity does not last. The virus has been isolated in primary fetal bovine kidney culture but cannot be serially propagated in continuous human cell lines. By electron microscopy the virus particles have typical poxvirus morphology.

BOVINE PUSTULAR STOMATITIS

Bovine pustular stomatitis virus (orf) causes watery papillomatous lesions on the cornea and mucous membranes of lambs. When humans are infected by close contact, a single lesion develops at the site of an abrasion. The lesion evolves into a hyperplastic nodular mass. The viral particles observed by electron microscopy are large, but instead of having the typical poxivrus brick shape, they are ovoid. None of these viruses provide any cross-immunity with the vaccinia or cowpox viruses.

REFERENCES

1. Fenner F, Henderson DA, Arita I, et al. Smallpox and Its Eradication. Geneva: World Health Organization; 1988:1288.
2. Postlethwaite R. Molluscum contagiosum. A review. Arch Environ Health 1970;21:432–52.
3. Fenner F, Henderson DA, Arita I, et al. Smallpox and Its Eradication. Geneva: World Health Organization; 1988:1317–18.
4. Katzman M, Carey JT, Elmets CA, et al. Molluscum contagiosum and the acquired immunodeficiency syndrome: Clinical and immunological details of two cases. Br J Dermatol. 1987;116:131–38.
5. Jezek Z. Arita I, Szczeniowski M, et al. Human tanapox in Zaire: Clinical and epidemiological observations on cases confirmed by laboratory studies. Bull WHO. 1985;63:1027–35.

Herpesviridae

117. INTRODUCTION TO HERPESVIRIDAE

STEPHEN E. STRAUS

The members of the Herpesviridae family are large, DNA-containing, enveloped viruses. Nearly 80 known herpesviruses infect a broad spectrum of the animal kingdom. Six human viruses are recognized (Table 1). Numerous herpesviruses infect new- or old-world monkeys, one of which is a rare cause of disease in humans. Well-characterized examples of other herpesviruses that do not infect humans include the channel catfish virus, Marek's disease virus of chickens, and several economically important viruses of horses, pigs, and cattle.[1–5]

CLASSIFICATION

The herpesviruses may be classified into three subfamilies according to virus host range and other biologic properties (Table 1). The α-herpesviruses grow rapidly in a wide range of tissues and efficiently destroy their host cells. The β-herpesviruses grow slowly and only in limited types of cells. Members of the γ-herpesvirus subfamily, almost without exception, grow slowly in or immortalize lymphoid cells of their natural hosts.

STRUCTURE

All herpesviruses are large particles (150–250 nm) that are composed of four fundamental structural elements (Fig. 1) that, moving inwardly, include a trilaminar outer envelope, the tegument, the nucleocapsid, and an internal core consisting of proteins and the viral genome.[7–10]

The envelope is derived from portions of the nuclear and cytoplasmic membranes that are pinched off as the developing particle traverses the nucleus into the cytoplasm and eventually exits the cell. In the process, viral glycoproteins that had been inserted into the cellular membranes are captured, with the end result that they project outward from the virion envelope.

The envelope glycoproteins of herpesviruses exhibit a number of biologic properties, some obvious and some obscure.[11] Certain of the glycoproteins such as glycoproteins B and D of herpes simplex viruses 1 and 2 are probably responsible for the binding and penetration of virions into cells.[11,12] Others, such as the herpes simplex virus 1 and 2 glycoproteins E, are Fc receptors, while glycoprotein C has C3b-binding activity.[13,14] The cell surface receptors to which herpesvirus glycoproteins must bind to initiate infection are generally not known except for Epstein-Barr virus, which binds to the cellular C3d complement receptor.[15] Antibodies to most herpesvirus envelope glycoproteins neutralize virus infectivity, presumably by interfering with receptor binding.

The virion tegument consists of a seemingly amorphous assemblage of one or more virus-encoded proteins that may be important for initiating the viral replicative cycle within susceptible cells.

Herpesvirus nucleocapsids are approximately 100 nm in diameter and consist of 162 discrete protein capsomeres in an icosapentahedral array with 5:3:2 symmetry. The nucleocapsids contain viral DNAs that for all herpesviruses are linear double-stranded DNA molecules. Herpesvirus DNAs are structurally organized into a variety of complicated patterns depending upon the relative number, size, and position of repeated sequences. For example, herpes simplex viruses 1 and 2 possess two major, virtually uninterrupted expanses of unique DNA sequences. Each of these unique sequences is flanked by repeated sequences[16] (Fig. 2). For some herpesviruses the unique sequences can be inverted, one relative to the other, during the course of replication. Each virion contains one of the possible isomeric forms of the genome. All isomers of herpesvirus DNAs appear to be infectious. Although many herpesvirus DNAs are similarly organized, most show little sequence homology. By DNA hybridization, herpes simplex viruses 1 and 2 can be shown to share long stretches of homologous DNA (>50 percent overall relatedness). Most of the other viruses possess only scattered regions of DNA homology such that there is a weak (<5 percent) overall sequence relatedness that can be demonstrated only by using relatively nonstringent DNA hybridization conditions.

As herpesviruses spread serially through the community, minor mutations gradually accrue in their DNA sequences. Ultimately, these minor changes can be detected by sensitive molecular techniques such as restriction endonuclease cleavage analysis. The virus strain recovered from one person is generally indistinguishable from that of the person from whom the virus was acquired. Viruses from individuals who have not been in contact with one another are readily distinguished by endonuclease analysis. This powerful molecular epidemiologic tool has aided in our understanding of herpesvirus spread and reactivation.

Herpesvirus DNA sequences are used very efficiently, expressing sufficient numbers of RNAs to encode 70 to over 100 distinct proteins. The viral RNAs are transcribed from both strands of the genome in a generally nonoverlapping manner, with very few noncoding regions.

VIRUS REPLICATION

Herpesvirus replication is a carefully regulated, multistep process.[17] Shortly after infection a small number of genes is tran-

TABLE 1. Classification and Structure of Herpesviridae That Infect Humans

Common Name	Other Designation	Subfamily	Genome Size (MW × 106)	No. of Genome Isomers	Genome Type[a]	Guanine-Plus-Cytosine Content (%)
Human viruses						
Herpes simplex virus type 1	Human herpesvirus 1	α	96	4	1	67
Herpes simplex virus type 2	Human herpesvirus 2	α	96	4	1	69
Varicella-zoster virus	Human herpesvirus 3	α	80	2	2	46
Epstein-Barr virus	Human herpesvirus 4	γ	114	1	3	59
Cytomegalovirus	Human herpesvirus 5	β	145	1	1	57
B-lymphotropic virus	Human herpesvirus 6	γ	~115	?	?	46
Simian viruses						
Herpes B virus	Herpesvirus simiae	α	~105	?	?	74

Abbreviation: MW: molecular weight.
[a] Genomic arrangements are shown in Figure 2.

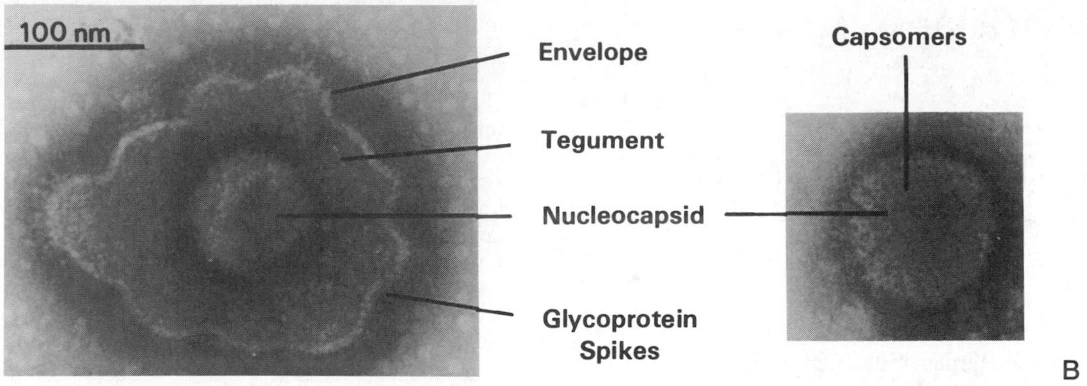

FIG. 1. Electron micrographs of varicella-zoster virus negatively stained with phosphotungstic acid. (×40,000) **(A)** The complete enveloped virion. **(B)** A purified viral nucleocapsid. (From Straus,[6] with permission.)

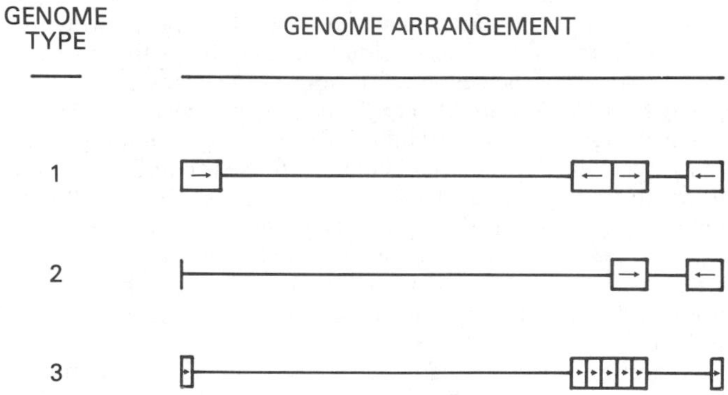

FIG. 2. Organization of three genome types of human herpesviruses. The large boxes denote major repeat elements, between or adjacent to which are unique sequences. The arrows denote the relative directions of the repeated sequences. Isomers of genomes are generated by the inversion of the unique sequences and their flanking inverted repeats. For example, varicella-zoster virus DNA (genome type 1) occurs primarily in two isomeric forms that differ solely in the reversal of the shorter unique sequence.

scribed. These "immediate-early" genes encode proteins that regulate their own synthesis and stimulate the synthesis of a second, larger wave of proteins from the "early" genes of the virus. Herpesvirus early proteins are involved in genome replication. The best characterized of these include the deoxypyrimidine (thymidine) kinases, DNA polymerases, ribonucleotide reductases, exonucleases, etc.

The precise manner in which herpesvirus DNA is replicated is not known, but the existence of terminal repeat sequences implies that circularization of the genome may be involved. There is evidence with some herpesviruses that progeny DNA molecules are generated continuously by a rolling circle mechanism.[18] Newly synthesized multimers of the genome are then cleaved appropriately and packaged.

After DNA replication the bulk of herpesvirus genes are expressed. These "late" gene products are incorporated into or aid in the assembly of progeny virions. New particles bud out of their host cells and promptly infect contiguous susceptible cells.

TROPISM

Herpesviruses vary widely in their abilities to infect different types of cells, a feature that is considered in classifying the virus into subfamilies (Table 1). For example, herpes simplex viruses grow readily in epithelial cells and fibroblasts of humans, monkeys, rabbits, mice, and many other animals. Varicella-zoster virus grows best in human epithelial cells and fibroblasts. In cell culture cytomegalovirus grows well only in human fibroblasts. Epstein-Barr virus can be cultivated only in B-lymphocytes.

The relative breadth of a herpesvirus' host range, however, is of more than taxonomic importance; it is highly predictive of the tissues that are clinically infected by the virus. Thus, the diseases associated with the lymphotropic herpesviruses are predominantly lymphoproliferative ones. In contrast, the herpesviruses that replicate readily in tissues of epithelial origin are primarily associated with mucocutaneous infections.

LATENCY

All herpesviruses induce lifelong latent infection in their natural hosts. The process of virus latency is still incompletely understood, but some of the key questions regarding its nature have been resolved in the past few years. It is clear that for any herpesvirus latency occurs within small numbers of very specific types of cells (Table 2). Latent herpes simplex viruses and Epstein-Barr virus genomes are carried extrachromosomally.[19,20] Integrated copies of the genome also exist for some viruses such as Epstein-Barr virus.[21]

There had been a long-standing debate as to whether latent herpesvirus genomes are totally quiescent or whether viral genes are expressed. Compelling data from studies of Epstein-Barr virus in lymphoid cell lines and of herpes simplex virus within ganglion neuronal cells indicate that the latent state is characterized by a vigorous expression of selected viral genes. Up to six Epstein-Barr virus genes are expressed as proteins displayed on the cell surface or within the nucleus of virus-immortalized cell lines.[22] A single region of the herpes simplex virus genome was recently shown to be active in latently infected ganglia.[23] Analyses of the selected herpesvirus genes that remain active suggest that they are regulatory in nature and may be serving to maintain the virus in its latent state.

TRANSFORMATION

Another biologic attribute of most herpesviruses is the ability to transform cells. Some of the viruses transform only cells of animals different from their natural hosts, while others transform their hosts' cells as well. The relevance of transformation that is observed to occur only in laboratory-derived model systems is uncertain. Thus, the ability of herpes simplex virus type 1 or 2, cytomegalovirus, or parts of their genomes to transform cells in culture may be clinically meaningless.[24] In fact, there remains no definitive evidence linking these herpesviruses to

TABLE 2. Features of Productive, Latent, and Transforming Herpesvirus Infections of Humans

Virus	*Typical Primary Infections*	*Typical Recurrent Infections*	*Infection in the Compromised Host*	*Sites of Latency*	*Association with Human Cancers*
Herpes simplex virus 1	Gingivostomatitis Keratoconjunctivitis Cutaneous herpes Genital herpes Encephalitis	Herpes labialis Keratoconjunctivitis Cutaneous herpes Encephalitis	Gingivostomatitis Keratoconjunctivitis Cutaneous herpes Esophagitis Pneumonitis Hepatitis, etc.	Sensory nerve ganglia	Squamous carcinoma of the oropharynx??
Herpes simplex virus 2	Genital herpes Cutaneous herpes Gingivostomatitis Meningoencephalitis Neonatal herpes	Genital herpes Cutaneous herpes	Genital herpes Cutaneous herpes Disseminated infection	Sensory nerve ganglia	Cervical cancer?
Varicella-zoster virus	Varicella	Dermatomal zoster	Disseminated infection	Sensory nerve ganglia	None
Cytomegalovirus	Mononucleosis Hepatitis Congenital cytomegalic inclusion disease	?	Hepatitis Retinitis Pneumonitis Encephalitis Colitis, etc.	Monocytes? Neutrophils? Lymphocytes?	Kaposi sarcoma?
Epstein-Barr virus	Mononucleosis Hepatitis Encephalitis	?	Lymphoproliferative syndromes	B lymphocytes, salivary glands	African-type Burkitt's lymphoma Nasopharyngeal carcinoma
Human herpesvirus type 6	?	?	?	Lymphocytes?	Rare B cell lymphomas?
Simian herpes B virus	Mucocutaneous lesions Encephalitis	?	?	Sensory nerve ganglia?	?

cancer. An active search for the effects of related virus sequences in human neoplasms should continue nonetheless.

To date, only lymphotropic herpesviruses are proved to be tumorigenic; most lead to lymphoproliferative malignancies.[25] Epstein-Barr virus, however, is also associated with naospharyngeal carcinoma and rare other carcinomas as well. Viral gene expression in cell lines transformed by lymphotropic herpesviruses is closely regulated but may differ from that typical of latent infection. In vivo, specific mechanisms must be engaged to prevent completion of the virus replicative cycle and to foil immune surveillance of virally induced tumors.

EPIDEMIOLOGY AND TRANSMISSION

Herpesviruses are fragile and do not survive for prolonged periods in the environment. As such, transmission generally requires the inoculation of a virus-containing fresh body fluid of an infected person directly into the susceptible tissues of a previously uninfected person. Susceptible sites include oral, ocular, genital, or anal mucosa, the respiratory tract, and the blood stream. Herpesviruses do not penetrate keratinized skin efficiently.

The six herpesviruses whose modes of transmission to humans are understood are acquired predominantly by intimate contact (Table 3). Direct contact with infected lesions transfers herpes simplex, varicella-zoster, and herpes B viruses.[26] Sexual intercourse and oral–genital contact transmit herpes simplex viruses and cytomegalovirus.[27] The major vehicle for Epstein-Barr virus is probably infected saliva; however, the recent identification of this virus in exfoliated cervical cells suggests that it may also be sexually transmitted.[28–30]

Given the prolonged intimate contact between mother and baby during pregnancy and delivery, it is not surprising that all of the human herpesviruses cause congenital and neonatal infections; those associated with cytomegalovirus are the most prevalent.[27] Some herpesviruses can be transmitted without person-to-person contact. For example, varicella can result from inhalation of infectious aerosols.[31] Cytomegalovirus and Epstein-Barr virus can also be transmitted by blood transfusion and transplantation.[27,29]

Herpesviruses are ubiquitous, and few humans escape being infected by them. Behaviors that promote the exchange of body fluids increase the risk of acquiring every herpesvirus (Table 3). The viruses are transmitted by individuals in whom active virus replication is occurring either during the course of their own primary infections or during reactivation infections. Some of those who transmit herpesviruses are symptomatic, but many are asymptomatic.

Except for the varicella-zoster virus infections, most herpesvirus infections are transmitted asymptomatically. Over the course of a lifetime, episodes of asymptomatic shedding of herpesviruses probably exceed those of symptomatic shedding, and thus there may be more opportunities to transmit these viruses asymptomatically than symptomatically. With herpes simplex viruses, asymptomatic reactivation and shedding of virus occurs on about $\frac{1}{2}$–1 percent of days.[26] Epstein-Barr virus shedding rates are much higher, exceeding 20 percent of the days in normal seropositive individuals.[31]

The likelihood of transmission depends on the quantity of virus shed. There are indications that the titer of virus recoverable during symptomatic infections greatly exceeds that of asymptomatic infections. The net result of these factors is that both symptomatic and asymptomatic infections contribute substantially to rates of herpesvirus transmission. The best data are available for genital herpes infections. Between one-half to three-fourths of infections are acquired from asymptomatic sexual partners.[32] It is likely that an even greater proportion of Epstein-Barr virus infections are transmitted asymptomatically.

PATHOGENESIS

Herpesviruses induce disease in three manners: by direct destruction of tissues, by provoking immunopathologic responses, and by facilitating neoplastic transformation.

Mucocutaneous herpes simplex virus, varicella-zoster virus, and herpesvirus simiae infections represent the direct consequences of tissue destruction by replicating virus. Visceral infections with these viruses or with cytomegalovirus, such as encephalitis, pneumonitis, retinitis, and hepatitis, also reflect virus-induced cytopathogenicity.

Certain complications of herpesvirus infections, however, such as erythema multiforme, hemolytic anemia, and thrombocytopenia are primarily immune mediated.[33,34] Whether the neurologic complications of varicella and zoster are also im-

TABLE 3. Transmission and Seroepidemiology of Herpesviruses That Infect Humans.

	Modes of Transmission				*Seroprevalence (%) (United States)*		
Virus	*Perinatal*	*Blood Products*	*Intimate Contact*	*Aerosol*	*Normal Children*	*Normal Adults*	*Groups or Activities with Higher Risk of Infection*
Herpes simplex virus 1	+	−	+	−	20–40	50–70	Frequent intimate contact
Herpes simplex virus 2	+	−	+	−	0–5	20–50	Frequent intimate contact
Varicella-zoster virus	+	−	+	+	50–75	85–95	Children in day care
Cytomegalovirus	+	+	+	−	10–30	40–70	Children in day care Promiscuous gay men Transplant or blood recipients
Epstein-Barr virus	+	+	+	−	10–30	60–90	Frequent intimate contact
Human herpesvirus type 6	?	?	?	?	10–60?	20–80?	Cellular immune deficiency states
Simian herpes B	?	−	+	−	0	<1	Monkey handlers

Abbreviations: +: well-recognized association; −: rare or no association; ?: inadequate data.

TABLE 4. Clinical Syndromes Associated with Herpesviruses

Syndrome	*Herpes Simplex Virus 1*	*Herpes Simplex Virus 2*	*Varicella-Zoster Virus*	*Cytomegalovirus*	*Epstein-Barr Virus*	*Herpesvirus Simiae*
Gingivostomatitis	+	+				+
Genital lesions	+	+	+			+
Cutaneous lesions	+	+	+			+
Keratoconjunctivitis	+	+	+			+
Retinitis	+			+		
Esophagitis	+	+	+	+		
Pneumonitis	+	+	+	+	+	
Hepatitis	+	+	+	+	+	
Myopericarditis			+	+	+	
Meningitis		+	+			
Encephalitis	+	+	+	+	+	+
Myelitis	+	+	+			+
Erythema multiforme	+	+	+			
Arthritis			+		+	
Hemolytic anemia			+	+	+	
Leukopenia			+	+	+	
Thrombocytopenia			+	+	+	
Mononucleosis				+	+	
Lymphoma					+	

TABLE 5. Available Means to Prevent or Treat Herpesvirus Infections

Virus	*Host*	*Indication*	*Prevention*	*Treatment*
Herpes simplex virus 1	Any	Primary mucocutaneous infection	Avoid contact	None or po acyclovir
	Normal	Recurrent mucocutaneous infection	Avoid UV exposure	None
	Immune compromised	Any syndrome	None	iv or po acyclovir
	Any	Visceral infection	None	iv acyclovir
Herpex simplex virus 2	Any	Primary mucocutaneous infection	Avoid contact	po or iv acyclovir
	Any	Recurrent mucocutaneous infection	None	po or iv acyclovir
	Neonate	Visceral infection	Avoid contact	iv acyclovir
Varicella-zoster virus	Normal	Varicella	Vaccine?	None
	Immune compromised		Varicella-Zoster immune globulin Vaccine	iv acyclovir
	Normal	Zoster	None	None, or po acyclovir
	Immune compromised		None	po or iv acyclovir or none
Cytomegalovirus	Normal	Any syndrome	None	None
	Immune compromised	Visceral infection	Seronegative donor tissues and blood Specific immune globulin?, acyclovir?	Ganciclovir?
Epstein-Barr virus	Normal	Infectious mononucleosis	None	None, steroids in selected cases
	Immune compromised	Any infection	None	None, or acyclovir?
Human herpesvirus type 6	Any	Any infection	?	?
Herpesvirus simiae	Any	Any infection	Avoid infected monkeys	Acyclovir?, ganciclovir?

mune mediated has been widely debated. Because encephalitis, transverse myelitis, and cranial nerve palsies typically arise as the cutaneous component of varicella-zoster infection is resolving, these neurologic problems are often considered to be immune mediated.[35] Isolated instances in which the virus or its constituents have been detected in the involved central nervous system tissues, however, suggest that the virus itself can directly contribute to neurologic disease in some settings.[36]

It is very likely that most of the clinical manifestations of Epstein-Barr virus infection, including the hematologic and neurologic complications, are immunopathologically mediated. Except in the setting of severe congenital or acquired cellular immune deficiency disorders, only a minute fraction of the cells that infiltrate the lymph nodes, liver, and spleen during primary Epstein-Barr virus infection are actually virus-infected B lymphocytes.[37] Most represent reactive T cells of diverse types. It is for this reason that corticosteroids have a role in the management of some severe complications of Epstein-Barr virus infection and, conversely, that the potent antiviral drug acyclovir is not useful in the treatment of acute infectious mononucleosis.[38,39]

While the association of Epstein-Barr virus with certain B-cell lymphomas and nasopharyngeal carcinoma is well known, the role this virus plays in tumorigenesis is not. Most recent hypotheses assume Epstein-Barr virus to confer growth advantages on cells, thereby increasing opportunities for spontaneous chromosomal translocations or other potentially transforming events to occur and to allow tumor cells to escape immune surveillance.[40]

DIAGNOSIS

Most herpesvirus infections can be diagnosed clinically, but there are several situations in which specific tests are helpful. Laboratory confirmation of a herpesvirus infection helps to exclude other similar illnesses, may allay anxiety, guides counseling and treatment, and can be used to identify drug-resistant viruses.

A practical example of the value of confirmatory testing is genital herpes, the diagnosis of which often implies recurrent discomfort and chronic psychological and social distress. It would be unfair and inappropriate to casually render this diagnosis, recommend behavioral modification, and prescribe acyclovir. Another example of the value of testing is recurrent zosteriform eruptions, which are frequently misdiagnosed as repeated zoster outbreaks rather than as recurrent cutaneous herpes simplex virus infections.[41] Timely proof of the diagnosis in herpes simplex encephalitis, neonatal herpes, cytomegalovirus pneumonia, and other life-threatening infections permits the most efficient use of clinical resources and avoids the hazards and expense of ceaseless empiricism.

Acute herpes simplex virus, varicella-zoster virus, and herpesvirus simiae infections are best diagnosed by isolation of the virus in culture.[42–44] Serologic tests for these viruses are predominantly used to confirm recent or past infections. Diagnoses of Epstein-Barr virus infections, however, are most often confirmed serologically, isolation methods being too cumbersome or expensive for routine use.[45] Cytomegalovirus infections are often diagnosed serologically, but there is an increased effort to detect the virus in clinical specimens, particularly with relatively rapid methods.[46] Once a diagnosis has been made, serial serologic determinations are of little value in considering chronic or recurrent virus activity.

CLINICAL SYNDROMES

Herpesviruses cause a wide spectrum of clinical disease (Table 4). These can be grouped into mucocutaneous, visceral, central nervous system, and reactive syndromes. These infections are covered in detail in Chapters 118, 119, 120, and 121. Human infections with two other viruses warrant a more thorough review here.

Herpesvirus simiae infections are too rare to define their full spectrum. This virus is enzootic in macaques. Of rhesus monkeys in captivity, 30–80 percent are seropositive and experience recurrent symptomatic and asymptomatic infections that closely resemble those caused in humans by herpes simplex viruses. During periods of stress, as in handling or shipping, rhesus monkeys show high rates of virus shedding.[47] Monkey handlers bitten or scratched by infectious animals are at risk of acquiring the virus. Fortunately such infections have been documented rarely. As of 1988 only about 30 symptomatic human infections were recorded. Over two-thirds developed progressive mucocutaneous disease and fatal encephalitis. A recent outbreak involving four cases of symptomatic infection was particularly instructive in revealing that human-to-human transmission occurs via direct contact and that acyclovir suppresses mild infections.[48] Continued surveillance of the survivors of that outbreak revealed evidence of periodic asymptomatic reactivation and shedding of herpesvirus simiae.

Herpesvirus type 6 infection has not as yet been firmly linked to specific disease entities. Preliminary data suggest that it may be associated with exanthem subitum (roseola infantum) and a mononucleosis-like illness.[49] Herpesvirus type 6 is recovered from peripheral blood mononuclear cells by cocultivation in human umbilical cord blood lymphocytes.[50] Virus is most readily recovered from patients with lymphoproliferative malignancies and the acquired immunodeficiency syndrome (AIDS). It grows in B and T lymphocytes and in a few special nonlymphoid cell lines as well.[51] Unlike Epstein-Barr virus, infected lymphocytes are destroyed rather than immortalized. However, herpesvirus type 6 DNA has been detected by hybridization in B-cell lymphomas arising in immunocompromised individuals. Herpesvirus type 6 infections are common; most healthy children and adults possess antibodies to this virus.

PREVENTION AND TREATMENT

Rapid progress has been made over the last few years in the prevention and treatment of some herpesvirus infections (Table 5). A live varicella vaccine has been proved efficacious and is currently under consideration for licensure.[53,54] Varicella-zoster immune globulin is now widely available, albeit expensive.[55] Studies of cytomegalovirus-specific immune globulin, plasma, and vaccines are underway.[56,57]

Acyclovir is the major antiviral drug in use today and has proven indications for the treatment of several mucocutaneous and visceral herpesvirus infections.[58–60] Ganciclovir, a more toxic analogue of acyclovir, is being evaluated for the treatment of life-threatening cytomegalovirus infections in immunocompromised patients.[61] Its efficacy for arresting sight-threatening cytomegalovirus retinitis in patients with AIDS is already evident.[62]

REFERENCES

1. Roizman B, Batterson W. Herpesviruses and their replication. In: Fields BN, Knipe, DM, Chanock RM, et al., eds. Virology. New York: Raven Press; 1985:497–526.
2. Roizman B, ed. The Herpesviruses. v. 1. New York: Plenum; 1982.
3. Roizman B, ed. The Herpesviruses. v. 2. New York: Plenum; 1983.
4. Roizman B, ed. The Herpesviruses. v. 3. New York: Plenum; 1985.
5. Roizman B, Lopez C, eds. Immunobiology and Prophylaxis of Human Herpesvirus Infections. New York: Plenum; 1984.
6. Straus SE, Ostrove JM, Inchauspe G, et al. Varicella zoster virus infections: Biology, natural history, treatment, and prevention. Ann Intern Med. 1988;108:221.
7. Wildy P, Russell WC, Horne RW. The morphology of herpes virus. Virology. 1960;12:204.
8. Epstein MA. Observations on the mode of release of herpes virus from infected HeLa cells. J Cell Biol. 1962;12:589.
9. Ben-Porat T, Kaplan AS. Studies on the biogenesis of herpesvirus envelope. Nature. 1972;235:165.

10. Roizman B, Furlong D. The replication of herpesviruses. In: Fraenkel-Conrat H, Wagner RR, eds. Comprehensive Virology. v. 3. New York: Plenum; 1974:229–403.
11. Spear P. Herpesviruses. In: Blough HA, Tiffany JM, eds. Cell Membranes and Viral Envelopes. v. 2. New York: Academic Press; 1980:709–750.
12. Highlander SL, Sutherland SL, Gage PJ, et al. Neutralizing monoclonal antibodies specific for herpes simplex vires glycoprotein D inhibit virus penetration. J Virol. 1987;61:3356.
13. Baucke RB, Spear PG. Membrane proteins specified by herpes simplex virus. V. Identification of an Fc-binding glycoprotein. J Virol. 1979;32:779.
14. Friedman HM, Cohen GH, Eisenberg RJ, et al. Glycoprotein C of HSV-1 functions as a C3b receptor on infected endothelial cells. Nature. 1984;309:633.
15. Frade R, Barel M, Ehlin-Henriksson B, et al. gp140, the C3d receptor of human B lymphocytes, is also the Epstein-Barr virus receptor. Proc Natl Acad Sci USA. 1985;82:1490.
16. Roizman B. The structure and isomerization of herpes simplex virus genomes. Cell. 1979;16:481.
17. Jones PC, Roizman B. Regulation of herpesvirus macromolecular synthesis. VIII. The transcription program consists of three phases during which transcription and accumulation of RNA in the cytoplasm are regulated. J Virol. 1979;31:299.
18. Ben-Porat T, Tokazewski S. Replication of herpesvirus DNA. II. Sedimentation characteristics of newly synthesized DNA. Virology. 1977;79:292.
19. Mellerick DM, Fraser NW. Physical state of the latent herpes simplex virus genome in a mouse model system: Evidence suggesting an episomal state. Virology. 1987;158:265.
20. Adams A, Lindahl T. Epstein-Barr virus genomes with properties of circular DNA molecules in carrier cells. Proc Natl Acad Sci USA. 1975;72:1477.
21. Adams A, Lindahl T, Klein G. Linear associations between cellular DNA and EBV DNA in a human lymphoblastoid cell line. Proc Natl Acad Sci USA. 1973;70:2888.
22. Dambaugh T, Hennessy K, Fennewald S, et al. The virus genome and its expression in latent infections. In: Epstein MA, Achong BG, eds. The Epstein-Barr Virus: Recent Advances. v. 1. London: William Heinemann; 1986:13–46.
23. Stevens JG, Wagner EK, Devi-Rao GB, et al. RNA complementary to a herpes virus α gene mRNA is prominent in latently infected neurons. Science. 1987;235:1056.
24. Tevethia MJ. Transforming potential of herpes simplex viruses and human cytomegalovirus. In: Roizman B, ed. The Herpesviruses. v. 3. New York: Plenum; 1982:257–314.
25. Magrath I. Infectious mononucleosis and malignant neoplasia. In: Schlossberg D, ed. Infectious Mononucleosis. New York: Praeger Publishers; 1983:225–77.
26. Whitley RJ. Epidemiology of herpes simplex viruses. In: Roizman B, ed. The Herpesviruses. v. 3. New York: Plenum; 1982:1–44.
27. Naraqi S. Cytomegaloviruses. In: Belshe RB, ed. Textbook of Human Virology. Littleton, MA: PSG Publishing; 1984:887–928.
28. Chang RS, Lewis JP, Abildgaard CF. Prevalence of oropharyngeal excretors of leukocyte transforming agents among a human population. N Engl J Med. 1973;289:1325.
29. Fleisher GR. Epidemiology and pathogenesis. In: Schlossberg D, ed. Infectious Mononucleosis. New York: Praeger Publishers; 1983:15–47.
30. Sixbey JW, Lemon SM, Pagano JS. A second site for Epstein-Barr virus shedding: The uterine cervix. Lancet. 1986;2:1122.
31. Leclair JM, Zaia JA, Levin MJ, et al. Airborne transmission of chickenpox in a hospital. N Engl J Med. 1980;302:450.
32. Mertz GJ, Schmidt O, Jourden JL, et al. Frequency of acquisition of first-episode genital infection with herpes simplex virus from symptomatic and asymptomatic source contacts. Sex Transm Dis. 1985;12:33.
33. Oorton PW, Huff JC, Tonnesen MG, et al. Detection of a herpes simplex viral antigen in skin lesions of erythema multiforme. Ann Intern Med. 1984;101:48.
34. Harris AI, Meyer RJ, Brody EA. Cytomegalovirus-induced thrombocytopenia and hemolysis in an adult. Ann Intern Med. 1975;83:670.
35. Johnson R, Milbourne PE. Central nervous system complications of chickenpox. Can Med Assoc J. 1970;102:831.
36. Ryder JW, Croen K, Kleinschmidt-DeMasters BK, et al. Progressive encephalitis three months after resolution of cutaneous zoster in a patient with AIDS. Ann Neurol. 1985;19:182.
37. Rocchi G, DeFelici A, Ragona G, et al. Quantitative evaluation of Epstein-Barr virus infected mononuclear peripheral blood leukocytes in infectious mononucleosis. N Engl J Med. 1972;296:132.
38. Bender DE. The value of corticosteroids in the treatment of infectious mononucleosis. JAMA. 1967;199:529.
39. Andersson J, Britton S, Ernberg I, et al. Effect of acyclovir on infectious mononucleosis: A double-blind placebo-controlled study. J Infect Dis. 1986;153:283.
40. Erikson J, Finan J, Nowell PC, et al. Translocation of immunoglobulin V_H genes in Burkitt's lymphoma. Proc Natl Acad Sci USA. 1982;79:5611.
41. Kalman CM, Laskin OL. Herpes zoster and zosteriform herpes simplex virus infections in immunocompetent adults. Am J Med. 1986;81:775.
42. Straus SE, Rooney JF, Sever JL, et al. Herpes simplex virus infection: Biology, treatment, and prevention. Ann Intern Med. 1985;103:404.
43. Straus SE, Ostrove JM, Inchauspe G, et al. Varicella-zoster virus infections: Biology, natural history, treatment, and prevention. Ann Intern Med. 1988;108:221.
44. Kalter SS, Hilliard JK, Heberling RL. The differential diagnosis of herpesvirus infections in man and animals. Dev Biol Stand. 1982;52:101.
45. Henle W, Henle GE, Horwitz CA. Epstein-Barr virus specific diagnostic tests in infectious mononucleosis. Hum Pathol. 1974;5:551.
46. Gleaves CA, Smith RF, Shuster EA, et al. Comparison of standard tube and shell vial cell culture techniques for the detection of cytomegaloviruses in clinical specimens. J Clin Microbiol. 1985;21:217.
47. Palmer AE. B-virus, herpesvirus simiae: Historical perspective. J Med Primatol. 1987;16:99.
48. Centers for Disease Control. B-virus infection in humans. Pensacola, Florida. MMWR. 1987;36:209.
49. Yamanishi K, Okuno T, Shiraki K, et al. Identification of human herpesvirus type-6 as a causal agent for exanthan subitum. Lancet; 1988;1:1005.
50. Salahuddin SZ, Ablashi DV, Markham PD, et al. Isolation of a new virus, HBLV, in patients with lymphoproliferative disorders. Science. 1986;234:596.
51. Ablashi DV, Salahuddin SZ, Josephs SF, et al. Human B-lymphotropic herpesviruses (HBLV) in human cell lines. Nature. 1987;329:207.
52. Josephs SF, Buchbinder A, Streicher HZ, et al. Detection of human B-lymphotropic virus (human herpesvirus 6) sequences in B cell leukemia. Leukemia. 1988;2:132.
53. Weibel RE, Neff BJ, Kuter BJ, et al. Live attenuated varicella virus vaccine: Efficacy trial in healthy children. N Engl J Med. 1984;310:1409.
54. Gershon AA, Steinberg SP, Gelb L. Live attenuated varicella vaccine use in immunocompromised children and adults. Pediatrics. 1986;78:757.
55. Centers for Disease Control. Varicella-zoster immune globulin for the prevention of chickenpox: Recommendations of the Immunization Practices Advisory Committee. Ann Intern Med. 1984;100:859.
56. Winston DJ, Pollard RB, Winston GH, et al. Cytomegalovirus immune plasma in bone marrow transplant recipients. Ann Intern Med. 1982;97:11.
57. Starr SF, Glazer JP, Friedman HM, et al. Specific cellular and humoral immunity after immunization with live Towne strain cytomegalovirus vaccine. J Infect Dis. 1981;143:585.
58. Mitchell CD, Bean B, Gentry SR, et al. Acyclovir therapy for mucocutaneous herpes simplex infections in immunocompromised patients. Lancet 1981;1:1389.
59. Corey L, Fife KH, Benedetti JK, et al. Intravenous acyclovir for the treatment of primary genital herpes. Ann Intern Med. 1983;98:914.
60. Straus SE, Takiff HE, Seidlin M, et al. Suppression of frequently recurring genital herpes: A placebo-controlled double-blind trial of oral acyclovir. N Engl J Med. 1984;310:1545.
61. Masur H, Lane HC, Palestine A, et al. Effect of 9-(1,3-dihydroxy-2-propoxymethyl) guanine on serious cytomegalovirus disease in eight homosexual men. Ann Intern Med. 1986;104:41.
62. Collaborative DHPG Treatment Study Group. Treatment of serious cytomegalovirus infections with 9-(1,3-dihydroxy-2-propoxymethyl) guanine in patients with AIDS and other immunodeficiencies. N Engl J Med. 1986;314:801.

118. HERPES SIMPLEX VIRUS

MARTIN S. HIRSCH

Herpes simplex virus (HSV) infections are among the most common maladies affecting humans. Often they are annoying and troublesome; occasionally they are life-threatening. The term *herpes* is derived from the Greek word meaning to creep, and clinical descriptions of herpes labialis go back to the time of Hippocrates.[1] Astruc, physician to the king of France, is credited with the first description of genital herpes in 1736.[2] Between 1910 and 1920, the infectious nature of herpes lesions was demonstrated by producing corneal lesions in rabbits with material derived from herpes keratitis and labialis.[3] As techniques for isolating and characterizing the virus became more simplified and serologic procedures were developed, our understanding of the HSV clinical spectrum has greatly expanded. Studies during the past two decades have brought insights into the molecular biology of HSV,[4,5] the mechanisms of HSV latency and recurrence,[6–9] and the first successful approaches to therapy for certain types of HSV infections.[10,11]

DESCRIPTION OF THE PATHOGEN

Herpes simplex virus (herpesvirus hominis) shares many properties with other members of the herpesvirus groups, which in humans includes varicella-zoster, cytomegalovirus, Epstein-Barr virus, and human herpesvirus type 6. The members of this group have an internal core containing double-stranded DNA, an icosahedral capsid with 162 hollow capsomeres, and a lipid-containing laminated membrane or envelope. The overall diameters of enveloped herpesviruses are 150–200 nm. Replication occurs primarily within the cell nucleus and is completed by the addition of protein envelopes as the virus passes through the nuclear membrane. Complete virus replication is associated with lysis of the productive cell. All members of the human herpesvirus group can also establish latent states within certain types of cells they infect, although the physical nature of the viruses during periods of latency is unclear.

The most commonly used means of separating HSV from other members of the herpesvirus group are antigenic analyses and definition of biologic properties, for example, host range and types of cytopathologic changes. Herpes simplex virus may also be differentiated by neutralization kinetics, polypeptide analysis, DNA base composition, or molecular hybridization characteristics.[12]

Within recent years, further subdivision of HSV into specific types has become possible (Table 1). Although the most readily apparent differences between HSV-1 and HSV-2 are in their clinical and epidemiologic patterns, they can also be separated by a variety of biochemical and biologic characteristics. Among these are the pock size on chick embryo chorioallantoic membranes, the ability to form plaques in chick embryo cultures, the ability to induce syncytial giant cells in cell cultures, neurotropism in mice, sensitivity to heparin or temperature change in cell culture, and the base composition of their DNA.[12,13–15]

The development of monoclonal antibody and restriction enzyme technologies have permitted an even finer definition of variations among individual HSV isolates.[16–20] It is now clear that HSV-1 and HSV-2 share certain glycoprotein antigens (e.g., gB) and differ with respect to others (e.g., gG). Serologic differentiation between HSV-1 and HSV-2 infections can be readily made by detection of type-specific gG antibodies. Moreover, recognition of ever more subtle differences among isolates by DNA analysis has introduced a new field of medical investigation, that of molecular epidemiology.[16–18]

EPIDEMIOLOGY

Herpes simplex viruses have a worldwide distribution. Even remote Brazilian Indian tribes are infected with these agents.[21] There are no known animal vectors for HSV, and although experimental animals can easily be infected, humans appear to be the only natural reservoir. Direct contact, with transmission through infected secretions, is the principal mode of spread. HSV-1 is transmitted primarily by contact with oral secretions and HSV-2 by contact with genital secretions. Transmission can occur both from overtly infected persons or from asymptomatic excretors, although virus titers are higher in persons with active lesions and thus transmissability may be greater. Approximately 0.65–15 percent of the adults may be excreting HSV-1 or HSV-2 at any given time depending on the population studied.[22–25] For example, since shedding of HSV-2 is related to sexual activity, prostitutes may have unusually high rates of excretion.[25]

There does not appear to be a marked seasonal or sexual variation in the incidence of overt infection, but rates of infection are inversely related to socioeconomic status.[26–28] Only 30–50 percent of the adults in higher socioeconomic groups have HSV antibodies, whereas in lower socioeconomic groups, the rates are 80–100 percent, probably reflecting more crowded living conditions among the latter populations. The age-related patterns of infection are different for HSV-1 and HSV-2. HSV-1 antibodies rapidly rise during childhood. By puberty, nearly all members of lower socioeconomic groups have been infected; the incidence in higher socioeconomic groups is somewhat lower. In contrast, the major period of infection with HSV-2 follows puberty and is related to venereal transmission between the ages of 14–29. The frequency of HSV-2 antibodies among populations varies from approximately 3 percent in nuns to 70 percent in prostitutes.[25,27]

Spread of HSV-1 infection from oral secretions to other skin areas is a hazard of certain occupations such as dentists, respiratory care unit personnel, and wrestlers.[29,30] Laboratory-acquired and nosocomial outbreaks in hospital personnel or in neonatal nurseries have been reported.[16,31,32] Transmission of HSV-2 to other skin sites can occur among infants born to mothers having genital infections. Anal and perianal infections with HSV-2 are common among sexually active male homosexual populations.[33,34] Autoinoculation from genital areas to other sites including hands, thighs, and buttocks is not uncommon. With changing sexual mores and increasing oral–genital contact, some studies have reported an increasing incidence of genital HSV-1 and oral HSV-2 infections.[35,36]

Recurrent infection occurs frequently with both HSV-1 and HSV-2. Most recurrences are secondary to the endogenous reactivation of virus rather than exogenous reinfection[37] and occur despite the presence of circulating antiviral antibodies. Recurrent infections of the lips or perioral areas occur in 20–40 percent of the population.[38,39] HSV-2 oral–labial lesions recur less frequently than do HSV-1 lesions.[40] Recurrences vary in frequency from more than one attack per month (5–25 percent) to less than one attack every 6 months (10–65 percent).[39,41] The precipitating factors may be stereotyped for any given person and yet vary considerably among individuals. They include sunlight, fever, local trauma, trigeminal nerve manipulation, menstruation, and emotional stress. Recurrent HSV keratitis is less common; it has been estimated that 5 percent of all people attending ophthalmologic clinics have ocular HSV infections; of these, 25–50 percent have a recurrence within 2 years.[42,43] The frequency of genital recurrences depends on a variety of factors including sex, HSV type, and both the presence and titer of neutralizing antibody.[44] HSV-1 genital lesions recur less frequently than do HSV-2 lesions, and recurrences develop more frequently in men than in women. Overall recurrence rates approximate 60–90 percent of those with initial episodes. Although most recurrences are related to reactivation, reinfection accounts for occasional episodes.[37]

TABLE 1. Differences between HSV-1 and HSV-2[a]

Characteristics	*HSV-1*	*HSV-2*
Urogenital infections	−(10–30%)	+(70–90%)
Nongenital infections		
Labialis	+(80–90%)	−(10–20%)
Keratitis	+	−
Whitlow (hand)	+	+
Encephalitis (adult)	+	−
Neonatal infection	−(~30%)	+(~70%)
Transmission	Primarily nongenital	Primarily genital
Mice–genital or intramuscular	Less neurotropic	More neutropic
Pock size on chorioallantoic membranes	Small	Large
Plaques in chick embryo monolayers	−	+
Temperature sensitivity (40°C)	−	+
Heparin sensitivity	+	−
Syncytium formation in human embryonic kidney cells	−	+

[a] Antigenic differences between HSV-1 and HSV-2 can be detected by a variety of serologic techniques including immunofluorescence, immunoperoxidation, microneutralization, and enzyme-linked immmunoadsorption.

PATHOGENESIS

On entry into skin sites, HSV replicates locally in parabasal and intermediate epithelial cells, which results in the lysis of infected cells and the instigation of a local inflammatory response.

This series of events results in the characteristic lesion of superficial HSV infection, that is, a thin-walled vesicle on an inflammatory base. Multinucleated cells are formed with ballooning degeneration, marked edema, and characteristic Cowdry type A intranuclear inclusions. Such lesions are indistinguishable from those caused by varicella-zoster virus. Lymphatics and regional lymph nodes draining the site of primary infection become involved. Further virus replication may result in viremia and visceral dissemination, depending on the immune competence of the host. In murine models the maturity of macrophages at the site of local infection helps determine whether virus remains localized or disseminates.[45] Subsequently, other host defense mechanisms, for example, the production of interferons, natural killer cells, protective antibodies, and sensitized killer lymphocytes, are elicited to prevent the spread of infection.[46,47] It is unclear whether similar mechanisms operate in humans, although infants with immature immune mechanisms as well as immunosuppressed or malnourished children and adults are more likely to disseminate their infections. Depression of cell-mediated immune mechanisms appears to be more closely associated with severe HSV infections than does alteration in humoral immunity.[48] Viremia can be demonstrated in malnourished children with widespread infection, in certain immunosuppressed adults, and occasionally in immunologically intact persons.[49–52] Viremic spread may result in the infection of multiple visceral organs including the liver, lung, and central nervous system.

After primary infection, HSV may become latent within sensory nerve ganglion sites via travel along sensory nerve pathways.[6–9] Once within the ganglion, viral DNA and possibly some mRNA transcripts can be localized within neurons, although the intracellular form of the HSV DNA is unclear. Various immunologic and biochemical theories of HSV latency and reactivation have been proposed but remain unproven.[8,9,11,53,54] Reactivated virus or viral genetic information appears to spread peripherally by sensory nerves as well. The neuron appears to be unique in that production of fully infectious virus does not result in cell lysis. It is possible that only early viral products are produced within the neuron and that the final viral replicative assembly takes place in epithelial cells. Once HSV has traveled to cutaneous sites, further spread is from cell to cell, and limitation of spread results from the activation of humoral and cellular immune mechanisms, perhaps acting through the local production of interferon.[46,47]

Latency has been demonstrated in humans within trigeminal, sacral, and vagal ganglia.[67,55,56] Reactivation depends on the integrity of the anterior root and peripheral nerve pathways. A curious observation is that all areas supplied by a latently infected nerve are not equally involved and that recurrences usually develop in the vicinity of the primary infection. However, latent infections have not been demonstrated at skin sites themselves.[57] It is possible that other sites of HSV latency will be uncovered since intermittent oral or genital secretion and leukocyte carriage have been demonstrated.

A variety of humoral and cell-mediated immune mechanisms are recruited in response to primary and recurrent HSV infections including the production of various types of antibodies, the production of interferon, the activation of macrophages, the induction of T-lymphocyte–mediated reactivity, and the development of both natural killer cell and antibody dependent lymphocyte cytotoxicity. The relative roles of these mechanisms in the limitation of HSV infection are unclear.

CLINICAL MANIFESTATIONS

Primary Infections

Primary HSV-1 infection is frequently asymptomatic but may present as gingivostomatitis and pharyngitis most commonly in children under the age of 5 years but occasionally in older persons. Incubation periods range from 2 to 12 days and are followed by fever and sore throat with pharyngeal edema and erythema. Shortly after its onset, small vesicles develop on the pharyngeal and oral mucosa; these rapidly ulcerate and increase in number, often involving the soft palate, buccal mucosa, tongue, and floor of the mouth. Gums are tender and bleed easily, and lesions may extend to the lips and cheeks (Fig. 1). Fever and toxicity may persist for many days, and the patient complains of severe mouth pain. Breath is fetid, and cervical adenopathy is present. In children, dehydration may result from poor intake, drooling, and fever. In college-aged persons, primary HSV infection often presents as a posterior pharyngitis or tonsilitis.[58] Included in the age-related differential diagnosis are streptococcal or diphtheritic pharyngitis, herpangina, aphthous stomatitis, Stevens-Johnson syndrome, Vincent's infection, and infectious mononucleosis. The severe systemic symptoms, diffuse intraoral involvement, and the lack of other mucous membrane lesions usually cause little problem in recognizing the disease in children. The disease generally runs its course in 10–14 days with no sequelae, although cervical adenopathy may persist for several weeks. Autoinoculation of other sites, particularly the fingers in young children, is not uncommon.

Herpes simplex virus infections of the eye are usually caused by HSV-1.[59,60] Primary infections may be manifested by a unilateral follicular conjunctivitis with regional adenopathy and/or a blepharitis with vesicles on the lid margin. Photophobia, chemosis, excessive tearing, and edema of the eyelids may be present. Some patients develop dendritic figures (Fig. 2) or coarse, punctate, epithelial opacities. If disease is limited to the conjunctiva, healing takes place within 2–3 weeks. However, if systemic symptoms and signs of stromal involvement are

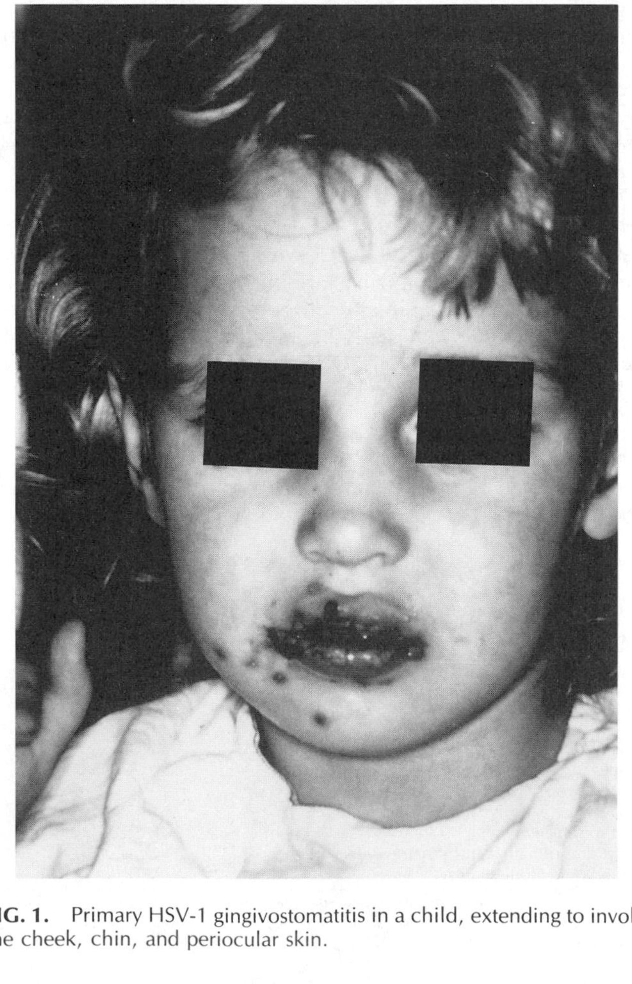

FIG. 1. Primary HSV-1 gingivostomatitis in a child, extending to involve the cheek, chin, and periocular skin.

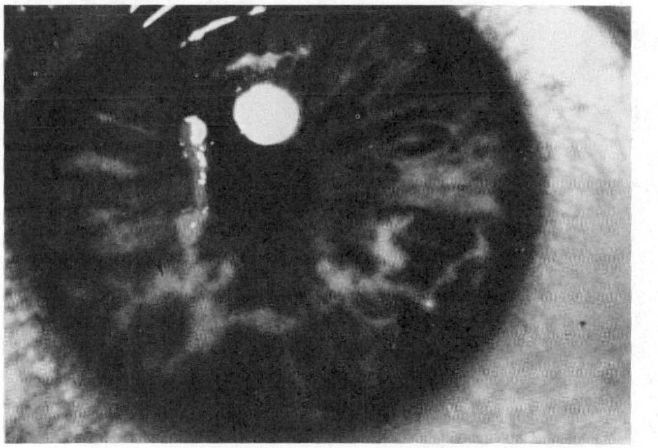

FIG. 2. HSV-1 dendritic keratitis. (From Pavan-Langston,[61] with permission.)

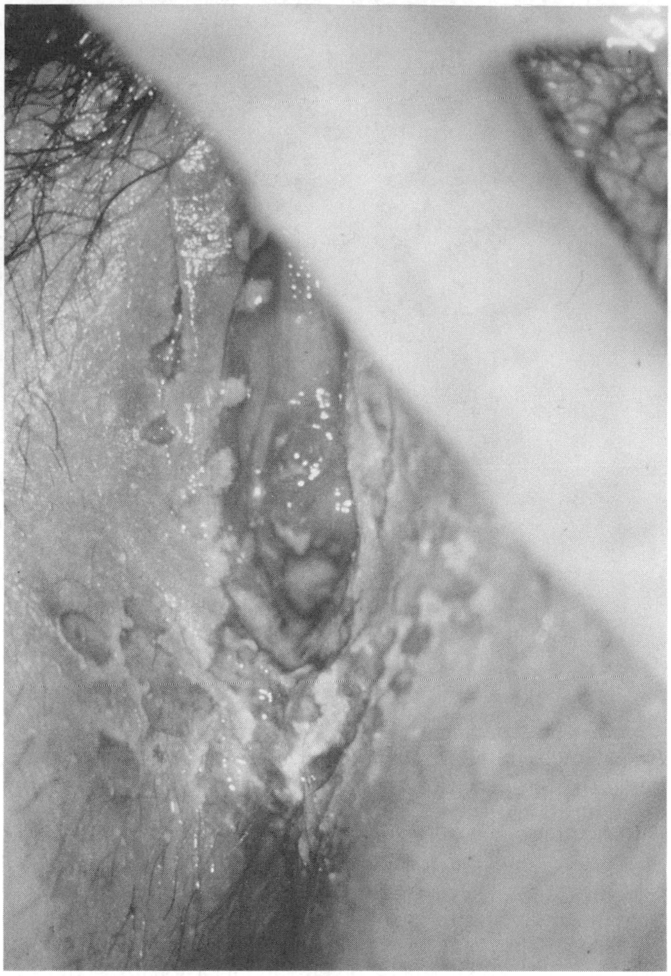

FIG. 3. Herpes (HSV-2) of the vulva.

present, the healing phase may be delayed. Spontaneous healing of the conjunctiva and cornea is usually complete.

Primary genital infection is most common in adolescents and in young adults and is usually (in 70–95 percent of the cases) caused by HSV-2. Incubation periods are 2–7 days. In men, vesicular lesions on an erythematous base usually appear on the glans penis or the penile shaft. In the female, lesions may involve the vulva, perineum, buttocks, cervix, and vagina and are frequently accompanied by a vaginal discharge (Fig. 3). Extragenital lesions occur during the course of primary infection in 10–20 percent of patients.[44] Primary infection in both sexes may be associated with fever, malaise, anorexia, and tender bilateral inguinal adenopathy. Although vesicular lesions may persist for several days in men, in women they rapidly ulcerate and become covered by a grayish white exudate. Such lesions may be exquisitely tender, and urethral involvement may result in dysuria or urinary retention. Herpetic sacral radiculomyelitis accompanying genital infection may also lead to urinary retention, neuralgias, and obstipation; in such patients a loss of anal tone, diminished bulbocavernosus reflex, and cystometrographic evidence of lower motor neuron dysfunction can sometimes be demonstrated.[62] Lesions of primary genital herpes may persist for several weeks before healing is complete. Previous HSV-1 infection may reduce the severity and duration of a first episode of genital herpes. In the diagnosis of genital herpes, other venereal infections such as chancroid or syphilis, erosions secondary to excoriation, genital manifestations of Behçet syndrome or erythema multiforme, and local moniliasis must all be distinguished.

Although primary infections are usually in perioral, ocular, or genital areas, any skin site may be initially involved. Primary HSV skin infections may be extensive and mimic herpes zoster, although a dermatomal distribution is not usually maintained and the pain is less severe. Primary finger infections (whitlows) may be misdiagnosed as pyogenic paronychiae and may be unnecessarily incised. Usually only one digit is involved, initially with intense itching or pain, and is followed by one or many deep vesicles that may coalesce (Fig. 4). Systemic complaints and intense local pain are frequently present, and neuralgia and axillary adenopathy may occur. If not incised, healing gradually takes place over a period of 2–3 weeks; if incised, secondary bacterial infection may develop and delay healing. Among medical, paramedical, or dental personnel, whitlows are commonly caused by HSV-1, whereas in the general community they are more commonly secondary to infection with HSV-2.[63]

Primary perianal and anal HSV-2 infection is becoming increasingly well recognized, particularly in male homosexuals.[34] Pain is the primary symptom, with itching, tenesmus, and discharge also noted. Systemic complaints of fever, chills, malaise, headache, difficulty in urinating, and sacral paresthesias may be present. On examination, vesicles and ulcerations may be seen in perianal and sometimes in anal areas. They may become confluent and result in a grayish ulcerating cryptitis surrounded by a red edematous mucosa. Bilateral inguinal adenopathy is common. The course is generally self-limited unless bacterial infection supervenes, with healing occurring in 1–3 weeks. However, in the setting of the acquired immunodeficiency syndrome (AIDS), herpes proctitis may be prolonged and progressive.[33]

Recurrent Infections

Recurrent herpes labialis is frequently heralded by prodromal symptoms (pain, burning, tingling, or itching) generally lasting for less than 6 hours but occasionally as long as 24–48 hours.[39,41] Vesicles appear most commonly at the vermillion border of the outer lip and are associated with considerable pain. The lower lip is more frequently involved, although individual patients may have stereotyped lesions at similar sites during each recurrence. The lesion area is usually less than 100 mm^2, and lesions progress from the vesicle to the ulcer/crust stage within 48 hours. Pain is most severe within the first 24 hours after the appearance of lesions. Healing is generally complete within 8–10 days. Rarely, recurrences may occur in the mouth or on the nose, chin, or cheek. Systemic complaints do not usually accompany recurrent herpes labialis, although local adenopathy may occur.

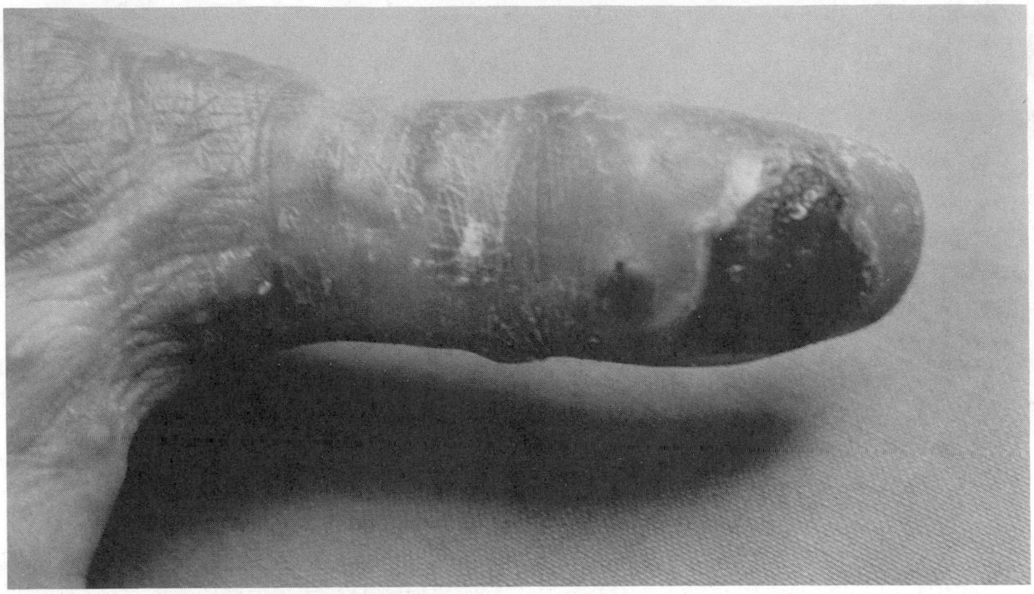

FIG. 4. Ulcerated herpetic whitlow in a respiratory care nurse. Her uncovered thumb had been used on a suction device to remove secretions from the mouth of a patient with herpes labialis. Secondary vesicles are seen at the base of the thumb.

Ocular infection may recur as keratitis, blepharitis, or keratoconjunctivitis. Recurrent keratitis is usually unilateral but is rarely (in 2–6 percent of the cases) bilateral. Two main types of keratitis may develop: dendritic ulceration or stromal involvement. Branching dendritic ulcers that stain with fluorescein are virtually diagnostic (Fig. 1) and are often accompanied by a loss in corneal sensation. Visual acuity may be decreased because the ulcers frequently involve the pupillary portion of the cornea. They may be accompanied by minimal anterior opacification or deep stroma involvement. Occasionally, extensive ameboid corneal ulcers may evolve, particularly if topical steroids have been applied. Superficial keratitis usually heals, but recurrent infection may lead to deep stromal involvement and uveitis, which may in part be mediated by hypersensitivity reactions to viral or altered cellular antigens.[64] A gradual diminution in visual acuity takes place, and individual attacks may last for several months with the formation of dense scars, corneal thinning, and neovascularization. Permanent visual loss may result, and rarely, rupture of the globe develops.

Recurrent genital lesions in both sexes are generally associated with less severe systemic symptoms and less extensive local involvement than are primary attacks. A prodrome of tenderness, itching, burning or tingling is often noted for several hours before a recurrence. Lesions in women are most often noted on the labia minora, labia majora, and perineum and less commonly on the mons pubis or buttocks.[65] Lesions in men are most often found on the glans or penile shaft. In women recurrences tend to be more severe.[44] Healing generally occurs in 6–10 days.[65,66] Virus shedding diminishes more slowly in women and can occur between recurrences in both sexes.[66,67] Occasionally, genital recurrences are associated with headache and even with aseptic meningitis.[68] Urethral stricture and labial fusion have also been reported after recurrent genital infections.

Recurrent HSV-1 or HSV-2 infections may develop on extremities; occasionally such lesions are associated with severe local neuralgia.[69,70] Local edema and lymphangitis may also occur during recurrences on extremities.

Complications

Encephalitis. Herpes simplex encephalitis is a rare complication of herpetic infection and yet is one of the most common acute sporadic viral diseases of the brain in the United States.[71–74] Estimates of its frequency range from several hundred to several thousand cases per year. Beyond the neonatal period, HSV-1 is the principal causal agent. Although little is known about the pathogenesis of HSV-1 encephalitis in humans, the virus is believed to spread by neural routes into the brain during either primary or recurrent infection.[18,74,75] Temporal lobes are the principal target areas of the virus, and a necrotizing hemorrhagic encephalitis results.

Herpes simplex encephalitis occurs at all ages, in both sexes, and in all seasons. The clinical course may begin suddenly or after a brief influenza-like prodrome. Headache, fever, behavioral disorders, speech difficulties, and focal seizures are prominent features; olfactory hallucinations may be present. Cerebrospinal fluid examination is variable but frequently shows a moderate pleocytosis with mononuclear and polymorphonuclear leukocytes; protein levels are slightly elevated, and glucose is generally normal. Infectious virus is rarely present in cerebrospinal fluid during encephalitis, and brain biopsy with appropriate histologic and cultural techniques is currently the most reliable way to make the diagnosis.[70–73] Although various antibody and antigen assays may provide adjunctive information,[74,76] they are not sensitive enough to provide a sufficiently early diagnosis. Herpes simplex virus encephalitis must be distinguished from other forms of viral encephalitis, tuberculous and fungal meningitis, brain abscesses, cerebrovascular accidents, and brain tumors. It is often helpful to identify the involved brain area by electroencephalography (EEG), magnetic resonance imaging (MRI), or computerized axial tomography so that biopsies can be appropriately localized. Of these, MRI and EEG may provide the earliest evidence of localization.[73,77] The course in untreated patients is usually one of rapid deterioration over several days that progresses to coma and death. Mortality in untreated biopsy-proven cases is 60–80 percent, and fewer than 10 percent of the patients are left without significant neurologic sequelae.[70–72]

Neonatal Infections. Involvement of the newborn with HSV can range from a mild localized infection to a fatal disseminated one. The incidence of neonatal HSV infection has been estimated to be between 1 in 2500 and 1 in 10,000 live births and is higher in premature than in full-term infants.[77–79] Most infections result from the retrograde spread of HSV-2 secondary to maternal genital infection or via passage of the infant through an infected maternal genital tract. The use of fetal monitor scalp electrodes may increase the risk of transmission.[80] The overall risk of serious neonatal infection has been estimated to be 40–50 percent after primary maternal infection and ≤8 percent after recurrent infection.[78] Primary infection during pregnancy may also lead to abortion, premature labor, skin lesions, chorioretinitis, microcephaly, or uterine growth retardation.[79] Both primary and recurrent infections during pregnancy may be asymptomatic with unsuspected viral shedding.[81] Rarely, nosocomial nursery infection may occur.[16,31,32]

Congenital infection may be recognized at birth along with jaundice, hepatosplenomegaly, a bleeding diathesis, central nervous system anomalies such as microcephaly or microphthalmia, seizures, irritability, temperature instability, chorioretinitis, and skin vesicles. In the absence of vesicles, congenital HSV infection may be difficult to distinguish from similar syndromes caused by rubella, cytomegalovirus, or *Toxoplasma*. In contrast, neonatal infection appears several days to several weeks after birth and may mimic neonatal sepsis. Often, infection occurs in the setting of prematurity. Vesicles may or may not be present, and conjunctivitis may be the first observed abnormality. Neurologic signs often predominate; seizures, cranial nerve palsies, lethargy, and coma may develop. The neurologic morbidity associated with neonatal HSV-2 infection is greater than that with HSV-1 infection.[82] A cerebrospinal fluid pleocytosis with increased protein and normal glucose levels is observed. Although some children with relatively localized disease apparently recover without significant sequelae, many develop severe complications such as destructive encephalitis or disseminated intravascular coagulation. Hepatic and adrenal necrosis may occur in fatal cases. The mortality of untreated neonatal infections is related to the type of illness, disseminated disease having the highest mortality (approximately 85 percent) and localized disease of the skin, eye, or mouth having virtually no mortalities.

Compromised Host. Patients compromised by immunodeficiency or immunosuppression, by malnutrition, or by disorders of skin integrity (e.g., burns, eczema) are at greater risk of developing severe HSV infections.

The renal, cardiac, or bone marrow transplant recipient frequently excretes HSV-1 in throat washings during the first few weeks after grafting.[48,83–86] Often these infections are asymptomatic, but occasionally they are particularly severe and persist for weeks to months (Fig. 5); they may spread down the respiratory or gastrointestinal tracts and result in tracheobronchitis, pneumonia, or esophagitis.[87] It appears that such severe infections are related to iatrogenic suppression of cell-mediated immunity early after transplantation.[49,85,86] Patients with hematologic and lymphoreticular neoplasms and children with congenital thymic disorders also may develop unusually severe, chronic, or progressive mucocutaneous HSV infection.[88,89] HSV infection during pregnancy[90,91] or in geriatric populations[92] may on rare occasions be associated with disseminated disease involving visceral organs, particularly the liver. Such disseminated disease is perhaps secondary to relative T-lymphocyte immunodeficiency states that occur with aging or during pregnancy. Instrumentation of debilitated patients with devices such as nasogastric tubes appears to facilitate spread. Herpetic esophagitis has been found to occur in approximately 25 percent of unselected autopsied patients, most of whom had nasogastric tubes in place shortly before death.[93] Herpetic esophageal ulcers are sometimes asymptomatic but may be associated with odynophagia, gastrointestinal bleeding, and diffusely scattered shallow ulcers on double-contrast esophagograms.[94]

Severe HSV infections are a prominent feature of AIDS.[33] Progressive HSV perianal ulcers, colitis, esophagitis, pneumonia, and a variety of neurologic disorders have been observed in patients with AIDS.

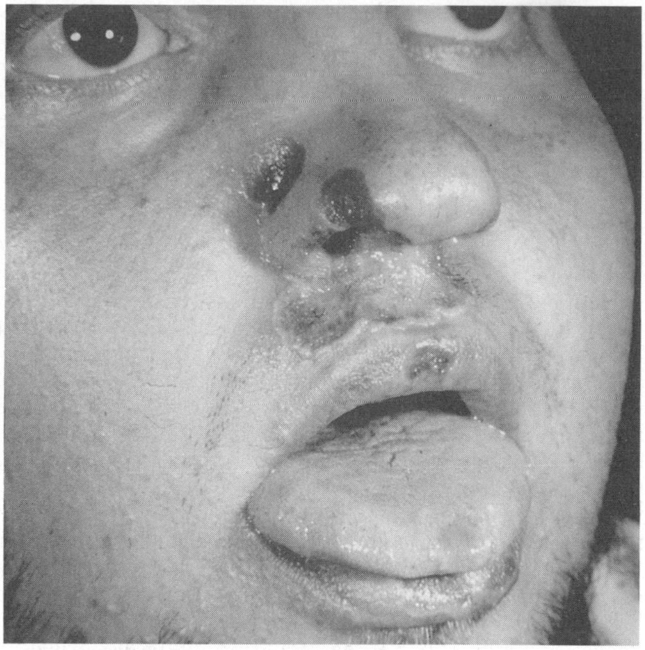

FIG. 5. Progressive HSV-1 infection of a renal transplant patient involving lip, tongue, and nose. The infection spread to involve trachea and lungs, resulting in fatal hemorrhagic pneumonitis.

Burn wound infections with HSV are becoming increasing well recognized.[95] Erosive, discolored, or vesicular areas in partially healing burns are suspicious of herpes simplex infection and should be cultured, or biopsies should be done. Occasionally HSV in burn patients disseminates to other skin areas, to the upper and lower respiratory tract, or to visceral organs. Patients with a variety of other skin disorders, for example, eczema, pemphigus, Darier's disease, or Sézary syndrome may also be unable to effectively localize their infections, thereby resulting in widespread cutaneous spread (eczema herpeticum, Kaposi varicelliform eruption).[96–98] These infections may recur and disseminate to visceral organs.[98]

Relationship to Other Diseases

Erythema Multiforme. Allergic cutaneous and mucous membrane disorders may accompany or follow acute HSV infections.[99–102] Up to 75 percent of all cases of erythema multiforme are regularly preceded by an attack of herpes simplex. Both HSV-1 and HSV-2 may be involved, and the cutaneous manifestations range from mild to severe (Stevens-Johnson syndrome) and may be recurrent. Inactivated HSV antigens injected intradermally into persons subject to erythema multiforme have induced such attacks,[99] and HSV antigen has been identified in skin biopsy specimens from affected lesions.[102]

Cancer. Many series, although not all, have indicated that patients with cervical carcinoma have a higher incidence and higher titers of HSV-2 antibodies than do matched controls.[103,104] These findings may reflect an earlier age of first intercourse and multiple sexual partners. Attempts to demonstrate infectious virus, viral antigens, or viral DNA sequences in cervical carcinoma cells have given contradictory results.[105,106]

Idiopathic Neurologic Syndromes. Herpes simplex virus infections have been implicated as possible factors involved in the pathogenesis of various neurologic disorders of unknown etiology including idiopathic facial paralysis (Bell's palsy), multiple sclerosis, atypical pain syndromes, ascending myelitis, trigeminal neuralgia, and temporal lobe epilepsy.[56,107–111] The associations are based on the known predilection of HSV for nerve tissue, on serologic studies, and on the occasional observations of temporal relationships between attacks of herpes labialis or genitalis and attacks of the neurologic syndrome.

DIAGNOSIS

Although experimental animals and embryonated eggs are both susceptible to infection with HSV strains, tissue cultures have largely replaced these hosts for diagnostic purposes. Primary human embryonic kidney, rabbit kidney, and human amnion cells readily support the replication of HSV. Continuous cell strains or cell lines of human diploid origin and certain continuous monkey kidney cell lines also support HSV replication, but to a lesser extent. Cytopathic effects usually appear rapidly, within 24–48 hours if the virus inoculum is high. Cells become rounded and clump, with rapid progression of cytopathic effects throughout the cell monolayer. Ballooning degeneration and the formation of multinucleated syncytial giant cells may be observed, particularly with HSV-2 isolates. Vesicles contain their highest titers of virus within the first 24–48 hours,[41] and specimens should be collected early and promptly inoculated into tissue cultures. If a delay is unavoidable, specimens can be stored in appropriate carrying medium at 4–9°C for a few hours, but for longer periods they should be stored at −70°C. Typing of isolates can be accomplished by using a variety of serologic techniques including immunofluorescence or microneutralization[112,113] or by certain biologic properties, for example, temperature or heparin sensitivity.[14,15] When tissue specimens such as neural ganglia are being studied for the presence of virus, tissue explantation or cell cocultivation techniques have proved useful in facilitating virus isolation.

The recent development of monoclonal antibodies to individual herpes virus antigens should allow for the more precise identification and typing of HSV isolates.[19,20,114,115] HSV-1 and HSV-2 have both type-specific and cross-reactive antigens that are useful for both grouping and type discrimination. Moreover, the cloning of herpes DNA fragments in recombinant bacteria may permit the production of probes to identify herpes genomes in the absence of infectious virus.[115]

For a rapid diagnosis of skin or mucous membrane lesions, scrapings from suspect lesions may be smeared, fixed with ethanol or methanol, and stained with Giemsa or Wright preparation. The presence of multinucleated giant cells indicates infection with HSV or varicella-zoster virus (Fig. 6). When using cytologic techniques, e.g., the Papanicolaou cervicovaginal stain or the Paragon multiple stain, intranuclear inclusions may also be seen.[116] Alternatively, such material can be examined for herpes antigens by immunofluorescent techniques or for virus particles by electron microscopy.

Serologic techniques may be helpful in diagnosing primary HSV infections but are rarely of value in recurrent infections. A variety of assays have been used including neutralization, complement fixation, passive hemagglutination, indirect immunofluorescence, radioimmunoassay, complement-mediated cytolysis, and antibody-dependent cellular cytolysis. During primary infections, a fourfold or greater rise in titer is observed between acute and convalescent sera. In recurrent infections such rises may or may not be observed.

Measurement of IgM HSV antibodies in infants may be helpful in the diagnosis of neonatal infection.[117] Such antibodies usually appear within the first 4 weeks of life in infected infants and persist for many months. Measurement of IgM antibodies in older persons has not proved useful in separating primary from recurrent infections.

Approaches to detect specific HSV antigens or antibodies to them by immunoblotting techniques in cerebrospinal fluid are under study. Such techniques may circumvent the need for invasive procedures such as brain biopsy to make the diagnosis of herpes encephalitis.[76,118]

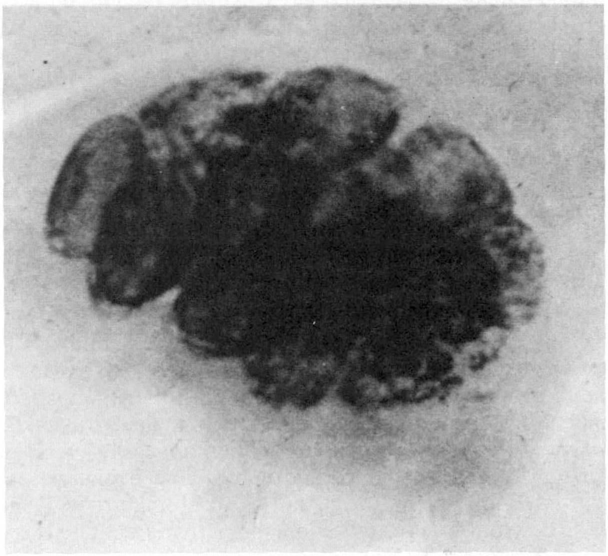

FIG. 6. Scraping of a vesicle base, stained with Giemsa preparation (Tzanck smear), showing a multinucleated giant cell indicative of infection with herpes simplex or varicella-zoster virus.

Studies of cell-mediated immunity in HSV infection are still in their infancy. Some observers have noted diminished lymphocyte proliferation to herpes virus antigens and a reduced production of certain lymphokines in association with recurrences.[49,119–121] However, these assays have not yet reached the stage of clinical usefulness.

PREVENTION AND TREATMENT

A number of nucleoside derivatives interfere with the synthesis of HSV DNA. Some of these (idoxuridine, trifluorothymidine, vidarabine) are useful in and licensed for the topical treatment of herpes keratitis[122] (see also Chapters 34 and 99). Vidarabine and acyclovir are also useful for systemic HSV infections. None of these agents affects latent virus.

Vidarabine (9-β-D-arabinofuranosyladenine) has shown efficacy in both herpes simplex encephalitis and neonatal herpes infection. In herpes encephalitis, placebo-controlled double-blind studies indicate that vidarabine, in intravenous doses of 15 mg/kg/day for 10 days, can reduce both mortality and morbidity.[71,72] The age and level of consciousness at entry are important variables in determining the outcome; patients under the age of 30 with higher levels of consciousness do better.

Controlled trials also indicate that vidarabine can lower the mortality from neonatal HSV infections.[123] In infants with central nervous system or disseminated disease, fatalities were reduced from 74 to 38 percent. Subsequent studies suggest that newborns tolerate higher doses of vidarabine than do older people and that progression from localized skin involvement to central nervous system disease is less when doses of 30 mg/kg/day for 10 days are employed. Topical vidarabine is also effective for the treatment of herpes simplex keratitis[124] but not for therapy for cutaneous infections.[125,126]

The most common adverse effects of intravenous vidarabine have been gastrointestinal and neurologic. Tremors, paresthesias, ataxia, and seizures may appear several days after the onset of therapy but are usually reversible. Pre-existing renal or hepatic disease may predispose patients to vidarabine neurotoxicity. The drug should be used cautiously in patients with renal insufficiency, with dose reductions of at least 25 percent.

The development of acyclovir, 9-(2-hydroxyethoxy methyl) guanine, represents a major advance in antiherpes therapy. Infection of cells with HSV results in the induction of a viral thymidine kinase that phosphorylates acyclovir to a monophosphate form. This is subsequently converted to acyclovir triphosphate by cellular enzymes. Acyclovir triphosphate is a potent inhibitor of HSV DNA polymerase and has little cellular toxicity.

Acyclovir is available in three formulations in the United States—a topical 5% ointment, an intravenous form, and an oral form. All three preparations are useful in the treatment of primary genital herpes.[127–131] The oral formulation is recommended for most uses (200 mg five times daily for 10 days). Acyclovir has only a modest effect on recurrent genital herpes attacks and does not appear to influence subsequent recurrences[132]; it is thus not recommended for therapy for most episodes of recurrent herpes in the immunologically competent host. In individuals subject to frequent and severe recurrences, suppression or prophylaxis with oral acyclovir may be indicated.[133,134] In patients whose recurrences are associated with severe complications such as erythema multiforme, recurrent aseptic meningitis, or eczema herpeticum, suppression is also of benefit. Oral administration appears safe and effective when used continuously for up to 1 year. Daily suppressive regimens (200 mg three to four times a day) are more effective than are intermittent regimens.[135,136]

The use of acyclovir in oral–labial HSV infections has been less extensively studied. Anecdotal reports suggest its use in primary attacks, but it is not generally recommended for recurrent herpes labialis.

In the immunocompromised host, acyclovir is useful as both treatment and suppression of recurrent mucocutaneous HSV lesions.[136–142] For the treatment of acute episodes, virus shedding, local symptoms, e.g., pain, and time to healing can be reduced by intravenous or oral regimens (e.g., 400 mg five times per day). Acyclovir is also useful in the prevention of herpetic recurrences in immunocompromised hosts including transplant recipients, leukemics undergoing induction chemotherapy, and patients with AIDS. Regimens of 200–400 mg two to five times per day have been satisfactory in preventing recurrences among seropositive patients.

Parenteral acyclovir is indicated for disseminated or central nervous system HSV infections. In patients with biopsy-proven HSV encephalitis, acyclovir was compared with vidarabine and found to be superior in reducing mortality (54 vs 28 percent, $p = .008$). Acyclovir in a dose of 10 mg/kg every 8 hours is recommended.[143] In newborns with disseminated HSV infections, acyclovir and vidarabine appear equivalent (R. J. Whitley, unpublished observations).

Acyclovir has little acute toxicity. Drug-related neurotoxicity (disorientation, hallucinations, tremors, ataxia, seizures) has been described rarely, and reversible renal dysfunction may follow a rapid bolus infusion.

A concern with respect to chronic acyclovir treatment is the possible development of resistant mutants of HSV. Mutants may have thymidine kinase with altered substrate specificity, lack thymidine kinase, or have DNA polymerase with altered substrate specificity.[144] Thymidine kinase–deficient (TK-) mutants have been isolated from immunocompromised patients, both in the presence and in the absence of acyclovir. Most of these have not been associated with progressive disease. However, acyclovir-resistant pathogenic isolates are becoming increasingly associated with progressive disease,[145,146] and it is possible that resistance will become a major problem in the years ahead. A number of other agents have received attention in the treatment of HSV infections including interferons and phosphonoformate, but none of these agents has been licensed for use in herpes infections. These agents may be useful for the treatment of infections resulting from TK-, acyclovir-resistant mutants.[147]

Experimental vaccines against HSV have shown promise in animal models,[148] and some are undergoing human trials. It is unlikely, however, that a human HSV will be generally available in the near future.

Attempts at prophylaxis have also been directed toward avoiding contact with infected lesions. Medical and dental personnel should be strongly encouraged to avoid direct contact with potentially infectious lesions by wearing gloves. Patients with extensive herpetic lesions, for example, eczema herpeticum, should be isolated. The use of condoms is recommended to prevent genital spread when one sexual partner has active lesions or a history of recurrent genital infections.

The prevention of neonatal disease in the offspring of mothers with genital infection presents special problems.[78–80] Although sufficient data have not yet been accumulated, it appears that if clinically apparent cervical infection is detected at parturition before membrane rupture, cesarean section is recommended. However, if membrane rupture has occurred, it is doubtful whether cesarean section is safer than vaginal delivery is, although rapid delivery by either route is clearly indicated to lessen the exposure of the infant. If clinical examination is negative at parturition, vaginal delivery appears safe. However, close monitoring of infants born to seropositive women is essential, with early intervention if illness develops during the first weeks of life.

REFERENCES

1. Wildy P. Herpes: History and classification. In: Kaplan AS, ed: The Herpesviruses. New York: Academic Press; 1973:1.
2. Hutifield DC. History of herpes genitalis. Br J Vener Dis. 1966;42:263.
3. Lowenstein A. Aetiologische untersuchungen uber den fieberhaften Herpes. Munch Med Wochenschr. 1919;66:768.
4. Roizman B. The structure and isomerization of herpes simplex virus genomes. Cell. 1979;16:481.
5. Schaffer PA. Molecular genetics of herpes simplex viruses. In: Nahmias AJ, Dowdle WR, Schinazi RF, eds. The Human Herpesviruses: An Interdisciplinary Approach. New York: Elsevier Science Publishing; 1981:55.
6. Bastian FO, Rabson AS, Yee CL, et al. Herpesvirus hominis: Isolation from human trigeminal ganglion. Science. 1972;178:306.
7. Baringer JR, Swoveland P. Recovery of herpes-simplex virus from human trigeminal ganglions. N Engl J Med. 1973;288:648.
8. Stevens JG, Wagner EK, Dovi-Rao GB, et al. RNA complementary to a herpesvirus and gene in RNA is prominent in latently infected neurons. Science. 1987;236:1056.
9. Openshaw H, Sekizawa T, Wohlenberg C, et al. The role of immunity in latency and reactivation of herpes simplex viruses. In: Nahmias AJ, Dowdle WR, Schinazi RF, eds. The Human Herpesviruses: An Interdisciplinary Approach. New York: Elsevier Science Publishing; 1981:289.
10. Hirsch MS, Schooley RT. Treatment of herpes virus infections. N Engl J Med. 1983;309:963,1034.
11. Corey L, Spear PG. Infections with herpes simplex viruses. N Engl J Med. 1986;314:686,749.
12. Gentry GA, Randal CC. The physical and chemical properties of the herpesviruses. In: Kaplan AS, ed. The Herpesviruses. New York: Academic Press; 1973:45.
13. Nahmias AJ, Josey WE. Epidemiology of herpes simplex viruses 1 and 2. In: Evans A, ed. Viral Infections of Humans: Epidemiology and Control. 2nd ed. New York: Plenum; 1982:351.
14. Nordlund JJ, Anderson C, Hsiung GD. The use of temperature sensitivity and selective cell culture systems for differentiation of herpes simplex virus types 1 and 2 in a clinical laboratory. Proc Soc Exp Biol Med. 1977;155:118.
15. Marks-Hellman S, Ho M. Use of biological characteristics to type herpesvirus hominis types 1 and 2 in diagnostic laboratories. J Clin Microbiol. 1976;3:277.
16. Buchman TG, Roizman B, Adams G, et al. Restriction endonuclease fingerprinting of herpes simplex virus DNA: A novel epidemiological tool applied to a nosocomial outbreak. *J Infect Dis.* 1978;138:488.
17. Hammer SM, Buchman TG, D'Angelo LJ, et al. Temporal cluster of herpes simplex encephalitis: Investigation by restriction endonuclease cleavage of viral DNA. J Infect Dis. 1980;141:436.
18. Whitley R, Lakeman AD, Nahmias A, et al. DNA restriction-enzyme analysis of herpes simplex virus isolates obtained from patients with encephalitis. N Engl J Med. 1982;307:1060.
19. Showalter SD, Zweig M, Hampar B. Monoclonal antibodies to herpes simplex virus type 1 proteins, including the immediate early protein ICP 4. Infect Immun. 1981;34:684.
20. Pereira L, Dondero DV, Gallo D, et al. Serological analysis of herpes simplex virus types 1 and 2 with monoclonal antibodies. Infect Immun. 1982;35:363.
21. Black FL. Infectious diseases in primitive societies. Science. 1975;187:515.

22. Douglas RG Jr, Couch RB. A prospective study of chronic herpes simplex virus infection and recurrent herpes labialis in humans. J Immunol. 1970;104:289.
23. Centifanto YM, Drylie DM, Deardourff SL, et al. Herpes type 2 in the male genitourinary tract. Science. 1972;178:318.
24. Bolognese RJ, Corson SL, Fuccillo DA, et al. Herpesvirus hominis type II infections in asymptomatic pregnant women. Obstet Gynecol. 1976;48:507.
25. Duenas A, Adam E, Melnick JL, et al. Herpesvirus type 2 in a prostitute population. Am J Epidemiol. 1972;95:483.
26. Buddingh GJ, Schrum DI, Lanier JC, et al. Studies on the natural history of herpes simplex infection. Pediatrics. 1953;11:595.
27. Nahmias AJ, Josey WE, Naib AM, et al. Antibodies to herpesvirus hominis types 1 and 2 in humans. I. Patients with genital herpetic infections. Am J Epidemiol. 1970;91:539.
28. Rawls WE, Campione-Piccardo J. Epidemiology of herpes simplex virus type 1 and type 2 infections. In: Nahmias AJ, Dowdle WR, Schinazi RF, eds. The Human Herpesviruses: An Interdisciplinary Approach. New York: Elsevier Science Publishing; 1981:137.
29. Rosato FE, Rosato EF, Plotkin SA. Herpetic paronychia: An occupational hazard of medical personnel. N Engl J Med. 1970;283:804.
30. Selling B, Kibrick S. An outbreak of herpes simplex among wrestlers (herpes gladiatorum). N Engl J Med. 1964;270:979.
31. Hale BD, Rendtorff RC, Walker LC, et al. Epidemic herpetic stomatitis in an orphanage nursery. JAMA. 1963;183:1068.
32. Francis DP, Herrmann KL, MacMahon JR, et al: Nosocomial and maternally acquired herpesvirus hominis infections. Am J Dis Child. 1975;129:889.
33. Siegal FP, Lopez C, Hammer GS, et al. Severe acquired immunodeficiency in male homosexuals manifested by chronic perianal ulcerative herpes simplex lesions. N Engl J Med. 1981;305:1439.
34. Goodell SE, Quinn TC, Mkrtichian E, et al. Herpes simplex virus proctitis in homosexual men. Clinical, sigmoidoscopic, and histopathological features. N Engl J Med. 1983;308:868.
35. Chang TW. Genital herpes and type 1 herpesvirus hominis. JAMA. 1977;238:155.
36. Wolontis S, Jeanson S. Correlation of herpes simplex virus type 1 and 2 with clinical features of infection. J Infect Dis. 1977;135:28.
37. Buchman TG, Roizman B, Nahmias AJ. Demonstration of exogenous genital reinfection with herpes simplex virus type 2 by restriction endonuclease fingerprinting of viral DNA. J Infect Dis. 1979;140:295.
38. Embil JA, Stephens RG, Manuel FR. Prevalence of recurrent herpes labialis and aphthous ulcers among young adults on six continents. Can Med Assoc J. 1975;113:627.
39. Young SK, Rowe NH, Buchanan RA. A clinical study for the control of facial mucocutaneous herpes virus infections. 1. Characteristics of natural history in a professional school population. Oral Surg. 1976;41:498.
40. Lafferty WE, Coombs RW, Benedetti J, et al. Recurrences after oral and genital herpes infection and viral type. N Engl J Med. 1987;316:1444.
41. Spruance SL, Overall JC Jr, Kern ER, et al. The natural history of recurrent herpes simplex labialis: Implications for antiviral therapy. N Engl J Med. 1977;297:69.
42. Kaufman HE, Brown DC, Ellison ED. Herpes virus in the lacrimal gland, conjunctiva, and cornea of man: A chronic infection. Am J Ophthalmol. 1968;65:32.
43. Carroll JM, Martola EL, Laibson PR, et al. The recurrence of herpetic keratitis following idoxuridine therapy. Am J Ophthalmol 1967;63:103.
44. Corey L, Adams H, Brown Z, et al. Genital herpes simplex virus infections: Clinical manifestations, course, and complications. Ann Intern Med. 1983;98:958.
45. Hirsch MS, Zisman B, Allison AC. Macrophages and age-dependent resistance to herpes simplex virus in mice. J Immunol. 1970;104:1160.
46. Notkins AL. Interferon as a mediator of cellular immunity in viral infections. In: Notkins AL, ed. Viral Immunology and Immunopathology. New York: Academic Press; 1975:149.
47. Lopez C. Resistance to herpes simplex virus–type 1 (HSV-1). Curr Top Microbiol Immunol. 1981;92:15.
48. Hirsch MS. Herpesgroup virus infections in the compromised host. In: Rubin RH, Young LS, eds. Clinical Approach to Infection in the Immunocompromised Host. 2nd ed. New York: Plenum; 1988:347.
49. Rand KH, Rasmussen LE, Pollard RB, et al. Cellular immunity and herpesvirus infections in cardiac-transplant patients. N Engl J Med. 1977;296:1372.
50. Becker WB, Kipps A, McKenzie D. Disseminated herpes simplex virus infection—its pathogenesis based on virological and pathological studies in 33 cases. Am J Dis Child. 1968;115:1.
51. Naraqi S, Jackson GG, Jonasson OM. Viremia with herpes simplex type 1 in adults: Four nonfatal cases, one with features of chicken pox. Ann Intern Med. 1976;85:165.
52. Craig C, Nahmias A. Different patterns of neurologic involvement with herpes simplex virus types 1 and 2: Isolation of herpes simplex virus type 2 from the buffy coat of two adults with meningitis. J Infect Dis. 1973;127:365.
53. Galloway DA, Fenoglio C, Shevchuk M, et al. Detection of herpes simplex RNA in human sensory ganglia. Virology. 1979;95:265.
54. Puga A, Cantin EM, Wohlenberg C, et al. Different sizes of restriction endonuclease fragments from the terminal repetitions of the herpes simplex type 1 genome latent in trigeminal ganglia of mice. J Gen Virol. 1984;65:347.
55. Baringer JR. Recovery of herpes simplex virus from human sacral ganglions. N Engl J Med. 1974;291:828.
56. Warren KG, Gilden DH, Brown SM, et al. Isolation of herpes simplex virus from human trigeminal ganglia, including ganglia from one patient with multiple sclerosis. Lancet. 1977;2:637.
57. Rustigian R, Smulow JB, Tye M, et al. Studies on latent infection of skin and oral mucosa in individuals with recurrent herpes simplex. J Invest Dermatol. 1966;47:218.
58. Glezen WP, Fernald GW, Lohr JA. Acute respiratory disease of university students with special reference to the etiologic role of herpesvirus hominis. Am J Epidemiol. 1975;101:111.
59. Binder PA. Herpes simplex keratitis. Surv Ophthalmol. 1977;21:313.
60. Ostler HB. Herpes simplex: The primary infection. Surv Ophthalmol. 1976;21:91.
61. Pavan-Langston D, ed. Ocular Viral Disease. v. 15. Boston: Little, Brown; 1975;19–36.
62. Caplan LR, Kleeman FJ, Berg S. Urinary retention probably secondary to herpes genitalis. N Engl J Med. 1977;297:920.
63. Glogau R, Hanna L, Jawetz E. Herpetic whitlow as part of genital virus infection. J Infect Dis. 1977;136:689.
64. O'Connor GR. Recurrent herpes simplex uveitis in humans. Surv Ophthalmol. 1976;21:165.
65. Guinan ME, MacCalman J, Kern ER, et al. The course of untreated recurrent genital herpes simplex infections in 27 women. N Engl J Med. 1981;304:759.
66. Vontver LA, Reeves WC, Rattray M, et al. Clinical course and diagnosis of genital herpes simplex virus infection and evaluation of topical surfactant therapy. Am J Obstet Gynecol. 1979;133:548.
67. Adam E, Dreesman GE, Kaufman RH, et al. Asymptomatic virus shedding after herpes genitalis. Am J Obstet Gynecol. 1980;137:827.
68. Hevron JE JR. Herpes simplex virus type 2 meningitis. Obstet Gynecol. 1977;49:622.
69. Layzer RB. Neuralgia in recurrent herpes simplex. Arch Neurol. 1974;31:233.
70. Hinthorn DR, Baker LH, Romig DA. Recurrent conjugal neuralgia caused by herpesvirus hominis type 2. JAMA. 1976;236:587.
71. Whitley RJ, Soong S-J, Dolin R, et al. Adenine arabinoside therapy of biopsy-proved herpes simplex encephalitis. NIAID collaborative antiviral study. N Engl J Med. 1977;297:289.
72. Whitley RH, Soong S-J, Hirsch MS, et al. Herpes simplex encephalitis. Vidarabine therapy and diagnostic problems. N Engl J Med. 1981;304:313.
73. Whitley RJ, Soong S-J, Linneman C Jr, et al. Herpes simplex encephalitis. Clinical assessment. JAMA. 1982;247:317.
74. Nahmias AJ, Whitley RJ, Visintine AM, et al. Herpes simplex virus encephalitis: Laboratory evaluations and their diagnostic significance. J Infect Dis. 1982;145:829.
75. Ojeda V. Fatal herpes simplex encephalitis with demonstration of virus in the olfactory pathway. Pathology. 1980;12:429.
76. Lakeman FD, Koga J, Whitley RJ. Detection of antigen to herpes simplex virus in cerebrospinal fluid from patients with herpes simplex encephalitis. J Infect Dis. 1987;155:1172.
77. Schroth G, Gawehn J, Thron A, et al. Early diagnosis of herpes simplex encephalitis by MRI. Neurology (NY). 1987;37:179.
78. Brown ZA, Vontver LA, Benedetti J, et al. Effects on infants of first episode of genital herpes during pregnancy. N Engl J Med. 1987;317:1246.
79. Hulto C, Arvin A, Jacobs R, et al. Intrauterine herpes simplex virus infections. J Pediatr. 1987;110:97.
80. Kaye EM, Dooling EC. Neonatal herpes simplex meningoencephalitis associated with fetal monitor scalp electrodes. Neurology (NY). 1981;31:1045.
81. Prober CG, Hensleigh PA, Boucher FD, et al. Use of routine viral cultures at delivery to identify neonates exposed to herpes simplex virus. N Engl J Med. 1988;318:887.
82. Corey L, Whitley RJ, Stone EF, et al. Difference between herpes simplex virus type 1 and type 2 neonatal encephalitis in neurological outcome. Lancet. 1988;1:1.
83. Montgomerie JZ, Croxson MC, Becroft DMO, et al. Herpes simplex virus infection after renal transplantation. Lancet. 1969;2:867.
84. Korsager B, Spencer ES, Mordhorst CH, et al. Herpes virus hominis infections in renal transplant recipients. Scand J Infect Dis. 1975;7:11.
85. Pass RF, Whitley RJ, Whelchel JD, et al. Identification of patients with increased risk of infection with herpes simplex virus after renal transplantation. J Infect Dis. 1979;140:487.
86. Meyers JD, Fluornoy N, Thomas ED. Infection with herpes simplex virus and cell-mediated immunity after marrow transplant. J Infect Dis. 1980;142:338.
87. Ramsey PG, Fife KH, Hackman RC, et al. Herpes simplex virus pneumonia: Clinical, virologic, and pathologic features in 20 patients. Ann Intern Med. 1982;97:813.
88. Muller SA, Herrmann EC Jr, Winkelmann RD. Herpes simplex infections in hematologic malignancies. Am J Med. 1972;52:102.
89. Buss DH, Scharyj M. Herpes virus infection of the esophagus and other visceral organs in adults: Incidence and clinical significance. Am J Med. 1979;66:457.
90. Young EJ, Killam AP, Greene JF Jr. Disseminated herpesvirus infection: Association with primary genital herpes in pregnancy. JAMA. 1976;235:2731.
91. Hillard P, Seeds J, Cefalo R. Disseminated herpes simplex in pregnancy: Two cases and a review. Obstet Gynecol Surv. 1982;37:449.

92. Eron L, Kosinski K, Hirsch MS. Hepatitis in an adult caused by herpes simplex virus type 1. Gastroenterology. 1976;71:500.
93. Nash G, Ross JS. Herpetic esophagitis: A common cause of esophageal ulceration. Hum Pathol. 1974;5:339.
94. Agha FP, Lee HH, Nostrant TT. Herpetic esophagitis; a diagnostic challenge in immunocompromised patients. Am J Gastroenterol. 1986;8:246.
95. Foley FD, Greenwald KA, Nash G, et al. Herpesvirus infection in burned patients. N Engl J Med. 1970;282:652.
96. Pugh RCB, Dudgeon JA, Bodian M. Kaposi's varicelliform eruption (eczema herpeticum) with typical and atypical visceral necrosis. J Pathol Bacteriol. 1955;69:67.
97. Hazen PG, Bennett-Eppes R. Eczema herpeticum caused by herpesvirus type 2. A case in a patient with Darier disease. Arch Dermatol. 1977;113:1085.
98. Orenstein JM, Castadot MJ, Wilens SL. Fatal herpes hepatitis associated with pemphigus vulgaris and steroids in an adult. Hum Pathol. 1974;5:489.
99. Shelley WB. Herpes simplex virus as a cause of erythema multiforme. JAMA. 1967;201:153.
100. Bean SF, Quezada RK. Recurrent oral erythema multiforme: Clinical experience with 11 patients. JAMA. 1983;249:2810.
101. Britz M, Sibulkin D. Recurrent erythema multiforme and herpes genitalis (type 2). JAMA. 1975;233:812.
102. Orton PW, Huff JC, Tonnesen MG, et al. Detection of a herpes viral antigen in skin lesions of erythema multiforme. Ann Intern Med. 1984;101:48.
103. Rawls WE, Garfield CH, Seth P, et al. Serological and epidemiological considerations of the role of herpes simplex virus type 2 in cervical cancer. Cancer Res. 1976;36:829.
104. Nahmias AJ, Josey WE, Oleske JM. Epidemiology of cervical cancer. In: Evans A, ed. Viral Infections of Humans: Epidemiology and Control. New York: Plenum; 1975:501.
105. Aurelian L, Kessler II, Rosenshein NB, et al. Viruses and gynecologic cancers: Herpesvirus protein (ICP 10/AG-4), a cervical tumor antigen that fulfills the criteria for a marker of carcinogenicity. Cancer. 1981;48:455.
106. Galloway DA, McDougall JK. The oncogenic potential of herpes simplex viruses: Evidence for a "hit and run" mechanism. Nature. 1983;302:21.
107. Finelli PF. Herpes simplex virus and the human nervous system: Current concepts and review. Milit Med. 1975;140:765.
108. Ellison GW. Multiple sclerosis: A fever blister of the brain. Lancet. 1974;2:664.
109. Krohel GB, Richardson JR, Farelli DF. Herpes simplex neuropathy. Neurology (NY). 1976;26:596.
110. Adour KK, Hilsinger RL Jr, Byl FM. Herpes simplex polyganglionitis. Otolaryngol Head Neck Surg. 1980;88:270.
111. Vahlne A, Edström S, Arstila P, et al. Bell's palsy and herpes simplex virus. Arch Otolaryngol. 1981;107:79.
112. Hanna L, Keshishyan H, Jawetz E, et al. Diagnosis of herpesvirus hominis infections in a general hospital laboratory. J Clin Microbiol. 1975;1:318.
113. Corey L. Laboratory diagnosis of herpes simplex virus infections. Principles guiding the development of rapid diagnostic tests. Diag Microbiol Infect Dis. 1986;4:1115.
114. Goldstein LC, Corey L, McDougall JK, et al. Monoclonal antibodies to herpes simplex viruses: Use in antigenic typing and rapid diagnosis. J Infect Dis. 1983;147:829.
115. Goldin AL, Sandri-Goldin RM, Levine M, et al. Cloning of herpes simplex virus type 1 sequences representing the whole genome. J Virol. 1981;38:50.
116. Barr RJ, Herten J, Graham JH. Rapid method for Tzanck preparation. JAMA. 1977;237:119.
117. Nahmias AJ, Dowdle WR, Josey WE, et al. Newborn infection with herpesvirus hominis types 1 and 2. J Pediatr. 1970;17:185.
118. Kahlon J, Chatterjee S, Lakeman FD, et al. Detection of antibodies to herpes simplex virus in the cerebrospinal fluid of patients with herpes simplex encephalitis. J Infect Dis. 1987;155:38.
119. Kirchner H, Schwenteck M, Northoff H, et al. Defective in vitro lymphoproliferative responses to herpes simplex virus in patients with frequently recurring herpes infections during disease-free intervals. Clin Immunol Immunopathol. 1978;11:267.
120. Arvin AM, Pollard RB, Rasmussen LE, et al. Cellular and humoral immunity in the pathogenesis of recurrent herpes viral infections in patients with lymphoma. J Clin Invest. 1980;65:869.
121. Sheriden JF, Donnenberg AD, Aurelian L, et al. Immunity to herpes simplex virus type 2. IV. Imparied lymphokine production during recrudescence correlates with an imbalance in T lymphocyte subsets. J Immunol. 1982;129:326.
122. Pavan-Langston D. Herpetic diseases. In: Smolin G, Thoft R, eds. The Cornea—Scientific Foundations and Clinical Practice. Boston: Little, Brown; 1983:178.
123. Whitley RJ, Nahmias AJ, Soong SJ, et al. Vidarabine therapy of neonatal herpes simplex virus infection. Pediatrics. 1980;66:495.
124. Pavan-Langston D, Buchanan RA. Vidarabine therapy of simple and IUD-complicated herpetic keratitis. Trans Am Acad Ophthalmol Otolaryngol. 1976;81:813.
125. Goodman EL, Luby JP, Johnson MT. Prospective double-blind evaluation of topical adenine arabinoside in male herpes progenitalis. Antimicrob Agents Chemother. 1975;8:693.
126. Adams HG, Benson EA, Alexander ER. Genital herpetic infection in men and women: Clinical course and effect of topical application of adenine arabinoside. J Infect Dis. 1976;133(Suppl):151.
127. Corey L, Nahmias AJ, Guinan ME, et al. A trial of topical acyclovir in genital herpes simplex virus infections. N Engl J Med. 1982;306:1313.
128. Reichman RC, Badger GJ, Guinan ME, et al. Topically administered acyclovir in the treatment of recurrent herpes simplex genitalis: A controlled trial. J Infect Dis. 1983;147:336.
129. Mindel A, Adler MW, Sutherland S, et al. Intravenous acyclovir treatment for primary genital herpes. Lancet. 1982;1:697.
130. Nilsen AE, Aasen T, Halsos AM, et al. Efficacy of oral acyclovir in treatment of initial and recurrent genital herpes. Lancet. 1982;2:571.
131. Bryson YJ, Dillon M, Lovett M, et al. Treatment of first episodes of genital herpes simplex virus infection with oral acyclovir. A randomized double-blind controlled trial in normal subjects. N Engl J Med. 1983;308:916.
132. Reichman RC, Badger GJ, Mertz GJ, et al. Treatment of recurrent genital herpes simplex infections with oral acyclovir: A controlled trial. JAMA. 1984;251:2103.
133. Straus SE, Takiff HE, Seidlin M, et al. Suppression of frequently recurring genital herpes: A placebo-controlled trial of oral acyclovir. N Engl Med. 1983;310:1545.
134. Douglas JM, Critchlow C, Benedetti J, et al. Prevention of recurrent genital herpes simplex infection with daily oral acyclovir: A double-blind trial. N Engl J Med. 1984;310:1551.
135. Straus SE, Seidlin M, Takiff HE, et al. Double-blind comparison of weekly and daily regimens of oral acyclovir for suppression of recurrent genital herpes. Antiviral Res. 1986;6:151.
136. Gold D, Corey L. Acyclovir prophylaxis for herpes simplex virus infection. Antimicrob Agents Chemother. 1987;31:361.
137. Saral R, Burns WH, Laskin OL, et al. Acyclovir prophylaxis of herpes-simplex-virus infections: A randomized, double-blind controlled trial in bone-marrow-transplant recipients. N Engl J Med. 1981;305:63.
138. Wade JC, Newton B, McLaren C, et al. Intravenous acyclovir to treat mucocutaneous herpes simplex virus infection after marrow transplantation. Ann Intern Med. 1982;96:265.
139. Meyers JD, Wade JC, Mitchell CD, et al. Multicenter collaborative trial of intravenous acyclovir for treatment of mucocutaneous herpes simplex virus infection in the immunocompromised host. Am J Med. 1982;73(1A):229.
140. Whitley RJ, Levin M, Barton N, et al. Infections caused by herpes simplex virus in the immunocompromised host: Natural history and topical acyclovir therapy. J Infect Dis. 1984;150:323.
141. Shepp DH, Newton BA, Dandliker PS, et al. Oral acyclovir therapy for mucocutaneous herpes simplex virus infections in immunocompromised marrow transplant recipients. Ann Intern Med. 1985;102:783.
142. Conant MA. Prophylactic and suppressive treatment with acyclovir and the management of herpes in patients with acquired immunodeficiency syndrome. J Am Acad Dermatol. 1988;18:186.
143. Whitley RJ, Alford CA, Hirsch MS, et al. Vidarabine versus acyclovir therapy in herpes simplex encephalitis. N Engl J Med. 1986;314:144.
144. Crumpacker C. Resistance of herpes viruses to nucleoside analogues—mechanisms and clinical importance. In: Mills J, Corey L, ed. Antiviral Chemotherapy—New Directions for Clinical Application and Research. New York: Elsevier Science Publishing; 1986:226.
145. Erlich KS, Mills J, Chatis P, et al. Acyclovir resistant herpes simplex virus infections in patients with the acquired immunodeficiency syndrome. N Engl J Med. 1989;320:293.
146. Mirsch MS, Schooley RT. Resistance to antiviral drugs: The end of innocence. N Engl J Med. 1989;320:313.
147. Chatis PA, Miller CH, Schrager LE, et al. Successful treatment with foscarnet of an acyclovir-resistant mucotaneous infection with herpes simplex virus in a patient with acquired immunodeficiency syndrome. N Engl J Med. 1989;320:297.
148. Rooney JF, Wohlenberg C, Cremer KJ, et al. Immunization with a vaccinia virus recombinant expressing herpes simplex virus type I glycoprotein D: Long-term protection and effect of revaccination. J Virol. 1988;62:1530.

119. VARICELLA-ZOSTER VIRUS

RICHARD J. WHITLEY

Varicella-zoster virus (VZV) causes two distinct clinical diseases. Varicella, or more commonly chickenpox, is the primary infection and results from exposure of a susceptible individual to the virus. Chickenpox is ubiquitous and extremely contagious, but for the most part, it is a benign illness characterized by a generalized exanthematous rash. It occurs seasonally and in epidemics. Recurrence of infection results in the more localized phenomenon known as herpes zoster, often referred to as shingles, a common infection among the elderly. As of this date, there is no licensed vaccine for the prevention of chickenpox in the United States, although a promising candidate is under review of the Bureau of Biologics. Infection caused by VZV remains of medical significance. It is estimated that between 300,000 and 500,000 individuals seek medical care for chickenpox, with nearly half of these patients requiring a second office appointment. Similarly, it is estimated that herpes zoster accounts for over 1.5 million physician visits per year and that most of these individuals require follow-up medical care.

HISTORY

Shingles has been recognized since ancient times as a unique clinical entity because of the dermatomal vesicular rash; however, chickenpox was often confused with smallpox.[1] In 1875, Steiner successfully transmitted VZV by inoculation of the vesicular fluid from an individual suffering from chickenpox to "volunteers."[2] The infectious nature of VZV was further defined by von Bokay, who observed chickenpox in individuals who had close contact with others suffering from herpes zoster.[3,4] He correctly described the mean incubation period for the development of chickenpox in susceptible patients as well as the average range in days. Kundratitz in 1925 showed that the inoculation of vesicular fluid from patients with herpes zoster into susceptible individuals resulted in chickenpox.[5] Similar observations were reported by Bruusgaard[6] and others,[7] and in 1943 Garland suggested that herpes zoster was the consequence of the reactivation of latent VZV.[8]

Since early in the twentieth century, similarities in the histopathologic findings of skin lesions and in epidemiologic and immunologic studies indicated that varicella and herpes zoster were caused by the same agent.[9,10] Tyzzer described the histopathology of skin lesions resulting from VZV infections and noted the development of intranuclear inclusions and multinucleated giant cells.[11] These descriptions came from histologic studies performed on serial skin biopsy specimens that were obtained over the first week of illness. The histopathologic descriptions were amplified by Lipschutz in 1921 for herpes zoster.[12]

Isolation of VZV in 1958 permitted a definition of the biology of this virus.[10] Viral isolates from patients with chickenpox and herpes zoster demonstrated similar alterations in tissue culture, specifically the appearance of eosinophilic intranuclear inclusions and multinucleated giant cells. These findings are virtually identical to those encountered with clinically available biopsy material. Taken together these data provided a universal acceptance that both diseases were caused by VZV. By 1958, Weller and colleagues had been able to establish that there were no differences between the viral agents isolated from patients with these two clinical entities from either a biologic or immunologic standpoint.[10,13–15]

Later studies proved their identity by rigorous biochemical methods.[16] More recently, viral DNA from a patient with chickenpox who subsequently developed herpes zoster was examined by restriction endonuclease analyses, and the molecular identity of these two viruses was verified.[17,18]

PATHOGEN AND REPLICATION

Varicella-zoster virus is a member of the Herpesviridae and shares structural characteristics with other members of the family. The virus has icosahedral symmetry containing centrally located double-stranded DNA with a surrounding envelope. The total size of the virus is approximately 150–200 nm and has a lipid-containing envelope with glycoprotein spikes.[17] The naked capsid has a diameter of approximately 90–95 nm.[19–21] The DNA contains 125,000 base pairs or approximately 80 megadaltons and encodes approximately 75 proteins. The organization of the viral genome is similar to other herpesviruses. There are unique long (U_l)—105 kilobases—and unique short (U_s)—5.2 kilobases—regions of the viral genome. Each unique sequence contains terminal repeat sequences. With replication, the U_s region can invert upon itself and result in two isomeric forms, as recently reviewed.[22]

Five families of VZV glycoproteins (gp) have been identified, gp I, gp II, gp III, gp IV, and gp V. Viral infectivity can be neutralized by monoclonal antibodies directed against gp I, gp II, and gp III. These glycoproteins have been the subject of intense investigative interest because they represent the primary marker for both humoral and cell-mediated immunity.

Only enveloped virions are infectious; this may account for the lability of VZV. Furthermore, the envelope is sensitive to detergent, ether, and air drying.

Varicella-zoster virus is highly cell associated and spreads from cell to cell by direct contact. Virus can be isolated in a variety of continuous and discontinuous cell culture systems of human and simian origin. Approximately 8–10 hours after infection, virus-specific immunofluorescence can be detected in the cells immediately adjacent to the initial focus of infection. This parallels the microscopic observation of the radial spread of cytopathology.[23,24] Electron microscopic studies demonstrate the appearance of immature viral particles within 12 hours of the onset of infection. As with herpes simplex, the naked capsids acquire their envelope at the nuclear membrane, being released into the perinuclear space where large vacoules are formed.[19,25] Infectious virus is then spread to adjacent cells after fusion of plasma membranes.

EPIDEMIOLOGY OF VARICELLA-ZOSTER VIRUS INFECTIONS

Chickenpox

Humans are the only known reservoir for VZV. Chickenpox follows exposure of the susceptible or seronegative individual to VZV and represents the primary form of infection. Although it is assumed that the virus is spread by the respiratory route and replicates in the nasopharynx or upper respiratory tract, retrieval of virus from individuals incubating VZV has been uncommon. Chickenpox is a common infection of childhood and involves both sexes equally and individuals of all races. To a certain extent the virus is endemic in the population at large; however, it becomes epidemic among susceptible individuals during seasonal periods, namely, late winter and early spring. It is estimated that 3 million cases occur each year.[26] Intimate contact appears to be the key determinant for transmission. Overall, chickenpox is a disease of childhood because 90 percent of cases occur in children less than 3 years of age. Typically, the virus is introduced into the susceptible school-age or preschool child. In a study by Wells and Holla, 61 of 67 susceptible children in kindergarten through the fourth grade contracted chickenpox.[27] Approximately 10 percent of individuals over the age of 15 years are considered susceptible to VZV infection. The incubation period of chickenpox, namely, the time interval between exposure of a susceptible person to an infected individual, the index case, and the development of a vesicular rash in generally regarded as 14–15 days, but disease can appear within a range of 10–20 days.[28,29] Secondary attack rates in susceptible siblings within a household are defined as between 70 and 90 percent.[30] Patients are infectious for a period of approximately 48 hours before the period of vesicle formation and generally 4–5 days therefore until all vesicles are crusted.

While chickenpox exists worldwide in children, it should be noted that it occurs more frequently in adults resident in tropical regions than in other geographic areas. Stokes noted a higher incidence of chickenpox among soldiers during World War II where the incidence was 1.41 and 2.27 per 1,000 individuals annually. These data contrast with the United States where the rates were approximately one-half.[31]

Herpes Zoster

The epidemiology of herpes zoster is somewhat different. Varicella-zoster virus characteristically becomes latent after primary infection. It is presumed that VZV establishes latency within the dorsal root ganglia. Reactivation leads to herpes zoster, a sporadic disease. Histopathologic examination of the nerve route after infection with VZV demonstrates characteristics indicative of VZV infection. In those individuals who die after recent herpes zoster infection, an examination of the dorsal root ganglia reveals satellitosis, lymphocytic infiltration in the nerve route, and degeneration of the ganglia cells.[32,33] Intranuclear inclusions can be found within the ganglia cells. Although it is possible to demonstrate the presence of VZV by electronmicroscopy, it is not possible to isolate this virus in cultures, usually from explant dorsal root ganglia, as has been done after herpes simplex virus infection. The biologic mechanism by which VZV establishes latency remains a mystery at this time.

Herpes zoster is a disease that occurs at all ages, but it will afflict about 10 percent or more of the population overall, mainly among the elderly.[34,35] Herpes zoster, known also as shingles, occurs in individuals who are seropositive for VZV or, more specifically, in individuals who have had prior chickenpox. Reactivation appears dependent upon a balance between virus and host factors. Most patients who develop herpes zoster have no history exposure to other individuals with VZV infection at the time of the appearance of lesions. The highest incidence of disease varies between 5 and 10 cases per 1000 for individuals over the sixth decade of life.[13] It has been recognized that approximately 4 percent of patients will suffer a second episode of herpes zoster. Notably, a rare patient will even experience a third episode. In a 7-year study performed by McGregor the annualized rate of herpes zoster was 4.8 per 1000 patients, with three-fourths of those patient being over the age of 45 years.[36] Individuals who are immunocompromised have a higher incidence of both chickenpox and shingles.[37–40]

Herpes zoster has occurred within the first 2 years of life in children born to women who have had chickenpox during pregnancy. These particular cases likely reflect in utero chickenpox with reactivation early in life.

PATHOGENESIS

The pathogenesis of VZV infection that results in chickenpox reflects the natural history of the disease. It occurs in susceptible individuals who are exposed to virus after intimate contact. The appearance of a diffuse vesicular rash has been well studied from a pathologic standpoint. Histopathologic findings in human VZV infection, whether chickenpox or herpes zoster, are virtually identical. The vesicles involve the corium and dermis. As viral replication progresses, the epithelial cells undergo degenerative changes characterized by ballooning, with the subsequent appearance of multinucleated giant cells and prominent eosinophilic intranuclear inclusions, as noted previously from early reports of the disease. Under unusual circumstances, necrosis and hemorrhage may appear in the upper portion of the dermis. As the vesicle evolves, the collected fluid becomes cloudy as a consequence of the appearance of polymorphonuclear leukocytes, degenerated cells, and fibrin. Ultimately, the vesicles either rupture and release the infectious fluid or gradually become reabsorbed.

Transmission is likely by the respiratory route, followed by localized replication at an undefined site, which leads to seeding of the reticuloendothelial system and, ultimately, viremia. The occurrence of viremia in patients with chickenpox is supported by the diffuse and scattered nature of the skin lesions and can be verified in selected cases by the recovery of virus from the blood.[41] As noted, the mechanism of the reactivation of VZV that results in herpes zoster is unknown.

CLINICAL MANIFESTATIONS

Chickenpox

The medical importance of chickenpox should be stressed. There are approximately 100 deaths per year in the United States from this infection. For the normal child, mortality is less than 2 per 100,000 cases. This risk increases by over 15-fold for adults. Chickenpox presents with a rash, low-grade fever, and malaise. A prodrom of symptoms may occur 1–2 days before the onset of the exanthem in a few patients. For the most part, chickenpox in the immunocompetent child is a benign illness associated with lassitude and a temperature of 100–103°F of only 3–5 days' duration. Constitutional symptoms that develop after the onset of rash include malaise, pruritus, anorexia, and listlessness. These symptoms gradually resolve as the illness abates. The skin manifestations, the hallmark of infection, consist of maculopapules, vesicles, and scabs in varying stages of evolution. The lesions initially contain clear vesicular fluid, but over a very short period of time they pustulate and scab. Most lesions are small, having an erythematous base with a diameter of 5 mm to as large as 12–13 mm. The lesions can be round or oval, with central umbilication occurring as healing progresses. The lesions themselves have often been referred to as "dew drop-like" during the early stages of formation. If they do not rupture within a few hours, the contents will rapidly become purulent in appearance. The lesions appear on the trunk and face and rapidly spread centripally to involve other areas of the body. Successive crops of lesions generally appear over a period of 2–4 days. Thus early in the disease, the hallmark of the infection is the appearance of lesions at all stages, as noted previously. The lesions can also be found on the mucosa of the oropharynx and even the vagina; however, these sites are less common overall. It is customary for the crust to completely fall off within 1–2 weeks after the onset of infection and leave a slightly depressed area of skin.

Immunocompromised children, particularly those with leukemia, have more numerous lesions, often with a hemorrhagic base. Healing takes nearly three times longer in this population.[37] These children are at greater risk for visceral complications, which occur in 30–50 percent of cases and can be fatal in as many as 15 percent of cases. A notable complication of cutaneous lesions is secondary bacterial infection—often in association with gram-positive organisms. Infection in the neutropenic host can be systemic.

Noncutaneous sites of involvement after chickenpox most frequently involve the central nervous system and are manifested as acute cerebellar ataxia or encephalitis.[26,42,43] Cerebellar ataxia has been estimated to occur in 1 in 4,000 cases for children less than 15 years of age. Cerebellar ataxia can appear as late as 21 days after the onset of rash. It is more common, however, for acute cerebellar ataxia to present within a week of the onset of the exanthem. An extensive review of Underwood of 120 cases demonstrated that ataxia, vomiting, altered speech, fever, vertigo, and tremor were all common on physical examination.[44] Cerebrospinal fluid from these patients often demonstrates lymphocytosis and elevated levels of cerebrospinal fluid protein. This is usually a benign complication in children, and resolution occurs within 2–4 weeks.

A more serious central nervous system complication is encephalitis, which can be life-threatening in adults. Encephalitis is reported to occur in 0.1–0.2 percent of individuals suffering from the disease.[45] Underwood's review reveals this illness to be characterized by depression in the level of consciousness with progressive headaches vomiting, altered thought patterns, fever, and frequent seizures.[44] The duration of disease in these patients is at least 2 weeks. Some patients suffer from progressive neurologic deterioration leading to death. Mortality in these patients has been estimated to vary between 5 and 20 percent, and neurologic sequelae have been detected in as many as 15 percent of survivors.

A neurologic complication of note is the late appearance of cerebral angiitis after zoster ophthalmicus. This problem has been noted in several patients and defined to be progressive, with mortality being exceedingly high. Other nervous system manifestations of chickenpox include meningitis, transverse myelitis, and Reye syndrome.

A serious and life-threatening complication is the appearance of varicella pneumonitis, a complication that occurs more commonly in adults and in the immunocompromised host.[26,42,46] In adults, it is estimated to occur in 1 in 400 cases of infection and, not infrequently, in the absence of clinical symptoms. It generally appears 3–5 days into the course of illness and is associated with tachypnea, cough, dyspnea, and fever. Chest radiographs usually reveal nodular or interstitial pneumonitis.

In a prospective study of male military personnel, radiographic abnormalities were detected in nearly 16 percent of enlisted men who developed varicella, yet only one-quarter of these individuals had evidence of cough.[47] Only 10 percent of those with radiographic abnormalities developed evidence of tachypnea, thus indicating that asymptomatic pneumonitis may exist more commonly than was initially predicted. Other non-cutaneous and non-neurologic sites of involvement include the appearance of myocarditis, nephritis, bleeding diatheses, and hepatitis.

Perinatal varicella is associated with a high death rate when maternal disease develops 5 days before delivery or 48 hours postpartum.[48,49] In large part, this is the consequence of the newborn not receiving protective transplacental antibodies and the immaturity of the immune system. It has been reported that under such circumstances the mortality is as high as 30 percent. These children have been reported to have progressive disease involving visceral organs, especially the lung. The outcome in these children has been summarized by Brunell.[50] Congenital varicella with clinical manifestations at birth is uncommon, but it has been characterized by skin scarring, hypoplastic extremities, eye abnormalities, and evidence of central nervous system impairment.[51]

It should be noted that varicella has been associated epidemiologically with the development of Reye syndrome.[52] The syndrome begins in the later stages of varicella with vomiting, followed by restlessness, irritability, and a progressive decrease in the level of consciousness, all associated with progressive cerebral edema. The encephalopathy is associated with elevated levels of ammonia, a bleeding diathesis, hyperglycemia, and elevated transaminase levels.[53] The recent association between the administration of aspirin as an antipyretic and the development of Reye syndrome would indicate a statistical association between these two entities. Therefore, aspirin is contraindicated for individuals with varicella infection.

Chickenpox in the Immunocompromised Patient. Chickenpox in the immunocompromised child or adult poses significant hazards of morbidity and mortality. As noted previously, the duration of healing of cutaneous lesions can be extended by a minimum of threefold. However, a more important problem is the progressive involvement of visceral organs. Data from a variety of immunocompromised patient populations indicate a broad spectrum of disease in individuals with lymphoproliferative malignancies and solid tumors vs. bone marrow transplant recipients. In studies at St. Jude's by Feldman and colleagues, approximately one-third of children developed progressive disease with involvement of multiple organs, including the lungs, liver, and central nervous system.[54] Most of these children, 20 percent of all of those who acquire chickenpox, developed pneumonitis within the first week after the onset of infection. Mortality in this patient population has been thought to approximate 15–18 percent.[54–56] Those individuals with lymphoproliferative malignancies who require continuous chemotherapy appear to be at the greatest risk for visceral involvement.

In individuals undergoing bone marrow transplantation, the incidence of VZV infections over the first year has been estimated to be 30 percent by 1 year post-transplant. Eighty percent of these infections occurred within the first 9 months after transplantation, and 45 percent of these patients had cutaneous or visceral dissemination. Overall, 23 deaths occurred in one prospective series.[57] Risk factors identified for the acquisition of VZV infection included an age between 10 and 29 years, a diagnosis other than chronic myelogenous leukemia, the post-transplant use of anti-thymocyte globulin, allogenic transplant, and acute or chronic graft-vs.-host disease. Notably, graft-vs.-host disease increases the probability of visceral dissemination significantly.

Herpes Zoster

Herpes zoster, or shingles, is characterized by a unilateral vesicular eruption with a dermatomal distribution. Thoracic and lumbar dermatomes are most commonly involved; however, the ophthalmic branch of the trigeminal nerve can lead to zoster ophthalmicus, a sight-threatening complication. Generally, the onset of disease is heralded by pain within the dermatome that precedes the lesions by 48–72 hours. Early in the disease course erythematous, macropapular lesions will appear that rapidly evolve into a vesicular rash. Vesicles may coalesce to form bullous lesions. In the normal host, these lesions continue to form over a period of 3–5 days, with the total duration of disease being 10–15 days. However, it may take as long as 1 month before the skin returns to normal.

Unusual cutaneous manifestations of herpes zoster, in addition to zoster ophthalmicus, include the involvement of the maxillary or mandibular branch of the trigeminal nerve, which results in intraoral involvement with lesions of the pallet, tonsillar fossa, floor of the mouth, and tongue. When the geniculate ganglion is involved, the Ramsay Hunt syndrome may occur, with pain and vesicles in the external auditory meatus, loss of taste in the anterior two-thirds of the tongue, and ipsilateral facial palsy.

No known factors are responsible for the precipitation of the events of herpes zoster. If herpes zoster occurs in the child, the course is generally benign and not associated with progressive pain or discomfort. In the adult, systemic manifestations include those mainly associated with pain, as noted below.

The most significant clinical manifestations of herpes zoster is the associated acute neuritis and, later, post-herpetic neuralgia. Post-herpetic neuralgia, while uncommon in young individuals, may occur in as many as 25–50 percent of patients over the age of 50 years.[58–60] It is estimated that as many as 50 percent of individuals over 50 years of age will have pain considered debilitating that persists for over 1 month.

Extracutaneous sites of involvement include the central nervous system with the appearance of meningoencephalitis or encephalitis. The clinical manifestations are similar to that of other viral infections of the central nervous system. However, a rare manifestation of central nervous system involvement by herpes zoster is gramulomatous angiitis, usually involving the internal carotid artery. It should be noted that involvement of the central nervous system with cutaneous herpes zoster probably is more common than is recognized clinically. Invariably, patients who undergo cerebrospinal fluid examination for other reasons during episodes of shingles are found to have evidence of pleocytosis without elevated cerebrospinal fluid protein levels. These patients are without signs of meningeal irritation and infrequently complain of headaches.

Classically, VZV infection involves dorsal root ganglia. Motor paralysis can occur as a consequence of the involvement of the anterior horn cells in a manner similar to that encountered with polio. Patients with involvement of the anterior horn cells are particularly prone to excruciating pain. Other neuromuscular disorders associated with herpes zoster include transverse myelitis[61] and myositis.[62,63]

Herpes zoster in the immunocompromised host is more severe than in the normal individual. Lesion formation continues for up to 2 weeks, and scabbing may not take place until 3–4 weeks into the disease course.[40] Patients with lymphoproliferative malignancies are at risk for cutaneous dissemination and visceral involvement, including varicella pneumonitis, hepatitis, and meningoencephalitis. However, even in the immunocompromised patient disseminated herpes zoster is rarely fatal.

It should be noted that a new clinical manifestation of herpes zoster has become apparent in recent years. Chronic herpes zoster may also occur in the immunocompromised host, particularly those individuals with a diagnosis of human immunodeficiency virus infection. Individuals have sustained new lesion formation with an absence of healing of the existing lesions. These syndromes can be particularly debilitating and, interestingly, have been associated with the isolation of a VSV isolate resistant to acyclovir.

DIAGNOSIS

The diagnosis of both chickenpox and shingles is usually made by history and physical examination. In the latter part of the twentieth century, the differential diagnosis of varicella and herpes zoster is less confusing than it was 20–30 years ago. Smallpox or disseminated vaccinia were confused with varicella because of the similar appearance of the cutaneous lesions. Now with the worldwide eradication of smallpox and the discontinuation of vaccination, these disease entities no longer confuse the clinical diagnosis. For the most part, the characteristic skin rash with evidence of lesions in all stages of development provide the clinical diagnosis of infection. The presence of pruritus, pain, and low-grade fever are sufficient to establish a diagnosis of chickenpox. The localization of a vesicular rash makes the diagnosis of herpes zoster highly likely; however, other viral infections can masquerade as this disease.

Impetigo and varicella can be confused clinically. While impetigo is usually caused by the group A β-hemolytic streptococcus, it will follow an abrasion of the skin or inoculation of bacteria at the site of the skin break and lead to small vesicles in the surrounding area. There may or may not be systemic signs of disease unless the skin affliction is associated with progressive cellulitis or secondary bacteremia. Unroofing of these lesions and careful Gram staining of the scraping of the base of the lesion should reveal evidence of gram-positive cocci in chains, which is suggestive of the streptococcus, or gram-positive cocci in clusters, which is suggestive of staphylococcus, a less common cause of vesicular skin lesions. Obviously, the treatment modality for these diseases are distinctly different from that used in the management of chickenpox and would require the administration of an appropriate antibiotic.

In a smaller number of cases, disseminated vascular lesions can be caused by herpes simplex virus. In these children, disseminated herpes simplex virus infection usually is a consequence of an underlying skin disease such as atopic dermatitis or eczema. In this situation an unequivocal diagnosis can only be confirmed by isolation of the offending pathogen in an appropriate tissue culture system.

More recently, it has been recognized that disseminated enteroviral infections, particularly those caused by group A coxsackievirus, can provide widespread distal vesicular lesions. These rashes are more commonly morbilliform in nature with a hemorrhagic component rather than a vesicular or vesiculopustular appearance. Generally these diseases occur during late summer and early fall and are associated with lesions of the oropharynx, palms, and soles. This latter finding is most helpful in distinguishing enteroviral disease.

Unilateral vesicular lesions in the dermatomal pattern should immediately lead the clinician to suspect a diagnosis of shingles. It has been reported that herpes simplex virus infections and coxsackievirus infections can masquerade as dermatoma vesicular lesions. In such situations, diagnostic viral cultures remain the best method for determining the etiology of infection. Confirmation of the diagnosis is possible through the isolation of VZV in susceptible tissue culture cell lines or by the demonstration of either seroconversion or seroboosting when using standard antibody assays and employing both acute and convalescent specimens. A Tzanck smear, performed by scraping the base of the lesion, may demonstrate multinucleated giant cells. Direct immunofluorescence staining of cells from the skin base or the detection of viral antigens by other assays can be used, although most of these procedures are only performed by research groups at the present time. Useful antibody assays include immune adherence hemagglutination, fluorescence antibody to membrane antigen (FAMA) or enzyme-linked immunoabsorbent assays (ELISA).[64]

THERAPY

The medical management of chickenpox and shingles in the normal host is directed toward avoiding known complications. For chickenpox, hygiene is important including bathing, astringent soaks, and closely cropped fingernails to avoid a source for secondary bacterial infection associated with the pruritic skin lesions. Pruritus can be decreased with topical dressing or the administration of antipruritic drugs. Aluminum acetate or Burrow solution soaks for the management of herpes zoster can be both soothing and cleansing. Acetaminophen should be used to reduce fever in the child suffering from chickenpox because of the association between aspirin and the appearance of Reye syndrome.

At the present time, the treatment of chickenpox and herpes zoster in the normal host does not entail the administration of either antiviral drugs or corticosteroids. The latter has been suggested to be useful for decreasing both acute neuritis and the frequency of post-herpetic neuralgia; however, these data are controversial. In the immunocompromised host or with the appearance of visceral complications in the normal host such as varicella pneumonitis, the deployment of either acyclovir or vidarabine may be of value.[65–68] Although commonly believed to be superior, acyclovir is not licensed for use in VZV infections. Vidarabine has been extensively studied for the treatment of both chickenpox and herpes zoster in the immunocompromised host. In studies of vidarabine for chickenpox therapy in immunosuppressed children at a dosage of 10 mg/kg/day of body weight given intravenously over a period of 12 hours the duration of lesion formation was decreased from 5.6 to 3.8 days, and the frequency of visceral complications decreased from 8 of 13 to 1 of 8. Furthermore, there were two study deaths in the placebo recipients. Both the duration of lesion formation and the decreased frequency of visceral dissemination were statistically superior in the treated group as compared with the counterpart placebo recipients. In two studies of vidarabine therapy for localized and disseminated zoster in the immunocompromised host, it was possible to demonstrate slowing of new lesion formation and clearance of virus from lesions as well as a decreased time to total healing. Visceral complications were decreased from 58 to 14 in placebo recipients and from 63 to 5 in treated patients, with a parallel decrease in visceral complications from 11 to 3 patients in each of the respective groups. These outcome events were statistically significantly accelerated for treated as compared with placebo recipients. Furthermore, there was a suggestion from these studies that improvement of both acute pain and resolution of chronic pain were enhanced in the treated as compared with the placebo recipients. The dosage is 10 mg/kg/day administered once daily intravenously over a period of 12 hours at a concentration of 0.5 mg of standard intravenous fluids.

More recently, acyclovir has been evaluated in controlled studies for all herpesvirus infections. Acyclovir is a guanine derivative that was a degree of selectivity for the inhibition of VZV replication that is predicated on its selected phosphorylation and activation by virus-coded thymidine kinase and, then, its selective inhibition of the viral DNA polymerase. It is estimated that the concentration of acyclovir required to inhibit VZV replication in vitro varies between 2.1 and 6.3 μM, a concentration easily achieved after the intravenous administration of medication.[69] It should be noted, however, that such concentrations are not easily achieved after even high-dose administration of oral acyclovir. Studies of acyclovir administered at 500 mg/m^2 every 8 hours vs. placebo indicate acceleration of healing in adults with localized infection as evidenced by the decreased frequency of visceral disease. However, it was not apparent from the original controlled study that the value of acyclovir would be unequivocal for the management of zoster in targeted patient populations.

One controlled study has indicated that acyclovir appears to be superior for therapy for localized zoster in bone marrow transplant patients when compared with vidarabine.[70] The decreased frequency of complications when acyclovir is used has led to its deployment by many physicians, even though it is not licensed for therapy for VZV infections in the immunocompromised host at the present time. The recommended dosage for acyclovir is from 5 to 10 mg/kg administered every 8 hours or, as suggested by some, 500 mg/m^2 every 8 hours, especially for children.

Management of varicella pneumonitis and other complications requires excellent supportive nursing care in addition to evaluating, on an individual basis, the potential for antiviral therapy. The management of acute neuritis and/or post-herpetic neuralgia can be particularly problematic. It requires the judicious use of analgesics ranging from non-narcotic to narcotic derivatives and may include the deployment of such drugs as amitriptyline hydrochloride and fluphenazine hydrochloride.

PREVENTION

In the normal host, prophylaxis and treatment of chickenpox are of little relevance since the disease is usually benign. Transmission of infection can be prevented by isolation of the infected patient (see Chapter 277). It is important to recognize that patients who require hospitalization because of varicella are a source of nosocomial infection within the hospital environment. Because approximately 10 percent of adults are seronegative, the risks in the medical care environment can be extremely high. Those most likely to become infected are nurses and medical personnel providing care to the infected individuals. Airflow can be documented as a means of transmission of infection from one area to another in the hospital environment.

In the immunocompromised host who has not been previously exposed to chickenpox, the deployment of varicella immune globulin (VZIG) and varicella-zoster immune plasma (ZIP) have been shown to be useful for both prevention and/or amelioration of symptomatic chickenpox is high-risk individuals.[71–74] VZIG should be administered to the immunodeficient patient under 15 years of age who has a negative or unknown history of chickenpox, who has not been vaccinated against VZV, or who has had contact in the household with a playmate or in a shared hospital room for more than 1 hour. It should also be administered to the newborn whose mother had an onset of chickenpox less than 5 days before delivery or 48 hours postpartum. The use of VZIG for susceptible individuals over 15 must be evaluated on an individual basis.

A vaccine is being developed for the prevention of chickenpox in the immunocompromised and normal hosts.[75–81] Although licensed in Japan, this vaccine remains experimental in the United States and is under review by the Bureau of Biologics. Studies performed to date indicate a high probability of protection after vaccination.

The Oka strain of VZV has been developed by Takahashi and colleagues in Japan and studied as a vaccine extensively in both the normal and leukemic child. In immunocompromised children, serologic evidence of host response after vaccination has been achieved in between 89 and 100 percent of vaccinated individuals. These studies now have encompassed well over 1000 patients. Vaccine-induced rash, however, is not uncommon and occurs in varied percentages of patients from approximately 6 percent to as high as 47 percent. The factor most predictive of the appearance of rash is the degree of immunosuppression. Specifically, for children with acute lymphoblastic leukemia, the likelihood of rash can be as high as 40–50 percent. The subsequent occurrence of natural varicella after community exposure is decreased in the larger control studies and averaging 8–16 percent. The occurrence of herpes zoster after vaccination does not seem to pose a major risk at the present time.

Similar studies have been performed in normal children, with total numbers well in excess of 1000 individuals as recently reviewed.[22] In these studies the appearance of antibody responses was higher than in the immunocompromised host and varied between 94 and 100 percent. Vaccine-induced rash was far less common in these individuals and occurred at a frequency of 0.5 percent to approximately 19 percent overall, with the subsequent appearance of varicella after community exposure averaging between 1 and 5 percent. Theoretically, this vaccine might be useful for boosting immunity in older individuals as a mechanism to prevent herpes zoster infection; however, this hypothesis remains to be tested. It should be noted that the subsequent development of herpes zoster is not increased in vaccine recipients.[82]

REFERENCES

1. Gordon JE, Meader FM. The period of infectivity and serum prevention of chickenpox. JAMA. 1929;93:2013.
2. Steiner P. Zur Inokulation der Varicellen. Wein Med Wochenschr. 1875;25:306.
3. von Bokay J. Das Auftreten der Schafblattern uter besonderen Umstanden. Unger Arch Med. 1892;1:159.
4. von Bokay J. Uberden atiologischen zusammenhang der varizellen mit gewissen fallen von herpes zoster. Wein Klin Wochenschr. 1909;22:1323.
5. Kundratitz K. Experimentelle ubertragungen von herpes zoster auf menschen und die beziehungen von herpes zoster zu varicellen. Z Kinderheilkd. 1925;39:379.
6. Brunsgaard E. The mutual relation between zoster and varicella. Br J Dermatol Syph. 1932;44:1.
7. School Epidemics Committee of Great Britian. Epidemics in Schools. Medical Research Council. Special Report Series, No. 227. London: His Majesty's Stationery Office; 1938.
8. Garland J. Varicella following exposure to herpes zoster. N Engl J Med. 1943;228:336.
9. Seiler HE. A study of herpes zoster particularly in its relationship to chickenpox. J Hyg. 1949;47:253–62.
10. Weller TH, Witton HM. The etiologic agents of varicella and herpes zoster: Serologic studies with the viruses as propagated in vitro. J Exp Med. 1958;228:336–7.
11. Tyzzer EE. The histology of the skin lesions in varicella. Philippine J Sci. 1906;1:349.
12. Lipschutz B. Untersuchengen uber die Atiologies der Krankheiten der Herpesgruppe (Herpes Zoster, Herpes Genitalis, Herpes Febrilis). Arch Dermatol Syph. 1921;136:428.
13. Weller TH. Serial propagation in vitro of agents producing inclusion bodies derived from varicella and herpes zoster. Proc Soc Exp Biol Med. 1953;83:340–6.
14. Weller TH, Coons AH. Fluorescent antibody studies with agents of varicella and herpes zoster propagated in vitro. Proc Soc Exp Biol Med. 1954;86:789.
15. Weller TH, Stoddard MB. Intranuclear inclusion bodies in cultures of human tissue inoculated with varicella vesicle fluid. J Immunol. 1952;68:311.
16. Davison AJ, Scott JE. The complete DNA sequence of varicella-zoster virus. J Gen Virol. 1986;67:1759–816.
17. Sawyer MH, Ostrove JM, Felser JM, et al. Mapping of the varicella zoster virus deoxypyrimidine kinase gene and preliminary identification of its transcript. Virology. 1986;149:1–9.

18. Dumas AM, Geelen JL, Mares W, et al. Infectivity and molecular weight of varicella-zoster virus DNA. J Gen Virol. 1980;47:233–5.
19. Achong BC, Meurisse EV. Observations on the fine structure and replication of varicella virus in cultivated human amnion cells. J Gen Virol. 1968;3:305.
20. Almeida JD, Howatson AF, Williams MG. Morphology of varicella (chickenpox) virus. Virology. 1962;16:353.
21. Tournier P, Cathala F, Bernhard W. Ultrastructure et developpement intracellulaire du virus de la varicelle. Observe ou microscope electronique Presse Med. 1957;65:1229.
22. Straus SE, Ostrove JM, Inchauspe G. Varicella-zoster virus infections: Biology, natural history, treatment and prevention. Ann Intern Med. 1988;108:221–37.
23. Rapp F, Vanderslice D. Spread of zoster virus in human embryonic lung cells and the inhibitory effect of idoxyuridine. Virology. 1964;22:321.
24. Vaczi L, Geder L, Koller M, et al. Influence of temperature on the multiplication of varicella virus. Acta Microbiol Acad Sci Hung. 1963;10:109.
25. Grose C, Perrotta DM, Brunell PA, et al. Cell-free varicella-zoster virus in cultured human melanoma cells. J Gen Virol. 1979;43:15.
26. Preblud SR. Varicella: Complications and costs. Pediatrics. 1986;78:728–35.
27. Wells MW, Holla WA. Ventilation in the flow of measles and chickenpox through a community. JAMA. 1950;142:1337.
28. Preblud SR, Orenstein WA, Bart KJ. Varicella: Clinical manifestations, epidemiology, and health impact in children. Pediatr Infect Dis. 1984;3:505–9.
29. Hope-Simpson RE. Infectiousness of communicable diseases in the household (measles, chickenpox, and mumps). Lancet. 1952;2:549.
30. Ross AH. Modification of chicken pox in family contacts by administration of gamma globulin. N Engl J Med. 1962;267:369–76.
31. Strokes J Jr. Chickenpox. Communicable diseases transmitted chiefly through respiratory and alimentary tracts. In: Preventive Medicine in World War II. v. 4. Washington, DC: Department of the Army;1958:55.
32. Bastain FO, Rabson AS, Yee CL, et al. Herpesvirus varicellae: Isolated from human dorsal root ganglia. Arch Pathol. 1974;97:331.
33. Esiri MM, Tomlinson AH. Herpes zoster; Demonstration of virus in trigeminal nerve and ganglion by immunofluorescence and electron microscopy. J Neurol Sci. 1972;15:35.
34. Ragozzino MW, Melton LJ III, Kurland LT, et al. Population-based study of herpes zoster and its sequelae. Medicine (Baltimore). 1982;51:310–6.
35. Hope-Simpson RE. The nature of herpes zoster: A long-term study and a new hypothesis. Proc R Soc Med. 1965;58:9.
36. McGregor RM. Herpes zoster, chickenpox, and cancer in general practice. Br Med J.1957;1:84.
37. Feldman S, Hughes WT, Daniel CB. Varicella in children with cancer; Seventy-seven cases. Pediatrics. 1975;56:388–97.
38. Arvin AM, Pollard RB, Rasmussen LE, et al. Cellular and humoral immunity in the pathogenesis of recurrent herpes viral infections in patients with lymphoma. J Clin Invest. 1980;68:869–78.
39. Locksley RM, Flournoy N, Sullivan KM, et al. Infection with varicella zoster virus after marrow transplantation. J Infect Dis. 1985; 152:1172–81.
40. Whitley RJ. Varicella-zoster infections. In: Galasso G, Merigan T, Buchanan R, eds. Antiviral Agents and Viral Infections of Man. New York: Raven Press; 1984:517–41.
41. Asano Y, Itakura N, Hiroishi Y, et al. Viremia is present in incubation period in nonimmunocompromised children with varicella. J Pediatr. 1985;106:69–71.
42. Fleisher G, Henry W, McSorley M, et al. Life-threatening complications of varicella. Am J Dis Child. 1981;135:896–9.
43. Johnson R, Milbourne PE. Central nervous system manifestations of chickenpox. Can Med Assoc J. 1970;102:831–4.
44. Underwood EA. The neurological complications of varicella: A clinical and epidemiological study. Br J Child Dis. 1935;32:83,177,241.
45. Johnson R, Milbourn PE. Central nervous system manifestations of chickenpox. Can Med J 1970;102:831.
46. Triebwasser JH, Harrie RE, Bryant RE, et al. Varicella pneumonia in adults: Report of seven cases and a review of literature. Medicine (Baltimore). 1967;46:409–23.
47. Ward JR, Bishop B. Varicella arthritis. JAMA. 1970;212:1954.
48. Brunell PA. Fetal and neonatal varicella zoster infections. Semin Perinatol. 1983;7:47–56.
49. Preblud SR, Bregman DJ, Vernon LL. Deaths from varicella in infants. Pediatr Infect Dis. 1985;4:503–7.
50. Brunell PA. Placental transfer of varicella-zoster antibody. Pediatrics. 1966;38:1034.
51. Paryani SG, Arvin AM. Intrauterine infection with varicella zoster virus after maternal varicella. N Engl J Med. 1986;314:1542–6.
52. Linnemann CC, Shea L, Partin JC, et al. Reye's syndrome: Epidemiologic and viral studies. Am J Epidemiol. 1975;101:517.
53. Hilty MD, Romshe CA, Delamater PV. Reye's syndrome and hyperaminoacidemia. J Pediatr. 1974;84:362.
54. Feldman S, Hughes WT, Daniel CB. Varicella in children with cancer. Seventy-seven cases. Pediatrics. 1975;56:388.
55. Arvin AM, Kushner JH, Feldman S, et al. Human leukocyte interferon for treatment of varicella in children with cancer. N Engl J Med. 1982;306:761.
56. Whitley RJ, Soong SJ, Dolin R, et al. Early vidarabine therapy to control the complications of herpes zoster in immunosuppressed patients. N Engl J Med. 1982;307–971.
57. Loxley RM, Flournoy N, Sullivan KM, et al. Infection with varicella-zoster virus after marrow transplantation. J Infect Dis. 1985;6:1172–81.
58. deMoragas JM, Kierland RR. The outcome of patients with herpes zoster. Arch Dermatol. 1957;73:193–6.
59. Watson PN, Evans RJ. Postherpetic neuralgia; A review. Arch Neurol. 1986;43:836–40.
60. Esmann V, Kroon S, Petersblund NA, et al. Prednisolone does not prevent post-herpetic neuralgia. Lancet. 1987;2:126–9.
61. Hogan EL, Krigman MR. Herpes zoster myelitis. Arch Neurol. 1973;29:309.
62. Norris FH, Dramov B, Calder CD, et al. Virus-like particles in myositis accompanying herpes zoster. Arch Neurol. 1969;21:25.
63. Rubin D, Fusfeld RD. Muscle paralysis in herpes zoster. Calif Med. 1965;103:261.
64. Forghani B, Schmidt NJ, Dennis J. Antibody assays for varicella-zoster virus; comparison of enzyme immunoassay with neutralization, immune adherence hemagglutination and complement fixation. J Clin Microbiol. 1978;8:545–52.
65. Whitley RJ, Hilty M, Haynes R, et al. Vidarabine therapy of varicella in immunosuppressed patients. J Pediatr. 1982;101:125–31.
66. Prober CG, Kirk LE, Keeney RE. Acyclovir therapy of chickenpox in immunosuppressed children: A collaborative study. J Pediatr. 1982;101:622–5.
67. Whitley RJ, Chien LT, Dolin R, et al. Adenine arabinoside therapy of herpes zoster in immunosuppressed patients. N Engl J Med. 1982;307:971–5.
68. Balfour HH Jr, Bean B, Laskin OL, et al. Acyclovir halts progression of herpes zoster in immunocompromised patients. N Engl J Med. 1983;308:1448–53.
70. Shepp DH, Dandliker PS, Meyers JD. Treatment of varicella zoster virus infection in severely immunocompromised patients: A randomized comparison of acyclovir and vidarabine. N Engl J Med. 1986;314:208–12.
71. Brunell PA, Ross A, Miller H, et al. Prevention of varicella by zoster immune globulin. N Engl J Med. 1969;280:1191–4.
72. Gershon AA, Steinberg S, Brunell PA. Zoster immune globulin: A further assessment. N Engl J Med. 1969;280:1191–4.
73. Zaia JA, Levin MJ, Preblud SR, et al. Evaluation of varicella zoster immune globulin: Protection of immunosuppressed children after household exposure to varicella. J Infect Dis. 1983;147:737–43.
74. Centers for Disease Control. Varicella zoster immune globulin for the prevention of chickenpox: Recommendations of the immunization practices advisory committee. Ann Intern Med. 1984;100:859–65.
75. Takahashi M, Otsuka T, Okuno Y, et al. Live vaccine used to prevent the spread of varicella in children in hospital. Lancet. 1974;2:1288–90.
76. Gershon AA, Steinberg SP, Gelb L. Live attenuated varicella vaccine use in immunocompromised children and adults. Pediatrics. 1986;78:757–62.
77. Takahashi M. Clinical overview of varicella vaccine: Development and early studies. Pediatrics. 1986;78:736–41.
78. Yabuuchi H, Baba K, Tsuda N, et al. A live varicella vaccine in a pediatric community. Biken J. 1984;27:43–9.
79. Horiuchi K. Chickenpox vaccination of healthy children: Immunological and clinical responses and protective effect in 1978–1982. Biken J. 1984;27:37–8.
80. Weibel RE, Neff BJ, Kutter BJ, et al. Live attenuated varicella virus vaccine: Efficacy trial in healthy children. N Engl J Med. 1984;310:1409–15.
81. Asano Y, Nagai T, Miyata T, et al. Long-term protective immunity of recipients of the OKA strain of live varicella vaccine. Pediatrics. 1985;75:667–71.
82. Lawrence R, Gershon AA, Holzman R, et al. The risk of zoster after vaccination in children with leukemia. N Engl J Med. 1988;318:543–8.

120. CYTOMEGALOVIRUS

MONTO HO

Cytomegalovirus (CMV) causes a number of protean disease syndromes in pediatric and adult medicine. It exemplifies a characteristic of many infectious agents. Infection is common and reaches most of the population, while associated disease is a relatively exceptional event. In newborns it causes a congenital syndrome that may at times be fatal. In normal immunocompetent subjects, it is a recognized cause of CMV mononucleosis. But it is among various groups of the immunosuppressed such as the immature neonate, the recipients of organ transplants, and in acquired immunodeficiency syndrome (AIDS) that CMV causes its most significant disease syndromes. Infection and diseases caused by CMV are still relatively refractory to both prevention and therapy.

CMV shares with other herpesviruses the unique capacity to remain latent in tissues after recovery of the host from an acute infection. "Once infected, always infected." Hence they are "opportunists" par excellence because they are frequently already in hosts waiting to be activated when they become immunosuppressed. But immunosuppression alone does not explain all aspects of CMV disease. Why do some apparently normal people get CMV mononucleosis instead of the usual asymptomatic infection? We now know that most perinatal as well as congenital infections are also asymptomatic. Occasionally, though, a baby born with CMV will present with the fulminant congenital disease. Others may develop subtle disabilities later in life. Why is this?

The distinction between primary and secondary infections should be clearly understood. The first occurs in the seronegative immunologic "virgin," while secondary infection represents activation of a latent infection or reinfection or a seropositive "immune" person. Secondary infection is not a problem with virus infections that do not become latent or when acquired immunity is almost absolute. Clinical disease may result from either primary or secondary infection by CMV, although primary infections usually cause more severe disease.

In this chapter, emphasis is placed on up-to-date developments and clinical relevance. To understand the diseases caused by the virus, virologic, epidemiologic, and pathogenetic aspects are discussed first. For more details, Ho's monograph[1] may be consulted.

DESCRIPTION OF THE PATHOGEN

The Agent and Its History

In 1881 Ribbert[2] first noted large "protozoan-like" cells in the kidney of a stillborn. By 1932, 25 cases of cytomegalic inclusion disease were described. Farber and Wolbach[3] found by postmortem examination that 12 percent of the submaxillary glands from 183 infants who died of various causes had intranuclear and cytoplasmic inclusions, thus suggesting that the infection was not a rare event.

The modern virologic era began with the isolation of murine CMV in mouse cell culture by Smith.[4] Later, the isolation of human CMV was accomplished independently by Smith,[5] Rowe et al.,[6] and Weller et al.[7]

The term *cytomegalovirus* was coined by Weller et al.[8] to replace *salivary gland virus* or *cytomegalic inclusion disease virus*. Klemola and Kaariainen[9] first described recognizable CMV infection and disease in a normal, healthy adult. Later it was found that CMV mononucleosis can occur sporadically and also after blood[10] and leukocyte transfusions.[11]

The site of latency of CMV is not precisely known, but it probably includes at least the circulating peripheral mononuclear and possibly polymorphonuclear leukocyte.[12,13] In normal seropositive individuals lymphocytes have been found when using an immediate early antigen probe, to be abortively infected by CMV by in situ hybridization.[14] These infected cells do not ordinarily produce virus. This finding may explain why blood and organs have been found to transmit CMV, although we still do not understand how an abortive infection is triggered into a productive cycle.

One unproven characteristic of human CMV is its possible oncogenicity. All members of the herpesvirus group are candidate oncogenic agents, but the evidence for Epstein-Barr virus (EBV) is the strongest. The association of CMV with Kaposi's sarcoma is based on the epidemiologic finding that CMV infection is more common in African patients with Kaposi's sarcoma,[15] and the finding by some investigators that low copy numbers of CMV genomes are present in cells of Kaposi's sarcoma.[16]

Laboratory Diagnosis

The diagnosis of CMV infection in children and adults and in healthy or immunosuppressed persons requires laboratory confirmation and cannot be made on clinical grounds alone.

The first useful laboratory test was reported by Fetterman,[17] who found large, inclusion-bearing cells in the urine sediment. This test is diagnostic when positive but may be falsely negative in viruric patients. It is less valuable after the newborn period.

The laboratory diagnosis of CMV infection depends on either isolation of the virus or demonstration of a serologic rise. The sensitivity and precision of both approaches is generally good.

More recent technical developments include the use of monoclonal antibodies to early antigens to detect infected cells in tissue specimens[18] and the use of labeled, cloned, viral nucleic acid probes to detect virus DNA or RNA in specimens by nucleic acid hybridization.[19,20] The main advantage of these techniques is rapidity. Hybridization methods have been applied to both the clinical specimens such as buffy coat, or tissue specimens. So far they are adjunctive methods and have not supplanted cultural methods.

Cultivation of Cytomegalovirus

Human CMV cannot be readily grown in any experimental animal.[21] It, however, is easily cultured on human fibroblast cultures. The one drawback is the time needed to develop cytopathology. Ordinarily this may take 1–4 weeks, but the time required has also been shortened to 48 hours by the use of cytospin and monoclonal antibody to detect cytopathology before it becomes visible.[22] The typical cytopathology of CMV is usually sufficiently characteristic for identification in the laboratory without further serologic confirmation. When in doubt, antigen may be prepared from the virus for identification by the complement fixation (CF) test using known antiserum.[21]

When present, CMV may be readily isolated from urine, mouth swabs, buffy coat, cervical swabs, or other tissues obtained from biopsies or at postmortem examination. Virus is demonstrable in patients even if they have circulating neutralizing antibodies.

Ordinarily, CMV is not detectable in normal adults. The exceptions are females who may carry the virus in the cervix and males, particularly homosexual males, who may carry CMV in semen. The presence of CMV in the throat, urine, and blood by culture is usually abnormal. It is, however, important to note additional circumstances under which CMV may be chronically carried. Anyone who is recovering from an acute infection may carry CMV in the urine, throat, and occasionally blood for months. Patients with congenital or perinatal infection and immunosuppressed patients with transplants or human immunodeficiency virus (HIV) infection and AIDS are often chronic virus carriers for years. The meaning of isolating the virus from such patients requires careful interpretation.

Serology of Cytomegalovirus

Like herpes simplex virus, strains of CMV have enough genomic variation so that they may be "fingerprinted" after digestion with restriction endonucleases. There is, however, still enough DNA homology among different strains to suggest that, for diagnostic purposes, only one serotype of human CMV exists. The problem is more complex in understanding immunity to CMV since serologic distinctions on the basis of neutralization or other biologically meaningful measures may be present. The CF antigen of AD169 is more broadly reactive than are antigens of other strains and has been extensively used in epidemiologic and clinical studies. The CF test itself is no longer widely used because of its relative lack of sensitivity.

Compared with the CF test, the indirect fluorescent antibody (IFA) and the anti-complement immunofluorescent (ACIF) tests are more sensitive.[23,24] In primary infections, titers by IFA and ACIF tests are higher and become positive earlier than do the corresponding CF titers, at times by as much as 1–2 months. The ACIF test is superior because there is less nonspecific fluorescence.[23]

Many other tests are on the market, largely because fluorescence microscopy is cumbersome. These are the indirect hemagglutination test, radioimmunoassay, latex agglutination, automated immunofluorescence, and various versions of the enzyme-linked immunosorbent assay (ELISA). By and large the same antigens are used as in the older CF and fluorescence tests. Each one must be checked out against the reliable older ones. At times, the lower level of sensitivity (i.e., whether a test is positive or negative) is unknown or unreliable. This information may be essential to evaluate the immune and risk status before pregnancies and organ transplantation. A diagnosis of infection by serology requires either an elevation of antibody titer or its conversion from negative to positive. Samples of serum before and after an illness are essential. When they are not available, the presence of IgM antibody against CMV is a useful but not completely reliable indication of an acute infection. IgM titers may not be positive during an active infection (false-negative), or they may persist for such a long time that it may not be diagnostic (false-positive). For example IgM titers has been found to be elevated in asymptomatic homosexuals.

EPIDEMIOLOGY OF CYTOMEGALOVIRUS INFECTIONS

Incidence and Prevalence of Infections

Studies of the prevalence of antibody against CMV in sera of the general population show that infection with this virus is widespread and usually inapparent. Depending on the socioeconomic condition of the population, the prevalence of antibodies in adults ranges from 40 to 100 percent.[25] It is lower in Europe, Australia, and parts of North America, while it is significantly higher in developing areas such as Africa and Southeast Asia. There is a wide range in various parts of the United States. For example, it is 45 percent in Albany, NY, and 79 percent in Houston.

Analysis of studies on age-related incidence rate of infection suggests that there is at least one and perhaps two periods of increased infection during a life span. The first is the perinatal period. In some countries, such as Japan, Thailand, Guatemala, and Finland (a mix of economically advanced and developing countries), perinatal infection as demonstrated by viruria during the first year of life is 36–56 percent.[1] Infection increases slowly throughout childhood after the first year. The second major spurt, particularly in countries with more susceptible seronegative subjects, is during the reproductive ages and is presumably accounted for by sexual activity (see below). Babies and children become infected in a number of ways. One source of infection is passage through a contaminated uterine cervix during birth. A second mechanism is transmission from human milk by breast-feeding or from banked milk.[26] CMV has been found in the milk of seropositive women.[27] A third mechanism of infection is transmission from other children in the newborn nursery,[28] in day care centers,[29] and probably among children within the family.[30] Infected children tend to carry the virus for long periods of time in the respiratory tract and in urine.[31] Other adults in the family are probably negligible sources of virus since healthy adults usually do not shed virus in the urine or respiratory tract.

Transmission by Blood

Kaariainen et al.[10] implicated blood transfusions in the transmission of CMV. Henle et al.[32] suggested that the risk was proportional to the number of units transfused, estimated as 5–12 percent per unit. Prince et al.[33] found that 31 of 152 patients who received 1269 units of blood subsequently seroconverted. They estimated an overall risk of 2.4 seroconversions per 100 units transfused. The risk of infection may also be estimated by primary infection (seroconversion or virus isolation) in children receiving blood. Armstrong et al.[34] studied a group of 93 seronegative children undergoing open heart surgery who received a mean of 3.9 units. Nine (9.7 percent) of this group subsequently became infected with CMV. This infection rate is consistent with a model of transmission by blood transfusion with a risk not greater than 2.7 percent per unit of blood, which is consistent with the findings of a number of other studies before 1980.[1] However, more recent studies evaluating large numbers of seronegative transfusion recipients show significantly less CMV infection.[35] Infection is usually asymptomatic, but symptomatic infection in well children and adults is a definite hazard with multiple transfusion after trauma or invasive surgery. It may also occur after the transfusion of granulocytes.[11] The risk of infection is decreased by using cryopreserved blood, leukocyte-poor blood, or blood from seronegative donors.[1]

The seronegative neonate who is immature at birth is at markedly greater risk for developing significant CMV disease from as little as 100 ml blood. Fifty percent of primary infections may be serious or fatal. CMV infection in such infants has been prevented by using blood from seronegative donors.[36]

Attempts to culture CMV from blood donors despite a clear indication that it must be present is usually unsuccessful.[1] The explanation is that CMV genomes are latently present in blood leukocytes but remain unexpressed in normal healthy seropositive individuals.[14] Presumably they are activated when transfused to a recipient, particularly if immunologically immature or deficient. Chou and colleagues[37] reported that if the recipient is HLA matched with the donor activation occurs much more frequently, perhaps because of better survival of infected cells.

Transmission by Sex

Two potential sources of venereal transmission of CMV are virus in the uterine cervix and in semen. The frequency of CMV infection of the cervix varies with age, socioeconomic class, sexual promiscuity, and parity. About 1–2 percent of women having routine medical examinations in private practice in this country carry the virus in the cervix.[1] In Taiwan, however, 18 percent of a nonpromiscuous female population carried the virus.[38] The cause of this marked discrepancy is unclear, and it is unknown how women acquire the virus at this site. On the other hand in a study of 347 young women attending a sexually transmitted disease (STD) clinic in Seattle, 34 percent of seropositive women over 21 years of age shed CMV in the cervix. The frequency of colonization was positively correlated with the number of sex partners and younger age of first sexual intercourse.[39] There is no direct evidence that virus in the cervix comes from sexual intercourse or that it can be transmitted by sexual intercourse. However, these data suggest that the uterine cervix is either constantly reinfected by sexual intercourse or that cervical carriage established at an early age persists. The role of pregnancy is discussed below. Indirect evidence of transmission by heterosexual sex comes from small outbreaks of CMV mononucleosis among sex partners in a university community. In one report, two males were presumably infected by a woman who was carrying the virus in the uterine cervix.[40]

CMV may also be found in high titers in the semen of both heterosexual and homosexual males.[41] How the virus gets there and the reasons for its persistence, just as in the case of the virus in the uterine cervix, is also unknown. Possibly, semen may carry CMV for only short periods after an active infection unless repeated infection takes place or chronic infection is facilitated by early age of infection or by immunosuppression. While there are no comparable data from heterosexual males, sperm carriage in homosexual males has been shown to be a reflection of sexual activity. CMV could be isolated from asymptomatic homosexual males, most frequently from semen, in 35–42 percent of the cases irrespective of whether they were HIV-positive.[42] The presence of CMV has been correlated with younger age of the subject (≤24), passive anal sex, and large numbers of sex partners.

Most homosexual males in this country have been infected with CMV. Those who are not become rapidly infected when followed prospectively.[43] What is even more striking, however, is that past infections continue to be active. Although CMV is carried in many other body fluids (urine, saliva, and blood), the high carriage frequency in semen in the healthy homosexual and its association with passive anal intercourse and the number of partners suggests that, as in the case of HIV infection,[44] CMV may be readily transmitted by infected sperm during anal intercourse.

Cervical Infection during Pregnancy and Perinatal Transmission

CMV in the uterine cervix is not only a potential source of venereal transmission to a sexual partner but also to a neonate during passage through the birth canal. Numazaki et al.[45] first reported from Japan an increased rate of cervical infection in the later stages of pregnancy. Similar results were found by Montgomery et al.[46] and by the Alabama group.[47]

The three studies covering 987 pregnant women are summarized in Table 1. All three found an increasing prevalence of infection progressing from the first (0–2 percent) to the second (6–10 percent) and third trimesters (11–28 percent). The three groups represent different populations. The Japanese group represents a nonpromiscuous middle-class population that was 85 percent CMV-seropositive. The Alabama group was also a high prevalence group (89 percent seropositive), but it was a young sexually promiscuous group with a 10 percent rate of gonorrhea. Montgomery et al.[46] studied 125 middle-class white and black pregnant women and 71 Navaho Indians.

High cervical CMV excretion during the third trimester of pregnancy suggests that the neonate is at risk during the process of birth. Reynolds et al.[48] showed this clearly. Only 2 (4 percent) of 50 babies born of nonsecretors became infected. In contrast, 12.5 percent of babies born to mothers who secreted CMV from the cervix only during the first or second trimester became infected, and 37 percent of the babies born of third-trimester excretors became infected. The infection rate of babies whose mothers shed virus postpartum and who were presumably shedding at birth rose to 57 percent. None of the babies of urine shedders were infected. About 5 percent of all live births in the Alabama population from a low socioeconomic stratum were perinatally infected.

Perinatal infection is usually diagnosed in a neonate who does not show evidence of infection at birth but becomes viruric 4–8 weeks after birth when the virus acquired during birth has replicated. Perinatal infections are usually asymptomatic, and no late deleterious effects have been described. They may be difficult to distinguish from infections acquired during birth, particularly if the child is first seen some months after birth.

TABLE 1. Cervical CMV Infection during Pregnancy

Source	Infection in Trimester: First	Second	Third	Overall Infection
Numazaki et al.[45]	0/30[a] (0%)	6/62 (9.7%)	17/61 (27.9%)	23/153 (15.0%)
Montgomery et al.[46]	1/43 (2%)	6/83 (7.2%)	6/49 (12.2%)	13/175 (7.4%)
Stagno et al.[47]	3/183 (1.6%)[b]	22/359 (6.1%)	42/371 (11.3%)	63/659 (9.6%)
Total infected/tested	4/256	34/504	65/481	99/987
Percentage infected	1.6	6.7	13.5	10.0

[a] Represents number of positive patients per number of patients tested.
[b] Number infected per number of specimens tested.

Congenital Infections in Infants of Nonimmune Mothers. Intrauterine or congenital infection by CMV occurs in between 0.5 and 2.2 percent of all live births.[49] Although less frequent than perinatal infection, congenital or intrauterine infections are important because most serious CMV disease syndromes in the neonate may be attributed to this type of infection. The diagnosis of congenital infection is most reliably demonstrated by viruria within the first week after birth. The presence of IgM-type antibodies against CMV in the cord serum is helpful but neither completely sensitive or specific.

The majority of clinically apparent congenital infections have occurred in infants of primiparous mothers who had a primary infection during pregnancy.[1] Such infections may be diagnosed by a change in antibody titer against CMV from negative to positive or by an IgM antibody test. The radioimmune IgM assay is reportedly both *sensitive* and *specific*.[50] The risk of intrauterine infection after primary infections can only be documented in large prospective studies in which mothers are followed throughout pregnancy. A number of such studies are summarized in Table 2.

Monif et al.[51] followed 664 pregnant women whose CF titers were less than 1:8 at bimonthly intervals. Two primary infections were documented in the second trimester. They were associated with two infants with elevated IgM in their cord serum, viruria, and multiple stigmata of congenital infection. Two cases of seroconversion occurred during the third trimester. Both mothers produced infants with elevated IgM in cord serum and viruria at birth. They were otherwise healthy. In this study, there was 100 percent correlation between primary CMV infection in the mother and congenital infection in the baby.

Stern and Tucker[52] studied 1040 pregnant women in London; 56 percent of the white and 90 percent of the Asian women were seropositive. Primary infection detected by the CF test occurred in 8 (3 percent) of 254 whites and 3 (19 percent) of 16 Asian women. About 45 percent of the offspring (5 of 11) had viruria at birth. One mentally retarded child was infected during the second trimester. Nankervis et al.[53] identified a total of 8 primary infections among over 3000 pregnant women. Four infected babies were produced; all were viruric but clinically healthy. Stagno et al.[54] followed 3712 pregnant women from both upper and lower socioeconomic strata from Alabama. Of 21 primary infections among 1382 seronegative mothers, there were 11 congenital infections, of whom 3 were symptomatic. These reports indicate that intrauterine infection after primary CMV infection is high (24 of 44, 55 percent). The rate of primary infection did not vary significantly with the socioeconomic status or immune status of the population. In these series, it was 0.52 percent. The rate of intrauterine CMV infection (24 in 8416 pregnancies) resulting from primary infections was 0.3 percent, of whom 25 percent (6 of 44) were symptomatic. It appears that primary infection at any stage of pregnancy presents a risk, but Stagno and Whitley[55] believe that infection during the first half of pregnancy produces more disease.

Congenital Infection of Infants of Immune Mothers. Stagno et al.[54] also reported 20 (0.5 percent) babies with congenital infections from 2330 mothers who were immune or seropositive. This type of congenital infection occurred more frequently in mothers of the lower socioeconomic group, who had a high prevalence of past infection. However, none of the 20 babies was symptomatic, although other workers have found that symptomatic congenital infection may occasionally result from infection in an immune mother.[56] There are also scattered reports of congenital disease in consecutive pregnancies, but as expected, these too are rare.[1] There seems no doubt, however, that immunity in the mother protects the baby from the disease.

Summarizing the above, it appears that several natural mechanisms exist in a population of immune mothers that facilitate CMV infections in the newborn, most or all of which are asymptomatic in nature and may be considered a form of natural live

TABLE 2. Risk of Congenital CMV Infection after Primary Infection of Mothers during Pregnancy

Authors	Number Pregnancies	Trimester	Primary Infection in Mothers Number	Primary Infection in Mothers Percentage[a]	Congenital Infection in Babies Number	Congenital Infection in Babies Percentage[b]	Symptomatic Babies Number	Symptomatic Babies Percentage[c]
Monif et al.[51]	664	1st	0	0	0		0	
		2nd	2	0.3	2	100	2	100
		3rd	2	0.3	2	100	0	0
Stern and Tucker[52]	1040	1st	2	0.19	2	100	0	100
		2nd	4	0.38	2	50	1	50
		3rd	5	0.48	1	20	0	0
Nankervis et al[53]	3000	1st	1	0.03	0	0	0	
		2nd	4	0.13	1	25	0	0
		3rd	3	0.1	3	100	0	0
Stagno et al.[54]	3712	All	21	0.57	11	52	3	27
Total	8416		44	0.52	24	55	6	25

[a] Percentage of primary infection in the total number of pregnancies.
[b] Percentage of congenital infections in offspring after primary infection in mothers.
[c] Percentage of congenital infections in offspring who showed stigmata of disease.

immunization. A small number of these infections arise transplacentally, and significant numbers are perinatal infections from CMV carried in the cervix during the later stages of pregnancy and perinatal infection from CMV in breast milk. The baby is protected from hazards of this "live immunization" by antibodies passively transferred from the mother and is rarely symptomatic. The noenate who gets CMV disease is one whose mother is not immune. Such infants are at particular risk if their mothers get a primary infection during pregnancy.

Cytomegalovirus Infection in the Immunosuppressed (Transplant Group)

It is remarkable that after organ transplantation most if not all patients develop CMV infection. This has been shown in all types of major transplantations such as renal, liver, heart, heart–lung, and bone marrow transplants (see also Chapters 290, 291, 292). For example, in 15 studies of 1145 patients the rate of infections after renal transplants as determined by serologic rise or isolation of the virus from the blood, urine, or throat varies from 52 to 100 percent with a mean of 71 percent.[1] The infection rate was significantly higher in those who were seropositive before organ transplantation (85 percent) and lower in seronegative recipients (53 percent).

For the development of primary infection, exposure to a source of virus is necessary. Theoretically, the virus may come from a contaminated environment such as intensive care units or dialysis centers or from infected contacts. In fact, the most important sources are transplanted tissues or organs and, to a lesser degree, transfused blood. In contrast, secondary infection may occur in anyone who is seropositive and latently infected.

Donated Organ or Tissue as a Source of Infection. As in the case of blood, attempts to isolate CMV from organs have failed; still, CMV may be transmitted by any major transplant. There are two types of evidence for this. The first type is epidemiologic. In the case of kidney transplantations, Ho et al.[57] and Betts et al.[58] noted that primary infections developed in 83 percent of seronegative recipients who received kidneys from seropositive donors, while very few of those who received kidneys from seronegative donors became infected. Besides incriminating the donated organ as the vehicle of infection, such data suggest that primary infection may be largely prevented if one uses organs from seronegative donors. This type of evidence is also available for heart, bone marrow, and liver transplantation (for details, see Chapters 291 and 292).

Role of Immunosuppressive Drugs. The most important factor accounting for reactivations of CMV infections is the iatrogenic immunosuppression essential for maintenance of the graft.[59] Cytotoxic drugs such as cyclophosphamide or azathioprine alone can reactivate a latent CMV infection but do not produce disease.[60] Corticosteroids play a subsidiary role. They continue to be used with all types of immunosuppressive regimes in moderate doses. It has been pointed out that CMV disease has decreased when compared with the time when corticosteroids were used in much higher doses as an adjunct to azathioprine.[61] Corticosteroids alone, which were used before the introduction of cytotoxic drugs, were insufficient to enhance CMV infection.

The addition of anti-lymphocyte serum to a combination of azathioprine and prednisone has reportedly been shown to increase the morbidity due to CMV infection.

Since 1981 cyclosporine has gradually supplanted azathioprine as the primary immunosuppressive agent. Its superiority has made possible a marked increase in the number and types of transplant operations. A controlled study in which renal transplant patients received either azathioprine and prednisone or cyclosporine and prednisone showed that infection and morbidity from CMV was comparable in both groups.[62] We also showed that, besides immunosuppression, the type of transplantations was also important in determining CMV morbidity. Liver, heart, and heart–lung transplant recipients had more morbidity due to CMV than did kidney recipients.[63,64]

Immunosuppression may be complicated in the future by the introduction of new agents or the use of multiple agents in an attempt to reduce the toxicity of cyclosporine due to excess or prolonged use. Each novel regimen will have to be evaluated for its effect on CMV infection. This includes the anti-lymphocyte serums and azathioprine. Polyclonal and monoclonal anti-lymphocyte serums have also been used for the treatment of rejections in addition to classic steroids. We showed, for example, that the OKT3 antiserum used to treat rejection in liver transplant patients increased the frequency of severe CMV diseases such as hepatitis and dissemination.[65]

Usually, immunosuppression does not inhibit the development of CMV antibodies. Rarely, in very severe infections, antibody production is inhibited.[66]

Effect of Allograft Reactions. Two types of allograft reactions may occur after organ transplantation, the host-vs.-graft (HvG) reaction and the graft-vs.-host (GvH) reaction. Depending on genetic compatibility and the transplant involved, one or both reactions may occur. Both reactions have been shown in experimental animals to affect virus infections. After C3H mice chronically infected with murine CMV received skin allografts from histoincompatible BALB/c donors, which produced an HvG reaction, CMV titers were increased in the spleen and kidneys.[67] Mouse CMV infection was also enhanced in the same model of infection under stimulation of a GvH reaction brought on by the administration of multiple doses of parental splenocytes to F_1(DBA/2 × C3H/he) recipients.[68]

One sees the most severe and lethal form of CMV disease, interstitial pneumonia, after bone marrow transplantation. Meyers et al.[69] showed that after patients who had leukemia or aplastic anemias were given *bone marrow transplants* those undergoing a GvH reaction were associated with CMV infection. GvH disease was significantly more common among patients with (82 percent) than among those without (27 percent) CMV interstitial pneumonia. Of patients with GvH disease 66 percent (27 of 41) developed interstitial pneumonia as compared with only 14 percent (6 of 44) of patients without GvH disease. Thus GvH reaction, of which a target organ may be the lung, is an important cofactor for CMV disease. The precise immunopathologic reaction underlying CMV interstitial pneumonia in marrow transplant recipients is still unknown, but its existence is underscored by the failure of antiviral therapy in this condition.[69a]

The evidence that an HvG reaction enhances CMV infection in humans is less clear-cut. CMV pneumonia is more common after heart–lung transplantation than after heart or renal transplantation.[64] Severe CMV hepatitis is a special problem after liver transplantation.[70] In both cases, the target organ of CMV disease is a cadaver allograft in which tissue mismatching is common and varying degrees of allograft reactions are expected to be present (see Chapter 292).

Cytomegalovirus Infection in the Immunosuppressed (Malignancies)

The frequency and morbidity of CMV infection in patients with malignancies is not as high as after major organ transplantation. Even patients with immunosuppressive malignancies (such as Hodgkin's lymphoma) or who are receiving immunosuppressive chemotherapy are not sufficiently immunosuppressed for a long enough period to get in trouble from a reactivation infection. Also, the primary complication of chemotherapy, neutropenia, does not appear to be a major risk factor for CMV infection. Finally, unless transfused many times, the patient with cancer does not have a ready outside source of virus for a primary infection.

That patients with malignancies may be infected by CMV may be documented in many ways. In early studies, evidence of increased infection was found in postmortem studies; by cultures of urine, throat, or blood; or by serologic studies. Before 1965, CMV disease in adults was primarily described in patients with chronic debilitating diseases, especially hematologic malignancies.[71] Since then, with the advent of chemotherapy, particularly in leukemias, CMV infections have been more frequently described. For example, Bodey et al.[72] report from the National Cancer Institute that, before 1962, 3 percent of autopsies on patients with acute leukemias showed CMV disease but, in 1962–1963, 15 percent of such patients were similarly afflicted. Some reports indicate higher CMV infection in leukemic children as measured by virurias.[1]

The significance of this is difficult to evaluate in children without controls. Henson et al.[73] followed 88 leukemic children of a mean age of 7.3 years for a mean period of 8.2 months. Evidence of infection over this time period was seen in 24 patients (27 percent) as measured by repeated urine and throat cultures. No serologic rise was observed in 16 of the virus excretors. Some had disseminated disease, and they had serologic rises. Infected patients had more pneumonitis and fever than did uninfected patients. Other findings coincident with a serologic rise were parotitis, prostatitis, upper respiratory infection, and hepatitis. Thus, in an individual patient, it is difficult to determine the etiologic role of CMV for such manifestations. Frequently infection occurred without clinical manifestations. More epidemiologic and clinical follow-up studies are needed in adults and in patients with other types of malignancies.

Cytomegalovirus Infection in the Immunosuppressed (AIDS and HIV Infection)

There is an intimate relationship between CMV and HIV infection. With progressive immunosuppression as a result of HIV infection, CMV activity increases. As stated above, 30–40 percent of homosexuals actively shed CMV in semen or urine irrespective of whether they are HIV-positive.[42] Of those infected, 95 percent have at one time or another elevated IgM titers against CMV, which suggests active infection. Such infection probably represents both activation of latent infections by one or more endogenous strains as well as superinfection by additional strains from repeated exposure.[74] Viremia usually remains absent in asymptomatic HIV-infected individuals,[75] while in progressive AIDS-related complex (ARC) patients and all patients with AIDS (Kaposi's sarcoma and/or opportunistic infections) viremia was present. As in the case of transplant recipients,[63] viremia is usually present in symptomatic CMV disease.

Since active CMV infection is present in most advanced HIV infections irrespective of whether CMV produces any symptoms, laboratory diagnosis of significant infection or disease is difficult. Serology is not helpful since primary infections are unusual and many have persistent IgM antibodies. Culturing the virus in urine, throat, semen, or even blood may not help. A sine qua non for the attribution of a clinical syndrome to CMV is the demonstration of local pathology characteristic of CMV infection or isolation or demonstration of the virus or viral activity at a local site. Even so, if CMV is present with other microbial agents such as *Pneumocystis carinii, Mycobacterium avium-intracellulare*, or HIV, which may be the actual cause of local pathology, the pathogenic role of the CMV may not be ascertained.

CLINICAL MANIFESTATIONS

Disease in Children

As already pointed out, symptoms occur in less than a quarter of the congenitally infected. The classic fulminant congenital cytomegalic inclusion disease (CID) is characterized by jaundice, hepatosplenomegaly, a petechial rash, and multiple system and organ involvement.[1] Microcephaly, motor disability, chorioretinitis, and cerebral calcifications are also seen.[76] The involvement of the central nervous system, the inner ear, and the choroid of the eye appears to be unique for congenital infection.

Clinically, immediately at birth or shortly thereafter, there is an onset of lethargy, respiratory distress, and convulsive seizures. The patient may die at any time from a few days to a few weeks. Most of the patients described in the earlier literature expired shortly after birth. Infants were later found to survive. Hemorrhagic phenomena, jaundice, and hepatosplenomegaly may subside after a variable period. However neurologic sequelae such as microcephaly, mental retardation, and motor disability may become apparent only later and are also the least likely to clear.

A large number of extraneural organ defects have also been associated with congenital infection. It should be noted, however, that most of the disease manifestations in congenital infection are associated with direct and active inflammation secondary to virus invasion or possibly immunologic reactions. Indirect interference with organ development, well documented in the case of rubella, is not evident in most cases of CMV infection.

The picture of postnatally acquired CMV disease is different from CID. Diffuse visceral or central nervous system involvement is rarely observed. When clinical manifestations are apparent, they may resemble some aspect of CMV mononucleosis. Mononucleosis itself may be absent, although it may occur, even in very young children.[9] Serious disease, however, can result from exchange transfusions.[36] Outbreaks of CMV infection have been described in neonatal intensive care units, where the seronegative, poorly developed infant may be at particular risk.[28]

Infants may also demonstrate prolonged respiratory disease such as pharyngitis, bronchitis, pneumonia, and croup. The association of CMV with pertussus is evident from the older literature. Olson and associates[30] noted that children with respiratory infection more frequently carried CMV in the upper respiratory tract. It is difficult to distinguish the precise etiologic role of CMV in such cases.

Subtle Sequelae of Neonatal Infections

Both perinatal and intrauterine CMV infections may be completely asymptomatic. So far no immediate or long-term abnormalities have been described in perinatally infected children. However, they may not have been followed long enough in sufficient numbers to rule out development of subtle abnormalities. In contrast, there is ample documentation of subtle sequelae after inapparent intrauterine infections.

In 8644 neonates from a higher socioeconomic class Hanshaw et al.[77] identified 53 with IgM antibodies against CMV in cord blood (1 in 163, 0.6 percent). One was stillborn, and one had clinical disease and died at 48 hours. Forty-four were evaluated at 3.5–7.0 years of age. The mean IQ of the group was 103, which was lower than matched controls. The predicted school failure rate, based on IQ and behavioral, neurologic, and auditory data, was 2.7 times that of controls matched for socioeconomic status. Five of forty (13 percent) had severe bilateral hearing loss, and three had profound deafness. This would go far to explain the estimated 1 in 1000 incidence of unexplained profound deafness in children. A more recent prospective controlled study showed that in the absence of hearing loss a lower IQ is not a late sequela of congenital infection.[78]

Stagno et al.[79] reported from Alabama on the incidence of sensorineural hearing loss in neonatal CMV infection in three types of neonatal CMV infection. There were 59 patients with congenital or intrauterine infection, 8 of whom were symptomatic at birth. Twenty-one had perinatal CMV infection, none of whom developed hearing loss. Late-onset hearing loss developed in 17 percent of all congenital and 14 percent of all subclinical congenital CMV infections. Pathologic studies in two patients showed virus in cells of the organ of Corti and in neurons of the spiral ganglia. Rare cells with typical intranuclear inclusions were seen in the cochlea. A third patient studied at postmortem examination had disseminated symptomatic disease but no evidence of viral infection in the inner ear.

The insidious nature of this problem was that (*1*) hearing loss could not be predicted by the severity of infection or the height of IgM levels at birth; (*2*) it may be progressive, and estimates so far may be minimal; and (*3*) the subtlety of the defect makes evaluation of preventive measures such as the use of vaccines difficult. Possibly an immune mechanism underlies its pathogenesis.

In contrast, eye pathology corresponds roughly to the severity of infection. It was found in 8 of 43 patients with congenital CMV infection. Five of the eight patients (63 percent) who were symptomatically infected had lesions. None with perinatal infections had pathologic eye changes.

Cytomegalovirus-Induced Mononucleosis and Disease Manifestations in Normal Adults

CMV-induced mononucleosis is clinically difficult to distinguish from infectious or EBV-induced mononucleosis. Fever is usually a dominant problem. There is relative and absolute lymphocytosis with abundant atypical lymphocytes. These may appear relatively late in the course of the disease, at times 1–2 weeks after the onset of fever. Relative well-being and paucity of findings are characteristic. CMV mononucleosis should be suspected in any case of mononucleosis in which the heterophile–agglutinin test is negative and in patients with fever of unknown origin. The prognosis is usually excellent.

Like EBV-induced mononucleosis, CMV mononucleosis may occur sporadically without any traceable source. The most important identifiable source is blood. In older children and adults, the probability of being infected by a unit of blood is around 3 percent or less.[34,35] Hence a large number of units transfused may present a proportionately greater risk. CMV is a cause of postoperative pyrexia. It should be considered along with other causes of postoperative sepsis, especially when large amounts of blood have been transfused.

Sexual or intimate contact with an infected person is undoubtedly important in the transmission of the virus. A history of such contact, however, is rarely obtained in an individual case.

The clinical features of this disease are described in a 8-year prospective study of 494 cases of mononucleosis by the Finnish group.[80] Most (79 percent) had positive heterophile–agglutinins and had EBV infection. Among 73 patients over 15 years of age with a negative response, 33 (45 percent) had CMV infection. When the first serum was taken 3–20 days after the onset of disease, 11 of 19 such patients were seronegative ($\leq$1:4) and developed a rise in CF antibodies. Peak titers were reached 4–7 weeks after the onset. Viruria was present in 10 of 12 tested. From this it appears that CMV mononucleosis usually represents primary infections in previously seronegative persons.

The age range was 18–66, the median age being 29, which is higher than is the susceptible age for EBV-induced mononucleosis. All patients were febrile, with fever lasting from 9 to 35 days with a mean of 19 days. Lymphocytosis varied from 55 to 86 percent, with 12–55 percent of the total leukocytes being atypical lymphocytes. Tonsillitis or pharyngitis is rare.

Enlargement of lymph nodes and the spleen is usually not striking but may occur. Mild elevations of liver function test results are a regular feature and an important aid to diagnosis. However, severe hepatitis or jaundice is unusual although chemical hepatitis is common.

In both CMV- and EBV-induced mononucleosis, there may be laboratory evidence of transient immunologic aberrations. For example, the appearance of mixed cryoglobulins, cold agglutinins, rheumatoid factor, and antinuclear and anticomplementary activity has been described.[80]

Most sporadic symptomatic cases represent primary infection in healthy subjects. However, secondary or reactivation infections may cause mononucleosis in the immunosuppressed, although it has been noted that atypical lymphocytosis per se is less apparent in such patients.

A number of complications or associated findings may occur more or less uncommonly with CMV infections, occasionally as the presenting syndrome, even in immunocompetent subjects.

Interstitial pneumonitis, a hallmark of CMV disease in the transplant patient may occur in CMV-induced mononucleosis. In the Finnish series, it was found in 2 of 33 patients.[81] These are primarily radiographic findings that eventually clear. This is in striking contrast to the life-threatening pneumonitis one sees in the immunosuppressed (see below). They may be different pathogenetically.

Hepatitis may be an initial asymptomatic sign of CMV infection. Symptomatic hepatitis occurs only rarely in immunocompetent subjects. Carter[82] described a 21-year-old immunocompetent man suspected of infectious hepatitis who had an enlarged and tender liver. Atypical lymphocytes were not seen. CMV was isolated from the urine, and there was a rise in CF antibodies.

Granulomatous hepatitis may also occasionally occur in healthy adults as an initial problem or accompanying mononucleosis.[83] There may be malaise, nausea, vomiting, and up to 50 percent atypical lymphocytes in the peripheral blood smear. CMV may be isolated from the throat, and there is an appropriate serologic rise. A percutaneous liver biopsy specimen shows resolving hepatitis, mononuclear infiltrates in portal areas, and scattered microscopic granulomas with giant cells. The patient usually recovers completely. These are important cases because one does not usually think of CMV when granulomas are found in the liver.

The *Guillain-Barré* syndrome is now a well-recognized and not uncommon complication of CMV-induced mononucleosis. Leonard and Tobin[84] described 9 patients with polyneuritis characterized by sensory and motor weakness in the extremities. Cranial nerve involvement was common, and 4 patients had to be treated in the respiratory unit. Sensation recovered before motor impairment, and complete recovery took about 3 months. There is no indication that immunosuppressed patients are more prone to this complication.

Schmitz and Enders[85] detected 10 cases of CMV infection in a series of 94 cases of Guillain-Barré syndrome (about 10 percent). They point out that the CF antibody titer is frequently already elevated by the time the patient is first seen within 1 week after onset and that no further diagnostic rise is observed. On the other hand, the IgM immunofluorescent antibody titer was high in 9 of 10 patients in the initial specimen, and all 10 showed a diagnostic decline at discharge. Six patients had to be cared for in the respiratory unit, but all recovered. The spinal fluids showed typically elevated protein levels and few cells. All patients had atypical lymphocytes.

Meningoencephalitis has been described in some cases of CMV infection in the immunocompetent.[86] It is usually associated with CMV-induced mononucleosis. These patients may have sensory and motor weaknesses that may be difficult to distinguish from polyradiculopathy. However, there may be severe headaches, photophobia, and pyramidal tract signs, and the spinal fluid may show mild mononuclear pleocytosis. It is not known whether this picture of "aseptic" meningoencephalitis is directly due to viral invasion or due to an allergic reaction.

Myocarditis has been described as a complication of CMV-induced mononucleosis. Tiula and Leinikki[87] reported that, in three of eight cases of mononucleosis, inversion of T waves was found in several leads by ECG examination. They described a 14-year-old boy with serologic evidence of CMV infection who died with evidence of hepatitis, myocarditis, and consumptive coagulopathy. Virus was found in the lungs at autopsy. Waris et al.[88] described a 43-year-old previously healthy woman who developed myocarditis, heart failure, encephalitis, hepatitis, and adrenal insufficiency. Evidence of CMV was found in the adrenals at autopsy. In general, myocardial involvement is rare in congenital CMV disease.

Thrombocytopenia and *hemolytic anemia* are well recognized in congenital CMV disease. They may also occur as a complication of CMV-induced mononucleosis in adults. Chanarin and Walford[89] described a 33-year-old man with CMV-induced mononucleosis who had generalized purpura and bleeding gums. His platelet count was 500/mm^3; hemoglobin, 3.6 g/dl; and reticulocyte count, 1.2 percent. There was serologic evidence of CMV infection and viruria. The patient recovered after treatment with prednisone.

Harris et al.[90] described a 26-year-old man with CMV infection who in addition to thrombocytopenia and purpura had red cells whose life span was decreased and an elevated reticulocyte count.

Petechial rashes may be observed in congenital CMV diseases. Rubelliform or maculopacular rashes may occur in CMV-induced mononucleosis with or without the administration of ampicillin.[91] Vesicular lesions are distinctly unusual in congenital or acquired CMV infection. Muller-Stamou et al.[92] described an unusual case of a 40-year-old man who developed generalized epidermolysis 8 weeks after the onset of hepatitis. He had viruria and viremia.

Clinical Aspects of Cytomegalovirus Infection in the Immunosuppressed

CMV infection is frequently asymptomatic, even in the immunosuppressed, but it may also produce protean clinical manifestations. A febrile mononucleosis indistinguishable from the disease in the nonsuppressed appears to be the most common clinical presentation. But in other immunosuppressed patients more extensive organ involvement, rarely seen in the healthy subjects, may be evident. Knowledge of the diverse pathologic spectrum due to CMV in adults has significantly increased since the discovery of AIDS. CMV can cause pneumonitis, hepatitis, gastrointestinal ulcerations, retinitis, encephalopathy, and endocrine disturbances. These are described below. Very often the precise role of CMV and other competing pathogens is difficult to ascertain. There is clear indication in AIDS that the degree of morbidity and its extensiveness is determined by the degree of suppression of CD4 lymphocytes.

In the *transplant recipient*, two factors determine the degree of morbidity due to CMV. The first is the degree and type of immunosuppression. Deaths due to CMV infection may be related to the use of anti-thymocyte globulin.[93] The second is the type of organ transplantation. Morbidity due to CMV is lowest in kidney transplantation and highest in bone marrow transplantation (see Chapters 291 and 292).

Suwansirikul et al.[94] and Betts et al.[95] reported the clinical and laboratory findings on a total of 154 renal transplant patients with CMV infection. Primary infections were significantly more symptomatic, but only 19 percent of the secondary infections were febrile. In the series of Suwansirikul et al.,[94] 13 of 18 primary infections were associated with at least two of the following: fever, leukopenia, atypical lymphocytes, lymphocytosis, hepatosplenomegaly, myalgia, or arthralgia.

Betts et al.[95] found elevations of hepatic enzyme (SGOT) levels in 10 of 16 (63 percent) primary infections. Five had pneumonia. A striking feature of their series was that primary infections occurred mainly in younger recipients who received parental kidneys. They also found that rejection occurred in 4 of 16 patients with primary infection. Twenty-four seronegative patients who received kidneys from seronegative donors and remained uninfected did not reject them. This is one of the few studies that shows clearly that CMV infection may increase rejection.

An important indirect effect of primary CMV infection is an increase in both serious fungal and bacterial infections after renal and cardiac transplantation.[96] This is the clinical significance of the known nonspecific immunosuppressive effect of CMV infection.[97]

Interstitial Pneumonia. Next to fever and mononucleosis, the most common manifestation of CMV infection in the compromised host is pneumonitis. It has been described in the immunocompetent host but is more common in the immunosuppressed.[1] The pneumonitis is more likely to show an interstitial rather than alveolar pattern, but nodules or cavities may be seen on x-ray films. Association with pneumocystis may be striking. This is particularly true in the case of AIDS. CMV pneumonia may range from asymptomatic virus shedding to rapidly fatal pneumonia. Respiratory complaints were present usually less than 2 weeks. Consistently, fever, nonproductive cough, and dyspnea associated with hypoxia were observed. Hypoxia is a poor prognostic sign. Most who required respiratory assistance expired. The severity and lethality of CMV pneumonia probably varies in different types of patients and varying degrees of immunosuppression. This has been best studied in interstitial pneumonia after bone marrow transplantation and where the lung may be a target for a GvH reaction. Eighty-four percent died.[98] In a much smaller series of renal transplant patients, 48 percent died.[99]

Hepatitis. CMV infection in its mildest symptomatic form is usually associated with chemical hepatitis and elevation of serum hepatic enzyme levels. Jaundice and hyperbilirubinemia are distinctly unusual. We have rarely seen clinically significant CMV hepatitis in patients after renal transplantation. However, this has been described in other centers, perhaps as a complication of more severe immunosuppression from using anti-lymphocyte globulin. Aldrete et al.[100] reported gastrointestinal and hepatic complications affecting 126 patients after renal transplantation. Hepatic dysfunction occurred in 22 percent of the patients. Severe hepatitis was seen in seven, from all of whom CMV was isolated in the blood, urine, sputum, or feces. Autopsies on five of these patients revealed evidence of CMV in the liver.

However, even in centers where it is not seen in renal and other types of transplantations, CMV hepatitis has become an important general problem after liver transplantation in both adults and children.[70,101] Like most other severe CMV diseases in transplant recipients, it is more common after primary infection. It is also associated with grafting a liver from a CMV-seropositive donor.[65] Recognition of this is partly due to the frequent practice of protocol liver biopsy to manage rejection in the first months after transplantation. However, it is not just a matter of recognition because all cases had clinical hepatitis characterized by prolonged fever, bilirubinemia, and elevated enzyme concentrations. Liver failure due to CMV hepatitis requiring retransplantation has also been seen. The most important management problem is to distinguish between rejection and CMV hepatitis. This differential diagnosis can only be made by a study of the biopsy specimen.[101] It is important to make this differential diagnosis because rejection is treated by increasing immunosuppression while CMV infection may be helped by decreasing immunosuppression and instituting antiviral therapy.

Cytomegalovirus Disease of the Gastrointestinal Tract. The etiologic role of CMV is frequently difficult to evaluate because CMV may be a fellow-traveling "opportunist." This is particularly true of CMV in the gastrointestinal tract. CMV has, for example, been suspected to play a role in acute idiopathic ulcerative colitis[102] and in gastric ulcers occurring in a patient with CMV mononucleosis.[103] The evidence for a causal relationship is often weak.

In contrast to the above and despite the difficult of diagnosis, there is little doubt now that CMV may cause important and at times lethal gastrointestinal syndromes in the immunosuppressed. Transplant patients may develop gastrointestinal hemorrhages or perforation that may be traced to submucosal ulcerations anywhere in the gastrointestinal tract from the esophagus to the rectum.[1,99] Patients with AIDS and CMV colitis may present with explosive watery diarrhea. Occasionally there may also be hematochezia. Fever is common, and other intestinal pathogens such as cryptosporidia or *Mycobacterium avium-intracellulare* may be present at the same time. By endoscopy, there may be plaquelike pseudomembranes, multiple erosions and serpigenous ulcers,[104] or lesions resembling Kaposi's sarcoma.[105] Perforation and gangrene has been described, although CMV may not be the sole cause. CMV may be demonstrated by a culture of specimens or biopsy material, or there may be typical inclusion bodies in the submucosal endothelium[105] or mucosal crypts.[104]

Besides the gastrointestinal tract itself, CMV is known to involve both the acinar and islet components of the pancreas,[1] and it can be seen in acute pancreatitis in an AIDS patient.[106] Cholecystitis has been associated with finding CMV in the bile duct, the gall bladder, and the biliary tree.[106,107]

Cytomogalovirus Retinitis. Chorioretinitis is a well-recognized finding in congenital CMV infections. It is usually not acquired postnatally in children, and it is quite rare in immunocompetent subjects. Foerster[108] described CMV retinitis in an enucleated eye of a 59-year-old woman with no apparent underlying disease or immunosuppression. CMV retinitis is usually a manifestation of severe immunosuppression. It is seen in transplant patients, in cancer patients receiving immunosuppressive drugs,[109] and particularly in patients with AIDS.[110] In the transplant recipient, unlike the acute infection that usually occurs regularly 2–6 months after organ transplantation, CMV retinitis may occur at any time. It is in AIDS that we see the full scope of the devastating effects of CMV retinitis.

Nonspecific complaints of blurred vision, scotoma, and decreased visual activity are the most frequent ophthalmologic symptoms. Visual impairment is usually progressive and irreversible, particularly with central retinal involvement. Blindness in one or both eyes is the expected result. The disease, however, may also be asymptomatic or discovered only at autopsy.

CMV retinitis has a characteristic funduscopic and pathologic appearance (Fig. 1). Initially, white granular necrotic patches develop that may be superimposed with patches of flame-shaped intraretinal hemorrhages. Pathologic examination shows extensive necrosis and disruption of all layers of the sensory retina and pigment epithelium. Wyhinny et al.[111] pointed out that in adult CMV retinitis the lesions are restricted by Bruch's membrane and do not extend to the choroid.

Retinitis is often a sign of active systemic infection, frequently of disseminated nature. The diagnosis may be made on the basis of the distinctive ophthalmologic picture and laboratory evidence of CMV systemic infection. The virus has been cultured from the aqueous or vitreous humor,[112] although this is not essential for the diagnosis.

Meningoencephalitis and Encephalopathy. The most devastating component of congenital CID is its destructive effect

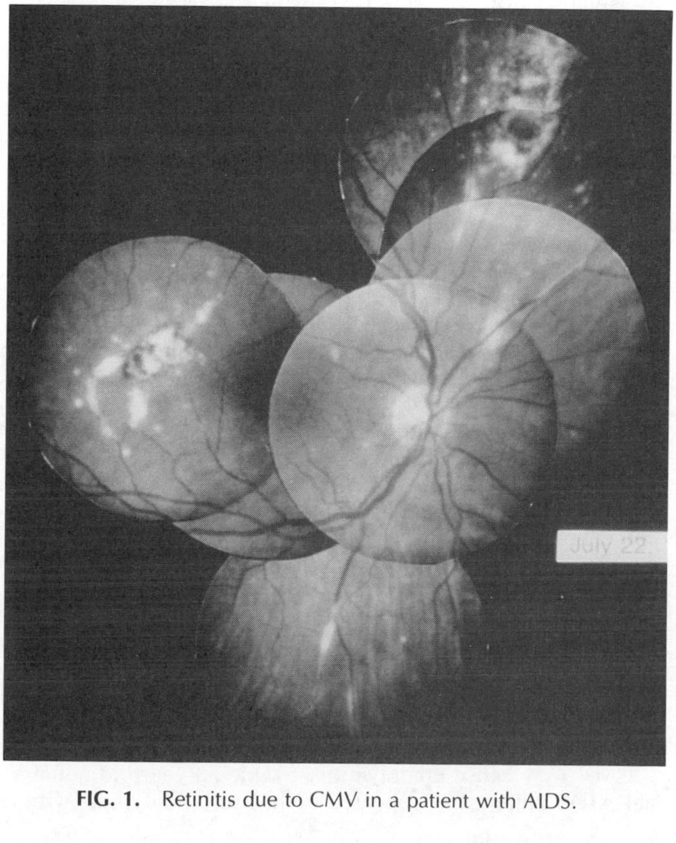

FIG. 1. Retinitis due to CMV in a patient with AIDS.

on the central nervous system. The severely brain-damaged infant may have periventricular calcifications, microcephaly, seizures, and spastic quadriplegia. About half of symptomatic congenital infections have some degree of central nervous system disease.[1] Asymptomatic ones may suffer late neurologic sequelae, the most important being neurosensory deafness (see above).

However, in postnatal life, the affinity of CMV for the central nervous system is much reduced, even in the immunosuppressed. When it has been found, its pathogenetic role is not always clear-cut. Rare cases of meningoencephalitis in immunocompetent individuals have been described. In two cases described by Phillips et al.,[113] the virus was isolated from a brain biopsy specimen and cerebrospinal fluid (CSF) as well as from urine. Both had headaches and minor CSF pleocytosis. Microglial and astrocyte proliferation with satellitosis of neurons and focal neuronal degeneration was found. Both patients recovered. Occasional cases of CMV encephalopathy have also been described in immunosuppressed transplant patients. The characteristic lesion is also microglial nodules, at times associated with cells that rarely have intranuclear inclusions.[114] However, it is in HIV infection and in AIDS that CMV has presented many neurologic complications, many of which remain to be clarified.

About 40 percent of patients with AIDS develop neurologic signs and symptoms. At postmortem examination, even more (78 percent) have pathologic changes in the central nervous system.[115–117] However, very likely the most common clinical central nervous system syndrome is due to HIV itself and is now subsumed under the term *AIDS dementia complex*.[117,118] This complex includes much of the pathology earlier ascribed to CMV such as the "subacute encephalitis" described by some authors.[115] The role of CMV in AIDS dementia complex is probably secondary.[118] The complex is associated with confusion, progressive dementia, and often, weakness and paresis. It is, however, possible that some cases are due to CMV, although when both HIV and CMV are present in the same lesion, it will be difficult to sort them out.

Other pathologic processes attributed to CMV and supported by isolation of CMV from CSF or neural tissues are CMV-induced demyelinating lesions associated with microglial nodules and lymphocyte infiltration in the brain[119] or spinal cord.[120] Clinically these cases would be difficult to distinguish from the HIV dementia and encephalitis complex, except for patients with radiculomyelitis, ascending myelitis, and necrotizing spinal lesions,[116] which may be more uniquely attributed to CMV.

Endocrinopathies and Glandular Involvement. The involvement of various endocrine organs as a part of disseminated CMV infection is well known, but clinical endocrinopathies were rare until the advent of AIDS. Diabetes mellitus may occur after congenital infection[121] and perhaps secondary to pancreatitis in an adult.[122] A case of acute CMV pancreatitis with histologic proof was described in a transplant patient.[123] A case of adrenal insufficiency in a healthy subject without pathologic proof is mentioned above.[88] Adrenalitis due to CMV is a common finding in AIDS patients. Of 41 autopsy cases, 21 showed cortical as well as medullary lesions.[124] However, no definite clinical evidence of adrenal cortical insufficiency was available even though hypotension and hyponatremia were common findings.

We have seen an AIDS patient who had CMV in his blood and CSF, who had CMV retinitis, and who developed adrenal insufficiency proven by a lack of adrenocorticotropic hormone (ACTH) stimulation. He also had diabetes insipidus controlled with vasopressin. I am not aware of any report of pathologic evidence of involvement of the posterior pituitary gland.

CMV may cause epididymitis.[125] One 33-year-old homosexual AIDS patient had repeated unilateral epididymitis with fevers that was resistant to antibiotics and treated with epididymectomy. Intracytoplasmic inclusions were seen in ductal epithelial cells.

Other related involvement by CMV in immunosuppressed adults includes a number of pathologic findings without clear clinical involvement: CMV oophoritis[126,127] and infection of the thyroid.[128] Two AIDS patients were described to have hypercalcemia, suppressed parathyroid activity, and disseminated CMV.[129]

TREATMENT AND PREVENTION OF CYTOMEGALOVIRUS INFECTIONS

Treatment

Specific treatment of systemic virus diseases until recently has been largely experimental. Putative antivirals were frequently not effective enough or too toxic. With the development of a series of promising nucleosides, specific therapy for infection with the herpesviruses is now an achievable goal. Unfortunately, CMV seems to be an unusually recalcitrant member of this group of viruses and is much more difficult to treat than is herpes simplex or varicella-zoster virus.

The treatment of a chronic viral infection in the immunosuppressed presents special problems. As in bacterial infections where the efficacy of certain antibiotics may be depressed because of the lack of critical host defenses essential for optimum effect of the drug, antivirals may have diminished effectiveness or may only be virus suppressive as long as they are administered. When they are removed, the infection reappears. Concurrent infections from other causes may complicate the picture. Compromised renal or other organ function may alter pharmacodynamics. The frequent bone marrow-suppressive or immunosuppressive properties of an antiviral agent itself may also complicate already considerable toxicity.

Interferon, a natural cytokine previously made in human leukocytes but now available as a recombinant product, can suppress CMV but is of questionable clinical usefulness. Hirsch et al.[130] reported that 3×10^6 units of α-interferon administered two to three times per week for 14 weeks after renal transplantation did not reduce infectivity, but morbidity among the infected was 5 percent (1/20) in the treated group while it was 32 percent (7/22) in the controls. This is a marginal benefit. α-Interferon was not effective for prophylaxis against CMV in bone marrow recipients.[131] It was also without therapeutic effect either alone or with other antivirals in the treatment of CMV pneumonia after bone marrow transplantation.[132]

Neither adenine-arabinoside (ara-A, vidarabine), or acyclovir, two FDA-approved nucleoside antivirals effective against herpes simplex and varicella-zoster viruses, can cure CMV infections.[133] However, high dose acyclovir (1500 mg/m^2 per day) was recently reported to reduce prophylactically CMV infections and disease in marrow recipients.[133a]

Ganciclovir. Ganciclovir is 10–100 times more effective than is acyclovir against herpes simplex and CMV infections.[134] Clinical trials in patients with CMV retinitis are encouraging. For example, one study involved 8 patients where 14 of 16 eyes showed active retinitis. When given 5 mg/kg intravenously two to three times a day for 3 weeks, 8 of 14 eyes with retinitis showed better than 90 percent resolution.[135,136] Blood and urine cultures for CMV became negative 1–4 weeks after the onset of therapy. However, all patients relapsed clinically and virologically 2–5 weeks after the cessation of therapy.

The response of other types of serious CMV disease was varied. If treatment was started early and if the patient survived long enough to benefit from treatment, efficacy was observed. For example, 30 of 40 patients with CMV gastrointestinal infection improved clinically, and a virologic response was seen in 32. Those who did not respond included eight who died within

4 weeks of treatment. Patients who responded relapsed as in the case of CMV retinitis. Early experience with ganciclovir in CMV pneumonia was discouraging. It did not have any effect in reducing mortality in bone marrow recipients.[137] Of 10 treated patients, 9 died, and the 10th showed no clinical improvement.

More recent data on the treatment of CMV pneumonia and other systemic disease due to CMV are somewhat more encouraging. For example, Erice et al.[138] report that 17 (55 percent) of 31 immunosuppressed patients with various types of CMV disease who received 2.5 mg/kg iv every 8 hours improved clinically during ganciclovir therapy. Viremia ceased in 93 percent (14/15) of the patients after a mean of 4.7 days of therapy. Unfortunately, it is difficult to document convincing efficacy in these anecdotal trials in which a control group is not available for comparison. A rigorous controlled trial may not be forthcoming because many clinicians believe that ganciclovir therapy is effective and, given a potentially lethal disease, it may not be possible to withhold ganciclovir. In view of the fact that interstitial CMV pneumonia in the marrow recipient may have an immunopathologic as well as viral element,[69a] recent reports indicate possible efficacy combining ganciclovir and immune globulin.[138a]

Passive Immune Prophylaxis

Large doses of γ-globulin may now be administered intravenously for therapeutic and prophylactic purposes with little toxicity. It has been used to decrease the frequency of CMV disease. Studies of hyperimmune plasma or globulin in bone marrow transplant recipients[139] and in kidney recipients[140] have demonstrated the efficacy of high-titered immune globulin in reducing disease, although not in preventing infection, in seronegative transplant recipients.

Winston et al.,[139] for example, illustrate one of many studies in marrow recipients. An equivalent of 1.0 g/kg immune globulin was administered to 38 recipients once weekly until day 120 after marrow transplantation; 37 were controls. Total CMV infection rates in the treated and control groups (47 and 57 percent) were not significantly different, but primary infections were significantly reduced by immune globulin (25 vs. 52 percent). Symptomatic CMV infection rates (21 vs. 46 percent), interstitial pneumonia due to CMV (16 vs. 32 percent), and deaths due to interstitial pneumonia (6 vs. 14 percent) were all significantly reduced. Most of the subjects in this study (63/75, or 84 percent) were negative for CMV antibodies before marrow transplantation. The CMV antibody titer of the preparation used in this study was 1:6400 by ELISA and 1:64 by neutralization. It should be pointed out that the best antibody test to titer immune serum is still unknown.

Besides marrow recipients, other transplant recipients are also being studied. Snydman et al.[140] elected to study only seronegative renal transplant recipients, of whom 24 were treated and 35 were controls. Those treated were given 150 mg/kg hyperimmune globulin within 72 hours of transplantation and 50–100 mg/kg every 2 weeks up to 16 weeks after kidney transplantation. CMV infection was not reduced when compared with controls (71 vs. 77 percent), but the rate of symptomatic disease was reduced significantly (21 and 60 percent). There was one death due to CMV in the treated and five in the control groups. This group of renal transplant patients seemed to have an unusually high rate of symptomatic CMV disease and deaths due to CMV, possibly related to the use of anti-thymocyte globulin. In summary, the prophylactic efficacy of immune globulin is probably best demonstrated in primary CMV infections and in situations where the morbidity of such infections is high. This is best illustrated in marrow transplantation. Morbidity, however, is not uniformly high in other transplant situations or under all immunosuppressive regimes. Whether immune globulin should be routinely used in kidney and other types of transplantations requires further studies and cost/benefit analyses.

Active Immunization

Though imperfect, active immunity develops after natural CMV infection and is an important part of humans' acquired immunity. The beneficial role of acquired immunity is attested to by the fact that most problems with CMV occur when it is absent in the host. Thus, congenital CMV disease follows primary infection in the mother when she has no acquired immunity, and in transplant patients, most severe symptomatic disease is also a consequence of primary infection in transplant patients. The efficacy of passive immunization in reducing CMV disease in seronegative transplant patients is further indirect proof of the importance of acquired immunity. Hence there is ample justification for the development of acquired immunity of active immunization. Two primary target populations may be considered for protective active immunization: the seronegative mother and the seronegative transplant recipient.

There have been a number of objections to the concept of using live CMV vaccine.[141] There are unanswered questions about strain variability of CMV isolates—and hence a possible lack of efficacy of a vaccine strain—and questions about the efficacy of humoral and cellular immunity developed by a vaccine. Live CMV vaccines may have troublesome long-term toxicity related to its persistence, latency, and potential transmissibility. CMV and other herpesviruses are also potentially oncogenic. Tests of the Towne strain of cell culture attenuated vaccine developed by Plotkin and his colleagues[142] seem to show that fears about its toxicity, persistence, and transmissibility are largely unfounded. Efficacy and cost-effectiveness in the immunosuppressed transplant patient, however, has not yet been conclusively proved. So far one live attenuated vaccine has been tested clinically in renal transplant recipients.[143,144] The rationale and strategy of immunizing seronegative mothers has not yet been worked out. The Towne attenuated vaccine produced an asymptomatic self-limited infection that resulted in the production of detectable antibodies and the development of a CMV-specific lymphocyte proliferative response in almost all healthy volunteers.[142] However, in a controlled clinical trial of 91 renal transplant recipients, 24 percent of the seronegative patients who received the vaccine failed to produce antibodies, and 5 of 6 also failed to develop a specific positive lymphocyte response while all 8 normal controls responded. The frequency of primary infection in seronegative recipients who received seropositive kidneys was similar in vaccinees and the placebo-treated subjects (15/16 or 94 percent vs. 11/14 or 78 percent). Also, the proportion of those infected who were symptomatic was not significantly different (60 vs. 91 percent). However, the degree of morbidity in the vaccines measured according to a quantitative scoring system was significantly lower (2.7 vs. 5.7).

The modest reduction in morbidity of CMV by the vaccine was not confirmed in a parallel study employing the same vaccine in Minnesota.[144] A total of 117 received the vaccine (6.6×10^3 viral infectious plaques), and 119 received placebo. Seventy-six percent of 63 seronegative subjects converted their antibody status after being immunized. Seropositive subjects also had a boost in their antibody titers.

Of the 236 study subjects, 47 (20 percent) developed CMV disease. There was a suggestion of protection by the vaccine among seronegative subjects who were given a seropositive kidney. Two of eight vaccinees with CMV disease had severe or lethal disease, while five of six placebo subjects with CMV disease experienced severe or lethal illness. This suggests that CMV disease was ameliorated, although the frequency of CMV disease in the vaccinated and placebo groups (38 and 43 percent) was not changed.

In summary, the Towne vaccine may have at best a marginal effect in preventing CMV disease due to primary infection. Future developments should aim at improving the immunogenicity of the vaccine in recipients. Other types of vaccines such as subunit and recombinant vaccines remain to be developed.

REFERENCES

1. Ho M. Cytomegalovirus: Biology and Infection. New York: Plenum; 1982:309.
2. Ribbert H. Ueber proozoanartige Zellen in der Niere eines syphilitischen Neugeborenen und in der Parotis von Kindern. Zentrabl Allg Pathol 1904;15:945–8.
3. Farber S, Wolbach SB. Intranuclear and cytoplasmic inclusions (protozoan-like bodies) in the salivary glands and other organs of infants. Am J Pathol. 1932;8:123–35.
4. Smith MG. Propagation of salivary gland virus of the mouse in tissue cultures. Proc Soc Exp Biol Med. 1954;86:435–40.
5. Smith MG. Propagation in tissue cultures of a cytopathogenic virus from human salivary gland virus (SGV) disease. Proc Soc Exp Biol Med. 1956;92:424–30.
6. Rowe WP, Hartley JW, Waterman S, et al. Cytopathogenic agent resembling human salivary gland virus recovered from tissue cultures of human adenoids. Proc Soc Exp Biol Med. 1956;92:418–24.
7. Weller TH, Macauley JC, Craig JM, et al. Isolation of intranuclear inclusion producing agents from infants with illnesses resembling cytomegalic inclusion disease. Proc Soc Exp Biol Med. 1957;94:4–12.
8. Weller TH, Hansahw JB, Scott DE. Serologic differentiation of viruses responsible for cytomegalic inclusion disease. Virology. 1960;12:130–2.
9. Klemola E, Karriaien L. Cytomegalovirus as a possible cause of a disease resembling infectious mononucleosis. Br Med J. 1965:1099–102.
10. Kaariainen L, Klemola E, Paloheimo J. Rise of cytomegalovirus antibodies in an infectious-mononucleosis–like syndrome after transfusion. Br Med J. 1966;2:1270–2.
11. Winston DJ, Ho WG, Howell CL, et al. Cytomegalovirus infections associated with leukocyte transfusions. Ann Intern Med. 1980;93:671–5.
12. Rinaldo CR, Black PH, Hirsch MS. Interactions of cytomegalovirus with leukocytes from patients with mononucleosis due to cytomegalovirus. J Inf Dis. 1977;136:667–678.
13. Rice GPA, Schrier RD, Oldstone MBA. Cytomegalovirus infects human lymphocytes and monocytes: Virus expression is restricted to immediate early antigen products. Proc Nat Acad Sci. 1984;81:6134–8.
14. Schrier RD, Nelson JA, Oldstone MBA. Detection of human cytomegalovirus in peripheral blood lymphocytes in a natural infection. Science. 1985;230:1048–51.
15. Giraldo G, Beth E, Coeur P, et al. Kaposi's sarcoma: A new model in the search for viruses associated with human malignancies. JNCI. 1972;49:1495–507.
16. Spector DH, Shaw SB, Hock LJ, et al. Association of human cytomegalovirus with Kaposi's sarcoma. In: Gottleib MS, Groopman JE, eds. Acquired Immune Deficiency Syndrome. New York: Alan R. Liss; 1984:109–26.
17. Fetterman GH. A new laboratory aid in the clinical diagnosis of inclusion disease of infancy. Am J Clin Pathol. 1952;22:424–5.
18. Martin WJ, Smith TJ. Rapid detection of cytomegalovirus in bronchoalveolar lavage specimens by a monoclonal antibody method. J Clin Microbiol. 1986;23:1006–8.
19. Chou S, Merigan TC. Rapid detection and quantitation of human cytomegalovirus in urine through DNA hybridization. N Engl J Med. 1983;308:921–5.
20. Churchill MA, Zaia JA, Forman SJ, et al. Quantitation of human cytomegalovirus DNA in lungs from bone marrow transplant recipients with interstitial pneumonia. J Infect Dis. 1987:155:501–9.
21. Lennette EH, Schmidt NJ. Diagnostic procedures for viral and rickettsial infections. 5th ed. New York: American Public Health Association; 1979:399–439.
22. Shuster EA, Beneke JS, Tegtmeier GE, et al. Monoclonal antibody for rapid laboratory detection of cytomegalovirus infections: Characterization and diagnostic application. Mayo Clinic Proc. 1985;60:577–85.
23. Rao N, Waruszewski DT, Ho M, et al. Evaluation of the anticomplement immunofluorescence test in cytomegalovirus infection. J Clin Microbiol. 1976;6:633–8.
24. Betts RF, George SD, Rundell BR, et al. Comparative activity of immunofluorescent antibody and complement-fixing antibody in cytomegalovirus infection. J Clin Microbiol. 1976;4:151–6.
25. Krech U. Complement-fixing antibodies against cytomegalovirus in different parts of the world. Bull WHO. 1973;49:103–6.
26. Stagno S, Reynolds DW, Pass RF, et al. Breast milk and the risk of cytomegalovirus infection. N Engl J Med. 1980;312:1073–4.
27. Hayes K, Danks DM, Gibas H, et al. Cytomegalovirus in human milk. N Engl J Med. 1972;287:177–8.
28. Gurevich I, Cunha BA. Nonparenteral transmission of cytomegalovirus in a neonatal intensive care unit. Lancet. 1981;2:222–4.
29. Pass RF, August AM, Dworsky M, et al. Cytomegalovirus infection in a day care center. N Engl J Med. 1982;307:477–9.
30. Olson LC, Ketusinha R, Mansuwan P, et al. Respiratory tract excretion of cytomegalovirus in Thai children. J Pediatr 1970;77:499–504.
31. Hanshaw JB, Steinfeld HJ, White CJ. Fluorescent-antibody test for cytomegalovirus macroglobulin. N Engl J Med. 1968;279:566–70.
32. Henle W, Henle G, Scriba M, et al. Antibody responses to the Epstein-Barr virus and cytomegaloviruses after open-heart and other surgery. N Engl J Med. 1970;282:1068–74.
33. Prince AM, Szmuness W, Millian SJ, et al. A serologic study of cytomegalovirus infections associated with blood transfusions. N Engl J Med. 1971;284:1125–31.
34. Armstrong JA, Tarr GC, Ho M, et al. Cytomegalovirus infection in children undergoing open-heart surgery. Yale J Biol Med. 1976;49:83–91.
35. Preiksaitis JK, Brown L, McKenzie M. The risk of cytomegalovirus infection in seronegative transfusion recipients not receiving exogenous immunosuppression. J Inf Dis. 1988;157:523–9.
36. Yeager AS, Grumet FC, Hafleigh EB, et al. Prevention of transfusion-acquired cytomegalovirus infections in newborn infants. J Pediatr. 1981;98:281–7.
37. Chou S, Kim DY, Norman DJ. Transmission of cytomegalovirus by pretransplant leukocyte transfusions in renal transplant candidates. J Infect Dis. 1987;155:565–7.
38. Alexander ER. Maternal and neonatal infection with cytomegalovirus in Taiwan (Abstract). Pediatr Res. 1967;1:210.
39. Chandler SH, Handsfield HH, McDougall JK. Isolation of multiple strains of cytomegalovirus from women attending a clinic for sexually transmitted diseases. J Infect Dis. 1987;155:655–60.
40. Chretien JH, McGinnis CG, Muller A. Veneral causes of cytomegalovirus mononucleosis. JAMA. 1977;238:1644–5.
41. Lang DJ, Kummer JF. Demonstration of cytomegalovirus in semen. N Engl J Med. 1972;287:756–8.
42. Collier AC, Meyers JD, Corey L, et al. Cytomegalovirus infection in homosexual men. Am J Med 1987;82:493–600.
43. Drew WL, Mills J, Levy J, et al. Cytomegalovirus infection and abnormal T-leukocyte subset ratios in homosexual men. Ann Intern Med. 1985;103:61–3.
44. Kingsley LA, Detels R, Kaslow R, et al. Risk factors for seroconversion to human immunodeficiency virus among male homosexuals. Lancet. 1987;2:345–9.
45. Numazaki Y, Yano N, Morizuka T, et al. Primary infection with human cytomegalovirus: Virus isolation from healthy infants and pregnant women. Am J Epidemiol. 1970;91:410–17.
46. Montgomery RL, Youngblood LA, Medearis DN Jr. Recovery of cytomegalovirus from the cervix in pregnancy. Pediatrics. 1972;49:524–31.
47. Stagno S, Reynolds D, Tsiantos A, et al. Cervical cytomegalovirus excretion in pregnant and non-pregnant women: Suppression in early gestation. J Infect Dis. 1975;131:522–7.
48. Reynolds DW, Stagno S, Hosty TS, et al. Maternal cytomegalovirus excretion and perinatal infection. N Engl J Med. 1973;289:1–5.
49. Stagno S, Pass RF, Dworsky ME, et al. Congenital and perinatal cytomegalovirus infections. Semin Perinatol. 1983;7:31–42.
50. Griffiths PD, Stagno S, Pass RF, et al. Infection with cytomegalovirus during pregnancy: Specific IgM antibodies as a marker of recent primary infection. J Infect Dis. 1982;145:647–53.
51. Monif GRG, Egan EA II, Held B, et al. The correlation of maternal cytomegalovirus infection during varying stages in gestation with neonatal involvement. J Pediatr. 1972;80:17–20.
52. Stern H, Tucker SM. Prospective study of cytomegalovirus infection in pregnancy. Br Med J. 1973;2:268–70.
53. Nankervis GA, Kumar ML, Gold E. Primary infection with cytomegalovirus during pregnancy. Pediatr Res. 1974;8:427.
54. Stagno S, Pass RF, Dworsky ME, et al. Congenital cytomegalovirus infection: The relative importance of primary and recurrent maternal infection. N Engl J Med. 1982;306:945–9.
55. Stagno S, Whitley RJ. Herpesvirus infections of pregnancy. Part I: Cytomegalovirus and Epstein-Barr virus infections. N Engl J Med. 1985;313:1270–4.
56. Ahlfors K, Harris S, Ivarsson S, et al. Secondary maternal cytomegalovirus infection causing symptomatic congenital infection. N Engl J Med. 1981;305:284.
57. Ho M, Suwansirikul S, Dowling JN, et al. The transplanted kidney as a source of cytomegalovirus infection. N Engl J Med. 1975;293:1109–12.
58. Betts RF, Freeman RB, Douglas RG Jr, et al. Transmission of cytomegalovirus infection with renal allograft. Kidney Int. 1975;8:387–94.
59. Ho M. Virus infections after transplantation in man. Arch Virol. 1977;55:1–24.
60. Dowling JN, Saslow AR, Ho M, et al. Cytomegalovirus infection in patients receiving immunosuppressive therapy for rheumatologic disorders. J Infect Dis. 1976;133:399–408.
61. Rubin RH. Infection in the renal transplant patient. In: Rubin, RH, Young, LS, eds. Clinical Approach to Infection in the Compromised Host. New York: Plenum; 1981:553–605.
62. Dummer JS, Hardy A, Poorsattar A, et al. Early infections in kidney, heart and liver transplant recipients on cyclosporine. Transplantation. 1983;36:259–67.
63. Ho M, Wajszczuk CP, Hardy A, et al. Infections in kidney, heart and liver transplant recipients on cyclosporine. Transplant Proc. 1983;15:2768–72.
64. Dummer JS, Montero CG, Griffith BP, et al. Infections in heart-lung transplant recipients. Transplantation. 1986;41:725–9.
65. Singh N, Dummer JS, Ho M, et al. Infections with cytomegalovirus and other herpesviruses in 121 liver transplant recipients: Transmission by donated organ and the effect of OKT3 antibodies. J Infect Dis. 1988;158:124–31.
66. Neiman P, Wasserman PB, Wentworth BB, et al. Interstitial pneumonia and cytomegalovirus infection as complications of human marrow transplantation. Transplantation. 1973;15:478–85.

67. Wu BC, Dowling JN, Ho M, et al. Enhancement of mouse cytomegalovirus infection during host versus graft reaction. Science. 1975;190:56–8.
68. Dowling JN, Wu BC, Ho M, et al. Enhancement of murine cytomegalovirus infection during graft versus host reaction. J Infect Dis. 1977;135:990–4.
69. Meyers JD, Spencer HC Jr, Watts JC, et al. Cytomegalovirus pneumonia after human marrow transplantation. Ann Intern Med. 1975;82:181–8.
69a. Grundy JE, Schanley JD, Griffiths PD. Is cytomegalovirus interstitial pneumonitis in transplant patients an immunopathological condition? Lancet. 1987;2:996–9.
70. Bronsther O, Makowka L, Jaffe R, et al. The occurrence of cytomegalovirus hepatitis in liver transplant patients. J Med Virol. 1988. In press.
71. Wong TW, Warner NE. Cytomegalic inclusion disease in adults. Arch Pathol. 1962;74:403–21.
72. Bodey GP, Wertlake PT, Douglas G, et al. Cytomegalic inclusion disease in patients with acute leukemia. Ann Intern Med. 1965;62:899–906.
73. Henson D, Siegel SE, Fuccillo DA, et al: Cytomegalovirus infections during acute childhood leukemia. J Infect Dis. 1972;126:469–81.
74. Spector SA, Hirata KK, Neuman TR. Identification of multiple cytomegalovirus strains in homosexual men with acquired immunodeficiency syndrome. J Infect Dis. 1984;6:953–6.
75. Fiala M, Cone LA, Chang CM. Cytomegalovirus viremia increases with progressive immune deficiency in patients infected with HTLV-III. AIDS Res. 1986;2:175–81.
76. Hanshaw JB. Developmental abnormalities associated with congenital cytomegalovirus infection. In: Wollam DHM, ed. Advances in Teratology. v. 4. New York: Academic Press; 1970:64.
77. Hanshaw JB, Scheiner AP, Moxley AW, et al. School failure and deafness after "silent" congenital cytomegalovirus infection. N Engl J Med. 1976;295:468–70.
78. Conboy TJ, Pass RF, Stagno S, et al. Intellectual development in school-aged children with asymptomatic congenital cytomegalovirus infection. Pediatrics. 1986;77:801–6.
79. Stagno S, Reynolds DW, Amos CS, et al. Auditory and visual defects resulting from symptomatic and sublinical congenital cytomegaloviral and toxplasma infections. Pediatrics. 1977;59:669–78.
80. Klemola E, von Essen R, Henle G, et al. Infectious-mononucleosis–like disease with negative heterophil agglutination test. Clinical features in relations to Epstein-Barr virus and cytomegalovirus and antibodies. J Infect Dis. 1970;121:608–14.
81. Klemola E, Stenstrom R, von Essen R. Pneumonia as a clinical manifestation of cytomegalovirus infection in previously healthy adults. Scand J Infect Dis. 1972;4:7–10.
82. Carter AR. Cytomegalovirus disease presenting as hepatitis. Br Med J. 1968;3:786.
83. Bonkowsky HL, Lee RV, Klatskin G. Acute granulomatous hepatitis: Occurrence in cytomegalovirus mononucleosis. JAMA. 1984;233:1284–8.
84. Leonard JC, Tobin JOH. Polyneuritis associated with cytomegalovirus infections. Q J Med. 1971;40:435–42.
85. Schmitz H, Enders G. Cytomegalovirus as a frequent cause of Guillain-Barré syndrome. J Med Virol 1977;1:21–7.
86. Klemola E, Kaariainen L, von Essen R, et al. Further studies on cytomegalovirus mononucleosis in previously healthy individuals. Acta Med Scand 1967;182:311–22.
87. Tiula E, Leinikki P. Fatal cytomegalovirus infection in a previously healthy boy with myocarditis and consumption coagulopathy as presenting signs. Scand J Infect Dis. 1972;4:57–60.
88. Waris E, Rasanen P, Kreus KE, et al. Fatal cytomegalovirus disease in a previously healthy adult. Scand J Infect Dis. 1972;4:61–7.
89. Chanarin I, Walford DM. Thrombocytopenic purpura in cytomegalovirus mononucleosis. Lancet. 1973;1:238–9.
90. Harris AI, Meyer RJ, Brody EA. Cytomegalovirus-induced thrombocytopenia and hemolysis in an adult. Ann Intern Med. 1975;83:670–1.
91. Klemola E. Hypersensitivity reactions to ampicillin in cytomegalovirus mononucleosis. Scand J Infect Dis. 1970;2:29–31.
92. Muller-Stamou A, Senn HJ, Emody G. Epidermolysis in a case of severe cytomegalovirus infection. Br Med J. 1974;3:609–10.
93. Ho M. Infection and organ transplantation. In: Gelman S, ed. Anesthesia and Organ Transplantation. Philadelphia: WB Saunders; 1987:49–60.
94. Suwansirikul S, Rao N, Dowling JN, et al. Primary and secondary cytomegalovirus infection. Arch Intern Med. 1977;137:1026–9.
95. Betts RF, Freeman RB, Douglas RG, et al. Clinical manifestations of renal allograft derived primary cytomegalovirus infection. Am J Dis Child. 1977;131:759–63.
96. Chatterjee SN, Fiala M, Weiner J, et al. Primary cytomegalovirus and opportunistic infections. Incidence in renal transplant recipients. JAMA. 1978;240:2446–9.
97. Carney WP, Rubin RH, Hoffman RA, et al. Analysis of T-lymphocyte subsets in cytomegalovirus mononucleosis. J Immunol. 1981;126:2114–6.
98. Meyers JD, Flournoy N, Thomas ED. Risk factors for cytomegalovirus infection after human marrow transplantation. J Infect Dis. 1986;153:478–88.
99. Petersen PK, Balfour HH Jr, Marker SC, et al. Cytomegalovirus disease in renal allograft recipients. A prospective study of the clinical features, risk factors and impact on renal transplantation. Medicine (Baltimore). 1980;59:283–300.
100. Aldrete JS, Sterling WA, Hathaway BM, et al. Gastrointestinal and hepatic complications affecting patients with renal allografts. Am J Surg. 1975;129:115–24.
101. Demetris AJ, Lasky S, Van Thiel DH, et al. Pathology of hepatic transplantation. Am J Pathol. 1985;116:151–61.
102. Powell RD, Warner NE, Levin RS. Cytomegalic inclusion disease and ulcerative colitis. Am J Med 1961;30:334–40.
103. Campbell DA, Piercey JRA, Schnika TK. Cytomegalovirus-associated gastric ulcer. Gastroenterology. 1977;72:533–5.
104. Knapp AB, Horst DA, Eliopoulos G, et al. Widespread cytomegalovirus gastroenterocolitis in a patient with acquired immunodeficiency syndrome. Gastroenterology. 1983;85:1399–402.
105. Meiselman MS, Cello JP, Margaretten W. Cytomegalovirus colitis. Report of the clinical, endoscopic, and pathologic findings in two patients with acquired immune deficiency syndrome. Gastroenterology. 1985;88:171–5.
106. Texidor HS, Honig CL, Norsoph E, et al. Cytomegalovirus infection of the alimentary canal: Radiologic findings with pathologic correlation. Radiology. 1987;163:317–23.
107. Blumberg RS, Kelsey P, Perrone T, et al. Cytomegalovirus- and cryptosporidium-associated acalculous gangrenous cholecystitis. Am J Med 1984;76:1118–23.
108. Foerster HW. Pathology of granulomatous uveitis. Surv Ophthalmol. 1959;4:296.
109. Egbert PR, Pillard RB, Gallagher JB, et al. Cytomegalovirus retinitis in immunosuppressed hosts. II. Ocular manifestations. Ann Intern Med. 1980;93:664–70.
110. Holland GN, Gottlieb MS, Yu RD, et al. Ocular disorders associated with a new severe acquired cellular immune deficiency syndrome. Am J Ophthalmol. 1982;93:393–402.
111. Wyhinny GJ, Apple DJ, Guastella FR. Adult cytomegalic incusion retinitis. Am J Ophthalmol. 1973;76:773–81.
112. Friedman AH, Orellana J, Freeman WR, et al. Cytomegalovirus retinitis: A manifestation of the acquired immune deficiency syndrome (AIDS). Br J Ophthalmol. 1981;67:372–80.
113. Phillips CA, Fanning WL, Gump DW, et al. Cytomegalovirus encephalitis in immunologically normal adults. Successful treatment with vidarabine. JAMA. 1977;28:2299–300.
114. Dorfman LJ. Cytomegalovirus encephalitis in adults. Neurology (NY). 1973;23:136–44.
115. Nielsen SL, Petito CK, Urmacher CD, et al. Subacute encephalitis in acquired immune deficiency syndrome: A postmortem study. Am J Clin Pathol. 1984;82:678–82.
116. Wiley CA, Schrier RD, Denaro FJ, et al. Localization of cytomegalovirus proteins and genome during fulminant central nervous system in an AIDS patient. Neuropathol Exp Neurol. 1986;45:127–39.
117. Morgello S, Cho ES, Nielsen, S. Cytomegalovirus encephalitis in patients with acquired immunodeficiency syndrome: An autopsy study of 30 cases and a review of the literature. Hum Pathol. 1987;289–97.
118. Navia BA, Jordon BD, Price RW. The AIDS dementia complex: I. Clinical features. Ann Neurol. 1986;19:517–24.
119. Munoz DG, Perl DP, Pendlebury WW. Comparison of cytomegalovirus infection of brain and lung in a patient with subacute encephalopathy of acquired immunodeficiency syndrome. Arch Pathol Lab Med. 1987;111:234–7.
120. Moskowitz LB, Gregorios JB, Hensley GT, et al. Cytomegalovirus–induced demyelination associated with acquired immune deficiency syndrome. Arch Pathol Lab Med. 1984;108:873–7.
121. Ward KP, Galloway WH, Auchterlonie IA. Congenital cytomegalovirus infection and diabetes. Lancet. 1979;1:497.
122. Leonard JC, Tobin JOH. Polyneuritis associated with cytomegalovirus infections. Q J Med. 1971;40:435–42.
123. Parham DM. Post-transplantation pancreatitis associated with cytomegalovirus (report of a case). Hum Pathol. 1981;12:663–5.
124. Glasgow BJ, Steinsapir KD, Anders K, et al. Adrenal pathology in the acquired immune deficiency syndrome. Am J Clin Pathol. 1985;84:594–7.
125. Randazzo RF, Hulette CM, Gottlieb MS, et al. Cytomegaloviral epididymitis in a patient with the acquired immune deficiency syndrome. J Urol. 1986;1095–7.
126. Subietas, A, Deppisch LM, Astarloa J. Cytomegalovirus oophoritis: Ovarian cortical necrosis. Hum Pathol. 1977;8:285–92.
127. LiVolsi VA, Merino MJ. Cytomegalovirus infection of ovarian thecoma. Arch Pathol Lab Med. 1979;103:653–4.
128. Frank TS, LiVolsi VA, Connor AM. Cytomegalovirus infection of the thyroid in immunocompromised adults. Yale J Biol Med. 1987;60:1–8.
129. Zaloga GP, Chernow B, Eil C. Hypercalcemia and disseminated cytomegalovirus infection in the acquired immunodeficiency syndrome. Ann Intern Med. 1985;102:331–3.
130. Hirsch MS, Schooley RT, Cosimi AB, et al. Effects of interferon-alpha on cytomegalovirus reactivation syndromes in renal-transplant recipients. 1983;308:1489–93.
131. Meyers JD, Mcguffin RW, Bryson YJ, et al. Treatment of cytomegalovirus pneumonia after marrow transplant with combined vidarabine and human leukocyte interferon. J Infect Dis. 1982;146:80–2.
132. Meyers JD, Flournoy N, Sanders JE, et al. Prophylactic use of human leukocyte interferon after allogeneic marrow transplantation. Ann Intern Med. 1987;107:809–16.
133. Shepp DH, Newton BA, Meyers JD. Intravenous lymphoblastoid interferon and acyclovir for treatment of cytomegaloviral pneumonia. J Infect Dis. 1984;150:776–77.
133a. Meyers JD, Reed EC, Shepp DH, et al. Acyclovir for prevention of cy-

tomegalovirus infection and disease after allogenic marrow transplantation. New Engl J Med. 1988;318:70–75.
134. Mar EC, Cheng YC, Huang ES. Effect of 9-(1,3-dihydroxy-2-propoxymethyl) guanine on human cytomegalovirus replication in vitro. Antimicrob Agents Chemother. 1984;24:518–21.
135. Masur H, Lane HC, Palestine A, et al. Effect of 9-(1,3-dihydroxy-2-propoxymethyl) guanine on serious cytomegalovirus disease in eight immunosuppressed homosexual men. Ann Intern Med. 1986;104:41–4.
136. Palestine AG, Rodrigues MM, Macher AM, et al. Ophthalmic involvement in acquired immunodeficiency syndrome. Ophthalmology. 1984;91:1092–9.
137. Shepp DH, Dandliker PS, de Miranda P, et al. Activity of 9-(2-hydroxy-1-(hydroxymethyl)ethoxymethyl) guanine in the treatment of cytomegalovirus pneumonia. Ann Intern Med. 1985;103:368–73.
138. Erice A, Jordon MC, Chase BA, et al. Ganciclovir treatment of cytomegalovirus disease in transplant recipients and other immunocompromised hosts. JAMA. 1987;257:3082–7.
138a. Reed EC, Bowden RA, Dandliker PS, et al. Treatment of cytomegalovirus pneumonia with ganciclovir and intravenous cytomegalovirus immunoglobulin in patients with bone marrow transplants. Ann Intern Med. 1988;109:738–88.
139. Winston DJ, Ho WG, Lin CH, et al. Intravenous immune globulin for prevention of cytomegalovirus infection and interstitial pneumonia after bone marrow transplantation. Ann Intern Med. 1987;106:12–8.
140. Snydman DR, Werner BG, Heinze-Lacey B, et al. Use of cytomegalovirus immune globulin to prevent cytomegalovirus disease in renal-transplant recipients. N Engl J Med. 1987;317:1049–54.
141. Osborn JE. Cytomegalovirus: Pathogenicity, immunology, and vaccine initiatives. J Infect Dis. 1981;143:618–30.
142. Plotkin SA, Farquhar J, Hornberger E. Clinical trials of immunization with the Towne 125 strain of human cytomegalovirus. J Infect Dis. 1976;134:470–5.
143. Plotkin SA, Smiley ML, Friedman HM, et al. Towne-vaccine–induced prevention of cytomegalovirus disease after renal transplants. Lancet. 1984;1:528–30.
144. Balfour HH Jr, Welo PK, Sach GW. Cytomegalovirus vaccine trial in 400 renal transplant candidates. Transplant Proc. 1985;17:81–3.

121. EPSTEIN-BARR VIRUS (INFECTIOUS MONONUCLEOSIS)

ROBERT T. SCHOOLEY
RAPHAEL DOLIN

Epstein-Barr virus (EBV) is a ubiquitous member of the human herpesvirus group. Infection with EBV is common, worldwide in distribution, and largely subclinical in early childhood. EBV has been established as the etiologic agent of heterophile-positive infectious mononucleosis, which occurs most frequently in late adolescence or early adulthood. In addition, an association between EBV and African Burkitt's lymphoma as well as between EBV and nasopharyngeal carcinoma has been suggested by seroepidemiologic data and by the detection of the EBV genome in cells from both tumors. However, the potential etiologic relationship between EBV and these tumors remains to be established.

HISTORY

Historical accounts of infectious mononucleosis often ascribe the initial description of the disease to Filatov or Pfeiffer who nearly simultaneously at the end of the nineteenth century described an illness characterized by malaise, fever, hepatosplenomegaly, lymphadenopathy, and abdominal discomfort.[1,2] This illness came to be known as Drusenfieber (glandular fever) and occurred in family outbreaks. However, without specific techniques with which to establish the diagnosis, the concept of Drusenfieber as a clinical entity fell into disrepute. Between 1910 and 1920 a number of observers reported cases of apparent spontaneous remission of leukemia, with a clinical course that is consistent with the spontaneous resolution of infectious mononucleosis.[3,4] The establishment of infectious mononucleosis as a clinical entity is credited to Sprunt and Evans who in 1921 described six cases of fever, lymphadenopathy, and prostration occurring in previously healthy young adults.[5] The authors pointed out the mononuclear lymphocytosis that developed in each of the patients and contrasted the "pathologic" appearance of these lymphocytes to the uniform lymphocyte morphology observed in children with other infections. Two years later, Downey and McKinlay described additional cases of infectious mononucleosis and provided a more detailed morphologic description of the atypical lymphocyte.[6] The recognition of atypical lymphocytosis as a hematologic marker for the disease led to more accurate descriptions of the clinical manifestations of illness.

A major advance occurred in 1932 when Paul and Bunnell, investigating immunologic mechanisms in serum sickness, unexpectedly encountered high titers of spontaneously occurring sheep red blood cell agglutinins in the sera of patients with infectious mononucleosis.[7] Davidsohn later enhanced the specificity of detection of this heterophile antibody by differential absorption of serum with guinea pig kidney and with beef erythrocytes.[8]

During the 1940s and 1950s, substantial efforts were made to detect an etiologic agent for infectious mononucleosis. Attempts to culture etiologically related bacteria and viruses from patients with infectious mononucleosis proved unsuccessful. The disease could not be transmitted to animals. Interpretation of experimental attempts to transmit the disease to humans was hindered by the failure to appreciate the widespread occurrence of asymptomatic infection in preadolescents as well as the absence of a serologic marker of immunity.[9–11]

The identification of EBV followed the description by Burkitt in 1958 of an unusual lymphoma with a predilection for the head and neck.[12] The geographic distribution of this tumor paralleled that of certain mosquito-borne diseases in Africa, and a search for an etiologically related arbovirus was undertaken. Epstein and associates in 1964 described the presence of particles that resembled herpesviruses in tissue cultures of biopsy specimens from patients with Burkitt's lymphoma.[13] However, attempts to propagate the virus in conventional tissue cultures were unsuccessful. An indirect immunofluorescent antibody technique to this virus, now called Epstein-Barr virus, was developed by Werner and Gertrude Henle,[14] and high titers of this antibody were detected in patients with Burkitt's lymphoma. Additional studies revealed that 90 percent of American adults had demonstrable EBV antibodies as well.[14] The development of infectious mononucleosis in a technician in the Henles' laboratory on whom sequentially obtained sera were analyzed for EBV antibody suggested that acute EBV infection may be associated with this illness.[15] Large-scale epidemiologic studies[16–19] demonstrated that heterophile-positive infectious mononucleosis occurred in patients without pre-existing EBV antibody and, conversely, heterophile-positive infectious mononucleosis was always accompanied by acquisition of EBV antibodies. These epidemiologic studies indicated that subclinical EBV infection also occurred. With specific antibody tests for EBV, it became apparent that 10–20 percent of the cases of mononucleosis, of which most are heterophile-negative, were caused by other agents, of which the most frequent was cytomegalovirus (CMV). This chapter deals primarily with EBV-induced infectious mononucleosis.

DESCRIPTION OF EPSTEIN-BARR VIRUS

Physical Properties

Epstein-Barr virus has the characteristic morphology of the herpesvirus group of viruses of which it is a member. By electron microscopy, individual virions are 180–200 nm in diameter and appear as hexagonal nucleocapsids surrounded by a complex envelope. Enveloped virus has a buoyant density of 1.186 g/cm^3 in CsCl. The nucleocapsids are 100 nm in diameter and consist of an orderly array of capsomeres with the 5:3:2 symmetry seen in the herpesvirus group.[20] Acrylamide gel electrophoresis of purified EBV preparations has identified more than 30 polypeptides with molecular weights from 2.8×10^4 to 2.9×10^5.[21] EBV DNA is double stranded with a molecular weight of $101 \pm 3 \times 10^6$ and a buoyant density of 1.718 g/cm^3 in CsCl.[22] This buoyant density corresponds to a guanosine-plus-cytosine content of 58 percent.

Biologic Properties

The host range of the virus is quite limited. In vitro cultivation of the virus has been described only in B lymphocytes and nasopharyngeal epithelial cells of humans and certain nonhuman primates.[23] The virus generally does not produce cytopathic effects in infected cells. After infection by the virus, cells that contain the EBV genome are capable of continuous in vitro cultivation, and are termed *transformed* or *immortalized*. EBV has been confirmed as the transforming agent by the detection of viral antigens by indirect immunofluorescence within the nuclei of transformed cells or by hybridization of cellular DNA with purified EBV DNA.

Epstein-Barr virus receptors are demonstrable on B lymphocytes and nasopharyngeal epithelial cells of humans and certain nonhuman primates.[24,25] EBV receptors are also present on a smaller proportion of complement receptor–bearing, non-B, non-T lymphocytes.[26–28] The EBV receptor has recently been identified as the receptor for the d region of the third component of complement.[29,30] The C3d receptor (also known as CR2 or CD21), a 145 kD glycoprotein, is encoded by a member of a multiple gene family that specifies a number of cell membrane molecules.

After attachment to the receptor, the virus gains entry to susceptible B lymphocytes. Before the detection of virus-directed protein synthesis, Epstein-Barr nuclear antigens (EBNA) are demonstrable in nuclei of infected cells.[31] At high multiplicities of infection up to 25 percent of EBV-exposed B lymphocytes express EBNA.[32] Viral DNA synthesis is initiated with the production of multiple copies of the EBV genome. In transformed cells from patients with infectious mononucleosis or Burkitt's lymphoma, some viral DNA may be incorporated into the DNA of the host cell, although most of the DNA remains in a circular nonintegrated form as an episome. Linear integration of EBV DNA into host cell DNA may be enhanced by stimulation of the host cells by B-cell mitogens such as bacterial lipopolysaccharide at the time of transformation.[33] The host cell gains the property of immortality whether the virus is present in integrated, in episomal, or in a combination of the two forms.[33] The recent application of molecular biologic techniques to the study of immortalization has provided insights into the roles played by EBNAs in cellular transformation events.[34–39] These nuclear antigens include at least five different nuclear proteins. Expression of EBNA2 in the nucleus of transformed B lymphocytes is associated with induction of the B-cell activation antigen CD23.[40–42] Under most culture conditions 10 percent or fewer of EBV-exposed B lymphocytes form continuous cell lines.[32] After transformation, the host cell replicates, and the progeny cells contain several EBV genocopies in latent form. Viral expression in transformed cells is dependent on both intra- and extracellular regulatory phenomena. In addition to viral antigens. EBV-transformed B lymphocytes produce and/or secrete immunoglobulin.[43–46] Although most polyclonally transformed lines produce immunoglobulin of the IgM class, studies of clonally transformed B lymphocytes indicate that EBV is capable of induction of the synthesis of immunoglobulin of the IgG, IgA, or IgM classes.[47]

Cell lines that contain EBV genomes are characterized as producer or nonproducer lines. In producer lines, a variable proportion of cells contains viral capsid antigen (VCA) and releases mature virions. VCA is not demonstrable in the cytoplasm of nonproducer cell lines. Growth in the presence of 5′-bromodeoxyuridine (BUdR) or 5-iodo-2-deoxyuridine (IUDR) or in arginine-free medium induces expression of EBV early antigens.[48] Early antigens may also be induced by superinfection of nonproducer cell lines by EBV capable of lytic infection.[49] Most of the time EBV remains in latent form both in vitro in established cell lines and in vivo in circulating lymphocytes.

EPIDEMIOLOGY

Serum Antibody Prevalence

Antibodies to EBV have been found in all population groups studied, and most studies have shown no predilection for either sex. Antibodies are acquired earlier in life in tropical than in industrialized countries, but by adulthood 90–95 percent of most populations have demonstrable EBV antibodies.[50,51] In the United States and in Great Britain, EBV seroconversion occurs before the age of 5 in about 50 percent of the population.[51–53] A second wave of seroconversion occurs midway through the second decade of life. EBV seroconversion may occur at a younger average age in the southern United States than in other areas of the country.[54] Lower socioeconomic groups have a higher EBV antibody prevalence than do more affluent age-matched controls. The reported increased prevalence of EBV antibodies among blacks probably reflects this socioeconomic distribution.

Incidence of Infection

Clinically apparent infectious mononucleosis occurs most frequently in populations in which primary EBV exposure is delayed until the second decade of life. The disease is diagnosed most frequently among adolescents of higher socioeconomic groups in industrialized countries.[55] The incidence of infectious mononucleosis in a large epidemiologic study in this country was 45.2 cases/100,000/yr.[56] The incidence was highest in the 15- to 24-year-old age group. The incidence was the same for women as for men, but the peak age-specific incidence occurred 2 years earlier in women. The incidence of infectious mononucleosis was 30 times higher for whites than for blacks. The infrequency of infectious mononucleosis among blacks, noted as early as 1940, is probably a reflection of earlier primary EBV infection and the higher frequency of subclinical infections in children.[57–59] No clear seasonal incidence has been noted.

Methods of Spread

Low titers of EBV are present in throat washings of those with infectious mononucleosis.[60–62] Susceptible roommates of students with infectious mononucleosis or with inapparent EBV infection experience EBV seroconversion no more frequently than the general susceptible college population does.[18,54] Only 6 percent of those with infectious mononucleosis cite previous contact with another case of infectious mononucleosis.[56] The virus persists in the oropharynx of patients with infectious mononucleosis for up to 18 months after clinical recovery.[63] It can be cultured from throat washings from 10 to 20 percent of normal healthy adults, from 50 percent of renal transplant recipients, and from greater proportions of those critically ill with leukemia or lymphoma (Table 1).[64–66] EBV sequences and/or antigens have also been identified in parotid duct and uterine cervical epithelia, although the implications of this distribution are unclear with respect to viral transmission.[67,68]

EBV, like other herpesviruses, is relatively labile in the laboratory, and the virus has not been recovered from environ-

TABLE 1. Frequency of EBV Shedding

Population Description	Oropharyngeal Shedding Rate (%) (Range)	Reference
EBV-seronegatives	0	61
Seropositive healthy adults	12–25	61, 64–66
Solid tumor patients	27	65, 66
Renal transplant recipients	56–70	64, 66
Infectious mononucleosis patients	50–100	60–63
Critically ill leukemia or lymphoma patients	74–92	65, 66

mental sources, including fomites. These data suggest that EBV is a widespread agent of low contagiousness and that most cases of infectious mononucleosis are probably contracted by intimate contact between susceptibles and asymptomatic shedders of EBV. Among young adults spread of the virus may be facilitated by the transfer of saliva with kissing.[69,70] Serologic evidence suggests that the virus may also be spread among susceptible siblings within families.[71] Infectious mononucleosis has also been spread by blood transfusion and after open heart surgery as the "postpump perfusion" syndrome.[72] Most "postpump perfusion" infectious mononucleosis is, however, attributable to CMV.

Although several apparent epidemics of infectious mononucleosis have been described, these reports have not been substantiated with EBV serologic data and have lacked rigorous epidemiologic, clinical, or laboratory support. Some of these have resulted from errors in the performance of Monospot tests.[73] On the basis of the previously discussed information, it is unlikely that true epidemics of infectious mononucleosis occur.

Public Health Impact

College and military populations experience the highest morbidity from infectious mononucleosis, although cases occur in other groups as well. Infectious mononucleosis accounted for 5 percent of all hospitalizations of University of Wisconsin students, with an incidence of 450 admissions per 100,000 students per year. Other American universities have reported similar incidences.[74,75] Approximately 12 percent of susceptible college students undergo EBV seroconversion yearly.[18,19] Many of these infections are subclinical (see below).[18,54] Although primary EBV infection may only be clinically apparent in about 10 percent of military cases, infectious mononucleosis ranked fourth as the cause of days lost due to illness in army personnel.[76,77] Detailed information on the impact of infectious mononucleosis on the general population is not available since infectious mononucleosis is not a reportable disease in most states. However, it is likely that morbidity from infectious mononucleosis is generally underestimated since a specific diagnosis may not be made and the nonspecific illness can be attributed to a variety of other causes.

PATHOGENESIS

Histopathologic Findings

The usually benign course of infectious mononucleosis has limited pathologic examination to tissues obtained from fatal cases or from cases with atypical features from which biopsy specimens were obtained for diagnostic evaluation. During the acute phase of the illness, lymph nodes throughout the body are moderately enlarged. Individual nodes reveal increased numbers of enlarged, moderately active lymphoid follicles. Germinal centers are also enlarged with cores containing blast cells, histiocytes, and lymphocytes. Although the reticulin framework remains intact, invasion by the hyperplastic pulp makes its borders less distinct.[78] In studies of spleens obtained at autopsy or at surgery after rupture, the organ is usually two to three times its normal weight.[79] The splenic capsule and trabeculae are edematous, thinned, and invaded by lymphoid cells. Most of the increased splenic size is the result of hyperplasia of the red pulp. Throughout the red pulp, pleomorphic blast cells are evident. The spleen is often congested with focal, particularly subcapsular, hemorrhages. The white pulp is relatively normal. Tonsillar biopsy specimens obtained during the course of mononucleosis reveal intense proliferation with numerous mitoses.[80] Bone marrow aspirate and biopsy specimens are often strikingly normal when compared with the florid changes noted in peripheral blood. Biopsy specimens are usually normocellular to mildly hypercellular. Small granulomas may be present, but these are not specific for mononucleosis and have no prognostic significance.[81,82]

Changes in hepatic histology are usually mild. Hepatocytes demonstrate minimal swelling and vacuolization. Pleomorphic lymphocytic and monocytic portal infiltration is usually evident. Bile ducts may be minimally swollen, but frank biliary stasis is rare.[83,84] A number of histopathologic changes have been reported in the nervous system of fatal cases of infectious mononucleosis.[80,85,86] These changes include neuronal degeneration, perivascular cuffing, perivascular hemorrhage, and astrocytic hyperplasia. Little mononuclear infiltration may be present despite demonstrable degenerative changes in the neurons of the cortex, basal ganglia, cerebellum, or spinal cord.

Humoral and Cell-Mediated Immune Responses

On the basis of the available evidence, the likely route of initial EBV infection is via the oropharynx. Cytohybridization studies have demonstrated EBV DNA within oropharyngeal epithelial cells. The virus presumably infects susceptible B lymphocytes within lymphoid tissue of the pharynx either simultaneously or subsequently.[87] During the 30–50 day incubation period, viral replication and dissemination occurs throughout the lymphoreticular system. The immune response to EBV-infected transformed lymphocytes is complex and involves both humoral and cell-mediated immune mechanisms.[88]

Epstein-Barr virus–induced infectious mononucleosis results in the synthesis of circulating antibodies directed against viral antigens as well as against unrelated antigens found on sheep, horse, and beef red cells. These latter are the so-called heterophile antibodies, which are detected as sheep and horse red cell agglutinins and beef cell hemolysins. The role of these antibodies in the pathogenesis or in recovery from the illness is unclear. Heterophile antibodies are a heterogeneous group of predominantly IgM antibodies that may be separated by affinity chromatography into antibody populations with either Paul-Bunnell or Forssman specificity.[89] Heterophile antibodies do not cross react with antibodies specific for EBV.[90] Immunization with sheep erythrocytes elicits sheep red cell agglutinins but has no effect on pre-existing antibodies to EBV.[91,92] There is no good correlation between the heterophile titer and the severity of the illness. Specific antibodies directed against EBV capsid antigen and often against other EBV antigens are demonstrable in most patients with infectious mononucleosis. These EBV-specific antibodies are discussed in detail under "Laboratory Diagnosis." In addition, a number of antibodies with other specificities have been detected during primary EBV infection. Among these are antibodies that bind platelets, neutrophils, lymphocytes, nuclear antigens, and ampicillin.[93–101] The potential role of these antibodies in some of the complications of infectious mononucleosis is not yet clear.

Non-EBV-specific cell-mediated immune functions are depressed early in the course of the illness, as measured by cutaneous anergy and decreased proliferative responses to mitogens and antigens.[102] During the first few weeks of clinical illness, a mononuclear lymphocytosis is present. Although earlier studies have suggested that an increase in B lymphocytes may occur as well, most of the increased numbers of lymphocytes have T-cell markers.[103–105] Studies using monoclonal antibodies have demonstrated an increase in both the relative and absolute number of T lymphocytes expressing surface antigens that have been associated with suppressor/cytotoxic function in vitro.[106–108] At the height of the illness, 0.005–0.5 percent of circulating mononuclear cells are capable of forming continuous cell lines in vitro.[109] Up to 20 percent of peripheral blood non-T lymphocytes may express EBNA during the first week of illness.[110]

The cellular immune response to EBV is complex and well integrated and includes both T lymphocytes and natural killer cells.[111–114] T lymphocytes from adults with immunity to EBV or from patients who are recovering from infectious mononucleosis have the capacity to suppress the outgrowth of autologous EBV-infected B lymphocytes. T lymphocytes with cytotoxic properties for EBV-containing cell lines have also been demonstrated in patients with infectious mononucleosis.[115,116] Recent studies have identified at least one region of the EBV latent membrane protein that serves as a target for EBV-specific cytotoxic T lymphocytes.[88]

During the acute phase of infectious mononucleosis, T lymphocytes capable of suppression of immunoglobulin synthesis are demonstrable in the peripheral blood.[117,118] Blastogenic responses and migration inhibitory factor are produced in response to soluble antigens extracted from EBV-containing cell lines.[119] These latter functions appear after the peak of the atypical lymphocytosis and well after recovery from illness has occurred.

With recovery from illness, the atypical lymphocytosis gradually resolves. Functional and surface phenotypic abnormalities of circulating T lymphocytes also subside. Despite clinical recovery and the presence of both humoral and cell-mediated immune functions specific for EBV, the virus is not eliminated from the host. Thus, EBV shares the property of latency or persistence with other members of the herpesvirus group. The virus can be cultivated from oropharyngeal washings for up to 12–18 months after recovery from infectious mononucleosis and can be recovered from the oropharynx and blood intermittently from both healthy and immunosuppressed people.[63,66] Although asymptomatic shedding of EBV by healthy people does not appear to be associated with demonstrable immunologic abnormalities, reactivation of EBV by immunosuppressive drugs may be associated with a return of the abnormal distribution of T-lymphocyte surface phenotypes.[120]

Animal Models

No entirely satisfactory animal models for EBV infection are currently available. Primate models have generally led either to inapparent EBV infection or to neoplasia. The administration of autologous EBV-transformed lymphocytes to squirrel monkeys has resulted in the transient appearance of heterophile antibodies and VCA antibodies but failed to induce either clinical illness or persistent EBV antibodies.[121] Lymphoblastoid cell lines successfully transplanted to neonatal or immunosuppressed rodents have produced tumor masses but have not elicited EBV antibodies.[122] Malignant lymphoma has been induced by the administration of either continuous EBV-containing cell lines or cell-free virus to several other primates including owl monkeys and cotton top marmosets.[123,124] None of these models has, however, reproducibly induced an illness similar to infectious mononucleosis in humans.

CLINICAL MANIFESTATIONS

Spectrum of Illness

EBV induces a broad spectrum of illness in humans. Classic or typical infectious mononucleosis is an acute illness characterized clinically by sore throat, fever, and lymphadenopathy; serologically by the transient appearance of heterophile antibodies; and hematologically by a mononuclear leukocytosis that consists, in part, of atypical lymphocytes (Table 2). An individual case may have most but not necessarily all the aforementioned characteristics. Specific serologic tests for EBV infection indicate that infection results in a spectrum of clinical manifestations. Attempts to exclude cases that fail to meet the classic criteria for infectious mononucleosis result in artificial and often misleading distinctions.

The age of the patient has a profound influence on the clinical expression of EBV infection. In children, primary EBV infection is often asymptomatic. Young children may be more likely to exhibit rashes, neutropenia, or pneumonia than might individuals undergoing primary EBV infection at an older age.[125] Clinically apparent infections in very young children are heterophile-negative in about one-half of the cases.[126] The ratios of clinically apparent to inapparent disease and of EBV-induced heterophile-positive to heterophile-negative cases increase with age. By 4 years of age, 80 percent of children undergoing primary EBV infection are heterophile antibody–positive.[127]

In patients of college age, the ratio of clinically apparent to inapparent EBV infection ranges from 1:3 to 3:1.[18,54] In military recruits, this ratio has been as low as 1:10.[77] Because of previously existing immunity, the disease is less common in older patients. When it does occur, however, clinical and serologic manifestations are similar to those found in adolescents.[128] During the course of the illness, 90 percent of the adolescents with clinically apparent infectious mononucleosis should be heterophile-positive. Therefore, EBV infection is generally inapparent or is a self-limited illness lasting 2 or 3 weeks. In rare cases the disease can be devastating and can be accompanied by severe prostration, major complications, and even death,[129] as is discussed below.

Symptoms

In the vast majority of cases, the clinical manifestation of infectious mononucleosis is that of the clinical triad of sore throat, fever, and lymphadenopathy (Table 3). The onset may be abrupt, but often several days of prodromal symptomatology can

TABLE 2. Manifestations of EBV-Induced Infectious Mononucleosis

Clinical	
	Fever
	Sore throat
	Lymphadenopathy
Hematologic	
	More than 50 percent mononuclear cells
	More than 10 percent atypical lymphocytes
Serologic	
	Transient appearance of heterophile antibodies
	Permanent emergence of antibodies to EBV

TABLE 3. Symptoms of Infectious Mononucleosis

Symptom	*Rate*	*Percentage*	*Range (%)*
Sore throat	409/502	82	70–88
Malaise	243/426	57	43–76
Headache	216/426	51	37–55
Anorexia	117/546	21	10–27
Myalgias	66/326	20	12–22
Chills	54/326	16	9–18
Nausea	18/156	12	2–17
Abdominal discomfort	37/426	9	2–14
Cough	3/56	5	5
Vomiting	3/56	5	5
Arthralgias	1/56	2	2

(Data from Evans,[74] Cameron et al.,[130] Hoagland,[131] and Mason et al.[132])

be elicited, including chills, sweats, feverish sensations, anorexia, and malaise. Loss or taste for cigarettes is common early in the illness but is not specific for infectious mononucleosis. Retro-orbital headaches, myalgias, and feelings of abdominal fullness are other common prodromal symptoms. The most frequent complaint is sore throat, which may be the most severe the patient has experienced.[130,131] Other patients seek medical attention because of prolonged fever or malaise and less frequently because of incidentally encountered lymphadenopathy. Rarely, the first manifestation of illness is one of the complications of infectious mononucleosis described below.

Signs

The signs of infectious mononucleosis are summarized in Table 4. Fever is present in over 90 percent of the patients with infectious mononucleosis. The fever usually peaks in the afternoon with temperatures of 38–39°C, although a temperature as high as 40°C is not uncommon. In most cases fever resolves over a 10- to 14-day period. A rash, which may be macular, petechial, scarlatinaform, urticarial, or erythema multiforme-like, is present in about 5 percent of patients. The administration of ampicillin produces a pruritic, maculopapular eruption in 90–100 percent of the patients, and this rash may appear after cessation of treatment with the drug.[134,135] Periorbital edema has been reported in up to one-third of the cases in some series,[131] but it has been less frequently observed in others.[132] Tonsillar enlargement is usually present, occasionally with tonsils meeting at the midline. The pharynx is erythematous with an exudate in about one-third of the cases. Palatal petechiae may be seen in 25–60 percent of the cases but are not diagnostic of infectious mononucleosis. The petechiae are usually multiple, 1–2 mm in diameter, occur in crops lasting 3–4 days, and are usually seen at the junction of the hard and soft palate.[136] Cervical adenopathy, usually symmetric, is present in 80–90 percent of the patients. Posterior adenopathy is most common, but submandibular and anterior adenopathy are quite frequent as well, and axillary and inguinal adenopathy also occur. Individual nodes are freely movable, are not spontaneously painful, and are only mildly tender to palpation. The results of examination of the lungs and heart are usually normal. Abdominal examination may detect hepatomegaly in 10–15 percent of the cases, although mild tenderness to fist percussion over the liver is present somewhat more frequently.[130,132] Jaundice is present in approximately 5 percent of the cases.[131] Splenomegaly is present in about one-half of the cases if sought carefully over the course of the illness. The splenomegaly is usually maximal at the beginning of the second week of illness and regresses over the next 7–10 days. The results of neurologic examination are generally normal, although occasional complications may occur (see below).

Complications

The vast majority of patients with infectious mononucleosis recover uneventfully. Complications that occur occasionally have been extensively reported in the literature, but even these complications have generally resolved fully, although there have been rare fatalities.

TABLE 4. Signs of Infectious Mononucleosis

Sign	*Rate*	*Percentage*	*Range (%)*
Lymphadenopathy	495/526	94	93–100
Pharyngitis	444/526	84	69–91
Fever	399/526	76	63–100
Splenomegaly	244/470	52	50–63
Hepatomegaly	34/370	12	6–14
Palatal enanthem	18/156	11	5–13
Jaundice	37/426	9	4–10
Rash	49/470	10	0–15

(Data from Cameron et al.,[130] Hoagland,[131] Mason et al.,[132] and Joncas et al.[133])

Hematologic. Autoimmune hemolytic anemia occurs in 0.5–3 percent of the patients with infectious mononucleosis.[137,138] Cold agglutinins, almost always of the IgM class, are present in 70–80 percent of the cases.[139] Anti-i specificity has been reported in 20–70 percent of the cases.[98,140] Most but not all cases of autoimmune hemolytic anemia in infectious mononucleosis are mediated by antibodies of this specificity.[141–144] The hemolysis usually becomes clinically apparent during the second or third week of illness and subsides over a 1- to 2-month period.[145] Corticosteroids may hasten recovery in some cases.

Mild thrombocytopenia is common in infectious mononucleosis. Platelet counts below 140,000/mm^3 were noted in 50 percent of the patients with uncomplicated infectious mononucleosis in one series.[146] Profound thrombocytopenia with bleeding occurs rarely,[147] but platelet counts below 1000/mm^3 and deaths from intracerebral bleeding have been reported.[148,149] The mechanism for the thrombocytopenia is not known. The presence of normal or increased numbers of megakaryocytes in the marrow coupled with reports of antiplatelet antibodies suggest that peripheral destruction of platelets may be occurring, possibly on an autoimmune basis.[99,100,143] Corticosteroids have been reported to be beneficial for the thrombocytopenia in some but not all cases.[147–150] For retractory cases splenectomy may be indicated.[99] Mild neutropenia is seen rather frequently in uncomplicated infectious mononucleosis. The neutropenia is usually mild and self-limiting, although deaths associated with bacterial sepsis and/or pneumonia have been reported.[101,151–157] Anaerobic sepsis without associated granulocytopenia, presumably of pharyngeal origin, has also been reported.[158]

Splenic Rupture. Splenic rupture is a rare but dramatic complication of infectious mononucleosis. Lymphocytic infiltration of the capsule, trabeculae, and vascular walls coupled with rapid splenic enlargement predisposes the organ to rupture. The incidence of rupture is highest in the second or third week of illness but may be the first sign of infectious mononucleosis. Abdominal pain is uncommon in infectious mononucleosis,[159] and splenic rupture must be strongly considered whenever abdominal pain occurs. The onset of this pain may be insidious or abrupt. Pathologic examination of some of the ruptured spleens has revealed subcapsular hematomas that suggest that rupture may be preceded by intermittent subcapsular bleeding. The pain, usually in the left upper quadrant, may radiate to the left scapular area. Left upper quadrant tenderness to palpation, with or without rebound tenderness, is usually present along with peritoneal signs or shifting dullness. In rare cases, splenic rupture is unaccompanied by pain and is manifested as shock. Laboratory findings include a falling hematocrit and, in some cases, an elevated left hemidiaphragm. The abdominal catastrophe may reverse the usual differential count of infectious mononucleosis and evoke a neutrophilia. Confirmatory findings should not be awaited if splenic rupture is suspected. Prompt splenectomy is the treatment of choice, although nonoperative observation and splenorrhaphy have a role in the management of selected patients with subcapsular splenic hematoma.[160,161] Since a history of trauma may be elicited in about one-half the cases of splenic rupture,[162] elimination of contact sports, attention to constipation, and caution in splenic palpation are prudent measures in the first few weeks after diagnosis.

Neurologic. Neurologic complications, which occur in fewer than 1 percent of the cases, can dominate the clinical presentation[163] (Table 5). On occasion, these neurologic signs can be the first or only manifestation of infectious mononucleosis. In many cases, the heterophile antibody determination is negative, atypical lymphocytes may be low in number or delayed in appearance, and the diagnosis must be made by

TABLE 5. Neurologic Complications of Infectious Mononucleosis

Neurologic Complication	*Reference*
Encephalitis	164–168
Meningitis	164
Myelitis	169
Guillain-Barré syndrome	169
Optic neuritis	170
Retrobulbar neuritis	171
Cranial nerve palsies	169
Mononeuritis multiplex	172
Brachial plexus neuropathy	173
Seizures	164, 168
? Subacute sclerosing panencephalitis	174
Transverse myelitis	175
Psychosis	176

changes in EBV-specific antibodies.[163,164,169] The encephalitis seen with infectious mononucleosis may be acute in onset and rapidly progressive and severe but is usually associated with a complete recovery. The encephalitis is commonly manifested as a cerebellitis but may also be global.[165–167] The clinical presentation may also resemble aseptic meningitis. In both encephalitis and meningitis, changes in the spinal fluid are mild. The opening pressure is normal or slightly elevated. A predominantly mononuclear pleocytosis may be present, with most cell counts well below 200/mm^3. Atypical lymphocytes have been seen in the cerebrospinal fluid in a number of cases. The protein level is usually normal to mildly elevated, and the glucose concentration is usually normal. Low titers of EBV VCA can be found in the cerebrospinal fluid.[168] Cases of Guillain-Barré syndrome, Bell's palsy, and transverse myelitis have been reported in primary EBV infection.[169] Although neurologic complications are the most frequent cause of death in infectious mononucleosis, the benign outcome of the vast majority of these episodes should be emphasized.[177] Eighty-five percent of the patients with neurologic complications recover completely.[163]

Hepatic. Hepatic manifestations levels, consist largely of self-limited elevations of hepatocellular enzyme levels, which are present in 80–90 percent of the cases of infectious mononucleosis.[178] Reported cases of infectious mononucleosis leading to cirrhosis or other chronic sequelae are poorly documented.

Cardiac. Clinically significant cardiac disease is very uncommon. Electrocardiographic (ECG) abnormalities, usually confined to ST-T wave abnormalities, were reported in 6 percent of the cases in one series.[179] Pericarditis and fatal myocarditis have also been observed.[180,181]

Pulmonary. Pulmonary manifestations of infectious mononucleosis are quite rare.[182–184] Early studies reported the presence of interstitial infiltrates in 3–5 percent of the cases. However, systematic examination for other causes of nonbacterial pneumonias, e.g., *Mycoplasma*, were not carried out in these studies, and it is not clear that these infiltrates were related to EBV infection. The attribution of pulmonary lesions to EBV infection should be made only after other pathogens have been carefully excluded.

Death. Death from infectious mononucleosis is rare.[177,185] Death may occur either as a result of overwhelming EBV infection or from complications of the disease. Overwhelming infection with demonstrable virus in lymph nodes, spleen, thymus, and other organs may occur in apparently healthy persons, but a familial syndrome of immunodeficiency and EBV infection has also been described.[186] This immunodeficiency syndrome is passed in an X-linked recessive pattern and has acquired the name of the originally described affected kindred (Duncan).[187,188] Within families with this syndrome, individual cases may end in overwhelming infection and death during the acute phase of the illness, or agammaglobulinemia or lymphoma may develop over a several-year period after infectious mononucleosis.[189–194] The immunologic defect in this syndrome is not yet defined, but disordered immunoregulation after the induction of anomalous killer cells has been postulated.[194]

Neurologic complications of the illness, splenic rupture, or upper airway obstruction are the most frequent causes of death from infectious mononucleosis in otherwise apparently healthy persons. Deaths from complications associated with granulocytopenia, thrombocytopenia, hepatic failure, and myocarditis have also been reported.[144,155,177,181,195,196]

Clinical Course

The vast majority of cases of infectious mononucleosis resolve spontaneously over a 2- to 3-week period. The sore throat is usually maximal for 3–5 days and then gradually resolves over the course of a week to 10 days. Patients remain febrile for 10–14 days, but in the last 5–7 days, the fever is usually low grade and associated with little morbidity. The prostration associated with infectious mononucleosis is generally more gradual in its resolution. As the illness resolves, patients often have days of relative well-being that alternate with recrudescence of the symptoms.

Chronic or Persistent Epstein-Barr Virus Infection

It has been suggested that persistent EBV infection is a frequent cause of fatigue and malaise in young and middle-aged adults.[197–200] This speculation has arisen from reports of a syndrome characterized by fatigue, sore throat, mild cognitive dysfunction, and myalgias initially noted in association with an apparent increase in antibody titers to the EBV early antigen complex[197,198] (See "Laboratory Diagnosis," below). These reports have included primarily young adults, usually with a female preponderance, who develop a nonspecific symptom complex more reminiscent of the prodrome of infectious mononucleosis than of the syndrome itself (often known as "chronic mononucleosis syndrome" or "chronic fatigue syndrome"). These patients have been noted either sporadically[197,198,201] or in epidemic clusters.[200] The initial suggestion that the syndrome is attributable to EBV has become untenable on the basis of serologic and epidemiologic observations.[200,202] Investigation of the syndrome has been hampered by the vagueness of the symptoms and the absence of objective laboratory diagnostic criteria. Recently a concensus case definition has emerged that focuses on fatigue rather than on EBV as the central feature of the syndrome.[203] Although this case definition is likely to provide a useful working case definition for epidemiologic studies, it is less useful in its application to the evaluation of an individual patient.

At this point no etiologic agent(s) for the syndrome have been clearly identified. In addition, the potential role of a neuropsychiatric contribution to the pathogenesis of the syndrome is under investigation. Patients with the rather nonspecific symptom complex should be evaluated for other potential etiologies for fatigue. There is no role for routine EBV-specific serologic testing in the clinical evaluation of such patients.[199,204] Although a number of therapeutic agents such as acyclovir and intramuscular or intravenous immunoglobulin have been advocated by some clinicians, no randomized double-blind studies support the use of antiviral agents in this syndrome.[205] The most effective management consists of supportive reassurance and encouragement to modulate activities during periods of greatest fatigue.

In contrast to patients with the nonspecific syndrome just noted, rare patients have been identified in which EBV appears to be playing a direct role in ongoing objective organ system dysfunction.[206–210] These patients may present with fever, pulmonary parenchymal involvement, pancytopenia, or ophthalmologic or neurologic abnormalities. Such patients may be distinguished from those with the chronic fatigue syndrome by the presence of objective symptoms and signs and by extremely abnormal EBV-specific serologic findings. Temporary partial or complete responses to acyclovir have been reported in occasional patients.

Association with Burkitt's Lymphoma, Other Lymphomas, and Nasopharyngeal Carcinoma

Virtually all African patients with Burkitt's lymphoma and most patients with nasopharyngeal carcinoma possess high antibody titers to EBV. Viral capsid antibody titers are 10- to 15-fold higher in patients with these tumors than in matched controls.[50,211] DNA hybridization studies have demonstrated the presence of the EBV genome in biopsy specimens from both Burkitt's lymphoma and nasopharyngeal carcinoma.[212] Epstein-Barr nuclear antigen is demonstrable in the nuclei of cells in Burkitt's lymphoma biopsy specimens, and the virus can be recovered from tissue cultures of biopsy specimens of Burkitt's lymphoma. In contrast, evidence for the association of EBV with histologically identical tumors in the American population has been lacking.[213] The geographic restriction of Burkitt's lymphoma in Africa and the apparent predilection of nasopharyngeal carcinoma for certain ethnic groups suggests that genetic and/or environmental factors (including other viruses) may also play a role in tumor development.

Increasing evidence suggests that EBV may also be related to neoplasia in several other settings. Uncontrolled EBV-induced lymphoproliferation may occur in patients with the X-linked lymphoproliferative syndrome (see above).[186–193] Occasional sporadic cases of primary EBV infection evolve into uncontrolled lymphoproliferative syndromes.[214,215] In the setting of immunodeficiency, EBV may play more of a role in the induction of B-cell lymphomas than was previously appreciated.[216] Recently, fatal T-cell lymphomas have been reported in three patients with chronic EBV infection.[217]

EBV-related lymphoproliferative syndromes have been observed after renal and bone marrow transplantation and in association with the acquired immunodeficiency syndrome (AIDS).[218–223] Epstein-Barr virus–related lymphoproliferative syndromes associated with immunosuppression may be a particular problem for patients treated with cyclosporine A.[221] The EBV genome has been detected in a tumor from a patient with a primary central nervous system (CNS) B-cell lymphoma without the presence of overt immunosuppression, which suggests a possible association between EBV and lymphoma in that setting.[224] More widespread application of DNA hybridization techniques should help more fully delineate the spectrum of malignancy associated with EBV.[216]

LABORATORY DIAGNOSIS

Hematologic Findings

The central hematologic manifestation of the illness is the circulating lymphocytosis. At presentation, a relative and absolute mononuclear lymphocytosis is found in about 70 percent of the cases. The lymphocytosis peaks during the second or third week of illness, and monocytes and lymphocytes account for 60–70 percent of the total white cell counts of 12,000–18,000/mm^3. However, higher white cell counts are not uncommon, and occasional cases manifest 30,000–50,000 leukocytes/mm^3. Atypical lymphocytes are the hematologic hallmark of infectious mononucleosis and account for about 30 percent of the differential count at the height of the atypical lymphocytosis.[131,132] The wide range in the atypical lymphocytosis is well recognized, and some cases show none or only a few atypical lymphocytes, while 90 percent or more of the circulating lymphocytes may be atypical in other cases. However, atypical lymphocytes are not pathognomonic for infectious mononucleosis (Table 6). They are also noted in other syndromes, including CMV infection, viral hepatitis, toxoplasmosis, rubella, mumps, and roseola as well as in drug reactions.[225,226] The atypical lymphocyte is generally larger than is the mature lymphocyte encountered in peripheral blood. The cytoplasm is often vacuolated and basophilic, and its edges have a rolled-up appearance. Nuclei are often lobulated and are eccentrically placed. Although the cells may appear quite immature, the heterogeneity of morphologic and tinctoral characteristics of such cells helps to distinguish atypical lymphocytes from the more uniform lymphoblasts of acute lymphocytic leukemia.[6,225]

A relative and absolute neutropenia is evident in 60–90 percent of the cases, and neutrophils that remain in circulation exhibit a mild left shift.[151,152] In most cases, the neutropenia is mild, with total granulocyte counts of 2000–3000/mm^3, although profound granulocytopenia has also been reported.[101,153–157,190,227] The neutropenia is usually self-limited, and counts rise gradually toward normal by a month after presentation.[151]

Thrombocytopenia is also common, and 50 percent of the patients in one series manifested platelet counts of <140,000/mm^3.[146] Although cases of profound thrombocytopenia with bleeding are reported,[147–150] these are quite rare and contrast markedly with the generally benign course of the common, mild thrombocytopenia.

Heterophile Antibodies

Heterophile antibodies, originally described by Paul and Bunnell[7] as sheep erythrocyte agglutinins, are present in about 90 percent of the cases at some point during the illness. Beef erythrocyte hemolysins and agglutinating antibodies to horse, goat, and camel erythrocytes are also demonstrable in infectious mononucleosis. The classic heterophile antibody titer is reported as the highest serum dilution at which sheep erythrocytes are agglutinated after absorption of the test serum by guinea pig kidney (Table 7). The differential absorption permits a distinction between naturally occurring Forssman antibodies, the antibodies of serum sickness, and heterophile antibodies of infectious mononucleosis. Beef red cell hemolysins do not require differential absorption for interpretation. Although titers may vary depending on laboratory techniques, a titer of 40 or greater after guinea pig absorption along with a compatible clinical presentation is strong evidence for infectious mononucleosis.

Heterophile antibodies may be demonstrable at the onset of illness or may appear later in the course of the illness. A delayed appearance of heterophile antibodies may be associated with a

TABLE 6. Syndromes in Which Atypical Lymphocytosis May Be Found

Epstein-Barr virus–induced infectious mononucleosis
Cytomegalovirus infections
Toxoplasmosis
Acute viral hepatitis
Rubella
Roseola
Mumps
Drug reactions

TABLE 7. Heterophile Antibodies: Effect of Absorption

		After Absorption with	
Source of Serum	*Unabsorbed*	*Guinea Pig Kidney*	*Beef Red Cells*
Infectious mononucleosis	+ + + +	+ + +	0
Serum sickness	+ + +	0	0
Normal serum (Forssman antibody)	+	0	+

more prolonged convalescence.[228] Horse red cell agglutination is more sensitive than are tests for sheep red cell agglutination or beef red cell hemolysis. Horse red cell agglutinins persist for a year after diagnosis in 75 percent of the cases[229] while sheep cell agglutinins fall to titers of less than 40 by a year in 70 percent of cases. False-positive titers greater than 40 of sheep and horse erythrocyte agglutinins have been found in 12 and 6.7 percent of sera, respectively.[229] Recently, commercial, generally specific and sensitive spot kits for the demonstration of heterophile antibodies have become available. The correlation between the results obtained by the use of these kits and by the classic tube heterophile method is quite good, although the sensitivity of the spot and slide tests is slightly greater than that of the classic tube heterophile test. Occasional false-positive Monospot test responses have been reported in patients with lymphoma or hepatitis, but the rarity of this event makes confirmation of a positive Monospot test result by classic sheep cell agglutination unnecessary.[230–232]

Epstein-Barr Virus–Specific Antibodies

In addition to the transient heterophile antibodies, infection with EBV results in the development of virus-specific antibodies. A determination of EBV-specific antibodies is rarely necessary for the diagnosis of infectious mononucleosis since 90 percent of the cases are heterophile-positive and few false-positive results are obtained if the test if properly performed (see above). For heterophile-negative cases and for diagnosis in atypical cases, a determination of EBV antibodies may help to establish an etiology[223] (Table 8).

Antibodies to viral capsid antigen (VCA) as measured by immunofluorescence arise early in the course of the illness and are demonstrable at presentation in most cases. IgG antibodies to VCA are usually present at titers of 80 or greater on the first visit to a physician. Since these initially detected levels are close to peak VCA titers, a fourfold rise in titer is demonstrable in only 10–20 percent of the cases. After recovery, detectable titers of VCA IgG antibody are maintained for life. Thus, IgG VCA antibody titers may be of little help in the establishment of the diagnosis of infectious mononucleosis. On the other hand, IgM antibodies to VCA are sensitive and specific for infectious mononucleosis but are difficult to measure. Antibody titers of >5 as measured by indirect immunofluorescence are demonstrable in 90 percent of the cases early in illness. Titers fall rapidly thereafter, and in only 10 percent of the cases are titers of >5 retained by 4 months after diagnosis.[229,234] IgM VCA antibodies are not demonstrable in the general population, and thus their presence is virtually diagnostic of acute EBV infection.

Serum antibodies to early antigens are also demonstrable by indirect immunofluorescence, and two distinct patterns of fluorescence emerge.[233,235] Certain sera stain both nuclei and cytoplasm diffusely (anti-D), while others stain cytoplasmic aggregates (anti-R). Anti-D antibody is found in about 70 percent of the patients with acute infectious mononucleosis (Table 8). Anti-D titers arise later in the course of illness than do those to VCA and disappear after recovery. Anti-D antibodies may be found in the sera of patients with advanced nasopharyngeal carcinoma but are absent from the general population. The appearance of anti-D antibodies in a patient with IgG VCA antibodies suggests recent EBV infection. Unfortunately, only 70 percent of EBV-induced cases manifest anti-D antibodies. The presence and titer of anti-D antibodies correlate with the duration and severity of clinical illness.[235] Anti-R antibodies are only occasionally seen in infectious mononucleosis (Table 8). They are present more often in protracted or atypical cases, arise after the anti-D antibodies peak, and remain detectable for up to 2 years.[236] Anti-R antibodies are also present in higher titers in patients with African Burkitt's lymphoma and occasionally in healthy persons who also possess high VCA titers.[237]

Antibodies to EBNA appear late in the course of all cases of infectious mononucleosis and persist for life.[238] The appearance of EBNA antibodies in a patient who was previously VCA-positive and EBNA-negative is strong evidence of recent EBV infection. The recent resolution of a number of distinct EBNAs has provided an additional serologic tool that might provide useful insights into EBV pathogenesis.[210] Neutralizing antibodies to EBV also appear late in the course of infectious mononucleosis and reach maximal levels 6–7 weeks after the onset of illness.[239] Neutralizing antibodies persist at stable titers (mean of 40) for life. The appearance or a rise in titer of neutralizing antibodies to EBV also indicates recent EBV infection. Neutralizing antibodies are, however, difficult to measure, and tests for them are not routinely available. Complement-fixing antibodies to soluble antigens (anti-S) appear in infectious mononucleosis in a time course similar to the appearance of EBNA antibodies.[240] A fourfold rise in titer of anti-S antibody suggests recent EBV infection. Anti-S antibody persists for life.

Detection of Epstein-Barr Virus

Epstein-Barr virus may be cultured from orpharyngeal washings or from circulating lymphocytes of 80–90 percent of the patients with infectious mononucleosis.[60–63,69,109] Cultivation of the

TABLE 8. Antibodies to EBV

Antibody Specificity	*Time of Appearance in Infectious Mononucleosis*	*Percentage of EBV-Induced Mononucleosis Cases with Antibody*	*Persistence*	*Comments*
Viral capsid antigens				
IgM VCA	At clinical persentation	100	4–8 wk	Highly sensitive and specific but difficult to perform
IgG VCA	At clinical presentation	100	Lifelong	High titer at presentation and lifelong persistence make IgG VCA more useful as epidemiologic tool than in diagnosis of individual case
Early antigens				
Anti-D	Peaks at 3–4 wk after onset	70	3–6 mon	Correlated with severe disease; also seen in nasopharyngeal carcinoma
Anti-R	2 wk to several months after onset	Low	2 mon to > 3 yr	Occasionally seen with unusually severe or protracted illness; also seen in African Burkitt's lymphoma
Epstein-Barr nuclear antigen	3–4 wk after onset	100	Lifelong	Late appearance helpful in diagnosis of heterophile-negative cases
Soluble complement-fixing antigens (anti-S)	3–4 wk after onset	100	Lifelong	Late appearance helpful in diagnosis of heterophile-negative cases
Neutralizing antibodies	3–4 wk after onset	100	Lifelong	Technically difficult to perform

virus is, however, not routinely available in most diagnostic virology laboratories. This, coupled with the ubiquity of virus shedding in both healthy persons and in those with unrelated illnesses, renders cultivation of the virus of little clinical use (Table 1). Rapid diagnostic techniques based on DNA hybridization or monoclonal antibody techniques are currently under development.[216,241,242]

Other Laboratory Abnormalities

Liver function test results are abnormal in almost all cases of infectious mononucleosis.[178,243,244] The hepatocellular enzyme (serum glutamic oxaloacetic transaminase [SGOT], serum glutamic pyruvic transaminase [SGPT], and lactic dehydrogenase [LDH]) levels are the most commonly elevated, and one of the three is abnormal in about 90 percent of the cases. Elevations are usually mild, with individual values in the range of two to three times the upper limit of normal. Elevation to more than 10 times the upper limit of normal requires a search for another diagnosis.[178] The alkaline phosphatase level is elevated in about 60 percent of the cases.[243,244] Mild elevation of the bilirubin level is noted in approximately 45 percent of the cases, although frank jaundice occurs in only about 5 percent. Elevations are maximal in the second week of illness and decline gradually over a 3- to 4-week period.

Cryoproteins are present in modest amounts in 90–95 percent of patients.[140,245] The cryoproteins are generally mixed cryoglobulins of IgG and IgM classes. When the cryoglobulins are dissociated, antibody of anti-i, anti-I, or both specificities is usually demonstrable.[245,246]

Differential Diagnosis

In most cases, the diagnosis of infectious mononucleosis is straightforward. The clinical manifestations of sore throat, fever, lymphadenopathy, and malaise coupled with atypical lymphocytosis and a positive heterophile test result establish the diagnosis of EBV-induced infectious mononucleosis. Difficulties arise, however, when the clinical manifestations are less striking, particularly when the heterophile test response is negative.

Heterophile-negative infectious mononucleosis may be caused by several different agents. Attention to the clinical manifestations of the illness and proper use of the laboratory will provide an etiologic diagnosis in 85–90 percent of all cases of infectious mononucleosis. The frequency with which heterophile-negative infectious mononucleosis is seen depends largely on three factors: (*1*) age of the patient population—EBV-induced infectious mononucleosis tends to be a milder illness and is more often heterophile-negative in pediatric populations than in young adults; (*2*) sensitivity of the heterophile test—heterophile antibodies are more often demonstrable by horse red cell agglutination than by beef red cell hemolysis or by sheep red cell agglutination; and (*3*) diligence with which heterophile antibodies are sought—typical cases of infectious mononucleosis may be heterophile-negative on presentation but, if retested later in the course of the illness, may become heterophile-positive.

The most frequent cause of heterophile-negative infectious mononucleosis in most populations is CMV.[247] While differentiation of individual cases of EBV- vs. CMV-induced infectious mononucleosis may be difficult, certain features are more common in CMV infections. CMV more frequently follows transfusion and is more frequently manifested as a typhoidlike syndrome without sore throat and lymphadenopathy. Splenomegaly may be slightly more prominent with CMV-induced disease, while the atypical lymphocytosis is usually less intense in CMV-induced infectious mononucleosis. In age-matched controls, the results of liver function tests are less elevated when the agent is CMV. Cryoglobulins are demonstrable in both EBV- and CMV-induced disease, but anti-i specificity is not seen in CMV-induced mononucleosis.[246] The illness may be attributed to CMV if there is serologic evidence of acute CMV infection and no evidence of acute EBV infection.

Heterophile-negative infectious mononucleosis may also be caused by EBV. As previously noted, this is not uncommon in the pediatric age group.[126,127] The diagnosis rests on the demonstration of appropriate changes in specific EBV serologic tests (Table 8).

Viral hepatitis may result in fever, lymphadenopathy, malaise, and an atypical lymphocytosis. Generally, the atypical lymphocytosis is of lesser magnitude, and atypical lymphocytes account for fewer than 10 percent of the leukocytes. In viral hepatitis, hepatocellular enzyme levels are usually markedly elevated at the initial visit, in contrast to infectious mononucleosis in which the results of liver function tests are only mildly elevated initially and rise gradually over a 1- to 2-week period. In addition, specific serologic tests are currently available for the detection of infection with hepatitis A and B viruses.

Acute toxoplasmosis may also give rise to an infectious mononucleosis-like illness. Usually the degree of the lymphocytosis is mild, and a diagnosis can be made by serologic tests for *Toxoplasma*. Rubella may also occasionally be manifested by fever, lymphadenopathy, and a mild atypical lymphocytosis, but the appearance of the exanthem and the clinical course of the illness are generally not confused with those of infectious mononucleosis. A serologic diagnosis of recent rubella infection can be obtained if the diagnosis remains in doubt. Infectious lymphocytosis of childhood is a disease of uncertain etiology that is characterized by fever, lymphadenopathy, occasionally diarrhea, and a lymphocytosis that consists almost exclusively of small mature lymphocytes. The disease is most common in the pediatric mature lymphocytes. The disease is most common in the pediatric age group, may occur in epidemics, and is not associated with EBV infection.[248]

A streptococcal sore throat may also mimic infectious mononucleosis clinically. Adenopathy is generally submandibular and anterior cervical, and splenomegaly is absent in streptococcal sore throat. Culture of group A β-hemolytic streptococci from the throat is supportive but not conclusive evidence for this diagnosis since colonization with the organism is common in this patient population. Serologic tests for recent infection with group A streptococci may help to establish the etiology.

TREATMENT

Treatment of infectious mononucleosis is largely supportive since more than 95 percent of the patients recover uneventfully without specific therapy. The level of activity is generally tailored to what the individual patient can comfortably tolerate. Contact sports or heavy lifting should be avoided during the first 2–3 weeks of illness, especially if splenomegaly is present. Aspirin or acetaminophen are helpful in relieving the sore throat and in suppressing the fever. Sore throat may be further alleviated by gargling warm salt water. If constipation is present, it should be treated with a gentle laxative.

Corticosteroids are often advocated, but their use in uncomplicated illness is still controversial. Most infectious disease consultants prefer not to administer corticosteroids in this self-limited disease in the absence of certain specific indications. Corticosteroids are generally used in the following situations: (*1*) impending airway obstruction, (*2*) severe thrombocytopenia, or (*3*) hemolytic anemia. Some also advocate the use of corticosteroids for CNS involvement, myocarditis, or pericarditis. If corticosteroids are administered in these situations, treatment should be initiated in doses equivalent to 60–80 mg of prednisone per day given in a split daily regimen. The response is usually rapid, and the dosage can be tapered over a 1- to 2-week period. In selected cases of severe or prolonged prostration, a short tapering course of lower doses of prednisone may be of benefit. In these situations, an initial dose equivalent to 40 mg of prednisone is usually sufficient to produce the desired effect.

Specific antiviral chemotherapy against EBV infection is nearing clinical application. Phosphonoacetic acid (PAA), adenine arabinoside (ara-A), acyclovir, and interferons have been demonstrated to inhibit EBV in vitro.[249–260] Acyclovir did not appear to benefit two patients with X-linked lymphoproliferative syndrome but did appear to induce a temporary remission of a polyclonal B-cell lymphoproliferative disorder observed in a patient after renal transplantation and in two patients with EBV-associated fever and interstitial pneumonitis.[206,217,261,262]

A small study of patients with infectious mononucleosis treated with intravenous acyclovir resulted in interruption of virus shedding in the throat but had a minimal clinical effect.[263] Interferon-α decreased the incidence of shedding of EBV by renal allograft recipients in a prophylactic placebo-controlled study, but it has not been widely used for therapy for ongoing infection.[264] The role of antiviral chemotherapy in the management of EBV infections is likely to broaden as new agents are developed. The latter compound has demonstrated clinical utility in other herpesvirus infections, and administration of ara-A or other relatively nontoxic antiviral compounds may eventually play a role in the management of serious EBV-induced disease.

PREVENTION

Public Health Measures

Since the spread of virus requires intimate contact, isolation of patients with infectious mononucleosis is not necessary. Because virocytemia is demonstrable for several months after recovery, consideration should be given to postponement of blood donation by patients with infectious mononucleosis for at least 6 months after the onset of illness.

Immunization against EBV, particularly of high-risk groups such as susceptible students or military populations, has been considered in the past. Immunization with sheep red cells gives rise to heterophile antibodies, but these are neither persistent nor protective.[90,91] Cell lines that produce large quantities of virus are available, and the possibility exists that an inactivated vaccine could be produced. However, additional data on the risk of administration of inactivated EBV need to be gathered before trials in humans can be contemplated. The potential oncogenicity of EBV requires that this hazard be carefully evaluated in any potential vaccine. Recent progress in the purification of individual EBV polypeptides and cloning of the EBV genome may reduce or eliminate such hazards, but further information is required on the immunogenicity of these polypeptides, and on the antibody directed against these subunits.[21,265–267]

Novel vaccine approaches such as those that use recombinant vaccinia virus to present relevant EBV antigens have begun to show promise in animal studies, but large-scale human studies are not yet warranted.[268]

REFERENCES

1. Filatov NF. Lektuse ob ostrikh infektsion Nikh Lolieznyak (Lectures on Acute Infectious Disease of children). Moscow: U. Deitel; 1885.
2. Pfeiffer E. Drusenfieber. Jahrb f Kinderheilk. 1889;29:257.
3. Türk W. Septische Erkrankungen bei Verkümmerung des Granulozytensystems. Wein Klin Wochenschr. 1907;20:157.
4. Hall AJ. A case resembling acute lymphatic leukaemia, ending in complete recovery. Proc R Soc Med. 1915;8:15.
5. Sprunt TP, Evans FA. Mononuclear leukocytosis in reaction to acute infections ("infectious mononucleosis"). Johns Hopkins Hosp Bull. 1921;31:410.
6. Downey H, McKinlay CA. Acute lymphadenosis compared with acute lymphatic leukemia. Arch Intern Med. 1923;32:82.
7. Paul JR, Bunnell W. The presence of heterophile antibodies in infectious mononucleosis. Am J Med Sci. 1932;183:90.
8. Davidsohn I. Serologic diagnosis of infectious mononucleosis. JAMA. 1937;108:289.
9. Evans AS. Experimental attempts to transmit infectious mononucleosis to man. Yale J Biol Med. 1947;20:19.
10. Evans AS. Further experimental attempts to transmit infectious mononucleosis to man. J Clin Invest. 1950;29:508.
11. Niederman JC, Scott RB. Studies on infectious mononucleosis: Attempts to transmit the disease to human volunteers. Yale J Biol Med. 1965;38:1.
12. Burkitt D. A sarcoma involving the jaws in African children. Br J Surg. 1958;46:218.
13. Epstein MA, Achong BA, Barr YM. Virus particles in cultured lymphoblasts from Burkitt's lymphoma. Lancet. 1964;1:702.
14. Henle G, Henle W. Immunofluorescence in cells derived from Burkitt lymphoma. J Bacteriol. 1966;91:1248.
15. Henle G, Henle W, Diehl V. Relation of Burkitt's tumor associated herpes-type virus to infectious mononucleosis. Proc Natl Acad Sci USA. 1968;59:94.
16. Niederman JC, McCollum RW, Henle G, et al. Infectious mononucleosis: Clinical manifestations in relation to EB virus antibodies. JAMA. 1968;203:205.
17. Evans AS, Niederman JC, McCollum RW. Seroepidemiologic studies of infectious mononucleosis with EB virus. N Engl J Med. 1968;279:1123.
18. Sawyer RN, Evans AS, Niederman JC, et al. Prospective studies of a group of Yale University freshmen. I. Occurrence of infectious mononucleosis. J Infect Dis. 1971;123:263.
19. University Health Physicians and PHLS Laboratories. A joint investigation of infectious mononucleosis and its relationship to EB virus antibody. Br Med J. 1971;4:643.
20. Miller S, Lipman M. Release of infectious Epstein Barr virus by transformed marmoset leukocytes. Proc Natl Acad Sci USA. 1973;70:190.
21. Dolyniuk M, Pritchett R, Kieff E. Proteins of Epstein Barr virus. I. Analysis of the polypeptides of enveloped Epstein Barr virus. J Virol. 1976; 17:935.
22. Pritchett RF, Hayward SD, Kieff E. DNA of Epstein Barr virus. Comparative studies of the DNA of Epstein Barr virus from HRI and B95-8 cells: I. Size, structure, and relatedness. J Virol. 1975;15:556.
23. Sixbey JW, Vesterinen EH, Nedrud JG, et al. Replication of Epstein Barr virus in human epithelial cells infected in vitro. Nature. 1983;306: 480–3.
24. Young LS, Sixbey JW, Clark D, et al. Epstein-Barr virus receptor on human pharyngeal epithelia. Lancet. 1986;1:240–2.
25. Sixbey JW, Davis DS, Young LS, et al. Human epithelial cell expression of an Epstein Barr virus receptor. J Gen Virol. 1987;68:805–11.
26. Jondal M, Klein G. Surface markers on human B and T lymphocytes. II. Presence of Epstein Barr virus receptors on B lymphocytes. J Exp Med. 1973;138:1365.
27. Yefenof E, Bakacs T, Einhorn L, et al. Epstein Barr virus receptors, complement receptors and EBV infectibility of different lymphocyte fractions of human peripheral blood. I. Complement receptor distribution and complement binding by separated lymphocyte subpopulations. Cell Immunol. 1978;35:34.
28. Einhorn L, Steinitz M. Yefenof E, et al. Epstein Barr virus receptors, complement receptors and EBV infectibility of different lymphocyte fractions of human peripheral blood. II. Epstein Barr virus studies. Cell Immunol. 1978;35:43.
29. Fingeroth JD, Weiss JJ, Tedder TF, et al. Epstein-Barr virus receptor of human B lymphocytes is the C3d receptor CR2. Proc Natl Acad Sci USA. 1984;81:4510–4.
30. Frade R, Barel M, Ehlin-Eriksson B, et al. gp140, the C3d receptor of human B lymphocytes, is also the Epstein-Barr virus receptor. Proc Natl Acad Sci USA. 1985;82:1490–3.
31. Robinson J, Smith D. Infection of human B lymphocytes with high multiplicities of Epstein-Barr virus: Kinetics of EBNA expression, cellular DNA synthesis, and mitosis. Virology. 1981;109:336.
32. Henderson E, Miller G, Robinson J, et al. Efficiency of transformation of lymphocytes by Epstein-Barr virus. Virology. 1977;76:152.
33. Andersson-Anvret M, Falk L, Lindahl T. Integration of EBV DNA. In: Proceedings of the Third International Symposium on Oncogenesis and Herpesviruses. Boston, July 25–29. Lyons, France: IARC Press; 1977:46.
34. Hennessy K, Kieff E. A second nuclear protein is encoded by Epstein-Barr virus in latent infection. Science. 1984;227:1238–40.
35. Mueller-Lantzsch N, Lenoir GM, Sauter M, et al. Identification of the coding region for a second Epstein-Barr virus nuclear antigen (EBNA 2) by transfection of cloned DNA fragments. EMBO. 1985;4:1805–11.
36. Hennessy K, Fennewald S, Kieff E. A third viral nuclear protein in lymphoblasts immortalized by Epstein-Barr virus. Proc Natl Acad Sci USA. 1985;82:5944–8.
37. Hennessy K, Wang F, Bushman EW, et al. Definitive identification of a member of the Epstein-Barr virus nuclear protein 3 family. Proc Natl Acad Sci USA. 1986;83:5693–7.
38. Killner J, Kallin B, Alexander H, et al. An Epstein-Barr virus (EBV)-determined nuclear antigen (EBNA5) partly encoded by the transformation-associated *Bam* WYH region of EBV DNA: Preferential expression in lymphoblastoid cell lines. Proc Natl Acad Sci USA. 1986;83:6641–5.

39. Petti L, Sample J, Wang F, et al. A fifth Epstein-Barr virus nuclear protein (EBNA3C) is expressed in latently infected growth-transformed lymphocytes. J Virol. 1988;62:1330–8.
40. Swendenman S, Thorley-Lawson DA. The activation antigen BLAST-2, when shed, is an autocrine BCGF for normal and transformed B cells. EMBO 1987;6:1637–42.
41. Calender A, Billaud M, Aubry JP, et al. Epstein-Barr virus (EBV) induces expression of B-cell activation markers on in vitro infection of EBV-negative B-lymphoma cells. Proc Natl Acad Sci USA. 1987;84:8060–4.
42. Wang F, Gregory CD, Rowe M, et al. Epstein-Barr virus nuclear antigen 2 specifically induces expression of the B-cell activation antigen CD23. Proc Natl Acad Sci USA. 1987;84:3452–6.
43. Rosen A, Gergely P, Jondal M, et al. Polyclonal Ig production after Epstein-Barr virus infection of human lymphocytes in vitro. Nature. 1977;267:52.
44. Luzzatti AL, Hengartner H, Schrier MH. Induction of plaque-forming cells by combined action of antigen and Epstein-Barr virus. Nature. 1977;269:419.
45. Kirchner H, Tosato G, Blaese M, et al. Polyclonal immunoglobulin in secretion by human B-lymphocytes exposed to Epstein-Barr virus in vitro. J Immunol. 1979;122:1310.
46. Schooley RT, Haynes BF, Payling-Wright CR, et al. Mechanisms of Epstein-Barr virus induced human B-lymphocyte activation. Cell Immunol. 1980;56:518.
47. Brown NA, Miller G: Immunoglobulin expression by human B lymphocytes clonally transformed by Epstein Barr virus. J Immunol. 1982;28:24.
48. Sugawara K, Mizuno F, Osto T. Epstein Barr virus associated antigens in non-producing clones of human lymphoblastoid cell lines. Nature. 1972;239:242.
49. Henle W, Henle G, Zajac BA, et al. Differential reactivity of human serums with early antigens induced by Epstein-Barr virus. Science. 1970;169:188.
50. Henle G, Henle W, Clifford P, et al. Antibodies to Epstein-Barr virus in Burkitt's lymphoma and control groups. JNCI. 1969;43:1147.
51. Pereira MS, Blake JM, Macrae AD. EB virus antibody at different ages. Br Med J. 1969;4:526.
52. Porter DD, Wimberly I, Benyesh-Melnick M. Prevalence of antibodies to EB virus and other herpesviruses. JAMA. 1969;208:1675.
53. Gerber P, Rosenblum EN. The incidence of complement fixing antibodies in sera of human and non-human primates to viral antigens derived from Burkitt's lymphocyte cells. Proc Nat Acad Sci USA. 1967;58:478.
54. Hallee TJ, Evans AS, Niederman JC, et al. Infectious mononucleosis at the United States Military Academy. A prospective study of a single class over 4 years. Yale J Biol Med. 1974;47:182.
55. Nye FJ. Social class and infectious mononucleosis. J Hyg (Lond). 1973;71:145.
56. Heath CW Jr, Brodsky AL, Potolsky AI. Infectious mononucleosis in a general population. Am J Epidemiol. 1972;95:46.
57. Bernstein A. Infectious mononucleosis. Medicine (Baltimore). 1940;19:85.
58. Henle G, Henle W. Observations on childhood infections with the Epstein-Barr virus. J Infect Dis. 1970;121:303.
59. Tamir D, Benderly A, Levy J, et al. Infectious mononucleosis and Epstein-Barr virus in childhood. Pediatrics. 1974;53:330.
60. Chang RS, Golden HD. Transformation of human leukocytes from throat washings from infectious mononucleosis patients. Nature. 1971;234:359.
61. Gerber P, Nonoyama M, Lucas S, et al. Oral excretion of Epstein Barr virus by healthy subjects and patients with infectious mononucleosis. Lancet. 1972;2:988.
62. Niederman JC, Miller G, Pearson HA, et al. Infectious mononucleosis: Epstein Barr virus shedding in saliva and the oropharynx. N Engl J Med. 1976;294:1355.
63. Miller G, Niederman JC, Andrews LL. Prolonged oropharyngeal excretion of Epstein Barr virus after infectious mononucleosis. N Engl J Med. 1973;288:229.
64. Strauch B, Siegel N, Andrews LL, et al. Oropharyngeal excretion of Epstein Barr virus by renal transplant recipients and other patients treated with immunosuppressive drugs. Lancet. 1974;1:234.
65. Chang RS, Lewis JP, Abildgaard CF. Prevalence of oropharyngeal excreters of leukocyte transforming agents among a human population. N Engl J Med. 1973;289:1325.
66. Chang RS, Lewis JS, Reynolds RD, et al. Oropharyngeal excretion of Epstein Barr virus by patients with lymphoproliferative disorders and by recipients of renal homografts. Ann Intern Med. 1978;88:34.
67. Wolf H, Haus M, Wilmer E. Persistence of Epstein Barr virus in the parotid gland. J Virol. 1984;51:795–8.
68. Sixbey JW, Lemon SM, Pagano JS. A second site for Epstein-Barr virus shedding: The uterine cervix. Lancet 1986;2:122–4.
69. Lipman M, Andrews L, Niederman J, et al. Direct visualization of enveloped Epstein-Barr herpesvirus in throat washing with leukocyte transforming activity. J Infect Dis. 1975;132:520.
70. Hoagland RS. The transmission of infectious mononucleosis. Am J Med Sci. 1955;229:262.
71. Fleisher GR, Pasquariello PS, Warren WS, et al. Intrafamilial transmission of Epstein-Barr virus infections. J Pediatr. 1981;98:16.
72. Gerber P, Walsh JH, Rosenblum EN, et al. Association of EB virus infection with the post perfusion syndrome. Lancet. 1969;1:593.
73. Herbert JT, Feorino P, Caldwell GG. False-positive epidemic infectious mononucleosis. Am Fam Physician. 1977;115:119.
74. Evans AS. Infectious mononucleoses in University of Wisconsin students. Report of a 5 year investigation. Am J Hyg. 1960;71:342.
75. Evans AS. Epidemiology and pathogenesis of infectious mononucleosis. In: Proceedings of the International Infectious Mononucleosis Symposium. Evanston, IL: American College Health Association; 1967:40.
76. Evans AS. Infectious mononucleosis in the Armed Forces. Milit Med. 1970;135:300.
77. Lehane DE. A seroepidemiologic study of infectious mononucleosis. The development of EB virus antibody in a military population. JAMA. 1970;212:2240.
78. Downey H, Stasney J. The pathology of the lymph nodes in infectious mononucleosis. Folia Haematol (Leipz). 1936;54:417.
79. Smith EB, Custer RP. Rupture of spleen in infectious mononucleosis: Clinicopathologic report of 7 cases. Blood. 1946;1:317.
80. Custer RP, Smith EB. The pathology of infectious mononucleosis. Blood. 1948;3:830.
81. Hovde RF, Sundberg RD. Granulomatous lesions in the bone marrow in infectious mononucleosis. Blood. 1950;5:209.
82. Pease GL. Granulomatous lesions in bone marrow. Blood. 1956;11:720.
83. Nelson RS, Darragh JH. Infectious mononucleosis hepatitis. A clinicopathologic study. Am J Med. 1956;21:26.
84. Sullivan BH, Irey NS, Pieggi VJ, et al. The liver in infectious mononucleosis. Am J Dig Dis. 1957;2:210.
85. Bergin JD. Fatal encephalopathy in glandular fever. J Neurol Neurosurg Psychiatry. 1960;23:69.
86. Ambler M, Stoll J, Tzamaloukas A, et al. Focal encephalomyelitis in infectious mononucleosis. A report with pathologic description. Ann Intern Med. 1971;75:579.
87. Lemon SM, Hutt LM, Li J-LH, et al. Replication of Epstein Barr virus occurs in epithelial cells during infectious mononucleosis. In: Proceedings of the Third International Symposium on Oncogenesis and Herpesviruses. Boston, July 25–29. Lyons, France: IARC Press; 1977:98.
88. Thorley-Lawson DA, Israelsohn ES. Generation of specific cytotoxic T cells with a fragment of the Epstein-Barr virus–encoded p63/latent membrane protein. Proc Natl Acad Sci USA. 1987;84:5384–8.
89. Langhorne J, Feizi T. Studies on the heterophile antibodies of infectious mononucleosis. I. Separation of four antibody populations, one of which contains lymphocytotoxic activity. Clin Exp Immunol. 1977;30:354.
90. Henle W, Henle G, Hewetson J, et al. Failure to detect heterophile antigens in Epstein Barr virus infected cells and to demonstrate interaction of heterophile antibodies with Epstein Barr virus. Clin Exp Immunol. 1974;17:281.
91. Leikola J, Aho K. Experimentally induced mononucleosis-like heterophile antibodies in man. Clin Exp Immunol. 1969;5:67.
92. Mangi RJ, Niederman JC, Kelleher JE, et al. Depression of cell mediated immunity during acute infectious mononucleosis. N Engl J Med. 1974;291:1149.
93. Stevens DL, Everett ED, Boxer LA, et al. Infectious mononucleosis with severe neutropenia and opsonic antineutrophil activity. South Med J. 1979;72:519.
94. Carter RL. Antibody formation in infectious mononucleosis. II. Other 19S antibodies and false positive serology. Br J Haematol. 1966;12:268.
95. Kaplan ME, Tan EM. Antinuclear antibodies in infectious mononucleosis. Lancet. 1968;1:561.
96. McKenzie, Pavat D, White RG. IgM and IgG antibody levels to ampicillin in patients with infectious mononucleosis. Clin Exp Immunol. 1976;26:214.
97. Chartlesworth JA, Quin JW, MacDonald GJ, et al. Complement, lymphocytotoxins, and immune complexes in infectious mononucleosis: Serial studies in uncomplicated cases. Clin Exp Immunol. 1978;34:241.
98. Jenkins WJ, Koster HG, Marsh WL, et al. Infectious mononucleosis: An unsuspected source of anti-i. Br J Haematol. 1965;11:480.
99. Ellman L, Carvalho A, Jacobson BM, et al. Platelet autoantibody in a case of infectious mononucleosis presenting as thrombocytopenic purpura. Am J Med. 1973;55:723.
100. Kernoff LM. Demonstration of increased platelet bound IgG in infectious mononucleosis complicated by severe thrombocytopenia. Scand J Infect Dis. 1980;12:67.
101. Schooley RT, Densen P, Harmon D, et al. Antineutrophil antibodies in infectious mononucleosis. Am J Med. 1984;76:85.
102. Haider S, Coutinho M de L, Emond RTD, et al. Tuberculin anergy and infectious mononucleosis. Lancet. 1973;2:74.
103. Papamichail M, Sheldon PJ, Holborow EJ. T- and B-cell subpopulations infectious mononucleosis. Clin Exp Immunol. 1974;18:1.
104. Engberg RN, Eberle BJ, Williams RC. T- and B-cells in peripheral blood during infectious mononucleosis. J Infect Dis. 1974;130:104.
105. Pattengale PK, Smith RW, Perlin E. Atypical lymphocytes in acute infectious mononucleosis. Identification by multiple T and B markers. N Engl J Med. 1974;291:1145.
106. DeWaele M, Thielemans C, Van Camp BKG. Characterization of immunoregulatory T-cells in EBV induced infectious mononucleosis by monoclonal antibodies. N Engl J Med. 1981;304:460.
107. Reinherz EL, O'Brien C, Rosenthal P, et al. The cellular basis for viral-induced immunodeficiency: Analysis by monoclonal antibodies. J Immunol. 1980;125:1269.
108. Reinherz EL, Schlossman SF. The differentiation and function of human T-lymphocytes. Cell. 1980;19:821.
109. Rocchi G, DeFelici A, Ragona G, et al. Quantitative evaluation of Epstein-Barr virus infected mononuclear peripheral blood leukocytes in infectious mononucleosis. N Engl J Med. 1977;296:132.
110. Robinson JE, Smith D, Niederman J. Plasmacytic differentiation of circu-

lating Epstein-Barr virus infected B-lymphocytes during acute infectious mononucleosis. J Exp Med. 1981;153:235.
111. Blazar B, Patarroyo M, Klein E, et al. Increased sensitivity of human lymphoid lines to natural killer cells after induction of the Epstein-Barr viral cycle by superinfection or sodium butyrate. J Exp Med. 1980;151:614.
112. Rickinson AB, Crawford D, Epstein MA. Inhibition of the in vitro outgrowth of Epstein-Barr virus transformed lymphocytes by thymus dependent lymphocytes from infectious mononucleosis patients. Clin Exp Immunol. 1977;28:72.
113. Thorley-Lawson DA, Chess L, Strominger JA. Suppression of in vitro Epstein Barr virus infection: A new role for the adult human T lymphocyte. J Exp Med. 1977;146:495.
114. Schooley RT, Haynes BF, Payling-Wright CR, et al. Development of suppressor T-lymphocytes for Epstein-Barr virus induced B-lymphocyte outgrowth: Assessment by two quantitative systems. Blood. 1981;57:510.
115. Svedmyr E, Jondal M. Cytotoxic effector cells specific for B cell lines transformed by Epstein Barr virus are present in patients with infectious mononucleosis. Proc Natl Acad Sci USA. 1975;72:1622.
116. Hutt LM, Huang VT, Dascomb HE, et al. Enhanced destruction of lymphoid cell lines by peripheral blood leukocytes taken from patients with acute infectious mononucleosis. J Immunol. 1975;115:243.
117. Haynes BF, Schooley RT, Payling-Wright CR, et al. Emergence of suppressor cells of immunoglobulin synthesis during acute Epstein-Barr virus–induced infectious mononucleosis. J Immunol. 1979;123:2095.
118. Tosato G, Magrath I, Koski I, et al. Activation of suppressor T cells during Epstein-Barr virus–induced infectious mononucleosis. N Engl J Med. 1979;301:1133.
119. Lai PK, Alpers MP, MacKay-Scollay EM. Development of cell-mediated immunity to Epstein-Barr herpesvirus in infectious mononucleosis as shown by leukocyte migration inhibition. Infect Immun. 1977;17:28.
120. Schooley RT, Hirsch MS, Colvin RB, et al. Association of herpesvirus infections with T-lymphocyte subset alterations, glomerulopathy, and opportunistic infections after renal transplantation. N Engl J Med. 1983;308:313.
121. Shope T, Miller G. Epstein Barr virus: Heterophile responses in squirrel monkeys inoculated with virus-transformed autologous leukocytes. J Exp Med. 1973;137:140.
122. Adams RA, Hellerstein EE, Pathier L, et al. Malignant potential of a cell line isolated from the peripheral blood in infectious mononucleosis. Cancer. 1971;27:651.
123. Miller G. The oncogenicity of Epstein-Barr virus. J Infect Dis. 1974;130:187.
124. Miller G, Shope T, Coope D, et al. Lymphoma in cotton-top marmosets after inoculation with Epstein Barr virus, tumor incidence, histologic spectrum of antibody responses, demonstration of viral DNA, and characterization of virus. J Exp Med. 1977;145:948.
125. Sumaya CV, Ench Y. Epstein-Barr virus infectious mononucleosis in children. I. Clinical and general laboratory findings. Pediatrics. 1985;75:1003–10.
126. Schmitz H, Volz D, Krainick-Riechert CH, et al. Acute Epstein-Barr virus infections in children. Med Microbiol Immunol. 1972;158:58.
127. Sumaya CV, Ench Y. Epstein-Barr virus infectious mononucleosis in Children. II. Heterophil antibody and viral-specific responses. Pediatrics. 1985;75:1011–9.
128. Horwitz CA, Henle W, Henle G, et al. Clinical and laboratory evaluation of elderly patients with heterophile antibody positive infectious mononucleosis. Report of seven patients ages 40 to 78. Am J Med. 1976;61:333.
129. Britton S. Andersson-Anvret M, Gergely P, et al. Epstein Barr virus immunity and tissue distribution in a fatal case of infectious mononucleosis. N Engl J Med. 1978;298:89.
130. Cameron D, MacBear LM. A Clinical Study of Infectious Mononucleosis and Toxoplasmosis. Baltimore: Williams & Wilkins; 1973:8.
131. Hoagland RJ. Infectious mononucleosis. Am J Med. 1952;13:158.
132. Mason WR Jr, Adams EK. Infectious mononucleosis. An analysis of 100 cases with particular attention to diagnosis, liver function tests, and treatment of selected cases with prednisone. Am J Med Sci. 1958;236:447.
133. Joncas J, Chaisson JP, Turcotte J, et al. Studies on infectious mononucleosis. III. Clinical data, serologic and epidemiologic findings. Can Med Assoc J. 1968;98:848.
134. Pullen H, Wright N, Murdock J McC. Hypersensitivity reactions to antibacterial drugs in infectious mononucleosis. Lancet. 1967;2:1176.
135. Patel BM. Skin rash with infectious mononucleosis and ampicillin. Pediatrics. 1967;40:910.
136. Caird FI, Holt PR. The enanthem of glandular fever. Br Med J. 1958;1:85.
137. Karzon DT. Infectious mononucleosis. Adv Pediatr. 1976;22:231.
138. Hoagland RJ. Infectious Mononucleosis. New York: Grune & Stratton; 1967:64.
139. Horwitz CA, Moulds J, Henle W, et al. Cold agglutinins in infectious mononucleosis and heterophile antibody negative mononucleosis like syndromes. Blood. 1977;50:195.
140. Capra JD, Dowling P, Cook S, et al. An incomplete cold reactive γ G antibody with i specificity in infectious mononucleosis. Vox Sang. 1969;16:10.
141. Bowman HS, Marsh WL, Schumacher HR, et al. Auto anti-N immunohemolytic anemia in infectious mononucleosis. Am J Clin Pathol. 1974;61:465.
142. Troxel DB, Innella F, Cohen RJ. Infectious mononucleosis complicated by hemolytic anemia due to anti-i. Am J Clin Pathol. 1966;46:625.
143. Wilkinson LS, Petz LD, Garraty G. Reappraisal of the role of anti-i in haemolytic anemia in infectious mononucleosis. Br J Haematol. 1973;25:715.
144. Rosenfield RE, Schmidt PJ, Calvo RC, et al. Anti-i, a frequent cold agglutin in infectious mononucleosis. Vox Sang. 1965;10:631.
145. Worlledge SM, Dacie JV. Hemolytic and other anemias in infectious mononucleosis. In: Carter RL, Penman HG, eds. Infectious Mononucleosis. Oxford: Blackwell Scientific Publishing; 1969:82.
146. Carter RL. Platelet levels in infectious mononucleosis. Blood. 1965;25:817.
147. Clark BF, Davies SH. Severe thrombocytopenia in infectious mononucleosis. Am J Med Sci. 1964;248:703.
148. Radel EG, Schorr JB. Thrombocytopenic purpura with infectious mononucleosis. J Pediatr. 1963;63:46.
149. Goldstein E, Porter DY. Fatal thrombocytopenia with cerebral hemorrhage in mononucleosis. Arch Neurol. 1969;20:533.
150. Grossman LA, Wolff SM. Acute thrombocytopenic purpura in infectious mononucleosis. JAMA. 1959;171:2208.
151. Carter RL. Granulocyte changes in infectious mononucleosis. J Clin Pathol. 1966;19:279.
152. Cantow EK, Kostinas JE. Studies on infectious mononucleosis. iv. Changes in the granulocytic series. Am J Clin Pathol. 1966;46:43.
153. Wulff HR. Acute agranulocytosis following infectious mononucleosis. Report of a case. Scand J Haematol. 1965;2:180–82.
154. Habib MA, Babka JC, Burningham RA. Case Report. Profound granulocytopenia associated with infectious mononucleosis. Am J Med Sci. 1973;265:339–46.
155. Neel EU. Infectious Mononucleosis. Death due to agranulocytosis and pneumonia. JAMA. 1976;236:1493–4.
156. Eriksson KF, Holmberg L, Gustafbergstrand C. Infectious Mononucleosis and Agranulocytosis. Scand J Infect Dis. 1979;11:307–9.
157. Hammond WP, Harlan JM, Steinberg SE. Severe neutropenia in infectious mononucleosis. West J Med. 1979;131:92–7.
158. Dagan P, Powell KR. Postanginal sepsis following infectious mononucleosis. Arch Intern Med. 1987;147:1581–3.
159. Hoagland RJ, Henson HM. Splenic rupture in infectious mononucleosis. Ann Intern Med. 1957;46:1184.
160. Peters RM, Gordon LA. Nonsurgical treatment or splenic hemorrhage in an adult with infectious mononucleosis. Am J Med. 1986;80:123–5.
161. McLean ER, Diehl W, Edoga JK, et al. Failure of conservative management of splenic rupture in a patient with mononucleosis. J Pediatr Surg. 1987;22:1034–5.
162. Smith EB. The anatomic pathology of infectious mononucleosis and its complications. In: Proceedings of the International Infectious Mononucleosis Symposium. Washington, DC: American College Health Association; 1967:109.
163. Bernstein TC, Wolff HG. Involvement of the nervous system in infectious mononucleosis. Ann Intern Med. 1950;33:1120.
164. Silverstein A, Steinberg S, Nathanson M. Nervous system involvement in infectious mononucleosis. The heralding and/or major manifestation. Arch Neurol. 1972;26:353.
165. Bennett DR, Peters HA. Acute cerebellar syndrome secondary to infectious mononucleosis in a 52 year old man. Ann Intern Med. 1961;55:147.
166. Gilbert JW, Culebras A. Cerebellitis in infectious mononucleosis. JAMA. 1972;220:727.
167. Bejada S. Cerebellitis in glandular fever. Med J Aust. 1976;1:153.
168. Joncas JH, Chicoine L, Thivierge R, et al. Epstein-Barr virus antibodies in the cerebrospinal fluid. Am J Dis Child. 1974;127:282.
169. Grose C, Henle W, Henle G, et al. Primary Epstein Barr virus infections in acute neurologic diseases. N Engl J Med. 1975;292:392.
170. Tanner OR. Ocular manifestations of infectious mononucleosis. Arch Ophthalmol. 1954;51:229.
171. Shechter FR, Lipsius EI, Rasansky HN. Retrobulbar neuritis. Am J Dis Child. 1955;89:58.
172. Gautier-Smith PC. Neurological complications of glandular fever (infectious mononucleosis). Brain. 1965;88:323.
173. Watson P, Ashby P. Brachial plexus neuropathy associated with infectious mononucleosis. Can Med Assoc J. 1976;114:758.
174. Feorino PM, Humphrey D, Hochberg F, et al. Mononucleosis associated subacute sclerosing panencephalitis. Lancet. 1975;2:530.
175. Cotton PB, Webb-Peploe MM. Acute transverse myelitis as a complication of glandular fever. Br Med J. 1966;1:654.
176. Raymond RW, Williams RL. Infectious mononucleosis with psychosis. Report of a case. N Engl J Med. 1948;239:542.
177. Penman HG. Fatal infectious mononucleosis: A critical review. J Clin Pathol. 1970;23:765.
178. Finkel M, Parker GW, Fanselau HA. The hepatitis of infectious mononucleosis: Experience with 235 cases. Milit Med. 1964;129:533.
179. Hoagland RJ. Mononucleosis and heart disease. Am J Med Sci. 1964;248:1.
180. Shapiro SC, Dimich I, Steier M. Pericarditis as the only manifestation of infectious mononucleosis. Am J Dis Child. 1973;126:662.
181. Frishman W, Kraus ME, Zabkar J, et al. Infectious mononucleosis and fatal myocarditis. Chest. 1977;72:535.
182. Mundy GR. Infectious mononucleosis with pulmonary parenchymal involvement. Br Med J. 1972;1:219–20.
183. Offit PA, Fleisher GR, Koven NI, et al. Severe Epstein-Barr virus pulmonary involvement. J Adolesc Health Care. 1981;2:121–5.
184. Andiman WA, McCarthy P, Markowitz RI, et al. Clinical, virologic, and serologic evidence of Epstein-Barr virus infection in association with childhood pneumonia. J Pediatr. 1981;99:880–6.

185. Lukes RJ, Cox FH. Clinical and morphologic findings in 30 fatal cases of infectious mononucleosis. Am J Pathol. 1958;34:586.
186. Bar RS, Delor CJ, Clausen KP, et al. Fatal infectious mononucleosis in a family. N Engl J Med. 1974;290:363.
187. Purtilo DT, Cassel CK, Yang JPS, et al. X-linked recessive progressive combined variable immunodeficiency (Duncan's disease). Lancet. 1975;1:935.
188. Purtilo DT, Cassel CK, Yang JPS. Fatal infectious mononucleosis in familial lymphohistiocytosis. N Engl J Med. 1974;291:736.
189. Purtilo DT, Bhawan J, Hutt LM, et al. Epstein-Barr virus infections in the X-linked recessive lymphoproliferative syndrome. Lancet. 1978;1:798.
190. Provisor AJ, Iacuone JJ, Chilcote RR, et al. Acquired agammaglobulinemia after a life-threatening illness with clinical and laboratory features of infectious mononucleosis in three related male children. N Engl J Med. 1975;293:62.
191. Purtilo DT, Yang JP, Cassel CK, et al. X-linked recessive progressive combined variable immunodeficiency. Lancet. 1975;1:935.
192. Hamilton JK, Paquin L, Sullivan J, et al. X-linked lymphoproliferative syndrome registry report. J Pediatr. 1980;96:669.
193. Purtilo DT, DeFloria D Jr, Hutt L, et al. Variable phenotypic expression of an X-linked expressive lymphoproliferative syndrome. N Engl J Med. 1977;297:1077.
194. Sullivan JL, Byron KS, Brewster FE, et al. X-linked lymphoproliferative syndromes: Natural history of the immunodeficiency. J Clin Invest. 1983;71:1765.
195. Allen UR, Bass BH. Fatal hepatic necrosis in glandular fever. J Clin Pathol. 1963;16:337.
196. Dorman JM, Glick TH, Shannon DC, et al. Complications of infectious mononucleosis: A fatal case in a 2-year-old child. Am J Dis Child. 1974;128:239.
197. Jones JF, Ray CG, Minnich LL, et al. Evidence for active Epstein Barr virus infection in patients with persistent, unexplained illnesses: Elevated anti-early antigen antibodies. 1985;102:1–7.
198. Straus SE, Tosato G, Armstrong G, et al. Persisting illness and fatigue in adults with evidence of Epstein-Barr virus infection. Ann Intern Med. 1985;102:7–16.
199. Straus SE. The chronic mononucleosis syndrome. J Infect Dis. 1988;157:405–12.
200. Holmes GP, Kaplan JE, Stewart JA, et al. A cluster of patients with a chronic mononucleosis-like syndrome. JAMA. 1987;257:2297–302.
201. Buchwald D, Sullivan JL, Komaroff AL. Frequency of "chronic active Epstein-Barr virus infection" in a general medical practice. JAMA. 1987;257:2303–7.
202. Horwitz CA, Henle W, Henle G, et al. Long-term serological follow-up of patients for Epstein-Barr virus after recovery from infectious mononucleosis. J Infect Dis. 1985;151:1150–3.
203. Holmes GP, Kaplan JE, Gantz NM, et al. Chronic fatigue syndrome: A working case definition. Ann Intern Med. 1988;108:387–9.
204. Hellinger WC, Smith TF, Van Scoy RE, et al. Chronic fatigue syndrome and the diagnostic utility of antibody to Epstein-Barr virus early antigen. JAMA. 1988;260:971–3.
205. Straus SE, Dale JK, Tobi M, et al. Acyclovir treatment of the chronic fatigue syndrome: Lack of efficacy in a placebo controlled trial. N Engl J Med. 1989. 1988;319:1692–8.
206. Schooley RT, Carey RW, Miller G, et al. Chronic Epstein-Barr virus infection associated with fever and interstitial pneumonitis. Ann Intern Med. 1986;104:636–43.
207. Snydman DR, Rudders RA, Daquest P, et al. Infectious mononucleosis in an adult progressing to fatal immunoblastic lymphoma. Ann Intern Med. 1982;96:737–42.
208. Virelizier J-L, Lenoir G, Griscelli C. Persistent Epstein-Barr virus infection in a child with hypergammaglobulinaemia and immunoblastic proliferation associated with a selective defect in immune interferon secretion. Lancet 1978;2:231–4.
209. Kuis W, Roord JJ, Zegers BJM, et al. Heterogeneity of immune defects in three children with a chronic active Epstein-Barr virus infection. J Clin Immunol. 1985;5:377–85.
210. Miller G, Grogan E, Rowe D, et al. Selective lack of antibody to a component of EB nuclear antigen in patients with chronic active Epstein-Barr virus infection. J Infect Dis. 1987;156:26–35.
211. Henle W, Henle G, Ho HC, et al. Antibodies to Epstein-Barr virus in nasopharyngeal carcinoma, other head and neck neoplasms, and control groups. JNCI. 1970;44:225.
212. Zur Hausen H, Schulte-Holthausen H, Klein G, et al. EBV DNA in biopsies of Burkitt's tumors and anaplastic carcinomas of the nasopharynx. Nature. 1970;228:1056.
213. Pagano JS, Huang CH, Levine P. Absence of Epstein Barr viral DNA in American Burkitt's lymphoma. N Engl J Med. 1973;289:1395.
214. Robinson J, Brown N, Andiman W, et al. Diffuse polyclonal B-cell lymphoma during primary infection with Epstein-Barr virus. N Engl J Med. 1980;302:1293.
215. Snydman DR, Rudders RA, Daoust P, et al. Infectious mononucleosis in an adult progressing to fatal immunoblastic lymphoma. Ann Intern Med. 1982;96:737.
216. Andiman W, Gradonville L, Heston L, et al. Use of cloned probes to detect Epstein-Barr viral DNA in tissues of patients with neoplastic and lymphoproliferative disease. J Infect Dis. 1983;148:967.
217. Jones JF, Shurin S, Abramowsky C, et al. T cell lymphomas containing Epstein-Barr viral DNA in patients with chronic Epstein-Barr virus infections. N Engl J Med. 1988;318:733–41.
218. Hanto DW, Frizzera G, Gajl-Peczalska KJ, et al. Epstein-Barr virus induced B-cell lymphoma after renal transplantation. Acyclovir therapy and transition from polyclonal to monoclonal B-cell proliferation. N Engl J Med. 1982;306:913.
219. Frizzera G, Hanto DW, Gajl-Peczalska J, et al. Polymorphic diffuse B-cell hyperplasias and lymphomas in renal transplant recipients. Cancer Res. 1981;41:4262.
220. Hanto DW, Frizzera G, Gajl-Peczalska J, et al. The Epstein-Barr virus in the pathogenesis of post-transplant lymphoma. Transplant Proc. 1981;13:756.
221. Crawford DH, Thomas JA, Janossy G, et al. Epstein-Barr virus nuclear antigen positive lymphoma after cyclosporin: A treatment in a patient with a renal allograft. Lancet. 1980;1:1355.
222. Zeigler JL, Miner RC, Rosenbaum E, et al. Outbreak of Burkitt's-like lymphoma in homosexual men. Lancet. 1982;2:631.
223. Ho M, Jaffe R, Miller G, et al. The frequency of Epstein-Barr virus infection and associated lymphoproliferative syndrome after transplantation and its manifestations in children. Transplantation. 1988;45:719–27.
224. Hochberg FG, Miller G, Schooley RT, et al. Central nervous system lymphoma related to Epstein-Barr virus. N Engl J Med. 1983;309:745.
225. Wood TA, Frenkel EP. The atypical lymphocyte. Am J Med. 1967;42:923.
226. Chin TDY. Diagnosis of infectious mononucleosis. South Med J. 1976;69:654.
227. Penman HG. Extreme neutropenia in glandular fever. J Clin Pathol. 1968;21:48.
228. Chretien JH, Esswein JG, Holland WG, et al. Predictors of the duration of infectious mononucleosis. South Med J. 1977;70:437.
229. Evans AS, Niederman JC, Cenabre LC, et al. A prospective evaluation of heterophile and Epstein Barr virus specific IgM antibody tests in clinical and subclinical infectious mononucleosis. Specificity and sensitivity of the tests and persistence of antibody. J Infect Dis. 1975;132:546.
230. Basson V, Sharp AA. Monospot: A differential slide test for infectious mononucleosis. J Clin Pathol. 1969;22:324.
231. Seitanidis B. A comparison of the Monospot with the Paul-Bunnell test in infectious mononucleosis and other diseases. J Clin Pathol. 1969;22:321.
232. Wolf P, Dorfman R, McClenahan J, et al. False-positive infectious mononucleosis spot test in lymphoma. Cancer. 1970;25:626.
233. Henle W, Henle G, Horwitz CA. Epstein-Barrr virus specific diagnostic tests in infectious mononucleosis. Hum Pathol. 1974;5:551.
234. Schimitz H, Scherer M. IgM antibodies to Epstein Barr virus in infectious mononucleosis. Arch Gesamte Virusforsch. 1972;37:332.
235. Henle W, Henle G, Niederman JC, et al. Antibodies to early antigens induced by Epstein Barr virus in infectious mononucleosis. J Infect Dis. 1971;124:58.
236. Horwitz CA, Henle W, Henle G, et al. Clinical evaluation of patients with infectious mononucleosis and development of antibodies to the R component of the Epstein-Barr virus induced early antigen complex. Am J Med. 1975;58:330.
237. Reedman BM, Klein G. Cellular localization of an Epstein Barr virus associated complement fixing antigen in producer and nonproducer lymphoblastoid cell lines. Int J Cancer. 1973;11:499.
238. Henle G. Henle W, Horwitz CA. Antibodies to Epstein Barr virus associated nuclear antigen in infectious mononucleosis. J Infect Dis. 1974;130:231.
239. Hewetson JF, Rocchi S, Henle W, et al. Neutralizing antibodies to Epstein Barr virus in healthy populations and patients with infectious mononucleosis. J Infect Dis. 1973;128:283.
240. Benyesh-Melnick M, Lewis RT, Wimberly I. Some properties of the soluble (S) antigen of cultured lymphoblastoid cell lines. Arch Gesamte Virusforsch. 1970;31:113.
241. Thorley-Lawson DA, Schooley RT, Bhan AK, et al. Epstein-Barr virus superinduces a new human B cell differentiation antigen (B-LAST 1) expressed on transformed lymphoblasts. Cell. 1982;30:415.
242. Diaz-Mitoma F, Preiksaitis JK, Leung WC, et al. DNA-DNA dot hybridization to detect Epstein-Barr virus in throat washings. J Infect Dis. 1987;155:297–303.
243. Baron DN, Bell JL, Demmett WN. Biochemical studies on hepatic involvement in infectious mononucleosis. J Clin Pathol. 1965;18:209.
244. Rosalki SB, Jones TG, Verney AF. Transaminase and liver function studies in infectious mononucleosis. Br Med J. 1960;1:929.
245. Kaplan ME. Cryoglobulinemia in infectious mononucleosis: Quantitation and characterization of the cryoproteins. J Lab Clin Med. 1968;71:754.
246. Horwitz CA, Moulds J, Henle W, et al. Cold agglutinins in infectious mononucleosis and heterophil-antibody-negative mononucleosis-like syndromes. Blood. 1977;50:195.
247. Horwitz CA, Henle W, Henle G, et al. Heterophile negative infectious mononucleosis and mononucleosis-like illness. Laboratory confirmation of 43 cases. Am J Med. 1977;63:947.
248. Blacklow NR, Kapikian AZ. Serological studies with EB virus in infectious lymphocytosis. Nature. 1970;226:647.
249. Thorley-Lawson D, Strominger JL. Transformation of human lymphocytes by Epstein-Barr virus is inhibited by phosphonoacetic acid. Nature. 1976;263:332.
250. Nyormoi O, Thorley-Lawson DA, Elkington J, et al. Differential effect of phosphonoacetic acid on the expression of Epstein-Barr viral antigens and virus production. Proc Natl Acad Sci USA. 1976;78:1745.

251. Summers WC, Klein G. Inhibition of Epstein-Barr virus DNA synthesis and late gene expression by phosphonoacetic acid. J Virol. 1976;18:151.
252. Rickinson AB, Epstein MA. Sensitivity of the transforming and replicative functions of Epstein-Barr virus to inhibition by phosphonoacetate. J Gen Virol. 1978;40:409.
253. Thorley-Lawson DA, Strominger JL. Reversible inhibition by phosphonoacetic acid of human B-lymphocyte transformation by Epstein-Barr virus. Virology. 1978;86:423.
254. Coker-Vann M, Dolin R. Effect of adenine arabinoside on Epstein Barr virus in vitro. J Infect Dis. 1977;135:447.
255. Colby BM, Shaw JE, Elion GB, et al. Effect of acyclovir [9-(2-hydroxyethoxymethyl)guanine] on Epstein-Barr virus DNA replication. J Virol. 1980;34:560.
256. Colby BM, Shaw JE, Datta AK, et al. Replication of Epstein-Barr virus DNA in lymphoblastoid cells treated for extended periods with acyclovir. Am J Med. 1982;73:77.
257. Pagano JS, Datta AK. Perspectives on interactions of acyclovir with Epstein-Barr and other herpes viruses. Am J Med. 1982;73:18.
258. Adams A, Strander H, Cantell K. Sensitivity of the Epstein-Barr virus transformed human lymphoid cell lines to interferon. J Gen Virol. 1975;28:207.
259. Thorley-Lawson DA. The transformation of adult but not newborn lymphocytes by Epstein-Barr virus and phytohemagglutinin is inhibited by interferon: The early suppression by T-cells of Epstein-Barr infection is mediated by interferon. J Immunol. 1981;126:829.
260. Garner JG, Hirsch MS, Schooley RT. Prevention of Epstein-Barr virus–induced β-cell outgrowth by interferon-alpha. Infect Immun. 1984;43:920.
261. Sullivan JL, Byron KS, Brewster FE, et al. Treatment of life-threatening Epstein-Barr virus infections with acyclovir. Am J Med. 1982;73:262.
262. Sullivan JL, Baker JN, Byron KS, et al. Failure of acyclovir to inhibit polyclonal Epstein-Barr virus induced lymphoproliferation. Fed Proc. 1983;42:458.
263. Andersson J, Britton S, Ernberg I, et al. Effect of acyclovir on infectious mononucleosis: A double-blind, placebo-controlled study. J Infect Dis. 1986;153:283–90.
264. Cheeseman SH, Henle W, Rubin RH, et al. Epstein-Barr virus infection in renal transplant recipients: Effects of anti-thymocyte globulin and interferon. Ann Intern Med. 1980;93:39.
265. Dolyniuk M, Wolff E, Kieff E. Proteins of Epstein-Barr virus. II. Electrophoretic analysis of the polypeptides of the nucleocapsid and the glucosamine-and-polysaccharide–containing components of enveloped virus. J Virol. 1976;18:289.
266. Skare J, Strominger JL. Cloning and mapping of BAM H1 endonuclease fragments of DNA from the transforming B95-8 strain of Epstein-Barr virus. Proc Natl Acad Sci USA. 1980;77:3860.
267. Hummel M, Kieff E. Mapping of polypeptides encoded by the Epstein-Barr virus genome in productive infection. Proc Natl Acad Sci USA. 1982;79:5698.
268. Mackett M, Arrand JR. Recombinant vaccinia virus induces neutralizing antibodies in rabbits against Epstein-Barr virus membrane antigen gp340. EMBO. 1985;4:3229–34.

Adenoviridae

122. ADENOVIRUS

STEPHEN G. BAUM

Adenoviruses are most important clinically because of their capacity to cause acute infections of the respiratory system and conjunctivae. The current intense biologic interest in these viruses derives from their ability to cause tumors in animals, their propensity for latent infection in several types of host cells, and their ability to interact with another virus (simian virus 40 [SV40]) to form hybrid viruses with unique biologic properties. These varied capacities are exhibited by a virus with a relatively simple genetic composition, which offers the promise of resolving the mechanisms of a number of important biologic phenomena.

The adenoviruses were discovered in 1953 by Rowe and his colleagues who noted that adenoidal tissue removed at the time of surgery spontaneously underwent a characteristic degeneration when the tissues were maintained in culture for several weeks.[1] An agent was isolated from these degenerating tissues, and this agent, called *adenovirus* to denote its origin, could be serially passed in epithelial cells and lead to the typical cytopathic changes that have come to be attributed to the adenovirus group (Fig. 1). Over the next few years several adenovirus serotypes were isolated from adenoidal tissues in which the virus appeared to cause a latent infection.[2] Other serotypes were isolated from pulmonary secretions of young adults suffering from acute respiratory disease, and still other types were isolated from the eyes of patients with conjunctivitis. In the dozen years after the initial adenovirus isolation, 31 human serotypes were isolated and characterized; several new serotypes have recently been described to bring the total to about 41 or 42. Although many serotypes have been shown to be the cause of specific syndromes, a role in causing human disease remains obscure for over half of the known types.

In the past few years adenovirus types 2, 5, 7, and 12 have been the subject of intensive physical and biochemical analysis. The genetic maps of these viruses have been constructed, and functions have been assigned to most of the regions of the DNA viral genome.

Viruses similar to human adenoviruses are found in many animal classes including monkey, bovine, bird, and lower mammals. With the exception of avian adenoviruses, these agents all share a cross-reacting group-specific antigen. All adenoviruses have similar morphology and nucleic acid composition and produce characteristic cytopathic changes in susceptible cells. The adenoviruses of lower animals play no known role in the etiology of human disease.

DESCRIPTION OF THE PATHOGEN

Human adenoviruses have DNA as their genetic material. The outer covering of the virus is a protein coat, or capsid, containing 252 subunits called *capsomeres*. These capsomeres are arranged in an icosahedral structure that has 20 sides and 12 vertices (Fig. 2). The capsid subunits are of three morphologic types. *Hexons*, which account for 240 of the capsomeres, have six nearest neighbors, while the 12 vertices are occupied by *pentons*, which as the name implies, have five nearest neighbors. Rodlike structures with knobs at the ends project from the penton base capsomeres. These rods are called *fibers*. The hexons, pentons, and fibers differ from one another immunologically as well as morphologically. The hexon appears to have some antigenic sites that are common to all human adenoviruses and other sites that show type specificity. Fiber antigen seems

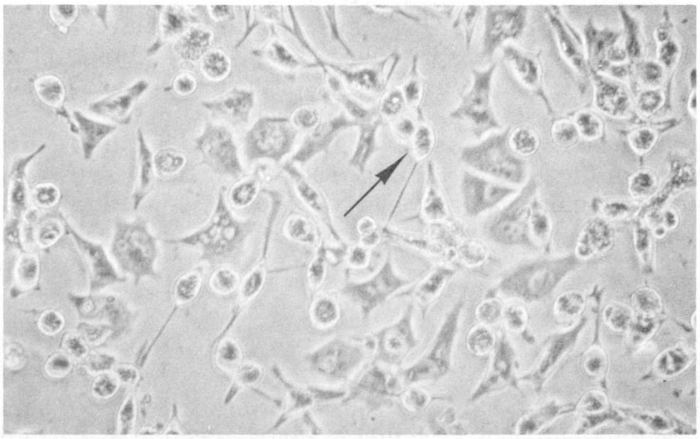

FIG. 1. Typical cytopathogenic effect (CPE) seen in human epithelial cell tissue cultures 2–5 days after infection with adenovirus. Note the enlarged rounded cells (arrow) with strands connecting them to one another and to cells that have not yet begun to show CPE. (Phase contrast, ×400)

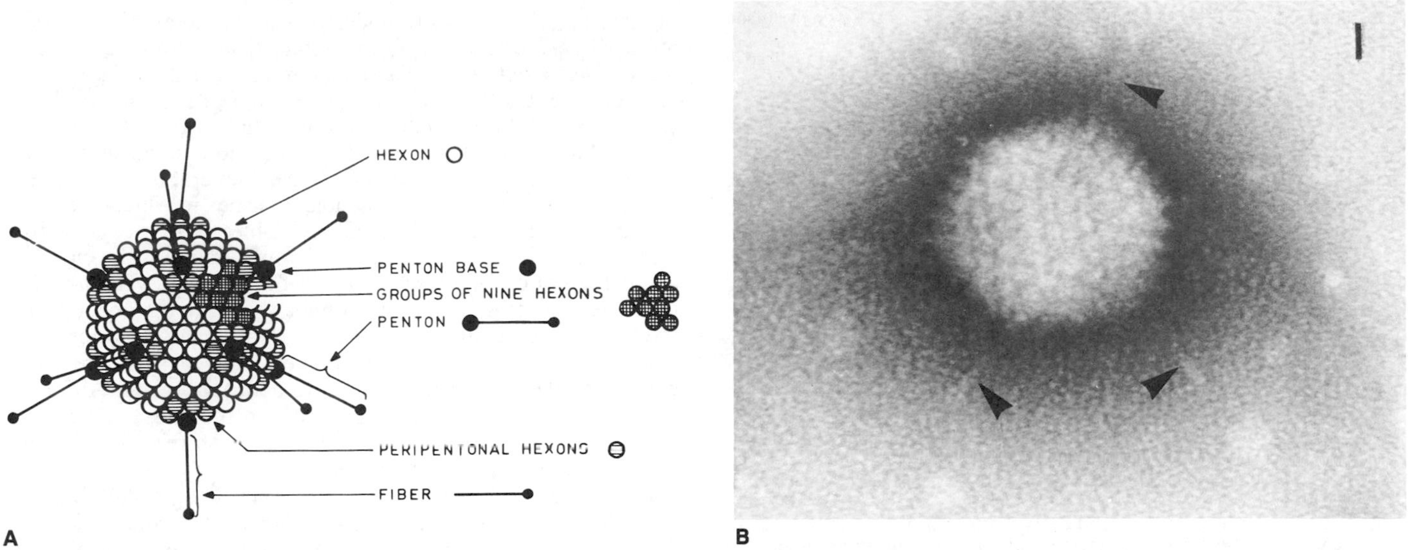

A B

FIG. 2. **(A)** Drawing of an adenovirion and its components. (From Philipson et al.,[17] with permission.) **(B)** Electron micrograph of type 5 adenovirus negatively stained. (Arrows indicate fibers; the bar represents 10 nm.)

to be primarily type specific with some group specificity, while the penton base antigen is common to the adenovirus family.[3] Neutralizing antibody is directed at the hexon type-specific antigen.

In addition to these surface structural proteins, there are a number of internal proteins surrounding the DNA in the adenovirion. These core proteins have been identified electrophoretically[4] and may play a role in maintaining the integrity of the DNA genome. Adenovirus DNA is double stranded and linear and has a molecular weight of about 23×10^6. The DNA represents 10–15 percent of the mass of the virus, and the intact virion has a diameter of about 70 nm, which places it in the middle-sized range of animal viruses.[5]

In the three decades since their discovery, the adenoviruses have been classified in a number of different ways depending on the viewpoint of the taxonomist and on the state of knowledge in virology at the time. The interrrelationship of some of these classifications is given in Table 1. Of particular note is the relationship of a high oncogenic potential with a low guanine and cytosine (G + C) content in the virus DNA. Recently, the adenovirus family has been divided into two genera: adenoviruses of mammals (mastadenoviruses), and those of birds (aviadenoviruses). Mastadenoviruses of humans have been further subdivided (see Table 1) on the basis of antigenicity into subgenera and serotypes that bear a letter h (for human) and a number, for example, mastadenovirus h 7.[6]

As stated earlier, the DNA of adenoviruses is currently being mapped, and functions are being assigned to different regions of the genome. The regions coding for the three capsid proteins have been identified, and the oncogenic potential of these viruses appears to reside in a small area comprising less than 10 percent of the genome near one end. A complete discussion of adenovirus molecular biology is outside the scope of this chapter. Recent reviews by Philipson and colleagues,[17] Wold and coworkers,[18] and Horwitz[19] provide detailed information on this facet of adenovirology.

PATHOGENESIS

Adenoviruses appear to be capable of at least three types of interaction with cells. The first is a lytic infection in which the virus goes through an entire replicative cycle.[9] Lytic infection occurs in human epithelial cells and results in cell death and in the production of 10,000–1 million progeny viruses per cell, of which 1–5 percent are infectious. The second interaction is a latent or chronic infection. This usually involves lymphoid cells, as in the case of the tonsillar infection from which the virus was first isolated.[1,2] Studies have shown that monkey epithelial cells can also undergo latent infection with human adenoviruses.[20] During latent infection only small numbers of viruses may be released, and cell death may be outstripped by cell multiplication, thereby resulting in inapparent infection. The mechanisms of latency are not clearly established.

The third significant virus–cell interaction occurring with adenoviruses is that of oncogenic transformation.[21,22] In this situation, only the early steps in virus replication occur. The viral DNA is apparently integrated into and replicated with the cell's DNA, but no infectious virions are produced. In all three types of infection, virus-specific proteins, the so-called T antigens, are synthesized.[20,23] These antigens give evidence of adenoviral presence even in the absence of infectious virus. The T antigens are detected either by complement fixation or by immunofluorescence assays using serum from hamsters bearing tumors induced by adenovirus. The tumor cells contain large amounts of virus-specific T antigen to which the hamster makes antibody. Figure 3 shows the typical pattern of adenovirus T antigen as shown by immunofluorescence of human cells infected with adenovirus.

EPIDEMIOLOGY

Human adenovirus infections are ubiquitous, although there are slight variations in serotypes causing various syndromes in different parts of the world. Primary infection with an adenovirus usually takes place in the first few years of life, and most of the population has experienced infection with one or another adenovirus serotype by the end of the first decade.[24] The serotype of adenovirus that tends to infect and the disease caused when infection occurs depend a great deal on the age of the patient.

Types 1, 2, 5, and 6 are frequently isolated from the in situ tonsils and adenoids of young children. The children may be asymptomatic or may have upper respiratory infection at the time of isolation, and it is clear from the work of Rowe et al.,[1] Schlesinger,[25] and others that the virus may remain latent in lymphoepithelial tissue in the nasopharynx and elsewhere. Types 3, 4, and 7 are most frequently isolated from young adult patients with acute upper and lower respiratory disease.[24] Military recruits seem particularly prone to colonization and infection by these agents, as they are to infection by mycoplasmal

TABLE 1. Classification Schemes for Adenoviruses of Humans (*Mastadenovirus* h)

Subgenus[a]	Hemagglutination Groups[b]	Serotypes	Oncogenic Potential[c]: Tumors in Animals	Oncogenic Potential[c]: Transformation in Tissue Culture	Percentage of G + C in DNA	Syndromes in Humans Associated with Some Members of a Group
A	IV (little or no agglutination)	12, 18, 31	High	Moderate	48–49	Meningoencephalitis (T12)
B	I (complete agglutination of monkey erythrocytes)	3, 7	Moderate	Moderate	50–52	Pharyngitis, tracheobronchitis, pneumonia, pharyngoconjunctival fever, meningoencephalitis
		11, 21				Hemorrhagic cystitis in children
		14, 16 34, 35[d]				Pneumonia and urinary tract infection in immunocompromized
C	III (partial agglutination of rat erythrocytes)	1, 2, 5, 6	Low or none	Low	57–59	Respiratory infection in children, intussusception
D	II (complete agglutination of rat erythrocytes)	8, 19, 37[e] 9, 10, 13, 15, 17, 42[f] 19, 20, 22–30 32, 33, 36,[g] 38,[h] 39[i]	Low or none	Moderate	57–61	Epidemic keratoconjunctivitis
E	III	4	Low or none	Low	57–59	Respiratory infection in children and closed populations
Fastidious (no genus assigned)		40, 41[j]	Unknown			Enteritis and pneumonia in children

[a] According to Matthews.[6]
[b] According to Rosen.[7]
[c] Derived from Freeman et al.[8] and Ginsberg.[9]
[d] Stalder et al.[10]
[e] Keenlyside et al.[11]
[f] Wigand et al.[12]
[g] Wigand et al.[13]
[h] de Jong et al.[14]
[i] Hierholzer et al.[15]
[j] de Jong et al.[16]

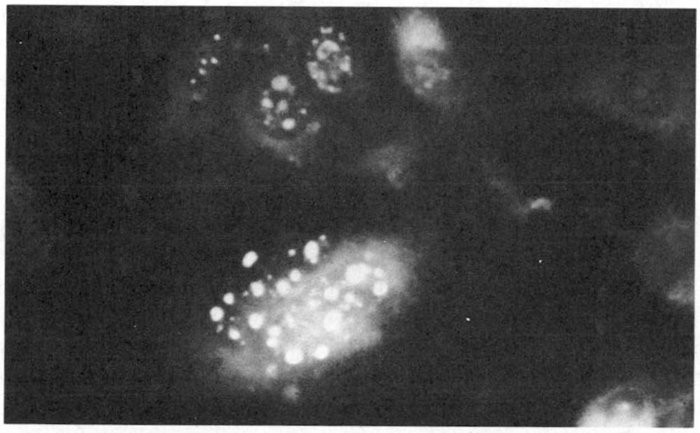

FIG. 3. Adenovirus T antigen detected by immunofluorescence assay of human epithelial cells infected 24 hours earlier with adenovirus, type 7. (×500)

ane meningococcal organisms. The common denominator leading to increased infection rates is probably the crowding of a susceptible population. Infection in these cases seems to be spread by aerosols. Adenovirus type 8 and 19 have frequently been isolated from eye infections in adults,[26,27] and types 11 and 21 have been linked to infections of the lower urinary tract in children.[28]

Two major viral epidemiologic studies have been carried out in this country in the last 20 years.[29,30] Both studies have sought to establish the prevalence of various viruses in clinical and subclinical infections over an extended period in a large population. In each study, adenovirus represented the largest number of isolates in children. Types 1, 2, 3, and 5 were most commonly isolated, and the stool rather than the respiratory secretions was the most common source. It was estimated that 5 percent of all infectious illness in infants and 3 percent in children aged 2–4 years was caused by adenovirus. If seroconversion rather than virus isolation were the criterion, the proportion of illness caused by adenovirus was even higher.

CLINICAL SYNDROMES (Table 2)

Respiratory Infection

In nonepidemic circumstances such as in the general population, at least half of the infections by adenovirus do not lead to clinically significant illness.[24] On the other hand, serologic surveys have shown that about 10 percent of all respiratory diseases in children are caused by adenoviruses.[31]

When respiratory disease in children does result from infection with adenovirus, the illness usually takes the form of mild pharyngitis or tracheitis. In infants, adenovirus type 7 may cause fulminant bronchiolitis and pneumonia.[32] In addition, some investigators have implicated adenovirus as the cause of whooping cough syndrome when *Bordetella pertussis* cannot

TABLE 2. Diseases Caused by Adenoviruses

Group Affected	Syndromes	Common Causal Adenovirus Serotypes
Infants	Coryza, pharyngitis (most asymptomatic)	1, 2, 5
Children	Upper respiratory disease	1, 2, 4–6
	Pharyngoconjunctival fever	3, 7
	Hemorrhagic cystitis	11, 21
	Diarrhea	2, 3, 5, 40, 41
	Intussusception	1, 2, 4, 5
	Meningoencephalitis	2, 6, 7, 12
Young adults	Acute respiratory disease and pneumonia	3, 4, 7
Adults	Epidemic keratoconjunctivitis	8, 19, 37
Immunocompromised	Pneumonia with dissemination, urinary tract infection	5, 34, 35, 39
	CNS disease including encephalitis	7, 12, 32

be incriminated. The virus has also been isolated in cases where this bacterium is cultured.[33] Adenoviruses have been isolated more commonly than have any other nonbacterial pathogen from patients with this syndrome, although a causal relationship has not been clearly established.

The first isolation of adenoviruses from diseased patients occurred in a study of military recruits in 1954.[34] The patients had a variety of influenza-like syndromes grouped under the term *acute respiratory disease* (ARD), and up to one-fifth of these patients required hospitalization. Most of the recruits had tracheobronchitis. It was recognized that the isolates from these patients were similar to those first described by Rowe in 1953 and further characterized by Huebner and colleagues as adenoidal-pharyngeal-conjunctival (APC) viruses.[2] Serum specimens saved from patients having similar syndromes in World War II were later shown to contain antibodies against these viruses. Volunteer studies showed the incubation period to be 4–5 days.

Cough, fever, sore throat, and rhinorrhea are the most common symptoms and usually last 3–5 days. These symptoms are confirmed by physical examination where findings of pharyngitis, rales, and rhonchi are common. X-ray films of the chest in patients with pneumonia show patchy interstitial infiltrates primarily in the lower lung fields. The correlation between physical and radiographic findings in adenoviral pneumonia seems to be better than it is in *Mycoplasma*-induced pneumonia. In this latter condition, the extent of infiltrates on the roentgenogram is surprising because physical findings in the chest examination are minimal.

Other infectious agents that cause a similar syndrome of "atypical" pneumonia in this population are influenza and parainfluenza viruses and *Mycoplasma pneumoniae*. Of the 40 percent of all atypical pneumonia cases that are caused by adenoviruses, types 4 and 7 are most often isolated. The disease is self-limited, and superinfection and death are rare.

Pharyngoconjunctival Fever

In children, the best described syndrome attributed to adenoviruses is the so-caled pharyngoconjunctival fever. This disease occurs in small epidemics and is one of the most common syndromes seen by physicians at children's summer camps. It is characterized by conjunctivitis, pharyngitis, rhinitis, cervical adenitis, and temperatures to 38°C. The onset is acute, and the fever and other symptoms last 3–5 days. Bulbar and palpebral conjunctivitis may be the only finding, and the palpebral conjunctivae usually have a granular appearance. Although the onset is frequently monoculor, the other eye usually becomes involved. There is little bacterial superinfection and no permanent damage to the eye.

Early reports of this syndrome in the 1950s mentioned meningismus as a prominent symptom in one-sixth of the cases. At that time, this finding led to some diagnostic confusion with poliomyelitis. Today, other enteroviral infections and infectious mononucleosis should be considered in young patients with conjunctivitis and pharyngitis.

Respiratory involvement in this syndrome usually does not progress to the bronchi or lungs, and bacterial superinfection is rare. Contaminated swimming pools and ponds have been implicated as the source of spread in this disease, and several of the most complete studies of this syndrome have shown type 3 adenovirus to be the causative agent.[35]

Epidemic Keratoconjunctivitis

Keratoconjunctivitis occurring in epidemic form in adult populations was first ascribed to adenovirus infection by Jawetz and coworkers in 1955.[26] They showed that eyes of shipyard workers that had sustained minor trauma due to paint and rust chips were frequently infected with adenovirus type 8. Other serotypes have caused sporadic cases, but the only other serotypes that have been involved in major epidemics are types 19 and 37.[11] An epidemic involving both types simultaneously has also been reported.[27] Infection in one epidemic was through the use of a roller towel for drying hands and faces.[36] Contaminated ophthalmic solutions have also provided a vector.[11]

The incubation period may be 4–24 days, and the conjunctivitis may last 1–4 weeks. The onset of conjunctivitis is insidious and frequently bilateral, and preauricular adenopathy is common. Keratitis begins as the conjunctivitis wanes, and the cornea may remain involved for several months and produce visual disturbance. There is secondary spread to household contacts in about 10 percent of the cases, with a higher incidence of secondary cases occurring with increased duration of the index case.[27] Virus can be isolated readily for at least 9 days after the onset of symptoms.[37]

Hemorrhagic Cystitis

A recent review of cases of hemorrhagic cystitis in Japanese and American children showed that 23–51 percent of these children had adenoviruria. Adenovirus types 11 and 21 were isolated more frequently than was any other single bacterial or viral agent. Boys were much more commonly affected than were girls (2–3 : 1), whereas in bacterial hemorrhagic cystitis girls predominated. The average duration of gross hematuria was 3 days. Microscopic hematuria, dysuria, and urinary frequency persisted for several days longer.[28]

The duration and severity of the disease were increased in the Japanese as compared with the American children. There was no seasonal preponderance. Serologic studies indicated a large proportion of subclinical infections with adenovirus type 11 in children.

No structural abnormalities were discovered in the sick children, and this fact plus the predominance in boys made it likely that the cystitis was not due to retrograde spread from the urethra. However, no viremia was demonstrated.

Infantile Diarrhea

There has been recent intense interest and investigative activity into the viral etiology of infantile diarrhea. Much of the progress in this area has resulted from the use of electron microscopy and immune electron microscopy to identify virus particles morphologically and immunologically. These studies have shown that rotaviruses (Chapter 129) and adenoviruses are the predominant pathogens in this disease.[38,39] These adenoviruses are readily seen in large numbers but are not culturable on standard human tissue culture cells. They are defective and require either cells that are transformed by adenovirus[39] or Chang conjunctival cells.[38] These have also been called "enteric" or "uncultivatable" adenovirus, but they have recently been serotyped and are now known as types 40 and 41 (Table 1).

The defect in their replication seems to be a step before DNA synthesis.[40]

Intussusception

Another intestinal syndrome in which adenoviruses have been etiologically implicated is intussusception in children. In one recent study, adenoviruses were the most commonly isolated agent, representing 41 percent of all cases and 80 percent of all isolates. Serotypes 1, 2, 3, and 5 predominated, and many of the patients had preceding or concurrent respiratory infection.[41] Viral isolations were, however, rarely accompanied by type-specific rises in antibody.

Central Nervous System Infection

Encephalitis and meningoencephalitis cases occurring sporadically have been caused by adenoviruses. In addition, epidemics of central nervous system (CNS) infection have occurred as complications of respiratory epidemics. Serotype 7 has been most commonly found,[42] but serotypes 1, 6, and 12 have also been found regularly. Pneumonia is a frequent finding in cases of adenovirus CNS disease. Spinal fluid findings are quite variable, and the values for cell count and protein and glucose levels are not helpful in establishing a diagnosis. Chronic meningoencephalitis with serotypes 7, 12, and 32 is well documented in hypogammaglobulinemic patients.

Other Diseases Infrequently Attributed to Adenoviruses

Adenoviruses have at one time or another been implicated as the cause of pericarditis,[43] chronic interstitial fibrosis,[44] rubelliform illness,[45] and congenital anomalies.[46] Although adenovirus may be involved in these syndromes, it is unproved and unlikely that these viruses commonly play an etiologic role in any of these illnesses.

Disseminated disease due to adenovirus has been described in bone marrow and renal transplant recipients.[47,48]

Among the immunocompromized patients from whom adenoviruses have been cultured are a number of patients with the acquired immunodeficiency syndrome (AIDS). Adenovirus type 35 has been recovered from the urine of these patients. This is an uncommon isolate in nonimmunocompromised people, and the reservoir for this virus is unknown.[49]

DIAGNOSIS

A diagnosis of adenoviral infection is frequently made in the proper setting on clinical criteria alone. A definitive diagnosis rests on visualization of the virus by electronmicropscopy,[50] isolation of the virus in tissue culture, demonstration of adenovirus antigens in infected cells, or demonstration of fourfold rises in antibodies to adenovirus during the course of the illness.

Adenoviruses may be cultured from pharynx, sputum, stool, and conjunctival scrapings and fresh urine in the appropriate syndromes. Viral culture is performed in monolayers of human epithelial cells, and depending on the amount of virus in the inoculum, typical cytopathogenic changes occur in 2–7 days. Isolated adenovirus can be grouped by hemagglutination (Table 1) and then specifically serotyped. Virus isolation is successful in 50–70 percent of serologically confirmed cases of respiratory disease or conjunctivitis.

Adenovirus antigens have been demonstrated in exfoliated cells in cases of epidemic keratoconjunctivitis, pharyngoconjunctival fever, and hemorrhagic cystitis. The indirect immunofluorescence technique has been used and has correlated very well with virus isolation. This technique is much quicker and cheaper than is virus culture, and it can be used to demonstrate both T and capsid antigens in infected cells.[28,51]

Serologic diagnosis of adenovirus infection involves the demonstration of a fourfold rise in antibodies that will fix complement, neutralize the virus, or prevent adenoviral hemagglutination or that can be detected in an enzyme-linked immunosorbent assay (ELISA) or radioimmunoassay (RIA) test. Complement-fixing antibodies are group specific, while neutralizing and hemagglutination-inhibiting antibodies are type specific.

The rise in antibodies begins about 1 week after infection. As in other viral infections, complement-fixing antibodies are the earliest to fall and disappear by 1 year after infection. Neutralizing antibodies may persist for a decade or more in relatively undiminished titer. Heterotypic reinfection may be responsible for repeated boosts of these long-lived antibodies.

Mufson and Belshe have reported that a single determination of neutralizing antibodies to adenovirus types 11 or 21 at a titer of greater than 1:32 in a patient with hemorrhagic cystitis may be taken as a confirmatory evidence of adenovirus disease.[28]

TREATMENT

There are no specific drugs or therapeutic measures available for the treatment of adenovirus infections. Fortunately, most of the syndromes are self-limited, and death is extremely rare.

PREVENTION

Because of the ubiquity and severity of adenovirus respiratory disease in certain populations, vaccines were developed to prevent the disease. Although these live and inactivated virus vaccines were reasonably effective, the findings that adenoviruses were oncogenic and could combine with simian virus 40 to produce an even more oncogenic hybrid virus curtailed the use of parenteral vaccines. Vaccines have also been produced by using capsid components free of DNA. These vaccines have been effective in volunteer studies but are not currently available for general administration.[24]

Oral vaccines have been developed for use in military recruit populations. These vaccines contain live adenovirus types 4 and 7 in an enteric-coated capsule. These viruses are not attenuated, but advantage is taken of the fact that inoculation of adenovirus into the gastrointestinal tract does not result in illness, in contrast to inoculation into the respiratory tract. Their efficacy and safety have been well established in the past 10 years, and the problem of acute respiratory disease in recruits has been markedly diminished.[52] It will be interesting to see whether other adenovirus serotypes or nonviral infectious agents increasingly appear as causes of acute respiratory disease in this population.

ADENO-ASSOCIATED VIRUSES

Adenovirus preparations are often contaminated with a 2 nm icosahedral virus that has been called *adeno-associated virus* (AAV).[53] The AAV are defective in that they require adenovirus coinfection of cells to replicate. Herpesvirus and vaccinia can also provide a helper function for these viruses.[54] AAV contain single-stranded DNA that is not homologous to adenovirus DNA and has a molecular weight of 1.4×10^6. AAV are unique among DNA animal viruses in that complementary strands of viral DNA are made within the cell and either strand may enter the virus particle to give rise to some virions with DNA of one polarity and some with the complementary strand.[55] The presence of AAV in an adenovirus preparation diminishes the infectivity of the adenovirus by an unknown mechanism.[53]

There are four serotypes of AAV, and although they have not been implicated in any human disease, the viruses have been isolated from human pharyngeal secretions and stool, and most people have antibodies to one or another AAV serotype by 10 years of age.[56] A closely related parvovirus (B19) has been proved to cause erythema infectiosum (fifth disease) in both children and adults and causes aplastic crises in patients with hemoglobinopathies[57,58] (Chapter 125).

ADENOVIRUS–SV40 HYBRID VIRUSES

During the course of vaccine development adenovirus stocks became contaminated with SV40, which was indigenous in the monkey cells in which the adenovirus was propagated. The SV40 actually enabled the human adenovirus to grow in monkey cells, which are otherwise nonpermissive for adenovirus.[11,59] Contaminating SV40 virus was eliminated by multiple passages in the presence of antiserum to SV40. However, dual selective pressures existed that gave rise to a hybrid virus: the monkey cells were nonpermissive for adenovirus growth, and antibody to SV40 inhibited the growth of SV40 alone. The resulting hybrid virion contained partial genomes of adenovirus and SV40 linked to one another within a normal adenovirus capsid.[60,61] This hybrid virus could grow in monkey cells and had increased oncogenic potential over that of the adenovirus alone.[62] Hybrid viruses exist between SV40 and adenovirus types 1 through 7 and 12.[63] Many of the hybrid viruses are defective and require coinfection of cells with nonhybrid adenovirus to allow replication. However, some involving type 2 adenovirus are nondefective.[64]

These viruses have not been implicated in human disease, although they were used as vaccine agents before their true character and animal oncogenicity was appreciated. Their unique molecular composition, however, has provided an invaluable tool for investigations of the genetics of adenovirus and SV40 infection. Knowledge of these hybrid viruses offers a fascinating model for the consideration of viral pathogenesis, vaccine development, and oncogenesis. The independent existence of adenovirus and SV40 viruses was recognized before the emergence of the hybrids. Had this not been the case, the true molecular nature of the hybrids and the fact that hybrids can form at all would not have been appreciated. The potential for one virus to pick up genetic material from another, thereby changing host range and oncogenicity, must now be taken into account in the development of live virus vaccines and may be a factor in the emergence of new syndromes.

REFERENCES

1. Rowe WP, Huebner RJ, Gillmore LK, et al. Isolation of a cytopathogenic agent from human adenoids undergoing spontaneous degeneration in tissue culture. Proc Soc Exp Biol Med. 1953;84:570.
2. Huebner RJ, Rowe WP, Ward TG, et al. Adenoidal-pharyngeal-conjunctival agents: A newly recognized group of common viruses of the respiratory system. N Engl J Med. 1954;251:1077.
3. Norby E. The structural and functional diversity of adenovirus capsid components. J Gen Virol. 1969;5:14.
4. Anderson CW, Baum PR, Gesteland RF. Processing of adenovirus 2-induced proteins. J Virol. 1973;12:241.
5. Green M, Pina M, Kimes R, et al. Adenovirus DNA. I. Molecular weight and conformation. Proc Natl Acad Sci USA. 1967;57:1302.
6. Matthews REF. The classification and nomenclature of viruses: Summary of results of meetings of the international committee on taxonomy of viruses in Strasbourg, August 1981. Intervirology. 1981;16:53.
7. Rosen L. Hemagglutination by adenoviruses. Virology. 1958;5:574.
8. Freeman AE, Black PH, Vanderpool EA, et al. Transformation of primary rat embryo cells by adenovirus type 2. Proc Natl Acad Sci USA. 1967;58:1205.
9. Ginsberg HS. Adenoviruses. In: Davis BD. Dulbecco R, Eisen HN, et al, eds. Microbiology. Hagerstown, MD: Harper & Row; 1980:1047.
10. Stalder H, Hierholzer JC, Oxman MN. New human adenovirus (candidate adenovirus type 35) causing fatal disseminated infection in a renal transplant recipient. J Clin Microbiol. 1977;6:257.
11. Keenlyside RA, Hierholzer JC, D'Angelo LJ. Keratoconjunctivitis associated with adenovirus type 37: An extended outbreak in an ophthalmologist's office. J Infect Dis. 1983;147:191.
12. Wigand R, Adrian T, Bricout F. A new human adenovirus of subgenus D: Candidate adenovirus type 42. Arch Virol. 1987;94:283–6.
13. Wigand R, Gelderblom H, Wadell G. New human adenovirus (candidate adenovirus 36): A novel member of subgroup D. Arch Virol. 1980;64:225.
14. de Jong JC, Wigand R, Adrian T, et al. Adenovirus 38: A new human adenovirus species of subgenus D. Intervirology. 1984;22:164–9.
15. Hierholzer JC, Kemp MC, Gary W Jr, et al. New human adenovirus associated with respiratory illness: Candidate adenovirus type 39. J Clin Microbiol. 1982;16:15.
16. de Jong JC, Wigand R, Kidd AH, et al. Candidate adenoviruses from human infant stool. J Med Virol. 1983;11:215.
17. Philipson L, Pettersson U, Lindberg U. Molecular Biology of Adenoviruses. Virology Monographs 14. New York: Springer Publishing; 1975.
18. Wold WSM, Green M, Büttner W. Adenoviruses. In: Nayak PP, ed. Molecular Biology of Animal Viruses. v. 2. New York: Marcel Dekker; 1978:673.
19. Horwitz MS. Adenoviruses. In: Fields BN, Melnick JL, Chanock R, et al, eds. Human Viral Diseases. New York: Raven Press; 1985:477–95.
20. Baum SG. Persistent adenovirus infections of nonpermissive monkey cells. J Virol. 1977;23:412.
21. Huebner RJ, Rowe WP, Lane WT. Oncogenic effects in hamsters of human adenoviruses types 12 and 18. Proc Natl Acad Sci USA. 1962;48:2051.
22. Trentin JJ, Yabe Y, Taylor G. The quest for human cancer viruses. Science. 1962;137:835.
23. Pope JH, Rowe WP. Immunofluorescent studies of adenovirus 12 tumors and of cells transformed or infected by adenovirus. J Exp Med. 1964;120:577.
24. Knight V, Kasel JA. Adenoviruses. In: Knight V, ed. Viral and Mycoplasmal Infections of the Respiratory Tract. Philadelphia: Lea & Febiger; 1973:65.
25. Schlesinger RW. Adenoviruses: The nature of the virion and controlling factors in productive or abortive infection and tumorigenesis. Adv Virus Res. 1969;14:1.
26. Jawetz E, Kimura S, Nicholas AN, et al. New type of APC virus from epidemic keratoconjunctivitis. Science. 1955;122:1190.
27. Guyer B, O'Day DM, Hierholzer JC, et al. Epidemic keratoconjunctivitis: A community outbreak of mixed adenovirus type 8 and type 19 infection. J Infect Dis. 1975;132:142.
28. Mufson MA, Belshe RB. A review of adenoviruses in the etiology of acute hemorrhagic cystitis. J Urol. 1976;115:191.
29. Fox JP, Brandt CD, Wasserman FE, et al. The virus watch program: A continuing surveillance of viral infections in metropolitan New York families. Am J Epidemiol. 1969;89:25.
30. Fox JP, Hall CE, Cooney M. The Seattle virus watch. VII. Observations of adenovirus infections. Am J Epidemiol. 1977;105:362.
31. Brandt CD, Hyun WK, Vargosko AJ, et al. Infections in 18,000 infants and children in a controlled study of respiratory tract disease. I. Adenovirus pathogenicity in relation to serologic type and illness syndrome. Am J Epidemiol. 1969;90:484.
32. Angella JJ, Connor JD. Neonatal infection caused by adenovirus type 7. J Pediatr. 1968;72:474.
33. Olson LC. Pertussis. Medicine (Baltimore). 1975;54:427.
34. Hilleman MR, Werner JH. Recovery of a new agent from patients with acute respiratory illness. Proc Exp Biol Med. 1954;85:183.
35. Sobel G, Aronson B, Aronson S, et al. Pharyngoconjunctival fever. Am J Dis Child. 1956;92:596.
36. Sprague JB, Hierholzer JC, Currier RW II, et al. Epidemic keratoconjunctivitis: A severe industrial outbreak due to adenovirus type 8. N Engl J Med. 1973;289:1341.
37. Koc J, Wigand R, Weil M. The efficacy of various laboratory methods for the diagnosis of adenovirus conjunctivitis. Zentralbl Bakteriol Mikrobiol Hyg [A]. 1987;263:607–15.
38. Kidd AH, Cosgrove BP, Brown RA, et al. Faecal adenoviruses from Glasgow babies. J Hyg (Camb). 1982;88:463.
39. Yolken RH, Lawrence F, Leister F, et al. Gastroenteritis associated with enteric type adenovirus in hospitalized infants. J Pediatr 1982;101:21.
40. Takiff HE, Straus SE. Early replicative block prevents the efficient growth of fastidious diarrhea-associated adenovirus in cell culture. J Med Virol. 1982;9:93.
41. Nicolas JC, Ingrand D, Fortier B, et al. A one-year virological survey of acute intussusception in childhood. J Med Virol. 1982;9:267.
42. Simila S, Jouppila R, Salmi A, ert al. Encephalomeningitis in children associated with an adenovirus type 7 epidemic. Acta Paediatr Scand. 1970;59:310.
43. Rahal JJ, Millian SJ, Noriega ER. Coxsackie and adenovirus infection. Association with acute febrile and juvenile rheumatoid arthritis. JAMA. 1976;235:2496.
44. Kawai T, Fujiwara T, Aoyama Y, et al. Diffuse interstitial fibrosing pneumonitis and adenovirus infection. Chest. 1976;69:692.
45. Gutekunst RR, Heggie AD. Viremia and viruria in adenovirus infection: Detection in patients with rubella and rubelliform illness. N Engl J Med. 1961;264:374.
46. Evans TN, Brown GC. Congenital anomalies and virus infection. Am J Obstet Gynecol. 1963;87:749.
47. Keller EW, Rubin RH, Black PH, et al. Isolation of adenovirus type 34 from a renal transplant recipient with interstitial pneumonia. Transplantation. 1977;23:188.
48. Shields AF, Hackman RC, Fife KH, et al. Adenovirus infections in patients undergoing bone marrow transplantation. N Engl J Med. 1985;312:529–33.
49. Flomenberg PR, Chen M, Munk G, et al. Molecular epidemiology of adenovirus type 35 infections in immunocompromised hosts. J Infect Dis. 1987;155:1127–34.
50. Madely CR, Cosgrove BP, Bell EJ, et al. Stool viruses in babies in Glasgow. J Hyg (Lond). 1977;78:261.
51. Schwartz HS, Vastine DW, Yamashiroya H, et al. Immunofluorescent detection of adenovirus antigen in epidemic keratoconjunctivitis. Invest Ophthalmol. 1976;15:199.
52. Dudding BA, Top FH Jr, Winter PE, et al. Acute respiratory disease in military trainees. The adenovirus surveillance program 1966–1971. Am J Epidemiol. 1973;97:187.
53. Hoggan MD, Blacklow NR, Rowe WP. Studies of small DNA viruses found in various adenovirus preparations: Physical, biological and immunological characteristics. Proc Natl Acad Sci USA. 1966;55:1467.
54. Schlehofer JR, Ehbar M, zur-Hausen H. Vaccinia virus, herpes simplex virus and carcinogens induce DNA amplification in a human cell line and support replication of helper virus dependent parvovirus. Virology. 1986;152:110–17.
55. Berns KI, Rose JA. Evidence for a single-stranded adenovirus associated virus genome: Isolation and separation of complementary single strands. J Virol. 1970;5:693.
56. Parks WP, Boucher DW, Melnick JL, et al. Seroepidemiological and ecological studies of the adenovirus associated satellite viruses. Infect Immun. 1970;2:716.
57. Anderson MJ. Human paravovirus infections. J Virol Methods. 1987;17:175–81.
58. Conrad MR, Studdard H, Anderson LJ. Aplastic crisis in sickle cell disorders: Bone marrow necrosis and human parvovirus infection. Am J Med Sci. 1988;95:212–5.
59. O'Connor GT, Rabson AS, Berezesky IK, et al. Mixed infection with simian virus 40 and adenovirus 12. JNCI. 1963;31:903.
60. Rowe WP, Baum SG. Evidence for a possible genetic hybrid between adenovirus type 7 and SV40 viruses. Proc Natl Acad Sci USA. 1964;52:1340.
61. Rapp F, Melnick JL, Butel JS, et al. The incorporation of SV40 genetic ma-

terial into adenovirus 7 as measured by intranuclear synthesis of SV40 tumor antigen. Proc Natl Acad Sci USA. 1964;52:1348.
62. Huebner RJ, Chanock RM, Rubin BA, et al. Induction by adenovirus type 7 of tumors in hamsters having the antigenic characteristics of SV40 virus. Proc Natl Acad Sci USA. 1964;52:1333.
63. Lewis AM, Baum SG, Prigge KO, et al. Occurrence of adenovirus-SV40 hybrids among monkey kidney cell adapted strains of adenovirus. Proc Soc Exp Med Biol. 1966;122:214.
64. Lewis AM Jr, Levine AS, Crumpacker CS, et al. Studies of nondefective adenovirus 2 simian virus 40 hybrid viruses. V. Isolation of additional hybrids which differ in their simian virus 40–specific biologic properties. J Virol. 1973;11:655.

Papovaviridae

123. PAPILLOMAVIRUSES

RICHARD C. REICHMAN
WILLIAM BONNEZ

Human papillomaviruses (HPVs) are widespread throughout the population, produce epithelial tumors of the skin and mucous membranes, and have been closely associated with genital tract malignancies. Papillomaviruses have been detected in a variety of vertebrates, although the viruses are highly species specific and cross-species infections occur rarely, even under experimental conditions. The infectious nature of human warts was initially demonstrated in the late nineteenth century when human wart extracts were shown to produce warts when injected into humans. Ciuffo was the first to suggest that the infectious agent of warts was a virus when he transmitted the infection, using cell-free filtrates, in 1907.[1] Despite these early observations, HPVs have not been studied using standard virologic techniques because they have not been propagated successfully in tissue culture or in standard laboratory animals. As recently as 15 years ago, it was generally thought that all warts were caused by a single papillomavirus and that differences among warts were due to local anatomic factors. As a result of recent advances in molecular biology, it has been shown that a large number of HPVs exist. In addition, these techniques have led to an understanding of the genomic organization of HPVs and of the functions of different viral genes. Detailed reviews of these advances have recently been published.[2–4]

VIROLOGY

Animal and human HPVs are members of the A genus of the Papovaviridae family.[5] They are nonenveloped viruses 55 nm in diameter, with an icosahedral capsid composed of 72 capsomers enclosing a double-stranded, circular DNA genome. Virion particles contain at least two capsid proteins. The major capsid protein constitutes 80 percent of the virion by weight and has a molecular weight of about 56,000. The minor capsid protein has a molecular weight of approximately 76,000.

The antigenic characteristics of intact viral particles have not been studied extensively. However, broadly cross-reactive, genus-specific antigenic determinants, probably located in the middle of the major capsid protein,[6] can be prepared by denaturing viral particles with detergents and reducing agents. Antisera prepared against this papillomavirus *common antigen* have been used widely in the immunocytochemical diagnosis of HPV infections[7] (see below under "Diagnosis").

The HPV genome consists of approximately 7900 base pairs. All putative coding sequences (open reading frames, or ORFs) are arranged on one DNA strand. The genomic organization of all well-studied papillomaviruses is similar.[8] Specific protein products appear to be derived from these ORFs. However, analyses of viral messenger RNA (mRNA) transcripts suggest that most viral proteins derive from splicing of more than one ORF-specific mRNA. The genome is functionally divided into three regions. An "early" region of 5–7 ORFs (E1–7) codes for proteins responsible for transformation and replication functions. ORFs L1 and L2 constitute the "late" region and code for the major and minor capsid proteins, respectively. A third, noncoding region is essential for regulatory functions of the genome.[8]

Although several papillomaviruses have been shown to transform tissue culture preparations, in vitro replication of complete virion particles has not been achieved. However, HPV type 11 has been successfully propagated in human neonatal foreskin implants placed under the renal capsule of nude mice.[9] Virions of most HPV types cannot be purified from naturally occurring lesions in significant quantities, and well-characterized, type-specific antigens are not available. Thus, types are determined according to the degree of nucleic acid homology, rather than by serologic techniques. DNA of unique HPV types cross hybridize less than 50 percent with DNAs of other types.[8] Over 60 different HPV types have now been identified. HPVs are host specific, and each type is, to a large extent, associated with a distinct histopathologic process (Table 1).

EPIDEMIOLOGY

Incidence and Prevalence

The epidemiology of HPV infections is poorly understood. Few systematically conducted studies have been carried out, techniques for seroepidemiologic investigation remain inadequate, and diagnoses have been based primarily on physical examination alone. However, several generalizations regarding the epidemiology of some HPV infections can be made.

Three types of cutaneous HPV infections are widespread throughout the general population and demonstrate little gender preference. Common warts occur frequently among school-age children, with prevalence rates as high as 50 percent. Although less common, plantar warts are observed frequently among adolescents and young adults. Juvenile or flat warts are the least common of the three types and occur predominantly in children. Another group at high risk for the development of cutaneous warts includes butchers, meatpackers, and fish handlers.[10–13] Epidermodysplasia verruciformis is a rare, probably autosomal

TABLE 1. HPV Types and Their Disease Association

Disease	*Associated HPV Types*[a]
Deep plantar warts	1; 2, 4[b]
Common warts	2,1; 4, 41
Common warts of meat handlers	7
Flat warts	3, 10; 27, 41
Intermediate warts	10, 26, 28
Epidermodysplasia verruciformis	5*[c], 8*, 9, 12, 14, 15, 17, 19–25, 36, 46, 47
Condyloma acuminatum	6, 11; 10, 40–44, 45, 51
Intraepithelial neoplasias, unspecified	33*, 35, 42–45, 51, 52
Bowen's disease	16*, 31
Bowenoid papulosis	16*, 34, 39, 42
High-grade dysplasias	16*, 18*
Low-grade dysplasias	6, 11; 31, 45
Laryngeal papillomas	6, 11, 30*
Focal epithelial hyperplasia of Heck	13; 32
Conjunctival papillomas	6, 11
Others[d]	37, 38

[a] Types 29, 48–50, 52–60 have also been identified but not published (data supplied by Ethel-Michele de Villiers; HPV Reference Center, Heidelberg, FRG).
[b] HPV types to the left of the semicolon are those most frequently encountered.
[c] The asterisk indicates those types believed to have a high malignant potential.
[d] Keratoacanthoma and malignant melanoma, respectively.

recessive condition, characterized by the appearance early in life of disseminated cutaneous warts and frequent malignant transformation.[14,15]

Condyloma acuminatum, or anogenital warts, is a common sexually transmitted disease (STD) that appears to be increasing rapidly in incidence. Using data collected by the National Disease and Therapeutic Index, the Centers for Disease Control estimated that the number of patient–physician interactions in the private sector increased from 169,000 in 1966 to 1,150,000 in 1984 in the United States.[16] In an STD clinic setting in the United Kingdom, the annual incidence of genital warts per 100,000 population was estimated to have increased from about 30 in 1971 to 50 in 1978.[17] Smaller studies in better-defined patient populations have also shown dramatic increases in the prevalence of this disease in recent years.[18,19] HPV infection of the cervix gives rise to the most common cause of squamous cell abnormalities on Papanicolaou smears.[20–23]

Recurrent respiratory papillomatosis is an uncommon disease with a bimodal age distribution. Symptoms occur in pre-school-age children, as well as in adults. An estimated 1500 new cases occur annually in the United States.[24]

Transmission

Close personal contact is assumed to be important for the transmission of most cutaneous warts, although strong epidemiologic evidence for this assumption is lacking. Minor trauma at the site of inoculation may also be important, as suggested by the high frequency of disease among meat handlers. The role of fomites in the transmission of HPV infection is uncertain.

Evidence that anogenital warts are sexually transmitted includes the observation that the age of onset is similar to that of other STDs and that approximately two-thirds of sexual contacts of patients with anogenital warts will go on to develop the disease.[25,26] In addition, these patients often have other concomitant STDs or a history of such infections. Also, as outlined in Table 1, particular HPV types are associated with these lesions. These types are rarely found at other sites.

Recurrent respiratory papillomatosis in young children is thought to be acquired by passage through an infected birth canal. This hypothesis is based upon the observation that similar HPV types are related to both respiratory papillomatosis and anogenital warts, and that a large percentage of the mothers of these children have a history of genital tract HPV disease. However, cases of laryngeal papillomatosis have been documented at birth, even after cesarian section.[24,27–29] The mode of transmission of recurrent respiratory papillomatosis in adults is unknown. The disease may be a late complication of perinatal infection or may be acquired by oral-genital contact.

Association between HPV and Malignancies

Several different epidemiologic observations suggest a strong link between HPV lesions and genital tract malignancies. For example, studies have demonstrated that women with a history of genital warts may be four times more likely to develop cervical carcinoma in situ than women without such a history.[30] Case–control studies have also shown an increased risk of developing cervical carcinoma in patients with a history of genital warts.[18] Also of interest is the observation that women married to men who developed cancer of the penis are significantly more likely to develop cervical cancer than are other women.[31] In addition, nuns rarely develop cervical cancer.[32]

An additional strong piece of evidence linking HPV with cervical cancer is the observation that more than 90 percent of these lesions contain HPV DNA, usually of types 16, 18, 31.[33] Other evidence suggesting the importance of HPV types 16 and 18 in the pathogenesis of cervical neoplasias derives from limited longitudinal studies that indicate that dysplastic lesions associated with these types are much more likely to progress to severe forms of dysplasia than lesions that contain the HPV types associated with benign condylomas (types 6 and 11).[34] However, one recent large comparative study failed to show a direct association between the prevalence of HPV types 16 and 18 in cervical smears and the incidence of cervical cancer.[35]

Although a significant amount of information suggesting a close association between HPV and genital tract malignancies exists, the epidemiologic studies have been criticized for flaws in design such as small sample sizes, biased selection of study subjects, lack of established criteria for histologic or molecular diagnosis, and inadequate statistical techniques.[36]

PATHOGENESIS

The incubation period of HPV disease was established experimentally by inoculation of human subjects with extracts of cutaneous warts.[1,37] Most often, warts developed within 3–4 months, although lesions occasionally developed as early as 6 weeks or as long as 2 years after inoculation. A similar incubation period was observed for genital warts among wives of American soldiers returning from the Korean War.[38] All types of squamous epithelium may be infected by HPV, but other tissues appear to be relatively resistant. Gross histologic appearances of individual lesions vary with the site of infection and the virus type. Figure 1 is a schematic diagram of a typical exophytic, cutaneous wart. Although nothing is known about the first stage of HPV infection, it is assumed that the virus life cycle begins with the entry of particles into the stratum germinativum, since viral DNA has been detected in the nuclei of the basal cells.[39] As the basal cells differentiate and progress to the surface of the epithelium, HPV DNA replicates and transcribes, and viral particles are assembled in the nucleus. Ultimately, complete virions are released when dead keratinocytes are shed. Viral replication is associated with excessive proliferation of all of the epidermal layers except the basal layer. This process produces acanthosis, parakeratosis, and hyperkeratosis. There is also, where normally present, a deepening of the rete ridges, producing typical papillomatous cytoarchitecture. This hyperproliferation of tissue may be indirectly mediated, since many cells in a wart do not appear to harbor HPV DNA.[39] Some infected cells undergo the characteristic transformation of koilocytosis. Koilocytes (from the Greek *koilos*, meaning cavity) are large, usually polygonal squamous cells with a shrunken nucleus lodged inside a large cytoplasmic vacuole. Cytoplasmic keratohyalin inclusion bodies may also be observed.

It is important to note that normal-appearing epithelium may contain HPV DNA[40,41] and that the presence of residual DNA after the treatment of warts may lead to recurrent disease.

In benign lesions caused by HPV, viral DNA is located extrachromosomally in the nuclei of infected cells. However, when HPV DNA is detected in severe dysplasias and cancers, it is generally integrated.[42] Integration of HPV DNA into malignant cells occurs at specific sites within the viral genome, although integrated viral DNA is found randomly in host cell chromosomes. Similar observations have been made in several continuous cell lines that have been demonstrated to contain HPV DNA.[42]

Host defense responses to HPV infection are poorly understood. Nevertheless, several clinical observations suggest that an effective immune system is important in the resolution of HPV infection. HPV diseases occur frequently and are often severe in patients with both primary and secondary immunodeficiencies. Such patients include those with the Wiskott-Aldrich syndrome and common variable immunodeficiency.[43] Severe, frequent HPV disease is also seen in patients with human immunodeficiency virus (HIV) infections and in those with lymphoproliferative disorders.[43,44] Immunosuppressive therapy, notably in renal allograft recipients, has also been associated with high rates of extensive HPV infection.[45–47] Another clinical

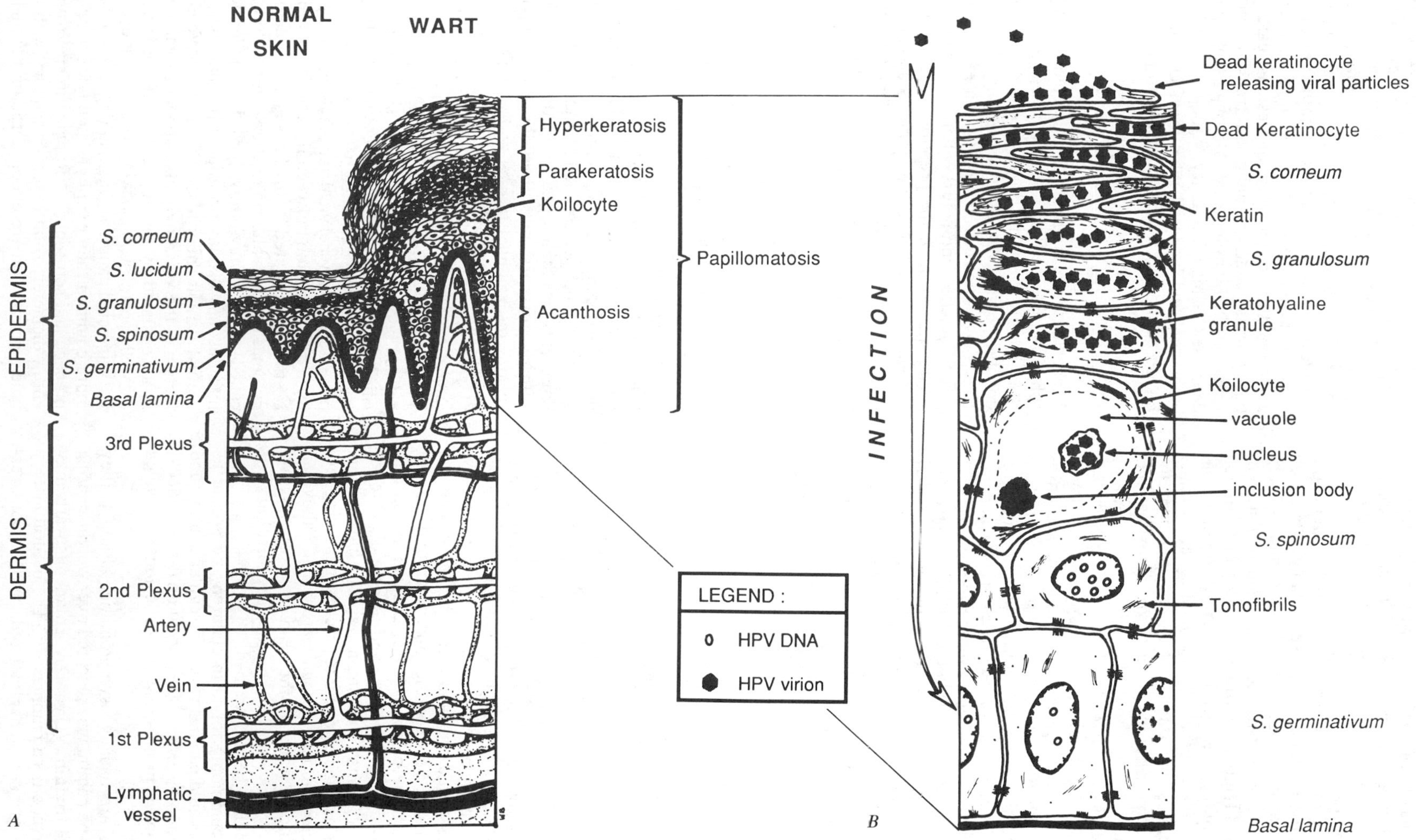

FIG. 1. Exophytic cutaneous wart—HPV pathogenesis. **(A)** Histologic features; **(B)** cytologic features (see text for details).

observation suggesting the potential importance of the immune system in the resolution of HPV disease is that when one wart regresses, other lesions also frequently resolve. This common clinical observation has been confirmed statistically in one recent study.[48] Also of interest is the observation that pregnancy appears to be associated with an apparently increased incidence and severity of HPV diseases.[26,49,50]

A variety of alterations in the immune system, including the presence of circulating immune complexes, changes in T-cell numbers, T-cell helper/suppressor subset ratios, and NK cell function, as well as depressed responses to dinitrochlorobenzene sensitization and lymphocyte transformation or migration inhibition assays to mitogens, have been described among patients with several HPV diseases.[43] The significance of many of these observations is uncertain, and a consistent immune defect has not been demonstrated to be present in most patients with HPV infection.

Although some serologic studies have suggested that the appearance of specific IgG antibodies may be associated with wart regression, the importance of type-specific immune responses has not been adequately evaluated.[51] In addition, rates of lesion recurrence after spontaneous resolution of disease, and correlations between development of recurrent disease and immune responses to HPV, have not been described.

Of interest are a variety of morphologic studies suggesting that macrophages located within the skin may be important in the spontaneous resolution of HPV infections.[52] These observations, along with the well-localized nature of HPV disease, suggest that skin (or mucous membrane)-associated lymphoid tissue may be more relevant to the pathogenesis and resolution of HPV infections than circulating peripheral blood mononuclear leukocytes.

CLINICAL MANIFESTATIONS

Cutaneous Warts

Cutaneous warts include deep plantar warts, common warts, and plane or flat warts.[14,53]

Deep plantar warts, also called *myrmecia* (from the Greek meaning ant hill), affect mostly adolescents and young adults. The lesions characteristically appear as raised bundles of soft keratotic fibers 2 mm to 1 cm in diameter, and shaving reveals punctate, bleeding blood vessels. These lesions are often painful and may also be located on the palms of the hands.

Common warts appear as well-demarcated, exophytic, hyperkeratotic papules with a rough surface. They may occur on the dorsum of the hand, between the fingers, around the nail (periungual warts), on the palms or soles, and, rarely, on mucous membranes. Warts may coalesce and reach a diameter of 1 cm. Morphologic variants of common warts include mosaic warts, which appear as cobblestone-like patches measuring several square centimeters in diameter and barely rising above an indurated base. Filiform warts on the head or vegetating, hyperproliferative warts on the hands of butchers or meatpackers[11] have also been described.

Plane warts are commonly found in children and appear as multiple, slightly elevated papules with an irregular contour and distribution and a smooth surface. They occur on the face, neck, and hands. When more protuberant, these lesions are called *intermediate warts*.

Cutaneous warts are usually asymptomatic, although they may bleed, and can be painful when located over weight-bearing surfaces or points of friction. Very rarely, cutaneous warts may degenerate into verrucous carcinomas.[54,55] The natural history of cutaneous warts is poorly characterized. Spontaneous resolution appears to occur in 50 percent of children within a year,[56] but persistence for many years is not uncommon.

Epidermodysplasia verruciformis

Lesions are associated with a large array of HPV types (Table 1), most of which are specific for epidermodysplasia verruciformis (EV).[14,15] These warts have several morphologic variants. They resemble flat warts but most commonly are similar to pityriasis versicolor, covering the torso and upper extremities. Over extensor surfaces these warts may become hypertrophic and coalescent. In the majority of patients, warts appear in the first decade of life. Beginning in young adulthood, in about one-third of patients, the lesions, particularly in sun-exposed areas, undergo malignant transformation into invasive squamous cell carcinomas. Although these patients may have depressed cellular immunity,[57] they have normal resistance to other viral and bacterial infections. Of note is that lesions of EV do not appear to be contagious to normal contacts.

Anogenital Warts

Anogenital warts are flesh- to gray-colored, hyperkeratotic, exophytic papules, either sessile on the skin or, more frequently, attached by a short, broad peduncle. Lesions range from smooth, pearly papules to more jagged, acuminate growths. They range in size from less than a millimeter in diameter to several square centimeters when they merge into plaques. In uncircumcised men, the preputial cavity is involved in 85–90 percent of cases.[26,58] In the United States, where about 85 percent of the male population is circumcised, the penile shaft is the most common site of lesions.[18,59] In 1 percent to a quarter of patients, the urethral meatus is also involved.[26,58–61] Urethral warts are clearly visible by inversion of the meatus or with the use of a pediatric nasal speculum. They are mostly confined to the fossa navicularis or, less frequently, to the distal 3 cm of the urethra. Involvement of the bladder or proximal urethra is exceptional.[59,61–63] Involvement of the perianal area varies according to sexual practice, from very high among homosexual men to low among heterosexual men.[59,64,65] The scrotum, perineum, groin, and pubic area are involved only occasionally.

In women, the vast majority of lesions are distributed over the posterior introitus and, to a lesser degree, over the labia majora and minora and the clitoris. In order of decreasing frequency, the perineum, vagina, anus, cervix, and urethra each represents less than a quarter of the sites of involvement.[18,26]

In recent years, with the help of the colposcope and prior soaking of examined tissues with 3–5 percent acetic acid, the clinical spectrum of anogenital warts, particularly those caused by HPV types 16 and 18, has expanded. This technique initially revealed the existence of flat condylomas on the uterine cervix. Typically, these lesions are shiny, white patches with poorly defined borders and an irregular surface containing characteristic capillary loops.[66] The presence of external genital warts may indicate the existence of cervical flat condylomas, which often accompany cervical intraepithelial neoplasia.[67] Morphologic differentiation between the two is not reliable, and biopsy is strongly indicated.[68] In the vagina, in addition to flat condylomas, small white nodosities centered on a capillary loop, called *spiked condylomas*, have been identified.[69] The vulvar introitus may display prominent papillae that, although often a normal variant, may also reflect HPV infection.[70,71] HPV infection of the vulva may also appear as white patches revealed or accentuated by the application of acetic acid.[60,72,73] In men as well, acetic acid soaking and/or colposcopy have shown HPV-infected papules (Fig. 2) and macules to be up to two times more common than exophytic condylomas, particularly on the prepuce and scrotum.[59,74] Ranging in size from minuscule to 1 cm in diameter, round, sessile papules with a brown to slate blue pigmentation are encountered on the male and female external genitalia. These lesions are important to recognize because they may represent either HPV 6- or 11-infected benign

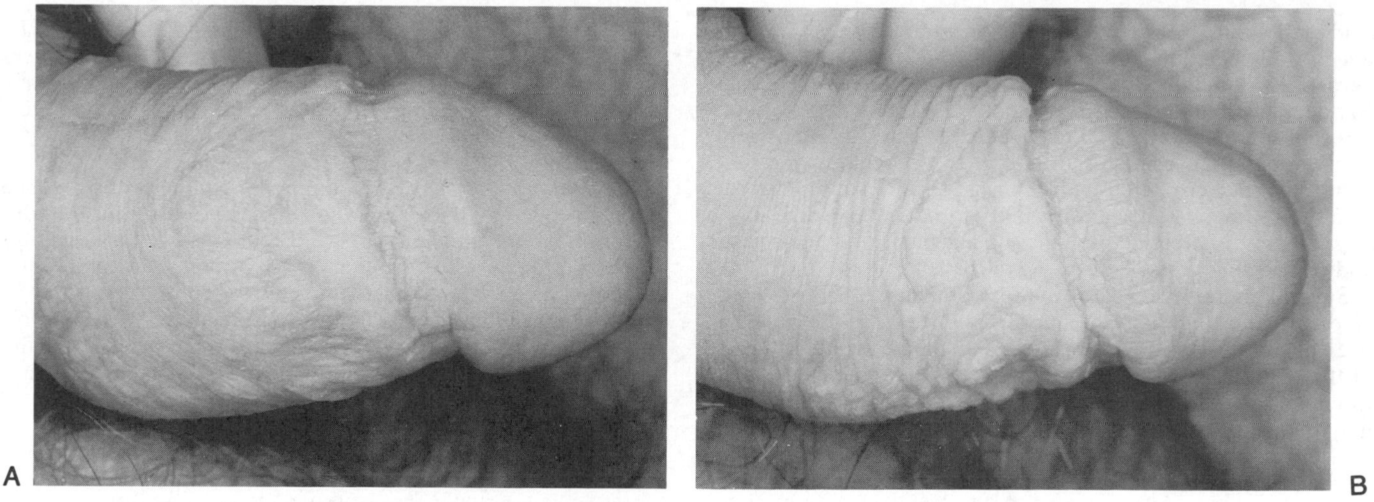

FIG. 2. Aceto-whitening of an HPV-induced flat papule of the penile shaft before **(A)** and after **(B)** application of 3% acetic acid for 5 minutes.

condyloma,[75] seborrheic keratoses,[60] or intraepithelial neoplasia (bowenoid papulosis) with HPV type 16 or 18 infection.[60]

About three-quarters of the patients with anogenital warts are asymptomatic.[18] However, itching and burning, as well as pain and tenderness, are encountered frequently.[18,70] The natural history of genital warts, particularly of subclinical HPV disease, is poorly understood, but spontaneous remission may occur, as demonstrated by the results of recently conducted, randomized, placebo-controlled therapeutic trials, which indicate a 20 percent spontaneous remission rate in untreated lesions over a 3- to 4-month period.[48,76–78]

Exophytic genital warts rarely transform into invasive squamous cell carcinomas, including verrucous carcinoma.[79] They may also reach considerable size, particularly during pregnancy or immunosuppression. When large condylomas reveal histologic features of local destructive invasion without metastases, they may be called *Buschke-Lowenstein tumors, condylomatous carcinomas*, or *giant condylomas*.[80] Genital HPV infections may also belong to the spectrum of penile, vulvar, vaginal, and cervical intraepithelial neoplasias (PIN, VIN, VAIN, and CIN, respectively). Pigmented papules of the external genitalia may histologically demonstrate condylomatous cytoarchitecture with evidence of intraepithelial neoplasia. This clinicopathologic entity is called *bowenoid papulosis*.[81] Bowenoid papulosis can evolve to Bowen's disease, a flat, red to brown plaque with well-demarcated borders and a scaly, irregular surface.[82] On the glans penis the lesion is known as *erythroplasia of Queyrat*. Histologically, carcinoma in situ is present. HPV 16 and 18 have been recovered from bowenoid papulosis and Bowen's disease.[83] The natural history of intraepithelial neoplasias is best understood in cervical lesions.[84,85] It is clear that the outcome (regression, no change, or progression) is highly variable and depends upon the histologic grade of the tumor, the HPV type, and the method of diagnosis (conization, punch biopsy, or scraping).

Perianal warts are common among homosexual men, and up to two-thirds of patients with external anal warts also have internal lesions.[86] Although malignant transformation of anal condyloma has been described,[87] only in recent years has the association between anorectal dysplasia or cancer and HPV infections been recognized in homosexual men.[88–90] Passive anal intercourse carries a high risk of anal cancer in homosexual men, and heterosexual men and women with a history of genital warts have a 30-fold increased risk of disease compared to control populations.[91] During pregnancy, condylomas may become so large as to impair normal delivery mechanically.[26,50] Anogenital warts in young children strongly raise the possibility of sexual abuse.[92,93]

Respiratory Papillomatosis

Patients present with hoarseness or, in infants, with an altered cry. Sometimes these symptoms may be accompanied by respiratory distress and stridor. The disease may spread to the trachea and lungs, leading to obstruction, infection, and respiratory failure. In young children, rapid growth of lesions often threatens the upper respiratory tract and frequently requires surgical excision to avoid asphyxiation. In adults, the course of the disease is usually less aggressive. Lesions may, however, undergo malignant transformation, particularly in patients who have received radiation therapy.[24,27–29]

Other Warts

Focal epithelial hyperplasia of the oral cavity (Heck's disease) is caused by HPV 13 and tends to regress spontaneously. Other HPV infections may also occur in the oral cavity.[94] Conjunctival HPV-related papillomas[95] and nasal warts in cocaine snorters have been described as well.[96]

TREATMENT

Safe, effective treatment for most HPV infections is not currently available. Most therapeutic modalities consist of physical or chemical destruction of grossly visible lesions. Few rigorously controlled therapeutic trials have been conducted for HPV infections. Such trials are needed because of the variable natural history of the disease and the lack of a suitable in vitro or animal model system with which to evaluate different therapeutic modalities.

Cutaneous Warts

Because of the benign, usually self-limited nature of cutaneous warts, treatment should be individualized. On the basis of several randomized, non-placebo-controlled comparative trials, Bunney et al.[97] have proposed several treatment approaches, usually involving paring of the wart. For hand warts, self-application of salicylic and lactic acid paint (salicylic acid, lactic acid, collodion, 1:1:4; SAL) daily for up to 12 weeks has produced a 69 percent cure rate. About the same cure rate (67 percent) was obtained with cryotherapy given every 3 weeks. For deep plantar warts, SAL paint cured 84 percent of patients, a response comparable to the 81 percent cure rate in patients with podophyllin resin. About half of the patients with mosaic plantar warts were cured with SAL paint, 10% glutaraldehyde, or 5-fluorouracil. Flat warts usually do not require treatment. Cryotherapy is preferred for the management of eyelid, nasal, and periungual warts.[98,99]

Several alternative treatments for cutaneous warts are available.[98,99] Curettage may be appropriate for partial removal of deep plantar warts. Wedge resection should be avoided because of the resulting painful scarring. Electrosurgery includes electrocautery, electrocoagulation, and electrodesiccation. The last may be useful for removal of flat or filiform warts of the face, as well as other well-localized warts. Scarring is a potential complication.

Anogenital Warts

Because anogenital warts are sexually transmitted and associated with genital tract dysplasias and malignancies, there is general agreement that they should be treated. However, optimal methods of treatment have not been established, and the effects of currently available therapies on transmissibility of infection or development of neoplasias are unknown. In addition, evaluations of treatment modalities have generally not taken into account the subclinical or multifocal characteristics of the disease.

Podophyllin, a resin extract from the rhizome of *Podophyllum peltatum* (podophyllum resin, USP) or *P. emodi* has been the principal mode of therapy for many years.[100] The active molecules are lignans, particularly podophyllotoxin. Although podophyllin is a mitotic poison, its mode of action in warts is unknown. The compound is usually applied as a 10% solution in benzoin, directly on the wart, once weekly. Washing of lesions within 12 hours is recommended to minimize local reactions. Lack of regression after four applications suggests the need for alternative therapies. Although initial reports of podophyllin therapy suggested almost complete efficacy, more recent observations demonstrate cure rates ranging from 20 to 40 percent.[58,100,101] Side effects are both local and systemic.[100,102] Chemical burns are seen in one-third to one-half of the patients. Transient pseudoneoplastic histopathologic changes have also been reported. Allergic sensitization, neurologic, hematologic, and febrile complications, sometimes leading to death, have been associated with administration of topical podophyllin. The drug is contraindicated in pregnancy. The use of podophyllotoxin circumvents the problem of the variable potency of podophyllin preparations. In addition, the efficacy of podophyllotoxin may be equivalent, if not superior, to that of podophyllin.[58,102,103] The self-administration of 0.5% podophyllotoxin topically twice daily for 3 consecutive days per week for up to 4 weekly cycles appears to be a well-tolerated and effective regimen in men.[58,103] Side effects are similar to those of podophyllin. Relapses with both podophyllin and podophyllotoxin are common.

Many other compounds, with an uncertain mode of action, have been employed in the treatment of external anogenital warts. 5-Fluorouracil, used topically as a 5% cream applied daily, has been reported to have cure rates of 30–95 percent; the best results have been obtained with intraurethral warts.[58,62,104] In a comparative trial in men, 5-fluorouracil appeared to be equivalent in efficacy to podophyllin.[105] In addition, prophylactic activity of 5-fluorouracil has been reported for vulvar warts.[106] The drug often produces pain, ulceration, and, if applied in the urethra, dysuria.[58] Like other antimetabolites, 5-fluorouracil is contraindicated during pregnancy. Trichloracetic acid and, to a lesser extent, bichloracetic acid have been used in the treatment of genital warts.[107] Trichloracetic acid in a 10–50% solution is used topically at weekly intervals. The application is painful. In one comparative trial, trichloracetic acid therapy appeared to be equivalent to cryotherapy, with cure and relapse rates of 81 and 36%, respectively.[108]

Cryotherapy, along with podophyllin, is one of the regimens recommended by the Centers for Disease Control for the treatment of external genital warts.[109] Liquid nitrogen is most often used. Lesions are frozen every 1 or 2 weeks. Cryotherapy is regarded as an effective treatment, with cure rates in the 50–100% range, and is safe even during pregnancy.[108,110] One comparative study suggested that cryotherapy is more effective than podophyllin.[111] Side effects are tolerable. They include burning, which resolves within a few hours, and ulceration, which heals in 7–10 days with little or no scarring.

Various surgical techniques for the treatment of anogenital warts have also been used. Conventional surgery offers the advantage of providing immediate eradication of visible lesions. This technique has been reserved mainly for the treatment of perianal warts. Approximately a third of patients have recurrences, and scarring is a common complication.[112,113] Electrosurgical techniques have often been applied for the treatment of external genital warts, with results similar to those of cryotherapy.[114] Cure rates of 80–90% have been reported with CO_2 laser therapy.[115–117] In a comparative assessment, however, laser therapy was not deemed superior to conventional surgery.[118] Although this study was criticized for its poor laser technique,[117] no precise agreement exists regarding optimal technique. In addition, laser therapy is expensive, often requires general anesthesia, and is often accompanied by pain and scarring. Infrared coagulation has also been employed.[119]

Immunotherapy has been directed predominantly at the treatment of recalcitrant warts. Autogenous vaccination with an extract of the patient's own condyloma appeared promising in initial studies but was not effective in a subsequent controlled trial.[120–122] Dinitrochlorobenzene skin sensitization is a tedious, protracted, and painful approach that has been claimed to be effective.[123,124] Proper comparative studies have not been conducted.

Interferons have antiviral, immunomodulatory, and antiproliferative properties. Encouraging in vitro and preliminary clinical studies were confirmed by four randomized, double-blind trials that demonstrated the efficacy of intralesionally administered α- and β-interferons compared to placebo.[48,76–78] In these studies, 1 million units of interferon were generally administered per wart, three times per week for 3–4 weeks; 35–60 percent of interferon-injected warts resolved compared to 20 percent of placebo-injected lesions. Parenterally administered interferons have also been evaluated for treatment of condyloma acuminatum. Although in one trial β-interferon gave results far superior to those of a placebo,[125] a more recent study of various α-interferons revealed more modest effects in comparison to a placebo.[126] Interferon, in the doses used, has been well tolerated. Side effects (influenza-like symptoms, neutropenia, and thrombocytopenia) are usually mild and are seen more frequently with higher doses.

Because internal genital warts are often associated with genital dysplasias and malignancies, and because of the special skills and technical resources required for proper diagnosis and management, patients with internal lesions should be referred to a qualified specialist. Warts of the urinary meatus can be treated by careful application of podophyllin, podophyllotoxin,[58] or 5-fluorouracil.[58,127] Laser therapy[59] and cryotherapy[128] are alternative forms of treatment. These therapeutic modalities are applicable to intraurethral warts, as are 5-fluorouracil, thiotepa, and colchicine.[104,129,130] Anal and rectal warts may be treated with cryotherapy[131] or laser treatment.[132] For vaginal warts, 5-fluorouracil has been used both therapeutically[133] and prophylactically.[106] Laser therapy[134,135] and cryotherapy[110] have the advantage of being relatively safe during pregnancy, and may be used for treatment of cervical warts as well.

Other Warts

The lesions of EV should be carefully observed and any malignant changes treated by surgical techniques or 5-fluorouracil ointments.[14] Oral retinoids and intralesional interferon improve but do not cure the lesions of EV.[15]

Laryngeal papillomatosis is managed by endoscopic cryotherapy or, more often, laser therapy.[24,27,29] Tracheostomy should be avoided because of the possible risk of spreading disease to the distal respiratory tree. Similarly, radiotherapy is contraindicated in view of the risk of malignant transformation.[24] A recent large study has indicated that the benefit of α-interferon as an adjunctive treatment is probably limited to the first 6 months of treatment.[136] α-Interferon does not eradicate HPV DNA from involved tissues.[41]

In the oral cavity, verruca vulgaris can be treated by 20% podophyllin in ethanol solution or cryotherapy, and condyloma acuminatum by cryotherapy, electrosurgery, or surgical excision.[94] Because of its benign natural history, focal epithelial hyperplasia should not be treated.

DIAGNOSIS

The diagnosis of warts is usually made clinically. Exophytic warts have a characteristic appearance. Deep plantar warts may be confused with calluses, but paring of these warts usually reveals the typical punctated, thrombosed capillaries. Nevi, seborrheic keratoses, acrochordons, acanthomas, molluscum contagiosum, lichen planus, syringomas, and dermofibromas may be confused with cutaneous warts. Lesions of EV may be similar to those of flat warts or pityriasis versicolor. However, the patient's history will clarify the diagnosis.

Condyloma acuminatum of the external anogenital tract should rarely be confused with other STDs such as condyloma latum of syphilis, nodular scabies, genital herpes, lymphogranuloma venereum, chancroid, or granuloma inguinale. Nevertheless, molluscum contagiosum, particularly in its more atypical presentations, may be difficult to distinguish from anogenital warts. In contrast to condyloma acuminatum, molluscum contagiosum lesions tend to predominate over the pubis and are rarely pedunculated, but rather appear as very smooth, sessile domes with a depressed center out of which cheesy material can be expressed. In men, a normal anatomic variant of the corona, hirsutoid papillomatosis (pearly coronal papules, papillae corona glandis), may be extremely difficult to differentiate from small warts. A similar anatomic presentation exists in the vulvar introitus and may appear identical to that of HPV-related vulvar papillomatosis. On the keratinized vulva, hidradenoma papilliferum may be confused with a large wart. On the scrotum, epidermoid cysts and angiokeratomas should be easy to identify. Small and flat HPV lesions sometimes may be difficult to distinguish from lichen planus, lichen sclerosus et atrophicus, lichen nitidus, or syringomas, even with the help of the colposcope and acetic acid application. Finally, pigmented HPV lesions may be confused with nevi and seborrheic keratoses.

Although initially designed for the evaluation of the female internal genital tract, colposcopy with prior application for 3–5 minutes of a 3–5% acetic acid solution has become an important diagnostic tool for other HPV infections as well (Fig. 2). In studies of male partners of women with either cervical condylomas or dysplasias, biopsy-proven genital condylomas were detected in 65–88 percent of the patients. More significantly, 43–73 percent of the lesions were seen only with a colposcope, while aceto-whitening alone made the diagnosis in 22 percent of patients.[74,137,138] The same technique applied to the vulva revealed subclinical papillomavirus infection in 96 percent and 80 percent of women who, respectively, had vulvar warts or were the partners of men with penile warts.[139]

Lesions of the external genitalia that are pigmented, appear as plaques, bleed, or are large in size should be biopsied in order to establish the diagnosis. Biopsy is also indicated to confirm the diagnosis of EV and of lesions of the oral cavity or upper airways.

Anoscopic examination is encouraged in every patient with genital warts, particularly when they harbor perianal lesions or have a history of anal receptive intercourse. Most intra-anal lesions are below the pectinate line, and sigmoidoscopy is not routinely indicated.[140,141]

Appropriate evaluation of the vagina and cervix requires colposcopy and acetic acid application, and should seek to rule out invasive cancer. Women with a history of anogenital HPV disease, or whose sexual partners have had anogenital HPV disease, should have a cytologic examination of a cervical smear (Pap smear). Koilocytes on a cytologic smear are the hallmark of HPV infection. More importantly, diagnoses of dysplasia and cancer can also be made from the smear.[142] Depending on the patient's age and the location and nature of the HPV infection, the sensitivity of the Pap smear in detecting HPV infection ranges from 30 to 90 percent.[143,144] Cytology has also been applied with success to the diagnosis of intra-anal HPV infection.[88]

The general histopathologic features of HPV infection are usually characteristic (see above under "Pathogenesis"). Whenever indicated, biopsy is therefore the routine and standard confirmatory mode of diagnosis. It can also identify the presence of dysplastic or malignant changes.

To enhance the sensitivity and specificity of cytohistopathology, several techniques are available in research settings. They rely on either the demonstration of the papillomavirus common antigen or the detection of HPV nucleic acids in biopsy specimens. The papillomavirus common antigen is detected by peroxidase-antiperoxidase immunocytochemical staining. It is present in about half of HPV lesions, although less frequently in HPV 16- or 18-infected tissues.[7] Various techniques exist for the detection and typing of HPV DNA.[145] They are all based on the demonstration, under controlled conditions, of the ability of the nucleic acid being tested to reassociate with a probe (i.e., a known HPV DNA labeled with either radioisotopes or chemically reactive ligands). If hybridization occurs, the hybrid can be detected by an autoradiogram or a colored reaction. Hybridization methods are not standardized and vary in sensitivity, specificity, cost, and convenience. The sensitivity of nucleic acid detection techniques can be enhanced by DNA amplification with the polymerase chain reaction.[146] The usefulness of the recently licensed Virapap kit in the management of patients with HPV infections has not been established.

Virus cultivation and reliable serologic techniques are not yet available for diagnosis of HPV infections.

PREVENTION

At present, no effective methods of prevention are available for warts other than avoiding contact with infectious lesions. Barrier methods of contraception may be helpful in preventing the transmission of HPV infection of the genital tract, although studies have given conflicting results.[147,148] Sexual partners of patients with anogenital warts should be evaluated and treated if necessary. Effective vaccines are not currently available.[149]

ACKNOWLEDGMENTS

This chapter was supported in part by contracts NO1-AI-32510 and NOI-AI-82509 and grant ROI-AI-23418 from the National Institutes of Health, Bethesda, MD. Dr. Bonnez is the recipient of a Wilmot Cancer Research Fellowship.

REFERENCES

1. Ciuffo G. Imnesto positivo con filtrato di verruca volgare. Giorn Ital Mal Venereol. 1907;48:12–7.
2. Jablonska S, Orth G. Warts/human papillomaviruses. Clin Dermatol. 1985;3(4):1–220.
3. Reid R. Human papillomaviruses. Obstet Gynecol Clin North Am. 1987;14(2):329–614.
4. Sryjanen K, Gissmann L. Koss LG. Papillomaviruses and Human Disease. Berlin: Springer Verlag; 1987.
5. Melnick JL, Allison AC, Butel JS, et al. Paporaviridae. Intervirology. 1974;3:106–20.
6. Strike DG, Bonnez W, Rose RC, Reichman RC. Expression in *Escherichia coli* of seven DNA segments comprising the complete L1 and L2 open reading frames of human papillomavirus type 6b and localization of the "comon antigen" region. J Gen Virol. 1989;70:543–55.
7. Jenson AB, Kurman RJ, Lancaster WD. Detection of papillomavirus common antigens in lesions of skin and mucosa. Clin Dermatol. 1985;3(4):56–63.
8. Broker TR. Structure and genetic expression of papillomaviruses. Obstet Gynecol Clin North Am. 1987;14:329–48.
9. Kreider JW, Howett MK, Leure-Dupree AE, et al. Laboratory production in vivo of infectious human papillomavirus type 11. J Virol. 1987;61:590–3.
10. De Peuter M, De Clercq B, Minette A, et al. An epidemiological survey of virus warts of the hands among butchers. Br J Dermatol. 1977;96:427–31.
11. Jennings LC, Ross AD, Faoagali JL. The prevalence of warts on the hands of workers in a New Zealand slaughterhouse. N Z Med J. 1984;97:473–6.
12. Rudlinger R, Bunney MH, Grob R, et al. Warts in fish handlers. Br J Dermatol. 1989;120:375–80.
13. Taylor SWC. A prevalence study of warts on the hands in a poultry processing and packing station. J Soc Occup Med. 1980;30:20–3.
14. Grussendorf-Conen E-I. Papillomavirus-induced tumors of the skin: Cutaneous warts and epidermodysplasia verruciformis. In: Syrjanen K, Gissmann L, Koss LG, eds. Papillomaviruses and Human Disease. Berlin: Springer Verlag; 1987:158–81.
15. Lutzner MA, Blanchet-Bardon C. Epidermodysplasia verruciformis. Curr Probl Dermatol. 1985;13:164–85.
16. Becker TM, Blount JF, Guinan ME. Trends in genital herpes infections among private practitioners in the United States, 1966–1981. JAMA. 1985;253:1601–3.
17. Chief Medical Officer, Department of Health and Social Security, United Kingdom. Sexually transmitted diseases. Br J Vener Dis. 1983;59:134–7.
18. Chuang T, Perry HO, Kurland LT, et al. Condyloma acuminatum in Rochester, Minn., 1950–1978. I. Epidemiology and clinical features. Arch Dermatol. 1984;120:469–75.
19. Becker TM. Genital human papillomavirus infection: An epidemiological perspective. In: Norrby SR, ed. New Antiviral Strategies. Edinburgh: Churchill Livingstone; 1988;44–9.
20. de Villiers E-M, Schneider A, Miklaw H, et al. Human papillomavirus infections in women with and without abnormal cytology. Lancet. 1987;2:703–6.
21. Ludwig ME, Lowell DM, Li Volsi VA. Cervical condylomatous atypia and its relationship to cervical neoplasia. Am J Clin Pathol. 1981;76:255–62.
22. Meisels A, Fortin R, Roy M. Condylomatous lesions of the cervix. II. Cytologic, colposcopic, and histopathologic study. Acta Cytol. 1977;21:379–90.
23. Garrido JL. Pathological incidence study of human papilloma virus (HPV) carried out on 1,439 patients between 1982–1985 in Panama. Eur J Gynaecol Oncol. 1988;9:144–8.
24. Mounts P, Shah KV. Respiratory papillomatosis: Etiological relation to genital tract papillomaviruses. Prog Med Virol. 1984;29:90–114.
25. Campion MJ, Singer A, Clarkson PK, et al. Increased risk of cervical neoplasia in consorts of men with penile condylomata acuminata. Lancet. 1985;1:943–6.
26. Oriel JD. Natural history of genital warts. Br J Vener Dis. 1971;47:1–13.
27. Kashima HK, Shah K. Recurrent respiratory papillomatosis. Clinical overview and management principles. Obstet Gynecol Clin North Am. 1987;14:581–8.
28. Steinberg BM, Abramson AL. Layngeal papillomas. Clin Dermatol. 1985;3(4):130–8.
29. Chuang T, Perry HO, Kurland LT, et al. Condyloma acuminatum in Rochester, Minnesota, 1950–1978. Arch Dermatol. 1984;120:469–75.
30. Franchesci S, Doll R, Gallwey J, et al. Genital warts and cervical neoplasm: An epidemiological study. Br J Cancer. 1983;48:621–8.
31. Graham S, Priore R, Graham M, et al. Genital cancer in wives of penile cancer patients. Cancer. 1979;44:1870–4.
32. Fraumeni JF, Lloyd JM, Smith EM, et al. Cancer mortality among nuns: Role of the marital status in etiology of neoplastic disease in women. J Natl Cancer Inst. 1969;42:455:68.
33. zur Hausen H. Genital papillomavirus infections. Prog Med Virol. 1985;32:15–21.
34. Campion MU, Cuzick J, McCance DJ, et al. Progressive potential of mild cervical atypia: Prospective cytological, colposcopic, and virological study. Lancet. 1986;2:237–40.
35. Kjaer SK, de Villiers E-M, Haugaard BJ, et al. Human papillomavirus, herpes simplex virus and cervical cancer incidence in Greenland and Denmark. A population-based cross-sectional study. Int J Cancer. 1988;41:518–24.
36. Munoz N, Bosch X, Kaldor JM. Does human papillomavirus cause cervical cancer? The state of the epidemiological evidence. Br J Cancer. 1988;57:1–5.
37. Goldschmidt H, Klingman AM. Experimental inoculation of humans with ectodermotropic viruses. J Invest Dermatol. 1958;31:175–82.
38. Barrett TJ, Silbar JD, McGinley JP. Genital warts—A venereal disease. JAMA. 1954;154:333–4.
39. Stoler MH, Broker TR. In situ hybridization detection of human papillomavirus DNAs and messenger RNAs in genital condylomas and a cervical carcinoma. Hum Pathol. 1986;17:1250–8.
40. Ferenczy A, Mitao M, Nagai N, et al. Latent papillomavirus and recurring genital warts. N Engl J Med. 1985;313:784–8.
41. Steinberg BM, Gallagher T, Stoler M, et al. Persistence and expression of human papillomavirus during interferon therapy. Arch Otolaryngol Head Neck Surg. 1988;114:27–32.
42. Howley PM. The role of papillomaviruses in human cancer. In: de Vita V, Hellman S, Rosenberg SA, eds. Important Advances in Oncology, 1987. Philadelphia: Lippincott; 1987:55–73.
43. Kirchner H. Immunobiology of human papillomavirus infection. Prog Med Virol. 1986;33:1–41.
44. Matis WL, Triana A, Shapiro R, et al. Dermatologic findings associated with human immunodeficiency virus infection. J Am Acad Dermatol. 1987;17:746–51.
45. Boyle J, Briggs JD, Mackie RM, et al. Cancer, warts, and sunshine in renal transplant patients. A case-control study. Lancet. 1986;1:702–5.
46. Rudlinger RM, Smith IW, Bunney MH, et al. Human papillomavirus infections in a group of renal transplant recipients. Br J Dermatol. 1986;115:681–92.
47. Sillman F, Stanek A, Sedlis A, et al. The relationship between human papillomavirus and lower genital intraepithelial neoplasia in immunosuppressed women. Am J Obstet Gynecol. 1984;150:300–8.
48. Reichman RC, Oakes D, Bonnez W, et al. Treatment of condyloma acuminatum with three different interferons administered intralesionally. A double-blind, placebo-controlled trial. Ann Intern Med. 1988;108:675–9.
49. Schneider A, Hotz M, Gissmann L. Increased prevalence of human papillomaviruses in the lower genital tract of pregnant women. Int J Cancer. 1987;40:198–201.
50. Young RL, Acosta AA, Kaufman RH. The treatment of large condylomata acuminata complicating pregnancy. Obstet Gynecol. 1973;41:65–73.
51. Matthews RS, Shirodaria PV. Study of regressing warts by immunofluorescence. Lancet. 1973;1:689–91.
52. Oguchi M, Komura J, Tagami H, et al. Ultrastructural studies of spontaneously regressing plane warts. Macrophages attack verruca-epidermal cells. Arch Dermatol Res. 1981;270:403–11.
53. Jablonska S, Orth G, Obalek S, et al. Cutaneous warts. Clinical, histologic, and virologic correlations. Clin Dermatol. 1985;3(4):71–82.
54. Goette DK. Carcinoma in situ in verruca vulgaris. Int J Dermatol. 1980;19:98–101.
55. Swanson NA, Taylor WB. Plantar verrucous carcinoma. Arch Dermatol. 1980;116:794–7.
56. Massing AM, Epstein WL. Natural history of warts. A two year study. Arch Dermatol. 1963;87:306–10.
57. Jablonska S, Orth G, Lutzner MA. Immunopathology of papillomavirus-induced tumors in different tissues. Springer Semin. Immunopathol. 1982;5:33–53.
58. von Krogh G. Podophyllotoxin for condylomata acuminata eradication. Clinical and experimental comparative studies on *Podophyllum lignans*, colchicine and 5-fluorouracil. Acta Dermato-Venereol. 1981;(Suppl 98):1–48.
59. Rosemberg SK, Jacobs H, Fuller T. Some guidelines in the treatment of urethral condylomata with carbon dioxide laser. J Urol. 1982;127:906–8.
60. Gross G, Ikenberg H, Gissmann L, et al. Papillomavirus infection of the anogenital region: Correlation between histology, clinical picture, and virus type. Proposal of a new nomenclature. J Invest Dermatol. 1985;85:147–52.
61. Sand PK, Bowen LW, Blischke SO, et al. Evaluation of male consorts of women with genital human papilloma virus infection. Obstet Gynecol. 1986;68:679–81.
62. de Benedictis JT, Marmar JL, Praiss DE. Intraurethral condylomata acuminata: Management and a review of the literature. J Urol. 1977;118:767–9.
63. Masse S, Tosi-Kruse A, Carmel M, et al. Condyloma acuminatum of the bladder. Urology. 1981;17:381–2.
64. Goorney BP, Waugh MA, Clarke J. Anal warts in heterosexual men. Genitourin Med. 1987;63:216.
65. Oriel JD. Anal warts and anal coitus. Br J Vener Dis. 1971;47:373–6.
66. Reid R, Laverty CR, Coppleson M, et al. Noncondylomatous cervical wart virus infection. Obstet Gynecol. 1980;55:476–83.
67. Walker PG, Colley NV, Grubb C, et al. Abnormalities of the uterine cervix in women with vulvar warts. Br J Vener Dis. 1983;59:120–3.
68. Vayrynen M, Syrjanen K, Castren O, et al. Colposcopy in women with papillomavirus lesions of the uterine cervix. Obstet Gynecol. 1985;65:409–15.
69. Roy M, Meisels A, Fortier M, et al. Vaginal condylomata: A human papillomavirus infection. Clin Obstet Gynecol. 1981;24:461–83.
70. Growdon WA, Fu YS, Lebherz TB, et al. Pruritic vulvar squamous papillomatosis. Evidence for human papillomavirus etiology. Obstet Gynecol. 1985;66:564–8.

71. Manoharan V, Sommerville JM. Benign squamous papillomatosis: Case report. Genitourin Med. 1987;63:393–5.
72. McCance DJ, Singer A. The importance of HPV infections in the male and female genital tract and their relationship to cervical neoplasia. In: Peto R, zur Hausen H, eds. Viral Etiology of Cervical Cancer. Banbury Report 21. New York: Cold Spring Harbor Laboratory; 1986:311–9.
73. Reid R, Greenberg M, Jenson AB. Sexually transmitted papillomaviral infections: I. The anatomic distribution and pathologic grade of neoplastic lesions associated with different viral types. Am J Obstet Gynecol. 1987;156:212–22.
74. Barrasso R, de Brux J, Croissant O, et al. High prevalence of papillomavirus-associated penile intraepithelial neoplasia in sexual partners of women with cervical intraepithelial neoplasia. N Engl J Med. 1987;317:916–23.
75. Campion MJ. Clinical manifestations and natural history of genital human papillomavirus infection. Obstet Gynecol Clin North Am. 1987;14:363–88.
76. Eron LJ, Judson F, Tucker S, et al. Interferon therapy for condylomata acuminata. N Engl J Med. 1986;315:1059–64.
77. Friedman-Kien A, Eron LJ, Conant M, et al. Natural interferon alpha for the treatment of condylomata acuminata. JAMA. 1988;259:533–8.
78. Vance JC, Bart BJ, Hansen RC, et al. Intralesional recombinant alpha-2 interferon for the treatment of patients with condyloma acuminatum or verruca plantaris. Arch Dermatol. 1986;122:272–7.
79. Shafeek MA, Osman NI, Hussein MA. Carcinoma of the vulva arising in condylomata acuminata. Obstet Gynecol. 1979;54:120–3.
80. Becker FT, Walder HJ, Larson DM. Giant condylomata acuminata. Buschke-Lowenstein tumor. Arch Dermatol. 1969;100:184–6.
81. Wade TR, Kopf AW, Ackerman AB. Bowenoid papulosis of the penis. Cancer. 1978;42:1890–903.
82. DeVillez RL, Stevens CS. Bowenoid papules of the genitalia. A case progressing to Bowen's disease. J Am Acad Dermatol. 1980;3:149–52.
83. Ikenberg H, Gissmann L, Gross G, et al. Human papillomavirus type 16-related DNA in genital Bowen's disease and in bowenoid papulosis. Int J Cancer. 1983;32:563–5.
84. Buckley CH, Butler EB, Fox H. Vulvar intraepithelial neoplasia and microinvasive carcinoma of the vulva. J Clin Pathol. 1984;37:1201–11.
85. Syrjanen KH. Papillomavirus infection and cancer. In: Syrjanen K, Gissmann L, Koss LG, eds. Papillomaviruses and Human Diseases. Berlin: Springer Verlag; 1987:467–503.
86. Schlappner OLA, Schaffer EA. Anorectal condylomata acuminata: A missed part of the condyloma spectrum. Can Med Assoc J. 1978;118:172–3.
87. Prasad ML, Abcarian H. Malignant potential of perianal condyloma acuminatum. Dis Colon Rectum. 1980;23:191–7.
88. Frazer IH, Crapper RM, Meddley G, et al. Association between anorectal dysplasia, human papillomavirus, and human immunodeficiency virus infection in homosexual men. Lancet. 1986;2:657–60.
89. Gal AA, Meyer PR, Taylor CR. Papillomavirus antigens in anorectal condyloma and carcinoma in homosexual men. JAMA. 1987;257:337–40.
90. Nash G, Allen W, Nash S. Atypical lesions of the anal mucosa in homosexual men. JAMA. 1986;256:873–6.
91. Daling JR, Weiss NS, Hislop TG, et al. Sexual practices, sexually transmitted diseases, and the incidence of anal cancer. N Engl J Med. 1987;317:973–7.
92. deJong AR. Sexually transmitted diseases in sexually abused children. Sex Trans Dis. 1986;13:123–6.
93. Schachner L, Hankin DE. Assessing child abuse in childhood condyloma acuminatum. J Am Acad Dermatol. 1985;12:157–60.
94. Syrjanen SM. Human papillomavirus infections in the oral cavity. In: Syrjanen K, Gissmann L, Koss LG, eds. Papillomaviruses and Human Disease. Berlin: Springer Verlag; 1987:104–37.
95. Lass JH, Grove AS, Papale JJ, et al. Detection of human papillomavirus DNA sequences in conjunctival papilloma. Am J Ophthalmol. 1983;96:670–4.
96. Schuster DS. Snorter's warts. Arch Dermatol. 1987;123:571.
97. Bunney MH, Nolan MW, William DA. An assessment of methods of treating viral warts by comparative treatment trials based on a standard design. Br J Dermatol. 1976;94:667–9.
98. Bunney MH. Viral Warts: Their Biology and Treatment. Oxford: Oxford University Press; 1982.
99. Rees RB. The treatment of warts. Clin Dermatol. 1985;3(4):179–84.
100. Miller RA. Podophyllin. Int J Dermatol. 1985;24:491–8.
101. Simmons PD. Podophyllin 10% and 25% in the treatment of ano-genital warts. A comparative double-blind study. Br J Vener Dis. 1981;57:208–9.
102. Beutner KR. Podophyllotoxin in the treatment of genital human papillomavirus infection: A review. Semin Dermatol. 1987;6:10–8.
103. Edwards A, Atma-Ram A, Thin RN. Podophyllotoxin 0.5% v podophyllin 20% to treat penile warts. Genitourin Med. 1988;64:263–5.
104. Dretler SP, Klein LA. The eradication of intraurethral condyloma acuminata with 5 per cent 5-fluorouracil cream. J Urol. 1975;113:195–8.
105. Wallin J. 5-Fluorouracil in the treatment of penile and urethral condylomata acuminata. Br J Vener Dis. 1977;53:240–3.
106. Krebs H-B. Prophylactic topical 5-fluorouracil following treatment of human papillomavirus-associated lesions of the vulva and vagina. Obstet Gynecol. 1986;68:837–41.
107. Richart RM, Kaufman RM, Woodruff JD. Advances in managing condylomas. Contemp Ob/Gyn. 1982;20:164–93.
108. Godley MJ, Bradbeer CS, Gellan M, et al. Cryotherapy compared with trichloracetic acid in treating genital warts. Genitourin Med. 1987;63:390–2.
109. 1985 STD Treatment Guidelines. Morbid Mortal Week Rep. 1985;34(Suppl 4S).
110. Matsunaga J, Bergman A, Bhatia NN. Genital condylomata acuminata in pregnancy: Effectiveness, safety and pregnancy outcome following cryotherapy. Br J Obstet Gynaecol. 1987;94:168–72.
111. Bashi SA. Cryotherapy versus podophyllin in the treatment of genital warts. Int J Dermatol. 1985;24:535–6.
112. Jensen SL. Comparison of podophyllin application with simple surgical excision in clearance and recurrence of perianal condylomata acuminata. Lancet. 1985;2:1146–8.
113. McMillan A, Scott GR. Outpatient treatment of perianal warts by scissor excision. Genitourin Med. 1987;63:114–5.
114. Simmons PD, Langlet F, Thin RNT. Cryotherapy versus electrocautery in the treatment of genital warts. Br J Vener Dis. 1981;57:273–4.
115. Baggish MS. Improved laser techniques for the elimination of genital and extragenital warts. Am J Obstet Gynecol. 1985;153:545–50.
116. Fuselier HA, McBurney EI, Brannan W, et al. Treatment of condylomata acuminata with carbon dioxide laser. Urology. 1980;15:265–6.
117. Reid R. Physical and surgical principles governing expertise with the carbon dioxide laser. Obstet Gynecol Clin North Am. 1987;14:513–35.
118. Duus BR, Philipsen T, Christensen JD, et al. Refractory condylomata acuminata: A controlled clinical trial of carbon dioxide laser versus conventional surgical treatment. Genitourin Med. 1985;61:59–61.
119. Bekassy Z, Westrom L. Infrared coagulation in the treatment of condyloma acuminata in the female genital tract. Sex Transm Dis. 1987;14:209–12.
120. Abcarian H, Sharon N. Long-term effectiveness of the immunotherapy of anal condyloma acuminatum. Dis Colon Rectum. 1982;25:648–51.
121. Malison MD, Morris R, Jones LW. Autogenous vaccine therapy for condyloma acuminatum. A double-blind controlled study. Br J Vener Dis. 1982;58:62–5.
122. Powell LC Jr. Condyloma acuminatum: Recent advances in development, carcinogenesis, and treatment. Clin Obstet Gynecol. 1978;21:1061–79.
123. Dunagin WG, Millikan LE. Dinitrochlorobenzene immunotherapy for verrucae resistant to standard treatment modalities. J Am Acad Dermatol. 1982;6:40–5.
124. Sanders BB, Smith KW. Dinitrochlorobenzene immunotherapy of human warts. Cutis. 1981;27:389–92.
125. Schonfeld A, Schattner A, Crespi M, et al. Intramuscular human interferon-beta injections in treatment of condylomata acuminata. Lancet. 1984;1:1038–42.
126. Reichman RC, Farchione A, Whitley R, et al. A placebo-controlled trial of three different interferon preparations administered parenterally for condyloma acuminatum. Abstract 1430. 28th Interscience Conference on Antimicrobial Agents and Chemotherapy. Los Angeles; October 23–26, 1988.
127. Ng N, Vuignier BI, Hart LL. Fluorouracil in condyloma acuminatum. Drug Intel Clin Pharmacol. 1987;21:175–6.
128. Sand PK, Shen W, Bowen LW, et al. Cryotherapy for the treatment of proximal urethral condyloma acuminatum. J Urol. 1987;137:874–6.
129. Halverstadt DB, Parry WL. Thiotepa in the management of intraurethral condylomata acuminata. J Urol. 1969;101:729–31.
130. Gigax JH, Robison JR. The successful treatment of intraurethral condyloma acuminata with colchicine. J Urol. 1971;105:809–11.
131. Dodi G, Infantino A, Moretti R, et al. Cryotherapy of anorectal warts and condylomata. Cryosurgery. 1982;19:287–8.
132. Billingham RP, Lewis RG. Laser versus electrical cautery in the treatment of condylomata acuminata of the anus. Surg Gynecol Obstet. 1982;155:865–7.
133. Krebs HB. Treatment of vaginal condylomata acuminata by weekly topical application of 5-fluorouracil. Obstet Gynecol. 1987;70:68–71.
134. Ferenczy A. Treating genital condyloma during pregnancy with the carbon dioxide laser. Am J Obstet Gynecol. 1984;148:9–12.
135. Wertheimer A. Indirect colposcopy and laser vaporization in the management of vaginal condylomata. J Reprod Med. 1986;31:39–42.
136. Healy GB, Gelber RD, Trowbridge AL, et al. Treatment of recurrent respiratory papillomatosis with human leukocyte interferon. N Engl J Med. 1988;319:401–7.
137. Sedlacek TV, Cunnane M, Carpiniello V. Colposcopy in the diagnosis of penile condyloma. Am J Obstet Gynecol. 1986;154:494–6.
138. Krebs H-B, Schneider V. Human papillomavirus-associated lesions of the penis: Colposcopy, cytology, and histology. Obstet Gynecol. 1987;70:299–304.
139. Singer A, Campion MJ, Clarkson PK, et al. Recognition of subclinical human papillomavirus infection of the vulva. J Reprod Med. 1986;31:985–6.
140. McMillan A. Sigmoidoscopy—A necessary procedure in the routine investigation of homosexual men? Genitourin Med. 1987;63:44–6.
141. Parker BJ, Cossart YE, Thompson CH, et al. The clinical management and laboratory assessment of anal warts. Med J Aust. 1987;147:59–63.
142. Saigo PE. Cytology of the uterine cervix. Semin Diagn Pathol. 1986;3:204–10.
143. Purola E, Savia E. Cytology of gynecologic condyloma acuminatum. Acta Cytol. 1977;21:26–31.
144. Syrjanen KJ, Heinonen U-M. Kauraniemi T. Cytologic evidence of the association of condylomatous lesions with dysplastic and neoplastic changes in the uterine cervix. Acta Cytol. 1981;25:17–22.
145. Schneider A. Methods of identification of human papillomaviruses. In: Syrjanen K. Gissmann L, Koss LG, eds. Papillomaviruses and Human Disease. Berlin: Springer Verlag; 1987:19–39.

146. Shibata DK, Arnheim N, Martin WJ. Detection of human papilloma virus in paraffin-embedded tissue using the polymerase chain reaction. J Exp Med. 1988;167:225–30.
147. Syrjanen K, Vayrynen M, Castren O, et al. Sexual behaviour of women with human papillomavirus (HPV) lesions of the uterine cervix. Br J Vener Dis. 1984;60:243–8.
148. Richardson AC, Lyon JB. The effect of condom use on squamous cell cervical intraepithelial neoplasia. Am J Obstet Gynecol. 1981;140:909–13.
149. Schreier AA, Allen WP, Laughlin C, et al. Prospects for human papillomavirus vaccines and immunotherapies. J Natl Cancer Inst. 1988;80:896–9.

124. JC, BK, AND OTHER POLYOMAVIRUSES (PROGRESSIVE MULTIFOCAL LEUKOENCEPHALOPATHY)

JAMES R. LEHRICH

Progressive multifocal leukoencephalopathy (PML) is a rare, subacute, and progressive demyelinating disease of the central nervous system (CNS) that appears in immunosuppressed adults. It was first identified and given its name in 1958 by Aström et al.,[1] who reported two cases in patients with lymphocytic leukemia, one in a patient with Hodgkin's disease and five additional cases found on review of the literature. Because of the presence of intranuclear inclusion bodies in oligodendrocytes and the association of PML with immunologic incompetence, a viral etiology was proposed by Cavanaugh[2] and by Richardson.[3] In 1965, Zu Rhein and Chou[4] used the electron microscope to study formalin-fixed brain tissue from PML patients and observed papovavirus-like particles in distended oligodendroglial nuclei. These findings were confirmed in fresh autopsy material by Silverman and Rubenstein.[5] The viral particles were studied under the electron microscope by negative staining methods[6,7] and were shown to be similar structurally to virions of the SV40-polyoma type, rather than to the larger human papilloma (wart) virus. In spite of these data pointing to a papovavirus etiology for PML, numerous attempts to isolate a virus were unsuccessful until 1971; Padgett and coworkers[8] recovered a virus that they called *JC virus* from primary cultures of human fetal glial cells inoculated with homogenized PML brain tissue. This agent appears to differ from all previously known papovaviruses. In 1972, Weiner et al.,[9] using different methodology, isolated agents that appeared to be identical to SV40 virus from the brains of two patients with PML. Numerous subsequent viral isolations from PML brain tissue have all been of the JC virus type.

DESCRIPTION OF THE PATHOGEN

The papovavirus family Papovaviridae[10] has been divided into two genera: papillomavirus (which includes the human wart virus; see Chapter 123) and polyomavirus (including polyoma virus and SV40 virus [Simian vacuolating agent-40]). The name *papova* is derived from the first two letters of *pa*pilloma, *po*lyoma, and *va*cuolating agent. These are small, naked icosahedral virions (papillomaviruses 52–54 nm in diameter, polyomaviruses 45 nm in diameter) containing double-stranded, cyclic DNA of molecular weight 3–5 × 10^6 daltons. The viruses replicate in the cell nucleus. Most are potentially oncogenic. Polyoma virus causes lysis (lytic infection) of mouse cells in tissue culture but causes transformation (temperate infection) of hamster and rat cells. SV40 virus is lytic in monkey cells and temperate in mouse cells; isolated SV40 DNA is capable of infecting and transforming susceptible cells.

JC Virus[11,12]

All but two of the viruses successfully isolated or identified by electron microscopic agglutination (EMA) in PML have been strains of JC virus. Although more than 10^{10} viral particles can be present in each gram of brain,[13] recovery of the virus has required inoculation of infectious material onto primary human fetal glial (PHFG) cell cultures containing a preponderance of spongioblasts.[8] Cytopathic effects (CPE) appear after 10–12 days and consist of loss of contact inhibition, cells in mitosis, necrotic cells, intranuclear inclusion bodies, destruction of spongioblasts, and enlarged, multinucleate astrocytes. Electron microscopy of these infected cells has shown papovavirus-like particles with an average diameter of 42.5 nm in many of the spongioblast nuclei. The viral particles occur both singly and in crystalline arrays. The virus does not multiply or produce CPE in a variety of other human, monkey, rabbit, and mouse cells that have been tested. There are differences in JC virus genomes derived from infected brain tissue from different patients with PML.[14]

As Walker et al.[11] have observed, the size, structure, stability, lack of essential lipid, and intranuclear multiplication of JC virus place it in the polyomavirus genus of Papovaviridae (Table 1). Unlike SV40, JC agglutinates human, guinea pig, and chicken erythrocytes, and it does not multiply in monkey cells. There are some minor antigenic similarities between JC and SV40, since some hyperimmune anti-SV40 sera have low levels of antibody to JC virus. Unlike human papilloma (wart) virus, JC is smaller, has a hemagglutinin, and shows no antigenic cross-reactivity. Immunofluorescence studies of JC-infected PHFG cells have shown staining with antiserum to JC virus, but not with SV40, human papilloma, polyoma, or BK (see below) antisera. Frozen sections of brain from a patient from whom JC virus was isolated showed nuclear fluorescence in cells in white matter when stained using JC antiserum, but no staining with antisera to SV40 or BK.[15] EMA tests have identified JC virus particles in extracts from most of the PML brains studied; only minimal agglutination has been found with SV40 antisera.[16]

There is evidence that the JC virus may be present outside the CNS. It has been cultured from urine of PML and renal transplant recipient patients; epithelial cells containing viral inclusions may be seen in the urine.[17,18] JC virus DNA has been detected in spleen, lymph node, liver, and lung, and in mononuclear cells in bone marrow and brain perivascular spaces.[19,20] Inoculation of the virus into experimental animals has induced a variety of nervous system tumors, including glioma, medulloblastoma, meningioma, pineocytoma, meningeal sarcoma, and neuroblastoma.[21] There has been no multifocal demyeli-

TABLE 1. Human Polyomaviruses

	JC	*SV40-PML*	*BK*
Size	39–42.5 nm	34–16 nm	43.6 nm
Nucleic acid	DNA	DNA	DNA
Envelope	None	None	None
Multiplication site	Nucleus	Nucleus	Nucleus
Site of infection in patient	Brain	Brain	Ureter
Hemagglutinin	Yes	No	Yes
Multiplication in human fetal glial cells	Good	Moderate	Good
Multiplication in human kidney cells	No	Poor	Good
Multiplication in monkey kidney cells	No	Poor	Moderate
Antigenic relationship to SV40	Slight	Strong	Slight
Oncogenicity in brain	Strong	Moderate	Weak
Oncogenicity in other tissues	Moderate	Strong	Weak

(Data from Walker et al.,[11] Walker,[12] and Weiner et al.[15])

nating disease resembling PML induced in an animal model. Transgenic mice that contain the early region of JC virus in all cells show defective myelination, which suggests that JC virus T antigens may arrest the maturation of oligodendrocytes and inhibit myelination.[22]

SV40-PML Viruses

Weiner et al.[9] have isolated viruses very closely related to SV40 from the brains of two patients with PML, using the method of explant culture of cells from brain biopsy specimens and subsequent fusion to primary African green monkey kidney cells. The SV40-like virus was also reisolated[23] in a later study by inoculating brain homogenates from one of the two patients onto PHFG cell cultures, using the method that Padgett et al.[8] had used to isolate JC virus. These SV40-like agents were demonstrated to be similar antigenically to SV40 by means of neutralization tests, fluorescent antibody staining of infected monkey kidney cells and brain sections from one of the patients, and EMA with SV40 antiserum—but not with antisera to JC, BK, or polyoma viruses.[15] Later studies using hyperimmune rabbit sera have shown some cross-reactivity among JC, SV40-PML, and BK viruses at low serum dilutions. Like prototype SV40 virus, the SV40-PML viruses cause a productive lytic infection of monkey kidney cells, with induction of T and V antigens; they are capable of inducing tumors in neonatal hamsters. Some minor differences in nucleic acid and plaque morphology in infected monkey kidney cells have been found when the two SV40-PML viruses were compared with prototype SV40 strains.[15]

The two patients from whom the SV40-PML viruses were isolated each survived for more than 1 year, which is unusually long for PML. Such cases have been described, however, including one in which the JC virus was identified. In other respects, the SV40-PML cases were clinically and histologically typical. One of the patients showed an eightfold rise in serum antibody to SV40 during the course of her illness; there was no serum SV40 antibody in the other patient.[9]

Since Weiner's report in 1972,[9] SV40 virus has been recovered from only one other PML patient.[24] It has been suggested that these isolates might be genetic recombinants of a human papovavirus, such as JC, with simian viruses in the monkey kidney cell cultures used in the recovery procedure.[25] In Weiner's cases, evidence against that possibility includes reisolation of SV40 in human fetal glial cells, direct identification by EMA of particles extracted from PML brain, and production of antibody to SV40 in rabbits immunized with particles extracted directly from PML brain.[15]

BK Virus

This virus has not been found in association with PML but is noteworthy in that it is the only well-characterized human polyomavirus and because it has been carefully compared with the JC and SV40-PML viruses. Since 1971, when Gardner et al.[26] first isolated this new papovavirus from urine of an immunosuppressed renal allograft recipient, there have been several isolations from immunoincompetent patients. In Gardner's case, virus-like particles were seen in urine and in ureteral lining cells; the virus was isolated after inoculation of urine onto the Vero line of African green monkey kidney cells. Human fetal glial cells and human embryonic lung cells are also susceptible to infection with BK. Under the electron microscope, the particles have the appearance of papovaviruses and a diameter of 43.6 nm. BK virus agglutinates human type 0 erythrocytes, as does JC but not SV40 (see Table 1). There is some antigenic similarity to SV40 virus, as indicated by EMA, immunofluorescence, and neutralization antibody tests, but little cross-reaction with JC. The complete DNA sequence of BK virus has been determined, and it shares 70 percent homology with SV40; this suggests a close evolutionary relationship.[27] BK virus is not known to cause clinical disease. It has been isolated from the urine of children with the Wiskott-Aldrich syndrome[28] and from a reticulum cell sarcoma from the brain of one such child.[29] BK virus DNA has been detected in brain tumors and other neoplasms in humans.[30] It is less oncogenic than the JC and SV40-PML viruses, but it can induce choroid plexus papillomas, ependymomas, and insulinomas in experimental animals.[31–33]

EPIDEMIOLOGY

PML is an extremely rare disease of worldwide distribution. The majority of patients are adults between 40 and 70 years of age, although a 5-year-old patient and an 18-year-old patient have been reported. Most cases have occurred in hypergic persons, often as a late complication of a preexisting generalized, chronic systemic disease. More than half of the patients have had lymphoproliferative or myeloproliferative neoplasms, with Hodgkin's disease and chronic lymphocytic leukemia being the two largest groups. The disease has also been associated with carcinoma in various sites, sarcoid, tuberculosis, Whipple's disease, and systemic lupus erythematosus (SLE). Many cases have occurred in patients with acquired immunodeficiency syndrome (AIDS).[34,35] As many as 16 percent of PML patients have AIDS as the underlying disorder,[12] and 2–4 percent of AIDS patients with neurologic complications have developed PML.[34–36,51] There have also been case reports of PML in renal transplant recipients and in other patients who have received immunosuppressive treatment. A few cases have been reported in persons without any apparent associated systemic disease or immunologic deficit, but this is decidedly uncommon.

Surveys of serum antibodies have shown that papovavirus infections without known illness must be common. Hemagglutination-inhibition antibodies to JC virus have been found in about 70 percent of adults. The prevalence of positive sera rises with increasing age; the highest rate of conversion to seropositivity occurs during the first 14 years of life (0–4 years, 10 percent; 10–14 years, 65 percent; and 50–59 years, 75 percent).[37] BK virus antibodies also are present in 60–70 percent of adults, appear first in early childhood, and increase in prevalence with increasing age.[38] Although antibodies to JC and BK viruses have similar prevalence, there appears to be an independent experience with the two viruses in the several population groups studied.[38] SV40 antibodies, which are much less common, have been found in 3 percent of children born since inactivated poliovirus vaccines were cleared of SV40 contamination and in about 20 percent of sera from persons who had received one or more doses of potentially contaminated vaccine (during 1955–1960).[39] Neither of the two PML patients from whom SV40 was isolated had a history of exposure to monkeys or to contaminated poliovirus vaccine.[9] Brown et al.[38] have found a significantly higher prevalence of neutralization antibodies to SV40 in BK-antibody-positive sera than in BK-negative sera. They have suggested that infection with BK or a closely related virus may be responsible for SV40 antibody activity when it is present in humans who have not been exposed to either contaminated vaccines or monkeys. However, SV40 infection does not appear to stimulate heterologous antibody response to BK virus.[40] In some PML patients, there are serum antibodies directed against the virus identified in the brain; however, the antibody response has been variable—a finding that might be explained by the disordered cell-mediated and humoral immunity of these patients. As noted previously, one PML patient showed an eightfold rise in antibodies to SV40 virus during the course of her illness.[9] There has been no evidence to indicate that PML is a contagious disease.

PATHOGENESIS

Antibody surveys suggest that infection with the JC (and BK) papovaviruses must be quite common, although it is not known whether such antibodies were present in a given patient with PML before the onset of disease. The antibody data do not explain why PML is so rare, even among immunologically compromised persons. As noted above, most PML patients have had underlying diseases that are associated with immunologic impairment or have had documented defects in humoral and cell-mediated immunity, and this association must play an important role in pathogenesis. It has been postulated that PML results from activation of latent virus in brain or other tissue when the immune response becomes impaired. As an alternative explanation, PML may occur as a primary infection in a person who fails to acquire immunity to the virus during childhood and who becomes immunologically compromised in adult life.

PML is a demyelinating disease; that is, there is selective destruction of myelin, with relative preservation of axons and other CNS tissue elements. As distinct from multiple sclerosis (see Chapter 69), however, there is little inflammation in the lesions of PML, and the myelin destruction appears to result from infection and destruction of oligodendrocytes by the virus, rather than being lymphocyte-mediated, as in multiple sclerosis. CNS myelin sheaths are, in fact, multilayered wrappings of oligodendrocyte cell membranes around axons. Destruction of these cells would be a direct cause of demyelination.

The bizarre neoplastic-appearing astrocytes (see below) that are also found in PML have an uncertain role in its pathogenesis. They are probably related to the oncogenic potential of the papovaviruses and may indicate temperate infection and neoplastic transformation of these cells; this can be demonstrated in vitro with the SV40, JC, and BK viruses.[12,41,42] Thus, in PML, the same virus may cause latent infection of astrocytes and lytic infection of oligodendrocytes. As noted previously, inoculation of JC and SV40-PML viruses into experimental animals results in brain tumors,[17] rather than in a demyelinating disease. However, a PML-like disease caused by SV40 virus has developed spontaneously in monkeys.[43,44] PML has rarely occurred in patients with brain tumors. It is not a neoplastic disease per se, although a case has been reported in which multiple gliomas were found in areas of PML demyelination.[45,46]

PATHOLOGIC FINDINGS[47]

There are multiple discrete foci of myelin destruction, with relative preservation of axons (demyelination). The foci tend to become confluent, producing large plaques (Fig. 1). Involvement is asymmetric, without preferential localization to any one region of the CNS, although lesions are infrequent in the spinal cord. Oligodendrocytes in and around the lesions often show characteristic nuclear enlargement, with loss of the regular chromatin pattern and intranuclear inclusions that may be basophilic, eosinophilic, or amphophilic. Giant astrocytes are found in most cases, particularly in late lesions. Nuclei of these astrocytes are pleomorphic and hyperchromatic, sometimes with mitotic figures, and may be indistinguishable from the malignant astrocytes seen in glioblastomas. Inflammatory cells are usually sparse or absent in these lesions. In rare cases, plasma cell infiltrates are found in the demyelinated foci.[48] Under the electron microscope, rounded papovavirus-like particles (28–40 nm in diameter in formalin-fixed tissue) are seen in the nuclei of affected oligodendrocytes and, rarely, in oligodendrocyte cytoplasm or in astrocye nuclei (Fig. 2). JC virus can also be identified in lesions by means of immunofluorescent, immunohistochemical, and in situ DNA hybridization techniques.[49,50]

CLINICAL MANIFESTATION

As noted above, the disease usually appears in hypergic adults. The evolution is rapid, typically 2–4 months from the appearance of the first neurologic symptom to death. Rare cases of remission or prolonged survival have been reported; these may

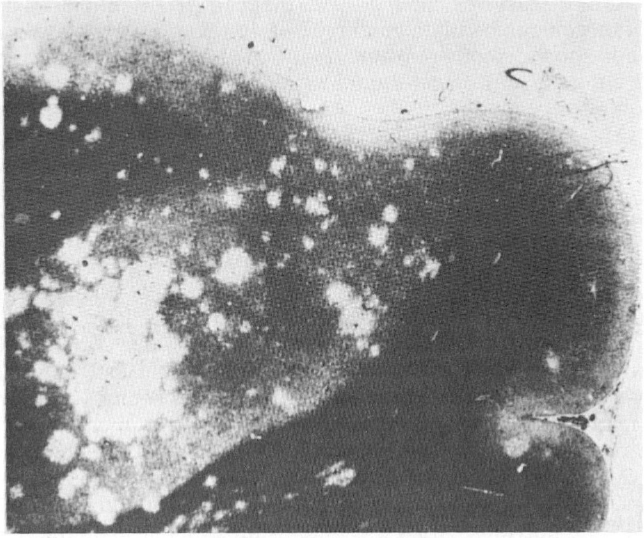

FIG. 1. Progressive multifocal leukoencephalopathy. A section of parietal lobe from a patient with chronic lymphocytic leukemia and PML. There are scattered lesions of demyelination in white and gray matter, some of which have merged to form a larger plaque. (Stained for myelin, ×3.25.) (Courtesy of Dr. K. E. Aström, Stockholm, Sweden.)

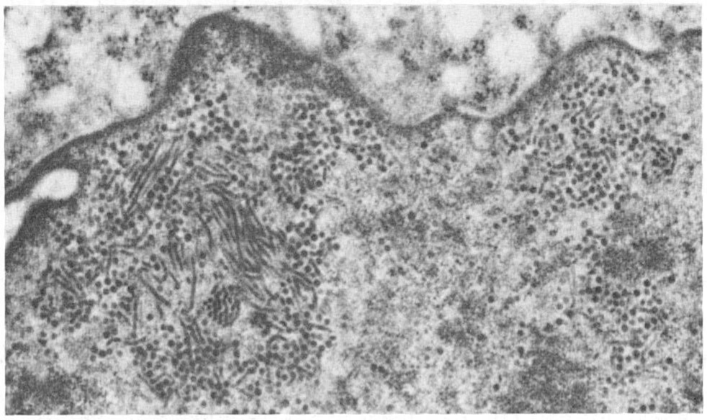

FIG. 2. Progressive multifocal leukoencephalopathy. Electron micrograph of viral inclusion in the nucleus of an oligodendrocyte in the brain. Polyomavirus-like particles are polyhedral bodies with a diameter of 35–40 nm and filaments with a slightly smaller diameter. The nuclear membrane is in the upper part of the figure. (×28,000.) (Courtesy of Dr. K. E. Aström, Stockholm, Sweden.)

be more common in AIDS-associated cases.[35] The clinical symptoms and signs are diverse, reflecting multiple foci of destruction of myelin, which may develop at any level of the CNS. In the early stages, there may be monoparesis or hemiparesis, personality change, mental impairment, ataxia, dysarthria, dysphasia, or cortical blindness. Later, quadriparesis, severe dementia, and coma often appear. Cases of transverse myelopathy have been reported but are quite rare. Headaches, convulsive seizures, and cerebellar ataxia are unusual. There is no evidence of increased intracranial pressure.

The diagnosis should be considered when a rapidly progressive neurologic illness develops in a person with impaired immunologic competence, especially if there is evidence of multiple sites of CNS damage. Because as many as 4 percent of AIDS patients with neurologic complications may have PML, it must be considered in the differential diagnosis, along with other CNS opportunistic infections (as with *Toxoplasma gondii,* fungi, mycobacteria, or cytomegalovirus), primary CNS lymphoma, and vascular disease (such as emboli from endocarditis and CNS hemorrhage in thrombocytopenic patients), as well as primary AIDS encephalopathy.[34–36,51] The reader is referred to Chapter 108 for a detailed discussion of the differential diagnosis of the neurologic complications of AIDS.

Computed tomography (CT) and magnetic resonance imaging (MRI) can be useful in localizing the demyelinative lesions; the lack of contrast enhancement of CT lesions in PML is usually helpful in distinguishing these lesions from those of toxoplasmosis.[34,36,51,52] The electroencephalogram (EEG) is usually diffusely and nonspecifically slow. Cerebrospinal fluid (CSF), radionuclide brain scans, and angiograms are usually normal. Serologic studies of serum and CSF are not helpful, since antibodies to JC virus are present in serum in most normal adults and are not found in CSF.[12]

PREVENTION AND TREATMENT

At present, nothing is known about prevention of PML. Several reported cases have been treated with adenine arabinoside,[17] cytosine arabinoside,[53,54] and transfer factor,[54] with variable responses, but there are as yet no controlled data establishing the effectiveness of any therapy.

REFERENCES

1. Aström KE, Mancall EL, Richardson EP Jr. Progressive multifocal leukoencephalopathy. Brain. 1958;81:930.
2. Cavanagh JB, Greenbaum D, Marshall AHE, et al. Cerebral demyelination associated with disorders of the reticuloendothelial system. Lancet. 1959;2:525.
3. Richardson EP Jr. Progressive multifocal leukoencephalopathy. N Engl J Med. 1961;265:815.
4. Zu Rhein GM, Chou SM. Particles resembling papovaviruses in human cerebral demyelinating disease. Science. 1965;148:1477.
5. Silverman L, Rubenstein LJ. Electron microscopic observations on a case of progressive multifocal leukoencephalopathy. Acta Neuropathol. 1965;5:215.
6. Howatson AF, Nagai M, Zu Rhein GM. Polyoma-like virions in a human demyelinating brain disease. Can Med Assoc J. 1965;93:379.
7. Schwerdt PR, Schwerdt CE, Silverman L, et al. Virions associated with progressive multifocal leukoencephalopathy. Virology. 1966;29:519.
8. Padgett BL, Walker DL, Zu Rhein GM, et al. Cultivation of papova-like virus from human brain with progressive multifocal leukoencephalopathy. Lancet. 1971;1:1257.
9. Weiner LP, Herndon RM, Narayan O, et al. Isolation of virus related to SV40 from patients with progressive multifocal leukoencephalopathy. N Engl J Med. 1972;286:385.
10. Fraenkel-Conrat H. Comprehensive Virology: Descriptive Catalogue of Viruses. v. 1. New York: Plenum Press: 1974.
11. Walker DL, Padgett BL, Zu Rhein GM, et al. Current study of an opportunistic papovavirus. In: Zeman W, Lennette E, eds. Slow Virus Disease. Baltimore: Williams & Wilkins; 1973:49.
12. Walker DL. Progressive multifocal leukoencephalopathy. In: Vinken PJ, Bruyn GW, Klawans HL, eds. Handbook of Clinical Neurology. v. 47. Amsterdam: Elsevier/North-Holland; 1985:503–24.
13. Dorries K, Johnson RT, ter Meulen V. Detection of polyoma virus DNA in PML-brain tissue by in situ hybridization. J Gen Virol. 1979;42:49.
14. Grinnell BW, Martin JD, Padgett BL, et al. Comparison of infectious JC virus DNS's cloned from human brain. J Virol. 1983;45:299–308.
15. Weiner LP, Narayan O: Virologic studies of progressive multifocal leukoencephalopathy. Prog Med Virol. 1974;18:229.
16. Narayan O, Penney JB, Johnson RT, et al. Etiology of progressive multifocal leukoencephalopathy. Identification of papovavirus. N Engl J Med. 1973;289:1278.
17. Rand KK, Johnson KP, Rubenstein LJ, et al. Adenine arabinoside in the treatment of progressive multifocal leukoencephalopathy: Use of virus-containing cells in the urine to assess response to therapy. Ann Neurol. 1977;1:458.
18. Hogan TF, Borden EC, McBain JA, et al. Human polyomavirus infections with JC virus and BK virus in renal transplant patients. Ann Intern Med. 1980;92:373.
19. Grinnell BW, Padgett BL, Walker DL. Distribution of nonintegrated DNA from JC papovavirus in organs of patients with progressive multifocal leukoencephalopathy. J Infect Dis. 1983;147:669–75.
20. Houff SA, Major EO, Katz DA, et al. Involvement of JC virus-infected mononuclear cells from the bone marrow and spleen in the pathogenesis of progressive multifocal leukoencephalopathy. N Engl J Med. 1988;318:301–5.
21. Zu Rhein GM. Studies of JC virus-induced nervous system tumors in the Syrian hamster: A review. Prog Clin Biol Res. 1983;105:205–21.
22. Trapp BD, Small JA, Pulley M, et al. Dysmyelination in transgenic mice containing JC virus early region. Ann Neurol. 1988;23:38–48.
23. Weiner LP, Herndon RM, Narayan O, et al. Further studies of a simian virus 40-like virus isolated from human brain. J Virol. 1972;10:147.
24. Scherneck S, Geissler E, Janisch W, et al. Isolation of a SV40-like virus from a patient with progressive multifocal leukoencephalopathy. Acta Virol. 1981;25:191.
25. Black PH, Hirsch MS. Viruses and progressive multifocal leukoencephalopathy. N Engl J Med. 1972;286:429.
26. Gardner SD, Field AM, Coleman DV, et al. New human papovavirus (BK) isolated from urine after renal transplantation. Lancet. 1971;1:12530.
27. Yang RC, Wu R. BK virus DNA: Complete nucleotide sequence of a human tumor virus. Science. 1979;206:456.
28. Takemoto KK, Rabson AS, Mullarkey MF, et al. Isolation of papovavirus from brain tumor and urine of a patient with Wiskott-Aldrich syndrome. J Natl Cancer Inst. 1974;53:1205.
29. Takemoto KK, Rabson AS, Mullarkey MF, et al. Isolation of papovaviruses from brain tumor and urine of a patient with Wiskott-Aldrich syndrome. J Natl Cancer Inst. 1974;53:1205.
30. Corallini A, Pagnani M, Viadana P, et al. Association of BK virus with human brain tumors and tumors of pancreatic islets. Int J Cancer. 1987;39:60–7.
31. Greenlee JE, Narayan O, Johnson RT, et al. Induction of brain tumors in hamsters with BK virus, a human papovavirus. Lab Invest. 1977;36:636.
32. Corallini A, Barbanti-Brodano G, Bortoloni W, et al. High incidence of ependymomas induced by BK virus, a human papovavirus: Brief communication. J Natl Cancer Inst. 1977;59:1561.
33. Bordi C, de Vita O, Ferrari C, et al. Histologic, immunofluorescence, and ultrastructural study of malignant islet-cell tumors of the pancreas induced in hamsters by BK human papovavirus. Am J Pathol. 1985;118:256–65.
34. Snider WD, Simpson DM, Nielson S, et al. Neurological complications of the acquired immunodeficiency syndrome: Analysis of 50 patients. Ann Neurol. 1983;14:403–18.
35. Berger JR, Mucke L. Prolonged survival and partial recovery in AIDS-associated progressive multifocal leukoencephalopathy. Neurology. 1988;38:1060–5.
36. Berger JR, Kaszovitz B, Post MJ, et al. Progressive multifocal leukoencephalopathy associated with human immunodeficiency virus infection. A review of the literature with a report of sixteen cases. Ann Intern Med. 1987;107:78–87.
37. Padgett BL, Walker DL. Prevalence of antibodies in human sera against JC virus, an isolate from a case of progressive multifocal leukoencephalopathy. J Infect Dis. 1973;127:467.
38. Brown P, Tsai T, Gajdusek C. Seroepidemiology of human papovaviruses. Am J Epidemiol. 1975;102:331.
39. Shah KV. Evidence for an SV40-related papovavirus infection of man. Am J Epidemiol. 1972;95:199.
40. Brown P, Morris JA. Serologic response to BK virus following human infection with SV40. Proc Soc Exp Biol Med. 1976;152:130.
41. Shein HM. Transformation of astrocytes and destruction of spongioblasts induced by a simian tumor virus SV40 in cultures of human fetal neuroglia. J Neuropathol Exp Neurol. 1967;26:60.
42. Oster-Granite ML, Narayan O, Johnson RT, et al. Studies of cultured human and simian fetal brain cells. III. Infections with human (BK) and simian (SV40) papovaviruses. Neuropathol Appl Neurobiol. 1978;4:443.
43. Gribble DH, Haden CC, Schwartz LW, et al. Spontaneous progressive multifocal leukoencephalopathy (PML) in macaques. Nature. 1975;254:602.
44. Holmberg CA, Gribble DH, Takemoto KK, et al. Isolation of simian virus 40 from rhesus monkeys (Macaca mulatta) with spontaneous progressive multifocal leukoencephalopathy. J Infect Dis. 1977;136:593.
45. Castaigne P, Rondot P, Escourolle R, et al: Leucoencephalopathie multifocale progressive at "gliomes" multiples. Rev Neurol. 1974;130:379.
46. Sima AA, Finkelstein SD, McLachlan DR. Multiple malignant astrocytomas in a patient with spontaneous progressive multifocal leukoencephalopathy. Ann Neurol. 1983;14:183–8.
47. Richardson EP Jr, Webster HD. Progressive multifocal leukoencephalopathy: Its pathological features. Prog Clin Biol Res. 1983;105:191–203.
48. Richardson EP, Johnson PC. Atypical progressive multifocal leukoencephalopathy with plasma-cell infiltrates. Acta Neuropathol. 1975;6(Suppl):247.
49. Aksamit AJ, Sever JL, Major EO. Progressive multifocal leukoencephalopathy: JC virus detection by in situ hybridization compared with immunohistochemistry. Neurology. 1986;36:499–504.
50. Itoyama Y, Webster H, Sternberger NH. Distribution of papovavirus, myelin-associated glycoprotein, and myelin basic protein in progressive multifocal leukoencephalopathy lesions. Ann Neurol. 1982;11:396–407.
51. Krupp LB, Lipton RB, Swerdlow ML, et al. Progressive multifocal leukoencephalopathy: Clinical and radiographic features. Ann Neurol. 1985;17:344–9.
52. Guilleux MH, Steiner RE, Young IR. MR imaging in progressive multifocal leukoencephalopathy. AJNR. 1986;7:1033–5.
53. Marriott PJ, O'Brien MD, Mackensie ECK, et al. Progressive multifocal leukoencephalopathy: Remission with cytarabine. J Neurol Neurosurg Psychiatry. 1975;38:205.
54. Horn GV, Bastian FO, Moake JL. Progressive multifocal leukoencephalopathy: Failure of response to transfer factor and cytarabine. Neurology. 1978;28:794.

Hepadnaviridae

125. HEPATITIS B VIRUS AND HEPATITIS DELTA VIRUS

WILLIAM S. ROBINSON

HISTORY

The first cases of *serum hepatitis* (acute hepatitis with a long incubation period after the percutaneous transfer of material containing human serum) to be recorded appear to be those that followed the administration of smallpox vaccine containing human lymph to shipyard workers in Bremen in 1833.[1] In the early and middle parts of this century, serum hepatitis was repeatedly observed after the use of contaminated needles and syringes, for example, in diabetic[2] and venereal disease clinics,[3–5] in plasma administration as for immunoprophylaxis in measles[6] and mumps,[7] in administration of vaccines containing human serum such as for yellow fever,[8,9] and in the transfusion of blood.[10,11] Although some of these cases may have been due to agents now referred to as *non-A, non-B hepatitis viruses*, most were undoubtedly due to the virus now known as *hepatitis B virus (HBV)*.

Serum hepatitis was not clearly distinguished from *infectious hepatitis* until the 1940s and 1950s, when apparent antigenic[12–16] and biologic[12,13,17–22] differences were demonstrated in experimental transmission studies in human volunteers. After the discovery of Australia antigen (now designated *hepatitis B surface antigen,* or *HBsAg*) in serum by Blumberg et al. in 1965[23] and its eventual association with serum hepatitis,[24–26] hepatitis B virus was identified and characterized. The development of serologic tests for HBV antigens and their respective antibodies led to the recognition that HBV has a worldwide distribution and that infection rates in some parts of the world, such as parts of Asia, Africa, and Oceania, are extremely high.[27] Serologic testing provided direct evidence that many serum hepatitis cases were associated with HBV infection and that HBV was distinct from the virus associated with most infectious hepatitis cases (hepatitis A virus).[28] It has also become clear that not all post-transfusion hepatitis is associated with HBV infection; additional agents (non-A, non-B hepatitis viruses) are responsible for many cases.[28–30]

HBV is now known to be a small DNA virus with unique ultrastructural, molecular, antigenic, and biologic features that distinguish it from members of all previously recognized virus families.[31,32] Recently, three other very similar viruses were found in woodchucks in the eastern United States,[33] ground squirrels in California,[34] and Peking ducks in China and the United States.[35] These viruses form a new virus family that has recently been formally named the Hepadnaviridae.[31,36] Among the unique molecular features of these viruses is their DNA structure (a very small, circular DNA that is partly single-stranded), their mechanism of replication, and the presence of an enzyme in virions with the property of reverse transcriptase. Among the notable biologic features of the viruses are their striking tropism for hepatocytes and their propensity to cause persistent infection (chronic carrier state), with high concentrations of viral antigen consisting of complete and incomplete viral forms remaining in the blood continuously for many months or years. In highly endemic areas of the world, chronic carrier rates can exceed 10 percent of the population, and it has been estimated that there are more than 170 million chronic carriers in the world today.[27] The name *serum hepatitis*, used for many years, indicated the first recognized common route of HBV transmission resulting from the continuous viremia, namely, by percutaneous transfer of serum. It is now clear that HBV is spread most commonly by routes that do not involve direct percutaneous transfer, such as by sexual contact and from mothers to their newborn infants. HBV infection is one of the most common causes of acute viral hepatitis. Persistent HBV infections are associated with a broad spectrum of disease, including chronic hepatitis, sometimes leading to cirrhosis, hepatocellular carcinoma, and immune complex disease taking forms such as polyarteritis and glomerulonephritis. HBV is a major (if not the most common) cause of chronic liver disease and hepatocellular carcinoma in the world today, and it is a major cause of necrotizing vasculitis (polyarteritis).

DISCOVERY AND NATURE OF VIRAL FORMS IN THE BLOOD

Hepatitis B viral forms in the blood of infected patients were identified and characterized after the discovery of the antigen on the surface of these particulate forms. HBsAg was discovered in 1965 by Blumberg et al.[23] while investigating human serum protein polymorphism. The antigen was first found in the serum of an Australian aborigine when a precipitin line formed in agar gel diffusion between that serum and the serum of a patient with hemophilia who had received multiple blood transfusions. Thus, the antigen was first named *Australia antigen*.[37] It was not immediately recognized to be a viral antigen. Several years of investigation led to its eventual association with acute hepatitis B[24–26]; it was then named *hepatitis-associated antigen (HAA)* and later given the current name, *hepatitis B surface antigen*. HBsAg in the blood remains the most useful marker of active HBV infection. It appears in the blood exclusively as a component of virion and incomplete particulate viral forms; no soluble or low molecular weight form has been detected.[38,39] The serum of infected patients has been a principal source of viral material for physical characterization of HBV and was originally used for vaccine production, since this virus has not been grown in tissue culture.

Small spherical particles, heterogeneous in size and appearance (diameters from approximately 16 to 25 nm and called *22-nm particles*), and filamentous or rod-shaped particles (approximately 22 nm wide and up to several hundred nanometers in length) (Fig. 1) were the first HBsAg particulate forms observed in electron micrographs by Bayer et al. in 1968.[39] These are the most numerous HBsAg-bearing particles in the serum of most HBV-infected patients; they consist of protein, carbohydrate, and lipid. No nucleic acid has been found in them, and they are now considered to be incomplete viral envelope particles. In 1970 a larger and more complex HBsAg-bearing particle was described by Dane et al.[40] Strong evidence indicates that this particle is the complete hepatitis B virion. The virion has a diameter of approximately 42 nm, with a lipid-containing outer layer or envelope approximately 7 nm in width and an electron-dense, 28-nm-diameter spherical internal core or nucleocapsid[40] (Fig. 2, left panel). The surface of the virion shares antigenic determinants (HBsAg) with the incomplete viral forms (22-nm spherical and filamentous particles).[40,41] The other envelope of the viron with HBsAg can be removed by treatment with nonionic detergents, leaving free core particles (Fig. 2, right panel) containing the virus-specified hepatitis B core antigen (HBcAg), which is antigenically distinct from HBsAg.[41] The viral core also contains the viral DNA[42] with a covalently attached polypeptide,[43] DNA polymerase activity,[44,45] protein kinase activity,[46] and the third antigen associ-

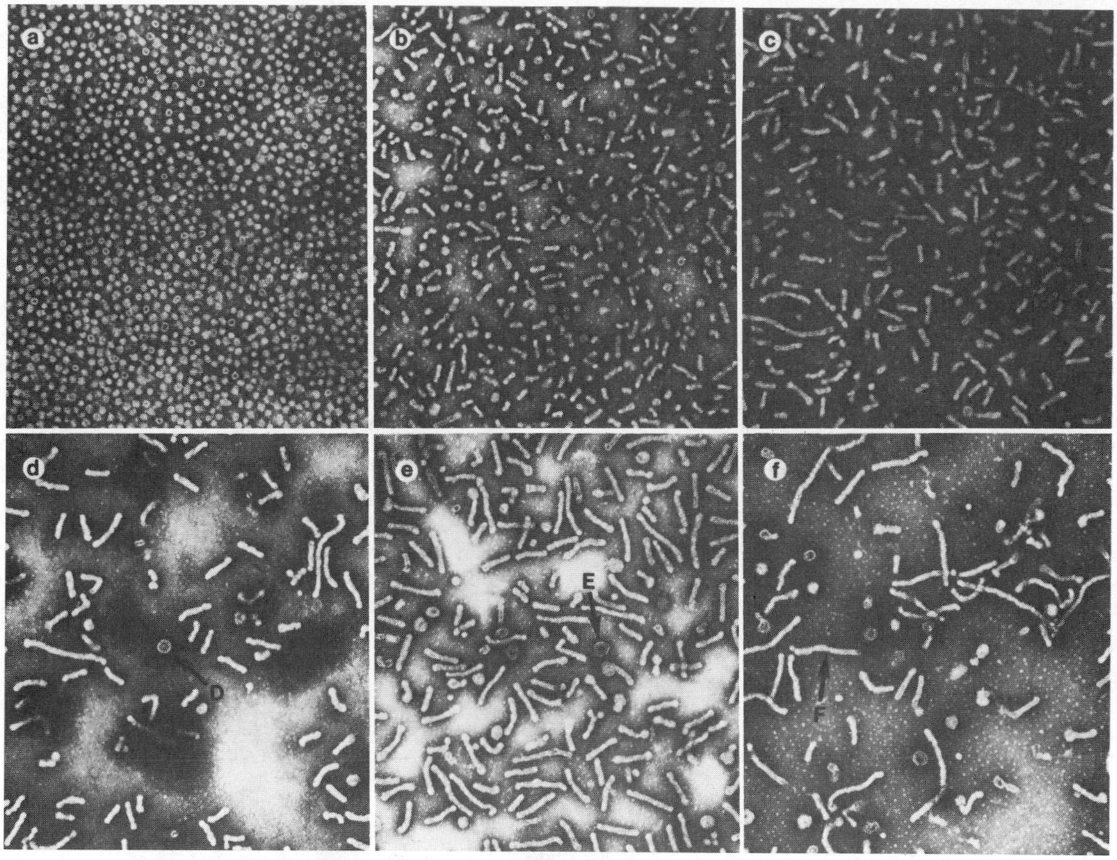

FIG. 1. Electron micrograph of hepatitis B viral forms in the blood of an infected patient. **(A–F)** Sucrose density gradient fractions after rate zonal sedimentation of particles. **(D)** indicates a virion with an electron-dense core, **(E)** shows an empty virion, and **(F)** indicates a filamentous form. (Experiment by John L. Gerin, Rockville, MD.)

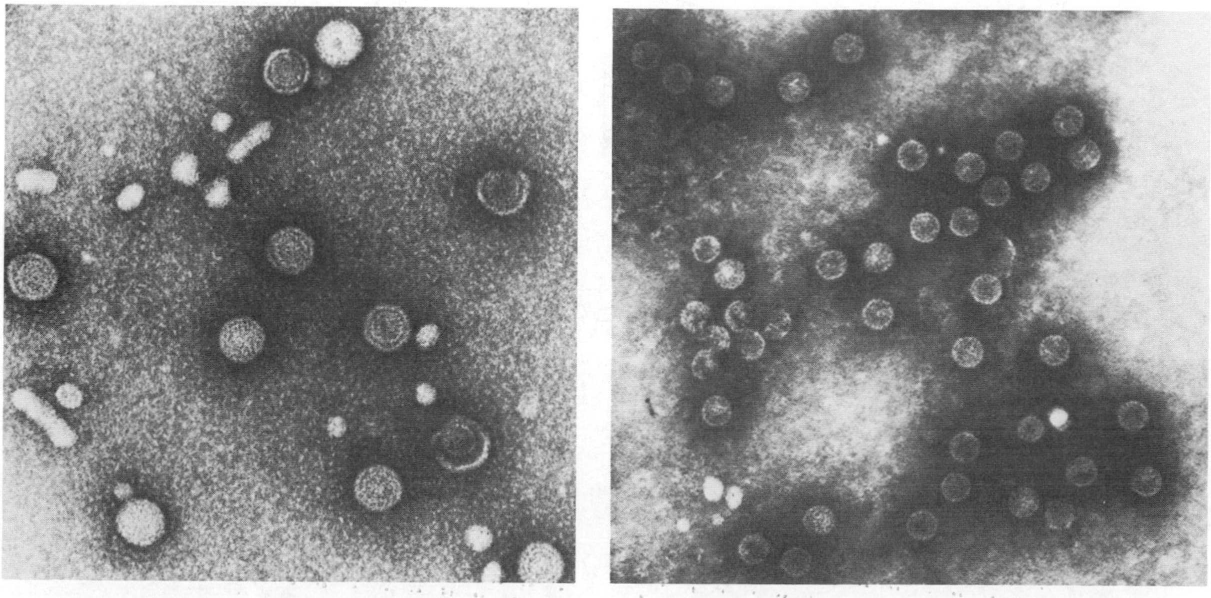

FIG. 2. Electron micrograph of virions (left) and virion cores (right) after detergent (NP-40) treatment of virions. (Experiment by June Almedia, London, UK.)

ated with hepatitis B virus infection, hepatitis B e antigen (HBeAg).[47] Figure 3 summarizes the viral structures found in the blood.

Some HBsAg-reactive sera have infected humans or chimpanzees in dilutions of up to 10^{-7}[48] or 10^{-8}[49,50] indicating that such patients circulate high concentrations of infectious virions. Other HBsAg-reactive sera have failed to infect chimpanzees when undiluted,[49] suggesting that some HBsAg carriers circulate only incomplete HBsAg particles and not complete virions. The concentrations of incomplete viral forms in serum usually greatly exceed the concentrations of complete virions. Concentrations of 10^{13} 22-nm spherical particles per milliter (approximately 500 mg/ml) or higher have been found in some sera,[51] and these particles outnumber virions by 10^4-fold or more in most sera.

HBV has been shown to retain infectivity of humans for 6 months when stored in serum at 30–32°C[52] and for 15 years when frozen at −20°C. All infectivity for human volunteers is not lost at 60°C for up to 4 hours,[53] but it is lost at 60°C after 10 hours when in albumin[54] although not completely in whole serum.[55,56] Infectivity in serum was destroyed at 90°C after 1[57] or 20 minutes.[58] Infectivity has also been destroyed by dry heat at 160°C after 1 hour.[59]

VIRUS STRUCTURE

Hepatitis B Surface Antigen

HBsAg is a complex antigen, and the antibody response to the antigen reflects this complexity. At least five antigenic specificities may be found on HBsAg particles. A group-specific determinant (*a*) is shared by all HBsAg preparations, and two pairs of subtype determinants (*d,y* and *w,r*) (the determinants of each pair are for the most part mutually exclusive and thus usually behave as alleles) have been demonstrated.[60,61] Antigenic heterogeneity of the *w* determinants and additional determinant such as *q* and *x* or *g* have also been described.[62,63] The eight HBsAg subtypes, ayw_1, ayw_2, ayw_3, ayw_4, *ayr*, adw_2, adw_4, and *adr*, have been identified.[63] Isolated and usually single cases from the Far East with unusual combinations of HBsAg subtype determinants, such as *awr*, *adwr*, *adyw*, *adyr*, and *adywr*, have been reported.[63] The subtype determinants in these cases are found on the same particles, suggesting that phenotypic mixing or unusual genetic recombinants have formed during mixed infections.

The S gene contains three regions—$preS_1$, $preS_2$, and S, each downstream of a separate inframe start codon. The major viral protein components of the envelope of virions and 22-nm

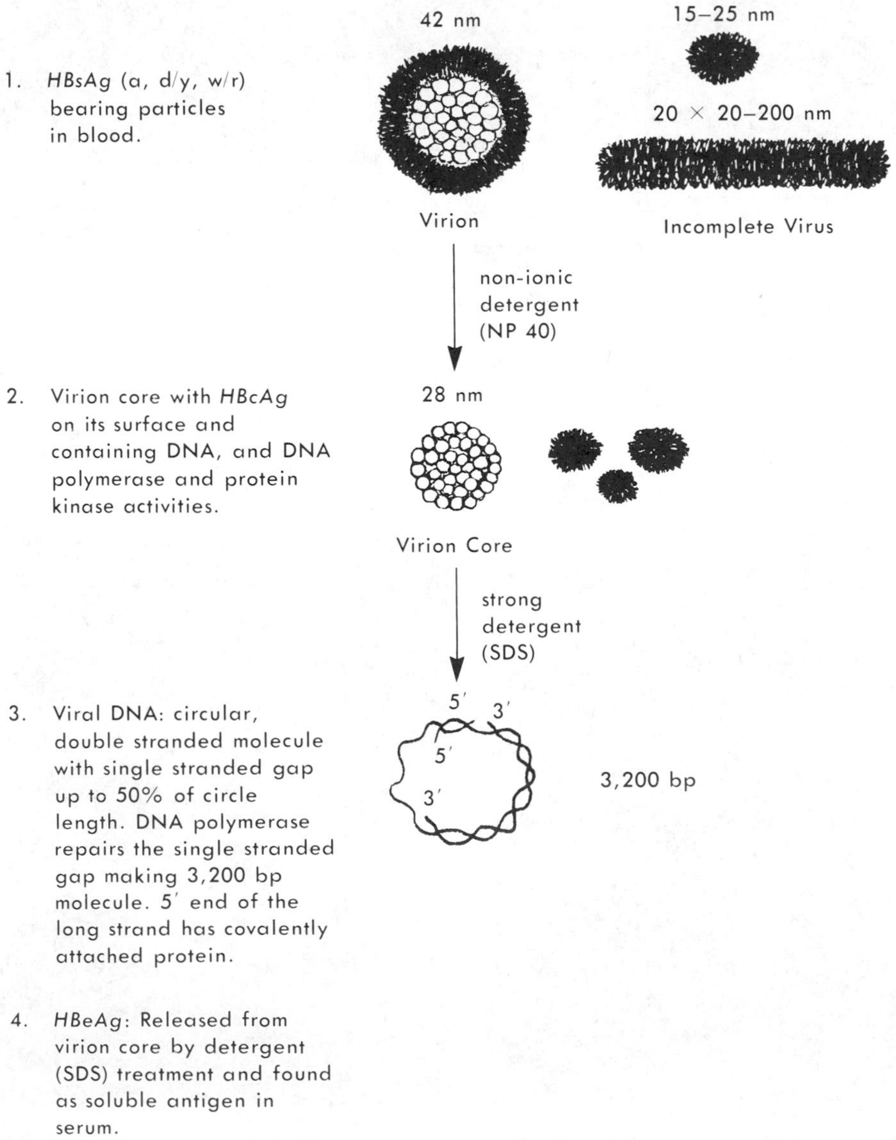

42 nm
15–25 nm
1. HBsAg (a, d/y, w/r) bearing particles in blood.
20 × 20–200 nm
Virion
Incomplete Virus
non-ionic detergent (NP 40)
28 nm
2. Virion core with HBcAg on its surface and containing DNA, and DNA polymerase and protein kinase activities.
Virion Core
strong detergent (SDS)
5′
3′
5′
3′
3,200 bp
3. Viral DNA: circular, double stranded molecule with single stranded gap up to 50% of circle length. DNA polymerase repairs the single stranded gap making 3,200 bp molecule. 5′ end of the long strand has covalently attached protein.
4. HBeAg: Released from virion core by detergent (SDS) treatment and found as soluble antigen in serum.

FIG. 3. Schematic representation of hepatitis B viral forms found in the blood of infected patients.

HBsAg particles are 226 amino acid polypeptides (24 kD and 27 kD, representing, respectively, nonglycosylated and glycosylated forms) encoded by the S region and containing the group *a* and subtype HBsAg determinants. Less abundant polypeptides include middle-sized polypeptides (33 and 36 kD) containing the 55 amino acid $preS_2$ sequence at the N-terminus of the S polypeptide) and large polypeptides (39 and 42 kD) consisting of an additional 165–221 amino acids (the size differing in different HBsAg subtypes) encoded by the $preS_1$ sequence at the N-terminus of preS- and S-encoded sequences. The large polypeptides containing $preS_1$-encoded sequences are found in higher abundance in virions and filaments than in the 22-nm spherical particles, while the middle-sized and small proteins are more abundant in the spherical particles.[65] Many epitopes contained in $preS_1$, $preS_2$, and S peptide sequences are present on the surfaces of these particles and epitopes in the $preS_1$,[66] $preS_2$,[67] and S[68] regions appear able to elicit protective immune responses.

The Viral Core

The virion core or nucleocapsid (Figs. 2B and 3) bears the HBcAg and is found in the blood only as an internal component of virions; no free HBcAg has been detected in serum. Highly purified Dane particle cores and liver-derived HBcAg particles contain a single predominant polypeptide with an apparent weight of approximately 19,000 daltons[69,70] encoded by the viral C gene. The protein kinase activity in cores phosphorylates the major 19,000-dalton polypeptide of core particles but not other polypeptides.[46] Although the antigenic specificity of HBcAg from different sources has not been carefully compared, no antigenic heterogeneity or variation has been described.

Hepatitis B e Antigen

Hepatitis B e antigen (HBeAg), discovered in 1972, is physically and antigenically distinct from HBsAg and HBcAg.[71] It was found as a soluble antigen in serum often complexed with immunoglobulin.[72] HBeAg is contained in a 17,500-dalton cleavage product of the viral core structural polypeptide and is thus encoded by the same viral gene (C gene). HBeAg is released when virion cores are disrupted with detergents,[47,73–75] and the isolated major polypeptide of core particles (19,000 daltons) appears to react with anti-HBe.[47] Thus, the polypeptides of Dane particle cores manifest different antigenic specificities before (HBcAg) and after (HBeAg) detergent treatment.

There is a high correlation between the presence of the HBeAg in sera of HBV-infected patients and high concentrations of physical virions[76–79] and infectious HBV,[49,50] indicating that HBeAg and virions are produced together by hepatocytes during infection.

The Viral DNA

Hepatitis B virions contain small, circular DNA molecules[42] that are partially double-stranded (schematically illustrated in Fig. 4). The single-stranded portion varies in length from approximately 15 to 60 percent of the circle length in different molecules.[80–82] The DNA polymerase activity in the virion repairs the single-stranded region in the viral DNA to make fully double-stranded molecules of approximately 3200 base pairs. DNA synthesis is initiated for this reaction at the 3′ end of the short strand. DNA synthesis is terminated when the uniquely located 5′ end of the short strand is reached. The long strand is not a closed circle, but a nick exists at a unique site approximately 300 bp from the 5′ end of the short strand.[80,83,84] A polypeptide is covalently attached to the 5′ end of the long strand of the DNA isolated from virions.[43] This protein appears to function as a primer for synthesis of the viral minus DNA strand during DNA replication.[85] This DNA structure is shared by the other hepadna viruses and is unique to this virus family.

HBV DNA has been cloned in bacterial cells, and the complete nucleotide sequence has been determined.[85–87] Four open reading frames have been identified in the complete or long DNA strand, which is therefore the minus strand (by convention a viral DNA plus strand has the same nucleotide sequence as the viral messenger RNA, and the minus strand is complementary to messenger RNA). Open reading frame S (Fig. 4) contains the nucleotide sequence specifying the major surface antigen reactive polypeptide. Open reading frame C (Fig. 4) contains the nucleotide sequence that specifies the major polypeptide of the virion core (HBcAg) and of HBeAg. The largest open reading frame (P), which overlaps the S gene, appears to encode the viral DNA polymerase. The smallest open reading frame (X) encodes a protein that can transactivate some heterologous viral and cell transcriptional control sequences, but its role in HBV replication is unclear.

VIRUS REPLICATION

The earliest studies of HBV in infected hepatocytes revealed that HBcAg could be detected only in nuclei of hepatocytes by immunofluorescent staining, and HBsAg in cytoplasm and on cell surfaces.[88–90] Consistent with this, electron microscopy demonstrated particles with the appearance of virion cores exclusively in hepatocyte nuclei.[91–93] During persistent infection, a variable number of cells contain detectable viral antigens by immunofluorescent staining (from less than 1 percent to virtually all hepatocytes in different patients).[88–90] Interestingly, the pattern of viral antigen expression appears to be different in different cells of the same chronically infected liver. Commonly, most positive cells stain only for HBsAg, fewer cells have only detectable HBcAg, and even fewer ones contain both HBsAg and HBcAg. In the liver of some chronic carriers, HBsAg is the only detectable viral antigen. In all chronic carriers producing relatively high concentrations of viral DNA and DNA polymerase containing virions, significant numbers of HBcAg-positive cells can be found. The different patterns of viral antigen synthesis in individual cells of the same chronically infected liver indicate that individual viral genes are expressed differently in different cells.

Studies of DHBV-infected duck liver[94,95] and HBV-infected human liver[96,97] indicate that hepadna virus DNA replication involves a reverse transcriptase step that is unique for DNA viruses. Hepadna viruses and cauliflower mosaic virus are the only DNA viruses known to use a reverse transcriptase (RNA copied into DNA) step in their replication, a mechanism previously known only for RNA tumor viruses or retroviruses. This replication mechanism and the nucleotide sequence homology between HBV and retroviruses[98] indicate a phylogenetic relationship between these two virus families. In addition to episomal replicating viral DNA forms, viral DNA sequences integrated into cellular DNA are present in at least some HBV-infected livers[97,99] and HBsAg, but apparently no other viral genes may be expressed by such integrated viral sequences.

TISSUE TROPISM

For some time, hepatocytes were considered to be the only cell type infected by HBV,[100–102] and permanent eradication of HBV infection after liver transplantation in one case[103] was taken as evidence that the liver was the only site of infection in that case. However, high concentrations of HBsAg found in the pancreatic juice of some patients[104] raised the question of whether HBV may occasionally also infect pancreatic cells. HBsAg and HBcAg have been detected by immunofluorescent staining in pancreatic cells in 18 and 6, respectively, of 30 HBV-infected human cases and not in uninfected controls.[105] High concentrations of DHBV DNA have been detected in the pan-

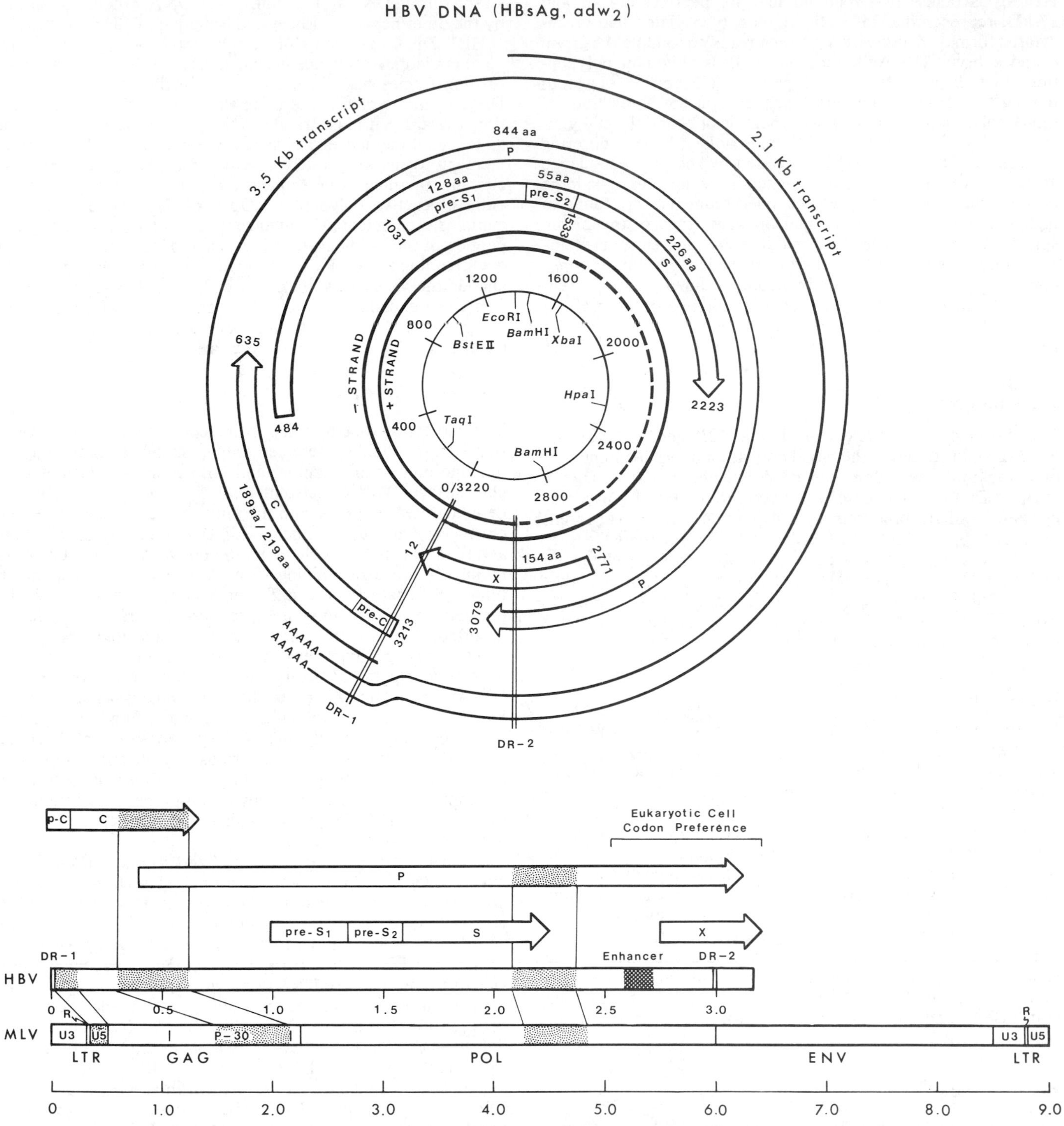

FIG. 4. Physical and genetic map of HBV DNA. The broken line in the + DNA strand represents the region in which the 3′ end of this strand may occur in different molecules, and the corresponding region of the − strand is that which may be single-stranded in different molecules. Regions of sequence homology with a murine retrovirus are indicated by the shaded areas.

creas of infected Peking ducks,[35] suggesting that the pancreas of that species may be infected by another hepadna virus closely related to HBV. HBV DNA has also been found in some circulating leukocytes.[106,107] Thus, some pancreatic cells and leukocytes may become infected and support limited HBV replication, but the liver is most regularly and extensively infected and hepatocytes are the most permissive cell for HBV.

VIRUS HOST RANGE

HBV has a narrow host range that is probably restricted to humans and some other primates. Tests for HBsAg in the sera of captive nonhuman primates have revealed infection in chimpanzees,[108–111] gibbons,[109,110] orangutans,[111] African green monkeys,[108,111] and squirrel monkeys.[108,111] Testing for anti-

HBs has revealed evidence of past infection in the same species,[111,112] as well as in baboons, Celebes, apes, macaques, and some other Old World and some New World monkeys.[111] Only negative tests have been found in numerous other primate species. These studies do not indicate clearly whether HBV infection occurred in any of the nonhuman primates in their natural habitat or whether the virus was always acquired in captivity by exposure to humans. It seems likely that natural infection with HBV or a cross-reactive virus analogous to woodchuck hepatitis virus (WHV) and ground squirrel hepatitis virus (GSHV) may occur at least in some of these species.

HBV has also been experimentally transmitted to chimpanzees,[88–113,114] which are highly susceptible and demonstrate patterns of infection like those in humans (see the next section), except for less severe liver disease. Experimental infection has also been reported in gibbons,[115] African green monkeys,[116] rhesus monkeys,[117] and woolly monkeys.[118] The latter three species appear to be much more resistant to infection than chimpanzees and humans, because much higher virus doses are required, infection is irregular and very transient when it occurs, and little or no liver disease is seen. For these reasons, these monkeys are unsuitable as animal models for HBV infection and for infectivity titrations. No successful infections of subprimate species have been reported.

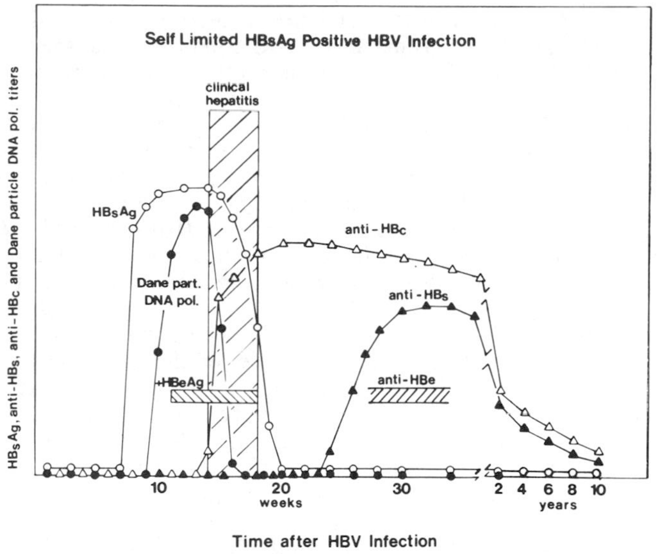

FIG. 5. Schematic representation of viral markers in the blood throughout the course of self-limited, HBsAg-positive primary HBV infection.

COURSE OF THE VIRUS INFECTION

Studies of natural HBV infections in humans and experimental infections in humans and chimpanzees have defined several patterns of infection with this virus. Most primary infections in adults are self-limited and resolve completely within 6 months of onset. Most infections also appear to be subclinical and are detected only by serologic testing and other methods. A fraction of infections fail to resolve, become persistent, and may continue for many years. A unique feature of infections with HBV is the presence of viral forms continuously in the blood during active infection in almost all patients. These forms are most commonly detected by their antigenicity (e.g., HBsAg). Tests for HBsAg essentially detect the incomplete viral forms described above (22-nm particles and filaments), which greatly outnumber complete virions in most patients. Although most persistently infected patients appear to have complete infectious virus in the blood as well as incomplete viral forms, some such patients appear to have no infectious virus. The presence of viral forms in the blood that can be detected by serologic testing and other methods and the immune responses to the viral antigens offer markers that can be used to follow the course of HBV infections. Several patterns of infection that define the spectrum of responses to this virus will be described here in detail.

Self-Limited HBsAg-Positive Primary Infection

This pattern, in which HBsAg can be detected transiently in the blood, is the most common pattern of primary HBV infection in adults. HBsAg is usually the first viral marker to appear in the blood after HBV infection (Fig. 5). The presence of this antigen is considered to be synonymous with active infection. HBsAg can be detected as early as 1[119] or 2[120] weeks and as late as 11 or 12 weeks[120] after exposure to HBV when very sensitive assays are used. Evidence of hepatitis was found to follow the appearance of HBsAg by an average of 4 weeks (usual range, 1–7 weeks)[121] and after at least 3–6 weeks[120] in different studies. In self-limited infections, HBsAg was found to remain detectable by complement fixation in the blood for 1–6 weeks in most patients,[121] although it may persist for up to 20 weeks.[120] Patients who remain HBsAg positive for less than 7 weeks rarely appear to develop symptomatic hepatitis.[120] The severity of hepatitis, as measured by bilirubin elevation has been roughly correlated with the duration of HBsAg positivity in patients with self-limited experimental infections.[120] As symptoms and jaundice clear, the HBsAg titer usually falls and HBsAg becomes undetectable in most symptomatic patients several weeks after resolution of hepatitis. However, in experimental transmission studies, 9 percent of patients had become HBsAg negative even before the onset of symptoms, and 28 percent were negative by the time symptoms had resolved.[120]

HBeAg is another regular and early marker of HBV infection, as depicted in Figure 5. Highly sensitive assays such as passive hemagglutination[122,123] and radioimmunoassay (RIA)[124–127] have demonstrated that HBeAg appears simultaneously or within a few days of the appearance of HBsAg in all or almost all primary infections, and its titer peaks and then declines in parallel with that of HBsAg. The prevalence of HBeAg declines constantly over the first 10 weeks after the onset of symptoms.[127] It usually disappears just before the disappearance of HBsAg in self-limited infections. Patients who remain HBeAg positive for 10 weeks or longer appear likely to become persistently infected.[126] Anti-HBe appears in most patients at the time HBeAg becomes undetectable or shortly thereafter. Anti-HBe persists for 1–2 years after resolution of HBV infection.[119]

The third viral marker in order of appearance is DNA and DNA polymerase-containing virions. These particles, detected by their DNA polymerase activity or by hybridization for viral DNA, appear in the blood of most patients soon after the appearance of HBsAg, rise to high concentrations during the late incubation period of hepatitis B, and fall with the onset of hepatic disease,[128,129] as shown in Figure 5.

A fourth marker of infection, which appears in virtually all patients and before the onset of hepatic injury in most, is anti-HBc, the antibody directed against the internal antigen of virions. Anti-HBc can usually be detected 3–5 weeks after the appearance of HBsAg in the blood and before the onset of clinically apparent hepatitis,[119,120,129] as shown in Figure 5. Anti-HBc titers usually rise during the period of HBsAg positivity, level off, and eventually fall after HBsAg becomes undetectable. The highest titers of anti-HBc appear in the patients with the longest period of HBsAg positivity.[129] Anti-HBc titers fall three- to fourfold in the first year after acute infection and then drop more slowly.[130] Anti-HBc can still be detected by immunoelectroosmophoresis 5–6 years after acute infection in most patients.[119,130] The high correlation between the prevalence of anti-HBc detected by immunoelectroosmophoresis[131] or RIA[120] and anti-HBs detected by RIA indicates that the two antibodies persist for a similar time after acute self-limited infections.

Although most of the anti-HBc activity is in the IgG class, IgM anti-HBc has been found in almost all patients with acute hepatitis B.[132–135] Using a sensitive enzyme-linked immunosorbent assay (ELISA) test, anti-HBc IgM was found to decline rapidly in titer after the disappearance of HBsAg in only 40 percent of cases with self-limited acute hepatitis B. In the remainder the decline was slow, with 20 percent of patients still positive after 2 years.[136]

Antibody to HBsAg (anti-HBs) has been shown to appear during antigenemia and before the onset of clinically apparent hepatitis in the 10–20 percent of patients who develop arthritis and rash associated with immune complex formation.[136] HBsAg–anti-HBs complexes have also been detected in a significant fraction of acute hepatitis B cases without well-recognized immune complex disease.[137–139] In most patients with self-limited HBV infection, however, anti-HBs can be detected only after HBsAg disappears from the blood,[17,119–121,129,140] as illustrated in Figure 5. Anti-HBs cannot be detected even by the most sensitive tests in many patients immediately after HBsAg disappears. There is a time interval of up to several months between the disappearance of detectable HBsAg and the appearance of anti-HBs in approximately one-half of the patients with self-limited infections.[120,129] In approximately 10 percent of the patients with transient antigenemia, anti-HBs never appears when tested for by the most sensitive assays.[120] In patients with measurable anti-HBs responses, the antibody titer rises slowly during recovery and may still be rising 6–12 months after the disappearance of HBsAg.[120,121] In contrast to the anti-HBc response, the highest titers of anti-HBs appear in those patients with the shortest period of antigenemia.[120] This antibody may persist for years after HBV infection and is associated with protection against reinfection.[17,141–143]

In contrast to the extensive studies of viral markers in the blood early in the course of primary HBV infection, only a few investigators have examined the state of virus in liver cells at this early time. During the late incubation period and early in the acute disease, almost all hepatocytes have been reported to be positive by immunofluorescent staining for HBsAg and HBcAg.[88–90] During acute hepatitis B, the state of viral DNA in liver has not been adequately studied, although evidence for integrated viral DNA has been reported for two patients.[144] However, the forms of virus in blood and antigen expression in liver suggest that almost all hepatocytes are replicating complete virions during the early stages of primary infection.

Self-Limited Primary Infections without Detectable Serum HBsAg

A significant fraction of patients with evidence of acute, self-limited primary HBV infection apparently never have detectable HBsAg in the blood. Anti-HBs usually appears 4–12 weeks after exposure to HBV (at about the time HBsAg appears in patients with detectable antigen), and the titer typically rises rapidly to high levels and is sustained,[120] as depicted in Figure 6. An anti-HBc response is also detected, but the antibody usually appears only in low titer and may not persist as long as it does in patients manifesting antigenemia.[120] IgM anti-HBc is probably found regularly in these patients, since it was detected in each of 31 patients with apparent acute hepatitis B who were HBsAg negative from the time of their admission to the hospital.[135] Although some of the patients in this study may have been HBsAg positive before testing began, others undoubtedly represented HBsAg-negative primary infections. Infections associated with a primary antibody response without detectable HBsAg in the blood are usually accompanied by asymptomatic disease with only minor elevations in serum transaminase activity.[129,141,145] Although the patterns of anti-HBs and anti-HBc response differ in order and relative magnitude compared with the responses of patients with detectable antigenemia, the fact that both antibodies (including IgM anti-HBc) and liver function abnormalities appear after a length of time consistent with the incubation period of HBV infection indicates that actual infection with HBV has taken place. DNA polymerase-containing virions and HBeAg have not been studied in such cases. No studies have been done to assess the state of virus in liver cells during infection of this kind.

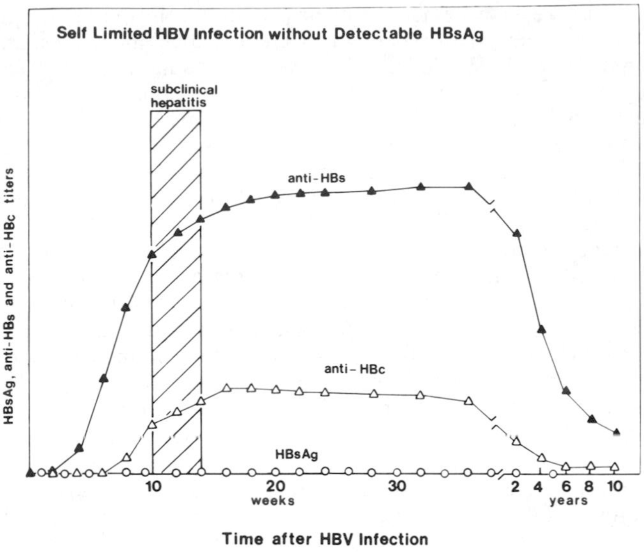

FIG. 6. Schematic representation of the serologic response throughout the course of HBsAg-negative primary HBV infection.

In a large series of adult patients experimentally infected with HBV, 70 percent had self-limited infection with transient HBsAg positivity and 23 percent had no detectable antigenemia but primary anti-HBs and anti-HBc responses.[120] The frequency of each response after natural infections would probably depend on the dose of infecting virus and other factors that might differ for different populations.

HBsAg-Positive Persistent HBV Infection

Patients who remain HBsAg positive for 20 weeks or longer after primary infection are very likely to remain positive indefinitely and can be designated *chronic HBsAg carriers* (Fig. 7). Virions (Dane particles) can be detected by electron microscopy,[146] DNA polymerase activity,[147,148] HBcAg,[149] or virion DNA[150] in the blood of a significant fraction of persistently infected patients positive for HBsAg. By a sensitive assay for virion DNA polymerase, approximately 50 percent of persistently infected patients tested positive and 5–10 percent had very high levels.[147] All patients with detectable virion DNA polymerase in the blood have HBcAg detected by immunofluorescence in liver biopsies,[148] and when a highly sensitive assay for virions is used, all patients with HBcAg in liver have been found to have detectable virions in serum.[150]

Almost all persistently infected patients have high titers of anti-HBc in the blood,[120] as shown in Figure 7. The titers of this antibody are significantly higher during persistent infection than during most self-limited infections or in convalescence.[120] Interestingly, although most of the anti-HBc is undoubtedly in the IgG fraction, IgM anti-HBc continues to be made and can be detected indefinitely in the serum of most persistently infected patients.[135,151]

As described above, HBeAg can be detected in the serum of almost all patients early in primary HBV infection, and anti-

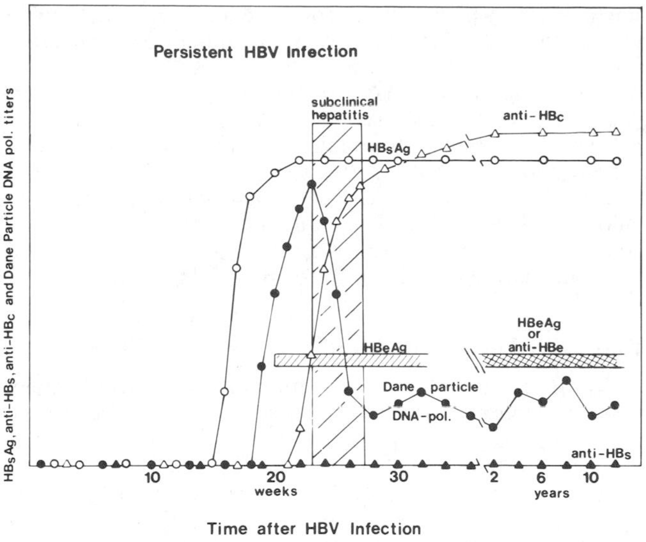

FIG. 7. Schematic representation of viral markers in the blood throughout the course of HBV infection that becomes persisent.

HBe appears in almost all of them during resolution of the infection. In persistent infection, on the other hand, sensitive assays such as RIA or passive hemagglutination have detected HBeAg in one-fourth to one-half of patients and anti-HBe in almost all of the remainder.[122,152] When less sensitive assays are used, neither marker may be detected in 50 percent or more of persistently infected patients.[153–156] The observation that the high molecular weight form of HBeAg in serum represents a complex between HBeAg and immunoglobulin[157,158] suggests that the anti-HBe may be produced by many or all HBeAg-positive patients, but is present exclusively as a complex with HBeAg, so that no free antibody can be detected. There is a very high correlation between the presence in serum of HBeAg and virions detected by electron microscopy[76] or by their DNA polymerase activity.[76–79,159]

There is a wide range of HBsAg titers in persistently infected patients. In general, those with the highest titers of infectious virus[141,145] and detectable virion DNA polymerase activity[160] and/or HBeAg[160–162] have the highest HBsAg titers.

The most sensitive assay for complete virions is undoubtedly infectivity titrations by inoculation into susceptible hosts such as humans or chimpanzees, because, as described above, infectious HBV can be demonstrated in some sera after dilution by as much as 10^{-8}.[49,50] Although most HBsAg carriers have high titers of infectious HBV in serum, some carriers appear to have no detectable infectious virus. The highest titers are found in patients with detectable HBeAg[49,50] and/or virion DNA polymerase activity[49] in serum, and those without these markers[50] or with anti-HBe have much lower titers. Recently, undiluted sera from six HBsAg carriers without detectable virion DNA polymerase or HBeAg failed to infect chimpanzees.[49] This was a direct demonstration that some persistently infected patients who continue to produce HBsAg do not produce detectable amounts of infectious HBV, and these would appear to be HBsAg carriers without detectable virion DNA polymerase or HBeAg. The fraction of HBsAg carriers who have no detectable infectious virus is not known. Patients with detectable virion DNA polymerase and HBeAg in their serum, but not those without them, appear to be highly contagious,[77,161,163] in agreement with the data on titers of infectious HBV in the blood. A few HBsAg carriers with HBeAg, and with DNA and DNA polymerase containing virions in the blood, have been shown to have free replicating forms of viral DNA (closed and relaxed circular and linear double-stranded, single-stranded, and DNA–RNA hybrids) and probably integrated viral DNA in the liver,[97,99,144,164] providing biochemical evidence that complete virus replication is proceeding in at least some cells. A variable number of liver cells in such patients appear to contain HBsAg and/or HBcAg by immunofluorescent staining. Such patients frequently but not always have chronic persistent or chronic active hepatitis.[159,165,166]

Investigation of a few HBsAg carriers with no detectable DNA and DNA polymerase containing virions or HBeAg in the blood has revealed evidence of integrated viral DNA sequences but no detectable free viral DNA forms or HBcAg in liver cells.[97,99,144,164] As described above, not all cells (and frequently only a small fraction of cells) are HBsAg positive by immunofluorescent staining. These findings and the infectivity studies cited above indicate that these patients are replicating complete virus at a very low level or not at all, and the only viral gene expressed appears to be the HBsAg gene in an integrated state. Many but not all of these patients appear to have little or no liver disease[89,158,185] and are considered to be healthy carriers.

Anti-HBs has been regularly detected as a complex with HBsAg in the serum of patients with certain extrahepatic disease syndromes such as HBV-associated polyarteritis nodosa and membranous glomerulous nephritis.[136] In addition, there is evidence for HBsAg–anti-HBs complexes in the serum of a significant fraction of persistently infected patients with chronic liver disease and in some healthy carriers,[137–139] indicating that in at least some patients, anti-HBs is made in the face of ongoing persistent infection and without significant associated disease. Standard assays for anti-HBs rarely detect this antibody in persistently infected subjects because of the great antigen excess in their serum. It is not known whether the anti-HBs response in these cases is quantitatively diminished; however, the frequent presence of this antibody, anti-HBc, and anti-HBe during persistent HBV infection would suggest that complete immunologic tolerance to these respective viral antigens does not account for the persistence of the infection.

Although the long-term natural history of persistent HBV infection is not completely defined, prolonged infection (e.g., for many years) appears to be the rule for most chronic carriers, and HBsAg positivity lasting for as long as 20 years has been documented.[166] The titers of HBsAg and virion DNA polymerase levels have been shown to be relatively stable over a period of weeks or even a few months,[148] but increasing evidence suggests that persistent HBV infections tend to decrease spontaneously over a period of many months to years, with HBsAg titers slowly falling and virion DNA polymerase and HBeAg titers falling below the level of detection with time. In one prospective study of persistently infected patients with significant levels of virion DNA polymerase activity in their sera, virion DNA polymerase levels spontaneously fell to below the level of detection in approximately 10 percent of patients per year, and a similar rate of disappearance of serum HBeAg was observed.[148] In a different group of patients with HBeAg, this antigen disappeared from the serum in 45 percent over a 2- to 7-year period.[167] Similar spontaneous disappearance of HBeAg and/or virion DNA polymerase activity has been shown in many other cases.[79,165,167–170] Anti-HBe can eventually be detected in most patients after they become HBeAg negative. In HBsAg carriers without virion DNA polymerase activity or HBeAg in serum, these markers have infrequently been observed to reappear spontaneously.[171,172] Although the time after the onset of infection when HBeAg and virion levels fall to below the level of detection appears to vary greatly in different individuals, and although these markers may remain detectable in persistently infected patients for years, the duration of infection is clearly an important factor that is strongly correlated with the presence of detectable HBeAg and virions. Spontaneous clearance of all viral markers of active HBV infection, although unusual, can occur at any time. HBsAg became undetectable at a rate of approximately 2 percent per year, using data combined from three different studies, including a total of 800 HBsAg-positive blood donors, most of whom were undoubtedly chronic carriers, and with individual follow-ups ranging from 2 to 44 months.[173–175] In another study of persistently infected patients, most of whom had chronic hepatitis, HBsAg became undetectable in 1.5 percent over a 10-month period.[160] Spontaneous disappearance of HBsAg in persistently infected patients has been observed in numerous other cases.[79,165,176] A number of factors that appear to influence the incidence of persistent infection, such as age, sex, immunologic status, and possibly race, may also influence rates of spontaneous remission, but preliminary evidence suggesting that persistent infections in females resolve at a faster rate than in males[177] is the only evidence bearing on these factors.

HBsAg-Negative Persistent HBV Infection

There is good evidence that some patients with persistent HBV infection do not have detectable HBsAg in their serum. Hoofnagle et al.[120] described a patient with persistent HBV infection with a high anti-HBc titer and an HBsAg titer that fluctuated just above and below the level of detection by RIA, so that at certain times the patient's serum was HBsAg negative by the most sensitive tests, although active infection apparently continued. A small but significant fraction of blood donors whose sera are HBsAg negative by the most sensitive tests transmit HBV infection to recipients of their blood.[178–180] Although some of these donors could be in the incubation period of hepatitis B before the appearance of detectable HBsAg, they probably are persistently infected, with HBsAg levels below the level of detection, because they have high titers of anti-HBc. Finally, cases of chronic hepatitis without detectable HBsAg have been ascribed to active HBV infection because of persistent high titers of anti-HBc.[181]

Exogenous Factors That May Alter the Course of Persistent HBV Infection

Corticosteroid therapy appears to regularly alter the course of persistent HBV infection. Initiation of approximately 20–30 mg prednisone per day has been shown to be rapidly and regularly followed by a rise in virion DNA polymerase activity and HBsAg titer in blood.[181] Occasional HBsAg-negative patients with anti-HBc[182] or anti-HBs[183] have been shown to become positive during immunosuppressive therapy. This suggests the possibility that HBV may be present in a latent state in some patients and that virus replication can be activated in such patients by immunosuppression. Withdrawal of the corticosteroid is usually associated with a fall in HBsAg titer and virion DNA polymerase level, the latter sometimes to below the level of detection.[184] The mechanism of the effects observed with corticosteroids is not understood, but suppression of the immune response may be involved. Corticosteroids, on the other hand, appear to have a direct stimulatory effect on the replication of some viruses,[185] independently of their effects on the immune system.

Certain antiviral agents, such as interferons and adenine arabinoside, have been shown to inhibit HBV replication in all persistently infected patients.[148,149,186,187] Experimental treatment with either antiviral agent or with the two together has been accompanied by a rapid reduction in the level of virions in the serum of all patients and a much more gradual reduction in HBsAg titers in only some patients, suggesting that these antiviral agents act primarily on a step involved in virion production and not on incomplete HBsAg particle production. In some patients the permanent disappearance of only virions and HBeAg, and in a few patients the disappearance of those markers as well as of HBsAg, have been observed (reviewed below under "Management of Hepatitis B"). Although these responses to antiviral treatment have been well documented, the frequency with which each response occurs can be determined only in carefully designed trials including placebo-treated controls.

Finally, several cases have been observed in which HBeAg and virion DNA polymerase levels have fallen to undetectable levels and HBsAg titers have fallen significantly in persistently infected patients during intercurrent infections with other agents such as hepatitis A virus (W. S. Robinson, unpublished results). Although these anecdotal cases are suggestive, more evidence is needed to establish a cause-and-effect relationship and to elucidate the mechanism for these observations.

PROTECTIVE IMMUNITY AGAINST HBV INFECTION

The presence of anti-HBs in the serum of convalescent patients appears to confer almost complete resistance to reinfection. The anti-HBs produced after primary HBV infection is primarily of anti-a specificity, although anti-d, anti-y, or another type-specific antibody appropriate to the subtype of the infecting virus may also appear.[188] Protection against reinfection with HBV of either the same or a different subtype has been shown,[141] suggesting that immunity is probably generally conferred by anti-a. In exceptional cases, however, a second infection with HBV in patients with anti-HBs has been reported,[189–191] and in some cases HBV of a different subtype infected an individual with an antibody of restricted (e.g., only subtype) specificity.[189] It has also been shown that chimpanzees can be reinfected when challenge doses are sufficiently large, even when the identical strain of HBV is used for the initial and challenge exposures.[141,192] Second infection with HBV overcoming immunity by either mechanism must be unusual, since individuals with multiple episodes of acute viral hepatitis have not been found to develop hepatitis B more than one time.[193–195]

Although evidence from primary immunization with purified HBsAg (after which anti-HBs but no anti-HBc appears)[142] and from passive immunization with high-titer anti-HBs[143] indicates that anti-HBs protects against reinfection, patients with anti-HBc and no detectable anti-HBs have also been shown to resist reinfection.[120] More recently, immunization of chimpanzees with HBcAg purified from infected liver[196] and HBcAg produced in bacterial cells transformed with a plasmid expression vector containing the HBcAg gene[197] led to protection against challenge with HBV. Anti-HBe also appears to be protective.[198] These results suggest a role of the immune response to HBcAg and HBeAg in protecting against HBV infection and raise the question of whether HBcAg as well as HBsAg could be used as a vaccine.

Cellular immune responses directed against HBsAg and HBcAg are described in the next section. The role of cellular immunity in resolution of HBV infection and protection against reinfection is undoubtedly important.

PATHOGENESIS OF DISEASES ASSOCIATED WITH HBV INFECTION

Acute and Chronic Hepatitis B

Acute and chronic hepatitis B represent syndromes of hepatocellular necrosis and inflammatory responses associated with HBV infection of hepatocytes. Primary HBV infection may be associated with little or no liver disease or with acute hepatitis varying in severity from mild to fulminant.[199] Persistent HBV infection is sometimes associated with a histologically normal or nearly normal liver and normal liver function, and sometimes with syndromes designated *chronic persistent hepatitis (CPH)* or *chronic active hepatitis (CAH)*.[199] CPH is not considered progressive, and CAH may be more severe and progress to cirrhosis. The mechanism of liver cell injury in hepatitis B has not been established, but there has been much conjecture about the role of the immune response (reviewed in Refs. 200 and

201). Several factors have been identified that appear to correlate with the severity of acute or chronic hepatitis B and that may provide clues to the pathogenesis. Among these is the infecting dose of virus, with high doses of HBV usually resulting in shorter incubation periods and more severe acute hepatitis than low doses.[48] A second factor appears to be age. Hepatitis B virus infections at very young ages are usually associated with very mild initial hepatitis.[202,203] Anecdotal cases suggest that HBV infections are associated with milder initial disease in immunologically impaired hosts than in immunologically healthy persons.[204,205] These observations raise the possibility that the immune response may influence the severity of acute hepatitis B.

During acute and chronic HBV infection, there is almost always a humoral immune response to HBcAg,[120] and frequently to HBsAg[137–139] and during chronic infection with HBeAg.[122,152,163] There is also evidence that humoral immunity to hepatic (host) antigens occurs in chronic hepatitis B (reviewed in Ref. 200). However, a role for the humoral immune response in hepatic injury would appear to be excluded by the observation that severe acute and chronic viral hepatitis can occur in the absence of an intact humoral immune response, such as in patients with agammaglobulinemia.[206]

Cellular immune responses directed against HBsAg and/or liver cell antigens in acute and chronic HBV infection have also been detected by numerous investigators (reviewed in Refs. 200 and 201). Specific cellular immune reactivity to HBsAg has been detected by leukocyte migration inhibition and lymphocyte transformation assays during acute hepatitis B, variably during chronic hepatitis B, and most strongly and regularly during recovery and early convalescence. Cellular sensitization to HBsAg by these assays is frequently undetectable or weak in HBsAg carriers without liver disease. No convincing evidence of lymphocyte cytotoxicity directed against cells bearing HBsAg has been reported, although optimum testing for such cytotoxic effector cell activity may not have been carried out.[207]

Cellular sensitization to host antigens in viral hepatitis has also been demonstrated by several investigators (reviewed in Ref. 201). Sensitization to a liver-specific hepatocyte surface membrane lipoprotein (liver-specific protein, or LSP) has been detected in approximately one-half of patients with acute hepatitis B, but is transient and has not been demonstrated after recovery.[208,209] Reactivity to the same antigen is also detectable in most patients with chronic active hepatitis (whether HBsAg positive or not). Suppressor T-cell activity is also depressed in the blood of patients with acute and chronic hepatitis B and returns to normal with recovery.[210]

Certain viral markers in the serum and liver of persistently infected patients appear to be present more often in the presence than in the absence of significant chronic hepatitis. HBeAg[153–159,211,212] and virion DNA polymerase activity[159] in serum, and HBcAg as well as HBsAg in the liver detected by immunofluorescent staining,[159] are often found in patients with CAH or CPH. There is little different between the prevalence of these markers, however, in CAH and CPH.[155–157, 159] In contrast, healthy carriers,[211–213] including those with little or no abnormality documented by liver biopsy,[159,214] appear most often to be HBeAg negative, virion DNA polymerase negative,[159] and frequently anti-HBe positive.[157,159,212–214] Further, liver biopsies reveal only HBsAg and no HBcAg by immunofluorescent staining.[89,90,159] These findings suggest that complete virus replication is more often proceeding in the liver cells of patients with chronic hepatitis B compared with those of carriers with little or no hepatitis, in whom most often the expression of only the HBsAg viral gene product can be detected. These findings raise the possibility that it is the cellular immune response directed at HBcAg or HBeAg rather than at HBsAg that is responsible for hepatic injury during HBV infection. Evidence for cytotoxicity of peripheral blood cells for autologous hepatocytes in chronic hepatitis B that is blocked by anti-HBc suggests that HBcAg may be the target antigen for cytotoxic T cells.[215,216]

The Hepatitis Delta Virus

A final mechanism for liver cell injury in some cases during HBV infection appears to be coinfection with a second cytopathic virus, the hepatitis delta (δ) virus (HDV). Delta antigen (HDAg) was discovered by immunofluorescent staining as a nuclear antigen distinct from HBsAg, HBcAg, and HBeAg in hepatocytes of some HBsAg carriers in Italy, the geographic area with the highest prevalence of HDAg.[217] Most patients with HDAg in liver have antibody to this antigen (anti-δ) in their sera. Surveys show a high prevalence of anti-δ in Italians residing in southern Italy[218] and in other Mediterranean populations,[219] and a particularly high prevalence in those living in North Africa.[220] Epidemics have been reported in parts of South America.[221] In the United States, the prevalence is low in the general population but high in some groups, such as intravenous drug users, and in polytransfused HBsAg carriers.[218] Although HDAg has not been found in HBsAg-negative patients, δ is found in low prevalence in polytransfused HBsAg-negative patients, but only in those with anti-HBs.

HDAg is contained in a 68,000-dalton protein encoded by the HDV genome, which is a small, single-stranded, circular RNA with features of viroids. Virions of HDV consist of a core of HDAg and RNA enclosed in an HBsAg-containing envelope.[222] Inoculation of HDV-containing sera into HBsAg carrier chimpanzees without hepatic HDAg resulted in the appearance of HDAg in the hepatocyte nuclei of these animals, the disappearance of HBcAg detected by immunofluorescent staining in liver, and a rise in serum alanine aminotransferase (ALT).[223] Thus HDV appears to be a defective virus; its replication requires coinfection with HBV; phenotypic mixing results in HDAg-containing particles with HBsAg-containing envelopes; and infection with the agent results in hepatic injury and suppression of HBV replication.

There is a higher incidence of HVD infection in HBsAg-positive patients with acute and chronic hepatitis compared with asymptomatic carriers.[218] Simultaneous infection with HBV and HDV may lead to severe or fulminant hepatitis more often than infection with HBV alone, and cases of fulminant hepatitis B positive for HDAg in populations with a high prevalence of δ agent have been observed.[221,224,225] In countries with a low prevalence of HDV infection, such as the United States[225] and Ireland,[226] HDAg appears to be present in only a small fraction of fulminant hepatitis B cases; thus, δ agent probably plays no role in most cases. HDV may play a more prominent role in chronic liver disease, especially in geographic areas where it is common, such as Italy, where 32 percent of HBsAg carriers with CAH and 52 percent of those with cirrhosis were found to be HDAg positive compared with HBsAg carriers with no liver disease, none of whom had detectable HDAg.[227,228] Exacerbations of hepatitis may occur in HBsAg carriers when they subsequently acquire HDV infection,[226,227] but how often this mechanism accounts for such exacerbations, and the precise impact of HDV on the severity of acute and chronic hepatitis B in the United States, remain to be determined. The mechanism of liver cell injury associated with HDV infection has not been studied.

Hepatocellular Carcinoma

A second disease associated with chronic HBV infection is hepatocellular carcinoma (HCC), and there is increasing evidence supporting an etiologic role for HBV. HCC has a worldwide distribution and, numerically, is one of the major cancers in the world today (reviewed in Ref. 27). Although HCC is rare in most parts of the world, it occurs commonly in sub-Saharan Africa, Southeast Asia, Japan, Oceania, Greece, and Italy. In certain areas of Asia and Africa, it is the most common cancer. Geographic areas with the highest incidence of HCC are also areas where hepatitis B virus infection is common and persistent HBV infections occur at the highest known frequencies. Within the limits of the available data, there appears to be a good correlation between the worldwide geographic distribution of HCC and active HBV infection, with the highest frequency of both occurring in sub-Saharan Africa and Southeast Asia.[27] In addition, active HBV infection occurs significantly more frequently in patients with HCC than in controls in both high- and low-HCC geographic areas.[27] A recent prospective study of HBsAg-positive and HBsAg-negative middle-aged men in Taiwan revealed an incidence of HCC over 300 times higher in the HBsAg-positive group than in the HBsAg-negative group.[229] Similar results have been obtained in Japan.[230]

The high incidence of persistent HBV infection in mothers of HCC patients, in contrast to that in fathers,[231] suggests that transmission from mothers to newborn or infant children may be a frequent mode and time of HBV infection in HCC patients. The finding of low serum HBsAg titers and absence of HBeAg, together with the rare occurrence of hepatic HBcAg in most HCC patients,[27,232] also suggest that the persistent infections in HCC patients are of long duration. If HBV infection does occur frequently at very early ages in HCC patients in high-HCC areas, the age distribution of patients with clinically recognized tumors would suggest that these tumors appear after a mean duration of approximately 35 years of HBV infection.[233] Very few cases of HCC occur in children.[233] Between 60 and 90 percent of HCC patients have coexisting cirrhosis,[229,233–236] suggesting that this lesion, in association with persistent HBV infection, may predispose a person to HCC, although clearly cirrhosis need not be present.

Hepatitis B virus infection in humans is not the only hepadna virus infection associated with HCC. In fact, a much higher incidence of HCC formation occurs in WHV-infected woodchucks[33,237] and GSHV-infected ground squirrels than in humans with HBV.

Immunofluorescent and immunoperoxidase staining of tumor tissue have demonstrated that in patients with HBsAg in the blood and in whom nontumorous liver cells are positive for HBsAg and/or HBcAg, tumor cells appear most often to be negative, although some studies have reported small numbers of HBsAg-positive cells in tumors (reviewed in Ref. 236). HBcAg has been detected even more rarely. HBV DNA integrations in a clonal pattern have been found in tumor DNA in 85–90 percent of HCC, and the cellular DNA site of viral integrations is different in each HCC.[238] At this time, there is no demonstrated difference between the state of integrated viral DNA in HCC and infected, nontumorous liver. The specific role of these viruses in HCC formation at the molecular level is not clear.

Extrahepatic Disease

Several additional syndromes with extrahepatic manifestations have been associated with HBV infection, and for some there is evidence that HBsAg–anti-HBs complexes play a role in pathogenesis (reviewed in Refs. 136 and 239). The serum sickness-like syndrome, consisting of fever, rash, urticaria, arthralgias, and sometimes acute arthritis, which occurs in 10–20 percent of patients during the incubation period of acute hepatitis B, is accompanied by HBsAg–antibody complexes and low levels of complement components in serum, synovial fluid, and synovial membranes from involved joints.[240,241]

In several series, one-third to one-half of patients with biopsy-proven polyarteritis nodosa have had persistent HBV infection (reviewed in Refs. 136 and 239). Among all HBsAg carriers, however, this syndrome occurs infrequently (1 out of 43 cases in one series).[242] Such patients have low serum complement levels and circulating HBsAg–anti-HBs complexes. Immune complexes and complement components have also been regularly detected in diseased vessels by immunofluorescent staining.[243,244]

A significant number of cases of membranous glomerulonephritis have been associated with chronic active hepatitis and persistent HBV infection (reviewed in Refs. 136 and 239). Immune complex deposits can be found along the subepithelial surfaces of glomerular basement membranes by electron microscopy, and nodular deposits of HBsAg, immune globulin, and C_3 in glomeruli have been observed by immunofluorescent staining in these cases.[245–249]

Several additional syndromes with unknown pathogenesis have also been associated with HBV infection. Infantile papular acrodermatitis appears to be frequently associated with persistent HBV infection in Mediterranean countries[250] and Japan.[251] In a series of 19 patients with essential mixed cryoglobulinemia, cryoprecipitates were shown to contain HBsAg in 6 cases and anti-HBs in 11,[252] suggesting that some cases of cryoglobulinemia may be related to HBV infection. This association, however, could not be confirmed in a subsequent study.[253] A significant number of cases of aplastic anemia have been observed after acute viral hepatitis.[254] Although in most cases the specific hepatitis virus has not been identified, in a few cases acute hepatitis B has been documented.[255,256] The basis of this apparent association is not yet clear. Further work is needed to clarify the pathogenesis of these syndromes and to determine whether HBsAg–antibody complexes or HBV infection in some other way plays an important role.

Clearly, infections with HBV and other hepadna viruses have protean manifestations, and different distinct pathogenetic mechanisms appear to be responsible for a number of different disease syndromes.

EPIDEMIOLOGY

Incidence of Primary HBV Infection

The Centers for Disease Control[257] has estimated that there are approximately 200,000 primary HBV infections per year in the United States. Most are in young adults, and approximately one-fourth are associated with acute icteric disease. More than 10,000 persons are hospitalized with hepatitis B each year, and 250 die with fulminant hepatitis B. Between 6 and 10 percent fail to resolve the infection and become persistently infected (chronic HBsAg carriers). The lifetime risk of HBV infection is estimated to be 5 percent for the whole U.S. population, but for certain high-risk groups it may reach nearly 100 percent.

Most acute hepatitis B cases in the United States, as previously mentioned, are in young adults, unlike the younger age distribution of hepatitis A.[177] The age distribution is related to the circumstances leading to transmission (see below). More cases occur in men than in women,[177] unlike hepatitis A, for which there is no apparent sex difference in incidence. The incidence of acute hepatitis B differs in different populations in the United States[257] (Table 1). Percutaneous drug users; patients receiving blood transfusions or other blood products and those requiring hemodialysis; laboratory personnel who work with human blood, serum, and blood products; homosexuals and others with frequent and different sexual contacts; and medical and dental personnel with frequent blood contacts are at greatest risk. Blood donor screening for HBsAg by the most sensitive tests, and a shift away from paid blood donors and the use of volunteer donors, greatly reduced but did not completely eliminate post-transfusion hepatitis B during the 1970s.[29,178–180,258] Recent studies of post-transfusion hepatitis indicate that 5–10 percent of cases are still hepatitis B. Most of these occur after transfusion of blood negative for HBsAg by the most sensitive tests available, indicating that this test does not detect every individual with infectious HBV in the blood.

TABLE 1. Prevalence of Serologic Markers of HBV Infection in Different Population Groups in the United States (Grouped According to Risk of Infection)

	Prevalence of Serologic Markers of HBV Infection	
	HBsAg (%)	*All Markers[a] (%)*
High risk		
Immigrants/refugees from areas of high HBV endemicity	13	70–85
Clients in institutions for the mentally retarded	10–20	35–80
Users of illicit parenteral drugs	7	60–80
Homosexually active males	6	35–80
Household contacts of HBV carriers	3–6	30–60
Patients of hemodialysis units	3–10	20–80
Intermediate risk		
Prisoners (male)	1–8	10–80
Staff of institutions for the mentally retarded	1	10–25
Health care workers, frequent blood contact	1–2	15–30
Low risk		
Health care workers, infrequent blood contact or none	0.3	3–10
Healthy adults (first-time volunteer blood donors)	0.3	35

[a] All markers include HBsAg, anti-HBs, and anti-HBc.
(Data from the Centers for Disease Control.[257])

The prevalence of serum antibody to HBsAg (anti-HBs), indicating past HBV infection (or, in recent years, vaccination) by the most sensitive techniques, has been shown to increase with age in the general U.S. population up to about ages 30–45, above which approximately 5–20 percent of people are positive in most studies.[177,259] The prevalence of serum anti-HBs also differs significantly in different U.S. populations, and the same groups described above that are at increased risk of acute hepatitis B have the highest prevalence of serum anti-HBs (see Table 1). Different socioeconomic groups also have different risks for infection. Cherubin et al.[260] found the frequency of anti-HBs to be 44, 18, and 10 percent for people over age 30 in New York City sections of Harlem, Staten Island, and Park Avenue, respectively.

Primary HBV infections occur at much higher frequencies, and at much earlier ages, in high-prevalence geographic areas of the world such as parts of Asia and Africa.[177] This is undoubtedly because the important routes of transmission (see below under "Routes of Transmission") are different than in the United States and most often appear to involve transmission from infected mothers to their children. In countries such as Senegal, Thailand, and Taiwan, infection rates are very high in infants and continue through early childhood, when the prevalence of HBsAg in serum may exceed 25 percent (reviewed in Ref. 177). In Panama, New Guinea, the Solomon Islands, Greenland, and the Alaskan Indians, infection rates in infants are relatively low and increase rapidly during early childhood (reviewed in Ref. 177). In all these populations, the prevalence of serum anti-HBs reaches a plateau, usually well above 50 percent, between ages 10 and 19 years.[177]

Although clinically apparent acute viral hepatitis, often severe, was the first manifestation of primary HBV infection to be recognized, it is now clear that this is probably not the most common response to infection, except possibly when infection involves iatrogenic routes of transmission to susceptible adults, such as by blood transfusion or other direct percutaneous transfer of virus-containing serum. In geographic areas of the world with very high infection rates at early ages and where routes of transmission that do not involve overt percutaneous transfer are the rule, primary infections most often appear to be clinically silent or mild, as is the persistent infection that appears to be a common outcome of primary infection in that setting. Similarly, the natural infections of woodchucks, ground squirrels, and ducks by the respective hepadna viruses that are related to HBV appear to be silent until late forms of disease (e.g., HCC) appear in some animals. Thus, much of the severe acute viral hepatitis that was first associated with primary HBV infection appears to be a manifestation of medical procedures and other practices (e.g., blood transfusions and illicit parenteral drug abuse) peculiar to technologically advanced cultures.

Persistent HBV Infections

Persistent or chronic HBV infection (usually designated the *HBsAg carrier state*) is one of the most common persistent viral infections in humans. It has been estimated that more than 170 million people in the world today are persistently infected with HBV.[27] A large fraction of them are found in East Asia and sub-Saharan Africa, where the prevalence of chronic infection is very high and the associated chronic liver disease and liver cancer are among the most important health problems. It is estimated that there are 400,000 to 800,000 chronic carriers in the United States and that as many as 25 percent of these may have chronic active hepatitis.[257] As many as 4000 persons per year may die from hepatitis B-related cirrhosis and 800 from liver cancer. Although a small number of long-established chronic carriers apparently terminate their active infection and become HBsAg negative (approximately 2 percent per year),[148,173–175] most chronic carriers remain infected for many years,[166] and infection for life appears to be common.

The HBsAg carrier rate varies from 0.1 to 20 percent in different populations.[27] The incidence of the HBsAg carrier state in various populations is related most importantly to the incidence and age of primary infection. However, there are also other host and viral factors that appear to increase the risk of developing persistent infection, and these may be important in establishing carrier rates for some epidemiologic groups. A genetic predisposition for persistent infection has been suggested by family studies in which the chronic carrier state appears to cluster in families, with a distribution consistent with possible segregation as an autosomal recessive trait.[261,262] An association between persistent infection and certain HLA types has also been reported.[263] Other studies, however, have failed to confirm either of these findings.[264,265] Some evidence suggests that after primary HBV infection, New York City residents of Chinese origin are more likely to become carriers than whites.[266] Whether this represents a genetic predisposition for persistent HBV infection remains to be determined.

Very young age appears to be one of the most important factors predisposing to persistent HBV infection. Although approximately 5–10 percent of adults with acute hepatitis B in the United States have been shown to become chronically infected,[120,242] persistent infection almost invariably follows acute neonatal hepatitis B, which is most commonly anicteric.[202,203] The HBsAg carrier state appears to be most common in young adults in the United States, and the frequency in men is several times that in women in this age group (reviewed in Ref. 177). The higher proportion of male carriers observed in many populations[177,267–269] is due at least in part to the greater probability that more men than women become persistently infected after primary infection, as well as to the apparently more rapid rate at which women terminate the carrier state.[177]

Anecdotal cases suggest that immunosuppression may be associated with milder initial disease and more frequent persistent infection than occurs in immunologic normals. For example, HBV infection in renal dialysis patients frequently becomes persistent.[270] Finally, the HBsAg carrier state appears to be more common in patients with certain diseases, such as Down syndrome, lepromatous leprosy, and chronic lymphocytic leukemia, than in the general population (reviewed in Refs. 268 and 269). Although the mechanism by which each of the above conditions leads to persistent infection is not clear, a common mechanism could be a modified or inadequate immune response so that the virus is not eliminated as it is after most acute infections.

The infecting virus dose and the severity of the initial disease also appear to correlate with the probability of developing persistent infection. Persistent infection occurs more frequently after initial anicteric hepatitis compared with initial icteric disease.[48,271] Survivors of fulminant hepatitis rarely become persistently infected, and HBsAg carriers frequently have no history of recognized acute hepatitis.[242] Experimental infections with different dilutions of infectious serum suggest that lower doses of virus result more often in long incubation periods, mild initial disease, and subsequent chronic infection compared with higher virus doses.[48] This relationship is so regular that the infecting dose can usually be estimated from the incubation period in experimental transmission studies.[48,50,141] There is no evidence that hepatitis B virus strains (e.g., HBsAg subtypes) have different virulence or propensity for persistent infection.

Striking differences occur in HBsAg carrier rates in different populations in the United States and other geographic areas. In most areas of the United States, less than 0.1 percent of volunteer blood donors have been found to be HBsAg positive (reviewed in Ref. 27). Almost all of them are chronic HBsAg carriers, whereas the carrier rate in paid donors is usually closer to 1 percent. Among certain populations, such as percutaneous drug abusers, patients in some hemodialysis centers, and certain homosexual populations, the carrier rate may be 1–5 percent (e.g., Ref. 272). These high rates appear to reflect the frequent exposure to the virus experienced by members of these groups. The carrier rates in most Western European countries are similar to those in the United States (reviewed in Ref. 27), but in other highly endemic areas of the world, such as many countries in Africa, Asia, and Oceania, the rate may be as high as 20 percent, and almost all HBsAg-negative adults are positive for anti-HBs and/or anti-HBc, indicating past infection.[27,177,268] The increased carrier rates in some underdeveloped countries may not only be related to poor sanitary conditions and increased exposure at very early ages; there may also be differences in the predisposition to chronic infection on a genetic, nutritional, or other basis in different populations. Transmission of virus from persistently infected mothers to newborn or young infants, who then usually develop persistent infection, has been estimated to account for 40 percent of the carriers in Taiwan.[273,274]

Among HBsAg carriers worldwide, there is an uneven geographic distribution of HBsAg subtypes. As described above, almost all antigens contain either determinants *d* or *y* and either *w* or *r*. The *d* determinant is common in the United States, Northern Europe, Asia, and Oceania, although the *y* determinant is found at a lower frequency in these regions.[275,276] The *d* determinant, to the near exclusion of *y*, is found in Japan. The *y* determinant (and rarely *d*) is found in Africa and in Australian aborigines. The *y* determinant is also found frequently in India and the Mediterranean region. The *w* determinant predominates in Europe, the United States, Africa, India, Australia, and Oceania. The *r* determinant predominates in Japan, China, and Southeast Asia. Subtypes *adw*, *ady*, and *adr* are each found in extensive geographic regions of the world. Subtype *ayr* is rarer, although it is commonly found in small populations in Oceania. The geographic distributions of subtypes probably reflect the locations of their origins (i.e., diversion from a common HBsAg ancestor) and the migrations of infected human populations.

Routes of HBV Transmission

It appears that the only important source or reservoir of virus for human infections is humanity itself. No important animal reservoir is known. Although some higher primates other than humans may be infected in nature (reviewed above under "Virus Host Range"), there is no evidence that they are important sources of human infections. If nonhuman primates are infected in nature, it is unlikely that they would infect humans, because transmission from infected individuals requires specific patterns of intimate contact such as those described below. Although some environmental surfaces, such as toothbrushes, razors, needles, and toys, may mediate person-to-person transmission of hepatitis A virus to large numbers of people. Hepatitis B virus does not often appear to be present in feces, and there is no evidence of fecal–oral transmission, as there is for hepatitis A virus. These features of HBV and the particular kinds of close contact required for transmission probably account for the infrequent epidemic pattern of spread, in contrast to many agents that are spread by enteric (e.g., hepatitis A virus) or respiratory routes. Persistent infections in which infectious HBV may be continuously present in blood and certain other body fluids for many years or for life represent a stable human reservoir of virus, so that HBV can be maintained indefinitely, even in small, isolated populations (e.g., those of some islands).

Although blood and blood products are the best-documented sources of infectious virus, HBsAg has also been found in feces, urine, bile, sweat, tears, saliva, semen, breast milk, vaginal secretions, cerebrospinal fluid, synovial fluid, and cord blood. Only serum (e.g., see Ref. 48), saliva,[115,277] and semen[277] have actually been shown to contain infectious HBV in experimental transmission studies. The report of transmission by the bite of an infected patient[278] is consistent with the presence of HBV in saliva. During the 1940s, more than 50 attempts to transmit serum hepatitis to human volunteers using feces from persons after experimental infections were unsuccessful (e.g., see Refs. 13 and 18), suggesting that infectious HBV probably enters feces infrequently in the absence of gastrointestinal bleeding, and thus that feces must not be a common source of virus for HBV infections acquired in the community. Other body fluids have not been tested for infectious virus. Often the concentrations of HBsAg in fluids other than the serum of infected patients are lower or not detectable at all. When present, antigen can sometimes be demonstrated only after concentration has occurred. When infectious virus is also present in such fluids, its concentration is undoubtedly lower than that in serum. Infectious HBV has also been shown to be present in blood without detectable HBsAg,[29,178–180,258] so that the failure to detect antigen does not exclude the presence of infectious virus.

Several specific routes of transmission appear to be well established. The most important routes of transmission in the United States are undoubtedly by percutaneous transfer, and probably by mucous membrane contact of blood and possibly other body fluids (e.g., saliva), and by heterosexual and homosexual contacts. Direct percutaneous inoculation of virus by needles can occur with contaminated blood or blood products, hemodialysis, tattooing, ear piercing, acupuncture, sharing needles during illicit drug use, or accidental needle sticks by hospital personnel. Clearly, HBV is commonly transmitted by routes other than these overt parenteral ones.[279] Infectious material contacting open skin breaks or mucous membranes such as that of the eye can also be expected to result in infection. Because HBV is quite stable, transmission by means of environmental surfaces that may contact mucous membranes or open skin breaks, such as toothbrushes, baby bottles, toys, eating utensils, razors,[280,281] or hospital equipment such as respirators, endoscopes,[282,283] or laboratory glassware and instruments,[284] can be expected. In households, transmission is more common from HBV-infected persons to sexual partners than to other kinds of household contacts.[162,285–287] Hepatitis B virus infection rates are unusually high among female prostitutes[288] and male homosexuals,[289,290] who are commonly exposed to many different sexual partners. Cases of apparent direct transmission from HBV-infected persons to susceptible individuals after sexual intercourse have been reported.[291] The exact route of transmission in these cases is not yet proven, but it seems likely that sexual contact is among the most common circumstances leading to HBV transmission in populations with high carrier rates. The demonstration of infectious virus in the semen and saliva of infected persons[277] supports the possibility of venereal transmission.

Health care personnel have been shown to be at greater risk for HBV infection than the general public,[292–294] undoubtedly due to their more frequent exposure to infected patients. The specific routes of transmission from patients to medical and dental workers are not known, although it appears that the greater the direct exposure to blood and serum (e.g., in surgeons[294,295] and workers in renal dialysis units[294]), the greater the frequency of HBV infection.

A few persistently infected physicians,[296] dentists,[297] and oral surgeons,[298,299] as well as acutely infected health care personnel,[300,301] have been implicated in the transmission of HBV infection to multiple patients, although most health care personnel who are carriers,[302] as well as those with acute infection,[302,303] appear to represent little risk to their patients. Transmission of infection from certain chronic HBsAg carrier women, but not others, to their newborn infants has also been observed.[161,273] Transmission of virus from chronic carriers via administration of their blood products or via accidental needle puncture in a medical setting has also been frequently observed. Although these are the best-documented instances of the spread of HBV infection from chronic carriers, transmission also appears to occur commonly from chronic carriers to sexual contacts,[287,289,291] to those taking illicit drugs by self-injection when needles are shared, and to individuals by other routes described above. However, proof of transmission from patients during the persistent phase of infection rather than during the acute phase has not been as clearly demonstrated for the latter routes of transmission.

Infection after oral intake of infectious material has been clearly demonstrated, although the dose of virus needed for successful infection by the oral route appears to be higher than that needed for parenteral infection.[17] That oral infection does not occur via the intestinal tract, but through small breaks postulated to exist regularly in the oral mucosa, was suggested by experiments in which two susceptible chimpanzees failed to be infected by infectious material placed directly in their stomachs but were infected by an oral spray of infectious material after their gums were lightly brushed with a toothbrush.[304] Evidence consistent with an intestinal phase of HBV infection is the occurrence of anti-HBs.[305] Surface antigens with HBcAg have not been detected by immunofluorescence in the cells of any tissue except liver, however, and further investigation will be required to establish whether intestinal or other mucosal surfaces actually contain cells susceptible to infection by HBV. Although food and water apparently are never sources of virus for HBV infections, HBsAg has been detected in clams from coastal waters into which untreated sewage has been drained.[306] Despite this finding, published outbreaks of shellfish-associated hepatitis have not been of type B. Although HBV can infect by the oral route, it is not clear how important this portal of entry is in community-acquired infections. There is no evidence that the fecal–oral route plays a significant role in HBV transmission.

Persistent viremia would appear to be a favorable condition for transmission by blood-feeding insects such as mosquitoes. Although some populations of wild mosquitoes and bedbugs caught in Africa[307–310] and the United States[310] have been shown to contain HBsAg, there has been no direct demonstration of transmission to humans by insect vectors. Unlike arboviruses, HBV probably does not infect insects, so that passive transfer would be required.

In areas of the world where HBV infection rates are much higher than in the United States, there would appear to be less opportunity for virus transmission by overt parenteral routes, and other routes of transmission appear to be much more important. In this setting, transmission from infected mothers to newborn infants or young children appears to account for a very large fraction of HBV infections. Neonatal transmission from chronic carrier mothers and mothers with acute hepatitis B in the third trimester or first 2 months postpartum has been clearly documented in the United States,[202,203] as well as in highly endemic populations,[161,273] and such infected infants commonly develop persistent infection. In Taiwan it has been estimated that 40–50 percent of HBsAg carriers acquired their infection in the perinatal period.[161] Only 5–10 percent of them appeared to be infected in utero; the others appeared to be infected at the time of delivery by exposure to infected maternal blood.[221] Many infants not infected perinatally are infected in the first few months or years of life, probably by contact with their infected mothers or siblings, although the exact routes of transmission are not known. Clustering of carriers in families in which mothers are infected[231–312] is consistent with this pattern of spread. The presence of HBsAg in maternal milk would suggest that breast-feeding might be an important route, although one study[313] suggests that this may not be the case. Mastication of food by mothers before feeding it to infants is common in some cultures and might be expected to lead to infection of infants in those populations. Other kinds of intimate contact between mothers and children, as well as between siblings, are undoubtedly important. Bedbugs, mosquitoes, or other blood-feeding insects would appear to offer an opportunity for transmission between individuals sharing the same household or bed, but there is little direct evidence supporting this possibility.

The presence of significant Dane particle concentrations and/or HBeAg in the blood has been correlated with the transmission of infection from carrier mothers to neonates,[161,162,203,230] from carriers to normal health care personnel accidentally inoculated with contaminated needles,[177,314] from carrier health care personnel to patient contacts, (W. S. Robinson, unpublished results), and among sexual partners in households.[163] The regular appearance of Dane particles in high concentrations and of HBeAg in the serum of patients during the late incubation period of acute hepatitis B[128,129] suggests that this is a time when the patients are probably highly contagious, as appear to be the few chronic HBsAg carriers with high concentrations of Dane particles and/or HBeAg in their blood. The very frequent transmission of infection from mothers with acute hepatitis B during the third trimester of pregnancy or the first 2 months postpartum[202,203] is consistent with this finding.

CLINICAL MANIFESTATIONS AND PROGNOSIS

Acute Hepatitis B

The incubation period of acute serum hepatitis (most cases of which were undoubtedly hepatitis B) was long ago established to be 4–28 weeks, but in most cases the interval is 60–110 days.[12,13,315–318] Among patients with acute icteric hepatitis B, 10–20 percent have a serum sickness-like illness with an erythematous maculopapular rash, urticaria, arthralgias, sometimes arthritis, and sometimes fever several days to weeks before the onset of clinically apparent liver disease.[136,239] Symmetric involvement of distal joints or large joints is the rule. The symptoms usually last for 2–10 days and clear without causing residual changes, although findings can persist for weeks or even months in unusual cases.

The clinical course of acute hepatitis B in individual cases is indistinguishable from that of acute hepatitis A. The severity varies widely, and many infections appear to be clinically inapparent.[319–321] Although inapparent hepatitis is not associated with symptoms or abnormal physical findings, most cases are accompanied by abnormal serum transaminase activity. Less commonly, HBV infection appears to occur without associated liver function abnormalities and is detected in these cases only by specific serologic tests for the virus.

Symptomatic acute hepatitis B can be mild and anicteric or more severe and associated with icterus. Typically, symptoms of headache, malaise, loss of appetite, nausea and occasional vomiting, moderate fever (temperatures of 37.5–39°C), and chills are initial symptoms and appear 2–7 days before the onset of jaundice in icteric cases. Loss of appetite is very common and is often characterized by actual distaste for or aversion to food and tobacco; the smell of food or tobacco may induce nausea. Abdominal discomfort or pain localized in the right upper quadrant is common. Urine becomes dark and stools light or clay-colored.

In icteric cases, symptoms may progress, persist unchanged, decrease in severity, or clear rapidly with the onset of jaundice. Scleral icterus can be observed when the serum bilirubin level exceeds 2.5 or 3.0 mg%. Mild pruritis lasting for only a few days occurs in one-half of these patients, but occasionally patients may have protracted or severe itching. Arthralgias may occur in 10–20 percent of patients.

Common physical findings include right upper quadrant tenderness; enlargement of the liver (up to a 15-cm increase in vertical breadth) with a rounded, tender edge; and scleral, mucous membrane, and cutaneous icterus. Massive hepatic enlargement is rare. The spleen can be palpated in 10–15 percent of patients. Mild enlargement of lymph nodes, particularly in the posterior cervical region, may be noted. Spider angiomas may develop and disappear after recovery. Transient gynecomastia occurs but is unusual. Children usually recover in 2 weeks and adults in 4–6 weeks.[322]

Laboratory tests may reveal normal or moderately reduced hematocrit and hemoglobin concentrations. Mild hemolysis is often observed. The total white cell count is usually normal and rarely exceeds 12,000 cells per cubic millimeter.[323] There may, however, be granulocytopenia and a relative lymphocytosis. Large, atypical lymphocytes are commonly present but rarely exceed 10 percent.[324] Mild proteinuria may occur. Urobilinogen and bilirubin are common in the urine before the onset of jaundice and decrease in amount as jaundice progresses. Transient steatorrhea may occur early in the illness.

Liver function abnormalities may include an increase in direct reacting serum bilirubin early when total bilirubin is normal. Total serum bilirubin usually increases for 10–14 days and does not exceed 10 mg% in most patients.[325] Occasional patients have high peak values. The bilirubin concentration usually falls gradually over 2–4 weeks. The hallmark of acute viral hepatitis is the striking elevation in serum transaminase (aminotransferase) activity.[326,327] Elevations may precede the onset of symptoms and usually peak in the first week of symptoms. Peak levels above 1000 units/ml are common, and SGPT levels usually exceed SGOT levels. The peak levels may correlate roughly with the extent of liver injury but are not a prognostic factor. The serum transaminase activity usually returns to normal as the illness subsides. Serum alkaline phosphatase activity may be normal or mildly elevated. Concentrations of serum albumin and globulins are usually normal, although in severe or protracted viral hepatitis, albumin levels may be decreased and γ-globulin increased up to two times the normal level. Glucose tolerance may be decreased during acute viral hepatitis, but fasting blood glucose levels may be low. Most patients with icteric acute hepatitis B eliminate the virus and have no residual disease.

Infrequently, severe depression; neurologic syndromes such as meningitis, Guillain-Barré syndrome, myelitis, or encephalitis; hematologic disorders such as agranulocytosis, thrombocytopenia, or aplastic anemia; and electrocardiographic abnormalities including arrhythmias may occur in association with or after acute viral hepatitis. The role of the viral infection in these problems is unclear.

Acute hepatitis B may be clinically indistinguishable from acute hepatitis A and from hepatitis caused by the so-called non-A, non-B hepatitis agents, Epstein-Barr virus, cytomegalovirus, yellow fever virus, leptospirosis, and, less commonly, other infectious agents. Toxic hepatitis caused by ethanol, numerous drugs (e.g., halothane), and numerous industrial chemicals (e.g., benzene) may also produce similar syndromes.

A number of variants of hepatitis B may occur. Fulminant hepatitis is a severe form accompanied by hepatic failure with encephalopathy. The mortality in such cases is exceedingly high.[328] Occasionally, death occurs before the onset of jaundice, one-half of the patients die within 10 days of the onset of symptoms, and three-fourths die within 3 weeks. Encephalopathy with hepatic failure is associated with hyperexcitability, impaired mentation, asterixis, confusion, obtundation, and eventually coma. Vomiting and seizures may also occur. Extensive hepatic necrosis may be associated with rapid reduction in the size of an enlarged liver, a fall in previously elevated serum transaminase activity and HBsAg, and progressive prolongation of the prothrombin time. Oliguria and azotemia, as well as edema and ascites, may develop. Primary infection with HBV-accompanied δ agent may carry a special risk of fulminant hepatitis.[221,224,225]

Other variant forms of viral hepatitis include prolonged acute hepatitis, in which abnormal laboratory findings, mild symptoms, and abnormal physical findings may persist beyond 3 or 4 months and sometimes up to 12 months or more. Probably only 3–5 percent of the cases of acute icteric viral hepatitis extend beyond 3 or 4 months.[318] The ultimate prognosis for patients with prolonged acute viral hepatitis is probably no different from that of patients with a more typical shorter course, but prolonged acute viral hepatitis may be difficult to distinguish from chronic forms of hepatitis, to be described subsequently, until they become HBsAg negative and the hepatitis resolves.

Relapsing hepatitis follows a course to recovery followed by one or more episodes similar to, although usually milder than, the initial acute illness. Relapses occur in a small proportion of cases and have been attributed to too early ambulation, consumption of alcohol, and treatment with corticosteroids during the acute illness in anecdotal cases. A relapse must be distinguished from a second episode of acute viral hepatitis with a different infectious agent.

Although most infections with HBV appear to result in anicteric initial disease, and although acute icteric hepatitis is usually a benign, self-limited disease, relative high fatality rates among icteric patients occur under certain circumstances. At least two factors are known to influence the severity of acute hepatitis B. One is age. In general, infants and young children have milder initial disease than older age patients,[202,329] and the older the patient, the longer the icteric phase.[242] Mortality in post-transfusion hepatitis appears to be related to age.[330] In patients with hepatic failure during acute hepatitis, mortality can also be correlated with age. Survival is rare in such patients over age 40 compared with the significant rate of survival in younger patients.[242] Severe or fulminant hepatitis appears to be uncommon in infants and young children, although it does occur.[331] It has been stated that the better prognosis of younger patients with severe hepatitis is due to their capacity for hepatocyte regeneration after hepatic necrosis in contrast to older patients.[242]

Another factor influencing the severity of disease is the virus dose. Experimental transmission studies have shown that the higher the dose, the shorter the incubation period and the more likely that icteric hepatitis will result.[48] The highest virus doses received by patients may be by transfusion of infectious blood. Mortality of transfusion-associated icteric hepatitis was 10 percent or more in many series before blood bank testing for HBsAg,[332] and most of the cases in these studies were undoubtedly hepatitis B. The poor prognosis in such patients may be related to the large virus dose resulting from blood transfusion and/or to the severity of the associated underlying disease. Since the advent of HBsAg testing, the mortality of post-transfusion hepatitis appears to be lower.[330] This may reflect, in part, the elimination of blood units with very high concentrations of HBV. The mortality of acute hepatitis B appears to be unusually high in patients with malignant disease or preexisting cirrhosis.[242]

A final factor that may be associated with severe acute hepatitis in some cases is coinfection with δ agent,[221,224,225] as described above under "Pathogenesis of Disease."

Persistent HBV Infection

In a 1- to 5-year follow-up study of 429 patients hospitalized with acute icteric hepatitis B, 90 percent became HBsAg negative and 10 percent became persistent HBsAg.[242] Of the latter group, 70 percent had chronic persistent hepatitis and 30 percent had chronic active hepatitis. One of these patients developed polyarteritis nodosa and one membranous glomerulonephritis. No persistent liver disease was found in any of the patients who became HBsAg negative after acute hepatitis. Persistent infection with HBV is most often asymptomatic. When associated with CPH, patients are generally in good health and have persistent or recurrent elevations of SGOT and SGPT without jaundice.[242] Persistent mild hepatomegaly is common, and splenomegaly is occasionally present. Long-term follow-up of such patients shows no evidence of progression, and complete resolution occurs in some cases. Late disappearance of HBsAg occurs rarely.[242]

CAH associated with persistent HBV infection is sometimes difficult to distinguish from prolonged acute viral hepatitis or CPH in the first 6 or 12 months on either clinical or histologic grounds, but in time the distinction can be made.[242] Patients with CAH may have chronic jaundice, intermittent episodes of jaundice, or no jaundice throughout their course. Episodes of jaundice are usually associated with significant transaminase elevations. The prognosis of patients who develop CAH is variable. Progression to cirrhosis occurs in many patients, and some may progress to cirrhosis, hepatic failure, and death within 1 year. Superinfections of HBsAg carriers with δ agent can lead to exacerbations of active hepatitis,[226,227] and persistent δ agent infection in HBsAg carriers may be commonly associated with chronic hepatitis,[227,228] as described above under "Pathogenesis of Disease."

MAKING A VIRAL DIAGNOSIS

A diagnosis of acute viral hepatitis can usually be made from the clinical findings, and the responsible viral agent can often be suspected from the epidemiologic setting and features such as the incubation period; however, only virus-specific tests can conclusively identify the infecting virus. Highly sensitive tests for HBsAg, anti-HBs, anti-HBc, anti-HBc IgM, HBeAg, anti-HBe, and anti-HDAg are specific for HBV, or HDV, diagnostically useful, and commercially available. Tests specific for Dane particles or DNA and DNA polymerase-containing virions, and for HDAg and HDV RNA in liver and serum, are available only in research laboratories. Table 2 shows typical serologic test findings at different stages of HBV infection and in convalescence. This table does not include all variations and does not convey the dynamic nature of the infection during which individual markers appear and/or disappear (not always in the same order in different patients) during the evolution of infection, as indicated in Figures 5, 6, and 7 and discussed above under "Course of the Virus Infection."

Tests for serum HBsAg, anti-HBs, anti-HBc, and anti-HBc IgM are important for clinical evaluation of patients for active and past HBV infection.[333,334] HBsAg is the most important and most commonly used marker for active infection because its presence in serum indicates active infection with HBV in almost all cases, the rare exception being after passive transfer of HBsAg (e.g., by blood transfusion). HBsAg can be detected in most cases, although, as described above under "Course of the Virus Infection," not all patients have infectious HBV in the blood.[120,178–180] Sera or other body fluids or secretions should be considered infectious when HBsAg is present.

When serum HBsAg is positive in patients with apparent acute hepatitis, acute hepatitis B is suggested, although superimposed hepatitis caused by another agent or acute exacerbations of chronic active hepatitis may give similar findings in a patient persistently infected with HBV. Falling titers of HBsAg and/or rising anti-HBc titers and positive anti-HBc IgM in such patients suggest acute hepatitis B (Fig. 5). As described above under "Course of the Virus Infection," in a fraction of patients with acute HBV infection, HBsAg can never be detected (e.g., Fig. 6); in some, HBsAg becomes undetectable before the end of the clinical disease; and in a few, it becomes negative even before the onset of disease. In such patients with acute hepatitis, HBV infection may only be established by the presence of anti-HBc IgM, a rising titer of anti-HBc, and/or the subsequent appearance of anti-HBs.

HBsAg in the absence of detectable anti-HBc suggests early infection (i.e., during the first few weeks after becoming HBsAg positive and before the appearance of anti-HBc) (Fig. 5). HBsAg can also occur alone in any infected patient unable to mount an antibody response (e.g., as in agammaglobulinemia). HBsAg in the presence of anti-HBc IgM suggests primary infection sometime after the above early period (Fig. 5), and a high titer of anti-HBc without anti-HBc IgM suggests persistent infection (Fig. 7). Anti-HBc titers are usually significantly higher during persistent infection than during or after self-limited infection.[120,333,334]

The presence of anti-HBs and anti-HBc in the absence of HBsAg and anti-HBc IgM indicates past infection with HBV and immunity.[120,333,334] In general, the more recent the infection, the higher the titers of these antibodies. The presence of either anti-HBs or anti-HBc alone in low titers most commonly occurs after infection in the distant past in individuals who have since lost the second antibody. Anti-HBc alone may be present in relatively high titer after the disappearance of HBsAg and before the appearance of anti-HBs (Fig. 5), thus indicating recent infection. Anti-HBc is the only antibody detected after self-limited infection in 10 percent of patients who never develop detectable anti-HBs.

Infrequently, blood containing high titers of anti-HBc but no detectable HBsAg has been shown to transmit HBV infection to recipients.[120] Such blood probably comes from persistently

TABLE 2. HBV Serologic Markers in Different Stages of Infection and Convalescence

			Anti-HBc			
Stage of Infection	*HBsAg*	*Anti-HBS*	*IgG*	*IgM*	*HBeAg*	*Anti-HBe*
Late incubation period of hepatitis B	+	–	–	–	+ or –	–
Acute hepatitis B	+	–	+	+	+	–
HBsAg-negative acute hepatitis B	–	–	+	+	–	–
Healthy HBsAg carrier	+	–	+ + +	+ or –	–	+
Chronic hepatitis B	+	–	+ + +	+ or –	+	–
HBV infection in recent past	–	+ +	+ +	+ or –	–	+
HBV infection in distant past	–	+ or –	+ or –	–	–	–
Recent HBV vaccination	–	+ +	–	–	–	–

infected patients or those with self-limited infection who have HBsAg titers too low for detection by even the most sensitive assays. Thus, blood containing anti-HBc alone, particularly in high titer, should be considered potentially infectious.

The presence of anti-HBs in the absence of anti-HBc and HBsAg indicates past HBV infection or past vaccination for HBV.[120,333,334] Low anti-HBs titers in patients without past HBV vaccination suggests infection in the distant past in patients in whom anti-HBc had fallen below the level of detection. High anti-HBs titers alone may occur after a secondary anti-HBs response after exposure to HBV and HBsAg (e.g., by receiving HBsAg-containing blood products or immunization with HBV vaccine) without reinfection, which would result in a rise in anti-HBc as well as anti-HBs. Blood containing detectable anti-HBs rarely if ever transmits HBV infection.[335,336]

Passive transfer of HBsAg, anti-HBs, and/or anti-HBc can produce any of the patterns described above after transfusion with blood containing the appropriate serologic activity.

Although analysis of a single blood sample may provide an accurate diagnosis in some cases, a second sample 1 month or more after the first or serial samples may be required to fully establish HBV infection and the stage of infection or convalescence in some patients. For example, falling HBsAg titers in serial blood samples suggest resolving acute infection (Fig. 5). A fourfold or greater rise in anti-HBc titer and anti-HBc IgM suggest ongoing infection (Figs. 5 and 6). Such a rise in anti-HBs suggests recent infection (Figs. 5 and 6), a secondary response after exposure to HBsAg without infection, or recent vaccination. Persistent infection (i.e., the chronic carrier state) usually cannot be established until HBsAg has been shown to be present for at least 6 months.

Assays for Dane particles, HBeAg, and anti-HBe in serum are also clinically useful for assessing patients with HBV infection. Dane particles detected by their DNA polymerase activity[147] or their viral DNA content by nucleic acid hybridization[150] and HBeAg are not found in serum without detectable HBsAg. High levels of Dane particle DNA polymerase activity and HBeAg appear regularly in the late incubation period of hepatitis B and their presence with HBsAg in sera of patients without anti-HBc suggests the early stage of infection (Fig. 5). The presence of Dane particles and HBeAg during acute or persistent infection may be used to identify patients more likely to transmit infection to others than infected patients without these markers. As described above under "Epidemiology," the presence of these activities correlates well with transmission of HBV infection from carriers via the percutaneous route,[77,325] from carrier pregnant women to their newborn infants,[161,162,203,273] from medical care personnel such as dentists to their patients (W. S. Robinson, unpublished results), and from persistently infected patients to their sexual contacts (W. S. Robinson, unpublished results). HBsAg carriers with anti-HBe in their serum appear to transmit infection by these routes much less frequently. These correlations are not absolute,[337] and some blood containing HBsAg and anti-HBe has been clearly shown to contain infectious HBV,[48,338] although in much lower titer than in blood containing HBeAg.[48] Thus, while these viral markers clearly distinguish infected patients who readily transmit infection from those unlikely to infect others, at least by certain routes of transmission, because the correlations are not absolute, the outcome of contacts with infected patients in individual cases cannot be predicted with certainty from knowledge of these viral markers.

MANAGEMENT OF HEPATITIS B

Acute Hepatitis B

No therapeutic measure has been proven to have a beneficial effect on the disease process in the liver after the onset of acute viral hepatitis. The benefit of bed rest and the harm of exercise have been much debated, and many of the opinions about physical activity have been based on uncontrolled observations.[339] It has been claimed that relapses and deaths may be increased by strenuous exercise or even early ambulation. However, several controlled studies have failed to confirm a deleterious effect of exercise.[340,341] Most of these studies have involved young, otherwise healthy adult patients with relatively mild disease. Under such circumstances, early ambulation or even light exercise is probably not harmful. For older patients and those with more severe disease, ambulation should be more gradual, and should be determined by the severity of the disease and by the patient's strength and sense of well-being. If evidence suggests that improvement in liver disease may have been halted or reversed by increasing physical activity, the level of activity can be reduced to determine whether this appears to have a beneficial effect. Because prolonged bed rest may be deleterious to a patient's overall condition, it should be avoided unless needed for sound medical reasons.

No specific dietary alterations appear to affect the outcome of acute viral hepatitis, with the exception of hepatic failure, for which protein and/or salt restriction may be indicated. The choice of foods should be dictated by palatability, by the tolerance of the individual patient, and by the attempt to maintain the best possible nutritional state. High carbohydrate, high protein or other special additions to the diet have not been shown to be of benefit.

Corticosteroids have been used by some physicians for severe acute viral hepatitis, but recent controlled trials in severe[342] and fulminant[343] hepatitis have shown either no difference or less favorable outcomes for patients so treated compared with controls. Exchange transfusions, hemodialysis, cross-perfusion, and γ-globulin containing high titers of anti-HBs[344] have not been shown to favorably affect the course of fulminant hepatitis.

Chronic Hepatitis B

The progression of chronic active hepatitis has been favorably altered by administration of corticosteroids and sometimes azothioprine in controlled trials.[345–347] Liver function returns toward normal, and cirrhosis appears to be prevented in some patients on these drugs. Women treated at an early stage in the disease appear to respond best. Recent studies indicate, however, that HBsAg-positive patients with CAH respond significantly less often than HBsAg-negative patients,[348] and HBsAg-positive patients with HBeAg may be particularly unresponsive.[349] In addition, corticosteroid therapy regularly appears to enhance HBV replication, with rises in the titers of HBsAg, HBeAg, and Dane particles, or induces the appearance of the latter markers in carriers without them.[182–184] This effect reverses the gradual winding down of the infection over months or years observed in many carriers. It has been recommended that corticosteroid therapy be used only for CAH patients who are symptomatic, HBsAg negative, and with severe histologic lesions in liver biopsies, and not for HBsAg-positive patients.[350] It remains to be determined whether or not CAH that appears to follow acute non-A, non-B hepatitis[351] is responsive to corticosteroid therapy. When indicated for CAH, prednisone in doses of 15–30 mg/day should be continued for at least 2 or 3 years. If troublesome side effects occur, the dose should be reduced to the minimum needed to maintain liver function tests near normal.

Transfer factor has been given to patients with CAH-B, with little evidence of an effect on the course of infection or liver disease.[352,353]

Two antiviral agents, human leukocyte (α) interferon (HLI)[148,149] and adenine arabinoside (ara A),[148,186] have been shown to regularly inhibit the production of Dane particles in persistently infected patients (HBsAg positive for more than 1 year) with chronic hepatitis. Three kinds of responses have been observed in uncontrolled trials. In a fraction of patients, all markers of infection in serum (HBsAg, HBeAg, virion DNA polymerase, and infectious HBV[49]) and liver (HBcAg and HBsAg) fall below the level of detection during treatment and remain so indefinitely after treatment is stopped (type I response). In other patients, HBeAg, virion DNA polymerase, and apparently infectious HBV[49] and HBcAg disappear from the serum and liver, respectively, during treatment and remain absent permanently after treatment is stopped, although serum and hepatic HBsAg persists (type II response). In still other patients, virion DNA polymerase levels are partially suppressed during treatment and return to pretreatment levels when treatment is stopped (type III response). Type I and type II responses appear to occur more frequently in women than in men, in patients with low virion DNA polymerase levels than in those with high levels, in patients with CAH than in those with CPH, and when both antiviral agents are given than when either is given alone. Type I and type II but not type III responses are associated with improvements in liver function and histology.[187] Both antiviral agents suppress white blood cell and platelet counts, and HLI causes fatigue, malaise, and, rarely, hair loss; these effects are immediately reversible when therapy is stopped. In addition, ara A leads to neurologic toxicity including agitation, mental confusion, hallucinations and seizure activity in rare cases; pain in lower limbs, probably due to peripheral neuropathy, which sometimes persists for weeks or months after treatment is stopped, is not uncommon after prolonged therapy. Further studies including controlled trials are necessary to establish the extent and frequency of the beneficial effects of these antiviral agents on persistent HBV infection and on the associated hepatic disease, and to determine whether the results can be improved and the side effects reduced by dosage adjustments and/or the use of other antiviral agents. Although these experimental studies are encouraging, until more conclusive data are available and because of the toxicity, it is unjustified to use either of these antiviral agents for the treatment of persistent HBV infection at this time, except in the context of studies designed to establish their efficacy and toxicity. Studies on the effects of antiviral agents in acute hepatitis B have been too limited to allow us to draw conclusions, and no efficacy has yet been demonstrated.[354]

In the management of HBsAg carriers, it is often useful for the patient to be aware of the course of certain serologic markers. As described above under "Routes of Transmission," the presence of serum HBeAg indicates a high level of contagiousness for contacts, and the absence of HBeAg and the presence of anti-HBe indicate low contagiousness. In HBeAg and the presence of anti-HBe indicate low contagiousness. In HBeAg-positive carriers, this test might be done at yearly intervals to make the patient aware of a seroconversion (which occurs in approximately 15 percent of HBe-Ag-positive carriers per year; see above under "Course of the Virus Infection") and the accompanying change in contagiousness. Similarly, periodic testing (every 1 or 2 years) for HBsAg would detect complete resolution of the infection (which occurs in 1–2 percent of carriers per year) with loss of contagiousness and the risk of HBV-associated liver disease.

The high risk of HCC formation in certain HBsAg carriers (as high as 3 percent per year in Chinese male carriers above age 50 and more than 12 percent per year for those with cirrhosis[229]) is a serious problem for these individuals. Several recent studies have shown that when serum α-fetoprotein (AFP) followed serially in HBsAg carriers rises significantly above the patient's own baseline (e.g., above 100 μg/ml), HCC can often be detected by liver scanning or ultrasound procedures at a stage when the tumor can be cured by surgical resection (e.g., Refs. 355 and 356). This suggests that many HBsAg carriers should have regular serial serum AFP determinations, although larger prospective studies are needed to better define the sensitivity, specificity, and predictive value of AFP screening and to better establish the indications for it. The interval between infection and HCC formation is usually many years, and the risk rises in proportion to the duration of infection.[229] Thus, in individuals infected in infancy or childhood, AFP testing and ultrasound examination at 6-month intervals might be done for those above age 35 or 40 years. It is recommended that all HBsAg carriers with cirrhosis have regular serum AFP testing and ultrasound examinations.

PREVENTION OF HBV INFECTION

Several measures have been successfully used to prevent the spread of HBV. These include application of environmental control measures to contain the virus and prevent exposure, and the use of passive and active immunization to render individuals or groups resistant to infection. The development of successful control measures has depended to a large extent on the growing understanding of the epidemiology and biology of this virus and on the availability of serologic assays to identify infected and immune individuals.

Immunization

Pre-Exposure Passive Immunization. Passive immunization with both hyperimmune serum globulin (HBIG) preparations that are positive for anti-HBs in dilutions approaching or exceeding 1:100,000 by sensitive tests such as phytohemagglutinin (PHA) or RIA, and standard immune serum globulin (ISG), preparations of which since 1970 have regularly been positive for anti-HBs in dilutions of 1:16 to 1:1000 by these tests,[357,358] have been shown to protect against HBV infection and/or disease under certain circumstances. Pre-exposure prophylaxis with HBIG was shown to provide protection for hemodialysis patients[359,360] and staff[361,362] and for institutionalized children in the 1970s. Several studies failed to show a difference in the incidence of hepatitis or HBsAg in the serum of patients treated with ISG containing measurable anti-HBs titers or with HBIG in these settings,[359,361,363] suggesting that HBIG was not superior to ISG containing anti-HBs for pre-exposure prophylaxis. In some studies,[362–364] there appeared to be a greater frequency of primary antibody response in the ISG-treated group than in those given HBIG. These results suggest that ISG might be superior to HBIG in producing passive-active immunity. If so, ISG could be more effective in providing long-term protection for persons at high risk for infection.

With the availability of an effective vaccine, there appears to be little or no indication for pre-exposure passive immunization, except in individuals who fail to respond to vaccine or with disorders that preclude a response (e.g., agammaglobulinemia), in which the risk of exposure remains high despite all environmental control measures designed to prevent infection. In such rare cases, HBIG is not indicated and standard ISG in doses of 5–10 ml intramuscularly every 4 months[359,360,365,366] might be used.

Pre-Exposure Immunization with Hepatitis B Vaccine. Plasma-derived vaccine (Heptavax-B; Merck, Sharpe and Dohme, licensed in the United States in November 1981) consists of HBsAg particles highly purified from plasma of HBsAg carriers and inactivated by treatment with pepsin at pH 2, 8 M urea and 1:4000 formalin, conditions that have been shown to inactivate non-A, non-B hepatitis virus[367,368] and the human immunodeficiency virus (HIV), and that should inactivate almost all known viruses,[369] except possibly spongiform encephalopathy agents such as the Kuru or Creutzfeldt-Jakob agents. A recombinant vaccine consisting of HBsAg particles expressed in yeast cells and highly purified (Recombivax-HB; Merck, Sharpe and Dohme) was licensed in the United States in July 1986. It is recommended that immunologically normal adults receive 1 ml (20 μg Heptavax-B and 10 μg Recombivax-HB) and children under age 10 years 0.5 ml intramuscularly at 0, 1, and 6 months.[257] Anti-HBs responses with these dosage schedules in experimental vaccine trials were good. Well over 90 percent of the patients in all age groups under age 60, including infants, had high antibody titers after the third vaccine dose.[370–375] Between 80 and 90 percent of those above age 60 had anti-HBs responses. Age is an important factor influencing the response to vaccine, with younger vaccinees, including newborn infants, having the highest rates of seroconversion in experimental trials. Older age, obesity, heavy smoking, and immunologic impairment have been associated with lower anti-HBS responses.[376,377] Significantly lower seroconversion rates (e.g., 50–75 percent) have been reported in some vaccination programs of healthy adults. Further investigation will be required to determine whether this represents the use of vaccine lots with low potency due to improper storage or to other factors. Although anti HBs titers fall with time after vaccination, 85 percent of homosexual men who responded to three doses of vaccine retained detectable anti-HBs 5 years after vaccination.[370,376] The higher the anti-HBs titer after vaccination, the longer anti-HBs persists.[376] Whether vaccines will require regular booster doses and at what time intervals remains to be determined. Immunologically impaired individuals such as those undergoing hemodialysis or those with organ transplants respond less well, and a higher vaccine dose (2 ml) is recommended.[257,378]

Simultaneous administration of ISG with high anti-HBs titers does not impair the anti-HBs response to vaccine.[379,380] Administration of vaccine to HBsAg carriers results in no recognizable ill effects and no alteration in the course of the infection.[381] Administration to individuals with serum anti-HBs results in a rise in the titer of this antibody and no recognizable ill effects. Although no special ill effects have been associated with vaccination of individuals with serum HBsAg or anti-HBs, such vaccination is of no value and is not indicated.

After administration to more than 19,000 individuals in clinical studies and many more for purposes of medical care, the only known side effects of Heptavax-B have been moderate soreness at the injection site in approximately 12 percent, mild fever in less than 2 percent, and other mild constitutional symptoms. In placebo-controlled trials, no difference in those side effects between recipients of vaccine and placebo was found.[371–375] Side effects with Recombivax-HB have been similar.

At this time, there is no evidence that more serious side effects have occurred in response to the current HBV vaccines. Although a few cases of Guillain-Barré syndrome or other neurologic disorders have been observed after Heptavax-B vaccination (e.g., Refs. 382 and 383), there is no evidence that the incidence is higher than that of sporadic disease in the general population. In controlled trials in homosexual men, the incidence of AIDS was the same in groups receiving vaccine and placebo.[384] No cases of non-A, non-B hepatitis have been reported after Heptavax-B administration. Hypersensitivity reactions to Recombivax-HB can be expected in some persons allergic to yeast antigens, and this vaccine is not recommended for such individuals.

In four prospective, double-blind, placebo-controlled trials with Heptavax-B carried out in homosexual men,[384–387] hemodialysis unit staff,[388] and hospital personnel,[380] more than 90 percent protection was shown. Almost all of the vaccinated individuals who were subsequently infected with HBV were among the small fraction of vaccine recipients who failed to seroconvert. Recombivax-HB has been shown to reduce significantly the rate of perinatal infection in babies of HBsAg-positive mothers. In summary, Heptavax-B and Recombivax-HB appear to be effective and safe vaccines to prevent HBV infection, and susceptible individuals with a significant risk of infection with HBV should be vaccinated.

Individuals with a high risk of exposure to HBV (see Table 1) include some health care workers, particularly those with frequent contact with blood or serum, such as laboratory technicians, phlebotomists, hemodialysis and cardiac catheterization staff, dental and other surgeons, emergency room and intensive care personnel with patient contact; homosexually active men and others with frequent and different sexual contacts; illicit parenteral drug users; hemodialysis patients; regular recipients of certain blood products such as factors VIII or IX; clients and staff of some institutions for the mentally retarded and inmates of some prisons; and household and sexual contacts of carriers. Although in general these groups are at greater risk for HBV infection than others in the population, individual circumstances must be considered in assessing the need for vaccination, since all members of all such groups are not at equal risk. For example, the risk of HBV infection for particular categories of hospital-based health care workers may be quite different in different hospitals because the prevalence of active HBV infection in different patient populations varies widely.

Before vaccination, the serum of individuals in high-risk groups may be tested for either anti-HBs or anti-HBc (the markers most likely to detect past infection)[385] in order to avoid unnecessary vaccination of those who are already immune. Serum anti-HBc will also be positive in HBsAg carriers, for whom vaccination is not beneficial. Some have recommended testing for anti-HBc in preference to anti-HBs because anti-HBc may be a more specific indicator of past HBV infection and appears to correlate with high anti-HBs titers,[385] and because rare patients with low anti-HBs titers that may or may not be nonspecific appear to remain susceptible to HBV infection.[189–191] After vaccination of seronegative individuals, testing for anti-HBs should be done to determine whether seroconversion has resulted. It is important for individuals to know when they have failed to seroconvert after vaccination because they remain susceptible to HBV infection and should receive ISG for appropriate future exposures to HBV. Such passive immunization is unnecessary for HBV exposure of those who successfully seroconvert after vaccination.

Revaccination (by the same three-dose schedule) of individuals who have no detectable anti-HBs response after receiving the third vaccine dose of a primary immunization series has been shown to lead to an anti-HBs response in more than 50 percent, but the titers tend to be lower and less persistent than in those who respond to the first vaccination series.[389] Several studies have shown that doses of 2–5 μg intradermally may give seroconversion rates similar to those achieved by 20- to 40-μg doses of the same HBV vaccine given intramuscularly. Larger studies are needed to confirm the effectiveness of intradermal administration before it can be generally used.

Postexposure Immunization. Krugman and Giles in 1973 showed that serum immunoglobulin preparations with high titers of anti-HBs, when given 4 hours after experimental inoculation of children with relatively high doses of infectious HBV, reduced the incidence of (although did not eliminate) infection in comparison with that of placebo-treated controls.[390] ISG with a low anti-HBs titer appeared to give a significant but lower level of protection.

Most prospective controlled trials of postexposure prophylaxis of adults since that time have compared HBIG with ISG rather than with a placebo. Significant protecting by HBIG has been shown in larger trials in hospital personnel with needle stick or mucous membrane exposure to blood containing HBsAg[143] and in spouses of acute hepatitis B patients.[391] A significant difference in protection between HBIG and ISG was not shown in a second similarly designed needle stick trial.[392,393] The rate of HBV infection in both the ISG- and HBIG-treated groups, however, was lower than anticipated for untreated patients in this study. The difference in the results of these studies appears to be due to a difference in the ISG employed. The ISG used in the first two trials contained no detectable anti-HBs, whereas that in the latter trial contained a significant anti-HBs titer. These studies suggest that HBIG provides protection when given after exposure to HBV. It also appears that ISG containing significant amounts of anti-HBs may provide similar protection, unlike ISG without anti-HBs, which is clearly inferior to HBIG.

The timing of HBIG doses necessary for the most effective postexposure prophylaxis has not been well defined. In most clinical trials, two doses at a 1-month interval were used. For this reason, the Public Health Service Advisory Committee on Immunization Practices currently recommends such a two-dose schedule.[394] It is not clear, however, that more than one dose offers more protection than a single dose. In some studies clearly demonstrating protection,[390,391] a single dose was employed, and in some trials employing two doses,[393] no protection by HBIG in comparison to ISG was shown. In one study,[366] a single dose of HBIG was compared directly with one-half of the same dose given at the time of exposure and repeated after 1 month; there was no statistically significant difference in the subsequent infection rate. Thus, a single dose given at the time of exposure appears to provide significant protection, and the addition of a second dose has not been clearly shown to increase the beneficial effect.

There is also little information about the effect of the interval after exposure when HBIG is first given on its protective effect. Because HBIG was given within 7 days of exposure in some studies showing protection,[143,392,393] administration of the first HBIG dose within this period has been recommended by the Public Health Service Advisory Committee on Immunization Practices.[394] An unexpected finding in one study,[391] however, was apparent protection even when HBIG was not given until several weeks after the postulated time of exposure. On the other hand, there is evidence that when HBIG or ISG is given within 48 hours of needle stick exposure, it is more effective than when given 3–7 days after exposure.[363] Thus, rapid administration of HBIG after exposure to HBV appears to be important for maximum protection.

The dose of HBIG required for effective postexposure treatment is not precisely known, but a dose shown to protect adults in two different controlled trials was 0.07 ml/kg.[143,391–393]

There is no evidence in the studies to date suggesting that ISG or HBIG can transmit HBV infection or can increase the rate at which subsequent primary infections become persistent.

Postexposure Immunization of Children and Adults. A major indication for HBIG is after a single acute, direct exposure to HBV, such as occurs with accidental needle stick, mucous membrane, or broken skin contact with blood or other body fluids known to contain HBsAg, or after sexual intercourse or oral exchange of saliva, such as by kissing or sharing a toothbrush with a partner who is HBsAg positive. If HBIG is not available, ISG containing detectable anti-HBs should be used after such exposure. Patients who are known to have serum anti-HBs or anti-HBc are resistant to infection and need not be given prophylaxis after exposure. Similarly, individuals who are HBsAg positive do not benefit. Because of the apparent benefit of immune globulin administration as soon as possible after exposure, a delay to test an exposed individual for anti-HBs is not recommended and ISG should be rapidly administered after an appropriate exposure to HBV. If test results later reveal that the exposed individual was susceptible to HBV (i.e., anti-HBs negative), administration of HBIG can be considered, although it probably offers little additional benefit if the ISG originally given contained a moderate anti-HBs titer. Similarly, to delay passive immunization after significant exposure to a patient with evidence of acute or chronic hepatitis of an unknown type in order to attempt to identify a viral agent by serologic testing is not recommended. Again, ISG should be rapidly given to the exposed individual. Such treatment should provide protection against HBV as well as HAV. If continued long-term exposure to HBV is expected for the exposed individual, active immunization with vaccine should be started in addition to ISG or HBIG administration.

Postexposure Immunization of Newborns. An important setting for postexposure immunization is in neonates born to HBsAg-positive mothers. Such infants are commonly infected, especially when the mothers are HBeAg positive, and 90 percent or more of infected infants appear to become chronic carriers.[161,162,395–397] Several studies have shown that rapid administration of high doses of HBIG after birth to infants with HBeAg-positive carrier mothers reduces the infection rate by 70–80 percent.[396–398] When low doses are administered and when the administration of the first dose is delayed beyond 48 hours, little or no protection is observed.[399] A significant fraction of infants protected by HBIG in the neonatal period are infected later when passive antibodies disappear.[396,400] The use of vaccine alone shortly after birth has been shown to give a similar level of protection.[401] Almost 100 percent of newborn infants have anti-HBs responses to the vaccine.[311,401]

When HBIG and vaccine were used together in the neonatal period, 94 percent protection was achieved.[311] One-half of the few infants who became chronic carriers in that study had moderate HBsAg titers in cord blood, suggesting intrauterine infection, a condition not likely to be reversed by immunization after birth. It is currently recommended that 0.5 ml HBIG be administered intramuscularly to infants in the delivery room after birth to an HBsAg-positive mother and that 0.5 ml Heptavax-B or Recombivax-HB be given intramuscularly at the same time or within the first week after delivery.[378] The second and third vaccine doses should be given at 1 and 6 months, respectively. Although the risk of infection is greatest when mothers are HBeAg positive, a small risk for infants of anti-HBe-positive carrier mothers remains, and these infants should be managed the same way. All pregnant women from groups with a high prevalence of HBV infection (e.g., those born in Asia or other high-prevalence geographic areas) should be routinely tested for HBsAg so that newborn infants of positive mothers can be appropriately immunized after birth.

Environmental and Other Control Measures

Among the most important and effective approaches to the control of HBV are the use of environmental barriers and personal hygiene, which effectively prevent virus transmission. As described above under "Epidemiology," the principal modes of transmission that must be interrupted in the United States appear to be (*1*) direct percutaneous inoculation of infective blood or serum (e.g., by administration of contaminated blood or blood products, tattooing, ear piercing, acupuncture, drug abuse, accidental needle sticks by hospital personnel); (*2*) contamination of mucosal surfaces by infective blood or serum (e.g., by mouth, pipetting, splashes in eyes or transfer from hands to eyes or mouth) or by other infective secretions (e.g., by sexual or other activity involving semen or saliva); and (*3*) transfer of such infective material via vectors or environmental surfaces into skin breaks or mucous membranes (e.g., by contaminated objects such as toothbrushes, toys, baby bottles, cups or glasses, rubber gloves, razors, towels, or hospital equipment). Feces and urine are not important sources of HBV in the absence of gastrointestinal bleeding. The ability to identify infected patients and susceptible individuals through serologic testing permits the application of containment measures in situations where the risk of transmission is recognized. Education of HBsAg-positive individuals and their contacts, and of high-risk populations such as health care personnel, about common sources of HBV, routes of transmission, and methods of preventing transmission are essential for the most effective prevention of infections through environmental and personal hygiene control measures. Disease surveillance and consistent case reporting are also important to permit recognition of changes in epidemiologic trends so that communitywide control measures can be rationally applied.

Several methods have been recommended for disinfection or sterilization of contaminated material.[402,403] Heat is the treatment of choice for materials that tolerate the required conditions. Boiling in water (100°C for 10 minutes), autoclaving at 121°C and 15 psi for 15 minutes, or dry heat (160°C) for 2 hours exceed the conditions known to inactivate HBV. Alternative methods presumed to be effective because they have been shown to destroy HBsAg antigenicity or are cidal for bacterial endospores (although not demonstrated to render HBV noninfective) are solutions of sodium hypochlorite, 0.5–1.0% (5,000 to 10,000 ppm chlorine) for 30 minutes, 40% aqueous formalin (16% aqueous formaldehyde) for 12 hours, or gas sterilization with ethylene oxide. Very active detergents such as sodium dodecyl sulfate (1% SDS), which completely disrupt Dane particles and are cidal for most viruses, are also undoubtedly cidal for HBV. Thorough mechanical cleaning of surfaces to remove adherent material that might interfere with chemical disinfection is also important.

The Committee on Viral Hepatitis, Division of Medical Sciences, National Academy of Sciences, the National Research Council, and the Public Health Service Advisory Committee on Immunization Practices have made recommendations for minimizing transmission in specific settings.[402]

Households. Spouses and other intimate contacts of HBsAg-positive patients with acute or persistent infection appear to be at greatest risk for infection in households. All household members should be informed about sources of HBV, routes of transmission, and methods of personal hygiene to prevent the spread of infection. The need for frequent handwashing; the proper disposal or decontamination of objects contaminated with blood, urine, feces, saliva, sputum, nasal secretions, and so on of infected patients; the importance of not sharing toothbrushes, thermometers, razors, eating utensils, towels, washcloths, food from the same dish, or other personal items; and the risk of direct contact with blood, saliva, semen, and other body fluids of the HBsAg-positive patient should be emphasized. Close (e.g., sexual) household contacts, including all children, who are anti-HBs negative should receive the HBV vaccine.

General Patient Care Hospital Areas. HBsAg-positive patients, whether acutely or persistently infected with HBV, need not be isolated or confined to hospital rooms. However, blood and other body fluids likely to be infective, as well as instruments, bed clothes, and other objects contaminated with potentially infective material, must be handled in a manner that prevents transmission and appropriately decontaminated. Gloves should be worn by personnel when drawing blood from HBsAg-positive patients or when handling potentially contaminated objects. Additional protective clothing such as gowns, masks, and glasses should be worn for procedures that could result in splashing of potentially infective material. Whether or not gloves are worn, careful handwashing should be done after any contact with HBsAg-positive patients or contaminated objects before contact with other patients. HBsAg-positive and HBsAg-negative patients should not share personal objects. Items such as tourniquets, blood pressure cuffs, marking pens used on the skin, antiseptics, skin care lotion, and so on should not be used on HBsAg-negative patients after use on HBsAg-positive patients unless they are first decontaminated. Potentially infective specimens such as blood from HBsAg-positive patients should be appropriately labeled to alert all who handle them of their infective nature. Bed linens, towels, and environmental surfaces in patient rooms, such as the tops of eating tables, should be decontaminated before being used for HBsAg-negative patients. Any spill of blood or other potentially infective material should be cleaned up immediately in a manner that contains and inactivates the virus. Susceptible (e.g., anti-HBs-negative) hospital personnel or others should be given HBIG only after a recognized episode of direct percutaneous or mucous membrane exposure, as described above. The above preventive measures should be discontinued only after patients become HBsAg negative, at which time they can be considered noninfective. The same general approaches should be used with HBsAg-positive patients in nursing homes and institutions for the mentally retarded.

Hospital Patient Care Areas with Special High Risk. Special hospital patient care areas where the risk of HBV infection is high for patients and staff, such as hemodialysis units, may require procedures in addition to those outlined for general patient care areas to control the spread of infection. Patient care personnel assigned to these hospital areas, as well as those assigned to care for HBsAg-positive patients in any hospital area, should be vaccinated, whether anti-HBs positive by virtue of past infection or HBsAg positive and not at risk for HBV infection. Education of patients and staff about sources of HBV, routes of transmission, and methods of preventing spread is particularly important in high-risk hospital units. Geographic separation of HBsAg-positive and HBsAg-negative patients has been quite successful in preventing the spread of HBV to staff and susceptible patients in many hemodialysis units. Use of separate wards and dialysis rooms, separate dialysis machines, and all other pieces of equipment, proper decontamination of nondisposable items of equipment, use of disposable equipment or materials when possible, use of separate nursing personnel for HBsAg-positive and -negative patient groups, and vaccination of susceptible patients with a high risk of infection may be necessary to eliminate the possibility of spread in certain high-risk areas.

Laboratory Processing of Infective Material. Clinical serology, chemistry, hematology, and pathology laboratories and research laboratories handling infective material should employ procedures that reduce the risk of HBV infection of personnel. Mouth pipetting, smoking, and eating should be forbidden in laboratories handling HBsAg-positive material. Gloves should be used to handle potentially infective material. In addition, gowns and masks should be used during any procedures in which splashing might occur (e.g., performing autopsies). HBsAg-positive specimens should be appropriately packaged, labeled, and confined to specified areas of the laboratory (e.g., benches, refrigerators, freezers) designated for infective material, and these areas should be thoroughly cleaned and disinfected regularly. None of the above procedures to contain HBV in the laboratory can substitute, however, for careful technique and appropriate personal habits (e.g., handwashing) to avoid spreading virus. Personnel working with potentially infective material in a laboratory should be vaccinated against HBV.

Management of Persistently Infected Persons with Special Risk for Transmission to Others

HBsAg-positive persons in certain occupations (e.g., health care personnel) and other circumstances may represent a special risk for transmission of HBV to contacts. To prevent transmission from such individuals with acute hepatitis B, it is desirable to restrict their activity and contact with others until they are HBsAg negative. Persistent HBV infection, on the other hand, is not necessarily a reason to restrict an individual's activities, although clearly personal precautions should be taken.

Health Care Personnel. Persistently infected health care personnel with direct patient contact, such as dentists, nurses, physicians, and some technicians, should not be restricted from patient contact unless transmission to patients is documented. As discussed above under "Epidemiology," most health care workers appear to represent little risk to patient contacts, although some appear to have spread infection to their patients. The presence of high blood concentrations of Dane particles and HBeAg appears to correlate with the risk of transmission. The potential for transmission by any carrier must be recognized, however. It is important that such persons understanding the sources of HBV and the routes of transmission, and personal procedures and practices should be used to reduce the chances of transmission. Scrupulous aseptic technique, avoidance of personal hand injuries, and use of gloves for minor surgery, blood drawing, dental procedures, wound dressing, and so on should be practiced. Persistently infected individuals should be tested for HBsAg at 6-month intervals, since they may become HBsAg negative (and thus no longer infective to others) at any time. Some surveillance of their patient contacts to determine whether virus transmission occurs is desirable. If they are implicated in transmission, some restrictive measures (e.g., limiting or eliminating some types of procedures or patient contact) may be required.

Food Handlers. Although no cases of virus transmission from HBV-infected food handlers have been documented, it is reasonable to educate any such persistently infected personnel about the sources of HBV, the routes of transmission, and the need to practice good personal hygiene, frequent handwashing, and avoidance of hand injuries. Food handlers with acute hepatitis B should be barred from work until they become HBsAg negative.

Elimination of Infective Blood Products

Among the most important ways of preventing hepatitis B is to eliminate infective blood used for transfusions and blood products. Since 1972 the U.S. Food and Drug Administration has required that blood banks test all blood donors for HBsAg. Although such testing eliminates much of the infective blood, evidence shows that even the most sensitive tests for HBsAg, such as RIA, do not identify a significant small number of blood donors whose blood transmits HBV to recipients.[178–180] The exclusive use of blood from volunteer donors also significantly reduces the incidence of post-transfusion hepatitis compared with the use of blood from paid donors (e.g., Ref. 404). The shift from paid to volunteer donors and HBsAg testing have reduced post-transfusion HBV infection by 80 percent or more in the past few years, and 80–90 percent of post-transfusion hepatitis now appears to be due to one or more of the undefined agents that make up non-A, non-B hepatitis.[148,179,404] Methods for eliminating the remaining blood units infective for HBV and not eliminated by the above measures must be developed.

REFERENCES

1. Lurman A. Eine icterus epidemic. Berl Klin Wochenscher. 1855;22:20.
2. Flaum A, Malmros H, Persson E. Eine nosocomiale icterus epidemic. Acta Med Scand. 1926;(Suppl 16):544.
3. Bigger JW, Dubi SD. Jaundice in syphilitics under treatment. Lancet. 1943;1:457.
4. MacCallum FO. Transmission of arsenotherapy jaundice by blood: Failure with feces and nasopharyngeal washings. Lancet. 1945;1:342.
5. McNatty AS. Great Britain Ministry Health Report of Chief Medical Officer, Annual Report. London;1937.
6. Propert SA. Hepatitis after prophylactic serum. Br Med J. 1938;2:677.
7. Beeson PB, Chesney G, McFarlan AM. Hepatitis following injection of mumps convalescent plasma. Lancet. 1944;1(24):814.
8. Findlay GM, MacCallum FO. Note on acute hepatitis and yellow fever immunization. Trans Soc Trop Med Hyg. 1937;31:297.
9. Anonymous. Jaundice following yellow fever vaccine. JAMA. 1942;119:1110.
10. Beeson PB. Jaundice occurring one to four months after transfusion of blood or plasma. JAMA. 1943;121:1332.
11. Morgan HW, Williamson DAJ. Jaundice following administration of human blood products. Br Med J. 1943;1:750.
12. Paul RJ, Havens WP, Sabin AB, et al. Transmission experiments in serum jaundice and infectious hepatitis. JAMA. 1945;128:911.
13. Neefe JR, Gellis SS, Stokes J Jr. Homologous serum hepatitis and infectious (epidemic) hepatitis: Studies in volunteers bearing on immunological and other characteristics of the etiological agents. Am J Med. 1946;1:3.
14. Krugman S, Giles JP, Hammon J. Infectious hepatitis: Evidence for two distinctive clinical, epidemiological and immunological types of infection. JAMA. 1967;200:365.
15. Havens WP. Experiment in cross immunity between infectious and homologous serum jaundice. Proc Soc Exp Biol Med. 1945;59:148.
16. Neefe JR, Stokes J, Gellis SS. Homologous serum hepatitis and infectious (epidemic) hepatitis: Experimental study of immunity and cross immunity in volunteers. Am J Med Sci. 1945;210:561.
17. Krugman S, Giles JP. Viral hepatitis: New light on an old disease. JAMA. 1970;212:1019.
18. Neefe JR, Stokes J Jr, Reinhold JG. Oral administration to volunteers of feces from patients with homologous serum hepatitis and infectious (epidemic) hepatitis. Am J Med Sci. 1945;210:29.
19. Havens WP. Period of infectivity of patients with homologous serum jaundice and routes of infection in this disease. J Exp Med. 1946;83:441.
20. Stokes J, Berk JE, Malamut LL. The carrier state of viral hepatitis. JAMA. 1954;154:1059.
21. Voegt H. Zur Aetiologie der Hepatitis Epidemica. Muchen Med Wochenschr. 1942;89:76.
22. Neefe RJ, Norris RF, Reinhold JG, et al. Carriers of hepatitis virus in blood and viral hepatitis in whole blood recipients: 1. Studies on donors suspected as carriers of hepatitis virus and as sources of post-transfusion viral hepatitis. JAMA. 1954;154:1066.
23. Blumberg BS, Alter HJ, Visnich S. A "new" antigen in leukemia sera. JAMA. 1965;191:541.
24. Blumberg BS, Gerstley JS, Hungerford DA, et al. A serum antigen (Australia antigen) in Down's syndrome leukemia and hepatitis. Ann Intern Med. 1967;66:924.
25. Okachi K, Murakami S. Observations on Australia antigen in Japanese. Vox Sang. 1968;15:374.
26. Prince AM. An antigen detected in the blood during the incubation period of serum hepatitis. Proc Natl Acad Sci USA. 1968;60:814.
27. Szmuness W. Hepatocellular carcinoma and the hepatitis B virus: Evidence for a causal association. Proc Med Virol. 1978;24:40.
28. Feinstone SM, Kapikian AZ, Purcell RH, et al. Transfusion associated hepatitis not due to viral hepatitis type A or B. N Engl J Med. 1975;282:767.
29. Knodell RG, Conrad ME, Dienstag JL, et al. Etiological spectrum of post-transfusion hepatitis. Gastroenterology. 1975;69:1278.
30. Alter HL, Purcell RH, Feinstone SM, et al. NonA/nonB hepatitis: A review and interim report of an ongoing prospective study. In: Vyas GN, Cohen SN, Schmid R, eds. Viral Hepatitis: A Contemporary Assessment of Etiology, Epidemiology, Pathogenesis and Prevention. Philadelphia: Franklin Institute Press; 1978:359.
31. Robinson, WS. Genetic variation among hepatitis B and related viruses. Ann NY Acad Sci. 1980;354:371–8.
32. Robinson WS, Marion PL, Feitelson M, et al. The hepadna virus group: Hepatitis B and related viruses. In: Szmuness W, Alter HJ, JE Maynard, eds. Viral Hepatitis. Philadelphia: Franklin Institute Press; 1982:57–68.
33. Summers J, Smolec JM, Snyder R. A virus similar to human hepatitis B virus associated with hepatitis and hepatoma in woodchucks. Proc Natl Acad Sci USA. 1978;75:4533–7.
34. Marion PL, Oshiro L, Regnery DC, et al. A virus in Beechey ground squirrels that is related to hepatitis B virus of man. Proc Natl Acad Sci USA. 1980;77:2941–5.
35. Mason WS, Seal G, Summers J. Virus of Pekin ducks with structural and biological relatedness to human hepatitis B virus. J Virol. 1980;36:829–36.
36. Gust ID, Burnell CJ, Coulepis AG, et al. Taxanomic classification of hepatitis B virus. Intervirology. Intervirol. 1986;25:14–29.
37. Alter HJ, Blumberg BS. Further studies on a "new human isoprecipitin system (Australia antigen). Blood. 1966;27:297.
38. LeBouvier GL, McCollum RW. Australia (hepatitis associated) antigen: Physicochemical and immunological characteristics. Adv Virus Res. 1970;16:357.
39. Bayer ME, Blumberg BS, Werner B. Particles associated with Australia antigen in the sera of patients with leukemia, Down's syndrome and hepatitis. Nature (Lond.) 1968;218:1057–9.
40. Dane DS, Cameron CH, Briggs M. Virus-like particles in serum of patients with Australia antigen associated hepatitis. Lancet. 1970;2:695–8.
41. Almeida JD, Rubenstein D, Stott EJ. New antigen antibody system in Australia antigen positive hepatitis. Lancet. 1971;2:1225–7.
42. Robinson WS, Clayton DA, Greenman RL. DNA of a human hepatitis B virus candidate. J Virol. 1975;14:384–91.
43. Gerlich W, Robinson WS. Hepatitis B virus contains protein attached to the 5′ terminus of its complete DNA strand. Cell. 1980;21:801.
44. Kaplan PM, Greenman RL, Gerin JL, et al. DNA polymerase associated with human hepatitis B antigen. J Virol. 1973;12:995–1005.
45. Robinson WS, Greenman RL. DNA polymerase in the core of the human hepatitis B virus candidate. J Virol. 1974;13:1231–6.

46. Albin C, Robinson WS. Protein kinase activity in hepatitis B virus. J Virol. 1980;34:297–302.
47. Takahashi K, Akahane Y, Gotanda T, et al. Demonstration of hepatitis e antigen in the core of Dane particles. J Immunol. 1979;122:275–9.
48. Barker LF, Murray R. Relationship of virus dose to incubation time of clinical hepatitis and time of appearance of hepatitis-associated antigen. Am J Med Sci. 1972;263:27.
49. Scullard G, Greenberg HB, Smith JL, et al. Antiviral treatment of chronic hepatitis B virus infection: Infectious virus cannot be detected in patient serum after permanent responses to treatment. Hepatology. 1982;2:39.
50. Shikata T, Karasawa T, Abe K, et al. Hepatitis B e antigens and infectivity of hepatitis B virus. J Infect Dis. 1977;136:571.
51. Kim, CY, Tilles JG. Purification and biophysical characterization of hepatitis B antigen. J Clin Invest. 1970;52:1176.
52. Redeker AG, Hopkins CE, Jackson B, et al. A controlled study of the safety of pooled plasma stored in the liquid state of 30–32°C for 6 months. Transfusion. 1968;8:60.
53. Murray R, Die Fenbach WC. Effect of heat on the agent of homolgous serum hepatitis. Proc Soc Exp Biol Med. 1953;84:230.
54. Gellis SS, Neefe JR, Stokes J Jr, et al. Chemical, clinical and immunological studies on the products of human plasma fractionation. XXXVI. Inactivation of the virus of homologous serum hepatitis in solution of normal serum albumin by means of heat. J Clin Invest. 1948;27:239.
55. Soulier JP, Blatix C, Courouce AM, et al. Prevention of virus B hepatitis (SH virus). Am J Dis Child.
56. Shikata T, Karasawa T, Abe K, et al. Incomplete inactivation of hepatitis B virus after heat treatment at 60°C for 10 hours. J Infect Dis. 1978;138:242–4.
57. Krugman S, Giles JP, Hammond J. Hepatitis virus: Effect of heat infectivity and antigenicity of MS-1 and MS-2 strains. J Infect Dis. 1970;122:432–6.
58. Wewalka F. Zur epidemiologie des ikterus bei der antisyphlitischen behandlung. Schweiz Z Allg Pathol. 1953;16:307–12.
59. Salaman MH, Williams DI, King AJ, et al. Prevention of jaundice resulting from antisyphilitic treatment. Lancet. 1944;2:7–8.
60. LeBouvier GL. The heterogenicity of Australia antigen. J Infect Dis. 1971;123:671–5.
61. Bancroft WH, Mundo FK, Russel PK. Detection of additional determinants of hepatitis B antigen. J Immunol. 1972;109:842–8.
62. Courouce-Pauty AM, Soulier JP. Further data on HBs antigen subtypes -geographical distribution. Vox Sang. 1974;27:533–49.
63. Courouce AM, Holland PV, Muller JY, et al. HBsAg antigen subtypes. Proceedings of the International Workshop on HBs antigen subtypes. Bibl Haematol. 1976;42:1–158.
64. Tiolais P, Pourcel C, de Jean A. Nature. 1985;317:489–95.
65. Heerman KH, Goldman U, Schwarts W, et al. J Virol. 1984;52:396.
66. Thornton GB, Moriarty AM, Milich D, et al. Protection of chimpanzees from hepatitis B virus infection after immunization with synthetic peptides. Cold Spring Harbor Vaccine Meeting. 1988.
67. Itoh Y, Taka E, Ohnuma H, et al. Proc Natl Acad Sci USA. 1986;83:9174–8.
68. Gerin JL, Alexander H, Shih J, et al. Proc Natl Acad Sci USA. 1983;80:2365.
69. Hruska JF, Robinson WS. The proteins of hepatitis B Dane particle cores. J Med Virol. 1977;1:119–31.
70. Budkowska A, Shih JWK, Gerin JL. Immunochemistry and polypeptide composition of hepatitis B core antigen (HBcAg). J Immunol. 1977;118:1300–50.
71. Magnius LO, Espmark JA. New specificities in Australia antigen-positive sera distinct from Le Bouvier determinants. J Immunol. 1972;109:1017–21.
72. Magnius LO. Characterization of a new antigen–antibody system associated with hepatitis B. Clin Exp Immunol. 1975;20:209–16
73. Neurath AR, Strick N. Association of hepatitis B e-antigen (HBeAg) determinants with the core of Dane particles. J Gen Virol. 1979;42:645–9.
74. Budkowska A, Kalinowska B, Nowoslowski A. Identification of two HBeAg subspecificities revealed by chemical treatment and enzymatic digestion of liver-derived HBcAg. J Immunol. 1979;123:1415–6.
75. Ohori H, Onodera S, Ishida N. Demonstration of hepatitis B e antigen (HBeAg) in association with intact Dane particles. J Gen Virol. 1979;43:423–7.
76. Hindman SH, Gravelle CR, Murphy BL, et al. "e" antigen, Dane particles, and serum DNA polymerase activity in HBsAg carriers. Ann Intern Med. 1976;85:458–60.
77. Alter HJ, Seeff LB, Kaplan PM, et al. Type B hepatitis: The infectivity of blood positive for e antigen and DNA polymerase after accidental needlestick exposure. N Engl J Med. 1976;295:909–13.
78. Takahashi K, Imai M, Tsuda F, et al. Association of Dane particles with e antigen in the serum of asymptomatic carriers of hepatitis B surface antigen. J Immunol. 1976;117:102–5.
79. Nordenfeldt E, Andren-Sandberg M. Dane particle associated DNA polymerase and e antigen: Relation to chronic hepatitis among carriers of hepatitis B surface antigen. J Infect Dis. 1976;134:85–9.
80. Summers JA, O'Connell A, Millman I. Genome of hepatitis B virus: Restriction enzyme cleavage and structure of DNA extracted from Dane particles. Proc Natl Acad Sci USA. 1975;72:4597–4601.
81. Landers TA, Greenberg, HB, Robinson WS. Structure of hepatitis B Dane particle DNA and nature of the endogenous DNA polymerase reaction. J Virol. 1977;23:368–76.
82. Hruska JF, Clayton DA, Rubenstein JLR, et al. Structure of hepatitis B Dane particle DNA before and after the Dane particle DNA polymerase reaction. J Virol. 1977;21:666–72.
83. Sattler F, Robinson WS. Hepatitis B viral DNA molecules have cohesive ends. J Virol. 1979;32:226–33.
84. Siddiqui A, Sattler FR, Robinson WS. Restriction endonuclease cleavage map and location of unique features of the DNA of hepatitis B virus, subtype adw_2. Proc Natl Acad Sci USA. 1979;76:4664–8.
85. Molnar-Kimber K, Summers J, Taylor J, et al. Protein covalently bound to minus-strand DNA intermediates of duck hepatitis B virus. J Virol. 1983;45:165.
86. Galibert F, Mandart E, Fitoussi F, et al. Nucleotide sequence of hepatitis B virus genome (subtype ayw) cloned in *E. coli*. Nature (Lond.) 1979;281:646–50.
87. Valenzuela P, Quiroga M, Zaldivar J, et al. The nucleotide sequence of the hepatitis B genome and the identification of the major viral genes. In: Fields B, Jaenisch R, Fox CF, eds. Animal Virus Genetics. New York: Academic Press; 1980:57–70.
88. Barker LF, Chisari F, McGrath PP, et al. Transmission of type B viral hepatitis to chimpanzees. J Infect Dis. 1973;127:648.
89. Gudat F, Bianchi O, Sonnabend W. Pattern of core and surface expression in liver tissue reflects state of specific immune response in hepatitis B. Lab Invest. 1975;32:1.
90. Ray MB, Desmet VI, Bradburne AF. Distribution patterns of hepatitis B surface antigen (HBsAg in liver of hepatitis patients). Gastroenterology. 1976;71:462.
91. Almedia JD, Watterson AP, Trowel JM, et al. The finding of virus-like particles in two Australia-antigen-positive human livers. Microbios. 1970;2:145–53.
92. Huang SA. Hepatitis associated antigen hepatitis: An electron microscopic study of virus-like particles in liver cells. Am J Pathol. 1971;64:783.
93. Camamia F, DeBac C, Ricci G. Virus-like particles within hepatocytes of Australia antigen carriers. Am J Dis Child. 1972;123:309.
94. Mason WS, Aldrich C, Summers J, et al. Asymmetric replication of duck hepatitis B virus DNA in liver cells (free minus-strand DNA). Proc Natl Acad Sci USA. 1982;79:3997–4001.
95. Summers J, Mason WS. Replication of the genome of a hepatitis B-like virus by reverse transcription of an RNA intermediate. Cell. 1982;29:403–15.
96. Miller R, Robinson WS. Hepatitis B virions from plasma and particles from liver of infected patients synthesize DNA of DNA-RNA hybrid molecules. Virology. In press.
97. Miller RH, Robinson WS. Hepatitis B viral DNA forms in infected liver. Virology. In press.
98. Miller RH, Robinson WS. Common evolutionary origin of hepatitis B virus and retroviruses. Proc Natl Acad Sci. USA. 1986;23:2531–5.
99. Kam W, Rall L, Smuckler E, et al. Hepatitis B viral DNA in liver and serum of asymptomatic carriers. Proc Natl Acad Sci USA. 1982;79:7522–6.
100. Nowoslawski A, Krawczyuski K, Brzosko WJ. Tissue localization of Australia antigen immune complexes in acute and chronic hepatitis and liver cirrhosis. Am J Pathol. 1972;68:31–48.
101. Shikata T. Australia antigen in liver tissue. Jpn J Exp Med. 1973;43:231–45.
102. Murphy BL, Peterson JM, Ebert JW. Immunofluorescent localization of hepatitis B antigens in chimpanzee tissues. Intervirology. 1975;6:207–11.
103. Johnson PJ, Wansbrough-Jones MH, Portmann B. Familial HBsAg positive hepatoma: Treatment with orthotopic liver transplantation and specific immunoglobulin. Br Med J. 1978;1:216.
104. Hoefs JC, Renner IG, Ashcavai M, et al. Hepatitis B surface antigen in pancreatic and biliary secretion. Gastroenterology. 1980;79:191–4.
105. Karasawa T, Tsukagoshi S, Yoshimura M, et al. Light microscopic localization of hepatitis B virus antigens in the human pancreas: Possibility of multiplication of hepatitis B virus in the human pancreas. Gastroenterology. 1981;81:998–1005.
106. Romet-Lemonne JL, McLane MF, Elfassi E, et al. Hepatitis B virus infection in cultured human lymphoblastoid cells. Science. 1983;221:667.
107. Lie-Injo LE, Balasegaram M, Lopez CG, et al. Hepatitis B virus DNA in liver and white blood cells of patients with hepatoma. DNA. 1983;2:301.
108. Blumberg BS, Sutnick AI, London WT. Hepatitis and leukemia: Their relation to Australia antigen. Bull NY Acad Med. 1968;44:1566.
109. Hirschman RJ, Shulman NR, Barker LF. Virus-like particles in sera of patients with infectious and serum hepatitis. JAMA. 1969;208:1667.
110. Maynard JE, Hartwell WV, Berquist KR. Hepatitis associated antigen in chimpanzees. J Infect Dis. 1971;126:660.
111. World Health Organization. Viral hepatitis: Report of a scientific group. WHO Tech Rep Ser. 1973;512.
112. Lichter EA. Chimpanzee antibodies to Australia antigen. Nature. 1969;224:810.
113. Prince AM. Infection of chimpanzees with hepatitis B virus. In: Vyas GN, Perkins HA, Schmid R, eds. Hepatitis and Blood Transfusions. New York: Grune and Stratton; 1972:403.
114. Markenson JH, Gerety RJ, Hoofnagle JH. Effects of cyclophosphamide on hepatitis B virus infection and challenge in chimpanzees. J Infect Dis. 1975;131:79.
115. Bancroft WH, Snitbhan R, Scott RM, et al. Transmission of hepatitis B virus to gibbons by exposure to human saliva containing hepatitis B surface antigen. J Infect Dis. 1977;135:79.
116. London TW, Milman I, Sutnick AI. Transmission, replication and passage

of Australia antigen in African green monkeys (vervets). Clin Res. 1970;18:636.
117. London WT, Alter HJ, Lander J. Serial transmission in rhesus monkeys of an agent related to hepatitis-associated antigen. J Infect Dis. 1972;125:382.
118. Barker LF, Maynard JE, Purcell RH, et al. Viral hepatitis, type B, in experimental animals. Am J Med Sci. 1975;270:189.
119. Krugman S, Overby LR, Mushahwar IK, et al: Viral hepatitis, type B: Studies on natural history and prevention reexamined. N Engl Med J. 1979;300:101–6.
120. Hoofnagle JH, Seeff LB, Bales ZB, et al. Serologic responses in hepatitis B. In: Vyas GN, Cohen SN, Schmid T, eds. Viral Hepatitis: A Contemporary Assessment of Etiology, Epidemiology, Pathogenesis and Prevention. Philadelphia: Franklin Institute Press; 1978:219–42.
121. Shulman RN. Hepatitis-associated antigen. Am J Med. 1971;49:669–92.
122. Takahashi K, Fukuda M, Baba K, et al. Determination of e antigen and antibody to e by means of passive hemagglutination method. J Immunol. 1977;119:1556–9.
123. Aikawa T, Sairenji H, Furuta S, et al. Seroconversion from hepatitis B e antigen to anti-HBe in acute hepatitis B virus infection. N Engl J Med. 1978;298:439–41.
124. Fields HA, Bradley DW, Davis C, et al. Radioimmunoassay for the detection of hepatitis B e antigen (HBeAg) and its antibody (anti-HBe). J Immunol. 1978;121:273.
125. Myakawa Y, Akahane Y, Gotand T. Application of microtiter solid phase radioimmunoassay to the determination of hepatitis B "e" antigen. J Immunol. 1979;122:273.
126. Ling C, Mushahwar IK, Overby LR, et al. Hepatitis B e-antigen and its correlation with other serologic markers in chimpanzees. Inf Immun. 1979;24:352–6.
127. Aldershvile J, Frosner GG, Nielsen JO, et al. Hepatitis B e antigen and antibody radioimmunoassay in acute hepatitis B surface antigen-positive hepatitis. J Infect Dis. 1980;141:293.
128. Kaplan PM, Gerin JL, Alter HJ. Hepatitis B-specific DNA polymerase activity during post-transfusion hepatitis. Nature. 1974;249:762.
129. Krugman S, Hoofnagle JH, Gerety RJ, et al. Viral hepatitis type B: DNA polymerase activity and antibody to hepatitis B core antigen. N Engl J Med. 1974;290:1331–5.
130. Hansson BG. Age and sex-related distribution of antibodies to hepatitis B surface and core antigens in Swedish population. Acta Pathol Microbiol Scand Sect B. 1976;84:342.
131. Hansson BG. Persistence of antibody to hepatitis B core antigen. J Clin Microbiol. 1977;6:209.
132. Brzosko WJ, Mikulska B, Cianciara J, et al. Immunoglobulin classes of antibody to hepatitis B core antigen. J Infect Dis. 1975;132:1–5.
133. Cohen BJ. The IgM antibody responses to the core antigen of hepatitis B virus. J Med Virol. 1978;3:141–50.
134. Neimeijer P, Gips CH. Antibodies and the infectivity of serum in hepatitis B. N Engl J Med. 1978;299:958.
135. Gerlich WH, Luer W, Thomssen R. Diagnosis of acute and inapparent hepatitis B virus infections by measurement of IgM antibody to hepatitis B core antigen. J Infect Dis. 1980;142:95–101.
136. Gocke DJ. Extrahepatic manifestations of viral hepatitis. Am J Med Sci. 1975;270:49–52.
137. Almeida JD, Waterson AP. Immune complexes in hepatitis. Lancet. 1969;2:983–6.
138. Madalinski L, Bragiel I. HBsAg immune complexes in the course of infection with hepatitis B virus. Clin Exp Immunol. 1979;36:371–8.
139. Lambert PH, Tribollet E, Celada A, et al. Quantitation of immunoglobulin associated HBs antigen in patients with acute and chronic hepatitis, in healthy carriers, and in polyarteritis nodosa. J Clin Lab Immunol. 1980;3:1–8.
140. Lander JJ, Giles JP, Purcell RH. Viral hepatitis type B (MS-2) strain): Detection of antibody after primary infection. N Engl J Med. 1970;283:303.
141. Barker LF, Maynard JE, Purcell RH, et al. Hepatitis B virus infection in chimpanzess: Titration of subtypes. J Infect Dis. 1975;132:451.
142. Purcell RH, Gerin JL. Hepatitis B subunit vaccine: A preliminary report of safety and efficacy tests in chimpanzees. Am J Med Sci. 1975;270:395–9.
143. Seef LB, Wright EC, Zimmerman HJ, et al. Type B hepatitis after needle-stick exposure: Prevention with hepatitis B immune globulin. A final report of the Veterans Administration Cooperative Study. Ann Intern Med. 1978;88:285.
144. Brechot C, Hadchouel M, Scotto J, et al. State of hepatitis B virus DNA in hepatocytes of patients with hepatitis B surface antigen-positive and -negative liver disease. Proc Natl Acad Sci. 1981;78:3906–10.
145. Hoofnagle JH. Hepatitis B surface antigen (HBsAg) and antibody (anti-HBs). In: Bianchi L, Gerok W, Sickinger K, et al, eds,. Virus and the Liver. Lancaster, UK: MTP Press; 1980:27.
146. Nielsen JO, Nielsen MH, Elling P. Differential distribution of Australia-antigen-associated particles in patients with liver disease and normal carriers. N Engl J Med. 1973;288:484.
147. Robinson WS. DNA and DNA polymerase in the core of Dane particles. Am J Med Sci. 1975;270:151.
148. Scullard GH, Pollard RB, Smith JL, et al. Antiviral treatment of chronic hepatitis B virus infection. I. Changes in viral markers with interferon combined with adenine arabinoside. J Infect Dis. 1981;143:772.
149. Greenberg HB, Pollard RB, Lutwixk LI, et al. Effect of human leukocyte interferon on hepatitis B virus infection in patients with chronic active hepatitis. N Engl J Med. 1976;295:517.
150. Bonino F, Hoyer B, Moriarty A, et al. Hepatitis B virus DNA in the sera of HBsAg carriers: A marker of active HBV replication in the liver. Gastroenterology. 1980;79:1009.
151. Kryger P, Mathiesen LR, Aldershvile J, et al. Presence and meaning of anti-HBc IgM as determined by ELISA in patients with acute type B hepatitis and healthy HBsAg carriers. Hepatology. 1981;1:233–7.
152. Aldershvile J, Skinhoj P, Frosner GG, et al. The expression pattern of hepatitis B e antigen and antibody in different ethnic and clinical groups of hepatitis B surface antigen carriers. J Infect Dis. 1980;142:18–22.
153. Eleftheriou N, Heathcoate J, Thomas HC, et al. Incidence and clinical significance of e antigen and antibody in acute and chronic liver diseases. Lancet. 1975;2:1171.
154. Smith JL, Murphy BL, Auslander MO, et al. Studies of the "e" antigen in acute and chronic hepatitis. Gastroenterology. 1976;71:208.
155. Nielsen JO, Dietrichson O, Juhl E. Incidence and meaning of the "e" determinant among hepatitis-B-antigen positive patients with acute and chronic liver diseases. Lancet. 1974;2:913–5.
156. Fay O, Tanno H, Ronocoroni M, et al. Prognostic implications of the e antigen of hepatitis B virus. JAMA. 1977;238:2501.
157. Takahashi K, Imai M, Miyakawa Y, et al. Duality of hepatitis B e antigen in serum of persons infected with hepatitis B virus: Evidence for non-identity of e antigen and immunoglobulin. Proc Natl Acad Sci USA. 1978;75:1952.
158. Takahashi K, Miyakawa Y, Gotanda T, et al. Shift from free "small" hepatitis B e antigen to IgG-bound "large" form in the circulation of human beings and a chimpanzee acutely infected with hepatitis B virus. Gastroenterology. 1979;77:1193.
159. Hess G, Arnold W, Shih JWK, et al. Expression of hepatitis B virus-specific markers in asymptomatic hepatitis B surface antigen carriers. Infect Immun. 1977;17:550–4.
160. Andres LL, Sawhney VK, Scullard GH, et al. Dane particle DNA polymerase and HBeAg: Impact on clinical, laboratory, and histologic findings in hepatitis B-associated chronic liver disease. Hepatology. 1981;1:583–5.
161. Okada K, Kainiyama I, Inometa M, et al. e Antigen and anti-e in the serum of asymptomatic carrier mothers as indicators of positive and negative transmission of hepatitis B virus in their infants. N Engl J Med. 1976;294:746.
162. Beasley RP, Trepo C, Stevens CE, et al. The e antigen and vertical transmission of hepatitis B surface antigen. Am J Epidemiol. 1977;105:94–8.
163. Perrillo RP, Gelb L, Campbell C, et al. Hepatitis B e antigen, DNA polymerase activity, and infection of household contacts with hepatitis B virus. Gastroenterology. 1979;76:1319–25.
164. Koshy R, Maupas P, Muller R, et al. Detection of hepatitis B virus-specific DNA in the genomes of human hepatocellular carcinoma and liver cirrhosis tissue. J Gen Virol. 1981;57:95.
165. Norkrans G, Nordenfeldt E, Hermodsson ES, et al. Long-term follow-up of chronic hepatitis patients with HBsAg, HBeAg and Dane particle associated DNA polymerase. Scand J Infect Dis. 1980;12:159.
166. Zuckerman AJ, Taylor PE. Persistence of the serum hepatitis (SH-Australia) antigen for many years. Nature. 1969;223:81.
167. Realdi G, Alberti A, Rugge M, et al. Seroconversion from hepatitis B e antigen to anti-HBe in chronic hepatitis B virus infection. Gastroenterology. 1980;79:195.
168. Aikawa T, Seirenji S, Furuta S, et al. Seroconversion from hepatitis B e antigen to anti-HBe in acute hepatitis B virus infection. N Engl J Med. 1978;298:439.
169. Alberti A, Diana S, Scullard GM, et al. Full and empty Dane particles in chronic hepatitis virus infection: Relationship to hepatitis B e antigen and presence of liver damage. Gastroenterology. 1978;75:869.
170. Hoofnagle JH, Seef LB, Dusheiko GM, et al. Seroconversion from hepatitis B e antigen to antibody during chronic type B hepatitis. Gastroenterology. 1980;79:1026.
171. Perrillo RP, Campbell CR, Saunders GE, et al. Spontaneous clearance and reactivation of HBV infection among male homosexuals with chronic type B hepatitis. Ann Intern Med. 1984;100:43.
172. Davis GL, Hoofnagle JH, Waggoner JG. Spontaneous reactivation of chronic hepatitis B virus infection. Gastroenterology. 1984; 86:230.
173. Szmuness W, Prince AM, Brotman B. Hepatitis B antigen and antibody in blood donors: An epidemiologic study. J Infect Dis. 1973;127:17.
174. Helske T. Carriers of hepatitis B antigen and transfusion hepatitis in Finland. Scand J Haematol. 1974;22(Suppl):1.
175. Sampliner RE, Hamilton FA, Iseri OA. The liver histology and frequency of clearance of the hepatitis B surface antigen in chronic carriers. Am J Med Sci. 1979;277:17.
176. Feinman SV, Cooter N, Sinclair JC, et al. Clinical and epidemiological significance of the HBsAg (Australia antigen): Carrier state. Gastroenterology. 1975;68:113.
177. Szmuness W, Harley EJ, Ikran H, et al. Sociodemographic aspects of the epidemiology of hepatitis B. In: Vyas GN, Cohen SN, Schmid R, eds. Viral Hepatitis: A Contemporary Assessment of Etiology, Epidemiology, Pathogenesis and Prevention. Philadelphia: Franklin Institute Press; 1978:297.
178. Hollinger FB, Werch J, Melnick JL. A prospective study indicating that double-antibody radioimmunoassay reduces the incidence of post-transfusion hepatitis B. N Engl J Med. 1974;290:1104–9.
179. Alter HJ, Holland PV, Purcell RH. The emerging pattern of post-transfusion hepatitis. Am J Med Sci. 1975;270:329.
180. Hoofnagle JH, Seeff LB, Bales ZB, et al. The Veterans Administration Hep-

atitis Cooperative Study Group. Type B hepatitis after transfusion with blood containing antibody to hepatitis B core antigen. N Engl J Med. 1978;298:1379–83.
181. Bories P, Coursaget P, Degott C, et al. Antibody to hepatitis B core antigen in chronic active hepatitis. Br Med J. 1978;1:396–7.
182. Nagington J, Cossart YE, Cohen BJ. Reactivation of hepatitis B after transplantation operations. Lancet. 1977;1:558.
183. Wands JR, Chura CM, Roll FJ, et al. Serial studies of hepatitis associated antigen and antibody in patients receiving anti-tumor chemotherapy for myeloproliferative and lymphoproliferative disorders. Gastroenterology. 1975;68:105.
184. Scullard GH, Smith CI, Merigan TC, et al. Effect of immunosuppressive therapy on viral markers in chronic active hepatitis B. Gastroenterology. 1981;81:978.
185. Ringold G, Yamamoto KR, Thompkins GM, et al. Dexamethasone-mediated induction of mouse mammary tumor virus RNA: A system for studying glucocorticoid action. Cell. 1975;6:299.
186. Pollard RB, Smith JL, Beal A, et al. Effect of vidarabine onchronic hepatitis B virus infection. JAMA. 1978;239:1648.
187. Scullard GH, Andres LL, Greenberg HB, et al. Antiviral treatment of chronic hepatitis B virus infection: Improvement in liver disease with interferon and adenine arabinoside. Hepatology. 1981;1:228.
188. Gold JWM, Alter HJ, Holland PV. Passive hemagglutination assay for antibody to subtypes of hepatitis B antigen. J Immunol. 1976;117:2260.
189. Koziol DE, Alter HJ, Dirchner JP. Development of HBsAg positive hepatitis despite previous existence of antibody to HBsAg. J Immunol. 117:1976.
190. Sherertz RJ, Spindel E, Hoofnagle JH. Antibody to hepatitis B surface antigen may not always indicate immunity to hepatitis B virus infection. N Engl J Med. 1983;309:1519.
191. Linnemann CC, Askey PA. Susceptibility to hepatitis B despite high titer anti-HBs antibody. Lancet. 1984;1:346.
192. Trepo CG, Prince AM. Absence of complete homologous immunity to hepatitis B infection after massive exposure. Ann Intern Med. 1976;85:427.
193. Karvountzis GG, Mosley JW, Redecker AG. Serologic characterization of patients with two episodes of acute viral hepatitis. Am J Med. 1975;58:815.
194. Mosley JW. Hepatitis types B and non-B: Epidemiologic background. JAMA. 1975;233:967.
195. Mosley JW, Redecker AG, Feinstone SM. Multiple hepatitis viruses in multiple attacks of acute viral hepatitis. N Engl J Med. 1977;296:75.
196. Tabor E, Gerety RJ. Possible role of immune response to hepatitis B core antigen in protection against hepatitis B infection. Lancet. 1984;1:172.
197. Murray K, Bruce SA, Hinnen A, et al. Hepatitis B virus antigens made in microbial cells immunise against viral infection. EMBO J. 1984;3:645–50.
198. Prince AM. Mechanism of protection against hepatitis B infection by immunization with hepatitis B virus cores. Lancet. 1984;1:512.
199. Peters RL. Viral hepatitis: A pathologic spectrum. Am J Med Sci. 1975;270:17.
200. Edgington TS, Chisari FV. Immunological aspects of hepatitis B infection. Am J Med Sci. 1975;270:213–27.
201. Dienstag JL, Khan AK, Klingenstein RJ, et al. Immunopathogenesis of liver disease associated with hepatitis B. In: Szmuness W, Alter HJ, Maynards JE, eds. Viral Hepatitis. Philadelphia: Franklin Institute Press; 1982:221–36.
202. Schweitzer IL, Dunn AEF, Peters RL, et al. Viral hepatitis in neonates and infants. Am J Med. 1973;55:762.
203. Tong MJ, Thursby M, Rakela J, et al. Studies of the maternal–infant transmission of the viruses which cause acute hepatitis. Gastroenterology. 1981;80:999.
204. London WT, di Figlia M, Sutnick AI, et al. An epidemic of hepatitis in a chronic hemodialysis unit. N Engl J Med. 1969;281:571–8.
205. Nordenfeldt E, Lindholm T, Dailquist E. A hepatitis epidemic in a dialysis unit: Occurrence and persistence of Australia-antigen among patients and staff. Acta Pathol Microbiol Scand Sect. B. 1970;78:692.
206. Good RA, Page AR. Fatal complications of virus hepatitis in two patients with agammaglobulinemia. Am J Med. 1960;29:804.
207. Dienstag JL, Bhan AK. Enchanced in vitro cell-mediated cytotoxicity in chronic hepatitis B virus infection: Absence of specificity for virus-expressed antigen on target cell membranes. J Immunol. 1980;125:2269.
208. Lee WM, Reed WD, Osman CG, et al. Immune responses to the hepatitis B surface antigen and liver-specific lipoprotein in acute type B hepatitis. Gut. 1977;18:250.
209. Moussouros A, Cochrane AMG, Thomson AD. Transient lymphocyte mediated hepatotoxicity in acute viral hepatitis. Gut. 1975;16:835.
210. Chisari FW, Castle KL, Xavier C, et al. Functional properties of lymphocyte subpopulations in hepatitis B virus infection: I. Suppressor cell control of T-lymphocyte responsiveness. J Immunol. 1981;126:38.
211. Trepo CG, Magnius LO, Schaefer RA, et al. Detection of e antigen and antibody: Correlations with hepatitis B surface and hepatitis B core antigen, liver disease, and outcome in hepatitis B infections. Gastroenterology. 1976;71:804.
212. Aldershvile J, Nielsen JO, Dietrichson O, et al. Long-term followup of e antigen (HBeAg) positive acute viral hepatitis. Scand J Gastroenterol. 1979;14:845.
213. Magnius LO, Lindholm A, Lundin P, et al. A new antigen–antibody system. Clinical significance in long term carriers of hepatitis B surface antigen. JAMA. 1975;231:356.
214. Reinicke V, Dybkjaer E, Poulsen H, et al. A study of Australia-antigen-positive blood donors and their recipients, with special reference to liver histology. N Engl J Med. 1972;286:867.
215. Eddleston ALWF, Mondelle M, Mieli-Vergani G, et al. Lymphocyte cytotoxicity to autologous hepatocytes in chronic hepatitis B virus infection. Hepatology. 1982;2:122s.
216. Naumov NW, Mondelli M, Alexander GJM, et al. Relationship between expression of hepatitis B virus antigens in isolated hepatocytes and autologous lymphocyte cytotoxicity in patients with chronic hepatitis B virus infection. Hepatology. 1984;4:13.
217. Rizzetto M, Canese MG, Arico S. Immunofluorescence detection of a new antigen system (delta/anti-delta) associated to the hepatitis B virus in the liver and the serum of HBsAg carriers. Gut. 1977;18:997.
218. Rizzetto M, Purcell RH, Gerin JL. Epidemiology of HBV-associated delta agent: Geographical distribution of anti-delta and prevalence of polytransfused HBsAg carriers. Lancet. 1980;1:1215.
219. Hadziyannis S, Hatzakis A, Karamanos B. Clinical features of chronic delta infection. In: Vyas GN, ed. Viral Hepatitis. Philadelphia: Franklin Institute Press. 1984:701.
220. Ponzetta, Forzani E, Shafi MS. Delta agent infection in Saudi Arabia: A general population study. In: Vyas, GN, ed. Viral Hepatitis. Philadelphia: Franklin Institute Press. 1984:615.
221. Hadler S, Monzon M, Ponzetto A, et al. Delta virus infection and serum hepatitis: An epidemic in the Yucpa Indians of Venezuela. Ann Intern Med. 1984;100:339.
222. Rizzetto M, Hoyer B, Canese MG, et al. Delta agent: The association of delta antigen with hepatitis B surface antigen and ribonucleic acid in the serum of delta-infected chimpanzees. Proc Natl Acad Sci USA. 1980;77:6124.
223. Rizzetto M, Canese MG, Gerin JL, et al. Transmission of the hepatitis B virus-associated delta antigen to chimpanzees. J Infect Dis. 1980;141:590.
224. Smedile A, Farci P, Verme G. Influence of delta infection on severity of hepatitis B. Lancet. 1982;2:945.
225. Tabor E, Ponzetto A, Gerin JL, et al. Does delta agent contribute to fulminant hepatitis? Lancet. 1983;1:765.
226. Shattock A, Morgan B, Peutherer J, et al. High incidence of delta antigen in serum. Lancet. 1983;2:104–5.
227. Columbo M, Cambieri R, Rumi M, et al. Long-term delta superinfection in hepatitis B surface antigen carriers and its relationship to the course of chronic hepatitis. Gastroenterology. 1983;85:235–9.
228. Rizzetto M, Verme G, Recchia S. Chronic hepatitis in carriers of hepatitis B surface antigen, with intrahepatic expression of delta antigen: An active and progressing disease unresponsive to immunosuppressive treatment. Ann Intern Med. 1983;98:437.
229. Beasley RP, Lin CC, Hwang LY, et al. Hepatocellular carcinoma and hepatitis B virus: A prospective study of 22,707 men in Taiwan. Lancet. 1981;2:1129–33.
230. Obata H, Hayashi N, Motoike Y. A prospective study of development of hepatocellular carcinoma from liver cirrhosis with persistent hepatitis B virus infection. Int J Cancer. 1980;25:741.
231. Larouze B, London WT, Saimot G, et al. Host responses to hepatitis-B infection in patients with primary hepatic carcinoma and their families: A case-control study in Senegal, West Africa. Lancet. 1976;2:534.
232. Nishioka K, Hirayama T, Sekine T, et al. Australia antigen and hepatocellular carcinoma. Gann Monogr Can Res. 1973;14:167.
233. Steiner PE. Cancer of the liver and cirrhosis in trans-Saharan Africa and the United States of America. Cancer. 1960;13:1085.
234. Trichopoulos D, Violaki M, Sparros L, et al. Epidemiology of hepatitis B and primary hepatic carcinoma. Lancet. 1975;2:1038.
235. Peters, RL. Pathology of hepatocellular carcinoma. In: Okuda K, Peters RL, eds. Hepatocellular Carcinoma. New York: Wiley; 1976:107.
236. Kew MD. Hepatoma and HBV. In: Vyas GM, Cohen SN, Schmid R, eds. Viral Hepatitis: A Contemporary Assessment of Etiology, Epidemiology, Pathogenesis and Prevention. Philadelphia: Franklin Institute Press; 1978:439.
237. Popper H, Shih JWK, Gerin JL, et al. Woodchuck hepatitis and hepatocellular carcinoma: Correlation of histologic with virologic observations. Hepatology. 1981;1:91.
238. Miller RH, Lee SC, Liaw YF, et al. Hepatitis B viral DNA in infected liver and hepatocellular carcinoma. J Infect Dis. 1985;151:1081–92.
239. Gocke JD. Immune complex phenomena associated with hepatitis. In: Vyas GN, Cohen SN, Schmidt R (eds). Viral Hepatitis: A Contemporary Assessment of Etiology, Epidemiology, Pathogenesis and Prevention. Philadelphia: Franklin Institute Press; 1978:277.
240. Schumacher HR, Gall EP. Arthritis in acute hepatitis and chronic active hepatitis: Pathology of the synovial membrane with evidence for the presence of Australia antigen in synovial membranes. Am J Med. 1974;57:655.
241. Wands JR, Mann EA, Isselbacher KJ. The pathogenesis of arthritis associated with acute hepatitis B surface antigen positive hepatitis. Complement activation and characterization of circulating immune complexes. J Clin Invest. 1975;55:930.
242. Redeker AG. Viral hepatitis: Clinical aspects. Am J Med Sci. 1975;270:9.
243. Gocke DJ, Hsu K, Morgan C, et al. Vasculitis in association with Australia antigen. J Exp Med. 1971;134:330s.
244. Fye KH, Becker MJ, Theofilopoulos AN, et al. Immune complexes in hepatitis B antigen associated polyarteritis nodosa: Detection by antibody dependent cell mediated cytotoxicity in Raji cell assay. Am J Med. 1977;62:783.
245. Combes B, Stastny P, Shorey J, et al. Glomerulonephritis with deposition

of Australia antigen–antibody complexes in glomerular basement membrane. Lancet. 1971;2:234.
246. Kohler PF, Croniln RE, Hammond WS. Chronic membranous glomerulonephritis caused by hepatitis B antigen–antibody immune complexes. Ann Intern Med. 1974;81:488.
247. Knieser WR, Jens EH, Howenthal DT, et al. Pathogenesis of renal disease associated with viral hepatitis. Arch Pathol. 1974;97:193.
248. Ozawa T, Levisohn P, Orsini E, et al. Acute immune complex disease associated with hepatitis. Arch Pathol Lab Med. 1976;100:484.
249. McIntosh RH, Koss MN, Gocke DJ. The nature and incidence of cryoproteins in hepatitis B antigen (HBsAg) positive patients. J Med. 1976;45:23.
250. Gianotti F. Papular acrodermatitis of childhood: An Australia antigen disease. Arch Dis Child. 1973;48:794.
251. Ishimaru Y, Ishimaru H, Toda G, et al. An epidemic infantile papular acrodermatitis in Japan associated with hepatitis B surface antigen subtype *ayw*. Lancet. 1976;1:707.
252. Levo Y, Gorevic PD, Kassab HJ, et al. Association between hepatitis B virus and essential mixed cryoglobulinemia. N Engl J Med. 1977;296:1501.
253. Popp JW, Dienstag JL, Wands JR, et al. Essential mixed cryoglobulinemia without evidence for hepatitis B virus infection. Ann Intern Med. 1980;92:383.
254. Hagler L, Pastore RN, Bergin JJ. Aplastic anemia following viral hepatitis. Medicine. 1975;54:139.
255. Nakamura S, Sato T, Maeda T, et al. Viral hepatitis B and aplastic anemia. Tohoku J Exp Med. 1975;116:101.
256. Casciato DA, Klein CA, Kaplowitz N, et al. Aplastic anemia associated with type B viral hepatitis. Arch Intern Med. 1978;138:1557.
257. Centers for Disease Control. Inactivated hepatitis B virus vaccine. Morb Mort Weekly Rep. 1982;31:318.
258. Holland PV. Available methods to further reduce post-transfusion hepatitis. In: Szmuness W, Alter HJ, Maynard JE, eds. Viral Hepatitis: 1981 International Symposium. Philadelphia: Franklin Institute Press; 1982:563.
259. Lander JJ, Holland PV, Alter HJ, et al. Antibody to hepatitis-associated antigen. Frequency and pattern of response as detected by radioimmunoprecipitation. JAMA. 1972;220:1079–81.
260. Cherubin CE, Purcell RH, Landers JJ, et al. Acquisition of antibody to hepatitis B antigen in three socioeconomically different medical populations. Lancet. 1972;2:149.
261. Blumberg BS, Friedlander JS, Woodside A, et al. Hepatitis and Australia antigen: Autosomal recessive inheritance of susceptibility to infection in humans. Proc Natl Acad Sci USA. 1969;62:1108.
262. Grossman RA, Benenson MW, Scott RM, et al. An epidemiologic study of hepatitis B virus in Bangkok, Thailand. Am J Epidemiol. 1975;101:144.
263. Hillis WD, Hillis A, Bias WB, et al. Association of hepatitis B surface antigenemia with HLA locus B specificities. N Engl J Med. 296:1310.
264. Stevens EC, Beasley RP. Lack of an autosomal recessive genetic influence in the vertical transmission of hepatitis B antigen. Nature. 1976;260:715.
265. Patterson MJ, Hourani MR, Mayor GH, et al. HLA antigens and hepatitis B virus. N Engl J Med. 1977;297:1124.
266. Szmuness W, Stevens CE, Ikram H, et al. Prevalence of hepatitis B virus infection and hepatocellular carcinoma in Chinese-Americans. J Infect Dis. 1978;137:822.
267. Mosley JW. Epidemiologic implications of changing trends in type A and type B hepatitis. In: Vyas GN, Perkins HA, Schmid R, eds. Hepatitis and Blood Transfusion. New York: Grune and Stratton; 1972:349.
268. Blumberg BS. Australia antigen: The history of its discovery with comments on genetic and family aspects. In: Vyas GN, Perkins HA, Schmid R, eds. Hepatitis and Blood Transfusion. New York: Grune and Stratton; 1972:63.
269. Blumberg BS, Sutnick AI, London WT, et al. Sex distribution of Australia antigen. Arch Intern Med. 1972;130:231.
270. London WT, Drew JS, Lustbader DE, et al. Host response to hepatitis B infection in patients in a chronic hemodialysis unit. Kidney Int. 1977;12:51.
271. Krugman S. Hepatitis B immune globulin. In: Vyas GN, Perkins HA, Schmid R, eds. Hepatitis and Blood Transfusion. New York: Grune and Stratton; 1972:349.
272. Szmuness W, Much WM, Prince AM, et al. On the role of sexual behavior in the spread of hepatitis B infection. Ann Intern Med. 1975;83:489.
273. Stevens CE, Beasley RP, Tsui V, et al. Vertical transmission of hepatitis B antigen in Taiwan. N Engl J Med. 1975;292:771.
274. Beasley RP, Hwang LY, Lin CC, et al. Incidence of hepatitis B virus infections in preschool children in Taiwan. J Infect Dis. 1982;147:185.
275. Mazzur S, Burget S, Blumberg BS. Geographical distribution of Australia antigen determinants *d*, *y* and *w*. Nature. 1974;247:38.
276. Bancroft WH, Holland PV, Mazzur S, et al. The geographical distribution of HBsAg subtypes. Bibl Haematol. 1976;42:42.
277. Alter JH, Purcell RH, Gerin JL. Transmission of hepatitis B to chimpanzees by hepatitis B surface antigen-positive saliva and semen. Infect Immun. 1977;16:928.
278. Centers for Disease Control. Hepatitis transmitted by a human bite. Morbid Mort Weekly Rep. 1974;23:24.
279. Prince AM, Hargrove RI, Szmuness W. Immunologic distinction between infectious and serum hepatitis. N Engl J Med. 1970;282:987.
280. Gocke DJ. Type B hepatitis—Good news and bad news. N Engl J Med. 1974;291:1409.
281. Pattison CP, Boyer KM, Maynard JE. Epidemic hepatitis in a clinical laboratory: Possible association with computer card handling. JAMA. 1974;230:854.
282. Morris IM, Cattle DS, Smits BJ. Endoscopy and transmission of hepatitis B. Lancet. 1975;2:1152.
283. McDonald GB, Silverstein FE. Can gastrointestinal endoscopy transmit hepatitis B to patients? Gastrointest Endosc. 1975;22:168.
284. Lauer JL, Van Drunen NA, Washburn JW, et al. Transmission of hepatitis B virus in clinical laboratory areas. J Infect Dis. 1979;140:513.
285. Mirick GS, Shank RE. An epidemic of serum hepatitis studied under controlled conditions. Trans Am Climatol Assoc. 1959;71:176.
286. Hersh T, Melnick JL, Goyal RK, et al. Nonparenteral transmission of viral hepatitis type B (Australia antigen-associated serum hepatitis). N Engl J Med. 1971;285:1363.
287. Heathcote J, Gateau P, Sherlock S. Role of hepatitis B antigen carriers in non-parenteral transmission of hepatitis B virus. Lancet. 1974;2:370.
288. Papaevangllon D, Trichopoulos D, Kemagtinon A, et al. Prevalence of hepatitis B antigen and antibody in prostitutes. Br Med J. 1975;2:256.
289. Szmuness W, Much WM, Prince AM. On the role of sexual behavior in the spread of hepatitis B infection. Ann Intern Med. 1975;83:489.
290. Dietzman DE, Harmisch JP, Ray CG, et al. Hepatitis B surface antigen (HBsAg) and antibody to HBsAg: Prevalence in homosexual and heterosexual men. JAMA. 1977;238:2625.
291. Wright RA. Hepatitis B and the HBsAg carrier: An outbreak related to sexual contact. JAMA. 1975;232:717.
292. Lewis TL, Alter HJ, Chalmers TC. A comparison of the frequency of hepatitis B antigen and antibody in hospital and non-hospital personnel. N Engl J Med. 1973;289:647.
293. Mosley JW, Edwards VM, Casey BS. Hepatitis virus infection in dentists. N Engl J Med. 1975;293:730.
294. Maynard JE. Viral hepatitis as an occupational hazard in the health care professional. In: Vyas GN, Cohen SN, Schmid R, eds. Viral Hepatitis: A Contemporary Assessment of Etiology, Epidemiology, Pathogenesis and Prevention. Philadelphia: Franklin Institute Press; 1978:321.
295. Rosenberg JL, Jones DP, Lipitz LR. Viral hepatitis: An occupational hazard to surgeons. JAMA. 1973;223:395.
296. Graf JP, Moeschlin P. Risk to contacts of a medical practitioner carrying HBsAg. N Engl J Med. 1975;293:197.
297. Levin ML, Maddrey CW, Wands JR. Hepatitis B transmission by dentists. JAMA. 1974;228:1139.
298. Goodwin D, Fannin SL, McCracker BB. An oral surgeon related hepatitis B outbreak. Calif Morb. California State Department of Health, April 16. Berkeley: 1976.
299. Rimland D, Parkin WE, Miller GB. Hepatitis B outbreak traced to an oral surgeon. N Engl J Med. 1977;296:153.
300. Syndmen DR, Hindman SH, Wineland MD. Nosocomial viral hepatitis B: A cluster among staff with subsequent transmission to patients. Ann Intern Med. 1976;85:573.
301. Garibaldi RA, Rasmussen CM, Holmes AW. Hospital acquired serum hepatitis: Report of an outbreak. JAMA. 1972;219:1577.
302. Alter HJ, Chalmer TC, Freeman BM. Health-care workers positive for hepatitis B surface antigen: Are their contacts at risk? N Engl J Med. 1975;292:454.
303. Williams SV, Pattison CP, Berquist KR. Dental infection with hepatitis B. JAMA. 1975;232:1231.
304. Centers for Disease Control. Hepatitis Surveillance Report. No. 41. September 1977.
305. Ogra PL. Immunologic aspects of hepatitis associated antigen and antibody in body fluids. J Immunol. 1974;110:1197.
306. Mohoney P, Gleischner G, Millman I. Australia antigen: Detection and transmission in shellfish. Science. 1974;183:80.
307. Prince AM, Metselaar D, Kapuko GW. Hepatitis B antigen in wild caught mosquitoes in Africa. Lancet. 1972;2:247.
308. Brotman B, Prince AM, Godfrey HK. Role of arthropods in transmission of hepatitis B virus in the tropics. Lancet. 1973;1:1305.
309. Wills W, Laroiuze B, London WT. Hepatitis B in bedbugs from Senegal. Lancet. 1977;2:217.
310. Dick SJ, Tamborro CH, Leevy CM. Hepatitis B antigen in urban caught mosquitoes. JAMA. 1974;229:1627.
311. Beasley RP, Hwang LY, Lee GC, et al. Prevention of perinatally transmitted hepatitis B virus infections with hepatitis B immunoglobulin and hepatitis B vaccine. Lancet. 1983;2:1099.
312. Ohbayashi A, Okochi K, Mayumi M, et al. Familial clustering of asymptomatic carriers of Australia antigen in patients with primary liver disease and primary liver cancer. Gastroenterology. 1972;62:618.
313. Beasley RP, Stevens CE, Shiao IS, et al. Evidence against breast feeding as a mechanism for vertical transmission of hepatitis B. Lancet. 1975;2:740.
314. Grady GF, Gitnick FL, Prince AM. Relation of e antigen to infectivity of HBsAg-positive inoculation among medical personnel. Lancet. 1976;2:492.
315. Oliphant JW. Jaundice following administration of human serum. Pub Health Rep. 1943;58:1233.
316. MacCallum FO, Bauer DJ. Homologous serum jaundice: Transmission experiments with human volunteers. Lancet. 1944;1:622.
317. Oliphant JW. Jaundice following administration of human serum. Bull NY Acad Med. 1944;20:429.
318. Havens WP. Properties of the etiologic agent of infectious hepatitis. Proc Soc Exp Biol Med. 1945;58:203.
319. DeRitis F, Mallucci L, Coltorti M, et al. Anicteric virus hepatitis in a closed environment as shown by serum transaminase activity. Bull WHO. 1959;20:589.

320. Shimizu Y, Kitamoto O. The incidence of viral hepatitis after blood transfusion. Gastroenterology. 1963;44:740.
321. Hampers CL, Prager D, Senior JR. Past transfusion anicteric hepatitis. N Engl J Med. 1964;271:747.
322. Galambos JT. Chronic persisting hepatitis. Am J Pathol. 1946;22:867.
323. Molner JG, Meyer KF. Jaundice in Detroit. Am J Public Health. 1940;30:509.
324. Litwins J, Leibowitz S. Abnormal lymphocytes in virus diseases other than infectious mononucleosis. Acta Haematol. 1951;5:223.
325. Swift WE, Gardner HT, Moore DJ, et al. Clinical course of viral hepatitis and the effect of exercise during convalescence. Am J Med. 1950;8:614.
326. Madsen S, Bang NU, Iverson K. Serum glutamic oxalactic transaminase in disease of the liver and biliary tract. Br Med J. 1958;1:543.
327. Schneider AJ, Mosley JW. Studies of variations of glutamic-oxalacetic transaminase in serum and infectious hepatitis. Pediatrics. 1959;24:367.
328. Lucke B, Mallory T. The fulminant form of epidemic hepatitis. Am J Pathol. 1946;22:867.
329. Merril DN, Dubois RS, Kohler PF. Neonatal onset of the hepatitis associated antigen carrier state. N Engl J Med. 1972;287:1280.
330. Goldfield M, Bill J, Colosimo F. The control of transfusion-associated hepatitis. In: Vyas GN, Cohen SN, Schmidt R, eds. Viral hepatitis: A Contemporary Assessment of Etiology, Epidemiology, Pathogenesis and Prevention. Philadelphia: Franklin Institute Press; 1978:405–14.
331. Dupuy JM, Frommel D, Alagille D. Severe viral hepatitis type B in infancy. Lancet. 1975;1:191.
332. Allen JG, Sayman WA. Serum hepatitis from transfusions of blood. JAMA. 1962;180:1079.
333. Hoofnagle JH. Type B viral hepatitis: Virology, serology and clinical course. Semin Liver Dis. 1981;1:7.
334. Overby LR, Ling CM, Decker RH, et al. Serodiagnostic profiles of viral hepatitis. In: Szmuness W, Alter HJ, Maynard JE, eds. Viral Hepatitis: 1981 International Symposium. Philadelphia: Franklin Institute Press; 1982:169.
335. Aach RD, Alter HJ, Hollinger FB, et al. Risk of transfusing blood containing antibody to hepatitis B surface antigen. Lancet. 1974;2:190.
336. Renton PH, Wadsworth LD. Infectivity of blood containing hepatitis B antibody. Lancet. 1975;1:736.
337. Schweitzer IL, Edwards VM, Brezina M. E antigen in HBsAg-carrier mothers. N Engl J Med. 1975;293:940.
338. Berquist KR, Maynard JE, Murphy BL. Infectivity of serum containing HBsAg and antibody to e antigen. Lancet. 1976;1:1026.
339. Kirkler DM, Zilberg B. Activity and hepatitis. Lancet. 1966;2:1046.
340. Chalmers TC, Eckhardt RD, Reynolds WD, et al. The treatment of infectious hepatitis: Controlled studies of the effects of diet, rest and physical reconditioning on the acute course of disease and the incidence of relapses and residual abnormalities. J Clin Invest. 1955;34:1163.
341. Repsher LH, Freebern RK. Effects of early and vigorous exercise on recovery from infectious hepatitis. N Engl J Med. 1969;281:1393.
342. Gregory PB, Knauer M, Hempson RL, et al. Steroid therapy in severe viral hepatitis: A double blind randomized trial of methy-prednisolone versus placebo. N Engl J Med. 1976;294:728.
343. Redeker AG, Schweitzer IL, Yamahiro HS, et al. Randomization of corticosteroid therapy in fulminant hepatitis. N Engl J Med. 1976;294:728.
344. Acute Hepatic Failure Study Group. Failure of specific immunotherapy in fulminant type hepatitis. Ann Intern Med. 1977;86:272.
345. Cook CG, Mulligan R, Sherlock S. Controlled prospective trial of corticosteroid therapy in active hepatitis. Q J Med. 1971;40:159.
346. Soloway RD, Summerskill WHJ, Baggenstoss AH, et al. Clinical, biochemical and histological remission of severe chronic active liver disease: A controlled study of treatments and early prognosis. Gastroenterology. 1972;63:820.
347. Murray-Lyon IM, Stern RB, Williams R. Controlled trial of prednisone and azothioprine in active chronic hepatitis. Lancet. 1973;1:735.
348. Schalm SW, Summerskill WHJ, Gitnick GL, et al. Contrasting features and responses to treatment of severe chronic active liver disease with and without hepatitis Bs antigen. Gut. 1976;17:781.
349. Vogten AJM, Summerskill WHJ, Gilnick GL, et al. Behavior of e antigen and antibody during chronic liver disease. Relation to HB antigen–antibody system and prognosis. Lancet. 1976;2:126.
350. Wright EC, Seef LB, Berk PD, et al. Treatment of chronic active hepatitis. Gastroenterology. 1977;73:1422.
351. Redeker AJ. Advances in clinical aspects of acute and chronic liver disease of viral origin. In: Vyas GN, Cohen SN, Schmidt R, eds. Viral Hepatitis: A Contemporary Assessment of Etiology, Epidemiology, Pathogenesis and Prevention. Philadelphia: Franklin Institute Press; 1978:425–30.
352. Tong MJ, Mystram JS, Redeker AG, et al. Failure of transfer factor therapy in chronic active type B hepatitis. N Engl J Med. 1976;295:209.
353. Shulman ST, Hutto JH, Ayoub EM, et al. Transfer factor in treating hepatitis B. N Engl J Med. 1976;295:898.
354. Robinson WS. Summary of workshop on antiviral therapy. In: Vyas GN, Cohen SN, Schmidt R, eds. Viral Hepatitis: A Contemporary Assessment of Etiology, Epidemiology, Pathogenesis and Prevention. Philadelphia: Franklin Institute Press; 1978:681–2.
355. Heyward WL, Lanier AP, Bender TR. Early detection of primary hepatocellular carcinoma by screening for alpha fetoprotein in high risk families. Lancet. 1983;2:1161.
356. Centers for Disease Control. Early detection of primary hepatocellular carcinoma-Alaska. Morb Mort Weekly Rep. 1984;33:53.
357. Hoofnagle JH, Gerety RI, Barker LF. Antibody to the hepatitis B surface antigen in immune serum globulin. Transfusion. 1975;15:408.
358. Grady GF, Rodman M, Larsen L. Hepatitis B antibody in conventional globulin. J Infect Dis. 1975;132:474.
359. Courouce-Pauty AM, Delons S, Soulier JP. Attempt to prevent hepatitis B by using specific anti-HBs immunoglobulin. Am J Med Sci. 1975;270:375.
360. Desmyter J, Bradbourne AF, Vermylen C, et al. Hepatitis B immunoglobulin in prevention of HBs antigenaemia in haemodialysis patients. Lancet. 1975;2:377.
361. Iwarson S, Ahlmen J, Erickson E, et al. Hepatitis B immune serum globulin and standard gamma globulin in prevention of hepatitis B infection among hospital staff: A preliminary report. Am J Med Sci. 1975;270:385.
362. Iwarson S, Ahlmen J, Erickson E, et al. Hepatitis B immune globulin in prevention of hepatitis B among hospital staff members. J Infect Dis. 1977;135:473.
363. Grady GF. Viral hepatitis passive prophylaxis with globulins: State of the art in 1978. In: Vyas GN, Cohen SN, Schmidt R, eds. Viral Hepatitis: A Contemporary Assessment of Etiology, Epidemiology, Pathogenesis and Prevention. Philadelphia: Franklin Institute Press; 1978:467–76.
364. Szmuness W, Prince AM, Goodman N, et al: Hepatitis B immune serum globulin in prevention of non-parenteral transmitted hepatitis B. N Engl J Med. 1974;290:701.
365. Ginsberg AL, Conrad ME, Bancroft WH, et al. Prevention of endemic HAA-positive hepatitis with gamma globulin. Use of a simple radioimmune assay to detect HAA. N Engl J Med. 1972;296:562.
366. Klein HG, Alter HA. Comparison of hepatitis B immune globulin given in single or divided doses for protection against hepatitis B virus infection. In: Vyas GN, Cohen SN, Schmidt R, eds. Viral Hepatitis: A Contemporary Assessment of Etiology, Epidemiology, Pathogenesis and Prrevention. Philadelphia: Franklin Institute Press; 1978.
367. Tabor E, Gerety RJ. Inactivation of an agent of human nonA, nonB hepatitis with formalin. 1980;142:767.
368. Yoshizawa H, Itoh Y, Iwakiri S. Non A, non B (type 1) hepatitis agent capable of inducing tubular ultrastructures in the hepatocyte cytoplasm of chimpanzees: inactivation by formalin and heat. Gastroenterology. 1982;82:502.
369. Gerety RJ, Tabor E. Newly licensed hepatitis B vaccine: Known safety and unknown risks. JAMA. 1983;249:745.
370. McLean AA, Buynak EB, Kuter BJ, et al. Clinical experience with hepatitis vaccine. In: Proceedings of the Symposium on Hepatitis B: The Virus, the Disease, the Vaccine. New York: Plenum Press. In press.
371. Szmuness W, et al. Hepatitis B vaccine: Demonstration of efficacy in a controlled clinical trial in a high-risk population in the United States. N Engl J Med. 1980;303:833.
372. Szmuness W, et al. A controlled trial on the efficacy of the hepatitis B vaccine (Heptavax B): A final report. Hepatology. 1982;1:377.
373. Dienstag JL, et al. Hepatitis B vaccine in health care personnel: A randomized, double-blind, placebo-controlled trial. Hepatology. 1982;2:696.
374. Francis DP, et al. The prevention of hepatitis B with vaccine. Report of the Centers for Disease Control multi-center trial among homosexual men. Ann Intern Med. 1982;97:362.
375. Szmuness W, et al. Hepatitis B vaccine in medical staff of hemodialysis units. Efficacy and subtype cross-protection. N Engl J Med. 1981;307:385.
376. Hadler SC, et al. Long term immunogenicity and efficacy of hepatitis B vaccine in homosexual men. N Engl J Med. 1986;315:209.
377. Horowitz MM, Ershler WB, Balliola RJ. Duration of immunity after hepatitis B vaccination: Efficacy of low dose booster vaccine. Ann Intern Med. 108:185–9.
378. Centers for Disease Control. Update on hepatitis B prevention. Mort Weekly Rep. 1987;36:353.
379. Deinhardt F. Aspects of vaccination against hepatitis B: Passive-active immunization schedules and immune responses in different age groups. Scand J Infect Dis. 1983;(Suppl):17.
380. Szmuness W, et al. Passive-active immunization against hepatitis B: Immunogenicity studies in adult Americans. Lancet. 1981;1:575.
381. Deinstag JL, Stevens CE, Bhan AK, et al. Hepatitis B vaccine administered to chronic carriers of hepatitis B surface antigen. Ann Intern Med. 1982;96:575.
382. Kreider SD, Lange WR. Hepatitis B vaccine. N Engl J Med. 1984;310:466.
383. Centers for Disease Control. The safety of hepatitis B vaccine. Morb Mort Weekly Rep. 1983;32:134.
384. Stevens CE. No increased incidence of AIDS in recipients of hepatitis B vaccine. N Engl J Med. 1983;308:1163.
385. Grady GF. Hepatitis B immunity in hospital staff targeted for vaccination: Role of screening tests in immunization programs. JAMA. 1982;248:2266.
386. Miller KD, Gibbs RD, Mulligan MM, et al. Intradermal hepatitis B virus vaccine: Immunogenicity and side effects in adults. Lancet. 1983;2:1454.
387. Zoulek G, Lorbeer B, Jilg W, et al. Antibody responses and skin reactivity after intradermal hepatitis B vaccine. Lancet. 1984;1:568.
388. Miyanohara A, Toh-E A, Nozaki C, et al. Expression of hepatitis B surface antigen gene in years. Proc Natl Acad Sci USA. 1983;80:1.
389. Hadler SC, Francis DP, Maynard, JE, et al. Long term immunogenicity and efficacy of hepatitis B vaccine in homosexual men. N Engl J Med. 1986;315:209–14.
390. Krugman S, Giles JP. Viral hepatitis, type B (MS-2 strain). Further observations on natural history and prevention. N Engl J Med. 1973;288:755.
391. Redeker AJ, Mosely JW, Gocke DJ, et al. Hepatitis B immune globulin as

a prophylactic measure for spouses exposed to acute type B hepatitis. N Engl J Med. 1975;293:1055.
392. Grady GF, Gitnick GL, Prince AM, et al. Hepatitis B immune globulin: Prevention of hepatitis from accidental exposure among medical personnel. N Engl J Med. 1975;293:1067.
393. Grady GF, Lee VA, Prince AM, et al. Hepatitis B immune globulin for accidental exposures among medical personnel. Final report of a multicenter controlled trial. J Infect Dis. 1978;137:131.
394. Centers for Disease Control. Immune globulins for protection against viral hepatitis. Morb Mort Weekly Rep. 1977;26:425.
395. Stevens CE, Neurath RA, Beasley RP, et al. HBeAg and anti-HBe detection by radioimmunoassay: Correlation with vertical transmission of hepatitis B virus in Taiwan. J Med Virol. 1979;3:237.
396. Beasley RP, Hwang LY, Lin CC, et al. Hepatitis B immunoglobulin (HBIG) efficacy in the interruption of perinatal transmission of hepatitis B virus carrier state. Lancet. 1981;2:388.
397. Beasley RP, Hwang YL, Stevens CE, et al. Efficacy of hepatitis B immune globulin (HBIG) for prevention of perinatal transmission of the HBV carrier state: Final report of a randomized double-blind placebo-controlled trial. Hepatitis. 1983;3:135.
398. Reesink HW, Reesink-Brongers EE, Lafeber-Schut BJT, et al. Prevention of chronic HBsAg carrier state in infants of HBsAg-positive mothers by hepatitis B immunoglobulin. Lancet. 1979;2:436.
399. Beasley RP, Stevens CE. Vertical transmission of HBV and interruption with globulin. In: Vyas GN, Cohen SN, Sched R, eds. Viral Hepatitis: A Contemporary Assessment of Etiology, Epidemiology, Pathogenesis and Prevention. Philadelphia: Franklin Institute Press; 1978:333.
400. Beasley RP, Hwant LY. Postnatal infectivity of HBeAg carrier mothers. J Infect Dis. 1983;147:185.
401. Beasley RP, Hwang LY, Lee CY, et al. Efficacy of HBV vaccine for the interruption of the perinatally transmitted hepatitis B virus carrier state. Lancet. 1983;2:1099–128.
402. Center for Disease Control. Perspectives on control of viral hepatitis, type B. Morb Mort Weekly Rep. 1976;25(17 Suppl):3.
403. Bond WW, Peterson NJ, Fauero MS. Viral hepatitis B: Aspects of environmental control. Health Lab Sci. 1977;14:235.
404. Aach RD, Lander JJ, Sherman LA, et al. Transfusion-transmitted virus: Interim analysis of hepatitis among transfused and non-transfused patients. In: Vyas GN, Cohen SN, Schmid R, eds. Viral Hepatitis: A Contemporary Assessment of Etiology, Epidemiology, Pathogenesis and Prevention. Philadelphia: Franklin Institute Press; 1978:383.

Parvoviridae

126. PARVOVIRUSES (ERYTHEMA INFECTIOSUM, APLASTIC CRISIS)

RAPHAEL DOLIN

Parvoviruses are small DNA viruses that infect a wide range of animal species including humans. Human parvoviruses had not been associated with disease until recently when a human parvovirus, designated "B19," was shown to be the cause of erythema infectiosum and of aplastic crises in patients with chronic hemolytic anemias. B19 infection has also been associated with erythroblastosis fetalis and with some arthropathies.[1]

PATHOGEN

Parvovirus B19 was originally discovered in the sera of asymptomatic blood donors who had false-positive results for hepatitis B surface antigen by counterimmunoelectrophoresis tests. Although B19 is antigenically unrelated to other animal or human parvoviruses, the physical properties of this virus are consistent with those of parvoviruses. B19 virus is 22–23 nm in diameter, nonenveloped, and relatively dense, with a buoyant density of 1.38–1.42 g/dl.[2] The virus contains three structural polypeptides of molecular weights of 48,000, 68,000, and 80,000 kD.[3] The genome consists of single-stranded DNA that is largely linear in organization, and approximately equal proportions of strands of positive and negative polarity are packaged in separate particles.[4] In vitro cultivation of the virus in conventional systems has not yet been achieved, although replication of virus in bone marrow cultures has been recently reported (see below).

PATHOGENESIS

The pathogenesis of infection with B19 virus was studied by Anderson and colleagues who challenged susceptible volunteers intranasally with serum that contained infectious virus.[5] Infection led to a transient viremia that was followed by virus-specific IgM and IgG antibody titer rises. Viremia, during which virus was detected in extremely high titers, was first noted 6–8 days after challenge and lasted for 4–7 days. At that time, virus was also found in respiratory tract secretions, but not in urine or stool specimens. The illness that was observed manifested a biphasic pattern. The first phase occurred at the time of the viremia and consisted of fever and mild systemic symptoms, including malaise, myalgia, and chills, that lasted 1–4 days. The second phase of the illness occurred 17–18 days after challenge and was manifested by a fine maculopapular rash accompanied by arthalgias and some joint swelling. The rash faded after 2–3 days, and the joint symptoms resolved 1 2 days thereafter. In addition, hematologic changes were noted at 1 week after the onset of the viremia. These changes consisted of a reticulocytopenia and a fall in hemoglobin concentration of approximately 0.2 g/dl/day for 7–10 days. Bone marrow samples taken at this time demonstrated a marked depletion of erythroid precursors. Peripheral lymphocyte, platelet, and neutrophil counts also dropped during this time by an as yet undefined mechanism. The observations in these volunteer experiments correlated well with the manifestations of naturally occurring illness after B-19 infection, which are described below.

ERYTHEMA INFECTIOSUM

Erythema infectiosum, also referred to as the fifth disease, is an acute, febrile, self-limited illness that was long presumed to be caused by an undetected viral agent.[6] The term *fifth disease* is derived from the common assignation of Roman numerals I–VI to exanthems of childhood in the late nineteenth century.[7] Erythema infectiosum appears to be worldwide in distribution and occurs most commonly during the spring and early summer.[1,8–10] It is seen in children between the ages of 5 and 14 years but can occur in adults as well, and there is no apparent sex predilection. Sporadic cases as well as outbreaks have been noted, and secondary attack rates have been estimated to be approximately 30 percent.[10] B19 virus was first clearly associated with erythema infectiosum in an outbreak in children attending an elementary school in London in which 582 cases were reported including 53 secondary cases in household contacts.[11] Serum specimens taken from 36 cases all contained anti-B19 IgM, as well as anti-B19 IgG, while none of the control children or well family contacts had anti-B19 IgM. Of 17 individuals who had family contact with erythema infectiosum cases but who remained well, 16 had serum anti-B19 IgG antibodies, which was consistent with previous infection and represented apparent immunity to the virus. Similar serologic findings were subsequently found in two outbreaks in Japan,[12] and multiple outbreaks as well as sporadic cases have been associated with B19 infection throughout the world.[1,13,14] Seroprevalence studies have indicated that approximately 60 percent of adults have serum antibody to B19.[15]

The clinical manifestations of erythema infectiosum in children are those of a mild, self-limited disease. The hallmark of illness is a rash that erupts on the face and may be preceded by a prodrome of low-grade fever. The rash has been most frequently described as having a "slapped-cheek" appearance. A rash on the extremities may appear simultaneously with the rash on the cheeks[9] or may be seen 1–4 days later.[16] The rash on the extremities is variable in appearance and can be morbilliform, annular, or confluent. As central clearing of lesions occurs, the rash may take on a lacelike appearance. It is uncommon for the rash to involve the trunk and even more rare to involve the palms and soles. The rash generally disappears within a week but may come and go late in illness, especially after exercise, bathing, thermal changes, or stress. Occasionally, an intermittently present rash may be noted for several weeks. Most children have few if any other signs or symptoms of illness associated with the rash, although up to 25 percent of cases may have mild fever, headache, sore throat, and abdominal discomfort.[10] Adenopathy, arthalgia, and arthritis may also occur but are seen more frequently in adults, in whom the disease is somewhat more severe, as is the case for most childhood exanthems. Arthritis associated with erythema infectiosum involves primarily the wrists and knees and is also generally mild. Easy fatiguability and listlessness lasting for several weeks after the acute illness have been noted in some cases in adults.[10,16] Complications associated with erythema infectiosum are extremely rare. Cases of encephalitis,[17] and pneumonia[18] have been reported.

APLASTIC CRISIS

Infection with B19 virus is now well established as a cause of aplastic crisis in patients with chronic hemolytic anemias.[1] This has been noted most frequently in patients with sickle cell anemia[19–21] but has also been reported in patients with hereditary spherocytosis,[22,23] pyruvate kinase deficiency,[24] and β-thalassameia intermedia.[21] B19 viremia has been detected in patients within 2 days of the onset of symptoms associated with aplastic crisis, and anti-B19 IgM antibody develops early in illness. Seroepidemiologic studies have revealed significantly higher rates of serum antibody to B19 in patients with chronic hemolytic anemias who have had aplastic crises as compared with those who have not had aplastic crises.[1] However, apparently asymptomatic infection with B19 in sicklers can also occur.[20] Whether B19 infection is invariably the principal cause of aplastic crisis in such patients is uncertain at present. The pathogenesis of the aplastic crisis appears to be related to the inhibition of bone marrow erythroid precursors by virus infection. Proliferation of erythroid precursors in vitro can be inhibited by the addition of purified B19 virus to bone marrow cultures.[25] Cytotoxic effects in the erythroid precursor cells can be seen, and intracellular viral particles as well as extracellular infectious virus can be detected in such cultures.[26,27]

FETAL INFECTION

The ability to cause fetal infections has been long recognized as an important property of animal parvoviruses. Fetal infection by B19 in humans has now been clearly demonstrated,[1,28,29] although the overall outcome of B19 infection in pregnancy is uncertain. In recent studies, 6 of 18 cases of infection in pregnancy resulted in hydrops fetalis and/or spontaneous abortions.[30–32] Large-scale prospective studies to determine the overall risk of B19 infection in pregnancy are currently underway.

ARTHROPATHY

As noted earlier, arthralgia and arthritis can accompany erythema infectiosum in children and is seen more frequently in adults. However, joint manifestations have also been associated with B19 infection in the absence of a rash.[33,34] These arthropathies have been observed preponderantly in women and most often present as an acute, symmetrically polyarthritis involving the hands, wrists, and/or knees. Arthritis usually resolves within 2–4 weeks, althouh occasionally cases with a prolonged duration of symptoms have been reported.[34] The overall epidemiology and frequency of B19-associated arthropathies are unknown, but considerable interest exists in the possible role of B19 and other parvovirus infections in arthritides of unknown etiology such as rheumatoid arthritis. However, seroprevalence rates of antibody to B19 in patients with seropositive rheumatoid arthritis are similar to those in healthy adults.[35]

DIAGNOSIS

Widely available diagnostic tests have not yet been developed for B19 infection, in part because the virus has not been successfully cultivated in conventional systems. Currently, the source of B19 antigen continues to be patients with viremia, although there has been considerable progress in cloning the viral genome.[4] Radioimmunoassay[36] and enzyme-linked immunosorbent assay (ELISA)[15] methods have been developed for the detection of both antibody and antigen, and methods for the detection of viral DNA are under development.[37] The most useful diagnostic test at present is the detection of anti-B19 IgM antibody, which is present early in illness, begins to decrese 1–2 months after the onset of illness, and is usually absent 2–3 months later.

TREATMENT AND PREVENTION

Erythema infectiosum is a mild, self-limited illness that generally requires no treatment, although antipyretics, analgesics, and anti-inflammatory agents can alleviate the symptoms in more severe cases. Treatment for aplastic crises is largely supportive, with the administration of blood transfusions as required. An effective vaccine or other means of immunoprophylaxis to prevent B19 infections is not available. Such a vaccine might be of significant benefit in patients with chronic hemolytic anemias and may be of potential interest in the prevention of fetal infections once the risk of B19 infection in pregnancy is better defined.

REFERENCES

1. Anderson MJ. Parvoviruses as agents of human disease. Prog Med Virol. 1987;34:55–69.
2. Cossart YE, Field AM, Cant B, et al. Parvovirus-like particles in human sera. Lancet 1985;1:72–3.
3. Clewley JP. Biochemical characterization of a human parvovirus. J Gen Virol. 1984;65:241–5.
4. Cotmore S, Tattersall P. Characterization and molecular cloning of a human parvovirus genome. Science. 1984;226:1161–6.
5. Anderson MJ, Higgins PG, Davis LR, et al. Experimental parvovirus infection in man. J Infect Dis. 1985;152:257–65.
6. Herrick TP. Erythema infectiosum: Clinical report of 74 cses. Am J Dis Child. 1962;31:486–95.
7. Shapiro L. The numbered diseases: First through sixth. JAMA. 1965;194:680–6.
8. Lauer BA, MacCormack JN, Wilfert C. Erythema infectiosum. An elementary school outbreak. Am J Dis Child 1976;130:252–4.
9. Ager EA, Chin TDY, Poland JD. Epidemic erythema infectiosum. N Engl J Med. 1966;275:1326–31.
10. Greenwald P, Bashe WJ. An epidemic of erythema infectiosum. Am J Dis Child. 1964;107:30–4.
11. Anderson MJ, Lewis E, Kidd IM, et al. An outbreak of erythema infectiosum associated with human parvovirus infection. J Hyg (Lond). 1984;93:85–93.
12. Okabe N, Kobiyashi S, Tatsuzawa O, et al. Detection of antibodies to human parvovirus in erythema infectiosum (fifth disease). Arch Dis Child 1984;59:1016–9.
13. Plummer FA, Hammond GW, Forward K, et al. An erythema infectiosum-like illness caused by human parvovirus infection. N Engl J Med. 1985;313:74–9.
14. Lefrere JJ, Courouce AM, Muller JY, et al. Human parvovirus and purpura. Lancet. 1985;1:730.
15. Cohen BJ, Mortimer PP, Pereira MS. Diagnostic assays with mononuclear

antibodies for the human serum parvovirus-like virus. J Hyg (Lond). 1983;91:113–30.
16. Balfour HH. Erythema infectiosum (fifth disease). Clin Pediatr (Phila) 1969;8:721–7.
17. Balfour HH, Schiff GM, Bloom JE. Encephalitis associated with erythema infectiosum. J Pediatr. 1970;77:133–6.
18. Bazemore JM. Discussion of Phillips, IE: Erythema infectiosum. South Med J. 1954;47:253.
19. Pattison JR, Jones SE, Hodgson J, et al. Parvovirus infections and hypoplastic crises in sickle-cell anaemia. Lancet 1981;1:664–5.
20. Serjeant GR, Mason K, Topley JM, et al. Outbreak of aplastic crisis in sickle cell anaemia associated with parvovirus-like agent. Lancet 1981;2:595–7.
21. Rao KRP, Patel AR, Anderson MJ, et al. Infection with a parvovirus-like virus and aplastic crisis in chronic haemolytic anaemia. Ann Intern Med 1983;98:930–2.
22. Kelleher JH, Luban NLC, Mortimer PP, et al. The human serum parvovirus. A specific cause of aplastic crisis in hereditary spherocytosis. J Pediatr. 1983;102:720–2.
23. Green DH, Bellingham AJ, Anderson MJ. Parvovirus infection in a family with aplastic crisis in an affected sibling pair with hereditary spherocytosis. J Clin Pathol. 1984;37:1144–6.
24. Duncan JR, Capellini MD, Anderson MJ, et al. Aplastic crisis due to parvovirus infection in pyruvate kinse deficiency. Lancet. 1983;2:14–6.
25. Mortimer PP, Humphries RK, Moore JG, et al. A human parvovirus-like virus inhibits haemopoietic colony formation in vitro. Nature 1983;302:426–9.
26. Young NS, Harrison M, Moore JG, et al. Direct demonstration of the human parvovirus in erythroid progenitor cells infected in vitro. J Clin Invest. 1984;74;2024–32.
27. Ozawa K, Kurtzman G, Young N. Productive infection by B19 parvovirus of human erythroid bone marrow cells in vitro. Blood. 1987;70:384–91.
28. Brown T, Anand A, Pitchie LD, et al. Intrauterine human parvovirus infection and hydrops foetalis. Lancet 1984;2;1033–4.
29. Knott PD, Welply GAC, Anderson MJ. Serologically proven intrauterine infection with parvovirus. Br Med J. 1984;289:1660.
30. Gray ES, Anard A, Brown T. Parvovirus infections in pregnancy. Lancet. 1986;1:208.
31. Mortimer PP, Cohen BJ, Buckley MM, et al. Human parvovirus and the fetus. Lancet. 1985;2;1012.
32. Anand A, Gray ES, Brown T, et al. Human parvovirus infection in pregnancy and hydrops fetalis. N Engl J Med. 1982;316:183–6.
33. Reid DM, Reid TMS, Brown T, et al. Human parvovirus-associated arthritis: A clinical and laboratory description. Lancet 1985;2:422–5.
34. White DG, Mortimer PP, Blake DR, et al. Human parvovirus arthropathy. Lancet 1985;1:982.
35. Lefrere JJ, Meyer O, Menkes CJ, et al. Human parvovirus and rheumatoid arthritis. Lancet 1985;1:982.
36. Anderson MJ, Davis LR, Jones SE, et al. The development of use of an antibody capture assay for specific IgM to a human parvovirus-like agent. J Hyg (Lond). 1982;83:309–24.
37. Clewley JP. Detection of human parvovirus using a molecularly cloned probe. J Med Virol. 1985;15:173–81.

RNA VIRUSES

Reoviridae

127. COLORADO TICK FEVER

THOMAS P. MONATH

Colorado tick fever (CTF), formerly known as "mountain fever," is the only human orbiviral disease in the United States. The disease was described as early as 1850, but differentiation from Rocky Mountain spotted fever and tularemia was not made until the 1930s. In 1944 Florio et al.[1] transmitted the disease by serial passage in human volunteers and isolated the virus from *Dermacentor andersoni* ticks. A comprehensive review of CTF has been published by Emmons.[2]

The orbivirus genus belongs to the family Reoviridae. Colorado tick fever virions are 50–60 nm particles with double-stranded RNA genomes containing 12 segments. Colorado tick fever virus is related to Eyach virus isolated from *Ixodes* ticks in France and West Germany. Antigenic variants of CTF virus occur in the United States.

Colorado tick fever occurs in mountainous areas within the range of *D. andersoni* ticks (Colorado, Wyoming, Montana, Idaho, Utah, and parts of South Dakota, New Mexico, California, Oregon, Washington, Alberta, and British Columbia). During the spring and summer, the virus is amplified in a cycle involving larval and nymphal *D. andersoni* ticks and ground squirrels and chipmunks, which develop prolonged viremias lasting weeks or even months. Hibernating nymphal and adult ticks carry the virus through the winter months, and infected nymphs reinitiate the cycle by feeding on rodents the next spring. Human infection is acquired through the bite of adult ticks.

Several hundred human cases are recorded annually in the United States,[3,4] but the actual incidence of the disease is probably 10-fold higher. A history of tick exposure is elicited in 90 percent of patients. Young adult male residents with outdoor exposures are at highest risk: campers, foresters, hunters, telephone linesmen, and so forth. The peak incidence is between late May and early July. Truly asymptomatic infections are rare. Long-lasting immunity follows infection, although in at least one instance two laboratory-confirmed clinical episodes were recorded in one person. Viremia is erythrocyte associated and may persist for prolonged periods; one instance of blood transfusion–induced CTF has been described. Peak viremia titers are found during the second and third weeks after onset. Approximately one-half of the infected persons are viremic 4 weeks after the onset of illness.[4]

The incubation period, approximately 3–6 days, is followed by a sudden onset of fever, chills, lethargy, prostation, headache, myalgia, ocular pain, photophobia, abdominal pain, nausea, and vomiting. The duration of the acute illness is usually 7–10 days. Fever is biphasic ("saddle-backed") in about 50 percent of the cases; the initial 2–3 days of fever is followed by a remission of similar duration and, in turn, by another febrile period.

Physical examination may reveal conjunctival injection. Rash is noted in 5–12 percent of the cases and has been described as macular, maculopapular, or rarely, petechial, without any characteristic distribution. Meningoencephalitis is a potentially serious complications in children, with an incidence of 3–7 percent.[3,5] A hemorrhagic syndrome has been described in two children with fatal infections[6] and is characterized by purpura, petechiae, and gastrointestinal hemorrhage, possibly associated with disseminated intravascular coagulation (DIC). Other unusual complications include pericarditis, myocarditis, epididymo-orchitis, and atypical pneumonia; these findings generally occur late and may have an immunopathologic etiology. Congenital infection has been documented but has not been clearly associated with abortion or congenital anomalies.

There may be a prolonged convalescence with asthenia, especially in adults over 30 years. Residual paresis was noted in one patients who recovered from an acute CTF neurologic syndrome.

High interferon levels correlate with fever but not with the frequency or severity of symptoms. Leukopenia is present in a high proportion of cases early in the course of illness[7] and may be diagnostically helpful. Thrombocytopenia has been marked in cases with a bleeding diathesis, but mildly to moderately depressed platelet counts are also found in patients with typical CTF. In patients with neurologic signs, the cerebrospinal fluid (CSF) contains cells ($<500/mm^3$) that are predominantly lymphocytes.

A specific diagnosis depends on the isolation of CTF virus by inoculating suckling mice or cell cultures with suspensions of blood clot or erythrocytes washed free of plasma. CTF antigen can also be demonstrated in erythrocytes by the fluorescent antibody (FA) method.[8] Antibodies appear rather late; the IgM enzyme-linked immunosorbent (ELISA) and FA techniques provide the most sensitive and earliest serologic diagnosis.[9,10]

Colorado tick fever is best prevented by public education to avoid tick-infested areas and tick bites by use of protective clothing, repellents, and inspection to remove ticks before they attach and feed. In local areas (such as campgrounds), reduction of tick and/or rodent populations may be justified.

Treatment is supportive and symptomatic. In children, alernatives to aspirin as an antipyretic–analgesic may be advised because of the thrombocytopenia and possible bleeding diathesis. Antiviral compounds including ribavirin[11] are experimentally effective but have not been used in humans. Patients should not serve as blood donors for at least 6 months after recovery. Women who acquire infection during pregnancy should be followed carefully since information on fetal risk is lacking.

REFERENCES

1. Florio L, Steward MO, Mugrage ER. The experimental transmission of Colorado tick fever. J Exp Med. 1944;80:165.
2. Emmons RW: Colorado tick fever. In: Steele JH, ed. Handbook Series in Zoonoses. Section B. Viral Zoonoses. West Palm Beach, FL: CRC Press; 1981:113.
3. Spruance SL, Bailey A. Colorado tick fever. A review of 115 laboratory confirmed cases. Arch Intern Med. 1973;131:288.
4. Goodpasture HC, Poland JD, Francy DB, et al. Colorado tick fever: Clinical epidemiologic, and laboratory aspects of 228 cases in Colorado in 1973–1974. Ann Intern Med. 1978;88:303.
5. Draughn DE, Sieber OE Jr, Umlauf HJ Jr. Colorado tick fever encephalitis. Clin Pediatr (Phila). 1965;4:626.
6. Eklund CM, Kohls GM, Jellison WL, et al. The clinical and ecological aspects of Colorado tick fever. In: Proceedings of the 6th International Congress on Tropical Medicine and Malaria. V. 5. Rio de Janeiro: 1959;197.
7. Andersen RD, Entringe MA, Robinson WA. Virus-induced leukopenia: Colordo tick fever as a human model. J Infect Dis. 1985;151:449.
8. Emmons RW, Lennette EH. Immunofluorescent staining in the laboratory diagnosis of Colorado tick fever. J Lab Clin Md. 1966;68:923.
9. Emmons RW, Dondero DV, Devlin V, et al. Serologic diagnosis of Colorado tick fever. A comparison of complement-fixation, immunofluorescence, and plaque-reduction methods. Am J Trop Med Hyg. 1969;18:796.
10. Calisher CH, Poland JD, Calisher SB, et al. Diagnosis of Colorado tick fever virus infection by enzyme immunoassays for immunoglobulin M and G antibodies. J Clin Microbiol. 1985;22:84.
11. Smee DF, Sidwell RW, Clark SM, et al. Inhibition of bluetongue and Colorado tick fever orbiviruses by selected antiviral substances. Antimicrob Agents Chemother. 1981;20:533.

128. REOVIRUS AND ORBIVIRUS

THOMAS P. MONATH

The family Reoviridae includes three genera of nonenveloped, segmented, double-stranded RNA viruses causing human disease (orthoreovirus, orbivirus, and rotavirus (see also Chapters 127 and 129). The orthoreoviruses and most orbiviruses have 10 RNA segments; orbiviruses are distinguished from orthoreoviruses by arthropod transmission cycles, susceptibility to an acid pH, and protein structure. Orbiviruses are divded into 13 antigenically distinct serogroups.

Orthoreoviruses are ubiquitous agents that cause infections of all vertebrate classes. Three serotypes (types 1–3) are associated with mammalian infections. Reovirus infection of mice has been used as an elegant model of viral pathogenesis.[1] Human disease is rare, although infection is highly prevalent as determined by antibody surveys. Enteritis in infants and children and upper respiratory infections characterized by fever, pharyngitis, rhinitis, headache, and occasionally rash have been reported. An outbreak of reovirus type 1 in a nursery was associated with a brief (2-day) illness characterized by fever, rhinorrhea, and pharyngitis.[2] Adult volunteers experimentally infected with reovirus types 1 and 2 developed the latter syndrome, which lasted 4–7 days, whereas those given type 3 developed only mild rhinitis.[3] In infants, reovirus type 3 infection has been implicated in neonatal hepatitis and extrahepatic bilary atresia.[4] This association is of interest since type 3 virus produces chronic obstructive jaundice in mice.[5]

Isolated reports of other syndromes including encephalitis, pneumonia, and renal disease have suggested a role for reoviruses. In view of the ubiquity of human reovirus infections, these reports remain suspect. Reoviruses can induce a transient diabetic state in susceptible mouse strains, but a relationship to insulin-dependent diabetes in humans has not been shown.[6]

Among the orbiviruses (other than Colorado tick fever, Chapter 127), six agents have been implicated in human disease. Changuinola virus (prototype of a serogroup containing 13 viruses) was isolated from a single case of self-limited febrile illness in Panama. The virus is transmitted by *Phlebotomus* flies. Lebombo virus has been recovered from a febrile child in Nigeria and from mosquitoes in Nigeria and South Africa. Three tick-borne viruses of the Kemerovo serogroup (Kemerovo, Lipovnik, Tribec) have been associated with or suspected to cause meningoencephalitis[7] or polyradiculitis and other neuropathies in the Soviet Union and eastern Europe. Orungo virus, an antigenically ungrouped mosquito-borne virus, is widely present in sub-Saharan Africa, and the prevalence of human infection is very high. Most infections are asymptomatic or mild, but Orungo virus occasionally causes undifferentiated febrile illness[8] and has been implicated in a case of encephalitis.[9] The transmission cycle may involve monkey and sylvatic *Aedes* mosquitoes (similar to yellow fever), with secondary interhuman transmission by *Anopheles*. Although outbreaks and severe disease have been blamed on this virus, convincing evidence for an etiologic role is lacking.

REFERENCES

1. Tyler KL, Fields BN. Reoviruses and its replication. In: Fields BN, ed. Virology. New York; Raven Press; 1985:823.
2. Rosen L, Hovis, JF, Mastrota FM, et al. An outbreak of infection with a type 1 reovirus among children in an institution. Am J Hyg. 1960;71:266.
3. Rosen L. Reovirus infection in human volunteers. Am J Hyg. 1963;77:29.
4. Glaser JH, Morecki R. Reovirus type 3 and neonatal cholestasis. Semin Liver Dis. 1987;7:100.
5. Papadimitriou JM. The biliary tract in acute murine reovirus 3 infection. Am J Pathol. 1968;52:595.
6. Toniolo A, Conaldi PG, Garzelli C, et al. Role of antecedent mumps and reovirus infections on the development of type 1 (insulin-dependent) diabetes. Eur J Epidemiol. 1985;1:172.
7. Chumakov MP, Karpovich LG, Sarmanova ES, et al. Report on the isolation from *Ixodes persulcatus* ticks and from patients in Western Siberia of a virus differing from the agent of tick-borne encephalitis. Acta Virol. 1963;7:82.
8. Saluzzo JF. Etude ecologique du virus Orungo en Afrique Centrale. Ann Virol (Paris). 1983;134:327.
9. Familusi JB, Moore DL, Fomufud AR, et al. Virus isolates from children with febrile convulsions in Nigeria. Clin Pediatr (Phila). 1972;11:272.

129. ROTAVIRUS

JOHN E. HERRMANN
NEIL R. BLACKLOW

Acute diarrheal diseases are of public health importance in both developed and developing countries, and they affect people in all age groups. Worldwide, they are the greatest single cause of morbidity and mortality. Infectious diarrhea in Asia, Africa, and Latin America has been estimated to result in 5 million or more deaths annually, with the highest mortality occurring in infants and young children. In developed countries, infectious diarrhea is also a major debilitating disease, and gastroenteritis due to rotavirus alone causes up to 50 percent of all pediatric hospitalizations during the winter months.

Several viruses have been associated with diarrheal disease, including rotaviruses, Norwalk and Norwalk-like viruses, enteric adenoviruses, caliciviruses, astroviruses, enteric coronavirus, and unclassified small round viruses of 27–32 nm diameter. The traditional rotaviruses (group A rotaviruses) are considered to be the major agents of gastroenteritis of infants and young children in most countries, and they are a major cause of infant mortality in many areas of the world. Non-group A rotaviruses, especially those in group B, have been detected far less frequently and have only been associated with epidemics of gastroenteritis in China. The age groups primarily affected by group B rotaviruses are older children and adults.

DESCRIPTION OF ROTAVIRUSES

The rotavirus virion contains double-stranded (ds) RNA enclosed in a double capsid (complete or double-shelled particles). Complete particles are approximately 70 nm in diameter and are infectious. Incomplete (or single-shelled) particles of approximately 55 nm in diameter are also found. The morphology of the intact particles, as seen by negative stain electron microscopy (Fig. 1), distinguishes the rotavirus genus of viruses from reoviruses and orbiviruses, the other members of the family Reoviridae, and the double capsid gives the virus a characteristic wheel (Latin: rota) shape. Double-shelled particles have a density of 1.36 g/cm^3 in cesium chloride and a sedimentation coefficient of 520–530 S. Single-shelled particles have a density of 1.38 g/cm^3 in cesium chloride.[1–6]

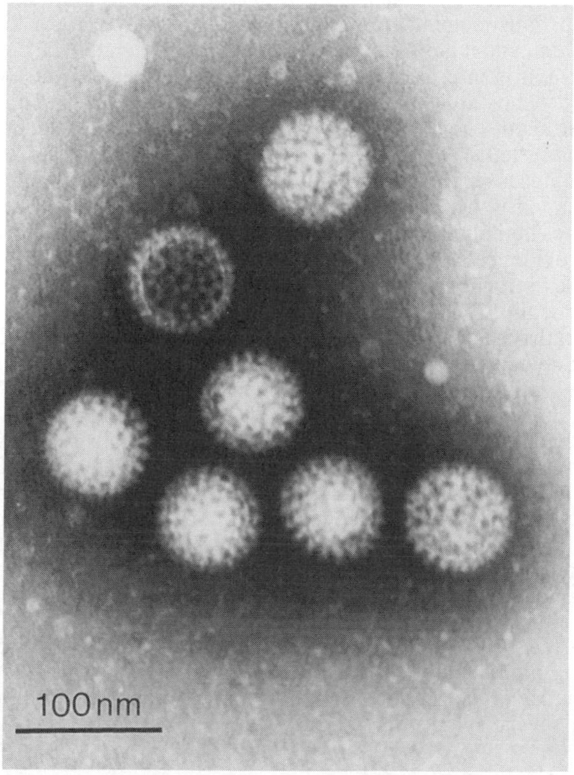

FIG. 1. Rotavirus particles observed by negative-stain electron microscopy in a stool suspension of child with diarrhea. (Courtesy of Dr. W.D. Cubitt, London, UK.)

The viral genome is comprised of 11 segments of double-stranded RNA, as shown by electrophoretic analysis. The molecular weights of the segments range from 2×10^5 to 2.2×10^6 daltons, with estimated total weights of 1.1×10^7 to 1.4×10^7 daltons.[7] Strains of rotaviruses can be distinguished by differences in the migration patterns of the RNA segments by polyacrylamide gel electrophoresis (PAGE), and the electropherotypes obtained can be used to investigate rotavirus epidemiology. The migration patterns of the RNA segments differ among the various human and animal rotavirus strains as well. Those rotaviruses, both animal and human, that do not share the rotaviral common antigen also show distinctive RNA patterns by PAGE.[8–13] These non-group A rotaviruses have also been referred to as atypical rotaviruses, groups B or C rotaviruses, or pararotaviruses. Details concerning the rotavirus genome and the molecular epidemiology of rotaviruses have been reviewed.[7,14]

Group A viruses, which are the ones that have been traditionally classified as rotaviruses, all contain a group-specific common antigen (VP6, the inner capsid protein). The more recently recognized non-group A rotaviruses, which include groups B, C, and possibly more, also contain 11 segments of dsRNA and are morphologically the same as other rotaviruses but lack VP6. These antigenically atypical rotaviruses have been detected in humans,[8,12] pigs,[10,11] calves,[13] chickens,[15] and lambs.[13] Among the group A human rotaviruses there are also four well-defined serotypes, based on outer capsid protein (VP7) differences, and two subgroups, based on antigenic differences in VP6. Possible new serotypes have also been described.[16,17] Table 1 summarizes the various human and animal rotavirus classifications. The outer capsid proteins (VP3, product of gene 4, and VP7, product of gene 8 or 9) are the major antigens that give rise to neutralizing antibody. In addition to these antigenic classifications, there are numerous electropherotypes based on migration of rotaviral RNA segments in gels.

In regard to virus stability, a simian rotavirus strain has been shown to retain infectivity at pH 3.5 or pH 10.0 and is not inactivated by ether, chloroform, fluorocarbons, proteases, or freeze-thawing.[14] It loses infectivity after incubation or freezing in 2 M $MgCl_2$, $CaCl_2$; EDTA, and also after heating in NaCl for 15 minutes at 50°C. Human rotaviruses are also inactivated by chelating agents. The most effective disinfectant for rotaviruses has been shown to be 95% ethanol.[19] Formalin and Lysol are also effective.[20] Sodium hypochlorite may[21] or may

TABLE 1. Summary of Human and Animal Rotavirus Serotypes and Strains

Species	*Serotype*[a]	*Subgroup*[b]	*Strains*
Human	1	2	Wa, KU, K8, DB
	2	1	DS-1, S2, KUN, HN-126, 390
	3	2	M, P, YO, McM2, MO, Ito, Walk 57/14, 15
	4	1	St. Thomas 3 and 4, Hochl, Hosokawa
Animal	1		None described
	2		None described
	3	1	Simian SA11, MMU 18806, canine CU-1, feline (Taka)
		—[c]	Equine H-2
	4	1	Porcine SB-2
		2	Porcine SB-1A, Gottfried
	5	1	Porcine OSU, EE, A580, equine H-1
	6	1	Bovine NCDV, UK, B641, B720, B14, II-2
	7	—[c]	Bovine B223, chicken Ch 2
	8	—[c]	Turkey Ty1, Ty3
	9	—[c]	Chicken Ch 1

[a] Serotypes are based on virus neutralization.
[b] Subgroups are based on VP6 antigenic relationships determined by ELISA, complement fixation, or other assays.
[c] Not subgrouped.
(Data from refs. 7, 14, and 18.)

not[20] be effective. Rotavirus has also been shown to survive standard chlorine treatment in a community water supply.[22]

PATHOGENESIS

The mechanism of rotavirus-induced diarrhea is not completely known. The major mechanism appears to be decreased absorption of salt and water related to selective infection of the absorptive intestinal villous cells, resulting in net fluid secretion. Impaired D-xylose absorption has been observed,[23] and some patients have depressed levels of disaccharidases.[24] Pale, fatty stools are occasionally associated with rotaviral diarrhea, which suggests that rotavirus infection may impede digestion of fats.[25] Histopathologic studies in rotavirus infections have revealed villous shortening, reticular cell enlargement, mitochondrial swelling, lymphocyte infiltration of the villous lamina propria, and irregular microvilli.

There do not appear to be any major differences in the pathogenesis of the non-group A rotaviruses studied thus far. Mature enterocytes become infected and exfoliate, which results in shortened villi and subsequent decreased absorption, as for the group A rotaviruses.[26] The occurrence of syncytia on the surface of villi, with fusion of up to 20 enterocytes, has been detected in a number of animal species and may be a pathognomonic lesion for the non-group A rotaviruses.[26]

EPIDEMIOLOGY

Gastroenteritis induced by group A rotavirus usually occurs in infants and young children, although outbreaks in adult populations have been reported. In temperate climates, rotavirus infection may be responsible for close to half of the hospitalizations of infants during the winter months, whereas in tropical climates, infections tend to occur year round. Transmission of the virus is thought to be primarily by the fecal-oral route, although transmission through food and water has been suggested. The estimated incubation period of rotavirus diarrhea in clinical studies is less than 2 days, and in adult volunteers, 2–4 days.[7] In stools, the maximal viral shedding occurs from 2 to 5 days after the onset of diarrhea, although there may be no correlation observed between the maximal amount of virus excreted in the stools and the severity of the diarrhea.[27] Virus-specific IgA has been detected in pharyngeal secretions of patients with rotavirus gastroenteritis[27] and rotavirus antigen has been detected in respiratory secretions of children with pneumonia,[28] which suggest the possibility of transmission via a respiratory route or by ingestion of virus aerosols.

Infant mortality due to diarrheal diseases is high in developing countries, and rotavirus is thought to be of major importance. In developed countries, mortality due to rotavirus infection is infrequent but has been reported.[29] Chronic disease is not usually found, but may be seen in immunodeficient children and in patients immunosuppressed for bone marrow transplantation.

Rotavirus infection may also be asymptomatic, especially in newborn children. In one study, 62 (57 percent) of 108 children examined were found to shed rotavirus during the first few days of life, whereas only 4 (6 percent) of these children had diarrhea.[30] In another study, rotavirus was found in 83 (29 percent) of 283 children under 2 years old, with 40 (48 percent) of these asymptomatic.[31] The likelihood of symptoms being associated with rotavirus increases with the age of the child. In neonates, virus shedding was associated with diarrhea in 29 percent, in children aged 1 to 6 months 50 percent, and in 7–24-month-old children 74 percent.[31] Infection in adults is also usually asymptomatic. In one study comparing rotavirus infections of children and adults in families, the attack rate was 32 percent in children, compared with 17 percent for adults.[32] Seventy percent of infected children were symptomatic, whereas only 40 percent of the infected adults were symptomatic.[32] Thus it appears that asymptomatic rotaviral infection is most frequent in neonates, and that the recovery of virus from stools of patients with diarrhea, while not always of diagnostic significance, is usually associated with symptomatic disease in children above the age of 6 months. In one study, there did not appear to be any differences in the strains that infect newborns asymptomatically, compared with the strains causing illness in older infants.[33]

Rotavirus infections are also a major cause of diarrhea in young farm animals worldwide, especially cows,[34,35] horses,[36,37] pigs,[38] and sheep,[39] and rotaviruses have been identified in a number of species including monkeys and apes,[40–42] dogs,[43,44] cats,[45] rabbits,[46] mice,[47] chickens and turkeys,[48,49] goats,[50] antelopes,[51] and deer.[52] There is no evidence that natural virus transmission from man to animals or animals to man occurs, although administration of rhesus monkey rotavirus vaccine to children causes mild symptoms in some of the recipients, as discussed below under "Prevention." Experimental infection of newborn animals, especially gnotobiotic ones, with human strains of rotavirus may result in symptomatic infection.[53]

CLINICAL MANIFESTATIONS

The clinical spectrum of rotavirus infections varies from asymptomatic to severe, fatal disease. Common clinical findings usually include vomiting, abdominal distress, diarrhea, and mild dehydration. Fever and vomiting frequently precede diarrhea. In one study, fever of 37.9°C–39°C was present in 46 percent of children with gastroenteritis and confirmed rotavirus infection; fever of more than 39°C was found in 31 percent of these patients.[54] Associated clinical findings may include irritability and pharyngeal or tympanic membrane erythema. Stools are typically watery and usually do not contain blood or leukocytes. Vomiting and dehydration occur more frequently in children hospitalized for rotavirus diarrhea than in those hospitalized for other infectious diarrheas.[54] The course of rotavirus disease is generally 3 to 9 days, and the mean time of hospitalization, when required due to severe dehydration, is 4 days.[55] The highest frequency of disease occurs in the 6–24-month-old age group. Nosocomial infections in hospital wards are a known problem, and it has been reported that approximately 20 percent of rotavirus infections in hospitals were considered nosocomial.[56,57] Thus appropriate infection control measures should be undertaken when patients with suspected viral gastroenteritis are admitted.

Numerous case reports have associated rotavirus infection with a variety of conditions such as intussusception, Reye syndrome, hemolytic uremic syndrome, and Kawasaki syndrome. The evidence for a disease association with rotavirus seems to be strongest for some cases of neonatal necrotizing enterocolitis.[58]

Deaths are not unusual in developing countries and typically are due to severe dehydration and resultant electrolyte imbalance. Fatalities are rare in developed countries; in a report from Canada, 21 deaths were reported over a 5-year period, and nearly all children were known to be previously healthy.[29] Chronic symptomatic diarrhea with prolonged fecal shedding and antigenemia may occur in patients with primary immunodeficiency diseases, and severe disease may also occur in those who are immunosuppressed for bone marrow transplantation.

Rotavirus infections in adults are usually asymptomatic and accompanied by a seroconversion to the virus. Symptomatic infections in adults are usually mild, but severe illness has been reported both in elderly patients[59] and in apparently normal young adults.[60] Infections due to non-group A rotaviruses in China have been reported to cause epidemics of gastroenteritis with severe symptoms in adults.[8]

DIAGNOSIS

Prior to the development of antigen-detecting immunoassays for rotavirus, electron microscopy (EM) was the major technique used and is still useful for standardizing new detection techniques as they are developed. Human rotaviruses can also now be identified by isolation from stool samples in primary monkey kidney (MK) cells or the simian continuous cell line MA104, with the aid of proteolytic enzymes. Treatment of the virus with trypsin prior to infection, incorporation of trypsin in the maintenance medium, and the use of roller tube cultures all enhance virus propagation. For isolation of rotavirus from clinical materials, the use of primary African green MK or cynomolgous MK cells appears to be more effective than MA104 cells,[61–63] but isolation of human strains is still considered to be inefficient, and the methods are time-consuming.

Among the various tests that have been developed for diagnosis of rotavirus infection, antigen detection by enzyme-linked immunosorbent assay (ELISA) is now the preferred method because it has been found equivalent in sensitivity to EM, is simpler to perform, and does not require an electron microscope or other specialized equipment. It is also more rapid and cheaper than isolation procedures. The earlier commercially produced tests used polyclonal sera, which can lead to occasional false-positive results, especially in stool samples from neonates.[64,65] The use of monoclonal antibody to the rotaviral group antigen has been found to give results that are higher in sensitivity than polyclonal antibody, and it eliminates the problems of nonspecificity.[66] Both polyclonal antibody and monoclonal antibody ELISA tests are commercially available in kit form from a number of manufacturers. For non-group A rotaviruses, an ELISA test has been developed[67] but is not widely available. Whether routine testing for the non-group A rotaviruses will become necessary will depend on future epidemiologic studies. At present, routine testing is not warranted.

Latex agglutination tests for detection of rotavirus antigen in stool samples are also available from several commercial sources. To date, they all use polystyrene particles sensitized with polyclonal antibody, although monoclonal antibody-based tests have been reported.[68] The agglutination tests can usually be done more rapidly than ELISA tests, but may be far less sensitive than the better ELISA assays.[69–71] They are, however, convenient to use and can be easily applied to on-site testing of patients' samples.

A number of different specimens can be used for viral antigen detection, such as anal swabs, soiled diapers from infants, or other stool-containing materials, if the preferred specimen, a freshly collected undilute stool sample, is not available. Samples to be assayed for rotavirus antigen may be shipped on wet ice and stored for a few days at 4°C. The preferred method for handling virus samples is to send them on dry ice, with subsequent storage at −70°C, especially if virus isolation in cell culture is to be attempted.

Rapid detection of rotavirus in stools by analysis of viral nucleic acid after gel electrophoresis can also be accomplished,[72] and we have found this method equal in sensitivity to ELISA and to EM (unpublished data). Although it is more cumbersome than ELISA and is unnecessary for routine diagnosis, the method is useful for determining the nucleic acid patterns ("electropherotyping") in epidemiologic studies. It is also the only method widely available for diagnosis of non-group A rotavirus infections, if these are suspected.

Nucleic acid probes have been applied to rotavirus identification as well.[73,74] For routine clinical diagnosis, as is true for the diagnosis of a number of infectious agents,[75,76] there is no advantage at present of probes compared with monoclonal or polyclonal antibody-based assays for detection of rotavirus in gastroenteritis. The sensitivity is similar, but the probe techniques as now configured are considerably more complex and require more time to obtain results than antibody-based ELISA tests.

If a definitive diagnosis cannot be obtained with commercially produced or other rotavirus assays, it may be necessary to use additional tests for confirmation. The best method is the use of gel electrophoresis; EM or immune EM can also be used, if available. If an ELISA was used for the initial assay, a blocking ELISA can be used,[77] or a test that uses preimmune serum as capture antibody can be done. In the latter test, the solid phase used in the ELISA (wells of microtiter plates, tubes, or beads) is coated with preimmune serum for comparison with results obtained with immune serum (capture antibody). The immune serum should give ELISA values that are at least twice that of values obtained with preimmune serum to be considered positive. Because the reagents necessary for these confirmatory ELISA tests are unlikely to be available for commercially produced assays, the preferred confirmatory test is gel electrophoresis done directly on the stool sample, or after isolation in cell cultures if such cultures are available.

Diagnosis of rotaviruses as to specific subgroup and serotype is not routinely done or required, and preparation of specific antisera is difficult. However, the availability of monoclonal antibodies to subgroup antigens[78,79] and to specific serotypes[80,81] should facilitate classification of rotavirus isolates for epidemiologic studies. Direct serotyping of rotaviruses in stool samples by monoclonal antibody-based ELISA has also been accomplished, but it is not as sensitive as EM or other tests for detecting virus in unconcentrated stools.[80,81]

TREATMENT

Specific antiviral therapy for rotaviral infection is not presently available. Ribavirin has been shown to inhibit animal rotaviruses in vitro[82,83] but was not effective against murine rotavirus infection in vivo.[82,83]

Therapy, therefore, is directed at prevention of severe dehydration and electrolyte imbalance. Intravenous fluids are well established as an effective therapy, but an oral rehydration salts solution has been shown in recent years to be an equally effective therapy for mild to moderately severely dehydrating rotavirus gastroenteritis in ambulatory and hospital settings.[84,85] Oral rehydration of patients can be achieved using glucose or sucrose solutions containing electrolytes, such as the standard World Health Organization formula that consists of (per liter of water) glucose 20 g, sodium chloride 3.5 g, sodium bicarbonate 2.5 g, and potassium chloride 1.5 g. Ready-to-use oral electrolyte solutions are commercially available. Intravenous therapy must be administered if oral rehydration is not successful in replacing fluids and electrolytes, or if the patient is in shock or is severely dehydrated.

Oral administration of rotavirus antibody to two immunodeficient patients with chronic diarrhea was effective in reducing symptoms,[86] but was not effective in treating infants and children with rotavirus diarrhea who had no apparent underlying immune dysfunction.[87]

PREVENTION

Because of the importance of gastroenteritis as a cause of infant morbidity and mortality in many areas of the world, and the substantive role that rotaviruses have in this disease syndrome, considerable effort has been directed toward its prevention. The principal approach taken in recent years has been active immunization with orally administered animal strains of rotavirus.

The use of animal strains for human rotavirus vaccines is based on the finding that there is cross-protection among animals with both homotypic and heterotypic animal rotaviruses, and with animal and human rotaviruses.[88,89] Two vaccines have been used the most extensively in field trials. One uses the Nebraska calf diarrhea virus (NCDV) strain of bovine rotavirus, and the other uses a rhesus rotavirus strain. The NCDV bovine strain, designated RIT 4237, was attenuated by 147 tissue culture passages in primary bovine kidney cells and produced at passage 154 in primary monkey kidney cells.[90]

The rhesus monkey rotavirus strain RRV-1, also designated

MMY-18006, was originally isolated from the stool of an infant rhesus monkey with acute diarrhea.[91] The strain was passaged nine times in primary monkey kidney cells and seven times in a diploid monkey kidney cell line.[92]

Preliminary tests with the RIT 4237 vaccine did not give uniform seroconversion in that 5 of 17 seronegative children aged 2 years or less did not show definite seroconversion after receiving that vaccine.[93] However, these studies did show that the attenuated bovine vaccine stimulated an immune response in most of the susceptible children, and there were no apparent side effects. Field trials in Finland with this vaccine indicated that a high level of protection was afforded. In two studies of infants aged 6 to 12 months at the time of vaccination or placebo administration, only 7 of 254 vaccinees had rotavirus diarrhea over a 5-month observation period, compared with 44 of 252 placebo recipients.[94,95] Seroconversion occurred in approximately 50 percent of the vaccine recipients.

Studies in Butare, Rwanda with the same vaccine, however, did not show any protective effect.[96] Furthermore, there were no significant differences in the rates of seroconversion among the 122 vaccine and 123 placebo recipients. A similar lack of protection was found in a study of Gambian children, which involved 170 vaccine and 83 placebo recipients.[97] There were no clear reasons for the failure of the vaccine in these studies, although interference by other enteric viruses might be a factor.[96,98] It has also been surmised that breast-feeding could interfere with vaccines due to antirotavirus antibody and nonspecific rotavirus inhibitors.[98–101] In the Finnish studies, there was no apparent interference of breast-feeding with oral vaccination.[102]

To avoid these political problems, which may be more important in developing countries than in others, vaccination of neonates might be a better means to provide immunity. This approach was investigated by Vesikari et al.,[103] who administered RIT 4237 vaccine to 119 newborn infants and placebo to 120 others in Finland. The age of the infants in each group was approximately 5 days. Over a 16-month observation period, the vaccine gave no protection against rotavirus infection. The vaccine did, however, appear to significantly lessen the severity of the diarrheal episodes. Whether the same finding would be obtained in developing countries remains to be determined.

It has also been noted that natural neonatal rotavirus infection does not confer immunity against reinfection but does protect against development of severe disease,[104] as was found in a vaccine study.[103] In two consecutive naturally occurring outbreaks among 44 young children exposed once or twice to rotavirus type 3 in Japan, protection against gastroenteritis seemed to be serotype-specific and to be related to levels of neutralizing antibody against the homotypic virus.[105] This study suggests that a rotavirus vaccine may need to contain all 4 of the known, medically important serotypes to produce sufficient clinical protection against group A rotaviruses.

In view of the failure of the RIT 4237 vaccine to provide protection against rotaviral disease in developing countries,[96–99] clinical studies with this vaccine are no longer being undertaken. Clearly, a successful rotavirus vaccine will need to be effective with the population groups at greatest risk for developing severe rotavirus illness—infants and young children in developing countries.

Clinical trials with the rhesus rotavirus vaccine have not been as extensive as those with the NCDV vaccine. In a limited study[106] involving 14 vaccinees and 10 controls receiving placebo, 3 control children developed rotavirus diarrhea over an approximate 1.5-year period compared with none of the controls ($p < 0.059$). In a somewhat larger study involving 24 vaccinees and 25 control children, it was reported that there was no significant differences in the incidence of rotavirus diarrhea among vaccine or placebo recipients observed over the course of the first winter after vaccination.[107] The vaccine has also been evaluated in Venezuela,[108] where it was found over a 1-year surveillance period that there were 5 episodes of rotavirus diarrhea in the 123 vaccinated infants, compared with 16 episodes in the 124 infants who had received placebo ($p = 0.013$). The rhesus rotavirus vaccine and the NCDV vaccine have not been directly compared for efficacy in preventing rotavirus diarrhea, but the rhesus rotavirus vaccine has been tested in Finland in a setting comparable with the one used for the bovine rotavirus vaccine trials.[102] Of 100 children receiving vaccine, there were two episodes of rotavirus diarrhea compared with six in the 100 receiving placebo. The authors concluded that the degree of protection was similar to that obtained with the bovine rotavirus vaccine. It has been noticed in this study and others[92,109] that the rhesus rotavirus vaccine may cause side effects symptomatic of natural rotavirus infection and therefore has to be given at 100–1000-fold lower infective doses than the bovine strain. This finding has led Vesikari et al.[102] to conclude that the bovine strains may be overattenuated and the rhesus rotavirus vaccine too little attenuated for use in humans.

The rhesus rotavirus vaccine also has been shown to replicate to titers of more than 10^3 infectious units per ml of 10 percent stool suspension,[107] which is well beyond the dose of human rotavirus required to cause infection.[110] There is no evidence, however, that secondary transmission occurs in situations such as day care centers, where transmission would be likely.[104]

A number of other vaccines have been proposed, including other bovine rotavirus vaccines and vaccines based on reassortant viruses,[98,111,112] but whether these will be an improvement over the RIT 4237 bovine rotavirus vaccine or the rhesus rotavirus vaccine remains to be determined. There is evidence that reassortant porcine rotaviruses are effective immunogens and confer immunity to challenge in gnotobiotic piglets.[112] Reassortant rotavirus vaccines containing gene segments coding for neutralization proteins for either serotypes 1, 2, or 4 have been administered in human trials for determining safety and immunogenicity[113] but not as yet for studying protection against infection. It was found that the vaccines were immunogenic in 70 percent or more of the recipients without a high pre-existing antibody titer and caused detectable side effects (low-grade fever) only in the serotype 2 vaccine recipients. Whether multivalent vaccines will result in interference with or enhancement of immunity remains to be determined. As to the present vaccine situation, there are sufficient reports available to conclude that the bovine RIT 4237 and the rhesus rotavirus vaccines are effective in preventing severe rotavirus diarrhea (but not necessarily infection) in developed, temperate zone countries, but that no vaccine has been shown to be effective in developing countries.

In addition to the question of efficacy, there are a number of other issues that will need to be resolved before a rotavirus vaccine can become commonplace. The most important of these is whether a rotavirus vaccine could be given concomitantly with oral poliovirus without interference with either vaccine. This would be the most convenient approach to facilitate widespread vaccination, but studies to date indicate that both the number of vaccinees responding and the intensity of the response to rotavirus are decreased when given simultaneously with oral poliovirus vaccine.[114] The immune response to the poliovirus vaccine did not appear to be affected. Some other issues that are also unresolved are whether repeated vaccinations are of any value,[98,102] or what the optimal age is for maximum effectiveness of vaccination. Finally, there are ancillary issues in vaccine trials such as uniform standards for grading severity of illness and the most effective vehicle for vaccine administration.[98]

Passive immunization has also been investigated. It is known that human breast milk contains rotavirus-specific IgA, and that this IgA can be transferred to neonates and detected in the neonates' feces.[115] This fact is likely to account, at least in part, for the protective, anti-infective influences of breast milk.[116] Passive immunization by artificial means has been successfully demonstrated to prevent rotavirus illness in animals, as has oral administration of rotavirus-specific antibodies to neonates[117] or children.[87] Current interest in prevention, however, has been concentrated on vaccine development and testing rather than better means of passive immunization.

The mechanism of immunity as a result of either vaccination or natural infection appears to involve more than virus-neutralizing antibody production, and the degree of immunity may be strain-related. It was found by Bishop et al.[104] that natural neonatal rotavirus infection did not protect infants from subsequent infections with heterotypic strains, but did lessen the severity of illness. This immunity was assumed to be due to local IgA production in the intestinal mucosa or to cellular immune mechanisms. Immune responses examined in children who had received rhesus rotavirus vaccine lend some support to the concept of mucosal immunity. In a comparison of rotavirus-specific serum antibody and coproantibody IgA, it was found that the serum neutralization response, primarily homotypic as compared with a heterotypic response in adult volunteers,[118] occurred in 91 percent (31/34) of children, and there were fecal IgA responses in 69 percent (11/16). However, two children who did not show a serum neutralizing antibody response did have serum and fecal IgA responses.[119]

REFERENCES

1. Bridger JC, Woode GN. Characterization of two particle types of calf rotavirus. J Gen Virol. 1976;31:245–50.
2. Kapikian AZ, Kalica AR, Shih JW, et al. Buoyant density in cesium chloride of the human reovirus-like agent of infantile gastroenteritis by ultracentrifugation, electron microscopy, and complement fixation. Virology. 1976;70:564–69.
3. Tam JS, Szymanski MT, Middleton PJ, et al. Studies on the particles of infantile gastroenteritis virus (orbivirus group). Intervirology. 1976;7:181–91.
4. Rodger SM, Schnagl R, Holmes IH. Further biochemical characterization, including the detection of surface glycoproteins, of human, calf, and simian rotaviruses. J Virol. 1977;24:91–8.
5. Elias MM. Separation and infectivity of two particle types of human rotavirus. J Gen Virol. 1977;37:191–4.
6. Palmer E, Martin ML. Further observations on the ultrastructure of human rotavirus. J Gen Virol. 1982;62:105–11.
7. Kapikian AZ, Chanock RM. Rotavirus. In: Fields BN, ed. Virology. New York: Raven Press; 1985:863–906.
8. Hung T, Chen G, Wang C, et al. Waterborne outbreak of rotavirus diarrhoea in adults in China caused by a novel rotavirus. Lancet. 1984;1:1139–42.
9. Pedley S, Bridger JC, Brown JF, et al. Molecular characterization of rotaviruses with distinct group antigens. J Gen Virol. 1983;64:2093–2101.
10. Bohl EH, Saif LJ, Theil KW, et al. Porcine pararotavirus: detection, differentiation from rotavirus, and pathogenesis in gnotobiotic piglets. J Clin Microbiol. 1982;15:312–9.
11. Bridger JC, Clarke IN, McCrae MA. Characterization of an antigenically distinct porcine rotavirus. Infect Immun. 1982;35:1058–62.
12. Espejo RT, Puerto F, Soler C, et al. Characterization of human pararotavirus. Infect Immun. 1984;44:112–6.
13. Snodgrass DR, Herring AJ, Campbell JM, et al. Comparison of atypical rotaviruses from calves, piglets, lambs and man. J Gen Virol. 1984;65:909–14.
14. Estes MK, Palmer EL, Obijeski JF. Rotaviruses: a review. Curr Top Microbiol Immunol. 1983;105:123–84.
15. McNulty MS, Allan GM, Todd D, et al. Isolation from chickens of a rotavirus lacking the group antigen. J Gen Virol. 1981;55:405–13.
16. Matsuno S, Hasegawa G, Mukoyama A, et al. A candidate for a new serotype of human rotavirus. J Virol. 1985;54:623–4.
17. Clark HF, Hoshino Y, Bell LM, et al. Rotavirus isolate WI61 representing a presumptive new human serotype. J Clin Microbiol. 1987;25:1757–62.
18. Estes MK, Graham DY, Petrie BL. Antigenic structure of rotaviruses. In: van Regenmortel MHV, Neurath AR, eds. Immunochemistry of Viruses. The Basis for Serodiagnosis and Vaccines. Amsterdam: Elsevier Science Publishers; 1985:389–405.
19. Tan JA, Schnagl RD. Inactivation of a rotavirus by disinfectants. Med J Aust. 1981;1:19–23.
20. Snodgrass DR, Herring JA. The activity of disinfectant on lamb rotavirus. Vet Rec. 1977;101:81.
21. Tan JA, Schnagl RD. Rotavirus inactivated by a hypochlorite-based disinfectant: a reappraisal. Med J Aust. 1983;1:550.
22. Smith EM, Gerba CP. Development of a method for detection of human rotavirus in water and sewage. Appl Environ Microbiol. 1982;43:1440–50.
23. Mavromichalis J, Evans N, McNeish AS, et al. Intestinal damage in rotavirus and adenovirus gastroenteritis assessed by D-xylose malabsorption. Arch Dis Child. 1977;52:589–91.
24. Bishop RF, Davidson GP, Holmes IH, et al. Virus particles in epithelial cells of duodenal mucosa from children with viral gastroenteritis. Lancet. 1973;2:1281–3.
25. Thomas MEM, Luton P, Matimer JY. Virus diarrhoea associated with pale fatty faeces. J Hyg. 1981;87:313–9.
26. Hall GA. Comparative pathology of infection by novel diarrhoea viruses. In: Novel Diarrhoea Viruses. Ciba Foundation Symposium. 1987;128:218–31.
27. Stals F, Walther FJ, Bruggeman CA. Faecal and pharyngeal shedding of rotavirus and rotavirus IgA in children with diarrhoea. J Med Virol. 1984;14:333–9.
28. Santosham M, Yolken RH, Quiroz E, et al. Detection of rotavirus in respiratory secretions of children with pneumonia. J Pediatr. 1983;103:583–5.
29. Carlson JAK, Middleton PJ, Szymanski M, et al. Fatal rotavirus gastroenteritis: an analysis of 21 cases. Am J Dis Child. 1978;132:477–9.
30. Perez-Schael I, Daoud G, White L, et al. Rotavirus shedding by newborn children. J Med Virol. 1984;14:127–36.
31. Champsaur H, Questiaux E, Prevot J, et al. Rotavirus carriage, asymptomatic infection, and disease in the first years of life. I. Virus shedding. J Infect Dis. 1984;149:667–74.
32. Wenman WM, Hinde D, Feltham S, et al. Rotavirus infection in adults: result of a prospective family study. N Engl J Med. 1979;301:303–6.
33. Vial PA, Kotloff KL, Losonsky GA. Molecular epidemiology of rotavirus infection in a room for convalescing newborns. J Infect Dis. 1988;157:668–73.
34. Fernelius AL, Ritchie AE, Classick LG, et al. Cell culture adaption and propagation of a reovirus-like agent of calf diarrhea from a field outbreak in Nebraska. Arch Ges Virusforsch. 1972;37:114–30.
35. Mebus CA, Kono M, Underdahl NR, et al. Cell culture propagation of neonatal calf diarrhea (scours) virus. Can Vet J. 1971;12:69–72.
36. Flewett TH, Bryden AS, Davies H. Virus diarrhea in foals and other animals. Vet Rec. 1975;96:477.
37. Tzipori S, Walker M. Isolation of rotavirus from foals with diarrhea. Aust J Exp Biol Med Sci. 1978;56:453–7.
38. Rodger SM, Craven JA, Williams I. Demonstration of reovirus-like particles in intestinal contents of piglets with diarrhoea. Aust Vet J. 1975;51:536.
39. Snodgrass DR, Smith W, Gray EW, et al. A rotavirus in lambs with diarrhea. Res Vet Sci. 1976;20:113–4.
40. Malherbe HH, Strickland-Cholmley M. Simian virus SA-11 and the related "O" agent. Arch Ges Virusforsch. 1967;22:235–45.
41. Stuker G, Oshiro LS, Schmidt NJ, et al. Virus detection in monkeys with diarrhea: the association of adenoviruses with diarrhea and the possible role of rotaviruses. Lab Anim Sci. 1979;29:610–6.
42. Ashley CR, Caul EO, Clark SKR, et al. Rotavirus infection of apes. Lancet. 1978;2:477.
43. Roseto A, Lema F, Sitbon M, et al. Detection of rotavirus in dogs. Soc Occup Med. 1979;7:478.
44. England JJ, Poston RP. Electron microscopic identification and subsequent isolation of a rotavirus from a dog with fatal neonatal diarrhea. Am J Vet Res. 1980;41:782–3.
45. Snodgrass DR, Angus KW, Gray EW. A rotavirus from kittens. Vet Rec. 1979;104:222–3.
46. Bryden AS, Thouless ME, Flewett TH. A rabbit rotavirus. Vet Rec. 1976;99:323.
47. Much D, Zajac I. Purification and characterization of epizootic diarrhea of infant mice virus. Infect Immun. 1972;6:1019–24.
48. Jones RC, Hughes CS, Henry RR. Rotavirus infection in commercial laying hens. Vet Rec. 1979;104:22.
49. McNulty MS, Allan GM, Todd D, et al. Isolation and cell culture propagation of rotaviruses from turkeys and chickens. Arch Virol. 1979;61:13–21.
50. Scott AC, Luddington J, Lucas M, et al. Rotavirus in goats. Vet Rec. 1978;103:145.
51. Reed DE, Daley CA, Shave HJ. Reovirus-like agents associated with neonatal diarrhea in pronghorn antelope. J Wildl Dis. 1976;12:488–91.
52. Tzipori S, Caple IW, Butler R. Isolation of a rotavirus from deer. Vet Rec. 1976;99:398.
53. Wyatt RG, Mebus CA, Yolken RH, et al. Rotaviral immunity in gnotobiotic calves: heterologous resistance to human virus induced by bovine virus. Science. 1975;203:548–50.
54. Rodriguez WJ, Kim HW, Arrobio JO, et al. Clinical features of acute gastroenteritis associated with human reovirus-like agent in infants and young children. J Pediatr. 1977;90:188–93.
55. Middleton PJ, Szymanski MT, Petric M. Viruses associated with acute gastroenteritis in young children. Am J Dis Child. 1977;131:733–7.
56. Ryder RW, McGowan JE, Hatch MH, et al. Reovirus-like agent as a cause of nosocomial diarrhea in infants. J Pediatr. 1977;90:698–702.
57. Black RE, Merson MH, Rahman ASMM, et al. A two-year study of bacterial, viral and parasitic agents associated with diarrhea in rural Bangladesh. J Infect Dis. 1980;142:660–4.
58. Rotbart HA, Nelson WL, Glode MP, et al. Neonatal rotavirus associated necrotizing enterocolitis: case control study and prospective surveillance during an outbreak. J Pediatr. 1988;112:87–93.
59. Marrie TJ, Lee SHS, Faulkner RS, et al. Rotavirus infection in a geriatric population. Arch Intern Med. 1982;142:313–6.
60. Echeverria P, Blacklow NR, Cukor G, et al. Rotavirus as a cause of severe gastroenteritis in adults. J Clin Microbiol. 1983;18:663–7.
61. Hasegawa A, Matsuno S, Inouye S, et al. Isolation of human rotaviruses in

primary cultures of monkey kidneys cells. J Clin Microbiol. 1982;16:387–90.
62. Ward RL, Knowlton DR, Pierce MJ. Efficiency of human rotavirus propagation in cell culture. J Clin Microbiol. 1984;19:748–53.
63. Naguib T, Wyatt RG, Mohieldin MS, et al. Cultivation and subgroup determination of human rotaviruses from Egyptian infants and young children. J Clin Microbiol. 1984;19:210–12.
64. Krause PJ, Hyams JS, Middleton PJ, et al. Unreliability of rotazyme ELISA test in neonates. J Pediatr. 1983;103:259–62.
65. Chrystie IL, Totterdell BM, Banatvala JE. False positive rotazyme tests on faecal samples from babies (Letter). Lancet. 1983;2:1028.
66. Herrmann JE, Blacklow NR, Perron DM, et al. Monoclonal antibody enzyme immunoassays for the detection of rotavirus in stool specimens. J Infect Dis. 1985;152:830–2.
67. Brown DWG, Beards GM, Guang-Mu C, et al. Prevalence of antibody to group B (atypical) rotavirus in humans and animals. J Clin Microbiol. 1987;25:316–9.
68. Pothier P, Limone F, Kohli E, et al. Development and preliminary evaluation of a latex agglutination test using a monoclonal antibody for rotavirus detection in stool specimens. Ann Inst Pasteur. 1987;138:523–6.
69. Morinet F, Ferchal F, Colimon R, et al. Comparison of six methods for detecting human rotavirus in stools. Eur J Clin Microbiol. 1984;3:136–40.
70. Knisley CV, Bednarz-Prashad AJ, Pickering LK. Detection of rotavirus stool specimens with monoclonal and polyclonal antibody-based assay systems. J Clin Microbiol. 1986;23:897–900.
71. Doern GV, Herrmann JE, Henderson P, et al. Detection of rotavirus with a new polyclonal antibody enzyme immunoassay (rotazyme II) and a commercial latex agglutination test (Rotalex): comparison with a monoclonal antibody enzyme immunoassay. J Clin Microbiol. 1986;23:226–9.
72. Theil KW, McCloskey CM, Saif LJ, et al. Rapid, simple method of preparing rotaviral double-stranded ribonucleic acid for analysis by polyacrylamide gel electropheresis. J Clin Microbiol. 1981;14:273–80.
73. Flores J, Boeggeman E, Purcell RH, et al. A dot hybridization assay for detection of rotavirus. Lancet. 1983;1:555–9.
74. Dimitrov DH, Graham DY, Estes MK. Detection of rotaviruses by nucleic acid hybridization with cloned DNA of simian rotavirus SAll genes. J Infect Dis. 1985;162:293–300.
75. Herrmann JE, Armstrong AS, Edberg SC. Rapid methods for the immunodiagnosis of infectious diseases: recent developments. Yale J Biol Med. 1985;58:412–5.
76. Edberg SC. Principles of nucleic acid hybridization and comparison with monoclonal antibody technology for the diagnosis of infectious diseases. Yale J Biol Med. 1985;58:425–42.
77. Brandt CD, Kim HW, Rodriguez WJ, et al. Comparison of direct electron microscopy, immune electron microscopy, and rotavirus enzyme-linked immunosorbent assay for detection of gastroenteritis viruses in children. J Clin Microbiol. 1981;13:976–81.
78. Lambert KP, Marbehant P, Marissens D, et al. Monoclonal antibodies directed against different antigenic determinants of rotavirus. J Virol. 1984;51:47–51.
79. Taniguchi K, Urasawa T, Urasawa S, et al. Production of subgroup-specific monoclonal antibodies against human rotaviruses and their application to an enzyme-linked immunosorbent assay for subgroup determination. J Med Virol. 1984;14:115–25.
80. Coulson BS, Unicomb LE, Pitson GA, et al. Simple and specific enzyme immunoassay using monoclonal antibodies for serotyping human rotaviruses. J Clin Microbiol. 1987;25:509–15.
81. Taniguchi K, Urasawa T, Morita Y, et al. Direct serotyping of human rotaviruses in stools by an enzyme-linked immunosorbent assay using serotype 1-, 2-, 3-, and 4-specific monoclonal antibodies to VP7. J Infect Dis. 1987;155:1159–66.
82. Schoub BD, Prozesky DW. Antiviral activity of ribavirin in rotavirus gastroenteritis in mice. Antimicrob Agents Chemother. 1977;12:543–4.
83. Smee DF, Sidwell RW, Clark SM, et al. Inhibition of rotavirus by selected antiviral substances: mechanisms of viral inhibition in vivo activity. Antimicrob Agents Chemother. 1982;21:66–73.
84. Santosham M, Daun RS, Dillman L, et al. Oral rehydration therapy of infantile diarrhea. A controlled study of well-nourished children hospitalized in the United States and Panama. N Engl J Med. 1982;306:1070–3.
85. Santosham M, Burns B, Nadkarni V, et al. Oral rehydration therapy for acute diarrhea in ambulatory children in the United States: a double-blind comparison of four different solutions. Pediatrics. 1985;76:159–63.
86. Saulsbury FT, Winkelstein JA, Yolken RH. Chronic rotavirus infection in immunodeficiency. J Pediatr. 1980;97:61–5.
87. Ebina T, Sato A, Umezu K, et al. Prevention of rotavirus infection by cow colostrum containing antibody against human rotavirus. Lancet. 1983;2:1029–30.
88. Zissis G, Lambert JP, Marbehant P, et al. Protection studies in colostrum-deprived piglets of a bovine rotavirus vaccine candidate using human rotavirus strains for challenge. J Infect Dis. 1983;148:1061–8.
89. Wyatt RG, Mebus CA, Yolken RH, et al. Rotaviral immunity in gnotobiotic calves: heterologous resistance to human virus induced by bovine virus. Science. 1979;203:548–50.
90. Delem A, Lobmann M, Zygraich N. A bovine rotavirus developed as a candidate for use in humans. J Biol Stand. 1984;12:443–5.
91. Stuker G, Oshiro L, Schmidt NL. Antigenic comparisons of two new rotaviruses from rhesus monkeys. J Clin Microbiol. 1980;11:202–3.
92. Rennels MB, Losonsky GA, Shindledecker CL, et al. Immunogenicity and reactogenicity of lowered doses of rhesus rotavirus vaccine strain MMU 18006 in young children. Pediatr Infect Dis J. 1987;6:260–4.
93. Vesikari T, Isolauri E, Delem A, et al. Immunogenicity and safety of live attenuated bovine rotavirus vaccine strain RIT 4237 in adults and young children. Lancet. 1983;2:807–11.
94. Vesikari T, Isolauri E, D'Hondt E, et al. Protection of infants against rotavirus diarrhoea by RIT 4237 attenuated bovine rotavirus strain vaccine. Lancet. 1984;1:977–81.
95. Vesikari T, Isolauri E, Delem A, et al. Clinical efficacy of the RIT 4237 live attenuated bovine rotavirus vaccine in infants vaccinated before a rotavirus epidemic. J Pediatr. 1985;189–94.
96. DeMol P, Zissis G, Butzler JP, et al. Failure of live, attenuated oral rotavirus vaccine. Lancet. 1986;2:108.
97. Hanlon P, Marsh V, Shenton F, et al. Trial of an attenuated bovine rotavirus vaccine (RIT 4237) in Gambian infants. Lancet. 1986;1:1342–5.
98. Edelman R. Perspective on the development and deployment of rotavirus vaccine. Pediatr Infect Dis J. 1987;6:704–10.
99. Albert MJ. Failure of live, oral vaccine in developing countries. J Infect Dis. 1987;155:1350.
100. McLean BS, and Holmes IH. Effects of antibodies, trypsin and trypsin inhibitors on susceptibility of neonates to rotavirus infection. J Clin Microbiol. 1981;13:22–29.
101. Berger R, Hadziselimovic F, Just M, et al. Influence of breast milk on nosocomial rotavirus infection in infants. Infection. 1984;12:171–4.
102. Vesikari T, Isolauri E, Ruuska T, et al. Clinical trials of rotavirus vaccines. In: Novel Diarrhoea Viruses. Ciba Foundation Symposium. 1987;128:218–31.
103. Vesikari T, Isolauri E, Delem A, et al. Clinical efficacy of the RIT 4237 live attenuated bovine rotavirus vaccine in infants vaccinated before a rotavirus epidemic. J Pediatr. 1985;107:189–94.
104. Bishop RF, Barnes GL, Cipriani E, et al. Clinical immunity after neonatal rotavirus infection. A prospective longitudinal study in young children. N Engl J Med. 1983;309:72–6.
105. Chiba S, Yokoyama T, Nakata S, et al. Protective effect of naturally acquired homotypic and heterotypic rotavirus antibodies. Lancet. 1986;2:417–21.
106. Rennels MB, Losonsky GA, Levine MM, et al. Preliminary evaluation of rhesus rotavirus vaccine strain MMU 18006 in young children. Pediatr Infect Dis J. 1986;5:587–8.
107. Wright PF, Tajima T, Thompson J, et al. Candidate rotavirus vaccine (rhesus rotavirus strain) in children: an evaluation. Pediatrics. 1987;80:473–80.
108. Flores J, Gonzalez M, Perez M, et al. Protection against severe rotavirus diarrhoea by rhesus rotavirus vaccine in Venezuelan infants. Lancet. 1987;1:882–4.
109. Vesikari T, Kapakian AZ, Delem A, et al. A comparative trial of rhesus monkey (RRV-1) and bovine (RIT 4237) oral rotavirus vaccines in young children. J Infect Dis. 1986;153:832–9.
110. Ward RL, Bernstein DI, Young EL, et al. Human rotavirus studies in volunteers: determinations of infectious dose and serological response to infection. J Infect Dis. 1986;154:871–80.
111. Midthun K, Greenberg HB, Hoshino Y, et al. Reassortment rotaviruses as potential live rotavirus vaccine candidates. J Virol. 1985;53:949–54.
112. Hoshino Y, Saif LJ, Sereno MM, et al. Infection immunity of piglets to either VP3 or VP7 outer capsid protein confers resistance to challenge with a virulent rotavirus bearing the corresponding antigen. J Virol. 1988;62:744–8.
113. Halsey NA, Anderson EL, Sears SD, et al. Human-rhesus reassortment vaccines: safety and immunogenicity in adults, infants, and children. J Infect Dis. 1988;158:1261–7.
114. Vodopija I, Baklaic Z, Vlatkovic R, et al. Combined vaccination with live oral polio vaccine and the bovine rotavirus RIT 4237 strain. Vaccine. 1986;4:223–6.
115. Rahmen MM, Yamauchi M, Hanada N, et al. Local production of rotavirus-specific IgA in breast tissue and transfer to neonates. Arch Dis Child. 1987;62:401–5.
116. Welsh JK, May TT. Anti-infective properties of breast milk. J Pediatr. 1979;94:1–9.
117. Barnes GL, Doyle LW, Hewson PH, et al. A randomized trial of oral gamma globulin in low-birth weight infants infected with rotavirus. Lancet. 1983;1:1371–3.
118. Kapikian AZ, Wyatt RG, Levine MM, et al. Oral administration of human rotavirus to volunteers: induction of illness and correlates of resistance. J Infect Dis. 1983;147:95–106.
119. Losonsky G, Rennels MB, Lim Y, et al. Systemic and mucosal immune responses to rhesus rotavirus vaccine MMU 18006. Pediatr Infect Dis J. 1988;7:388–93.

Togaviridae

130. ALPHAVIRUS (EASTERN, WESTERN, AND VENEZUELAN EQUINE ENCEPHALITIS)

THOMAS P. MONATH

Three alphaviruses are causative agents of human disease in the United States: eastern equine encephalitis (EEE), western equine encephalitis (WEE), and Venezuelan equine encephalitis (VEE).

HISTORY

Western equine encephalitis and EEE virus recovered from the brains of horses with encephalitis in California (1930) and New Jersey (1933), respectively, were established as etiologic agents of human encephalitis in humans in 1938.[1–3] Venezuelan equine encephalitis virus was first isolated from the brains of horses with encephalitis during an epidemic in Venezuela in 1938.[4] Human disease was recognized in 1943 as a result of laboratory infections; naturally acquired human illness was first reported from Colombia in 1952 in association with an epizootic disease in equines.[5] In 1968, human disease due to VEE was first reported in the United States.[6]

PATHOGENS

The alphaviruses (former group A arboviruses) comprise a genus of the family Togaviridae, which is characterized by enveloped virions 50–60 nm in diameter and infectious single-stranded linear RNA. The structure, morphogenesis, and replication strategy of alphaviruses have been recently reviewed.[7] Other medically important alphaviruses include chikungunya (in Africa, Asia), O'nyong-nyong (Africa), Mayaro (South America), Ross River (Australia, Oceania), and Sindbis (Africa, Scandanavia, Soviet Union, Asia), all of which produce epidemic denguelike human disease.

Alphaviruses share antigenic relationships revealed by complement fixation (CF) and hemagglutination inhibition (HI) tests. Serologically defined subtypes and geographic varieties have important epidemiologic and clinical distinctions. North and South American subtypes of EEE virus are recognized anigenic variants. In the eastern United States, a virus (Highlands J) closely related to WEE is less virulent and rarely causes disease. Venezuelan equine encephalitis virus comprises 5 subtypes. Subtype I occurs in tropical America and is medically most important; this subtype is further divided into five geographic variants. Variants IAB and IC are associated with equine epizootics and human epidemics. Variants ID and IE and subtype II (Everglades virus) have been implicated in sporadic cases of human central nervous system (CNS) disease in Central America and Florida, respectively.

EPIDEMIOLOGY

Eastern equine encephalitis is a summertime disease of low incidence, with fewer than 15 human cases occurring annually along the Gulf and Atlantic States. Children and the elderly are most susceptible to severe illness.[8] The disease in horses and humans is often geographically focal. The case fatality rate is 50–70 percent. The virus is maintained in a cycle involving many species of wild birds and a principal mosquito vector, *Culiseta melanura*, that breeds in freshwater swamps. Infection with EEE virus has no adverse effect on most wild avian species, but a viremia is produced of sufficient magnitude to infect vector mosquitoes. Mosquitoes may transmit the virus tangentially to penned exotic birds (e.g., pheasants), horses, and humans, all of which suffer clinical disease; horses and humans have low viremias and are dead-end hosts. Species other than *C. melanura*, including salt-marsh mosquitoes, play a role in epizootics/epidemics.

Western equine encephalitis occurs as a summertime disease of horses and humans in states west of the Mississippi and in corresponding Canadian provinces. Since 1955 the annual incidence has varied between 0 and 200 cases, the latter in years of epizootic/epidemic activity (e.g., 1965, 1975, 1977). Infants are most susceptible to severe disease. Risk factors for the acquisition of infection include rural residence, outdoor employment in farming, and male sex. The case fatality rate is 3–5 percent. The principal vector of WEE virus is *Culex tarsalis*, which is especially prevalent in irrigated areas. Wild avian species are the principal viremic vertebrate hosts. The mechanism(s) by which WEE and EEE viruses overwinter in temperate climates is an unsolved mystery.

Venezuelan equine encephalitis outbreaks in South and Central America have been associated with tens of thousands of both equine and human cases.[9] In Venezuela in 1962–1964 32,000 human cases were reported with a fatality rate of 0.6 percent. The spread of epidemic VEE into Texas in 1971 caused the loss of over 10,000 horses, and control programs were reported to cost over $20 million. Severe human disease with encephalitis is most frequent in children. Unlike EEE and WEE where equines play no important role in virus maintenance, equines infected with epidemic VEE strains (sutypes IAB and IC) manifest high viremias, sufficient to infect many species of mosqitoes. At least 10 species of five different genera (*Culex, Aedes, Mansonia, Psorophora, Deinocerites*) have been incriminated as probable epidemic vectors.[10]

The strain of VEE virus endemic in the southern United States (Everglades virus or subtype II) is a very rare cause of human illness; only three confirmed cases of encephalitis due to this endemic strain have been recognized.[6] The ID and IE variants have caused sporadic human disease including fatalities in Central America.[10] These viruses are maintained in transmission cycles involving rodent hosts and *Culex* (*Melanoconion*) spp. mosquitoes in freshwater swamp habitats.

PATHOGENESIS

Alphavirus infections of humans are initiated under natural conditions by the percutaneous deposition of virus in mosquito salivary secretions. Some alphaviruses, notably VEE, are also highly infectious by aerosol and have caused numerous infections in laboratory workers. The initial phase of an alphavirus infection involves virus replication in non-neural tissues that is manifested by a viremia and often a febrile response. Venezuelan equine encephalitis virus replicates in lymphoid tissues as well as in other organs, and virulent strains exhibit a marked lymphotoxic effect. Infections may be terminated by the host defense mechanisms after a clinically inapparent course or after a benign febrile illness; however, viral invasion of the CNS with consequent encephalitis may follow the viremic phase. When invasion of the CNS occurs, EEE, WEE, and VEE viruses replicate extensively in the involved tissues and cause cell destruction and a severe inflammatory response. Pathologic manifestations at autopsy include focal areas of neuronal necrosis with polymorphonuclear and microglial cell infiltrates, vascular lesions, and perivascular cuffing. In both EEE and WEE, infectious lesions may be widespread throughout the brain and cord; often the cerebral cortex and basal ganglia are most severely involved. Venezuelan equine encephalitis virus is pancreatropic and produces glucose intolerance in experimental animals (not shown in humans). Transplacental infections with WEE and VEE have resulted in severe encephalitis of newborn infants.[8,9] Neurologic sequelae may follow recovery from acute alphaviral encephalitis, but chronic, persistent infections have not been documented.

CLINICAL MANIFESTATIONS

The initial symptoms of EEE nd WEE include headache, fever, chills, nausea, and vomiting. Mental confusion and somnolence occur within a day or two of onset and may progress to a profound coma. Convulsions are common in infants and children. The temperature is usually elevated to 102–104°F. Neurologic findings are variable and may include a stiff neck, bulging fontanelles (infants), depressed or hyperactive reflexes, tremors, muscle twitching, and spastic paralysis. A leukocytosis is usually present. The cerebrospinl fluid (CSF) shows an increased protein level and cell count, usually 50–500/mm^3 (WEE) and 600–2000/mm^3 (EEE), with a predominance of lymphocytes; however, early examination of the CSF may show a preponderance of polymorphonuclear cells. Neurologic sequelae including mental retardation, behavioral changes, convulsive disorders, and paralysis occur in 30 and 70 percent of infants recovering from WEE nd EEE, respectively. Sequelae are less frequent in older persons. Parkinsonism may follow WEE in adults.

Human infections due to VEE virus may result in subclinical infection, a benign influenza-like illness, or in approximately 4 percent of cases, a febrile disease with severe encephalitis.[9,11] The most common clinical manifestation is a febrile illness with headache, myalgia, vomiting, diarrhea, lethargy, somnolence, pharyngitis, and leukopenia. Encephalitis usually appears after a few days or a week of febrile illness. In most cases uneventful recovery occurs in 3–5 days, but prolonged neurasthenia is common. Although the overall case fatality rate in VEE is less than 1 percent, approximately 20 percent of patients with full-blown encephalitis succumb. Sequelae include personality changes and paralysis.

DIAGNOSIS

Alphavirus encephalitis may mimic herpes simplex virus encephalitis and other treatable infections. Establishing the diagnosis of an alphavirus infection depends on suspecting the etiology on clinical and epidemiologic grounds and on obtaining appropriate specimens for virologic and serologic tests. Serologic confirmation in nonfatal cases depends on a demonstration of a rise in antibody titer by immunoflorescence, HI, CF, virus neutralization, or IgM immunoassay. Obtaining early acute-phase and convalescence-phase serum is necessary. Virus may be isolated from the CSF (rarely) or from CNS tissues obtained by biopsy[8] or at autopsy. In VEE cases, virus may be isolated from the blood and from pharyngeal swab specimens.

TREATMENT AND PREVENTION

There is no specific therapy for alphavirus infections. Supportive measures, relief of symptoms, and intensive nursing care are indicated as with other forms of encephalitis. Prevention of EEE and WEE in humans is entirely dependent on surveillance and control of the vectors by public health authorities. Since transmission of epidemic strains of VEE depends upon viremic horses, equine immunization prevents human infection. Commercial EEE, WEE, and VEE vaccines are available for use in equines. Experimental vaccines developed by the U.S. Army are used to protect laboratory workers from EEE, WEE, and VEE.

ACKNOWLEDGMENT

This chapter is based in part on a chapter in the previous edition by Phillip K. Russell.

REFERENCES

1. Howitt BE. Recovery of the virus of equine encephalomyelitis from the brain of a child. Science. 1938;88;455.
2. Webster LT, Wright FH. Recovery of eastern equine encephalomyelitis virus from brain tissue of human cases of encephalitis in Massachusetts. Science. 1938;88;305.
3. Fothergill LD, Dingle JH, Farber S, et al. Human encephalitis caused by a virus of eastern variety of equine encephalomyelitis. N Engl J Med. 1983;219:411.
4. Beck CE, Wyckof RWG. Venezuelan equine encephalomyelitis. Science. 1938;88:530.
5. SanMartin-Barberi C, Groot H, Osborno-Mesa E. Human epidemic in Colombia caused by the Venezuelan equine encephalomyelitis virus. Am J Trop Med Hyg. 1954;3:283.
6. Ehrenkranz NJ, Ventura AK. Venezuelan equine encephalitis virus infection in man. Annu Rev Med. 1974;25:9.
7. Schlesinger S, Schlesinger MJ, eds. The Togaviridae and Flaviviridae. New York: Plenum; 1986.
8. Tsai TF, Monath TP. Viral diseases in North America transmitted by arthropods or from vertebrate reservoirs. In: Feigin RD, Cherry JD, eds. Textbook of Pediatric Infectious Diseases. 2nd ed. Philadelphia: WB Saunders; 1988:1417.
9. Groot H. The health and economic impact of Venezuelan equine encephalitis. In: Venezuelan Encephalitis, Proceedings of the Workshop-Symposium on Venezuelan Encephalitis Virus. Washington, DC: Pan American Health Organization; 1972:244.
10. Johnson KM, Martin DH: Venezuelan equine encephalitis. Adv Vet Sci Comp Med. 1974;18:79.
11. Bowen GS. Human disease—USA. In: Venezuelan Encephalitis, Proceedings of the Workshop-Symposium on Venezuelan Encephalitis Virus. Washington, DC: Pan American Health Organization; 1972:231.

131. RUBELLA VIRUS (GERMAN MEASLES)

ANNE A. GERSHON

Rubella is an acute exanthematous viral infection of children and adults. The clinical illness is characterized by rash, fever, and lymphadenopathy and resembles a mild case of measles (rubeola). While many infections with the agent are subclinical, this virus has the potential to cause fetal infection with resultant birth defects and, rarely in adults, various forms of arthritis.

Rubella virus was first isolated in 1962 by Parkman, and colleagues[1] and by Weller and Neva.[2] Rubella virus is now classified in the Togaviridae family[3,4] on the basis of its RNA genome, icosahedral capsid, and lipoprotein envelope. Rubella virus is thought to be closely related to the alphaviruses, but unlike alphaviruses, no vector is required for transmission of rubella, and it is serologically distinct from alphaviruses.[4] Therefore, rubella virus has been placed in a separate genus, *Rubivirus*.

On electron microscopy rubella virus is roughly spherical. Its envelope, which has short surface projections, has a diameter of about 60 nm. The envelope surrounds the nucleocapsid, which has a diameter of about 30 nm; it is composed of a helix of protein and RNA. Rubella virus matures by budding from the cell membrane.[5]

The rubella virus is relatively unstable, and it is inactivated by lipid solvents, trypsin, formalin, ultraviolet light, extremes of pH and heat, and amantadine.[6] In tissue culture the virus does not always produce cytopathic effects. In such instances the virus may be demonstrated by interference techniques, that is, failure of another virus to multiply in cells that have already been infected with rubella virus.[6]

The known antigens of rubella virus consist of a hemagglutinin[7] present on the envelope of the virion, a complement-fixing antigen,[8] and two precipitins, termed *theta* and *iota*.[9]

EPIDEMIOLOGY

Rubella was not distinguished from certain other exanthematous infections clinically until the late nineteenth century. It was at one time termed *third* disease, measles and scarlet fever being *first* and *second,* respectively.[10] Since postnatal rubella is such a mild illness, the disease was considered to be of only minor importance for many years. However, in 1941 when Gregg[11] recognized the link between maternal rubella and certain congenital defects, a more complete picture of disease due to rubella virus began to emerge.

The incidence of clinical cases of rubella is highest in the spring, and it has been traditionally recognized to be most common in children 5–9 years of age.[12] There is, however, some evidence to suggest that rubella is now being seen with increasing frequency in an older age group because of the widespread use of rubella vaccine.[13] Rubella is only a moderately contagious illness in contrast to measles. Thus, in the prevaccine era only 80–90 percent of adults were immune to rubella, while 98 percent were immune to measles.[12]

Epidemics of rubella of minor proportions used to occur in the prevaccine era every 6–9 years, with major epidemics occurring at intervals of up to 30 years. The most recent major epidemic in the United States occurred in 1964, during which some 12,500,000 persons were infected.[14] Since the licensure of a live attenuated rubella vaccine in 1969, there have been no subsequent large rubella epidemics in countries where the vaccine is widely used. Limited outbreaks have continued to occur, however, in settings such as schools and military camps where groups of susceptibles have close contact with each other.[13]

Spread of Rubella

Rubella virus is spread in droplets that are shed from the respiratory secretions of infected persons. Patients are most contagious when the rash is erupting, but they may shed virus from the throat from 10 days before the onset of the rash to 15 days after its onset. Patients with subclinical cases of illness may also transmit the infection to others.[6]

Infants with congenital rubella shed large quantities of virus from body secretions for many months. They may thus transmit the infection to those who care for them. These babies continue to excrete rubella virus despite high titers of neutralizing antibody, a puzzling phenomenon that has yet to be explained.[15]

Persons who have received rubella vaccine do not transmit rubella to others, although the virus may be isolated from the pharynx. It may be that the quantity of virus shed is too small to be infectious.[16–18]

Maintenance of Immunity to Rubella

After an attack of rubella, lifelong protection against the disease develops in most persons. However, the factors responsible for this protection are not precisely understood. It is known that antibody titers to rubella virus develop, but whether these antibody titers decline significantly with time remains unclear. Cell-mediated immunity to rubella virus has also been detected in in vitro assays[19]; this may be detected years after an attack of rubella. The persistence of humoral and cellular immunity to rubella in a group of cloistered nuns who had no opportunity for reexposure to rubella virus has been documented.[20] The persistence of specific antibody as long as 14 years after immunization has also been demonstrated.[21,22]

Nevertheless, despite the presence of specific immunity to rubella virus, it appears that reinfection with rubella virus can occur. This had been long suspected on clinical grounds alone.[23,24] More recently rubella reinfections have been documented by detection of a significant boost in rubella antibody titer in naturally immune persons after reexposure to the virus. The overwhelming majority of reinfections are asymptomatic.[25] It is likely that the virus can multiply locally in the upper respiratory tract but that viremia occurs infrequently because the host's immune response eradicates the virus before it can invade the blood. However, occasionally, patients with documented rubella reinfection years after natural rubella and with symptoms indicative of viremia such as arthritis and rash have been described.[26]

Rubella reinfection some months or years after the receipt of rubella vaccine has also been observed. Several investigators have documented reinfections in up to 80 percent of persons who had received rubella vaccine previously and who were subsequently exposed to rubella during an epidemic.[25,27,28] Most of these reinfections have not been characterized by clinical illness but only by a boost in antibody titer. Viremia is probably extremely rare in this situation,[27,29,30] although rubella virus has been recovered from throat secretions in reinfections.[25,29] In one study of eight seronegative adult vaccinees who were experimentally challenged with wild-type rubella virus, replication in the respiratory tract was found in seven and viremia was present in two.[31] These subjects, however, also experienced only a mild illness or remained asymptomatic.[31]

Reinfections have been more common in vaccinees than in those who had natural rubella, and reinfections are most common in persons with hemagglutination inhibitions (HAI) antibody titers of 1:64 or less.[25,27,29] It has been suggested that there may also be qualitative differences in antibody between those with vaccine and natural immunity since, in one study, even with similar HAI titers vaccinees were 10 times more likely to be reinfected than were those with natural immunity to rubella.[25]

Whether rubella reinfection that occurs during pregnancy can transmit the virus to the fetus has been the subject of much debate. Several case reports in the older literature ascribing fetal defects to maternal rubella reinfection were actually primary maternal infections in all likelihood.[32–34] Viremia has been documented, however, in one woman with detectable rubella antibody before immunization.[35] Boué followed a small number of women with documented subclinical cases of rubella reinfection during pregnancy who carried their babies to term, and all the babies were normal.[36] Finally there have been five case reports of rubella reinfection during pregnancy in which the infant, carried to term, had symptoms suggestive of congenital rubella.[37–41] Most of these reinfections occurred years after the natural infection, although one occurred some years after immunization.[41] However, these are acknowledged to be extremely rare events, particularly as reflected by the exceedingly low incidence of rubella in the United States today (see below).

In summary, it appears that persons immune to rubella, by virtue either of having had the natural infection or having received rubella vaccine, may be reinfected when reexposed. However, this infection is usually asymptomatic and detectable only by serologic means. Viremia in reinfection appears, fortunately, to be a rare event.

It was at one time hoped that large numbers of immune people in a community could prevent rubella epidemics from occurring, so-called herd immunity. However, it has been documented that herd immunity does not decrease the spread of rubella.[42]

PATHOGENESIS

The incubation period of rubella ranges from 12 to 23 days, with an average of 18 days. As in measles (Chapter 136), a primary and secondary viremia are believed to accompany rubella. Rubella virus has been detected in leukocytes of patients as long as 1 week before the onset of symptoms.[43] Again, as in measles, the rubella rash appears as immunity develops and the virus disappears from the blood,[6] thus suggesting that the rash is immunologically mediated. While circulating immune complexes occur during rubella, they do not seem to contribute to the development of rash.[44,45] Rubella virus has been isolated from involved skin,[46] but this does not preclude the concept that the rash is secondary to an immune response to the virus.

CLINICAL MANIFESTATIONS

Age is the most important determinant of the severity of rubella. Postnatally acquired rubella is generally an innocuous infection, and as is true for many viral illnesses, children are apt to have milder disease than are adults. In contrast, thc fctus is at high risk to develop severe rubella with long-lasting sequelae if infected transplacentally during maternal rubella in early pregnancy.

Postnatal Rubella

Many if not most cases of these infections are subclinical.[14,47] Of those patients who are symptomatic, children do not experience a prodromal phase, but adults may have a prodrome of malaise, fever, and anorexia for several days. The major symptoms of postnatal rubella are adenopathy, which may last several weeks, and rash. The lymph nodes involved include the posterior auricular, posterior cervical, and suboccipital chains; on occasion splenomegaly also occurs.[48] These symptoms are not specific for rubella, and they may accompany other infections such as measles and toxoplasmosis.

The rash of rubella begins on the face and moves down the body. It is maculopapular but not confluent, may desquamate during convalescence, and may be absent in some cases. An enanthem consisting of petechial lesions on the soft palate (Forscheimer spots) has been described for rubella, but unlike Koplik spots in measles, this enanthem is not diagnostic for rubella. The rash may be accompanied by mild coryza and conjunctivitis. Usually the rash lasts 3–5 days. Fever, if present, rarely lasts beyond the first day of rash.

Complications of Postnatal Rubella. In contrast to measles (rubeola), complications of postnatal rubella are uncommon. Bacterial superinfection after rubella is rare.

Arthritis or arthralgia has been reported in as many as one-third of women with rubella; interestingly, this complication is less frequent in children and men.[49] This arthritis tends to involve the fingers, wrists, and knees, and it occurs either as the rash is appearing or soon afterward. It may be rather slow to resolve and take as long as a month. Rarely does chronic arthritis develop.

The pathogenesis of rubella arthritis is not entirely understood. The frequency of detection and the quantity of circulating immune complexes is higher in rubella vaccinees reporting joint complaints than in those with no joint involvement.[44,50] Rubella virus has been isolated from joint effusions in cases of acute and recurrent rubella arthritis associated either with previous natural infection or vaccination.[51–59] Rubella virus has also been isolated from peripheral blood mononuclear cells in patients with chronic arthritis.[58,60] A persistent rubella virus infection of human synovial cells cultured in vitro has also been reported, which has been advanced as an explanation for the pathogenesis of chronic forms of rubella arthritis.[61]

Hemorrhagic manifestations occur as a complication in approximately 1 of 3000 cases of rubella.[48,62] In contrast to other complications of rubella, this occurs more often in children than in adults. This complication may be secondary to both thrombocytopenia and vascular damage, and it is probably immunologically mediated.[62] It has been proposed that mild thrombocytopenia often goes undetected in apparently "uncomplicated" rubella.[63] Thrombocytopenia may last from weeks to months and may cause serious problems if bleeding into vital areas such as the brain, kidney, or eye occurs.[48] Thrombocytopenic purpura as the single clinical manifestation of rubella in children has also been reported.[62]

Encephalitis is an extremely uncommon complication of rubella; it has been reported, during an epidemic, to occur in 1 of 5000 cases. It occurs more frequently in adults than in children, and it is associated with a mortality of 20–50 percent.[48,64,65] A 2-month-old who died of rubella encephalitis whose mother had rubella in the last week of pregnancy has been reported.[66]

Mild hepatitis has been described as an unusual complication of rubella.[67]

Congenital Rubella

Rubella can be a disastrous disease in early gestation and lead to fetal death, premature delivery, and an array of congenital defects.

The incidence of congenital rubella in a given population is quite variable, depending on the number of susceptibles, the circulation of virus in the community, and in recent times, the use of rubella vaccine. The rubella epidemic of 1964 left 30,000 affected infants in its wake. Between 1969 and 1979, however, an average of 39 cases per year was reported to the Centers for Disease Control (CDC).[68,69] Since then, an all-time low of only an average of eight cases per year has been reported in the United States.[69]

The effects of rubella virus on the fetus are, to a large extent, dependent on the time of infection; generally the younger the fetus when infected, the more severe the illness. During the first 2 months of gestation the fetus has a 40–60 percent chance of being affected, with an outcome of either multiple congenital defects and/or spontaneous abortion. Rubella during the third month of fetal life has been associated with a 30–35 percent chance of developing a single defect such as deafness or congenital heart disease. Fetal infection during the fourth month carries a 10 percent risk of a single congenital defect. Occasionally fetal damage (deafness alone) is seen if rubella occurs up to the 20th week of gestation.[70]

The specific symptoms of congenital rubella may be classified as temporary such as low birth weight, permanent such as deafness, and developmental such as myopia.[68] The most common manifestations are deafness, cataract or glaucoma, congenital heart disease, and mental retardation; a comprehensive list of the myriad of known sequelae is shown in Table 1.[68]

Prospective studies of the congenital rubella syndrome suggest that it should not be thought of as a static disease. Some children whose mothers had rubella during pregnancy and who, at birth, were considered normal have been found to have manifestations of congenital rubella on reaching school age.[71,72] Diabetes millitus appearing in late childhood has also been observed more frequently in children with congenital rubella than in the normal population.[73] Insulin-dependent diabetes has been reported in 40 percent of adult survivors of congential rubella from the 1942 epidemic.[74] Interestingly, in another follow-up study of 242 children with congenital rubella syndrome, rubella virus-induced diabetes was found to have similar genetic and immunologic features to other forms of insulin-dependent diabetes: the frequency of HLA-DR3 was increased and that of HLA-DR2 was decreased.[75] Antibodies to pancreatic islet cells or cytotoxic surface antibodies were present in 80 percent of the patients with abnormalities of serum glucose.[75] In congenital rubella patients at autopsy, the virus has also been isolated from the pancreas, which has been noted to have a subnormal number of glandular cells.[75] Progressive encephalopathy resembling

TABLE 1. Congenital Rubella: Transient (T), Permanent (P), and Developmental (D) Manifestations

Common		*Uncommon or Rare*	
Low birth weight	(T)	Jaundice	(T)
Thrombocytopenic purpura	(T)	Dermatoglyphic "abnormality"	(P)
Hepatosplenomegaly	(T)	Glaucoma	(P)
Bone "lesions"	(T)	Cloudy cornea	(T)
Large anterior fontanelle	(T)	Severe myopia	(P, D)
Meningoencephalitis	(T)	Myocardial abnormalities	(P)
Hearing loss	(P, D)	Hepatitis	(T)
Cataract (and microphthalmia)	(P)	Generalized lymphadenopathy	(T)
Retinopathy	(P)	Hemolytic anemia	(T)
Patent ductus arteriosus	(P)	Rubella pneumonitis	(T)
Pulmonic stenosis	(P, D)	Diabetes mellitus	(P, D)
Mental retardation	(P, D)	Thyroid disorders	(D, P)
Behavior disorders	(P, D)	Seizure disorders	(D)
Central language disorders	(P, D)	Precocious puberty	(D)
Cryptorchidism	(P)	Degenerative brain disease	(D)
Inguinal hernia	(P)		
Spastic diplegia	(P)		
Microcephaly	(P)		

(From Cooper,[68] with permission.)

subacute sclerosing panencephalitis (SSPE) has been observed in children with congenital rubella.[76,77]

Infants with congenital rubella develop high titers of neutralizing antibody that may persist for years.[78] However, these children may eventually lose their antibody.[79] Reinfection with rubella has also been documented in some of these children.[80] Impairment of cell-mediated immunity to rubella antigen has been found in some children with congenital rubella.[81]

A number of pathologic mechanisms have been proposed to explain certain manifestations of congenital rubella. It has been suggested that persistent infection with rubella virus leads to a mitotic arrest of cells, which in turn causes inhibition of cellular growth and thus retarded organ growth.[82] Additional hypotheses put forth to explain the growth retardation seen in congenital rubella are that infection leads to angiopathy with placental and fetal vasculitis that compromises growth[83] and that tissue necrosis without inflammation or fibrotic damage leads to cellular damage.[84] Human fibroblasts infected with rubella virus in vitro have been found to produce a growth inhibitor, which might also account for fetal growth retardation.[85] It has also been found that there is an increased frequency of chromosomal breakage in cultured cells from children with congenital rubella as compared with cells from healthy children.[86] It has been postulated that lymphocyte abnormalities in patients with the congenital rubella syndrome may predispose them to organ-specific autoimmunity.[87]

DIAGNOSIS

Since rubella is usually a mild disease with nonspecific symptoms, it is often difficult to diagnose clinically. The disease has been confused with other infections such as scarlet fever, mild measles, infectious mononucleosis, toxoplasmosis, roseola, erythema infectiosum, and certain enteroviral infections.[88,89] Routine laboratory studies are not helpful for diagnosis since they may reveal only a leukopenia and atypical lymphocytes; therefore more specific laboratory diagnostic techniques are usually necessary.

Virus isolation from throat swabs, urine, or other body secretions is an acceptable method for diagnosis. However, this technique is time-consuming, often not available, and expensive, so it is therefore reserved for special circumstances such as the diagnosis of congenital rubella.[6,90] The diagnosis of congenital rubella has been made in vitro by isolation of virus from amniotic fluid.[91]

The laboratory diagnosis of rubella is most often made serologically. At one time HAI was the preferred means to measure rubella antibody titers, but this technique has been supplanted by simpler more accurate methods of similar sensitivity.[6,7,90,92–96] These include enzyme-linked immunosorbent assays (ELISA), passive latex agglutination, and radial hemolysis. In the latex agglutination test latex particles are coated with rubella antigens that are then reacted with the serum being tested; agglutination indicates the presence of rubella antibodies. Most of these tests may be used to measure either IgG or IgM antibodies. A demonstration of specific IgG on one serum sample is evidence of immunity to rubella. Acute rubella infection may be diagnosed either by a demonstration of specific IgM in one serum sample or by a fourfold or greater increase in rubella antibody titer in two serum specimens performed in the same test. Results of many of these tests are available within a matter of minutes or hours and yield prompt useful information.

For a serologic diagnosis of congenital rubella in the neonatal period, antibody to rubella virus should be measured in both infant and maternal sera. It may be necessary to perform several antibody determinations on serum from the infant to detect whether the titer of rubella antibody is falling, indicative of passively acquired maternal antibody, or rising, suggesting rubella infection. If rubella IgM is detected in a newborn infant's serum, it is indicative that transplacental rubella infection has occurred. Congenital rubella has been diagnosed by placental biopsy at 12 weeks, demonstration of rubella antigen with monoclonal antibody, and detection of RNA by in situ hybridization.[97] It may also be diagnosed by the presence of specific IgM in fetal blood, but this may not be present until as late as 22 weeks' gestation.[98]

TREATMENT

Since postnatal rubella is such a mild infection in most instances, no treatment is indicated. There is no specific therapy, but for patients with fever and arthritis and/or anthralgia, the treatment of symptoms is indicated.

At one time immune globulin (IG) was advocated for the prevention or modification of rubella in susceptible pregnant women who were exposed to the infection. However, it was discovered that while IG might suppress symptoms it would not necessarily prevent viremia.[99] Therefore, indications for the use of IG for rubella prophylaxis are few. Possibly IG may be used if a pregnant susceptible woman is exposed to rubella and refuses to have an abortion should she develop rubella. Fortunately with the advent of rubella vaccine, it is now possible to immunize susceptible women of childbearing age against rubella before they become pregnant.

VACCINATION AGAINST RUBELLA

Rubella virus was isolated in 1962[1,2] and attenuated in 1966[100,101]; the live attenuated vaccine was licensed for use in this country in 1969. The rationale for use of the vaccine is to prevent congenital rubella by controlling postnatal rubella. In the United States the major thrust at first was to vaccinate prepubertal children, to minimize exposure of susceptible pregnant women to clinical cases of rubella. More recently there has also been an emphasis on immunizing rubella-susceptible women of childbearing age who are not pregnant. Often this is done just after delivery of an infant; nursing mothers who are so vaccinated do not cause harm to their infants. In some other countries the approach has been to vaccinate girls against rubella as they approach puberty.

Immunization programs in the United States have reduced the transmission of rubella in young children and prevented major epidemics of rubella. There have been no major epidemics of rubella during the past 20 years, a phenomenon never observed previously in the United States. In 1986, only 551 cases of postnatal rubella were reported to the CDC, which represents a 99 percent decline in incidence as compared with the prevaccine era.[69] There has been little alteration of the incidence of rubella immunity in women of childbearing age, 80–90 percent, however. This has been apparent from mini-outbreaks of rubella in colleges, the military, places of employment, and hospitals. Thus there is a continued need to emphasize the importance of immunization of women of childbearing age who are not pregnant and hospital employees as well as infants.[101]

At present the only rubella vaccine available in the United States is RA 27/3. This vaccine has been widely used in Europe and is more immunogenic than the previously used vaccines, HPV 77 DE5 and Cendehill, without an increase in side effects. RA 27/3 vaccine also stimulates the production of secretory as well as humoral IgA, which may account for its increased immunogenic potency.[102–104]

Complications of Vaccination

Rubella vaccine may cause viremia,[105,106] and thus the main complications are fever, adenopathy, arthritis, and arthralgia. All the complications are more common in adults than children and most common in women over 25 years of age.[107–110] In one study, up to 40 percent of such vaccinees developed joint complications[110]; however, all reactions were transient. It is uncommon for children to develop complications. In general, the incidence of joint complications even in adults is less after vaccination than after natural rubella.[13,106]

Efficacy of Vaccination

Since the introduction of rubella vaccine the number of reported cases of clinical rubella has declined progressively. The vaccines available today, when properly administered, produce a seroconversion rate of approximately 95 percent.[13] Since antibody titers are lower after vaccination than after natural disease, the question has been raised whether the antibody titer years after vaccination will remain high enough to prevent clinical rubella. Only time and continued surveillance will provide an answer to this question, but at this time there is no evidence of waning immunity,[21,22] again reflected by the low incidence of rubella in the United States. Booster injections of rubella vaccine are therefore not routinely indicated.

Effects of Rubella Vaccine on the Fetus

Since rubella vaccine was licensed in 1969, the CDC has followed the outcome of women who were reported to have been inadvertently immunized against rubella during early pregnancy. As of late 1987, 812 such women who carried their infants to term had been reported to the CDC, but no cases of the congenital rubella syndrome were attributed to rubella vaccine.[111] The observed risk of congenital rubella after immunization thus is reported as zero; however, the theoretic maximum risk could be as high as 2 percent. This is in contrast to a 30 percent or greater risk after maternal rubella in the first trimester.[111] Interestingly, it is known that the vaccine-type virus can cross the placenta; rubella virus has been isolated from both decidua and fetal tissue at abortion after inadvertent vaccination of pregnant women.[112–115] Rubella virus has been isolated from a fetus of a woman given rubella vaccine 7 weeks before conception.[116] It is therefore advised that women vaccinated against rubella not become pregnant for at least 3 months after the vaccine has been administered. While it is not recommended that rubella vaccine be administered to women who are pregnant, the currently recognized minimal fetal risk does not mandate automatic termination of a pregnancy. Many if not most such vaccinated women may wish to carry the infant to term.

REFERENCES

1. Parkman PD, Buescher EC, Artenstein MS. Recovery of rubella virus from army recruits. Proc Soc Exp Biol Med. 1962;111:225.
2. Weller TH, Neva FA. Propagation in tissue culture of cytopathic agents from patients with rubella-like illness. Proc Soc Exp Biol Med. 1962;111:215.
3. Andrewes CH. Generic names of viruses of vertebrates. Virology. 1970;40:1070.
4. Horzinek M, Maess J, Laufs R. Studies on the substructure of togaviruses. II Analysis of equine arteritis, rubella, bovine viral diarrhea, and hog cholera viruses. Arch Gesamte Virusforsch. 1971;33:306.
5. Murphy FA, Halomen PE, Harrison AK. Electron microscopy of the development of rubella virus in BHK-21 cells. J Virol. 1968;2:1223.
6. Rubella virus. In: Lennette EH, Schmidt NJ, eds. Diagnostic Procedures for Viral and Rickettsial Infections, ed 5. New York: American Public Health Association; 1979:725–66.
7. Stewart GL, Parkman PD, Hopps HE, et al. Rubella-virus hemagglutinin-inhibition test. N Engl J Med. 1967;276:554.
8. Sever JL, Hubner RJ, Castellano GA, et al. Rubella complement fixation test. Science. 1965;148:385.
9. Le Bouvier GL. Physiochemical characteristics of rubella antigens theta and iota. Nature. 1969;221:78.
10. Shapiro L. The numbered diseases: First through sixth. JAMA. 1971;194:680.
11. Gregg NM. Congenital cataract following German measles in the mother. Trans Ophthalmol Soc Aust. 1941;3:35.
12. Witte JJ, Karchmer AW, Case G, et al. Epidemiology of rubella. Am J Dis Child. 1969;118:107.
13. Krugman S. Present status of measles and rubella immunization in the United States: A medical progress report. J Pediatr. 1977;90:1.
14. Horstmann DM. Rubella: The challenge of its control. J Infect Dis. 1971;123:640.
15. Cooper LZ, Green RH, Krugman S, et al. Neonatal thrombocytopenic purpura and other manifestations of rubella contracted in vitro. Am J Dis Child. 1965;110:416.
16. Halstead SB, Diwan AR. Failure to transmit rubella vaccine virus. JAMA. 1971;215:634.
17. Scott HD, Byrne EB. Exposure of susceptible pregnant women to rubella vaccines. JAMA. 1971;215:609.
18. Fleet WF, Schaffner W, Lefkowitz LB, et al. Exposure of susceptible teachers to rubella vaccinees. Am J Dis Child. 1972;123:28.
19. Steele RW, Hensen SA, Vincent MM, et al. A ^{51}Cr microassay technique for cell-mediated immunity to viruses. J Immunol. 1973;110:1502.
20. Rossier E, Phipps PH, Weber JM, et al: Persistence of humoral and cell-mediated immunity to rubella virus in cloistered nuns and in schoolteachers. J Infect Dis. 1981;144:137–41.
21. Horstmann D, Schluederberg A, Emmons JE, et al. Persistence of vaccine-induced immune responses to rubella: Comparison with natural infection. Rev Infect Dis. 1985;7(Suppl):80–5.
22. Plotkin S, Buser F. History of RA27/3 rubella vaccine. Rev Infect Dis. 1985;7(Suppl):77–8.
23. Hillenbrand FKM. Rubella in a remote community. Lancet. 1956;2:64.
24. Fry J, Dillane JB, Fry L. Rubella 1962. Br Med J. 1962;2:833.
25. Horstmann DM, Liebhaber H, Le Bouvier GL, et al. Rubella: Reinfection of vaccinated and naturally immune persons exposed in an epidemic. N Engl J Med. 1970;283:771.
26. Wilkins J, Leedom JM, Salvatore MA, et al. Clinical rubella with arthritis resulting from reinfection. Ann Intern Med. 1972;77:930.
27. Davis WJ, Larson HE, Simsarian JP, et al. A study of rubella immunity and resistance to infection. JAMA. 1971;215:600.
28. Chang TW, Des Rosiers S, Weinstein L. Clinical and serologic studies of an outbreak of rubella in a vaccinated population. N Engl J Med. 1970;283:246.
29. Wilkins J, Leidom JM, Portnoy B, et al. Reinfection with rubella virus despite live vaccine-induced immunity. Am J Dis Child. 1969;118:275.
30. Forrest JM, Menser MA, Honeyman MC, et al. Clinical rubella eleven months after vaccination. Lancet. 1972;2:399.
31. Schiff G, Young B, Stefanovic, et al. Challenge with rubella virus after loss of detectable vaccine-induced immunity. Rev Infect Dis. 1985;7(Suppl):156–63.
32. Northrop RL, Gardner WM, Guttmann WF. Rubella reinfection during early pregnancy. A case report. Obstet Gynecol (NY). 1972;39:524.
33. Banatvala JE, Best JM. Rubella infections. Lancet. 1973;1:1452.
34. Biano S, Cochran W, Herrmann KL, et al. Rubella reinfection during pregnancy. Am J Dis Child. 1975;129:1353.
35. Balfour HH, Groth KE, Edelman CK. Rubella viraemia and antibody responses after rubella vaccination and reimmunization. Lancet. 1981;1:1078.
36. Boue A, Nicolas A, Montagron B. Reinfection with rubella in pregnant women. Lancet. 1971;1:2151.
37. Eilard T, Strannegard O. Rubella reinfection in pregnancy followed by transmission to the fetus. J Infect Dis. 1974;129:594.
38. Levine JB, Berkowitz CD, St. Geme JW. Rubella virus reinfection during pregnancy leading to late-onset congenital rubella syndrome. J Pediatr. 1982;100:589.
39. Fosgren M, Carlson G, Strongert K. Case of congenital rubella after maternal reinfection. Scand J Infect Dis. 1979;11:81–93.
40. Partridge JW, Flewett TH, Whitehead JEM. Congenital rubella affecting an

infant whose mother had rubella antibodies before conception. Br Med J. 1981;282:187–8.
41. Bott LM, Eizenberg DH. Congenital rubella after successful vaccination. Med J Aust. 1982;1:514–5.
42. Klock LE, Rachelfsky GS. Failure of rubella herd immunity during an epidemic. N Engl J Med. 1973;288:69.
43. Heggie AD, Robbins FC. Rubella in naval recruits. N Engl J Med. 1964;271:231.
44. Coyle PK, Wolinsky JS, Buimovici-Klein E, et al. Rubella-specific immune complexes after congenital infection and vaccination. Infect Immun. 1982;36:498–503.
45. Ziola B, Lund G, Meurman O, et al. Circulating immune complexes in patients with acute measles and rubella virus. Infect Immun. 1983;41:578–89.
46. Heggie AD. Pathogenesis of Rubella exanthem. Isolation of rubella virus from skin. N Engl J Med. 1971;285:664.
47. Buescher EL. Behavior of rubella virus in adult populations. Arch Gesamte Virusforsch. 1965;16:470.
48. Heggie AD, Robbins FC. Natural rubella acquired after birth. Am J Dis Child. 1969;118:12.
49. Johnson RE, Hall AP. Rubella arthritis. N Engl J Med. 1958;258:743.
50. Vergani D, Morgan-Capner P, Davies ET, et al. Joint symptoms, immune complexes and rubella. Lancet. 1980;1:321–2.
51. Hildebrandt HM, Maassab HF. Rubella synovitis in a one-year-old patient. N Engl J Med. 1966;274:1428.
52. Phillips CA, Behbehani AM, Johnson LW, et al. Isolation of rubella virus: an epidemic characterized by rash and arthritis. JAMA. 1965;191:615.
53. Ogra PL, Herd JK, Arthritis associated with induced rubella infection. J Immunol. 1971;107:810–3.
54. Smith CA, Petty RE, Tingle AJ. Rubella virus and arthritis. Rheum Dis Clin North Am. 1987;13:265–74.
55. Grahame R, Armstrong R, Simmons NA, et al. Isolation of rubella virus from synovial fluid in five cases of seronegative arthritis. Lancet. 1981;2:649–51.
56. Grahame R, Armstrong R, Simmons NA, et al. Chronic arthritis associated with the presence of intrasynovial rubella virus. Ann Rheum Dis. 1983;42:2–13.
57. Fraser JR, Cunningham AL, Hayes K, et al. Rubella arthritis in adults. Isolation of virus, cytology, and other aspects of synovial infection. Clin Exp Rheumatol. 1983;1:287–93.
58. Chantler JK, Tingle AJ, Petty RE. Presistent rubella virus infection associated with chronic arthritis in children. N Engl J Med. 1985;313:1117–23.
59. Chantler JK, da Roza DM, Bonnie ME, et al. Sequential studies on synovial lymphocyte stimulation by rubella antigen, and rubella virus isolation in an adult with persistent arthritis. Ann Rheum Dis. 1985;44:564–68.
60. Chantler JK, Ford DK, Tingle AJ. Persistent rubella infection and rubella-associated arthritis. Lancet. 1982;1:1323–5.
61. Cunningham AL, Fraser JRE. Persistent rubella virus infection of human synovial cells cultured in vitro. J Infect Dis. 1985;151:638–45.
62. Ozsoyla S, Kanra G, Savas G. Thrombocytopenic purpura related to rubella infection. Pediatrics. 1978;62:567.
63. Boyer WL, Sherman FE, Michaels RH, et al. Purpura in congenital and acquired rubella. N Engl J Med. 1965;273:1362.
64. Steen E, Torp KH. Encephalitis and thrombocytopenic purpura after rubella. Arch Dis Child. 1956;31:470.
65. Sherman FE, Michaels RH, Kenny FM. Acute encephalopathy (encephalitis) complicating rubella. JAMA. 1965;192:675.
66. Sheinis M, Sarov I, Maor E, et al. Severe neonatal rubella following maternal infection. Pediatr Infect Dis J. 1985;4:202–3.
67. Zeldis JB, Miller JG, Dienstag JL. Hepatitis in an adult with rubella. Am J Med. 1985;79:515–6.
68. Cooper LZ. Congenital rubella in the United States. In: Krugman S, Gershon A, eds. Infections of the Fetus and the Newborn Infant. New York: Alan R. Liss; 1975:1.
69. CDC. Rubella and congenital rubella—United States, 1984–1986. MMWR 1987;36:664–6.
70. Marshall WC. Rubella: Current problems and recent developments. Br J Clin Pract. 1976;30:56.
71. Menser MA, Forrest JM. Rubella: High incidence of defects in children considered normal at birth. Med J Aust. 1974;1:123.
72. Peckham CS. Clinical and laboratory study of children exposed in utero to maternal rubella. Arch Dis Child. 1972;47:571.
73. Forrest JM, Menser M, Burgess JA: High frequency of diabetes mellitus in young adults with congenital rubella. Lancet. 1971;2:332.
74. Menser MA, Forrest JM, Honeyman MC, et al. Diabetes, HLA antigens and congenital rubella. Lancet. 1974;2:1508–9.
75. Ginsberg-Felner F, Witt ME, Fedun B, et al. Diabetes mellitus and autoimmunity in patients with the congenital rubella syndrome. Rev Infect Dis. 1985;7(Suppl):170–6.
76. Townsend JJ, Baringer JR, Wolinsky JS, et al. Progressive rubella panencephalitis: Late onset after congenital rubella. N Engl J Med. 1975;292:990.
77. Weil MC, Itabashi HH, Cremer NE, et al. Chronic progressive panencephalitis due to rubella virus simulating subacute sclerosing panencephalitis. N Engl J Med. 1975;292:994.
78. Alford CA, Neva FA, Weller TH. Virologic and serologic studies on human products of conception after maternal rubella. N Engl J Med. 1964;271:1275.
79. Hardy JB, Sever JL, Gilkeson MR. Declining antibody titers in children with congenital rubella. J Pediatr. 1969;75:213.
80. Doege TC, Kim KK. Studies of rubella and its prevention with gamma globulin. JAMA. 1967;200:584.
81. Fuccillo DA, Steele RW, Hensen SA, et al. Impaired cellular immunity to rubella virus in congenital rubella. Infect Immun. 1974;9:81.
82. Naeye RL, Blanc W. Pathogenesis of congenital rubella. JAMA. 1965;194:1277.
83. Driscoll SG. Histopathology of gestational rubella. Am J Dis Child. 1969;118:49.
84. Tondury G, Smith DW. Fetal rubella pathology. J Pediatr. 1966;68:867.
85. Plotkin SA, Vaheri A. Human fibroblasts infected with rubella virus produce a growth inhibitor. Science. 1967;154:659.
86. Nusbacher J, Hirschhorn K, Cooper LZ. Chromosomal abnormalities in congenital rubella. N Engl J Med. 1967;276:1409.
87. Rabinowe SL, George KL, Loughlin R, et al. Congenital rubella. Monoclonal antibody–defined T cell abnormalities in young adults. Am J Med. 1986;81:779–82.
88. Cherry JD. Newer viral exanthems. Prog Med Virol. 1973;16:269.
89. Bell EF, Ross CA, Grist NR. ECHO 9 infection in pregnant women with suspected rubella. J Clin Pathol. 1975;28:267.
90. Meyer HM, Parkman PD, Hopps HE. The clinical application of laboratory diagnostic procedures for rubella and measles (rubeola). Am J Clin Pathol. 1972;57:803.
91. Levin MJ, Oxman MN, Moore MG, et al. Diagnosis of congenital rubella in utero. N Engl J Med. 1974;290:1187.
92. Chernesky M, Wyman L, Mahoney J, et al. Clinical evaluation of the sensitivity and specificity of a commercially available enzyme immunoassay for detection of rubella virus–specific immunoglobulin M. J Clin Microbiol. 1984;20:400–4.
93. Field PR, Gong CM. Diagnosis of postnatally acquired rubella by use of three enzyme-linked immunoadsorbent assays for specific immunoglobulins G, and M and single radial hemolysis for specific immunoglobulin G. J Clin Microbiol. 1944;20:951–8.
94. Wittenburg RA, Roberts M, Elliott L, et al. Comparative evaluation of commercial rubella virus antibody kits. J Clin Microbiol. 1985;21:161–3.
95. Hedman K, Salonen E, Keski-Oja J, et al. Single-serum radial hemolysis to detect recent rubella infection. J Infect Dis. 1986;154:1018–23.
96. Ferraro MJ, Kallas WM, Welch KP, et al. Comparison of a new, rapid enzyme immunoassay with a latex agglutination test for qualitative detection of rubella antibodies. J Clin Microbiol. 1987;25:1722–4.
97. Terry GM, Ho TL, Warren RC, et al. First trimester prenatal diagnosis of congenital rubella: A laboratory investigation. Br Med J. 1986;292:930–3.
98. Daffos F, Forestier F, Grangeot-Keros L, et al. Prenatal diagnosis of congenital rubella. Lancet. 1984;2:1–3.
99. Schiff GM. Titered lots of immune globulin. Efficacy in the prevention of rubella. Am J Dis Child. 1969;118:322.
100. Parkman PD, Meyer HM, Kirschstein RL, et al. Attenuated rubella virus I. Development and laboratory characterization. N Engl J Med. 1966;275:569.
101. Preblud SR, Serdula MK, Frank JA, et al. Rubella vaccination in the United States: A ten-year review. Epidemiol Rev. 1980;2:171.
102. Plotkin SA, Farquhar JD, Katz M, et al. Attenuation of RA 27/3 rubella virus in W1-38 human diploid cells. Am J Dis Child. 1969;118:178.
103. LeBouvier GL, Plotkin SA. Precepitin responses to rubella vaccine RA 27/3. J Infect Dis. 1971;123:220.
104. Ogra PL, Kerr-Grant D, Umana G, et al. Antibody response in serum and nasopharynx after naturally acquired and vaccine-induced infection with rubella virus. N Engl J Med. 1971;285:1333.
105. Modlin JF, Branding-Bennett AD, Witte JJ, et al. A review of 5 years' experience with rubella vaccine in the United States. Pediatrics. 1975;55:20.
106. Tingle AJ, Chantler JK, Pot KH, et al. Postpartum rubella immunization: Association with development of prolonged arthritis, neurological sequellae, and chronic rubella viremia. J Infect Dis. 1985;152:606–12.
107. Cooper LZ, Ziring PR, Weiss HJ, et al. Transient arthritis after rubella vaccination. Am J Dis Child. 1969;118:218.
108. Horstmann DM, Liebheber H, Kohorn EI. Postpartum vaccination of rubella-susceptible women. Lancet. 1970;2:1003.
109. Monto AS, Cavallero JJ, Whale EH. Frequency of arthralgia in women receiving one of three rubella vaccines. Arch Intern Med. 1970;126:635.
110. Lerman ST, Nankervis GA, Heggie AD, et al. Immunologic response, virus excretion and joint reactions with rubella vaccine. A study of adolescent girls and young women given live attenuated virus vaccine (HPV-77 DE5). Ann Intern Med. 1971;74:67.
111. CDC. Rubella vaccination during pregnancy 1971–1986. MMWR 1987;36:457–61.
112. Phillips CA, Maeck JVS, Rogers WA, et al. Intrauterine rubella infection following immunization with rubella vaccine. JAMA. 1970;213:624.
113. Vahieri A, Vesikari T, Oker-Blum N, et al. Isolation of attenuated rubella-vaccine virus from human products of conception and uterine cervix. N Engl J Med. 1972;286:1071.
114. Wyll SA, Herrmann K. Inadvertent rubella vaccination of pregnant women. Fetal risk in 215 cases, JAMA. 1973;225:1472.
115. Modlin JF, Herrmann K, Brandling-Bennett DA, et al. Risk of congenital abnormality after inadvertent rubella vaccination of pregnant women. N Engl J Med. 1976;294:972.
116. Fleet WF, Benz EW, Karzon DT, et al. Fetal consequences of maternal rubella immunization. JAMA. 1974;227:621.

Flaviviridae

132. FLAVIVIRUS (YELLOW FEVER, DENGUE, AND ST. LOUIS ENCEPHALITIS)

THOMAS P. MONATH

The family Flaviviridae (or group B arboviruses) includes 66 viruses, most of them arthropod borne and grouped on the basis of serologic cross-reactions. Twenty-two viruses cause infections of medical importance (Table 1).

HISTORY

Yellow fever was first recognized as a disease in the seventeenth century. Viral etiology and mosquito transmission was proved in 1900, and the virus was first isolated in 1927. The 17D yellow fever vaccine was deployed in 1937. Yellow fever remains an important epidemic disease in the South American and African tropics.

The first definite clinical report of dengue (''breakbone fever'') is attributed to Benjamin Rush in 1789. The viral etiology and mosquito transmission were established during the first two decades of the twentieth century. During World War II, Sabin defined the existence of multiple serotypes.[1] A severe form, dengue hemorrhagic fever was described in the early 1950s and is now an important epidemic disease in southeast Asia[2] (see Chapter 143).

St. Louis encephalitis virus was isolated in 1933 during an epidemic in St. Louis, Missouri. A mosquito vector was suspected by Lumsden in 1933 but was not proved until the early 1940s. St. Louis encephalitis has caused periodic outbreaks with up to 2000 cases in the United States, Canada, and Mexico.[3]

PATHOGENS

Flaviviruses are small (40 nm diameter) enveloped viruses with single-stranded, positive-sense RNA genomes approximately 11,000 nucleotides in length. Virions form on the endoplasmic reticulum of infected cells and are released by exocytosis or cell lysis. The replication strategy and gene structure have been recently reviewed.[4] Flaviviruses are readily inactivated by heat (56°C, 10 minutes), detergents, ultraviolet irradiation, trypsin digestion, formaldehyde, and chlorine and phenolic disinfectants.

TABLE 1. Flaviviruses (Group B Togaviruses) Known to Cause Human Disease

Epidemiologic Characteristics	Virus	Clinical Syndrome(s)	Primary Transmission Cycle: Principal Vector(s)	Primary Transmission Cycle: Host(s)	Geographic Distribution
Mosquito-borne, epidemic	Yellow fever	Hepatitis; gastrointestinal hemorrhage	*Aedes aegypti* (urban)	Humans	South America, Africa
			Aedes sp. (sylvan)	Simian sp.	South America, Africa
	Dengue (types 1–4)	Febrile illness with rash; hemorrhagic fever (HF)	*Aedes aegypti*	Humans	Worldwide; HF in SE Asia, Caribbean
	West Nile	Febrile illness (rash); encephalitis	*Culex univittatus*	Birds	Africa, Asia, Middle East, Europe
	St. Louis encephalitis	Encephalitis	*Culex tarsalis, C. pipiens, C. nigripalpus*	Birds	Western Hemisphere
	Rocio	Encephalitis	? *Aedes scapularis*	? Birds	Sao Paulo State, Brazil
	Japanese encephalitis	Encephalitis	*Culex tritaeniorhynchus*	Pigs, birds	Japan, Korea, China, SE Asia, India
	Murray Valley encephalitis	Encephalitis	*Culex annulirostris*	Birds	Australia
Mosquito-borne, rare or sporadic	Banzi	Febrile illness	*Culex rubinotus*	Rodents	Southern and East Africa
	Bussuquara	Febrile illness	*Culex* sp.	Rodents	Brazil, Colombia, Ecuador, Panama
	Ilheus	Febrile illness; encephalitis	?*Psorophora* sp.	Birds	South, Central America
	Sepik	Febrile illness	?	?	New Guinea
	Spondweni	Febrile illness	*Aedes circumluteolus*	?	Southern and West Africa
	Usutu	Febrile illness (rash)	? *Culex* spp.	Birds	Africa
	Wesselsbron	Febrile illness	*Aedes* sp.	Cattle, sheep	Africa, Thailand
	Zika	Febrile illness	*Aedes* sp.	? Monkeys	Africa, Malaysia
Tick-borne, epidemic and endemic	Tick-borne encephalitis	Encephalitis	*Ixodes persulcatus, I. ricinus*	Rodents, birds, goats, cattle (transmission to humans also by vehicle of unpasteurized goat's milk)	USSR, Central Europe, Scandanavia
	Kyasanur Forest disease	Hemorrhagic fever	*Haemaphysalis* sp.	Rodents, monkeys	Karnataka State, India
	Omsk hemorrhagic fever	Hemorrhagic fever	*Dermacentor, Ixodes* spp.	Rodents	Siberia
Tick-borne, rare or sporadic	Powassan	Encephalitis	*Ixodes cookei, I. marxi*	Rodents	US, Canada
	Louping ill	Encephalitis	*Ixodes ricinus*	Rodents, sheep	Great Britain
	Negishi	Encephalitis	?	?	Japan, China
No arthropod vector, rare or sporadic	Rio Bravo	Febrile illness	None	Bats	US, Mexico

The viruses replicate in a variety of vertebrate and arthropod cells in culture with or without producing cytopathic effects. Most of the flaviviruses also cause lethal infections in infant mice inoculated intracerebrally. Infant mice are insensitive hosts for the isolation of unadapted dengue viruses.

Extensive serologic relatedness, due to shared group-specific antigens, links members of the family; in general, crossing is most extensive by hemagglutination inhibition, intermediate by complement fixation, and least by neutralization tests.

EPIDEMIOLOGY

Yellow Fever

For a detailed description of yellow fever ecology, see Monath.[5] The virus is present in tropical areas of South America and Africa but has never appeared in Asia. Up to 1000 human cases are officially reported annually, but the true incidence may be 200 times greater. The case fatality rate is 20–50 percent in patients developing jaundice and approximately 5 percent overall. The virus is maintained in a forest transmission cycle between monkeys and tree-hole breeding mosquitoes (in Africa, *Aedes* spp.; in South America, *Haemagogus* spp.) Humans exposed to these vectors may acquire jungle yellow fever. In South America such infections are closely related to clearing forest for agriculture, and adult males are at highest risk. In savanna habitats of Africa, tree-hole breeding *Aedes* may sustain an intense epidemic spread of virus from monkeys to humans and between humans. The sex ratio of cases is nearly equal, and both children and adults are at risk. In urban environments and areas with low rainfall, the domestic mosquito vector, *Aedes aegypti* may be present at high density by breeding in artificial containers used to store water. This epidemic vector may transmit yellow fever virus from human to human (so-called urban yellow fever).

Dengue

Dengue is endemic and epidemic in tropical America, Africa, and Asia where the principal vector *Aedes aegypti* is continuously present. The transmission cycle is similar to urban yellow fever. Viremic air travellers may rapidly spread the disease over long distances, thereby resulting in explosive epidemics. Cross-immunity between the four dengue serotypes lasts only a few weeks, and individuals may thus sustain multiple sequential infections. All ages and both sexes are susceptible, but in endemic areas a high prevalence of immunity in adults may limit outbreaks to children. Classic dengue fever is a self-limited nonfatal disease.

Dengue hemorrhagic fever (DHF) has caused large outbreaks in southeast Asian cities that have resulted in over 1.5 million cases and 33,000 deaths since 1950.[6] Epidemic DHF appeared in the New World (Cuba) in 1981, with over 116,000 hospitalized cases. The case fatality rate in patients receiving good medical care is 1–3 percent; in untreated or inadequately treated patients, it is as high as 50 percent.

St. Louis Encephalitis

Summertime St. Louis encephalitis epidemics occur at approximately 10-year intervals with varying severity.[3] The case fatality rate is 5–15 percent; elderly persons are at the highest risk of overt clinical infection and severe disease. The virus circulates between wild birds by the agency of *Culex* mosquitoes. Birds develop viremic infections without illness. Mosquito vectors thereby infected may transmit the virus to humans, which may fall ill but do not sustain viremias sufficiently high to infect mosquitoes.

PATHOGENESIS

Yellow Fever

The yellow fever virus is mainly viscerotropic in humans and causes damage to the liver, kidney, heart, and gastrointestinal tract.[7] Necrosis of the midzonal portion of the liver lobule is associated with the formation of intracellular hyaline deposits (Councilman bodies) and an absence of inflammatory cell infiltrate. Healing is complete in patients who recover. The kidneys show cloudy swelling and fatty degeneration of the proximal tubules. Experimental studies in monkeys suggest that the oliguria in yellow fever is the result of circulatory collapse and progression from prerenal failure to acute tubular necrosis.[8] When the heart is involved, it is usually flabby and pale, with scattered pericardial petechial hemorrhages. Microscopically, there is degeneration of myocardial fibers. Clinically, these patients may have bradycardia and electrocardiographic (ECG) abnormalities; the contribution of direct cardiac damage to hypotension is uncertain. Late deaths have been attributed to arrhythmia.

The classic gastrointestinal sign of yellow fever is "black vomit" or hematemesis from constantly oozing petechial hemorrhages of the stomach and duodenum. Decreased synthesis of vitamin K dependent coagulation factors by the diseased liver is the principal cause, but disseminated intravascular coagulation may also occur.

The brain may be edematous and show petechial hemorrhages.

Dengue

Increased vascular permeability, bleeding, and possibly intravascular coagulation constitute the major pathophysiologic changes in DHF.[6,9] These abnormalities may be mediated by circulating dengue antibody–antigen complexes, activation of complement, and release of vasoactive amines. Dengue hemorrhagic fever usually occurs during second dengue infections in persons with pre-existing actively or passively (maternally) acquired immunity to a heterologous dengue virus serotype. The phenomenon of *immune enhancement* has been invoked to explain these observations.[10] Virus complexed with pre-existing non-neutralizing antibodies to a heterologous dengue serotype gains access to monocyte-macrophages via Fc receptors, thereby enhancing virus replication. In the process of immune elimination of infected cells, proteases and lymphokines may be released and activate complement, coagulation cascades, and vascular permeability factors. Virulence differences between dengue strains may also determine the clinical spectrum of dengue.

St. Louis Encephalitis

After inoculation of the virus, peripheral sites of viral replication such as lymphatic tissue, muscle, or endothelium initiate and maintain viremia. The mode of viral penetration into the human central nervous system is unknown but is generally thought to be via the hematogenous route.[11] In laboratory rodents, the olfactory neuroepithelium, infected by blood-borne virus, is a site of early virus replication and spread via olfactory axons to the brain[12]; the virus then spreads throughout the neuraxis.

The neuropathology of fatal human St. Louis encephalitis viral infection[13] is characterized by leptomeningeal mononuclear cell infiltration and parenchymal lesions consisting of lymphocytic and reactive microglial cell perivascular infiltrates and cellular nodules. Neuronal degeneration is encountered near cellular nodules. Lesions are most prevalent in selected gray matter nuclei, especially the substantia nigra and thalamic nuclei.

CLINICAL MANIFESTATIONS

Yellow Fever

After a 3- to 6-day incubation period the classic syndrome starts with an abrupt onset of chills and fever followed by headache, backache, generalized pain, nausea, and vomiting, a flush face, conjunctival injection, and leukopenia. This period of infection (during which virus is present in the blood) is followed in approximately 3 days by a period of remission lasting several hours to a day. The patient then enters a period of intoxication with reappearance of fever, jaundice, hemorrhages, especially hematemesis (black vomit), albuminuria, and oliguria. The Faget sign (bradycardia inappropriate for the fever) is often present in the period of infection and intoxication. Death generally occurs in the 7th–10th day after the onset of symptoms following a terminal period characterized by delirium, agitation, shock, and coma.

Dengue

Classic dengue fever is characterized by an incubation period of 5–8 days followed by fever, chilly sensations, headache, retro-orbital pain, backache, arthralgia, anorexia, weakness, prostration, nausea, vomiting, epigastric discomfort, cutaneous hyperesthesia, and altered taste sensation.[14] The fever of dengue lasts 5–7 days. Early in the disease the face and neck may appear flushed, and a generalized transient macular rash may be evident that blanches on pressure. Shortly after defervescence, a maculopapular rash appears that lasts 1–5 days, spares the palms and soles, and occasionally is followed by desquamation. Fever may reappear with this rash, with a resulting "saddle-back" fever curve. Lymphadenopathy and minor hemorrhagic manifestations (petechiae, epistaxis) may occur. Unusual complications attributed to dengue include myocarditis and encephalopathy. Convalescence may be prolonged, with weakness and mental depression.

The diagnosis of DHF is made in the presence of (*1*) fever, (*2*) hemorrhagic manifestations (positive tourniquet test response with or without spontaneous bleeding: petechiae, purpura, epistaxis, gum bleeding, gastrointestinal bleeding), and (*3*) thrombocytopenia and hemoconcentration (hematocrit increased by ≥20 percent).[15] Hepatomegaly is an inconstant finding. The chest roentgenogram often shows pleural effusions. In severe cases hypotension, narrowed pulse pressure and circulatory failure (dengue shock syndrome) develop with a mortality of 1–3 percent (treated) to 50 percent (untreated). Biochemical abnormalities include decreased serum protein and sodium concentrations; acidemia; rising blood urea nitrogen levels; a reduction in fibrinogen and clotting factor V, VII, IX, and X concentrations; and the appearance of fibrin split products in the plasma. Reductions in serum complement (C3, C4, C5, Clq, C3 proactivator) are proportional to the severity of illness.

St. Louis Encephalitis

Three clinical syndromes are associated with St. Louis encephalitis viral infection: (*1*) fever and headache, (*2*) aseptic meningitis, and (*3*) encephalitis. Increased severity and a higher incidence of encephalitis occur with advancing age. The onset of illness follows an incubation period of 4–21 days and is characterized by a variable period of nonspecific symptoms (malaise, fever, headache, myalgia) and then by acute meningeal or neuroparenchymal signs or both. In patients with encephalitis, an altered level of consciousness is the most frequent finding; tremors of the extremities, face, and tongue and pathologic reflexes are present in about 50 percent of the patients. Cranial nerve abnormalities and paresis are less common, and sensory deficits are rare. Convulsions occur in about 10 percent of the patients and are a grave prognostic sign. Signs of bladder or renal dysfunction have been described. A mild syndrome of inappropriate secretion of antidiuretic hormone occurs in about one-third of the patients. Laboratory findings include moderate peripheral leukocytosis; cerebrospinal fluid (CSF) pleocytosis (<500 cells/mm^3, with early polymorphonuclear and later lymphocytic cell preponderance); elevated CSF protein concentration; and variably elevated glutamic-oxaloacetic transaminase (GOT) and serum creatine phosphokinase (CPK) levels. The electroencephalogram shows diffuse generalized slowing and amorphous delta wave activity. The brain scan findings are normal. Neuresthenic complaints are common after clinical recovery, but objective neurologic residua are relatively infrequent.

DIAGNOSIS

Yellow Fever

The differential diagnosis of severe yellow fever includes hepatitis, malaria, typhoid, leptospirosis, and other viral hemorrhagic fevers (dengue, Rift Valley fever, Lassa fever, Marburg-Ebola virus disease, Congo-Crimean hemorrhagic fever).

A specific diagnosis depends upon virus isolation, serologic test results, or histologic examination of liver. The yellow fever virus may be isolated from blood, especially during the first 4 days of illness. Viral antigen may be detected in blood or liver tissue by enzyme-linked immunosorbent assay (ELISA), which provides a rapid diagnosis. Serologic diagnosis is achieved by IgM antibody-capture ELISA, hemagglutination inhibition (HI), complement fixation (CF), or neutralization. IgM, HI, and neutralizing antibodies appear within 5 days after onset, and CF antibodies appear within 7–14 days. Cross-reacting antibodies (particularly HI and CF antibodies) to other flaviviruses may complicate serologic interpretation.

Dengue

The differential diagnosis of classic dengue fever includes malaria, scrub typhus, and a wide variety of viral infections including those caused by influenza, chikungunya, Mayaro fever, West Nile, Sindbis, and Ross River viruses. Dengue hemorrhagic fever must be differentiated from malaria, bacterial sepsis (including meningococcemia), leptospirosis, rickettsioses, and other viral hemorrhagic fevers.

A specific diagnosis is achieved by virus isolation from blood or by serology. Virus isolation is best achieved by inoculation of mosquito cells (or adult mosquitoes) and serotype-specific identification by immunofluorescence using monoclonal antibodies.[16] Serologic methods are as described for yellow fever.

St. Louis Encephalitis

This disease must be distinguished from other infectious causes of meningoencephalitis and from noninfectious acute disorders of the central nervous system. Because of its occurrence in the elderly, St. Louis encephalitis has been misdiagnosed as stroke.

Virus isolation from blood or CSF is rarely successful. The virus has been recovered from brain tissue and viral antigen demonstrated by immunofluorescence in frozen sections of brain. St. Louis encephalitis is most often diagnosed by serologic methods; the IgM ELISA is especially useful and may be applied to serum as well as CSF.

PREVENTION AND TREATMENT

Yellow Fever

Patients should be protected from mosquito bites. Acetaminophen may be used to reduce fever and headache. Antacids and cimetidine may be used to reduce the risk of gastric bleeding. Oxygen should be administered to severely ill patients, and they should be monitored closely for signs of oliguria, hypotension, and blood gas and electrolyte imbalance. Blood replacement or the use of alternative volume expanders may be indicated in case of severe hemorrhage or shock. Heparin therapy may be considered only if there are clear indications from hematologic tests of disseminated intravascular coagulopathy. Patients with renal failure may benefit from dialysis. No specific antiviral therapy is currently available.

Yellow fever control has been achieved by the destruction of mosquito vectors and by vaccination. Live 17D yellow fever vaccine affords long-lasting (probably lifelong) protection. Neurologic accidents are extremely rare; most have occurred in infants under 6 months, who should not receive the vaccine. On theoretic grounds, the vaccine should not be administered to pregnant women or to persons who are immunologically compromised.

Dengue

The principal means of preventing dengue and controlling epidemics is by reducing *Aedes aegypti* vector populations. Live attenuated vaccines against all four dengue serotypes are under development. The treatment of patients with classic dengue fever is symptomatic. Patients with DHF require careful observation for early signs of shock. If shock appears, immediate replacement of the existing plasma loss is essential, with careful monitoring of hematocrit and central venous pressure. Electrolyte and blood gas abnormalities should be corrected. Corticosteroids are of no benefit, and no specific antiviral therapy is available.

St. Louis Encephalitis

Surveillance of St. Louis encephalitis viral activity in vectors and avian hosts is useful in defining the risk of an impending human outbreak and as a guide for preventive measures to reduce vector mosquito populations. Epidemics of St. Louis encephalitis are controlled by the use of insecticides to kill infected adult mosquitoes. No vaccine is available. Treatment is supportive.

REFERENCES

1. Sabin AB. Research on dengue during World War II. Am J Trop Med Hyg. 1952;1:30.
2. Halstead SB. Mosquito-borne hemorrhagic fevers of South and South-East Asia. Bull WHO. 1966;35:3–15.
3. Monath TP. St. Louis Encephalitis. Washington, DC: American Public Health Association; 1980.
4. Rice CM, Strauss EG, Strauss JH. Structure of the flavivirus genome. In: Schlesinger S, Schlesinger MJ, eds. The Togaviridae and Flaviviridae. New York: Plenum; 1986:279.
5. Monath TP. Yellow fever. In: Monath TP, ed. The Arboviruses: Epidemiology and Ecology. Boca Raton, FL: CRC Press; 1988.
6. Halstead SB. Pathogenesis of dengue: Challenges to molecular biology. Science. 1988;239:476.
7. Monath TP. Yellow fever: A medically neglected disease. Report on a seminar. Rev Infect Dis. 1987;9:165.
8. Monath TP, Brinker KR, Chandler FW, et al. Pathophysiologic correlations in a rhesus monkey model of yellow fever. Am J Trop Med Hyg. 1981;30:431.
9. Halstead SB. Dengue haemorrhagic fever: A public health problem and a field for research. Bull WHO. 1980;58:1.
10. Halstead SB. Immunopathology in viral disease: Immune enhancement of dengue virus infection. In: Olson LC, ed. Virus Infections: Modern Concepts and Status. New York: Marcel Dekker; 1982:41.
11. Nathanson N. Pathogenesis. In: Monath TP, ed. St. Louis Encephalitis. Washington, DC: American Public Health Association; 1980:201.
12. Monath TP, Cropp CB, Harrison AK. Mode of entry of a neurotropic arbovirus into the central nervous system. Reinvestigation of an old controversy. Lab Invest. 1983;48:399.
13. Gardner JJ, Reyes M. Human pathology of St. Louis encephalitis. In: Monath TP, ed. St. Louis Encephalitis. Washington, DC: American Public Health Association; 1980:551.
14. Sabin AB. Dengue. In: Rivers TM, Horsfall FL Jr, eds. Viral and Rickettsial Infections of Man. Philadelphia: JB Lippincott; 1959:361.
15. Dengue Haemorrhagic Fever: Diagnosis, treatment and control. Geneva; World Health Organization; 1986.
16. Gubler DJ, Kuno G, Sather GE, et al. Use of mosquito cell cultures and specific monoclonal antibodies for routine surveillance of dengue viruses. Am J Trop Med Hyg. 1984;33:158.

Coronaviridae

133. CORONAVIRUS

KENNETH McINTOSH

In 1965 Tyrrell and Bynoe were able to passage a virus obtained from the respiratory tract of an adult suffering from a common cold by serially culturing nasal wash fluids in human embryonic tracheal organ cultures.[1] The medium from these cultures consistently produced colds in volunteers. The agent involved, however, failed to grow in tissue culture. It was ether sensitive but not related to any of the known myxo- or paramyxoviruses. Subsequently, electron microscopy of fluids from infected organ cultures revealed particles that resembled the infectious bronchitis virus of chickens.[2] The particles were medium sized (80–150 nm), pleomorphic, membrane coated, and covered with widely spaced club-shaped surface projections. At about the same time Hamre and Procknow recovered a cytopathic agent in secondary human embryonic kidney tissue culture from medical students with colds.[3] This agent also was unrelated to known myxo- and paramyxoviruses and was ether sensitive. Subsequent electron microscopy revealed similar or identical particles.[2]

After this, McIntosh and others reported the recovery of multiple strains of ether-sensitive agents from the human respiratory tract, all of which had the typical morphology of infectious bronchitis virus.[4] At much the same time a number of previously unclassified animal viruses including mouse hepatitis virus and transmissible gastroenteritis virus of swine were shown to have the same characteristic morphology by electron microscopy.[5,6] Very shortly thereafter an international ad hoc committee was assembled and recommended that this group of viruses receive separate classification; the name *coronaviruses* (the prefix "corona" denoting the crownlike appearance of the surface projections) was chosen to signify the new genus.[7,8]

The number and importance of animal coronaviruses quickly grew, with the eventual inclusion of viruses causing diseases, often of great economic importance, in rats, mice, chickens, turkeys, calves, dogs, cats, and pigs. A brief and probably incomplete list of animal coronaviruses and the diseases they cause is shown in Table 1. It is clear that the variety of animal species infected and the multiplicity of organ systems involved have made this one of the most important veterinary viral genera.

In view of the prominance of enteric coronaviruses in animal diseases, it is not surprising that coronavirus-like particles have also been described in human fecal materials. During the past 5–10 years reports of such particles have been numerous, and the existence of this new family as well as their likely involvement in gastrointestinal disease has gained credibility. It has been difficult to grow them reproducibly in vitro, and knowledge about them is limited. Much of what is said below concerns the better-characterized human respiratory coronaviruses, but information about enteric coronaviruses is included wherever possible.

Because even the respiratory coronaviruses have been difficult to recover from clinical specimens, most of our knowledge

TABLE 1. Members of the Coronavirus Genus

Animal Host	Virus Species	Disease Association
Human	Human coronavirus	Common cold, ? pneumonia
Chicken	Infectious bronchitis virus	Infectious bronchitis, nephrosis, uremia
Pig	Transmissible gastroenteritis virus	Gastroenteritis
Pig	Hemagglutinating encephalomyelitis virus	Encephalitis, vomiting, and wasting disease
Turkey	Turkey bluecomb coronavirus	Infectious diarrhea (bluecomb disease)
Cattle	Bovine coronavirus	Diarrhea in newborn calves
Mouse	Mouse hepatitis virus	Hepatitis and encephalitis
Rat	Rat coronavirus	Pneumonia in newborns
Rat	Sialodacryoadenitis virus	Sialodacryoadenitis
Cat	Feline infectious peritonitis virus	Peritonitis
Dog	Canine coronavirus	Enteritis

about their epidemiology derives from serologic surveys. In such surveys only two antigenic strains have been used, those for which antigens of adequate potency are available. There may be other antigenically distinct strains that grow only in organ culture and whose epidemiology is not known. For this reason, it may be that the description outlined below is incomplete.

DESCRIPTION OF THE PATHOGEN

The coronavirus nucleic acid is RNA, and the viral particle contains three protein species: a surface glycoprotein found in the surface projections that is probably responsible for the stimulation of neutralizing antibody; a membrane glycoprotein contained within the trilamellar membrane; and a nucleocapsid protein complexed with the RNA.[9] The RNA is of positive sense, single-stranded, polyadenylated, and infectious, and it has a molecular weight of about 6×10^6.[10] The strategy of replication of coronaviruses is unique in that all messenger RNAs form a nested set with common polyadenylated 3′ ends, with only the unique portion of the 5′ end being translated.[11]

All coronaviruses develop exclusively in the cytoplasm of infected cells. They appear to bud into cytoplasmic vesicles from membranes of the endoplasmic reticulum. These virus-filled vesicles then are either extruded by reverse pinocytosis or released from the cell when the cell is destroyed.[12] The resultant virus particles have a diameter of 60–220 nm and are pleomorphic, with widely spaced, petal-shaped projections 20 nm long. Viral antigens appear on the surface of the cell during replication.[13]

The important human coronavirus strains are shown in Table 2 along with some of their laboratory characteristics. Two antigenic strains, 229E and OC43, are best studied because of their successful adaptation to growth in tissue culture or animals. Most of the strains isolated from the human respiratory tract are antigenically related to one or the other of these strains.[14] The two strains are antigenically distinct[15] but may be distantly related. It appears likely, moreover, that there are complex antigenic interrelationships between the other human coronavirus serotypes. Some volunteers infected with several of the types for which serologically useful antigens are not available develop antibody titer rises to both 229E and OC43.[16]

Coronavirus strain 229E and some closely related strains grow in human diploid cell lines (Figs. 1 and 2). Recovery from clinical specimens is difficult and often requires blind subpassage. The resultant cytopathic effect is nonspecific and resembles the natural degeneration of the cell monolayer, particularly in early passages. All other human respiratory coronaviruses (including some strains antigenically similar to 229E) have been recovered from clinical specimens only in organ cultures from human embryonic trachea or nasal epithelium. Strains OC43 and OC38, antigenically identical to each other, were subsequently adapted first to growth in suckling mouse brain and then to tissue culture. Tissue culture-grown OC43 and 229E serve as antigens for serosurveys of disease and infection in various human populations.[17]

Enteric coronaviruses have also been difficult to cultivate in vitro. All but a few strains have been detected only by electron microscopy of human fecal material.[18–22] Some strains have been antigenically characterized by immune electron microscopy of particles in stool and found to be related to the respiratory coronavirus OC43.[23] Several strains have been propagated in intestinal organ culture.[24,25] Two strains obtained from an outbreak of necrotizing enterocolitis in Texas and passaged in intestinal organ cultures were found to contain four or five antigenically active proteins separable on polyacrylamide gels.[25] These proteins migrated with apparent molecular weights very similar to those of well-studied coronaviruses. Antigenic relatedness to OC43 or other coronaviruses was not, however, demonstrable. The accumulating evidence favors the view that these strains and strains antigenically related to OC43[23] are members of the genus *Coronaviridae*. The less well studied strains, characterized only by their distinctive morphology on electron microscopy and called, for lack of a better name, "coronavirus-like particles" (CVLPs), may also be coronaviruses, but the evidence is less compelling. A degree of uncertainty about all enteric human coronaviruses, however, compels a parallel uncertainty concerning their pathogenicity and the nature and epidemiology of the diseases associated with them.

CLINICAL MANIFESTATIONS

The human respiratory coronaviruses have been proved to cause colds in adults, and most strains were originally recovered from adults during upper respiratory tract illness. Almost all the antigenically distinct respiratory coronavirus strains have been administered to volunteers, and all these produce illness with similar characteristics.[14] A summary of these characteristics is shown in Table 3 where a comparison is made with colds produced by rhinoviruses in similarly inoculated volunteers. The incubation period of coronavirus colds was longer and their duration somewhat shorter, but the symptoms were very similar. Low-grade fever was present in about one volunteer in five, and malaise after coronavirus inoculation was frequent. Asymptomatic infection was sometimes seen and, indeed, has been a feature of serologic surveys of natural infection of children and adults.

It is likely that the colds produced in volunteers are similar to those produced in adults by natural infection. These details have been studied by several investigators. In one such survey the colds associated with antibody titer rise to 229E were distinguished by prominent nasal symptoms; in those accompanying a rise in OC43 antibody titer there was sore throat and cough in addition to rhinorrhea.[27]

More serious, lower respiratory tract illness is probably on occasion caused by coronavirus infection. Several strains resembling 229E have been recovered from infants with pneumonia,[28] and antibody titer rises also have been found with a frequency of 3–8 percent in this group.[28,29] However, an extensive survey of hospitalized children in England failed to uncover a single instance of coronavirus infection.[30] It seems likely, therefore, that, if indeed coronaviruses can produce more serious infections in infants, this is not a common event.

Coronavirus infection in marine recruits has been associated with pneumonia or pleural reaction in about one-third, and it is possible that lower respiratory tract disease can, under special circumstances, occur in adults.[31] An association of coronavirus infection with bouts of wheezing in asthmatic children has also been described.[32] Finally, three separate longitudinal serologic studies of adults with chronic pulmonary disease have each shown a significant association of coronavirus infection with exacerbations of respiratory symptoms.[33–35]

TABLE 2. Human Respiratory Coronaviruses

Strain and Original Description	*Tissues Useful for Growth of Virus from Patient Specimens*	*Tissues in Which Strains Have Been Adapted*	*Antigens Available for Clinically Useful Serologic Tests*	*Number of Serologically Identical Strains Known*
229E (Hamre and Procknow[3])	WI-38 Secondary human emb. kidney MA-177 HETOC[a]	HETOC[a]	CF, ELISA	Many
OC43 (McIntosh et al.[4])	HETOC[a]	Suckling mouse brain Rhesus monkey kidney Vero WI-38	CF, HI, ELISA	Many
B814 (Tyrrell and Bynoe[1])	HETOC[a] L-132	None	None	None
OC16 (McIntosh et al.[4])	HETOC[a]	None	None	None
OC37 (McIntosh et al.[4])	HETOC[a]	None	None	None

Abbreviations: CF: complement fixing; ELISA: enzyme-linked immunosorbent assay; HI: hemagglutination inhibiting.
[a] Human embryonic tracheal organ culture.

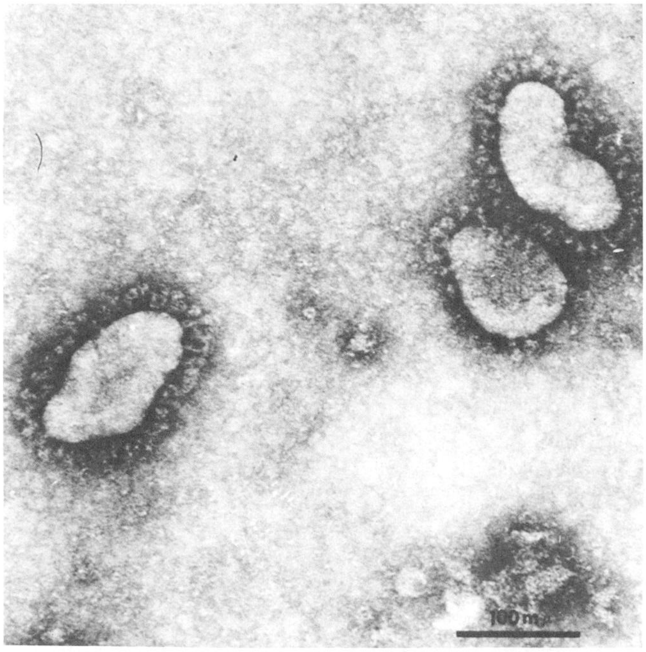

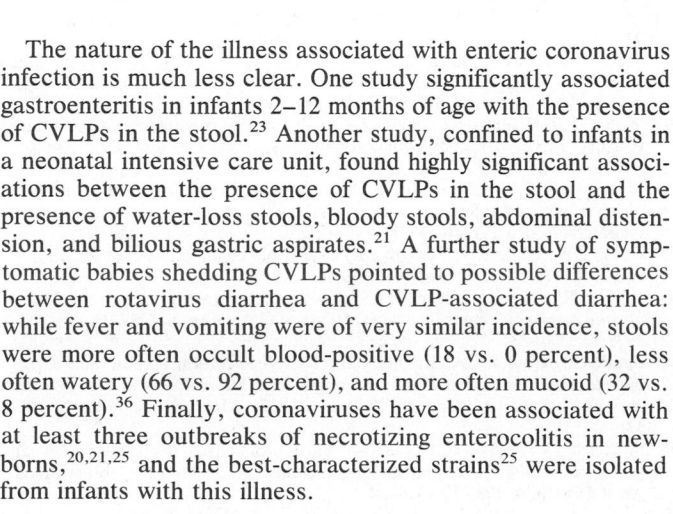

FIG. 1. Coronavirus, strain 229E, harvested from infected WI-38 cells. (Phosphotungstic acid stain)

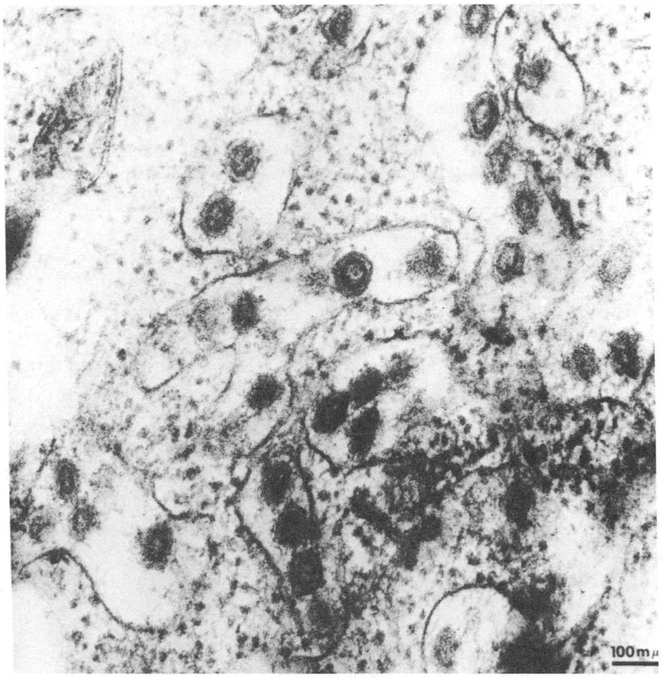

FIG. 2. Coronavirus strain 229E in WI-38 cells.

The nature of the illness associated with enteric coronavirus infection is much less clear. One study significantly associated gastroenteritis in infants 2–12 months of age with the presence of CVLPs in the stool.[23] Another study, confined to infants in a neonatal intensive care unit, found highly significant associations between the presence of CVLPs in the stool and the presence of water-loss stools, bloody stools, abdominal distension, and bilious gastric aspirates.[21] A further study of symptomatic babies shedding CVLPs pointed to possible differences between rotavirus diarrhea and CVLP-associated diarrhea: while fever and vomiting were of very similar incidence, stools were more often occult blood-positive (18 vs. 0 percent), less often watery (66 vs. 92 percent), and more often mucoid (32 vs. 8 percent).[36] Finally, coronaviruses have been associated with at least three outbreaks of necrotizing enterocolitis in newborns,[20,21,25] and the best-characterized strains[25] were isolated from infants with this illness.

EPIDEMIOLOGY

As with all other known respiratory viruses, coronavirus infections have been found wherever they have been sought. This includes North America, South America, Europe, and Asia.

In temperate climates, respiratory coronavirus infections occur more often in the winter and spring than in the summer and fall. The contribution of coronavirus infections to the total number of upper respiratory illnesses may be as high as 35 percent during times of peak virus activity. Overall, the proportion of adult colds produced by coronaviruses may be reasonably estimated at 15 percent.

In the United States, the two strains that have been extensively studied, OC43 and 229E, have demonstrated periodicity, with large epidemics occurring at 2- to 3-year intervals.[37] Strain 229E tends to be epidemic throughout the United States, whereas strain OC43 tends to appear in localized outbreaks. The proportion of those infected (as judged by a rise in antibody titer) who become ill is about one-half. Reinfection appears to

TABLE 3. Clinical Features of Colds Produced by Inoculating Four Viruses

Feature	Coronaviruses 229E	Coronaviruses B814	Rhinoviruses Type 2 (HGP or PK)	Rhinoviruses DC
No. of volunteers inoculated	26	75	213	251
No. getting colds	13(50%)	34(45%)	78(37%)	77(31%)
Incubation period (days)				
Mean	3.3	3.2	2.1	2.1
Range	2–4	2–5	1–5	1–4
Duration (days)				
Mean	7	6	9	10
Range	3–18	2–17	3–19	2–26
Maximum no. of handkerchiefs used daily				
Mean	23	21	14	18
Range	8–105	8–120	3–38	33–60
Malaise (%)	46	47	28	25
Headache (%)	85	53	56	56
Chill (%)	31	18	28	15
Pyrexia (%)	23	21	14	18
Mucopurulent nasal discharge (%)	0	62	83	80
Sore throat (%)	54	79	87	73
Cough (%)	31	44	68	56
No. of volunteers with colds of indicated severity				
Mild	10(77%)	24(71%)	63(80%)	36(47%)
Moderate	2(15%)	7(20%)	12(15%)	28(36%)
Severe	1(8%)	3(9%)	4(5%)	13(17%)

(From Bradburne et al.,[26] with permission.)

be common. Infection occurs at all ages but is most common in children.

Enteric coronaviruses (or CVLPs) have been most frequently associated with gastrointestinal disease in neonates and infants under 12 months of age. Particles have been found in the stools of adults with the acquired immunodeficiency syndrome (AIDS)[38] and have also been found in populations throughout the world. Asymptomatic shedding is common, particularly in tropical climates.[39] They are apparently shed for prolonged periods[19,21,36] and have little or no seasonality.[40]

PROSPECTS FOR PREVENTION AND AREAS IN WHICH FUTURE STUDIES ARE NEEDED

It seems unlikely that coronaviruses will become the target of a large preventive campaign as long as the traditional modes of immunoprophylaxis are used. Multiple antigenic strains exist, and reinfection is common. The prospects of control by immunization therefore appear dim. It is likely, however, that, because of their unique biology and their prominence in veterinary medicine, methods of control through chemotherapy will be developed. If these are sufficiently nontoxic, it may be possible to apply them to respiratory disease in humans.

The two areas in greatest need of research on human coronaviruses are in the development of superior techniques for the recovery of respiratory coronaviruses from clinical specimens and the better characterization of enteric coronaviruses.

REFERENCES

1. Tyrrell DAJ, Bynoe ML. Cultivation of a novel type of common-cold virus in organ cultures. Br Med J. 1965;1:1467–70.
2. Almeida JD, Tyrrell DAJ. The morphology of three previously uncharacterized human respiratory viruses that grow in organ culture. J Gen Virol. 1967;1:175–8.
3. Hamre D, Procknow JJ. A new virus isolated from the human respiratory tract. Proc Soc Exp Biol. 1966;121:190–3.
4. McIntosh K, Dees JH, Becker WB, et al. Recovery in tracheal organ cultures of novel viruses from patients with respiratory disease. Proc Nat Acad Sci USA. 1967;57:933–40.
5. McIntosh K, Becker WB, Chanock RM. Growth in suckling mouse brain of "IBV-like" viruses from patients with upper respiratory tract disease. Proc Nat Acad Sci USA. 1967;58:2268–73.
6. Witte KH, Tajima M, Easterday BD. Morphologic characteristic and nucleic acid type of transmissible gastroenteritis virus of pigs. Arch Ges Virusforsch. 1968;23:53.
7. Tyrrell DAJ, Almeida JD, Berry DM, et al. Coronaviruses. Nature. 1968;220:650.
8. McIntosh K. Coronaviruses: A comparative review. Curr Top Microbiol Immunol. 1974;63:85–129.
9. Schmidt OW, Kenny GE. Polypeptides and functions of antigens from human coronaviruses 229E and OC43. Infect Immun. 1982;35:515–22.
10. Tannock GA, Hierholzer JC. The RNA of human coronavirus OC43. Virology. 1983;78:500.
11. Sidell S, Wege H, Ter Meulen V. The biology of coronaviruses. J Gen Virol. 1983;64:761–6.
12. Becker WB, McIntosh K, Dees JH, et al. Morphogenesis of avian infectious bronchitis virus and a related human virus (strain 229E). J Virol. 1967;1:1019–27.
13. Gerna G, Battaglia M, Cereda PM, et al. Reactivity of human coronavirus OC43 and neonatal calf diarrhea coronavirus membrane-associated antigens. J Gen Virol. 1982;60:385–90.
14. Macnaughton MR, Madge MH, Reed SE. Two antigenic groups of human coronaviruses detected by using enzyme-linked immunosorbent assay. Infect Immun. 1981;33:734–7.
15. Schmidt OW. Antigenic characterization of human coronaviruses 229E and OC43 by enzyme-linked immunosorbent assay. J Clin Microbiol. 1984;20:175–80.
16. Bradburne AF, Somerset BA. Coronavirus antibody titres in sera healthy adults and experimentally infected volunteers. J Hyg (Camb). 1972;70:235–44.
17. Kraaifeveld CA, Reed SE, Macnaughton MR: Enzyme-linked immunosorbent assay for detection of antibody in volunteers experimentally infected with human coronavirus strain 229E. J Clin Microbiol. 1980;12:493–7.
18. Mathan M, Mathan VI, Swaminathan SP, et al. Pleomorphic virus-like particles in human faeces. Lancet. 1975;1:1068–9.
19. Baker SJ, Mathan M, Mathan VI, et al. Chronic enterocyte infection with coronavirus: One possible cause of the syndrome of tropical sprue? Dig Dis Sci. 1983;27:1039–43.
20. Chany C, Moscovici O, Lebon P, et al. Association of coronavirus infection with neonatal necrotizing enterocolitis. Pediatrics. 1982;69:209–14.
21. Vaucher YE, Ray CG, Minnich LL, et al. Pleomorphic, enveloped, virus-like particles associated with gastrointestinal illness in neonates. J Infect Dis. 1982;145:27–36.
22. Maass G, Baumeister HG, Freitag N. Viren als Ursache der akuten Gastroenteritis bei Sauglingen und Kleinkindern. Munch Med Wochenschr. 1977;119:1029.
23. Gerna G, Passarani N, Battaglia M, et al. Human enteric coronaviruses: Antigenic relatedness to human coronavirus OC43 and possible etiologic role in viral gastroenteritis. J Infect Dis. 1985;151:796–803.
24. Caul EO, Egglestone SI. Further studies on human enteric coronaviruses. Arch Virol. 1977;54:107–17.
25. Resta S, Luby JP, Rosenfeld CR, et al. Isolation and propagation of a human enteric coronavirus. Science. 1985;229:978–81.
26. Bradburne AF, Bynoe ML, Tyrrell DAJ. Effects of a "new" human respiratory virus in volunteers. Br Med J. 1967;3:767–9.
27. Hendley JO, Fishburne HB, Gwaltney JM Jr. Coronavirus infections in working adults: Eight-year study with 229E and OC43. Am Rev Respir Dis. 1972;105:805–11.
28. McIntosh K, Chao RK, Krause HE, et al. Coronavirus infections in acute lower respiratory tract disease in infants. J Infect Dis. 1974;130:502–7.
29. McIntosh K, Kapikian AZ, Turner HC, et al. Seroepidemiologic studies of coronavirus infection in adults and children. Am J Epidemiol. 1970;91:585–92.
30. McIntosh K, McQuillin J, Reed SE, et al. Diagnosis of human coronavirus infection by immune fluorescence: Method and application to respiratory disease in hospitalized children. J Med Virol. 1978;2:341–6.
31. Wenzel RP, Hendley JO, Davies JA, et al. Coronavirus infections in military recruits: Three-year study with coronavirus strains OC43 and 229E. Am Rev Respir Dis. 1976;109:621–4.
32. McIntosh K, Ellis EF, Hoffman LS, et al. The association of viral and bacterial respiratory infections with exacerbations of wheezing in young asthmatic children. J Pediatr. 1973;82:578–93.
33. Gump DW, Phillips A, Forsyth BR, et al. Role of infection in chronic bronchitis. Am Rev Respir Dis. 1976;113:465–74.
34. Buscho RO, Saxtan D, Shultz PS, et al. Infections with viruses and *Mycoplasma pneumoniae* during exacerbations of chronic bronchitis. J Infect Dis. 1978;137:377–83.
35. Smith CB, Golden CA, Kanner RE, et al. Association of viral and *Mycoplasma pneumoniae* infections with acute respiratory illness in patients with chronic obstructive pulmonary diseases. Am Rev Respir Dis. 1980;121:225–32.
36. Mortensen ML, Ray CG, Payne CM, et al. Coronaviruslike particles in human gastrointestinal disease. Epidemiologic, clinical, and laboratory observations. Am J Dis Child. 1985;139:928–34.

37. Monto AS. Medical reviews, coronaviruses. Yale J Biol Med. 1974;47:234–51.
38. Kern P, Muller G, Schmitz H, et al. Detection of coronavirus-like particles in homosexual men with acquired immunodeficiency and related lymphadenopathy syndrome. Klin Wocheschr 1985;63:68–72.
39. Marshall JA, Birch CJ, Williamson HG, et al. Coronavirus-like particles and other agents in the faeces of children in Efate, Vanuatu. J Trop Med Hyg. 1982;85:213–5.
40. Payne CM, Ray CG, Borduin V, et al. An eight-year study of the viral agents of acute gastroenteritis in humans: Ultrastructural observations and seasonal distribution with a major emphasis on coronavirus-like particles. Diagn Microbiol Infect Dis. 1986;5:39–54.

Paramyxoviridae

134. PARAINFLUENZA VIRUSES

J. OWEN HENDLEY

INTRODUCTION

The paramyxoviruses are a group of enveloped viruses that vary widely in size. In addition to the human paramyxoviruses that are discussed, there are a number of paramyxoviruses that infect animals.[1] The characteristics of the paramyxoviruses are as follows:

Nucleocapsids develop in the cytoplasm of infected cells.
A virion is a spherical enveloped particle with a diameter of 150–300 nm (range, 100–800 nm) that contains a nucleocapsid.
Hemagglutinin is present in envelope of the virion; some members of the group also have neuraminidase.
Members of group are antigenically stable; genetic recombination does not occur.

Paramyxoviruses that infect humans include parainfluenza viruses 1, 2, 3, and 4A and 4B, mumps virus, measles virus, and respiratory syncytial virus. Newcastle disease virus, which is a pathogen of the respiratory tract of chickens, may accidentally infect humans. The parainfluenza and mumps viruses are grouped together with the Newcastle disease virus under paramyxovirus because of very similar properties. Measles virus has a hemagglutinin but no neuraminidase and is grouped under morbillivirus. Nucleocapsids of measles virus are produced in the nucleus of the infected cell in addition to the cytoplasm. Respiratory syncytial virus has neither hemagglutinin nor neuraminidase and is placed under pneumovirus.

The infectious virion of a paramyxovirus has two components, the nucleocapsid and the envelope (schematically shown in Fig. 1). The nucleocapsid is a tubelike structure that measures 1 μm in length and 18 nm in diameter. It is composed of a linear molecule of RNA intimately associated with repeating protein subunits of the capsid that protect it from destruction by nucleases.[2] The nucleocapsid is encased in the envelope of the virion. Most envelopes contain one nucleocapsid; inclusion of more than one nucleocapsid increases the size of the virion. The envelope contains a lipid bilayer derived from the cytoplasmic membrane of the host cell in which the virus was synthesized. Two different glycoproteins (designated HN and F) of viral origin that are anchored in the lipid bilayer form spikelike projections (peplomers) from the surface of the envelope.[3] The HN protein of the paramyxovirus has both hemagglutinating and, in some members of the group, neuraminidase activity. In contrast, these two activities are present in two different glycoproteins in myxoviruses.[4] The F (fusion) glycoprotein is responsible for viral penetration into host cells by fusion of viral and cell membranes and for hemolysis and cell fusion. The lipid in the envelope makes it sensitive to disruption by organic solvents such as ether and chloroform. Disruption of the envelope renders the virion noninfectious.

Replication of the nucleocapsids of paramyxoviruses occurs in the cytoplasm of infected cells (Fig. 2) where the viral RNA associates with the protein of the capsid. A virus-coded protein (M protein) is associated with the inner surface of the cell membrane where it interacts with the spike glycoproteins that are inserted in the lipid bilayer and also serves as the recognition site for the nucleocapsid. The nucleocapsid is then aligned next to the segment of the cell membrane that contains the HN and F glycoproteins. The protein of this segment of cell membrane is replaced by virus-specific protein including hemagglutinin. The plasma membrane evaginates and produces a bud. The presence of buds containing hemagglutinin on the host cell surface is responsible for the hemadsorption of red blood cells by infected cells. The new virion is formed as the bud containing the nucleocapsid is pinched off the cell surface. Eosinophilic inclusion bodies in the cytoplasm (and in the nucleus with measles virus) of infected cells contain excess nucleocapsids that have not been incorporated into a virion.

The antigens of the paramyxovirus group are of importance in the serodiagnosis of infection in humans. There is no antigen common to the whole group. Each of the parainfluenza viruses and the mumps virus possess a hemagglutinin and a neuraminidase. All show some cross-reactions in complement fixation (CF) or neutralization tests with at least one other member of the group,[5] which suggests that there are some shared antigens. As a consequence, human infection with one parainfluenza virus is often followed by a heterotypic antibody response. Similarly, clinical mumps may be followed by an antibody titer rise to one of the parainfluenza viruses. Measles shows serologic cross-reactivity with animal paramyxoviruses (distemper in dogs and rinderpest of cattle),[6] while respiratory syncytial virus is serologically distinct from the other paramyxoviruses.

PARAINFLUENZA VIRUS

The parainfluenza viruses, which are members of the Paramyxoviridae family and the *Paramyxovirus* genus, are important causes of respiratory disease in infants and young children. They are the most common identifiable agents in the croup syndrome and are second only to respiratory syncytial virus as a cause of lower respiratory tract disease requiring hospitalization in infants.[7] The spectrum of disease due to the parainfluenza viruses ranges from a mild afebrile cold to croup, bronchiolitis, and pneumonia.

Description of the Pathogen

Biologic Characteristics. The parainfluenza viruses contain RNA in a nucleocapsid encased within an envelope derived from the host cell membrane (Table 1). Production of excess nucleocapsids may lead to the formation of cytoplasmic inclusions in infected cells. Parainfluenza virus will hemagglutinate the red blood cells of some animals due to the presence of hemagglutinin on the surface. In addition, infected mammalian cells in culture will hemabsorb red cells due to viral hemagglutinin on the surface of the cell.

Serotypes

The parainfluenza viruses can be separated into four antigenic types on the basis of CF and hemagglutinating antigens (Table

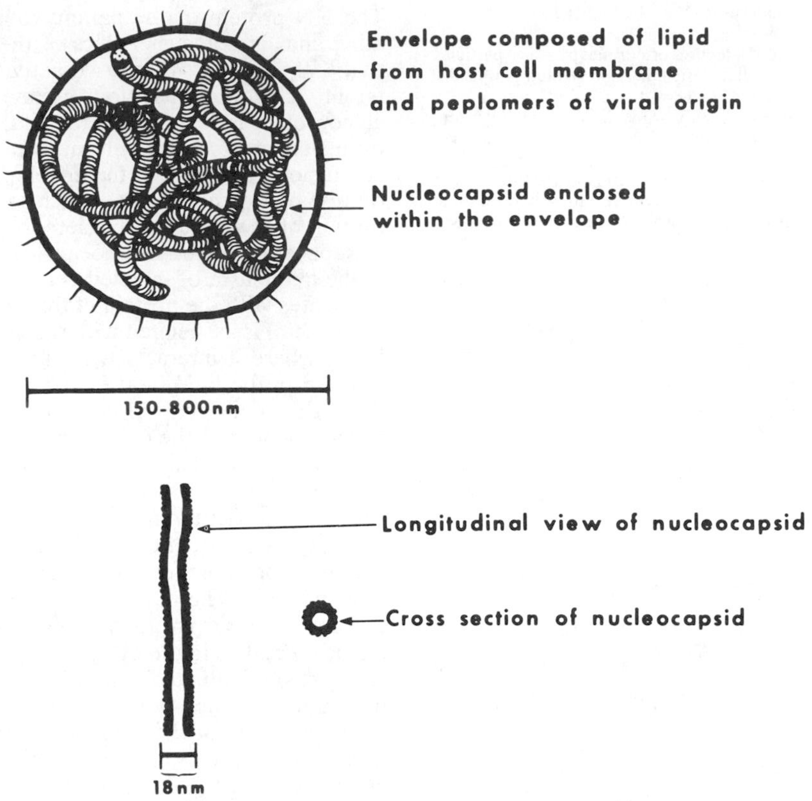

FIG. 1. Schema of paramyxovirus virion components.

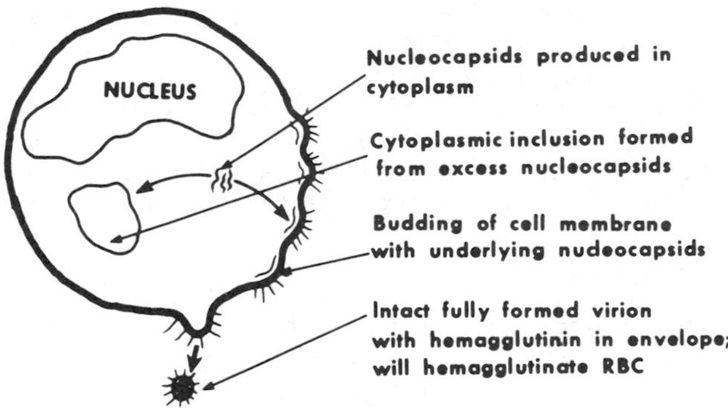

FIG. 2. Schematic view of paramyxovirus virion production in an infected cell.

TABLE 1. Biologic Characteristics of Parainfluenza Viruses

Size: 150–300 nm
The nucleocapsid contains RNA produced within the cytoplasm of an infected cell
The nucleocapsid is encased within an envelope derived from the cell membrane
The envelope has peplomers (projections) of hemagglutinin
Tissue culture cells infected with types 1–4 will hemadsorb
Hemolysin is present in types 1–3
Neuraminadase is present in types 1–3
They are sensitive to ether and acid (pH $<$ 3.0)
Viruses have been antigenically stable over 30 years of observation

2). In contrast to influenza viruses, the parainfluenza viruses have remained antigenically stable for 30 years of observations. Parainfluenza viruses similar to human types 1, 2, and 3 have been isolated from animals, but cross-infections between humans and animals do not occur. However, an antibody titer rise to an animal strain of parainfluenza virus frequently occurs in humans who are infected with a human virus, especially during reinfection.

TABLE 2. Serotypes of Parainfluenza Viruses

Human Type	*Original Designation*	*Animal Strain*
1	Hemadsorption type 2	Sendai virus from mice is antigenically similar
2	Croup associated	SV-5 and SV-41 from monkeys are antigenically similar
3	Hemadsorption type 1	SF-4 from cattle, which is economically important, is antigenically similar
4 A, B[a]		

[a] All type 4 viruses have common CF antigen. Subtypes A and B are distinguishable by hemagglutination inhibition and neutralizing antibody testing.

Detection of Infection in Humans

The most sensitive means for detecting infection with parainfluenza virus is by isolating the virus from a clinical specimen inoculated into primary or continuous[8] monkey kidney or human embryonic kidney tissue culture. Although some parainfluenza viruses can be adapted to grow in continuous tissue culture lines such as HeLa and HEp-2, these cell cultures are not sensitive for primary isolation from clinical specimens. Similarly, human embryonic lung fibroblasts (WI-38 strain) are not sensitive for primary isolation. Rapid viral diagnosis may be accomplished by detecting viral antigen in exfoliated epithelial cells in nasal secretions[9,10] by using commercially available fluorescent antibody for types 1–3.

For isolation of virus in tissue culture, pharyngeal secretions are collected on a swab and transferred to the laboratory in collecting medium containing protein. Inoculation of specimens before freezing provides the best results, but specimens can be stored at −60°C in collecting medium. Before inoculation, monkey kidney cell cultures previously incubated in the presence of antiserum against SV-5 virus are rinsed free of serum. The cultures are observed for cytopathic effect (CPE), although in primary passage only type 2 virus regularly produces CPE, which consists of syncytia. Parainfluenza viruses may be detected in infected cultures by hemadsorption of guinea pig red blood cells to the cell monolayer or by hemagglutination by virus in the culture fluid.[10] After the addition of the red cells, tubes are read for hemadsorption at 4°C and again after elution at 23°C.[11] Most strains of parainfluenza virus types 1–3 produce detectable hemadsorption by 10 days of incubation; type 4 virus may require 20 days or more for detection. Specimens containing parainfluenza virus obtained from adults who are undergoing reinfection usually require 15–20 days of incubation before hemadsorption in present. This delay is presumably related to a low titer of virus in respiratory secretions in the presence of antibody.[12,13] Hemadsorbing agents in tissue culture are identified as a parainfluenza virus with either hemadsorption inhibition, hemagglutination inhibition (HI) or CF using commercially available antisera.[14] Parainfluenza types 1–3 (but not type 4) may produce hemagglutination in the medium overlying the infected tissue culture cells.

Serologic evidence of infection with one of the parainfluenza viruses may be provided by the demonstration of a fourfold rise in antibody titer to the virus in a convalescent serum collected 3–4 weeks after infection. Titer rises may be demonstrated with a variety of techniques including CF, HI, and neutralization.[14] Detection of infection by testing for a rise in titer of HI antibody is as sensitive as testing for neutralizing antibody.

A major problem with the serologic diagnosis of parainfluenza virus infections is that infection with one serotype is frequently accompanied by heterotypic antibody responses, especially during reinfections.[15] As a consequence, the serotype causing infection cannot always be determined by serologic tests. On the other hand, an antibody titer rise to one or more of the parainfluenza viruses is a sensitive indicator of infection, especially in adults who may excrete only a small amount of virus for a short time.[13] A combination of viral isolation in tissue culture and serologic testing provides the most accurate estimate of the incidence of parainfluenza virus infections.

Epidemiology

The parainfluenza viruses are distributed worldwide. Types 1–3 have been isolated everywhere they have been sought with appropriate tissue culture techniques.[12] Type 4 virus has been isolated in the United States[16] and England[17]; serologic surveys suggest that it is also distributed worldwide.[18]

The epidemic behavior and age and sex distribution of severe illnesses caused by parainfluenza virus types 1 and 2 are different from those caused by type 3. The behavior of type 4 is not well characterized since disease due to this virus is so mild that it does not require medical attention. Parainfluenza types 1 and 2 characteristically cause epidemics of disease in the fall[19–21] that are associated with an epidemic of croup,[22] while type 3 virus produces disease year-round in some longitudinal surveys. In other studies types 1 and 2 may be endemic,[7,23] and parainfluenza type 3 may be episodic with a peak of infections in the spring after the yearly influenza epidemic.[24]

The behavior of the parainfluenza viruses is typical of the interference phenomenon in viral respiratory infections.[25,26] Glezen and Denny[25] pointed out that when the incidence of disease due to a major virus peaked in a community other viruses were absent. The result of this interference phenomenon was that total respiratory illness rates were relatively constant from year to year as successive waves of different viruses circulated in the community. Parainfluenza 3 may be an exception since it circulates most of the time regardless of the presence of other agents.

The age distribution of severe lower respiratory tract disease due to parainfluenza viruses 1 and 2 differs from that of parainfluenza virus 3. Passively transferred maternal antibody apparently influences the manifestations of infection with types 1 and 2 in the infant; severe disease due to those types is uncommon under the age of 4 months.[27] After 4–6 months of age, the incidence of lower respiratory tract disease, especially croup, due to these viruses increases and remains up until 4–6 years of age. After the age of 6, infections (usually reinfections) continue but with diminishing frequency and severity. In contrast, parainfluenza virus 3 may cause severe disease in young infants like respiratory syncytial virus does,[23] but transplacental maternal antibody may provide some protection during the first 4 months of life.[24] The severity of illness due to type 3 virus declines after the age of 3, although reinfections continue.

Boys are more likely than are girls to have severe disease due to parainfluenza types 1 and 2. However, this sex difference relates only to illnesses severe enough to require medical attention or hospitalization.[23] Rates of infection accompanied by minor illness were the same in children of both sexes followed longitudinally,[28] and acquisition of antibody was the same in girls and boys. Illness rates for severe disease due to parainfluenza 3 are similar in girls and boys.

Pathogenesis

Parainfluenza virus is transmitted from person to person, presumably by the transfer of respiratory tract secretions by direct contact or large droplets. Although type 3 virus in a small-particle aerosol (droplet nuclei) that was produced experimentally remained viable for 1 hour,[29] virus was recovered from only 1 of 30 air samples collected within 60 cm of patients with natural parainfluenza virus illnesses who were known to be shedding virus.[30] The high rate of infection in infants and young children and the frequency of reinfection suggest that these viruses spread readily and that a small inoculum is required to infect.[27] Spread of types 1–3 has been shown in a nursery[15] and in a day care center.[28] Type 3 has been shown to spread among hospitalized children.[31]

The sequence of events after implantation of a parainfluenza virus on the respiratory tract mucosa is not known. Local multiplication of virus in respiratory mucosa is probably sufficient for the production of disease, although viremia has been noted.[32] Parainfluenza virus has been demonstrated with fluorescent antibody in ciliated, columnar epithelial cells in respiratory secretions from ill children.[9] The histopathologic changes of parainfluenza disease in the lung in the small number of patients who have died are indistinguishable from those of other viral lower respiratory tract diseases.[33] Although the mechanism for the subglottic involvement with parainfluenza 1–3 in the croup syndrome is not known, the possibility that virus-specific IgE may play a role [34] and that patients with croup have a defect in T-cell suppressor function[35] has been suggested recently.

How parainfluenza virus infections are cleared is not known. Prolonged excretion of parainfluenza 3 has occurred in normal children[36] and adults[37,38]; persistent infection leading to death has been reported in children with deficient cell-mediated immunity.[39] Usually, however, excretion of virus is brief (Table 3). Interferon, which has been detected in nasal secretions during the acute illness,[41] might aid resolution. Alternatively, infection might be cleared by secretory IgA antibody against the virus that appears in nasal secretions within 1 week of the onset of illness.[42]

Clinical Manifestations

The spectrum of clinical manifestations due to parainfluenza virus infection in children varies from no illness to life-threat-

TABLE 3. Characteristics of Parainfluenza Virus Infections in Children

			Clinical Manifestations		
Virus Type	*Usual Age at Onset*	*Length of Time Virus Shed*	*Severe*	*Mild*	*Proportion with Fever*
Primary infections					
Types 1, 2	8–30 mon	3–12 days (range for type 1)	Croup	Cold, bronchitis	$\frac{1}{2}$–$\frac{2}{3}$
Type 3	1–24 mon	8 days (median); 3–16 days (range)	Croup, pneumonia, bronchiolitis	Cold	$\frac{3}{4}$
Types 4 A, B	<6 yr	NI	None	Cold	NI
Reinfections					
Types 1–3	Within a few months to several years after primary; may occur in adults	1–3 days (type 3)	Rare	Cold, bronchitis	$\frac{1}{3}$

Abbreviation: NI: no information.
(Data from Canchola et al.,[16] Gardner,[17] Downham et al.,[20] Glezen et al.,[27] and Chanock et al.[40])

ening croup or bronchiolitis. Factors that influcncc the clinical picture include the serotype of the virus causing the infection, the sex of the patient, and whether it is the primary or a reinfection with a particular serotype (Table 3). The most common syndrome associated with the parainfluenza viruses is a "cold," often accompanied by bronchitis. Colds and bronchitis due to parainfluenza viruses are seen in both children and adults. The croup syndrome, characterized by a barking cough and hoarseness with or without inspiratory stridor, is the predominant *severe* clinical manifestation of primary infection with one of the parainfluenza viruses (Table 4). One-quarter to one-half of the cases of croup syndrome in young children are associated with infection with one of the parainfluenza viruses. These viruses may also cause pneumonia.

Although the incubation period of parainfluenza virus infections is not definitely established, it probably ranges from 3 to 6 days.[20,44] The incubation period for reinfections in adults volunteers inoculated with parainfluenza virus varied from 3 to 8 days.[45]

Primary Infections. The first infection with parainfluenza types 1–3 commonly causes coryza, pharyngitis, and/or bronchitis. Most patients will have a temperature over 100°F for 2–3 days and rhinorrhea, pharyngeal erythema without cervical adenopathy, cough, and rhonchi on chest auscultation. The characteristic picture with parainfluenza virus type 4 infection is a mild upper respiratory tract illness.[12] Most children with a primary parainfluenza virus infection are not seen by a physician. In a longitudinal study,[27] two-thirds of 62 children followed for the first 2 years of life were infected by parainfluenza 3, as indicated by the presence of neutralizing antibody at the age of 2. One-half of the infected children had no discernible illness. Approximately 15 percent of the ill children had lower tract involvement, and only 2 percent were seen by a physician. Chanock and coworkers[15] noted that one-third of the patients in a welfare nursery with primary infection with type 3 and one-quarter of those with type 1 or 2 virus had associated lower tract involvement (bronchitis or pneumonitis). However, only 2 or 76 children with primary type 1 and 2 infections had croup, and both patients had mild disease not requiring hospitalization. Although primary infections with parainfluenza viruses are common, disease severe enough to necessitate medical attention is uncommon.

TABLE 4. Percentage of Lower Respiratory Illness in Children Due to Parainfluenza Viruses[a]

	Illness		
Virus Type	*Croup*	*Pneumonia*	*Bronchiolitis*
1	18–21	3	1–3
2	4–8	1	1
3	9–13	3–13	5–14
Total	31–42	7–17	7–18

[a] The diagnosis of parainfluenza infection is based on serologic test results of hospitalized patients[15] and on the results of viral isolation from outpatients.[43]
(Data from Chanock et al.[15] and Glenzen et al.[43])

Most children are infected at least once in the first 5 years of life with each of the four types of parainfluenza virus. By 6 years of age, 90–100 percent of children have antibody to type 3,[27] 75 percent have antibody to type 1, and 60 percent to type 2.[15] Surprisingly, 50 percent of 6-year-old children have antibody to type 4 virus, although infections are infrequently recognized.[17]

Consideration of primary infections from the vantage point of illnesses in patients seeking medical care provides a different picture of these agents. Infection with one of the parainfluenza viruses has been found in 31–42 percent of the patients with croup, in 7–17 percent of the patients with pneumonia, and in 7–18 percent of those with bronchiolitis (Table 4). The major severe manifestation of infection with types 1 and 2 is croup, while type 3 causes all three syndromes.[26] Croup caused by parainfluenza virus is not distinguishable from that caused by other viruses. However, an outbreak of croup in the fall involving children aged 6–30 months could be assumed to be due to parainfluenza type 1 or 2. Bronchiolitis occurring in an infant when respiratory syncytial virus was not active in the community might be due to parainfluenza type 3. A firm etiologic diagnosis, however, would have to be based on isolation of virus or on a rise in antibody titer to one of the parainfluenza viruses.

Reinfections. Reinfections with parainfluenza viruses are common, may be multiple, and may occur within 3 months of the primary infection[40] or years later. Reinfections are rarely associated with severe disease; most illnesses are indistinguishable from the common cold. However, infection with one parainfluenza type does not protect against lower respiratory tract involvement during subsequent infection with a different type.[46] Chanock and coworkers noted that in infants the presence of antibody to parainfluenza 3, denoting previous infection, protected against fever and severe lower tract involvement.[40] During reinfection, virus was shed only briefly. Virtually all parainfluenza virus illness in adults is due to reinfection.[13]

Treatment

There is no specific antiviral therapy for parainfluenza virus infections at present. The decision to hospitalize a patient with lower respiratory tract involvement for vigorous supportive measures should be based on the clinical evaluation of the patient. Management of patients with croup due to parainfluenza viruses includes the provision of humidified air to prevent the drying of secretions and to soothe the inflammed glottis. The need for insertion of an endotracheal tube or for a tracheostomy is based on the adequacy of the airway and the patient's course. Although corticosteroids have been used by some authors in the management of croup, it is not clear that they have a beneficial effect.[47] Nebulized racemic epinephrine is advocated by some authors for the treatment of croup.

Prevention

The parainfluenza viruses contribute to the "common cold"; they are common by virtue of their ability to reinfect. Since reinfection with a parainfluenza virus may occur within months of primary infection with wild virus, it is unlikely that illness due to these agents can be completely prevented. However, two features of parainfluenza infections suggest that some morbidity due to these viruses may be preventable. First, primary infection in a young child may produce severe lower respiratory tract disease with croup or pneumonia, whereas reinfection is associated with a coldlike illness even in young children.[40] A vaccine administered to infants that would convert the illness during the child's first encounter with wild virus to the milder, reinfection-type illness might be beneficial by reducing morbidity in spite of not preventing infection. Second, immunity to reinfection correlates with neutralizing antibody in nasal secretions[45,48] or high levels of serum antibody[49] in studies in adult volunteers. A live attenuated virus vaccine administered intranasally might prevent infection with parainfluenza viruses if it produced persistent levels of nasal secretory antibody. Such a vaccine has not been tested in young infants, which would be the appropriate target population.

A different approach to immunoprophylaxis has been undertaken after the characterization of two glycoproteins that form spikes that project from the surface of the envelope of paramyxoviruses. The HN (hemagglutinin-neuraminidase) glycoprotein is important in the attachment of virus to host cell receptors, while the F (fusion) glycoprotein is involved in the fusion of viral and host cell membranes that leads to the entry of virus into the cell. Antibody to either glycoprotein can prevent exogenous virus from infecting cells, but only antibody to the F glycoprotein can prevent the spread of virus from cell to cell by fusion.[50] The failure of inactivated parainfluenza virus vaccine to prevent disease[48,51] might be due to the stimulation of antibody to HN but not F glycoprotein.[50] The serum antibody response to the HN and F glycoproteins of parainfluenza type 3 after infection in infancy[52] and the development of a subunit vaccine[53] containing these glycoproteins are the initial steps in pursuing this approach to prevention.

REFERENCES

1. Melnick JL. Taxonomy of viruses, 1980. Prog Med Virol. 1980;26:224.
2. Fenner F, McAuslan BR, Mims CA, et al. The Biology of Animal Viruses. 2nd ed. New York: Academic Press; 1974:119.
3. Choppin PW, Scheid A. The functions and inhibition of the membrane glycoproteins of paramyxoviruses and myxoviruses and the role of the measles virus M protein in subacute sclerosing panencephalitis. J. Infect Dis. 1981;143:252.
4. Choppin PW, Scheid A. The role of viral glycoproteins in adsorption, penetration, and pathogenicity of viruses. Rev Infect Dis. 1980;2:40.
5. Cook MK, Andrews BE, Fox HH, et al. Antigenic relationships among the "newer" myxoviruses (parainfluenza). Am J Hyg. 1959;69:250.
6. DeLay PD, Stones SS, Karzon DT, et al. Clinical and immune response of alien hosts to inoculation with measles, rinderpest, and canine distemper viruses. Am J Vet Res. 1965;26:1359.
7. Monto AS. The Tecumseh study of respiratory illness. V. Patterns of infection with the parainfluenza viruses. Am J Epidemiol. 1973;97:338.
8. Frank AL, Couch RB, Griffis CA, et al. Comparison of different tissue cultures for isolation and quantitation of influenza and parainfluenza viruses. J Clin Microbiol. 1979;10:32.
9. Gardner PS, McQuillin J, McGuckin R, et al. Observations on clinical and immunofluorescent diagnosis of parainfluenza virus infections. Br Med J. 1971;2:7.
10. Wong DT, Welliver RC, Riddlesberger KR, et al. Rapid diagnosis of parainfluenza virus infection in children. J Clin Microbiol. 1982;16:164.
11. Herrmann EC Jr, Hable KA. Experiences in laboratory diagnosis of parainfluenza viruses in routine medical practice. Mayo Clin Proc. 1970;45:177.
12. Chanock RM, Parrott RH. Para-influenza viruses. In: Horsfall FL, Tamm I, eds. Viral and Rickettsial Infections of Man. 4th ed. JB Lippincott: Philadelphia; 1965:741–54.
13. Bloom HH, Johnson KM, Jacobson R, et al. Recovery of parainfluenza viruses from adults with upper respiratory illness. Am J Hyg. 1961;74:50.
14. Chanock RM. Parainfluenza viruses. In Lennette EH, Schmidt NJ, eds. Diagnostic Procedures for Viral and Rickettsial Infections. 5th ed. 1979:611–32.
15. Chanock RM, Parrott RH, Johnson KM, et al. Myxoviruses: Parainfluenza. Am Rev Respir Dis. 1963;88:152.
16. Canchola J, Vargosko AJ, Kim HW, et al. Antigenic variation among newly isolated strains of parainfluenza type 4 virus. Am J Hyg. 1964;79:357.
17. Gardner SD. The isolation of parainfluenza 4 subtypes A and B in England and serological studies of their prevalence. J Hyg (Camb). 1969;67:545.
18. Killgore GE, Dowdle WR. Antigenic characterization of parainfluenza 4A and 4B by the hemagglutination-inhibition test and distribution of HI antibody in human sera. Am J Epidemiol. 1970;91:308.
19. Brandt CD, Kim HW, Chanock RM, et al. Parainfluenza virus epidemiology. Pediatr Res. 1974;8:422.
20. Downham MAPS, McQuillin J, Gardner PS. Diagnosis and clinical significance of parainfluenza virus infections in children. Arch Dis Child. 1974;49:8.
21. Clarke SKR. Parainfluenza virus infections. Postgrad Med J. 1973;49:792.
22. Denny FW, Murphy TF, Wallace AC Jr, et al. Croup: An 11-year study in a pediatric practice. Pediatrics. 1983;71:871.
23. Mufson MA, Krause HE, Mocega HE, et al. Viruses, *Mycoplasma pneumoniae* and bacteria associated with lower respiratory tract disease among infants. Am J Epidemiol. 1970;91:192.
24. Glezen WP, Frank AL, Taber LH, et al. Parainfluenza virus type 3: Seasonality and risk of infection and reinfection in young children. J Infect Dis. 1984;150:851.
25. Glezen WP, Denny FW. Epidemiology of acute lower respiratory disease in children. N Engl J Med. 1973;288:498.
26. Denny FW, Clyde WA Jr. Acute lower respiratory tract infection in nonhospitalized children. J Pediatr. 1986;108:635.
27. Glezen WP, Loda FA, Denny FW. The parainfluenza viruses. In Evans AS, ed. Viral Infections of Humans. New York: Plenum; 1982:441–54.
28. Loda FA, Glezen W, Clyde WA Jr. Respiratory disease in group day care. Pediatrics. 1972;49:428.
29. Miller WS, Artenstein MS. Aerosol stability of three acute respiratory disease viruses. Proc Soc Exp Biol Med. 1967;125:222.
30. McLean DM, Bannatyne RM, Giban K. Myxovirus dissemination by air. Cana Med Assoc J. 1967;96:1449.
31. Mufson MA, Mocega HE, Krause HE. Acquisition of parainfluenza 3 virus infection by hospitalized children. I. Frequencies, rates, and temporal data. J Infect Dis. 1973;128:141.
32. Rocchi G, Arangro-Ruiz G, Giannini V, et al. Detection of viremia in acute respiratory disease of man. Acta Virol. 1970;14:405.
33. Zinserling A. Peculiarities of lesion in viral and mycoplasma infections of the respiratory tract. Virchows Arch [A]. 1972;356:259.
34. Welliver RC, Wong DT, Middleton E Jr, et al. Role of parainfluenza viruse-specific IgE in pathogenesis of croup and wheezing subsequent to infection. J Pediatr. 1982;101:889.
35. Welliver RC, Sun M, Rinaldo D. Defective regulation of immune responses in croup due to parainfluenza virus. Pediatr Res. 1985;19:716.
36. Frank AL, Taber LH, Wells CR, et al. Patterns of shedding of myxovirus and paramyxoviruses in children. J Infect Dis. 1981;144:433.
37. Gross PA, Green RH, Curnen MGM. Persistent parainfluenza type 3 virus in man. Am Rev Respir Dis. 1973;108:894.
38. Muchmore HG, Parkinson AJ, Humphries JE, et al. Persistent parainfluenza virus shedding during isolation at the South Pole. Nature. 1981;289:187.
39. Fishaut M, Tubergen D, McIntosh K. Cellular response to respiratory viruses with particular reference to children with disorders of cell-mediated immunity. J Pediatr. 1980;96:179.
40. Chanock RM, Bell JA, Parrott RH. Natural history of parainfluenza infection. In Pollard, ed. Perspectives of Virology II. New York: Harper & Row; 1960:126–39.
41. Hall CB, Douglas RG Jr, Simons RL, et al. Interferon production in children with respiratory syncytial, influenza, and parainfluenza virus infections. J Pediatr. 1978;93:28.
42. Yanagihara R, McIntosh K. Secretory immunological response in infants and children to parainfluenza virus types 1 and 2. Infect Immun. 1980;30:23.
43. Glezen WP, Loda FA, Clyde WA Jr, et al. Epidemiologic patterns of acute lower respiratory disease of children in a pediatric group practice. J Pediatr. 1971;78:397.
44. Rendtorff RC, Walker LC, Roberts AN. A parainfluenza 3 virus outbreak in an orphanage nursery. Am J Hyg. 1963;77:82.
45. Smith CB, Purcell RH, Bellanti JA, et al. Protective effect of antibody to parainfluenza type 1 virus. N Engl J Med. 1966;275:1145.
46. Welliver R, Wong DT, Choi TS, et al. Natural history of parainfluenza virus infection in children. J Pediatr. 1982;101:180.
47. Cherry JD. The treatment of croup: Continued controversy due to failure of recognition of historic, ecologic, etiologic and clinical perspectives. J Pediatr. 1979;94:352.
48. Smith CB, Bellanti JA, Chanock RM. Immunoglobulins in serum and nasal secretion following infection with type 1 parainfluenza virus and injection of inactivated vaccines. J Immunol. 1967;99:133.
49. Tremonti LP, Lin JSL, Jackson GG. Neutralizing activity in nasal secretions and serum in resistance of volunteers to parainfluenza virus type 2. Immunol. 1968;101:572.
50. Merz DC, Scheid A, Choppin PW. Importance of antibodies to the fusion glycoprotein of paramyxoviruses in the prevention of spread of infection. J Exp Med. 1980;151:275.
51. Vella PP, Weibal RE, Woodhour AF. Respiratory virus vaccines. VIII. Field evaluation of trivalent parainfluenza virus vaccine among preschool children in families, 1967–68. Am Rev Respir Dis. 1969;99:526.

52. Kasel JA, Frank AL, Keitel WA, et al. Acquisition of serum antibodies to specific viral glycoproteins of parainfluenza virus 3 in children. J Virol. 1984;52:828.
53. Ray R, Brown VE, Compans RW. Glycoproteins of human parainfluenza virus type 3: Characterization and evaluation as a subunit vaccine. J Infect Dis. 1985;152:1219.

135. MUMPS VIRUS

STEPHEN G. BAUM
NATHAN LITMAN

Mumps is an acute generalized viral infection that occurs primarily in school-age children and adolescents. The most prominent manifestation of this disease is nonsuppurative swelling and tenderness of the salivary glands, with one or both parotid glands involved in most cases. The disease is benign and self-limited, one-third of the persons having subclinical infection. Meningitis and epididymo-orchitis represent the two most important of the less frequent manifestations of this disease. As is characteristic of many viral infections, mumps in the post-pubertal person is usually a more severe illness than in children and more commonly leads to extrasalivary gland involvement.

HISTORY

Hippocrates described mumps and its contagious characteristics in the fifth century BC. In the late 1700s Hamilton emphasized the occurrence of orchitis as a manifestation of mumps. The experimental production of the disease in monkeys by Johnson and Goodpasture in 1934[1] provided the evidence that a filterable virus was present in the saliva of patients with mumps. In 1945, Habel reported the cultivation of mumps virus in the chick embryo.[2] Enders and colleagues described the skin test and the development of complement-fixing (CF) antibodies after mumps in humans.[3] A killed virus vaccine used in the early 1950s on human subjects achieved limited success,[4] and in 1966 Buynak and Hilleman reported the development of an effective live virus vaccine.[5]

The etymology of the term *mumps* is unclear. It may arise from the English noun *mump* meaning a lump or the English verb *mump*, defined as to be sulky—a description of the characteristic facial expression. Alternatively, the term *mumps* has been ascribed to the mumbling speech pattern of the affected individual. In the older literature, mumps may be called epidemic parotitis.

THE AGENT

Mumps virus is a member of the Paramyxoviridae family, which includes the following genera: *Paramyxovirus* (mumps, parainfluenza, and Newcastle disease virus), *Morbillivirus* (measles), and *Pneumovirus* (respiratory syncytial virus). The complete mumps virion has an irregular spherical shape with a diameter ranging from 90 to 300 nm and averaging about 200 nm. The nucleocapsid is enclosed by an envelope that has three layers and is about 10 nm thick.[6] The external surface is regularly studded with glycoproteins possessing hemagglutinin, neuraminidase, and cell-fusion activity. The viral (V) antigen detected late in infection by the CF test is associated with this layer. The middle component of the envelope is a lipid bilayer that is acquired from the host cell as the virus buds off the cytoplasmic membrane. The innermost surface of the envelope is a nonglycosylated membrane protein that maintains the outer structure of the virus. The genome of the virus is contained in a nucleocapsid that is a helical structure composed of a continuous linear molecule of single-stranded RNA surrounded by symmetrically repeating protein subunits. The capsid protein carries RNA polymerase activity. The nucleocapsid represents the soluble (S) antigen detectable early in infection by the CF test. Only one serotype of mumps virus is known.

Mumps virus is ether sensitive by virtue of its lipid envelope. It is stable at 4°C for several days and at −65°C for months to years; however, repeated freezing and thawing may diminish viral activity.

The virus replicates in a variety of cell cultures as well as in embryonated hens' eggs.[7] In routine diagnostic virology, monkey kidney, human embryonic kidney, or HeLa cell cultures are used for primary isolation procedures. Cytopathic effects such as intracytoplasmic eosinophilic inclusions, rounding of cells, or the fusion of cells into giant multinucleate syncytia may occur.[8] The presence of mumps virus is usually confirmed by the hemadsorption inhibition (HAI) test that uses mumps convalescent serum to inhibit the adsorption of chick erythrocytes added to mumps-infected epithelial cells.

EPIDEMIOLOGY

Mumps is endemic throughout the world. In the United States before the licensing of live attenuated mumps vaccine in 1967, epidemics occurred every 2–5 years.[9] Although the disease occurs throughout the year, the peak incidence is between January and May.[10] Epidemics have been reported in military populations and other closed communities such as prisons, boarding schools, ships, and remote islands.[11,12] Meyer demonstrated that mumps is spread through the community by children in schools with secondary spread to family members.[13] There has been a greater than 95 percent decline in the annual U.S. incidence of mumps since the licensure of the mumps vaccine in 1967. However, a relative resurgence of mumps occurred in 1986 and 1987 when approximately three times as many cases were reported annually as compared with the average of the previous 5 years.[14]

Mumps is uncommon in infants less than 1 year of age. Resistance to infection in this age group is on the basis of passive immunity acquired by the placental transfer of maternal mumps antibody. In the prevaccine era, more than 50 percent of the cases occurred in the 5- to 9-year-old age group, and 90 percent of the disease occurred in children less than 14 years of age. In recent years, only 25 percent of the cases occur in the 5- to 9-year-old age group, and more than 50 percent of the disease occurs in the teenage years.[14] Of adults 20 years or older, 80–90 percent are immune to mumps as assessed by the presence of mumps-neutralizing antibody, although approximately 30 percent have no history of mumps.[15] Men and women have the same incidence of this disease with respect to the development of parotitis.[16]

Humans are the only known natural host; however, monkeys and other laboratory animals have been experimentally infected.[1] Although persistent infections in cultured cells are commonly established by mumps virus,[17] a carrier state is not known to exist in humans.

PATHOGENESIS

The virus is naturally transmitted via direct contact, droplet nuclei, or fomites and enters through the nose or mouth. More intimate contact is needed to transmit mumps than for either measles or varicella. The period of peak contagion is just before and at the onset of parotitis.

Experimental mumps infection has been produced in humans and monkeys by direct instillation of the virus into Stensen's duct.[1] However, the incubation period in this situation is shorter than in the naturally occurring disease, and this model fails to explain the fact that meningitis or other manifestations of mumps infection may occur before the onset of parotitis. An alternative hypothesis has therefore been proposed. This hypothesis suggests that during the incubation period the virus proliferates in the upper respiratory tract epithelium and that viremia ensues, with secondary dissemination and localization in glandular and neural tissue.[18,19]

PATHOLOGY

Salivary glands from patients infected with mumps are rarely available for pathologic examination because of the benign course of the great majority of the cases. When parotid glands have been examined, there is a diffuse interstitial edema and serofibrinous exudate consisting primarily of mononuclear leukocytes. Neutrophils and necrotic debris accumulate within the ductal lumen, and the ductal epithelium shows degenerative changes. The glandular cells are relatively spared, but they too may be involved secondary to edema and overflow of the inflammatory reaction from the interstitial tissues. The multinucleate syncytia and intracytoplasmic eosinophilic inclusions that are occasionally seen in mumps-infected cell culture are not present in vivo. When the pancreas or testis is involved, the microscopic picture is quite similar to that seen in the salivary glands, except that interstitial hemorrhage and polymorphonuclear leukocytes are more frequently noted in orchitis. Local areas of infarction may occur because the vascular supply is compromised by increased pressure due to edema developing within an inelastic tunica albuginea. When the process has been particularly severe, atrophy of the germinal epithelium may result and be accompanied by hyalinization and fibrosis.

The description of the brain in mumps encephalitis has most often been that of a postinfectious encephalitis characterized by perivenous demyelinization, perivascular mononuclear cuffing, and a generalized increase in microglial cells with relative sparing of neurons.[20] More recently, however, descriptions of what appears to be a primary mumps encephalitis have been reported that show widespread neuronolysis but without evidence of demyelinization.[21]

CLINICAL MANIFESTATIONS

The incubation period of mumps averages 16–18 days, with a range of 2–4 weeks. Characteristically, the prodromal symptoms are nonspecific and include low-grade fever, anorexia, malaise, and headache. Within a day, the nature of the illness becomes apparent when the patient complains of an earache, and tenderness can be elicited by palpation of the ipsilateral parotid. The involved gland is soon visibly enlarged, with progression to maximum size over the ensuing 2–3 days. The most severe pain accompanies the period of rapid enlargement. At its height, the parotitis results in lifting of the ear lobe upward and outward. Lesser degrees of enlargement can more readily be appreciated by viewing the patient from behind. The enlarged parotid gland obscures the angle of the mandible, whereas cervical adenopathy does not hide this anatomic landmark. Usually one parotid gland enlarges a couple of days after the other; however, mumps results in unilateral parotitis alone in one-quarter of patients with salivary gland involvement. The orifice of Stensen's duct is frequently edematous and erythematous. Trismus may result from the parotitis, and the patient may have difficulty with pronunciation and mastication. Ingestion of citrus fruits or juices typically exacerbates the pain. During the first 3 days of illness, the patient's temperature may range from normal to 40°C. After the parotid swelling has reached its peak, the pain, fever, and tenderness rapidly resolve, and the parotid returns to its normal size within a week. Complications of parotitis are rare but are reported to include sialectasia resulting in recurrent acute and chronic sialadenitis.[22]

Involvement of the other salivary glands may occur in conjunction with parotitis in up to 10 percent of the cases but is rare as the sole manifestation of mumps infection (Table 1).

TABLE 1. Incidence of Common Clinical Manifestations of Mumps Infection

Manifestation	*Incidence (%)*
Glandular	
Parotitis	60–70
Submandibular and/or sublingual sialadenitis	10
Epididymo-orchitis[a]	25 (postpubertal men)
Oophoritis[a]	5 (postpubertal women)
Neural	
CSF pleocytosis	50
Meningitis	1–10
Encephalitis	0.1
Transient high-frequency deafness	4
Other	
ECG abnormalities	5–15
Renal function abnormalities (mild)	>60

[a] Rare before puberty and usually unilateral.

Submandibular gland involvement mimics signs of anterior cervical lymphadenopathy. The sublingual glands are the least frequently inflamed during mumps infection; when involvement occurs, it is usually bilateral and may be associated with swelling of the tongue. Presternal pitting edema develops in 6 percent of patients with mumps, most commonly in those patients with submandibular adenitis.[23] The proposed mechanism for the involvement of the tongue and presternal area is obstruction of the lymphatic drainage of those regions by enlarged salivary glands.

Central nervous system involvement is the most common extrasalivary gland manifestation of mumps. As documentation of the remarkable neurotropism of this virus, Bang and Bang[24] reported the presence of cerebrospinal fluid (CSF) pleocytosis in 51 percent of 255 patients with mumps but without other evidence of meninigitis. Clinical meningitis occurs in 1–10 percent of the persons with mumps parotitis[25]; on the other hand, only 40–50 percent of the patients with mumps meningitis, confirmed by serology or viral isolation, have parotitis.[25–28] Meningeal symptoms, like any of the other manifestations of mumps infection, may occur before, during, after, or in the absence of parotitis. Its onset averages 4 days after the appearance of salivary gland involvement but may occur as early as 1 week before or as late as 2 weeks after parotitis.[24–27] Men are afflicted three times as often as women,[25–28] but the age distribution is the same as for uncomplicated mumps. Ritter noted that mumps meningitis with parotitis is most frequent in the spring whereas meningitis without parotitis is most frequent in summer.[26] The typical clinical features associated with viral meningitis are present, that is, headache, vomiting, fever, and nuchal rigidity. Lumbar puncture yields CSF containing 10–2000 WBC/mm^3, the predominating cells are usually lymphocytes, but 20–25 percent of the patients have a polymorphonuclear leukocyte predominance.[27] Protein levels are normal to mildly elevated, and 90–95 percent of the patients have a CSF protein content of less than 70 mg/100 ml.[27,28] Hypoglycorrhacia (CSF glucose concentration, <40 mg/100 ml) is reported in 6–30 percent of the patients[27–29] and appears to be more common than in other viral meningitides. These CSF abnormalities may persist for 5 weeks or longer.[26,29] The findings of a depressed CSF sugar level with a moderate to marked pleocytosis may cause the physician to consider bacterial meningitis in the differential diagnosis, especially if neutrophils predominate as they may early in the disease. In other cases with mononuclear cells prevailing, tuberculous and fungal etiologies should be considered.

Subsidence of fever by lysis and resolution of symptoms generally occur 3–10 days after the onset of illness. The meningitis is benign, with complete recovery and an absence of sequelae. Before the introduction of the live attenuated mumps vaccine in 1967, mumps accounted for approximately 10 percent of aseptic meningitis in the United States. Currently, 1 percent of aseptic meningitis is attributed to mumps.[30]

Encephalitis is reported to occur in from 1 in 6000[31] to 1 in 400[32] cases of mumps. The former ratio probably represents a more accurate estimate. There appears to be a bimodal distribution of the time of onset: an early group that coincides with the presence of parotitis and a larger late group that develops 7–10 days after the onset of parotitis. As already alluded to in the section on pathology, early-onset encephalitis represents damage to neurons directly due to viral invasion similar to the situation in herpes simplex encephalitis, whereas the late-onset disease is a postinfectious demyelinating process due to the host response to infection as is typical of measles encephalitis. These two processes probably merely represent the ends of a continuum of disease. Some patients die after the primary viral invasion of the brain, and some of those who survive produce antibodies to the virus and/or neural breakdown products and develop an "autoimmune" reaction. The clinical features are generally those of a nonfocal encephalitis; in addition to marked changes in the level of consciousness, neurologic findings may include convulsions, paresis, aphasia, and involuntary movements. Cerebrospinal fluid values are similar to those in uncomplicated meningitis. Fevers are quite high, characteristically with temperatures of 40–41°C. Neurologic symptoms and fever gradually resolve over a period of 1–2 weeks. Sequelae such as psychomotor retardation and convulsive disorders are reported,[26–28] but their frequency cannot be determined from the available data. Death occurs in 1.4 percent of the reported cases.[32]

Through the mid-1960s mumps was the leading etiology of viral encephalitis, being responsible for 20–30 percent of the cases. However, by 1981, it represented only 0.5 percent of nationwide cases of viral encephalitis and was the seventh most common cause.[32] The major factor accounting for this change was an effective mumps immunization program.

The term *meningoencephalitis* is frequently used when describing patients with various degrees of central nervous system involvement.[21,25,26,29,33] This term should be eliminated in reference to mumps since it confuses a common and essentially benign condition (meningitis) with a relatively uncommon and serious illness (encephalitis) that may result in neurologic residua or death. Clearly, many patients with mumps meningitis may have lethargy, as may a large percentage of persons with any viral infection such as influenza. However, the presence of profound changes in the level of consciousness or other findings suggestive of supratentorial involvement indicate the clear diagnosis of encephalitis as distinct from the ambiguous designation of meningoencephalitis. Although nuchal rigidity and CSF pleocytosis may be present in patients with encephalitis, the meningeal component is a trivial aspect of this illness.

Transient high-frequency-range deafness has been reported in 4.4 percent of the cases of mumps in a military population.[34] Permanent unilateral deafness occurs once per 20,000 cases of mumps.[35] The onset of otologic symptoms may be gradual or abrupt; vertigo is frequently present. On subsequent testing, vestibular function has been normal.

Other neurologic syndromes rarely associated with mumps include cerebellar ataxia,[36] facial palsy,[37] trasverse myelitis,[38] ascending polyradiculitis (Guillain Barré syndrome),[39] and a poliomyelitis-like syndrome.[40] There are now several well-documented cases of aqueductal stenosis and hydrocephalus developing after central nervous system infection due to mumps.[41,42] Experimental and clinical reports clearly implicate mumps as the probable etiology.[43,44]

Epididymo-orchitis is the most common extrasalivary gland manifestation in the adult man. It develops in 20–30 percent of postpubertal men undergoing mumps infection and is bilateral in one of six of those with testicular involvement.[45,46] Although it has been reported in infancy, it is rare before puberty. Two-thirds of cases occur during the first week of parotitis, and another one-quarter arise during the second week.[45] However, gonadal involvement may precede parotitis or occur as the only manifestation of mumps. The onset is abrupt, with temperatures in the range of 39–41°C, chills, headache, vomiting, and testicular pain. Genital examination reveals warmth, swelling, and tenderness of the involved testicle and erythema of the scrotum. Epididymitis is present in 85 percent of the cases and usually precedes the orchitis. The testis may be enlarged three to four times over its normal size. Constitutional complaints and fever generally parallel the severity of gonadal involvement. Fever resolves in 84 percent of the patients in 5 days or less. Pain and swelling resolve shortly after defervescence. However, tenderness may persist for longer than 2 weeks in 20 percent of the cases.[45] Early in convalescence, a loss of turgor may be appreciated. When testes are examined months to years later, 50 percent show some degree of atrophy.

The anxiety engendered by mumps orchitis is difficult to allay. The psychological fears of sexual impotence and sterility far outweigh the potential debility from testicular atrophy. Clearly, most men who have unilateral orchitis need fear nothing other than a possible cosmetic imbalance. Even those with bilateral involvement should be assured that impotence (other than psychogenic) is not a sequela and that sterility is rare. In large surveys of infertile men, mumps is infrequently implicated as the etiology. Twenty-eight cases of testicular malignancy after atrophy of the testis due to mumps orchitis have been reported.[47]

Oophoritis develops in 5 percent of postpubertal women with mumps. Symptoms include fever, nausea, vomiting, and lower abdominal pain. Impaired fertility and premature menopause have been reported as a consequence of ovarian involvement but must be considered rare.[48]

Joint involvement during mumps is noted infrequently in adults and rarely in children.[49,50] Migratory polyarthritis is the most frequently described clinical form. Monoarticular arthritis and arthralgia have also been reported; both large and small joints are involved. Symptoms most commonly start 10–14 days after the onset of parotitis and may last up to 5 weeks. The process spontaneously resolves without residual joint damage.

Pancreatitis is manifested by severe epigastic pain and tenderness accompanied by fever, nausea, and vomiting. It is uncommon as a severe illness; however, many people may complain of mild degrees of upper abdominal discomfort.

Electrocardiographic changes appear in up to 15 percent of the patients with mumps; the most common abnormalities are depressed ST segments, flattened or inverted T waves, and prolonged PR intervals.[51,52] Clinical myocarditis is rare; however, deaths have been reported both during the acute illness and after a chronically progressive deteriorating course.[51,52]

Utz et al.[53] prospectively evaluated the renal function in 20 young adult Navy servicemen admitted with mumps. They discovered transient mild to moderate abnormalities of urinary concentration, creatinine clearance, and phenosulfonphthalein excretion in most of this group. Hughes and associates have reported two deaths due to mumps-associated nephritis.[54]

A variety of other manifestations have accompanied mumps infection, but the following must be considered extremely rare: thyroiditis,[55] mastitis,[56] prostatitis,[57] hepatitis,[58] and thrombocytopenia.[59]

COMPLICATIONS

Gestational viral infections have been extensively investigated in a controlled cohort study by Siegel et al.[60–62] They observed excessive fetal deaths when mumps developed during the first trimester; second and third trimester mumps were not associated with increased fetal mortality.[60] Low birth weight (<2500 g) was identified in 7.7 percent of infants born to mumps-infected mothers as compared with 3.3 percent of a control group; this is not, however, a statistically significant difference. Although the number of cases was small, when the data were analyzed with respect to the onset of infection, the effect on birth weight was greatest when mumps occurred in the first trimester.[61] A variety of congenital malformations have been described in pregnancies complicated by maternal mumps[63]; however, these anomalies are described in single case reports without comparison with an uninfected control population. In Siegel's studies,[62] major congenital defects occurred with equal incidence in both mumps and control newborn populations; even when the data were analyzed by timester, no trends could be established. Similar results have been obtained by a British team in reviewing 500 pregnancies complicated by maternal mumps.[64]

St. Geme and others have suggested an "embryopathic" relationship between intrauterine mumps infection and endocardial fibroelastosis (EFE) on the basis of a high percentage of skin test reactivity to mumps antigen in the EFE group.[65] Experimentally induced infection of the chick embryo has added histopathologic support to this association.[66] Other observers dispute that mumps plays an etiologic role.[67] The controversy is unresolved.

A similar controversy exists over the possible role of mumps in the etiology of juvenile diabetes mellitus. Diabetes, either transient or permanent, developing soon after mumps has been the subject of a number of case reports.[68,69] However, coincidental occurrence has not been eliminated as a possibility. Epidemiologic studies have demonstrated a 7-year periodicity in the incidence of both mumps and childhood diabetes with a 3- to 4-year lag time between their respective peaks.[70] Coxsackievirus B4 has also been epidemiologically linked to diabetes.[71] However, there has not been an apparent decline in the frequency of either juvenile diabetes mellitus or EFE coincident with the decreasing incidence of natural mumps after the introduction of the mumps vaccine.

IMMUNOLOGY

After clinical or subclinical mumps infection, a variety of immunologic responses can be demonstrated. Complement-fixing antibodies directed against the S antigen appear rapidly; sometimes they are present at the onset of clinically apparent illness. Anti-V antibody titers rise more slowly and peak about 2–4 weeks after the beginning of disease.[72] However, anti-S antibody titers decline rapidly over a period of several months to undetectable levels, while anti-V antibody titers drop more slowly and persist for years. This pattern of response provides the possibility of a serologic diagnosis of mumps from a single serum specimen. An acute-phase serum demonstrating a high anti-S and a low anti-V or a high anti-S and a high anti-V titer can be interpreted as evidence of current or very recent infection. A serum having only anti-V antibodies would indicate a more remote infection with mumps.

Neutralizing antibodies appear during convalescence, and detectable titers persist for years. Although this is the most reliable test to determine a person's immune status to mumps, it is cumbersome and not routinely performed. Hemagglutination inhibition antibodies also develop after mumps. Although this is the simplest of the serologic studies, it is the least reliable due to cross-reactions with other paramyxoviruses. Enzyme-linked immunosorbent assays (ELISA) for antibody to mumps have been developed[73] and are becoming widely available.

Delayed hypersensitivity to an intradermally administered mumps skin test antigen develops between 3 weeks and 3 months after mumps.[3] The skin test was widely used as a measure of immunity to mumps as well as a test for competent general delayed hypersensitivity. The use of mumps skin test antigen to determine immunity to mumps has been abandoned for a number of reasons. Different lots of the skin test antigen have variable potency, and false-positive and false-negative results make this test an unreliable predictor of immune status to mumps.[74] Use of the skin test in a mumps-immune person was found to stimulate an anamnestic response of neutralizing, CF, and HAI antibodies,[75] and these results caused diagnostic confusion.

Interferon is produced during mumps infection.[76] The highest serum titers are found during the first 3 days of clinical illness but rapidly decline to undetectable levels beyond 7 days. Salivary levels parallel those in the blood.

Transplacental transfer of maternal mumps CF, HAI, and neutralization antibodies has been demonstrated.[77] Titers in maternal and cord serum are nearly identical. Neutralizing antibodies persist for several months and account for the rarity of mumps in young infants as well as the lack of response to immunization during this time period.

One attack of mumps, whether inapparent or evidenced by unilateral or bilateral parotitis or any of the other clinical manifestations, confers lifelong immunity. The V antigen CF test is the technique routinely used to determine immune status. It combines ease of performance with reliability.

DIAGNOSIS

In most instances, the diagnosis of mumps is made on the basis of a history of exposure and on the presence of parotid swelling and tenderness accompanied by mild to moderate constitutional symptoms.

The WBC and differential counts in mumps are normal, or there may be a mild leukopenia with a relative lymphocytosis. When meningitis, orchitis, or pancreatitis is present, leukocytosis with a shift to the left is most commonly encountered. The serum amylase level is elevated in the presence of parotitis and may remain abnormal for 2–3 weeks. This enzyme level may also be elevated in the absence of clinical salivary gland involvement. Mumps pancreatitis similarly increases amylase levels; differentiation from salivary gland involvement may be achieved by isoenzyme analysis or serum pancreatic lipase determinations.

The typical CSF findings in mumps meningitis have previously been described. Similar although less marked changes are present in half of the people with parotitis but without apparent central nervous system involvement. In a patient with aseptic meningitis, an elevated serum amylase level should suggest mumps as the etiologic agent.

Laboratory confirmation in typical mumps is unnecessary. However, when parotitis is absent or recurrent, when extrasalivary gland manifestations are prominent, or when documentation of a specific viral etiology is desired, a variety of diagnostic aids are available.

The definitive diagnosis of mumps depends on serologic studies or viral isolation. The demonstration of a fourfold rise between acute and convalescent sera in the CF, HAI, ELISA, or neutralization tests confirms the diagnosis. The HAI test in particulr suffers from the possibility of heterologous antibody response to parainfluenza virus infection. In view of reports of parotitis caused by parainfluenza 3,[78] serologic testing directed at this agent as well as attempts at virus isolation should be undertaken if the HAI test is to be used in the diagnosis of mumps.

Virus may be isolated from a number of sources. It is usually present in saliva for about 1 week, usually 2–3 days before and 4–5 days after the onset of parotitis. However, virus has been isolated from saliva as early as 6 days before and as late as 9 days after the fist signs of salivary gland involvement. In addition, virus may be recovered from the saliva of persons with inapparent infection or those manifesting only extrasalivary gland signs.[79] The virus is frequently isolated from the CSF in patients with clinical meningitis during the first 3 days of meningeal symptoms[25]; its presence has been documented as late as the sixth day of central nervous system disease. Viruria has been detected during the first 2 weeks of illness: 72 percent of urine specimens during the first 5 days of illness yielded a positive culture.[53] Viremia has rarely been detected and was found only on the first 2 days of illness.[18,19]

DIFFERENTIAL DIAGNOSIS

There are a variety of entities that may simulate mumps parotitis. Most of these conditions actually involve the parotid but can be easily differentiated from mumps on the basis of chronicity or associated symptoms.

Other infectious processes are most likely to be confused with mumps because of their acute onset and associated fever. Parainfluenza type 3, coxsackie-, and influenza type A viruses have been reported to cause acute parotitis.[78,80,81] These entities can be differentiated from mumps only by viral culture and/or serology. Suppurative parotitis, most often due to *Staphylococcus aureus*, usually occurs in the postoperative state, in premature newborns, or in debilitated patients with poor oral intake. The gland is warm, hard, and extremely tender; the overlying skin is erythematous. Massage of the parotid expresses purulent drainage from Stensen's duct.

Parotid enlargement caused by drugs or metabolic disorders is usually bilateral and asymptomatic. Phenylbutazone, thiouracil, iodides, and phenothiazines have been implicated in this condition.[57] Diabetes mellitus, malnutrition, cirrhosis, and uremia are among the metabolic disorders described as causing parotid swelling.[57]

Tumors, cysts, and obstruction due to stones or stricture are usually unilateral. Rare conditions that at the time of onset may mimic mumps include Mikulicz syndrome, Parinaud syndrome, uveoparotid fever of sarcoidosis, and Sjögren syndrome.

THERAPY

Therapy for mumps parotitis is limited to symptomatic and supportive measures. Treatment with an analgesic-antipyretic agent such as aspirin or acetaminophen relieves the pain caused by salivary gland inflammation and reduces fever. Topical application of warm or cold packs to the parotid may also ameliorate the discomfort of some patients. Intravenous fluid administration is indicated for those patients with meningitis or pancreatitis who have persistent vomiting. Lumbar puncture may relieve the headache associated with meningitis.

Management of orchitis is purely symptomatic. Bed rest, narcotic analgesics, support of the inflamed testis with a bridge, and ice packs make the patient feel more comfortable. An anesthetic block of the spermatic cord with 1% procaine hydrochloride may alleviate severe pain.[82] There is no convincing evidence that the use of steroids or diethylstilbestrol or incision of the tunica albuginea produces more rapid resolution of the orchitis or prevents subsequent atrophy.

Gellis[83] and colleagues have shown that 20 ml of mumps immune glublin administered intramuscularly to adult men with mumps reduces the incidence of orchitis from 27.4 to 7.8 percent. Mumps immune globulin is no longer commercially available.

PREVENTION

Recommendations for the management of patients with mumps generally include isolation until the parotid swelling has resolved to prevent the spread of infection to susceptibles. This measure may be of little value, particularly in closed populations such as schools or hospitals,[73] because virus is present in saliva days before clinically apparent parotitis and the persons with inapparent infection, although asymptomatic, are nonetheless contagious.

Passive protection to exposed susceptible persons may be afforded by the use of mumps immune globulin. However, Reed et al.[12] report that use of this product during an epidemic in Alaska neither reduced clinical parotitis and inapparent infection rates nor diminished the incidence of meningitis and orchitis.

Active immunization with a live attenuated mumps virus vaccine has been available in the United States since licensing in Dcember 1967. The vaccine is prepared in chick embryo cell culture.[5] A single subcutaneous inoculation produces protective levels of mumps-neutralizing antibody in more than 95 percent of vaccinees.[5] Although the antibody levels produced are lower than after natural infection, satisfactory titers are maintained for at least 10.5 years.[84] Adverse reactions to the vaccine are uncommon; transient suppression of tuberculin delayed hypersensitivity has been reported. Vaccine virus is not present in secretions of immunized children.

All children over 12 months of age should be immunized. In routine pediatric practice, administration takes place at 15 months of age in the form of the combined live measles-mumps-rubella viruses vaccine (MMR). Most states now require evidence of immunity to mumps (i.e., documented immunization, physician-diagnosed disease, or antibody studies) for school entrance and attendance. (see Chapter 296). Immunization should also be considered for male adolescents and adults without a history of mumps. Male medical personnel found to have no neutralizing antibodies to mumps should be immunized. Immunization after exposure may not provide protection from development of natural infection. However, if the current exposure did not result in infection, the vaccination will produce immunity to mumps.

As with most other live virus vaccines, mumps vaccine should not be administered to pregnant women, patients receiving immunosuppressive therapy, or those persons with a severe febrile illness, malignancy, or congenital or acquired immunodeficiency.

REFERENCES

1. Johnson CD, Goodpasture EW. An investigation of the etiology of mumps. J Exp Med. 1934;59:1.
2. Habel K. Cultivation of mumps virus in the developing chick embryo and its application to the studies of immunity to mumps in man. Pub Health Rep. 1945;60:201.
3. Enders JF, Cohen S, Kane LW. Immunity in mumps. II. The development of complement fixing antibody and dermal hypersensitivity in human beings following mumps. J Exp Med. 1945;81:119.
4. Habel K. Vaccination of human beings against mumps; vaccine administered at the start of an epidemic. I. Incidence and severity of mumps in vaccinated and control groups. Am J Hyg. 1951;54:295.
5. Buynak EB, Hilleman MR. Live attenuated mumps virus vaccine. I. Vaccine development. Proc Soc Exp Biol Med. 1966;123:768.
6. Choppin PW, Compans RW. Reproduction of myxoviruses. In: Fraenkel-Conrat H, Wagner RR, eds. Comprehensive Virology 4. New York: Plenum; 1975:95.
7. Deinhardt FW, Shramek GJ. Mumps virus. In: Lennette EH, Spaulding EH, Truant JP, eds. Manual of Clinical Microbiology. Washington, DC: American Society for Microbiology; 1974:703.
8. Henle G, Deinhardt F, Girardi A. Cytolytic effects of mumps virus in tissue cultures of epithelial cells. Proc Soc Exp Biol Med. 1954;87:386.
9. Centers for Disease Control. Mumps surveillance 1973. MMWR. 1974;23:431.
10. Centers for Disease Control. Reported morbidity and mortality in the United States, 1976. MMWR. 1977;25:51.
11. Philip RN, Reinhard KR, Lackman DB. Observations on a mumps epidemic in a "virgin" population. Am J Hyg. 1959;69:91.
12. Reed D, Brown G, Merrick R, et al. A mumps epidemic on St. George Island, Alaska. JAMA. 1967;199:967.
13. Meyer MG. An epidemiologic study of mumps; its spread in schools and families. Am J Hyg. 1962;75:259.
14. Cochi SL, Preblud SR, Orenstein WA. Perspectives on the relative resurgence of mumps in the United States. Am J Dis Child. 1988;142;499–507.
15. St. Geme JW, Yamauchi T, Eisenklam EJ, et al. Immunologic significance of the mumps virus skin test in infants, children and adults. Am J Epidemiol. 1975;101:253.
16. Centers for Disease Control. Mumps surveillance, Report No. 1. January 1968. Report No. 1. January 1968.
17. Truant AL, Hallum JV. A persistent infection of baby hamster kidney—21 cells with mumps virus and the role of temperature sensitive variants. J Med Virol. 1977;1:49.
18. Kilham L. Isolation of mumps virus from the blood of a patient. Proc Soc Exp Biol Med. 1948;69:99.

19. Overman JR. Viremia in human mumps infection. Arch Intern Med. 1958;102:354.
20. Donohue WL, Playfair FD, Whitaker L. Mumps encephalitis. J Pediatr. 1955;47:395.
21. Taylor FB, Toreson WE. Primary mumps meningo-encephalitis. Arch Intern Med. 1963;112:216.
22. Travis LW, Hecht DW. Acute and chronic inflammatory diseases of the salivary glands, diagnosis and management. Otolaryng Clin North Am 1977;10:329.
23. Gellis SS, Peters M. Mumps with presternal edema. Bull J Hopkins Hosp. 1944;75:241.
24. Bang HO, Bang J. Involvement of the central nervous system in mumps. Acta Med Scand. 1943;113:487.
25. McLean DM, Bach RD, Larke RPB, et al. Mumps meningoencephalitis, Toronto, 1963. Can Med Assoc J. 1964;90:458.
26. Ritter BS. Mumps meningoencephalitis in children. J Pediatr. 1958;52:424.
27. Levitt LP, Rich TA, Kinde SW, et al. Central nervous system mumps. Neurology (NY). 1970;20:829.
28. Johnstone JA, Ross CAC, Dunn M. Meningitis and encephalitis associated with mumps infection. Arch Dis Child. 1972;47:647.
29. Wilfert CM. Mumps meningoencephalitis with low cerebrospinal-fluid glucose, prolonged pleocytosis and elevation of protein. N Engl J Med. 1969;280:855.
30. Center for Disease Control. Aseptic meningitis surveillance report. Annual Summary 1976. January 1979.
31. Russell RR, Donald JC. The neurological complications of mumps. Br Med J. 1958;2:27.
32. Centers for Disease Control. Mumps surveillance, January 1977–December 1982. MMWR. 1984;
33. Azimi PH, Shaban S, Hilty MD, et al. Mumps meningoencephalitis prolonged abnormality of cerebrospinal fluid. JAMA. 1975;234:1161.
34. Vuori M, Lahikainen EA, Peltonen T. Perceptive deafness in connection with mumps. Acta Otolaryngol. 1962;55:231.
35. Everberg G. Deafness following mumps. Acta Otolaryngol. 1957;48:397.
36. Davis LE, Harms AC, Chin TDY. Transient cortical blindness and cerebellar ataxia associated with mumps. Arch Ophthalmol. 1971;85:366.
37. Beardwell A. Facial palsy due to the mumps virus. Br J Clin Pract. 1969;23:37.
38. Silverman AC. Mumps complicated by a preceding myelitis. N Engl J Med. 1949;241:262.
39. Ghosh S. Guillain-Barré syndrome complicating mumps. Lancet. 1967;1:895.
40. Lennette EH, Caplan GE, Magoffin RL. Mumps virus infection simulating paralytic poliomyelitis. Pediatrics. 1960;25:788.
41. Timmons GD, Johnson KP. Aqueductal stenosis and hydrocephalus after mumps encephalitis. N Engl J Med. 1970;283;1505.
42. Bray PF. Mumps: A cause of hydrocephalus? Pediatrics. 1972;49:446.
43. Johnson RT, Johnson KP. Hydrocephalus following viral infection. The pathology of aqueductal stenosis developing after experimental mumps virus infection. J Neuropathol Exp Neurol. 1968;27:591.
44. Herndon RM, Johnson RT, Davis LE, et al. Ependymitis in mumps virus meningitis. Arch Neurol. 1974;30:475.
45. Candel S. Epididymitis in mumps, including orchitis: Further clinical studies and comments. Ann Intern Med. 1951;34;20.
46. Lambert B. The frequency of mumps and of mumps orchitis. Acta Genet Stat Med. 1951;2(Suppl 1):1.
47. Kaufman JJ, Bruce PT. Testicular atrophy following mumps, a cause of testis tumour? J Urol. 1963;35:67.
48. Morrison JC, Givens JR, Wiser WL. Mumps oophoritis: A cause of premature menopause. Fertil Steril. 1975;26:655.
49. Appelbaum E, Kohn J, Steinman RE, et al. Mumps arthritis. Arch Intern Med. 1952;90:217.
50. Caranasos GJ, Felker JR. Mumps arthritis. Arch Intern Med. 1967;119:394.
51. Kussy JC, Fatal mumps myocarditis. Minn Med. 1974;57:285.
52. Roberts WC, Fox SM. Mumps of the heart, clinical and pathologic features. Circulation. 1965;32:342.
53. Utz JP, Houk VN, Alling DW. Clinical and laboratory studies of mumps. IV. Viruria and abnormal renal function. N Engl J Med. 1964;270:1283.
54. Hughes WT, Steigman AJ, Delong HF. Some implications of fatal nephritis associated with mumps. Am J Dis Child. 1966;111:297.
55. Eylan E, Zmucky R, Sheba C. Mumps virus and subacute thyroiditis: Evidence of a causal association. Lancet. 1957;1:1062.
56. Krugman S, Ward R, Katz SL. Mumps (epidemic parotitis). In: Infectious Disease of Children. 6th ed. St. Louis: CV Mosby; 1977:181.
57. Marcy SM, Kibrick S. Mumps. In: Hoeprich PD, ed. Infectious Diseases. 2nd ed. Hagerstown, MD: Harper & Row; 1977:621.
58. Petersdorf RG, Bennett IL. Treatment of mumps orchitis with adrenal hormones: Report of 23 cases with a note on the hepatic involvement in mumps. Arch Intern Med. 1957;99:222.
59. Graham DY, Brown CH, Benrey J, et al. Thrombocytopenia: A complication of mumps. JAMA. 1974;227:1162.
60. Siegel M, Fuerst HT, Peress NS. Comparative fetal mortality in maternal virus diseases: A prospective study on rubella, measles, mumps, chickenpox and hepatitis. N Engl J Med. 1966;274:768.
61. Siegel M, Fuerst HT. Low birth weight and maternal virus diseases: A prospective study of rubella, measles, mumps, chickenpox and hepatitis. JAMA. 1966;197:680.
62. Siegel MS. Congenital malformations following chickenpox, measles, mumps, and hepatitis. Results of a cohort study. JAMA. 1973;226:1521.
63. Young NA. Chickenpox, measles, and mumps. In: Remington JS, Klein JO, eds. Infectious Diseases of the Fetus and Newborn. Philadelphia: WB Saunders; 1976:521.
64. Manson MM, Logan WPD, Loy RM. Rubella and other virus infections in pregnancy. Reports on Public Health and Medical Subjects, No. 101. London: Ministry of Health; 1960.
65. St. Geme JW, Noren GR, Adams P. Proposed embryopathic relation between mumps virus and primary endocardial fibroelastosis. N Engl J Med. 1966;275:339.
66. St. Geme JW, Peralta H, Farias E, et al. Experimental gestational mumps virus infection and endocardial fibroelastosis. Pediatrics. 1971;48:821.
67. Gersony WM, Katz SL, Nadas AS. Endocardial fibroelastosis and the mumps virus. Pediatrics. 1966;37:430.
68. Dacou-Voutetakis C, Constantinidis M, Moschos A, et al. Diabetes mellitus following mumps: Insulin reserve. Am J Dis Child. 1974;127:890.
69. Hinden E. Mumps followed by diabetes. Lancet. 1962;1:1138.
70. Sultz HA, Hart BA, Zielezny M, et al. Is mumps virus an etiologic factor in juvenile diabetes mellitus. J Pediatr. 1975;86:654.
71. Gamble DR, Kinsley ML, Fitzgerald MG, et al. Viral antibodies in diabetes mellitus. Br Med J. 1969;3:627.
72. Henle G, Harris S, Henle W. The reactivity of various human sera with mumps complement fixation antigens. J Exp Med. 1948;88:133.
73. Nigro G, Nanni F, Midulla M. Determination of vaccine-induced and naturally acquired class-specific antibodies by two indirect ELISAs. J Virol Methods. 1986;13:91–106.
74. Brunell PA, Brickman A, O'Hare D, et al. Ineffectiveness of isolation of patients as a method of preventing the spread of mumps. N Engl J Med. 1968;279:1357.
75. Henle G, Burgoon JS, Bashe WJ, et al. Studies on the prevention of mumps. II. The effect of skin testing upon antibody level and resistance. J Immunol. 1951;66;551.
76. Waddell DJ, Wilbur JR, Merigan TC. Interferon production in human mumps infection. Proc Soc Exp Biol Med. 1968;127:320.
77. Hodes D, Brunell PA. Mumps antibody placental transfer and disappearance during the first year of life. Pediatrics. 1970;45:99.
78. Zollar LM, Mufson MA. Acute parotitis associated with parainfluenza 3 virus infection. Am J Dis Child. 1970;119:147.
79. Henle G, Henle W, Wendell KK, et al. Isolation of mumps virus from human beings with induced apparent or inapparent infections. J Exp Med. 1948;88:223.
80. Howlett JG, Somlo F, Kalz F. A new syndrome of parotitis with herpangina caused by the coxsackie virus. Can Med Assoc J. 1957;77:5.
81. Brill SJ, Gilfillan RF. Acute parotitis associated with influenza type. A. N Engl J Med. 1977;296:1391.
82. Lyon RP, Bruyn HB. Mumps epididymo-orchitis: Treament by anesthetic block of the spermatic cord. JAMA. 1966;196:736.
83. Gellis SS, McGuiness AC, Peters M. A study on the prevention of mumps orchitis with gamma globulin. Am J Med Sci. 1945;210:661.
84. Weibel RE, Buynak EB, McLean AA, et al. Persistence of antibody in human subjects following administration of combined live attenuated measles, mumps, and rubella vaccines. Proc Soc Exp Biol Med. 1980;165:260.

136. RESPIRATORY SYNCYTIAL VIRUS

CAROLINE BREESE HALL

Were we but able to explain
  The fiefdom of the microbe—
Why one man is his serf,
  Another is his lord
When all are his domain. . . .

Respiratory syncytial virus (RSV) is the major cause of lower respiratory tract illness in young children.[1–5] Its presence may be witnessed in most communities in this country by the yearly upsurge of pneumonia, bronchiolitis, and tracheobronchitis in the very young. So effectively does RSV spread that essentially all persons have experienced infection with this agent within the first few years of life. Immunity, however, is not complete, and reinfection is common and causes upper respiratory tract illness and tracheobronchitis in older children and adults. Although life-threatening infections generally occur only during the first few years of life, there is growing concern that contracting bronchiolitis and lower respiratory tract illness during infancy may have sequelae that may contribute to the development of chronic lung disease in later life.[6–16]

HISTORY

Outbreaks of bronchiolitis occurring in the winter or spring have been noted for some time. But the major agent of the outbreaks was not discovered until 1956 when Morris and coworkers[17] isolated a new virus from 1 of 14 chimpanzees suffering from colds. They entitled this new agent "chimpanzee coryza agent" (CCA). Whether this agent was also able to infect humans was not then known but was suspected since one laboratory worker developed specific antibody to CCA. Subsequently, Chanock and his colleagues[18] confirmed that the agent was able to cause respiratory illness in humans when they obtained two isolates that were indistinguishable from CCA. These isolates were recovered from the throat swabs of a child with bronchopneumonia (Long strain) and from a child with laryngotracheobronchitis (Synder strain). Chanock and Finberg[19] subsequently detected rises of specific neutralizing antibody to CCA in children with respiratory illnesses and also discovered that such antibody was present in most children by the time they reached school age. It thus became apparent that it was inappropriate to call this virus "chimpanzee coryza agent." The virus was renamed "respiratory syncytial virus" to denote its clinical and laboratory manifestations. Proof soon accumulated that indicated RSV as the major agent causing outbreaks of lower respiratory disease in infants.[20–30]

DESCRIPTION

Classification

RSV belongs to the Paramyxoviridae family and to the genus *Pneumovirus*.[31] Since RSV has morphologic and biologic characteristics very similar to the pneumonia virus of mice (PVM) and bovine RSV, it has been suggested that these viruses should be classified together as a separate group and, because of their intermediate size, should be called metamyxoviruses.[32]

Characteristics

RSV is an enveloped single negative-strand RNA virus of medium size.[33] By sucrose density gradient centrifugation RSV has been estimated to have a diameter of 90–120 nm, and by negative stain the viral particles measure 120–300 nm.[18,34] Its inner helix appears to have a mean diameter of 13.5 nm, which is intermediate in size between the helix of the influenza viruses and that of the paramyxoviruses.[32] On electron microscopy the virus appears pleomorphic with both spherical and filamentous forms that range in diameter from 80 to 500 nm and range in length up to 2.5 μm.[32] The fringed envelope gives the virus the appearance of a thistle, with the glycoprotein spikes being 12 nm in length and 10 nm apart.[32] The indirect immunofluorescent technique has revealed RSV antigens only in the cytoplasm of cells, which may be observed in 8 hours.[32] Electron microscopy of ultrathin sections of infected tissue has revealed that RSV matures at the cytoplasmic membrane, with round or filamentous particles budding from the cytoplasmic membrane.[32]

The RSV genome encodes for at least 10 unique viral polypeptides ranging in size from 160,000 daltons (160 kD) to 9.5 kD.[35–40] Four of these proteins are associated with the envelope. Two are nonglycosylated: the M protein, a 26 kD matrix protein, and a 22–24 kD protein of unknown function.[35] The two glycosylated surface proteins, the F and G proteins, appear to be of particular importance in the infectivity and pathogenesis of the virus. The F protein is a 70 kD fusion protein consisting of two disulfide-linked fragments of 50 and 20 kD (F_1 and F_2).[39] The F protein appears to initiate viral penetration by fusing viral and cellular membranes and promote the spread of the virus by fusing infected to adjacent uninfected cells, thereby resulting in the characteristic syncytia. The largest glycoprotein, the 84–90 kD G protein, appears to mediate attachment of the virus to the host cells.[40] The other nonglycosylated proteins associated with the nucleocapsid are the 42 kD nucleocapsid protein (N), the 34 kD phosphoprotein (P), and the 160 kD polymerase (L). The nucleotide sequence of the mRNAs for each of the proteins, except for the polymerase, has been determined.[41–48]

RSV withstands changes in temperature and pH relatively poorly. Only 10 percent of RSV remained after exposing the virus to 55°C for 5 minutes.[49] At 37°C the virus was stable for 1 hour, but only 10 percent of the infectivity remained after 24 hours. At 25°C 10 percent infectivity was present after 48 hours, and at 4°C 1 percent of the infectivity remained after 7 days.[49] RSV tolerates slow freezing and thawing poorly. If the virus is slowly frozen at −30°C and then thawed, there is complete loss of infectivity.[21] When slowly frozen at −65°C, the infectivity titer fell by approximately 0.5 log.[49] RSV also withstands an acid medium poorly, and the optimal pH is 7.5.[49] The virus is quickly inactivated by ether, chloroform, and a variety of detergents such as 0.1% sodium deoxycholate, sodium dodecyl sulfate, and Triton X-100. Storage of RSV can be enhanced by flash freezing in an alcohol and dry ice bath and by adding glycerine or sucrose.[32]

At room temperature RSV in the secretions of patients may survive on nonporous surfaces such as countertops for 3–30 hours, depending on the humidity.[50] On porous surfaces such as cloth and paper tissue, survival is generally shorter, usually less than an hour. The infectivity of RSV on the hands is variable from person to person but is usually less than 1 hour. The survival of RSV in the environment appears to depend in part on the drying time as well as the humidity.[50,51]

Laboratory Propagation

RSV grows well in several human cell lines and may be adapted to a number of others. For primary isolation, human heteroploid cells such as HEp-2 and HeLa cells are usually preferred. Other cell lines that may be used but are usually less sensitive include human kidney, amnion, and diploid fibroblastic cells and monkey kidney cells.[21,52] The sensitivity of all these cell lines, including the heteroploid human lines, for the growth of RSV is variable and must be monitored.[52,53] The presence of RSV in infected cell cultures is detected by its characteristic syncytial appearance (Figs. 1 and 2). However, the degree of syncytial formation depends on the type of cell culture, the heaviness of the cell sheet, the medium, the strain of virus, the multiplicity of infection, and its laboratory adaptation.[54–57] On primary isolation in sensitive heteroploid cell cultures, the characteristic cytopathic effect of RSV may be first detected after an average 3–5 days.[58] With strains of RSV that are adapted to tissue culture, new infectious virus may first be detected 10–12 hours after inoculation, but the typical syncytia do not develop until 10–24 hours later.[59,60] The syncytia progress until the cell sheet is completely destroyed, which usually occurs within 4 days. A variable proportion of the cell sheet may also show rounding of the cells without fusion, especially in some primary cell lines.

About 90 percent of the inoculum is absorbed within 2 hours by standard sensitive cell lines. The virus enters an eclipse period of approximately 12 hours, with new virus appearing thereafter. The subsequent log phase of replication lasts approximately 10 hours.[51,61] By immunofluorescent techniques, viral antigen may be detected in the cytoplasm 7–10 hours after inoculation.[59] Cell-free virus may be subsequently demonstrated in the culture medium, but most remains cell associated. Even at the point when maximal titers of infectious virus are achieved, approximately half of the virus remains cell associated.[55,59,61] When the virus has been subjected to repeated high passage, persistent infection may occur.[62] The amount of cell-

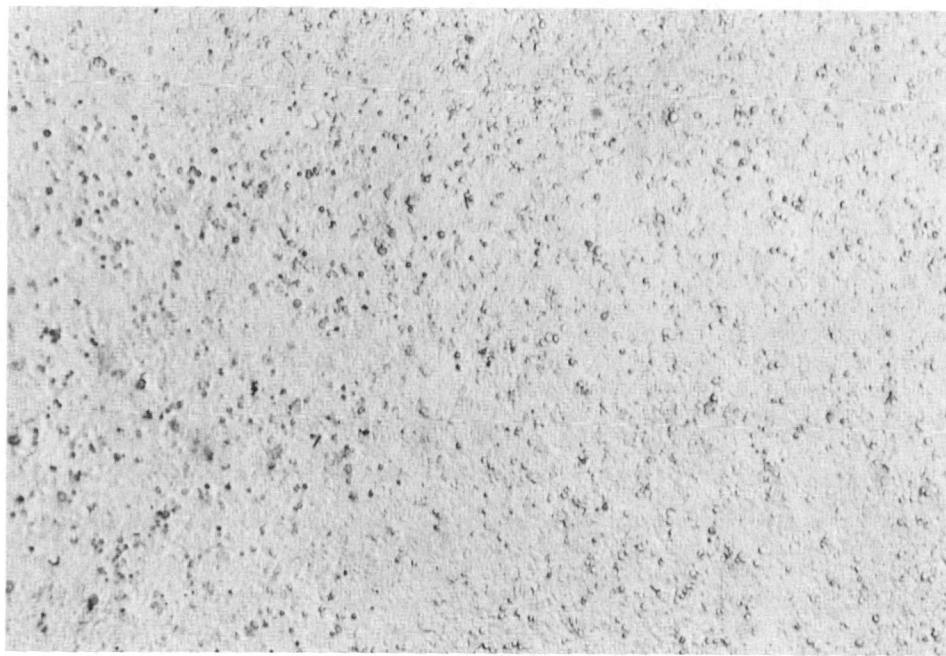

FIG. 1. Uninfected HEp-2 cell culture.

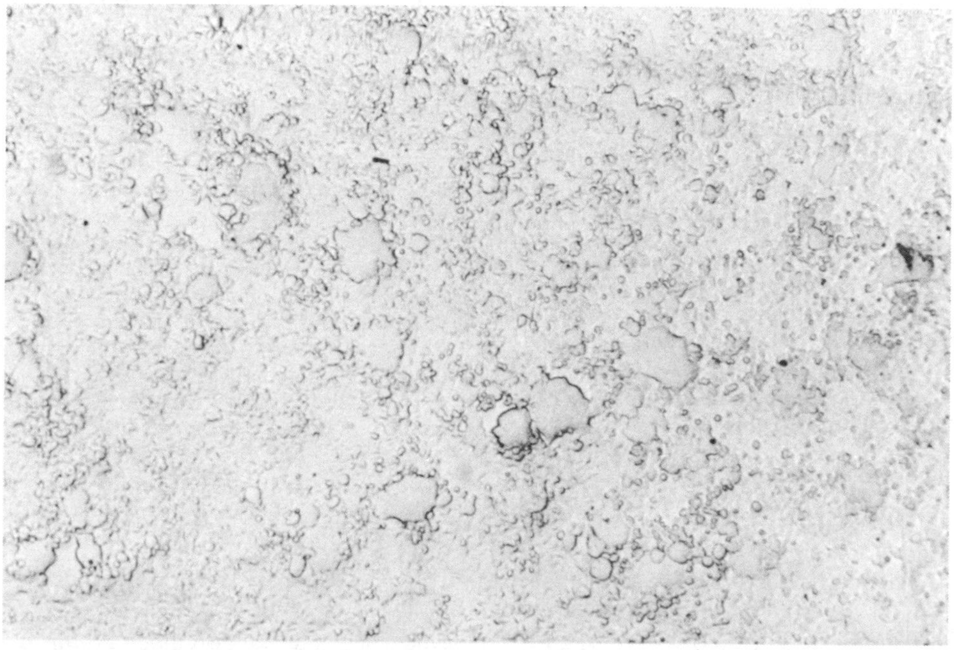

FIG. 2. HEp-2 culture 4 days after inoculation with a nasal wash from an infant hospitalized with pneumonia. Multiple foci of the characteristic refractile syncytial cytopathic effect of RSV are apparent.

free virus then diminishes, and the characteristic cytopathic effect is lost when persistent infection is established. Production of defective interfering particles, which is dependent on the multiplicity of infection, may also occur and results in less infectious virus and cytopathology.[57]

Antigenic Variation

Antigenic variation among strains of RSV has been thought to be minor and of little importance with RSV infections because minor antigenic differences were only detectable by neutralization tests with animal hyperimmune sera but not with human sera.[63–65] New knowledge about the surface glycoproteins of the virus, however, has shown that appreciable strain variation exists and results in two major subgroups of RSV designated group A or 1 and group B or 2.[66–76] The group A strains are represented by the prototype Long or A2 strains and group B by strain 18537. Characterization of strains from these groups by monoclonal and polyclonal antibodies reveals that the major antigenic differences reside on the G protein, while the F proteins are relatively similar.[71,72,75,76] The antigenic relatedness as measured by enzyme-linked immunosorbent assay (ELISA) antibody responses to the F proteins of the two subgroups is about 50% as compared with 5–7 percent for the G proteins.[75,76]

Strains of both groups circulate simultaneously, but the proportion of each may vary from year to year.[68,70,73,74] The epidemiologic and clinical implications of this strain variation are as of yet unclear.

Infection in Animals

A variety of species of animals may be experimentally infected with RSV, but natural infection is limited to humans and chimpanzees. Closely related bovine strains of RSV have been recovered from cows with respiratory illness.[77–81] Chimpanzees when infected with RSV develop respiratory illness and shed large quantities of virus, similar to babies, and thus have been proposed as a possible animal model for the study of RSV disease, but they do not develop lower respiratory tract disease.[17,82,83] The only animal model thus far found to develop pneumonia is the cebus monkey.[84] RSV infection in laboratory animals is generally asymptomatic, thus limiting the study of the immunopathology of RSV disease in animal models. Infection in ferrets, however, may be associated with some histopathologic changes in the upper respiratory tract and, in infant ferrets, in the lower respiratory tract.[85,86] Hamsters may be easily infected with RSV, but histopathologic changes in the respiratory tract are only occasionally present.[87] Other animals that may be asymptomatically infected with RSV include other primates, guinea pigs, minks, chinchillas, and mice.[82,85]

EPIDEMIOLOGY

Distribution

In every geographic area studied, evidence of infection with RSV has been found. In areas of widely differing climates RSV infection appears to have similar characteristics. It is common, and primary infection occurs in the very young.[3,5,29,30,88–93]

Seasonal Occurrence

Outbreaks of RSV infection occur yearly. Indeed, RSV is the only viral respiratory agent that may be relied on to produce a sizable crop of infection each year.[3–5,91,94] The outbreaks usually occur in the winter or spring. In Washington, D.C., and in Chapel Hill, North Carolina, the epidemics have been noted to occur in "long and short" cycles, alternating between appearances in the winter and spring.[1,3,4,95] In other areas with colder climates RSV has tended to appear at regular yearly intervals in the winter, with the peak prevalence falling in January to March.[91,96] Wherever the area, RSV appears to have an unusually predictable and regular pattern.[3,93,95,97,98] Also, when RSV takes a community's "center stage," it tends to be the sole actor. Rarely are other respiratory viral agents that occur in outbreaks concurrently present.[3,94,99] This "interference phenomenon" is often manifested by the disappearance of the parainfluenza viruses types 1 or 2 when RSV appears, and as RSV activity declines, influenza activity may rise.[3,94,96,99] Occasionally, however, overlapping outbreaks of RSV infection and influenza occur.[96,100,101]

Epidemiologic Manifestations

The spread of RSV infection within a community produces such characteristic ramifications that the presence of RSV may be detected without the aid of a viral laboratory. The characteristic fingerprints of RSV are a rise in the number of cases of bronchiolitis and pediatric pneumonia in the community and a rise in the number of hospital admissions of young children with acute lower respiratory tract disease.[4,29,95,96] The size of the outbreaks of RSV infection in general does not vary enough to change these barometers in most temperate climates, but occasionally a very mild outbreak is observed, frequently to be followed the next season by an outbreak of greater than usual severity.[4]

Acquisition of Infection According to Age

Experience with RSV is so universal at a young age that virtually all children have been infected before they enter school. All newborns passively receive specific neutralizing antibody and antibody to the major surface glycoproteins of the virus from their mothers.[5,102,103] Without natural infection the level of antibody falls over the next 6–7 months such that little is detectable.[5] By 1 year of age 25–50 percent of infants have specific antibody as a result of natural infection.[19,30,102] By 4–5 years of age most children have specific antibody.[19,26,30,102]

Prevalence and Incidence

The importance of RSV in causing respiratory illness in children is illustrated in Table 1. It is the major agent recovered from young children with pneumonia and bronchiolitis. The proportion of cases identified as being caused by RSV varies according to the population examined and the methods used. During the peak period of an epidemic, RSV may be isolated from up to 89 percent of the young children admitted to the hospital with acute lower respiratory tract disease.[58] In contrast, RSV is rarely isolated from children without respiratory disease[4,22] (Table 1).

Parrott and colleagues[1,4,5] have estimated from their studies in Washington, D.C., that about one-half of the infants they followed longitudinally were infected during their first RSV epidemic and that essentially all had become infected after experiencing two RSV epidemics. Furthermore, in 40 percent of these first infections a febrile pneumonitis developed. The yearly attack rate for RSV lower respiratory tract disease has been estimated as 23 per 1000 children less than 1 year of age in middle-income families in North Carolina and as 9 per 1000 in families in a Seattle prepaid medical practice.[95,98] During the second year of life the rates were approximately the same. In children 2–3 years of age the attack rates declined to 15 in Chapel Hill and 7 in Seattle. In 4- and 5-year-old children the yearly attack rate was estimated to be 8 and 5, respectively. Prospective studies suggest that the frequency of lower respiratory tract infection with RSV is actually much higher than even these rates show. In groups of infants followed closely the attack rate for RSV lower respiratory tract diseases varied from 15 to 50 percent.[95,107,112–114] Similarly, in a pediatric group practice in Chapel Hill, bronchiolitis has been estimated to occur each year in children under 2 years of age at a rate of 6 to 7 cases per 100 children.[104,112,115] Similar rates were observed for children under 6 months of age. However, the rates were phenomenally higher in the day care center in which the children were examined almost daily. Under these circumstances, which would detect the mildest illnesses, the rate in children 6 months of age or younger was 115 per 100 children per year.[104]

Age, sex, and socioeconomic factors appear to influence the expression of RSV disease. The most severe illness occurs in the youngest infants (Fig. 3). Boys appear to have a higher incidence of lower respiratory tract disease. In Chapel Hill, boys under 6 years of age had a rate of RSV lower respiratory tract

TABLE 1. Proportion of Respiratory Illnesses Caused by RSV in Children

Syndrome	*Percentage Caused by RSV*	*References*
Bronchiolitis	43–90	1,4,91,104,105,115
Pneumonia	5–40	1–3,22,94,106–111
Tracheobronchitis	10–30	4,107
Croup	3–10	3,4,21,91,94,107,109
Asymptomatic	0.3	4

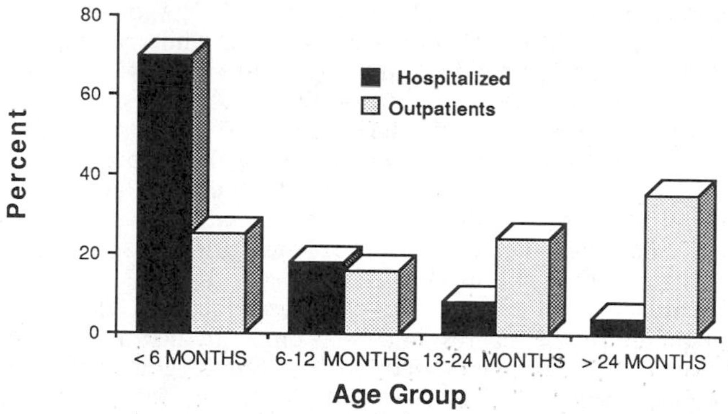

FIG. 3. The difference in the age distribution of inpatients and outpatients with RSV infection in Rochester, New York, illustrates the effect of age on the severity of infection. Seventy percent of infants requiring hospitalization were under 6 months of age. In comparison 25 percent of the children treated as outpatients were under 6 months of age, and 38 percent were over 2 years of age.

disease of 2.4 per 100 as compared with 1.5 per 100 for girls.[3,94] That boys get more severe disease is also suggested by the preponderance of boys admitted to the hospital with lower respiratory tract disease.[5,58] Also, a greater proportion of hospitalized children are from lower socioeconomic areas.[3,95,104] In a middle-income practice in Chapel Hill approximately 1 of every 1000 patients with RSV infection has required hospitalization.[94,95] In contrast, in a lower-income population in Washington, D.C., the need for hospitalization has been estimated to occur in 1 of every 100 RSV infections.[4,116] Sex and socioeconomic factors, however, do not appear to influence the attack rate but rather the severity of the infection.[95,104]

Incidence of Repeated Infections

Repeated infections with RSV are common, and no age group appears protected. In a Chapel Hill day care center 98 percent of children first exposed to RSV became infected.[117] Second exposure resulted in 74 percent of the children becoming infected, and a third exposure only reduced the attack rate to 65 percent. In urban Rochester, 44 percent of the families with young children became infected with RSV during the winter months when it was prevalent in the community.[118] Of the exposed family members, 46 percent became infected. Although the attack rate was highest in infants, between 38 and 47 percent of older children and adults acquired RSV infection. In the Houston family study in which children are followed from birth, the infection rate was 68.8 per 100 children in the first year of life, and during the second year at least half were reinfected.[114]

PATHOGENESIS

In adult volunteers experimental infection occurs after an average incubation of 5 days.[119,120] Most studies confirm this as the average incubation period with a range of 2–8 days.[24,121–123] Inoculation of the virus may occur through the nose or eye. The eye and nose appear to be equally sensitive portals of entry and the mouth, a much less sensitive means of inoculation.[124] RSV infection is generally confined to the respiratory tract, and spread of the virus may occur from the upper passageways to involve the entire lower respiratory tract.

Initially in bronchiolitis, the pathologic findings are a lymphocytic peribronchiolar infiltration with some edema of the walls and surrounding tissue.[28,91,125–128] Subsequently, the characteristic proliferation and necrosis of the epithelium of the bronchioles develop. The lumens of these small airways become obstructed from the sloughed epithelium and from the increased mucus secretion. Impedence to the flow of air occurs during both inspiration and expiration but is greater in the latter when the lumen is narrowed further by the positive expiratory pressure. Hyperinflation thus, results from the trapping of air peripheral to the sites of partial occlusion. Subsequently, with complete obstruction multiple areas of atelectasis develop. Thus, in the infant with bronchiolitis, an increase in lung volume and expiratory resistance occurs.[129–132]

Often infants with lower respiratory tract disease from RSV have pathologic evidence of both pneumonia and bronchiolitis. Pneumonia cases demonstrate an intersitital infiltration of mononuclear cells that is sometimes accompanied by edema and necrotic areas that lead to alveolar filling.[125]

Some histologic evidence of recovery is present in most cases of bronchiolitis within the first week of illness and is marked by the beginning regeneration of the bronchiolar epithelium.[125] However, ciliated cells may not be present for weeks, and other morphologic alterations may persist indefinitely.[9]

Theories of Pathogenesis

How RSV engenders these pathogenic findings remains mostly a mystery. RSV is the only respiratory pathogen that produces its most devastating illness at the time when specific antibody, maternally derived, is invariably and abundantly present. The severity of RSV infection in the very young infant and in those children with high levels of circulating antibody induced by an inactivated RSV vaccine has suggested that immunologic mechanisms may contribute to the pathogenesis of the disease in infants.[85,113,133,134]

Recently, increased interest and effort have been devoted to developing an animal model of the enhanced pathology that developed with natural infection in children who had previously received the inactivated RSV vaccine.[135–137] In cotton rats immunized with this formalin-inactivated RSV vaccine and subsequently challenged with live RSV, a similar enhancement of disease occurred with pulmonary pathology resembling an Arthus reaction.[135] The rats developed high levels of ELISA antibody to the F and G glycoproteins but relatively low levels of neutralizing antibody, thus suggesting that formalin inactivated the neutralizing epitopes. Similar antibody responses were found in the serum of the children who had received the inactivated vaccine.[138]

Chanock and colleagues[139,140] suggested some time ago that an immune complex reaction might occur between the virus and passively acquired IgG antibody in the lung of an infant who lacks the local defense of secretory antibody. The inactivated vaccine similarly engendered high levels of IgG antibody but not secretory antibody.[113,133,134] However, this theory of an immune complex (type III) reaction is not supported by levels of maternal antibody or complement being related to the severity of the disease in the infant.[5,141–144]

Chanock et al. and Kim and her coworkers[140,145] noted that the recipients of the inactivated vaccine also had a greater cell-mediated immune response. They thus suggested that a cell-mediated (type IV) immune reaction may occur in the lungs of infected infants.[145] Gardner and his associates[146] proposed that the immunopathologic changes in infants with bronchiolitis stem from an IgE-mediated (type I) response in the lungs of those babies who have previously been sensitized to RSV by natural infection. This theory is based on their observations that infants dying with bronchiolitis had only small amounts of RSV antigen detectable in their lungs by immunofluorescence as compared with infants dying with RSV pneumonia.[146] However, the temporal occurrence of bronchiolitis during an RSV epidemic does not tend to corroborate this concept. Furthermore, most infants with bronchiolitis do not have increased serum IgE levels, nor do they have an anamnestic serologic response.[1,147,148] More recent evidence, however, has suggested that IgE in the respiratory secretions may have a pathogenic role in some infants with RSV disease.[149–151] IgE bound to exfoliated nasopharyngeal epithelial cells has been found in most patients with acute RSV infection but appeared to persist for longer periods in those with wheezing.[149] Furthermore, the titers of RSV-specific IgE and the histamine content in the secretions was significantly higher in infants with RSV infection associated with wheezing.[150]

A fourth hypothesis contends that those infants most severely affected with RSV infection suffer from a developmental immunologic immaturity of imbalance. The young infant's serum antibody response to RSV infection is often poor and appears inversely related to the amount of passively transferred antibody.[141,147]

Furthermore, infants may be incapable of responding with adequate amounts of certain types of antibody. The G protein, being heavily glycosylated, appears to be a relatively poor immunogen in young children.[152] Murphy et al.[153,154] have shown that younger infants produced diminished antibody responses to both the F and G proteins and that most failed to produce serum or nasal wash neutralizing antibody. Passive antibody may also inhibit the specific cytotoxic T-cell response in the infant as suggested by the mouse model.[155]

Alternatively, severe RSV infection in infancy may be explained without involving any immunologic mechanism. Exposure to large doses of virus coupled with the anatomy of the infant's airway during that vulnerable stage of development may be sufficient to produce the severe disease seen in the young baby. Infection in the small peripheral airways of the infant produces greater physiologic changes than in the older child, and the developing lung is anatomically less able to compensate.[9,156]

Immunity

Naturally acquired immunity to RSV infection is incomplete. Repeated infections are common, but severe disease rarely occurs after the primary encounter. Lower respiratory tract involvement may occur with repeated infections, but it is generally confined to those at either end of the age spectrum.[104,114,117,157,158]

The role of serum antibody in immunity to RSV remains a conundrum. In general, the level of serum antibody has not been predictive of the risk of infection, severity of illness, or recovery in children or adults.[5,141,159] Clearly maternal antibody does not provide complete protection during infancy. However, several studies have suggested that high levels of maternal antibody correlate with lower infection rates[103,160–162] and with less severity of illness in some studies[142,161] but not in others.[5,141]

The recent deciphering of the antigenic cloak of RSV has engendered new interst in the role that antibody to the specific viral proteins might play in the cabal of RSV immunity. Monoclonal antibodies to the F and G proteins that were passively administered to rodents have resulted in nearly complete protection against RSV challenge of the lung but not upper respiratory tract.[163–165] Immunization of animals with F, G, and N proteins, either purified or in vaccinia vectors, has resulted in similar protection.[166–170] The immunity afforded by antibody to each of these specific viral proteins in humans is less clear. However, in adults who were repetetively challenged with RSV after a natural infection, the level of ELISA antibody to the F and G protein of the homologous strain correlated inversely with the rate of infection.[171] Protection against illness appeared to correlate most with antibody to the G protein and neutralizing antibody to the homologous strain.

An appreciable proportion of infected infants as well as adults may not produce a significant rise in serum antibody levels.[141,147,153,154,171] In part this is related to young age and inversely to the level of antibody before infection in all age groups. As noted previously, young infants generally have a diminished response to the F and G proteins, and a neutralizing antibody response may not be detectable.[153,154] Age particularly appears to affect the F antibody response, while passive antibody has the greatest effect on the response to the G protein.[153] The antibodies induced in infants by the F and G proteins appear to be primarily of the IgG1 and IgG3 subclasses, which suggests that it is the protein rather than the carbohydrate of these glycoproteins that is immunodominant in young children.[172] In some children specific IgE and IgG4 serum antibodies have been detected, especially in those whose infections are marked by wheezing.[173]

Whether strain variation is a significant factor in determining the immune or clinical response is as of yet unknown. However, in infants with primary infection, the homologous and heterologous antibody responses to the F proteins of the two major subgroups appear to be similar, but not to the G protein to which there is relatively little heterologous response.[76]

Local antibody production may be important in RSV infection since the virus spreads from cell to cell and in animal studies circulating antibody does not prevent viral replication in the nasal passage.[163–165] A number of studies have identified neutralizing activity in the nasal secretion of children with RSV infection, but a correlation with protection or severity of illness was often impossible.[113,139,141,174–176] The presence of this neutralizing activity in the secretions was associated with diminished viral shedding.[139,176,177] However, it was also present at the time of hospital admission in the secretions of infants suffering from primary infections.[175,176] McIntosh and his coworkers[176] have defined the nonspecific nature of this neutralizing activity and have demonstrated that a specific IgA antibody response does occur in infants recovering from RSV infection. Although this specific IgA antibody does not neutralize the virus, its presence is correlated with diminished titers of virus.

Gardner[178] has shown that, in the secretions of RSV-infected children of all ages, specific antibody develops that may be shown by immunofluorescence techniques to coat RSV-infected cells. This antibody is predominantly IgA and appears early in the course of illness. Specific IgM, IgG, and IgE antibodies may also be found in the secretions of children with RSV infections.[150,176,178] The IgM antibody tends to appear early and disappear, and the IgG appears later. Antibody-dependent cell-mediated cytotoxicity (ADCC), primarily associated with immunoglobulin G, has also been detected in the nasopharyngeal secretions of infected children.[179] The ADCC responses appear to peak 2–4 weeks after the onset of illness and are greater after secondary than primary infection.

Using a more sensitive assay, an ELISA with purified F and G protein, Murphy et al.[154] were able to show that the nasal antibody response of infants to the RSV surface glycoproteins was similar to their serum antibody response in that the youngest infants less frequently responded with a significant IgA or IgG nasal antibody to their F and G proteins.

Cell-mediated immunity is likely to be pivotal in the response to infection and recovery. This is supported by the observations that immunosuppressed children, especially those with congenital T-cell defects, as well as experimentally immunosuppressed animals have more severe disease and prolonged shedding.[180–183]

Lymphocytes from the cord blood of most infants demonstrate cell-mediated immunity toward RSV.[184] Specific lymphocyte transformation in the majority of infants with RSV infection has been detected in their convalescent sera.[184,185] A pathogenic role for this immune response has been suggested by the tendency for infants with more severe disease to develop greater cell-mediated immune responses.[145]

In mice, immunization with RSV proteins has been shown to induce memory cell populations of cytotoxic T cells aimed at the specific viral proteins.[186,187] Similarly, specific cytotoxic responses of lymphocytes from the peripheral blood of adults have also been demonstrated and from a few infants with RSV bronchiolitis who were under 4 months of age.[187–189]

CLINICAL MANIFESTATIONS

Infection in Young Children

Primary infections with RSV may be manifested as lower respiratory tract disease, pneumonia, bronchiolitis, tracheobronchitis, or upper respiratory tract illness often accompanied by fever and otitis media. Rarely is the infection asymptomatic.[4,22,25,107,117] The risk of lower respiratory tract involvement occurring with the first infection appears high. Pneumonia or bronchiolitis has been estimated to occur in 30–71 percent.[5,24,107,114,117] In closed populations of infants, the proportion developing lower respiratory tract disease may be even higher, up to 89 percent.[122,123] Even in previously healthy outpatients the proportion who develop lower respiratory tract disease is high (Fig. 4).

Of the lower respiratory tract syndromes, pneumonia and bronchiolitis are the most frequent in infants.[3,4,107,174] Croup is the least common form of clinical illness and usually accounts for less than 5–10 percent of the cases.[107] Pneumonia and bronchiolitis are often difficult to differentiate, and many infants may appear to have both syndromes. Wheezing, rhonchi, rales, and infiltrates on chest roentgenograms may be present in both syndromes.[91,95] In bronchiolitis, the infiltrates are due to atelectasis, but these often cannot be differentiated from the inflammatory shadows of pneumonia. In bronchiolitis the two classic signs of wheezing and hyperaeration of the lung must be present.

Lower respiratory tract disease is usually heralded by an upper respiratory tract infection with nasal congestion and often pharyngitis. Fever occurs in most young children, with temperatures ranging from 38° to 40°C. Usually fever is present for 2–4 days. The height or duration of the fever does not correlate with the severity of the disease and is frequently absent at the time of admission to the hospital.[89,123] Cough may be the most frequent and predominant sign. It may be paroxysmal and associated with vomiting, but not with a ''whoop'' typical of pertussis.[27,53,89,190] Laryngitis or hoarseness is not a common feature. Usually after several days of upper respiratory tract signs and a deepening cough, the lower respiratory tract involvement may become evident by the onset of dyspnea, an increased respiratory rate, and retractions of the intercostal muscles. In bronchiolitis expiration tends to be prolonged, and the respiratory rate may be remarkably elevated, often reaching 80 respirations per minute. Intercostal retractions are also particularly prominent in bronchiolitis, which emphasizes that there is inspiratory obstruction of the lower airway as well as the more obvious expiratory obstruction. On ascultation, the infant may have rales, rhonchi, and wheezing, which may be intermittently present and may fluctuate in intensity.[27,191,192]

The chest roentgenogram may show a variety of findings, most typically multiple areas of interstitial infiltration and hyperinflation of the lung.[193–195] Hyperaeration has been shown to be especially indicative of RSV infection and occurs in over half of the children hospitalized with RSV infection.[91,195] Hyperaeration was commonly present with peribronchial thickening, but in 15 percent hyperaeration was the only abnormality. Consolidation has been noted in about 20–25 percent of the children and most commonly is subsegmental in the right upper or middle lobe.[194,195]Pleural fluid is rarely demonstrated, although one study states its occurrence at 5 percent.[194] Thus, although certain signs such as hyperinflation and right upper or middle lobe consolidation may be indicative of RSV infection, roentgenographic differentiation from infection by other viruses and at times bacteria often is not possible.

Cyanosis is rarely evident in infants hospitalized with RSV lower respiratory tract disease despite hypoxemia that may be profound.[192,196,197] All infants hospitalized with RSV lower respiratory tract disease during one outbreak were examined, and all were hypoxemic.[196] On admission to the hospital their mean arterial oxygen saturation was 87 percent (equivalent to a PaO_2 of 53 mmHg) with a range of 74–95 percent (40–75 mmHg). The degree of hypoxemia and thus the severity of the illness were difficult to assess clinically. Moderate to severe degrees of hypoxemia were present without cyanosis. The degree of hypoxemia could be correlated with an increasing respiratory rate, but not with the severity of the wheezing, retractions, lethargy, or irritability. Abnormalities in the arterial oxygen saturation were prolonged beyond the time of discharge, which correlates with the prolonged viral shedding of these infants.[83,196] In most infants the duration of illness is 7–21 days, and hospitalization, if required, averages 4–7 days.[89,196,198,199]

Otitis Media

Otitis media is a common complication of RSV infection in young children.[24,27,89,118,200–205] It may accompany both primary and secondary infection, but it is most frequent in infants. In one series of nine infants hospitalized with RSV lower respiratory tract disease, the virus was recovered from an ear aspiration in all the infants.[201] RSV appeared to be the sole path-

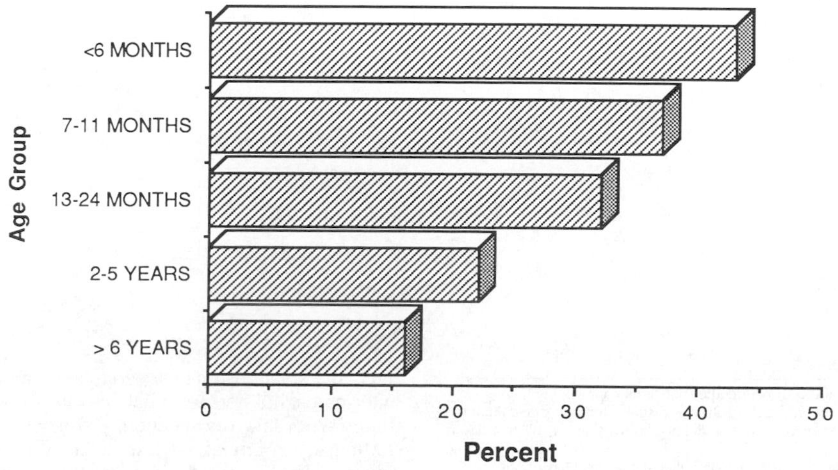

FIG. 4. The proportion of outpatients according to age in Rochester, New York, 1977–1987, who were infected with RSV and developed lower respiratory tract disease.

ogen, and bacteria were not simultaneously recovered. In other studies RSV was recovered alone and in conjunction with a bacterial pathogen, usually *Streptococcus pneumoniae*.[202–205] That RSV may have a primary as well as a secondary role in the development of otitis media has also been indicated by the demonstration that RSV may replicate within the middle ear of experimental animals.[89,200]

Infections in Older Children and Adults

Repeated or secondary infections occurring after the first 3 years of life are most commonly manifested as an upper respiratory tract illness or tracheobronchitis, or they may be asymptomatic.[107,114,118] Occasionally, however, lower respiratory tract illness may occur.[158,206,207]

When families infected with RSV have been studied, repeated infection was rarely found to be asymptomatic.[118] Most family members developed signs of upper respiratory tract infection, with nasal congestion and cough as the most common signs (Table 2). Fever and earache were more common in young children than in the older family members. Although RSV infections may mimic the common cold, they tend to be more severe and prolonged than are other upper respiratory tract infections.[118,208] Illnesses caused by RSV are associated with a greater frequency of fever and conjunctivitis in the acute phase of the illness and with more prolonged nasal congestion, cough, and earache (Table 2). One week after the start of their RSV illness only 32 percent of the family members had recovered as compared with 74 percent of those with respiratory illnesses not caused by RSV. The family members with RSV infection remained symptomatic for an average of 9 days and a range of 1–32 days.

TABLE 2. Frequency of Signs and Symptoms in 37 Illnesses Associated with Respiratory Syncytial Virus (RSV) and in 82 Illnesses Not Associated with RSV

Sign or Symptom	*RSV- Associated Illness (%)*	*RSV- Negative Illness (%)*	P *Value*[a]
Nasal congestion			
Acute[b]	91.9	83	NS
Late[c]	59.5	26	>.001
Cough			
Acute	81.1	78	NS
Late	45.9	21	<.01
Hoarseness			
Acute	35.1	26	NS
Late	2.7	4	NS
Sore throat			
Acute	32.4	37	NS
Late	2.7	5	NS
Fever			
Acute	27.0	13	>.05–<.10
Late	5.4	1	NS
Conjunctivitis			
Acute	24.3	12	>.05–<.10
Late	0.0	2	NS
Earache			
Acute	18.9	13	NS
Late	13.5	2	<.05
Rash			
Acute	8.1	4	NS
Late	5.4	1	NS
Asymptomatic			
Acute	—	—	NS
Late	32.4	74	<.001

[a] Probability is derived from the chi-square test; NS denotes not significant.

[b] Acute RSV illness is defined as occurring on the day RSV was first isolated plus one culture day before or after isolation; acute RSV-negative illness is defined as starting on the first day of symptoms plus the next culture day.

[c] Late RSV illness is defined as occurring on the first day after the acute phase until the first symptomatic day; late RSV-negative illness is defined as occurring on the first day after the acute phase to the first symptomatic day.

(From Hall et al.,[118] with permission.)

Natural RSV infection in adults has been studied most closely in hospital staff, who generally are young, healthy adults with close exposure to infected infants.[207,209–212] Most of these young adults were symptomatic with their RSV infection. In half, the illness was severe enough to cause some incapacitation. Viral shedding in these adults occurred for an average of 3–6 days, with a range of 1–2 days. In a proportion of these adults with moderate clinical symptoms, serial pulmonary function testing was performed. In all those tested total pulmonary resistance was elevated, and hyperreactivity of the airway to cholinergic stimulus was demonstrated for 8 weeks after the onset of illness (Fig. 5).[207] This prolonged hyperreactivity has been postulated as resulting from the epithelial inflammation and damage caused by the virus. With destruction of the normal epithelium, sensitization of the rapidly adapting sensory receptors of the airways may occur.

In adults with underlying diseases, RSV infections can involve both the upper and the lower respiratory tract and occasionally appear to have a spectrum of illness similar to that seen in infants. In adults with chronic bronchitis, RSV infection has been associated with an exacerbation of their bronchitis.[158,213,214] In hospitalized adults, RSV has been associated with bronchitis, pneumonia, and influenza-like illnesses.[158,206,214–217] In the elderly, outbreaks of RSV infection have been associated with a particularly high proportion developing bronchopneumonia.[158,215–217] In one study of hospitalized older patients (most over 70 years of age), two-thirds developed pneumonia. In a recent outbreak in a nursing home, 25 percent of the women and 5 percent of the men were infected. Pneumonia developed in 47 percent, 87 percent had fever.[217]

Uncommon Manifestations of RSV Infection

Respiratory syncytial virus infection has occasionally been associated with disease of the central nervous system. The role of the virus in producing these disorders is unclear. Nevertheless, RSV infection has been identified in patients with a variety of central nervous system disorders such as meningitis, myelitis, ataxia, and hemiplegia.[218,219] Although the infection could

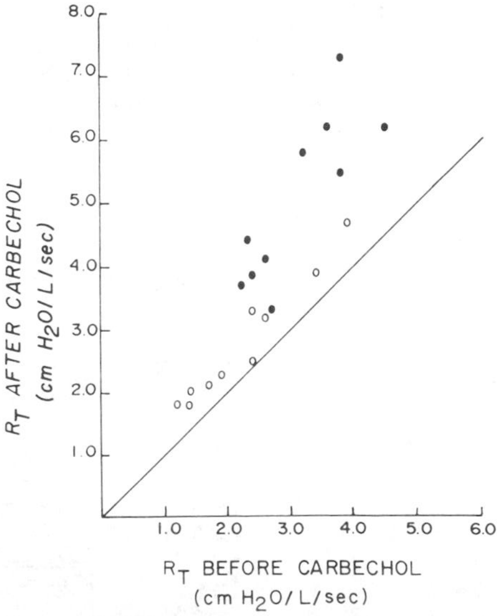

FIG. 5. Relationship between total pulmonary resistance (R_T) before and after carbachol aerosol inhalation in 10 normal adults with acute respiratory syncytial virus infection. Closed circles are values obtained at initial testing; open circles, at testing 16 weeks later. The line is the line of identity. The increased airway reactivity demonstrated on the initial testing was prolonged beyond the time of the clinical symptoms and lasted for at least 8 weeks. (Data from Hall et al.[207])

be coincidental, specific antibody to RSV was detected in the cerebrospinal fluid of several children with meningitis and myelitis.[218] RSV has also rarely been associated with the development of myocarditis and complete heart block.[28,220] A variety of exanthems involving the trunk and/or face have also occasionally been related to RSV infection.[221,222]

NOSOCOMIAL INFECTION

Respiratory syncytial viral infection nosocomially acquired has recently been recognized both in this country and in England as a frequent and concerning occurrence.[121,209–212,223–233] The following are reasons for the magnitude of the problem: (*1*) RSV is an ubiquitous and frequent infection. It regularly causes outbreaks affecting a very high proportion of young children, and a number of these children with lower respiratory tract disease are admitted to the hospital each year. (*2*) These infants are highly contagious and shed high titers of virus for prolonged periods.[83,198] Once the virus is introduced onto the ward, a susceptible population is always present. Repeated infections are common, and thus, any infant or member of the hospital staff is potentially susceptible. (*3*) Those children most at risk for the complications of RSV infection, young infants with underlying diseases, are apt to be grouped in an infants' ward.

In 1941 Adams[234] described an outbreak of pneumonia that affected young hospitalized infants and resulted in the death of 28 percent. This was probably the first description of a nosocomial outbreak of RSV infection, but only some 20 years later was RSV implicated as the cause when Adams and his coworkers[20,235] observed a similar outbreak of RSV illness in infants. Fortunately, the more recent nosocomial outbreaks of RSV have not been associated with such a high mortality. Nevertheless, fatal infection from nosocomial acquisition of RSV still does occur.[211,228,232,233] During one community outbreak of RSV infection, 45 percent of the infants not admitted with RSV infection became infected after 1 week in the hospital.[209] The risk of nosocomial infection increased with an increasing duration of hospitalization. The nosocomial infections acquired by infants are almost always symptomatic and range from a febrile upper respiratory tract illness to severe lower respiratory tract involvement and death.[209–211,232,233] Pneumonia or bronchiolitis is a common manifestation of nosocomial illness in infants and occurs in one-third to one-half of those affected.

How RSV spreads so effectively on infant wards is not entirely clear. However, adults caring for these infants appear to be important in the spread of the virus.[109–211,223–226,231–233] During these nosocomial outbreaks, close to one-half of the hospital personnel have acquired RSV infection.[209–211,223,224,232] Transmission of the virus appeared to occur not only through the staff becoming infected but also possibly by their spreading contaminated secretions from infected infants. This mode of spread appears feasible since RSV in the secretions of an infected infant may survive on countertops for 7 to over 24 hours and on hospital gowns, paper, tissues, and skin for 15–60 minutes.[50] Furthermore, infectious virus may be recovered from hands that have contacted these contaminated surfaces. A subsequent study on an infant ward during an RSV outbreak confirmed that fomite spread can occur.[231] Volunteers were exposed to infected infants in one of three ways that allowed spread to occur: (*1*) close contact, (*2*) fomites with subsequent self-inoculation, or (*3*) small-particle aerosol. Volunteers exposed by either of the first two but not the last method became infected. For infection control procedures, see the subsequent section on prevention.

COMPLICATIONS

Complicated RSV infection is most likely to occur in young infants and those with underlying diseases, especially those with cardiopulmonary and congenital disorders[28,89,180,182,199,229] (Fig. 6). It has been estimated that between one-quarter and two-thirds of the fatal RSV infections occur in children with such underlying diseases.[28,89,125–238,180,236] Infants in the first few months of life with congenital heart disease appear particularly at risk for severe or fatal RSV infection.[236] In one prospective study of hospitalized infants with congenital heart disease and RSV infection, the mortality rate was 37 percent.[236] If pulmonary hypertension complicated their cardiac lesions, 73 percent died from their RSV illness. Of note was that one-fifth of the infants had acquired their RSV infection nosocomially.

Immunosuppressed patients of all ages also appear at risk for complicated and sometimes fatal RSV infection.[180–182,237–241] These patients tend to have prolonged and intermittent shedding of the virus and severe lower respiratory tract disease even at older ages, including adulthood. In such patients, the mechanisms to control the spread of the virus appear greatly diminished, thus resulting in not only prolonged but also abundant shedding and sometimes multiplication of the virus beyond the respiratory tract to other organs.

The acute complications of RSV infection in infants include apnea, respiratory failure, and rarely secondary bacterial infection. Apnea has been demonstrated to occur in about 20 percent of the infants hospitalized with RSV infection.[196,242–244] Infants who appear particularly at risk for this complication are those in the first couple of months of life, those who were premature, and those developing moderate to severe hypoxemia.[196,242–244] RSV infection has also been associated with the sudden infant death syndrome, particularly in infants over 3 months of age.[126,127,229,245,246] Progressive hypercarbia, respiratory failure, and apnea are the major reasons leading to assisted ventilation. Although hypoxemia is very common in hospitalized infants, progressive hypercarbia is uncommon.[192,193,196] Secondary bacterial infection is unusual in RSV infection.[27,89,125,247,248] In a 9-year prospective study of infants hospitalized with RSV lower respiratory tract disease, secondary bacterial pneumonia occurred in less that 1 percent but appeared to be more frequent in infants who had been treated with broad-spectrum antibiotics.[247]

The long-term complications of RSV infection are difficult to delineate. Whether hypoxemia, prolonged or unrecognized, in infancy affects the infant's later development is unknown. However, evidence has recently been accumulated to suggest that pulmonary function may be affected later in life. Bronchiolitis in infancy has been associated with an increased chance of recurrent wheezing and asthma.[10–12] More recent evidence has suggested that, even in people without an allergic predisposition, bronchiolitis and other lower respiratory tract disease in infancy may be a major risk factor in the development of chronic obstructive airway disease in later life. The epide-

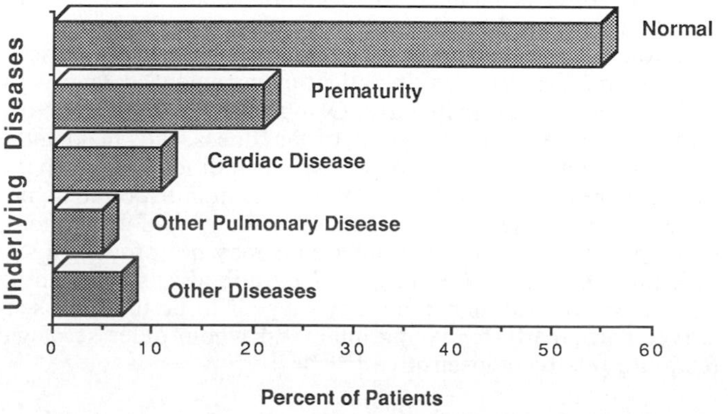

FIG. 6. Proportion of patients admitted with RSV infection to Strong Memorial Hospital, Rochester, New York, 1985–1987, who have underlying diseases.

miologic studies from Tucson[7,249] indicate that a history of childhood respiratory disease is associated with relatively mild impairment of pulmonary function in young adults but that in later years it is associated with an excessive decrease in ventilatory function, even in nonsmokers. In these studies the exact etiology of the childhood respiratory illness was not known. But in studies from Tyneside[250–252] children with RSV bronchiolitis in infancy were examined 8–10 years later. Approximately half the children had had subsequent, usually mild, episodes of wheezing. When compared with control children, those with RSV bronchiolitis in infancy had significantly greater exercise-induced bronchial lability and lower maximum expiratory flow rates at rest but no excess of atopy. These authors concluded that bronchiolitis and subsequent asthma were not closely related but that the link to later respiratory disease may be from the RSV infection, a genetic predisposition, and environmental factors.[250–252] Kattan and coworkers[13] have also followed children who as infants were hospitalized with bronchiolitis during a winter outbreak. Ten years after their hospitalization these children, who had been asymptomatic and free of all signs of allergy in the interim, received careful pulmonary function testing. The majority had an abnormal PaO_2, abnormal volume of isoflow, and an elevated ratio of the residual volume to total lung capacity. Thirty-one percent of these children, although asymptomatic, had all three of these pulmonary abnormalities, thus suggesting residual small airway disease. The relative contribution to the development of later chronic lung disease from RSV infection in infancy and from genetic and environmental factors is yet to be determined.

DIAGNOSIS

The diagnosis of RSV infection in infants with lower respiratory tract disease may often be made with reasonable accuracy on the basis of clinical and epidemiologic findings. Confirmation may be made by viral isolation or one of the new rapid diagnostic tests. A nasal wash is the preferred specimen to be obtained for viral isolation since it produces the highest rate of virus recovery.[58] Alternatively, a swab of the nasopharynx and one of the throat combined together in one vial of medium can be used. Since RSV is a relatively labile virus, the specimen should be inoculated onto the proper cell line as soon as possible. An appreciable decrease in the titer of the virus may occur if the specimens are subjected to freezing, thawing, or pH changes.[21,49,253] With proper handling of the specimens, the virus may be identified by its characteristic cytopathic effect within 3–7 days and often by the fourth day.[58,253]

A variety of rapid techniques for the identification of the viral antigen in clinical specimens are now commercially available, including direct and indirect immunofluorescent assays and ELISA.[254–256] In general, the immunofluorescent assays using monoclonal antibodies are somewhat more sensitive and specific, but for large numbers of specimens the ELISA offers the advantages of speed and objective readings.

Serologic diagnosis of RSV infection has been most useful for epidemiologic studies. In patient management, diagnosis by serologic tests is of limited use. Convalescent sera must be obtained 2–4 weeks after the onset of the illness, thus making the diagnosis in most cases retrospective. In addition, infants in the first 6 months of life, especially the first 3 months, often do not produce an adequate antibody response.[152–154] Furthermore, older patients with repeated infections may not produce a significant rise in antibody titer.[23,119,171] Antibody rises measured by ELISA or neutralization assays appear to be the most sensitive, particularly for young infants in whom older serologic tests are relatively insensitive.[153,154,257,258]

PREVENTION AND TREATMENT

Good supportive care is of the utmost importance in the management of severely ill infants. Alleviation of the hypoxemia and monitoring of the infant's respiratory status and blood gas levels are essential in the management. Since the hypoxemia is related to an unequal ratio of ventilation to perfusion, most infants respond to relatively low concentrations of inspired oxygen of about 40 percent.[196,197] Corticosteroids have been shown to be of no benefit in these lower respiratory tract infections.[259,260] Bronchodilating agents have generally not been of benefit in RSV lower respiratory tract disease and may have unwanted side effects in marginally compensated small infants.[130,261] However, a small subgroup of infants with hyperreactive airways may respond to a carefully monitored trial of aerosolized or parenteral bronchodilators.

Recently ribavirin, a synthetic nucleoside that is a broad-spectrum antiviral agent, was approved for the treatment of infants hospitalized with RSV lower respiratory tract disease.[262] The drug is administered as a small-particle aerosol into a tent, oxyhood, mask, or ventilator for a period of 12–18 hours each day, usually for 2–5 days, depending on the time to improvement. All the controlled studies to date have shown benefit in diminishing clinical severity and significantly improving the infants' arterial oxygen saturation.[263–272] Ribavirin is virustatic, and viral shedding may not be eradicated after a course of therapy. However, when it has been used in infants with severe combined immunodeficiency disease with overwhelming viral infection, shedding ceased within 24 hours but tended to recur once treatment was stopped, thus necessitating repeated courses.[273,274] The drug appears to be well tolerated by aerosol, and toxicity has not been repored. The long-term effects of ribavirin and whether it will affect the rate of subsequent pulmonary function abnormalities associated with RSV infection are unknown. Of interest, however, is the observation that ribavirin inhibits the RSV-specific IgE response in the nasal secretions that has been associated with the development of wheezing and hypoxia.[275] Aerosol administration for 8–20 hours gives drug levels in the secretions that are hundreds of times the median inhibitory concentration for RSV, but relatively little is systemically absorbed, and blood levels are low.[276]

Prevention

The search for a vaccine to prevent RSV infection in infancy has been underway for over a decade. The initial vaccines developed in the 1960s were alum precipitated and formalin inactivated. These vaccines produced excellent rates and levels of antibody response. Despite this, the vaccines were not protective and even predisposed the recipient to more exaggerated disease during subsequent natural infection.[113,133,134,142,277] Subsequently, a live attenuated vaccine has been sought.[139,278,279] One such vaccine, adapted to grow at 26°C, appeared promising in children and adults already possessing antibody.[280–282] In seronegative infants, however, the vaccine produced illness involving the lower respiratory tract.[281,282] Similarly, another attenuated vaccine developed from a temperature-sensitive mutant produced unacceptable degrees of illness in seronegative infants.[278,280–284] The search for more suitable live attenuated vaccines continues.[278] A recent avenue of approach has been to develop a subunit vaccine for RSV by using a purified surface glycoprotein, particularly the F protein.

Immunoglobulin has been administered to animals and been shown to afford protection against experimental RSV infection; it also appeared to be synergystic if administered with ribavirin.[285–287] In a subsequent double-blind, placebo-controlled study, intravenous immunoglobulin containing high titers of RSV neutralizing antibody was administered to children hospitalized with RSV infection and appeared to be beneficial.[288] Intravenous immunoglobulin given to high-risk infants on a monthly basis during the RSV season is now being explored as a possible means of prophylaxis.

Other methods of prevention or protection of the infant are as of yet mostly unexplored. Breast-feeding appears to offer the infant some protection against RSV lower respiratory tract infection. Epidemiologic studies have suggested that the risk of acquiring RSV infection requiring hospitalization is less in infants who are breast-fed.[95,229,289,290]

Prevention of infection through interruption of transmission of the virus is probably impossible at home. However, on hospital wards attempts to prevent spread of the virus are warranted. RSV may be spread by close contact and by direct inoculation of droplets of the secretions from an infected person. In addition, however, RSV may possibly be spread indirectly from the hands touching infectious secretions that contaminate surfaces in the environment.[50,209,210,231] Hence, careful handwashing by all personnel is of particular importance. The use of eye-nose goggles has been shown to appreciably decrease the nosocomial infection rate, assumedly by decreasing self-inoculation of the virus into the eyes and nose.[223,224] The use of gowns and masks has not been shown to be of further benefit in two studies.[212,291] However, in another study increased compliance with a policy of glove and gown isolation precautions significantly reduced the nosocomial infection rate.[225] Infected infants should be separated from the other infants on the ward, and staff with respiratory illness during RSV outbreaks should not care for those infants most at risk for complicated RSV infection.[210,232,233]

REFERENCES

1. Brandt CD, Kim HW, Arrobio JO, et al. Epidemiology of respiratory syncytial virus infection in Washington, DC. III. Composite analysis of eleven consecutive yearly epidemics. Am J Epidemiol. 1973;98:355–64.
2. Chanock RM, Parrott RH. Acute respiratory disease in infancy and childhood: Present understanding and prospects for prevention. Pediatrics. 1965;36:21–39.
3. Glezen WP, Denny FW. Epidemiology of acute lower respiratory disease in children. N Engl J Med. 1973;288:498–505.
4. Kim HW, Arrobio JO, Brandt CD, et al. Epidemiology of respiratory syncytial virus infection in Washington DC. I. Importance of the virus in different respiratory tract disease syndromes and temporal distribution of infection. Am J Epidemiol. 1973;98:216–25.
5. Parrott RH, Kim HW, Arrobio JO, et al. Epidemiology of respiratory syncytial virus infection in Washington, DC. II. Infection and disease with respect to age, immunologic status, race and sex. Am J Epidemiol. 1973;98:289–300.
6. Burrows B, Lebowitz MD, Knudson RJ. Epidemiologic evidence that childhood problems predispose to airways disease in the adult (an association between adult and pediatric respiratory disorders). Pediatr Res. 1977;11:218–20.
7. Burrows B, Knudson RJ, Lebowitz MD. The relationship of childhood respiratory illness to adult obstructive airway disease. Am Rev Respir Dis. 1977;115:751–60.
8. Chernick V. The vulnerable small airway. Pediatrics. 1977;59:783–4.
9. Reid L. Influence of the pattern of structural growth of lung on susceptibility to specific infectious diseases in infants and children. Pediatr Res. 1977;11:210–5.
10. Eisen AH, Bacal HL. The relationship of acute bronchiolitis to bronchial asthma. A 4- to 14-year follow-up. Pediatrics. 1963;31:859–61.
11. Rooney JC, Williams HE. The relationship between proved viral bronchiolitis and subsequent wheezing. J Pediatr. 1971;79:744–7.
12. Zweiman B, Schoenwetter WF, Hildreth EA. The relationship between bronchiolitis and allergic asthma. J Allergy. 1966;37:48–53.
13. Kattan M, Klens TG, Lapierre JG, et al. Pulmonary function abnormalities in symptom-free children after bronchiolitis. Pediatrics. 1977;59:683–8.
14. Gurwitz D, Mindorff C, Levison H. Increased incidence of bronchial reactivity in children with a history of bronchiolitis. J Pediatr. 1981;98:551–5.
15. Stokes GM, Milner AD, Hodges IGC, et al. Lung function abnormalities after acute bronchiolitis. J Pediatr. 1981;98:871–4.
16. Twiggs JT, Larson LA, O'Connell EJ, et al. Respiratory syncytial virus infection: Ten year follow-up. Clin Pediatr (Phila). 1981;20:187–90.
17. Morris JA, Blount RE, Savage RE. Recovery of cytopathogenic agent from chimpanzees with coryza. Proc Soc Exp Biol Med. 1956;92:544–9.
18. Chanock R, Roizman B, Myers R. Recovery from infants with respiratory illness of a virus related to chimpanzee coryza agent (CCA): I. Isolation, properties and characterization. Am J Hyg. 1957;66:281–90.
19. Chanock RM, Finberg L. Recovery from infants with respiratory illness of a virus related to chimpanzee coryza agent (CCA): II. Epidemiologic aspects of infection in infants and young children. Am J Hyg. 1957;66:291–300.
20. Adams JM, Imagawa DT, Zike K. Epidemic bronchiolitis and pneumonitis related to respiratory syncytial virus. JAMA. 1961;176:1037–9.
21. Beem M, Wright FH, Hamre D, et al. Association of the chimpanzee coryza agent with acute respiratory disease in children. N Engl J Med. 1960;263:523–30.
22. Chanock RM, Kim HW, Vargosko AJ, et al. Respiratory syncytial virus. I. Virus recovery and other observations during 1960 outbreak of bronchiolitis pneumonia, and minor respiratory diseases in children. JAMA. 1961;176:647–53.
23. Hamre D, Procknow JJ. Viruses isolated from natural common colds in the USA. Br Med J. 1961;2:1382–5.
24. Kapikian AZ, Bell JA, Mastrota FM, et al. An outbreak of febrile illness and pneumonia associated with respiratory syncytial virus infection. Am J Hyg. 1961;74:234–48.
25. McClelland L, Hilleman MR, Hamparian VV, et al. Studies of acute respiratory illnesses caused by respiratory syncytial virus. N Engl J Med. 1961;264:1169–75.
26. Parrott RH, Vargosko AJ, Kim HW, et al. Respiratory syncytial virus. II. Serologic studies over a 34-month period of children with bronchiolitis, pneumonia, and minor respiratory diseases. JAMA. 1961;176:653–7.
27. Reilly CM, Stokes J Jr, McClelland L, et al. Studies of acute respiratory illness caused by respiratory syncytial virus. 3. Clinical and laboratory findings. N Engl J Med. 1961;264:1176–82.
28. Gardner PS, Turk DC, Aherne WA, et al. Deaths associated with respiratory tract infection in childhood. Br Med J. 1967;4:316–20.
29. Grist NR, Ross CAC, Stott EJ. Influenza, respiratory syncytial virus, and pneumonia in Glasgow, 1962–1965. Br Med J. 1967;1:456–7.
30. Suto T, Yano N, Ikeda M, et al. Respiratory syncytial virus infection and its serologic epidemiology. Am J Epidemiol. 1965;82:211–24.
31. Fenner F. The classification and nomenclature of viruses. Summary of the results of the International Committee on Taxonomy of viruses in Madrid, September, 1975. Virology. 1976;71:371–8.
32. Berthiaume L, Joncas J, Pavilanis V. Comparative structure, morphogenesis, and biological characteristics of the respiratory syncytial (RS) virus and the pneumonia virus of mice (PVM). Arch Gesamte Virusforsch. 1974;45:39–51.
33. Lambert DM, Pons MW, Mbuy GN, et al. Nucleic acids of respiratory syncytial virus. J Virol. 1980;36:837–46.
34. Waterson AP, Hobson D. Relationship between respiratory syncytial virus and Newcastle disease parainfluenza group. Br Med J. 1962;2:1166–7.
35. Huang YT, Collins PL, Wertz GW. Characterization of the 10 proteins of human respiratory syncytial virus: Identification of a fourth envelope-associated protein. Virus Res. 1985;2:157–73.
36. Dickens LE, Collins PL, Wertz GW. Transcriptional mapping of human respiratory syncytial virus. J Virol. 1984;52:364–9.
37. Collins PL, Huang YT, Wertz GW. Identification of a tenth mRNA of respiratory syncytial virus and assignment of polypeptides to the 10 viral genes. J Virol. 1984;49:572–8.
38. Collins PL, Wertz GW. cDNA cloning and transcriptional mapping of nine polyadenylated RNAs encoded by the genome of human respiratory syncytial virus. Proc Natl Acad Sci USA. 1983;80:3208–12.
39. Walsh EE, Brandriss MW, Schlesinger JJ. Purification and characterization of the respiratory syncytial virus fusion protein. J Gen Virol. 1985;66:409–15.
40. Walsh EE, Schlesinger JJ, Brandreiss MW. Purification and characterization of GP90, one of the envelope glycoproteins of respiratory syncytial virus. J Gen Virol. 1984;65:761–7.
41. Satake M, Venkatesan S. Nucleotide sequence of the gene encoding respiratory syncytial virus matrix protein. J Virol. 1984;50:92–9.
42. Baybutt HN, Pringle CR. Molecular cloning and sequencing of the F and 22 K membrane protein genes of the RSS-2 strain of respiratory syncytial virus. J Gen Virol. 1987;68:2789–96.
43. Wertz GW, Collins PL, Huang YT, et al. Nucleotide sequence of the G protein gene of human respiratory syncytial virus reveals an unusual type of viral membrane protein. Proc Natl Acad Sci USA. 1985;82:4075–9.
44. Elango N, Satake M, Venkatesan S. mRNA sequence of three respiratory syncytial virus genes encoding two nonstructural proteins and a 22K structural protein. J Virol. 1985;55:101–10.
45. Collins PL, Wertz GW. Nucleotide sequences of the 1B and 1C nonstructural protein mRNAs of human respiratory syncytal virus. Virology. 1985;143:442–51.
46. Collins PL, Wertz GW. The 1A protein gene of human respiratory syncytial virus: Nucleotide sequence of the mRNA and a related polycistronic transcript. Virology. 1985;141:283–91.
47. Satake M, Elango N, Venkatesan S. Sequence analysis of the respiratory syncytial virus phosphoprotein gene. J Virol. 1984;52:991–4.
48. Collins PL, Anderson K, Langer SJ, et al. Correct sequence for the major nucleocapsid protein mRNA of respiratory syncytial virus. Virology. 1985;146:69–77.
49. Hambling MH. Survival of the respiratory syncytial virus during storage under various conditions. Br J Exp Pathol. 1964;45:647–55.
50. Hall CB, Geiman JM, Douglas RG Jr. Possible transmission by fomites of respiratory syncytial virus. J Infect Dis. 1980;141:98–102.
51. Rechsteiner J, Winkler KC. Inactivation of respiratory syncytial virus in aerosol. J Gen Virol. 1969;5:405–10.
52. Parrott RH, Kim HW, Brandt CD, et al. Respiratory syncytial virus. In: Lennette EH, Schmidt NJ, eds. Diagnostic Procedures for Viral Rickettsial and Chlamydial Infections. Washington, DC. American Public Health Association; 1979:695–708.
53. Tyrrell DAJ. Discovering and defining the etiology of acute respiratory disease. Am Rev Respir Dis. 1963;88:77–84.

54. Baldridge P, Senterfit LB. Persistent infection of cells in culture by respiratory syncytial virus (39286). Proc Soc Exp Biol Med. 1976;151:684–8.
55. Jordan WS Jr. Growth characteristics of respiratory syncytial virus. J Immunol. 1962;88:581–90.
56. Klein JD, Strangert K, Collier AM. Stability of respiratory syncytial virus in a new bentonite holding medium. J Clin Microbiol. 1975;1:534–5.
57. Treuhaft MW, Beem MO. Defective interfering particles of respiratory syncytial virus. Infect Immun. 1982;37:439–44.
58. Hall CB, Douglas RG Jr. Clinically useful method for the isolation of respiratory syncytial virus. J Infect Dis. 1975;131:1–5.
59. Kisch AL, Johnson KM, Chanock RM. Immunofluorescence with respiratory syncytial virus. Virology. 1962;16:177–89.
60. Bennett CR Jr, Hamre D. Growth and serological characteristics of respiratory syncytial virus. J Infect Dis. 1962;110:8–16.
61. Levine S, Hamilton R. Kinetics of the respiratory syncytial virus growth cycle in HeLa cells. Arch Gesamte Virusforsch. 1969;28:122–32.
62. Senterfit LB. Persistent infection of RSV. In: RSV Workshop. Washington, DC: National Institutes of Health. July 20–21, 1977.
63. Coates HV, Alling DW, Chanock RM. An antigenic analysis of respiratory syncytial virus isolates by a plaque reduction neutralization test. Am J Epidemiol. 1966;83:229–313.
64. Coates HV, Kendrick L, Chanock RM. Antigenic differences between two strains of respiratory syncytial virus (28221). Proc Soc Exp Biol Med. 1963;112:958–64.
65. Hierholzer JC, Hirsch MS. Croup and pneumonia in human infants associated with a new strain of respiratory syncytial virus. J Infect Dis. 1979;140:826–8.
66. Anderson LJ, Hierholzer JC, Tsou C, et al. Antigenic characterization of respiratory syncytial virus strains with monoclonal antibodies. J Infect Dis. 1985;151:626–33.
67. Mufson MA, Orvell C, Rafnar B, et al. Two distinct subtypes of human respiratory syncytial virus. J Gen Virol. 1985;66:2111–24.
68. Hendry RM, Talis AL, Godfrey E, et al. Concurrent circulation of antigenically distinct strains of respiratory syncytial virus during community outbreaks. J Infect Dis. 1986;153:291–7.
69. Norrby E, Mufson MA, Hooshmand S. Structural differences between subtype A and B strains of respiratory syncytial virus. J Gen Virol. 1986;67:2721–9.
70. Akerlind B, Norrby E. Occurrence of respiratory syncytial virus subtypes A and B strains in Sweden. J Med Virol. 1986;19:241–7.
71. Johnson PR, Spriggs MK, Olmsted RA, et al. The G glycoprotein of human respiratory syncytial viruses of subgroups A and B: Extensive sequence divergence between antigenically related proteins. Proc Natl Acad Sci USA. 1987;84:5625–9.
72. Walsh EE, Brandriss MW, Schlesinger JJ. Immunological differences between the envelope glycoproteins of two strains of human respiratory syncytial virus. J Gen Virol. 1987;68:2169–76.
73. Morgan LA, Routledge EG, Willcocks MM, et al: Strain variations of respiratory syncytial virus. J Gen Virol. 1987;68:2781–8.
74. Mufson MA, Belshe RB, Orvell C, et al. Respiratory syncytial virus epidemics: Variable dominance of subgroups A and B strains among children, 1981–1986. J Infect Dis. 1988;157:143–8.
75. Johnson PR, Olmsted RA, Prince GA, et al. Antigenic relatedness between glycoproteins of human respiratory syncytial virus subgroups A and B: Evaluation of the contributions of F and G glycoproteins to immunity. J Virol. 1987;10:3163–6.
76. Hendry RM, Burns JC, Walsh EE, et al. Strain-specific serum antibody responses in infants undergoing primary infection with respiratory syncytial virus. J Infect Dis. 1988;157:640–7.
77. Inabu Y, Tanaka Y, Sato K, et al. Bovine respiratory syncytial virus: Studies on an outbreak in Japan, 1968–1969. Jpn J Microbiol. 1972;16:373–83.
78. Mohanty SB, Lillie MG, Ingling AL. Effect of serum and nasal neutralizing antibodies on bovine respiratory syncytial virus infection in calves. J Infect Dis. 1976;134:409–13.
79. Paccaud MF, Jacquier CL. A respiratory syncytial virus of bovine origin. Arch Gesamte Virusforsch. 1970;30:327–42.
80. Van Den Ingh TSGAM, Verhoeff I, Van Nieuwstadt APKMI. Clinical and pathological observations on spontaneous bovine respiratory syncytial virus infections in calves. Res Vet Sci. 1982;33:152–8.
81. Baker JC, Werdin RE, Ames TR, et al. Study on the etiologic role of bovine respiratory syncytial virus in pneumonia of dairy calves. J Am Vet Med Assoc. 1986;189:66–70.
82. Belshe RB, Richardson LS, London WT, et al. Experimental respiratory syncytial virus infection of four species of primates. J Med Virol. 1977;1:157–62.
83. Hall CB, Douglas RG Jr, Geiman JM. Respiratory syncytial virus infections in infants: Quantitation and duration of shedding. J Pediatr. 1976;89:11–5.
84. Richardson LS, Belshe RB, Sly L, et al. Experimental respiratory syncytial virus pneumonia in Cebus monkeys. J Med Virol. 1978;2:45–59.
85. Coates HV, Chanock RM. Experimental infection with respiratory syncytial virus in several species of animals. Am J Hyg. 1962;76:302–12.
86. Prince GA, Porter DD. The pathogenesis of respiratory syncytial virus infection in infant ferrets. Am J Pathol. 1976;82:339–52.
87. Collier AM, Clyde WA Jr. Model systems for studying the pathogenesis of infections causing bronchiolitis in man. Pediatr Res. 1977;11:243–6.
88. Sung RYT, Murray HGS, Chan RCK, et al. Seasonal patterns of respiratory syncytial virus infection in Hong Kong: A preliminary report. J Infect Dis. 1987;156:527–8.
89. Berglund B. Studies on respiratory syncytial virus infection. Acta Paediatr Scand [Suppl] 1967;176:1.
90. Forbes JA, Bennett NM, Gray NJ. Epidemic bronchiolitis caused by respiratory syncytial virus: Clinical aspects. Med J Aust. 1961;2:933–5.
91. Gardner PS. How etiologic, pathologic, and clinical diagnoses can be made in a correlated fashion. Pediatr Res. 1977;11:254–61.
92. Morrell RE, marks MI, Champlin R, et al. An outbreak of severe pneumonia due to respiratory syncytial virus in isolated arctic populations. Am J Epidemiol. 1975;101:231–7.
93. Spence L, Barratt N. Respiratory syncytial virus associated with acute respiratory infections in Trinidadian patients. Am J Epidemiol. 1968;88:257–66.
94. Glezen WP, Loda FA, Clyde WA, et al. Epidemiologic patterns of acute lower respiratory disease of children in a pediatric group practice. J Pediatr. 1971;78:397–406.
95. Glezen WP. Pathogenesis of bronchiolitis-epidemiologic considerations. Pediatr Res. 1977;11:239–43.
96. Hall CB, Douglas RG Jr. Respiratory syncytial virus and influenza: Practical community surveillance. Am J Dis Child. 1976;130:615–20.
97. Mufson MA, Levine HD, Wasil RE, et al. Epidemiology of respiratory syncytial virus infection among infants and children in Chicago. Am J Epidemiol. 1973;98:88–95.
98. Foy HM, Cooney MK, Maletzky AJ, et al. Incidence and etiology of pneumonia, croup, and bronchiolitis in preschool children belonging to a prepaid medical care group over a four-year period. Am J Epidemiol. 1973;97:80–92.
99. Ånestad G. Interference between outbreaks of respiratory syncytial virus and influenza virus infection. Lancet. 1982;2:502.
100. Grist NR, Martin K, Pinkerton IW, et al. Double infections with respiratory syncytial virus and influenza. Lancet. 1970;2:1033.
101. Hoekstra RE, Herrmann EC, O'Connell EJ. Virus infections in children. Am J Dis Child. 1970;120:14–6.
102. Beem M, Egerer R, Anderson J. Respiratory syncytial virus neutralizing antibodies in persons residing in Chicago, Illinois. Pediatrics. 1964;34:761–70.
103. Ward KA, Lambden PR, Ogilvie MM, et al. Antibodies to respiratory syncytial virus polypeptides and their significance in human infection. J Gen Virol. 1983;64:1867–76.
104. Denny FW, Collier AM, Henderson FW, et al. The epidemiology of bronchiolitis. Pediatr Res. 1977;11:234–6.
105. Jackson GG, Muldoon RL. Viruses causing common respiratory infections in man. III. Respiratory syncytial viruses and coronaviruses. J Infect Dis. 1973;128:674–92.
106. Murphy TF, Henderson FW, Clyde WA Jr, et al. Pneumonia: An eleven-year study in a pediatric practice. Am J Epidemiol. 1981;113:12–21.
107. Denny FW, Clyde WA. Acute lower respiratory tract infections in nonhospitalized children. J Pediatr. 1986;108:635–46.
108. Coates HV, Chanock RM. Clinical significance of respiratory syncytial virus. Postgrad Med. 1964;35:460–5.
109. Loda FA, Clyde WA, Glezen WP, et al. Studies of the role of viruses, bacteria, and *M. pneumoniae* as causes of lower respiratory tract infections in children. J Pediatr. 1968;72:161–76.
110. Macasaet FF, Kidd PA, Bolano CR, et al. The etiology of acute respiratory infections. III. The role of viruses and bacteria. J Pediatr. 1968;72:829–39.
111. Maletzky AJ, Cooney MK, Luce R, et al. Epidemiology of viral and mycoplasmal agents associated with childhood lower respiratory illness in a civilian population. J Pediatr. 1971;78:407–14.
112. Loda FA, Glezen WP, Clyde WA Jr. Respiratory disease in group day care. Pediatrics. 1972;49:428–37.
113. Kim HW, Canchola JG, Brandt CD, et al. Respiratory syncytial virus disease in infants despite prior administration of antigenic inactivated vaccine. Am J Epidemiol. 1969;89:422–34.
114. Glezen WP, Taber LH, Frank AL, et al. Risk of primary infection and reinfection with respiratory syncytial virus. Am J Dis Child. 1986;140:543–46.
115. Henderson FW, Clyde WA, Collier AM, et al. The etiologic and epidemiologic spectrum of bronchiolitis in pediatric practice. J Pediatr. 1979;95:183–90.
116. Parrott RH, Kim HW, Brandt CD, et al. Respiratory syncytial virus in infants and children. Prev Med. 1974;3:473–80.
117. Henderson FW, Collier AM, Clyde WA Jr, et al. Respiratory syncytial virus infections, reinfections and immunity. A prospective, longitudinal study in young children. N Engl J Med. 1979;300:530–4.
118. Hall CB, Geiman JM, Biggar R, et al. Respiratory syncytial virus infections within families. N Engl J Med. 1976;294:414–9.
119. Johnson KM, Chanock RM, Rifkind D, et al. Respiratory syncytial virus. IV. Correlation of virus shedding, serologic response, and illness in adult volunteers. JAMA. 1961;176:663–7.
120. Kravetz HM, Knight V, Chanock RM, et al. Respiratory syncytial virus: III. Production of illness and clinical observations in adult volunteers. JAMA. 1961;176:657–63.
121. Gardner PS, Court SDM, Brocklebank JT, et al. Virus cross-infection in paediatric wards. Br Med J. 1973;2:571–5.
122. Lee GC-Y, Funk GA, Chen ST, et al. An outbreak of respiratory syncytial virus infection in an infant nursery. J Formosan Med Assoc. 1973;72:39–46.
123. Sterner G, Wolontis S, Bloth B, et al. Respiratory syncytial virus. An out-

break of acute respiratory illness in a home for infants. Acta Paediatr Scand. 1966;55:273–9.
124. Hall CB, Douglas RG Jr, Schnabel KC, et al. Infectivity of respiratory syncytial virus by various routes of inoculation. Infect Immun. 1981;33:779–83.
125. Aherne W, Bird T, Court SDM, et al. Pathological changes in virus infections of the lower respiratory tract in children. J Clin Pathol. 1970;23:7–18.
126. Downham MAPS, Gardner PS, McQuillin J, et al. Role of respiratory viruses in childhood mortality. Br Med J. 1975;1:235–9.
127. Ferris JAJ, Aherne WA, Locke WS, et al. Sudden and unexpected deaths in infants: Histology and virology. Br Med. J. 1973;2:439–42.
128. Urquhart GED, Gibson AAM. RSV infections and infant deaths. Br Med J. 1970;3:110.
129. Krieger I. Mechanics of respiration in bronchiolitis. Pediatrics. 1964;33:45–52.
130. Phelan PD, Williams HE, Freeman M. The disturbances of ventilation in acute viral bronchiolitis. Aust Paediat J. 1968;4:96–104.
131. Wohl MEB. Present capacity to evaluate pulmonary function relevant to bronchiolitis. Pediatr Res. 1977;11:252–3.
132. Wohl MEB, Stigol LC, Mead J. Resistance of the total respiratory system in healthy infants and infants with bronchiolitis. Pediatrics. 1969;43:495–509.
133. Fulginiti VA, Eller JJ, Sieber OF, et al. Respiratory virus immunization. I. A field trial of two inactivated respiratory virus vaccines; an aqueous trivalent parainfluenza virus vaccine, and an alum-precipitated respiratory syncytial virus vaccine. Am J Epidemiol. 1969;89:435–48.
134. Kapikian AZ, Mitchell RH, Chanock RM, et al. An epidemiologic study of altered clinical reactivity to respiratory syncytial (RS) virus infection in children previously vaccinated with an inactivated RS virus vaccine. Am J Epidemiol. 1969;89:405–21.
135. Prince GA, Jenson AB, Hemming VG, et al. Enhancement of respiratory syncytial virus pulmonary pathology in cotton rats by prior intramuscular inoculation of formalin-inactivated virus. J Virol. 1986;57:721–8.
136. Stott EJ, Taylor G, Ball LA, et al. Immune and histopathological response in animals vaccinated with recombinant vaccinia virus that express individual genes of human respiratory syncytial virus. J Virol. 1987;61:3855–61.
137. Piedra PA, Ogra PL. Modulation of mucosal immune response and immunopathology in experimentally induced infection with respiratory syncytial virus (RSV) in balb-c mice (Abstract 849). Pediatr Res. 1986;20:298.
138. Murphy BR, Prince GA, Walsh EE, et al. Dissociation between serum neutralizing antibody responses of infants and children who received inactivated respiratory syncytial virus vaccine. J Clin Microbiol. 1986;24:197–202.
139. Chanock RM. Control of acute mycoplasmal and viral respiratory tract disease. Science. 1970;169:248–56.
140. Chanock RM, Kapikian AZ, Mills J. Influence of immunological factors in respiratory syncytial virus disease of the lower respiratory tract. Arch Environ Health. 1970;21:347–55.
141. Bruhn FW, Yeager AS. Respiratory syncytial virus in early infancy. Am J Dis Child. 1977;131:145–8.
142. Lamprecht CL, Krause HE, Mufson MA. Role of maternal antibody in pneumonia and bronchiolitis due to respiratory syncytial virus. J Infect Dis. 1976;134:211–7.
143. Jacobs JW, Peacock DB, Corner BD, et al. Respiratory syncytial and other viruses associated with respiratory disease in infants. Lancet. 1971;1:871–6.
144. Ana PPS, Arrobio JO, Kim HW, et al. Serum complement in acute bronchiolitis. Proc Soc Exp Biol Med. 1970;134:499–503.
145. Kim HW, Leikin SL, Arrobio JO, et al. Cell-mediated immunity to respiratory syncytial virus induced by inactivated vaccine or by infection. Pediatr Res. 1976;10:75–8.
146. Gardner PS, McQuillin J, Court SDM. Speculation on pathogenesis in death from respiratory syncytial virus infection. Br Med J. 1970;1:327–30.
147. Ross CA, Pinkerton IW, Assaad FA. Pathogenesis of respiratory syncytial virus diseases in infancy. Arch Dis Child. 1971;46:702–4.
148. Polmar SH, Robinson LD Jr, Minnefor AB. Immunoglobin E in bronchiolitis. Pediatrics. 1972;50:279–84.
149. Welliver RC, Kaul TN, Ogra PL. The appearance of cell-bound IgE in respiratory-tract epithelium after respiratory-syncytial-virus infection. N Engl J Med. 1980;303:1198–202.
150. Welliver RC, Wong DT, Sun M, et al. The development of respiratory syncytial virus–specific IgE and the release of histamine in naso-pharyngeal secretions after infection. N Engl J Med. 1981;305:841–6.
151. Welliver RC, Sun M, Rinaldo D. Predictive value of respiratory syncytial virus (RSV) specific IGE titer for recurrent wheezing following bronchiolitis (Abstract 986). Pediatr Res. 1986;20:323.
152. Ward KA, Lambden PR, Ogilvie MM, et al. Antibodies to respiratory syncytial virus polypeptides and their significance in human infection. J Gen Virol. 1983;64:1867–76.
153. Murphy BR, Alling DW, Snyder MH, et al. Effect of age and preexisting antibody on serum antibody response of infants and children to the F and G glycoproteins during respiratory syncytial viral infection. J Clin Microbiol. 1986;24:894–8.
154. Murphy BR, Graham BS, Prince GA, et al. Serum and nasal-wash immunoglobulin G and A antibody response of infants and children to respiratory syncytial virus F and G glycoproteins following primary infection. J Clin Microbiol. 1986;23:1009–14.
155. Bangham CRM. Passively acquired antibodies to respiratory syncytial virus impair the secondary cytotoxic T cell response in the neonatal mouse. Immunology. 1986;59:37–41.
156. Hogg JC, Williams J, Richardson JB, et al. Age as a factor in the distribution of lower-airway conductance and in the pathologic anatomy of obstructive lung disease. N Engl J Med. 1970;282:1283–7.
157. Beem M. Repeated infections with respiratory syncytial virus. J Immunol. 1967;98:1115–22.
158. Fransen H, Sterner G, Forsgren M, et al. Acute lower respiratory illness in elderly patients with respiratory syncytial virus infection. Acta Med Scand. 1967;182:323–30.
159. Toms GL, Scott R. Respiratory syncytial virus and the infant immune response. Arch Dis Child. 1987;62:544–6.
160. Ogilvie MM, Vatheneo S, Radford M, et al. Maternal antibody and respiratory syncytial virus infection in infancy. J Med Virol. 1981;7:263–71.
161. Glezen WP, Paredes A, Allison JE, et al. Risk of respiratory syncytial virus infection for infants from low-income families in relationship to age, sex, ethnic group and maternal antibody level. J Pediatr. 1981;98:708–15.
162. Fernald GW, Almond JR, Henderson FW. Cellular and humoral immunity in recurrent respiratory syncytial virus infections. Pediatr Res. 1983;17:753–8.
163. Prince GA, Horswood RL, Chanock RM. Quantitative aspects of passive immunity to respiratory syncytial virus infection in infant cotton rats. J Virol. 1985;55:517–20.
164. Taylor G, Stott EJ, Bew M, et al. Monoclonal antibodies protect against respiratory syncytial virus infection in mice. Immunology. 1984;52:137–42.
165. Walsh EE, Schlesinger JJ, Brandriss MW. Protection from respiratory syncytial virus infection in cotton rats by passive transfer of monoclonal antibodies. Infect Imun. 1984;43:756–8.
166. Walsh EE, Hall CB, Briselli M, et al. Immunization with glycoprotein subunits of respiratory syncytial virus to protect cotton rats against viral infection. J Infect Dis. 1987;155:1198–203.
167. Olmsted RA, Elango N, Prince GA, et al. Expression of the F glycoprotein of respiratory syncytial virus by a recombinant vaccinia virus: Comparison of the individual contributions of the F and G glycoproteins to host immunity. Proc Natl Acad Sci USA. 1986;83:7462–6.
168. Wertz GW, Stott EJ, Young KKY, et al. Expression of the fusion protein of human respiratory syncytial virus from recombinant vaccinia virus vectors and protection of vaccinated mice. J Virol. 1987;61:293–301.
169. King AMQ, Stott EJ, Langer SJ, et al. Recombinant vaccinia viruses carrying the N gene of human respiratory syncytial virus: Studies of gene expression in cell culture and immune response in mice. J Virol. 1987;61:2885–90.
170. Stott EJ, Taylor G, BAll LA, et al. Immune and histopathological responses in animals vaccinated with recombinant vaccinia virus that express individual genes of human respiratory syncytial virus. J Virol. 1987;61:3855–61.
171. Hall CB, Walsh EE. Respiratory syncytial virus reinfections: Roles of antibody (ab) to fusion F and G proteins (AG,BG) of subgroups A and B (Abstract 1017). Pediatr Res. 1988;23:370.
172. Wagner DK, Graham BS, Wright PF, et al. Serum immunoglobulin G antibody subclass responses to respiratory syncytial virus F and G glycoproteins after primary infection. J Clin Microbiol. 1986;24:304–6.
173. Bui RHD, Molinaro GA, Kettering JD, et al. Virus-specific IgE and IgG_4 antibodies in serum of children infected with respiratory syncytial virus. J Pediatr. 1987;110:87–90.
174. Scott R, Gardner PS. Respiratory syncytial virus neutralizing activity in nasopharyngeal secretions. J Hyg (Camb) 1970;68:581–8.
175. Kaul TN, Welliver RC, Wong DT, et al. Secretory antibody response to respiratory syncytial virus infection. Am J Dis Child. 1981;135:1013–6.
176. McIntosh K, Masters HB, Orr I, et al. The immunologic response to infection with respiratory syncytial virus in infants. J Infect Dis. 1978;138:24–32.
177. Mills JV, Van Kirk JE, Wright PF, et al. Experimental respiratory syncytial virus infection of adults. Possible mechanisms of resistance to infection and illness. J Immunol. 1971;107:123–30.
178. Gardner PS. Immunologic studies of RS infections. In: Workshop of Respiratory Syncytial and Parainfluenza Viruses. Bethesda, MD: National Institutes of Health; July 21, 1977.
179. Kaul TN, Welliver RC, Ogra PL. Development of antibody-dependent cell-mediated cytotoxicity in the respiratory tract after natural infection with respiratory syncytial virus. Infect Immun. 1982;37:492–7.
180. Hall CB, Powell KR, MacDonald NE, et al. Respiratory syncytial virus infection in children with compromised immune function. N Engl J Med. 1986;315:77–81.
181. Fishaut M, Tubergen D, McIntosh K. Cellular response to respiratory viruses with particular reference to children with disorders of cell-mediated immunity. J Pediatr. 1980;96:179–86.
182. Ogra PL, Patel J. Respiratory syncytial virus infection and the immunocompromised host. Pediatr Infect Dis J. 1988;7:246–9.
183. Johnson RA, Prince GA, Suffin SC, et al. Respiratory syncytial virus infection in cyclophosphamide-treated cotton rats. Infect Immun. 1982;37:369–73.
184. Scott R, Kaul A, Scott M, et al. Development of in-vitro correlates of cell mediated immunity to respiratory syncytial infection in humans. J Infect Dis. 1978;137:810–7.
185. Cranage MP, Gardner PS. Systemic cell-mediated and antibody responses in infants with respiratory syncytial virus infections. J Med Virol. 1980;5:161–70.
186. Pemberton RM, Cannon MJ, Openshaw PJM, et al. Cytotoxic T cell specificity for respiratory syncytial virus proteins: Fusion protein is an important target antigen. J Gen Virol. 1987;68:2177–82.

187. Bangham CRM, Openshaw PJM, Ball LA, et al. Human and murine cytotoxic T cells specific to respiratory syncytial virus recognize the viral nucleoprotein (N), but not the major glycoprotein (G), expressed by vaccinia virus recombinants. J Immunol. 1986;137:3973–7.
188. Bangham CRM, McMichael AJ. Specific human cytotoxic T cells recognize B cell lines persistently infected with respiratory syncytial virus. Proc Natl Acad Sci USA. 1986;83:9183–7.
189. Isaacs D, Bangham CRM, McMichael AJ. Cell-mediated cytotoxic response to respiratory syncytial virus in infants with bronchiolitis. Lancet. 1987;2:769–71.
190. Gardner PS. Respiratory syncytial virus infections. Postgrad Med J. 1973;49:788–91.
191. Hilleman MR. Respiratory syncytial virus. Am Rev Respir Dis. 1963;88:181–97.
192. Wohl MEB. Bronchiolitis. Pediatr Ann. 1986;15:307–13.
193. Wohl MEB, Chernick V. Bronchiolitis. Am Rev Respir Dis. 1978;118:759–81.
194. Rice RP, Loda F. A roentgenographic analysis of respiratory syncytial virus pneumonia in infants. Radiology. 1966;87:1021–7.
195. Simpson W, Hacking PM, Court SDM, et al. The radiological findings in respiratory syncytial virus infection in children. II. The correlation of radiological categories with clinical and virological findings. Pediatr Radiol. 1974;2:155–60.
196. Hall CB, Hall WJ, Speers DM. Clinical and physiological manifestations of bronchiolitis and pneumonia: Outcome of respiratory syncytial virus. Am J Dis Child. 1979;133:798–802.
197. Reynolds EOR. Arterial blood gas tensions in acute disease of lower respiratory tract in infancy. Br Med J. 1963;1:1192–5.
198. Hall CB, Douglas RG Jr, Geiman JM. Quantitative shedding patterns of respiratory syncytial virus in infants. J Infect Dis. 1975;132:151–6.
199. McMillan JA, Tristram DA, Weiner LB, et al. Prediction of the duration of hospitalization in patients with respiratory syncytial virus: Use of clinical parameters. Pediatrics. 1988;81:22–6.
200. Berglund B, Kortekangas AE, Lauren P. Experimental inoculation of guinea pigs' middle ear with respiratory syncytial virus. Acta Otolaryngol (Stockh). 1966;224(suppl):268.
201. Berglund B, Salmivalli A, Toivanen P, et al. Isolation of respiratory syncytial virus from middle ear exudates of infants. Arch Dis Child. 1966;41:554–5.
202. Gronroos JA, Vihma L, Salmivalli A, et al. Co-existing viral (respiratory syncytial) and bacterial (pneumococcus) otitis media in children. Acta Otolaryngologica 1968;65:505–17.
203. Klein BS, Dollete FR, Yolken RH. The role of respiratory syncytial virus and other viral pathogens in acute otitis media. J Pediatr. 1982;101:16–20.
204. Henderson FW, Collier AM, Sanyal MA, et al. A longitundinal study of respiratory viruses and bacteria in the etiology of acute otitis media with effusion. N Engl J Med. 1982;306:1377–83.
205. Chonmaitree T, Howie VM, Truant AL. Presence of respiratory viruses in middle ear fluids and nasal wash specimens from children with otitis media. Pediatrics. 1986;77:698–702.
206. Finger R, Anderson LJ, Dicker RC, et al. Epidemic infections caused by respiratory syncytial virus in institutionalized young adults. J Infect Dis. 1987;155:1335–9.
207. Hall WJ, Hall CB, Speers DM. Respiratory syncytial virus infections in adults: Clinical, virologic and serial pulmonary function studies. Ann Intern Med. 1978;88:203.
208. Monto AS, Cavallaro JJ. The Tecumseh study of respiratory illness: II. Patterns of occurrence of infection with respiratory pathogens, 1965–1969. Am J Epidemiol. 1971;94:280–9.
209. Hall CB, Douglas RG Jr, Geiman JM, et al. Nosocomial respiratory syncytial virus infections. N Engl J Med. 1975;293:1343–6.
210. Hall CB, Geiman JM, Douglas RG Jr, et al. Control of nosocomial respiratory syncytial viral infections. Pediatrics. 1978;62:728–31.
211. Hall CB, Kopelman A, Douglas RG Jr. Neonatal respiratory syncytial viral infections. N Engl J Med. 1979;300:393–6.
212. Hall CB, Douglas RG Jr. Nosocomial respiratory syncytial virus infections: The role of gowns and masks on prevention. Am J Dis Child. 1981;135:512–5.
213. Carilli AD, Gohd RS, Gordon W. A virologic study of chronic bronchitis. N Engl J Med. 1964;270:123–7.
214. Sommerville RG. Respiratory syncytial virus in acute exacerbations of chronic bronchitis. Lancet. 1963;2:1247–8.
215. Mathur U, Bentley DW, Hall CB. Concurrent outbreaks of respiratory syncytial virus and influenza A/Texas/77 infection in the institutionalized elderly and chronically ill. Ann Intern Med. 1980;93:49–52.
216. Garvie DG, Gray J. Outbreak of respiratory syncytial virus infection in the elderly. Br Med J. 1980;281:1253–4.
217. Centers for Disease Control. Respiratory syncytial virus—Missouri. MMWR. 1977;26:351–2.
218. Cappel R, Thirty L, Clinet G. Viral antibodies in the CSF after acute CNS infections. Arch Neurol. 1975;32:629–31.
219. Wallace SJ, Zealley H. Neurological, electroencephalgraphic, and virological findings in febrile children. Arch Dis Child. 1970;45:611–23.
220. Giles TD, Gohd RS. Respiratory syncytial virus and heart disease. JAMA. 1976;236:1128–30.
221. Berkovich S, Kibrick S. Exanthem associated with respiratory syncytial virus infection. J Pediatr. 1964;65:368–70.
222. Moss PD. Serological studies with respiratory syncytial virus. Lancet. 1963;1:298–300.
223. Gala CL, Hall CB, Schnabel KC, et al. The use of eye-nose goggles to control nosocomial respiratory syncytial virus infection. JAMA. 1986;256:2706–8.
224. Agah R, Cherry JD, Garakian AJ, et al. Respiratory syncytial virus (RSV) infection rate in personnel caring for children with RSV infections. Am J Dis Child. 1987;141:695–7.
25. Leclair JM, Freeman J, Sullivan BF, et al. Prevention of nosocomial respiratory syncytial virus infections through compliance with glove and gown isolation precautions. N Engl J Med. 1987;317:329–34.
226. Snydman DR, Greer C, Mesner HC, et al. Prevention of nosocomial transmission of respiratory syncytial virus in a newborn nursery. Infect Control Hosp Epidemiol. 1988;9:105–8.
227. Ditchburn RK, McQuillin J, Gardner PS, et al. Respiratory syncytial virus infection in hospital cross-infection. Br Med J. 1971;3:671–3.
228. Hall CB. The shedding and spreading of respiratory syncytial virus. Pediatr Res. 1977;11:236–9.
229. Sims DG, Downham MAPS, McQuillin J, et al. Respiratory syncytial virus infection in north-east England. Br Med J. 1976;2:1095–8.
230. Sims DG, Downham MAPS, Webb JKG, et al. Hospital cross-infection on children's wards with respiratory syncytial virus and the role of adult carriage. Acta Paediatr Scand. 1975;64:541–5.
231. Hall CB, Douglas RG Jr. Modes of transmission of respiratory syncytial virus. J Pediatr. 1981;99:100–3.
232. Hall CB. Nosocomial viral respiratory infections: Perennnial weeds on pediatric wards. Am J Med. 1981;70:670–6.
233. Hall CB: The nosocomial spread of respiratory syncytial virus infections. Annu Rev Med. 1983;34:311–9.
234. Adams JM. Primary virus pneumonitis with cytoplasmic inclusion bodies; a study of an epidemic involving thirty-two infants with nine deaths. JAMA. 1941;116:925–33.
235. Adams JM, Imagawa DT, Zike K. Relationship of pneumonitis in infants to respiratory syncytial virus. Lancet. 1961;81:502–6.
236. MacDonald NE, Hall CB, Suffin SC, et al. Respiratory syncytial viral infection in infants with congenital heart disease. N Engl J Med. 1982;307:397–400.
237. Bruce E, Reid MM, Craft AW, et al. Multiple virus isolations in children with acute lymphoblastic leukaemia. J Infect. 1979;1:243–48.
238. Brugman S, Hutter JJ. Respiratory syncytial virus (RSV) pneumonitis in acute leukemia. Am J Hematol Oncol. 1980;2:371–4.
239. Craft AW, Reid MM, Gardner PS, et al. Virus infections in children with acute lymphoblastic leukemia. Arch Dis Child. 1979;54:755–69.
240. Crane LR, Kish JA, Ratanatharathorn V, et al. Fatal syncytial virus pneumonia in a laminar airflow room. JAMA. 1981;246:366–8.
241. Levenson RM, Kantor OS. Fatal pneumonia in an adult due to respiratory syncytial virus. Arch Intern Med. 1987;147:791–2.
242. Bruhn FW, Mokrohisky ST, McIntosh K. Apnea associated with respiratory syncytial virus infection in young infants. J Pediatr. 1977;90:382–6.
243. Anas NG, Boettrich C, Hall CB, et al. The association of apnea and respiratory syncytial virus infection in infants. J Pediatr. 1982;101:65–8.
244. Church NR, Anas NG, Hall CB, et al. Respiratory syncytial virus–related apnea in infants: Demographics and outcome. Am J Dis Child. 1984;138:247–50.
245. Williams AL, Uren EC, Bretherton L. Respiratory viruses and sudden infant death. Br Med J. 1984;288:1491–3.
246. Southall DP. Role of apnea in the sudden infant death syndrome: A personal view. Pediatrics. 1988;81:73–84.
247. Hall CB, Powell KR, Schnabel KC, et al. The risk of secondary bacterial infection in infants hospitalized with respiratory syncytial viral infection. J Pediatr. 1988;113:266–71.
248. Berkovich S. Acute respiratory illness in the premature nursery associated with respiratory syncytial virus infections. Pediatrics. 1964;34:753–60.
249. Lebowitz MD, Burrows B. The relationship of acute respiratory illness history to the prevalence and incidence of obstructive lung disorders. Am J Epidemiol. 1977;105:544–54.
250. Sims DG, Downham MAPS, Gardner PS, et al. Study of 8-year-old children with a history of respiratory syncytial virus bronchiolitis in infancy. Br Med J. 1978;1:11–4.
251. Sims DG, Gardner PS, Weightman D, et al. Atopy does not predispose to RSV bronchiolitis or post bronchiolitic wheezing. Br Med J. 1981;282:2086–8.
252. Pullan CR, Hey EN. Wheezing, asthma and pulmonary disfunction 10 years after infection with respiratory syncytial virus in infancy. Br Med J. 1982;284:1665–9.
253. Walsh EE, Hall CB. Respiratory syncytial virus. In: Lennette EH, Schmidt NJ, eds. Diagnostic Procedures for Viral and Rickettsial Infections. New York: American Public Health Association, Inc; 1989. In press.
254. Hughes JH, Mann DR, Hamparian VV. Detection of respiratory syncytial virus in clinical specimens by viral culture, direct and indirect immunofluorescence and enzyme immunoassay. J Clin Microbiol. 1988;26:588–91.
255. Chonmaitree T, Bessette-Henderson BJ, Hepler RE, et al. Comparison of three rapid diagnostic techniques for detection of respiratory syncytial virus from nasal wash specimens. J Clin Microbiol. 1987;25:746–7.
256. Minnich LL, Shehab ZM, Ray CG. Application of pooled monoclonal antibodies for one hour detection of respiratory syncytial virus antigen in clinical specimens. Diagn Microbiol Infect Dis. 1987;7:137–41.
257. Kaul TN, Welliver RC, Ogra PL. Comparison of fluorescent-antibody, neu-

tralizing-antibody, and complement-enhanced neutralizing-antibody assays for detection of serum antibody to respiratory syncytial virus. J Clin Microbiol. 1981;13:957–62.
258. Anderson LJ, Hierholzer JC, Bingham PG, et al. Microneutralization test for RSV based on an enzyme immunoassay. J Clin Microbiol. 1985;22:1050–2.
259. Stecenko AA. Treatment of viral bronchiolitis: Do steroids make sense? Contemp Pediatr 1987;4:121–30.
260. Leer JA Jr, Green JL, Heimlich EM, et al. Corticosteroid treatment in bronchiolitis. Am J Dis Child. 1969;117:495–503.
261. Rutter N, Milner AD, Hiller EJ. Effect of bronchodilators on respiratory resistance in infants and young children with bronchiolitis and wheezy bronchitis. Arch Dis Child. 1975;50:719–22.
262. Knight V, Gilbert BE. Chemotherapy of respiratory viruses. Adv Intern Med 1986;31:95–118.
263. Hall CB, McBride JT, Walsh EE, et al. Aerosolized ribavirin treatment of infants with respiratory syncytial virus infection: A randomized double-blind study. N Engl J Med. 1983;308:1443–7.
264. Taber LH, Knight V, Gilbert BE, et al. Ribavirin aerosol treatment of bronchiolitis due to respiratory syncytial virus infection in infants. Pediatrics. 1983;72:613–8.
265. Hall CB, Walsh EE, Hruska JF, et al. Ribavirin aerosol treatment of experimental respiratory syncytial viral infection in young adults: A controlled double-blind study. JAMA. 1983;249:2666–70.
266. Rodriquez WJ, Kim HW, Brandt CD, et al. Aerosolized ribavirin in the treatment of patients with respiratory syncytial virus disease. Pediatr Infect Dis J. 1987;6:159–63.
267. Conrad DA, Christenson JC, Waner JL, et al. Aerosolized ribavirin treatment of respiratory syncytial virus infection in infants hospitalized during an epidemic. Pediatr Infect Dis J. 1987;6:152–8.
268. Caramia G, Palazzini E. Efficacy of ribavirin aerosol treatment for respiratory syncytial virus bronchiolitis in infants. J Int Med Res. 1987;15:227–33.
269. Barry W, Cockburn F, Cornall R, et al. Ribavirin aerosol for acute bronchiolitis. Arch Dis Child. 1986;61:593–4.
270. Frankel LR, Wilson CW, Demers RR, et al. A technique for the administration of ribavirin to mechanically ventilated infants with severe respiratory syncytial virus. Crit Care Med. 1987;15:1051–4.
271. Demers RR, Parker J, Frankel LR, et al. Administration of ribavirin to neonatal and pediatric patients during mechanical ventilation. Respir Care. 1986;31:1188–96.
272. Outwater KM, Meissner C, Peterson MB. Ribavirin administration to infants receiving mechanical ventilation. Am J Dis Child. 1988;142:512–5.
273. Gelfand EW, McCurdy D, Rao P, et al. Ribavirin treatment of viral pneumonitis in severe combined immunodeficiency disease. Lancet. 1983;2:732–33.
274. McIntosh K, Kurachek SC, Cairns LM, et al. Treatment of respiratory viral infection in an immunodeficient infant with ribavirin aerosol. Am J Dis Child. 1984;138:305–8.
275. Rosner IK, Welliver RC, Edelson PJ, et al. Effect of ribavirin therapy on respiratory syncytial virus-specific IgE and IgA responses after infection. J infect Dis. 1987;155:1043–7.
276. Connor JD, Hintz M, Van Dyke R, et al. Ribavirin pharmacokinetics in children and adults during therapeutic trials. In: Smith RA, Knight V, Smith JAD, eds. Clinical Applications of Ribavirin. Orlando, FL: Academic Press; 1984:107–23.
277. Chin J, Magoffin RL, Shearer LA, et al. Field evaluation of a respiratory syncytial virus vaccine and a trivalent parainfluenza virus vaccine in a pediatric population. Am J Epidemiol. 1969;89:449–63.
278. Chanock RM, Richardson LS, Belshe RB, et al. Prospects for prevention of bronchiolitis caused by respiratory syncytial virus. Pediatr Res. 1977;11:264–7.
279. Wright PF, Belshe RB, Kim HW, et al. Administration of a highly attenuated live respiratory syncytial virus vaccine to adults and children. Infect Immun. 1982;37:397–400.
280. Friedewald WJ, Forsyth BR, Smith CB, et al. Low-temperature-grown RS virus in adult volunteers. JAMA. 1968;204:690.
281. Kim HW, Arrobio JO, Pyles G, et al. Clinical and immunological response of infants and children to administration of low-temperature adapted respiratory syncytial virus. Pediatrics. 1971;48:745–55.
282. Parrott RH, Kim HW, Brandt CD. Potential of attenuated respiratory syncytial virus vaccine for infants and children. Dev Biol Stand 1975;28:389–99.
283. Kim HW, Arrobio JO, brandt CD, et al. Safety and antigenicity of temperature sensitive (TS) mutant syncytial virus (RSV) in infants and children. Pediatrics. 1973;52:56–79.
284. McIntosh K, Arbeter AM, Stahl MK, et al. Attenuated respiratory syncytial virus vaccines in asthmatic children. Pediatr Res. 1974;8:689–90.
285. Prince GA, Hemming VG, Chanock RM: The use of purified immunoglobin in the therapy of respiratory syncytial virus infections. Pediatr Infect Dis. 1986;5:5201–6.
286. Prince GA, Hemming VG, Horswood RL, et al. Immunoprophylaxis and immunotherapy of respiratory syncytial virus infection in the cotton rat. Virus Res. 1985;3:193–206.
287. Gruber WC, Wilson SZ, Throop BJ, et al. Immunoglobulin administration and ribavirin therapy: Efficacy in respiratory syncytial virus infection in the cotton rat. Pediatr Res. 1987;21:270–4.
288. Hemming VG, Rodriguez W, Kim HW, et al. Intravenous immunoglobulin treatment of respiratory syncytial virus infections in infants and young children. Antimicrob Agents Chemother. 1987;31:1882–6.
289. Downham MAPS, Scott R, Sims DG, et al. Breast-feeding protects against respiratory syncytial virus infections. Br Med J. 1976;2:274–6.
290. Pullan CR, Toms GL, Martin AJ, et al. Breast feeding and respiratory syncytial virus infection. Br Med J. 1980;281:1034–1036.
291. Murphy D, Todd JK, Chao RR, et al. The use of gowns and masks to control respiratory illness in pediatric personnel. J Pediatr. 1981;99:746.

137. MEASLES VIRUS (RUBEOLA)

ANNE A. GERSHON

Measles is an acute infection caused by the rubeola virus. It is a highly contagious disease that is usually seen in children. The illness is characterized by cough, coryza, fever, and a maculopapular rash that begins several days after the initial symptoms. There is a characteristic enanthem, Koplik spots, that is specific for measles and that also precedes the onset of rash. Recovery from measles is the rule, but serious complications of the respiratory and central nervous systems may occur. Measles in the United States has been dramatically controlled since the introduction of live attenuated measles vaccine in 1963, but it remains a serious problem in developing countries.

Measles virus is a paramyxovirus that is closely related to canine distemper and rinderpest viruses; each causes a similar disease in humans, dogs, and certain cattle, respectively. The agents share certain antigens, and antiserum to each cross reacts with the other two.[1] Wild measles virus is pathogenic only for primates, and no strain differences have been identified.

DESCRIPTION OF THE PATHOGEN

Morphology

On electron microscopy, measles virions are pleomorphic spheres with a diameter of 120–250 nm. Virions consist of an inner nucleocapsid that is a coiled helix of protein and RNA and an envelope that bears short, surface projections.[2,3] Although the molecular weight of the single-stranded RNA has been reported to be $6.2–6.4 \times 10^6$ daltons,[4] more recently it has been thought to be 4.8×10^6.[5]

Chemical and Antigenic Composition

Measles virus is composed of six structural proteins. Three are complexed with RNA, and three are associated with the viral envelope.[6] The membrane envelope contains the M protein, a nonglycosylated protein associated with the inner lipid bilayer, and two glycoproteins designated H and F.[7] The H glycoprotein is responsible for the adsorption of virus to receptors on the host cell, the first step in infection, and it also constitutes the antigen that mediates hemagglutination. Hemagglutination of red blood cells from old-world Monkeys forms the major serologic test for measuring antibody to measles virus, the hemagglutination inhibition (HI) test. The F glycoprotein is responsible for the membrane fusion of virus and host cell, penetration of the virus into the host cell, and hemolysis, a property that is exploited in the HI test for antibodies to measles virus. Unlike many other paramyxoviruses, neuraminidase is not found on the envelope of measles virus.[8] The measles virus antigens and their now-recognized role in human disease[7,9] are discussed later.

Growth of Measles Virus in Tissue Culture

Measles virus was first successfully isolated in the laboratory by Enders and Peebles in 1954.[10] The virus was initially propagated in primary human renal cells, but later it was found that the virus could also be cultivated in kidney cell cultures of simian origin. Wild measles virus is rather difficult to propagate in vitro since it is slow growing and only a limited number of types of cell cultures are permissive for the virus. Laboratory and vaccine strains are easier to propagate than wild strains are because the yields of virus are greater and the spectrum of permissive cells is wider.[11]

Cytopathic effects (CPE) produced by measles virus in tissue culture are of two varieties. Multinucleate giant cells are characteristic of wild measles virus.[12] These giant cells are similar to the giant cells seen in pathologic specimens obtained from patients with clinical measles. The latter are referred to as Warthin-Finkeldey cells after the investigators who first described them[13,14]; these cells may be of epithelial or endothelial origin. In tissue culture, giant cells are associated with a high degree of infectivity and low interferon production.[12]

The other type of CPE associated with measles virus is termed *spindle cell transformation*. This CPE is typical of that produced by vaccine strains, and it is associated with low infectivity, high hemagglutination titers, and high interferon production.[12]

Host Range

Humans are the only natural host for wild measles virus, but monkeys may also be infected with the virus. In general the illness caused by measles virus in monkeys is milder than that in humans.[15] It has not been possible to infect small laboratory animals such as rodents with wild measles virus. However, newborn and suckling rodents may be infected with vaccine strains administered by the intracerebral route.[16,17]

Epidemiology

Measles has been recognized as a disease for some 2000 years, but the infectious nature of the illness was not recognized until about 145 years ago. In 1846 Panum[18] studied an epidemic of measles in the Faroe Islands and noted that the disease was contagious, that there was an incubation period of about 2 weeks, and that infection appears to lead to lifelong immunity.

The next major advance in the understanding of measles did not occur until 1954 when Enders and Peebles[10] reported their success in propagating wild measles virus in primary human renal tissue culture cells. Their success led directly to the development of live measles vaccine, which was licensed for use in the United States in 1963.

Measles is seen in every country in the world. Without the use of vaccine, epidemics of measles lasting 3–4 months would be predicted to occur every 2–5 years. Countries in which measles vaccine is widely used have experienced a marked decrease in the incidence of disease. For example, for many years 200,000–500,000 cases of measles were reported yearly in the United States. Since 1963 when the vaccine was licensed, the incidence of measles in the United States has decreased by over 95 percent.[19] This has been especially pronounced since the enactment of laws requiring proof of immunity to measles for school entry in the early 1980s. The yearly incidence of measles in the United States reached a nadir in 1983 when 1497 cases were reported to the Centers for Disease Control (CDC) in Atlanta. In 1986 the incidence increased; there were over 6000 reported cases of measles. More recently, however, there is a decreasing trend again; the number of reported cases for the first 26 weeks of 1987 was less than the comparable period in 1986. Therefore the upward trend in the incidence of measles in the United States appears to have been reversed. At present, about one-third of the reported cases of measles occur in persons who have previously been vaccinated. It is believed that most of these cases are due to primary vaccine failure and not the result of waning of immunity. Measles today in the United States is most often seen in individuals under 20 years of age, with the highest incidence in those between the ages of 5 and 19 years.[21] It is estimated that as many as 7 million young adults in the United States are susceptible to measles.[22] Miniepidemics of measles continue to be reported when large groups of susceptibles are congregated as occurs, for example, in colleges.[19,21,23] The major reasons that measles has not been eliminated from the United States include a failure to immunize all individuals who qualify for vaccination, primary vaccine failure, and importations of measles to the United States from other countries.[24,25]

Spread of Infection

The measles virion is a very labile agent that is sensitive to acid, proteolytic enzymes, strong light, and drying.[11] The virus, however, remains infective in droplet form in air for several hours, especially under conditions of low relative humidity. This latter fact may account for the increased incidence of measles in winter.[26]

Measles is spread by direct contact with droplets from respiratory secretions of infected persons. It is one of the most communicable of the infectious diseases. Patients with measles are most infectious during the late prodromal phase of the illness when cough and coryza are at their peak[15]; however, the disease is probably contagious from several days before the onset of rash to several days after the onset of rash. Measles virus has been isolated from respiratory secretions of patients with measles only up to 48 hours after the onset of rash.[27] Airborne spread of measles in physicians' offices has been observed.[28,29]

Additional Diseases Associated with Measles Virus

Diseases other than measles that have been associated with measles virus include subacute sclerosing panencephalitis (SSPE), multiple sclerosis (MS), and systemic lupus erythematosus (SLE). Subacute sclerosing panencephalitis is a chronic degenerative neurologic disease that occurs several to many years after an attack of measles, particularly in children who developed measles before 2 years of age. The disease was at one time more common in the rural southeast than in other areas of the United States. A few children who received measles vaccine and who had no prior history of measles have been observed to develop SSPE. However, it is unknown whether these children might have had a subclinical case of measles before receiving vaccine. Clearly the incidence of SSPE appears to have declined since the introduction of measles vaccine.[19,30]

Patients with SSPE have unusually high measles antibody titers both in their serum and in their cerebrospinal fluid (CSF).[31] A measleslike virus has been reported to have been isolated from the brain and lymph nodes of patients dying of SSPE, which suggests that the disease is caused by measles virus or a similar virus and that the infection is not limited to the nervous system.[32–35] There is some evidence that patients with SSPE may have deficiencies in their immune response to measles virus.[36–38] An alternative hypothesis is that SSPE results from the unchecked synthesis of some viral proteins in the brain.[7,9,39] This has been ascribed to the failure of certain brain cells to synthesize measles M protein, which plays a major role in assembly of virions. An abortive measles virus infection therefore occurs with a marked production of measles antigens other than M protein and corresponding immune stimulation as is seen in SSPE.

Multiple sclerosis and SLE have a much more tenuous etiologic link with measles virus than does SSPE. Statistically, persons with MS are found to have higher measles antibody titers than do patients without MS.[40] A similar phenomenon has been demonstrated in persons with SLE. In addition, tubular structures resembling myxovirus nucleocapsids have been observed in electron micrographs of renal biopsy specimens from patients with SLE.[41] The significance of this finding and the elevated measles antibody titers is unknown.

PATHOGENESIS

Measles virus infects by invasion of the respiratory epithelium. Studies on volunteers inoculated with live measles virus indicate that infection may occur from the instillation of virus at any point from the nose to lower parts of the respiratory tract.[42]

Based on Fenner's mousepox model for exanthems[43] and a monkey model of measles infection,[44] it has been suggested[15] that local multiplication at the respiratory mucosa leads to a primary viremia during which the virus spreads in leukocytes to the reticuloendothelial system. Due to necrosis of infected reticuloendothelial cells, an increased amount of virus is released, and reinvasion of leukocytes (secondary viremia) occurs.

Measles virus has been isolated from the leukocytes of patients with clinical cases of measles.[45] The virus has also been propagated in vitro in human T and B lymphocytes and in monocytes.[46] It has been postulated that the direct invasion of T lymphocytes in clinical cases of measles may account for the temporary depression of cell-mediated immunity that occurs with the disease. In measles this depression has not been associated with the activation of suppressor T cells as has been observed in varicella.[47,48]

After the secondary viremic phase of measles occurs, the entire respiratory mucosa becomes involved with the disease. This accounts for the cough and coryza that are classic signs of measles. In addition, measles may directly cause croup, bronchiolitis, and pneumonia. It has also been postulated that damage to the respiratory tract from, for example, edema and a loss of cilia, predisposes to secondary invasion resulting in such complications as bacterial otitis media and pneumonia.[15]

Within a few days after generalized involvement of the respiratory tract has occurred Koplik spots appear and are followed by the development of a rash. Both manifestations are believed to result from similar pathologic mechanisms. On microscopic examination of skin and mucous membranes, multinucleate giant cells as well as other similar histologic changes are observed in both the epidermis and the oral epithelium.[49]

It has long been recognized that the appearance of the measles rash coincides temporally with the appearance of serum antibody and the termination of communicability of the disease. Therefore, it has been postulated that the skin and mucous membrane manifestations of measles actually represent hypersensitivity of the host to the virus. Measles virus antigen has been demonstrated in the involved skin and mucous membranes by immunofluorescence, although it remains controversial whether endothelial or epithelial cells are involved.[49–51] Measles virus has also been isolated from the rash in its early stages.[44] If hypersensitivity is the actual cause of the rash, however, it is probably mediated by cellular rather than humoral immunity.[52] Thus patients with agammaglobulinemia who contract measles develop a rash. Patients with deficiencies in cell-mediated immunity may, on the other hand, develop measles giant cell pneumonia (Hecht's) without a rash after an exposure to measles or if measles vaccine is given.[53,54]

Immunity

Immunity to measles after an attack of the disease appears to be lifelong. After measles vaccination, immunity is similarly of many years' duration and probably lifelong.[19] It remains unknown why measles antibody persists for years after infection. One possible explanation is that measles virus becomes latent after the acute infection and, while latent, provides an immunologic stimulus to antibody formation. However, latent measles virus has not been demonstrated in humans or in experimental animals. An alternative explanation for the persistence of measles antibody is that reexposure to the virus results in an antigenic boost and continued antibody synthesis. It is known that reinfection with measles can occur and that reinfection is almost always asymptomatic although it is detectable by a boost in antibody titer.[55] Cellular immunity to measles virus probably also plays a role in the prevention of recurrent measles since patients with agammaglobulinemia do not develop multiple attacks of measles. A cell-mediated response to measles antigen in the absence of detectable measles antibody was reported in two physicians who developed no disease despite repeated exposures to measles.[56] Thus, when humoral antibodies to measles are absent or of low magnitude, cellular immunity to the virus may protect against subsequent illness.

CLINICAL MANIFESTATIONS

The incubation period of measles is 10–14 days; it is often somewhat longer in adults than in children. A prodromal phase lasting several days begins after the incubation period. This phase probably coincides with the secondary viremia.[15] It is manifested by malaise, fever, anorexia, conjunctivitis, and respiratory symptoms such as cough and coryza and may resemble a severe upper respiratory infection. Towards the end of the prodrome, just before the appearance of the rash, Koplik spots appear.

Koplik spots are pathognomonic of measles. First noted by Koplik in 1896,[57] they consist of bluish gray specks on a red base. They have also been likened to grains of sand, and without examination of the buccal mucosa in good light, they may be overlooked. Most often they appear on the mucosa opposite the second molars. However, in severe cases the entire mucous membrane of the mouth may be involved. This enanthem persists for several days and begins to slough as the rash appears.

The rash of measles usually begins on the face and proceeds down the body to involve the extremities last including the palms and soles (Fig. 1). During the healing phase the involved

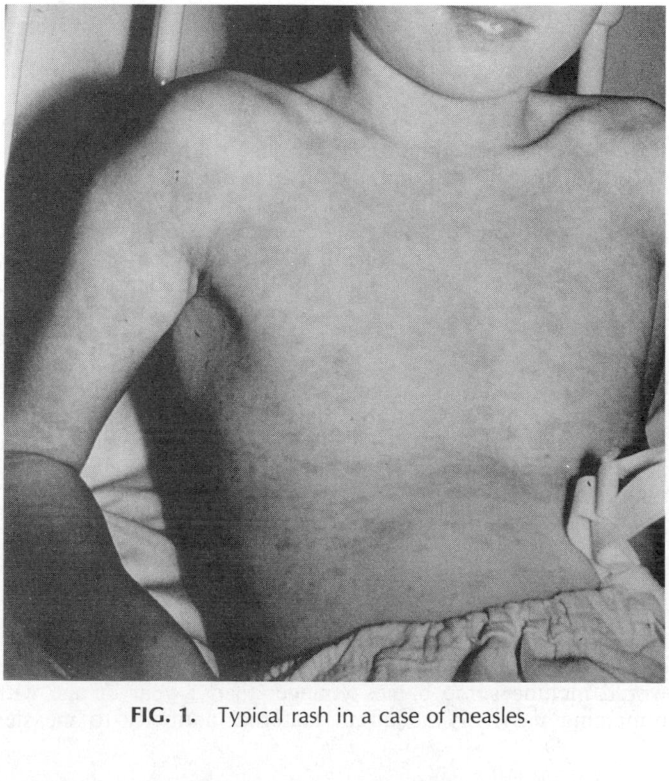

FIG. 1. Typical rash in a case of measles.

areas (except palms and soles) may desquamate. The rash is erythematous and maculopapular; as it progresses it becomes confluent, especially on the face and the neck. The rash usually lasts about 5 days and starts to clear on the skin that was first involved. The patient with measles is usually most ill during the first or second day of the rash. Several days after the appearance of the rash the fever abates, and the patient begins to feel better. The entire uncomplicated illness from late prodrome to resolution of the fever and rash lasts 7–10 days; cough may be the last symptom to disappear.

Complications

The most common complications of measles involve the respiratory tract and the central nervous system (CNS). Involvement of the respiratory tract is part of the virus infection itself. In addition, bacterial superinfection may occur in any area of the respiratory tract. Superinfection may be secondary to local tissue damage inflicted by the virus as well as depression of cellular immunity.[58] Thus, pneumonia accompanying measles may be due either to direct viral invasion of the lungs or to bacterial superinfection. Roentgenographic evidence of pneumonia is not uncommon even during apparently uncomplicated measles.[15] Pneumonia accounts for about 60 percent of deaths in infants dying of measles, whereas death due to the complication of acute encephalitis is more often observed in children aged 10–14 years.[59,60]

Encephalitis after measles may be acute or chronic as in SSPE. Acute measles encephalitis presents with a resurgence of fever during convalescence and frequently with headaches, seizures, and changes in the state of consciousness. Up to 50 percent of the patients with measles and no symptoms suggesting cerebral involvement may have abnormalities detected by electroencephalography (EEG),[61] so it is believed that viral invasion of the CNS is a common feature of measles. However, only 1 in 1000 to 1 in 2000 patients with measles develop clinical signs of encephalitis. Measles encephalitis ranges from mild to severe, with a high proportion of patients who recover being left with neurologic sequelae.

Measles virus has been reported to have been isolated from the brain of several persons dying of measles encephalitis.[62–65] However, virus isolation is uncommon and usually requires special virologic techniques such as cocultivation. It has therefore been suggested that acute measles encephalitis is due to hypersensitivity to virus in brain tissue. Viral antigens as well as host antigens are present on the surface of measles-infected cells in vitro.[66] Therefore the hypersensitivity may be directed against both viral and host (brain) antigens, thus accounting for the encephalitic symptoms. Demyelination, vascular cuffing, gliosis, and infiltration of fat-laden macrophages near blood vessel walls are noted on pathologic specimens of brain from patients with measles encephalitis.[11] In a laboratory study of serum and cerebrospinal fluid (CSF) from 19 patients with postinfectious measles encephalitis, similarities between experimental allergic encephalomyelitis such as immune responses to myelin basic protein and early destruction of myelin were demonstrated in about 50 percent. There was no evidence of intrathecal synthesis of antibody against measles virus, thus suggesting the importance of the immune response in the pathogenesis of measles encephalitis rather than viral multiplication.[67]

Transient hepatitis has been reported during acute measles.[68]

Modified Measles

An extremely mild form of measles has been observed in persons with some degree of passive immunity to the virus. This would include some babies younger than 1 year of age with remaining passively acquired, maternal antibody to measles virus and susceptible persons who have received γ-globulin after an exposure to measles.

The symptoms of modified measles are variable, and certain "classic" symptoms such as the prodromal period, conjunctivitis, Koplik spots, and rash may be absent. The incubation period may be prolonged. At times the infection may be subclinical, and with a great degree of passively acquired immunity the infection may be completely prevented.[55]

Atypical Measles

This syndrome has been described in persons who received killed measles vaccine (or killed vaccine followed soon afterward by live vaccine) and who, several years later, were exposed to wild measles virus.[69,70] In the face of an undetectable or a very low measles antibody titer, these patients have developed unusual manifestations of measles followed by the appearance of extremely high measles antibody titers (e.g., 1:100,000) in their serum.[71]

After a prodrome of fever and pain for 1–2 days, the rash appears. Unlike classic measles, it begins peripherally and may be urticarial, maculopapular, hemorrhagic, and/or vesicular. The disease may be misdiagnosed as varicella, Rocky Mountain spotted fever, Henoch-Schönlein purpura, drug eruptions, and toxic shock syndrome. The patient has a high fever, edema of the extremities, interstitial pulmonary infiltrates, hepatitis, and on occasion, a pleural effusion. The disease tends to be quite severe with a somewhat more prolonged course than regular measles has. At least one fatality has been reported. No specific therapy is available. Measles virus has not been isolated from these patients, and they do not appear to transmit measles to others.[70]

The pathogenesis of this syndrome is believed to be one of hypersensitivity to measles virus in a partially immune host. Whether cell-mediated or humoral immune mechanisms or both are involved remains controversial.[70,72,73]

One hypothesis concerning pathogenesis is that killed measles vaccine lacks the antigen that stimulates the antibody that is responsible for preventing the entry of measles virus into cells, thus allowing measles infection to occur in the face of partial immunity derived from killed vaccine.[74,75] Recently it has been shown that killed measles vaccine did not induce antibody to the F protein; an antigen that facilitates spread of the virus from one cell to another. This further explains the paradox of severe measles infection despite partial immunity.[7,75]

Recurrences of atypical measles have not been reported. Therefore it has been suggested that persons who received killed measles vaccine (or killed vaccine followed soon afterward by live vaccine) in the past be reimmunized with live measles vaccine. It is important that persons who have received killed vaccine be made aware that severe local reactions may follow an injection of live vaccine.[76–78] Usually the reaction consists of tenderness and erythema around the injection site. However, severe local edema and high fever may also occur. Although the opportunity for exposure to wild measles virus in the United States today is extremely low, immunization with live vaccine is recommended since the associated risk is lower than the risk of being exposed to the wild-type virus, especially if foreign travel is anticipated.[21]

Measles in Immunocompromised Patients

Severe measles may occur in persons with compromised or deficient cellular immunity such as those being treated for malignant disease and children with the acquired immunodeficiency syndrome (AIDS) or any form of congenital immunodeficiency.[53,79,80] Should such children be inadvertantly exposed to measles, they may develop giant cell pneumonia without evidence of a rash.[53,79] In such instances the clinical diagnosis of measles may be difficult or impossible to make. Since these children may also have poor antibody responses, virus isolation from infected tissue (or identification of measles antigen by immunofluorescence) may be the only means for diagnosis. A chronic form of encephalitis resembling SSPE, often with a concomitant pneumonia, has also been reported in persons with deficient cellular immunity.[36,37]

Malnourished children, especially in the developing countries, have also been reported to develop severe measles. This may possibly be related to poor cell-mediated immune responses secondary to malnutrition.[81] Intense exposure to the virus secondary to crowding may also play a role in the severity of measles in developing countries.[82,83]

Measles in Pregnant Women and Their Offspring

Measles (rubeola) during pregnancy, in contrast to German measles (rubella), is not known to cause congenital anomalies of the fetus.[84] However, measles in pregnancy has been associated with spontaneous abortions and premature delivery.[15] Measles in the offspring of mothers with measles ranges from mild to severe.[85,86] It is therefore recommended that infants born to women with active measles be passively immunized with immune globulin (IG) (see below).

Measles in Persons with Tuberculosis

It has long been thought that tuberculosis is aggravated in persons who contract natural measles, presumably secondary to a depression of cell-mediated immunity by measles virus.[58] For example, the tuberculin test has been reported to become negative for about 1 month after measles or measles vaccination.[15] Although the concept of depressed cell-mediated immunity tuberculosis secondary to measles has been questioned,[87] it seems prudent to defer measles vaccine in persons with known tuberculosis until antituberculous therapy is underway. In geographic areas and populations where tuberculosis is rare, it is no longer considered mandatory to perform a tuberculin test on an infant before administering measles vaccine.[88]

DIAGNOSIS

Classic measles with cough, coryza, conjunctivitis, Koplik spots, and a maculopapular rash beginning on the face is easily diagnosed clinically. Often there is a striking leukopenia, perhaps related to the infection and death of leukocytes. A laboratory diagnosis of measles is helpful when the clinician is unfamiliar with the illness due to the decline in cases of clinical measles since introduction of measles vaccine. A laboratory diagnosis may also be helpful in cases of possible atypical measles or when unexplained pneumonia and/or encephalitis occur in an immunocompromised patient.

Measles may be diagnosed in the laboratory by virus isolation, by the identification of measles antigen in infected tissues, and by the demonstration of a significant serologic response to measles virus. Virus isolation is technically difficult, and facilities for isolation are not always available. It is therefore useful only in a few situations such as in patients with fatal pneumonia or in patients with an immunodeficiency, people in whom an antibody response may be minimal. Immunofluorescent examination of cells from nasal exudates or from urinary sediment for the presence of measles antigen, if available, may be useful for a rapid diagnosis of measles.[11]

The most frequently used method of laboratory diagnosis, however, is the serologic response to the virus. A fourfold or greater increase in measles antibody titer in acute and convalescent serum specimens is considered diagnostic for measles. A number of methods are available, usually through state health department laboratories, including neutralization, complement fixation, and HI. Neutralization, which requires propagation of the virus in vitro, is technically difficult: Therefore, this test, while sensitive, is infrequently used. Complement fixation is not an overly sensitive technique, but it is adequate for the diagnosis of acute measles. It is not useful, however, for determining the immune status to measles.

Therefore, the most helpful laboratory method for measuring antibodies is the HI test. This test is slightly less sensitive than virus neutralization is, but generally there is good correlation between the two tests. Antibodies detectable by this test persist for many years, so immune status to measles may also be determined by HI. For the diagnosis of acute or atypical measles, two serum specimens, acute and convalescent, are required. Subacute sclerosing panencephalitis may also be diagnosed by the demonstration of high measles HI titers in serum and CSF in the presence of clinical evidence of the illness.[11]

An enzyme-linked immunosorbent assay (ELISA) has also been described that is more sensitive and more simple to perform than HI is.[89] This assay may also be adapted to measure specific IgM antibody, and it is therefore useful for the diagnosis of acute measles on one serum sample. An HI test that uses capillary blood collected on filter paper from finger- or heelstick specimens has also been described; it is used by some state health department laboratories and obviates the need for venipuncture.[90]

PREVENTION

Since the development and use of live measles vaccine, methods to prevent measles have changed dramatically. Prevention nowadays is ideally carried out long before an anticipated exposure to measles by the administration of live vaccine during the early part of the second year of life. However, there are rare occasions when passive immunization against measles with γ-globulin must be used.

Included in the group of persons for whom passive immunization is recommended are those who are at high risk to develop severe or fatal measles, who are susceptible, and who have been exposed to the infection. Such persons would include children with malignant disease, particularly if they are receiving chemotherapy and/or radiotherapy, and children with deficits in cell-mediated immunity. Babies less than 1 year of age (including newborns whose mothers have measles) are also at increased risk after an exposure to measles. To be effective, passive immunization must be given within 6 days after an exposure; administration after 6 days would not be expected to influence the course of the disease.

For a healthy infant less than 1 year of age who has been exposed to measles, the modifying dose of immune globulin (IG) is 0.25 ml/kg intramuscularly. An infant passively immunized in this fashion should be given live measles vaccine at the age of 15 months.[88] For immunocompromised, susceptible, exposed children, a larger dose of IG is required. These children should be administered IG, 0.5 mg/kg intramuscularly, with a maximum of 15 ml.[88] High-dose intravenous IG given at regular intervals is currently being evaluated to determine whether it will protect human immunodeficiency virus (HIV)-infected children against measles and other serious infections.[91]

Active immunization against measles was developed in the early 1960s. Live and killed measles vaccines were licensed for use in the United States in 1963. Killed vaccine was withdrawn from the market in 1968 after the recognition of atypical measles in recipients of this vaccine. The first marketed live measles vaccine was the Edmonston B strain. This vaccine was associated with a fairly high incidence of moderately severe side reactions such as rash and fever, and it was therefore often administered along with a dose of IG. Subsequently more attenuated vaccines were developed (Schwarz and Attenuvax), and since the incidence of vaccine reactions is low with these vaccines, IG is no longer given along with measles vaccine.

Since 1976 it has been recommended that all healthy children be administered live measles vaccine at 15 months of age.[88]

Properly administered measles vaccine has been associated with the persistence of immunity to measles for at least 16 years.[92,93] In one study, although measles HI antibodies were no longer detectable in some individuals, antibodies were demonstrated by neutralization, and revaccination was associated with a classic booster antibody response.[92] In the general population, 95 percent of properly immunized children can be expected to respond serologically to measles vaccine. Research on a measles vaccine that may be administered by aerosol and that induces an immune response in infants over 6 months of age is ongoing.[94]

Transient fever and rash develop about 1 week after vaccination in 5–15 percent of children.[88] In a 1986 study of 1162 twins who were given either mumps-measles-rubella (MMR) or placebo, there were side effects (fever, irritability, drowsiness, conjunctivitis) in 0.5–4 percent.[95] Symptoms of CNS dysfunction after measles vaccine are exceedingly rare. Since measles may be severe in adults,[96] immunization of adults who were not vaccinated previously, who have no history of measles, and who were born after 1956 is recommended by the CDC.[21] A 1986 Chicago study of hospital employees, however, indicated that only 1 of 266 (0.03 percent) was susceptible to measles; about one-third were born after 1957.[97]

A number of reasons for apparent "vaccine failures" of measles vaccine have been proposed.[19] These include improper storage of vaccine at temperatures exceeding 4°C, a failure to use the proper diluent for the lyophilized vaccine, exposure of the vaccine to light or heat, and vaccination in the face of low levels of passive antibody. The latter may occur when infants are immunized at 12 months of age or younger, i.e., when transplacental maternal measles IgG may not yet have been lost. It may also occur if children were vaccinated 1 or 2 months after receiving an injection of IG, if the more attenuated vaccines were given with IG, and if live measles vaccine was administered soon after killed measles vaccine. Reimmunization of children who received live measles vaccine before 12 months of age is recommended. No deleterious effects have been associated with measles revaccination. Although immunization between 12 and 14 months of age is a risk factor for the development of measles in epidemic situations,[98] routine reimmunization of persons who were vaccinated at this age is not recommended since most such individuals are immune to measles.[21] However, the CDC recommends that revaccination of such individuals under epidemic conditions be considered.[21] Although it is probably unusual, sustained transmission of measles has been reported in secondary schools even if 95 percent of the students are immune and over 99 percent have been immunized.[99,100]

Live measles vaccine is contraindicated in persons with deficits in cell-mediated immunity and in pregnant women. Fatal measles in children with AIDS has been reported.[80,101] Although the potential risks of measles vaccine in these children are unknown, they may be less than the disease itself. Theoretically the vaccine virus might multiply in these children in an uncontrolled fashion, or immune stimulation from the vaccine might include latent HIV infection to become active. It has been reported that 63 HIV-infected children have been immunized with measles vaccine, however, without apparent ill effects.[80] It is currently recommended that children with known asymptomatic HIV infection receive measles vaccine at the age of 15 months.[80,91] The use of measles vaccine should also be *considered* for children with known HIV infection who manifest symptoms including AIDS,[91] especially if they live in locations where there is transmission of measles such as certain inner-city areas.

Serious hypersensitivity reactions to measles vaccine in persons allergic to egg protein have been reported.[102] Individuals with a history of anaphylactic reactions after the ingestion of eggs should be vaccinated only with extreme caution.[88]

Susceptible persons who are exposed to measles, with the exception of young babies, pregnant women, and immunocompromised persons, may be given live measles vaccine to prevent disease. If the vaccine is given shortly after exposure, clinical cases of measles may be prevented since the incubation period of measles vaccine is about 7 days as compared with 10 days for clinical measles.[15]

TREATMENT

No specific treatment for measles is available. The patient should be given supportive therapy such as antipyretics and fluids as indicated. Bacterial superinfection should be promptly treated with appropriate antimicrobials, but prophylactic antibiotics to prevent superinfection are of no known value and are therefore contraindicated. Experimental therapies such as interferon and inosiplex have not been useful for treatment of measles or its complications.[103,104]

REFERENCES

1. Imagawa DT. Relationships among measles, canine distemper and rinderpest viruses. Prog Med Virol. 1968;10:160.
2. Waterson AP. Measles virus. Arch Ges Virusforsch. 1965;16:57.
3. Nakai M, Imagawa DT. Electron microscopy of measles virus replication. J Virol. 1969;3:187.
4. Hall WW, Martin SJ. Purification and characterization of measles virus. J Gen Virol. 1973;19:175.
5. Udem SA, Cook KA. Isolation and characterization of measles virus intracellular nucleocapsid RNA. J Virol. 1984;49:57–65.
6. Norrby E. Measles. In: Fields BN, ed. Virology. New York: Raven Press; 1985:1305–21.
7. Choppin PW, Richardson CD, Merz DC, et al. The functions and inhibition of the membrane glycoproteins of paramyxoviruses and myxoviruses and the role of the measles virus M protein in subacute sclerosing panencephalitis. J Infect Dis. 1981;143:352.
8. Howe C, Schluederberg A. Neuraminidase associated with measles virus. Biochem Biophys Res Commun. 1970;40:606.
9. Hall WW, Choppin PW. Measles-virus proteins in the brain tissue of patients with subacute sclerosing panencephalitis. Absence of the M protein. N Engl J Med. 1981;304:1152.
10. Enders JF, Peebles TC. Propagation in tissue cultures of cytopathogenic agents from patients with measles. Proc Soc Exp Biol Med. 1954;86:277.
11. Gershon A, Krugman S. Measles. In: Lennette E, Schmidt N, eds. Diagnostic Procedures for Viral and Rickettsial Infections. 5th ed. Washington, DC: American Public Health Association; 1979:665.
12. Enders JF. Measles virus, historical review, isolation and behavior in various systems. Am J Dis Child. 1962;103:282.
13. Warthin AS. Occurrence of numerous large giant cells in tonsils and pharyngeal mucosa in prodromal stage of measles. Report of four cases. Arch Pathol. 1931;11:864.
14. Finkeldey W. Über Riesenzellbefunde in den Gaumenmandeln. Zugleich ein Beitrag zur Histopathologie der Mandelverä-derungen im Maserninkubationsstadium. Virchows Arch. 1931;281:323.
15. Kempe CH, Fulginiti VA. The pathogenesis of measles virus infection. Arch Ges Virusforsch. 1965;16:103.
16. Burnstein T, Frankel JW, Jensen JH. Adaptation of measles virus to suckling hamsters. Fed Proc. 1958;17:507.
17. Imagawa DT, Adams JM. Propagation of measles virus in suckling mice. Proc Soc Exp Biol Med. 1958;98:567.
18. Panum P. Observations made during the epidemic of measles on the Faroe Islands in the year 1846. Med Classics. 1938–9;3:829.
19. Krugman S. Present status of measles and rubella immunization in the United States: A medical progress report. J Pediatr. 1977;90:1.
20. CDC. Measles—United States, first 26 weeks. 1987. MMWR. 1988;37:53–7.
21. CDC. Recommendations of the Immunization Practices Advisory Committee—Measles. MMWR. 1987;36:409–25.
22. CDC. Summary of the Second National Community Forum on Adult Immunization. MMWR. 1987;36:677–80.
23. CDC. Measles—United States, 1985. MMWR. 1986;35:366–70.
24. Frank JA, Orenstein WA, Bart KJ, et al. Major impediments to measles elimination. Am J Dis Child. 1985;39:881–8.
25. Bennish M, Arnow PM, Beem MO, et al. Epidemic measles in Chicago in 1983. Sustained transmission in the preschool population. Am J Dis Child. 1986;140:341–4.
26. De Jong JG. The survival of measles virus in air, in relation to the epidemiology of measles. Arch Ges Virusforsch. 1965;16:97.
27. Ruckle G, Rogers KD. Studies with measles virus II. Isolation of virus and immunologic studies in persons who have had the natural disease. J Immunol. 1957;78:341.
28. Bloch AB, Orenstein W, Ewing WM, et al. Measles outbreak in a pediatric practice: Airborne transmission in an office setting. Pediatrics. 1985;75:767–83.

29. Remington PL, Hall W, Davis IH, et al. Airborne transmission of measles in a physician's office. JAMA. 1985;253:1574–7.
30. Modlin JF, Jabbour JT, Witte JJ, et al. Epidemiologic studies of measles, measles vaccine, and subacute sclerosing panencephalitis. Pediatrics. 1977;59:505.
31. Connolly JH, Allen IV, Hurwitz LJ, et al. Measles-virus antibody and antigen in subacute sclerosing panencephalitis. Lancet. 1967;1:542.
32. Barbosa LH, Fuccillo DA, Sever JL, et al. Subacute sclerosing panencephalitis: Isolation of measles virus from a brain biopsy. Nature. 1969;221:974.
33. Kettyls GD, Dunn HG, Dombsky N, et al. Subacute sclerosing panencephalitis: Isolation of a measles-like virus in tissue culture of brain biopsy. Can Med Assoc J. 1970;103:1183.
34. Payne FE, Baublis JV, Itabashi HH. Isolation of measles virus from cell cultures of brain from a patient with subacute sclerosing panencephalitis. N Engl J Med. 1969;281:585.
35. Ueda A, Okuno Y, Hamamoto Y, et al. Subacute sclerosing panencephalitis (SSPE): Isolation of a defective variant of measles virus from brain obtained at autopsy. Biken J. 1975;18:113.
36. Aicardi J, Goutieres F, Arsenio-Nunes ML, et al. Acute measles encephalitis in children with immunosuppression. Pediatrics. 1977;59:232.
37. Breitfeld V, Hashida Y, Sherman FE, et al. Fatal measles infection in children with leukemia. Lab Invest. 1973;28:279.
38. Gerson KL, Haslam HA. Subtle immunologic abnormalities in four boys with subacute sclerosing panencephalitis. New Engl J Med. 1971;285:78.
39. Sever JL. Persistent measles infection of the central nervous system: subacute sclerosing panencephalitis. Rev Infect Dis. 1983;4:467–73.
40. Adams JM, Imagawa DT. Measles antibodies in multiple sclerosis. Proc Soc Exp Biol Med. 1962;111:562.
41. Tannenbaum M, Hsu K, Buda J, et al. Electron microscopic virus-like material in systemic lupus erythematosus: With preliminary immunologic observations on presence of measles antigen. J Urol. 1971;105:615.
42. Kress S, Schluederberg AE, Hornick RB, et al. Studies with live attenuated measles-virus vaccine. Am J Dis Child. 1961;101:701.
43. Fenner F. The pathogenesis of the acute exanthems. Lancet. 1948;2:915.
44. Sergiev PS, Ryazantseva NE, Shroit IG. The dynamics of pathological processes in experimental measles in monkeys. Acta Virol (Engl). 1960;4:265.
45. Gresser I, Chany C. Isolation of measles virus from the washed leucocytic fraction of blood. Proc Soc Exp Biol Med. 1963;113:695.
46. Joseph BS, Lampert PW, Oldstone MBA. Replication and persistence of measles virus in defined subpopulations of human leukocytes. J Virol. 1975;16:1638.
47. Arneborn P, Biberfeld G. T-lymphocyte subpopulations in relation to immunosuppression in measles and varicella. Infect Immun. 1983;39:29–37.
48. Greenstein JI, McFarland HF. Response of human lymphocytes to measles virus after natural infection. Infect Immun. 1983;40:198–204.
49. Suringa DWR, Bank LJ, Ackerman AB. Role of measles virus in skin lesions and Koplik's spots. N Engl J Med. 1970;283:1139.
50. Kimura A, Tosaka K, Nakao T. Measles rash I. Light and electron microscopic study of skin eruptions. Arch Virol. 1975;47:295.
51. Kimura A, Tosaka K, Nakao T. An immunofluorescent and electron microscopic study of measles skin eruptions. Tohoku J Exp Med. 1975;117:245.
52. Lackmann PJ. Immunopathology of measles. Proc R Soc Med. 1974;67:12.
53. Enders JF, McCarthy K, Mitus A, et al. Isolation of measles virus at autopsy in cases of giant cell pneumonia without rash. N Engl J Med. 1959;261:875.
54. Mitus A, Holloway A, Evans AE, et al. Attenuated measles vaccine in children with acute leukemia. Am J Dis Child. 1962;103:413.
55. Krugman S, Giles JP, Friedman H, et al. Studies on immunity to measles. J Pediatr. 1965;66:471.
56. Ruckdeschel JC, Graziano KD, Mardiney MR. Additional evidence that the cell-associated immune system is the primary host defense against measles (rubeola). Cell Immunol. 1975;17:11.
57. Koplik H. The diagnosis of the invasion of measles from a study of the exanthemata as it appears on the buccal mucous membranes. Arch Pediatr. 1896;13:918.
58. Smithwick EM, Berkovich S. In vitro suppression of the lymphocyte response to tuberculin by live measles virus. Proc Soc Exp Biol Med. 1966;123:276.
59. Barkin RM. Measles mortality: A retrospective look at the vaccine era. Am J Epidemiol. 1975;102:341–9.
60. Barkin RM. Measles mortality. Analysis of the primary cause of death. Am J Dis Child. 1975;129:307–9.
61. Gibbs FA, Gibbs EL, Carpenter PR, et al. Electroencephalographic changes in "uncomplicated" childhood diseases. JAMA. 1959;171:1050.
62. McLean DM, Best JM, Smith PA, et al. Viral infections of Toronto children during 1965: II. Measles encephalitis and other complications. Can Med Assoc J. 1966;94:905.
63. Meulen VT, Müller D, Käckell Y, et al. Isolation of infectious measles virus in measles encephalitis. Lancet. 1972;2:1172.
64. Scott TF. Postinfectious and vaccinial encephalitis. Med Clin North Am. 1967;51:701.
65. Shaffer MF, Rake G, Hodes HL. Isolation of virus from a patient with fatal encephalitis complicating measles. Am J Dis Child. 1942;64:815.
66. Drzenick R, Rott R. Host-specific antigens of lipid-containing RNA viruses. Viruses as a carrier of cell-specific antigens. Int Arch Allergy. 1969;36(Suppl):146.
67. Johnson RT, Griffin D, Hirsch R, et al. Measles encephalomyelitis—clinical and immunologic studies. N Engl J Med. 1984;310:137–41.
68. McLellan RK, Gleiner JA. Acute hepatitis in an adult with rubeola. JAMA. 1982;247:2000.
69. Rauh LW, Schmidt R. Measles immunization with killed virus vaccine. Am J Dis Child. 1965;109:232.
70. Fulginiti VA, Eller JJ, Downie AW, et al. Altered reactivity to measles virus. JAMA. 1967;202:1075.
71. Frey HM, Krugman S. Atypical measles syndrome: Unusual hepatic, pulmonary, and immunologic aspects. Am J Med. 1981;281:55.
72. Lennon RG, Isacson P, Rosales T, et al. Skin tests with measles and poliomyelitis vaccines in recipients of inactivated measles virus vaccine: Delayed dermal hypersensitivity. JAMA. 1967;200:275.
73. Bellanti JA, Sanga RL, Klutinis B, et al. Antibody responses in serum and nasal secretions of children immunized with inactivated and attenuated measles-virus vaccines. N Engl J Med. 1969;280:628.
74. Norrby E, Ruckle GE, Meulen VT. Differences in the appearance of antibodies to structural components of measles virus after immunization with inactivated and live virus. J Infect Dis. 1975;132:262.
75. Annunziato D, Kaplan M, Hall WW, et al. Atypical measles syndrome: Pathologic and serologic features. Pediatrics. 1982;70:203–9.
76. Scott TJ, Bonanno DE. Reactions to live-measles virus vaccine in children previously inoculated with killed-virus vaccine. N Engl J Med. 1967;277:248.
77. Fulginiti VA, Arthur JH, Pearlman DS, et al. Altered reactivity to measles virus: Local reactions following attenuated measles virus immunization in children who previously received a combination of inactivated and attenuated vaccines. Am J Dis Child. 1968;115:671.
78. Stetler HC, Gens RD, Seastrom GR. Severe local reactions to live measles virus vaccine following an immunization program. Am J Public Health. 1983;73:899–900.
79. Mitus A, Enders JF, Craig JM, et al. Persistence of measles virus and depression of antibody formation in patients with giant cell pneumonia after measles. N Engl J Med. 1959;261:882.
80. CDC. Recommendations of the Immunization Practices Advisory Committee (ACIP))—Immunization of children infected with human T-lymphotrophic virus type III/lymphadenopathy-associated virus. MMWR. 1986;35:595–606.
81. Katz M, Stiehm ER. Host defense in malnutrition. Pediatrics. 1977;59:490.
82. Aaby P, Bukh J, Lisse IM, et al. Measles mortality, state of nutrition, and family structure: A community study for Guinea-Bissau. J Infect Dis. 1983;147:693–701.
83. Aaby P, Bukh J, Hoff G, et al. High measles mortality in infancy related to intensity of exposure. J Pediatr. 1986;109:40–4.
84. Gershon A, Young N. Chickenpox, measles, and mumps. In: Remington J, Klein J, eds. Infectious Diseases of the Fetus and Newborn Infants. Philadelphia: WB Saunders; 1989. In press.
85. Bloch AB, Orenstein WA, Hinman AR. Comment. J Infect Dis. 1981;143:753–4.
86. Gazala E, Karplus M, Liberman JR, et al. The effect of maternal measles on the fetus. Pediatr Infect Dis J. 1985;4:203–4.
87. Flick JA. Does measles really predispose to tuberculosis? Am Rev Respir Dis. 1976;114:257–65.
88. Report of the Committee on Infectious Diseases. 20th ed. Evanston, IL: American Academy of Pediatrics ("The Red Book"); 1988.
89. Rice GPA, Casali P, Oldstone MBA. A new solid-phase enzyme-linked immunosorbent assay for specific antibodies to measles virus. J Infect Dis. 1983;147:1055–9.
90. Wassilak S, Bernier R, Herrmann K, et al. Measles seroconfirmation using dried capillary blood specimens in filter paper. Pediatr Infect Dis J. 1984;3:117–21.
91. CDC. Recommendations of the Immunization Practices Advisory Committee—Immunization of children infected with human immunodeficiency virus—supplementary ACIP statement. MMWR. 1988;37:181–3.
92. Krugman S. Further-attenuated measles vaccine: Characteristics and use. Rev Infect Dis. 1983;5:477–81.
93. Pederson IR, Mordhorst CH, Ewald T, et al. Long-term antibody response after measles vaccination in an isolated arctic society in Greenland. Vaccine. 1986;4:173–8.
94. Sabin A, Albrecht P, Takeda A, et al. High effectiveness of aerosolized chick embryo fibroblast measles vaccine in seven-month-old and older infants. J Infect Dis. 1985;152:1231–7.
95. Peltola H, Heinonen O. Frequency of true adverse reactions to measles-mumps-rubella vaccine. Lancet 1986;1:939–44.
96. Gremillion D, Crawford G. Measles pneumonia in young adults. An analysis of 106 cases. Am J Med. 1981;71:539–42.
97. Chou T, Weil D, Arnow P. Prevalence of measles antibodies in hospital personnel. Infect Cont. 1986;7:309–11.
98. Hull H, Montes J, Hays P, et al. Risk factors for measles vaccine failure among immunized students. Pediatrics. 1985;76:518–23.
99. Wassilak S, Orenstein W, Strickland P, et al. Continuing measles transmission in students despite a school-based outbreak control program. Am J Epidemiol. 1985;122:208–17.
100. Gustafson T, Lievens A, Brunell P, et al. Measles outbreak in a fully immunized secondary-school population. N Engl J Med. 1987;316:771–4.
101. CDC, Measles in HIV-infected children, United States MMWR 1988;37:183–186.
102. Herman JJ, Radin R, Schneiderman R. Allergic reactions to measles (rubeola) vaccine in patients hypersensitive to egg protein. J Pediatr. 1983;102:196.

103. Olding-Stenkvist E, Forsgren M, Henley D, et al. Measles encephalopathy during immunosuppression: Failure of interferon treatment. Scand J Infect Dis. 1982;14:1–4.
104. DuRant R, Dyken P, Swift A. The influence of inosiplex treatment on the neurological disability of patients with subacute sclerosing panencephalitis. J Pediatr. 1982;101:288–93.

138. MEASLES-LIKE VIRUS (SUBACUTE SCLEROSING PANENCEPHALITIS)

JAMES R. LEHRICH

This progressive inflammatory dementing illness of children and young adults was first described by Dawson[1] in 1934. In the past, it has been called *subacute inclusion body encephalitis*[1] and *subacute sclerosing leukoencephalitis*,[2] but *subacute sclerosing panencephalitis* (SSPE) is now the generally accepted descriptive term. Dawson[1] first suspected that this was a viral disease because of the inflammation and intranuclear inclusion bodies he observed in the brain tissue, but many attempts at animal transmission during the next three decades were unsuccessful. In 1965 the electron microscope revealed paramyxovirus-like nucleocapsids within inclusion bodies in brain cells (Fig. 1)[3,4]; these observations were followed by demonstration of elevated titers of antibodies to measles in serum and cerebrospinal fluid (CSF) samples from patients with SSPE[5,6] and of measles antigen in brain tissue.[5,6] However, because of the latent state of the virus, it was not until 1969 that infectious measles-like virus could be isolated from brain cells in cultures derived from SSPE patients.[7–9]

DESCRIPTION OF THE PATHOGEN

A paramyxovirus quite similar to measles virus has been isolated in several cases from explant cell cultures established from brain or lymphoid tissue derived from biopsy specimens or from recent autopsies.[7–10] For a description of measles virus, the reader is referred to Chapter 136. The viruses that have been isolated from SSPE brain tissue differ in a number of subtle ways from measles virus, and there are variations among strains of SSPE virus isolated from different patients.

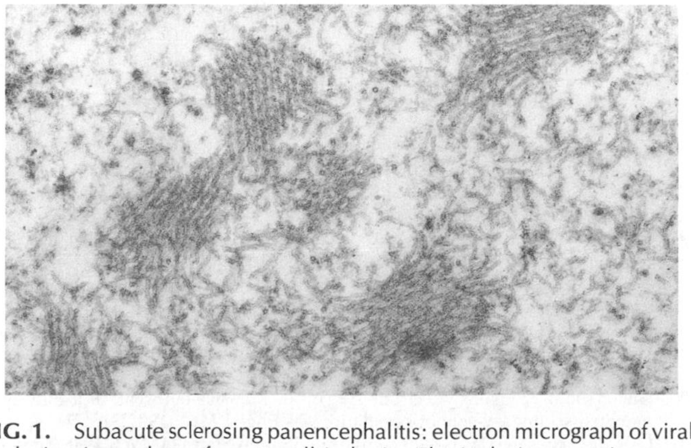

FIG. 1. Subacute sclerosing panencephalitis: electron micrograph of viral inclusion in nucleus of nerve cell in brain. The inclusion contains paramyxovirus-like nucleocapsid filaments with an outer diameter of 17 nm arranged singly and in aggregates. (×54,000) (Courtesy of Dr. K. E. Aström, Stockholm, Sweden.)

Some SSPE virus strains are capable of causing encephalitis in experimental animals[11,12]; measles virus can do so only after serial passage in animal brains. Measles and SSPE viruses behave differently in tissue culture, as judged by such criteria as plaque morphology, virus yield, and nuclear and cytoplasmic viral antigen formation.[13,14] It has also been reported that SV40-transformed cells and also cultured brain cells derived from non-SSPE persons are susceptible to measles virus but not to early-passage SSPE agents.[14] The SSPE viral RNA and structural polypeptides differ from those of measles virus.[15–17]

The appearance of the viruses under the electron microscope also differs.[18] In cells infected with SSPE virus, there are large intranuclear inclusions filled with smooth nucleocapsid filaments, filaments are not aligned under the cell membrane, and particles that bud from the cell membrane contain no nucleocapsids. Measles-infected cells contain small aggregates of smooth filaments in the nucleus, and buds from the cell membrane contain granular filaments that have been accumulated under the cytoplasmic membrane.

In SSPE virus infections, there is restricted synthesis of viral RNA and structural proteins, especially M (matrix) protein, and the quantities differ from patient to patient.[19–22] The deficiency of M protein has been shown in brain tissue from SSPE patients and in cell cultures infected with SSPE virus; it is especially characteristic of more virulent, nonbudding strains of SSPE virus.[19,20] Patients with SSPE show a relative lack of serum and CSF antibodies to M protein, in spite of high titers of antibodies to the other measles virus proteins.[23]

The differences between measles virus and the viruses isolated from SSPE tissue indicate that the SSPE virus is a variant of measles virus rather than a separate virus. Measles virus has been demonstrated to be labile and is susceptible to change as a result of serial passage in experimental animals or in tissue culture cells. Mutation of the virus might occur before infection or, as seems more likely, during a prolonged latent infection existent between the episode of clinical measles and the onset of SSPE. The increased genetic material in SSPE virus shown by RNA hybridization experiments suggests the possibility that the SSPE virus might arise as a result of recombination of measles virus with another as yet unknown second virus.[15,16]

The difficulty of isolating virus from patients with SSPE has been mentioned above. Virus has never been isolated from CSF or blood, and standard methods of inoculation of tissue extracts onto measles-susceptible cells in tissue culture have also been unsuccessful. Virus isolation has required establishment of explant cell cultures from fresh brain tissue obtained at biopsy or recent (usually less than 8 hours) autopsy.[7–9] Similar methods have also allowed isolation of the virus from lymph node biopsy specimens.[10] After 5–12 subcultivations (splits), these cells begin to show a cytopathic effect (CPE) of syncytia and multinucleate giant cell formation, similar to the CPE in measles-infected cells; these SSPE brain cells contain measles antigen demonstrable by immunofluorescent methods, as well as intranuclear and intracytoplasmic nucleocapsids that are visible under the electron microscope. Even at that stage, virus cannot be isolated unless the brain cell cultures are cocultivated or fused with susceptible cells (e.g., HeLa or monkey kidney cells). Not all SSPE-derived brain cell lines have yielded virus to these techniques; one group has reported only a 25 percent success rate.[24] These difficulties in virus detection and isolation indicate that measles virus is present in a latent or defective form in SSPE.

EPIDEMIOLOGY

SSPE is quite rare. Fewer than 40 new cases are reported each year in the United States. Reported incidence rates in different places have ranged from 0.12 to 1.4 per million, with some variation, probably related to differences in diagnosis and reporting.[25] The distribution is worldwide. Incidence rates have been stable or declining, with a dramatic decrease in the United States since 1970.[26] Most series of cases reported have shown a nonurban predominance, male/female ratios of 3:1 or greater, and more frequent occurrence in families of lower socioeconomic level. An association of SSPE with exposure to sick animals and the higher incidence in men from rural areas have suggested some form of zoonotic infection, perhaps with a second agent.[27,28] Although there have been reports of multiple cases of SSPE, it does not appear to be a contagious disease. SSPE may rarely occur after measles vaccination, but the overall impact of vaccination appears to have been to decrease the incidence of SSPE by preventing natural measles.[26,29,30]

Of considerable interest is the observation that a large proportion of patients with SSPE have had measles early in life; for example, in one case-control study, the patients with SSPE had measles (by history) at a mean age of 15 months, while the mean age was 48 months in the control group.[27] The interval between measles and the onset of SSPE ranges between 6 months and 18 years, with a mean of 7 years.[31]

PATHOGENESIS

Although a great deal has been learned about SSPE and its viral agent, the pathogenesis has not been explained. Almost the entire United States population has had measles or measles vaccination, but only one person in a million develops SSPE. There is evidence that the measles-like SSPE virus exists in a latent, defective form in the CNS and lymphoid tissues of patients; several intriguing hypotheses have been offered to explain how this causes the disease.

The defective nature of the virus is indicated by the difficulties encountered in its "rescue" from infected tissue, by the electron microscope evidence of incomplete viral maturation in infected cells, which results in defective bud formation,[18] and by the diminished synthesis of M protein. Moreover, dense oligoclonal IgG gamma globulin bands found in SSPE serum, CSF, and brain tissue extracts have been shown to contain antibodies to nucleocapsid and ribonucleoprotein antigens of measles virus, an observation that suggests persistent immunization of the host with defective, incompletely assembled, nonenveloped virus.[32]

The defective virus is present in large quantities in brains of SSPE patients, as demonstrated by electron microscope and by immunofluorescent antibody techniques, and an active humoral immune response is induced. High titers of antibodies to measles virus are found in serum and significant titers in CSF in most patients at some time during the course of the disease, and the titers may continue to rise as the disease progresses.[33] More than one-half the total CSF IgG may be measles-specific.[34] Both IgM and IgG antibodies are present in CSF and serum,[35] the IgM being another indication of persisting active infection. CSF flow studies with radioisotope-labeled IgG[36] and studies of oligoclonal IgG antibodies in CSF[32] have provided direct evidence that antibodies are synthesized within the CNS. Thus, the virus apparently replicates, and the disease progresses in spite of the high levels of humoral antibody present.

The disease could result from peculiarities of the SSPE virus (or viruses) itself. It is conceivable that the ways in which the SSPE virus differs from measles virus permit it to cause chronic CNS infection, but this remains to be proved. It is notable that the measles-like SSPE virus, but not measles virus itself, can produce subacute encephalitis in hamsters,[37] dogs,[38] calves,[39] lambs,[39] and ferrets.[40] A pathogenetic interaction between a papovavirus and measles virus has been postulated, based on electron microscope observation of papovavirus-like bodies in cells cultured from SSPE brains and on the epidemiologic data that suggest a zoonotic infection (see above).[27,28]

The defective production of viral RNA and M protein in SSPE virus-infected brain cells (see above) may indicate that the persistence of measles virus results from gene defects that prevent assembly of viral particles.[22] The deficiency of M protein may be particularly important in the pathogenesis of the disease,[19,20,23,41] since it is essential for attachment of nucleocapsids to the inner surface of the cell membrane. Its lack prevents budding of mature infectious virus, causing nucleocapsids to accumulate within the cell cytoplasm and nucleus, and viral glycoproteins to be exposed on the cell surface where they may stimulate production of high levels of antibodies.

It may be that the host immune response is more important in the causation of SSPE than is the virus itself. The high levels of measles antibody are not protective and might be harmful. Cells cultured from the brain of a patient with SSPE can be lysed in vitro by SSPE serum or CSF or measles antisera, in the presence of complement,[42] and a similar mechanism could cause tissue injury in vivo. Immune complexes of virus-IgG and complement have been found in renal glomeruli, muscle blood vessels, and brain cells,[43] but no pathogenetic role has been demonstrated for them. It has also been postulated that normal or exaggerated humoral immunity is accompanied by specific tolerance of thymus-dependent delayed hypersensitivity, so-called split tolerance.[44] No defect in cell-mediated immunity, similar to that found immediately after measles, has been demonstrated consistently in patients with SSPE.[45] A blocking factor that suppresses lymphocyte-mediated immunity to SSPE-measles virus has been described in SSPE CSF and plasma,[46] but other investigators have found that SSPE lymphocytes are cytotoxic to measles-infected target cells and that this cytotoxicity is actually enhanced by antimeasles antibodies.[47,48] Measles virus RNA sequences are found in circulating and brain perivascular lymphocytes in patients with SSPE, and it may be that infected lymphocytes play a role in the pathogenesis of the disease.[49] It is possible that virus-infected brain cells in SSPE patients are protected from immune attack by the clearance of surface viral antigens by measles antibody. As suggested by in vitro studies,[50] this antibody-induced antigenic modulation could prevent release and spread of enveloped viruses and allow accumulation of nucleocapsid and other viral proteins within the cell.

There are experimental animal models that appear to be relevant to the interaction of host immunity and viral latency in SSPE. In one model, hamster-adapted neurotropic (HNT) measles virus has been used to induce latent infection by means of intracerebral inoculation of newborn hamsters born of measles virus-immunized mothers.[51] This latent infection can be activated to produce an acute encephalitis by subsequent immunosuppression of the infected animals. In BALB-c mice inoculated intracerebrally with HNT virus, passive administration of measles antibody transforms an acute fatal encephalitis to a subacute encephalitis with persistent viral infection.[52] In another model, hamster-adapted SSPE virus causes a productive infection in weanling hamster brain, which later changes to a cell-associated or defective infection coincident with the appearance of high levels of measles antibodies in serum.[37]

It is intriguing to speculate that measles virus infection early in life, when passive maternal immunity is present and the host immune response is immature, may allow establishment of chronic infection and selection of cell-associated neurotropic mutants of measles virus, which eventually produce SSPE. However, at the present time the pathogenesis of SSPE remains to be elucidated.

PATHOLOGIC FINDINGS

This is a subacute encephalitis involving white and gray matter of cerebral hemispheres and brain stem, with perivascular and diffuse infiltrates of lymphocytes and plasma cells and with destruction of nerve cells. In more chronic cases, there is diffuse proliferation of microglia and astrocytes (gliosis) and degeneration of myelin. This is not a selective loss of myelin, since there is destruction of all brain tissue elements. Thus, SSPE should not be considered a demyelinating disease; the histopathologic changes resemble certain viral encephalitides of animals (e.g., visna and distemper) rather than multiple sclerosis (see Chapter 69) or postinfectious encephalomyelitis of humans (see Chapter 68).

Intranuclear eosinophilic inclusion bodies with surrounding halos (Cowdry type A) are seen in oligodendrocytes, astrocytes, and neurons. Intracytoplasmic inclusions are sometimes found in late stages of the disease. Histochemical and cytochemical studies have shown the inclusions to be composed of RNA and ribonucleoprotein (reviewed in Ref 53). Under the electron microscope, the inclusions are seen to contain tubular paramyxovirus-like nucleocapsids 17–19 nm in diameter[3,4] (Fig. 1). Immunofluorescence studies show measles antigen in inclusion bodies and also diffusely in nuclei and cytoplasm of neurons and glial cells.[5,6,53]

CLINICAL MANIFESTATION

SSPE is a progressive neurologic disease of children and young adults; rare cases have been reported in persons over 18 years of age. The average age of onset is between 7 and 8 years. Although there is a steady worsening of signs and symptoms of disease of gray and white matter of both cerebral hemispheres and of the brain stem, the illness may appear to evolve in stages. In the first of these, there is an insidious onset of intellectual decline, poor school performance, and abnormal behavior; this may seem to be a psychological problem. In the second stage, which develops after a period of weeks to months, the child may suddenly develop seizures, myoclonic jerks, apraxia, and visual impairment, accompanied by more severe intellectual deterioration. There may be cranial nerve palsies and chorioretinitis.[54] Fever and headache are not present. With further progression into the final stage, rigidity, hyperactive reflexes, extensor plantar responses, and further depression of consciousness develop, until the patient is reduced to a decorticate state, often with multifocal myoclonus. Death, usually a result of intercurrent infection, comes after a period of months (in children) to years (in adolescents). Rare patients die within a few weeks. Remissions are unusual, but occasional cases may stabilize or improve without treatment; such patients are usually severely impaired neurologically.

The CSF IgG gamma globulin level is increased and is accompanied by a first-zone colloidal gold curve; pressure, cell count, total protein, and glucose level are usually normal. Serum IgG is also increased. The CSF and serum immunoglobulins contain oligoclonal IgG M components of restricted heterogeneity, most of them with measles antibody activity[32,34]; these are not found in patients with measles. Antibodies to measles virus are found in serum and CSF in most patients at some time during the course of the disease, and titers may continue to rise as the disease progresses.[33] More than one-half of the total CSF IgG may be measles-specific.[34] The serum measles antibody levels are much higher than those found during or following measles or after measles vaccination. The antibodies in CSF are probably synthesized in the brain[36,32] and have not merely diffused passively from serum. The presence of significant titers of measles antibody in CSF is virtually diagnostic of SSPE, although low levels have been reported in multiple sclerosis (see Chapter 69).

The electroencephalogram (EEG) is diffusely slow early in the disease but eventually develops a periodic, synchronous burst-suppression pattern with high-voltage biphasic 1–4/second slow and sharp waves recurring every 3–10 seconds.[56] These waves may or may not be synchronous with myoclonic jerks. The isotope brain scan may be helpful in revealing lesions of both cortex and deeper structures.[57] Computed tomographic scans may show brain atrophy and areas of low attenuation in the white matter.[58]

PREVENTION AND TREATMENT

The incidence of SSPE after attenuated measles virus vaccination has been estimated to be $0.5–1.1/10^6$, as compared with an incidence of $5.2–9.7/10^6$ after natural measles,[29] so prophylactic immunization with measles vaccine should reduce the occurrence of the disease, as indicated by the declining incidence observed in the United States.[26]

There have been reports of small numbers of cases treated with a variety of antiviral and immunomodulatory agents, including bromodeoxyuridine, iododeoxyuridine, amantidine, corticosteroids, transfer factor, interferon, and plasma exchange, without convincing benefit. Reports of a beneficial effect of the antiviral and immunomodulatory drug inosiplex require confirmation.[59–61] Corticosteroid treatment has been ineffective. Supportive therapy, including treatment of seizures and proper care of the comatose patient, can help make the course of the illness smoother for the patient and his family.

REFERENCES

1. Dawson JR. Cellular inclusions in cerebral lesions of epidemic encephalitis. Arch Neurol Psychiatry. 1934;31:685.
2. Bogaert L van. Une leuco-encephalite sclérosante subaiguë. J Neurol Neurosurg Psychiatry. 1945;8:101.
3. Bouteille M, Fontaine C, Vedrenne C, et al. Sur un cas d'encéphalite subaiguë à inclusions. Étude anatomoclinique et ultrastructurale. Rev Neurol. 1965;113:454.
4. Tellez-Nagel J, Harter DH. Subacute sclerosing leucoencephalitis: ultrastructure of intranuclear and intracytoplasmic inclusions. Science. 1966;154:899.
5. Connolly JH, Allen IV, Hurwitz LJ, et al. Measles virus antibody and antigen in subacute sclerosing panencephalitis. Lancet. 1967;1:542.
6. Freeman JM, Magoffin RL, Lennette EH, et al. Additional evidence of the relation between subacute inclusion-body encephalitis and measles virus. Lancet. 1967;2:129.
7. Horta-Barbosa L, Sever J, Zeman W. Subacute sclerosing panencephalitis: isolation of measles virus from a brain biopsy. Nature. 1969;221:974.
8. Payne FE, Baublis JV, Itabashi HH. Isolation of measles virus from cell cultures of brain from a patient with subacute sclerosing panecephalitis. N Engl J Med. 1969;281:585.
9. Barbanti-Brodano G, Oyanagi S, Katz M, et al. Presence of two different viral agents in brain cells of patients with subacute sclerosing panencephalitis. Proc Soc Exp Biol Med. 1970;134:230.
10. Horta-Barbosa L, Hamilton R, Wittig B, et al. Subacute sclerosing panencephalitis: isolation of suppressed measles virus from lymph node biopsies. Science. 1971;173:840.
11. Katz M, Rorke LB, Masland WS, et al. Transmission of encephalitogenic agents from brains of patients with subacute sclerosing panencephalitis to ferrets. N Engl J Med. 1968;279:793.
12. Lehrich JR, Katz M, Rorke LB, et al. Subacute sclerosing panencephalitis. Encephalitis in hamsters produced by viral agents isolated from human brain cells. Arch Neurol. 1970;23:97.
13. Horta-Barbosa L, Fuccillo DA, Hamilton R, et al. Some characteristics of SSPE measles virus. Proc Soc Exp Biol Med. 1970;134:17.
14. Meulen V ter, Katz M, Käckell Y-M, et al. Subacute sclerosing panencephalitis: in-vitro characterization of viruses isolated from brain cells in culture. J Infect Dis. 1972;126:11.
15. Yeh J. Characterization of virus-specific RNA's from subacute sclerosing panencephalitis virus-infected CV-1 cells. J Virol. 1973;12:962.
16. Hall WW, Meulen V ter. RNA homology between subacute sclerosing panencephalitis and measles viruses. Nature. 1976;264:474.
17. Schluederberg A, Chavanich S, Lipman MB, et al. Comparative molecular weight estimates of measles and subacute sclerosing panencephalitis virus structural polypeptides by simultaneous electrophoresis in acrylamide gel slabs. Biochem Biophys Res Commun. 1974;58:647.
18. Oyanagi S, Meulen V ter, Katz M, et al. Comparison of subacute sclerosing panencephalitis and measles viruses: An electron microscope study. J Virol. 1971;7:176.
19. Lin FH, Thormar H. Absence of M protein in a cell-associated subacute sclerosing panencephalitis virus. Nature. 1980;285:490.
20. Hall WW, Choppin PW. Measles-virus proteins in the brain tissue of patients with subacute sclerosing panencephalitis. Absence of the M protein. N Engl J Med. 1981;304:1152.
21. Haase AT, Gantz D, Eble B, et al. Natural history of restricted synthesis and expression of measles virus genes in subacute sclerosing panencephalitis. Proc Natl Acad Sci USA. 1985;82:3020–24.
22. Baczko K, Liebert UG, Billeter M, et al. Expression of defective measles virus genes in brain tissues of patients with subacute sclerosing panencephalitis. J Virol. 1986;59:472–78.
23. Hall WW, Lamb RA, Choppin PW. Measles and subacute sclerosing panencephalitis virus proteins: lack of antibodies to the M protein in patients with subacute sclerosing panencephalitis. Proc Natl Acad Sci USA. 1979;76:2047.

24. Katz M, Koprowski H. The significance of failure to isolate infectious viruses in cases of subacute sclerosing panencephalitis. Arch Ges Virusforschung. 1973;41:390.
25. Brody JA, Gibbs CJ Jr. Chronic neurological diseases: subacute sclerosing panencephalitis, progressive multifocal leukoencephalopathy, kuru, Creutzfeldt-Jakob disease. In: Evans AS, ed. Viral Infections of Humans. New York: Plenum; 1976:519.
26. Modlin JF, Halsey NA, Eddins DL, et al. Epidemiology of subacute sclerosing panencephalitis. J Pediatr. 1979;94:231.
27. Detels R, Brody JA, McNew J, et al. Further epidemiologic studies of subacute sclerosing panencephalitis. Lancet. 1973;2:11.
28. Koprowski H. Interaction between papova-like virus and paramyxovirus in human cells: a hypothesis. Nature. 1970;225:1045.
29. Modlin JF, Jabbour JT, Witte JJ, et al. Epidemiologic studies of measles, measles vaccine, and subacute sclerosing panencephalitis. Pediatrics. 1977;59:505.
30. Halsey NA, Modlin JF, Jabbour JT, et al. The risk factors in subacute sclerosing panencephalitis: A case-control study. Am J Epidemiol. 1980;111:415.
31. Bellman MH, Dick G. Surveillance of subacute sclerosing panencephalitis. Br Med J. 1980;281:393–94.
32. Salmi AA, Noorby E, Panelius M. Identification of different measles virus-specific antibodies in the serum and cerebrospinal fluid from patients with subacute sclerosing panencephalitis and multiple sclerosis. Infect Immun. 1972;6:248.
33. Horta-Barbosa L, Krebs H, Ley A, et al. Progressive increase in cerebrospinal fluid measles antibody levels in subacute sclerosing panencephalitis. Pediatrics. 1971;47:782.
34. Mehta PD, Kane A, Thormar H. Quantitation of measles virus-specific immunoglobulins in serum, CSF, and brain extract from patients with subacute sclerosing panencephalitis. J Immunol. 1977;118:2254.
35. Connolly JH, Haire M, Hadden DSM. Measles immunoglobulins in subacute sclerosing panencephalitis. Br Med J. 1971;1:23.
36. Cutler RW, Merler E, Hammerstad JP. Production of antibody by the central nervous system in subacute sclerosing panencephalitis. Neurol. 1968;18(Pt 2):129.
37. Byington DP, Johnson KP. Experimental subacute sclerosing panencephalitis in the hamster: Correlation of age with chronic inclusion-cell encephalitis. J Infect Dis. 1972;126:18.
38. Nottermans SLH, Tijl WFJ, Willens FTC, et al. Experimentally induced subacute sclerosing panencephalitis in young dogs. Neurology. 1973;23:543.
39. Thien P, Mayr A, Meulen V ter, et al. Subacute sclerosing panencephalitis: Transmission of the virus to calves and lambs. Arch Neurol. 1962;27:540.
40. Mehta PD, Thormar H. Immunological studies of subacute measles encephalitis in ferrets: similarities to human sclerosing panencephalitis. J Clin Microbiol. 1979;9:601.
41. Choppin PW. Measles virus and chronic neurological diseases. Ann Neurol. 1981;9:17.
42. Oldstone MBA, Bokisch VA, Dixon FJ, et al. Subacute sclerosing panencephalitis: destruction of human brain cells by antibody and complement in an autologous system. Clin Immunol Immunopathol. 1975;4:52.
43. Dayan AD, Stokes MI. Immune complexes and visceral deposits of measles antigens in subacute sclerosing panencephalitis. Br Med J. 1972;2:374.
44. Burnet FM. Hypothesis: measles as an index of immunological function. Lancet. 1968;2:610.
45. Proceedings of the conference on cellular immunity and SSPE. Arch Neurol. 1975;32:488.
46. Ahmed A, Strong DM, Sell KW, et al. Demonstration of a blocking factor in the plasma and spinal fluid of patients with subacute sclerosing panencephalitis. J Exp Med. 1974;139:902.
47. Perrin LH, Tishon A, Oldstone MBA. Immunologic injury in measles virus infection. III. Presence and characterization of human cytotoxic lymphocytes. J Immunol. 1977;118:282.
48. Kreth HW, ter Meulen V. Cell-mediated cytotoxicity against measles virus in SSPE. J Immunol. 1977;118:291.
49. Fournier JG, Tardieu M, Lebon P, et al. Detection of measles virus RNA in lymphocytes from peripheral-blood and brain perivascular infiltrates of patients with subacute sclerosing panencephalitis. N Engl J Med. 1985;313:910–15.
50. Oldstone MBA, Tishon A. Immunologic injury in measles virus infection. IV. Antigenic modulation and abrogation of lymphocyte lysis of virus-infected cells. Clin Immunol Immunopathol. 1978;9:55.
51. Wear D, Rapp F. Latent measles virus infection of the hamster central nervous system. J Immunol. 1971;107:1593.
52. Rammohan KW, McFarland HF, McFarlin DE. Subacute sclerosing panencephalitis after passive immunization and natural measles infection: Role of antibody in persistence of measles virus. Neurology. 1982;32:390.
53. Meulen V ter, Katz M, Müller D. Subacute sclerosing panencephalitis. Curr Top Microbiol Immunol. 1972;57:1.
54. Robb RM, Watters GV. Ophthalmic manifestations of subacute sclerosing panencephalitis. Arch Opthalmol. 1970;83:426.
55. Panitch HS, Hooper CJ, Johnson KP. CSF antibody to myelin basic protein. Measurement in patients with multiple sclerosis and subacute sclerosing panencephalitis. Arch Neurol. 1980;37:206.
56. Gloor P, Kalabay O, Giard N. The electroencephalogram in diffuse encephalopathies: electroencephalographic correlates of grey and white matter lesions. Brain. 1968;91:779.
57. Dodson WE, Prensky AL, Siegel BA. Radionuclide imaging in subacute sclerosing panencephalitis. Neurology. 1979;29:749.
58. Krawiecki NS, Dyken Pr, Gammal T, et al. Computed tomography of the brain in subacute sclerosing panencephalitis. Ann Neurol. 1984;15:344–49.
59. Jones CE, Dyken PR, Huttenlocher PR, et al. Inosiplex therapy in subacute sclerosing panencephalitis. Lancet 1982;1:1034.
60. DuRant RH, Dyken PR. The effect of inosiplex on the survival of subacute sclerosing panencephalitis. Neurology. 1983;33:1053–55.
61. Noetzel MJ, Dodson WE. Progressive CT abnormalities despite clinical improvement in SSPE treated with inosiplex. Ann Neurol. 1983;13:457–60.

Rhabdoviridae

139. VESICULAR STOMATITIS VIRUS AND RELATED VIRUSES

MARK STOECKLE

Vesicular stomatitis virus (VSV) and related viruses commonly infect wild and domestic animals and occasionally are transmitted to humans, primarily to persons in close contact with infected animals. This chapter will describe the biology of VSV and related viruses and the clinical illnesses associated with infection in humans.

THE PATHOGEN

Vesicular stomatitis virus serotype Indiana is the prototype of the genus *Vesiculovirus*.[1] Vesiculoviruses are members of the family Rhabdoviridae, which includes rabies and related viruses (genus *Lyssavirus*). Like other rhabdoviruses, vesiculoviruses are enveloped RNA viruses with a single-stranded, negative-sense RNA genome and replicate in the cytoplasm of infected cells. The virions have a distinctive bullet-shaped appearance.

Vesiculoviruses are found in a wide variety of animal and insect species.[2] Seven of the characterized vesiculoviruses are thought to infect humans (Table 1). The original vesiculovirus isolates, VSV-New Jersey and VSV-Indiana, were obtained during outbreaks of vesicular stomatitis in livestock in 1925 and 1926.[6] The other vertebrate vesiculoviruses were identified only recently, and it is likely that additional vesiculoviruses will be discovered.

TABLE 1. Vesiculoviruses That Infect Humans

Virus Type	*Area of Endemic Virus Activity*	*Clinical Illness*
VSV-New Jersey	Southeastern United States, Central America, northern South America	Influenza-like
VSV-Indiana	Central America, northern South America	Influenza-like
VSV-Alagoas	Colombia, Brazil	Not known
Calchaqui	Argentina	Not known
Piry	Brazil	Influenza-like[a]
Chandipura	India	Influenza-like[a]
Isfahan	Iran	Not known

[a] Based on a small number of case reports.[3–5]

EPIDEMIOLOGY OF VSV-NEW JERSEY AND VSV-INDIANA

Disease activity in North America is limited to the two types that were first identified in the 1920s: VSV-New Jersey and VSV-Indiana. The range of VSV-New Jersey and VSV-Indiana extends into Central and South America. The reservoir for these viruses is thought to be wild animal populations in the southern United States and Central and South America. Transmission of VSV-New Jersey among wild swine in Georgia occurs during nonepidemic years,[7] and serologic studies in Central America suggest that both serotypes are enzootic in a wide variety of animal species ranging from porcupines to spider monkeys.[8]

Transmission of VSV among animals is thought to occur primarily through insect vectors. Vesicular stomatitis virus can be isolated from biting insects (including phlebotomine sandflies, midges, and black flies) in areas of endemic and epidemic disease activity.[9–11] Insects fed on infected animals can transmit VSV and other vesiculoviruses to uninfected animals in laboratory experiments.[12–14] Insects may be part of the reservoir cycle for VSV because these studies also indicate that virus can be maintained in sandflies by transovarial transmission.

Although insects are implicated as vectors in animal transmission, most cases of human infection in the United States are associated with direct contact with the oral secretions of infected animals.[15–18] The portal of entry is thought to be through abrasions on the skin or directly through oral mucosa. The infectivity of VSV for humans in these situations appears to be low. In one study 17 of 133 veterinarians and research workers (12.8 percent) who had been exposed to ill animals or to virus during an outbreak of VSV-New Jersey had neutralizing antibody to the virus as compared with 3 of 52 unexposed persons (5.8 percent).[18] A risk factor for seropositivity was a history of being sneezed upon by an infected animal. Seroconversion occurred in only 2 of 12 persons who had frequent contact with infected animals. The acquisition of VSV in a laboratory worker after the accidental injection of virus into the finger has also been described.[19]

The pattern of human infection with VSV is different in areas where VSV is enzootic. In Central America, 25–95 percent of persons in rural areas have neutralizing antibody to VSV-New Jersey, VSV-Indiana, or both and the prevalence of seropositivity increases with age.[8–10,20,21] A similar prevalence of seropositivity may be present in enzootic areas in the United States. One study found neutralizing antibody to VSV-New Jersey in 25 percent of persons living in rural Georgia.[22] The mechanism of transmission in enzootic areas is not known. It may be due to repeated close contact with infected animals or to transmission by insects.

In the United States, most recognized cases of human infection have developed during epidemics of vesicular stomatitis in horses and cattle.[6,17,18] Outbreaks of vesicular stomatitis have occurred at irregular intervals in the United States since the first established report in 1916. The most recent outbreak, in 1982, involved livestock in 14 western states. Disease activity is limited to the summer and fall (July–October) and is most frequent in three areas: in states bordering the Gulf of Mexico, in the upper Mississippi River valley, and in the Rocky Mountains.

EPIDEMIOLOGY OF OTHER VESICULOVIRUSES

The geographic ranges of the other vesiculoviruses are distinct (Table 1), but the patterns of transmission appear to be similar to that of VSV-New Jersey and VSV-Indiana. Serologic studies show a high prevalence of antibody in wild and domestic animals as well as in humans living in endemic areas, and virus has been isolated from biting insects in these areas.[3,4,23–25]

CLINICAL MANIFESTATIONS OF INFECTION WITH VSV-NEW JERSEY AND VSV-INDIANA

Vesicular stomatitis in horses and cattle is an acute febrile illness characterized by a vesicular exanthem of the mouth, tongue, and teats that may be clinically indistinguishable from foot-and-mouth disease. Vesicular stomatitis is rarely fatal in livestock, but economic losses may be significant, especially in dairy cattle in which decreased milk production after infection is common.

In humans, VSV produces an acute influenza-like febrile illness usually without clinical distinguishing features. The onset of illness occurs within 24–48 hours of exposure and is marked by fever, chills, general malaise, myalgias, nausea, vomiting, and pharyngitis. Oral vesicular lesions are reported in a few patients. The duration of illness is usually 4–7 days. Complications including pneumonia or meningitis have not been reported. The frequency of asymptomatic infection is not known but may be considerable. In one retrospective study, only 57 percent of persons with seroconversion to VSV-New Jersey or VSV-Indiana gave a history of clinical illness.[26]

CLINICAL MANIFESTATIONS OF INFECTION WITH OTHER VESICULOVIRUSES

Chandipura virus has been isolated from the blood in three patients in India with acute febrile illnesses including one child thought to have Reye syndrome,[5,17] and Piry virus infection has been reported in a laboratory worker.[4] Except for these reports, the clinical manifestations of human infection with the other vesiculoviruses are not known, although serologic studies suggest that human infection with VSV-Alagoas, Isfahan, Calchaqui, Piry, and Chandipura viruses is common in their respective endemic areas.[3,4,23–25]

DIAGNOSIS

The diagnosis of vesiculovirus infection rests on demonstrating seroconversion. Complement-fixing (CF) and neutralizing antibodies appear 10–14 days after the onset of illness. The titer of complement-fixing antibodies declines over a period of several months, but neutralizing antibodies persist for at least 1 year.[18,19] There is cross-reactivity between different vesiculoviruses, especially in CF immunofluorescence tests.[25,27] However, there is not enough cross-reactivity to reliably diagnose infection with a particular vesiculovirus unless type-specific antigens are used.

Although VSV-New Jersey and VSV-Indiana are readily cultured from oral lesions of infected animals, they have not been isolated from human cases, even when oral lesions were present. VSV-New Jersey was isolated from blood taken during the first 24 hours of illness in an infected laboratory worker,[16] but most other attempts to isolate virus from the blood of ill individuals have been negative.

TREATMENT

Human infection with VSV produces a self-limited illness of short duration for which symptomatic therapy is appropriate. A nucleotide analogue, carbocyclic 3-deazaadenosine, is very active against VSV in vitro (minimum inhibitory concentration, 0.2 μg/ml), and will protect mice against a lethal dose of VSV.[28] However, its usefulness in natural infection has not been established.

REFERENCES

1. Mathews REF. Classification and nomenclature of viruses: Fourth report of the international committee on taxonomy of viruses. Intervirology. 1982;17:109–14.

2. Shope RE, Tesh RB. The ecology of rhabdoviruses that infect vertebrates. In: Wagner RR, ed. *The Rhabdoviruses*. New York: Plenum; 1987:509–34.
3. Bhatt PN, Rodrigues FM. Chandipura: A new arbovirus isolated in India from patients with febrile illness. Indian J Med Res. 1967;55:1295–305.
4. Karabatsos N. International Catalogue of Arboviruses Including Certain Other Viruses of Vertebrates. 3rd ed. San Antonio: American Society of Tropical Medicine and Hygiene; 1985.
5. Rodrigues JJ, Singh PB, Dave DS, et al. Isolation of Chandipura virus from the blood in acute encephalopathy syndrome. Indian J Med Res. 1983;77:303–7.
6. Hanson RP. The natural history of vesicular stomatitis. Bacteriol Rev. 1952;16:179–204.
7. Stallknecht DE, Fletcher WO, Erickson GA, et al. Antibodies to vesicular stomatitis New Jersey type virus in wild and domestic sentinel swine. Am J Epidemiol. 1987;125:1058–65.
8. Tesh RB, Peralta PH, Johnson KM. Ecologic studies of vesicular stomatitis virus. Am J Epidemiol. 1969;90:255–61.
9. Shelodov A, Peralta PH. Vesicular stomatitis virus, Indiana type: An arbovirus infection of tropical sandflies and humans? Am J Epidemiol. 1967;86:149–57.
10. Tesh RB, Chaniotis BN, Peralta PH, et al. Ecology of viruses isolated from Panamanian phlebotomine sandflies. Am J Trop Med Hyg. 1974;23:258–69.
11. Walton TE, Webb PA, Kramer WL, et al. Epizootic vesicular stomatitis in Colorado, 1982. Epidemiologic and entomologic studies. Am J Trop Med Hyg. 1987;36:166–76.
12. Tao TR, Singh KRP, Dhanda V, et al. Experimental transmission of Chandipura virus by mosquitoes. Indian J Med Res. 1967;55:1306–10.
13. Tesh RB, Chaniotis BN, Johnson KM. Vesicular stomatitis virus (Indiana serotype): Transovarial transmission by phlebotomine sandflies. Science. 1972;175:1477–9.
14. Tesh RB, Modi GB. Growth and transovarial transmission of Chandipura virus (Rhabdoviridae: *Vesiculovirus*) in *Phlebotomus papatasi*. Am J Trop Med Hyg. 1983;32:621–23.
15. Hanson RP, Rasmussen AF, Brandly CA, et al. Human infection with the virus of vesicular stomatitis. J Lab Clin Med. 1950;36:754–8.
16. Fellowes ON, Dimopoullos GT, Callis JJ. Isolation of vesicular stomatitis virus from an infected laboratory worker. Am J Vet Res. 1955;16:623–6.
17. Fields BN, Hawkins K. Human infection with the virus of vesicular stomatitis during an epizootic. N Engl J Med. 1967;277:989–94.
18. Reif JS, Webb PA, Monath TP, et al. Epizootic vesicular stomatitis in Colorado, 1982: Infection in occupational risk groups. Am J Trop Med Hyg. 1987;36:17–82.
19. Johnson KM, Vogel JE, Peralta PH. Clinical and serologic response to laboratory-acquired human infection by Indiana type vesicular stomatitis virus (VSV). Am J Trop Med Hyg. 1966;15:244–6.
20. Brody JA, Fischer GF, Peralta PH. Vesicular stomatitis virus in Panama. Am J Epidemiol. 1967;86:158–61.
21. Cline BL. Ecological associations of vesicular stomatitis virus in rural Central America and Panama. Am J Trop Med Hyg. 1976;25:878–83.
22. Hanson RP, Karstad L. Feral swine as a reservoir of vesicular stomatitis virus in southeastern United States. Proc US Livestock Sanitary Assn. 1958;62:309–15.
23. Tesh R, Saidi S, Javadian E, et al. Isfahan virus, a new *Vesiculovirus* infecting humans, gerbils, and sandflies in Iran. Am J Trop Med Hyg. 1977;26:299–306.
24. Calisher CH, Monath TP, Sabattini MS, et al. A newly recognized vesiculovirus, Calchaqui virus, and subtypes of Melao and Maguari viruses from Argentina, with serologic evidence for infections of humans and horses. Am J Trop Med Hyg. 1987;36:114–9.
25. Tesh RB, Boshell J, Modi GB, et al. Natural infection of humans, animals, and phlebotomine sand flies with the Alagoas serotype of vesicular stomatitis virus in Columbia. Am J Trop Med Hyg. 1987;36:653–61.
26. Patterson WC, Mott LO, Jenney EW. Study of vesicular stomatitis in man. J Am Vet Med Assn. 1958;133:57–66.
27. Tesh RB, Travassos Da Rosa APA, Travassos Da Rosa JS. Antigenic relationship among rhabdoviruses infecting terrestrial vertebrates. J Gen Virol. 1983;64:169–76.
28. Clercq E, Montgomery JA. Broad-spectrum antiviral activity of the carbocyclic analog of 3-deazaadenosine. Antiviral Res. 1983;3:17–24.

140. RABIES VIRUS

KENNETH W. BERNARD
DANIEL B. FISHBEIN

Rabies is one of the oldest known and most feared of human diseases. It is caused by the rabies virus, which is 1 of over 100 rhabdoviruses currently recognized.[1] Only four (rabies, Mokola, Duvenhage, and vesicular stomatitis virus) are known to cause disease in humans. Rabies, almost always transmitted to humans by the bite of an infected mammal, was well recognized in early Middle Eastern civilizations including Egypt where it is mentioned in the Eshnunna Code dating to before 2300 BC. It was described in animals by Aristotle,[2,3] and rabies was well described by Celsus in 100 AD, who recognized hydrophobia as a symptom and recommended cautery of animal bites with a hot iron as a preventive measure.[4] Rabies appears to have been unrecognized in the New World before the arrival of Europeans and may have been introduced to North and South America by dogs accompanying conquistadors. It has always been known as a disease primarily affecting dogs, although it is now well recognized that major reservoirs occur in many wild animal species. In 1198, Moses Maimonides, the Talmudic scholar and physician, wrote in his *Treatise on Poisons and their Antidodes* that, "Everything in the literature against the bite of a mad dog is useful, if at all, only when applied before rabies sets in. When such is the case I have as yet seen nobody who escaped with his life."[5] The treatment of choice for rabid animal bites remained cautery until 1885 when Pasteur introduced a rabies vaccine.[6] Rabies remains a disease that is much more easily prevented than treated, although in the 1970s three patients with rabies recovered. Several excellent reviews of human and animal rabies are available.[7–10]

VIROLOGY

Classification

Rabies and rabies-related viruses belong to the family of viruses called Rhabdoviridae (Gk. *rhabdos,* rod) because of their bulletlike shape. This group of morphologically similar viruses consists of members that infect vertebrates, invertebrates, and plants. Within the animal rhabdoviruses, two genera have been designated on the basis of distinct antigenic and biologic characteristics[11–12]: *Lyssavirus* (Gk. *lyssa,* frenzy) and *Vesiculovirus* (L. *vesicula,* little bladder). The lyssaviruses include rabies virus and five rabies-related viruses (Table 1). Vesicular stomatitis virus and related vesiculoviruses, not covered in this chapter, cause disease in cattle, swine, horses, and a variety of other vertebrates. Humans are occasionally infected, usually asymptomatically and occasionally with a nonfatal, nonspecific, influenza-like viral syndrome.[13] Marburg and Ebola viruses, formally included within the Rhabdoviridae, are now classed in the family Filoviridae.[11]

Morphology and Antigenic Structure

Rabies virions measure approximately 180 by 75 nm and are cylindrical with one round or conical end and one flat end, giving each particle the shape of a bullet (Fig. 1). In cell cultures, bacilliform particles, some of which are short and some of which are long, commonly are seen, and it has been proposed that these shapes may be artifacts of preparation or staining procedures. The surface of the virus consists of a bilayered envelope derived primarily from host cell membranes. Regularly spaced knoblike spikes 6 to 7 nm long cover the surface of the virion except at the flat end where there is an axial depression.[1]

TABLE 1. Lyssaviruses

Name	Source
Rabies virus[a]	Most mammals
Duvenhage[a]	Insectivorous bats, humans
Lagos bat	Frugivorous bats
Mokola[a]	*Crocidura* shrews, humans
Kotonkan[b]	*Culicoides* midges
Obodhiang[b]	*Mansonia* mosquitoes

[a] Known to cause disease in humans.
[b] Distantly related to rabies virus only through serologic cross-reactions.

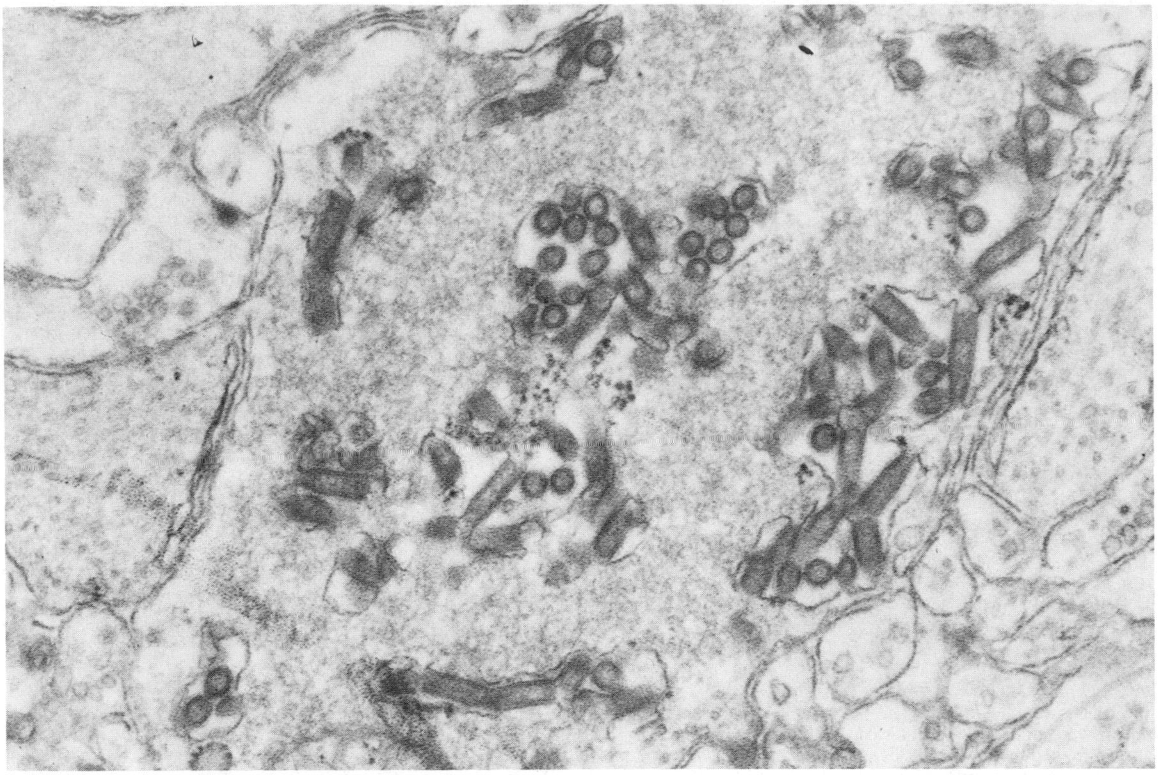

FIG. 1. Electron micrograph of CVS rabies virus from the brain of a mouse. The virus is bullet-shaped when viewed longitudinally and round when viewed transversely. (×67,000) (Courtesy of Dr. Carey S. Callaway.)

The envelope encloses an infectious 50 by 165 nm helical nucleocapsid consisting of 30–35 coils. The viral nucleic acid is a single molecule of noninfectious, negative-stranded RNA with a molecular weight of 4,600,000.

Five proteins have been identified from purified rabies virus: glycoprotein (G), nucleocapsid (N) protein, viral polymerase (large [L]), and two smaller proteins, NS(P), and M.[14] The glycoprotein (molecular weight, 67,000), the primary structural component of the surface spikes, is the antigen capable of inducing the virus-neutralizing antibody.[15] The N protein (molecular weight, 56,000) makes up the group-specific antigen common to all lyssaviruses.[16] Although antinucleocapsid antibody does not possess neutralizing activity, it is useful for detecting rabies-specific intracytoplasmic inclusions (Negri bodies) by immunofluorescence and indicates that these Negri bodies are composed primarily of nucleocapsid material. The NS(P) protein (molecular weight, 38,000) is associated with the nucleocapsid, while the M protein (molecular weight, 26,000) is associated with the lipoprotein viral envelope.[17]

Monoclonal antibodies directed against both nucleocapsid and glycoprotein antigens have been developed.[18] The use of monoclonal antibodies has not only allowed the rapid differentiation of rabies and rabies-related viruses but has also demonstrated substantial rabies virus strain variation suggesting antigenic specificity related to geographic area and animal origin.[19–21]

Environmental Stability

Rabies virus is unstable at pH ≤3 or pH ≥11. Virus suspended in 0.1% bovine serum albumin at neutral pH is inactivated with a half-life of about 24 hours at 4°C, 4 hours at 40°C, 30 minutes at 54°C, and 35 seconds at 60°C.[22] Rabies virus is stable for many years when frozen at −70°C or freeze-dried and held at 0–4°C. The virus is rapidly inactivated by desiccation, ultraviolet and x-irradiation, sunlight, trypsin, β-propiolactone, ether, and detergents.[23]

Rabies-Related Viruses

Five rhabdoviruses have been reported to be morphologically and serologically related to but distinct from rabies virus[8,20]: Mokola virus, Kotonkan virus, and Lagos bat virus were first isolated in Nigeria; Duvenhage virus was isolated from a person in South Africa with a fatal case of rabies-like encephalitis[24]; and Obodhiang virus was isolated in Sudan (Table 1). Although all six lyssaviruses are related through common complement fixation and immunofluorescent antigens, Obodhiang and Kotonkan viruses display only limited cross-reactivity with rabies virus and are more closely related to Lagos bat virus. The individual members of the *Lyssavirus* genus can be differentiated by monoclonal antibody techniques. Other than rabies, only Duvenhage and Mokola viruses have been isolated from humans. Clinically, the fatal illness with Mokola was a paralytic form of encephalitis without furious symptoms suggesting rabies.[25] The rabies-related viruses are known to occur naturally only in sub-Saharan Africa; only limited information is available on their epidemiology and clinical significance.

EPIDEMIOLOGY

Animal Rabies

Rabies is primarily a disease of animals, and the epidemiology of human rabies closely parallels the epizootiology of animal rabies.[7,26] In areas where domestic animal rabies has not been adequately controlled, dogs account for 90 percent or more of the reported human cases. In contrast, in areas where domestic animal rabies is well controlled such as the United States, Canada, and many western European countries, dogs account for fewer than 5 percent of the reported cases.

Domestic animals other than dogs account for 5–10 percent of all reported animal rabies worldwide. Cats and cattle account for most of these cases, but horses, sheep, and occasionally pigs and other farm animals also may develop rabies. Exotic pets such as skunks, racoons, and ferrets in recent years, have been confirmed as rabid and have resulted in many persons requiring rabies postexposure prophylaxis.

Most wild mammals can become infected with rabies including animals that are extremely susceptible to rabies infection such as foxes, coyotes, wolves, and jackals; those that have intermediate susceptibility to infection such as skunks, raccoons, bats, bobcats, mongooses, and monkeys; and those such as the opposum that are quite resistant to infection.[22] Principal wildlife vectors of rabies include the mongoose and jackal in Africa; the fox in Europe and the Arctic and sub-Arctic regions; the wolf in western Asia; the vampire bat in Latin America; and the striped skunk, raccoon, and insectivorous bat in the United States.[27] It is likely that rabies is maintained as an endemic illness in each of the aforementioned species by animal-to-animal bite transmission wherever the density of the population is sufficiently great.[7] Small rodents, birds, and reptiles are not known to serve as reservoirs of rabies in nature, although rodents and birds can be infected.[28]

As shown in Figure 2, domestic animal rabies was controlled in the United States by the early 1960s, and by 1975 only 2242 rabid animals were reported. However, in the late 1970s, wild animal epizootics occurred in several areas. Beginning in 1979 an increase was noted in the number of rabid skunks reported in the central region of the United States from Texas north to the Dakotas. By 1981, the number of rabid skunks reached a high of 4480, pushing the total number of confirmed rabid animals to 7211, the highest level since 1954.[29] Through 1988, skunks remained the most commonly reported rabid animal in the United States. Beginning in 1977 with a single rabid raccoon reported from West Virginia, an explosive epizootic of raccoon rabies swept through the mid-Atlantic states of Virginia, West Virginia, Maryland, Pennsylvania, and the District of Columbia. This epizootic was possibly started by the importation of rabid raccoons from northern Florida and southern Georgia for hunting purposes.[30]

Human Rabies

Human rabies has been acquired on all continents except Australia and the Antarctic. The largest number of cases occur in countries in which domestic animal rabies has not been adequately controlled, and although the worldwide incidence of human rabies is not known, in 1985, 25,000 deaths were reported to the World Health Organization (WHO).[31] Reporting to WHO is voluntary, and this number certainly underestimates the actual number of cases. Based on this reporting, rates of human disease in endemic countries range from less than 0.01/million/yr in the United States, to 28.8/million/yr in India.[32] Approximately 60 countries including the United Kingdom, Japan, Finland, Sweden, Norway, Portugal, many Caribbean islands, and most of Pacific Oceania including Australia are reported to be rabies free as a result of geographic isolation, animal control programs, and quarantine regulations.[31,33,34]

Of the 50 human rabies cases reported to the Centers for Disease Control (CDC) between 1960 and 1987, 19 (38 percent) occurred in persons under the age of 16 years, and 9 (18 percent) occurred in those older than age 55. This presumably reflects a greater likelihood of exposure, greater susceptibility, or a greater relative effect of a given quantity of virus in these age groups.[8,35] Seventy-two percent of rabies victims were men. Figure 3 illustrates the changing epidemiologic picture of human rabies in the United States since 1950. The number of human cases decreased from 20 in 1952 to between 0 and 5 per year since 1960. This decline parallels the marked decrease in reported cases of dog rabies associated with the development of domestic animal control programs in the 1950s. In 1987, dogs and cats accounted for only 6 percent of the laboratory-confirmed rabid animals in the United States; however, 55 percent of the estimated 20,000 persons undergoing rabies postexposure prophylaxis reported dog or cat exposures as the reason for treatment.[36] Most cases of human rabies in the United States are now caused by dog bites that occurred in countries that have not controlled rabies, or involve persons who have either an unknown exposure history or were bitten by wild animals (Fig. 3). Of the 50 human cases reported to the CDC from 1960 to 1987, 14 (28 percent) acquired their infections after bites from rabid dogs outside the United States. It has been estimated that, worldwide, the incidence of dog bites ranges between 200 and 800 bites per 100,000 population per year and is independent of the presence of rabies in dogs.

A small number of cases of ''nonbite human rabies'' have been reported in which there were exposures to environments containing rabies virus in extremely high concentration, including caves in which aerosolized rabies virus from bat secretions was present, and in laboratories working with infected tissues or aerosolized virus.[37–40] Experimental studies have shown that rabies can be produced by contact of the virus on conjunctiva, on mucous membranes, or on scratches, and in the United States 40 percent of persons obtaining postexposure prophylaxis report nonbite exposures.[36] Rabies has occurred in four persons who received corneal transplants from donors who

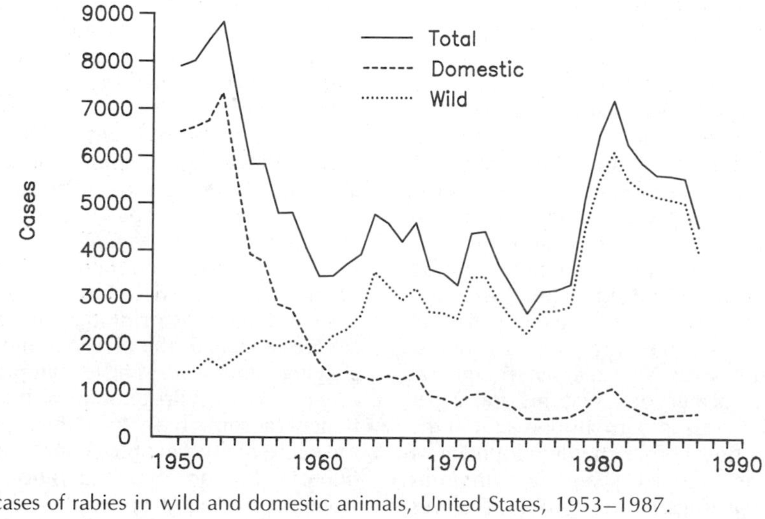

FIG. 2. Reported cases of rabies in wild and domestic animals, United States, 1953–1987.

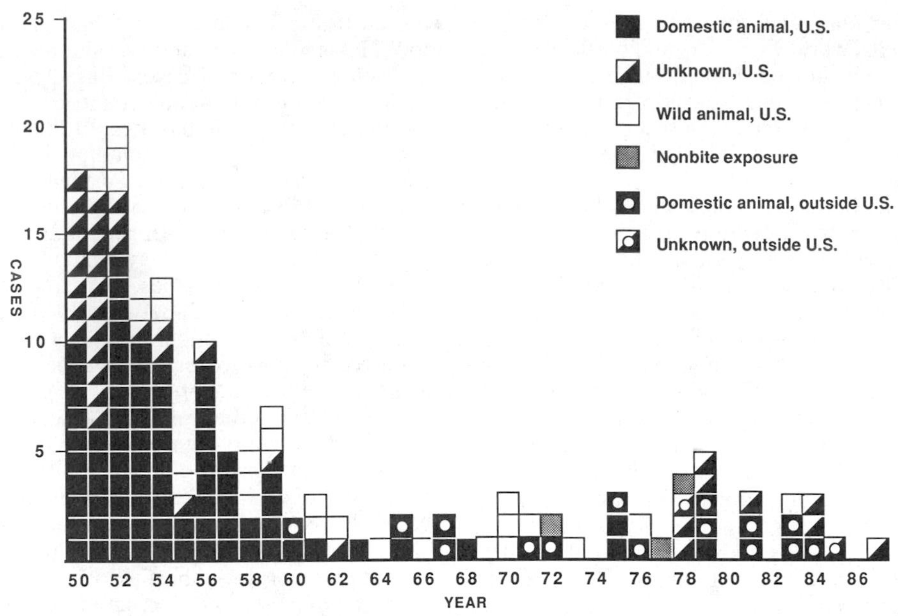

FIG. 3. Human rabies cases and source of exposure, United States, 1950–1987.

died of undiagnosed rabies encephalitis; all four recipients later died of rabies.[41–43] Despite these exceptions, rabies is usually always caused by bites of a rabid animal whose saliva contains the virus.

PATHOGENESIS AND CLINICAL MANIFESTATIONS

Incubation Period

The reported incubation period of rabies in the literature has varied from as short as 4 days to as long as 19 years.[9] Ninety-five percent of the cases have incubation periods less than 1 year, although several well-documented cases have occurred 1–5 years or more after exposure.[8,44–46] In some of these cases with long incubation periods, the possibility that secondary exposures had occurred was not ruled out (Fig. 4). The incubation period is usually between 20 and 90 days. It has been reported to be shorter when the site of the bite is on the head (25–48 days) than when it is on an extremity (46–78 days).[44] This difference may be related to the severity of the bite or to the quantity of virus inoculated.[46] Although it has been thought that vaccinated people have shorter incubation periods, a recent analysis of human rabies cases in the United States revealed no difference in the incubation period between persons who had received postexposure prophylaxis and those who received no treatment.[47] During the incubation period, the person is usually well except for symptoms related to local wound healing. Some reports suggest that acute stress or corticosteroid administration may terminate the incubation period and precipitate clinical disease, although these are generally anecdotal observations.[8] Steroids have been reported to increase rabies mortality in experimental animals and to decrease the immune response to vaccines.[48] Thus the use of steroids in treating persons exposed to rabies is not recommended.[49] During the incubation period the virus apparently remains localized near the site of the bite, possibly undergoing multiplication within the muscle cells.[50,51] After a latent period lasting from days to several weeks, months, or possibly years, the virus spreads via peripheral nerves to the spinal cord, central nervous system, and especially the limbic system.[7,51] The virus is normally present in the central nervous system in high titer before the development of systemic symptoms.[51,52] By the time the systemic symptoms occur, the virus has traveled centrifugally down efferent nerves to nearly every organ and tissue including, most importantly for the life cycle of the virus, the salivary glands.

Prodrome

The initial symptoms of clinical rabies most often are nonspecific and consist of malaise, fatigue, headache, anorexia, and fever. In approximately 50 percent of the patients, pain or paresthesia occurs at the site of the exposure and may be the first rabies-specific symptom. In the absence of local complaints the prodrome commonly is entirely nonspecific, although apprehension, anxiety, agitation, irritability, nervousness, insomnia, psychiatric disturbances, or depression may suggest neurologic involvement. Other nonspecific and common symptoms occur often during the prodrome including cough, chills, sore throat, abdominal pain, nausea, vomiting, or diarrhea. These symptoms often lead to an initial diagnosis of common respiratory or abdominal infections.[7,8,47,53]

Acute Neurologic Period

The prodrome normally lasts 2–10 days and merges with the acute neurologic period, which begins when the patient develops objective signs of central nervous system involvements. The initial neurologic signs may include hyperactivity, disorientation, hallucinations, seizures, bizarre behavior, nuchal stiffness, or paralysis. In most cases marked hyperactivity typically develops and lasts hours to days. Hyperactivity characteristically is intermittent, with 1- to 5-minute periods of agitation, thrashing, running, biting, or other bizzare behavior alternating with periods of calm.[8,9,53] The hyperactive episodes may occur spontaneously or may be precipitated by a variety of tactile, auditory, visual, or other stimuli. Between these episodes the patient commonly is cooperative and oriented, although he may remain anxious. In 50 percent or more of these cases attempts at drinking during this period are followed by severe spasms of the pharynx and larynx that produce choking, gagging, and fear. These symptoms may be precipitated by seeing water (hydrophobia) or by blowing air on the face of the patient (aerophobia).[54,55] Other symptoms and signs seen during the acute neurologic phase include fever, muscle fasciculations, hyperventilation, hypersalivation, focal or generalized convulsions, and rarely priapism.

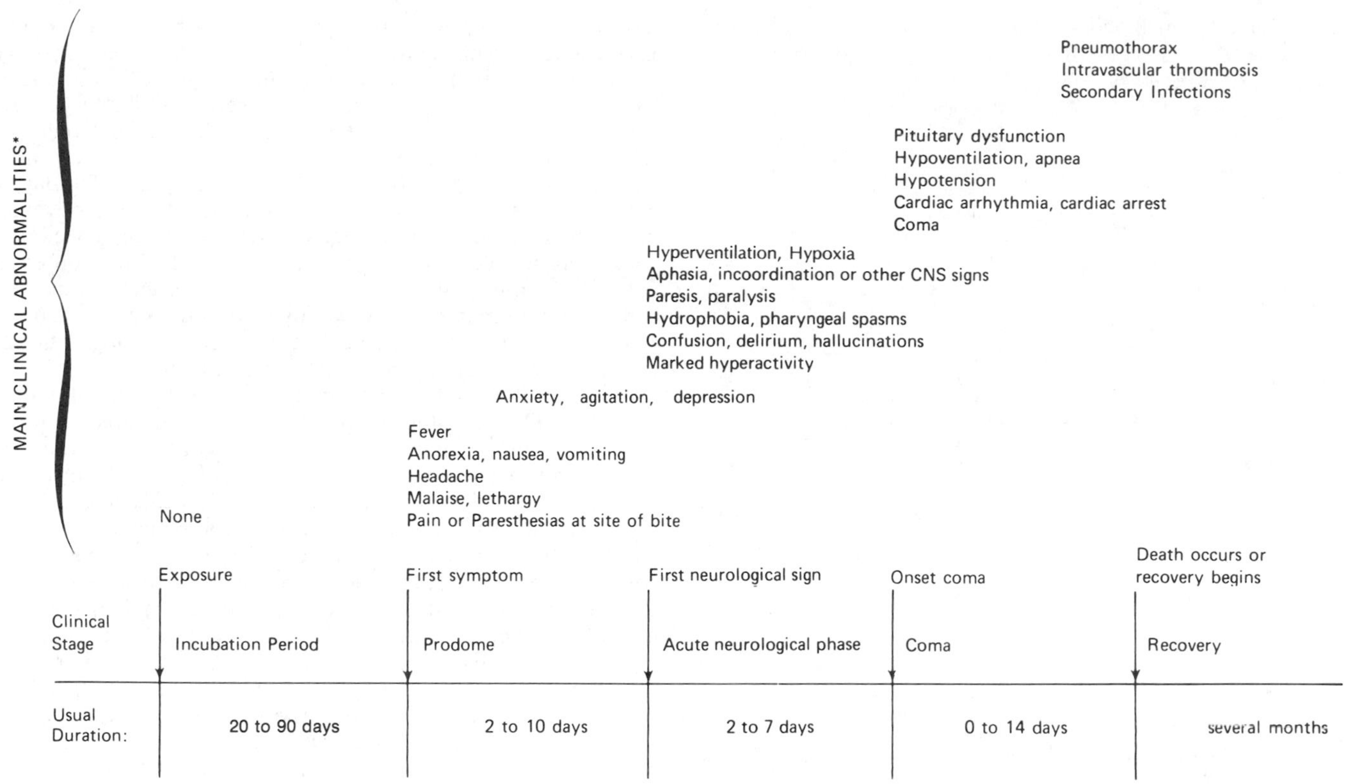

FIG. 4. The natural history of clinical rabies in humans. Hypothetical composite case. (All clinical abnormalities need not be present in each case.)

Unless the patient dies abruptly (usually from respiratory or cardiac arrest), paralysis develops and becomes the predominant neurologic problem. In approximately 20 percent of the patients, paralysis dominates the entire clinical course (paralytic rabies).[56–58] The paralysis may be maximal in the bitten extremity, diffuse and symmetric, or it may ascend as in the Guillain-Barré syndrome. Paralytic rabies apparently appears more frequently after exposures to rabid bats and after postexposure vaccination with nerve tissue-derived vaccines.

During the acute neurologic period the mental status gradually progresses from confusion to disorientation, stupor, and finally coma. Nuchal stiffness may be present. Cerebrospinal fluid (CSF) pressure may be normal or elevated, and CSF protein levels are most often normal. An increased number of leukocytes may be seen in the CSF during the first week of illness in approximately 70 percent of persons, and the differential count is highly variable.[47] The acute neurologic phase lasts 2–7 days, with longer durations in the paralytic forms. It ends either with an abrupt death or with the onset of coma. Throughout this period the mental status continues to fluctuate with periods of agitation or severe obtundation alternating with periods of relative normality.

Coma

Coma occurs 4–10 days after the onset of symptoms and may last for hours to months. In untreated patients, respiratory arrest usually occurs at or shortly after the onset of coma, and the patient dies. In patients in the United States not receiving intensive supportive care, the average duration of illness until death is 7 days. For those receiving intensive support, the duration of illness averages 25 days.[47] A variety of fatal or potentially fatal complications occurs during the coma phase as is discussed below. Death is usually the immediate result of one of these complications.

Recovery

Three cases of recovery from presumed rabies have now been reported.[38,59,60] In these nonfatal cases, each person had received either postexposure or pre-exposure prophylaxis before the onset of clinical illness. Several additional poorly documented cases of recovery from rabies had been reported previously in the medical literature. The first well-documented case occurred in a 6-year-old boy in 1970. In that case the coma lasted 7 days, and there was a progressive gradual improvement in symptoms that led to no detectable abnormalities 6 months after the onset.[59] The second nonfatal case was reported from Argentina in 1972 with encephalitic symptoms (without coma) lasting approximately 3 months and a slow recovery over a period of approximately 6 months.[60] The third case of rabies developed in a laboratory worker who had had pre-exposure immunization and was infected with a laboratory strain of virus. The coma lasted approximately 2 weeks, and gradual but incomplete improvement followed.[38] Although most of the rabies cases in the United States since 1970 have received intensive medical management, no other survivors have been reported.

Complications

A large number of complications have been documented in rabies, most of which occur during the coma phase (Table 2).[59,61] Neurologic complications reported in addition to those previously noted include increases in intracranial pressure that may occur during the late neurologic or coma phases, hypothalamic involvement producing inappropriate secretion of antidiuretic hormone and/or diabetes insipidus, and autonomic dysfunction leading to hypertension, hypotension, cardiac arrhythmias, or hypothermia. Seizures are common, may be generalized or focal, and may be accompanied by cardiac arrhythmias, cardiac arrest, or respiratory dysfunction. Respiratory complications occur in all cases. Hypoventilation and respiratory depression

TABLE 2. Clinical Complications of Human Rabies

Reported Problems	*Treatment*
Neurologic	
Hyperactive episodes	Phenothiazines, benzodiazepines
Hydrophobia	Nothing by mouth
Focal seizures	Carbamazepine, phenytoin
Localized neurologic signs	None
Cerebral edema	Mannitol, glycerol
Aerophobia	Avoid stimulation
Pituitary	
Inappropriate secretion of antidiuretic hormone	Fluid restriction
Diabetes insipidus	Fluid, vasopressin
Pulmonary	
Hyperventilation	None
Hypoxemia	Oxygen, ventilation, PEEP
Atelectasis	Artificial ventilation
Apnea	Artificial ventilation
Pneumonia	Physical therapy, antibiotics
Pneumothorax	Reexpansion
Cardiovascular	
Cardiac arrhythmia	Oxygen therapy, drugs as indicated
Hypotension	Fluid, drugs as indicated
Congestive heart failure	Restrict fluid, drugs as indicated
Arterial or venous thrombosis	Heparin
Superior vena caval obstruction	Prevention
Cardiac arrest	Resuscitation
Other	
Anemia	Transfusions
Gastrointestinal bleeding	H_2 blockers, transfusions
Hyperthermia	Cooling mattress
Hypothermia	Heat blankets
Hypovolemia–hypervolemia	Fluid balance
Paralytic ileus	Parenteral fluids
Urinary bladder paralysis	Catheterization
Acute renal failure	Hemodialysis
Pneumomediastinum	None

Abbreviation: PEEP: positive end-expiratory pressure.

develop routinely during the acute neurologic phase, although hyperventilation and respiratory alkalosis appear to be common, particularly during the prodrome and early neurologic phase.[59,61] Progressive hypoxia, which is not corrected by increasing the inspired oxygen concentration, and decreased pulmonary compliance develop later. Chest x-ray films are commonly normal early in the course but later may show diffuse or localized infiltrates secondary to aspiration, superinfection, congestive heart failure, pneumomediastinum or the adult respiratory distress syndrome. Cardiac supraventricular arrhythmias are common, and severe bradycardia and cardiac arrest may occur in association with hypoxia. Histologic evidence of myocarditis has been reported.[62,63] The hypotension that accompanies these problems aggravates pre-existing hypoxia, and death commonly follows rapidly. Hypotension may also develop as a result of congestive heart failure, fluid depletion, autonomic dysfunction, or intrinsic vascular dysfunction. Other major complications that have been reported include acute renal failure, thrombosis of the superior vena cava, secondary bacterial infection of the lungs or urinary tract, and gastrointestinal hemorrhage.[61,64,65] A transient skin rash has been reported. The white blood cell count typically ranges from 8000 to 13,000/mm^3 with 6–8 percent atypical monocytes. The platelet count is usually normal, and hematocrit and hemoglobin values gradually decrease during the clinical course. Albuminuria and an increased number of white cells in the urinary sediment are commonly seen.

Diagnosis

No tests are currently available to diagnose rabies in humans before the onset of clinical disease. The virus is immunologically protected, probably within myocytes or neurons near the exposure site, and does not usually stimulate antibody production until after invasion of the central nervous system. In human rabies cases reported in the United States between 1960 and 1979, rabies serum neutralizing antibody was detected at the earliest on the sixth day of clinical illness, and CSF antibodies were negative as long as 7 days after serum antibody was detected.[47] Of the patients in this series who had not received rabies postexposure prophylaxis, 50 percent had serum antibody titers by the 8th day and 100 percent by the 15th day of clinical illness. However, a 5-year-old girl who died of rabies in March 1983 and had been given steroids during her clinical course did not develop diagnostic titers until 28 days after its onset.[66] Another rabies patient who had probable immunosuppression from interferon therapy died 24 days after the onset of clinical symptoms without detectable neutralizing antibody in either the serum or CSF at the time of death.[67]

In the United States, the rapid fluorescent focus inhibition test (RFFIT) is the standard test for measuring rabies-neutralizing antibody.[68] The results from this in vitro cell culture neutralization test are available within 24 hours, and the test is as specific and sensitive as the in vivo mouse neutralization test, which can take as long as 14 days to complete. Neutralizing antibody titers are often expressed in international units (IU), which are derived from a comparison of the test serum titer with an international standard antiserum containing a fixed quantity of rabies-neutralizing antibody per milliliter (depending on the circumstances of the testing procedure, a titer of 1.0 IU is approximately equal to a reciprocal titer of 1:30–1:140). The WHO has determined that the conservative value of 0.5 IU is an adequate titer. The CDC considers complete neutralization at the 1:5 level by RFFIT an adequate titer. Although rabies-neutralizing antibody is frequently found in the serum of healthy dogs and wild carnivores, there has been only one well-documented report of an idiopathic rabies titer in a human who had neither received rabies vaccine nor had clinical disease.[69]

The magnitude of the titers may be helpful in making the clinical diagnosis of rabies in persons who have been vaccinated with either nerve tissue or duck embryo rabies vaccines because these vaccines usually elicit neutralizing antibody titers of under 10 IU and have not been reported to produce titers over 50 IU. Clinical rabies in humans has produced serum titers as high as 1:64,000 (approximately 640 IU).[59] Because human diploid cell rabies vaccine is immunologically more potent, vaccination usually produces titers higher than 10 IU, and titers as high as 868 IU have been reported.[70] In persons vaccinated with human diploid cell vaccine, CSF antibody levels may be useful in making the diagnosis because high CSF titers (usually 2–25 percent of serum titers) are only seen in clinical disease.[59,60,71,72]

Antemortem, rabies virus has been isolated from human saliva brain tissues, CSF, urine sediment, and tracheal secretions.[61,73–75] Brain biopsy material may yield the best isolation results, although negative viral recovery does not rule out the diagnosis. Postmortem isolations have been made from both central and peripheral nervous tissue, skin at the site of the bite, and many visceral organs including pericardium, adrenal gland, pancreas, liver, bladder, and many other organs.[67,76] Viral isolation is most successful within the first 2 weeks of clinical illness, i.e., before the development of neutralizing antibodies. Virus has not been recovered from stool, and except for a few anecdotal reports, virus has not been isolated from human blood or serum.

Rabies virus may also be demonstrated by immunofluorescent rabies antibody staining of brain biopsy tissue, skin biopsy tissue, corneal impressions, or other patient material, although these tests can also become negative after antibodies develop.[73,77–79] The most reliable and reproducible of the direct immunofluorescent studies that can aid in patient diagnosis is the neck skin biopsy. In this test, a 6 to 8 mm full-thickness wedge or punch biopsy specimen containing as many hair follicles as possible is obtained from the posterior aspect of the neck above the hair line. The specimen should be placed in a small vial with a piece of moist tissue but without formalin fixation and stored at −70°C until shipping instructions can be obtained from a laboratory familiar with the technique. This test is both more sensitive and more specific than is the corneal impression test, although false-negative results have occurred.[80,81]

Histologic examination of brain tissue from human rabies cases typically shows perivascular inflammation of the gray matter, various amounts of neuronal degeneration, and in many cases characteristic cytoplasmic inclusion bodies (Negri bodies). Negri bodies are absent in 20–30 percent of cases, particularly in persons who have received vaccine or who have survived several weeks. Negri bodies are sharply defined cytoplasmic inclusions that are round or oblong and vary in size from 2 to 10 μm.[82,82] They are particularly common in the hippocampus, in the horn of Ammon, and in the Purkinje cells of the cerebellum but less frequently can be found in the motor area of the cerebral cortex or spinal ganglia. One or more may be found in a single cell. They are eosinophilic and Feulgen-negative, usually contain basophilic spots, and consist of viral nucleocapsid proteins.[82,83] Histologic staining with rabies fluorescent antibodies may be needed to demonstrate the inclusions.

Differential Diagnosis

The diagnosis of rabies is not difficult when a patient is known to have been bitten by a potentially rabid animal and presents clinically with hyperactivity and hydrophobia. However, a history of possible rabies exposure has been obtained in only 71–84 percent of rabies patients in several published series.[44,47] Hydrophobia and aerophobia are virtually pathognomonic of rabies when present. In the absence of an exposure history or hydrophobia, there is little to initially differentiate rabies from other viral encephalitides such as those caused by herpesviruses and arboviruses.

Although occasionally confused with rabies, the muscular rigidity of tetanus differs from rabies in that the contractions are more prolonged and frequently involve the masseter muscles and back. In addition, the CSF is invariably normal, and hydrophobia is not present in tetanus.

One must distinguish between true rabies and rabies hysteria, a psychological reaction seen in persons exposed to an animal that they believe might have rabies. Persons with rabies hysteria have an acute onset of bizarre behavior, agitation, anxiety, and often behavior resembling or indistinguishable from convulsions. These patients are frequently uncooperative—often attempting to bite medical personnel—in contrast to patients with true rabies who are most often cooperative between episodes of agitation and hyperactivity. The patient with hysteric rabies will refuse to attempt to drink water, while the true rabies patient is often thirsty and initially will accept liquids and attempt to drink, which leads to pharyngeal spasms after the liquid comes into contact with the oral cavity.

It is perhaps more difficult to distinguish paralytic rabies from other paralytic neurologic diseases. Paralytic rabies is occasionally mistaken for poliomyelitis, although in poliomyelitis sensory disturbances are usually absent and fever is often absent after the onset of neurologic symptoms. Other diseases commonly in the differential diagnosis of paralytic rabies include Guillain-Barré syndrome and transverse myelitis.

A particularly difficult problem is distinguishing clinical rabies from postvaccinial encephalomyelitis, which occurs in 1:200–1:1,600 persons immunized with adult animal nerve tissue rabies vaccines (Semple type).[84–87] In the absence of supporting laboratory tests such as viral isolation, the distinction may be difficult or impossible. Timing may be helpful because postvaccinial encephalomyelitis usually begins 2 weeks after the first dose of vaccine, an unusually short incubation period for rabies. Treatment is supportive, and there is a case fatality rate of approximately 15 percent.

Other diagnoses that have been mentioned in the literature and must be excluded in a suspected case of rabies include an intracranial mass, cerebrovascular accident, epilepsy, and poisoning with atropine-like compounds.

Treatment of Clinical Human Rabies

Specific chemotherapy for clinical rabies is not available, and treatment consists of intensive supportive care concentrating particularly on maintaining respiratory and cardiovascular support.[8,9,59,60] Isolation of the patient is essential both to prevent secondary bacterial infection of the patient and to prevent exposure of the hospital staff to rabies virus, which may be present in saliva, tears, urine, or other body fluids or tissues.[8,47,75] Face masks, gloves, and gowns are sufficient to protect the staff, and postexposure or pre-exposure rabies prophylaxis is not required unless persons sustain a bite or have clear contamination of mucous membranes by the patient's saliva, urine, or other body tissues (such as might occur in mouth-to-mouth resuscitation). Since the virus may be present in saliva and other body fluids including CSF, tears, and urine, these should be treated with careful sterilization procedures. Virus has not been recovered from human blood,[75] however, and standard blood handling precautions are sufficient.

Basic patient therapy consists of supportive care with particular attention paid to treatment of each of the potentially fatal complications noted in Table 2. The most important clinical problems appear to be hypoxia, cardiac arrhythmias, fluid imbalance, hypotension, cerebral edema, and iatrogenic complications. Regular monitoring of arterial blood gases, cardiac monitoring, and monitoring of neurologic function are essential, and abnormalities should be treated with standard measures. Steroids should be avoided in the treatment of cerebral edema if it occurs.

As noted earlier, three persons who received either preexposure or postexposure prophylaxis have survived. In two of these, full recovery has been reported. In persons who have received no immunotherapy before the onset of clinical illness, intensive supportive care alone may not be sufficient for recovery.[64,88] High-dose passive rabies immune globulin has been used in several cases with no clear effect.[88,89] The administration of vaccine after the onset of clinical illness has not been successful, and rabies antibody may, in fact, contribute to the disease pathology.[90] Only limited experience with antiviral agents exists. Interferon has been noted to have activity against rabies virus in tissue culture. Based on encouraging results in animal studies,[91,92] human leukocyte interferon has been administered both peripherally and intrathecally to five human rabies patients in several countries 2–14 days after the onset of clinical disease.[93] All five patients progressively deteriorated and died. In the two patients treated in the United States, virus was isolated for many days after the institution of α-interferon therapy, and rabies-neutralizing antibody titers were either absent or minimal at the time of death. Clearly, the interferon had a nonbeneficial immune-modulating effect.[76,93]

PREVENTION

Once disease symptoms occur, rabies has the highest case fatality rate of any known human infection (close to 100 percent); it is a disease better prevented than cured. Because rabies is a zoonosis, the cornerstone of prevention is the control of rabies in animals (especially domestic animals), which results in a decrease in human contact with the virus. However, with the advent of modern biologics, rabies in humans can almost always be prevented if exposures are recognized and appropriate postexposure treatment is initiated.

Postexposure Prophylaxis

Rationale of Treatment. Often the most difficult question confronting physicians is whether or not to initiate treatment at all. Figure 5 illustrates an algorithm for determining whether postexposure prophylaxis is necessary. The first consideration is, of course, whether the person was actually exposed to the virus.[94] Rabies is transmitted to humans by either a *bite* or a *nonbite* exposure. A *bite* exposure is defined as any penetration of the skin by teeth and resultant contamination of the wound with potentially infectious saliva. A *nonbite* exposure is the contamination of scratches, abrasions, open wounds, or mucous membranes with saliva or other potentially infectious materials such as brain tissue from a rabid animal. Casual contact such as petting a rabid animal (without a bite or nonbite exposure as described above) does not constitute an exposure and is not an indication for prophylaxis.[49] As previously mentioned, unusual and extremely uncommon nonbite exposures have included corneal transplantation and breathing aerosolized rabies virus in laboratories or in a cave infested with rabid bats.

In addition, a decision on treatment requires knowledge of whether rabies is present in the animal species in the geographic area in which the exposure occurred. Exposures by certain animals such as bats routinely require postexposure prophylaxis unless the animal has been proved by laboratory examination to be nonrabid. Small rodents (including squirrels, hamsters, guinea pigs, gerbils, chipmunks, rats, and mice) and lagomorphs (including rabbits and hares) are rarely found to be infected with rabies and have not been known to cause human rabies; their bites almost never call for postexposure prophylaxis.[28,95] If rabies is present in wild terrestrial animals in an area, bites by dogs or cats that are not available for quarantine or examination usually justify treatment.[96] In some areas where effective surveillance has existed for many years and no rabies has been found in domestic animals, public health officials no longer recommend routine postexposure prophylaxis for bites from escaped dogs and cats.[97] At present these "rabies-free areas" are generally urban areas such as New York City and Philadelphia, or isolated areas such as Hawaii. Consultation with local or state health officials is necessary to determine whether postexposure prophylaxis is indicated after the exposure to a species in a particular geographic area.

Other considerations may help the health official decide whether prophylaxis is necessary. Unusual behavior such as the loss of normal fear of humans by a skunk or fox or daylight activity by a nocturnal animal may suggest rabies. Furious behavior, classically associated with rabies, may be observed in only about one-half of animals with clinical disease.[7] An unprovoked attack is more likely than a provoked attack is to indicate that the animal is rabid. Unfortunately, what constitutes provocation is questionable, especially in the case of wild animals. Bites inflicted on a person attempting to handle or feed an apparently healthy animal can generally be regarded as provoked. In most other circumstances, the distinction offers little help. If the exposure was from a vaccinated dog or cat, rabies transmission is unlikely but has occurred, especially outside the United States. From 1981 through 1987, four of the eight Americans known to have died of rabies were bitten by rabid dogs outside the United States; two of the four rabid dogs had a history of recent rabies vaccination.[67,76]

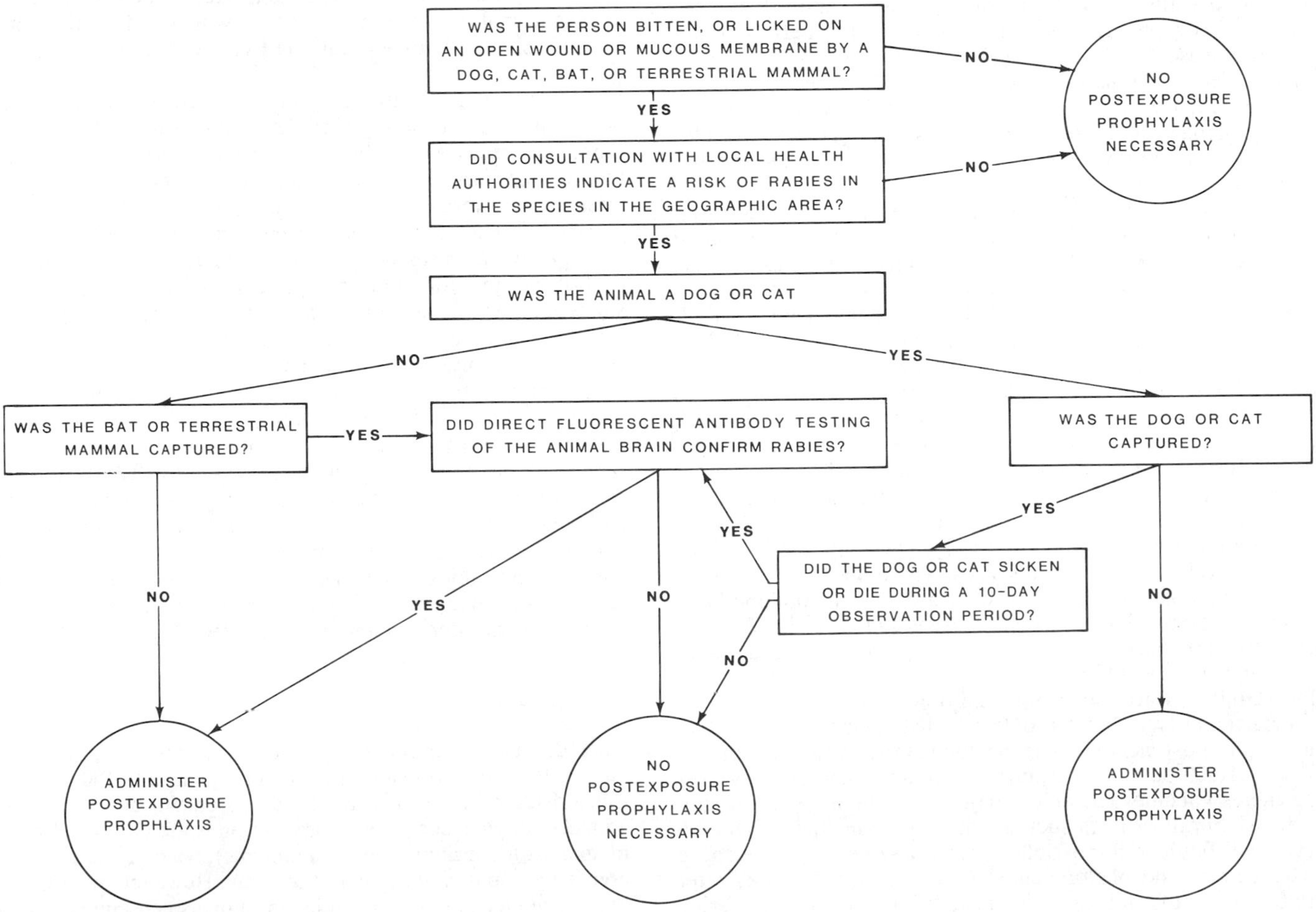

FIG. 5. Algorithm for human rabies postexposure prophylaxis. In highly suspect animals or in cases of severe exposure, treatment should be started immediately and discontinued if fluorescent antibody testing of the animal brain is negative.

As illustrated in Figure 5, only domestic dogs and cats should be quarantined and observed as an alternative to sacrificing the animal and examining the brain for rabies. Studies done during the 1960s demonstrated that the virus could not be isolated from the saliva of a rabid cat more than 1 day before the onset of clinical rabies and could not be isolated from a rabid dog more than 3 days before onset.[98,99] Because the median duration of illness in a cat was shown to be 5 days and in a dog 3 days, it was decided that if a dog or cat remained healthy for a 10-day quarantine period it would not have had rabies virus in its saliva at the time of the exposure. In a recent study in which 22 dogs were challenged with a strain of rabies virus obtained from a Mexican dog, 10 (45 percent) excreted virus in their saliva 1–7 days before the signs of clinical disease were observed. The incubation period ranged from 12 to 69 days, and the duration of illness was 1–5 days. When challenged with an Ethiopian strain of virus, dogs excreted virus for up to 13 days before the signs of illness were observed.[100] There have been a few reports of long periods of symptom-free virus excretion in dogs infected with rabies viruses from Ethiopia and from India, although the significance of these reports is unclear.[8,101] Despite these findings, no cases of human rabies have been reported after proper adherence to a 10-day quarantine period. Skunks have been shown to excrete virus for 8 days before becoming ill, raccoons for 1 day, and insectivorous bats for as long as 12 days.[7,102] Because data are less complete for these species, accurate safe observation periods cannot be determined, and quarantine is therefore not appropriate.

Biologics

Vaccines. The first antirabies vaccine was prepared by Louis Pasteur from a virus strain isolated from the brain of a rabid cow in 1882 and subsequently passaged in rabbits. The "Pasteur" treatment, first used in 1885, consisted of multiple injections of a suspension prepared from dessicated, infected rabbit spinal cords and contained variable amounts of live rabies virus.[6] Modifications of this original nerve tissue vaccine were introduced during the succeeding 50 years. Semple-type phenol-inactivated adult animal nerve tissue vaccine (NTV) is still used in many developing countries in Africa and Asia because it is inexpensive and relatively easy to produce. The efficacy of NTV has been much disputed, and only one study has shown it to be more effective than is local wound treatment alone.[103] In addition, NTV produces an unacceptable rate of postvaccination neurologic complications such as encephalomyelitis and peripheral neuropathy, which occur in approximately 1:200–1:1600 vaccinees; death from postvaccinial encephalomyelitis occurs in approximately 14 percent of affected people.[84–86]

Two newer rabies vaccines were developed in an attempt to circumvent the occurrence of neurologic complications by eliminating myelin basic protein and other foreign tissue proteins believed to be responsible for the immunologically mediated neurologic reactions.[104–106] Suckling mouse brain (SMB) vaccine, developed in 1955, is derived from suckling mouse brain tissue that has not yet developed myelin. It is a potent and effective vaccine, although neurologic complications have been recorded with an incidence of approximately 1:8,000 vaccinees.[107] A duck embryo vaccine (DEV), the vaccine used in the United States from 1958 until 1980, was prepared from rabies-infected duck embryos. The potency of this DEV is low, with 23 subcutaneous abdominal injections failing to produce antibody in 10–20 percent of recipients,[108] and treatment failures were reported. This vaccine was associated with a 35 percent incidence of minor local reactions, a 30 percent incidence of transient systemic reactions (fever, myalgia), and a neurologic complication rate of approximately 1:24,000.[109] Only two vaccine-associated fatalities have been reported after the use of this DEV, and both may have in fact been due to rabies. DEV is no longer produced in the United States.

The successful adaptation of rabies virus to WI-38 human diploid cell culture in 1963 led to the development of the safe and immunologically potent human diploid cell rabies vaccine (HDCV).[110–112] Its efficacy was dramatically demonstrated in Iran in 1975 and 1976 when 45 persons exposed to rabid dogs or wolves were vaccinated with HDCV and mule antirabies serum. Although the interval between bite and vaccination varied from 32 hours to 14 days, all persons developed antibodies, and none died of rabies.[70]

The HDCV generally available in the United States is manufactured in France by the Merieux Institute and contains inactivated whole virions. Another rabies vaccine produced in rhesus monkey diploid cells (rabies vaccine, adsorbed [RVA]) has recently been licensed in the United States but is not currently widely available.[113]

For postexposure rabies prophylaxis, the Immunization Practices Advisory Committee (ACIP) of the U.S. Public Health Service recommends that HDCV be administered as five 1 ml im doses given over a 1-month period. A sixth dose, given 90 days after the first dose, was previously recommended by the WHO but is now considered optional.[114] No cases of human rabies developed in over 500 persons who were bitten by laboratory-confirmed rabid animals and treated in the United States with a regimen of only five doses of HDCV, local wound treatment, and human rabies immune globulin (CDC, unpublished information).

Unfortunately, there have been two documented cases of human rabies occurring outside the United States in people given both HDCV and rabies immune globulin.[115,116] In both cases the HDCV was administered in the gluteal area—not the recommended deltoid site. Vaccine administered in the gluteal region may not be sufficiently immunogenic to confer protection.[117] In addition, there have been two other reported cases of rabies in persons given HDCV alone without rabies immune globulin.[118,119] It is apparent that vaccine alone, even vaccine as immunologically potent as HDCV, is not sufficient to offer complete protection in all cases. Postexposure recommendations *must* be followed exactly to provide maximum protection.

With nearly 5 million doses of HDCV used worldwide from 1974 to 1988, no deaths resulting from adverse reactions to the vaccine have been reported. Reported adverse reactions to HDCV include systemic reactions such as headache, malaise, fever, local or generalized lymphadenopathy, nausea, abdominal pain in 20–50 percent of recipients, and local reactions such as swelling, pain, or induration at the site of injection in 50–80 percent of vaccinees. There have been two reports of neuroparalytic illness temporally associated with administration of the vaccine. Both patients had a Guillain-Barré type of illness; both recovered without sequellae, and a cause-and-effect relationship was not demonstrated.[120,121] Rarely, a severe reaction has required hospitalization and close monitoring of the patient during subsequent vaccine injections. Occasionally, urticaria or other allergic reactions have been seen, but fatal anaphylactic reactions have not been reported.

In 1–20 percent of persons given booster doses of Merieux HDCV after primary immunization with the same vaccine, nonfatal systemic allergic reactions have been reported. These reactions, consisting primarily of hives and associated angioedema, occur 2–14 days after the booster dose. Respiratory distress is uncommon.[122,123] Recent studies have demonstrated that the responsible antigen is a human albumin component of the vaccine that has been modified by β-propiolactone, the viral inactivating agent.[124]

Steroids should not be used to treat adverse reactions to rabies vaccine unless the reaction is life-threatening. Immunosuppression, either resulting from a disease process or from drugs such as steroids, reduces the neutralizing antibody response in rabies vaccine recipients. It is essential, therefore, that immunosuppressed patients who must receive rabies prophylaxis be monitored closely, with antibody titers determined when the last dose of vaccine is given and additional doses of vaccine administered if necessary.

Because HDCV is an inactivated virus preparation, its use is not specifically contraindicated during pregnancy. Although no controlled clinical trials have been performed, a number of pregnant women have been vaccinated with HDCV with no reported untoward effects for either mother or fetus.

A number of new rabies vaccines are under various stages of development and licensure in the United States and around the world (Table 3). In general, when compared with HDCV, these vaccines are either less expensive to produce, more purified, or both. The licensure of these new vaccines should increase the availability of safe and effective cell culture vaccines in countries where the cost of currently available vaccines limit their use. Modern genetic engineering techniques have been applied to the experimental production of vaccines consisting of the specific viral antigens capable of producing immunologic protection without adverse reactions. These vaccines show great promise for the future.[125]

Immune Globulin. Although the administration of rabies antiserum for human postexposure prophylaxis has been practiced since 1889, it was not until 1954 that its efficacy was dramatically illustrated when 29 persons were bitten in Iran by a rabid wolf. In this instance, only 1 of 17 patients treated with the combination of nerve tissue vaccine and one or more doses of antiserum died of rabies, whereas 3 of 12 persons who received vaccine alone died.[126] Other studies completed since that time have supported the increased efficacy of combined vaccine and antiserum for postexposure prophylaxis.[127] The use of passive antibody administration in the form of heterologous antiserum of equine origin poses several difficulties. In one study, 16 percent of all persons given equine antirabies serum (ARS) developed serum sickness, with 45 percent of those over the age of 15 becoming ill.[128] The use of purified equine rabies immune globulin has recently been demonstrated to greatly decrease the frequency of serum sickness reactions.[129] The administration of passive antibody simultaneously with vaccine can interfere with the development of active antibody, especially with the less potent nerve tissue and avian-origin vaccines.[130,131] With HDCV, standard doses do not interfere with the production of antibody.[132]

The production of human rabies immune globulin (HRIG) from serum obtained from rabies-immunized human donors provided an antiserum that was both potent and free of the risk of anaphylaxis and serum sickness.[133] Since its licensure in the United States in 1975, there have been no reports of hepatitis or other virus transmission (including human immunodeficiency virus) and no significant adverse reactions after its use. When given as a single dose of 20 IU/kg, HRIG has been shown to cause minimal interference with the development of active antibody from HDCV.[132,134] Experimental animal studies have shown that serum infiltration in the exposure site is significantly more protective than systemic injection is alone.[135] It is recommended, therefore, that a portion of the HRIG be infiltrated locally at the site of the bite. In countries where HRIG is unavailable, the decision to use ARS depends on the individual skin test sensitivity to the antiserum and the severity of the exposure. Experimental work done in animal models has demonstrated the efficacy of using interferon or interferon inducers instead of rabies antiserum in an attempt to eliminate interference with active antibody development and thereby reduce the total number of doses of vaccine necessary for postexposure prophylaxis.[91,92]

TABLE 3. Newer Rabies Vaccines Currently under Evaluation or in Use in Various Countries of the World

Rabies vaccine (human diploid cell, [HDCV]), (Institute Merieux)[a]
Rabies vaccine, adsorbed (RVA), (Michigan Department of Health)[a]
Rabies vaccine, inactivated (diploid cell origin), dried, (Connaught Laboratories)
Purified vero rabies vaccine (Institute Merieux)
Purified chick embryo cell culture vaccine (Behringwerke AG)
Fetal bovine kidney cell vaccine (FBKCV) (Institute Pasteur)
Primary hamster kidney cell rabies vaccine (Wuhan Institute, China)
Purified duck embryo vaccine (Swiss Serum and Vaccine Institute)

[a] Licensed for use in the United States in 1988.

Postexposure Therapy

It is essential that, for maximum effectiveness, all three components of postexposure prophylaxis be performed, including (*1*) local wound treatment, (*2*) passive antibody administration, and (*3*) vaccine administration. The only exception involves persons who have been previously immunized with a licensed tissue culture vaccine or have a previously documented adequate rabies titer (see below).

In the United States, the median delay between exposure to a confirmed rabid animal and the institution of postexposure prophylaxis is 5 days.[36] There is ample time, therefore, to completely evaluate the exposure incident before starting therapy.

Local Wound Treatment. It has been demonstrated in experimental animals that thorough and vigorous cleansing to the depth of the wound with a 20% soap solution can reduce the risk of rabies by up to 90 percent, especially if the wound is superficial.[135] Agents such as nitric acid or viricidal agents such as quaternary ammonium compounds are not more effective than a 20% soap solution is and are not recommended.[136] Local wound treatment also includes infiltration of HRIG whenever possible.

Passive Antibody Administration. Passive immunization with HRIG provides protection for the initial 1–2 weeks before the vaccine elicits an active antibody response and should only be omitted if rabies pre-exposure or postexposure prophylaxis with HDCV has been *previously* administered. Human rabies immune globulin should be given regardless of the age of the patient, the species of the exposing animal, the location or severity of the bite, or whether the exposure was a bite or nonbite type[49] and is administered as a single dose of 20 IU/kg body weight (1 ml of HRIG contains 150 IU of neutralizing antibody). As much as 50 percent of the calculated HRIG dose should be infiltrated around the wound site; if the anatomic site of the wound is small such as the nose or finger, the amount infiltrated at the site should be reduced appropriately. The remainder of the calculated dose of HRIG should be given im in the upper outer quadrant of the buttocks or the anterolateral aspect of the thigh. If HRIG is unavailable and ARS or other animal-derived globulin product must be used, it should be given as a single dose of 40 IU/kg at the time of the first vaccine dose. If a significant delay of days or weeks has occurred between exposure and administration of postexposure prophylaxis, it is still recommended that HRIG be given at the time the first dose of vaccine is administered to provide immediate protection against rabies virus until antibody can be developed. If passive antibody administration was omitted at the time of the initial vaccine dose, it should be given any time within the first 7 days after the initial dose of vaccine. After that time, it is likely the vaccine will have elicited an active antibody response, and additional passive antibody would be unnecessary.

Vaccine Administration. Human diploid cell rabies vaccine should be administered as five 1 ml im doses, the first dose given as soon as reasonable after exposure and an additional dose given on each of days 3, 7, 14, and 28 after the first dose. Other volumes or routes of administration (intradermal, for example) have been evaluated for postexposure prophylaxis[137,138] but have not been approved for use in the United States. Vaccine should not be given by the same syringe or in the same im site as the immune globulin. Outside the United States, HDCV should be used whenever available; however, if circumstances prevent its use, other available vaccines should be administered according to recommendations of local health officials.

Infants and small children should receive the same quantity and number of vaccine doses as adults. Because of the proven immunologic potency of HDCV, routine serologic testing is not recommended for persons who have received a five-dose intramuscular postexposure regimen.[139] Persons who are immunosuppressed, either secondary to a disease process or the administration of immunosuppressant drugs, should have serum drawn for antibody determination at the time of the last dose of vaccine. Antibody titers should also be determined after immunization with NTV, DEV, and SMB vaccines.

If a person has been previously immunized with a tissue culture vaccine (as defined above) or has had a documented adequate antibody response to pre-exposure immunization with another rabies vaccine, postexposure prophylaxis consists only of thorough wound cleansing followed by two 1 ml im doses of HDCV given one each on days 0 and 3.[49]

If aberrant schedules of rabies vaccine have been given, especially in persons whose treatment was begun in another country, a decision should be made whether the treatment should be repeated or an antibody titer determined. This decision can be best made after consulting knowledgeable public health authorities.

Pre-exposure Prophylaxis

Pre-exposure prophylaxis should be offered to persons at high risk for exposure to rabies such as veterinarians, veterinary students, certain laboratory worker, spelunkers (people who explore or study caves), and persons living in or visiting countries for more than 30 days where rabies is a constant threat. Pre-exposure immunization provides protection for persons at unusually high risk and for persons whose postexposure therapy might be delayed, and also provides the basis for a rapid anamnestic antibody response when booster doses of the vaccine are given. In addition, it eliminates the need for passive immunization with HRIG and reduces the number of doses of vaccine needed should later postexposure treatment be necessary. The dose schedule for HDCV consists of three 1.0 ml im doses given one each on days 0, 7, and 21 or 28.[49,140] The rabies vaccine produced by the Merieux Institute has been evaluated and shown to be effective and safe for pre-exposure use when given as three 0.1 ml intradermal (id) doses one each on days 0, 7, and 28 in the skin over the deltoid area.[141–143] The ACIP recommends that three pre-exposure doses be given because this ensures both seroconversion and adequate duration of protective antibody.[144] Serologic testing is not required after a three-dose regimen by either the im or id route.

Chloroquine phosphate (given for malaria chemoprophylaxis) and unidentified factors (that may include multiple concurrent vaccinations) may interfere with the antibody response to rabies vaccine in persons traveling to developing countries.[145,146] The im dose/route of pre-exposure prophylaxis provides a sufficient margin of safety in this setting. In persons receiving pre-exposure prophylaxis in preparation for travel to a rabies-endemic area, the id dose/route should be initiated early enough to allow the three-dose series to be completed 30 days before departure. If this is not possible, the im dose/route should be used.[144]

Persons at continuing risk of exposure should have titers determined every 2 years, and if inadequate, should receive a booster dose, either 1.0 ml im or 0.1 ml id. Persons who work with live rabies virus in virus research laboratories or vaccine production facilities and are at risk of inapparent exposure should have their rabies antibody titer determined every 6 months; booster doses of vaccine should be given as needed to maintain an adequate titer. Other tissue culture rabies vaccines have been shown to be safe and immunogenic and have been used for pre-exposure prophylaxis.[147–149]

REFERENCES

1. Wagner RR. Rhabdovirus biology and infection, an overview. In: Wagner RR, ed. The Rhabdoviruses. New York: Plenum; 1987:9–74.
2. Steele JH. History of rabies. In: Baer G, ed. The Natural History of Rabies. v.1. New York: Academic Press; 1975:1.
3. Tierkel ES. Historical review of rabies in Asia. In: Nagano Y, Davenport FM eds. Rabies. Tokyo: University of Tokyo Press; 1971:3.
4. Jeunhomme P. A propos la rage vieille histoire. Presse Med. 1924;73:1551.
5. Muntner S, Moses Maimonides; Treatise on Poisons and their Antidodes. Philadelphia: JB Lippincott; 1966:39.
6. Pasteur L. Methode pour prevenir la rage apres morsure. CR Acad Sci (Paris). 1885;101:765.
7. Baer GM, ed. The Natural History of Rabies. v. 1 and 2. New York: Academic Press; 1975.
8. Hattwick MAW. Human rabies. Public Health Rev. 1974;3:229.
9. Kaplan C, Turner GS, Warrell DA. Rabies: The Facts. Oxford: Oxford University Press; 1986.
10. Kaprowski H, Plotkin S, eds. World's Debt to Pasteur. New York: Alan R Liss; 1985.
11. Fourth Report of the International Committee on Taxonomy of Viruses, Matthews REF, ed. Classification and nomenclature of viruses. Intervirology. 1982;17(Suppl 1–3):109.
12. Brown F, Bishop DHL, Crick J, et al. Rabdoviridae. Intervirology. 1979;12:1.
13. Fields BN, Hawkins K. Human infection with the virus of vesicular stomatitis during an epizootic. N Engl J Med. 1967;277;989–94.
14. Wunner WH, Dietzschold B, Wiktor TJ. Antigenic structure of Rabdoviruses. In: Van Regenmortel MHV, Neurath AR, eds. Immunochemistry of Viruses: the Basis for Serodiagnosis and Vaccines. Amsterdam: Elsevier North Holland; 1985:367–88.
15. Wiktor TJ, Gijorgy E, Schlumberger, et al. Antigenic properties of rabies virus components. J Immunol. 1973;110:269.
16. Schneider LG, Dietzschold B, Dierks RE, et al. Rabies group-specific ribonucleoprotein antigen and a test system for grouping and typing of rhabdoviruses. J Virol. 1963;2:748.
17. Wunner WH. Structure of rabies viruses. In: Kaprowski H, Plotkin S, eds. World's Debt to Pasteur. New York: Alan R Liss; 1985;171–86.
18. Wiktor TJ, Flamond A, Koprowski H. Use of monoclonal antibodies in diagnosis of rabies virus infections and differentiation of rabies and rabies related viruses. J Virol Methods. 1980;1:33.
19. Sureau P, Rollin P, Wiktor TJ. Epidemiologic analysis of antigenic variations of street rabies virus: Detection by monoclonal antibodies. Am J Epidemiol. 1983;117:605.
20. Smith JS, Sumner JW, Roumillat LF, et al. Antigenic characteristics of isolates associated with a new epizootic of raccoon rabies in the United States. J Infect Dis. 1984;149:769–74.
21. Smith JS, Reid-Sanden FL, Roumillat LF, et al. Demonstration of antigenic variation among rabies virus isolates by using monoclonal antibodies to nucleocapsid proteins. J Clin Microbiol. 1986;24:573–80.
22. World Health Organization Expert Committee on Rabies. Sixth report. Geneva: World Health Organization Technical Report Series No. 523; 1973:12.
23. Johnson HN. Rabies virus. In: Horsfall FL, Tamm I, eds. Viral and Rickettsial Infections of Man. Philadelphia: JB Lippincott; 1965:814.
24. Meredith ED, Rossouw AP, Koch HVR. An unusual case of human rabies thought to be of chiropteran origin. S Afr Med J. 1971;45:767.
25. Familusi JB, Osunkoya BO, Moore DL, et al. A fatal case of infection with mokola virus. Am J Trop Med Hyg. 1972;921:959.
26. Chadli A. La rage en Tunisie: Analyse des résultats des 34 dernières années. Arch Inst Pasteur Tunis. 1986;63:15–33.
27. Kaplan MM, Koprowski H. Rabies... Sci Am. 1980;242:120.
28. Fishbein DB, Beloto AJ, Pacer RE. Rabies in rodents and lagomorphs in the United States, 1971–1984: Increased cases in the woodchuck (*Marmota monax*) in mid-Atlantic states. J Wildl Dis. 1986;22:151–5.
29. Centers for Disease Control. Rabies—United States, 1981. MMWR. 1982;31:379.
30. Jenkins S, Winkler W. Descriptive epidemiology from an epizootic of racoon rabies in the Middle Atlantic states. Am J Epidemiol. 1987;126:429–37.
31. World Health Organization. World Survey of Rabies XXII (for Years 1984/85). Geneva: World Health Organization; 1987:33.
32. Bögel K, Motschwiller E. Incidence of rabies and post-exposure treatment in developing countries. Bull WHO. 1986;64:883–7.
33. World Health Organization Collaborating Centre for Rabies Surveillance and Research. Rabies Bull Eur. 1987;11:1.
34. Pan American Zoonoses Center. Epidemiological surveillance of rabies for the Americas. 1987;18:1.
35. Cerughino JJ, Osterud HT, Pinnas JL, et al. Rabies: A rare disease but a serious pediatric problem. Pediatrics. 1970;45:839.
36. Helmick CG. The epidemiology of human rabies postexposure prophylaxis, 1980–81. JAMA. 1983;250:1990.
37. Winkler WG, Fashinell TR, Leffingwell L, et al. Non-bite transmitted rabies in a laboratory worker. JAMA. 1973;226:1219.

38. Centers for Disease Control. Rabies in a laboratory worker, New York. MMWR. 1977;26:183.
39. Constantine DG. Rabies transmission by the non-bite route. Public Health Rep. 1962;77:287.
40. Humphry GL, Kemp GE, Wood EG. A fatal case of rabies in a woman bitten by an insectivorous bat. Public Health Rep. 1960;75:317–26.
41. Houff SA, Burton RC, Wilson RW, et al. Human-to-human transmission of rabies virus by corneal transplant. N Engl J Med. 1979;300:603.
42. Centers for Disease Control. Human-to-human transmission of rabies via a corneal transplant—France. MMWR. 1980;29:25.
43. Centers for Disease Control. Human-to-human transmission of rabies via corneal transplant—Thailand. MMWR. 1981;30:473.
44. Held JR, Tierkel ES, Steele, JH. Rabies in man and animals in the United States, 1946–1965. Public Health Rep. 1967;82:1009.
45. Rubin RH, Gregg MB, Sikes RK. Rabies in citizens of the United States, 1963–1968: Epidemiology, treatment, and complications of treatment. J Infect Dis. 1969;120:268.
46. Nikolitsch M. Virus concentration and incubation period. Trop Dis Bull. 1958;55:395.
47. Anderson LJ, Nicholson KG, Tauxe RV, et al. Human rabies in the United States, 1960–1979: Epidemiology, diagnosis, and prevention. Ann Intern Med. 1984;100:728–35.
48. Enright JB. The effects of corticosteroids on rabies in mice. Can J Microbiol. 1974;16:667.
49. Recommendation of the Immunization Practices Advisory Committee of the U.S. Public Health Service. Rabies prevention—United States, 1984. MMWR. 1984;33:393–402,407–8.
50. Murphy FA. Rabies pathogenesis: Brief review. Arch Virol. 1975;54:279.
51. Murphy FA. The pathogenesis of rabies virus infection. In: Kaprowski H, Plotkin S, eds. World's Debt to Pasteur. New York: Alan R Liss; 1985:153–69.
52. Schneider IG, Hamann I. Rabies pathogenesis in mice. III. Centrifugal virus spread and virus generalization in the organism. Zentrabl Bakteriol Mikrobiol Hyg [A]. 1969;212:13.
53. Babes V. Traite de la Rage. Paris: JV Bailliere; 1912:81.
54. Wilson JM, Hettiarachchi J, Wijesuriya IM. Presenting features and diagnosis of rabies. Lancet. 1975;2:1139.
55. Warrell DA. The clinical picture of rabies in man. Trans R Soc Trop Med Hyg. 1976;70:188.
56. Chopra JS, Banerjee AK, Murthy MK, et al. Paralytic rabies: A clinicopathologic study. Brain. 1980;103:789.
57. Love SV. Paralytic rabies: Review of the literature and report of a case. J Pediatr. 1944;24:312.
58. Varma K, Maheshwari MC, Chawdhary C, et al. Acute ascending motor paralysis due to rabies: A clinical pathological report. Eur Neurol. 1985;24:160.
59. Hattwick MAW, Weiss TT, Stechshulte J, et al. Recovery from rabies: A case report. Ann Intern Med. 1972;76:931.
60. Porras C, Barbozajj, Fuenzalida E, et al. Recovery from rabies in man. Ann Intern Med. 1976;85:44.
61. Bhatt DR, Hattwick MAW, Gerdsen R, et al. Clinical rabies: Diagnosis, management, and complications. Am J Dis Child. 1974;127:862.
62. Cheetham HD, Hart J, Coghill HF, et al. Rabies with myocarditis: Two cases in England. Lancet. 1970;2:921.
63. Araujo MF, Brito RD, Machada CG. Myocarditis in human rabies. Rev Inst Med Trop (Sao Paulo). 1971;13:99.
64. Gode GR, Raju AV. Intensive care in rabies therapy. Lancet. 1976;2:6.
65. Thiodet J, Forrier A, Syergeol. Tentatives therapeutiques de la rage declarce chez l'homme. Presse Med. 1963;71:172.
66. Centers for Disease Control. Human rabies—Michigan. MMWR. 1983;32:159.
67. Centers for Disease Control. Human rabies acquired outside the United States from a dog bite. MMWR. 1981;30:538.
68. Smith JS, Yager PA, Baer GM. A rapid reproducible test for determining rabies neutralizing antibody. Bull WHO. 1973;48:535.
69. Laboratory Center for Disease Control. Idiopathic rabies titre—Ontario. Can Dis Week Rep. 1982;8:23.
70. Bahmanyar M, Faydy A, Nour-Salehi S, et al. Successful protection of humans exposed to rabies infection: Post-exposure treatment with the new human diploid cell rabies vaccine and antirabies serum. JAMA. 1976;236:2751.
71. Arko RJ, Schneider LG, Baer GM. Nonfatal canine rabies. Am J Vet Res. 1973;34:937.
72. Bell JF, Sancho MF, Diaz AM, et al. Non-fatal rabies in an enzootic area: Results of a survey and evaluation of techniques. Am J Epidemiol. 1972;95:190.
73. Emmons RW, Leonard LL, Degenaro F, et al. A case of human rabies with prolonged survival. Intervirology. 1973;1:60,72.
74. Sulkin SE, Hartford CG. Concerning infectivity of saliva in human rabies. Ann Intern Med. 1943;19:256.
75. Helmick CG, Tauxe RV, Vernon AA. Is there a risk to contacts of patients with rabies? Rev Infect Dis. 1987;9:511.
76. Centers for Disease Control. Imported human rabies. MMWR. 1983;32:78.
77. Goldwasser RA, Kissling RE. Fluorescent antibody staining of street and fixed rabies virus antigens. Proc Soc Exp Bio Med. 1958;98:219.
78. Rubin RH, Sullivan L, Summers R, et al. A case of human rabies in Kansas: Epidemiologic, clinical and laboratory consideration. J Infect Dis. 1970;122:318.
79. Schneider LG. The cornea test: A new method for the intra vitam diagnosis of rabies. Zentrabl Veterinarmed [B] 1969;16:24.
80. Smith WB, Blendon DC, Fuh TH, et al. Diagnosis of rabies by immunofluorescent staining of frozen sections of skin. J Am Vet Med Assoc. 1972;161:1495.
81. Blenden C, Creech W, Torres-Anjel MJ. Use of immunofluorescence examination to detect rabies virus antigen in skin of humans with clinical encephalitis. J Infect Dis. 1986;154:698.
82. Sung JH, Hayano M, Mastri AR, et al. A case of human rabies and ultrastructure of the Negri body. J Neuropathol Exp Neurol. 35(5), 541, 1976;35:541.
83. Dupont JR, Earle KM. Human rabies encephalitis. Neurology (Minneapolis). 1966;15:1023.
84. Abdussalem M, Bogel K. The problem of antirabies vaccination. International Conference on the Application of Vaccines Against Viral, Rickettsial, and Bacterial Diseases of Man. PAHO Sci Publ. 1971;226:54.
85. Appelbaum E, Greenberg H, Nelson J. Neurologic complications following antirabies vaccine. JAMA. 1953;151:188.
86. Hemachudha T, Phanuphak P, Johnson RT, et al. Neurologic complications of Semple-type rabies vaccine: Clinical and immunologic studies. Neurology (NY). 1987;37:550–6.
87. Hemachudha T, Griffin E, Johnson RT, et al. Immunologic studies of patients with chronic encephalisis induced by post-exposure Semple rabies vaccine. Neurology (NY). 1988;38:42–4.
88. Maton PN, Pollard JD, Davis JN. Human rabies encephalomyelitis. Br Med J. 1976;1:1038.
89. Hattwick MAW, Corey L, Creech WB. Clinical use of human globulin immune to rabies virus (Abstract). J Infect Dis. 1976;133(Suppl):266.
90. Smith JS, McClelland CL, Reid FL, et al. Dual role of the immune response in street rabies virus infection of mice. Infect Immun. 1982;35:213.
91. Baer GM, Shaddock JH, Moore SA, et al. Successful prophylaxis against rabies in mice and rhesus monkeys: The interferon system and vaccine. J Infect Dis. 1977;136:286.
92. Baer GM, Moore SA, Shaddock JH, et al. An effective rabies treatment in exposed monkeys: A single dose of interferon inducer and vaccine. Bull WHO. 1979;57:807.
93. Merigan TC, Baer GM, Winkler WG, et al. Human leukocyte interferon administration to symptomatic rabies and suspect rabies patients. Ann Neurol. 1984;16:82–7.
94. Mann JM. Systematic decision-making in rabies prophylaxis. Pediatr Infect Dis. 1983;2:162.
95. Winkler WG. Rodent rabies in the United States. J Infect Dis. 1972;126:565.
96. Kappus K. Canine rabies in the United States, 1971–1973. Am J Epidemiol. 1976;103:242.
97. Marr JS, Beck AM. Rabies in New York City, with new guidelines for prophylaxis. Bull NY Acad Med. 1976;52:605.
98. Vaughn JB, Gerhardt P, Newell KW. Excretion of street rabies virus in saliva of dogs. JAMA. 1965;193:363.
99. Vaughn JB, Gerhardt P, Paterson J. Excretion of street rabies virus in saliva of cats. JAMA. 1963;184:705.
100. Fekadu M, Shaddock JH, Baer GM. Excretion of rabies virus in the saliva of dogs. J Infect Dis. 1982;145:715.
101. Fekadu M, Shaddock JH, Baer GM. Intermittent excretion of rabies virus in the saliva of a dog two and six months after it had recovered from experimental rabies. Am J Trop Med Hyg. 1981;30:1113.
102. Sikes RK. Pathogenesis of rabies in wildlife, I. Comparative effect of varying doses of rabies virus inoculated into foxes and skunks. Am J Vet Res. 1962;23:1041.
103. Veeraraghavan N. Annual Report, Director, Pasteur Institute of Southern India. Madras, India: Coonoor, Diocesan Press; 1970.
104. Hemachudha T, Griffin E, Giffels JJ, et al. Myelin basic protein as an encephalitogen in encephalomyelitis and polyneuritis following rabies vaccine. N Engl J Med. 1987;316:369–74.
105. MacFarlane JO, Culbertson CG. Attempted production of allergic encephalomyelitis with duck embryo suspensions and vaccines. Can J Public Health. 1954;45:28.
106. Patterson PY. Experimental allergic encephalomyelitis and autoimmune disease. Adv Immunol. 1966;5:131.
107. Held JR, Lopez Adaros H. Neurological disease following administration of suckling mouse brain antirabies vaccine. Bull WHO. 1972;46:321.
108. Hattwick MAW, Corey L, Creech WB. Clinical use of human globulin immune to rabies virus (Abstract). J Infect Dis. 1976;133:266.
109. Rubin RH, Hattwick MAW, Jones S, et al. Adverse reactions to duck embryo rabies vaccine range and incidence. Ann Intern Med. 1973;78:643.
110. Plotkin SA, Wiktor TJ. Rabies vaccine prepared in human cell cultures: Progress and perspectives. Rev Infect Dis. 1978;2:433.
111. Anderson LJ, Sikes RK, Langkop CW et al. Post-exposure trial of a human diploid cell strain rabies vaccine. J Infect Dis. 1980;142:133.
112. Anderson LJ, Winkler WG, Hafkin B et al. Clinical experience with a human diploid cell rabies vaccine. JAMA. 1980;244:781.
113. Centers for Disease Control. Rabies vaccine adsorbed: A new rabies vaccine for use in humans. MMWR. 1988;37:217–8.
114. World Health Organization. WHO Expert Committee on Rabies—Seventh Report. Technical report series 709. Geneva: World Health Organization; 1984.

115. Shill M, Baynes RD, Miller SD. Fatal rabies encephalitis despite appropriate post-exposure prophylaxis: A case report. N Engl J Med. 1987;20:1257–8.
116. Centers for Disease Control. Human rabies despite treatment with rabies immune globulin and human diploid cell rabies vaccine—Thailand. MMWR. 1987;36:759–60.
117. Fishbein DB, Sawyer LA, Reid-Sanden FL, et al. Administration of human diploid cell rabies vaccine in the gluteal area (Letter). N Engl J Med. 1987;318:124–5.
118. Devriendt J, Staroukine M, Costy F et al. Fatal encephalitis apparently due to rabies: Occurrence after treatment with human diploid cell vaccine but not rabies immune globulin. JAMA. 1982;248:2304.
119. Wattanasri S, Boonthai P, Thongcharoen P. Human rabies after late administration of human diploid cell vaccine without hyperimmune serum (Letter). Lancet. 1982;2:870.
120. Böe E, Nyland H. Guillain-Barré syndrome after vaccination with human-diploid cell rabies vaccine. Scand J Infect Dis. 1980;12:231.
121. Bernard KW, Smith PW, Kader FJ et al. Neuroparalytic illness and human diploid cell rabies vaccine. JAMA. 1982;248:3136.
122. Centers for Disease Control. Systemic allergic reactions following immunization with human diploid cell rabies vaccine. MMWR. 1984;33:185.
123. Dreesen DW, Bernard KW, Parker RA, et al. Immune complex-like disease in 23 persons following a booster dose of rabies human diploid cell vaccine. Vaccine. 1986;4:45–9.
124. Anderson MC, Baer H, Frazier J, et al. The role of specific IgE and beta-propiolactone in reactions resulting from booster doses of human diploid cell rabies vaccine. J Allergy Clin Immunol. 1987;80:861–8.
125. Kieny MP, Desmettre P, Soulebot J-P, et al. Rabies vaccine: Traditional and novel approaches. Prog Vet Microbiol Immun. 1987;3:73–111.
126. Baltazard M, Bahmanyar M, Ghodssin, et al. Essai pratique du serum antirabique chez les mordus par loyps enrages. Bull WHO. 1955;13:747.
127. Fang-tao L, Shu-beng C, Guan-Fu W, et al. Study of the protective efficacy of primary hamster kidney cell rabies vaccine. J Infect Dis. 1986;154:1047–8.
128. Karliner JS, Belaval GS. Incidence of reactions following administration of antirabies serum: A study of 562 cases. JAMA. 1965;193:359.
129. Wilde H, Chomchey P, Prakongsri S, et al. Safety of equine rabies immune globulin (Letter). Lancet. 1987;2:1275.
130. Wiktor RJ. Inhibitory effect of passive antibody on active immunity induced against rabies by vaccination. Bull WHO. 1971;45:747.
131. Corey L, Hattwick MAW. Serum neutralizing antibodies after rabies post-exposure prophylaxis. Ann Intern Med. 1976;85:170.
132. Helmick CG, Johnstone C, Sumner J, et al. A clinical study of Merieux human rabies immune globulin. J Biol Stand. 1982;10:357–67.
133. Loofbourow JC, Cabasso VJ, Roby RE, et al. Rabies immune globulin (human): Clinical trials and dose determination. JAMA. 1971;217:1825.
134. Hafkin B, Alls ME, Baer GM. Human rabies globulin and human diploid vaccine dose determinations. Dev Biol Stand. 1978;40:121.
135. Dean DJ, Baer GM, Thompson WR. Studies on the local treatment of rabies infected wounds. Bull WHO. 1963;28:477.
136. Anderson LJ, Winkler WG. Aqueous quaternary ammonium compounds and rabies treatment. J Infect Dis. 1979;139:494.
137. Warrell MJ, Suntharasamai P, Nicholson KG, et al. Multisite intradermal and multi-site subcutaneous rabies vaccination: Improved economical regimens. Lancet. 1984;1:874–6.
138. Warrell MJ, Nicholson KG, Warrell DA, et al. Economical multiple-site intradermal immunization with human-diploid-cell strain vaccine is effective for post-exposure rabies prophylaxis. Lancet. 1985;1:1059–62.
139. Recommendation of the Immunization Practices Advisory Committee of the United States Public Health Service. Supplementary statement on rabies vaccine and serologic testing. MMWR. 1981;30:535.
140. Tint H, Rosanoff EI. Clinical responses to T(n)BP-disrupted HDCS (Wi-38) rabies vaccine. Dev Biol Stand. 1977;37:287.
141. Nicholson KG, Turner GS, Aolsi FY. Immunization with a human diploid cell strain of rabies virus vaccine: Two year results. J Infect Dis. 1978;137:783.
142. Bernard KW, Roberts MA, Sumner I, et al. Human diploid cell rabies vaccine: Effectiveness of immunization with small intradermal or subcutaneous doses. JAMA. 1982;247:1138.
143. Bernard KW, Mallonee J, Wright JC, et al. Preexposure immunization with intradermal human diploid cell rabies vaccine: Risks and benefits of primary and booster vaccination. JAMA. 1987;257:1059–63.
144. Recommendation of the Immunization Practices Advisory Committee of the U.S. Public Health Service. Supplementary statement on the preexposure use of human diploid cell rabies vaccine by the intradermal route. MMWR. 1986;35:767–8.
145. Bernard KW, Fishbein DB, Miller KD, et al. Pre-exposure rabies immunization with human diploid cell rabies vaccine: Decreased antibody responses in persons immunized in developing countries. Am J Trop Med Hyg. 1985;34:633–47.
146. Pappaioanou M, Fishbein DB, Dreesen DW et al. Antibody response to preexposure human diploid-cell rabies vaccines given concurrently with chloroquine. N Engl J Med. 1986;314:280–4.
147. Fangtao L, Fanzhen Z, Longmu L, et al. The primary hamster kidney cell rabies vaccine: Adaption of viral strain, production of vaccine, and pre- and postexposure treatment. J Infect Dis. 1983;147:467.
148. Nicholson KG, Farrow PR, Bijok U, et al. Preexposure studies with purified chick embryo cell culture rabies vaccine and human diploid cell vaccine: Serological and clinical responses in man. Vaccine. 1987;5:208–10.
149. Vodopija I, Sureau P, Lafon M, et al. An evaluation of second generation tissue culture rabies vaccines for use in man: A four-vaccine comparative immunogenicity study using a preexposure vaccination schedule and an abbreviated 2-1-1 postexposure schedule. Vaccine. 1986;4:245–8.

Filoviradae

141. MARBURG AND EBOLA VIRUSES

KARL M. JOHNSON

The Marburg virus was discovered as the result of an outbreak of severe human disease in Marburg, Germany, in 1967. The morphologically related Ebola virus was initially described during a study of clinically similar outbreaks in Sudan and Zaire in 1976. Originally classified as members of the rhabdovirus family, these agents are now considered to be members of a distinct virus group.[1–3]

VIROLOGY

Marburg and Ebola viruses are bacilliform rods 65 nm by 800–900 nm that contain a negative-sense RNA genome.[4] Virions contain seven proteins, one of which is glycosylated and forms characteristic surface spikes 10 nm in length.[5,6] Nucleotide sequences at the 3′ end of the virus genome were conserved for Marburg and Ebola viruses and differed from their closest relatives, the Rhabdoviridae and Paramyxoviridae.[7] These properties have been judged sufficiently distinct to define a new virus family, the Filoviridae (International Committee on Taxonomy of Viruses, 1987, unpublished). The viruses can be isolated from blood and tissue specimens by inoculation of guinea pigs or Vero cell cultures. Virions in such specimens can often be visualized directly by electron microscopy, and viral antigens can be detected by indirect immunofluorescence (IFA). Complement-fixing and IFA antibodies develop in infected humans and animals and serve to confirm the diagnosis and distinguish Marburg from Ebola virus. No antigenic relationship has yet been found between the two agents.[8] The viruses can be inactivated by heating at 60°C for 1 hour, by acid treatment at pH 4 or lower, and by organic solvents such as ether.[9] Because of the highly hazardous properties of these agents suspect materials should be referred to the Centers for Disease Control, Atlanta, for diagnosis.

EPIDEMIOLOGY

The natural reservoirs of Marburg and Ebola viruses remain unknown. The animal source for the original Marburg outbreak was a group of several hundred African green monkeys (*Cercopithecus aethiops*) imported from Uganda to Germany and Yugoslavia for use in vaccine preparation. At least 13 of these animals were infected at the time of arrival in Germany, and the disease was uniformly fatal in these animals. Subsequent work has strongly suggested that this monkey does not serve as a natural virus reservoir because all animals infected with even tiny amounts of Marburg virus succumb and because evidence for presence of virus-specific antibodies in wild monkeys from Uganda was not found.[10,11] A similar problem exists with Ebola virus; despite entensive study of wild vertebrates in Sudan and Zaire, no convincing clue to the identity of the presumed reservoir has emerged.

Humans serve as the only known source of infection, with transmission resulting from contact with blood, body fluids, and possibly urine or respiratory secretions. The virus concentration in the blood of patients is very high (up to 10^6 infectious units/ml) and typically persists until death or resolution of the clinical crisis.[12] In addition, virus may persist in certain tissues weeks or months after acute disease. Marburg virus was recovered from liver biopsy specimens after 31 and 73 days and from the interior chamber of the eye 3 months after the onset of disease. Additionally, Marburg and Ebola viruses have been isolated from semen up to 3 months after illness, and in one instance, semen was the documented source of transmission of infection from a husband to his wife.[13]

There were 31 Marburg illnesses during the initial 1967 outbreaks in Germany and Yugoslavia. Twenty-five were primary cases, all of whom had contact with infected monkey kidneys or tissue cultures. Interestingly no infection occurred among laboratory animal care staff, and there was no secondary spread among monkeys in these facilities. Six secondary human cases were documented, all among persons having direct contact with patients. There were seven deaths among primary infections, none in the secondary cases.[14]

Since that time, there have been six reported cases of Marburg disease: three in South Africa, 1975; two in Kenya, 1980; and one in South Africa, 1982.[15,16] In the first two episodes, a fatal index case was followed by transmission to one or more persons, usually medical attendants who were unaware of the diagnosis. In the last instance, South African medical authorities, fully sensitized to this disease, immediately instituted isolation procedures that prevented the spread of infection. A thorough investigation of the movements and activities of all three index cases failed to identify a natural source of infection.

Ebola virus epidemiology is equally obscure. Present knowledge is based on major disease outbreaks in Sudan and Zaire in 1976, a sporadic case in Zaire in 1977, and another Sudan outbreak in 1979.[12,17–19] Index cases all acquired disease in unknown ways (all were dead when investigations commenced), and outbreaks were centered in rural hospitals and nearby villages. More than 500 cases were registered in 1976, and the mortality was about 70 percent making this, after rabies, the most lethal virus disease of humans. In Zaire, much transmission was traced to contaminated syringes and needles at a hospital, and all such patients died. Secondary transmission from patients cared for in the home ranged from 4 to 11 percent, and simple isolation procedures interrupted virus spread, which suggests that blood and body fluids rather than respiratory droplets or aerosols were the principal sources of transmission. During the 1979 Sudan outbreak, most patients were managed at home, and a careful study of the type and duration of exposure of family members was made to determine the pattern of secondary transmission. A 30 percent rate was found for persons who were primary care givers or who prepared bodies for funeral, with virtually no spread to any others in the family.[19] This result strengthens the concept that contact rather than aerosol is the principal mode of person-to-person transmission of these viruses. Although Ebola virus was first recognized in 1976, there is retrospective evidence for its presence in Zaire as early as 1972. In that year a missionary physician performed an autopsy on a young student nurse at his institution who died of "yellow fever." He lacerated a finger during the procedure and 11 days later experienced a severe febrile illness having all the features of Ebola disease save hemorrhage. In 1977, he was the only person among 50 residents and workers at the hospital who had Ebola virus antibodies.[18] Antibodies to Ebola virus were subsequently found in about 9 percent of the persons in the region. If specific, and this is not yet certain, these antibody data suggest that infection by Marburg and Ebola viruses or closely related agents is much more common than was originally believed and clinically much less virulent.

It was initially thought that the 1976 Ebola outbreaks were caused by the same virus. The epidemics began about 2 months apart, and human contacts across the intervening 500 miles were established.[17] Subsequent studies, however, disclosed that viruses from Sudan and Zaire had distinctive differences in antigens, peptide digests, and endonuclease RNA maps.[20–22] In addition, it was found that monkeys infected with the Sudan variant generally survived while the Zaire agent caused uniformly lethal infection.[23] The independent occurrence of two first outbreaks of a human disease within the observed frame off time and geography represents a striking biologic coincidence.

CLINICAL MANIFESTATIONS

After an incubation period of 4–16 days, Marburg and Ebola diseases may have a sudden or insidious onset of fever, headache, myalgia, and conjunctival suffusion (Table 1). Within 2–3 days nausea, vomiting, and significant diarrhea appear together with thrombocytopenia and leukopenia. Leukocyte numbers remain within normal limits in some patients. Proteinuria, a maculopapular rash over the trunk, and hemorrhages from the intestines, nose, and vagina appear 1–2 days later. There are marked increases in serum glutamic oxaloacetic transaminase (SGOT) and serum glutamic pyruvic transaminase (SGPT) levels without increase in bilirubin or evidence of clinical jaundice.[25] Chemical and symptomatic pancreatitis may occur. Patients exhibiting hemorrhage usually pursue an inexorable course to death with shock and occasionally encephalitis. Abnormalities in coagulation parameters including the appearance of fibrin split products indicate that disseminated intravascular coagulation occurs and may be the proximate cause of death, which most often takes place 7–10 days after the onset of illness. At autopsy, the liver shows major but random hepatocellular necrosis with little or no inflammatory reaction.

Although Ebola infections are more often marked by chest pain and cough, both diseases are clinically similar in all important features. Differentiation of these entities from many other African fevers, particularly in the absence of hemorrhage, is difficult or impossible clinically, a fact that surely accounts for the failure to recognize them for so many decades.[13,26] Among the acute hemorrhagic diseases of Africa, Marburg and Ebola infections most resemble the hemorrhagic form of Rift Valley fever,[27] although individual cases of Lassa fever and nonicteric yellow fever could readily be confused with them. Specific virologic diagnostic tests are required to document each of these diseases (Table 2).

PREVENTION AND TREATMENT

In the absence of critical information, it is not possible to prevent primary infection with these viruses. Secondary transmission among humans is definitely preventable by isolating patients and by the institution of enteric precautions including the use of gloves, gowns, eye protection, and reliable measures for decontamination and disposal of all fomites.[28] Laboratory work must be done very carefully and, if possible, should be carried out in high-containment facilities because the viruses have been shown experimentally to be highly infectious via the respiratory route.

Treatment of these diseases is also difficult. One patient with a laboratory-acquired Ebola infection was treated with 6 million units of leukocyte interferon daily for 14 days and 450 ml of plasma from convalescent patients. Viremia levels decreased dramatically after therapy was initiated, and the patient survived.[29] Subsequent studies of both interferon and passive antibodies in monkeys, however, were disappointing; all animals

TABLE 1. Clinical and Epidemiologic Characteristics of Viral Hemorrhagic Fever

Characteristic	*Lassa Fever*	*Ebola Hemorrhagic Fever*	*Marburg Virus Disease*	*Crimean-Congo Hemorrhagic Fever*
Endemic areas	West Africa (Guinea to Central Africa)	East Africa (Zaire, Sudan, Central African Republic, Kenya)	East Africa, South Africa	Eastern Europe, Asia, Africa
Etiologic agent classification	Arenaviridae	Filoviridae	Filoviridae	Bunyaviridae
Reservoir in nature	Rodents (*Mastomys natalensis*)	Not known	Not known	Ticks (*Hyalomma* genus and others), wild and domesticated mammals
Modes of transmission	Rodent to human (virus excreted in urine); person to person	Not known; person to person	Not known; person to person	Tick bite; person to person
Incubation period (days)	6–21	2–21	3–9	3–6
Symptoms (% of cases)				
Headache	50–75	75–100	75–100	75–100
Myalgia	25–50	75–100	50–75	50–75
Sore throat	75–100	75–100	50–75	25–50
Cough	50–75	25–50	5–25	25–50
Dysphagia	5–25	5–25	25–50	—
Vomiting	75–100	50–75	75–100	75–100
Diarrhea	25–50	75–100	75–100	25–50
Chest pain	25–50	50–75	5–25	5–25
Abdominal pain	50–75	75–100	5–25	75–100
Signs (% of cases)				
Fever	75–100	75–100	75–100	75–100
Conjunctivitis	25–50	50–75	25–50	5–25
Pharyngitis	75–100	25–50	5–25	25–50
Cervical lymphadenopathy	25–50	—	25–50	—
Abdominal tenderness	50–75	25–50	—	25–50
Skin rash (macular)	5–25	50–75	75–100	—
Hemorrhage (skin or gastrointestinal)	25–50	75–100	25–50	75–100
Shock	25–50	25–50	25–50	50–75
Laboratory findings (% of cases)				
Leukopenia	25–50	5–25	75–100	50–75
Thrombocytopenia	—	—	75–100	75–100
Proteinuria	50–75	50–75	—	50–75
Disseminated intravascular coagulation	—	—	5–25	5–25

(From Centers for Disease Control.[24])

TABLE 2. Global Viral Hemorrhagic Fevers

Disease	*Virus*	*Virus Group*	*Geography*
Marburg disease	Marburg	Filoviridae	Africa
Ebola disease	Ebola	Filoviridae	Africa
Argentine HF	Junin	Arenaviridae	Argentina
Bolivian HF	Machupo	Arenaviridae	Bolivia
Lassa fever	Lassa	Arenaviridae	West Africa
Yellow fever	Yellow fever	Togaviridae: Flavivirus	Africa-South America
Dengue HF	Dengue	Togaviridae: Flavivirus	SE Asia, Oceania, tropical Americas
Omsk HF	Omsk	Togaviridae: Flavivirus	USSR
Kyasanur Forest disease	KFD	Togaviridae: Flavivirus	India
Congo-Crimean HF	C-CHF	Bunyaviridae	USSR, central-west Asia, Africa
Rift Valley fever	RVF	Bunyaviridae	Africa
HF with renal syndrome	Hantaan	Bunyaviridae	Northern Eurasia

Abbreviation: HF: hemorrhagic fever.

died.[30] Indeed it has not been possible to detect neutralizing antibodies in convalescent sera, which brings into question the role of antibodies in survival from infection.

Supportive therapy is extremely difficult. Secondary bacterial infection may occur, and there are major problems in acid-base and electrolyte management. Hypoxia and shock must be aggressively combated. Once bleeding has begun, replacement of platelets and clotting factors is the best management strategy, although it has not been tried sufficiently to judge its merits. Intravenous heparin therapy, if begun *before* hemorrhage, may be effective. This approach was used in two contact Marburg infections in South Africa. Although seriously ill, both patients survived.

REFERENCES

1. Siegert R, Shu HL, Slenezka W, et al. On etiology of an unknown human infectious disease originating from monkeys. Dtsch Med Wochenschr 1967;92:2341.
2. Johnson KM, Webb PA, Lange JV, et al. Isolation and partial characterization of a new virus causing acute haemorrhagic fever in Zaire. Lancet. 1977;1:569.
3. Kiley MP, Bowen ETW, Eddy GA, et al. Filoviridae: A taxonomic home for Marburg and Ebola viruses? Intervirology. 1982;18:24.
4. Sanchez A, Kiley MP. Identification and analysis of Ebola virus proteins. Virology. 1987;157:414.
5. Elliott LH, Kiley MP, McCormick JB. Descriptive analysis of Ebola virus proteins. Virology. 1985;147:169.
6. Murphy FA, van der Groen G, Whitfield SG, et al. Ebola and Marburg virus morphology and taxonomy. In: Pattyn SR, ed. Ebola Virus Haemorrhagic Fever. Amsterdam: Elsevier North Holland; 1978:61.
7. Kiley MP, Wilusz J, McCormick JB, et al. Conservation of the 3′ terminal nucleotide sequences of Ebola and Marburg virus. Virology. 1986;149:251.
8. van der Groen G, Elliott LH. Lack of cross reactivity of rhabdovirus antibodies with Marburg and Ebola antigens in the indirect immunofluorescent antibody test. Ann Soc Belg Med Trop 1982;62:67.
9. Bowen ETW, Simpson DIH, Bright WF, et al. Vervet monkey disease: Studies on some physical and chemical properties of the causative agent. Br J Exp Pathol. 1969;50:400.
10. Simpson DIH, Bowen ETD, Bright WF. Vervet monkey disease: Experimental infection of monkeys with the causative agent and antibody studies in wild-caught monkeys. Lab Anim. 1968;2:75.
11. Slenczka W, Wolff G, Siegert R. A critical study of monkey sera for the presence of antibody against the Marburg virus. Am J Epidemiol. 1971;93:496.
12. Report of International Commission. Ebola haemorrhagic fever in Zaire, 1976. Bull WHO. 1978;56:271.
13. Wulff H, Conrad LJ. Marburg virus. In: Kurstak E, Kurstak C, eds. Comparative Diagnosis of Viral Disease. New York: Academic Press; 1977:3.
14. Martini GA. Marburg virus. Postgrad Med J. 1973;49:542.

15. Gear JSS, Cassel GA, Gear AJ, et al. Outbreak of Marburg virus disease in Johannesburg. Br Med J. 1975;4:489.
16. Smith DH, Johnson BK, Isaacson M, et al. Marburg-virus disease in Kenya. Lancet. 1982;1:816.
17. WHO International Study Team. Ebola haemorrhagic fever in Sudan, 1976. Bull WHO. 1978;56:247.
18. Heymann DL, Weisfeld JS, Webb PA, et al. Ebola hemorrhagic fever: Tandala, Zaire, 1977–1978. J Infect Dis. 1980;142:372.
19. Baron RC, McCormick JB, Zubeir OA. Ebola virus dissemination in southern Sudan: Hospital dissemination and intrafamilial spread. Bull WHO. 1983;61:997.
20. Richman DD, Cleveland PH, McCormick JB, et al. Antigenic analysis of strains of Ebola virus: Identification of two Ebola virus serotypes. J Infect Dis. 1983;147:268.
21. Buchmeier MJ, DeFries RU, McCormick JB, et al. Comparative analysis of the structural polypeptides of Ebola virus from Sudan and Zaire. J Infect Dis. 1983;147:276.
22. Cox NJ, McCormick JB, Johnson KM, et al. Evidence for two subtypes of Ebola virus based on oligonucleotide mapping of RNA. J Infect Dis. 1983;147:272.
23. Bowen ETW, Platt GS, Lloyd G, et al. A comparative study of strains of Ebola virus isolated from southern Sudan and Northern Zaire in 1976. J Med Virol. 1980;6:129.
24. Centers for Disease Control. Viral hemorrhagic fever: Initial management of suspected and confirmed cases. Ann Intern Med. 1984;101:73.
25. Martini GA. Marburg virus disease: The clinical syndrome. In: Martini GA, Siegert R, eds. Marburg Virus Disease. Berlin: Springer-Verlag, 1971:1.
26. Gear JS, Ryan J, Rossouw. A consideration of the diagnosis of dangerous infectious fevers in South Africa. S Afr Med J. 1978;53:235.
27. Laughlin LW, Meegan JM, Stransbaugh LJ, et al. Epidemic Rift Valley fever in Egypt: Observations of the spectrum of human illness. Trans R Soc Trop Med Hyg. 1978;73:630.
28. Clausen L, Bothwell TH, Isaacson M, et al. Isolation and handling of patients with dangerous infectious disease. S Afr Med J. 1978;53:238.
29. Emond RTD, Brandon E, Bowen ETW, et al. A case of Ebola virus infection. Br Med J. 1977;2:541.
30. Bowen ETW, Baskerville A, Cantell K, et al. The effect of interferon on experimental Ebola virus infection in rhesus monkeys. In: Pattyn SR, ed. Ebola Virus Haemorrhagic Fever. Amsterdam: Elsevier North Holland; 1978:245.

Orthomyxoviridae

142. INFLUENZA VIRUS

ROBERT F. BETTS
R. GORDON DOUGLAS, JR.

Influenza is an acute, usually self-limited, febrile illness caused by infection with influenza type A or B virus that occurs in outbreaks of varying severity almost every winter. The attack rates during such outbreaks may be as high as 10–40 percent over a 5- to 6-week period. The most common clinical manifestations are fever, myalgias, and cough, but infection with influenza virus may produce similar clinical syndromes to those resulting from infection with other respiratory viruses such as common colds, pharyngitis, croup, tracheobronchitis, bronchiolitis, or pneumonia. Conversely, any of the other respiratory viruses (e.g., respiratory syncytial virus, rhinovirus, adenovirus) may produce infections with clinical manifestations indistinguishable from those of the characteristic systemic illness with cough that results from influenza virus infection, but such infections do not occur in epidemics. The two most important features of influenza are the epidemic nature of the disease and the mortality that results in part from its pulmonary complications.

HISTORY

Influenza virus has been causing recurrent epidemics of febrile respiratory disease every 1–3 years for at least the past 400 years.[1,2] Although the disease is not associated with a characteristic manifestation such as rash, the high attack rate, the explosive nature of the epidemic, and the frequency of cough allow the identification of some past epidemics. For example, Syndenham's account of an outbreak that occurred in 1679 is a clear description of influenza.[3] Hirsch tabulated 299 outbreaks occurring at an average interval of 2.4 years between 1173 and 1875.[1] Epidemics of worldwide scope occur less often and are referred to as pandemics. The first pandemic that clearly fits the description of influenza occurred in 1580, although others may have occurred earlier. Since then 31 pandemics have been described. The greatest pandemic occurred in 1918–1919 when, during three "waves" of influenza, 21 million deaths were recorded worldwide, among them 549,000 in the United States.[4]

The modern era of understanding of influenza was ushered in by Smith and associates when they isolated influenza A virus in ferrets in 1933.[5] Influenza B virus was isolated by Francis in 1939[6] and influenza C virus by Taylor in 1950.[7] The discovery by Burnet in 1936, that influenza virus could be grown in embryonated hens' eggs has led to an intensive study of the properties of the virus and to the development of inactivated vaccines.[8] The phenomenon of hemagglutination, which was discovered by Hirst in 1941, led to simpler and inexpensive methods for the measurement of virus and specific antibody.[9] With the advent of cell culture systems in the 1950s, numerous additional methods for preparing virus stocks have been available. In the last decade, there has been an enormous explosion of information on virus structure and genetics.

Since 1940, viruses have been isolated annually from various parts of the world during epidemics and pandemics. Also, testing of serum specimens (serologic archeology) obtained at specified times from elderly persons who were alive during more distant outbreaks, for example, 1889–1890 or 1918–1919, has added a great deal of information about epidemics that occurred before 1940.[10,11]

Evidence of the protective efficacy of inactivated vaccines was developed in the 1950s.[12,13] Vaccines have been in widespread use in various parts of the world since, but usually only for selected segments of a population. The first attempt at immunization of an entire population was made in 1976 in the United States with the National Immunization Program against swine influenza, but it was not possible to estimate its efficacy since an epidemic did not occur. An effective chemotherapeutic agent, amantadine, was approved for use in the United States as a chemoprophylactic agent for influenza A2 virus (H2N2) infections in 1966, and the approval was expanded to include all influenza A viruses and therapy in 1976.

THE VIRUSES

Classification

Influenza viruses belong to the family Orthomyxoviridae, which contains two genera: influenza virus type A and influenza virus type B.[14] Influenza virus type C probably represents another genus, although it has not yet been officially so classified.

Morphologic Characteristics

The morphologic characteristics of all influenza virus types, subtypes, and strains are similar. Electron microscopic studies estimate their size to be in the medium range—80–120 nm in diameter—and show them to be enveloped viruses covered with surface projections or spikes.[15] They may exist as spherical or elongated filamentous particles as well (Figs. 1 and 2). The latter predominate in newly isolated strains, whereas most laboratory-adapted strains consist almost entirely of spherical parti-

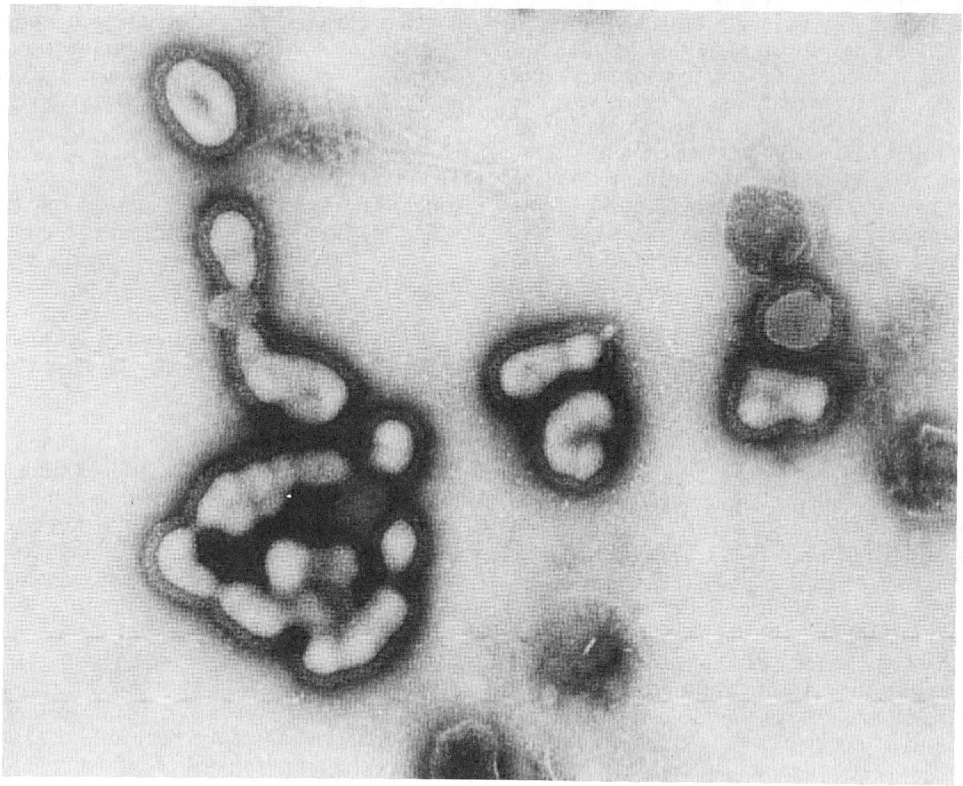

FIG. 1. Electron micrograph of influenza A/USSR/77 H1N1. (×189,000)

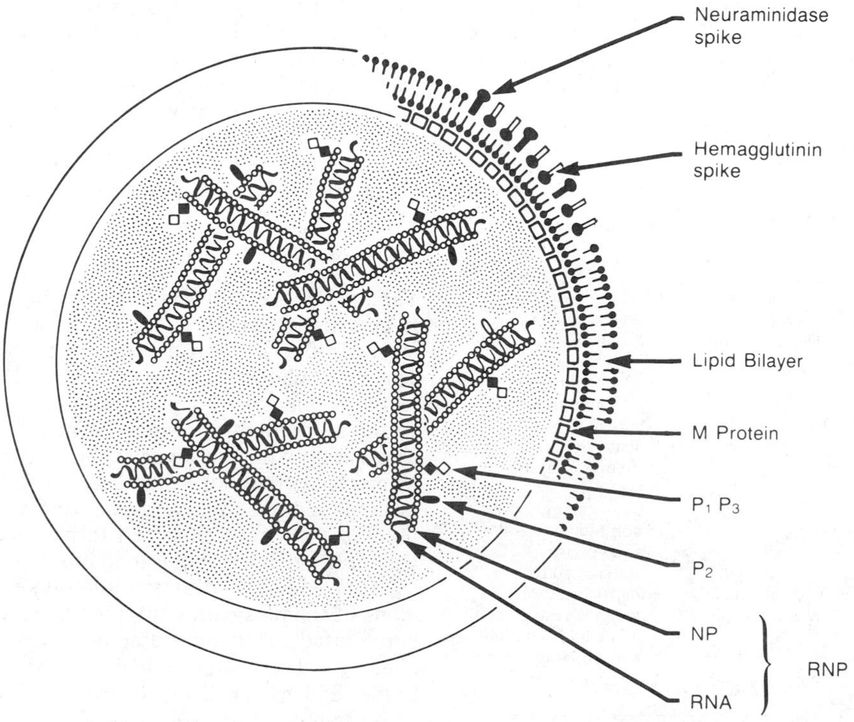

FIG. 2. Schematic model for the influenza virus virion. (Modified from Ginsberg,[16] with permission.)

cles. The filamentous forms vary in length but may be up to 400 nm long. Eight proteins have been identified in influenza viruses (Table 1).[20] The surface spikes are glycoproteins that process either hemagglutinin or neuraminidase activity.[21] The envelope is composed of a lipid bilayer on the inner surface of which is a layer of protein called matrix (M) protein.[22] This protein is believed to provide stability to the virion. Within the envelope are eight segmented pieces of nucleocapsid (Table 1).[23] The nucleocapsid is a double helix formed by a single species of protein, nucleoprotein (NP), and by pieces of the segmented single-stranded RNA genome. Three other proteins, polymerase (PB1, PB2, and PA) proteins, are also found within the viral envelope; these proteins appear to be involved in RNA transcriptase activity. Finally, there are two internal nonstructural (NS1, NS2) proteins of unknown function.

The Peplomers

Hemagglutinin. The rod-shaped hemagglutinin (HA) "spikes" of peplomers each measure 4 nm in diameter by 14 nm in length and are subdivided into HA_1 (molecular weight, 50,000) and HA_2 (molecular weight, 27,000). They can be removed from the intact virion by sodium dodecyl sulfate, by bromelain, or by chymotrysin. Each spike appears to be a trimer composed of three HA polypeptides with molecular weights of 75,000–80,000. They in turn form a trimer of molecular weight of approximately 224,640.[24] Each spike has a hydrophobic end and a hydrophilic end, the former being bound to the membrane. Antigenic sites and red cell and mammalian cell-binding sites reside in the hydrophilic region of the molecule. Peptide mapping studies reveal large differences in amino acid sequences in the HA among different subtypes of influenza A, whereas in closely related strains only small differences are observed.[25] Thus, it is clear that HA glycoproteins with markedly different amino acid sequences are capable of being functionally active and that the degree of difference may be related directly to degree of antigenic variation.

The HA spike is the site for the attachment of the virus to host cells to initiate infection or to erythrocytes, from which it derives its name.[24] The HA is one of the major antigens of the influenza virus. It contains common (to subtype) and strain-specific antigens and is the protein most frequently involved with antigenic variation. Specific antibody to the HA prevents the initiation of infection or hemagglutination. Influenza viruses attach to clusters of specific sialic acid-containing glycoproteins or glycolipids in red cell membranes, and the differences in charge between the cell membranes and the HA spike may be important in this interaction. The attachment of HA to host cells is also due to sialic acid residues.

There are two important steps in viral entry and replication. The first of these is proteolytic cleavage of the HA molecule,[26] which is carried out by trypsinlike proteases. The second, for which the first is a precondition, is the capacity of the HA to fuse with the cell membrane.[27] Clearly, the HA is essential for infection, but these two steps are physiologic requirements.

Neuraminidase. Neuraminidase (NA), like HA, is one of the important antigens of influenza virus. It contains antigens common to each subtype and also shows some antigenic variation within a subtype. Neuraminidase spikes are found in fewer numbers than are HA spikes on the envelope of an influenza virion. The NA spike is shaped like a mushroom rather than a rod (Fig. 2) and has a molecular weight of 240,000. These peplomers apparently consist of a tetramer of NA polypeptides, each with a molecular weight of 58,000. Red blood cells (RBCs) agglutinated with influenza virus disagglutinate spontaneously at 37°C. On the addition of fresh virus, they do not reagglutinate. The eluted virus, however, agglutinates fresh RBCs. This phenomenon, due to viral NA activity, results because the enzyme cleaves the bond between *N*-acetylneuraminic acid and the adjacent D-galactose or D-galactosamine on the erythrocyte. Several suggestions have been offered for the role of this enzyme in the pathogenesis of influenza infection.[17,28,29] Neuraminidase polypeptide probably directs the transport of proteins to apical cell surfaces. Neuraminidase may function to remove neuraminic acid from mucins present in the respiratory tract. The mucins are inhibitors of hemagglutination and might interfere with attachment of influenza virus to surface epithelial cells. A second possibility is that viral NA is not important in the early steps of viral replication but that it may play an important role in the release of mature virions from an infected cell. Specific anti-NA antibodies diminish the number of newly formed virions released from infected cells. In addition, NA may play a role in the prevention of virus aggregation. In infection with NA-defective mutants, mature virions form at cell surfaces, but they form aggregates of up to 500 particles rather than being released as individual virions.[18] The number of infectious units is decreased, and the infectivity titer is reduced accordingly. In this setting, viral NA presumably removes sialic acid residues from the envelope of the virion and, by so doing, eliminates receptors on the surface for HA that would cause the virus to aggregate and form conglomerates. Thus, NA appears to protect the virus from its own HA.

The Envelope

The lipid bilayer portion of the influenza virion envelope is derived from the host cell membrane.[30] Thus, its composition closely reflects that of the membrane from which it is derived. The hydrophobic ends of the NA and HA peplomers are attached to the outer layer of the lipid bilayer but do not penetrate within it. The matrix or membrane (M) protein is found in close association with the inner surface of the inner lipid layer. The M protein is the most abundant (33–46 percent of a total virion protein) and one of the smallest (molecular weight, 26,000) proteins of the virion. It is felt to play a major structural role in the viral envelope, but other functions have been ascribed to it.[31] For example, during assembly, M protein migrates to regions of the plasma membrane where viral peplomers have become attached to the outer lipid layer; nucleocapsid material aligns itself specifically beneath these areas of plasma membrane, and host cell proteins are specifically excluded. Thus, M protein creates a selective environment for the inclusion of virus-coded proteins that is important in the early assembly

TABLE 1. The Genes of Influenza A Virus and Their Protein Products of Influenza A Virus

RNA[a] Segment Number	Gene Product Description	Name of Protein	Proposed Fractions of Protein
1	PB1	Polymerase	RNA transcriptase
2	PB2	Polymerase	RNA transcriptase
3	PA	Polymerase	RNA transcriptase
4	HA	Hemagglutinin	Viral attachment to cell membranes; strain-specific antigen; common antigen to subtype
5	NA	Neuraminidase	Release from membranes; prevents aggregation; common antigen to subtype; strain-specific antigen
6	NP	Nucleoprotein	Encapsidates RNA
7	M	Matrix	Surrounds viral core; involved in assembly and budding
8	NS1 NS2	Nonstructural	Unknown

[a] Determined by polyacrylamide gel electrophoresis.
(Data from Palese et al.[17–19])

stage of viral replication. The M protein also serves as a type-specific antigen.

Nucleocapsid (Ribonucleoprotein)

The nucleocapsid of influenza virus exists in the form of discrete segments, each of which contains one molecule of viral RNA, multiple copies of the nucleoprotein (NP) polypeptides, and probably one or more polymerase (P) polypeptides.[19] The NP protein is the subunit of the helical nucleocapsid. It has a molecular weight of approximately 60,000.[32] It contains no carbohydrate and possesses the type-specific antigenicity on which the classification of influenza into A, B, and C types is based. Available data suggest that genome segments are incorporated randomly into mature virions, a process that might only rarely result in a virion containing all the genome segments required for infectivity but that could account for enhanced infectivity by the aggregation of influenza virions. In aggregates, complementation of two or more virus particles could occur, whereas if they presented singly and each lacked one or more RNA segments required for infectivity, infection might not occur. This random process would also account for the high frequency of reassortment of RNA segments between two influenza viruses that occurs when cells are simultaneously infected with two different influenza viruses. This mixing process may be of fundamental importance as a mechanism of antigenic variation.

EPIDEMIOLOGY

Antigenic Variation

One of the unique and most remarkable features of influenza virus is the frequency with which changes in antigenicity occur; these changes are referred to as antigenic variation. Antigenic variation is a frequent (almost annual) event with influenza A virus but occurs less frequently with influenza B virus and has not been associated with influenza C virus. Alteration of its antigen structure leads to infection with variants to which little or no resistance may be present in the population at risk. The phenomenon of antigenic variation helps explain why influenza continues to be a major epidemic disease of humans. This thesis assumes similar transmissibility and virulence characteristics of viruses that undergo antigenic variation.

Antigenic variation involves principally the two external glycoproteins of the virus, the HA and NA. However, virion structural proteins and even nonstructural protein may vary.[33–37] The HA is the most important since it is more frequently involved in antigenic variation than the NA is and also since antibody to this protein neutralizes infection. Antigenic variation is referred to as antigenic drift or antigenic shift, depending on whether the variation is great or small.

Antigenic Drift. Antigenic drift refers to relatively minor changes that occur frequently (every year or every few years) within an influenza subtype. Each subtype is named by its HA and NA. To date three hemagglutinins (H1, H2, and H3) and two neuraminidases (N1, N2) have been recognized. The former designations HO and HSW are now classified as variants of H1.[38] Each strain within the subtype is identified by the site and year of isolation of the virus. Thus, influenza A/Texas/77/H3N2 indicates an influenza type A virus of the H3N2 subtype isolated in 1977 in Texas. The original H3N2 variant was isolated in Aichi, Japan, in 1968; this strain is referred to as A/Aichi/68/H3N2. All isolates worldwide for the next 3 years were serologically identical. Subsequent antigenic drift resulted in the recovery of variants possessing minor differences: A/England/72/H3N2, A/Port Chalmers/73/H3N2, A/Scotland/74/H3N2, A/Georgia/74/H3N2, A/Victoria/75/H3N2, A/Texas/77/H3N2, and so on. It is generally accepted that antigenic drift results from mutation(s) affecting the RNA segment coding for either the HA or NA, but more commonly the former.[39] As a result, there is an alteration in protein structure involving one or a few amino acids. This leads to minor changes in antigenicity. Immunologic selection takes place, that is, the new virus is favored over the old for person-to-person transmission because of the less frequent presence of antibody in the population. Support for this thesis comes from experimental work demonstrating that antigenic variants (drift) can be produced in cell cultures in the presence of sublimiting amounts of antibody, and these variants have changes in a single amino acid sequence in one of three antigenic areas of the HA.[39,40] The complete nucleotide sequence of the HA of several H3 strains has been determined.[41,42] Additional common determinants remain constant within a given subtype.[42]

Antigenic drift occurs infrequently after the emergence of a new subtype; new variants appear more and more frequently as the end of an era approaches, and this was the pattern with the H3N2 viruses as described above. However, it is of interest that, in the second year (1978–1979) of the H1N1 era that began in 1977, most recovered viruses showed drift away from A/USSR/77/H1N1 to a new variant called A/Brazil/78/H1N1. Perhaps this occurred so rapidly because so large a portion of the population was already immune to H1N1 viruses.

Antigenic Shift. The major antigenic shifts that herald pandemic influenza presumably result from a different mechanism. These viruses are "new" viruses to which the population has no immunity. There is very little or no serologic relationship between the HA and/or NA antigens of the "old" and "new" virus; hence, in nomenclature, each receives a different designation. In this century, three "new" hemagglutinins and two "new" neuraminidases have appeared. For example, the new virus that appeared in 1957 is now given the designation H2N2 to distinguish it from previously prevalent strains of the H1N1 subtype, indicating that both the NA and HA of the 1957 virus bore no antigenic relationship to the H1N1 virus (Table 2). In 1968, the shift involved only the HA, hence the designation H3N2, and in 1977, it again involved both antigens but resembled a previously recognized virus—hence the designation H1N1.

Maps of tryptic peptide digests of HA subunits reveal marked changes of amino acid sequence among hemagglutinins obtained from H2- and H3-containing viruses.[43] Studies by polyacrylamide gel electrophoresis of the genomes of viruses of different subtypes reveal that RNA segments coding for the HA and NA from different types migrate to different positions on the gel, which indicates that segments of RNA coding for either the HA, NA, or both are markedly different for different subtypes.[19,44,45] The mechanism of antigenic shift with the introduction of a "new" segment of RNA resulting in a new surface glycoprotein has been shown to be most easily explained by genetic reassortment.

It is well recognized that genetic reassortment among influenza A viruses takes place frequently in eggs and in tissue culture.[46,47] It has been stated that recombinant influenza A viruses with the desired surface antigens, growth potential, or other biologic properties can be made "to order."[39] For example,

TABLE 2. Antigenic Subtypes of Influenza A Virus Associated with Pandemic Influenza

Year	Interval (yr)	Designation	Extent of Antigenic Change in Indicated Surface Protein[a]	Severity of Pandemic
1889	—	H3N2	?	Moderate
1918	29	H1N1[b]	H+ + +N+ + +	Severe
1957	39	H2N2	H+ + +N+ + +	Severe
1968	11	H2N2	H+ + +N−	Moderate
1977	9	H1N1	H+ + +N+ + +	Mild

[a] +: minor change; + +: moderate change; + + +: major change; −: no change.
[b] Former designation, Hsw1N1.[38]

annually for vaccine manufacturing purposes, a virus with currently relevant surface antigens and a second virus with A/PR8 H1N1 antigens that has the property of growth in eggs are used to infect eggs simultaneously.[48] This results in progeny possessing the relevant surface glycoproteins and high growth potential in eggs. Such a virus possessing both desired properties is then selected as the vaccine strain. Data have accumulated that indicate that genetic reassortment occurs in vivo in mixed infection in swine and turkeys.[49,50] Further support for the natural occurrence of genetic reassortment in vivo is provided by the finding that some influenza viruses of humans, lower mammals, and birds share similar surface antigens.[51] These observations suggest that new strains of influenza A can arise in nature by genetic reassortment in animal or avian hosts. Since there is a high level of immunity within the human population to the "old" strain and a lack of immunity to the "new" strain, a great advantage exists for the "new" strain. Provided it possesses other properties such as intrinsic virulence and transmissibility, such a new strain could produce pandemic influenza.

Epidemic Influenza

An epidemic is an outbreak of influenza confined to one location, be it city, town, or country. In a given community, epidemics of influenza A virus infection have a characteristic pattern. A graphic description of an epidemic due to an A/Victoria/75/H3N2-like virus that occurred in 1976 in Houston, Texas, is shown in Figure 3 and Table 3. Such localized epidemics begin rather abruptly, reach a sharp peak in 2–3 weeks, and last 5–6 weeks.[52] Reports of increased numbers of children with febrile respiratory illness are often the first indication of influenza in a community. This is usually soon followed by the occurrence of influenza-like illnesses among adults. The next event is increased hospital admissions for patients with pneumonia, exacerbation of chronic obstructive pulmonary disease, croup, and congestive heart failure. Increased school and industrial absenteeism also occur, but they are insensitive and late indicators of influenza in a community.[52] Although an increased number of deaths due to pneumonia and influenza is a highly specific indicator of influenza, it invariably lags behind the other indicators due to two factors: the time from the onset of illness to time of death and the delay involved in reporting deaths to public health officials.[53]

In tropical countries influenza can be isolated year round although epidemics seem to follow changes in weather patterns, e.g., monsoons in India. However, in temperate climates cooperative prospective studies of viral isolations from children with febrile respiratory diseases on a year-round basis show that a few influenza virus isolates are obtained in the several weeks preceding an epidemic.[52–54] After the first influenza isolate the number rapidly rises to a peak over a period of 2–3 weeks, which correlates with increased numbers of influenza-like cases (Fig. 3). The number of viruses recovered then rapidly falls over a 2- to 3-week period. A few isolates may be obtained in the ensuing several weeks. Then, mysteriously, during the remainder of the year influenza viruses are almost never recovered. Also appreciated from these prospective year-round surveillance activities are geographic differences in attack rates for different age groups for different outbreaks. For example, when H1N1 viruses reappeared in the late winter of 1977–78 after a 21-year period, influenza activity was almost exclusively restricted to college-aged populations. This occurred despite the fact that younger children were not immune and that most persons over 52 years of age possessed low antibody titers against H1N1 virus. When influenza A/USSR/77/H1N1 activity was detected again in the winter of 1978–79, much less activity was seen in college-age persons, and most disease was seen in children. It still appeared only rarely in elderly persons.

Epidemics occur almost exclusively in the winter months

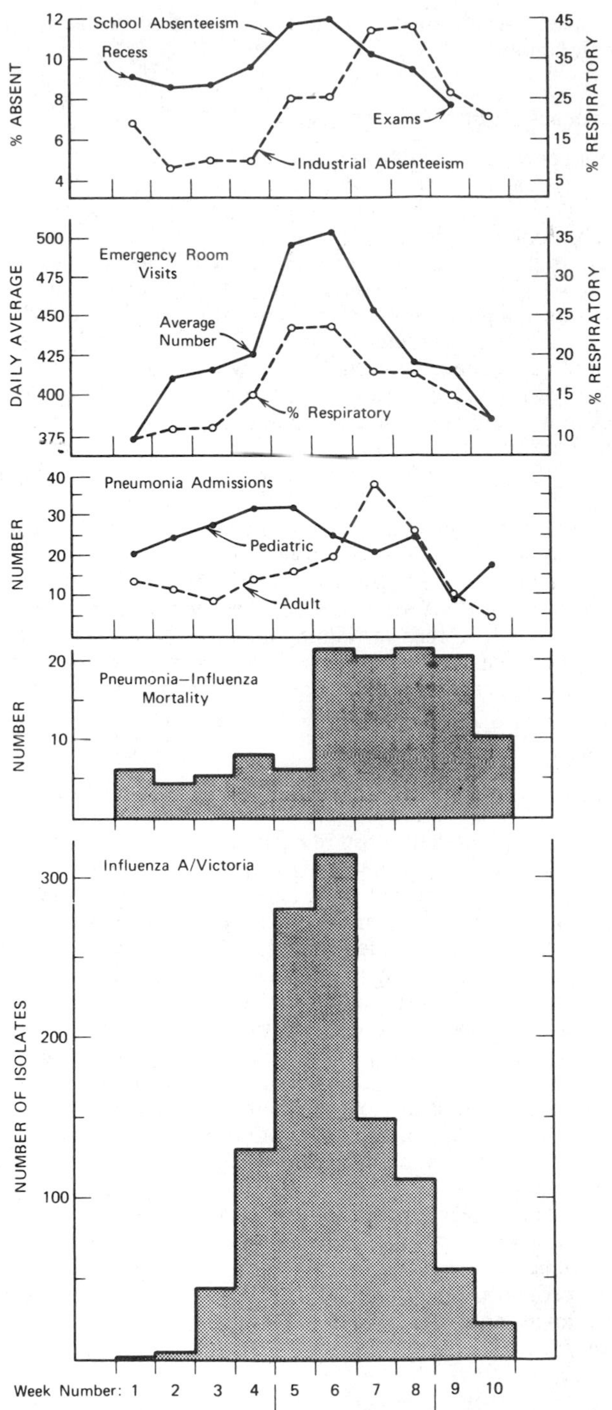

FIG. 3. Correlation of the nonvirologic indexes of epidemiologic influenza with the number of isolates of influenza A/Victoria virus according to week, Houston, 1976 (industrial absenteeism is indicated by the percentage with respiratory complaints). (From Glezen et al.,[52] with permission.)

(December to April) in the Northern hemisphere. If a new strain with a significantly different antigenic makeup appears, outbreaks may be detected as early as October (see Table 3, 1957–58 and 1968). In the Southern hemisphere, outbreaks occur May to September and may predict the type of virus that will occur in the Northern hemisphere the following winter.[55] When observed in large countries such as the United States or Australia, regional differences in the time occurrence of influenza outbreaks are apparent.[56] It is not uncommon to have major out-

TABLE 3. Influenza A Activity in the United States, 1957–1988

Year	*Season*	*A H1N1*	*A H2N2*	*A H3N2*	*B*	*Excess Mortality*
1957–58	Sep–Mar	0	A/Japan/57(99+)	0	0	69,800
1959	Feb–May	0	A/Japan/57(20)	0	B/Maryland/59(80)	7,900
1960	Jan–Mar	0	A/Japan/57(100)	0	0	38,000
1961–62	Nov–Mar	0	0	0	B/Maryland/59(100)	17,100
1963	Jan–Apr	0	A/Japan/62(100)	0	0	43,200
1964	Jan–Apr	0	A/Taiwan/64(100)	0	0	0
1965	Jan–Mar	0	A/Taiwan/64(80)	0	B/Maryland/59(20)	14,900
1966	Jan–Apr	0	A/Taiwan/64(40)	0	B/Massachusetts/66(60)	15,900
1967	Feb–Apr	0	A/Georgia/67(70)	0	B/Massachusetts/66(30)	0
1968–69	Oct–Feb	0	0	A/Hong Kong/68(60)	B/Massachusetts/66(40)	51,000
1970	Jan–Mar	0	0	A/Hong Kong/68(100)	0	32,000
1971	Jan–Mar	0	0	A/Hong Kong/68(20)	B/Massachusetts/66(80)	0
1971–72	Dec–Feb	0	0	A/Hong Kong/68(90)	B/Massachusetts/71(10)	32,000
1972–73	Dec–Feb	0	0	A/England/72(90)	B/Massachusetts/71(10)	29,000
1973–74	Dec–Apr	0	0	A/Port Chalmers/73(20)	B/Hong Kong/72(80)	5,830
1974–75	Nov–Mar	0	0	A/Port Chalmers/73(100)	0	15,000
1976	Jan–Apr	0	0	A/Victoria/75(70)[a]	B/Hong Kong/72(30)	26,000
1977	Jan–Apr	0	0	A/Victoria/75(5)	B/Hong Kong/72(95)	0
1977–78	Oct–Mar	A/USSR/77(26)	0	A/Texas/77(60)	B/Hong Kong/72(14)	32,000
1978–79	Oct–Mar	A/Brazil/78(98)	0	0	B/Hong Kong/72(2)	NA
1979–80	Oct–Mar	A/Brazil/78(1)	0	A/Bangkok/79(2)	B/Singapore/79(97)	NA
1980–81	Oct–Mar	A/Brazil/78(23)	0	A/Bangkok/79(77)	0	NA
1981–82	Oct–Mar	A/Brazil/78(24)	0	A/England/80(1)	B/Singapore/79(75)	NA
1982–83	Oct–Mar	A/Chile/83(10)	0	A/Philippines/82(79)	B/USSR/83(11)	NA
1984	Jan–May	A/Chile/83(50)	0	A/Philippines/82(5)	B/USSR/83(45)	NA
1984–85	Dec–Apr	0	0	A/Philippines/82(97)	B/USSR/83(3)	NA
1986	Jan–Apr	0	0	A/Mississippi/85(24)	B/Ann Arbor/86(76)	NA
1987–88	Oct–Apr	A/Taiwan/86(80)	0	0	B/Ann Arbor/86(20)	NA

Abbreviation: NA: not available. Numbers in parentheses are percentages of total isolates.
[a] A/New Jersey/76/Hsw1N1 was isolated from sporadic cases in 1976 and 1977.

breaks occurring in some communities or regions while others are experiencing no activity whatsoever. Often those communities so spared experience similar outbreaks at a later time, particularly if the prevalent virus demonstrates significant antigenic variation as compared with previously prevalent viruses. During epidemics, average overall attack rates are estimated to be 10–20 percent, but in selected populations or age groups, attack rates of 40–50 percent are not unusual.[57] Serologic evidence confirms the clustering of influenza activity during winter outbreaks when isolates are frequently obtained. Only rarely is evidence of infection obtained at other times of the year.[56]

For many years it had been thought that during an epidemic of influenza a single strain of influenza virus prevailed and that other respiratory viruses were diminished or disappeared.[57–59] However, with increasing surveillance in recent years it has been recognized that two different strains within a single subtype (A/Victoria/3/75/H3N2 and A/Texas/1/77/H3N2)[60,61] or that two differing influenza A subtypes (H1N1 and H3N2) cocirculate. Furthermore, concomitant outbreaks of influenza A and B or simultaneous outbreaks of influenza A and respiratory syncytial virus have been demonstrated.[59] In the 1987–88 influenza season, three different viruses circulated, A/Sichuan/87/H3N2, A/Taiwan/85/H1N1, and B/Ann Arbor/80. In some cities, all three viruses could be recovered in a single month and occurred in pockets. For example, A/Taiwan/85/H1N1 outbreaks were documented in a university, an A/Sichuan/88/H3N2 outbreak was observed in a nursing home, and B/Ann Arbor/86 was occurring in another nursing home and in patients being seen in emergency room visits, all simultaneously. Table 3 demonstrates that the pattern of influenza epidemics as well as minor strain variations changes from year to year in an unexplained manner. Note that the A subtype may be the most prevalent type one year, not be detected the next, and then reappear the following year at a reasonably high frequency (see A/Brazil/78). Note also that the B influenza strains tend to remain more stable antigenically and thus persist for a greater number of years (see Table 3) than influenza A does.

Glezen et al. have described a wave of influenza virus infections that occurs during the latter half of one epidemic period and heralds the epidemic virus for the following year.[61] Such a herald wave may be of obvious importance for vaccine composition.

Pandemic Influenza

Pandemics of influenza result from the emergence of a new virus to which the overall population possesses no immunity so that epidemics of influenza progress to involve all parts of the world. The association of different subtypes of influenza A with pandemic influenza for the past 88 years is shown in Table 2. The pandemics of 1957, 1968, and 1977 all began in mainland China and then spread both east and west, but primarily to the Soviet Union and western Europe, before reaching the American continent.[55] The interval between pandemics is quite variable and unpredictable, and this unpredictability, in part, led to the National Immunization Program against swine influenza when a small outbreak of A/New Jersey/76/Hsw1N1 (now designated as H1N1[38]) infection was detected at Fort Dix, New Jersey.[62]

The most severe pandemics have resulted when major alterations occurred in both of the major surface antigens.[55] The most striking exception to this generalization occurred when A/USSR/77/H1N1 did not cause a severe pandemic in spite of major shifts in both surface glycoproteins. In part, this discrepancy may be due to the fact that much of the world's population had been alive during the previous H1N1 era, that is, 1917–1957, and thus possessed protective immunity. Furthermore, it appears that transmissibility from person to person and intrinsic virulence (severity of the disease) are virus-coded functions that vary much as does antigenicity. For example the intrinsic virulence with H1N1 viruses since 1978 appears to be less than with H3N2 viruses.

Proposed Mechanism of Epidemic Behavior

A scheme is shown in Figure 4 that ties together the concepts of antigenic shifts and antigenic drifts in relation to population immunity. When a new virus, here called Ah*x*N*x*, is introduced into a population lacking antibody to it, pandemic influenza results. After one or more waves of pandemic influenza, the level of immunity in the population increases, which makes the setting for emergence of a variant showing antigenic drift fa-

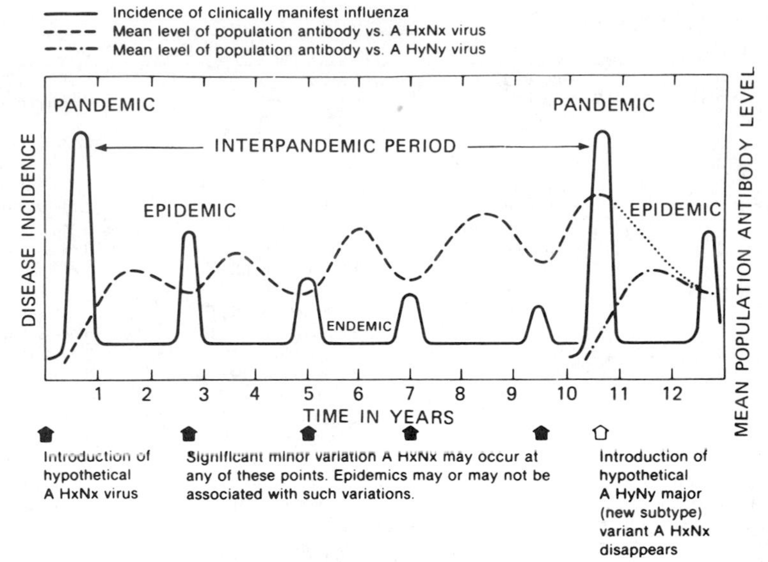

FIG. 4. Schema of the occurrence of influenza pandemics and epidemics in relation to the level of immunity in the population. AXxNx and AHyNy represent influenza viruses with completely different hemagglutinins and neuraminidases. (Modified from Kilbourne,[55] with permission.)

vorable since the level of immunity to it will be less than to the original strain. This phenomenon is repeated with subsequent epidemics due to strains of influenza AH*x*N*x* that probably exhibit some antigenic drift. After 10–30 years of circulation of variants with this given subtype, the level of immunity in the population to all variants within the subtype is very high, and the conditions for the spread of a new virus, AH*y*N*y*, are favorable. Such a virus arises by genetic reassortment. Thus it possesses a markedly different HA, NA, or both with respect to the AH*x*N*x* subtype, and the next pandemic occurs.

While the concepts of immunity of the population together with antigenic variation are important in understanding the epidemiology of influenza, they do not provide the entire explanation. For example, it is apparent that virus factors must contribute to virulence and transmissibility. If a virus does not possess these characteristics yet possesses new surface antigens, epidemic influenza will not occur. An example of this was the emergence of A/New Jersey/76/HswN1 (now H1N1[38]) at Fort Dix, New Jersey, in January 1976. Clearly it possessed the antigenic criteria for epidemic spread. Although it spread and caused death within the confines of a military base, it did not spread in civilian populations. It appeared to lack transmissibility in civilian populations.

Besides the development of new antigens, other factors must be important in the development of an epidemic, but it should be emphasized that other than the known association of influenza outbreaks with cold weather there is no explanation as to what allows an epidemic to develop. Furthermore, it is equally unclear what factors are responsible for "shutting off" an epidemic after 5–6 weeks when only a portion of susceptibles are infected. As noted previously, where the virus resides between epidemics is not understood. In prospective year-round surveillance studies of febrile children (Fig. 3), influenza viruses are only recoverable from ill children for a few weeks before and a few weeks after the 5- to 6-week epidemic.[52] Thus, there is a period of 9–10 months when influenza virus cannot be detected; during this period rare serologic responses are detected.[56] Possible explanations include infection with disease at a very low rate, asymptomatic or latent infection in humans, or transmission of the virus to swine, avian, or equine hosts. None of these postulates is supported by data, and none is entirely satisfactory in terms of explaining the disappearance of virus from human populations between epidemics.

Mortality

In addition to the enormous morbidity that accompanies epidemic or pandemic influenza, substantial mortality is also associated with such outbreaks.[55,56,64,65] The devastating mortality of the 1918–1919 swine influenza pandemic has been described previously. There have been recent changes in the methods used to calculate excess mortality in the United States by the Centers for Disease Control. Beginning with the H3N2 (A/Hong Kong) epidemic of 1968–1969, final estimates of excess mortality are based on time–series analysis of the National Center for Health Statistics (NCHS) final mortality data.[66–68] Earlier estimates were based on data from 121 or 122 cities. Pneumonia and influenza deaths fluctuate annually in a predictable fashion with peaks in the winter and troughs in the summer (Fig. 5).[67] When pneumonia and influenza deaths exceed the epidemic threshold, this is almost always due to influenza A virus activity or occasionally to influenza B virus activity. The estimated number of deaths together with an estimation of the extent of activity for both influenza A and B viruses from 1957 to 1988 is shown in Table 3. As noted, influenza activity was recorded in 26 of 28 winters and excess mortality in at least 15 of these winters.[66,67,69] Similar data plotted back to 1934 demonstrate the frequent occurrence of mortality due to influenza A virus (Fig. 6).[68] It occurs during interpandemic periods as well as during pandemic years. Influenza B has a lesser but definite contribution. It should be noted that the total interpandemic mortality exceeds that of the pandemic years.

Influenza of Other Species

Influenza A viruses commonly infect other species, most notably horses, swine, and avian species, but not primates.[51] The disease in swine is very similar to that in humans in that it produces a respiratory and systemic illness with low mortality and with occasional pulmonary bacterial superinfection. Equine influenza is a milder disease without complications, whereas the disease in water fowl varies from inapparent infection to a lethal infection involving primarily the gastrointestinal and central nervous systems and also the sinuses and the trachea. There are many antigenic relationships among avian influenza viruses and those isolated from humans.

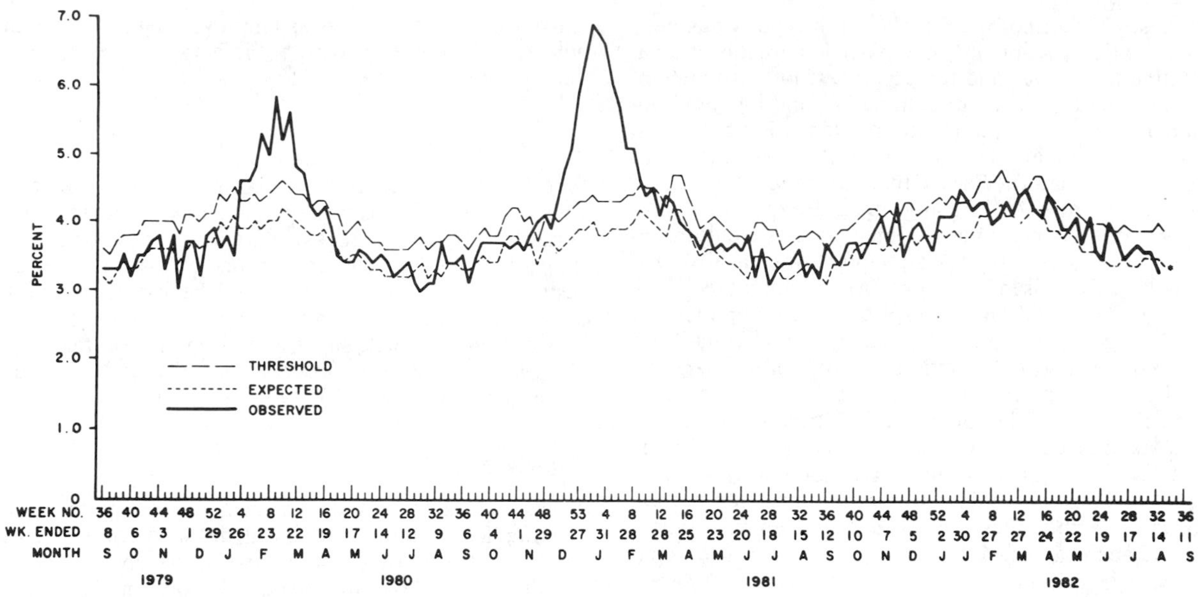

*FORECASTS ARE MADE AT 4-WEEK INTERVALS EXCEPT DURING EPIDEMIC PERIODS

FIG. 5. Pneumonia–influenza deaths. The observed and expected ratios of deaths attributed to pneumonia and influenza in 121 cities are presented as determined by the time–series method, September 1979 to August 1982. The mortality statistics for the 1981–1982 influenza season do not show a national increase in the ratio of deaths associated with pneumonia and influenza (P&I) beyond the expected seasonal variation. For the 1980–1981 season, the ratio of P&I total deaths was elevated for 13 weeks. (From the Centers for Disease Control.[67])

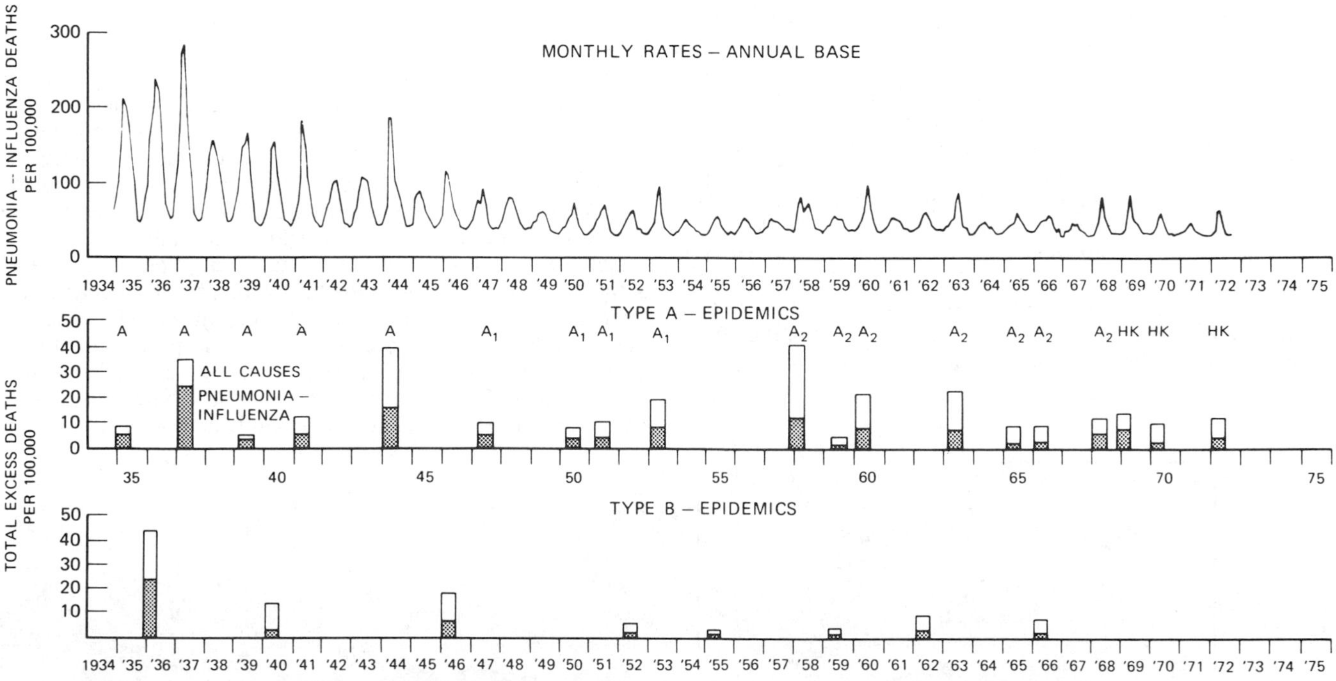

* FROM EPIDEMIOLOGY PROGRAM, CENTER FOR DISEASE CONTROL

FIG. 6. Pneumonia–influenza death rates by month and excess mortality during epidemic periods, United States, 1934–1972. (From Centers for Disease Control.[68])

PATHOPHYSIOLOGY

Transmission

Influenza virus infection is acquired by a mechanism involving the transfer of virus-containing respiratory secretions from an infected to a susceptible person.[70] A number of lines of evidence indicate that small-particle aerosols (<10 μm mass median diameter) may be of predominant importance in such person-to-person transmission. First, large amounts of virus are present in respiratory secretions of infected persons at the time of illness and are thus available for dispersion in small-particle aerosols created by sneezing, coughing, and talking.[70] Second, the explosive nature and simultaneous onset in many persons suggest that a single infected person can transmit virus to a large number of susceptibles. Furthermore, influenza virus type A has been shown to be relatively stable in small-particle aerosols at a variety of relative humidities and temperatures, but survival appears to be favored by low relative humidity and low environmental temperature.[71] In experimental influenza in volunteers, inoculation with small-particle aerosols produces an illness that more closely mimics natural disease than does inoculation with large drops into the nose.[72,73] Finally, in such experimental infections, doses of 137–300 times the median tissue culture infective dose ($TCID_{50}$) are required to infect via nasal drops, whereas 0.6–3.0 $TCID_{50}$ is infectious by the aerosol route.[72,74,75]

Once virus is deposited on the respiratory tract epithelium, it may attach to and penetrate columnar epithelial cells if not prevented from doing so by specific secretory antibody (IgA), by nonspecific nucleoproteins to which virus may attach, or by the mechanical action of the mucociliary apparatus. Once adsorption has taken place, the virion initiates a replication cycle. Studies in cell cultures indicate that the single cell replication cycle takes 4–6 hours.[76] Virus release continues for several hours before cell death ensues. Released virus then may initiate infection in adjacent and nearby cells, so within a few replication cycles, a large number of cells in the respiratory tract are releasing virus and dying due to virus replication. The duration of the incubation period to the onset of illness or the onset of virus shedding, which occurs in close proximity, varies from 18 to 72 hours depending in part on the inoculum dose.[70,77]

Virus Shedding

Quantitation of virus in respiratory tract specimens reveals a characteristic pattern (Fig. 7). Virus is first detected just before the onset of illness (within 24 hours), rapidly rises to a peak of 3.0–7.0 $\log_{10}$ $TCID_{50}$/ml, remains elevated for 24–48 hours, and then rapidly decreases to low titers.[78] Usually influenza virus is no longer detectable after 5–10 days of virus shedding. In young children, shedding at high titers of virus is prolonged.[79]

The severity of illness correlates temporally with quantities of virus shed in experimental influenza in volunteers, thus suggesting that a major mechanism in the production of illness is cell death resulting from viral replication.[70,74] It is not known whether such a correlation holds for natural influenza. However, some severely ill persons shed only small amounts of virus. In primary infection, neither serum nor secretory antibody is detectable at this time, thus indicating that immunologic mechanisms are not involved in production of illness. The occurrence of systemic illness and fever suggest dissemination of virus via the blood stream, but infectious virus in the blood has only rarely been detected.[80]

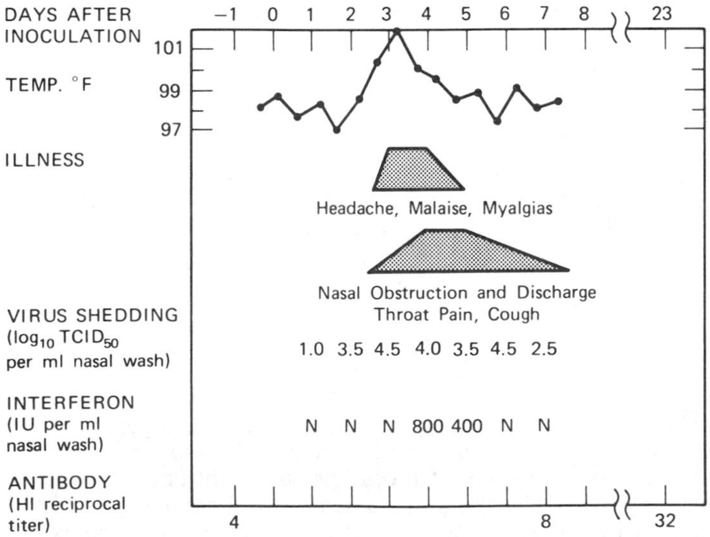

FIG. 7. A case report of a volunteer inoculated by nose drops with 300 $TCID_{50}$ A/Aichi/69/H3N2 (N: negative).

Interferon Response

Interferon is frequently detected in respiratory tract specimens and serum specimens from patients or volunteers with influenza virus infection and illness.[78,81] Usually shedding of virus precedes by 1–2 days the appearance of interferon in both nasal secretions and serum. The time of the appearance of interferon correlates with an improvement of symptoms and a decrease in virus titers, which suggests that interferon may be active in the recovery process between the third and sixth day before serum or secretory antibody is detected.

Pathologic Characteristics

Nasal and bronchial biopsy specimens from persons with acute uncomplicated influenza reveal desquamation of ciliated columnar epithelium into the lumen of the bronchus (Fig. 8). Individual cells show shrinkage, pyknotic nuclei, and a loss of cilia. The lungs in fatal influenza viral pneumonia, in addition to sloughing of epithelium in the tracheobronchial tree, show extensive hemorrhage, hyaline membrane formation, and a paucity of polymorphonuclear cell infiltration (Fig. 9). Patients with secondary bacterial pneumonia have the changes characteristic of bacterial pneumonia in addition to the tracheobronchial findings of influenza (Fig. 10).

Immunology

Neutralizing, hemagglutination-inhibiting (HAI), complement-fixing enzyme-linked immunosorbent assay (ELISA), and immunoflourescent antibodies develop in the serum of persons experiencing primary infection with influenza virus beginning the second week after exposure to antigen and reaching peak titers by 4 weeks. The antibody response is more rapid after reinfection. The development of anti-NA antibodies parallels that of HAI antibodies.[82] Hemagglutination-inhibiting and neutralizing antibodies, which are primarily directed against the HA antigen, persist for months to years with a gradual decline thereafter. Because of the cost and requirement for cell cultures for the neutralization test, the HAI test is the primary method of detecting antigenic relatedness among hemagglutinins of influenza viruses. Their classification into subtype and strain is based on this test. On the other hand, complement-fixing an-

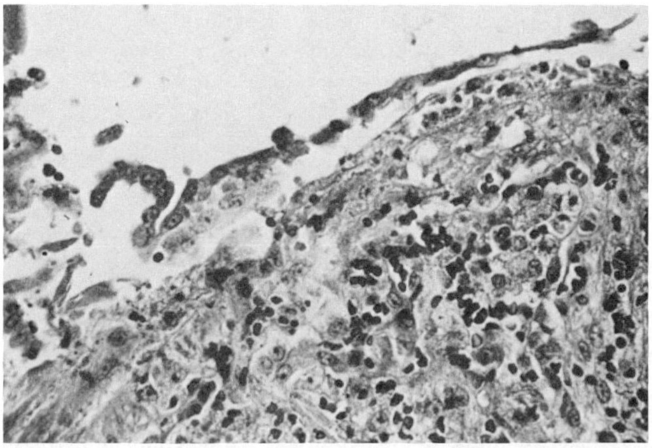

FIG. 8. A small bronchus in acute influenza A infection shows ulceration and attempted regeneration of epithelium. (H&E, ×100) (Courtesy of I.D. Stuard, Reading, PA.)

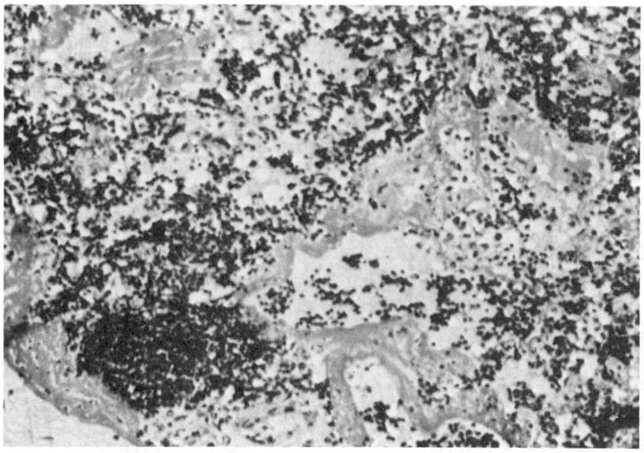

FIG. 9. Lung parenchyma in primary influenza viral pneumonia shows extensive hemorrhage, acellular hyaline membrane lining alveolar ducts and alveoli, and a paucity of inflammatory cells within the alveoli. (H&E, ×400) (Courtesy of I.D. Stuard, Reading, PA.)

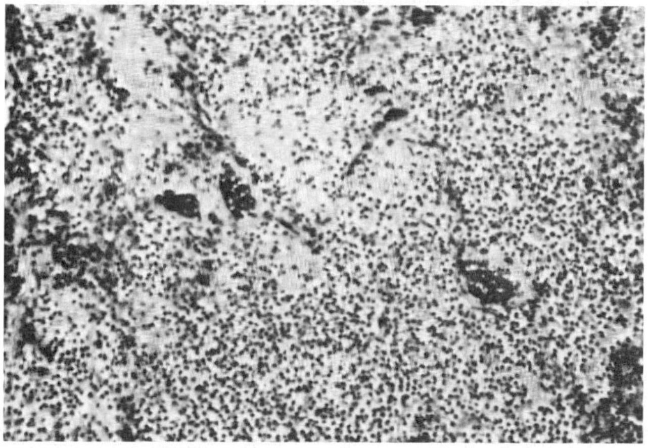

FIG. 10. Lung parenchyma in secondary bacterial infection (*Streptococcus pneumoniae*) complicating influenza A virus infection. Note the marked intra-alveolar polymorphonuclear cell exudate. (H&E, ×400) (Courtesy of I.D. Stuard, Reading, PA.)

tibodies are directed against the ribonucleoprotein and are type specific. They disappear much more rapidly (weeks to months) than do neutralizing, HAI, or anti-NA antibodies, primarily because they are predominantly IgM rather than IgG antibodies, and thus, they may be useful for clinical diagnosis.

Secretory antibodies develop in the respiratory tract after influenza infection and consist predominantly of IgA antibodies.[83–86] Near-peak titers are reached 14 days after the onset of infection. Secretory antibodies have been detected in saliva, nasal secretions, sputum, and tracheal washings.[83] They are usually measured by the neutralization test, for IgA does not fix complement, and nonspecific mucous inhibitors of HA found in the respiratory tract interfere with the HAI test. Although their appearance parallels that of serum antibodies, secretory antibodies do not persist as long, probably several months.

Protection against infection is afforded by the presence of substantial levels of antibody.[87,88] Although there is no exact correlation, serum HAI titers of 1:40 or greater or serum neutralizing titers of 1:8 or greater are associated with protection against infection in most subjects, whereas HAI titers of 1:20 or 1:10 are associated with lesser degrees of protection. Similarly, almost all persons with nasal neutralizing antibody titers of 1:4 or greater are protected against influenza.[87,88] Since both serum and secretory antibodies develop simultaneously in subjects naturally and experimentally infected and since the magnitude of antibody response in the two sites is directly related, it has not been possible to dissociate the role of the two. Available data suggest that optimal protection occurs when both are present.[86]

Antibody, if present in insufficient quantity, in the blood but not in nasal secretions, or directed against a heterologous strain of influenza, may only modify the severity of illness and may not prevent infection. On the other hand, protection in clinical studies has been shown to be strain specific as well as against strains showing antigenic drift within a subtype.[89,90] The degree of protection depends on the degree of drift. For example, Foy et al. showed that influenza A vaccine (A/Hong Kong/68/H3N2) induced protection 3 years later to natural infection with A/England/72/H3N2 virus.[89]

Studies in cell culture systems and in animal systems indicate that the primary role of anti-NA antibody is to decrease the amount of infectious virus released from infected cells and thus to reduce the magnitude of virus shedding in the infected animals.[91] Thus, it seems likely that, in humans, the primary role of anti-HA antibody may be to inhibit infection and that of anti-NA antibody to ameliorate illness. Support for this comes from studies of both natural and experimental influenza in humans in which it has been shown that anti-HA antibody protects against illness as well as against infection, that the presence of serum anti-NA antibody both protects against and shortens the duration of illness due to influenza A,[82,92] and that there are data that indicate that if anti-NA antibody is high titered there is protection against infection as well as against illness.[93]

CLINICAL FINDINGS

Uncomplicated Influenza

During an influenza outbreak there are individuals with respiratory disease with all degrees of severity. Presumably some with mild sore throats and minimal systemic symptoms are infected with influenza. However, many infected individuals have classic "flu," which is characterized by an abrupt onset after an incubation period of 1–2 days; many patients can pinpoint the hour of onset.[70,77,94–97] Initially, systemic symptoms predominate and include feverishness, chilliness, or frank shaking chills, headaches, myalgias, malaise, and anorexia. In more severe cases, prostration is observed. Usually, myalgias or headache are the most troublesome symptoms, and the severity of symptoms is related to the height of the fever. Myalgias may involve the extremities or the long muscles of the back, and arthralgias but not frank arthritis are commonly observed. Severe pain in the eye muscles can be elicited by gazing laterally. Other occular symptoms include tearing and burning. The systemic symptoms usually persist for 3 days, the usual duration of fever. Respiratory symptoms, particularly a dry cough and nasal discharge, are usually also present at the onset but are overshadowed by the systemic symptoms. Nasal obstruction, hoarseness, and a dry or sore throat may also be present, but these symptoms tend to appear as systemic symptoms diminish, and thus they become more prominent as the disease progresses.

Fever is the most important physical finding. The temperature usually rises rapidly to a peak of 100–104°F and occasionally to 106°F within 12 hours of the onset, concurrent with the development of systemic symptoms. Fever is usually continuous but may be intermittent, especially if antipyretics are administered. On the second and third days of illness, the temperature elevation is usually 0.5–1.0° lower than on the first day, and as the fever subsides, the systemic symptoms diminish. Classically, the duration of fever is 3 days, but it may last 4–8 days. In a small number of cases, a second fever spike occurs on the third or fourth day and results in a biphasic fever curve.

Early in the course of illness the patient appears toxic, the face is flushed, and the skin is hot and moist. The eyes are watery and reddened. A clear nasal discharge is common, but nasal obstruction is uncommon. The mucous membranes of the nose and throat are hyperemic, but exudate is not observed. Small, tender cervical lymph nodes are often present. Transient scattered rhonchi or localized areas of rales are found in fewer than 20 percent of the cases.

As systemic signs and symptoms diminish, respiratory complaints and findings become more apparent. Cough is the most frequent and troublesome of these symptoms and may be accompanied by substernal discomfort or burning. Nasal obstruction and discharge occur but not to the degree seen in rhinovirus common colds, and pharyngeal pain and injection are also common. Such symptoms and signs usually persist 3–4 days after the fever subsides. Cough commonly persists longer. A convalescent period of 1, 2, or more weeks to full recovery then ensues. Cough, lassitude, and malaise are the most frequent symptoms during this period.

Illness in Other Subtypes and Types of Influenza. The above description of illness occurs in any type or subtype of influenza A virus infection.[70] Available data suggest that illness associated with influenza B virus infection closely resembles that described for influenza A, although some have suggested that influenza B illness may be somewhat milder than influenza A illness is.[97,98] In contrast, influenza C infection, when it occurs, causes afebrile common colds and rarely, if ever, produces the influenza syndrome.[99] It does not occur in epidemics.

Relation of Age to Illness. As discussed previously, influenza attack rates are higher in children than in adults, although the incidence of pulmonary complications is lower. Maximal temperatures tend to be higher among children, and cervical adenopathy is more frequent among children than among adults.[77] Croup associated with influenza virus infection occurs only among children.[100–102] Among elderly persons, fever remains a very frequent finding, although the height of the febrile response may be lower than among children and young adults.

COMPLICATIONS OF INFLUENZA

Pulmonary Complications

Two manifestations of pneumonia that are associated with influenza are well recognized: primary influenza viral pneumonia and secondary bacterial infection (Table 4). In addition, less distinct and milder pulmonic syndromes often occur during an outbreak of influenza that may represent tracheobronchitis, localized viral pneumonias, or possibly mixed viral and bacterial pneumonias. Comparative features of these clinical syndromes are shown in Table 4.

Primary Influenza Viral Pneumonia. The syndrome of primary influenza viral pneumonia first became well documented in the 1957–1958 outbreak.[103–105] However, it is clear that many of the deaths in the 1918–1919 outbreak were due to the occurrence of this syndrome among young healthy adults. In outbreaks since 1918, primary influenza viral pneumonia has occurred predominantly among persons with cardiovascular disease, especially rheumatic heart disease with mitral stenosis, although cases occur in young healthy adults in every large outbreak. Other chronic disorders and pregnancy have been implicated as risk factors in some epidemics. After a typical onset of influenza, there is a rapid progression of fever, cough, dyspnea, and cyanosis. Physical examination and chest roentgenography reveal bilateral findings but no consolidation, findings consistent with the adult respiratory distress syndrome. Blood gas studies show marked hypoxia, a Gram stain of the sputum fails to reveal significant bacteria, and bacterial culture yields sparse growth of normal flora, whereas viral cultures yield high titers of influenza A virus. Such patients do not respond to antibiotics; the mortality is high. At autopsy, findings consist of tracheitis, bronchitis, diffuse hemorrhagic pneumonia, hyaline membranes lining alveolar ducts and alveoli, and a paucity of inflammatory cells within the alveoli (see Figs. 8 and 9).

Secondary Bacterial Pneumonia. Secondary bacterial pneumonia often produces a syndrome that is clinically distinguishable from that of primary viral pneumonia (Table 4).[105,106] The patients, who most often are elderly or who have chronic pulmonary, cardiac, and metabolic or other disease, have a classic influenza illness followed by a period of improvement lasting usually 4–14 days. Recrudescence of fever is associated with symptoms and signs of bacterial pneumonia such as cough, sputum production, and an area of consolidation detected on physical examination and chest roentgenography. Gram staining and the culture of sputum reveals a predominance of a bacterial pathogen, most often *S. pneumoniae, S. aureus,* or *H. influenzae* (Table 5). Such patients usually respond to specific antibiotic therapy.

During an outbreak of influenza many cases are observed that do not clearly fit into either of the aforementioned categories.[107] The disease is not relentlessly progressive, and yet the fever pattern may not be biphasic. These patients may have primary

TABLE 4. Comparative Features of Pulmonary Complications of Influenza

Feature	*A, Primary Viral Pneumonia*	*B, Secondary Bacterial Pneumonia*	*C, Mixed Viral–Bacterial Pneumonia*	*D, Localized Viral Pneumonia*
Setting	Cardiovascular disease Pregnancy Young adult (Hsw1N1)	Age >65 yrs Pulmonary disease	Any associated with A or B	? Normal
Clinical history	Relentless progression from classic 3-day influenza	Improvement, then worsening after 3-day influenza	Picture of A or B	Continuation of classic 3-day syndrome
Physical examination	Bilateral findings, no consolidation	Consolidation	Consolidation	Area of rales
Sputum bacteriology	Normal flora	*Pneumococcus* *Staphylococcus* *Haemophilus influenzae*	*Pneumococcus* *Staphylococcus* *H. influenzae*	Normal flora
Chest x-ray infiltrate	Bilateral findings	Consolidation	Consolidation	Segmental
White blood cell count	Leukocytosis with a shift to the left	Leukocytosis with a shift to the left	Leukocytosis with a shift to the left	Usually normal
Isolation of influenza virus	Yes	No	Yes	Yes
Response to antibiotics	No	Yes	Often	No
Mortality	High	Low	Variable	Very low

TABLE 5. Etiology of Bacterial Pneumonia during an Influenza A H3N2 Outbreak as Compared with the Preceding Year

	Number of Patients with Indicated Bacterial Etiology	
Bacterial Etiology	*During Influenza Outbreak[a] 1968–1969*	*Preceding Year[b] (No Influenza)*
Pneumococcus	52 (48%)	103 (62%)
Staphylococcus	21 (19%)	10 (6%)
Staphylococcus and others	7 (7%)	7 (4%)
Haemophilus influenzae	12 (11%)	14 (8%)
Other gram-negative species	16 (15%)	32 (20%)
Total	108	167

[a] Three-week period only.
[b] Twelve-month period.
(From Schwarzmann et al.,[105] with permission.)

viral, secondary bacterial, or mixed viral and bacterial infection of the lung (Table 6). Many patients respond to antibiotics. In addition, milder forms of influenza viral pneumonia involving only one lobe or segment have been described that do not invariably lead to death and that are more likely to be confused with pneumonia due to *Mycoplasma pneumoniae* than to that produced by bacterial infection (Table 5).

In children, pneumonia may occur, but it is less common than in adults. Bronchiolitis may also occur due to influenza A or B virus infection, but respiratory syncytial virus and parainfluenza virus type 3 are more important causes of bronchiolitis.

Other Pulmonary Complications

In addition to pneumonia, other pulmonary complications are recognized.

Croup. Significant numbers of cases of croup occur in influenza A and B outbreaks, and that associated with influenza A virus appears to be more severe but less frequent than that associated with parainfluenza virus types 1 or 3 or respiratory syncytial virus infections[100,101] (see Chapter 45).

Exacerbation of Chronic Obstructive Pulmonary Disease. In adults with chronic obstructive pulmonary disease, influenza A or B virus infection may lead to primary viral or to secondary bacterial pneumonia but also may lead to an acute exacerbation of chronic bronchitis, a phenomena that is associated with other respiratory viruses and bacteria.[108–110] Studies by Monto and Ross have shown that such infections result in a permanent loss of pulmonary function.[111] Another major process that is exacerbated is asthma. Often, stable asthmatics will worsen to status asthmaticus due to influenza.[112,113]

Frequency of Pulmonary Involvement. Although the vast majority of patients with influenza do not have clinically detectable pneumonia, pulmonary function abnormalities frequently occur, even in the course of nonpneumonic influenzal infections. Such abnormalities include gas exchange and peripheral airway dysfunction, and these persist well beyond clinical illness.[114–117] These findings suggest that viral invasion of the lower respiratory tract is common in uncomplicated influenza and may help to explain the relatively long convalescence. The frequency of overt involvement of the respiratory tract has been answered in part by Fry[118–120] (Table 6). In five successive epidemics, he showed the overall rate of chest complications (tracheobronchitis or pneumonia) to be 9.5 percent of cases. From the ages of 5–50, the rate was low (4–8 percent), but it increased progressively after the age of 60 to a level of 73 percent in those over 70 years of age. Foy et al. studied seven successive epidemics of influenza A infection and showed the six of the seven were associated with at least a doubling of pneumonia rates among adults.[121]

Nonpulmonary Complications

Most of the complications of influenza have been evaluated in years when there were sizable outbreaks.[64–66,103] However, as antigenic variation of a subtype evolves and as the exposure of the population to vaccine and to virus occurs, the full-blown influenza syndrome becomes a less frequent manifestation. Nonetheless, infection rates may remain high, and consequences of infection in severely compromised elderly patients remain significant. In the 1982–1983 outbreak in Rochester, New York, two nursing home populations were carefully monitored for evidence of influenza infection. Culture-proven attack rates were high in each institution and averaged between 10 and 20 percent. There were 12 deaths among residents with culture-documented influenza, and an additional 15 residents died who did not have cultures performed or who were culture-negative. The number of deaths was six during the same period for these two institutions in the previous year in the absence of an influenza outbreak. Most of the people who died did not have pulmonary complications but simply did not recover from what initially seemed like a rather mild influenza-like illness. In general, those who died had been, before the outbreak, more incapacitated than were other residents within the institution.

Myositis

Myositis and myogloblinuria with tender leg muscles and elevated serum creatine phosphokinase (CPK) levels have been reported mostly in children after influenza A or influenza B infection, most commonly after the latter.[122–126] Symptoms may be sufficiently severe to prevent walking, but neurologic changes are not evident.

Cardiac Complications

Both myocarditis and pericarditis have been rarely associated with influenza A or B virus infection. Some investigators have associated influenza with myocardial infarction. However, neither myocarditis nor pericarditis are commonly observed at autopsy among those who died of primary influenza viral pneumonia.[103,127–132] In patients with cardiac disease, the acquisition of influenza provides a significant risk of death.[133]

TABLE 6. Distribution of Chest Complications in Persons with Influenza in a General Practice

	Age									
Distribution	*0–4*	*5–9*	*10–19*	*20–29*	*30–39*	*40–49*	*50–59*	*60–69*	*70*	*Total*
Lobar pneumonia[a]	—	—	—	—	1	1	1	3	1	7
Segmental pneumonia[b]	3	9	6	3	2	3	5	6	6	43
Acute bronchitis	6	1		1	2	3	4	6	7	30
Total	9	10	6	4	5	7	10	15	14	80
Percentage of all cases of influenza	12	8	4	4	4	7	10	36	73	9.5

[a] X-ray evidence of pneumonia.
[b] Persistent rales.
(Data from Fry.[118–120])

Toxic Shock Syndrome

In recent outbreaks of influenza B, toxic shock-like syndrome has occurred in previously healthy children or adults presumably because viral infection changed colonization and replication characteristics of the toxin-producing staphylococcus. An association between influenza and pulmonary infection with staphylococcus has been recognized previously. In this instance, the *S. aureus* strain involved has the capability of producing the specific toxin[134] and hence toxic shock.

Central Nervous System Complications

Guillain-Barré syndrome has been reported to occur after influenza A infection, as it has after numerous other infections, but no definite etiologic relationship has been established.[135,136] In addition, cases of transverse myelitis and encephalitis have occurred rarely.[132,137] Influenza B in adults is more commonly linked with an encephalitis that appears to be a severe encephalopathy afflicting both brain stem and higher system function.[132,137,138] An etiologic association of these syndromes with influenza virus infection has only infrequently been proved, and influenza infection may account for only a small proportion of cases of each of these syndromes.

Reye Syndrome

Epidemiology. Reye syndrome, first described in 1963, is now a frequently recognized hepatic and central nervous system (CNS) complication of influenza A and, less commonly, influenza A virus infection. This syndrome occurs almost exclusively in children,[139] most often between the ages of 2 and 16 years, and has a high mortality of 10–40 percent.[140] Because of the epidemic nature of the occurrence of influenza A or B virus infection, Reye syndrome also has an epidemic occurrence. Many other viruses have been associated with Reye syndrome: adenovirus, coxsackie A, coxsackie B, Epstein-Barr virus, echovirus, poliovirus, parainfluenza viruses, retrovirus, rubella virus, measles virus, varicella-zoster virus, and herpes simplex virus.[140–142] However, most of these associations are single cases occurring sporadically and year-round in young children (median age, six years), except for those associated with varicella-zoster virus infection. Far more important, however, were the large outbreaks (nine since 1967) in the United States that were associated with influenza B virus infection and the one that occurred in the 1978–1979 influenza A/Brazil/78/H1N1 outbreak.[140–142] In addition to the epidemiologic clustering, these cases occur more frequently in older children (median age, 11 years) than do the sporadically occurring cases.[140,141]

Reye syndrome can occur several days after a typical upper respiratory, gastrointestinal, or chickenpox infection.[140,141,143–145] In 1974 in the United States, 316 of 379 total cases for the year occurred in a 2-month period and were associated with an outbreak of influenza B/Hong Kong/5/72 virus infection.[140,141] Although appropriate specimens were only obtained from a few patients, laboratory evidence of influenza B virus infection was obtained in 17 percent. Ninety percent of the patients had an antecedent upper respiratory infection, and the mean duration between the onset of illness and hospitalization was 5.7 days (range, 1–17 days). The period from onset of antecedent varicella or gastrointestinal illness to hospitalization for Reye syndrome is similar, usually 4–6 days (range, 1–14 days). A particularly well documented clustering of cases occurred during the winter of 1978–1979 when 85 cases occurred in association with influenza A H1N1 activity.[142] This was the first association of epidemic Reye syndrome with influenza A virus infection. There is also a strong epidemiologic link between aspirin usage and Reye syndrome.[146–148] This has led to warnings being inserted on the labels of aspirin products and to recommendations that another antipyretic be used in children with fever due to varicella or influenza.

Clinical Picture. The classic manifestation of Reye syndrome is a change in mental status.[140,141,143] Manifestations range from lethargy to delirium, obtundation, seizures, and respiratory arrest (Table 7). In three-quarters of the cases, CNS manifestations are preceded by nausea and vomiting lasting 1–2 days before hospitalization. The children are usually afebrile and have hepatomegaly but are not jaundiced. Mortality is related to the stage of coma on admission and ranges from a high of approximately 40 percent[139,140,142–144,149,150] to a low of 10 percent.[150] Lumbar puncture reveals normal protein values and cell counts confirming the presence of encephalopathy rather than encephalitis or meningoencephalitis. The most frequent laboratory abnormality is elevation of the blood ammonia value, which occurs in almost all patients. Hypoglycemia is present most often in patients with antecedent varicella or gastrointestinal illness (37 percent) as compared with upper respiratory illness (15 percent). Serum glutamic oxaloacetic transaminase (AST), serum glutamic pyruvic transaminase (ALT), and bilirubin values are commonly elevated as are CPK and lactic dehydrogenase (LDH) levels. The prothrombin time is usually increased. Coma (stage 4 or 5) on admission is evidence of increased intracranial pressure, and a blood ammonia level greater than 300 μg/dl is significantly associated with mortality. Among survivors, 30 percent of those who developed either decerebrate posturing or seizures during hospitalization had serious neurologic sequelae.

Pathologic Findings. The striking feature is the absence of inflammatory changes.[143,144] The gross appearance of the liver on biopsy specimens is usually pale yellow, and on microscopic examination the chief features are fatty filtration of hepatocytes consisting of multiple small droplets of lipids uniformly distributed throughout the cells. The main ultrastructural finding is alteration of the hepatocyte mitochondria including swelling and pleomorphism. The pathologic findings most often detected in the brain have been cerebral edema, anoxic neuronal degeneration, but no gross inflammation.

Pathophysiology. The pathophysiology of Reye syndrome is uncertain, but the association with the virus infection may act merely as a triggering mechanism for a toxin since the pathologic processes more closely resemble the effects of a toxin than an infection. Aflatoxins have been suspected since the disease

TABLE 7. Reye Syndrome: Clinical Characteristics

Characteristic	*Percentage of Patients with Indicated Condition*
Antecedent illness[a]	89% Upper respiratory tract illness
	7% Varicella
	4% Gastrointestinal illness
Central nervous system manifestations	
Stage of coma on admission	
0	2% Alert
1	26% Lethargy, follows verbal commands
2	42% Stupor, combativeness, conjugate deviation
3	17% Coma, decortication
4	10% Coma, decerebration, loss of oculocephalic reflexes
5	3% Coma, absent pupillary reaction, flaccidity
Laboratory data	
Blood glucose	15% 50 mg/dl
Blood ammonia	98% 48 μg/dl (upper limit of normal)
	76% 100 μg/dl
	46% 200 μg/dl
	13% 500 μg/dl
Cerebrospinal fluid	Protein: normal; cells: 8 mononuclears/mm^3

[a] Interval between onset of the antecedent illness and hospitalization (mean, 5.7 days).
[b] Percentage of patients whose serum ammonia concentration is greater than concentration indicated. All of these numbers pertain to ammonia, not to protein and cells.
(Data from Corey et al.[141] and Concensus Development Conference.[149]

has a high incidence in Thailand where, during the rainy season, there is a high rate of contamination of foodstuffs with aflatoxins. Such toxins have not been found in the food or environment of patients who develop Reye syndrome outside of Thailand.[144]

Several other pathophysiologic mechanisms have been postulated[146,147,151–154] including hepatic injury leading to hypoglycemia and acidosis, excessive fatty acid mobilization with fatty acids acting as endogenous toxins, hyperammonemia leading to encephalopathy, and most recently, transient dysfunction of hepatic urea-cycle mitochondrial enzymes. Assays of urea-cycle enzymes in liver tissue from patients with Reye syndrome reveal decreased ornithine transcarbamylase activity and decreased carbamyl phosphate synthetase levels.[152,153] Thus it is postulated that the hyperammonemia of Reye syndrome apparently results from excess waste nitrogen that overwhelms the abilities of reduced ornithine transcarbamylase and occasionally carbamyl phosphate synthetase to detoxify the ammonia load.[154] The decreased activity of these enzymes explains the absent plasma citrulline, the product of ornithine transcarbamylase, and the increased blood ammonia, the substrate of carbamyl phosphate synthetase. Ammonia is taken up by the brain of patients with Reye syndrome, and the amount fixed correlates with increased cerebral lactate production; the magnitude of these changes parallels the amount of central neurologic hyperventilation.

On the other hand, there are a number of arguments that all the CNS dysfunction cannot be explained by excess blood ammonia levels. Smith has postulated that Reye syndrome is a result of generalized acute mitochondrial damage induced by viral illness.[154] All organs, except for the brain, appear to recover uneventfully from the transient interference with mitochondrial function. Since most patients receive aspirin therapy for their antecedent illness, aspirin has been suspected, and a recent study reported that children who received aspirin for fever related to influenza had an excess frequency of Reye syndrome.[146–148] Therefore, the American Academy of Pediatrics has recommended that another antipyretic agent be substituted for aspirin in children with fever due to influenza or varicella.[148,155]

A number of modes of therapy directed at the biochemical abnormalities have been suggested, and the survival rate has apparently improved with some of them. General supportive measures are important, with careful attention to fluid and electrolyte balance and the provision of assistance for ventilation when needed. Intravenous glucose is infused to correct hypoglycemia. Hemodynamic monitoring is important. Intubation should be elective. Efforts such as dialysis and amino acid and phosphate and insulin infusions to correct specific metabolic abnormalities have not altered the outcome.[149,156,157] Since the major cause of death is cerebral edema, therapy directed at lowering increased intracranial pressure (such as mannitol and glycerol) and at monitoring intracranial pressure by means of a cerebral ventricular catheter is indicated.[158]

DIAGNOSIS

Virus Isolation

The specific methods of viral diagnosis are discussed in Chapter 14. It should be noted that the detection of infectious virus or viral antigen in respiratory secretions is optimal for clinical purposes since serologic tests, although sensitive and specific, do not yield data at a clinically relevant time due to the requirement for convalescent sera.[159] Virus can be isolated readily from nasal swab specimens, throat swab specimens, nasal washes, or sputum. If the patient is producing sputum, this is perhaps the best specimen.[159] If not, a combination nose and throat swab specimen or a nasal wash is ideal. Such swabs should be thrust into containers of viral transport medium and transported to the laboratory as soon as possible. Specimens for influenza are inoculated onto rhesus monkey kidney, cynomologus monkey kidney, or Madin-Darby canine kidney cell cultures where virus is detected by examining for cytopathic effect or hemadsorption. About two-thirds of the positive cultures can be detected within 3 days of inoculation and the remainder by 5–7 days. Many hospital viral diagnostic laboratories and most state health laboratories can detect influenza virus by these cell culture techniques or by the inoculation of embryonated hens' eggs.

Serology

For serologic diagnosis, complement-fixing antibody tests are most commonly used. Paired serum specimens, including an acute and a convalescent serum obtained 10–20 days after the acute-phase serum specimen, should be submitted for testing. Fourfold or greater rises or falls in titer are considered diagnostic of infection, and a high convalescent titer, when only a single convalescent serum specimen is available, suggests recent infection.[159]

Epidemiology

A diagnosis can also be made on epidemiologic grounds. That is, when influenza virus is confirmed in a region or community by the local or state health department or by the Centers for Disease Control, persons with fever, muscle aches, and cough most likely have influenza. In fact, several studies have shown the association to be as high as 85 percent.[160–166] It is also likely that those people with minor respiratory symptoms also are infected with influenza virus during such periods.[96]

TREATMENT

Uncomplicated Influenza

Amantadine is approved in the United States for the treatment of influenza (see Chapter 34). It has been shown to reduce the duration of signs and symptoms of clinical influenza by approximately 50 percent.[160–166] Its major drawback is the association of minor, reversible, CNS side effects such as insomnia, dizziness, or difficulty in concentrating. However, in controlled studies, the reduction of influenza symptoms is greater than is the occurrence of drug side effects, so the net benefit to the patient is substantial. The one group for which amantadine appears to have particular risk are individuals with known seizure disorders. An increased frequency of seizures occurs even if anticonvulsant therapy is maintained.[166] For healthy subjects with normal renal function the usual dose is 200 mg po initially and 100 mg bid thereafter. Recently 100 mg/day was shown to be equally effective to 100 mg bid.[165] For persons over 65 years of age, the dose should not exceed 100 mg/day. The duration is for 3–5 days for patients with influenza-like illness and temperatures over 100°F that occur in the winter and at the time when Centers for Disease Control or the state or local health department has reported influenza in or near the community.

Although not yet approved for use, rimantadine, a drug that is closely related structurally to amantadine, appears to be of equal efficacy to amantadine in uncomplicated influenza.[160,164] Because side effects may be somewhat less frequent[96,164] with rimantadine, it may eventually replace amantadine. The dosage is 100 mg bid. The emergence of resistance to rimantadine in children receiving therapy has been recognized.[167] Resistance development seems to occur only in young children who shed high titers of virus. It is likely that resistance to amantadine would develop in children treated with amantadine as well as with rimantadine.

Other measures involve symptomatic relief. The acutely ill febrile patient should be at bed rest, and fluid intake should be adequate. Acetylsalicylic acid, 0.6–0.9 g every 3–4 hours is effective in reducing fever.[165] However, antipyretics other than aspirin are recommended for children.[155] Nasal obstruction may be benefited by phenylephrine (0.25%) or oxymetazoline hydrochloride (0.05%; 0.025% in young children) nasal sprays or drops, and cough may be reduced with cold water vaporization or guaifenesin cough syrup containing dextromethorphan, 1–3 teaspoons every 3–4 hours (lower dose in young children).

Pulmonary Complications

There have been no controlled studies of amantadine treatment of influenza viral pneumonia, so its use in this condition is based on extrapolation from anecdotal case reports of benefit and on data indicating an effect of amantadine on peripheral airways resistance in uncomplicated influenza.[117,168]

Supportive care is important, including fluid and electrolyte management. Supplemental oxygen, intubation, tracheostomy, assisted ventilation, and the use of positive end-expiratory pressure may have a role depending on the severity of the illness.[169,170]

For patients with proven or suspected bacterial suprainfection, appropriate antibiotics should be administered, and a discussion of this therapy can be found in the respective chapters. Because of the rapidly advancing nature of many cases of pneumonia occurring during an influenza epidemic, therapy to "cover" the potential pathogens, most importantly *S. aureus, S. pneumoniae,* and *H. influenzae*, is indicated if an etiologic diagnosis cannot be made from a Gram stain of the sputum or transtracheal aspirate.

Other Complications

There is no specific therapy for the cardiac, CNS, or other complications. A discussion of the treatment of Reye syndrome is presented in the section dealing with that illness.

PREVENTION

Vaccine

The mainstay for the prevention of influenza since the late 1940s has been inactivated virus vaccines. A number of trials in military and civilian populations have demonstrated the efficacy of inactivated, parenterally administered influenza vaccines in the prevention of naturally occurring outbreaks of H1N1, H2N2, and H3N2 viruses.[171–178] Efficacy rates have varied between 67 and 92 percent. Careful studies suggest that the frequency of severe illness is reduced to a greater degree than is the frequency of infection. Similar observations have been made in the elderly.[179,180]

Each year, the Public Health Advisory Committee on Immunization Practices makes recommendations with regard to the composition of the vaccine. The composition of some of these recent vaccines is given in Table 8. In general, vaccines have contained both an A and a B virus, usually the types isolated in the previous winter's influenza season. In recent years where two influenza A subtypes have circulated (1978–1987), both have been included in the vaccine because of a lack of reliable methods of predicting the type of influenza to be encountered. Since 1940, numerous improvements and changes have been made in the vaccines. In an effort to improve antibody responses, the antigenic mass was increased in vaccines for the 1972–1973 through the 1975–1976 influenza seasons.[87] More recently (1981–1987), the dose of antigen was doubled in an effort to improve response rates and to provide antibody that had greater cross-reactivity.[181–183] In recent studies, doubling the dose of antigen administered has enhanced antibody response in the elderly,[184] but this has not been a consistent finding.

A major advance in the use of influenza vaccines has been the standardization of antigenic mass. Influenza virus vaccines are made from allantoic fluid harvests from embryonated hens' eggs infected with a strain of influenza A or B virus. Virus is inactivated with formalin treatment and is purified to remove egg proteins. Some preparations are further treated with lipid solvents to yield so-called subvirion or split-product vaccines. Those not so treated are called "whole-virion" or "whole-virus" vaccines. The antigenic mass is currently measured by immunodiffusion, a method that yields microgram quantities of hemagglutinin rather than chick cell agglutination (CCA) units. The measurement of CCA units was imprecise and hard to reproduce, so that measure did not give reliable, comparable data for subvirion and whole-virus preparations.

TABLE 8. Influenza Vaccine Composition in Recent Years

Year	Type	Antigens	Quantity of Antigen (μg)
1983–84[a,b]	Trivalent	A/Brazil/78 H1N1	15
		A/Philippines/82 H3N2	15
		B/Singapore	15
1984–85[a,b]	Trivalent	A/Chile/83 H1N1	15
		A/Philippines/82 H3N2	15
		B/USSR/1/83	15
1985–86[a,b]	Trivalent	A/Chile/1/83 H1N1	15
		A/Philippines/82 H3N2	15
		B/USSR/83	15
1986–87[a,b]	Trivalent	A/Chile/1/83 H1N1	15
		A/Mississippi/1/85 H3N2	15
		B/Ann Arbor/1/86	15
	Monovalent		15
1987–88[a,b]	Trivalent	A/Taiwan/1/85 H1N1	15
		A/Mississippi/1/85 H3N2	15
		B/Ann Arbor/1/86	15
1988–89[a,b]	Trivalent	A/Taiwan/1/86 H1N1	15
		A/Sichuan/2/87 H3N2	15
		B/Victoria/2/87	15

[a] Subviron vaccine for those <2 years.
[b] Two doses for those <12 years unless one dose of any influenza was given in any year from 1978 to 1983.

The vaccine is associated with side effects.[181–183, 185] One-quarter to one-half of the vaccine recipients feel some discomfort at the vaccine site 8–24 hours after vaccination, but only about 5 percent have moderately severe, transient, local reactions. Fever or other systemic reactions may be present in 1–2 percent. Systemic reactions are less frequent in older persons and more frequent in young children where the rate of occurrence of fever may be as high as 24–40 percent, but this can be reduced by decreasing the antigenic mass. Data obtained in the 1976 vaccination trials indicated that, for equivalent antigenic mass in CCA units, whole-virus products were more reactogenic and antigenic than were subvirion vaccines, hence the recommendation for the exclusive use of subvirion vaccines in children under 12 years of age. In the 1978 vaccine trials, the antigenic mass was determined by immunodiffusion, and when this was done, both types of vaccine appeared to be equivalent in terms of the rate of reaction and the frequency and magnitude of antibody responses. It does appear, however, that some degree of reactogenicity is a necessary associate of an effective inactivated vaccine.

During the 1976 National Immunization Program against swine influenza, 45 million persons received influenza vaccine. In the first 4–6 weeks after vaccination, an excess rate of Guillain-Barré syndrome occurred among vaccinees as compared with persons who did not receive the vaccine.[186] The estimated risk of acquiring Guillain-Barré syndrome during that vaccination program was 1 in 100,000 vaccinations; the mortality for those with Guillain-Barré was five percent, and another 5–10 percent had some residual neurologic abnormality. Since this is the only known fatal complication of influenza vaccination, the mortality of vaccination can be calculated to be 1 in 2 million. It is noteworthy that since 1976 Guillain-Barré syndrome has not been associated with influenza vaccination despite the use of 15–18 million doses annually.

It has been claimed that influenza vaccination can be associated with severe drug toxicity in patients taking warfarin or theophylline due to vaccine-induced depression of the metabolic activity of the hepatic cytochrome P-450 enzyme system.[187] However, two different approaches to this question failed to support the initial observations. A prospective study of residents (155 taking theophylline, 48 taking warfarin) in 52 nursing homes during the 1982–1983 influenza season failed to reveal evidence of warfarin or theophylline toxicity in the 30-day period after vaccination.[188] Similar findings were documented elsewhere.[189,190]

In 1984, the strategy for vaccine usage changed from a general recommendation to immunize persons over the age of 65 and those with chronic underlying conditions to specific guidelines to more effectively vaccinate those at highest risk.[191] Three levels of risk have been established.[191] First, adults and children undergoing regular medical care or who were hospitalized in the past year for chronic pulmonary or cardiac conditions and residents of nursing homes and other chronic care facilities should be given the highest priority for vaccination. The next level includes healthy individuals over the age of 65; those with other chronic underlying diseases such as diabetes mellitus, renal dysfunction, anemia, immunosuppression, or asthma; and children and teenagers receiving chronic aspirin therapy. Efforts should be made to vaccinate at least 80 percent of individuals in the first two risk categories. Finally, physicians, nurses, and other personnel who have extensive contact with high-risk patients as well as providers of home care to high-risk persons should be vaccinated.[192]

Recommendations for Vaccine Use. The only contraindication to vaccination is hypersensitivity to hens' eggs. Generally, if persons can eat eggs or egg-containing products, vaccination is safe.

Special attention needs to be given to the timing of vaccine administration in those who are receiving cytotoxic drugs. Studies both in children[193] and in adults[194] who are receiving treatment for malignancy show that a significantly lower proportion of patients produce antibody (50 percent of adults or children) when vaccine is administered simultaneously with chemotherapy than when vaccine is administered at the nadir of the white count response or when no chemotherapy is given. Over 95 percent of the adults or children with malignancies responded to A/New Jersey/76 if chemotherapy was not being administered at the time vaccine was given.[193,194] For patients with chronic renal failure, the response rate may be somewhat lower[195] or the same[196–198] as normal persons. Patients undergoing hemodialysis respond similarly to normal persons.[196–199] Patients who have undergone renal allotransplantation, on the other hand, respond less well than control subject do.[200–202] The blunted response may be related to the degree of renal malfunction.[200] Although studies are limited, there is some indication that the antibody response may be blunted by cyclosporine but not by azathioprine.[203] Importantly, adverse effects from vaccine are no more frequent than are those that occur in control subjects, and renal function is not adversely affected.

A number of studies have been carried out that compare response rates in patients with systemic lupus erythematosus to determine whether vaccine will produce adverse effects in this group with abnormal immune responses.[204–207] Single doses of vaccine are well tolerated. Although repeated vaccine administration to healthy persons has no deleterious effects,[208] further studies are required before it is clear that repeated vaccine is well tolerated in patients with lupus. Studies of other groups at risk for pulmonary complications of influenza but who might have a greater potential to develop side effects from vaccine administration (e.g., patients with neurologic disease) are not generally available. One study in patients with multiple sclerosis[209] showed no deleterious effects and response rates comparable with those for healthy persons. Elderly patients respond well to vaccine with minimal side effects.[179,180,184,210] Patients with human immunodeficiency virus (HIV) infection, with the acquired immunodeficiency syndrome (AIDS) related complex, and with AIDS respond poorly to influenza vaccines. Zidovudine partially corrects this deficit[211] (see Table 9).

Pregnancy presents a special situation. There are good data to show that influenza vaccine is not harmful to either mother or fetus; yet it is prudent to limit the use of biologics in pregnancy.[212] In the 1918–1919 and 1957–1958 epidemics, pregnancy was associated with increased mortality. None has been observed since that time. Thus, it is recommended that pregnant women with chronic disease should receive influenza vaccine whereas others should not.

The overall risk of dying of influenza is approximately 1 in 5,000 to 1 in 10,000 per year. The risk is higher among elderly persons and persons with chronic disease than among normal young persons. It is obviously higher in years of large epidemics and is negligible in the absence of an epidemic. Since epidemics are not predictable, the overall risk is used in the calculation of the risk–benefit ratio. If this risk is compared with the risk of vaccination (1 death in 2 million vaccinations during the swine influenza vaccination program),[186] the benefit–risk ratio for mortality is between 200 and 400 in favor of vaccination.

Currently, much work is in progress to develop improved inactivated vaccines that may contain only one or two antigens such as the HA or NA or to develop live attenuated vaccines that may lead to increased efficacy.

Live Influenza Vaccine. Two factors have stimulated the development of live influenza vaccine. First, with other viruses, inactivated vaccine is less effective than live vaccine is. Second, although inactivated vaccine for influenza has been effective, it does not completely prevent infection. Furthermore, according to Hoskins and coworkers, vaccine postpones infection until a later year but does not eliminate clinical illness.[213]

To develop live vaccine, markers for attenuation are essential. For influenza vaccines, restriction of growth at temperature above 37.8°C has correlated with attenuation.[214] One vaccine developed by Maassab and coworkers[215] that was selected for cold adaptation is designated CA. Another approach taken by Murphy and coworkers was the use of avian recombinants.[216] Both approaches took advantage of the capacity for influenza to undergo genetic reassortment in vitro. For CA vaccine, coinfection of cultures with attenuated virus and wild-type virus allowed the selection for daughter virions with the capacity to replicate to high titer in eggs that carried the marker for attenuation and that possessed the surface antigen of currently circulating strains. The vaccine viruses thus selected are not only temperature sensitive and cold adapted but also markedly reduced in their virulence for ferrets, hamsters, and humans, and they grow to high titers for vaccine production.[217,218] Avian human reassortants appeared to have similar characteristics.

Numerous studies have been carried out in young, healthy volunteers in experimental challenge studies,[214] and some studies have been conducted in children,[214] in the elderly,[219] and in the field.[214] At doses of either type of vaccine that infect 90–95 percent of susceptible volunteers, reactogenicity is minimal or very mild. Fever is unusual but does occur occasionally and is short lived. Mild respiratory symptoms occur in some recipients. There is no transmission to serosusceptibles in close contact with vaccine recipients. Nasal and serum antibodies are produced, and even though serum antibody levels are not of the same titer as those produced by inactivated vaccine, volunteers challenged 1–5 months after receiving live vaccine are protected against both infection and illness.[214,220] Protection against experimental challenge is greater than that produced by inactivated vaccine.[220] In extensive studies conducted to date, the CA vaccine has not reverted to wild type.[214]

TABLE 9. Serum Hemagglutination-Inhibition Antibody Responses to Monovalent and Trivalent Inactivated Influenza Vaccines (Antibody Geometric Mean Titers and Percentage with Fourfold or Greater Rises by Indicated Hemagglutinatin Antigen)

	A/Taiwan/86 H1N1					A/Mississippi/85 H3N2					B/Ann Arbor/86				
Groups	No.	(%)[a]	Before	After	With Rise (%)	No.	(%)[a]	Before	After	With Rise (%)	No.	(%)[a]	Before	After	With Rise (%)
HIV-seronegative															
Heterosexual	16	(94)	7	274	88	16	(94)	6	223	94	14	(93)	10	79	86
Homosexual	22	(95)	17	256	86	22	(95)	15	256	86	21	(71)	14	56	43
HIV-seropositive[b]	27	(52)	4	56	78	27	(89)	9	111	85	22	(32)	6	18	32
AIDS-related complex	14	(36)	5	20	57	14	(29)	6	21	50	13	(15)	5	11	31
Patients with AIDS															
Not receiving zidovudine	15	(13)	5	23	13	15	(13)	5	11	27	10	(20)	6	11	30
Receiving zidovudine	10	(40)	7	18	60	10	(50)	10	49	60	6	(17)	4	7	17

[a] Percentage with protective level.
[b] Subjects were seropositive but had no symptoms or only had lymphadenopathy syndrome.
(From Nelson et al.,[211] with permission.)

Field trials necessary to demonstrate superior efficacy in natural infections have yet to be completed, but the current results are certainly encouraging. Most promising is the low rate of vaccine-associated reactions in a large number of recipients. It is hoped that some of the shortcomings of inactivated vaccine may be overcome with these biologic products.

Chemoprophylaxis

Amantadine. Amantadine is approved for use as a prophylactic agent against influenza. Its level of efficacy is about 75–90 percent, similar to that of vaccine.[63,96,221–229] It is additive to that of vaccine. In a recent study evaluating prophylaxis against influenza, rimantadine was compared with amantadine and placebo.[96] There was no significant difference between amantadine and rimantadine, and both were significantly more effective in preventing clinical influenza than was placebo. The major difference between rimantadine and amantadine was that the former yielded a lower incidence of toxic side effects. In fact, side effects in rimantadine recipients were similar in frequency to those in placebo recipients. More recently, rimantadine administered prophylactically to 60 people over the age of 65 was as well tolerated as placebo and yielded a lower incidence of clinical influenza than did placebo.[227] Taken together, these data support the replacement of amantadine with rimantadine. Because of the requirement to take two 100 mg capsules each day for 5–6 weeks, its cost, side effects, and the requirements for surveillance to detect the beginning of an influenza epidemic in a given community, prophylaxis is not recommended for general use. Currently, amantadine is recommended as short-term (5–7 weeks) prophylaxis during a presumed outbreak of influenza A for persons who did not receive vaccine.[174,191] In such situations it may be used for 2 weeks only if vaccine is given simultaneously. It may also be used to supplement protection offered by vaccine in patients who might be expected to respond poorly to vaccine and as chemoprophylaxis throughout the influenza season (winter months) in lieu of vaccine when vaccine is contraindicated in a high-risk patient. Household contacts of an index case may be given prophylaxis. Finally, staff and patients in hospitals or institutions may be given prophylaxis to prevent an outbreak.[63,226,228,229]

Others

Nosocomial influenza has produced major problems in several epidemics in the past. This is not surprising since hospitals include a concentration of patients at risk for excess mortality. Thus, special attention to the prevention of nosocomial spread of influenza should be undertaken when an epidemic is identified in the community.

Factors that seem appropriate include encouragement of vaccine supplemented with a prophylactic agent for the hospital staff.[63,192,226,229] If staff members develop illness, they should, if at all possible, be required to stay home from work. Visitors with any illness should be restricted. Patients with acute illness should be isolated in single rooms or cohorted, and staff should be cohorted to care for only ill or only well patients. It may be prudent to place special emphasis on prophylaxis for staff caring for acutely ill patients. Gowns, masks, and handwashing are a logical part of the isolation procedure for influenza. It may also be wise to control elective surgery when nosocomial influenza is apparent since anesthesia may add to the risk of pulmonary complication developing with influenza. The value of these procedures has not been documented. However, nosocomial influenza has produced disastrous consequences, and reasonable and logical efforts to curtail it seem justified.[63,192,226,228,229]

REFERENCES

1. Hirsch A. Handbook of Geographical and Historical Pathology. v. 1. Translated from the second German edition by Charles Creighton. London: New Sydenham Society; 1883:7.
2. Thomson D, Thomson R. Influenza. Ann Pickett-Thomas Res Lab. 1933;9:4.
3. Sydenham T. Influenza: Of the epidemic diseases. In: Major RH, ed. Classical Descriptions of Disease. Springfield, IL: Charles C Thomas; 1955:201.
4. Crosby AW. Epidemic and Peace, 1918. part IV. Westport, CT: Greenwood Press; 1976:203.
5. Smith W, Andrews CH, Laidlaw PP. A virus obtained from influenza patients. Lancet. 1933;2:66.
6. Francis T Jr. A new type of virus from epidemic influenza. Science. 1940;92:405.
7. Taylor RM. A further note on 1233 (''influenza C'') virus. Arch Gesamte Virusforsch. 1951;4:485.
8. Burnet FM. Influenza virus on the developing egg. I. Changes associated with the development of an egg-passage strain of virus. Br J Exp Pathol. 1936;17:282.
9. Hirst GK. The agglutination of red cells by allantoic fluid of chick embryos infected with influenza virus. Science. 1941;94:22.
10. Nasurel, N, Marine WM. Recycling of Asian and Hong Kong influenza A virus hemagglutinins in man. Am J Epidemiol. 1973;97:44.
11. Marine WM, Workman WM. Hong Kong influenza immunologic recapitulation. Am J Epidemiol. 1969;901:406.
12. Francis T Jr. Vaccination against influenza. In: Influenza World Health Organization Monograph Series 20. Geneva: WHO; 1954:125.
13. Francis T Jr. The current status of the control of influenza. Ann Intern Med. 1955;45:534.
14. Fenner F. The classification and nomenclature of viruses. Summary of results of meeting of the International Committee on Toxonomy of Viruses in Madrid, September, 1975. Virology. 1976;71:371.
15. Dowdle WR, Noble GR, Kendal AP. Orthomyxovirus-influenza: Comparative diagnosis unifying concept. In: Krustak E, Krustak C, eds. Comparative Diagnosis of Viral Diseases. New York: Academic Press; 1977:447.
16. Ginsberg HS. Orthomyxoviruses. In: Davis BD, Dulbecco R, Eisen HN, et al., eds. Orthomyxoviruses in Microbiology. 3rd ed. Hagerstown, MD: Harper & Row; 1980:1119–38.
17. Palese P, Schulman JL, Bodo G, et al. Inhibition of influenza and parainfluenza virus replication in tissue culture by 2-deoxy-2,3-dehydro-*N*-trifluoracetylneuraminic acid (FANA). Virology. 1974;59:490.
18. Palese P, Tobita K, Ueda M, et al. Characterization of temperature sensitive influenza virus mutants defective in neuraminidase. Virology. 1974;61:397.
19. Palese P, Schulman JL. RNA pattern of ''swine'' influenza virus isolated

from man is similar to those of other swine influenza viruses. Nature. 1976;263:528.
20. Choppin PW, Compans RW. The structure of influenza virus. In: Kilbourne ED, ed. The Influenza Viruses and Influenza. New York: Academic Press; 1975:15.
21. Schulze IT. Structure of the influenza virion. In: Lauffer MA, Bang TB, Maramorosh K, et al., eds. Advances in Virus Research. v. 18. New York: Academic Press; 1973:1.
22. Kendal AP, Galphin JC, Palmer EL. Replication of influenza virus at elevated temperatures: Production of virus-like particles with reduced matrix protein content. Virology. 1977;76:186.
23. Pons MW. Influenza virus RNA(s). In: Kilbourne ED, ed. The Influenza Viruses and Influenza. New York: Academic Press; 1975:145.
24. Wilson IA, Skehel JJ, Wiley DG. Structure of the hemagglutinin membrane glycoprotein of influenza virus at 3^0 A resolution. Nature. 1981;289:366.
25. Webster PG. On the origin of pandemic influenza viruses. Curr Top Microbiol Immunol. 1972;59:75.
26. Klink H-D, Garten W, Bosch FX, et al. The role of the hemagglutinin as a determinant for the pathogenicity of avian influenza viruses. In: Potter EW, ed. The Molecular Virology and Epidemiology of Influenza. London: Academic Press; 1984:195.
27. White J, Matlin K, Helenius A. Cell fusion by Semliki Forrest, influenza and vesicular stomatitis viruses. J Cell Biol. 1981;89:674.
28. Jones LV, Compans RW, Davis AR, et al. Surface expression of influenza virus neuraminadase and aminoterminally anchored viral membrane glycoproteins in polarized epithelial cells. Mol Cell Biol. 1985;5:2189.
29. Kilbourne ED. Recombination of influenza A viruses of human and animal origin. Science. 1968;160:74.
30. Kates M, Allison AC, Tyrrell DA, et al. Lipids of influenza virus and their relation to those of the host cell. Biochim Biophys Acta. 1961;52:455.
31. Compans RW, Choppin PW. Reproduction of myxoviruses. In: Fraenkel-Conrat H, Wagner RR, eds. Comprehensive Virology. v. 4. New York: Plenum Press; 1975:179.
32. Pons MW, Schulze IT, Hirst GK. Isolation and characterization of the ribonucleoprotein of influenza virus. Virology. 1969;39:250.
33. Webster RG, Laver WG, Air GM. Antigenic variation among type A influenza viruses. In: Palese P, Kinepbury DW, eds. Genetics of Influenza Viruses. New York: Springer-Verlag; 1983:127.
34. Wiley DC, Wilson IA, Skehel JJ. Structure identification of the antibody binding sets of Hong Kong influenza hemagglutinin and their involvement in antigenic variation. Nature. 1987;289:323.
35. Shaw MW, Lamon EW, Compans RW. Immunologic studies of the influenza A virus non-structural protein NA-1. J Exp Med. 1982;156:243.
36. Martinez C, DelRio L, Portela A, et al. Evolution of influenza virus neuraminadase gene during drift of the N2 subtype. Virology. 1983;130:539.
37. Zhinov OP. The host origin of influenza A viruses can be assessed by the intracellular cleavage of the viral nucleocapsid protein. Arch Virol. 1988;99:277.
38. Schild GC, Newman RW, Webster RG, et al. Antigenic analysis of influenza A virus surface antigens: Consideration for the nomenclature of influenza virus. Arch Virol. 1980;63:171.
39. Webster RG, Laver WG, Air GM, et al. The mechanism of antigenic drift in influenza viruses: Analysis of Hong Kong (H3N2) variants with monoclonal antibodies to the hemagglutinin molecule. Ann NY Acad Sci. 1980;354:142.
40. Lai CJ, Markoff LJ, Sveda MM, et al. Genetic variation of influenza A viruses as studied by recombinant DNA techniques. Ann NY Acad Sci. 1980;354:162.
41. Hauptmann R, Clarke LD, Mountford RC, et al. Nucleotide sequence of the hemagglutinin gene of influenza virus A/England/321/77. J Gen Virol. 1983;64:215.
42. Webster RG, Laver WG. Determination of the number of nonoverlapping antigenic areas on Hong Kong (H2N2) influenza virus hemagglutinin with monoclonal antibodies and the selection of variants with potential epidemiological significance. Virology. 1980;104:39.
43. Laver WG, Webster RG. Selection of antigenic mutants of influenza viruses. Isolation and peptide mapping of their hemagglutination proteins. Virology. 1968;34:193.
44. Scholtissek C, Von Hoyningen V, et al. Genetic relatedness between the new 1977 epidemic strains (H1N1) of influenza and human influenza strains isolated between 1947 and 1957. Virology. 1978;89:613.
45. Hinshaw VS, Bean WJ, Webster RG, et al. The prevalence of influenza viruses in swine and the antigenic and genetic relatedness of influenza viruses from man and swine. Virology. 1978;84:51.
46. Kilbourne ED, Schulman JL. The induction of broadened (multitypic) immunity with doubly antigenic influenza virus recombinants. Trans Assoc Am Physicians. 1965;78:323.
47. Easterday BC, Laver WG, Pereira HG, et al. Antigenic composition of recombinant virus strains produced from human and avian influenza A viruses. J Gen Virol. 1968;5:83.
48. Kilbourne ED, Schulman JL, Schild GD, et al. Correlated studies of a recombinant influenza-virus vaccine. I. Derivation and characterization of virus and vaccine. J Infect Dis. 1971;124:449.
49. Webster RG, Campbell CH, Granoff A. The "in vivo" production of "new" influenza A viruses. 3. Isolation of recombinant influenza viruses under simulated conditions of natural transmission. Virology. 1973;51:149.
50. Webster RG, Campbell CH, Granoff A. The "in vivo" production of "new" influenza A viruses. I. Genetic recombination between avian and mammalian influenza viruses. Virology. 1971;44:317.
51. Easterday BC. Animal influenza. In: Kilbourne ED, ed. Influenza Viruses and Influenza. New York: Academic Press; 1975:449.
52. Glezen WP, Couch RB. Interpandemic influenza in the Houston area, 1974–76. N Engl J Med. 1978;298:587.
53. Glezen WP, Payne AA, Snyder DN, et al. Mortality and influenza. J Infect Dis. 1982;146:313.
54. Marine WM, McGowan JE Jr, Thomas JE. Influenza detection: A prospective comparison of surveillance methods and analysis of isolates. Am J Epidemiol. 1976;116:589.
55. Kilbourne ED. Epidemiology of influenza. In: Kilbourne ED, ed: Influenza Viruses and Influenza. New York: Academic Press; 1975:483.
56. Centers for Disease Control. Influenza–Respiratory Disease Surveillance. Report No. 90. US Department of Health, Education and Welfare, Public Health Service, February 1976.
57. Monto AS, Kioumehr F. The Tecumseh study of respiratory illness. IX. Occurrence of influenza in the community, 1966–1971. Am J Epidemiol. 1975;102:553.
58. Epidemiology of influenza: Summary of influenza workshop IV, National Institutes of Health. J Infect Dis. 1973;128:361.
59. Hall CB, Douglas RG Jr. Respiratory syncytial virus and influenza. Am J Dis Child. 1976;130:615.
60. Kendal AP, Schieble J, Cooney MK, et al. Co-circulation of two influenza A (H3N2) antigenic varients detected by virus surveillance in individual communities. Am J Epidemiol. 1978;108:308.
61. Glezen WP, Couch RB, Six HR. The influenza herald wave. Am J Epidemiol. 1982;116:589.
62. Schoenbaum SC, McNeil BJ, Kavet J. The swine-influenza decision. N Engl J Med. 1976;295:759.
63. Douglas RG Jr. Respiratory diseases. In: Galasso GJ, Merigan TC, Buchanan R, eds: Antiviral Agents and Viral Diseases of Man. New York: Raven Press; 1984:320–45.
64. Barker WH, Mulloohy JP. Pneumonia and influenza deaths during epidemics: Implications for prevention. Arch Intern Med. 1982;142:85.
65. Tillett HE, Smith JWG, Clifford RE. Excess morbidity and mortality associated with influenza in England and Wales. Lancet. 1980;1:793.
66. Choi K, Thacker SB. Mortality during influenza epidemics in the United States, 1967–1978. Am J Public Health. 1982;72:1280.
67. Centers for Disease Control. Annual summary. MMWR. 1982;30:117.
68. Centers for Disease Control. Influenza-Respiratory Disease Surveillance Report No. 88. U.S. Department of Health, Education and Welfare, Public Health Service. 1973.
69. Alling DW, Blackwelder WG, Stuart-Harris CH. A study of excess mortality during influenza epidemics in the United States, 1968–1976. Am J Epidemiol. 1981;113:30.
70. Douglas RG Jr. Influenza in Man. In: Kilbourne ED, ed. Influenza Viruses and Influenza. New York: Academic Press; 1975:395.
71. Hemmes JH, Winkler KC, Kool SM. Virus survival as a seasonal factor in influenza and poliomyelitis. Nature. 1960;188:430.
72. Alford RH, Kasel JA, Gerone PJ, et al. Human influenza resulting from aerosol inhalation (31255). Proc Soc Exp Biol Med. 1966;122:800.
73. Little JW, Douglas RG Jr, Hall WJ et al. Attenuated influenza produced by experimental intranasal inoculation. J Med Virol. 1979;3:177.
74. Couch RB, Douglas RG, Jr, Fedson DS, et al. Correlated studies of a recombinant influenza virus vaccine. III. Protection against experimental influenza in man. J Infect Dis. 1971;124:473.
75. Couch RB, Kasel HA, Gerin JL, et al. Induction of partial immunity to influenza by a neuraminidase-specific vaccine. J Infect Dis. 1974;129:411.
76. Scholtissek C, Rott R, Klenk H-D. Two different mechanisms of the inhibition of the multiplication of enveloped viruses of glucosamine. Virology. 1975;63:191.
77. Jordan WS, Denny FW, Badger GF, et al. A study of illness in a group of Cleveland families. XVII. The occurrence of Asian influenza. Am J Hyg. 1958;68:190.
78. Murphy BR, Baron S, Chelhub EG, et al. Temperature sensitive mutants of influenza virus. IV. Induction of interferon in the nasopharynx by wild-type and a temperature-sensitive recombinant virus. J Infect Dis. 1973;128:488.
79. Hall CB, Douglas RG Jr. Nosocomial influenza infection as a cause of intercurrent fevers in infants. Pediatrics. 1975;55:673.
80. Stanley ED, Jackson GG. Viremia in Asian influenza. Trans Assoc Am Physicians. 1966;79:376.
81. Jao RL, Wheelock EF, Jackson GG. Production of interferon in volunteers infected with Asian influenza. J Infect Dis. 1970;121:419.
82. Murphy BR, Kasel JA, Chanock RM. Association of serum antineuraminidase antibody with resistance to influenza in man. N Engl J Med. 1972;286:1329.
83. Mann JJ, Walderman RH, Toga Y, et al. Antibody response in respiratory secretions of volunteers given live and dead influenza virus. J Immunol. 1968;100:725.
84. Alford RH, Rossen RD, Butler WT, et al. Neutralizing and hemagglutination inhibiting activity of nasal secretions following experimental human infection with A2 influenza virus. J Immunol. 1967;98:724.
85. Waldman RH, Mann JJ, Small PA. Immunization against influenza: Prevention of illness in man by aerosolized inactivated vaccine. JAMA. 1969;207:520.
86. Couch RB, Douglas RG Jr, Rossen R, et al. Role of secretory antibody in

influenza. In: Dayton DH Jr, Small PA Jr, Chanock RM, et al., eds. The Secretory Immunologic System. Washington, DC: US GPO; 1969:93.
87. Wenzel RP, Hendley JO, Sande MA, et al. Revised (1972–1973) bivalent influenza vaccine: Serum and nasal antibody responses to parenteral vaccination. JAMA. 1973;226:435.
88. Kilbourne ED, Butler WT, Rossen RD. Specific immunity in influenza—summary of influenza workshop III. J Infect Dis. 1973;127:220.
89. Foy HM, Cooney MK, McMahan R, et al. Single-dose monovalent A_2/Hong Kong influenza vaccine. Efficacy 14 months after immunization. JAMA. 1971;217:1067.
90. Meiklejohn G, Eickhoff TC, Graves P, et al. Antigenic drift and efficacy of influenza virus vaccines, 1976–1977. J Infect Dis. 1978;138:618.
91. Schulman JL, Khakpour M, Kilbourne ED. Protective effects of hemagglutinin and neuraminidase antigens on influenza virus: Distinctiveness of hemagglutinin antigen of Hong Kong-68 virus. J Virol. 1968;2:778.
92. Monto AS, Kendal AP. Effect of neuraminidase antibody on Hong Kong influenza. Lancet. 1973;1:623.
93. Douglas RG Jr, Markoff LJ, Murphy BR, et al. Live victoria/75-ts-1(E) influenza A virus vaccines in adult volunteers. Role of hemagglutinin immunity in protection against illness and infection caused by influenza A virus. Infect Immun. 1979;26:274.
94. Stuart-Harris CH. Twenty years of influenza epidemics. Am Rev Respir Dis. 1961;83:54.
95. Kilbourne ED, Loge JP. Influenza A prime: A clinical study of an epidemic caused by a new strain of virus. Ann Intern Med. 1950;33:371.
96. Dolin R, Reichman RC, Madore HP, et al. A controlled trial of amantadine and rimantadine in the prophylaxis of influenza A infection. N Engl J Med. 1982;307:580.
97. Nigg C, Ecklund CM, Wilson DE, et al. Study of epidemics of influenza B. Am J Hyg. 1942;35:265.
98. Taylor RM, Parodi AS, Fernandez RB, et al. Un estudio sobroe la etiologia de la influenza ocurrida en la Argentina durante 1941; comparacion de la epidemiologia de influenza A ya B. Rev Inst Vacterial Dep Nac Hig (Argent). 1942;11:44.
99. Mogabgab WJ. Virus association with upper respiratory illnesses in adults. Ann Intern Med. 1963;59:306.
100. Glezen WP, Loda FA, Clyde WA Jr, et al. Epidemiologic patterns of acute lower respiratory disease of children in a pediatric group practice. J Pediatr. 1971;48:394.
101. Howard JB, McCracken GH Jr, Luby JP. Influenza A2 virus as a cause of croup requiring tracheotomy. J Pediatr. 1972;81:1148.
102. Glezen WP, Paredes A, Taber LH. Influenza in children. JAMA. 1980;243:1345.
103. Louria DB, Blumenfeld HL, Ellis JT, et al. Studies on influenza in the pandemic of 1957–1958. II. Pulmonary complications of influenza. J Clin Invest. 1959;38:213.
104. Martin LM, Kunin CM, Gottlieb LS, et al. Asian influenza A in Boston, 1957–1958. II. Severe staphylococcal pneumonia complicating influenza. Arch Intern Med. 1959;103:532.
105. Schwarzmann SW, Adler JL, Sullivan RJ, et al. Bacterial pneumonia during the Hong Kong influenza epidemic of 1968–1969. Arch Intern Med. 1971;127:1037.
106. Bisno AL, Griffin JP, VanEpps KA. Pneumonia and Hong Kong influenza: A prospective study of the 1968–1969 epidemic. Am J Med Sci. 1971;261:251.
107. Kaye D, Rosenbluth M, Hook EW, et al. Endemic influenza 1, 2. II. The nature of the disease in the post-pandemic period. Am Rev Respir Dis. 1962;85:9.
108. Carilli AD, Gohd RS, Gordon W. A virologic study of chronic bronchitis. N Engl J Med. 1964;270:123.
109. Stark JE, Heath RB, Curwen MP. Infection with influenza and parainfluenza viruses in chronic bronchitis. Thorax. 1965;20:124.
110. Stenhouse AC. Rhinovirus infection in acute exacerbations of chronic bronchitis: A controlled prospective study. Br Med J. 1967;3:461.
111. Monto AS, Ross HW. The Tecumseh study of respiratory illness. Am J Epidemiol. 1978;107:57.
112. Clementsen P, Jensen CB, Hannoun C, et al. Influenza A virus potentiates basophil histamine release caused by endotoxin induced complement activation. Allergy. 1988;43:93.
113. Lin C-Y, Kuo Y-C, Liu W-T, et al. Immunomodulation of influenza virus infection in the precipitating asthma attack. Chest. 1988;93:1234.
114. Johanson WG Jr, Pierce AK, Sanford JP. Pulmonary function in uncomplicated influenza. Am Rev Respir Dis. 1969;100:141.
115. Horner GJ, Gray FD Jr. Effect of uncomplicated presumptive influenza on the diffusing capacity of the lung. Am Rev Respir Dis. 1973;108:866.
116. Hall WJ, Douglas RG Jr, Hyde RW, et al. Pulmonary mechanics following uncomplicated influenza A infection. Am Rev Respir Dis. 1976;113:141.
117. Little JW, Hall WJ, Douglas RG Jr, et al. Airway hyperreactivity and peripheral airway dysfunction in influenza A infection. Am Rev Respir Dis. 1978;118:295.
118. Fry J. Lung involvement in influenza. Br Med J. 1951;2:1374.
119. Fry J. Influenza A (Asian) 1957: Clinical and epidemiological features in a general practice. Br Med J. 1958;1:259.
120. Fry J. Influenza, 1959: The story of an epidemic. Br Med J. 1959;2:135.
121. Foy HM, Cooney MK, Allen I, et al. Rates of pneumonia during influenza epidemics in Seattle, 1964 to 1975. JAMA. 1979;241:253.
122. Middleton PJ, Alexander RM, Szymanski MT. Severe myositis during recovery from influenza. Lancet. 1970;2:533.
123. Simon NM. Acute myoglobulinuria associated with type A-2 influenza. JAMA. 1970;212:1704.
124. Dietzman DE, Schaller JG, Ray CG, et al. Acute myositis associated with influenza B infection. Pediatrics. 1976;57:255.
125. Minow RA, Gorbach S, Johnson BL, et al. Myoglobinuria associated with influenza A infection. Ann Intern Med. 1974;80:359.
126. Greco TP, Askenase PW, Kashgarian M. Postviral myositis: Myxovirus-like structures in affected muscle. Ann Intern Med. 1977;86:193.
127. Bainton D, Jones GR, Hole D. Influenza and ischemic heart disease: A possible trigger for acute myocardial infarction. Int J Epidemiol. 1978;7:231.
128. Finland M, Parker F, Barnes M, et al. Acute myocarditis in influenza A infections. Am J Med Sci. 1945;207:455.
129. Woodward TE, McCrumb FR, Carey TN, et al. Viral and rickettsial causes of cardiac disease, including the coxsackie virus etiology of pericarditis and myocarditis. Ann Intern Med. 1960;53:1130.
130. Hildebrandt HM, Maassab HF, Willis PW. Influenza virus pericarditis. Am J Dis Child. 1962;104:179.
131. Adams CW. Post viral myopericarditis associated with influenza virus: Report of eight cases. Am J Cardiol. 1959;4:56.
132. Edelen JS, Bender TR, Chin TDY. Encephalopathy and pericarditis during an outbreak of influenza. Am J Epidemiol. 1974;100:79.
133. Glezen WB, Decker M, Perrotta DM. Survey of underlying conditions of persons hospitalized with acute respiratory disease during influenza epidemics in Houston 1978–81. Am Rev Respir Dis. 1987;136:550.
134. Sperber SJ, Francis JB. Toxic shock during an influenza outbreak. JAMA. 1987;257:1086.
135. Wells CEC, James WRL, Evans AD. Guillain-Barré syndrome and virus of influenza A (Asian strain). Arch Neurol Psychiatry. 1959;81:699.
136. Leneman F. The Guillain-Barré syndrome. Arch Intern Med. 1966;118:139.
137. Wells CEC. Neurologic complications of so-called influenza: A winter study in southeast Wales. Br Med J. 1971;1:369.
138. Bayer WH. Influenza B encephalitis. West J Med. 1987;147:466.
139. Varma RR, Riedel DR, Komorouski RA, et al. Reye's syndrome in nonpediatric age groups. JAMA. 1979;242:1373.
140. Corey L, Rubin RJ, Hattwick MA, et al. A nationwide outbreak of Reye's syndrome: Its epidemiologic relationship to influenza B. Am J Med. 1976;61:615.
141. Corey L, Rubin RJ, Bregman D, et al. Diagnostic criteria for influenza B-associated Reye's syndrome: Clinical vs. pathologic criteria. Pediatrics. 1977;60:602.
142. Centers for Disease Control. Reye syndrome—United States. MMWR. 1979;28:97.
143. Chaves-Carballo E, Gomez MR, Sharbrough FW. Encephalopathy and fatty infiltration of the viscera (Reye-Johnson syndrome): A 17-year experience. Mayo Clin Proc. 1975;50:209.
144. Schiff GM. Reye's syndrome. Annu Rev Med. 1976;27:447.
145. Corey L, Rubin RJ, Hatwick MAW. Reye's syndrome: Clinical progression and evaluation of therapy. Pediatrics. 1977;60:708.
146. Waldman RJ, Hall WN, McGee H, et al. Aspirin as a risk factor in Reye's syndrome. JAMA. 1982;247:3089.
147. Halpin RJ, Holtzhauer FJ, Campbell RJ, et al. Reye's syndrome and medication use. JAMA. 1982;248:687.
148. Starks KM, Ray G, Dominguez LB. Reye's syndrome and salicylate use. Pediatrics. 1980;66:859.
149. Consensus Development Conference. Diagnosis and treatment of Reye's syndrome. JAMA. 1981;246:2441.
150. Lichtenstein PK, Heubi JE, Daugherty CC, et al. Grade I Reye's syndrome: A frequent cause of vomiting and liver dysfunction after varicella and upper-respiratory-tract infection. N Engl J Med. 1983;309:133.
151. Daniels SR, Greenberg RS, Ibrahim MA. Scientific uncertainties in the studies of salicylate use and Reye's syndrome. JAMA. 1983;249:1311.
152. Brown T, Hug G, Lansky L, et al. Transiently reduced activity of carbamyl phosphate synthetase and ornithine transcarbamylase in livers of children with Reye's syndrome. N Engl J Med. 1976;294:861.
153. Snodgrass PJ, DeLong GR. Urea-cycle enzyme deficiencies and an increased nitrogen load producing hyperammonemia in Reye's syndrome. N Engl J Med. 1976;294:855.
154. Smith AL. Ammonia disposal in Reye's syndrome. N Engl J Med. 1976;294:897.
155. Fulginiti VA and the Committee on Infectious Diseases. Special report: Aspirin and Reye's syndrome. Pediatrics. 1982;69:810.
156. Hottenlocher PR. Reye's syndrome: Relation of outcome to therapy. J Pediatr. 1970;80:845.
157. Trey C, Burns DG, Saunder SJ. Treatment of hepatic coma by exchange blood transfusion. N Engl J Med. 1966;294:473.
158. Kindt GW, Waldman J, Kohl S, et al. Intracranial pressure in Reye's syndrome; monitoring and control. JAMA. 1975;231:822.
159. Schild GC, Dowdle WR. Influenza virus characterization and diagnostic serology. In: Kilbourne ED, ed. The Influenza Viruses and Influenza. New York: Academic Press; 1975:315.
160. Wingfield WL, Pollack D, Grunert RR. Therapeutic efficacy of amantadine HCl and rimantadine HCl in naturally occurring influenza A2 respiratory illness in man. N Engl J Med. 1969;281:579.
161. Knight V, Fedson D, Baldini J, et al. Amantadine therapy of epidemic influenza A2 (Hong Kong). Infect Immun. 1970;1:200.
162. Galbraith AW, Oxford JS, Schild GC, et al. Therapeutic effect of I-ada-

mantanamine hydrochloride in naturally occurring influenza A2/Hong Kong infection. Lancet. 1971;2:113.
163. Rabinovich S, Baldini JT, Bannister R. Treatment of influenza. The therapeutic efficacy of rimantadine HCl in naturally occurring influenza A2 outbreak. Am J Med Sci. 1969;257:328.
164. Van Voris LP, Betts RF, Hayden FG, et al. Successful treatment of naturally occurring influenza A/USSR/77 H1N1. JAMA. 1981;245:1128.
165. Younkin SW, Betts RF, Roth FK, et al. Reduction in fever and symptoms in young adults with aspirin or amantadine. Antimicrob Agents Chemother. 1983;23:577.
166. Atkinson WL, Arden NH, Patriarca PA, et al. Amantadine prophylaxis during an institutional outbreak of type A (H1N1) influenza. Arch Intern Med. 1986;146:1751.
167. Hall CB, Dolin R, Gala C, et al. Children with influenza A infection: Treatment with rimantadine. Pediatrics. 1987;80:275.
168. Little JW, Hall WJ, Douglas RG, et al. Amantadine effect on peripheral airways abnormalities in influenza. Ann Intern Med. 1976;85:177.
169. Winterbauer RH, Ludwig WR, Hammer SP. Clinical course, management, and long-term sequelae of respiratory failure due to influenza viral pneumonia. Johns Hopkins Med J. 1977;141:148.
170. Lefrak EA, Stevens PM, Pitha J, et al. Extracorporeal membrane oxygenation for fulminant influenza pneumonia. Chest. 1974;66:385.
171. Monto AS, Davenport FM, Napier JA, et al. Modification of an outbreak of influenza in Tecumseh, Michigan, by vaccination of school children. J Infect Dis. 1970;122:16.
172. Gundelfinger BF, Stille WT, Bell HA. Effectiveness of influenza vaccines during an epidemic of Asian influenza. N Engl J Med. 1958;259:1005.
173. Edmondson WP Jr, Rothenberg R, White PW, et al. A comparison of subcutaneous, nasal, and combined influenza vaccination. II. Protection against natural challenge. Am J Epidemiol. 1971;93:480.
174. Arden NH, Patriarca PA, Fasano MB, et al. The role of vaccination and amantadine prophylaxis controlling an outbreak of influenza A (H3N2) in a nursing home. Arch Intern Med. 1988;148:865.
175. Ruben FL, Johnson F, Streiff EJ. Influenza in a partially immunized aged population: Effectiveness of killed Hong Kong vaccine against infection with the England strain. JAMA. 1974;230:863.
176. Hoskins TW, Davies JR, Allchin A, et al. Controlled trial of inactivated influenza vaccine containing the A/Hong Kong strain during an outbreak of influenza due to the A/England/42/72 strain. Lancet. 1973;2:116.
177. Stiver HG, Graves P, Eickhoff TC, et al. Efficacy of Hong Kong vaccine in preventing England variant influenza A in 1972. N Engl J Med. 1973;289:1267.
178. Beutner KR, Chow T, Rubi E, et al. Evaluation of a neuraminidase-specific influenza A virus vaccine in children: Antibody responses and effects of two successive outbreaks of natural infection. J Infect Dis. 1979;140:844.
179. Gross PA, Quinnan GV, Rodstein M, et al. Association of influenza immunization with reduction in mortality in an elderly population. A prospective study. Arch Intern Med. 1988;148:562.
180. Keitel WA, Cate TR, Couch RB. Efficacy of sequential annual vaccination with inactivated influenza virus vaccine. Am J Epidemiol. 1988;127:353.
181. Cate TR, Couch RB, Kasel JA, et al. Clinical trials of monovalent influenza A/New Jersey/76 virus vaccines in adults: Reactogenicity, antibody response, and antibody persistence. J Infect Dis. 1977;136(Suppl):450.
182. Betts RF, Douglas RG Jr. Comparative study of reactogenicity and immunogenicity of influenza A/New Jersey/8/76 (Hsw 1N1) virus vaccine in normal volunteers. J Infect Dis. 1977;136(Suppl):433.
183. Gross PA: Reactogenicity and immunogenicity of bivalent influenza vaccine in one- and two-dose trials in children: A summary. J Infect Dis. 1977;136(Suppl):616.
184. Gross PA, Quinnan GV Jr, Webster ME, et al. Immunization of elderly people with high doses of influenza vaccine. J Am Geriat Soc. 1988;36:209.
185. Barry DW, Mayner RE, Hockstein HD, et al. Comparative trial of influenza vaccines. II. Adverse reactions in children and adults. Am J Epidemiol. 1976;104:47.
186. Center for Disease Control. Follow-up on Guillain-Barré syndrome—United States. MMWR. 1977;26:52.
187. Kramer P, McClain CJ. Depression of aminopyrine metabolism by influenza vaccination. N Engl J Med. 1981;305:1262.
188. Patriarca PA, Kendal AP, Stricof RL, et al. Influenza vaccination and warfarin or theophylline toxicity in nursing-home residents. N Engl J Med. 1983;308:1601.
189. Hannan SE, May JJ, Pratt DS, et al. The effect of whole virus influenza vaccination on theophylline pharmacokinetics. Am Rev Respir Dis. 1988;137:903.
190. Bussey HJ, Saklad JJ. Effect of influenza vaccine on chronic warfarin therapy. Drug Intell Clin Pharm. 1988;22:198.
191. Centers for Disease Control. Prevention and Control of Influenza. MMWR. 1988;37:361.
192. Weingarten S, Staniloff H, Ault M, et al. Do hospital employees benefit from influenza vaccine? J Gen Intern Med. 1988;3:32.
193. Gross PA, Lee H, Wolff HA, et al. Influenza immunization in immunosuppressed children. J Pediatr. 1978;92:30.
194. Ortbals DW, Liebhaber H, Presant CA, et al. Influenza immunization of adult patients with malignant diseases. Ann Intern Med. 1977;87:522.
195. Pabico RC, Douglas RG Jr, Betts RF, et al. Influenza vaccination of patients with glomerular diseases. Ann Intern Med. 1974;81:171.
196. Osanloo EO, Berline BS, Popli S, et al. Antibody responses to influenza vaccination in patients with chronic renal failure. Kidney Int. 1978;14:614.
197. Ortbals DW, Marks ES, Liebhaber H. Influenza immunization in patients with chronic renal disease. JAMA. 1978;239:2562.
198. Seth KJ, Freeman ME, Eisenberg C, et al. Influenza virus immunization antibody response and adverse effects in children with renal disease. JAMA. 1978;239:2559.
199. Jordon MC, Rousseau WE, Tegtmier GT, et al. Immunogenicity of inactivated influenza virus vaccine in chronic renal failure. Ann Intern Med. 1973;79:790.
200. Pabico RC, Douglas RG Jr, Betts RF, et al. Antibody response to influenza vaccination in renal transplant patients. Ann Intern Med. 1976;85:431.
201. Stiver HG, Graves P, Meiklejohn G, et al. Impaired serum antibody response to inactivated influenza A and B vaccine in renal transplant recipients. Infect Immun. 1977;16:738.
202. Kumar SS, Ventura AK, VanderWerf B. Influenza vaccination in renal transplant recipients. JAMA. 1978;239:840.
203. Versluis DJ, Beyer WEP, Masurel N, et al. Impairment of the immune response to influenza vaccination in renal transplant recipients by cyclosporin but not azathioprine. Transplantation. 1986;42:370.
204. Williams GW, Steinberg AD, Reinerstein JL, et al. Influenza immunization in systemic lupus erythematosus: A double-blind trial. Ann Intern Med. 1978;88:729.
205. Brodman R, Gilfillan R, Glass B, et al. Influenza vaccine response in systemic lupus erythematosus. Ann Intern Med. 1978;88:735.
206. Ristow SC, Douglas RG Jr, Condemi JJ. Influenza vaccination of patients with systemic lupus erythematosus. Ann Intern Med. 1978;88:786.
207. Louie JS, Nies KM, Shaji KT, et al. Clinical and antibody responses after influenza immunization in systemic lupus erythematosus. Ann Intern Med. 1978;88:790.
208. White CS III, Adler WH, McGann VG. Repeated immunization: Possible adverse effects. Ann Intern Med. 1974;81:594.
209. Sibley WA, Bamford CR, Laguna JF. Influenza vaccination in patients with multiple sclerosis. JAMA. 1976;236:1965.
210. Brandriss MW, Betts RF, Mathur U, et al. Responses of elderly subjects to monovalent A/USSR/77 (H1N1) and trivalent A/USSR/77 (H1N1)–A/Texas/77 (H3N2)–B/Hong Kong/72 vaccines. Am Rev Respir Dis. 1981;124:681.
211. Nelson KE, Clements ML, Miotti P, et al. The influence of human immunodeficiency virus (HIV) infection on antibody responses to influenza vaccines. Ann Intern Med. 1988;109:383.
212. Centers for Disease Control. Recommendation of the Public Health Service Advisory Committee on Immunization Practices. MMWR. 1983;32:333.
213. Hoskins TW, Davies JR, Smith AJ, et al. Assessment of inactivated influenza A vaccine after three outbreaks of influenza A at Christ's Hospital. Lancet. 1979;1:33.
214. Wright PF, Karzan DT. Live attenuated influenza vaccine. Prog Med Virol. 1987;24:70.
215. Maassab HG, Francis T Jr, Davenport FM, et al. Laboratory and clinical characteristics of attenuated strains of influenza virus. Bull WHO. 1969;41:589.
216. Murphy BR, Clements, ML, Tierney EL, et al. Dose response of influenza A/Washington/897/80 (H3N2) avian-human reassortant virus in adult volunteers. J Infect Dis. 1985;152:225.
217. Maassab AF. Biologic and immunologic characteristics of cold adapted influenza virus. J Immunol. 1969;102:728.
218. Murphy BR, Sky DL, Tierney EL, et al. Reassortant virus derived from avian and human influenza A viruses in attenuated and immunogenic monkeys. Science. 1982;218:1330.
219. Douglas RG Jr, Bentley DW, Betts RF, et al. Evaluation of a temperature sensitive influenza virus in elderly and chronically ill subjects. Am Rev Respir Dis. 1976;113:293.
220. Clements ML, Betts RF, Murphy BR. Advantage of live attenuated cold-adapted influenza A virus over inactivated vaccine for A/Washington/80/H3N2 wild type virus infection. Lancet. 1984;1:705.
221. Monto AS, Gunn RA, Bandyk MG, et al. Prevention of Russian influenza by amantadine. JAMA. 1979;241:1003.
222. Jackson GG, Muldoon RL, Akers LW. Serological evidence for prevention of influenza infection in volunteers by an anti-influenzal drug amantadine hydrochloride. In: Sylvester JC, ed. Antimicrobial Agents and Chemotherapy—1963. Ann Arbor, MI: American Society for Microbiology; 1963:703.
223. Togo Y, Hornick RB, Dawkins AT Jr. Studies on induced influenza in man. I. Double-blind studies designed to assess prophylactic efficacy of amantadine hydrochloride against A2/Rockville/1/65 strain. JAMA. 1968;203:1089.
224. Smorodintsev AA, Zlydnikov DM, Kiseleva DM, et al. Evaluation of amantadine in artificially induced A2 and B influenza. JAMA. 1970;213:1448.
225. Smorodintsev AA, Karpuchin GI, Zlydnikov DM, et al. The prospect of amantadine for prevention of influenza A2 in humans (effectiveness of amantadine during influenza A2/Hong Kong epidemics in January-February, 1969, in Leningrad). Ann NY Acad Sci. 1970;173:44.
226. O'Donoghue JM, Ray CG, Terry DW Jr, et al. Prevention of nosocomial influenza infection with amantadine. Am J Epidemiol. 1973;97:276.
227. Betts RF, Treanor JJ, Graman PS, et al. Antiviral agents to prevent or treat influenza in the elderly. J Respir Dis. 1987;8(Suppl):56.
228. Douglas RG, Betts RF, Hruska JF, et al. Epidemiology of nosocomial viral infections. In: Weinstein L, ed. Seminars in Infectious Disease. New York: Stratton; 1979:98–144.
229. Dolin R. Antiviral chemotherapy and chemoprophylaxis. Science. 1985;227:1296.

Bunyaviridae

143. CALIFORNIA ENCEPHALITIS AND BUNYAVIRAL HEMORRHAGIC FEVERS

KARL M. JOHNSON

California encephalitis (CE) viruses are a major cause of mosquito-borne encephalitis in the United States and second in importance to St. Louis encephalitis in recent years. Cases reported annually to the Centers for Disease Control (CDC) range from 60–130, and the actual number is undoubtedly much greater. A number of antigenically related viruses compose the CE group,[1] and five of these have been recognized as medically significant pathogens. Although not important in North America, at least three other members of the 160-member Bunyaviridae family, Rift Valley fever (RVF), Congo–Crimean hemorrhagic fever (CCHF), and Hantaan (HTN) viruses, cause serious and fatal acute disease with hemorrhagic manifestations on other continents.[2–4] In addition, close relatives of HTN virus, isolated initially in Korea in 1978,[5] are present in wild rodents in the United States[6,7]; limited work discloses evidence for infection of humans but, to date, no documentation of significant disease.[8,9] These viruses are members of four distinct genera within the Bunyaviridae and are distinguished by morphologic,[10] biochemical,[11] and immunologic characteristics. Salient features of these agents including genus placement, and associated diseases are summarized in Table 1. Emphasis in the following presentation is given primarily to CE and HTN viruses with comparative properties for RVF and CCHF where appropriate.

VIRUS CHARACTERIZATION

Structure, Genetics, Antigenic Relationships

Bunyaviridae are spherical, membrane-bound viruses 90–100 nm in diameter that have hexagonally arranged surface projections. These agents are negative-sense RNA viruses having tripartite genomes with sedimentation coefficients of 32S, 26S, and 16S. The small RNA codes for a viral nucleoprotein of about 22,000 daltons and the middle RNA for two glycosylated envelope polypeptides of 38–110,000 (G1) and 32–55 (G2) daltons as well as a nonstructural protein of 20,000 daltons.[11] The large RNA is thought to encode a viral polymerase. The G1 and G2 proteins are responsible for virus neutralization,[12] fusion of infected cells,[13] and hemagglutination,[14] while the nucleocapsid protein is thought to largely account for immunologic relationships observed within and across genera of the family. California encephalitis viruses share antigens as revealed by complement fixation and hemagglutinin inhibition (HI) methods.[1] Immunofluorescent techniques are used to define antigenic members of the *Hantavirus* genus. Virus neutralization is regarded as definitive for the designation of biologic immunotypes for both CE and HTN agents, although the HI method gives similar results for the latter genus.[15]

Morphogenesis

Viral morphogenesis occurs intracellularly, usually in association with intracytoplasmic membranes.[11] The NS protein of RVF, however, was found to accumulate in nuclei of infected cells.[16] Maturation of virions takes place by budding from the Golgi complex and endoplasmic reticulum into vesicles,[11] and viral lipid envelope has a phospholipid composition that is clearly host cell derived. An exception is RVF virus, which also buds through the outer cell membrane of hepatocytes.[17]

EPIDEMIOLOGY

Basic Ecology and Distribution

California Encephalitis Viruses. LaCrosse virus (LAC) is medically the most significant CE virus in the United States, although it now appears likely that Jamestown Canyon virus is more important than was previously recognized.[18] The principal vector of LAC virus is *Aedes triseriatus*, a forest-dwelling, tree-hole–breeding mosquito of the north-central and northeastern regions of the country. LaCrosse virus is maintained in this mosquito by transovarial transmission supplemented by intraspecific venereal transmission and amplification during summer by mosquito feeding on viremic chipmunks, squirrels, foxes, and woodchucks.[19,20]

Female mosquitos infected by any of these mechanisms are capable of transmitting virus by bite. The virus survives during the winter in mosquito eggs.[21] A related mosquito, *Aedes atropalpus*, appears to be of increasing importance. Normally a northern rock-pool breeder, it shares the essential LAC biology manifested by *A. triseriatus*, is as efficient a vector, and effectively competes with the latter species for breeding sites in

TABLE 1. Some Characteristics of Severe Diseases Caused by Bunyaviridae

Disease	*Agents*	*Ecology and Transmission*	*Disease Pattern/Annual Incidence*	*Major Clinical Features*
California encephalitis (CE)	Bunyaviruses (4) LaCrosse Jamestown Canyon	*Aedes triseriatus*; Transovarial infection; mosquito bite	Summer–fall; Northern US: 60–130 cases	Epileptiform meningoencephalitis, disorders after acute seizure
Hemorrhagic fever with renal syndrome (HFRS)	Hantaviruses (3) Hantaan Puumula Seoul	Chronic infection in rodents; (*Apodemus, Clethrionomys, Rattus*) Infectious aerosols from rodent excreta	Endoepidemic; Fall–winter; Asia, Europe: 100,000 cases	Acute interstitial nephritis, thrombocytopenia, capillary leak syndrome, minor hemorrhage
Rift Valley fever (RVF)	Phleboviruses (1) RVF virus	*Aedes* mosquitos; Transovarial infection, mosquito bite, contact with infected domestic animals	Infrequent epidemics; Heavy rains promote; Africa: 50–100,000 cases	Retinitis, encephalitis, fulminant hemorrhagic hepatitis
Congo–Crimean hemorrhagic fever (CCHF)	Nairoviruses (1) CCHF virus	*Hyalomma* ticks; Hares, domestic animals; tick bite, contact with blood of man or domestic animals	Spring–summer; USSR, Middle East, Africa: 50–200 cases	Hepatitis with major blood loss

abandoned tires, a man-made ecologic perturbation of increasing importance in the epidemiology of CE.[22,23] LaCrosse virus and human encephalitis occur principally in the upper Mississippi and Ohio River valleys. Most cases have been reported from Wisconsin, Minnesota, Iowa, Indiana, Ohio, and Illinois.[24] During 1987, however, 19 encephalitis cases were recorded in West Virginia,[25] and 8 cases were reported from Georgia in 1982.[26]

Other CE viruses have distinct ecologic cycles, although all are known or thought to be based on the property of transovarial transmission in mosquitos. In particular, Jamestown Canyon virus, which is distributed widely across North America, is transmitted by *Culiseta inornata* and several species of *Aedes* mosquitos. White-tailed deer may play a role in the vertebrate amplification of Jamestown Canyon virus.

Hantaan viruses. These agents are fundamentally parasites of wild rodents and insectivores.[27] As such, hantaviruses are the exception to the general rule that Bunyaviridae members are arthropod-borne viruses. Although many rodent species worldwide have been shown to harbor antibodies, antigens, and/or infectious viruses, the four presently recognized immunotypes each have a single or several closely related rodent host species. Hantaan virus, the cause of severe hemorrhagic fever with renal syndrome (HFRS) in Korea, China, the eastern Soviet Union, and southeast Europe, is found principally in the striped field mouse *Apodemus agrarius*.[5] These rodents become chronically infected despite a competent immune response and excrete virus in urine and saliva for weeks or months. Mechanisms of intraspecific transmission have not been elucidated but may depend largely on horizontal transmission between sexually mature animals. *Apodemus agrarius* is found in or near cultivars of humans and has both seasonal spring and fall and cyclic population peaks occurring at 2- to 4-year intervals.

Voles of the genus *Clethrionomys*, principally *C. glareolus*, are the reservoir–vectors of Puumula virus, cause of a milder form of HFRS termed nephropathia epidemica (NE), in Scandinavia, the Soviet Union west of the Ural Mountains, and northwestern Europe. These small rodents are found in forests and agricultural hedgerows, have highly cyclic populations, and disperse into rural and suburban gardens and dwellings in the fall and winter of years when their populations reach peaks.[28,29]

Another HTN virus (Seoul) is found worldwide in *Rattus norvegicus* and *R. rattus*. The ecology of this agent appears to be similar to that of HTN virus. Continuous intraspecific transmission of the virus during a 5-year period has been documented in Baltimore, Maryland.[30] A fourth HTN immunotype, Prospect Hill, has been identified as a parasite of *Microtus pennsylvanicus* in the United States.

Rift Valley Fever and Congo–Crimean Hemorrhagic Fever. Rift Valley fever virus is now believed to be maintained in eastern and southern Africa by transovarial transmission in certain *Aedes* mosquitos, notably *A. linneatopenis*.[31] Infected eggs can remain dormant but viable in soil for years while awaiting heavy rains for subsequent hatching. Other mosquitos are important during epizootics and epidemics; large vertebrates such as sheep, cattle, wild ungulates, and humans serve as amplifiers because they experience high viremia during infection.[32] Rift Valley fever is widely distributed on the African continent and would likely become epidemic if introduced into North America.

Congo–Crimean hemorrhagic fever virus is transmitted by ticks. The principal vectors belong to the genus *Hyalomma*. Immature stages feed on hares, hedgehogs, and ground feeding birds, while adults parasitize larger wild and domestic animals. The virus is not transovarially transmitted but is passed from immature ticks infected on viremic small mammals to adult ticks during molting. This virus is widely distributed in the southwestern Soviet Union, the Balkans, the Middle East, and Africa.[3]

Transmission to Man

California Encephalitis Viruses. Transmission occurs through the bite of female mosquitos that have virus infection of their salivary glands. Human infection occurs mainly during the summer and early fall in persons entering forested areas for recreation or those living near forests.[33] *Aedes triseriatus* will range considerable distances from forest across open terrain in search of a blood meal.[34]

Hantaan Viruses. Dusty aerosols contaminated by infectious rodent urine are thought to represent the principal vehicle for the transmission of HTN viruses; transmission by the bite of infected rodents (saliva) also has been documented.[35] *Apodemus*- and *Celthrionomys*-associated virus infections are acquired principally by persons visiting or working in forests and on farms. The incidence of transmission is highest in the fall and early winter and maximum in "high-rodent" years, when suburban residents may be exposed to dispersing infecting rodents.[28] The prevalence of Puumula virus in *C. glareolus* in Finland was shown to vary directly with rodent density, which contributes significantly to the concordance of a high rodent population and human disease years.[36]

The HTN virus of *Rattus* is presumed to be transmitted in a manner not different from its more rural relatives. Human infection may occur on farms, and in residential areas. Cases of HFRS were thus traced to nonmobile residents of urban Seoul, Korea, and Osaka, Japan.[37,38] *Rattus*-borne disease has a striking seasonal prevalence (winter–spring) in China.[39] In addition, infection, human disease, and even death have been linked to infected laboratory rats in Korea, Japan, Belgium, France, and the United Kingdom. The United States apparently is spared this problem because rat stocks imported for research are caesarean delivered and barrier maintained.

Rift Valley Fever and Congo–Crimean Hemorrhagic Fever. Before a major epidemic in Egypt in 1977, which was largely mosquito transmitted, RVF in Africa was principally a disease of farmers, veterinarians, and abattoir workers who have direct contact with sick domestic livestock and carcasses infected with high concentrations of virus. Transmission to humans is mainly epidemic, with infrequent years of heavy precipitation on otherwise dry savannahs triggering the dormant transovarial virus cycle. Congo–Crimean hemorrhagic virus is transmitted to humans principally by the bite of adult *Hyalomma* ticks. Milkers and shepherds are the frequent victims. This virus also has caused several alarming nosocomial hospital outbreaks with fatalities in medical personnel. Highly infectious blood was the principal vehicle for transmission in settings where the correct diagnosis of the index case was not suspected.[40,41]

CLINICAL MANIFESTATIONS

California Encephalitis Viruses

Infection of humans by these viruses is most commonly asymptomatic. After an incubation period of 3–7 days, however, individuals may suffer mild febrile illness, encephalitis, or meningoencephalitis. More than 90 percent of acute central nervous system (CNS) disease caused by LAC virus occurs in children less than 15 years of age[25]; males are affected more often than females are, and the mortality in acute CNS disease is about 1 percent. Clinically and pathologically, it is difficult to distinguish CE from other acute viral infections of the CNS. Fever, headache, nausea, and vomiting are present in most patients. Lethargy, aphasia, incoordination, and focal motor abnormalities, even paralysis, may be present, but the outstanding serious finding is convulsion, which occurs in about one-half of cases. A stiff neck may be the major clinical sign in mild CNS infection. The spinal fluid generally shows a modest pleocytosis (<100 WBCs/mm^3) that may be largely granulocytic and exhibits normal or slightly increased protein concentrations. Peripheral leukocytosis in excess of 15,000 WBCs/mm^3 is not uncommon.[42,43] Although most patients make uneventful recoveries, 75 percent of patients have abnormal electroencephalographic (ECG) findings 1–5 years later, emotional lability is persistent in 10 percent, and epilepsy is a chronic problem in 6–10 percent of all diagnosed cases. Thus, CE is a much more serious disease than is generally appreciated.

Jamestown Canyon

Jamestown Canyon virus encephalitis occurs more frequently in adults. Although recorded cases are few, this may be largely due to a failure to include this agent in routine viral CNS diagnostic tests.[18]

Hantaan Viruses

The hallmarks of clinical infection by members of this genus are fever, thrombocytopenia, and acute renal insufficiency, pathologically typical of acute interstitial nephritis. The incubation period may vary from 9 to 35 days. In the severe Asian form of HFRS, patients who survive progress through febrile (toxic), hypotensive, oliguric, and polyuric clinical stages and may require weeks or months to recover from general asthenia. There are no chronic sequelae of infection.

In the toxic phase, patients complain of headache, abdominal and lower back pain, dizziness, and in about half of the cases, blurred vision.[44] Conjunctival injection and petechiae occur over the upper trunk and soft palate. An erythematous flush that blanches on pressure is characteristically seen on the torso and face. Leukocytes may exceed 20,000/mm^3, and platelets frequently are reduced to 30,000/mm^3 or less. At the end of the toxic febrile period (4–7 days), many patients experience severe clinical shock. Those surviving then must endure varying grades of renal insufficiency including a complete shutdown, mucosal bleeding diathesis, electrolyte and acid-base abnormalities, hypertension, and pneumonitis complicated by pulmonary edema. After 3–10 days, oliguria gives way to polyuria with its attendant stresses on fluid and electrolyte balance. The fatality rate in Asian HFRS averages about 6 percent: one-third during the shock phase and two-thirds (cerebrovascular accidents and pulmonary edema) during the renal phases of illness.[45] Hemodynamic pathogenesis is based on a massive acute capillary leak syndrome of uncertain specific etiology, and the renal lesions, predominantly in medullary proximal tubules, are possibly related to antigen–antibody complexes either deposited from circulation or engendered locally at the site of virus-infected tubules.[46,47]

The milder NE form of HFRS is rarely hemorrhagic and fatal in fewer than 1 percent of clinical cases. There is strong evidence that up to 90 percent of Puumula virus infections are asymptomatic. In this disease proteinuria, creatinine elevation, and leukocytosis, although common, are much less severe than for Asian HFRS.

Rift Valley Fever and Congo–Crimean Hemorrhagic Fever

Rift Valley fever infection in humans causes undifferentiated febrile disease in the great majority of instances. However, 10–20 percent of patients experience macular and perimacular retinitis and vasculitis that may cause a permanent loss of vision. In as much as 1 percent of infections, fulminant hepatitis with jaundice and hemorrhage may develop at the end of a 4- to 6-day febrile episode. Most of these patients die. Others experience acute, severe, frequently fatal encephalitis directly related to viral invasion of the CNS.

Congo–Crimean hemorrhagic fever is a severe hemorrhagic fever. There is acute icteric hepatitis, major compromise of coagulation function, disseminated intravascular coagulation (DIC), major loss of erythrocytes, and severe thrombocytopenia. Mortality ranges from 20 to 50 percent.

DIAGNOSIS

The diagnosis of CE is immunologic because virus is not present in blood or secretions during the phase of clinical CNS disease. The diagnosis can be rapidly and specifically achieved by enzyme-linked immunosorbent assay (ELISA) tests for antivirus IgM antibodies in blood and cerebrospinal fluid. Many patients are positive at the time of admission.[48,49] A similar situation exists for Asian HFRS. Virtually all patients have both IgM and IgG HTN antibodies when admitted to the hospital.[5,50] The agent also can be recovered with difficulty by the inoculation of concentrated blood leukocytes that contain infected monocytes[51] into cell cultures or suckling mice or rats. In contrast, only about two-thirds of NE patients develop such antibodies within 10 days of the onset of illness. Except for leptospirosis, however, the clinical and epidemiologic features of this disease are sufficient to make the diagnosis in at least 75 percent of subsequently confirmed cases.[52] Rift Valley fever and CCHF viruses are readily recovered from the blood of acutely ill patients by using cell cultures, suckling mice, or adult hamsters. Antibodies detectable by a variety of methods generally appear within 10–14 days of onset. ELISA detection of IgM antibodies is a reliable definitive method.[53] Because of the aerosol hazard to laboratory personnel, however, attempts to isolate these two agents should be restricted to facilities with maximum containment.

PREVENTION AND TREATMENT

With the exception of RVF for which there is an experimental inactivated vaccine of probable efficacy,[54] prevention of these diseases is only accomplished by personal means (mosquito and tick repellents) and perhaps in the case of CE by elimination of man-made containers of mosquito breeding together with aerial spraying of slow-release insecticides over forested areas of known high *A. triseriatus* reproduction.[55]

Ribavirin (Virazole) has been found effective in the treatment of suckling mice infected with HTN virus, and clinical trials are in progress in China for the treatment of HFRS by using the intravenous dosing regimen established for Lassa fever (Chapter 144). Studies in vitro and in laboratory animals suggest that ribavirin also might be effective in the treatment of severe RVF disease.[56] The use of convalescent human plasma may have reduced disease severity in a recent nosocomial outbreak of CCHF.[57]

Effective supportive medicine is important in all of the severe *Bunyavirus* diseases. Careful management of seizures is important in CE patients; there is danger in too vigorous use of phenobarbitol in children with status epilepticus. Phenytoin, 15 mg/kg loading dose, not to exceed a total daily dose of 1 g, is a preferred regimen.[58]

Patients with Asian HFRS may require one or two lifesaving treatments of hemodialysis or peritoneal dialysis during the oliguric phase, and plasma protein and/or whole blood may be required during hemorrhagic/shock phases of this and the other two hemorrhagic fevers. Heparin is not recommended for the treatment of presumptive or incipient DIC. Patients with NE rarely require dialysis; the mean peak creatinine values range from 5 to 7 mg/dl and seldom exceed 10 mg/dl.[28]

REFERENCES

1. Karabatsos N, ed. International Catalogue of Arboviruses. 3rd ed. San Antonio, TX: American Society of Tropical Medicine and Hygiene; 1985:1147.
2. Swartz TA, Klingberg MA, Goldblum N, eds. Rift Valley Fever. Contributions to Epidemiology and Biostatistics J. Basel: S Karger AG; 1981:196.
3. Hoogstraal H. The epidemiology of tick-borne Crimean–Conge hemorrhagic fever in Asia, Europe, and Africa. J Med Entomol. 1979;15:304.
4. Haemorrhagic fever with renal syndrome: Report of a Working Group. Manila; WHO: 1982.
5. Lee HW, Lee PW, Johnson KM. Isolation of the agent of Korean hemorrhagic fever. J Infect Dis. 1978;137:298.
6. LeDuc JW, Smith GA, Johnson KM. Hantaan-like viruses from domestic rats captured in the United States. Am J Trop Med Hyg. 1984;33:992.
7. Lee PW, Amyx HL, Yanagihara R, et al. Partial characterization of Prospect Hill virus isolated from meadow voles in the United States. J Infect Dis. 1985;152:826.
8. Yanagihara R, Gajdusek GC, Gibbs CJ Jr, et al. Prospect Hill virus: Serologic evidence for infection in mammalogists. N Engl J Med. 1984;310:1325.
9. Yanagihara R, Chin C-T, Weiss MB, et al. Serological evidence of Hantaan infection in the United States. Am J Trop Med Hyg. 1985;34:396.
10. Martin ML, Lindsey-Regnery H, Sasso DR, et al. Distinction between Bunyaviridae genera by surface structure and comparison with Hantaan virus using negative stain electron microscopy. Arch Virol. 1985;86:17.
11. Bishop DHL, Calisher CH, Casals J, et al. Bunyaviridae. Intervirology. 1980;14:125.
12. Pensiero MN, Jenning GB, Schmaljohn CS, et al. Expression of the Hantaan virus M genome segment by using a vaccinia virus recombinant. J Virol. 1988;62:696.
13. Gonzales-Scarano F, Janssen RS, Najjar JA, et al. An avirulent G1 glycoprotein variant of LaCrosse bunyavirus with defective fusion function. J Virol. 1985;54:757.
14. Dantas JR Jr, Okuno Y, Asada H, et al. Characterization of glycoproteins causing hemorrhagic fever with renal syndrome (HFRS) using monoclonal antibodies. Virology. 1986;151:379.
15. Dantas JR Jr, Okuno Y, Tanishita O, et al. Viruses of hemorrhagic fever with renal syndrome (HFRS) grouped by immunoprecipitation and hemagglutination inhibition. Intervirology. 1987;27:161.
16. Struthers JK, Swanepoel R. Identification of a major non-structural protein in the nuclei of Rift Valley fever virus–infected cells. J Gen Virol. 1982;60:381.
17. Anderson DW Jr, Smith JF. Immunoelectron microscopy of Rift Valley fever viral morphogenesis in primary rat hepatocytes. Virology. 1987;161:91.
18. Deibel R, Srihongse S, Grayson MA, et al. Jamestown Canyon virus: The etiologic agent of an emerging human disease? In: Calisher CH, Thompson WH, eds. California Serogroup Viruses, Proceedings of an International Symposium. New York: Alan R Liss; 1983:313.
19. Thompson WH: Vector–virus relationships. In: Calisher CH, Thompson WH, eds. California Serogroup Viruses, Proceedings of an International Symposium. New York: Alan R Liss; 1983:57.
20. Yuill TM. The role of mammals in the maintenance and dissemination of LaCrosse virus. In: Calisher CH, Thompson WH, eds. California Serogroup Viruses, Proceedings of an International Symposium. New York: Alan R Liss; 1983:77.
21. Watts DM, Thompson WH, Yuill TM, et al. Overwintering of LaCrosse virus in *Aedes triseriatus*. Am J Trop Med Hyg. 1974;23:694.
22. Freier JE, Beier JC. Oral and transovarial transmission of LaCrosse virus by *Aedes atropalpus*. Am J Trop Med Hyg. 1984;33:708.
23. DeFoliart GR, Lisitza MA. Activity of *Aedes triseriatus* in open terrain. Mosq News. 1980;26:373.
24. Centers for Disease Control. Viruses of the california serogroup. MMWR. 1985;34:291.
25. Centers for Disease Control. La Crosse encephalitis in West Virginia. MMWR. 1988;37:79.
26. Sikes RK, Calisher CH, Smith JD. Human infections with LaCrosse virus in Georgia, 1982. South Med J. 1984;77:972.
27. LeDuc JW, Smith GA, Childs JE, et al. Global survey of antibody to Hantaan-related viruses among peridomestic rodents. Bull WHO. 1986;64:139.
28. Nystrom K. The incidence and prevalence of endemic benign (epidemic) nephropathy in AC county, Sweden, in relation to population density and prevalence of small rodents. Acta Med Scand [Suppl] 1977;609:1.
29. Korpela H, Lähdevirta J. The role of small rodents and patterns of living in the epidemiology of nephropathia epidemica. Scand J Infect Dis. 1978;10:303.
30. Childs JE, Korch GW, Glass GE, et al. Epizootiology of *Hantavirus* infections in Baltimore: Isolation of a virus from Norway rats, and characteristics of infected rat populations. Am J Epidemiol. 1987;126:55.
31. Linthicum KJ, Davies FG, Kairo A, et al. Rift Valley fever virus (family Bunyaviridae, genus *Phlebovirus*). Isolations from Diptera collected during an interepizootic period in Kenya. J Hyg (Camb). 1985;95:197.
32. Easterday BC. Rift Valley fever. Adv Vet Sci. 1965;10:65.
33. Henderson BE, Coleman PH. The growing importance of California arboviruses in the etiology of human disease. Prog Med Virol. 1971;13:404.
34. Mather TN, DeFoliart GR. Disperson of gravid *Aedes triseriatus* (Diptera: Culcicidae) from woodlands into open terrain. J Med Entomol. 1984;21:384.
35. Kawamata J, Yamanouchi T, Dohmae K, et al. Control of laboratory acquired hemorrhagic fever with renal syndrome (HFRS) in Japan. Lab Anim Sci. 1987;37:431.
36. Brummer-Korvenkontio M, Henttonen H, Vahera A. Hemorrhagic fever with renal syndrome in Finland: Ecology and virology of nephropathia epidemica. Scand J Infect Dis [Suppl]. 1982;36:88.
37. Lee HW, Baek LJ, Johnson KM. Isolation of Hantaan virus, the etiologic agent of Korean hemorrhagic fever, from wild urban rodents. J Infect Dis. 1982;146:638.
38. Tamura M. Occurrence of epidemic hemorrhagic fever in Osaka City: First cases found in Japan with characteristic feature of marked proteinuria. Biken J. 1964;7:79.
39. Chen HX, Qiu FX, Dong BJ, et al. Epidemiological studies on hemorrhagic fever with renal syndrome in China. J Infect Dis. 1986;154:394.
40. Burney MI, Ghafoor A, Saleen M, et al. Nosocomial outbreak of viral hemorrhagic fever caused by Crimean hemorrhagic fever–Congo virus in Pakistan, January 1976. Am J Trop Med Hyg. 1980;29:941.
41. Van Eeden PJ, Joubert JR, van de Wal BW, et al. A nosocomial outbreak of Crimean–Congo haemorrhagic fever at Tygerberg hospital. I. Clinical features. S Afr Med J. 1985;68:711.
42. Young DJ. California encephalitis virus. Report of three cases and review of the literature. Ann Intern Med. 1966;65:419.
43. Johnson KP, Lepow ML, Johnson RT. California encephalitis. I. Clinical and epidemiologic studies. Neurology (NY). 1968;89:250.
44. Lee JS, Cho BY, Lee MC, et al. Clinical features of serological proven Korean hemorrhagic fever patients. Seoul J Med. 1980;21:163.
45. Lee M. Korean hemorrhagic fever. Seoul: Seoul National University Press; 1981:146.
46. Penttinen K, Lähdevirta J, Kekomäki R, et al. Circulating immune complexes, immunoconglutinins, and rheumatoid factors in nephropathia epidemia. J Infect Dis. 1981;143:15.
47. Collan Y, Lähdevirta J, Jokinen EJ. Electron microscopy of nephropathia epidemia. Renal tubular basement membrane. Am J Pathol. 1978;92:167.
48. Dykers TI, Brown KL, Gunderson CB, et al. Rapid diagnosis of LaCrosse encephalitis: Detection of specific immunoglobulin M in cerebrospinal fluid. J Clin Microbiol. 1985;22:740.
49. Calisher CH, Pretzman CI, Muth DJ, et al. Serodiagnosis of LaCrosse virus infections in humans by detection of immunoglobulin M class antibodies. J Clin Microbiol. 1986;23:667.
50. Tsai TF, Tang YW, Hu SL, et al. Hemagglutination-inhibiting antibody in hemorrhagic fever with renal syndrome. J Infect Dis. 1984;150:895.
51. Nagai T, Tanishita O, Takahashi Y, et al. Isolation of hemorrhagic fever with renal syndrome virus from leucocytes of rats and virus replication in cultures of rat and human macrophages. J Gen Virol. 1985;66:1271.
52. Lähdevirta J, Savola J, Brummer-Korvenkontio M, et al. Clinical and serological diagnosis of nephropathia epidemica, the mild type of haemorrhagic fever with renal syndrome. J Infect. 1984;9:230.
53. Saluzzo JF, LeGuenno B. Rapid diagnosis of human Crimean–Congo hemorrhagic fever and detection of the virus in naturally infected ticks. J Clin Microbiol. 1987;25:922.
54. Niklasson B, Peters CJ, Bengtsson E, et al. Rift Valley fever virus vaccine trial: Study of neutralizing antibody response in humans. Vaccine. 1985;3:123.
55. Francy DB. Mosquito control for prevention of California (LaCrosse) encephalitis. In: Calisher CH, Thompson WH, eds. California Serogroup Viruses. Proceedings of an International Symposium. New York: Alan R Liss; 1983:365.
56. Peters CJ, Reynolds JA, Slone TW, et al. Prophylaxis of Rift Valley fever with antiviral drugs, immune serum, an interferon inducer, and a macrophage activator. Antiviral Res. 1986;6:285.
57. Shepherd AJ, Swanepoel R, Shepherd SP, et al. A nosocomial outbreak of Crimean–congo haemorrhagic fever at Tygerberg hospital. V. Virological and serological observations. S Afr Med J. 1985;68:733.
58. Deering WM. Neurologic aspects and treatment of LaCrosse encephalitis. In: Calisher CH, Thompson WH, eds. California Serogroup Viruses. Proceedings of an International Symposium. New York: Alan R Liss; 193:187.

Arenaviridae

144. LYMPHOCYTIC CHORIOMENINGITIS VIRUS, LASSA VIRUS (LASSA FEVER), AND OTHER ARENAVIRUSES

KARL M. JOHNSON

The arenaviruses are a family possessing single-stranded RNA, a unique morphology, and a predilection for rodents as basic virus reservoirs. They include lymphocytic choriomeningitis virus (LCM), Lassa virus, and the new-world antigenically related Tacaribe group of viruses (Tacaribe, Junin, Machupo, Amapari, Tamiami, Pichinde, Parana, Latino, and Flexal). The old-world members (LCM and Lassa) as well as two new-world members (Junin and Machupo) cause significant human disease. The family prototype, LCM, was first isolated in 1933 during serial monkey passage of human material obtained from a fatal infection in the first documented epidemic of St. Louis encephalitis.[1] Junin, Machupo, and Lassa viruses were first recovered during investigations of human disease in 1958,[2] 1963,[3] and 1969,[4] respectively.

VIRUS CHARACTERIZATION

Virions are round, oval, or pleomorphic particles averaging about 110–130 nm in diameter but ranging from 50 to 300 nm.[5] The viral envelope is formed by budding through the host cell unit membrane, and it consists of the three layers normally attributed to that structure. Hollow club-shaped projections are present on the virion surface. These are about 10 nm long and are similar to surface glycoproteins found in other membrane-bound RNA viruses. The interior of the virion apparently is structureless except for the presence of a variable number of dense granules 20–25 nm in diameter, which have been shown to be host cell ribosomes (Fig. 1). These unique structures resembling grains of sand are responsible for the family name (L. *arenosus*, sandy). This character is so typical that the first electron micrograph of Lassa virus immediately classified this unknown cause of serious human disease and indicated the direction for successful elucidation of the important epidemiologic variables of the disease.[4]

Arenaviruses contain a segmented RNA genome of negative, noninfectious sense. The respective strands are 31S and 22S.[6] Host ribosomal RNA of 28S, 18S, and 4–6S is also present but apparently is not biologically functional.[7] The molecular weights of L and S viral RNA have been estimated at 2.6 and 1.4×10^6 daltons.[8]

The S RNA of arenaviruses codes for three virionic proteins[9,10] in a unique manner.[11,12] The nucleocapsid core protein (N) is read first in a conventional negative sense and is followed by the production of a glycoprotein precursor polypeptide (GP-C) that is constructed from genomic positive-sense mRNA. This pattern has been termed "ambisense."[11] The GP-C protein is then cleaved and glycosylated to form structural units G1 and G2. Molecular weights of the virionic polypeptides are about 75,000, 54,000, and 38,000, respectively.[13] The G1 protein is thought to represent the surface projections of the virus, while G2 is believed to be a membrane-embedded protein that may be partially expressed on the virus surface. Studies with monoclonal antibodies to LCM proteins indicate that GP-1 is dominant in arenavirus neutralization, and recent work with this agent shows that portions of the GP-C molecule are also important for elucidation of T-cell–mediated cytolysis of virus-infected cells.[14–16]

Arenavirus L RNA codes for a viral polymerase of about 200,000 daltons and perhaps other as yet unidentified proteins.[17] The large genome also was found to code for the virulence of LCM in guinea pigs.[18]

EPIDEMIOLOGY AND EPIZOOTOLOGY

Arenaviruses are parasites of rodents. They exhibit high species specificity such that one or occasionally two rodents are reservoirs for a given agent. Chronic virus infection with the release of virus into excreta, especially urine, is the basis for both intraspecific virus maintenance and transmission to humans. Thus, human arenaviral disease is determined by virus pathogenicity, by the geographic distribution of a particular reservoir rodent, and by rodent–human ecologic factors that permit contact with excreted virus.

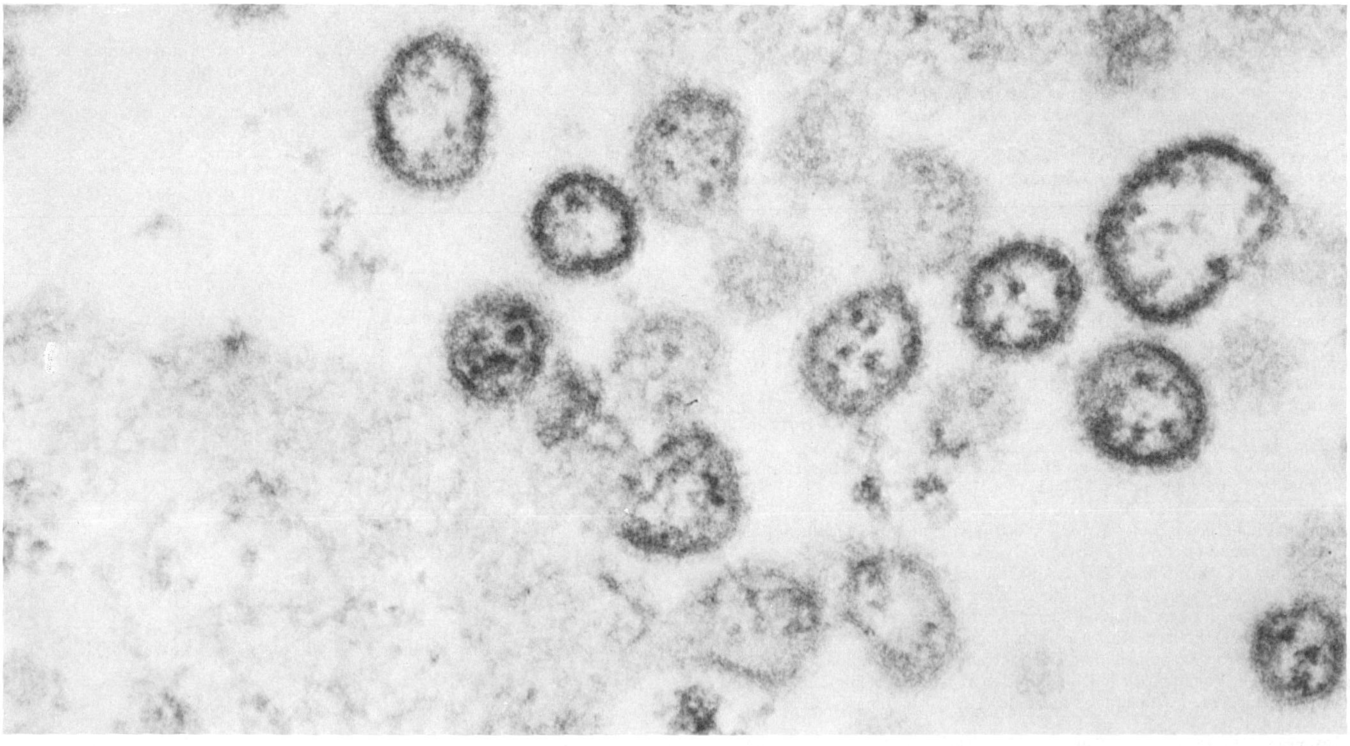

FIG. 1. Electron micrograph of Lassa virus in the first Vero cell passage envelope, and electron-dense interior granules can be seen. (×121,000).

Lymphocytic Choriomeningitis

Although LCM virus infection may occur worldwide, it has been demonstrated so far only in Europe and the Americas.[19] Moreover, in regions where the virus is known to exist, infection in *Mus musculus*, the definitive reservoir, is highly focal. Studies conducted in Boston and Washington, D.C., several decades ago revealed a spotty distribution of virus-positive mice in houses.[20] Similarly, more recent studies in the Federal Republic of Germany disclosed much higher murine infection rates in the west-central than in the southern or northern portions of the country.[21]

Human cases of LCM are least common during the summer. It is not clear whether this pattern is the result of seasonal population densities of rodents, movement of mice into homes and barns, seasonal variation in infection rates of *Mus*, or differential survival of excreted virus related to the temperature and relative humidity. It has been shown, however, that aerosolized arenaviruses survive better at lower humidity.[22]

Most human LCM infections occur among young adults, although persons of all ages have been affected. There are no sex or racial differences in attack frequency. Laboratory workers, particularly those handling mice or hamsters, have an increased risk of infection.

The mode of transmission in most sporadic human infections is not definitely known; however, experimental and epidemiologic observations implicate aerosols,[23] direct contact with rodents, and rodent bites in that order as the most likely vehicles.[20] The incubation period of human LCM disease is variable, but it most often ranges from 5 to 10 days. Patients not seeking medical care for the nonspecific febrile illness that begins at this time but who may later present with acute meningitis generally are found to have been exposed 2–3 weeks before the onset of nervous system signs.

While most sporadic LCM cases are attributed to contact with infected mice, outbreaks of disease have been traced without exception to infected Syrian hamsters (*Mesocricetus auratus*). Several of these were the result of the introduction of LCM virus into hamsters through infected tumor cell lines.[23–26] Other outbreaks in the United States and Europe resulted from exposure in the home to pet hamsters obtained from breeders with infected stock.[27,28]

Lassa Fever

Lassa fever is a disease of West Africa; however, with the contemporary ease of international travel, it may occur anywhere in the world. This disease is distinguished from other arenaviral diseases by its occasional ability to spread from person to person. Lassa fever was initially recognized in a Nigerian hospital where three nurses developed illness successively.[29] Since then, at least six nosocomial outbreaks have been reported from Nigeria, Liberia, and Sierra Leone. Lassa virus has been recovered from patients in Guinea, and serologic studies have shown its presence in every country of West Africa from Nigeria to Senegal. West Africa, however, represents only a small part of the range of *Mastomys natalensis*, which is the virus reservoir rodent found throughout the continent south of the Sahara Desert. Recent work showing that *Mastomys* rodents have distinct karyotypes and probably species that are geographically separate[30–31]—together with the isolation of Lassa-like viruses presumably nonpathogenic for humans from some of these and related rodents [32–34]—provides an attractive partial explanation for the observed regional boundaries of Lassa fever.

Most of the nonsocomial outbreaks of Lassa fever have occurred during the dry season (January to April). Endemic transmission occurs throughout the year, with more cases during dry than wet periods.[35,36] All ages and both sexes are infected equally; in Sierra Leone, infection rates in villages may reach 10–20 percent per year. Thus, there are about 20 mild or inapparent infections for each hospitalized case. Serologic studies suggest that clinically inapparent reinfection may occur.[37] In contrast, retrospective studies among white missionaries suggest but do not yet prove that moderately severe or even fatal illness nearly invariably follows infection.[38] Outbreaks typically include health care workers because of their direct exposure to patients and their infectious excreta. Pregnant women often experience severe disease, and abortion is a common complication.

The modes of Lassa virus transmission are not precisely known, but they are almost certainly multiple. Endemic transmission is related to infected rodents by aerosol and direct contact and most probably to person-to-person spread (contact) in homes. A *Mastomys* control campaign in a village in Sierra Leone resulted in a fourfold reduction but not the elimination of transmission to the residents (J. B. McCormick, P. A. Webb, K. M. Johnson, Centers for Disease Control, unpublished observations). During nosocomial outbreaks, parenteral inoculation of body fluids (e.g., surgery or autopsy accidents), contact with infected body fluids, and aerosols generated by patients have all been incriminated.[35] Tertiary and quaternary cases in outbreaks are less numerous than are secondary cases, which suggests that only the unusual patient is infectious. Virologic parameters of Lassa fever to be described under the section in this chapter on "Clinical Manifestations" support this concept.

The incubation period varies from 3 to 16 days (usually 7–12) when transmitted from person to person. It is assumed to be similar in rodent-transmitted infection.

Argentine and Bolivian Hemorrhagic Fevers

These diseases are caused by Junin and Machupo viruses. The principal reservoir rodents are *Calomys musculinus* and *Calomys callosus*.[39,40] The pattern of virus transmission to humans for both agents is endemic–epidemic, which is a phenomenon related to the 3- to 5-year cyclic population pattern of the rodents.[41] This pattern, in turn, may well be linked to fetal death observed in *Calomys* females chronically infected with Junin or Machupo virus.[42] Argentine hemorrhagic fever (AHF) occurs mostly in the rich agricultural pampa of northern Buenos Aires provice. *Calomys* populations reach their highest density in the cornfields during the austral fall (February to May); the disease thus affects principally adult males engaged in harvesting corn. Roughly 200–2000 cases are reported annually, and the numbers have not changed substantially despite more than a 10-fold reduction in persons exposed, which was occasioned by the conversion from manual to mechanized harvesting techniques. Infectious aerosols and direct contact of abraded fingers with blood and tissues of rodents crushed by machinery and impaled on screens are thought to be the most likely modes of transmission.

Bolivian hemorrhagic fever (BHF) is restricted to the tropical savannah province of Beni in northeastern Boliva. *Calomys callosus* freely enters homes and gardens in this region, and most infections are house acquired. The incidence of cases is greatest from April to July (late rainy and early dry season), but the dominant feature of the epidemiologic pattern is that of small outbreaks in different villages and ranches with several years of quiescence thereafter.

All ages and both sexes are equally affected. Transmission is thought to occur by aerosol contact or by contact with food contaminated by infectious rodent urine.

The incubation period of AHF after parenteral inoculation may be as short as 2 days. The estimated interval after natural exposure to both Junin and Machupo viruses, however, ranges from 5 to 19 days, with a mode of 7–12 days.

PATHOGENESIS

Rodents

Arenavirus infection of reservoir rodent hosts usually is chronic but clinically rather benign. Laboratory-manipulated strains of LCM virus exhibit different pathogenicity for inbred strains of albino laboratory mice. The route of infection and age of the host are important variables. The unnatural intracerebral inoculation of adult mice produces an acute fatal choriomeningitis that has been shown to be mediated by immune cytotoxic T cells. Infection of newborn mice, in contrast, results in chronic viremic infection in which T-cell immunity is suppressed and in which antiviral antibodies are complexed with viral antigens; this eventually leads to development of chronic glomerulonephritis.[43] Although there is widespread infection of tissues including brain, little or no inflammation occurs outside the kidncy.

Rather similar patterns are observed in *Calomys* rodents experimentally infected with Junin or Machupo virus.[44,45] The differences are that lethal infection is not inducible by any route at any age, that antigen–antibody complexes are not demonstrable (nor antibodies of any type), and that some adult rodents develop chronic infection exactly like that typical for very young mice. In addition, chronic infection with Machupo virus induces a microcytic–hemolytic anemia (Coombs-negative) that results in chronic splenomegaly and eventual iron storage disease.

Mastomys rodents infected with Lassa virus similarly show no acute signs, do not develop inflammatory responses, and exhibit chronic infection or a self-limited response depending on age.[46] Chronic infection is marked by persistent immunofluorescent antibodies, but no observations regarding possible late immune complex disease have been made.

Arenavirus infection of nonreservoir rodents results either in benign, self-limited infection and immunity or in severe acute disease. Inbred strains of guinea pigs, in particular, respond in a manner somewhat similar to that of primates.

Primates

Monkeys provide good but not perfect models for the pathogenesis of arenavirus infection in humans. Cynomolgus monkeys infected by the inhalation of LCM virus exhibit both hilar lymph node and pulmonary replication of virus within 48 hours followed by viremia and wide dissemination to other organs.[19] There may be focal necrosis of the liver—at times with hemorrhage and splenic and lymph node hyperplasia—and interstitial and perivascular infiltration of mononuclear cells in the kidney, heart, skeletal muscle, adrenal, epididymis, and other organs. Lymphocytic meningitis is a common lesion.

Lassa virus infection of squirrel or rhesus monkeys also produces viremia and disseminated infection.[46,47] At about 1 week postinoculation, necrosis of the secondary follicles of lymph nodes is a conspicuous lesion. Hepatic, adrenal, and splenic red pulp necrosis ensue. Lassa virus induced a similar fatal disease in rhesus monkeys infected by small-particle aerosols.[22]

Meningoencephalomyelitis, skeletal muscle myositis, pulmonary vasculitis, and widespread systemic arthritis are generally evident at death. Despite the appearance of anti-Lassa antibodies before death, the vascular infiltrates are uniformly mononuclear, which suggests that this condition does not have a classic immune complex etiology.

Machupo virus also produces a viremic, usually fatal infection in rhesus, cynomolgus, or African green monkeys. Infection is marked by a macular rash, mild hemorrhage from mucosal surfaces, lymphadenopathy, and necrosis of hepatic, adrenal, splenic, and lymph node parenchyma.[48] Necrotizing enteritis is a common lesion. Animals surviving acute disease develop meningoencephalomyelitis and a severe diffuse lymphocytic vasculitis, and they usually die of central nervous system (CNS) disturbances 30–80 days after inoculation.

The outcome of Junin virus infection depends on both the virus strain and monkey species. The marmoset *Callithrix jacchus* usually suffers a fatal infection similar to that caused by Machupo virus in rhesus monkeys but without late vasculitis in survivors.[49] Strains of Junin virus vary widely in pathogenicity for rhesus monkeys, but some produce fatal hemorrhagic disease.[50] Squirrel monkeys, by contrast, exhibit no clinical signs at all, a pattern previously documented for Machupo virus in several new-world primates.

Few data are available regarding terminal events in human LCM infection, which is almost never lethal. Two fatal cases associated with early studies of the virus in monkeys displayed hemorrhagic necrosis much more typical of the other arenaviruses[51]; they arc rcgarded as aberrant human responses to this agent. Fatal Lassa virus infection in humans differs from that of monkeys chiefly in the virtual absence of pulmonary vasculitis, systemic arteritis, and also myositis, so typical of the lower primates. Variable necrosis with little or no inflammatory response has been observed in liver, spleen, and adrenal,[52] but in no instance was hepatic pathology sufficient to cause death.[53] Recent studies in rhesus monkeys suggest that platelet and endothelial cell dysfunction, directly or indirectly virus mediated, may lead to shock and death after infection with Lassa virus.[54] Thus, the search for understanding arenavirus pathogenesis in monkeys and humans must be molecular and biochemical rather than descriptively pathologic.

Patients dying of AHF or BHF have few prominent findings. There is no vasculitis, virtually no inflammatory response in any organ, and a pattern of small focal hemorrhages (primarily in mucosal surfaces). Hepatic necrosis, on the average, is more severe in Lassa than in Junin or Machupo infections, but Councilman-like bodies are readily discernible in all three diseases. Bronchopneumonia, either primary viral or secondary bacterial, is a common finding in these diseases as well.

Argentine hemorrhagic virus patients exhibit extremely high concentrations of circulating endogenous α-interferon that reach a maximum at 6–12 days of illness. Highest levels were observed in fatal cases.[55] Experimental and clinical studies support the concept that interferons may prove to be detrimental rather than beneficial in arenavirus infections and certain other diseases.[56]

Virus can be recovered from the blood of acutely ill patients in all arenavirus infections, but titers are highest in Lassa fever and lowest in BHF. The viremic interval ranges from 3 to 20 days, with Lassa fever being the most persistent. Throat swabs are frequently positive as well, and late shedding (second to third week) into urine is observed in LCM and Lassa infection. Lymphocytic choriomeningitis and Lassa patients who exhibit meningeal signs have increased protein, leukocytes, and virus in spinal fluids.

At autopsy, tissues of monkeys and humans infected by Lassa, Junin, or Machupo viruses contain large amounts of virus, viral antigen, and in some instances (Lassa—liver) virions. Spleen, nodes, and bone marrow are major replication sites for Junin and Machupo viruses, while Lassa virus is found in many viscera and, notably, in the placentas of pregnant women.

CLINICAL MANIFESTATIONS

Clinically apparent infections with all the arenaviruses are similar in presenting manifestations. Fever is typically insidious in onset and is accompanied by headache and significant myalgia and malaise. Relative bradycardia is common, as is dysesthesia, particularly hyperesthesia of the skin. Thereafter, the various diseases pursue different courses.

Lymphocytic Choriomeningitis Virus

Lymphocytic choriomeningitis virus infections are most commonly "grippelike." After 3–5 days of nonspecific illness, occasionally with lymphadenopathy and a maculopapular rash, the fever subsides, but it frequently recurs in 2–4 days with several days of even more severe headache. A minority of patients exhibit frank meningitis during this second febrile period. There may be papilledema; cerebrospinal fluid (CSF) pressure usually is elevated, the protein concentration ranges from 50 to 300 mg/dl,and several hundred lymphocytes/mm^3 are commonly observed. Hypoglycorrhachia is found in less than one-third of cases. Encephalomyelitis may present as encephalitis lethargica, psychosis, paraplegia, or disturbances of cranial, sensory, or autonomic nerve function. There are unconfirmed reports of perinatal disease comprising meningitis, chorioretinitis, and even hydrocephalus.

Occasional patients develop orchitis, myopericarditis, arthritis, or alopecia. Orchitis develops 1–3 weeks after the onset of illness; it is usually unilateral and painful and resolves within 2 weeks. Myopericarditis is revealed by electrocardiographic (ECG) changes and labile tachycardia during and after the second febrile period. Pericardial effusion has been noted in a few patients. Arthritis occurs during convalescence, principally affects the metacarpophalangeal and proximal interphalangeal joints, and is marked by minimal swelling and redness. It generally resolves within a few weeks. Alopecia, most common among patients having high fevers more than 4 days, also occurs during convalescence and persists for 2–4 months maximum. This finding is also highly common during convalescence after clinical infection with other arenaviruses.

Clinical pathologic patterns observed in LCM infection are given in Table 1. The second febrile episode as well as some of the complications of convalescence have long been thought to represent an immunopathologic phenomenon. Immunofluorescent antibodies appear at about this time; therefore, this notion is at least possible, although no patient studies directed toward this hypothesis have yet been reported.

Lassa Fever

Most Lassa virus infections in Africans are mild or subclinical.[37] Severe multisystem disease occurs in only 5–10 percent of infections. Case fatality rates in hospitalized patients average 15–25 percent.[36,57]

In a case-control (306–339 patients) study of Lassa fever in Sierra Leone, the frequencies of selected findings (percentages) on the admission of adult Lassa patients were retrosternal chest pain, 74; sore throat, 60; back pain, 62; cough, 62; abdominal pain, 50; vomiting, 49; diarrhea, 26; conjunctivitis, 25; facial edema, 10; and proteinuria, 43. The frequency of some of these increased during the course of the illness; however, mucosal bleeding at any time was noted in just 17 percent of patients. These findings were present in many febrile non-Lassa patients, which rendered a clinical diagnosis in many instances impossible. A combination of fever, pharyngitis, retrosternal pain and proteinuria correctly predicted 70 percent of laboratory-confirmed Lassa fever cases and 80 percent, by exclusion, of the control illnesses.[58]

Lassa virus infection also causes serious disease and death in children, although manifestations may be even more protean or clinically confusing than among adults.[50] Four cases (three fatal) of a distinctive "swollen-baby" syndrome consisting of severe generalized edema, abdominal distension, and bleeding were recorded in children less than 2 years old in Liberia.[60]

Concentrations of virus and SGOT in the blood at admission are highly reliable, objective predictors of the outcome of infection. This situation (see Table 1) is virtually unique in human viral disease. Patients having at least 10^3 times the median tissue culture infective dose ($TCID_{50}$)/ml of virus and 150 IU/liter of SGOT experienced 78 percent mortality, while 83 percent of those with neither value survived.[61,62] The clinical manifestations associated with death, however, generally occur during the second week of illness. These consist of hypovolemic hypotension, vasoconstriction, reduced urinary output, facial and pulmonary edema, and in some cases pleural effusions and ascites. These events, often accompanied by minor hemorrhages from mucosal surfaces, strongly suggest a lesion of diffuse capillary leakage. Myocarditis and an element of congestive heart failure may contribute to the basic defect.

Patients who do not develop a capillary leak syndrome may experience other complications during the second or third week of illness. Chief among these is eighth-nerve deafness, which may be unilateral or bilateral, is usually permanent, and has a frequency of 5–8 percent. About 3–5 percent of male patients suffer auscultatory pericarditis that resolves clinically in 7–10 days; all such patients survive. Less common complications include uveitis and orchitis. Many hospitalized Lassa fever patients undergo some degree of transient alopecia during convalescence.

TABLE 1. Clinical Laboratory Findings in Human Arenaviral Disease

	Virus			
			Lassa	
Parameter	*LCM*	*Junin–Machupo*	*Fatal*	*Not Fatal*
Leukopenia	+ + +	+ + +	±	±
Thrombocytopenia	+ + +	+ + +	0	0
Hemoconcentration	0	+ + +	+ +	0
Coagulation changes	ND	Bleeding time ± factor II, VII, X ↓	Bleeding time + PTT ↑	N
Proteinuria	±	+ + +	+ + +	+ + +
BUN-creatinine	N	N	+ ↑	N
CPK	ND	N to 150 IU	> 1200 IU	to 500 IU
SGOT	N to 250 IU	N to 250 IU	av. 985 IU	av. 175 IU
LDH	N to 350 IU	N to 650 IU	N to 900 IU	N to 500 IU

Abbreviations: N: normal; ND: no data; ↑: increased value; ↓: decreased value; 0: absence of finding; ± to + + +: frequency and severity of finding; BUN: blood urea nitrogen; CPK: creatine phosphokinase; SGOT: serum glutamic oxaloacetic acid; LDH: lactic dehydrogenase.

South American Hemorrhagic Fevers

Argentine and Bolivian hemorrhagic fevers are remarkably similar clinically, and the mortality rate in each is about 10–20 percent. The onset of illness is insidious, with progressive fever, malaise, and myalgia often centered over the lower back. There may be epigastric pain, retro-orbital pain, dizziness, photophobia, and constipation. Conjunctival injection, flushing of the face and upper portion of the trunk, and orthostatic hypotension also are common. An enanthem consisting of petechiae and/or small vesicles on the palate and fauces is present in most patients, as are skin petechiae, particularly in the axilla, and generalized lymphadenopathy.[63]

Fever is unremittant, and despite the lack of evidence of significant hepatitis (see Table 1), some patients become progressively ill with one or a combination of syndromes of vascular or neurologic disease. Vascular disease consists of (*1*) increasing evidence of a capillary leak syndrome; (*2*) proteinuria, rising hematocrit, an onset of gingival gastrointestinal, nasal, and other membrane hemorrhages; (*3*) narrowing pulse pressure; and (*4*) vasoconstriction and clinical shock.[64] There may be signs of pulmonary exudation due to a vascular leak and/or to secondary bacterial infection, which is a common complication. Such patients are extremely difficult to manage. Plasma expanders may precipitate refractory pulmonary edema. Neurologic disease is heralded by development of hyporeflexia followed by station abnormalities, palmomental reflex, tremors of the tongue and upper extremities, and other cerebellar signs. If these changes are followed by clonic seizures and coma, the prognosis is extremely grave. This form of the disease causes more fatalities in AHF than does the bleeding–shock crisis.

Convalescence requires several weeks but is without sequelae. Alopecia and nail furrows are very common, as is postural hypotension for 1–2 weeks.

DIAGNOSIS

The diagnosis of past infection (i.e., epidemiologic studies) with arenaviruses is best done with cell culture plaque reduction neutralization because this method is sensitive and specific and antibodies endure for many years. The diagnosis of acute illness, by contrast, has features unique to each agent. In the case of LCM, blood and spinal fluid are usually virus-positive for nearly 1 week. The most sensitive test is to inoculate young adult mice in the brain and then challenge them 7 days later with endotoxin, which promotes illness if they are infected. Immunofluorescent antibody (IFA) tests of inoculated cell cultures should reveal virus sooner in most instances.

Lassa virus is easily isolated from blood during the first 7–10 days of illness by using cell cultures.[61] Junin virus was recovered from 96 percent of patients by cocultivation of patient blood mononuclear cells with Vero cell cultures, whereas cell cultures or suckling mice were only about 50 percent positive when unconcentrated blood was tested.[65] Isolation of Machupo virus is difficult, but the improved Junin virus technique has not been evaluated. Throat swabs may be positive in some patients with each arenavirus disease, and urine may contain virus up to 67 days in LCM and Lassa patients.[66] Biopsy or autopsy specimens of lymphoid tissues, marrow, and liver (Lassa) usually yield virus, often in concentrations greatly exceeding those found in blood.[52]

Serodiagnosis of Lassa fever by IFA or enzyme-linked immunosorbent assay (ELISA) detection of IgM antibodies is rapid and quite sensitive.[67,68] In Sierra Leone, 75 percent of patients were IFA-positive on admission (mean duration of illness, 8.5 days).[61] Detection of Lassa virus antigenemia should permit an early diagnosis for many patients before the appearance of such antibodies.[68] Antibodies detectable by IFA appear about 2 weeks after the onset of LCM illness. Antibodies to Junin and Machupo viruses, however, may not develop until 3–4 weeks after clinical illness.

PREVENTION AND TREATMENT

Arenavirus infection may be prevented by interdicting transmission from rodents to humans, from person to person, and from infected specimens to laboratory workers or by passive or active immunization. Community rodent control completely halted a major outbreak of BHF[69]; elimination of infected laboratory hamsters controlled LCM outbreaks.[23] A household rodent control study of Lassa infection, however, gave disappointing results.[70] Community-wide control programs suggest that this approach is less successful than for BHF.

Person-to-person spread within hospitals has been a problem with Lassa fever. In endemic situations such as Sierra Leone, partial spatial isolation of patients and the use of ''enteric precautions'' such as gloves, gowns, and careful disposal of patient wastes and fomites has generally served to prevent the spread of infection. Segregation of patients on the basis of the risk of death and likely content of virus in blood and body fluids by measuring SGOT levels is of major value. Some hospital outbreaks, particularly in Nigeria, appear to have been caused by infectious aerosols. Thus, wherever practical, it is advisable to place patients in single rooms with isolated negative-pressure airflow, to provide medical staff with goggles and filter masks (e.g., Custom Comfo Respirator, type A ultrafilter cartridge, Mine Safety Applicance Co.), and to double-bag all potentially contaminated refuse or specimens and rinse the outer bag with 0.6% sodium hydrochlorite before removal from the patient's room. Isolation of patients should continue until three consecutive blood and urine specimens are virus-negative. Outside Africa, however, surveillance of contacts of Lassa fever patients has failed to disclose a single instance of person-to-person transmission.

Laboratory-acquired infection is a major problem because all arenaviruses are infectious as aerosols. Several infections, some fatal, have occurred in laboratory workers. Thus, it is imperative that work (isolation or scientific manipulation) with all agents except LCM be conducted in special laboratories having maximum biologic containment. Clinical pathologic tests, particularly with Lassa fever patients, also present problems. Aerosols must be minimized or contained, and acid treatment will inactivate virus, so it is appropriate for leukocyte counts and blood smears; heating serum at 60°C for 1 hour is feasible for measuring heat-stable substances such as electrolytes, urea nitrogen, and creatinine.[71]

There are no licensed arenavirus vaccines. However, preliminary phase 1 tests of Junin attenuated vaccine were successful, and field trials for efficacy are in progress. A nucleocapsid Lassa gene inserted into vaccinia virus has protected guinea pigs against fatal Lassa infection.[72] More work will be required to determine whether N, G, or both are required to effectively immunize monkeys and humans.

Convalescent human plasma was proved effective in the treatment of AHF (16 percent placebo vs. 1 percent treated mortality) provided therapy was begun before the ninth day of illness.[73] The total dose of neutralizing antibody in plasma is important.[74] Cerebellar signs, usually transient and possibly the result of restricted virus multiplication, occurred in 10 percent of those receiving this treatment. Immune plasma treatment of Lassa fever has not been as successful,[75] and experiments in animals suggest that this may be related to the fact that neutralizing antibodies after Lassa virus infection are generally of low titer and avidity.[76]

Ribavirin, a purine nucleoside having broad-spectrum antiviral properties, was found to be lifesaving for lethally infected monkeys.[47] The intravenous administration of this compound to patients admitted to the hospital in Sierra Leone with SGOT elevations of at least 150 IU reduced the mortality from 55 to 5 percent if treatment was begun before day 7 of the disease.[62] A positive effect on survival was achieved, however, at all stages of infection. After a 1 g loading dose, patients were given 1 g ribavirin 4 times daily for 4 days and then 0.5 g 3 times daily for 6 additional days. Reversible anemia never requiring a transfusion was the only adverse effect associated with treatment.

Supportive care may be lifesaving in arenavirus infection. Careful monitoring for and early correction of the capillary leak syndrome is of cardinal importance. Fluid balance should be maintained per os as long as posible. Protein replacement therapy should be started before the appearance of clinical shock, and appropriate therapy for myocarditis and electrolyte imbalance (usually metabolic acidosis) should be maintained.

REFERENCES

1. Armstrong C, Lillie RD. Experimental lymphocytic choriomeningitis of monkeys and mice produced by a virus encountered in studies of the 1933 St. Louis encephalitis epidemic. Public Health Rep. 1934;49:1019.
2. Parodi AS, Greenwya DJ, Rugiero HR, et al. Sobre la etiologia del brote epidemico de Junin. Diagn Med. 1958;30:2300.
3. Johnson KM, Wiebenga NG, Mackenzie RB, et al. Virus isolations from human cases of hemorrhagic fever in Bolivia. Proc Soc Exp Biol Med. 1965;118:113.
4. Buckley SM, Casals J. Lassa fever, a new virus disease of man from East Africa. III. Isolations and characterization of the virus. Am J Trop Med Hyg. 1970;19:680.
5. Murphy FA, Whitfield SG. Morphology and morphogenesis of arenaviruses. Bull WHO. 1975;52:408.
6. Pederson IR. Lymphocytic choriomeningitis virus RNA's. Nature. 1971; 234:112.
7. Carter MF, Biswal N, Rawls WE. Characterization of the nucleic acid of Pichinde virus. J Virol. 1973;11:61.
8. Auperin DD, Compans RW, Bishop DHL. Nucleotide sequence conservation

at the 3′ termini of the virion RNA species of New World and Old World arenaviruses. Virology. 1982;121:200.
9. Harnish DG, Dimock K, Bishop DHL, et al. Gene mapping in Pichinde virus. Assignment of viral polypeptides to genomic L and S RNAs. J Virol. 1983;46:638.
10. Rivière Y, Ahmed R, Southern PJ, et al. The S RNA segment of lymphocytic choriomeningitis virus codes for the nucleoprotein and glycoproteins 1 and 2. J Virol. 1985;53:966.
11. Auperin D, Romanowski V, Galinsky M, et al. Sequencing studies of Pichinde virus sRNA indicate a novel coding strategy, an ambisense viral sRNA. J Virol. 1984;52:897.
12. Fuller-Pace FV, Southern PJ. Temporal analysis of transcription and replication during acute infection with lymphocytic choriomeningitis virus. Virology. 1988;162:260.
13. Howard CR, Simpson DIH. The biology of arenaviruses. J Gen Virol. 1980;51:1.
14. Parekh BS, Buchmeier MJ. Proteins of lymphocytic choriomeningitis virus: Antigenic topography of the viral glycoprotein. Virology. 1986;153:168.
15. Whitton JL, Southern PJ, Oldstone MB. Analyses of the cytotoxic T-lymphocyte responses to glycoprotein and nucleoprotein components of lymphocytic choriomeningitis virus. Virology. 1988;162:321.
16. Whitton JL, Gebhard JR, Lewicki H, et al. Molecular definition of a major cytotoxic T-lymphocyte epitope in the glycoprotein of lymphocytic choriomeningitis virus. J Virol. 1988;62:687.
17. Singh MK, Fuller-Pace FV, Buchmeier MJ, et al. Analysis of the genomic L RNA segment from lymphocytic choriomeningitis virus. Virology. 1987; 16:448.
18. Rivière Y, Ahmed R, Southern PJ, et al. Genetic mapping of lymphocytic choriomeningitis virus pathogenicity: Virulence in guinea pigs is associated with L RNA segment. J Virol. 1985;55:704.
19. Lehmann-Grube F. Lymphocytic Choriomeningitis Virus. New York: Springer Publishing; 1971.
20. Farmer TW, Janeway CA. Infection with the virus of lymphocytic choriomeningitis. Medicine (Baltimore). 1942;21:1.
21. Ackermann R, Bloedhorn H, Kupper B, et al. Uber die Verbreitung des Virus der lymphocytaren Choriomeningitis unter den Mausen in Westdeutschland. I. Untersuchungen uberwiegend an Hausmausen (*Mus musculus*). Zentrabl Bakteriol. 1964;194:407.
22. Stephenson EH, Larson EW, Dominik JW. Effect of environmental factors on aerosol induced Lassa virus infection. J Med Virol. 1984;14:295.
23. Hinman AR, Fraser DW, Douglas RG, et al. Outbreak of lymphocytic choriomeningitis virus infections in medical center personnel. Am J Epidemiol. 1975;101:103.
24. Bowen GS, Calisher CH, Winkler WG, et al. Laboratory studies of a lymphocytic choriomeningitis virus outbreak in man and laboratory animals. Am J Epidemiol. 1975;102:233.
25. Baum SG, Lewis AM Jr, Rowe WP, et al. Epidemic nonmeningitic lymphocytic-choriomeningitis-virus infection. N Engl J Med. 1966;274:934.
26. Armstrong D, Fortner JG, Rowe WP, et al. Meningitis due to lymphocytic choriomeningitis virus endemic in a hamster colony. JAMA. 1969;209:265.
27. Biggar RJ, Woodall JP, Walter PD, et al. Lymphocytic choriomeningitis outbreak associated with pet hamsters: Fifty-seven cases from New York State. JAMA. 1975;232:494.
28. Ackermann R, Stille W, Blumenthal W, et al. Syrische Goldhamster als Ubertrager von Lymphozytarer Choriomeningitis. Dtsch Med Wochenschr. 1972;97:1725.
29. Frame JD, Baldwin JM Jr, Gocke DJ, et al. Lassa fever, a new virus disease of man from West Africa. I. Clinical description and pathological findings. Am J Trop Med Hyg. 1970;19:670.
30. Green CA, Gordon DH, Lyons NF. Biological species in *Praomys (Mastomys) natalensis* (Smith), a rodent carrier of Lassa virus and bubonic plague in Africa. Am J Trop Med Hyg. 1978;27:627.
31. Robbins CB, Krebs JW Jr, Johnson KM. *Mastomys* (Rodentia: Muridae) species distinguished by hemoglobin pattern differences. Am J Trop Med Hyg. 1983;32:624.
32. Wulff H, McIntosh BM, Hamner DG, et al. Isolation of an arenavirus closely related to Lassa virus from *Mastomys natalensis* in south-east Africa. Bull WHO. 1977;55:441.
33. Johnson KM, Taylor P, Elliott LH, et al. Recovery of a Lassa related arenavirus in Zimbabwe. Am J Trop Med Hyg. 1981;30:1291.
34. Gonzalez JP, McCormick JB, Saluzzo JF, et al. An arenavirus isolated from wild caught rodents (*Praomys* species) in the Central African Republic. Intervirology. 1983;19:105.
35. Monath TP. Lassa fever: Review of epidemiology and epizootiology. Bull WHO. 1975;52:577.
36. McCormick JB. Clinical, epidemiologic, and therapeutic aspects of Lassa fever. Med Microbiol Immunol (Berl). 1986;175:153.
37. McCormick JB, Webb PA, Krebs JW, et al. A prospective study of the epidemiology and ecology of Lassa fever. J Infect Dis. 1987;155:437.
38. Frame JD. Surveillance of Lassa fever in missionaries stationed in West Africa. Bull WHO. 1975;52:593.
39. Sabattini MS, Maiztegui JI. Fiebre Hemorrhagica argentina. Medicina (Buenos Aires). 1970;30(Suppl):111.
40. Johnson KM, Kuns ML, Mackenzie RB, et al. Isolation of Machupo virus from wild rodent *Calomys callosus*. Am J Trop Med Hyg. 1966;15:103.
41. Crespo JA, Sabattini MS, Piantanida MJ, et al. Estudios ecologicos sobre reodores silvestres. Min Bienestar Social Argent. 1970; p 45.
42. Johnson KM, Webb PA, Justines G. Biology of Tacaribe-complex viruses. In Lehmann-Grubb F, ed. Lymphocytic Choriomeningitis Virus and Other Arenaviruses. New York: Springer Publishing; 1973:241.
43. Oldstone MBA, Dixon FJ. Pathogenesis of chronic disease associated with persistent lymphocytic choriomeningitis infection. II. Relationship of the anti-lymphocytic choriomeningitis immune response to tissue injury in chronic lymphocytic choriomeningitis disease. J Exp Med. 1970;131:1.
44. Webb P, Justines G, Johnson KM. Infection of wild and laboratory animals with Machupo and Latino viruses. Bull WHO. 1975;52:493.
45. Vitullo AD, Hodara VL, Merani MS. Effect of persistent infection with Junin virus on growth and reproduction of its natural reservoir, *Calomys musculinus*. Am J Trop Med Hyg. 1987;37:663.
46. Walker DH, Wulff H, Lange JV, et al. Comparative pathology of Lassa virus infection in monkeys, guinea pigs, and *Mastomys natalensis*. Bull WHO. 1975;52:523.
47. Jahrling PB, Hesse RA, Eddy GA, et al. Lassa virus infection of rhesus monkeys: Pathogenesis and treatment with ribavirin. J Infect Dis. 1980;141:580.
48. Kastello MD, Eddy GA, Kuehne RW. A rhesus monkey model for the study of Bolivian hemorrhagic fever. J Infect Dis. 1976;133:57.
49. González PH, Laguens RP, Frigerio MJ, et al. Junin virus infection of *Callithrix jacchus*: Pathologic features. Am J Trop Med Hyg. 1983;32:417.
50. McKee KT Jr, Mahlandt BG, Maiztegui JI, et al. Experimental Argentine hemorrhagic fever in rhesus monkeys: Viral strain-dependent clinical response. J Infect Dis. 1985;152:218.
51. Smadel JE, Green RH, Paltauf RM, et al. Lymphocytic choriomeningitis: Two human fatalities following an unusual febrile illness. Proc Soc Exp Biol. Med. 1942;49:683.
52. Walker DH, McCormick JB, Johnson KM, et al. Pathologic and virologic study of fatal Lassa fever in man. Am J Pathol. 1982;107:349.
53. McCormick JB, Walker DB, King IJ, et al. Lassa virus hepatitis: A study of fatal Lassa fever in humans. Am J Trop Med Hyg. 1986;35:401.
54. Fisher-Hoch SP, Mitchell SW, Sasso DR, et al. Physiological and immunologic disturbances associated with shock in a primate model of Lassa fever. J Infect Dis. 1987;155:465.
55. Levis SC, Saavedra MC, Ceccoli C, et al. Correlation between endogenous interferon and the clinical evolution of patients with Argentine hemorrhagic fever. J Interferon Res. 1985;5:383.
56. Vilček J. Adverse effects of interferon in virus infections, autoimmune diseases and acquired immunodeficiency. Prog Med Virol. 1984;30:62.
57. Monson MH, Frame JD, Jahrling PB, et al. Endemic Lassa fever in Liberia. I. Clinical and epidemiological aspects at Curran Lutheran Hospital, Zorzor, Liberia. Trans R Soc Trop Med Hyg. 1984;78:549.
58. McCormick JB, King IJ, Webb PA, et al. A case-control study of the clinical diagnosis and course of Lassa fever. J Infect Dis. 1987;155:445.
59. Webb PA, McCormick JB, King IJ, et al. Lassa fever in children in Sierra Leone, West Africa. Trans R Soc Trop Med Hyg. 1986;80:577.
60. Monson MH, Cole AK, Frame JD, et al. Pediatric Lassa fever: A review of 33 Liberian cases. Am J Trop Med Hyg. 1987;36:408.
61. Johnson KM, McCormick JB, Webb PA, et al. Clinical virology of Lassa fever in hospitalized patients. J Infect Dis. 1987;155:456.
62. McCormick JB, King IB, Webb PA, et al. Lassa fever: Effective therapy with ribavirin. N Engl J Med. 1986;314:20.
63. Maiztegui JI. Clinical and epidemiological patterns of Argentine haemorrhagic fever. Bull WHO. 1975;52:567.
64. Stinebaugh BJ, Schloeder FX, Johnson KM, et al. Bolivian hemorrhagic fever: A report of four cases. Am J Med. 1966;40:217.
65. Ambrosio AM, Enria DA, Maiztegui JI. Junin virus isolation from lymphomononuclear cells of patients with Argentine hemorrhagic fever. Intervirology. 1986;25:97.
66. Emond RTD, Bannister B, Lloyd G, et al. A case of Lassa fever: Clinical and virological findings. Br Med J. 1982;285:1001.
67. Niklasson BS, Jahrling PB, Peters CJ. Detection of Lassa virus antigens and Lassa virus-specific immunoglobulins G and M by enzyme-linked immunosorbent assay. J Clin Microbiol. 1984;20:239.
68. Jahrling PB, Niklasson BS, McCormick JB. Early diagnosis of human Lassa fever by ELISA; detection of antigen and antibody. Lancet. 1985;1:250.
69. Mackenzie RB. Epidemiology of Machupo virus infection. I. Pattern of human infection, San Joaquin, Bolivia, 1962–1965. Am J Trop Med Hyg. 1965;14:808.
70. Keenlyside RA, McCormick JB, Webb PA, et al. Case-control study of *Mastomys natalensis* and humans in Lassa virus-infected households in Sierra Leone. Am J Trop Med Hyg. 1983;32:829.
71. Mitchell SW, McCormick JB. Physicochemical inactivation of Lassa, Ebola, and Marburg viruses and effect on clinical laboratory analyses. J Clin Microbiol. 1984;20:486.
72. Clegg JCS, Lloyd G. Vaccinia recombinant expressing Lassa-virus internal nucleocapsid protein protects guinea pigs against Lassa fever. Lancet. 1987;2:186.
73. Maiztegui JI, Fernandez NJ, de Damilano AJ. Efficacy of immune plasma in treatment of Argentine hemorrhagic fever and association between treatment and a late neurological syndrome. Lancet. 1979;2:1216.
74. Enria DA, Briggiler AM, Fernandez NJ, et al. Importance of dose of neutralizing antibodies in treatment of Argentine haemorrhagic fever with immune plasma. Lancet. 1984;2:255.
75. Peters CJ, Jahrling PB, Liu CT, et al. Experimental studies of arenaviral hemorrhagic fevers. Curr Top Microbiol Immunol. 1987;134:5.
76. Jahrling PB, Peters CJ. Passive antibody therapy of Lassa fever in cynom-

olgus monkeys: Importance of neutralizing antibody and Lassa virus strain. Infect Immun. 1984;44:528.

Retroviridae

145. INTRODUCTION—TYPE C ONCOVIRUSES INCLUDING HUMAN T-CELL LEUKEMIA VIRUS TYPES I AND II

MARK STOECKLE

The discovery in 1911 by Rous of a virus that caused sarcomas in chickens[1] was followed by the identification of a number of viruses that produce solid tumors or leukemias in animals. Most of these oncogenic viruses were found to belong to a single virus family, the Retroviridae. However, there was no conclusive evidence for any human retrovirus until 1980 when investigators in Gallo's laboratory reported the isolation of a type C retrovirus, now called human T-cell leukemia virus type I (HTLV-I), from a patient with a T-cell malignancy.[2] Since then three additional human retroviruses have been characterized, and a remarkably complex picture of human retroviral disease has emerged. This section will describe the laboratory and clinical findings associated with the human type C oncoviruses HTLV-I and HTLV-II.

Two key discoveries laid the groundwork for the isolation of HTLV-I and other human and primate retroviruses. The first was the finding of reverse transcriptase in RNA tumor viruses, which was reported independently by Temin and Mizutani[3] and by Baltimore in 1970.[4] Based on this finding, sensitive assays of reverse transcriptase activity were designed that could be used to detect small amounts of virus. The second was the development of culture techniques for maintaining T lymphocytes in culture by using T-cell growth factor, now called interleukin-2.[5] Using these techniques Poiesz et al. isolated a novel retrovirus, now known as HTLV-I, from cultured T lymphocytes from a 28-year-old male with a cutaneous T-cell lymphoma.

In parallel with work in Gallo's laboratory, Japanese investigators had been studying a clinically distinct T-cell malignancy that was largely confined to persons born in the islands of southern Japan.[6] The striking geographic clustering of cases suggested that this disorder might be due to an infectious agent. In 1981 Japanese workers reported finding type C retrovirus particles in cell lines from patients with adult T-cell leukemia (ATL), and they named the putative agent adult T-cell leukemia virus (ATLV).[7] Retrospective analysis of the U.S. cases from which HTLV-I was isolated indicated that they were clinically indistinguishable from Japanese ATL. Subsequent work from many laboratories rapidly demonstrated that HTLV-I and ATLV are the same virus, that HTLV-I is the etiologic agent of ATL, and that HTLV-I infection is endemic in many scattered populations throughout the world.[8]

In 1982 Gallo and co-workers isolated a related but antigenically distinct type C retrovirus, designated HTLV-II, from patient with a T-cell variant of hairy cell leukemia.[9] A second isolate of HTLV-II from a patient with a similar variant form of hairy cell leukemia has been described, thus suggesting an etiologic role for HTLV-II in this particular disorder.[10]

After the discovery of HTLV-I and the role of the virus in ATL, an unexpected association with chronic neurologic disease was uncovered. In 1985 Gessain and colleagues reported that a large proportion of patients with tropical spastic paraparesis (TSP) in Martinique, where HTLV-I infection is endemic, had high levels of antibody to HTLV-1.[11]

THE PATHOGEN

HTLV-I and HTLV-II are type C oncoviruses, members of the family Retroviridae (Table 1). The virions are spherical, 100 nm in diameter, and are composed of an internal core of structural proteins (nucleocapsid, capsid, and matrix proteins [previously named p15, p24, and p19 *gag* proteins]) surrounding the viral RNA and polymerase and an outer layer of viral envelope glycoprotein (surface and transmembrane glycoprotein [previously named gp46 and gp41]) anchored in a lipid membrane.[8]

HTLV-I and -II contain several genes that are not present in most other retroviruses. These genes encode proteins that appear to regulate the expression of other viral genes.[12,13] The best characterized of these, designated *tax* (previously named *tat*-1), markedly enhances viral replication by increasing the transcription of viral RNA. HTLV-1 *tax* protein appears to be unrelated in structure and function to HIV-1 *tat* proteins.[14]

HTLV-1 is very similar to simian T-cell lymphotropic virus (STLV).[15] However, the human and primate viruses are clearly distinct, and there is no evidence that monkeys serve as a reservoir for human infection. HTLV-II is relatively divergent, with approximately 70 percent amino acid sequence identity to HTLV-I.[16,17] HTLV-I and -II are more distantly related to the human and simian immunodeficiency viruses (HIV-1 and -2 and SIV).

TABLE 1. Human Retroviruses

Oncoviruses
- Human T-cell leukemia virus type I (HTLV-I)
  - *Former names*: Human T-cell lymphotropic virus type I or adult T-cell leukemia virus (ATLV)
  - *Epidemiology*: Highest prevalence in southern Japan and the Caribbean basin (including blacks in SE U.S.). Transmission occurs through the same routes as HIV-1
  - *Clinical illness*: Approximately 1% of persons infected in childhood develop adult T-cell leukemia–lymphoma (ATLL) as adults. HTLV-I infection is also associated with an illness known as tropical spastic paraparesis (TSP) or HTLV-I–associated myelopathy (HAM)
- Human T-cell leukemia virus type II
  - *Epidemiology*: Unknown
  - *Clinical illness*: Unknown. Possible etiologic role in atypical T-cell hairy cell leukemia

Lentiviruses
- Human immunodeficiency virus type 1 (HIV-1)
  - *Former names*: Human T-cell lymphotropic virus type III (HTLV-III) or lymphadenopathy-associated virus (LAV, LAV-1)
  - *Epidemiology*: Now distributed worldwide. The prevalence of infection and the patterns of transmission vary widely in different areas
  - *Clinical illness*: A large proportion of HIV-1–infected persons develop acquired immunodeficiency syndrome (AIDS) or AIDS-related illnesses. The time from acquisition of infection to clinical illness is usually several years
- Human immunodeficiency virus type 2 (HIV-2)
  - *Former names*: Human T-cell lymphotropic virus type IV (HTLV-IV) or lymphadenopathy-associated virus type 2 (LAV-2)
  - *Epidemiology*: Limited to West Africa with a few cases in Europe and the U.S.
  - *Clinical illness*: Possibly less pathogenic than HIV-1, but can cause AIDS

Spumaviruses
- Human foamy virus
  - *Other names*: Human spumaretrovirus, human syncytium-forming virus
  - *Epidemiology*: Unknown
  - *Clinical illness*: Unknown. Isolates have been obtained from patients with a variety of inflammatory and neoplastic diseases, but no pathogenic role has been established

EPIDEMIOLOGY OF HTLV-I

Geographic Distribution

At present, HTLV-I infection is largely confined to a few scattered populations. The two best-studied areas are the islands of southwestern Japan where approximately 20 percent of the adult population is seropositive,[18] and the Caribbean basin, where 2–5 percent of black adults are seropositive. The endemic areas in the Caribbean basin include the West Indies[8,19–21] (cases reported from Jamaica, Trinidad, and the Lesser Antilles), northern South America[8,22] (cases reported from Venezuela, Ecuador, Peru, Columbia, Guyana, Surinam, Brazil), and the southeastern United States[23–25] (cases reported from Florida, Georgia, Alabama, North Carolina, Texas). HTLV-1 infection is also found in immigrant populations from the following areas: in West Indians living in England,[26] in natives of southern Japan living in Hawaii,[27] and in blacks from southern United States in New York City.[28]

In addition to these well-studied populations, serologic surveys indicate the presence of HTLV-I in other areas including Africa,[29–31] the Middle East,[32] the Arctic,[33] and islands of the Indian Ocean[34] and the south Pacific.[35] However, some of these findings have been questioned.[36–38] At present the distribution and prevalence of HTLV-I in many populations, especially in Africa, is not well understood.

HTLV-I is rare in the general population in the United States. From a serologic study of adults who received multiple blood products in New York City in 1976–1983, it was calculated that 2.3 units per 10,000 carried HTLV-I.[39] A nearly identical result was obtained in a study of sera of 39,898 U.S. blood donors in which 10 were seropositive for HTLV-I (2.5 per 10,000).[40] HTLV-I infection is also rare in Europe, although a focus of infection has been reported in a native population in southern Italy.[41] HTLV-I seropositivity has been reported in occasional male homosexuals in Europe and the United States[42,43] as well as in 15 percent of male homosexuals in an endemic area.[44] In addition, 18–49 percent of intravenous drug users are reported to be seropositive, with the highest prevalence in black drug abusers in the United States.[45–47]

The prevalence of seropositivity increases with age in endemic populations.[18] It has been suggested that this is due to a historical change in the transmission of HTLV-I,[48] to the acquisition of disease in adulthood by undefined routes,[35] or to delayed seroconversion in persons with latent infection.[27]

Transmission

HTLV-I is transmitted from mother to child, by sexual contact from male to female and male to male, by blood transfusion, and by contaminated needles. In endemic areas, seropositives are clustered in families, which probably reflects the predominance of mother–child and male–female transmission. All studies indicate that infection persists for life. Virus is consistently isolated from seropositive persons regardless of their clinical status.

Mother to Child. Most infections that are acquired in childhood can be traced to a seropositive mother. In one study 27 percent of the children with a seropositive mother and a seropositive father were seropositive, whereas 0 of 82 children with a seronegative mother and a seropositive father was seropositive.[49] Thus, infection was transmitted exclusively from mother to child, irrespective of the father's status. Breast milk is thought to be an important vehicle of transmission of HTLV-I because seroconversion is unusual in infants who are not breast-fed.[50] In addition, virus-positive lymphocytes are abundant in the breast milk of seropositive mothers,[51] and infection can be transmitted to animals by feeding infected breast milk.[52] Abstaining from breast feeding may break the cycle of endemicity in some populations.

Maternal anti–HTLV-I IgG is present in the cord blood of virtually all infants born to seropositive mothers, but anti–HTLV-I IgM and virus-positive lymphocytes are not found, which suggests the absence of prenatal transmission.[53] Maternal antibody persists until 3–6 months of age in a small minority of cases. Seroconversion and virus-positive lymphocytes are not detected until 9–18 months,[53,54] which is thought to reflect delayed postnatal transmission.

Heterosexual. Sexual transmission from husband to wife, but infrequently from wife to husband, is inferred from the epidemiologic data. In a study in Japan, the probability of husband-to-wife transmission was calculated to be 61 percent over a period of 10 years; that from wife to husband was less than 1 percent over the 10-year period.[49] Virus-positive mononuclear cells have been detected in the semen of a seropositive man.[55] This finding together with the observation that female-to-male transmission is very low suggests that semen is the major vehicle of sexual transmission. The use of condoms may prevent the sexual transmission of HTLV-I.

Homosexual. Given what is known about HIV-1, it is not surprising that HTLV-I seropositivity is more prevalent in male homosexuals than in the general population. In a study of male homosexuals in Trinidad, seroprevalence for HIV-1 was three times higher than that for HTLV-I (40 vs. 15 percent) which suggests that HTLV-I is less efficiently transmitted by homosexual contact than HIV-1 is.[44]

Blood Products. Whole blood, packed cells, and platelet concentrates from seropositive donors will transmit infection. In one study, 26 of 41 (63 percent) of recipients of 1 or 2 units of such blood products demonstrated seroconversion.[56] Anti–HTLV-I IgM and IgG antibodies were first detected at 3 to 6 weeks. On the other hand, 0 of 14 patients who received 1 unit of fresh frozen plasma from an infected donor showed seroconversion, which suggests that the titer of virus is low in cell-free blood products. In support of this, HTLV-I seroconversion has not been detected in hemophiliacs who received pooled clotting factor concentrates prepared in the United States.[57,58] However, experience with pooled clotting factors prepared from seropositive donors has not been reported, so the risk of transmission cannot be confidently said to be zero.

HTLV-I transmission from a seronegative donor has not been described. However, virus has been isolated from a seronegative individual.[59] On the other hand, the risk of transmission from mother to child is proportional to the mother's anti–HTLV-I titer,[60] thus suggesting that virus-positive persons with low or undetectable antibody levels are at low risk for transmission.

EPIDEMIOLOGY OF HTLV-II

The distribution of HTLV-II is not known. Only four cases of HTLV-II infection have been documented by virus isolation: two U.S. whites with a T-cell variant of hairy cell leukemia, 1 patient with the acquired immunodeficiency syndrome (AIDS), and 1 hemophilia A patient with pancytopenia.[9,10] Increased HTLV-II seropositivity is reported in intravenous drug users in New York City (10 of 56 positive)[46] and in England (3 of 113 positive).[42] However, current serologic studies are confounded by cross-reaction with HTLV-I antigens.

ADULT T-CELL LEUKEMIA–LYMPHOMA

Evidence That HTLV-I Is the Etiologic Agent of Adult T-Cell Leukemia–Lymphoma

The evidence indicating that HTLV-I is the etiologic agent of adult T-cell leukemia–lymphoma (ATLL) can be summarized as follows: (*1*) virtually all cases of ATLL are seropositive for HTLV-I; (*2*) HTLV-I provirus is present in leukemic cells but not in other cells from patients with ATLL; and (*3*) HTLV-1 provirus is monoclonally integrated in leukemic cells, which indicates that infection preceded the development of malignancy.[61,62] In addition, STLV, which is closely related to HTLV-I, is associated with leukemia in monkeys.[63]

Incidence of ATLL

Adult T-cell leukemia–lymphoma develops in a small minority of HTLV-I carriers. In Japan, the annual incidence of ATLL among 1000 HTLV-I carriers older than 40 years is estimated to be 1 in females and 2 in males.[64] It is thought that more women than men acquire infection through sexual transmission. This may explain the difference in incidence since women who acquire infection as adults from infected husbands have less time for ATLL to develop. Alternatively, it is suggested that a prerequisite for ATLL may be the establishment of infection in childhood or the introduction of infection by the mother–child route. Interestingly, no case of ATLL has been traced to blood transfusion, which may also be due to the late acquisition of infection since most transfusions are administered to adults.

Clinical Illness

Adult T-cell leukemia–lymphoma is a malignant proliferation of HTLV-I–infected mature T cells. Adult T-cell leukemia–lymphoma may produce a smoldering leukemia that is present for years or a fulminant illness progressing to death within a few months. The disease has been well described in Japan,[6,65–69] the United States,[23,70,71] and the Caribbean[26,72,73] and is similar in all areas except that ATLL is seen in younger persons in the United States than in Japan (mean age at presentation, 34 years and 55 years, respectively).

The most common physical findings at presentation are lymphadenopathy, skin lesions, hepatomegaly, and splenomegaly. Rapid development of diffuse peripheral lymphadenopathy without mediastinal involvement is typical. The skin lesions seen in ATLL are varied and include localized or diffuse nodules and papules, localized erythema and plaques, and generalized erythroderma (Fig. 1). Recurrent superficial fungal infections are a frequent finding and may be the presenting complaint.

An elevated WBC count of 10,000–100,000 cells/mm^3 that consists of abnormal lymphocytes and normal neutrophils is present in most patients, but a lymphomatous presentation without circulating leukemic cells occurs in up to one-third of cases. Circulating lymphocytes with indented nuclei are highly suggestive of ATLL (Fig. 2). A biopsy of skin lesions usually reveals dermal or epidermal infiltration of malignant cells. In lymph nodes, diffuse infiltration of pleomorphic lymphocytes is found. The phenotype of malignant cells present in blood and tissues is that of activated mature helper T cells; CD4+, CD8-, TdT-, E-rosette–positive, Tac antigen–positive. Southern analysis reveals a monoclonal integration of HTLV-I proviral DNA.[74] Patients with smoldering leukemia typically have a normal WBC count with a small percentage of leukemic cells and have minimal skin and organ involvement. A progressive wasting illness in a patient with chronic ATL has also been described.[71]

Elevated serum calcium levels are seen in most patients with aggressive disease and may be accompanied by diffuse lytic lesions detected on bone x-ray. The cause of hypercalcemia is not known. A biopsy of the lytic lesions reveals activated osteoclasts without lymphoma cells. Levels of parathyroid hormone, vitamin D osteoclast activating factor, and serum phosphorus are usually normal.

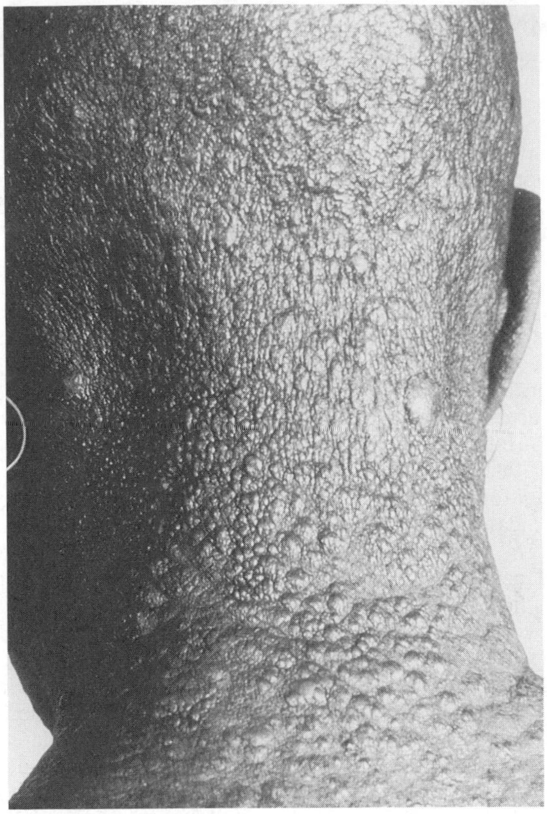

FIG. 1. Skin lesions in an adult patient with ATLL. (Courtesy of Dr. Samuel Broder, National Cancer Institute, Washington DC.)

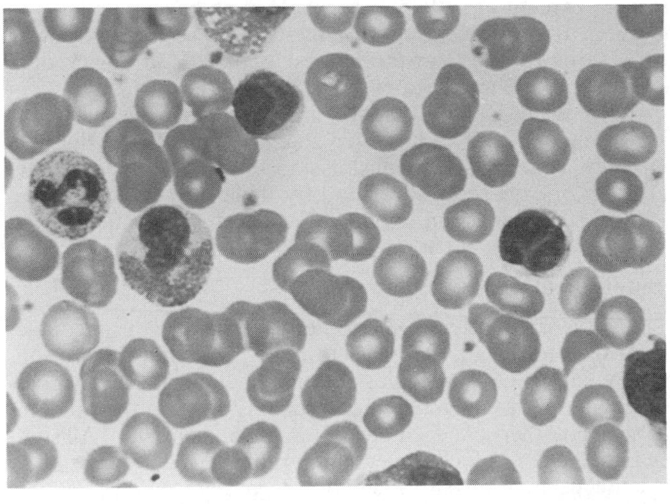

FIG. 2. A blood smear of a patient with ATLL shows an atypical lymphocyte with an indented nucleus. (Courtesy of Dr. Samuel Broder, National Cancer Institute, Washington DC.)

Infectious Complications

Opportunistic infections are frequent in patients with ATLL. The spectrum of infectious agents is similar to that seen in AIDS, including protozoans (*Pneumocystis carinii* pneumonia), fungi (*Cryptococcus neoformans* meningitis, candidal esophagitis), and viruses (cytomegalovirus [CMV] pneumonia, herpes zoster, generalized herpes simplex) as well as bacterial infections related to chemotherapy-induced neutropenia.

Immunity may also be impaired in HTLV-I–infected persons in the absence of extensive malignant disease. Dermatophyte infections are a frequent presenting complaint in patients with chronic ATLL.[66,67] Carriage of *Strongyloides stercoralis* is reported to be more frequent in apparently healthy HTLV-I seropositives than in seronegative controls.[75]

Pathogenesis

The mechanisms of oncogenesis in ATLL are not known. The *tax* protein of HTLV-I can activate cellular genes and is oncogenic in animals, which suggests that it may be important in pathogenesis.[76]

Diagnosis

Adult T-cell leukemia–lymphoma should be suspected in any adult patient with a T-cell malignancy who is from a population with endemic infection. The presence of skin lesions, hypercalcemia, and abnormal circulating lymphocytes are highly suggestive. The diagnosis of ATLL should be considered in patients who are thought to have other cutaneous T-cell malignancies including mycosis fungoides, Sézary syndrome, and cutaneous T-cell lymphoma. Adult T-cell leukemia–lymphoma patients with a lymphomatous presentation are often initially classified as having non-Hodgkin's lymphoma. The diagnosis can be confirmed by testing for anti-HTLV-I antibody and identification of monoclonal integration of proviral DNA in the malignant cells.

Treatment

Most patients with acute presentations will respond to chemotherapy for non-Hodgkin's lymphoma, but the duration of remission is usually short. Although a few cases of prolonged survival have been reported, the median survival in patients with acute presentations is 6 months. Nucleotide analogues will inhibit HTLV-I in vitro[77] and might be useful at some stage in HTLV-I disease. However, viral RNA and protein are not detected in fresh lymphocytes from patients with ATLL,[78] which suggests that antiviral therapy would not be effective at this stage.

NEUROLOGIC COMPLICATIONS OF HTLV-I INFECTIONS

HTLV-I is linked to some cases of neurologic disease with slowly progressive spastic paraparesis and mild sensory involvement.[11,79–82] Various clinical diagnoses have been applied to these patients including tropical spastic paraparesis (TSP), HTLV-I–associated myelopathy (HAM), and chronic progressive myelopathy (CPM). The evidence for the involvement of HTLV-I in these syndromes is (*1*) the occurrence of disease in areas endemic for HTLV-I, (*2*) high-titer anti-HTLV-I antibodies in the serum and cerebrospinal fluid (CSF) of affected patients, and (*3*) the demonstration of viral DNA and proteins and the isolation of virus from the CSF.[82,83] However, only 60–80 percent of patients with TSP or CPM are seropositive for HTLV-I, which suggests that these clinical diagnoses include diseases of differing etiology. The onset of myelopathy after a blood transfusion is reported, with a mean interval between transfusion and symptoms of 2 years (range, 6 months to 8 years).[84]

The mean age at the onset of symptoms is 40–50 years, and the usual complaints are bilateral weakness and stiffness of the lower extremities. Other symptoms are peripheral numbness or dysesthesia, back pain, and urinary symptoms of frequency, urgency, and incontinence. Neurologic examination reveals spastic paraparesis with hyperactive deep tendon reflexes. Mild sensory changes may be noted. Cerebrospinal fluid examination may be normal or may show slight elevations of protein levels and mononuclear cell counts. Abnormal lymphocytes similar to those seen in ATLL may be present in the CSF or peripheral blood. Oligoclonal banding of the CSF is also described. A favorable response to steroids has been described in Japanese patients.[80]

INTERACTIONS WITH OTHER RETROVIRUSES

Co-infection with HIV-1 and HTLV-I is described in clinically well individuals and in patients with AIDS,[85,86] but the consequences of dual infection are not established. In one small study in Trinidad, the rate of progression to AIDS was higher in persons seropositive for HIV-1 and HTLV-I as compared with persons seropositive for HIV-1 alone.[87] One patient infected with HIV-1 and HTLV-I had an unusual CD8+ T-cell malignancy.[88]

OTHER ILLNESSES ASSOCIATED WITH HTLV-I

In endemic areas, the seroprevalence of HTLV-I is higher in patients with B-cell chronic lymphocytic leukemia (CLL) than in the general population.[89] Two seropositive patients with B-cell CLL were found to have anti-HTLV-I immunoglobulin on the malignant cells, which suggests that chronic antigenic stimulation by HTLV-I played a role in the development of disease.[90]

Increased seroprevalence is also reported in patients with polymyositis.[91] In addition, some studies have suggested a role for HTLV-I or a related retrovirus in multiple sclerosis,[92] but these findings have not been replicated in other studies.[38,93]

REFERENCES

1. Rous P. A sarcoma of the fowl transmissible by an agent separable from the tumor cells. J Exp Med. 1911;13:397–411.
2. Poiesz BJ, Ruscetti FW, Gazdar AF, et al. Detection and isolation of type C retrovirus particles from fresh and cultured lymphocytes of a patient with cutaneous T-cell lymphoma. Proc Natl Acad Sci USA. 1980;77:7415–19.
3. Temin HM, Mizutani S. RNA-dependent DNA polymerase in virions of Rous sarcoma virus. Nature. 1970;226:1211–3.
4. Baltimore D. RNA-dependent DNA polymerase in virions of RNA tumor viruses. Nature. 1970;226:1209–11.
5. Morgn DA, Ruscetti FW, Gallo R. Selective in vitro growth of T lymphocytes from normal human bone marrows. Science. 1976;193:1006–7.
6. Uchiyama T, Yodoi J, Sagawa K, et al. Adult T-cell leukemia: Clinical and hematologic features of 16 cases. Blood. 1977;50:481–92.
7. Hinuma Y, Nagata K, Hanaoka M, et al. Adult T-cell leukemia: Antigen in an ATL cell line and detection of antibodies to the antigen in human sera. Proc Natl Acad Sci USA. 1981;78:6474–80.
8. Wong-Staal F, Gallo RC. Human T-lymphotropic retroviruses. Nature. 1985;317:395–403.
9. Kalyanaraman VS, Sarngadharan MG, Robert-Guroff M, et al. A new subtype of human T-cell leukemia virus (HTLV-II) associated with a T-cell variant of hairy cell leukemia. Science. 1982;218:571–3.
10. Rosenblatt JD, Golde DW, Washsman W, et al. A second isolate of HTLV-II associated with atypical hairy-cell leukemia. N Engl J Med. 1986;315:372–7.
11. Gessain A, Barin F, Vernant JC, et al. Antibodies to human T-lymphotropic virus type-I in patients with tropical spastic paralysis. Lancet. 1985;2:407–9.
12. Nagashima K, Yoshida M, Seiki M. A single species of pX mRNA of human T-cell leukemia virus type I encodes trans-activator p40x and two other phosphoproteins. J Virol. 1986;60:394–9.
13. Rosenblatt JD, Cann AJ, Slamon DJ, et al. HTLV-II transactivation is regulated by the overlapping *tax/rex* nonstructural genes. Science. 1988;240:916–9.
14. Siekevitz M, Josephs SF, Dukovich M, et al. Activation of the HIV-1 LTR by T cell mitogens and the trans-activator protein of HTLV-I. Science. 1987;238:1575–8.
15. Watanabe T, Seiki M, Tsujimoto, H, et al. Sequence homology of the simian retrovirus genome with human T-cell leukemia virus type I. Virology. 1985;144:59–65.
16. Sodroski J, Patarca R, Perkins D, et al. Sequence of the envelope glycoprotein gene of type II human T lymphotropic virus. Science. 1984;225:421–4.
17. Haseltine WA, Sodroski, J, Patarca R, et al. Structure of the 3′ terminal region of type II human T lymphotropic virus: Evidence for new coding region. Science. 1984;225:419–21.
18. Hinuma Y, Komoda H, Chosa T, et al. Antibodies to adult T-cell leukemia-virus–associated antigen (ATLA) in sera from patients with ATL and controls in Japan: A nation-wide seroepidemiologic study. Int J Cancer. 1982;29:631–5.
19. Schupbach J, Kalyanaraman VS, Sarngadharan MG, et al. Antibodies against

three purified proteins of the human type C retrovirus, human T-cell leukemia-lymphoma virus, in adult T-cell leukemia-lymphoma patients and healthy blacks from the Caribbean. Cancer Res. 1983;43:886–91.
20. Schaffar-DesHayes H, Chavance M, Monplaisir N, et al. Antibodies to HTLV-I p24 in sera of blood donors, elderly people and patients with hemopoietic diseases in France and in French West Indies. Int J Cancer. 1984;34:667–70.
21. Miller GJ, Pegram SM, Kirkwood BR, et al. Ethnic composition, age and sex, together with location and standard of housing as determinants of HLTV-I infection in an urban Trinidadian community. Int J Cancer. 1986;38:801–8.
22. Roman G. The neuroepidemiology of tropical spastic paralysis. Ann Neurol. 1988;23(Suppl):113–20.
23. Bunn Jr PA, Schechter GP, Jaffe E, et al. Clinical course of retrovirus-associated adult T-cell lymphoma in the United States. N Engl J Med. 1983;309:257–64.
24. Blayney DW, Blattner WA, Robert-Guroff M, et al. The human T-cell leukemia-lymphoma virus in the southeastern United States. JAMA. 1983;250:1048–52.
25. Centers for Disease Control. Adult T-celll leukemia/lymphoma associated with human T-lymphotropic virus type I (HTLV-I) infection—North Carolina. MMWR. 1987;36:804–12.
26. Catovsky D, Greaves MF, Rose M, et al: Adult T-cell lymphoma-leukaemia in blacks from the West Indies. Lancet. 1982;1:639–43.
27. Blattner WA, Nomura A, Clark JW, et al. Modes of transmission and evidence for viral latency from studies of human T-cell lymphotrophic virus type I in Japanese migrant populations in Hawaii. Proc Natl Acad Sci USA. 1986;83:4895–8.
28. Dosik H, Anandakrishman A, Denic S, et al. Adult T cell leukemia/lymphoma. A cluster in Brooklyn, a new endemic area (Abstract). Blood. 1985; 66(Suppl):187.
29. Hunsmann G, Schneider J, Schmitt J, et al. Detection of serum antibodies to adult T-cell leukemia virus in non-human primates and in people from Africa. Int J Cancer. 1983;32:329–32.
30. Saxinger W, Blattner WA, Levine PH, et al. Human T-cell leukemia virus (HTLV-I) antibodies in Africa. Science. 1984;225:1473–6.
31. Biggar RJ, Saxinger C, Gardiner C, et al. Type-I HTLV antibody in urban and rural Ghana, West Africa. Int J Cancer. 1984;34:215–9.
32. Ben-Ishai A, Haas M, Triglia D, et al. Human T-cell lymphotropic virus type-I antibodies in Falashas and other ethnic groups in Israel. Nature. 1985;315:665–6.
33. Robert-Guroff M, Clark J, Lanier AP, et al. Prevalence of HTLV-I in arctic regions. Int J Cancer. 1985;36:651–5.
34. Roman GC, Schoenberg BS, Madden DL, et al. Human T-lymphotropic virus type I antibodies in the serum of patients with tropical spastic paraparesis in the Seychelles. Arch Neurol. 1987;44:605–7.
35. Kazura JW, Saxinger WC, Wenger J, et al. Epidemiology of human T cell leukemia virus type I infection in East Sepik Province, Papua New Guinea. J Infect Dis. 1987;155:1100–7.
36. Karpas A, Maayan S, Raz R. Lack of antibodies to adult T-cell leukaemia virus and to AIDS virus in Israeli Falashas. Nature. 1986;319:794.
37. Weiss RA, Cheingsong-Popov R, Clayden S, et al. Lack of HTLV-I antibodies in Africans. Nature. 1986;319:794–5.
38. Karpas A, Malik K, Lida J. Studies of human retroviruses in relation to adult T-cell leukaemia, acquired immune deficiency syndrome and multiple sclerosis. Arch Virol. 1987;95:237–49.
39. Minamoto GY, Gold JWM, Scheinberg DA, et al. Infection with human T-cell leukemia virus type I in patients with leukemia. N Engl J Med. 1988;318:219–22.
40. Williams AE, Fang Chyang CT, Slamon DJ, et al. Seroprevalence and epidemiological correlates of HTLV-I infection in U.S. blood donors. Science. 1988;240:643–6.
41. Manzari V, Gradilone A, Barillari G, et al. HTLV-I is endemic in southern Italy: Detection of the first infectious cluster in a white population. Int J Cancer. 1985;36:557–9.
42. Tedder RS, Shanson DC, Jeffries DJ, et al. Low prevalence in the UK of HTLV-I and HTLV-II infection in subjects with AIDS, with extended lymphadenopathy, and at risk of AIDS. Lancet. 1984;2:125–7.
43. Robert-Gurofff M, Blayney DW, Safai B, et al. HTLV-1-specific antibody in AIDS patients and others at risk. Lancet. 1984;2:128–30.
44. Bartholomew C, Saxinger WC, Clark JW, et al. Transmission of HTLV-I and HIV among homosexual men in Trinidad. JAMA. 1987;257:2605–8.
45. Gradilone A, Zani M, Barillari G, et al. HTLV-I and HIV infection in drug addicts in Italy. Lancet. 1986;2:753–4.
46. Robert-Guroff M, Weiss SH, Giron JA, et al. Prevalence of antibodies to HTLV-I, -II and -II in intravenous drug abusers from an AIDS endemic region. JAMA. 1986;255:3133–7.
47. Weiss SH, Ginzburg HM, Saxinger WC, et al. Emerging high rates of human T-cell lymphotropic virus type I (HTLV-I) and HIV infection among U.S. drug aubsers (Abstract). Proceedings of the Third International Conference on AIDS, 1987.
48. Sugiyama H, Doi H, Yamaguchi K, et al. Significance of postnatal mother-to-child transmission of human T-lymphotropic virus type-I on the development of adult T-cell leukemia/lymphoma. J Med Virol. 1986;20:253–60.
49. Kajiyama W, Kashiwagi S, Ikematsu H, et al. Intrafamilial transmission of adult T cell leukemia virus. J Infect Dis. 1986;154:851–7.
50. Ando Y, Nakano S, Saito K, et al. Transmission of adult T-cell leukemia retrovirus (HTLV-I) from mother to child: Comparison of bottle-fed with breast-fed babies. Jpn J Cancer Res. 1987;78:322–4.
51. Kinoshita K, Amagasaki T, Hino S, et al. Milk-borne transmission of HTLV-I from carrier mothers to their children. Jpn J Cancer Res. 1987;78:674–80.
52. Uemura Y, Kotani S, Yoshimoto S, et al. Oral transmission of human T-cell leukemia virus type I in the rabbit. Jpn J Cancer Res. 1986;77:970–3.
53. Hino S, Yamaguchi K, Katamine S, et al. Mother-to-child transmission of human T-cell leukemia virus type-I. Jpn J Cancer Res. 1985;76:474–80.
54. Nakano S, Ando Y, Saito K, et al. Primary infection of Japanese infants with adult T-cell leukaemia-associated retrovirus (ATLV): Evidence for viral transmission from mothers to children. J Infect. 1986;12:205–12.
55. Nakano S, Ando Y, Ichijo M, et al. Search for possible routes of vertical and horizontal transmission of adult T-cell leukemia virus. Jpn J Cancer Res. 1984;75:1044–5.
56. Ocochi K, Sato H, Hinuma Y. A retrospective study on transmission of adult T cell leukemia virus by blood transfusion: Seroconversion in recipients. Vox Sang. 1984;46:245–53.
57. Chorba TL, Jason JM, Ramsey RB, et al. HTLV-I antibody status in hemophilia patients treated with factor concentrates prepared from U.S. plasma sources, and in hemophilia patients with AIDS. Thromb Haemost. 1985;53:180–2.
58. Jason JM, McDougal JS, Cabradilla C, et al. Human T-cell leukemia virus (HTLV-I) p24 antibody in New York City blood product recipients. Am J Hematol. 1985;20:129–37.
59. Sarin PS, Aoki T, Shibata A, et al. High incidence of human type-C retrovirus (HTLV) in family members of a HTLV-positive Japanese T-cell leukemia patient. Proc Natl Acad Sci USA. 1983;80:2370–4.
60. Hino S, Doi H, Yoshikuni H, et al. HTLV-I carrier mothers with high-titer antibody are at high risk as a source of infection. Jpn J Cancer Res. 1987;78:1156–8.
61. Yoshida M. Human leukemia virus associated with adult T-cell leukemia. Jpn J Cancer Res. 1983;74:777–89.
62. Kuefler PR, Bunn Jr PA. Adult T cell leukemia/lymphoma. Clin Haematol. 1986;15:695–726.
63. Tsujimoto H, Noda Y, Ishikawa K, et al. Development of adult T-cell leukemia-like disease in African green monkey associated with clonal integration of simian T-cell leukemia virus type I. Cancer Res. 1987;47:269–74.
64. Tajima K, Kamura S, Ito S, et al. Epidemiologic features of HTLV-I carriers and incidence of ATL in an ATL-endemic island: A report of the community-based co-operative study in Tsushima, Japan. Int J Cancer. 1987;40:741–6.
65. Kinoshita K, Kamhira S, Ikeda S, et al. Clinical, hematologic, and pathologic features of leukemia T-cell lymphoma. Cancer. 1982;50:1554–62.
66. Yamaguchi K, Nishimura H, Kohrogi H, et al. A proposal for smoldering adult T-cell leukemia: A clinicopathological study of five cases. Blood. 1983;62:758–66.
67. Kawano F, Yamaguchi K, Nishimura H, et al. Variation in the clinical courses of adult T-cell leukemia. Cancer. 1985;55:851–6.
68. Clark JW, Robert-Guroff M, Ikehara O, et al. Human T-cell leukemia-lymphoma virus type 1 and adult T-cell leukemia-lymphoma in Okinawa. Cancer Res. 1985;45:3849–52.
69. Kinoshita K, Amagasaki T, Ikeda S, et al. Preleukemic state of adult T cell leukemia: Abnormal T lymphocytosis induced by human adult T cell leukemia-lymphoma virus. Blood. 1985;66:120–7.
70. NIH Conference. T-cell lymphoproliferative syndrome associated with human T-cell leukemia/lymphoma virus. Ann Intern Med. 1984;100:543–57.
71. Ratner L, Griffith RC, Marselle L, et al. A lymphoproliferative disorder caused by human T-lymphotropic virus type I. Am J Med. 1987;83:953–8.
72. Blattner WA, Gibbs WN, Saxinger C, et al. Human T-cell leukaemia/lymphoma virus-associated lymphoreticular neoplasia in Jamaica. Lancet. 1983;2:61–4.
73. Gibbs WB, Lofters WS, Campbell M, et al. Non-Hodgkin lymphoma in Jamaica and its relation to adult T-cell leukemia-lymphoma. Ann Intern Med. 1987;106:361–8.
74. Yoshida M, Seiki M, Yamaguchi K, et al. Monoclonal integration of human T-cell leukemia provirus in all primary tumors of adult T-cell leukemia suggests causative role of human T-cell leukemia virus in the disease. Proc Natl Acad Sci USA. 1984;81:2534–7.
75. Nakada K, Kohakura M, Komoda H, et al. High incidence of HTLV antibody in carriers of *Strongyloides stercoralis*. Lancet. 1984;1:683.
76. Nerenberg M, Hinrichs SH, Reynolds RK, et al. The *tat* gene of human T-lymphotropic virus type 1 induces mesenchymal tumors in transgenic mice. Science. 1987;237:1324–9.
77. Matsushita S, Mitsuya H, Reitz MS, et al. Pharmacologic inhibition of in vitro infectivity of human T lymphotropic virus type I. J Clin Invest. 1987;80:394–400.
78. Franchini G, Wong-Staal F, Gallo RC. Human T-cell leukemia virus (HTLV-I) transcripts in fresh and cultured cells of patients with adult T-cell leukemia. Proc Natl Acad Sci USA. 1984;81:6207–11.
79. Osame M, Usuku K, Izumo S, et al. HTLV-I associated myelopathy, a new clinical entity. Lancet. 1986;1:1031–2.
80. Osame M, Matsumoto M, Usuku K, et al. Chronic progressive myelopathy associated with elevated antibodies to human T-lymphotropic virus type I and adult T-cell leukemialike cells. Ann Neurol. 1988;21:117–22.
81. Vernant JC, Maurs L, Gessain A, et al. Endemic tropical spastic paralysis associated with human T-lymphotropic virus type I: A clinical and seroepidemiologic study of 25 cases. Ann Neurol. 1988;21:123–30.
82. Bhagavati S, Ehrlich G, Kula RW, et al. Detection of human T-cell lymphoma/

leukemia virus type I DNA and antigen in spinal fluid and blood of patients with chronic progressive myelopathy. N Engl J Med. 1988;318:1141–7.
83. Jacobson S, Raine CS, Mingioli ES, et al. Isolation of an HTLV-1-like retrovirus from patients with tropical spastic paraparesis. Nature. 1988;331:540–3.
84. Osame M, Izumo S, Igata A, et al. Blood transfusion and HTLV-I associated myelopathy. Lancet. 1986;2:104–5.
85. Getchell JP, Heath JL, Hicks DR, et al. Detection of human T cell leukemia virus type I and human immunodeficiency virus in cultured lymphocytes of a Zairian man with AIDS. J Infect Dis. 1987;155:612–6.
86. Kanner SB, Parks ES, Scott GB, et al. Simultaneous infections with human T cell leukemia virus type I and the human immunodeficiency virus. J Infect Dis. 1987;155:617–25.
87. Bartholomew C, Blattner W, Cleghorn F. Progression to AIDS in homosexual men co-infected with HIV and HTLV-I in Trinidad. Lancet. 1987;2:1469.
88. Harper ME, Kaplan MH, Marselle LM, et al. Concomitant infection with HTLV-I and HTLV-III in a patient with T8 lymphoproliferative disease. N Engl J Med. 1986;315:1073–8.
89. Fleming AF, Maharajan R, Abraham M, et al. Antibodies to HTLV-I in Nigerian blood-donors, their relatives and patients with leukaemias, lymphomas and other diseases. Int J Cancer. 1986;38:809–13.
90. Mann DL, DeSantis P, Mark G, et al. HTLV-I-associated B-cell CLL: Indirect role for retrovirus in leukemogenesis. Science. 1987;236:1103–6.
91. Mora CA, Garruto RM, Brown P, et al: Seroprevalence of antibodies to HTLV-I in patients with chronic neurological disorders other than tropical spastic paraparesis. Ann Neurol. 1988;23(Suppl):192–5.
92. Koprowski H, DeFreitas EC, Harper ME, et al. Multiple sclerosis and human T-cell lymphotropic retroviruses. Nature. 1985;318:154–60.
93. Madden DL, Mundon FK, Tzan NR, et al. Antibody to human and simian retrovirus, HTLV-I, HTLV-II, HIV, STLV-II, and SRV-I not increased in patients with multiple sclerosis. Ann Neurol. 1988;23(Suppl):171–3.

146. LENTIVIRUSES

ASHLEY T. HAASE

A little more than a half century ago, epidemic diseases of the lungs and central nervous system (CNS), called maedi and visna respectively, ravaged the sheep populations in Iceland. Bjorn Sigurdsson investigated these afflictions, demonstrated their transmissibility, and discovered the long incubation period that defines a slow infection, a concept he introduced in 1954. In the ensuing two decades, rare examples of slow infections in humans were recognized (see Chapter 69), and the virus or viruslike agents were more fully characterized. These analyses of structure and replication documented properties (Fig. 1) that placed the visna–maedi agents in the family of retroviruses as a subfamily with distinct biologic behavior (Fig. 2). Lentiviruses fuse and kill cells in culture and cause slow infections; oncornaviruses generally transform cells in culture and cause tumors in their hosts, and the spumaviruses induce vacuolation in cells in culture and cause inapparent infections.[2] The discovery that the acquired immunodeficiency syndrome (AIDS) is a slow infection caused by the human immunodeficiency virus (HIV), which is related, albeit distantly, to the agents of visna and maedi,[3,4] has greatly stimulated research on lentiviruses and expanded the subfamily to include agents causing slow diseases in other ungulates,[5,6] cats,[7] and primates.[8]

This chapter discusses the general principles and themes that govern, dominate, and distinguish lentivirus infections; these are drawn largely from the experience with animal models. As such, it should serve to set the stage for the detailed treatment of HIV (Chapter 146) and the problems of unprecedented difficulty lentiviruses present with respect to control.

RESTRICTED VIRAL GENE EXPRESSION AND PERSISTENCE

One of the striking features of lentivirus infection is the persistence of virus despite the host's immune response. A number

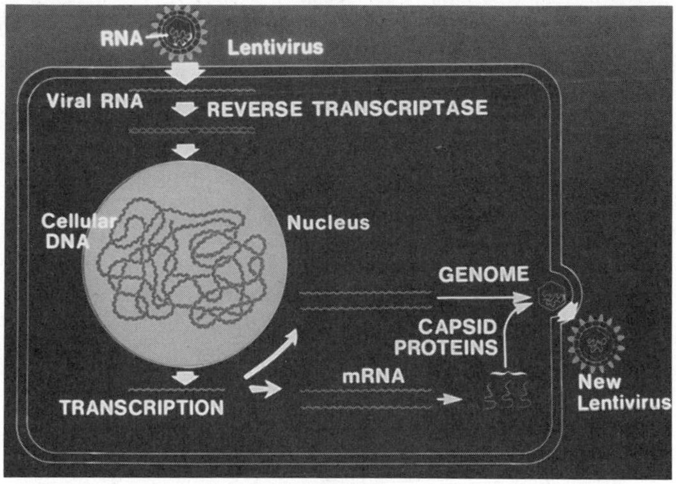

FIG. 1. Lentivirus life cycle. Lentiviruses, like other retroviruses, are enveloped viruses with RNA genomes. Knoblike structures on the virion surface that are composed of the *env* gene product attach the particle to specific receptors (e.g., CD4 on T cells for HIV). After entry and uncoating, the virion-associated reverse transcriptase synthesizes a double-stranded DNA copy of virion RNA. In cells infected with visna virus, this is predominantly a linear duplex molecule with a gap in one strand. Supercoiled circular DNA and integrated proviruses have been demonstrated in infected cells, but accumulation of extrachromosomal DNA is characteristic of cells infected with lentiviruses, and this DNA may serve as template for virion RNA synthesis.[1] Translation and processing of viral mRNAs and their products is followed by assembly and budding of mature progeny from the infected cell membrane.

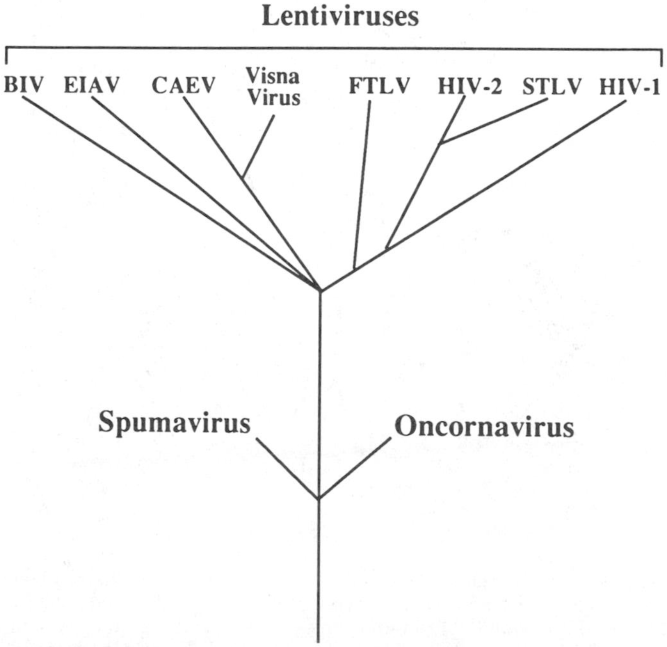

FIG. 2. Taxonomy. Three subfamilies make up the family of retroviruses: oncornaviruses, spuma viruses, and lentiviruses. The members of the latter are shown in detail: BIV: bovine immunodeficiency virus; EIAV: equine infectious anemia virus; CAEV: caprine arthritis and encephalitis virus; FTLV: feline lymphotropic lentivirus; STLV: simian lymphotropic virus; HIV: human immunodeficiency virus.

of explanations have been advanced for why virus is not eliminated by antibodies and cellular immunity, but the most important is the covert nature of infection. In animal lentivirus infections, viruses pass from cell to cell and are harbored in a state where gene expression is reduced by about two orders of magnitudes as compared with productive infections.[9,10] Few if any viral particles are produced, and viral antigens are undetectable by the most sensitive contemporary assays. It is in this immunologically silent state that infection is perpetuated.

INTRACELLULAR HAVEN IN THE MONOCYTE AND DISSEMINATION BY A TROJAN HORSE MECHANISM

Lentiviruses also spread in and between infected individuals despite humoral and cellular immunity, again in large measure because of restricted gene expression in cells in blood and tissue fluids, which act as an intracellular haven and reservoir. It has been known for some time that the principal mobile cell in which lentiviruses spread in animals is the monotyce (Fig. 3),[12–14] and it is now clear that this cell also plays an important role in HIV infections.[15,16] Viral replication in monocytes varies from low levels to production of virus confined inside the cell to high levels of replication in activated cells. This mechanism of disguising virus in monocytes and protecting it from host defense mechanisms has been termed "Trojan horse."

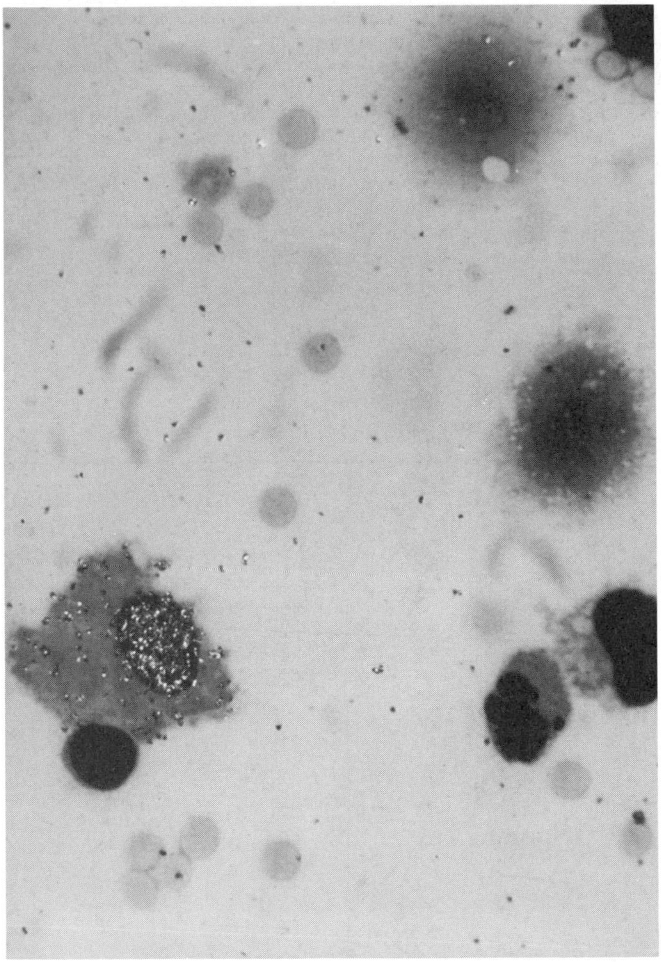

FIG. 3. Lentivirus genes in a monocyte. In situ hybridization has been used to reveal the RNA of visna virus in the nucleus of a monocyte in CSF. To detect viral RNA, a radioactive probe specific for viral genes has been hybridized to the cells.[11] In the developed radioautograph, the grains over the nucleus represent signal generated by the probe and indicate the presence of viral RNA. The infected cell contains low concentrations of viral RNA and antigen and consequently is not neutralized by antibody or reactive T cells present in blood and CSF. These findings fulfill the prediction of the Trojan horse model for viral dissemination. (×360). (From Peluso et al.,[14] with permission.)

ORGAN SANCTUARY: REFUGE AND DISEASE IN THE CENTRAL NERVOUS SYSTEM

The frequent spread of lentiviruses to the CNS provides an additional mechanism for persistence, with the blood-brain barrier acting in this instance to put the virus beyond the reach of the immune system. The infected monocyte probably plays a critical role both in bringing virus into the CNS and in the ensuing pathologic process. In lentivirus infections of animals such as visna, infection of oligodendrocytes and the attendant mononuclear cell inflammatory response primarily in white matter results in extensive destruction eventually manifested as a progressive paralytic disease.[17] In HIV infections, cells in the monocyte-macrophage lineage probably play an even more central role in neurologic disease. Infected monocytes may convey virus to the CNS where enhanced replication accompanying differentiation is associated with pathologic changes in white matter. These alterations in subcortical areas ultimately give rise to the AIDS dementia complex.[18]

THE PARADOX OF PERSISTENCE AND DISEASE: A SPECTRUM OF STATES OF VIRAL GENE EXPRESSION AND IMMUNOPATHOLOGY

If persistence depends in large measure on sequestration of viral genes in cells where the level of expression is too low for efficient detection and destruction by immune surveillance, why should lentiviral infections eventually evolve into overt illness? This apparent paradox is resolved by thinking of gene expression (Fig. 4) as a spectrum in which the latent or dormant infection subtends one end of the spectrum and the acute destructive–productive infection of tissue culture marks the other end. In the intermediate regions are the infected cells in which viral antigens and particles are produced to provoke and sustain the immune and inflammatory response. In animal lentivirus infections, this response has pathologic consequences ranging from the interstitial inflammatory pneumonitis of maedi to immunopathologic diseases of the CNS (visna), joints (caprine arthritis), or hematopoietic system (equine infectious anemia). The rate of accumulation of these pathologic changes is proportional to the extent of gene expression and is quite slow because of the constraints in replication in most of the infected cell population.

The extent to which immunopathology contributes to the manifestations of HIV infection has not been fully defined, but it is clear that the concept of a spectrum of replicative states is applicable to this human lentivirus infection as an explanation for the "iceberg" distribution of seropositive individuals, with most in the category of asymptomatic chronically infected individuals and decreasing numbers with AIDS-related complex (ARC) syndromes or frank AIDS. There are also analogies in vitro in which HIV infections may be latent, persistent and noncytocidal or productive with cytopathic effects.[19]

THE IMPORTANCE AND COMPLEXITY OF LENTIVIRUS GENE EXPRESSION

The extent of lentivirus gene expression is the major determinant of persistence, "slowness" (the length of the incubation period to the point where cumulative pathologic damage becomes manifested clinically), and the proportion of infected individuals who will eventually become ill. For this reason, understanding the control of gene expression is and has been a central preoccupation in research on lentiviruses. These investigations have uncovered a surprising complexity of regulation.

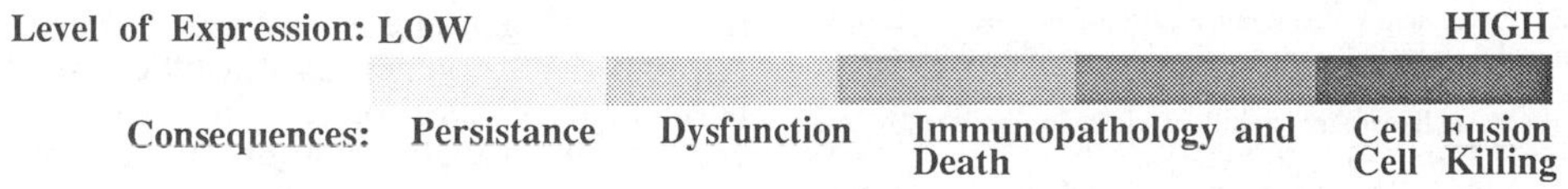

FIG. 4. The spectrum of lentivirus gene expression and its consequences. The complex regulation of lentivirus gene expression results in a spectrum of states from fully productive to dormant infections, which are characteristic of tissue culture and persistent infections, respectively. In the intermediate range are cells that provoke and sustain pathologic processes. These directly or indirectly kill cells and ultimately result in disease at a slow tempo commensurate with the minor fraction of cells in this state.

In addition to the genes whose products are required to form the viral particle (*gag* and *env* genes) and replicate the genome (*pol* genes), there are additional genes largely clustered in the center of the genome that affect the steady-state level and translatability of viral mRNAs. There is also a gene in HIV at the 3′ end whose product represses gene expression.[20] All of the products of the regulatory genes act on the 5′ long terminal repeat (LTR) of the provirus, which has sequence elements that respond as well to proteins produced in stimulated T cells (by mitogens, antigens, or human T-leukemia/lymphoma virus 1 [HTLV-1]) or coinfected with other viruses.[21–23] Understanding the molecular rules governing gene expression promises to shed considerable light on the pathogenesis of lentivirus infections and open new avenues to interventions to control or eradicate infection.

BIOLOGY AND GENETICS OF VARIABILITY

One additional common theme that emerges from studies of lentiviruses is their variability. In biologic terms this is expressed in the variability in the outcome of infections and incubation periods. In visna, for example, depending on the strain of the virus and host, clinical disease may develop from 3 months to 8 years after direct inoculation into the brain, and in natural infections, persistent inapparent infection is the rule, with disease in only about a third of seropositive animals.[24]

Polymorphism is manifested in the sequence diversity of different isolates of HIV[25] and antigenic variants of animal lentiviruses.[26,27] Although these variants provide a potential mechanism for escape from natural or vaccine-induced immunity, fortunately, from the standpoint of vaccine development, such a mechanism appears to play a minor role, if any, in animal lentivirus infections.[28–30] What is likely to prove more important are strain variations that alter the host range of the virus or its replicative efficiency since these changes may determine the ability of the virus to cause disease in general and, specifically, in the CNS.[31,32]

LENTIVIRUSES AS FORMIDABLE ADVERSARIES IN THE QUEST FOR CONTROL

To summarize, the particular features of lentivirus infection that make control by conventional vaccine approaches unusually problematic include their ability to enter host cells more rapidly than they are neutralized[33] and establish a persistent infection in which too little antigen is presented for efficient detection and destruction by immune surveillance. The persistently infected population acts both as reservoir and mechanism to perpetuate and transmit infections to new sites and new hosts. At the same time, restrictions in gene expression diminish or eliminate the deleterious effects of viral replication on the host cell or the immunopathologic response to infection. Thus, if this state could be maintained by blocking the replication of virus with drugs like azidothymidine (AZT) and by other novel approaches, it should be possible to limit or prevent the pathologic sequelae of infection. Similarly, effective vaccines that induce effective humoral and cellular immunity to neutralize extracellular virus and eliminate productively infected cells should decrease the aggregate burden of infection and slow or prevent progression to overt disease. Approaches that already are effective or appear promising for the control of lentivirus infection are considered in depth in the next chapter.

REFERENCES

1. Harris JD, Blum H, Scott J, et al. Slow virus visna: Reproduction in vitro of virus from extrachromosomal DNA. Proc Natl Acad Sci USA. 1984;81:7212–15.
2. Haase AT. Pathogenesis of lentivirus infections. Nature. 1986;332:130–6.
3. Gonda MA, Wong-Staal F, Gallo RC, et al. Sequence homology and morphologic similarity of HTLV-III and visna virus, a pathogenic lentivirus. Science. 1985;227:173–7.
4. Sonigo P, Alizon M, Staskus K, et al. Nucleotide sequence of the visna lentivirus: Relationship to the AIDS virus. Cell. 1985;42:369–82.
5. Chiu IM, Yaniv A, Dahlberg JE, et al. Nucleotide sequence evidence for relationship of AIDS retrovirus to lentiviruses. Nature. 1985;317:366–8.
6. Gonda MA, Braun MJ Carter SG , et al. Characterization and molecular cloning of a bovine lentivirus related to human immunodeficiency virus. Nature. 1987;330:388–91.
7. Pedersen NC, Ho EW, Brown ML, et al. Isolation of a T-lymphotropic virus from domestic cats with an immunodeficiency-like syndrome. Science. 1987;235:790–3.
8. Daniel MD, Letvin NL, King NW, et al. Isolation of T-cell tropic HTLV-III-like retrovirus from macaques. Science. 1985;228:1201–4.
9. Haase AT, Stowring LS, Narayan O, et al. The slow persistent infection caused by visna virus: Role of host restriction. Science. 1977;195:175–7.
10. Brahic M, Stowring L, Ventura P, et al. Gene expression in visna virus infection. Nature. 1981;292:240.
11. Haase AT. Analysis of viral infections by in Situ hybridization. In: Valentino K, Roberts J, Barchas J, eds. In Situ Hybridization—Applications to Neurobiology. Symposium Monograph, Fairlawn, NJ; Oxford University Press; 1986;197–219.
12. Klevjer-Anderson P, Anderson LW. Caprine arthritis-encephalitis virus infection of caprine monocytes. J Gen Virol. 1982;58:195–8.
13. Narayan O, Wolinsky JS, Clements JE, et al. Slow virus replication: The role of macrophages in the persistence and expression of visna viruses of sheep and goats. J Gen Virol. 1982;59:345–56.
14. Peluso R, Haase A, Stowring L, et al. A Trojan horse mechanism for the spread of visna virus in monocytes. Virology. 1985;147:369–82.
15. Gartner S, Markovits P, Markovitz DM, et al. The role of mononuclear phagocytes in HTLV-III/LAV infection. Science. 1986;233:215–9.
16. Koenig S, Gendelman HE, Orenstein JM, et al. Detection of AIDS virus in macrophages in brain tissue from AIDS patients with encephalopathy. Science. 1986;233:1089–94.
17. Stowring L, Haase AT, Petursson G, et al. Detection of visna virus antigens and RNA in glial cells in foci of demyelination. Virology. 1985;141:311–8.
18. Price RW, Brew B, Sidtis J, et al. The brain in AIDS: Central nervous system HIV-1 infection and AIDS dementia complex. Science. 1988;239:586–592.
19. Folks T, Powell DM, Lightfoote MM, et al. Induction of HTLV-III/LAV from a nonvirus-producing T-cell line: Implications for latency. Science. 1986;231:600–2.
20. Chen ISY, Regulation of AIDS virus expression. Cell. 1986;47:1–2.
21. Folks TM, Justement J, Kinter A, et al. Cytokine-induced expression of HIV-1 in a chronically infected promonocyte cell line. Science. 1987;238:800–2.
22. Tong-Starksen SE, Luciw PA, Peterlin BM. Human immunodeficiency virus long terminal repeat responds to T-cell activation signals. Proc Natl Acad Sci USA. 1987;84:6845–9.
23. Mosca JD, Bednarik DP, Raj NBK, et al. Herpes simplex virus type-1 can reactivate transcription of latent human immunodeficiency virus. Nature. 1987;325:67–70.
24. Nathanson N, Georgsson G, Palsson PA, et al. Experimental visna in Icelandic sheep: The prototype lentiviral infection. Rev Infect Dis. 1985;7:75–83.
25. Hahn BH, Gonda MA, Shaw GM, et al. Genomic diversity of the acquired immune deficiency syndrome virus HTLV-III: Different viruses exhibit greatest divergence in their envelope genes. Proc Natl Acad Sci USA. 1985;82:4813–7.

26. Kono Y, Kobayashi K, Fukunaga Y. Antigenic drift of equine infectious anemia virus in chronically infected horses. Arch Ges Virusforschung. 1973;41:1–10.
27. Narayan O, Griffin DE, Chase J. Antigenic shift of visna in persistently infected sheep. Science. 1977;197:376–8.
28. Lutley R, Petursson G, Palsson PA, et al. Antigenic shift in visna: Virus variation during long-term infection of Icelandic sheep. J Gen Virol. 1983;64:1433–40.
29. Thormar H, Barshatzky MR, Arnesen K, et al. The emergence of antigenic variants is a rare event in long-term visna virus infection in vivo. J Gen Virol. 1983;64:1427–32.
30. Carpenter S, Evans LH, Sevoian M, et al. Role of the host immune response in selection of equine infectious anemia virus variants. J Virol. 1987;12: 3783–9.
31. Asjo B, Morfeldt-Manson L, Albert J, et al. Replicative capacity of human immunodeficiency virus from patients with varying severity of HIV infection. Lancet. 1986;9:660–3.
32. Koyanagi Y, Miles S, Mitsuyasu R, et al. Dual infection of the central nervous system by AIDS viruses with distinct cellular tropisms. Science. 1987; 236:819–22.
33. Kennedy-Stoskopf S, Narayan O. Neutralizing antibodies to visna lentivirus: Mechanism of action and possible role in virus persistence. Virol. 1986;59:37–44.

147. HUMAN IMMUNODEFICIENCY VIRUS

MARVIN S. REITZ, JR.
ROBERT C. GALLO

The disease known as acquired immunodeficiency syndrome (AIDS) was first recognized in the early 1980s. Its apparent sexual transmission among homosexuals and, more tellingly, its transmission to hemophiliacs and other persons receiving transfusion with blood products suggested the involvement of an infectious agent. This agent was identified as a retrovirus within several years of the identification of the disease. The rapid identification of the AIDS agent was made possible by use of knowledge and techniques amassed from earlier work on retroviruses that had been undertaken to explore the relationship between these viruses and human cancers. This has led to a relatively complete understanding of the etiology of the disease and the routes of transmission. It has aided diagnosis immeasurably. It has also resulted in the development of antiviral therapies that, while not completely successful, do have significant effects in the treatment and management of the disease. While it has not yet lead to the development of a protective vaccine, it assisted in the design of different approaches to vaccine development, some of which may prove to lead to fully protective vaccines in the future. Obviously, much remains to be done. This chapter attempts to summarize some of the progress to date as well as identify some of the most critical areas for present and future research.

BACKGROUND

Leukemia, lymphoma, and other related hematopoietic disorders are widely distributed in animal species and occur not only in humans and other mammals but also in birds, reptiles, fish, and even molluscs. In most cases where the etiology of these diseases as they naturally occur has been worked out, the proximal cause is infection with a retrovirus. Retroviruses are enveloped viruses that contain a genomic plus strand RNA; a DNA copy of the RNA is transcribed by the viral DNA polymerase or reverse transcriptase (Fig. 1). This process gives this group of viruses their name. Integration of the viral DNA into the host cell genome is necessary to establish infection. Since retroviruses are generally not lytic, infection thus tends to be permanent. Virus propagation from the infected cell can proceed either through virion production, followed by infection of a new cell (horizontal transmission), or passively by replication of infected cells (vertical transmission). If a retrovirus infects the germ line of a species and is unbiquitously transmitted vertically, it is called an endogenous virus. Endogenous viruses appear to play very little role in naturally occurring disease, although they can recombine with retroviruses that are transmitted from one host to another by horizontal transmission (exogenous viruses) to make hybrid viruses with altered biologic properties such as host range or pathogenicity. All naturally occurring pathogenic retroviruses identified thus far are of the exogenous type.

In addition to hematopoietic neoplasms, which are proliferative in nature, retroviruses also cause ablative diseases of the hematopoietic system, including anemia and immune disorders. In some cases, retroviruses also appear to be able to infect cells of the nervous system and thereby cause neurologic disorders such as paralysis. This may be due to similarities in cell surface receptors and transcriptional and translation control signals between hematopoietic cells and cells of the nervous system.

Retroviruses were first discovered in chickens in the early part of this century by Ellerman and Bang from leukemias[1] and by Rous from sarcomas.[2] Rous demonstrated that the sarcoma could be transmitted by cell-free filtrates. This was the first report of an oncogenic virus. Many other avian retroviruses have since been described, and the diseases with which they are associated include lymphoma, myeloblastosis, erythroblastosis, and osteopetrosis. Many avian retroviruses are defective recombinants that have recombined with host cell DNA and thus acquired cell-derived oncogenes, genes that endow the virus with the ability to induce transformation of tissue culture. The recombination process alters the structure of the cellular protooncogene and thereby converts it to a gene with the ability to directly transform target cells. This results in an acutely transforming virus that can transform all infected cells and that gives a polyclonal tumor. Rous sarcoma virus is of this type. Most of these viruses are laboratory creations resulting possibly from the high multiplicities of infection generally used during in vitro passage. Most field isolates, in contrast, are complete, replication-competent viruses that fail to directly transform cells. Their oncogenic potential is expressed relatively slowly and inefficiently and is thought to be mediated by insertional mutagenesis of host cell protooncogenes by integration of viral DNA.[3,4] Since the integration site is not specific, this results in monoclonal tumors originating from the rare infected cell that by chance has the relevant integration event. In addition, since some oncogenes immortalize cells and others eliminate contact inhibition and since both properties are necessary for malignant transformation, secondary event(s) not necessarily related to the virus may be critical for tumorigenesis. Consequently, these slowly transforming viruses cause disease very inefficiently and generally only after a long latent phase.

The next important findings, which linked retroviruses with leukemia in mammals, were in the early 1950s when Ludwik Gross[5] established that murine leukemia virus, a retrovirus first isolated from inbred strains of laboratory mice, induced leukemia in neonate mice. Since then, many different types of related murine leukemia viruses have been identified. Some are endogenous to inbred laboratory strains of mice, others are endogenous to all mice, and others are not endogenous but rather are horizontally transmitted. Many of the horizontally transmitted viruses are recombinants that have acquired part of their genomes from endogenous viruses. All pathogenic murine leukemia viruses are horizontally transmitted (although recombination during infection with endogenous viruses may be a required step in leukemogenesis). Wild mice also harbor retroviruses, including horizontally transmitted viruses that can

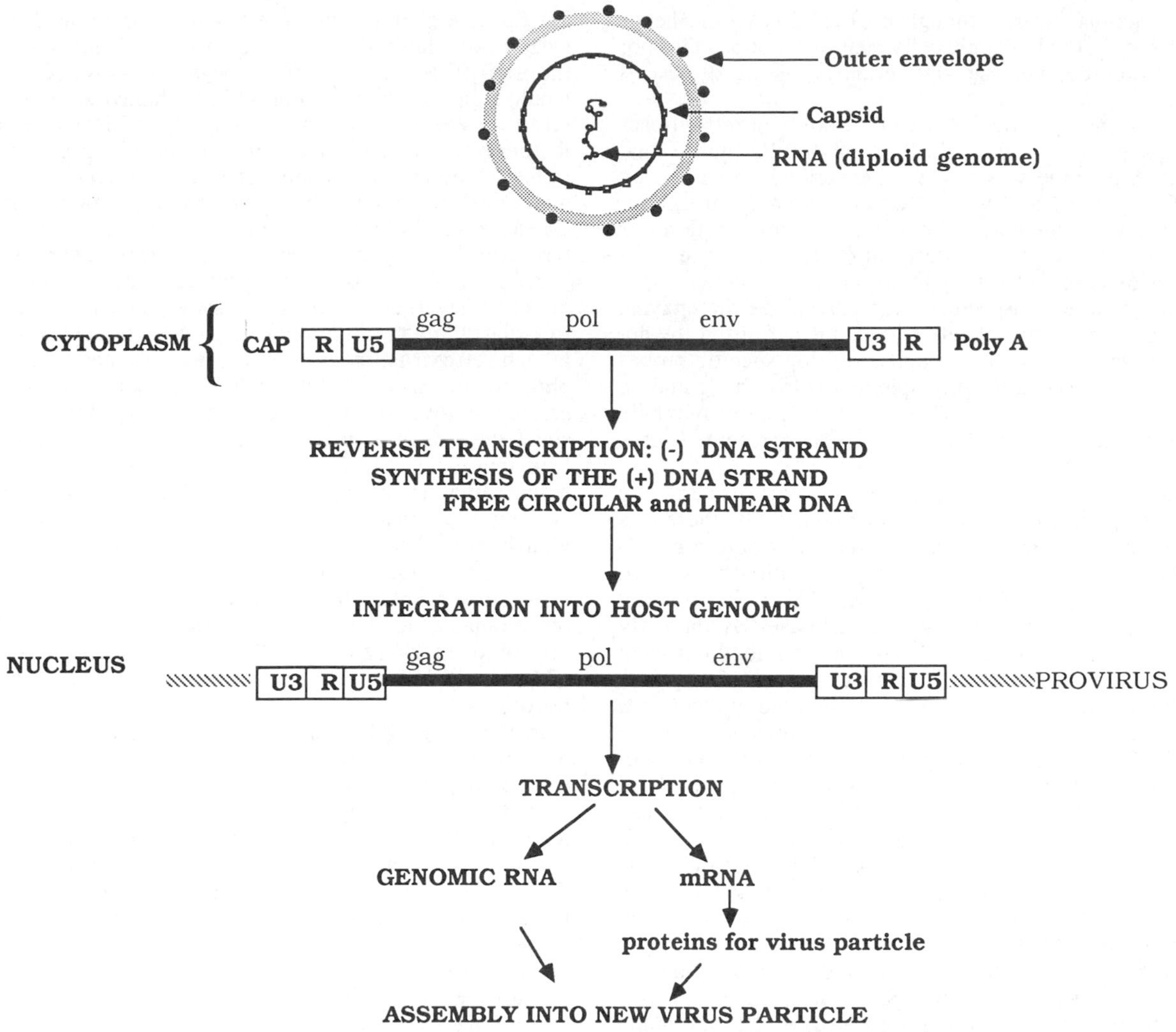

FIG. 1. Life cycle of a retrovirus. As shown above, the retroviral particle, or virion, shown at the top of the figure attaches to and penetrates the surface of the target cell. The RNA genome is uncoated in the cytoplasm and reverse transcribed into linear double-stranded viral DNA. This is transported to the nucleus where it is circularized and integrated into the host genome. The integrated viral DNA is the provirus. This is transcribed into viral RNA, which can either be used for the virion genomic RNA or be used for mRNAs, which are translated into the virion proteins.

cause lymphoma and a paralytic neurologic disease. The mechanisms by which leukemogenic murine retroviruses cause neoplasia are not understood, but oncogene capture or activation by insertional mutagenesis may be involved in some cases. In addition, recombinant envelope proteins derived from two different parental viruses, as with Friend and Rauscher murine leukemia viruses, can result in acutely pathogenic viruses. In this case, it may be that the envelope can insert into or bind to the cell membrane so as to cause an inappropriate signal to a surface receptor involved in the regulation of growth or differentiation.

The next findings involving retroviruses and leukemia was the work in the mid-1960s of W. Jarrett and his colleagues who discovered that naturally occurring lymphosarcoma in outbred populations of cats was caused by feline leukemia virus, a horizontally transmitted retrovirus of cats.[6] This was the first indication that transmission of leukemogenic retroviruses occurs in nature. As is the case with other naturally occurring retroviruses, feline leukemia virus is not acutely transforming and induces leukemia only after a long latent phase and only in a small percentage of infected cats. As with other similar viruses, the basic mechanism is not clear, although evidence for insertional mutagenesis of protooncogenes has been reported in some cases. In this mechanism, integration of viral genome into the host cell genome results in mutagenesis and activation of host-coded genes. The virus also appears to have a relatively high tendency to recombine with different oncogenes and create acutely transforming viruses, possibly because of a high replication rate in infected animals. Various strains of feline leukemia virus frequently cause a variety of other diseases, including immune deficiency syndrome, anemia, and spontaneous abortion. Different diseases may be virus strain specific. Cats also contain endogenous virus-related sequences that can recombine with the infecting virus and create new viruses during the course of infection.

All of the aforementioned retrovirus-induced leukemias involve abundant virus replication. This led to the expectation that this would invariably be the case in other animals. Lymphoma in cattle, however, had long been suspected to be of viral etiology because of the occurrence of disease clusters within herds, but no virus was identified until the late 1960s. Only after tumor cells could be successfully grown was bovine leukemia virus discovered.[7] It was shown to be the etiologic agent of the lymphomas by seroepidemiology. It was now evident that leukemia could have a retroviral etiology even with a lack of detectable virus in the leukemic animal. In the case of bovine leukemia virus, although proviral DNA (and hence virus) is present in the leukemic cells, neither viral proteins nor RNA are expressed, yet the viral etiology of the disease is established.

A significant finding in the history of the study of retroviruses was the discovery by Temin and Mizutani[8] and Baltimore[9] that the viral RNA genome was reverse transcribed into DNA by the viral DNA polymerase, which they called reverse transcriptase. The reversal of the normal flow of genetic information was unprecedented and led to the designation of the viruses that used it as retroviruses. One very important consequence of the discovery of reverse transcriptase was that (since the enzyme is a necessary component of retroviruses) it permitted the detection of low levels of virus without requiring specific probes such as antibodies. Thus, in principle any retrovirus could be detected by its reverse transcriptase activity. The retroviral life cycle and the role of reverse transcriptase are presented schematically in Figure 1.

Table 1 lists the leukemogenic animal retroviruses. Because of the retroviral etiology of many animal leukemias, there was considerable expectation that human leukemia would prove to have a similar etiology, and much effort was directed toward the isolation of comparable human viruses. This was especially true after the discovery of reverse transcriptase. By the early 1970s examples of leukemias with retroviral etiology has even been found in the gibbon apes,[10–12] which increased expectations that human leukemia viruses would be readily identified. This turned out to not be the case for several reasons. For one thing, much of this research was predicated on the studies with the previously described animal systems where high levels of virus replication and viremia were usually the case. This has definitely not been true for any human retroviruses described to date. Additionally, as mentioned before in the case of bovine leukemia virus, some retroviruses remain in a latent state even after the onset of disease unless the infected cells are grown in culture. The virus must also be able to be transmitted to a proper target cell for isolation. Since previously described animal retroviruses could be grown in fibroblasts, it seemed as if this would also be the case for human retroviruses. Despite much effort, only suggestive evidence was obtained for the presence of human retroviruses. This included the occasional detection of cell-associated reverse transcriptase-like activity by various laboratories including our own[13,14] and the detection of apparently exogenous (and by implication, viral) DNA sequences in some human leukemias by Baxt and Speigleman.[15] No convincing isolation of a biologically active human retrovirus was achieved, however, when using the available cell cultures systems.

Since it was increasingly evident that growth of the infected cells (i.e., hematopoietic cells) would be necessary for the successful detection of human retroviruses and that the target cell systems available for virus isolation were not appropriate, in the mid-1970s our laboratory began to look for factors that would support the growth of different hematopoietic cells. This effort succeeded with the discovery by Morgan et al.[16] of a factor present in media from phytohemagglutinin-stimulated peripheral blood cells that supported the long-term growth of large quantities of human T cells. We used this factor (first called T-cell growth factor [TCGF] but now more commonly called interleukin-2 [IL-2]) to establish cultures from a variety of human T-cell neoplasias.[17] By using these cultures in conjunction with sensitive reverse transcriptase assays, Poiesz et al. were able to isolate human T-lymphotropic virus I (HTLV-I), the first human retrovirus, from several cases of cutaneous T-cell lymphoma/leukemias.[18,19] Although these neoplasms were first described as mycosis fungoides and Sézary syndrome, in retrospect they were actually the disease now called adult T-cell leukemia (ATL). In fact, the discovery of HTLV-I helped to define ATL as a distinct disease. HTLV-I was shown to be horizontally transmitted and not detectably related to other previously described retroviruses.[20,21]

Using techniques similar to those used for the isolation of HTLV-I and antibodies to HTLV-I proteins as a probe, Kalyanaraman et al.[22] shortly thereafter isolated a virus distantly related to HTLV-I from T cells of a patient with a T-cell variant of hairy cell leukemia. This was HTLV-II, the second human retrovirus.

In the early 1980s a new and fatal epidemic disease, which we now know as AIDS, was first noted.[23,24] Several features were strongly suggestive of an infectious etiology. These included case clustering, apparent sexual transmission, and most tellingly, apparent transmission by blood products. Several findings made retroviruses seem a likely possibility. For one, AIDS was a T-cell disease, and the known human retroviruses were T-cell tropic. Second, animal retroviruses, notably feline leukemia virus, are commonly associated with immunosuppressive disorders[25] (so, for that matter, is HTLV-I[26]). Third, the disease had a delayed onset after presumptive transmission that is consistent with a retrovirus. Fourth, since the agent was still present in filtered blood products, it could not be a bacterium or other larger organism.

Our initial hypothesis was that a strain of HTLV-I was the AIDS agent. Despite some suggestive early data, this turned out to not be the case. By using IL-2 for T-cell cultures and looking for retroviruses by reverse transcriptase, however, Barre-Sinoussi et al.[27] were able to identify a presumptive retrovirus that ultimately proved to be the AIDS agent. The virus, however, was highly cytotoxic for T cells and consequently could not be grown in quantity. In fact, it was not initially certain that it was in fact a retrovirus. Clearly it was not related to HTLV-I. A detailed characterization became possible with the identification of replication-permissive T-cell lines able to at least partially resist the cytotoxicity of the virus.[28,29] (This virus has been variously called lymphodenopathy-associated virus [LAV] and HTLV-III, but it is now by general agreement called human immunodeficiency virus 1 [HIV-1].) It was then possible to show that this was indeed the cause of AIDS.

By this use of similar techniques and using probes for HIV-1, distantly related viruses were identified in African monkeys[30,31] and in humans in western Africa.[32,33] The latter virus is now called HIV-2. Although it, too, appears to be associated with an AIDS-like disease, it appears far less pathogenic than HIV-1 does. HIV-1 and -2 are the third and fourth human retroviruses to be discovered.

TABLE 1. Representative Diseases for Which Retroviruses Are the Etiologic Agent

Virus	*Representative Diseases*
Avian leukosis virus	Bursal lymphoma
Murine leukemia virus	Thymic lymphoma, erythroleukemia, paralytic neurologic disease
Feline leukemia virus	T- and B-cell lymphoma, anemia, spontaneous abortion, immunodeficiency (FAIDS)
Gibbon ape leukemia virus	Lymphoid and granulocytic leukemia
Bovine leukemia virus	Lymphoma, persistent lymphocytosis
HTLV-I	Adult T cell leukemia, immunosuppression, tropical spastic paraparesis
HTLV-II	Hairy cell leukemia (?)
HIV-1, HIV-2	AIDs
SIV	AIDS-like disease in macaques

Abbreviations: HTLV: human T-lymphotrophic virus; HIV: human immunodeficiency virus; SIV: simian immunodeficiency virus.

THE PATHOGEN

HIV-1 is in many respects typical of all retroviruses. Its morphology on electron micrographs (shown in Fig. 2) is most like

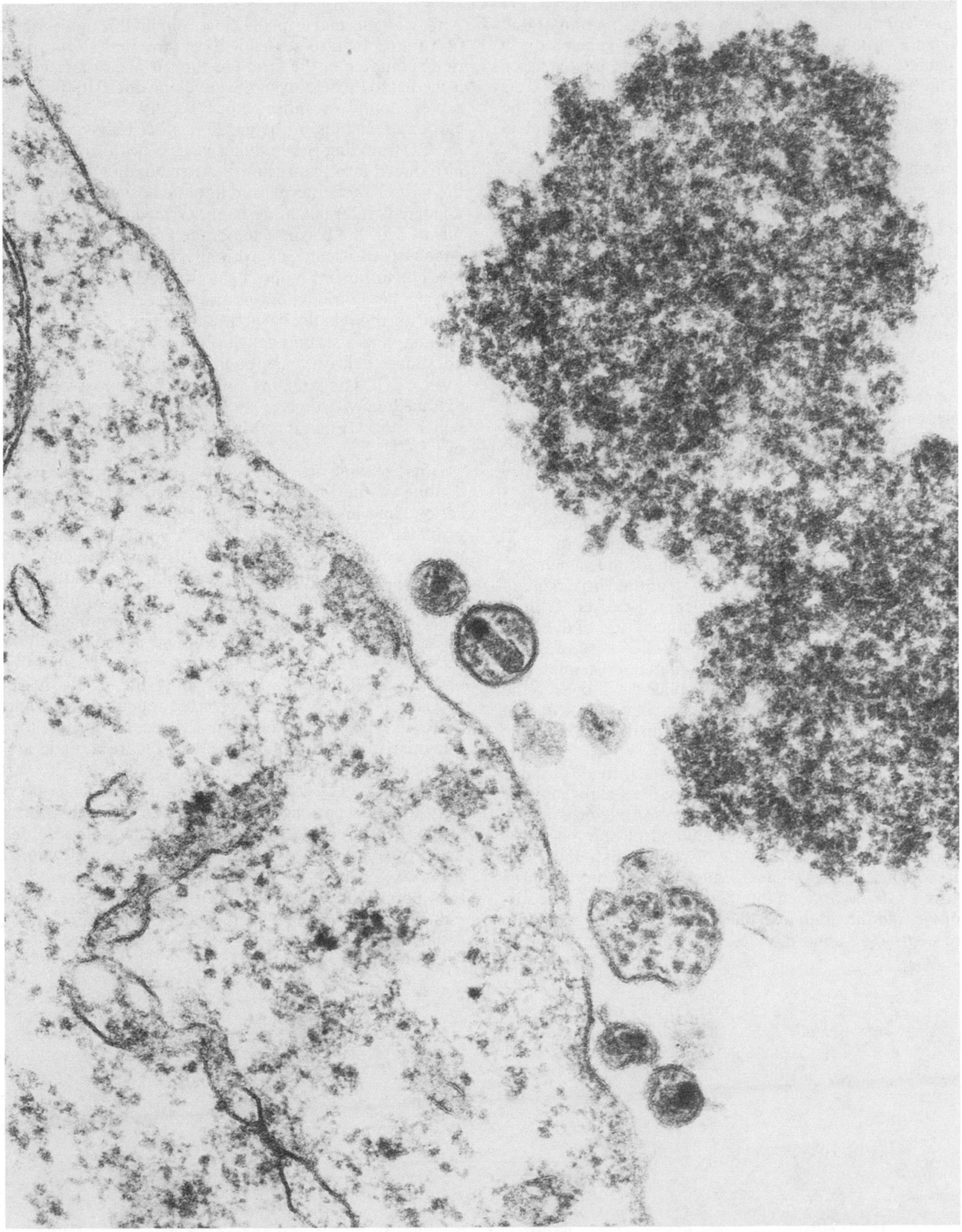

FIG. 2. Electron micrograph of HIV-1. Shown is the typical appearance of HIV-1 by electron microscopy. (Courtesy of Bernhard Kramarsky, Electronucleonics, Inc., Silver Spring, MD.)

that of the ungulate lentiviruses, although it shares only a distant relatedness by DNA sequence similarity.[34–37] Like other retroviruses, as represented in Figure 3, the genome contains *gag*, *pol*, and *env* genes in the order 5′ to 3′. However, unlike many other retroviruses such as murine leukemia virus, the HIV-1 genome also contains other genes and open reading frames that do not code for structural proteins. Some of these gene products help to regulate or modulate virus replication, and are discussed below. The function of others, if any, is not understood. This was quite surprising for a retroviral genome, although the HTLV-I genome had been shown previously to also contain extra open reading frames.[38] A second surprising aspect of the HIV-1 genome was that different isolates of the virus displayed substantial heterogeneity in their DNA sequence. The genomic variability is not evenly distributed, however, and much of it is clustered within the *env* gene, particularly the coding region for the gp120 or large external glycoprotein.[39–42] Even within the *env* gene, regions of hypervariability are separated by highly conserved regions. The latter must represent parts of the envelope protein that are critical for envelope function and whose sequence may not therefore be substantially altered without losing virus viability. The heterogeneity of the hypervariable regions is a consequence not only of point mutations but also of small duplications and deletions that occur in multiples of three nucleotides and preserve the integrity of the downstream reading frame. These regions may represent noncritical regions for which heterogeneity has been selected by the immune system of the host.

AIDS is characterized by a profound depletion of CD4-positive T cells, most of which are helper T cells. It is interesting, therefore, that in culture the virus has a strong tropism for CD4-positive T cells and is profoundly cytotoxic for the same cells. In fact, this cytotoxicity precluded growth of the virus in quantity or detailed study until partially resistant T-cell tumor lines could be identified.[28,29] Once the successful culture of the virus was achieved, it was quickly shown to be the cause of AIDS by seroepidemiology. This is covered in detail in Chapter 106. The reason for the partial resistance of some T-cell lines to the cytopathic effects of HIV-1 is not clear, but low levels of expression of the CD4 cell surface protein is one possible reason.[43]

The molecular cloning of the virus[44,45] was also made possible by the availability of stable producer lines. This allowed other studies, among which was the demonstration of virus in the brain of infected individuals.[46] The method of entry of virus into the brain was not clear, but the discovery that HIV-1 can infect macrophages[47] as well as T cells suggests that the virus may be carried to the brain in infected macrophages.[48] The discovery of virus in the brain also helped to explain the moderate to severe neurologic abnormalities that are a frequent clinical manifestation of HIV-1 infection and are described in Chapter 108.

ESTABLISHMENT OF INFECTION

After gaining entry to the host, either through parenteral exposure to blood or sexual activity, the first step in virus infection is binding of the virion to the surface of a target cell. This is mediated by binding of the envelope gp120 to the CD4 surface protein found on most helper T cells.[49,50] A region near the carboxy terminus of the gp120 has been shown to be required for CD4 binding by studying viruses with different mutations introduced into this region.[51] After binding to the cell surface, the virus is then internalized into the host cell where it becomes uncoated. Internalization is either mediated through envelope fusion with the plasma membrane of the target cell[52] or within endocytosed vacuoles.[53] Although binding to CD4 is necessary, it is not sufficient; mouse cells expressing human CD4 on their surface bind virions, but no productive infection occurs.[52] The block is thought to be at the stage of internalization or uncoating, and a second cell surface protein found on human but not mouse cells may be required in addition to CD4. A soluble form of CD4, containing only the outermost domains of the extracellular portion of the protein, blocks virus infection, which suggests that this fragment contains the virus binding site of CD4.[54–58]

After binding to the receptor and internalization and uncoating of the virus particle, the viral RNA is reverse transcribed into linear double-stranded viral DNA in the cytoplasm of infected cells by the viral DNA polymerase and then transported to the nucleus where it is first circularized and then integrated into the host cell. Integration is mediated by the viral endonuclease or integrase, which is coded within the *pol* gene, as shown in Figure 4. The viral large terminal repetitive sequences (LTRs), present at each end of the linear viral DNA, themselves contain a short inverted repeat present at both ends of each LTR. Circularization joins the LTRs head to tail, thereby joining two of the inverted repeats and forming a palindrome. The palindrome forms the recognition site for the viral integrase.[59] This is summarized in Figure 4. It is an unusual characteristic of HIV-1 that infected cells contain a great deal of unintegrated DNA,[45] and integrated viral DNA only becomes easy to detect in long-term cultures of infected cells. It is not clear, therefore, that HIV-1 needs to integrate in order to replicate or express viral proteins, but by analogy with other retroviruses, it is likely that it does. After integration, cells are thus persistently infected, and the only way an infected individual can eliminate the virus is by the elimination of all infected cells.

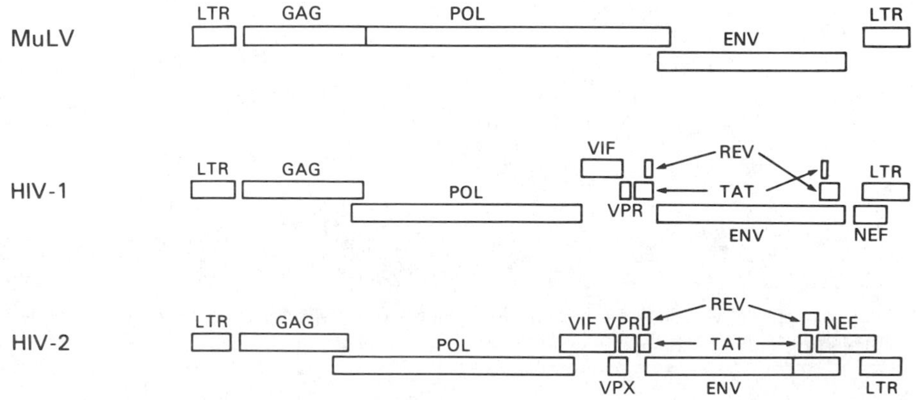

FIG. 3. Retroviral genome organization. Shown above are the major reading frames for viral proteins for the indicated viruses. MuLV: Moloney murine leukemia virus; HIV: human immunodeficiency virus.

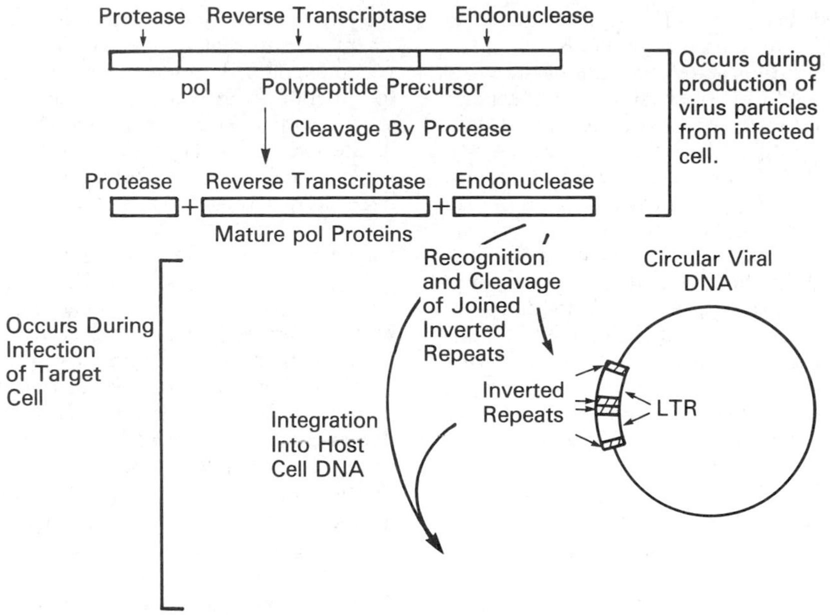

FIG. 4. Integration of retroviral DNA. The *pol* gene products are synthesized as a polyprotein that is cleaved by the protease of the *pol* gene. The endonuclease (or integrase) of the *pol* gene recognizes and cleaves the circular unintegrated viral DNA. The recognition site is formed by the junction of the inverted repeat sequences of the long terminal repeats (LTRs), which form a palindrome. The viral DNA is then integrated into the host genome.

PRODUCTION OF VIRUS FROM INFECTED CELLS

The integrated viral DNA, or provirus, is transcribed into full-length RNA by the host cell RNA polymerase II. Transcriptional rates are regulated, however, by the viral promoter, enhancer, and negative regulatory elements contained in the upstream viral LTR. The downstream LTR contains transcriptional termination and polyadenylation signals. The product of the *tat* gene appears to increase the steady-state levels of viral RNA, perhaps acting in concert with tissue-specific cellular proteins.[60–65] The activity of the viral RNA polymerase promoter also seems to be increased by T-cell activation signals.[66] The full-length RNA transcript can serve one of three functions. It can be packaged within virus particles to serve as the genome of progeny virus. It can serve as an mRNA for the synthesis of the viral *gag* and *pol* gene products. Finally, it can be spliced to form mRNAs for the *env* gene products and the products of the various regulatory genes. Splicing is presumably carried out by cellular components, but one of the regulatory genes (previously called *trs*/*art* but now called *rev*[67]) exerts a negative regulatory effect on the relative levels of spliced RNA.[61,68,69] HIV-1 has a pattern of splicing that is unusually complex for a retrovirus and includes double splicing for formation of the regulatory gene mRNAs. In the absence of the *rev* gene product, most of the viral RNA appears as the doubly spliced mRNAs.

The viral mRNAs are next translated into viral polypeptide precursors. A second function of the *tat* protein appears to be to increase the translation rate of viral proteins.[60,61,70] The *gag* and *pol* precursor polypeptides are cleaved to their proper proteins by the viral protease encoded within the *pol* gene. The *env* precursor polypeptide is cleaved to remove the membrane insertion signal peptide and generate the final proteins and is glycosylated. These steps are carried out by cellular enzymes. The viral structural components are assembled at the cell surface around a dimer of genomic RNA. The virion then buds from the cell surface and is ready to infect another cell. HIV-1 also induces the fusion of cells into syncytia; infected cells can fuse with uninfected cells as long as the uninfected cells are expressing CD4 on their surface.[71] In this way the virus may be transmitted directly from cell to cell, thus protecting the virus from the humoral immune system.

The function of *tat* and *rev* are at least partially understood, but the other (presumably) regulatory genes are not. The 3′ *orf* (now called *nef*) is not necessary for viral replication.[72] In fact, ablation of *nef* increases the viral replication rate somewhat, and it is possible that it has a negative regulatory effect important in latency. *Nef* has been reported to possess a protein kinase activity.[73] *Vif*, previously called *sor*, seems to be necessary to form free virions that can infect cells without cell-to-cell contact; in its absence only infection by cell-to-cell contact occurs.[74,75] *Vpr*, formerly *R*, is translated into protein *in vivo* since infected individuals make antibodies to it.[76] Its function is completely unknown.

PATHOGEN–HOST RELATIONSHIPS

One of the prime manifestations of HIV-1 infection is a profound depletion of CD4+ T cells, which is reflected in vitro by the cytotoxicity of HIV-1 for cultured CD4+ T cells. The basis for this cytotoxic effect is not completely understood. One aspect appears to involve the formation of multicellular syncytia that is dependent on the expression of the envelope proteins on the surface of infected cells and CD4 on the surface of other cells, which need not be infected.[71,77] The fusogenic regions of the envelope have been mapped by mutagenesis.[78] Thus, by formation of syncytia, one infected cell can account for the death of many noninfected cells. It has recently been reported,[43,79] however, that infected cells are also killed in the absence of syncytia formation, and it appears that there is at least one mechanism for CD4+ T-cell depletion in addition to syncytium formation. Infected macrophages, in contrast to T cells, do not appear to be highly susceptible to HIV-1-mediated cell killing.

The basis for the neuropathy frequently evident in AIDS is not clear, even though HIV-1-infected cells are found in the brain. The rapid improvement in neurologic symptoms that has been reported after administration of azidodeoxythymidine[80] suggests that the neurologic effects are mediated by some generalized factor produced directly or indirectly by the virus rather than as the result of structural damage.

There is considerable interest in the relationship of the virus with the immune system since this is the basis for any vaccine. Infected individuals generally have serum antibodies that neutralize viral infectivity,[81,82] but their presence does not seem to afford long-term protection. Infection also elicits a cytotoxic T-cell response[83] that also apparently fails to achieve long-term protection. It has been postulated that the hypervariable regions of the envelope are the result of cumulative selection of variants by the host immune system. It has been shown that transmission and growth of a molecularly cloned virus in the continuous presence of neutralizing antiserum from a healthy infected individual can result in the emergence of neutralization-resistant variants.[84] Surprisingly, the change resulting in the resistant phenotype was a single amino acid substitution within a highly conserved region of the gp41 transmembrane protein.[85] This result indicates that immunoselection can occur and that extremely small changes in the *env* gene can result in large differences in the neutralizability of HIV-1.

RELATED VIRUSES

In 1985 a virus was discovered in captive macaques with immune deficiency that was immunologically cross-reactive with HIV-1.[30,31] The cross-reaction was primarily due to the major core protein p24. A similar virus was soon found in healthy wild African green monkeys and related species.[86] This virus was first called simian T-lymphotropic virus III (STLV-III) but is now known as simian immunodeficiency virus (SIV). Speculation that it could have served as an immediate ancestor to HIV-1 was shown to be incorrect by DNA sequence analyses[87–89]; although SIV and HIV-1 have the same genomic organization and are clearly related (see Fig. 3), the overall DNA sequence identity is only 40–60 percent. By using antigens from this virus, however, a closely related virus was soon discovered in healthy humans[32] and in humans with immunodeficiency.[33] This virus, first called HTLV-IV and LAV-2 but now known as HIV-2, is endemic to western Africa. Even though prevalence rates are extremely high for this region, the rate of AIDS is low, and the degree to which HIV-2 can cause the disease is not certain. It is likely that it has the pathogenic ability to cause AIDS, but at a far lower efficiency than does HIV-1. Sequence analyses of HIV-2 isolates indicate that their genetic divergence is similar in kind and degree to that of different isolates of HIV-1.[90,91] Moreover, HIV-2 is much more closely related to SIV than it is to HIV-1; in fact, different HIV-2 isolates are almost as closely related to SIV as they are to each other, which suggests that divergence from a common ancestor has been rather recent indeed. It is probably only a matter of time before HIV-2 becomes established in the United States and Europe.

ANTIVIRAL STRATEGIES

The only currently effective means of controlling HIV-1 is to avoid infection in the first place. Education is important in persuading people to avoid high-risk behavior such as intravenous drug abuse and promiscuity. Screening blood for antibodies to HIV-1 has almost eliminated transfusion-mediated transmission of the virus. However, many people are already infected, and many will continue to be at risk, so other strategies are also needed.

High on the list of priorities is a protective vaccine against HIV-1, but there are many serious obstacles to the development of such a vaccine. One problem presented is the high degree of envelope heterogeneity seen among different strains of HIV-1. Since the envelope proteins are the main target for neutralizing antibodies, any candidate vaccine will have to be highly polyvalent, that is, it will have to include many serotypes of the virus. Moreover, as mentioned earlier, even small changes in the *env* gene can have large consequences for neutralizability. There are no really good animal systems with which to test vaccines; only chimpanzees have been shown to be susceptible to infection,[92] and these are large, expensive to maintain, and scarce. Obviously, humans who have been injected with candidate vaccines cannot be challenged with a lethal virus.

One vaccine that has been tested in chimpanzees has already been shown to not be protective against different strains of HIV-1.[93] A recombinant vaccine comprised of the *env* gene spliced into vaccinia virus has been tested on human volunteers[94] and shown to elicit neutralizing antibodies and a cytotoxic T-cell response. There is no possible way to tell whether this response would be protective, however. As mentioned earlier, infected humans who have these responses go on to develop AIDS in spite of their presence, thus suggesting that it may be impossible for many humans to mount a protective response to this virus. The hope is that if the levels of such activities were higher and were already established when the first virus exposure occurred then protection against the establishment of infection would occur.

For the many persons who are already infected, therapies to limit virus spread are the only possibility. One of these, treatment with azidodeoxythymidine, has proved to be of some success, although it is not without serious side effects.[80] One of the problems with antiviral drugs is that the viral life cycle is so intimately connected with cellular processes that selectivity is made very difficult. There are some steps in the viral life cycle that are unique, however, and these may be amenable to selective inhibition. The first step is binding of the virus to its cellular receptor. Interference with this binding should inhibit infection. In fact, truncated, soluble forms of CD4, as mentioned earlier, have been shown to inhibit virus infection[53–57] without interfering detectably with T-cell function. Perhaps peptides based on the CD4 molecule could be used therapeutically. This may also be the stage at which neutralizing antibodies work. Dextran sulfate has also been reported to block infection by inhibiting binding to CD4.[95,96]

Inhibition of the reverse transcription of viral RNA is another possibility for antiviral activity. This in fact is the step at which azidodeoxythymidine and other derivatives of DNA precursors that lack a 3′ hydroxyl group act. The compound is incorporated into the growing DNA chain, and the lack of a 3′ hydroxyl group effectively terminates chain elongation.[97] Integration is another possible step that could by used to inhibit infection, although it is not certain that HIV-1 needs to integrate in order to replicate.

Many of the steps in the expression of virus from infected cells such as transcription and translation of viral mRNA, glycosylation of the envelope proteins, and myristylation of the gag polypeptide precursor are carried out by cellular components. There are a few possible viral targets, however, that are unique to the virus. *Tat* and *rev*, for example, do not appear to have cellular homologues and are absolutely necessary for virus replication. It may be possible to find a way to selectively inhibit either or both of these proteins. The viral proteins are assembled at the cell surface around the packaging recognition site on the viral RNA. Recognition of this site is another potential step for antiviral intervention. The gag and pol precursor polypeptides are proteolytically processed by the protease encoded by the viral *gag* gene; without this cleavage, the virus would not be active. Perhaps this process could be selectively inhibited.

Although there are many potential ways to interfere with virus infection, expression, and spread, it is unlikely that any single method will be sufficient, and many different approaches will be needed. Since several approaches have shown either promise or actual success, however, it is highly possible that such a combination of approaches will enable us to ultimately contain and control the human immunodeficiency viruses.

REFERENCES

1. Ellerman V, Bang O. Experimentelle Leukamie bei Huhnern. Centralbl Bakteriol. 1908;46:595–605.
2. Rous P. Transmission of a malignant new growth by means of a cell-free filtrate. JAMA. 1911;56:198–204.
3. Hayward WS, Neel BG, Astrin SM. Induction of lymphocytic leukosis by avian leukosis virus: Activation of a cellular "onc" gene by promoter insertion. Nature. 1981;290:475–79.
4. Neel BG, Hayward WS, Robinson HL, et al. Avian leukosis virus-induced tumors have common proviral integration sites and synthesize discrete new RNAs: Oncogenesis by promoter insertion. Cell. 1981;23:323–34.
5. Gross L. "Spontaneous" leukemia developing in C3H mice following inoculation in infancy with AK-leukemic extracts, or AK-embryos. Proc Soc Exp Biol Med. 1951;78:27–39.
6. Jarrett W, Crawford E, Martin W, et al. Leukemia in the cat. A virus-like particle associated with leukaemia (lymphosarcoma). Nature. 1964;202:567–8.
7. Miller J, Miller L, Olson C, et al. Virus-like particles in phytohemagglutinin-stimulated lymphocyte cultures with reference to bovine lymphosarcoma. JNCI. 1969;43:1297–303.
8. Temin H, Mizutani S. RNA-dependent DNA polymerase in virions of Rous sarcoma virus. Nature. 1970;226:1211–3.
9. Baltimore D. Viral RNA-dependent DNA polymerase. Nature. 1970;226:1209–11.
10. Kawakami TG, Huff SO, Buckley PM, et al. Isolation and characterization of a C-type virus associated with gibbon lymphosarcoma. Nature. 1972; 235:170–2.
11. Theilen GH, Gould D, Fowler M, et al. C-type virus in tumor tissue of a woolly monkey (*Lagothrix* spp.) with fibrosarcoma. JNCI. 1971;47:881–6.
12. Wolfe WG, Deinhardt F, Theilen GH, et al. Induction of tumors in marmoset monkeys by simian sarcoma virus type-C (*Lagothrix*): A preliminary report. JNCI. 1971;47:1115–9.
13. Goodenow RS, Kaplan HS. Characterization of the reverse transcriptase of a type C virus produced by a human lymphoma cell line. Proc Natl Acad Sci USA. 1979;76:4971–5.
14. Sarngadharan MG, Sarin PS, Reitz MS, et al. Reverse transcriptase activity of human acute leukemic cells: Purification of the enzyme, response to AMV 70S RNA, and characterization of the DNA product. Nature. 1972;240:67–9.
15. Baxt WG, Spiegleman S. Nuclear DNA sequences present in human leukemic cells and absent in normal leukocytes. Proc Natl Acad Sci USA. 1973;71:1309–13.
16. Morgan DA, Ruscetti FL, Gallo RC. Selective in vitro growth of T-lymphocytes from normal human bone marrow. Science. 1976;193:1007–10.
17. Poiesz BJ, Ruscetti FW, Mier JW, et al. T-cell lines established from human T-lymphocytic neoplasias by direct response to T-cell growth factor. Proc Natl Acad Sci USA. 1980;77:6815–9.
18. Poiesz BJ, Ruscetti FW, Gazdar AF, et al. Detection and isolation of type C retrovirus particles from fresh and cultured lymphocytes of a patient with cutaneous T-cell lymphoma. Proc Natl Acad Sci USA. 1980;77:7415–9.
19. Poiesz BJ, Ruscetti FW, Reitz MS, et al. Isolation of a new type-C retrovirus (HTLV) in primary uncultured cells of a patient with Sézary T-cell leukaemia. Nature. 1981;294:268–71.
20. Gallo RC, Mann DL, Broder S, et al. Human T-cell leukemia-lymphoma virus (HTLV) is in T- but not B-lymphocytes from a patient with cutaneous T-cell lymphoma. Proc Natl Acad Sci USA. 1982;79:4680–4.
21. Reitz MS, Poiesz BJ, Ruscetti FW, et al. Characterization and distribution of nucleic acid sequences of a novel type C retrovirus isolated from neoplastic human T lymphocytes. Proc Natl Acad Sci USA. 1981;78:1887–91.
22. Kalyanaraman VS, Sarngadharan MG, Robert-Guroff M, et al. A new subtype of human T-cell leukemia virus (HTLV-II) associated with a T-cell variant of hairy cell leukemia. Science. 1982;218:571–5.
23. Gottlieb MS, Schroff R, Schanker HM, et al. *Pneumocystis carinii* pneumonia and mucosal candidiasis in previously healthy homosexual men: Evidence of a new acquired cellular immunodeficiency. N Engl J Med. 1981;305:1425–31.
24. Masur H, Michelis MA, Greene JB, et al. An outbreak of community-acquired *Pneumocystis carinii* pneumonia: Initial manifestation of cellular immune dysfunction. N Engl J Med. 1981;305:1431–8.
25. Anderson LJ, Jarrett WF, Jarrett O, et al. Feline leukemia virus infection of kittens: Mortality associated with atrophy of the thymus and lymphoid depletion. JNCI. 1971;47:807–17.
27. Barre-Sinoussi F, Chermann JC, Rey F, et al. Isolation of a T-lymphotropic retrovirus from a patient at risk for acquired immune deficiency syndrome (AIDS). Science. 1983;220:868–70.
28. Gallo RC, Salahuddin SZ, Popovic M, et al. Frequent detection and isolation of cytopathic retroviruses (HTLV-III) from patients with AIDS and at risk for AIDS. Science. 1984;224:500–4.
29. Popovic M, Sarngadharan MG, Read E, et al. Detection, isolation, and continuous production of cytopathic retroviruses (HTLV-III) from patients with AIDS and pre-AIDS. Science. 1984;224:500–4.
30. Daniel MD, Letvin NL, King NW, et al. Serologic identification and characterization of a macaque T-lymphotropic retrovirus closely related to HTLV-III. Science. 1985;228:1201–3.
31. Kanki PJ, McLane MF, King NW, et al. Serologic identification and characterization of a macaque T-lymphotropic retrovirus closely related to HTLV-III. Science. 1985;228:1199–201.
32. Clavel F, Guetard F, Brun-Vezinet F, et al. Isolation of a new human retrovirus from West African patients with AIDS. Science. 1986;233:343–6.
33. Kanki PJ, Barin F, M'Boup M, et al. New human T-lymphotropic retrovirus related to simian T-lymphotropic virus type III (STLV-III). Science. 1986;232:238–40.
34. Ratner L, Haseltine W, Patarca R, et al. Complete nucleotide sequence of the AIDS virus, HTLV-III. Nature. 1985;313:277–84.
35. Sanchez-Pescador R, Power MD, Barr PJ, et al. Nucleotide sequence and expression of an AIDS-associated retrovirus (ARV-2). Science. 1985;227:484–92.
36. Sonigo P, Alizon M, Staskus K, et al. Nucleotide sequence of the visna lentivirus: Relationship to the AIDS virus. Cell. 1985;42:369–82.
37. Wain-Hobson S, Sonigo P, Danos O, et al. Nucleotide sequence of the AIDS virus, LAV. Cell. 1985;40:9–17.
38. Seiki M, Hattori S, Hirayama Y, et al. Human adult T-cell leukemia virus: Complete nucleotide sequence of the provirus genome integrated in leukemia cell DNA. Proc Natl Acad Sci USA. 1983;80:3618–22.
39. Alizon M, Wain-Hobson S, Montagnier L, et al. Genetic variability of the AIDS virus: Nucleotide sequence analysis of two isolates from African patients. Cell. 1986;46:63–74.
40. Gurgo C, Guo H, Franchini G, et al. Envelope sequences of two new United States HIV-1 isolates. Virology. 1988;164:531–6.
41. Starcich BR, Hahn BH, Shaw GM, et al. Identification and characterization of the conserved and variable regions in the envelope gene of HTLV-III/LAV, the retrovirus of AIDS. Cell. 1986;45:637–48.
42. Willey RL, Rutledge RA, Dias S, et al. Identification of conserved and divergent domains within the envelope gene of the acquired immunodeficiency syndrome retrovirus. Proc Natl Acad Sci USA. 1986;83:5038–42.
43. Stevenson M, Meier C, Mann AM, et al. Envelope glycoprotein of HIV induces interference and cytolysis resistance in CD4+ cells: Mechanism for persistence in AIDS. Cell. 1988;53:483–96.
44. Hahn BH, Shaw GM, Arya SK, et al. Molecular cloning and characterization of the HTLV-III virus associated with AIDS. Nature. 1984;312:166–9.
45. Shaw GM, Hahn BH, Arya SK, et al. Molecular characterization of human T-cell leukemia (lymphotropic) virus type III in the acquired immune deficiency syndrome. Science. 1984;226:1165–71.
46. Shaw GM, Harper ME, Hahn BH, et al. HTLV-III infection in brains of children and adults with AIDS encephalopathy. Science. 1985;227:177–82.
47. Gartner S, Markovits P, Markovitz DM, et al. The role of mononuclear phagocytes in HTLV-III/LAV infection. Science. 1986;233:215–9.
48. Gartner S, Markovits P, Markovitz DM, et al. Virus isolation from and identification of HTLV-III/LAV-producing cells in brain tissue from a patient with AIDS. JAMA. 1986;256:2365–71.
49. Dalgleish AG, Beverley PC, Clapham PR, et al. The CD4 (T4) antigen is an essential component of the receptor for the AIDS retrovirus. Nature. 1985;312:763–7.
50. Klatzmann D, Champagne E, Chamaret S, et al. T-lymphocyte T4 molecule behaves as the receptor for human retrovirus LAV. Nature. 1985;312:767–8.
51. Lasky LA, Nakamura G, Smith DH, et al. Delineation of a region of the human immunodeficiency virus type 1 gp120 glycoprotein critical for interaction with the CD4 receptor. Cell. 1987;50:975–85.
52. Stein BS, Gowda SD, Lifson JD, et al. pH-independent HIV entry into CD4-positive T cells via virus envelope fusion to the plasma membrane. Cell. 1987;49:659–68.
53. Maddon PJ, Dalgleish AG, McDougal JS, et al. The T4 gene encodes the AIDS virus receptor and is expressed in the immune system and the brain. Cell. 1986;47:333–48.
54. Deen KC, McDougal JS, Inacker R, et al. A soluble form of CD4 (T4) protein inhibits AIDS virus infection. Nature. 1988;331:82–4.
55. Fisher RA, Bertonis JM, Meier W, et al. HIV infection is blocked in vitro by recombinant soluble CD4. Nature. 1988;331:76–8.
56. Hussey RE, Richardson NE, Kowalski M, et al. A soluble CD4 protein selectively inhibits HIV replication and syncytium formation. Nature. 1988;331:78–81.
57. Smith DH, Byrn RA, Marsters SA, et al. Blocking of HIV-1 infectivity by a soluble, secreted form of the CD4 antigen. Science. 1987;238:1704–7.
58. Traunecker A, Luke W, Karjalainen K. Soluble CD4 molecules neutralize human immunodeficiency virus type 1. Nature. 1988;331:84–6.
59. Panganiban AT, Temin HM. The retrovirus pol gene encodes a product required for DNA integration: Identification of a retrovirus *int* locus. Proc Natl Acad Sci USA. 1984;81:7885–9.
60. Cullen BR. Trans-activation of human immunodeficiency virus occurs via a bimodal mechanism. Cell. 1986;46:973–82.
61. Feinberg M, Jarrett RF, Aldovini A, et al. HTLV-III expression and production involve complex regulation at the levels of splicing and translation of viral RNA. Cell. 1986;46:807–17.
62. Kao SY, Calman AF, Luciw PA, et al. Anti-termination of transcription within the long terminal repeat of HIV-1 by *tat* gene product. Nature. 1987:330:489–93.
63. Muesing MA, Smith DH, Capon DJ. Regulation of mRNA accumulation by a human immunodeficiency virus trans-activator protein. Cell. 1987;48:691–701.
64. Sodroski J, Patarca R, Rosen C, et al. Location of the trans-activating region on the genome of human T-cell lymphotropic virus type III. Science. 1985;229:74–7.
65. Sodroski J, Rosen C. Wong-Staal F, et al. Trans-acting transcriptional reg-

ulation of human T-cell leukemia virus type III long terminal repeat. Science. 1985;227:171–3.
66. Tong-Starksen SE, Luciw PA, Peterlin BM. Human immunodeficiency virus long terminal repeat responds to T-cell activation signals. Proc Natl Acad Sci USA. 1987;84:6845–9.
67. Gallo RC, Haseltine WA, Montagnier L, et al. Revised nomenclature of human retroviral genes. Nature. 1988. In press.
68. Rosen CA, Terwilliger E, Dayton A, et al. Intragenic cis-acting *art* gene-responsive sequences of the human immunodeficiency viruses. Proc Natl Acad Sci USA. 1988;85:2071–5.
69. Sodroski J, Goh WC, Rosen C, et al. A second post-transcriptional trans-activator gene required for HTLV-III replication. Nature. 1986;321:412–7.
70. Rosen C, Sodroski J, Goh WC, et al. Post-transcriptional regulation accounts for the trans-activation of the human T-lymphotropic virus type III. Nature. 1986;319:555–9.
71. Lifson JC, Feinberg MB, Reyes GR, et al. Induction of CD4-dependent cell fusion by the HTLV-III/LAV envelope glycoprotein. Nature. 1986;323:725–8.
72. Luciw, PA, Cheng-Mayer C, Levy JA, et al. Mutational analysis of the human immunodeficiency virus: The *orf*-B region down-regulates virus replication. Proc Natl Acad Sci USA. 1987;84:1434–8.
73. Guy B, Kieny MP, Riviere Y, et al. HIV F/3′ *orf* encodes a phosphorylated GTP-binding protein resembling an oncogene product. Nature. 1987;330:266–9.
74. Fisher AG, Ensoli B, Ivanoff L, et al. The *sor* gene of HIV-1 is required for efficient virus transmission in vitro. Science. 1987;237:888–93.
75. Strebel K, Daugherty D, Clouse K, et al. The HIV 'A' (*sor*) gene product is essential for virus infectivity. Nature. 1987;328:728–30.
76. Wong-Staal F, Chanda PK, Ghrayeb J. Human immunodeficiency virus: The eighth gene. AIDS Res Hum Retroviruses. 1987;3:33–9.
77. Sodroski J, Goh WC, Rosen C, et al. Role of the HTLV-III/LAV envelope in syncytium formation and cytopathicity. Nature. 1986;322:470–4.
78. Kowalski M, Potz J, Basiripour L, et al. Functional regions of the envelope glycoprotein of human immunodeficiency virus type 1. Science. 1987; 237:1351–5.
79. Somasundaran M, Robinson HL. A major mechanism of human immunodeficiency virus-induced cell killing does not involve cell fusion. J Virol. 1987;61:3114–9.
80. Surbone A, Yarchoan R, McAtee N, et al. Treatment or the acquired immune deficiency syndrome (AIDS) and AIDS-related complex with a regimen of 3′-azido-2′,3′-dideoxythymidine (azidothymidine or zidovudine). Ann Intern Med. 1988;108:534–40.
81. Robert-Guroff M, Brown M, Gallo RC. HTLV-III-neutralizing antibodies in patients with AIDS and AIDS-related complex. Nature. 1985;316:72–4.
82. Weiss RA, Clapham PR, Cheingsong-Popov R, et al. Neutralization of human T-lymphotropic virus type III by sera of AIDS and AIDS-risk patients. Nature. 1985;316:69–72.
83. Walker BD, Chakrabarti S, Moss B, et al. HIV-specific cytotoxic T lymphocytes in seropositive individuals. Nature. 1987;328:345–8.
84. Robert-Guroff M, Reitz MS, Robey WG, et al. In vitro generation of an HTLV-III variant by neutralizing antibody. J Immunol. 1986;137:3306–9.
85. Reitz MS, Wilson C, Naugle C, et al. Generation of a neutralization-resistant variant of HIV-1 is due to selection for a point mutation in the envelope gene. Cell. 1988;54:57–63.
86. Kanki PJ, Alroy J, Essex M. Isolation of a T-lymphotropic retrovirus related to HTLV-III/LAV from wild-caught African green monkeys. Science. 1985;230:951–4.
87. Chakrabarti L, Guyader M, Alizon M, et al. Sequence of simian immunodeficiency virus from macaque and its relationship to other human and simian retroviruses. Nature. 1987;328:543–7.
88. Franchini G, Gurgo C, Guo H, et al. Sequence of simian immunodeficiency virus and its relationship to the human immunodeficiency viruses. Nature. 1987;328:539–43.
89. Hirsch V, Riedel N, Mullins JI. The genome organization of STLV-3 is similar to that of the AIDS virus except for a truncated transmembrane protein. Cell. 1987;49:307–19.
90. Guyader M, Emerman M, Sonigo P, et al. Genome organization and transactivation of the human immunodeficiency virus type 2. Nature. 1987; 326:662–9.
91. Zagury JF, Franchini G, Reitz M, et al. The genetic variability between HIV-2 isolates is comparable to the variability among HIV-1. Proc Natl Acad Sci USA. 1988;85:5941–5.
92. Fultz PN, McClure HM, Swenson RB, et al. Persistent infection of chimpanzees with human T-lymphotropic virus type III/lymphadenopathy-associated virus: A potential model for acquired immunodeficiency syndrome. J Virol. 1986;58:116–24.
93. Matthews TJ, Langlois AJ, Robey WG, et al. Restricted neutralization of divergent human T-lymphotropic virus type III isolates by antibodies to the major envelope glycoprotein. Proc Natl Acad Sci USA. 1986;83:9709–13.
94. Zagury D, Bernard J, Cheynier R, et al. A group specific anamnestic immune reaction against HIV-1. Nature. 1988;332:728–31.
95. Mitsuya H, Looney DJ, Kuno S, et al. Dextran sulfate suppression of viruses in the HIV family: Inhibition of virion binding to CD4+ cells. Science. 1988; 240:646–9.
96. Ueno R, Kuno S. Dextran sulphate, a potent anti-HIV agent in vitro having synergism with zidovudine (letter). Lancet. 1987;1:1379.
97. Mitsuya H, Jarrett RF, Matsukura M, et al. Long-term inhibition of human T-lymphotropic virus type III/lymphadenopathy-associated virus (human immunodeficiency virus) DNA synthesis and RNA expression in T cells protected by 2′,3′-dideoxynucleosides in vitro. Proc Natl Acad Sci USA. 1987;84:2033–7.

Picornaviridae

148. INTRODUCTION

JOHN F. MODLIN

CHARACTERISTICS OF PICORNAVIRUSES

The sigla of the coined word ''picornavirus'' (*pico*, very small; *RNA*, nucleic acid type) describe the hallmarks of this large family of animal viruses.[1] Picornaviruses are icosahedral, 20–30 nm in diameter, and nonenveloped. The virion capsid is composed of 60 structural subunits that are synthesized from four polypeptides with an aggregate molecular weight of 80,000–140,000. The capsid encloses a linear, single-stranded RNA genome with a molecular weight of 2.6×10^6 (~7.5 kilobases). The RNA is infectious and either may serve as a template for the synthesis of additional RNA or may be encapsidated to form progeny virions. The RNA also functions as a monocistronic messenger whose translational product, a ''polyprotein'' of molecular weight 250,000, is coded for by a single, open reading frame involving about 90 percent of the entire genome. The polyprotein subsequently undergoes specific cleavages to form the structural polypeptides, a virus-coded RNA replicase, proteases, and other additional polypeptides necessary for intracellular replication.

Lacking a lipid envelope, picornaviruses are resistant to ether, chloroform, and alcohol. However, they are readily inactivated by ionizing radiation, formaldehyde, and phenol.[1]

Classification of Picornaviruses

A classification of picornaviruses is given in Table 1. Two genera commonly infect humans: (*1*) the genus *Enterovirus*, which has 67 recognized species (serotypes) and (*2*) the genus *Rhinovirus*, with more than 100 human species.[1] In addition there are other enteroviruses and rhinoviruses whose natural hosts are monkeys, cattle, equines, rodents, birds, fish, and possibly insects. Two examples are the agent of foot-and-mouth disease, a virus closely related to rhinoviruses and an important cause of economic loss in the cattle industry, and encephalomyocarditis virus, which is capable of infecting and producing disease in many species including (rarely) humans.[2,3]

A number of clinical, epidemiologic, and biophysical properties distinguish enteroviruses, which are found throughout the gastrointestinal tract, from rhinoviruses, which inhabit the upper respiratory tract. Enteroviruses are stable at pH 3–10, while rhinoviruses are unstable below pH 6. After initial replication in the oropharynx, enteroviruses therefore can survive transit through the acidic environment of the stomach and reach the lower intestinal tract where they replicate more extensively. The buoyant density of enteroviruses in cesium chloride is 1.32–1.35 g/cm^3, while that of rhinoviruses is 1.39–1.45 g/cm^3. The optimal temperature for the replication of enteroviruses is 37°C; in contrast, the 33°C optimum for rhinoviruses possibly reflects their adaptation to the lower temperatures of the nasal passages. The stability of enteroviruses at ambient temperatures exceeds

TABLE 1. Classification of Family Picornaviridae

Genus	Species (Serotypes)	Experimental Host Range		
		Primates	Suckling Mice	Cell Cultures
Enterovirus	Polioviruses 1–3	+ +	– –[a]	+ +
	Coxsackieviruses A 1–24[b]	– –[c]	+ +	±[d]
	Coxsackieviruses B 1–6	– –	+ +	+ +
	Echoviruses 1–34[e]	– –	– –	+ +[f]
	Enteroviruses 68–72[g]	Variable	Variable	+ +
	Enteroviruses of lower animals[h]			
Rhinovirus	1A, 1B, 2–89	– –	– –	+ +
	Rhinoviruses of lower animals[i]			

[a] Rare strains, e.g., Lansing strain of poliovirus 2, have been adapted to mice.
[b] Coxsackievirus A23 has been reclassified as echovirus 9, which leaves 23 coxsackieviruses in group A. Coxsackieviruses A13 and A18 are interrelated.
[c] Coxsackievirus A7 is pathogenic for the CNS of primates.
[d] Most coxsackievirus serotypes of group A are not readily isolated in cell cultures, but exceptions exist, e.g., types A9 and A16; additional serotypes have been adapted to cell cultures.
[e] Echoviruses 1 and 8 are identical; echovirus 10 has been reclassified as reovirus 1 and echovirus 28 as rhinovirus 1A. Echovirus 34 is a variant of coxsackievirus A24; a total of 30 serotypes of echovirus therefore remain from the original 34.
[f] Except echovirus 21.
[g] Hepatitis A virus has been classified as enterovirus 72.
[h] Examples include cardioviruses (e.g., encephalomyocarditis virus, Mengo virus), murine encephalomyelitis virus; bovine, simian, and porcine enteroviruses.
[i] Examples include foot-and-mouth disease virus, equine and bovine rhinoviruses.

that of rhinoviruses and can be further enhanced by the presence of molar concentrations of $MgCl_2$. As a consequence enteroviruses may frequently be isolated from unrefrigerated specimens, and live poliovirus vaccines stabilized by $MgCl_2$ may maintain potency even when refrigeration is suboptimal or unavailable.

Subclassification of Enteroviruses

Enteroviruses historically have been subdivided primarily on the basis of antigenic relationships and differences in host range into polioviruses, groups A and B coxsackieviruses, and echoviruses (Table 1). There were 72 enterovirus types originally identified, but this number has been reduced to 67 distinct serotypes because some were mistakenly classified or redundantly numbered. Several enteroviruses have biologic properties bridging these major groups, which makes it impossible to categorize them unambiguously (see below). Newly recognized enteroviruses, from type 68 upward, have therefore been sequentially numbered and classified simply as enteroviruses.[4] The distinctive characteristics of the major enterovirus subgroups are outlined below.

Polioviruses. Polioviruses replicate only in primates or primate cell cultures. Rare strains such as the type 2 Lansing strain have been adapted to rodents. Although polioviruses multiply in the alimentary tract of some subhuman primates, the hallmark of these viruses is the characteristic histopathologic lesions produced by direct inoculation of the central nervous system. Three serotypes are recognized by cross-neutralization tests.

Coxsackieviruses. Coxsackieviruses, unlike polioviruses, produce paralysis and death in experimentally infected suckling mice. This property enabled their recognition as a distinct class of agents when they were first recovered in 1948 from the feces of two children suffering from a poliomyelitis-like syndrome in the town of Coxsackie, New York.[5] When additional serologically distinct agents were discovered, it was soon recognized that some (group A coxsackieviruses) produced generalized myositis of skeletal muscle that resulted in flaccid paralysis of suckling mice, while others (group B coxsackieviruses) produced focal myositis but a more generalized infection of the myocardium, brown fat, pancreas, and central nervous system that resulted in spastic paralysis.[6] Moreover the group B agents, like polioviruses, usually could also be propagated by the newly discovered technique of inoculation of cultured primate cells, while most of the group A coxsackieviruses grew poorly or not at all in cell cultures. Eventually 23 serotypes of group A and 6 serotypes of group B were recognized.

Echoviruses. After the development of cell culture techniques, additional viruses were discovered in fecal specimens of healthy children.[7,8] They produced cytopathic effects in primate cell cultures but were immunologically distinct from polioviruses and generally nonpathogenic for suckling mice or for the central nervous system of primates. Initially unassociated with any disease state, these "orphan" viruses were named ECHO (*e*nteric *c*ytopathic *h*uman *o*rphan) viruses, subsequently simplified to echoviruses. Thirty serotypes of echoviruses are now recognized.

Newer Enteroviruses. Several of the first 63 numbered serotypes defied precise classification, although they had all the physiochemical properties of enteroviruses. For example, coxsackievirus A9 could regularly be isolated in cultured primate cells, although its pathogenicity for mice was typical of group A coxsackieviruses. Some isolates of echovirus 9 were discovered that were antigenically identical to the prototype strain but were pathogenic for mice. Because of these biologic and serologic ambiguities, newly recognized human enterovirus serotypes are designated by serial numbers only.[4] Since adoption of this simplified taxonomic scheme in 1970, four new serotypes have been discovered (enteroviruses 68–71). Hepatitis A virus has recently been classified as enterovirus 72.

Despite some overlap in the types of illness produced by virus groups of the original classification, the association of a particular group with a specific syndrome (for example, group B coxsackieviruses with myocarditis and pericarditis) is sufficiently distinctive to justify the continued use of the older scheme for the first 63 serotypes. Moreover, comparisons of the genomes of polioviruses, coxsackieviruses, and echoviruses by nucleic acid hybridization support the validity of this classification.[12] About 5 percent of the nucleotide sequences are common to all human enteroviruses so far examined, but relationships within groups are much closer. Different serotypes of echoviruses share approximately half their nucleotide sequences, while coxsackieviruses of group A share fewer than 20 percent of their sequences with group B viruses or echoviruses.[9]

Molecular Biology of Enteroviruses and Their Replication

The RNA genomes of several strains of naturally occurring and attenuated polioviruses have been fully sequenced, and the replication of polioviruses within primate cells has been studied in great detail.[1,10] Furthermore, poliovirus RNA has been reverse transcribed and the complementary DNA sequences cloned.[11] Transfection of monkey cells with the vector containing these sequences results in progeny polioviruses.[12] While the molecular biology of the nonpolio enteroviruses has not been studied as closely, representative strains of coxsackieviruses B1 and B3 have been sequenced.[13,14] The molecular structure and intracellular replicative events are thought to be very similar for all of the human enteroviruses.[1]

Sequencing of the enterovirus genome reveals approximately 7450 nucleotides divided into three regions; a 5′ end region of 743 nucleotides, a continuous coding region of about 6625 nucleotides, and a 3′ poly (A) end region of variable length. The 5′ terminus is covalently linked to a small virus-coded protein of approximately 7000 daltons (VPg) that is involved in the initiation of RNA synthesis. Removal of the poly (A) 3′ terminus renders the RNA noninfectious. Capsid proteins are encoded on the 5′ end of the open reading frame. The remainder of the open reading frame codes for nonstructural proteins whose known functions include promotion of viral RNA synthesis, proteolytic cleavage of the translation products, and inhibition of host cell protein synthesis. Sequencing data indicates that the most conserved regions of the genome are those coding for the VPg protein, the RNA polymerase, and the 5′ noncoding region.[15] The genes coding for the structural proteins are less conserved. There is considerable genomic variation within the regions of the VP1 gene that code for neutralizing antibody epitopes.

The four structural proteins VP1, VP2, VP3, and VP4 are present in equimolar amounts, with 60 copies of each in the virion. For polioviruses, VP1 is the dominantly exposed protein and contains at least two epitopes that induce neutralizing antibodies including the type-specifying antigenic determinant(s).[16,17] VP3 and VP2 are also partially exposed proteins that are antigenic in the native virion; VP4 is an internal protein closely associated with the viral RNA.

At the cellular level, enterovirus infection is initiated by attachment to a specific cell membrane receptor. Recent studies point to the presence of separate families of enterovirus receptors on primate cells.[18] For example, the three poliovirus serotypes share a common receptor on HeLa cells that does not bind coxsackievirus B5 or echovirus 30,[19] while other HeLa cell receptor(s) have been found that bind group B coxsackieviruses 1, 3, and 5 but not the polioviruses or certain other enterovirus serotypes.[18,20] The gene for the poliovirus receptor, which has been mapped to human chromosome 19, induces susceptibility to poliovirus infection when transfected into normally nonsusceptible mouse cells.[21]

Penetration, uncoating, and release of the nucleic acid into the cytoplasm occurs within minutes at 37°C. RNA synthesis begins about 30 minutes after infection and results in the exponential increase of complementary and progeny RNA until 2.5 hours after infection when there is a switch to a linear accumulation of mainly progeny RNA. Each cell synthesizes about 2×10^5 molecules of progeny RNA, 50 percent of which is used as messenger RNA by the cell. The regulation of RNA synthesis involves the synthesis of a viral RNA-dependent RNA polymerase. Initiation is primer dependent. The 22 amino acid protein covalently linked to RNA may be a primer.

The RNA translation product is a large polyprotein with a molecular weight of about 250,000 daltons. Production of both virion and nonstructural proteins and virion assembly proceeds by a series of discrete steps in which large polypeptides are cleaved by proteolytic enzymes to smaller proteins.

Host protein and RNA synthesis are severely compromised by 3 hours after infection. After about 6–7 hours virions are visible by electron microscopy within the cytoplasm, and they are subsequently released by lysis of the cell, which results in a yield of approximately 10^5 particles per cell.

PATHOGENESIS AND IMMUNITY IN ENTEROVIRAL INFECTIONS

Pathogenesis

The pathogenesis of infection is best understood for polioviruses, which have been extensively investigated both in primates experimentally infected with neurovirulent strains and in humans infected with vaccine strains.[22–26] Although comparable data are not available for the nonpolio enteroviruses, available information supports the essential similarity of the pathogenetic events except for the principal target organs affected after viremia. Studies of coxsackievirus infection in subprimate mammals, principally mice, have produced much information on the influence of various host and environmental factors on the ability of the virus to replicate in target organs and on the mechanism of vertical transmission of enteroviruses from infected pregnant animals to their offspring.

Enteroviruses infect humans primarily as a result of the ingestion of fecally contaminated material. Ingested virus implants and replicates in susceptible tissues of the pharynx or distal part of the gut. Whether initial replication takes place in mucosal epithelial cells or cells of the lamina propria has not been established, but further replication in lymphoid tissue of the gut, especially tonsils and Peyer's patches of the ileum, is detectable 1–3 days after the ingestion of virus. Humans ingesting $>10^6$ times the median tissue culture infective dose ($TCID_{50}$) of attenuated poliovirus regularly shed virus in both oropharyngeal secretions and feces, while lower infecting doses ($<10^5$ $TCID_{50}$) result only in fecal shedding.[23] Moreover, the quantity of virus recoverable from the tonsils is much less than in Peyer's patches where it may reach 10^7–10^8 $TCID_{50}$/g. The maximal duration of viral excretion is 3–4 weeks from the pharynx and 5–6 weeks or even longer in the feces. These observations suggest that polioviruses replicate most efficiently in the lower intestines, especially the distal portion of the small bowel.

After multiplication in submucosal lymphatic tissues, enteroviruses pass to regional lymph nodes (cervical, mesenteric) and give rise to a "minor viremia" that is transient, of small magnitude, and not usually detectable. The virus may spread hematogenously to distinct reticuloendothelial tissue such as the liver, spleen, bone marrow, and deep lymph nodes. In subclinical infections, which are the most common, viral replication at this point ceases or is contained by host defense mechanisms. However, in a minority of infected persons, further replication of virus occurs in these reticuloendothelial sites and causes a heavy, sustained shedding into the blood stream ("major viremia") that coincides with the "minor illness" of poliomyelitis and probably the nonspecific febrile illnesses associated with other enterovirus infections. Prodromal viremia has been demonstrated with wild strains of poliovirus[26,27] and echovirus 9[28] but is uncommon with Sabin vaccine strains except for type 2.[29]

The major viremia results in dissemination to target organs such as the meninges, heart, and skin. In these tissues necrosis and inflammatory lesions are observed, while histopathologic lesions are generally not seen in the gut and lymphoreticular tissues associated with earlier replicative events. In target organs, the degree of inflammatory change and tissue necrosis corresponds with the titer of infectious virus present. The severity of infection in experimental animals can be enhanced by induced exercise, cold exposure, malnutrition, pregnancy, and immunosuppression with corticosteroids or radiation.

Mutation of Enteroviruses during Natural Infection

Enteroviruses undergo a high rate of mutation during replication in the human gastrointestinal tract. Point mutations frequently occur within several days after feeding attenuated polioviruses to young children, an event that is thought responsible for the reversion of the type 3 Sabin strain to a neurovirulent state.[30,31] Recombination between the genomes of different serotypes has also been demonstrated to be a common event. Oligonucleotide fingerprinting of serial polio vaccine virus and nonpolio enterovirus isolates from children with agammaglobulinemia demonstrates that these viruses undergo continuous genetic variation during replication in the gastrointestinal tract over a period of months to years.[32,33]

IMMUNITY AND THE IMMUNE RESPONSE

Immunity to enterovirus infections is type specific. Antibody-mediated immune mechanisms operate both in the alimentary tract to prevent implantation of virus and in the blood stream to prevent dissemination to the target organs.

Circulating antibodies play the most important role in preventing enteroviral *disease* as opposed to infection. Even trace amounts of type-specific neutralizing antibodies prevent poliovirus viremia and paralysis in experimentally infected primates.[34] Passive immunity to paralytic disease in humans can be achieved by the administration of immune serum globulin before exposure to neurovirulent polioviruses.[35,36] After the onset of signs of central nervous system infection, parenterally administered immune globulin does not modify the outcome since at this late stage of illness patients invariably have circulating antibodies. Immune globulin therefore has no role in the treatment of established disease.[37]

IgA antibody appears in nasal secretions 2–4 weeks after the administration of live, attenuated, oral poliovirus vaccine (OPV) and persists for at least 15 years.[25] The intranasal administration of inactivated poliovirus vaccine (IPV) induces low, transient secretory IgA levels. Alimentary immunity is relative. On reexposure to infection virus, high titers of IgA antibodies either prevent the implantation of virus or are associated with only evanescent shedding of small quantities of virus. With lower titers of IgA antibodies, there is more extensive oropharyngeal replication of virus and more prolonged shedding.[25] A similar inhibition of viral replication by IgA antibodies has been shown in the distal gut. The elaboration of virus-specific IgA antibodies by the lower intestine appears to depend on *local* immunocompetent tissues, not those of the pharynx. This principle was elegantly demonstrated by experiments in which infants with double-barrel colostomies were fed live, attenuated poliovirus through the colostomy. Although they developed serum IgA, IgG, and IgM antibodies to poliovirus, secretory IgA antibodies were elaborated only in the distal loop of the colostomy and not in the pharynx or proximal loop. When subsequently challenged with OPV orally, they shed virus from the pharynx but not from the distal segment of the bowel and then proceeded to develop IgA antibodies in pharyngeal secretions.[38]

Antibodies to enteroviruses are present in the colostrum and milk of immune women and may interfere with replication of virus when breast-fed babies are given OPV, thus preventing a vaccine "take."[39,40] Maternal antibodies passively acquired either transplacentally or via milk have also been postulated to exert a possible modifying role on enterovirus infections of early infancy either by preventing infection or by causing subclinical but nonetheless immunizing infection.[41]

In the serum both IgM and IgG humoral antibodies are produced as early as 1–3 days after enterovirus challenge. IgM antibodies predominate during the first month and disappear 2–3 months after immunization.[25] IgG antibody is mostly of the IgG1 and IgG3 subtypes [42] The IgA response in serum, detectable at 2–6 weeks, is generally low and not present in all persons. Neutralizing IgG antibodies in serum persist for life after natural infection with enteroviruses.

Antibodies appear to have an important role in the *recovery* from enterovirus infection. Perhaps the best evidence of the importance of humoral antibodies is found in the patients with isolated agammaglobulinemia who have persistent enterovirus infections.[43] Nonetheless, there is both clinical and laboratory evidence that humoral antibody alone is not sufficient to limit enterovirus replication in target organs. Data from several laboratories indicate that macrophage function is also a critical component of the immune response to enterovirus infection.[44,45] Selective ablation of macrophage function in experimental animals markedly enhances the severity of coxsackievirus B infections,[44] while inhibition of T-lymphocyte function has little effect.[46]

Even though T lymphocytes do not contribute to the inhibition of enterovirus replication, there is growing evidence that certain immunopathologic events after enterovirus infection are mediated by T-cell activity. In the murine model of coxsackievirus B3 induced myocarditis, a late phase of the inflammatory response appears to be secondary to virus-induced, cytotoxic T-cell destruction of myocytes, a process that is partially controlled by the major histocompatibility genetic locus in the mouse.[47]

EPIDEMIOLOGY OF ENTEROVIRUS INFECTIONS

Endemic and Epidemic Behavior

Enteroviruses are Distributed Worldwide. Infection rates vary dramatically with the season, geography, and age and socioeconomic status of the population sampled. Enterovirus infections occur throughout the year, but in temperate climates infections are strikingly more prevalent in the summer and autumn months (June to October in the Northern Hemisphere).[48,49] This seasonal periodicity, which has never been satisfactorily explained, is repeatedly observed each year in cites of the northern United States but is less pronounced in Atlanta and Miami and disappears altogether in the tropics where enterovirusees are endemic the year round. Climate also affects the frequency and abundance of enteroviruses isolated from the feces of heatlhy children. For example, several surveys of southern and southwestern cities of the United States have indicated that 7–15 percent of children sampled during the year excreted enteroviruses while comparable populations in New York, Buffalo, and Minneapolis had annual excretion rates less than 5 percent.[50]

Young infants have the highest rates of infection. During the annual peak period of enterovirus transmission in Rochester, NY, the incidence of infection was found to be 12.8 percent during the first month of life.[51] Rates of symptomatic enterovirus infection drop after the second month of life (J. F. Modlin and L. Berlin, unpublished observations) but remain higher for infants and toddlers as compared with older children and adults. Enterovirus infections are more prevalent among lower socioeconomic class children than among children of the upper or middle classes, a fact probably explained by crowding, poor hygiene, and opportunities for fecal contamination. Simultaneous infection by more than one serotype is common under these circumstances. A study of infants in Karachi, Pakistan, revealed that 80 percent yielded rectal swabs with at least one enterovirus. Of the positives, nearly half yielded two enteroviruses and occasional subjects as many as four.[52]

The frequency with which particular serotypes of enteroviruses are observed varies markedly. Polioviruses circulating in developed countries are almost exclusively vaccine strains, while in developing countries most are virulent natural strains. Generally all three poliovirus serotypes cocirculate simultaneously, although one or two strains may predominate briefly within a given locality. In urban areas of the United States, usually one to three nonpolio enterovirus serotypes predominate each season, and these vary from one city to another. Some enteroviruses are isolated with low frequency in the same locality in sequential years, while others have produced epidemics only to disappear the following season and for years thereafter. Occasional epidemics are almost global, such as the one caused by echovirus 9 in the late 1950s and the explosive pandemic of acute hemorrhagic conjunctivitis due to enterovirus 70 that began in 1969. During the 14-year period 1970–1983, the 15 most common serotypes of nonpolio enterovirus isolates submitted from state and local public health laboratories to the Enterovirus Surveillance Program of the Centers for Disease Control accounted for 65–89 percent of all isolates within a given year.[53] Echoviruses represent slightly more than half of these clinical isolates and group B coxsackieviruses represent about one-fourth (Table 2).[49,53] It is likely that group A coxsackieviruses are considerably underrepresented in these data because only a few serotypes such as A9 and A16 grow readily in cell culture.[54] Among the frequently isolated serotypes, echovirus types 3, 4, 6, 7, 9, and 11 and coxsackievirus B5 occurred in seasonal epidemics within a 2-year period, while the remaining agents caused sporadic, endemic activity annually without evidence of epidemic behavior.[49] Some serotypes, such as coxsackievirus B6 and the newer enteroviruses 68, 69, and 71 have been recognized only rarely.

Why particular serotypes of enteroviruses appear and dis-

TABLE 2. Most Common Nonpolio Enterovirus Serotypes Isolated in United States 1970–1983

Serotype	*Percentage*
Echovirus 11	12.2
Echovirus 9	11.3
Coxsackievirus B5	8.7
Echovirus 4	6.3
Echovirus 6	5.5
Coxsackievirus B2	4.8
Coxsackievirus B4	4.6
Coxsackievirus A9	4.5
Coxsackievirus B3	4.5
Echovirus 3	3.2
Echovirus 7	3.0
All others	31.4

(Data from Strikas et al.[53])

appear and the reasons for endemic vs. epidemic behavior are not well understood. some epidemic strains such as echovirus 9 may spread rapidly and exhaust susceptibles in the population beyond a "critical mass" necessary for continued transmission, while those strains appearing endemically over several years may be less contagious. Periodic reappearances of the same serotype are sometimes marked by strain variation as measured by differences in neutralization kinetics, by immune sera or by various molecular markers (see below). Variation among strains of the same serotype, which has been demonstrated with several enterovirus serotypes including echovirus 30, poliovirus 3,[56,57] and coxsackievirus B5,[58] may also affect the secular trends of infection.

Molecular Epidemiology

In recent years, powerful new molecular genetic techniques have been applied to the study of the epidemiology of enterovirus infections. Two-dimensional oligonucleotide gel electrophoresis ("fingerprinting"), RNA sequencing, and labeled complementary DNA (cDNA) probe analysis have each been used to unambiguously differentiate vaccine and naturally occurring poliovirus strains.[59] These methods have also been useful in tracing the routes of spread of poliovirus type 1[60] and enterovirus 70[61,62] by determining the degree of genetic relatedness among epidemiologically distinct isolates.

RNA sequencing of the genome has proved the most adept in characterizing the evolutionary relationships among poliovirus isolates of the same serotype. "Genotypes" are distinguished from one another by the divergence of more than 15 percent among the RNA nucleotides in the homologous portions of the genome that are sequenced.[59] Current data suggest that several different poliovirus type 1 genotypes exist in the Western Hemisphere, each with geographically distinct origins and patterns of transmission.[59] In addition, Hamby and colleagues have recently used RNA fingerprinting to demonstrate the reemergence of an epidemic coxsackievirus B5 strain in 1983 in the United States that had remained epidemiologically dormant over a period of 16 years.[58]

Transmission

Enterovirus transmission among humans is not fully understood. Because viral shedding from the gastrointestinal tract is more prolonged than is shedding from the upper respiratory tract, the fecal–oral route is thought to be the predominant mode of transmission. Notable exceptions to this pattern occur, however. Coxsackievirus A21, which especially causes upper respiratory infections, is probably spread by respiratory secretions, while enterovirus 70, the agent of acute hemorrhagic conjunctivitis, appears to be spread by fomites, fingers, and ophthalmologic instruments contaminated with virus in tears. Respiratory–oral spread has been postulated to play a role in the transmission of poliovirus among upper socioeconomic class persons and also in the spread of coxsackieviruses, which are frequently shed simultaneously from both the upper and lower ends of the alimentary canal.[63]

Direct spread of enteroviruses from person to person is postulated, but mechanisms of transmission by direct or indirect contact have not been studied under experimental conditions. Vigorous washing with soap and water reduces but does not eliminate infectious poliovirus from the hands.[64] Although enteroviruses have been isolated from flies, cockroaches, food exposed to naturally infected flies, and dog feces, transmission by these vehicles has never been demonstrated. Sampling of sewage in most cities, especially in summer months, usually yields several enterovirus serotypes.[65] Clams in seawater polluted by sewage concentrate enteroviruses 10- to 60-fold. Nevertheless water-borne epidemics attributed to shellfish ingestion have never been demonstrated.

Longitudinal studies have shown clustering of enterovirus infections in families.[63] Once the virus has been introduced into the household, secondary attack rates for infection among susceptible family members (those lacking type-specific antibody) are 90–100 percent for wild polioviruses[66] and 76 percent for coxsackieviruses.[63] Secondary attack rates for echoviruses are less than 50 percent, probably because these viruses tend to be shed only in feces and for shorter periods. Asymptomatic infants shedding virus in the feces are the most efficient disseminators of infection. Mothers and infant siblings are at greater risk of acquiring infection than are fathers and teenagers.[63] For all enteroviruses, the period of maximum contagiousness corresponds to the period of maximum virus excretion in the feces.

Reinfections (virus excretion by a person with pre-existing antibodies to a given serotype) are rare, but when they occur, they are not associated with illness. The duration of excretion of virus is shorter (usually only a few days) than in the primary infection.[63,66]

Incidence of Infection and Illness

Approximately 95 percent of infections due to wild polioviruses and at least 50–80 percent of nonpolio enteroviral infections are completely asymptomatic. Even symptomatic infections usually produce undifferentiated febrile illnessses lasting but a few days, often accompanied by symptoms of upper respiratory tract infection.[67] These illnesses may be caused by virtually any enterovirus serotype and are clinically indistinguishable from infection by many other viral agents. Disease syndromes considered characteristic of enteroviruses such as aseptic meningitis or pericarditis are in fact unusual manifestations of infection; a 4-year longitudinal family-based study in New York City detected 291 enterovirus infections, none with "characteristic" illnesses, and only 6 with exanthems.[63]

Age and sex are important factors in enteroviral infections. World Health Organization data indicate that approximately three-quarters of the reported enteroviral infections, most of them symptomatic, occur in children less than 15 years old. Attack rates for both infection and illness with nonpolio enteroviruses are highest in infants 1 year of age or younger.[50,68] However, the risk of certain enterovirus-related clinical syndromes seems to vary with age. For example, aseptic meningitis is most commonly recognized in very young infants, while some other illnesses such as pleurodynia and myopericarditis are recognized predominantly in adolescents and young adults. Symptomatic enteroviral infections in the elderly are very uncommon. Among young children, boys are at greater risk of illness (but not infection) than are girls.[68] Aseptic meningitis and poliomyelitis occur nearly twice as often in boys. After puberty the reverse is true, perhaps because adult women have greater exposure than do men to children shedding virus.[63,69] Pregnancy also appears to enhance the severity of enterovirus infections. The incidence of paralytic poliomyelitis was two to three times higher in pregnant women than in age-matched nonpregnant women in Boston before the control of poliomyelitis.[70] There are also clinical and epidemiologic data that suggest that enteroviral illnesses are more frequent[71] and more severe[72] in persons who exercise vigorously before the onset of symptoms. Although these data are anecdotal, they are supported by considerable evidence in laboratory animals that exercise enhances the severity of coxsackievirus B infection.

Although the incidence and prevalence of nonpolio enterovirus infections have been accurately measured in selected populations and they are undeniably common, the overall incidence in the United States is unknown. Virus isolations tend to be reported only from patients with symptomatic illness, especially the "characteristic" syndromes, for which reporting is incomplete. Serologic surveys encompassing all 67 enteroviral serotypes are not feasible. Antibody prevalence rates measured for a few serotypes indicate that, after the decline of passively acquired maternal antibodies after the age of 6 months, the fraction of immune persons in the population rises progressively with age until 15–90 percent of the adult population have type-specific neutralizing antibodies for each serotype tested, depending on the serotype and the socioeconomic class of the population surveyed.[63,68]

Incubation Period and Period of Communicability

The incubation period for illness due to enteroviral infections can rarely be determined precisely. Because the source of infection is often an asymptomatic person who transmits virus as readily as one who is ill, the time of exposure is usually unknown. While the incubation period may range from 2 days to 2 weeks, it is usually 3–5 days. Patients with enteroviral illnesses typically excrete virus in throat secretions or feces for several days before the onset of symptoms and continue to excrete virus in feces for several weeks thereafter. The period of communicability is therefore potentially long. However the period of maximum communicability is believed to be early in illness, when viral shedding is greatest.

LABORATORY DIAGNOSIS OF ENTEROVIRAL INFECTIONS

Virus isolation in cell culture remains the mainstay of diagnosis of enterovirus infection, although serologic tests are sometimes useful in certain cases and several rapid diagnostic techniques have been developed in recent years. Isolation of virus from feces or from throat secretions is not definitive proof of the etiology of temporally associated illness because intercurrent enteroviral infections etiologically unrelated to the observed illness may be present. However such evidence is strong presumptive evidence of etiologic association. The most definitive etiologic evidence is provided by virus isolation from sources such as cerebrospinal fluid, pericardial fluid, or skin lesions as dictated by the clinical syndrome. In young infants with nonlocalized febrile illnesses, enteroviruses can often be recovered from whole blood or serum specimens.[73]

The most useful information is obtained when cultures are obtained from multiple sites, which should include throat secretions and feces because virus is often not present simultaneously in all specimens. Echoviruses, for example, are often recovered from the cerebrospinal fluid of patients with aseptic meningitis when they are not present in the alimentary tract.[74] Conversely, late in the course of enteroviral illnesses, viral cultures of feces are useful because the lower intestine may be the only site from which the agent is still being excreted.

In most instances the diagnosis is accomplished most quickly and economically by virus isolation. With the use of three or four appropriately chosen cell lines, a presumptive diagnosis of enterovirus infection can be reported by the laboratory within 2–5 days in most cases,[75] although specific serotyping of the isolate will take longer. The primary monkey kidney cell lines and the human embryonic fibroblast cell lines used routinely in diagnostic virology laboratories will support the growth of most polioviruses, group B coxsackieviruses, and echoviruses. The inclusion of buffalo green monkey kidney cells and human rhabdomyosarcoma (RD) cells will enhance the recovery of group B coxsackieviruses and echoviruses, respectively.[75] Only a few serotypes of the group A coxsackieviruses (e.g., A9, A16) grow readily in routinely used cell lines. Although the use of specialized cell lines such as RD,[76] human amnion,[77] guinea pig embryo,[78] or human colonic carcinoma[79] may aid the recovery of some group A coxsackieviruses in cell culture, inoculation of newborn mice remains the method of choice for recovery of this class of enteroviruses.[54]

Serologic testing has limited usefulness in the diagnosis of nonpolio enteroviral infections, principally because it is not feasible to test for antibodies to each of the 67 virus serotypes that would be required, for example, in the case of aseptic meningitis. It is generally practical only to determine antibody titers against the patient's own virus isolate or against one or two serotypes known to be prevalent in the community at that time. Possible exceptions to this rule are the use of serologic tests to diagnose enteroviral syndromes usually caused by only a few serotypes such as hand-foot-and-mouth disease due to coxsackievirus A16 or myopericarditis due to coxsackieviruses B1–5. The neutralization test is the established standard method for the determination of serotype-specific antibodies in sera. While a microneutralization technique is widely employed, methods based on neutralization are relatively insensitive, poorly standardized, labor intensive, and expensive. Immunoassay techniques have been demonstrated to be a type-specific and sensitive means of detection of antibodies to enteroviruses.[80] Because immunoassays offer a potential versatility not found in the neutralization method, they may become the preferred method of enterovirus antibody assay in the future. Paired acute and convalescent phase sera collected as early in the illness as possible and 2–4 weeks later are desirable since even high, stable antibody titers do not exclude infection in the remote past. A variety of new techniques have been employed in an attempt to diagnose enterovirus infections more rapidly, but none have yet achieved the sensitivity and specificity of virus isolation in cell culture. Antigen detection methods such as counterimmunoelectrophoresis and enzyme immunoassay fail to detect the picogram amounts of viral antigen that are present in cerebrospinal fluid or stool specimens from infected patients.[81,82] Nucleic acid hybridization methods have been developed in which labeled complementary DNA and RNA probes react with the genomes of many enterovirus serotypes; each of the methods reported lack sufficient sensitivity to be clinically useful.[83–85] Serum IgM antibody to the group B coxsackieviruses can often be detected early in the course of illness, but positive test results are not serotype specific and may occur during infections with enteroviruses of other classes.[86] In contrast, a highly serotype specific IgM assay to enterovirus 70 has been described.[87]

Evidence for group B coxsackievirus infection of the heart has been obtained by immunofluorescent staining of myocardial tissue[88] and with the use of labeled DNA probes,[89] but the sensitivity and specificity of these methods are unknown, and they have not gained wide acceptance.

TREATMENT AND PREVENTION OF ENTEROVIRAL INFECTIONS

Although a variety of antiviral and immunomodulating agents have been tested against enteroviruses in the laboratory, effective drug therapy is not available to the clinician for the treatment of enterovirus infections.[90–93] The single exception to this dictum may be the successful management of persistent enterovirus infections in some immunocompromised patients with immune globulin (see Chapter 150).

The pre-exposure administration of immune globulin is known to reduce the risk of paralytic poliomyelitis.[36] It is very likely that immune globulin would also prevent nonpolio enterovirus disease as well, but this strategy is rarely applicable to clinical practice. The successful vaccine approach against paralytic poliomyelitis is detailed in Chapter 149. In the setting of a community epidemic or a patient hospitalized with enteroviral illness, simple hygienic measures such as handwashing and careful disposal or autoclaving of potentially infected feces and secretions should be practiced. Gown and mask procedures or isolation of the patient except in the newborn nursery are unwarranted. Pregnant women, especially those near term, should be advised to avoid contact with patients suspected of having enteroviral illness.

ACKNOWLEDGMENT

This chapter is based in part on a chapter in the second edition coauthored by Alice S. Huang.

REFERENCES

1. Melnick JL. Portraits of viruses: The picornaviruses. Intervirology. 1983;20:61–100.
2. Dick GWA, Best AM, Haddow AJ, et al. Mengo encephalomyelitis, a hitherto unknown virus affecting man. Lancet. 1948;2:286.
3. Tesh RB. The prevalence of encephalomyocarditis virus neutralizing antibodies among various human populations. Am J Trop Med Hyg. 1978;27:144.
4. Rosen L, Melnick JL, Schmidt NJ, et al. Subclassification of enteroviruses and ECHO virus type 34. Arch Ges Virusforsch. 1970;30:89.
5. Dalldorf G, Sickles GM. An unidentified, filtrable agent isolated from the feces of children with paralysis. Science. 1948;108:61.
6. Melnick JL, Shaw EW, Curnen EC. A virus from patients diagnosed as nonparalytic poliomyelitis or aseptic meningitis. Proc Soc Exp Biol Med. 1949;71:344.
7. Melnick JL, Agren K. Poliomyelitis and coxsackie viruses isolated from normal infants in Egypt. Proc Soc Exp Biol Med. 1952;81:621.
8. Ramos-Alvarez M, Sabin AB. Characteristics of poliomyelitis and other enteric viruses recovered in tissue culture from healthy American children. Proc Soc Exp Biol Med. 1954;87:655.
9. Young NA. Polioviruses, coxsackieviruses, and echoviruses: Comparison of the genomes by RNA hybridization. J Virol. 1973;11:832.
10. Levintow L. Reproduction of picornaviruses. In: Fraenkel-Conrat H, Wagner RR eds. Comprehensive Virology. V. 2. New York: Plenum; 1974;109.
11. Racaniello VR, Baltimore, D. Molecular cloning of poliovirus cDNA and determination of the complete nucleotide sequence of the viral genome. Proc Natl Acad Sci USA. 1981;78:4887.
12. Racaniello VR, Baltimore D. Cloned poliovirus complementary DNA is infectious in mammalian cells. Science. 1981;214:916.
13. Iizuka N, Kuge S, Nomoto A. Complete nucleotide sequence of the genome of coxsackievirus B1. Virology. 1987;156:64–73.
14. Lindberg AM, Stalhandske PO, Pettersson U. Genome of coxsackievirus B3. Virology. 1987;156:50–63.
15. Werner G, Rosenwirth B, Bauer E, et al. Molecular cloning and sequence determination of the genomic regions encoding protease and genome-linked protein of three picornaviruses. J Virol. 1986;57:1084–93.
16. Emini EA, Jameson BA, Lewis AJ, et al. Poliovirus neutralizing epitopes: Analysis and localization with neutralizing monoclonal antibodies. J Virol. 1982;43:997.
17. Minor PD, Schild GC, Bootman J, et al. Location and primary structure of a major antigenic site for poliovirus neutralization. Nature. 1983;301:674.
18. Crowell RL, Field AK, Schlief WA, et al. Monoclonal antibody that inhibits infection of HeLa and rhabdomyosarcoma cells by selected enteroviruses through receptor blockade. J Virol. 1986;57:438–45.
19. Nobis P, Zibirre R, Meyer G, et al. Production of a monoclonal antibody against an epitope on HeLa cells that is the functional poliovirus binding site. J Gen Virol. 1985;66:2563–9.
20. Mapoles JE, Krah DL, Crowell RL. Purification of a HeLa cell receptor protein for group B coxsackieviruses. J Virol. 1985;55:560–6.
21. Mendelsohn C, Johnson B, Lionetti KA, et al. Transformation of a human poliovirus receptor gene into mouse cells. Proc Natl Acad Sci USA. 1986;83:7845–9.
22. Bodian D. A reconsideration of the pathogenesis of poliomyelitis. Am J Hyg. 1952;55:414.
23. Sabin AB. Behavior of chimpanzee-avirulent poliomyelitis viruses in experimentally infected human volunteers. Am J Med Sci. 1955;230:1.
24. Sabin AB. Pathogenesis of poliomyelitis: Reappraisal in light of new data. Science. 1956;123:1151.
25. Ogra PL, Karzon DT. Formation and function of poliovirus antibody in different tissues. Prog Med Virol. 1971;13:157.
26. Horstmann DM, McCollum RW. Poliomyelitis virus in human blood during the "minor illness" and the asymptomatic infection. Proc Soc Exp Biol Med. 1953;82:434.
27. Davis DC, Melnick JL. Two additional examples of viremia in asymptomatic poliomyelitis infection. Pediatrics. 1957;20:975.
28. Yoshioka I, Horstmann DM. Viremia in infection due to ECHO virus type 9. N Engl J Med. 1960;262:224.
29. Horstmann DM, Opton EM, Klemperer R, et al. Viremia in infants vaccinated with oral poliovirus vaccine (Sabin). Am J Hyg. 1964;79:47.
30. Jameson BA, Bonin J, Wimmer E, et al. Natural variants of the Sabin type 1 vaccine strains of poliovirus and correlation with a poliovirus neutralization site. Virology. 1985;143:337–41.
31. Minor PD, John A, Ferguson M, et al. Antigenic and molecular evolution of the vaccine strain of type 3 poliovirus during the period of excretion by a primary vaccinee. J Gen Virol. 1986;67:693–706.
32. O'Neil KM, Pallansch MA, Winkelstein JA, et al. Chronic group A coxsackievirus infection in agammaglobulinemia: Demonstration of genomic variation of serotypically identical isolates persistently excreted by the same patient. J Infect Dis. 1988;157:183–86.
33. Yoneyama T, Hagiwara A, Hara M, et al. Alteration in oligonucleotide fingerprint patterns of the viral genome in poliovirus type 2 isolated from paralytic patients. Infect Immun. 1982;37:46–53.
34. Bodian D, Nathanson N. Inhibitory effect of passive antibody on virulent poliovirus excretion and on immune response in chimpanzees. Bull Johns Hopkins Hosp. 1960;107:143.
35. Stevens KM. Estimate of molecular equivalent of antibody required for prophylaxis and therapy of poliomyelitis. J Hyg (Camb). 1959;57:198.
36. Hammon WMcD, Coriell LI, Stokes J. Evaluation of Red Cross gamma globulin as a prophylactic agent for poliomyelitis. I. Plan of controlled field tests and results of 1951 pilot study in Utah. JAMA. 1952;150:739–56.
37. Bahlke AM, Perkins JE. Treatment of preparalytic poliomyelitis with gamma globulin. JAMA. 1945;129:1146.
38. Ogra PL, Karzon DT. Distribution of poliovirus antibody in serum, nasopharynx, and alimentary tract following segmental immunization of lower alimentary tract with poliovaccine. J Immunol. 1969;102:1423.
39. Athreya BH, Coriell LI, Charney J. Poliomyelitis antibodies in human colostrum and milk. J Pediatr. 1964;6:79.
40. Warren RJ, Lepow ML, Bartsch GE, et al. The relationship of maternal antibody, breast feeding, and age to the susceptibility of newborn infants to infection with attenuated poliovirus. Pediatrics. 1964;34:4.
41. Modlin, JF, Polk BF, Horton P, et al. Perinatal echovirus infection: Risk of transmission during a community outbreak. N Engl J Med. 1981;305:368.
42. Torfason EG, Reimer CB, Keyserling HL. Subclass restriction of human enterovirus antibodies. J Clin Microbiol. 1987;25:1376–9.
43. McKinney RE Jr, Katz SL, Wilfert CM. Chronic enteroviral meningoencephalitis in agammaglobulinemic patients. Rev Infect Dis. 1987;9:334–56.
44. Roger-Zisman B, Allison AC. The role of antibody and host cells in the resistance of mice against infection by coxsackie B-3 virus. J Gen Virol. 1973;19:329.
45. Woodruff JF. Lack of correlation between neutralizing antibody production and suppression of coxsackie B-3 replication in target organs: Evidence for involvement of mononuclear inflammatory cells in host defense. J Immunol. 1979;123:31.
46. Woodruff JF, Woodruff JJ. Involvement of T lymphocytes in the pathogenesis of coxsackievirus B3 heart disease. J Immunol. 1974;113:1726.
47. Rose NR, Wolfgram LJ, Herskowitz A, et al. Postinfectious autoimmunity: Two distinct phases of coxsackievirus B3-induced myocarditis. Ann NY Acad Sci. 1986;475:146–56.
48. Miller SA, Wald ER, Bergman I, et al. Enteroviral meningitis in January with marked cerebrospinal fluid pleocytosis. Pediatr Infect Dis. 1986;5:706–7.
49. Moore M. Enteroviral disease in the United States, 1970–1979. J Infect Dis. 1982;146:103.
50. Gelfand HM, Holgium AH, Marchetti GE, et al. A continuing surveillance of enterovirus infections in healthy children in six United States cites. I. Viruses isolated during 1960 and 1961. Am J Hyg. 1963;78:358.
51. Jenista JA, Powell KR, Menegus MA. Epidemiology of neonatal enterovirus infection. J Pediatr. 1984;104:685–90.
52. Parks WP, Queiroga LT, Melnick JL. Studies of infantile diarrhea in Karachi, Pakistan. II. Multiple virus isolations from rectal swabs. Am J Epidemiol. 1967;85:469.
53. Strikas RA, Anderson LJ, Parker RA. Temporal and geographic patterns of isolates of nonpolio enteroviruses in the United States. J Infect Dis. 1986;153:346–51.
54. Lipson SM, Walderman R, Costello P, et al. Sensitivity of rhabdomyosarcoma and guinea pig embryo cell cultures to field isolates of difficult-to-cultivate group A coxsackieviruses. J Clin Microbiol. 1988;26:1298–303.
55. Matsumoto K, Kobayashi T, Kimura Y. Seroepidemiological studies of echovirus type 30 infection. Microbiol Immunol. 1986;30:935–8.
56. Huovilainen A, Hovi T, Kinnunen L, et al. Evolution of poliovirus during an outbreak: Sequential type 3 poliovirus isolates from several persons show shifts of neutralization determinants. J Gen Virol. 1987;68:1373–8.
57. Hovi T, Cantell K, Huovilainen A, et al. Outbreak of paralytic poliomyelitis in Finland: Widespread circulation of antigenically altered poliovirus type 3 in a vaccinated population. Lancet. 1986;1:1427–32.

58. Hamby BB, Pallansch MA, Kew OM. Reemergence of an epidemic coxsackievirus B5 genotype. J Infect Dis. 1987;156:288–92.
59. Kew OM. Applications of molecular epidemiology to the surveillance of poliomyelitis. Proceedings of the National Academy of Medicine, Institute of Medicine Conference "Poliomyelitis Vaccines: Re-evaluating Policy Options." Washington DC: National Academy of Sciences; January 1988.
60. Hatch MH, Marchetti GE, Nottay BK, et al. Strain characterization studies of poliovirus type 1 isolates from poliomyelitis cases in the United States in 1979. Dev Biol Stand. 1981;47:307–15.
61. Takeda N, Miyamura K, Ogino T, et al. Evolution of enterovirus type 70: Oligonucleotide mapping analysis of RNA genome. Virology. 1984;134:375–88.
62. Miyamura K, Tanimura M, Takeda N, et al. Evolution of enterovirus 70 in nature: All isolates were recently derived from a common ancestor. Arch Virol. 1986;89:1–14.
63. Kogon A, Spigland I, Frothingham TE, et al. The virus watch program. A continuing surveillance of viral infections in metropolitan New York families. Am J Epidemiol. 1969;89:51.
64. Schurmann W, Eggers HJ: An experimental study on the epidemiology of enteroviruses: Water and soap washing of poliovirus 1—contaminated hands, its effectiveness and kinetics. Med Microbiol Immunol. 1985;174:221–36.
65. Horstmann DM, Emmons J, Gimpel L, et al. Enterovirus surveillance following a community-wide oral poliovirus vaccination program: A seven-year study. Am J Epidemiol. 1973;97:173.
66. Fox JP. Epidemiology of poliomyelitis in populations before and after vaccination with inactivated viruses. In: Poliomyelitis. Papers and Discussions Presented at the Fourth International Poliomyelitis Conference. Philadelphia. JB Lippincott; 1958;136.
67. Johnson KM, Bloom, HH, Forsyth B, et al. The role of enteroviruses in respiratory disease. Am Rev Respir Dis. 1963;88:240.
68. Froeschle JE, Feorino PM, Gelfand HM. A continuing surveillance of enterovirus infection in healthy children in six United States cities. II. Surveillance enterovirus isolates 1960–1963 and comparison with enterovirus isolates from cases of acute central nervous system disease. Am J Epidemiol. 1966;83:455.
69. Siegel M, Greenberg M, Bodian J. Presence of children in the household as a factor in the incidence of paralytic poliomyelitis in adults. N Engl J Med. 1957;257:958.
70. Weinstein L, Aycock L, Feenster RF. The relation of sex, pregnancy and menstruation to susceptibility to poliomyelitis. N Engl J Med. 1951;245:54.
71. Baron RC, Hatch MHH, Kleeman K, et al. Aseptic meningitis among members of a high school football team. An outbreak associated with echovirus 16 infection. JAMA 1982;248:1724.
72. Josselson J, Pula T, Sadler JH. Acute rhabdomyolysis associated with an echovirus 9 infection. Arch Intern Med. 1980;140:1671.
73. Dagan R, Jenista JA, Prather SL, et al. Viremia in hospitalized children with enterovirus infections. J Pediatr. 1985;106:397–401.
74. Lepow ML, Carver DH, Wright HT Jr. A clinical, epidemiologic and laboratory investigation of aseptic meningitis during the four-year period, 1955–1958. N Engl J Med. 1962;266:1181.
75. Dagan R, Menegus MA. A combination of four cell types for rapid detection of enteroviruses in clinical specimens. J Med Virol. 1986;19:219–228.
76. Schmidt NJ, Ho HH, Lennette EH. Propagation and isolation of group A coxsackieviruses in RD cells. J Clin Microbiol. 1975;2:183.
77. Wenner H, Lenahan MF. Propagation of group A coxsackieviruses in tissue culture. II. Some interactions between virus and mammalian cells. Yale J Biol Med. 1961;34:421.
78. Landry ML, Madore HP, Fong CKY, et al. Use of guinea pig embryo cell cultures for isolation and propagation of group A coxsackieviruses. J Clin Microbiol. 1981;13:588.
79. Reigel F. Isolation of human pathogenic viruses from clinical material on $CaCo_2$ cells. J Virol Methods. 1985;12:323–7.
80. Dorries R, ter Meulen V. Detection of enterovirus specific IgG and IgM antibodies in humans by an indirect solid phase radioimmunoassay. Med Microbiol Immunol. 1980;168:159.
81. Bromberg K, Shank PR, Zinner SH, et al. Inability of counterimmunoelectrophoresis to detect echovirus in cerebrospinal fluid. Am J Clin Pathol. 1983;80:383–385.
82. Ukkonen P, Huovilainen A, Hovi T. Detection of poliovirus antigen by enzyme immunoassay. J Clin Microbiol. 1986;24:954–8.
83. Rotbart HA, Levin MJ, Villarreal LP, et al. Factors affecting the detection of enteroviruses in cerebrospinal fluid with coxsackievirus B3 and poliovirus 1 cDNA probes. J Clin Microbiol. 1985;22:220–4.
84. Tracy S. Comparison of genomic homologies in the coxsackievirus B group by use of cDNA:RNA dot-blot hybridization. J Clin Microbiol. 1985;21:371–4.
85. Newman C, Modlin JF, Yolken RH, et al. Monoclonal solution hybridization assay for detection of enteroviruses. Proceedings of the 27th Interscience Conference on Antimicrobial Agents and Chemotherapy. New York: American Society for Microbiology; September, 1987.
86. Pattison JR. Tests for coxsackie B virus-specific IgM. J Hyg (Lond). 1983;90:327–32.
87. Wulff H, Anderson LJ, Pallansch MA, et al. Diagnosis of enterovirus 70 infection by demonstration of IgM antibodies. J Med. Virol. 1987;21:321–7.
88. Burch GE, Sun SC, Colcolough HL, et al. Coxsackie B viral myocarditis and valvulitis identified in routine autopsy specimens by immunofluorescent techniques. Am Heart J. 1967;74:13.
89. Easton AJ, Eglin RP. The detection of coxsackievirus RNA in cardiac tissue by in situ hybridization. J Gen Virol. 1988;69:285–91.
90. McKinlay MA, Steinberg BA. Oral efficacy of WIN 51711 in mice infected with human poliovirus. Antimicrob Agents Chemother. 1986;29:30–2.
91. Korant BD, Towatari T, Ivanoff L, et al. Viral therapy: Prospects for protease inhibitors. J Cell Biochem 1986;32:91–5.
92. Matsumori A, Crumpacker CS, Abelmann WH. Prevention of viral myocarditis with recombinant human leukocyte interferon alpha A/D in a murine model. J Am Coll Cardiol. 1987;9:1320–5.
93. Stansfield SK, de la Pena W, Koenig S, et al. Human leukocyte interferon in the treatment and prophylaxis of acute hemorrhagic conjunctivitis. J Infect Dis. 1984;149:822–3.

149. POLIOVIRUS

JOHN F. MODLIN

Polioviruses are the cause of poliomyelitis, a systemic infectious disease of widely varying severity that prominently affects the central nervous system and sometimes is complicated by paralysis. The name of the disease (polios, gray; myelos, marrow or spinal cord), now commonly shortened to *polio*, is descriptive of the pathologic lesions that involve neurons in the gray matter, especially in the anterior horn of the spinal cord. Older, less commonly used names for the disease include *infantile paralysis* and *Heine-Medin disease*.

HISTORY

The history of poliomyelitis has been recorded in detail by John Paul, who made major contributions to the understanding of the epidemiology of the disease.[1] The clinical features of poliomyelitis were described as early as 1840, but the epidemic nature of the disease remained largely unknown until 1890, when Medin, a Swedish pediatrician, characterized the natural history of acute poliomyelitis and the neurologic complications during outbreaks in Scandinavia. In 1894 Caverly described 132 cases of poliomyelitis in Vermont, the largest outbreak recorded up to that time. Major progress in understanding poliomyelitis was signaled by the conclusive demonstration of its infectious nature by Landsteiner and Popper, who in 1908 transmitted the disease to monkeys by inoculation of human spinal cord homogenates. Serial passages of the agent in the central nervous system (CNS) of primates led to the concept of strict neurotropism. Although the virus was known to be present in the feces of patients with poliomyelitis, the notion that the infection might occur primarily in the alimentary tract rather than in the central nervous system fell into oblivion. Progress remained limited until the landmark discovery in 1949 by Enders, Weller, and Robbins that poliovirus could be propagated in vitro in cultures of human embryonic tissues of non-neural origin.[2] This discovery was the keystone that facilitated experimental investigation of the pathogenesis of the disease and later the development of vaccines. Bodian first recognized that there were three distinct serotypes of poliovirus.[3] By 1952, Bodian and Horstmann independently had discovered that viremia occurred early in infection, possibly explaining the systemic phase of the illness and spread of the virus to the central nervous system by non-neural pathways.[4–6] Salk reported in 1953 that human subjects could be successfully immunized with formalin-inactivated poliovirus,[7] which rapidly led to extensive field trials and licensure of vaccines in 1955. The dramatic decline in paralytic poliomyelitis, which immediately ensued, has rightfully been hailed as one of the great accomplishments of medical science. Meanwhile, Sabin, Koprowski, Melnick, and others developed live, attenuation poliovirus vaccines,[8] which led to still further reductions in disease incidence after their licensure in 1962.

Polio vaccines have so successfully prevented disease in developed countries that virtually all discussion regarding poliomyelitis relate to vaccines and vaccine public policy rather than the primary disease. In the developing world, where vaccines reach only a fraction of children, poliomyelitis continues to be a major cause of lameness.

INFECTIOUS AGENTS

Polioviruses are members of the genus *Enterovirus*, family Picornaviridae, whose properties are described in Chapter 148.

Antigenic Properties

There are three serotypes of polioviruses that are distinguished from one another by neutralization tests. Before the introduction of oral polio vaccine, most paralytic disease was caused by type 1.[9,10] Type-specific, lifelong immunity to disease follows both natural infection and (probably) infection with attenuated polio vaccine viruses. Occasional second attacks of paralysis occur with infection by heterologous serotypes.[11]

Host Range and Virulence

Humans are the only natural host and reservoir of polioviruses, although experimental infections and disease can be produced in other primates and polioviruses can be adapted to replicate in subprimate mammals. Naturally occurring strains vary over a 10 million-fold range in neurovirulence.[12] Evolution among primates is inversely correlated with susceptibility of their neurons to polioviruses and is directly correlated with susceptibility of their alimentary tract. Thus, most polioviruses readily paralyze rhesus or cynomolgus monkeys, while much higher doses or more virulent strains are required to paralyze chimpanzees and humans. In contrast, polioviruses are more infectious for the human gut than for the gut of lower primates.

Characteristics of Vaccine Strains

Vaccine strains occasionally are able to paralyze rhesus and cynomolgus monkeys only when injected in high doses directly into the CNS. In addition to their low neurovirulence, vaccine strains can often be distinguished from naturally occurring wild strains by their temperature sensitivity and by subtle antigenic differences. However, these tests are not completely reliable because strains of vaccine origin may undergo mutation in the gastrointestinal tract resulting in biologic properties that are intermediate between those of reference vaccine strains and natural poliovirus strains.[13] Applied molecular biologic techniques such as oligonucleotide fingerprinting, cDNA hybridization, genomic sequencing, and more reliable means of distinguishing vaccine strains from naturally occurring strains. Genomic sequencing has recently proved to be the most powerful of these methods.[14]

PATHOGENESIS

The early events in the pathogenesis of poliomyelitis and other enterovirus infections, described in Chapter 148, include implantation and replication of virus in the gut and adjacent lymphoid tissues. After spread to deep lymph nodes, a "minor viremia," may disseminate virus to susceptible reticuloendothelial tissues. In asymptomatic infections, the virus is contained at this point and elicits the formation of type-specific antibodies. In a few persons, however, replication in the retriculoendothelial system gives rise to a "major viremia," which corresponds temporally with the "minor illness" also known as abortive poliomyelitis. Viremia also may result in seeding of the leptomeninges, causing aseptic meningitis.

At this point, the course of poliomyelitis deviates from other enteroviral infections in the capacity of polioviruses to cause extensive necrosis of neurons in the gray matter of the brain and spinal cord. How the virus reaches the central nervous system in cases of paralytic poliomyelitis remains somewhat controversial. The preponderance of the evidence supports the view that dissemination to the CNS is hematogenous.[15,16] Viremia is known to precede paralysis in humans, and experimental viremia produces paralysis in chimpanzees.[16] The precise route by which virus passes from the blood to the CNS is unknown. Not only viremia but also the virulence of the virus strain are important factors in the production of disease. There is experimental evidence that neurotropism of polioviruses is related in part to their ability to bind to cell membranes of neuronal tissue in vitro.[17] Neuropathologic studies and animal experiments suggest that spread is neural once the virus reaches the CNS.[18,19]

Pathologic Features

Poliovirus principally affects motor and autonomic neurons. Destruction of neurons is accompanied by an inflammatory infiltrate of polymorphonuclear leukocytes, lymphocytes, and macrophages. The most characteristic feature of the histopathology of poliomyelitis is the distribution of the lesions; the main sites of attack are the gray matter of the anterior horn of the spinal cord and the motor nuclei of the pons and medulla.[20] Involved less severely are neurons of the mesencephalon, cerebellar roof nuclei, and precentral gyrus of the cerebral cortex. Clinical symptoms depend on the severity of lesions rather than on their distribution, which is similar in essentially all cases; almost all fatal cases have involvement of both the spinal cord and the cranial nerve nuclei and brain stem, even in the absence of bulbar signs. The dorsal root ganglia are commonly involved pathologically, but this does not result in sensory deficits. The quantity of virus in the spinal cord is maximal during the first few days after onset of paralysis and generally is undetectable by one week, but inflammatory lesions may persist for months.

EPIDEMIOLOGY

Epidemiologic features of poliovirus infections are similar to those caused by other enteroviruses (Chapter 148), but certain features of poliomyelitis are distinctive. The disease was predominantly sporadic before the late 1800s, when epidemics were first recognized in Scandinavia and Western Europe, followed by the United States. In the developed countries, the first half of the twentieth century witnessed sporadic epidemic disease occurring every few years without regular periodicity. By the late 1940s and early 1950s, epidemic polio occurred regularly in the United States with 15,000–21,000 cases of paralytic disease reported annually. Accompanying the increased incidence was a shift in the affected age groups. In 1920, 90 percent of the cases occurred in infants under 5 years of age ("infantile paralysis"), in the early 1950s the peak incidence was in 5- to 9-year-olds; more than one-third of the cases occurred in persons over 15 years of age. Abundant epidemiologic evidence supports the explanation that in the endemic period before 1900, polioviruses were ubiquitous and resulted in mostly inapparent infections that conferred widespread immunity in early childhood; with rising standards of hygiene in the twentieth century, infection frequently was delayed until a later age, when the pool of susceptible people was large enough to permit an epidemic. This concept presupposes that the appearance of epidemics of paralytic poliomyelitis was a result of a higher ratio of paralysis to inapparent infections in older age groups, a widely,[21] but not universally,[22] held theory.

The introduction of inactivated vaccines (IPV) in 1955 and live, attenuated oral vaccines (OPV) in 1962 produced sudden, dramatic reductions in the incidence of paralytic poliomyelitis in the developed countries of the world. In the United States, the attack rate fell from 17.6 cases of poliomyelitis (paralytic and nonparalytic) per 100,000 population in 1955 to 0.4 cases per 100,000 in 1962. Since 1972, the rate has been less than 0.01 cases per 100,000, or fewer than 10 cases annually. In some underdeveloped countries, an endemic pattern similar to that seen in the nineteenth century United States is now observed, with virtually all children over the age of 4 years being immune. Lameness surveys in some locations attest to high rates of endemic paralytic poliomyelitis in the underdeveloped world.[23] However, increasing use of OPV under the World Health Organization's Expanded Program on Immunization is beginning to have an impact on the incidence of poliomyelitis in many underdeveloped countries.

Poliomyelitis in the Postvaccine Era

Widespread use of OPV in the United States has resulted in the disappearance of circulating wild poliovirus strains, despite the fact that many preschool children remain unimmunized and as many as 21 percent of young adults remain susceptible to at least one poliovirus type.[24] This "fadeout" of naturally occurring strains may have occurred because the proportion of susceptibilites in the population is too low to allow perpetuation of the virus during periods when transmission is low (i.e., winter and spring[22]). Epidemic disease no longer exists in the United States, although outbreaks have occurred in isolated groups of unvaccinated persons as recently as 1979.[25] The last known sporadic case of endemic poliomyelitis also occurred in 1979, indicating that indigenous transmission of naturally occurring polioviruses has completely ceased in the United States.[26] With the eradication of naturally occurring poliomyelitis, virtually all of the 5–10 cases that occur in the United States annually are associated with the use of OPV.[27] Vaccine associated disease is seen in two groups: (*1*) recipients of the vaccine and (*2*) their contacts. Recipient cases occur predominantly in children less than 4 years old, approximately 15 percent of whom have some form of immune deficiency. Most recipient cases occur 7–21 days after oral administration of vaccine. In contrast, disease in contacts occurs mostly in young adults, with onset usually 20–29 days after vaccine administration. More than 80 percent of both recipient and contact cases are associated with first dose of OPV.[27] OPV virus types 3 and 2 are more common causes of vaccine associated paralysis than type 1; however, more than one type has been isolated from clinical specimens in some cases.[27] The overall risk of OPV related disease is estimated to be 1 case per 2.6 million doses of OPV distributed.[27] Mortality from vaccine associated poliomyelitis has been 10 percent overall, but much higher in immune-deficient recipients.

CLINICAL FEATURES

Incubation Period

Best estimates of the incubation period of poliomyelitis are 9–12 days (range: 5–35 days) measured from presumed contact until onset of the prodrome, and 11–17 days (range: 8–36 days) until onset of paralysis.[28] The lower limits of these ranges are suspect, because even in instances of *presumed* single exposures, both the presumed index case and the contact may have had prior exposure to other asymptomatically infected persons. Poliovirus has been detected in the feces 19 days before the onset of paralysis.[29]

Clinical Manifestations of Infection

The manifestations of infection by polioviruses range from inapparent illness to severe paralysis and death. Usual estimates of the ratio of inapparent to clinically recognized polio infection vary between 60:1 and 1000:1.[22,30] Figure 1 depicts the time of onset for the various clinical manifestations of poliovirus infection. At least 95 percent of infections are asymptomatic or inapparent and can be recognized only by the isolation of poliovirus from feces or oropharynx or by a rise in antibody titer. In *abortive poliomyelitis*, which occurs in 4–8 percent of infections, there is fever, headache, sore throat, listlessness, anorexia, vomiting, and abdominal pain. The neurologic examination is normal. The illness lasts only a few hours to 2–3 days. Abortive poliomyelitis is not clinically distinguishable from many other viral infections and can only be suspected clinically during an epidemic. *Nonparalytic poliomyelitis* differs from abortive poliomyelitis by the presence of signs of meningeal irritation. The disease is clinically indistinguishable from aseptic meningitis with other enteroviruses. The systemic manifestations of nonparalytic poliomyelitis are generally more severe than in abortive poliomyelitis.

Spinal Paralytic Poliomyelitis.

Frank paralysis occurs in roughly 0.1 percent of all poliovirus infections. In children there frequently is a biphasic course with "minor" and "major" illnesses.[31] The minor illness, coinciding with viremia, corresponds with the symptoms of abortive poliomyelitis and lasts 1–3 days. The patient then appears to be recovering and remains symptom-free for 2–5 days before the generally abrupt onset of the major illness. The preparalytic symptoms of the major illness are meningitic, with headache, fever, malaise, vomiting, neck stiffness, and central spinal fluid (CSF) pleocytosis. The temperature is generally 37–39°C, which often is accompanied by chilliness, but rarely by rigors. This biphasic pattern (seen in perhaps one-third of the children) rarely is observed in adults, who usually have a single phase but a more prolonged prodrome of symptoms before the more gradual onset of paralysis.[31,32] Very rarely, paralysis is almost the first manifestation of illness.

Characteristic of the onset of the major illness, especially in older persons, is the occurrence of spontaneous muscle pain. The pain may involve one muscle or several, most commonly those of the neck or lumbar region, but also those of the flank, abdomen, or limbs. It is relieved by motion; the patient sometimes paces nervously to "work it off." Localized cutaneous hyperesthesia, paresthesias, involuntary muscle spasm, and muscular fasciculations occasionally are observed during this phase.

The meningitic phase of the major illness and accompanying muscle pain generally are present for 1–2 days before frank weakness and paralysis ensue. The severity of the disease varies from weakness of a single portion of one muscle to complete quadriplegia. The paralysis is flaccid; stretch reflexes, which were initially hyperactive, become absent. *The most characteristic feature of the paralysis is its asymmetric distribution*, which affects some muscle groups while sparing others. Proximal muscles of the extremities tend to be more involved than distal muscles, the legs are more commonly involved than the arms, and the large muscle groups of the hand are at greater risk than the small ones. Any combination of limbs may be paralyzed, but the most common pattern is involvement of one leg, followed by one arm, or both legs and both arms. Quadriplegia is almost never observed in infants.[32] While occasional cases progress from onset of weakness to complete quadriplegia and bulbar involvement in a few hours, more commonly the paralysis extends over 2–3 days. Progression of paralysis almost invariably halts when the patient becomes afebrile.[31] Paralysis of the bladder usually is associated with paralysis of the legs. It occurs in about one-quarter of the adults, but is uncommon in children. Sensory loss in poliomyelitis is very rare,[33] and its occurrence should strongly suggest some other diagnosis (e.g., Guillain-Barré syndrome).

Bulbar Paralytic Poliomyelitis. In bulbar poliomyelitis, there

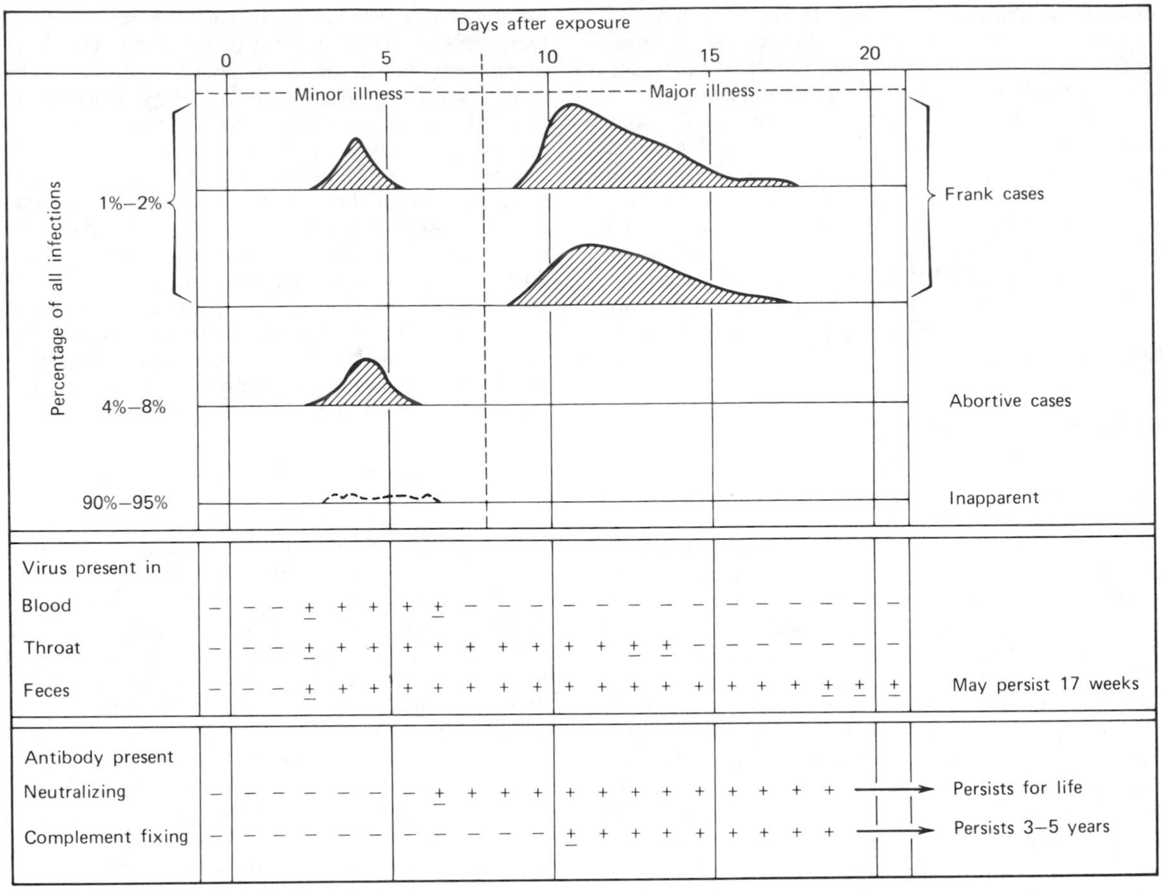

FIG. 1. Schema of the clinical and subclinical forms of poliomyelitis, showing presence of virus and antibodies in relation to the development and persistence of the infection. (From Paul,[21] with permission.)

is paralysis of muscle groups innervated by cranial nerves, especially those of the soft palate and pharynx, and less often the larynx. Bulbar paralysis results in dysphagia, nasal speech, and sometimes dyspnea. The prognosis becomes ominous when there is involvement of the circulatory and respiratory centers of the medulla. The frequency of the bulbar form of the disease has varied in different epidemics from 5 to 35 percent of paralytic cases. It is more common in adults.[32] Mixed bulbospinal involvement is common, with pure bulbar poliomyelitis accounting for not more than about 10 percent of paralytic poliomyelitis.

The ninth and tenth cranial nerves are by far the most frequently involved,[34] and pharyngeal paralysis often is the only obvious sign. Pooling of secretions occurs, and patients usually are extremely anxious and agitated about their inability to swallow and breathe. Respiratory difficulties resulting from aspiration of secretions, or less commonly from spasm of the glottis or larynx, soon become dominant.[34] Other cranial nerve nuclei frequently are involved but rarely pose a threat to life. Ocular palsies and pupillary disturbances occur in 11 percent. Fifth nerve involvement is uncommon and causes difficulty in chewing; it is important when it results in trismus, which may prevent adequate removal of secretions by suction. Paresis of the facial nerve occurs in approximately 50 percent of the patients; however, unlike in Bell's palsy, it tends to be segmental, resulting in weakness only of muscles supplying the forehead, the cheek, or the lips. Bilateral deafness and vestibular disturbances are rare. Paralysis of the sternomastoid and trapezius muscles is not uncommon, but its importance is overshadowed by difficulties in swallowing and airway obstruction produced by combined involvement of the tenth, eleventh, and twelfth cranial nerves.

Bulbar poliomyelitis involving the respiratory and vasomotor centers is less common than paralysis of the cranial nerve nuclei. Lesions of the respiratory center produce irregularities of the rhythm and depth of respiration despite an adequate airway and intact respiratory musculature. Usually a rapid pulse and some elevation in blood pressure are associated with hypoxia.[35] Progression leads to Cheyne-Stokes respiration with associated confusion, delirium, coma, and usually death. Vasomotor involvement is manifested by severe circulatory collapse, occasionally in the absence of cranial nerve palsy or respiratory involvement.[34,36] Disturbances of cardiac rhythm occur, most commonly sinus tachycardia, bradycardia, or prolongation of the Q–T interval.[36] Autonomic manifestations (e.g., flushing, cutaneous vasoconstriction with hyperthermia, or severe hypertension) may be seen.[35,36]

Polioencephalitis. Encephalitis, manifested primarily by confusion and disturbances of consciousness, is an uncommon form of poliomyelitis occurring principally in infants. It is the only type of poliomyelitis in which seizures are common. In contrast to spinal paralytic polio, there may be spastic paralysis, which reflects the presence of an upper motor neuron lesion. The illness is not clinically distinguishable from many other infectious causes of encephalitis, and it usually is suspected only in an epidemic.

Complications

The most important complications of paralytic poliomyelitis involve the respiratory tract. *Respiratory failure* may be caused by paralysis of the respiratory muscles, by airway obstruction from involvement of the cranial nerve nuclei, or by lesions of the respiratory center.[37] Paralysis of the respiratory muscles may involve the diaphragm and the intercostal muscles. These patients have rapid, shallow breathing, which often is difficult to evaluate because of superimposed anxiety. With intercostal muscle paralysis, the chest wall is partially or completely immobile, and the accessory respiratory muscles may be in use. Patients with diaphragmatic paralysis are unable to sniff vigorously. Advanced paralysis of the respiratory muscles causes a weak—but otherwise normal—cough, because the patient is unable to take a deep breath. In contrast, the patient with pharyngeal paralysis blows rather than coughs, because of inability to close off the glottis. Pharyngeal paralysis typically results in noisy respirations because of pooling of secretions. Nonparalytic respiratory complications also are seen in poliomyelitis; they include *aspiration pneumonia* and *pulmonary edema* associated with bulbar disease, and *pulmonary embolism* promoted by venous stasis in paralyzed limbs.[35]

Myocarditis has been documented by virus isolation and histologic lesions at autopsy,[35,38] but it rarely is diagnosed clinically. Electrocardiographic disturbances are common but usually nonspecific; even when accompanied by heart failure, tachycardia, and vasomotor collapse, they are difficult to separate from signs produced by involvement of the bulbar regulatory centers.

Gastrointestinal complications include *hemorrhage, paralytic ileus*, and *gastric dilatation*.[39] These generally occur acutely. *Urinary calculi* are a common late complication resulting from catheter associated urinary infections and resorption of calcium from bone in immobilized patients with residual spinal paralysis.[40]

Risk Factors

A number of provocative or risk factors are known to influence the likelihood that an individual, once infected with poliovirus, will develop paralysis.

Age, Sex, and Pregnancy. Before puberty, poliovirus infections occur equally in boys and girls, although paralysis is more common in boys.[41] Among adults, women are at greater risk of infection but are not necessarily at greater risk of paralysis.[41,43] Clinical data suggest that both incidence and severity of poliomyelitis may be increased in pregnant women.[42–44] Not only are women of childbearing age more likely to be exposed to infections in young children,[43] but late pregnancy may also induce a state of relative immunosuppression and increased susceptibility to more serious illness.

Immune Deficiency States. Currently about 14 percent of reported paralytic poliomyelitis cases in the United States occur among OPV recipients or contacts of OPV recipients who are immune-deficient.[27] Most patients have had either isolated B-cell immunodeficiency or severe combined immune deficiency syndrome.[45–49] The majority of infections in immunocompromised children and adults have been associated with type 2 OPV virus, although it is presumed that all live vaccine and naturally occurring polioviruses represent an increased risk.[45] The risk of OPV related paralytic disease in patients with hereditary immunodeficiencies is estimated to be 10,000 times that in normal children.[46] However, the risk is relative: although most children with X-linked agammaglobulinemia receive OPV, only about 2.5 percent develop poliomyelitis.[48] Children with severe combined immunodeficiency syndrome have received OPV without any ill effects.[47] Poliomyelitis in children with hereditary immunodeficiencies differs from the classic disease in several respects. The incubation period after ingestion of OPV is unusually long, ranging from 30 to 120 days. The illness is protracted, and it may be associated with progression of paralysis over several weeks, chronic meningitis, and progressive neurologic dysfunction that includes both upper and lower motor neuron signs.[46,49] In addition to the characteristic histopathologic lesions of poliomyelitis, there are unusual changes, such as microcystic degeneration and heavy involvement of unusual areas such as the basal ganglia.[46,49] Chronic fecal excretion of virus in these cases is characteristic.

Strenuous Exercise. Fatigue and strenuous exercise substantially increase both incidence and severity of paralytic poliomyelitis. These effects have been amply documented both clinically[50,51] and experimentally.[52] Exercise during the minor illness or the prodrome has no effect, but it is detrimental when it occurs during the first 3 days of the major illness.[51] Strict bed rest has a sparing effect on paralysis and, therefore, is mandatory in the management of acute poliomyelitis.

Injections or Trauma. Paralytic poliomyelitis tends to localize in a limb that has been the site of an intramuscular injection within 2 weeks before onset of infection[53,54] or in a limb injured by fracture, operative trauma, or other factors. Observations in experimental poliomyelitis confirm this association and suggest that the mechanism of the provoking effect of trauma (and possibly also exercise) is not viral spread from the periphery along neural pathways, but rather a reflex effect on blood vessels in the corresponding portion of the spinal cord; this allows access of virus from the circulating blood.[55,56]

Tonsillectomy. Tonsillectomized people have a risk of acquiring bulbar poliomyelitis that is approximately eight times the risk in those people with intact tonsils. At risk are individuals with onset of infection shortly before or after tonsillectomy and those whose tonsillectomy was performed in the remote past.[57,58] Since the ninth and tenth cranial nerves supply the fauces, spread of virus from damaged nerve endings may explain the acute effect, or it may be due to vascular effects on the medulla.[58] The remote effect alternatively may be due to loss of immunocompetent tissues from the tonsils, which is known to be associated with greater and more prolonged replication of poliovirus in the oropharynx.[59]

Genetic Factors. Paralytic poliomyelitis occurs with high frequency among families whose members may be attacked many years apart. These and other observations suggest that genetic factors may play a role in susceptibility to *paralysis* beyond the likelihood of acquiring *infection* from another family member excreting virus.[60] At the cellular level susceptibility to poliovirus infection is conferred by a gene carried on human chromosome 19.[61] In addition, there is evidence that genetically determined histocompatibility antigens influence the risk of *paralytic* infection.[62,63]

Differential Diagnosis

Many diseases may mimic the nonspecific signs and symptoms of abortive poliomyelitis. Also, the aseptic meningitis caused by polioviruses is clinically indistinguishable from meningitis due to many other viral causes (see Chapters 66 and 150).

Few diseases, however, are likely to be confused with paralytic poliomyelitis. The most important is the *Guillain-Barré syndrome* (GBS). The patient with poliomyelitis is febrile, has signs of meningeal irritation, and appears acutely ill. The paralysis is characteristically asymmetric and virtually never accompanied by sensory loss. In contrast, in GBS there is symmetrical, ascending paralysis with loss of sensation in approximately 80 percent of the cases. Facial diplegia occurs in about half of patients with GBS, but is very uncommon even in bulbar poliomyelitis. In poliomyelitis, continued extension of paralysis beyond 3–4 days is unusual, whereas in GBS the paralysis may spread in successive stages over a period of up to 2 weeks. Paresthesias are uncommon in poliomyelitis but common in GBS. Characteristics of the CSF are useful in distinguishing the two conditions. In poliomyelitis, pleocytosis and minimally elevated protein concentration are present, whereas in GBS the protein is elevated with absent or minimal pleocytosis (albuminocytologic dissociation). The CSF may be less helpful 2 or 3 weeks into the illness, when (in poliomyelitis) the cell count has returned to normal, but the protein elevation may persist.

In *acute transverse myelitis*, the findings are motor and sensory deficits at a particular level of the spinal cord and spastic paralysis characteristic of an upper motor neuron lesion; prominent sphincter disturbances are also seen. Other diagnoses that may be considered include paralytic disease due to *nonpolio enteroviruses* (Chapter 150), *hysteria*, neuropathies caused by *diphtheria* and *botulism*, *tick paralysis*, *pseudoparalysis* in children with arthritis or osteomyelitis of the long bones, and *encephalitis* with paralysis.

Laboratory Diagnosis

The peripheral white blood cell count may be normal or elevated. Abnormalities of the CSF are not distinguishable from other viral causes of aseptic meningitis.

General aspects of the laboratory diagnosis of enteroviral infections are discussed in Chapter 148. Polioviruses usually can be isolated from throat secretions in the first week of illness, and from feces often for several weeks. However, unlike many other enteroviruses causing aseptic meningitis, polioviruses rarely are isolated from the CSF. In sporadic cases of poliomyelitis occurring in areas of very low incidence such as the United States and other developed nations, it is important to characterize virus isolates as either wild type (naturally occurring strains) or vaccine-like; this methodology is currently available only through public health reference laboratories.[19] Isolations from CSF (or brain and spinal cord in fatal cases), although uncommon, are especially valuable in evaluating vaccine associated disease, because recovery of fecal virus is expected in this situation and only a CNS virus isolate with vaccine markers provides conclusive evidence of etiologic association.

In the absence of a virus isolate, the diagnosis of poliovirus infection can be established serologically by testing paired acute and convalescent sera against antigens of the three serotypes. The neutralization test, which is type-specific, remains the most widely used assay and is the standard to which other methods are compared. Solid phase immunoassays employing whole virus antigens are not sufficiently type-specific for general use, but technical improvements to these methods can be expected. Complement fixation tests are rarely used now.

Prognosis

The overall mortality of paralytic poliomyelitis in epidemics of the past was 5–10 percent but is substantially higher in some forms of the disease. In bulbar poliomyelitis, especially when combined spinobulbar paralysis, mortality is 20–60 percent.[64] Most deaths occur in the first week after onset of paralysis. The prognosis in polioencephalitis is particularly poor; death is the rule. The mortality in spinal paralytic polio is very low unless respiratory assistance is required, in which case it is 20–50 percent.[64,65]

Full return of function is less likely in severely paralyzed muscles than in mildly paralyzed ones, and some degree of permanent damage is observed in about one-third of victims of poliomyelitis. Those requiring mechanical ventilation because of spinal respiratory paralysis rarely recover without some sequelae. Curiously, although bulbar poliomyelitis causes the greatest threat to life in the first week of illness, it rarely is responsible for permanent damage in surviving patients. Recovery from pharyngeal paralysis usually is evident by 10 days and eventually complete. Muscular paralysis in poliomyelitis usually progresses or extends for only 1–3 days after its onset, but occasionally for as long as 1 week.[66] Some estimate of the eventual outcome can be made after 1 month, when most reversible damage will have disappeared. Very little additional return of function can be expected beyond 9 months, although surviving muscles can be reeducated to perform additional tasks. New onset of neuromuscular weakness occurring several decades after acute paralytic poliomyelitis has been described in some patients. Weakness recurs mostly in muscle groups involved after the acute poliovirus infection and progresses very gradually. Infectious and immunologic mechanisms do not appear to be operative in the postparalytic paralysis syndrome; instead it may be caused by a gradual deterioration in motor neurons that survive the initial paralytic episode.[67]

Management

Specific antiviral agents for the treatment of poliomyelitis are not available. Management, therefore, is supportive and symptomatic.

In the acute phase of paralytic poliomyelitis, patients should be hospitalized. Bed rest is essential to prevent augmentation or extension of paralysis. A board under the mattress is helpful in relieving severe back pain caused by muscle spasm; in cases involving paralyzed legs, placing the feet against a board at right angles to the mattress is useful in preventing a foot-drop deformity. Hot moist packs applied to muscles are very helpful in relieving pain and spasm. Frequent testing of muscular strength in the acute phase of the illness causes discomfort; it should be performed only two or three times per week. Physical therapy should be initiated once progression of paralysis has ceased.

The greatest challenge is the management of problems threatening the respiratory tract. Paralysis of the respiratory muscles necessitates mechanical ventilation before hypoxia develops, generally, when the vital capacity falls to less than 50 percent. Tank respirators used in the past to treat this form of paralysis are available in few hospitals at present; despite their advantage of preventing tracheal intubation, they have been replaced by positive pressure ventilators, which permit easier access to the patient. Pooling of secretions in the pharynx in mild bulbar poliomyelitis, if it is unaccompanied by spinal respiratory paralysis, can be managed with postural drainage and suction. Severe bulbar paralysis necessitates tracheal intubation. Weakness or paralysis of the bladder may necessitate catheterization.

Management of chronic aspects and sequelae of paralytic poliomyelitis is beyond the scope of this book. Management of psychiatric complications, both acutely and during convalescence, is of supreme importance in the total care of these patients. The reader is referred to excellent older references on these topics.[68,69]

PREVENTION: VACCINES

Both inactivated poliovirus vaccines (IPV) and live, attenuated oral poliovirus vaccines (OPV) have been used effectively for more than 30 years in controlling paralytic poliomyelitis. The introduction of Salk IPV in 1955 led to an immediate and dramatic reduction in both epidemic and endemic poliomyelitis. The IPV available for the first several years possessed relatively low potency, accounting for the observation that as many as 17 percent of children with paralytic poliomyelitis in 1959 had received three or more doses of IPV.[70] Meanwhile live, attenuated oral poliovirus vaccine strains were developed by multiple passage of polioviruses in monkey kidney cell culture and selection of mutants with low virulence for primates.[71] Successful field trials of the Sabin OPV vaccine strains were carried out in the United States and many foreign countries from 1955 to 1959, and OPV was introduced for routine use in 1962 as separate monovalent vaccines; the trivalent product became available in 1964. OPV was quickly accepted by the pediatric and public health community because of several preceived advantages, including superior immunogencity; lower cost; ease of administration; spread of vaccine virus to unimmunized, susceptible persons; and induction of gastrointestinal immunity. The nearly exclusive use of OPV since 1969 has resulted in total eradication of indigenous naturally occurring polioviruses in the United States.[26] However, the decline in countries such as Finland, Sweden, and the Netherlands, which use only IPV, has been equally dramatic. The successful use of OPV has engendered the paradoxical situation in which the risk of very rare OPV related paralytic disease exceeds the risk of disease due to naturally occurring polioviruses.[72] The litigation attending these few OPV related cases has driven up the cost of OPV dramatically in the past several years.[73] There has always been controversy over the relative merits of IPV and OPV. However, now because of the increased social and legal costs of OPV and because of the recent licensure of a more potent IPV formulation,[74] polio vaccine policy in the United States is now undergoing active review by national expert committees.[75]

IPV is prepared by formalin inactivation of well characterized poliovirus seed strains that are now produced in continuous monkey kidney or human diploid cells grown in microcarrier cultivation systems. The resulting "enhanced potency" IPV preparations, which have largely supplanted the older, less potent IPV, are formulated to contain 40, 8, and 32 D antigen units for types 1, 2, and 3, respectively. They are more immunogenic than OPV, producing antibodies to all three types in 99 percent of recipients after two doses and a significant boost in antibody titer after a third dose.[76,77] Neutralizing antibody persists at protective levels for at least 5 years.[78] There are few data regarding vaccine efficacy of enhanced potency IPV; however, a case control study in Senegal indicated lower than expected protection rates of 36 and 89 percent for recipients of one and two doses, respectively.[79] The recommended primary series for enhanced potency IPV is the same as for OPV (i.e., three doses administered at 2 months, 4 months, and 12–18 months of age).[74] IPV is the preferred poliomyelitis vaccine for persons who are immunodeficient and for previously unvaccinated adults.[74]

Trivalent OPV contains 800,000, 100,000, and 500,000 median tissue culture dose ($TCID_{50}$) of attenuated, Sabin strain poliovirus types 1, 2, and 3, respectively. Two doses given at 2 months and 4 months of age produce antibodies in more than 90 percent of infants,[77,80] type 2 OPV virus's producing the highest seroconversion rates and highest mean antibody titer. Type 3 OPV is the least immunogenic strain at the current formulation. A third dose given at 12–18 months of age results in neutralizing antibody to all three types in more than 97 percent of infants.[77] Detectable antibodies persist for at least 5 years in 84–98 percent after primary immunization.[81] Reinfection with either naturally occurring polio viruses or vaccine strains undoubtedly plays a role in reinforcing OPV induced humoral immunity.[82,83] The efficacy of OPV has never been tested under controlled conditions of exposure to natural polioviruses in the United States. During a type 1 poliovirus outbreak in Taiwan, vaccine efficacy for OPV was estimated to be 82, 96, and 98 percent for one, two, and three or more doses, respectively.[84] Complete immunization requires a primary series of three doses of trivalent OPV, which are normally administered at 2, 4, and 12–18 months of age; a booster dose is also recommended at 4–6 years of age prior to grade school entry.[85]

Both IPV and OPV have excellent records of safety and efficacy when used according to published recommendations. Different economic, social, and epidemiologic conditions in various countries tend to favor the use of one vaccine over the other. IPV has been very effective in developed countries capable of achieving nearly universal vaccination, but outbreaks of poliomyelitis may occur in these locations among small pockets of unimmunized persons[86] or it IPV of low potency is used.[87] Underdeveloped nations use OPV almost exclusively because of lower cost, less demanding storage conditions, and ease of administration. In addition, the transmission of vaccine virus to unimmunized persons is considered a major advantage in settings where only a fraction of the population may receive the recommended number of polio vaccine doses, and the secretory immunity induced in the gastrointestional tract by OPV may reduce transmission of naturally occurring polioviruses in the household and in the community. The Expanded Program on Immunization of the World Health Organization recommends a dose of OPV at birth and three additional doses of OPV in the first year of life, spaced by at least 2 months.[88]

For reasons that are poorly understood, OPV fails to elicit serum antibodies in a high proportion of recipients in some warm climate countries.[89–91] Intercurrent enterovirus infections do not appear to be responsible for the diminished seroconversion rates observed.[90] An increase in the OPV type 3 content may improve OPV immunogenicity in tropical climates somewhat, but unknown factors other than vaccine formulation reduce the chance that vaccine virus of all three types will replicate in the gastrointestinal tract.[90,91] Enhanced potency IPV is highly immunogenic in these same tropical areas when used alone[92] or simultaneously with OPV.[93]

School immunization laws and public health vaccine initiatives have resulted in improved immunization rates in the United States compared to the low rates prevalent in the 1970s, but low levels of immunity persist among pre-school-age children, particularly those from disadvantaged backgrounds.[73] It is largely for this reason that trivalent OPV remains the preferred vaccine for routine poliomyelitis immunization in the United States.[72,85] However, poliomyelitis immunization public policy will continue to undergo periodic examination.[75] The most recent recommendations of the immunization advisory committees should be reviewed for current information.[74,85,94]

REFERENCES

1. Paul JR. A History of Poliomyelitis. New Haven: Yale University Press; 1971.
2. Enders JF, Weller TH, Robbins FC. Cultivation of the Lansing strain of poliomyelitis virus in cultures of various human embryonic tissues. Science. 1949;109:85.
3. Bodian D, Morgan IM, Howe HA. Differentiation of three types of poliomyelitis virus: III. The grouping of fourteen strains into three immunological types. Am J Hyg. 1949;49:234.
4. Horstmann DM. Poliomyelitis in the blood of orally infected monkeys and chimpanzees. Proc Soc Exp Biol Med. 1952;79:417.
5. Bodian D. Pathogenesis of poliomyelitis in normal and passively immunized primates after virus feeding. Fed Proc. 1952;11:462.
6. Horstmann DM, McCollum RW. Poliomyelitis virus in human blood during the "minor illness" and the asymptomatic infection. Proc Soc Exp Biol Med. 1953;82:434.
7. Salk JE, Bennett BL, Lewis LJ, et al. Studies in human subjects on active immunization against poliomyelitis: I. A preliminary report of experiments in progress. JAMA. 1953;151:1081.
8. Live Poliovirus Vaccines. First and Second International Conferences on Live Poliovirus Vaccines. Washington, D.C.: World Health Organization; 1959:1960.
9. Shelokov A, Habel K, McKinstry DW. Relation of poliomyelitis virus types to clinical disease and geographic distribution: A preliminary report. Ann NY Acad Sci. 1955;61:998.
10. Centers for Disease Control. Neurotropic diseases surveillance. Annual Poliomyelitis Summary, 1971. Atlanta: CDC; 1973.
11. Bodian D. Second attacks of parlytic poliomyelitis in human beings in relation to immunity, virus types and virulence. Am J Hyg. 1951;54:174.
12. Sabin AB. Properties and behavior of orally administered attenuated polio virus vaccine. In: Poliomyelitis Papers and Discussions Presented at the Fourth International Poliomyelitis Conference. Philadelphia: JB Lippincott; 1958:124.
13. Minor PD, John A, Ferguson M, et al. Antigenic and molecular evolution of the vaccine strain of type 3 poliovirus during the period of excretion by a primary vaccinee. J Gen Virol. 1986;67:693–706.
14. Kew OM. Applications of molecular epidemiology to the surveillance of poliomyelitis. Presented to the National Academy of Medicine, Institute of Medicine Conference "Poliomyelitis Vaccines: Re-evaluating Policy Options." Washington D.C.: January 1988.

15. Bodian D. Emerging concepts of poliomyelitis infection. Science. 1955;122:105.
16. Bodian D. Viremia in experimental poliomyelitis: I. General aspects of infection after intravascular inoculation with strains of high and low invasiveness. Am J Hyg. 1954;60:339.
17. Holland JJ. Receptor affinities as major determinants of enterovirus tissue tropisms in humans. Virology. 1961;15:312.
18. Bodian D, Howe HA. An experimental study of the role of neurones in the dissemination of poliomyelitis virus in the nervous system. Brain. 1940;63:135.
19. Jubelt B, Gallez-Hawkins G, Narayan O, et al. Pathogeneis of human poliovirus infection in mice. II. Age dependency of paralysis. J Neuropathol Exp Neurol. 1980;39:149.
20. Bodian D. Histopathologic basis of the clinical findings in poliomyelitis. Am J Med. 1949;6:563.
21. Paul JR. Epidemiology of poliomyelitis. Poliomyelitis. World Health Organization Monograph Series, 1955;26:9.
22. Nathanson N, Martin JR. The epidemiology of poliomyelitis: Enigmas surrounding its appearance, periodicity, and disappearance. Am J Epidemiol. 1979;110:672.
23. Mabey DC. Paralytic poliomyelitis in the Gambia: Lameness in urban children. Ann Trop Pediatr. 1981;1:45–9.
24. Burke DS, Gaydos JC, Hodder RA, et al. Seroimmunity to polioviruses in U.S. Army recruits. J Infect Dis. 1979;139:225.
25. Schonberger LB, Kaplan J, Kim-Farley R, et al. Control of paralytic poliomyelitis in the United States. Rev Infect Dis. 1984;6:S424–6.
26. Kim-Farley RJ, Bart KJ, Schonberger LB, et al. Poliomyelitis in the USA: Virtual elimination of disease caused by wild virus. Lancet. 1984;2:1315–7.
27. Nkowane BM, Wassilak SCF, Orenstein WA, et al. Vaccine-associated paralytic poliomyelitis: United States: 1973 through 1984. JAMA. 1987;257:1335–40.
28. Horstmann DM, Paul JR. The incubation period in human poliomyelitis and its implications. JAMA. 1947;135:11.
29. Brown GC, Francis T Jr, Pearson HE. Rapid development of carrier state and detection of poliomyelitis virus in stool nineteen days before onset of paralytic disease. JAMA. 1945;129:121.
30. Melnick JL, Ledinko N. Social serology: Antibody levels in a normal young population during an epidemic of poliomyelitis. Am J Hyg. 1951;54:354.
31. Horstmann DW. Clinical aspects of acute poliomyelitis. Am J Med. 1949;6:592.
32. Weinstein L, Shelokov A, Seltser R, et al. A comparison of the clinical features of poliomyelitis in adults and in children. N Engl J Med. 1952;246:296.
33. Plum F. Sensory loss with poliomyelitis. Neurology. 1956;6:166.
34. Baker AB. Bulbar poliomyelitis: Its mechanism and treatment. Am J Med. 1949;6:614.
35. Weinstein L. Cardiovascular disturbances in poliomyelitis. Circulation. 1957;15:735.
36. Spencer WA, Jackson RR, Vallbona C, et al. Circulatory disturbances in life-threatening poliomyelitis. Am Heart J. 1960;59:384.
37. Ibsen B. The clinical diagnosis and evaluation of respiratory problems in patients with acute poliomyelitis. In: Poliomyelitis: Papers and Discussions Presented at the Fourth International Poliomyelitis Conference. Philadelphia: JB Lippincott; 1958:483, 487.
38. Galpine JF, Wilson WCM. Occurrence of myocarditis in paralytic poliomyelitis. Br Med J. 1959;2:1379.
39. Neu HN. Gastro-intestinal complications in poliomyelitis. In: Poliomyelitis: Papers and Discussions Presented at the Fourth International Poliomyelitis Conference. Philadelphia: JB Lippincott; 1958:546.
40. Plum F. Prevention of urinary calculi after paralytic poliomyelitis. JAMA. 1958;1302–6.
41. Abramson H, Greenberg M. Acute poliomyelitis in infants under one year of age: Epidemiological and clinical features. Pediatrics. 1955;16:477.
42. Weinstein L, Aycosk WL, Feemster RF. Relation of sex, pregnancy, and menstruation to susceptibility in poliomyelitis. N Engl J Med. 1951;245:54.
43. Siegel M, Greenberg M, Bodian J. Presence of children in the household as a factor in the incidence of paralytic poliomyelitis in adults. N Engl J Med. 1957;257:958.
44. Anderson GW, Anderson G, Skaar A, et al. Poliomyelitis in pregnancy. Am J Hyg. 1952;55:127.
45. Wright PF, Hatch MH, Kasselberg AG, et al. Vaccine-associated poliomyelitis in a child with sex-linked agammaglobulinemia. J Pediatr. 1977;91:408.
46. Wyatt HV. Poliomyelitis in hypogammaglobulinemics. J Infect Dis. 1973;128:802.
47. Lopez C, Biggar WD, Park BH, et al. Nonparalytic poliovirus infections in patients with severe combined immunodeficiency disease. J Pediatr. 1974;84:497–502.
48. Wyatt HV. Risk of live poliovirus in immunodeficient children. J Pediatr. 1975;87:152.
49. Davis LE, Bodian D, Price D, et al. Chronic progressive poliomyelitis secondary to vaccination of an immunodeficient child. N Engl J Med. 1977;297:241.
50. Russell WR. Paralytic poliomyelitis: The early symptoms and the effect of physical activity on the course of the disease. Br Med J. 1949;1:465.
51. Horstmann DM. Acute poliomyelitis. Relation of physical activity at the time of onset to the course of the disease. JAMA. 1950;142:236.
52. Levinson SO, Milzer A, Lewin P. Effect of fatigue, chilling, and mechanical trauma on resistance to experimental poliomyelitis. Am J Hyg. 1945;42:204.
53. Hill AB, Knowelden J. Inoculation and poliomyelitis: A statistical investigation in England and Wales in 1949. Br Med J. 1950;2:1.
54. Greenberg M, Abramson H, Cooper HM, et al. The relation between recent injections and paralytic poliomyelitis in children. Am J Public Health. 1952;42:142.
55. Bodian D. Viremia in experimental poliomyelitis: II. Viremia and the mechanism of the "provoking" effect of injections or trauma. Am J Hyg. 1954;60:358.
56. Trueta J, Hodes R. Provoking and localizing factors in poliomyelitis: An experimental study. Lancet. 1954;1:998.
57. Eley RC, Flake CG. Acute anterior poliomyelitis following tonsillectomy and adenoidectomy: With special reference to the bulbar form. J Pediatr. 1938;13:63.
58. Paffenbarger RS Jr. The effect of prior tonsillectomy on incidence and clinical type of acute poliomyelitis. Am J Hyg. 1957;66:131.
59. Ogra P. Effect of tonsillectomy and adenoidectomy on nasopharyngeal antibody response to poliovirus. N Engl J Med. 1971;284:59.
60. Aycock WL. Familial aggregation in poliomyelitis. Am J Med Sci. 1942;203:456.
61. Miller DA, Miller OJ, Dev VG, et al. Human chromosome 19 carries a poliovirus receptor gene. Cell. 1974;1:167.
62. Pietsch MC, Morris PJ. An association of HL-A3 and HL-A7 with paralytic poliomyelitis. Tissue Antigens. 1974;4:50.
63. van Eden W, Persijn GG, Bijkerk H, et al. Differential resistance to paralytic poliomyelitis controlled by histocompatibility leukocyte antigens. J Infect Dis. 1983;147:422.
64. Ferris BG Jr, Auld PAM, Cronkhite L, et al. Life threatening poliomyelitis, Boston, 1955. N Engl J Med. 1960;262:371.
65. Lassen HCA. Statistical considerations of mortality and prognosis of patients with respiratory distubances. In: Poliomyelitis. Papers and Discussions Presented at the Fourth International Poliomyelitis Conference. Philadelphia: JB Lippincott; 1958:472.
66. Russell WR, Fischer-Williams M. Recovery of muscular strength after poliomyelitis. Lancet. 1954;1:330.
67. Dalakas MC, Elder G, Hallett M, et al. A long-term follow-up study of patients with post-poliomyelitis neuromuscular symptoms. N Engl J Med. 1986;314:959–63.
68. Weinstein L: Diagnosis and treatment of poliomyelitis. Med Clin North Am. 1948;32:1377.
69. Bennett RI. Care of the after effects of poliomyelitis. Am J Med. 1949;6:620.
70. Melnick JL. Advantages and disadvantages of killed and live poliomyelitis vaccines. Bull WHO. 1978;56:21.
71. Sabin AB. Oral poliovirus vaccine: History of its development and use and current challenge to eliminate poliomyelitis from the world. J Infect Dis. 1985;151:420–6.
72. Hinman AR, Koplan JP, Orenstein WA, et al. Live or inactivated poliovirus vaccine: An analysis of the benefits and risks. Am J Public Health 1988;78:291–5.
73. McBean AM, Modlin JF. Rationale for the sequential use of inactivated poliovirus vaccine and live attenuated poliovirus vaccine for routine use in the United States. Pediatr Infect Dis J. 1987;6:881–7.
74. Centers for Disease Control. Poliomyelitis prevention: Enhanced-potency inactivated poliomyelitis vaccine—supplementary statement. MMWR. 1987;36:795–8.
75. Institute of Medicine, National Academy of Sciences. An Evaluation of Poliomyelitis Vaccine Policy Options. Washington, D.C.: National Academy of Sciences; 1988.
76. Simoes EA, John TJ. The antibody response of seronegative infants to inactivated poliovirus vaccine of enhanced potency. J Biol Stand. 1986;14:127–31.
77. McBean AM, Thoms ML, Albrecht P, et al. The serologic response to oral polio vaccine and enhanced potency inactivated polio vaccines. Am J Epidemiol. 1988;128:615–28.
78. Swartz TA, Roumiantzeff M, Peyron L, et al. Use of a combined DTP-polio vaccine in a reduced schedule. Dev Biol Stand. 1986;65:159–66.
79. Robertson SE, Traverso HP, Drucker JA, et al. Clinical efficacy of a new, enhanced-potency, inactivated poliovirus vaccine. Lancet. 1988;1:897–9.
80. Hardy GE, Hopkins CC, Linneman, et al. Trivalent oral poliovirus vaccine: A comparison of two infant immunization schedules. Pediatrics. 1970;45:444–8.
81. Krugman RD, Hardy GE, Sellers C. Antibody persistence after primary immunization with trivalent oral poliovirus vaccine. Pediatrics. 1977;60:80–2.
82. Bass JW, Halstead SB, Fischer GW, et al. Oral polio vaccine: Effect of booster vaccination one to 14 years after primary series. JAMA. 1978; 239:2252–5.
83. Nishio O, Ishihara Y, Sakae K, et al. The trend of acquired immunity with live poliovirus vaccine and the effect of revaccination: Follow-up of vaccinees for ten years. J Biol Stand. 1984;12:1–10.
84. Kim-Farley RJ, Rutherford G, Lichfield P, et al. Outbreak of paralytic poliomyelitis, Taiwan. Lancet. 1984;2:1322–4.
85. Centers for Disease Control. Recommendations of the Immunization Practices Advisory Committee: Poliomyelitis prevention. MMWR. 1982;31:22–6, 31–4.
86. Schaap GJP, Bijkerk H, Coutinho RA, et al. The spread of wild poliovirus in the well-vaccinated Netherlands in connection with the 1978 epidemic. Prog Med Virol. 1984;29:124–40.
87. Kinnunen E, Hovi T, Stenvik M. Outbreak of poliomyelitis in Finland in 1984:

Description of nine cases with persisting paralysis. Scand J Infect Dis. 1986;18:15–8.
88. Katona P, Jones TS. Operational aspects of the use of oral poliovirus vaccine in developing countries. In: Halsey NA, de Quadros CA, eds. Recent Advances in Immunization. Washington, D.C.: Pan American Health Organization; 1983:18–19.
89. John TJ: Oral polio vaccination of children in the tropics: II. Antibody response in relation to vaccine virus infection. Am J Epidemiol. 1975;102:414.
90. John TJ, Christopher S. Oral polio vaccination of children in the topics: III. Intercurrent enterovirus infections, vaccine virus take and antibody response. Am J Epidemiol. 1975;102:422.
91. Patriarca PA, Laender F, Palmeira G, et al. Randomised trial of alternative formulations of oral poliovaccine in Brazil. Lancet. 1988;1:429–33.
92. Simoes EA, John TJ. The antibody response of seronegative infants to inactivated poliovirus vaccine of enhanced potency. J Biol Stand. 1986;14:127–31.
93. Lasch EE, Abed Y, Marcus O, et al. Combined live and inactivated poliovirus vaccine to control poliomyelitis in a developing country—five years after. Dev Biol. Stand. 1986;65:137–43.
94. Committee on Infectious Diseases. Amercian Academy of Pediatrics. Report of the Committee on Infectious Diseases. 20th ed. Elk Grove Village, Ill.: American Academy of Pediatrics; 1986:283–91.

150. COXSACKIEVIRUSES, ECHOVIRUSES, AND NEWER ENTEROVIRUSES

JOHN F. MODLIN

As members of the genus *Enterovirus*, coxsackieviruses and echoviruses share many characteristics with polioviruses, such as their structure, physicochemical properties, and mode of replication. The pathogenesis and epidemiology of infections with these viruses (described in Chapter 148) are also remarkably similar. More than 90 percent of infections caused by each group either are asymptomatic or result only in undifferentiated febrile illnesses.[1] Aseptic meningitis is commonly caused by each of these three *Enterovirus* groups, but the coxsackieviruses and echoviruses also produce a variety of distinctive clinical syndromes. The protean manifestations of illness vary with the age, sex, and immune status of the host (see Chapter 148) and with the serotype and the intratypic strain of coxsackievirus or echovirus responsible for the illness. The mechanisms responsible for the diversity of clinical manifestations are unknown.

Some clinical syndromes are highly, but not exclusively, associated with certain enterovirus groups or serotypes; for example, herpangina is largely caused by the group A coxsackieviruses and myopericarditis is most commonly associated with the group B coxsackieviruses. There are also a large and diverse number of clinical syndromes that have been causally linked to enterovirus infection with varying degrees of supportive evidence. However, the role of enterovirus infection in each syndrome remains undefined. The clinical spectrum of coxsackievirus and echovirus infections is presented in Table 1.

Five new enteroviruses, serotypes 68–72, have been recognized since adoption of the simplified classification scheme described in Chapter 148. The known geographic distribution of these viruses and the illnesses associated with them are listed in Table 2. Enterovirus 68, recovered from the stool of an asymptomatic child, has yet to be associated with a disease and is therefore considered an "orphan" virus.[2] Enterovirus 69 has been isolated from throat secretions of infants with bronchiolitis and pneumonia.[3] These two viruses, of which there are only a handful of isolates from California and Mexico, have been little studied. Enterovirus 70 is recognized as the major cause of acute hemorrhagic conjunctivitis, a new and distinctive infection affecting persons in warm, humid coastal areas in many parts of the world. Enterovirus 71, initially recognized as the cause of outbreaks of aseptic meningitis and encephalitis in California between 1969 and 1972,[4] has subsequently been recovered in Sweden, Australia, Japan, Hong Kong, Bulgaria, Hungary, France, and the states of New York, Alaska, Arkansas, and Pennsylvania. Most recognized infections have been in patients with aseptic meningitis or hand–foot–and–mouth disease.[5–9] However, a significant proportion of patients with enterovirus 71 infections have had more serious CNS complications, especially acute paralytic manifestations similar to poliomyelitis.[10–16] Recently hepatitis A virus has been designated enterovirus 72 on the basis of the biologic characteristics of the virus.[17,18] Hepatitis A infection is discussed in Chapter 151.

ILLNESSES CAUSED BY MANY ENTEROVIRAL SEROTYPES

Acute Aseptic Meningitis

Acute aseptic meningitis is a syndrome characterized by signs and symptoms of meningeal irritation cerebrospinal fluid (CSF) pleocytosis, and an absence of pyogenic bacteria or fungi. There are many infectious and noninfectious causes of aseptic meningitis, but enteroviruses account for more than 90 percent of cases in which an etiologic agent is identified. Aseptic meningitis and its etiologies other than enteroviruses are further described in Chapter 66.

Etiologic Agents. Approximately 80 percent of coxsackievirus and echovirus serotypes have been incriminated as causes of aseptic meningitis. Echoviruses are the most common, especially types 4, 6, 9, 11, 16, and 30, all of which have been responsible for both outbreaks and sporadic cases. The coxsackievirus serotypes most frequently implicated are B2–B5, A7, and A9.

Clinical Manifestations. The attack rates for enteroviral aseptic meningitis are highest in children less than 1 year old. The disease is also seen in older children and young adults, but enteroviral aseptic meningitis after the age of 40 is unusual.[19] The onset may be gradual or abrupt. Typically, the patient feels chilly and has fever and headache for only a few hours before frank signs of miningitis are present. Nausea and vomiting are common, especially in children. Pharyngitis and other symptoms of upper respiratory tract infections are often present. The illness is sometimes biphasic, as in poliomyelitis; in these patients, fever and myalgia are present for a few days, followed by defervescence and absence of symptoms for 2–10 days before the sudden reappearance of fever and headache signal the onset of meningitis. The severity of meningeal symptoms and other signs of neurologic disease varies widely. In infants less than 1 year of age, signs of meningeal irritation are absent altogether. Even in older children and adults, meningismus usually is mild. Stiffness of the neck and back, sometimes with muscle spasm, is the only neurologic sign in most cases. Kernig's and Brudzinski's signs are present in only about one-third of the cases. In 5–10 percent of ominous neurologic signs such as seizures, lethargy, coma, sensory deficit, or movement disorders develop.

Laboratory Diagnosis. PERIPHERAL BLOOD. The white blood cell count may be normal, elevated, or depressed, with a normal differential count or slight left shift.

CHARACTERISTICS OF CEREBROSPINAL FLUID. The CSF is clear and under normal or mildly increased pressure. The total cell count is usually 10–500/mm^3, but occasionally may exceed 1000. Cell counts less than 10/mm^3 may occur in a substantial minority of cases.[20–23] Conversely, pleocytosis and virus iso-

TABLE 1. Clinical Spectrum of Infection with Coxsackieviruses and Echoviruses[a]

	Coxsackieviruses Group A	*Coxsackieviruses Group B*	*Echoviruses*
Illness associated with many enteroviruses	Asymptomatic infection Febrile illness with or without respiratory symptoms Aseptic meningitis (1–11,14,16–18,22,24) Encephalitis (2,5,6,7,9) Paralysis (4,6,7,9,11,14,21)	Asymptomatic infection Febrile illness with or without respiratory symptoms Aseptic meningitis, (1–6) Encephalitis (1–3,5,6) Paralysis (1–6)	Asymptomatic infection Febrile illness with or without respiratory symptoms Aseptic meningitis (all except 24,26,29,32) Encephalitis (2–4,6,7,9,11,14,17–19,25) Paralysis (1–4,6,7,9,11,14,16,18,19,30)
Illness more characteristic of particular groups or serotypes	Herpangina (2–6,8,10,22) Hand–foot–and–mouth syndrome (5,7,9,10,16) Lymphonodular pharyngitis (10) Exanthem (2,4,5,9,16) Epidemic conjunctivitis (24)	Exanthem (1,3,4,5) Pleurodynia (1–5) Pericarditis (1–5) Myocarditis (1–5) Generalized disease of newborn (1–5)	Exanthem (especially 9,16 but also 1–8,11,14,18,19,25,30,32,33) Generalized disease of newborn (6,9,11,14,19,31) Neonatal diarrhea (11,14,18) Chronic meningoencephalitis in agammaglobulinemics (2,3,5,9,11,19,24,25,30,33)
Etiologic role undefined or uncertain	Diarrhea Hemolytic–uremic syndrome (4) Myositis (9) Guillain-Barré syndrome (2,5,9) Reye syndrome Mononucleosis-like syndrome (5,6) Infectious lymphocytosis	Diarrhea Myositis (2,6) Diabetes mellitus Hemolytic–uremic syndrome (2,4) Mononucleosis-like syndrome (5) Reye syndrome	Diarrhea Hemolytic–uremic syndrome (22) Reye syndrome Myositis (9,11) Guillain-Barré syndrome (6,22) Infectious lymphocytosis (25)

[a] Implicated serotypes designated in parentheses.

TABLE 2. Illnesses Associated with Newer Enteroviruses

	Immunotype			
Characteristic	*68*	*69*	*70*	*71*
Known geographic distribution	California	Mexico	Global except Australia	California New York Sweden Australia Japan Bulgaria Hungary France
Type of infection or illness				
Asymptomatic	+	+	+	+
Fever and respiratory disease	+		+	+
Meningitis/encephalitis			+	+
Paralysis			+	+
Acute hemorrhagic conjunctivitis			+	
Hand–foot–mouth disease				+
Maculopapular exanthem				+
Myopathy				+

lation from the CSF may occur without signs of meningeal irritation.[21] Differential cell counts of the CSF typically reveal a predominance of lymphocytes; however, during the early phase of the illness, polymorphonuclear leukocytes may outnumber lymphocytes. In general, the CSF glucose concentration is normal and CSF protein content is normal or slightly elevated (but not greater than 100 mg/dl percent). However, because the CSF glucose concentration is depressed to less than 50 percent of the blood glucose in 18–33 percent of cases,[24–26] and because rare cases have been observed in which the differential CSF white blood cell count is 90–100 percent polymorphs have been observed,[21] it is occasionally difficult to exclude bacterial meningitis on initial evaluation. In some cases, the CSF findings may closely mimic those of tuberculous meningitis.[27]

VIROLOGIC DIAGNOSIS. Echoviruses and coxsackieviruses can often be isolated from the CSF in the first few days after onset of meningitis and (rarely) after the first week.[28,29] While in certain echovirus epidemics (types 9 and 18) up to 80 percent of CSF specimens from patients with meningitis have yielded the virus,[21,22,30] substantially lower rates of isolation are usual in sporadic disease or epidemics due to other agents.[31–34] Echovirus 9 can often be recovered from CSF when cultures from the alimentary tract are negative,[21,32] in contrast, coxsackieviruses are almost always present in throat washings or feces when the agent is recovered from CSF.[32] Specimens for virus isolation from all three sites are therefore desirable in suspected cases of enteroviral aseptic meningitis.

Because of the multiplicity of serotypes, serologic diagnosis is rarely practical in the diagnosis of enteroviral aseptic meningitis (see Chapter 148).

Differential Diagnosis. Partially treated bacterial meningitis is the most important condition to be distinguished from enteroviral aseptic meningitis. It is commonly taught that *bacterial meningitis* incompletely treated with antimicrobials mimics viral aseptic meningitis when therapy has been instituted prior to lumbar puncture. However, several studies have demonstrated that pretreatment of bacterial meningitis alters the CSF minimally; even when some parameters are altered by therapy (i.e., change from polymorphonuclear to lymphocytic pleocytosis), others continue to indicate bacterial disease (i.e., low glucose or high protein).[35–37]

Mumps virus, the arboviruses, lymphocytic choriomeningitis virus (LCM), and leptospirosis account for virtually all remaining cases of aseptic meningitis occurring in the absence of other clinical manifestations. Before the widespread use of mumps virus vaccine in the United States, mumps infection was a common cause of aseptic meningitis. Mumps infections occur commonly in late winter and early spring; enteroviruses exhibit peak activity in the late summer and early autumn. Aseptic meningitis associated with parotitis or orchitis is strongly suggestive of mumps. However, approximately 20–50 percent of patients with mumps aseptic meningitis do not have parotitis.[38] Moreover, orchitis,[39–43] and parotitis[44] have also been reported with enterovirus infections. While the signs and symptoms of meningeal irritation due to mumps and enteroviruses are usually indistinguishable, disturbances of consciousness suggestive of encephalitis are more characteristic of mumps or arbovirus infections. CSF abnormalities also are usually similar; however, the early preponderance of polymorphs common in enteroviral meningitis is rare in mumps[29,45] and not seen in *lymphocytic chriomeningitis*.[46] Profound hypoglycorrhachia (CSF glucose less than 30 mg/dl) occurs in occasional patients with mumps meningitis[45] and lymphocytic choriomeningitis[46–48] but is very rare in enteroviral aseptic meningitis. Poliovirus aseptic meningitis is clinically indistinguishable from meningitis caused by coxsackieviruses and enteroviruses (Chapter 148).

Aseptic meningitis occurs with many other infectious and noninfectious diseases (Chapter 66) where the etiology usually is apparent because of the presence of characteristic systemic signs and symptoms.

Management and Prognosis. While hospitalization is not necessary for all cases of aseptic meningitis during summer epidemics of enterovirus infections, it is advisable for sporadic cases or when the presence of disturbances of consciousness, muscle weakness, or a petechial rash suggests the possibility of a more serious illness, such as encephalitis, poliomyelitis, or meningococcemia. Pyogenic bacterial meningitis should be excluded by lumbar puncture and tests for bacterial polysaccharide antigens in blood, urine, and CSF. In cases in which partially treated bacterial meningitis cannot be excluded or the CSF reveals a high cell count with greater than 90 percent polymorphonuclear leukocytes or low glucose concentration, administration of appropriate antimicrobials is advisable after performing Gram stains and bacterial cultures. Viral cultures may provide a presumptive diagnosis in as little as 48 hours; therefore, they can be useful in deciding whether continued administration of antimicrobials is indicated (Chapter 66).

The patient with aseptic meningitis with headache and photophobia generally wishes to be left alone in bed in a darkened room. In most cases treatment consists only of relief of symptoms. Because the syndrome of inappropriate secretion of antidiuretic hormone has been demonstrated in 9 percent of children with aseptic meningitis, it is advisable to assess the serum Na concentration early in the course of the illness.[49] Fever and signs of meningeal irritation subside in a few days to 1 week. Cerebrospinal fluid pleocytosis may persist for 1 week or more after fever and signs of meningeal irritation have resolved.[29] When the diagnosis is not in doubt and the patient is recovering satisfactorily, repeated lumbar punctures are unnecessary and more likely to cause worry because of persisting abnormalities of the CSF than they are to aid in management. The great majority of older children and adults recover uneventfully without sequelae, but lassitude and easy fatigability occasionally persist for weeks to months after the acute illness. In one study of enteroviral aseptic meningitis, subtle disturbances of motor function have been observed during convalescence, such as limitation of passive motion, muscle spasm, and poor coordination.[50] These abnormalities slowly resolve and are rarely detectable 1 year after infection.

The long-term prognosis for young infants with enteroviral meningitis is less clear. Several studies have suggested that enteroviral meningitis in the first year of life may result in permanent neurologic sequelae, such as spasticity, diminished head circumference, and impaired intellectual functions in a minority of cases,[51–53] while other studies have found no evidence of CNS sequelae.[54] The definitive study of neurologic outcome of aseptic meningitis remains to be performed.

Encephalitis

Frank encephalitis is a well-described, though unusual manifestation of central nervous system (CNS) infection with coxsackieviruses and echoviruses. Symptoms of encephalitis sometimes complicate the course of aseptic meningitis. Rarely, full-blown encephalitis dominates the clinical illness in the presence or absence of meningeal involvement. The enteroviruses, including poliovirus, account for only 11–22 percent of all cases of encephalitis that are proven to be viral; this ranks behind arboviruses, herpes simplex virus, and LCM.[55,56] Numerous serotypes have been implicated as causes of encephalitis (see Table 1); coxsackievirus types A9, B2, and B5, and echovirus types 6 and 9 are the serotypes reported most often. The evidence linking each of these serotypes to encephalitis is highly variable. In a minority of cases, a specific etiology has been proved by isolating virus from brain tissue or CSF; in others, the cause of encephalitis has been inferred by isolating virus from a non-neurologic site or by serology.

In perinatally acquired enterovirus infection, encephalitis may be one manifestation of generalized viral infection. Beyond the neonatal period, children and young adults have been most frequently affected. Clinical manifestations have ranged from lethargy, drowsiness, and personality change to seizures, paresis, and coma. Although the clinical features of most cases of coxsackievirus and echovirus encephalitis suggest generalized cerebral involvement, it is clear that focal encephalitis does occur.[57–60] Patients with focal encephalitis have presented with partial motor seizures, hemichorea, and acute cerebellar ataxia. The CSF findings in enteroviral encephalitis are similar to those found in aseptic meningitis. Abnormalities on an electroencephalogram (EEG) usually reflect the extent and severity of brain involvement. The majority of patients with coxsackievirus and echovirus encephalitis beyond the neonatal period recover fully, although static neurologic sequelae and rare deaths occur.[56,58,61,62] Residual endocrine abnormalities also have been observed after coxsackievirus B5 encephalitis involving the hypothalamic–pituitary axis.[63]

The differential diagnosis includes encephalitis due to other viruses—especially arboviruses, herpes simplex virus, LCM and mumps, postinfectious encephalitis after measles, rubella, varicella or pertussis, Reye syndrome, Lyme disease, and toxic encephalopathies (e.g., lead poisoning). In cases of focal encephalitis, management decisions may be more complicated because herpes simplex infection (the most common and treatable cause of focal encephalitis) only can be diagnosed reliably by a brain biopsy specimen. Prospective studies of encephalitis diagnosed by brain biopsy have shown that coxsackievirus infection occasionally mimics the clinical features of herpes simplex encephalitis.[64]

Paralysis and Other Neurologic Complications of Coxsackievirus and Echovirus Infections

Sporadic cases of flaccid motor paralysis have been associated with coxsackievirus and echovirus infections. Etiologic evidence in most of these cases consists of isolation of virus from feces, sometimes accompanied by rising antibody titers to the infecting virus, and absence of evidence of simultaneous infection with a poliovirus. Few cases have been documented by isolation of a nonpolio enterovirus from CSF, brain, or spinal cord. Only coxsackievirus A7, which is neuropathogenic in monkeys, has caused paralytic disease with sufficient frequency to be recognized as the etiologic agent of small outbreaks in Scotland and the USSR.[65,66] Coxsackievirus A9 was found to be the etiology of 3.1 percent of poliomyelitis cases in New Delhi, India, over a period of 7 years.[67] In sporadic cases, the serotypes that are most often implicated have been coxsackieviruses A7, A9, and B1–5, and echoviruses 6 and 9. Less frequently implicated serotypes are coxsackieviruses A4, A5, and A10 and echoviruses 1–4, 7, 11, 14, 16–18, and 30.[68–71]

The disease is milder than poliomyelitis. Paralysis, which is less common than muscle weakness, is usually not permanent. Cranial nerve involvement has occasionally resulted in complete unilateral oculomotor palsy.[72] Rare cases of fatal bulbar involvement have been reported.[73]

Guillain-Barré syndrome has been reported in a small number of patients associated with coxsackievirus serotypes A2, A5, and A9, and with echovirus serotypes 6 and 22.[32,74–77] In a few cases, the implicated virus has been isolated from CSF or brain stem.[74] Transverse myelitis has been reported in one patient who had a rise in neutralizing antibody to coxsackievirus B4,[77] and in another who had echovirus 5 recovered from the CSF.[78] Systemic coxsackievirus B2 disease has been reported with many of the clinical features of *Reye syndrome*.[79] Furthermore, several children with well-documented Reye syndrome have had a variety of enteroviruses isolated concurrently from multiple sites, including brain and CSF[80,81]; however, a clear etiologic or epidemiologic link between enterovirus infection and Reye syndrome has not been established. Opsoclonus–myoclonus, or the "dancing eyes" syndrome, has been reported in two children with concurrent coxsackievirus B3 infection.[82]

Exanthems

Coxsackieviruses and echoviruses cause a variety of exanthems, which sometimes are associated with enanthems. With the exception of hand–foot–and–mouth disease, these rashes are not sufficiently distinctive to permit reliable etiologic diagnosis on clinical grounds alone. The pathogenesis of the eruptions is poorly understood. Virus can be isolated from the vesicular lesions of hand–foot–and–mouth disease, which therefore appears to be a direct result of viral invasion of the skin after viremia. There are no reports of attempted virus isolation from the skin in cases of maculopapular and petechial exanthems; consequently, it is not known whether these lesions also are caused by the virus directly or by immunopathologic mechanisms. Laboratory evidence supporting a diagnosis of enteroviral exanthem, at present, rests on isolation of virus from vesicles, blood, feces, or throat secretions (Chapter 14).

Enteroviral exanthems themselves cause little morbidity. They are important as sentinels of the prevalence of coxsackieviruses and echoviruses in the community, and because they are often confused with other infective exanthems, some of which have more serious implications. Therefore, rashes caused by enteroviruses may be grouped according to the type of exanthem that they mimic: (*1*) rubelliform or morbilliform, (*2*) roseoliform, (*3*) vesicular, and (*4*) petechial. Some overlap between these types of exanthems often is observed in different patients infected with the same enterovirus or even among different lesions in the same patient.

Rubelliform or Morbilliform Exanthems. Fine maculopapular rashes resembling rubella, but occurring during summer epidemics, have been reported most often with echoviruses. Thousands of cases and high attack rates have been caused by echovirus 9, which is by far the most common serotype associated with rubelliform rash. In one epidemic, 57 percent of persons less than 5 years old with illness due to echovirus 9 had rash, 41 percent of those 5–9 years old, but only 6 percent of those older than 10 years.[30] The rash characteristically occurs simultaneously with fever and begins on the face, which is involved in all cases. It then spreads to the neck (75 percent), chest (64 percent), and extremities (56 percent). Usually, there are innumerable faint pink macules, 1–3 mm in diameter, which do not itch or desquamate. The exanthem is most likely to be confused with rubella,[83] but helpful distinguishing features include the summertime occurrence and absence of pruritis and lymphadenopathy in the posterior cervical and postauricular regions.[84] In occasional patients with an enanthem resembling Koplik's spots and a blotchy eruption, the disease may be confused with measles, but the coryza and conjunctivitis characteristic of that disease are absent.[85]

Rubelliform rashes may be seen with many echovirus serotypes in addition to type 9. Echoviruses 2, 4, 11, 19, and 25 have each been associated with small outbreaks. Coxsackievirus A9 eruptions may be maculopapular and begin on the face and trunk. Lesions on the limbs are most numerous on the distal parts and extensor surfaces, although the palms and soles are occasionally involved.[84] There are generally also fever and malaise. Posterior cervical or occipital lymphadenopathy similar to that seen in rubella has been present in about half the patients with rash due to coxsackievirus A9.[84]

Roseoliform Exanthems. The enterovirus exanthems are distinctive not in their appearance, but in their timing; as in roseola, the rash does not appear until defervescence. The prototype is the "Boston exanthem," the first of the enterovirus exanthems to be recognized and now known to be caused by echovirus 16.[86,87] Multiple cases often occur sequentially in families, with as many as one-quarter of the children in a household developing a rash. The mean age of those affected is 3 years. Most children are mildly ill, but infants often appear ill enough to be suspected initially of having sepsis.[88] The temperature is 38–39°C, and there may be pharyngitis without cough or coryza. The fever lasts 24–36 hours. As it declines discrete, nonpruritic, salmon-pink macules and papules (0.5–1.5 cm) appear first on the face and upper chest. Less commonly, the extremities are involved. The duration of the lesions is 1–5 days. Although the temporal sequence described above is characteristic, it is by no means absolute; also, rashes due to echovirus 16 are occasionally observed simultaneously with fever rather than after defervescence.[88]

In contrast to enterovirus exanthems, roseola is a sporadic, nonseasonal disease that usually occurs without known contact in children under 3 years of age. In addition to echovirus 16, other serotypes (coxsackievirus B1, B5, and echoviruses 11, 25) also occasionally have been associated with roseola-like illness.[88–90]

Herpetiform Exanthems. Coxsackievirus A16 (less commonly A5, A7, A9, A10, B2, and B5) is the etiologic agent of a distinctive vesicular eruption known as hand–foot–and–mouth (HFM) disease or vesicular stomatitis with exanthem.[91–93] Numerous cases of this syndrome, which occurs predominantly in children under 10 years of age, have been reported from Canada, Great Britain, the United States, Sweden, and Germany. Disease involving multiple family members is common. Most children complain of sore throat or mouth or refuse to eat. Fever of 38–39°C lasts 1–2 days and is accompanied in essentially all cases by vesicles in the oral cavity. These occur chiefly on the buccal mucosa and tongue. Several lesions may coalesce to form bullae, which frequently ulcerate by the time they are seen by a physician. Cutaneous lesions are less constant, occurring in 75 percent of the patients.[94] Unlike the rubelliform and roseoliform eruptions, which are characteristically central, the exanthem of HFM disease is peripherally distributed. Lesions are most common on the hands and feet, where either the extensor surfaces or the palms and soles may be involved. Less commonly, lesions occur more proximally on the extremities or buttocks and rarely on the genitalia. More extensively disseminated lesions have been described in an infant with preexisting atopic eczema and have been given the sobriquet "eczema coxsackium" by analogy, with eczema herpeticum and eczema vaccinatum.[95] The skin lesions of HFM disease are tender and consist of mixed papules and clear vesicles with a surrounding zone of erythema. The cutaneous lesions of HFM diesease are located subepidermally and are accompanied by mixed lymphocytic and polymorphonuclear inflammation and extensive acantholysis of the overlying epidermis.[96] Eosinophilic nuclear inclusions and intracytoplasmic picornavirus particles can be seen microscopically within cells surrounding dermal vessels.[97]

The vesicular lesions of HFM disease superficially resemble those caused by herpes simplex or varicella-zoster viruses. Patients with HFM disease invariably have lesions of the oral mucosa. In contrast, oral lesions are less common in patients with chickenpox; moreover, they generally appear more ill, and their cutaneous lesions are more extensive and centrally distributed, generally with sparing of the palms and soles. Patients with primary herpetic gingivostomatitis also usually appear more ill and have higher fever and cervical lymphadenopathy; lesions are usually confined to the oral cavity and do not involve the extremities. The enanthem of herpangina also resembles HFM disease, but it occurs more posteriorly and typically involves the fauces and soft palate. Enterovirus 71 also causes HFM syndrome, sometimes in association with central nervous system disease (see Chapter 150).

Generalized vesicular eruptions are reported to be caused by coxsackievirus A9[98] and echovirus 11.[99] Those eruptions caused by coxsackievirus A9 are similar to the lesions of HFM disease, but they occur in crops on the head, trunk, and extremities. Unlike chickenpox, the vesicles do not evolve to form pustules and scabs. The vesicular eruptions caused by echovirus 11 have occurred in immunocompromised adult patients.[99] An acute eruption resembling dermatomal zoster in which echovirus 6 was isolated from the bullous lesions[100] has been reported.

Petechial Exanthems and Other Cutaneous Manifestations. Petechial and purpuric rashes have been described with echovirus 9[30,101] and coxsackievirus A9[102] infections. When these rashes with a hemorrhagic component occur, the illness is easily confused with meningococcal disease, especially if aseptic meningitis occurs simultaneously. Occasionally, cutaneous eruptions of coxsackievirus A9 disease have a urticarial nature.[98] One child has been reported to have papular acrodermatitis (Gianotti-Crosti syndrome) that was secondary to coxsackievirus A16 infection.[103]

Acute Respiratory Disease

Undifferentiated febrile illnesses ("summer grippe") caused by most enterovirus serotypes are sometimes accompanied by upper respiratory symptoms, such as sore throat and occasionally cough or coryza. These illnesses are not clinically distinguishable from similar disease caused by other agents, such as rhinoviruses, parainfluenza viruses, and adenoviruses. In experimentally infected volunteers, and occasionally in individuals with naturally acquired disease, some coxsackieviruses and echoviruses appear capable of causing lower respiratory tract disease. However, the role of enteroviruses in lower respiratory illness is not clearly defined; at present, they must be considered rare causes of nonbacterial pneumonia when compared with respiratory syncytial virus, parainfluenza viruses, and influenza viruses, *Mycoplasma pneumoniae*, and adenoviruses.

The best characterized enteroviral respiratory pathogens are coxsackieviruses A21 and A24, which produce illness resembling the common cold except (perhaps) for a higher incidence of fever.[104,105] Outbreaks of coxsackievirus A21 illness have occurred predominantly in military populations. Although epidemics in civilians have not been recognized, sporadic infections presumably account for antibody prevalence rates of 70 percent in persons over 50 years of age.[105] Unlike most other enteroviruses, coxsackievirus A21 is more readily recovered from throat swabs than feces. In volunteers receiving small-particle aerosols of the virus, illness has included not only coryza and sore throat, but also tracheobronchitis and pneumonia.[106]

Among echovirus, type 11 is the most firmly established and (possibly) the most common cause of respiratory disease,[105] although types 4, 8, 9, 20, 22, and 25 appear to be responsible for similar illnesses. Echovirus 11 produces sore throat, coryza, cough, and sometimes fever. It also has been associated with croup.

Group B coxsackieviruses have been associated with a variety of respiratory illnesses, especially in infants and children, but their etiologic role in most of these illnesses is not firmly established. The spectrum of disease includes coryza, laryngotracheobronchitis, bronchiolitis, and pneumonia.[77,107] The pneumonia, which may be interstitial or a patchy bronchopneumonia, has occurred in children[108] and rarely in adults[109] it is documented by virus isolation from lung.

ILLNESSES USUALLY CHARACTERISTIC OF PARTICULAR GROUPS OR SEROTYPES OF COXSACKIEVIRUSES AND ECHOVIRUSES

Herpangina

Herpangina (*herpes*, vesicular eruption; *angina*, quinsy, or inflammation of the throat) is a specific infectious disease characterized by a vesicular enanthem of the fauces and soft palate accompanied by fever, sore throat, and pain on swallowing.

The disease primarily affects children between the ages of 3 and 10 years, but occasionally attacks teenagers and young adults. Summer outbreaks of herpangina have been reported more commonly than sporadic, interepidemic illness. Transmission in families usually produces inapparent infections, but one child after another may contact the sore throat at intervals of 2–10 days. Isolated cases without known source are numerous during outbreaks.

Etiologic Agents. Coxsackieviruses of group A (types 1–10, 16, and 22) are the etiologic agents in the great majority of cases. Other enteroviruses that have been isolated far less commonly from persons with herpangina include coxsackievirus B1–5 and echoviruses 3, 6, 9, 16, 17, 25, and 30.[110]

Clinical Manifestations. The illness begins suddenly with fever of 37.7–40.5°C. Vomiting, myalgia, and headache are common at the onset but generally do not persist. Sore throat and pain on swallowing are the most prominent symptoms and precede the appearance of the enanthem by several hours to 1 day. Casual inspection of the throat reveals erythema and mild exudate of the tonsils, which leads to a diagnosis of pharyngitis or tonsillitis if the characteristic enanthem is missed. The enanthem begins as punctate macules, which evolve over a 24-hour period to 2- to 4-mm erythematous papules that vesiculate, then ulcerate centrally. The lesions, usually two to six but rarely 1 dozen, are moderately painful. They are located on the soft palate, most frequently on the free-hanging margin between the tonsils and the uvula. Less commonly, they are on the tonsils, the posterior pharyngeal wall, or the buccal mucosa. Fever subsides in 2–4 days, but the ulcers may persist up to 1 week.

A variant of the syndrome, *acute lymphonodular pharyngitis*, has been described in association with coxsackievirus A10 infection.[111] Lesions occur in the same distribution as herpangina, but consist of tiny nodules of packed lymphocytes that eventually recede without undergoing vesiculation or ulceration. There is no compelling reason for separating these two entities.

The patient with herpangina does not appear very ill and requires only symptomatic treatment for sore throat. Antimicrobial therapy is not indicated. Prompt recovery occurs in all cases.

Differential Diagnosis. The disease most often is confused with bacterial tonsillitis or other viral causes of pharyngitis, but these infections do not produce vesicular lesions. Herpangina is a disease of the posterior oral cavity, while other vesicular enanthems such as primary herpetic gingivostomatitis or hand–foot–and–mouth disease characteristically occur in the front of the mouth, especially on the inner aspects of the lip, the anterior buccal mucosa, and the tongue. Gingivitis, prominent systemic toxicity, and cervical lymphadenitis are additional features of primary herpes simplex infection that are not seen in herpangina. In hand–foot–and–mouth disease, lesions also occur on the extremities in most cases. Aphthous stomatitis is characterized by larger, ulcerative lesions of the lips, tongue, and buccal mucosa; there is a history of multiple recurrences, and the disease usually occurs in older children and adults.

Laboratory Diagnosis. The white blood cell and differential counts are normal. Smears of scrapings of the lesions do not reveal the giant cells or intranuclear inclusions that are characteristic of herpes simplex. Typical cases can be diagnosed confidently on clinical grounds, but confirmation may be obtained by isolation of the etiologic agent from the throat or feces.

Epidemic Pleurodynia

Epidemic pleurodynia is an acute infectious disease characterized by fever and sharp, spasmodic pain in the chest or upper abdomen. The name pleurodynia (*pleura*, rib or side; *odyne*, pain) calls attention to the common symptom of a "stitch" in the intercostal region and does not connote disease of the pleura.

History. Pleurodynia was first described in 1872 by Daae and by Homann during an outbreak of "acute muscular rheumatism spread by contagion" in Norway. Other reports subsequently appeared in Scandinavia; in particular, Ejnar Sylvest, a Danish general practitioner, in 1933 described his experiences with the disease on the island of Bornholm in the Baltic Sea. His classic monograph received worldwide attention after it was translated into English in 1934.[112] Over the years, many synonyms for the disease have been used; among them are epidemic myalgia, epidemic benign dry pleurisy, devil's grippe, Drangedal disease, Bamle disease, Bornholm disease, and Sylvest's disease. Little has been added to Sylvest's descriptions of the disease and its epidemiology, pathogenesis, and complications. The etiologic role of coxsackieviruses was established in 1949.[113,114]

Etiologic Agents. Group B coxsackieviruses are the most important cause of epidemic pleurodynia. Other agents rarely implicated in pleurodynia include echoviruses 1, 6, 9, 16, and 19 and coxsackieviruses A4, 6, 9, and 10.[68,69,115,116]

Epidemiology. Persons with pleurodynia are somewhat older than those with most other diseases caused by coxsackieviruses and echoviruses. Multiple family members may be attacked almost simultaneously or in rapid succession separated by several days. Major epidemics have been reported at infrequent intervals, often 10–20 years apart, in contrast to the annual occurrence of outbreaks of enteroviral aseptic meningitis. Attack rates during epidemics of pleurodynia have been higher in sparsely populated areas than in cities. It is probable that the disease occurs worldwide, but published reports have come primarily from Europe and North America.

Pathogenesis. Pleurodynia is a disease of muscle, not of the pleura or peritoneum. Tenderness mimicking spontaneously occurring pain can be elicited by pressure on affected muscles in most cases; also, palpable, often visible, muscle swelling is a subtle finding in some cases.[112] A pleural friction rub has been rare or absent in most epidemics, although this sign occasionally has been noted in 7 percent or more of those afflicted.[117,118]

Although pleurodynia probably results from direct viral invasion of muscles after viremia, direct virologic evidence supporting this hypothesis is lacking.

Clinical Manifestations

Signs and Symptoms. Pleurodynia usually has no prodrome and begins with the abrupt onset of spasmodic pain, typically over the lower rib cage or upper abdomen. Fever of 38–39.5°C reaches its peak within 1 hour after the onset of each paroxysm and subsides as the pain recedes. Sore throat and headache may occur, but cough and catarrhal symptoms are notably absent.

Intensity of the pain varies considerably. It is variously described as sticking, a "stitch" in the side, lancinating, stabbing, constricting, or vise-like. Patients asked to localize the pain are likely to indicate a broad area with the palm of the hand, rather than a specific point with the finger. The most common location is the vicinity of the costal margin on one or both sies, or occasionally the subxiphoid region. Approximately half the patients, especially adults, have pain primarily in muscles of the thorax, especially the intercostals, trapezius, and occasionally the erector spinae or pectoralis major. In the other half, pain is primarily in the upper abdomen, especially the hypochondrium (internal and external obliques and transversus abdominis) or the epigastrium (rectus abdominis). Periumbilical pain and pain in the lower abdominal quadrants are also seen, especially in children in whom abdominal localization of pain is the rule.[104,117] A few patients experience pain in neither the chest nor the abdomen, but instead in the neck or limbs[119]; in these cases, the diagnosis can only be made by association with other typical cases in the family. Whatever the localization of the pain, it is usual for the individual patient to experience this pain in only one or two areas of the body.

Although the location and severity vary, *it is the spasmodic and paroxysmal character of the pain that is its hallmark.* If the pain is mild and the patient ambulatory, he or she stoops forward or leans to the side, splinting the chest. With more severe pain, the patient lies still in bed and appears acutely ill and apprehensive. Chest pain limits deep inspiration, so that respirations are shallow and rapid. Auscultation of the chest reveals no abnormalities. Motion also produces pain, and patients resist being turned in bed.

Pain can be elicited by pressure on the involved muscles in most patients. Swelling is seen or felt only occasionally and by careful, sequential observations; it is detected most readily when there is involvement of the rectus abdominis or erector spinae. Involvement of the muscles of the hypochondrium does not cause discrete swelling, but spasm of these muscles leads to loss of the upper superficial abdominal reflexes.

COURSE. Most patients are ill for 4–6 days (range: 12 hours to 3 weeks). Children, in whom the disease tends to be milder, may not even be confined to bed. The first paroxysm is the most severe, and subsequent paroxysms are shorter and accompanied by less fever. Although dull aching of involved muscles usually persists between bouts of sharp pain, the patient may look and feel entirely healthy between paroxysms. About one-quarter of patients experience multiple recurrences, often after they have been pain-free for 1 day or more and have felt well enough to return to work or school.[112,119] In about half of these persons, the recurrence of pain is at the same site; in the remainder a new site is attacked. Late relapses occur in some patients after they have been symptom-free for 1 month or more.[119]

ASSOCIATED ILLNESS. *Aseptic meningitis* occurred in 3–6 percent of the cases in the Oxford epidemic, generally 4 or 5 days after the onset of the disease.[119] *Orchitis*, which has been recorded in many outbreaks,[112,119,120] occurs in less than 5 percent of postpubertal males with epidemic pleurodynia. *Pericarditis* and *pneumonia* are rare.[118]

Diagnosis. The severity, location, and other characteristics of the pain are so protean that the disease is readily confused with many other illnesses. Pain in the chest may mimic pneumonia, pulmonary infarction, myocardial ischemia, and the preeruptive phase of zoster. Abdominal pain in epidemic pleurodynia may resemble a variety of causes of acute abdomen. During the Birmingham epidemic of 1951, children were admitted to surgical wards as commonly as to medical wards, and 9 of 49 of these children underwent laparotomy with negative findings before it was realized that they had pleurodynia. Normal auscultatory examination of the chest, together with the characteristic spasmodic and relapsing character of the pain, are helpful in excluding pneumonia. A negative chest radiographic film also is helpful, although rare pleural effusions may be present.

The white blood cell and differential cell counts usually are normal.[112,117] Virologic diagnosis can be achieved in most cases by isolating a group B coxsackievirus from throat washings or feces early in the illness or by demonstrating rising antibody titers to one of these agents in paired acute and convalescent sera.

Management and Prognosis. Salicylates and application of heat to affected muscles are useful in relieving pain[112] in most cases, but opiate analgesics are recommended for severe pain unless an acute abdomen is suspected. Despite the distressing tendency of the disease to relapse, all patients eventually recover completely. Debility out of all proportion to the apparent severity of the illness is occasionally observed for several months during convalescence.[112,120]

Myopericarditis

Coxsackieviruses rarely, if ever, attack the pericardium alone without involving pathologically the subepicardial myocardium; the term *myopericarditis* therefore best describes the disease caused by these viruses.[121] Clinically, however, the signs of either myocarditis or pericarditis often predominate. In older children and adults, the severity of myopericarditis varies from asymptomatic cardiac involvement to fulminant disease with intractable heart failure and death. The myopericarditis that occurs with generalized enterovirus infection in the newborn is discussed separately below in the section on neonatal infections.

Etiologic Agents. The evidence linking a given enterovirus serotype with myopericarditis is quite variable. Proof of causation exists for all group B coxsackievirus serotypes, group A coxsackievirus types 4 and 16, and echovirus types 9 and 22 by demonstration of infectious virus or viral antigen in myocardium or pericardial fluid.[69,122–126] There is less substantive evidence for group A coxsackievirus types 1, 2, 5, 8, and 9, and echovirus types 1–4, 6–8, 11, 14, 19, 25, and 30.[122,124,125,127–135] In most cases, these latter serotypes have been recovered from noncardiac sources during an episode of acute myopericarditis, some with a significant increase in antibody titer to the homotypic virus. Group B coxsackievirus types 2–5 are the most common etiologic agents. They account for about one-third to one-half of cases of sporadic myopericarditis[136–140] and virtually all cases during epidemics.[141] In cases of "pure" pericarditis, evidence of recent group B coxsackievirus infection has been found in 7–13 percent of the patients[138,142] with a range of 4–43 percent, depending on the stringency of the diagnostic criteria in different series.[137,138,142,143] Thus, group B coxsackieviruses are the most important recognized agents in myocarditis but appear to play a lesser role in pericarditis. Because serologic diagnosis is feasible for group B viruses, but not normally for group A or echoviruses unless a specific serotype is suspected, it is possible that the true contribution of the non-group B enteroviruses is actually higher.

Epidemiology. Epidemic disease was noted in Finland in the autumn of 1965, when 18 cases of coxsackievirus B5 myopericarditis were admitted to a single hospital.[141] Epidemic myopericarditis appears to be exceptional, however, and most reported cases beyond the neonatal period have been sporadic. This is probably because involvement of the heart is a relatively uncommon manifestation of illness even during substantial enterovirus epidemics. Only 3 percent of group B coxsackievirus isolates reported to the World Health Organization were associated with predominantly cardiac manifestations[68]; even this figure undoubtedly represents an overestimate because of selective reporting of more severe disease.

Pathogenesis and Pathologic Features. Group B coxsackieviruses and other enteroviruses reach the heart during the viremia that follows replication in the gastrointestinal tract or respiratory tract (Chapter 148). Experimental studies in a murine model strongly suggest that virus replication occurs in myofibers, resulting initially in scattered necrosis of myofibers and later in focal infiltration of inflammatory cells, including polymorphonuclear leukocytes, lymphocytes, plasma cells, and macrophages.[123] A chronic inflammatory response persists for several weeks when replicating virus is no longer present in the heart. Healing is accompanied by a variable degree of interstitial fibrosis and evidence of loss of myofibers. The role of myocardial injury produced directly by the virus or by immunopathologic mechanisms is discussed at length in Chapter 148.

Clinical Manifestations. Enteroviral myocarditis occurs at all ages but has a special predilection for adolescents and active young adults. The incidence in males is at least twice that in females.[136,140] In two-thirds of cases, an upper respiratory tract illness precedes the onset of cardiac manifestations by 7–14 days.[136] The most common symptoms are dyspnea, chest pain, fever, and malaise, each of which occurs in about 60–90 percent of the cases.[136,137,141,144,145] Pain in the precordial area is usually dull, but it may resemble angina pectoris or be sharp, pleuritic, and aggravated by recumbency when there is pericarditis. A pericardial friction rub, often transient, has been observed in 35–80 percent of the cases. Enlargement of the cardiac silhouette on chest radiograph films, present in about 50 percent, may be due to either pericardial effusion or cardiac dilatation. A gallop rhythm and other signs of frank congestive heart failure are observed in roughly 20 percent.[137,145]

Electrocardiographic abnormalities are invariably present. With pericarditis or mild myocarditis, which are the most common, these consist of S–T segment elevations or nonspecific S–T- and T-wave abnormalities. More severe myocardial disease may lead to the development of Q waves, ventricular tachyarrhythmias, and all degrees of heart block. Serum levels of myocardial enzymes and the white blood cell count are frequently elevated. Other clinical manifestations of systemic enteroviral disease sometimes occur with myopericarditis, including aseptic meningitis, pleurodynia, hepatitis, and orchitis.

Course and Prognosis. Most children and adults recover uneventfully. Fatalities during the acute disease occur in only 0–4 percent of the cases and are essentially restricted to those in whom severe myocarditis predominates over pericarditis. One or more recrudescences of myopericarditis occurring several weeks to more than 1 year after the initial illness have been observed in approximately 20 percent of the people. Persistent electrocardiographic abnormalities (10–20 percent), cardiomegaly (5–10 percent), and chronic congestive heart failure indicate that permanent myocardial injury sometimes occurs.[136,137,145] Idiopathic cardiomyopathy may, in some instances, be a sequel of unrecognized coxsackievirus infections. Chronic constrictive pericarditis has occurred after intervals of 5 weeks to 1 year.[146–148]

Management. Supportive treatment of pericardial pain, effusions, arrhythmias, and heart failure is similar regardless of etiology. Bed rest is recommended during the acute stage, because evidence in experimentally infected mice indicates that exercise augments the mortality of coxsackievirus myocarditis (see Chapter 148). Although corticosteroids are recommended by some investigators, there is experimental evidence that this may be harmful during the acute illness, when virus is still present in the myocardium. Controlled studies on the effects of steroid treatment have not been made; the collective experience reported so far fails to show either clear-cut benefit or harm from steroid therapy for myopericarditis.

Older children and adults with suspected coxsackievirus myopericarditis do not require isolation. Appropriate control measures are those recommended for enterovirus infections in general (see Chapter 148).

Diagnosis and Differential Diagnosis. Many other viruses have been associated with myopericarditis, although influenza A virus,[149] mumps virus,[150] and vaccinia virus[151] are the only nonenterovirus agents to be recovered directly from pericardial fluid or myocardial tissue. The weight of clinical evidence suggests that Epstein-Barr virus, adenovirus, varicella virus, and measles virus also can cause myopericarditis. Cardiac disease caused by most of these agents can be distinguished from enteroviral myopericarditis on the basis of associated epidemiologic and clinical features. *Acute myocardial infarction* is an important cause of chest pain, arrhythmias, and congestive heart failure that may be difficult to distinguish from myopericarditis. Focal myocardial necrosis has been demonstrated in myopericarditis caused by coxsackievirus B5.[152] Prospective studies of patients with the clinical picture of acute myocardial infarction have shown that 5–20 percent have evidence of concurrent group B coxsackievirus infection[153–155]; however, that proportion may not differ significantly from the background incidence of infection in controls.[154,156]

Although coxsackieviruses have been isolated on numerous occasions from pericardial fluid or heart muscle at autopsy[140] or by open biopsy procedure,[157,158] in practice these specimens are rarely available. Diagnosis by virus isolation from myocardium obtained by percutaneous, transvenous biopsy procedure of the right ventricle is theoretically feasible but has not yet been reported. In the absence of isolation of virus from heart tissues, the diagnosis rests on circumstantial evidence provided by recovery of the agent from the oropharynx or feces and/or serologic evidence of recent infection by a group B coxsackievirus. Even serologic diagnosis is difficult; it is often impossible to demonstrate seroconversion, because many patients already have high, stable titers of neutralizing antibodies within a few days of onset of illness. High, stable antibody titers may persist for years in some persons and are of less diagnostic significance than seroconversion. Serodiagnosis of echoviruses and group A coxsackieviruses is not practical (see Chapters 14 and 148). Criteria for establishing an etiologic diagnosis of enteroviral myopericarditis that weight the significance of various laboratory tests (high-, moderate-, and low-order associations; see Chapter 148) have been proposed.

Coxsackievirus and Echovirus Disease in the Newborn Infant

The human neonate is uniquely susceptible to coxsackievirus and echovirus disease. While many enterovirus serotypes cause the same self-limited clinical syndromes in neonates as they do in older persons (e.g., aseptic meningitis, exanthems, hand–foot–and–mouth syndrome), some serotypes are capable of producing fulminant, frequently fatal disease in the newborn infant. The group B coxsackievirus serotypes 2–5 and echovirus 11 are most frequently associated with overwhelming, systemic neonatal infections. Other echovirus serotypes (i.e., 4, 6, 7, 9, 12, 14, 19, 21, and 31) have been reported to cause sporadic cases.[159–163] Rare cases of serious neonatal disease are reported with group A coxsackievirus serotypes 3, 9, and 16.[164–166]

Epidemiology. Although most neonatal enteroviral infections are acquired directly from the mother, some infections are transmitted nosocomially. The initial descriptions of group B coxsackievirus disease in newborn infants followed outbreaks occurring in newborn nurseries in South Africa, Rhodesia, and the Netherlands.[167] Numerous nursery outbreaks of neonatal echovirus infection have been recorded; the severity of neonatal disease varies according to serotype or serotypic strain.[159] Nosocomial outbreaks of neonatal enteroviral infection usually have been traced to infected mothers or hospital personnel. Infant to infant spread within nurseries probably occurs via the hands of personnel engaged in mouth care, gavage feeding, and other activities requiring close direct contact.[168]

The majority of neonatal enteroviral infections are perinatally acquired from an infected mother. Thus, the incidence and severity of neonatal enteroviral infection tend to reflect the occurrence of enteroviral disease in the community. Many cases occur sporadically, usually during the enterovirus season. Clusters of vertically transmitted neonatal infection also have been recorded during community outbreaks with a single enterovirus serotype.[169,170]

Clinical Manifestations. Most serious neonatal coxsackievirus and echovirus illnesses have onset of symptoms between 3 and 7 days of life.[159,171] In some cases, manifestations of infection have been present in the delivery room or developed within the first 1–2 days of life[159,171]; conversely, fatal infection has been documented in infants as old as 3 months.[172] Male and premature infants are overrepresented among infants with serious illness. Early symptoms generally are mild and nonspecific, including listlessness, anorexia, and transient respiratory distress. Fever may or may not be present. Approximately one-third of cases have a biphasic illness with a period of 1–7 days of apparent well-being interspersed between the initial symptoms and the appearance of more serious manifestations.

Generalized enterovirus disease in the newborn usually occurs as one of two characteristic syndromes. In the first syndrome, myocarditis and frequently encephalitis are the dominant clinical features. The encephalomyocarditis syndrome generally is caused by the group B coxsackievirus types 1–5[69,167]; however, echovirus 11 also has been reported as a cause of neonatal myocarditis.[133,173] The second syndrome is characterized by hypotension, profuse hemorrhage, and frequently massive hepatic necrosis. Echovirus 11 has been responsible for more than one-half of the reported cases of hemorrhage–hepatitis syndrome, and echovirus types 4, 6, 7, 9, 12, 14, 19, 21, and 31 are responsible for the remainder of the well-documented cases.[159–163]

The encephalomyocarditis syndrome is generally heralded by the onset of heart failure. This is manifest as respiratory distress, tachycardia often exceeding 200 beats/min, cardiomegaly, systolic murmur, and electrocardiographic evidence of myocardial injury. Pericarditis, clinical or electrocardiographic, is not a feature of the disease in neonates.

Severely affected infants rapidly develop cyanosis and circulatory collapse. In fatal cases, there is often disseminated viral infection involving other organs in a pattern resembling that seen in experimentally infected suckling mice; these organs, in order of frequency, are the central nervous system, liver, pancreas, and adrenal gland. Most affected neonates are lethargic, but the presence of convulsions, bulging fontanelles, and cerebrospinal fluid pleocytosis points to meningoencephalitis. Enlargement of the liver, in which there is predominantly centrolobular necrosis, is more often due to congestive heart failure and hypoxia than to viral hepatitis.

Although initial reports suggested that most cases of neonatal coxsackievirus myocarditis ended fatally, accumulated experience now indicates that the mortality is less than 50 percent. Death usually occurs within 1 week of onset, but a fulminant course with death in less than 24 hours is sometimes seen. In survivors, myocardial function improves rapidly after defervescence, generally by 1 week, although in a few infants convalescence is prolonged for several weeks.

The initial symptoms of the hemorrhage–hepatitis syndrome are lethargy, poor feeding, and increasing jaundice. These nonspecific symptoms usually lead to a work-up for bacterial sepsis and initiation of systemic antibiotic therapy. However, within 1–2 days, the jaundice progresses, the infant develops ecchymoses and bleeding from puncture sites, and signs of metabolic acidosis develop. From this stage, most infected infants progress rapidly downhill with uncontrollable hemorrhage, hepatic failure, acute renal failure, and generalized seizures.

Hepatic transaminase levels rise rapidly to extremely high

levels, reflecting the overwhelming hepatitis. Thrombocytopenia generally is profound; markedly prolonged prothrombin times and partial thromboplastin times are indicative of extensive diffuse intravascular coagulation. The white blood cell count is surprisingly normal or close to normal, considering the dramatic nature of the illness. Cultures of blood and CSF for bacteria are invariably sterile.

At least 80–90 percent of infants with the hemorrhage–hepatitis syndrome die within 2–6 days after onset of symptoms, despite therapy with blood products and intensive supportive care. A few fatal cases have persisted for up to 3 weeks.[169] Occasional infants have recovered,[174–176] but the long-term prognosis for survivors is not known.

There are several reports of cases of pneumonia occurring in the first few days of life, all of them fatal, caused by echovirus types 6,[177] 9,[178] and 11[179] and group A coxsackievirus type 3.[165]

Management. The management of neonatal enteroviral disease is supportive. Infants in congestive heart failure require judicious fluid management and administration of digoxin and diuretics. The profuse bleeding and coagulopathy of the hemorrhage–hepatitis syndrome necessitate frequent replacement therapy with packed red blood cells, platelets, and fresh-frozen plasma. Vitamin K should be administered intravenously in pharmacologic doses.

Diagnosis and Differential Diagnosis. The diagnosis of neonatal coxsackievirus and echovirus infection is most rapidly made by isolating the virus in an appropriate cell line or animal host (Chapter 14). Virus is usually present in the infected neonate in high titer so that recovery from oropharyngeal secretions, feces, and urine is relatively rapid; virus is often recovered from blood, CSF, ascitic fluid, and multiple tissues obtained at biopsy or autopsy. Because infected infants make humoral antibody to the virus, the diagnosis can also be made by serologic means when a particular serotype is suspected.

Neonatal myocarditis is sometimes mistaken for congenital heart disease, because in both conditions there may be murmurs and evidence of congestive heart failure. However, fever and electrocardiographic evidence of acute myocardial injury are absent in congenital heart disease. The early features of both the encephalomyocarditis syndrome and the hemorrhage–hepatitis syndrome resemble those of bacterial sepsis. Because of liver and CNS involvement with either syndrome, visceral dissemination with perinatally acquired herpes simplex virus (HSV) in the absence of cutaneous lesions may be suspected. Most cases of neonatal HSV infection have their onset at a slightly older age (>7 days) than that of infants with systemic enterovirus infection (<7 days).

Pathology. At postmortem examination, infants with myocarditis have enlarged dilated hearts; extensive myocardial necrosis with variable degrees of inflammation is present histologically. Inflammation may also be found in the brain, meninges, lungs, liver, pancreas, and adrenal glands. The predominant postmortem finding in infants who die after the hemorrhage–hepatitis syndrome is extensive hemorrhage into the cerebral ventricles, pericardial sac, renal medullae, and interstitial spaces of multiple organs. Extensive tissue necrosis and inflammation are generally limited to the liver and adrenal glands, with sparing of other organs including the brain, meninges, and heart.

Pathophysiology. Most newborns with life-threatening enterovirus disease become infected via vertical transmission from the infected mother in the perinatal period.[159,180] Approximately 60–70 percent of women who bear infected infants have a febrile illness during the last week of pregnancy.[159,181] Ample experimental evidence indicates that the fetus is relatively protected during maternal infection by the placenta,[182,183] but the parturient newborn has a high risk of infection,[184,185] perhaps as a result of exposure to either virus-positive cervical secretions[174,186] or viremic maternal blood.[187] While most vertically transmitted enterovirus infections are probably acquired during delivery, some infants are infected before delivery as evidenced by the recovery of virus from cord blood[174] and the development of disease within the first 2 days of life.[159,171]

Once the newborn infant is infected, it is presumed that enteroviruses spread systemically via the blood stream. Tropism for, and replication within, specific organs of the neonatal host appear to depend on both virus and host factors. Experimental evidence suggests that some neonatal tissues are innately more susceptible to infection with some enteroviruses than the corresponding tissues from an adult host.[188] In addition, the immune response of the neonatal host may be insufficient to control the replication and spread of virulent enteroviruses adequately. Although both premature and full-term human infants are fully capable of responding to enterovirus infection with humoral antibody,[189] impaired macrophage function may be responsible for the inadequate neonatal immune response.[190,191]

The outcome of neonatal infection is heavily influenced by the virulence of the particular enterovirus serotype, mode of transmission, and presence or absence of passively acquired maternal antibody. Humoral IgG antibody transferred from the mother before delivery does not prevent infection but appears to protect the newborn from the development of severe diseases.[169,182,185,192]

Chronic Meningoencephalitis in Agammaglobulinemic and Other Immunocompromised Patients

Enteroviruses have been responsible for persistent, sometimes fatal, infections of the central nervous system, gastrointestinal tract, and skeletal muscle in patients with agammaglobulinemia. The illness is commonly associated with a dermatomyositis-like syndrome.

Etiologic Agents. Most cases have been caused by echoviruses; single cases caused by group A coxsackievirus serotypes 4, 11, and 15 and by group B coxsackievirus serotypes 2 and 3 are recorded.[193,194]

Clinical Manifestations. The disease is characterized by chronic meningoencephalitis in patients with hereditary or acquired defects in B-lymphocyte function; most of the patients have been children with X-linked agammaglobulinemia.[193] More than half of the patients also have a dermatomyositis-like syndrome, and many have evidence of chronic hepatitis. Nervous system manifestations may be totally absent, or there may be mild nuchal rigidity, headache, lethargy, papilledema, seizure disorders, motor weakness, tremors, and ataxia. These neurologic abnormalities may fluctuate in severity, disappear, or steadily progress. The CSF exhibits lymphocytic pleocytosis and a higher protein concentration than is usually seen in cases of acute enteroviral aseptic meningitis. An enterovirus can be repeatedly recovered from the CSF over a period of months to years, usually in high titer. In some cases, virus is isolated only intermittently from the CSF. For unknown reasons, it is typically more difficult to find virus in the feces than in the CSF. Enteroviruses have been recovered from many other sites in these patients, including brain, lung, liver, spleen, kidney, myocardium, pericardial fluid, skeletal muscle, and bone marrow.[193] Some patients have been infected with more than one enterovirus serotype, either concurrently[195] or sequentially.[193,194] The etiology of the chronic muscle and soft tissue inflammation is not fully understood, but recovery of echovirus from muscle in one case suggests a role for direct virus infection.[196] Although these patients presumably have intact T-lymphocyte function before infection, some patients have developed profound depression of T-lymphocyte transformation during the course of persistent echovirus infection.[196,197]

In many persons, possibly a majority, the disease ends fatally. Autopsy findings have included chronic leptomeningitis and encephalitis, with lymphocytic perivascular cuffing, focal loss of neurons, and gliosis of both gray and white matter. However, widespread destruction of motor neurons such as that seen in poliomyelitis, has not been observed.

Prophylaxis and Therapy. Periodic administration of γ-globulin appears not to prevent the disease, since most children have been receiving this therapy regularly at the time they develop CNS infection. Use of intravenous immune globulin with a high titer of type-specific antibody has been ineffective, perhaps because of poor penetration into the CSF. Some, but not all, patients have experienced improvement when immune globulin has been injected directly into the ventricles.[193]

Infections in Bone Marrow Transplant Patients. Bone marrow allograft recipients have profoundly suppressed immunologic responses during the immediate post-transplant period, including the ability to mount a humoral immune response. Townsend et al. have observed considerable morbidity and mortality during an outbreak of coxsackievirus A1 diarrheal illness in a bone marrow transplantation unit.[198] During this outbreak, viral induced diarrhea was difficult to distinguish from graft-host enteropathy.

ACUTE HEMORRHAGIC CONJUNCTIVITIS

Acute hemorrhagic conjunctivitis (AHC) is a contagious ocular infection characterized by pain, swelling of the eyelids, and subconjunctival hemorrhages, which generally resolve spontaneously within a week. Epidemic or pandemic disease has now occurred in most parts of the world.

Etiologic Agents

Enterovirus 70 has been responsible for tens of millions of cases of AHC since 1969. A variant of coxsackievirus A24 causes a similar, but geographically more restricted, disease that has afflicted hundreds of thousands of persons. Some epidemics of conjunctivitis in the Far East have involved both viruses sequentially or concurrently. Although the relative etiologic contribution of these two agents has not always been defined, it is clear that enterovirus 70 has accounted for greater total morbidity.

Epidemiology

Global Dissemination of AHC. Since the emergence of AHC as an apparently new disease in 1969, its explosive, pandemic spread has been without parallel among viral infections other than influenza. The disease was first recognized almost simultaneously in Ghana and Indonesia, and from these two foci it rapidly spread.[199] During 1970–1972, the epidemic reached westward and northward along the coast of Africa to Liberia, Sierra Leone, Morocco, and Egypt; southeastward to Nigeria; and ultimately to Zaire and South Africa. In Europe, small outbreaks in 1971–1973 occurred in England, the USSR, Holland, France, and Yugoslavia. Enterovirus 70 was the cause of these epidemics[200,201] but an antigenically distinct virus, subsequently shown to be a variant of coxsackievirus A24, was identified as the etiologic agent of more than 60,000 cases of AHC in Singapore in 1970.[202–204] During the following summer, 1971, the disease again appeared in Singapore, but this time the epidemic was caused by enterovirus 70. Smaller outbreaks due to enterovirus 70 continued in Singapore until 1974–1975, when coxsackievirus A24 once again emerged as the epidemic strain. During at least two epidemics (Hong Kong, 1971, and India, 1975) both viruses circulated simultaneously.[205,206] AHC has since been epidemic in most of the Far East and India. Enterovirus 70 was responsible in 1971 alone for an estimated 1 million cases in Calcutta[207] and 500,000 in Bombay.[208] Other regions of Asia and the Far East where AHC has been epidemic include Vietnam, Bangladesh, Thailand, Sri Lanka, Taiwan, the Philippines, American Samoa, and Japan.

Thus far, the western hemisphere has been spared the widespread epidemic disease experienced in Asia and Africa. Most disease in the West has been confined to seasonal outbreaks in Central America and the Caribbean. AHC did not appear in the United States until September 1981, when enterovirus 70 disease was first noted in Key West, Florida. Within weeks, approximately 2500 cases occurred, largely among disadvantaged blacks in Miami.[209] However, this outbreak was brief, and AHC activity has not been noted in the United States since 1981, with the exception of a few imported cases.[210] Coxsackievirus A24 AHC cases first appeared in the Western Hemisphere in Trinidad, Jamaica, St. Croix, Panama, and Mexico in 1986.[211] Approximately 31,000 cases occurred in Puerto Rico in 1987.[212]

Although the geographic distribution of AHC is wide, large-scale epidemics have occurred predominantly in crowded coastal areas of tropical countries during the hot, rainy season.[213] Outbreaks in economically developed countries and temperate climates have been much more limited.

Patterns of Transmission. Unlike most other enterovirus infections, AHC is probably transmitted primarily from fingers or fomites directly to the eye rather than by respiratory secretions or fecal contamination. Both enterovirus 70 and coxsackievirus A24 can be recovered regularly from the conjunctiva early in the illness but only infrequently from throat secretions or feces. Both appear to be naturally occurring, temperature-sensitive viruses, whose optimal replication at 33–35°C probably reflects their adaptation to the temperature of the conjunctiva.[214,215] Not only is virus shedding quantitatively greater from the eye than from the gut, but rapid serial transmissions at approximately 24-hour intervals are more consistent with direct spread of virus from hand to eye rather than with fecal–oral spread, because fecal shedding would probably be delayed for several days after implantation of virus.

AHC is highly contagious and spreads rapidly. During a 1980 enterovirus 70 outbreak in Singapore, the secondary attack rate within affected households was 72.6 percent.[216] Contagion is favored by crowding and unsanitary living conditions. AHC occurs substantially more often among the poor than among others living in the same country.[217,218] Reuse of water for bathing and sharing of towels are implicated as factors contributing to the spread of infection. Limited outbreaks of AHC in Europe have been primarily nosocomial, particularly in ophthalmology clinics, where infection appears to have been spread directly by physicians' fingers or by instruments.

Seroepidemiology and Origins of AHC. Postepidemic antibody prevalence rates of nearly 50 percent have been observed in Ghana and Indonesia but only 6 percent in affected populations of Japan. These findings are consistent with less explosive spread of AHC in economically developed regions. Antibody prevalence rates are highest in children under 10 years of age, while attack rates for clinical disease are greatest in young adults, indicating that many infections in children must be inapparent or mild.[219,220]

In sera from the United States or from Japan collected before 1969, neutralizing antibodies to enterovirus 70 have been detected only rarely and in low titer, even among the elderly.[213,219] These antibodies may not be specific, and it seems likely that AHC has not previously been epidemic in the twentieth century. The occurrence of neutralizing substances in the serum of many horses and cattle has led to speculation that enterovirus

70 is a new human pathogen that emerged from an animal reservoir of infection.[213,219,221]

Clinical Manifestations

Acute hemorrhage conjunctivitis begins abruptly, and the illness reaches its peak on the first day. It usually occurs first in one eye and then a few hours later in the other. The main symptoms are a burning, foreign body sensation; ocular pain; photophobia; swelling of the eyelids; and watery discharge.[215] Constitutional symptoms such as fever, malaise, and headache are observed in 20 percent of the cases. The most distinctive sign is subconjunctival hemorrhage, which is present in 70–90 percent of the patients with AHC due to enterovirus 70[220] but is much less frequent in cases caused by coxsackievirus A24.[202,204,206] The hemorrhages may be pinpoint or occupy the entire bulbar conjunctiva and are precipitated by everting the upper lid or by rubbing the eyes (Fig. 1). Conjunctival edema is said to be more common in the elderly; hemorrhage is more profuse in young patients.[220] Small follicles appear on the tarsal conjunctiva after 3–5 days in 90 percent of patients. Corneal erosions or a fine punctate epithelial keratitis, clearly seen only by slit lamp examination after staining with fluorescein, is also present in most cases. The ocular discharge is serous or seromucoid and contains abundant polymorphonuclear leukocytes in the first 24 hours. Preauricular lymph nodes are often enlarged and tender by the second day of illness. Recovery is usually noticeable by the second or third day and is complete in most cases in 10 days. Discoloration from old hemorrhages sometimes persists for many days after pain and inflammation have subsided.

Complications

Ocular. In severe cases of AHC, keratitis occasionally persists for several weeks but almost never leads to permanent scarring. Iritis has not been reported. Conjunctivitis may be complicated by secondary bacterial infection.

Neurologic. Motor paralysis occurs in persons who have recently recovered from AHC. Although more than 200 cases of this important complication have now been reported from India, Thailand, Formosa, and Senegal,[208,222–225] paralysis is rare compared with the enormous number of cases of AHC. The disease is clinically indistinguishable from poliomyelitis except for its occurrence almost exclusively in persons more than 20 years old and its temporal association with AHC, which it generally follows by 2–5 weeks (range 5–60 days). A "minor illness" with fever and constitutional symptoms usually precedes the onset of neurologic manifestations by 1–3 days. Radicular pain and paresthesias are prominent early symptoms preceding the onset of asymmetric paralysis of the limbs. Bulbar paralysis complicates as many as one-half of cases; respiratory failure has been observed rarely. The cerebrospinal fluid abnormalities are those of aseptic meningitis.

The evidence that the paralysis is caused by enterovirus 70 is mostly epidemiologic and circumstantial. Neurologic complications of AHC have been reported only during epidemics due to enterovirus 70 and not those caused by coxsackievirus A24. Patients with AHC-associated paralysis have no serologic evidence of recent poliovirus infection. Enterovirus 70 has not been recovered from the CSF and only once from feces.[223] However, high titers of specific neutralizing antibody to enterovirus 70 have been demonstrated in the CSF in virtually all patients with motor paralysis but not in patients with AHC alone.[224] Neutralizing antibodies to this virus are also present in the serum of patients with AHC-associated paralysis, although seroconversion has only rarely been documented, because titers are already stably elevated at the onset of the neurologic illness. The neuroparalytic potential of enterovirus 70 is supported by reproduction of poliomyelitis clinically and pathologically after inoculation of the agent into the CNS of monkeys.[226]

Differential Diagnosis

Acute hemorrhage conjunctivitis is not likely to be confused with other causes of conjunctivitis during major epidemics.

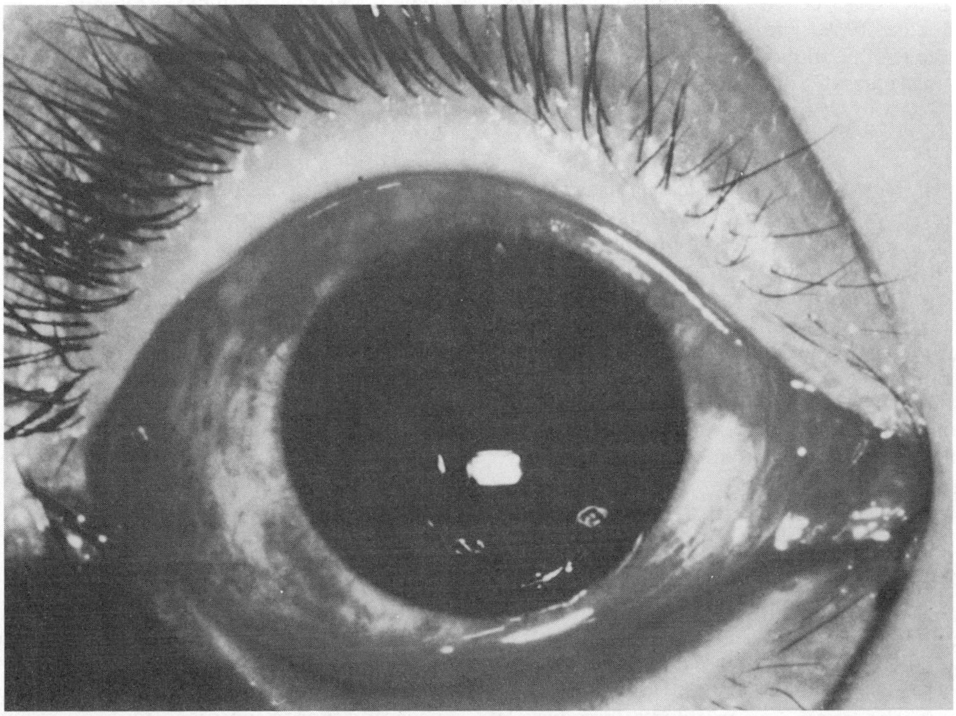

FIG. 1. Acute hemorrhagic conjunctivitis due to enterovirus 70. (From Kono et al.,[220] with permission.)

Small outbreaks or sporadic cases may be mistaken for adenovirus infection which causes epidemic keratoconjunctivitis (EKC). The incubation period of EKC is longer, usually 5–7 days, compared with 1 day for AHC. In AHC the conjunctivitis reaches its peak several hours after onset and lasts less than 1 week, whereas symptoms from EKC are maximal after several days and sometimes last for 2 or 3 weeks. Early in the illness pain and subconjunctival hemorrhage are characteristic of AHC but are uncommon in EKC. Follicular deposits on the conjunctiva are much more prominent in EKC, as are subepithelial corneal opacities persisting after conjunctivitis has subsided.

Bacterial and chlamydial causes of conjunctivitis generally do not cause extensive outbreaks with abrupt onset after a short incubation period.

AHC-associated paralysis and poliomyelitis cannot be distinguished on clinical grounds alone.

Laboratory Diagnosis

Enterovirus 70 and coxsackievirus A24 can be recovered from conjunctival swabs or scrapings of patients with AHC during the first 3 days of illness.[201,227] Isolation rates exceeding 90 percent from conjunctival scrapings have been reported for coxsackievirus A24, but recovery rates for enterovirus 70 have been somewhat lower.[217] Less than 5 percent of fecal specimens or throat swabs have been positive for either virus. Rising antibody titers can be demonstrated in paired sera from patients with conjunctivitis.

Treatment and Prevention

Treatment of conjunctivitis is symptomatic. Antimicrobial agents are not indicated unless there is bacterial suprainfection. Contagion can be prevented by careful handwashing, use of separate towels, and sterilization of ophthalmologic instruments.

ENTEROVIRUS 71 INFECTIONS

Enterovirus 71 is the most recently discovered human enterovirus serotype. The virus is known to have been reponsible for clusters of cutaneous and CNS disease in scattered locations throughout the world since 1969. The prime interest in enterovirus 71 is because the first nonpolio enterovirus with the potential to cause epidemic paralytic disease.

Etiologic Agent

Enterovirus 71 is a heat-stable, acid-stable picornavirus that is pathogenic for suckling mice, producing a myositis characteristic of the group A coxsackieviruses. A poliomyelitis-like disease can be produced by oral or parenteral challenge in cynomolgus monkeys.[228,229] Neurovirulence in monkeys appears related to the ability of enterovirus 71 strains to replicate at higher temperatures, but characterization by two-dimensional oligonucleotide electrophoresis and by separation of virion proteins with gel electrophoresis does not distinguish neurovirulent strains.[230] The antigenic relatedness of several strains isolated in different parts of the world has been demonstrated by cross-neutralization testing.[231]

Epidemiology

The first isolations of enterovirus 71 were from young children with encephalitis and aseptic meningitis in California in 1969.[4] This serotype was not isolated outside California until 1972, when enterovirus 71 CNS infections were diagnosed nearly simultaneously in the state of New York[232] and in Melbourne, Australia.[6] In both locations, cutaneous manifestations were a prominent feature of the illness in many patients. Subsequently, clusters of enterovirus 71 disease have been reported from diverse temperate climate locations. [5–16,233,234] The largest outbreaks of serious CNS disease occurred in Bulgaria and Hungary, where significant numbers of poliomyelitis-like cases and numerous deaths were noted.[10,13,235]

Enterovirus 71 has been reponsible for localized outbreaks of disease involving small numbers of patients over several years[4,11,14] and also for regional epidemics involving hundreds to thousands of persons within a single season.[7,8,15] The mode of transmission is presumed to be similar to that of most enterovirus serotypes, that is, predominantly fecal–oral spread. Most symptomatic infections occur in children less than 6 years old, and very young children have a disproportionately high number of cases of encephalitis and motor paralysis.

Clinical Manifestations

Because the literature contains few data from individual patients,[11] only a general summary of the clinical features of enterovirus 71 infection can be given. Furthermore, most reports of enterovirus 71 infections have come from central reference virus laboratories; thus, cases that have only mild or nonspecific symptoms or signs are likely to be underrepresented in the literature. Regardless, it is apparent that the spectrum of clinical illness has varied considerably among outbreaks of infection reported from different locations. During outbreaks of enterovirus 71 infection in Australia, Sweden, and Japan, most patients had either typical hand–foot–and–mouth disease or aseptic meningitis, usually after a prodrome of 1–3 days of fever[5–7,9]; serious CNS disease was not observed. In contrast, hand–foot–and–mouth disease was not seen in the 1975 Bulgarian epidemic of enterovirus 71 aseptic meningitis.[13] However, 21 percent of recognized Bulgarian cases developed an acute paralytic syndrome indistinguishable from poliomyelitis. Paralytic complications tended to develop rapidly, often within 10–30 hours after onset of symptoms. Approximately one-half of those with paralysis had evidence of encephalitis or cranial nerve involvement (bulbar syndrome). The overall mortality for those with documented infection was 6.2 percent, including 29.5 percent of patients with paralytic disease and 65 percent of patients witth bulbar involvement.[13]

The occurrence of hand–foot–and–mouth syndrome and serious CNS disease is not mutually exclusive since both features of enterovirus 71 infection have been noted during outbreaks in Rochester, New York,[11] Japan,[12] Hong Kong,[14] and Australia.[14] Other less common manifestations attributed to enterovirus 71 infection include generalized maculopapular rash,[6] myocarditis,[13] infection polyneuritis,[6] and upper respiratory tract disease.[6,13] Serologic evidence of enterovirus 71 infection in a neonate has been associated with a myopathy.[236]

Differential Diagnosis

Infections caused by enterovirus 71 may be clinically indistinguishable from infections caused by certain other enterovirus serotypes. The principal cause of hand–foot–and–mouth disease is coxsackievirus A16, although a variety of other enterovirus serotypes may also be responsible (Chapter 150). Epidemic paralytic disease has virtually always been attributed to the polioviruses, although rare cases of sporadic motor paresis or paralysis have been caused by other enterovirus serotypes.

Laboratory Diagnosis

Enterovirus 71 has been isolated from a number of clinical specimens, including vesicle fluid, feces, oropharyngeal secretions, urine, and CSF. Isolation rates are highest from vesicle swabs and lowest from the CSF.[10,13,15] Primary isolation has been most successful in African green monkey kidney cell culture and in suckling mice. Even under optimal conditions, cytopathic effect may take 5–8 days to become visible, progressing slowly and incompletely.[10,11] Because standard enterovirus antiserum pools do not contain antiserum to enterovirus 71, isolates of this serotype may be reported as "nontypable enterovirus."

Treatment and Prevention

Treatment of enterovirus 71 infection is symptomatic and supportive. Widespread distribution of oral polio vaccine during the Bulgarian epidemic was postulated to have dampened spread of enterovirus 71 disease by virtue of gastrointestinal interference, but proof of a significant effect of OPV is lacking. A killed enterovirus 71 vaccine was prepared for use during this epidemic but not employed in humans.

ILLNESSES IN WHICH THE ETIOLOGIC ROLE OF ENTEROVIRUSES IS UNCERTAIN OR UNDEFINED

Coxsackieviruses and echoviruses, possibly as a result of their habitat in the gut, are frequently cited as causes of nonbacterial *diarrhea* or *gastroenteritis*. However, conflicting results have been obtained in several studies that compare rates of enteroviral isolations from children with acute diarrheal illness with matched healthy control subjects.[69,237,239] The census of these investigations is that there is a variable, generally small, excess of enteroviral infections in subjects with diarrhea. Evidence is somewhat stronger that certain echoviruses, particularly types 11, 14, and 18, have occasionally been responsible for epidemic diarrhea of young infants.[69,239,240] Most of these studies were performed before the discovery of toxigenic *Escherichia coli,* rotaviruses, and the Norwalk-like agents now established as major causes of diarrheal illness. In light of this new knowledge, additional epidemiologic investigations encompassing all these agents will be required before the contribution of enteroviruses to diarrheal diseases can be accurately assessed. Nonetheless, their role probably is minor.

The hemolytic–uremic syndrome has been temporally associated with coxsackieviruses A4, B2, and B4 and with echovirus 22.[241–243] Similarly, coxsackievirus B5 has been reported in association with acute renal failure in five patients.[244] Although it has been speculated that immune complexes or a nonimmunologic Schwartzman-like reaction are triggered by the virus, an etiologic relationship has not been established.

Enteroviruses have been reported as causing *acute myositis* in several patients.[172,245–252] although the diagnosis has rarely been proved virologically. Echovirus 11 has been recovered from clinically involved skeletal muscle of a 3-month-old infant with a fatal systemic infection.[172] In other cases, coxsackievirus A9, group B coxsackievirus types 2 and 6, and echovirus 9 have been etiologically linked to myositis on the basis of serology, recovery of virus from throat or feces, or demonstration of viral antigen in muscle by immunofluorescence. Both generalized polymyositis and focal myositis have been noted, the latter sometimes localized to the thighs. Clinical myositis presents with fever, chills, weakness, hypotonia, tenderness, and edema of the involved muscle groups. Myoglobinemia, myoglobinuria, and an elevated creatine–phosphokinase level often are demonstrated by laboratory tests. Most reported patients have recovered rapidly.

The possible relationship between group B coxsackievirus infections and *chronic cardiomyopathy* is discussed under the section on myopericarditis in this chapter. Viral *endocarditis*[253,254] and *aortitis*[255] also have been claimed, primarily on the basis of demonstration of coxsackievirus antigens in tissues by immunofluorescence. Confirmation of these results by other techniques in independent laboratories is required.

Hepatitis has been associated with enterovirus infections, especially group B coxsackieviruses. Generally, hepatitis has been part of severe multisystem disease in neonates or, rarely, in adults.[256–261] An etiologic association between coxsackievirus infection and isolated hepatitis has not been established.

Pancreatitis has occurred in patients with group B coxsackievirus and echovirus infections.[262–265] Prospective studies of acute pancreatitis have demonstrated a concurrent enterovirus infection in 2–20 percent of cases.[264,265] Group B coxsackievirus types 1–5 and echovirus types 6, 11, 22, and 30 are the serotypes that have been recovered from patients with pancreatitis. *Orchitis* has been observed in adolescent boys during infection with coxsackievirus A9, group B coxsackieviruses 2, 4, and 5, and echovirus 6,[39–41,43] which includes coxsackievirus B5 isolation from a testicular biopsy specimen in one case (22). A relationship of these viruses to juvenile-onset *diabetes mellitus* has been claimed, but evidence accumulated so far is inconclusive.[263,266–268] In mice, certain strains of a related picornavirus, encephalomyocarditis virus, cause specific destruction of beta cells in the islets of Langerhans. Because human coxsackievirus infections are common, but juvenile-onset diabetes is rare, it has been postulated that susceptibility of human beta cells to coxsackieviruses is genetically determined or that the disease is caused only by certain strains of virus.

Lymphadenopathy has been described in a few outbreaks of illness due to coxsackieviruses and echoviruses, but it has not been prominent.[69] Splenomegaly and a heterophile-negative, *mononucleosis-like syndrome* have also been reported.[69] Echoviruses have been associated with acute arthritis; echovirus 11 was recovered from synovial fluid in one case.[269,270] In separate case reports, echovirus 25[271] and an untyped enterovirus resembling a group A coxsackievirus[272] have been recovered from the gastrointestinal tracts of children with *infectious lymphocytosis*; however, further evidence of an etiologic association is lacking.

REFERENCES

1. Kogon A, Spigland I, Frothingham TE, et al. The virus watch program: A continuing surveillance of viral infections in metropolitan New York families: VII. Observations on viral excretion, seroimmunity, intrafamilial spread and illness association in coxsackie and echovirus infections. Am J Epidemiol. 1969;89:51.
2. Rosen L, Schmidt NJ, Kern J. Toluca-1, a newly recognized enterovirus. Arch Ges Virusforsch. 1973;40:132.
3. Schieble JH, Fox VL, Lennette EH. A probable new human picornavirus associated with respiratory disease. Am J Epidemiol. 1967;85:297.
4. Schmidt NJ, Lennette EH, Ho HH. An apparently new enterovirus isolated from patients with disease of the central nervous system. J Infect Dis. 1974;129:304.
5. Bloomberg J, Lycke E, Ahlfors K, et al. New enterovirus type associated with epidemic of aseptic meningitis and/or hand, foot, and mouth disease. Lancet. 1974;2:112.
6. Kennett ML, Birch CJ, Lewis FA, et al. Enterovirus type 71 infection in Melbourne, Bull WHO. 1974;51:609.
7. Hagiwara A, Tagaya I, Yoneyama T. Epidemic of hand, foot, and mouth disease associated with enterovirus 71 infection. Intervirology. 1978;9:60.
8. Miwa C, Ohtani M, Watanabe H, et al. Epidemic of hand, foot and mouth disease in Gifu prefecture in 1978. Jpn J Med Sci Biol. 1980;33:167.
9. Tagaya I, Takayama R, Hagiwara A. A large-scale epidemic of hand, foot and mouth disease associated with enterovirus 71 infection in Japan in 1978. Jpn J Med Sci Biol. 1981;34:191.
10. Chumakov MP, Voroshilova MK, Shindarov L, et al. Enterovirus 71 isolated from cases of poliomyelitis-like disease in Bulgaria. Arch Virol. 1979;60:329.
11. Chonmaitree T, Menegus MA, Schervish-Swierkosz EM, et al. Enterovirus 71 infection: Report of an outbreak with two cases of paralysis and a review of the literature. Pediatrics. 1981;67:489.
12. Ishimaru Y, Nakano S, Yamaoka K, et al. Outbreak of hand, foot, and mouth disease by enterovirus 71: High incidence of complication disorders of central nervous system. Arch Dis Child. 1980;55:583.
13. Shindarov LM, Chumakov MP, Voroshilova MK, et al. Epidemiological, clinical, and pathomorphological characteristics of epidemic poliomyelitis-like disease caused by enterovirus 71. J Hyg Epidemiol Microbiol Immunol. 1979;23:284.
14. Samuda GM, Chang WK, Yeung CY, et al. Monoplegia caused by Enterovirus 71: An outbreak in Hong Kong. Pediatr Infect Dis J. 1987;6:206–8.
15. Gilbert GL, Dickson KE, Waters M-J, et al. Outbreak of enterovirus 71 infection in Victoria, Australia, with a high incidence of neurologic involvement. Pediatr Infect Dis J. 1988;7:484–8.
16. Centers for Disease Control. Case of paralytic illness associated with enterovirus 71 infection. MMWR. 1988;37:107–8, 113–4.

17. Matthews REF. Fourth report of the International Committee on Taxonomy of Viruses. Interviology. 1982;17:1.
18. Ticehurst JR, Racaniello VR, Baroudy BM, et al. Molecular cloning and characterization of hepatitis A virus cDNA. Proc Natl Acad Sci USA. In press.
19. Centers for Disease Control. Enteric and neurotropic viral diseases surveillance. Enterovirus Surveillance, 1971–1975. Atlanta: CDC; 1977.
20. Lake AM, Lauer BA, Clark JC, et al. Enterovirus infections in neonates. J Pediatr. 1976;89:787.
21. Haynes RE, Cramblett HG, Kronfol HJ. Echovirus 9 meningoencephalitis in infants and children. JAMA. 1969;208:1657.
22. Wilfert CM, Lauer BA, Cohen M, et al. An epidemic of echovirus 18 meningitis. J Infect Dis. 1975;131:75.
23. Wenner HA, Abel D, Olson LC, et al. A mixed epidemic associated with echovirus types 6 and 11. Am J Epidemiol. 1981;114:369.
24. Avner E, Satz J, Plotkin SA. Hypoglycorrhachia in young infants with viral meningitis. J Pediatr. 1975;87:883.
25. Sumaya CV, Corman LI. Enteroviral meningitis in early infancy: Significance in community outbreaks. Pediatr Infect Dis. 1982;1:151.
26. Singer JI, Maur PR, Riley JP, et al. Management of central nervous system infections during an epidemic of enteroviral aseptic meningitis. J Pediatr. 1980;96:559.
27. Malcom BS, Eiden JJ, Hendley JO. Echovirus type 9 meningitis simulating tuberculous meningitis. Pediatrics 1980;65:725.
28. Portnoy B, Leedom JM, Hanes B, et al. Factors affecting ECHO-9 virus recovery from cerebrospinal fluid. Am J Med Sci. 1964;248:521.
29. Gray JA, Moffatt MAJ, Sangster G. Viral meningitis: A 10 year study. Scott Med J. 1969;14:234.
30. Sabin AB, Krumbiegel ER, Wigand R. ECHO type 9 virus disease. AMA J Dis Child. 1958;96:197.
31. Lennette EH, Magoffin R, Knouf EG. Viral central nervous system disease: An etiologic study conducted at the Los Angeles County General Hospital. JAMA. 1962;179:687.
32. Lepow ML, Carver DH, Wright HT Jr, et al. A clinical epidemiologic and laboratory investigation of aseptic meningitis during the four-year period, 1955–1958: I. Observations concerning etiology and epidemiology. N Engl J Med. 1962;266:1181.
33. Torphy DE, Ray CG, Thompson RS, et al. An epidemic of aseptic meningitis due to echovirus type 30: Epidemiologic features and clinical and laboratory findings. Am J Public Health. 1970;60:1447.
34. Marier R, Rodriguez W, Chloupek RJ, et al. Coxsackievirus B5 infection and aseptic meningitis in neonates and children. Am J Dis Child. 1975;129:321.
35. Dalton HP, Allison MJ. Modification of laboratory results by partial treatment of bacterial meningitis. Am J Clin Pathol. 1968;49:410.
36. Converse GM, Gwaltney JM Jr, Strasburg DA, et al. Alteration of cerebrospinal fluid findings by partial treatment of bacterial meningitis. J Pediatr. 1973;83:220.
37. Mandal BK. The dilemma of partially treated bacterial meningitis. Scand J Infect Dis. 1976;8:185.
38. Azlmi PH, Cramblett HG, Haynes RE. Mumps meningoencephalitis in children. JAMA. 1969;207:509.
39. Craighead JE, Mahoney EM, Carver DH, et al. Orchitis due to coxsackie virus group B, type 5. N Engl J Med. 1962;267:498.
40. Ager EA, Felsenstein WC, Alexander ER, et al. An epidemic of illness due to coxsackie virus group B, type 2. JAMA. 1964;187:251.
41. Murphy AM, Simmul R. Coxsackie B4 virus infections in New South Wales during 1962. Med J Aust. 1964;2:443.
42. Willems WR, Hornig C, Bauer H, et al. A case of coxsackie A9 virus infection with orchitis. J Med Virol. 1978;3:137–40.
43. Welliver RC, Cherry JD. Aseptic meningitis and orchitis associated with echovirus 6 infection. J Pediatr. 1978;92:239.
44. Howlett JG, Somlo F, Kalz F. A new syndrome of parotitis with herpangina caused by the coxsackie virus. Can Med Assoc J. 1957;77:5.
45. Wilfert CM. Mumps meningoencephalitis with low cerebrospinal fluid glucose, prolonged pleocytosis, and elevation of protein. N Engl J Med. 1969;280:855.
46. Green WR, Sweet LK, Pritchard RW. Acute lymphocytic choriomeningitis. J Pediatr. 1949;35:688.
47. Biggar RJ, Woodall JP, Walter PD, et al. Lymphocytic choriomeningitis outbreak associated with pet hamsters: Fifty-seven cases from New York State. JAMA. 1975;232:494.
48. Vanzee BE, Douglas RG Jr, Betts RF, et al. Lymphocytic choriomeningitis in university hospital personnel. Clinical features. Am J Med. 1976;58:803.
49. Chemtob S, Reece ER, Mills EL. Syndrome of inappropriate secretion of antidiuretic hormone in enteroviral meningitis. Am J Dis Child. 1985;139:292–4.
50. Lepow ML, Coyne N, Thompson LB, et al. A clinical, epidemiologic and laboratory investigation of aseptic meningitis during the four-year period, 1955–1958: II. The clinical disease and its sequelae. N Engl J Med. 1962;266:1188.
51. Sells CJ, Carpenter RL, Ray CG. Sequelae of central-nervous-system enterovirus infections. N Engl J Med. 1975;293:1.
52. Farmer K, MacArthur BA, Clay MM. A follow-up study of 15 cases of neonatal meningoencephalitis due to coxsackie virus B5. J Pediatr. 1975;87:568.
53. Wilfert CM, Thompson RJ, Sunder TR, et al. Longitudinal assessment of children with enteroviral meningitis during the first three months of life. Pediatrics. 1981;67:811.
54. Bergman I, Painter MJ, Wald ER, et al. Outcome in children with enteroviral meningitis during the first year of life. J Pediatr. 1987;110:705–9.
55. Meyer HM, Johnson RT, Crawford IP, et al. Central nervous system syndromes of viral etiology. A study of 713 cases. Am J Med. 1960;29:334.
56. Lennette EH, Magoflin RL, Knouf EG. Viral central nervous system disease. JAMA. 1962;179:687.
57. Roden VJ, Cantor HE, O'Connor DM, et al. Acute hemiplegia of childhood associated with coxsackie A9 viral infection. J Pediatr. 1975;86:56.
58. Chalhub E, Devivo D, Siegel BA, et al. Coxsackie A9 focal encephalitis associated with acute infantile hemiplegia and porencephaly. Neurology. 1977;27:574.
59. Peters ACB, Vielvoye GJ, Verstey J, et al. Echo 25 focal encephalitis and subacute hemichorea. Neurology. 1979;29:676.
60. Morens DM. Enteroviral disease in early infancy. J Pediatr. 1978;92:374.
61. Price RA, Garcia JH, Rightsel WA. Choriomeningitis and myocarditis in an adolescent with isolation of coxsackie B-5 virus. Am J Clin Pathol. 1970;53:825.
62. Klapper PE, Bailey AS, Longson M, et al. Meiningo-encephalitis caused by coxsackievirus group B type 2: Diagnosis confirmed by measuring intrathecal antibody. J Infect. 1984;8:227–31.
63. Hagg E, Ostrom L, Steen L. Persistent hypothalamic-pituitary insufficiency following acute meningoencephalitis. Acta Med Scand. 1978;203:231.
64. Whitley RJ, Soong S-J, Hirsch MS, et al. Herpes simplex encephalitis: Vidarabine therapy and diagnostic problems. N Engl J Med. 1981;304:313.
65. Voroshilova MK, Chumakov MP. Poliomyelitis-like properties of AB-IV-coxsackie A7 group of viruses. Progr Med Virol. 1959;2:106.
66. Grist NR, Bell EJ. Enteroviral etiology of the paralytic poliomyelitis syndrome. Arch Environ Health. 1970;21:382.
67. Santhanam S, Choudhury DS. Coxsackie A-9 in the etiology of poliomyelitis-like diseases. Indian J Pediatr. 1985;52:405–8.
68. Assaad F, Cockburn WC. Four year study of WHO virus reports on enteroviruses other than poliovirus. Bull WHO. 1972;46:329.
69. Kibrick S. Current status of coxsackie and ECHO viruses in human disease. Progr Med Virol. 1964;6:27.
70. Grist N, Bell EJ, Reid D. The epidemiology of enteroviruses. Scott Med J. 1975;20:27.
71. Godtfredsen A, Hansen B. A case of mild paralytic disease due to ECHO virus type 11. Acta Pathol Microbiol Scand. 1961;53:111.
72. Hertenstein JR, Sarnat HB, O'Connor DM. Acute unilateral oculomotor palsy associated with ECHO 9 viral infection. J Pediatr. 1976;89:79.
73. Steigman AJ, Lipton MM. Fatal bulbospinal paralytic poliomyelitis due to ECHO 11 virus. JAMA. 1960;174:178.
74. Geer J. Coxsackie virus infections in Southern Africa. Yale J Biol Med. 1961;34:289.
75. Karzon DT, Hayner NS, Winkelstein W Jr, et al. An epidemic of aseptic meningitis syndrome due to ECHO virus type 6: II. A clinical study of ECHO 6 infection. Pediatrics. 1962;29:418.
76. Parker W, Wilt JC, Dawson JW, et al. Landry-Guillain-Barré syndrome—the isolation of an echovirus type 6. Can Med Assoc J. 1960;82:813.
77. Dery P, Marks MI, Shapera R: Clinical manifestations of coxsackievirus infections in children. Am J Dis Child. 1974;128:464.
78. Barak Y, Schwartz JF. Acute transverse myelitis associated with ECHO type 5 infection (Letter). Am J Dis Child. 1988;142:128.
79. Kaul A, Cohen ME, Broffman G, et al. Reye-like syndrome associated with coxsackie B2 virus infection. J Pediatr. 1979;94:67.
80. Brunberg JA, Bell WE. Reye syndrome. Arch Neurol. 1974;30:304.
81. Alvira MM, Mendoza M. Reye's syndrome: A viral myopathy? N Engl J Med. 1975;292:1297.
82. Kuban KC, Ephros MA, Freeman RL, et al. Syndrome of opsoclonus–myoclonus caused by Coxsackie B3 infection. Ann Neurol. 1983;13:69–71.
83. Bell EJ, Ross CAC, Grist NR. Echo 9 infection in pregnant women with suspected rubella. J Clin Pathol. 1975;28:267.
84. Lerner AM, Klein JO, Levin HS, et al. Infections due to coxsackie virus group A, type 9, in Boston, 1959, with special reference to exanthems and pneumonia. N Engl J Med. 1960;263:1265.
85. Annunziato D. Koplik spots and echo 9 virus (Letter). NY State J Med. 1987;87:667.
86. Neva FA, Femster RF, Gorbach IJ. Clinical and epidemiological features of an unusual epidemic exanthem. JAMA. 1954;155:544.
87. Neva FA. A second outbreak of Boston exanthem disease in Pittsburgh during 1954. N Engl J Med. 1956;254:838.
88. Hall CB, Cherry JD, Hatch MH, et al. The return of Boston exanthem: Echovirus 16 infections in 1974. Am J Dis Child. 1977;131:323.
89. Cherry JD, Lerner AM, Klein JO, et al. Coxsackie B5 infections with exanthems. Pediatrics. 1963;31:455.
90. Moritsugu Y, Sawada K, Hinohara M, et al. An outbreak of type 25 echovirus infection with exanthem in an infant home near Tokyo. Am J Epidemiol. 1968;87:599.
91. Robinson CR, Doane FW, Rhodes AJ. Report of an outbreak of febrile illness with pharyngeal lesions and exanthem. Can Med Assoc J. 1958;79:615.
92. Lindenbaum JE, Van Dyck PC, Allen RG. Hand, foot and mouth disease associated with coxsackievirus group B. Scand J Infect Dis. 1975;7:161.
93. Hughes RO, Roberts C. Hand, foot, mouth disease associated with coxsackie A9 virus. Lancet. 1972;2:751.
94. Adler JL, Mostow SR, Mellin II, et al. Epidemiologic investigation of hand,

foot, and mouth disease: Infection caused by coxsackievirus A16 in Baltimore, June through September 1968. Am J Dis Child. 1970;120:309.
95. Nahmias AJ, Froeschle JE, Feorino PM, et al. Generalized eruption in a child with eczema due to coxsackievirus A16. Arch Dermatol. 1968;97:147.
96. Miller GD. Hand–foot–and–mouth disease. JAMA. 1968;203:827.
97. Kimura A, Abe M, Nakao T. Light and electron microscopic study of skin lesions in patients with hand, foot, and mouth disease. Tohoku J Exp Med. 1977;122:237.
98. Cherry JD, Lerner AM, Klein JO, et al. Coxsackie A9 infections with exanthems with particular reference to urticaria. Pediatrics. 1963;31:819.
99. Deseda-Tous J, Byatt PH, Cherry JD. Vesicular lesions in adults due to echovirus 11 infections. Arch Dermatol. 1977;113:1705.
100. Meade RH, Chang TW. Zoster-like eruption due to echovirus 6. Am J Dis Child. 1979;133:283–4.
101. Frothingham TE. ECHO virus type 9 associated with three cases simulating meningococcemia. N Engl J Med. 1958;259:484.
102. Cherry JD, Jahn CL. Virologic studies of exanthems. J Pediatr. 1966;68:204.
103. James WD, Odom RB, Hatch MH. Gianotti-Crosti-like eruption associated with coxsackievirus A16 infection. J Am Acad Dermatol. 1982;6:862.
104. Johnson KM, Bloom HH, Forsyth B, et al. The role of enteroviruses in respiratory disease. Am Rev Resp Dis. 1963;88:240.
105. Jackson GG, Muidoon RL. Viruses causing common respiratory infections in man: II. Enteroviruses and paramyxoviruses. J Infect Dis. 1973;128:387.
106. Couch RB, Cate TR, Gerone PJ, et al. Production of illness with a small particle aerosol of coxsackie A-21. J Clin Invest. 1965;44:535.
107. Eckert HL, Portnoy B, Salvatore MA, et al. Group B coxsackie virus infection in infants with acute lower respiratory disease. Pediatrics. 1967;39:526.
108. Flewett TH. Histological study of two cases of coxsackie B virus pneumonia in children. J Clin Pathol. 1965;18:743.
109. Jahn CL, Felton OL, Cherry JD. Coxsackie B1 pneumonia in an adult. JAMA. 1964;189:236.
110. Cherry JD, Jahn CL: Herpangina. The etiologic spectrum. Pediatrics. 1965;36:632.
111. Steigman AJ, Lipton MM, Braspennickx H. Acute lymphonodular pharyngitis: A newly described condition due to coxsackie A virus. J Pediatr. 1962;61:331.
112. Sylvest E. Epidemic Myalgia: Bornholm Disease. London: Oxford University Press; 1934:1–155.
113. Curnen EC, Shaw EW, Melnick JL. Disease resembling nonparalytic poliomyelitis associated with virus pathogenic for infant mice. JAMA. 1949;141:894.
114. Weller TH, Enders JF, Buckingham M, et al. Etiology of epidemic pleurodynia: Study of two viruses isolated from typical outbreak. J Immunol. 1950;65:337.
115. Bell EJ, Grist NR. ECHO viruses, carditis, and acute pleurodynia. Am Heart J. 1971;82:133.
116. Madhaven HN, Bedninath S, Chanraseker S. A case of pleurodynia associated with coxsackie virus type A9. J Assoc Physicians India. 1977;25:491.
117. Disney ME, Howard EM, Wood BSB. Bornholm disease in children. Br Med J. 1953;1:1351.
118. Bain HW, McLean DM, Walker SJ: Epidemic pleurodynia (Bornholm disease) due to coxsackie B-5 virus: The interrelationship of pleurodynia, benign pericarditis, and aseptic meningitis. Pediatrics. 1961;27:889.
119. Warin JF, Davies JBM, Sanders FK, et al. Oxford epidemic of Bornholm disease, 1951. Br Med J. 1953;1:1345.
120. Gordon RB, Lennette EH, Sandrock RS. The varied clinical manifestations of coxsackie virus infections. AMA Arch Intern Med. 1959;103:63.
121. Smith WG. Adult heart disease due to the coxsackie virus group B. Br Heart J. 1966;28:204.
122. Lerner AM, Wilson FM: Virus myocardiopathy. Progr Med Virol. 1973;15:63.
123. Woodruff JF. Viral myocarditis. Am J Pathol. 1980;101:427.
124. Grist NR, Bell EJ. Coxsackieviruses and the heart. Am Heart J. 1969;77:295.
125. Meehan WF, Bertrand CA. Ventricular tachycardia associated with echovirus infection. JAMA. 1970;212:1701.
126. Russell SJM, Bell EJ. Echoviruses and carditis. Lancet. 1970;1:784.
127. Kanra G, Dogruel N, Tinaztepe K, et al. Myocarditis caused by echovirus 11 virus. Turk J Pediatr. 1978;20:24.
128. Schleissner LA, Fiala M, Imagawa DT, et al. Application of systolic time intervals to acute cardiomyopathy with echovirus 2. Chest. 1976;69:563.
129. Grist NR, Bell EJ. Coxsackie virus and heart diseases. Br Med J. 1968;3:556.
130. Grist NR, Bell EJ, Assaad F. Enteroviruses in human disease. Progr Med Virol. 1978;24:114.
131. Lewes D, Rainford DJ, Lane WF. Symptomless myocarditis and myalgia in viral and *Mycoplasma pneumoniae* infections. Br Heart J. 1974;36:924.
132. Van Loon GR, Masson AM. Viral pericarditis: A report of five cases. Can Med Assoc J. 1968;99:163.
133. Berkovich S, Rodriguez-Torres R, Lin J-S. Virologic studies in children with acute myocarditis. Am J Dis Child. 1968;115:207.
134. Bell EJ, Grist NR. Echoviruses, carditis and acute pleurodynia. Lancet. 1970;1:326.
135. Johnson RT, Portnoy B, Rogers NG, et al. Acute benign pericarditis: Virologic study of 34 patients. Arch Intern Med. 1961;108:823.
136. Sainani GS, Krompotic E, Slodki SJ. Adult heart disease due to the coxsackie virus B infection. Medicine. 1968;47:133.
137. Koontz CH, Ray CG. The role of coxsackie group B virus infections in sporadic myopericarditis. Am Heart J. 1971;82:750.
138. Grist NR, Bell EJ. A six-year study of coxsackievirus B infections in heart disease. J Hyg (Camb). 1974;73:165.
139. Ayuthya PSN, Jayavasu JJ, Pongpanich B. Coxsackie group B virus and primary myocardial disease in infants and children. Am Heart J. 1974;88:311.
140. Grist NR. Coxsackie virus infections of the heart. In: Waterson AP, ed. Recent Advances in Clinical Virology. no. 1. Edinburgh: Churchill Livingstone; 1977:141.
141. Helin M, Savola J, Lapinleimu K. Cardiac manifestations during a coxsackie B5 epidemic. Br Med J 1968;2:97.
142. Lau RC. Coxsackie B virus infections in New Zealand patients with cardiac and non-cardiac diseases. J Med Virol. 1983;11:131–7.
143. Johnson RT, Portnoy B, Rogers NG, et al. Acute benign pericarditis: Virologic study of 34 patients. Arch Intern Med. 1961;108:823.
144. Sainani GS, Dekate MP, Rao CP. Heart disease caused by coxsackievirus B infection. Be Heart J. 1975;37:819.
145. Smith WG. Coxsackie B myopericarditis in adults. Am Heart J. 1970;80:34.
146. Gibbons JE, Goldbloom RB, Dobell ARC. Rapidly developing pericardial constriction in childhood following acute nonspecific pericarditis. Am J Cardiol. 1965;15:863.
147. Howard EJ, Maier HC. Constrictive pericarditis following acute coxsackie viral pericarditis. Am Heart J. 1968;75:247.
148. Matthews JD, Cameron SJ, George M. Constrictive pericarditis following coxsackie virus infection. Thorax. 1970;25:624.
149. Hildebrandt HM, Massab HF, Willis PW. Influenza virus pericarditis. Am J Dis Child. 1962;104:579.
150. Fatal mumps myocarditis in England. MMWR. 1980;27:425.
151. Caldera R, Sarrut S, Mallet R, et al. Existe-t-il des complications cardiaques de la vaccine? Sem Hop Paris. 1961;37:1281.
152. Desaneto A, Bullington JD, Bullington RH, et al. Coxsackie B5 heart disease. Demonstration of inferolateral wall myocardial necrosis. Am J Med. 1980;68:295.
153. Woods JD, Nimmo MJ, MacKay-Scollay EM. Acute transmural myocardial infarction associated with active coxsackie virus B infection. Am Heart J. 1975;89:283.
154. Griffiths PD, Hannington G, Booth JC. Coxsackie B virus infection and myocardial infarction. Lancet. 1980;1:1387.
155. Lau RC. Coxsackie B virus-specific IgM responses in coronary care unit patients. J Med Virol. 1986;18:193–8.
156. Hannington G, Booth JC, Bowes RJ, et al. Coxsackie B virus-specific IgM antibody and myocardial infarction. J Med Microbiol. 1986;21:287–91.
157. Sutton GC, Tobin JR, Fox RT, et al. Study of the pericardium and ventricular myocardium: Exploratory mediastinoscopy and biopsy in unexplained heart disease. JAMA. 185:786, 1963.
158. Sutton GC, Harding HB, Truehart RP, et al. Coxsackie B4 myocarditis in an adult: Successful isolation of virus from ventricular myocardium. Aerospace Med. 1967;38:66.
159. Modlin JF. Perinatal echovirus infection: Insights from a literature review of 61 cases of serious infection and 16 outbreaks in nurseries. Rev Infect Dis. 1986;8:918–26.
160. Spector SA, Straube RC. Protean manifestations of perinatal enterovirus infections. West J Med. 1983;138:847–51.
161. Georgieff MK, Johnson DE, Thompson TR, et al. Fulminant hepatic necrosis in an infant with perinatally acquired echovirus 21 infection. Pediatr Infect Dis J. 1987;6:71–3.
162. Speer ME, Yawn DH. Fatal hepatoadrenal necrosis in the neonate associated with echovirus types 11 and 12 presenting as a surgical emergency. J Pediatr Surg. 1984;19:591–3.
163. Wreghitt TG, Gandy GM, King A, et al. Fatal neonatal echo 7 virus infection (Letter). Lancet. 1984;2:465.
164. Wright HT, Landing BH, Lennette EH, et al. Fatal infection in an infant associated with coxsackie virus group A, type 16. N Engl J Med. 1963;268:1041.
165. Talsma M, Vegting M, Hess J. Generalized Coxsackie A9 infection in a neonate presenting with pericarditis. Br Heart J. 1984;52:683–5.
166. Baker DA, Phillips CA. Maternal and neonatal infection with coxsackievirus. Obstet Gynecol. 1980;55:12S–15S.
167. Gear JHS, Measroch V. Coxsackievirus infections of the newborn. Progr Med Virol. 1973;15:42.
168. Kinney JS, McCray E, Kaplan JE, et al. Risk factors associated with echovirus 11 infection in a newborn nursery. Pediatr Infect Dis J. 1986;5:192–7.
169. Modlin JF. Fatal echovirus 11 disease in premature neonates. Pediatrics. 1980;6:775.
170. Piraino FF, Sedmak G, Raab K. Echovirus 11 infections of newborns with mortality during the 1979 enterovirus season in Milwaukee, Wis. Public Health Rep. 1982;97:346.
171. Kaplan MH, Klein SW, McPhee J, et al. Group B coxsackie-virus infections in infants younger than three months of age: A serious childhood illness. Rev Infect Dis. 1983;5:1019–32.
172. Halfon N, Spector SA. Final echovirus type 11 infections. Am J Dis Child. 1981;135:1017.
173. Drew JH. Echo 11 virus outbreak in a nursery associated with myocarditis. Aust J Pediatr. 1973;9:90.
174. Jones MJU, Kolb M, Votava HJ, et al. Intrauterine echovirus type 11 infection. Mayo Clin Proc. 1980;55:509.
175. Gillam GL, Stokes KB, McLellan J, et al. Fulminant hepatic failure with

intractable ascites due to an echovirus 11 infection successfully managed with a peritoneo-venous (LeVeen) shunt. J Pediatr Gastroenterol Nutr. 1986;5:476–80.
176. Manning D, Gorman WA, Hillary IB. Neonatal echovirus type 17 infection in twins. Ir J Med Sci. 1983;152:316–7.
177. Boyd MT, Jordan SW, Davis LE. Fatal pneumonitis from congenital echovirus type 6 infection. Pediatr Infect Dis J. 1987;6:1138–9.
178. Cheeseman SH, Hirsch MS, Keller EW, et al. Fatal neonatal pneumonia caused by echovirus type 9 (Letter). Am J Dis Child. 1977;131:1169.
179. Toce SS, Keenan WJ. Congenital echovirus 11 pneumonia in association with pulmonary hypertension. Pediatr Infect Dis J. 1988;7:360–2.
180. Modlin JF, Kinney JS. Perinatal Enterovirus Infections. In: Aronoff SC, Hughes WT, Kohl S, et al. eds. Advances in Pediatric Infectious Diseases. v. 2. Chicago: Year Book Medical; 1987.
181. Lake AM, Lauer BA, Clark JC, et al. Enterovirus infections in neonates. J Pediatr. 1976;89:787–91.
182. Modlin JF, Bowman M. Perinatal transmission of coxsackie B3 virus in a murine model. J Infect Dis. 1987;156:21–5.
183. Abzug MJ, Rotbart HA, Levin MJ. The placental barrier to fetal enterovirus infection: Characterization by *in situ* hybridization. Presented to the Society for Pediatric Research, Washington, D.C., May 1988.
184. Cherry JD, Soriano F, Jahn CL. Search for perinatal virus infection. Am J Dis Child. 1968;116:245–50.
185. Modlin JF, Polk BF, Horton P, et al. Perinatal echovirus infection: Risk of transmission during a community outbreak. N Engl J Med. 1981;305:368.
186. Reyes MP, Ostrea EM, Roskamp J, et al. Disseminated neonatal echovirus 11 disease following antenatal maternal infection with a virus-positive cervix and virus negative gastrointestinal tract. J Med Virol. 1983;12:155–9.
187. Yoshioka I, Horstmann DM. Viremic infection due to echovirus type 9. N Engl J Med. 1960;262:224–8.
188. Kunin CM. Virus–tissue union and the pathogenesis of enterovirus infections. J Immunol. 1962;88:556.
189. Eichenwald HF, Kotsevalov O. Immunologic responses of premature and full-term infants to infection with certain viruses. Pediatrics. 1960;25:829.
190. Rager-Zisman B, Allison AC. The role of antibody and host cells in the resistance of mice against infection by coxsackie B-3 virus. J Gen Virol. 1973;19:329.
191. Woodruff JF. Lack of correlation between neutralizing antibody production and suppression of coxsackievirus B-3 replication in target organs: Evidence for involvement of mononuclear inflammatory cells in host defense. J Immunol. 1979;123:31.
192. Berry PJ, Nagington J. Fatal infection with echovirus 11. Arch Dis Child. 1982;57:22.
193. McKinney RE, Katz SL, Wilfert CM. Chronic enteroviral meningoencephalitis in agammaglobulinemic patients. Rev Infect Dis. 1987;9:334–56.
194. O'Neil KM, Pallansch MA, Winkelstein JA, et al. Chronic group A coxsackievirus infection in agammaglobulinemia: Demonstration of genomic variation or serotypically identical isolates persistently excreted from the same patient. J Infect Dis. 1988;157:183–6.
195. Webster ADB. Echovirus disease in hypogammaglobulinaemic patients. Clin Rheum Dis. 1984;10:189–203.
196. Mease PJ, Ochs HD, Wedgwood RJ. Successful treatment of echovirus meningoencephalitis and muositis-fasciitis with intravenous immune globulin therapy in a patient with X-linked agammaglobulinemia. N Engl J Med. 1981;304:1278.
197. Ziegler JB, Penny R. Fatal echo 30 virus infection and amyloidosis in X-linked hypogammaglobulinemia. Clin Immunol Immunopathol. 1975;3:347.
198. Townsend TR, Bolyard EA, Yolken RH, et al. Outbreak of coxsackie A1 gastroenteritis: A complication of bone-marrow transplantation. Lancet. 1982;1:820.
199. Kono R. Apollo 11 disease or acute hemorrhagic conjunctivitis: A pandemic of a new enterovirus infection of the eyes. Am J Epidemiol. 1975;101:383.
200. Kono R, Sasagawa A, Ishii K, et al. Pandemic of new type of conjunctivitis. Lancet. 1972;2:1191.
201. Mirkovic RR, Kono R, Yin-Murphy M, et al. Enterovirus type 70: The etiologic agent of pandemic acute hemorrhagic conjunctivitis. Bull WHO. 1973;49:341.
202. Yin-Murphy M, Lim KH. Picornavirus epidemic conjunctivitis in Singapore. Lancet. 1972;2:857.
203. Mirkovic RR, Schmidt NJ, Yin-Murphy M, et al. Enterovirus etiology of the 1970 Singapore epidemic of acute conjunctivitis. Intervirology. 1974;4:119.
204. Yin-Murphy M, Lim KH, Yo YM. A coxsackievirus type A24 epidemic of acute conjunctivitis. Southeast Asian J Trop Med Public Health. 1976;7:1.
205. Higgins PG, Scott RJ, Davies PM, et al. A comparative study of viruses associated with acute hemorrhagic conjunctivitis. J Clin Pathol. 1974;27:292.
206. Christopher S, Theogaraj S, Godbole S, et al. An epidemic of acute hemorrhagic conjunctivitis due to coxsackievirus A24. J Infect Dis. 1982;146:16–9.
207. Ray I, Roy IS, Sarkhar JK, et al. Laboratory investigations of an epidemic of conjunctivitis in Calcutta: A preliminary report. Bull Calcutta Sch Trop Med. 1972;20:1.
208. Kono R, Miyamura K, Tajiri E, et al. Neurologic complications associated with acute hemorrhagic conjunctivitis virus infection and its serologic confirmation. J Infect Dis. 1974;129:590.
209. Sklar VE, Patriarca PA, Onorato IM, et al. Clinical findings and results of treatment in an outbreak of acute hemorrhagic conjunctivitis in southern Florida. Am J Ophthalmol. 1983;95:45.
210. Kuritsky JN, Weaver JH, Bernard KW, et al. An outbreak of acute hemorrhagic conjunctivitis in central Minnesota. Am J Ophthalmol. 1983;96:449–52.
211. Centers For Disease Control. Acute hemorrhagic conjunctivitis caused by coxsackievirus A24—Caribbean. MMWR. 1987;36:245–51.
212. Centers For Disease Control. Acute hemorrhagic conjunctivitis caused by coxsackie A24 variant—Puerto Rico. MMWR. 1988;37:123–4.
213. Hierholzer JC, Hilliard KA, Esposito JJ. Serosurvey for "acute hemorrhagic conjunctivitis" virus (enterovirus 70) antibodies in the southeastern United States, with review of the literature and some epidemiologic implications. Am J Epidemiol. 1975;102:533.
214. Miyamua K, Yamazaki S, Tajiri E, et al. Growth characteristics of acute hemorrhagic conjunctivitis (AHC) virus in monkey kidney cells. Intervirology. 1974;4:279.
215. Stanton GJ, Langford MP, Baron S. Effect of interferon, elevated temperature, and cell type on replication of acute hemorrhagic conjunctivitis viruses. Infect Immun. 1977;18:370.
216. Goh KT, Doraisingham S, Yin-Murphy M: An epidemic of acute conjunctivitis caused by enterovirus-70 in Singapore in 1980. Southeast Asian J Trop Med Public Health. 1981;12:473
217. Arnow PM, Hierholzer JC, Higbee J, et al. Acute hemorrhagic conjunctivitis: A mixed virus outbreak among Vietnamese refugees on Guam. Am J Epidemiol. 1977;105:68.
218. Onorato IM, Morens DM, Schonberger LB, et al. Acute hemorrhagic conjunctivitis caused by enterovirus type 70: An epidemic in American Samoa. Am J Trop Med Hyg. 1985;34:984–91.
219. Kono R, Sasagawa A, Miyamura K, et al. Serologic characterization and seroepidemiologic studies on acute hemorrhagic conjunctivitis (AHC) virus. Am J Epidemiol. 1975;101:444.
220. Kono R, Uchida Y. Acute hemorrhagic conjunctivitis. Ophthalmol Dig. 1977;39:14.
221. Kono R, Sasagawa A, Yamazaki S. Seroepidemiologic studies of acute hemorrhagic conjunctivitis virus (enterovirus type 70) in West Africa: III. Studies with animal sera from Ghana and Senegal. Am J Epidemiol. 1981;114:362.
222. Hung TS, Sung SM, Liang HC, et al. Radiculomyelitis following acute hemorrhagic conjunctivitis. Brain. 1976;99:771.
223. Kono R, Miyamura K, Tajiri E, et al. Virological and serological studies of neurological complications of acute hemorrhagic conjunctivitis in Thailand. J Infect Dis. 1977;135:706.
224. Wadia NH, Katrak SM, Misra VP, et al. Polio-like motor paralysis associated with acute hemorrhagic conjunctivitis in an outbreak in 1981 in Bombay, India: Clinical and serologic studies. J Infect Dis. 1983;147:660.
225. Katiyar BC, Misra S, Singh RB, et al. Adult polio-like syndrome following Enterovirus 70 conjunctivitis (natural history of the disease). Acta Neurol Scand. 1983;67:263–74.
226. Kono R, Uchida N, Sasagawa A, et al. Neurovirulence of acute-hemorrhagic-conjunctivitis virus in monkeys. Lancet. 1973;1:61.
227. Yin-Murphy M. Simple tests for the diagnosis of picornavirus epidemic conjunctivitis (acute haemorrhagic conjunctivitis). Bull WHO. 1976;54:675.
228. Hashimoto I, Hagiwara A, Kodama H. Neurovirulence in cynomolgus monkeys of enterovirus 71 isolated from a patient with hand, foot and mouth disease. Arch Virol. 1978;56:257.
229. Hashimoto I, Hagiwara A. Pathogenicity of a poliomyelitis-like disease in monkeys infected orally with enterovirus 71. Neuropathol Appl Neurobiol. 1982;8:149.
230. Hagiwara A, Yoneyama T, Takami S, et al. Genetic and phenotypic characteristics of enterovirus 71 isolates from patients with encephalitis and with hand, foot and mouth disease. Arch Virol. 1984;79:273–83.
231. Melnick JL, Schmidt NJ, Minkovic RR, et al. Identification of Bulgarian strain 258 of enterovirus 71. Intervirology. 1980;12:297.
232. Deibel R, Gross LL, Collins DN. Isolation of a new enterovirus. Proc Soc Exp Biol Med. 1975;148:203.
233. Sohier R. Enterovirus type 71 surveillance: France. WHO Wkly Epidemiol Rec. 1979;54:219.
234. Moses EB, Narian JP, Hatch MH, et al. Isolation of echovirus type 11 and enterovirus type 71 in a day care winter outbreak. J Arkansas Med Soc. 1987;83:469–71.
235. Nagy G, Takatsy S, Kukan E, et al. Virological diagnosis of enterovirus type 71 infections: Experiences gained during an epidemic of acute CNS diseases in Hungary in 1978. Arch Virol. 1982;71:217.
236. Hansson O, Kristensson K, Lycke E, et al. Generalized myopathy and cerebral malformations possibly related to an enteroviral infection. Acta Paediatr Scand. 1975;64:881.
237. Ramos-Alvarez M, Olarte J. Diarrheal diseases of children. Am J Dis Child. 1964;107:218.
238. Yow DM, Melnick JL, Blattner JR, et al. Enteroviruses in infantile diarrhea. Am J Hyg. 1963;77:283.
239. Steinhoff MC. Viruses and diarrhea—a review. Am J Dis Child. 1978;132:302.
240. Patel JR, Daniel J, Mathan VI. An epidemic of acute diarrhoea in rural southern India associated with echovirus type 11 infection. J Hyg (Lond). 1985;95:483–92.
241. Glasgow LA, Balduzzi P. Isolation of coxsackie virus group A, type 4, from a patient with hemolytic-uremic syndrome. N Engl J Med. 1965;273:754.

242. Ray CG, Tucker VL, Harris DJ, et al. Enteroviruses associated with the hemolytic–uremic syndrome. Pediatrics. 1970;46:378.
243. Oregan S, Robitaille P, Mongeau JG, et al. The hemolytic–uremic syndrome associated with echo 22 infection. Clin Pediatr. 1980;19:125.
244. Aronson MD, Phillips CA. Coxsackievirus B5 infections in acute oliguric renal failure. J Infect Dis. 1975;132:303.
245. Fukuyama Y, Ando T, Yokota J. Acute fulminant myoglobinuric polymyositis with picornavirus-like crystals. J Neurol Neurosurg Psychiatr. 1977;40:775.
246. Gyorkey F, Cabral GA, Gorkey PK, et al. Coxsackievirus aggregates in muscle cells of polymyositis patient. Intervirology. 1978;10:69.
247. Schiraldi O, Iandolo E. Polymyositis accompanying coxsackie virus B2 infection. Infection. 1978;6:32.
248. De Renck J, De Coster W, Inderadjaja N. Acute viral polymyositis with predominant diaphragm involvement. J Neurol Sci. 1977;33:453.
249. Josselson J, Pula T, Sadler JH. Acute rhabdomylysis associated with echovirus 9 infection. Arch Intern Med. 1980;140:1671.
250. Jehn UW, Fink MK. Myositis, myoglobinemia, and myoglobinuria associated with enterovirus echo 9 infection. Arch Neurol. 1980;33:457.
251. Bowles NE, Dubowitz V, Sewry CA, et al. Dermatomyositis, polymyositis, and coxsackie-B-virus infection. Lancet. 1987;1:1004–7.
252. Kuroda Y, Neshige R, Oda K, et al. Chronic polymyositis: Presence of coxsackievirus A9 antigen in muscle. Jpn J Med. 1986;25:191–4.
253. Burch GE, DePasquale NP. Viral endocarditis. Am Heart J. 1964;67:721.
254. Burch GE, DePasquale NP, Sun SC, et al. Experimental coxsackievirus endocarditis. JAMA. 1966;196:349.
255. Burch GE, Harb JM, Hiramoto Y, et al. Viral infection of the aorta of man associated with early atherosclerotic changes. Am Heart J. 1973;86:523.
256. O'Shaughnessey WJ, Buechner HA. Hepatitis associated with a coxsackie B5 virus infection during late pregnancy. JAMA. 1962;179:71.
257. Morris JA, Elisberg BL, Pond WL, et al. Hepatitis associated with coxsackie virus group A, type 4, N Engl J Med. 1962;267:1230.
258. Sun NC, Smith VM. Hepatitis associated with myocarditis: Unusual manifestation of infection with coxsackie virus group B, type 3. N Engl J Med. 1966;274:190.
259. Leggiadro RJ, Chwatsky DN, Zucker SW. Echovirus 3 infection associated with anicteric hepatitis. Am J Dis Child. 1982;136:744.
260. Gregor GR, Geller SA, Walker GF, et al. Coxsackie hepatitis in an adult with ultrastructural demonstration of the virus. Mt Sinai J Med. 1975;42:575.
261. Lansky LL, Krugman S, Huq G. Anicteric coxsackie B hepatitis. J Pediatr. 1979;94:64.
262. Ursing B. Acute pancreatitis in coxsackie B infection. Br Med J. 1973;3:524.
263. Craighead JE. The role of viruses in the pathogenesis of pancreatic disease and diabetes mellitus. Progr Med Virol. 1975;19:162.
264. Arnesjo B, Eden T, Ihse I, et al. Enterovirus infections in acute pancreatitis—a possible etiologic connection. Scand J Gastroenterol. 1976;11:645.
265. Imrle CW, Ferguson JC, Sommerville RG. Coxsackie and mumps virus infection in a prospective study of acute pancreatitis. Gut. 1977;18:53.
266. Notkins AL: Virus-induced diabetes mellitus. Arch Virol. 1977;54:1.
267. Yoon JW, Austin M, Onodera T, et al. Isolation of a virus from the pancreas of a child with diabetic ketoacidosis. N Engl J Med. 1979;300:1173–9.
268. Barrett-Connor E. Is insulin-dependent diabetes mellitus caused by coxsackievirus B infection? A review of the epidemiologic evidence. Rev Infect Dis. 1985;7:207–15.
269. Blotzer JW, Myers AR. Echovirus associated polyarthritis. Report of a case with synovial fluid and synovial histologic characterization. Arthritis Rheum. 1978;21:978.
270. Kujala G, Newman JH. Isolation of echovirus type 11 from synovial fluid in acute monocytic arthritis. Arthritis Rheum. 1985;28:98–9.
271. Van der Sar A. Acute infectious lymphocytosis with echovirus type 25. West Indian Med J. 1979;28:185.
272. Norwitz MS, Moore GT. Acute infectious lymphocytosis: An etiologic study of an outbreak. N Engl J Med. 1968;279:399.

151. HEPATITIS A VIRUS

F. BLAINE HOLLINGER
ALAN PAUL GLOMBICKI

HISTORY

Early accounts of contagious jaundice were recorded by the Chinese several millennia ago (reviewed by Zuckerman[1]). In the past four hundred years, increasingly frequent reports of icterus, affecting both military and civilian populations, were recorded in wartime chronicles as *campaign jaundice*. The disease complex included acute onset of malaise, transient fever, myalgia, nausea, anorexia, abdominal pain, and darkening of the urine. After the discovery of leptospira by Weil[2] in 1886, the term *infectious jaundice* was reserved for this disease, with the milder, more transmissible form of icterus thereafter labeled *epidemic catarrhal jaundice*. Subsequent epidemiologic investigations by Cockayne[3] in 1912 distinguished another entity, *acute yellow atrophy*, from epidemic catarrhal jaundice. Acute yellow atrophy was more fulminant and had a relatively high mortality rate in pregnant women. It is postulated[4] that this form of hepatitis, which was recorded in greater frequency in Southern Europe and the Mediterranean, may have been caused by enterically transmitted non-A, non-B hepatitis, a recently discovered disease. Conversely, the milder epidemic or endemic form of hepatitis that was more common in Northern Europe, Greenland, and North America probably resulted from infection with hepatitis A virus.

In 1923, Blumer[5] reviewed 63 epidemics of hepatitis that occurred in the United States over 110 years and identified several key epidemiologic features of a form of viral hepatitis now known as viral hepatitis type A. The peak incidence of this disease occurred in the fall and winter among young adults and children, and the infection appeared to be transmitted largely by person-to-person contact after a brief period of exposure to a jaundiced patient. By the 1940s, hepatitis agents were shown to have a size consistent with that of viruses.[6,7]

During the ensuing three decades, the existence of at least two agents associated with the viral hepatitis syndrome was appreciated from studies of natural infections and experimental transmission studies in human volunteers.[8,9] These agents, designated infectious hepatitis, or hepatitis A virus (HAV), and serum hepatitis, or hepatitis B virus (HBV), could be distinguished by differences in incubation period,[7,9–18] antigenic differences demonstrated in cross-protection transmission studies,[7,9,11,19,20] the regular presence of HAV and never HBV in feces of infected patients,[7,11,21,22] and the chronic carriage of HBV and never HAV in the blood.[23,24] Fecal–oral or contact transmission was associated with the sporadic and epidemic patterns of HAV infection, and HBV appeared to be primarily transmitted percutaneously by blood and blood products resulting in different epidemiologic features.

The reports by Deinhardt et al.,[25–27] starting in 1967, of successful infection of marmosets with HAV, and the detection of hepatitis A virions by immune electron microscopy in the feces of patients infected with HAV by Feinstone et al.[28] in 1973 ultimately led to the development of methods for detecting infectious virus, viral antigen, and viral antibody, and for diagnosing HAV infections. Infection of chimpanzees with HAV was documented in 1975.[29,30] This was followed by the successful propagation of marmoset-adapted HAV in primary explant cultures of marmoset liver and in a fetal rhesus monkey kidney cell line by Provost and Hilleman in 1979.[31] These developments led to further characterization of the agent and to a more complete understanding of the epidemiology and course of HAV infection.

HAV infection is common throughout the United States and the rest of the world. Infection is usually subclinical in children, but in adults it may be associated with acute hepatitis, which may vary in severity from a mild illness to severe and rarely fulminant hepatitis. HAV does not cause persistent infection or chronic liver disease. Although HAV has some distinguishing epidemiologic features, hepatitis A in individual cases usually cannot be distinguished from acute hepatitis caused by other viruses on clinical grounds alone.

THE ETIOLOGIC AGENT OF HEPATITIS A

Almost 40 years ago the agent causing infectious hepatitis in human volunteers was shown to pass through a Seitz filter, which retains bacteria,[6,7] indicating that the agent has a size smaller than that of bacteria. In 1973 Feinstone and colleagues[28] described virus-like particles in the feces of patients experimentally infected with HAV. The particles were immunoprecipitated by serum from patients in the convalescent phase but not the preillness phase of infection, a result considered to indicate the appearance of antibody directed against these particles during the illness. Similar particles were observed during natural infections, and their presence in feces was temporally associated with the illness.

Biophysical Properties

Both full and empty particles have been observed. The virions are nonenveloped (naked), spherical, and 27 to 32 nm in diameter; fine structural analysis has demonstrated icosahedral symmetry[28,32] (Fig. 1). Similar particles also have been found in liver extracts, bile, and serum of HAV infected *Saguinus mystax*.[33] Full particles of HAV purified from infected human[31,35] and chimpanzee[36,37] feces and from marmoset liver[33] have a primary buoyant density in CsCl of 1.32 to 1.34 g/cm^3 and a sedimentation coefficient of 156 to 160S in neutral sucrose solutions.[33–42] Empty particles appear at a density of 1.29–1.31 g/cm^3 with sedimentation coefficients from 50 to 90S.[35–37,43,44] These are usually detected in fecal extracts during the early stages of infection[35,37,39,43–45] but are also observed as a minor population in cell culture.[41] They are believed to represent premature, defective virions. Another less well-defined "heavy" population of HAV is found in feces at buoyant densities of 1.40 to 1.48 g/cm^3.[34,35,38,39,44] Their density is believed to result from the penetration and binding of cesium to the viral capsid. The size and appearance of the particles in electronmicrographs and the multiple buoyant densities and sedimentation coefficients are similar to those of other picornaviruses. The complete virions and the alternative forms display the same major surface antigens.[46]

Biochemical Characteristics

HAV has a linear, single-stranded RNA genome of 7.48 kb in length, a low content of guanidine + cytosine (38% G + C), and a capsid containing redundant copies of three or four proteins.[33,38,40,42,47–51] Analysis of iodinated HAV genomic material[49] has demonstrated that HAV RNA sediments at 33S with a buoyant density of 1.64 g/cm^3 and a molecular weight of 2.25×10^6. The HAV genome has a poly(A) sequence[42,49] localized to the 3′ terminus of the RNA strand[52] suggesting that HAV is a positive-stranded virus (i.e., virions contain the messenger RNA strand) that follows the same translation strategy as the monocistronic genome of other picornaviruses. Cells can be infected with RNA isolated from intact HAV[49,53] or with RNA transcribed from cloned HAV cDNA,[54,55] and HAV RNA has been translated in vitro.[56]

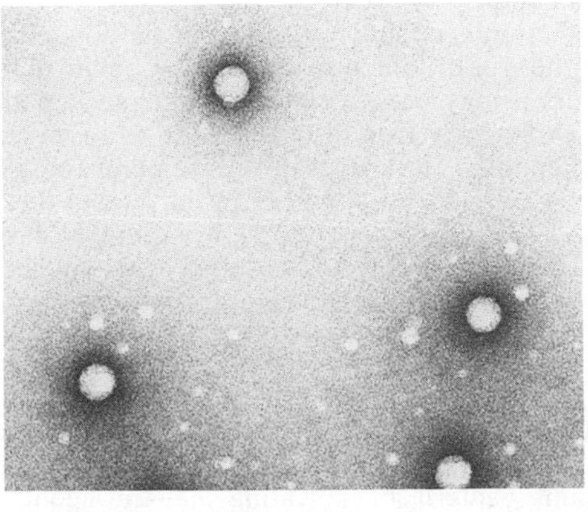

FIG. 1. Electron micrograph of HAV particles highly purified from human feces.

Some molecular similarities of HAV to other picornaviruses include the existence of a 22S double-stranded RNA replicative intermediate and a genome that can be divided in three parts: (*1*) a 5′ noncoding segment, (*2*) a single open reading frame that encodes all of the viral proteins, and (*3*) a short 3′ noncoding region. Sequences from human HAV strains collected from various geographic regions of the world exhibit remarkable conservation (~90 percent sequence homology).[57–61]

Polyacrylamide gel electrophoresis has been used to identify the three major HAV capsid proteins: VP1 (or 1D, the major surface protein: 30,000–33,000 kDa), VP2 (or 1B: 24,000–25,000 kDa), and VP3 (or 1C: 21,000–27,000 kDa).[42,45,47,50,62–65] A fourth protein (VP4 or 1A) has not been conclusively documented. However, VPO, a presumptive uncleaved precursor of VP2 and VP4,[66] has been detected[42,62,65,67] as has an additional structural protein, VPg, which is linked to the 5′ terminus of the genome.[68] Resistance of HAV to incubation at 60°C and to disoxaril suggests that the HAV capsids are structurally dissimilar to other picornaviruses.[69–71]

Antigenic Composition

A single HAV serotype has been detected among human strains isolated in different parts of the world.[72–75] Global protection of individuals by immune globulin prepared in different parts of the world[76,77] supports the concept that HAV is antigenically similar throughout the world. Reactivity of virus isolates to monoclonal antibodies also is similar.[73,78] In addition, nucleotide and amino acid sequences of these strains are highly conserved (>90 percent and >98 percent identity, respectively.[79] Isolated HAV proteins are immunologically distinct from antigens associated with the intact viral particles, presumably on the basis of tertiary structure. Monoclonal antibodies against HAV have detected several epitopes on intact virions, but do not bind to isolated capsid proteins.[80] No nucleotide similarity or serologic cross-reactivity has been observed between HAV and other agents causing viral hepatitis including the virus of enterically transmitted non-A, non-B hepatitis.[81]

Stability of Virus to Physical and Chemical Treatments

Assessment of the stability of HAV after exposure to a myriad of physicochemical conditions has been facilitated by reproducible assays such as the radioimmunofocus assay[82] and the in situ radioimmunoassay.[83] HAV is stable at pH 3.0 for 3 hours at 25°C and resists organic solvents such as ether, chloroform, dichlorodifluoromethane (Freon), and trichlorotrifluoroethane (Arklone, Genetron).[6,33,84] Thus, lipid is not an essential component of the virion.

HAV is relatively resistant to heat especially when compared with other picornaviruses.[85] The virus has survived 60°C for 1 hour[86] and was only partially inactivated after 10 to 12 hours.[85,87] Drying and storage of HAV at 25°C and 42 percent humidity fails to inactive the virus for a minimum of 1 month,[88] while survival is effectively maintained for years at −20°C. Experimentally contaminated freshwater, seawater, wastewater, soils, marine sediment, live oysters, creme-filled cookies, and dried feces on polystyrene surfaces have been demonstrated to harbor infective organisms for days to months.[89] Conversely, HAV infectivity for human volunteers is destroyed at 98 to 100°C for 1 minute.[33,90] HAV also is inactivated by autoclaving (121°C for 20 minutes), by ultraviolet irradiation (1.1 watts at a depth of 0.9 cm for 1 minute or 197 μW/cm^2 for 4 minutes), by formalin (1:4000 for 72 hours at 37°C, or 3% for 5 minutes and 8% for 1 minute at 25°C), by iodine (3 mg/L for 5 minutes), and by β-propiolactone (0.03% for 72 hours at 4°C). Although recent data suggest that HAV may be more resistant to chlorination than other picornaviruses,[91] the virus will be completely inactivated by 10 to 15 ppm residual chlorine concentration after 30 minutes, a free residual chlorine concentration of 2.0 to 2.5 mg/L for 15 minutes, or contact with sodium hypochlorite, 3 to 10 mg/L at 20°C for 5 to 15 minutes providing the organic content of the solution to be decontaminated is not excessive.[32,33,91–93] Exposure to 70% ethanol at 25°C for 3 minutes or 60 minutes will reduce infectivity 2.25 logs and 5.5 logs, respectively.[50] Chemicals that interfere with HAV replication include ribavirin, amantadine, and 2-deoxy-D-glucose.[94,95]

Host Range

HAV, like HBV, has a very restricted host range. In 1961, Hillis,[96,97] and subsequently others,[98] described the occurrence of a hepatitis A-like illness in animal caretakers after close exposure to chimpanzees. In subsequent investigations, HAV was shown to experimentally infect several species of *Saguinus* South American marmoset (tamarin) monkeys,[25–27,99–103] chimpanzees (*Pan troglodytes*),[29,30,104] owl monkeys (*Aotus trivirgatus*),[105,106] cynomolgous monkeys (*Macaca* spp.),[107,109] and Patas monkeys.[110] Although the disease resembles that in humans, it is usually milder. Nevertheless, virions and viral antigen can be detected in feces, serum, and bile and hepatic tissue after infection, and serologic responses are virtually identical.

In 1979, Provost and Hilleman[31] first reported the successful propagation of HAV in tissue culture cells. They used virus passaged 31 times in marmosets to infect fetal rhesus monkey kidney cells and primary explants of *S. labiatus* marmoset liver. Since then, several investigators have successfully infected different cell types, including human hepatoma cell lines,[111,112] and primary African green monkey cells (AGMK),[113] with HAV directly from feces of naturally infected humans. After adaptation, other cell types have been shown to support the growth of HAV including primary human fibroblast cells, continuous human diploid (MRC-5) cells, and cell lines derived from AGMK (B-SC-1, Vero, and BGMK).[83,111,113–117] Persistent infection of these AGMK cell lines is readily achieved.

HAV appears to be mostly cell-associated and produces little or no cytopathic effect in cell culture.[31,112] Accumulation of clusters of virus within cytoplasmic vesicles are seen ultrastructurally.[118–120] In some studies,[111,113] a long (e.g., 4 weeks) eclipse period between inoculation of the culture and appearance of viral antigen in the cells has been observed,[117,121] and in others HAV antigen has appeared more rapidly (e.g., 4 days). Some variants of HAV have been found to be cytolytic for specific cell lines.[61,122–126]

Tissue and Cellular Sites of Viral Antigen Synthesis

HAV antigen has been detected by direct immunofluorescence in the liver tissue of experimentally infected chimpanzees[127] and marmosets.[128] Specific staining was distributed diffusely throughout the liver as a finely granular pattern in the cytoplasm of hepatocytes but not in the nucleus. This cytoplasmic localization of HAV antigen is supported by the finding of 27-nm particles in vesicles within the hepatocyte cytoplasm of experimentally infected chimpanzees.[37] Such particles are indistinguishable from those found in feces. The cytoplasmic location of HAV antigen is consistent with the cellular site of synthesis of other small RNA viruses such as polio.[129–131] No evidence of viral antigen synthesis in other tissues, including large and small bowel, has been detected.[127,128,132] It seems likely, however, that some cells in the gastrointestinal tract are susceptible to HAV infection, since infections in humans occur so readily by the oral route.

Relationship of HAV to Picornaviridae

Although HAV shares some biophysical and biochemical characteristics with the enteroviruses or other Picornaviridae, a number of differences exist: (*1*) the predicted lengths of several HAV proteins and their amino acid sequences are unlike those of other picornaviruses; (*2*) the virus is difficult to isolate and propagate in cell culture, replicates slowly, and is usually not cytopathic; (*3*) HAV is resistant to temperatures and chemicals that inactivate other picornaviruses; and (*4*) only one serotype is known to exist with an immunodominant neutralization site. Because of these unique features, HAV should be classified as a separate genus within the family Picornaviridae.

EPIDEMIOLOGY

HAV, like hepatitis B virus (HBV), has a worldwide distribution.[133] The epidemiology of HAV differs from that of HBV because of several significant differences in the biologic behavior of the two viruses. Persistent infection with continuous viremia does not occur with HAV as with HBV. Thus transmission by blood via parenteral routes, which is common for HBV, is unusual with HAV.[134]

HAV, unlike HBV, is found in feces of all infected patients, and it spreads readily by the fecal–oral route, frequently by food or water contaminated with feces. Because no form of persistent infection has been documented for HAV and no animal or other reservoir is known, this virus must be maintained in a population by serial transmission from acute cases to susceptibles. Recurrent epidemics are a prominent feature of the disease. Three distinct age-specific anti-HAV profiles have been identified.[135] In developing countries most children develop subclinical, anicteric HAV infections within the first decade of life with nearly universal seroconversion occurring by adulthood. Developed countries generally have a low anti-HAV prevalence in children and young adults while a high frequency of antibody may be found in the elderly, a pattern reflecting distant historical exposures. The third, much rarer, profile consists of a low seroprevalence of anti-HAV in children but the universal presence of antibody in adults. This pattern is observed principally in isolated populations of limited size, where HAV has actually been found to disappear after an epidemic that followed its introduction from outside and then reappear years later when again brought in from the outside.[136–139] This behavior in small, isolated populations is similar to that of measles, mumps, rubella, and poliomyelitis viruses,[140] which do not commonly cause persistent infection in humans and for which no reservoir outside of humans is known.

Surveillance Data for Hepatitis A

The total number of cases of hepatitis A in the United States is not precisely known because not all cases of viral hepatitis are evaluated by specific HAV serology. The contribution of HAV to *hospitalized adult* hepatitis cases in two urban populations has been assessed. Approximately 20 percent of the cases appeared to be associated with HAV, 50 percent with HBV, and the remainder were neither type A nor type B hepatitis.[141,142] In 1988, 54,011 cases of hepatitis were reported to the Centers for Disease Control, of which 49 percent were categorized as hepatitis A.[143] Thus, the reported incidence of hepatitis A in the United States is approximately 11 cases per 100,000 population. The actual number of HAV infections is probably several times higher, since most primary infections are subclinical[144] and physicians report fewer than 15 percent of the hospitalized cases they diagnose.[145,146] The highest incidence of reported cases has been in adolescents and young adults,[147] with a relatively even distribution between males and females.[144,147] In temperate zones, a minor peak is observed each year in the fall and winter whereas an additional cyclic phase is seen every 6 to 10 years.

HAV infection rates are high in circumstances of poor sanitation and/or crowded living conditions such as in institutions for the developmentally disabled, military facilities, prisons, etc.[144] Other high-risk groups in the United States include the children and staff of day care centers[148,149] and homosexual men,[150,151] groups in which close physical contact appears to promote spread of enterically transmitted infections. The risk of hepatitis A in day care centers is greatest when care is provided for large numbers of diapered children under the age of 2. Infection in the children is usually asymptomatic, and spread from infected children to household contacts provides the majority of recognized cases. Secondary attack rates are high in members (particularly children) of households with an index case. The high rate of acquisition of HAV reported in homosexual males was strongly associated with an oral–anal pattern of sexual contact.

The prevalence of antibody to HAV (anti-HAV) as serologic evidence of past infection varies among different populations in the United States. Seroepidemiologic studies also have revealed striking differences in the prevalence of anti-HAV in different areas of the world.[133,144] In general, the highest rates of HAV infection are in economically developing countries that have the lowest living standards, the highest density of people, and the poorest hygiene and sanitation. This includes Central and South America, Africa, the Mediterranean area, and Asia. In such areas, antibody appears at very early ages, and most infection at these ages appears to be subclinical and anicteric.[133] Thus, although HAV infections are worldwide, they are not evenly distributed.

Modes of HAV Transmission

Transmission by the Fecal–Oral Route through Close Personal Contact. The most common mode of HAV transmission is through close person-to-person contact, usually by the fecal–oral route. On numerous occasions, HAV has been shown to infect humans when given by mouth in experimental transmission studies.[16,22,152–156] Epidemiologic data on the spread of HAV in households[157,158] and institutions[159,160] and after transmission from primary cases via drinking water[161] or food[162–164] indicate that most secondary cases occur approximately one incubation period after onset of symptoms in the index case, suggesting that patients are most infectious in the late incubation period or about the time symptoms begin. Table 1 summarizes the results of several experimental human and animal studies that document the presence of HAV in stool specimens collected as early as 2 to 3 weeks before and up to 8 days after the onset of jaundice. No infectivity has been found 4 weeks or more before[156,165] or 19 days or more after the onset of jaundice.[21,152,156,166] These results probably define the time limits for successful transmission of HAV to a susceptible host, bearing in mind that communicability is lowest near the conclusion of virus shedding when larger quantities of fecal contamination would be required for infection to occur.

Infectivity of feces closely parallels detection of HAV-like particles in the fecal extracts of infected patients by immune electron microscopy or radioimmunoassay. The maximum numbers of particles have been found in the late incubation period and at the time symptoms develop.[157,167–177] In most studies, excretion of particles appears to end before the peak serum transaminase activity is reached or the onset of jaundice occurs,[157,167–174] although some studies have detected low levels of hepatitis A antigen up to 16 days after the onset of icterus.[169,173,174] These data on fecal infectivity, viral antigen shedding, and natural transmission are consistent and indicate that the period during which transmission occurs in most cases is around the time of onset of symptoms and before the onset of jaundice.

Unequivocal transmission of HAV has not been documented more than 2 to 3 weeks after the development of icteric liver disease[21,22,152] regardless of whether transaminase levels remain elevated.[22,178] Epidemiologic evidence also suggests that persistent HAV excretion probably does not occur. The disappearance of hepatitis A in small isolated populations after introduction of HAV from the outside[136–138] and the pattern of periodic reintroduction of HAV after long intervals in institutions for the mentally handicapped[179–182] are consistent with the view that long-term intestinal carriers probably do not exist. However, many more cases of infection must be studied by methods that specifically identify HAV to establish finally whether or not persistent infection ever occurs.

Transmission by Fecally Contaminated Food and Water. Besides spread of HAV by close personal contact, water and food have clearly been documented as vehicles for transmission of HAV.[183–187] Between 1958 and 1965, water-borne epidemics in the United States numbered over 50 but constituted less than 1 percent of all reported cases.[188] Although private water supplies contaminated with sewage have most often been the reported sources of water-borne disease,[189,190] public water sys-

TABLE 1. Detection of Infectious Hepatitis A Virus in Feces of Infected Patients[a]

Time of Fecal Collection			Tests of Infectivity			
Days After Experimental Infection	*Days After Onset of Symptoms*	*Days Before (−) or After (+) Onset of Jaundice*	*Infectivity*	*Ratio (Infected/ Inoculated)*	*Test System*	*Reference*
7		−34	−	(0/6)	M	165
11		Pool −28 to −35	−	(0/8)	H	156
25		Pool −14 to −21	+	(4/11)	H	156
33		−8	+	(2/6)	M	165
38		−3	+	(6/6)	M	165
29	5	−1	+	(2/3)	H	166
		+1	+		H	153
		Pool +1 to +5	+	(7/18)	H	213
		+3	+		H	153
	Pool 1 to 8		+	(2/3)	H	166
	Pool 3 to 10		+		C	17
47		+6	+	(4/6)	M	165
		Pool +1 to +8	+	(16/37)	H	156
		+8	+		H	153
		+19	−		H	166
		+20	−		H	166
	Pool 25 to 29		−		H	166
		Pool +19 to +33	−	(0/10)	H	152
		+32	−		H	152
		+33	−		H	21
		+43	−		H	156

KEY: M: marmoset; H: human subject; C: chimpanzee.
[a] Pooled fecal samples are from 3 to 7 patients.

tems also have been implicated.[184,191,192] With rare exceptions, water-borne HAV epidemics typically exhibit low attack rates.[193]

Numerous examples of epidemic and endemic hepatitis A have been associated with shellfish ingestion.[194–201] Sewage-contaminated raw clams have been implicated most often, but oysters,[195,199,201] mussels,[200] and improperly steamed clams[198] also have been a source of infection. Their assumed role has been that of virus concentrators of water polluted by sewage rather than propagators of virus by replication in shellfish. Nonbivalve mollusks, such as lobster or shrimp, do not impart the same risk for transmitting HAV.

Milk-borne hepatitis A has been described[202,203] and is thought to occur after the use of contaminated water to wash milk containers and equipment. Transmission via other food and drink has been reported on numerous occasions,[170,195,204–212] and in some instances a food handler with hepatitis A has been implicated as the source.[204,205,207–210]

Transmission After Exposure to Nonfecal Sources of HAV. Transmission of HAV through contact with body fluids other than feces is believed to occur infrequently as evidenced by the paucity of clinical and experimental reports. However, precise interpretation of risk is impeded because susceptibility of volunteers is unknown in studies conducted prior to the availability of serologic assays for HAV. Regardless, infectivity for human volunteers was reported in 2 of 33 subjects who were inoculated with nasopharyngeal washings from patients in various stages of acute HAV disease.[166,213,214] Transmission of HAV by the aerosol route also was suggested in at least one epidemiologic study.[215] More recently, saliva from an infected patient was shown to cause HAV in two chimpanzees.[132] These results suggest that respiratory secretions may rarely contain infectious HAV and lead to transmission by contact or aerosol via such secretions.

Urine collected just before or at the time of onset of jaundice appears to contain low levels of infectious HAV in some patients. Three of six subjects in one study[155] and one of twelve in another[154] were infected by urine samples. On the other hand, three other studies have reported failure to infect a total of 29 subjects with the urine of patients with clinically diagnosed hepatitis A.[166,213,214] In another study, urine and semen were not infectious for chimpanzees although the serum and feces from the same donor were capable of transmitting HAV to other animals.[132] Thus, although urine has been implicated as a possible source of contamination of food in at least one epidemic,[207] it seems unlikely that urine is commonly involved in infections in the community.

No cases of intrauterine infection with HAV have been reported. In 6 cases of acute hepatitis A followed prospectively in pregnant women (3 occurring at the time of delivery), there was no evidence of infection in the newborn infants.[216] Presumably, sufficient IgG anti-HAV is transported across the placenta to protect the newborn infant. Transmission of HAV by externally contaminated, coprophagous insects, or by biting insects, is conceivable but remains unconfirmed.

Viremia and Percutaneous Transmission. Although transient viremia has been documented after HAV infection,[16,134,156,166,217–220] percutaneous transfer of blood or serum appears to be an infrequent route of transmission. Data on the period when infectious virus is present in the blood are less complete than for fecal virus. Table 2 summarizes the results of several studies documenting blood-borne HAV. Virus has been found in blood during the latter half of the incubation period, but the time when viremia is terminated in most patients is not well established. The data in Table 2 suggest that the period of viremia may vary in different patients, although the negative infectivity tests in human subjects must be interpreted with the knowledge that the susceptibility of the subjects used for testing was unknown. In most instances, viremia precedes the development of clinical symptoms by 7 to 10 days, often reaching its maximum prior to peak ALT levels. Rarely, viremia may be present during the early stages of jaundice.[156] The period of antigenemia in experimentally infected chimpanzees also has been found to be transient and present exclusively during the late incubation period of hepatitis A.[177] These results suggest that viremia is present for a limited period, probably most often during the late incubation period of hepatitis A. Because the data on infectivity in blood and on antigenemia are quite limited, more investigation with improved methods are needed to establish conclusively the frequency, duration, and precise time limits of viremia on HAV infection in humans.

Because the incubation period of hepatitis A and the period of viremia are much shorter than for hepatitis B, and because persistent infection does not occur, the period for potential percutaneous transmission of HAV from asymptomatic patients is clearly less than for HBV. Epidemiologic evidence supports this view. Although multiply transfused children have been found to have a much higher frequency of anti-HBs than nontransfused populations, the frequency of anti-HAV has been found to be the same.[221] Similarly, patients and staff of hemodialysis centers have been found to have no higher incidence of anti-HAV (unlike anti-HBs) than expected for groups of similar demography.[222] Most studies of post-transfusion hepatitis have failed to reveal cases of hepatitis A by specific serologic testing,[223–227] but exceptions exist.[134,218,219,228–230] The reasons for these sporadic occurrences include the short-lived period of viremia, the low virus burden present in the blood, the absence of a carrier state, the probability that anti-HAV would be present in other units of blood administered to the patient resulting in neutralization of the virus, and the likelihood that the recipient is already immune.

Transmission After Exposure to Nonhuman Primates. Many cases of hepatitis have been reported after contact with chimpanzees and a few other nonhuman primates.[96,98,231–234] More recently, such cases have been confirmed serologically to be type A hepatitis.[235,236] In all cases, animals in captivity with previous contact with humans have been involved. It is most likely that the animals in these cases were first infected by contact with humans. The infection is associated with subclinical illness in nonhuman primates.

CLINICAL MANIFESTATIONS AND THE COURSE OF INFECTION

Although hepatitis A is generally less severe than hepatitis B, and certain clinical differences have been described, it is usually impossible to distinguish acute hepatitis A from acute hepatitis B or non-A, non-B hepatitis in individual cases. As with infection with other hepatitis agents, HAV infection can be associated with anicteric or icteric hepatitis. In addition, many infections are inapparent (subclinical) and thus are without symptoms or jaundice. Such patients only can be recognized by examining their blood for biochemical or serologic alterations. In general, the illness in children is milder and has a shorter course than in adults. Estimates of the ratio of anicteric to icteric cases in several studies have ranged from 12:1 in experimentally infected young children,[237] 9:1 in young adults and children in Alaska,[136] 2:1 in Holy Cross College football players[238] and mental institution patients aged 13 to 31 in New England,[239] 1.1:1 in institutionalized handicapped children in Los Angeles,[240] 1:1.7 in a community outbreak,[241] 1:2 in an institution for the mentally retarded in Virginia,[181] and 1:3.5 in U.S. Navy recruits.[167] Although age appears to influence the severity of hepatitis A,[149,242,243] the infecting dose of virus and other factors also may be important.

The incubation period after experimental infection or common-vehicle exposure (that is, the time between exposure and

TABLE 2. Detection of Infectious Hepatitis A Virus in Blood of Infected Patients

Time of Blood Collection				*Tests for Infectivity*			
Days After Experimental Infection	*Days Before (−) or After (+) Onset of Symptoms*	*Days Before (−) or After (+) Rise in SGOT*	*Days Before (−) or After (+) Onset of Jaundice*	*Infectivity*	*Ratio (Infected/ Inoculated)*	*Test System*	*Reference*
			Pool −21 to −28	−	(0/8)	H	152
12			−25	+	(1/6)	H	154
18			−23	−	(0/11)	H	152
25			Pool −14 to −21	+	(6/12)	H	152
13	−11		−17	−	(0/3)	H	166
	−11			+		H	219
29		−8		−	(0/10)	H	16
			−7	+	(1/1)	H	134
	−3			+		H	218
30		+6	−1	+	(5/10)	H	16
28	+4		−2	+	(3/6)	H	166
33 and 40			Pool −3 and −7	+	(7/9)	H	152
		Rising SGOT		+	(4/5)	M	204
		Peak SGOT		+	(3/5)	M	204
	Pool +1 to +8			+	(3/3)	H	166
43			+3	+	(1/10)	H	152
55	+31		+25	−	(0/3)	H	166

KEY: M: marmoset; H: human subject.

the onset of symptoms) was found to be between 10 and 50 days with a mode of 1 month regardless of the route of infection. However, the greater the dose of virus, the shorter is the incubation period.[152] During an outbreak, cases that occur less than 14 days apart suggest a coprimary rather than a secondary case.[7,11,189,206,208,212,244–247]

There are four studies of serologically verified HAV infections, involving either experimental transmission to volunteers[16,152] or single-source outbreaks,[167,238] that best define the clinical findings and course of hepatitis A in humans. The first clinical symptoms are usually fever (100°F to 103°F) with malaise, fatigue, myalgia, headache, anorexia, nausea, and vomiting. Interferon induction may be responsible for many of these symptoms,[248] which often occur abruptly (within 24 hours). Weight loss of 2 to 10 pounds is common due to anorexia and disordered taste and smell.[249,250] Epigastric and/or right upper quadrant pain often accompany these symptoms. Children may have diarrhea, which is uncommon in adults.[69] Cough, coryza, and sore throat have been common symptoms in some outbreaks.[167] Arthralgias and/or transient rash have been observed in up to 14 percent of patients during or immediately before the acute illness in some outbreaks.[167] Arthritis and vasculitis have been observed only rarely,[251] and a diffuse mild endothelial and mesangeal proliferative glomerulonephritis has been described in a patient who died following hepatitis A infection.[134] Meningoencephalitis associated with HAV infection has been reported[252] but must be rare. Hepatomegaly and splenomegaly, when they occur, usually precede the onset of jaundice by several days. Dark, golden-brown urine precedes jaundice by 1 to several days, and during the icteric phase pruritis and acolic stools may be present. Generalized adenopathy is not a component of hepatitis A, but often is present in cases of CMV- or EBV-related hepatitis.

Most infections are associated with acute, self-limited icteric or anicteric illness. However, some patients develop hepatic encephalopathy or fulminant hepatitis.[134,141,253–255] In one study,[255] 23 of 73 (31.5 percent) cases of fulminant hepatitis were due to HAV and 57 percent of these hepatitis A patients died. Relapsing hepatitis, occurring 1 to 4 months after recovery from hepatitis A, occasionally has been observed.[251,256–260] Clinical symptoms usually recur and are accompanied by biochemical abnormalities of liver dysfunction. Total serum antibody to HAV may increase[257,260] and IgM anti-HAV either persists or rises in titer.[251,256–258,260] No documented HAV infections have been reported to be followed by chronic hepatitis, and evidence of HAV infection has not been found in cases of chronic active hepatitis.[253]

Serum alanine aminotransferase (ALT) activity is usually the first liver function test to become abnormal within a few days of the onset of symptoms. This is usually 2 days to 2 weeks before the first elevated bilirubin. The ALT test is the most specific biochemical marker associated with viral hepatitis. Levels of this enzyme are significantly higher than the aspartate aminotransferase (AST) enzyme, resulting in a low AST/ALT ratio (<0.7) in almost all cases of uncomplicated acute viral hepatitis. The ALT level usually reaches its peak before the onset of jaundice. In children, the aminotransferase levels were found to return to normal within 2 to 3 weeks of onset of the illness. Conversely, hepatitis is usually more prolonged in adults and the icteric phase may last for a month or more. Among infected college students, 20 percent had an elevated AST value for 20 weeks after exposure and 15 weeks after acute illness,[238] and 50 percent of naval recruits were found to still have an elevated AST level 3 to 4 weeks after the onset of symptoms and 8 percent after 14 weeks.[167]

Most patients have a relative lymphocytosis.[261] Occasionally, hemolytic anemia occurs, usually in association with glucose-6-phosphate dehydrogenase deficiency.[262–264] Rarely patients with acute hepatitis A will present with agranulocytosis,[265] thrombocytopenia,[266] pancytopenia,[263,267] or aplastic anemia.[268–271]

Several virologic markers of HAV infection can be detected well before the onset of symptoms or evidence of liver disease. The first evidence of viral infection in nonhuman primates is the appearance of hepatitis A viral antigen and 27-nm particles in the liver 1 to 2 weeks after infection as determined by immunocytochemical staining or electron microscopy[37,101,127,272–275] (Fig. 2). This antigen may remain detectable in the liver for a period of 4 to 5 weeks, persisting even after the ALT has normalized.[127] Hepatitis A antigen also has been detected in the blood before the onset of disease,[127,134,276] but the time of its appearance and duration in the blood are not well defined serologically.

Shortly after its appearance in the liver, hepatitis A antigen can be detected in feces[127,277] and bile[37,277] by immune electron microscopy and radioimmunoassay. In human subjects, fecal hepatitis A antigen has been detected several days before the liver enzymes become abnormal, and usually reaches a peak when the ALT begins to rise.[157,168,171] In one study, the antigen persisted in two-thirds of the patients for up to 7 days after the onset of bilirubinuria and for 8 to 16 days in the remainder.[173] In another study, hepatitis A antigen was detected in fecal extracts 5 to 10 days after onset of jaundice.[169,170] These observations correlate with studies measuring fecal infectivity (see

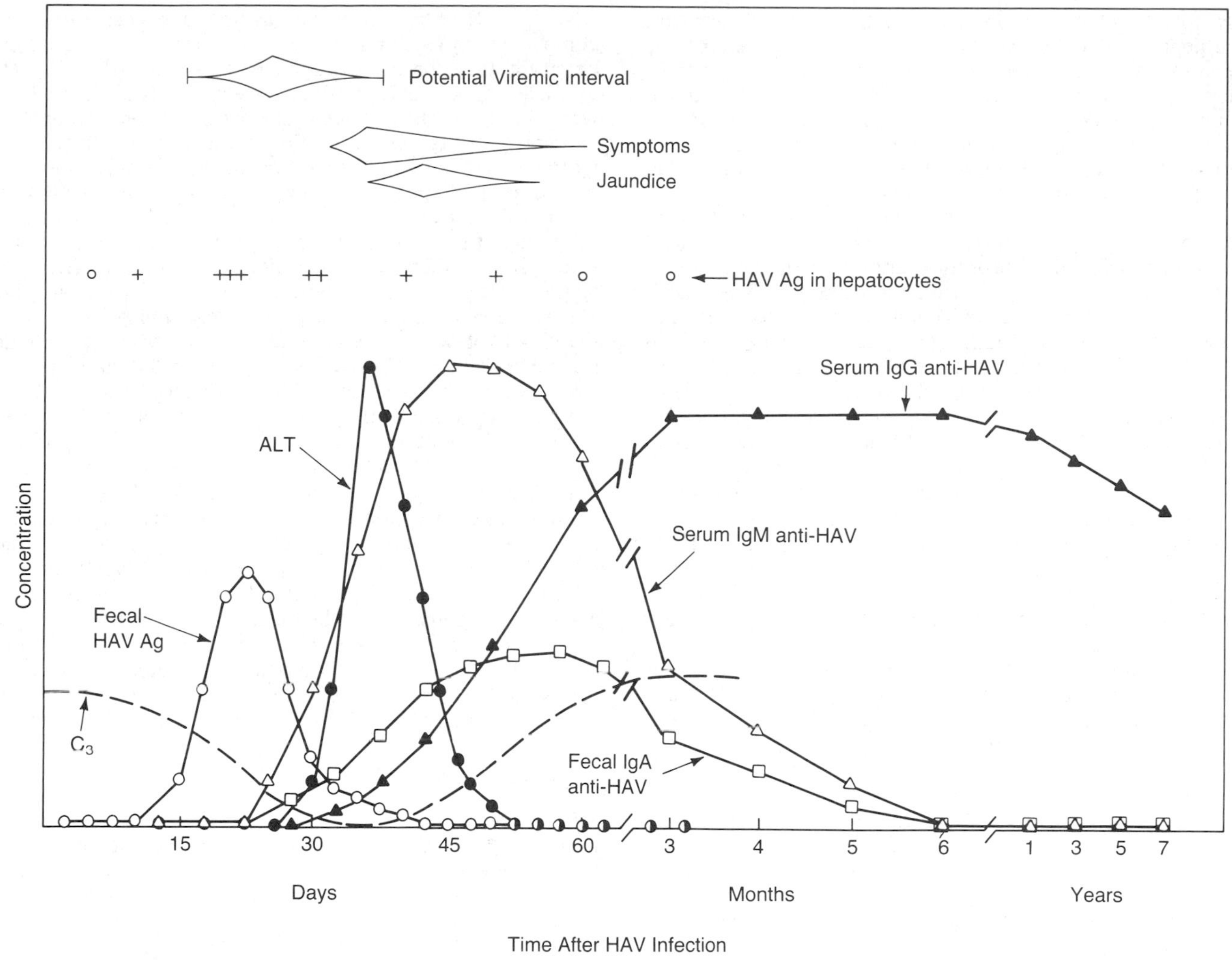

FIG. 2. Course of hepatitis A infection.

Table 1). There appears to be a rough correlation between the severity of hepatitis A and the concentration of hepatitis A antigen in the feces, and many patients with anicteric hepatitis A apparently have no detectable antigen by serologic assays.[167,169] Bile may be the major source of fecal antigen since hepatitis A antigen has not been detected in intestinal mucosa after infection of chimpanzees or marmosets by parenteral or oral routes.[37,127,128,132,277]

PATHOGENESIS AND PATHOLOGY

The sequence of events involved in the pathogenesis of hepatitis A after natural infection with HAV is poorly understood. For HAV to cause hepatitis after ingestion it must penetrate the mucosal barrier and spread within the host to the liver where disease can occur. Although the specific site of entry is not known, an early replicative event in the oropharynx or salivary glands similar to that which is observed with poliovirus is suspected.[103,150,278] However, the infrequent identification of HAV antigen and RNA in the intestinal mucosa also may implicate this site.[128,273,279–281] In this regard, it is noteworthy that intestinal reinfection with excretion of virus may occur in immune individuals.[282]

Coproantibodies of the IgA class have been detected in the feces of patients with acute viral hepatitis A.[282–285] They apparently lack neutralizing activity[289] but are capable of forming immune complexes with fecal antigen.[168,280,282,286–288] The role that such antibody plays in the curtailment of communicability or in resistance to reinfection is not proved, but it may be important by analogy with immunity that occurs with other viruses that infect by the enteric route.

HAV infection appears to result in solid immunity, and reinfections, if they occur, must be rare.[282] Experimental transmission of infectious hepatitis virus (or HAV) to human volunteers and subsequent rechallenge has shown resistance to reinfection by the same virus and no resistance to serum hepatitis virus (or HBV).[7,9,289] Studies of multiple episodes of apparent viral hepatitis by natural routes of transmission have not discovered individuals with more than a single episode of HAV infection, although HAV infection can follow HBV and vice versa.[290–292] These studies indicate that homologous immunity develops during the first infection with HAV and, not unexpectedly, no heterologous immunity to HBV infection is apparent. Protection of people by passive immunization in areas of the world different from the source of the immune globulin used to prevent HAV[76,77] indicates that this virus is antigenically similar in different regions of the world.

The histopathologic changes seen in acute hepatitis A are qualitatively similar to those described for hepatitis B and the agents of non-A, non-B hepatitis. As a general rule, liver tissue from patients with acute hepatitis A have less conspicuous parenchymal changes (including focal necrosis, Kupffer cell proliferation, acidophilic bodies, and ballooning degeneration) than tissue from hepatitis B patients, but portal inflammation is more prominent than is seen in biopsies from patients with non-A, non-B hepatitis. In addition, the limiting plate is more likely to be disrupted, and periportal inflammation may simulate chronic active hepatitis. Cholestasis, when it occurs, is more common in hepatitis A. Illness and histopathologic changes tend to be more severe in human cases of acute hepatitis A than in experimentally infected nonhuman primates.[293] Regardless, chronic hepatitis is not a complication of this disease.

Virus-induced cytopathology may not be responsible for the pathologic changes seen in HAV infection. Cellular injury is unimpressive during the early phase of maximal viral replication[67,128,294,295] and in vitro cytopathic effects are minimal when examined by light microscopy, although cellular organelle damage can be detected by electron microscopy.[119] These findings suggest that host-mediated immune responses and other host defense factors may contribute to the pathogenesis of hepatitis A. The concurrent appearance of hepatitis with IgM anti-HAV, immune complexes, and reduced levels of serum complement may be coincidental or relevant to the clinical pathology observed.[251,296–299] Lysis of HAV-infected target cells in vitro by natural killer cells and by cytolytic T lymphocytes has been observed.[300,301] If this occurred in vivo, progeny virus production would be curtailed. Increased levels of interferon also have been observed in the sera of HAV-infected patients.[302–304] This may result in the inhibition of virus production by virus-infected cells and may augment natural killer cell activity. Additional studies will be required to place these isolated events into their proper perspective.

Although transient arthralgias and occasionally arthritis and rash occur during the incubation period of hepatitis A,[167] these are apparently less frequent than in hepatitis B. The pathogenesis of the joint and skin involvement associated with HAV infection has not been as extensively studied as that with HBV. However, hepatitis A antigen and anti-HAV have been detected in the same serum,[128] anti-complementary activity occurs during the incubation period of hepatitis A,[305] and low C_3 levels are found during acute hepatitis A.[298] All of these events are consistent with immune complex formation, but the role of these changes in HAV-associated disease has not been proved.

IMMUNODIAGNOSIS

The most useful approach for making the diagnosis of acute hepatitis A is to test serum or plasma for IgM-specific anti-HAV by radioimmunoassay (RIA) or enzyme immunoassay (EIA).[296,306–309] Virtually all patients are positive for IgM anti-HAV by the time of onset of symptoms although a rare individual will be slow to seroconvert. In most patients, the antibody becomes nondetectable by 3 to 6 months[310] (Fig. 2), although it persists for more than 200 days in 10 to 15 percent.[311] The liver enzymes will be normal in more than 85 percent of the patients before or at the time IgM anti-HAV antibodies disappear. Thus, a normal ALT level in the presence of IgM anti-HAV is indicative of the late convalescent stage of HAV.

IgM anti-HAV should be accompanied by a positive test in the assay that measures total specific anti-HAV (IgG and IgM). In the absence of IgM anti-HAV, clinicians can assume that the antibody being detected by the total anti-HAV test is of the IgG immunoglobulin type. The IgG anti-HAV antibody persists for years after infection,[138] and indicates that the patient has had a previous infection with HAV and is protected against reinfection.

Correct interpretation of serologic results requires that the clinician exclude the potentially confounding consequences of recent transfusions, immune globulin administration, or a maternal antibody source within the previous 6 months. This latter source of antibody is more of an issue for IgG anti-HAV than for IgM anti-HAV, which does not cross the placental barrier.

Several other approaches for documenting an HAV infection are available only in a few research laboratories at this time. One such approach is to test fecal specimens for hepatitis A viral antigen or virus-like particles by IEM,[157,167,168,171,172] EIA,[312] or RIA.[312,313] However, as previously described, HAV components in feces rise and reach a maximum concentration about the time the ALT first becomes abnormal[157,168,172] (Fig. 2), then decline precipitously. In one study, HAV-like particles were found by IEM in fecal specimens of only 17 of 44 (39 percent) patients during the first week of hospitalization with icteric hepatitis A, and no specimens were positive more than 2 days after the peak of jaundice.[167] No positive results were found in 13 anicteric cases.

Testing of feces by RIA[167,312] and EIA[312] appear to be technically simpler than by immune electron microscopy (IEM), and some investigators have advocated their use for the clinical diagnosis of HAV infection. However, examining feces early in the course of acute icteric hepatitis A by these methods does not ensure that HAV particles will be detected, and a negative result is probable late in the illness in icteric cases (e.g., after the ALT level has peaked) and at any time after the onset of symptoms in anicteric cases. In a clinical setting, probably less than one-third of hepatitis A cases can be identified by examining feces for hepatitis A antigen by RIA or EIA.

Immunofluorescent staining of liver biopsy specimens from HAV infected chimpanzees indicates that hepatitis A antigen can be detected in liver for approximately 2 weeks after the ALT level begins to fall[127] (Fig. 2). If the same is true in humans, a specific diagnosis might be made by liver biopsy much later in the course of the illness than is possible by examination for antigen in the feces. However, the opportunity to make a diagnosis in this way does not arise frequently, since liver biopsy often is not clinically indicated during acute viral hepatitis.

THERAPY

Because of the relatively mild nature of the disease, especially in children, therapy is supportive and aimed at maintaining comfort and adequate nutritional balance. No specific treatment is currently being utilized. In general, bed rest is used prudently, being tailored to the severity of the patient's illness. Prolonged inactivity is not recommended[314,315] and hospitalization is not usually indicated.

The diet should supply adequate protein (1 g/kg) and calories (30 to 35 cal/kg). Restriction of fats is not essential and their utilization may ensure adequate caloric intake. Intravenous glucose with sodium and potassium chloride should be given to patients hospitalized for severe anorexia, nausea, and vomiting. Because patients with severe hepatitis may have difficulties excreting a water load, the use of 10% glucose, rather than 5%, is preferred. Phenergan or metoclopramide may be given for protracted vomiting. Adrenocortical steroids, immune globulin, or antibiotics are of no value in acute, uncomplicated viral hepatitis.[316–320] Patients who are taking oral contraceptives do not need to discontinue their use during the course of the disease.[321] Alcoholic beverages should not be consumed during acute hepatitis because of the direct hepatotoxic effect of ethanol.

Patients who are being followed for fulminant hepatitis should be closely monitored in a medical intensive care unit. The treatment of this entity generally has been unsatisfactory and mortality rates remain high. Conventional therapy for impending coma or the coma stage of encephalopathy includes the reduction of protein intake accompanied by the use of cleansing enemas to reduce the formation of ammonia and related compounds. Lactulose retention enemas (30 to 60 minutes) given every 4 to 6 hours is recommended. Blood or fresh frozen plasma (750 cc/day) should be administered to correct any significant clotting abnormalities. Seizures may be controlled with small, repeated doses of oxazepam, diazepam, or lorazepam. Lorazepam and oxazepam may be preferred since they are conjugated with glucuronic acid to inactive metabolites, a process that is not restricted to hepatic microsomes. Because hypoglycemia is often prominent in patients with fulminant hepatitis, the glucose level should be monitored twice daily and maintained with intravenous glucose (16 cal/kg). During this interval, vitamin B complex with thiamine should be supplied parenterally.[322] Electrolyte disturbances also should be corrected. These are common because sodium and free water clearance are impaired, especially in patients receiving blood products for coagulation abnormalities, osmotic diuretics for cerebral edema, or glucose in water for nutritional support.[323]

PREVENTION OF HEPATITIS A

General Measures

As with HBV, prevention of HAV infection and disease depends on halting transmission of virus and/or rendering susceptibles resistant to infection by active or passive immunization. Since the principal mode of spread of HAV is by the fecal–oral route, the most effective control measures must provide for prevention of fecal contamination of food, water, or other sources by infected individuals. Therein lies the problem, since maximum shedding of virus occurs before clinical disease becomes apparent and this correlates with increased communicability.[324] Thus, curtailment of virus spread depends in large measure on the hygienic practices of the patients. Nevertheless, the importance of careful handwashing by medical personnel contacting patients and laboratory workers handling infective specimens cannot be overemphasized. Because the personal hygiene of young children is often difficult to control, they should be restrained from maintaining close contact with their susceptible playmates during the first 2 weeks of illness or for at least 2 weeks after the onset of jaundice.

Strict isolation of patients with hepatitis A in households is not necessary since other household members almost always have been fully exposed by the time of onset of symptoms. Sharing of personal objects such as eating utensils, toothbrushes, razors, toys, etc., should be avoided; however, frequent handwashing, as described above, and careful handling and decontamination of objects contacted by the patients (particularly objects soiled with feces or blood) should be carried out. Patients should not prepare or handle food for others. Thorough washing with soap and hot water, with or without bleach, are probably sufficient to prevent transmission from utensils, clothes, bed clothes, or other contaminated objects in households. Surfaces such as those used to change diapers or hold clothes or other potentially soiled objects from patients with hepatitis A can be disinfected with solutions of household bleach (5.25% sodium hypochlorite) diluted 1:10 to 1:50.

Several seroprevalence or surveillance studies have shown that transmission of hepatitis A from adult patients to staff or from one patient to another is an unlikely event.[222,324,325] Indeed the risk of acquiring hepatitis A by health care professionals is no greater than that found outside the hospital environment.

Correspondingly, considering the low order of infectivity that is present during the icteric stage of disease, strict enteric precautions of hospitalized adult patients with hepatitis A is not necessary,[326] although measures to prevent spread of virus from feces and blood should be adhered to until 2 weeks after the onset of jaundice or peak ALT level. Conversely, enteric precautions are definitely recommended for infected newborn infants, young children, or fecally incontinent patients.

Hepatitis A patients should not be allowed to share personal objects with others while in the hospital. Objects that come in direct contact with patients such as eating utensils, bedclothes, thermometers, medical instruments, bedpans, and urinals should be decontaminated appropriately before being used for other patients. Hepatitis A patients need not be confined to their rooms and visitors need not be excluded, although contact with contaminated objects should be avoided by visitors. Responsibility for curtailing transmission resides with the patient who can avert transmission of HAV with scrupulous handwashing after a bowel movement.

Patient care personnel should wear gloves for blood drawing and for handling feces or soiled objects. Gown and mask should be used for procedures that may involve splashing of infectious material. Most important is conscientious handwashing after direct patient contact or the handling of potentially contaminated objects. Blood, feces, and other possibly infectious specimens should be labeled as infectious and handled appropriately. Hepatitis A patients with diarrhea or fecal incontinence appear to represent a significantly greater risk to hospital personnel than patients without these disorders.[327] They should be housed in single rooms, and increased precautions, including gown and gloves, should be instituted for any patient contact.

Newly imported chimpanzees or higher order primates that may be a source of HAV should be quarantined for at least 60 days during which time contact should be restricted to the care and feeding of the animals. Animal handlers should wear protective clothing and gloves when taking care of such animals, and should wash their hands when finished with their work. Routine immune globulin may be indicated for susceptible individuals who regularly contact newly imported animals in facilities where transmission of hepatitis A to humans has occurred and where other control measures have been unsuccessful.

Transmission via food can be decreased by good personal hygiene (e.g., regular handwashing) on the part of food-handlers, and by minimizing the extent to which food, particularly that to be eaten without further cooking, is touched. Food-handlers with hepatitis A should be prohibited from preparing food to be eaten by others until their illness has completely resolved. When food is implicated as the source of HAV and no source of contamination, such as an infected food-handler, can be identified, contaminated water used to wash the food should be suspected. Food should be protected from flies or other vectors carrying feces or sewage. The risk of raw shellfish-associated hepatitis A can be reduced by obtaining bivalve mollusks from waters known to be free from raw sewage.

The standard water sanitation practices in the United States provide water free of infectious HAV, but water-borne hepatitis A may result from inadvertent or unrecognized contamination of drinking water with sewage. Contamination may end before hepatitis cases occur or it may persist. In either case, the contaminated source of water must be identified as quickly as possible to avoid additional cases.

Passive Immunization with Immune Globulin

The effectiveness of immune globulin (Ig) for modifying or preventing hepatitis A has long been established.[328] Stokes and Neefe[329] in 1945 first reported that Ig dramatically reduced the incidence of icteric disease in a common source epidemic when compared with untreated controls. Numerous studies since have documented the effectiveness of Ig for pre-exposure and postexposure prophylaxis.[330–334] Most often the effect has been to completely suppress or markedly attenuate *clinical* hepatitis A in 80 to 90 percent of the participants, although the overall rate of *infection* often remains unchanged when compared to controls.[180,237,241] In such instances, active immunity appears to follow the mild infections.[324,332] Such "passive–active" immunity is clearly desirable because it results in long-term protection.

Immune globulin is effective when given up to 6 days prior to the onset of illness, and doses as low as 0.01 mL/kg have been found to be protective.[330,331] Larger doses of Ig may provide protection lasting a few more weeks, but, more importantly, passive–active responses are curtailed leaving a larger percentage of susceptibles available for infection after another exposure[324,332,335] (Table 3). It has been suggested that widespread use of Ig in hepatitis A outbreaks might result in enhanced spread of infection since many subclinical infections not recognized as sources for spread of virus would occur.[336] How-

TABLE 3. Effect of Immune Globulin (Ig) on Hepatitis A Virus Infection among Exposed Residents of a Custodial Institution

Ig Dose (mL/lb)	*No. of Susceptibles*	*No. with Infection*		*Seroconversion Only*	*Percentage Remaining Susceptible*
		Clinical	*Subclinical*		
None	19	8	4	4	16
0.02	15	1	3	3	53
0.08	10	0	0	2	80

(From Hall et al.,[335] with permission.)

ever, it has been shown that Ig clearly inhibits spread of HAV in both Ig recipients and those not receiving Ig in closed populations.[337]

Although all lots of Ig contain significant levels of anti-HAV, there has been significant differences in the titers of individual lots.[338,339] As fewer persons contract hepatitis A, the anti-HAV concentration in pooled plasma (and immune globulin) will continue to diminish.[340] Thus, recommended dosages may no longer be valid for protection. The safety of Ig given intramuscularly is well established. Within the United States, no instance of hepatitis or HIV infection has been attributed to intramuscular Ig correctly prepared by the Cohn ethanol fractionation procedure even when made from plasma known to be infectious for hepatitis B.[341] This observation, and the finding that fraction II of the Cohn ethanol procedure is free of HBsAg,[342] suggest that HBV is removed during Ig preparation. Adverse side effects may consist of discomfort at the injection site, slight elevation in temperature, myalgia, and lethargy. Hematoma formation is a risk in patients with bleeding or coagulation abnormalities. Anaphylactic reactions are extremely rare and appear most often with inadvertent intravenous administration.

Pre-exposure Prophylaxis. Suppression of disease clearly results from administration of Ig before exposure to hepatitis A. Table 4 lists the dosage of Ig and duration of protection found in several studies evaluating long-term protection of people in highly endemic settings. The variation in the duration of protection with dose may be related to the variation in anti-HAV concentration found in different lots of commercial Ig.[338,339] Pre-exposure prophylaxis is indicated most often for susceptible people residing in highly endemic areas for prolonged, but finite, intervals. Studies of American missionaries and their dependents have shown rates of viral hepatitis of around 0.5 percent per year in Japan; 1 to 2 percent per year in Southern Africa, India, and Southeast Asia; 2 to 3 percent per year in Central and South America; and 3 to 8 percent per year in North Africa and the Middle East.[339,343–348] Significant reductions in the incidence of viral hepatitis with the regular administration of Ig have been shown in Swedish soldiers stationed in the Middle East[333] and Peace Corps workers living in highly endemic areas.[76] The duration of protection depends on the dosage of Ig, and 0.06 mL/kg (or 5.0 mL for adults) appears to provide protection for up to 6 months. This dose should be given at 4 to 6 month intervals to susceptible people residing in these endemic areas. People should be tested for anti-HAV before instituting long-term repeated prophylaxis, since Ig need not be given to immune individuals. Similarly, those people receiving long-term Ig who become infected and seroconvert no longer require prophylaxis. Other indications for long-term pre-exposure Ig prophylaxis would be in institutions, such as those for the mentally impaired, or in primate facilities where a high risk of hepatitis A is shown to continue despite extensive environmental control measures.

TABLE 4. Pre-exposure Prophylaxis of Hepatitis A with Immune Globulin (Ig)

Ig Dose	*Duration of Protection (Months)*	*Type of Exposure*	*Reference*
0.02 mL/kg	5–8	Epidemics in closed institutions, 1951	332
0.01 or 0.02 mL/kg	2	Epidemics in closed institutions, 1954	180
0.12 mL/kg	5–12	Endemic disease in institutions, 1960	237
0.04 mL/kg 0.12 mL/kg	3 5	Endemic disease in institutions, 1963	349
0.10 mL/kg	4	Endemic disease in Peace Corps workers, 1969	76
2, 5 or 10 mL	6	Endemic disease in U.S. troops in Korea, 1971	77

Evidence indicates that short-term travelers to high-risk areas that are not outside the ordinary tourist routes usually have a very low risk of developing icteric viral hepatitis,[349,350] and Ig is not recommended for such sojourns. As with any enteric disease, the best system to prevent hepatitis A in these areas is to avoid potentially contaminated water and food by drinking bottled water, using it for brushing the teeth, and eschewing salads. In contrast, travelers to highly endemic areas outside ordinary tourist routes may be at increased risk. These individuals might be given 0.02 to 0.04 mL/kg Ig (or 2.0 mL for adults) if the anticipated exposure is for less than 2 months.

Postexposure Prophylaxis. Studies of household contacts have shown that Ig can reduce the attack rate of clinical hepatitis A by 80 to 90 percent. A dose of 0.01–0.02 mL/kg appears to offer as much protection as larger doses.[180,343] The earlier Ig is given after exposure the more likely that protection will result.[334,344] However, little or no protection is usually observed 2 weeks or more after exposure.[334] In view of the need for early Ig administration and its intrinsic safety and low cost, delay of administration to determine the anti-HAV status of the exposed individual is not recommended. The World Health Organization[351] and the Centers for Disease Control[345] recommend that 0.02 mL/kg Ig be administered intramuscularly to individuals within 2 weeks of an exposure carrying a significant risk of transmission. Simplified guidelines are shown in Table 5. Postexposure prophylaxis is not indicated for exposed people known to be immune (i.e., anti-HAV positive) because Ig would offer no benefit. Specific indications for immune globulin are listed in Table 6.

Active Immunization

Repeated exposure to HAV makes perpetual prophylaxis with Ig costly and impractical. Developing countries that are im-

TABLE 5. Guidelines for Immune Globulin (Ig) Prophylaxis against Hepatitis A

Person's Weight (lb)	*Immune Globulin Dose (mL)*	
	Routine	*High Risk[a] (Prolonged Exposure)*
<50	0.5	1.0
50–100	1.0	2.5
>100	2.0	5.0

[a] Within limits, larger doses of Ig provide longer-lasting but not necessarily more protection. Therefore, more Ig is prescribed in high-risk situations where continuous exposure is anticipated (i.e., institutional contacts, travelers to foreign countries).

TABLE 6. Recommendations for Immune Globulin (Ig) Prophylaxis for Hepatitis A

Pre-exposure prophylaxis

Travelers to foreign countries where the risk of acquiring hepatitis A is enhanced due to living conditions, the prevalence of HAV in the area, and the length of stay.

Postexposure prophylaxis

Close personal contact: all household and sexual contacts of persons with hepatitis A.

Day care centers: staff, attendees, and all members of households whose diapered children attend.

Schools, preschools, and institutions for custodial care: not generally warranted unless an institutional- or classroom-centered outbreak is identified.

Hospitals: not routinely indicated for hospital personnel. Instead, sound hygienic practices should be emphasized.

Offices and factories: not indicated under usual working conditions for persons exposed to a fellow worker with hepatitis A.

Common-source exposure: not warranted once cases have begun to appear. When a foodhandler with hepatitis A is identified, Ig should be given to other kitchen employees and may be considered for patrons if (a) the infected person is directly involved in handling foods that are not to be cooked, or handle cooked foods before they are eaten; (b) the hygienic practices of the worker are deficient; and (c) consumers can be identified and treated within 2 weeks of exposure.

proving their public sanitation systems may begin to experience epidemics as infection is delayed to adulthood, where symptomatic disease is more common. A recent epidemic affecting 292,000 people in Shanghai is a good example of this phenomenon.[352] By evoking an active immune response after administration of an infectious agent or one of its component parts, epidemics and sporadic cases of HAV might be prevented or ameliorated. Groups that might benefit from a more durable level of immunity achieved through vaccination include the military, children and staff of day care centers (or the parents of the children), male homosexuals, travelers to endemic areas, the patients and staff of closed institutions, and consumers of bivalve mollusks (oysters, clams, mussels).

Inactivated Vaccines. In 1978, Provost and Hilleman described the development of a formalin-treated HAV vaccine produced from infected marmoset liver that protected marmosets against subsequent HAV challenge.[353] These promising results stimulated further research that culminated in the successful propagation of HAV in cell culture,[31] a source more appropriate for vaccine production. Since then, several investigators have produced crude cell lysates of HAV-infected cells that have been inactivated with formalin or β-propiolactone. Binn, Sjogren, and their coworkers[354–356] have extensively characterized prototype formalin-inactivated vaccines prepared in B-SC-1 cells and in human diploid MRC-5 cells after infection with the HAV strain HM-175. Monkeys developed neutralizing antibody to several HAV strains from diverse geographic areas and resisted challenge to live HAV. No excretion of virus was observed in these animals either after vaccination or the live virus challenge. Eight human volunteers immunized with the vaccine derived from infected MRC-5 cells developed high titers ($\geq$1:160) of neutralizing antibodies to HAV that persisted for more than 12 months. Additional inactivated vaccines have been prepared from purified material. These studies confirm the feasibility of producing an inactivated vaccine. Improved cell culture techniques and the use of microcarriers or other specialized apparatus will be evaluated for their ability to increase virus yield.[83,357,358]

Attenuated Vaccines. HAV strains were adapted to growth in cell culture and, in the process, sometimes became attenuated.[103,294,359–362] These attenuated HAV variants have induced immune responses in primates, often without biochemical evidence of hepatitis or histopathologic changes in liver tissue. When hepatitis occurs, fecal antigen can occasionally be detected transiently. Challenge with wild-type HAV does not result in infection.

At least two of these variants have been administered to humans[361] by Provost and coworkers. Variant F was immunogenic in 17 of 20 humans but caused biochemical evidence of mild hepatitis in 5 subjects. Variant F′ was more attenuated in that none of 12 individuals developed biochemical evidence of hepatitis. Nevertheless, all but one of the human subjects made antibodies. Development of a safe and efficacious attenuated HAV vaccine is feasible but will require a better understanding of the interrelationship that exists between the host, the virus, and the route of inoculation.

Molecular Engineering and Subunit Vaccines. Hughes and Stanton isolated microgram quantities of HAV proteins VP1, VP2, and VP3 by electroelution from SDS polyacrylamide gels.[63] Neutralizing antibody was produced in animals inoculated with VP1 or VP3 but not with VP2. However, antibody titers were significantly lower than those observed in experimentally infected animals. Attempts to produce highly immunogenic proteins from cloned HAV cDNA have been disappointing, probably because antigenic determinants are conformationally expressed on the intact virion. Antibodies against recombinant constructs of VP1 generally do not exhibit neutralizing activity, although the proteins react with anti-HAV.[363–365] Conversely, Balayan and colleagues have elicited high titers of neutralizing anti-HAV in selected animals using similar constructs.[366] A combined immunization using synthetic VP1 epitopes of poliovirus type 1 followed by a subimmunogenic injection of purified HAV has resulted in the development of neutralizing antibodies without an IgM response.[367] Whether subunit vaccines, prepared by recombinant DNA technology, will play a role in HAV immunization efforts remains to be determined.

REFERENCES

1. Zuckerman AJ. The history of viral hepatitis from antiquity to the present. In: Viral Hepatitis: Laboratory and Clinical Science. Deinhardt F, Deinhardt J, eds. New York: Marcel Dekker; 1983:3–32.
2. Weil A. Uber eine eigentumliche, mit Milztumor. Ikterus und Nephritis einhergehende, akute Infections-Krankeit. Dtsch Arch Klin Med. 1886;39:209–32.
3. Cockayne EA. Catarrhal jaundice, sporadic and epidemic and its relation to acute yellow atrophy of the liver. Q J Med. 1912;6:1–28.
4. Purcell RH, Ticehurst JR. Enterically transmitted non-A, non-B hepatitis: Epidemiology and clinical characteristics. In: Zuckerman AJ, ed. Viral Hepatitis and Liver Disease. New York: Alan R Liss Inc; 1988:131–37.
5. Blumer G. Infectious jaundice in the United States. JAMA. 1923;81:353–58.
6. Havens WP, Jr. Properties of the etiologic agent of infectious hepatitis. Proc Soc Exp Biol Med. 1945;58:203–4.
7. Neefe JR, Gellis SS, Stokes J, Jr. Homologous serum hepatitis and infectious (epidemic) hepatitis: Studies in volunteers bearing on immunological and other characteristics of the etiological agents. Am J Med. 1946;1:3–22.
8. Murray R. Viral hepatitis. Bull NY Acad Med. 1955;31:341–58.
9. Krugman S, Giles JP, Hammond J. Infectious hepatitis: Evidence for two distinctive clinical, epidemiological, and immunological types of infection. JAMA. 1967;200:365–73.
10. Voegt H. Zur aetiologie der hepatitis epidemica. Munch Med Wochenschr. 1942;89:76–9.
11. Paul JR, Havens WP, Sabin AB, et al. Transmission experiments in serum jaundice and infectious hepatitis. JAMA. 1945;128:911–15.
12. Havens WP, Jr. The etiology of infectious hepatitis. JAMA. 1947;134:653–55.
13. Medical Research Council. Infective hepatitis: Studies in East Anglia during the period 1943–47. London: HMSO; Special Report Series, No. 273.
14. MacCallum FO, Bradley WH, van Rooyen CE, et al. Infective hepatitis and allied conditions. In: Cope Z, ed. History of the Second World War, Medicine and Pathology. vol. 2. London: HMSO; 1952:257–67.
15. Havens WP, Jr. Viral hepatitis. Postgrad Med J. 1963;39:212–23.
16. Boggs JD, Melnick JL, Conrad ME, et al. Viral hepatitis: Clinical and tissue culture studies. JAMA. 1970;214:1041–46.
17. Krugman S, Giles JP. Viral hepatitis: New light on an old disease. JAMA. 1970;212:1019–29.
18. Melnick JL, Boggs JD. Human volunteer and tissue culture studies of viral hepatitis. Can Med Assoc J. 1972;106:461–67.
19. Havens WP. Experiment in cross immunity between infectious hepatitis and homologous serum jaundice. Proc Soc Exp Biol Med. 1945;59:148–50.
20. Neefe JR, Stokes J, Gellis SS. Homologous serum hepatitis and infectious

(epidemic) hepatitis: Experimental study of immunity and cross immunity in volunteers. Am J Med Sci. 1945;210:561–75.
21. Neefe JR, Stokes J, Jr, Reinhold JG. Oral administration to volunteers of feces from patients with homologous serum hepatitis and infectious (epidemic) hepatitis. Am J Med Sci. 1945;210:29–32.
22. Havens WP, Jr. Period of infectivity of patients with homologous serum jaundice and routes of infection in this disease. J Exp Med. 1946;83:441–47.
23. Stokes J, Berk JE, Malamut LL, et al. The carrier state of viral hepatitis. JAMA. 1954;154:1059–65.
24. Neefe RJ, Norris RF, Reinhold JG, et al. Carriers of hepatitis virus in the blood and viral hepatitis in whole blood recipients: I. Studies on donors suspected as carriers of hepatitis virus and as sources of post-transfusion viral hepatitis. JAMA. 1954;154:1066–71.
25. Deinhardt F, Holmes AW, Capps RB, et al. Studies on the transmission of human viral hepatitis to marmoset monkeys. I. Transmission of disease, serial passages, and description of liver lesions. J Exp Med. 1967;125:673–88.
26. Holmes AW, Wolfe L, Rosenblate H, et al. Hepatitis in marmosets: Induction of disease with coded specimens from a human volunteer study. Science. 1969;165:816–17.
27. Holmes AW, Wolfe L, Deinhardt F, et al. Transmission of human hepatitis to marmosets: Further coded studies. J Infect Dis. 1971;124:520–21.
28. Feinstone SM, Kapikian AZ, Purcell RH. Hepatitis A: Detection by immune electron microscopy of a viruslike antigen associated with acute illness. Science. 1973;182:1026–28.
29. Maynard JE, Bradley DW, Gravelle CR, et al. Preliminary studies of hepatitis A in chimpanzees. J Infect Dis. 1975;131:194–96.
30. Dienstag JL, Feinstone SM, Purcell RH, et al. Experimental infection of chimpanzees with hepatitis A virus. J Infect Dis. 1975;132:532–45.
31. Provost PJ, Hilleman MR. Propagation of human hepatitis A virus in cell culture in vitro. Proc Soc Exp Biol Med. 1979;160:213–21.
32. Siegl G. Structure and biology of hepatitis A virus. In: Szmuness W, Alter HJ, Maynard JE, eds. Viral Hepatitis. Philadelphia: Franklin Institute Press; 1982:13–20.
33. Provost PJ, Wolanski BS, Miller WJ, et al. Physical, chemical and morphologic dimensions of human hepatitis A virus strain CR326. Proc Soc Exp Biol Med. 1975;148:532–39.
34. Moritsugo Y, Dienstag JL, Valdesuso J, et al. Purification of hepatitis A antigen from feces and detection of antigen and antibody by immune adherence hemagglutination. Infect Immun. 1976;13:898–908.
35. Siegl G, Frosner GG. Characterization and classification of virus particles associated with hepatitis A. I. Size, density, and sedimentation. J Virol. 1978;26:40–7.
36. Bradley DW, Hornbeck CL, Gravelle CR, et al. CsCl banding of hepatitis A-associated virus-like particles. J Infect Dis. 1975;131:304–6.
37. Schulman AN, Dienstag JL, Jackson DR, et al. Hepatitis A antigen particles in liver, bile, and stool of chimpanzees. J Infect Dis. 1976;134:80–4.
38. Bradley DW, Fields HA, McCaustland KA, et al. Biochemical and biophysical characterization of light and heavy density hepatitis A virus particles: Evidence that HAV is an RNA virus. J Med Virol. 1978;2:175–87.
39. Bradley DW, McCaustland KA, Schroeder MT, et al. Multiple buoyant densities of hepatitis A virus in cesium chloride gradients. J Med Virol. 1977;1:219–26.
40. Coulepis AG, Locarnini SA, Westaway EG, et al. Biophysical and biochemical characterization of hepatitis A virus. Intervirology. 1982;18:107–27.
41. Lemon SM, Jansen RW, Newbold JE. Infectious hepatitis A virus particles produced in cell culture consist of three distinct types with different buoyant densities in CsCl. J Virol. 1985;54:78–85.
42. Siegl G, Frosner GG, Gauss-Mueller V, et al. The physicochemical properties of infectious hepatitis A virions. J Gen Virol. 1981;57:331–41.
43. Feinstone SM, Kapikian AZ, Gerin JL, et al. Buoyant density of the hepatitis A virus-like particle in cesium chloride. J Virol. 1974;13:1412–14.
44. Bradley DW, Gravell CR, Cook EH, et al. Cyclic excretion of hepatitis A virus in experimentally infected chimpanzees. J Med Virol. 1977;1:133–38.
45. Tratschin JD, Siegl G, Frösner GG, et al. Characterization and classification of virus particles associated with hepatitis A. III. Structural proteins. J Virol. 1981;38:151–56.
46. Dienstag JL, Schulman AN, Gerety RJ, et al. Hepatitis A antigen isolated from liver and stool: Immunologic comparison of antisera prepared in guinea pigs. J Immunol. 1976;117:876–81.
47. Feinstone SM, Moritsugu Y, Shih JW-K, et al. Characterization of HAV. In: Vyas GN, Cohen SN, Schmid R, eds. Viral Hepatitis: Etiology, Epidemiology, Pathogenesis and Prevention. Philadelphia: Franklin Institute Press; 1978:41–8.
48. Siegl G, Frosner GG. Characterization and classification of virus particles associated with hepatitis A. II. Type and configuration of nucleic acid. J Virol. 1978;26:48–53.
49. Coulepis AG, Tannock GA, Locarnini SA, et al. Evidence that the genome of hepatitis A virus consists of single-stranded RNA. J Virol. 1981;37:473–77.
50. Coulepis AG, Locarnini SA, Ferris AA, et al. The polypeptides of hepatitis A virus. Intervirology. 1978;10:24–31.
51. Coulepis AG, Locarnini SA, Gust ID. Iodination of hepatitis A virus reveals a fourth structural polypeptide. J Virol. 1980;35:572–74.
52. Ticehurst JR, Racaniello VR, Baroudy BM, et al. Molecular cloning and characterization of hepatitis A virus cDNA. Proc Natl Acad Sci USA. 1983;80:5885–89.
53. Anderson DA, Locarnini SA, Ross BC, et al. Single-cycle growth kinetics of hepatitis A virus in BSC-1 cells. In: Brinton MA, Rueckert RR, eds. Positive Strand RNA Viruses. New York: Alan R. Liss: 1987:497–507.
54. Cohen JI, Rosenblum B, Feinstone S, et al. Use of infectious hepatitis A virus cDNA to study viral attenuation. In: Chanock RM, Lerner RA, Brown F, Ginsburg H, eds. Modern Approaches to New Vaccines Including Prevention of AIDS. New York: Cold Spring Harbor Laboratory: 1988:133–7.
55. Cohen JI, Rosenblum B, Ticehurst JR, et al. Complete nucleotide sequence of an attenuated hepatitis A virus: Comparison with wild-type virus. Proc Natl Acad Sci USA. 1987;84:2497–501.
56. Gauss-Müller V, von der Helm K, Deinhardt F. Translation in vitro of hepatitis A virus RNA. Virology. 1984;137:182–84.
57. Anderson BN, Ross BC, Gust ID. Sequence changes in capsid proteins of high-passage hepatitis A virus HM175. In: Zuckerman AJ, ed. Viral Hepatitis and Liver Diseases. New York: Alan R. Liss: 1988:55–8.
58. Linemeyer DL, Menke JG, Martin-Gallardo A, et al. Molecular cloning and partial sequencing of hepatitis A viral cDNA. J Virol. 1985;54:247–55.
59. Ovchinnikov IA, Sverdlov ED, Tsarev SA, et al. Sequence of 3372 nucleotide units of RNA of the hepatitis A virus, coding the capsid VP4-VP1 and some non-structural proteins. Dokl Akad Nauk SSSR. 1985;285:1014–18.
60. Robertson BH, Brown VK, Bradley DW. Nucleic acid sequence of the VP1 region of attenuated MS-1 hepatitis A virus. Virus Res. 1987;8:309–16.
61. Venuti A, Di Russo C, Del Grosso N, et al. Isolation and molecular cloning of a fast-growing strain of human hepatitis A virus from its double-stranded replicative form. J Virol. 1985;56:579–88.
62. Gauss-Müller V, Lottspeich E, Deinhardt F. Characterization of hepatitis A virus structural proteins. Virology. 1986;155:732–36.
63. Hughes JV, Stanton LW. Isolation and immunizations with hepatitis A viral structural proteins: Induction of antiprotein, antiviral, and neutralizing responses. J Virol. 1985;55:395–401.
64. Siegl G. The biochemistry of hepatitis A virus. In: Gerety RJ, ed. Hepatitis A. New York: Academic Press; 1984:9–32.
65. Wheeler CM, Robertson BH, Van Nest G, et al. Structure of the hepatitis A virion: Peptide mapping of the capsid region. J Virol. 1986;58:307–13.
66. Arnold E, Luo M, Vriend G, et al. Implications of the picornavirus capsid structure for polyprotein processing. Proc Natl Acad Sci USA. 1987;84:21–5.
67. Gust ID, Feinstone SM. Hepatitis A. Boca Raton, FL: CRC Press; 1988.
68. Weitz M, Baroudy BM, Maloy WL, et al. Detection of a genome-linked protein (VPg) of hepatitis A virus and its comparison with other picornaviral VPgs. J Virol. 1986;60:124–30.
69. Lemon SM. Type A viral hepatitis: New developments in an old disease. N Engl J Med. 1985;313:1059–67.
70. Smith TJ, Kremer MJ, Luo M, et al. The site of attachment in human rhinovirus 14 for antiviral agents that inhibit uncoating. Science. 1986;233:1286–93.
71. Widell A. Hepatitis A. Epidemiological and Virological Studies (Doctoral thesis). Malmö, Sweden: University of Lund; 1988.
72. Lemon SM, Binn LN. Antigenic relatedness of two strains of hepatitis A virus determined by cross-neutralization. Infect Immun. 1983;42:418–20.
73. Lemon SM, Chao S-F, Jansen RW, et al. Genomic heterogeneity among human and non-human strains of hepatitis A virus. J Virol. 1987;61:735–42.
74. Siegl G. Virology of hepatitis A. In: Zuckerman AJ, ed. Viral Hepatitis and Liver Disease. New York: Alan R Liss; 1988:3–7.
75. Zahn J, Vallbracht A, Flehmig B. Hepatitis A virus in cell culture. V. Neutralizing antibodies against hepatitis A virus. Med Microbiol Immunol. 1984;173:9–17.
76. Woodson RD, Clinton JJ. Hepatitis prophylaxis abroad: Effectiveness of immune serum globulin in protecting Peace Corps volunteers. JAMA. 1969;209:1053–8.
77. Conrad ME, US Army Medical Research and Development Command Immunization Team. Prophylactic gamma globulin for prevention of endemic hepatitis: Effects of US gamma globulin upon the incidence of viral hepatitis and other infectious diseases in US soldiers abroad (A cooperative study). Arch Intern Med. 1971;128:723–38.
78. Stapleton JT, Lemon SM. Neutralization escape mutants define a dominant immunogenic neutralization site on hepatitis A virus. J Virol. 1987;61:491–98.
79. Ticehurst J, Cohen JI, Feinstone SM, et al. Replication of hepatitis A virus: New ideas from studies with cloned cDNA. In: Semler BL, Ehrenfeld E, eds. Molecular Aspects of Picornavirus Infection and Detection. Washington, DC: American Society for Microbiology; (In press).
80. Hughes JV, Stanton LW, Tomassini JE, et al. Neutralizing monoclonal antibodies to hepatitis A virus: Partial localization of a neutralizing antigenic site. J Virol. 1984;52:465–73.
81. Arankalle VA, Ticehurst J, Sreenivasan MA, et al. Etiologic association of a virus-like particle with enterically-transmitted non-A, non-B hepatitis. Lancet. 1988;1:550–54.
82. Lemon SM, Binn LN, Marchwicki RH. Radioimmunofocus assay for quantitation of hepatitis A virus in cell cultures. J Clin Microbiol. 1983;17:834–39.
83. Siegl G, de Chastonay J, Kronauer G. Propagation and assay of hepatitis A virus in vitro. J Virol Methods. 1984;9:53–67.
84. Frosner GG. Zuchtung des Hepatitis A Virus in Gewebekultur: Moglichkeit zur Virusproducktion fur Impfstoffe und Testzwecke, zur Untersuchung von

Patienten auf Infektiositat und zur Prufung von Desinfektionsmitteln. Off Gesundheitswes. 1982;44:370–73.
85. Parry JV, Mortimer PP. The heat sensitivity of hepatitis A virus determined by a simple tissue culture method. J Med Virol. 1984;14:277–83.
86. Provost PJ, Ittensohn OL, Villarejos VM, et al. Etiologic relationship of marmoset-propagated CR326 hepatitis A virus to hepatitis in man. Proc Soc Exp Biol Med. 1973;142:1257–67.
87. Siegl G, Weitz M, Kronauer G. Stability of hepatitis A virus. Intervirology. 1984;22:218–26.
88. McCaustland KA, Bond WW, Bradley DW, et al. Survival of hepatitis A virus in feces after drying and storage for one month. J Clin Microbiol. 1982;16:957–58.
89. Sobsey MD, Shields PA, Hauchman FS, et al. Survival and persistence of hepatitis A virus in environmental samples. In: Zuckerman AJ, ed. Viral Hepatitis and Liver Disease. New York: Alan R Liss; 1988;121–24.
90. Krugman S, Giles JP, Hammond J. Hepatitis virus: Effect of heat on the infectivity and antigenicity of the MS-1 and MS-2 strain. J Infect Dis. 1970;122:423–36.
91. Peterson DA, Hurley TR, Hoff JC, et al. Effect of chlorine treatment on infectivity of hepatitis A virus. Appl Environ Microbiol. 1983;45:223–27.
92. Neefe JR, Stokes J, Jr, Baty JB, et al. Disinfection of water containing causative agent of infectious (epidemic) hepatitis. JAMA. 1945;128:1076–80.
93. Scheid R, Deinhardt F, Frosner G, et al. Inactivation of hepatitis A and B viruses and risk of iatrogenic transmission. In: Szmuness W, Alter HJ, Maynard JE, eds. Viral Hepatitis—1981 International Symposium. Philadelphia: Franklin Institute Press; 1982:627–28.
94. Passagot J, Biziagos E, Crance JM, et al. Effect of antiviral substances on hepatitis A virus replication. In: Zuckerman AJ, ed. Viral Hepatitis and Liver Disease. New York: Alan R Liss; 1988:953–55.
95. Widell A, Hansson BG, Oberg B, et al. Influence of twenty potentially antiviral substances on in vitro multiplication of hepatitis A virus. Antiviral Res. 1986;6:103–12.
96. Hillis WD. An outbreak of infectious hepatitis among chimpanzee handlers at a United States Air Force base. Am J Hyg. 1961;73:316–28.
97. Hillis WD. Viral hepatitis associated with sub-human primates. Transfusion. 1963;3:445–53.
98. Mosley JW, Reinhardt HP, Hassler FR. Chimpanzee-associated hepatitis: An outbreak in Oklahoma. JAMA. 1967;199:695–97.
99. Lorenz D, Barker L, Stevens D, et al. Hepatitis in the marmoset: *Saguinus mystax*. Proc Soc Exp Biol Med. 1970;135:348–54.
100. Mascoli CC, Ittensohn DL, Villarejos VM, et al. Recovery of hepatitis agents in the marmoset from human cases occurring in Costa Rica. Proc Soc Exp Biol Med. 1973;142:276–82.
101. Provost PJ, Villarejos VM, Hilleman MR. Suitability of the Rufiventer marmoset as a host animal for human hepatitis A virus. Proc Soc Exp Biol Med. 1977;155:283–6.
102. Purcell RH, Dienstag JL. Experimental hepatitis A virus infection. In: Oda T, ed. Hepatitis Viruses. Tokyo: Univ of Tokyo Press; 1978:3–12.
103. Purcell RH, Feinstone SM, Ticehurst JR, et al. Hepatitis A virus. In: Vyas GN, Dienstag JL, Hoofnagle JH, eds. Viral Hepatitis and Liver Disease. Orlando, FL: Grune & Stratton; 1984:9–22.
104. Maynard JE, Lorenz D, Bradley DW, et al. Review of infectivity studies in nonhuman primates with virus-like particles associated with MS-1 hepatitis. Am J Med Sci. 1975;270:81–5.
105. LeDuc JW, Lemon SM, Keenan CM, et al. Experimental infection of the new world owl monkey (*Aotus trivirgatus*) with hepatitis A virus. Infect Immun. 1983;40:766–72.
106. Lemon SM, LeDuc JW, Binn LN, et al. Transmission of hepatitis A virus among recently captured Panamanian owl monkeys. J Med Virol. 1982;10:25–36.
107. Andzhaparidze AG, Kazachkov YuA, Balayan MS, et al. Hepatitis A in *Macaca fascicularis* and *Macaca arctoides* infected with the Java monkey-55 strain of hepatitis A virus. Vopr Virus. 1987;2:440–8.
108. Burnell JM, Dawborn JK, Epstein RB, et al. Acute hepatic coma treated by cross-circulation or exchange transfusion. N Engl J Med. 1967;276:935–43.
109. Mao JS, Go YY, Huang HY, et al. Susceptibility of monkeys to human hepatitis A virus. J Infect Dis. 1981;144:55–60.
110. Bearcroft WGC. Studies on the transmission of the agent of infectious hepatitis to patas monkeys. J Med Microbiol. 1968;1:1–21.
111. Frosner GG, Deinhardt F, Scheid R, et al. Propagation of human hepatitis A virus in a hepatoma cell line. Infection. 1979;7:303–5.
112. Alexander JJ, Macnab G, Saunders R. Studies on in vitro production of hepatitis A surface antigen by a human hepatoma cell line. Perspect Virol. 1978;10:103–17.
113. Daemer RJ, Feinstone SM, Gust ID, et al. Propagation of human hepatitis A virus in African green monkey kidney cell culture: Primary isolation and serial passage. Infect Immun. 1981;32:388–93.
114. Binn LN, Lemon SM, Marchwicki RH, et al. Primary isolation and serial passage of hepatitis A virus strains in primate cell cultures. J Clin Microbiol. 1984;20:28–33.
115. Flehmig B. Hepatitis A-virus in cell culture. I. Propagation of different hepatitis A-virus isolates in a fetal rhesus monkey kidney cell line (Frhk-4). Med Microbiol Immunol. 1980;168:239–48.
116. Flehmig B. Hepatitis A virus in cell culture. II. Growth characteristics of hepatitis A virus in Frhk-4/R cells. Med Microbiol Immunol 1981;170:73–81.
117. Locarnini SA, Coulepis AG, Westaway EG, et al. Restricted replication of human hepatitis A virus in cell culture: Intracellular biochemical studies. J Virol. 1981;37:216–25.
118. Asher LVS, Binn LN, Marchwicki RH. Demonstration of hepatitis A virus in cell culture by electron microscopy with immunoperoxidase staining. J Virol Methods. 1987;15:323–8.
119. Asher LVS, Binn LN, Marchwicki RH, et al. Electron microscopy and immunoelectron microscopy of hepatitis A virus in cell culture. In: Zuckerman AJ, ed. Viral Hepatitis and Liver Disease. New York: Alan R Liss; 1988:19–23.
120. Kiernan RE, Marshall JA, Coulepis AG, et al. Cellular changes associated with persistent hepatitis A infection in vitro. Arch Virol. 1987;94:81–95.
121. Balayan MS, Andzhaparidze AG, Tol'skaia EA, et al. Possibility of reproducing hepatitis A virus infection in cell systems. Vopr Virus. 1979;6:675–6.
122. Wu S, Ju L, Shao H, et al. Strain of hepatitis A virus causing cytopathic effects isolated in A549 cell line. Chinese Med J. 1986;99:387–92.
123. Cromeans T, Fields HA, Sobsey MD. Kinetic studies of a rapidly replicating, cytopathic hepatitis A virus. In: Zuckerman AJ, ed. Viral Hepatitis and Liver Disease. New York: Alan R Liss; 1988:24–6.
124. Anderson DA. Cytopathology, plaque assay, and heat inactivation of hepatitis A virus strain HM-175. J Med Virol. 1987;22:35–44.
125. Anderson DA, Locarnini SA, Gust ID. Replication of hepatitis A virus. In: Zuckerman AJ, ed. Viral Hepatitis and Liver Disease. New York: Alan R Liss; 1988:8–11.
126. Nasser AM, Metcalf TG. Production of cytopathology in FRhK-4 cells by BS-C-1-passaged hepatitis A virus. Appl Environ Microbiol. 1987;53:2967–71.
127. Mathiesen LR, Feinstone SM, Purcell RH, et al. Detection of hepatitis A antigen by immunofluorescence. Infect Immun. 1977;18:524–30.
128. Mathiesen LR, Drucker J, Lorenz D, et al. Localization of hepatitis A antigen in marmoset organs during acute infection with hepatitis A virus. J Infect Dis. 1978;138:369–77.
129. Franklin RM, Rosner J. Localization of ribonucleic acid synthesis in mengovirus-infected L-cells. Biochem Biophys Acta. 1962;55:240–1.
130. Franklin RM, Baltimore D. Patterns of macromolecular synthesis in normal and virus-infected mammalian cells. Cold Spring Harbor Symposia on Quant Biol. 1962;27:175–95.
131. Dales S, Eggers HJ, Tamm I, et al. Electron microscopic study of the formation of poliovirus. Virology. 1965;26:379–89.
132. Feinstone SM, Purcell RH. New methods for the serodiagnosis of hepatitis A. Gastroenterology. 1980;78:1092–4.
133. Szmuness W, Dienstag JL, Purcell RH, et al. The prevalence of antibody to hepatitis A antigen in various parts of the world. Am J Epidemiol. 1977;106:392–8.
134. Hollinger FB, Khan NC, Oefinger PE, et al. Posttransfusion hepatitis type A. JAMA. 1983;250:2313–7.
135. Gust ID. Comparison of the epidemiology of hepatitis A and B. In: Szmuness W, Alter HJ, Maynard JE, eds. Viral Hepatitis—1981 International Symposium. Philadelphia: Franklin Institute Press; 1982:129–43.
136. Maynard JE. Infectious hepatitis at Fort Yukon, Alaska—report of an outbreak, 1960–61. Am J Public Health. 1963;53:31–9.
137. Skinhoj P, McNair A, Andersen ST. Hepatitis and hepatitis B-antigen in Greenland. Am J Epidemiol. 1974;99:50–7.
138. Skinhoj P, Mikkelsen F, Hollinger FB. Hepatitis A in Greenland: Importance of specific antibody testing in epidemiologic surveillance. Am J Epidemiol. 1977;105:140–7.
139. Wong DC, Purcell RH, Rosen L. Prevalence of antibody to hepatitis A and hepatitis B viruses in selected populations of the South Pacific. Am J Epidemiol. 1979;110:227–36.
140. Black FL, Hierholzer WJ, de Pinheiro F, et al. Evidence for persistence of infectious agents in isolated human population. Am J Epidemiol. 1974; 100:230–50.
141. Dienstag JL, Alaama A, Mosley JW, et al. Etiology of sporadic hepatitis B surface antigen-negative hepatitis. Ann Intern Med. 1977;87:1–6.
142. Hoofnagle JH, Ponzetto A, Mathiesen LR, et al. Serological diagnosis of acute viral hepatitis. Dig Dis Sci. 1985;30:1022–7.
143. Centers for Disease Control. Summary—cases of specified notifiable diseases, United States. MMWR. 1989;37:797.
144. Dienstag JL, Szmuness W, Stevens CE. Hepatitis A virus infection: New insights from seroepidemiologic studies. J Infect Dis. 1978;137:328–40.
145. Koff R, Chalmers T, Culhane PO, et al. Underreporting of viral hepatitis. Gastroenterology. 1973;64:1194–5.
146. Marier R. The reporting of communicable diseases. Am J Epidemiol. 1977;105:587–90.
147. Centers for Disease Control: Hepatitis Surveillance Report Number 48, 1982.
148. Centers for Disease Control. Hepatitis A outbreak in a day-care center—Texas. MMWR. 1980;29:565–7.
149. Hadler SC, Webster HM, Erben JJ, et al. Hepatitis A in day-care centers: A community-wide assessment. N Engl J Med. 1980;302:1222–7.
150. Corey L, Holmes KK. Sexual transmission of hepatitis A in homosexual men: Incidence and mechanism. N Engl J Med. 1980;302:435–8.
151. Fawaz KA, Matloff DS. Viral hepatitis in homosexual men. Gastroenterology. 1981;81:537–8.
152. Krugman S, Ward R, Giles JP. The natural history of infectious hepatitis. Am J Med. 1962;32:717–28.
153. Havens WP, Ward R, Drill VA, et al. Experimental production of hepatitis by feeding icterogenic materials. Proc Soc Exp Biol Med. 1944;57:206–8.

154. Giles JP, Liebhaber H, Krugman S, et al. Early viremia and viruria in infectious hepatitis. Virology. 1964;24:107–8.
155. Findlay GM, Willcox RR. Transmission of infective hepatitis by faeces and virus. Lancet. 1945;1:212.
156. Krugman S, Ward R, Giles JP, et al. Infectious hepatitis: Detection of virus during the incubation period and in clinically inapparent infection. N Engl J Med. 1959;261:729–34.
157. Rakela J, Mosley JW. Fecal excretion of hepatitis A virus in humans. J Infect Dis. 1977;135:933–8.
158. Ward R, Krugman S, Giles JP, et al. Infectious hepatitis: Studies of its natural history and prevention. N Engl J Med. 1958;258:407–16.
159. Knight V, Drake ME, Belden EA, et al. Characteristics of spread of infectious hepatitis in schools and households in an epidemic in a rural area. Am J Hyg. 1954;59:1–16.
160. Batten PJ, Runte VE, Skinner HG. Infectious hepatitis: Infectiousness during the presymptomatic phase of the disease. Am J Hyg. 1963;77:129–36.
161. Mosley JW, Smither WW. Infectious hepatitis: Report of an outbreak probably caused by drinking water. N Engl J Med. 1957;257:590–5.
162. Leger RT, Boyer KM, Pattison CP, et al. Hepatitis A: Report of the common-source outbreak with recovery of a possible etiologic agent. I. Epidemioilogic studies. J Infect Dis. 1975;131:163–6.
163. Dull HB, Doege TC, Mosley JW. An outbreak of infectious hepatitis associated with a school cafeteria. South Med J. 1963;56:475–80.
164. Denes AE, Smith JL, Hindman SH, et al. Foodborne hepatitis A infection: A report of two urban restaurant-associated outbreaks. Am J Epidemiol. 1977;105:156–62.
165. Deinhardt F, Peterson D, Cross G, et al. Hepatitis in marmosets. Am J Med Sci. 1975;270:73–80.
166. Havens WP. Period of infectivity of patients with experimentally induced infectious hepatitis. J Exp Med. 1946;83:251–8.
167. Routenberg JA, Dienstag JL, Harrison WO, et al. A food borne outbreak of hepatitis A: Clinical and laboratory features of acute and protracted illness. Am J Med Sci. 1979;278:123–37.
168. Dienstag JL, Feinstone SM, Kapikian AZ, et al. Faecal shedding of hepatitis-A antigen. Lancet. 1975;1:765–7.
169. Frosner GG, Overby LR, Flehmig B, et al. Seroepidemiological investigation of patients and family contacts in an epidemic of hepatitis A. J Med Virol. 1977;1:163–73.
170. Dienstag JL, Routenberg JA, Purcell RH, et al. Foodhandler-associated outbreak of hepatitis type A: An immune electron microscopic study. Ann Intern Med. 1975;83:647–50.
171. Flehmig B, Frank H, Frosner GG, et al. Hepatitis A-virus particles in stools of patients from a natural hepatitis outbreak in Germany. Med Microbiol Immunol (Berl). 1977;163:209–14.
172. Hopkins R, Scott TG. Hepatitis-A antigen in Edinburgh. Lancet. 1976;2:206.
173. Locarnini SA, Gust ID, Ferris AA, et al. A prospective study of acute viral hepatitis with particular reference to hepatitis A. Bull WHO. 1976;54:199–206.
174. Mao JS, Yu PH, Ding ZS, et al. Patterns of shedding of hepatitis A virus antigen in feces and of antibody responses in patients with naturally acquired type A hepatitis. J Infect Dis. 1980;142:654–9.
175. Coulepis AG, Locarnini SA, Lehmann NI, et al. Detection of hepatitis A virus in the feces of patients with naturally acquired infections. J Infect Dis. 1980;141:151–6.
176. Hall WT, Bradley DW, Madden DL, et al. Comparison of sensitivity of radioimmunoassay and immune electron microscopy for detecting hepatitis A antigen in fecal extracts. Proc Soc Exp Biol Med. 1977;155:193–8.
177. Hollinger FB, Bradley DW, Dreesman GR, et al. Detection of viral hepatitis type A. Am J Clin Pathol. 1976;65:854–65.
178. Neefe JR, Stokes J, Jr, Garber RS, et al. Studies on the relationship of the hepatitis virus to persistent symptoms, disability, and hepatic disturbance ("chronic hepatitis syndrome") following acute infectious hepatitis. J Clin Invest. 1947;26:329–38.
179. Ashley A. Use of gamma globulin for control of infectious hepatitis in an institution for the mentally retarded. N Engl J Med. 1955;252:88–91.
180. Drake ME, Ming C. Gamma globulin in epidemic hepatitis: Comparative value of two dosage levels, apparently near the minimal effective level. JAMA. 1954:155:1302–5.
181. Matthew EB, Dietzman DE, Madden DL, et al. A major epidemic of infectious hepatitis in an institution for the mentally retarded. Am J Epidemiol. 1973;98:199–215.
182. Horstmann DM, Havens WP, Deutsch J. Infectious hepatitis in childhood: Report of two institutional outbreaks and comparison of disease in adults and children. J Pediatr. 1947;30:381–87.
183. Melnick JL, Hollinger FB, Dreesman GR. Recent advances in viral hepatitis. South Med J. 1976;69:468–75, 634–41.
184. Morse LJ, Bryan JW, Hurley JP, et al. The Holy Cross College football team hepatitis outbreak. JAMA. 1972;219:706–8.
185. Mosley JW. Water-borne infectious hepatitis. N Engl J Med. 1959;261:703–8, 748–53.
186. Taylor FB, Eagen JH, Smith HFD Jr, et al. The case for water-borne hepatitis. Am J Public Health. 56:2093–105.
187. Tihen WS, Mailloux JR. A hospital-based outbreak of hepatitis-A—Vermont. MMWR. 1974;23:79–80.
188. Mosley JW. Transmission of viral diseases by drinking water. In: Berg G, ed. Transmission of Viruses by the Water Route. New York: John Wiley and Sons; 1967:5–23.
189. Tucker CB, Owen WH, Farrell RP. Outbreak of infectious hepatitis apparently transmitted through water. South Med J. 1954;47:732–40.
190. Rindge ME, Mason JO, Elsea WR. Infectious hepatitis: Report of an outbreak in a small Connecticut school, due to water-borne transmission. JAMA. 1962;180:33–7.
191. Mosley JW, Schrack WD, Jr, Densham TW, et al. Infectious hepatitis in Clearfield County, Pennsylvania. I. A probable water-borne epidemic. Am J Med. 1959;26:555–8.
192. Poskanzer DC, Beadenkopf WG. Water-borne infectious hepatitis epidemic from a chlorinated municipal supply. Public Health Rep. 1961;76:745–51.
193. Bowen GS, McCarthy MA. Hepatitis A associated with a hardware store water fountain and a contaminated well in Lancaster County, Pennsylvania, 1980. Am J Epidemiol. 1983;117:695–705.
194. Roos B. Hepatitis epidemic conveyed by oysters. Svenska Tkar. 1956;53:989.
195. Mason JO, McLean WR. Infectious hepatitis traced to the consumption of raw oysters: An epidemiologic study. Am J Hyg. 1962;75:90–111.
196. Dougherty WJ, Altman R. Viral hepatitis in New Jersey 1960–61. Am J Med. 1962;32:704–16.
197. Ruddy SJ, Johnson RF, Mosley JW, et al. An epidemic of clam-associated hepatitis. JAMA. 1969;208:649–55.
198. Koff RS, Sear HS. Internal temperature of steamed clams. N Engl J Med. 1967;276:737–9.
199. Portnoy BL, Mackowiak PA, Caraway CT, et al. Oyster-associated hepatitis: Failure of shellfish certification programs to prevent outbreaks. JAMA. 1975;233:1065–75.
200. Dienstag JL, Gust ID, Lucas CR, et al. Mussel-associated viral hepatitis, type A: Serological confirmation. Lancet. 1976;1:561–3.
201. Mackowiak PA, Caraway CT, Portnoy BL. Oyster-associated hepatitis: Lessons from the Louisiana experience. Am J Epidemiol. 1976;103:181–91.
202. Murphy WJ, Petrie LM, Work SD. Outbreak of infectious hepatitis, apparently milk-borne. Am J Public Health. 1946;36:169–73.
203. Raska K, A milk-borne infectious hepatitis epidemic. J Hyg Epidemiol Microb Immunol. 1966;10:413–28.
204. Barker JF, Dienstag JL, Lorenz DE, et al. Serologic and animal inoculation studies of a communal outbreak of viral hepatitis, type A. Am J Med Sci. 1977;274:247–53.
205. Read MR, Bancroft H, Doull JA, et al. Infectious hepatitis—presumably food-borne outbreak. Am J Public Health. 1946;36:367–70.
206. Ballance GA. Epidemic of infective hepatitis in an Oxford college. Br Med J. 1954;1:1071–4.
207. Joseph PR, Millar JD, Henderson DA. An outbreak of hepatitis traced to food contamination. N Engl J Med. 1965;273:188–94.
208. Philip JR, Hamilton TP, Albert TJ, et al. Infectious hepatitis outbreak with mai tai as the vehicle of transmission. Am J Epidemiol. 1973; 97:50–54.
209. Levy BS, Fontaine RE, Smith CA, et al. A large food-borne outbreak of hepatitis A: Possible transmission via oropharyngeal secretions. JAMA. 1975;234:289–94.
210. Meyers JD, Romm FJ, Tihen WS, et al. Food-borne hepatitis A in a general hospital: Epidemiologic study of an outbreak attributed to sandwiches. JAMA. 1975;231:1049–53.
211. Schoenbaum SC, Baker O, Jezek Z. Common-source epidemic of hepatitis due to glazed and iced pastries. Am J Epidemiol. 1976;104:74–80.
212. Eisenstein AB, Aach RD, Jacobsohn W, et al. An epidemic of infectious hepatitis in a general hospital: Probable transmission by contaminated orange juice. JAMA. 1963;185:171–4.
213. MacCallum, FO, Bradley WH. Transmission of infective hepatitis to human volunteers. Lancet. 1944;2:228.
214. Neefe JR, Stokes J, Jr. An epidemic of infectious hepatitis apparently due to a water-borne agent. JAMA. 1945:128:1063–75.
215. Aach RD, Evans J, Losoc J. An epidemic of infectious hepatitis possibly due to airborne transmission. Am J Epidemiol. 1968;87:99–109.
216. Tong MJ, Thursby M, Rakela J, et al. Studies of the maternal-infant transmission of the viruses which cause acute hepatitis. Gastroenterology. 1981;80:999–1004.
217. Boggs JD, Capps RB, Weiss CF, et al. Status report on tissue-culture cultivated hepatitis virus. II. Clinical trials. JAMA. 1961;177:678–82.
218. Francis T, Jr, Frisch AW, Quilligan JJ, Jr. Demonstration of infectious hepatitis virus in presymptomatic period after transfer by transfusion. Proc Soc Exp Biol Med. 1946;61:276–80.
219. Harden AG, Barondess JA, Parker B. Transmission of infectious hepatitis by transfusion of whole blood. N Engl J Med. 1955; 253:923–5.
220. Ward R, Krugman S. Etiology, epidemiology and prevention of viral hepatitis. Prog Med Virol. 1982;4:87–118.
221. Stevens CE, Silbert JA, Miller DR, et al. Serologic evidence of hepatitis A and B virus infections in thalassemia patients: A retrospective study. Transfusion. 1978;18:356–60.
222. Szmuness W, Dienstag JL, Purcell RH, et al. Hepatitis A and hemodialysis: A seroepidemiologic study in 15 U.S. centers. Ann Intern Med. 1977;87:8–12.
223. Feinstone SM, Kapikian AZ, Purcell RH, et al. Transfusion-associated hepatitis not due to viral hepatitis type A or B. N Engl J Med. 1975;292:767–70.
224. Knodell RG, Conrad ME, Dienstag JL, et al. Etiologic spectrum of post-transfusion-associated hepatitis. Gastroenterology. 1975;69:1278–85.

225. Alter HJ, Purcell RH, Holland PV, et al. Clinical and serological analysis of transfusion-associated hepatitis. Lancet. 1975;2:838–41.
226. Dienstag JL, Feinstone SM, Purcell RH, et al. Non-A, non-B post-transfusion hepatitis. Lancet. 1977;1:560–2.
227. Hollinger FB, Mosley JW, Szmuness W, et al. Non-A, non-B hepatitis following blood transfusion: Risk factors associated with donor characteristics. In: Szmuness W, Alter HJ, Maynard JE, eds. Viral Hepatitis—1981 International Symposium, Philadelphia: Franklin Institute Press; 1982:361–76.
228. Barbara JAJ, Howell DR, Briggs M, et al. Post-transfusion hepatitis A. Lancet. 1982;1:738.
229. Hollinger FB, Dreesman GR, Fields H, et al. HBcAg, anti-HBc, and DNA polymerase activity in transfused recipients followed prospectively. Am J Med Sci. 1975;270:343–8.
230. Seeberg S, Brandberg A, Hermodsson S, et al. Hospital outbreak of hepatitis A secondary to blood exchange in a baby. Lancet. 1981;1:1155–6.
231. Davenport FM, Hennessy AV, Christopher N, et al. A common source multi-household outbreak of chimpanzee-associated hepatitis in humans. Am J Epidemiol. 1966;83:146–51.
232. Ruddy SJ, Mosley JW, Held JR. Chimpanzee-associated viral hepatitis in 1963. Am J Epidemiol. 1967;86:634–40.
233. Friedmann CTH, Dinnes MR, Bernstein JF, et al. Chimpanzee-associated infectious hepatitis among personnel at an animal hospital. J Am Vet Med Assoc. 1971;159:541–5.
234. Centers for Disease Control. Hepatitis surveillance. II. Sub-human primate-associated hepatitis. no. 34. September 1971;8, 10–4.
235. Dienstag JL, Davenport FM, McCollum RW, et al. Nonhuman primate-associated viral hepatitis type A: Serologic evidence of hepatitis A viral infection. JAMA. 1976;236:462–4.
236. Pattison CP, Maynard JE, Bryan JS. Subhuman primate-associated hepatitis. J Infect Dis. 1975;132:478–80.
237. Krugman S, Ward R, Giles JP, et al. Infectious hepatitis: Studies on the effect of gamma globulin on the incidence of inapparent infection. JAMA. 1960;174:823–30.
238. Wacker WEC, Riodan JF, Snodgrass PJ, et al. The Holy Cross hepatitis outbreak: Clinical and chemical abnormalities. Arch Intern Med. 1972;130:357–60.
239. Hindman SH, Maynard JE, Bradley DW, et al. Simultaneous infection with type A and B hepatitis viruses. Am J Epidemiol. 1977;105:135–9.
240. Rakela J, Nugent E, Mosley JW. Viral hepatitis: Enzyme assays and serologic procedures in the study of an epidemic. Am J Epidemiol. 1977;106:493–501.
241. Schneider AJ, Mosley JW. Studies of variations of glutamic-oxaloacetic transaminase in serum in infectious hepatitis. Pediatrics. 1959;24:367–77.
242. Benenson MW, Takafuji ET, Bancroft WH, et al. A military community outbreak of hepatitis type A related to transmission in a child care facility. Am J Epidemiol. 1980;112:471–81.
243. Lednar WM, Lemon SM, Kirkpatrick JW, et al. Frequency of illness associated with epidemic hepatitis A virus infection in adults. Am J Epidemiol. 1985;122:226–33.
244. Paul JR, Havens WP. Recent advances in the study of infectious hepatitis and serum jaundice. Trans Assoc Am Physicians. 1946;59:133–41.
245. Wallace EC. Infectious hepatitis: Report of an outbreak, apparently waterborne. Med J Aust. 1958;1:101–2.
246. Havens WP. Infectious hepatitis. Medicine. 1948;27:279–326.
247. MacCallum FO. Infective hepatitis: Studies in East Anglia during the period 1943–47. Medical Res Council Special Rep Series. no. 273. London: HMS Office; 1951.
248. Pignatelli M, Waters J, Brown D, et al. HLA Class I antigens on the hepatocyte membrane during recovery from acute hepatitis B virus infection and during interferon therapy in chronic hepatitis B virus infection. Hepatology. 1986;6:349–53.
249. Henkin RI, Smith FR. Hyposmia in acute viral hepatitis. Lancet. 1971;1:823–6.
250. Smith FR, Henkin RI, Dell RB. Disordered gustatory acuity in liver disease. Gastroenterology. 1976;70:568–71.
251. Inman RD, Hodge M, Johnston MEA, et al. Arthritis, vaculitis and cryoglobulinemia associated with relapsing hepatitis A virus infection. Ann Intern Med. 1986;105:700–3.
252. Bromberg K, Newhall N, Peter G. Hepatitis A and meningoencephalitis. JAMA. 1982;247:815.
253. Rakela J, Redeker AG, Edwards VM, et al. Hepatitis A virus infection in fulminant hepatitis and chronic active hepatitis. Gastroenterology. 1978;74:879–82.
254. Rakela J, Mosley JW, Redeker AG. The role of hepatitis A virus in fulminant hepatitis. Gastroenterology. 1975;69:854.
255. Gimson AES, White YS, Eddleston ALWF, et al. Clinical and prognostic differences in fulminant hepatitis type A, B and non-A non-B. Gut. 1983; 24:1194–8.
256. Gruer LD, McKendrick MW, Beeching NJ, et al. Relapsing hepatitis associated with hepatitis A virus. Lancet. 1982;2:163.
257. Cornu C, Lamy ME, Geubel A, et al. Persistence of immunoglobulin M antibody to hepatitis A virus and relapse of hepatitis A infection. Eur J Clin Microbiol. 1984;3:45–6.
258. Jacobson IM, Nath BJ, Dienstag JL. Relapsing viral hepatitis type A. J Med Virol. 1985;16:163–9.
259. Gocke DJ. Hepatitis A revisited. Ann Intern Med. 1986;105:960–1.
260. Sjogren MH, Tanno H, Fay O, et al. Hepatitis A virus in stool during clinical relapse. Ann Intern Med. 1987;106:221–6.
261. Havens WP, Jr, Marck RE. The leukocytic response of patients with experimentally induced infectious hepatitis. Am J Med Sci. 1946;212:129–38.
262. Choremis C, Kattamis CA, Kyriazakou M, et al. Viral hepatitis in G-6-PD deficiency. Lancet. 1966;1:269–70.
263. Kivel RM. Hematologic aspects of acute viral hepatitis. Am J Dig Dis. 1961;6:1017–31.
264. Salen G, Goldstein F, Haurani F, et al. Acute hemolytic anemia complicating viral hepatitis in patients with glucose-6-phosphate dehydrogenase deficiency. Ann Intern Med. 1966;65:1210–20.
265. Nagaraju M, Weitzman S, Baumann G. Viral hepatitis and agranulocytosis. Am J Dig Dis. 1973;18:247–56.
266. Alt HL, Swank RL. Thrombopenic purpura associated with catarrhal jaundice: Report of a case. Ann Intern Med. 1937;10:1049–54.
267. Deller JJ, Jr, Cirksena WJ, Marcarelli J. Fatal pancytopenia associated with viral hepatitis. N Engl J Med. 1962;266:297–9.
268. Hagler L, Pastore RA, Bergin JJ. Aplastic anemia following viral hepatitis: Report of two fatal cases and literature review. Medicine (Baltimore). 1975;54:139–64.
269. Levy RN, Sawitsky A, Florman AL, et al. Fatal aplastic anemia after hepatitis. N Engl J Med. 1965;273:1118–23.
270. Parker ML. Aplastic anaemia and infectious hepatitis. Lancet. 1971;2:261–2.
271. Wilson HA, McLaren GD, Dworken HJ, et al. Transient pure red-cell aplasia: Cell-mediated suppression of erythropoiesis associated with hepatitis. Ann Intern Med. 1980;92:196–8.
272. Huang S-N, Lorenz D, Gerety RJ. Electron and immunoelectron microscopic study on liver tissues of marmosets infected with hepatitis A virus. Lab Invest. 1979;1:63–71.
273. Mathiesen LR, Moller AM, Purcell RH, et al. Hepatitis A virus in the liver and intestine of marmosets after oral inoculation. Infect Immun. 1980;28:45–8.
274. Murphy BL, Maynard JE, Bradley DW, et al. Immunofluorescence of hepatitis A virus antigen in chimpanzees. Infect Immun. 1978;21:663–5.
275. Shimizu YK, Mathiesen LR, Lorenz D, et al. Localization of hepatitis A antigen in liver tissue by peroxidase-conjugated antibody method: Light and electron microscopic studies. J Immunol. 1978;121:1671–9.
276. Hollinger FB, Bradley DW, Maynard JE, et al. Detection of hepatitis A viral antigen by radioimmunoassay. J Immunol. 1975;115:1464–66.
277. Bradley DW, Hollinger FB, Hornbeck CL, et al. Isolation and characterization of hepatitis A virus. Am J Clin Pathol. 1976;65:876–89.
278. Dulbecco R, Ginsberg HS, eds. Virology. Philadelphia: Harper and Row: 1980:1096–117.
279. Karayiannis P, Jowett T, Enticott M, et al. Hepatitis A virus replication in tamarins and host immune response in relation to pathogenesis of liver cell damage. J Med Virol. 1986;18:261–76.
280. Karayiannis P, McGarvey MJ, Fry MA, et al. Detection of hepatitis A virus RNA in tissues and faeces of experimentally infected tamarins by cDNA-RNA hybridisation. In: Zuckerman AJ, ed. Viral Hepatitis and Liver Disease. New York: Alan R Liss; 1988:117–20.
281. Krawczynski KK, Bradley DW, Murphy BL, et al. Pathogenetic aspects of hepatitis A virus infection in enterally inoculated marmosets. Am J Clin Path. 1981;76:698–706.
282. Villarejos VM, Hu R, Visona KA. Persistence and reinfection with hepatitis A virus. In: Zuckerman AJ, ed. Viral Hepatitis and Liver Disease. New York: Alan R Liss; 1988:111–2.
283. Locarnini SA, Coulepis AG, Kaldor J, et al. Coproantibodies in hepatitis A: Detection by enzyme-linked immunosorbent assay and immune electron microscopy. J Clin Microbiol. 1980;11:710–6.
284. Sikuler E, Keynan A, Hanuka N, et al. Detection and persistence of specific IgA antibodies in serum of patients with hepatitis A by capture radioimmunoassay. J Med Virol. 1983;26:40–7.
285. Yoshizawa H, Itoh Y, Iwakiri S, et al. Diagnosis of type A hepatitis by fecal IgA antibody against hepatitis A antigen. Gastroenterology. 1980;78:114–8.
286. Stapleton JT, LeDuc JW, Binn LN, et al. Lack of neutralizing activity in fecal extracts following experimental hepatitis A virus (HAV) infection in man and owl monkeys. J Med Virol. 1987;21:17A.
287. Bradley DW, McCaustland KA, Cook EH, et al. Dissociation of hepatitis A virus antigen-anti-HAV antibody complexes by 2-mercaptoethanol and dithiothreitol. J Med Virol. 1982;9:311–25.
288. Tassopoulus NC, Papaevangelou GJ, Ticehurst JR, et al. Faecal excretion of Greek strains of hepatitis A in patients with hepatitis A and experimentally infected chimpanzees. J Infect Dis. 1986;154:231–7.
289. Havens WP, Jr. Experiment in cross immunity between infectious hepatitis and homologous serum jaundice. Proc Soc Exp Biol Med. 1945;59:148–50.
290. Karvountzis GG, Mosley JW, Redeker AG. Serologic characterization of patients with two episodes of acute viral hepatitis. Am J Med. 1975;58:815–22.
291. Mosley JW. Hepatitis types B and non-B: Epidemiologic background. JAMA. 1975;233:967–9.
292. Mosley JW, Redeker AG, Feinstone SM, Purcell RH. Multiple hepatitis viruses in multiple attacks of acute viral hepatitis. N Engl J Med. 1977;296:75–8.
293. Dienstag JL, Popper H, Purcell RH. The pathology of viral hepatitis types A and B in chimpanzees. Am J Pathol. 1976;83:131–48.

294. Karron RA, Daemer R, Ticehurst J, et al. Studies of prototype live hepatitis A virus vaccines in primate models. J Infect Dis. 1988;157:338–45.
295. Ticehurst J, Feinstone SM, Chestnut T, et al. Detection of hepatitis A virus by extraction of viral RNA and molecular hybridization. J Clin Microbiol. 1987;25:1822–9.
296. Bradley DW, Maynard JE, Hindman SH, et al. Serodiagnosis of viral hepatitis A: Detection of acute-phase immunoglobulin M anti-hepatitis A virus by radioimmunoassay. J Clin Microbiol. 1977;5:521–30.
297. Thomas HC, de Villiers D, Potter B, et al. Immune complexes in acute and chronic liver disease. Clin Exp Immunol. 1978;31:150–7.
298. Baer GM, Walker JA. Studies of an outbreak of acute hepatitis A. I. Complement level fluctuation. J Med Virol. 1977;1:1–7.
299. Margolis HS, Nainan OV. Identification of hepatitis A viral capsid proteins in immune complexes isolated during hepatitis A infection. J Med Virol. 1987;22:20A.
300. Kurane I, Binn LN, Bancroft WH, et al. Human lymphocyte responses to hepatitis A virus-infected cells: Interferon production and lysis of infected cells. J Immunol. 1985;135:2140–4.
301. Vallbracht A, Hoffmann L, Wurster KG, et al. Persistent infection of human fibroblasts by hepatitis-A virus. J Gen Virol. 1984;65:609–15.
302. Davis GL, Hoofnagle JH, Waggoner JG. Acute type A hepatitis during chronic hepatitis B virus infection: Association of depressed hepatitis B virus replication with appearance of endogenous alpha interferon. J Med Virol. 1984;14:141–7.
303. Levin S, Hahn T. Interferon system in acute viral hepatitis. Lancet. 1982;1:592–4.
304. Zachoval R, Abb J, Zachoval V, et al. Circulating interferon in patients with acute hepatitis A. J Infect Dis. 1986;153:1174–5.
305. Provost PJ, Ittensohn OL, Villarejos VM, et al. A specific complement-fixation test for human hepatitis A employing CR326 virus antigen: Diagnosis and epidemiology. Proc Soc Exp Biol Med. 1975;148:962–9.
306. Locarnini SA, Coulepis AG, Stratton AM, et al. Solid-phase enzyme-linked immunosorbent assay for detection of hepatitis A-specific immunoglobulin M. J Clin Microbiol. 1979;9:459–65.
307. Frosner GG, Scheid R, Wolf H, et al. Immunoglobulin M anti-hepatitis A virus determination by reorienting gradient centrifugation for diagnosis of acute hepatitis A. J Clin Microbiol. 1979;9:476–8.
308. Flehmig B, Ranke M, Berthold H, et al. A solid-phase radioimmunoassay for detection of IgM antibodies to hepatitis A virus. J Infect Dis. 1979;140:169–75.
309. Duermeyer W, Wielaard F, van der Veen J. A new principle for the detection of specific IgM antibodies applied in an ELISA for hepatitis A. J Med Virol. 1979;4:25–32.
310. Roggendorf M, Frosner GG, Deinhardt F, et al. Comparison of solid phase test systems for demonstrating antibodies against hepatitis A virus (anti-HAV) of the IgM-class. J Med Virol. 1980;5:47–62.
311. Kao HW, Ashcavai M, Redeker AG. The persistence of hepatitis A IgM antibody after acute clinical hepatitis A. Hepatology. 1984;4:933–6.
312. Locarnini SA, Garland SM, Lehmann NI, et al. Solid-phase enzyme-linked immunosorbent assay for detection of hepatitis A virus. J Clin Microbiol. 1978;8:277–82.
313. Coursaget P, Maupas P, Hibon P, et al. Hepatitis A diagnosis in man: Radioimmunoassay for hepatitis A antigen detection in faeces. J Med Virol. 1980;6:53–60.
314. Chalmers TC, Eckhardt RD, Reynolds WE, et al. The treatment of acute infectious hepatitis: Controlled studies of the effects of diet, rest, and physical reconditioning on the acute course of the disease and on the incidence of relapses and residual abnormalities. J Clin Invest. 1955;34:1163–235.
315. Repsher LH, Freebern RK. Effects of early and vigorous exercise on recovery from infectious hepatitis. N Engl J Med. 1969;281:1393–6.
316. Blum AL, Stutz R, Haemmerli VP, et al. A fortuitously controlled study of steroid therapy in acute viral hepatitis. I. Acute disease. Am J Med. 1969;47:82–92.
317. Evans AS, Sprinz H, Nelson RS. Adrenal hormone therapy in viral hepatitis. I. The effect of ACTH in the acute disease. Ann Intern Med. 1953;38:1115–33.
318. Evans AS, Sprinz H, Nelson RS. Adrenal hormone therapy in viral hepatitis. II. The effect of cortisone in the acute disease. Ann Intern Med. 1953;38:1134–47.
319. Evans AS, Nelson RS, Sprinz H, et al. Adrenal hormone therapy in viral hepatitis. IV. The effect of gamma globulin and oral cortisone in the acute disease. Am J Med. 1955;19:783–9.
320. Gallis SS, Stokes J, Jr, Forster HW, Jr, et al. The use of human immune serum globulin (gamma globulin) in infectious (epidemic) hepatitis in the Mediterranean theater of operations. II. Studies on treatment in an epidemic of infectious hepatitis. JAMA. 1945;128:1158–9.
321. Schweitzer IL, Weiner JM, McPeak CM, et al. Oral contraceptives in acute viral hepatitis. JAMA. 1975;233:979–80.
322. Rossouw JE, Labadarios D, McConnell JB, et al. Plasma pyridoxal phosphate levels in fulminant hepatic failure and the effects of parenteral supplementation. Scand J Gastroenterol. 1977;12:123–7.
323. Wilkinson SP, Blendis LM, Williams R. Frequency and type of renal and electrolyte disorders in fulminant hepatic failure. Br Med J. 1974;1:186–9.
324. Mosley JW. Epidemiology of HAV infection. In: Vyas GN, Cohen SN, Schmid R, eds. Viral Hepatitis. Philadelphia: Franklin Institute Press; 1978:85–104.
325. Maynard JE. Viral hepatitis as an occupational hazard in the health care profession. In: Vyas GN, Cohen SN, Schmid R, eds. Viral Hepatitis. Philadelphia: Franklin Institute Press; 1978:321–32.
326. Favero MS, Maynard JE, Leger RT, et al. Guidelines for the care of patients hospitalized with viral hepatitis. Ann Intern Med. 1979;91:872–6.
327. Goodman RA, Carder CC, Allen JR, et al. Nosocomial hepatitis A transmission by an adult patient with diarrhea. Am J Med. 1982;73:220.
328. Cossart YE. Virus Hepatitis A And Its Control. Tindall, London: Bailliere; 1977:294.
329. Stokes J, Jr, Neefe J. The prevention and attenuation of infectious hepatitis by gamma globulin. JAMA. 1945;127:144–5.
330. Gellis SS, Stokes J, Jr, Brother GM, et al. The use of human immune serum globulin (gamma globulin) in infectious (epidemic) hepatitis in the Mediterranean theater of operations. I. Studies on prophylaxis in two epidemics of infectious hepatitis. JAMA. 1945;128:1062–3.
331. Havens WP, Jr, Paul JR. Prevention of infectious hepatitis with gamma globulin. JAMA. 1945;129:270–2.
332. Stokes J, Jr, Farquhar JA, Drake ME, et al. Infectious hepatitis: Length of protection by immune serum globulin (gamma globulin) during epidemics. JAMA. 1951;147:714–9.
333. Kluge T. Gamma-globulin in the prevention of viral hepatitis: A study on the effect of medium-size doses. Acta Med Scand. 1963;174:469–77.
334. Mosley JW, Reiser DM, Braholl D, et al. Comparison of two lots of immune serum globulin for prophylaxis of infectious hepatitis. Am J Epidemiol. 1968;85:539.
335. Hall WT, Madden DL, Mundon FK, et al. Protective effect of immune serum globulin (ISG) against hepatitis A infection in a natural epidemic. Am J Epidemiol. 1977;106:72–5.
336. Noble HB, Peterson DR. Evaluation of immune serum globulin for control of infectious hepatitis. Public Health Rep. 1965;80:173–7.
337. Paktoris EA. Aktual'nye voprosy epidemiologii i profilaktiki bolezhi Botkina. Vestn Akad Med Nauk SSSR. 1963;18:55–66.
338. Miller WJ, Provost PJ, McAleer WJ, et al. Specific immune adherence assay for human hepatitis A antibody. Application to diagnostic and epidemiologic investigations. Proc Soc Exp Biol Med. 1975;149:254–61.
339. Frosner GG, Haas H, Holtz G. Hepatitis-A antibody in commercial lots of immune serum globulin. Lancet. 1977;1:432–3.
340. Stapleton JT, Jansen R, Lemon SM. Neutralizing antibody to hepatitis A virus in immune serum globulin and in sera of human recipients of immune serum globulin. Gastroenterology. 1985;89:637–42.
341. Murray R, Ratner F. Safety of immune serum globulin with respect to homologous serum hepatitis. Proc Soc Exp Biol Med. 1953;83:554–5.
342. Holland PV, Alter H, Purcell R, et al. Hepatitis-associated antigen and antibody in cold ethanol fractionates of human blood. Vox Sang. 1971;20:464–5.
343. Fowinkle EW, Guthrie N. Comparison of two doses of gamma globulin in prevention of infectious hepatitis. Public Health Rep. 1964;79:634–7.
344. Krasna V, Radkovsky J. Evaluation of the effectiveness of gamma globulin in the prevention of infectious hepatitis in Prague in 1953–56. J Hyg Epidemiol Microb Immunol. 1962;6:295.
345. Centers for Disease Control. Immunoglobulins for protection against viral hepatitis. MMWR. 1981;30:423.
346. Kendrick MA. Viral hepatitis in American missionaries abroad. J Infect Dis. 1974;129:227–9.
347. Frame JD. Hepatitis among missionaries in Ethiopia and Sudan: Susceptibles at high risk. JAMA. 1968;203:819–26.
348. Woodson RD, Cahill KN. Viral hepatitis abroad: Incidence in Catholic missionaries. JAMA. 1972;219:1191–3.
349. Kendrick MA. Study of illness among Americans returning from international travel, July 11–August 24, 1971 (preliminary data). J Infect Dis. 1972;126:684–5.
350. Kendrick MA. Summary of study on illness among Americans visiting Europe, March 31, 1969–March 30, 1970. J Infect Dis. 1972;126:685–7.
351. Clinical Immunology Committee of the International Union of Immunological Societies and WHO. Appropriate uses of human immunoglobulin in clinical practice: Memorandum from an IUIS/WHO meeting. Bull WHO. 1982;60:43–7.
352. Weekly Epidemiological Record (WHO). 1988;63:91–2.
353. Provost PJ, Hilleman MR. An inactivated hepatitis A virus vaccine prepared from infected marmoset liver. Proc Soc Exp Biol Med. 1978;159:201–3.
354. Binn LN, Bancroft WH, Eckels KH, et al. Inactivated hepatitis A virus vaccine produced in human diploid MRC-5 cells. In: Zuckerman AJ, ed. Viral Hepatitis and Liver Disease. New York: Alan R Liss: 1988:91–3.
355. Binn LN, Bancroft WH, Lemon SM, et al. Preparation of a prototype inactivated hepatitis A-virus vaccine from infected cell cultures. J Infect Dis. 1986;153:749–56.
356. Sjogren MH, Eckels KH, Binn LN, et al. Safety and immunogenicity of an inactivated hepatitis A vaccine. In: Zuckerman AJ, ed. Viral Hepatitis and Liver Disease. New York: Alan R Liss; 1988:94–6.
357. Robertson BH, Khanna B, Brown VK, et al. Large scale production of hepatitis A virus in cell culture: Effect of type of infection on virus yield and cell integrity. J Gen Virol. 1988;69:2129–34.
358. Widell A, Hansson BG, Nordenfelt E. A microcarrier cell culture system for large scale production of hepatitis A virus. J Virol Methods. 1984;8:63–71.
359. Provost PJ, Bishop RP, Gerety RJ, et al. New findings in live, attenuated hepatitis A vaccine development. J Med Virol. 1986;20:165–76.
360. Provost PJ, Buynak EB, McLean AA, et al. Progress toward a live atten-

uated human hepatitis A vaccine. In: Vyas GN, Dienstag JL, Hoofnagle JH, eds. Viral Hepatitis and Liver Disease. Orlando, FL: Grune & Stratton; 1984:467–75.
361. Provost PJ, Emini EA, Lewis JA, et al. Progress toward the development of a hepatitis A vaccine. In: Zuckerman AJ, ed. Viral Hepatitis and Liver Disease. New York: Alan R Liss; 1988:83–6.
362. Feinstone SM, Daemer RJ, Gust ID, et al. Live attenuated vaccine for hepatitis A. In: Papaevangelou G, Hennessen W, eds. Viral Hepatitis: Standardization in immunoprophylaxis of infections by hepatitis viruses. Basel: Karger; 1983:429–32.
363. Harmon SA, Johnston JM, Ziegelhoffer T, et al. Expression of hepatitis A virus capsid sequences in insect cells. Virus Res. 1988;10:273–80.
364. Ostermayr R, von der Helm K, Seelmair S, et al. Expression of HAV VP1 antigen as recombinant protein in *Escherichia coli*. In: Zuckerman AJ, ed. Viral Hepatitis and Liver Disease. New York: Alan R Liss; 1988:59–61.
365. Ross BC, Anderson BN, Gust ID. Expression of the hepatitis A virus genome as beta-galactosidase fusion proteins in *Escherichia coli*. In: Zuckerman AJ, ed. Viral Hepatitis and Liver Disease. New York: Alan R Liss; 1988:62–4.
366. Balayan MS. Experimental development of vaccines against hepatitis A. Vopr Virus. 1988;1:5–11.
367. Emini EA, Hughes JV, Parlow DS, et al. Induction of hepatitis A virus-neutralizing antibody by a virus-specific synthetic peptide. J Virol. 1985;55:836–9.

152. RHINOVIRUS

JACK M. GWALTNEY, JR.

Since antiquity, people have been plagued with colds; however, it was only in 1914 that the first direct evidence of the infectious nature of colds was reported by Kruse. He produced colds in volunteers by intranasal instillation of bacterial-free filtrates of secretions from cold sufferers.[1] In the 1940s and 1950s, Dingle et al.[2] and a British research team headed by Andrewes[3] examined many facets related to the etiology and epidemiology of colds. At a later date, the nasal secretions used by Andrewes et al. for human transmission studies were shown to contain rhinoviruses.

Pelon et al.[4] and Price[5] independently isolated a new virus in 1956, which later was designated rhinovirus 1A. Another significant advance in the isolation and characterization of a number of rhinoviruses was the use by Ketler et al.[6] of the highly sensitive human embryonic lung cells developed by Hayflick and Moorehead.[7] By 1963, the number of known immunotypes had increased so rapidly that no single laboratory could characterize the rhinovirus group. Beginning in 1967, a collaborative program directed by Kapikian et al.[8] established a uniform classification system for the known rhinovirus immunotypes 1–55. In 1971 other immunotypes were added, bringing the total to 89,[9] and in 1986, the addition of 11 new immunotypes increased the number to 100.[10] The identification of the nucleotide sequence of the viral genome[11–13] and of the amino acid composition of the viral shell[14] has made rhinovirus one of the best characterized mammalian viruses.

Epidemiologic studies have now shown that rhinoviruses are the major known cause of the common cold.[15–17] There is also evidence that they may play a role in acute sinus infections,[18] exacerbations of chronic bronchitis,[19–21] and attacks of asthma.[22,23] The discovery of the rhinoviruses established that the common cold is an enormously complex syndrome produced by a large number of antigenically distinct viruses, and that controlling colds will be a difficult problem.

DESCRIPTION OF THE PATHOGEN

Classification

Rhinoviruses are one of the four genera of the picornavirus family (Table 1).[24] Although the group shares basic properties with enteroviruses, rhinoviruses are distinguished by their susceptibility to inactivation by exposure to an acid environment and a higher density in cesium chloride gradients.[25,26]

TABLE 1. Characteristics of Rhinovirus

Size: 20–27 nm
Shape: nonenveloped capsid with icosahedral symmetry constructed from 60 repeated protomers
Molecular weight: 8.16×10^6 daltons
Density: higher in cesium chloride gradient than other members of the picornavirus group, suggesting more open capsid structure
Nucleic acid: single-stranded RNA with positive polarity containing approximately 7,000 nucleotides
Optimal growth temperature: 33–35°C; growth restricted at 37°C
Replication: virus synthesis and maturation in cell cytoplasm
Antigenicity: type-specific

Morphology and Structure

The overall size of the virus is 20–27 nm.[25,26] Like other picornaviruses, rhinovirus contains four structural proteins (VP_1, VP_2, VP_3, and VP_4), which form a nonenveloped capsid with icosahedral symmetry. The high degree of cesium binding suggests that the capsid structure is less densely packed than other picornaviruses. Examination of the atomic structure of the viral shell has revealed that it is composed of 60 repeated subunits (protomers) containing the four viral proteins. A deep cleft exists on the viral surface that separates the five VP_1 subunits clustered about a pentamer axis from the adjacent VP_2 and VP_3 subunits. This cleft, the structure of which is highly conserved among immunotypes, is believed to be the site of viral attachment to the cellular receptor. The rhinovirus genome contains approximately 7,000 nucleotides and is organized in an essentially identical way to that of poliovirus. The virus is ether-resistant but labile in an acid environment of pH 3–5. Virus synthesis and maturation occurs in the cytoplasm.

Biologic Characteristics

Native human rhinovirus will only infect humans and higher primates and grows in cell cultures derived from these species. The optimal temperature for rhinovirus replication, 33–35°C, corresponds to the temperature found in the nose and large airways.[27] At core body temperature of 37°C, virus yields fall by as much as 90 percent of maximum.[28] The relatively low temperature range for optimal rhinovirus growth may explain why generalized infection as manifested by viremia has not been observed with rhinovirus.[29,30] Also, temperature may be one of the factors inhibiting viral replication in the intestinal tract. Gastrointestinal secretions may also have an adverse effect on virus survival.[31] In humans, the growth of rhinovirus takes place primarily in the cells of the upper airway.[32] Recent evidence suggests that the adenoidal area may be an important location for initiation of infection.[33] In some patients, the virus may also replicate in the large airways.[27] Rhinovirus survives on skin and environmental surfaces for at least several hours after contamination of these sites.[34]

Antigenic Characteristics

There are four major immunogenic neutralization sites within each rhinovirus protomer.[25,26] Rhinoviruses have been numbered 1–100 and subtype 1A on the basis of these surface antigens.[8–10] Identification is based on neutralization of viral growth with hyperimmune animal antiserum containing 20 units of antibody. The native antigenic structure of the virus can be altered by exposure to pH 5 at 56°C or to 2 M urea.[35] The configurational change in the capsid, which apparently results from such treatments, produces an altered state of antigenicity in which reactivity with heterologous rhinovirus types occurs. The altered, or C-antigenic state does not stimulate protective antibody.

With antisera against the 100 numbered rhinovirus immunotypes, it has been possible to identify most strains recovered in recent field studies.[36,37] Thus, it does not appear that new immunotypes of rhinovirus are emerging at a rapid rate. However, antigenic differences have been found in strains of the same type recovered several years apart[38,39]; also intertypes have been discovered,[40] suggesting that some antigenic drift of rhinoviruses does take place.

EPIDEMIOLOGY

Distribution and Prevalence

Rhinoviruses have a worldwide distribution. In a given geographic area, the different antigenic types circulate in a random fashion with no pattern other than for current types to be slowly replaced by strains of different antigenic types.[41] Infections begin to occur in early childhood and continue throughout life.[42–44] Studies of the prevalence of rhinovirus antibody show rapid acquisition of antibody during childhood and adolescence, with a peak prevalence in young adults,[45] probably reflecting their exposure to young children. Antibody prevalence then declines slightly and remains relatively constant throughout adulthood. A slight decrease in prevalence of antibody in older adults probably results from lessened viral exposure. Rhinoviruses are also encountered in military populations where they are a cause of respiratory disease in military recruits.[46–48]

Seasonal Pattern of Infection

In temperate climates, rhinoviruses have a well-established seasonal pattern, with fall and spring peaks of infection. Most characteristic in the United States is an early fall outbreak of rhinovirus colds, which annually initiates the respiratory disease season.[16,49] In adults with colds in the eastern United States, rhinovirus infection rates are highest in September. In some years, however, the fall rhinovirus outbreak is not evident. A second less prominent peak of rhinovirus infection occurs in March, April, and May. Rhinoviruses also account for a relatively high proportion of summer colds. In the winter months, rhinovirus activity is low; coronaviruses and possibly undiscovered agents are thought to account for most colds at that time. In tropical areas, rhinovirus outbreaks have been encountered in the rainy season,[42] and in the arctic during cold weather.[50] The reasons for the seasonal pattern of rhinovirus infection are not known. Volunteers exposed to thermal cold have not shown increased susceptibility to experimental rhinovirus colds.[51] Seasonal changes in living conditions, such as opening of schools and crowding indoors, may be important in initiating fall rhinovirus outbreaks.

Infection and Illness Rates

Rhinovirus colds are one of the most common infections in humans. Infection rates range from 1.2 infections per person-year in children under the age of 1 year[52] to 0.7 in young adults.[16,53] Infection rates in men and women are similar. In illness surveillance studies at the work place, not only in persons seeking medical care, cigarette smokers had rhinovirus illness rates similar to those of nonsmokers, although their illnesses were more severe.[16,54] From 70 to 88 percent of rhinovirus infections are associated with symptomatic respiratory illness, giving an apparent to inapparent infection ratio of approximately 3 : 1.[16,47,53,55,56]

Transmission

The major site for rhinovirus transmission is the home,[57–59] and the most frequent introducer of infection is a schoolchild. Secondary infections are most common in young siblings and mothers. Two to five-day intervals are seen between onsets of cases occurring in families. Secondary attack rates in family members have ranged from 25 to 70 percent and have varied with the immune status of the exposed person to the invading virus. An equally important location for rhinovirus spread is in schools.[60,61] In some outbreaks, up to 77 percent of children in a nursery school became infected, when a new serotype was introduced into the classroom.[62] Mixing of different rhinovirus types in a school population provides an efficient way for the virus to be disseminated in a community.

Epidemiologic observations suggest that efficient rhinovirus transmission depends on some type of close contact that allows exposure to infectious secretions over a short distance. Studies in volunteers have shown that spread of infectious nasal secretions from hand to hand, followed by autoinoculation of the nasal and conjunctival mucosa, is an efficient means of viral transmission.[63] Contamination of the hands with nasal secretions containing rhinovirus is a common occurrence in people with natural colds. These individuls may then pass virus on to the hands of others with whom they have contact. Finger-to-nose and finger-to-eye contact occur frequently in the course of normal behavior, providing a means for accidental self-inoculation of susceptible persons. Also, rhinovirus has been recovered from objects in the homes of persons with colds,[63] and infection has been transmitted to volunteers by means of contaminated plastic tiles.[64] In one field study employing regular treatments of the hands with a virucidal lotion, persons using the active treatments had fewer rhinovirus colds than did those using a placebo lotion.[65] The findings of that study provide direct evidence supporting the hand contamination/self-inoculation route of rhinovirus transmission.

Experimental rhinovirus infection has also been transmitted through the air in either large or small particle aerosols.[66] The development of a reliable aerosol model demonstrates the feasibility of that route of rhinovirus transmission. Further studies designed to interrupt spread of natural infection by the different routes are needed to determine their relative importance.[32]

PATHOGENESIS

Under experimental conditions, less than one tissue culture mean infective dose ($TCID_{50}$) of rhinovirus placed in the nose will lead to infection and illness.[67] Virus can be recovered in nasal secretions of a volunteer approximately 24 hours after nasal inoculation.[29,67] Viral shedding increases to peak levels on the second and third day, at which time nasal secretions contain 10–1000 $TCID_{50}$/ml of virus. Clinical manifestations of illness appear on the second day and reach a peak on the third and fourth days.[67,68] During the acute illness, large quantities of protein are released from the mucous membrane of the nose. Also at this time, ciliated epithelial cells containing rhinovirus antigen are present in nasal mucus, but their numbers are low and do not correlate with severity of illness in the individual case.[69]

The specific mechanisms by which rhinovirus produces disease have only recently been investigated. Histologic examination of nasal biopsy specimens from volunteers with experimental infections have failed to show consistent pathologic changes.[68,70] These studies suggest that damage to the epithelium is slight and that the infection might serve as a trigger for the release of chemical mediators, which are the ultimate cause of the clinical illness. Supporting this hypothesis is the recent finding of high concentrations of bradykinin and lysylbradykinin in nasal washes of persons with experimental rhinovirus colds.[71] In contrast, histamine levels were not elevated in the nasal wash specimens.

IMMUNITY

Rhinovirus infection stimulates the appearance of serum-neutralizing antibody in up to 80 percent of persons with natural colds.[54,72] The neutralizing activity is associated with serum fractions containing IgA and IgG.[73,74] After recent experimental infections, rhinovirus-neutralizing activity has also been associated with serum IgM. In addition, neutralizing activity is present in nasal secretions, where it is associated primarily with IgA in 9S and 11S fractions.[75] During rhinovirus colds, there is transudation of considerable amounts of serum immunoglobulin into nasal secretions.[76,77]

After an infection in which antibody has been stimulated, most persons appear to be immune to reinfection.[54,58,78] Longitudinal studies have shown the persistence of serum antibody for years,[43] and it is probable that most rhinovirus colds confer long-lasting immunity. Antibody responses do not follow all infections, however. Also, in volunteers, protection associated with pre-existing antibody can be overcome by a large virus challenge.[79] Therefore, it is evident that recurrent infections with the same rhinovirus type do occur.

It has been suggested that the primary immune mechanism in rhinovirus infection is the neutralizing antibody present in nasal secretions, rather than that in serum. Since nasal and serum antibody are found in close association,[73,80,81] it has been difficult to provide a definite answer to this question.[81–83]

CLINICAL MANIFESTATIONS

Signs and Symptoms of Rhinovirus Colds

Rhinoviruses produce a typical common cold. The median length of illness in young adults is 7 days, but symptoms last up to 2 weeks in one-quarter of the cases.[54] Complaints fall into nasal, pharyngeal, lower respiratory tract, and general categories. As observed in a group of patients, the symptoms of rhinovirus colds have a consistent pattern (Fig. 1). However, wide variations occur in the individual patient, and it is not possible to distinguish rhinovirus infections from other causes of upper respiratory illness on clinical grounds alone.

In an adult with an uncomplicated rhinovirus cold, fever is uncommon, and other systemic complaints are of low-grade severity. In most cases, rhinorrhea and nasal obstruction are the most prominent complaints. Sore or scratchy throat is also frequently present. Cough and hoarseness occur in approximately 30 percent and 20 percent of cases, respectively. In cigarette smokers, the frequency and duration of cough is prolonged. In the average case, nasal and pharyngeal symptoms subside rapidly during the third and fourth day of illness.

On examination, the end of the nose may have a red color, and clear or mucoid nasal secretions are frequently present. Nasal obstruction is often more obvious to the patient than to the physician, unless special methods are used to measure resistance to nasal airflow. A glistening appearance of the nasal membrane is often seen. The pharyngeal mucosa may show mild edema and erythema, but marked inflammation or exudate do not occur. Rhonchi may be heard on examination of the chest. In many patients with a moderate degree of subjective discomfort, the nose and throat show few objective changes at the time of examination.

Rhinoviruses also cause a common cold in children. Available evidence is conflicting on the role of rhinoviruses in viral pneumonia, croup, and bronchiolitis. The prevailing opinion is that rhinoviruses do not commonly cause these illnesses in children.[84–87] Rhinovirus infections are associated with a modest

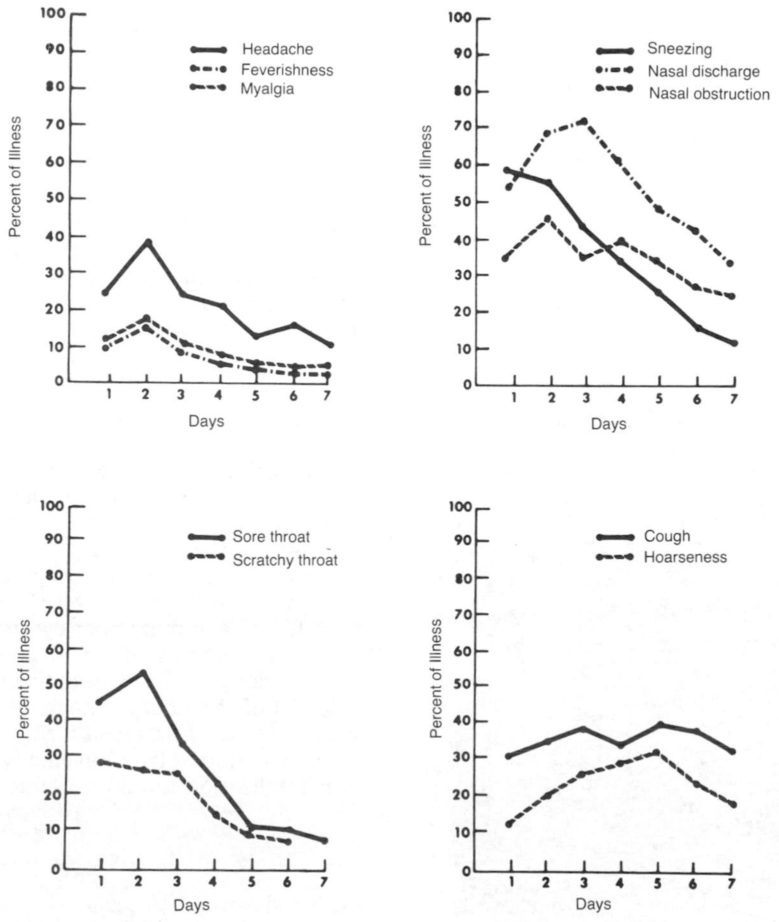

FIG. 1. Rhinovirus cold symptoms (139 adults with natural infection).

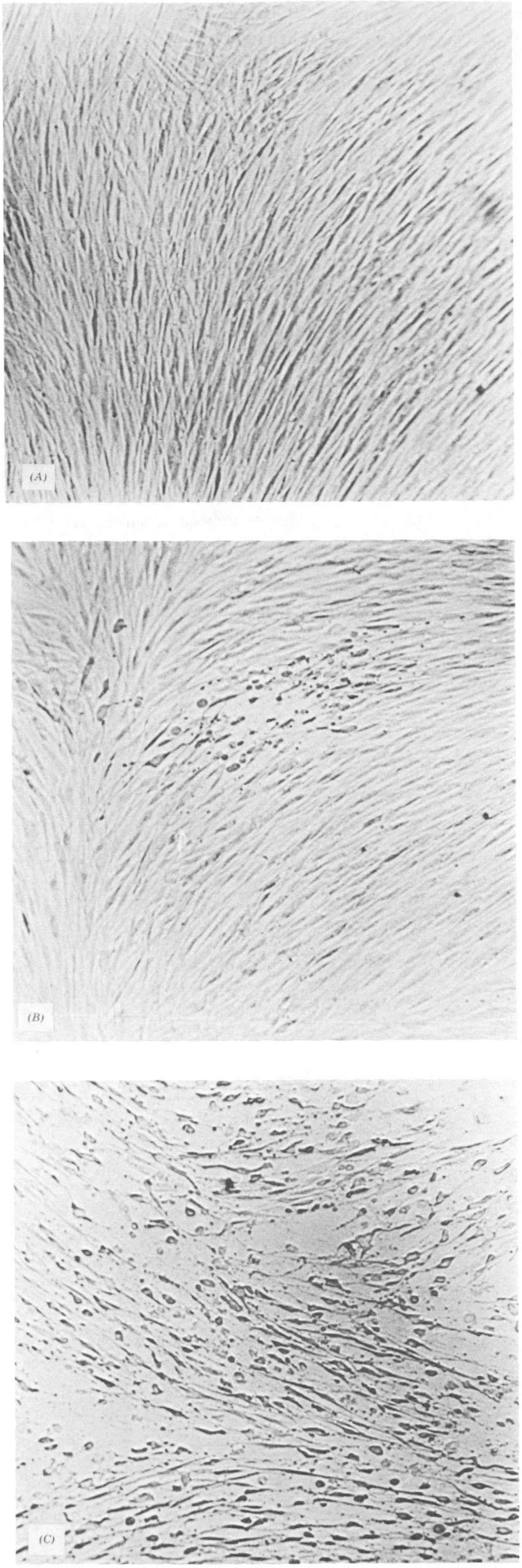

increase in circulating neutrophils and a moderate elevation of the erythrocyte sedimentation rate.[78]

Complications of Rhinovirus Colds

Sinusitis. Sinusitis has been reported to complicate 0.5 percent of common respiratory diseases.[2] In studies in adults with acute sinusitis, rhinovirus has been recovered from aspirates obtained by direct puncture of the maxillary sinus.[18] In some cases, virus was obtained alone, but in most cases bacterial pathogens, including *Streptococcus pneumoniae* and unencapsulated strains of *Haemophilus influenzae*, were also recovered. Presumably, the virus first gains entrance to the sinus cavity and initiates an infection that impairs the normal clearance mechanisms, allowing secondary bacterial infection to develop.

Otitis Media. Two percent of common respiratory disease is complicated by otitis media.[2] Respiratory viruses have been implicated in the pathogenesis of this disease by creating inflammatory obstruction of the eustachian tube. Also, respiratory viruses, including one rhinovirus, have been recovered directly from middle ear fluids of patients with otitis media.[88] In some cases, bacteria were recovered in combination with the virus. Experimental rhinovirus infection has recently been shown to produce abnormalities in eustachian tube function and middle ear pressure.[89]

Acute Infectious Episodes in Patients with Chronic Bronchitis. Rhinoviruses have been implicated in acute infectious exacerbations in patients with chronic bronchitis.[19–21] It is not known if rhinovirus invades the bronchial tree directly, but a study[27] using a sampling device designed to minimize upper airway contamination of specimens suggests that this can occur. Mild alterations in ventilation have been reported in some chronic bronchitics with rhinovirus infection.[90] Secondary bacterial infection may also play a role in this condition.

Precipitation of Asthma. Asthmatic children appear to experience a significantly greater number of viral respiratory infections than do nonasthmatic control subjects.[91] The most common cause of their infections is the rhinoviruses that have been recovered from these patients at the onset of an asthmatic attack, suggesting that the virus may be an initiating factor in the illness.[22,23] Experimental rhinovirus infection leads to a decrease in FEV_1 and an increase in histamine sensitivity in some, but not all, young adults with mild-to-moderate asthma.[92]

Diagnosis

Viral Isolation. Rhinoviruses grow well in several cell culture systems, particularly human embryonic lung (WI-38 and MRC-5 strains) and M-HeLa cells. However, unexplained variations in the sensitivity of these cells can cause problems in testing if they are not recognized.[93,94] Viral growth is optimum at 33–34°C, and cultures must be incubated in a roller drum to achieve maximum cytopathic change. Rhinovirus cytopathic effect is usually evident in 2–6 days (Fig. 2). Because the specificity of the viral antigen of each type prevents serologic identification of members of the group as a whole, culture remains the only practical method of diagnosis.

Identification of the antigenic type of an unknown rhinovirus by neutralization requires a large battery of antisera, and it is

FIG. 2. Rhinovirus cytopathic effect in human embryonic lung cells (WI-38). (**A**) Uninfected cell cultures (× 160). (**B**) Cytopathic effect of rhinovirus type 39 at 48 hours. (**C**) Cytopathic effect at 72 hours.

best accomplished with a system of intersecting antiserum pools.[95] A microtitration system can be used for a preliminary identification.[96,97] Final proof of antigenic type is demonstrated by neutralization of $TCID_{10-300}$ of virus by 20 units of antibody, using monovalent hyperimmune animal serum.

Serology. A neutralization test can be used for serodiagnosis of rhinovirus infection if the infecting type is known. However, the multiplicity of rhinovirus types prevents the use of serologic techniques for routine diagnosis. For measuring neutralizing antibody in human serum, it is necessary to use small doses of virus ($TCID_{3-30}$) if the test is to have satisfactory sensitivity.[98]

TREATMENT AND PREVENTION

Symptomatic Therapy (see Chapter 42)

Only symptomatic treatment is available for rhinovirus colds at present. Penicillin and other antibiotics have no place in therapy, since they neither ameliorate the viral illness nor reduce the frequency of bacterial complications.

Rest, hydration, nasal decongestants, saline gargles, and cough suppressants remain the mainstay of treatment. Constitutional symptoms are not usually prominent with rhinovirus infection, but will respond to aspirin when present. Nasal decongestants should be used on a regular basis during the acute stage of illness. The regular application of a petrolatum-based ointment helps prevent painful maceration of the nares. Patients with secondary bacterial sinusitis or otitis media require appropriate antimicrobial therapy.

Prospects for Vaccines and Antivirals

Studies of the molecular structure of the rhinovirus shell[25,26] confirm that rhinovirus is not a good candidate for vaccine development. The most conserved region of the viral capsid lies in the bottom of the surface cleft, where it is inaccessible to antibody. Experimental rhinovirus vaccines made against one immunotype of virus have reduced the rate of symptomatic illness and of viral shedding, but not the overall rate of infection of volunteers given an experimental challenge with rhinovirus.[80,99,100] Some hope for the eventual success of a vaccine approach comes from a study showing antigenic relationships among some of the numbered rhinoviruses.[101] Also, volunteers given multivalent rhinovirus vaccines have shown antibody responses to several antigenic types in the vaccine.[102] Another aspect of the problem of vaccine development is the suspected role of nasal antibody in immunity to rhinovirus. Experimental vaccines have been prepared with live attenuated strains of rhinovirus in hopes of more effectively stimulating antibody production in the upper respiratory tract.[103]

There has been a continuing discovery of chemical compounds with in vitro activity against rhinovirus.[104] However, most of those reaching the stage of testing in humans have, unfortunately, shown little, if any, effectiveness. The most promising results have been obtained with recombinant α_2-interferon applied topically in the nose. Given prophylactically in doses of approximately 5,000,000 units or greater a day, α_2-interferon has been highly effective in preventing experimental infection and/or illness.[105] When used for contact prophylaxis in two field studies in families, topical α_2-interferon reduced the overall rate of colds in treated persons by 40 percent and virtually eliminated colds due specifically to rhinovirus.[106,107] When used for treatment of experimental rhinovirus colds, α_2-interferon reduced viral shedding substantially but had only a modest effect on symptomatic illness.[105] Also, after administration for several days, topical α_2-interferon causes local side effects consisting of nasal irritation and stuffiness and pinpoint mucosal ulcerations, thus limiting its use to short-term administration, as in contact prophylaxis.

Environmental Measures to Control Infection

If the hand contact/self-inoculation route is one means by which rhinovirus spreads under natural conditions, persons can protect themselves by handwashing and avoiding finger-eye and finger-nose contact. Until further knowledge is gained on this question, it seems expedient to take such precautions, particularly when a member of the household has a respiratory illness. It may be possible to develop additional approaches to hand[65] and environmental[64] disinfection, which might be effective in interrupting spread of rhinovirus colds if the natural route of spread is by this means. Because aerosol spread may be another route of rhinovirus transmission,[66] covering coughs and sneezes with disposable nasal tissues is also recommended.

REFERENCES

1. Kruse W. Die Erreger von Husten and Schupfen. Munchen Med Worchenschr. 1914;61:1547.
2. Dingle JH, Badger GF, Jordan WS Jr. Illness in the Home. A Study of 25,000 Illnesses in a Group of Cleveland Families. Cleveland: The Press of Western Reserve University; 1964.
3. Andrewes C. The Common Cold. New York: WW Norton & Co; 1965.
4. Pelon W, Mogabgab WJ, Phillips IA, et al. A cytopathogenic agent isolated from naval recruits with mild respiratory illness. Proc Soc Exp Biol Med. 1957;94:262.
5. Price WH. The isolation of a new virus associated with respiratory clinical disease in humans. Proc Natl Acad Sci USA. 1956;42:892.
6. Ketler A, Hamparian VV, Hilleman MR. Characterization and classification of ECHO 28-rhinovirus-coryzavirus agents. Proc Soc Exp Biol Med. 1962;110:821.
7. Hayflick L, Moorhead PS. The serial cultivation of human diploid cell strains. Exp Cell Res. 1961;25:585.
8. Kapikian AZ, Conant RM, Hamparian VV, et al. Rhinoviruses: a numbering system. Nature. 1967;213:761.
9. Kapikian AZ, Conant RM, Hamparian VV, et al. A collaborative report: rhinoviruses—extension of the numbering system. Virology. 1971;43:524.
10. Hamparian VV, Colonno RJ, Cooney MK, et al. A collaborative report: rhinoviruses—extension of the numbering system from 89 to 100. Virology. 1987;159:191.
11. Callahan PL, Mizutani S, Colonno RJ. Molecular cloning and complete sequence determination of RNA genome of human rhinovirus 14. Proc Natl Acad Sci USA. 1985;82:732.
12. Stanway G, Hughes PJ, Mountford RC, et al. The complete nucleotide sequence of a common cold virus: human rhinovirus 14. Nucleic Acids Res. 1984;12:7859.
13. Skern T, Sommergruber W, Blaas D, et al. Human rhinovirus 2: complete nucleotide sequence and proteolytic processing signals in the capsid protein region. Nucleic Acids Res. 1985;12:2111.
14. Rossmann MG, Arnold E, Erickson JW, et al. The structure of a human common cold virus (rhinovirus 14) and its functional relations to other picornaviruses. Nature. 1985;317:145.
15. Hamre D, Procknow JJ. Viruses isolated from natural common colds among young adult medical students. Am Rev Respir Dis. 1963;88:277.
16. Gwaltney JM Jr, Hendley JO, Simon G, et al. Rhinovirus infections in an industrial population. I. The occurrence of illness. N Engl J Med. 1966; 275:1261.
17. Monto AS, Ullman BM. Acute respiratory illness in an American community: the Tecumseh study. JAMA. 1974;227:164.
18. Evans FO, Sydnor JB, Moore WEC, et al. Sinusitis of the maxillary antrum. N Engl J Med. 1975;293:735.
19. Eadie MB, Stott EJ, Grist RN. Virological studies in chronic bronchitis. Br Med J. 1966;2:671.
20. McNamara MJ, Phillips IA, Williams OB. Viral and *Mycoplasma pneumoniae* infections in exacerbations of chronic lung disease. Am Rev Respir Dis 1969;100:19.
21. Stenhouse AC. Rhinovirus infection in acute exacerbations of chronic bronchitis: a controlled prospective study. Br Med J. 1967;3:461.
22. Hilleman MR, Reilly CM, Stokes J Jr, et al. Clinical epidemiologic findings in coryzavirus infections. Am Rev Respir Dis. 1963;88(Suppl):274.
23. Minor TE, Dick EC, DeMeo AN, et al. Viruses as precipitants of asthmatic attacks in children. JAMA. 1974;227:292.
24. Wildy P. Classification and nomenclature of viruses. In: Melnick JL, ed. Monographs in Virology. Basel: Karger; 1971.
25. Couch RB. Rhinoviruses. In: BN Fields, DM Knipe, RM Chanock, et al, eds. Virology. New York: Raven Press; 1985:795.
26. Gwaltney JM Jr, Colonno RJ, Hamparian VV, et al. Rhinovirus. In: NJ Schmidt, R Emmons, eds. Diagnostic Procedures for Viral, Rickettsial and Chlamydial Infections. 6th ed. Washington, DC: American Public Health Association. March 1989:579.
27. Halperin SA, Eggleston PA, Hendley JO, et al. Pathogenesis of lower respiratory tract symptoms in experimental rhinovirus infection. Am Rev Respir Dis. 1983;128:806.

28. Stott EJ, Killington RA. Rhinoviruses. Ann Rev Microbiol. 1972;26:503.
29. Douglas RG Jr, Cate TR, Gerone PJ, et al. Quantitative rhinovirus shedding patterns in volunteers. Am Rev Respir Dis. 1966;94:159.
30. Douglas RG Jr, Rossen RD, Butler WT, et al. Rhinovirus neutralizing antibody in tears, parotid saliva, nasal secretions and serum. J Immunol. 1967;99:297.
31. Cate TR, Douglas RG Jr, Johnson KM, et al. Studies on the inability of rhinovirus to survive and replicate in the intestinal tract of volunteers. Proc Soc Exp Biol Med. 1967;124:1290.
32. Gwaltney JM Jr. Epidemiology of the common cold. Ann NY Acad Sci. 1980;353:54.
33. Winther B, Gwaltney JM Jr, Mygind N, et al. Sites of rhinovirus recovery after point inoculation of the upper airway. JAMA. 1986;256:1763.
34. Hendley JO, Wenzel RP, Gwaltney JM Jr. Transmission of rhinovirus colds by self-inoculation. N Engl J Med. 1973;288:1361.
35. Lonberg-Holm K, Yin FH. antigenic determinants of infective and inactivated human rhinoviruses type 2. J Virol. 1973;12:114.
36. Krilov L, Pierik L, Keller E, et al. The association of rhinoviruses with lower respiratory tract disease in hospitalized patients. J Med Virol. 1986;19:345.
37. Monto AS, Bryan ER, Ohmit S. Rhinovirus infections in Tecumseh, Michigan: illness frequency and number of serotypes. J Infect Dis. 1987;156:43.
38. Schieble JH, Lennette EH, Fox VL. Antigenic variation of rhinovirus type 22. Proc Soc Exp Biol Med. 1970;133:329.
39. Stott EJ, Walker M. Antigenic variation among strains of rhinovirus type 51. Nature. 1969;224:1311.
40. Halfpap LM, Cooney MK. Isolation of rhinovirus intertypes related to either rhinoviruses 12 and 78 or 36 and 58. Infect Immun. 1983;40:213.
41. Hamre D. Rhinoviruses. In: Melnick JL, ed. Monographs in Virology 1. Basel: Karger; 1968.
42. Monto AS, Johnson KM. A community study of respiratory infections in the tropics. II. The spread of six rhinovirus isolates within the community. Am J Epidemiol. 1968;88:55.
43. Taylor-Robinson D. Studies on some viruses (rhinoviruses) isolated from common colds. Arch Ges Virusforsch. 1963;13:281.
44. Tyrrell DAJ. Rhinoviruses. In: Gard S, Hallauer C, Myer KF, eds. Virology Monographs 2. New York: Springer-Verlag; 1968.
45. Hamparian VV, Conant RM, Thomas DC. Rhinovirus Reference Laboratory, Annual Contract Progress Report to the National Institute of Allergy and Infectious Diseases. National Institutes of Health, Bethesda, MD, Contract No. 69-2062, Dec 1, 1969–Nov 30, 1970.
46. Forsyth BR, Bloom HH, Johnson KM, et al. Patterns of illness in rhinovirus infection of military personnel. N Engl J Med. 1963;269:602.
47. Johnson KM, Bloom HH, Forsyth BR, et al. Relationship of rhinovirus infection to mild upper respiratory disease. II. Epidemiologic observations in male military trainees. Am J Epidemiol. 1965;81:131.
48. Rosenbaum MJ, DeBerry P, Sullivan EJ, et al. Epidemiology of the common cold in military recruits with emphasis on infections by rhinovirus type 1A, 2, and two unclassified rhinoviruses. Am J Epidemiol. 1971;93:183.
49. Monto AS, Cavallaro JJ. The Tecumseh study of respiratory illness. II. Patterns of occurrence of infection with respiratory illness pathogens, 1965–1969. Am J Epidemiol. 1971;94:280.
50. Wulff H, Noble GR, Maynard JE, et al. An outbreak of respiratory infection in children associated with rhinovirus types 16 and 29. Am J Epidemiol. 1969;90:304.
51. Douglas RG Jr, Lindgren KM, Couch RB. Exposure to cold environment and rhinovirus common cold: failure to demonstrate effect. N Engl J Med. 1968;279:743.
52. Cooney MK, Hall CE, Fox JP. The Seattle virus watch. III. Evaluation of isolation methods and summary of infections detected by virus isolations. Am J Epidemiol. 1972;96:286.
53. Hamre D, Connelly AP Jr, Procknow J. Virologic studies of acute respiratory disease in young adults. IV. Virus isolations during four years of surveillance. Am J Epidemiol. 1966;83:238.
54. Gwaltney JM Jr, Hendley JO, Simon G, et al. Rhinovirus infections in an industrial population. II. Characteristics of illness and antibody response. JAMA. 1967;202:494.
55. Fox JP, Hall CE, Cooney MK, et al. The Seattle virus watch. II. Objectives, study population and its observation, data processing and summary of illnesses. Am J Epidemiol. 1972;96:270.
56. Mufson MA, Bloom HH, Forsyth BR, et al. Relationship of rhinovirus to mild upper respiratory disease. III. Further epidemiologic observations in military personnel. Am J Epidemiol. 1966;83:379.
57. Dick EC, Blumer CR, Evans AS. Epidemiology of infections with rhinovirus types 43 and 55 in a group of University of Wisconsin student families. Am J Epidemiol. 1967;86:386.
58. Hendley JO, Gwaltney JM Jr, Jordan WS Jr. Rhinovirus infections in an industrial population. IV. Infections within families of employees during two fall peaks of respiratory illness. Am J Epidemiol. 1969;89:184.
59. Monto AS. A community study of respiratory infections in the tropics. III. Introduction and transmission of infections within families. Am J Epidemiol. 1968;88:69.
60. Periera MA, Andrews BE, Gardner SD. A study on the virus aetiology of mild respiratory infections in the primary school child. J Hyg. 1967;64:475.
61. Kendall EJC, Bynoe ML, Tyrrell DAJ. Virus isolations from common colds occurring in a residential school. Br Med J. 1962;2:82.
62. Beem MO. Acute respiratory illness in nursery school children: a longitudinal study of the occurrence of illness and respiratory viruses. Am J Epidemiol. 1969;90:30.
63. Gwaltney JM Jr, Moskalski PB, Hendley JO. Hand to hand transmission of rhinovirus colds. Ann Intern Med. 1978;88:463.
64. Gwaltney JM Jr, Hendley JO. Transmission of experimental rhinovirus infection by contaminated surfaces. Am J Epidemiol. 1982;116:828.
65. Hendley JO, Gwaltney JM Jr. Mechanisms of transmission of rhinovirus infections. Epidemiol Rev. 1988;10:242
66. Dick EC, Jennings LC, Mink KA, et al. Aerosol transmission of rhinovirus colds. J Infect Dis. 1987;156:442.
67. Douglas RG Jr. Pathogenesis of rhinovirus common colds in human volunteers. Ann Otol Rhinol Laryngol. 1970;79:563.
68. Douglas RG Jr, Alford BR, Couch RB. Atraumatic nasal biopsy for studies of respiratory virus infection in volunteers. Antimicrob Agents Chemother. 1968;8:340.
69. Turner RB, Hendley JO, Gwaltney JM Jr. Shedding of infected ciliated epithelial cells in rhinovirus colds. J Infect Dis. 1982;145:849.
70. Winther B, Farr B, Turner RB, et al. Histopathologic examination and enumeration of polymorphonuclear leukocytes in the nasal mucosa during experimental rhinovirus colds. Acta Otolaryngol [Suppl] (Stockh). 1984;413:19.
71. Naclerio RM, Proud D, Lichtenstein LM, et al. Kinins are generated during experimental rhinovirus colds. J Infect Dis. 1988;157:133.
72. Gwaltney JM Jr, Jordan WS Jr. Rhinoviruses and respiratory disease. Bacteriol Rev. 1964;28:409.
73. Cate TR, Rossen RD, Douglas RG Jr, et al. The role of nasal secretion and serum antibody in the rhinovirus common cold. Am J Epidemiol. 1966; 84:352.
74. Rossen RD, Douglas RG Jr, Cate TR, et al. The sedimentation behavior of rhinovirus neutralizing activity in nasal secretion and serum following the rhinovirus common cold. J Immunol. 1966;97:532.
75. Knopf HLS, Perkins JC, Bertran DM, et al. Analysis of the neutralizing activity in nasal wash and serum following intranasal vaccination with inactivated type 13 rhinovirus. J Immunol. 1970;104:566.
76. Butler WT, Waldmann TA, Rossen RD, et al. Changes in IgA and IgG concentrations in nasal secretions prior to the appearance of antibody during viral respiratory infection in man. J Immunol. 1970;105:584.
77. Rossen RD, Kasel JA, Couch RB. The secretory immune system: Its relation to respiratory viral infection. In Melnick JL, ed. Progress in Medical Virology. Basel: Karger; 1971:194.
78. Cate TR, Couch RB, Johnson KM. Studies with rhinoviruses in volunteers: production of illness, effect of naturally acquired antibody, and demonstration of a protective effect not associated with serum antibody. J Clin Invest. 1964;43:56.
79. Hendley JO, Edmondson WP Jr, Gwaltney JM Jr. Relation between naturally acquired immunity and infectivity of two rhinoviruses in volunteers. J Infect Dis. 1972;125:243.
80. Mufson MA, Ludwig WM, James HD Jr, et al. Effect of neutralizing antibody on experimental rhinovirus infection. JAMA. 1963;186:578.
81. Perkins JC, Tucker DN, Knopf HLS, et al. Comparison of protective effect of neutralizing antibody in serum and nasal secretions in experimental rhinovirus type 13 illness. Am J Epidemiol. 1969;90:519.
82. Perkins JC, Tucker DN, Knopf HLS, et al. Evidence for protective effect of an inactivated rhinovirus vaccine administered by the nasal route. Am J Epidemiol. 1969;90:319.
83. Gwaltney JM Jr. Rhinoviruses. In: Evans AS, ed. Viral Infections of Humans: Epidemiology and Control. New York: Plenum; 1976:383.
84. Bloom HH, Forsyth BR, Johnson KM, et al. Relationship of rhinovirus infection to mild upper respiratory disease. 1. Results of a survey in young adults and children. JAMA. 1963;186:38.
85. Glezen WP, Loda FA, Clyde WA, et al. Epidemiologic patterns of acute lower respiratory disease of children in a pediatric group practice. J Pediatr. 1971;78:397.
86. Mufson MA, Krause HE, Mocega HE, et al. Viruses, *Mycoplasma pneumoniae* and bacteria associated with lower respiratory tract disease among infants. Am J Epidemiol. 1970;91:192.
87. Portnoy B, Eckert HL, Salvatore MA. Rhinovirus infection in children with acute lower respiratory disease: Evidence against etiological importance. Pediatrics. 1965;35:899.
88. Gwaltney JM Jr. Virology of middle ear. Ann Otol Rhinol Laryngol. 1971; 80:365.
89. Doyle WJ, McBride TP, Skoner DP, et al. A double-blind placebo-controlled clinical trial of the effect of chlorpheniramine on the response of the nasal airway, middle ear and eustachian tube to provocative rhinovirus challenge. Pediatr Infect Dis J. 1988;7:222.
90. Smith CB, Kanner RE, Golden CA, et al. Effect of viral infections on pulmonary function in patients with chronic obstructive pulmonary diseases. J Infect Dis. 1980;141:271.
91. Minor TE, Baker JW, Dick EC, et al. Greater frequency of viral respiratory infections in asthmatic children as compared with their nonasthmatic siblings. J Pediatr. 1974;85:472.
92. Halperin SA, Eggleston PA, Beasley P, et al. Exacerbations of asthma in adults during experimental rhinovirus infection. Am Rev Respir Dis. 1985;132:976.
93. Brown PK, Tyrrell DAJ. Experiments on the sensitivity of strains of human fibroblasts to infection with rhinovirus. Br J Exp Pathol. 1964;45:571.
94. Gwaltney JM Jr, Edmondson WP Jr. Etiology and Epidemiology of Acute Respiratory Disease. Annual Progress Report to the Commission on Acute

Respiratory Disease of the Armed Forces Epidemiological Board, Contract No. DADA 49-007-MD-1000, Sept. 15, 1968.
95. Kenny GE, Cooney MK, Thompson DJ. Analysis of serum pooling schemes for identification of large numbers of viruses. Am J Epidemiol. 1970;91:439.
96. Gwaltney JM Jr. Micro-neutralization test for identification of rhinovirus serotypes. Proc Soc Exp Biol Med. 1966;122:1137.
97. Kriel RL, Wulff H, Chin TDY. Micro-neutralization test for determination of rhinovirus and coxsackievirus A antibody in human diploid cells. Appl Microbiol. 1969;17:611.
98. Douglas RG Jr, Fleet WF, Cate TR, et al. Antibody to rhinovirus in human sera. I. Standardization of a neutralization test. Proc Soc Exp Biol Med. 1968;127:497.
99. Andrewes C, Tyrrell DAJ, Stones PB, et al. Prevention of colds by vaccination against a rhinovirus: a report by the scientific committee on common cold vaccines. Br Med J. 1965;1:1344.
100. Douglas RG Jr, Couch RB. Parenteral inactivated rhinovirus vaccine: minimal protective effect. Proc Soc Exp Biol Med. 1972;139:899.
101. Cooney MK, Wise JA. Heterotypic Stimulation of Rhinovirus Antibodies in Rabits. Abstracts of the Annual Meeting of the American Society for Microbiology, May 6–11, 1973:114.
102. Hamory BH, Hamparian VV, Conant RM, et al. Human responses to two decavalent rhinovirus vaccines. J Infect Dis. 1975;132:623.
103. Douglas RG Jr, Couch RB. Attenuation of rhinovirus type 15 for humans. Nature. 1969;223:213.
104. Sperber SJ, Hayden FG. Minireview. Chemotherapy of rhinovirus colds. Antimicrob Agents Chemother. 1988;409.
105. Hayden FG. Use of interferons for prevention and treatment of respiratory viral infections. In: J Mills, L Corey, eds. Antiviral Chemotherapy: New Directions for Clinical Application and Research. Elsevier Science Publishing; New York: 1986:28.
106. Hayden FG, Albrecht JK, Kaiser DL, et al. Prevention of natural colds by contact prophylaxis with intranasal alpha$_2$-interferon. N Engl J Med. 1986;314:71.
107. Douglas RM, Moore BW, Miles HB, et al. Prophylactic efficacy of intranasal alpha$_2$-interferon against rhinovirus infections in the family setting. N Engl J Med. 1986;314:65.

Caliciviridae

153. CALICIVIRUSES AND ASTROVIRUSES

RAPHAEL DOLIN

Caliciviruses and astroviruses are small RNA viruses that have been associated with gastroenteritis in humans. Information regarding the molecular virology and epidemiology of these agents is at an early stage of development, and these viruses are the objects of considerable investigation at present.

CALICIVIRUSES

Caliciviruses were formerly classified as a genus within the family of picornaviruses but are now recognized as a separate family and have been reported to infect a wide variety of animal species.[1] Caliciviruses are nonenveloped, icosahedral viruses 31–35 nm in diameter. The name *calicivirus* is derived from the characteristic appearance of the viral particles under the electron microscope, which consists of a scalloped border with "cup-like" indentations on its surface (Fig. 1) from which the Latin name *chalice* or *calyx* is derived.[2,3] In contrast to animal caliciviruses, which are readily propagated in tissue culture, human caliciviruses have been difficult to cultivate in vitro and relatively little biochemical information is available regarding their replication. Caliciviruses contain a single, plus-stranded RNA genome with a 3′ poly (A) tail. The virion has a single major structural protein of approximately 60 kD in mass.[1]

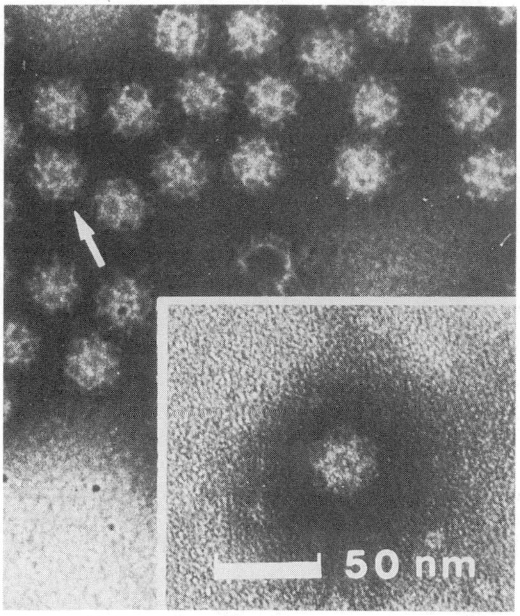

FIG. 1. Calicivirus particles (arrow) in a fecal extract from a child with gastroenteritis. (Inset is higher magnification of particle indicated by arrow.) (From Chiba et al.,[2] with permission.)

Calicivirus-like particles were first described in the stools of children with gastroenteritis in 1976[4] and have subsequently been detected in community-wide and nosocomial outbreaks of gastroenteritis in children as well as in sporadic cases in various parts of the world.[3–8] Seroepidemiologic studies of human caliciviruses carried out in Japan and in the United Kingdom indicate that antibody is acquired in early childhood and can be detected in up to 90 percent of older children and adults.[9,10] Infection with human caliciviruses also appears to be widely prevalent in Southeast Asia.[11] Currently, four or five serologic types of human caliciviruses have been described that apparently do not cross react with known animal caliciviruses.[10] Of interest, serologic cross-reactions have been noted between the Norwalk agent and some human calicivirus infections.[10] This observation as well as the presence of a single structural protein of similar molecular weight (60 kD) in the Norwalk-like agents suggests a potential relatedness between human caliciviruses and the Norwalk-like agents (see Chapter 155).

Little is known regarding the pathogenesis of calicivirus-induced illness. Calicivirus infections of animals have been associated with atrophy of the small intestinal mucosa along with a mild inflammatory infiltrate in the lamina propria.[12,13] Most outbreaks of gastrointestinal illness that have been associated with human caliciviruses have occurred in young children.[3–8] Disease has been generally mild and self-limited and consisted of vomiting and/or diarrhea, abdominal cramps, and low-grade fever. The estimated incubation period for this illness has been 24–72 hours, and disease manifestations have generally lasted from 1 to 3 days. The parameters of immunity to caliciviruses in humans have not been well studied. In a study of an outbreak that occurred in an orphanage in Japan, the presence of pre-existing serum antibody was associated with a lower likelihood of developing illness.[14]

ASTROVIRUSES

Astroviruses are also small RNA viruses that are found in a wide variety of animal species including humans.[15–18] Astroviruses are 28–30 nm in diameter and are nonenveloped with a cubic symmetry. Under the electron microscope, the particles have a characteristic morphology that consists of round smooth edges with multiple triangular electron-lucent areas and an electron-dense center, which results in the appearance of a five or six-pointed star from which the virus derives its name (Fig. 2).[15,16,19] Astroviruses have been difficult to cultivate in vitro, although the serial passage of human astroviruses in tissue culture has been recently reported.[20] Astroviruses have a density of 1.35–1.37 g/cc in CsCl, contain a positive single-stranded 35 S RNA genome with a poly (A) tail, and have two to four structural polypeptides.[21] In contrast to other recently described viral agents of gastroenteritis, astroviruses are often shed in large amounts in stool and can be readily detected by electron microscopy even without immune aggregation. Detection of astroviruses in tissue culture has been carried out by immune electron microscopy or by immunofluorescence, and an enzyme-linked immunosorbent asssay (ELISA) has been recently reported.[22] At least five serotypes of human astroviruses have been recognized in the United Kingdom,[22,23] and these appear to be serologically unrelated to Norwalk-like viruses with which they have been compared. Seroprevalence studies in the United Kingdom have shown that 75 percent of children between 3 and 4 years of age have detectable serum antibody,[24] but systematic studies of the epidemiology of astrovirus infections in humans have not been carried out.

The pathogenesis of astrovirus-induced illness is not well understood. Astrovirus infections in animals have been associated with small intestinal villus shortening and with mild inflammatory infiltrates in the lamina propria.[12,25] In humans, astroviruses have been detected in diarrheal stools from school outbreaks among young children, in pediatric wards, and from nursing homes outbreaks.[15,16,20,21] Stool filtrates that contain astroviruses readily infect volunteers after oral administration but induce illness very infrequently,[26] which suggests that astroviruses may be less "pathogenic" in adults than Norwalk-like agents are.

Illness attributed to astroviruses consists primarily of diarrhea, headache, malaise, and nausea, while vomiting appears to be less common. Low-grade fever is frequently present. The incubation period of illness has been estimated to be 3–4 days, and disease manifestations usually last only 2–3 days but occasionally can be longer in duration.

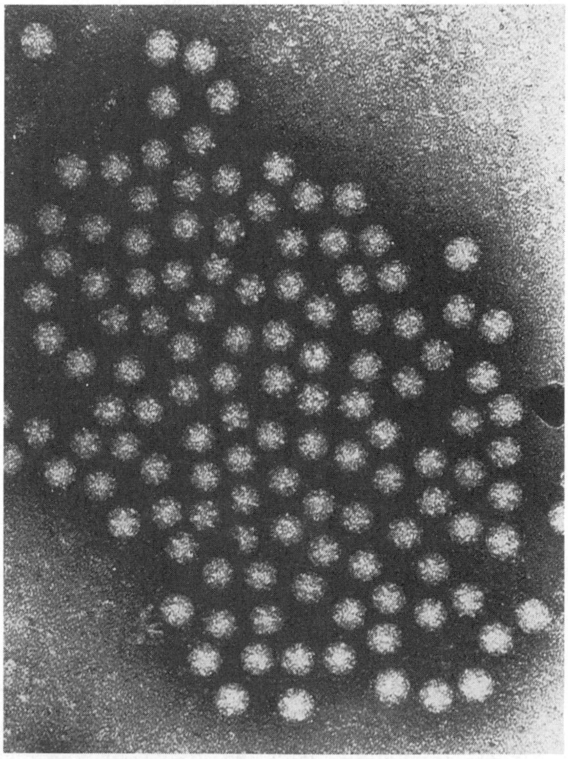

FIG. 2. Astrovirus in the intestinal contents of gnotobiotic lambs. Particles are 30 nm in diameter. (From Snodgrass et al.,[19] with permission.)

Diagnosis and Treatment

Laboratory diagnostic tests are research procedures that are not widely available at present. Caliciviruses and astroviruses can be detected in stool specimens by electron microscopy. A radioimmunoassay[27] has been recently developed for caliciviruses, and an ELISA has been reported for astroviruses,[22] and astroviruses can also be detected in tissue culture by using immunofluorescence techniques.[23] Illness associated with these agents is generally self-limited, and treatment is supportive, if required at all, and is directed at maintaining hydration and electrolyte balance.

REFERENCES

1. Schaffer FL, Bachrach HL, Brown F, et al. Caliciviridae. Intervirology. 1980;14:1–6.
2. Chiba S, Sakuma Y, Kogasaka R, et al. Fecal shedding of virus in relation to the days of illness in infantile gastroenteritis due to calicivirus. J Infect Dis. 1980;142:247–9.
3. Chiba S, Sakuma Y, Kogasaka R, et al. An outbreak of gastroenteritis associated with calicivirus in an infant home. J Med Virol. 1979;4:249–54.
4. Madeley CR, Cosgrove BP. Caliciviruses in man (Letter). Lancet. 1976;1;199–200.
5. Flewett TH, Davies H. Caliciviruses (Letter). Lancet. 1976;1:311.
6. Kjeldsberg E. Small spherical viruses in faeces from gastroenteritis patients. Acta Pathol Microbiol Immunol Scand 1977;85:351–4.
7. Spratt HC, Marks MI, Gomersall M, et al. Nosocomial infantile gastroenteritis associated with minirotavirus and calicivirus. J Pediatr. 1978;93:922–6.
8. Oishi I, Maeda A, Yamazaki K, et al. Calicivirus detected in outbreaks of acute gastroenteritis in school children. Biken J. 1980;23:163–8.
9. Sakuma Y, Chiba S, Kogasaka R, et al. Prevalence of antibody to human calicivirus in general population of Northern Japan. J Med Virol. 1981;7; 221–5.
10. Cubitt WD, Blacklow NR, Herrmann JE. Antigenic relationships between human caliciviruses and Norwalk virus. J Infect Dis. 1987;156:806–14.
11. Nakata S, Chiba S, Terashima H, et al. Prevalence of antibody to human calicivirus in Japan and Southeast Asia determined by radioimmunoassay. J Clin Microbiol. 1985;22:519–21.
12. Woode GN, Bridger JC. Isolation of small viruses resembling astroviruses and caliciviruses from acute enteritis of calves. J Med Microbiol. 1978;11:441–52.
13. Saif LJ, Bohl EH, Theil KW, et al. Rotavirus-like, calicivirus-like, and 23-nm virus-like particles associated with diarrhea in young pigs. J Clin Microbiol. 1980;12:105–11.
14. Nakata S, Chiba A, Terashima H, et al. Humoral immunity in infants with gastroenteritis caused by human calicivirus . J Infect Dis. 1985;152:274–9.
15. Madeley CR, Cosgrove BP. 28 nm particles in faeces in infantile gastroenteritis (Letter). Lancet. 1975;2:451.
16. Ashley CR, Caul EO, Paver WK. Astrovirus-associated gastroenteritis in children. J Clin Pathol. 1978;31:939–43.
17. Kurtz JB, Lee TW, Pickering D. Astrovirus associated gastroenteritis in a children's ward. J Clin Pathol. 1977;30:948–52.
18. Konno T, Suzuki H, Ishida N, et al. Astrovirus-associated epidemic gastroenteritis in Japan. J Med Virol. 1982;9:11–7.
19. Snodgrass DR, Gray W. Detection and transmission of 30 nm virus particles (astroviruses) in the faeces of lambs with diarrhoea. Arch Virol. 1977;55:287–91.
20. Lee TW, Kurtz JB. Serial propagation of astrovirus in tissue culture with the aid of trypsin. J Gen Virol. 1981;57:421–4.
21. Herring AJ, Gray EW, Snodgrass DR. Purification and characterization of bovine astrovirus. J Gen Virol 1981;53:47–55.
22. Herrmann JE, Hudson RW, Perron-Henry DM, et al. Antigen characterization of cell-cultivated astrovirus serotypes and development of astrovirus-specific monoclonal antibodies. J Infect Dis 1988;158:182–5.
23. Kurtz JB, Lee TW. Human astrovirus serotypes (Letter). Lancet 1984;2:1405.
24. Kurtz J, Lee T. Astrovirus gastroenteritis age distribution of antibody. Med Microbiol Immunol (Berl). 1978;166:227–30.
25. Snodgrass DR, Angus KW, Gray EW, et al. Pathogenesis of diarrhoea caused by astrovirus infection in lambs. Arch Virol. 1979;60:217–26.
26. Kurtz JB, Lee TW, Craig JW, et al. Astrovirus infection in volunteers. J Med Virol. 1979;3:221–30.
27. Nakata S, Chiba S, Terashima H, et al. Microtiter solid-phase radioimmunoassay for detection of human calicivirus in stools. J Clin Microbiol. 1983;17:198–201.

UNCLASSIFIED VIRUSES

154. NON-A, NON-B HEPATITIS, INCLUDING HEPATITIS C AND HEPATITIS E VIRUSES

STEPHEN M. FEINSTONE

HISTORY

The existence of non-A, non-B (NANB) hepatitis was first recognized after sensitive serologic tests for hepatitis B[1,2] and then hepatitis A[3] were developed. The early tests for Australia antigen, now called hepatitis B surface antigen (HBsAg) only marginally reduced the incidence of transfusion-associated hepatitis, and antibody tests (anti-HBs) could identify only a fraction of people who had been infected by the hepatitis B virus (HBV). When sensitive radioimmunoassay (RIA) tests for HBsAg were introduced for screening blood donors, the expected elimination of transfusion-associated hepatitis did not occur.[4] In studies carried out at the National Institutes of Health, it was felt that the major reduction of transfusion-associated hepatitis observed after introduction of the RIA test for HBsAg was due to the simultaneous elimination of commercial sources of donor blood.[5] Serologic analysis of these transfusion-associated hepatitis patients with highly sensitive tests for anti-HBs revealed that many of them did not seem to have been exposed to HBV. While some thought that hepatitis A virus (HAV) might have caused these cases of post-transfusion hepatitis, the epidemiology and clinical presentation of this disease did not fit with what had been described for type A hepatitis. Volunteer studies had demonstrated that HAV could be transmitted parenterally by serum. However, the viremic phase of hepatitis A was known to be relatively short, there was no evidence for a chronic carrier state, and the usual mode of transmission was fecal–oral.[6,7] In addition, secondary cases of hepatitis, as would expected for hepatitis A, were generally not reported in close contacts of these non-B transfusion-associated hepatitis cases. In 1974 Prince and colleagues reported a group of patients with transfusion-associated hepatitis who had incubation periods clearly longer than the 3–6 weeks that was accepted as the typical incubation period for hepatitis A.[8] The first specific test for hepatitis A was developed in 1973,[9] and one of the first applications was to analyze cases of non-B transfusion-associated hepatitis.[10] Out of 17 cases of well-documented non-B transfusion-associated hepatitis, none could be serologically associated with HAV infections. Thus the existence of a different form of transmissible, presumably viral hepatitis was demonstrated. While diagnostic tests for hepatitis A and B are now commonly available in most clinical laboratories, there is no specific diagnostic test for NANB hepatitis presently available. At this time the diagnosis of NANB hepatitis depends on the clinical and epidemiologic situation and the serologic exclusion of the known causes of viral hepatitis.

Because a specific diagnostic test has only recently been developed and is not yet widely available, research into the nature of the causative agent, the epidemiology, the clinical expression, as well as the prevention and treatment has necessarily been retarded. The most pressing problem of NANB hepatitis remains how to eliminate it from the blood supply, but many other important questions require answers such as the relationship of NANB viral hepatitis to chronic liver disease, cirrhosis, and hepatocelluular carcinoma. Many of these questions have answers or partial answers due to slow and methodical studies of dedicated researchers. However, confidence in our present knowledge is limited by our experience with the other hepatitis agents. While some concepts remained intact, many others had to be altered when specific diagnostics for hepatitis A and B were developed.

THE PATHOGEN

The most controversial aspect of NANB hepatitis has been the nature of the causative agent. There has been extensive searches made in many laboratories around the world for the agent of NANB hepatitis. Numerous serologic tests have been described, virus-like particles have been reported, viral-like enzymes have been detected, and nucleic acids have been detected and even cloned. While any one of these past reports may eventually prove to be correct, no test of any sort had been able to reliably detect the virus, any specific viral product, or antibody to any viral antigen. While it is not definitively known at this time how many different agents are responsible for NANB hepatitis or if there are different serotypes of these agents, it appears that at least one of the viruses, and probably the most important one, of NANB hepatitis is now being characterized by molecular and serologic techniques (see below).

What little is known about the NANB hepatitis virus(es) has been learned primarily from chimpanzee inoculation studies. It is not clear how many agents cause NANB hepatitis. Multiple bouts of NANB hepatitis have been recognized, especially in drug addicts and multiply transfused patients such as hemophiliacs.[9–11] It is not known whether these multiple attacks are new infections or exacerbations of chronic infections. Cross-challenge studies in chimpanzees have yielded confusing results. Two immunologically distinct agents seem to have been transmitted to chimpanzees.[12–16] These agents provide homologous but not heterologous immunity, and one causes the typical cytoplasmic tubules (see below) in hepatocytes while the other does not, and one is sensitive to extraction with chloroform and the other is not. However, Brotman and colleagues have been able to produce disease in chimpanzees by reinoculating a large dose of the identical material used to produce the initial infection.[17] Therefore second cases of NANB hepatitis may be either reinfection with the original agent, reactivation of a chronic or latent infection, or infection with a serologically and perhaps virologically distinct agent.

NANB hepatitis infectivity was shown to pass a 220 nm filter by Prince and associates in 1978.[18] This observation was extended by Bradley and colleagues who showed that the agents passed an 80 nm filter[19] and by He and colleagues who found that the agent passed a 50 but not a 30 nm filter.[20] The virus was shown to contain essential lipids, presumably in a lipid-containing envelope, by extracting infectious plasma with chloroform and demonstrating that this treated plasma had lost its infectivity.[21] Bradley and coworkers, however, have reported that one form of NANB hepatitis is caused by a chloroform-sensitive agent while another is caused by a chloroform-resistant virus.[16,19] The picture of a small (less than 50 nm) lipid-containing agent leaves very few possibilities among the known groups of viruses. These include the hepadnaviruses, the delta hepatitis agent, and the togaviruses.

The most intriguing of these possibilities is a hepatitis B related virus. Several reports have suggested a relationship between HBV and the causative agent of NANB hepatitis. The NANB hepatitis agent could be a variant of HBV expression or perhaps an entirely different hepadnavirus related to HBV in the same way that the duck or woodchuck hepatitis B viruses are to related to HBV. A hepadnavirus etiology for NANB hepatitis fits with the limited information on the physical and chemical properties of the virus. In addition, hepatitis B and NANB hepatitis share some epidemiologic and clinical features (see below). Antigens that cross react with hepatitis B surface (HBsAg), core (HBcAg) and e antigen (HBeAg) have been reported in patients with putative NANB hepatitis.[22–24] Wands and colleagues have developed monoclonal antibodies against HBsAg and used these antibodies to construct RIAs for HBsAg that they claim are more sensitive than are conventional RIAs based on polyclonal antibodies.[25] Using this RIA, Wands et al. found some patients who had been diagnosed as having NANB hepatitis to have HBsAg in their serum.[26] In addition to the possible serologic relationship between NANB and type B hepatitis, there are also reports of a genetic relationship. Both patients believed to have NANB hepatitis and chimpanzees experimentally infected with human blood derivatives thought to contain the NANB hepatitis agent have been studied for the presence of DNA in either their serum or in liver biopsy specimens that hybridize with specific HBV DNA probes. Such hybridizable sequences have been detected in both serum and liver often in association with the antigen detected by the Wands monoclonal antibody.[26–28] Thus it seems likely that some cases of NANB hepatitis are actually misdiagnosed HBV infections. In contrast, other laboratories have reported no HBV hybridizable sequences in NANB hepatitis specimens.[29–32] Nonetheless, it may also be possible that some NANB hepatitis may be caused by a replication-deficient HBV. Such a virus must be capable of growing only to low titers and expressing little if any excess HBsAg. In addition, the anti-HBc response in these patients and animals must be either limited or the core antigen toward which the antibody is directed must be poorly cross-reactive with the standard HBcAg. The studies of transfusion-associated hepatitis as well as the chimpanzee inoculations that have been performed seem to contradict the relatedness between HBV and common NANB hepatitis. In these studies there was no protection in HBV-seropositive patients or chimpanzees against infection by the NANB hepatitis agent whether the anti-hepatitis B was secondary to an HBV infection or vaccination. HBV-seropositive chimpanzees did not express an antibody booster response after NANB hepatitis infection (Fields et al.,[33] Feinstone et al.,[34] and Feinstone, unpublished observations). This possible similarity of NANB hepatitis to HBV will be resolved by isolation, cloning, and sequencing the genome of the NANB hepatitis agent that cross reacts with HBV.

In 1984 Seto and colleagues reported the detection of reverse transcriptase activity in the serum of patients with NANB hepatitis.[35] According to their report, this enzyme activity was associated with a particle that had some of the physical characteristics of a retrovirus. This report was followed by the detection of particles in infected chimpanzee hepatocyes that were said to resemble retroviruses[36] and the detection and purification of a glycoprotein with a molecular weight of about 77,000.[37] There is only one report confirming the reverse transcriptase reactivity,[38] but many laboratories have not been able to reproduce these results.[39] The proof of these findings depends on their utility in identifying patients with NANB hepatitis, and to this date neither the reverse transcriptase nor the glycoprotein tests have been shown to have such utility.

A Chiron Corporation group led by Michael Houghton reports that they have been successful in obtaining at least partial complementary DNA clones of the NANB hepatitis virus RNA genome. They have sequenced these clones and expressed a peptide from one of them that is reactive with antibody in the serum of patients convalescent from NANB hepatitis and, more importantly, in patients who are chronically infected by the virus either as inapparent carriers or with chronic disease. Therefore this antibody test may be useful for screening blood donors. Characterization of this RNA genome has revealed that it is approximately 10,000 bases in length, plus (message) sense, and it has a single open reading frame.[39a] This finding appears to be the most important yet reported and may finally lead to a fuller understanding of the virus, the disease, and its clinical and epidemiologic characteristics. It would seem that a specific test for diagnostics as well as screening blood donors is at hand (see Chapter 102).

EPIDEMIOLOGY

Many of the epidemiologic features of NANB hepatitis resemble hepatitis B in general ways, but there are important differences. Chronic infections and chronic disease have been demonstrated, and there must also be a chronic carrier state in people who have little if any overt disease that allows for the transmission of the virus by seemingly healthy blood donors. The carrier rate in blood donors has been estimated in several large studies of transmission-associated hepatitis in the United States. The attack rates among recipients of single-unit blood transfusions varied between 1 and 11.5 percent in the various centers of the Transfusion Transmitted Viruses Study (TTVS) and was approximately 1 percent for volunteer and 5.4 percent for commercial blood recipients in the Veterans Administration (VA) cooperative study.[40,41] It is estimated that there are 150,000 cases of transfusion-associated hepatitis in the United States each year and at least 95 percent are NANB hepatitis.

Many plasma derivatives that are made from large pools of plasma from perhaps thousands of donors are nearly universally contaminated with the NANB hepatitis virus. Factor VIII and IX products are particularly dangerous, and the rate of chronic liver disease among hemophiliacs is distressingly high.[42–45] Measures to eliminate the NANB hepatitis virus as well as HBV and the human immunodeficiency virus by both specific screening of donors and inactivation of remaining viruses are currently being applied (see "Prevention"), and it is hoped that these vital biologic products can rendered noninfectious.

Routes of Infection

While NANB hepatitis has been best recognized in association with transfusion of blood or blood products, it should be recognized that the vast majority of cases must occur without overt exposure to blood. It has been estimated that 1–7 percent of blood donors are carriers of the NANB hepatitis virus. Very few of these donors have ever had a blood transfusion or other parenteral exposure to blood or blood products. These patients must have acquired their infections by other mechanisms, most likely close personal contact in much the same ways as hepatitis B is acquired. It has been speculated that sporadic, community-acquired NANB hepatitis is a different disease from transfusion-associated hepatitis, that this form of the disease does not progress to chronic hepatitis, and that it probably is caused by the agent responsible for the enterically transmitted NANB hepatitis (see below). However, in an ongoing study of viral hepatitis in four sentinal counties being conducted by the Centers for Disease Control, Alter and colleagues reported that, among 131 patients diagnosed as having NANB hepatitis, 43 percent had a history of exposure including 20 percent transfused and 23 percent with iv drug use. Of the remainder, 3 percent were health care workers, and 2 percent were household contacts of patients with NANB hepatitis. Persistently elevated liver enzyme levels were observed in 66 (50 percent) of the 131 patients. There was no significant difference in the proportion of patients with chronic hepatitis among patients with a known exposure to blood as compared with patients who had only a known contact with patients with NANB hepatitis and patients who had no known exposure of any kind.[46,47] On the basis of these results there is no reason to suspect that the hepatitis related to blood transfusion and that acquired by unknown community exposure were caused by different agents.

NANB hepatitis does not seem to be as easily transmitted as hepatitis B by personal contact. This may be due to the relatively lower titer of infectious virus in NANB hepatitis as compared with hepatitis B. Secondary cases of hepatitis have been recognized in sexual contacts and family members of patients with parenteraly acquired NANB hepatitis, but this is not commonly observed.[48] The mild expression of acute disease may result in a low rate of recognitiion of secondary cases, but it is also likely that the low titers of the virus in the patient's blood and presumably in other body fluids result in infrequent transmission between family members. In the controlled trial of hepatitis B vaccine in homosexual men, a NANB hepatitis annual attack rate of 2.9 percent was observed.[49] However, the importance of sexual transmission or other possible modes of nonpercutaneous transmission in maintaining NANB hepatitis in the community are not clear. Certainly the epidemiology of NANB hepatitis does not follow either a respiratory or an oral mode of spread.

Maternal infant transmission has been suggested in one study in which it was found that six of nine infants of mothers with NANB hepatitis in the third trimester but none of these infants born to mothers in the second trimester had mild elevations in liver enzyme levels.[50] The full extent of maternal transmission will be better understood when a specific diagnostic test becomes available. It is also important to know whether NANB hepatitis acquired at a young age leads more commonly to chronic infections and what the consequences of this might be.

Since NANB hepatitis is known to be spread by the percutaneous route and there is recent information that the virus might be a member of the togavirus family, the possibility of an insect vector must be considered. At this time there is no direct evidence for this mode of transmission.

Population Groups

Very few data exist on relative rates of infection in various population groups or in geographic areas. It seems that NANB hepatitis can be found in any part of the world where it is carefully looked for, but the relative incidences of A, B and NANB hepatitis in various parts of the world is quite variable. The Transfusion Transmitted Viruses Study seems to indicate that blood donors from lower socioeconomic areas were more likely to transmit NANB hepatitis than were donors from more affluent areas.[40] It was also recognized very early that the elimination of commercial sources of blood significantly reduced both B and NANB transfusion-associated hepatitis.[1,41]

Incubation Period

The incubation period of NANB hepatitis in the setting of transfusion-associated hepatitis has been shown to have a rather broad range of less than 2 weeks and up to 6 months with a mean of about 7–8 weeks. Very short incubation periods of as little 4 days have been reported in some hemophiliac patients receiving factor VIII concentrate.[51,52] It has been speculated that this short-incubation hepatitis is caused by a virus different from the transfusion-associated hepatitis agent. This is not likely because when this factor VIII material is inoculated into chimpanzees the disease induced is identical to the disease in chimpanzees that is produced by whole blood plasma including the typical histologic markers of NANB hepatitis in chimpanzees (see below).[53] In addition, it would be hard to understand that there is a virus in a plasma fraction that is not in whole blood. It remains possible that the wide range of incubation periods is due to multiple etiologies of NANB hepatitis. When infectious plasma was titered by incoulating serial 10-fold dilutions into champanzees, there was essentially no change in the incubation period with the dose of the inoculum.[53] This is in contrast to both HAV and HBV infection in which the incubation periods were shown to be both reproducible and inversly related to the dose.

PATHOGENESIS

There is essentially nothing known about the pathogenesis of NANB hepatitis. The low viral titers found in clinical samples may indicate that the disease is not a result of a direct attack of the virus on hepatocytes. Immune complexes have been reported to be associated with NANB hepatitis, but again there is no information on their makeup or their role in pathogenesis.[54]

CLINICAL MANIFESTATIONS

The important clinical features of NANB hepatitis are that the acute infection tends to be mild relative to hepatitis A and B but that NANB hepatitis has a high propensity to produce chronic infections and disease. However, there are no specific clinical features that can distinguish an individual case of NANB hepatitis from A or B hepatitis. Acute hepatitis with complete recovery, acute fulminant hepatitis, relapsing disease, chronic inapparent infections, and chronic active hepatitis with cirrhosis have all been reported.[42–44,55,56]

Acute Hepatitis

In transfusion-associated NANB hepatitis the alanine aminotransferase (ALT) levels typically range between 200 and 600 units/L. Only about a quarter of these patients are icteric, and other signs and symptoms of acute viral hepatitis are less prominant in NANB hepatitis than in hepatitis B. Fulminant hepatitis cases have been diagnosed as NANB, but on the basis of the prospective transfusion-associated hepatitis studies, the proportion of NANB hepatitis cases that result in fulminant disease is not thought to be high. Among 20 fulminant hepatitis cases in Denmark, 4 were diagnosed as hepatitis A, 9 were hepatitis B, 1 was mixed hepatitis A and B, and 6 were thought to be NANB.[56] In other studies as many as 44 percent of fulminant cases were thought to be type NANB,[57] but without specific tests it is not possible to know whether all these cases were indeed NANB viral hepatitis or were acute hepatic failure caused by some nonviral etiology.

Relapsing Hepatitis

When patients with acute NANB hepatitis are followed carefully, they may seem to recover only to relapse either clinically or biochemically. This relapsing nature of the disease is one of its most typical features that occurs much less frequently in hepatitis B. Rarely have single relapses been reported to occur shortly after acute hepatitis A.[58] Whether these relapses represent exacerbations of chronic infections, reappearance of latent infections, or less likely, reinfection with the same or different NANB hepatitis virus is not known at this time.

Chronic Hepatitis

If NANB hepatitis caused only acute hepatitis, it would only be considered a highly unpleasant nuisance. However, the most troublesome aspect of this infection is that it frequently causes chronic infections and serious chronic liver disease. The proportion of NANB infections that become chronic is not known because many of those infected may not have overt liver disease and the only method at this time for demonstrating the presence of virus is champanzee inoculation. Nonetheless chronic infections in both humans and experimentally infected chimpanzees have been demonstrated.[59,60] In studies of transfusion-associated NANB hepatitis, chronic hepatitis rates between 10 and 70 percent have been reported.[61] In 75 carefully followed patient at the National Institutes of Health (NIH), Hoofnagle and Alter found that 68 percent had elevations in ALT levels that persisted for more than 1 year after transfusion.[62] In a recent report of 676 consecutive transfused patients from Milan, Italy, in which blood donors with elevated ALT levels were excluded, 96 patients developed hepatitis, and 92 were diagnosed as having type NANB.[63] Even though the hepatitis was completely asymptomatic in 68 of these patients, 60 percent had elevated ALT levels 1 year after the onset of the acute disease.

Long-term prospective follow-up studies have not been performed, so the natural history of chronic NANB hepatitis is not completely known. A number of patients have undergone biopsies to determine the nature of their chronic liver disease.[61] The important finding of these studies is that all ranges of histologic lesions of chronic hepatitis have been observed from chronic persistent hepatitis to chronic active hepatitis to cirrhosis with and without portal hypertension. Although patients who had biopsy samples taken in these studies probably represented the more severe end of the spectrum of the chronic patients, the severity of their lesions could not be predicted on clinical findings.

Di Bisceglie and associates performed biopsies on 50 patients who were referred to the NIH for a treatment trial.[64] The duration of hepatitis in these patients ranged between 6 months and 20 years, with a mean of 3.9 years. Twelve patients (24 percent) had cirrhosis, and most of these patients had their disease for several years. Three patients developed cirrhosis with clinical signs of portal hypertension within 12 months of the onset of their disease after blood transfusion. These three were 58, 63, and 68 years old, while the mean age of the group was 43 and the mean age of all the 12 patients with cirrhosis was 49.8. Thus serious chronic liver disease is a common finding in NANB hepatitis, and cirrhosis seems to correlate with the duration of the infection and the age of the patient. Older patients are perhaps more likely to experience the rapid onset of cirrhosis.

Extrahepatic Manifestations

It is not known whether the NANB hepatitis virus replicates outside the liver, but there is little evidence of extrahepatic pathology. Cases of agrnulocytosis and aplastic anemia with hepatitis have often been classified as type NANB,[65] but other than the rare occurrence of prodromal arthritis, the extrahepatic manifestations frequently seen in HBV infections have not been reported in NANB hepatitis.

Hepatocellular Carcinoma

The relationship of chronic HBV infection to hepatocellular carcinoma is well established,[66] although the mechanism of oncogenesis is not understood. Since NANB hepatitis may lead to chronic liver disease including cirrhosis, it is possible that NANB hepatitis is an important cause of hepatocellular carcinoma not related to HBV infections. Kiyosawa et al. reported a case of hepatocellular carcinoma that developed in a man 18 years after he conrtraced NANB hepatitis from a blood transfusion.[67] During this 18-year period he had five liver biopsies, and his course from acute to chronic hepatitis to cirrhosis and finally to hepatocellular carcinoma was well documented. Okuda and colleagues performed a retrospective analysis of 113 patients with non-alcohol-related chronic liver disease and hepatocellular carcinoma. Of these patients, 23 had no HBV markers and were therefore diagnosed as having NANB hepatitis, while 35 were HBsAg-positive, and 55 had serologic evidence of past HBV infections. Okuda et al. speculated that NANB infections may have played an important role either directly or indirectly through the induction of cirrhosis not only in the 23 NANB patients but also in at least a portion of the 55 patients with serologic evidence of past HBV infections.[68] The exact importance of NANB hepatitis in hepatocellular carcinoma will await the availability of specific tests.

DIAGNOSIS

Numerous serologic tests have been described to detect antigens and antibodies associated with NANB hepatitis. None of these tests have proved useful for diagnosing patients with the disease or for screening blood donors who may be asymptomatic carriers and will not be discussed. The recent announcement of the cloning of specific viral complementary DNA sequences and the expression of a peptide antigen recognized by antibody in the serum of patients in late acute, chronic, or convalescent stages of NANB hepatitis may quickly lead to the availability of specific diagnostic tests. For the present the diagnosis is still based on the clinical and epidemiologic situation and the exclusion of other forms of viral hepatitis by serologic testing (see the chapters on hepatitis A and B). It should be remembered that cytomegalovirus (CMV) has been implicated in transfusion-associated hepatitis and hepatitis is a frequent occurrence in Epstein-Barr virus (EBV) infections. It is important to exclude these two viruses as well as nonviral causes of hepatitis if the clinical situation warrants before a presumptive diagnosis of NANB hepatitis can be made.

Surrogate tests, ALT serum levels, and the presence of anti-HBc are now being used in an attempt to screen out high-risk blood donors (see below). These tests seem to have value in reducing the rate of transfusion-associated hepatitis, but they cannot be considered diagnostic tests for individual patients, epidemiologic studies, or even research applications.

Histopathologic changes characteristic of NANB hepatitis have been described that may aid in the diagnosis of patients with chronic liver disease but not with acute hepatitis because liver biopsy is rarely performed on these patients in the United States. Two typical lesions have been observed by light microscopy in liver biopsy specimens from patients with either acute or chronic NANB hepatitis.[69,70] First was an eosinophilic alteration of hepatocytes that was associated with a large number of acidophilic bodies. Second was an activation of the sinusoidal lining cells. Portal and periportal inflammation was observed but was mild relative to the degree of parenchymal reaction. The lesions were similar in both the acute and chronic cases although changes in the chronic hepatitis including cirrhosis have been observed.

In chimpanzees with acute and chronic NANB hepatitis a characteristic electron microscopic change has been regularly observed (Fig. 1). Cytoplasmic tubules (cylindrical confronting cisternae) consisting of double-unit membranes presumably

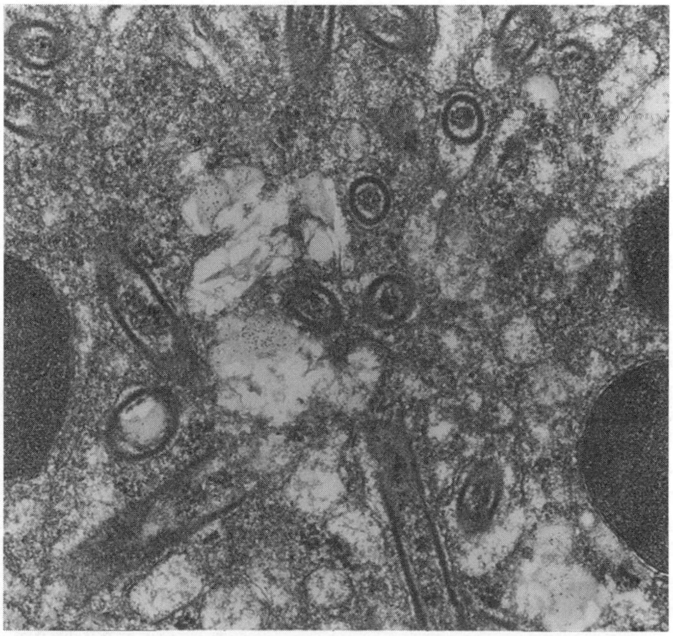

FIG. 1. An electron micrograph of a hepatocyte from a chimpanzee biopsied during acute NANB hepatitis. The typical membrane-bound tubules (cylindrical confronting cisternae) are seen in both cross and longitudinal section. (×60,000) (Courtesy of Dr. Terry Popkin, Bethesda, MD.)

formed from rolled and fused rough endoplasmic reticulum are seen in correlation with the disease state.[71,72] These structures have also been seen in human biopsy specimens[73] but at a much lower frequency than in chimpanzees where they can be seen in almost every hepatocyte during active disease. Precisely the same structures have been observed in chimpanzees with delta hepatitis (coexisting with HBV infection) but not in HAV- or HBV-infected chimpanzees.[71,74] In addition, similar structures have been observed in lymphocytes from patients with acquired immunodeficiency syndrome (AIDS).[75] The exact nature of these structures and what role they have in the replication of the NANB hepatitis virus is not known, but recent data suggest that these structures are a response to interferon.[76]

Shimizu and colleagues have developed monoclonal antibodies from EBV-immortalized peripheral blood lymphocytes from chimpanzees and humans convalescent from NANB hepatitis. They were able to select antibodies that reacted with acute-phase liver biopsy samples but not preinfection specimens in an indirect immunofluorescence assay.[77] Using immunoelectron microscopy, she found that these antibodies were directed against clusters of microtubular of filamentous structures that were seen commonly in chimpanzee hepatocytes during NANB hepatitis. Like the cytoplasmic fused membrane tubules, this structural antigen was also seen in liver biopsy specimens from chimpanzees with delta but not type A or B hepatitis.[78] Again it has been difficult to see this reactivity in humans, but by using immunoperoxidase Shimizu has been able to see what is likely to be the same antigen in human biopsy material (Shimizu, personal communication). The nature of the antigen is not completely known at this time, but it has been shown to be a host-coded antigen. Preliminary data further seem to indicate that the appearance of this antigen is also related to interferon. While increased levels of plasma interferon in NANB hepatitis have not been reported, it is possible that the NANB virus is a potent inducer of local interferon in the liver. It is curious that patients with NANB hepatitis make antibody to a host-coded antigen that seems to be produced in response to interferon. Whether this host response plays a role in pathogenesis can only be a matter for speculation at this time.

PREVENTION

Until this time efforts at preventing NANB hepatitis have focused primarily on the elimination of high-risk people as blood donors and inactivation of the NANB hepatitis virus in pooled plasma products such as factor VIII concentrate. With a specific test on the horizon it may be possible to identify carriers with a high degree of accuracy. In addition, the expression of an antigen associated with the NANB hepatitis virus will allow for a better understanding of the immune response in this disease and the possible preparation of a vaccine.

At present, all blood for transfusion is tested for either elevated levels of ALT or the presence of anti-HBc. These two tests together with the elimination of commercial blood donors has greatly reduced the risk of transfusion-associated hepatitis. The increased risk of hepatitis in transfused patients who received at least 1 unit of blood that had an elevated level of ALT was first recognized in the Transfusion Transmitted Viruses Study.[79] While hepatitis risk increased with the number of units received that had elevated ALT levels, the risk was also noted to be increased in recipients of single-unit transfusions when that unit had an elevated ALT content. It was calculated that exclusion of the blood units with elevated ALT levels would have resulted in a 30 percent reduction in the number of hepatitis cases. In an analysis of the multiply transfused heart surgery patients who had been followed prospectively at the NIH, Alter and associates found that elimination of blood with elevated ALT levels would have reduced hepatitis about 29 percent with a 1.6 percent loss in donors.[80]

In these same studies of transfusion-associated hepatitis it was shown that there was an association between the presence of anti-HBc in donor blood and the development of hepatitis in the recipient. Stevens et al. reported that the rate of NANB hepatitis was about threefold higher in recipients of anti-HBc-positive blood than in patients who received only anti-HBc-negative blood.[81] Studies by Alter at the NIH have confirmed the Transfusion Transmitted Viruses Study findings.[82] Although anti-HBc may predict high-risk blood donors, there is no evidence for a specific antigenic cross-reactivity between HBV and NANB hepatitis. Recipients of this anti-HBc-positive blood did not develop anti-HBc after NANB hepatitis. Alter has estimated that elimination of anti-HBc-positive blood would reduce transfusion-associated hepatitis approximately 40 percent with a loss of donors of 2–4 percent.[82] specific tests for the NANB hepatitis virus will eliminate the need for these surrogate tests and eliminate much of the cost of time, money, and lost donors. If, however, there proves to be more than one NANB hepatitis virus, surrogate tests may have a continuing role in screening blood donors until specific tests for all the viruses are established.

Methods are now being introduced to inactivate several viral agents that are known to contaminate cell-free blood products. These viruses include not only the NANB hepatitis agent but also HBV, hepatitis delta virus (HDV), human immunodeficiency virus (HIV), human T-cell lymphotropic virus I (HTLV-I), CMV, EBV, and the human parovarius. The methods include the use of heat, ultraviolet light with β-propiolactone, various organic solvents, and purification.[83,84] The most common method in use at this time is heat, which has been used either on the dry lyophylized product or as a pasteurization process while the product is still in aqueous solution.[85] The wet heating process seems to be somewhat more effective, but neither has been uniformly successful in eliminating all viral agents.[86,87]

Since most of the viruses that contaminate blood products have lipid envelopes, lipid solvents have been used to inactivate them. Chloroform has been shown to be a very effective inactivating agent but has not been widely used on blood products.[21,88] Ether has been used in combination with the detergent Tween 80, but the combination of tri-(*n*-butyl) phosphate with Tween 80 for factor IX or with sodium cholate for factor VIII seem to be highly effective.[84]

While a specific test for NANB hepatitis carriers may soon be available, the experience with HBV indicates that transmission of this virus to chronic users of plasma products made from large pools of plasma is still a problem and inactivation procedures may still be necessary. The ultimate solution may come from the use of synthetic plasma products produced through recombinant DNA technology.[89]

Studies have been performed on the efficacy of passive immunoprophylaxis by immune serum globulin (ISG) for the prevention of transfusion-associated hepatitis with mixed results, and at this time its use is not recommended. Kuhns and associates reported that ISG administered on the 7th and 30th days after transfusion was not effective in reducing NANB hepatitis.[90] In contrast, Knodell and colleagues reported that ISG administered before cardiac surgery reduced the incidence of both acute and chronic transfusion-associated hepatitis.[91,92] Seeff et al. found no significant difference in the rate of transfusion-associated hepatitis in recipients of ISG (9.8 percent) or placebo (12.1 percent), but icteric hepatitis was reduced from 1.8 to 0.8 percent; however, this effect was most pronounced in recipients of commercial blood, and elimination of this source of blood would have been much more effective in reducing all forms of hepatitis than would the use of ISG.[93]

THERAPY

Therapy for NANB hepatitis remains supportive. Chronic NANB hepatitis can be a serious, even life-threatening disease.

Therefore, the development of effective therapy would have clinical importance.

The use of corticosteroids in viral hepatitis is generally not recommended and does not appear to benefit patients with NANB hepatitis.[94] In a recent preliminary report, Hoofnagle and colleagues at the NIH treated 10 patients with human α-interferon and observed surprisingly good results.[95] Using various dosage schedules and durations of treatment the elevated serum levels of ALT declined to normal or near normal. The ALT levels quickly returned to pretreatment levels in two patients in whom treatment was stopped after 4 months, but they declined again when treatment was reinstituted at a lower dosage level. Three of the patients who were treated for 12 months underwent follow-up liver biopsy, which showed a marked improvement when compared with pretreatment specimens. These results will have to be confirmed in a larger, controlled trial, and presumably other antiviral agents will be studied.

The recent cloning and expression of the genome of the NANB hepatitis virus will put such treatment trials on much more objective virologic grounds. As the nature of the virus is revealed, it may be possible to design specific antiviral compounds.

ENTERICALLY TRANSMITTED NON-A, NON-B HEPATITIS

In the winter of 1955–1956 a large outbreak of hepatitis occurred in Delhi, India, in which an estimated 29,300 people were jaundiced and as much as 68 percent of the population was affected.[96] Epidemiologic investigations revealed that the outbreak was due to contamination of the water supply by raw sewage. The occurrence of a large outbreak of hepatitis was recognized as unusual in India because hepatitis B is endemic in India and is not commonly associated with large epidemics. Hepatitis A is usually a childhood infection in India, and the adult population is nearly universally immune. This outbreak involved primarily young adults. When tests for hepatitis B became available, Pavri et al. showed that the epidemic was not serologically related to HBV infections.[97] Later Wong and colleagues used the IgM anti-hepatitis A test as well as tests for HBV infections to show that the Delhi outbreak as well as a similar outbreak that occurred in Ahmedabad and endemic cases that were occurring in Pune were not caused by either HAV or HBV[98]; using a similar approach, Khuroo showed that an outbreak of hepatitis in Kashmir was NANB.[99] Therefore these hepatitis cases were thought to be caused by a NANB hepatitis agent that could be transmitted orally through contaminated water.

The epidemiology and some of the clinical characteristics of these cases seemed to distinguish them from the parenterally transmitted form of NANB hepatitis. The possibility that these cases were caused by a distinct serotype of HAV could not be ruled out.

Epidemiology

Enterically transmitted NANB (ET-NANB) hepatitis has now been reported from many parts of the world including India, Pakistan, Nepal, Burma, Soviet Asia, North Africa, and recently Mexico.[100] There have been no documented outbreaks of ET-NANB hepatitis in the United States, but imported cases have been reported.[101] In addition to the large outbreaks of hepatitis, the agent is endemic in certain parts of India where it is the major cause of sporadic hepatitis.[102]

Epidemiologic data have shown that the incubation period of ET-NANB hepatitis varies between 2 to 9 weeks, with a mean of about 6 weeks. It is not known what factors determine the incubation period, but viral dose may be important.

One of the features of ET-NANB hepatitis is a low secondary attack rate relative to hepatitis A. There may be a relatively high prevalence of subclinical disease to account for this observation, and that the young adult population seems to be the most affected may indicate that the disease is frequently inapparent in children. It must be appreciated that only jaundiced cases are commonly being diagnosed in the areas of the world where this disease is most prevalent. When Khuroo and associates studied household contacts of index cases of ET-NANB hepatitis in Kashmire, they found that 20 percent had abnormal liver function test results, thus indicating that the true rate of secondary cases may be higher than is generally observed by looking only for jaundiced patients.

ET-NANB hepatitis does not cause chronic infections or chronic liver disease.[102] Thus the disease is not spread by chronic carriers. While most epidemics have been related to contaminated water, the mode of spread in the sporadic cases not associated with an outbreak is not known. Immunity to ET-NANB hepatitis seems to be long lasting and is probably lifelong. Second attacks of this disease have not been reported, and the highest attack rates in epidemics are among the 15- to 39-year-old age group. Since the attack rate in the older population was relatively low, lifelong immunity seems likely. The recent development of serologic tests for antibody to the agent of ET-NANB hepatitis will show exactly the immune status of various population groups.

Clinical Manifestations

ET-NANB hepatitis resembles type A hepatitis in many respects. It causes only acute and not chronic hepatitis. Cholestasis is frequently associated with both diseases but is probably a more prominent feature of ET-NANB hepatitis. Fulminant hepatitis seems to be more common in ET-NANB hepatitis than in hepatitis A, and this is largely due to the severe disease in pregnant women, especially those in the third trimester. Case fatality rates of 1–2 percent of hospitalized patients and 10–20 percent in pregnant women have been reported, while in hepatitis A only about 1 out of 1000 hospitalized patients die, with essentially no difference in pregnant women.[103]

Causative Agent

The first successful transmission of ET-NANB hepatitis was reported in 1983 by Balayan et al. who collected material from an outbreak in Tashkent in Soviet Asia.[104] Five weeks after self-administration of a fecal extract, he developed hepatitis. Since he knew that he already had serum antibodies to HAV it became clear that the agent with which he was infected was not HAV. He identified a 27 to 30 nm particle in his acute-phase stool by immune electron microscopy and showed that he had a specific immune response to that particle by testing his pre-exposure and convalescent serum for their ability to aggregate the particles in his acute-phase stool (Fig. 2). This group subsequently inoculated the acute-phase particle–containing stool into two cynomolgus monkeys. The monkeys developed evidence of mild liver disease 4–5 weeks after inoculation and shed virus into their stools as detected by immune electron microscopy.

This particle has been confirmed by several other groups, and antigenic relatedness of outbreaks from different parts of the world has been established by immune electron microscopy using this 27 nm particle as the antigen.[105,106]

Bradley and colleagues at the Centers for Disease Control have begun to characterize the ET-NANB hepatitis virus. They believe that the virus is 27–34 nm in diameter and appears to have some surface structure that resembles a calicivirus or the Norwalk gastroenteritis virus more than a picornavirus like HAV, which has less apparent surface structure.[105] Balayan et al. found that the particle had a buoyant density in CsCl of approximately 1.35 g/cc,[104] and Bradley and associates found that it sedimented at about 183S as compared with 157S for HAV.[105]

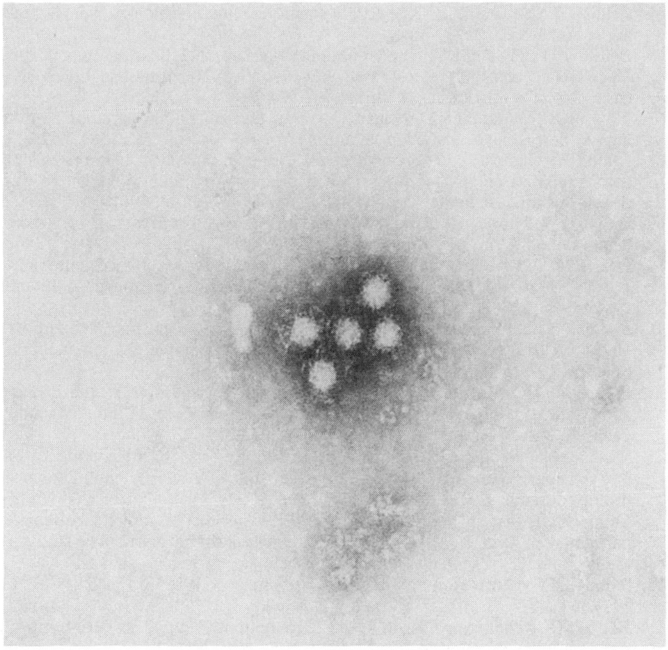

FIG. 2. An immune electron micrograph of a negatively stained preparation of a stool from a patient with ET-NANB hepatitis. The particles are covered with antibody, but some surface structure can be seen that resembled a calicivirus. (×125,000) (Courtesy of Dr. John Ticehurst, Washington, DC.)

There is little doubt that this 27–34 nm particle is the virus of ET-NANB hepatitis, but the agent still has not been grown in cell culture and fully characterized. In addition the immune response and seroepidemiology have not been fully studied because of difficulties in developing a rapid, simple serologic assay for either antigen or antibody.

SUMMARY

Two distinct forms of NANB hepatitis have been described in this chapter. The first resembles hepatitis B in many respects in that it is transmitted by percutaneous exposure and presumably by close personal contact. It causes chronic infections and chronic liver disease including cirrhosis and possibly hepatocellular carcinoma. Recent molecular cloning experiments indicate that the virus contains a positive-sense RNA genome. Expression of a portion of this genome produces a peptide to which most people who are either convalescent from NANB hepatitis or are chronically infected make antibody. This test may soon be in use for the diagnosis of patients and screening of blood donors. It should also be known in a short time whether there is a second agent of parenteral NANB hepatitis.

The second form of NANB hepatitis resembles hepatitis A in many respects. It is transmitted orally, often through contaminated water, and it causes only acute infections but has a relatively high case fatality rate, especially among pregnant women in their third trimester. It is probably caused by a small virus that grossly resembles HAV but is likely to be in a distinct virus group based on morphologic and physical characteristics.

Since these two agents have now been identified in specific ways, it is finally proper to drop the non-A, non-B hepatitis nomenclature and begin to refer to agents as hepatitis C virus (HCV) for the agent of the parenteral disease and hepatitis E virus (HEV) for the agent of ET-NANB hepatitis. The delta agent is now refered to as hepatitis D virus (HDV). Thus, what was classically a relatively simple situation of two forms of viral hepatitis caused by two viruses has now become five distinct diseases and viruses with the possibility of more to come.

REFERENCES

1. Alter HJ, Holland PV, Purcell RH, et al. Posttransfusion hepatitis after exclusion of the commercial and hepatitis B antigen positive donors. Ann Intern Med. 1972;77:691.
2. Hollinger FB, Werch J, Melnick JL. A prospective study indicating that double-antibody radioimmunoassay reduces the incidence of post-transfusion hepatitis B. N Engl J Med 1974;290:1104.
3. Feinstone SM, Kapikian AZ, Purcell RH. Hepatitis A: Detection by immune electron microscopy of a virus-like antigen associated with acute illness. Science. 1973;182:1026.
4. Feinstone SM, Kapikian AZ, Purcell RH, et al. Transfusion associated hepatitis not due to viral hepatitis type A or B. N Engl J Med. 1975;292:454.
5. Alter HJ, Purcell RH, Holland PV, et al. Clinical and serological analysis of transfusion-associated hepatitis. Lancet. 1975;2:838.
6. MacCallum FO. Early studies of viral hepatitis. Br Med Bull. 1972;28:105.
7. Krugman S, Giles JP, Hammond J. Infectious hepatitis: Evidence for two distinctive clinical epidemiological, and immunological types of infection. JAMA. 1967;200:365.
8. Prince AM, Brotman B, Grady GF, et al. Long-incubation post-transfusion hepatitis without serological evidence of exposure to hepatitis B virus. Lancet. 1974;2:241.
9. Havens WP Jr. Viral hepatitis: Multiple attacks in a narcotic addict. Ann Intern Med. 1956;44:199.
10. Mosley JW, Redeker AG, Feinstone SM, et al. Multiple hepatitis viruses in multiple attacks of acute viral hepatitis. N Engl J Med. 1977;296:75.
11. Norkrans G, Frosner G, Hermodsson S, et al. Multiple hepatitis attacks in drug addicts. JAMA. 1980;243:1056.
12. Bradley DW, Maynard JE, Cook EH, et al. Non-A, non-B hepatitis in experimentally infected chimpanzees: Cross-challenge and electron microscopic studies. J Med Virol. 1980;6:185.
13. Yoshizawa H, Itoh Y, Iwakiri S, et al. Demonstration of two different types of non-A, non-B hepatitis by reinjection and cross-challenge studies in chimpanzees. Gastroenterology. 1981;81:107.
14. Yoshizawa H, Itoh Y, Iwakiri S, et al. Non-A, non-B (type 1) hepatitis agent capable of inducting tubular ultrastructures in the hepatoocyte cytoplasm of chimpanzees: Inactivation by formalin and heat. Gastroenterology. 1982;82:502.
15. Hollinger FB, Mosley JW, Szmuness W, et al. Transfusion-transmitted viruses study. Experimental evidence for two non-A, non-B hepatitis agents. J Infect Dis. 1980;142:400.
16. Bradley DW, Maynard JE, Popper H, et al. Posttransfusion non-A, non-B hepatitis: Physicochemical properties of two distinct agents. J Infect Dis. 1983;148:254.
17. Brotman B, Prince AM, Huima T. Non-A, non-B hepatitis: Is there more than a single blood-borne strain? J Infect Dis. 1985;151:168.
18. Prince AM, Brotman B, Van Den Ende MC, et al. Non-A, non-B hepatitis. Identification of a virus specific antigen and antibody. A preliminary report. In: Vyas GN, Cohen SN, Schmid R, eds. Viral Hepatitis. Philadelphia: Franklin Institute Press; 1978:613.
19. Bradley DW, McCaustland KA, Cook EH, et al. Posttransfusion non-A, non-B hepatitis in chimpanzees: Physicochemical evidence that the tubule-forming agent is a small, enveloped virus. Gastroenterology. 1985;88:773.
20. He LF, Alling D, Popkin T, et al. Determining the size of non-A, non-B hepatitis by filtration. J Infect Dis. 1987;156:636.
21. Feinstone SM, Mihalik KB, Kamimura T, et al Inactivation of hepatitis B virus and non-A, non-B hepatitis by chloroform. Infect Immun. 1983;41:816.
22. Trepo C, Vitvitski L, Hantz O, et al. Identification and detection of virus specific core and e Ag/Ab across reacting with those of hepatitis B in non-A, non-B hepatitis (NANBH). Gastroenterology. 1980;79:1060.
23. Trepo C, Vititski L, Hantz O, et al. Detection by immunofluorescence of a new "core-like" Ag/Ab system in liver and serum of patients with NANB hepatitis. Liver. 1981;1:191.
24. Hantz O, Vitvitski L, Trepo C. Non-A, non-B hepatitis: Identification of hepatitis-B-like virus particles in serum and liver. J Med Virol. 1980;5:73.
25. Wands JR, Carlson RI, Schoemaker H, et al. Immunodiagnosis of hepatitis B with high-affinity IgM monoclonal antibodies. Proc Natl Acad Sci USA. 1981;78:1214.
26. Wands JR, Lieberman HM, Muchmore E, et al. Detection and transmission in chimpanzees of hepatitis B virus-related agents formerly designated "non-A, non-B" hepatitis. Proc Natl Acad Sci USA. 1982;79:7552.
27. Wands JR, Fujita YK, Isselbacher KJ, et al. Identification and transmission of hepatitis B virus-related varients. Proc Natl Acad Sci USA. 1986;83:6608.
28. Figus A, Blum HE, Vyas GN, et al. Hepatitis B viral nucleotide sequences in non-A, non-B or hepatitis B virus-related chronic liver disease. Hepatology. 1984;4:364.
29. Brechot C, Degos F, Lugassy C, et al. Hepatitis B virus DNA in patients with chronic liver disease and negative tests for hepatitis B surface antigen. N Engl J Med. 1985;312:270.
30. Fowler MJF, Monjardino J, Weller IV, et al. Failure to detect nucleic acid homology between some non-A, non-B viruses and hepatitis B virus DNA. J Med Virol. 1983;12:205.
31. Yap SH, Hellings JA, Rijntjes PJM, et al. Absence of detectable hepatitis B virus DNA in sera and liver of chimpanzees with non-A, non-B hepatitis. J Med Virol. 1985;15:343.
32. Tassopoulos NC, Papaevangelou GJ, Roumeliotou-Karayannis A, et al.

Search for hepatitis B virus DNA in sera from patients with acute type B or non-A, non-B hepatitis. J Hepatol. 1986;2:410.
33. Fields HA, Berninger M, Nath N, et al. Unrelatedness of factor VIII derived non-A, non-B hepatitis and hepatitis b virus. J Med Virol. 1983;11:59.
34. Feinstone SM, Alter HJ, Dienes HP, et al. Non-A, non-B hepatitis in chimpanzees and marmosets. J Infect Dis. 1981;144:588.
35. Seto B, Coleman WG, Iwarson S, et al. Detection of reverse transcriptase activity in association with the non-A, non-B hepatitis agent(s). Lancet. 1984;2:941.
36. Iwarson S, Schaff Z, Seto B, et al. Retrovirus-like particles in hepatocytes of patients with transfusion-acquired non-A, non-B hepatitis. J Med Virol. 1985;16:37.
37. Seto B, Gerety RJ: A glycoprotein associated with the non-A, non-B hepatitis agent(s): Isolation and immunoreactivity. Proc Natl Acad Sci USA. 1985;82:4934.
38. Casoli C, Tremolada F, Lori F, et al. Reverse transcriptase activity in post-transfusion non-A, non-B hepatitis: Characterisation and association with retrovirus particles in serum. Serodiagn Immunother Infect Dis. 1987;1:339.
39. Itoh Y, Iwakiri S, Kitajima K, et al. Lack of detectable reverse transcriptase activity in human and chimpanzee sera with a high infectivity for non-A, non-B hepatitis. J Gen Virol. 1986;67:777.
39a. Choo Q-L, Kuo G, Weiner AJ, et al. Isolation of a cDNA clone derived from a blood-borne non-A, non-B viral hepatitis genome. Science. 1989;244:359–62.
40. Hollinger FB, Mosley JW, Szmuness W, et al. Non-A, non-B hepatitis following blood transfusion: Risk factors associated with donor characteristics. In: Szmuness W, Alter HJ, Maynard JE, eds. Viral Hepatitis. Philadelphia: Frankling Institute Press; 1982:361.
41. Seeff LB, Wright EC, Zimmerman HJ, et al. VA cooperative study of post-transfusion hepatitis incidence and characteristics of hepatitis and responsible risk factors. Am J Med Sci. 1975;270:355.
42. Hashiba UW, Spero JA, Lewis JH. Chronic liver dysfunction in multitransfused hemophiliacs. Transfusion. 1977;17:490.
43. Spero JH, Lewis JH, Fisher SE, et al. The high risk of chronic liver disease in multitransfused juvenile hemophiliac patients. J Pediatr. 1979;94:875.
44. Preston FE, Triger DR, Underwood JCE, et al. Percutaneous liver biopsy and chronic liver disease in hemophiliacs. Lancet. 1978;2:592.
45. Hay CRM, Preston FE, Triger DR, et al. Progressive liver disease in hemophilia: An understated problem? Lancet. 1985;1:1495.
46. Alter MJ, Gerety RJ, Smallwood LA. Sporadic non-A, non-B hepatitis: Frequency and epidemiology in an urban U.S. population. J Infect Dis. 1982;145:886.
47. Alter MJ, Margolis HS, Krawczynski K, et al. The role of transfusions in the chronic disease burden associated with non-A, non-B hepatitis in the United States. (Abstract). Transfusion Associated Infections and Immune Response. 1988;III.4:15.
48. Dienstag JL, Stevens CE, Szmuness W. The epidemiology of non-A, non-B hepatitis: Emerging patterns. In: gerety RJ, ed. Non-A, non-B Hepatitis. New York: Academic Press; 1981:119.
49. Szmuness W, Stevens CE, Harley EJ, et al. Demonstration of efficacy in a controlled clinical trial in a high-risk population in the United States. N Engl J Med. 1980;303:833.
50. Tong MJ, Thursby M, Rakela J, et al. Studies on the maternal infant transmission of the viruses which cause acute hepatitis. Gastroenterology. 1981;80:999.
51. Craske J, Dilling N, Stern D. An outbreak of hepatitis associated with intravenous injection of factor-VIII concentrate. Lancet. 1975;2:221.
52. Hruby MA, Schauf V. Trausfusion-related short-incubation hepatitis in hemophilic patients. JAMA. 1978;240:1355.
53. Feinstone SM, Alter HJ, Dienes H, et al. Non-A, non-B hepatitis in chimpanzees and marmosets. J Infect Dis. 1981;144:588.
54. Dienstag JL, Bahn AK, Alter HJ, et al. Circulating immune complexes in non-A, non-B hepatitis. Lancet. 1979;1:1265.
55. Norkrans G, Frösner G, Hermodsson S, et al. Clinical epidemiological and prognostic aspects of hepatitis "non-A, non-B"; a comparison with hepatitis A and B. Scand J Infect Dis. 1979;11:259.
56. Mathiesen LR, Skinhoj P, Hardt F, et al. The Copenhagen Hepatitis Acuta Programme. Epidemiology and clinical characteristics of acute hepatitis types, A, B, and non-A, non-B. Scand J Gastroenterol. 1979;14:849.
57. Goldfield M, Bill J, Colosimo F. The control of transfusion associated hepatitis. In: Vyas GN, Cohen SN, Schmid R, eds. Viral Hepatitis. Philadelphia: Franklin Institute Press; 1979:405.
58. Sjogren MH, Tanno H, Fay O, et al. Hepatitis A virus in stool during clinical relapse. Ann Intern Med. 1987;106:221.
59. Tabor E, Seeff LB, Gerety RJ. Chronic non-A, non-B hepatitis carrier state. N Engl J Med. 1980;303:140.
60. Burk KH, Dreesman GR, Cabral GA, et al. Long-term sequelae of non-A, non-B hepatitis in experimentally infected chimpanzees. Hepatology. 1984;4:808.
61. Dienstag JL, Non-A, non-B hepatitis. I. Recognition, epidemiology, and clinical features. Gastroenterology. 1983;85:439.
62. Hoofnagle JH, Alter HJ. Chronic viral hepatitis. In: Vyas GN, Dienstag JL, Hoofnagle JH, eds. Viral Hepatitis and Liver Disease. Orlando, FL: Grune & Stratton; 1984:97.
63. Colombo M, Oldani S, Donata MF, et al. A multicenter, prospective study of posttransfusion hepatitis in Milan. Hepatology. 1987;7:709.
64. Di Bisceglie AM, Kassianides C, Lisker-Melman M, et al. Development of cirrhosis following chronic non-A, non-B hepatitis (Abstract). Gastroenterology. 1988;94:535.
65. Zeldis JB, Dienstag JL, Gale RP: Aplastic anemia and non-A, non-B hepatitis. Am J Med. 1983;74:64.
66. Beasley RP, Hwang LY. The edpimiology of hepatocellular carcinoma. In: Vyas GN, Dienstag JL, Hoffnagle JH, eds. Viral Hepatitis and Liver Disease. Orlando, FL: Grune & Stratton; 1984:209.
67. Kiyosawa K, Akahane Y, Nagata A, et al. Hepatocellular carcinoma after non-A, non-B posttransfusion hepatitis. Am J Gastroenterol. 1984;79:777.
68. Okuda H, Obata H, Motoike Y, et al. Clinicopathological features of hepatocellular carcinoma—comparison of seropositive and seronegative patients. Hepatogastroenterology. 1984;31:64.
69. Dienes HP, Popper H, Arnold W, et al. Histologic observations in human hepatitis non-A, non-B. Hepatology. 1982;2:562.
70. Omata M, Iwama S, Sumida M, et al. Clinicopathologic study of acute non-A, non-B hepatitis: Histologic features of liver biopsies in acute phase. Liver. 1981;1:201.
71. Shimizu YK, Feinstone SM, Purcell RH, et al. Non-A, non-B hepatitis: Ultrastructural evidence for agents in experimentally infected chimpanzees. Science. 1979;205:197.
72. Pfeifer V, Thomssen R, Legler K, et al. Experimental non-A, non-B hepatitis: Four types of cytoplasmic alterations in hepatocytes of infected chimpanzees. Virchows Arch [Cell Pathol]. 1980;33:233.
73. Watanabe S, Reddy KR, Jeffers L, et al. Electron microscopic evidence of non-A, non-B hepatitis markers and virus-like particles in immunocompromised humans. Hepatology. 1984;4:628.
74. Canese MG, Rizzetto M, Novara R, et al. Experimental infection of chimpanzees with the HBsAg-associated delta agent: An ultrastructural study. J Med Virol. 1984;13:63.
75. Sidhu GS. Ultrastructure of AIDS lymph nodes. N Engl J Med. 1983;309:1188.
76. Bockus D, Remington F, Luu J, et al. Induction of cylindrical confronting cisternae (AIDS inclusions) in Daudi lymphoblastoid cells by recombinant alpha-interferon. Hum Pathol. 1988;19:78.
77. Shimizu YK, Oomura M, Abe K, et al. Production of antibody associated with non-A, non-B hepatitis in a chimpanzee lymphoblastoid cell line established by in vitro transformation with Epstein-Barr virus. Proc Natl Acad Sci USA. 1985;82:2138.
78. Shimizu YK, Purceel RH, Gerin JL, et al. Further studies by immunofluorescence of the monoclonal antibodies assiciated with experimental non-A, non-B hepatitis in chimpanzees and their relation to D hepatitis. Hepatology. 1988;6:1329.
79. Aach RD, Szmuness W, Mosley JW, et al. Serum alanine aminotransferase of donors in relation to the risk of non-A, non-B hepatitis in recipients: The transfusion-transmitted viruses study. N Engl J Med. 1981;304:989.
80. Alter HJ, Purcell RH, Holland PV, et al. Donor transaminase and recipient hepatitis. JAMA. 1981;246:630.
81. Stevens CE, Aach RD, Hollinger FB, et al. Hepatitis B virus antibody in blood donors and the occurrence of non-A, non-B hepatitis in transfusion recipients: An analysis of the trasufsion-transmitted viruses study. Ann Intern Med. 1984;101:733.
82. Alter HJ. Posttransfusion hepatitis: Clinical features, risk and donor testing. In: Dodd RY, Barker LF, eds. Infections Immunity and Blood Transfusions. New York, Alan R Liss; 1985:47.
83. Gomperts EH. Procedures for the inactivation of viruses in clotting factor concentrates. Am J Hematol. 1986;23:295.
84. Prince AM, Horowitz B, Horowitz MS, et al. The development of virus-free labile blood derivatives—a review. Eur J Epidemiol. 1987;3:103.
85. Horowitz B, Wiebe M, Lippin A, et al. Inactivation of viruses in labile blood derivatics II. Physical methods. Transfusion. 1985;25:523.
86. Schimpf K, Mannucci PM, Kreutz W, et al. Absence of hepatitis after treatment with a pasteurized factor VIII concentrate in patients with hemophilia and no previous transfusions. N Engl J Med. 1987;316:918.
87. Colombo M, Mannucci PM, Carnelli V, et al. Transmission of Non-A, non-B hepatitis by heat-treated factor VIII concentrate. Lancet. 1985;2:1.
88. Quinnan GV, Wells MA, Wittek AE, et al. Inactivation of human T lymphotropic virus, type III (HTLV-III) by heat, chemicals and irradiation. Transfusion. 1986;26:481.
89. Eaton DL, Hass PE, Riddle L, et al. Characterization of recombinant human factor VIII. J Biol Chem. 1987;262:3285.
90. Kuhns WJ, Prince AM, Brotman B, et al. A clinical and laboratory evaluation of immune serum globulin from donors with a history of hepatitis: Attempted prevention of post-transfusion hepatitis. Am J Med Sci. 1976;272:255.
91. Knodell RG, Conrad ME, Ishak KG. Development of chronic liver disease after acute non-A, non-B post-transfusion hepatitis: Role of gamma-globulin prophylaxis in its prevention. Gastroenterology. 1977;72:902.
92. Knodell RG, Conrad ME, Ginsberg AL, et al. Efficacy of prophylactic gamma-globulin in preventing non-A, non-B post-transfusion hepatitis. Lancet. 1976;1:557.
93. Seeff LB, Zimmerman HJ, Wright EC, et al. A randomized, double blind controlled trial of the efficacy of immune serum globulin for the prevention of post-transfusion hepatitis: A Veterans Administration Cooperative Study. Gastroenterology. 1977;72:111.
94. Hoofnagle JH. Chronic hepatitis: The role of corticosteroids. In Szmuness W, Alter HJ, Maynard JE, eds. Viral Hepatitis. Philadelphia: Franklin Institute Press; 1982:573.
95. Hoofnagle JH, Mullen KD, Jones DB, et al. Treatment of chronic non-A, non-B hepatitis with recombinant human alpha interferon. N Engl J Med. 1986;315:1575.

96. Viswanathan R. Infectious hepatitis in Delhi (1955–56): A critical study; epidemiology. Indian J Med Res. 1957;45(Suppl):1.
97. Pavri KM, Niphadkar KB, Sheikh BH. Retrospective studies on Australia antigen in sera collected during the epidemic of viral hepatitis at Delhi in 1956. Indian J Med Res. 1972;60:1575.
98. Wong DC, Purcell RH, Sreenivasan MA, et al. Epidemic and endemic hepatitis in India: Evidence for a non-A, non-B hepatitis virus aetiology. Lancet. 1980;2:876.
99. Khuroo MS. Study of an epidemic of non-A, non-B hepatitis. Possibility of another human hepatitis virus distinct from post-transfusion non-A, non-B type. Am J Med. 1980;68:818.
100. Bradley DW, Krawczynski K, Cook EH, et al. Enterically transmitted non-A, non-B hepatitis: Etiology of disease and laboratory studies in nonhuman primates. In: Zuckerman AJ, ed. Viral Hepatitis and Liver Disease. New York: Alan R Liss; 1988:138.
101. Khuroo MS, Duermeyer W, Ahanger MA, et al. Acute sporadic non-A, non-B hepatitis in India. Am J Epidemiol. 1983;118:360.
102. Khuroo MS, Saleem M, Teli MR, et al. Failure to detect chronic liver disease after epidemic non-A, non-B hepatitis (Letter). Lancet. 1980;2:97.
103. Khuroo MS, Teli MR, Skidmore S, et al. Incidence and severity of viral hepatitis in pregnancy. Am J Med. 1981;70:252.
104. Balayan MS, Andzhaparidze AG, Savinskaya SS, et al. Evidence for a virus in non-A, non-B hepatitis transmitted via the fecal-oral route. Intervirology. 1981;20:23.
105. Bradley DW, Krawczynski K, Cook EH, et al. Enterically transmitted non-A, non-B hepatitis: Serial passage of disease in cynomolgus macaques and tamarins and recovery disease-associated 27- to 34-nm viruslike particles. Proc Natl Acad Sci USA. 1987;84:6277.
106. Arankalle VA, Ticehurst J, Sreenivasan MA, et al. Aetiological association of a virus-like particle with enterically transmitted non-A, non-B hepatitis. Lancet. 1988;1:550.

155. NORWALK AND RELATED AGENTS OF GASTROENTERITIS

RAPHAEL DOLIN

Acute gastrointestinal disease is an exceedingly common and widespread illness throughout the world. According to the National Health Interview Survey in the United States, such disease occurs with an incidence of 11.2 percent per year, with an estimated 23.7–26.0 days lost from work or school per 100 persons annually.[1] While the etiology of much of this disease remains unknown, recent evidence suggests that many cases result from viral infections with newly described agents.[2–3] In a survey of families in the Cleveland area, acute "nonbacterial" or viral gastroenteritis was second in frequency only to the common cold as a disease among families.[4] Worldwide, it has been estimated that acute diarrheal disease accounts for nearly 5 million deaths in children less than 5 years of age.[5] The group of viruses to be discussed here, the "Norwalk-like agents," accounts for an as yet unspecified portion of acute gastroenteritis. However, as is discussed below, recent data suggest that these agents may be important causes of acute gastroenteritis.

HISTORY

The failure to isolate causative agents, bacterial or viral, from apparently infectious outbreaks of diarrhea and/or vomiting led to the widely held assumption that undetected viruses were responsible for such disease. In 1945, Reimann and coworkers[6] transmitted disease to volunteers by administering bacteria-free filtrates of throat washings and/or stool filtrates from naturally occurring cases. Gordon et al.[7] and Jordan et al.[8] induced disease in normal volunteers with bacteria-free material. These studies described two transmissible agents of subbacterial size, the Marcy and FS agents, that appeared to be antigenically distinct. However, these workers were unable to detect viral agents in vitro with techniques available at that time. Despite extensive virologic investigations in laboratories throughout the world, relatively little progress was made in this area until 1972 when the Norwalk agent, the prototype of this "group," was described and partially characterized.[9,10] This agent was obtained from an outbreak of disease (primarily vomiting) in Norwalk, Ohio, that involved students in an elementary school and family contacts. Since that time, additional agents with apparently similar properties have been described: Hawaii,[11] MC,[12] Taunton,[13] and Snow Mountain.[14] It is likely that additional agents will emerge from ongoing studies.

DESCRIPTION OF NORWALK-LIKE AGENTS

The term *Norwalk-like agents* refers to a group of viral agents detected in stools from patients with acute gastroenteritis. These agents have been named most often for the location of the outbreak of the illness from which they have been derived.[2,11–14] The Norwalk-like agents have not been cultivated in vitro but share certain physical properties that have been determined by electron microscopic visualization (Fig. 1) and/or physicochemical manipulation of infectious inocula. The biophysical properties of these agents are presented in Table 1. The Norwalk-like agents are 26–34 nm in diameter, have cubic symmetry, lack envelopes, and have a buoyant density in CsCl of 1.34–1.41 g/ml. When examined, thesc agents appear to be relatively heat and acid stable and ether resistant.[9] The number and molecular weight of the polypeptides associated with the Norwalk and Snow Mountain agents suggested a similarity to those associated with caliciviruses.[15,16] However, nucleic acid

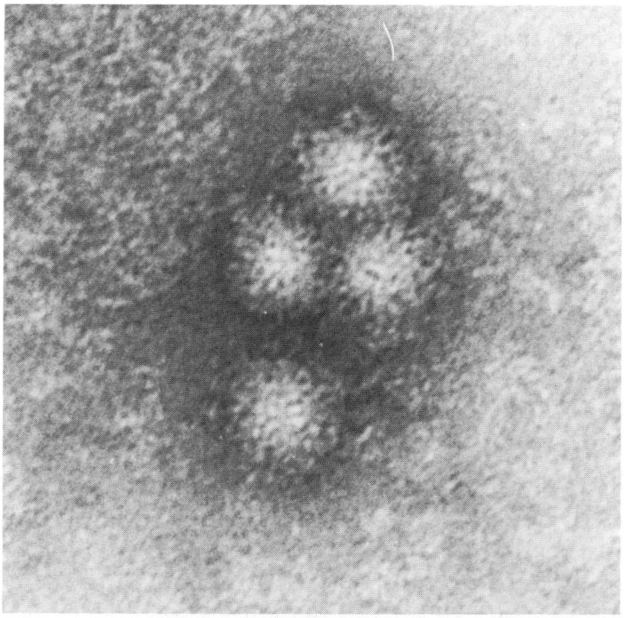

FIG. 1. Snow Mountain agent in stool filtrate from a volunteer with experimentally induced disease as visualized by immune electron microscopy. Particles are 27 nm in diameter and are stained with 2% phosphotungstic acid.

TABLE 1. Biophysical Properties of Norwalk-Like Agents

Agent	*Size (nm)*	*Buoyant Density (g/ml)*[a]
Norwalk	27–32	1.38–1.41
Hawaii	26–29	1.37–1.41
MC	27–32	1.37–1.41
Taunton	32–34	1.36–1.41
Snow Mountain	27–32	1.34

[a] In CsCl.

has not been extracted from these agents, and definitive classification awaits further characterization.

Antigenic relationships among these agents have only partly been determined by cross-challenge studies in normal volunteers,[17] by serum antibody analysis by immune electro microscopy (IEM),[12,14] and by radioimmunoassay (RIA).[18,19] Norwalk, Hawaii, and Snow Mountain agents appear to be antigenically distinct, while Norwalk and MC are antigenically related. The antigenic relationship of Taunton to the other agents is unknown. Thus, several antigenic types exist among these agents, although the precise nature of the antigenic relationships within this group of agents is not fully worked out.

EPIDEMIOLOGY

Until very recently, diagnostic tests that would be suitable for large-scale seroepidemiologic surveys of infection with Norwalk-like agents have not been available (see below). Thus, little has been known about the epidemiology of these agents. However, the clinical syndromes in which they have been implicated appear to be exceedingly widespread and common. These include winter vomiting disease,[20] epidemic diarrhea, viral gastroenteritis,[22] and acute infectious nonbacterial gastroenteritis.[23] Disease can occur throughout the year and affects all age groups in both open and closed populations. The precise method of spread remains unknown, although the experimental induction of illness in normal volunteers suggests the fecal–oral route. Many outbreaks have been associated with a common-source origin, including food-borne and waterborne outbreaks.[2,14] Explosive outbreaks with documented person-to-person transmission as well as sporadic cases have been described.

The recent development of RIA's for Norwalk and Snow Mountain antigen and antibody[18,19] have indicated that serum antibody is noted first at ages 3–4 in 11–20 percent of subjects and antibody prevalence gradually rises to greater than 50 percent by the fifth decade of life. In a study of more than 70 outbreaks off acute gastroenteritis of unknown etiology, 34–42 percent have been etiologically associated with the Norwalk agent as detected by RIA,[24,25] which indicates that this or related agents are major causes of this type of disease. Detailed investigation of the epidemiology of the other Norwalk-like agents has not been carried out, although the Snow Mountain agent has been associated with at least six outbreaks in various parts of the United States.[26]

PATHOGENESIS

Because of the unavailability of animal models for gastroenteritis induced by the Norwalk-like agents, information about the pathogenesis of this illness is based largely on studies of experimentally induced disease in normal volunteers. Gastrointestinal illness has been transmitted to normal volunteers after the oral administration of Norwalk, Hawaii, and Snow Mountain agents. Acute infection with Norwalk and Hawaii agents results in a reversible histopathologic lesion in the jejunum,[11,27–29] with apparent sparing of the stomach[30] and rectum (Fig. 2). The villi are blunted, but the mucosa is otherwise intact. Round cells and polymorphonuclear leukocytic infiltration are seen in the lamina propria. By electron microscopy, the epithelial cells are similarly intact, microvilli are shortened, and widened intercellular spaces are noted (Fig. 3). These histopathologic changes appear within 24 hours after virus challenge, are present at the height of illness, and persist for a variable period of time after the illness. The histopathologic changes have generally cleared within 2 weeks after the onset of illness, although some jejunal changes have been noted as late as 6 weeks after challenge. Histopathologic changes have been described in both clinical and subclinical cases of infection[28,29] and appear to be

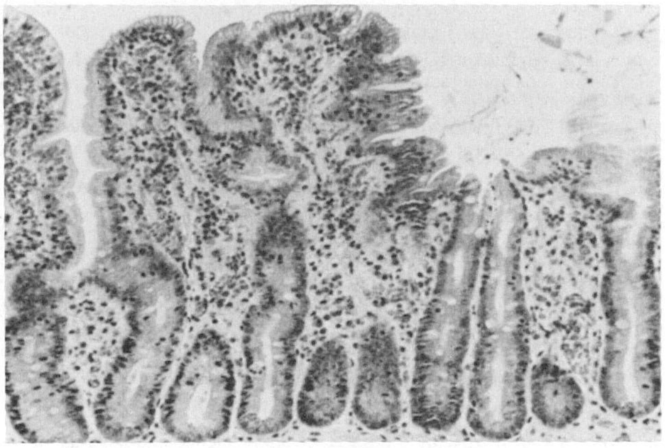

FIG. 2. Light micrograph of a jejunal mucosal biopsy specimen from a volunteer with Hawaii-induced disease 48 hours after challenge. Blunted villi and inflammatory cell infiltrate in the lamina propria are present. (Hematoxylin-eosin, ×140)

indistinguishable between Norwalk- and Hawaii-induced disease.

Diarrhea induced by the Norwalk agent is associated with a transient malabsorption of D-xylose and fat[23] and with decreased activity of brush-border enzymes including alkaline phosphatase and trehalase.[27] Absorption and brush-border enzyme levels returns to normal values within 2 weeks after challenge. During acute illness, a variable amount of intestinal fluid is produced, but infection with Norwalk and Hawaii agents has not been associated with detectable enterotoxin production. Adenylate cyclase levels in jejunal biopsy specimens appear to be normal during infection.[31] Thus, the precise mechanism of viral-induced diarrhea and/or vomiting remains unknown at present.

IMMUNE RESPONSES

Serum antibody to the Norwalk-like agents can be detected by several techniques (see below), and significant antibody titer rises occur 10–21 days after infection. The parameters of immunity, however, are poorly understood. Resistance to reinfection with the homologous agent persists for at least 6–14 weeks, although infection with antigenically distinct (heterologous) agents does not confer such protection.[17] In some persons, resistance wanes 24–42 months after challenge, and on occasion even short-term immunity may not develop.[32] In others, a poorly defined long-term resistance has been noted.[32] Infection and illness induced by Norwalk-like agents occur in the presence of a wide range of pre-existing serum antibody levels, which thus correlate poorly with protection. These findings suggest that such protection may be related to other host defense factors such as a local antibody that is produced in the gut in a manner analogous to the role played by secretory IgA in poliovirus infections.[33] Jejunal IgA synthesis has been shown to be elevated in biopsy specimens obtained 2 weeks after challenge with the Norwalk agent.[34] However direct measurements of intestinal antibody have failed to show a correlation with protection from Norwalk-induced illness.[24]

Limited studies of cell-mediated immune responses in these infections indicate that acute illness is associated with a transient lymphopenia that involves thymus-derived, bone marrow-derived, and null cell subpopulations.[35] The lymphocytes that remain in the circulation respond normally or even supranormally to mitogenic stimulation with phytohemagglutinin and concanavalin A.

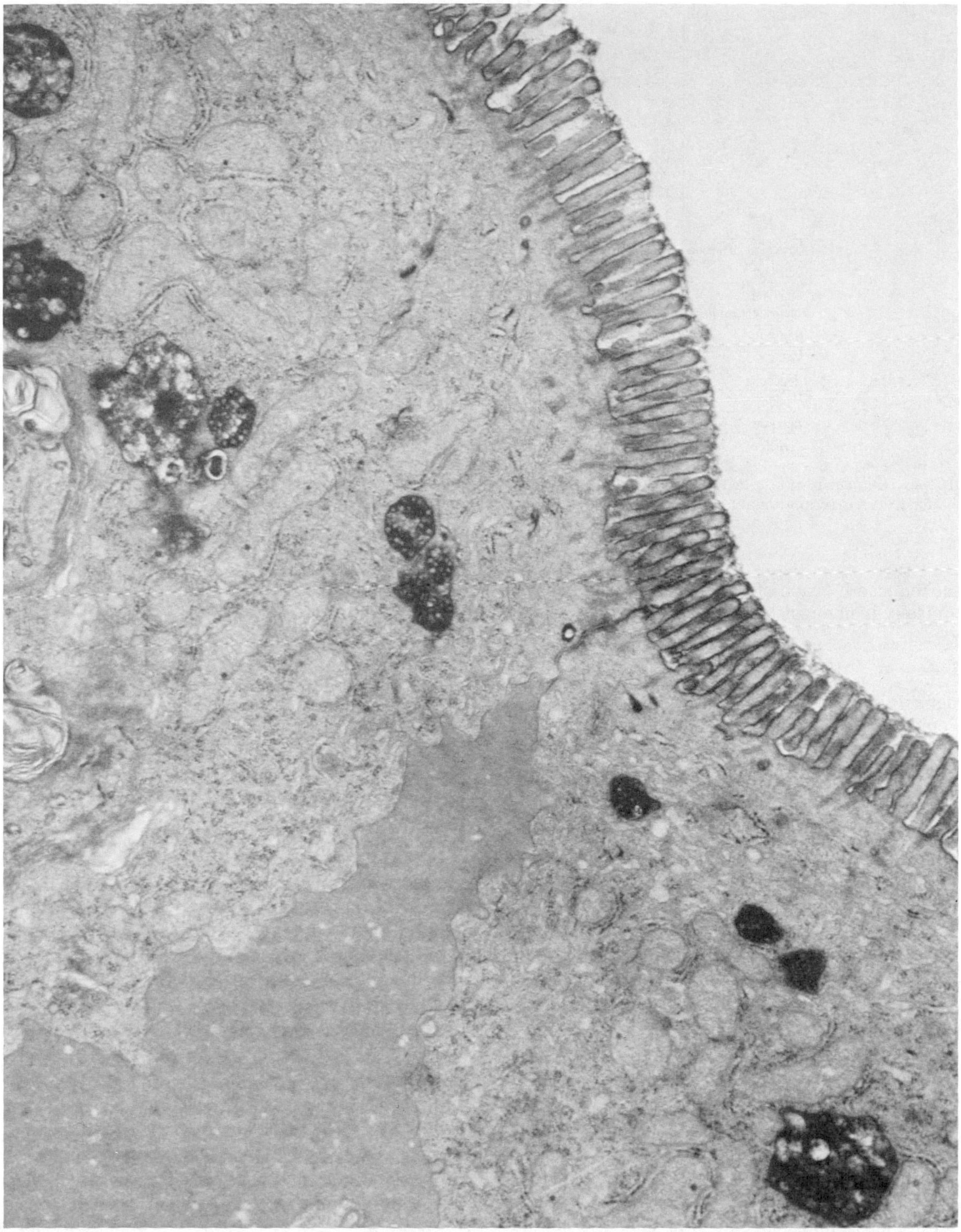

FIG. 3. Electron micrograph of a jejunal biopsy specimen taken 48 hours after inoculation with the Hawaii agent. Note the shortened and distorted microvilli and widening of the intercellular spaces. (Lead citrate stain, ×24,000)

CLINICAL MANIFESTATIONS

Clinical characteristics of illness induced by the Norwalk agent appear to be similar in both naturally occurring and experimentally induced disease (Fig. 4). Incubation periods are generally 24–48 hours, although ranges from 18 to 72 hours have been observed. The onset of symptoms can be either gradual or abrupt, and most persons complain first of abdominal cramps and/or nausea. Generally both vomiting and diarrhea occur, although either can be present alone. Myalgias, malaise, and occasional headaches are also seen. Low-grade fever (with temperatures of 101–102°F) occurs in approximately half the cases. Disease manifestations generally last 48–72 hours and remit without sequelae.

Diarrheal stool is generally moderate in amounts, with 4–8 stools being produced over a period of 24 hours. Stools are characteristically nonbloody, lack mucus, and may be loose to watery. Fecal leukocytes are not seen in Norwalk-induced dis-

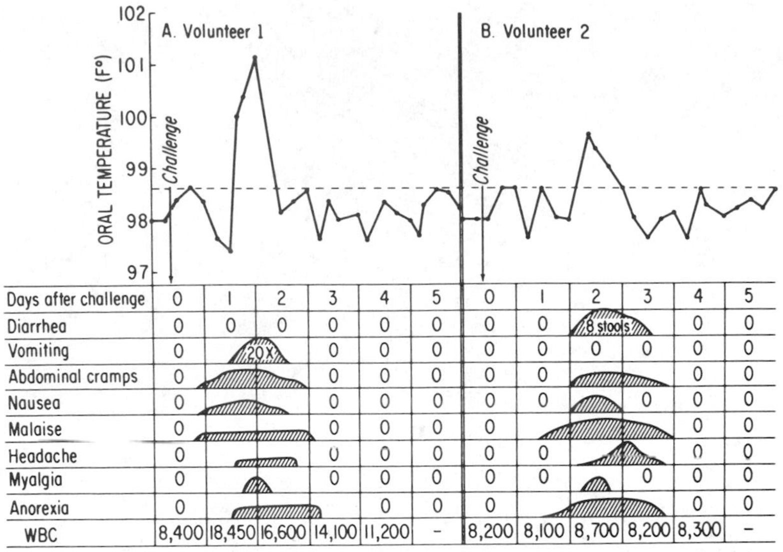

FIG. 4. Clinical response to two normal volunteers after the oral administration of the Norwalk agent. The height of the shaded curve is proportional to the severity of the sign or symptom. (From Dolin et al.,[2] with permission.)

ease. Illnesses induced by each of the Norwalk-like agents appear to be clinically indistinguishable.

DIAGNOSIS

A clinical diagnosis of Norwalk-like illness can be suspected on the basis of epidemiologic information and on the absence of other documented pathogens. However, the signs and symptoms of illness as described before are not sufficiently characteristic to enable a diagnosis to be made on clinical grounds alone, and a specific diagnosis requires laboratory confirmation, which is currently available only as a research technique. Since these agents currently cannot be cultivated in vitro, detection is based on the visualization of particles in stool specimens by IEM.[14,36] This technique uses immune sera to aggregate suspected particles in stool suspensions (Fig. 1) and cannot be used conveniently for the routine screening of stool specimens. The recent availability of an RIA for the detection of Norwalk[18] and Snow Mountain[19] particles and enzyme-linked immunosorbent assay (ELISA) techniques for the detection of Norwalk,[37] Snow Mountain,[38] and Hawaii agents should facilitate examination of stools.[39] Virus shedding as detected by IEM is maximal within the first 24–48 hours of Norwalk-like illness and is infrequently detected beyond 72 hours after its onset.[40]

The recent development of assays for the detection of antibody to the Norwalk, Hawaii, and Snow Mountain agents provides practical methods for a serologic diagnosis of infection. Serum antibody titer rises can be detected within 10–14 days after the onset of illness, and a specific viral diagnosis can thus be established. However, these assays use antigen present in stool and depend on the availability of such material from experimentally induced or naturally occurring cases.

Routine laboratory tests are generally not helpful in making a specific diagnosis of Norwalk-like infection. Peripheral white blood cell counts are normal or slightly elevated with a relative polymorphonuclear leukocytosis and lymphopenia but with otherwise unremarkable white cell morphology. The results of liver function tests, blood urea nitrogen (BUN) and creatinine determinations, and urinalysis are generally within normal limits. The absence of fecal leukocytes, as determined by microscopic examination of stools stained with methylene blue,[41] is a useful tool with which to exclude infection with enteroinvasive pathogens such as *Shigella*.

TREATMENT AND PREVENTION

Disease induced by the Norwalk-like agents is generally self-limited and resolves without specific treatment and without sequelae, although occasionally the disease may be somewhat more severe in debilitated hosts. Oral fluid replacement with isotonic liquids as tolerated by the patient is generally adequate to replace fluid losses. Rarely, parenteral iv therapy may be required if severe vomiting and diarrhea develop. Symptomatic treatment of headache, myalgias, and nausea with analgesics and antiemetics may provide relief. Recently, the administration of bismuth subsalicylate reduced gastrointestinal symptoms in Norwalk-induced disease in normal volunteers but had no effect on the number or character of stools or on virus shedding.[42] Although antiperistaltic agents are frequently prescribed to control diarrhea, their effect on the disease course and on excretion of virus has not been rigorously evaluated. Hospitalized patients are generally subjected to enteric precautions, but the efficacy of such measures has similarly not been demonstrated.

Attempts to develop suitable measures with which to prevent illness induced by the Norwalk-like agents face several obstacles. Since several antigenic types exist and immunity may be relatively short-lived, the development of effective vaccines appears to be difficult. Such vaccines may have to induce local rather than systemic immunity. The aforementioned illnesses appear to be reasonable targets for the application of broadly protective antiviral measures such as antiviral chemoprophylaxis and/or therapy. The efficacy of chemoprophylaxis against these infections has not been evaluated, although early efforts in the application of antivirals to in vitro intestinal organ culture systems appear to be promising.[43,44] Since several outbreaks of the aforementioned illnesses appear to be associated with waterborne or food-borne spread, efforts to reduce potential sources of contamination may also represent important control measures.

REFERENCES

1. National Center for Health Statistics, US Department of Health, Education and Welfare. Current estimates from the Health Interview Survey, United States—1972. Vital and Health Statistics, Publication No. (HRA) 74–1512, Series 10, No. 85. 1973. Washington, DC.
2. Dolin R, Treanor, J. Madore HP. Novel agents of viral enteritis in humans. J Infect Dis. 1987;155:365–75.

3. Blacklow NR, Culor G. Viral gastroenteritis. N Engl J Med. 1981;304:397–406.
4. Dingle JH, Badger GF, Feller AE, et al. A study of illness in a group of Cleveland families. I. A plan of study and certain general observations. Am J Hyg. 1953;58:16–37.
5. Snyder SD, Merson MH. The magnitude of the global problem of acute diarrheal disease: A review of active surveillance data. Bull WHO. 1982;60:605–13.
6. Reimann HA, Price AH, Hodges, et al. The cause of epidemic diarrhea, nausea, and vomiting (viral dysentery). Proc Soc Exp Biol Med. 1945;58:8–9.
7. Gordon I, Ingraham HS, Korns RF. Transmission of epidemic gastroenteritis to human volunteers by oral administration of fecal filtrate. J Exp Med. 1947;86:409–22.
8. Jordan WS, Gordon I, Dorrance WR. A study of illness in a group of Cleveland families. VII. Transmission of acute nonbacterial gastroenteritis to volunteers: Evidence for two different etiologic agents. J Exp Med. 1953;98:461–75.
9. Dolin R, Blacklow NR, DuPont H, et al. Biological properties of Norwalk agent of acute infectious nonbacterial gastroenteritis. Proc Soc Exp Biol Med. 1972;140:578–63.
10. Kapikian AZ, Gerin JL, Wyatt RG, et al. Density in cesium chloride of the termination by ultracentrifugation and immune electron microscopy. Proc Soc Exp Biol Med. 1973;142:874–7.
11. Dolin R, Levy AG, Wyatt RG, et al. Viral gastroenteritis induced by the Hawaii agent: Jejunal histopathology and serologic response. Am J Med. 1975;59:768–71.
12. Thornhill TS, Wyatt RG, Kalica AR, et al. Detection by immune electron microscopy of 26–27 nm virus-like particles associated with two family outbreaks of gastroenteritis. J Infect Dis. 1977;138:20–7.
13. Caul EO, Ashley C, Pether JVS. Norwalk-like particle in epidemic gastroenteritis in the U.K. Lancet. 1979;2:1292.
14. Dolin R, Reichman RC, Roessner KD, et al. Detection by immune electron microscopy of the Snow Mountain agent of acute viral gastroenteritis. J Infect Dis. 1982;146:184–9.
15. Greenberg HB, Valdesuso J, Kalica AR. Proteins of Norwalk virus. J Virol. 1981;37:994–9.
16. Madore HP, Treanor J, Dolin R. Characterization of the Snow Mountain agent of viral gastroenteritis. J Virol. 1986;58:487–92.
17. Wyatt RG, Dolin R, Blacklow NR, et al. Comparison of three agents of acute infectious nonbacterial gastroenteritis by virus challenge in volunteers. J Infect Dis. 1974;129:709–14.
18. Greenberg HB, Wyatt RG, Valdesuso, et al. Solid phase microtiter radioimmunoassay for detection of the Norwalk strain of acute non-bacterial epidemic gastroenteritis virus and its antibodies. J Med Virol. 1978;2:97–108.
19. Dolin R, Roessner KD, Treanor J, et al. Radioimmunoassay for detection of Snow Mountain agent of viral gastroenteritis. J Med Virol. 1986;19:11–18.
20. Zahorsky J. Hyperemesis hiemis or the winter vomiting disease. Arch Pediatr. 1929;46:391–5.
21. Hargreaves ER. Epidemic diarrhea and vomiting. Br Med J. 1929;46:391–5.
22. Cheever FS. Viral agents in gastrointestinal disease. Med Clin North Am. 1967;51:637–41.
23. Blacklow NR, Dolin R, Feson DS, et al. Acute infectious nonbacterial gastroenteritis: Etiology and pathogenesis. Ann Intern Med. 1972;76:993–1000.
24. Greenberg HB, Wyatt RG, Kalica AR, et al. New insights in viral gastroenteritis. Perspect Virol. 1981;11:163–87.
25. Kaplan JE, Gary GW, Barron RC, et al. Epidemiology of Norwalk gastroenteritis and the role of Norwalk virus in outbreaks of acute nonbacterial gastroenteritis. Ann Intern Med. 1982;96:756–61.
26. Brondum J, Spitalny KC, Vogt RL, et al. Snow Mountain agent associated with an outbreak of gastroenteritis in Vermont. J Infect Dis. 1985;152:834–7.
27. Agus SG, Dolin R, Wyatt RG, et al. Acute infectious nonbacterial gastroenteritis: Intestinal histopathology. Ann Intern Med. 1973;79:18–25.
28. Schreiber DS, Blacklow NR, Trier JS. The mucosal lesion of the proximal small intestine in acute infectious nonbacterial gastroenteritis. N Engl J Med. 1973;288:1318–23.
29. Schreiber DS, Blacklow, NR, Trier JS. The small intestinal lesion induced by Hawaii agent acute infectious nonbacterial gastroenteritis. J Infect Dis. 1974;129:705–8.
30. Widerlite L, Trier JS, Blacklow NR, et al. Structure of the gastric mucosa in acute infectious nonbacterial gastroenteritis. Gastroenterology. 1975; 60:425–30.
31. Levy AG, Widerlite, L. Schwartz CJ, et al. Jejunal adenylate cyclase activity in human subjects during viral gastroenteritis. Gastroenterology. 1976; 70:321–5.
32. Parrino TA, Schreiber DS, Trier JS, et al. Clinical immunity in acute gastroenteritis caused by Norwalk agent. N Engl J Med. 1977;291:86–9.
33. Ogra PL, Karzon DT. Formation and function of poliovirus antibody in different tissues. Prog Med Virol. 1971;13:156–93.
34. Agus SE, Falchuk ZM, Sessoms CS, et al. Increased jejunal IgA synthesis in vitro during acute infectious nonbacterial gastroenteritis. Am J Dig Dis. 1974;19:127–31.
35. Dolin R, Riechman RC, Fauci AS. Lymphocyte populations in acute viral gastroenteritis. Infect Immun. 1976;14:422–8.
36. Kapikian Z, Wyatt RG, Dolin R, et al. Visualization of a 27 nm particle associated with acute infectious nonbacterial gastroenteritis. J Virol 1972; 10:1075–81.
37. Herrmann JE, Nowak NA, Blacklow NR. Detection of Norwalk virus in stools by immunoassay. J Med Virol. 1985;17:127–33.
38. Madore HP, Treanor JJ, Pray KA, et al. Enzyme-linked immunosorbent assays for Snow Mountain and Norwalk agents of viral gastroenteritis. J Clin Microbiol. 1986;24:456–9.
39. Treanor JJ, Madore HP, Dolin R. Development of an enzyme immunoassay for the Hawaii agent of viral gastroenteritis. J Med Virol Methods. 1988;22:207–214.
40. Thornhill TS, Kalica AR, Wyatt RG, et al. Pattern of shedding of the Norwalk particle in stools during experimentally induced gastroenteritis in volunteers as determined by immune electron microscopy. J Infect Dis. 1975;132:28–34.
41. Harris JC, DuPont HL, Hornick RB. Fecal leukocytes in diarrheal illness. Ann Intern Med. 1972;76:697–703.
42. Steinhoff MC, Douglas RG Jr, Greenberg HB, et al. Bismuth subsalycylate therapy of viral gastroenteritis. Gastroenterology. 1980;78:1495–9.
43. Albright DJ, Whalen RA, Blacklow NR. Sensitivity of human fetal intestine to interferon. Nature. 1974;247:218–20.
44. Dolin R, Smith HA. Antiviral activity of adenine arabinoside and iododeoxyuridine in human fetal intestinal and tracheal organ cultures. J Infect Dis. 1975;132:287–95.

156. PRIONS

KENNETH L. TYLER

In 1982 Prusiner proposed the name *prion* for the agent responsible for a group of chronic progressive central nervous system (CNS) disorders that share similar pathologic features and are caused by a transmissible agent with unconventional biologic properties.[1] This group of disorders now includes the human diseases kuru, Creutzfeldt-Jakob disease, and Gerstmann-Straussler syndrome as well as the animal diseases scrapie, transmissible mink encephalopathy, chronic wasting disease of elk and deer, and bovine spongiform encephalopathy (see Chapter 69).

The emphasis of this chapter will be on reviewing the current status of "prions" and their relationship to the etiology of the transmissible spongiform encephalopathies. The term *prion* was initially chosen to emphasize the hypothesis that the causative agents of these disorders were *pro*teinaceous *in*fectious particles that could be distinguished from viruses and viroids by their apparent lack of a nucleic acid.[1] More recent definitions of the term have been more flexible. As currently employed by Prusiner and his colleagues, prion designates "a small infectious pathogen containing protein; it is resistant to procedures that modify or hydrolyze nucleic acids. Whether or not prions contain nucleic acid remains to be established."[2] Nonetheless, because the "prion hypothesis" remains unproven, many investigators have preferred to avoid the term "prion." However, many other commonly employed designations such as the terms "unconventional viruses"[3,4] or "virino"[5] also suffer from various unproven presuppositions concerning the general nature of this group of transmissible agents and are therefore equally unsatisfactory. Perhaps the least perjorative usage is simply to refer to the "scrapie agent," "kuru agent," etc. Obviously when the nature of these agents is conclusively established, more appropriate designations can be adopted.

The diseases caused by these agents share a number of fundamental properties (Chapter 69). First, their major pathologic manifestations are confined almost exclusively to the CNS. Second, the diseases typically have long incubation times that, at least in the case of kuru, may even exceed 30 years. Third, the diseases all appear to be progressive with an inexorably fatal outcome. Fourth, the pathologic hallmarks of the disease are strikingly similar. There is always a reactive astrocytosis in the CNS with no associated inflammatory response. Small vacuoles (spongiform change) and larger cavities (status spongiosus) within the neuropil are common but not invariable features. Finally, the unusual biochemical and biophysical properties of the inciting agents seem to set them apart from conventional viruses or viroids.

PROPERTIES OF THE SCRAPIE AGENT

The bulk of investigations of the molecular and biologic properties of this group of agents have involved the scrapie agent, which can be taken as the unofficial prototype for the group. Systematic studies of the resistance and susceptibility of the scrapie agent to a wide variety of physical and chemical agents have been undertaken in an effort to glean information concerning its fundamental composition and structure.[1,6] The agent is extraordinarily resistant to inactivation by agents that disrupt nucleic acids including nucleases (micrococcal nuclease; nuclease P, DNase I and II, RNase A, H, and T_1, phosphodiesterases I and II), ultraviolet (UV) irradiation at 254 nm, psoralen photoreaction, and chemical modification by nucleophiles such as hydroxylamine (NH_2OH). Infectivity is not significantly reduced by sonication for prolonged periods of time or by the use of divalent cations ($Zn(NO_3)_2$, $MgCl_2$).[7,8] There are three plausible explanations for these types of results. First, the scrapie agent does not contain a nucleic acid; second, the nucleic acid must be extremely small (e.g., <50 nucleotides); and third, the nucleic acid is enclosed within a densely packed protein shell in a fashion that does not allow for the penetration of enzymes, psoralens, nucleophiles, or divalent cations.

In contradistinction to the difficulty encountered in inactivating the scrapie agent with manipulations that alter or hydrolyze nucleic acids is the agent's comparative sensitivity to agents that digest, denature, or chemically modify proteins.[6] The infectivity of the scrapie agent can be reduced by proteolysis with proteinase K, trypsin, papain, and pronase. Agents such as diethylpyrocarbonate (DEP), which carbethoxylates amino acids, and butanedione, which modifies arginine, histidine, and lysine residues, also reduce infectivity. Several protein-denaturing agents including detergents (e.g., sodium dodecyl sulfate [SDS]), organic solvents (e.g., phenol), chaotropic salts, and urea have a similar effect. These studies suggest that protein(s) are an integral component of the scrapie agent and that its infectivity depends on their presence.

ASSAYS OF INFECTIVITY

Initial attempts to characterize the scrapie agent further were severely hampered by the lack of a suitable small animal model of scrapie and by the difficulties involved in conducting bioassays to measure scrapie infectivity. In 1961, a major breakthrough occurred when Chandler suceeded in transmitting scrapie to mice.[9] Before that time investigations were conducted exclusively on sheep and goats. Subsequently the disease was transmitted to Syrian golden hamsters,[10] which have become the experimental animal of choice for many investigations.

A bioassay of scrapie infectivity depends on either end-point titrations or the incubation time interval assay. The latter test is based on an inverse relationship between the titer of the scrapie agent in infected material and the incubation time (i.e., delay between inoculation and the development of illness or death) after the inoculation of this material into test animals.[11,12] Although a number of efforts have been made to establish the accuracy of this method in determining scrapie infectivity titers because of its obvious advantages in terms of both time and number of animals required to titrate samples,[12] there is still controversy concerning its validity.[13,14]

The ability to eliminate bioassays entirely in favor of in vitro tests would represent a major step forward. The use of enzyme-linked immunosorbent assays (ELISA) or Western immunoblots depends on the availability of polyclonal and monoclonal antibodies against protein components of the scrapie agent. Both polyclonal[15] and monoclonal[16] antibodies against the major protein component of prions have been generated. Unfortunately these antibodies do not distinguish between the normal and scrapie isoforms of this protein (see later), which limits their use as diagnostic reagents.

PURIFICATION OF THE SCRAPIE AGENT

Purification of the scrapie agent or related disease agents depends on the ability to demonstrate that a specific biochemical manipulation has resulted in higher infectivity (i.e., an increase in the median infective dose [ID_{50}] or the median lethal dose [LD_{50}]) per unit amount of material. Since measuring infectivity depends on time-consuming and difficult bioassay techniques, the problems of designing purification strategies is made even more complex.[17–19]

One current large-scale purification procedure[19] involves making homogenates of infected hamster brains and extracting them with detergent (Triton X-100) and sodium deoxycholate followed by precipitation with polyethylene glycol (PEG 8000). The resulting material is then digested with micrococcal nuclease and proteinase K and extracted with Sarkosyl and sodium cholate. This material is precipitated with ammonium sulfate and then reextracted with triton X-100 and SDS. The resulting material is then centrifuged through a sucrose gradient by using a zonal rotor. A slightly modified procedure has also been used to purify the scrapie agent from as little as 1 g of infected brain material. The large-scale procedures are reported to result in a 3000- to 10,000-fold purification in terms of specific infectivity (ID_{50} units/mg protein) as compared with the starting material.

By using purification strategies similar to that outlined above, as well as newer immuno-affinity purification techniques, Prusiner and his colleagues have made substantial progress in characterizing the nature of the material they have purified, which they believe represents the major component of the scrapie agent. They initially showed that the major component of their purified preparations was a hydrophobic protein and that this was apparently required for the infectivity of the scrapie agent.[20,21] This protein was subsequently shown to have a molecular weight of 27–30 kD and was designated PrP 27–30 (prion protein; molecular weight, 27–30 kD).[22,23] PrP 27–30 was subsequently shown to be a sialoglycoprotein that possesses N-linked oligosaccharides.[24] The C-terminus of the mature protein, which is quite hydrophobic, also appears to be removed during maturation and a phosphatidylinositol glycolipid added.[25] It polymerizes into rodlike structures with the characteristics of amyloid.[26] A protein of similar molecular weight to PrP has also been identified in scrapie-infected hamster brain by other investigators using different purification strategies.[17,18,27,28]

ANTIBODIES AGAINST THE SCRAPIE AGENT

Several groups have produced polyclonal antibodies directed against the entire PrP[15,27,29] or by using specific peptide fragments as immunogens.[30] Anti-PrP monoclonal antibodies have also been described.[16] It is important to recognize that, indistinction to these results when using specially immunized animals, under normal circumstances infection with the scrapie agent (or related disease agents) does not induce an agent-specific humoral immune response in the host. In addition, there is no evidence to suggest that infected animals develop disease-specific alterations in any component of the cellular immune response.

In Western immunoblots of preparations of infected brain material, anti-PrP antibodies identify PrP 27–30 as well as several lower-molecular-weight bands. Anti-PrP antibodies can also be used for immunochemical staining of fixed brain material. By using anti-PrP antisera it has been shown that the prion rods that are isolated from purifications of the scrapie agent contain PrP 27–30. In addition, the amyloid plaques that are a prominent feature in many scrapie-infected hamster brains also stain with anti-PrP antisera.[15,31] This suggests that PrP is a component of the amyloid plaques found in scrapie-infected hamster brains. These antisera also appear to stain the amyloid plaques found in human brain material from patients who died of Creutzfeldt-Jakob disease (CJD), Gerstmann-Straussler syndrome, and kuru.[32–34]

MORPHOLOGIC CHARACTERISTICS (SCRAPIE-ASSOCIATED FIBRILS AND PRION RODS)

Identifying the morphologic chharacteristics of the scrapie agent has proved to be as elusive a problem as definitively determining its biochemical composition. In 1981, Merz and colleagues desribed filamentous structures, referred to as scrapie-associated fibrils (SAFs), in electron micrographs of sodium phosphotungstate–stained, detergent-treated membrane extracts prepared from scrapie-infected mouse brains.[35,36] The SAFs were 4–6 nm in diameter and varied between 50 and 400 nm in length. They typically appeared as either helically intertwined doublets or tetramers. Scrapie-associated fibrils have also been described in preparations of brain tissue from human CJD.[37] Controversy continues concerning the relationship between SAFs and the rod-shaped structures that are identifiable in purified preparations of scrapie-infected brains after detergent solubilization of membranes. The major protein component of SAFs has a molecular weight similar to that of PrP 27–30,[38] its N-terminal amino acid sequence is identical to that of PrP,[39] and antisera to the prion protein react with SAFs,[40] which would certainly suggest that SAFs are closely related if not identical structures. The prion rods appear to be composed of aggregates of PrP 27–30. They are typically around 25 nm in width and 50–200 nm in length and appear to share a number of properties with purified amyloids.[26,41,42] Similar rod-shaped particles have been isolated from the brains of patients with CJD.[33]

MOLECULAR BIOLOGY OF THE SCRAPIE AGENT

In an effort to characterize PrP 27–30 further, the sequence of its last seven N-terminal amino acids was determined.[19] By using this sequence a series of icosameric oligonucleotide probes were created that contained possible nucleotide sequences that could code for the identified heptapeptide. These probes were used to screen a cDNA library containing about 150,000 colonies that was derived from scrapie-infected hamster brain. A single cDNA colony (1.9 kilobases [kb] in size) was found. This colony contained coding sequences for the original heptapeptide of PrP 27–30 as well as for a number of additional PrP 27–30 peptides that were generated by cyanogen bromide cleavage of PrP 27–30.[43] Subsequently a larger cDNA clone (2096 nucleotides) was identified that encompassed the original clone.[44] Additional cDNA clones from hamsters, rats, and humans have subsequently been identified.[45–47]

Analysis of the cDNA clone and the amino acid sequence it encodes has provided a great deal of information concerning the organization of the gene encoding the PrP 27–30 protein and the nature of the protein itself. The gene begins with a GC (guanine, cytosine)-rich region that resembles certain types of viral and cellular gene promoters. After a 10-kb intron there are two possible initiation (ATG) codons. The first of these two sites appears to be the initiation site and conforms to Kozak's rules for eukaryotic initiation codons. Assuming that this ATG is indeed the initiation site, there is a long open reading frame (ORF) contained within a single exon that would potentially encode a 254 amino acid protein. The N-terminus of this protein contains a 22 amino acid putative signal sequence that is presumably cleaved by host cell proteases. The amino acid sequence of protein PrP 27–30 is contained within this larger protein, which has subsequently been designated PrP 33–35. An even larger (54 kD) protein has also been proposed as the normal cellular precursor of PrP 27–30.[48] PrP 27–30 is presumably derived from the larger protein during purification by proteolytic removal of the first 67 amino acids.

It has been suggested that the PrP protein has a N-terminal hydrophilic extracellular domain composed of about 122 amino acids followed by a 23 amino acid transmembrane stretch. There is then a highly charged region of about 20 amino acids that may serve to "stop" membrane transfer of the protein. There is a long cytoplasmic domain followed by a hydrophobic C-terminus.[46] An alternative model in which PrP spans the cell membrane twice has also been proposed.[49] As discussed earlier, the hydrophobic C-terminus may be replaced by a phosphatidylinositol glycolipid that could serve to anchor PrP to the cell membrane.[25] It has been suggested that PrP is primarily a transmembrane protein that is found on the surface of cells, particularly neurons.[49,50]

There is no known amino acid sequence similarity between PrP 33–35 or PrP 27–30 and any other known proteins. The PrP cDNA has also been used as a probe in an attempt to detect complementary nucleic acid sequences within the scrapie agent. When this technique was used no PrP nucleic acids were found, again suggesting that PrP is not encoded by a gene carried within the scrapie agent.[43]

The initial expectation was that the gene encoding PrP 33–35 (and therefore also PrP 27–30) would be found in scrapie-infected brain material but not in normal uninfected animals. This was not found to be the case. When the chromosomal DNA of normal uninfected and scrapie-infected hamster brains was analyzed by Southern blotting using the cDNA described earlier as a probe, a single gene with the same restriction map was found in both cases.[43] Subsequently, related genes have been found in human DNA and in the DNA of a large number of organisms including nematodes, *Drosophila*, and yeast.[51] These studies clearly indicate that PrP is encoded by a host cell gene.

The fact that a gene encoding what is putatively the major protein of the scrapie agent can be found in the genomes of both uninfected and infected animals and in a wide variety of species not currently known to develop transmissible encephalopathies but not within the scrapie agent itself has a number of possible explanations. First, it is possible that the strategy used to purify the scrapie agent led instead to the inadvertent purification of a CNS neuronal or neuron-related protein. This protein could be a pathologic product that is copurified with the scrapie agent.[52,53] Second, it is possible that scrapie could result from differences in the transcription or translation of this gene in normal and infected animals.

Prusiner and his colleagues contend that PrP is a component of the scrapie agent and not merely an "innocent bystander" caught in their purification protocol.[50] The major lines of evidence are as follows: (*1*) PrP 27–30 is the most abundant macromolecule in purified preparations of the scrapie agent. (*2*) The concentration of PrP 27–30 is proportional to the scrapie agent titer in infected material. (*3*) Procedures that degrade PrP 27–30 also result in the loss of scrapie infectivity. (*4*) PrP 27–30 and scrapie agent infectivity partition together in many different forms including detergent-lipid-protein complexes that are apparently free of contaminating material.[54] (*5*) The gene encoding PrP ("Prn-p") is closely linked to a gene known to influence scrapie incubation times in infected mice ("Prn-i").[55] No one of these pieces of information provides conclusive evidence of the identity of PrP and the scrapie agent; the claim that PrP is inseparable from infectivity of the scrapie agent has been particularly contentious.[56] However, the accumulating weight of evidence does indicate that PrP is not simply a purification artifact.

In order to determine whether differences in transcription or translation of the PrP gene in normal and infected animals could provide an explanation for disease induction, a number of studies have been conducted. The levels of PrP mRNA are identical in normal and scrapie-infected hamster brains[43,57] and do not appear to increase during the course of scrapie infection. This would seem to exclude differences in gene transcription as an explanation for disease induction. Interestingly, PrP mRNA can be detected in a wide variety of non-neural tissues that are not known to be the site of pathologic alterations in scrapie or related diseases (e.g., heart, lung, kidney, pancreas, spleen, testes).[45,57] Within the CNS, mRNA levels appear to be significantly higher in neurons (about 50 copies per cell) than in glia (<3 copies per cell).[58] Differences in the fine structure of the mRNAs for PrP transcribed in normal and infected brains cannot be excluded as a potential difference in the two situations. However, the fact that the ORF is contained within a single exon of the PrP gene suggests that gross alterations such as differences in the pattern of mRNA splicing would be unlikely.

Having excluded differences in gene transcription as a likely cause to explain disease production in scrapie-infected animals, one is left with the possibility that, even though equal amounts of PrP mRNA are present in infected and normal animals, the proteins encoded differ with respect to post-translational modifications. It is possible that the presence of differences in post-translation processing of the PrP could be related to disease induction. According to Prusiner and his colleagues the PrP isolated from the brains of normal animals is sensitive to proteinase K digestion and fails to polymerize into rods. The PrP from scrapie-infected animals is digested into PrP 27–30 but then resists further proteinase K digestion. This material also polymerizes on exposure to detergents to form amyloid-like rods and filaments.[59] These results do suggest that there are differences in the PrP present in normal and scrapie-infected brains.

The levels of PrP appear to be significantly higher in infected brains as compared with normal brains. It is possible that this accumulation of PrP could somehow in itself be toxic. The mechanism for this accumulation remains unclear.

HOST FACTORS AND STRAINS OF THE SCRAPIE AGENT

One of the more interesting and less understood aspects of scrapie pathogenesis is the role played by different "strains" of the scrapie agent and by host factors in determining both the nature and outcome of infection. The susceptibility of the host to scrapie infection, the time interval between inoculation of the agent and the development of disease ("incubation time"), and the nature and distribution of neuropathologic changes (e.g., the degree and distribution of vacuolation and the presence or absence of amyloid plaques) are all influenced by host factors and apparently by differences in the nature of the agent itself.[27]

Dickinson and colleagues showed that different strains of inbred mice have marked variations in scrapie incubation times.[60] They coined the name "Sinc" (scrapie incubation) for the gene controlling this phenomena and identified several putative alleles of this gene in different strains of inbred mice. In 1983 a second gene, "Pid-1" (prion incubation determinant), was identified that influenced the susceptibility of mice to scrapie infection. This gene maps within the D subregion of the murine histocompatibility locus (H-2) on chromosome 17.[61] A third gene, "Prn-i" (prion incubation), that influences scrapie incubation times in mice was subsequently identified. Prn-i may in fact be identical to Sinc, although evidence on this point is still incomplete.[5,53] Prn-i appears to be closely linked to the structural gene (Prn-p) on murine chromosome 2 that encodes the prion protein.[55,62] In humans, PrP is encoded by a gene on the short arm of chromosome 20.

As noted earlier, not only do host factors appear to determine the features of disease development after the inoculation of animals with the scrapie agent, but there appear to be variations in the nature of the agent itself.[5,53,63] The existence of different strains of the scrapie agent has been used as evidence that the agent must contain an intrinsic genome.[5,53,64]

There appears to be general agreement that repeated passage of a particular strain of the scrapie agent within hosts of the same species results in a progressive diminution of the disease incubation time. Conversely, on first inoculating a strain of the scrapie agent into a new species there is a marked increase in incubation time. In addition, specific strains of inbred mice appear to show reproducible differences in incubation time after inoculation with different strains of the scrapie agent. Western immunoblot studies of CJD agent proteins suggest that there may be host species-specific epitopes on these proteins,[65] but their exact nature remains to be determined. Sequencing of the prion protein gene (Prn-P) from two strains of inbred mice that exhibit long (I/Ln) and short (NZW) disease incubation times indicated that the encoded proteins differ in two amino acids at positions 108 and 189. The Prp in I/Ln mice would be predicted to have a phenylalanine-from-leucine change (codon 108) and a valine-from-threonine change (codon 189) when compared with the PrP in NZW mice.[62] This result provides the first evidence at a molecular level for differences in the nature of different "strains" of the scrapie agent and suggests that differences in the nature of the PrP may directly influence disease incubation time. This result has been extended by the recent discovery that patients with Gerstmann-Straussler syndrome have a missense variant in the PrP gene that results in the substitution of a leucine for a proline at PrP codon 102.[67]

CONCLUSION

There are substantial gaps in our current knowledge of scrapie pathogenesis and, by analogy, our knowledge of related diseases.[66] First, the exact nature of the scrapie agent remains shrouded in controversy. Whether or not it contains nucleic acid remains an unresolved issue, although attempts to demonstrate its presence have not to date been successful. If a nucleic acid is present, its size and the nature of what it encodes are obviously still completely unknown. the scrapie agent is able to replicate itself, yet the process by which this occurs remains totally mysterious. Solving this mystery will be all the more interesting if PrP is indeed the major component of the scrapie agent in that this protein is encoded in host DNA rather than by nucleic acid contained in the agent itself. The scrapie agent is clearly capable of spreading within the host and between cells. The mechanism of this spread remains to be identified, although evidence has accumulated that suggests that it may be through nerves and may involve slow axonal transport.[63] Obviously infection of neurons leads ultimately to the clinical and pathologic manifestations of transmissible encephalopathy, yet the mechanisms by which the scrapie agent alters cellular function remain unknown. If this alteration involves changes in a normal protein constituent of neuronal membranes, it may have implications for a number of neurologic disorders. It will be important to identify the role of the normal cellular product of the PrP gene. Finally, evidence exists that there are different strains of the scrapie agent and that these strains differ in their biologic properties. The nature of these strain differences needs to be clarified further and their basis better understood.

REFERENCES

1. Prusiner SB. Novel proteinaceous infectious particles cause scrapie. Science. 1982;216:136–44.
2. Prusiner SB. Terminology. In: Prusiner SB, McKinley MP, eds. Prions. San Diego: Academic Press; 1987;37–53.
3. Gajdusek DC. Unconventional viruses and the origin and disappearance of kuru. Science. 1977;197:943–60.
4. Gajdusek DC. Unconventional viruses causing subacute spongiform encephalopathies. In: Fields BN, ed. Virology. New York: Raven Press; 1985;1519–57.
5. Hope J, Kimberlin RH. The molecular biology of scrapie: The last two years. Trends Neurosci 1987;10:149–51.
6. Prusiner SB. The prion hypothesis. In: Prusiner SB, McKinley MP, eds. Prions. San Diego: Academic Press; 1987:17–36.

7. Bellinger-Kawahara C, Diener TO, McKinley MP, et al. Purified scrapie prions resist inactivation by procedures that hydrolyze, modify, or shear nucleic acids. Virology. 1987;160:271–4.
8. Bellinger-Kawahara C, Cleaver JE, Diener TO, et al. Purified scrapie prions resist inactivation by UV irradiation. J Virol. 1987;61:159–66.
9. Chandler RL. Encephalopathy in mice produced with scrapie brain material. Lancet. 1961;1:1378–9.
10. Manuelidis EE, Angelo JN, Gorgacz EJ, et al. Transmission of Creutzfeldt-Jakob disease to syrian hamsters. Lancet. 1977;1:479.
11. Prusiner SB, Groth DF, Cochran SP, et al. Molecular properties, partial purification and assay by incubation time period measurements of the hamster scrapie agent. Biochemistry. 1980;19:4883–91.
12. Prusiner SB, Cochran SP, Groth DF, et al. Measurement of the scrapie agent using an incubation time interval assay. Ann Neurol. 1982;11:353–8.
13. Lax AJ, Millson GC, Manning EJ. Can scrapie titres be calculated accurately from incubation periods? J Gen Virol. 1983;64:971–3.
14. Somerville RA, Carp RI. Altered scrapie infectivity estimates by titration and incubation period in the presence of detergents. J Gen Virol. 1983;64:2045–50.
15. Bendheim PE, Barry RA, DeArmond SJ, et al. Antibodies to a scrapie prion protein. Nature. 1984;310:418–21.
16. Barry RA, Prusiner SB. Monoclonal antibodies to the cellular and scrapie prion proteins. J Infect Dis. 1986;154:518–21.
17. Diringer H, Hilmert H, Simon D, et al. Towards purification of the scrapie agent. Eur J Biochem. 1983;134:555–60.
18. Marsh RF, Dees C, Castle BE, et al. Purification of the scrapie agent by density gradient centrifugation. J Gen Virol. 1984;65:415–21.
19. Prusiner SB, Groth DF, Bolton DC, et al. Purification and structural studies of a major scrapie prion protein. Cell. 1984;38:127–34.
20. Prusiner SB, McKinley MP, Groth DF, et al. Scrapie agent contains a hydrophobic protein. Proc Natl Acad Sci USA. 1981;78:6675–9.
21. McKinley MP, Masiarz FR, Prusiner SB. Reversible chemical modification of the scrapie agent. Science. 1981;214:1259–61.
22. McKinley MP, Bolton DC, Prusiner SB. A protease resistant protein is a structural component of the scrapie prion. Cell. 1983;35:57–62.
23. Bolton DC, McKinley MP, Prusiner SB. Molecular characteristics of the major scrapie prion protein. Biochemistry. 1984;23:5898–905.
24. Bolton DC, Meyer RK, Prusiner SB. Scrapie PrP 27–30 is a sialoglycoprotein. J Virol. 1985;53:596–606.
25. Stahl N, Borchelt DR, Hsiao K, et al. Scrapie prion contains a phosphatidylinositol glycolipid. Cell. 1987;51:229–40.
26. Prusiner SB, McKinley MP, Bowman KA, et al. Scrapie prions aggregate to form amyloid-like birefringent rods. Cell 1983;35:349–58.
27. Carp RI, Merz PA, Kascsak RJ et al. Nature of the scrapie agent: Current status of facts and hypotheses. J Gen Virol. 1985;66;1357–68.
28. Castle BE, Dees C, German TL, et al. Effects of different methods of purification on aggregation of scrapie infectivity. J Gen Virol. 1987;68:225–31.
29. Diringer H, Rahn HC, Bode L. Antibodies to protein of scrapie-associated fibrils. Lancet. 1984;2:345.
30. Barry RA, Kent SB, McKinley MP, et al. Scrapie and cellular prion proteins share polypeptide epitopes. J Infect Dis. 1986;153:848–54.
31. DeArmond SJ, McKinley MP, Barry RA, et al. Identification of prion amyloid filaments in scrapie-infected brain. Cell. 1985;41:221–35.
32. Bendheim PE, Bockman JM, McKinley MP, et al. Scrapie and Creutzfeldt-Jakob disease prion proteins share physical properties and antigenic determinants. Proc Natl Acad Sci USA. 1985;82:997–1001.
33. Bockman JM, Kingsbury DT, McKinley MP, et al. Creutzfeldt-Jakob disease prion proteins in human brain. N Engl J Med. 1985;312:73–8.
34. Manuelidis L, Valley S, Manuelidis EE. Specific proteins associated with Creutzfeldt-Jakob disease and scrapie share antigenic and carbohydrate determinants. Proc Natl Acad Sci USA. 1985;82:4263–7.
35. Merz PA, Somerville RA, Wisniewski HM, et al: Abnormal fibrils from scrapie-infected brains. Acta Neuropathol (Berl). 1981;54:63–74.
36. Merz PA, Rohwer RG, Kascsak R, et al. Infection specific particle from the unconventional slow virus diseases. Science. 1984;225:437–40.
37. Merz PA, Somerville RA, Wisniewski HM, et al. Scrapie-associated fibrils in Creutzfeldt-Jakob disease. Nature. 1983;306:474–6.
38. Diringer H, Gelderbloom H, Hilmert H, et al. Scrapie infectivity, fibrils, and low molecular weight protein. Nature. 1983;306:476–8.
39. Hope J, Morton LJ, Farquhar CF, et al. The major polypeptide of scrapie-associated fibrils (SAF) has the same size, charge distribution and N-terminal protein sequence as predicted for the normal brain protein (PrP). EMBO J. 1986;5:2591–7.
40. Merz PA, Kascsak RJ, Rubenstein R, et al. Antisera to scrapie-associated fibril protein and prion protein decorate scrapie-associated fibrils. J Virol. 1987;61:42–9.
41. McKinley MP, Braunfeld MB, Bellinger CG, et al. Molecular characteristics of prion rods purified from scrapie-infected hamster brains. J Infect Dis. 1986;154:110–20.
42. McKinley MP, Braunfeld MB, Prusiner SB. Scrapie prion ultrastructure. In: Prusiner SB, McKinley MP, eds. Prions. San Diego: Academic Press; 1987;197–237.
43. Oesch B, Westaway D, Walachi M, et al. A cellular gene encodes scrapie PrP 27–30 protein. Cell. 1985;40:735–46.
44. Basler K, Oesch B, Scott M, et al. Scrapie and cellular PrP isoforms are encoded by the same chromosomal gene. Cell. 1986;46:417–28.
45. Robakis NK, Sawh PR, Wolfe GC, et al. Isolation of a cDNA clone encoding the leader peptide of prion protein and expression of the homologous gene in various tissues. Proc Natl Acad Sci USA. 1986;83:6377–81.
46. Liao Y-C, Tokes Z, Lim E, et al. Cloning of rat "prion related protein" cDNA. Lab Invest. 1987;57:370–4.
47. Liao Y-C, Lebo RV, Clawson GA, et al. Human prion protein cDNA: Molecular cloning, chromosomal mapping, and biological implications. Science. 1986;233:364–7.
48. Bendheim PE, Bolton DC. A 54-kDa normal cellular protein may be the precursor of the scrapie agent protease-resistant protein. Proc Natl Acad Sci USA. 1986;83:2214–18.
49. Hay B, Barry RA, Lieberburg I, et al. Biogenesis and transmembrane orientation of the cellular isoform of the scrapie prion protein. Mol Cell Biol. 1987;7:914–20.
50. Prusiner SB. Prions and neurodegenerative diseases. N Engl J Med. 1987;317:1571–81.
51. Westaway D, Prusiner SB. Conservation of the cellular gene encoding the scrapie prion protein. Nucleic Acids Res. 1986;14:2035–44.
52. Manuelidis L, Manuelidis EE. Recent developments in scrapie and Creutzfeldt-Jakob disease. Prog Med Virol. 1986;33:78–98.
53. Kimberlin RH, Hope J. Genes and genomes in scrapie. Trends Genet. 1987;3:117–8.
54. Gabizon R, McKinley MP, Prusiner SB. Purified prion proteins and scrapie infectivity copartition into liposomes. Proc Natl Acad Sci USA. 1987;84:4017–21.
55. Carlson GA, Kingsbury DT, Goodman PA, et al. Linkage of prion protein and scrapie incubation time genes. Cell. 1986;46:503–11.
56. Manuelidis L, Sklaviadis T, Manuelidis EE. Evidence suggesting that PrP is not the infectious agent in Creutzfeldt-Jakob disease. EMBO J. 1987;6:341–7.
57. Chesebro B, Race R, Wehrly K, et al. Identification of scrapie prion protein-specific mRNA in scrapie-infected and uninfected brain. Nature. 1985;315:331–3.
58. Kretzschmar HA, Prusiner SB, Stowring LE, et al. Scrapie prion proteins are synthesized in neurons. Am J Pathol. 1986;122;1–5.
59. Meyer RK, McKinley MP, Bowman KA, et al. Separation and properties of cellular and scrapie prion proteins. Proc Natl Acad Sci USA. 1986;83:2310–4.
60. Dickinson AG, Fraser H. Scrapie pathogenesis in inbred mice: An assessment of host control and response involving many strains of agent. In: ter Meulen V, Katz M, eds. Slow Virus Infections of the Central Nervous System. New York: Springer Publishing; 1977:3–14.
61. Kingsbury DT, Kasper KC, Stites DP, et al. Genetic control of scrapie and Creutzfeldt-Jakob disease in mice. J Immunol. 1983;131:491–6.
62. Westaway D, Goodman PA, Mirenda CA, et al. Distinct prion proteins in short and long scrapie incubation period mice. Cell. 1987;51:651–62.
63. Kimberlin RH: Scrapie: How much do we really understand? Neuropathol Appl Neurobiol. 1986;12:131–47.
64. Bruce ME, Dickinson G. Biological evidence that scrapie agent has an independent genome. J Gen Virol. 1978;68:79–89.
65. Bockman JM, Prusiner SB, Tateishi J, et al. Immunoblotting of Creutzfeldt-Jakob disease prion proteins: Host species-specific epitopes. Ann Neurol. 1987;21:589–95.
66. Fields BN. Powerful prions? N Engl J Med. 1987;317:1597–8.
67. Hsiao K, Baker HF, Crow TJ, et al. Linkage of a prion protein variant to Gerstmann-Straussler syndrome. Nature. 1989;338:342–5.

SECTION B. CHLAMYDIAL DISEASES

157. INTRODUCTION

WILLIAM R. BOWIE
KING K. HOLMES

The chlamydiae are obligate prokaryotic parasites of eukaryotic cells. For many years they were considered to be viruses, but since they have many of the characteristics of bacteria, they are now considered to be a special type of bacteria.[1] They differ from viruses because they contain both DNA and RNA, are susceptible to antibiotics, have a cell wall like that of gram-negative bacteria, divide by binary fission, synthesize protein independently, and contain ribosomes. They are unable to replicate extracellularly. They cannot synthesize ATP and can be considered energy parasites.[2]

In the past, the generic names of *Miyagawanella* and *Bedsonia* were suggested for these agents, but it is now accepted that because of their unique developmental cycle they belong to a separate order, Chlamydiales, with one family, Chlamydiaceae, containing one genus, *Chlamydia*.[3] There are three species, *C. trachomatis* and *C. psittaci*, which are distinguished by two criteria, and the recently described TWAR agent.[4] *Chlamydia trachomatis* is sensitive to sulfonamides and forms inclusions containing glycogen, which allows detection of the agent by iodine staining of infected cell cultures (Fig. 1). *Chlamydia psittaci* is resistant to sulfonamides and does not produce glycogen. In addition. *C. trachomatis* usually produces a single inclusion that displaces the nucleus, while *C. psittaci* inclusions rupture early and are thus distributed around the nucleus and do not displace it. In addition to the traditional differentiation by glycogen staining and inclusion morphology, species and subspecies can now also be readily distinguished by using monoclonal antibodies.[4]

Chlamydia trachomatis and *C. psittaci* have an identical group-reactive lipopolysaccharide antigen[5] and have a similar small genome size (660×10^6 daltons, about 500 structural genes for *C. trachomatis*),[6] but there is only about 10 percent DNA homology between *C. trachomatis* and *C. psittaci*.[7] DNA homology is high within species except for the mouse pneumonitis agent, which is classified as *C. trachomatis* but shows low homology with both *C. trachomatis* and *C. psittaci*. The TWAR agent, which was initially considered to be a strain of *C. psittaci*, lacks appreciable DNA homology with either *C. trachomatis* or *C. psittaci* and has different restriction endonuclease patterns, and unlike all strains of *C. trachomatis* and most strains of *C. psittaci*, 0 of 8 TWAR strains contained extrachromosomal DNA.[8,9] Thus, TWAR represents a third species, and the name *C. pneumoniae* has been proposed for the TWAR agent.

Chlamydiae have a unique developmental cycle with two distinct forms[2] (Fig. 2). One, the elementary body, is adapted for extracellular survival and for establishing infection but does not replicate. Elementary bodies are usually round, but that of the TWAR strains is pleomorphic but typically pear shaped.[11] Elementary bodies reach new susceptible cells locally within the host, by transmission of infected exudates by vectors, or by mucosa-to-mucosa contact (e.g., sexual transmission). On contact with new susceptible cells it attaches to the surface of the host cell and is actively ingested by endocytosis. Chlamydiae

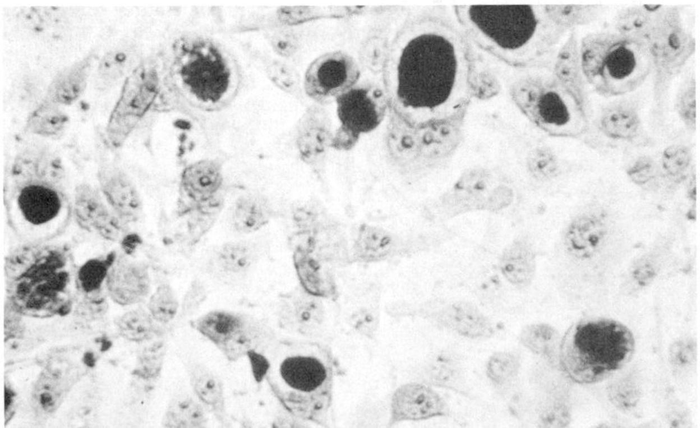

FIG. 1. Irradiated McCoy cell monolayer with glycogen-containing *C. trachomatis* inclusions, which stain darkly with iodine.

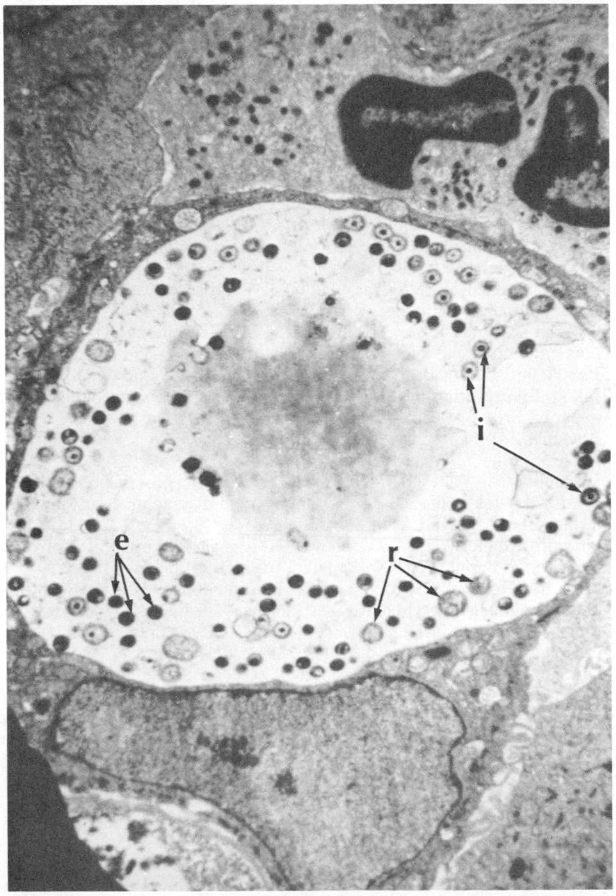

FIG. 2. Uterine cervical biopsy specimen showing all stages of the growth cycle of *C. trachomatis* within an inclusion in a columnar epithelial cell. The larger, lightly staining forms are reticulate bodies (r), which divide by binary fission. These condense to "intermediate forms" (i), which have dark centers resembling a target, and finally to the smaller darkly staining elementary bodies (e), which are the infectious particles adapted for extracellular survival. (Uranyl acetate, lead citrate; ×12,000) (From Swanson et al.,[10] with permission.)

appear to induce their own phagocytosis by normally nonphagocytic cells (induced phagocytosis). Within 6–8 hours after entering the host cell, the elementary body is reorganized into a metabolically active reticulate (initial) body that divides continuously by binary fission within a membrane-bound vacuole. The reticulate bodies are adapted for intracellular function. They have limited synthetic capacity, do not survive extracellularly, and cannot infect new cells. By 18–24 hours after infection, reticulate bodies begin to reorganize into elementary bodies. Depending on the strain, the vacuoles usually release their contents 48–72 hours after infection has commenced. The components of chlamydiae that control attachment, endocytosis, replication, and release and the factors controlling the host cell–chlamydiae balance are poorly understood.

The chlamydiae illustrate one of several intriguing mechanisms by which intracellular parasites can resist being killed by phagocytes. Chlamydiae, like *Toxoplasma gondii* and plasmodia, grow within the phagosome, somehow preventing lysosomal fusion. In contrast, *Trypansoma cruzii, Babesia*, and vaccina virus are thought to survive by rupturing the phagosomal membrane, thereby escaping the phagosome. Other organisms such as mycobacteria, *Listeria, Brucella abortus*, reovirus, and perhaps *Leishmania* survive and grow within the fused phagolysosome.

Chlamydial infections are ubiquitous in birds and mammals including humans.[12] There are many different biotypes of *C. psittaci* that cause natural infection in a wide range of nonprimate mammals in which respiratory disease, placental infection and abortion, arthritis, and enteritis are frequent manifestations. Humans become infected by zoonotic spread.[13] The differences between mammalian and avian strains of *C. psittaci* may eventually prove sufficient to divide them into separate species. It appears that the primary and possibly only means of spread of TWAR (*C. pneumoniae*) is from humans to humans. It has been implicated, usually by serology, in up to 5 percent of community-acquired pneumonias. *Chlamydia pneumoniae* pneumonia apparently affects adults of all ages and so far has had no uniquely distinctive clinical features. *Chlamydia pneumoniae* has also been identified in association with pharyngitis and bronchitis,[8] and outbreaks of pneumonia in military personnel have also been described.[14] Infection by TWAR strains likely accounts for much of the previously inadequately explained rise in serum antibody seen in children and young adolescents.[15]

Humans are the only known natural host for all strains of *C. trachomatis* except the mouse pneumonitis agent. The clinical spectrum and organ specificity of *C. trachomatis* infections are determined partly by the method of transmission and partly by the properties of the infecting strain. Microimmunofluorescence is used to classify *C. trachomatis* into serotypes A through L.[16] Types A through K infect epithelial cells and are variously associated with infections of the conjunctivae, pharynx, lower respiratory tract, urethra, endocervix, fallopian tubes, and the gastrointestinal tract. Types L1, L2, and L3 cause a systemic disease, lymphogranuloma venereum (LGV). These LGV strains differ from serotypes A through K in that LGV strains grow more rapidly in cell cultures, apparently use different cell receptors, and are more virulent for mice inoculated intracerebrally. The differences between mouse, LGB, and non-LGV strains are considerable. The 1984 edition of *Bergey's Manual* separates *C. trachomatis* into three biovars: mouse, LGV, and trachoma (serotypes A–K).[7]

The characteristic syndromes known or thought to be caused by the chlamydiae are outlined in Table 1.

The serum and local immunofluorescent antibody response to *C. trachomatis* infections have been extensively characterized, and the antigenic determinants are being clarified. The function of antibody in chlamydial infection is uncertain, although monoclonal antibody to certain outer membrane antigens has neutralizing activity in vitro. Similarly, the role of cellular immunity in limiting chlamydial infection or in contributing to immunopathology remains undefined. Long-term persistence of both *C. psittaci* and *C. trachomatis* is well documented in healthy animal and human carriers, but the mechanism of microbial persistence of these agents is unknown.

TABLE 1. Human Diseases Caused by Chlamydiae

Diseases	*Method of Transmission*	*Serotypes*
Chlamydia trachomatis		
Endemic trachoma	Fingers, fomites, flies	A, B, Ba, C
Inclusion conjunctivitis Infant pneumonia ? Otitis media	Perinatal	D, E, F, G, H, I, J, K
Nongonococcal urethritis	Sexually transmitted	D, E, F, G, H, I, J, K
Postgonococcal urethritis	Sexually transmitted	
Epididymitis	Sexually transmitted	
Proctitis	Sexually transmitted	
Mucopurulent cervicitis	Sexually transmitted	
Endometritis	Sexually transmitted	
Salpingitis	Sexually transmitted	
Fitz-Hugh-Curtis syndrome	Sexually transmitted	
Urethral syndrome	Sexually transmitted	
Reiter syndrome	Sexually transmitted	
Conjunctivitis	Sexually transmitted	
? Chorioamnionitis	Sexually transmitted	
? Pharyngitis	Sexually transmitted	
? Community-acquired pneumonia	?	
Lymphogranuloma venereum	Sexually transmitted	L1, L2, L3
Chlamydia psittaci		
Psittacosis	Zoonosis, from avians	
Abortion	Zoonosis, from animals	
TWAR (*C. pneumoniae*)		
Community-acquired pneumonia	? aerosol	

REFERENCES

1. Moulder JW. The relation of the *psittacosis* group (chlamydia) to bacteria and viruses. Annu Rev Microbiol. 1966;20:107–30.
2. Moulder, JW. A primer for chlamydiae. In: Mardh PA, Holmes KK, Oriel JD, et al. Chlamydial Infections. Amsterdam: Elsevier Biomedical; 1982;3–14.
3. Page LA. Proposal for the recognition of two species in the genus *Chlamydia* Jones, Rake, and Stearns 1945. Int J Syst Bacteriol. 1968;18:51–66.
4. Kuo CC, Chen HH, Wang SP, et al. Characterization of TWAR strains, a new group of *Chlamydia psittaci*. In: Oriel D, Ridgway G, Schachter J, et al., eds. Chlamydial Infections. Cambridge: Cambridge University Press; 1986:321–4.
5. Dhir SP, Hakomori S, Kenny GE, et al. Immunochemical studies on chlamydial group antigen. (Presence of a 2-keto-3-deoxycarbohydrate as immunodominant group.) J Immunol. 1972;109:116–22.
6. Sarov I, Becker Y. Trachoma agent DNA. J Mol Biol. 1969;42:581–9.
7. Moulder JW, Hatch TP, Kuo C-C, et al. Chlamydia. In: Krieg NR, ed. Bergey's Manual of Systematic Bacteriology. V. 1. Baltimore: Williams & Wilkins; 1984;729–39.
8. Grayston JT, Kuo C-C, Wang S-P, et al. A new *Chlamydia psittaci* strain, TWAR, isolated in acute respiratory tract infections. N Engl J Med. 1986;315:161–8.
9. Campbell LA, Kuo C-C, Grayston JT. Characterization of the new *Chlamydia* agent, TWAR, as a unique organism by restriction endonuclease analysis and DNA-DNA hybridization. J Clin Microbiol. 1987;25:1911–6.
10. Swanson J, Eschenbach DA, Alexander ER, et al. Light and electron microscopic study of *Chlamydia trachomatis* infection of the uterine cervix. J Infect Dis. 1975;131:678–87.
11. Chi EY, Kuo CC, Grayston JT. Unique ultrastructure in the elementary body of *Chlamydia* sp. strain TWAR. J Bacteriol. 1987;169:3757–63.
12. Meyer KF. The host spectrum of psittacosis-lymphogranuloma venereum (PL) agent. Am J Ophthalmol. 1967;63:1225–46.
13. Storz J. *Chlamydia* and *Chlamydia*-induced Diseases. Springfield, IL: Charles C Thomas; 1971.
14. Saikku P, Visakorpi R, Kleemola M, et al. *Chlamydia psittaci* TWAR-strains as a frequent cause of military pneumonia epidemics in Finland. In: Oriel D, Ridgway G, Schachter J, et al., eds. Chlamydial Infections. Cambridge: Cambridge University Press; 1986:333–6.
15. Schachter J. Human *Chlamydia psittaci* infection. In: Oriel D, Ridgway G, Schachter J, et al., eds. Chlamydial Infections. Cambridge: Cambridge University Press; 1986:311–20.

16. Grayston JT, Wang SP. New knowledge of chlamydiae and the diseases they cause. J Infect Dis. 1975;132:87–105.

158. CHLAMYDIA TRACHOMATIS (TRACHOMA, PERINATAL INFECTIONS, LYMPHOGRANULOMA VENEREUM, AND OTHER GENITAL INFECTIONS)

WILLIAM R. BOWIE
KING K. HOLMES

Chlamydia trachomatis has been called the LGV-TRIC (Lympho-Granuloma Venereum-TRachoma-Inclusion Conjunctivitis) agent; however, with advances in laboratory diagnosis and in association with the increasing incidence of sexually transmitted diseases (STDs), *C. trachomatis* has also been recognized as a major cause of nongonococcal urethritis (NGU) and epididymitis in men, cervicitis and acute pelvic inflammatory disease in women, and inclusion conjunctivitis and a distinctive form of interstitial pneumonia in infants. Except for the mouse pneumonitis agent, humans are the only known natural host for *C. trachomatis*. In the United States, there are estimated to be 3–4 million new cases of chlamydial infection annually,[1] and it has been estimated that the direct and indirect costs are $1.4 billion annually.[2]

Trachoma has been recognized since antiquity, and intracytoplasmic inclusions characteristic of *C. trachomatis* infections were recognized in conjunctival epithelial cells in 1907. In 1910, Lindner described epithelial inclusions in the cervix of the mother of an infant with typical inclusion conjunctivitis, and he also demonstrated epithelial inclusions in the cervix of the woman partner of a man with inclusion-positive NGU. Lymphogranuloma venereum (LGV) was described in 1912. *Chlamydia trachomatis* was initially isolated in the yolk sac of embryonated eggs in 1938. Cell culture techniques were introduced by Gordon and Quan in 1965[3] for *C. trachomatis* isolation, and the microimmunofluorescent method for the detection of antibody and for immunotyping was introduced by Wang and Grayston in 1970.[4] These developments made it possible both to confirm the etiologic role of *C. trachomatis* in NGU and cervicitis by case–control studies and to explore the role of this agent in other syndromes of unknown cause.

MORPHOLOGIC CHARACTERISTICS AND DEVELOPMENTAL CYCLE

Chlamydiae have two major forms: the infective, nondividing elementary body that survives extracellularly and the noninfective reticulate body that divides intracellularly by binary fission.[5–7] The elementary body is a spherical, electron-dense coccus 300 nm in diameter with numerous ribosomes surrounded by a rigid trilaminar wall. There are patches of regular arrays of hemispheric projections on its surface.[8] It has a hemagglutinin on the surface and an equal DNA and RNA content, is relatively resistant to sonication and trypsin, and is relatively impermeable. By contrast, the reticulate body is larger (up to 1000 nm), has nonrigid walls and lacks a hemagglutinin. It has three to four times more RNA than DNA, is relatively sensitive to sonication and trypsin, and is more permeable.

After attachment, chlamydiae are endocytosed by the host cell, perhaps in response to prostaglandin-mediated changes in host cell membrane fluidity.[9] Once endocytosed,[7,10] the elementary body loses infectivity and begins to undergo morphologic and molecular changes associated with transition to the reticulate body. Continued development occurs with a cytoplasmic vacuole bounded by a host cell membrane, which continues to increase in size even though protein synthesis in the host cell is inhibited. Endocytosis and growth within the vacuole do not incite phagolysosomal fusion. The reticulate body divides by binary fission; after 8–12 hours, there are 4–16 reticulate bodies present within the vacuole. The reticulate bodies continue to divide, and the size of individual bodies diminishes. After 20 hours, in some of the particles there is central condensation of the cytoplasmic contents that is associated with the synthesis of protein–carbohydrate complexes. These particles are typical elementary bodies. At this stage, an iodine-stainable, glycogen-containing material forms within the inclusion, and the inclusion begins to displace the nucleus. After 48–60 hours, the remaining reticulate bodies have reorganized into approximately 100 or more infectious elementary bodies within the cytoplasmic vacuole, which ruptures extracellularly to release the particles. The process of release may be initiated by a chlamydiae-specified proteinase.

The developmental cycle is dependent on the ability of the host cell to generate energy and other intermediates; chlamydiae must compete for them with the host cell. Chlamydial replication might be controlled by the nutritional state of the host cell.[6] Replication is inhibited by interferon[12] and lymphokine-altered macrophages.[12] Chlamydiae have a system for trading one molecule of their own ADP for one molecule of host ATP, but they do not generate their own ATP.[6] Chlamydiae possess a DNA-dependent RNA polymerase; but for RNA synthesis, there is an obligatory need for the host cell's nucleoside triphosphates. Similarly, although chlamydiae-specified proteins are synthesized throughout the developmental cycle, there is an obligatory need for some amino acids that *C. trachomatis* is unable to synthesize. Differential amino acid requirements of different strains may correlate with the site of infection.[13]

CHEMICAL COMPOSITION

The complete circular genome of *C. trachomatis* is 600×10^6 daltons (11×10^5 nucleotide pairs).[7] The guanine-plus-cytosine content is 42.5 percent. Chlamydiae contain 23S, 16S, and 5S ribosomal RNA as 50S and 30S subunits. Several enzymes, including DNA-dependent RNA polymerase, a polynucleotide phosphorylase, two enzymes that metabolize glucose-6-phosphate, glycogen synthetase, and a transaminase have all been found. *Chlamydia trachomatis* has two rRNA operons that differ from other prokaryotes.[14] Chlamydial lipids and carbohydrates are not well characterized.[15]

ANTIGENS

There are 15 known serovars of *C. trachomatis* that are distinguishable by microimmunofluorescence.[16] Types A, B, Ba, and C are primarily isolated from patients with ocular disease in areas of endemic trachoma. Types D, E, F, G, H, I, J, and K are primarily isolated from genital infections or neonatal infections acquired from the mother's cervix during birth, but they also cause ocular infections in adults in developed countries. Most non-LGV genital infections are caused by serovars D, E, F, and G.[17] Differences have been described in the relative prevalence of serovars between the cervix and the rectum of homosexual men.[18] Types L_1, L_2, and L_3 are isolated amost exclusively from patients with LGV. The 15 immunotypes can be grouped into two subspecies serogroups: the B complex (B, Ba, D, E, L_1, and L_2) and the C complex (C, J, H, I, and A). Types G and F are related to the B complex, while K and L_3 are related to the C complex but bridge both the C and B complexes. Thus, antigens can be classified according to reactivity: genus (or "group"), species, subspecies (or serogroup), and serotype (also known as serovar).

Chlamydiae possess numerous proteins, of which most of the recognized ones are surface constituents.[19] Chlamydiae also contain a lipopolysaccharide that resembles the Re chemotype of enterobacterial lipopolysaccharide but, in addition, has a unique antigenic determinant.[20,21] The major outer membrane protein has a molecular weight of approximately 40 kD. The subunit molecular weight is the same within serovars but differs slightly between serovars.[22] Gene sequence studies indicate that this diversity is due to clustered nucleotide substitutions for closely related serovars and insertions or deletions for distantly related serovars.[23] Peptidoglycan is not present in chlamydiae; the rigidity is due to covalent disulfide linkages among outer membrane proteins.[24] Antibody to the major outer membrane neutralizes *C. trachomatis* infectivity in vitro. In addition to the 40 kD major protein, numerous other proteins elicit a serum antibody response that correlates well with past or present *C. trachomatis* infection.[25] Many groups have cloned genes coding for proteins.

Monoclonal antibodies have clarified the nature of some antigenic determinants.[26] Serovars are antigenically interrelated, which accounts for considerable cross-reactivity. The 40 kD major outer membrane protein possesses genus-, species-, subspecies-, and serovar-specific determinants.[16,25,27] Low-molecular-weight (14–15 kD) cysteine-rich outer membrane proteins have determinants that are biovar and species specific.[28] The species-, subspecies-, and serovar-specific antigens are heat-stable, pronase-sensitive, and periodate-resistant proteins.

All chlamydiae have a group-reactive (genus-specific) antigen detectable in the supernatant of lysates. The antigen is a heat-stable, lipoprotein–carbohydrate complex with an immunodominant 2-keto-3-deoxyoctanoic acid.[29] Antibody to this antigen is detectable by complement fixation and immunofluorescence. By double immunodiffusion, there are three heat-stable group antigens common to *C. trachomatis* and *C. psittaci* and four heat-labile species-specific antigens.[30] Triton X solubilized strains revealed 16 distinct antigenic components for *C. psittaci* and 19 for an LGV *C. trachomatis* strain. Only one of these antigens was cross-reactive between species. Among *C. trachomatis* strains, there was marked homogeneity of antigen patterns.[31,32]

PATHOGENESIS AND IMMUNITY

To establish and perpetuate infection chlamydiae must attach to cells, induce their uptake, avoid lysosomal fusion, change from the nonreplicating elementary body into the replicating reticulate body, replicate, return to the elementary body stage, and then leave the host cell, all the while avoiding the lethal effects of the host response.[6,7,33] There are many differences between LGV and non-LGV strains in clinical virulence in humans, and these are correlated with differences in many of the stages of infection and with differences in cell culture and in experimental animal infections. Attachment of LGV and non-LGV strains is thought to involve different cell receptors. Attachment and endocytosis of non-LGV strains, but not LGV strains, are enhanced by pretreatment of tissue cells with diethylaminoethyl (DEAE) dextran and are blocked by neuraminidase; this suggests involvement of sialic acid cell receptors.[34] Centrifugation of the inoculum enhances the infectivity of non-LGV strains significantly, but only marginally for LGV. Mild heat or pretreatment of the host cell with trypsin inhibits the uptake of LGV but not non-LGV strains. Attachment of non-LGV strains is blocked by preincubation of tissue cells with killed non-LGV strains, but not by preincubation with killed LGV strains; this suggests receptor specificity. Some of these differences between LGV and non-LGV strains may be due to differences in surface properties such as hydrophobicity and negative surface charge.[35]

In vivo, chlamydiae have a marked tendency to persist for prolonged periods of time. Persistent infection in cell cultures is well known for *C. psittaci* but has now been established with non-LGV *C. trachomatis*. This produces a cycling between periods of massive host cell destruction by chlamydia and periods of host cell proliferation.[36] Infection appears to be maintained by cell-to-cell transfer, and there is no evidence for the cryptic form postulated for *C. psittaci*. With *C. trachomatis*, levels of endogenous cyclic AMP may be important in the switch from latent to overt infection.[37]

Uptake of chlamydiae in cell culture is abolished by incubation of host cells with trypsin and other proteases, and regeneration of the protein-sensitive component is inhibited by cycloheximide. This suggested that the cell surface receptor might be a protein or glycoprotein.[37a] Wheat germ agglutinin, a lectin specific for the monosaccharide N-acetyl-D-glucosamine, inhibits chlamydial attachment; N-acetyl-D-glucosamine decreases the inhibition caused by wheat germ agglutinin.[38]

Several mechanisms may contribute to cell damage. Intravenous injection of massive doses of elementary bodies kills mice within 24 hours despite antibiotic administration to prevent growth of the organism. Passive immunization of mice with antiserum to elementary body envelope or active immunization with formalinized organisms provides type-specific protection. Intravenous injection of heated elementary bodies or of unheated reticulate bodies are nontoxic for mice. When macrophages or established cell lines ingest viable or ultraviolet-inactivated elementary bodies at a high multiplicity of infection, immediate cytotoxicity is also demonstrable.[39,40] This toxic activity is also heat labile and is blocked by type-specific antibody. At a lower multiplicity of infection, cell death requires the growth of chlamydiae and may be partly related to competition for host cellular metabolism. Moulder and colleagues[39] have speculated that a single, still unidentified factor is responsible for mouse toxicity, for the cytotoxicity of phagocytosing cells in vitro, and for the inhibition of phagolysosomal fusion.

In macrophages that have ingested *C. trachomatis*, extralysosomal acid phosphatase increases and is released as the macrophages die.[41] This type of release of lysosomal enzymes may contribute to the inflammatory response in chlamydial infection. Human polymorphonuclear leukocytes, however, rapidly inactivate *C. trachomatis*.[42] Oxygen-dependent antimicrobial systems, including the myeloperoxidase systems, are not essential for the inactivation.[42] Lyzozyme has a significant inhibitory effect on *C. trachomatis*.[43] LGV serovars are more resistant than are other serovars to the antimicrobial activities of human mononuclear phagocytes.[44]

The immune response probably contributes to the pathogenesis of inflammation and scarring in *C. trachomatis* infection. The influence of the immune response has been studied by experimental active vaccination of animals and humans, by analysis of the course of repeated experimental infections, by passive transfer of antibody or mononuclear cells in animals, by analysis of the effects of immunosuppressive agents on experimental infection, and by histopathologic studies of human infections. In a salpingitis model in pig-tailed macaques, repeated but not initial infection caused extensive scarring and obstruction.[45] When using egg-grown killed vaccines, alterations in dose, immunotype, route of administration, and timing of administration can either reduce the risk of subsequent infection or result in more acute, more severe, and more prolonged infections in vaccinated people. In general, the use of a single vaccine dose, a small dose, or a vaccine immunotype heterologous to the subsequent infecting strain has been associated with more severe infection at a later date.[46] The immune response to natural or experimental active infection may influence subsequent infectious challenges in ways that differ from the influence of killed vaccine. In cynomolgus monkeys, repeated inoculation of the conjunctivae produced reinfection of reduced duration, but it eventually caused chronic follicular disease typical of trachoma.[47] In this model, a soluble triton extract rapidly reproduced inflammation, which suggests that a labile product released by living organisms may be particularly important in producing inflammation.[48] Passive transfer of serum antibody to *C. trachomatis* did not protect these monkeys from experimental conjunctival infection with homologous *C. trachomatis*.[49] However, passive transfer of serum or of spleen cells from immunized mice has resulted in attenuated courses of subsequent experimental infection in various murine models of *C. trachomatis* infections. The appearance of local antibody has been temporally associated with a disappearance of cultivable *C. trachomatis* in certain experimental infections, and the development of secretory IgA antibody in cervical secretions correlated with a striking decrease in the recovery of *C. trachomatis* from the cervix in women.[50]

Further studies are required to evaluate the possible protective or deleterious effects of antibodies to selected chlamydial antigens in humans. Antibody to the 57 kD antigen was associated with tubal damage and infertility in one study,[51] whereas the absence of antibody to the same antigen was associated with increased susceptibility to postabortal chlamydial salpingitis in another.[52]

The influence of immunosuppressive agents also suggests that cell-mediated immunity has an important protective role in animal models. In the *C. trachomatis* mouse pneumonia model, cortisone treatment inhibited the migration of peritoneal exudate cells, but not serum antibody production.[53] The cortisone treatment resulted in prolonged infection and reactivation of *C. trachomatis* infection. A similar prolongation of infection was noted with cyclophosphamide.

However, serum antibody is clearly compatible with active mucosal infection in humans, including the development of complications such as salpingitis. Women with chronic, asymptomatic cervical infection with *C. trachomatis* often have local cervical antibody demonstrable by indirect immunofluorescence. Peripheral blood lymphocytes from men and women with acute or chronic genital *C. trachomatis* infection usually undergo blastogenesis when exposed to *C. trachomatis* antigens in vitro.[54,55] Thus the presence of serum and local antibody (as detected by indirect immunofluorescence) and of sensitized blood lymphocytes is consistent with both the persistence of mucosal infection and the development of complications in humans. Thus far, the cellular immune response to *C. trachomatis* infection in humans has been characterized extensively by analysis of the peripheral blood lymphocyte transformation response and by characterization of mononuclear cellular infiltrates in experimental chlamydial infections. During pregnancy, the response in infected women was significantly depressed,[55] and it is speculated that this might lead to the reactivation of chlamydial infection in pregnancy. Among men with Reiter syndrome, blood lymphocyte transformation during exposure to *C. trachomatis* in vitro was significantly greater in those with "venereal" Reiter syndrome than in postdiarrheal Reiter syndrome, non-Reiter arthritis, and men with NGU without Reiter syndrome.[56] Another group had similar results with synovial lymphocytes.[57]

Despite abundant evidence that the immune response does not provide complete protection against infection with *C. trachomatis*, prior infection may reduce the risk of subsequent infection. Men and women with a history of an STD are less likely to have *C. trachomatis* isolated with a subsequent episode of urethritis or contact to urethritis.[58] Among women infected with *C. trachomatis*, the proportion with symptoms and the proportion developing pelvic inflammatory disease decrease with increasing age.

The histopathology of cervical and ocular infection with non-LGV strains of *C. trachomatis* shows inclusions in mucosal epithelial cells, patchy inflammation consisting mainly of mononuclear cells in chronic infections, shallow mucosal erosions with epithelial cellular metaplasia, and submucosal germinal centers. Colposcopy of the cervix or microscopic examination of the conjunctivae in chronic infections show edema, vascular dilatation, metaplasia, and eventually cicatrization. The exudate consists of a mixture of polymorphonuclear leukocytes, plasma cells, transformed lymphocytes, and histiocytes. The histopathology of LGV shows prominent granuloma formation, thus indicating the greater importance of cellular immunity in the immune response to LGV strains of *C. trachomatis*.

LABORATORY DIAGNOSIS

In all but classic trachoma, the diagnosis of *C. trachomatis* infection requires laboratory evaluation. The important procedures are direct examination for typical intracytoplasmic inclusions or *C. trachomatis* antigen, isolation of the organism, and detection of humoral or local antibody. The development of two new methods for the detection of chlamydial antigens in exudate represents the most important development in the laboratory diagnosis of chlamydial infection during the past decade.

Direct Examination of Cell Scrapings and Exudate

At present, the only feasible method for the laboratory diagnosis of *C. trachomatis* infection in many areas of the world is direct microscopic examination of Giemsa-stained cell scrapings. Giemsa stain shows inclusions in a high proportion of patients with papillary or follicular trachoma,[59] but is less sensitive in patients with less active ocular disease. As shown in Table 1, Giemsa stain is useful for the diagnosis of neonatal inclusion conjunctivitis, but is quite insensitive for the diagnosis of other infections.[60] Iodine staining for glycogen-containing inclusions is less sensitive than Giemsa stain is and is unreliable because glycogen is only present in a portion of the development cycle and because squamous cells normally contain glycogen. Giemsa stain is of little value in demonstrating inclusions in pus aspirated from patients with LGV.

Antigen Detection Systems Not Requiring Culture

The use of species-specific fluorescein-conjugated monoclonal antibodies to detect chlamydiae in direct smears has been a major advance in the diagnosis of chlamydial infections[1] that has made the laboratory diagnosis of chlamydial infection much more widely available than in the past. These antibodies show that cell-free elementary bodies are found much more often than are intracellular inclusion bodies in urethral, cervical, conjunctival, and nasopharyngeal specimens[61] (Fig. 1). Early experience with the detection of antigen in biopsy specimens is also promising. With training, a high degree of specificity can be achieved in identifying elementary bodies despite their small size. Immunofluorescence microscopy is required.

Enzyme-linked immunosorbent (immunoenzyme) assay (ELISA) techniques, with reading of specimens by spectrophotometry, also allow identification of *C. trachomatis* more quickly than culture does.[1] Many laboratories prefer this diagnostic system because it allows processing of large numbers of specimens by less intensively trained personnel. Although published results are very confusing, the general consensus is that this technique is both less sensitive and less specific than are cultures or fluorescence microscopy using monoclonal antibodies. Although more evaluation is required, its use is not currently recommended for specimens from sites other than the cervix and urethra.

TABLE 1. Usefulness of Laboratory Tests for the Diagnosis of *C. trachomatis* Infection

	Direct Stain		*Serum Antibody*				
	Giemsa	*Fluorescein-Conjugated Monoclonal Antibody*	*CF*	*Micro-IF*	*Local Antibody*	*Cell Culture*	*Enzyme Immunoassay*
Ocular infection							
Neonate	+	++	−	±	+	++	?
Adult	±	++	−	±	+	++	?
Trachoma	+[a]	++[a]	−	±	+	++[a]	?
Urethritis	±	++	−	±	?	++	++
Epididymitis	−	?	−	±	?	++	−
Proctitis (non-LGV)	−	?	−	±	?	++	−
Cervicitis	±	++	−	±	?	++	++
Salpingitis	−	++	−	+	−	++	++
Infant pneumonia	−	+	−	++	−	++	−
LGV	−	?	+	++	−	+	−

[a] Sensitive for active trachoma, but less sensitive for late trachoma.

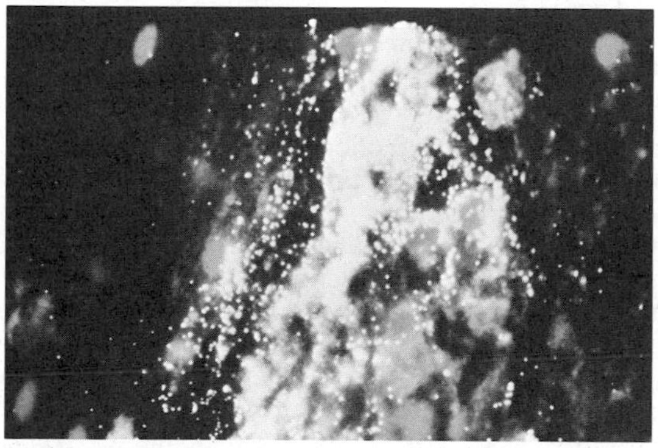

FIG. 1. Elementary bodies of *Chlamydia trachomatis* in cervical exudate as demonstrated by staining with fluorescein-conjugated, species-specific monoclonal antibody. (Fluorescence microscopy, ×1000)

Immunoenzyme assays can also be used to identify inclusions in specimens by microscopy. These are effective in cell cultures[62] but have not been adequate for the direct detection of elementary bodies on slides.

DNA hybridization is also being evaluated, usually by using a probe directed at the cryptic plasmid found in all isolates of *C. trachomatis*.[63]

Isolation in Cell Culture

Chlamydiae grow in the yolk sac of embryonated eggs, but tissue cell cultures are more convenient. Isolation in cell culture remains the gold standard for the diagnosis of chlamydial infection. LGV strains grow well in many cell lines, but non-LGV strains are more fastidious. The most common cell lines used are McCoy cells, a mouse heteroploid line, and HeLa 229 cells. With McCoy cells, pretreatment of the cells with irradiation, 5-iodo-2-deoxyuridine, or cytochalasin B or the addition of cycloheximide to the culture to inhibit tissue cell replication allows *C. trachomatis* to compete for cell nutrients and permits easier recognition of inclusions.[64] With both cell lines, pretreatment of the cells with DEAE dextran (a positively charged molecule that may neutralize electrostatic repulsion between the tissue cells and elementary bodies) and centrifugation of the inoculum onto the cell monolayer improve recovery of non-LGV strains but not of LGV ones. Between 40 and 70 hours after inoculation, depending on the cell line and immunotype, intracytoplasmic inclusions can be detected by Giemsa, Macchiavelli, or Gimenez stains or by immunofluorescence in either cell line, and iodine stain can be used to detect inclusions in McCoy cells. Inexperienced laboratories may have false-positive results, especially with iodine stains. Typical inclusions that can be serially passed are considered to be chlamydiae. Lymphogranuloma venereum strains spread in the monolayer, but non-LGV strains produce only a single inclusion for each viable elementary body that is endocytosed.

Cultures performed in vials are more sensitive than are cultures in microtiter trays for the detection of a small number of infectious particles; however, microtiter cultures are cheaper and better suited for clinical laboratories that perform a large number of cultures. Immunofluorescent staining with monoclonal antibodies is the most sensitive method for the detection of inclusions in primary cultures. The use of this method reduces the need for the traditional blind passage of cells that do not show inclusions after primary inoculation with the clinical specimen.

The rates of isolation are higher from adult or neonatal conjunctivitis or active trachoma than from mild or chronic ocular disease.[65] Isolation is the most sensitive procedure for genital infection. Approximately 10–15 percent of the men with NGU who have negative cultures for *C. trachomatis* may develop seroconversion or serum IgM antibody to *C. trachomatis*, which is indicative of recent *C. trachomatis* infection.[66] False-negative cultures arise from sampling the urethral meatus rather than the endourethra, the use of toxic swabs, inappropriate transport media, a delay in transit, or contamination. Contamination of cell cultures is an occasional problem with rectal and cervical cultures. In infants with pneumonia or asymptomatic upper respiratory tract infection, the rates of isolation are higher from the nasopharynx than from the conjunctiva.[67,68] In LGV, *C. trachomatis* is isolated from approximately 30 percent of bubo pus and occasionally from the cervix, male urethra, or systemic sites. *Chlamydia trachomatis* has been isolated from the urethra, semen, expressed prostatic secretions, and/or epididymal aspirates from men with acute epididymitis and also from the endocervix, fallopian tube biopsy specimens, or lumenal swabs from women with salpingitis, but rarely from culdocentesis fluid.

SEROLOGIC DIAGNOSIS

The usefulness of serologic tests depends on the site of infection, duration of disease, infecting serovars of *C. trachomatis*, and previous exposure to chlamydial antigens. The major tests used are the complement fixation (CF) and the microimmunofluorescent (micro-IF) tests.[69] The CF test uses a group-reactive antigen, and its only present value probably is in the diagnosis of psittacosis and LGV. There are no known cross-reactions with other organisms; however, because the antigen is group reactive and because *C. trachomatis* is ubiquitous, there is a significant background level of CF seropositivity in patients without active psittacosis or LGV. In addition, because LGV has a long latent period and clinical diagnosis is often delayed, antibody is usually present by the time acute serum is obtained, and fourfold rises in antibody titer often cannot be documented. Consequently, even though CF titers above 1:8 or 1:16 represent antibody to chlamydiae, a single or stable titer of at least 1:64 or greater is recommended for the diagnosis of LGV or psittacosis. These titers have been detected in 80 percent of patients with LGV, in 77 percent of patients with psittacosis, in 9 percent of adults with inclusion conjunctivitis, in 18 percent of women with uncomplicated *C. trachomatis* cervical infection, and in 0 of 60 men with *C. trachomatis* urethritis.[69] Thus a high titer supports the diagnosis of psittacosis or LGV, particularly in men. As a corollary, however, the CF test is of little value in diagnosing urethral infection.

The micro-IF test is more sensitive than is the CF test, is serovar specific, can be used to measure IgG and IgM antibody, and will detect serum, tear, and other local antibody. Unfortunately, there is a higher prevalence of seropositivity in culture-negative individuals than for the CF test. Titers of 1:8 or greater are considered positive but are detected in up to 10 percent of pediatric patients, in 20–25 percent of men and 50–70 percent of women attending STD clinics, and in over 80 percent of trachoma-endemic populations.[16] Consequently, serologic diagnosis of recent *C. trachomatis* infection by means of the micro-IF test requires a demonstration of seroconversion or a fourfold rise in titer to a specific serovar. The detection of IgM antibody by micro-IF also indicates recent infection and is particularly helpful in infants where detection of high levels of IgM antibody by micro-IF ($\geq$1:32) in a single serum may be the method of choice for the diagnosis of pneumonia in infants.[70] Reinfection with a homologous serovar results only in an anamnestic rise in IgG antibody without stimulating IgM antibody, whereas reinfection with a new serovar (e.g., F) in a person previously infected with a heterologous serovar (e.g., D) results in an IgM antibody response to the new serovar (F) as well as an anamnestic IgG antibody rise to the previous type (D). Since most ocular and genital infections in developed countries are caused by either the closely related types D/E or the closely related types F/G, reinfections with homologous serovars commonly occur with negative IgM micro-IF test results.

In LGV patients, micro-IF titers are usually very high (e.g., $\geq$1:512); such titers are very rare in men with genital infections with non-LGV strains. The exception is proctitis, where CF titers >1:16 and micro-IF titers >1:1000 may occur with non-LGV strains.[71] Women occasionally develop titers >1:512 with non-LGV *C. trachomatis* infection, especially with salpingitis and perihepatitis. In LGV, titers are often highest against serovars L_{1-3}, which is diagnostic of LGV. However, since L_{1-3} are "junior" *C. trachomatis* antigens, sera from LGV patients often react broadly with other serovars; this precludes the diagnosis of LGV solely on the basis of serovar specificity in many cases.

The detection of tear antibody by micro-IF is considered by some authors to be diagnostic of ocular infection, although this is debated. The titer correlates with disease activity.[72] Detection of tear antibody is more sensitive than culture is. Testing for local antibody at other sites requires further evaluation.

ELISA using whole elementary bodies as the antigen can also be used to detect antibody to *C. trachomatis*.[73] It is probably at least as sensitive as micro-IF, but its real value is uncertain. It may be difficult to establish a diagnosis on the basis of changes in amount of antibody in individual patients, although ELISA may be of considerable use for epidemiologic studies. Other antigens in the ELISA system or other systems also may prove useful in the future, but so far no serologic test other than the IgM micro-IF antibody test has been shown to correlate with recent or active infection.

Intradermal inoculation of LGV-infected yolk sac (the Frei test) has been used in the past to detect a delayed-type hypersensitivity reaction. However, the antigen is group reactive and, thus, is also positive with psittacosis and occasionally with oculogenital *C. trachomatis* infection. Conversely, a negative Frei test result does not exclude the diagnosis of LGV. The CF and micro-IF tests are more sensitive than the Frei test is, and the Frei test is no longer used.[74]

CLINICAL MANIFESTATIONS

Chlamydia trachomatis infections can be divided epidemiologically into three categories: (*1*) classic trachoma occurring in trachoma-endemic countries where the reservoir is chronic ocular infection and transmission typically occurs among children via fingers, fomites, and probably flies[75]; (*2*) sexually transmitted genital infection of adults including LGV, which has become rare in developed countries, and the non-LGV infections, which constitute most recognized *C. trachomatis* infections in adults in developed countries; and (*3*) perinatal infant eye and respiratory infections, which are acquired during birth from the mother's infected cervix. The resulting clinical syndromes and serovars associated with each syndrome are summarized in Chapter 157, Table 1.

Chlamydia Trachomatis Ocular Infections

Ocular *C. trachomatis* infections can be divided into separate categories: infant inclusion conjunctivitis, adult inclusion conjunctivitis with or without subepithelial keratitis, and trachoma.[75] While some ophthalmologists reserve the term *trachoma* for characteristic infections that occur in trachoma-endemic regions, others have observed a continuum in the clinical spectrum up to and including trachoma in nonendemic areas. Furthermore, progression from inclusion conjunctivitis to classic trachoma has been observed in persons followed prospectively with persistent or recurrent ocular *C. trachomatis* infection.[72,76]

Trachoma

Classic trachoma is characterized by chronic follicular keratoconjunctivitis that is followed by conjunctival scarring and pannus formation (invasion of vessels into the cornea). Trachoma has in the past been the greatest single cause of blindness in the world. It was estimated in 1973 that 400 million people had trachoma, with blindness occurring in 2 million.[77] Since World War II, the endemic regions have been significantly reduced, but trachoma remains of tremendous importance in the Middle East, North Africa, and in northern India in areas with inadequate public sanitation and poor personal hygiene. In endemic areas, acute conjunctivitis of adults or infants is seldom recognized, although most children become chronically infected within a few years of birth. Where present, however, active disease in adults over 20 years of age is three times as frequent in women as in men, presumably because of closer contact with children.

Trachoma usually begins abruptly with inflamed palpebral and bulbar conjunctivae. A mixed inflammatory cell exudate appears; within a few weeks, lymphocytes and macrophages coalesce to form soft or necrotic follicles beneath the conjunctival surface. In the absence of reinfection, the disease at this stage may spontaneously heal completely. With repeated infection, however, vascularization of the cornea begins—usually at the upper limbus—and progresses. Simultaneous scarring of the conjunctiva also occurs, which in the late stages results in trichiasis and entropion. Bacterial infection, specially when repetitive, contributes to scarring. The combination of pannus, scarring of the conjunctiva, trichiasis, and bacterial infection can result in blindness.

Inclusion Conjunctivitis

In developed countries where trachoma is not endemic but sexually transmitted genital *C. trachomatis* infection is epidemic,

C. trachomatis eye infections have been documented in approximately one-third of infants given ophthalmic silver nitrate prophylaxis and whose mothers had cervical chlamydial infection at term. Thus, where the prevalence of prenatal chlamydial infections is high, neonatal chlamydial conjunctivitis has been seen in 2–6 percent of newborn infants.[68,76] In North America and Europe, neonatal chlamydial conjunctivitis is many times more common than gonococcal ophthalmia neonatorum is. However, most infants with conjunctivitis have neither organism. Inclusion conjunctivitis appears 2–25 days after birth (earlier when membranes rupture long before delivery); it is manifested by acute, copious mucopurulent discharge and inflamed and edematous conjunctiva. Conjunctival follicles may appear with chronic or relapsing infection. Without therapy, these manifestations usually resolve spontaneously over several months without sequelae, although Mordhorst[76] reported the development of mild trachoma in 50 percent of infected infants.

Inclusion conjunctivitis in adults is usually manifested relatively acutely with a foreign body sensation, photophobia, mucopurulent discharge, and follicular conjunctivitis—often with keratitis. In the absence of reinfection, the lesions tend to heal over a period of several months to 2 years. Among adults presenting to STD clinics with chlamydial infections, chlamydial conjunctivitis is very infrequent; but among those with chlamydial conjunctivitis presenting to ophthalmologists, genital chlamydial infection in the patient or the sexual partner(s) is frequent.[78]

Diagnosis of Eye Infections

In infants, the principal, differential diagnostic concern is gonococcal conjunctivitis, which usually has an incubation period of only 1–5 days and can be confirmed by smears and cultures for *Neisseria gonorrhoeae*. In the older child or adult, the differential diagnosis includes many other infective and noninfective causes of conjunctivitis and keratoconjunctivitis. The specific diagnosis of *C. trachomatis* infection in acute disease can be made by direct immunofluorescence, Giemsa stain, detection of tear antibody by micro-IF, and culture. In chronic disease, tear antibody detection may be the most sensitive diagnostic test.

Treatment of Eye Infection

Without therapy, the initial episode of infection usually will not result in significant residual damage. Topical therapy often will suppress signs of infection but will not necessarily eradicate the organism. This is of particular concern in infants, who may be at risk for developing pneumonia caused by *C. trachomatis*. Erythromycin (e.g., erythromycin, 12.5 mg/kg four times daily for 14 days) can be used in neonates, although experience is limited.[79] Systemic therapy with a tetracycline (e.g., doxycycline, 100 mg twice daily, or tetracycline, 500 mg four times daily) for 3 weeks is preferred in adults. In chronic trachoma, therapy has been more difficult. The most effective regimen in these patients has been doxycycline (2.5–4 mg/kg once daily) over a 40-day period.[80] In holoendemic areas, improved health standards probably have a much greater effect than antimicrobial therapy does.[77,81] Surgical intervention to correct lid deformities will help considerably in the prevention of blindness.

LYMPHOGRANULOMA VENEREUM

Lymphogranuloma venereum is the only chlamydial infection that produces multisystem involvement and constitutional manifestations. Lymphogranuloma venereum has a primary phase with a transient lesion, a secondary stage with suppurative regional lymphadenopathy and prominent constitutional symptoms, and a late phase with sequelae related to fibrotic changes and abnormal lymphatic drainage. Lymphogranuloma venereum is endemic in Asia, Africa, and South America, but as many as 500 cases per year have been reported in the United States since 1965. In many of these cases, the diagnosis is based on low-titer CF seropositivity and cannot be confirmed by micro-IF testing. In the United States, LGV has been reported three times as frequently in men as in women, with the highest occurrence in persons of low socioeconomic status living in the Southeast, in homosexual men, and in persons returning from endemic regions outside the United States. Transmission by fomites and by laboratory accidents caused by aerosolization of LGV strains without biosafety precautions has resulted in pneumonitis, pleural effusions, and/or mediastinal or hilar lymphadenopathy. However, LGV is primarily sexually transmitted. The reservoirs have not been ascertained but probably are persons with asymptomatic or ignored symptomatic urethral, cervical, or anorectal infection.

Within 3 days to 3 weeks after exposure, a small painless herpetiform vesicle or a nonindurated papule or ulcer may develop. These are noted on the penis of one-third or fewer of men with inguinal LGV and even less frequently on the labia, fourchette, or posterior vagina of women. Because the lesion heals quickly, does not scar, and antedates the lymphadenopathy, LGV is not usually diagnosed at this stage. In homosexual men and occasionally in women, a primary anorectal—rather than a primary genital—infection may occur. With anorectal infection, the initial manifestations may be an anal ulcer or diarrhea, tenesmus, and a bloody or mucopurulent anal discharge associated with diffuse or discrete ulcerations in the rectosigmoid colon. Fever and other constitutional symptoms are common, and inguinal or perirectal lymphadenopathy occur. Rectal biopsy shows diffuse inflammation, mucosal ulceration, crypt abscesses, and granuloma formation.

A study conducted in Swaziland and South Africa described a different presentation of LGV.[82] *Chlamydia trachomatis* (presumed but not proved to be LGV) was isolated from genital ulcers of 10 men and 2 women. Most had micro-IF antibody to *C. trachomatis*. Inguinal lymphadenopathy was present in only 50 percent, usually was unilateral, and was fluctuant in only one study subject. The lesions were unlike the typically described transient lesion. They were deep and 4–6 mm in diameter, had elevated edges, and had a purulent or indurated base. The mean duration of illness was 72 days, with a median of 45 days.

Within 2–6 weeks after the initial exposure to LGV, regional lymphadenopathy develops. The location varies with the initial site of involvement: (*1*) inguinal and femoral nodes with penile, vulvar, and occasionally anal infection; (*2*) hypogastric and deep iliac nodes with rectal infection; and (*3*) obturator and iliac nodes with upper vaginal or cervical infection. The most characteristic manifestation is the inguinal syndrome, with unilateral or bilateral (one-third of cases) painful inguinal lymphadenopathy frequently associated with palpable iliac and femoral nodes on the ipsilateral side. The nodes are initially discrete, but because of extensive periadenitis, the nodes become matted, and the overlying skin becomes fixed and inflamed (Fig. 2). Histologically, the nodes initially show characteristic, small stellate abscesses surrounded by histiocytes. The abscesses eventually coalesce, thus becoming necrotic and fluctuant. The overlying skin becomes thin, and the nodes eventually suppurate with multiple draining fistulas. The fistulas heal over a period of several months, but scars and masses persist. Complications of anorectal infection at this stage include fistula in ano; perirectal abscesses; and rectovaginal, rectovesical, and ischiorectal fistulas.

Systemic symptoms usually are present in the second stage. Fever, chills, anorexia, headache, meningismus, myalgias, and arthralgias are common. Less common are aseptic meningitis, meningoencephalitis, conjunctivitis, hepatitis, erythema nodosum, and arthritis with a sterile effusion. Leukocytosis, an elevated erythrocyte sedimentation rate, and abnormal liver

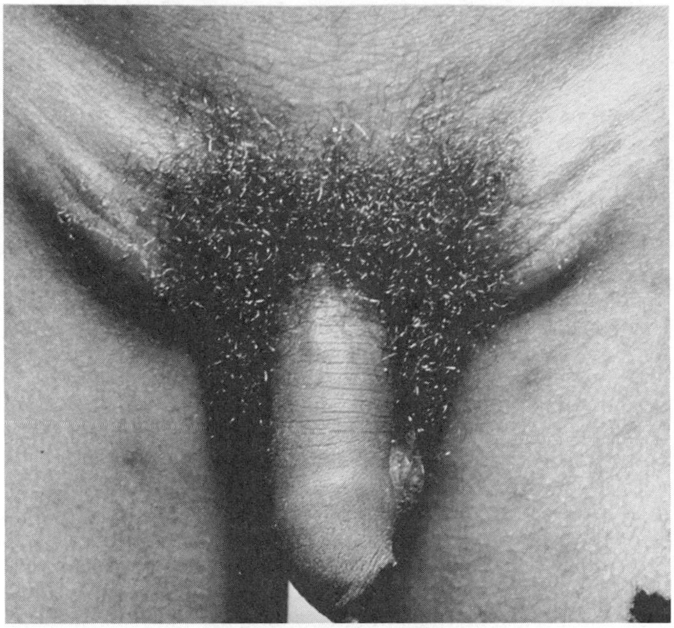

FIG. 2. Inguinal adenopathy above and below Poupart's ligament in a patient with lymphogranuloma venereum (LGV). This is the "sign of the groove" that is strongly suggestive but not diagnostic of LGV.

function test findings are common. Hyperglobulinemia, increased IgA, IgG, and IgM, rheumatoid factor, and mixed cryoglobulins have been reported. In addition, positive serologic tests for syphilis have been reported, but in these patients, the diagnosis of syphilis should be strongly considered.

Disease may progress, or complications may develop into a third stage. Approximately 5 percent of the men with genital LGV have chronic and progressive ulcerative or infiltrative involvement of the penis, urethra, or scrotum with fistulas, ulcers, and urethral strictures that especially involve the posterior urethra. Late complications are also related to fibrosis and abnormal lymphatic drainage. Rectal strictures may develop 2–6 cm from the anorectal junction. Polypoid swelling of the skin and keloid formation in the genitalia in association with induration and lymphedema may clinically resemble granuloma inguinalc or genital tuberculosis. Uncommonly, the induration and lymphedema may produce genital elephantiasis, with enlargement of the penis or vulva. Chronic ulcerations of the vulva (esthiomene) and smooth pedunculated perianal growths (lymphorrhoids) may also occur.

Diagnosis of LGV

The differential diagnosis of primary or secondary genital LGV usually includes syphilis, genital herpes, and chancroid. Syphilis is differentiated by the induration of the chancre, the absence of tenderness of the inguinal lymphadenopathy, the presence of a secondary rash, a positive darkfield examination, and a positive serologic test for syphilis. Herpes simplex virus infection is differentiated by the painful tender vesicles or ulcers, nonsuppurative nature of the regional lymphadenopathy, history of previous episodes, and demonstration of herpes simplex virus by cytology or culture. In chancroid, the ulcer is more prominent, systemic symptoms are usually absent, and *Haemophilus ducreyi* can be isolated from the ulcer and/or inguinal nodes.

The differential diagnosis of anorectal LGV in homosexual men includes (*1*) the infectious causes of anal ulceration (especially syphilis, herpes, and chancroid); (*2*) the infective causes of proctitis (gonorrhea, herpes, syphilis, and non-LGV strains of *C. trachomatis*); (*3*) the infectious causes of protocolitis (*Campylobacter* species, *Shigella* species, *Entamoeba histolytica,* and *Clostridium difficile*); and (*4*) the noninfective causes of proctitis or proctocolitis (especially Crohn's disease and idiopathic ulcerative colitis). Because anorectal LGV often causes inguinal adenopathy, fever, and other constitutional symptoms, it can closely resemble anorectal herpes clinically. Because rectal LGV produces a granulomatous proctocolitis, it can closely resemble Crohn's disease histopathologically.

The definitive diagnosis of LGV is best established by the isolation of an LGV serovar from a bubo, from an ulcer, or from the rectum, cervix, or urethra. Unfortunately, bubo aspirates are culture-positive in only about 30 percent of the suspected cases. A CF test with a fourfold increase in titer or a single titer of 1:64 or over is very suggestive. High micro-IF antibody titer (e.g., ≥1:512) to one of the LGV immunotypes is both more sensitive and more specific than the CF test is.

Treatment of LGV

Fluctuant buboes should be aspirated through normal skin with an 18 gauge or larger needle as often as required to prevent rupture. If a genital lesion is present, three darkfield microscopic examinations should be obtained before initiating therapy unless an antimicrobial that does not suppress *Treponema pallidum* is used (for example, a sulfonamide). Sulfonamides, tetracyclines, erythromycin, and rifampin are very active in vitro against *C. trachomatis*.[79] The recommended antimicrobial regimen for LGV is tetracycline, 500 mg four times daily for at least 14 days.[83] Alternative regimens are at least 14 days of doxycycline (100 mg orally twice daily), erythromycin (500 mg four times daily), or sulfamethoxazole (1 g twice daily or another sulfonamide in equivalent dosage). These regimens often have a rapid effect on constitutional symptoms but have only a limited effect on the duration of healing of buboes.[84] Late complications do not respond to antimicrobials alone, and surgical procedures often are required to improve strictures, fistulas, and elephantiasis.

OTHER GENITAL INFECTIONS

The clinical spectrum of sexually transmitted or perinatal *C. trachomatis* infections is remarkably similar to the spectrum of gonococcal infections (Table 2). These *C. trachomatis* infections include urethritis and epididymitis in men and cervicitis and acute pelvic inflammatory disease in women. Because the incidence of NGU has continued to rise dramatically over the last quarter century[85] and because *C. trachomatis* has been consistently isolated from 30–50 percent of the men with NGU, the incidence of sexually transmitted *C. trachomatis* genital infections has undoubtably also been rising during this period.

TABLE 2. Similarity of Usual Clinical Manifestations of Infections Caused by *Neisseria gonorrhoeae* and *Chlamydia trachomatis*

Site of Infection	N. gonorrhoeae	C. trachomatis
Male		
Urethra	Urethritis	Urethritis
Epididymis	Epididymitis	Epididymitis
Rectum	Proctitis	Proctitis
Systemic	Disseminated gonococcal infection	(?) Reiter syndrome
Female		
Uterus	Cervicitis, endometritis, salpingitis	Cervicitis, endometritis, salpingitis
Urethra	Urethritis	Urethral syndrome
Rectum	Proctitis	Proctitis
Infant		
Eye	Conjunctivitis	Conjunctivitis
Other	Disseminated gonococcal infection	Pneumonia

Despite anticipated changes in sexual behavior during the acquired immunodeficiency syndrome (AIDS) era, the reported number of cases of NGU in men in England and Wales (where surveillance in STD clinics is good) has continued to increase through 1986, even though reported gonorrhea in men has declined steadily for more than a decade.[85]

Chlamydia trachomatis may be less contagious than gonococcal infections are. In one study, when index patients had both *C. trachomatis* and *N. gonorrhoeae, C. trachomatis* was isolated from 45 percent of female and 28 percent of male partners while *N. gonorrhoeae* was isolated from 64 percent and 77 percent, respectively.[86] However this difference in rates of isolation of *C. trachomatis* and *N. gonorrhoeae* from patients could be explained by a greater sensitivity of cultures for *N. gonorrhoeae* rather than by greater transmissibility of *N. gonorrhoeae*.

Chlamydia trachomatis was isolated more often from partners of index patients with both *C. trachomatis* and *N. gonorrhoeae* than from partners of index patients with *C. trachomatis* alone. This study also showed that 38 percent of women whose partners only had gonococcal infection had double infection with *C. trachomatis* and *N. gonorrhoeae*. Perhaps, in some cases *C. trachomatis* is activated by some other stimulus such as gonococcal infection.[87] Alternatively, risk factors that lead to infection with one STD pathogen may lead to infection with other pathogens as well, or inflammation of the urethra or cervix might increase shedding of *C. trachomatis* from these sites.

Urethritis

Etiology of Nongonococcal and Postgonococcal Urethritis. *Chlamydia trachomatis* has been isolated from 0–11 percent of asymptomatic sexually active men.[66,88,89] Among men with urethral gonorrhea, concurrent urethral infection with *C. trachomatis* has been found in approximately 20 percent of heterosexual men and approximately 5 percent of homosexual men.[88,90] If the gonorrhea is treated with a single dose of penicillin, ampicillin, ceftriaxone, or aminocyclitol—which does not eradicate *C. trachomatis*—most of these men will develop postgonococcal urethritis.[88,90,91] *Chlamydia trachomatis* is isolated from 30–50 percent of men with NGU.[66,88,91] Since NGU is twice as frequent as gonorrhea in STD clinics and is probably three to four times more frequent in private practice, *C. trachomatis* urethritis is more frequent than gonococcal urethritis is. Furthermore, the prevalence of urethral infection with *C. trachomatis* is much greater than with *N. gonorrhoeae* among men without urethritis,[89] which suggests that a higher proportion of chlamydial infections are asymptomatic.

The causal role of *C. trachomatis* in urethritis has been further established by serology, therapeutic trials, and experimental inoculation.[91] Seroconversion, a fourfold titer rise, or the presence of IgM micro-IF humoral antibody was seen in 17 of 20 NGU patients from whom *C. trachomatis* was isolated but in only 3 of 39 patients from whom *C. trachomatis* was not isolated.[66] *Chlamydia trachomatis*-positive NGU responds significantly better than does *C. trachomatis*-negative NGU to tetracyclines and sulfonamides, but it does not respond to aminocyclitols, to which *C. trachomatis* organisms are resistant.[63,93,94] Intraurethral inoculation of *C. trachomatis* into primates produces urethral inflammation.[95]

Clinical Manifestations and Diagnosis of Nongonococcal Urethritis. Nongonococcal urethritis generally causes less dysuria and less profuse, less purulent urethral exudate than gonorrhea does; however, in an individual patient, NGU cannot be differentiated clinically from gonorrhea. Symptoms include urethral discharge, itching, or dysuria. Signs include meatal erythema and tenderness and a urethral discharge, which often is demonstrable only in the morning after stripping the urethra. Commonly in an apprehensive patient with symptoms but no signs of urethritis, it is necessary to differentiate between true urethritis and venereophobia. Although the absence of urethritis does not exclude the presence of *C. trachomatis* or *N. gonorrhoeae*, the diagnosis of NGU requires documentation of a leukocytic exudate as well as exclusion of urethral gonorrhea by Gram stain and culture. The presence of four or more polymorphonuclear leukocytes per oil-immersion field on a Gram stain of an intraurethral swab specimen or 15 or more leukocytes per high-power field in the sediment of the first 10–15 ml of urine examined under a coverslip is consistent with urethritis. In adolescent males, a recently developed screening strategy involves testing the first-voided urine for the detection of pyuria by microscopy[96] or with leukocyte esterase strips. This appears to be a promising and cost-effective way to select those at increased risk for urethritis associated with sexually transmitted pathogens.

Epididymitis

Chlamydia trachomatis and *Neisseria gonorrhoeae* are the usual causes of epididymitis in sexually active young men. The relative proportion of cases of epididymitis caused by one or the other of these two agents depends upon their relative incidence in the population studied. Where gonorrhea is uncommon, *C. trachomatis* is the major cause. It has been isolated from epididymal aspirates.[97] Coliform bacteria and *Pseudomonas aeruginosa* are the most common causes of epididymitis in men over 35 years of age. The presence of a urethral discharge in association with epididymitis suggests the diagnosis of chlamydial or gonococcal epididymitis, whereas the presence of midstream pyuria and bacteriuria in an older patient without urethral discharge suggest coliform or *Pseudomonas* infection.

Proctitis and Proctocolitis

Among homosexual men, non-LGV serovars of *C. trachomatis* have been associated with proctitis (inflammation limited to the rectum), while LGV serovars seemed, in a small number of cases studied, to be associated with either proctitis or proctocolitis.[98,99] Other rectal pathogens often are present concurrently. With non-LGV serovars, symptoms include mid-to-moderate rectal discharge, mild anorectal pain, tenesmus, and constipation; also, the rectal mucosa is erythematous and bleeds easily when swabbed, and biopsy specimens show a polymorphonuclear leukocyte infiltrate in the lamina propria. In contrast, with LGV serovars, symptoms are more severe; the rectal mucosa shows hemorrhages and ulcers, fever and inguinal lymphadenopathy may occur, and rectal biopsy specimens may be consistent with Crohn's disease.[98,99]

Reiter Syndrome

In several recent studies, *C. trachomatis* has been recovered from the urethra from up to 70 percent of men with untreated Reiter syndrome who have associated urethritis.[100] Men with *C. trachomatis*-associated "venereal" Reiter syndrome were also significantly more likely than were those with postdiarrheal Reiter syndrome to have urethritis for longer than 7 days before the onset of the arthritis.[56] Men with "venereal" Reiter syndrome are also more likely to demonstrate high titers of antibodies to *C. trachomatis*,[56,100] and in some cases, synovial fluid lymphocytes demonstrate a significant proliferative response to *C. trachomatis* antigens.[57] Almost all studies have failed to isolate *C. trachomatis* from synovial fluid or tissue.[100] However, in one recent study employing micro-IF with monoclonal antibody, typical chlamydial elementary bodies were detected in joint material from several men with sexually acquired reactive arthritis, but not from those with effusions due to other causes.[101] In our own unpublished study where men presenting with NGU without arthritis were treated with a tetracycline, Reiter syndrome did not subsequently arise in HLA-B27–positive men with or without *C. trachomatis* infection. When comparing men with NGU and men with Reiter syndrome, even by immunoblotting, there was no pattern of humoral immune response that was specific for either Reiter syndrome or HLA-B27 positivity.[102] Thus, the data are not conclusive but generally suggest that chlamydial urethritis—especially if untreated—may be a risk factor for the development of Reiter syndrome in genetically predisposed populations.

Infertility with Genital Infection with Chlamydia trachomatis in Men

In contrast to chlamydial infection in women, infertility is not an established consequence of chlamydial infection in men. Unilateral epididymitis has not been proved to result in infertility. In a study of infertile couples where there did not appear to be a female factor, the frequency of antibody to *C. trachomatis* was low, and presence of antibody was not significantly associated with abnormalities in the male.[103] Other studies have also failed to show an association.[104]

Prostatitis

Although *C. trachomatis* can be isolated from the prostatic fluid of men with chlamydial urethritis and has reportedly been isolated from prostatic biopsy material, there is still no convincing evidence for a role of *C. trachomatis* in either acute or chronic prostatitis.[91] Further studies employing histologic and microbiologic studies of prostatic tissue from symptomatic men are needed.

Genital Chlamydia trachomatis Infection in Women

As with gonococcal infection, *C. trachomatis* infection probably is more prevalent in women than in men, but it often escapes detection clinically. *Chlamydia trachomatis* has been isolated from the cervix of 30–60 percent of women with gonorrhea or those who have a history of contact with a partner with gonorrhea or NGU, from 10–20 percent of women attending STD clinics who do not have a history of contact with a partner with urethritis, and from about 5–10 percent of U.S. college students or young women attending gynecology clinics, family planning clinics, or prenatal clinics in most recent studies.[1] Rates of detection are generally higher in sexually active teenagers, especially those attending adolescent clinics or who are pregnant. In most studies done in settings other than STD clinics, *C. trachomatis* has been several times more prevalent than *N. gonorrhoeae*; in one study of relatively asymptomatic women, *C. trachomatis* was isolated from the cervix nine times as often as *N. gonorrhoeae*.[105] The prevalence of cervical *C. trachomatis* infection, like that of gonorrhea, is related to young age, single or divorced marital status, black race, low socioeconomic status, urban residence, and number of sexual partners.[1,106] The prevalence of *C. trachomatis* infection has been increased in oral contraceptive users in most studies.[107]

Chlamydial genital infections in women are important not only because of their frequency but also because of their consequences. Among women with genital infection, an estimated 10 percent have symptoms and signs of acute salpingitis. Since clinically inapparent endometrial infection is very frequent[108] and a high proportion of women with involuntary infertility secondary to bilateral tubal damage do not give a history suggestive of prior pelvic infection, it is likely that the proportion with significant ascending infection is much greater than 10 percent. Among those with ascending infection major sequelae include infertility due to tubal occlusion, ectopic pregnancy, and chronic pelvic pain. Most women infected at term will transmit infection to their infants after vaginal infection.

MUCOPURULENT CERVICITIS

In a recent study of STD clinic patients, mucopurulent cervicitis was more common than NGU was. Over 80 percent of women with cervical chlamydial infection had mucopurulent cervicitis, and approximately two-thirds of women with mucopurulent cervicitis had chlamydial infection.[109] Thus, empirical treatment of mucopurulent cervicitis with a tetracycline is recommended for women at high risk for STDs, just as NGU in men is treated empirically if confirmatory tests for *C. trachomatis* are not available. However, the predictive value of clinical evidence of mucopurulent cervicitis for *C. trachomatis* infection may be lower in women in other clinical settings where there is a lower risk of chlamydial infection. Although many women with *C. trachomatis* cervical infection have a normal cervix or only nonspecific changes, there is a significant correlation of this infection with mucopurulent endocervical discharge and with the presence of increased numbers of polymorphonuclear leukocytes per oil-immersion field in a Gram-stained smear of endocervical mucous (obtained after first cleansing the ectocervix with large swabs to remove vaginal leukocytes).[109,110] It is more difficult to quantitate polymorphonuclear leukocytes in cervical exudates than in urethral exudates. Although an earlier study[109] found that ≥10 polymorphonuclear leukocytes per 1000-power field in strands of cervical mucus was best correlated with chlamydial infection, we currently use a cutoff of ≥30 polymorphonuclear leukocytes per 1000-power field in mucus to achieve a higher predictive value for chlamydial or gonococcal infection. Mucopus is defined as a yellow or creamy yellow appearance of endocervical secretions, especially when viewed on a cotton-tipped swab.[110] Bleeding of the cervical columnar epithelium often can be induced with a cotton swab; edema and erythema of the zone of cervical ectopy are also common. The changes resolve with therapy.[110,111] The presence of mucopurulent endocervicitis, as defined by the above criteria, suggests the presence of *C. trachomatis*. Most but not all studies in STD and student health service clinics have confirmed these observations.[112] In a study in an adolescent clinic, five or more polymorphonuclear leukocytes on a smear correlated with the presence of *C. trachomatis*, but clinical findings did not.[113] Herpes simplex virus causes inflammation and ulceration of the ectocervix. Pathologically, *C. trachomatis* cervical infection often is associated with an intense polymorphonuclear leukocytic inflammatory reaction in the epithelial and subepithelial areas and lymphocytic and plasma cell infiltration in the stroma, occasionally with follicular aggregation of lymphocytes.[114] As with postgonococcal urethritis in men, women with gonorrhea and concurrent *C. trachomatis* infection who receive antimicrobials only active against *N. gonorrhoeae* often have persistent postgonococcal chlamydial cervicitis.[115,116]

The use of the aforementioned clinical features plus selected demographic and behavioral characteristics can improve the cost-effectiveness of laboratory testing for chlamydial infection. In one recent study in two family planning clinics, by screening 65 percent of the women, 90 percent of chlamydial infections would have been identified if testing had been restricted to all women with two or more of the following: age 24 years or less, intercourse with a new partner within the preceding 2 months, purulent or mucopurulent cervical exudate on examination, induced mucosal bleeding, and the use of a nonbarrier or no method of contraception.[106]

Endometritis, Salpingitis, and Perihepatitis

Chlamydia trachomatis is a frequent cause of acute endometritis and acute salpingitis, and it can lead to salpingitis after intrauterine device insertion, curettage, and hysterosalpingography and in the postpartum and postabortal period. Salpingitis has been produced by *C. trachomatis* in primate models, and it has been found in the cervix, endometrium, or fallopian tube of about one-third of women with laparoscopically verified acute pelvic inflammatory disease in Sweden[117] and in Seattle.[118] Similarly, *C. trachomatis* has been isolated from the cervix or urethra from about one-third of Canadian women who presented with clinical evidence of salpingitis such as a recent history of low abdominal pain, pain on sexual intercourse, or abnormal vaginal bleeding who additionally were found to have pain on movement of the cervix or palpation of the adnexa but who did not undergo laparoscopy.[119] Serologic data further suggest that as many as 50–60 percent of women with salpingitis in Seattle and Sweden have chlamydial infection. *Chlamydia trachomatis* appears to be more common than *N. gonorrhoeae* is among Scandinavian patients with salpingitis; it is about as common as *N. gonorrhoeae* among women with salpingitis in the Pacific Northwest. Clinically, the symptoms and signs of chlamydial endometritis or salpingitis are usually mild. However, the clinical impression is deceiving; at laparoscopy, women with chlamydial salpingitis have disease as severe as women with gonococcal salpingitis.[120] In keeping with the relatively asymptomatic spread of infection to the upper genital tract, women without symptoms of abdominal pain who have chlamydial cervicitis will often have a plasma cell endometritis.[108] A related development is serologic demonstration of IgM antibody seroconversion or high IgG titers to *C. trachomatis*, which is suggestive of recent infection with *C. trachomatis*, in 20 of 23 women with acute peritonitis and/or perihepatitis (Fitz-Hugh Curtis syndrome).[121] Variations of intraperitoneal spread of infection include chlamydial periappendicitis and perisplenitis.

Women with salpingitis are at considerable risk for developing involuntary infertility due to tubal occlusion. The risk rises with the number and severity of episodes. Overall, the risk is about 10 percent with one episode, 30 percent with two episodes, and greater than 50 percent with three or more. The risks, as they relate to chlamydial salpingitis, need to be further elucidated, but they appear to be at least as frequent as with salpingitis overall. The prevalence of antibody to *C. trachomatis* is higher among women with infertility and tubal occlusion than in comparison groups. One group in France has frequently isolated *C. trachomatis* from tubal or peritubal specimens from infertile women with tubal obstruction.[122] Others have not yet confirmed this.

Other Infections

Not surprisingly, *C. trachomatis* has now been implicated in the dysuria–pyuria (urethral) syndrome in women.[123] Among women with urethral or cervical *C. trachomatis* infection, about 50 percent have positive cultures from the cervix and urethra, about one-third from the cervix alone, and about one-sixth from the urethra alone. Among women presenting with genital symptoms, most with *C. trachomatis* in the urethra do not have urinary tract symptoms.[124] In contrast, *C. trachomatis* infection is relatively common among young women presenting with an acute onset of dysuria and frequency. In one study of such women, two-thirds of those with pyuria who had sterile bladder urine had *C. trachomatis* infection.[123]

Chlamydia trachomatis has also been isolated from the rectum of 10 percent of women with *C. trachomatis* genital infection and from pus expressed from Bartholin's gland in association with bartholinitis. It is not a cause of vaginitis in adult women.

Complications in Pregnancy

Data on the importance of *C. trachomatis* as a cause of spontaneous abortions, stillbirths, chorioamnionitis, premature rupture of membranes, premature delivery, and neonatal deaths are conflicting. In four separate case–control studies in Seattle, isolation of *C. trachomatis* from pregnant women has been associated with preterm delivery and other pregnancy morbidity.[125] Two studies have shown an association with these complications only in the small subset of women who also demonstrated an IgM antibody response to *C. trachomatis* and who presumably had recently acquired the infection.[126] Several studies found no relationship of perinatal chlamydial infection to prematurity, but some of these did not look for IgM antibody or certain other infections linked to premature delivery.[127] It is hoped that a large multicenter National Institutes of Health (NIH) study, now in progress, of vaginal and cervical infections in pregnancy will help clarify the relationship of chlamydial infection to pregnancy morbidity.

There are conflicting data on the influence of prior chlamydial infection on the success of in vitro fertilization, with some investigators showing a significantly poorer outcome in those with antibody to *C. trachomatis* as compared with those without antibody,[128] while others found no effect.[129]

Cervical Cytologic Manifestations of Chlamydial Infection

"Reactive" atypias of metaplastic cells and columnar cells have been significantly correlated with the isolation of *C. trachomatis* from the cervix, as has colposcopic evidence of a typical metaplasia of the cervix. The relationship of chlamydial infection to cervical dysplasia or cervical cancer is uncertain.[130] In addition to the atypias of metaplastic and endocervical cells, a characteristic pattern of inflammatory changes—including polymorphonuclear leukocytes, plasma cells, transformed lymphocytes, and histiocytes in cervical mucus—can be identified by cytopathologists, who can suggest further confirmatory tests for *C. trachomatis* on the basis of such findings.[131] Large cytoplasmic inclusions within vacuoles also can be seen, but they are an insensitive and nonspecific index of this infection.

Therapy for Genital Chlamydia trachomatis Infection

Tetracyclines and, to a lesser extent, erythromycins are the most important antimicrobials for the treatment of chlamydial infections.[1,83,132] Although isolates of *C. trachomatis* that are relatively resistant to erythromycin have been described, no isolates have been shown to be resistant to tetracyclines. Therapy for chlamydial urethritis is more effective than is therapy for other forms of NGU.[79,93] *Chlamydia trachomatis* is eradicated from the urethra by 7 days of treatment with tetracycline HCl (500 mg four times daily), minocycline (100 mg once or twice daily), or doxycycline (100 mg once or twice daily). Any of these tetracycline regimens is preferred for the treatment of NGU. Other effective regimens are erythromycin (500 mg twice daily for 14 days or 500 mg four times daily for 7 days) and sulfisoxazole (500 mg four times daily for 10 days). Although a 6- to 10-day treatment with rifampin, chloramphenicol, or even ampicillin or amoxicillin in high oral dosage has also been effective in some reports, these are not considered to be first-line antimicrobials for chlamydial infections.[79,93,94] *Chlamydia trachomatis* is not reliably eradicated by single-dose therapy with any antimicrobial agent. Tetracycline (500 mg orally four times daily for 5 days) and trimethoprim-sulfamethoxazole (720–300 mg once daily for 3 days) eradicates some but not all *C. trachomatis* infections.[133] Eradication of *C. trachomatis* from the cervix has been demonstrated with tetracycline, doxycycline, and sulfisoxazole in doses similar to those described above.[79] In one study, erythromycin base, 500 mg four times daily, was poorly tolerated, but 250 mg four times daily for 7 days was tolerated and effective in women. The optimal treatment for *C. trachomatis* in pregnancy is not yet clear, but an erythromycin regimen (using base, stearate, or ethylsuccinate, but not estolate) probably is the best choice. The equivalent of 500 mg base four times daily for 1 week or 250 mg four times daily for 2 weeks has been recommended.[1,83,134] We advocate the higher dosage schedule for up to 2 weeks if tolerated. For those who cannot tolerate erythromycin in pregnancy, sulfonamides can be used in the first and second trimester, and amoxicillin has been used successfully in many patients later in pregnancy, generally in doses of 500 mg orally four times daily for 10–14 days.

For complicated chlamydial infections, a minimum of 10 days of doxycycline, 100 mg twice daily, or tetracycline, 500 mg four times daily, is required.[1,83] For outpatient treatment of pelvic inflammatory disease or epididymitis in the young adult, this should be given in combination with a single dose of ceftriaxone, 250 mg intramuscularly, to eradicate *N. gonorrhoeae*. Since the clinical diagnosis of pelvic inflammatory disease may be incorrect and serious illnesses such as acute appendicitis or ectopic pregnancy may be missed, it is mandatory that a woman who is treated as an outpatient have a follow-up assessment, if only by phone, 48–72 hours into treatment. A failure to improve should usually result in hospitalization and a laparoscopy. For inpatient management, intravenous cefoxitin, 2 g q6h, plus intravenous or oral doxycycline, 100 mg twice daily, is the preferable choice. Alternatively and especially where there is a possibility of a tubal or adnexal abscess or the infection arose after pelvic surgery other than a therapeutic abortion, intravenous therapy with clindamycin, 900 mg q8h, plus full-dose aminoglycoside (for example, gentamicin) can be given. With both regimens the combination is continued for at least 4 days or until the woman has improved for 48 hours, if that takes longer. The woman can than be placed on a regimen of oral doxycycline, 100 mg twice daily, with the first approach or oral clindamycin, 450 mg four times daily, with the second approach to complete 14 days of total therapy. The clindamycin-aminoglycoside regimen has not been extensively studied for efficacy against *C. trachomatis* and *N. gonorrhoeae*,[118] so some Canadian authorities suggest the addition of doxycycline to that regimen.[135] Therapy with cephalosporins alone is not adequate since they rarely eradicate *C. trachomatis* even though there may be clinical improvement.[136]

The search continues for alternative antimicrobials for use in pregnancy and for an antimicrobial that has activity against *C. trachomatis*, all types of *N. gonorrhoeae*, and the genital mycoplasmas. The new quinolones are highly active against *N. gonorrhoeae*, and a few of the quinolones, especially ofloxacin, have considerable activity in vivo against *C. trachomatis*, but further evaluation is required.

Other Measures for the Prevention of Chlamydia trachomatis Infection in Adults

Until recently, no meaningful effort to prevent chlamydial infections has been undertaken in any country. Measures now being used effectively include public health education, emphasizing the use of barrier contraceptives, and avoiding promiscuity for the prevention of AIDS and other STDs; selective use of diagnostic tests for *C. trachomatis*, which are now less expensive and more widely available since the introduction of direct fluorescent antibody slide tests and ELISA tests; clinical recognition of syndromes commonly caused by *C. trachomatis* (NGU, epididymitis, mucopurulent cervicitis, and pelvic inflammatory disease) and treatment of these with an antichlamydial antimicrobial[83]; treatment of gonorrhea with a regimen active against coexisting chlamydial infection; and identification and treatment of sex partners exposed to individuals with presumptive or proven chlamydial infection.

The effectiveness of barrier contraceptives against chlamydial and gonococcal infection in women is suggested by the fact that women who have used barrier contraceptives and spermicides have lower rates of tubal infertility.[137] Prostitutes using nonoxynol-9–impregnated contraceptive sponges were partially protected against infection with both *C. trachomatis* and *N. gonorrhoeae*.[138]

The cost-effectiveness of diagnostic testing for *C. trachomatis* is highest when patients are selected who have the highest prevalence of infection.[139,140] It is most useful to test sexually active young women, particularly those who have cervicitis or pelvic inflammatory disease or who are adolescent and single, inner-city residents.[106] In practice, it is becoming common to perform a test for *C. trachomatis* whenever testing for *N. gonorrhoeae*. Screening in pregnancy is particularly useful to prevent perinatal transmission to the infant and postpartum endometritis in the mother. The potential benefit of treating chlamydial infection in pregnancy to prevent pregnancy morbidity such as prematurity remains to be evaluated.

Treatment of sexual partners of patients with presumptive or proven chlamydial infection is supported by the frequent occurrence of symptomatic or asymptomatic *C. trachomatis* infection in partners of infected individuals. One large study has shown that approximately 50 percent of infected male or female partners of men or women with *C. trachomatis* infection are asymptomatic.[141] Results were very similar with respect to gonorrhea. As a general guide, when one person is treated for a syndrome compatible with *C. trachomatis* infection, it is usually prudent to treat the partner with a regimen that is also active against *C. trachomatis*. Where treatment of the partner could not be arranged, in one series 55 percent of women with chlamydial cervicitis became reinfected within 8 weeks after treatment.[117] At least in one study, field follow-up by trained investigators was both the most efficient and the most cost-effective method of identifying individuals with *C. trachomatis* infection or a significant risk of infection.[142] In Seattle–King County where a chlamydial control program encompassing most of the above features has been in place for a decade, the incidence of chlamydial infection has in fact been falling—like that of gonorrhea.

Prospects for developing an effective vaccine are presently remote.[46,143]

Chlamydia trachomatis Infections in Infants

Between 2 and 6 percent of pregnant women have had *C. trachomatis* genital infection in several North American studies, and maternal *C. trachomatis* infection is transmitted to 60–70 percent of exposed infants after vaginal delivery.[68] Infection also has been well documented after cesarian section, even when performed before rupture of membranes, but is less common than after vaginal delivery. Among infected infants, positive cultures are infrequent in the first few days of life; however, after 1–2 weeks positive cultures are frequently detected in the conjunctiva and shortly after in the nasopharynx. The rate of isolation from the conjunctiva begins to fall by 5–6 weeks, but infection of various sites, including the nasopharynx, conjunctiva, rectum, and vagina, can be detected—usually without signs of infection—for many months and, in a few infants followed without treatment, for a year or more. In a compilation of studies of 189 exposed infants, 37 percent had positive cultures or smears, and 67 percent had serologic evidence of *C. trachomatis* infection. Of those infants with positive cultures or cytology, 77 percent developed conjunctivitis, 19 percent had pneumonia, and 13 percent had neither disease.

Infant Pneumonia. The interstitial pneumonia described by Beem and Saxon is distinctive.[67] Its onset is gradual, with a range of onset from 2 weeks to 3 months (peak, 3–6 weeks). Infants are always afebrile, but the course is protracted. The initial manifestation often is rhinitis with nasal obstruction, usually without nasal discharge. Approximately one-half of infants who develop pneumonia have or have had conjunctivitis. A distinctive cough eventually develops (a series of closely spaced staccato coughs, with each separated by a brief inspiration), with tachypnea, rales, hyperinflation, diffuse interstitial involvement, slight eosinophilia, and elevated serum immunoglobulin levels. Clinical illness lasts several weeks, while inspiratory rales and radiologic signs may persist for months. Harrison and colleagues showed that 30 percent of human infants between 1 and 6 months of age who were admitted to the hospital with pneumonitis had *C. trachomatis* infection.[144] A much higher proportion of infants with afebrile interstitial pneumonia had *C. trachomatis* infection. Today, such infants are now often recognized early by pediatricians and treated as outpatients.

Between asymptomatic infection, on the one hand, and the interstitial pneumonia, on the other, are presentations that are also compatible with *C. trachomatis* infection; however, supporting evidence is more circumstantial.[145] These include nasopharyngitis, secretory otitis media (with positive cultures from middle ear aspirates in a portion), bronchitis, and pneumonia associated with pulmonary infection by *C. trachomatis* together with other pathogens. In one study[146] of infants who would fit the general picture of *C. trachomatis* pneumonia, cytomegalovirus, *Pneumocystis carinii,* and *Ureaplasma urealyticum* infections were as frequent as *C. trachomatis* infection. A follow-up evaluation indicated that, irrespective of the initial etiology, a high proportion of infants showed residual clinical, radiologic, and pulmonary function abnormalities.[147] It is highly probable as well that a mild form of pneumonitis that is not clinically apparent also exists. No gastrointestinal disease has been recognized as a consequence of infant rectal shedding. There have been several cases of sudden infant deaths in infants infected with *C. trachomatis*, but a link has not been proved.

The diagnosis of infection in infants may be made by demonstrating chlamydiae by direct immunofluorescent staining or Giemsa stain in conjunctival smears, by ELISA of conjunctival exudate, by isolation of *C. trachomatis* from the nasopharynx or conjunctiva, or by demonstration of tear antibody. Diagnosis of pneumonia is further supported by isolation from tracheal secretions (frequent) or lung tissue (rare) and by elevated IgM antibodies to *C. trachomatis*.[70] The few infants with pneumonia studied had greatly enhanced antibody production from peripheral blood mononuclear cells.

Therapy for Chlamydia trachomatis Infections in Infants. Therapy for inclusion conjunctivitis with topical tetracycline or sulfonamide for 2–3 weeks frequently does not eradicate conjunctival or nasopharyngeal carriage of *C. trachomatis*.[79] Instead, conjunctival colonization persists up to at least 40 weeks, and nasopharyngeal colonization persists for up to 18 months or more in spite of topical therapy. Therefore, systemic treatment of neonatal inclusion conjunctivitis is indicated to eradicate eye infection as well as to prevent pneumonia and perhaps upper respiratory infection. Erythromycin or, in older infants, sulfonamides probably are the drugs of choice, but data are needed on the optimal dosage and duration of therapy. Treatment of infants with pneumonia with sulfisoxazole (150 mg/kg/day) or erythromycin estolate or ethyl-succinate (50 mg/kg/day) for 2–3 weeks has resulted in both symptomatic improvement in 5–7 days and negative cultures after 9 days in one study.[148] The latter regimens also seem to be relatively effective for neonatal conjunctival and nasopharyngeal infections when compliance with therapy is good. Most infants remained culture-negative after cessation of therapy. However, the use of lower doses of erythromycin for 10–14 days has resulted in high rates of failure.[79] Further data are needed.

The best prevention of infection in infants will require diagnosis and treatment of infection in parents. At birth, ocular prophylaxis with silver nitrate does not prevent the transmission of *C. trachomatis* to infants, although silver nitrate has not been compared with placebo in this regard. In one small study, single-dose ocular prophylaxis with erythromycin provided greater protection than silver nitrate did against chlamydial conjunctivitis but did not significantly decrease the overall acquisition of *C. trachomatis*.[149] Subsequent experience suggests that when the application of erythromycin to the infants' eyes is delayed to allow maternal–infant eye-to-eye "bonding" the prophylaxis is not effective.

OTHER INFECTIONS

It is highly likely that associations between *C. trachomatis* and other illnesses will be described. Recent experience shows that these reports must be interpreted cautiously because of spurious identification of chlamydiae in inexperienced laboratories and technical difficulties in the past with differentiating antibody to the different species of *Chlamydia*. For example, in previous studies, antibody thought to be directed against *C. trachomatis* was identified in a large proportion of children,[150,151] and so-called acute antibody (i.e., high-titer, changing-titer, or IgM antibody) was found in 9 percent of those 10 years or older with a recent history of pneumonia. It now seems that the TWAR strain (*C. pneumoniae*) accounts for much of this antibody, and it has been isolated from some of the individuals with illness.[152]

Numerous groups have evaluated the role of *C. trachomatis* as a cause of pharyngitis. Outside of STD clinic populations, initial serologic studies apparently showing an association between *C. trachomatis* infection and pharyngitis[153] can now likely be attributed to infection with the TWAR strain.[154] In STD clinic populations, although most groups have not recovered *C. trachomatis* from the pharynx, some groups have isolated it infrequently.[155]

Despite the observation that some men with LGV proctitis have biopsy specimen findings compatible with Crohn's disease, other data do not support an association between *C. trachomatis* and Crohn's disease.[156] A case of meningoencephalitis with exceedingly high antibody titer to *C. trachomatis* has been described.[157] Four cases of myocarditis in children aged 1–6 years had increasing or high stable antibody titers to *C. trachomatis*.[158] One fatal case of *C. trachomatis* endocarditis in a pregnant woman has been described.[159] Evidence of *C. trachomatis* as one cause of pneumonia has been described for adult community-acquired pneumonia in normal hosts[160] and for pneumonia arising in compromised hosts.[161] In the latter category, concurrent infection with cytomegalovirus was frequent. In normal hosts, some of the cases of apparent *C. trachomatis* infection distant from mucosal sites are probably due to LGV rather than non-LGV strains. A recent example is a report of laboratory-acquired LGV infections in normal hosts where LGV caused systemic illness with mediastinal and supraclavicular lymphadenitis and interstitial pneumonia with pleural effusions.[162]

REFERENCES

1. Centers for Disease Control. *Chlamydia trachomatis* infections: Policy guidelines for prevention and control. MMWR. 1985;34(Suppl 3):53–74.
2. Washington AE, Johnson RE, Sanders LL Jr. *Chlamydial trachomatis* infections in the United States: What are they costing us? JAMA. 1987; 257:2070–2.
3. Gordon FB, Quan AL. Isolation of the trachoma agent in cell culture. Proc Soc Exp Biol Med. 1965;354:354–9.
4. Wang S-P, Grayston JT. Immunologic relationship between genital TRIC, lymphogranuloma venereum, and related organisms in a new microtiter indirect immunofluorescence test. Am J Ophthalmol. 1970;70:367–74.
5. Manire GP. Biological characteristics of chlamydiae. In: Hobson D, Holmes KK, eds. Nongonococcal Urethritis and Related Infections. Washington, DC: American Society for Microbiology; 1977:167–75.
6. Moulder JW. A primer for chlamydiae. In: Mårdh P-A, Holmes KK, Oriel JD, et al., eds. Chlamydial Infections. Amsterdam: Elsevier Biomedical; 1982:3–14.
7. Becker Y. The chlamydia: Molecular biology of procaryotic obligate parasites of eucaryocytes. Microbiol Rev. 1978;42:274–306.
8. Gregory WW, Gardner M, Byrne G, et al. Arrays of hemispheric surface projections on *Chlamydia psittaci* and *Chlamydia trachomatis* observed by scanning electron microscopy. Infect Immun. 1979;138:241–4.
9. Ward ME, Salari HS. Control mechanisms governing the infectivity of *Chlamydia trachomatis* for HeLa cells: Mechanisms of endocytosis. J Gen Microbiol. 1982;128:639–50.
10. Kramer MJ, Gordon FB. Ultrastructural analysis of the effects of penicillin

and chlortetracycline on the development of a genital tract Chlamydia. Infect Immun. 1971;3:333–41.

11. Rothermel CD, Byrne GI, Havell EA. Effect of interferon on the growth of *Chlamydia trachomatis* in mouse fibroblasts (L cells). Infect Immun. 1983;39:362–70.
12. Byrne GI, Kreuger DA. Lymphokine-mediated inhibition of *Chlamydia* replication in mouse fibroblasts is neutralized by anti-gamma interferon. Infect Immun. 1983;42:1152–8.
13. Allan I, Pearce JH. Amino acid requirements of strains of *Chlamydia trachomatis* and *C. psittaci* growing in McCoy cells: Relationship with clinical syndrome and host origin. J Gen Microbiol. 1983;129:2001–7.
14. Engel JN, Ganem D. Chlamydial rRNA operons: Gene organization and identification of putative tandem promotors. J Bacteriol. 1987;169:5678–85.
15. Larsson L, Jimenez J, Odham G, et al. Preliminary studies on cellular lipids of *Chlamydia trachomatis* using capillary gas chromatography. In: Mårdh P-A, Holmes KK, Oriel JD, et al., eds. Chlamydial Infections. Amsterdam: Elsevier Biomedical; 1982;37–40.
16. Wang S-P, Grayston JT. Microimmunofluorescence antibody responses in *Chlamydia trachomatis* infection, a review. In: Mårdh P-A, Holmes KK, Oriel JD, et al., eds. Chlamydial Infections. Amsterdam: Elsevier Biomedical; 1982;301–16.
17. Kuo C-C, Wang S-P, Holmes KK, et al. Immunotypes of *Chlamydia trachomatis* isolates in Seattle, Washington. Infect Immun. 1983;41:865–8.
18. Barnes RC, Rompalo AM, Stamm WE. Comparison of *Chlamydia trachomatis* serovars causing rectal and cervical infections. J Infect Dis. 1987;156:953–8.
19. Allan I. Chlamydial antigenic structure and genetics. In: Oriel D, Ridgway G, Schachter J, et al., eds. Chlamydial Infections. Cambridge: Cambridge University Press; 1986:73–80.
20. Nurminen M, Rietschel ET, Brade H. Chemical characterization of *Chlamydia trachomatis* lipopolysaccharide. Infect Immun. 1985;48:573–5.
21. Caldwell HD, Hitchcock PJ. Monoclonal antibody against a genus-specific antigen of *Chlamydia* species. Location of the epitope on chlamydial lipopolysaccharide. Infect Immun. 1984;44:306–14.
22. Caldwell HD. Structural analysis of the major outer membrane proteins of *Chlamydia* spp. In: Mårdh P-A, Holmes KK, Oriel JD, et al., eds. Chlamydial Infections. Amsterdam: Elsevier Biomedical; 1982:45–50.
23. Stephens RS, Sanchez-Pescador R, Wagar EA, et al. Diversity of *Chlamydia trachomatis* major outer membrane protein genes. J Bacteriol. 1987;169:3879–85.
24. Newhall WJ V. Biosynthesis and disulfide cross-linking of outer membrane components during the growth cycle of *Chlamydia trachomatis*. Infect Immun. 1987;55:162–8.
25. Jones RB, Batteiger B, Newhall WJ V. Cross-reactive antigenic determinants in the major surface proteins of *Chlamydia trachomatis*. In: Mårdh P-A, Holmes KK, Oriel JD, et al., eds. Chlamydial Infections. Amsterdam: Elsevier Biomedical; 1982:261–4.
26. Stephens RS, Tam MR, Kuo C-C, et al. Monoclonal antibody to *Chlamydia trachomatis*: Antibody specificities and antigen characterization. J Immunol. 1982;128:1083–9.
27. Batteiger BE, Newhall WJ V, Terho P, et al. Antigenic analysis of the major outer membrane protein of *Chlamydia trachomatis* with murine monoclonal antibodies. Infect Immun. 1986;53:530–3.
28. Zhang YX, Watkins NG, Stewart S, et al. The low-molecular-mass, cysteine-rich outer membrane protein of *Chlamydia trachomatis* possesses both biovar- and species-specific epitopes. Infect Immun. 1987;55:2570–3.
29. Dhir SP, Hakomori S, Kenny GE, et al. Immunochemical studies on chlamydial antigen. (presence of a 2-keto-3-deoxycarbohydrate as immunodominant group.) J Immunol. 1972;109:116–22.
30. Kuo C-C, Kenny GE, Wang S-P. Trachoma and psittacosis antigens in agar gel double immunodiffusion. In: Nichols RL, ed. Trachoma and Related Disorders Caused by Chlamydial Agents. Amsterdam: Excerpta Medica; 1971:113–23.
31. Caldwell HD, Kuo C-C, Kenny GE. Antigenic analysis of chlamydiae by two-dimensional immunoelectrophoresis. I. Antigenic heterogeneity between *C. trachomatis* and *C. psittaci*. J Immunol. 1975;115:963–8.
32. Caldwell HD, Kuo C-C, Kenny GE. Antigenic analysis of chlamydiae by two-dimensional immunoelectrophoresis. II. A trachoma-LGV specific antigen. J Immunol. 1975;115:969–75.
33. Ward ME. Outstanding problems in chlamydial cell biology. In: Oriel D, Ridgway G, Schachter J, et al., eds. Chlamydial Infections. Cambridge: Cambridge University Press; 1986:3–14.
34. Lee CK. Interaction between a trachoma strain of *C. trachomatis* and mouse fibroblasts (McCoy) cells in the absence of centrifugation. Infect Immun. 1981;31:584–91.
35. Soderlund G, Kihlstrom E. Physicochemical surface properties of elementary bodies from different serotypes of *Chlamydia trachomatis* and their interaction with mouse fibroblasts. Infect Immun. 1982;36:893–9.
36. Lee CK, Moulder JW. Persistent infection of mouse fibroblasts (McCoy cells), with a trachoma strain of *Chlamydia trachomatis*. Infect Immun. 1981;32:822–9.
37. MacDonald AB, Than KA, Stuart ES. Persistent infection of BHK cells with *Chlamydia trachomatis* can be switched to an overt infection by treatment with cyclic nucleotides. In: Oriel D, Ridgway G, Schachter J, et al., eds. Chlamydial Infections. Cambridge: Cambridge University Press; 1986:67–70.
38. Levy NJ. Wheat germ agglutinin blockage of chlamydial attachment sites: Antagonism by *N*-acetyl-D-glucosamine. Infect Immun. 1979;25:946–53.
39. Moulder JW, Hatch TP, Byrne GL, et al. Immediate cytotoxicity of high multiplicities of *Chlamydia psittaci* for mouse fibroblasts (L cells). Infect Immun. 1976;14:277–89.
40. Kuo C-C. Immediate cytotoxicity of *Chlamydia trachomatis* for mouse peritoneal macrophages. Infect Immun. 1978;20:613–8.
41. Taverne J, Blyth WA, Ballard RC. Interactions of TRIC agents with macrophages: Effects on lysosomal enzymes of the cell. J Hyg. 1974;72:297–309.
42. Yong EC, Klebanoff SJ, Kuo C-C. Toxic effect of human polymorphonuclear leukocytes on *Chlamydia trachomatis*. Infect Immun. 1982;37:422–6.
43. Register KB, Davis CH, Wyrick PB, et al. Nonoxidative antimicrobial effects of human polymorphonuclear leukocyte granular proteins on *Chlamydia* spp. in vitro. Infect Immun. 1987;55:2420–7.
44. Yong EC, Chi EY, Kuo CC. Differential antimicrobial activity of human mononuclear phagocytes against the human biovars of *Chlamydia trachomatis*. J Immunol. 1987;139:1297–302.
45. Patton DL, Kuo CC, Wang SP, et al. Distal tubal obstruction induced by repeated *Chlamydia trachomatis* salpingeal infection in pig-tailed macaques. J Infect Dis. 1987;155:1292–9.
46. Grayston JT, Wang S-P. The potential for vaccine against infection of the genital tract with *Chlamydia trachomatis*. Sex Transm Dis. 1978;5:73–7.
47. Taylor HR, Prendergast RA, Dawson CR, et al. Animal model of trachoma: III. The necessity of repeated exposure to live chlamydia. In: Mårdh P-A, Holmes KK, Oriel JD, et al., eds. Chlamydial Infections. Amsterdam: Elsevier Biomedical; 1982:387–90.
48. Taylor HR, Johnson SL, Schachter J, et al. Pathogenesis of trachoma: The stimulus for inflammation. J Immunol. 1987;138:3023–7.
49. Orenstein NS, Mull JD, Thompson SE III. Immunity to chlamydial infections of the eye. V. Passive transfer of antitrachoma antibodies to owl monkeys. Infect Immun. 1973;7:600–3.
50. Brunham RC, Kuo C-C, Cles L. Correlation of host immune response with quantitative recovery of *Chlamydia trachomatis* from the human endocervix. Infect Immun. 1983;39:1491–4.
51. Brunham RC, Maclean IW, Binns B. *Chlamydia trachomatis*: Its role in tubal infertility. J Infect Dis. 1985;152:1275–82.
52. Brunham RC, Peeling R, Maclean I, et al. Postabortal *Chlamydia trachomatis* salpingitis: Correlating risk with antigen-specific serologic responses with neutralization. J Infect Dis. 1987;155:749–55.
53. Stephens RS, Chen W-J, Kuo C-C. Effects of corticosteroids and cyclophosphamide on a mouse model of *Chlamydia trachomatis* pneumonitis. Infect Immun. 1982;35:680–4.
54. Brunham RC, Martin DH, Kuo C-C, et al. Cellular immune response during uncomplicated genital infection with *Chlamydia trachomatis* in humans. Infect Immun. 1981;34:98–104.
55. Brunham RC, Martin DH, Hubbard TW, et al. Depression of the lymphocyte transformation response to microbial antigens and to phytohemagglutinin during pregnancy. J Clin Invest. 1983;72:1629–38.
56. Martin DH, Pollack S, Kuo C-C, et al. Urethral chlamydial infection in men with Reiter's syndrome. In: Mårdh P-A, Holmes KK, Oriel JD, et al., eds. Chlamydial Infections. Amsterdam: Elsevier Biomedical; 1982:107–10.
57. Ford DK, da Roza DM, Schulzer M. The specificity of synovial mononuclear cell responses to microbiological antigens in Reiter's syndrome. J Rheumatol. 1982;9:561–7.
58. Katz BP, Batteiger BE, Jones RB. Effect of prior sexually transmitted disease on the isolation of *Chlamydia trachomatis*. Sex Transm Dis. 1987;14:160–4.
59. Hanna L. Microscopic demonstration of chlamydial inclusions by Giemsa, iodine, or immunofluorescence stains. In: Hobson D, Holmes KK, eds. Nongonococcal Urethritis and Related Infections. Washington, DC: American Society for Microbiology; 1977:266–71.
60. Schachter J, Dawson CR. Comparative efficiency of various diagnostic methods for chlamydial infection. In: Hobson D, Holmes KK, eds. Nongonococcal Urethritis and Related Infections. Washington, DC: American Society for Microbiology; 1977:337–41.
61. Tam MR, Stamm WE, Handsfield HH, et al. Culture-independent diagnosis of *Chlamydia trachomatis* using monoclonal antibodies. N Engl J Med. 1984;310:1146–50.
62. Mahony JB, Sellors J, Chernesky MA. Detection of chlamydial inclusions in cell culture or biopsy tissue by alkaline phosphatase–anti-alkaline phosphatase staining. J Clin Microbiol. 1987;25:1864–7.
63. Horn JE, Hammer ML, Falkow S, et al. Detection of *Chlamydia trachomatis* in tissue culture and cervical scrapings by in situ DNA hybridization. J Infect Dis. 1986;153:1155–9.
64. Ripa KT, Mardh P-A. New simplified culture technique for *Chlamydia trachomatis*. In: Hobson D, Holmes KK, eds. Nongonococcal Urethritis and Related Infections. Washington, DC: American Society for Microbiology; 1977:323–7.
65. Darougar S, Woodland RM, Forsey T, et al. Isolation of chlamydia from ocular infections. In: Hobson D, Holmes KK, eds. Nongonococcal Urethritis and Related Infections. Washington, DC: American Society for Microbiology; 1977:295–8.
66. Bowie WR, Wang S-P, Alexander ER, et al. Etiology of nongonococcal urethritis: Evidence for *Chlamydia trachomatis* and *Ureaplasma urealyticum*. J Clin Invest. 1977;59:735–42.
67. Beem MO, Saxon EM. Respiratory tract colonization and a distinctive pneu-

monia syndrome in infants infected with *Chlamydia trachomatis*. N Engl J Med. 1977;296:306–10.
68. Beem MO, Saxon EM. *Chlamydia trachomatis* infection of infants. In: Mardh P-A, et al., eds. Chlamydial Infections. Amsterdam: Elsevier Biomedical; 1982:199–212.
69. Schachter J. Chlamydiae. In: Rose NR, Friedman H, eds. Manual of Clinical Immunology. Washington, DC: American Society for Microbiology; 1976: 494–9.
70. Schachter J, Grossman M, Azimi PH. Serology of *Chlamydia trachomatis* in infants. J Infect Dis. 1982;146:530–5.
71. Schachter J. Confirmatory serodiagnosis of lymphogranuloma venereum proctitis may yield false-positive results due to other chlamydial infections of the rectum. Sex Transm Dis. 1981;8:26–8.
72. Grayston JT, Yeh LJ, Wang S-P, et al. Pathogenesis of ocular *Chlamydia trachomatis* infections in humans. In: Hobson D, Holmes KK, eds. Nongonococcal Urethritis and Related Infections. Washington, DC: American Society for Microbiology; 1977:113–25.
73. Levy NJ, McCormack WM. Detection of serum antibody to chlamydia with ELISA. In: Mårdh P-A, Holmes KK, Oriel JD, et al., eds. Chlamydial Infections. Amsterdam: Elsevier Biomedical; 1982:341–4.
74. Schachter J, Smith DE, Dawson R, et al. Lymphogranuloma venereum. I. Comparison of the Frei test, complement fixation test, and isolation of the agent. J Infect Dis. 1969;120:372–5.
75. Dawson CR. Eye disease with chlamydial infections. In: Oriel D, Ridgway G, Schachter J, et al., eds. Chlamydial Infections. Cambridge: Cambridge University Press; 1986:135–44.
76. Mordhorst CH. Clinical epidemiology of oculogenital chlamydia infection. In: Hobson D, Holmes KK, eds. Nongonococcal Urethritis and Related Infections. Washington, DC: American Society for Microbiology; 1977:126–34.
77. Tarizzo M, ed. Field Methods for the Control of Trachoma. Geneva: World Health Organization; 1973:9.
78. Ronnerstam R, Persson K. Chlamydial conjunctivitis in a Swedish population. In: Mårdh P-A, Holmes KK, Oriel JD, et al., eds. Chlamydial Infections. Amsterdam: Elsevier Biomedical; 1982:87–90.
79. Bowie WR. Treatment of chlamydial infections. In: Mårdh P-A, Holmes KK, Oriel JD, et al., eds. *Chlamydial Infections*. Amsterdam: Elsevier Biomedical Press; 1982;231–44.
80. Hoshiwara I, Oster B, Hanna L, et al. Doxycycline treatment of chronic trachoma. JAMA. 1973;224:220–3.
81. Taylor HR. Strategies for the control of trachoma. Aust NZ J Ophthalmol. 1987;15:139–43.
82. Piot P, Ballard RC, Fehler HG, et al. Isolation of *Chlamydia trachomatis* from genital ulcerations in Southern Africa. In: Mårdh P-A, Holmes KK, Oriel JD, et al., eds. Chlamydial Infections. Amsterdam: Elsevier Biomedical; 1982:115–8.
83. Centers for Disease Control. 1985 STD treatment guidelines. MMWR. 1985;34(Suppl 4):75–108.
84. Greaves AB, Hilleman MR, Taggart SRT, et al. Chemotherapy in bubonic lymphogranuloma venereum. A clinical and serological evaluation. Bull WHO. 1957;16:277–89.
85. Stamm W, Holmes KK. *Chlamydia trachomatis* infections in the adult. In Holmes KK, Mårdh P-A, Sparling PF, et al., eds. Sexually Transmitted Diseases. 2nd ed. New York: McGraw-Hill; 1989.
86. Lycke E, Lowhagen G-B, Hallhagen G, et al. The risk of transmission of genital *Chlamydia trachomatis* infection is less than that of genital *Neisseria gonorrhoeae* infection. Sex Transm Dis. 1980;7:6–10.
87. Oriel JD, Ridgway GL. Studies of the epidemiology of chlamydial infections of the human genital tract. In: Mårdh P-A, Holmes KK, Oriel JD, et al., eds. Chlamydial Infections. Amsterdam: Elsevier Biomedical; 1982:425–8.
88. Holmes KK, Handsfield HH, Wang S-P, et al. Etiology of nongonococcal urethritis. N Engl J Med. 1975;292:1199–205.
89. Podgore JK, Holmes KK, Alexander ER. Asymptomatic urethral infections due to *Chlamydia trachomatis* in male U.S. military personnel. J Infect Dis. 1982;146:828.
90. Oriel JD, Reeve P, Thomas BJ, et al. Infection with chlamydia group A in men with urethritis due to *Neisseria gonorrhoeae*. J Infect Dis. 1975; 131:376–82.
91. Oriel D. Infection of the male genital tract. In: Mårdh P-A, Holmes KK, Oriel JD, et al., eds. Chlamydial Infections. Amsterdam: Elsevier Biomedical; 1982:93–106.
92. Gale J, Hinds MW. Male urethritis in King County, Washington, 1974–75: I. Incidence. Am J Public Health. 1978;68:20–5.
93. Handsfield HH, Alexander ER, Wang S-P, et al. Differences in the therapeutic response of chlamydia-positive and chlamydia-negative forms of nongonococcal urethritis. J Am Vener Dis Assoc. 1975;2:5–9.
94. Bowie WR, Alexander ER, Floyd JF, et al. Differential response of chlamydial and ureaplasma-associated urethritis to sulfafurazole (sulfisoxazole) and aminocyclitols. Lancet. 1976;2:1276–8.
95. Taylor-Robinson D, Purcell RH, London WT, et al. Microbiological, serological, and histopathological features of experimental *Chlamydia trachomatis* urethritis in chimpanzees. Br J Vener Dis. 1981;57:36–40.
96. Shafer MA, Schachter J, Vaughan E, et al. Evaluation of the first catch urinalysis as a screening tool for detection of urethritis among adolescent males attending teen clinics, in Oriel D, Ridgway G, Schachter J, et al., eds. Chlamydial Infections. Cambridge: Cambridge University Press; 1986:255–8.
97. Berger RE, Alexander ER, Monda GD, et al. *Chlamydia trachomatis* as a cause of acute "idiopathic" epididymitis. N Engl J Med. 1978;298:301–4.
98. Quinn TC, Goodell SE, Mkrtichian E, et al. *Chlamydia trachomatis* proctitis. N Engl J Med. 1981;305:195–200.
99. Quinn TC, Stamm WE, Goodell SE, et al. The polymicrobial origin of intestinal infections in homosexual men. N Engl J Med. 1983;309:576–82.
100. Keat A, Thomas BJ, Taylor-Robinson D. Chlamydial infection in the aetiology of arthritis. Br Med Bull. 1983;39:168–74.
101. Keat A, Thomas B, Dixey J, et al. *Chlamydia trachomatis* and reactive arthritis: The missing link. Lancet. 1987;1:72–4.
102. Inman RD, Johnston ME, Chiu B, et al. Immunochemical analysis of immune response to *C. trachomatis* in Reiter's syndrome and nonspecific urethritis. Clin Exp Immunol. 1987;69:246–54.
103. Close CE, Wang SP, Roberts PL, et al. The relationship of infection with *Chlamydia trachomatis* to the parameters of male fertility and sperm autoimmunity. Fertil Steril. 1987;48:880–3.
104. Auroux MR, De Mouy DM, Acar JF. Male fertility and positive chlamydial serology. A study of 61 fertile and 82 subfertile men. J Androl. 1987;8:197–200.
105. Schachter J, Hanna L, Hill EC, et al. Are chlamydial infections the most prevalent venereal disease? JAMA. 1975;231:1252–5.
106. Handsfield HH, Jasman LL, Roberts PL, et al. Criteria for selective screening for *Chlamydia trachomatis* infection in women attending family planning clinics. JAMA. 1986;255:1730–4.
107. Washington AE, Gove S, Schachter J, et al. Oral contraceptives, *Chlamydia trachomatis* infection, and pelvic inflammatory disease: A word of caution. JAMA. 1985;253:2246–50.
108. Paavonen J, Kiviat N, Brunham RC, et al. Prevalence and manifestations of endometritis among women with cervicitis. Am J Obstet Gynecol. 1985;152:280–6.
109. Brunham RC, Paavonen J, Stevens CE, et al. Mucopurulent cervicitis: The ignored counterpart of urethritis in men. N Engl J Med. 1984;311:1–6.
110. Rees E, Tait IA, Hobson D, et al. Chlamydia in relation to cervical infection and pelvic inflammatory disease. In: Hobson D, Holmes KK, eds. Nongonococcal Urethritis and Related Infections. Washington, DC: American Society for Microbiology; 1977:67–76.
111. Brunham RC, Kuo C-C, Stevens CE, et al. Therapy of cervical chlamydial infection. Ann Intern Med. 1982;97:216–9.
112. Paavonen J, Critchlow CW, DeRouen T, et al. Etiology of cervical inflammation. Am J Obstet Gynecol. 1986;154:556–64.
113. Moscicki B, Shafer M-A, Millstein SG, et al. The use and limitations of endocervical Gram stains and mucopurulent cervicitis as predictors for *Chlamydia trachomatis* in female adolescents. Am J Obstet Gynecol. 1987; 157:65–71.
114. Kiviat N, Paavonen J, Wolner-Hanssen P, et al. Histologic manifestations of chlamydial cervicitis. In: Oriel D, Ridgway G, Schachter J, et al., eds. Chlamydial Infections. Cambridge: Cambridge University Press; 1986:209–12.
115. Arya OP, Mallinson H, Pareek SS, et al. Post-gonococcal cervicitis and post-gonococcal urethritis. Br J Vener Dis. 1981;57:395–9.
116. Rees E, Davies JA, Bradley MG, et al. *Chlamydia trachomatis* in relation to post-gonococcal cervicitis. In: Mårdh P-A, Holmes KK, Oriel JD, et al., eds. Chlamydial Infections. Amsterdam: Elsevier Biomedical Press; 1982:147–50.
117. Mardh P-A, Ripa T, Svensson L, et al. *Chlamydia trachomatis* infection in patients with acute salpingitis. N Engl J Med. 1977;296:1377–9.
118. Wasserheit JN, Bell TA, Kiviat NB, et al. Microbial causes of proven pelvic inflammatory disease and efficacy of clindamycin and tobramycin. Ann Intern Med. 1986;104:187–93.
119. Bowie WR, Jones H. Acute pelvic inflammatory disease in outpatients: Association with *Chlamydia trachomatis* and *Neisseria gonorrhoeae*. Ann Intern Med. 1981;95:685–8.
120. Svensson L, Westrom L, Ripa KT, et al. Differences in some clinical and laboratory parameters in acute salpingitis related to culture and serologic findings. Am J Obstet Gynecol. 1980;138:1017–21.
121. Wang S-P, Eschenbach DA, Holmes KK, et al. *Chlamydia trachomatis* in the Fitz-Hugh-Curtis syndrome. Am J Obstet Gynecol. 1980;138:1034–8.
122. Henry-Suchet J, Catalan F, Loffredo V, et al. *Chlamydia trachomatis* associated with chronic inflammation in abdominal specimens from women selected for tuboplasty. Fertil Steril. 1981;36:599–605.
123. Stamm WE, Wagner KF, Amsel R, et al. Causes of the acute urethral syndrome in women. N Engl J Med. 1980;303:409–415.
124. Johannisson G. Studies on *Chlamydia trachomatis* as a cause of lower urogenital tract infection. Acta Dermatovener. 1981;93(Suppl).
125. Hillier SL, Martius J, Krohn M, et al. A case–control study of chorioamnionic infection and chorioamnionitis in prematurity. N Engl J Med. 1988;319:972–8.
126. Sweet RL, Landers DV, Walker C, et al. *Chlamydia trachomatis* infection and pregnancy outcome. Am J Obstet Gynecol. 1987;156:824–33.
127. Lamont RF, Taylor-Robinson D, Wigglesworth JS, et al. The role of mycoplasmas, ureaplasmas, and chlamydiae in the genital tract of women presenting in spontaneous early preterm labour. J Med Microbiol. 1987;24: 253–7.
128. Rowland GF, Forsey T, Moss TR, et al. Failure of in vitro fertilization and embryo replacement following infection with *Chlamydia trachomatis*. J In Vitro Fert Embryo Transfer. 1985;2:151–5.

129. Torode HW, Wheeler PA, Saunders DM, et al. The role of chlamydial antibodies in an in vitro fertilization program. Fertil Steril. 1987;48:987–90.
130. Paavonen J, Kiviat N, Koutsky L. Sexually transmitted diseases and genital and anal neoplasias. In: Holmes KK, Mårdh P-A, Sparling PF, et al., eds. Sexually Transmitted Diseases. 2nd ed. New York: McGraw-Hill; 1989.
131. Kiviat NB, Peterson M, Kinney-Thomas E, et al. Cytologic manifestations of cervical and vaginal infections. II. Confirmation of *Chlamydia trachomatis* infection by direct immunofluorescence using monoclonal antibodies. JAMA. 1985;253:997–1000.
132. Sanders LL, Harrison HR, Washington AE. Treatment of sexually transmitted chlamydial infections. JAMA. 1986;255:1750–6.
133. Stamm WE, Guinan ME, Johnson C, et al. Effect of treatment regimens for *Neisseria gonorrhoeae* on simultaneous infection with *Chlamydia trachomatis*. N Engl J Med. 1984;310:545–9.
134. Schachter J, Sweet RL, Grossman M, et al. Experience with the routine use of erythromycin for chlamydial infections in pregnancy. N Engl J Med. 1986;314:276–9.
135. MacDonald N, Bowie WR, Read S, eds. 1988 Canadian guidelines for the treatment of sexually transmitted diseases in neonates, children, adolescents and adults. Can Dis Weekly Rep 1988;14(Suppl 2):1–20.
136. Sweet RL, Schachter J, Robbie MO. Failure of beta-lactam antibiotics to eradicate *Chlamydia trachomatis* in the endometrium despite apparent clinical cure of acute salpingitis. JAMA. 1983;250:2641–5.
137. Cramer DW, Goldman MB, Schiff I, et al. The relationship of tubal infertility to barrier method and oral contraceptive use. JAMA. 1987;257:2446–50.
138. Rosenberg MJ, Rojanapithayakorn W, Feldblum PJ, et al. Effect of contraceptive sponge on chlamydial infection, gonorrhea, and candidiasis: A comparative clinical trial. JAMA. 1987;257:2308–12.
139. Nettleman MD, Jones RB, Roberts SC, et al. Cost-effectiveness of culturing for *Chlamydia trachomatis*: A study in a clinic for sexually transmitted diseases. Ann Intern Med. 1986;105:189–96.
140. Phillips RS, Aronson MD, Taylor WC, et al. Should tests for *Chlamydia trachomatis* cervical infection be done during routine gynecologic visits? An analysis of the costs of alternative strategies. Ann Intern Med. 1987;107:188–94.
141. Thelin I, Wennstrom A-M, Mardh P-A. Contact tracing in patients with genital chlamydial infections. Br J Vener Dis. 1980;56:259–62.
142. Katz BP, Danos CS, Quinn TS, et al. Efficiency and cost-effectiveness of field follow-up for patients with *Chlamydia trachomatis* infection in a sexually transmitted disease clinic. Sex Transm Dis. 1988;15:11–6.
143. Schachter J. Overview of *Chlamydia trachomatis* infection and the requirements for a vaccine. Rev Infect Dis. 1985;7:713–6.
144. Harrison HR, English MG, Lee CK, et al. *Chlamydia trachomatis* infant pneumonitis. Comparisons with matched controls and other infant pneumonitis. N Engl J Med. 1978;298:702–8.
145. Harrison HR. Chlamydial infection in neonates and children. In: Oriel D, Ridgway G, Schachter J, et al., eds. Chlamydial Infections. Cambridge: Cambridge University Press; 1986:283–92.
146. Stagno S, Brasfield DM, Brown MB, et al. Infant pneumonitis associated with cytomegalovirus, chlamydia, pneumocystis, and ureaplasma: A prospective study. Pediatrics. 1981;68:322–9.
147. Brasfield DM, Stagno S, Whitley RJ, et al. Infant pneumonitis associated with cytomegalovirus, *Chlamydia, Pneumocystis,* and *Ureaplasma:* Follow-up. Pediatrics. 1987;79:76–83.
148. Beem MO, Saxon E, Tipple MA. Treatment of chlamydial pneumonia of infancy. Pediatrics. 1979;63:198–203.
149. Hammerschlag MR, Chandler JW, Alexander ER, et al. Erythromycin ointment for ocular prophylaxis of neonatal chlamydial infection. JAMA. 1980;244:2291–3.
150. Black SB, Grossman M, Cles L. et al. Serologic evidence of chlamydial infection in children. J Pediatr. 1981;98:65–7.
151. Grayston JT, Wang S-P, Foy HM, et al. Seroepidemiology of *Chlamydia trachomatis* infection. In: Mårdh P-A, Holmes KK, Oriel JD, et al., eds. Chlamydial Infections. Amsterdam: Elsevier Biomedical; 1982:405–19.
152. Grayston JT, Kuo C-C, Wang S-P, et al. A new *Chlamydia psittaci* strain, TWAR, isolated in acute respiratory tract infections. N Engl J Med. 1986;315:161–8.
153. Komaroff AL, Aronson MD, Pass TM, et al. Serologic evidence of chlamydial and mycoplasmal pharyngitis in adults. Science. 1983;222:927–9.
154. Schachter J. Human *Chlamydia psittaci* infection. In: Oriel D, Ridgway G, Schachter J, et al., eds. Chlamydial infections. Cambridge, Cambridge University Press, 1986, 311–20.
155. Jones RB, Rabinovitch RA, Katz BP, et al. *Chlamydia trachomatis* in the pharynx and rectum of heterosexual patients at risk for genital infection. Ann Intern Med. 1985;102:757–62.
156. Mardh P-A, Ursing B, Sandgren E. Lack of evidence for an association between infection with *Chlamydia trachomatis* and Crohn's disease, as indicated by microimmunofluorescence antibody tests. Acta Pathol Microbiol Scand [B]. 1980;88:57–9.
157. Myhre EB, Mardh P-A. *Chlamydia trachomatis* infection in a patient with meningoencephalitis. N Engl J Med. 1981;304:910.
158. Grayston JT, Mordhorst CH, Wang S-P. Childhood myocarditis associated with *Chlamydia trachomatis* infection. JAMA. 1981;246:2823–7.
159. van der Bel-Kahn JM, Watanakunakorn C, Menefee MG, et al. *Chlamydia trachomatis* endocarditis. Am Heart J. 1978;95:627–36.
160. Komaroff AL, Aronson MD, Schachter J. *Chlamydia trachomatis* in adults with community-acquired pneumonia. JAMA. 1981;245:1319–22.
161. Tack KJ, Peterson PK, Rasp FL, et al. Isolation of *Chlamydia trachomatis* from the lower respiratory tract of adults. Lancet. 1980;1:116–20.
162. Bernstein DI, Hubbard T, Wenman WM, et al. Mediastinal and supraclavicular lymphadenitis and pneumonitis due to *Chlamydia trachomatis* serovars L_1 and L_2. N Engl J Med. 1984;311:1543–6.

159. CHLAMYDIA PSITTACI (PSITTACOSIS)

WILLIAM SCHAFFNER

Psittacosis (parrot fever) is an infectious disease of birds that is transmissible to humans. Although first described in association with parrots and parakeets, it is now well recognized in many avian species. For this reason some authors prefer the more general designation *ornithosis*, but the colorful term *psittacosis* is securely rooted in both the literature and clinical parlance.

HISTORY

Ritter in Switzerland described several cases of unusual pneumonia associated with exposure to tropical birds in 1879. Morange in Paris investigated an outbreak in 1894 and concluded that parrots were the source of infection. He named the illness after the Greek word for that bird, *psittakos*. The disease occurred only rarely in this country and Europe until the ownership of pet tropical birds became fashionable. Outbreaks in many countries occurred in 1929–1930 after the large-scale importation of infected South American birds to Europe and the United States as vividly described by Meyer.[1] Bedson isolated the filterable agent from human and avian tissues in 1930 while investigating an epidemic at the London Zoo. Rivers and his colleagues studied the infection in laboratory animals and showed that the probable route of human infection was by the upper respiratory tract due to the inhalation of dried excreta of birds shedding the agent. Burnet investigated the ecology of the infection in wild bird species in Australia and demonstrated that fledglings acquired infection in the nest from asymptomatic parent birds.

THE PATHOGEN

Chlamydia psittaci is an obligate intracellular parasite whose genome contains both DNA and RNA. The agent is capable of limited independent metabolism and has a cell wall. Reproduction is by growth and binary fission, which can be inhibited by certain antibiotics. It may be seen in cells as a large cytoplasmic inclusion (0.3–1.0 μm in diameter) that is glycogen-negative. The special mixture of viral and bacterial properties that charaterize *Chlamydia* has led to both taxonomic and terminologic confusion. Long classified as viruses, *Chlamydia* organisms now are considered specialized bacteria.

EPIDEMIOLOGY

The distribution of psittacosis is worldwide. Virtually any species of bird can serve as host for the organism. Psittacine birds are considered the major reservoir, but human cases have been associated with canaries, pigeons, sparrows, ducks, cockatiels, and occasionally mammals. Fowl, especially turkeys, recently have been the source of several outbreaks of disease among employees of poultry processing plants.

Psittacosis in humans is usually a sporadic disease[2]; 40–60 cases are reported annually in the United States. Owners of pet birds constitute approximately one-half of the cases. The disease must be considered an occupational hazard of pet shop employees, pigeon fanciers, zoo workers, veterinarians, and others who work with birds. In recent years outbreaks of psittacosis have occurred only in turkey processing plants, particularly among workers who eviscerated carcasses and those who killed birds and removed the feathers.

Three factors are thought to have contributed to the striking decline in cases over the past two decades: (*1*) the use of tetracycline-mediated poultry feed, (*2*) the requirement that commercially imported psittacine birds be medicated for 30 days before entry into this country, and (*3*) the striking growth of the domestic parakeet-breeding industry. Although medication may not eliminate infection in birds completely, it greatly reduces transmission of the agent. Domestic and imported birds are often comingled in commerce. Because birds rapidly become infectious under such conditions of crowding and stress, there is no assurance that domestic birds are psittacosis free. The disease is seemingly more common in Great Britain where budgerigars are favored cage birds and importation regulations are more lenient.

Chlamydia psittaci is present in the blood, tissues (especially the liver, spleen, and kidneys), excreta, and feathers of infected birds. Birds may be obviously ill and die of the infection but more often manifest only minor symptoms such as anorexia, diarrhea, lethargy, and ruffled feathers, thus bringing the concerned owner into closer contact with the bird. Asymptomatic birds and birds that have recovered from infection may shed the agent for months.

Humans usually are infected via the airborne route by the inhalation of dried bird excreta in which the agent can survive for long periods. Handling contaminated plumage or tissues also has led to infection as have bird bites. Mouth-to-beak intimacies have resulted in transmission of the agent. Person-to-person spread is very rare but is said to result in more severe disease. Whether this is due to strain virulence, a dose effect, or chlamydia adaptation through human "passage" remains speculative. Close or prolonged contact with birds is not necessary for the acquisition of infection. Indeed, cases have been recorded where the patient had only momentary contact with an environment in which an infected bird had been present previously. Such fleeting exposures may account for the 20 percent of patients with psittacosis who can provide no history of bird contact. There is no record of infection acquired by handling dressed, eviscerated birds or eating poultry products or game birds. Second cases in humans, especially pet shop employees, have been described.

PATHOGENESIS

Chlamydia psittaci produces systemic disease in humans, but the lung is the organ involved most prominently. After entering the body via the respiratory tract, the organism is transported to the reticuloendothelial cells of the liver and spleen. It replicates in these sites and then invades the lung and other organs by hematogenous seeding. This two-stage process accounts for the rather long incubation interval. This is contrasted with the short incubation periods of certain respiratory pathogens such as the influenza virus that replicate directly at the site of implantation on the respiratory mucosa.

The inflammatory response is predominantly lymphocytic and occurs in both the alveolar and interstitial spaces, particularly in the dependent lobes. These areas become edematous, thickened, and necrotic. Small hemorrhages may occur, which accounts for the occasional hemoptysis seen clinically. Mucus plugs of bronchioles occur and contribute to the cyanosis and anoxia of severe illness. Macrophages containing cytoplasmic inclusions are characteristic of psittacosis. The epithelium of the bronchial tree usually remains intact. Enlargement of hilar nodes, spleen, and liver may be present, with focal necrosis within the latter organs. In fatal cases, changes in the heart, pericardium, meninges, brain, and adrenals also have been noted.

CLINICAL MANIFESTATIONS

The clinical course of psittacotic infection can vary widely.[3–5] The incubation period ranges from 7 to 15 days or even longer. The disease often starts suddenly with chills and high fever (38–40.5°C), but it may be ushered in over a period of 2–4 days with gradually increasing fever and malaise. As with certain other intracellular infections (e.g., brucellosis, typhoid) the pulse rate may be slow relative to the height of the fever. Headache is a quite constant symptom; severe and usually diffuse, it is often among the patient's chief complaints. Malaise, anorexia, and painful myalgias (particularly of the back and neck) and arthralgias are common. A pale macular rash (Horder spots) reminiscent of the rose spots of typhoid fever has been seen.

A persistent cough is prominent. Often dry and hacking, it may be productive of small amounts of mucoid sputum with occasional blood streaking. The cough may be present from the onset or appear only several days into the course of illness. Pleuritic pain is rare. The respiratory rate is elevated proportional to the severity of the disease; dyspnea and cyanosis reflect extensive pulmonary involvement.

Changes in mentation may occur toward the end of the first week of disease and usually are associated with hypoxia. Lethargy, confusion, and delirium may progress to stupor and coma. A minority of the patients have gastrointestinal complaints including nausea, vomiting, abdominal bloating, and diarrhea. Jaundice is seen only in the severely ill. Some patients also have a mild sore throat or epistaxis.

The physical findings may belie the extent of pulmonary involvement revealed by chest x-ray films. Fine, crepitant rales may be heard over localized areas of the lower lung fields. The classic percussion and auscultatory changes indicative of true consolidation are not present in most patients but do occur occasionally.[3–5] Pleural and pleuropericardial friction rubs and pleural effusions may be present. Nontender hepatomegaly occurs frequently. Palpable splenomegaly has been seen in 10–70 percent of patients. When splenomegaly is present in a patient with a puzzling pneumonitis, the diagnosis of psittacosis should be entertained.

Secondary bacterial infections are rare and usually are nosocomial infections complicating the technology of treating acute pulmonary insufficiency in the seriously ill.

LABORATORY FINDINGS

Routine laboratory studies are of scant assistance in establishing the diagnosis. The white blood cell count is often within the normal range, but modest leukopenia or leukocytosis may occur. A few patients develop anemia during the course of illness. Proteinuria is often detected when the illness is most acute. Although hepatomegaly is rather common, disturbances of liver function are not. The cerebrospinal fluid is usually normal. Microscopic examination of sputum shows no organisms and few leukocytes.

Roentgenographic findings are as variable as are the clinical manifestations (Fig. 1). They usually consist of soft patchy infiltrates radiating out from the hilum, particularly in the lower lung fields. However, the lesions may appear atelectatic, miliary, or nodular. It is important to recognize that the classic infiltrates of lobar consolidation usually attributed to pyogenic infection have been recognized in psittacosis[3,4] and should not "rule out" the diagnosis.

The diagnosis can be confirmed either by the isolation of *C. psittaci* or by serologic studies. Isolation is hazardous to laboratory personnel, so this service is available only from specialized laboratories. Specimens from humans or birds may be

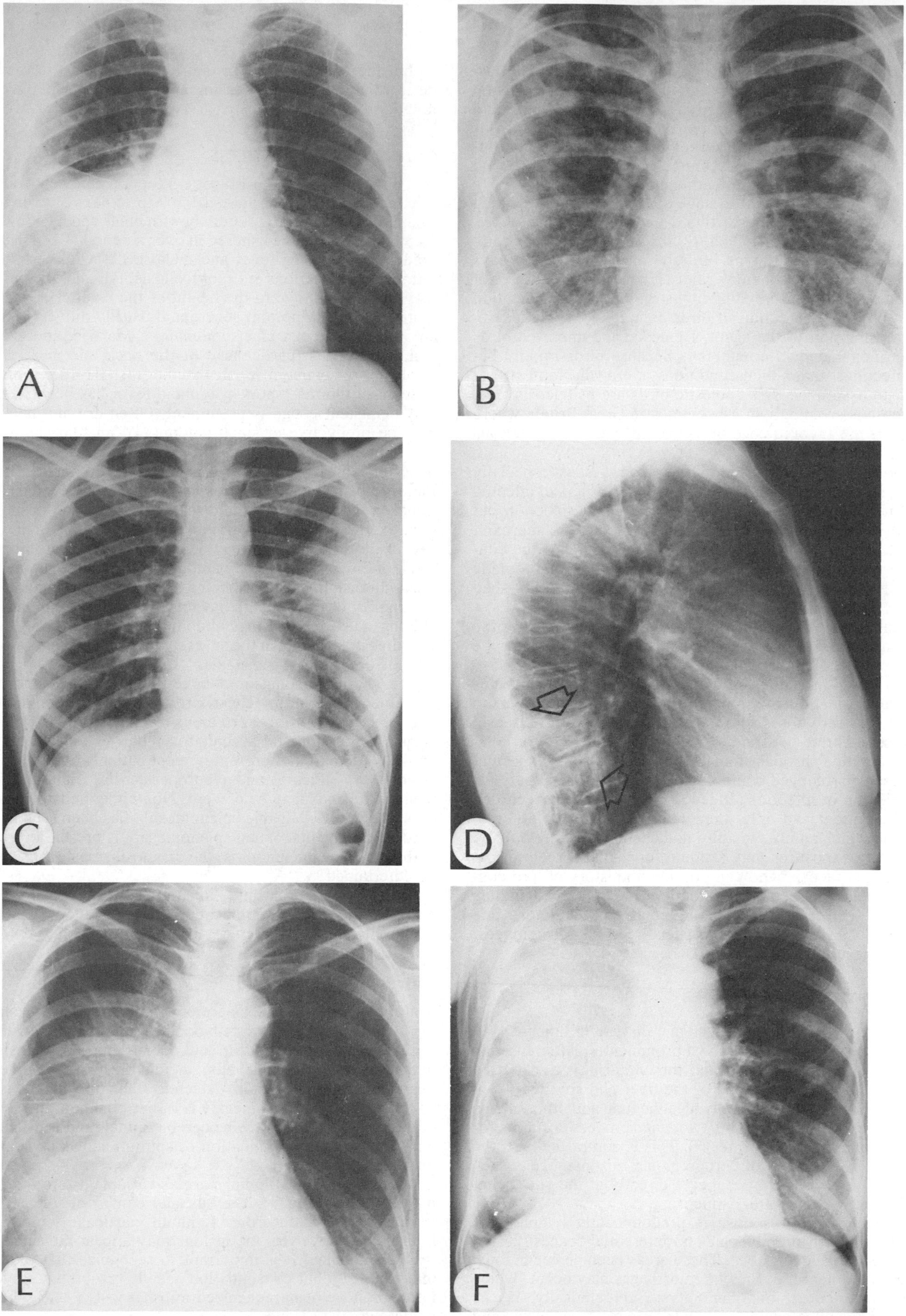

FIG. 1. Various x-ray film presentations of psittacosis. (**A**) Right middle-lobe consolidation in a pet shop employee. There was a marked inspiratory lag of the right hemithorax. (**B**) A patchy interstitial infiltrate symmetrically distributed throughout both lung fields, especially the lower portions. Only a few dry late inspiratory rales were heard on auscultation. (**C**) Infiltrate in the superior segment of the left lower lobe. A pleuropericardial friction rub was heard. (**D**) Mottled infiltrates in the posterior segments of the right lower lobe. There was dullness to percussion over this area with diminished breath sounds and rales. (E) Right lower-lobe consolidation that progressed to involve the entire right lung (F) in a profoundly ill patient.

submitted to the Centers for Disease Control, Atlanta, Georgia. Serologic diagnosis is the usual method used. A fourfold rise in complement-fixing antibodies in acute and convalescent serum specimens is diagnostic. Antibody titers generally rise by the end of the second week of illness. A single titer of 1:32 in a patient with a compatible illness is presumptive evidence of psittacosis. Early treatment with tetracycline can delay the appearance of antibody for several weeks. Thus, final confirmation of the diagnosis may depend on serum specimens drawn during follow-up visits after the patient has been discharged from the hospital. False-positive titer rises are uncommon but have occurred in some patients with legionnaires' disease.

DIFFERENTIAL DIAGNOSIS

Because of its varying clinical presentation, the diagnosis of psittacosis can be difficult. All patients with pneumonitis should be queried about contact with birds, for it may be the major clue to the diagnosis. Repeated questioning of the patient and family may be necessary to elicit this information. Nevertheless, approximatelly 20 percent of patients cannot recall any prior contact with birds. The syndrome of pneumonia with a persistent high fever, unusually severe headache, myalgia, and a pulse–temperature dissociation should suggest the diagnosis. When present, splenomegaly is a helpful finding. Infectious disease consultants often are requested to see patients with pneumonia who have not responded to several days of penicillin therapy (''penicillin-resistant'' pneumonia). In addition to psittacosis, a short list of diseases that can produce this syndrome includes *Mycoplasma* infection, tularemia, tuberculosis, fungal infection, legionnaires' disease, and bacterial infection behind a bronchial obstruction. If pulmonic symptoms are less prominent, psittacosis can be confused with brucellosis, infectious mononucleosis, hepatitis, and disseminated tuberculosis among others.

TREATMENT

The tetracyclines are considered the most effective antimicrobial agents. Therapy with 2–3 g of tetracycline daily usually results in improvement within 48–72 hours, although the response may be slow. Thus, a ''therapeutic trial'' with tetracycline cannot be relied on as a means of supporting a clinical impression of psittacosis. Relapses are common,[6] and treatment should be continued for 10 days to 2 weeks after defervescence to minimize recurrence.

The prognosis is good. Case fatality ratios of 20–40 percent were recorded before the era of antimicrobial therapy; the current figure is about 1 percent. All cases should be reported promptly to local public health authorities.

ENDOCARDITIS

Physicians from the British Isles have reported destructive aortic and mitral valve endocarditis caused by *C. psittaci*[7]; rare cases have been reported from the United States.[8] The diagnosis was established by serologic means as well as by histopathologic evidence of *C. psittaci* infection found in the heart valves removed at surgery or autopsy. Most of the patients have had evidence of rheumatic heart disease or congenital valvular abnormality, but one patient without prior cardiac disease has been reported. Although these findings should be regarded as preliminary, patients with suspected endocarditis and persistently negative blood cultures might benefit from a serologic test for *C. psittaci* antibody.

REFERENCES

1. Meyer KF. The ecology of psittacosis and ornithosis. Medicine (Baltimore). 1942;21:175–206.
2. Potter ME, Kaufmann AK, Plikaytis BD. Psittacosis in the United States 1979. CDC Surveillance Summaries. MMWR. 1983;32(Suppl 1):27–31.
3. Seibert RH, Jordan WS, Dingle JH. Clinical variations in the diagnosis of psittacosis. N Engl J Med. 1956;254:925–30.
4. Schaffner W, Drutz DJ, Duncan GW, et al. The clinical spectrum of endemic psittacosis. Arch Intern Med. 1967;119:433–43.
5. Yung AP, Grayson ML. Psittacosis—a review of 135 cases. Med J Aust. 1988;148:228–33.
6. Bowman P, Wilt JC, Sayed H. Chronicity and recurrence of psittacosis. Can J Pub Health 1973;64:167–73.
7. Jariwalla AG, Davies BH, White J. Infective endocarditis complicating psittacosis: Response to rifampin. Br Med J. 1980;280:155.
8. Jones RB, Priest JB, Kuo C. Subacute chalmydial endocarditis. JAMA. 1982;247:655–8.

160. TWAR

WILLIAM SCHAFFNER

TWAR is a recently identified *Chlamydia* that causes both upper and lower respiratory tract infection including pneumonia. Its unusual designation was constructed by combining the laboratory identifiers from the first two isolates, TW-183 and AR-39. A proposal has been made to give the organism the formal name of *Chlamydia pneumoniae*.

HISTORY

The original strain (TW-183) was isolated in 1965 from the eye of a child in Taiwan with a trachoma-like illness. The first isolate from the respiratory tract (AR-39) was from the pharynx of a college student in the United States with an upper respiratory infection. TWAR is fastidious and difficult to isolate in tissue culture. The use of fluorescein-conjugated TWAR monoclonal antibody to identify TWAR inclusions in cell culture has substantially enhanced investigations of the role of this organism in disease.

THE PATHOGEN

TWAR now is recognized as a *Chlamydia* strain that is distinct from both *C. trachomatis* and *C. psittaci*. When TWAR was first isolated, the morphology of the characteristic intracytoplasmic inclusions was relied upon to differentiate between the chlamydial species. The TWAR inclusions were glycogen-negative and seemed to resemble those of *C. psittaci*; for a time the organism was thought to be a variant strain of that agent. Subsequently, electron microscopic studies have shown that TWAR elementary bodies are typically pear shaped, quite different from those of other *Chlamydia*. TWAR strains are also immunologically distinct and lack cross-reactivity when exposed to monoclonal antibodies to strains of *C. trachomatis* and *C. psittaci*. Furthermore, molecular techniques have confirmed the distinctiveness of TWAR. Unlike all *C. trachomatis* strains and most strains of *C. psittaci*, plasmid DNA has not been found in TWAR, restriction endonuclease patterns were not shared, and there was no substantial DNA homology between TWAR and other *Chlamydia*.[1]

EPIDEMIOLOGY

No bird or animal reservoirs for TWAR have been found. Spread appears to be from person to person, although the mode of transmission is not yet known. Serologic studies in several countries have shown that antibody prevalence is low during childhood but rises rapidly during the teenage years. In adults, the prevalence of TWAR antibody ranges from 25 to over 50 percent. The persistence of antibody into old age raises the possibility of repeated infection with periodic boosts in antibody. Men generally exhibit a higher prevalence of antibody than do women.

Although the first isolate of TWAR was from a conjunctival swab, no further association with ocular disease has been found. Retrospective serologic surveys have shown that TWAR was the major cause of several outbreaks of puzzling pneumonia among both military recruit and civilian populations in Scandinavia. Included among these was an epidemic of "ornithosis" that had swept across northern Europe in the early 1980s.[2]

Such retrospective surveys soon were followed by prospective investigations of the role of TWAR in respiratory infections among college students in the state of Washington[3] as well as community-acquired pneumonia in Nova Scotia.[4] These observations demonstrated that TWAR could produce infections with a wide spectrum of symptoms.

A provocative recent report has demonstrated greater levels of TWAR antibody among patients with acute myocardial infarction and chronic coronary heart disease than among a comparable group of healthy persons.[5] These preliminary results are sure to stimulate further inquiry into the possible role of TWAR in coronary heart disease.

PATHOGENESIS

Knowledge of the pathogenesis of TWAR infections still is almost nonexistent because the organism has only recently been identified. There are, as yet, no animal models of infection, and the generally mild nature of the illness has precluded autopsy studies.

CLINICAL MANIFESTATIONS

TWAR can cause a variety of relatively mild respiratory infections that lack any distinctive clinical presentation. To date, pneumonia has been the illness most often associated with TWAR infection. Among college students, TWAR caused 13 percent of clinically diagnosed pneumonias[3]; among older adults in Nova Scotia, 6 percent of community-acquired pneumonitis was attributed to TWAR.[4] Fever, cough, and sore throat are common symptoms. A few patients have had a biphasic illness; an episode of pharyngitis and laryngitis that resolves spontaneously followed in 2 or 3 weeks by bronchitis and pneumonia.

Many pneumonic illnesses in young adults are sufficiently mild that the patients are not hospitalized. Elderly adults may become more gravely ill, but the severity is accounted for more by their underlying disease than by the TWAR pneumonia.

Rales are almost invariably present; signs of consolidation are less common. Chest x-ray films usually reveal modest-sized single pneumonic infiltrates.

LABORATORY FINDINGS

The laboratory is of little help in establishing a diagnosis. Young people with mild pneumonia usually have a normal white blood cell and differential counts; older adults with more severe disease are more likely to have a leukocytosis. The erythrocyte sedimentation rate is predictably elevated. Two patterns of TWAR antibody response occur. In the first, thought to represent primary infection, complement fixation antibody appears early, followed in 10 days to a month by IgM antibody measured by the microimmunofluorescence test. IgG usually does not appear before 6 weeks after the illness. The second pattern is attributed to reinfection. Complement-fixing antibody does not appear, IgM antibody occurs at low titers if at all, and IgG antibody appears more promptly after infection. At present these TWAR-specific antibody tests are performed only in research laboratories.

DIFFERENTIAL DIAGNOSIS

Because the clinical syndrome of pneumonitis caused by TWAR is not distinctive, the array of agents producing generally mild pneumonia is included in the differential diagnosis. Among young adults, the most common pathogen producing a similar illness is *Mycoplasma pneumoniae*.

TREATMENT

No studies of antibiotic therapy for TWAR infections have been performed. Limited clinical experience suggests that erythromycin may not be adequate and results in continuing symptoms or relapses. Based on experience with other *Chlamydia* infections, tetracycline, 2 g/day for 10 to 14 days, is suggested.

REFERENCES

1. Campbell LA, Kuo C-C, Grayston JT. Characterization of the new *Chlamydia* agent, TWAR, as a unique organism by restriction endonuclease analysis and DNA-DNA hybridization. J Clin Microbiol. 1987;26:1911–6.
2. Mordhorst CH, Wang SP, Grayston JT. Epidemic "ornithosis" and TWAR infection, Denmark 1976–85. In: Oriel D, Ridgway G, Schachter J, et al., eds., Chlamydial Infections. Cambridge, England: Cambridge University Press; 1986;325–8.
3. Grayston JT, Kuo C-C, Wang S-P, et al. A new *Chlamydia psittaci* strain, TWAR, isolated in acute respiratory tract infections. N Engl J Med. 1986;315:161–8.
4. Marrie TJ, Grayston JT, Wang S-P, et al. Pneumonia associated with the TWAR strain of *Chlamydia*. Ann Intern Med. 1987;106:507–11.
5. Saikku P, Leinonen M, Mattila K, et al. Serological evidence of an association of a novel chlamydia, TWAR, with chronic coronary heart disease and acute myocardial infarction. Lancet. 1988;2:983–6.

SECTION C. MYCOPLASMA DISEASES

161. INTRODUCTION

ROBERT B. COUCH

The mycoplasmas are the smallest free-living organisms. They are distinct from true bacteria in lacking a cell wall and the ability to synthesize cell wall precursors; they are distinct from viruses in their ability to grow on cell-free media. The mycoplasmas are ubiquitous as saprophytes and/or parasites of the animal and plant kingdom. A variety of plant and animal diseases are caused by the mycoplasmas, and many of the organisms and diseases have served as models for evaluating the role of mycoplasmas in a variety of human diseases of uncertain etiology. However, only *Mycoplasma pneumoniae, Ureaplasma urealyticum*, and *Mycoplasma hominis* have been clearly shown to be pathogenic for humans. *Mycoplasma pneumoniae* is a major cause of acute respiratory disease including pneumonia, and it may also be a significant cause of disease at other sites. *Ureaplasma urealyticum, M. hominis*, and possibly *Mycoplasma genitalium* cause urogenital tract disease.

HISTORY

The first mycoplasma was isolated by Nocard and Roux[1] from cattle with contagious bovine pleuropneumonia in 1898. Two years later Dujardin-Beaumetz[2] described the colonial morphologic feature that is considered typical of these organisms, that is, a tendency to grow down into agar and produce a dark center and light periphery—the so-called fried egg appearance. Using gradacol filters, Elford[3] in 1929 showed the existence of viable 125 to 150 nm organisms. At that time size was a major criterion for viruses, so many considered the organism to be a virus despite its ability to grow on artificial media.

Because the original isolation of a mycoplasma was from bovine pleuropneumonia, the organism was called the *pleuropneumonia organism*, and subsequent isolations of organisms with similar colonial morphologic features from a variety of animals were designated pleuropneumonia-like organisms (PPLO). Classification of these organisms has now been systematized.[4] They are called *mycoplasmas* and have been placed in the class Mollicutes. Some confusion has arisen by considering colonial morphologic features as characteristic since most L-phase variants of bacteria produce colonies that exhibit the "fried egg" appearance. Such organisms are not considered mycoplasmas. It is tempting to speculate whether the mycoplasmas represent the natural evolutionary occurrence of stable L-phase variants of bacteria, and some evidence to support such an origin has been provided.[5]

Mycoplasmas have been isolated from almost all animals, from a variety of environmental circumstances, and from plants.[4] The first isolate of a mycoplasma from humans was reported by Dienes and Edsall in 1937.[6] The isolate was from a Bartholin's gland abscess. Subsequent contemporary reports of the isolation of mycoplasmas from a variety of urogenital sites and diseases failed to prove any were causally related to a human disease. In 1954 Shepard[7] described the isolation of mycoplasmas that produced "tiny colonies" on agar from men with nongonococcal urethritis. These organisms were shown to differ from the other mycoplasmas in their ability to metabolize urea and have been placed in a separate genus, *Ureaplasma*.

The first clearly proven instance of a mycoplasma as the cause of a human disease was provided by Chanock and colleagues in a series of reports[8–12] that culminated in the isolation of a mycoplasma that was shown to cause most cases of atypical pneumonia in military recruits. The organism was named *Mycoplasma pneumoniae*[13] and was subsequently shown to be a significant cause of respiratory disease in school-age children as well.

TAXONOMY AND PROPERTIES

The mycoplasmas are classified under the class Mollicutes (soft skin).[4] The major properties of the class Mollicutes, order Mycoplasmatales, are shown in Table 1. The taxonomy of the class is shown in Table 2, where only the human species are listed.

The mycoplasmas differ in some properties from true bacteria but are markedly different from viruses. It is not inappropriate to think of them as small gram-negative bacteria with no cell wall. Most are facultative anaerobes and divide by binary fission. Division of the genome and cytoplasm may be synchron-

TABLE 1. Major Properties of the Mycoplasmatales

Procaryotic
Small (200 nm) and pleomorphic
Small genome (500–1000 kD)
Low guanine + cytosine content (usually 25–34 mol/dl)
Bounded by single triple-layered membrane
Gram-negative
Susceptible to lipolytic agents
Grow on artificial media
Metabolism is mainly fermentative
Most are facultative anaerobes
Divide by binary fission
Resistant to penicillin
Susceptible to antibody

TABLE 2. Taxonomy of the Mycoplasmas

Taxonomic Category	*Primary Distinguishing Feature*
Class: Mollicutes	Procaryotic cells bound by a single membrane
Order: Mycoplasmatales	Procaryotic cells bound by a single membrane
Family: Mycoplasmataceae	Require sterol for growth
Genus: *Mycoplasma*	Most metabolize glucose or arginine
Species (human):	Serologic differences
M. pneumoniae	
M. salivarium	
M. orale	
M. buccale	
M. faucium	
M. lipophilum	
M. primatum	
M. fermentans	
M. hominis	
M. genitalium	
Genus: *Ureaplasma*	Metabolize urea
Species (human):	Only one human species described
U. urealyticum	
Family: Acholeplasmataceae	Do not require sterol for growth
Genus: *Acholeplasma*	Do not require sterol for growth
Species (human): *A. laidlawii*	
Family: Spiroplasmataceae	Helical; require sterol for growth
Genus: *Spiroplasma*	Helical; require sterol for growth
Species (human): None	
Family: Anaeroplasmataceae	Strict anaerobes
Genus: *Anaeroplasma*	Some require sterol for growth
Species (human): None	

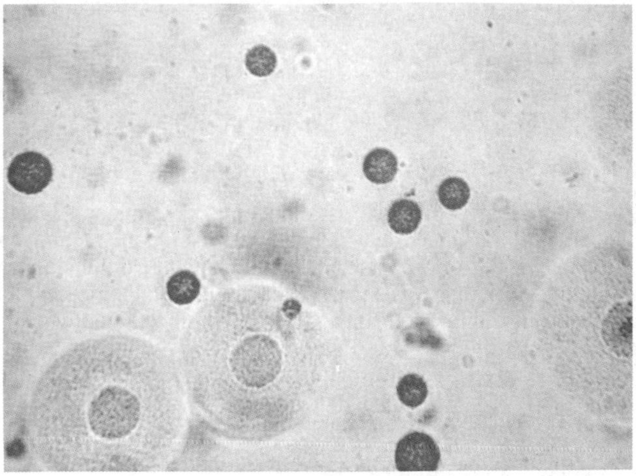

FIG. 1. Mixture of *M. hominis* and *U. urealyticum* colonies on differential agar medium A7: unstained, natural appearance. Colonies of *U. urealyticum* are unmistakably identified by their deep golden brown color on this A7 medium, whereas colonies of *M. hominis* are unreactive. (×100) (From Shepard et al.,[15] with permission.)

ous, so development of multinucleate filaments that transform into chains of cocci may precede the appearance of single cells.[5] The genome of mycoplasmas and ureaplasmas is about 500 kD, while those of acholeplasmas and spiroplasmas are about 1000 kD.[14] These are the smallest genomes described for self-replicating microorganisms. They are usually nonmotile, and no resting stage is known. Growth is inhibited by antibody, and because they lack a cell wall, they are resistant to cell wall-active antibiotics such as the penicillins. Because of the plasticity of the mycoplasmas, they all have a tendency to grow down into solid media and produce the characteristic "fried egg" appearance. Colonies shown in Figure 1 depict the typical appearance of a "large-colony" mycoplasma and that of a "tiny-colony" (T-strain) mycoplasma. Mature large colonies are generally 100–300 μm in diameter, and the "tiny" colonies are usually 10–25 μm in diameter, although colonies of both types of mycoplasmas exhibit a considerably wider variation in size with different cultural conditions. The mycoplasmas require sterols for growth, and most metabolize glucose or arginine.

Species of the genus *Mycoplasma* were described by serologic methods, although they are best distinguished by analyses of DNA homology.[5,16] There are ten accepted human species, and only *M. pneumoniae* has been clearly proved to produce disease in humans (Chapter 161). *Mycoplasma salivarium* and *Mycoplasma orale* are common inhabitants of the oropharynx, particularly if oral hygiene is poor. *Mycoplasma buccale, Mycoplasma faucium, Mycoplasma primatum*, and *Mycoplasma lipophilum* are uncommon inhabitants of the oropharynx, and *Mycoplasma fermentans* has on rare occasions been recovered from the oropharynx and from the genital tract. *Mycoplasma hominis* causes disease on occasion and like *U. urealyticum* is a genital mycoplasma (Chapter 163). *Mycoplasma genitalium* is a recently described genital mycoplasma that may cause nonspecific urethritis (Chapter 163).

The genus *Ureaplasma* currently contains only one species that is a human pathogen, *U. urealyticum* (Chaper 163), but there are many serotypes. These organisms do not metabolize either glucose or arginine but do metabolize urea.

REFERENCES

1. Nocard E, Roux ER. Le microbe de la péripneumoniae. Ann Inst Pasteur (Paris). 1898;12:240.
2. Dujardin-Beaumetz E. Le microbe de la péripneumonie et sa culture, (thesis). Paris, 1900.
3. Elford WJ. Ultrafiltration methods and their application in bacteriological and pathological studies. Br J Exp Pathol. 1929;10:126.
4. Freundt EA. The Mycoplasmas. In Buchanan RE, Gibbons NE, eds. Bergey's Manual of Determinative Bacteriology. 8th ed. Baltimore: Williams & Wilkins; 1974:929.
5. Razin S. Molecular biology and genetics of mycoplasmas (Mollicutes). Microb Rev. 1985;49:419.
6. Dienes L, Edsall G. Observations on L-organisms of Klieneberger. Proc Soc Exp Biol Med. 1937;36:740.
7. Shepard MC. The recovery of pleuropneumonia-like organisms from Negro men with and without nongonococcal urethritis. Am J Syph. 1954;38:113.
8. Chanock RM, Mufson MA, Bloom HH, et al. Eaton agent pneumonia. JAMA. 1961;175:213.
9. Kingston JR, Chanock RM, Mufson MA, et al. Eaton agent pneumonia. JAMA. 1961;176:118.
10. Mufson MA, Manko MA, Kingston JR, et al. Eaton agent pneumonia—clinical features. JAMA. 1961;178:369.
11. Rifkind D, Chanock R, Kravetz H, et al. Ear involvement (myringitis) and primary atypical pneumonia following inoculation of volunteers with Eaton agent. Am Rev Respir Dis. 1962;35:479.
12. Chanock RM, Hayflick L, Barile MF. Growth on artificial medium of an agent associated with atypical pneumonia and its identification as a PPLO. Proc Natl Acad Sci USA. 1962;48:41.
13. Chanock RM, Dienes H, Eaton MD, et al. *Mycoplasma pneumoniae*: Proposed nomenclature for atypical pneumonia organism (Eaton agent). Science. 1963;140:662.
14. Razin S, Barile MF, Harasawa R, et al. Characterization of the *Mycoplasma* genome. Yale J Biol Med. 1983;56:357.
15. Shepard MC, Lunceford CD. Differential agar medium (A7) for identification of *Ureaplasma urealyticum* (human T mycoplasmas) in primary cultures of clinical material. J Clin Microbiol. 1976;3:613.
16. Gobel UB, Geiser A, Stanbridge EJ. Oligonucleotide probes complementary to variable regions of ribosomal RNA discriminate between *Mycoplasma* species. J Gen Microbiol. 1987;133:1969.

BIBLIOGRAPHY

Barile MF, Razin S, Smith PF. eds. Current topics in mycoplasmology. Rev Infect Dis. 1982;4(Suppl):1–279.

Barile MF, Razin S, Tully JG, et al., eds. Cell biology. In: The Mycoplasmas. v. 1. Human and animal mycoplasma. In: The Mycoplasmas. v. 2. New York: Academic Press; 1979.

Barile MF, Razin S, Tully JG, et al., eds. Mycoplasma pathogenicity. The Mycoplasmas. v. 4. New York: Academic Press; 1985.

Buchanan RE, Gibbons NE. eds. Bergey's Manual of Determinative Bacteriology. 8th ed. Baltimore: Williams & Wilkins; 1984.

Maramorosch K. ed. Mycoplasma and mycoplasma-like agents of human, animal, and plant diseases. Ann NY Acad Sci. 1973;225:1.

Razin S, Tully JG. eds. Mycoplasma characteristics. In: Methods in Mycoplasmology. v. 1. Diagnostic Mycoplasmology. In: Methods in Mycoplasmology. v. 2. New York: Academic Press; 1983.

Workshop on the Mycoplasmatales as Agents of Disease: National Institutes of Health, Bethesda MD, March 29–30, 1971. J Infect Dis. 1973;127(Suppl):1–92.

162. MYCOPLASMA PNEUMONIAE (PRIMARY ATYPICAL PNEUMONIA)

ROBERT B. COUCH

Mycoplasma pneumoniae is a pathogen of humans that primarily produces acute respiratory disease including pneumonia. Serious disease is seen principally in older children and young adults, although milder disease occurs in infants and small children. It occurs sporadically in all seasons and in epidemics that may last months or years. Spread involves close contact and is extensive in families. Pneumonia responds to treatment with the tetracyclines and erythromycin. Recovery is the rule, although convalescence may be prolonged.

HISTORY

In 1938, Reimann[1] applied the name *primary atypical pneumonia* to a group of pneumonias unlike the typical pneumonias caused by known microorganisms. The fortuitous identification of high titers of cold hemagglutinins in the sera of patients with this disease in 1943[2] provided a diagnostic test for the syndrome. At a later time the occurrence of agglutinins for the MG streptococcus was also noted.

During and after World War II, the Armed Forces Commission on Acute Respiratory Disease defined many of the clinical features of the disease.[3] The transmission of the disease to healthy volunteers by filtered secretions reproduced the disease and led to the opinion that atypical pneumonia was caused by a virus. In 1944 Eaton and associates[4] reported the production of pneumonia in cotton rats and hamsters with filtered secretions from naturally occurring cases of the disease and the prevention of the disease with prior administration of convalescent antiserum.

In 1957 Liu[5] used immunofluorescence to show the growth and localization of Eaton's agent on the surface of the bronchial epithelium of the chick embryo. Using the test described by Liu, Chanock and associates[6] presented definitive evidence in 1961 that Eaton's agent caused a majority of nonbacterial pneumonias and practically all cold agglutinin-positive pneumonias in military recruits. Clyde and Goodburn and Marmion[7,8] had earlier shown the bronchial epithelial fluorescence to be attributable to small coccobacillary bodies and suggested Eaton's agent might be a mycoplasma, but Chanock and colleagues[9] reported the successful growth of the agent on agar in 1962, which provided definitive proof that the organism was a mycoplasma.

Koch's postulates for a role in human respiratory disease were fulfilled by studies in volunteers by Rifkind et al.,[10] and numerous subsequent reports have confirmed the significance of *M. pneumoniae* as a cause of disease in humans.

DESCRIPTION OF THE PATHOGEN

Properties

Mycoplasma pneumoniae possesses all the properties listed for Mycoplasmatales (Chapter 161, Table 1) except that it is not a facultative anaerobe. Additional properties of *M. pneumoniae* are shown in Table 1. The organism is filamentous, about 10 × 200 nm in size,[11] and somewhat motile.[12] One end of the filamentous form exhibits an electron-dense core that represents the attachment site to host cell membranes.[13] Analysis of microorganism proteins has indicated that attachment is mediated by a 168,000 molecular weight (MW) protein (P1).[14–16] It appears to be contained in surface projections morphologically similar to viral peplomers.[14] Attachment to host cell membranes is via these P1-containing projections and neuraminic acid-containing glycoproteins at the cell membrane surface.[17–20] The presence of this receptor on red blood cells accounts for the phenomenon of hemadsorption to colonies on agar.

Growth of the Organism

Mycoplasma pneumoniae requires yeast extract and supplementary serum for growth,[21] a feature whose discovery resulted in the first successful cultivation. The essential growth factors provided by these supplements have not been identified. An enriched medium developed by Tully[22] for the isolation and study of spiroplasmas appears to promote better growth than the original medium does. Unlike most mycoplasmas, *M. pneumoniae* grows equally well in an aerobic and anaerobic environment, and growth is slow.[23] The mean generation time for organisms adapted to growth in artificial media is 6 hours.[24] On solid media, colonies of organisms are usually homogeneously granular in contrast to the "fried egg" appearance of other mycoplasmas, although a central more dense area is frequently discernible.

Mycoplasma pneumoniae is resistant to cell wall-active antibiotics such as penicillin and to thallium acetate.[25] These features were used to design a selective medium, with the two additives included for the inhibition of bacteria and fungi in specimens. Methylene blue was described as a useful additive that would prevent the growth of other *Mycoplasma* species and thus provide a highly selective media[26]; however, more recent data have indicated that this additive may be inhibitory for many strains of *M. pneumoniae* and that it should not be used in isolation media.[22] Since *M. pneumoniae* ferments glucose, inclusion of glucose and a pH indicator permits an indication of acid formation to be used for the presumptive isolation of *M. pneumoniae*. When prepared with an agar and a liquid phase (diphasic medium), the indicator change is apparent in the agar phase.

Mycoplasma pneumoniae is inactivated by treatment with lipid solvents, formalin, and a variety of antiseptics. Stability of saline suspensions is enhanced by the addition of horse serum.[27] Strains adapted to growth in artificial media survive repeated freeze-thaw cycles without significant loss,[27] but practice has indicated that recovery of the organisms from human secretions may be difficult after freeze-thaw. Growth of all *M. pneumoniae* strains is inhibited by the tetracyclines and erythromycin.[28] Although some other antimicrobials also inhibit growth to a variable extent, erythromycin and tetracycline are the most commonly used antimicrobials for human disease.

TABLE 1. Major Properties of *Mycoplasma pneumoniae*

Requires yeast extract and supplementary serum for growth
Grows slowly
Grows equally well in aerobic or anaerobic atmospheres
Colonies are usually homogeneously granular
Ferments glucose
Produces a peroxide hemolysin
Exhibits hemadsorption
Resistant to penicillin and thallium acetate
Inhibited by tetracycline, erythromycin, and specific antisera

Antigenic Composition and Serologic Responses

Analysis of several strains of *M. pneumoniae* by a variety of techniques designed to evaluate homology revealed that all strains were identical, and an antigenic analysis of strains isolated over a 10-year period did not reveal any antigenic variation.[29,30] Immunization of animals with *M. pneumoniae* organisms has resulted in the development of antibodies with a variety of specificities. Glycolipids serve as essential structural components of the mycoplasmal membrane, and in association with protein they constitute the major antigenic components of membranes.[31] An abundance of protein is present, but studies have suggested that only a small number (about six) are located external to the lipid.[32] Recent, more specific studies on these proteins led to identification of the P1 protein that mediates attachment.[14] Radioimmunoprecipitation in conjunction with gel electrophoresis and fluorography of convalescent human sera revealed a specific immune response to the P1 and P2 proteins, thus suggesting their possible use as antigens for diagnosis and as immunogens for the prevention of attachment.[33] Also, recent studies on the carbohydrates of *M. pneumoniae* have indicated the presence of a fraction that crossreacts with antibody to *Streptococcus pneumoniae* types 23 and 32 and that stimulates a protective response in hamsters to challenge with virulent *M. pneumoniae*.[34,35] Growth inhibition is accomplished with an antiserum to a lipid-containing extract of *M. pneumoniae* membrane, and this growth inhibition is blocked by a glycolipid.[36–38] Lysis of organisms occurs in the presence of antibody and complement, and glycolipids have been conclusively shown to be the surface site for this reaction.[39]

Glucose- and galactose-containing glycolipid antigens similar to those in mycoplasmal membranes are present in a variety of substances including normal mammalian tissue, bacteria, and spinach. Kenny and Newton[40] have shown trigalactosyl diglyceride extracted from spinach to react in complement fixation tests of convalescent sera from human infections as well as *M. pneumoniae*-derived glycolipid antigen. This may account for the detection of antibody in some animal sera and in the sera of some infants and young children. The glycolipids in the membrane presumably also account for the so-called nonspecific reactions seen among persons infected with *M. pneumoniae*. A phospholipid produced by *Mycoplasma*, while distinct from cardiolipin, is capable of fixing complement in tests of some Wasserman-positive sera,[31] and a positive serologic test finding for syphilis sometimes develops after infection with this organism. Cross-reactions with glucosyl glycerides from streptococcus MG may account for the occasional rise in antibody level in this organism,[31] and a glycolipid-containing extract of the organism has been shown to inhibit the cold hemagglutinin reaction that may accompany *M. pneumoniae* infection.[41] Recent studies with I and i erythrocyte antigen have indicated that both glycoproteins and glycolipids may serve as receptors for *M. pneumonia* provided they contain 2,3-sialylated, poly-*N*-acetyllactosamine sequences.[42] This interaction could elicit the cold hemagglutinin autoantibody. Other reported autoimmune antibodies that may have similar derivations include antibody to lung, brain, smooth muscle, and human lymphocytes.[43–45] Except for a probable role of the cold hemagglutinin antibody in the occasional occurrence of intravascular hemolysis in association with *M. pneumoniae* pneumonia, the significance of these various antibodies in the pathogenesis of disease is unknown.

EPIDEMIOLOGY

Patterns of Occurrence

Mycoplasma pneumoniae infections occur worldwide, although they are best documented as a significant cause of respiratory disease in temperate climates.[46–52] The infection is continually present in large population groups throughout the year without any evidence of seasonality. In summer *M. pneumoniae* may cause up to 50 percent of all pneumonias.[49] There is a suggestion that epidemics occur at intervals of 4–8 years, and when this has occurred in both civilian and military populations, disease was most prevalent in late summer and fall.[47–49,53] "Epidemic periods" have exhibited a slow onset and a duration of up to 2 years.[48,49,53,54] During these periods the incidence of infection may be three to five times that seen during other periods and is most apparent in older children and young adults.[48–54] Localized outbreaks may, however, occur in small populations or in localized segments of large populations at any time.[49,53]

The contribution of *M. pneumoniae* to the total occurrence of pneumonia has varied with the population studied. Frequencies have varied from 4 percent in an indigent civilian hospitalized population[55] to as high as 44 percent in a population of young airmen.[56] In an extensive community survey in Seattle, Washington, 15 percent of all pneumonias were associated with *M. pneumoniae* infection.[49] A more recent survey in Britain revealed a frequency of 18 percent.[57] It is probable that comparable frequencies occur in communities in the United States.

The mildness of *M. pneumoniae* is indicated in low hospitalization frequencies. Only 2 percent of patients in the Seattle survey were hospitalized; although other estimations are somewhat higher, it seems clear that less than 5 percent of cases of pneumonia are severe enough to warrant hospitalization.

Age Relationship

Infection rates with *M. pneumoniae* are greatest in school-age children and young adults. Shown in Figure 1 are the rates for

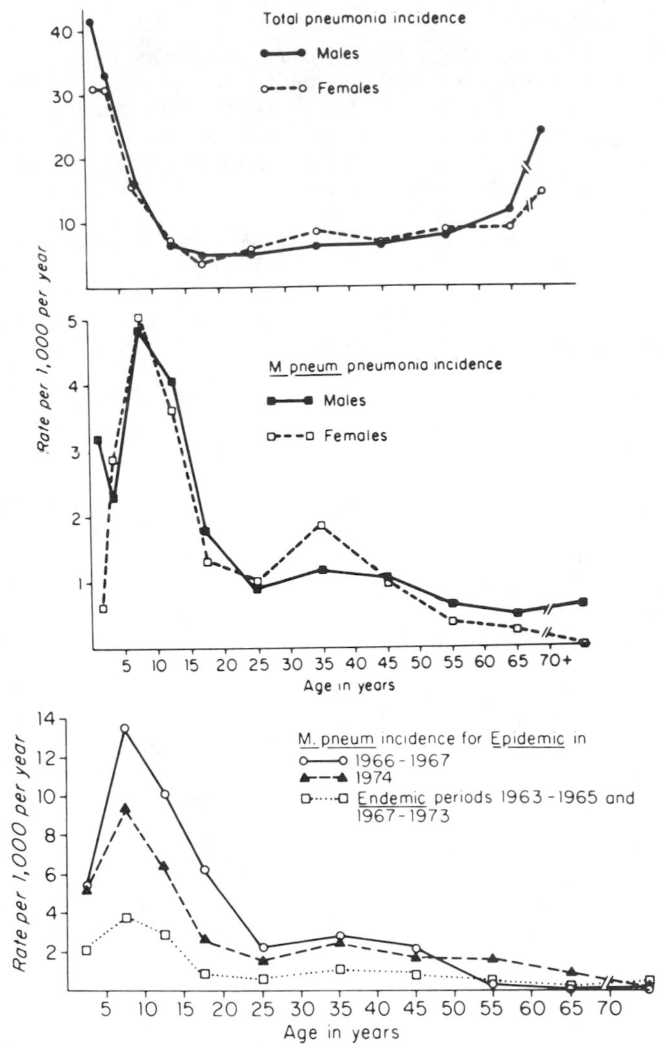

FIG. 1. Incidence of *Mycoplasma pneumoniae* pneumonia by age, sex, and epidemiologic period. Group Health Cooperative (Seattle), December 1, 1963, through February 28, 1975. (From Foy et al.,[49] with permission.)

all pneumonias and for those associated with *M. pneumoniae* in the Seattle study. *Mycoplasma pneumoniae* was most commonly encountered as a cause of pneumonia in the 5- to 15-year age group, and rates during the epidemic period were disproportionately increased in these age groups. For the age range 5–20 years, *M. pneumoniae* caused 30–60 percent of all pneumonias, and the proportion was highest in the 15- to 19-year age group. Although rates of *M. pneumoniae* pneumonia are low for adults, the organism is an important cause of pneumonia throughout the remaining years of life.

In a long-term study of lower respiratory illness among children attending a private practice, *M. pneumoniae* was considered the cause of 51 percent of cases of pneumonia among children 5–9 years of age and 74 percent among those aged 9–15.[52] In addition, it was the most common cause of tracheobronchitis and lower respiratory illness with wheezing in these same age groups.[50,51] A survey of a rural practice in Canada reported that *M. pneumoniae* was the presumed cause of 48 percent of instances of acute respiratory disease that caused persons to seek health care in a 1-year period and that 41 percent of these had pneumonia.[58] While the age group was 2–59 years, 60 percent of patients were between 5 and 20 years old. Finally, *M. pneumoniae* was detected in 37 percent of adult (15–69 years old) outpatients with pneumonia in a study in Sweden.[59]

Pneumonia is slightly more common in boys than in girls, and illnesses tend to be somewhat more severe in boys.[49] The exception is a higher frequency among women aged 30–39 years, an age range containing many mothers of school-age children. Family studies and studies of day care nurseries have indicated that infection with *M. pneumoniae* is common in children under 5 years of age, and although conflicting reports exist, most infections are apparently symptomatic.[60–62] These illnesses tend to be mild, with coryza and wheezing without fever being common findings. Although not well documented radiologically, these illnesses frequently occur without pneumonia even when severe enough to warrant hospitalization.[63]

TRANSMISSION

The usual sequence of the spread of *M. pneumoniae* appears to be first between school-age children and then within families after its introduction by a school-age child.[60,64] Spread in schools and in institutionalized populations is slow and apparently requires close contact with an ill person.[48,65] The study of a community outbreak in the Seattle area led Foy et al.[54] to conclude that spread between playmates was more important than between classmates in a school.

Once infection is introduced into a family, slow but extensive spread occurs. Attack rates have varied between 64 percent and 81 percent among children and between 17 and 58 percent among adults. The major limiting factor in the acquisition of infection by an exposed family member appears to be pre-existing immunity. An example of a family outbreak is shown in Figure 2. Although infection was introduced by the mother, introduction by a school-age child is more common. The family involvement eventually included all members, and the incubation period between cases was about 3 weeks. A similar high frequency of spread has also been noted in military barracks and in college populations, situations that presumably involve close contact comparable to the family.[65–68] The apparent low communicability of *M. pneumoniae* outside a close contact situation in combination with a long incubation period causes spread in the community to be slow and the infection to exhibit a smoldering endemic behavior. Nevertheless, rapid progression of epidemics may occur, and point-source outbreaks that lack a close and prolonged exposure have been described,[66,67,69] which suggests that transmission via small particle aerosols may occur.

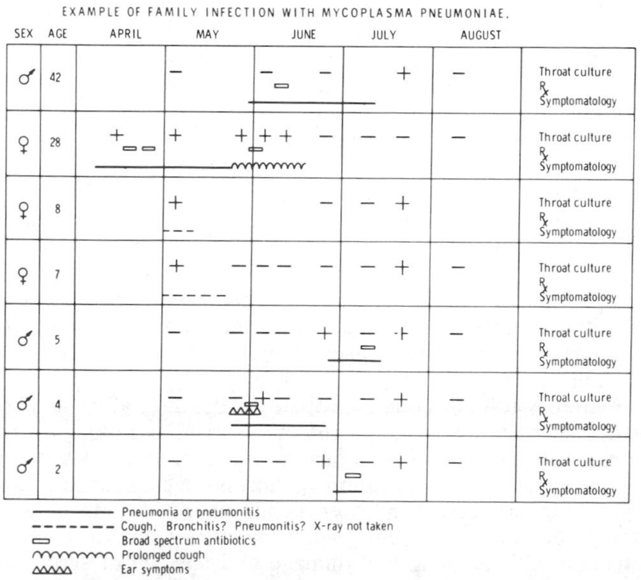

FIG. 2. Example of a family epidemic of *M. pneumoniae* infection. Infection was introduced by the mother, although schoolchildren are more commonly responsible. Subsequent cases in the family occurred at approximately 3-week intervals, and three separate cycles of cases were seen. Pneumonia occurred in five of seven family members, and a 4-month period elapsed before this family became free of *M. pneumoniae* infection. (From Foy et al.[60] with permission.)

ILLNESS RISK

The risk of clinically apparent illness with *M. pneumoniae* infection is low among those less than 5 years old, high for those 5–20 years of age, and then reduced among adults. However, when it occurs, illness is frequently more severe among middle-aged and elderly persons. Reports in military populations indicated that no more than 5 percent of infections were manifested by pneumonia.[70] Comparable estimates for clinically apparent pneumonia in the Seattle studies were 10 percent for children and 5 percent for teenagers and young adults.[49] Using a signs and symptoms definition of pneumonia, studies in children at Chapel Hill, North Carolina, revealed that 46 percent of infected children over 5 years of age with a lower respiratory illness had pneumonia,[52] and a similar frequency was seen in a Canadian rural practice.[58] These latter findings are similar to those for family studies that indicated that about one-third of the infected persons exhibit pneumonia and 70–80 percent exhibit lower respiratory illness.[54,62,64,70] Pharyngitis alone may occur, and infants may exhibit mild respiratory syndromes. Carefully performed evaluations of families indicate that asymptomatic infection is not common and, in combination with the low incidence of clinically apparent pneumonia, emphasize the mild nature of illnesses.

PATHOGENESIS

Mechanisms for Injury

Mycoplasma pneumoniae is a primary pathogen of the respiratory tract. The organism is acquired from an infected person by means of infected respiratory secretions, and evidence indicates that transmitters are generally ill with lower respiratory disease.[48] Studies on volunteers revealed a 50 percent human infectious dose (HID_{50}) of laboratory-passaged strains of about one colony forming unit (cfu) by small-particle aerosol and about 100 cfu by intranasal instillation.[71] Sequential studies revealed the onset of mycoplasmal shedding in respiratory secretions 2–8 days preceding the onset of clinical symptoms.[71] Concentrations of organisms in secretions progressively increased and was highest near the onset of illness. Numbers then progressively decreased after a 2- to 4-day interval of maximal titers but persisted in low titer for protracted periods. In naturally occurring infections this has occurred for up to 10–14 weeks.[72]

The reasons for the predilection of *M. pneumoniae* for the lower respiratory tract and the manner in which it reaches that site are unknown. Nevertheless, many of the events that precede and are associated with the occurrence of cell injury have been elucidated. In a series of studies Collier and associates[11,13,73–79] described the filamentous nature of the organism in organ culture and the apparent attachment to the respiratory mucosal cell through the differentiated terminal structure with an electron-dense core. The attachment factor has been identified as a 168,000 MW protein (P1) and the cell receptor as a glycoprotein.[14–20,42] The gliding motility exhibited by *M. pneumoniae* may aid in penetration through respiratory secretions and between cilia and lead to the required orientation of the terminal structure for production of disease. As shown in Figure 3, the organism remains extracellular during infection and is positioned parallel to the cilia. Organisms are also found in intercellular spaces, thus indicating that some penetration of the mucosal layer occurs.[80] Recent studies have described a role for oxidants produced by the organism in cellular injury. *Mycoplasma pneumoniae* produces H_2O_2 and superoxide.[81] Super-

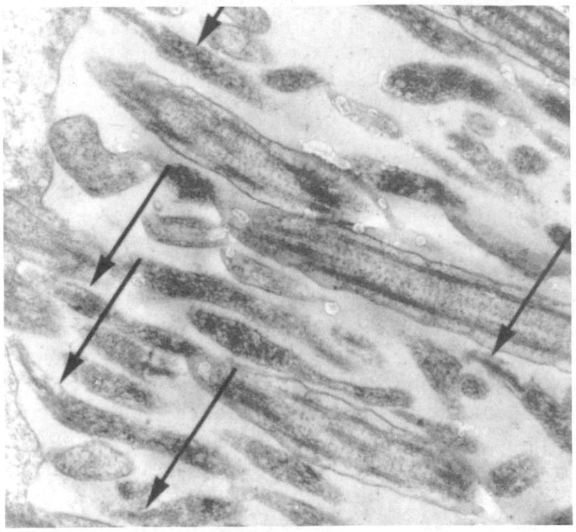

FIG. 3. Electron micrograph of human fetal tracheal tissue infected in organ culture with *M. pneumoniae* for 48 hours. Mycoplasmal cells appear as pleomorphic electron-dense structures at the cell surface and between cilia. The differentiated portion of the organism with an electron-dense core is noted by arrows. (From Collier et al.,[11] with permission.)

oxide anions penetrate the cell membrane and inhibit intracellular catalase.[81] Intracellular peroxides then accumulate and, in combination with superoxide, inhibit superoxide dismutase and further perpetuate the destructive process. As a consequence of damage, membranes leak, and a rapid and quantitative alteration in cellular nucleic acid and energy metabolism occurs.[81–84]

Cellular injury of mucosal cells is accompanied by ciliostasis and followed by the development of cytopathic effects and extrusion of superficial epithelial cells.[80] Ciliostasis in organ culture has been associated with a loss of the normal organization of ciliary necklace particles.[78] Extrapulmonary spread has been detected in a small number of cases.[85–89]

The apparent high prevalence of infection and the mild nature of disease in infected infants and small children[61,90] and the occurrence of more severe disease with infection at a later age has led to the hypothesis that severe disease is primarily a result of immunologic responses to reinfection. A variety of antigens to which the host may be responding have been described,[30] but a precise mechanism for a deleterious effect has not been identified. In any event, antigen–antibody interactions locally and/or the cell-mediated immune response could account for disease at the time of reinfection.

Disease may appear at distant sites (central nervous system [CNS], myocardial and pericardial, skin, joint, and vascular). As noted earlier, *M. pneumoniae* has been isolated from these distant sites on occasion, but such attempts are usually unsuccessful. Although elaboration of toxins has been postulated and presence of hypercoagulability may have special significance for CNS complications,[91] concepts of the disease process suggest that some of these complications have an immunologic basis. The description of the development of antibodies for normal tissues during *M. pneumoniae* infection[43–45] provides a basis for autoimmune reactions. A number of features of *M. pneumoniae* and *M. pneumoniae* infection provide support for this possibility. The organism stimulates a proliferative response by T lymphocytes in vitro; the loss of tuberculin reactions among infected persons suggests significant suppressor T-cell activity.[86,92,93] *Mycoplasma pneumoniae* is also a B-cell mitogen polyclonal activator.[86,92–93] In combination with altered host cell surfaces, these immunologic aberrations could enhance occurrence of autoimmune reactions. Alternatively, antibody or sensitized lymphocytes could develop to the glucose- and galactoside-containing glycolipids shared with normal tissue and mediate cell injury. However, the absence of a uniform relationship between the presence of anti-tissue antibodies and the occurrence of disease at those sites suggest that other factors must also be involved. Circulating antigen–antibody complexes during acute illness have been described, but the antigen has not been identified.[94,95] Such complexes could also be responsible for local or distant disease.

Pathologic Characteristics

Descriptions of the pathologic changes in human cases are limited because of the benign nature of most infections. Fatal cases have exhibited patchy areas of lung infiltration grossly and bronchitis, bronchiolitis, and interstitial and alveolar pneumonitis in microscopic sections.[96,97] Mucosal linings of airways are thickened due to edema, congestion, and cellular infiltration. The characteristic cellular infiltrate is a peribronchiolar occurrence of lymphocytes and plasma cells. Macrophages and neutrophils are present in the peribronchial tissue and lumen and may be prominent if cellular necrosis is present. Tissue from open lung biopsy revealed a similar histology, with hyperplasia of type II pneumocytes and peribronchiolar septal widening.[98] That this cellular response is primarily an immune reaction and that it accounts for the pneumonia seen on x-ray films is suggested by the occurrence of severe disease in hypogammaglobulinemic patients without x-ray evidence of pneumonia.[99]

Histologic findings in a death from encephalitis revealed a leukoencephalitis type of pathology with demyelination and edema and hemorrhage in the white matter.[100] Histology in deaths accompanying carditis and renal failure revealed nonspecific inflammatory changes.

Immunity

Recovery from infection appears to be primarily a consequence of a local accumulation of antibody, and both IgG and IgA antibody appear locally.[101,102] Potential mechanisms described for an antibody effect are antibody-complement–mediated lysis of organisms,[90] antibody-mediated inhibition of attachment,[11] and phagocytosis and destruction of opsonized organisms by polymorphonuclear leukocytes and macrophages.[103] Phagocytes appear to have poor ability to engulf and kill *M. pneumoniae* in the absence of antibody.[104] Data on clinical resolution of infiltrates on x-ray films and cessation of cough indicate that the recovery process is prolonged.[53,105]

Both challenge experiments in volunteers[10] and responses in persons exposed to naturally occurring disease[6] indicate that resistance to infection may occur. This immunity is associated with the presence and magnitude of serum antibody to the organism.[70] A variety of techniques including immunofluorescence, complement fixation, indirect hemagglutination, growth inhibition, mycoplasmacidal, and radioimmunoprecipitation techniques have been used for demonstration of this relationship.[70,102,106]

Secretory IgA antibody is probably short-lived after infection as has been shown for other infectious agents, although it has been demonstrated in secretions, and its presence has been associated with an amelioration of illness in challenged volunteers.[102] IgG is present in lower respiratory secretions remotely after infection, but usually in low quantities.[102] However, an infection with minimal cell damage and leakage of serum antibodies into the lumen of bronchi and bronchioles might be sufficient to abort infection before illness occurs or to hasten recovery and result in occurrence of a minor illness.

Thus, immune mechanisms are postulated to prevent the occurrence of infection as well as induce clinical manifestations of disease in infected persons. A unified concept for these contradictions requires that an imbalance or an insufficient quantity of the pertinent resistance mechanism(s) exist in those persons who develop pneumonia after exposure to *M. pneumoniae*, whereas those persons with a full complement of the pertinent mechanism(s) resist infection and disease entirely. Although attractive, this concept must be regarded as unproven.

The duration of immunity is unknown. The occurrence of second infections and second episodes of pneumonia is well documented.[107] However, Foy and colleagues provided data indicating that persons whose initial episode of disease included pneumonia appeared more likely to resist a second exposure than did those whose initial illness episode was mild.[108]

CLINICAL MANIFESTATIONS

The incubation period to disease onset is about 3 weeks, with most cases occurring in 15–25 days after exposure.[60] Disease is generally insidious in onset; constitutional symptoms consisting of fever, malaise, and headache are usually present 2–4 days before localization of disease.

Three disease syndromes have been clearly attributed to infection with *M. pneumoniae*: pneumonia, tracheobronchitis, and pharyngitis. A variety of complications in association with these syndromes has been described. In addition, it has been suggested that some cases of otitis media, erythema multiforme and some other skin diseases, myocarditis and pericarditis, and neurologic disease may be caused by *M. pneumoniae* infection without accompanying respiratory disease. The clinical spectrum of diseases and complications reported in persons with *M. pneumoniae* infection is shown in Table 2.

Pneumonia

Pneumonia is the best described syndrome caused by *M. pneumoniae*. It is generally mild, and hospitalization is usually not required. Fever, cough, and malaise are the most commonly reported symptoms. The frequency of these and other manifestations in cases occurring in a large urban area are shown in Table 3. The onset of disease is insidious, with headache, malaise, and occasionally fever as initial manifestations. Headache is more prominent in adults and teenagers than in children. These symptoms generally increase in severity over a course of 2–4 days, and cough then appears. Cough becomes a prominent manifestation, and its absence makes a diagnosis of *M. pneumoniae* pneumonia unlikely. Cough is usually nonproductive, although small amounts of purulent or mucoid sputum occasionally containing flecks of blood may be seen. A report of diffuse or substernal soreness in the chest that increases with inspiration is common, but frank pleuritic pain is rare. Mild coryza, sore throat, hoarseness, and earache may be present. Severe sore throat and severe ear pain because of the occurrence of hemorrhagic bullous myringitis may occasionally be seen. Maximal fever varies with temperature elevations between 100° and 104°F, although the daily elevation is usually less than 102°F. Chilly sensations are commonly reported in febrile patients, but frank shaking chills are rare.

On physical exxamination patients usually do not appear seriously ill. Tachypnea, dyspnea, and cyanosis are seen only in rare cases with extensive infiltration. Fever is sustained unless altered in pattern by the use of antipyretics. Some coryza is frequently present, and examination of the ears may reveal injection of the tympanic membrane. Frank myringitis occurs in about 15 percent of the cases, and an occasional one of these will subsequently develop blebs or bullae. When present, hemorrhage into the bleb or bulla usually occurs within 1–2 days. Vascular congestion and some erythema of the posterior portion of the pharynx and enlarged, tender, anterior cervical nodes commonly occur. If patients exhibit paroxysmal coughing, they will report a tender trachea on lateral movement.

Findings in the chest are usually limited to auscultation. Wheezes, rhonchi, and occasional moist rales may be heard over the involved area; however, examination of the chest may be entirely negative. Lobar consolidation occurs occasionally,[109] and these patients will exhibit dullness on percussion over the consolidated area and bronchial breathing, bronchophony, and rales.

Muscle tenderness is common, and arthralgias, anorexia, nausea, and vomiting may occur. Skin rashes are seen in about 15 percent of the cases a few days after onset. Most are maculopapular in nature, although vesicular and vesiculobullous eruptions may also be seen.[53,110–114] Since most patients are

TABLE 2. Spectrum of Diseases Related to *Mycoplasma pneumoniae* Infection

Primary Diseases			*Complications of Respiratory Disease*	
Definitely Related	*Possibly Related*	*Reported*	*Definitely or Probably Related*	*Reported*
Pneumonia	Myringitis Otitis media	Arthritis	Relapse of primary disease Respiratory insufficiency	Pleural abnormality Pneumatocele
Tracheobronchitis		Pancreatitis	Pleural effusion Atelectasis	Lung Abscess Bronchiolitis obliterans Bronchiectasis Secondary bacterial infection Cavitation
Wheezing in infants and older children	Erythema multiforme (major and minor)	Fever only	Sinusitis	Nephritis IgA neuphropathy
Pharyngitis	Myocarditis and pericarditis		Otitis media Myringitis	Hepatitis
Rhinitis	Meningoencephalitis Mono- and polyneuritis Meningitis		Maculopapular rashes Vesicular rashes Urticaria Erythemia multiforme Erythema nodosum	Pancreatitis
			Intravascular hemolysis Intravascular coagulation Raynaud's phenomenon	Thrombocytopenic purpura Pelger-Huët abnormality Hemophagocytosis
			Myocarditis and pericarditis Arthritis Meningoencephalitis Mono- and polyneuritis Meningitis Cerebellar ataxia "Toxic" psychosis	Transverse myelitis Postinfectious leukoencephalitis Cerebrovascular accident Optic neuritis Sensorineural hearing loss Polymyositis Benign myositis in children

TABLE 3. Symptoms and Findings in Group Health Cooperative Patients with *Mycoplasma pneumoniae* Pneumonia

Symptom/Finding	*Total*	*Percentage*
Coryza	365	29
Sore throat	364	54
Hoarseness	355	37
Malaise	366	89
Headache	348	66
Earache (subjective)	326	31
Ear infections (objective)	263	21
Cough	379	99
Sputum	353	45
Chills	356	58
Temperature ≥100°F (37.8°C)	378	94
Temperature ≥102°F (38.9°C)	378	77
Diarrhea	360	15
Nausea and/or vomiting	361	29
Skin rash	319	17
Pleuritis	286	2
WBC count ≥15,000/mm^3	238	5
WBC count ≥10,000/mm^3	238	27
Pre-existing disease	371	14
Recurrent pneumonia	315	22
Cigarette smokers (adults only)	51	29
Family size ≥4 persons	363	91
Hospitalization	385	2

(From Foy et al.,[60] with permission.)

receiving drug therapy when rashes appear, the relationship of the rashes to infection is uncertain.

Roentgenographic Changes. X-ray examination of the chest usually reveals a unilateral segmental bronchopneumonia of a lower lobe[53,105,115–117]; however, multiple-lobe involvement is not unusual, and lobar involvement may occur. Small pleural effusions may be seen in about 25 percent of the cases,[118] but significant pleural effusion is rare.

Laboratory Findings. Peripheral leukocytes are usually within the normal range, although, as shown in Table 3, counts greater than 10,000/mm^3 are common and counts greater than 15,000/mm^3 may occur. Leukocyte differential counts usually reveal 60–85 percent neutrophils with a few band forms. Erythrocyte sedimentation rates are generally increased, sometimes to a striking level.

When available, a Gram stain of sputum reveals mononuclear and polymorphonuclear cells but no predominant organism. Sputum or throat cultures for bacteria reveal a pattern of normal respiratory tract flora, and blood cultures are negative.

Urinalyses are within normal limits except for the occasional occurrence of albuminuria, which is attributable to fever. Other abnormal test results are attributable to a complication of the disease or to an underlying condition.

A number of nonspecific serologic responses have been described in association with *M. pneumoniae* disease, and some are helpful in diagnosis. The best-known and best-studied reaction is the development of cold hemagglutinins. This antibody is an IgM that usually exhibits specificity for the I antigen of red cells.[42,119,120] It is best detected at 4°C but, when present in high titer, is detectable at 25 and 37°C. The antibody usually develops toward the end of the first week of illness or early in the second week of illness. Fifty percent of marine recruits with *M. pneumoniae* infection developed the antibody,[6,106] and other studies indicate that it develops more often in patients with more severe illnesses. About 30 percent of the patients develop antibody to the MG streptococcus[121]; this is also more common in more severely ill patients and tends to occur in the same patients who develop cold hemagglutinins. Some patients develop a false-positive serologic test response to syphilis, some develop a positive direct Coombs test reaction in association with cold hemagglutinins, and an occasional patient develops antinuclear antibody.

Clinical Course. The course of *M. pneumoniae* pneumonia is variable, although recovery is the rule. Death has occurred, but it is rare. In the untreated case, fever may last from 2 days to 2 weeks; it usually subsides by lysis, and slow but progressive improvement in symptoms ensues. Malaise, cough, and x-ray abnormalities frequently persist for 2–6 weeks.[53,105,116] Clinically inapparent sinusitis is common[122]; the duration of disease in naval recruits with and without this complication is shown in Figure 4.

Complications. Reports of hospitalized patients have emphasized the severe manifestations pneumonia may exhibit and the occurrence of a variety of nonrespiratory complications. These latter complications reportedly occur in 2–10 percent of hospitalized patients, but frequencies may be higher in referral hospitals.[123,124] Community studies indicate that about 2 percent of children and 10 percent of adults with *M. pneumoniae* are hospitalized.[49] Thus, although the frequency of cases of *M. pneumoniae* with severe disease or a complication is low, the high frequency of this disease leads to the common recognition of such cases. Similarly, because of the high frequency of *M. pneumoniae* infection, coincidental but unrelated diseases may be seen. Finally, the sometimes uncertain specificity of the *M. pneumoniae* complement fixation test using glycolipid antigen (see earlier) further complicates assignment of diseases to *M. pneumoniae*. The extensive variety of diseases reported in association with *M. pneumoniae* or evidence of *M. pneumoniae* infection is shown in Table 2. It seems probable or possible that many of these diseases are etiologically related to *M. pneumoniae*, although some of the designations in Table 2 must be regarded as uncertain.

The most common complications of *M. pneumoniae* infection are pulmonary. Extensive involvement and lobar consolidation may produce respiratory insufficiency.[109,125–127] Transient atelectasis and significant pleural effusion may occur as complications of mild cases. The occurrence of severe disease and significant pleural effusion in patients with sickle cell disease has been emphasized.[128,129] Clinical relapse apparently occurs in up to 10 percent of the cases[130] and may be accompanied by an infiltrate noted on x-ray examination in the same segment originally involved or in another segment of the same or other lung.[109] When relapse occurs, it is usually within 2–3 weeks of the initial acute illness. Residual pleural abnormality, pneumatocele development, lung abscess, bronchiolitis obliterans, secondary bacterial infection, bronchiectasis, and cavitation have all been reported, although the significance of the organism in their occurrence is uncertain.

Clinically inapparent sinusitis frequently occurs, and myringitis may also be seen.[10,122] Secondary bacterial infections of the middle ear may occur,[131] and this is more common in younger age groups.

In addition to maculopapular and sometimes vesicular skin rashes, *M. pneumoniae* disease may be complicated by urticaria, erythema multiforme, and erythema nosodum. Erythema multiforme is apparently the more common of these three skin manifestations, and occurrence of the severe form (erythema multiforme major or Stevens-Johnson syndrome) may be of special significance since it is usually preceded by respiratory symptoms and may be accompanied by pneumonia.[89,110,111]

Significant intravascular hemolysis in association with serum cold hemagglutinins generally occurs only in patients with high titers,[132] although clinically inapparent hemolysis may be more common.[133] Titers at 4°C in patients with clinical hemolysis are usually greater than 1:500 and are demonstrable at 37°C. Such hemolysis usually occurs late in the illness and may coincide with the return of body temperature to normal or when chilling of peripheral tissues occurs. Other hematologic complications include intravascular coagulation and Raynaud's phenomenon.

Various neurologic complications of *M. pneumoniae* have recently been emphasized; reported frequencies in hospitalized

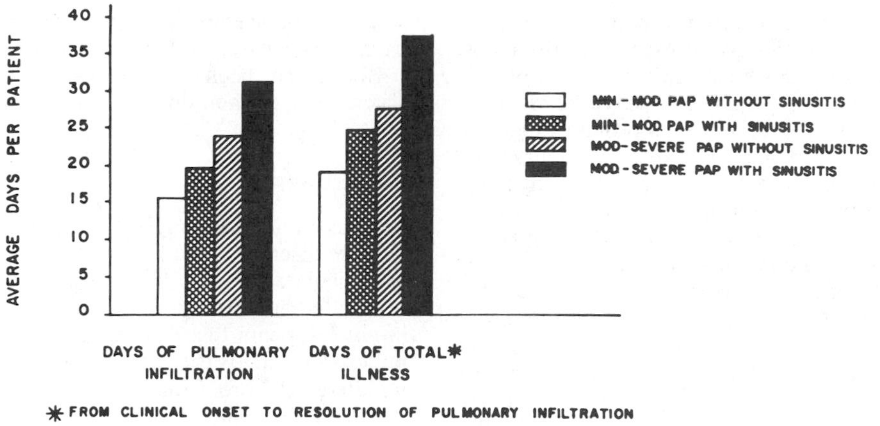

FIG. 4. Duration of disease in 80 patients with primary atypical pneumonia: combined effect of maxillary sinusitis and extent of pneumonia. (From Griffin et al.,[122] with permission.)

patients are up to 10 percent.[86,123] Encephalitis, meningoencephalitis, mono- or polyneuritis, and meningitis are most commonly seen, although cerebrovascular accidents, cerebellar ataxia, "toxic" psychosis, transverse myelitis, and a variety of mononeuropathies including cranial nerve palsies, phrenic nerve paralysis, and sudden deafness have been reported.[86,123,125,134–139] Meningoencephalitis has exhibited a variable number and type of cells in cerebrospinal fluid, although mononuclear cells are prominent. Protein levels are elevated and the CSF sugar content is usually normal, but a low sugar concentration has been reported.[140,141]

Reports of myocardial and pericardial involvement have varied from clinically inapparent alterations in electrocardiograms[142] to significant myocarditis and pericarditis with marked pericardial effusion.[85,123,143–145] Prominent arthralgias are common, but arthritis is rare.[146] Hepatitis, pancreatitis, benign myositis in children, polymyositis, nephritis, IgA nephropathy, disseminated intravascular coagulation, thrombocytopenic purpura, hemophagocytosis, and the Pelger-Huët abnormality have been reported.[86,123,125,138,147–151]

Diagnosis. During the acute stage of disease diagnosis must be made by clinical means.[109] *M. pneumoniae* pneumonia should be considered when a patient exhibits the features of an atypical pneumonia[109]; these include marked headache in adults, definite occurrence of nasopharyngeal findings, and the presence of nonproductive or minimally productive cough. An absence of the usual features of acute bacterial pneumonia such as a toxic appearance, shaking chills, significant pleural pain, purulent or bloody sputum with a predominant organism detected by Gram stain, and a peripheral leukocytosis with neutrophilia is important supporting evidence. Nevertheless, it is important to remember that *M. pneumoniae* pneumonia may be severe and may exhibit each of these findings.

Other causes of atypical pneumonia include Q fever, psittacosis, TWAR pneumonia (*Chlamydia* species), legionnaires' disease, and the respiratory viruses. A history of exposure for the former two should be sought; age and epidemiologic circumstance are most helpful for diagnosis of the latter (see appropriate chapters for details). Other causes of pulmonary infiltrates such as tuberculosis, mycotic infection, pulmonary infarction, and malignancy must also be considered.

If the patient is between 5 and 30 years of age, the case is occurring during summer or early fall, and similar cases are occurring in the family, a diagnosis of *M. pneumoniae* pneumonia is more certain.

The test for cold hemagglutinins is generally available. It is useful, particularly for hospitalized patients, since it is more commonly positive in more seriously ill patients. Only a minority of cases of "cold hemagglutinin-positive nonbacterial pneumonia" are caused by *M. pneumoniae*; however, most infections with titers ≥1:128 are caused by *M. pneumoniae*. A "bedside" test for cold hemagglutinins[152] may be useful since a positive test result indicates a serum titer of ≥1:64. For the test, 1 ml of blood is mixed with an anticoagulant and immersed for 1–2 minutes in ice. Hemagglutination is apparent on microscopic examination and usually on macroscopic examination as well. Confirmation is provided by the disappearance of hemagglutination on warming to 37°C. When a negative or low titer of cold hemagglutinins is obtained, the test should be repeated in 3–5 days since a rise in titer is most meaningful. The test for MG streptococcus agglutinins is not useful since they develop less commonly than do cold hemagglutinins and usually in the same patients.

Definitive diagnosis requires demonstration of the organism or a rise in concentration of specific antibody. Isolation of the organism is best accomplished from sputum, but a throat swab specimen is acceptable. The SP-4 medium developed by Tully et al.[22] is best for isolation tests.[153] Both the diphasic medium (broth over agar) and agar plates are acceptable; ideally both should be simultaneously inoculated. A comparison of these two media for isolation suggested that the former was more sensitive.[154]

A color change of the phenol red indicator in diphasic media after day 3 of incubation is usually caused by acid production by *M. pneumoniae* (occasional bacterial overgrowth will produce a similar color change in the first day or 2 of incubation). A change in color of diphasic cultures tends to occur 1–2 days after the appearance of characteristic colonies on agar cultures, but in both systems at least 5 days of incubation and sometimes 14–21 days is required for evidence of growth. Acceptable clinical confirmation of *M. pneumoniae* isolation is provided by subculture of positive diphasic cultures to agar with testing for hemolysis or hemadsorption with guinea pig red blood cells[155] or by performing the latter tests directly on the agar isolation plate. Reaction of the organism with specific antiserum is, however, required for definitive identification. This is best accomplished by inhibition of growth on agar around an antiserum-impregnated disk.[156] Although identification of *M. pneumoniae* in sputum by immunofluorescence has been reported,[157] the technique has not been used for the diagnosis of human cases.

Specific DNA probes have recently been proposed as useful for the rapid diagnosis of *M. pneumoniae* infection.[158,159] A kit for this purpose is available commercially, and it appears to be useful clinically.[159a]

A variety of serologic procedures have been described for demonstrating a rise in specific antibodies to *M. pneumoniae* between acute and convalescent sera. Complement fixation is the most available procedure, and reports indicate that a rise in titer may be detected in as high as 80 percent of the cases, although as low as 50 percent has been reported. *Mycoplasma pneumoniae* glycolipid and protein antigens have been shown to cross react with those of *M. genitalium*, a probable cause of urethritis. Thus, although serologic overlap may occur, there is no overlap among diseases for which a serologic diagnosis might be attempted. Growth inhibition and mycoplasmacidal tests are more sensitive assays for antibody, but they require experience with cultivation techniques that are not generally available.[106] Use of recently described enzyme-linked immunoadsorbant assays (ELISA) should become more prevalent[160–161]; this test has the advantage of permitting separate detection of IgM and IgG antibody. Thus far it appears that ELISA tests utilizing whole lysed organisms have about the same sensitivity as the complement fixation test and suffer from the same problems with specificity described earlier.[162,163] An ELISA assay utilizing the purified adhesion P1 protein appears to carry adequate sensitivity and a high degree of specificity.[164–166]

Tracheobronchitis

Tracheobronchitis is the most common clinical syndrome resulting from infection with *M. pneumoniae*.[60,64] Although tracheitis with frequent paroxysmal coughing and substernal discomfort may be prominent, bronchitis with frequent cough usually predominates. A similar illness in infants and older children is commonly accompanied by wheezing; in fact, a predominance of lower respiratory illness with wheezing among older children is an indication that *M. pneumoniae* infection is prevalent in the community.[51] The occurrence of wheezing suggests the presence of bronchiolitis. The onset and clinical picture of these cases of tracheobronchitis are similar to those for pneumonia. As indicated earlier, the basic pathologic characteristic of *M. pneumoniae* infection is bronchitis. Thus, when the peribronchial infiltrate is sufficiently extensive, chest x-ray findings are abnormal, and the diagnosis is pneumonia. This relationship is emphasized by the fact that most cases of pneumonia are clinically diagnosed as tracheobronchitis and that chest x-ray films reveal an infiltrate. These cases with negative chest x-ray films tend to have fewer and milder systemic symptoms and a shorter duration of fever and cough and tend to exhibit a lower frequency of rises in levels of serum cold hemagglutinins. The complications described for *M. pneumoniae* also occur in cases of tracheobronchitis, but it is not known whether they occur at a lower frequency.

Diagnosis is complicated by the high proportion of cases of tracheobronchitis caused by viruses. The epidemiologic circumstances described for pneumonia and the occurrence of ear disease may aid in a clinical diagnosis of *M. pneumoniae* tracheobronchitis. Definitive diagnosis requires demonstration of the organism or a rise in specific antibody levels.

Pharyngitis and Rhinitis

Pharyngitis frequently accompanies lower respiratory disease caused by *M. pneumoniae*, but it may occur as the predominant manifestation of disease.[60,64] The onset is usually insidious with fever and headache, but sore throat appears early and becomes the predominant symptom. Cough and coryza may also be present. On examination, the posterior pharynx is diffusely erythematous, and pharyngeal and tonsillar exudates may be seen. Tender anterior cervical lymph nodes are common, and when accompanied by mild or no pharyngeal infection, a primary diagnosis of cervical adenitis is more appropriate. A clinical diagnosis of *M. pneumoniae* pharyngitis is not possible since cases are indistinguishable from cases of pharyngitis caused by viruses and group A streptococci.[167,168]

Rhinitis has been described as a major finding in infants under 1 year of age when infected with *M. pneumoniae*.[63]

Ear Disease

Bullous myringitis may occur as a complication of *M. pneumoniae* disease of the respiratory tract and has also been seen as an isolated disease.[123] A former assumption that most cases of isolated bullous myringitis were probably caused by *M. pneumoniae* appears to be incorrect.[169,170] Although proposed that bullous myringitis is a manifestation of bacterial infection of the middle ear,[169] proof for such a pathogenesis is not available.[170] It seems clear that *M. pneumoniae* can cause isolated bullous myringitis, although most cases probably have another cause. Patients with this disease complain of ear pain that on occasion may be severe. *Mycoplasma pneumoniae* has been reported as a cause of otitis media,[171] but attempts to further define the occurrence of this disease have been unrewarding.

Other Reported Diseases

Although *M. pneumoniae* infection has been reported in association with a variety of nonrespiratory disease states, it has been most prominently, although not definitively, implicated in meningoencephalitis, meningitis, mono- and polyneuritis, myocarditis and pericarditis, and erythema multiforme. Each disease is reported as a complication of respiratory disease, so it is possible that some cases without apparent respiratory disease may occur.

An evaluation of aseptic meningitis revealed *M. pneumoniae* as a possible cause in up to 6–8 percent of cases,[172] and an evaluation of hospitalized cases of *M. pneumoniae* infection has regularly revealed a number of cases of meningitis, meningoencephalitis, and neuritis that were neither preceded by nor accompanied by apparent respiratory disease.[123,135,173] The course of illness is not well described, but death and residual neurologic deficits have been reported.[123,135,174] CSF findings usually exhibit mononuclear pleocytosis; isolation of the organism from CSF has been reported.[87,88,175]

Erythema multiforme major (Stevens-Johnson syndrome) may be primarily caused by *M. pneumoniae*,[89,110,111] although preceding or associated respiratory disease usually exists. Lyell and associates[176] reported 13 cases of erythema multiforme minor without associated respiratory disease, although in a subsequent report for 17 patients[177] no evidence of *M. pneumoniae* infection was found. They also reported isolation of the organism from vesicular lesions of the two most severely ill patients.[176] Since these findings have not been reproduced, the suggestion that *M. pneumoniae* may cause erythema multiforme minor without associated respiratory disease must remain in question.

Evidence of myocarditis and pericarditis have been detected by electrocardiographic testing in typical cases,[125,142] and a death was reported with recovery of the organism from blood and pericardial fluid at autopsy.[85] A retrospective analysis by Sands et al.[143] has suggested that myocarditis and pericarditis without associated respiratory disease may be caused by *M. pneumoniae* infection. Of their 13 patients 7 did not have associated respiratory disease, and no other cause for the pericarditis or perimyocarditis was detected. Although two deaths occurred in patients with an underlying disease and associated pneumonia, a complete recovery ensued in all cases without an underlying disease.

Polyarthritis and Reiter syndrome have been reported in association with evidence of *M. pneumoniae* infection, and *M.*

pneumoniae was isolated from joint fluid of a hypogammaglobulinemic patient with chronic arthritis.[178] Antibody responses may be detected in up to one-third of cases of acute pancreatitis.[179,180] In one study this antibody was shown to be an IgM antibody, and no transition to an IgG antibody occurred; the authors proposed that the response was nonspecific.[179]

TREATMENT

Tetracycline and its derivatives and erythromycin are effective in the treatment of *M. pneumoniae* pneumonia.[181] In controlled trials both antimicrobials were shown to hasten the disappearance of clinical manifestations and infiltrates on chest x-ray films.

Until rapid diagnostic tests are proved to be useful, decisions on antimicrobial therapy must be made on clinical grounds. Both tetracycline and erythromycin are recommended for therapy. A basis for preferring erythromycin over tetracycline exists in the absence of effect on teeth in children, the fact that standard doses give higher blood levels and good diffusion into respiratory secretions, and in the demonstration of greater sensitivity of the organism in vitro.[28] However, both antimicrobials are equally effective in clinical studies. Tetracyclines have the additional advantage of a proven effectiveness against psittacosis and Q fever and probably against the TWAR agent, but erythromycin has a proven effectiveness in legionnaires' disease. Clinical resistance to tetracycline with a response to erythromycin and resistance to erythromycin with a response to tetracycline have both been reported.

Patients presumed to have *M. pneumoniae* pneumonia should be treated with erythromycin or tetracycline in doses of 0.5 g q8h. Among infants and children the following schedules are recommended: erythromycin, 30–50 mg/kg/day for those weighing less than 25 kg and 1 g/day for those above 25 kg. Reports on therapy with these antimicrobials have usually indicated a treatment duration of 6–8 days. These short courses of treatment clearly reduce the intensity of infection, but it appears to increase again in many cases after antimicrobial withdrawal.[182] Moreover, results with these short courses frequently indicate incomplete relief of cough and occasional clinical relapse. Although not studied, it seems probable that prolonged treatment would improve results, and therefore a 2- to 3-week course of treatment is recommended. The additional use of antipyretics, antitussives, assisted ventilation, oxygen, and the like is determined by individual needs.

Treatment of patients with pharyngitis and tracheobronchitis on a routine basis is not recommended unless a diagnosis is certain because these illnesses are indistinguishable by clinical techniques from the great majority of acute respiratory illnesses caused by viruses. However, if protracted illness occurs and *M. pneumoniae* infection has been proved, the aforementioned antimicrobials may be used. An effect of antimicrobial therapy on the nonrespiratory complications of *M. pneumoniae* infections has not been shown; indeed, the occasional occurrence of these complications during adequate antimicrobial therapy raises questions about the role of the organism in their causation.

PREVENTION

No method has been established as being effective for the prevention of *M. pneumoniae* infection and disease. Patients should probably be isolated, and attempts should be made in the home to prevent close contact with ill persons. Antimicrobial therapy apparently does not alter transmission rates.[48]

The prophylactic use of oxytetracycline therapy for 10 days in family members exposed to an ill family member was reported as effective.[171] A significantly lower occurrence of illness in a treated group but no difference in infection rates between treated and placebo groups was seen. This suggests that the antimicrobial was either ineffective for the prevention of infection and only reduced the intensity or that it was most commonly given during the incubation period before illness developed, thus constituting early treatment. No repeat of this important study has been reported.

Vaccine trials have involved both inactivated and live attenuated agents. Early trials with inactivated vaccines indicated that a high frequency of serologic conversion could be obtained. In large field trials in the military with two inactivated vaccine preparations, one of which appeared optimally potent, only about 50 percent protection against pneumonia and 30 percent against bronchitis was obtained.[183,184] In both studies a harmful effect of vaccination as suggested by an earlier study[185] was sought, and none was detected. It thus appears that inactivated whole-organism *M. pneumoniae* vaccines cannot be made sufficiently potent to advise general use, particularly since data suggest that immunity is relatively short.[107]

Live attenuated vaccines have also been tested in humans.[186,187] Using the hamster model, Fernald and Clyde[188] convincingly demonstrated that this approach was more likely to be successful than was the inactivated vaccine approach. Early studies in humans with material passaged in artificial media[186] indicated that attenuation occurred but that an associated reduction in infectivity limited this approach. Although still of interest, the indications that disease is mediated by immune responses, that immunity is short-lived, and that potentially serious extrapulmonary disease may result from *M. pneumoniae* infection has caused reduced interest in the live vaccine approach to the prevention of *M. pneumoniae* disease.

Recent interest in vaccine development for *M. pneumoniae* has focused on the identification and use of purified material.[189] The most prominent candidate at present is the adhesin protein that mediates attachment to the cell membrane.[15,16]

REFERENCES

1. Reimann HA. An acute infection of the respiratory tract with atypical pneumonia. A disease entity probably caused by a filterable virus. JAMA. 1938;111:2377.
2. Peterson OL, Han TH, Finland M. Cold agglutinins (autohemagglutinins) in primary atypical pneumonias. Science. 1943;97:167.
3. Commission on Acute Respiratory Diseases: Fort Bragg, North Carolina. Transmission of primary atypical pneumonia to human volunteers. I. Experimental method, II. Results of inoculation, III. Clinical features, IV. Laboratory studies. Bull Johns Hopkins Hosp. 1946;79:97.
4. Eaton MD, Meiklejohn G, van Herick W. Studies on the etiology of primary atypical pneumonia. A filterable agent transmissible to cotton rats, hamsters, and chick embryos. J Exp Med. 1944;79:649.
5. Liu C. Studies on primary atypical pneumonia. I. Localization, isolation, and cultivation of virus in chick embryos. J Exp Med. 1957;1006:455.
6. Chanock RM, Mufson MA, Bloom HH, et al. Eaton agent pneumonia. JAMA. 1961;175:213.
7. Clyde WA Jr. Demonstration of Eaton's agent in tissue culture. Proc Soc Exp Biol Med. 1961;107:715.
8. Goodburn GM, Marmion BP. Study of properties of Eaton's primary atypical pneumonia organism. J Gen Microbiol. 1962;29:271.
9. Chanock RM, Hayflick L, Barile MF. Growth on artificial medium of an agent associated with atypical pneumonia and its identification as a PPLO. Proc Natl Acad Sci USA. 1962;48:41.
10. Rifkind D, Chanock R, Kravetz H, et al. Ear involvement (myringitis) and primary atypical pneumonia following inoculation of volunteers with Eaton agent. Am Rev Respir Dis. 1962;35:479.
11. Collier AM, Clyde WA. Relationships between *Mycoplasma pneumoniae* and human respiratory epithelium. Infect Immun. 1971;3:694.
12. Bredt W. Motility and multiplication of *Mycoplasma pneumoniae*, a phase contrast study. Pathol Microbiol. 1968;32:321.
13. Powell DA, Hu PC, Wilson M, et al. Attachment of *Mycoplasma pneumoniae* to respiratory epithelium. Infect Immun. 1976;13:959.
14. Hu PC, Cole RM, Huang YS, et al. *Mycoplasma pneumoniae* infection: Role of a surface protein in the attachment organelle. Science. 1982;216:313.

15. Trevino LB, Haldenwang WG, Baseman JB: Expression of *Mycoplasma pneumoniae* antigens in *Escherichia coli*. Infect Immun. 1986;53:129.
16. Su CJ, Tryon VV, Baseman JB. Cloning and sequence analysis of cytadhesin P1 gene from *Mycoplasma pneumoniae*. Infect Immun. 1987;55:3023.
17. Manchee RJ, Taylor-Robinson D. Studies on the nature of receptors involved in attachment of tissue culture cells to mycoplasmas. Br J Exp Pathol. 1969;50:66.
18. Cabridge MG, Taylor-Robinson D. Interaction of *Mycoplasma pneumoniae* with human lung fibroblasts: Role of receptor sites. Infect Immun. 1979;24:455.
19. Chandler DKF, Grabowski MW, Barile MF. *Mycoplasma pneumoniae* attachment: Competitive inhibition by mycoplasmal binding component and by sialic acid-containing glycoconjugates. Infect Immun. 1982;38:598.
20. Geary SJ, Gabridge MG: Characterization of a human lung fibroblast receptor site for *Mycoplasma pneumoniae*. Isr J Med Sci. 1987;23:462.
21. Hayflick L. Fundamental biology of the class Mollicutes, order Mycoplasmatales. In: Hayflick L, ed. The Mycoplasmatales and the L-Phase of Bacteria. New York: Appleton-Century-Crofts; 1969:15.
22. Tully JG, Rose DL, Whitcomb RF, et al. Enhanced isolation of *Mycoplasma pneumoniae* from throat washings with a newly modified culture medium. J Infect Dis. 1979;139:478.
23. Clyde WA Jr. Studies on nature and properties of Eaton's agent (*Mycoplasma pneumoniae*) (Abstract). Bacteriol Proc. 1964;M60:54.
24. Furness G, Pipes FJ, McMurtrey MJ. Analysis of the life cycle of *Mycoplasma pneumoniae* by synchronized division and by ultraviolet and X irradiations. J Infect Dis. 1968;118:7.
25. Grayston JT, Foy HM, Kenny GE. The epidemiologyof mycoplasma infections of the human respiratory tract. In: Hayflick L, ed. The Mycoplasmatales and the L-Phase of Bacteria. New York: Appleton-Century-Crofts; 1969:651.
26. Kraybill WH, Crawford YE. Comparison of two agar media for the isolation of mycoplasmas from the human oropharynx. Ann NY Acad Sci. 1967;143:401.
27. Kim KS, Clyde WA Jr, Denny FW. Physical properties of human mycoplasma species. J Bacteriol. 1966;92:214.
28. Jeo RL, Finland M. Susceptibility of *Mycoplasma pneumoniae* to 21 antibiotics in vitro. Am J Med Sci. 1967;253:639.
29. Chandler DKF, Razin S, Stephens EB, et al. Genomic and phenotypic analyses of *Mycoplasma pneumoniae* strains. Infect Immun. 1982;38:604.
30. Vu AC, Foy HM, Cartwright FD, et al. The principal protein antigens of isolates of *Mycoplasma pneumoniae* as measured by levels of immunoglobulin G in human serum are stable in strains collected over a 10-year period. Infect Immun. 1987;55:1830.
31. Plackett P, Marmion BP, Shaw EJ, et al. Immunochemical analysis of *Mycoplasma pneumoniae*. 3. Separation and chemical identification of serologically active lipids. Aust J Exp Biol Med Sci. 1969;47:171.
32. Kahane I, Marchesi VT. Studies on the orientation of proteins in mycoplasma and erythrocyte membranes. Ann NY Acad Sci. 1973;225:38.
33. Leith DK, Trevino LB, Tully JG, et al. Host discrimination of *Mycoplasma pneumoniae* proteinaceous immunogens. J Exp Med. 1983;157:502.
34. Allen PZ, Prescott B. Immunochemical studies on a *Mycoplasma pneumoniae* polysaccharide fraction: Cross-reactions with type 23 and 32 antipneumococcal rabbit sera. Infect Immun. 1978;20:421.
35. Brunner H. Protective efficacy of *Mycoplasma pneumoniae* polysaccharides. Isr J Med Sci. 1981;17:678.
36. Pollack JD, Somerson NL, Senterfit LB. Isolation, characterization, and immunogenicity of *Mycoplasma pneumoniae* membranes. Infect Immun. 1970;2:326.
37. Razin S, Prescott B, Caldes G, et al. Role of glycolipids and phosphatidylglycerol in the serological activity of *Mycoplasma pneumoniae*. Infect Immun. 1970;1:408.
38. Razin S, Prescott B, Caldes G, et al. Production and properties of antisera to membrane glycolipids of *Mycoplasma pneumoniae*. Infect Immun. 1971;3:420.
39. Brunner H, Razin S, Kalica AR, et al. Lysis and death of *Mycoplasma pneumoniae* by antibody and complement. J Immunol. 1971;106:907.
40. Kenny GE, Newton RM. Close serological relationship between glycolipids of *Mycoplasma pneumoniae* and glycolipids of spinach. Ann NY Acad Sci. 1973;225:54.
41. Costea N, Yakulis VJ, Heller P. Inhibition of cold agglutinins by *M. pneumoniae* antigens. Proc Soc Exp Biol Med. 1972;139:476.
42. Loomes LM, Uemura K, Feizi T. Interaction of *Mycoplasma pneumoniae* with erythrocyte glycolipids of I and i antigen types. Infect Immun. 1985;47:15.
43. Biberfeld G, Sterner G. Smooth muscle antibodies in *Mycoplasma pneumoniae* infection. Clin Exp Immunol. 1976;24:287.
44. Biberfeld G. Antibodies to brain and other tissues in cases of *Mycoplasma pneumoniae* infection. Clin Exp Immunol. 1971;8:319.
45. Biberfeld G, Biberfeld P, Wigzell H. Antibodies to surface antigens of lymphocytes and lymphoblastoid cells in cold-agglutinin-positive sera from patients with *Mycoplasma pneumoniae* infection. Scand J Immunol. 1976;5:87.
46. Fleming PC, Kreiger E, Turner JAP, et al. Febrile mucocutaneous syndrome with respiratory involvement, associated with isolation of *Mycoplasma pneumoniae*. Can Med Assoc J. 1967;97:1458.
47. Grayston JT, Foy HM, Kenny GE. The epidemiology of mycoplasma infections of the human respiratory tract. In: Hayflick I, ed. The Mycoplasmatales and the L-Phase of Bacteria. New York: Appleton-Century-Crofts; 1969:651.
48. Foy HM, Alexander ER. *Mycoplasma pneumoniae* infections in childhood. Adv Pediatr. 1969;16:301.
49. Foy HM, Kenny GE, Cooney MK, et al. Long-term epidemiology of infections with *Mycoplasma pneumoniae*. J Infect Dis. 1979;139:681.
50. Chapman RS, Henderson FW, Clyde WA Jr, et al. The epidemiology of tracheobronchitis in pediatric practice. Am J Epidemiol. 1981;114:786.
51. Henderson FW, Clyde WA Jr, Collier AM, et al. The etiologic and epidemiologic spectrum of bronchiolitis in pediatric practice. J Pediatr. 1979;98:183.
52. Murphy TF, Henderson FW, Clyde WA Jr, et al. Pneumonia: An eleven-year study in a pediatric practice. Am J Epidemiol. 1981;113:12.
53. Foy HM, Kenny GE, McMahan R, et al. Mycoplasma pneumoniae pneumonia in an urban area. JAMA. 1970;214:1666.
54. Foy HM, Kenny GE, McMahan R, et al. *Mycoplasma pneumoniae* in the community. Am J Epidemiol. 1971;93:55.
55. Mufson MA, Chang V, Gill V, et al. The role of viruses, mycoplasmas and bacteria in acute pneumonia in civilian adults. Am J Epidemiol. 1967;86:526.
56. Mogabgab WJ. *Mycoplasma pneumoniae* and adenovirus respiratory illnesses in military and university personnel. 1959–1966. Am Rev Respir Dis. 1968;97:345.
57. Community-acquired pneumonia in adults in British hospitals in 1982–83: A survey of aeiology, mortality, prognostic factors, and outcome. From the Research Committee of the British Thoracic Society and the Public Health Laboratory Service. Q J Med. 1986;62:195.
58. Dular R, Lambert M, Bruce BW, et al. *Mycoplasma pneumoniae* infections in a rural setting in Canada. Can Med Assoc J. 1987;136:1271.
59. Berntsson E, Lagergard T, Strannegard O, et al. Etiology of community-acquired pneumonia in out-patients. Eur J Clin Microbiol. 1986;5:446.
60. Foy HM, Grayston JT, Kenny GE, et al. Epidemiology of *Mycoplasma pneumoniae* infection in families. JAMA. 1966;197:859.
61. Fernald GW, Collier AM, Clyde WA Jr. Respiratory infections due to *Mycoplasma pneumoniae* in infants and children. Pediatrics. 1975;55:327.
62. Hanukoglu A, Hebroni S, Fried D. Pulmonary involvement in *Mycoplasma pneumoniae* infection in families. Infection. 1986;14:1.
63. Mok JYQ, Inglis JM, Simpson H. *Mycoplasma pneumoniae* infection. Acta Paediatr Scand. 1979;68:833.
64. Balassanian N, Robbins FC. *Mycoplasma pneumoniae* infection in families. N Engl J Med. 1967;277:719.
65. Steinberg P, White RJ, Fuld SL, et al. Ecology of *Mycoplasma pneumoniae* infections in Marine recruits at Parris Island, South Carolina. Am J Epidemiol. 1969;89:62.
66. Evatt BL, Dowdle WR, Johnson M, et al. Epidemic mycoplasma pneumonia. N Engl J Med. 1971;285:374.
67. Sande MA, Gadot F, Wenzel RP. Point source epidemic of *Mycoplasma pneumoniae* infection in a prosthodontics laboratory. Am Rev Respir Dis. 1975;112:213.
68. Cordero L, Cuadrado R, Hall CB, et al. Primary atypical pneumonia: An epidemic caused by *Mycoplasma pneumoniae*. J Pediatr. 1967;71:1.
69. Broome CV, LaVenture M, Kaye HS, et al. An explosive outbreak of *Mycoplasma pneumoniae* infection in a summer camp. Pediatrics. 1980;66:884.
70. Chanock RM. *Mycoplasma infections of man*. N Engl J Med. 1965;273:1199.
71. Couch RB. Unpublished information.
72. Grayston JT, Kenny GE, Foy HM, et al. Epidemiological studies of *Mycoplasma pneumoniae* infections in civilians. Ann NY Acad Sci. 1967;143:436.
73. Collier AM, Baseman JB. Organ culture techniques with mycoplasmas. Ann NY Acad Sci. 1973;225:277.
74. Collier AM, Clyde WA Jr. Appearance of *Mycoplasma pneumoniae* in lungs of experimentally infected hamsters and sputum from patients with natural disease. Am Rev Respir Dis. 1974;110:765.
75. Hu PC, Collier AM, Baseman JB. Alterations in the metabolism of hamster tracheas in organ culture after infection by virulent *Mycoplasma pneumoniae*. Infect Immun. 1975;11:704.
76. Hu PC, Collier AM, Baseman JB. Interaction of virulent *Mycoplasma pneumoniae* with hamster tracheal organ cultures. Infect Immun. 1976;14:217.
77. Carson JL, Collier AM, Clyde WA Jr. Ciliary membrane alterations occurring in experimental *Mycoplasma pneumoniae* infection. Science. 1979;206:349.
78. Carson JL, Collier AM, Hu SS. Ultrastructural observations on cellular and subcellular aspects of experimental *Mycoplasma pneumoniae* disease. Infect Immun. 1980;29:1117.
79. Hu PC, Collier AM, Baseman JB. Surface parasitism by *Mycoplasma pneumoniae* of respiratory epithelium. J Exp Med. 1977;145:1328.
80. Denny FW. Atypical pneumonia and the Armed Forces epidemiological board. J Infect Dis. 1981;143:305.
81. Almagor M, Kahane I, Yatziv S. Role of superoxide anion in host cell injury induced by *Mycoplasma pneumoniae* infection. J Clin Invest. 1984;73:842.
82. Upchurch S, Gabridge MG. De Novo purine synthesis, purine salvage, and DNA synthesis in normal and Lesch-Nyhan fibroblasts infected with *Mycoplasma pneumoniae*. Infect Immun. 1983;39:164.
83. Gabridge MG, Stahl YDB. Role of adenine in the pathogenesis of *Mycoplasma pneumoniae* infections of tracheal epithelium. Med Microbiol Immunol. 1978;165:43.
84. Gabridge MG. Metabolic consequences of *Mycoplasma pneumoniae* infection. Isr J Med Sci. 1987;23:574.

85. Naftalin JM, Wellisch G, Kahana Z, et al. *Mycoplasma pneumoniae* septicemia. JAMA. 1974;228:565.
86. Cassell GH, Cole BC. Mycoplasmas as agents of human disease. N Engl J Med. 1981;304:80.
87. Kasahara I, Otsubo Y, Yanase T, et al. Isolation and characterization of *Mycoplasma pneumoniae* from cerebrospinal fluid of a patient with pneumonia and meningoencephalitis. J Infect Dis. 1985;152:823.
88. Abramovitz P, Schvartzman P, Harel D, et al. Direct invasion of the central nervous system by *Mycoplasma pneumoniae*: A report of two cases. J Infect Dis. 1987;155:482.
89. Stutman HR. Stevens-Johnson syndrome and *Mycoplasma pneumoniae*: Evidence for cutaneous infection. J Pediatr. 1987;111:845.
90. Brunner H, Prescott B, Greenberg H, et al. Unexpectedly high frequency of antibody to *Mycoplasma pneumoniae* in human sera as measured by sensitive techniques. J Infect Dis. 1977;135:524.
91. Mulder LJMM, Spierings ELH. Stroke in a young adult with *Mycoplasma pneumoniae* infection complicated by intravascular coagulation. Neurology (NY). 1987;37:1430.
92. Fernald GW. Immunologic interactions between host cells and mycoplasmas: An introduction. Rev Infect Dis. 1982;4(Suppl):201.
93. Fernald GW. Humoral and cellular immune responses to mycoplasmas. In: Tully JG, Whitcomb RF, eds. The Mycoplasmas. v. 2. New York: Academic Press; 1979:399.
94. Biberfeld G, Norbeg R. Circulating immune complexes in *Mycoplasma pneumoniae* infection. J Immunol. 1974;112:413.
95. Mizutani H, Mizutani H. Circulating immune complexes in patients with *Mycoplasma pneumoniae*. Am Rev Respir Dis. 1984;130:627.
96. Jordan WS, Dingle JH. *Mycoplasma pneumoniae* infections. In: Dubos RJ, Hirsch JG, eds. Bacterial and Mycotic Infections of Man. Philadelphia: JB Lippincott; 1965:810.
97. Maisel JC, Babbit LH, John TJ. Fatal *Mycoplasma pneumoniae* infection with isolation of organisms from lung. JAMA. 1967;202:287.
98. Rollins S, Colby T, Clyton F. Open lung biopsy in *Mycoplasma pneumoniae* pneumonia. Arch Pathol Lab Med. 1986;110:34.
99. Foy HM, Ochs H, Davis SD, et al. *Mycoplasma pneumoniae* infections in patients with immunodeficiency syndromes: Report of four cases. J Infect Dis. 1973;127:388.
100. Fisher RS, Clark AW, Wolinsky JS, et al. Postinfectious leukoencephalitis complicating *Mycoplasma pneumoniae* infection. Arch Neurol. 1983;40:109.
101. Biberfeld G, Sterner G. Antibodies in bronchial secretions following natural infection with *Mycoplasma pneumoniae*. Acta Pathol Microbiol Scand. 1971;79:620.
102. Brunner H, Greenberg HB, James WD, et al. Antibody to *Mycoplasma pneumoniae* in nasal secretions and sputa of experimentally infected human volunteers. Infect Immun. 1973;8:612.
103. Powell DA, Clyde WA Jr, Fernald GW. Interactions between alveolar macrophages and *Mycoplasma pneumoniae* (Abstract). J Reticuloendothel Soc. 1974;15:36.
104. Erb P, Bredt W. Interaction of *Mycoplasma pneumoniae* with alveolar macrophages: Viability of adherent and ingested mycoplasmas. Infect Immun. 1979;25:11.
105. Mufson MA, Manko MA, Kingston JR, et al. Eaton agent pneumonia—clinical features. JAMA. 1961;178:369.
106. Brunner H, Horswood RL, Chanock RM. More sensitive methods for detection of antibody to *Mycoplasma pneumoniae*. J Infect Dis. 1973; 127(Suppl):52.
107. Foy HM, Kenny GE, Sefi R, et al. Second attacks of pneumonia due to *Mycoplasma pneumoniae*. J Infect Dis. 1977;135:673.
108. Foy HM, Kenny GE, Cooney MK, et al. Naturally acquired immunity to pneumonia due to *Mycoplasma pneumoniae*. J Infect Dis. 1983;147:967.
109. Couch RB. Diagnosis and treatment of *M. pneumoniae* disease in man. In: Hayflick L, ed. The Mycoplasmatales and the L-Phase of Bacteria. New York: Appleton-Century-Crofts; 1969:683.
110. Fleming PC, Krieger E, Turner JAP, et al. Febrile mucocutaneous syndrome with respiratory involvement, associated with isolation of *Mycoplasma pneumoniae*. Can Med Assoc J. 1967;97:1458.
111. Foy HM, Kenny GE, Koler J. *Mycoplasma pneumoniae* in Stevens-Johnson's syndrome. Lancet. 1967;2:550.
112. Lascari AD, Garfunkel JM, Mauro DG. Varicella-like rash associated with *Mycoplasma* infection. Am J Dis Child. 1974;128:254.
113. Teisch JA, Shapiro L, Walzer RA. Vesiculopustular eruption with *Mycoplasma* infection. JAMA. 1970;211:1694.
114. Cherry JD, Hurwitz ES, Welliver RC. *Mycoplasma pneumoniae* infections and exanthems. J Pediatr. 1975;87:369.
115. George RB, Weill H, Rasch JR, et al. Roentgenographic appearance of viral and mycoplasmal pneumonias. Am Rev Respir Dis. 1967;96:1144.
116. Finnegan OC, Fowles SJ, White RJ. Radiographic appearances of mycoplasma pneumonia. Thorax. 1981;35:469.
117. Brolin I, Wernstedt L. Radiographic appearance of mycoplasmal pneumonia. Scand J Respir Dis. 1978;59:179.
118. Fine NL, Smith LR, Sheedy PF. Frequency of pleural effusions in mycoplasma and viral pneumonias. N Engl J Med. 1970;283:790.
119. Dacie JV. The haemolytic anemias. In: The Auto-Immune Haemolytic Anemias. 2nd ed. Part 2. New York: Grune & Stratton; 1962:493.
120. Janney FA, Lee LT, Howe C. Cold hemagglutinin cross-reactivity with *Mycoplasma pneumoniae*. Infect Immun. 1978;22:29.
121. Clyde WA Jr, Denny FW Jr. Etiology and therapy of atypical pneumonia. Med Clin North Am. 1963;47:1201.
122. Griffin JP, Klein EW. Role of sinusitis in primary atypical pneumonia. Clin Med. 1971;78:23.
123. Ponka A. The occurrence and clinical picture of serologically verified *Mycoplasma pneumoniae* infections with emphasis on central nervous system, cardiac, and joint manifestations. Ann Clin Res. 1979;24:1.
124. Ponka A. Clinical and laboratory manifestations in patients with serological evidence of *Mycoplasma pneumoniae* infection. Scand J Infect Dis. 1978;10:271.
125. Murray HW, Masur H, Senterfit LB, et al. The protean manifestations of *Mycoplasma pneumoniae* infection in adults. Am J Med. 1975;58:229.
126. Fraley DS, Ruben FL, Donnelly EJ. Respiratory failure secondary to *Mycoplasma pneumoniae* infection. South Med J. 1979;72:437.
127. Koletsky RJ, Weinstein AJ. Fulminant *Mycoplasma pneumoniae* infection. Am Rev Respir Dis. 1980;122:491.
128. Shulman ST, Bartlett J, Clyde WA, et al. The unusual severity of *Mycoplasma* pneumonia in children with sickle-cell disease. N Engl J Med. 1972;287:164.
129. Solanki DL, Berdoff RL. Severe *Mycoplasma* pneumonia with pleural effusions in a patient with sickle cell-hemoglobin C (SC) disease. Am J Med. 1979;66:707.
130. Watson GI. *Mycoplasma pneumoniae* in general practice. J Coll Gen Pract. 1967;13:174.
131. Halsted C, Lepow ML, Balassanian N, et al. Otitis media. Am J Dis Child. 1968;115:542.
132. Jacobson LB, Longstreth GF, Edgington TS. Clinical and immunologic features of transient cold agglutinin hemolytic anemia. Am J Med. 1973;54:514.
133. Feizi T. Cold agglutinins, the direct Coombs' test and serum immunoglobulins in *Mycoplasma pneumoniae* infection. Ann NY Acad Sci. 1967;143:801.
134. Taylor MG, Burrow GN, Strauch B, et al. Meningoencephalitis associated with pneumonitis due to *Mycoplasma pneumoniae*. JAMA. 1967;199:149.
135. Ponka A. Central nervous system manifestations associated with serologically verified *Mycoplasma pneumoniae* infection. Scand J Infect Dis. 1980;12:175.
136. Shanon E, Zikk D, Redianu C, et al. Sudden deafness due to infection by *Mycoplasma pneumoniae*. Ann Otol. 1982;91:163.
137. Warren P, Fischbein C, Mascoli N. Poliomyelitis-like syndrome caused by *Mycoplasma pneumoniae*. J Pediatr. 1978;93:451.
138. Rothstein TL, Kenny GE. Cranial neuropathy, myeloradiculopathy, and myositis. Arch Neurol. 1979;36:476.
139. Westenfelder GO, Akey DT, Corwin SJ, et al. Acute transverse myelitis due to *Mycoplasma pneumoniae* infection. Arch Neurol. 1981;38:317.
140. Klimek JJ, Russman BS, Quintiliani R. *Mycoplasma pneumoniae* meningoencephalitis and transverse myelitis in association with low cerebrospinal fluid glucose. Pediatrics. 1976;58:133.
141. Maida E, Kristoferitsch W. Cerebrospinal fluid findings in *Mycoplasma pneumoniae* infections with neurological complications. Acta Neurol Scand. 1982;65:524.
142. Lewes D, Rainford DJ, Lane WF. Symptomless myocarditis and myalgia in viral and *Mycoplasma pneumoniae* infections. Br Heart J. 1974;36:924.
143. Sands MG, Satz JE, Turner WE, et al. Pericarditis and perimyocarditis associated with active *Mycoplasma pneumoniae* infection. Ann Intern Med. 1977;86:544.
144. Sands MJ, Rosenthal R. Progressive heart failure and death associated with *Mycoplasma pneumoniae* pneumonia. Chest. 1982;81:763.
145. Ponka A. Carditis associated with *Mycoplasma pneumoniae* infection. Acta Med Scand. 1979;206:77.
146. Jones MC. Arthritis and arthralgia in infection with *Mycoplasma pneumoniae*. Thorax. 1970;25:748.
147. Kanayama Y, Shiota K, Kotumi K, et al. *Mycoplasma pneumoniae* associated with IgA nephropathy. Scand J Infect Dis. 1982;14:231.
148. Pasternack A, Helin H, Vantitinen T, et al. Acute tubulointerstitial nephritis in a patient with *Mycoplasma pneumoniae* infection. Scand J Infect Dis. 1979;11:85.
149. Belardi C, Roberge R, Kelly M, et al. Myalgia cruris epidemica (benign acute childhood myositis) associated with a *Mycoplasma pneumoniae* infection. Ann Emerg Med. 1987;16:579.
150. Van Hook L, Spivack C, Duncanson FP. Acquired Pelger-Huët anomaly associated with *Mycoplasma pneumoniae* pneumonia. Am J Clin Pathol. 1985;84:248.
151. Gill K, Marrie TJ. Hemophagocytosis secondary to *Mycoplasma pneumoniae* infection. Am J Med. 1987;82:668.
152. Griffin JP. Rapid screening for cold agglutinins in pneumonia. Ann Intern Med. 1969;70:701.
153. Senterfit LB. Laboratory diagnosis of *Mycoplasma* infections. Isr J Med Sci. 1984;20:905.
154. Craven RB, Wenzel RP, Calhoun AM, et al. Comparison of the sensitivity of two methods for isolation of *Mycoplasma pneumoniae*. J Clin Microbiol. 1976;4:225.
155. Purcell RH, Chanock RM. Mycoplasma of human origin. In: Lennette EH, Schmidt NJ, ed. Diagnostic Procedures for Viral and Rickettstal Infections. 4th ed. New York: American Public Health Association; 1969:786.
156. Stanbridge E, Hayflick L. Growth inhibition test for identification of *Mycoplasma* species utilizing dried antiserum impregnated paper discs. J Bacterial. 1967;93:1392.

157. Hers JFP, Masurel M. Infection with *Mycoplasma pneumoniae* in civilians in the Netherlands. Ann NY Acad Sci. 1967;143:447.
158. Hyman HC, Yogev D, Razin S. DNA probes for detection and identification of *Mycoplasma pneumoniae* and *Mycoplasma genitalium*. J Clin Microbiol. 1987;25:726.
159. Razin S, Hyman HC, Nur I, et al. DNA probes for detection and identification of mycoplasmas (mollicutes). Isr J Med Sci. 1987;23:735.
159a. Dular R, Kajioka R, Kasatiya S. Comparison of Gen-Probe commercial kit and culture technique for the diagnosis of *Mycoplasma pneumoniae* infection. J Clin Microbiol. 1988;26:1068.
160. Busolo F, Tonin E, Conventi L. Enzyme-linked immunosorbent assay for detection of *Mycoplasma pneumoniae* antibodies. J Clin Microbiol. 1980;12:69.
161. Dussaix E, Slim A, Tournier P. Comparison of enzyme-linked immunosorbent assay (ELISA) and complement fixation test for detection of *Mycoplasma pneumoniae* antibodies. J Clin Pathol. 1983;35:228.
162. van Griethuysen AJA, de Graaf R, van Druten JAM, et al. Use of the enzyme-linked immunosorbent assay for the early diagnosis of *Mycoplasma pneumoniae* infection. Eur J Clin Microbiol. 1984;3:116.
163. Raisanen SM, Suni JI, Leinikko PO. Serological diagnosis of *Mycoplasma pneumoniae* infection by enzyme immunoassay. J Clin Pathol. 1980;33:836.
164. Jacobs E, Bennewitz A, Bredt W. Reaction pattern of human anti-*Mycoplasma pneumoniae* antibodies in enzyme-linked immunosorbent assays and immunoblotting. J Clin Microbiol. 1986;23:517.
165. Jacobs E, Fuchte K, Bredt W. A 168-kilodalton protein of *Mycoplasma pneumoniae* used as antigen in a dot enzyme-linked immunosorbent assay. Eur J Clin Microbiol. 1986;5:435.
166. Jacobs E, Buchholz A, Kleinmann B, et al. Use of adherence protein of *Mycoplasma pneumoniae* as antigen for enzyme-linked immunosorbent as antigen for enzyme-linked immunosorbent assay (Elisa). Isr J Med Sci. 1987;23:709.
167. Clyde WA Jr, Denny FW Jr. *Mycoplasma* infections in childhood. Pediatrics. 1967;40:669.
168. Glezen WP, Clyde WA Jr, Senior RJ, et al. Group A streptococci, mycoplasmas, and viruses associated with acute pharyngitis. JAMA. 1967;202:455.
169. Robert DB. The etiology of bullous myringitis and the role of mycoplasmas in ear disease: A review. Pediatrics. 1980;65:761.
170. Wetmore SJ, Abramson M. Bullous myringitis with sensorineural hearing loss. Otolaryngol Head Neck Surg. 1979;87:66.
171. Jensen KE, Senterfit LB, Scully WE, et al. *Mycoplasma pneumoniae* infections in children: An epidemiological appraisal in families treated with oxytetracycline. Am J Epidemiol. 1967;86:419.
172. Sköldenberg B. On the role of viruses in acute infectious diseases of the central nervous system. Clinical and laboratory studies on hospitalized patients. Scand J Infect Dis. 1972;3(Suppl):48.
173. Lind K, Zoffmann H, Larsen SO, et al. *Mycoplasma pneumoniae* infection associated with affection of the central nervous system. Acta Med Scand. 1979;205:325.
174. Dorff B, Lind K. Two fatal cases of meningoencephalitis associated with *Mycoplasma pneumoniae* infection. Scand J Infect Dis. 1976;8:49.
175. Fleischauer P, Huben U, Mertens H, et al. Nachweis von *Mycoplasma pneumoniae* in Liquor bei akuter Polyneuitis. Dtsch Med Wochenschr. 1972;97:678.
176. Lyell A, Gordon AM, Dick HM, et al. Mycoplasmas and erythema multiforme. Lancet. 1967;2:1116.
177. Lyell A, Gordon AM, Dick HM, et al. The role of *Mycoplasma pneumoniae* infection in erythema multiforme. Proc R Soc Med. 1968;61:1330.
178. Johnston CLW, Webster ADB, Talor-Robinson D, et al. Primary late-onset hypogammaglobulinaemia associated with inflammatory polyarthritis and septic arthritis due to *Mycoplasma pneumoniae*. Ann Rheum Dis. 1983;442:108.
179. Leinikki PO, Panzar P, Tykka H. Immunoglobulin M antibody response against *Mycoplasma pneumoniae* lipid antigen in patients with acute pancreatitis. J Clin Microbiol. 1978;8:113.
180. Freeman R, McMahon MJ. Acute pancreatitis and serological evidence of infection with *Mycoplasma pneumoniae*. Gut. 1978;19:367.
181. Shames JM, George RB, Holliday WB, et al. Comparison of antibiotics in the treatment of mycoplasmal pneumonia. Arch Intern Med. 1970;125:680.
182. Smith CB, Friedewald WT, Chanock RM. Shedding of *Mycoplasma pneumoniae* after tetracycline and erythromycin therapy. N Engl J Med. 1967;276:1172.
183. Mogabgab WJ. Protective effects of inactive *Mycoplasma pneumoniae* vaccine in military personnel. Am Rev Respir Dis. 1968;97:359.
184. Wenzel RP, Craven RB, Davies JA, et al. Field trial of an inactivated *Mycoplasma pneumoniae* vaccine. I. Vaccine efficacy. J Infect Dis. 1976;134:571.
185. Smith CB, Friedwald WT, Chanock RM. Inactivated *Mycoplasma pneumoniae* vaccine. JAMA. 1967;199:353.
186. Couch RB, Cate TR, Chanock RM. Infection with artificially propagated Eaton agent (*Mycoplasma pneumoniae*). JAMA. 1964;187:442.
187. Greenberg H, Helms CM, Brunner H, et al. Asymptomatic infection of adult volunteers with a temperature sensitive mutant of *Mycoplasma pneumoniae*. Proc Nat Acad Sci USA. 1974;71:4015.
188. Fernald GW, Clyde WA Jr. Protective effect of vaccines in experimental *Mycoplasma pneumoniae* disease. Infect Immun. 1970;1:559.
189. Barile MF. Immunization against *Mycoplasma pneumoniae* disease: A review. Isr J Med Sci. 1984;20:912.

163. UREAPLASMA UREALYTICUM (T-STRAIN MYCOPLASMA) AND MYCOPLASMA HOMINIS

DAVID TAYLOR-ROBINSON

CHARACTERISTICS, ISOLATION, AND IDENTIFICATION

Of the seven mycoplasma species isolated from the human genital tract (Table 1), *Ureaplasma urealyticum* and *Mycoplasma hominis* are found most frequently. *Ureaplasma urealyticum* is one of three species in the genus *Ureaplasma*, and *M. hominis* is one of 77 species in the genus *Mycoplasma*, within the family Mycoplasmataceae and the class Mollicutes (see Chapter 162). The general properties noted in Table 1 of Chapter 161 for the mycoplasmas are also exhibited by *U. urealyticum* organisms (referred to as ureaplasmas) and *M. hominis*. Properties that distinguish these two microorganisms from each other, in addition to those they share with other mycoplasmas that are found less frequently in the genital tract, are presented in Table 1.

Detection of mycoplasmas in the genital tract depends on culturing specimens on appropriate media and identifying the isolates.[1] The medium most often used, as for other mycoplasmas, comprises a beefheart infusion broth, available commercially as pleuropneumonia-like organism (PPLO) broth, supplemented with fresh yeast extract (10 percent vol/vol; 25 percent wt/vol) and horse serum (20 percent vol/vol). However, the recovery of *M. hominis* may be improved by using a medium[2] developed originally for the isolation of spiroplasmas and used subsequently for the isolation of *Mycoplasma genitalium*. Genital mycoplasmas grow well in broth medium under atmospheric conditions, but on agar, colonies develop best in an atmosphere of 95 percent N_2 and 5 percent CO_2. The metabolic activity of mycoplasmas is used to detect their growth in broth medium. Clinical material is added to separate vials of broth-containing phenol red (0.002 percent) and 0.1 percent urea, arginine, or glucose. Ureaplasmas grow best at pH 6.0 or less and possess a urease that breaks down urea to ammonia, thus raising the pH level of the medium so that the color changes from yellow to red. *Mycoplasma hominis* metabolizes arginine to ammonia; thus a similar color change is produced in medium initially at pH 7.0. Glucose-fermenting mycoplasmas cause a decrease in the pH value of the medium that initially is set at 7.5 to 7.8. Aliquots of medium from cultures in which these color changes have occurred are subcultured onto agar medium. Use of this liquid-to-agar technique provides the most sensitive method for the isolation of both ureaplasmas and *M. hominis*.[1] Culturing ureaplasmas takes no more than 1 to 2 days, and M. hominis takes up to about 1 week. However, 1 to 2 months or more may be required to culture *M. genitalium*, the mycoplasma most recently discovered in the genital tract[3] and the respiratory tract.

Ureaplasmas were originally termed *T strains* or *T mycoplasmas* (T for tiny) because they produce very small colonies ranging from 15 to 60 μm in diameter. Colonies of *M. hominis* are about 200 to 300 μm in diameter and have a characteristic "fried egg" appearance (Fig. 1, Chapter 161). Colony size and morphology are, however, not fully reliable as means of identification because increasing the volume of agar and buffering the medium have been shown to increase ureaplasmal colony size, and crowded *M. hominis* colonies may be small and uncharacteristic. On blood agar, *M. hominis*, but not ureaplasmas,

TABLE 1. Properties of Mycoplasmas Found in the Genital Tract

Mycoplasma	Frequency of Isolation	Metabolism of	Preferred Atmosphere	pH	Hemadsorption	Susceptibility to Thallium	Susceptibility to Erythromycin	Susceptibility to Lincomycin
U. urealyticum	Common	Urea	Anaerobic	6.0	Serotype 3 only	Yes	Yes	No
M. hominis	Common	Arginine	Aerobic	7.0	No	Yes	No	Yes
M. fermentans	Rare	Glucose and arginine	Anaerobic	7.5	No	No	Yes	Yes
M. genitalium	?	Glucose	Anaerobic	7.5	Yes	Yes	Yes	Yes
M. pneumoniae	Very rare	Glucose	Aerobic	7.5	Yes	No	Yes	Yes
M. primatum	Rare	Arginine	Anaerobic	7.0	No	No	Yes	Yes
M. salivarium	Rare	Arginine	Anaerobic	7.0	No	No	Yes	Yes

produces nonhemolytic pinpoint colonies, and it also grows in most routine blood culture media without changing their appearance. A blind subculture onto blood agar can be used in a diagnostic bacteriology laboratory to diagnose bloodstream invasion with *M. hominis*.[4]

Antibacterial agents, such as penicillin and thallous acetate, are usually added to mycoplasmal media to inhibit bacterial growth. However, since ureaplasmas, *M. genitalium*, and to a lesser extent *M. hominis* are sensitive to thallous acetate,[1,2] it should be omitted from the media when these organisms are being sought. Because erythromycin is far more active against ureaplasmas than against *M. hominis*, and lincomycin has the reverse effect, they may be used to separate the genital mycoplasmas in culture.

Serotyping

There are 14 or more serotypes of *U. urealyticum* and at least seven serotypes of *M. hominis*. Although the data are scanty, none of the work to date has suggested that a particular serotype is convincingly associated with a particular disease.

EPIDEMIOLOGY

Colonization of Infants and Children

Infants usually become colonized with genital mycoplasmas during passage through the infected birth canal; infants delivered by cesarian section are colonized far less often than those delivered vaginally. Ureaplasmas have been isolated from the genitalia of up to one-third of infant girls and *M. hominis* from a smaller proportion.[5,6] The mucosa of the male genital tract is probably less exposed, and this is reflected in the less frequent recovery of mycoplasmas from the genital tract of infant boys.[6] Mycoplasmas, mainly ureaplasmas, have been isolated from the nose and throat of about 15 percent of infants of both sexes.[5] The figures mentioned are estimates and vary from one population to another, depending on the proportion of pregnant women who are colonized.

Neonatal colonization tends not to persist beyond 2 years of age.[6] When mycoplasmas do persist, they do so more often in girls. Thus, genital mycoplasmas have seldom been recovered from prepubertal boys, whereas in one study[7] as many as one-fifth of prepubertal girls were colonized with ureaplasmas and 6 percent with *M. hominis*. In sexually abused children, the organisms are found even more frequently.[8]

Colonization of Adults

After puberty, colonization with genital mycoplasmas occurs primarily as a result of sexual contact.[9,10] This may be deduced from the fact that sexually mature people who have no history of sexual contact are infrequently colonized, whereas colonization among those who are sexually experienced increases in relation to the number of sexual partners. Genital mycoplasmas have been isolated more often from black men and women than from white men and women, but the extent to which these differences are due to differing sexual experience is not clear.

Genital mycoplasmal colonization is also related to socioeconomic status. In Boston, *M. hominis* was isolated from about one-half of the clinic patients at a municipal hospital and ureaplasmas from three-quarters of them, compared to one-fifth and one-half respectively, of the patients visiting private obstetricians and gynecologists in the same area.[11] Whether this apparent socioeconomic difference is a reflection of a difference in sexual experience or whether other factors are involved is unknown. These may include contraception, menstruation, pregnancy, and menopausal changes and have been discussed elsewhere.[12] Genital mycoplasmas appear to be isolated more frequently from pregnant than from nonpregnant women and are isolated less frequently after the menopause, so that the sex hormones may have an influence on colonization.

CLINICAL MANIFESTATIONS

Ureaplasmas and *M. hominis* have been associated with a large variety of clinical conditions,[12,13] as summarized in Table 2, but are considered a cause of only a few conditions.

Nongonococcal Urethritis

There have been numerous studies concerned with the role of large-colony-forming mycoplasmas in nongonococcal urethritis (NGU).[12,13] It is clear that most of them (Table 1) cannot be considered as significant causes of NGU because they are isolated so rarely from the genitourinary tract in either healthy or diseased states. *Mycoplasma genitalium* has been detected by a DNA probe in about one-quarter of men with persistent or recurrent NGU and may account for some of these cases.[14] Although *M. hominis* may be isolated from up to 30 percent of patients, the results of numerous studies have failed to implicate it as a cause of the disease.[12,13] On the other hand, several lines of investigation, discussed below, indicate that ureaplasmas are one of the causes of NGU. Their significance has to be evaluated in relation to other microorganisms, particularly *Chlamydia trachomatis* organisms (chlamydiae), which are an undoubted cause.

Isolation Studies. The selection of inappropriate subjects as controls has probably contributed most to the differences among the results of various investigations. NGU patients have been found to harbor ureaplasmas significantly more often than subjects apparently free from disease in about one-half the investigations, whereas the rate of isolation for the NGU and healthy groups has been about the same in the other studies. It is the recovery of ureaplasmas from healthy persons that has been the main source of contention. Most studies have been qualitative, and if ureaplasmas are involved in the pathogenic process, it would be reasonable to expect them to be present in larger numbers than if they were behaving only as commensals. A few workers[15–18] have provided quantitative data to support this idea.

TABLE 2. Association of *Ureaplasma urealyticum* and *Mycoplasma hominis* with Genitourinary and Reproductive Diseases

	Evidence Suggesting an Association between Indicated Mycoplasma and Disease		*Evidence Indicating That Mycoplasma Is a Cause of Disease*			
Disease	U. urealyticum	M. hominis	U. urealyticum	M. hominis	*Reference Number*	*Comments on the Relationship and Proportion of Disease Attributable to Mycoplasmas*
Nongonococcal urethritis	++++	−	++++	−	3, 12–22, 25, 56	The proportion of NGU caused by ureaplasmas is unknown.
Urethroprostatitis	+++	+	++	−	3, 12, 13, 16	Ureaplasmas may cause some acute disease, but there is no evidence that they or *M. hominis* cause chronic disease.
Epididymitis	+++	−	+++	−	12, 13, 46	One case due to ureaplasmas has been described.
Urinary calculi	++	−	++	−	13, 47	Experimentally, ureaplasmas cause bladder calculi in male rats, and evidence for a cause of natural human disease is increasing.
Pyelonephritis	+	++++	−	++++	13, 26, 27	*M. hominis* causes some cases of acute pyelonephritis and exacerbations.
Reiter's disease	+	−	−	−	12, 13, 22, 36	The significance of ureaplasmas should be assessed further.
Abscess of Bartholin's gland	−	+	−	−	12, 13	Doubtful whether *M. hominis* is involved.
Vaginitis, vaginosis, and cervicitis	−	++	−	−	12, 13	*M. hominis* is associated with vaginosis, but a causal relation is unproved.
Pelvic inflammatory disease	+	++++	−	+++	12, 13, 28–31	*M. hominis* probably causes some cases, but the proportion is unknown.
Postabortal fever	−	++++	−	++++	13	*M. hominis* is responsible for some cases, but the proportion is unknown.
Postpartum fever	++	++++	++	++++	4, 13, 32, 33	*M. hominis* may be a major cause.
Involuntary infertility	++	−	+	−	13, 48, 49, 59	Ureaplasmas are associated with reduced sperm motility and with infertility in women associated with a male factor.
Repeated spontaneous abortion and stillbirth	++	−	−	−	3, 13, 50, 51	Maternal and fetal infections associated with spontaneous abortion, but a causal relation is unproved.
Chorioamnionitis	++	−	++	−	13, 52	Increasing evidence in some cases.
Low birth weight	++	+	+	−	13, 59	An association exists in some studies, but a causal relation is unproved.

Key: ++++: strong; +++: good; ++: moderate; +: weak; −: none.

Antibody Studies. Attempts by most workers to detect antibody responses to ureaplasmal infection have not been very successful.[12] However, responses have been detected in about 50 percent of patients by using a large number of serotypes in the metabolism-inhibition test or by employing the enzyme-linked immunosorbent assay (ELISA).[19]

Antibiotic Studies. Some antibiotic studies have been helpful in assessing the role of ureaplasmas in NGU.[12,13] For example, (*1*) in a placebo-controlled trial of minocycline,[20] there was a significant association between minocycline therapy and the resolution of symptoms and signs in patients from whom only ureaplasmas had been isolated. The association was only a little less convincing than that seen between therapy and resolution of disease in patients from whom only chlamydiae had been isolated; in a further study,[21] the best clinical response (96 percent cure rate) to short-term minocycline therapy was seen in men who were experiencing their first attack of NGU and who harbored ureaplasmas only. (*2*) Urethritis in men who harbor chlamydiae and ureaplasmas was unaffected by treatment with differential antibiotics, namely streptomycin and spectinomycin, which eradicate ureaplasmas only; similarly, the disease was unaffected by treatment with sulfafurazole, which eliminates chlamydiae only.[15] Furthermore, more patients responded to minocycline (effective against both microorganisms) than to rifampicin (effective against chlamydiae only), and those infected with ureaplasmas failed to respond to rifampicin significantly more often than those who were not infected.[22] (*3*) About 10 percent of ureaplasmas are resistant to tetracyclines,[17,23,24] and the urethritis of some patients infected by these ureaplasmas is cured only by treatment with antibiotics, such as erythromycin, to which the organisms are susceptible.

Animal and Human Inoculation Studies. Some ureaplasma strains, unpassaged in the laboratory, have produced urethritis and an antibody response in chimpanzees inoculated intraurethrally. In addition, three investigators inoculated themselves intraurethrally, and each developed urethritis. Two of them[25] received 5×10^4 ureaplasmas of serotype 5, which had been isolated from patients with NGU who had no other detectable pathogenic microorganisms. The first subject developed urethritis characterized by dysuria, urinary frequency, urethral discomfort, and pyuria. Ureaplasmas were isolated consistently from urine, but they and the associated symptoms and signs disappeared during treatment with minocycline. The second subject also had evidence of mild urethritis and, like the first, a transient antibody response. The predominant feature, however, was the appearance of urinary threads, containing polymorphonuclear leucocytes, which persisted for at least 6 months after treatment with minocycline had eliminated the organisms from meatal, urine, and semen samples.

These various findings suggest that ureaplasmas as well as chlamydiae cause NGU, and, indeed, they would be difficult to explain if ureaplasmas were not involved at all. However, because ureaplasmas may be found in healthy persons, it is important to emphasize that at the present time there is no virtue in subjecting patients with NGU to tests for ureaplasmas on a qualitative routine basis, since positive results, so easy to obtain, are difficult for the clinician to interpret and use in patient management.

Pyelonephritis

Mycoplasma hominis has been isolated, sometimes in pure culture, from the upper urinary tract of almost 10 percent of patients with acute pyelonephritis and antibody to *M. hominis*, measured by the indirect hemagglutination test, has been demonstrated in the serum and urine of some of them. In contrast, recovery has not been achieved from the upper urinary tract of patients with noninfectious urinary diseases, nor has antibody been detected in their urine. Overall, the data[26] suggest that *M. hominis* causes a few cases of acute pyelonephritis or acute exacerbations of chronic pyelonephritis. Ureaplasmas have been recovered very occasionally in the same circumstances and also from aspirates of scarred and renal tissue in patients with reflux nephropathy[27] but their role is not clear.

Pelvic Inflammatory Disease

Like NGU, nongonococcal pelvic inflammatory disease (PID) does not have a single cause. Numerous investigators[12,13] have considered that infection by genital mycoplasmas might be one cause of PID, and three types of study indicate their involvement.

Isolation Studies. *Mycoplasma hominis* has been prominent among more than a dozen reports of the isolation of large-colony-forming mycoplasmas from inflamed fallopian tubes, tuboovarian abscesses, and pelvic abscesses or fluid. The most revealing studies of PID, however, have been those of Swedish workers[28] who used laparoscopy to confirm the diagnosis and collect specimens. *Mycoplasma hominis* was isolated directly from the fallopian tubes of about 10 percent of women with acute salpingitis, but not from those of women without signs of the disease. Similar observations were made in the United Kingdon in 1986 (CM Stacey, PE Munday, D Taylor-Robinson, unpublished data).

Ureaplasmas have been studied less intensively, but have been isolated directly from the fallopian tubes of only a very small proportion of patients with acute salpingitis, from pelvic fluid, and from a tuboovarian abscess. The significance of these findings is unclear, but it seems that if ureaplasmas have any importance, it is much less than that of *M. hominis*.

Antibody Studies. Complement-fixing antibody to *M. hominis* has been found in greater titers in the sera of some patients with salpingitis than in those of others serving as controls. Swedish workers[29] used the more sensitive indirect hemagglutination technique and found antibody to *M. hominis* in about one-half of their patients with salpingitis but in only 10 percent of healthy women. Furthermore, a significant rise or fall in antibody titer occurred during the course of the disease in more than one-half of the women who had *M. hominis* in the lower genital tract. Other workers[30] found that patients with gonococcal PID were more likely to respond serologically to *M. hominis* than those without such disease: they suggested that damage caused by the other organisms was a factor in the response and questioned the primary role of *M. hominis*.

Antibody responses to ureaplasmas in patients with PID have been detected less often than responses to *M. hominis*. This is consistent with the impression that ureaplasmas are less important than *M. hominis* in this disease, although the greater difficulty of detecting ureaplasmal antibody responses must not be forgotten.

Organ Culture and Animal Inoculation Studies. The effect of microorganisms on cells may be examined in organ cultures in which tissues can be maintained almost as in vivo. In fallopian tube organ culturres, *Neisseria gonorrhoeae* rapidly destroys the epithelium, causing complete loss of ciliary activity, whereas *M. hominis*, although multiplying, usually produces little more than swelling of some of the cilia. No damage by ureaplasmas of human origin has been detected.[12,13] This decreasing grade of effect may be a true reflection of the pathogenicity of these microorganisms in vivo, but lack of damage in organ culture does not mean necessarily that the organisms are avirulent. The host immune systems, absent in organ culture, may contribute to pathogenesis, and studies in intact animals may be helpful. It is of interest, therefore, that the introduction of *M. hominis* into grivet monkey oviducts has resulted in a self-limiting acute salpingitis and parametritis with an antibody response,[31] whereas ureaplasmas have had no effect.

The various data strongly suggest that *M. hominis* has a role in causing some cases of acute PID, although the extent to which it behaves as a primary pathogen is still not clear.

Postabortal and Postpartum Fever

Mycoplasma hominis has been isolated from the blood of about 10 percent of women who have fever after abortion, but not from afebrile women who have abortions or from normal pregnant women. In addition, a rise in the titer of *M. hominis* antibody has been detected in about one-half of the women who become febrile, but in only a small proportion of those who have abortions and remain afebrile. Thus, the evidence[13] indicates that *M. hominis* causes some cases of postabortal fever. There is, however, no evidence to suggest that ureaplasmas do likewise. The patients usually recover rapidly without appropriate antimycoplasmal treatment.

After normal vaginal delivery, genital mycoplasmas may be found almost immediately and transiently in the blood of less than 10 percent of women, unassociated with postpartum fever. However, there have been many reports[13] of individual patients with postpartum fever from whose blood *M. hominis* has been isolated a day or more after delivery and in whom an antibody response has been detected.[4] It seems that the organisms may be isolated from the blood of about 5 to 10 percent of such women. Since genital mycoplasmas seldom are recovered from the blood of afebrile women one or more days after delivery, it appears that *M. hominis* induces postpartum fever, presumably by causing endometritis.[32] As in postabortal fever, the patients have a low-grade fever for a day or two after delivery, are not severely ill, and usually recover uneventfully without antibiotic therapy.[4] The role of ureaplasmas is less clear, but they may also be involved.[33]

Hypogammaglobulinemia and Immunosuppression

Some hypogammaglobulinemic patients have developed a chronic urethrocystitis that seemed to be caused by a persistent ureaplasmal and/or *M. hominis* infection, other microorganisms not being isolated.[34] In one case of chronic NGU, the very large number of ureaplasmas recovered persistently from the urethra suggested a causal relationship.[35] Easier to establish is the mycoplasmal etiology of arthritis seen in some patients with hypogammaglobulinemia.[36] This possibility should be considered in any such patient who develops an abacterial septic arthritis. Ureaplasmas and *M. hominis* have been isolated from synovial fluids of a small proportion of these patients, and *M. hominis* has been isolated very occasionally after childbirth in otherwise normal mothers who develop arthritis of sudden onset.[36] The arthritis responds to tetracyclines or other antibiotics to which the organisms are sensitive, a further indication that they are a cause of the disease.

Immunosuppression may lead to proliferation of mycoplasmas, and septicemia,[37] and peritonitis[38] due to *M. hominis* have been recorded.

Other Diseases

The few reported cases of neonatal meningitis or brain abscess in which *M. hominis* has been isolated from cerebrospinal fluid[39–41] or abscess[42,43] have resulted presumably from infection in utero or from colonization at birth with subsequent infection. The same comment applies to the recovery of ureaplasmas from cerebrospinal fluid.[41] The possibility should be considered in cases of neonatal central nervous system disease in which the results of bacteriologic staining and culture are negative. Apart from fever following abortion or normal childbirth, fever associated with burns and trauma has also been attributed to *M. hominis* infection,[37,44] and this mycoplasma has also been implicated in some wound infections.[45]

Conditions of Rare or Equivocal Mycoplasmal Etiology

As shown in Table 2, there are various conditions, such as epididymitis, urinary calculi, Reiter disease, infertility, spontaneous abortion, chorioamnionitis, and low birth weight, with which ureaplasmas, in particular, have been associated. In some instances the association is rare, and in others there is insufficient proof or no proof that the organisms are a cause. Recent observations indicate that ureaplasmas are a rare cause of acute nonchlamydial epididymitis, the organisms having been recovered from the epididymis in association with an antibody response.[46] Furthermore, the results of studies on ureaplasmas in urinary calculi,[47] infertility,[48] particularly among a subgroup of infertile women whose problem is associated with a male factor,[49] abortion,[50,51] chorioamnionitis,[52] and respiratory disease in the newborn,[53] including the respiratory distress syndrome,[54] and chronic lung disease[55] are provocative and should stimulate further work to define their role.

MANAGEMENT AND TREATMENT

Since culturing for mycoplasmas is not generally available to clinicians, management depends on recognizing clinical syndromes for which mycoplasmas could be responsible and providing therapy that would be adequate to eliminate them.

The weight of accumulated evidence suggests that both *C. trachomatis* and *U. urealyticum* cause NGU. Patients should receive a tetracycline, for example doxycycline, 100 mg twice daily for 7 days. However, about 10 percent of ureaplasmas are resistant to tetracyclines,[17,23,24] and patients with NGU due to resistant organisms often have no clinical response to the administration of a tetracycline.[56] In this circumstance, the patients should be examined for tetracycline-resistant ureaplasmas if laboratory facilities are available. Meanwhile, they should be treated with erythromycin, 0.5 g four times daily for 7 days, since most tetracycline-resistant ureaplasmas are sensitive to this antibiotic.

It would be advisable to treat PID with a tetracycline in areas where a substantial proportion of the disease is nongonococcal, since tetracyclines are active against most strains of *M. hominis* as well as against *C. trachomatis*, which also causes PID. However, the emergence of tetracycline-resistant strains of *M. hominis*[36,40,57] means that other antibiotics, such as lincomycin or clindamycin, may need to be considered. If *M. hominis*-induced fever following abortion or vaginal delivery does not settle rapidly, tetracycline therapy should be instituted while keeping tetracycline resistance in mind. The latter assumes greater importance in other clinical situation, such as arthritis and neonatal disease, where *M. hominis* is considered to be responsible.

Antibiotic treatment for infertility,[58] spontaneous abortion,[50] or low birth weight[59] is obviously legitimate on a research basis. However, for these and other conditions in which a mycoplasmal etiology has not been proved, it is difficult to justify either examination for the organisms or treatment directed against them on a routine basis. Culture of genital specimens from adults with an idiopathic disorder results in the isolation of either ureaplasmas or *M. hominis*, or both, from about one-half of them. To consider the organisms a cause of the disorder on the basis of such a predictable microbiologic finding is not warranted, and to provide routine antibiotic therapy aimed at the mycoplasmas in such instances would seem as unethical as not initiating effective treatment when the etiology is understood.

REFERENCES

1. Taylor-Robinson D, Furr PM. Recovery and identification of human genital tract mycoplasmas. Isr J Med Sci. 1981;17:648.
2. Tully JG, Taylor-Robinson D, Rose DL, et al. Evaluation of culture media for the recovery of *Mycoplasma hominis* from the human urogenital tract. Sex Transm Dis. 1983;10:256.
3. Taylor-Robinson D, Tully JG, Furr PM, et al. Urogenital mycoplasma infections of man: A review with observations on a recently discovered mycoplasma. Isr J Med Sci. 1981;17:524.
4. Wallace RJ Jr, Alpert S, Brown K, et al. Isolation of *Mycoplasma hominis* from blood cultures in patients with postpartum fever. Obstet Gynecol. 1978;51:181.
5. Klein JO, Buckland D, Finland M. Colonization of newborn infants by mycoplasmas. N Engl J Med. 1969;280:1025.
6. Foy HM, Kenny GE, Levinsohn EM, et al. Acquisition of mycoplasmata and T-strains during infancy. J Infect Dis. 1970;121:579.
7. Hammerschlag MR, Alpert S, Rosner I, et al. Microbiology of the vagina in children: Normal and potentially pathogenic organisms. Pediatrics. 1978; 62:57.
8. Hammerschlag MR, Doraiswamy B, Cox P, et al. Colonization of sexually abused children with genital mycoplasmas. Sex Transm Dis. 1987;14:23.
9. McCormack WM, Lee Y-H, Zinner SH. Sexual experience and urethral colonization with genital mycoplasmas. A study in normal men. Ann Intern Med. 1973;78:696.
10. McCormack WM, Almeida PC, Bailey PE, et al. Sexual activity and vaginal colonization with genital mycoplasmas. JAMA. 1972;221:1375.
11. McCormack WM, Rosner B, Lee Y-H. Colonization with genital mycoplasmas in women. Am J Epidemiol. 1973;97:240.
12. Taylor-Robinson D, Csonka GW. Laboratory and clinical aspects of mycoplasmal infections of the human genitourinary tract. In Harris JRW, ed. Recent Advances in Sexually Transmitted Diseases. London: Churchill Livingstone; 1981:151.
13. Taylor-Robinson D, McCormack WM. Medical progress: The genital mycoplasmas. N Engl J Med. 1980;302:1003–63.
14. Hooton TM, Roberts MC, Roberts PL, et al. Prevalence of *Mycoplasma genitalium* determined by DNA probe in men with urethritis. Lancet. 1988;1:266.
15. Bowie WR, Wang S-P. Alexander ER, et al. Etiology of nongonococcal urethritis: Evidence for *Chlamydia trachomatis* and *Ureaplasma urealyticum*. J Clin Invest. 1977;59:735.
16. Weidner W, Brunner H, Krause W, et al. Zur Bedeutung von *Ureaplasma urealyticum* bei unspezifischer Prostato-urethritis. Quantitative Untersuchungen am 312 Patienten. Dtsch Med Wochenschr. 1978;103:465.
17. Hawkins DA, Taylor-Robinson D, Evans RT, et al. Unsuccessful treatment

of non-gonococcal urethritis with rosoxacin provides information on the aetiology of the disease. Genitourin Med. 1985;61:51.
18. Ahmed-Jushuf IH, Pratt BC, Arya OP. Incidence of *Ureaplasma urealyticum* in endourethral swabs compared with first voided urine from men. Genitourin Med. 1988;64:78.
19. Brown MB, Cassell GH, Taylor-Robinson D, et al. Measurement of antibody to *Ureaplasma urealyticum* by an enzyme-linked immunoassay and detection of antibody responses in patients with nongonococcal urethritis. J Clin Microbiol. 1983;17:288.
20. Prentice MJ, Taylor-Robinson D, Csonka GW. Non-specific urethritis: A placebo-controlled trial of minocycline in conjunction with laboratory investigations. Br J Vener Dis. 1976;52:269.
21. Taylor-Robinson D, Evans RT, Coufalik ED, et al. Effect of short term treatment of non-gonococcal urethritis with minocyline. Genitourin Med. 1986; 62:19.
22. Coufalik ED, Taylor-Robinson D, Csonka GW. Treatment of nongonococcal urethritis with rifampicin as a means of defining the role of *Ureaplasma urealyticum*. Br J Vener Dis. 1979;55:36.
23. Evans RT, Taylor-Robinson D. The incidence of tetracycline-resistant strains of *Ureaplasma urealyticum*. J. Antimicrob Chemother. 1978;4:57.
24. Taylor-Robinson D, Furr PM. Clinical antibiotic resistance of *Ureaplasma urealyticum*. Pediatr Infect Dis. 1986;5:S335.
25. Taylor-Robinson D, Csonka GW, Prentice MJ. Human intra-urethral inoculation of ureaplasmas. Q J Med. 1977;46:309.
26. Thomsen AC. Mycoplasma infections in the upper urinary tract. Dan Med Bull. 1982;29:309.
27. Birch DF, Fairley KF, Pavillard RE: Unconventional bacteria in urinary tract disease. *Ureaplasma urealyticum*. Kidney Int. 1981;19:58.
28. Weström L, Mårdh P-A. Acute salpingitis. Aspects on aetiology, diagnosis, and prognosis. In: Danielsson D, Juhlin L, Mårdh P-A, eds. Genital Infections and Their Complications. Stockholm: Almqvist and Wiksell;1975:157.
29. Mårdh P-A, Weström L. Antibodies to *Mycoplasma hominis* in patients with genital infections and in healthy controls. Br J Vener Dis. 1970;46:390.
30. Lind K, Kristensen GB, Bollerup AC, et al. Importance of *Mycoplasma hominis* in acute salpingitis assessed by culture and serological tests. Genitourin Med. 1985;61:185.
31. Møller BR, Freundt EA, Black FT, et al. Experimental infection of the genital tract of female grivet monkeys by *Mycoplasma hominis*. Infect Immun. 1978;20:248.
32. Platt R, Lin J-SL. Warren JW, et al. Infection with *Mycoplasma hominis* in postpartum fever. Lancet. 1980;2:1217.
33. Eschenbach DA. *Ureaplasma urealyticum* as a cause of postpartum fever. Pediatr Infect Dis. 1986;5:S258.
34. Webster ADB, Taylor-Robinson D, Furr PM, et al. Chronic cystitis and urethritis associated with ureaplasmal and mycoplasmal infection in primary hypogammaglobulinaemia. Br J Urol. 1982;54:287.
35. Taylor-Robinson D, Furr PM, Webster ADB. *Ureaplasma urealyticum* causing persistent urethritis in a patient with hypogammaglobulinaemia. Genitourin Med. 1985;61:404.
36. Taylor-Robinson D, Thomas BJ, Furr PM, et al. The association of *Mycoplasma hominis* with arthritis. Sex Transm Dis. 1983;10:341.
37. DeGirolami PC, Madoff S. *Mycoplasma hominis* septicemia. J Clin Microbiol. 1982;16:566.
38. Mokhbat JE, Peterson PK, Sabath LD, et al. Peritonitis due to *Mycoplasma hominis* in a renal transplant recipient. J Infect Dis. 1982;146:713.
39. Gewitz M, Dinwiddle R, Rees L, et al. *Mycoplasma hominis*. A cause of neonatal meningitis. Arch Dis Child. 1979;54:231.
40. Hjelm E, Jonsell G, Linglöv T, et al. Meningitis in a newborn infant caused by *Mycoplasma hominis*. Acta Paediatr Scand. 1980;69:415.
41. Waites KB, Rudd PT, Crouse DT, et al. Chronic *Ureaplasma urealyticum* and *Mycoplasma hominis* infections of central nervous system in preterm infants. Lancet. 1988;1:17.
42. Siber GR, Alpert S, Smith AL, et al. Neonatal central nervous system infection due to *Mycoplasma hominis*. J Pediatr. 1977;90:625.
43. Payan DG, Seigal N, Madoff S. Infection of a brain abscess by Mycoplasma hominis. J Clin Microbiol. 1981;14:571.
44. Ti TY, Dan M, Stemke GW, et al. Isolation of *Mycoplasma hominis* from the blood of men with multiple trauma and fever. JAMA. 1982;247:60.
45. Steffenson DO, Dummer JS, Granick MS, et al. Sternotomy infections with *Mycoplasma hominis*. JAMA. 1987;106:204.
46. Jalil N, Doble A, Gilchrist C, et al. Infection of the epididymis by *Ureaplasma urealyticum*. Genitourin Med. 1988;64:367.
47. Pettersson S, Brorson JE, Grenabo L, et al. *Ureaplasma urealyticum* in infectious urinary tract stones. Lancet. 1983;1:526.
48. Taylor-Robinson D. Evaluation of the role of *Ureaplasma urealyticum* in infertility. Pediatr Infect Dis. 1986;5:S262.
49. Cassell GH, Younger JB, Brown MB, et al. Microbiologic study of infertile women at the time of diagnostic laparoscopy. Association of *Ureaplasma urealyticum* with a defined subpopulation. N Engl J Med. 1983;308:502.
50. Quinn PA, Schewchuk AB, Shuber J, et al. Efficacy of antibiotic therapy in preventing spontaneous pregnancy loss among couples colonized with genital mycoplasmas. Am J Obstet Gynecol. 1983;145:239.
51. Quinn PA, Shewchuk AB, Shuber J, et al. Serologic evidence of *Ureaplasma urealyticum* infection in women with spontaneous pregnancy loss. Am J Obstet Gynecol. 1983;145:245.
52. Cassell GH, Waites KB, Gibbs RS, et al. Role of *Ureaplasma urealyticum* in amnionitis. Pediatr Infect Dis. 1986;5:S247.
53. Rudd PT, Waites KB, Duffy LB, et al. *Ureaplasma urealyticum* and its possible role in pneumonia during the neonatal period and infancy. Pediatr Infect Dis. 1986;5:S288.
54. Gallo D, Dupuis KW, Schmidt NJ, et al. Broadly reactive immunofluorescence test for measurement of immunoglobulin M and G antibodies to *Ureaplasma urealyticum* in infant and adult sera. J Clin Microbiol. 1983;17:614.
55. Cassell GH, Waites KB, Crouse DT, et al. Association of *Ureaplasma urealyticum* infection of the lower respiratory tract with chronic lung disease and death in very low birth weight infants. Lancet. 1988;2:240.
56. Stimson JB, Hale J, Bowie WR, et al. Tetracycline-resistant *Ureaplasma urealyticum*: A cause of persistent nongonococcal urethritis. Ann Intern Med. 1981;94:192.
57. Koutsky LA, Stamm WE, Brunham RC, et al. Persistence of *Mycoplasma hominis* after treatment with different antimicrobials. Sex Transm Dis. 1983;10:374.
58. Toth A, Lesser ML, Brooks C, et al. Subsequent pregnancies among 161 couples treated for T-mycoplasma genital-tract infection. N Engl J Med. 1983;308:505.
59. Kass EH, McCormack WM, Lin J-S, et al. Genital mycoplasmas as a cause of excess premature delivery. Trans Assoc Am Phys. 1981;94:261.

SECTION D. RICKETTSIOSIS

164. INTRODUCTION

ALFRED J. SAAH

The family of microbes Rickettsiaceae is maintained in nature through a cycle involving reservoirs in mammals and insect vectors. The public health impact on lives or productivity lost is largely unmeasured, but it is suspected to be quite high worldwide.[1] Humans are incidental hosts and are not useful in propagating the organism in nature. An exception is louse-borne typhus where humans are the principal reservoir and the human body louse is the vector, thereby creating a cycle that involves humans alone. However, even louse-borne typhus may also prove to be a zoonotic disease. Data have been reported implicating the flying squirrel as a reservoir of the agent that produces louse-borne typhus,[2,3] and serologic evidence in humans suggests that louse-borne typhus occurs indigenously in the United States[4,5] (see Chapter 168).

DESCRIPTION OF THE PATHOGEN

Rickettsiae are fastidious bacterial organisms that are obligate, intracellular parasites. The organisms are small, pleomorphic coccobacilli. Coccal forms usually are 0.3 μm in diameter, while bacillary forms measure 0.3 μm × 1.0–2.0 μm. The bacterial nature of these organisms is now well established[6]; they multiply by binary fission, contain both RNA and DNA, and have both synthetic and energy-producing enzyme systems. In addition, typhus and spotted fever group rickettsiae contain endotoxins; an exception is the scrub typhus pathogen where current evidence suggests that it is lacking.

With the exception of *Coxiella burnetii* (Q fever), the rickettsiae survive only briefly outside of a host (reservoir or vector). *Coxiella burnetii* is a hearty organism that resists desiccation, heat, and sunlight and is transmitted primarily by the airborne route. Based on antigenic similarities and intracellular growth characteristics, the rickettsiae have been broadly divided into spotted fever and typhus groups (Table 1).

If isolation of rickettsial organisms is attempted, it should be done only in a reference laboratory that is skilled in handling rickettsiae. Blood cells are sufficient for isolation attempts; the cells should be separated from serum immediately after clotting. The clot should be quick-frozen in dry ice and alcohol and kept at −70°C continuously (including shipment) until thawed for injection into laboratory animals.[6]

EPIDEMIOLOGY

The etiologic agents of Rocky Mountain spotted fever (RMSF), murine typhus, scrub typhus, and rickettsialpox (*Rickettsia rickettsii, R. typhi, R. tsutsugamushi*, and *R. akari*, respectively) exist in a classically commensal fashion with their insect vectors. Three of these organisms (*R. rickettsii, R. tsutsugamushi*, and *R. akari*) are transmitted transovarially to progeny of their vectors. *Rickettsia prowazekii* (louse-borne typhus) causes the death of its vector (human body louse) in 1–3 weeks. The zoonotic reservoirs of the rickettsiae are quite varied but generally are composed of small mammals and livestock (Table 1).

In the United States,[7] RMSF, Q fever, and murine typhus are endemic; rickettsialpox and epidemic typhus also may occur. In addition, recrudescent louse-borne typhus (Brill-Zinsser disease) still occurs—predominantly in immigrants who were living in eastern Europe during World War II.

PATHOLOGIC CHARACTERISTICS

Except for Q fever, the pathogenesis of both spotted fever and typhus group organisms is vasculitis caused by the proliferation of organisms in the endothelial lining of small arteries, veins, and capillaries. Evidence for a rickettsial toxin has been shown in experimental animals, but its relationship to human disease is undefined. The organisms can be seen in histopathologic specimens in the cytoplasm and—in the case of RMSF—in the nuclei of cells as well. The organisms do not stain well with Gram stain but are stained effectively by Giemsa or Gimenez stain.

The direct immunofluorescent technique identifies specific organisms and has proved to be useful in identifying *R. rickettsii* in ticks[8] and histopathologic specimens.[9] This method has also been shown to aid in the early diagnosis of RMSF through skin biopsy specimens.[10]

CLINICAL MANIFESTATIONS AND DIAGNOSIS

During the appropriate season—generally spring and summer—the triad of fever, headache, and rash should alert the physician to consider a rickettsial etiology. Historic features should be sought such as tick attachment, recent camping, or occupational exposure. Differential diagnoses are included in the chapters that follow.

The diagnosis of a rickettsial illness is most often confirmed by serologic testing. Serologic methods were first used in Poland in 1915 when Weil and Felix found that serum from patients with typhus agglutinated certain strains of *Proteus vulgaris*. Familiarity and ease of the Weil-Felix reaction has led to its widespread and continued use; the Centers for Disease Control in Atlanta, Georgia, have downgraded the Weil-Felix reaction in the diagnosis of RMSF.[11] A case with positive titers by Weil-Felix reaction is only considered a probable (formerly confirmed) case of RMSF. More specific tests such as complement fixation (CF), indirect hemagglutination,[12] direct[10] and indirect[13,14] immunofluorescence tests, and others[15–18] have been developed. However, except for the CF and direct immunofluorescent tests, these procedures are used primarily by reference laboratories.

Serologic evidence of infection occurs no earlier than the second week of illness in any of the rickettsial diseases; therefore, therapy must be instituted on clinical grounds. In RMSF, the direct immunofluorescence test on skin lesions[10] identifies organisms and allows the diagnosis to be made when the rash appears (3–5 days).

RECENT DEVELOPMENTS

There have been numerous rickettsial strains isolated from ticks in many countries. Some of these strains may be associated with the various clinical types of spotted fever that have been iden-

TABLE 1. Synopsis of Certain Epidemiologic and Clinical Features of Selected Rickettsioses

			Hosts			
Disease	*Organism*	*Geographic Area*	*Arthropods*	*Vertebrates*	*Rash Distribution*	*Eschar*
Spotted fever group						
RMSF	*R. rickettsii*	Western hemisphere	Tick	Wild rodents, dogs	Extremities to trunk	No
Boutonneuse	*R. conorii*	Africa, Mediterranean, India	Tick	Wild rodents, dogs	Trunk, extremities, face	Yes
Queensland tick typhus	*R. australis*	Australia	Tick	Wild rodents, marsupials	Trunk, extremities, face	Yes
North Asian tick typhus	*R. sibirica*	Siberia, Mongolia	Tick	Wild rodents	Trunk, extremities, face	Yes
Rickettsialpox	*R. akari*	USA, USSR, Korea, Africa	Mite	Mouse	Vesicular; trunk, extremities, face	Yes
Typhus group						
Epidemic typhus	*R. prowazekii*	Highland areas of South America, Africa, Asia, ? USA	Body louse	Humans, flying squirrel	Trunk to extremities	No
Brill-Zinsser	*R. prowazekii*	Worldwide based upon immigration	None	Humans (Recurrence years after primary attack)	Trunk to extremities (may be absent)	No
Murine typhus	*R. typhi*	Worldwide in pockets	Flea	Small rodents	Trunk to extremities	No
Scrub typhus	*R. tsutsugamushi*	South Pacific, Asia, Australia	Mite	Wild rodents	Trunk to extremities	Yes
Others						
Q fever	*C. burnetii*	Worldwide	? Ticks	Cattle, sheep, goats (Inhalation of organism)	None	No
Trench fever	*Rochalimaea quintana*	Highly focal	Lice	Humans	Transient or none	No

tified in Asia and Africa. In North America, *R. canada* was isolated from *Haemaphysalis leporispalustris* ticks in Canada in 1963.[19] It was shown by high cross-reacting of antibody to possess antigens in common with *R. typhi* and *R. prowazekii*, which placed it in the typhus group. However, its growth pattern includes intranuclear growth, which mimics characteristics of the spotted fever group.[20] Human infection with *R. canada* is supported by serologic evidence,[21] but confirmation awaits fulfillment of Koch's postulates.

An interesting development involves *R. prowazekii*, its reservoir in the southern flying squirrel, and the serologic evidence that disease (epidemic typhus) in humans is occurring in the United States[2–5] (see Chapter 168).

Another interesting discovery is that an *Ehrlichia canis*-like organism produces naturally acquired infection and disease in humans.[22] The organism seems to be transmitted to humans by ticks and produces an illness similar to RMSF but does not produce a rash (see Chapter 171).

REFERENCES

1. WHO Working Group on Rickettsial Diseases. Rickettsioses: A continuing disease problem. Bull WHO. 1982;60:157–64.
2. Bozeman FM, Masiello SA, Williams MS, et al. Epidemic typhus rickettsiae isolated from flying squirrels. Nature. 1975;255:545–7.
3. Sonenshine DE, Bozeman FM, Williams MS, et al. Epizootiology of epidemic typhus (*Rickettsia prowazekii*) in flying squirrels. Am J Trop Med Hyg. 1978;27:339–49.
4. McDade JE, Shepard CC, Redus MA, et al. Evidence of *Rickettsia prowazekii* infections in the United States. Am J Trop Med Hyg. 1980;29:277–84.
5. Duma RJ, Sonenshine DE, Bozeman FM, et al. Epidemic typhus in the United States associated with flying squirrels. JAMA. 1981;245:2318–23.
6. Ormsbee RA. Rickettsiae. In: Lennette EH, Balows A, Hausler WJ Jr, et al., eds. Manual of Clinical Microbiology. 3rd ed. Washington, DC: American Society for Microbiology; 1980:922.
7. Woodward TE. Rickettsial diseases in the United States. Med Clin North Am. 1959;43:1507–35.
8. Burgdorfer W, Lackman D. Identification of *Rickettsia rickettsii* in the wood tick, *Dermacentor andersoni*, by means of fluorescent antibody. J Infect Dis. 1960;107:241.
9. Burgdorfer W. Evaluation of the fluorescent antibody technique for the detection of Rocky Mountain spotted fever rickettsia in various tissues. Pathol Microbiol (Basel). 1961;24(Suppl):27.
10. Woodward TE, Pedersen CE, Oster CN, et al. Prompt confirmation of Rocky Mountain spotted fever: Identification of rickettsia in skin tissues. J Infect Dis. 1976;134:297–301.
11. Centers for Disease Control: Rickettsial Disease Surveillance Report No. 2 Summary: 1979. Issued May 1981.
12. Shirai A, Dietel JW, Osterman JV. Indirect hemagglutination test for human antibody to typhus and spotted fever group rickettsiae. J Clin Microbiol. 1975;2:430–7.
13. Goldwasser RA, Shepard CC. Fluorescent antibody methods in the differentiation of murine and epidemic typhus sera: Specificity changes resulting from previous immunization. J Immunol. 1959;82:373–80.
14. Goldwasser RA, Shepard CC, Jordan ME, et al. The specificity of antibody response in typhus fever. Its alteration during murine typhus infection as a result of previous exposure to epidemic typhus antigen. J Immunol. 1959;83:491–5.
15. Philip RN, Casper EA, Ormsbee RA, et al. Microimmunofluorescence test for the serological study of Rocky Mountain spotted fever and typhus. J Clin Microbiol. 1976;3:51–61.
16. Philip RN, Casper EA, MacCormack JN, et al. A comparison of serologic methods for diagnosis of Rocky Mountain spotted fever. Am J Epidemiol. 1977;105:56–67.
17. Ormsbee R, Peacock M, Philip R, et al. Serologic diagnosis of epidemic typhus fever. Am J Epidemiol. 1977;105:261–71.
18. Kaplan JE, Schonberger LB. The sensitivity of various serologic tests in the diagnosis of Rocky Mountain spotted fever. Am J Trop Med Hyg. 1986;35:840–4.
19. McKiel JA, Bell EJ, Lackman DB. *Rickettsia canada*: A new member of the typhus group of rickettsiae isolated from *Haemaphysalis leporispalustris*. Can J Microbiol. 1967;13:503–10.
20. Burgdorfer W, Brinton LP. Intranuclear growth of *Rickettsia canada*, a member of the typhus group. Infect Immun. 1970;2:112–4.
21. Bozeman FM, Elisberg BL, Humphries JW, et al. Serologic evidence of *Rickettsia canada* infection of man. J Infect Dis. 1970;121:367–71.
22. Maeda K, Markowitz N, Hawley RC, et al. Human infection with *Ehrlichia canis*, a leukocytic rickettsia. N Engl J Med. 1987;316:853–6.

165. RICKETTSIA RICKETTSII AND OTHER SPOTTED FEVER GROUP RICKETTSIAE (ROCKY MOUNTAIN SPOTTED FEVER AND OTHER SPOTTED FEVERS)

D. RAOULT
D. H. WALKER

The spotted fevers comprise a large group of tick- and mite-borne zoonotic infections that are caused by closely related rickettsiae. They include Rocky Mountain spotted fever, boutonneuse fever, North Asian tick typhus, Queensland tick typhus, and rickettsialpox. These diseases have a broad spectrum of severity; the most virulent, Rocky Mountain spotted fever, has a fatality-to-case ratio of 20 percent unless treated early and appropriately. Even young and previously healthy people may die with Rocky Mountain spotted fever. In recent years the wide distribution and potential severity of the other spotted fevers have been recognized, especially in southern Europe, Africa, China, and Japan. Establishing an early diagnosis remains deceptively difficult.

ROCKY MOUNTAIN SPOTTED FEVER

The Pathogen

Rocky Mountain spotted fever (RMSF) was first described in Idaho in the late nineteenth century.[1] Ricketts established the infectious nature of the illness and demonstrated the role of ticks as the vector in western Montana in 1906.[2] Wolbach in 1919 clearly identified the etiologic rickettsiae within endothelial cells.[3]

The etiologic agent, *Rickettsia rickettsii*, belongs to the spotted fever group of rickettsiae, which are genetically related but differ from one another in their surface antigenic proteins.[4] Some presumably nonpathogenic rickettsiae also belong to this group. Spotted fever group rickettsiae are obligate intracellular bacteria that reside in the cytosol and less often in the nucleus of their host cells. The rickettsiae are small, measuring approximately 0.3 μm by 1.0 μm. The cell wall has the ultrastructural appearance of a gram-negative bacterium and contains lipopolysaccharide (LPS). Rickettsiae are difficult to stain with ordinary bacterial stains but are conveniently stained by the Gimenez method or with acridine orange. They have not been cultivated in cell-free medium. Growth requires living host cells such as the yolk sac of embryonated eggs, experimental animals (e.g., guinea pigs), or cell culture (e.g., Vero cells, L cells, and chick embryo cells). Rickettsiae are not a defective or degenerate life form but rather are highly adapted for intracellular survival with effective transport systems and metabolic enzymes.[5] Among the protein antigens of *R. rickettsii*, two surface proteins (155 kD and 120 kD) contain heat labile epitopes that seem critical to immunity.[6,7] Some epitopes of these proteins are species specific, and others are shared among the members of the group. The LPS of spotted fever group rickettsiae contains highly immunogenic antigens that are strongly cross-reactive among all members of the group, cross react to a lesser extent with *R. typhi* and *R. prowazekii*, and are responsible for the cross-reactivity of spotted fever group rickettsiae with *Proteus* and *Legionella*. However, monoclonal antibodies to LPS do not confer passive protection against experimental infection of animals.

Epidemiology

The role of a tick bite in the transmission of RMSF was demonstrated by McCalla and Brereton[1]; a tick obtained from a patient suffering from RMSF transmitted the disease to two volunteers. The seasonal distribution of RMSF mirrors tick activity. The tick is both the vector and the main reservoir.[8] *Dermacentor variabilis*, the American dog tick, is the prevalent vector in the eastern United States; *D. andersoni*, the Rocky Mountain wood tick, in the western states; *Rhipicephalus sanguineus*, in Mexico; and *Amblyoma cajennense*, in Central and South America. (See Chapter 272 for illustrations of ticks.) Causes for the variation in infection rates among populations of ticks are not clear, although humidity, climatic variations, human activities altering the vegetation and fauna, and the use of insecticides have been suspected to play a role in the fluctuation of the prevalence of human rickettsiosis.

Rickettsia rickettsii is transmitted trans-stadially and transovarially in ticks, thus maintaining the agent in nature. The likelihood of low-level attrition of the infected ticks owing to rickettsial injury implies that horizontal transmission would also be necessary for the maintenance of *R. rickettsii*. In fact, in most mammals rickettsemia is of very short duration and allows for infection of ticks only rarely.[8] Of the three tick stages, larva, nymph, and adult, only the adult *Dermacentor* ticks feed on humans. The prevalence of pathogenic rickettsiae in various populations of ticks is variable. Many nonpathogenic rickettsiae have been isolated and characterized in the United States including *R. bellii, R. montana, R. rhipicephali*, and *R. parkeri*.[4,9] These rickettsiae may compete for the ecologic niche by an interference mechanism that inhibits the establishment of infection of ticks with *R. rickettsii*.[10]

The tick transmits the disease to humans during feeding. The bite is painless and frequently unnoticed. After the attached tick has fed for 6–10 hours, rickettsiae are released from the salivary glands. An even longer period may be required for reactivation of rickettsial virulence in unfed ticks. Humans may also be infected by exposure to infective tick hemolymph during the removal of ticks from humans or domestic animals, especially when the tick is crushed between the fingers.

Although *R. rickettsii* has rarely been recovered from feral animals, serum antibodies are detected in many of these animals, and the prevalence of antibodies in dogs correlates with the prevalence of human cases in the particular area.

Laboratory-acquired infection[11] transmitted by infectious aerosols or parenteral inoculation of *R. rickettsii* may be prevented by careful technique, biohazard containment hoods, and masks and gloves.

The considerable fluctuation in the annual number of patients with RMSF in the United States (Fig. 1)[12] may reflect cyclic changes in the ecology of the tick–rickettsia relationship. The increase in the infection rate that occurred between 1969 and 1977 may have several hypothetical explanations: an increase in the infected tick population or tick contact, an increase of interest of physicians in the disease, and the development of more sensitive, specific serologic tools. The fall in incidence in 1949 followed the introduction of effective antibiotics, and the increased incidence of the 1970s coincided with a decline in the use of tetracycline as a first-choice antibiotic for many other infections. These correlations imply a substantial occurrence of undiagnosed cases aborted by early treatment.

From the 1870s until 1931, RMSF was only recognized to exist in the western United States. At present, the prevalence of the disease is higher in the South Atlantic states (0.83 per 100,000 inhabitants) and in the west south central region (0.53 per 100,000) than in the Rocky Mountain states (Fig. 2). The local prevalence in highly endemic areas such as North Carolina is as high as 14.59 per 100,000.[14] Moreover, while the incidence of infection may be decreasing in one area, it may be increasing simultaneously in another region. The recent discovery of a focus in the South Bronx emphasizes that the ecologic conditions permitting the establishment of RMSF are widely distributed.[15] Most cases are diagnosed during late spring and summer. However, especially in the southern states a few cases also occur during the winter.[16]

In the southern states, the incidence is highest among children and patients who are known to be exposed more often to ticks than are matched controls.[14] In the western states owing to transmission by the wood tick *D. andersoni*, a higher proportion of adult males contract the disease because of occupational factors. The case-to-fatality ratios are significantly higher for nonwhites than for whites, for males than for females, and for patients older than 30 years than for persons younger than 30.[17]

Serosurveys of humans have been conducted to evaluate the prevalence of the disease. The specificity of the assays has been questioned because of cross-reactivity of *R. rickettsii* with nonpathogenic rickettsiae and other bacteria, some of the methods employed, and the selection of minimal significant titers.

Pathogenesis

Rickettsiae introduced into the skin apparently spread via lymphatics and small blood vessels to the systemic and pulmonary circulation where they attach to and enter their target cells, the vascular endothelium, to establish numerous disseminated foci of infection.[18] After entry by induced phagocytosis, the rickettsiae escape from the phagosome into the cytoplasm and less frequently the nucleus. Rickettsiae proliferate intracellularly by binary fission and are released from the infected cells via long thin cell projections. The presence of large quantities of rickettsiae in damaged cells supports the concept of direct cell injury.[19,20] The major pathophysiologic effect of endothelial cell injury is increased vascular permeability, which in turn results in edema, hypovolemia, hypotension, and hypoalbuminemia. Hyponatremia seems to be caused by secretion of antidiuretic hormone as a response to hypovolemia. High quantities of rickettsiae infecting the pulmonary microcirculation increase the vascular permeability and cause noncardiogenic pulmonary edema. Vascular injury and the subsequent host mononuclear leukocytic response correspond to the distribution of rickettsiae and include interstitial pneumonia, interstitial myocarditis, perivascular glial nodules of the central nervous system, and similar vascular lesions in the rash, gastrointestinal tract, pancreas, liver, skeletal muscles, and kidneys. Severe vascular injury may lead to hemorrhage. Platelets are consumed locally in numerous foci of infection; subsequently thrombocytopenia is observed in 32–52 percent of patients.[21,22] Increased adherence of platelets to infected endothelial cells has also been demonstrated in vitro.[23] Although the coagulation mechanism and platelets are activated,[24] true disseminated intravascular coagulation occurs only rarely. *R. rickettsii* infection is also associated with the classic acute-phase response, activation of the kallikrein-kinin system, and an immune response to rickettsiae. T-lymphocyte-mediated host defenses including γ-interferon seem to be most important in combating infection with rickettsiae.[25]

Plaque formation in vitro as well as the pathologic findings indicate that rickettsiae directly injure the infected cells. There are no convincing data to support endotoxin or exotoxin as a pathogenic mechanism; immunopathology and coagulation do not appear to be pathogenic mechanisms.

Clinical Manifestations

The incubation period ranges from 2 to 14 days, with a median of 7 days.[26] Variation in the incubation time may be related in part to the inoculum size. The disease usually begins with fever,

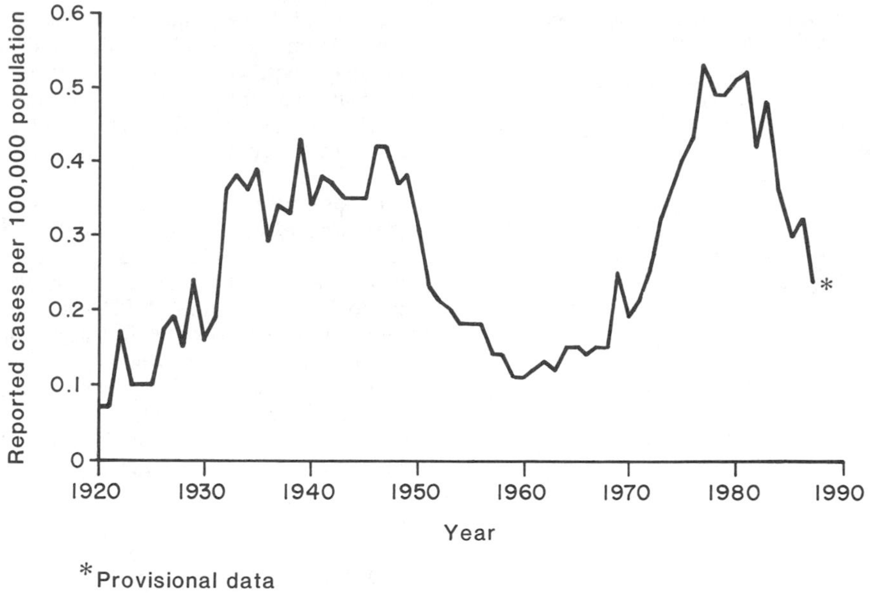

FIG. 1. Rocky Mountain spotted fever rates, by year—United States, 1920–1987. (Courtesy of Dr. Daniel B. Fishbein, Centers for Disease Control, Atlanta, GA.)

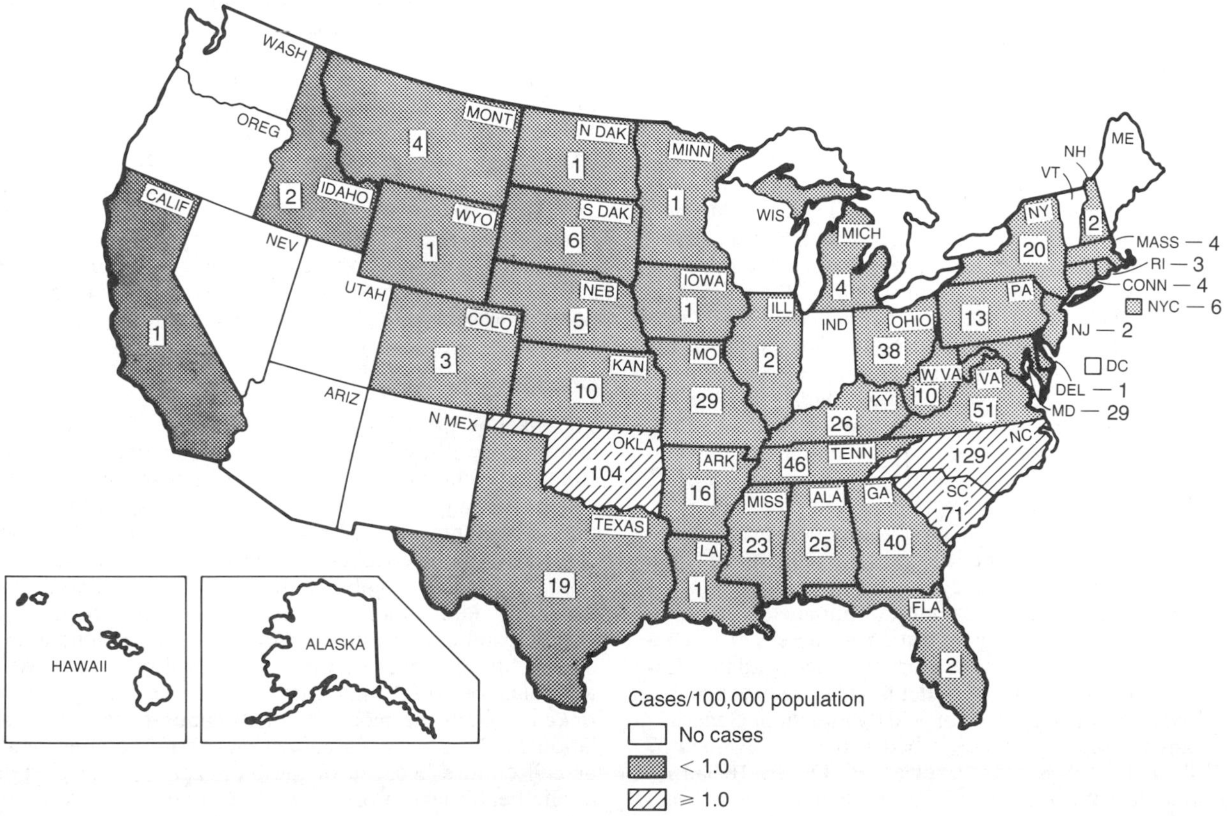

FIG. 2. Reported Rocky Mountain spotted fever cases and rates, by state—United States, 1986. (From Centers for Disease Control.[13])

myalgia, and headache (Table 1). The temperature is greater than 102°F in 63 percent during the first 3 days and in 90 percent later.[21] The variable incidence of reported headache and myalgias in different series may be related to the proportion of young children who may not complain of pain. Other signs and symptoms are frequently prominent early in the course before the onset of rash. Gastrointestinal involvement with nausea, vomiting, abdominal pain, diarrhea, and abdominal tenderness occurs in substantial portions of patients and may suggest gastroenteritis or an acute surgical abdomen.

The rash, the major diagnostic sign, appears in a small fraction of patients on the first day of the disease and in 49 percent during the first 3 days, usually appearing 3–5 days after the onset of fever and occurring in 84–91 percent of patients overall.

TABLE 1. Symptoms, Signs, and Laboratory Data in Rocky Mountain Spotted Fever (RMSF) and Boutonneuse Fever (BF).

Feature	*RMSF (%)*	*BF (%)*
Fever	99–100	100
Headache	79–91	56
Rash	88–90	97
Tache noire	0	72
Myalgia	72–83	36
Nausea/vomiting	56–60	
Abdominal pain	34–52	
Petechial rash	45–49	10
Conjunctivitis	30	9
Lymphadenopathy	27	
Stupor	21–26	10
Diarrhea	19–20	
Edema	18–20	
Ataxia	5–18	
Meningismus	18	11
Splenomegaly	14–16	6
Hepatomegaly	12–15	13
Pneumonitis	12–17	
Cough	33	10
Dyspnea		21
Coma	9–10	
Jaundice	8–9	2
Seizures	8	
Shock/hypotension	7–17	
Decreased hearing	7	
Arrhythmia	7–16	
Myocarditis	5–26	11
Death	4–8	2.5
Increased SGOT level	37–62	39
Thrombocytopenia	32–52	35
Anemia	5–24	
Hyponatremia	19–56	25
Azotemia	12–14	6

Abbreviations: RMSF: Rocky Mountain Spotted Fever; BF: boutonneuse fever.
(Data from Helmick et al.,[21] Kaplowitz et al.,[22] and Raoult et al.[27])

Rocky Mountain ''spotless'' fever occurs more often in older patients and in black patients.[21] A delay in diagnosis is at times associated with the absence or late onset of rash. The rash typically begins around the wrists and ankles but may start on the trunk or be diffuse at the onset. Involvement of the palms and soles is considered characteristic, yet occurs in only 36–82 percent of patients who have a rash and often appears late in the course (Figs. 3 and 4). Skin necrosis or gangrene develops in 4 percent of cases as a result of rickettsial damage to the microcirculation.[21] Gangrene involves the digits or limbs and occasionally requires amputation. A careful initial examination seldom reveals an eschar at the site of the tick bite in RMSF.[28] Headache is usually quite severe. Focal neurologic deficits, transient deafness, meningismus, and photophobia may suggest meningitis or meningoencephalitis. The cerebrospinal fluid (CSF) contains increased leukocytes in one-third of the patients, with either lymphocytic or polymorphonuclear predominance.[22]; the CSF protein concentration is increased in one-third of the patients. However, the glucose concentration is low in the CSF of only 8 percent of patients. The electroencephalogram (EEG) may show diffuse cortical dysfunction. Generally neurologic involvement portends a bad prognosis. Among 37 patients followed for 1–8 years after acute RMSF, 21 had residual neurologic abnormalities.[29] These sequelae were headache and other subjective findings, but 12 had EEG abnormalities. These sequelae occur less often in patients with early antibiotic treatment. On funduscopic examination, retinal vein engorgement, arterial occlusion, flame hemorrhages, and papilledema without increased CSF pressure have been noted. These changes may reflect retinal vasculitis with increased permeability and focal thrombosis. Renal failure is an important problem in severe RMSF.[30] Prerenal azotemia related to hypovolemia responds to intravenous hydration; however, acute tubular necrosis may require hemodialysis. Pulmonary involvement is suggested by cough and radiologic changes including alveolar infiltrates, interstitial pneumonia, and pleural effusion.[31] Pulmonary edema with impairment of pulmonary function may require oxygen therapy and ventilatory assistance. Echocardiographic studies reveal minimal myocardial dysfunction,[32] and normal pulmonary capillary wedge pressure measurements document the noncardiogenic nature of the pulmonary edema.

In classic RMSF, death occurs 8–15 days after the onset of symptoms when appropriate therapy is not given in a timely manner. In fulminant RMSF death occurs within the first 5 days. Several features account for the extreme difficulty in the diagnosis of fulminant RMSF: the course is rapid, the rash develops shortly before death if at all, antibodies to *R. rickettsii* do not have time to develop, and the pathologic lesions even appear different, containing more thrombi and lacking the characteristic lymphohistiocytic component.[33] Fulminant RMSF is more often observed in black males with glucose-6-phosphate dehydrogenase (G6PD) deficiency. Other risk factors for a lethal outcome include older age, male sex, and possibly alcoholism.

Characteristic laboratory data may support the clinical diagnosis of classic RMSF but are relatively nonspecific.[21,22] The white blood cell count is generally normal, but increased quantities of immature myeloid cells occur frequently. Anemia is observed in 5–30 percent. Thrombocytopenia occurs in the more severe cases, but also in some patients with mild disease. Actually, coagulopathy with prolonged coagulation times and decreased concentrations of fibrinogen and other clotting factors occurs infrequently. Hyponatremia is observed in half of patients with RMSF. Increased concentrations of serum lactate dehydrogenase, creatine kinase, and other enzymes are related to diffuse tissue injury including multifocal rhabdomyonecrosis.

The prognosis in RMSF is largely related to the timeliness of initiation of appropriate therapy. The intervals between onset of the disease and appearance of the rash, clinical diagnosis, and effective antibiotic treatment are significantly longer in patients dying than in patients surviving.[17,21] Fatal cases more frequently have hepatomegaly, jaundice, stupor, and renal insufficiency and report less often a history of tick exposure. Patients who survive RMSF have solid immunity to *R. rickettsii.*

Diagnosis

The diagnosis of RMSF before the onset of the rash is clinical and epidemiologic. The differential diagnosis at the first consultation includes nonspecific viral illness, fever of unknown origin, typhoid fever, measles, rubella, respiratory tract infection, gastroenteritis, acute surgical abdomen, viral meningoencephalitis, meningococcemia, disseminated gonococcal infection, secondary syphilis, leptospirosis, immune complex vasculitis, idiopathic thrombocytopenic purpura (ITP), thrombotic thrombocytopenic purpura (TTP), infectious mononucleosis, drug reaction, and other rickettsial diseases. The laboratory diagnosis of RMSF may be achieved by isolation of *R. rickettsii* from the blood.[34,35] Few laboratories undertake isolation of *R. rickettsii* in guinea pigs, embryonated hen's eggs, or cell culture because of the biohazard. Some hospitals and public health laboratories are able to demonstrate *R. rickettsii* in cutaneous biopsy specimens by direct immunofluorescence, the only timely diagnostic method during the acute phase.[35–37] Serology, the usual method for confirmation of the diagnosis, is retrospective, serum antibodies becoming detectable during convalescence.[37–39] The Weil-Felix test using *Proteus* OX-19 and OX-2 agglutination is not to be relied upon. This method lacks sensitivity and specificity. Four methods for the detection of antibodies to specific rickettsial antigens are indirect hemagglutination, indirect immunofluorescence, latex agglutination, and complement fixation. The diagnostic titers are 1:16 for the complement fixation test, 1:128 for indirect hemagglu-

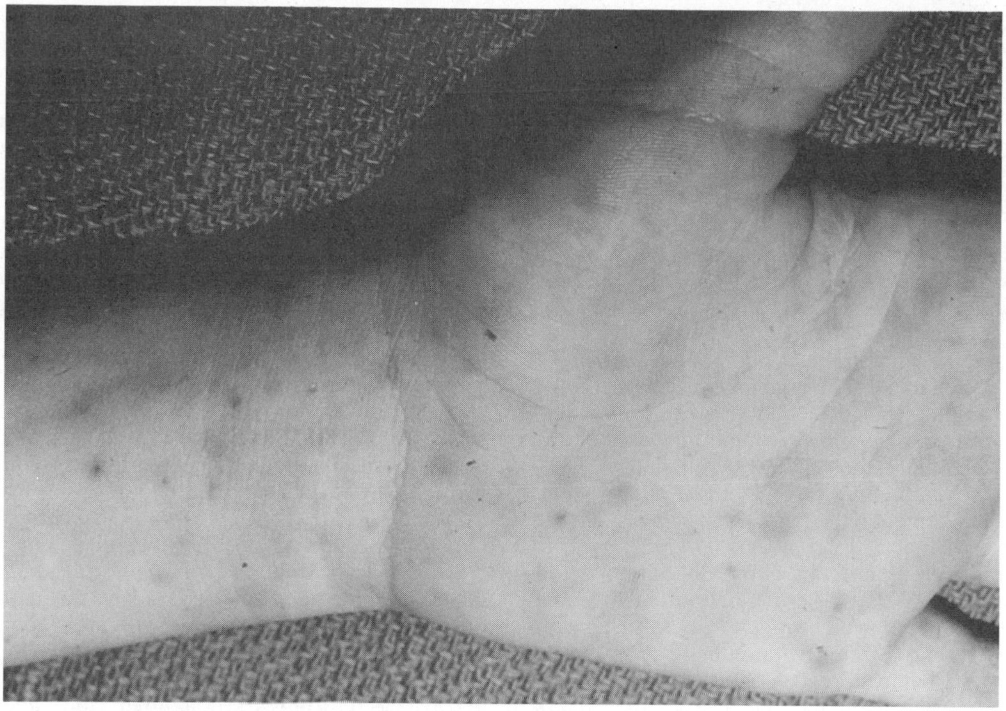

FIG. 3. The wrist and palm manifest the rash of Rocky Mountain spotted fever with central petechiae in some of the maculopapules.

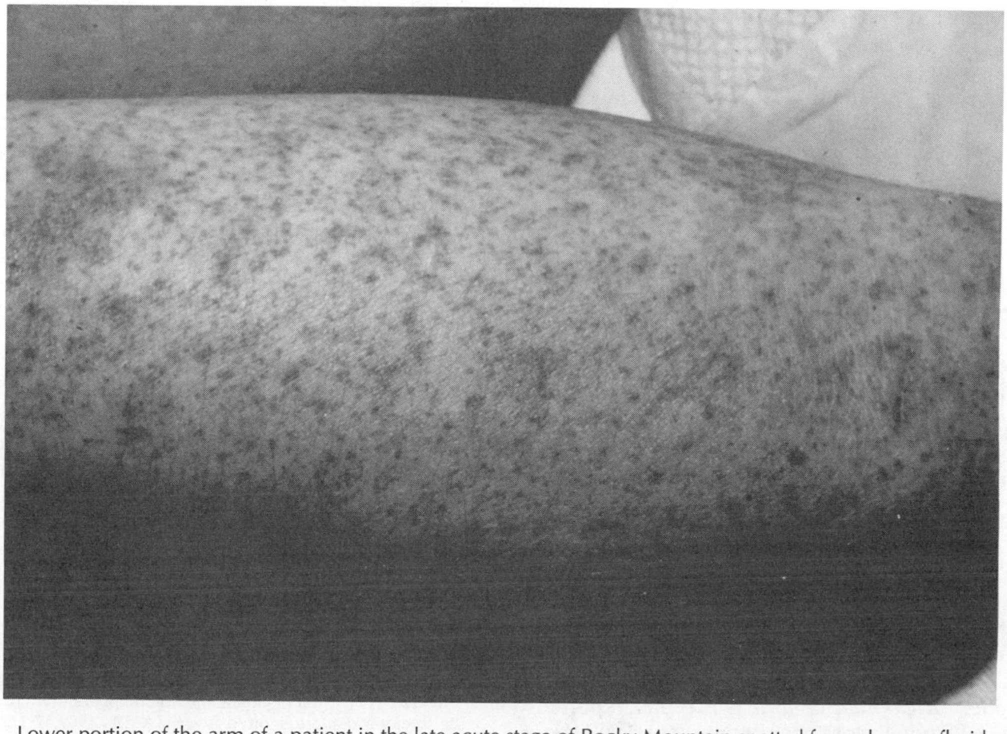

FIG. 4. Lower portion of the arm of a patient in the late acute stage of Rocky Mountain spotted fever shows a florid petechial rash.

tination, and 1:64 for microimmunofluorescence and latex agglutination. Indirect hemagglutination and indirect immunofluorescence are the most sensitive and specific. Complement fixation is much less sensitive. Latex agglutination has the major advantage of commercially available reagents. Early clinical diagnosis remains essential for this life-threatening disease.

Treatment

Since the introduction of chloramphenicol and the tetracyclines, including doxycycline, the lethality of the disease decreased dramatically to 3–7 percent. In vitro and in ovo, *R. rickettsii* is susceptible to chloramphenicol, tetracycline, rifampin,[40] and some new quinolone compounds such as ciprofloxacin[41] and pefloxacin.[42] The organism is resistant to β-lactam antibiotics, aminoglycosides, and trimethoprim-sulfamethoxazole. Erythromycin has minimal inhibitory concentration (MIC) of 3–8 μg/ml and is not effective.[43]

RMSF responds to treatment with oral tetracycline (25–50 mg/kg/day) or chloramphenicol (50–75 mg/kg/day) given in four divided doses. Doxycycline, 100 mg given every 12 hours, is quite effective. The selected antibiotic is usually administered for 7 days, continuing until 2 days after the patient has become afebrile. Treatment should be given intravenously in cases with nausea and vomiting. Doxycycline or another tetracycline is considered by many to be the drug of choice, but chloramphenicol is preferred during pregnancy because of the effects of tetracycline on fetal bones and teeth. Tetracyclines are also avoided in young children when staining the teeth is a concern. Severely ill patients require intensive supportive care. Fluid maintenance is critical in order to maintain organ perfusion. Because of the vascular permeability and the risk of extravasation of fluid into pulmonary alveoli, a Swan-Ganz catheter may be needed to monitor the hemodynamics in some patients. Glucocorticosteroids are sometimes given to severely ill patients, but there has been no documentation of efficacy.

Prevention

Although no vaccine is available currently, the immunodominant surface proteins have been identified, and recently McDonald et al.[44] cloned the genes for the 155 and 120 kD species-specific protein antigens of *R. rickettsii*. Further development of an effective vaccine should lead to immunization of high-risk patients in highly endemic areas.

Currently the best means of prevention remains the avoidance of contact with ticks by the use of repellents and protective clothing. In the hot weather often associated with the tick season, these techniques are often impractical. Regular checks of the body including scalp, pubic, and axillary hair allow removal of the tick before rickettsial transmission. To remove an attached tick, one may use forceps to detach the intact tick without leaving any mouth parts in the skin. The tick bite should be cleansed. Although tick control is theoretically possible, long-term eradication of ticks from the environment has not been achieved.

OTHER SPOTTED FEVER GROUP RICKETTSIOSES

Among the four other spotted fever group rickettsial species known to be pathogenic for human (*R. conorii, R. sibirica, R. australis*, and *R. akari*), the first three are transmitted by tick bite. The last, *R. akari*, is discussed in Chapter 166. *Rickettsia conorii* infection has been designated by many geographic names, Marseilles fever, Mediterranean spotted fever, Kenya tick typhus, South African tick bite fever, Israel tick typhus, and Indian tick typhus. *Rickettsia conorii* is a typical spotted fever group rickettsia, having more than 90 percent DNA homology with *R. rickettsii*. There are also cross-reactive protein and LPS antigens, and cross-protection is shared among *R. conorii, R. sibirica*, and *R. rickettsii*. The heat-sensitive epitopes on the surface proteins of *R. conorii* and *R. sibirica* also appear to be important for immunity.

During the 1970s and 1980s, an increased incidence of spotted fever rickettsioses was noticed in many parts of the world, particularly in Spain, France, Italy, and Israel. Spotted fever rickettsioses have also been described recently in China[45] and Japan.[46] Historically boutonneuse fever was first described by Conor and Bruch in 1909 in Tunisia; in Marseilles in 1923 Olmer and Pieri described the "tache noire," the eschar at the site of the tick bite. *Rickettsia conorii* has been identified in India, Pakistan, Israel, Ethiopia, Kenya, South Africa, Morocco, and southern Europe. *Rickettsia sibirica* has been documented in the USSR, China, Mongolia, and Pakistan. *Rickettsia australis* is limited to northern Australia. The etiologic rickettsial species of the spotted fever rickettsiosis of Japan appears to be a new species; however, the spotted fever group rickettsia of southeastern Asia has yet to be determined. The epidemiology of boutonneuse fever and ecology of *R. conorii* are closely related to ticks, particularly *Rhipicephalus sanguineus* as well as various other species of *Dermacentor, Haemaphysalis, Amblyomma, Hyalomma*, and *Ixodes*. *Rickettsia conorii* is maintained transovarially in ticks and is transmitted to humans by tick bite. Cases occur mainly in warm months with the peak incidence in July, August, and September in many Mediterranean locations. A substantial number of imported cases occurs in travelers returning to the United States and northern Europe from Africa and southern Europe. In northern China *R. sibirica* has been isolated from humans and ticks. Spotted fever group rickettsiae have been isolated from six species of ticks in northern Asia as well as from wild mammals. Transovarial transmission is an important mechanism of survival of *R. sibirica* in nature.

The pathogenic basis for tissue injury in the spotted fevers is well elucidated in the tache noire (black spot) or eschar at the site of the infective tick bite. Dermal and epidermal necrosis and perivascular edema are the consequences of endothelial injury by *R. conorii*.[47] Necropsies of fatal cases of boutonneuse fever reveal disseminated vascular infection and injury by *R. conorii* including meningoencephalitis and vascular lesions in kidneys, lungs, gastrointestinal tract, liver, pancreas, heart, spleen, and skin.[48] Hepatic biopsy specimens reveal focal hepatocellular necrosis. In contrast with the reputation of boutonneuse fever as a benign illness, recent reanalysis of the disease in France,[49] Spain, and Israel demonstrated a death rate ranging from 1.4 to 5.6 percent, similar to that of RSMF in the antibiotic era. After a mean incubation period of 7 days, fever, myalgias, and headache characterize the onset[27] (Table 1). A careful clinical examination may reveal a tache noire, which facilitates the clinical diagnosis. Severe disease resembling RMSF occurs in patients with underlying diseases such as diabetes or cardiac insufficiency, alcoholism, old age, and G6PD deficiency. The disease is milder in children. The diagnosis as for RMSF may be established by immunofluorescent demonstration of *R. conorii* in skin biopsy material.[47,50] During the convalescent phase, production of antibodies to spotted fever group rickettsiae is demonstrated by using microimmunofluorescence, latex agglutination, or complement fixation.[51] Successfuul treatment is achieved with doxycycline (200 mg/day), tetracycline (25 mg/kg/day), chloramphenicol, or ciprofloxacin.[52]

REFERENCES

1. Weiss E. History of Rickettsiology. In: Walker DH, ed. Biology of Rickettsial Diseases. V. 1. Boca Raton, FL: CRC press; 1988:15–32.
2. Ricketts HT. A micro-organism which apparently has a specific relationship to Rocky Mountain spotted fever. JAMA. 1909;52:379–80.
3. Wolbach SB. Studies on Rocky Mountain spotted fever. J Med Res. 1919;41:2–197.
4. Weiss E, Moulder JW. The rickettsias and chlamydias. In: Kreig NR, Holt

JG, eds. Bergey's Manual of Systematic Bacteriology. Baltimore: Williams & Wilkins; 1984:687–739.
5. Austin FE, Winkler HH. Relationship of rickettsial physiology and composition to the rickettsia–host cell interactions. V. 2. In: Walker DH, ed. Biology of Rickettsial Diseases. Boca Raton, FL: CRC Press; 1988:29–49.
6. Anacker RL, McDonald GA, List RH, et al. Neutralizing activity of monoclonal antibodies to heat-sensitive and heat-resistant epitopes of *Rickettsia rickettsii* surface proteins. Infect Immun. 1987;55:825–7.
7. Lange JV, Walker DH. Production and characterization of monoclonal antibodies to *Rickettsia rickettsii*. Infect Immun. 1984;46:289–94.
8. Burgdorfer W. Ecological and epidemiological considerations of Rocky Mountain spotted fever and scrub typhus. In: Walker DH, ed. Biology of Rickettsial Diseases. V. 1. Boca Raton, FL: CRC Press; 1988:33–50.
9. Philip RN, Casper EA, Anacker RL, et al. *Rickettsia bellii* sp. nov.; a tick borne rickettsia, widely distributed in the United States, that is distinct from the spotted fever and typhus biogroups. Int J Syst Bacteriol. 1983;33:94–106.
10. Burgdorfer W, Hayes SF, Mavros AJ. Nonpathogenic rickettsiae in *Dermacentor andersoni*: A limiting factor for the distribution of *Rickettsia rickettsii*. In: Burgdorfer W, Anacker RL, eds. Rickettsiae and Rickettsial Diseases. New York: Academic Press; 1981:585–94.
11. Johnson JE, Kadull PJ. Rocky Mountain spotted fever acquired in a laboratory. N Engl J Med. 1967;227:842–6.
12. Hattwick MAW, O'Brien RJ, Hanson BF. Rocky Mountain spotted fever; epidemiology of an increasing problem. Ann Intern Med. 1976;84:732–9.
13. Centers for Disease Control. Rocky Mountain spotted fever—United States, 1986. MMWR. 1987;36:314.
14. Wilfert CM, McCormack JN, Kleeman K, et al: Epidemiology of Rocky Mountain spotted fever as determined by active surveillance. J Infect Dis. 1984;150:469–79.
15. Salgo MP, Telzak EE, Currie B, et al. A focus of Rocky Mountain spotted fever within New York City. N Engl J Med. 1988;318:1345–8.
16. Lange JV, Walker DH, Wester TB. Documented Rocky Mountain spotted fever in wintertime. JAMA. 1982;247:2403–4.
17. Hattwick MAW, Retailliau H, O'Brien RJ, et al. Fatal Rocky Mountain spotted fever. JAMA. 1979;240:1499–503.
18. Walker DH. Pathology and pathogenesis of the vasculotropic rickettsioses. In: Walker DH, ed. Biology of Rickettsial Diseases. V. 1. Boca Raton, FL: CRC Press, 1988:115–38.
19. Walker DH, Cain BG. The rickettsial plaque. Evidence for direct cytopathic effect of *Rickettsia rickettsii*. Lab Invest. 1980;43:388–96.
20. Walker DH, Firth WT, Edgell CJS. Human endothelial cell culture plaques induced by *Rickettsia rickettsii*. Infect Immun. 1982;37:301–6.
21. Helmick CG, Bernard KW, D'Angelo LJ. Rocky Mountain spotted fever: Clinical, laboratory, and epidemiological features of 262 cases. J Infect Dis. 1984;150:480–6.
22. Kaplowitz LG, Fischer JJ, Sparling PF. Rocky Mountain spotted fever: A clinical dilemma. In: Remington JB, Swartz HN, eds. Current Clinical Topics in Infectious Diseases. V. 2. New York: McGraw-Hill; 1981:89–108.
23. Silverman DJ. Adherence of platelets to human endothelial cells infected by *Rickettsia rickettsii*. J Infect Dis. 1986;153:694–700.
24. Rao AK, Schapira M, Clements ML, et al. A prospective study of platelets and plasma proteolytic systems during the early stages of Rocky Mountain spotted fever. N Engl J Med. 1988;318:1021–8.
25. Jerrells TR. Mechanisms of immunity to *Rickettsia* species and *Coxiella burnetii*. In: Walker DH, ed. Biology of Rickettsial Diseases. V. 2. Boca Raton, FL: CRC Press; 1988:79–100.
26. Walker DH, Lane TW. Rocky Mountain spotted fever: Clinical signs, symptoms and pathophysiology. In: Walker DH, ed. Biology of Rickettsial Diseases. v. 1. Boca Raton, FL: CRC Press; 1988:63–78.
27. Raoult D, Weiller PJ, Chagnon A, et al. Mediterranean spotted fever: Clinical, laboratory and epidemiological featurs of 199 cases. Am J Trop Med Hyg. 1986;35:845–50.
28. Walker DH, Gay RM, Valdes-Dapena M. The occurrence of eschars in Rocky Mountain spotted fever. J Am Acad Dermatol. 1981;4:571–6.
29. Rosenblum MJ, Masland RL, Harrell GT. Residual effects of rickettsial disease on the central nervous system. Arch Intern Med. 1952;90:444–5.
30. Walker DH, Mattern WD. Acute renal failure in Rocky Mountain spotted fever. Arch Intern Med. 1979;139:443–8.
31. Donohue JF. Lower respiratory tract involvement in Rocky Mountain spotted fever. Arch Intern Med. 1980;140:223–7.
32. Feltes TF, Wilcox WD, Feldman WE, et al. M-Mode echocardiographic abnormalities in Rocky Mountain spotted fever. South Med J. 1984;787:1130–2.
33. Walker DH, Hawkins HL, Hudson P. Fulminant Rocky Mountain spotted fever. Its pathologic characteristics associated with glucose-6-phosphate dehydrogense deficiency. Arch Pathol Lab Med. 1983;107:121–5.
34. Walker DH, Peacock MG. Laboratory diagnosis of rickettsial diseases. In: Walker DH, ed. Biology of Rickettsial Diseases. V. 2. Boca Raton, FL: CRC Press; 1988:135–155.
35. Kaplowitz LG, Lange JV, Fischer JJ, et al. Correlation of rickettsial titers, circulating endotoxin, and clinical features in Rocky Mountain spotted fever. Arch Intern Med. 1983;143:1149–51.
36. Woodward TE, Pedersen CE, Oster CN, et al. Prompt confirmation of Rocky Mountain spotted fever: Identification of rickettsiae in skin tissues. J Infect Dis. 1976;134:297–301.
37. Walker DH, Burday JD, Folds MS. Laboratory diagnosis of Rocky Mountain spotted fever. South Med J. 1980;73:1443–7.
38. Kaplan JE, Schonberger LB. The sensitivity of various serologic tests in the diagnosis of Rocky Mountain spotted fever. Am J Trop Med Hyg. 1986;35:840–4.
39. Hechemy KE, Michaelson EE, Anacker RL, et al. Evaluation of latex-*Rickettsia rickettssii* test for Rocky Mountain spotted fever in 11 laboratories. J Clin Microbiol. 1983;18:938–46.
40. Spicer AJ, Peacock MG, Williams JC. Effectiveness of several antibiotics in suppressing chick embryo lethality during experimental infections by *Coxiella burnetii, Rickettsia typhi* and *R. rickettsii*. In: Burgdorfer W, Anacker RL, eds. Rickettsiae and Rickettsial Diseases. New York: Academic Press; 1981;375–83.
41. Raoult D, Roussellier P, Vestris G, et al. In vitro antibiotic susceptibility of *Rickettsia rickettsii* and *Rickettsia conorii*: plaque assay and microplaque colorimetric assay. J Infect Dis. 1987;155:1059–62.
42. Raoult D, Roussellier P, Vestris G, et al. Susceptibility of *Rickettsia conorii* and *R. rickettsii* to pefloxacin, in vitro and in ovo. J Antimicrob Chemother. 1987;19:303–5.
43. Raoult D, Roussellier P, Tamalet J. In vitro evaluation of josamycin, spiramycin, and erythromycin against *Rickettsia rickettsii* and *Rickettsia conorii*. Antimicrob Agents Chemother. 1988;32:255–6.
44. McDonald GA, Anacker RL, Garjian K. Cloned gene of *Rickettsia rickettsii* surface antigen: Candidate vaccine for Rocky Mountain spotted fever. Science. 1987;235:83–5.
45. Fan MY, Walker DH, Yu SR, et al. The epidemiology and ecology of rickettsial diseases in the People's Republic of China. Rev Infect Dis. 1987;9:823–40.
46. Uchida T, Tashiro F, Funato T, et al. Isolation of a spotted fever group rickettsia from a patient with febrile exanthematous illness in Shikoku, Japan. Microbiol Immunol. 1986;30:1323–6.
47. Montenegro MR, Mansueto S, Hegarty BC, et al. The histology of "taches noires" of boutonneuse fever and demonstration of *Rickettsia conorii* in them by immunofluorescence. Virchows Arch [A] 1983;400:309–17.
48. Walker DH, Gear JM. Correlation of the distribution of *Rickettsia conorii*, microscopic lesions, and clinical features in South African tick bite fever. Am J Trop Med Hyg. 1985;34:361–71.
49. Raoult D, Zuchelli P, Weiller PJ, et al. Incidence, clinical observations and risk factors in the severe form of Mediterranean spotted fever among patients admitted to hospital in Marseilles 1983–1984. J Infect. 1986;12:111–6.
50. Raoult D, De Micco C, Gallais H, et al. Laboratory diagnosis of Mediterranean spotted fever by immunofluorescent demonstration of *Rickettsia conorii* in cutaneous lesions. J Infect Dis. 1985;150:145–8.
51. Hechemy KE, Raoult D, Eisemann C, et al. Detection of antibodies to *Rickettsia conorii* with a latex agglutination test in patients with Mediterranean spotted fever. J Infect Dis. 1986;153:132–5.
52. Raoult D, Gallais H, De Micco C, et al. Ciprofloxacin therapy in Mediterranean spotted fever. Antimicrob Agents Chemother. 1986;30:606–7.

166. RICKETTSIA AKARI (RICKETTSIALPOX)

ALFRED J. SAAH

Rickettsialpox is a nonfatal, zoonotic, and febrile disease caused by *Rickettsia akari*. Since the disease was first characterized in 1946,[1] it has been recognized in other urban areas of the United States and in South Africa, Korea, and in parts of Russia.

ETIOLOGY

Rickettsia akari is a small, coccobacillary intracellular bacterium. It is best seen in tissue by the Giemsa stain. The organism is in the spotted fever group of rickettsia and has prominent serologic cross-reactivity with these agents (e.g., *Rickettsia rickettsii*).

EPIDEMIOLOGY

Rickettsialpox is a zoonotic disease. The organism seems to be transmitted among mice (*Mus musculus*) by mouse ectoparasites, and it is transmitted to humans by mouse mites (*Allodermanyssus sanguineus*). This mite is very small and colorless, and its bite is painless.

A reported outbreak from New York[2] reaffirms the importance of continued vigilance for this disease as a marker for excessive proliferation of mice and mites. Adequate control of mice and their ectoparasites prevents disease in humans.

PATHOLOGY AND PATHOGENESIS

After the bite of an infected mite, *R. akari* proliferates locally in the skin. A papule develops and then ulcerates to form the eschar. Seeding of peripheral sites occurs during rickettsemia near the time of onset of clinical symptoms. The rash lesions of rickettsialpox show epidermal infiltration by mononuclear cells. As in other rickettsial diseases, blood vessels are prominently involved and show extravasated erythrocytes and fibrin thrombi.[2,3]

CLINICAL MANIFESTATIONS

The incubation period of rickettsialpox is 9–14 days (range, 7–21 days). A painless papule that ulcerates and forms the eschar occurs in most cases. The eschar is formed 3–7 days before onset; it is approximately 0.5–3.0 cm in diameter. Regional lymphadenopathy is usually present, but it is nontender or minimally so.[4]

The onset of symptoms is sudden. Chills, fever, and headache are most common at onset. Other symptoms that may be present include myalgia, especially backache, and photophobia. Because of the hectic fever, many patients have rigors and profuse sweating.

Within 2–3 days after onset (range, hours to 9 days), a generalized papulovesicular rash appears. Lesions usually begin as firm erythematous papules that are 2–10 mm in diameter. After the lesions form vesicles, they heal by crusting.

The disease is mild; complications or death is very rare. Untreated illness resolves in 2–3 weeks, but residual headache and lassitude may persist for 1–2 weeks.

DIAGNOSIS

Routine laboratory tests are nonspecific. Early in disease, a mild leukopenia can be seen. The Weil-Felix test is negative for all antigens. Complement fixation (CF) tests can be used for diagnosis, but the indirect fluorescent antibody test is more sensitive as a rule. Because of the cross-reactivity with other spotted fever group organisms, initial screening of sera can be done by using *R. rickettsii* antigen. A cross-absorption technique similar to that described under "Diagnosis" in Chapter 169 can be performed by using *R. rickettsii* and *R. akari* antigens.

As in other rickettsial diseases, antibiotic treatment blunts and delays the antibody response. Convalescent serum specimens should be obtained 6–8 weeks after onset in treated patients if earlier specimens are negative.

DIFFERENTIAL DIAGNOSIS

Any rickettsial disease that produces an eschar should be considered in the differential diagnoses. These include scrub typhus, Mediterranean spotted fever (boutonneuse fever), Siberian tick typhus, and Queensland tick typhus.

The viral disease that is most like rickettsialpox is chickenpox. Lesions in chickenpox are more vesiculated than in rickettsialpox, which are more papular with a central vesicle. Other diseases that should be considered include certain enterovirus infections, gonococcemia, and infectious mononucleosis.

TREATMENT AND PREVENTION

Symptoms resolve within 48 hours after antirickettsial therapy is begun. Tetracycline, 15 mg/kg/day in four divided doses, is effective when given for 3–5 days. Relapse is very uncommon.

Adequate control of mice and their ectoparasites is effective in preventing infection in humans.[5]

REFERENCES

1. Huebner RJ, Stamps P, Armstrong A. Rickettsialpox—a newly recognized rickettsial disease. 1. Isolation of the etiologic agent. Public Health Rep. 1946;61:1605.
2. Brettman LR, Lewin S, Holzman RS, et al. Rickettsialpox: Report of an outbreak and a contemporary review. Medicine. 1981;60:363–72.
3. Dolgopol VB. Histologic changes in rickettsialpox. Am J Pathol (Baltimore). 1948;24:119.
4. Greenberg M. Rickettsialpox in New York City. Am J Med. 1948;4:866–74.
5. Lackman DB. A review of information on rickettsialpox in the United States. Clin Pediatr (Phila). 1963;2:296–301.

167. COXIELLA BURNETII (Q FEVER)

THOMAS J. MARRIE

Q fever is an acute (on occasion chronic) febrile illness that occurs worldwide. The most common animal reservoirs for this zoonosis are cattle, sheep, and goats. These domestic ungulates, when infected, shed the desiccation-resistant organisms in urine, feces, milk, and especially in birth products. The placenta of infected sheep contains up to 10^9 organisms per gram of tissue. Humans are infected by inhalation of contaminated aerosols and after an incubation period of 20 days (range, 14–39 days) become ill with severe headache, fever, chills, fatigue, and myalgia. Other symptoms depend upon the organs that are involved. In contrast to other rickettsial infections, rash almost never occurs in acute Q fever. The rash in chronic Q fever (endocarditis) is that of palpable purpura due to an immune-complex vasculitis. Other differences between Q fever and other rickettsial infections are the aerosol route of infection and the lack of cross-reacting antibodies to *Proteus* X strains (the Weil-Felix reaction).

THE PATHOGEN

Coxiella burnetii, the etiologic agent of Q fever, is a highly pleomorphic coccobacillus with a gram-negative cell wall. It measures 0.3 × 1 μm,[1] but unlike true rickettsiae, it enters the cell by a passive mechanism. Within host cells it survives within the phagolysosome—the low pH of this environment is necessary for the metabolic functioning of *C. burnetii*. Large and small cell variants exist, and a spore stage has been described.[2] This spore stage probably explains the ability of *C. burnetii* to withstand harsh environmental conditions.[3] It survives for 7–10 months on wool at 15–20°C, for more than 1 month on fresh meat in cold storage, and for more than 40 months in skim milk at room temperature.[4] While it is destroyed by 2% formaldehyde, the organism has been isolated from infected tissues stored in formaldehyde for up to 4–5 months. It has also been isolated from fixed "paraffinized" tissues. Lysol, 1%, or 5% hydrogen peroxide will kill *C. burnetii*.

Coxiella burnetii undergoes "phase" variation.[4,5] In nature and in laboratory animals it exists in the "phase I" state in which organisms react with late (45 days) convalescent guinea pig sera and only slightly with early (21 days) sera.[4] Repeated passage of phase I virulent organisms in embryonated chicken eggs leads to gradual conversion to phase II avirulent forms. There is no morphologic difference between the two phases, although they differ in the sugar composition of their lipopolysaccharides (LPS),[6] in their buoyant density in cesium chloride, and in their affinity for hematoxylin and basic fuchsin dyes. *Coxiella burnetii* LPS are nontoxic to chicken embryos at doses of over 80 μg per embryo, in contrast to *Salmonella typhimurium* smooth-and-rough-type LPS, which are toxic in nanogram amounts.[7]

Plasmids have been found in both phase I and phase II cells.[8] Three different plasmid types varying in length from 36 to 45 kilobases have been isolated.[3] To date their function is unknown.

Coxiella burnetii is extremely infectious for humans—a single viable organism is enough to cause an infection.[3]

EPIDEMIOLOGY

Coxiella burnetii has been identified in arthropods, fish, birds, rodents, marsupials, and livestock.[1] Worldwide, the most common animal reservoirs are cattle, sheep, and goats.[9] A variety of other animals may be infected by *Coxiella burnetii* including horses, dogs, swine, camels, water buffalo, pigeons, ducks, geese, turkeys, several species of wild birds, squirrels, deer mice, harvest mice, cats, and rabbits. The epidemiology of *C. burnetii* varies from country to country. For example, collared doves have been suspected of carrying *C. burnetii* from Western Europe to Ireland. In Nova Scotia exposure to infected parturient cats has resulted in several outbreaks of Q fever.[10,11] Humans become infected by inhalation of small particle aerosols containing *C. burnetii*. The resulting illness has been termed Q fever. Derrick, a medical officer of health in Queensland, Australia, in 1935 investigated a febrile illness that affected 20 of 800 employees of a Brisbane meat works.[12] He coined the term *Q* (or query) *fever*. Burnet and Freeman[13] showed that the organism isolated from the blood and urine of these patients was a rickettsia. At about the same time Davis and Cox[14] isolated a microorganism from ticks (*Dermacentor andersoni*) collected near Nine Mile Creek, Montana. Later Dyer[15,16] showed that *Rickettsia burnetii* (Burnet and Freeman's organism) was the same as *R. diaporica* (Cox's organism)—it is now known as *Coxiella burnetii*. Q fever has been reported from at least 51 countries on five continents.[5] It is usually an occupational disease affecting those with direct contact with infected animals such as farmers, veterinarians, and abbatoir workers.[5] However, indirect contact with infected animals has resulted in outbreaks of Q fever as in Switzerland when over 350 persons who lived along a road over which sheep travelled from mountain pastures developed Q fever.[17] Exposure to contaminated straw, manure, or dust from farm vehicles caused Q fever in residents who lived along a road in Britain.[18] Exposure may be even more indirect as in the case of laundry workers who developed Q fever after handling contaminated laundry.[19]

Ingesting contaminated raw milk,[20] being exposed to infected parturient cats,[10] and skinning infected wild rabbits are also ways in which Q fever may be acquired.

Coxiella burnetii has also been isolated from human milk[21] and human placentas.[22]

Laboratory exposure to *C. burnetii*[23] and transport of infected sheep through hospitals to research laboratories have resulted in large outbreaks of Q fever.[24,25]

Rarely Q fever has been transmitted via blood transfusion.[26] Transmission has occurred during an autopsy[27] but has not been documented during the clinical care of infected patients. There is one report of apparent human-to-human transmission of Q fever among members of a household.[28]

PATHOGENESIS

The most likely sequence of events in the cycle of transmission of *C. burnetii* to humans is that the organism is maintained in ticks or other arthropods. These ectoparasites infect domestic and other animals including a variety of small mammals. Infected domestic ungulates are usually asymptomatic, although abortion or stillbirth may result. The heavily infected placenta contaminates the environment at the time of parturition. Air samples are positive for up to 2 weeks after parturition, and viable organisms are present in the soil for periods of up to 150 days.[29–31] Humans are infected by the inhalation of contaminated aerosols. The microorganisms proliferate in the lung(s), and rickettsemia follows. This results in the onset of systemic symptoms and a variety of clinical manifestations depending upon the dose of the microorganism inhaled and likely the characteristics of the infecting strain.

CLINICAL MANIFESTATIONS

Humans are the only animals known to regularly develop illness as a result of *C. burnetii* infection.[32] There are several clinical syndromes.

1. A self-limited febrile illness (2–14 days)
2. Pneumonia
3. Endocarditis
4. Hepatitis
5. Osteomyelitis
6. Q fever in the immunocompromised host
7. Q fever in infancy
8. Neurologic manifestations—encephalitis, aseptic meningitis, toxic confusional states, dementia, extrapyramidal disease, manic psychosis

Self-Limited Febrile Illness

This is probably the most common form of Q fever. In many areas 11–12 percent of individuals have antibodies to *C. burnetii*—most do not recall pneumonia or other severe illness.[33] It is likely that the age at which infection occurs and the dose of the agent determine whether or not Q fever is a mild self-limited febrile illness.[34,35] There is also a suggestion that some infections may be totally asymptomatic.[36] The proportion of all Q fever infections that represent "asymptomatic" seroconversion is unknown.

Pneumonia

There are three presentations of this form of Q fever: atypical pneumonia, rapidly progressive pneumonia, and pneumonia as an incidental finding in a patient with a febrile illness. This latter presentation is probably the most common form of Q fever pneumonia.

Atypical pneumonia[37] is a clinical term used to describe pneumonia occurring in a young adult and is characterized by a dry nonproductive cough and blood and sputum cultures negative for conventional bacterial pathogens. Cough is a symptom in only 28 percent of patients with radiographically confirmed Q fever pneumonia. This illness may be of gradual or sudden onset.[38] Fever occurs in all patients. A severe headache is present in about 75 percent of patients and is a useful clue to the diagnosis. Other symptoms and the frequency with which they occur are fatigue, 98 percent; chills, 88 percent; sweats, 84 percent; myalgia, 68 percent; nausea, 49 percent; vomiting, 25 percent; pleuritic chest pain, 28 percent; and diarrhea, 21 percent. On occasion diarrhea may be a presentation of Q fever.[39]

Physical examination of the chest is often unremarkable. The most common physical finding is inspiratory crackles.[38] Patients with rapidly progressive pneumonia usually have the physical signs of pulmonary consolidation. About 5 percent of patients have splenomegaly. Fever and severe headache suggest central nervous system (CNS) infection, and lumbar puncture is often performed. The spinal fluid is usually normal; however, *C. burnetii* has been isolated from the spinal fluid under such circumstances.[40] The rapidly progressive form of Q fever pneumonia mimics legionnaires' disease, the pneumonic form of tularemia, and indeed, all the causes of rapidly progressive pneumonia enter the differential diagnosis.

The radiographic picture of Q fever pneumonia is variable. Subsegmental and segmental pleural-based opacities are common.[41–43] Multiple rounded opacities are very suggestive of Q fever that follows exposure to infected cat placentas.[32] Pleural effusion is found in 35 percent of cases, is usually small, but on occasion may be large.[42] Atelectasis, an increase in reticular markings, and hilar adenopathy may occur. In one series the resolution time ranged from 10 to 70 days with a mean of 30 days.[42]

Coxiella burnetii pneumonia is rarely fatal, and in such instances there is usually a coexisting condition that contributes to the mortality.[43] Information regarding the histology of this form of pneumonia in humans is limited. Pierce et al.[44] found small coccobacilli within alveolar macrophages on transbronchial biopsy. A fatal case of pneumonia in a 43-year-old male was characterized by severe intra-alveolar hemorrhagic, focal necrotizing pneumonia with associated necrotizing bronchitis. Histiocytes, lymphocytes, and plasma cells were in the alveoli. This was felt to be Q fever pneumonia on the basis of organisms seen on a modified Giemsa stain.[45] A resolving *C. burnetii* pneumonia lesion was characterized by an inflammatory pseudotumor—a lung mass composed of mixtures of macrophages (foam cells, plasma cells, lymphocytes). The bronchiolar epithelium was focally absent, regenerated, or hyperplastic.[46] The lesions that result from the inoculation of the lungs of rhesus monkeys resemble those reported for humans. The resulting nodular consolidation is peribronchial or peribronchiolar.[47] The interstitial infiltrate has more lymphocytes than monocytes.

The white blood cell count is usually normal, but one-third of patients have an increased count. A slight elevation (two to three times normal) of the hepatic transaminase levels occurs in almost all patients. The serum bilirubin is usually normal, but jaundice may occur. Rarely the syndrome of inappropriate secretion of antidiuretic hormone occurs.[48]

The treatment of choice for *C. burnetii* pneumonia is tetracycline.[49] Chloramphenicol has been used to treat Q fever.[44] Yeaman et al.[50] performed antibiotic susceptibility testing of *C. burnetii* by using persistently infected L929 fibroblast cells. The most effective agents were quinolones (difloxacin, ciprofloxacin, oxolinic acid) and rifampin. Chloramphenicol, doxycycline, and trimethoprim were somewhat effective, while tetracycline, gentamicin, streptomycin, erythromycin, sulfamethoxazole, penicillin G, and polymyxin B were ineffective. Erythromycin is usually the drug of choice for the treatment of atypical pneumonia. While others have reported an apparent response of *C. burnetii* pneumonia to erythromycin therapy,[51,52] we have observed that all of our severe cases have failed to respond to this therapy despite dosages of up to 4 g/day. The addition of rifampin, 600 mg bid po, resulted in cure.

The diagnosis of Q fever (*C. burnetii*) pneumonia is confirmed serologically since most laboratories do not have the facilities required to isolate *C. burnetii*.[53] The microagglutination,[54] complement fixation (CF),[55] and microimmunofluorescence tests[56] as well as the enzyme-linked immunosorbent assay[57] have all been used in the serologic diagnosis of this illness. The CF test is most commonly used. A fourfold rise in titer between the acute and convalescent samples is diagnostic of Q fever. To date no cross-reactions have been reported between antibodies to other microorganisms and antibodies to *C. burnetii*.[58] Some authors have advocated using the indirect immunofluorescent test to detect antibodies to IgM so that a single serum specimen may be used in the diagnosis of acute Q fever.[59] However, IgM antibodies may persist for up to 678 days,[60] and in one study,[61] 3 percent of 162 patients still had a significant IgM antibody level 1 year after the infection.

Endocarditis

Endocarditis is the prime manifestation of "chronic" Q fever.[62–79] Usually abnormal or prosthetic cardiac valves are affected[80]; however any part of the vascular tree may become infected[79] including clot in a left ventricular aneurysm. Such patients have a defective cell-mediated immune response to *C. burnetii*.

The incidence of Q fever endocarditis is increasing, but this may reflect increased recognition of this entity. Turck et al.[62] reported 16 cases of chronic Q fever diagnosed between 1968 and 1973; their review of the world's literature yielded 55 cases. From 1975 to 1980, 79 cases of Q fever endocarditis were reported to the Public Health Laboratory Service Communicable Disease Surveillance Center in England.[75] Indeed, from 1975 to 1981 *C. burnetii* accounted for 3 percent of all cases of endocarditis reported in England and Wales.[74] The clinical presentation is that of culture-negative endocarditis; however, fever is frequently absent. Q fever endocarditis is rare in children.[78] The manifestations are the same as those in adults.

Marked clubbing of the fingers and hyperglobulinemia are frequently present. Splenomegaly and hepatomegaly are found in slightly more than half the patients. A purpuric rash due to leukocytoclastic vasculitis occurs in about 20 percent. The erythrocyte sedimentation rate is usually >100 mm/hr; anemia and microscopic hematuria are also found. Arterial emboli complicate the course of one-third of the patients.

The confirmation of the diagnosis in most instances is serologic. A CF titer of ≥1:200 to phase I antigen is said to be diagnostic of chronic Q fever, although not all patients in the series of Turck et al.[62] had this titer. In acute Q fever CF antibody titers to phase I antigen do not reach this level.

With the microimmunofluorescence test, phase I titers are much higher in Q fever endocarditis than they are in acute Q fever—although for this test no single titer has been suggested as diagnostic of chronic Q fever; this is due to the fact that titer end points vary considerably from laboratory to laboratory.[60,76] One study[81] reported high titers of IgA antibodies to phase I antigen in chronic Q fever (endocarditis and granulomatous hepatitis), while another[60] found that patients with acute Q fever also produced IgA antibodies to phase I antigen, albeit in low titer. Antibody titers fall slowly with treatment.

There is no agreement on type and duration of antimicrobial therapy for Q fever endocarditis.[62,63] Some authorities recommend that treatment be continued indefinitely.[62] We have used tetracycline in combination with trimethoprim-sulfamethoxazole or rifampin for 2 years. Antibody titers should be determined every 6 months during therapy and every 3 months for the first 2 years after therapy. Successful therapy is accompanied by a falling erythrocyte sedimentation rate, correction of anemia, and hyperglobulinemia. Valve replacement is frequently necessary but should be dictated by the patient's hemodynamic status.

Hepatitis

There are three presentations of Q fever hepatitis[82–89]:

1. An infectious hepatitis-like picture
2. Fever of unknown origin with characteristic granulomas on liver biopsy
3. As an incidental finding in a patient with acute Q fever pneumonia

In patients with fever of unknown origin due to Q fever, the typical "doughnut granuloma" is seen on liver biopsy.[84,85] This is a granuloma with a dense fibrin ring surrounded by a central lipid vacuole. These granulomas are highly suggestive of Q fever but may be seen in Hodgkin's disease and infectious mononucleosis. *Coxiella burnetii* has been isolated from the liver of patients with Q fever hepatitis, but the organism has not been visualized within the hepatic parenchyma.[62] Antibiotic treatment for 2 weeks is probably sufficient.

Neurologic Manifestations

Severe headache is the most common manifestation[90–92] and probably represents CNS infection, although little evidence of serious brain involvement occurs in Q fever.[90] Aseptic meningitis and encephalitis do occur. A variety of other manifestations including extrapyramidal disease and dementia have been reported, although the evidence that these manifestations were due to *C. burnetii* is not conclusive.

Other Manifestations of Q Fever

Vertebral osteomyelitis[93] and infection in the immunocompromised host[94] are uncommon manifestations of Q fever. Q fever may also occur in infancy[95] where it has caused pneumonia, febrile seizures, pyrexia of unknown origin, malaise, and meningeal irritation. Hematologic manifestations include bone marrow necrosis,[96] histiocytic hemophagocytosis,[97] and hemolytic anemia,[98] and on occasion this disease may simulate lymphoma.[99] Other hematologic manifestations include transient hypoplastic anemia,[100] reactive thrombocytosis, and rarely thrombocytopenia. Optic neuritis[101] and erythema nodosum[102] have also rarely been reported in association with *C. burnetii* infection. There is also a suggestion that Kawasaki disease may be a variant of Q fever.[103,104]

PREVENTION

Vaccination of those at risk for infection (e.g., abbatoir workers and veterinarians) should be carried out as soon as a safe vaccine is available.[105,106] Using only seronegative sheep in research facilities will prevent outbreaks in these institutions. Because of the lack of person-to-person spread there is no need to isolate patients hospitalized with Q fever.[107] Simple measures like consumption of only pasteurized milk serves to eliminate cases of Q fever that are transmitted in this manner. In Cyprus the incidence of Q fever among sheep and goats was reduced by a program in which aborted material was destroyed, affected dams isolated, and the premises disinfected.[108] Control of ectoparasites on cattle, sheep, and goats is also important in the control of Q fever.

REFERENCES

1. Baca OG, Paretsky D. Q fever and *Coxiella burnetii*: A model for host–parasite interaction. Microbiol Rev. 1983;47:127–49.
2. McCaul TF, Williams JC. Development cycle of *Coxiella burnetii*: Structure and morphogenesis of vegetative and sporogenic differentiations. J Bacteriol. 1981;147:1063–76.
3. Sawyer LA, Fishbein DB, McDade JE. Q fever: Current Concepts. Rev Infect Dis. 1987;9:935–46.
4. Q fever. In: Christie AB. Infectious Diseases, Epidemiology and Clinical Practice. Churchill Livingstone: Edinburgh; 1974:876–91.
5. Leedom JM. Q fever: An update. In: Remington JS, Schwartz MN, eds. Current Clinical Topics in Infectious Diseases. New York: McGraw-Hill; 1980:304–31.
6. Schramek S, Mayer H. Different sugar compositions of lipopolysaccharides isolated from phase I and pure phase II cells of *Coxiella burnetii*. Infect Immun. 1982;38:53–7.
7. Hackstadt T, Peacock MG, Hitchcock PJ, et al. Lipopolysaccharide variation in *Coxiella burnetii*: Intrastrain heterogenicity in structure and antigenicity. Infect Immun. 1985;48:359–65.
8. Samuel JE, Frazier ME, Mallavia LP. Correlation of plasmid type and disease caused by *Coxiella burnetii*. Infect Immun. 1985;49:775–77.
9. Babudieri B. Q fever: A zoonosis. Adv Vet Sci. 1959;5:81–181.
10. Langley JM, Marrie TJ, Covert A, et al. Poker players' pneumonia. An urban outbreak of Q fever following exposure to a parturient cat. N Engl J Med. 1988;319:354–6.
11. Marrie TJ, Durant H, Williams JC, et al. Exposure to parturient cats: A risk factor for acquisition of Q fever in maritime Canada. J Infect Dis. 1988;158:101–8.
12. Derrick EH. "Q" fever, new fever entity: Clinical features, diagnosis and laboratory investigation. Med J Aust. 1937;2:281–99.
13. Burnet FM, Freeman M. Experimental studies on virus of "Q" fever. Med J Aust. 1937;2:299–305.
14. Davis G, Cox HR. A filter-passing infectious agent isolated from ticks: Isolation from *Dermacentor andersoni*, reactions in animals, and filtration experiments. Public Health Rep. 1938;5:2259–67.
15. Dyer RE. A filter-passing infectious agent isolated from ticks. IV. Human infection. Public Health Rep. 1939;53:2277–83.
16. Dyer RE. Similarity of Australian Q fever and a disease caused by an infectious agent isolated from ticks in Montana. Public Health Rep. 1939;54:1229–37.
17. Q fever outbreak—Switzerland. MMWR. 1984;33:355–61.
18. Salmon MM, Howells B, Glencross EJG, et al. Q fever in an urban area. Lancet. 1982;1:1002–4.
19. Oliphant JW, Gordon DA, Meis A, et al. Q fever in laundry workers presumably transmitted from contaminated clothing. Am J Hyg. 1949;49:76–82.
20. Bell JA, Beck MD, Huebner RJ. Epidemiologic studies of Q fever in Southern California. JAMA. 1950;142:868–72.
21. Kumar A, Yadav MP, Kakkar S. Human milk as a source of Q fever infection in breast-fed babies. Indian J Med Res. 1981;73:510–12.
22. Syrucek L, Sobeslavsky O, Gutvirth I. Isolation of *Coxiella burnetii* from human placentas. J Hyg Epidemiol Microbiol Immunol. 1958;2:29–35.
23. Johnson JE II, Kadull PJ. Laboratory-acquired Q fever. Am J Med. 1966;41:391–403.
24. Hall CJ, Richmond SJ, Caul EO, et al. Laboratory outbreak of Q fever acquired from sheep. Lancet. 1982;1:1004–6.
25. Meiklejohn G, Reimer LG, Graves PS, et al. Cryptic epidemic of Q fever in a medical school. J Infect Dis. 1984;144:107–14.
26. Editorial comment on Q fever transmitted by blood transfusion—United States. Can Dis Wkly Rep 1977;3:210.
27. Harman JB. Q fever in Great Britain. Lancet. 1949;2:1028–30.
28. Mann JS, Douglas JG, Inglis JM, et al. Q fever: Person to person transmission within a family. Thorax. 1986;41:974–5.
29. Welsh HH, Lennette EH, Abinanti FR, et al. Air-borne transmission of Q fever: The role of parturition in the generation of infective aerosols. Ann NY Acad Sci. 1958;528–40.
30. Lennette EH, Welsh HH. Q fever in California. X. Recovery of *Coxiella burnetii* from the air of premises harboring infected goats. Am J Hyg. 1951;54:44–9.
31. Welsh HH, Lennette EH, Abinanti FR, et al. Q fever studies XXI. The recovery of *Coxiella burnetii* from the soil and surface water of premises harboring infected sheep. Am J Hyg. 1959;70:14–20.
32. Stoker MGP, Marion BP. The spread of Q fever from animals to man. The natural history of a rickettsial disease. Bull WHO. 1955;13:781–806.
33. Clark WH, Romker MS, Holmes MA, et al. Q fever in California VIII. An epidemic of Q fever in a small rural community in Northern California. Am J Hyg. 1951;54:25–34.
34. Gonder JC, Kishimoto RA, Kastello MF, et al. Cynomolgus monkey model for experimental Q fever infection. J Infect Dis. 1979;139:191–6.
35. Tigertt WD, Benenson AS, Goscheneur WS. Airborne Q fever. Bacteriol Rev. 1961;25:285–93.
36. Luoto L, Casey ML, Pickens EG. Q fever studies in Montana. Detection of asymptomatic infection among residents of infected dairy premises. Am J Epidemiol. 1965;81:356–69.
37. Cunha BA, Quintiliani R. The atypical pneumonias. A diagnostic and therapeutic approach. Postgrad Med. 1979;66:95–102.
38. Feinstein M, Yesner R, Marks JL. Epidemic of Q fever among troops returning from Italy in the spring of 1945. 1. Clinical aspects of the epidemic at Fort Patrick Henry, Virginia. Am J Hyg. 1946;44:72–87.
39. Lim KCL, Kang JYU. Q fever presenting with gastroenteritis. Med J Aust. 1980;1:327.
40. Robins FC. Q fever in the Mediterranean area: Report of its occurrence in allied troops. Am J Hyg. 1946;51–71.
41. Gordon JD, MacKeen AD, Marrie TJ, et al. The radiographic features of epidemic and sporadic Q fever pneumonia. J Can Assoc Radiol. 1984;35:293–6.
42. Millar JK. The chest film findings in 'Q' fever—a series of 35 cases. Clin Radiol. 1978;29:371–5.
43. Perin TL. Histopathologic observations in a fatal case of Q fever. Arch Pathol. 1949;47:361–5.
44. Pierce TH, Yucht SC, Gorin AB, et al. Q fever pneumonitis: Diagnosis by transbronchoscopic lung biopsy. West J Med. 1979;130:453–5.
45. Urso FP. The pathologic findings in rickettsial pneumonia. Am J Clin Pathol. 1975;64:335–42.
46. Janigan DT, Marrie TJ. An inflammatory pseudotumor of the lung in Q fever pneumonia. N Engl J Med. 1983;30:86–8.
47. Lillie RD, Perrin TL, Armstrong C. An institutional outbreak of pneumonitis. III. Histopathology in man and rhesus monkeys in the pneumonitis due to the virus of "Q: fever. Public Health Rep. 1941;56:1419–25.
48. Biggs BA, Douglas JG, Grant IWB, et al. Prolonged Q fever associated with inappropriate secretion of anti-diuretic hormone. J Infect. 1984;8:61–63.
49. Turck WPG. Q fever. In: Braude AL, Davis CE, Fierer J, eds. Medical Microbiology and Infectious Diseases. Philadelphia: WB Saunders; 1981:932–7.
50. Yeaman MR, Mitscher LA, Baca OG. In vitro susceptibility of *Coxiella*

burnetii for antibiotics, including several quinolones. Antimicrob Agents Chemother. 1987;31:1079–84.
51. D'Angelo LJ, Hetherington R. Q fever treated with erythromycin. Br Med J. 1979;2:305–6.
52. Ellis ME, Dunbar EM. In vivo response of acute Q fever to erythromycin. Thorax. 1982;37:867–8.
53. Huebner RJ, Jellison WL, Beck MD. Q fever, a review of current knowledge. Ann Intern Med. 1949;30:495–509.
54. Fiset P, Ormsbee RA, Silberman R, et al. A microagglutination technique for detection and measurement of rickettsial antibodies. Acta Virol. 1969;13:60–6.
55. Murphy AM, Field PR. The persistence of complement-fixing antibodies to Q fever (*Coxiella burnetii*) after infection. Med J Aust. 1970;2:1148–50.
56. Field PR, Hunt JG, Murphy AM. Detection and persistence of specific IgM antibody to *Coxiella burnetii* by enzyme-linked immunosorbent assay: A comparison with immunofluorescence and complement fixation tests. J Infect Dis. 1983;148:477–87.
57. Péter O, Dupuis G, Burgdorfer W, et al. Evaluation of the complement fixation and indirect immunofluorescence test in the early diagnosis of primary Q fever. Eur J Clin Microbiol. 1985;4:394–96.
58. Péter O, Dupuis G, Peacock MG, et al. Comparison of enzyme-linked immunosorbent assay and complement fixation and indirect antibody tests for detection of *Coxiella burnetii* antibody. J Clin Microbiol. 1987;25:1063–67.
59. Hunt JG, Field PR, Murphy AM. Immunoglobulin responses to *Coxiella burnetii* (Q fever): Single-serum diagnosis of acute infection using an immunofluorescence technique. Infect Immun. 1983;39:977–81.
60. Worswick D, Marmion BP. Antibody responses in acute and chronic Q fever and in subjects vaccinated against Q fever. J Med Microbiol. 1985;19:281–96.
61. Dupuis G, Péter O, Peacock M, et al. Immunoglobulin responses in acute Q fever. J Clin Microbiol. 1985;;22:484–7.
62. Turck WPG, Howitt G, Turnberg LA, et al. Chronic Q fever. Q J Med. 1976;45:193–217.
63. Wilson HG, Neilson GH, Galea EG, et al. Q fever endocarditis in Queensland. Circulation. 1976;53:680–4.
64. Grist NR. Q fever endocarditis. Am Heart J. 1968;75:846–9.
65. Robson AO, Shimmin CDGL. Chronic Q fever. I. Clinical aspects of a patient with endocarditis. Br Med J. 1959;2:980–3.
66. Varma MPS, Adgey AJ, Connolly JH. Chronic Q fever endocarditis. Br Heart J. 190;43:695–9.
67. Tobin MJ, Cahill N, Gearty G, et al. Q fever endocarditis. Am J Med. 1982;72:396–400.
68. Kimbrough RC II, Ormsbee RA, Peacock M. Q fever endocarditis in the United States. Ann Intern Med. 1979;91:400–2.
69. Ross PJ, Jacobson J, Muir JR. Q fever endocarditis of porcine xenograft valves. Am Heart J. 1983;105:151–3.
70. Wiley RF, Matthews MB, Peutherer JF, et al. Chronic cryptic Q fever infection of the heart. Lancet. 1979;2:270–2.
71. Subramanya NI, Wright JS, Khan MAR. Failure of rifampicin and co-trimoxazole in Q fever endocarditis. Br Med J. 1982;203:342–3.
72. Marmion BP. Subacute rickettsial endocarditis: An unusual complication of Q fever. J Hyg Epidemiol Microbiol Immunol. 1962;6:79–84.
73. Applefeld MM, Bellingsley LN, Tucker HG, et al. Q fever endocarditis: A case occurring in the United States. Am Heart J. 1977;903:669–70.
74. Palmer SR, Young SEJ. Q fever endocarditis in England and Wales, 1975–81. Lancet. 1982;2:1448–49.
75. Chronic Q fever (Editorial). J Infect. 1984;8:1–4.
76. Haldane EV, Marrie TJ, Faulkner RS, et al. Endocarditis due to Q fever in Nova Scotia: Experience with five patients in 1981–1982. J Infect Dis. 1983;148:978–85.
77. Raoult D, Etienne J, Massip P, et al. Q fever endocarditis in the south of France. J Infect Dis. 1987;155:570–3.
78. Laufer D, Lew PD, Oberhansli I, et al. Chronic Q fever endocarditis with massive splenomegaly in childhood. J Pediatr. 1986;108:535–9.
79. Raoult D, Piquet PH, Gallais H, et al. *Coxiella burnetii* infection of a vascular prosthesis. N Engl J Med. 1986;315:1358–9.
80. Tellez A, Sainz C, Echevarria C, et al. Q fever in Spain: Acute and chronic cases, 1981–1985. Rev Infect Dis. 1988;10:198–202.
81. Peacock MG, Philip RN, Williams JC, et al. Serological evaluation of Q fever in humans: Enhanced phase I titers of immunoglobulins G and A are diagnostic for Q fever endocarditis. Infect Immun. 1983;41:1089–98.
82. Hofmann CER, Heaton JW Jr. Q fever hepatitis. Clinical manifestations and pathological findings. Gastroenterology. 1982;83:474–9.
83. Dupont HL, Hornick EV, Levin HA, et al. Q fever hepatitis. Ann Intern Med. 1971;74:198–206.
84. Qizilbash AH. The pathology of Q fever as seen on liver biopsy. Arch Pathol Lab Med. 1983;107:364–7.
85. Travis LB, Travis WD, Li C-Y, et al. Q fever. A clinicopathologic study of five cases. Arch Pathol Lab Med. 1986;110:1017–20.
86. Weir WRC, Bannister B, Chambers S, et al. Chronic Q fever associated with granulomatous hepatitis. J Infect. 1980;8:56–60.
87. Pellegrin M, Delsol G, Auvergnat JC, et al. Granulomatous hepatitis in Q fever. Hum Pathol. 1980;11:51–7.
88. Voigt JJ, Delsol, Fabre J. Liver and bone marrow granulomas in Q fever. Gastroenterology. 1983;84:887–8.
89. Alkan WJ, Ewenchik Z, Eschar J. Q fever and infectious hepatitis. Am J Med. 1965;38:54–61.
90. Harrell GT. Rickettsial involvement of the central nervous system. Med Clin North Am. 1953;395–422.
91. Gomez-Aranda F, Diaz JKP, Acebol MR, et al. Computed tomographic brain scan findings in Q fever encephalitis. Neuroradiology. 1984;26:329–32.
92. Marrie TJ. Pneumonia and meningo-encephalitis due to *Coxiella burnetii*. J Infect. 1985;11:59–61.
93. Ellis ME, Smith CC, Moffatt MAJ. Chronic or fatal Q-fever infection: A review of 16 patients seen in north-east Scotland (1967–1980). Q J Med. 1983;205:54–66.
94. Heard SR, Ronalds CJ, Heath RB. *Coxiella burnetii* infection in immunocompromised patients. J Infect. 1985;11:15–18.
95. Richardus JH, Duma AM, Huisman J, et al. Q fever in infancy: A review of 18 cases. Pediatr Infect Dis. 1985;4:369–73.
96. Brada M, Bellingham AJ. Bone marrow necrosis and Q fever. Br Med J. 1980;210:1108–9.
97. Estrov Z, Bruck R, Shtalrid M, et al. Histiocytic hemophagocytosis in Q fever. Arch Pathol Lab Med. 1984;108:7.
98. Cardellach F, Font J, Agusti AGN, et al. Q fever and hemolytic anemia. J Infect Dis. 1983;148:769.
99. Ramos HS, Hodges RE, Meroney Wh. Q fever: Report of a case simulating lymphoma. Ann Intern Med. 1957;47:1030–5.
100. Hitchins R, Cobcroft RG, Hocker G. Transient severe hypoplastic anemia in Q fever. Pathology. 1986;18:254–5.
101. Schuil J, Richardus JH, Baarsma GS, et al. Q fever as a possible cause of bilateral optic neuritis. Br J Ophthalmol. 1985;69:580–3.
102. Conget I, Mallolas J, Mensa J, et al. Erythema nodosum and Q fever. Arch Dermatol. 1987;123:867.
103. Swaby ED, Fisher-Hoch S, Lambert HP, et al. Is Kawasaki disease a variant of Q fever? Lancet. 1980;2:146.
104. Weir WRC, Bouchet VA, Mitford E, et al. Kawasaki disease in European adult associated with serological response to *Coxiella burnetii*. Lancet. 1985;2:504.
105. Ascher MS, Berman MA, Ruppaner R. Initial clinical and immunologic evaluation of a new phase I Q fever vaccine and skin test in humans. J Infect Dis. 1983;148:214–224.
106. Marmion BP, Ormsbee RA, Kyrkou M, et al. Vaccine prophylaxis of abbatoir-associated Q fever. Lancet. 1984;2:1411–14.
107. Grant CG, Ascher MS, Bernard KW, et al. Q fever and experimental sheep. Infect Control. 1985;6:122–3.
108. Polydorou K. Q fever in Cyprus—recent progress. Br Vet J. 1985;141:427–30.

168. RICKETTSIA PROWAZEKII (EPIDEMIC OR LOUSE-BORNE TYPHUS)

ALFRED J. SAAH

Louse-borne typhus is the prototype of the typhus group of rickettsial diseases. The primary illness and its recrudescent form (Brill-Zinsser disease) are caused by *Rickettsia prowazekii*. Louse-borne typhus is also known as epidemic typhus, classic typhus, typhus exanthematicus, tarbardillo, fleckfieber, and jail fever.

The primary illness was distinguished from typhoid fever by Gerhard in 1836. In 1910, Brill described an illness that was similar to typhus but was milder and not accompanied by body lice. In 1934, Zinsser postulated its pathogenesis as being recurrent louse-borne typhus; this was subsequently confirmed.

The occurrence of typhus in this century parallels the history of war and famine. An astonishing 30 million cases occurred in the Soviet Union and Eastern Europe during 1918–1922, with an estimated 3 million deaths.

During World War II, typhus struck heavily in concentration camps in Eastern Europe and in North Africa. Its reputation as a military medical problem was cleverly used to protect residents of occupied areas from deportation to concentration camps for slave labor. The German army avoided epidemic areas of louse-borne typhus by using the Weil-Felix reaction for diagnosis. Knowing this fact, certain physicians used formalin-killed *Proteus* OX-19 strain organisms as a vaccine to create an artificial "epidemic area" of typhus in Poland. Persons would be unwittingly vaccinated (thinking they were receiving a rejuvenating protein suspension) when they were seen by the physicians with any symptom remotely suggestive of typhus. The scheme worked quite effectively, and much later was made public by Lazowski and Matulewicz.[1]

ETIOLOGY

The etiologic agent is *Rickettsia prowazekii*, an obligate intracellular bacterium that is closely related antigenically to the agent that causes murine typhus (*Rickettsia typhi*). The organism is coccobacillary but has inconstant morphologic characteristics. Reproduction is by binary fission, and diplobacilli are produced that are frequently seen in tissue sections. Special staining, Giemsa or Gimenez, provides good visualization of the organisms in the cytoplasm of cells. If isolation of the organism by animal inoculation is attempted, it should be done by experienced personnel and only in specially designed, full-containment facilities. Storing a blood clot from a patient at −70°C will maintain viability of the organism for years. Isolation attempts also can be made from blood clots that have been stored in a refrigerator for no longer than several days.

EPIDEMIOLOGY

Louse-borne typhus is transmitted from person to person by the body louse (*Pediculus humanus corporis*). The cycle is thought to be initiated by a human case of recrudescent typhus or by a recently introduced case of primary louse-borne typhus. The louse feeds on an infected, rickettsemic person. The organism in the louse infects its alimentary tract and results in large numbers of organisms in its feces within about 1 week. Close personal or clothing contact is usually required to transmit lice to others. When the louse takes a blood meal, it defecates. The irritation causes the host to scratch the site, thereby contaminating the bite wound with louse feces. Human infection might also occur by mucous membrane inoculation with contaminated louse feces.

Human conditions that foster the proliferation of lice are especially common during winter and during war or natural disasters—wherein clothing is not changed, crowding occurs, and bathing is very infrequent.

Rickettsia prowazekii and the louse do not coexist harmoniously; the louse dies of its infection (from obstruction of its alimentary tract) in 1–3 weeks and does not transmit the organism to its offspring.

A reservoir of *R. prowazekii* other than humans apparently exists in the southern flying squirrel *Glaucomys volans*.[2] This squirrel is distributed over the eastern United States from southern Maine to Florida and westward to the center of the United States (Minnesota to eastern Texas). Transmission among these rodents is suspected to be by squirrel lice and/or fleas.[3]

Fifteen reported human cases of indigenously acquired epidemic typhus have been diagnosed serologically in the eastern United States.[4,5] Evidence has been presented that implicates the flying squirrel as the probable source of infection,[5] but the mode of transmission is unclear. Confirmation of the etiology still requires isolating the organism from humans; however, it should be noted that very few appropriately obtained clinical specimens have been evaluated as of this writing.

Of the 15 reported patients with epidemic typhus, 14 resided in rural or suburban settings, 12 were white, 3 were black, and 8 were female. The median age for males was 24 years (range, 17–35 years) and for females, 44 years (range, 11–81 years). Twelve cases had onset during the colder months (November through March). All seven patients in one report[5] and two in the other[4] had direct or indirect contact with flying squirrels; however, such exposure is difficult to interpret without a comparison group. There was no evidence for person-to-person transmission.

PATHOGENESIS AND PATHOLOGIC CHARACTERISTICS

After local proliferation at the site of the louse bite, the organism presumably spreads hematogenously. *Rickettsia prowazekii*, as with most rickettsiae, produces a vasculitis by infecting the endothelial cells of capillaries, small arteries, and veins. The process results in fibrin and platelet deposition and then occlusion of the vessel. Perivascular infiltration with lymphocytes, plasma cells, histiocytes, and polymorphonuclear leukocytes occurs with or without frank necrosis of the vessel. The angiitis is most marked in the skin, heart, central nervous system, skeletal muscle, and kidneys.[6,7] If local thrombosis is extensive, gangrene of skin and/or distal portions of the extremities occurs.

Effects of rickettsial toxins have been shown in rodents, but their relationship to human illness and pathologic findings is unclear.

CLINICAL MANIFESTATIONS

Signs and Symptoms

After an incubation period of approximately 1 week, an abrupt onset with intense headache, chills, fever, and myalgia is characteristic. There is no eschar. The fever worsens quickly (102–104°F) and becomes unremitting, and the patient is soon prostrated by the illness. A rash begins in the axillary folds and upper part of the trunk on about the fifth day of illness and spreads centrifugally. Initially, the rash consists of nonconfluent, pink macules that fade on pressure. Within several days, the rash becomes maculopapular, darker, petechial, and confluent and involves the entire body but spares the face, palms, and soles.

Some manifestations of louse-borne typhus that occur with varying frequency include a nonproductive cough with x-ray evidence of pulmonary infiltrates, deafness, and tinnitus.

Indigenously acquired epidemic typhus is also characterized by abrupt onset and high fever. Overall, however, the illness seems to be milder than classic louse-borne typhus, but life-threatening illness has occurred. Where signs and symptoms are known as in the 15 reported cases, 9 of 13 patients had headache, 4 of 8 had myalgia, and 8 of 15 had rash. The rash was typical in distribution, but it frequently was evanescent. Signs of central nervous system involvement (other than headache) were found in six patients. The signs ranged from meningismus in one patient, confusion or delirium in three patients, to coma in two patients. One patient with confusion had cerebrospinal fluid (CSF) lymphocytic pleocytosis.

Course

In untreated, uncomplicated louse-borne typhus, the fever lyses after 2 weeks of illness; recovery of normal mentation is rapid, but recovery of strength usually requires a prolonged convalescence (2–3 months). Overall mortality is quite variable, but it has been reported to be as high as 40 percent under adverse conditions. Age-specific mortality rates are highest among those over 60 years of age. It is a mild illness in children. Specific treatment results in prompt recovery.

Response to antirickettsial agents in indigenously acquired epidemic typhus was reported to have usually occurred within 24 hours, with recovery in most patients after 48 hours. Three of the four patients who did not receive specific therapy recovered in 14 days. The remaining patient developed renal failure, required dialysis, and recovered. The etiology of this patient's renal failure, however, is unclear.[8]

Louse-borne typhus in a vaccinated person produces a mild

illness that closely mimics murine typhus clinically (see the section in this chapter on diagnosis).

Diagnosis

In the proper setting of cold weather, infrequent bathing and changing clothes, crowded conditions, and the presence of lice, the clinical symptomatology described before is compelling evidence for the presence of louse-borne typhus. The progression of rash serves to distinguish the disease from Rocky Mountain spotted fever (RMSF), which progresses centripetally, beginning on the wrists and ankles.

In the United States, diagnosis requires a high index of suspicion because of the great variability in presenting symptoms. It is important to examine the axillary folds repeatedly for evidence of rash. During the colder months of November through March, if RMSF is suspected from the clinical picture, this should be a clue in considering the diagnosis of epidemic typhus.[9]

The Weil-Felix reaction is the same as in murine typhus; special serologic methods are used to differentiate louse-borne typhus from murine typhus. These topics as well as suggestions for handling clinical specimens for attempted isolation of the organism are described in Chapter 169.

Nonrickettsial infections that, at some time during their course, may mimic louse-borne typhus include meningococcemia, measles, typhoid fever, bacterial meningitis, secondary syphilis, leptospirosis, relapsing fever, infectious mononucleosis, and rubella.

TREATMENT AND PREVENTION

Treatment

Chloramphenicol and tetracycline both are effective against typhus. The recommended dose for tetracycline is 25 mg/kg of body weight per day in four equally divided oral doses. The dosage for chloramphenicol is 50 mg/kg of body weight per day also in four equally divided oral doses. If the patient is too severely ill to take drugs orally, an iv preparation of chloramphenicol or tetracycline in the dosage described is recommended for use. If renal function is impaired, chloramphenicol or doxycycline (100 mg bid) should be used. Therapy should be continued for 2–3 days after defervescence.

In louse-borne typhus only, a single dose of doxycycline, 100 mg orally, is curative.[10] Conventional, multidose therapy is recommended for indigenously acquired epidemic typhus and murine typhus.

Treatment before serious complications occur virtually eliminates fatal illness. When antimicrobial therapy begins very early after onset (within 48 hours), an occasional patient will relapse. The recurrent illness responds to a second course of therapy.

Prevention

Control of the human body louse and the conditions that foster its proliferation is the mainstay in preventing louse-borne typhus. A vaccine is also available, but its widespread use is subordinate to delousing the affected population. Delousing should be done with an insecticide shown to be lousicidal for the infesting lice. Usually, dichlorodiphenyltrichloroethane (DDT) or lindane in powder form is effective. If the lice are not susceptible to these insecticides, then malathion or carbaryl may be used.

Typhus vaccine is prepared from formaldehyde-inactivated *Rickettsia prowazekii* grown in embryonated eggs. Typhus vaccination is suggested only for the following special risk groups[11]: (*1*) such persons as scientific investigators (e.g., anthropologists, archaeologists, or geologists), oil field and construction workers, missionaries, and some government workers who live in or visit foreign areas where typhus cases actually occur and who will be in close contact with the indigenous population; (*2*) medical personnel, including nurses and attendants, who provide care for patients in foreign areas in which louse-borne typhus occurs; and (*3*) laboratory personnel who work with *R. prowazekii*.

At present, no specific action can be recommended to prevent the suspected occurrence of indigenously acquired epidemic typhus.

BRILL-ZINSSER DISEASE

Brill-Zinsser disease (BZD) occurs as a recrudescence of previous infection with *R. prowazekii*. It occurs in the United States primarily in immigrants from Eastern Europe whose initial infection was during World War II. Its pathogenesis is unknown, but recurrence is presumed to be precipitated by stress or a waning immune system.

Manifestations and Diagnosis

The illness is similar to louse-borne typhus, but it is usually milder and more closely resembles murine typhus. Serologically, the Weil-Felix reaction is usually negative, but a low titer to OX-19 may be present. The differentiation of primary louse-borne or murine typhus from BZD is made by showing that the antibody produced is IgM (murine or primary louse-borne) or IgG (BZD).[12]

Treatment and Prevention

Therapy is the same as for primary louse-borne typhus. There is no known method of preventing BZD other than preventing primary infection.

REFERENCES

1. Lazowski ES, Matulewicz S. Serendipitous discovery of artificial positive Weil-Felix reaction used in '''private immunological war.'' ASM News. 1977;43:300–2.
2. Bozeman FM, Masiello SA, Williams MS, et al. Epidemic typhus rickettsiae isolated from flying squirrels. Nature. 1975;255:545–7.
3. Sonenshine DE, Bozeman FM, Williams MS, et al. Epizootiology of epidemic typhus (*Rickettsia prowazekii*) in flying squirrels. Am J Trop Med Hyg. 1978;27:339–49.
4. McDade JE, Shephard CC, Redus MA, et al. Evidence of *Rickettsia prowazekii* infections in the United States. Am J Trop Med Hyg. 1980;29:277–84.
5. Duma RJ, Sonenshine DE, Bozeman FM, et al. Epidemic typhus in the United States associated with flying squirrels. JAMA. 1981;245:2318–23.
6. Wolbach SB, Todd JL, Palfrey FW. The Etiology and Pathology of Typhus. Cambridge, MA: Harvard University Press; 1922.
7. Committee on Pathology, Division of Medical Sciences, National Research Council. Pathology of epidemic typhus. JAMA. 1953;56:397, 512.
8. Eastman J. Personal communication. Lancaster General Hospital, Lancaster, PA.
9. Kaplan JE, McDade JE, Newhouse VF. Suspected Rocky Mountain spotted fever in the winter—epidemic typhus? (Letter). N Engl J Med. 1981;305:1648.
10. Perine PL, Krause DW, Awoke A, et al. Single-dose doxycycline treatment of louse-borne relapsing fever and epidemic typhus. Lancet. 1974;2:742–4.
11. Centers for Disease Control: Typhus vaccine. MMWR. 1978;27:189.
12. Ormsbee R, Peacock M, Philip R, et al. Serologic diagnosis of epidemic typhus fever. Am J Epidemiol. 1977;105:261–71.

169. RICKETTSIA TYPHI (ENDEMIC OR MURINE TYPHUS)

ALFRED J. SAAH

In 1926, Maxcy inferred from epidemiologic studies that the reservoir for typhus in the United States was the rat, and he postulated its transmission to humans by the flea, mite, or possibly the tick. In Baltimore, Dyer and others substantiated Maxcy's hypothesis in 1931 by isolating rickettsiae from the brain of rats and from rat fleas.[1]

ETIOLOGY

The etiologic agent of murine typhus is *Rickettsia typhi* (formerly *R. mooseri*), an obligate intracellular bacterium that shares common soluble antigens with *Rickettsia prowazekii* (see the section in this chapter on diagnosis). The organism is less pleomorphic than *R. prowazekii* is; mostly coccobacillary forms can be seen in the cytoplasm of infected cells when using Giemsa or Gimenez stain.[2,3]

EPIDEMIOLOGY

Murine typhus is found in all parts of the world. The disease occurs in those people whose occupation or living conditions brings them into close contact with rats and therefore the ectoparasites of these rodents. The rat flea *Xenopsylla cheopis* is the primary vector that causes human infection. Illness in humans is a peripheral occurrence to the natural transmission of the organism in rodents.

Murine typhus continues to occur in the United States, although its reported incidence has declined sharply since its peak in the mid-1940s. Figure 1 shows the number of reported cases from 1955–1985. The early decline is attributable to intensive efforts aimed at controlling ectoparasite and rat populations. At present, reported cases occur predominantly in the southeastern United States and in the Gulf Coast port states; however, reporting is very uneven. The disease is probably extremely underreported. Murine typhus primarily occurs in urban settings, but it can occur in rural settings as well,[5] especially in persons working in granaries or food storage areas. One report[6] indicates that in 1979 most cases in Texas occurred in residential areas and primarily affected children and the elderly. A more recent report[7] confirms the high occurrence of murine typhus in persons older than 40 years and documents the high incidence in Hispanics in south Texas. The months of peak incidence in south Texas were April to June. Elsewhere in the United States, typhus is seen more often in late summer and early autumn.

Worldwide outbreaks and sporadic disease occur[8] where conditions favor the proliferation of rats and where inadequate ectoparasite control exists.

In the rat, the disease is nonfatal. It is transmitted rat to rat

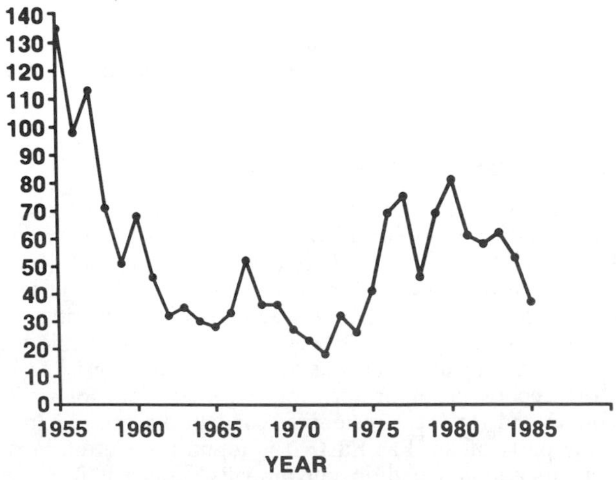

FIG. 1. Typhus fever, flea-borne (endemic, murine). Reported cases by year in the United States, 1955–1985. (From the Centers for Disease Control,[4] and supplemental surveillance data.)

by the rat flea (*X. cheopis*) and possibly by the rat louse *Polypax spinulosis* or other insects.[9] In the flea, the organism multiplies in the cells of the digestive tract without harm to the insect. *Rickettsia typhi* is now thought to be transmitted transovarially in the flea.[9a]

When the flea takes a blood meal, it defecates. Its feces is heavily contaminated with organisms and produces infection in humans by soiling the bite wound. Infection may also occur by mucous membrane (conjunctivae or nasal mucosa) contamination with flea feces or by aerosol in laboratory personnel.[10]

PATHOGENESIS AND PATHOLOGIC CHARACTERISTICS

Descriptions of the anatomic pathology of murine typhus are few because the disease is rarely fatal. A fatal case of murine typhus that occurred in an 81-year-old woman from Texas was recently reported.[11] Necropsy showed interstitial pneumonia, alveolar hemorrhages, cerebral petechiae, interstitial myocarditis, multifocal interstitial nephritis and hemorrhages, splenomegaly, portal triaditis, and mucosal hemorrhages in the urinary tract. *Rickettsia typhi* was demonstrated in the lungs, brain, kidney, liver, and heart. The histopathologic features that are described show the fatal illness to be quite similar to louse-borne typhus (see section on pathologic characteristics in Chapter 168).

CLINICAL MANIFESTATIONS

Signs and Symptoms

After an incubation period of 1–2 weeks, the illness is characterized by headache, myalgia, and fever. Its onset is variable, being gradual less often than sudden. There is no eschar. Frequently, a nonproductive cough occurs early in the course. Although the illness is infrequently prostrating, those stricken are nonetheless unable to work because of headache and myalgia.

Rash occurs in 60–80 percent of the patients, and it first becomes evident on the third to fifth day of illness.[7,12] The rash is initially macular and occurs on the upper thorax and abdomen, and it remains central in distribution. This distribution is quite distinct from the primarily peripheral (ankles, wrists, and face) distribution of spotted fever. Later, the rash of murine typhus becomes maculopapular and remains for 4–8 days. The rash may vary greatly in duration and intensity, and it may be quite evanescent.

In the untreated adult, temperature between 38.9°C (102°F) and 40°C (104°F) usually lasts 12–16 days. With antirickettsial antimicrobial therapy, the patient defervesces in 2–3 days. In either situation, convalescense is rapid. The disease is very mild in young children.

Diagnosis

The Weil-Felix reaction to OX-19 is positive (fourfold rise in titer or single titer of ≥1/320) during the second week of illness in the vast majority of untreated cases; also, OX-2 shows variable reactivity, and the reaction to OX-K is negative. The complement fixation (CF) test becomes positive several days later than the Weil-Felix reaction does. The antigen used in the CF test is usually the soluble antigen, which is common to both *R. typhi* and *R. prowazekii*, and it cross-reacts readily with serum from patients with either infection. Differentiating murine typhus (*R. typhi*) from Brill-Zinsser disease (recrudescent *R. prowazekii*) is discussed in Chapter 168.

Differentiating murine typhus from primary louse-borne typhus (in those vaccinated and not vaccinated against louse-borne typhus) is necessary under certain circumstances in the United States (see the section "Diagnosis" in Chapter 168). If the situation should occur, confirmation can be obtained by using the indirect immunofluorescent antibody (IFA) test after cross-absorption of the patient's serum with specially prepared antigens from *R. prowazekii* and *R. typhi*[13,14] or by isolating the organism. Rickettsial isolation is quite dangerous, and it requires special containment facilities and experience in handling the organism. However, obtaining and storing the clinical specimen (usually a clot of blood) for the isolation attempt poses no special hazard.

It is important to obtain blood for isolating the organism before antimicrobial treatment is begun. The blood should be allowed to clot, the serum removed, and the clot preferably frozen at −70°C or held in the refrigerator for 24–48 hours while arrangements are made for shipment on dry ice. Further information should be sought from the state health department laboratory or state epidemiologist.

Murine typhus and Rocky Mountain spotted fever (RMSF) are distinguishable by three criteria: (*1*) epidemiologically, murine typhus is primarily an urban disease that occurs in late summer and autumn, whereas RMSF occurs in rural or wooded settings during the spring and summer. A history of exposure to ticks is frequently obtained in RMSF, even though tick attachment may be denied. (*2*) The rash distribution in each disease is distinctive. The rash of RMSF occurs with greater frequency, begins on the ankles and wrists, and moves centrally. When rash occurs in murine typhus, it is central, and it infrequently extends to the distal parts of the extremities. (*3*) Serologically, the CF test for RMSF and murine typhus is helpful, although some cross-reaction occurs. If the need should arise, more specialized serologic tests are available through the state health department laboratory.

Differential Diagnoses

Differential diagnoses are given in Chapter 168. Mortality is very uncommon in murine typhus. Recovery is complete; in untreated cases, immunity is solid.

TREATMENT AND PREVENTION

Therapy with tetracycline or chloramphenicol produces defeverescence in 2 days. The doses and course of therapy are described in Chapter 168. Rarely, relapse occurs if treatment is instituted very early in the course of disease. However, repeating the course of antimicrobial therapy suffices.

The occurrence of murine typhus indicates the failure of effective ectoparasite and rodent control. Public health officials should be notified when the disease is suspected. The occurrence of murine typhus implies a situation that would facilitate the transmission of other flea- and rodent-borne diseases if introduced (e.g., plague). It is important to remember that simply killing rats, without first controlling their ectoparasites, can lead to epidemics in humans.[15]

REFERENCES

1. Woodward TE. A historical account of rickettsial diseases with a discussion of unsolved problems. The first Maxwell Finland lecture. J Infect Dis. 1973;127:583.
2. Ormsbee RA. Rickettsiae. In: Lennette EH, Balows A, Hausler WJ Jr, et al., eds. Manual of Clinical Microbiology. 3rd ed. Washington, DC: American Society for Microbiology; 1980:922.
3. Horsfall FL, Tamm I, eds. Viral and Rickettsial Infections in Man. 4th ed. Philadelphia: JB Lippincott; 1965:1059.
4. Centers for Disease Control. Annual summary 1981: Reported morbidity and mortality in the United States. MMWR. 1982;30(Suppl 54):97.
5. Gastel B, Charness ME, Murphy PA, eds. Murine typhus, clinical conferences at the Johns Hopkins Hospital. Johns Hopkins Med J. 1977;141:303–14.
6. Centers for Disease Control. Rickettsial Disease Surveillance Report No. 2 Summary: 1979. Issued May 1981.
7. Taylor JP, Betz TG, Rawlings JA. Epidemiology of murine typhus in Texas. 1980 through 1984. JAMA. 1986;255:2173–6.
8. World Health Organization Working Group on Rickettsial Diseases. Rickettsioses: A continuing disease problem. Bull WHO. 1982;60:157–64.
9. Traub R, Wisseman CL Jr, Farhang-Azad A. The ecology of murine typhus—a critical review. Trop Dis Bull. 1978;75:237–317.

9a. Farhang-Azad A, Traub R, Baqar S. Transovarial transmission of murine typhus rickettsiae in *Xenopsylla cheopis* fleas. Science. 1985;277:543–4.

10. Centers for Disease Control. Laboratory acquired endemic typhus—Maryland. MMWR. 1978;27:215.
11. Walker DH, Betz TG, Taylor JP, et al. Histopathology and immunohistologic demonstration of the distribution of *Rickettsia typhi* in fatal murine typhus. Seventh national meeting of the American Society for Rickettsiology and Rickettsial Diseases, Santa Fe, NM, April 16, 1988.
12. Al-Awadi AR, Al-Kazemi N, Ezzat G, et al. Murine typhus in Kuwait in 1978. Bull WHO. 1982;60:283.
13. Goldwasser RA, Shepard CC. Fluorescent antibody methods in the differentiation of murine and epidemic typhus sera: The differentiation of murine and epidemic typhus sera: Specificity changes resulting from previous immunization. J Immunol. 1959;82:373.
14. Goldwasser RA, Shepard CC, Jordan ME, et al. The specificity of antibody response in typhus fever. Its alteration during murine typhus infection as a result of previous exposure to epidemic typhus antigen. J Immunol. 1959;83:491.
15. Centers for Disease Control. Outbreak of murine typhus—Texas. MMWR. 1983;32:131–2.

170. RICKETTSIA TSUTSUGAMUSHI (SCRUB TYPHUS)

ALFRED J. SAAH

Scrub typhus is an acute, febrile illness of humans that is caused by *Rickettsia tsutsugamushi* (*R. orientalis*); it is transmitted to humans by the bite of larval-stage trombiculid mites (chiggers). Naturally occurring disease in humans occurs only in the Far East, but imported cases to the United States have been recognized.

ETIOLOGY

Rickettsia tsutsugamushi is an obligate intracellular bacterium that grows free in the cytoplasm of infected cells, that is, has no vacuolar membrane. The organism can best be seen in tissue by using the Giemsa stain. It is rather unusual among rickettsiae because of its large number of serotypes. However, there are three major serotypes (Karp, Gilliam, and Kato) that have sufficient cross-reactivity with antigens from other strains to be useful diagnostically by the indirect microimmunofluorescent test.[1]

Preliminary work has been done to improve discrimination between strains by using electrophoretic and fluorographic analysis of extracted proteins.[2]

EPIDEMIOLOGY

Scrub typhus occurs over a wide area of eastern Asia and the western Pacific region, from Korea to Australia, and from Japan to India and Pakistan. It gets its name from the type of vegetation that harbors the vector, that is, scrub or secondary vegetation in transitional terrain between forest and clearings. The name scrub is not altogether accurate because endemic areas are known from sandy beaches to semiarid locations.[3]

Scrub typhus is important, both as a problem for military personnel and for local residents. Civilian disease is endemic in many parts of the Far East. It is found most often in rural inhabitants and is usually occupationally acquired.[4,5]

Scrub typhus is a zoonotic disease in which humans are accidental hosts. The vector of the organism to humans is the larval stage (chigger) of trombiculid mites (*Leptotrombidium deliense* and others). These mites probably also represent the major reservoir of the organism because of the extraordinarily high rates of transovarial transmission and because most chiggers feed only once, whether on humans or on rodents. Studies have shown that 90–100 percent of individual or pooled offspring from infected female mites are capable of transmitting the organism to white mice.[6] Because of these unique characteristics of the mites and chiggers and because chiggers stay within several meters of where they hatch, highly focal "islands of infection" are created in endemic areas.

PATHOGENESIS AND PATHOLOGIC CHARACTERISTICS

When an infected chigger feeds, it inoculates the host with the etiologic agent of scrub typhus. The infection begins by local multiplication at the site of the bite. This produces a papule that later ulcerates. The ulcer forms a black crust, which is the eschar. Regional lymphadenopathy also occurs at this time and is followed by generalized lymphadenopathy in the next 4–5 days. Rickettsemia begins before the onset of symptoms.

CLINICAL MANIFESTATIONS

Signs and Symptoms

Clinical symptoms occur 6–18 days (often 10–12 days) after the bite of an infected chigger. The onset is usually sudden and is characterized by fever, severe headache, and myalgia. There is usually tender lymphadenopathy in the region of the bite wound or eschar. Temperatures usually rise quickly in the first several days of disease to 104°F or 105°F (40–40.5°C). Early in the course of illness, the pulse is relatively slow. Other symptoms at this time may include ocular pain, conjunctival injection, nonproductive cough, and apathy. The severity of symptoms vary widely, depending on the susceptibility of the host and/or the virulence of the infecting strain. After about 5 days of illness, rash occurs on the trunk and spreads to the extremities; it begins as a macular rash and may become papular. It is sometimes evanescent. At this time, there is generalized lymphadenopathy and splenomegaly.

In a small proportion of patients, tremors, delirium, nervousness, slurred speech, deafness, or nuchal rigidity may develop in the second week of illness. Cerebrospinal fluid (CSF) from such patients is either normal or has low numbers of mononuclear cells.

Eighty-seven American soldiers who became infected in South Vietnam all had fever and headache.[7] Of 74 soldiers, 36 (46 percent) had an eschar, and only 30 of 87 (34 percent) had rash. Lymphadenopathy was the most common sign and occurred in 85 percent (74/84) of patients. A common misdiagnosis in this series was infectious mononucleosis.

In untreated patients, fever subsides after an illness of about 2 weeks. Specific antirickettsial therapy shortens the illness considerably and reduces mortality to essentially nil. Mortality rates have ranged from 0 to 30 percent in untreated patients. Death is usually due to heart failure and circulatory collapse or pneumonia.

Routine laboratory studies are of no diagnostic value. Leukopenia may occur early. Lymphocytosis occurred later in 70 percent of the 87 American soldiers. Albuminuria was also common. No consistent liver enzyme abnormality was found.

New episodes of disease occur because of the many different serotypes of *R. tsutsugamushi*. Immunity to homologous strains is very good, but it is short-lived to heterologous strains.

Diagnosis

The Weil-Felix slide agglutination test is not very sensitive, but it is easy to do in less developed areas of the world. Antibodies to *Proteus* OX-K are found in roughly 50 percent of cases during the second week of illness. (*Proteus* OX-2 and OX-19 tests are negative.) The test is rather specific but does cross react in patients with leptospirosis. Criteria for a positive test are either one determination ≥1/320 or a fourfold rise in titer starting from 1/50. The indirect microimmunofluorescent test is similar to the Weil-Felix test in sensitivity and specificity. The diagnostic capability of these tests improved markedly when both were considered together in evaluating a Malaysian hospital population.[8] A modification of the fluorescent antibody test, the immunoperoxidase test, has recently been reported to be simpler to perform than the fluorescent test is and yet yields equivalent results.[9] Treatment in the first several days of illness may blunt or delay the serologic response.

Because of the susceptibility of white mice to *R. tsutsugamushi*, intraperitoneal injection of patient's blood can be used diagnostically. Autopsy of the mouse reveals rickettsiae in tissues. Complement fixation (CF) tests are now infrequently used for diagnosis.

DIFFERENTIAL DIAGNOSIS

The clinical picture of scrub typhus is nonspecific unless an eschar and regional lymphadenopathy are present in a person who was exposed in an endemic area. Eschars may occur in less than half of cases, but it is very helpful in diagnosis when present. Symptoms are like other forms of typhus (severe headache or myalgia). When rash occurs in this setting, the physician should consider a rickettsial infection.

The differential diagnosis includes typhoid fever, brucellosis, leptospirosis, infectious mononucleosis, toxoplasmosis, and flavivirus infection such as dengue.

TREATMENT

Tetracycline or chloramphenicol are both effective in treating scrub typhus; fever dissipates in less than 24 hours in most patients. Tetracycline (25 mg/kg/day in four divided doses) can be used for 3–7 days, or chloramphenicol (50 mg/kg/day in four divided doses) can be used. Tetracycline may be more effective in rapidly ameliorating symptoms.[10] Ciprofloxin may prove to be an effective agent against human scrub typhus.[11]

Relapse may occur, especially when treatment is begun before the fourth or fifth day of illness. Treatment for up to 2 weeks reduces the likelihood of relapse. Evidence is accumulating that shows single-dose doxycycline therapy to be effective in treating scrub typhus and in preventing relapse. In two recent studies,[12,13] a single 200 mg oral dose of doxycycline given at presentation was nearly as effective as 7 days of tetracycline or two doses (days 1 and 7) of doxycycline in preventing relapse. However, the numbers of subjects in these studies are relatively small to have demonstrated equivalent efficacy with reasonable confidence.

PREVENTION

Individuals who are traversing endemic areas should wear protective clothing and use insect repellants to avoid chigger bites.

An effective vaccine for humans has not been developed, mainly due to the serotypic heterogeneity of the organism.

Studies of chemoprophylaxis using doxycycline (200 mg orally weekly) have been evaluated for intensively exposed troops in the field[14] and in experimental infection.[15] Results are encouraging but preliminary; more work in this area is needed.

REFERENCES

1. Robinson DM, Brown GW, Gan E, et al. Adaptation of microimmunofluorescent test to the study of human *Rickettsia tsutsugamushi* antibody. Am J Trop Hyg. 1976;25:900–5.

2. Hanson B, Wisseman CL Jr. Heterogeneity among *Rickettsia tsutsugamushi* isolates: A protein analysis. In: Burgdorfer W, Anacker RL, eds. Rickettsiae and Rickettsial Diseases. New York: Academic Press; 1981:503.
3. Traub R, Wisseman CL Jr. The ecology of chigger-borne rickettsiosis (scrub typhus). J Med Entomol. 1974;11;237.
4. Olson JG, Bourgeois AL. Changing risk of scrub typhus in relation to socioeconomic development in the Pescadores Islands of Taiwan. Am J Epidemiol. 1979;109:236–43.
5. Brown GW, Robinson DM, Huxsoll DL, et al. Scrub typhus: A common cause of illness in indigenous populations. Trans R Soc Trop Med Hyg. 1976;70:444–8.
6. Roberts LW, Robinson DM. Efficiency of transovarial transmission of *Rickettsia tsutsugamushi* in *Leptotrombidium arenicola*. J Med Entomol. 1977;13:493.
7. Berman SJ, Kundin WD. Scrub typhus in South Vietnam, a study of 87 cases. Ann Intern Med. 1973;79:26–30.
8. Brown GW, Shirai A, Rogers C, et al. Diagnostic criteria for scrub typhus: Probability values for immunofluorescent antibody and *Proteus* OX-K agglutinin titers. Am J Trop Med Hyg. 1983;32:1101.
9. Kelly DJ, Wong PW, Gan E, et al. Comparative evaluation of the serodiagnosis of rickettsial disease. Am J Trop Med Hyg. 1988;38:400–6.
10. Sheehy TW, Hazlett D, Turk RE. Scrub typhus, a comparison of chloramphenicol and tetracycline in its treatment. Arch Intern Med. 1973;132:77–80.
11. McClain JB, Joshi B, Rice R. Chloramphenicol, gentamicin, and ciprofloxacin against murine scrub typhus. Antimicrob Agents Chemother. 1988;32:285–6.
12. Brown GW, Saunders JP, Singh S, et al. Single dose doxycycline therapy for scrub typhus. Trans R Soc Trop Med Hyg. 1978;72:412.
13. Olson JG, Fang RCY, Dennis DT. Risk of relapse associated with doxycycline therapy for scrub typhus. In: Burgdorfer W, Anacker, eds. Rickettsiae and Rickettsial Diseases. New York: Academic Press; 1981:201.
14. Olson JG, Bourgeois AL, Fang RCY, et al. Prevention of scrub typhus, prophylactic administration of doxycycline in a randomized double blind trial. Am J Trop Med Hyg. 1980;29:989–97.
15. Twartz JC, Shirai A, Selvaraju G, et al. Doxycycline prophylaxis for human scrub typhus. J Infect Dis. 1982;146:811–8.

171. EHRLICHIA SPECIES (HUMAN EHRLICHIOSIS)

ALFRED J. SAAH

Rickettsiaceae is a family of microorganisms that includes genera such as *Rickettsia* and *Coxiella*. Essentially all are zoonotic infections, some of which cause disease in humans. Besides the genera familiar to physicians, another such genus is *Ehrlichia*, a genus of intraleukocytic bacteria. *Ehrlichia sennetsu* is a human pathogen that was isolated in 1954 from a patient in Japan.[1] The patient had an illness clinically similar to infectious mononucleosis. Recently, an organism that is identical or closely related to *Ehrlichia canis*, which is known to produce pancytopenia in dogs, was morphologically and serologically identified as causing infection and illness in humans.[2,3]

ETIOLOGY

Ehrlichia is a genus of leukocytic rickettsiae that contains five species pathogenic for humans or animals. These organisms are obligate intracellular parasites that parasitize peripheral blood leukocytes; they resemble *Chlamydia* in their formation of intracellular morulae or inclusion bodies measuring 2–5 μm. These inclusion bodies are, in turn, made up of a variable number of elementary bodies measuring 0.2–0.8 μm.[4] Inclusion bodies are best seen with Giemsa or Leishman stain (Fig. 1).

Epidemiology

Ehrlichia canis is a tick-borne infection of dogs and wild canids that occurs worldwide. During U.S. involvement in Vietnam, a severe epizootic of canine ehrlichiosis occurred.[4] The disease became known as tropical canine pancytopenia because of severe and often fatal hematologic manifestations including hemorrhage from thrombocytopenia. The vector of *E. canis* for dogs is the brown dog tick *Rhipicephalus sanguineus*. While transstadial transmission in the tick of *E. canis* is documented, transovarial transmission apparently does not occur. The source(s) for continued tick infection is not known.

Human infection was recognized in 1986[2] in a patient who had had tick exposure in Arkansas. Additional patients have been reported who have had fourfold or greater antibody rises to *E. canis* after a characteristic febrile illness (see below) (Table 1). The Centers for Disease Control report[8] that cases occurred in 11 states, most of which are in the southeastern and south central areas of the United States. Illness occurred between March and October. The incubation period is estimated to be approximately 12–14 days. Controversy exists over the vector for humans because *R. sanguineus* reportedly does not normally feed on humans in North America.[9]

PATHOGENESIS AND PATHOLOGIC CHARACTERISTICS

Intraleukocytic inclusions were seen in the first human case report.[2] Parasitized cells included lymphocytes, atypical lymphocytes, band neutrophils, segmented neutrophils, and monocytes. Identification of organisms in the peripheral blood of the dog is uncommon,[4] and its significance in this case report is unclear. Inclusions were not seen in the published series[3] but were not specifically sought.

In the canine model, pathology in fatal cases is characterized by plasmacyte invasion of organs and by perivascular cuffing by plasma cells in the lung, meninges, spleen, and kidneys[4] and by hemorrhage.

CLINICAL MANIFESTATIONS

Signs and Symptoms

A prodrome is reported from one series.[3] Malaise was the most common prodrome; others included low back pain and nausea and vomiting. All patients had a sudden onset of high fever. Fever is often accompanied by relative bradycardia (<90 beats per minute). Headache is characteristically present. A history of tick attachment, the epidemiologic picture, and the clinical picture strongly suggests the diagnosis of Rocky Mountain spotted fever; however, rash is almost always *absent* in human ehrlichiosis. The remainder of the physical examination findings are normal.

Laboratory findings may provide useful clues to the diagnosis. In the report by Fishbein et al.,[3] the most common hematologic abnormality at presentation was absolute lymphopenia, i.e., <1500/μL. It occurred in all patients. The median absolute lymphocyte count was 408/μL (range, 234–1365/μL). The median WBC count was 3000/μL, and the WBC count was less than 4000/μL in five of six patients.

Thrombocytopenia was noted in the four patients in whom platelets were measured. Thrombocytopenia worsened in these four patients during the first week of hospitalization and reached a median level of 68,000/μL (range, 49,000–75,000/μL). Liver function abnormalities were noted in all four patients who were hospitalized; hepatitis A and B were ruled out. Peak aspartate aminotransferase (SGOT, AST) levels occurred approximately 1 week after onset, with a median level of 335 units/liter (range 90–538 units/liter). Similar abnormalities were noted in other reports.[5–7]

Course

Fishbein et al.[3] reported a median hospitalization of 7 days. Tetracycline resulted in defervescence in 1–2 days. Recovery was complete in all seven patients including two who were not given tetracycline.

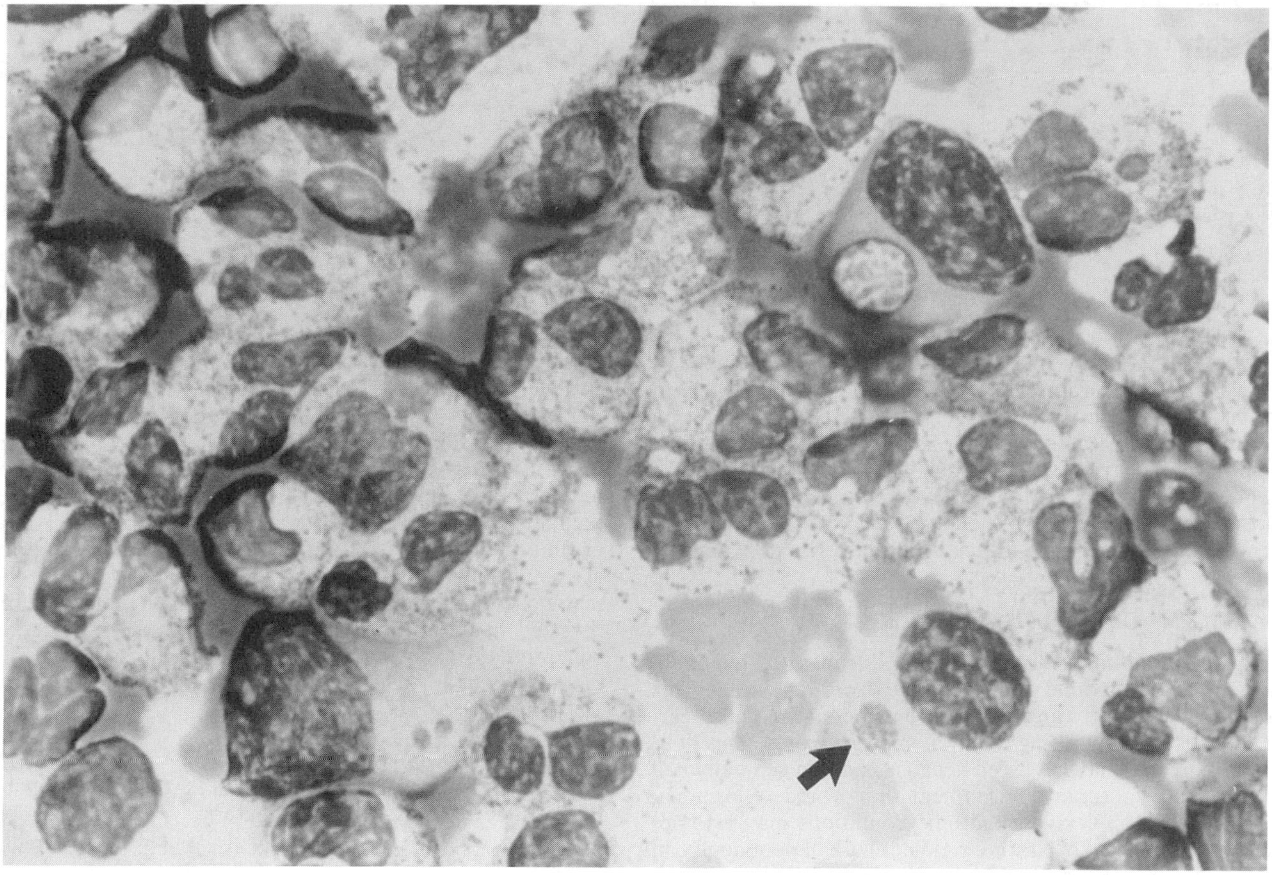

FIG. 1. Peripheral blood smear (buffy coat preparation) showing inclusions (arrows) in atypical lymphocytes. (Leishman stain, ×202). (From Maeda et al.,[2] with permission.)

TABLE 1. Summary of Published Series of Human Ehrlichiosis

Report	*n*	*Male*	*Age (yr)*	*Race*	*Tick Bite*
Maeda et al.[2]	1	1	51	White	1
Fishbein et al.[3]	6	5	26–59	White	6
Taylor et al.[5,6]	9	7	2–71	White	NR
Fishbein et al.[7]	7	5	59[a]	NR	4

Abbreviation: NR: not reported.
[a] Median age

DIAGNOSIS

The indirect fluorescent antibody (IFA) test, which is commonly used for diagnosing rickettsial infections, is the preferred test for human ehrlichiosis. The test is presently performed in a few reference laboratories including the Centers for Disease Control. Information on having sera tested may be obtained from the communicable disease office of your state or local health department. Both acute and convalescent serum specimens should be submitted for testing at the same time. Optimal timing for collecting convalescent specimens is not known, but 2–4 weeks after onset seems prudent.

DIFFERENTIAL DIAGNOSIS

The differential diagnosis includes any tick-borne febrile illness such as Rocky Mountain spotted fever, tularemia (*Francisella tularensis*), babesiosis, and Lyme disease (*Borrelia burgdorferi*). Murine typhus and Q fever should also be considered.

TREATMENT AND PREVENTION

From preliminary reports on humans and from experience in dogs, tetracycline or an analogue is effective in hastening defervescence and recovery. Tetracycline, 25 mg/kg of body weight per day in four equally divided doses, or doxycycline, 100 mg twice daily, may be used, but experience is limited. Therapy should be continued for at least 3 days after defervescence. Because leukopenia and thrombocytopenia are prominent features of human ehrlichiosis and because clinical efficacy has not been demonstrated, chloramphenicol is not recommended.

Prevention is best accomplished by frequently checking for ticks and removing them.

REFERENCES

1. Misao T, Kobayashi. Studies on infectious mononucleosis (glandular fever). I. Isolation of etiologic agent from blood, bone marrow, and lymph node of a patient with infectious mononucleosis by using mice. Kyushu J Med Sci. 1955;6:145–52.
2. Maeda K, Markowitz N, Hawley RC, et al. Human infection with *Ehrlichia canis*, a leukocytic *Rickettsia*. N Engl J Med. 1987;316:853–6.
3. Fishbein DB, Sawyer LA, Holland CJ, et al. Unexplained febrile illnesses after exposure to ticks. Infection with an *Ehrlichia*? JAMA. 1987;257:3100–4.
4. Ristic M. Pertinent characteristics of the leukocytic rickettsiae of humans and animals. In: Leive L, ed. Microbiology 1986. Washington, DC: American Society for Microbiology; 1986;182–7.
5. Taylor JP, Betz TG, Fishbein DB, et al. Serological evidence of possible human infection with *Ehrlichia* in Texas. J Infect Dis. 1988;158:217–20.
6. Taylor J. Human infection with *Ehrlichia canis* in Texas. Seventh National meeting of the American Society for Rickettsiology and Rickettsial Diseases, Santa Fe, NM, April 16, 1988.
7. Fishbein D. Active surveillance of human ehrlichiosis in hospitalized patients, southeast Georgia. Seventh National meeting of the American Society for Rickettsiology and Rickettsial Diseases, Santa Fe, NM, April 16, 1988.
8. Centers for Disease Control. Human erhlichiosis-United States. MMWR. 1988;37:270–7.
9. Ewing SA, Johnson DV, Kocan KM. Human infection with *Ehrlichia canis* (Letter). N Engl J Med. 1987;317:899–900.

SECTION E. BACTERIAL DISEASES

172. INTRODUCTION

DENNIS L. KASPER

A most useful method of classifying bacteria was developed in 1884 by Christian Gram. He observed that certain bacteria (gram-positive) retain a crystal violet dye after decolorization while others (gram-negative) do not. This staining trait is related to the differential structure of the cell wall of gram-positive and gram-negative bacteria. Both types of bacteria contain distinct, important, cell surface constituents, but also share other constituents found on the cell surface of all bacteria.[1]

THE ANTIGENS OF GRAM-NEGATIVE BACTERIA

Two phospholipid bilayer-type membranes separated by a peptidoglycan layer surround gram-negative bacteria (Fig. 1). This complex cell wall structure differs from the surface of eucaryotic cells where only a single-unit membrane exists. This double membrane may have evolved because bacteria generally had to adapt to a hypotonic environment that would lyse animal cells. The need to survive hypotonic conditions may also account for the presence of a rather rigid network of peptidoglycan located between the two double membranes of the bacteria.

The outer membrane of gram-negative bacteria is located external to the peptidoglycan layer.[2] This membrane serves as a barrier to the external environment. Functionally, it is thought to prevent toxic compounds from entering the cell. This barrier function may allow gram-negative bacteria to survive in the intestinal flora, by protecting the cytoplasmic membrane and the cytoplasm from direct exposure to bile salts that otherwise would lyse the organism. Host cells have the greatest contact with outer membrane constituents, and antibacterial immunity is developed most effectively to these structures. This membrane consists of a lipid bilayer composed of proteins, phospholipids and lipopolysaccharide (LPS). Most pathogenic bacteria also have capsular polysaccharides attached to the outer membrane, perhaps through small terminal lipids inserted into the membrane itself.[3] Many gram-negative bacteria contain pili or fimbriae that project outward from the outer membrane and are important for mucosal or epithelial attachment. Finally, many bacteria produce potent toxins and enzymes that are synthesized in the cytoplasm or periplasm and extruded. These cell products contribute to the pathogenic potential of these organisms.

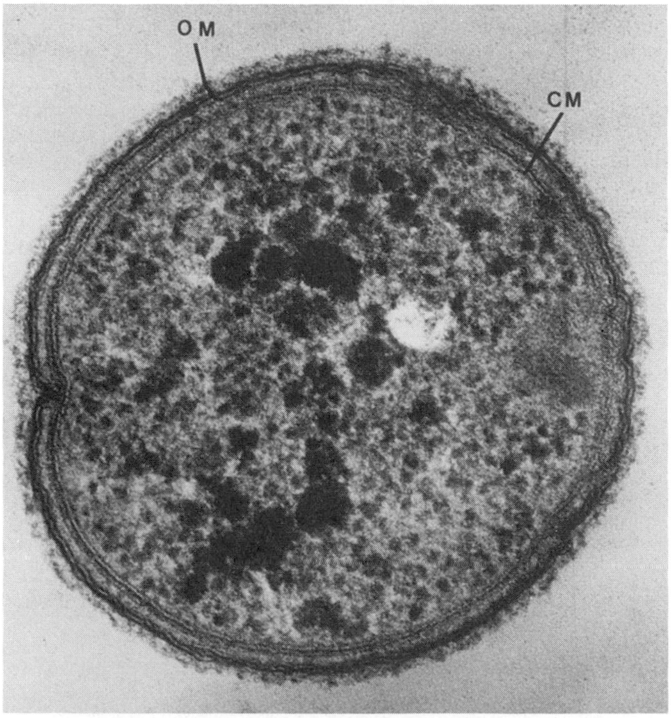

FIG. 1. Electron micrograph of a morphologically typical gram-negative rod, *Bacteroides vulgatus*. The well-defined double-membrane structure is clearly seen. The outer membrane (OM) and cytoplasmic membrane (CM) are separated by the periplasmic space containing the peptidoglycan layer.

PILI

Pili or fimbriae are hairlike structures that project outward from the surface of gram-negative bacteria.[4] Pili are actually polymers of proteins, primarily a single species called pilin. It is thought that these structures are important for mucosal or epithelial cell attachment. In several gram-negative bacteria these structures have been demonstrated to be important in contributing to bacterial virulence. For example, nonpiliated *Neisseria gonorrhoeae* do not attach well to tissue culture cell lines and do not adhere well to fallopian tube epithelium in organ cultures.[5] Piliated goncococci do adhere. Mutants of *Vibrio cholera* have been constructed by transposon mutagenesis.[6] These mutants lack the "toxin-coregulated pilus" (TCP) and have been shown to be defective in colonization of the intestinal mucosa. When using hybridization techniques, nonclinical isolates of *Vibrio cholera* were reported to lack the TCP genome, which suggests that these strains, without TCP, lack colonization properties.

In *Escherichia coli* two main types of pili are found: those that induce agglutination of guinea pig and other erythrocytes and are inhibited by D-mannose (type 1) and adhesins inducing agglutination of human and other erythrocytes and are unaffected by D-mannose (type 2).[7] It is believed that the mannose-resistant pili mediate attachment to human uroepithelial cells.[8] Evidence to date indicates that pili are complex proteins that have constant and variable regions and that these differences in structure may explain the affinity of some organisms for different cell surface receptors.[9] The strong adhesive function of mannose-sensitive (type 1) pili appears to be due to the concerted action of many of the thousand or so pilus proteins that make up pilus rods. Genetic evidence suggests that auxiliary pilus proteins also are required for adhesion. Three integral minor proteins have been identified on the type 1 pilus. The one located at the pilus tip is the receptor-binding adhesin.[10] Glycolipid molecules on the host cell membrane to which pili bind with specificity seem to serve as the primary receptor site for type 2 pili.[11] For an in-depth discussion see Chapter 195.

OUTER MEMBRANE PROTEINS

The proteins on the surface of gram-negative bacteria serve a variety of functions. These proteins play a role in the functional integrity of the membrane, act as receptor sites for bacteriophages and colicins, and are involved in the processes of cell division and conjugation.[12] Outer membrane proteins also function as nonspecific passive diffusion pores. They allow the passage of low-molecular-weight nutrients but also help protect against the loss of hydrolytic enzymes and nutrient-binding proteins that reside in the periplasmic region.[13] These proteins are also able to form gating channels in lipid membranes and have been designated *porins*. Outer membrane proteins appear to play a role in the virulence of organisms and in immunity to certain bacterial infections. Porins may be able to insert themselves in eukaryotic membranes and form gating channels for the entrance of the organism into the host cell.[14] Outer membrane proteins of several gram-negative bacteria including gonococci, *Neisseria meningitidis, Haemophilus influenza*, and *E. coli* have been demonstrated to induce antibodies during natural infection with these organisms.

LIPOPOLYSACCHARIDES

Lipopolysaccharide or endotoxin is an essential component of the outer membrane of gram-negative bacteria (see Chapters 59 and 195). This molecule is responsible for a variety of biologic effects on the host and is the major constituent of the outer membrane of gram-negative bacteria. Lipid A, the endotoxin moiety, is the lipid end of the LPS molecule and anchors the LPS to the membrane. Polysaccharide or oligosaccharide chains (''O'' antigens) extend outward from lipid A and represent a major immunodeterminant. ''Smooth'' LPS contains a repeating-unit O side chain polysaccharide linked by glycoside to the core oligosaccharide, whereas ''rough'' LPS lacks these saccharides. O side chains on a given organism vary in length as a function of the number of oligosaccharide repeating units that have been attached during biosynthesis. This variability can be seen as a ''step ladder'' pattern on polyacrylamide gels (Fig. 2).

The chemical composition and hence immunologic reactivity of the O side chain is serotype specific. Antibody to O side chain is protective against some bacterial species. Many gram-negative rods share a structurally similar region of a ''core'' oligosaccharide that bridges lipid A and the O side chain and extending for 8–10 sugar residues. The structure of the core oligosaccharide of the LPS molecule differ only in fine architectual detail among gram-negative species.[15] The core oligosaccharide consists of the same overall general structure with an outer core region composed of a branched hexose pentasaccharide and an inner core region containing phosphorylated heptose and 2-keto,3-deoxyoctonate (KDO). Evidence suggests the most complex portion of the core structure resides in the region of KDO that likely represents the linkage portion between the polysaccharide and the lipid A component of LPS. Even *Bacteroides* organisms, which were previously thought to lack KDO, have recently been found to contain an altered phosphorylated form of this sugar.[16,16a]

The lipid A portion of the LPS molecule is a phospholipid composed of a glucosamine disaccharide backbone, with the hydroxyl groups substituted by either KDO or various fatty acids.[17] Lipid A is the toxic portion of LPS, but also serves as the building block of the outer membrane where it plays a primary role in the structural integrity of this membrane.

Historically, *endotoxin* was defined as a molecule remaining attached to the bacterium during infection, whereas *exotoxins* were secreted to exert effects at a site distant from the organism. A more modern view of these terms might be that endotoxins are structurally integrated into the cell wall, although they are released, to some extent, from the bacterium during growth. A number of important activities are attributed to lipid A, including fever, hypothermia, local Shwartzman reaction, decreases and increases in white blood cell count, induction of prostaglandin synthesis in macrophages, mitogenesis for B lymphocytes, lethal toxicity in experimental animals, enhancement of monocyte migration, interferon induction, adjuvant activity, and tumor suppression.[18] Interleukin-1 and tumor necrosis factor production are linked directly to lipid A, and these are the major known mediators of LPS toxicity.[19,20]

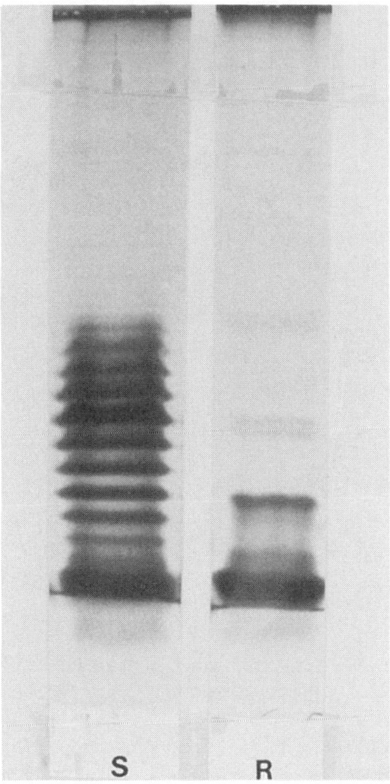

FIG. 2. Sodium dodecyl sulfate–polyacrylamide gel electrophoresis of rough (R) and smooth (S) lipopolysaccharides (LPS) from gram-negative bacteria. Note the ''step-ladder'' appearance in the smooth LPS that is the repeating subunit of the O side chain. (Courtesy of Dr. James Breeling.)

Antibodies to lipid A occur naturally in the serum of healthy humans and many animal species. These antibodies also have been demonstrated in patients with infection due to gram-negative bacteria. Antibodies to lipid A have been demonstrated to provide protection in experimental models of infection. Since these antibodies are broadly reactive among aerobic and facultative gram-negative bacteria, they are of interest for their vaccine potential. These antibodies can opsonize *E. coli* for subsequent phagocytosis in mice, and they can protect mice from infection with *Salmonella typhimurium*.[21] Antibodies to lipid A have been shown to prevent or inhibit development of the local Shwartzman reaction and suppress pyrogenicity in rabbits. Active immunization with lipid A or passive transfer of antibodies, however, fails to protect mice from the lethal effects of LPS.

In humans, individuals suffering from gram-negative sepsis who received serum taken from volunteers immunized with the J5 mutant of *E. coli* (galactose epimerase deficient and thus deficient in the outer portion of the core and the complete O side chain) were found to have a greater survival rate than had individuals receiving preimmunization serum.[22] Further testing of this approach is currently underway in several centers.

ANTIGENS UNIQUE TO GRAM-POSITIVE BACTERIA

The cell wall of gram-positive bacteria is depicted schematically in Figure 3. The innermost constituent is the cytoplasmic or protoplasmic membrane. Surrounding this membrane is a peptidoglycan layer that accounts for more than 40 percent of the cellular mass. In addition, other nonpeptidoglycan polymers frequently form part of the cell wall in gram-positive bacteria,

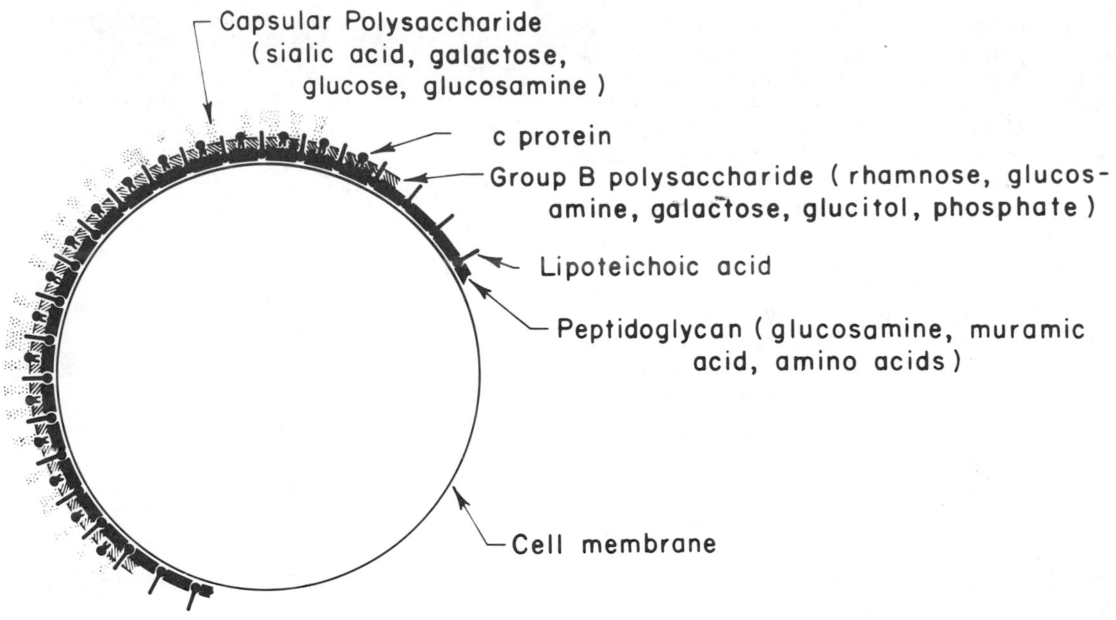

FIG. 3. Schematic diagram of the cell wall structure of a gram-positive bacteria (group B *Streptococcus*). (Adapted from Kasper et al.,[1] with persmission.)

including teichoic acids (phosphodiester-linked polymers containing sugar alcohols), teichuronic acids, and neutral or acidic polysaccharides. These structures frequently are covalently linked to the peptidoglycan. In addition, it is possible to delineate other structures not covalently linked. Capsular polysaccharides may be similar or identical in composition to non-peptidoglycan-linked polymers. External crystalline-like structures that are thought to be proteins have been observed on the surface of a variety of gram-positive species. Finally, lipoteichoic acids, which are cell membrane-associated, may be in intimate contact with the cell wall but may not be covalently linked.

In gram-positive bacteria the peptidoglycan is responsible for the rigidity, strength, and shape of the cell wall.[23] This polymer consists of repeating units of *N*-acetylglucosamine and *N*-acetylmuramic acid. The carbohydrate polymers are cross-linked through carboxyl groups of terminal D-alanine residues on tetrapeptides. The carbohydrate portion of peptidoglycan is well conserved in most gram-positive species; however, the structure of the peptide cross-bridge varies. Because of the conserved carbohydrate portion, extensive immunologic cross-reactivity can be demonstrated among peptidoglycans of various gram-positive bacteria. Biologically, peptidoglycans share a number of properties with the endotoxin or LPS of gram-negative bacteria. Peptidoglycans are pyrogenic in rabbits and initiate shock and death in experimental models. Peptidoglycan has been shown to produce a necrotic skin lesion in rabbits after local injection, and like endotoxin, this substance provokes a localized Shwartzman reaction.[24] Streptococcal peptidoglycan can produce carditis in rabbits when administered intravenously and is capable of lysing red blood cells and platelets.[25,26] Peptidoglycans of some species activate the complement system but there appears to be strain variability in this function.

Major polymers covalently linked to the peptidoglycan are the teichoic acids and group carbohydrates of the streptococci. The group carbohydrate of group A *Streptococcus* consists of *N*-acetylglucosamine and rhamnose.[27] The group carbohydrate of group B *Streptococcus* recently has been characterized structurally and is composed of rhamnose, glucosamine, and glucitol-containing oligosaccharides that are phosphodiester linked.[28] The fact that this material has both sugar alcohol and phosphodiester bonds suggests that the group B streptococcal cell wall carbohydrate is teichoic acid-like in composition.

SURFACE PROTEINS

Many pathogenic gram-positive cocci have important proteins on their surface such as the M protein in group A streptococci. These proteins have been linked to the virulence of these organisms.[29] There are other proteins on streptococcal cell surfaces that have not been associated with virulence and have been used only as epidemiologic markers.[30] Streptococcal M proteins vary immunologically from type to type but maintain similar biologic effects. For effective phagocytosis of M protein-positive strains opsonic antibody is required. M-positive bacteria activate the alternative complement pathway less efficiently in the absence of antibody than do M-negative strains.[31] M-positive bacteria also inhibit neutrophil chemotaxis. Much recent work has focused on the structural and genetic analysis of streptococcal M proteins. The amino acid sequenced displays seven-residue periodicity, or "heptad repeats" (hydrophobic and hydrophilic amino acids), which is consistent with an α helical structure.[32] The heptal repeat structure of M proteins is homologous to some other proteins such as myosin. It has been proposed that this structural similarity between M protein and heart muscle accounts for cardiac tropism in some cases of poststreptococcal rheumatic fever. The carboxy terminus of M proteins displays homology with other M-protein types and also with similar surface proteins of other streptococci such as the G protein of group G *Streptococcus*.[33] This similar carboxy region may explain why some immunologic cross-reactions are observed between different streptococcal M serotypes.

Other bacteria have proteins on their surface that bind to immunoglobulin. The best known of these is the protein A of *Staphylococcus aureus* that binds to the Fc fragment of IgG. The surface protein G purified from groups C and G streptococci has been demonstrated to have more general IgG-binding characteristics than protein A has, with avidity toward immunoglobulins to which protein A fails to react.[34] Another protein has been found on the surface of group B streptococci that binds IgA.[34a] Protein A from *S. aureus* and protein G from group G *Streptococcus* have been useful diagnostic and research reagents; however, their role in the pathogenesis of infection is unclear.

ANTIGEN COMMON TO GRAM-NEGATIVE AND GRAM-POSITIVE BACTERIA CAPSULAR POLYSACCHARIDES

The surface of most invasive gram-positive and gram-negative bacteria that are pathogenic for humans is covered with a capsular polysaccharide (Fig. 4). This carbohydrate structure plays a role in the pathogenicity of the bacterial cell, serving as an antiphagocytic function that allows the organism to evade normal host defense mechanisms.[35] To counteract the ability of the encapsulated organism to withstand nonspecific host clearance mechanisms requires specific antibody for opsonization and subsequent phagocytosis. Capsular polysaccharides are found in both gram-positive and gram-negative bacteria, and their role seems to be similar in both type of organisms. These polysaccharides serve a useful diagnostic function as well since, as organisms grow, the capsule tends to be sloughed into the surrounding fluids and may be detected in soluble form as free antigens in the cerebrospinal fluid, blood, and urine of infected patients.[36,37] Capsules are extremely hydrophilic structures that, in gram-negative bacteria, have been shown to have small lipid terminal ends that insert into the outer membrane. In gram-positive bacteria there is some suggestion, although not definitively proven, that the capsular polysaccharides may be cross-linked to the peptidoglycan.[38]

The chemical structures of capsular polysaccharides of many pathogenic bacteria have been identified. They are high-molecular-weight polymers composed of sugar constituents. Occasionally these sugars will contain polypeptides or single amino acids. A great immunologic diversity can be generated by simple sugars that is based on linkage and conformational differences. For example, a simple oligosaccharide consisting of three hexoses has 1056 different possible arrangements because each one of the monosaccharides can link to any one of six carbons on the adjacent hexose unit and each sugar can be in either an α or β configuration. In contrast, a simple peptide consisting of three amino acids has only six possible variations. In sugars specific linkages add the possibility of antigenic diversity. The structural diversity of pneumococcal capsules has made it difficult to devise vaccines against all serotypes. There are interesting examples of bacterial capsules in which only single linkages differ, and yet these polysaccharides are not immunologically cross-reactive. Such is the case with the groups B and C meningococcal polysaccharides. These two polysaccharides are homopolymers of sialic acid.[39] The specific chemical structure of the polysaccharide also seems to relate to tissue tropism. For example, *E. coli* strains that have a K-1 capsule seem to have a propensity for causing meningitis in neonates. Similarly, group B streptococci of serotype III cause more than 80 percent of the cases of meningitis due to this organism, yet type III group B streptococci account for only approximately one-third of strains causing pneumonia or bacteremia without meningitis, or one-third of all colonizing strains.

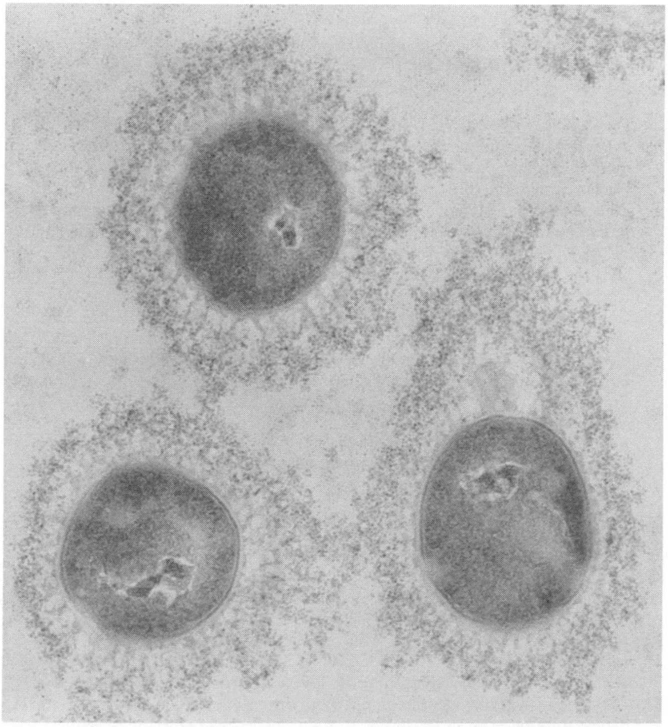

FIG. 4. Electron micrograph of type Ia group B *Streptococcus* demonstrating the capsular polysaccharide exterior to the cell wall. These bacteria were strained with specific antibodies coupled to particles to demonstrate the capsular polysaccharide.

TOXINS AND ENZYMES

Some bacteria produce disease by elaboration of exotoxins (see Chapter 1). An important example of this disease mechanism is the potent enterotoxin produced by *Vibrio cholera* (see Chapter 192).[40] This enterotoxin acts upon the luminal surface of mucosal cells in the small intestine and causes hypersecretion of electrolytes. The cholera toxin acts by activation of cell membrane adenylylcyclase, which results in a large increase in the cyclic AMP concentrations. The toxin is a complex of an A-subunit polypeptide and five copies of B-subunit polypeptides. The B-subunit peptides are responsible for binding of the cholera toxin to intestinal ganglioside GM_1. After enzymatic cleavage of the α-chain, the A1 fragment of the chain enters the cell where it transfers adenosine diphosphate ribose enzymatically from NAD to a covalent linkage with the regulatory "G" protein, which in turn is complexed with the cellular enzyme adenylylcyclase. ADP-ribosylated G protein causes persistent activation of adenylylcyclase, thereby resulting in an increased level of cyclic AMP that stimulates the secretion of ions and fluid into the intestinal lumen.

Not all exotoxins act locally. *Corynyebacterium diphtheriae* produces an exotoxin that is responsible for many of the clinical manifestations of disease[41] (see Chapter 183). This protein consists of a single polypeptide chain cross-linked by two disulfide bridges. This toxin has the ability to damage a variety of animal cells. A cleavage fragment, A, also functions as an NAD-dependent ADP ribosyltransferase. However, in contrast to cholera toxin, the target of diphtheria toxin is not the G protein of adenylylcyclase. Diphtheria toxin fragment A stops protein synthesis by covalently linking an ADP ribose moiety of NAD to the eukaryotic cells' elongation factor (EF-2). The toxin may fix to sensitive animal cells by its carboxy terminus, and proteolytic and reductive steps occur near the cell surface that liberate fragment A. Once inside the cell, fragment A inactivates EF-2. Inactivation of EF-2 stops protein synthesis and leads to cell death. The toxic manifestations of this exotoxin involve primarily the heart, kidneys, and peripheral nerves.

Some *Staphylococcus aureus* strains produce exotoxins that appear to be largely responsible for clinical syndromes such as toxic shock syndrome. The major mechanism of action of the toxin responsible for most cases (TSST-1) is through release of monokines, which are important mediators of inflammation (IL-1, TNF, etc.)[41a]

A number of enzymes are also produced by bacteria that interfere with the immune response. An IgA protease is produced

TABLE 1. Some Pathogenic Extracellular and Facultative Intracellular Bacteria

Extracellular Bacteria	*Facultative Intracellular Bacteria*
Gram-negative rods	Gram-negative rods
Escherichia coli	*Yersinia* species
Klebsiella species	*Francisella* species
Enterobacter species	*Salmonella typhi*
Serratia marcescens	*Salmonella paratyphi*
Proteus species	*Treponema pallidum*
Salmonella species (except *S. typhi* and *S. paratyphi*)	*Legionella pneumophila*
	Brucella species
Pseudomonas species and other nonfermenters	Gram-positive rods
Bacteroides fragilis	*Mycobacterium tuberculosis*
Haemophilus influenzae	*Mycobacterium leprae*
Vibrio species	*Listeria monocytogenes*
Gram-negative cocci	
Neisseria species	
Branhamella catarrhalis	
Gram-positive cocci	
Pneumococci	
Streptococci	
Staphylococci	
Gram-positive rods	
Actinomyces	
Bacillus species	
Clostridium species	

(Modified from Kasper et al.,[1] with permission.)

by a number of pathogenic bacteria including the *Neisseria* species. This protease cleaves the IgA of human serum that belongs to the IGA1 subclass.[42] Cleavage generates Fab and Fc fragments. This enzyme may enhance the pathogenicity of the infecting organism by decreasing the antibody activity of IgA in human secretions. Inactivation of IgA could result in enhanced attachment of bacteria to mucosal surfaces.

BACTERIAL INTERACTIONS WITH HOST DEFENSE

Bacteria are often divided into organisms that survive and replicate intracellularly and those that replicate extracellularly. An incomplete list of these organisms is provided in Table 1. Typically, those organisms living intracellularly may induce granulomas, whereas extracellular organisms, when localized in tissues, cause abscess formation. Either class of organism is capable of causing bacteremia. It is clear from experimental models that both abscess and granuloma formation are T-cell–dependent phenomena. The assumption has been that immunity to intracelluar bacteria is mediated by T cells and immunity to extracelluar bacteria is mediated through the humoral systems discussed earlier. However, it is now clear that even extracellular bacteria are capable of initiating T-cell responses, some of which are essential for immunity. A series of experiments using *Listeria monocytogenes* infection in inbred mice has clarified the nature of the cellular immune response to many intracellular organisms.[43,44] Immune spleen cells and not immune serum could transfer immunity to *Listeria*. These immune T cells function by activating macrophages. T-cell memory is antigen specific, but the activated macrophage is nonspecific in its killing action. The T cell activates macrophages by releasing soluble lymphokines such as γ-interferon.

Another form of T-cell immunity has been described for *Bacteroides fragilis*, an extracellular pathogen.[45] In a model system of intra-abdominal infection, it has been shown that T lymphocytes play an integral role in both induction of abscesses and immunity to abscess formation.[46]

REFERENCES

1. Kasper DL, Finberg RW. The Bacteria. In: Samter M, Talmage DW, Frank MM, et al., eds. Immunological Diseases. Boston: Little, Brown; 1988:803–32.
2. Inouye M. What is the outer membrane? In: Inouye M, ed. Bacterial Outer Membranes, Biogenesis and Functions. New York: John Wiley & Sons; 1979:1–12.
3. Gotschlich EC, Fraser BA, Nishimura O, et al. Lipid on capsular polysaccharide of gram-negative bacteria. J Biol Chem. 1981;256:8915–21.
4. Swanson J, Kraus SJ, Gotschlich EC. Studies on gonococcus infection: I. Pili and zones of adhesion: Their relation to gonococcal growth patterns. J Exp Med. 1971;134:886–906.
5. McGee ZA, Johnson AP, Taylor-Robinson D. Pathogenic mechanisms of *Neisseria gonorrhea*: Observations on damage to human fallopian tubes in organ culture by gonococci of colony type 1 and 4. J Infect Dis. 1981;143:413–22.
6. Mekalanos JJ. Cholera toxin: Genetic analysis, regulation, and role in pathogensis. Current Top Microbiol Immunol. 1985;118:97–118.
7. Ørskov I, Ørskov F, Birch-Andersen A, et al. Protein attachment factors: Fimbriae in adhering *Escherichia coli* strains. In: Robbins JB, Hill JC, Sadoff JC, eds. Seminars in Infectious Diseases, Bacterial Vaccines. vol. 4. New York: Thieme-Stratten; 1982:97–103.
8. Ørskov I, Ørskov F, Birch-Andersen A. Comparison of *Escherichia coli* fimbriae antigen F7 with type I fimbriae. Infect Immun. 1980;27:657–66.
9. Schoolnik GK, Fernandez R, Tai JY, et al. Gonococcal pili: Primary structure and receptor binding domain. J Exp Med. 1984;159:1351–70.
10. Hansen MS, Brinton CC Jr. Identification and characterization of *E. coli* type 1 pilus tip adhesion protein. Nature. 1988;332:265–8.
11. Kallenius G, Svenson S, Mollby R, et al. Structure of carbohydrate part of receptor on human uroepithelial cells for pyelonephritogenic *Escherichia coli*. Lancet. 1981;2:604–6.
12. Koninsky J. Specific transport systems and receptors for colicins and phages. In: Inouye M, ed. Bacterial Outer Membranes. Biogenesis and Functions. New York: John Wiley & Sons; 1979:319–60.
13. Nikaido H. Non-specific transport through the outer membrane. In: Inouye M, ed. Bacterial Outer Membranes, Biogenesis and Functions. New York: John Wiley & Sons; 1979:361–408.
14. Young JD, Blake M, Mauro A, et al. Properties of the major outer membrane protein from *N. gonorrhoeae* incorporated into model lipid membranes. Proc Natl Acad Sci USA. 1983;80:3831–5.
15. Galanos C, Luderitz O, Rietschel ET, et al. Newer aspects of the chemistry and biology of bacterial lipopolysaccharides, with special reference to their lipid A component. In: Goodwin TW, ed. Biochemistry of Lipids II. Baltimore: University Park Press; 1977:239–335.
16. Kasper DL. Chemical and biological characterization of the lipopolysaccharide of *Bacteroides fragilis*. subspecies *fragilis* J Infect Dis. 1976;134:59–66.
16a. Lindberg AA, Weintraub A, Zähringer U, et al. Structure-activity relationships in *Bacteroides fragilis* lipopolysaccharides. Rev Infect Dis. (In press).
17. Rietschel ET, Wollenweber HW, Russa R, et al. Concepts of the chemical structure of lipid A. Rev Infect Dis. 1984;6:432–8.
18. Morrison DC, Alving CR, eds. Molecular concepts of lipid A. Rev Infect Dis. 1984;6:427–31.
19. Michie HR, Manogue KR, Spriggs DR, et al. Detection of circulatory tumor necrosis factor after endotoxin administration. N Engl J Med. 1988;318:1481–5.
20. Dinarello CA, Mier JW. Lymphokines. N Engl J Med. 1987;317:940–5.
21. Galanos C, Freudenberg MA, Hase S, et al. Biological activities and immunological properties of lipid A. In: Schlessinger D, ed. Microbiology. Washington DC: American Society for Microbiology; 1977:269–76.
22. Ziegler EJ, McCutchan JA, Fierer J, et al. Treatment of gram-negative bacteremia and shock with human antiserum to a mutant *E. coli*. N Engl J Med. 1982;397:1225–30.
23. Glavert AM, Thornley MJ. The topography of the bacterial cell wall. Annu Rev Microbiol. 1969;23:159–93.
24. Rotta J. Endotoxin-like properties of the peptidoglycan. Z Immunitaetsforsch. 1975;149:230–44.
25. Heymer B. Biological properties of peptidoglycan. Z Immunitaetsforsch. 1975;149:245–57.
26. Spika JS, Peterson PK, Wilkinson BJ, et al. The role of peptidoglycan from *Staphylococcus aureus* in leukopenia, thrombocytopenia and complement activation associated with bacteremia. J Infect Dis. 1982;146:227–34.
27. Krause RM, McCarty M. Studies on the chemical structure of the streptococcal cell wall: I. The identification of a mucopeptide on the cell walls of groups A and A variant streptococci. J Exp Med. 1961;114:127–39.
28. Michon F, Brisson JR, Dell A, et al. Multiantennary group-specific polysaccharide of group B streptococcus. Biochemistry. 1988;27:5341–51.
29. Wiley GG, Bruno PN. The M antigens: Variations and interrelationships. In: Wannamaker LW, Matsen JM, eds. Streptococci and Streptococcal Diseases. New York: Academic Press; 1972:235–50.
30. Maxted WR, Widdowsen JP. The protein antigens of group A streptococci. In: Wannamaker LW, Matsen JM, eds. Streptococci and Streptococcal Diseases. New York: Academic Press; 1972:251–67.
31. Bisno AL. Alternate complement pathway activation by group A streptococci: Role of M protein. Infect Immun. 1979;26:1172–6.
32. Fishetti VA, Manjula BN. Biologic and immunologic implications of the structural relationship between streptococcal M protein and mammalian tropomysin. In: Robbins JB, Hill JC, Sadoff JC, eds. Seminars in Infectious Diseases. New York: Thieme-Stratton; 1982:411–8.
33. Fahnestock SR, Alexander P, Nagle J, et al. Gene for an immunoglobular binding protein from a group G *Streptococcus*. J Bacteriol. 1986;167:870–80.

34. Björck L, Kronwall G. Purification and some properties of streptococcal protein G, a novel IgG-binding reagent. J Immunol. 1984;133:969–74.
34a. Russell-Jones GJ, Gotschlich EC. Identification of protein antigens of group B streptococci with special reference to the Ibc antigens. J Exp Med. 1984;160:1476–1484.
35. Kasper DL. Bacterial capsule—old dogmas and new tricks. J Infect Dis. 1986;153:407–15.
36. Baker CJ, Webb BJ, Jackson CV, et al. Countercurrent immunoelectrophoresis in the evaluation of infants with group B streptococcal disease. Pediatrics. 1980;65:1110–4.
37. Kenny GE, Wentworth BB, Beasley RR, et al. Correlation of circulating capsular polysaccharide with bacteremia in pneumococcal pneumonia. Infect Immun. 1972;6:431–7.
38. DeCuenick BJ, Shockman GD, Swenson RM. Group B streptococcal cell wall composition and structure revealed through endo-*N*-acetylmuramic catalyzed hydrolysis. Infect Immun. 1982;35:572–81.
39. Jennings HJ, Bhattacharjee AK, Bundle DR, et al. Structures of the capsular polysaccharides of *Neisseria meningitidis* as determined by ^{13}C nuclear magnetic resonance spectroscopy. J Infect Dis. 1977;136(Suppl):78–83.
40. Moss J, Vaughan M. Activation of adenylate cyclase by choleragen. Annu Rev Biochem. 1979:581–600.
41. Pappenheimer AM Jr. Diphtheria in Bacterial Vaccines. In: Germanier R, ed. London: Academic Press; 1984:1–36.
41a. Parsonnet J. Mediators in the pathogenesis of toxic shock syndrome: overview. Rev Infect Dis. 1989;11:S263–S269.
42. Plaut AG, Gilbert JV, Artenstein MS, et al. *Neisseria gonorrhoeae* and *Neisseria meningitidis:* Extracellular enzyme cleaves human immunoglobulin A. Science. 1975;190:1103–5.
43. MacKaness MB. The influence of immunologically committed lymphoid cells on macrophage activity in vivo. J Exp Med. 1969;130:973–92.
44. Lane FC, Unanue ER. Requirement of thymus (T) derived lymphocytes for resistance to listeriosis. J Exp Med. 1972;135:1104–12.
45. Zaleznik DF, Finberg RW, Shapiro ME, et al. A soluble suppressor T cell factor protects against experimental intraabdominal abscesses. J Clin Invest. 1985;75:1023–7.
46. Shapiro ME, Kasper DL, Zaleznik DF, et al. Cellular control of abscess formation: The role of T cells in the regulation of abscesses formed in response to *Bacteroides fragilis*. J Immunol. 1986;137:341–6.

GRAM-POSITIVE COCCI

173. STAPHYLOCOCCUS AUREUS (INCLUDING TOXIC SHOCK SYNDROME)

FRANCIS A. WALDVOGEL

Staphylococci are among the hardiest nonspore-forming bacteria, and they can survive many nonphysiologic environmental conditions. They can be cultured from dried clinical material after several months, are relatively heat resistant, and can tolerate high salt media. Therefore, it is not surprising that despite the availability of potent antimicrobial agents and improved public health conditions, *Staphylococcus aureus* has remained a major human pathogen that colonizes and infects both hospitalized patients with decreased host defenses and healthy, immunologically competent people in the community.

The natural history of *S. aureus* infections can be summarized as follows: many neonates, and most children and adults, will become intermittently colonized by *S. aureus* by harboring the organism either in their nasopharynx or on their skin and clothing, or more rarely in the vagina. From these sites, *S. aureus* can contaminate any site on skin or mucous membrane, or other subjects by interpersonal transfer, by air or direct contact. The mucous membranes and the skin, although favoring the adhesion of *S. aureus*, offer a very efficient mechanical barrier against its local tissue invasion. If this barrier is breached due to trauma or surgery, *S. aureus* may gain access to the underlying tissue, creating its characteristic local abscess lesion (Figs. 1A,B), this consists of necrotic tissue, fibrin, and a large number of live and dead polymorphonuclear leukocytes (PMNs). Toxin liberation to skin and other organs can cause various types of skin rashes and general symptoms, as exemplified by the toxic shock syndrome. At any time, multiplying bacteria can overcome the local phagocytic mechanisms and gain access to the lymphatic channels and the blood stream. The ensuing staphylococcal septicemia is a dreaded complication, and it can lead to metastatic infections (e.g., endocarditis, pneumonia, or osteomyelitis) and to the patient's demise.

MICROBIOLOGY

Morphology

The term *Staphylococcus* is derived from the Greek expression *staphyle* (bunch of grapes), and it reflects its characteristic microscopic arrangement in clusters.

Microscopically, S. aureus is a gram-positive organism, characterized by individual cocci with a diameter of 0.7–1.2 μm (Fig. 2).These cocci occur singly, in pairs, in short chains, and have a strong tendency to form clusters, because cell division occurring in the three perpendicular planes does not lead to full separation of the daughter cells. Cluster formation is favored by culturing the organism on solid media. These properties,

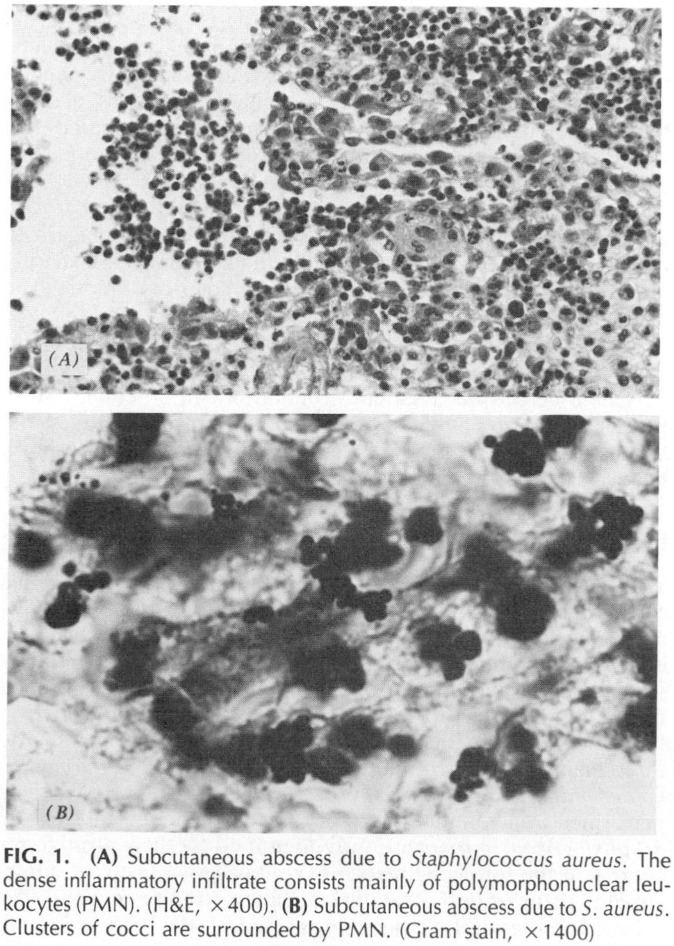

FIG. 1. **(A)** Subcutaneous abscess due to *Staphylococcus aureus*. The dense inflammatory infiltrate consists mainly of polymorphonuclear leukocytes (PMN). (H&E, ×400). **(B)** Subcutaneous abscess due to *S. aureus*. Clusters of cocci are surrounded by PMN. (Gram stain, ×1400)

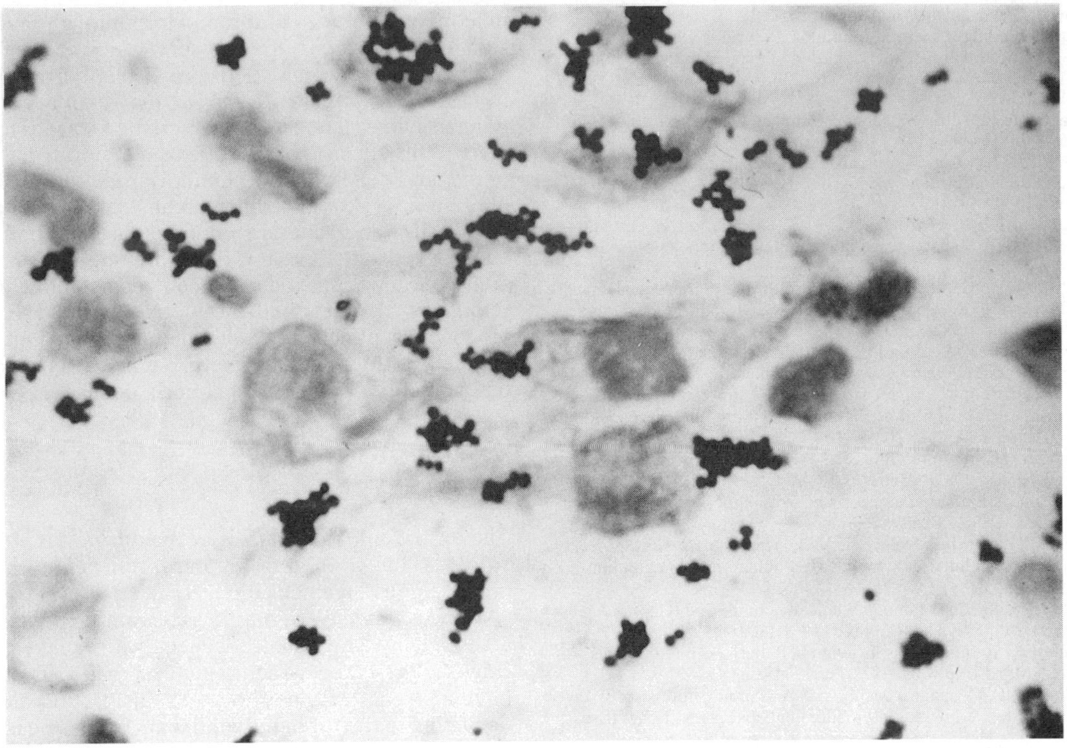

FIG. 2. Expectorated sputum with gram-positive cocci in clumps from a patient with staphylococcal pneumonia.

although most often present in laboratory strains, sometimes are missing in clinical specimens and can lead to erroneous diagnoses; thus, cells in stationary phase or ingested by phagocytes occasionally appear as gram-negative on smear; clustering can be very limited in liquid media. Formation of short chains has also been described but never exceeds four to five cocci. Since staphylococcal infections are characterized by abscess formation, most microbiologic specimens of clinical importance should contain additionally a large number of polymorphonuclear leukocytes—except in neutropenic patients.[1]

Macroscopically, S. aureus is characterized by rapid growth under both aerobic and anaerobic conditions on blood agar and other nonselective solid media. Individual colonies are sharply defined, smooth, and convex, with a diameter of 1–4 mm. The classic golden pigmentation, due to carotenoids, may not be readily apparent under certain conditions (e.g., growth under anaerobic conditions or in liquid medium) and may be visible only as a beige hue. Pigment production can be enhanced by further incubation at room temperature for 24–48 hours. Most strains of *S. aureus* produce hemolysis within 24–36 hours on horse, sheep, or human blood agar plates.[2]

Identification

Within the family Micrococcaceae, the human pathogenic genus *Staphylococcus* can be separated from the nonpathogenic genus *Micrococcus* by various tests, including: (*1*) anaerobic acid production from glucose, (*2*) sensitivity to 200 μg/ml of lysostaphin, and (*3*) production of acid from glycerol in the presence of 0.4 μg/ml of erythromycin, all three tests being positive in the case of staphylococci. Further subclassification into the three main species is of clinical importance (i.e., *S. aureus, S. epidermidis*, and *S. saprophyticus*). The most important tests performed in a routine laboratory are summarized in Table 1. *Staphylococcus aureus* are fully identified by their positive reactions in the following tests[2]: (*1*) catalase—a test that differentiates them from the catalase-negative streptococci and that is based on the catalytic decomposition of H_2O_2 in the presence of Fe^{3+}; (*2*) coagulase—a test allowing differentiation between *S. aureus* and *S. epidermidis,* which is coagulase-negative. It is based on the action of either a cell-bound bacterial enzyme acting directly on fibrinogen or on the action of an extracellular enzyme on a modified thrombin molecule in rabbit plasma—the complex reacts in turn with fibrinogen to produce a fibrin clot in the absence of Ca^{2+}; (*3*) mannitol fermentation—which most often allows differentiation between *S. aureus* (always positive) and *S. epidermidis* (rarely positive). The reaction is based on the property of *S. aureus* that degrades the polyhydric alcohol mannitol into acid compounds under anaerobic conditons; and (*4*) deoxyribonuclease test—most *S. aureus* give a positive reaction, as opposed to *S. epidermidis*. The test is based on the differential solubilization of whole DNA, or fragments thereof, in acid. Finally, novobiocin resistance allows identification of *S. saprophyticus*.

TABLE 1. Major Tests for the Differentiation of Human Staphylococci

Test	S. aureus	S. epidermidis	S. saprophyticus
Coagulase	+	−	−
Acid production by mannitol fermentation	+	−	+(−)[a]
DNAse (endonuclease)	+	−	−
Novobiocin resistance	−	−	+[b]
Anaerobic growth	+	+	(−)[c]
Hemolysis	+	−(+)[d]	−

[a] Usually positive; occasional negative result.
[b] Growth in the presence of ≤ 1.6 μg/ml novobiocin.
[c] *Staphylococcus saprophyticus* does not grow under anaerobic conditions, or grows only slowly.
[d] Usually negative; occasional positive result.

ANTIBIOTIC SUSCEPTIBILITY OF S. AUREUS

Historical Aspects

The interaction between pathogenic organisms and antibiotics is well illustrated by the history of the resistance of *S. aureus* toward the penicillins. Shortly after penicillin G became available, Spink reported the isolation of a resistant *S. aureus* strain, which produced a beta-lactamase (penicillinase) that inactivated the antibiotic.[3] Although initially a sporadic occurrence, this type of resistance rapidly spread to many *S. aureus* isolates, stimulating the development of semisynthetic penicillinase-resistant compounds; methicillin, the isoxazolyl penicillins (oxacillin, cloxacillin, etc.) and nafcillin were produced between 1960 and 1964. They solved the resistance problem only temporarily, since the isolation of methicillin-resistant strains was reported by Barber as early as 1961.[4] Although these organisms were initially associated with infections only in Europe, they have now been identified throughout the world.

Sensitivity and Resistance Patterns of S. aureus Toward β-Lactam Antibiotics

Sensitivity to Penicillin G. Only a very limited percentage of hospital strains and no more than 20–30 percent of community strains do not produce a β-lactamase and, therefore, are sensitive to penicillin G. Such strains usually are also sensitive to the β-lactamase stable compounds, although their minimum inhibitory (bacteriostatic) and bactericidal concentration (MIC and MBC) toward these drugs and usually higher. Thus, in case of infections with a penicillinase-negative strain, penicillin G remains the drug of choice.

Resistance of *S. aureus* to β-lactam antibiotics is a major clinical problem. At present, the distinction is made between three different types of resistance.[5]

β-LACTAMASE-MEDIATED RESISTANCE. In this case, the microorganism produces an extracellular enzyme that inactivates the antibiotic by opening its β-lactam ring before it has caused irreversible changes in the bacterium itself. This mutual time-dependent interaction implies that the presence of a large number of microorganisms will outweigh the effect of the antibiotic and accelerate its destruction, a phenomenon called the inoculum effect.The greatest stability is observed with methicillin and nafcillin, followed by oxacillin, cloxacillin, and dicloxacillin, and ending obviously with penicillin G. Cephalosporins show variable stabilities, depending on their structure.

There probably are three different types of β-lactamases in *S. aureus,* as evidenced by immunologic, substrate, and inhibitor characterization.[6] The enzymes are usually inducible and occasionally constitutive. Most often, they are coded for by plasmids, which carry other important genes such as those determining resistance to heavy metals, to erythromycin, and to other antibiotics. A few staphylococcal strains have been reported to harbor chromosomal genes for penicillinase production.[6]

INTRINSIC RESISTANCE. This form of resistance, inappropriately called methicillin resistance, encompasses all β-lactam antibiotics, including the cephalosporins.[5] Intrinsic resistance, defined as an MIC above 20 μg/ml of methicillin by the broth dilution method, can be missed in the diagnostic laboratory, if sensitivity testing is performed by a standard disk diffusion method or with an automated device. This is due to the fact that methicillin-resistant cells grow more slowly and encompass only 10^{-5}–10^{-6} cells of the total cell population when cultured at 37°C. Phenotypic expression can be enhanced by several methods; the simplest one is incubation at 30°C, where phenotypic expression is almost complete and growth can be observed in the near vicinity of the antibiotic disk. Incubation of antibiotic disk sensitivity plates for *S. aureus* at 30°C and 37°C (or of a single plate at 35°C) with a potent methicillin or oxacillin disk, therefore, should be performed in all diagnostic laboratories.[6]

Other characteristics of the intrinsically resistant *S. aureus* include microscopic heterogeneity and penicillinase production. Despite initial reports to the contrary, they possess a full armamentarium of pathogenic factors that include protein A, coagulase, and DNAase; catalase seems to be present in enhanced amounts.[7] They are as pathogenic in mice, and as sensitive to phagocytosis, as their methicillin-sensitive congeners.[8] Finally, they are associated with a high morbidity and mortality in human infections.[9]

Intrinsic resistance to β-lactam antibiotics is transmitted chromosomally. It is generally accepted that this type of resistance is due to a penicillin-binding protein (PBP) with reduced affinity for the β-lactamase-resistant penicillins, called PBP 2a.[10] This protein is inducible and confers resistance to all β-lactam antibiotics. Its genetic basis has been established by transductional mapping and identified in a 3.5 kb segment of the chromosomal genome.[11] Most of these strains are resistant to a multitude of antibiotics but often sensitive to rifampin, fusidic acid, and the quinolones. They are invariably sensitive to vancomycin,[5] which remains the drug of choice.

TOLERANCE TO THE KILLING ACTION OF β-LACTAM ANTIBIOTICS. Whereas the two mechanisms of resistance described above are well defined and uniformly accepted, there is still some dispute regarding the significance of the tolerance phenomenon. A tolerant *S. aureus* isolate is defined as a strain exhibiting a striking dissociation between the MIC and MBC of the β-lactam antibiotic that is tested in a standard dilution test, with the MBC being more than 32 times higher than the MIC.[5] In practice, most *S. aureus* strains will be nontolerant, that is, will show an MIC:MBC ratio of 1:4, whereas tolerant strains will give MIC:MBC ratios far in excess of 1:32, ranging up to 1:2000. The phenomenon, when observed in a given strain for one β-lactam antibiotic, is usually reproducible with the other β-lactam antibiotics—including the cephalosporins—and sometimes even with vancomycin.[5] The trait tends to disappear in the laboratory on subculture. Based on work performed on other species, it is presently assumed that β-lactam compounds fail to activate the autolytic enzymes in tolerant *S. aureus* strains.[12] Tolerance of *S. aureus* was associated, in some studies, with poor clinical response to β-lactam antibiotics in septicemia and endocarditis.[13] These clinical observations have been contradicted by experimental animal studies that show a similar behavior of tolerant and nontolerant strains.[14] Despite this controversy, it has been recommended that all *S. aureus* responsible for a severe infection be tested as to their MIC and MBC and that treatment be readjusted if necessary.[5]

Sensitivity and Resistance Patterns of S. aureus Toward Other Antibiotics

Staphylococcus aureus possesses a remarkable number of mechanisms for resisting antibacterial action.[6] Thus, depending on the local epidemiologic conditions, 5–20 percent of the isolates are resistant to antibacterial agents commonly used in staphylococcal infections such as erythromycin, lincomycin, and clindamycin. This percentage seems to be lower for fusidic acid, although the clinical experience with this drug is limited. Aminoglycoside-resistant strains have been described with increasing frequency. Rifampin, which is remarkably active against *S. aureus*, cannot be used as a single agent because of the high one-step mutation rate of 10^{-7}–10^{-8} to resistance.[15] Finally, no strain has been described so far as being fully resistant to vancomycin, which nevertheless should be used sparingly if its remarkable clinical usefulness is to be preserved.

Transfer of Resistance in S. aureus. Antibiotic resistance in *S. aureus* may be mediated by chromosomes or plasmids.[16] Staphylococci are probably exchanging genetic material by various mechanisms, including transduction and cell-to-cell contact.[17] Recent evidence is accumulating in favor of transfer of plasmids between *S. aureus* and *S. epidermidis,*[18] a worrisome observation indeed, if one considers the numerical importance of these saprophytes.

Phage Susceptibility of S. aureus[19]

Phage typing has been a popular technique to further subspecify *S. aureus* isolates. Although it provides remarkably useful information regarding the epidemiology (e.g., nosocomial infections) or the pathogenesis (e.g., scalded skin syndrome) of *S. aureus* infections, its complexity and cost in time and personnel has precluded its wide application for diagnostic and clinical purposes.

Practically, the solutions of typing phages, which are divided into five lytic groups (1–5) and five antigenic groups, are added to agar plates heavily seeded with the staphylococcal strain to be tested; lysis is detected by the appearance of clear zones after appropriate incubation. Sources of uncertainty include nonspecific lysis by phage suspensions, activation of latent prophages, and spontaneous variations in phage susceptibility.

EPIDEMIOLOGY

Carriers

The epidemiology of *S. aureus* infections is best depicted by observing the dynamics of human colonization throughout life. Shortly after birth, many neonates are colonized by their immediate human surroundings; the sites include the umbilical stump, the perineal area, the skin, and sometimes the gastrointestinal tract. *Staphylococcus aureus* can also contaminate the clothing and the linen, from which the organism can be shed to further contaminate the atmosphere. Later in life, children and adults can become carriers, but their reservoir is now most often the anterior nasal vestibule, where adherence of organisms seems to be mediated by their teichoic acid content.[20] At any given time, the nasal carriage rate in adults is estimated at about 20–40 percent, depending on seasonal and local epidemiologic factors.[21] Expressed longitudinally, about 30 percent of the population will be prolonged and 50 percent will be intermittent carriers of *S. aureus*, whereas 20 percent will never be colonized.[21] The incidence of toxic shock syndrome in the female population has led to an evaluation of the vaginal carriage rate in adult premenopausal women; the reported values are close to 10 percent, with an increase in carriage rate and bacterial counts during the menses.[22]

Some groups of individuals seem to be particularly prone to colonization with *S. aureus*. Thus, physicians, nurses, and hospital ward attendants may be nasopharyngeal carriers in a higher percentage of cases (50, 70, and 90 percent, respectively) than the general population (33 percent).[23] Diabetic patients receiving insulin injections, patients on chronic hemodialysis, and users of illicit intravenous (IV) drugs have a higher carriage rate than the general population.[24–26]

From the anterior nares, carriers will transfer the organisms to their skin, although there is usually resistance to colonization of the intact skin. Trauma, however, will provide a portal of entry to the organism with subsequent local and possibly generalized infection. It follows that, in case of infection, the offending organism is often of endogenous origin when submitted to phage or antibiotic typing—whereas in rare cases, it will be shown that it is transmitted by the hospital personnel or a family member.

The carrier state is clinically important, since carriers undergoing surgery or sustaining exudative skin conditions will experience more infections than noncarriers, usually caused by the same strain that colonized the patient on admission.

Methicillin-Resistant S. aureus

Despite their theoretic selective advantage, these organisms have shown a decline in Europe since 1970.[27] In general, the carriage rate in the community has been low, as has been their infection rate. Clustering of cases and epidemic occurrence have been recently described with increasing frequency in the United States mostly in large tertiary care referral hospitals.[28] Here again, the role of the house staff and of the personnel–patient transfer circuit has been emphasized.[29]

Epidemiologic Control Measures

Interruption of the interpersonal transfer of *S. aureus* by physical means and by various topical agents is an effective strategy against transmission from carriers to susceptible people and against intrahospital spread of the microorganism.

Careful, repeated, and compulsive hand-washing should be a daily routine for hospital personnel and is of utmost importance. In nurseries for the newborn, several strategies have helped prevent infections in the infants: cohort nursing, individual care by a limited number of people, cord care, arm and hand washing of the staff with chlorhexidine or an iodophor, and wearing of clean gowns by the staff.

Interference by artificial colonization with a "nonpathogenic" strain of *S. aureus*, strain 502A, has been used with limited success and is no longer advocated.[29] Another attempt to avoid *S. aureus* transmission has been the elimination of the nasal carriage state by local treatment (e.g., bacitracin) or by oral rifampin. The latter treatment has been shown to be effective in reducing shunt infections in dialysis patients.[30]

In summary, strategies for the prevention of *S. aureus* transmission include many preventive measures, none of which is fail proof. In this respect, the currently proposed measures for prevention of the spread of methicillin-resistant *S. aureus*—although partly disputed—should provide the clinician with useful guidelines when strict epidemiologic rules have to be decreed (Table 2).[28]

INFECTIONS DUE TO S. AUREUS: MICROBIOLOGIC DETERMINANTS

For the sake of clarity, our present knowledge regarding microbiologic determinants of *S. aureus* is classified here according to cellular locations, it should be considered an oversimplification of the complex structure of the organism.

Important Cell Wall Constituents

The basic component of the cell wall of *S. aureus*, which confers shape and stability to the organism and represents 50 percent of cell wall weight, is the *peptidoglycan*.[1] It is a polysaccharidic polymer composed of unbranched, β-linked (1 → 4) chains containing alternating subunits of *N*-acetylmuramic acid and *N*-acetylglucosamine. Pentapeptide side chains are linked to the muramic acid residue and are cross-linked by a pentaglycine bridge attached to L-lysine of one chain and D-alanine on the other chain (Fig. 3A). The basic polysaccharidic polymer is

TABLE 2. Measures to Prevent Spread of *S. aureus* among Hospitalized Patients

Accurate and timely identification of nosocomial strain (antibiotic sensitivity pattern, or phage typing)
Culture surveillance (with microbiologic criteria described above) of staff and patients in involved areas to define reservoir
Establishment of barrier precautions or strict isolation techniques for infected patients
Assignment of employees with dermatitis and positive cultures (same epidemic strain) to nonclinical duties
Reinforcement of hand-washing regulations and disinfection procedures in areas contaminated by epidemic strain
Discharge of patients infected with epidemic strain as soon as medically feasible
Clear notation of the presence of the epidemic strain in the medical record to take necessary precautions in case of readmission
In case of clear association with a particular instrumentation, careful review of sterilization procedures and nursing techniques

(Adapted from Haley et al.,[28] with permission.)

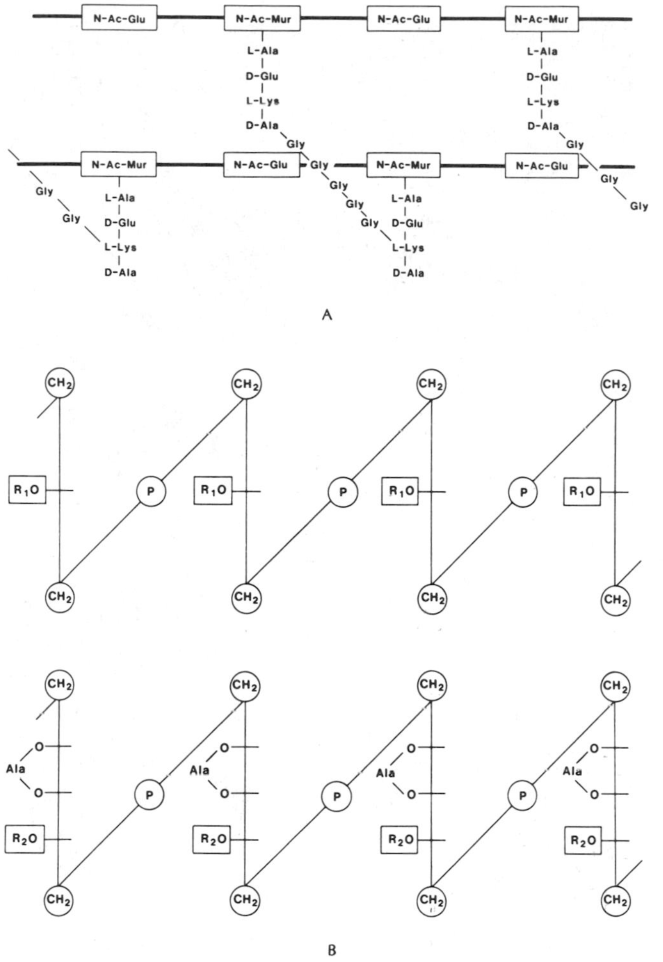

FIG. 3. (A) Peptidoglycan structure of *Staphylococcus aureus*.[31] The basic polymer is composed of 10 to 12 alternating units of *N*-acetylglucosamine (*N*-Ac-Glu) and *N*-acetylmuramic acid (*N*-Ac-Mur). Side chains are linked to the muramic acid (L-alanine, D-glutamine, L-lysine, D-alanine), and are cross-linked by a pentaglycine bridge (Gly-Gly . . .). **(B)** The two types of teichoic acids in *Staphylococcus aureus*.[33] Above: glycerol teichoic acid, with a basic structure of glycerol and phosphate. R_1 is gentobiose or alanine. This teichoic acid is bound covalently to the cell membrane (membrane teichoic acid). Below: Ribitol teichoic acid, with a basic structure of ribitol and phosphate. R_2 is *N*-acetylglucosamine or *N*-acetylgalactosamine. This teichoic acid is bound covalently to the peptidoglycan (cell wall teichoic acid).

found in many other organisms as well, whereas the pentaglycine cross-linking chain seems to be specific for *S. aureus*.[31] The peptidoglycan has important biologic properties: it elicits the production of endogenous pyrogen from human monocytes, induces a local Swartzmann reaction, is capable of attracting PMNs, has endotoxinlike activity, activates complement, and elicits the production of opsonic antibodies.[32]

Other important cell wall constituents include a group of phosphate-containing polymers called *teichoic acids,* which contribute about 40 percent of cell wall weight.[33] Some of these are covalently bound to the peptidoglycan and are called cell wall teichoic acids. Others are linked to the lipid of the bacterial cell membrane hence their name, membrane teichoic acids. The backbone of cell wall teichoic acid is an alternating sequence of ribitolphosphate. Side chains include single addition of *N*-acetylglucosamine and *N*-acetylgalactosamine (Fig. 3B).[32,33] Cell membrane teichoic acids have a very simple backbone made of glycerol–phosphate in repeating units. The side chain on the second C-atom of the glycerol molecule is an unusual disaccharide gentobiose—exceptionally alanine (Fig. 3B). Both teichoic acis are bound covalently to the peptidoglycan or to the lipid membrane of the microorganism.

In addition, *S. aureus* incorporates covalently into its outer peptidoglycan layer a protein with a molecular weight of 42,000 daltons, *protein A*. This compound is present in various amounts in most strains *S. aureus,* and it is also recovered in the supernatant of actively growing cultures. Although it can activate complement under well-defined conditions, its major interaction with host mechanisms consists of binding to the Fc terminal of all human immunoglobulin G subclasses except IgG3.[34] Most *S. aureus* also contains a *clumping factor* or bound coagulase on their outer surface, which binds to fibrinogen by a nonenzymatic reaction and causes the microorganisms to aggregate.[35]

Finally, many *S. aureus* strains are coated with an external polysaccharidc layer, meeting the definition of a capsule or a loosely associated slime layer.[36] Thus, the cell surface of *S. aureus* may best be viewed as a mosaic of different domains, represented by these various components, which can interact with the host.

Important Enzymes and Toxins

Staphylococcus aureus produces and secretes a number of enzymes and toxins, which have been variously implicated as possible pathogenic factors. The problem of their pathogenicity is compounded by the fact that the purification of many of these enzymes and toxins is technically difficult due to their instability. Therefore, their individuality, as well as their specificity, are often disputed.

Enzymes. CATALASE. Hydrogen peroxide is produced by all staphylococcal strains and is converted into nontoxic H_2O and O_2 by the action of catalase. Since staphylococcal phagocytic killing is mediated by toxic oxygen radicals produced by PMN, it has been proposed and shown that catalase production, by counteracting host defense mechanisms, correlates with pathogenicity.[37]

COAGULASE. These enzymes, which are either cell-bound or soluble, cause plasma to clot by activating the final steps of the coagulation cascade through mechanisms that differ from the human physiologic ones. Bound coagulase is also called the clumping factor and has been extensively studied.[38] It interacts with the D fragment of fibrinogen, resulting in conformational changes and clumping. The clumping factor also activates complement. Investigations regarding the pathogenic role of the two coagulases are still inconclusive.

HYALURONIDASE. This enzyme hydrolyzes hyaluronic acids, a group of acid mucopolysaccharides present in the acellular matrix of connective tissue. Its role in the pathogenicity of *S. aureus* is as yet unsolved.

β-LACTAMASES. Most of them are plasmid-mediated. Their physiologic role in the cellular metabolism in the absence of β-lactam antibiotics is unknown. Their role in antibiotic resistance has been reviewed above.

OTHER ENZYMES. *Staphylococcus aureus* produces a nuclease that is tested on a DNA substrate for taxonomic purposes, but in fact is a phosphodiesterase with both exo- and endonuclease activity that cleaves nucleic acids into 3′-phosphomononucleotides. In addition, *S. aureus* produces several lipases that are thought to play a disseminating role during infection.

Toxins. *Staphylococcus aureus,* in addition, produces a variety of extracellular products, which are defined as toxins because they affect host cell function and/or morphology, although some of them will express their detrimental effect by enzymatic action.

α-Toxin. Of the five membrane-damaging toxins produced by *S. aureus*, this is the most extensively studied. Electrophoretically a heterogeneous protein, it acts on a wide variety of cell membranes (e.g., erythrocytes, leukocytes, platelets, fibroblasts, and HeLa cells), but not on bacterial cytoplasmic membranes. Erythrocytes are the most sensitive target cells of the biologic action of *S. aureus*, and they display a species-specific external binding capacity that correlates with their sensitivity to hemolysis. The toxin, when injected subcutaneously, is also dermonecrotic.[39]

β-Toxin. This toxin displays its cytotoxic effect by degrading sphingomyelin. Therefore, it is active on a great variety of cells, including human erythrocytes, leukocytes, and fibroblasts. Its effects have been extensively investigated in erythrocytes, where the hemolytic activity depends on the sphingomyelin contents and/or distribution on the membrane surface of the erythrocytes.[39]

γ-Toxin. Its presence has now been firmly established by purification from strain 5R, which produces this toxin as its major cytolysin. It lyses erythrocytes from many species, including humans, by unknown mechanisms.[39]

δ-Toxin. This extracellular product is electrophoretically heterogeneous and dissociates into subunits in nonionic detergents; this explains why the reported molecular weights range from 68 to 200 kD. Some of its unique characteristics include hydrophobicity and thermostability. The molecule is strongly surface active, and it disrupts biologic membranes by a detergentlike action. Another interesting property of the δ-toxin is its inhibition of water absorption and simultaneous stimulation of cyclic AMP production in the rabbit and guinea pig ileum, which suggests a role in the pathogenesis of acute diarrhea in some staphylococcal infections.[39]

LEUKOCIDIN. This toxin, consisting of two components, apparently exerts an exclusive action on human and rabbit phagocytic cells. A single injection of leukocidin produces deep reversible granulocytopenia. Its direct membrane-damaging effect can be followed microscopically within 60 minutes. Both components of the toxin act synergistically at the phagocyte membrane level by forming pores, which leads to increased permeability to cations.[39]

EXFOLIATIN. Exfoliatin or exfoliative toxin is a group of, at least, two serologically and biologically distinct proteins responsible for the major dermatologic findings of the staphylococcal scalded skin syndrome. Exfoliatin A is a chromosomal gene product, is thermostable (after 20 minutes at 100°C), and is inactivated by EDTA whereas exfoliatin B, with the same molecular weight, is of plasmidic origin, is inactivated after incubation at 60°C for 20 minutes, and is stable in EDTA. Although exfoliatin production has been associated with phage group 2 staphylococci in the United States, no such correlation could be found, for example, in Japan. Individual strains, when examined, produce either none, one, or both toxins, and no clear relationship has been found between the phage group and the type of toxin produced.[39]

Exfoliatins produce dramatic changes in the epidermis of neonates, which are characterized by extensive scalding (Figs. 4 and 5). An identical phenomenon can be observed after injection of the toxin into newborn mice; under normal conditions, epidermal cells are cemented together by a matrix of mucopolysaccharides, and individual granular cells are linked to each other by specialized membrane structures called the desmosomes. Injection of exfoliatin at a distant site leads to splitting of the desmosome in the stratum granulosum, and it also most probably affects the intercellular matrix.[40]

The crucial pathogenic role of exfoliatins in the scalded skin syndrome is demonstrated by the fact that specific antibodies are protective and neutralizing in both humans and mice. An age factor implying maturation of the intercellular anchoring mechanisms is also of critical importance, since the disease is rare in adults and nonreproducible in adult mice.[39]

TOXINS ASSOCIATED WITH THE TOXIC SHOCK SYNDROME. Toxic shock syndrome (TSS), characterized by fever, desquamative skin rash, hypotension, and multisystem involvement, occurs in patients who harbor *S. aureus* strains that elaborate either toxic shock syndrome toxin 1 (TSST-1), or other related, as yet not totally identified, exotoxins.[41–44] There have also been reports of this syndrome with infections caused by coagulase-negative *Staphylococcus* and *Streptococcus pyogenes*.[45,46]

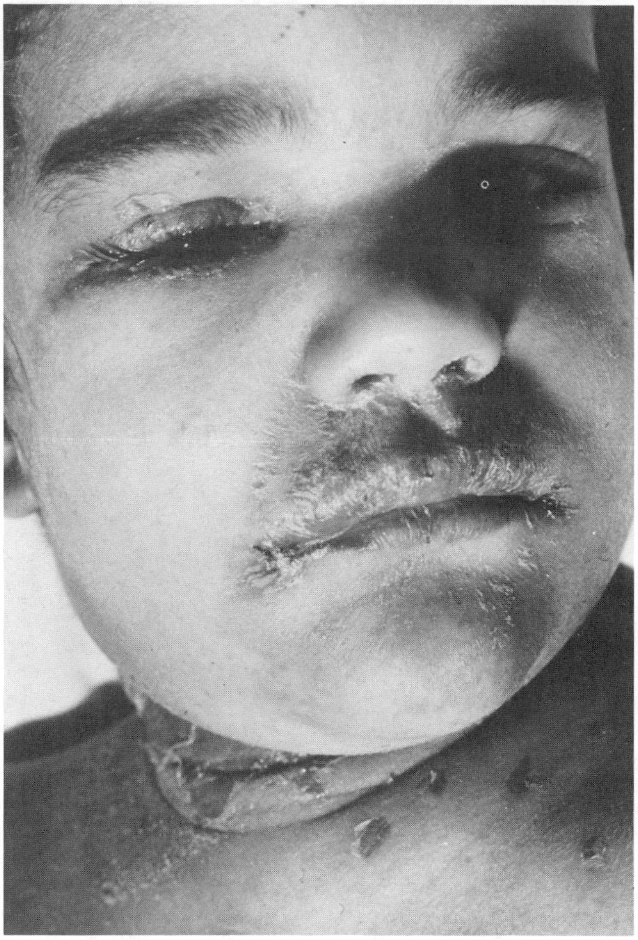

FIG. 4. Child with the staphylococcal scalded skin syndrome (SSSS) due to phage group 2 *Staphylococcus aureus*-producing exfoliative toxin. Note purulent conjunctivitis and the perioral flaky desquamation, whereas newer lesions (probably at the vesicular stage) are just starting to peel on the neck.

TSST-1 is protein that, upon injection into rabbits, produces fever and enhanced susceptibility to lethal shock. The toxin exerts a variety of biologic effects on other systems, such as suppression of IgM antibody synthesis in splenocyte culture systems, an effect that is accentuated by addition of endotoxin to the cell cultures. It increases the skin reactivity of rabbits sensitized to purified protein derivative and decreases, when injected with endotoxin, the reticuloendothelial clearance of colloidal carbon.[47] Above all, TSST-1 and related enterotoxins have been shown to be strong inducers of interleukin 1 in monocyte cultures.[44,48]

ENTEROTOXINS. About half of all isolated strains of *S. aureus* produce enterotoxins, of which there are presently five (A–E) serologically distinct types. They are a major cause of food poisoning. In addition, enterotoxin F and possibly others have been implicated in TSS. These remarkably heat-stable toxins have an unknown mode of action, but definitely increase intestinal peristalsis, possibly by sympathetic activation. A central nervous system effect is also suggested by the intensity of vomiting in food poisoning. Suggestive evidence also exists for interleukin-1 induction (see above).

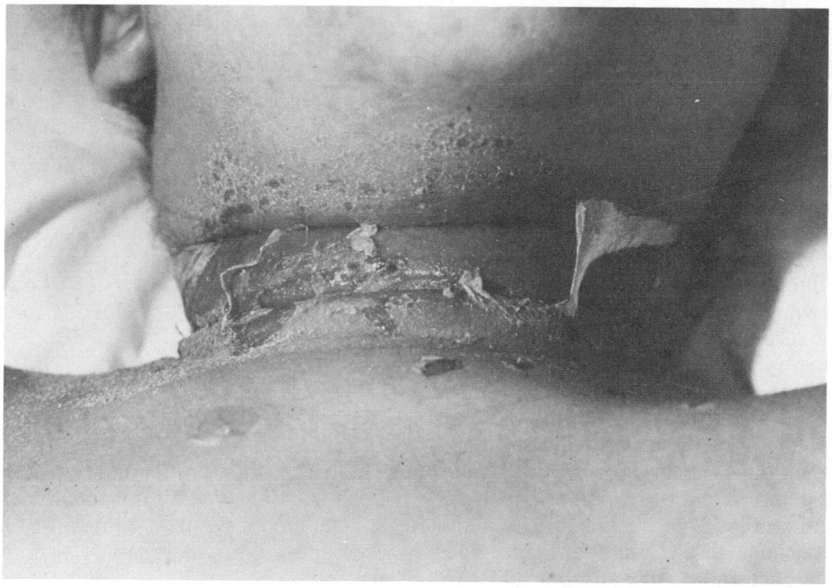

FIG. 5. Same child as in Figure 4 showing, at a later stage, an extensive exfoliation of the epidermis due to the toxin-induced cleavage through the stratum granulosum.

Summary of Pathogenic Factors

It has been difficult to ascribe a defined pathogenic effect to specific staphylococcal products because of problems linked with isolation, purification, specificity, and inadequate in vivo assays. Nevertheless, some components have clearly identified roles such as the epidermolytic toxins, the enterotoxins, the TSST-1; others are indirectly important by increasing adherence, or interfering with host defense mechanisms, such as peptidoglycan, protein A, teichoic acids, and catalase; the precise role of soluble coagulase and clumping factor, hyaluronidase, lipase, nuclease, and hemolysins is as yet ill defined.

INFECTIONS DUE TO S. AUREUS: HOST DETERMINANTS

Invasion of the human organism by *S. aureus* implies a series of interactions of the microorganism with a variety of host structures and mechanisms; these can be subdivided into adhesion, invasion, chemotaxis of PMN, ingestion, and intracellular killing by PMN.

Adhesion of S. aureus

Colonization by *S. aureus* requires its initial adherence to host cells. Three types of adherence must be considered; adherence to nasal mucosal cells is mediated by the teichoic acid component of *S. aureus*[20] and is increased in chronic staphylococcal carriers and after vaccination or infection with influenza A.[49,50]

Attachment of *S. aureus* to traumatized or disrupted skin, to foreign surfaces, and to endothelial structures involves interaction with four different proteins, i.e., fibrinogen,[35] fibronectin,[51] laminin,[52] and possibly collagen IV.[53] The interactions studied in most detail involve fibronectin and fibrinogen, in which the active domains of the host proteins have been characterized and their coating shown to modulate *S. aureus* adherence.[54]

Attachment of *S. aureus* to endothelial cells during septicemia is a complex event, where again the endothelial cell itself, fibronectin, and laminin play an important role. Postadherent events are here of additional importance, such as phagocytosis of *S. aureus* by endothelial cells—an extension of normal pinocytic activity[55]—and induction of tissue factor procoagulant activity.[56]

All these mechanisms provide solid anchoring systems of *S. aureus*, thus promoting bacterial settling.

Invasion

Invasion of the host after colonization requires penetration of the microorganism through the epithelial or mucosal surface, but little is known regarding the biologic mechanisms subtending it.

Chemotaxis

Once *S. aureus* has penetrated through the mucosal or epithelial layer, ingestion and killing by PMN, as well as by the monocyte–macrophage system, become the major line of defense. Mobilization of phagocytic cells at the site of bacterial growth requires the elaboration of microbial and host-specific signals. Among the former, cell wall-associated and extracellular products of *S. aureus* such as peptidoglycan, teichoic acids, and protein A are certainly involved. The major host signals result from the activation of the complement system; all cell wall components identified thus far can trigger this reaction, by producing among others C5a.[57]

Opsonization

Recognition of *S. aureus* by phagocytes is mediated by their receptors for the Fc fragment of IgG immunoglobulins, by their receptors for the activated subunit of the third component of the complement system C3b, and possibly by other complement receptors. This recognition process implies that *S. aureus*, in order to be ingested, has to be coated by C3b and/or IgG molecules—a process called opsonization. There is marked heterogeneity among various *S. aureus* strains as to their opsonic requirements; a strain such as *S. aureus* Wood 46, for example, is fully opsonized by the presence of complement only, while others require predominantly specific IgG.

In normal serum obtained from healthy *nonimmune* subjects, complement activation via either the classic or alternate pathways provides the major part of the opsonic activity.[58] However, this normal serum also will contain small amounts of antipeptidoglycan antibodies, which result from previous exposure to staphylococci or to other organisms. In vitro study of complement-dependent opsonization, therefore, would require the total elimination of IgG from normal serum; however, from a practical point of view this finite, but modest IgG opsonization is largely overridden by the complement system. In striking contrast, opsonization in hyperimmune subjects occurs predominantly by IgG molecules. However, the peptidoglycan present in *S. aureus* can also activate to some extent the complement system, as will the IgG molecules bound to the bacterial surface. This complex sequence of events involving complement is usually overshadowed by the IgG opsonization mechanism of the hyperimmune serum.[58]

The peptidoglycan matrix is presently considered to be a major determinant of opsonization; in the absence of antibody, peptidoglycan may trigger opsonization by activating the classical and even the alternative complement pathway. In hyperimmune rabbit serum, a direct opsonic effect of peptidoglycan-specific antibodies can be demonstrated.[59,60] There is still debate as to whether these antibodies are specific for the peptidoglycan from *S. aureus*; because at least three antigenic sites can be distinguished on this bacterial matrix and because peptidoglycan structures are ubiquitous in the bacterial world, a highly specific group of antibodies seems unlikely.[61] Although teichoic acids also elicit the production of antibodies against their two moieties, as demonstrated in patients with protracted *S. aureus* infections, their role in opsonization is debated and is probably indirect via activation of the complement cascade. In contrast, protein A probably plays a triple antiphagocytic role in the bacteria–cell recognition process by virtue of its binding to the Fc portion of IgG. First, extracellular, soluble protein A can react with the Fc terminal of IgG molecules of human serum, thereby producing immune aggregates that consume complement. Second, extracellular protein A can bind to the Fc portion of specific antistaphylococcal antibodies coating the microorganism by their Fab fragment, thereby preventing further interaction of the complex with the Fc receptor of phagocytes. Third, cell-bound protein A binds to the Fc fragment of any IgG molecule in its neighborhood, thereby eliminating nonspecific and specific antibodies.[58] The capsule of *S. aureus*, which may be present in up to 50 percent of human isolates, impairs the phagocytic process—probably by a steric hindrance mechanism. Specific anticapsular antibodies are required for opsonization of such strains.

Intracellular Killing

After being phagocytized, most intracellular staphylococci are rapidly killed and degraded within the phagocytic vacuole, but prolonged survival of a minority of organisms can be demonstrated by various techniques that possibly explain the high recurrence rate of some *S. aureus* infections.[61,62] The major staphylocidal role played by the oxygen-dependent bactericidal mechanisms, such as the production of O_2^-, H_2O_2, and other highly reactive radicals, has been repeatedly demonstrated. *Staphylococcus aureus* also possesses its own mechanism to escape the intraphagocytic killing action of oxidants, such as H_2O_2, by its own production of catalase. Oxygen-independent staphylocidal systems include the low pH prevailing in the phagocytic vacuoles, lactoferrin, and granular cationic proteins.

Humoral and Cell-Mediated Immunity

During a staphylococcal infection, a number of antibodies are produced against various cell wall antigens, as well as against various toxins of the organisms. At present, none of these antigens has been capable of inducing full protection against *S. aureus* infection. Each *S. aureus* strain, therefore, has to be conceptualized as an individual mosaic of various soluble and cell-bound antigens, modulating the clinical picture and outcome of the disease.

A cellular immune response to *S. aureus* can also be demonstrated experimentally and in patients with recurrent infections. Its specific role and mechanism of action are difficult to assess, since induction of delayed-type hypersensitivity also implies activation of the humoral response. In some experimental models, macrophage-activating lymphokines have been released by appropriately sensitized splenic lymphocytes and could possibly promote phagocytosis; in other systems, cell-mediated immunity has been shown to be detrimental to the host by increasing the extent of staphylococcal necrotic skin lesions.[58]

INFECTIONS DUE TO S. AUREUS: PREDISPOSING FACTORS

The list of underlying conditions conducive to *S. aureus* infections is extensive and nonspecific. In the following discussion, special emphasis will be given to those clinical conditions that predispose particularly to *S. aureus* infections.[63,64]

Chemotaxis Defects

Impairment of directional movement has been found in a group of patients previously described as having *Job syndrome,* or recurrent eczema with repeated skin infections and cold abscesses. Many of these patients have very high IgE levels, often exceeding 5000 ng/ml, and decreased chemotactic response of their PMN.[65] Other conditions with decreased chemotaxis include the Chédiak-Higashi syndrome, defined clinically by albinism and recurrent *S. aureus* infections, and cytologically by the presence of giant granules in the phagocytes and other cells as well; the Wiskott-Aldrich syndrome; and Down syndrome. Examples of acquired chemotactic defects include severe bacterial infections, rheumatoid arthritis, and decompensated acidotic diabetes mellitus.

Opsonization Defects

None of the opsonization defects described thus far prediposes specifically to *S. aureus* infections. Opsonic defects secondary to a variety of congenital and acquired, selective, or combined agammaglobulinemias, and due to several defects in complement levels (particularly of C3 and C5), therefore, will favor pyogenic infections due to a variety of bacterial species including *S. aureus*.[63,64]

Staphylocidal Defects of Polymorphonuclear Leukocytes

The major condition in which a staphylocidal defect of phagocytic cells has been clearly identified is chronic granulomatous disease (CGD), a group of diseases discussed elsewhere (see Chapter 7). Polymorphonuclear leukocytes from patients with CGD are unable to activate the plasmalemma-bound oxidase, which results in an almost total absence of superoxide and hydrogen peroxide generation within the phagocytic vacuoles. A defect in staphylococcal killing has also been shown in lymphoblastic leukemia, as well as in acute and chronic myelogenous leukemia.[63,64]

Integration of Predisposing Factors: S. aureus Infection in Diabetic Patients—Foreign Body Infections

As opposed to congenital defects, acquired phagocytic defects are often due to multiple factors acting in concert, diabetes mellitus and foreign body infections being two cases in point. In diabetes mellitus,[66] there is still controversy as to whether *S.*

aureus infections occur at an increased frequency, but it seems that once they occur, they may be severe and protracted. Nasopharyngeal colonization with *S. aureus* occurs at an increased frequency in diabetic patients on insulin therapy. Mild diabetic decompensation does not seem to induce deleterious changes in the phagocytic system when tested with conventional methods. Severe diabetic decompensation in vivo and its reproduction in vitro are associated with poor chemotaxis, ingestion, and killing by PMN, although part of these effects might be produced by the hyperosmolar state.

The role of a foreign body as an important factor favoring infections has been well known for years; it has recently received increased attention because of the growing use of intravascular devices and prosthetic material. The majority of these infections are due to *S. aureus*; some are due to other gram-positive organisms such as *S. epidermidis*. Most foreign body infections occur shortly after trauma or surgery and result from local contamination during penetration or implantation of the foreign material. Once established, foreign body infection cannot be eradicated by antibiotics alone, although the organism apparently remains sensitive to the drug used. Once the foreign material is eliminated, infection can be easily cured with a course of the same antibiotics.

Elek and Conen,[67] in their classic experiments, have shown that a subcutaneous injection of $>10^6$ cfu of *S. aureus* was easily controlled by the host defense mechanisms, whereas 3×10^2 cfu of the same organism invariably led to infection in the presence of a suture. Such stitch abscesses were characterized histologically by the presence of myriads of microorganisms and PMN. Recently, new experimental approaches have suggested at least three mechanisms conducive to foreign body infections. First, various organisms, including most strains of *S. epidermidis,* and many strains of *S. aureus*, have been shown to produce after several hours or days in contact with the foreign body surface a glycocalix that protects them possibly from the environment.[68,69] Second, the resident phagocytic population in the vicinity of noninfected implanted foreign bodies has been shown to be incapable of killing an *S. aureus* strain.[70,71] Finally, as mentioned above, firm anchoring of *S. aureus* on fibrinogen and fibronectin coating foreign surfaces provides another pathogenic mechanism. The interaction of these mechanisms has been recently reviewed.[72]

CLINICAL MANIFESTATIONS

General Aspects

The basic anatomic lesion induced by *S. aureus* is a pyogenic exudate or an abscess. In addition, extracellular toxins under certain circumstances dominate this clinical picture (e.g., food poisoning or TSS). Finally, any localized infection—even the most benign-appearing wound infection—occasionally can become the seeding point of a potentially lethal bacteremia, with development of metastatic foci. Consequently, the clinical descriptions that follow should not be taken as well-defined entities, since they often are intertwined and may have reciprocal effects on each other—provided that septicemic spread has occurred.

Infections of the Skin and Its Appendages

Localized Infections.[73] Skin infections due to *S. aureus* are best subdivided into local pyogenic infections without rash and localized infections with a diffuse skin rash characterized by general desquamation. Local pyogenic infections are favored by poor personal hygiene, minor traumas such as friction, maceration, and underlying skin diseases such as eczema and juvenile acne. Most of them are clustered around the hair follicle.

FOLLICULITIS. This is the most benign infection and is defined as a pyoderma involving the hair follicle and its immediate surroundings (Fig. 6). It presents clinically as a series of raised, often painful reddish lesions with an indurated basis, each of them being centered on a hair follicle. Extensive folliculitis of the bearded area of the face is called *sycosis barbae*. Constitutional symptoms are absent, and folliculitis responds well to local antiseptic measures in most cases.

FURUNCLES AND CARBUNCLES. Furuncles (boils) represent the extension of the infectious process involving the hair follicle. They are defined as a deep-seated infection in and around the hair follicle. They are located by definition on the hairy areas of the body, with a predilection for the face, neck, axillae, and buttocks. The disease starts as a painful red nodule and evolves in a few days into a hot, very painful, raised, and indurated lesion with a diameter of 1–2 cm. Its later evolution is characterized by the appearance of a yellowish area in its center and by fluctuance. On spontaneous rupture or surgical incision, it liberates a small amount of yellowish, creamy, and purulent discharge and of necrotic material. The signs of inflammation subside rapidly thereafter, but satellite lesions and new furuncles appearing at distant sites—secondary to autoinoculation—are frequent. General symptoms are usually absent, although mild fever and malaise often are reported in diffuse furunculosis.

Carbuncles are even more serious deep-seated infections of several hair follicles; they result from the coalescence and spreading of the infectious process into the depth of inclastic subcutaneous tissue usually located at the base of the neck. Multipole sinus tracts are frequently present (Fig. 7). The disease leads to the development of a central necrotic crater, which heals by progressive granulation and by the development of a

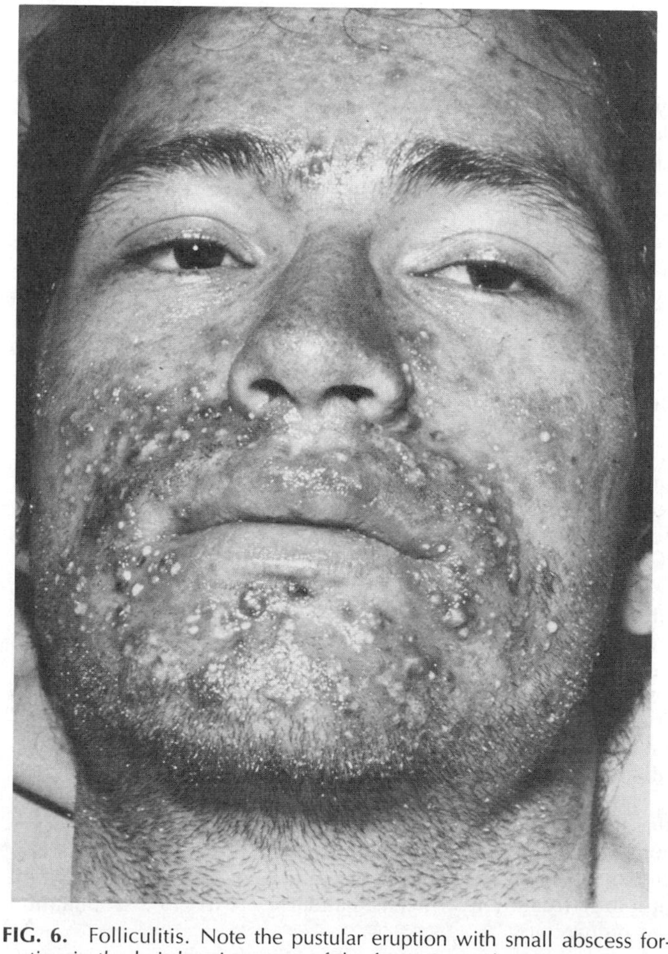

FIG. 6. Folliculitis. Note the pustular eruption with small abscess formation in the hair-bearing areas of the face. General symptoms usually are absent.

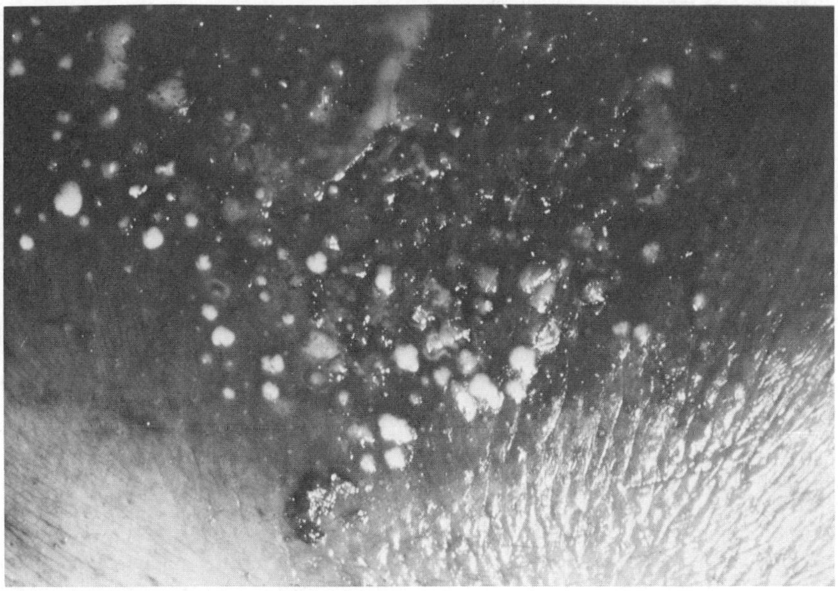

FIG. 7. Carbuncle. Close-up view showing the multiple purulent drainage sites that correspond to the spreading of the infectious process to adjacent follicles.

hard hypertrophic violaceous scar. The development of carbuncles is associated with general symptoms, such as fever and malaise. Chills and spiking fevers are more frequent in carbuncles than in boils, and they should raise the possibility of an incipient staphylcoccal septicemia or of a septic thrombophlebitis of the intracerebral veins, secondary to a deep-seated infection of the nares or the upper lip.

Recurrent furunculosis, characterized by repeated bouts of pyoderma extending over several months or years, is a difficult clinical problem that has not been adequately solved. Young patients with such disorders, particularly if suppurative lymph nodes coexist, should be investigated for the usual underlying general conditions conducive to recurrent infections—including phagocytic dysfunction and metabolic abnormalities. More importantly, however, the patient and his or her intimate contacts should be investigated for nasal staphylococcal carriage, since most cases are due to recurrent colonization from a family reservoir.

IMPETIGO. This is a very superficial staphylococcal skin infection affecting mostly children, usually on exposed areas of the body, i.e., on the face and the legs (Fig. 8). While a majority of these infections are due to *S. aureus*, about 10 percent are due to *Streptococcus pyogenes*; another 10 percent will yield both organisms on culture, the two or possibly three diseases being clinically indistinguishable without microbial identification.

The disease usually starts as a red macule, which evolves into a vesicle containing cloudy fluid based on an area of erythema. The vesicle rapidly ruptures, leaving a yellowish, thick, and wet crust with a diameter often exceeding 1 cm and surrounded by erythema. Most affected children present with multiple lesions of different ages. The infectious process heals without scarring. General symptoms are absent, but local inflammatory lymph node reaction is the rule.

The diagnosis can present some problems at the early vesicular stage of the first lesion, and it includes other vesicular eruptions such as herpes simplex and varicella. Gram stain and culture of a lesion will clarify the situation and suggest general antibiotic treatment, which is mandatory to avoid dissemination and recurrence.

HYDRADENITIS SUPPURATIVA. This is a recurrent pyogenic infection of the apocrine sweat glands often due to *S. aureus*. It presents clinically as crops of "furuncles" developing in the axillary, perineal, and/or genital areas. The lesions usually drain spontaneously, with the formation of many sinus tracts and with hypertrophic scarring. Differential diagnosis presents no problem when the axillary regions are involved, but it can be difficult if the disease affects the genital areas only, where it can mimic lymphogranuloma venereum.

Local treatment with moist dressings and incision if the lesion becomes fluctuant is usually effective, and an oral antistaphylococcal agent for 7–10 days is indicated only if general symptoms are present. Radical excision of hypertrophic scars has sometimes to be resorted to for esthetic reasons or in case of recurrences.

MASTITIS.[74] Of all nursing mothers, 1–3 percent will develop, most commonly during the second or third week of the puerperium, various forms of staphylococcal breast infections that encompass the spectrum from a painful erythematous nodule to frank canalicular abscess formation. General symptoms are absent in the former presentation, but are definitely present in the latter. *Staphylococcus aureus* is usually isolated from the mother and the infant.

Besides topical treatment, acute mastitis mandates the use of a general antibiotic treatment with a β-lactamase-stable penicillin. If abscess formation occurs, incision and drainage will rapidly control the infection. There is still disagreement whether nursing should be discontinued.

WOUND INFECTION. Staphylococcal postsurgical infections are characterized by the progressive appearance of edema, erythema, and pain around the surgical incision 2 or more days after surgery, when the signs of acute inflammation due to the intervention should normally be subsiding. Mild constitutional symptoms and fever are frequently present. Removal of one or two stitches and gentle pressure applied on one of the edges of the incision will produce a small amount of cloudy, odorless, and slightly hemorrhagic drainage, which on Gram stain and culture reveals the offending organism.

The specific management of wound infections has to be adapted to each case, since many variables need to be evaluated, such as the severity of underlying diseases affecting host defense mechanisms, the extension of the infection, the severity of the constitutional symptoms, the presence of foreign material, the potential contamination of deeper host or prosthetic

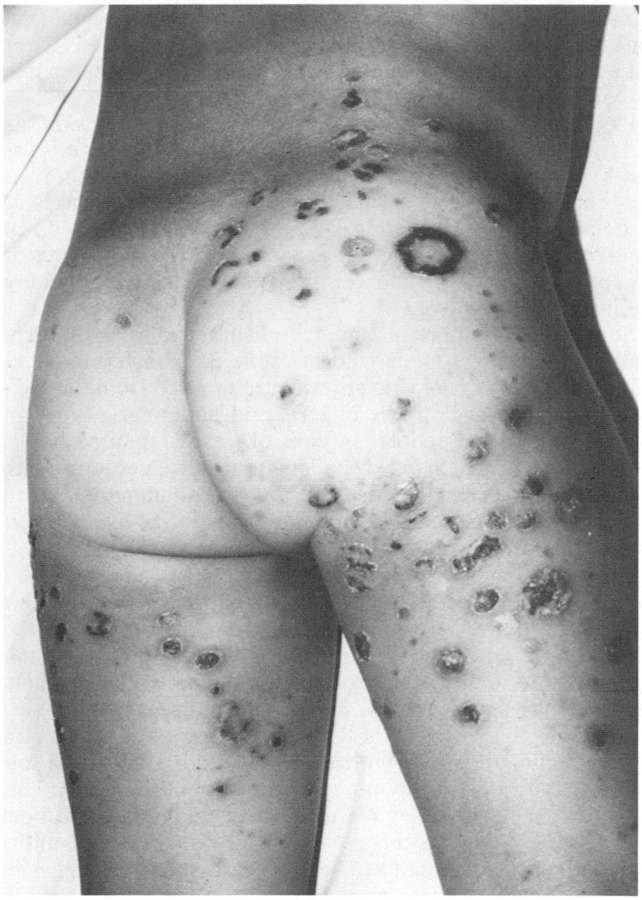

FIG. 8. Impetigo due to *Staphylococcus aureus* in a child. Note the multiple, very superficial lesions, with formation of large vesicopustules and secondary rupture. The same clinical picture can be produced by group A β-hemolytic streptococci.

structures, and so on. The most useful approach is a pragmatic one. First, the wound must be explored to determine the depth of the infection. If deeper structures are not involved, the release of the stitches and repeated cleansing of the wound under general antistaphylococcal coverage of 7–10 days is usually curative. If the incisional infection is minor and constitutional symptoms are absent, antibiotics probably are dispensable. If the infection involves deeper structures (e.g., bone) or foreign material (e.g., prosthetic devices), parenteral antibiotics should be given for 4–6 weeks and should be associated with local cleansing of the wound, which has to be packed open. Even with this optimized therapy, recurrence of infection has to be expected.

SPREADING PYODERMAS. All primary, localized skin infections due to *S. aureus* are characterized by rapid spread to the soft tissues; thus cellulitis, lymphangitis with lymphadenitis, and even necrotizing fasciitis can be caused by *S. aureus*. These infections are indistinguishable from those produced by group A streptococci on a clinical basis; presence of creamy pus, of isolated cocci or clumps of microorganisms on Gram stain should raise the possibility of the presence of *S. aureus* and mandate appropriate antibiotic coverage.

MANAGEMENT OF LOCALIZED SKIN INFECTIONS. Local care is of paramount importance in localized *S. aureus* pyoderma. Hair should be removed, repeated cleansing with an antiseptic nonirritant solution should alternate with the application of moist dressings, and the infected area should be covered with a sterile dressing. All material used for local care should be considered highly contagious, and hand-washing after a dressing change should be reinforced. Surgical incision and drainage is indicated whenever the lesion becomes fluctuant.

The decision whether to use systemic antibiotics in localized *S. aureus* skin infections is controversial and requires common sense. Empirically, local infections generally are not an indication for systemic antibiotics in th absence of fever. Antibiotics are necessary in some cases to avoid further spread of the infection, such as in impetigo, hydradenitis, and diffuse or recurrent furunculosis; a semisynthetic penicillinase-resistant penicillin that is reliably absorbed (e.g., cloxacillin or dicloxacillin) should be given in an oral dose of 30–40 mg/kg per day in four equal portions. Erythromycin (15–20 mg/kg per day in four equal portions) can be used in penicillin-allergic patients, and penicillin V (15–20 mg/kg per day in four equal doses) is still the drug of choice for the rare penicillin G-sensitive organism. Duration of treatment is poorly defined, but it definitely should not exceed 7–10 days. The same antibiotics at the same dosages are strongly indicated in case of pyoderma accompanied by constitutional symptoms, the decision to give them orally or parenterally depending on their severity, the risk of hematogenous spread, and the compliance of the patient. The same indication prevails before incision and drainage of a fluctuant lesion, but duration of treatment probably can be reduced to 3 days. Finally, ''bacteremic'' treatment with high doses of a parenteral penicillinase-resistant penicillin, such as nafcillin, should be instituted if the patient presents with chills, if the infection is severe and involves the face, or if bacteremic spread would have catastrophic consequences.

Localized Infections with Diffuse Skin Rash. The two disease entities characterized by skin rash include the staphylococcal scalded skin syndrome (SSSS) or Ritter disease when it occurs in neonates, and the toxic shock syndrome.

STAPHYLOCOCCAL SCALDED SKIN SYNDROME (SSSS). In 1878, Ritter von Rittershain described an exfoliative dermatitis in a large group of infants in a foundling home in Prague, Czechoslovakia. The disease was characterized by the appearance of large bullae and by the separation of extended areas of the epidermis, leaving behind well-delineated denuded areas. The disease was subsequently shown to be of staphylococcal etiology and to involve children and, in exceptional cases, adults. Besides being called Ritter's disease, it also became known as the staphylococcal scalded skin syndrome (SSSS). Some confusion occurred in 1956, when Lyell[75] and Lang[76] independently described a toxic epidermal necrolysis (TEN) in adults, which mimicked the SSSS in many ways. This entity, called Lyell's disease, was soon differentiated into two subtypes. One occurred essentially in older children and adults, secondary to drug hypersensitivity (barbiturates, sulfonamides and pyrazolone derivatives); the other occurred in infants infected with *S. aureus* and represented what was formerly known as Ritter's disease. The two subtypes also could be differentiated histologically, since Ritter's disease is characterized by intraepithelial splitting at the stratum granulosum level, whereas Lyell's disease (or TEN) is characterized by splitting at the dermoepidermal junction.

Staphylococcal scalded skin syndrome usually starts rather abruptly with perioral erythema and with a sunburnlike, tender rash, which spreads over the entire body in 2–3 days. At this stage bullae will appear rapidly, leading to partial or total desquamation. Gentle friction of apparently healthy skin will cause it to wrinkle and be displaced (Nikolsky sign). The flaccid bullae will slough off, leaving extended denuded areas that are red, raw, and wet. Hair and nails can sometimes shed. The exfoliated areas will eventually dry, with a flaky desquamation lasting 3–5 days. Within 10 days after onset, new epidermis has usually replaced the denuded areas; recovery is complete, provided that complications such as hypovolemia and secondary infections have been prevented. Staphylococci usually can be isolated from the nasopharynx and skin, but rarely from blood.

The early differential diagnosis of the SSSS includes, besides

TEN, other bullous lesions and TSS, which occurs in a different epidemiologic setting. Finally, Kawasaki mucocutaneous disorder is characterized by a negative Nikolsky's sign and negative bacterial cultures of the skin lesions.

The great majority of the SSSS in the United States is due to phage group II *S. aureus*, with 75 percent of them belonging to phage type 71,[77] but such an association is less clear in other countries. As demonstrated by Melish and Glasgow,[40] sublethal doses of *S. aureus* isolated from patients with SSS and injected either subcutaneously or intraperitoneally into neonatal mice simulate the human disease remarkably from a clinical and histologic point of view. SSSS-producing strains elaborate epidermolytic exotoxins called exfoliatin, epidermolysin, or more recently exfoliative toxin (as discussed above).

TOXIC SHOCK SYNDROME (TSS). In 1978, Todd and coworkers described an infectious syndrome in seven children ages 8–17 years, with the common clinical features of high fever, profound and refractory hypotension, profuse diarrhea, erythroderma, mental confusion, and renal failure.[78] Five of these patients were colonized with phage group I *S. aureus*. The entity was named toxic shock syndrome (TSS) and was later considered to be synonymous with staphylococcal scarlet fever, a sporadic disease entity known since 1927. In January, 1980, it suddenly became apparent that this multisystem disease was frequently observed in women, with onset mainly during menstruation.[79] The disease reached epidemic proportions in 1980 and 1981, and probably was favored by the introduction on the market of new hyperabsorbable tampons.[80] Since their removal from the market, the incidence of the disease has decreased only moderately; it is presently estimated at 3–15 per 100,000 women of menstrual age/year. The case fatality ratio, which was initially high at 5.6 percent, has now decreased to 3.3 percent.[81,82]

A retrospective analysis has shown that from 1970 to 1982, close to 1700 cases have been reported to the Centers for Disease Control, with 96 percent involving women and 92 percent having their onset during menstruation. Variant female cases of TSS have been associated with vaginal or Caesarean section deliveries, or with prolonged diaphragm use. In recent years, a variety of nonfemale cases of TSS have been described, linked to local *S. aureus* infections such as abscesses, osteomyelitis, postsurgical infections, and postinfluenza pneumonia.[83]

Clinical Manifestations. The clinical profile of a patient with TSS is a young woman between 15 and 25 years of age using tampons during her menstrual periods. The disease usually starts abruptly during her menses, and the clinical manifestationsl involve many organ systems as summarized in Table 3.[79] Prominent initial symptoms and signs include intense myalgias, fever, vomiting, and diarrhea. The patient is usually listless and confused, but presents without focal neurologic nor meningeal signs. Severe hypotension ensues rapidly with hypovolemic shock due to loss of colloids and fluid. An erythematous, deep-red, "sunburn" rash develops within a few hours, accompanied by conjunctival inflammation.[79,82]

Physical examination usually discloses, besides the skin rash and hypotension, erythematous mucosal surfaces; there is vaginal hyperemia and often vaginal discharge from which *S. aureus* can be recovered. In male, pediatric, or female cases not associated with menstruation, *S. aureus* has been isolated from focal lesions of skin, bone, lung, and stool. Blood cultures are exceptionally positive and cerebropsinal fluid (CSF) cultures are invariably negative.

Some of the important findings observed during the acute phase of TSS are summarized in Table 3.[79] Rash and shock, being part of the diagnostic criteria, are omitted from the table. Renal failure is of both the oliguric and nonoliguric type, and it most often is reversible. In case of death, main pathologic alterations have included desquamation and ulceration of the vaginal and cervical mucosa, periportal inflammation in the liver, acute tubular necrosis, and the formation of hyaline membranes that are characteristic of shock lung.[84]

Criteria for the diagnosis of TSS are presented in Table 4. Toxic shock syndrome is probable when three or more major criteria are met in the presence of desquamation, or more than five are met in its absence. In cases not associated with menstruation, the primary focus of infection can be inconspicuous, despite being positive for *S. aureus* on culture.

Although full recovery is the rule, with intense scaling and desquamation of the skin with a predilection for palms and soles (Fig. 9A,B) and with the mortality now about 3 percent, complications and sequelae have to be expected. Repeated bouts of TSS with fever, myalgias, vomiting, diarrhea, and diffuse rash with desquamation have been described in a nonnegligible number of cases. They tended to occur on the same day of the menses, to decrease in intensity, and to occur preferentially in patients not previously treated with appropriate antibiotics. Main sequelae include persistent neuropsychologic alterations, such as memory loss, an abnormal electroencephalogram (EEG), mild renal failure, late onset rash, and cyanotic extremities.[85]

Pathogenic Factors Involved in TSS. The arguments in favor of the crucial role played by *S. aureus* in the pathogenesis of TSS are overwhelming; they include (*1*) a vaginal isolation rate of 98 percent in appropriately cultured menses-associated TSS, as opposed to a carriage rate in various normal controls of 8–10 percent[22]; (*2*) isolation of *S. aureus* from other sites in all nonmenses-associated cases of TSS[86]; and (*3*) the low recurrence rate in females receiving antistaphylococcal antibiotics during the initial episode. A unique toxin—TSST-1—has been identified as being associated almost invariably with menstrually related TSS and in at least half of the patients with nonmenstrually related cases. TSST-1 corresponds to the toxins identified by Bergdoll[42] and Schlievert,[41] and its putative mode

TABLE 3. Frequency of Signs, Symptoms, and Laboratory Abnormalities in 52 Patients with Toxic-shock Syndrome[e]

Clinical sign or Symptom	%	*Laboratory Finding*	%
Diarrhea	98	Elevated serum creatinine	69
Myalgia	96	Thrombocytopenia[a]	59
Vomiting	92	Hypocalcemia[b]	58
Temperature ≥ 40°C	87	Azotemia	57
Headache	77	Hyperbilirubinemia	54
Sore throat	75	Elevated hepatic enzymes	50
Conjunctival hyperemia	57	Leukocytosis[c]	48
Decreased sensorium	40	Abnormal urinary sediment[d]	46
Vaginal hyperemia	33	Elevated CPK[f]	41
Vaginal discharge	28	Immature leukocytes ≥ 50%	36
Rigors	25		

[a] Platelet count < 100,000 per millimeter.
[b] Serum calcium ≤ 7.5 mg/dl.
[c] White blood cell count ≥ 15,000 per cubic millimeter.
[d] At least five white blood cells per high-power field, ≥ two red blood cells per high-power field, or presence of red blood cells casts.
[e] Rash and shock, being part of the definition, are omitted from the table.
[f] CPK, creatine phosphokinase.
(From Davis et al.,[79] with permission.)

TABLE 4. Criteria for the Diagnosis of TSS

Temperature >38.9°C
Systolic blood pressure <90 mmHg
Rash with subsequent desquamation, especially on palms and soles
Involvement of ≥3 of the following organ systems:
- Gastrointestinal: vomiting, profuse diarrhea
- Muscular: severe myalgias or >fivefold increase in CPK[a]
- Mucous membranes (vagina, conjunctivae, or pharynx): frank hyperemia
- Renal insufficiency: BUN[b] or creatinine at least twice the upper limit of normal, with pyuria in the absence of urinary tract infection
- Liver; hepatitis: bilirubin, SGOT, SGPT at least twice the upper limit of normal
- Blood: thrombocytopenia <100,000 per mm³
- Central nervous system: disorientation without focal neurologic signs

Negative results of the serologic tests for Rocky Mountain Spotted Fever, leptospirosis, and measles

[a] CPK, creatine phosphokinase.
[b] BUN, blood urea nitrogen.

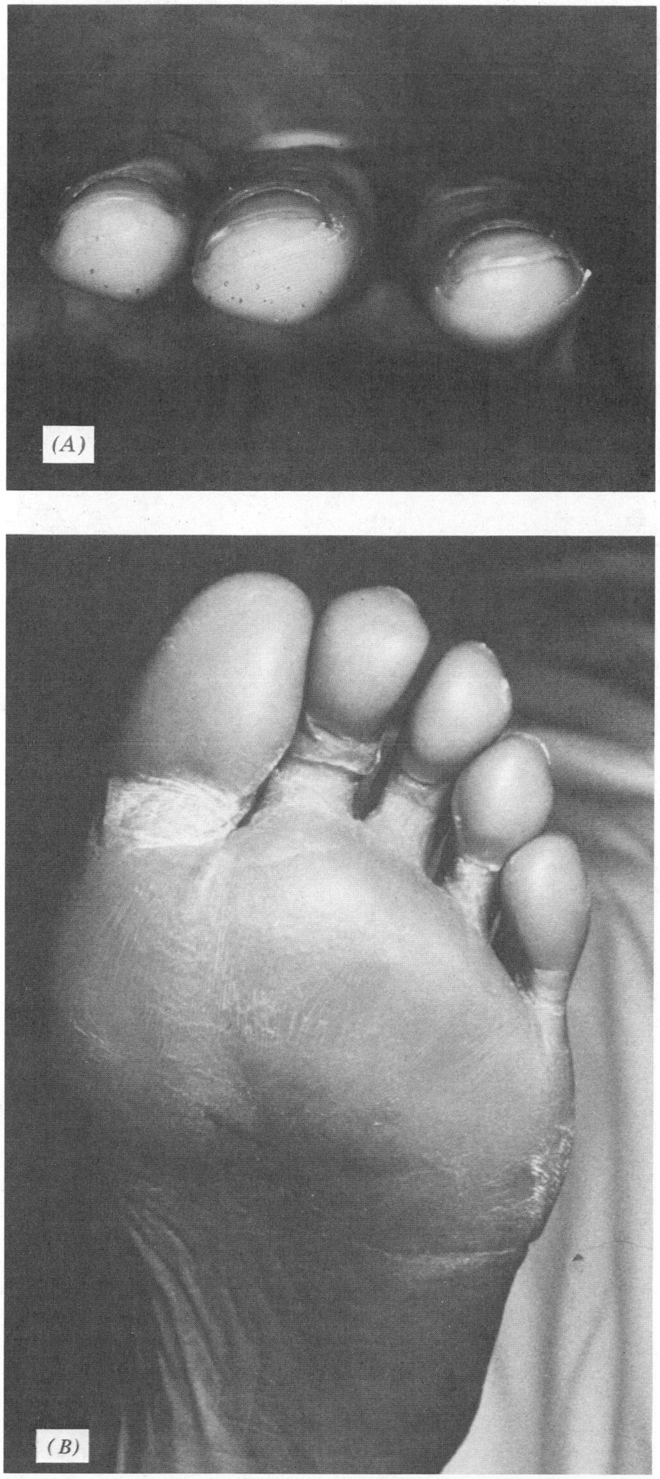

FIG. 9. Toxic shock syndrome **(A & B)**. Late desquamation of skin around fingernails and overlying toes. As opposed to the scalded skin syndrome, in which the area under the desquamation is not denuded, but still covered by a thin epithelium.

of action has been discussed previously.[44,48] It should be underscored that many factors prevailing in the vagina in the presence of hyperabsorbable tampons will favor the production of TSST-1, such as O_2 tension, appropriate CO_2 tension, and low Mg concentration.

The prevalence of antibodies against TSST-1 is above 90 percent in the general population. Practically all patients with menstruation-associated TSS had undetectable antibodies against TSST-1 at onset of the disease. All these data strongly favor the important role of TSST-1 in the development of TSS.

A significant percentage of non-menstruation-related TSS–*S. aureus*—close to 40 percent—do not produce TSST-1. In a recent study,[44] most of these strains were shown to produce various enterotoxins, and to be strong interleukin-1 inducers in a monocyte in vitro system. Thus, there is growing evidence in favor of the crucial role of TSST-1 and other, related enterotoxins in production of TSS.

The 1980–1981 epidemic in the United States of TSS and, by extension, the many sporadic cases throughout the world[81,82] have been statistically linked to the use of hyperabsorbable tampons. The present epidemiologic data can be summarized as follows. Toxic shock syndrome is exceptional in the pediatric population, in males, and in nonmenstruating females; it occurs only as a secondary event linked to a local staphylococcal infection. In contrast, menstruating women are particularly at risk for developing either primary or recurrent TSS. This risk is increased by the use of any tampons during the menstrual periods. Hyperabsorbable tampons introduced since 1977 on the U.S. market have even further increased this risk[59]; their withdrawal from the market has been paralleled by a decreased prevalence of TSS.

Management and Prevention of TSS. Acute management of a patient with TSS first requires aggressive fluid replacement with saline and/or colloid. Vaginal cxamination should be performed immediately thereafter, with removal of any tampon and with vaginal as well as cervical culturing for *S. aureus*. In variant TSS, cultures of the infectious focus should be obtained. A β-lactamase-resistant antistaphylococcal antibiotic such as oxacillin or nafcillin should be administered intravenously at a dosage of 8–10 g/day. Exacerbation of the skin rash is sometimes difficult to differentiate from a possible allergic reaction to the β-lactam antibiotic. In the absence of complications such as bacteremic spread or of a primary focus such as osteomyelitis, the treatment period should not exceed 10–15 days.

Prevention of recurrences includes parenteral antibiotic treatment of the first episodes as described, education of the patient, and avoidance of tampons. Prevention of first episodes probably requires minimal use of high-absorbancy tampons, educating the population at risk as to the use of other catamenial products, and a better identification of the factors associated with nonmenstrual cases.

Septicemia and Endocarditis

Epidemiological Aspects; Predisposing Factors. The clinical spectrum of staphylococcal septicemia and its outcome have been recently modified by several factors, such as a patient population with an increasing number of underlying diseases and the emergence of new social habits such as the use of illicit IV drugs. A very careful study performed in Denmark, encompassing 2000 cases of bacteremia observed in various hospitals, showed that epidemic strains can be replaced by new ones, with altered phage susceptibilities and new antibiotic resistance patterns.[87] Before the availability of antibiotics, the clinical manifestations of *S. aureus* bacteremia were remarkably uniform[88]; patients tended to be young, without underlying disease in 70 percent of the cases, and disseminated infection usually led to the establishment of metastatic foci and to death in 82 percent of the cases. In contrast, a more recent study of 185 consecutive patients identified two patient populations at high risk: those below the age of 10 and beyond the age of 60 with mortality rates of 28 percent and 63 percent, respectively. Of the patients studied, 75 percent had significant associated illnesses, including chronic renal insufficiency, kidney transplant, chronic active hepatitis, decompensated diabetes mellitus, metastatic cancer, heroin addiction, cardiovascular disease, leukemia, and various forms of dermatitis.[89]

Clinical Manifestations. In most cases, *S. aureus* septicemia is the consequence of a local infection, which has gained access to the blood stream, favored by one or several conditions such as trauma, surgery, foreign bodies of various types (including intravascular and intraperitoneal catheters), and so on. Musher and McKenzie have conveniently subdivided these infected foci into extravascular foci (cellulitis, ulcers, burns, osteomyelitis, and pneumonia), intravascular foci (IV access devices), and presumed intravascular foci (heroin addiction).[90] In about one-third of the cases of septicemia, no initial focus of infection can be detected.

In its classical presentation, the disease starts with several chills and sometimes with frank rigors. The patient often is obtunded, complains of joint pain, and more rarely of pleuritic chest pain. In a hospitalized patient, these symptoms associated with the presence of an IV catheter will mandate its removal and culture, the drawing of blood cultures, and the prompt initiation of antibacterial therapy. In nonhospitalized patients, the disease usually evolves untreated for several days before admission.

Physical examination usually reveals an acutely ill, often listless, and slightly obtunded patient. Careful examination of the skin sometimes will provide major diagnostic clues such as petechiae on the digits and extremities, subconjunctival hemorrhages, and a full spectrum of larger skin lesions extending from necrotic to necropurulent and hemorrhagic lesions; gangrenous, symmetric involvement of the extremities has also been described (Fig. 10). Funduscopic examination will sometimes disclose classic Roth spots and more often small punctiform hemorrhages.

Examination of the heart reveals tachycardia and often additional gallop sounds. Murmurs are difficult to interpret at this stage of the disease; a loud pansystolic murmur may reflect a rapidly developing mitral insufficiency or a tricuspid insufficiency, if accentuated during inspiration and accompanied by a wide jugular pulse. Diastolic murmurs, whether faint or loud, are indicative of aortic valve endocarditis with development of aortic regurgitation. A pericardial friction rub occasionally can be heard, and it can be replaced by frank signs of pericardial effusion.

The diagnosis of active endocarditis carries an ominous prognosis; the mortality of the disease varies from 40–60 percent. The morbidity due to annular and myocardial abscesses, and to central nervous system complications, is also considerable. Hemodynamic deterioration due to valve incompetence, myocardial involvement, and uncontrolled infection often warrants surgical intervention. In two series of 293 and 200 patients with endocarditis who were treated surgically, 18 percent and 45 percent respectively were due to *S. aureus*, with a mortality rate close to 50 percent, as opposed to a 15 percent mortality rate of streptococcal endocarditis treated surgically.[91,92]

Pulmonary examination is of utmost importance, particularly when right-sided endocarditis is suspected. Pleural friction rubs are frequently heard, and a purulent pleural effusion often develops. Pulmonary intraparenchymatous lesions are rarely heard on auscultation and mandate repeated chest radiographs.

The spleen is often slightly enlarged on percussion. Involvement of one or several joints is heralded by the development of exquisite pain and is followed by erythema and fluid accumulation in the joint space. Osteomyelitis usually presents with intense pain in a metaphyseal area, with normal overlying skin. Spondylitis can supervene at any stage of the disease, and its initial symptom is usually back pain accompanied by paravertebral spasm. Frank meningeal signs are usually absent, and focal neurologic deficits are an exception, unless embolization from an acute endocarditis is a prominent feature. Finally, rectal examination should be performed in all males, since in our experience it sometimes can demonstrate the presence of a prostatic abscess, which can be the initial focus of dissemination.

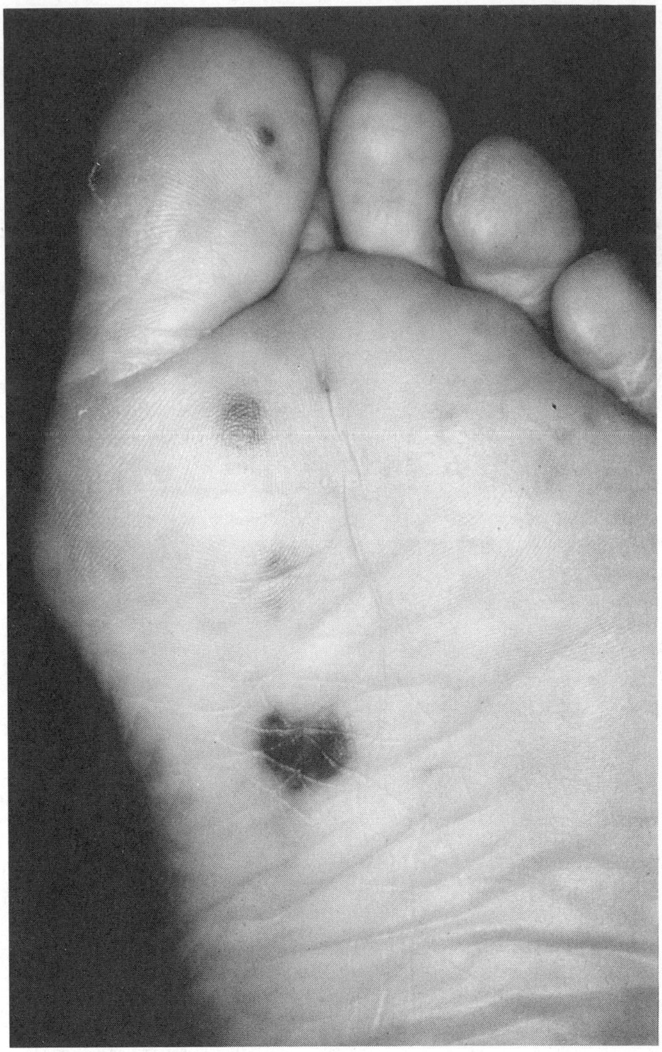

FIG. 10. Janeway lesions in a patient with *Staphylococcus aureus* endocarditis. (From Hook et al.,[131] with permission.)

Laboratory Investigations. Four blood cultures obtained at timed intervals and cultures of skin lesions, purulent exudates, and urine should be obtained; the latter specimen often shows less than 10^5 bacteria per ml on culture.[90] Routine hematologic tests often show a mild anemia. The white blood cell count can be either high with a marked shift to the left, or low; toxic granulations are often present. Thrombocytopenia is frequently observed; this suggests the possibility of disseminated intravascular coagulation—an early, exceptional, but often fatal complication of *S. aureus* septicemia. Mild renal insufficiency is frequently encountered and reflects either hypotension or intrinsic renal disease; *S. aureus* septicemia can produce either pyelonephritis, multiple cortical abscesses, or focal or diffuse glomerulonephritis.[93–95] The urine, therefore, can contain white blood cells, granular casts, red blood cells, or red blood cell casts. At present, none of these renal alterations is known to require specific treatment besides antibiotics, and renal biopsy, therefore, is rarely justified.

The choice of other laboratory investigations will depend on the clinical problems encountered. Electrocardiographic (ECG) abnormalities suggest myocarditis or pericarditis. Bone scans performed with Tc-phosphonate will help to identify a focus of osteomyelitis, but they often are difficult to interpret during the early stages of the disease due to multiple areas of skeletal uptake. Finally, computed tomography (CT) is of great help in selected cases, where local signs point towards a well-delineated secondary focus of metastatic infection amenable to surgical drainage.

The Clinical Dilemma of Positive Blood Cultures: Septicemia or Endocarditis? Despite more recent studies reporting an overall incidence of endocarditis of 10 percent or less, long-term parenteral antibiotic treatment has remained the standard practice in many centers, since early studies reported a risk of endocarditis of 60 percent. Recent observations make it possible in many cases of *S. aureus* septicemia to predict those with and those without endocarditis. These parameters, which are summarized in Table 5, should not be taken as absolute criteria, but as guidelines allowing the clinician to make a probabilistic decision on the management of each individual case.

CLINICAL PATTERNS. Nolan and Beaty have shown that patients with staphylococcal bacteremia can be differentiated into two groups.[96] The first group had a recognizable primary site of infection, was older, was likely to have significant underlying disorders, and was hospitalized when bacteremia developed. Only 10 percent of these patients developed secondary foci of infection, and only 3 percent developed clinically recognizable endocarditis. They had their primary site of infection easily removed, were treated for less than 2 weeks in most cases, and had a relapse rate of less than 2 percent. In contrast, patients of the second group tended to be younger, to have no identifiable site of primary infection, and to have acquired their septicemia in the community, often by use of illicit IV drugs. In this second group, 93 percent developed metastatic foci of infection, and 57 percent developed endocarditis. Despite parenteral therapy of more than 3 weeks, a sizeable number of these patients relapsed, further attesting to the presence of a metastatic focus and/or endocarditis. These results have been confirmed by Ianini et al.,[97] who successfully treated 29 patients falling into the low-risk group for 15 days without any recurrence.

ECHOCARDIOGRAPHY. Echocardiographic exploration of the heart valves occasionally can be of help in the positive diagnosis of endocarditis. A negative exploration does not rule out the diagnosis, since all the valvular structures cannot be examined in detail, the technique is not sensitive enough to detect small vegetations, and their development probably requires more than 10 days of evolution. The demonstration of vegetations by M-mode echocardiography further correlates with mortality (21 percent), surgical valve replacement (74 percent), and embolization (32 percent).[98]

IMMUNE COMPLEXES. Sustained intravascular infections are associated with the development of rheumatoid factor, of cryoglobulins, and of circulating immune complexes (CIC). Recent studies suggest that CIC can be detected in 50 percent of the patients with *S. aureus* endocarditis, as opposed to patients with septicemia who have undetectable levels of CIC.[99] Although useful, these determinations are not infallible; particularly since the antigenic determinants of the CIC are, as yet, unknown and are not necessarily of staphylococcal origin. Moreover, it is conceivable that early in the course of *S. aureus* endocarditis, the development of antibodies has not reached the level at which CIC are formed.

SEROLOGY OF S. AUREUS INFECTIONS. Starting with the hypothesis that a metastatic infection or endocarditis due to *S. aureus* may be a constant immunologic challenge to the host, several investigators have tried to document and correlate its presence with the levels and/or fluctuation of antistaphylococcal antibodies. Basically, three antigenic systems have been used: (*1*) *S. aureus* peptidoglycan (serum antibodies determined by ELISA[100] or by RIA[101]; (*2*) whole cell sonicates (serum antibodies determined by solid phase RIA[102]; (*3*) teichoic acids (serum antibodies determined by agar gel diffusion,[103] by CIE, by RIA,[104] and by ELISA). Of the three antigenic systems described, (*1*) the peptidoglycan seems to be presently the least specific and reproducible. A large amount of information is available regarding (*2*) antiteichoic acid antibodies, which are most conveniently detected by an agar diffusion method, whereas CIE and RIA techniques are more sensitive but cumbersome to perform. When a sensitive technique is used, close to 90 percent of patients with endocarditis will show positive results, but 20–40 percent of patients with bacteremia without metastatic foci will also have detectable antibody titers; 0–60 percent of patients with localized *S. aureus* infection without bacteremia will react positively. Thus it has been advocated to perform teichoic acid antibody assays early in the course of endocarditis, and at the end of an initial 2-week course of antibiotic treatment.[105] Finally, (*3*) a solid-phase RIA aimed at measuring antibodies directed against *S. aureus* Wood 46 sonicates also seems to provide discrimination between endocarditis (87 percent positivity), complicated bacteremia (77 percent positivity), and uncomplicated *S. aureus* bacteremia (0 percent positivity).[102,104]

In summary, whole cell extracts and teichoic acids seem to be the most suitable antigenic preparations, and they can be used in various immunologic tests to detect serum antibodies directed against *S. aureus*. Whereas antibodies can be demonstrated in almost all cases of endocarditis or bacteremias with metastatic foci, they are also present in a sizable number of uncomplicated septicemias. If these tests are to be adopted in the decision-making process concerning an individual patient, the immunologic procedure used and the up-to-date statistics of its sensitivity and specificity should be known to put the patient's results into proper perspective.

TABLE 5. Criteria Discriminating Between *S. aureus* Septicemia with or without Endocarditis

Criteria	*Septicemia without Endocarditis*	*Septicemia with Endocarditis*	*Comments*
Clinical			
Older patients Presence of underlying diseases Recognizable primary infection Hospitalized patients	Probable	Improbable	Primary focus is easily drained/removed
Younger patients Community acquired infection (illicit drugs)	Improbable	Most probable	Presence of metastatic foci + + +
Laboratory			
Endocardial vegetations demonstrated by echocardiography	Improbable	Confirmed	Absence of vegetation does not rule out endocarditis
Presence of circulating immune complexes	Improbable	Probable	Negative test does not rule out endocarditis
Presence of antistaphylococcal antibodies (see text)	Improbable	Probable and/or presence of metastatic foci	Predictive value depends on test used
Therapeutic			
Short-term treatment (2–3 weeks) effective)	Probable	Improbable	Short-term treatment only justified if all clinical and laboratory criteria are fulfilled to rule out endocarditis
Long-term treatment (4–6 weeks) necessary	Improbable	Probable	

Management of Bacteremia and Endocarditis. The mainstay of the treatment is the parenteral administration of a potent antistaphylococcal antibiotic, preferably of the penicillin family. As initial therapy, a semisynthetic IV penicillinase-resistant penicillin is recommended, such as nafcillin (1.5 g q4h) or methicillin or oxacillin (2.0 g q4h). If the microorganism has been shown by adequate laboratory methods to be unable to produce a penicillinase, treatment can be switched to penicillin G at a dosage of 4×10^6 units q4h intravenously.[106]

Whether an aminoglycoside should be combined with the β-lactam antibiotic is a question dealt with in Chapter 61. In brief, whereas aminoglycosides act synergistically with β-lactam antibiotics on most *S. aureus* strains in vitro, they only moderately improve the outcome of experimental endocarditis and do not show any significant effect in clinically documented endocarditis.[106]

In case of a benign penicillin allergy, several alternatives can be considered, such as a first- or second-generation cephalosporin at a dosage of 1.5 g q3h IV. A better possibility is vancomycin at a dosage of 0.5 g q6h IV, given as a slow infusion and with careful monitoring of the blood levels in patients with renal impairment. This is also the drug of choice in case of a methicillin-resistant *S. aureus* infection. Despite the fact that a sizeable number of isolates shows the phenomenon of in vitro tolerance, this problem does not seem to warrant other antibiotic strategies.[107]

The second question concerns the duration of therapy. If the criteria previously discussed undoubtedly point toward uncomplicated bacteremia, 2 weeks of treatment will usually suffice, but the patient should be followed very carefully for possible recurrence.[96,97] Short-term treatment has also been recommended for right-sided endocarditis in heroin addicts. In all other cases (i.e., those with septicemia complicated by metastatic infections or cases of endocarditis), patients should receive a full 4-week course of antibiotic therapy. In case of endocarditis occurring on prosthetic devices, a 6-week course of an adequately chosen penicillin with an aminoglycoside is the recommended schedule.

The third question is whether the determination of in vitro minimum bacteriostatic and bactericidal concentrations is of any help in monitoring therapy. It would seem prudent to select antibiotics that result either individually or, when necessary, in combination in a serum trough level of at least 1:8.[106]

Finally, various forms of adjuvant therapy and the place of surgery should be briefly discussed. Neither steroid nor anticoagulant administration is indicated. Development of valvular incompetence occasionally precipitates a patient into acute cardiac failure and may require early surgical valve replacement. Other surgical interventions should be aimed at draining suppurative exudates, such as purulent pericarditis, pleural empyema, or a perinephric abscess. Splenic or renal abscesses, if confirmed by CT scan, are also an indication for surgery, provided that the patient does not defervesce under optimal antibiotic management. If the initial focus of infection is an IV access device, it should be removed under all circumstances. If the septicemia originated from a septic thrombophlebitis, strong consideration should be given to the ligation and surgical removal of the vein.

A note of caution should be made regarding the prognosis of *S. aureus* endocarditis; a recent study[107] on a homogeneous population of 119 cases observed over a 5-year period has confirmed the severity of the disease by showing an overall mortality of 71 percent, favored by acquisition in hospital, age over 50 years, and delay in treatment.

Organ Infection

Since the two major modes of *S. aureus* spread are either by skin colonization and local spread or by hematogenous dissemination, it follows that any organ can occasionally be infected by *S. aureus*, either secondary to local invasion (surgery or trauma) or during disseminated infection (septicemia or endocarditis).

Pericarditis. Purulent pericarditis usually results from hematogenous spread as often as from perforating injury to the chest wall (trauma or surgery). A recent autopsy study has shown that 22 percent of pericarditides were due to *S. aureus*[108] and that myocardial abscesses and/or endocarditis were frequent concomitant findings. Aseptic pericardial effusions of various etiologies, including postoperative, postinfarction and uremic pericarditis, represent predisposing conditions.[109]

The diagnosis of purulent pericarditis is difficult, and antemortem diagnostic rates as low as 20 percent are still reported. During septicemia or endocarditis, sudden chest pain, a pericardial friction rub, uncontrolled heart failure, or cardiogenic shock even in the absence of cardiac enlargement on chest x-ray films should alert the clinician to perform repeated echocardiograms in the search for a pericardial effusion, which often amounts to less than 300 cc. Soon after thoracic surgery, pericarditis may be associated with severe mediastinitis that requires reoperation and drainage, or it may appear a few months later, mimicking Dressler syndrome.

As soon as the diagnosis is suspected, emergency diagnostic measures should be undertaken to confirm the diagnosis, that is, conventional chest x-ray films, echocardiography, and CT scan. Antibiotic therapy has to be instituted immediately as delineated for endocarditis, and diagnostic exploration of the pericardium should be undertaken. This can be accomplished by pericardial aspiration in hematogenous disease, but it often will require a thoracotomy after surgery because of anterior mediastinal adhesions. If the diagnosis is confirmed, radical exploration of the pericardial sac is usually required.

Pulmonary Infections. *Staphylococcus aureus* pneumonia can result either from aspiration or hematogenous spread. In both cases, the pulmonary infection can lead to local complications (e.g., abscesses and pleural empyema), or it can produce a secondary bacteremia with its well-known complications.

INHALATION PNEUMONIA. The disease often strikes a few days after the onset of influenza and has a mortality of 30–50 percent. Emergence of a few cases of communnity-acquired *S. aureus* pneumonia raises the suspicion of an outbreak of an influenza epidemic, whereas within the hospital setting, *S. aureus* pneumonia is favored by intubation and aspiration.[110,111] *Staphylococcus aureus* is also observed distal to a bronchogenic carcinoma, represents a distinct possibility in an immunocompromised host developing a fever and chest infiltrate. Finally, *S. aureus* is one of the pathogens infecting bronchiectases.

There are neither clinical nor radiologic features that are typical of *S. aureus* inhalation pneumonia. X-ray films can show a continuous spectrum from local consolidation or abscess formation to multiple patchy infiltrates, multiple abscesses of various sizes and wall thickness, and to a miliary pattern of small nodules. Factors that should raise the suspicion of a staphylococcal etiology include any of the previously mentioned predisposing factors, poor response to therapy aimed at treating pneumococcal pneumonia, rapid cavitation of a bronchopneumonia (25 percent) appearance of multiple areas of pulmonary consolidation (Fig. 11A–C), and development of a pleural empyema (10 percent).[110,111] Microbiologic confirmation requires either positive blood or empyema cultures or identification of *S. aureus* in a sputum culture. If doubt exists, transtracheal aspiration or bronchoscopy are indicated. Appropriate therapy implies the administration of IV nafcillin, oxacillin, or methicillin as described for bacteremia, for about 2 weeks, and will usually lead to complete clearing of the lung lesions if instituted promptly.

In pediatric patients, staphylococcal pneumonia presents as a highly febrile illness with nonproductive cough. Chest aus-

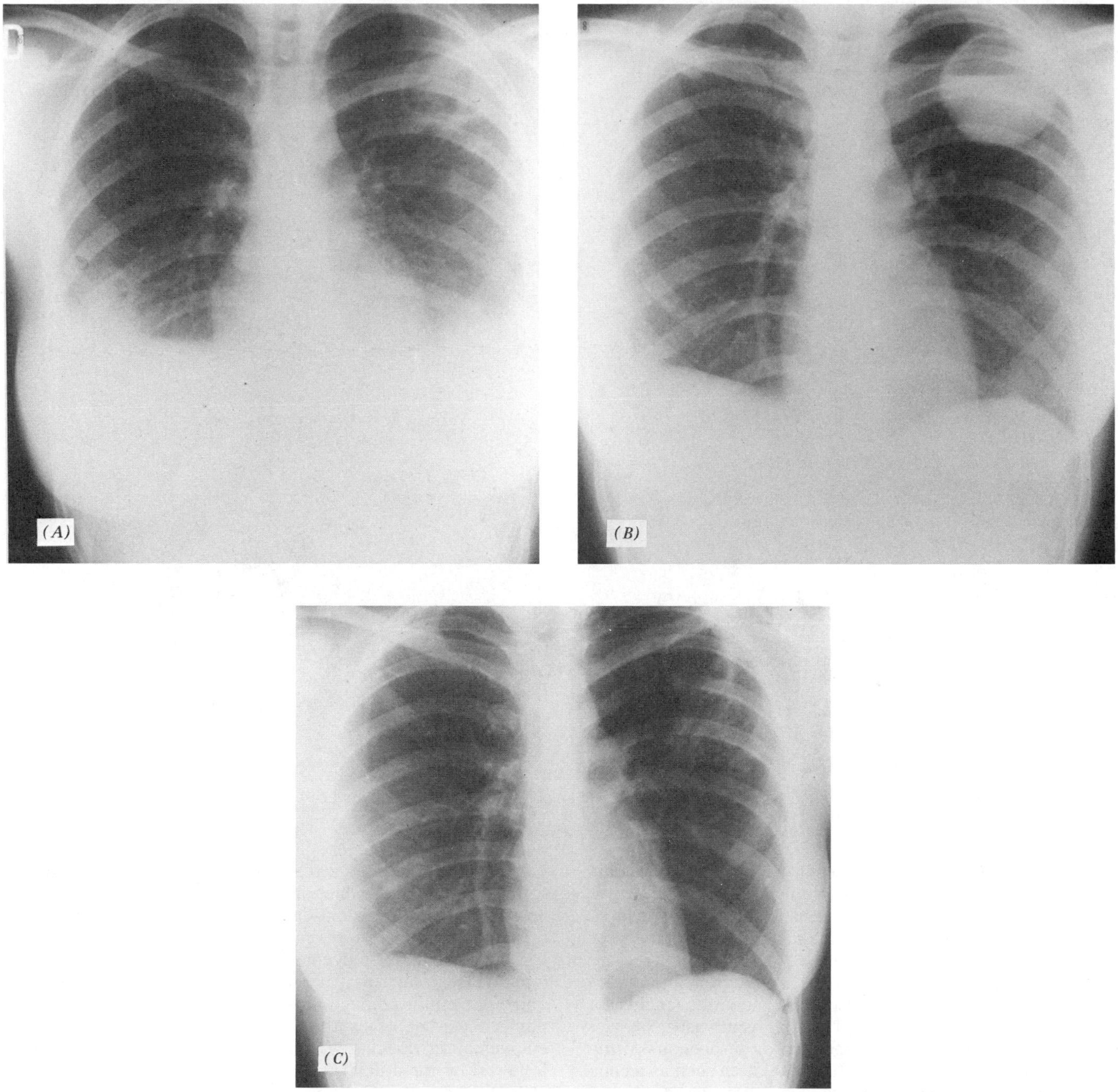

FIG. 11. X-ray films, of probably airborne staphylococcal pneumonia in a young girl. **(A)** Early abscess formation in the right lower and left upper lobe. **(B)** Evolution 2 weeks later, showing fluid accumulation in the left upper lobe abscess. **(C)** Another 2 weeks later—progressive clearing of the abscesses on antistaphylococcal treatment.

cultation may be normal initially, but x-ray films will soon show multiple, thin-walled abscesses, so-called pneumatoceles. Development of air–fluid levels ensues and pleural empyema can occur at any time. In most cases, blood cultures are negative, and treatment has to be started on an empiric basis. *Staphylococcus aureus* also is frequently isolated from bronchial secretions in children and young adults with cystic fibrosis. Although it has been suggested that aggressive antistaphylococcal treatment paves the way for superinfection with *Pseudomonas aeruginosa*, the current consensus is to treat these patients with a parenteral β-lactamase-resistant penicillin, if they show acute deterioration.

HEMATOGENOUS PNEUMONIAS. These usually are due to the release of infected thrombotic material from the venous system or from infected tricuspid vegetations, with subsequent septic infarction. Infection of the venous system is usually suggested by a patient's history or physical examination; many patients are heroin addicts,[112] others are on chronic hemodialysis and show evidence of an infected access device,[113] and still others have received prolonged IV therapy.[114] Physical examination discloses various combinations of localized skin infection, septic phlebitis, right-sided endocarditis, and bilateral pneumonitis. Chest x-ray films usually show multiple discrete, small pulmonary infiltrates; some of them become cavitary within a few days (Fig. 12A,B). Although it has been initially suggested that all of these patients have right-sided endocarditis, the rapid response to short-term antibiotic treatment casts doubt on this conclusion.

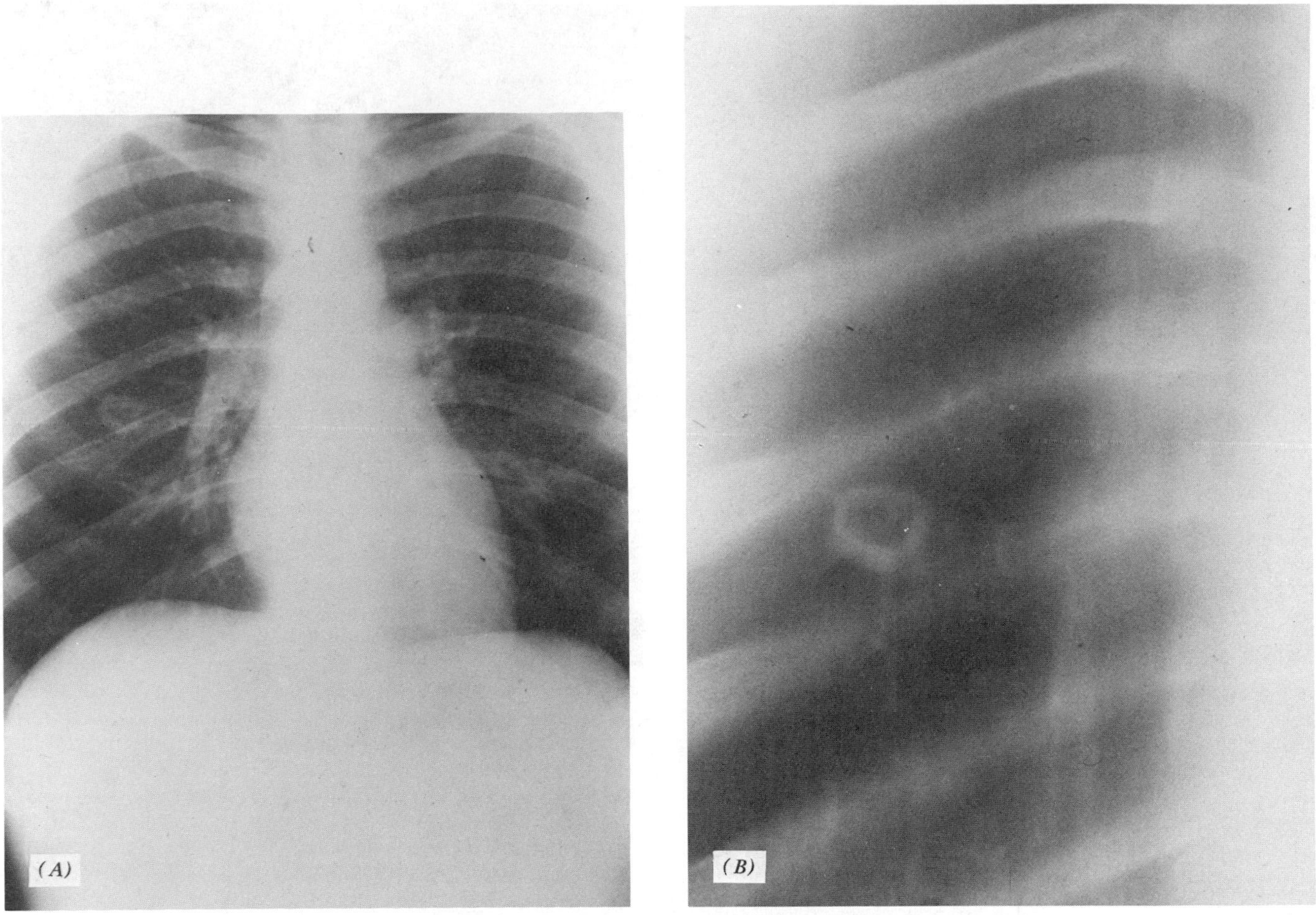

FIG. 12. X-ray film **(A)** and tomogram **(B)** of a septic embolus during right-sided endocarditis in a drug addict.

Treatment implies administration of a semisynthetic penicillin as delineated for septicemia. A short-term 2-week treatment is probably adequate if clinical response is prompt, no complication supervenes, and left- or right-sided endocarditis can be ruled out with reasonable probability.

PLEURAL EMPYEMA. *Staphylococcus aureus* remains one of the common causes of pleural empyema and still accounts for about one-third of the cases.[115] Acute empyema usually arises by direct extension from hematogenous or aerogenous *S. aureus* pneumonia or lung abscess. It is also often seen as a complication of thoracic surgery, particularly after resection of a bronchogenic carcinoma. Direct seeding of the pleural space during septicemia and/or endocarditis can also occur in rare instances.

Here again, the clinical manifestations are initially overshadowed by the underlying condition (pneumonia, lung abscess, endocarditis, or thoracic surgery). Development of pleural empyema is characterized by recurrence of chest pain and fever, shortness of breath, tachycardia, and signs of a pleural effusion. In postsurgical cases, inspection of the wound shows increased signs of inflammation from which cloudy material can sometimes be expressed. Conventional chest x-ray films and decubitus films can confirm the diagnosis of pleural effusion and give important information regarding loculation, a feared evolution particularly frequent in *S. aureus* infections. Finally, the demonstration of a pleural air–fluid level in the absence of a previous thoracocentesis suggests a bronchopleural fistula, another feared complication of *S. aureus* infections. This diagnosis requires confirmation by bronchoscopy and instillation of either methylene blue or a radioopaque dye, which will be recovered in the pleural space or in the chest tube.

The key to the etiologic diagnosis is the bacteriologic analysis of the pleural fluid, which in case of *S. aureus* empyema can be either cloudy or frankly purulent, but always odorless. Microscopic examination reveals sheets of PMNs and cocci.

Management of empyema implies recognition of its underlying causes, such as (*1*) a bronchopleural fistula, which requires carefully planned surgery; (*2*) treatment with antistaphylococcal agents by the IV route; and (*3*) drainage of the empyema. In rare cases, drainage by repeated aspirations is followed by rapid defervescence; in most cases, insertion of a chest tube is necessary and should lead to improvement of the clinical condition in a few days. In the more chronic cases not responding to these drainage attempts, surgical drainage by thoracotomy is necessary.[116]

Osteomyelitis, Septic Arthritis, Septic Bursitis, and Pyomyositis. Bone and joint infections can occur as complications of *S. aureus* septicemia (hematogenous osteomyelitis), but result most of the time from an infection secondary to local trauma or injury (osteomyelitis secondary to a contiguous focus of infection).[117]

OSTEOMYELITIS. *Hematogenous osteomyelitis* due to *S. aureus* occasionally is seen in neonates, where it usually affects the lower extremities as a consequence of an infected umbilical catheter. In children, hematogenous osteomyelitis is characterized by the sudden onset of high fever and pain in the metaphyseal area of a long bone. On physical examination, the overlying skin is normal and the adjacent joints can be freely moved, but pain is barely tolerable when the affected bone is palpated. Laboratory values usually are of little help. The sedimentation rate is high, and there is a leukocytosis with a left shift. X-ray films of the affected bone are initially normal and usually require 10–14 days to show typical changes (i.e., periosteal elevation or a radiolucent and mottled area of bone lysis). In contrast, ^{99m}Tc-phosphonate scanning is of great help in the detection of early bone lesions. Although the majority of hematogenous osteomyelitides in this age group are due to *S. aureus*, microbiologic confirmation of the infection remains mandatory. Blood cultures are positive in about 50 percent of the cases. If no positive bacteriologic information is available after 2–3 days of evolution and the patient is still febrile, a direct bone biopsy procedure for decompression, culture, and histology should be performed.[118]

In adults, *S. aureus* bacteremia only rarely leads to osteomyelitis of long bones, but vertebral osteomyelitis has been increasingly recognized as a frequent complication. In a large survey of 150 cases of vertebral osteomyelitis with an adequate bacteriologic work-up, *S. aureus* (and in small part *S. epidermidis*) accounted for 60 percent of infections.[119] The disease usually starts as a febrile episode with an excruciating back pain—most often in the lower dorsal, lumbar, and lumbosacral spine. Percussion over the affected vertebral bodies usually elicits intense pain. Neurologic signs are absent, but can supervene at any stage of the disease as the clinical expression of an epidural abscess. They mandate immediate neuroradiologic exploration of the spinal canal and neurosurgical decompression. X-ray films of the spine are of little help at the onset of the disease, but show a narrowing of the intervertebral disc space after 10–20 days, with mottling of the two adjacent vertebral plateaus (Fig. 13). Anterior bridging occurs within several weeks of evolution under antibiotic therapy. Early bone scanning with ^{99m}Tc-phosphonate is the preferred diagnostic

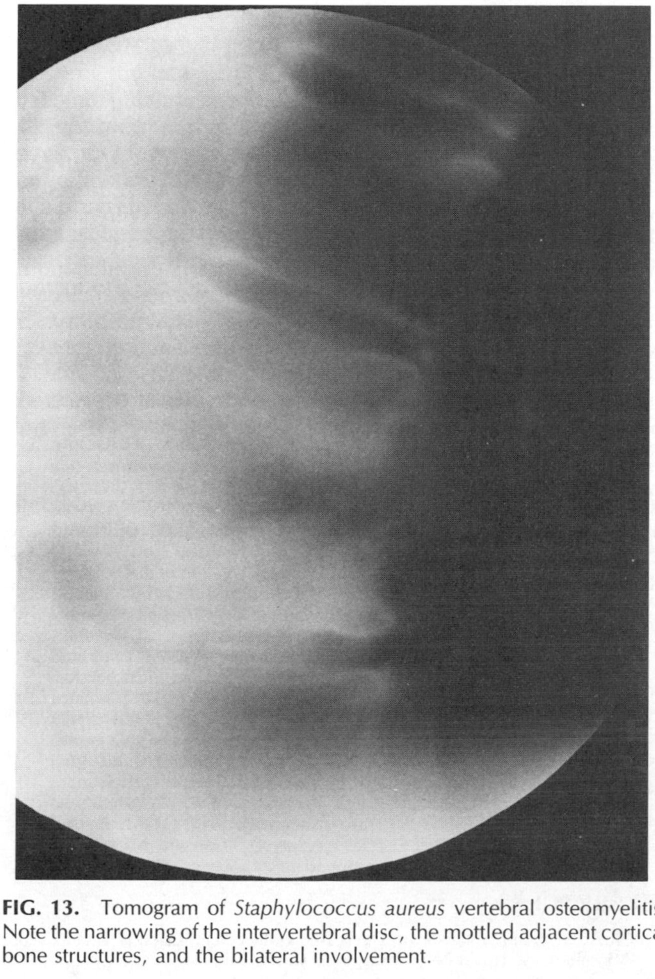

FIG. 13. Tomogram of *Staphylococcus aureus* vertebral osteomyelitis. Note the narrowing of the intervertebral disc, the mottled adjacent cortical bone structures, and the bilateral involvement.

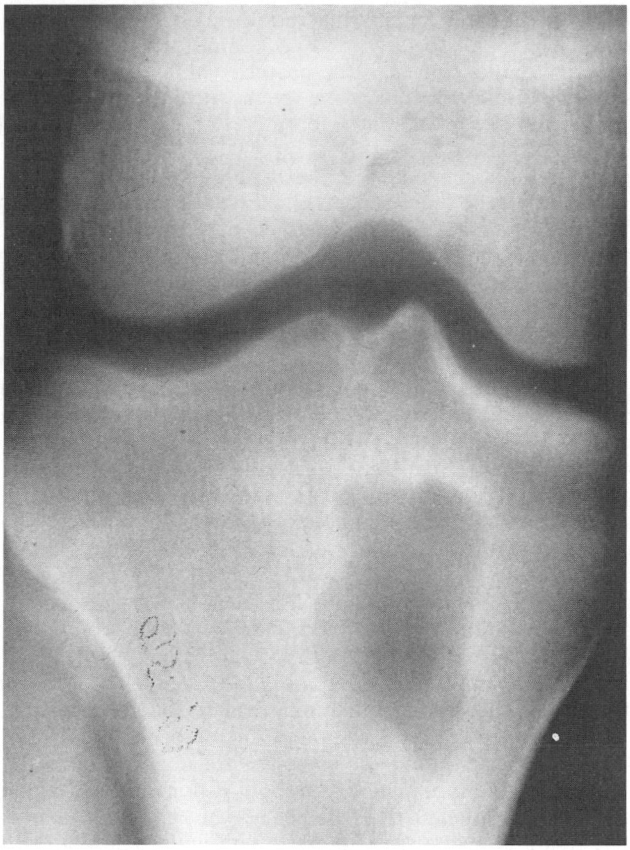

FIG. 14. *Staphylococcus aureus* Brodie's abscess of tibia. Note the radiolucent irregularly shaped area, with no adjacent osteoblastic reaction.

test. Since it does not give any clue as to the offending organism, direct needle aspiration is necessary in most cases.

Other rare clinical presentations of hematogenous *S. aureus* osteomyelitis should be mentioned briefly. A young patient will occasionally consult because of pain on walking without fever, and an x-ray film will show a well-delineated translucent area in the corresponding metaphysis (Fig. 14). Such lesions should be biopsied to exclude various types of benign or malignant tumors, but the possibility of Brodie's abscess due to *S. aureus* should also be entertained. *Staphylococcus aureus* osteomyelitis of the sternoclavicular area usually follows a septic thrombosis of the upper extremity.

The prognosis of adequately treated *S. aureus* hematogenous osteomyelitis is good; present cure rates are close to 90 percent. Patients should rest, particularly in case of vertebral osteomyelitis. A β-lactamase-resistant semisynthetic penicillin is the drug of choice, and it should be administered intravenously as described in the section in this chapter on *S. aureus* septicemia. Therapeutic alternatives include vancomycin in allergic patients if a methicillin-resistant organism has been isolated or, in case of a penicillin rash, other alternatives include a cephalosporin of the first or second generation, erythromycin, or clindamycin. Antibiotic treatment should be continued for 4 weeks. Surgery is indicated in case of medullary or periosteal abscess formation, persistence of fever, presence of a sequestrum, or doubts as to the offending organism. Vertebral osteomyelitis, because of the risk of paraplegia (10 percent) and paravertebral abscess formation, deserve special attention. These patients should be put on strict bed rest and observed daily for the appearance of neurologic signs.[119]

Short-term antibiotic therapy (i.e., 5–9 days of IV therapy) followed by 14–26 days of oral therapy has been shown to give an immediate cure rate of 95 percent in children whose infections were well documented bacteriologically, who responded promptly to initial therapy, had no complications, were compliant, and had adequate serum bactericidal levels on repeated testing.[120] Similar results have been recently reported for adults[121] and are interesting alternatives to long-term hospital treatment.

Osteomyelitis secondary to a contiguous focus of infection occurs most of the time as a complication of orthopedic surgery or trauma. Generally, this form of osteomyelitis does not present major diagnostic problems, since inspection of the operative site shows all signs of acute infection—including the early formation of a sinus tract. Isolation of *S. aureus* from the fistulous exudate most often reflects deep-seated infection due to the same organism. In case of doubt, or if multiple organisms have been isolated, a deep bone biopsy procedure is indicated.

Osteomyelitis due to *S. aureus* presents major diagnostic problems in deep-seated prosthetic infection after total hip or knee replacement. Such patients usually complain of increasing pain on ambulation. Physical examintion often is normal and x-ray film changes are compatible with both postsurgical bone remodeling and/or infection. Sequential ^{99m}Tc- and ^{67}Ga bone scannings allow, in some cases, the diagnosis of infection; Ga is concentrated in highly inflammatory lesions. In case of doubt, direct bone aspiration performed under strictly aseptic conditions will provide a solution to this diagnostic dilemma.

Antibiotic management of *S. aureus* osteomyelitis after surgery follows the recommendations established for hematogenous disease. In contrast with acute hematogenous infection, postsurgical or posttraumatic osteomyelitis always requires the collabortion of an orthopaedic surgeon. If bone union is stable, orthopaedic fixation devices should be kept in place. Removal of the fixation device after consolidation under antibiotic coverage will most often lead to bacteriologic cure. If bone union is unstable, all foreign material including sequestra should be removed at the site of infection and replaced, when possible, by an external fixation device. Infected hip or knee protheses should be removed with excision of the adjacent infected tissue, and a new prosthesis should be inserted either as a one-step or two-step procedure.

Finally, symptomatic improvement can be achieved by oral therapy in patients suffering from chronic *S. aureus* postsurgical osteomyelitis, if intravenous antibiotics are contraindicated; long-term oral treatment with cloxacillin, 2–4 g/day for many months or years, will decrease the number of flare-ups of the disease.[122]

SEPTIC ARTHRITIS. *Staphylococcus aureus* remains the main etiologic agent of septic arthritis in the prepubertal age group.[123] *Staphylococcus aureus* septic arthritis also occurs occasionally as a complication of septicemia in adults and in patients with rheumatoid arthritis. Therefore, a febrile patient with underlying arthritis who complains of acute pain in a single joint should have it aspirated and its fluid examined for bacteriologic growth. Clinical examination shows a hot, swollen, and painful joint, which is tender on palpation and on mobilization. Predilected joints in bacteremic *S. aureus* arthritis include, by order of frequency, the knee, hip, elbow, shoulder, and interphalangeal joints. The diagnosis is confirmed by joint aspiration, which yields a cloudy, sometimes purulent exudate that contains usually more than 50,000 granulocytes per mm^3 and gram-positive extracellular cocci on smear.[124]

The prognosis of *S. aureus* hematogenous septic arthritis in children is identical to osteomyelitis, that is, good. In adults, hematogenous septic arthritis has the prognosis of the underlying systemic infection (i.e., of septicemia or endocarditis). After reconstructive surgery, the foreign material most often will preclude complete bacteriologic cure unless it is removed.

Medical management in all cases of septic arthritis requires the same antibiotic regimen as for hematogenous osteomyelitis. Repeated joint aspirations will alleviate pain, allow bacteriologic monitoring, and probably reduce joint damage. Open joint drainage generally is unnecessary or even harmful, except for hip infections in children, where it seems to prevent aseptic necrosis of the femoral head.[125]

SEPTIC BURSITIS. This is an acute infection involving the periarticular bursae, and it is most often located in pressure areas such as the olecranon and in the prepatellar area.[126] It presents clinically as an acute juxtaarticular inflammation. As opposed to osteomyelitis and arthritis, the overlying skin is usually hot, bright red, and edematous, but the underlying joint can be moved freely. The portal of entry is probably local. Ninety percent of the cases are due to *S. aureus*, and bursal fluid contains usually more than 1000 granulocytes per mm^3. The prognosis is good, if an antistaphylococcal antibiotic is given for 2–3 weeks and if the bursa is aspirated repeatedly. Surgical excision of the bursa is recommended in case of recurrence.

PYOMYOSITIS. This is a purulent infection of skeletal muscles due to *S. aureus*, found in tropical climates[127] or among emigrants from tropical countries.[128] The disease starts with fever and muscle pain. The involved muscle is tender, swollen, and woody-hard. It contains numerous *S. aureus* and PMN, readily seen on aspiration and drainage. Surgical incision and antistaphylococcal antibiotics are highly effective.

STAPHYLOCOCCAL FOOD POISONING. Acute staphylococcal food poisoning occurs in epidemics. It results from the ingestion of heat-stable enterotoxin B that is preformed by a toxigenic strain of *S. aureus* growing in contaminated food.[129] The mechanisms by which the enterotoxin produces intestinal fluid loss have not yet been delineated.

The disease is the second most commonly reported cause of acute food poisoning in the United States. It accounts annually for 20 percent of outbreaks due to contaminated food. The epidemiology of staphylococcal food poisoning is characterized by person-to-person transmission. The responsible organism usually can be isolated from a person involved in the preparation of the meal. Any food product promoting growth of *S. aureus* has been implicated as the inanimate vector, in particular, custard-filled bakery goods, canned food, processed meat, potato salad, and ice cream. The food often has been only partially cooked and put back into the refrigerator until used and is normal in its aspect, odor, and taste.[129]

Staphylococcal food poisoning starts abruptly as an outbreak with acute salivation, nausea, and vomiting; it is followed by abdominal cramps and diarrhea. The disease most often affects almost all members of a group who have attended a common meal, and it has an incubation period of 2–6 hours, depending on the amount of toxin ingested.[130] The diarrhea is usually watery, but it can occasionally contain mucus and blood. Physical examination shows dehydration and hypotension commensurate with the fluid loss, but the patient is otherwise normal. In particular, there is no skin rash, and the temperature is normal. Although deep prostration may be present, neurologic examination is normal.

The diagnosis is often missed in individual cases, but it is suggested by community outbreaks of acute vomiting and diarrhea, a short incubation period, and an absence of fever and neurologic findings. Potentially contaminated food should be examined by Gram stain and culture and tested for the presence of enterotoxin B, since partial cooking may have killed the organism.

The prognosis of staphylococcal food poisoning is good, and symptoms usually disappear in 8 hours. Management implies a close monitoring of the fluid and electrolyte losses and their replacement. Antibiotics are unnecessary. The disease can be prevented by excluding patients with staphylococcal skin infections from food handling, rapid refrigeration of partially cooked food to temperatures below 4°C, and rapid serving when kept at room temperature.

REFERENCES

1. Norse SI. Staphylococci. In: Davis BD, Dulbecco R, Eisen HN, et al., eds. Microbiology. Hagerstown; Harper & Row; 1980:624.

2. Yu PKW, Washington JA II. Identification of aerobic and facultatively anaerobic bacteria. In: Washington JA, ed. Laboratory Procedures in Clinical Microbiology. 2nd ed. New York: Springer-Verlag; 1985:131–250.
3. Spink WW, Ferris V. Quantitative action of penicillin inhibitor from penicillin-resistant strains of staphylococci. Science. 1945;102:221.
4. Barber M. Methicillin-resistant staphylococci. J Clin Pathol. 1961;14:385.
5. Sabath LD. Mechanisms of resistance of beta-lactam antibiotics in strains of *Staphylococcus aureus*. Ann Intern Med. 1982;97:339.
6. Lacey RW. Antibiotic resistance plasmids of *Staphylococcus aureus* and their clinical importance. Bacteriol Rev. 1975;39:1.
7. Peacock JE, Moorman DR, Wenzel RP, et al. Methicillin-resistant *Staphylococcus aureus*: microbiologic characteristics, antimicrobial susceptibilities, and assessment of virulence of an epidemic strain. J Infect Dis. 1981;144:575.
8. Vaudaux P, Waldvogel FA. Methicillin-resistant strains of *Staphylococcus aureus*: relation between expression of resistance and phagocytosis by polymorphonuclear leukocytes. J Infect Dis. 1979;139:547.
9. Klimek JJ, Marsik FJ, Bartlett RC, et al. Clinical, epidemiologic and bacteriologic observations of an outbreak of methicillin-resistant *Staphylococcus aureus* at a large community hospital. Am J Med. 1976;61:340.
10. Hartman BM, Tomasz A. Low-affinity penicillin binding protein associated with beta-lactam resistance in *Staphylococcus aureus*. J Bacteriol. 1984;158:513.
11. Beck WD, Berger-Bachi B, Kayser FH. Additional DNA in methicillin-resistant *Staphylococcus aureus* and molecular cloning of mec-specific DNA. J Bacteriol. 1986;165:373–8.
12. Tomasz A. From penicillin-binding proteins to the lysis and death of bacteria: a 1979 view. Rev. Infect Dis. 1979;1:434.
13. Rajashekaraiah KR, Rice T, Rao VS, et al. Clinical significance of tolerant strains of *Staphylococcus aureus* in patients with endocarditis. Ann Intern Med. 1980;93:796.
14. Goldman PL, Petersdorf RG. Significance of methicillin tolerance in experimental staphylococcal endocarditis. Antimicrob Agents Chemother. 1979;15:802.
15. Moorman DR, Mandell GL. Characteristics of rifampin-resistant variants obtained from clinical isolates of *Staphylococcus aureus*. Antimicrob Agents Chemother. 1981;20:709.
16. Lacey RW. Antibiotic resistance plasmids of *Staphylococcus aureus* and their clinical importance. Bacteriol Rev. 1975;39:1–32.
17. Schaberg DR, Clewell DB, Glatzer L. Conjugative transfer of R-plasmids from *Streptococcus faecalis* to *Staphylococcus aureus*. Antimicrob Agents Chemother. 1982;22:204–7.
18. Cohen MI, Wong ES, Falkow S. Common R-plasmids in *Staphylococcus aureus* and *Staphylococcus epidermidis* during a nosocomial *Staphylococcus aureus* outbreak. Antimicrob Agents Chemother. 1982;21:210–5.
19. Blair JE, Carr M. The techniques and interpretation of phage typing of staphylococci. J Lab Clin Med. 1960;55:650.
20. Aly R, Shinefield HR, Litz C, Maibach HI. Role of teichoic acid in the binding of *Staphylococcus aureus* to nasal epithelial cells. J Infect Dis. 1980;141:463–5.
21. Fekety FR Jr. The epidemiology and prevention of staphylococcal infection. Medicine. 1964;43:593.
22. Martin RR, Buttram V, Besch P, et al. Nasal and vaginal *Staphylococcus aureus* in young women: quantitative studies. Ann Intern Med. 1982;96(Part 2):951.
23. Godfrey ME, Smith IM. Hospital hazards of staphylococcal sepsis. JAMA. 1958;166:1197.
24. Tuazon CU, Perez A, Kishaba T, et al. *Staphylococcus aureus* among insulin-injecting diabetic patients. An increased carriage rate. JAMA. 1975;231:1272.
25. Kirmani N, Tuazon CU, Murray HW, et al. *Staphylococcus aureus* carriage rate of patients receiving long-term hemodialysis. Arch Intern Med. 1978;138:1657.
26. Tuazon CU, Sheagren JN. Increased rate of carriage of *Staphylococcus aureus* among narcotic addicts. J Infect Dis. 1974;129:725.
27. Kayser FH. Methicillin resistant staphylococci 1965–1975. Lancet 1975;2:650.
28. Haley RW, Hightower AW, Khabbaz RF, et al. Emergence of methicillin-resistant *Staphylococcus aureus* infections in United States hospitals. Ann Intern Med. 1982;97:297.
29. Drutz DJ, Van Way MH, Schaffner W, et al. Bacterial interference in the therapy of recurrent staphylococcal infections. Multiple abscesses due to the implantation of the 502A strain of staphylococcus. N Engl J Med. 1966;275:1161.
30. Yu VL, Goetz A, Wagener M, et al. *Staphylococcus aureus* nasal carriage and infections in patients on hemodialysis. Efficacy of antibiotic prophylaxis. N Engl J Med. 1986;2:91–6.
31. Schleifer KH, Kandler O. Peptidoglycan types of bacterial cell walls and their taxonomic implications. Bacteriol Rev. 1972;36:407.
32. Kaplan MH, Tenenbaum MJ. Staphylococcus aureus: cellular biology and clinical application. Am J Med. 1982;72:248.
33. Knox KW, Wicken AJ. Immunological properties of teichoic acids. Bacteriol Rev. 1973;37:215.
34. Forsgren A, Sjoguist J. "Protein A" from *Staphylococcus aureus* I. Pseudo immune reaction with human globulin. J Immunol. 1966;97:822.
35. Hawiger J, Timmons S, Strong DD, et al. Identification of a region of human fibrinogen interacting with staphylococcal clumping factor. Biochemistry. 1982;21:1407.
36. Wilkinson BJ. Staphylococcal capsules and slime. In: Easmon CSF, ed. Staphylococci and Staphylococcal Disease. New York: Academic Press; 1983.
37. Mandell GL. Catalase, superoxide dismutase, and virulence of *Staphylococcus aureus*. In vitro and in vivo studies with emphasis on staphylococcal-leukocyte interaction. J Clin Invest. 1975;55:561.
38. Espersen F. Interactions between human plasma proteins and cell wall components of *Staphylococcus aureus*. Danish Med Bull. 1987;34:59–69.
39. Rogolsky M: Nonenteric toxins of *Staphylococcus aureus*. Microbiol Rev. 1979;43:320.
40. Melish ME, Glasgow LA. The staphylococcal scalded skin syndrome: development of an experimental model. N Engl J Med. 1970;282:1114.
41. Schlievert PM, Shands KN, Dan BB, et al. Identification and characterization of an exotoxin from *Staphylococcus aureus* associated with toxic-shock syndrome. J Infect Dis. 1981;143:509.
42. Bergdoll MS, Crass B, Reiser RF, et al. A new staphylococcal enterotoxin, enterotoxin F, associated with toxic-shock syndrome. *Staphylococcus aureus* isolates. Lancet. 1981;1:1017.
43. Garbe PL, Arka RJ, Reingold AL, et al. *Staphylococcus aureus* isolates from patients with nonmenstrual toxic shock syndrome. JAMA. 1985;253:2538–42.
44. Parsonnet J, Gillis ZA, Pier GB. Induction of interleukin-1 by strains of *Staphylococcus aureus* from patients with nonmenstrual toxic shock syndrome. J Infect Dis. 1986;154:55–63.
45. Cone LA, Woodward DR, Schlievert PM, et al. Clinical and bacteriologic observations of a toxic shock-like syndrome due to *Streptococcus pyogenes*. N Engl J Med. 1987;317:146–9.
46. Kahler RC, Boyce JM, Bergdoll MS, et al. Case report: toxic shock syndrome associated with TTST-1 producing coagulase-negative staphylococci. Am J Med Sci. 1986;292:310–2.
47. Schlievert PM. Alteration of immune function by staphylococcal pyrogenic exotoxin type C: possible role in toxic-shock syndrome. J Infect Dis. 1983;147:391.
48. Ikejima T, Dinarello CA, Gill DM, et al. Induction of human interleukin-1 by a product of *Staphylococcus aureus* associated with toxic shock syndrome. J Clin Invest. 1984;73:1312–20.
49. Davison VE, Sanford BA. Factors influencing adherence of *Staphylococcus aureus* to influenza A virus-infected cell cultures. Infect Immunol. 1982;37:946.
50. Fainstein V, Musher DM, Cate TR. Bacterial adherence to pharyngeal cells during viral infection. J Infect Dis. 1980;141:172.
51. Kuusela P. Fibronectin binds to *Staphylococcus aureus*. Nature. 1978;276:718.
52. Lopes JD, Dos Reis M, Brentani RR. Presence of laminin receptors in *Staphylococcus aureus*. Science. 1985;229:275–7.
53. Vercellotti GM, Lussenhop D, Peterson PK, et al. Bacterial adherence to fibronectin and endothelial cells: a possible mechanism for bacterial tissue tropism. Lab Clin Med. 1984;103:34.
54. Vaudaux P, Suzuki R, Waldvogel FA, et al. Foreign body infection: role of fibronectin as a ligand for the adherence of *Staphylococcus aureus*. J Infect Dis. 1984;150:545–53.
55. Hamill RJ, Vann JM, Proctor RA. Phagocytosis of *Staphylococcus aureus* by cultured bovine aortic endothelial cells: model for postadherence events in endovascular infections. Infect Immun. 1986;54:833–6.
56. Drake TA, Pang M. *Staphylococcus aureus* induces tissue factor expression in cultured human cardiac valve endothelium. J Infect Dis. 1988;157:749–56.
57. Wilkinson PC. Leukocyte locomotion and chemotaxis: effects of bacteria and viruses. Rev Infect Dis. 1980;2:293.
58. Creger WP, Coggins CH, Hancock EW. Annual Review of Medicine. v. 32. Palo Alto: Annual Reviews, Inc; 1981:624.
59. Peterson PK, Wilkinson BJ, Kim Y, et al. The key role of peptidoglycan in the opsonization of *Staphylococcus aureus*. J Clin Invest. 1978;61:597.
60. Verbrugh HA, Van Dijk WC, Peters P, et al. Opsonic recognition of staphylococci mediated by cell wall peptidoglycan: antibody-independent activation of human complement and opsonic activity of peptidoglycan antibodies. J Immunol. 1980;124:1167.
61. Schliefer KH, Kandler O. Peptidoglycan types of bacterial cell walls and their taxonomic implications. Bacteriol Rev. 1972;36:407.
62. Melly MA, Thomison JB, Rogers DB. Fate of staphylococci within human leukocytes. J Exp Med. 1960;112:1121.
63. Quie PG, Hill HR, Davis AT. Defective phagocytosis of staphylococci. Ann NY Acad Sci. 1974;236:233.
64. Clark RA. Disorders of granulocyte chemotaxis. In: Gallin JI, Quie PG, eds. Leukocyte Chemotaxis: Methods, Physiology and Clinical Complication. New York: Raven Press; 1978:329.
65. Schöpfer K, Douglas SD, Wilkinson BJ. Immunoglobulin E antibodies against *Staphylococcus aureus* cell walls in the sera of patients with hyperimmunoglobulinemia E and recurrent staphylococcal infections. Infect Immunol. 1980;27:563.
66. Allen JC. The diabetic as a compromised host. In: Allen JC, ed. Infection and the Compromised Host. 2nd ed. Baltimore: Williams & Wilkins; 1981:229.
67. Elek SD, Conen PE. The virulence of *Staphylococcus pyogenes* for man. A study of the problems of wound infection. Br J Exp Pathol. 1957;38:573.

68. Peters G, Locci R, Pulverer G. Adherence and growth of coagulase-negative staphylococci on surfaces of intravenous catheters. J Infect Dis. 1982;146:479.
69. Falcieri E, Vaudaux P, Huggler E, et al. Role of bacterial exopolymers and host factors on adherence and phagocytosis of *Staphylococcus aureus* in foreign body infection. J Infect Dis. 1987;155:524–31.
70. Zimmerli W, Waldvogel FA, Vaudaux P, et al. Pathogenesis of foreign body infection: description and characteristics of an animal model. J Infect Dis. 1982;146:487.
71. Zimmerli W, Lew PD, Waldvogel FA. Pathogenesis of foreign body infection. Evidence for a local granulocyte defect. J Clin Invest. 1984;73:1191–200.
72. Bisno AL, Waldvogel FA, eds. Infections Associated with Foreign Bodies: Pathogenesis, Clinical Features, and Management. American Society of Microbiology; Washington, D.C.: 1988. In press.
73. Swartz MN, Weinberg AN. Infections due to gram-positive bacteria. In: Fitzpatrick TB, Arndt KA, Clark WH, et al., eds. Dermatology in General Medicine. 3rd ed. New York: McGraw-Hill; 1987:2100–21.
74. Novy MJ. The puerperium. In: Benson RC, ed. Current Obstetric and Gynecologic Diagnosis and Treatment. Los Altos: Lange Medical Publications; 1980:781.
75. Lyell A. Toxic epidermal necrolysis: an eruption resembling scalding of the skin. Br J Dermatol. 1956;68:355.
76. Lang R, Walker J. An unusual bullous eruption. S Afr Med J. 1956;30:97.
77. Parker MT, Tomlinson AJH, Williams REO. Impetigo contagiosa. The association of certain types of *Staphylococcus aureus* and *Streptococcus pyogenes* in superficial skin infections. J Hyg Camb. 1955;53:458.
78. Todd J, Fishaut M. Toxic-shock syndrome associated with phage-group-I staphylococci. Lancet. 1978;2:1116.
79. Davis JP, Chesney PJ, Wand PJ, et al. Toxic-shock syndrome. N Engl J Med. 1980;303:1429.
80. Kass EH, Parsonnet J. On the pathogenesis of toxic shock syndrome. Rev Infect Dis. 1987;9:S482–9.
81. Osterholm MT, Davis JP, Gibson RW, et al. Tri-state toxic-shock syndrome study. I. Epidemiologic findings. J Infect Dis. 1982;145:431.
82. Davis JP, Osterholm MT, Helms CM, et al. Tri-state toxic-shock syndrome study. II. Clinical and laboratory findings. J Infect Dis. 1982;145:441.
83. Reingold AL, Hargrett NT, Dan BB, et al. Nonmenstrual toxic shock syndrome. A review of 130 cases. Ann Intern Med. 1982;96:871–4.
84. Paris AL, Herwaldt LA, Blum D, et al. Pathologic findings in twelve fatal cases of toxic shock syndrome. Ann Intern Med. 1982;96:852.
85. Rosene KA, Copass MK, Kastner LS, et al. Persistent neuropsychological sequelae of toxic shock syndrome. Ann Intern Med. 1982;96:865.
86. Bartlett P, Reingold AL, Graham DR, et al. Toxic shock syndrome associated with surgical wound infections. JAMA. 1982;247:1448.
87. Jessen O, Rosendal K, Bülow P, et al. Changing staphylococci and staphylococcal infections. A ten-year study of bacteria and cases of bacteremia. N Engl J Med. 1969;281:627.
88. Skinner D, Keefer CS. Significance of bacteremia caused by *Staphylococcus aureus*. A study of one hundred and twenty two cases and a review of the literature concerned with experimental infection in animals. Arch Intern Med. 1941;68:851.
89. Cluff LE, Reynolds RC, Page DL, et al. Staphylococcal bacteremia and altered host resistance. Ann Intern Med. 1968;69:859.
90. Musher DM, McKenzie SO. Infections due to *Staphylococcus aureus*. Medicine. 1977;56:383.
91. Jung JY, Saab SB, Almond CH. The case for early surgical treatment of left-sided primary infective endocarditis: A collective review. J Thorac Cardiovasc Surg. 1975;70:509.
92. Karchmer AW, Stinson EB. The role of surgery in infective endocarditis. In: Remington JS, Swartz MN, eds. Current Clinical Topics in Infectious Diseases. New York: McGraw-Hill; 1980:124.
93. Gutman RA, Striker GE, Gillilard BC, et al. The immune complex glomerulonephritis of bacterial endocarditis. Medicine. 1972;51:1.
94. Levy RL, Hong R. The immune nature of subacute bacterial endocarditis (SBE) nephritis. Am J Med. 1973;54:645.
95. Tu WH, Shearn MA, Lee JC. Acute diffuse glomerulonephritis in acute staphylococcal endocarditis. Ann Intern Med. 1969;71:335.
96. Nolan CM, Beaty HN. *Staphylococcus aureus* bacteremia. Current clinical patterns. Am J Med. 1976;60:495.
97. Iannini PB, Grossley K. Therapy of *Staphylococcus aureus* bacteremia associated with a removable focus of infection. Ann Intern Med. 1976;84:558.
98. Freedman LR. Infective Endocarditis and Other Intravascular Infections. New York: Plenum Press; 1982:243.
99. Bayer AS, Theofilopoulos AN, Tillman DB, et al. Use of circulating immune complex levels in the serodifferentiation of endocarditic and nonendocarditic septicemias. Am J Med. 1979;66:58.
100. Verbrugh HA, Peters R, Rozenbert-Arska M, et al. Antibodies to cell wall peptidoglycan of *Staphylococcus aureus* in patients with serious staphylococcal infections. J Infect Dis. 1981;144:1.
101. Wheat LJ, Wilkinson BJ, Kohler RB, et al. Antibody response to peptidoglycan during staphylococcal infections. J Infect Dis. 1983;147:16.
102. Wheat LJ, Luft FC, Tabbarah Z, et al. Serologic diagnosis of access device-related staphylococcal bacteremia. Am J Med. 1979;67:603.
103. Tuazon CU, Sheagren JN, Choa MS, et al. *Staphylococcus aureus* bacteremia: Relationship between formation of antibodies to teichoic acid and development of metastatic abscesses. J Infect Dis. 1978;137:57.
104. Wheat LJ, Kohler RB, White A. Solid-phase radioimmunoassay for immunoglobulin G *Staphylococcus aureus* antibody in serious staphylococcal infection. Ann Intern Med. 1978;89:467.
105. Sheagren JN. *Staphylococcus aureus*: the persistent pathogen. N Engl J Med. 1984;310(2 PT 2):1437–42.
106. Sande MA, Scheld WM. Combination antibiotic therapy of bacterial endocarditis. Ann Intern Med. 1980;92:390.
107. Frimodt-Moller N, Espersen F, Rosdahl VT. Antibiotic treatment of *Staphylococcus aureus* endocarditis. A review of 119 cases. Acta Med Scand. 1987;222:175–82.
108. Klacsmann PG, Bulkley BH, Hutchins GM. The changed spectrum of purulent pericarditis. An 86 year autopsy experience in 200 patients. Am J Med. 1977;63:666.
109. Rubin RH, Moellering RC Jr. Clinical, microbiologic and therapeutic aspects of purulent pericarditis. Am J Med. 1975;59:68.
110. Rebhan AW, Edwards HE. Staphylococcal pneumonia: a review of 329 cases. Can Med Assoc J. 1960;82:513.
111. Lindsay MI Jr, Herrmann EC Jr, Morrow GW Jr, et al. Hong Kong influenza: clinical, microbiologic, and pathologic features in 127 cases. JAMA. 1970;214:1825.
112. Tuazon CU, Cardella TA, Sheagren JN. Staphylococcal endocarditis in drug users. Clinical and microbiologic aspects. Arch Intern Med. 1975;135:1555.
113. Cross AS, Steigbigel RT. Infective endocarditis and access site infections in patients on hemodialysis. Medicine. 1976;55:453.
114. Maki DG, Goldman DA, Rhame FS. Infection control in intravenous therapy. Ann Intern Med. 1973;79:867.
115. Weese WC, Shindler ER, Smith IM, et al. Empyema of the thorax then and now. Arch Intern Med. 1973;131:516.
116. Varkey B, Rose HD, Kutty PK, et al. Empyema thoracis during a ten-year period. Analysis of 72 cases and comparison to a previous study (1952 to 1967). Arch Intern Med. 1981;141:1771.
117. Waldvogel FA, Medoff G, Swartz MN. Osteomyelitis: a review of clinical features, therapeutic considerations and unusual aspects I: hematogenous osteomyelitis. II. osteomyelitis secondary to a contiguous infection and secondary to vascular insufficiency. III. unusual organisms and unusual locations. N Engl J Med. 1970;282:198, 260, 316.
118. Dich VQ, Nelson JD, Haltalin DC. Osteomyelitis in infants and children: A review of 163 cases. Am J Dis Child. 1975;129:1273.
119. Waldvogel FA, Vasey H. Osteomyelitis: the past decade. N Engl J Med. 1980;303:360.
120. Tetzlaff TR, McCracken GH, Nelson JD. Oral antibiotic therapy for skeletal infections of children. J Pediatr. 1978;92:485.
121. Black J, Hunt TL, Godley PJ, et al. Oral antimicrobial therapy for adults with osteomyelitis or septic arthritis. J Infect Dis. 1987;155:968–72.
122. Bell SM. Further observations on the value of oral penicillins in chronic staphylococcal osteomyelitis. Med J Aust. 1976;2:591.
123. Goldenberg DL, Cohen AS. Acute infectious arthritis. A review of patients with nongonococcal joint infections (with emphasis on therapy and prognosis). Am J Med. 1976;60:369.
124. Krey PR, Bailen DA. Synovial fluid leukocytosis. A study of extremes. Am J Med. 1979;67:436.
125. Waldvogel FA. Treatment of osteomyelitis and septic arthritis. Bull NY Acad Med. 1982;58:733.
126. Ho G, Tice AD, Kaplan SR. Septic bursitis in the prepatellar and olecranon bursae. An analysis of 25 cases. Ann Intern Med. 1978;89:21.
127. Brown JD, Wheeler B. Pyomyositis. Report of 18 cases in Hawaii. Arch Intern Med. 1984;144:1749–51.
128. Levin MJ, Gardner P, Waldvogel FA. Tropical pyomyositis: an unusual infection due to *Staphylococcus aureus*. N Engl J Med. 1971;284:196–8.
129. Breckinridge JC, Bergdoll MS. Outbreak of foodborne gastroenteritis due to a coagulase-negative enterotoxin-producing staphylococcus. N Engl J Med. 1971;284:541.
130. Effersoe P, Kjerulf K. Clinical aspects of outbreak of staphylococcal food poisoning during air travel. Lancet. 1975;2:595.
131. Hook EW, et al. Current Concepts of Infectious Diseases. New York: John Wiley & Sons; 1977.

174. STAPHYLOCOCCUS EPIDERMIDIS AND OTHER COAGULASE-NEGATIVE STAPHYLOCOCCI

GORDON L. ARCHER

Staphylococcus epidermidis and other coagulase-negative staphylococci, often previously dismissed as culture contaminants, are assuming greater importance as true pathogens (Table 1). Infections caused by these organisms involve indwelling foreign bodies and are increasing as the number of catheters and artificial devices inserted through the skin become more numerous. These infections are characterized by their indolence but may necessitate the removal of the catheter or device. Resistance of infecting isolates to mulciple antibiotics may further complicate therapy. The importance of coagulase-negative staphylococci as nosocomial pathogens has prompted more interest in their detailed characterization through speciation, genetics, and antimicrobial susceptibility. A working knowledge of these differences may be necessary to distinguish infecting from contaminating isolates and to devise appropriate therapy.

MICROBIOLOGY

Identification

All staphylococci are members of the family Micrococcaceae. They are gram-positive cocci that produce catalase and divide in irregular clusters to produce packets of cells. In the clinical microbiology laboratory, staphylococci are differentiated primarily by their capacity to produce or not produce an enzyme (coagulase) that congeals rabbit plasma. Coagulase-positive staphylococci also ferment mannitol and produce heat-stable thermonucleases, characteristics shared by few coagulase-negative staphylococci. However, while human coagulase-positive staphylococci compose a fairly uniform species (*Staphylococcus aureus*), human coagulase-negative staphylococci have been subdivided into 11 species.[1] The relatedness of all staphylococci at the genus level has been confirmed by their similar DNA content of guanine-plus-cytosine; their divergence into separate species has been ascertained by examination of specific DNA sequence homology. Using restrictive criteria for DNA-DNA hybridization studies, groups of staphylococci with less than 50 percent DNA homology have been designated as separate species.[2] Certain species are more related to one another than others and form species groups. The current species grouping of coagulase-negative staphylococci relevant to humans is shown in Table 2.

Kloos and Schleifer devised a scheme by which coagulase-negative staphylococci could be easily differentiated into species by using biochemical characteristics.[3] Biochemical characterization was further simplified by the marketing of miniaturized kits that facilitated rapid identification of staphylococci.[4] The value of routine speciation of all staphylococci from clinical specimens is unclear, however. Speciation would be of potential clinical value if it could be used for biotyping or if there were clear associations of certain species with specific infections or antibiotic susceptibility patterns. However, to date only *Staphylococcus epidermidis* and *Staphylococcus saprophyticus* have been identified as being consistently pathogenic for humans; the latter can be reliably differentiated from other species by its resistance to novobiocin and nalidixic acid.[5] As further speciation is performed, the role of other coagulase-negative species in human infection may be clarified.

TABLE 1. Well-Documented Infections Caused by *Staphylococcus epidermis* and Other Coagulase-Negative Staphylococci

Urinary tract infections
Hospital acquired (*S. epidermidis*)
Outpatient women (*S. saprophyticus*)
Osteomyelitis
Sternal wound
Hematogenous
Native valve endocarditis
Bacteremia in immunosuppressed patients
Endophthalmitis after ocular surgery
Infections of indwelling foreign devices
Intravenous catheters
Hemodialysis shunts and grafts
Cerebrospinal fluid shunts
Peritoneal dialysis catheters
Pacemaker wires and electrodes
Prosthetic joints
Vascular grafts
Prothetic cardiac valves

Ecology

Coagulase-negative staphylococci are resident bacteria, indigenous to mammalian hosts, and are natural inhabitants of human skin.[2] *Staphylococcus epidermidis* is the most prevalent and persistent species on human glabrous skin and mucous membranes, comprising from 65 to 90 percent of all staphylococci recovered; *S. hominis* is the next most frequent species recovered. *Staphylococcus saccharolyticus* (formerly *Peptococcus saccharolyticus*) is the only strictly anaerobic staphylococcus comprising resident skin flora; its prevalence has not yet been evaluated. Other species are either less frequent members of the resident population (*S. haemolyticus, S. warneri*), found only transiently on skin (*S. xylosus, S. simulans, S. cohnii*), or found only in specific niches (*S. capitis* [head], *S. auricularis* [ear canal], *S. saprophyticus* [genitourinary skin]). The type and location of coagulase-negative species can be altered by antibiotic therapy[6] and the presence on mucous membranes of competing *S. aureus*.[2]

Genetics and Virulence Factors

Plasmid DNA is abundant in all species of coagulase-negative staphylococci,[7] but the function of only a few plasmids has been ascertained. Resistance to such antibiotics as penicillin, macrolides, lincosamides, tetracyclines, chloramphenicol, trimethoprim, and aminoglycosides has all been associated with specific plasmids; plasmid-mediated resistance has been confirmed by transfer of these plasmids to suitable plasmid-free recipients. Of considerable epidemiologic significance is the demonstration that certain aminoglycoside-resistance plasmids found in *S. epidermidis* can be transferred by conjugation to other *S. epidermidis* and to *S. aureus*.[8–10] These conjugative plasmids encode resistance to penicillin, trimethoprim, and disinfectants (quarternary ammonium compounds) and can mo-

TABLE 2. Human Coagulase-Negative Staphylococcal Species Groups

S. epidermidis[a]	*S. saprophyticus*[a]	*S. simulans*	*S. auricularis*
S. capitis	*S. xylosus*		
S. warneri	*S. cohnii*		
S. haemolyticus			
S. hominis			
S. saccharolyticus[b]			

[a] Species shown to be consistently pathogenic for humans.
[b] Formerly *Peptococcus saccharolyticus*; strict anaerobe.

bilize the transfer of plasmids encoding resistance to macrolides, lincosamides, and chloramphenicol. Conjugative resistance transfer may help explain the rapid increase in resistance seen among hospital-associated *S. epidermidis* isolates.[11,12]

Factors produced by coagulase-negative staphylococci that contribute to the pathogenesis of foreign body infections are being actively investigated. *Staphylococcus epidermidis* produces an exopolysaccharide ("slime") that may be one factor responsible for the adherence of these organisms to plastic surfaces,[13] their resistance to phagocytosis,[14] and the failure of antimicrobial therapy.[14,15] Production of this material is spontaneously lost and regained in vitro and may undergo true phase variation.[16] Some *S. epidermidis* also produce a toxin, similar to the *S. aureus* Δ-toxin, that has been implicated in the pathogenesis of neonatal necrotizing enterocolitis.[17]

EPIDEMIOLOGY

With the exception of natural valve endocarditis and some infections of peritoneal dialysis catheters, virtually all *S. epidermidis* infections are hospital acquired. In contrast, *S. saprophyticus* infections (urinary tract infections) are all acquired outside the hospital.[5,18] Hospital-associated *S. epidermidis* isolates are multiply antibiotic resistant, probably reflecting the selection pressure of widespread antibiotic use in the hospital.[6] Colonization of patients and hospital staff with antibiotic-resistant *S. epidermidis* precedes infection with these organisms. Thus, patients and personnel constitute the hospital reservoir for *S. epidermidis*. The organisms probably gain access to foreign bodies by direct inoculation during the insertion of the device.

Epidemiologic investigations of coagulase-negative staphylococci have been hampered by the absence of reliable markers with which to fingerprint isolates. Antibiotic susceptibility determinations, phage typing, and biotyping all suffer from a lack of sensitivity and specificity,[19] although they may be more helpful when they are used in concert.[20] The molecular analysis of the abundant plasmid DNA in coagulase-negative staphylococci has been used successfully in outbreak investigations[19,21] and in differentiating infecting from contaminating culture isolates.[22] However, the loss, gain, and rearrangement of plasmid DNA by coagulase-negative staphylococci in their native environment over time diminishes the power of this technique for longitudinal studies.[12,19] Techniques that identify more stable markers such as specific chromosomal DNA sequences and proteins of different electrophoretic mobility hold promise for the future.

ANTIBIOTIC SUSCEPTIBILITY

Coagulase-negative staphylococci from nosocomial infections, particularly *S. epidermidis* and *S. haemolyticus*, are usually resistant to multiple antibiotics, with more than 80 percent resistant to methicillin.[23,24] Resistance to methicillin in coagulase-negative staphylococci exhibits the same heterotypic expression, altered by changes in culture or environmental conditions, as do methicillin-resistant *S. aureus*.[25] In addition, DNA probes prepared from the *S. aureus* methicillin-resistance gene hybridize with chromosomal DNA from methicillin-resistant *S. epidermidis* and *S. haemolyticus*.[26] Therefore, coagulase-negative staphylococci that are found to be resistant to methicillin should be considered cross-resistant to all β-lactam antibiotics, as are methicillin-resistant *S. aureus*. Animal studies support cross-resistance even though routine antimicrobial susceptibility testing may suggest susceptibility to certain β-lactams.[27–29]

In addition to β-lactams, antimicrobials to which more than 50 percent of *S. epidermidis* and *S. haemolyticus* nosocomial isolates are resistant include erythromycin, clindamycin, chloramphenicol, and tetracycline.[24] Resistance to trimethoprim and gentamicin is high in some hospitals but may be low in others. *Staphylococcus haemolyticus* is the first staphylococcus to demonstrate resistance to vancomycin.[26,30] As with *S. aureus*, virtually all *S. epidermidis* produce β-lactamase.

Antimicrobials to which most coagulase-negative staphylococci are susceptible in vitro include vancomycin, rifampin, and ciprofloxacin. The former two agents are the mainstay of the treatment of deep-seated coagulase-negative staphylococcal foreign body infections (see below); the efficacy of ciprofloxacin in the treatment of these infections has yet to be adequately determined.

INFECTIONS

Nosocomial Bacteremia

Coagulase-negative staphylococci are the most common cause of nosocomial bacteremia, particularly in areas of the hospital where the use of indwelling vascular catheters is common.[31,32] However, these organisms are also the most common blood culture contaminants.[33] It is important, therefore, to obtain multiple blood cultures from separate venipuncture or access sites and to use rigorous criteria for defining true bacteremia.

Endocarditis of Native and Prosthetic Valves

Infections of native cardiac valves with coagulase-negative staphylococci are uncommon, accounting for only about 5 percent of all cases of infective endocarditis.[34] The infection presumably arises as a result of the seeding of damaged cardiac valves and endocardium with the organism following transient bacteremia, in a manner similar to infection with viridans streptococci. In fact, the subacute nature of the disease resembles that of infective endocarditis caused by viridans streptococci. However, in one study 67 percent of 21 patients with native valve endocarditis had complicated courses (systemic embolization, congestive heart failure, or new conduction abnormalities).[35] As many as one-half of the infecting isolates in this study were coagulase-negative staphylococcal species other than *S. epidermidis*. More than 80 percent of these isolates were susceptible to penicillinase-resistant semisynthetic penicillins, but most produced inducible β-lactamase and were, therefore, resistant to penicillin G.

In contrast to the low frequency with which coagulase-negative staphylococci infect native cardiac valves, they are the single most common cause of infections of prosthetic cardiac valves. *Staphylococcus epidermidis* was implicated as the cause of approximately 40 percent of the cases of prosthetic valve endocarditis at two large medical centers.[36,37] Furthermore, coagulase-negative staphylococci other than *S. epidermidis* are rarely implicated.[38] More than 80 percent of patients who develop prosthetic valve endocarditis due to *S. epidermidis* have a complicated infection.[38] That is, there is evidence of prosthetic valve dysfunction or persistent fever during therapy. Complicated prosthetic valve endocarditis results from infection of the valve sewing ring as opposed to infection of the working components or leaflets. Complications arising from infection of the sewing ring are valve dehiscence, dysrhythmia owing to extension of an abscess into the conducting system, or obstruction of the valve orifice owing to overgrowth of vegetative material. Dehiscence and dysrhythmia are more common with aortic prostheses, whereas obstruction is the commonest complication of infected mitral prostheses. Fever persists during therapy because the valve-ring abscess is relatively protected from antibiotics. The indolent nature of the infection and the extravascular location of the valve-ring abscesses characteristic of *S. epidermidis* prosthetic valve endocarditis also result in the absence of such classic endocarditis findings as peripheral emboli and multiple positive blood cultures. Valve dysfunction and fever are often the only findings associated with an infected valve.

Virtually all cases of prosthetic valve endocarditis caused by *S. epidermidis* that occur in the first year following surgery are probably caused by inoculation of organisms at the time of surgery. The usual postsurgical interval of 2 months that designates early (surgically acquired) from late (nonsurgically acquired) prosthetic valve endocarditis caused by other organisms is probably not appropriate for *S. epidermidis* infections.[37,38] This is based on several observations. First, most of the infections that occur in the first year are complicated, involving the sewing ring. Bacteremic seeding of this area after discharge from the hospital would be unlikely. Second, 87 percent of cases of *S. epidermidis* prosthetic valve endocarditis occurring in the first year following surgery are caused by methicillin-resistant organisms.[38] This multiresistant phenotype is associated with hospital-acquired organisms; patients out of the hospital are colonized with antibiotic-susceptible staphylococci.[6] Third, two patients known to have acquired *S. epidermidis* prosthetic valve endocarditis during an outbreak associated with cardiopulmonary bypass pump contamination had incubation periods of 8 and 13 months before the appearance of symptoms of infection.[21] Thus, patients infected at the time of surgery with *S. epidermidis* can have long latency periods before their disease becomes apparent.

Diagnosis of *S. epidermidis* prosthetic valve endocarditis is based on a high level of suspicion. In a patient with a prosthetic cardiac valve, fever, and even a few blood cultures positive for *S. epidermidis*, every effort should be made to detect valve dysfunction. This should include serial electrocardiograms, two-dimensional echocardiography, and, if necessary, angiography. Multiple blood isolates can also be examined for specific markers in an attempt to differentiate contamination from infection. Repetitive blood isolates with different markers are unlikely to have arisen from a single infected focus.

Therapy of *S. epidermidis* prosthetic valve endocarditis is usually both medical and surgical. The mainstay of antibiotic therapy for methicillin-resistant organisms is vancomycin. However, cure rates have been improved in both animals[39] and humans[38,40] by the addition of gentamicin, rifampin, or both to vancomycin. Antibiotics alone are often not adequate for cure, however, and surgical intervention may be crucial. In one series, 30 of 32 patients with complicated *S. epidermidis* prosthetic valve endocarditis who were cured required surgery.[38] Surgical removal of the infected valve should be attempted in any patient with valve dysfunction after stabilization on antibiotics or in any patient who is hemodynamically unstable as a result of a poorly functioning valve. Antibiotics are presumed to be important for sterilizing the perivalvular tissue around an infected prosthesis before implantation of a new valve. The relative roles of antibiotics and surgical débridement in preventing infection of the replacement prosthesis are unknown.

The role that antibiotic prophylaxis plays in preventing *S. epidermidis* prosthetic valve endocarditis is unclear. Antibiotic prophylaxis has been shown to increase the hospital reservoir for resistant organisms.[6] Patients then become infected with *S. epidermidis* resistant to the antibiotics used as prophylaxis.[6] Cephalosporins are the antibiotics most widely used and recommended for prophylaxis although they are ineffective in preventing experimental methicillin-resistant *S. epidermidis* endocarditis when animals are challenged with a high bacterial inoculum.[41] However, cephalosporin prophylaxis may decrease the number of infections with methicillin-sensitive *S. epidermidis*.

Intravenous Catheter Infections

Staphylococcus epidermidis is reported to be the single most common organism infecting intravenous catheters as defined by semi-quantitative culture techniques.[42] Studies evaluating central hyperalimentation catheters,[43–45] peripheral intravenous lines,[46] subclavian catheters for plasmapheresis or hemodialysis,[47] Hickman or Broviac central lines in infants[48] or cancer patients[49,50] and Swan-Ganz catheters[51] have all reported *S. epidermidis* to be the most common infecting organism. From 12 to 37 percent of all inserted catheters have become infected; *S. epidermidis* accounted for from 50 to 75 percent of organisms cultured. Along with the increase in catheter-associated infections has been an increase in the incidence of catheter-associated bacteremia due to *S. epidermidis* with a consequent marked increase in the number of cases of nosocomial *S. epidermidis* bacteremia. In some hospitals, this increase has resulted in gram-positive bacteria supplanting gram-negative bacteria as the leading cause of hospital-acquired bacteremia.

The reasons for the increase are not entirely clear, but there are various proposed explanations. These explanations include the operative insertion of central lines, resulting in a decrease in contamination with gram-negative bacteria and fungi and an increase in contamination with usual skin bacteria; the decreased use of antibiotics for long-term indwelling catheters, resulting in a decrease in candidal overgrowth; the long period of time that lines stay in place, increasing their chance of contamination with skin bacteria; the increasing resistance of *S. epidermidis* to antibiotics, prolonging their survival on the skin of seriously ill patients receiving multiple antibiotics; and the selection of a more catheter-adherent population of colonizing organisms.

The increase in true *S. epidermidis* bacteremias due to the increasing use of long-term indwelling intravenous catheters poses new problems for the clinician faced with positive blood cultures from a patient who does not appear clinically ill. Infected catheters may be present without gross evidence of purulence or erythema, and bacteremia may occur with few symptoms.[46,52] It seems prudent to regard as significant all percutaneous blood cultures that grow *S. epidermidis* and are obtained from patients who have indwelling catheters. Repeat blood cultures and careful examination of the catheter site would then be warranted. Serious complications, including lung abscesses and death, have been attributed to catheter-related *S. epidermidis* bacteremia.[43]

Therapy for *S. epidermidis* catheter infections would include removal of the catheter, if this is feasible. If the catheter cannot be removed, antibiotic therapy alone has been successful.[46] Vancomycin would be the most logical choice based on the high percentage of isolates from catheter-associated bacteremia that are reported to be methicillin-resistant.[43]

Cerebrospinal Fluid Shunt Infections

Staphylococcus epidermidis is the most common organism causing infection of cerebrospinal fluid shunts. In one series, 27 percent of 289 hydrocephalic patients developed shunt infections over a 10-year period; more than 50 percent of infections were caused by *S. epidermidis*.[53] *Staphylococcus epidermidis* is also a common cause of infections of ventriculostomy tubes inserted for drainage of cerebrospinal fluid in patients with head trauma and of indwelling cerebrospinal fluid catheters in patients receiving cancer chemotherapy for neoplastic meningitis.[54,55]

Infections usually occur within 2 weeks of implantation, revision, or manipulation of the shunt. In many cases usual physical findings of meningitis may be absent, with low-grade temperature, shunt malfunction, or wound infection as the only findings. Cerebrospinal fluid pleocytosis is almost always present but may be modest. Fluid obtained through the shunt may have different cellular findings from that obtained by way of lumbar puncture, but both should be obtained to optimize diagnosis. Cerebrospinal fluid glucose is often only mildly low. A rare complication of prolonged bacteremia associated with ventriculoatrial shunts is glomerulonephritis caused by deposition of immune complexes in the kidney.[56]

Because the infections are hospital acquired, infecting *S. epidermidis* should be assumed to be methicillin resistant. Therapy usually involves a combination of systemic and intraventricular administration of antibiotics, with vancomycin, rifampin, and gentamicin the drugs of choice,[57–59] Vancomycin and gentamicin can be given intraventricularly. This is the preferred route of administration.[59,60] Rifampin achieves adequate cerebrospinal fluid concentrations following systemic administration.[58] Patients with methicillin-sensitive *S. epidermidis* infections should receive a semisynthetic, penicillinase-resistant penicillin systemically. Some cerebrospinal fluid shunt infections have been successfully treated without shunt removal,[59,60] but removal is often required.[61] Antibiotic prophylaxis during shunt insertion has not been shown to be of benefit in preventing subsequent infections.[62,63]

Peritoneal Dialysis Catheter-Associated Peritonitis

The development of chronic ambulatory peritoneal dialysis (CAPD) as an alternative to hemodialysis for patients with chronic renal failure has been a remarkable breakthrough in the management of these patients. However, as many as 40 percent of these patients may develop peritonitis during the first year, with the overall incidence ranging from 0.6 to 6.3 episodes per patient-year.[64,65] The criteria for diagnosis are not uniform among various studies but include some combination of abdominal pain, cloudy fluid, more than 100 white blood cells/mm^3 with the majority polymorphonuclear leukocytes, and a positive culture. Gram stains of peritoneal fluid are usually negative.[66] The organism most frequently isolated from patients with peritonitis is *S. epidermidis*, which is recovered from the peritoneal fluid of from 17 to 50 percent of patients.[66,67] However, routine culture of small volumes of fluid may not yield an organism, and more sensitive techniques may be required. These techniques include inoculation and subculture of broth and the filtration or culture of large volumes (more than 100 ml) of peritoneal fluid.[66,68,69] Because these techniques detect very small numbers of organisms, there is obviously the possibility that some episodes of *S. epidermidis* peritonitis represent procurement contamination of sterile peritoneal fluid.

Antibiotic therapy of *S. epidermidis* peritonitis in patients on chronic ambulatory peritoneal dialysis is generally successful without catheter removal. Many treatment regimens have been used with approximately equal success. These include semisynthetic penicillinase-resistant penicillins, cephalosporins, sulfamethoxazole-trimethoprim, gentamicin, or vancomycin.[66,68,70–72] Parenteral antibiotics alone, parenteral plus oral, oral alone, or intraperitoneal antibiotics have all been effective routes of administration. In contrast to most *S. epidermidis* infections, 75 percent or more of the isolates recovered from patients with peritonitis are susceptible to methicillin.[67,73] This probably explains cure rates of 80 percent or greater with conventional therapy.[66,71,72] Infections caused by methicillin-resistant isolates have been successfully treated with weekly injections of vancomycin.[71] Treatment failures require retreatment or catheter removal.

Urinary Tract Infections

Two distinct populations of patients develop urinary tract infections with coagulase-negative staphylococci (Table 3). *Staphylococcus saprophyticus* is a coagulase-negative staphylococcus that is cultured infrequently from the genitourinary mucosa of young women. However, there is a high correlation between colonization with the organism and subsequent development of urinary tract infection.[18] This organism is readily identified by the clinical microbiology laboratory owing to its resistance to a 5-μg novobiocin disk. Novobiocin resistance is rarely found among even multiply resistant coagulase-negative staphylococci of other species that are grown from the urine.[5] *Staphylococcus saprophyticus* is a true urinary tract pathogen causing both upper and lower urinary tract disease.[74] Symptoms of a urinary tract infection are present in more than 90 percent of women from whom *S. saprophyticus* is cultured, and pyuria is present in from 70 to 85 percent of these women; the organism is a culture contaminant only 5 percent of the time. Conversely, 95 percent of all coagulase-negative staphylococci cultured from the urine of symptomatic female outpatients are *S. saprophyticus*.[5,18] Signs, symptoms, and urinalyses of women infected with this organism are indistinguishable from those of women infected with enteric bacteria. It is clearly an organism predominantly infecting young, sexually active women. Almost 70 percent of women in one study gave a history of sexual intercourse within the 24 hours preceding the onset of symptoms of their urinary tract infection.[18] Studies of female outpatients in Sweden and at the Universities of Florida and Washington found *S. saprophyticus* to be the cause of 32, 30, and 11 percent of urinary tract infections, respectively, second only to *Escherichia coli*, the cause of from 65 to 80 percent of infections.[18,74,75] Unlike infections with enteric bacteria, however, there appears to be a seasonal predilection for *S. saprophyticus* urinary tract infections, with the incidence rising in late summer and early fall.[74–76] Furthermore, since urine colony counts for *S. saprophyticus* are often lower than those for enteric bacteria ($<10^5$ cfu/ml) this staphylococcus has been implicated as one cause of the dysuria/pyuria syndrome (acute urethral syndrome or abacteriuric pyuria[77]).

Therapy is usually effective with most urinary tract antimicrobial agents including norfloxacin.[76] However, therapeutic failures have been reported with sulfonamides and nitrofurantoin, and the organism is uniformly resistant to nalidixic acid.[75] Relapse is uncommon, but the infection may recur in 10 percent or more of patients.

In contrast, other coagulase-negative staphylococci rarely infect the urine. Of non-*S. saprophyticus* coagulase-negative staphylococci cultured from the urine in significant numbers (10^4 cfu/ml), *S. epidermidis* is the predominant species, accounting for 80–90 percent of the isolates.[5] It is cultured almost exclusively from the urine of hospitalized patients with complications of the urinary tract. Half of these patients have an indwelling urinary catheter and nearly all have such complications as recent urinary tract surgery, renal transplantation, neurogenic bladder, stone disease, or obstructive uropathy.[5,78] Coagulase-negative staphylococci are recovered from less than 5 percent of all of the urine specimens from hospitalized patients

TABLE 3. Urinary Tract Infections Caused by Coagulase-Negative Staphylococci

Characteristics of Infections	*Organism* S. epidermidis	S. saprophyticus
Age and sex of affected patients	Men and women equal Usually older than 50	Women 95% 16 to 35 years old
Population at risk	Hospitalized patients with urinary tract complications	Healthy outpatients
Incidence	Uncommon—3.5% or less of all urinary tract infections in hospitalized patients	Common—20% or more of all urinary tract infections in this age group
Presentation	90% asymptomatic	90% symptomatic; indistinguishable from *E. coli* urinary tract infections
Therapy	Often resistant to multiple antibiotics	Responds readily to urinary tract antimicrobials except nalidixic acid
Outcome	Bacteriuria often persists after therapy	Relapse rare; occasional reinfection

from whom a significant number of bacteria are grown.[78] Furthermore, when it is present in the urine, it is associated with pyuria and a clinically significant urinary tract infection only about 10 percent of the time.[78,79] Men and women are equally affected, and most patients are 50 years of age or older. The causative organisms are multiply antibiotic resistant in at least 50 percent of the episodes.[5] When treatment is necessary, antibiotic therapy should be tailored to the susceptibility of the organism.

Bacteremia in Immunocompromised Patients

Staphylococcus epidermidis was not usually considered to be an important pathogen in immunosuppressed patients until reports from two large cancer centers in the United States[52,80] identified it as the most common cause of bacteremia among patients receiving immunosuppressive therapy in their hospitals. Investigators at the Baltimore Cancer Research Center identified *S. epidermidis* as the single most common cause of bacteremia in their patients between 1977 and 1979.[80] The majority of patients were neutropenic and heavily colonized with the organism in their rectum. The addition of oral vancomycin to the oral regimen of antibiotics for gut sterilization decreased both gastrointestinal colonization with *S. epidermidis* and bacteremia in these patients. Thus, these investigators considered the gastrointestinal tract to be the source for these *S. epidermidis* bacteremias. In contrast, investigators at the UCLA Center for the Health Scientists felt that infected Hickman or Broviac central intravenous catheters were the source for *S. epidermidis* bacteremias in their patients.[52] Between 1977 and 1980, *S. epidermidis* accounted for 26 percent of bacteremias in their patients, most of whom were also profoundly neutropenic.

Subsequent studies have more consistently implicated long-term indwelling catheters as the source of bacteremia in patients with hematologic malignancies and bone marrow transplants; insertion of long-term catheters in these patients has become standard practice. As noted above (see ''Intravenous Catheter Infections''), gram-positive bacteria, particularly *S. epidermidis*, account for 50 ot 80 percent of the organisms causing catheter-related bacteremia in this population.[50,81–83] Furthermore, *S. epidermidis* bacteremia has been documented to be a prominent source of morbidity and even mortality[84] in immunocompromised patients.

These studies illustrate several important points. First, colonization of the gut and skin with antibiotic-resistant *S. epidermidis* can follow the intensive use of oral and systemic antimicrobials.[6] Bacteremia originating from these sites can result from a compromise in both general and local defense mechanisms in severely immunocompromised patients. Second, *S. epidermidis* can be a lethal pathogen in neutropenic patients and should not be dismissed when it is grown from blood cultures that are appropriately obtained.

Osteomyelitis

Most reports that attempt to implicate *S. epidermidis* as an important cause of chronic osteomyelitis are not convincing. The organism is usually grown from sinus tracts as one of several potential pathogens. However, three infections meet valid criteria that establish *S. epidermidis* as the cause of some infections of bone. These are sternal oteomyelitis resulting from infection of the median sternotomy wound after cardiothoracic surgery,[85–87] infection of bone surrounding a prosthetic joint,[88] and hematogenous osteomyelitis resulting from infections of hemodialysis shunts.[89]

Sternal osteomyelitis is an uncommon but serious complication of cardiothoracic surgery, occurring in from 1 to 4.5 percent of operations in several series.[85–87] *Staphylococcus epidermidis* was the cause of 16 to 45 percent of the infections. Whenever the deep sternal wound becomes infected, osteomyelitis is assumed to be present, and surgical débridement is necessary. However, diagnosis may be difficult with fever, minimal wound erythema, and persistant costochondral pain as the only symptoms. If these symptoms occur within 30 days of surgery, aggressive diagnostic studies should be undertaken, including computed axial tomography scanning of the chest, needle aspiration of the wound for Gram stain and culture, and, if necessary, exploratory surgery. Advanced infection may require multiple reoperations, delayed secondary closure, and grafting. Complicated infections may have a mortality as high as 75 percent.[85] For this infection, antibiotics serve only as an adjunct to appropriate surgical débridement.

Osteomyelitis can result from infections of prosthetic joints and is discussed below. Hematogenous osteomyelitis can conceivably result from any bacteremic *S. epidermidis* infection but is surprisingly uncommon given the number of patients with bacteremia caused by this organism.

Infections of Prosthetic Joints

Although infection rates for implanted hip and knee prostheses are generally 2 percent or less,[90,91] such infections are devastating. Infected prostheses usually must be removed, and in only 13 to 20 percent of patients is reimplantation of a new prosthesis successful.[90] Coagulase-negative staphylococci have been reported to cause from 20 to 40 percent of these infections. While they ranked second to *S. aureus* as an etiologic agent in older series,[88,91] they were the leading cause in a more recent report.[92] In the latter study, 56 percent of the *S. epidermidis* infections were diagnosed more than a year after surgical implantation of the device and in all but two the organism was felt to be surgically acquired.

The diagnosis is most often suggested by pain in the hip; fever, swelling, joint dislocation, and drainage are seen in fewer than half of the patients. The erythrocyte sedimentation rate is usually elevated, and radiolucencies may be seen at the bone–cement interface in two-thirds of patients.[92] Definitive diagnosis is made by Gram stain and culture of infected material obtained by needle aspiration, bone biopsy, or at surgery.

Therapy is surgical in all cases with removal of the infected prosthesis and débridement of infected bone; osteomyelitis is invariably present. Long-term antimicrobial therapy directed at the multiresistant infecting organisms is usually required. The disastrous consequences of infection have led to a great deal of attention being paid to its prevention. Laminar flow operating suites, antimicrobial prophylaxis, and antibiotic-impregnated bone cement have all been used with apparent success, but their relative merits are unclear.[93,94]

Infection of Vascular Grafts

Staphylococcus aureus and coagulase-negative staphylococci are the most common cause of vascular graft infections. However, while most of the *S. aureus* infections occur in the early postoperative period, coagulase-negative staphylococcal infections are diagnosed months to years following surgery.[95,96] In one series, *S. epidermidis* caused 18 of 30 (60 percent) aortofemoral graft infections diagnosed over a 10-year period; the mean interval from surgery to infection was 41 months with a range of 14 to 80 months.[96] Most of the infections are probably acquired at the time of surgery as suggested by the multiresistant nature of infecting isolates[96] and the frequent perioperative isolation of contaminating *S. epidermidis* from the implanted graft.[97,98] The incidence of all graft infections is highest in aortofemoral and femoropopliteal grafts in which the surgical incision is made in the groin area; it is lowest in aortoiliac grafts.

Clinical findings suggesting late graft infection with *S. epidermidis* include anastomotic aneurysm and pseudoaneurysm formation, the development of inguinal sinus tracts, and vasculoenteric fistulas with gastrointestinal bleeding. Fever and leukocytosis are often absent.[96]

Surgical replacement of the graft and drainage of local abscesses is always required. Antibiotic therapy is necessary to prevent infection of the replacement graft and should be devised to treat methicillin-resistant bacteria. As with prosthetic cardiac valve infections, vancomycin, rifampin, and gentamicin are most likely to be effective against susceptible organisms. Antibiotic prophylaxis is recommended during initial graft implantation to (prevent infection, and a well-designed, controlled clinical trial has documented its efficacy, particularly in abdominal aortic resection and femoral-lower leg bypass surgery.[99]

Pediatric Infections

There has been a dramatic increase in coagulase-negative staphylococcal bacteremia in neonatal intensive care units. The incidence of bacteremia in this area alone has been a major reason for the increase in hospital-wide nosocomial coagulase-negative staphylococcal bacteremia.[31,32] One longitudinal study conducted over 2.5 years found that 73 percent of all nosocomial bacteremias in a neonatal intensive care unit were caused by coagulase-negative staphylococci; 22 percent of all low-birth-weight infants admitted to this unit became bacteremic with these organisms.[100] Bacteremia in neonates is associated with low birth weight, the presence of indwelling peripheral or umbilical catheters, and mechanical ventilation. The coagulase-negative staphylococcal isolates from these infants are typically *S. epidermidis* and are resistant to multiple antibiotics.[101]

An additional intriguing observation has been the association of coagulase-negative staphylococci colonizing the gut of neonates in intensive care units with necrotizing enterocolitis.[17,102] A toxin isolated from one necrotizing enterocolitis-associated *S. epidermidis* isolate produced hemorrhagic necrosis in the bowels of infant rats, and its presence in the stool of neonates was strongly associated with development of the syndrome.[17] Whether or not gut colonization with coagulase-negative staphylococci proves to be the cause of necrotizing enterocolitis, it provides another source for the development of bacteremia.[102]

Ocular Infections

Staphylococcus epidermidis is rapidly becoming the most common cause of endophthalmitis after ocular surgery, especially cataract extraction or lens implantation.[103–105] Diagnosis of endophthalmitis is made by physical and ocular examination, often with the aid of echography. The etiologic organism is determined by needle aspiration of the vitreous with Gram stain and culture of the fluid.[103] While the prognosis for maintaining sight in the affected eye used to be grim, new aggressive use of antibiotics has improved the outlook markedly. One study reported that visual acuity was preserved in 7 of 10 cases of *S. epidermidis* endophthalmitis by using combined systemic and intravitreal antibiotic administration without vitrectomy.[103] The penicillins, cephalosporins, aminoglycosides, and vancomycin penetrate the vitreous poorly after systemic administration, but all have been injected safely into the vitreous of either rabbits with experimental endophthalmitis or infected patients and shown to produce therapeutic vitreal levels.[103,106] Rifampin penetrates the vitreous well after systemic administration.

Miscellaneous Infections

Additional foreign bodies that have been associated with infection by *S. epidermidis* include pacemaker wires and power packs,[107] hemodialysis shunts,[89] and breast implants.[108] As the number of indwelling foreign devices that are implanted increases, the list of foreign bodies associated with *S. epidermidis* infection should also increase. More innovative strategies may have to be devised to prevent these infections in the future.

Although isolated reports of well-documented pneumonias, intra-abdominal abscesses, and wound infections caused by *S. epidermidis* have appeared, most of these infections do not meet strict criteria implicating the organism as a pathogen. The organism is usually isolated in mixed culture with other potential pathogens, is cultured only once or intermittently, and is never reported to have been seen on Gram stain or in pathologic specimens. Because the opportunity for contamination of a culture with *S. epidermidis* is present whenever intact skin is crossed, the interpretation of cultures growing the organism must be cautious. Stricter criteria for infection must be met than with traditional pathogens. However, the growing list of infections in which *S. epidermidis* has been conclusively implicated as the etiologic agent increases the difficulty with culture interpretation. Careful culture collection and Gram stain of infected material are thus more important than ever in these situations.

REFERENCES

1. Kloos WE. Coagulase-negative staphylococci. Clin Microbiol Newslett. 1982;4:75–9.
2. Kloos WE. Natural populations of the genus *Staphylococcus*. Annu Rev Microbiol. 1980;34:559–92.
3. Kloos WE, Schleifer KH. Simplified scheme for routine identification of human *Staphylococcus* species. J Clin Microbiol. 1975;1:82–8.
4. Kloos WE, Wolfshohl JF. Identification of *Staphylococcus* species with the API STAPHIDENT System. J Clin Microbiol. 1982;16;509–16.
5. Nicolle LE, Hoban SA, Harding GKM. Characterization of coagulase-negative staphylococci from urinary tract infections. J Clin Microbiol. 1983;17:267–70.
6. Archer GL, Armstrong BC. Alteration of staphylococcal flora in cardiac surgery patients receiving antibiotic prophylaxis. J Infect Dis. 1983;147:642–9.
7. Kloos WE, Orban BS, Walker DD. Plasmid composition of *Staphylococcus* species. Can J Microbiol. 1981;27:271–8.
8. Archer GL, Johnston JL. Self-transmissible plasmids in staphylococci that encode resistance to aminoglycosides. Antimicrob Agents Chemother. 1983;24:70–7.
9. Forbes BA, Schaberg DR. Transfer of resistance plasmids from *Staphylococcus epidermidis* to *Staphylococcus aureus*: Evidence for conjugative exchange of resistance. J Bacteriol. 1983;153:627–34.
10. McDonnell RW, Sweeney HM, Cohen S. Conjugational transfer of gentamicin resistance plasmids intra- and interspecifically in *Staphylococcus aureus* and *Staphylococcus epidermidis*. Antimicrob Agenst Chemother. 1983;23:151–60.
11. Allen JR, Hightower AW, Martin SM, et al. Secular trends in nosocomial infections: 1970–1979. Am J Med. 1981;70:389–92.
12. Archer GL, Dietrick DR, Johnston JL. Molecular epidemiology of transmissible gentamicin resistance among coagulase-negative staphylococci in a cardiac surgery unit. J Infect Dis. 1985;151:243–51.
13. Quie PG, Belani KK. Coagulase-negative staphylococcal adherence and persistence. J Infect Dis. 1987;156:543–7.
14. Peters G, Locci R, Pulverer G. Adherence and growth of coagulase-negative staphylococci on surfaces of intravenous catheters. J Infect Dis. 1982;146:479–82.
15. Diaz-Mitoma F, Harding GKM, Hoban DJ, et al. Clinical significance of a test for slime production in ventriculoperitoneal shunt infections caused by coagulase-negative staphylococci. J Infect Dis. 1987;156:555–60.
16. Christensen GD, Baddour LM, Simpson WA. Phenotypic variation of *Staphylococcus epidermidis* slime production in vitro and in vivo. Infect Immun. 1987;55:2870–7.
17. Scheifele DW, Bjornson GL, Dyer RA, et al. Delta-like toxin produced by coagulase-negative staphylococci is associated with neonatal necrotizing enterocolitis. Infect Immun. 1987;55:2268–73.
18. Jordan PA, Iravani A, Richard GA, et al. Urinary tract infection caused by *Staphylococcus saprophyticus*. J Infect Dis. 1980;142:510–5.
19. Parisi JT. Coagulase-negative staphylococci and the epidemiologic typing of *Staphylococcus epidermidis*. Microbiol Rev. 1985;49:126–39.
20. Christensen GD, Parisi JT, Bisno AL, et al. Characterization of clinically significant strains of coagulase-negative staphylococci. J Clin Microbiol 1983;18:258–69.
21. Archer GL, Vishniavsky N, Stiver G. Plasmid pattern analysis of *Staphylococcus epidermidis* isolates from patients with prosthetic valve endocarditis. Infect Immun. 1982;627–32.
22. Archer GL, Karchmer AW, Vishniavsky N, et al. Plasmid pattern analysis for the differentiation of infecting from non-infecting *Staphylococcus epidermidis*. J Infect Dis. 1985;145:913–22.
23. Archer GL. Molecular epidemiology of multiresistant *Staphylococcus epidermidis*. J Antimicrob Chemother. 1988;21(Suppl):133–8.
24. Archer GL. Antibiotic resistance in coagulase-negative staphylococci. In:

Mardh P-A, Schleifer KH, eds. Coagulase Negative Staphylococci. Stockholm: Almquist and Wiksell International; 1986:93–101.
25. Coudron PE, Jones DL, Dalton HP, et al. Evaluation of laboratory tests for detection of methicillin-resistant *Staphylococcus aureus* and *Staphylococcus epidermidis*. J Clin Microbiol. 1986;24:764–9.
26. Froggatt JW, Johnston JL, Galetto DW, et al. Antimicrobial resistance in nosocomial isolates of *Staphylococcus haemolyticus*. Antimicrob Agents Chemother. 1989;33:460–6.
27. Vazquez GJ, Archer GL. Antibiotic therapy of experimental *Staphylococcus epidermidis* endocarditis. Antimicrob Agents Chemother. 1980;17:280–5.
28. Lowy FD, Wexler WA, Steigbigel NH. Therapy of methicillin-resistant *Staphylococcus epidermidis* experimental endocarditis. J Lab Clin Med. 1982;100:94–8.
29. Berry A, Johnston JL, Archer GL. Imipenem therapy of experimental *Staphylococcus epidermidis* endocarditis. Antimicrob Agents Chemother. 1986;29:748–52.
30. Schwalbe RS, Stapleton JT, Gilligan PH. Emergence of vancomycin resistance in coagulase-negative staphylococci. N Engl J Med. 1987;316:927–31.
31. Centers for Disease Control. Nosocomial infection surveillance, 1984. Surveillance Summaries 1985;35(No. 1SS):17SS–29SS.
32. Ponce de Leon S, Wenzel R. Hospital-acquired bloodstream infection with *Staphylococcus epidermidis*, review of 100 cases. Am J Med. 1984;77:639–44.
33. Kirchoff LV, Sheagren JN. Epidemiology and clinical significance of blood cultures positive for coagulase-negative staphylococcus. Infect Control. 1985;6:479–86.
34. Kaye D. Infecting microorganism. In: Kay D, ed. Infective Endocarditis. Baltimore: University Park Press; 1976:43–54.
35. Caputo GM, Archer G, Calderwood SB, et al. Native valve endocarditis due to coagulase-negative staphylococci: Clinical and microbiologic features. Am J Med. 1987;83:619–25.
36. Ivert TSA, Dismukes WE, Cobbs CG, et al. Prosthetic valve endocarditis. Circulation. 1984;69:223–31.
37. Calderwood SB, Swinski LA, Waternaux CM, et al. Risk factors for the development of prosthetic valve endocarditis. Circulation. 1985;72:31–7.
38. Karchmer AW, Archer GL, Dismukes WE. *Staphylococcus epidermidis* prosthetic valve endocarditis: Microbiological and clinical observations as guide to therapy. Ann Intern Med. 1983;98:447–55.
39. Kobasa WD, Kaye KL, Shapiro T, et al. Therapy for experimental endocarditis due to *Staphylococcus epidermidis*. Rev Infect Dis. 1983;5:S533–S537.
40. Massanari RM, Donta ST. The eficacy of rifampin as adjunctive therapy in selected cases of staphylococcal endocarditis. Chest. 1978;73:371–5.
41. Archer GL, Vazquez GJ, Johnston JL. antibiotic prophylaxis of experimental methicillin-resistant *Staphylococcus epidermidis* endocarditis. J Infect Dis. 1980;142:725–31.
42. Maki DG, Weise CE, Sarafin HW. A semi-quantitative culture method for identifying intravenous catheter-related infection. N Engl J Med. 1977;296:1305–9.
43. Christensen GD, Bisno AL, Parisi JT, et al. Nosocomial septicemia due to multiply antibiotic-resistant *Staphylococcus epidermidis*. Ann Intern Med. 1982;96:1–10.
44. Liñares J, Sitges-Serra A, Garau J, et al. Pathogenesis of catheter sepsis: A prospective study with quantitative and semiquantitative cultures of catheter hub and segments. J Clin Microbiol. 1985;21:357–60.
45. Snydman DR, Murray SA, Kornfeld SJ, et al. Total parenteral nutrition-related infections; prospective epidemiologic study using semiquantitative methods. Am J Med. 1982;73:695–9.
46. Moyer MA, Edwards LD, Farley L. Comparative culture methods on 101 intravenous catheters: Routine, semiquantitative, and blood cultures. Arch Intern Med. 1983;143:66–9.
47. Shererty RJ, Falk RJ, Huffman KA, et al. Infections associated with subclavian Udall catheters. Arch Intern Med. 1983;143:52–6.
48. Chessbrough JS, Finch RG, Burden RP. A prospective study of the mechanisms of infection associated with hemodialysis catheters. J Infect Dis. 1986;154:579–89.
49. Raucher HS, Hyatt AC, Barzilai A, et al. Quantitative blood cultures in the evaluation of septicemia in children with Broviac catheters. J Pediatr. 1984;104:29–33.
50. Press OW, Ramsey PG, Larson EB, et al. Hickman catheter infections in patients with malignancies. Medicine. 1984;63:189–200.
51. Cooper GL, Hopkins CC. Rapid diagnosis of intravascular catheter-associated infection by direct gram-staining of catheter segments. N Engl J Med. 1985;312:1142–7.
52. Winston DJ, Dudnick DV, Chapin M, et al. Coagulase-negative staphylococcal bacteremia in patients receiving immunosuppressive therapy. Arch Intern Med. 1983;143:32–6.
53. Schoenbaum SC, Gardner P, Shillito J. Infections of cerebrospinal fluid shunts: Epidemiology, clinical manifestations, and therapy. J Infect Dis. 1975;131:543–52.
54. Mayhall CG, Archer NH, Lamb A, et al. Ventriculostomy-related infections: A prospective epidemiologic study. N Engl J Med. 1984;310:553–9.
55. Trump DL, Grossman SA, Thompson G, et al. CSF infections complicating the management of neoplastic meningitis: Clinical features and results of therapy. Arch Intern Med. 1982;142:583–6.
56. Dobrin RS, Day NK, Quie PG, et al. The role of complement, immunoglobulin, and bacterial antigen in coagulase-negative staphylococcal shunt nephritis. Am J Med. 1975;59:660–73.
57. Gombert ME, Landesman SH, Corrado ML, et al. Vancomycin and rifampin therapy for *Staphylococcus epidermidis* meningitis associated with CSF shunts. Report of three cases. J Neurosurg. 1981;55:633–6.
58. Archer GL, Tenenbaum MJ, Haywood HB III. Rifampin therapy of *Staphylococcus epidermidis*: Use in infections from indwelling foreign devices. JAMA. 1978;240:751–3.
59. Wald SL, McLaurin RL. Cerebrospinal fluid antibiotic levels during treatment of shunt infections. J Neurosurg. 1980;52:41–6.
60. Frame PT, McLaurin RL. Treatment of CSF shunt infections with intrashunt plus oral antibiotic therapy. J Neurosurg. 1984;60:354–60.
61. James HE, Walsh JW, Wilson HD, et al. Prospective randomized study of therapy in cerebrospinal fluid shunt infection. Neurosurgery. 1980;7;459–63.
62. Wang EEL, Prober CG, Hendrick BE, et al. Prophylactic sulfamethoxasole and trimethoprim in ventriculoperitoneal shunt surgery. JAMA. 1984;251:1174–7.
63. Slight PH, Gundling K, Plotkin SA, et al. A trial of vancomycin for prophylaxis of infections after neurosurgical shunts. N Engl J Med. 1985;312:921.
64. Oreopoulos DG, Khanna R, Williams P, et al. Continuous ambulatory peritoneal dialysis—1981. Nephron. 1982;30:293–303.
65. Gokal R. Peritonitis in continuous ambulatory peritoneal dialysis. J Antimicrob Chemother. 1982;9:417–9.
66. Rubin J, Rogers WA, Taylor HM, et al. Peritonitis during continuous ambulatory peritoneal dialysis. Ann Intern Med. 1980;92:7–13.
67. West TE, Walshe JJ, Krol CP, et al. Staphylococcal peritonitis in patients on continuous peritoneal dialysis. J Clin Microbiol. 1986;23:809–12.
68. Knight KR, Polak A, Crump J, et al. Laboratory diagnosis and oral treatment of CAPD peritonitis. Lancet. 1982;3:1301–4.
69. Dawson MS, Harford AM, Garner BK, et al. Total volume culture technique for the isolation of microorganisms from continuous ambulatory peritoneal dialysis patients with peritonitis. J Clin Microbiol. 1985;22:391–4.
70. DePaepe M, Belpaire F, Bogaert M, et al. Gentamicin for treatment of peritonitis in continuous ambulatory peritoneal dialysis. Lancet. 1981;2:424–5.
71. Krothapalli RK, Senekjian HO, Ayus JC. Efficacy of intravenous vancomycin in the treatment of gram-positive peritonitis in long-term peritoneal dialysis. Am J Med. 1983;75:345–8.
72. Boeschoten EW, Pietra PJGM, Krediet RT, et al. CAPD peritonitis: A prospective randomized trial of oral versus intraperitoneal treatment with cephradine. J Antimicrob Chemother 1985;16:789–97.
73. Baddour LM, Smalley DL, Kraus AP Jr, et al. Comparison of microbiologic characteristics of pathogenic and saprophytic coagulase-negative staphylococci from patients on continuous ambulatory peritoneal dialysis. Diagn Microbiol Infect Dis. 1986;5:197–205.
74. Latham RH, Running K, Stamm WE. Urinary tract infections in young adult women caused by *Staphylococcus saprophyticus*. JAMA. 1983;250:3063–6.
75. Wallmark G, Arremark I, Telander B. *Staphylococcus saprophyticus*: A frequent cause of acute urinary tract infection among female outpatients. J Infect Dis. 1978;138:791–7.
76. The Urinary Tract Infection Study Group. Coordinated multicenter study of norfloxacin versus trimethoprim-sulfamethoxasole treatment of symptomatic urinary tract infections. J Infect Dis. 1987;155:170–7.
77. Stamm WE, Wagner KF, Amsel R, et al. Causes of the acute urethral syndrome in women. N Engl J Med. 1980;303:409–15.
78. Lewis JF, Brake SR, Anderson DJ, et al. Urinary tract infection due to coagulase-negative staphylococcus. Am J Clin Pathol. 1982;77:736–9.
79. Sewell CM, Claridge JE, Young EJ, et al. Clinical significance of coagulase-negative staphylococci. J Clin Microbiol. 1982;16:236–9.
80. Wade JC, Schimpff SC, Newman KA, et al. *Staphylococcus epidermidis*: An increasing cause of infection in patients with granulocytopenia. Ann Intern Med. 1982;97:503–8.
81. Sanz MA, Such M, Rafecas FJ, et al. *Staphylococcus epidermidis* infections in acute myeloblastic leukemia patients fitted with Hickman catheters. Lancet. 1983;ii:1191–2.
82. Lowder JN, Lazarus HM, Herzig RH. Bacteremias and fungemias in oncologic patients with central venous catheters. Arch Intern Med. 1982;142:1456–9.
83. Pirsch JD, Maki DG. Infectious complications in adults with bone marrow transplantation and T-cell depletion of donor marrow. Ann Intern Med. 1986;104:619–31.
84. Bender JW, Hughes WT. Fatal *Staphylococcus epidermidis* sepsis following bone marrow transplantation. Johns Hopkins Med J. 1980;146:13–5.
85. Grossi EA, Culliford AT, Krieger KH, et al. A survey of 77 major infectious complications of median sternotomy: A review of 7,949 consecutive operative procedures. Ann Thorac Surg. 1985;40:214–23.
86. Bor HB, Rose RM, Modlin JF, et al. Mediastinitis after cardiovascular surgery. Rev Infect Dis. 1983;5:885–97.
87. Miholic J, Hudec M, Domanig E, et al. Risk factors for severe bacterial infections after valve replacement and aortocoronary bypass operations: Analysis of 246 cases by logistic regression. Ann Thorac Surg. 1985;40:224–8.
88. Fitzgerald RH, Nolan DR, Ilstrup DM, et al. Deep wound sepsis following total hip arthroplasty. J Bone Joint Surg [Am]. 1977;59-A:847–55.
89. Parker MA, Tuazon C. Cervical osteomyelitis: Infection due to *Staphylococcus epidermidis* in hemodialysis patients. JAMA. 1978;240:50–1.

90. Hunter G, Dandy D. The natural history of the patient with an infected total hip replacement. J Bone Joint Surg [Am]. 1977;59-B:293–7.
91. Salvati EA, Robinson RP, Zeno SM, et al. Infection rates after 3175 total hip and total knee replacements performed with and without a horizontal unidirectional filtered air-flow system. J Bone Joint Surg [Am]. 1982;64-A:525–35.
92. Inman RD, Gallegos KV, Brause BD, et al. Clinical and microbial features of prosthetic joint infection. Am J Med. 1984;77:47–53.
93. Fitzgerald RH, Bechtol CO, Eftekhar N, et al. Reduction of deep sepsis after total hip arthroplasty. Arch Surg. 1979;114:803–4.
94. Norden CW. A critical review of antibiotic prophylaxis in orthopedic surgery. Rev Infect Dis. 1983;5:928–32.
95. Goldstone J, Moore WS. Infection in vascular prostheses: Clinical manifestations and surgical management. Am J Surg. 1974;128:225–33.
96. Bandyk DF, Berni GA, Thiele BL, et al. Aorto-femoral graft infection due to *Staphylococcus epidermidis*. Arch Surg. 1984;119:102–8.
97. Wooster DL, Louch RE, Krajden S. Intraoperative bacterial contamination of vascular grafts: A prospective study. Can J Surg. 1985;28:407–9.
98. Bunt TJ. Sources of *Staphylococcus epidermidis* at the inguinal incision during peripheral revascularization. Am Surg. 1986;52:472–3.
99. Kaiser AB, Clayson KR, Mulherin JL, et al. Antibiotic prophylaxis in vascular surgery. Ann Surg. 1978;188:283–9.
100. Anday EK, Talbot GH. Coagulase-negative staphylococcus bacteremia—a rising threat in the newborn infant. Ann Clin Lab Sci. 1985;15:246–51.
101. Weinstein RA, Kabins SA, Nathan C, et al. Gentamicin-resistant staphylococci as hospital flora: epidemiology and resistant plasmids. J Infect Dis. 1982;145:374–82.
102. Gruskay JA, Abbasi S, Anday E, et al. *Staphylococcus epidermidis*-associated enterocolitis. J Pediatr. 1986;109:520–4.
103. Diamond JG. Intraocular management of endophthalmitis; a systematic approach. Arch Ophthalmol. 1981;99:96–9.
104. Puliafito CA, Baker As, Haaf J, et al. Infectious endophthalmitis. Review of 36 cases. Ophthalmology. 1982;89:921–9.
105. Weber DJ, Hoffman KL, Thoft RA, et al. Endophthalmitis following intraocular lens implantation: Report of 30 cases and review of the literature. Rev Infect Dis. 1986;8:12–20.
106. Peyman GA, Sanders DR. Treatment of endophthalmitis. In: Peyman GA, Sanders DR, eds. Advances in Uveal Surgery, Vitreous Surgery, and the Treatment of Endophthalmitis. East Norwalk, CT: Appleton-Century-Crofts; 1975:179.
107. Wohl B, Peters RW, Carliner N, et al. Late unheralded pacemaker pocket infection due to *Staphylococcus epidermidis*: A new clinical entity. PACE 1982;5:190–5.
108. Burkhardt BR, Fried M, Schnur PL, et al. Capsules, infection, and intraluminal antibiotics. Plast Reconstr Surg 1981;68:43–9.

175. CLASSIFICATION OF STREPTOCOCCI

ALAN L. BISNO

Streptococci are spherical or ovoid bacteria that grow in pairs or chains of varying lengths. Most are facultatively anaerobic, although some are obligate anaerobes. Streptococci are gram-positive, non-spore forming, catalase-negative, and ordinarily nonmotile. They have complex but variable nutritional requirements. Taxonomically, these organisms belong to the genus *Streptococcus*, of which there are over 20 identified species.[1] Some of these species are pathogenic for humans, most notably *Streptococcus pyogenes* and *Streptococcus pneumoniae*.

No single system of classification suffices to differentiate this heterogeneous group of organisms. Instead, classification depends on a combination of features including patterns of hemolysis observed on blood agar plates, antigenic composition, growth characteristics, biochemical reactions, and, more recently, genetic analyses.

When streptococci are cultivated on blood agar plates, notable differences in the surface morphologic characteristics (e.g., colony size, opacity) among individual strains are evident. Moreover, colonies of certain strains are surrounded by clear colorless zones within which the red cells in the medium have been completely lysed (Fig. 1). This pattern is designated β-hemolysis and is of considerable importance since it is exhibited by *S. pyogenes* and many of the other streptococci pathogenic for humans. A second group of organisms produces partial or α-hemolysis. Careful observation of α hemolytic strains under the microscope reveals an inner zone of unhemolyzed cells and an outer zone of hemolysis. α-Hemolytic colonies also produce a greenish discoloration in the medium. This greening reaction, which varies with the type of blood in the medium and the duration of incubation, gives rise to the term *viridans streptococci*, frequently applied to α-hemolytic strains. Pneumococci are α-hemolytic, as are many of the other streptococcal strains that normally inhabit the upper respiratory and gastrointestinal tract of humans. Finally, the term γ-hemolysis has been used to designate strains producing no hemolysis, although the term *nonhemolytic streptococci* is to be preferred.

More precise identification of the β-hemolytic streptococci was accomplished by Lancefield[2] who succeeded in differen-

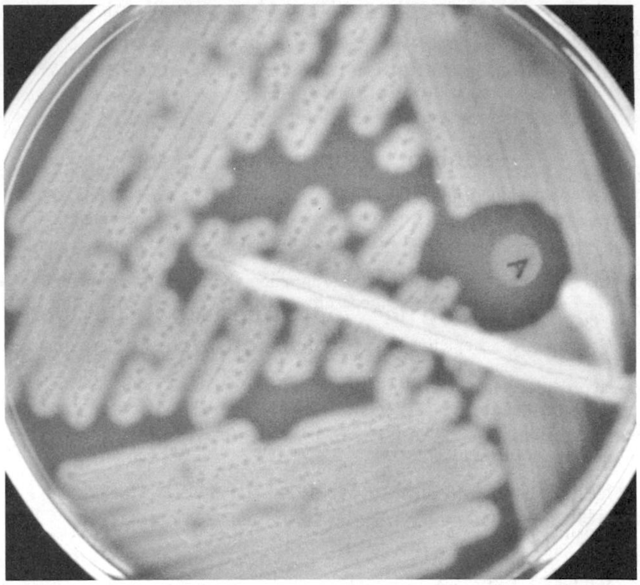

FIG. 1. Group A streptococci growing in pure culture on a sheep blood agar plate. Individual colonies are surrounded by zones of complete (β) hemolysis. Subsurface hemolysis (agar stab) is due in part to the action of streptolysin O, which is oxygen labile. The zone of inhibition around a low-potency bacitracin disk is a presumptive test for group A organisms.

TABLE 1. Streptococcal Serogroups Most Frequently Involved in Human Disease

Serogroup	*Group Specific Cell Wall Antigen*	*Usual Clinical Features*
A	Rhamnose-*N*-acetylglucosamine polysaccharide	Pharyngitis, tonsillitis, otitis media, sinusitis, scarlet fever, erysipelas, cellulitis, impetigo, pneumonia, endometritis, septicemia Delayed nonsuppurative sequelae: acute rheumatic fever, acute glomerulonephritis
B	Rhamnose-glucosamine polysaccharide	Chorioamnionitis, puerperal sepsis, neonatal sepsis and meningitis
C	Rhamnose-*N*-acetylgalactosamine polysaccharide	Upper respiratory infections
D	Glycerol teichoic acid	Genitourinary tract infections, wound infections, endocarditis
G	Rhamnose-galactosamine polysaccharide	Upper respiratory infections, cellulitis, septicemia, deep-tissue infections

tiating these organisms into serogroups by means of antigenic differences in cell wall carbohydrates. Group-specific antigens are readily extracted from streptococcal cell walls and identified by precipitin reactions using specific antisera. To date, serogroups A to H and K to V have been designated. Groups A, B, C, D, and G are those most commonly found in humans (Table 1); groups E, L, P, U, and V are isolated from humans rarely if at all.

Although the Lancefield grouping system was initially devised for the identification of β-hemolytic streptococci, certain α-hemolytic and nonhemolytic strains also contain group-specific antigen. Notable among these are group D streptococci, including the so-called enterococci, most strains of which fail to exhibit β-hemolysis. It has recently been proposed, however, that the enterococci be recognized as a separate genus.[3] The enterococci, which are significant causes of human disease, are discussed in detail in Chapter 179.

Streptococci that lack a recognizable group antigen are identified by physiologic tests that include fermentation reactions, growth at 10°C and 45°C, and growth in broth containing a high salt content. Three species of anaerobic streptococci and three species of microaerophilic streptococci are recognized in the most recent revision of *Bergey's Manual*. Hemolytic reactions of the organisms are variable. No satisfactory method of classification has been devised. These organisms are at times associated with human infections, particularly infections occurring in necrotic tissues (see also Chapter 224).

REFERENCES

1. Hardie JM. Genus *Streptococcus* Rosenbach 1884, 22[AL]. In: Holt JG, Sneath P, eds. Bergey's Manual of Systemic Bacteriology. v. 2. Baltimore: Williams & Wilkins; 1986:1043–71.
2. Lancefield RC. A serological differentiation of human and other groups of hemolytic streptococci. J Exp Med. 1933;57:571–95.
3. Schleifer KH, Kilpper-Balz R. Transfer of *Streptococcus faecalis* and *Streptococcus faecium* to the genus *Enterococcus* nom. rev. as *Enterococcus faecalis* comb. nov. and *Enterococcus faecium* comb. nov. Int J Syst Bacteriol. 1984;34:31–34,220–223.

176. STREPTOCOCCUS PYOGENES

ALAN L. BISNO

Streptococcus pyogenes (group A streptococcus) is one of the most important bacterial pathogens of humans. This ubiquitous organism is the most frequent bacterial cause of acute pharyngitis, and it also gives rise to a variety of cutaneous and systemic infections. Its unique place in medical microbiology stems from its propensity to initiate two nonsuppurative sequelae: acute rheumatic fever (ARF) and poststreptococcal acute glomerulonephritis (AGN). The former malady has been responsible for suffering, disability, and mortality in all parts of the world.

HISTORY

Streptococci were demonstrated in cases of erysipelas and wound infections by Billroth in 1874 and in the blood of a patient with puerperal sepsis by Pasteur in 1879. Fehleisen, in 1883, isolated chain-forming organisms in pure culture from erysipelas lesions and then demonstrated that these organisms could induce typical erysipelas in humans. Rosenbach applied the designation *Streptococcus pyogenes* to these organisms in 1884. Nevertheless, a variety of other appellations, now obsolete, such as *Streptococcus erysipelatos, Streptococcus scarlatinae*, and *Streptococcus hemolyticus* were applied from time to time.

Initial progress toward a rational classification of streptococci dates from the description by Schötmuller in 1903 of the blood agar technique for differentiating hemolytic from nonhemolytic streptococci. In 1919 J. H. Brown[1] made a systematic study of patterns of hemolysis and introduced the terms α-, β-, and γ-hemolysis (see Chapter 175).

Lancefield's classification of β-hemolytic streptococci into distinct serogroups in 1933[2] was a major turning point in our understanding of the epidemiology of streptococcal infections. Most strains pathogenic for humans were found to belong to serogroup A (*S. pyogenes*). Systems of serotyping group A streptococci were developed on the basis of M-protein precipitin reactions (Lancefield) or T-protein agglutination reactions (Griffith). In addition, Lancefield established the critical role of M protein in streptococcal virulence and the type-specific nature of protective immunity to group A streptococcal infection. Studies by Dochez and collaborators and by the Dicks in the 1920s established the relationship of scarlet fever to hemolytic streptococcal infection. A few years later, Todd's description of the method for titration of anti-streptolysin O (ASO) in serum added still another important tool to the armamentarium available for study of the immunology and epidemiology of streptococcal disease. Such tools were used by a number of investigators including Coburn, Collis, Rammelkamp, Stollerman, and Wannamaker to establish the relationship of group A streptococcal infection to ARF and AGN. Much of our modern knowledge of the detailed epidemiology of streptococcal infections and of ARF derives from the pioneering studies performed at Warren Air Force Base, Wyoming, during the years 1949–1951 by Rammelkamp, Wannamaker, and Denny.[3–5]

DESCRIPTION OF THE PATHOGEN

Group A streptococci grow as spherical or ovoid cells 0.6–1.0 μm in diameter and occur as pairs or as short to moderate-sized chains in clinical specimens. When growing in broth media enriched with serum or blood, long chains are frequently formed, and many strains produce capsules of hyaluronic acid. The organisms are gram-positive, nonmotile, non-spore forming, catalase-negative, and facultatively anaerobic. Group A streptococci are nutritionally fastidious and are usually cultivated in complex media, often supplemented with blood or serum.

When cultivated on blood agar plates, *Streptococcus pyogenes* appears as white to gray colonies 1 to 2 mm in diameter surrounded by zones of complete ("β") hemolysis. (Strains that fail to produce surface hemolysis occur but are rare.) Strains that produce copious amounts of the hyaluronate capsular material appear mucoid, at times resembling a water drop on the plate. Less mucoid strains assume a crinkled, so-called *matt* appearance. Small opaque colonies of organisms that lack capsules and detectable M protein are termed *glossy*.

A large number of somatic constituents and extracellular products of group A streptococci have been identified. The most important of these are indicated in the following sections.

Somatic Constituents

Figure 1 is a schematic representation of the group A streptococcal cell. The organism is enveloped in a hyaluronic acid capsule that serves as an accessory virulence factor in retarding phagocytosis by polymorphonuclear leukocytes and macrophages of the host. The cell wall is a complex structure containing many different antigenic substances. The group-specific carbohydrate of group A strains is a dimer of rhamnose and *N*-acetylglucosamine in a ratio of approximately 2:1. The mucopeptide (peptidoglycan) layer provides rigidity to the cell wall; it is composed of polymers of repeating subunits of *N*-acetyl-

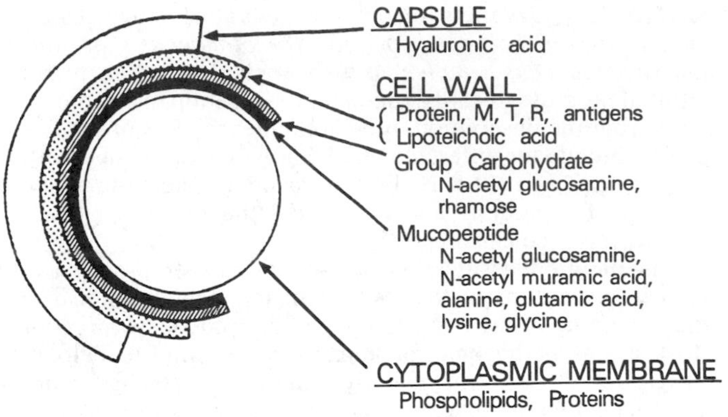

FIG. 1. Schema of group A streptococcal cell indicates somatic constituents of major biologic interest. (Modified from Krause,[6] with permission.)

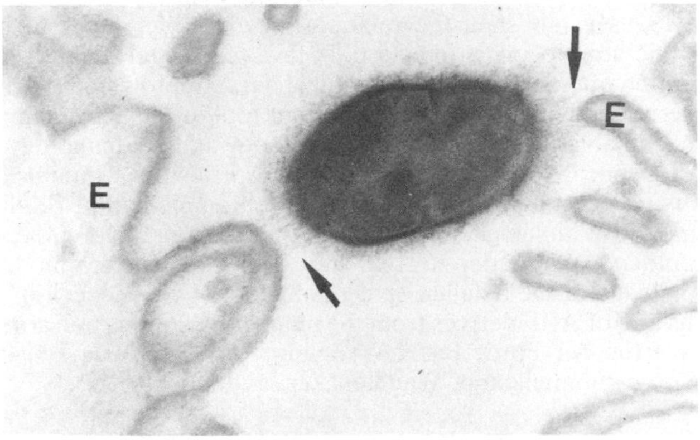

FIG. 2. Electron micrograph of group A streptococcus. Surface fibrils contain type-specific, antiphagocytic epitopes of M protein. Fibrils also participate in attachment of the streptococcal cell to the membrane (arrows) of a human oral epithelial cell (E). (×67,500) (From Beachey EH et al.,[8] with permission.)

glucosamine and *N*-acetylmuramic acid connected by amino acid side chains.

M protein is the major virulence antigen of group A streptococci. Strains rich in this protein are resistant to phagocytosis by polymorphonuclear leukocytes, multiply rapidly in fresh human blood, and are capable of initiating disease. Strains lacking M protein are avirulent.[7] Group A streptococci may be divided into serotypes on the basis of antigenic differences in M-protein molecules. Over 80 such serotypes are currently recognized. Acquired human immunity to streptococcal infection is based on the development of opsonic antibodies directed against the antiphagocytic moiety of M protein. Such immunity is type specific and quite durable, lasting for many years and perhaps indefinitely. In some instances, cross-protection by antibody to one type against organisms of a heterologous type has been demonstrated.

The M-protein molecule penetrates the cell wall; this configuration localizes the type-specific moiety on the tips of hair-like fibrils protruding from the cell surface (Fig. 2). The manner in which M protein exerts its antiphagocytic effect is under current investigation. The protein prevents interaction of the streptococcal cell with complement components,[9] an effect that is enhanced by the ability of M protein to precipitate fibrinogen directly onto the bacterial surface.[10] This protective effect is nullified by the presence of adequate concentrations of type-specific antibody.

In addition to unique type-specific antigens, the M-protein molecule also contains common antigens (non-type-specific M antigens [NTSM], M-associated protein antigens [MAP]) shared by a wide variety of different M serotypes. Another protein antigen very closely associated with the M-protein molecule is the so-called serum opacity factor (OF). This factor is an α-lipoproteinase, which is detected by its ability to opacify horse serum. Strains of 16 of the currently identified M types are OF-positive, but the rest do not elaborate this antigen. All strains of OF-positive serotypes produce this substance, and OF is readily demonstrated in such strains even if they should lose their ability to produce detectable amounts of M protein. OF itself is antigenic and type specific, that is, its ability to opacify serum can be specifically inhibited by antiserum raised against homologous but not heterologous M types. This substance is of importance for two reasons. First, it is a useful epidemiologic marker that assists in classifying streptococci even when they are not identifiable by M type. Second, type-specific and non-type-specific immune responses to streptococcal M protein are generally weaker after pharyngeal infection with OF-positive than with OF-negative serotypes.[7]

Many group A streptococcal strains cannot be serotyped by precipitin reactions using anti-M sera, either because they lack detectable M protein or because they belong to undesignated types for which antisera are not available. The latter situation pertains particularly in the case of many of the strains associated with pyoderma. Non-M-typable strains may frequently be identified by a subsidiary typing system using slide agglutination reactions and based on antigenic differences in T proteins. While T protein has proved to be a useful epidemiologic marker, it has no known role in streptococcal virulence.

Another cell wall constituent, lipoteichoic acid (LTA), is an important virulence factor in group A streptococci. This substance, which has a marked affinity for binding to biologic membranes, is responsible for the first step in colonization, namely, adherence of *S. pyogenes* to fibronectin on the surface of a human epithelial cell.[11] A recently characterized cell-bound peptidase cleaves the C5a component of complement and inhibits neutrophil chemotaxis in vitro and in vivo.[12]

Extracellular Products

During the course of growth in vitro or in vivo, group A streptococci elaborate numerous extracellular products, only a limited number of which have been well characterized. Streptococcal pyrogenic exotoxin, formerly known as erythrogenic toxin, is responsible for the rash of scarlet fever. Experimentally, this substance exhibits a variety of other toxic properties including pyrogenicity, cytotoxicity, and enhancement of susceptibility to the lethal effects of endotoxin. Toxin production is induced by lysogeny with a temperate bacteriophage. There are three serologically distinct toxins (A–C), the effects of which may be neutralized by antibody.

Two distinct hemolysins are elaborated. Streptolysin O derives its name from its oxygen lability. It is reversibly inhibited by oxygen and irreversibly inhibited by cholesterol. In addition to its effect on erythrocytes, it is toxic to a variety of cells and cell fractions including polymorphonuclear leukocytes, platelets, tissue culture cells, lysosomes, and isolated mammalian and amphibian hearts. Streptolysin O is produced by almost all strains of *S. pyogenes* (as well as many group C and G organisms) and is antigenic. Measurement of ASO antibodies in human sera has proved exceedingly useful as an indicator of recent streptococcal infection.

Streptolysin S is a hemolysin produced by streptococci growing in the presence of serum (hence the "S") or in the presence of a variety of other substances such as serum albumin, α-lipoprotein, ribonucleic acid, or detergents such as Tween. Streptolysin S is nonantigenic, or at least no antibody to it has been detected that will neutralize its hemolytic activity. Streptolysin S shares with streptolysin O the capacity to damage the membranes of polymorphonuclear leukocytes, platelets, and subcellular organelles. Unlike streptolysin O, it is not inactivated by oxygen, but it is quite thermolabile. Most strains of *S. pyogenes* produce both hemolysins. Hemolysis on the surface of blood agar plates is due primarily to streptolysin S, whereas streptolysin O exerts its hemolytic effect best in subsurface colonies (Fig. 1, Chapter 175), in pour plates, or in anaerobic cultures. An occasional strain may produce only one of the two hemolysins. Rarely, strains are encountered that lack both hemolysins.

Several extracellular products may, theoretically, serve to facilitate the liquefaction of pus and the spreading of streptococci through tissue planes. These include (*1*) four antigenically distinct enzymes that participate in the degradation of deoxyribonucleic acid (DNases A, B, C, and D); (*2*) hyaluronidase, which enzymatically degrades hyaluronic acid found in the ground substance of connective tissue; and (*3*) streptokinase, which promotes the dissolution of clots by catalyzing the conversion of plasminogen to plasmin. Still other known extracellular products are nicotinamide adenine dinucleotidase (NADase), proteinase, amylase, and esterase. Most of the substances just enumerated are antigenic. Antibodies to five of the extracellular products have been used in the serodiagnosis of streptococcal infection. These are ASO, anti-DNase B, antihyaluronidase, anti-NADase, and antistreptokinase.

The two most frequent clinical manifestations of streptococcal infection, pharyngitis and pyoderma, differ markedly in their epidemiologic, clinical, and bacteriologic characteristics.[13] Therefore, they are discussed separately.

STREPTOCOCCAL PHARYNGITIS

Epidemiology

Streptococcal sore throat is among the most common bacterial infections of childhood. Group A streptococci are responsible for the great majority of such infections, but strains of other serogroups, especially groups C and G, may be occasionally involved. The disease occurs primarily among children 5–15 years of age, with the peak incidence occurring during the first few years of school. All age groups are susceptible, however, and severe epidemics are common in military training facilities. There is no sex predilection. The disease is ordinarily spread by direct person-to-person contact, most likely via droplets of saliva or nasal secretions. Crowding such as occurs in schools or barracks favors interpersonal spread of the organism (Fig. 3) and may also enhance its virulence by processes of natural selection analagous to those that occur during mouse passage in the laboratory. The effect of crowding in facilitating transmission may account in part for the increased incidence of streptococcal pharyngitis in northern latitudes during the colder months of the year.

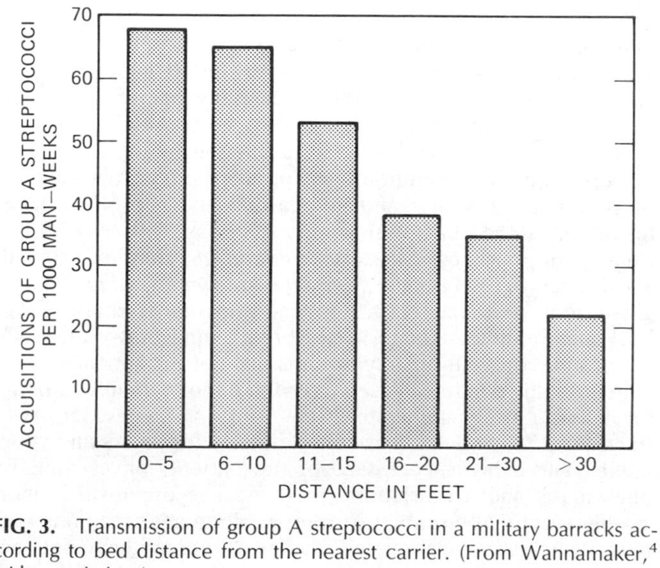

FIG. 3. Transmission of group A streptococci in a military barracks according to bed distance from the nearest carrier. (From Wannamaker,[4] with permission.)

Explosive food- or water-borne outbreaks are also well documented. Contamination of dust, clothing, blankets, or other fomites does not play a significant role in contagion.

Group A streptococci frequently colonize the throats of asymptomatic persons. Pharyngeal carriage rates among normal schoolchildren vary with geographic location and season of the year. Carriage rates of 15–20 percent have been noted in several studies. The carriage rate among adults is considerably lower.

Studies of experimentally induced human infections and of transmission within military barracks have shed considerable light on the variables involved in interpersonal spread. During the acute phase of tonsillopharyngeal infection, M-typable group A streptococci are frequently present in large numbers in both the nose and throat. In untreated infections, organisms may persist for many weeks, although the signs and symptoms of illness abate within a few days. During convalescence, the organisms decrease in numbers, and they tend to disappear from the anterior nares sooner than from the throat. In addition, the M-protein content and virulence of persisting organisms gradually decline. The result of these qualitative and quantitative changes is that convalescent carriers are much less likely to transmit the organism to close contacts than are acutely infected persons (Fig. 4).

In patients who do not receive effective antibiotic therapy, type-specific antibodies are frequently detectable in the serum between 4 and 8 weeks after the infection. These opsonic antibodies protect against subsequent infection with organisms of the same M type, but the person remains susceptible to infection by heterologous types. Prompt and effective antibiotic therapy ablates the type-specific immune response.

Clinical Manifestations

The usual incubation period of streptococcal pharyngitis is 2–4 days. The onset of illness is heralded by the rather abrupt onset of sore throat accompanied by malaise, feverishness, and headache. Nausea, vomiting, and abdominal pain are common in children. Prominent physical findings include redness, edema, and lymphoid hyperplasia of the posterior portion of the pharynx; enlarged, hyperemic tonsils studded with grayish white exudate; enlarged, *tender* lymph nodes at the angles of the mandibles; and a temperature of 101°F or higher. In the absence of the aforementioned symptoms and signs, simple coryza, hoarseness, cough, or conjunctivitis do not suggest the

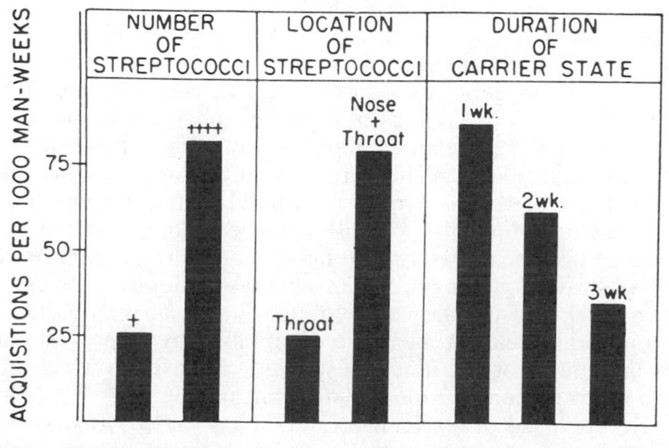

FIG. 4. Characteristics of individuals colonized with group A streptococci that influence communicability. Data were obtained in studies of military recruit populations. (From Rammelkamp,[3] with permission.)

presence of streptococcal infection. Laboratory findings include a positive throat culture for β-hemolytic streptococci and a total white blood cell count usually exceeding 12,000/mm^3 with increased numbers of polymorphonuclear leukocytes. The test for C-reactive protein is usually positive.

Not all patients with streptococcal pharyngitis have the full-blown syndrome just described. Endemically occurring infections in open populations manifest a wide spectrum of clinical severity. For example, only about half such patients with sore throats and positive throat cultures will have tonsillar or pharyngeal exudates. Patients who have undergone tonsillectomy tend to experience a milder clinical syndrome. In infants, the response to streptococcal infection is much less sharply focalized to the lymphoid tissue of the faucial and posterior pharyngeal area. Rhinorrhea, suppurative complications, low-grade fever, and a more protracted course tend to characterize infections at this age. Exudative pharyngitis in children less than 3 years of age is rarely streptococcal in etiology.

In the absence of suppurative complications, the disease is self-limited. Fever abates within 3–5 days. Virtually all acute signs and symptoms subside within a week, although several additional weeks may be required for tonsils and lymph nodes to return to their usual size. Penicillin shortens the period of fever and toxicity. Given the rather brief time course of untreated disease, however, such shortening of the clinical syndrome may not be striking unless therapy is initiated within the first 24 hours of illness.

Scarlet Fever. Scarlet fever results from infection with a streptococcal strain that elaborates streptococcal pyrogenic exotoxin (erythrogenic toxin). Although this disease is usually associated with pharyngeal infections, it may follow streptococcal infections at other sites such as wound infections or puerperal sepsis. Toxin production is dependent on lysogeny of the infecting streptococcus by a temperate bacteriophage. The clinical syndrome is similar in most respects to that associated with nontoxigenic strains, save for the scarlatinal rash. The latter must be differentiated from viral exanthems, drug eruptions, and particularly the rashes of toxic shock syndrome and Kawasaki disease.

The rash usually appears on the second day of clinical illness as a diffuse red blush with many points of deeper red that blanches on pressure. It is often first noted over the upper part of the chest and then spreads to the remainder of the trunk, neck, and extremities. The palms, soles, and usually the face are spared. Intradermal injection of scarlet fever antitoxin specifically neutralizes the toxin and causes blanching of the rash. This procedure (Schultz-Charlton reaction) is not used for diagnosis at the present time. Skin folds in the neck, axillae, groin, elbows, and knees appear as lines of deeper red (Pastia's lines). There are scattered petechiae, and the Rumpel-Leeds test of capillary fragility is positive. Occlusion of sweat glands imparts a sandpaper texture to the skin, a particularly helpful finding in dark-skinned patients.

The face appears flushed except for marked circumoral pallor. In addition to findings of exudative pharyngitis and tonsillitis, patients display an enanthem characterized by small, red, hemorrhagic spots on the hard and soft palate. The tongue is initially covered with a yellowish white coat through which may be seen the red papillae ("white strawberry tongue"). Later the coating disappears, and the tongue is beefy red in appearance ("red strawberry tongue"). The skin rash fades over the course of a week and is followed by extensive desquamation lasting for several weeks. A modest eosinophilia may be present early in the course of the illness, especially in cases in which both the rash and constitutional symptoms are slight.

Severe forms of scarlet fever, either associated with local and hematogenous spread of the organism (septic scarlet fever) or with profound toxemia (toxic scarlet fever), are characterized by high fever and marked systemic toxicity. The course may be complicated by arthritis, jaundice, and very rarely, hydrops of the gallbladder. Such severe forms of the disease are quite infrequent in the antibiotic era.

Intracutaneous administration of erythrogenic toxin in humans elicits local erythema (positive Dick test). No reaction occurs in persons with acquired immunity to the toxin. This test is not used clinically at the present time.

Recent reports have suggested the existence of a toxic shock-like syndrome due to *Streptococcus pyogenes*. The cases have occurred in adults, and in several instances the focus of infection has been a localized cellulitis or soft tissue infection. Patients have manifested a diffuse erythroderma, hypotension, mental status changes, and dysfunction of multiple organs including kidneys, liver, lungs, and heart.[14] The recent demonstration of an amino acid homology of nearly 50 percent between streptococcal pyrogenic exotoxin A and staphylococcal enterotoxin B, a putative mediator of nonmenstrual toxic shock syndrome, may explain the similarities in the syndromes caused by the two organisms.

Suppurative Complications. Inflammation in the faucial area induced by acute streptococcal infection may give rise to peritonsillar cellulitis, peritonsillar abscess, or retropharyngeal abscess. The abscesses themselves, however, frequently contain a variety of other oral flora including oral anaerobes, with or without group A streptococci. Direct extension of streptococci into adjacent structures may give rise to acute otitis media or acute sinusitis, which are among the most common suppurative complications of streptococcal pharyngitis. Suppurative cervical lymphadenitis may also occur. Extension up the cribriform plate of the ethmoid or via the mastoid bone may cause meningitis, brain abscess, or thrombosis of the intracranial venous sinuses. Streptococcal pneumonia, another potential suppurative complication, is discussed later.

Finally, bacteremic spread of the streptococci may result in a variety of metastatic foci of infection, for example, suppurative arthritis, endocarditis, meningitis or brain abscess, osteomyelitis, liver abscess, and so forth. Such complications are extremely rare since the advent of effective chemotherapy.

Nonsuppurative Complications. Nonsuppurative complications of streptococcal pharyngitis, ARF and AGN, are discussed in Chapter 177. The role of streptococci vis-à-vis other infectious and noninfectious agents in initiating certain other acute inflammatory disorders such as erythema nodosum and anaphylactoid purpura remains unresolved.

Diagnosis

Pharyngitis and tonsillitis may be due to a variety of infectious agents other than *Streptococcus pyogenes* (Chapter 43). *Corynebacterium diphtheriae*, the other major bacterial pathogen associated with exudative pharyngitis, is rare now, and when it occurs in classic form, it is differentiated by the appearance of the diphtheritic membrane, respiratory embarrassment, severe systemic toxicity, and myocardial and neurologic manifestations. Other bacterial agents such as *Neisseria gonorrhoeae* and, perhaps. *Neisseria meningitidis* may occasionally cause pharyngitis, as may *Mycoplasma pneumoniae*. Pharyngitis due to oral anaerobes (Vincent's angina) is characterized by a membranous exudate, fetid breath, and oral ulcerations. Fever and constitutional symptoms are not prominent.

Pharyngitis due to *Corynebacterium haemolyticum*, although rare, may closely mimic that due to *S. pyogenes*.[15] *Corynebacterium haemolyticum* affects primarily teenagers and young adults, and a high percentage of the patients have exudative pharyngitis and a scarlatiniform rash. The organism is more readily identified on rabbit or human blood agar than on sheep blood agar. Although detailed studies of therapy have not been carried out, *C. haemolyticum* pharyngitis appears to respond to benzathine penicillin G or oral erythromycin. Another rare cause of acute pharyngitis is *Yersinia enterocolitica*.[16] Patients infected with this organism may appear quite ill and may or may not have associated enteric symptoms. When *Y. enterocolitica* pharyngitis is associated with disseminated yersinosis, the mortality may be appreciable. Diagnosis depends upon clinical clues because the organism is unlikely to be detected on routine throat cultures and antistreptococcal therapy is unavailing (see Chapter 207).

Most throat infections are viral in etiology. Infectious mononucleosis and adenovirus infections frequently give rise to exudative pharyngitis and thus may closely mimic streptococcal sore throat. Even when careful microbiologic techniques are used to detect bacteria, *Mycoplasma*, and viruses, no etiologic agent can be detected in approximately one-half of all cases of acute sore throat.[17]

Approximately one–quarter to one-third of all children complaining of sore throat have a positive throat culture for group A streptococci. Of these, about one-half can be demonstrated to have immunologically significant infection, as judged by a significant rise in serum titer of one or more antistreptococcal antibodies. Most of the remainder probably represent asymptomatic carriers since the average carriage rate among school-age children during the winter months is approximately 15 percent. Such asymptomatic carriers are at no risk of developing suppurative or nonsuppurative complications and do not require antibiotic therapy. Thus, on the average, about 15 of every 100 children and adolescents with acute pharyngitis require treatment for streptococcal sore throat.

Numerous studies have tested the precision with which physicians may differentiate between streptococcal and nonstreptococcal sore throat by clinical criteria alone. In the presence of a scarlatinal rash or during a documented epidemic of streptococcal infections, such differentiation is easy. On the other hand, in the case of endemically occurring infections the problem is much more complex. Certain clinical findings, particularly tonsillopharyngeal exudate and *tender*, enlarged lymph nodes at the angles of the jaws, have a statistically significant correlation with the presence of positive throat cultures for group A streptococci.[18] Such findings are not diagnostic, however. For instance, only one-half of the patients with immunologically proven streptococcal sore throat have tonsillar exudate; conversely, one-half to three-quarters of all cases of exudative pharyngitis are nonstreptococcal in etiology. This percentage is even higher in children less than 3 years of age.

In two separate studies the presence of a positive throat culture was accurately predicted on clinical grounds alone in 55 percent and 75 percent of cases, respectively, while a negative throat culture was correctly predicted in 73 and 77 percent of cases.[19,20] Thus, even highly experienced clinicians using clinical impressions alone would fail to treat one-quarter to one-half of the patients with positive throat cultures and would needlessly treat one in four of the large number of persons who are neither infected nor colonized by group A streptococci. Algorithms using specific epidemiologic and clinical data have been devised to enhance the examiner's "batting average," but these remain less accurate than the culture.

For this reason, throat culture remains the preferred method for diagnosing streptococcal pharyngitis. Failure to isolate β-hemolytic streptococci in a carefully obtained and accurately interpreted throat culutre rules out the diagnosis of streptococcal sore throat for practical purposes. It is true that approximately 10 percent of negative throat cultures are weakly positive on reculture. While the significance of these false-negative cultures cannot be ascertained in a given patient, the phenomenon should not be a cause for undue concern. Most such cultures likely reflect streptococcal carriage rather than acute streptococcal infection. In cases where doubt exists as to the validity of a negative culture, it is usually preferable to repeat the culture than to treat empirically with antimicrobial agents.

While a negative culture eliminates the necessity for therapy, a positive culture does not differentiate between acute infection and asymptomatic carriage. Serum antibody titers do not rise until convalescence and are thus of no help in short-term management. Although the degree of positivity of the throat culture may assist in making this differentiation, it is best to assume that all positive cultures in patients with acute pharyngitis are significant and to treat accordingly, while recognizing that, even with the use of the throat culture, some degree of overtreatment is inevitable.

Detailed instructions for obtaining and processing a throat culture have been published by the American Heart Association.[21] Under direct visualization with good illumination, the cotton or Dacron swab should be rubbed over both tonsils, or tonsillar fossae, the oropharynx, and the nasopharynx posterior to the uvula. Care should be taken to avoid the tongue and buccal mucosa. After culturing, the swab should be rolled over a portion of the surface of a blood agar plate, and the inoculated plate should be streaked with a wire loop in a manner that will yield isolated colonies. A stab is made through the agar with the inoculation loop to permit subsurface growth. This allows observation of hemolysis due to the action of streptolysin O, which is oxygen labile.

Sheep blood agar is preferred because clear-cut patterns of hemolysis are obtained on this medium and because sheep blood inhibits the growth of *Haemophilus haemolyticus*, colonies of which appear similar to β-hemolytic streptococci on blood agar plates. Human blood from a blood bank is less desirable because the presence of type-specific antibodies, ASO antibodies, antibiotics, or high concentrations of citrate may inhibit the growth of streptococci or the expression of β-hemolysis. In regard to isolation of group A streptococci, there is controversy in the literature as to the relative merits of plain sheep blood agar plates vs. plates to which trimethoprim and sulfamethoxazole have been added to suppress competing normal pharyngeal flora. Similar controversy exists as to the optimal atmosphere of incubation: aerobic, aerobic in the presence of 5–10% carbon dioxide, or anaerobic.[22] If blood agar plates are not immediately available, the swab may be placed in a dry sterile tube for transportation to the laboratory. After overnight incubation at 35–37°C, culture plates from patients with streptococcal pharyngitis will show colonies surrounded by clear zones of hemolysis as well as β-hemolysis around the agar stab. Plates that are negative on first reading should be reexamined after an additional 24 hours of incubation. Serologic grouping of β-hemolytic streptococcal isolates may now be readily performed by using commercially available kits. A less expensive and highly serviceable screening procedure, the bacitracin sensitivity test, may be performed once the organism has been isolated in pure culture. This susceptibility procedure is based on the observation that greater than 95 percent of all group A streptococcal strains are inhibited by low-potency (0.04 units) bacitracin disks, while 80–90 percent of non-group A strains are resistant. Since no group A streptococci resistant to penicillin have yet been described, antibiotic testing is unnecessary if this drug is to be used. The same might be said for erythromycin since group A streptococci resistant to this drug are extremely rare in the United States at this time. The prevalence of erythromycin-resistant strains of *S. pyogenes* is higher in certain other parts of the world.[23]

Fluorescent antibody techniques provide excellent results and specifically identify group A organisms. No quantitative information is gained as to the degree of positivity of the culture. A variety of commercial kits are now available that use antibodies for the rapid detection of group A carbohydrate antigen directly from throat swabs. Indicator systems employed are latex agglutination or enzyme immunoassay, and the tests can be completed in a matter of minutes. Results obtained with the best of these kits are highly specific, so a positive reaction obviates the need for a throat culture. Unfortunately, the kits are somewhat less sensitive than are throat cultures,[22] and, therefore, immunologic tests may be negative in cases in which the conventional culture yields only a few streptococcal colonies. For this reason, physicians electing to use direct antigen tests should confirm negative test responses with a routine throat culture. This caveat applies with special force to epidemiologic settings in which the risk of acute rheumatic fever is appreciable (see Chapter 177).

Therapy

Therapy is directed toward the prevention of acute rheumatic fever and suppurative complications such as otitis media and acute sinusitis. Data on the preventability of poststreptococcal glomerulonephritis are less clear-cut. The drug of choice in the treatment of streptococcal infection is penicillin because its efficacy in the prevention of rheumatic fever is well established. Broader-spectrum, more expensive antibiotics such as ampicillin or amoxicillin are unnecessary.

Prevention of acute rheumatic fever requires eradication of the infecting streptococcus from the pharynx, an effect that depends on prolonged rather than high-dose penicillin therapy. This objective is efficientliy accomplished by the administration of a single injection of 1.2 million units of penicillin G benzathine. For children weighing less than 60 pounds, the dose is reduced to 600,000 units.[24] Many physicians elect to administer oral therapy. In this case, penicillin V, 250 mg three times a day, must be continued for a full 10 days. Even compliant patients, however, frequently find it difficult to remember to take the full course of oral therapy once they become asymptomatic.

In penicillin-allergic patients, erythromycin is the therapy of choice. Specific dosages vary somewhat with the preparation chosen but are in the range of 20–40 mg/kg/day divided into two to four equal doses, with the maximum daily dosage being 1 g. While twice-daily dosage appears satisfactory in children, data are lacking as to the efficacy of this dosage schedule in adults. Oral cephalosporins are effective in the treatment of streptococcal pharyngitis. They are useful in the penicillin-allergic patient whose allergy is not of the immediate type and who cannot tolerate oral erythromycin. The physician should bear in mind the possibility of an increased risk of allergic reactions to cephalosporins when treating penicillin-allergic patients.

Because tetracycline-resistant group A streptococci are prevalent in many areas, this drug is not recommended. Sulfonamides, which are highly effective in prophylaxis, are ineffective in the eradication of pharyngeal organisms or in the prevention of rheumatic fever when used as therapy for acute pharyngeal infections.

Treatment of group A streptococcal sore throat as long as 9 days after onset is still effective in the prevention of rheumatic fever.[25] Thus, if the patient is seen early in the course of his illness, the delay in initiation of therapy occasioned by obtaining a positive throat culture is not ordinarily a matter of concern. In the minority of patients, however, who are severely ill or toxic at presentation or who have evidence of sinusitis or otitis, antimicrobial therapy may be started at the initial visit after a throat culture has been obtained. Such therapy will reduce the period of infectivity and, if started early, shorten the duration of the clinical illness.[26] If oral therapy is prescribed, the throat culture serves as a guide to the necessity of completion of a full 10-day course or, alternatively, of recalling the patient for an injection of penicillin G benzathine. As discussed earlier, patients with signs and symptoms of acute pharyngitis and a positive test (properly performed and interpreted) for group A carbohydrate antigen should receive appropriate antimicrobial therapy.

Patients with more severe suppurative infections such as those involving the mastoid or ethmoid may require larger doses of penicillin (e.g., 600,000 units of penicillin G procaine intramuscularly once or twice a day or intravenous therapy with penicillin G). When streptococcal upper respiratory infection is complicated by the development of abscesses associated with suppurative cervical adenitis or in the peritonsillar or retropharyngeal soft tissues, incision and drainage are required.

Two aspects of therapy remain subject to debate. The first relates to the necessity for retreatment of "treatment failures." A variable percentage of patients, ranging from 5 to 30 percent, is found to harbor group A streptococci in the pharynx after completion of a course of penicillin. The incidence of failure is generally reported to be greater after oral than intramuscular therapy. Since prevention of rheumatic fever appears to require eradication of the streptococcus from the pharynx, such treatment failures are of concern. The causes for post-treatment culture positivity are multiple and include failure of compliance with oral medication schedules, reinfection with the same or different streptococcal types in the home or school environment, or true treatment failure. In everyday practice, it is usually impossible to differentiate between these alternatives.

True treatment failure is defined as reisolation of the original infecting streptococcal serotype shortly after completion of a full course of antibiotic therapy. It is sometimes associated with symptomatic relapse. Treatment failure occurs more frequently when the subject is a streptococcal carrier than it does among acutely infected individuals.[27] Recent reports suggest that the rate of treatment failure with oral and parenteral penicillin may be increasing somewhat. Proposed explanations for this phenomenon include the presence of β-lactamase-producing bacteria in the throat.[28] and the occurrence of penicillin tolerance among certain strains of group A streptococci.

The need for reculture of the throat after a course of antistreptococcal therapy is currently a matter of debate because the benefit–cost ratio of such cultures continues to decline in parallel with the incidence of acute rheumatic fever in developed countries. Certainly such cultures should be undertaken in high-risk circumstances (e.g., if the patient or a family member has a history of rheumatic fever) or when symptoms compatible with streptococcal infection persist or recur. Since 1985, rheumatic fever outbreaks have been reported in several areas of the United States in both civilian and military populations (see Chapter 177). In such areas, the approach to streptococcal infection must be particularly rigorous, and serious consideration should be given to routine performance of post-treatment cultures. Reculture is otherwise optional. If reculture is undertaken, only a single retreatment course is warranted for patients who still harbor group A streptococci.

The presence of persistently but weakly positive throat cultures after repeated courses of antibiotic therapy in an otherwise asymptomatic patient is not a cause for alarm. Such persons are streptococcal carriers[27] who are not at inordinate risk of developing rheumatic fever or of spreading their infection to others. Their most frequent problem is anxiety produced by multiple medical consultations and procedures associated with the streptococcal colonization. In the rare event in which, for medical or psychological reasons, eradication of chronic streptococcal carriage becomes highly desirable, recent data suggest that a combination of penicillin plus rifampin may be efficacious.[29,30]

A second unresolved issue relates to the management of family contacts of patients with streptococcal sore throat. Streptococcal acquisition rates of 25 percent or greater have been recorded in family contacts. Certainly, family contacts with symptoms of upper respiratory infection should be cultured and treated appropriately if positive. Asymptomatic family contacts should also be cultured in high-risk circumstances, e.g., the presence of a person in the family who has had rheumatic fever or known cases of rheumatic fever or poststreptococcal glomerulonephritis occurring in the general area. In situations of lesser risk, routine culture of asymptomatic family contacts is not recommended.[24]

There is no firm evidence to suggest that tonsillectomy reduces the incidence of rheumatic fever, either in healthy persons or in persons who have had rheumatic fever and faithfully maintained continuous antibiotic prophylaxis. In certain patients with recurrent bouts of tonsillopharyngitis, however, tonsillectomy may decrease the frequency of incapacitating acute infections. This potential benefit must be balanced against the possibility that tonsillectomized persons may be more likely to experience mild or subclinical infections that go unattended.

ERYSIPELAS

Erysipelas is an acute inflammation of the skin, with marked involvement of cutaneous lymphatic vessels, that is caused by group A streptococci. Occasionally group C strains are responsible. The disease, which occurs primarily in infants and in persons over 30 years of age, has become much less common in recent years. Erysipelas most often involves the face (Fig. 5), and in such cases there is usually a history of preceding streptococcal sore throat, although the exact mode of spread to the skin is unknown. When erysipelas involves the trunk or extremities, it often occurs at the site of a surgical incision or wound.

Clinically, the cutaneous inflammation is accompanied by chills, fever, and marked toxicity. The cutaneous lesion begins as a localized area of erythema and swelling and then spreads rapidly with advancing red margins, which are raised and well dermarcated from adjacent normal tissue. There is marked edema, often with bleb formation, and in facial erysipelas the eyes are frequently swollen shut. The lesion may demonstrate central resolution while continuing to extend on the periphery. Facial erysipelas most often resolves spontaneously in 4–10 days, whereas if untreated a lesion on the trunk or extremities may involve large areas of the body surface and terminate fatally. Treatment with penicillin is curative.

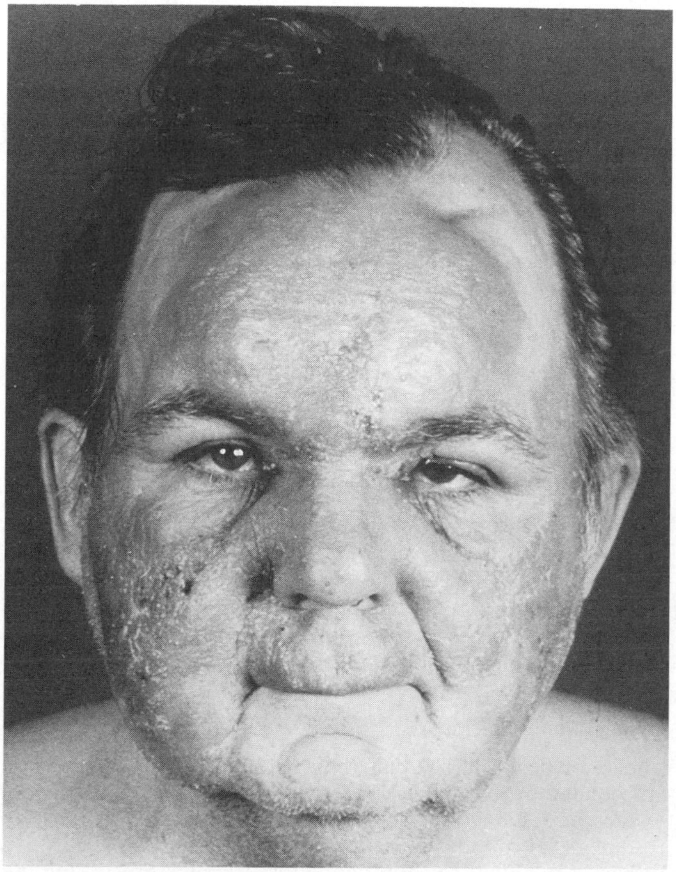

FIG. 5. Facial erysipelas. The lesion is well demarcated from surrounding skin and illustrates the typical "butterfly" distribution. (From Bisno,[31] with permission.)

STREPTOCOCCAL PYODERMA

Pyoderma is the term used collectively to denote localized purulent streptococcal infections of the skin. Some pyodermal lesions represent obvious secondary infections of wounds or burns. For the most part, however, the term is used synonymously with streptococcal impetigo or *impetigo contagiosa* to describe discrete purulent lesions that appear to be primary infections of the skin and that are extremely prevalent in many parts of the world.

Epidemiology

Pyoderma occurs most frequently among economically disadvantaged children dwelling in tropical or subtropical climates. It is also prevalent in northern climates during the summer months of the year in certain epidemiologic settings such as the American Indian reservations of Minnesota. The peak incidence of pyoderma is in children aged 2–5 years, as opposed to streptococcal pharyngitis, which occurs primarily in the 5- to 15-year-old age group. There is no sex predilection, and all races appear to be susceptible. The disease has been intensively studied, for example, among blacks in Mississippi and Alabama, American Indians in Minnesota, East Indians in Trinidad, and white military personnel in Vietnam.

The prevalence of pyoderma reaches extremely high levels in certain population groups. Among indigent black children attending Project Headstart classes during the summer in rural Mississippi, 40–50 percent were found to have identifiable pyodermal lesions in various stages of evolution. Eighty-five percent of children followed weekly throughout the summer had bacteriologically proven streptococcal impetigo[32]; most of these had multiple lesions. Recent reports from the United States and Europe have documented outbreaks of streptococcal pyoderma among workers in meat-packing plants who suffer numerous cutaneous cuts and abrasions.[33]

The prevalence of streptococcal pyoderma is markedly influenced by several factors, the most important of which appear to be climate and level of hygiene. Studies among Colombian school children[34] showed the lowest prevalence in Bogotà (8700 ft elevation, cool climate), intermediate prevalence in Medellin (5000 ft elevation, temperate climate), and highest incidence in Apartado (sea level, tropical climate). At each level of elevation, skin lesions were more frequent among persons with poor hygiene than among those with good hygiene (Fig. 6). Among Colombian military troops in the field, those conducting operations in humid tropical rain forests experienced a considerably greater incidence of pyoderma than those operating in the dry tropical savanna.

The mode of spread of streptococcal pyoderma is as yet poorly understood. Possible means of transmission include direct contact, environmental contamination, and arthropod vectors such as the *hippelates* fly, which has been shown to carry group A streptococci on its legs for periods of more than 24 hours.

Meticulous studies performed in children at Red Lake Indian Reservation, Minnesota[35] have demonstrated that the streptococci responsible for pyoderma initially colonize the unbroken skin, an observation that probably explains the influence of personal hygiene on disease incidence. Development of skin colonization with a given streptococcal type precedes the development of impetiginous lesions due to the same serotype by an average interval of 10 days (Fig. 7). The mechanism of production of skin lesions is unproved, but is most likely due to intradermal inoculation of surface organisms by abrasions, minor trauma, or insect bites. Lesions of scabies have also been

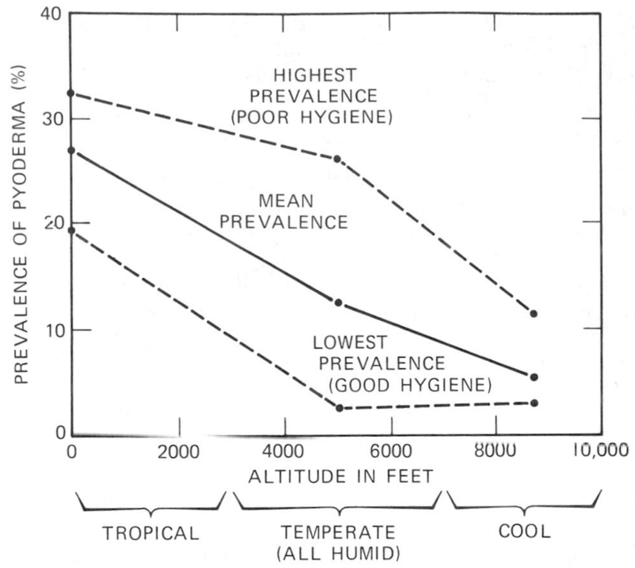

FIG. 6. Prevalence of pyoderma among lower socioeconomic class Colombian children in relation to altitude (climate) and level of hygiene. (From Taplin et al.,[34] with permission.)

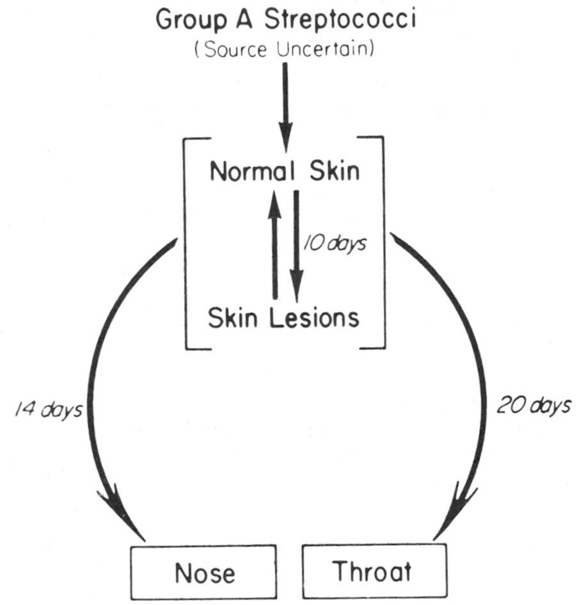

FIG. 7. Representative sequence of the spread of "pyoderma strains" of group A streptococci among different body sites. (From Ferrieri et al.,[35] with permission.)

demonstrated to harbor group A streptococci in Trinidad where epidemics of human scabies and of pyoderma-associated nephritis coexist. Frequently there is a transfer of the streptococcal strains from the skin and/or impetigo lesions to the upper respiratory tract. The interval between colonization of the skin and colonization of nose and/or throat averages 2–3 weeks (Fig. 7).

Bacteriologic Findings

Streptococci isolated from pyodermal lesions are primarily group A, but occasionally representatives of other serogroups such as C and G are responsible. Group A streptococci that cause impetigo differ in several respects from those usually associated with tonsillitis and pharyngitis. So-called skin strains belong to different M serotypes from the classic "throat strains"; since most have been identified in recent years, they tend to comprise the higher-numbered M types. There is a great multiplicity of M-protein types among the "skin strains," and many of these types have never been fully characterized and classified. As a result, many strains isolated from skin lesions are not typable with currently available batteries of M typing sera. Moreover, many pyodermal strains belong to "difficult" types that lose identifiable M protein rapidly on subculture in the laboratory and that are very weakly immunogenic in rabbits. Therefore, the M typing system is not entirely satisfactory for identifying "skin strains." This has led to increased use of the T-agglutination system. Unlike M protein, T antigen has no knnown biologic significance, but it is a stable, relatively easily measured epidemiologic marker by which the great majority of streptococcal strains can be categorized. Pyoderma streptococci are frequently not monotypic in their T typing reactions but tend to agglutinate several different typing sera, which gives rise to characteristic "pattern" reactions such as 3/13/B3264 and 8/25/imp 19. Each of these patterns may embrace several different M types, a fact that limits the utility of the T typing system at its current stage of development.

The well-known streptococcal M types that frequently give rise to exudative tonsillitis (e.g., types 1, 3, 5, 6, 12, 18, 19, 24, and others) are rarely found in skin lesions. On the other hand, as pointed out before, "skin strains" frequently colonize the throat. In populations in which pyoderma is hyperendemic, streptococcal carriage rates of 10–15 percent are seen during the warmer months, and most of these streptococci belong to "pyoderma" serotypes. For the most part, however, "skin strains" cause few or no symptoms when lodged in the throat. A relatively small number of serotypes seem capable of regularly initiating clinically apparent infection of both the skin and throat.[36]

Immunology

The ASO response after cutaneous streptococcal infection is weak. There is experimental evidence to suggest that this may be due to local inactivation of streptolysin O by skin lipids. Modest ASO responses are frequently observed when streptococcal pyoderma is accompanied by pharyngeal colonization. In contrast, the immune response to anti-DNase B is brisk; antihyaluronidase reactivity is also a useful test in the serodiagnosis of pyoderma.[37,38]

In uncomplicated pyoderma, type-specific opsonic antibodies are detectable 2–3 months after the development of infection. In one study[39] such antibodies were present in 12 percent of a small group of patients with pyoderma alone but in over half of the people who had concomitant pharyngeal carriage. In another study, type-specific antibodies were present in most patients convalescing from pyoderma-associated nephritis due to M type 55. It is not yet known whether such antibodies play a role in the prevention of reinfection analogous to that which has been established in pharyngeal infections. The existence of acquired immunity by whatever mechanism is suggested by the fact that, among American soldiers in Vietnam, pyoderma was more than 2.5 times as prevalent in whites as in blacks performing the same duties.

Clinical Manifestations

The lesion begins as a papule that rapidliy evolves into a vesicle surrounded by an area of erythema. The vesicular lesions are evanescent and rarely recognized clinically; they give rise to pustules that gradually enlarge and then break down over a period of 4–6 days to form characteristic thick crusts (Fig. 8). The lesions heal slowly and leave depigmented areas. A deeply ulcerated form of impetigo is known as *ecthyma*.

Streptococcal impetigo occurs on exposed areas of the body,

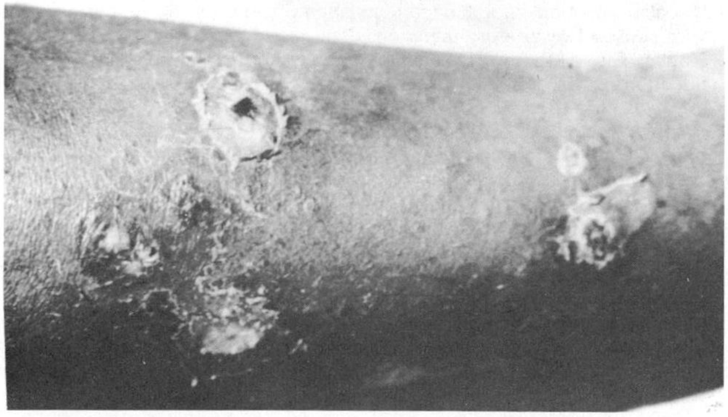

FIG. 8. Multiple pyoderma lesions on the lower extremities of rural Mississippi children. (Courtesy of Dr. K. Nelson, Baltimore, MD.)

most frequently on the lower extremities. The lesions remain well localized but are frequently multiple. Although regional lymphadenitis often occurs, systemic symptoms are not ordinarily present.

Adequate culture of crusted impetiginous lesions requires removal of the surface crusts and culture of the base of the lesions. If this is done, strongly positive cultures for group A streptococci are usually obtained, even from indolent-appearing lesions in later stages of healing. Staphylococci are often isolated as well but do not appear to be primary pathogens in this setting. The response to penicillin therapy is equally prompt whether or not the lesions contain penicillinase-producing staphylococci. Indeed, staphylococcal impetigo is a distinct entity that must be differentiated from that caused by *Streptococcus pyogenes*. Staphylococcal impetigo usually consists of bullous lesions that rupture and leave thin "varnishlike" crusts. Such bullae yield pure cultures of staphylococci, and often they are phage type 71.

Therapy and Prevention

Antibiotic treatment of streptococcal pyoderma is similar to that of pharyngitis. Intramuscular penicillin G benzathine, oral penicillin, or oral erythromycin all give excellent cure rates of 97 percent or higher. The exact duration of therapy is not firmly established; 10 days of treatment is advisable when oral regimens are used. Topical antibiotic or antiseptic preparations are much less effective and of course do not prevent the development of new lesions in untreated areas or terminate the frequently associated nasal and pharyngeal carrier state. A recent report indicating excellent clinical and bacteriologic results in clearing lesions with topical muciprocin awaits confirmation.[39a] Adherence to good regimens of personal hygiene, with special attention to frequent scrubbing with soap and water, is the most effective preventative measure currently available.

Complications

Although septicemia accompanies streptococcal impetigo on rare occasions, suppurative complications are on the whole most uncommon. For as yet unexplained reasons, rheumatic fever does not occur after streptococcal pyoderma (Chapter 177). On the other hand, cutaneous infections with nephritogenic strains of group A streptococci are the major antecedent of poststreptococcal glomerulonephritis in many areas of the world. There are as yet no conclusive data to indicate that treatment of an individual case of pyoderma will prevent the subsequent occurrence of nephritis in these patients. Such therapy is nevertheless important as an epidemiologic measure in eradicating nephritogenic strains from the environment.

OTHER STREPTOCOCCAL INFECTIONS

Streptococcal *cellulitis*, an acute, spreading inflammation of the skin and subcutaneous tissues, usually results from infection of burns or wounds. Recurrent episodes of cellulitis may occur in extremities in which lymphatic drainage has been impaired. Examples include patients with filariasis and women who have undergone radical mastectomy with axillary node dissection. Such episodes may be accompanied by high fever and prostration. Recurrent episodes of severe cellulitis have been reported in certain patients who have undergone coronary artery bypass grafts.[40] The cellulitis uniformly occurs in the extremity of the donor's saphenous vein, and patients with tinea pedis of the venectomy limb are particularly at risk.[41,42] Although pathogenic bacteria are difficult to recover during these episodes, the appearance of the lesions and the response to penicillin therapy suggest a streptococcal etiology. The few β-hemolytic streptococci that have been recovered and characterized belonged to serogroups other than group A.[43]

Lymphangitis may accompany cellulitis or may occur after clinically minor or inapparent skin infection. Lymphangitis is readily recognized by the presence of red, tender, linear streaks directed toward enlarged, tender regional lymph nodes. It is accompanied by systemic symptoms such as chills, fever, malaise, and headache. *Perianal cellulitis* or asymptomatic anal infection by group A streptococci has been the source of several reported outbreaks of hospital-acquired streptococcal infection. *Puerperal sepsis* follows abortion or delivery when streptococci colonizing the patient herself or transmitted from medical personnel invade the endometrium and surrounding structures, lymphatics, and blood stream. The resulting endometritis and septicemia may be complicated by pelvic cellulitis, septic pelvic thrombophlebitis, peritonitis, or pelvic abscess. This disease was associated with high mortality in the preantibiotic era. Although endocarditis due to *S. pyogenes* was relatively common in the preantibiotic era, it is now rarely seen.[44] Meningitis due to *S. pyogenes* usually follows upper respiratory infection and is indistinguishable clinically from other forms of acute pyogenic meningeal infection.[45]

Another rare but potentially life-threatening entity is streptococcal myositis.[46] It is characterized by severe pain and inflammation in the affected muscle, marked systemic toxicity, and elevated serum levels of creatine phosphokinase. Muscle compartment pressures may be elevated. Therapy includes aggressive surgical débridement and intravenous penicillin. Mortality in reported cases has been high. Streptococcal gangrene is discussed in Chapter 74.

Pneumonia due to *Streptococcus pyogenes* is now rare. When such cases do occur, they are frequently associated with preceding viral infections such as influenza, measles, or varicella or with chronic pulmonary disease. Numerous epidemics have been described in military recruit populations.[47] In one-third or fewer of the cases, there is a history of preceding streptococcal upper respiratory infection. The onset is typically abrupt, and the disease is characterized by chills, fever, dyspnea, cough productive of blood-streaked sputum, pleuritic chest pain, and in more severe cases, cyanosis. The pulmonary picture is that of bronchopneumonia with consolidation being uncommon. Empyema develops in 30–40 percent of the cases, tends to appear early in the disease, and typically consists of copious amounts of thin serosanguinous fluid. Bacteremia occurs in 10–15 percent of the cases. Complications include mediastinitis, pericarditis, pneumothorax, and bronchiectasis. Mortality is low with penicillin therapy and adequate drainage of empyema, but the clinical course of the disease is often prolonged.

REFERENCES

1. Brown JH. The Use of Blood Agar for the Study of Streptococci. New York: The Rockefeller Institute for Medical Research; 1919.

2. Lancefield RC. A serological differentiation of human and other groups of hemolytic streptococci. J Exp Med. 1933;57:571–95.
3. Rammelkamp CH Jr. Epidemiology of streptococcal infections. Harvey Lect. 1955–1956;51:113–42.
4. Wannamaker LW. The epidemiology of streptococcal infections. In: McCarty M, ed. Streptococcal Infections. New York: Columbia University Press; 1953:157–75.
5. Rammelkamp CH, Denny FW, Wannamaker LW. Studies on the epidemiology of rheumatic fever. In: Thomas L, ed. Rheumatic Fever. Minneapolis: University of Minnesota Press; 1952:72–89.
6. Krause RM. Antigenic and chemical composition of hemolytic streptococcal cell walls. Bacteriol Rev. 1963;27:369–80.
7. Widdowson JP, Maxted WR, Notley CM, et al. The antibody responses in man to infection with different serotypes of group A streptococci. J Med Microbiol. 1974;7:483–96.
8. Beachey EH, Ofek I. Epithelial cell binding of group A streptococci by lipoteichoic acid on fimbriae denuded of M protein. J Exp Med. 1976;143: 759–71.
9. Bisno AL. Alternate complement pathway activation of group A streptococci: Role of M protein. Infect Immun. 1979;26:1172–6.
10. Whitnack E, Beachey EH. Antiopsonic activity of fibrinogen bound to M protein on the surface of group A streptococci. J Clin Invest. 1982;69:1042–5.
11. Simpson WA, Courtney HS, Ofek I. Interactions of fibronectin with streptococci: The role of fibronectin as a receptor for *Streptococcus pyogenes*. Rev Infect Dis. 1987;9(Suppl):351–9.
12. O'Connor, Cleary SP. In vivo *Streptococcus pyogenes* C5a peptidase activity: Analysis using transposon- and nitrosoguanidine-induced mutants. J Infect Dis. 1987;156:495–504.
13. Wannamaker LW. Differences between streptococcal infections of the throat and of the skin. N Engl J Med. 1970;282:23–31, 78–85.
14. Cone LA, Woodard DR, Schlievert PM, et al. Clinical and bacteriologic observations of a toxic shock-like syndrome due to *Streptococcus pyogenes*. N Engl J Med. 1987;317:146–9.
15. Miller RA, Brancato F, Holmes KK. *Corynebacterium hemolyticum* as a cause of pharyngitis and scarlatiniform rash in young adults. Ann Intern Med. 1986;105:867–72.
16. Tacket CO, Davis BR, Carter GP, et al. *Yersinia enterocolitica* pharyngitis. Ann Intern Med. 1983;99:40–2.
17. Glezen WP, Clyde WA Jr, Senior RJ, et al. Group A streptococci, mycoplasmas, and viruses associated with acute pharyngitis. JAMA. 1967;202:455–60.
18. Kaplan EL, Top FH Jr, Dudding BA, et al. Diagnosis of streptococcal pharyngitis: Differentiation of active infection from the carrier state in the symptomatic child. J Infect Dis. 1971;123:490–501.
19. Breese BB, Disney FA. The accuracy of diagnosis of beta-streptococcal infections on clinical grounds. J Pediatr. 1954;44:670–3.
20. Siegel AC, Johnson EE, Stollerman GH. Controlled studies of streptococcal pharyngitis in a pediatric population. I. Factors related to the attack rate of rheumatic fever. N Engl J Med. 1961;265:559–66.
21. Rheumatic Fever Committee, American Heart Association. Throat Cultures for Rational Treatment of Sore Throat. New York: New York American Heart Association; 1972.
22. Kellogg JA, Manzella JP: Detection of group A streptococci in the laboratory or physician's office. JAMA. 1986;255:2638–42.
23. Maruyama S, Yoshioka H, Fujita K, et al. Sensitivity of a group A streptococci to antibiotics. Am J Dis Child. 1979;133:1143 5.
24. Committee on Rheumatic Fever, and Bacterial Endocarditis, and Kawasaki Disease. American Heart Association. Prevention of rheumatic fever. Circulation. 1988;78:1082–89.
25. Catanzaro FJ, Stetson CA, Morris AJ, et al. The role of the streptococcus in the pathogenesis of rheumatic fever. Am J Med. 1954;17:749–56.
26. Randolf MF, Garber MA, De Meokk, et al. Effect of antibiotic therapy on the clinical course of streptococcal pharyngitis. J Pediatr. 1985;106:870–5.
27. Kaplan EL, Gastanaduy AS, Huwe BB. The role of the carrier in treatment failures after antibiotic therapy for group A streptococci in the upper respiratory tract. J Lab Clin Med. 1981;98:326–35.
28. Brook I. The role of beta-lactamase-producing bacteria in the persistence of streptococcal tonsillar infection. Rev Infect Dis. 1984;6:601–7.
29. Tanz RR, Shulman ST, Barthel MJ, et al. Penicillin plus rifampin eradicates pharyngeal carriage of group A streptococci. J Pediatr. 1985;106:876–80.
30. Chaudhary S, Bilinsky SA, Hennessy JL, et al. Penicillin V and rifampin for the treatment of group A streptococcal pharyngitis: A randomized trial of 10 days penicillin with rifampin during the final 4 days of therapy. J Pediatr 1985;106:481–6.
31. Bisno AL. Cutaneous infections: Microbiologic and epidemiologic considerations. Am J Med. 1984;76(5A):172–9.
32. Nelson KE, Bisno AL, Waytz P, et al. The epidemiology and natural history of streptococcal pyoderma. An endemic disease of the rural southern United States. Am J Epidemiol. 1976;103:270–83.
33. Fehrs LJ, Flanagan K, Kline S, et al. Group A beta-hemolytic streptococcal skin infections in a U.S. meat-packing plant. JAMA. 1987;258:3131–4.
34. Taplin D, Lansdell L, Allen AM, et al. Prevalence of streptococcal pyoderma in relation to climate and hygiene. Lancet. 1973;1:501–3.
35. Ferrieri P, Dajani AS, Wannamaker LW, et al. Natural history of impetigo. I. Site sequence of acquisition and familial patterns of spread of cutaneous streptococci. J Clin Invest. 1972;51:2851–63.
36. Anthony BF, Kaplan EL, Wannamaker LW, et al. The dynamics of streptococcal infections in a defined population of children: Serotypes associated with skin and respiratory infections. Am J Epidemiol. 1976;104:652–66.
37. Kaplan EL, Anthony BF, Chapman SS, et al. The influence of the site of infection on the immune response to group A streptococci. J Clin Invest. 1970;49:1405–14.
38. Bisno AL, Nelson KE, Waytz P, et al. Factors influencing serum antibody response in streptococcal pyoderma. J Lab Clin Med. 1973;81:410–20.
39. Bisno AL, Nelson KE. Type-specific opsonic antibodies in streptococcal pyoderma. Infect Immun. 1974;10:1356–61.
39a. Melinn S. Topical muciprocin vs. systemic erythromycin treatment for pyoderma. Pediatr Infect Dis. 1988;7:785–90.
40. Baddour LM, Bisno AL. Recurrent cellulitis after saphenous venectomy for coronary bypass surgery. Ann Intern Med. 1982;97:493–6.
41. Greenberg J, DeSanctis R, Mills RM Jr. Vein-donor-leg cellulitis after coronary artery bypass surgery. Ann Intern Med. 1982;97:565–6.
42. Baddour LM, Bisno AL. Recurrent cellulitis after coronary bypass surgery: Association with superficial fungal infection in saphenous venectomy limbs. JAMA. 1984;251:1049–52.
43. Baddour LM, Bisno AL. Non-group A beta-hemolytic streptococcal cellulitis: Association with venous and lymphatic compromise. Am J Med. 1985;79:155–9.
44. Ramirez CA, Naraqi S, McCulley DJ. Group A beta-hemolytic streptococcus endocarditis. Am Heart J. 1984;108:1383–6.
45. Murphy DJ Jr. Group A streptococcal meningitis. Pediatrics. 1983;71:1–5.
46. Adams EM, Gudmundsson S, Yocum DE, et al. Streptococcal myositis. Arch Intern Med. 1985;145:1020–3.
47. Basiliere JL, Bistrong HW, Spence WF. Streptococcal pneumonia: Recent outbreaks in military recruit populations. Am J Med. 1968;44:580–9.

177. NONSUPPURATIVE POSTSTREPTOCOCCAL SEQUELAE: RHEUMATIC FEVER AND GLOMERULONEPHRITIS

ALAN L. BISNO

RHEUMATIC FEVER

Acute rheumatic fever (ARF) is a disease characterized by nonsuppurative inflammatory lesions involving primarily the heart, joints, subcutaneous tissues, and central nervous system. In its classic form, the disorder is acute, febrile, and largely self-limited. However, damage to heart valves may occur, and such damage may be chronic and progressive and lead to severe cardiac failure, total disability, and not infrequently, death many years after the acute attack. ARF is extremely variable in its manifestations; it remains, basically, a clinical syndrome for which no specific diagnostic test exists. Insofar as is known, all cases of ARF follow group A streptococcal upper respiratory tract infection, although the exact mechanisms mediating development of the disease remain speculative. Persons who have suffered an attack of ARF are particularly predisposed to recurrent episodes after subsequent group A streptococcal infections.

HISTORY

Guillaume de Baillou (1538–1616), also known as "Ballonius," first clearly distinguished acute arthritis from gout. Thomas Sydenham (1624–1689) described chorea but failed to associate this entity with other manifestations of ARF. Raymond Vieussens (1641–1715) published pathologic descriptions of mitral stenosis and aortic insufficiency. It remained, however, for William Charles Wells in 1812 to emphasize the association of rheumatism and carditis and to provide the first clear description of subcutaneous nodules. Jean-Baptiste Bouillard in 1836 and Walter B. Cheadle in 1889 published extensive studies of rheumatic arthritis and carditis that have come to be regarded as classic works in this field and form the basis for modern clinical concepts of ARF. The specific rheumatic lesion in the myocardium was described by Ludwig Aschoff in 1904.

J. K. Fowler pointed out the association of sore throat and rheumatic fever in 1880, and shortly after the dawn of the twentieth century, Bela Schick identified ARF as one of the "nachkrankheiten" of scarlet fever. The introduction of Rebecca Lancefield's grouping system for β-hemolytic streptococci allowed clarification of the epidemiology of the disease by a number of investigators in the United States and the United Kingdom, including Coburn, Collis, Rammelkamp, Wannamaker, Massell, and Stollerman. Finally, the widespread introduction of antibiotic agents after World War II resulted in the development of strategies for primary and secondary prevention of rheumatic fever.

ETIOLOGY AND PATHOGENESIS

ARF is a delayed nonsuppurative sequela of upper respiratory infection due to group A streptococci. Several lines of evidence firmly support this conclusion. There is a close temporal relationship between epidemics of streptococcal sore throat and scarlet fever and epidemics of ARF. Most patients with ARF give a history of preceding pharyngitis. Even in patients without such a clear-cut history, tests of antistreptococcal antibodies nearly always provide evidence of recent streptococcal infection. In prospective studies of primary and recurrent ARF, cases of this disease occur only after an immunologically significant streptococcal infection. Finally, continuous antimicrobial prophylaxis, when successful in preventing intercurrent streptococcal infections, also effectively prevents ARF recurrences in rheumatic persons.

An intriguing and as yet unexplained aspect of the host–parasite relationship is the fact that, insofar as is known, cutaneous streptococcal infections do not initiate ARF. This may indicate a requirement for the pharyngeal site, with its rich endowment of lymphoid tissue, for initiation of the disease process, or it may result from a lack of rheumatogenicity among the so-called pyoderma strains of group A streptococci.

The concept that group A streptococci may vary in their rheumatogenic potential has been a controversial one. This concept is, however, consistent with observed geographic and temporal variations in the incidence of ARF. Studies of outbreaks of streptococcal pharyngitis reveal that certain M serotypes are strongly epidemiologically associated with ARF[1] while others are not known to give rise to this sequela.[2] Investigations of endemic ARF cases in Trinidad[3] indicated that strains causing ARF belonged to different serotypes than those simultaneously causing acute glomerulonephritis (AGN) in the same population. It has been suggested[4] that opacity factor-negative streptococcal strains, which elicit high titers of antibodies to non-type-specific M antigens in humans and experimental animals (see Chapter 176), have the greatest potential for initiating attacks of rheumatic fever.

Although the group A streptococcus is known to be the causative agent of rheumatic fever, the exact mechanism by which this microorganism induces the disease remains unexplained. Several theories have been advanced. These include *(1)* direct tissue invasion by group A streptococci or by cell wall incomplete variants of this organism; *(2)* toxic effects of streptococcal products, particularly streptolysins S or O, which are known to be capable of inducting tissue injury; *(3)* serum sickness-like reaction mediated by antigen–antibody complexes, perhaps localized to sites of tissue injury; and *(4)* autoimmune phenomena induced by similarity or identity of certain streptococcal antigens to human tissue antigens.

Although none of these theories has been unequivocally proved or refuted, most attention in recent years has been focused on the concept of autoimmunity. Interest in this mechanism has been spurred by the identification of antibodies in the sera of patients with ARF or rheumatic heart disease that react with the human heart in a variety of test systems. These so-called heart-reactive antibodies (HRA) are also present, albeit in much lower titer, in sera of patients with uncomplicated streptococcal pharyngitis. The presence of bound immunoglobulin and complement in the myocardium of children dying of rheumatic carditis suggests that circulating HRA may have pathogenetic significance. On the other hand, HRA are also present in sera of persons with postcardiotomy and postmyocardial infarction syndromes and in endomyocardial fibrosis, and it is possible that they simply represent a secondary response to damaged myocardial tissue.

Heart-reactive antibodies in ARF sera are directed against several different antigenic specificities in heart tissue, and at least some of these moieties are cross-reactive with group A streptococcal antigens. Indeed, rabbit antisera raised against group A streptococci contain antibodies that bind to the sarcolemma and subsarcolemmal sarcoplasm in cardiac myofibers and skeletal muscle and to smooth muscle of vessel walls and endocardium. These reactions have been studied by immunofluorescence, and whole group A streptococci or fractions thereof have been shown to absorb the HRA. Streptococcal antigens cross-reactive with the human heart have been localized to the bacterial cell wall by some investigators[5] and to the cell membrane by others.[6,7] Epitopes of streptococcal M proteins have been identified that share antigenic determinants with cardiac myosin[8] and with sarcolemmal membrane proteins.[9] Goldstein et al.[10] have described a cross-reaction between group A polysaccharide and a structural glycoprotein isolated from human and bovine heart valves. Such a cross-reaction might explain the observation that serum levels of antibodies to group A carbohydrate appear to remain elevated for many years in patients with rheumatic valvulitis (but not in rheumatic patients without valvulitis)[11] and decline remarkably if valve resection is performed.

Chronic remittent nodular lesions have been observed in dermal connective tissue after injection into experimental animals of a streptococcal mucopeptide–polysaccharide cell wall complex.[12] Antibodies raised in rabbits against streptococcal hyaluronate cross react with human hyaluronate.[13] Many children with Sydenham's chorea have circulating antibodies that react both with neurons of the caudate and subthalamic nuclei and with group A streptococcal cell membranes.[14] Taken together, these cross-reactive and toxic phenomena could explain most of the individual manifestations of ARF. On the other hand, it should be emphasized that there exists no direct proof that these systems play any role in the pathogenesis of rheumatic fever.

Much of the work reviewed above, particularly that related to HRA and group A carbohydrate, has focused on humoral immune responses to streptococci. Indeed, serum antibody responses to streptolysin 0, non-type-specific M antigens, and virtually every other streptococcal antigen are on the average more vigorous in patients with ARF than in persons with uncomplicated streptococcal infections. However, the possible role of delayed hypersensitivity responses to streptococcal antigens in the etiology of ARF is currently under intensive study as well. Preparations of streptolysin S contain a nonspecific mitogen that is closely related but separable from the hemolytic activity. Rheumatic persons have a heightened lymphocyte reactivity to streptococcal cell walls and membranes, but the reactivity to membranes is more striking and persists for several years after an acute attack.[15] T lymphocytes from spleens of adult guinea pigs sensitized with streptococcal cells, cell walls, or protoplast membranes are cytotoxic for cultured guinea pig heart cells.[16]

A complete elucidation of the pathogenesis of ARF obviously

requires not only an understanding of the peculiarities of the etiologic agent but also of the nature of the susceptible host. The fact that, even in severe epidemics of exudative pharyngitis, rheumatic fever affects only a small proportion of infected persons, coupled with the known familial aggregation of ARF cases, has long suggested the possibility of a genetic predisposition to rheumatic attacks. Studies of the distribution of class I HLA antigens in rheumatics vs. controls have been inconclusive. On the other hand, the observation of a highly statistically significant association between the HL-A5 antigen and the degree of the blastogenic response of human lymphocytes to streptococcal extracellular products[17] suggests that immune responsiveness to certain streptococcal antigens may be under rather selective genetic control. Such control mechanisms might conceivably be important in determining who does and who does not develop ARF after an appropriate immunologic stimulus. Recently, a statistically significant association has been reported between certain of the class II HLA antigens (HLA-DR2 and HLA-DR4) and rheumatic fever.[18] A most intriguing potential link between the genetic constitution of the human host and susceptibility to ARF is the identification of certain alloantigens that are present on the circulating B lymphocytes of 75–90 percent of rheumatic subjects but only approximately 20 percent of normal controls.[19]

PATHOLOGIC FINDINGS

Rheumatic fever is characterized pathologically by exudative and proliferative inflammatory lesions of connective tissue, most notably the heart, joints, blood vessels, and subcutaneous tissue. In the early stages of the disease, there is fragmentation of collagen fibers, cellular infiltration that is predominantly lymphocytic, and fibrinoid deposition. This is followed shortly by the appearance of the myocardial Aschoff's nodule. Aschoff's nodule is a perivascular focus of inflammation that consists of an area of central necrosis surrounded by a rosette of large mononuclear and giant multinuclear cells. The nuclei of these cells may have a clear area just within the nuclear membrane ("owl-eyed nucleus") or present a serrated ("caterpillar") appearance depending on their orientation in microscopic cross section. Such cells are known as Anichkov's myocytes, although most authorities believe them to be of mesenchymal origin. Cardiac findings may include pericarditis, myocarditis, and/or endocarditis. Endocarditis involves the left side of the heart in most instances. A thickened and roughened area is frequently seen in the left atrium above the base of the posterior leaflet of the mitral valve ("MacCallum's patch"). Valvular lesions begin as edema and cellular infiltration of the leaflets and chordae with small verrucae along the line of closure. As healing occurs, the valves may become thickened and deformed, the chordae shortened, and the valve commissures fused, thereby resulting in valvular stenosis or insufficiency.

The joint lesions are characterized by fibrinous exudate over the synovial membrane and serous effusion without joint destruction. Histologic findings include cellular infiltration and fibrinoid degeneration. Subcutaneous nodules resemble Aschoff bodies in many features. They consist of a central zone of fibrinoid necrosis surrounded by histiocytes and fibroblasts; perivascular accumulations of lymphocytes and polymorphonuclear leukocytes are also apparent. Although scattered areas of arteritis and petechial hemorrhages have been found in the brain, their relationship to Sydenham's chorea remains uncertain.

EPIDEMIOLOGY

Acute rheumatic fever is most frequent among children in the 6- to 15-year-old group. Indeed, its relative rarity in infants and preschool-age children has led some observers to question whether repeated "primary" infections might be a prerequisite for the development of this disease. There is no clear-cut sex predilection, although there is a female preponderance in certain clinical manifestations, notably mitral stenosis and Sydenham's chorea when the latter occurs after puberty. In temperate climates rheumatic fever tends to occur during the cooler months of the year. The peak incidence along the northeastern seaboard of the United States is in March and April, while in the southeast the incidence tends to peak in the fall.

The attack rate of rheumatic fever after untreated streptococcal exudative tonsillitis in military recruit camps has been carefully studied and has been shown to be consistently around 3 percent.[20] The ARF attack rate is considerably lower after endemically occurring infections among open populations of schoolage children. Siegel et al.[21] studied 519 untreated children with pharyngitis associated with positive throat cultures for group A streptococci. The attack rate of ARF was 0.4 percent; among those patients with an immunologically significant infection, as judged by a rise in the serum titer of antistreptolysin O (ASO), the attack rate was 0.9 percent. In that study, ARF was only observed to occur among the group of 81 patients with exudative pharyngitis, positive throat cultures for group A streptococci, ASO titer rises, and prolonged convalescent streptococcal carriage. In this group, the ARF attack rate, 2.5 percent, approximated that seen in military recruit camps. These and other data suggest that ARF is *more likely* to occur after more severe forms of streptococcal throat infection, as judged by cclinical, bacteriologic, and immunologic criteria. Nevertheless, approximately one-third of the cases of ARF occur after asymptomatic streptococcal infection.

It is difficult for the physician trained in North America to comprehend the magnitude of the problem of ARF in the developing countires of the world. The disease is rampant, for example, in the Middle East, the Indian subcontinent, and selected areas of Africa and South America. It has been estimated that rheumatic heart disease accounts for 25–40 percent of all cardiovascular disease in much of the Third World.[22,23]

The overall incidence of ARF in the United States cannot be ascertained precisely because of inherent difficulties in diagnosing the disease and because most states no longer maintain operational rheumatic fever registries. Careful communitywide surveys of the incidence of ARF were performed during the 1960s in Baltimore, Maryland,[24] and Nashville, Tennessee.[25] ARF attack rates for school-age children were found to be in the range of 24–34 per 100,000. During this same period, the incidence among schoolchildren in the borough of Manhattan was approximately 61 per 100,000, with the highest rates, 78 to 79, occurring in the most congested Puerto Rican "ghetto" areas of Spanish Harlem.[26]

There is general agreement that the incidence of ARF and rheumatic heart disease has declined markedly over the course of the twentieth century in the United States and western Europe. The rate of decline appears to have been particularly steep during the 1960s and 1970s. Indeed, a survey in Memphis, Tennessee,[27] indicated that during 1977 through 1981 the incidence of ARF among white suburban schoolchildren was only 0.5 per 100,000 per year. Similar rates have been reported from many geographic areas of the United States.[28] Traditionally, ARF in the United States has been largely a disease of lower socioeconomic groups. The incidence has been much higher among blacks than whites, a fact that appears to relate to basic environmental conditions rather than to any genetic predisposition of the black race for the development of rheumatic fever. The major predisposing environmental condition that has been identified is crowding. The degree of crowding markedly influences the acquisition rate of group A streptococci (see Chapter 176) and hence the risk of development of ARF.

Recent events suggest the possibility of a resurgence of ARF in the United States. Beginning in early 1985, an epidemic of the disease occurred in Salt Lake City, Utah, and the surrounding intermountain area. By June 1986, 74 children had been admitted to the Primary Children's Medical Center in Salt Lake City.[28] Smaller clusters of ARF, ranging from 17 to 40 cases, were reported during approximately the same time period from Columbus and Akron, Ohio, and Pittsburgh, Pennsylvania.[29–31] A number of other communities in various parts of the country have also noted increases in the incidence of ARF, and for the first time in many years, outbreaks have occurred in military recruit camps.[32,32a]

Quite surprisingly the recently reported civilian cases have tended to occur among children of middle-class white families residing in suburban or rural settings. With only a few exceptions, the strains of group A streptococci responsible for the recent outbreaks either were not isolated or were discarded before they could be serologically characterized. In both the Salt Lake City and Columbus, Ohio, outbreaks, however, group A streptococci of M type 18, characterized by a highly mucoid colony morphology, were prevalent in the communities. There have been similar unpublished findings in a number of other communities in the United States. These observations are of interest because of the well-known associations of M-18[33] and of mucoid colonial forms[34] with ARF.

Persons who have suffered an initial attack of rheumatic fever have a marked predilection to develop recurrences after subsequent episodes of streptococcal pharyngeal infection. The risk of recurrence after streptococcal infection is highest within the first few years after the initial attack and then decclines. It is unclear whether this decline is duc to the length of time since the preceding attack or to the increasing age of the patient. Nevertheless, rheumatic patients remain at an increased risk of recurrence well into adult life. Two other factors positively correlated with a risk of rheumatic recurrences after streptococcal infection are the magnitude of the ASO response and the presence of pre-existing heart disease. In the classic studies conducted at Irvington House, New York,[35] for example, 56 percent of streptococcal infections occurring in persons with rheumatic heart disease and accompanied by four-tube or greater ASO titer rises induced ARF recurrences (Table 1).

CLINICAL MANIFESTATIONS

Rheumatic fever manifests itself as a variety of signs and symptoms that may occur singly or in combination. The most important of these, in terms of diagnosis, have been termed the *major manifestations* and include carditis, polyarthritis, chorea, subcutaneous nodules, and erythema marginatum. Certain additional findings that are frequently present in ARF but are nonspecific in nature constitute the so-called *minor manifestations*: fever, arthralgia, heart block, acute-phase reactants in the blood (C-reactive protein, elevation of the leukocyte count and erythrocyte sedimentation rate), and prior history of ARF or rheumatic heart disease.

The latent period between the onset of preceding streptococcal sore throat and the onset of ARF averages 19 days.[36] The range has been difficult to establish precisely but appears to be between 1 and 5 weeks. The average latent period is the same for recurrent attacks as for initial episodes.

The mode of onset is quite variable. If acute polyarthritis is the initial complaint, the disease may have a rather abrupt onset and may be marked by fever and toxicity. On the other hand, when isolated mild carditis is the initial manifestation, the onset of ARF may be insidious or even subclinical.

TABLE 1. Ratio of Rheumatic Recurrences to Streptococcal Infections Classified according to Cardiac Status before the Infection and to Magnitude of ASO Rise

ASO Rise in Number of Tube Dilutions	*Patients with Pre-existing Heart Disease*	*Patients without Pre-existing Heart Disease*
0–1	3/24 (13%)	1/79 (1%)
2	10/38 (26%)	3/50 (6%)
3	6/16 (38%)	5/34 (15%)
≧4	9/16 (56%)	9/26 (35%)

(From Taranta et al.,[35] with permission.)

Most attacks begin with polyarthritis, although occasionally this may be preceded by abdominal pain. Carditis, if it appears, usually does so early in the course of the disease. Overall, arthritis occurs in approximately 75 percent of first attacks of ARF, carditis in 40–50 percent, chorea in 15 percent, and subcutaneous nodules and erythema marginatum in fewer than 10 percent.[37] These incidences vary with age: carditis occurs most frequently when ARF strikes younger children, while the proportion of cases with arthritis increases with the age of the patients.

Carditis is the only manifestation of ARF that has the potential to cause long-term disability or death. Heart involvement in ARF is frequently a pancarditis involving the endocardium, myocardium, and pericardium. Nevertheless, in the absence of high fever or symptoms of acute pericarditis or congestive heart failure, it is usually asymptomatic. Carditis almost always manifests itself within the first 3 weeks of an attack of ARF if it is to appear at all. The clinical signs of carditis include the development of organic heart murmur(s) not previously present, cardiac enlargement, congestive heart failure, pericardial friction rubs, or signs of effusion.

Severe myocarditis may precipitate intractable heart failure and death in the acute phase of the disease, but fortunately, this occurrence is quite rare. On the other hand, chronic inflammatory changes involving the myocardium and endocardium may lead to the delayed development of chronic rheumatic rheumatic heart disease (Fig. 1). Endocarditis involves the mitral valve more frequently than it does the aortic valve. Characteristic murmurs of acute rheumatic carditis are three: a high-pitched blowing holosystolic apical murmur of mitral regurgitation, a low-pitched apical middiastolic flow murmur (Carey Coombs murmur), and a high-pitched decrescendo diastolic murmur of aortic regurgitation heard at the secondary and primary aortic areas. Murmurs of mitral and aortic stenosis are associated with chronic but not with acute rheumatic valvular disease. Delayed atrioventricular conduction, as manifested by a first-degree heart block, is a toxic phenomenon associated with ARF but not diagnostic of rheumatic carditis.

Joint involvement in ARF ranges from arthralgia without objective findings to frank arthritis characterized by heat, swelling, redness, and exquisite tenderness. There is an inverse relationship between the severity of joint involvement and the risk of development of carditis.[38] The most frequently involved joints are the knees, ankles, elbows, and wrists. The small joints of the hands are less frequently affected, and the spine is only rarely involved. When the course of the illness is not suppressed by anti-inflammatory drugs, multiple joints are usually involved; approximately 50 percent of the patients develop arthritis in more than six joints. Arthritis in ARF is classically migratory in nature, that is, the inflammation travels from joint to joint. Once a joint becomes involved, inflammation begins to subside within a few days to a week and disappears within 2 to 3 weeks. The evolution of arthritis in individual joints tends to overlap, so multiple joints may be inflamed at the same time. In most instances the entire bout of polyarthritis subsides within 4 weeks, leaving no residual articular damage. One possible exception to this has been claimed by several authors, who report the very rare occurrence of the so-called Jaccoud form of periarticular fibrosis after rheumatic arthritis.

Subcutaneous nodules usually are associated with severe carditis and tend to occur several weeks after its onset. They are firm and painless and vary in size from a few millimeters to 2.0 cm. Such nodules are usually found over bony surfaces or prominences and over tendons. Common sites are adjacent to elbows, knees, wrists, or ankles and over Achilles tendons, the occiput, or spinous processes of the vertebrae. Their number varies from one to a few dozen. They usually persist for a week

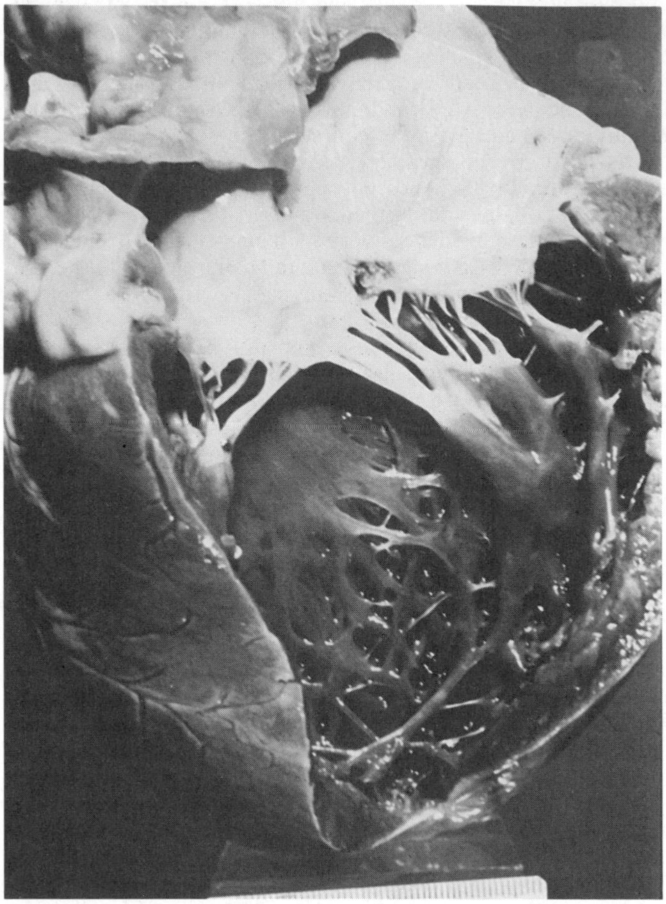

FIG. 1. Chronic rheumatic valvular heart disease. The mitral valve leaflets and chordae are thickened, fibrotic, and distorted; intercommissural adhesions are present. (Courtesy of Dr. L. Alvarez, VA Medical Center, Miami, Florida.)

or two. Somewhat similar but more persistent lesions are seen in rheumatoid arthritis.

Erythema marginatum is a nonpruritic, nonpainful erythematous eruption usually seen on the trunk or proximal aspects of the extremities. The individual lesions are evanescent, moving over the skin in serpiginous patterns that change before the observer's eyes and are often likened to smoke rings, with a tendency to advance at the margins while clearing in the center. The lesions may be macular or raised and appear to be more a vasomotor phenomenon than a manifestation of cutaneous pathologic changes. Individual lesions may come and go in minutes to hours, but the process may go on intermittently for weeks to months.

Sydenham's chorea ("St. Vitus dance") is a neurologic disorder characterized by emotional lability, muscular weakness, and rapid, incoordinated, involuntary purposeless movements. The choreiform movements disappear during sleep and may be partially suppressed by sedation. The nonrhythmic movements are most notable in the face, hands, and feet. Sensation remains intact. Detailed descriptions of the nature of the choreiform movements can be found elsewhere.[39,40] Individual attacks in hospitalized patients usually last 2–4 months.

Chorea may occur in relatively close association with other rheumatic manifestations or in isolated form ("pure chorea"). In cases of "pure chorea," laboratory evidences of acute inflammation (C-reactive protein, elevated erythrocyte sedimentation rate) or recent streptococcal infection (elevated levels of antistreptococcal antibodies) may be lacking. This observation, which led investigators in the past to question the relationship of ARF to "pure chorea," is now known to result from the fact that Sydenham's chorea often occurs with a longer latent period than do the other manifestations of ARF. Patients with "pure chorea" are found on follow-up to have a relatively high incidence of rheumatic heart disease.

Several clinical manifestations of ARF occur with some frequency but are not in themselves specific enough to be considered major manifestations. These include fever, which accompanies almost all ARF attacks at their onset, arthralgia, abdominal pain, and epistaxis. The pulmonary parenchyma in ARF may be involved by a variety of pathologic processes including pulmonary edema, atelectasis, pulmonary embolism, or thromboses. Many observers feel that in addition a specific rheumatic pneumonia occurs that has definable pathologic features. The issue remains unresolved.

The average duration of an attack, unaltered by anti-inflammatory therapy, is approximately 3 months. Less than 5 percent of the cases persist for longer than 6 months, justifying the designation of "chronic" rheumatic fever. Stollerman[39] lists the criteria for continuing clinical activity as follows: joint symptoms, new organic murmurs, changing heart size, congestive heart failure in the absence of long-standing valvular disease, subcutaneous nodules, sleeping pulse rate greater than 100 beats/min, erythema marginatum, chorea, positive C-reactive protein test findings, and a rectal temperature of 100.4°F or higher for 3 or more consecutive days.

DIAGNOSIS

Because ARF can have such diverse manifestations (acute polyarthritis, congestive heart failure, chorea, or combinations of these) and because there is no specific diagnostic test for the disease, the differential diagnostic possibilities in an individual case may be quite broad. Among the diseases that need most frequently to be differentiated are rheumatoid arthritis, juvenile rheumatoid arthritis, systemic lupus erythematosus, serum sickness, sickle cell crisis or cardiopathy, rubella arthritis, septic arthritis (especially gonococcal arthritis in adolescent patients), infective endocarditis, viral myocarditis, and early stages of Henoch-Schönlein purpura. Less frequent differential diagnostic considerations include gout, sarcoidosis, Hodgkin's disease, and leukemia.

Arriving at the correct diagnosis is particularly important in ARF, not only in terms of prescribing appropriate therapy for the acute attack and formulating an accurate prognosis but also because of the necessity for prescribing continuous antistreptococcal prophylaxis. To minimize over- and underdiagnosis, the criteria of T. Duckett Jones, as modified by a committee of the American Heart Association, have been generally accepted as the basis for reaching a diagnosis of ARF (Table 2).

The criteria are not infallable, particularly when the diagnosis rests on the presence of acute polyarthritis as the sole major criterion with supporting evidence of fever plus an elevated erythrocyte sedimentation rate or a positive test result for C-reactive protein. For this reason, it is important to recognize that evidence of recent streptococcal infection must be obtained to satisfy the revised Jones criteria. Such evidence might include a recently documented episode of streptococcal pharyngitis or scarlet fever, a positive throat culture for group A streptococci (although here the differentiation of infection from colonization presents a problem), or the demonstration of an elevated serum titer of antistreptococcal antibodies. In most cases, the latter criterion is relied on.

If a serum sample is obtained within 2 months of onset, approximately 80 percent of patients with ARF will have an ASO titer of greater than 200 Todd units/ml. If a second streptococcal antibody test is performed on the same serum specimen, the proportion of patients with ARF with at least one elevated titer will rise to 90 percent, and if a battery of three tests is performed, this figure exceeds 95 percent.[42] While an elevated an-

TABLE 2. Jones Criteria (Revised) for Guidance in the Diagnosis of Rheumatic Fever

Major Manifestations	*Minor Manifestations*
Carditis	Clinical
Polyarthritis	Previous rheumatic fever or rheumatic heart disease
Chorea	Arthralgia
Erythema marginatum	Fever
Subcutaneous nodules	Laboratory
	Acute-phase reactions: elevated erythrocyte sedimentation rate, C-reactive protein, leukocytosis
	Prolonged P-R interval
	PLUS

Supporting evidence of preceding streptococcal infection (increased ASO or other streptococcal antibodies; positive throat culture for group A streptococcus; recent scarlet fever

The presence of two major criteria or of one major and two minor criteria indicates a high probability of the presence of rheumatic fever if supported by evidence of a preceding streptococcal infection. The absence of the latter should make the diagnosis doubtful except in situations in which rheumatic fever is first discovered after a long latent period from the antecedent infection (e.g., Sydenham's chorea or low-grade carditis).

(From ad hoc committee report,[41] with permission.)

TABLE 3. Suggested Schedule of Anti-inflammatory Therapy in Rheumatic Fever

Clinical Severity	*Treatment*
Arthralgia or mild arthritis; no carditis	Analgesics only, such as codeine or propoxyphene
Moderate or severe arthritis; no carditis, or carditis *with or without* cardiomegaly, but without failure	Aspirin, 90–100 mg/kg/day for 2 weeks; increased if necessary; 60–70 mg/kg/day for the subsequent 6 weeks
Carditis with failure, with or without joint manifestations	Prednisone, 40–60 mg/day; increased, if necessary; methyl prednisone sodium succinate IV in fulminating cases; after 2–3 weeks, slow withdrawal to be completed in 3 more weeks. Aspirin to be continued for a month after discontinuation of prednisone

(From Stollerman,[39] with permission.)

tistreptococcal antibody titer is certainly not diagnostic of ARF, failure to demonstrate evidence of recent immunologically significant streptococcal infection by a battery of three serologic tests (e.g., ASO, anti-DNAse B, antihyaluronidase) makes the diagnosis of ARF very doubtful. An exception to this statement must be made for the patient with "pure" chorea whose antibody titers may have declined to the normal range due to the long latent period between the antecedent streptococcal infection and the onset of this manifestation. Likewise, the onset of isolated carditis may be difficult to date; if recognition of isolated carditis is delayed, immunologic evidence of recent streptococcal infection may have disappeared.

A simple slide hemagglutination test (Streptozyme, Carter-Wallace, Inc.) has been marketed for the detection of antibodies to streptococcal extracellular antigens.[43] Unfortunately, the exact nature of the antibodies assayed by this test has not been ascertained, and considerable lot-to-lot variability in the standardization of the reagent has been reported.[44] In view of these problems, the test is of limited use at the present time.

TREATMENT AND PROGNOSIS

The objectives of therapy in ARF are to quiet inflammation, decrease fever and toxicity, and control cardiac failure. The mainstays of treatment are salicylates and corticosteroids. Neither of these agents prevent or modify the development of chronic rheumatic heart disease. A suggested treatment schedule is outlined in Table 3. Analgesics only are recommended for patients with mild disease. This allows complete expression of the clinical manifestations to aid in diagnosis and also avoids post-therapeutic rebounds. Most patients require salicylates. Serum levels of 20 mg/100 ml or more are required to control the inflammatory response. If the high doses of salicylates required cannot be tolerated due to gastric irritation or if symptoms of salicylism develop, a reduction in the aspirin dosage or a change to corticosteroids is necessary. The more potent anti-inflammatory action of corticosteroids should be brought to bear whenever salicylates fail to control the inflammatory process or whenever carditis with congestive heart failure is present. The role, if any, for nonsteroidal anti-inflammatory agents in the management of ARF remains to be defined.

Reactivation of clinical or laboratory manifestations of rheumatic inflammation may occur after cessation of anti-inflammatory therapy. This "rebound" phenomenon is more frequent after therapy with corticosteroids than with aspirin. For this reason, therapy should be tapered rather than discontinued abruptly, and aspirin administration should be continued for a month after treatment with adrenal steroids is discontinued.

Bed rest should be enforced for 3 weeks for patients without carditis. For those with carditis without cardiomegaly or heart failure, bed rest should be continued for a month after carditis is detected. More prolonged periods of strict or modified bed rest are required for patients with cardiac enlargement or failure.[40] Heart failure should be treated in the usual way, with salt restriction and, as needed, oxygen, diuretics, and digitalis. Patients with chorea require a quiet, nonstimulatory environment and sedation.

The only long-term sequela of ARF is that of rheumatic heart disease. The prognosis is rheumatic patients has been greatly improved by our ability to prevent recurrent attacks with their concomitant threat of additional myocardial and valvular damage. The ultimate prognosis of an individual attack is rather directly related to the severity of cardiac involvement during the acute phase. This was best studied in the United Kingdom–United States Collaborative Study.[45] In that study, only 6 percent of the patients with no carditis or with only questionable carditis during their attack of ARF were found to have heart murmurs when reexamined 10 years later. Heart disease was present at follow-up in 30 percent of the patients initially found to have only apical systolic murmurs, in 40 percent of those with basal diastolic murmurs during the acute phase, and in 68 percent of those who initially suffered from congestive heart failure, pericarditis, or both. Patients with "pure" chorea appear to have a relatively high incidence of late development of rheumatic heart disease, even if carditis is not recognized at the time of the initial attack. It may be, however, that the initial findings of carditis are no longer prominent by the time that chorea (which often occurs after a long latent period) becomes apparent.

PREVENTION

Prevention of ARF in persons without a prior history of this disease depends on an accurate diagnosis and appropriate treatment of the antecedent streptococcal infection. This approach (so-called primary prevention) is outlined in Chapter 176. It is effective[46] but suffers from the limitation that a substantial proportion, probably about one-third, of ARF cases follow streptococcal infections that are either entirely subclinical or too mild to bring them to medical attention.

Rheumatic patients are at extremely high risk of developing recurrent ARF after immunologically significant streptococcal upper respiratory infections (Table 1). These persons require continuous prophylaxis to prevent intercurrent streptococcal infections. The preferred regimen[47] consists of a single injection of 1.2 million units of penicillin G benzathine administered every 4 weeks. In the most comprehensive study reported to date,[48] children following this regimen experienced a rheumatic fever recurrence rate of only 0.4 per 100 patient-years of observation (Table 4). Limited data suggest that, in those areas of the world where ARF and rheumatic heart disease remain very highly prevalent, ARF recurrence rates may be even lower when injections of penicillin G benzathine are administered every 3 weeks rather than every 4 weeks.[49] The possible benefits of such a regimen must be balanced against the potential decrease in patient compliance and increase in associated costs.

Oral sulfadiazine, 1 g/day for persons over 60 lb and 0.5 g/day for those weighing less than 60 lb, or penicillin V, 125 or 250 mg twice a day, are also acceptable prophylactic agents but are less effective than is penicillin G benzathine (Table 4). The lesser efficacy of oral regimens is due at least in part to the extreme difficulty of enforcing compliance. Patients allergic or intolerant to both penicillin and sulfa may be given erythromycin, 250 mg twice a day. Patients requiring protection for many years are often begun on a regimen of penicillin G benzathine, which is changed to oral prophylaxis later in life when the risk of recurrence is deemed to be lower.

The optimal duration of continuous antimicrobial prophylaxis remains unsettled. Some authorities recommend that prophylaxis be continued "indefinitely," presumably for life. On the other hand, the risk of streptococcal infection and ARF recurrences declines with age and becomes quite low in older adults without heart disease who are not in intimate contact with school-age children. In view of these facts, the Committee on Rheumatic Fever and Infective Endocarditis of the American Heart Association recognizes that "physicians may wish to make exceptions to maintaining prophylaxis indefinitely, especially in older individuals, on an individual basis. In making such decisions, the physician must carefully weigh a number of factors, including the patient's risk of acquiring a streptococcal infection, the anticipated recurrence rate per infection, and the consequences of recurrence."[47] In the author's opinion, even when all these factors are favorable, prophylaxis should never be discontinued until the patient has reached his early twenties and at least 5 years have elapsed since the most recent rheumatic attack.

In addition to prevention of recurrences of ARF, patients with residual rheumatic valvular disease must be protected from bacterial endocarditis whenever they undergo dental or surgical procedures that consistently evoke bacteremia or are known to be associated with the development of endocarditis. The antimicrobial regimens suggested for endocarditis prophylaxis are entirely distinct from those required for rheumatic fever prophylaxis. This concept is a frequent source of confusion both to physicians and to dentists. Regimens for the prevention of bacterial endocarditis are discussed in Chapter 63.

Investigative efforts are currently being directed toward the development of a safe, effective M-protein vaccine for the prevention of streptococcal infection and ARF. Such a vaccine would of necessity be polyvalent, as is that currently licensed for the prevention of *Streptococcus pneumoniae* infections. Efforts at vaccine development have been hampered, however, by the difficulty of separating those antigenic determinants that elicit type-specific protective immunity from closely related moieties that share antigenic determinants with human heart tissue.[50] Nevertheless, the considerable progress that has been made in recent years in elucidating the molecular structures of a number of M-protein serotypes may well foreshadow the solution to this problem.

TABLE 4. Prophylaxis and Attack Rates[a] of Streptococcal Infection and Rheumatic Fever Recurrences

	Parenteral Benzathine Penicillin	*Oral Penicillin*	*Oral Sulfadiazine*
Number of patient-years	560	545	576
Number and rate of all streptococcal infections, exclusive of the carrier state	24 (4.3)	101 (18.5	102 (17.7)
Number and rate of rheumatic recurrences	2 (0.4)	30 (5.5)	16 (2.8)

[a] Rates are listed in parentheses as number per 100 patient-years.
(From Wood et al.,[48] with permission.)

GLOMERULONEPHRITIS

Poststreptococcal acute glomerulonephritis (AGN) is an acute inflammatory disorder of the renal glomerulus that is characterized pathologically by diffuse proliferative glomerular lesions and clinically by edema, hypertension, hematuria, and proteinuria. The disease is a delayed nonsuppurative sequela of pharyngeal or cutaneous infection with certain "nephritogenic" group A streptococcal strains belonging to a limited number of serotypes.

HISTORY

Richard Bright (1789–1858) clearly differentiated cardiac from renal dropsy. He also noted the association between acute diseases, particularly scarlet fever, and AGN.[51] Subsequently, many investigators confirmed the relationship between β-hemolytic streptococcal infections and AGN. Schick[52] in 1907 commented on the similarity of the latent period in serum sickness to that in AGN, thus raising the possibility of an immunologic basis for the latter disease. Rammelkamp and Weaver[53] explained the puzzling variations in attack rate of AGN after group A streptococcal infection by proposing that only certain serotypes of *Streptococcus pyogenes* were nephritogenic. Detailed prospective studies of the epidemiology, bacteriology, immunology, and natural history of pyoderma-associated nephritis by Wannamaker[54] in Minnesota, Potter et al.[55] in south Trinidad, and Dillon and coworkers[56] in Alabama have added greatly to our understanding of this disease.

ETIOLOGY AND PATHOGENESIS

Poststreptococcal AGN follows infection with a limited number of group A streptococcal serotypes (Table 5). Type 12 is the most frequent M serotype causing AGN after pharyngitis or tonsillitis, while M-49 is the type most frequently related to pyoderma-associated nephritis. Not all streptococcal strains belonging to these serotypes are nephritogenic, however. As yet, there are no reliable biologic markers to differentiate nephritogenic from non-nephritogenic streptococci. Poststreptococcal AGN is almost always due to strains of serogroup A. There are, however, two well-documented outbreaks due to group C organisms.[57,58]

The precise mechanism by which streptococcal infection gives rise to AGN has not been delineated. The weight of evi-

TABLE 5. M Serotypes of Group A Streptococci Associated with Acute Glomerulonephritis[a]

Pharyngitis-Associated AGN	*Pyoderma-Associated AGN*
1	2
3	49[b]
4	55[b]
12	57
25	59
	60
	61

[a] This list represents the major serotypes known to be associated with AGN, but is not all inclusive. Other serotypes may at times be involved, and certain pyoderma strains potentially associated with AGN have not been assigned M-type designations.
[b] M-types 49 and 55 have also been reported on occasion to cause pharyngitis-associated AGN.

dence favors the view that the renal injury is immunologically mediated. Such evidence includes the latent period between infection and the development of AGN; the associated hypocomplementemia; and the fact that immunoglobulins, complement components, and antigens that react with streptococcal antisera are present in the renal glomerulus early in the course of the disease.[59–62] It is possible that antibodies elicited by nephritogenic streptococci react with normal or damaged renal antigens in such a way as to produce glomeruluar injury. Indeed, antigenic similarities between constituents of the streptococcus and the human kidney have been described.[63–65] On the other hand, the electron microscopic finding of nodular subepithelial "humps" in renal biopsy specimens from patients with AGN has led many investigators to hypothesize that the renal injury is more likely due to deposition of preformed complexes consisting of streptococcal antigen and host antibody within the glomerulus. Such a hypothesis seems highly plausible because such subepithelial nodular deposits are a characteristic feature of experimentally induced disease caused by circulating immune complexes. Several groups[66–68] have detected circulating immune complexes in AGN.

The identity of the streptococcal constituent(s) involved in the pathogenesis of AGN remains unknown. M protein is an obvious candidate because of the close association of nephritogenicity and the M serotype. Indeed, monoclonal antibodies raised against human glomeruli have been found to cross react with streptococcal M protein.[65] Moreover, in an animal model of nephritis induced by nephritogenic type 12 streptococci, Lindberg and Vosti[69] eluted bound glomerular antibodies and found them to be directed against type 12 M protein but not against other streptococcal and renal antigens. Others, however, have described cross-reactions between fragments of streptococcal cell membrane and human glomerular basement membrane[63] and produced proliferative glomerular lesions in rhesus monkeys by immunization with streptococcal membrane fragments or by intravenous injection of antibodies to these fragments.[70] Lange and associates[71] have described an antigen (termed *endostreptosin*) demonstrable in the glomerulus only during the initial phase of AGN that reacts in direct immunofluorescence tests with antibodies present in convalescent sera of AGN patients. An apparently identical antigen is found in a water-soluble fraction of nephritogenic streptococci and is most likely derived from streptococcal plasma membrane. Another nephritis-associated antigen, initially identified as an extracellular product of nephritogenic streptococci, has recently been characterized as a streptokinase.[72]

PATHOLOGIC CHARACTERISTICS

In the acute phase of illness, light microscopic examination of renal biopsy specimens demonstrates a marked increase in glomerular intracapillary cellularity due to endothelial and mesangial cell proliferation. These changes involve virtually all the glomeruli, which appear enlarged and bloodless, tending to fill the Bowman space.[73] In addition to this diffuse proliferative endocapillary process, a variable degree of polymorphonuclear leukocytic exudation is observed. Proliferation of parietal and visceral epithelial cells occurs to a modest degree only and is rarely extensive enough to give rise to well-developed crescent formation. Thin sectioning and special stains may reveal discrete deposits on the epithelial side of the basement membrane that correspond to the "humps" visible on electron microscopy. Focal degeneration, interstitial edema, and cellular infiltration also occur in the renal tubular cells, but these tubular changes are far less prominent than is the glomerulitis. Arterioles are normal or nearly so in most cases of AGN.

Immunofluorescence technique demonstrates considerable variability in the pattern of deposition of immunoglobulin and complement components. C3 and properdin are virtually always present in the glomeruli, and deposits of IgG are also frequently demonstrable. These substances are present in the form of discrete deposits similar in size and location to the subepithelial humps visualized under the electron microscope,[60,61] although deposits of C3 may also occur in an interrupted linear pattern along the basement membrane or in the mesangium.[61] Deposits of IgM, C1q, C4, and fibrin are found less commonly. The prominent deposition of C3 and properdin, in contrast to the rather weak and inconsistent deposition of early complement components, suggests that activation of the alternate complement pathway may play a role in the immunopathology of AGN.

EPIDEMIOLOGY

The epidemiologic characteristics of AGN largely reflect those of the antecedent group A streptococcal infection, that is, pharyngitis or pyoderma (Table 6). Thus, the classic streptococcal sore throat occurs primarily among school-age children during the cooler months of the year. Pyoderma is largely a disease of children aged 2–6 years and occurs, in temperate climates, during the summer and early fall. There are data to suggest that, given a skin infection with a nephritogenic strain, the attack rate of AGN is higher in children 6 or younger than in older children.[74] There are, however, some unexplained epidemiologic differences between cases of pyoderma nephritis and those associated with pharyngitis such as the fact that the sex distribution appears equal in the former while the literature suggests a male preponderance in the latter. The latent period of AGN is variable but averaged 10 days after pharyngeal infection in the classic studies of Stetson et al.[75]; prospective studies at Red Lake Indian Reservation in Minnesota indicate the usual latent period of pyoderma-associated AGN to be 3 weeks or longer.[74] While the attack rate of AGN after throat or skin infection with a nephritogenic strain is substantial (i.e., 10–15 percent),[71,74] the disease differs dramatically from acute rheumatic fever in that recurrences are rare. This is due at least in part to the relatively limited number of streptococcal serotypes that are nephritogenic and presumably also to the acquisition of type-specific protective immunity to the serotype that elicited the initial attack. Moreover, in contrast to rheumatic subjects, there is no evidence that AGN patients are unusually susceptible to recurrent attacks after reinfection with a potentially nephritogenic strain. When second attacks of AGN do occur, they are clinically and histologically indistinguishable from the initial attack.[76] A more commonly recognized phenomenon than recurrent AGN attacks is the propensity for streptococcal infections to precipitate exacerbations of chronic glomerulonephritis.[77] Such exacerbations often occur after a relatively brief latent period of 1–4 days.

The introduction of a highly nephritogenic strain into a family unit may result in multiple cases. For example, during the 1964–1966 epidemic of AGN in south Trinidad involving 720 patients, multiple cases occurred in 47 households.[78] Where systematic

TABLE 6. Epidemiologic Characteristics of Pharyngitis-Associated and Pyoderma-Associated Acute Nephritis

Feature	*Pharyngitis-Associated AGN*	*Pyoderma-Associated AGN*
Age	Early school age	Preschool age
Sex	M/F ratio approx. 2:1	Equally distributed
Season	Winter and spring	Late summer and early fall
Geographic distribution	North and South	Predominantly South
Familial occurrence	Common	Common
Latent period	10 days	3 weeks
Attack rate[a]	10–15%	10–15%
Serologic types	Limited types	Also limited, but different types
Recurrences	Rare	Rare

[a] After infection with known nephritogenic strain.
(From Wannamaker,[54] with permission.)

screening of sibling contacts for hypertension, urinary abnormalities, and serum complement levels has been performed, the incidence of proven and suspected cases of AGN in sibling contacts has been extremely variable,[79–81] with estimates ranging as high as 20 percent.[82]

CLINICAL AND LABORATORY FEATURES

The typical clinical features of AGN, as seen in children entering the hospital with this disease, include edema, hypertension, and smoky or rusty colored urine. Patients also exhibit pallor and may complain of lethargy, malaise, weakness, anorexia, headache, and dull back pain. Fever is not prominent.

Facial and periorbital edema are usually present, especially on arising in the morning, but edema also involves dependent areas such as feet and legs, scrotum, and sacrum. In severe cases, ascites or pleural effusions may occur. Another manifestation of fluid overload is circulatory congestion, which may give rise to dyspnea, orthopnea, rales at the lung bases, distended neck veins, and even frank pulmonary edema. Such findings are due solely to fluid accumulation and not to heart failure unless the patient has underlying cardiac disease. Manifestations of circulatory overload tend to be particularly prominent in the occasional cases of AGN occurring in older adults and, in such persons, may obscure the correct diagnosis if urinary findings are not properly interpreted.

Hypertension occurs in most patients but is usually of modest degree. Hypertensive retinopathy or heart failure do not ordinarly complicate the clinical picture. On the other hand, a small proportion of AGN patients, perhaps 5–10 percent, develop severe hypertension complicated by signs and symptoms of encephalopathy. These range from headache and vomiting to confusion, somnolence, and convulsions.

While the clinical features enumerated above are typical of hospitalized patients, many cases of AGN are so mild as to escape detection unless persons at risk are tested prospectively for urinary sediment abnormalities and serum complement levels. Two studies that included renal biopsy data have concluded that, in epidemic situations, as many as 50 percent of cases of AGN may be subclinical.[79,82] Whatever the exact proportion might be (and chances are this varies considerably in differing epidemiologic settings), it seems clear that subclinical episodes of AGN are by no means rare.

Laboratory findings include a mild normocytic normochronic anemia, elevated erythrocyte sedimentation rate, slight hypoproteinemia, and elevations of the blood urea nitrogen and serum creatinine concentrations. Hypercholesterolemia and hyperlipemia may also be present. Serum levels of total hemolytic complement and C3 complement are markedly reduced in the great majority of patients with clinically apparent AGN. Urine volume may be significantly diminished, and the urine itself is smoky, rusty, or brownish with a high specific gravity and positive test findings for protein and hemoglobin. Total urinary protein excretion is usually less that 3 g/day.[83] Microscopic examination of the urine reveals erythrocytes, leukocytes, and hyaline, granular, and red blood cell casts.

The pathologic findings in AGN urine must be distinguished from the mild hematuria and proteinuria that may be seen during the acute phase of acute streptococcal infection and other febrile illnesses. The relationship, if any, of these early urinary findings to the development of AGN is at present unknown.[84] Finally, diagnostic confusion is almost inevitable in the rare cases in which pronounced clinical manifestations of AGN occur in patients with minimal or no urinary sediment abnormalities.[85]

DIAGNOSIS

The diagnosis of AGN is based on the clinical history, physical findings, and confirmatory evidence of antecedent streptococcal infection. The latter may include a recent history of scarlet fever, isolation of group A streptococci from throat or skin lesions, or demonstration of elevated serum titers of streptococcal antibodies. Even in the absence of bacteriologic isolation of streptococci, the presence of skin lesions morphologically compatible with streptococcal impetigo is highly suggestive.

It is almost always possible to demonstrate an elevated level of streptococcal antibodies in AGN,[43] although, in cases with relatively short latent periods, serial bleedings may be necessary. It must be recalled that in pyoderma-associated nephritis ASO responses are weak and it is frequently necessary to perform serum titrations of anti-DNAse B and/or antihyaluronidase. Although anti-Streptozyme titers rise in pyoderma nephritis, technical problems limit the reliability of the test (see above). Finally, if renal biopsy is performed, the demonstration of diffuse proliferative glomerulonephritis with subepithelial electron-dense deposits is a very helpful confirmatory finding.

Poststreptococcal acute glomerulonephritis must be differentiated from a variety of other infectious process involving the kidney. It is, for example, often extremely difficult to differentiate an acute exacerbation of chronic glomerulonephritis, such as may be precipitated by streptococci or by a variety of other intercurrent infections, from a true attack of AGN. A short latent period of 1 to 4 days suggests that the episode is an exacerbation of pre-existing renal disease. Patients with subacute bacterial endocarditis tend to develop high serum levels of circulating immune complexes and may develop either diffuse proliferative or focal glomerulonephritis, both of which may be confused clinically with poststreptococcal nephritis. A variety of other bacterial and protozoan infections such as pneumococcal pneumonia, typhoid fever, leptospirosis, syphilis, toxoplasmosis, and *P. falciparum* malaria have been reported on occasion to be associated with nephritis. Viral infections such as hepatitis B, infectious mononucleosis, measles, mumps, and togaviral and enteroviral disease have likewise been implicated as causes of viruria, transient renal dysfunction, or actual glomerulonephritis.[86] Other entities that may at times mimic AGN are Henoch-Schönlein disease, systemic lupus erythematosus, polyarteritis nodosa, acute tubular necrosis, focal glomerulonephritis with hematuria, hereditary nephritis, rapidly progressive glomerulonephritis, idiopathic nephrotic syndrome, and malignant hypertension.

THERAPY

Because no form of treatment is known to alter the long-term prognosis of AGN, therapy is directed toward management of the acute problems. Bed rest is ordered, and attention is directed to what is ordinarily the most immediate problem, namely, circulatory overload. In most cases this is handled adequately by salt and fluid restriction alone, but at times diuretics are required. Digitalis is not ordinarily indicated since myocardial function is intact. In most instances, specific antihypertensive therapy is unnecessary, but in cases of severe hypertension and hypertensive encephalopathy, potent parenteral agents such as hydralazine or diazoxide are required. Patients developing acute pulmonary edema or severe and prolonged oliguria require measures conventionally used in these conditions. The reader is referred to other sources for detailed descriptions of the management of complications of AGN.

All nonallergic patients should receive penicillin, preferably penicillin G benzathine (see Chapter 176 for dosage schedule), to eradicate the nephritogenic streptococcal strain. Penicillin-allergic patients should receive erythromycin in the doses recommended for the treatment of streptococcal pharyngitis. In addition to urinalysis and serum C3 complement determination, family contacts should have cultures of throat and skin lesions. Persons with positive cultures for group A streptococci should be treated appropriately. Such treatment is for epidemiologic purposes only and will not modify the course of pre-existent

AGN nor, in all probability, abort the disease in persons who are within the latent period (see below).

With skillful use of the supportive measures outlined above, mortality during the acute phase of AGN is now rare. Perhaps 1 percent or fewer of patients develop severe and irreversible renal failure. In the remainder, signs and symptoms often begin to abate within a few days after admission. Serum complement levels return to normal within a month, but microscopic hematuria and cylinduria frequently persist for months despite the patient's general feeling of well-being.

PREVENTION

Although penicillin treatment of the antecedent streptococcal infection is highly efficacious in preventing acute rheumatic fever, the same does not appear to be the case in AGN. Stetson et al.,[75] studying in a controlled fashion an epidemic of pharyngitis-associated (type 12) AGN in a military population, found a small but not statistically significant[87] preventive effect of penicillin. Uncontrolled observations during an epidemic of nephritis in Israel[88] (both throat and skin infections due to M type 55) documented the occurrence of AGN in a number of subjects who had received prior antibiotic therapy according to a variety of different dosage regimens. Moreover, there was no difference in the clinical severity of AGN between subjects who had and those who had not received antibiotic therapy. Data presently available are not adequate to determine whether penicillin might have a small effect on the primary prevention of AGN, but such effect, at any rate, is not striking.[89]

As indicated above, penicillin is, nevertheless, effective in epidemiologic attempts to eradicate nephritogenic strains by treatment of AGN patients and their colonized family contacts. In appropriate high-risk settings during epidemics of AGN, universal penicillin prophylaxis of selected populations might be considered in a manner somewhat analogous to that formerly used in U.S. military recruit camps for rheumatic fever control. Such universal prophylaxis is rarely indicated and should be used only after careful consideration of the specific epidemiologic parameters involved.

Because recurrent episodes of AGN are so rare, continuous antistreptococcal prophylaxis, such as is used in the secondary prevention of rheumatic fever, is unnecessary.

PROGNOSIS

One of the most important and hotly debated issues relating to poststreptococcal glomerulonephritis is the frequency with which patients afflicted with the disease eventually develop chronic glomerulonephritis. It is well known that, in a certain group of AGN patients constituting only a small percentage of its victims, the acute attack is never resolved and the disease enters a subacute phase leading to a virtually complete loss of renal function within 6 months to 2 years. It is the ultimate fate of the remainder of the patients in whom the illness appears clinically to have resolved that remains controversial. Most observers now agree that the long-term prognosis in children is excellent. A 10-year follow-up of 61 patients involved in an epidemic at Red Lake, Minnesota,[90] revealed no cases of chronic glomerulonephritis. Moreover, in a 12- to 17-year follow-up of 534 Trinidadians convalescent from AGN,[91] only 3.5 percent of the subjects had persistent urine abnormalities, 3.7 percent were hypertensive, and none had serum creatinine values greater than 1.25 mg/dl. These figures are not in excess of what would be expected in surveys of normal populations. Almost all the Trinidadian patients had been children at the time of their attack of AGN. There was no difference in outcome of sporadic AGN cases as opposed to those associated with epidemics.

These data stand in sharp contrast to the findings of Baldwin,[92] who followed 168 subjects for periods up to 18 years and concluded that "irreversible renal damage has ensued in 50 percent of these patients, as evidenced by the presence of proteinuria and/or hypertension," although clinical uremia occurred in only 6 patients. Renal biopsy specimens from the subjects in Baldwin's series showed that proliferative changes had decreased while glomerulosclerosis of marked degree was present in over half of the specimens. Baldwin's study population contains a high proportion of adults, who are generally agreed to have a worse prognosis than do children.[93] Moreover, the results presented have been challenged because of the difficulty of sorting out exacerbations of chronic nephritis from true de novo attacks of AGN in studies of sporadically occurring disease[94] and because of the paucity of published data documenting the poststreptococcal etiology of the cases studied.[95]

Based on the bulk of currently available data, it seems likely that more than 90 percent of the children with AGN make an uneventful recovery and that this disease in the pediatric age group is not an important precursor of chronic glomerulonephritis or hypertension. The prognosis appears more guarded in adult patients, but the proportion who might be left with residual renal function impairment is at present unknown.

REFERENCES

1. Bisno AL. The concept of rheumatogenic and nonrheumatogenic group a streptococci. In: Read S, Zabriskie JB, eds. Streptococcal Diseases and the Immune Response. New York: Academic Press; 1980;789–803.
2. Kuttner AG, Krumwiede E. Observations on the effect of streptococcal upper respiratory infections on rheumatic children: A three-year study. J Clin Invest. 1941;20:273–87.
3. Potter EV, Svartman M, Mohammed I, et al. Tropical acute rheumatic fever and associated streptococcal infections compared with concurrent acute glomerulonephritis. J Pediatr. 1978;92:325–33.
4. Widdowson JP, Maxted WR, Notley CM, et al. The antibody responses in man to infection with different serotypes of group A streptococci. J Med Microbiol. 1974;7:483–96.
5. Kaplan MH, Meyeserian M. An immunological cross-reaction between group A streptococcal cells and human heart tissue. Lancet. 1962;1:706–10.
6. Zabriskie JB, Freimer EH. An immunological relationship between group A streptococcus and mammalian muscle. J Exp Med. 1966;124:661–78.
7. Van de Rijn I, Zabriskie JB, McCarty M. Group A streptococcal antigens cross-reactive with myocardium: Purification of heart reactive antibody and isolation and characterization of the streptococcal antigen. J Exp Med. 1977;146:579–99.
8. Dale JB, Beachey EH. Epitopes of streptococcal M proteins shared with cardiac myosin. J Exp Med. 1985;162:583–91.
9. Dale JB, Beachey EH. Protective antigenic determinant of streptococcal M protein shared with sarcolemmal membrane protein of human heart. J Exp Med. 1982;156:1165–76.
10. Goldstein I, Rebeyrotte P, Parlebas J, et al. Isolation from heart valves of glycopeptides which share immunological properties with *Streptococcus haemolyticus* group A polysaccharides. Nature. 1968;219:866–8.
11. Dudding BA, Ayoub EM. Persistence of streptococcal group A antibody in patients with rheumatic valvular disease. J Exp Med. 1968;128:1081–98.
12. Schwab JH, Cromartie WJ. Immunological studies on a C polysaccharide complex of group A streptococci having a direct toxic effect on connective tissue. J Exp Med. 1960;111:295–307.
13. Fillit HM, McCarty M, Blake M. Induction of antibodies to hyaluronic acid by immunization of rabbits with encapsulated streptococci. J Exp Med. 1986;164:762–76.
14. Husby G, van de Rijn I, Zabriskie JB et al. Antibodies reacting with cytoplasm of subthalamic and caudate nuclei neurons in chorea and acute rheumatic fever. J Exp Med. 1976;144:1094–110.
15. Read SE, Fischetti VA, Utermohlen V, et al. Cellular reactivity studies to streptococcal antigens: Migration inhibition studies in patients with streptococcal infections and rheumatic fever. J Clin Invest. 1974;54:439–50.
16. Yang LC, Soprey PR, Wittner MK, et al. Streptococcal-iinduced cell-mediated immune destruction of cardiac myofibers in vitro. J Exp Med. 1977;146:344–60.
17. Greenberg LJ, Gray ED, Yunis E. Association of HL-A5 and immune responsiveness in vitro to streptococcal antigens. J Exp Med. 1975;141:934–43.
18. Ayoub EM, Barrett DJ, Maclaren NK, et al. Association of class II human histocompatibility leukocyte antigens with rheumatic fever J Clin Investg. 1986;77:2019–26.
19. Zabriskie JB, Lavenchy D, Williams RC Jr, et al. Rheumatic-fever associated B-cell alloantigens as identified by monoclonal antibodies. Arthritis Rheum. 1985;28:1047–51.
20. Rammelkamp CH, Denny FW, Wannamaker LW. Studies on the epidemiology of rheumatic fever in the armed services. In: Thomas L, ed. Rheumatic Fever: A Symposium. Minneapolis: University of Minnesota Press; 1952:72–89.

21. Siegel AC, Johnson EE, Stollerman GH. Controlled studies of streptococcal pharyngitis in a pediatric population. I. Factors related to the attack rate of rheumatic fever. N Engl J Med. 1961;265:559–66.
22. Markowitz M. Observations on the epidemiology and preventability of rheumatic fever in developing countries. Clin Ther. 1981;4:240–51.
23. World Health Organization. Community control of rheumatic heart disease in developing countries. I. A major public health problem. WHO Chron. 1980;34:336–45.
24. Gordis L, Lilienfeld A, Rodriguez R. Studies in the epidemiology and preventability of rheumatic fever. I. Demographic factors and incidence of acute attacks. J Chronic Dis. 1969;21:645–54.
25. Quinn RW, Federspiel CF. The incidence of rheumatic fever in metropolitan Nashville, 1963–1969. Am J Epidemiol. 1974;99:273–80.
26. Brownell KD, Bailen-Rose F. Acute rheumatic fever in children: Incidence in a borough of New York City. JAMA. 1973;224:1593–7.
27. Land MA, Bisno AL. Acute rheumatic fever, a vanishing disease in suburbia. JAMA. 1983;249:895–8.
28. Veasy LG, Wiedmeier SE, Orsmond GS, et al. Resurgence of acute rheumatic fever in the intermountain area of the United States. N Engl J Med. 1987;316:421–7.
29. Hosier DM, Craenen JM, Teske DW, et al. Resurgence of acute rheumatic fever. Am J Dis Child. 1987;141:730–3.
30. Congeni B, Rizzo C, Congeni J, et al. Outbreak of acute rheumatic fever in northeast Ohio. J Pediatr. 1987;111:176–9.
31. Wald ER, Dashefsky B, Feidt C, et al. Acute rheumatic fever in western Pennsylvania and the tristate area. Pediatrics. 1987;80:371–4.
32. US Public Health Service, Centers for Disease Control. Acute rheumatic fever at a navy training center—San Diego, California. MMWR. 1988;37:101–4.
32a. US Public Health Service, Centers for Disease Control. Acute rheumatic fever among army trainees—Fort Leonard Wood, Missouri, 1987–1988. MMWR. 1988;37:519–22.
33. James L, McFarland RB. An epidemic of pharyngitis due to a nonhemolytic group A streptococcus at Lowrey Air Force Base. N Engl J Med. 1971;284:750–2.
34. Stollerman GH. The relative rheumatogenicity of strains of group A streptococci. Mod Concepts Cardiovasc Dis. 1975;44:35–40.
35. Taranta A, Kleunberg E, Feinstein AR, et al. Rheumatic fever in children and adolescents. V. Relation of the rheumatic fever recurrence rate per streptococcal infections to pre-existing clinical features of the patients. Ann Intern Med. 1964;60(Suppl 5):58–67.
36. Rammelkamp CH Jr, Stolzer BL. The latent period before the onset of acute rheumatic fever. Yale J Biol Med. 1961;34:386–98.
37. Sanyal SK, Thapar MK, Ahmed SH, et al. The initial attack of acute rheumatic fever during childhood in north India. Circulation. 1974;49:7–12.
38. Feinstein AR, Spagnuola M. The clinical pattern of acute rheumatic fever: A reappraisal. Medicine (Baltimore). 1962;41:279–305.
39. Stollerman GH. Rheumatic Fever and Streptococcal Infection. New York: Grune & Stratton; 1975.
40. Taranta A. Rheumatic fever: Clinical aspects. In: Hollander JL, McCarty DJ Jr, eds. Arthritis and Allied Conditions. 8th ed. Philadelphia: Lea & Febiger; 1972:764–820.
41. Ad hoc committee to revise the Jones criteria (modified) of the Council on Rheumatic Fever and Congenital Heart Disease of the American Heart Association: Committee report. Circulation. 1965;32:664–8.
42. Stollerman GH, Lewis AJ, Schultz I, et al. Relationship of the response to group A streptococci to the course of acute, chronic and recurrent rheumatic fever. Am J Med. 1956;20:163–9.
43. Bisno AL, Ofek I. Serologic diagnosis of streptococcal infection: Comparison of a rapid hemagglutination technique with conventional antibody tests. Am J Dis Child. 1974;127:676–81.
44. Kaplan EL, Kunde C. Quantitative evaluation of variation in composition of the streptozyme agglutination reagent for detection of antibodies to group A streptococcal extracellular antigens. J Clin Microbiol. 1981;14:678–80.
45. United Kingdom and United States Joint Report. The natural history of rheumatic fever and rheumatic heart disease: Ten year report of a cooperative clinical trial of ACTH, cortisone, and aspirin. Circulation. 1965;32:457–76.
46. Gordis L. Effectiveness of comprehensive care programs in preventing rheumatic fever. N Engl J Med. 1973;289:331–5.
47. Shulman ST, Amren DP, Bisno AL, et al. American Heart Association Committee Report. Prevention of rheumatic fever. Circulation. 1984;70:1118A–22A.
48. Wood HF, Feinstein AR, Taranta A, et al. Rheumatic fever in children and adolescents. III. Comparative effectiveness in three prophylaxis regimens in preventing streptococcal infections and rheumatic recurrences. Ann Intern Med. 1964;60(Suppl 5):31–46.
49. Lue HC, Wu MH, Hsieh KH, et al. Rheumatic fever recurrences: controlled study of 3-week versus 4-week benzathine penicillin prevention programs. J Pediatr. 1986;108:299–304.
50. Bronze MS, Beachey EH, Dale JB. Protective and heart cross-reactive epitopes located within the NH_2 terminus of type 19 streptococcal M protein. J Exp Med. 1988;167:1849–60.
51. Bright R. Cases and observations, illustrative of renal disease accompanied with the secretion of albuminous urine. Guys Hosp Rep. 1936;1:338–400.
52. Schick B. Die nachkrankheiten des Scharlach. J Kinderheilk. 1907;65:132–73.
53. Rammelkamp CH Jr, Weaver RS. Acute glomerulonephritis. The significance of the variations in the incidence of the disease. J Clin Invest. 1953;32:345–58.
54. Wannamaker LW. Differences between streptococcal infections of the throat and of the skin. N Engl J Med. 1970;282:23–31.
55. Potter EV, Ortiz JS, Sharrett AR, et al. Changing types of nephritogenic streptococci in Trinidad. J Clin Invest. 1971;50:1197–205.
56. Dillon HC, Derrick CW, Dillon MS. M-antigens common to pyoderma and acute glomerulonephritis. J Infect Dis. 1974;130:257–67.
57. Duca E, Teodorovici GR, Rudu C, et al. A new nephritogenic streptococcus. J Hyg (Lond). 1969;67:691–8.
58. Barnham M, Thornton TJ, Lange K. Nephritis caused by *Streptococcus zooepidemicus* (Lancefield group C). Lancet. 1983;1:945–8.
59. Seegal BC, Andres GA, Hsu KC, et al. Studies on the pathogenesis of acute and progressive glomerulonephritis in man by immunofluorescein and immunoferritin technique. Fed Proc. 1965;24(pt 1):100–8.
60. Michael AF Jr, Drummond KM, Good RA, et al. Acute poststreptococcal glomerulonephritis: Immune deposit disease. J Clin Invest. 1966;45:237–48.
61. Michael AF, Hoyer JR, Westberg NG, et al. Experimental models for the pathogenesis of acute poststreptococcal glomerulonephritis. In: Wannamaker LW, Masten JM, eds. Streptococci and Streptococcal Diseases. New York: Academic Press; 1972:481–500.
62. Zabriskie JB. The role of streptococci in human glomerulonephritis. J Exp Med. 1971;134(Suppl):180–92.
63. Lange CF. Chemistry of cross-reactive fragments of streptococcal cell membrane and human glomerular basement membrane. Transplant Proc. 1969;1:959–63.
64. Bisno AL, Wood JW, Lawson J, et al. An antigen in urine of patients with glomerulonephritis and in normal human serum which cross-reacts with group A streptococci: Identification and partial characterization. J Lab Clin Med. 1978;91:500–13.
65. Goroncy-Bermes P, Dale JB, Beachey EH, et al. Monoclonal antibody to human renal glomeruli cross-reacts with streptococcal M protein. Infect Immun. 1987;55:2416–9.
66. Ooi YM, Vallota EH, West CD. Serum immune complexes in membranoproliferative and other glomerulonephritides. Kidney Int. 1977;11:275–83.
67. Tung KSK, Woodroffe AJ, Ahlin TD, et al. Application of the solid phase Clq and Raji cell radioimmune assays for the detection of circulating immune complexes in glomerulonephritis. J Clin Invest. 1978;62:61–72.
68. Van de Rijn I, Fillit H, Brandeis WE, et al. Serial studies on circulating immune complexes in poststreptococcal sequelae. Clin Exp Immunol. 1978;34:318–25.
69. Lindberg LH, Vosti KL. Elution of glomerular bound antibodies in experimental streptococcal glomerulonephritis. Science. 1969;166:1032–3.
70. Markowitz AS, Horn D, Aseron C, et al. Streptococcal related glomerulonephritis. II. Glomerulonephritis in rhesus monkeys immunologically induced both actively and passively with a soluble fraction from nephritogenic streptococcal protoplasmic membranes. J Immunol. 1971;107:504–11.
71. Lange K, Ahmed U, Kleinberger H, et al. A hitherto unknown streptococcal antigen and its probable relation to acute poststreptococcal glomerulonephritis. Clin Nephrol. 1976;5:207–15.
72. Johnston KH, Zabriskie JB. Purification and partial characterization of the nephritis-strain associated protein from *Streptococcus pyogenes* group A. J Exp Med. 1986;163:697–712.
73. Lewy JE, Salinas-Madrigal L, Herdson PB, et al. Clinicopathologic correlations in acute poststreptococcal glomerulonephritis. Medicine (Baltimore). 1971;50:453–501.
74. Anthony BF, Kaplan EL, Wannamaker LW, et al. Attack rates of acute nephritis after type 49 streptococcal infection of the skin and of the respiratory tract. J Clin Invest. 1969;48:1697–704.
75. Stetson CA, Rammelkamp CH Jr, Krause RM et al. Epidemic acute nephritis: Studies on etiology, natural history, and prevention. Medicine (Baltimore). 1955;34:431–50.
76. Roy S III, Wall HP, Etteldorf JN. Second attacks of acute glomerulonephritis. J Pediatr. 1969;75:758–67.
77. Seegal D, Lyttle JD, Loeb EN, et al. On the exacerbation in chronic glomerulonephritis. J Clin Invest. 1940;19:569–89.
78. Poon-King T, Mohammed I, Cox R, et al. Recurrent epidemic nephritis in south Trinidad. N Engl J Med. 1967;277:728–33.
79. Kaplan EL, Anthony BF, Chapman SS, et al. Epidemic acute glomerulonephritis associated with type 49 streptococcal pyoderma. I. Clinical and laboratory findings. Am J Med. 1970;48:9–27.
80. Derrick CW, Reeves MS, Dillon HC Jr. Complement in overt and asymptomatic nephritis after skin infection. J Clin Invest. 1970;49:1178–87.
81. Sharrett AR, Poon-King T, Potter EV, et al. Subclinical nephritis in south Trinidad. Am J Epidemiol. 1971;94:231–45.
82. Dodge WF, Spargo BH, Travis LB. Occurrence of acute glomerulonephritis in sibling contacts of children with sporadic acute glomerulonephritis. Pediatrics. 1967;40:1029–30.
83. Schwartz WB, Kassirer JP. Clinical aspects of acute poststreptococcal glomerulonephritis. In: Strauss MB, Welt LG, eds. Diseases of the Kidney, ed 2. Boston: Little, Brown; 1971:419–62.
84. Freedman P, Meister HP, Lee HJ, et al. The renal response to streptococcal infection. Medicine (Baltimore). 1970;49:433–63.
85. Berman LB, Vogelsang P. Poststreptococcal glomerulonephritis without proteinuria. N Engl J Med. 1963;268:1275–7.
86. Smith RD, Aquino J. Viruses and the kidney. Med Clin North Am. 1971;55:89–106.

87. Kassirer JP, Schwartz WB. Acute glomerulonephritis. N Engl J Med. 1961;265:686–92.
88. Lasch EE, Frankel V, Vardy PA, et al. Epidemic glomerulonephritis in Israel. J Infect Dis. 1971;124:141–7.
89. Weinstein L, LeFrock J. Does antimicrobial therapy of streptococcal pharyngitis or pyoderma alter the risk of glomerulonephritis? J Infect Dis. 1971;124:229–31.
90. Perlman LV, Herdman RC, Kleinman H. Poststreptococcal glomerulonephritis. A ten-year follow-up of an epidemic. JAMA. 1965;194:63–70.
91. Potter EV, Lipschultz SA, Abidh S, et al. Twelve to seventeen-year follow-up of patients with poststreptococcal acute glomerulonephritis in Trinidad. N Engl J Med. 1982;307:725–9.
92. Baldwin DS. Poststreptococcal glomerulonephritis. A progressive disease? Am J Med. 1977;62:1–11.
93. Jennings RB, Earle DP. Poststreptococcal glomerulonephritis. Histopathologic and clinical studies of acute, subsiding acute and early chronic latent phases. J Clin Invest. 1961;40:1525–95.
94. Kurtzman NA. Does acute poststreptococcal glomerulonephritis lead to chronic renal disease? N Engl J Med. 1978;298:795–6.
95. Kaplan EL, Vernier RL. Progressive nephritis after strep infection questioned. Am J Med. 1978;64:910–911.

178. STREPTOCOCCUS PNEUMONIAE*

MAURICE A. MUFSON

Streptococcus pneumoniae, or the pneumococcus (previously designated *Diplococcus pneumoniae*), persists as a major respiratory tract pathogen of adults, especially of elderly persons, and of persons of all ages manifesting a distinctive susceptibility because of splenic dysfunction, asplenia, or other immune disorders. Pneumococcal disease ranks among the 10 leading causes of death in the United States, and case fatality rates with bacteremic infections are about 20–25 percent in pneumonia, and 30 percent in meningitis. The most common cause of community-acquired pneumonia, the pneumococcus, ranks as the second most common pathogen of bacterial meningitis, and it causes more than one-half of otitis media illnesses in children. An estimated 150,000–270,000 cases of pneumonia and 2600–6200 cases of meningitis occur annually (Table 1).[1] Notwithstanding that deaths from bacteremic pneumococcal disease occur much less often now than in the pre-antibiotic era, case fatality rates remain much higher than expected in view of the fact that nearly all isolates of pneumococcus are susceptible to penicillin and to several other antibiotics appropriate for the treatment of this infection. The emergence of penicillin-resistant strains and of multiple antibiotic-resistant strains, although uncommon and limited to a few capsular types, complicates the strategy for the treatment of pneumococcal infection.

HISTORICAL PERSPECTIVE

The elucidation of the biologic properties of *S. pneumoniae* and their relationship to clinical medicine has included some of the most fundamental contributions to biomedical science. In 1881, the pneumococcus was first identified from the saliva of a patient with rabies by Pasteur and from his own saliva by Sternberg. The association of the pneumococcus with lobar pneumonia was initially described by Friedlander and Talamon in 1883 and also by Frankel in 1884 and by Weichselbaum in 1886. Between 1900 and 1902, Neufeld discovered bile lysis by pneumococci, and the quellung reaction with homologous pneumococcal antisera was discovered by Neufeld. By 1910, Neufeld and Handel reported that antisera conferred type-specific immunity in mice, which formed the basis for type-specific antisera in the treatment of pneumococcal pneumonia. During this period, clinical observations of pneumococcal pneumonia were meticulously recorded by both Sir William Osler at Johns Hopkins Hospital and by Dr. Rufus Cole at The Rockefeller Hospital.

Over the next three decades, from 1915 to 1945, the chemical structure and antigenicity of the pneumococcal capsular polysaccharide and its association with virulence were elucidated. These elegant studies, which were the first to demonstrate the immunologic role of bacterial polysaccharides in human disease, were conducted for the most part in the laboratory of Dr. Oswald T. Avery at The Rockefeller Institute.[2] Avery's colleagues who contributed to studies of the pneumococcal polysaccharides included A.T. Dochez, M. Heidelberger, R. J. Dubos, W. Goebel, W.S. Tillett, T. Francis, Jr., and T.J. Abernathy. Although various pneumococcal vaccines were tested clinically over this period, the investigations by Avery and others formed the basis for the first successful field trial of a polyvalent polysaccharide vaccine for pneumococcal pneumonia in 1944–1945 by MacLeod and collaborators.[3] After the introduction of penicillin therapy for pneumococcal pneumonia by Dr. C. Keefer and others, many physicians felt the need neither to serotype isolates nor to administer vaccine. For the next 20 years, clinical and investigative interests in the pneumococcus were quiescent. It was largely through the singular efforts of Dr. R. Austrian during three decades starting in the 1950s that the medical community recognized the continuing importance of the pneumococcus as a major pathogen of serious pulmonary disease and the need for an effective polyvalent pneumococcal vaccine.[4] The development of a polyvalent polysaccharide vaccine for persons at high risk of serious pneumococcal disease began in 1967, and 10 years later a 14-valent vaccine was approved for clinical use in the United States. Subsequently, the 14-valent formulation was revised to include 23 capsular polysaccharides, and this polysaccharide vaccine was approved in 1983.

In addition to the immunochemical studies of pneumococcal polysaccharides, the transformation of pneumococcal types was a major contribution to biomedical science since it provided the basis on which molecular genetics was founded. In 1928, Griffith, although unaware of the implication of his observations at that time, postulated that rough pneumococci were not only reverted to smooth (encapsulated) cells of their parental type by heat-killed smooth cells of the same type but were also transformed to a different smooth type by heat-killed cells of that type.[5] In 1944, Avery and colleagues at The Rockfeller Institute succeeded in isolating the active transforming substance and identified it as deoxyribonucleic acid.[6]

TABLE 1. Occurrence of Serious Pneumococcal Disease in the United States

Category of Disease	Estimated Number of Cases (Thousands/yr)	Estimated Incidence (per 100,000 Population/yr)	Estimated Case Fatality Rate (%)
Pneumonia	150–570	68–260	5
Bacteremia	16–55	7–25	20
Meningitis	2.6–6.2	1.2–2.8	30

* The author has made extensive use of the excellent chapter by Richard Roberts, M.D., from the second edition of this text.

MICROBIOLOGY

Classification

Although the pneumococcus has been referred to as either *S. pneumoniae* or *D. pneumoniae*, the organism has been officially classified in the genus *Streptococcus*, and the former terminology should be used.[7] The similarities between the pneumococcus and other streptococci include the following characteristics:

1. *Morphology:* Pneumococci grow in short chains in broth cultures.

2. *Metabolism:* Streptococci, including the pneumococcus, are lactic acid bacteria, that is, they ferment glucose by the hexose monophosphate pathway to yield lactic acid.
3. *Antigenic structure:* Both pneumococci and streptococci contain a group-specific carbohydrate and M protein. The pneumococcal M protein, however, is not antiphagocytic. The peptide subunit structure of the cell wall peptidoglycan in both pneumococci and group a streptococci is similar.
4. *Deoxyribonucleic acid transformation:* Antibiotic resistance, type specificity, and other genetic markers have been transferred from one species to the other.
5. *Nucleic acid homology:* By chemical analysis, the guanine-plus-cytosine (G+C) content of DNA in 15 streptococcal species, including the pneumococcus, ranged from 33 to 42 mol percent.

Metabolism and Growth Requirements

Streptococcus pneumoniae is similar to the other species of streptococci in that metabolism is fermentative and lactic acid is the predominant end product. The concentration of glucose in culture media must not exceed 1%, or the pH of the media must be maintained above pH 7.0 due to lactic acid production during growth. Although inulin fermentation has been used in the past for the identification of pneumococci, it is no longer useful since many laboratory strains do not ferment inulin and other streptococcal species, especially *Streptococcus sanguis* and occasionally *Streptoccus mitior* ferment this sugar.

Pneumococci are facultative anaerobes in that oxygen or other hydrogen acceptors may alter the end products of carbohydrate metabolism. The organism lacks cytochromes and uses oxygen through a flavoprotein enzyme system. Hydrogen peroxide (H_2O_2) is the end product of this reaction and may accumulate since pneumococci do not produce catalase or peroxidase for H_2O_2 degradation. A source of catalase such as red blood cells must be incorporated into culture media, and prolonged incubation should be avoided.

Pneumococci are relatively fastidious organisms, and their viability is reduced if clinical specimens are allowed to dry at room temperature or are placed in sterile physiologic solution. Clinical specimens must be transported in nutrient broth and stored at 4°C. An enriched culture medium is necessary for isolation. For optimum growth, a pH of 7.8 (6.5–8.3) and a temperature of 37°C (25–42°C) is required. Since 5–10 percent of pneumococcal isolates require increased carbon dioxide for growth on agar medium, all cultures should be placed in this environment. Broth cultures tend to clear during prolonged incubation due to cell lysis (see autolysins).

Laboratory Identification

Direct Morphology. The pneumococcus is a gram-positive coccus that typically is lancet shaped and occurs in pairs (diplococcal) with the tapered ends in juxtaposition (Fig. 1). It may also occur singly or in short chains and may be spherical or oval in shape. Chain formation is more likely to occur in broth cultures and in the presence of type-specific antibody. After prolonged incubation, organisms may be gram-negative. Pneumococci are nonmotile and do not form spores.

Colonial Morphology. Colonies on blood agar appear smooth, glistening, and flat or dome shaped with a diameter of 0.5–1.5 cm. Encapsulated organisms, especially type 3, form mucoid colonies on agar. After 48 hours of incubation, the center of the colony collapses due to autolysis to produce a doughnut or umbilicated form. If incubated exceeds 72 hours, the remainder of the organism spontaneously lyses, and only a depression in the agar remains. Colonies produce a greenish discoloration on blood agar (α-hemolysis), although if incubated anaerobically, β-hemolysis occurs due to oxygen-sensitive pneumolysin O. Pneumococci tend to grow diffusely in blood broth and produce a greenish discoloration of the liquid medium.

Cultures suspected of containing pneumococci must be differentiated from other species of streptococci. Most diagnostic laboratories use the *optochin disk sensitivity test*. Paper disks impregnated with 5 μg or 1:400 optochin (ethyl hydrocupriene hydrochloride) are plated on agar on which a pure culture of organisms has been placed. Since optochin inhibits the growth of pneumococci but not other streptococcal species, a zone of inhibition occurs. Although the degree of growth inhibition may be less in the presence of CO_2, the test should be performed in a CO_2 environment to ensure adequate growth of all isolates.

Bile solubility may also differentiate pneumococci from other streptococcal species, but it is rarely used by diagnostic laboratories. This test is based on the presence of an autolytic amidase in pneumococci that cleaves the bond between alanine and muramic acid in the peptidoglycan, thereby causing lysis of the organism at a neutral pH. The amidase is activated by various surface-active agents such as bile and bile salts. The test is performed with 10% deoxycholate and a saline suspension of a viable, young culture of organisms. The test should not be performed on an agar surface because of false-positive results.

Quellung Reaction. The Neufeld quellung reaction, or capsular precipitin reaction, provides rapid identification of pneumococci in various clinical specimens including spinal fluid, sputum, and exudate or in broth culture. The procedure is to air-dry a suspension of the organism on a microscopic slide and resuspend it with a loopful of pneumococcal antiserum to which methylene blue has been added. After a few minutes, the slide is examined under oil immersion. If positive, the organism will be surrounded by a large capsule. The capsular appearance is probably due to both capsular swelling and greater refraction. Pneumococcal antisera for both the quellung reaction and serotyping are available from Statens Seruminstitut, Copenhagen, Denmark. Three kinds of antisera are available: (1) Omni-serum, which contains antisera to all 84 known pneumococcal types, (2) 9 pooled sera (lettered A through I), each pool containing 7 to 11 single or multiple types, and (3) individual antisera, which are numbered 1 to 48. These latter antisera may be of one type, for example, types 1, 2, 3, 4, 5, and 8, or of multiple types, for example, type 6 incorporates 6A and 6B, and type 7 contains 7A, 7B, 7C, and 7F. Reconstituted antisera may be stored at 4°C for 1–2 years. For rapid identification, the clinical specimen should be mixed with both Omni-serum and type 3 antiserum since a type 3 quellung reaction may not occur with Omni-serum. In addition, a false-negative test result may occur with types 3 and 37 antisera due to antigen excess (prozone phenomenon).

Animal Inoculation (Mouse Virulence Test). Intraperitoneal inoculation of mice with sputum from patients with pneumonia and the subsequent isolation of pneumococci from mouse heart blood 24 hours later was performed by many diagnostic laboratories before antimicrobial therapy. This procedure is rarely performed as a diagnostic test at the present time because it is expensive and time-consuming. Many research laboratories use this experimental model to test the virulence of a particular isolate or type. However, certain types, especially type 14, may not be virulent for mice.

Surface Antigens: Capsular Polysaccharides

Pneumococcal capsular substances are complex polysaccharides that form hydrophilic gels on the surface of the organism.[8] Capsular polysaccharides are antigenic and form the basis for classifying pneumococci by serotypes.

There are at present 84 known serotypes. Two systems of nomenclature, that is, American and Danish, have been de-

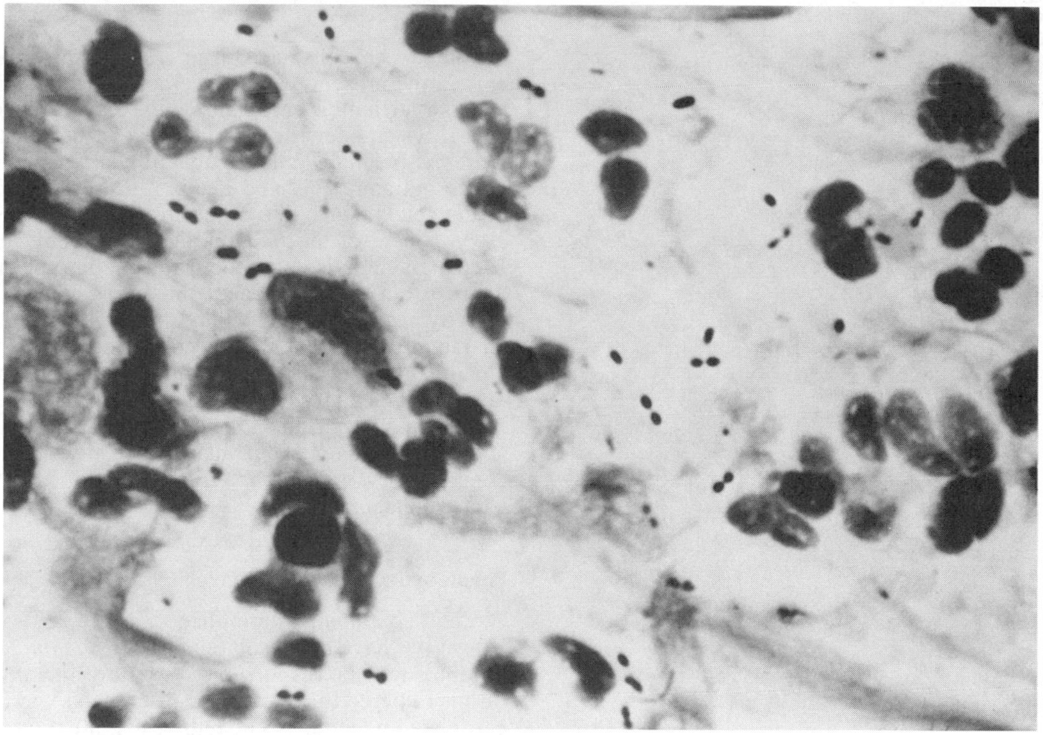

FIG. 1. Expectorated sputum with gram-positive, lancet-shaped diplococci from a patient with pneumococcal pneumonia.

veloped, due in part to classification of cross-reactions among certain types. Correlation of the two designations is summarized in Table 2. Although pneumococcal typing had been largely abandoned by routine diagnostic laboratories, since the advent of penicillin therapy for pneumococcal infections, the introduction of immunoprophylaxis with a 23-valent vaccine necessitates monitoring of pneumococcal types associated with systemic infections.

Capsular polysaccharides may be demonstrated by agglutination, by precipitation, by the quellung reaction, and by counterimmunoelectrophoresis. Capsular size is greatest during log-phase growth and is reduced in stationary-phase growth due to the diffusion of polysaccharide into the medium. Increasing concentrations of glucose stimulate capsule production but, as mentioned previously, are also toxic to the organism because of lactic acid production.

Cross-reactions of capsular polysaccharides exist between individual pneumococcal types as well as with other bacteria. Examples of the former include types 2 and 5, types 3 and 8, types 7 and 18, and types 15 and 30. Pneumococcal capsular polysaccharides also cross-react with polysaccharides from *Escherichia coli, Klebsiella pneumoniae, Salmonella* species, type b *Haemophilus influenzae*, and viridans streptococci. Type 14 polysaccharide cross reacts with type III group B streptococci and human ABO blood group isoantigens. The cross-reaction with A, B, H, and Le^a substances is probably related to *N*-acetyl-D-glucosamine, which is the common terminal end group shared by these polysaccharides.

The pathogenicity of pneumococci is related primarily to its capsular polysaccharide. Encapsulated organisms (S = smooth) are virulent for humans and experimental animals, whereas organisms without capsular polysaccharides (R = rough) are not. Active or passive immunization employing "smooth" pneumococci protects against subsequent infection by the homologous type in animals, and immunization of humans with purified capsular polysaccharides prevents subsequent bacteremic pneumonia by the same pneumococcal type. Certain pneumococcal types appear more virulent, such as types 1, 2, 3, 4, 7, 8, 12, and 14. The mechanism by which the capsular polysaccharide is responsible for the virulence of pneumococci is based on its antiphagocytic property.

C-Substance or C-Polysaccharide. This teichoic acid contains phosphocholine and galactosamine-6-phosphate and is a major constituent of the cell wall.[9] It is analogous to but antigenically distinct from the group-specific carbohydrate of hemolytic streptococci since it is species but not type specific. The C-substance forms a portion of the Forssman, or F, antigen. It consists also of techoic acid and covalently bound lipid.[9] F antigen is a specific inhibitor of homologous autolysin. It also precipitates with a serum β-globulin in the presence of calcium. This β-globulin, called C-reactive protein (CRP), is not an antibody but a protein that is present in low concentrations in normal blood and is elevated in patients with acute inflammatory diseases. The binding of CRP to C-polysaccharide can activate complement[10] and can mediate phagocytosis.

M-Protein Antigen. M-protein antigen is type rather than species specific and is therefore analogous to the M protein of group A streptococci. However, it is antigenically distinct from the latter protein and does not exert an antiphagocytic effect. The type-specificity of this antigen is independent of that associated with the pneumococcal capsular polysaccharide.

R-Protein Antigen. R-protein antigen was first isolated from rough pneumococci and is poorly characterized. It is localized on or near the cell surface and is antigenically similar to the C-polysaccharide in that it is species specific.

Toxins

The ability of pneumococci to produce disease is thought to be due to their resistance to phagocytosis and their subsequent invasion and multiplication in host tissue. However, the elaboration of toxic substances by these organisms is suggested by the following clinical observations: (*1*) abrupt onset of symp-

TABLE 2. Correlation of the American and Danish Serotype Designations

USA	Denmark	USA	Denmark
1	1	43	11A
2	2	44	18A
3	3	45	40
4	4	46	23A
5	5	47	35A
6	6A	48	7B
7	7A	49	9L
8	8	50	7C
9	9N	51	7F
10	10F	52	47F
11	11F	53	11C
12	12F	54	15B
13	13	55	18B
14	14	56	18C
15	15F	57	19A
16	16	58	19B
17	17	59	19C
18	18F	60	24B?
19	19F	61	35C
20	20	62	35A
21	21	63	22A
22	22F	64	23B
23	23F	65	24A
24	24F	66	35B
25	25	67	32A
26	6B	68	9V
27	27	69	39
28	28	70	33F
29	29	71	38
30	15A	72	45
31	31	73	46
32	32F	74	41A
33	9A	75	43
34	10A	76	11B
35	35F	77	15C
36	36	78	17A
37	37	79	28A
38	41F	80	42
39	33C	81	44
40	33A	82	48
41	34	83	12A
42	33B	84	47A

toms, (*2*) profound toxicity, and (*3*) fulminant clinical course with disseminated intravascular coagulation (DIC) in patients with splenectomy. Although the following pneumococcal toxins have been described, their pathogenic role remains to be elucidated.

Pneumolysin. This acidic protein is immunologically related to the oxygen-labile O hemolysins of hemolytic streptococci, *Clostridium tetani* and *Clostridium welchii*, and is responsible for the β-hemolysis when pneumococci are grown anaerobically. It is released during autolysis, has a molecular weight of 63,000, is destroyed by heat, and is inactive by oxygen. It has dermatoxic properties in experimental animals and may cause the hemolytic anemia observed in rabbits with pneumococcal bacteremia.

Purpura-Producing Principle. This substance causes purpura and dermal hemorrhage in experimental animals. It is associated with the mucopeptide of the cell wall and is released during autolysis. The purpuric activity appears to require intact β-1,4-glucosidic linkages.

Neuraminidase. This low-molecular-weight protein is produced by fresh isolates only during log-phase growth. Unlike the purpura-producing principle, it is antigenic and species specific. This enzyme is lethal for mice. Since cell membrane glycoproteins and glycolipids are substrates, this enzyme may contribute to the invasiveness of pneumococci in host tissue.

Autolysins

Pneumococcal cells lyse during prolonged incubation. Lysis occurs in the presence of surface-active agents and antimicrobial agents that inhibit cell wall synthesis. The basis for pneumococcal lysis under these conditions is the release of *N*-acetyl-muramyl-l-alanine amidase an autolysin that splits the bond between muramic acid and alanine in the peptidoglycan portion of the cell wall. Unlike other streptococcal species, choline is a component of the teichoic acid in pneumococcal cell walls. If ethanolamine is substituted for choline, pneumococcal cells are resistant to the amidase, and autolysis does not occur even in the presence of penicillin ("antibiotic tolerance"). Other characteristics of pneumococcal cells grown in the presence of ethanolamine include long-chain formation because cells fail to divide and the failure to undergo transformation. Pneumococcal autolysin is important not only in the activity of bacteriocidal antimicrobial agents but also in cell division and separation, competence for genetic transformation, and infection by bacteriophage.

Pneumococcal Bacteriophage

A lipid-containing diplophage (Dp1) and several omega phages[11,12] have been isolated from *S. pneumoniae*. Diplophage products may be responsible for autolysin activation, which in turn is required for the release of progeny virus particles.[13] Encapsulated pneumococcal cells resist infection by omega phage but have no effect on the release of infectious phage. Several lysogenic phages have been isolated from fresh encapsulated pneumococcal strains that were lytic for nonencapsulated organisms, thus suggesting a relationship between pneumococcal phage and capsule formation.[14] Dp4 phage can transfect the pneumococcus and provides a tool for the study of DNA after infection.[15,16]

Genetic Transformation

Genetic recombination by the introduction of deoxyribonucleic acid was discovered by Avery and associates in 1944.[6] Genetic markers that have been successfully transformed in vitro in pneumococci include (*1*) capsular polysaccharide type specificity, (*2*) the amount of capsular polysaccharide produced, (*3*) antimicrobial (penicillin, streptomycin, sulfonamides) and optochin resistance, (*4*) type specificity of somatic M proteins, (*5*) chain formation of rough and smooth mutants, and (*6*) the capacity to produce certain inducible enzymes. The frequency of transformation in nature is presently unknown.

EPIDEMIOLOGY OF PNEUMOCOCCAL PNEUMONIA

Incidence

Pneumococcal pneumonia is the most common community-acquired pneumonia. In the United States, pneumococcal pneumonia is not a reportable disease; the estimated incidence of pneumococcal pneumonia is 68–260 cases per 100,000 population per year (or 150,000–570,000 cases per year) (Table 1).[1] Bacteremia develops in about 20–25 percent of cases. Higher incidence rates have been observed in closed communities such as the military, in certain occupations including painters and welders, and in distinctive population groups such as American Indians residing on reservations and native miners in the Union of South Africa.[17] The highest incidence rates of pneumococcal pneumonia have been recorded among the native miners of South Africa's diamond and gold mines: 9000 cases per 100,000 population per year and higher. Pneumococcal pneumonia occurs more commonly in men than in women in all decades of life (3:2). Among persons older than 40 years of age, the incidence is three to four times greater as compared with persons under 30 years of age.

The incidence of pneumococcal pneumonia peaks during the winter and early spring months in temperate climates. Pneumococcal pneumonia is the most common secondary bacterial complication of influenza virus infections, and the increase in cases of pneumococcal pneumonia parellels the epidemic of influenza virus. Seasonal variation also occurs in other pyogenic bacterial infections such as *Neisseria meningitidis* and *Haemophilus influenzae*.

Endogenous and Exogenous Infections

Pneumococci are common inhabitants of the human upper respiratory tract and have been isolated from 5 to 70 percent of the normal adult population. The rate of asymptomatic carriage varies with age, environment, and the presence of upper respiratory tract infections.[18] Rates in urban families decline as age increases (30–35 percent from 6 to 11 years and 18–19 percent in adults). Only 5–10 percent of the adults without children are pneumococcal carriers. Rates in closed populations are higher than in the general urban population, that is, 27–58 percent in schools and orphanages and 50–60 percent in closed military installations. The duration of pneumococcal carriage also varies and is longer in children than in adults and in persons who have low antibody levels before colonization. Spread of the organism within a family is influenced by crowding, the season (fall and winter), and the presence of upper respiratory tract infections or pneumococcal disease such as pneumonia or otitis media.[19] The relationship of pneumococcal carriage to the development of natural immunity is poorly understood. A significant rise in type-specific antibody after colonization has been observed in over 50 percent of children but rarely in adults. Many adults have relatively high antibody levels before colonization, which may explain, in part, the lower rate and shorter duration of colonization.

Carrier strains in the normal population are often higher capsular types that are not commonly associated with clinical disease. On the other hand, the same serotypes responsible for pneumococcal disease such as pneumonia and otitis media can be recovered from the upper respiratory tract during acute infections. Community-acquired pneumococcal pneumonia is usually a sporadic disease in carriers who have an injury to various pulmonary defense mechanisms that result in interference with bacterial clearance. Since pneumococcal pneumonia is usually an endogenous infection, hospitalized patients do not require isolation.[20]

Epidemics of pneumococcal pneumonia, even in closed populations, are uncommon. During epidemic periods, person-to-person transmission occurs via droplets. Epidemics may be associated with either multiple types in large susceptible populations or rarely with one type in small closed populations.

Morbidity and Mortality

In the United States, of all infectious diseases only pneumonia-influenza ranks among the 10 leading causes of death. Annually an estimated 50,000 deaths occur from pneumococcal pneumonia. The disease carries a total case fatality rate of about 5 percent as compared with a rate of 30 percent in the pre-antibiotic era.

Case fatality rates in pneumococcal pneumonia increase sharply with bacteremia and especially when an extrapulmonary focus of infection also exists.[21,22] In bacteremic pneumococcal pneumonia, the total case fatality rate is about 20 percent, and with infection of the central nervous system the case fatality rate is about 60 percent.[21,22] These data underscore the importance of obtaining blood cultures in all patients with pneumonia whether or not complicated by extrapulmonary disease. The case fatality rate in pneumococcal pneumonia varies with increasing age, capsular type, and underlying condition. In normal children, the case fatality rate in bacteremic pneumococcal pneumonia is less than 1 percent, and the total case fatality rate in children with systemic pneumococcal disease is about 6 percent.[23] In young adults, the case fatality rate in bacteremic pneumococcal pneumonia is about 20 percent, in adults aged 50 and 69 years the rate is 25–40 percent, and in adults over 70 years the rate is 50–60 percent (Table 3).

The risk of death from pneumococcal disease is higher in persons with underlying disease including immunodeficiency syndromes, splenic dysfunction, persons who have had splenectomy, acute alcoholism, delirium tremens, Laennec cirrhosis, chronic obstructive pulmonary disease, congestive heart failure, and malignancy,[21,22,25,26] The case fatality rate may be higher with certain capsular types, for example, type 3 infection carries a higher rate as compared with other capsular types. The prognosis in pneumococcal disease is worsened by leukopenia, involvement of three or more lobes of the lungs, jaundice, and extrapulmonary complications.[21,22,26]

Pneumococcal Types

Of the 84 capsular types of pneumococcus that have been characterized (Table 2), usually the lower number types are most pathogenic for humans. In the pre-antibiotic era, the predominant capsular types were types 1, 2, and 3. These three serotypes caused about 75 percent of bacteremic disease.[27] During the past four decades, a different pattern of prevalent capsular types has emerged. Now 8–10 capsular types cause most serious bacteremic disease among adults (Table 4). Most often types 1, 3, 4, 7, 8, 9, 12, 14, and less often, types 6, 18, and 19 (not listed in rank order) as a group have been associated with most bacteremic cases.[21–23,25,28,29] An analysis of bacteremic cases among adults admitted to hospitals in five cities in the United States and the United Kingdom during 1952 to 1985 shows that the eight most common capsular types in each of those hospitals accounted for about 66 percent of cases. No one type predominated, and types that rarely occurred in the pre-antibiotic era occur regularly now. Among children with bacteremic disease, the spectrum of common capsular types shows differences from pneumococcal infections in adults. Capsular types 14, 6, 18, 19, 23, 1, 4, and 9 are associated with most of

TABLE 3. Case Fatality Rate by Age in Bacteremic Pneumococcal Disease in the Antibiotic Era[a]

Population Group, City and County (Study Interval)	*Age (yr)*	*Number in Group*	*Case Fatality Rate (%)*	*Reference*
Brooklyn, NY (1952–1962)	12–29	51	8	21
	30–49	205	12	
	50–69	179	29	
	70+	94	54	
Chicago, IL (1967–1970)	12–29	35	6	22
	30–49	156	19	
	50–69	111	41	
	70+	23	61	
Huntington, WV (1978–1981)	1–13	17	6	24
	14–49	16	9	
	50–70+	56	33	
London, UK (1970–1982)	0–9	26	15	25
	10–29	27	18	
	30–49	52	23	
	50–69	144	28	
	70+	76	41	
Jerusalem, Israel (1977–1985)	1–12	49	6	26
	13–30	12	16	
	31–50	6	0	
	51–70	12	42	
	71+	25	44	

[a] Pneumococcal disease includes pneumonia with bacteremia and extrapulmonary disease with or without pneumonia.

TABLE 4. Occurrence of Capsular Types among Adults or Children with Bacteremic Pneumococcal Disease in the Antibiotic Era[a]

Geographic Location, Interval	*Rank Order of Capsular Type (%)*								
	1st	*2nd*	*3rd*	*4th*	*5th*	*6th*	*7th*	*8th*	*Reference*
Adults:									
Brooklyn, NY 1952–1962 (*N* = 529)	1 (15)	7 (12)	8 (12)	3 (9)	4 (4)	12 (7)	5 (5)	14 (4)	21
Chicago, IL 1967–1970 (*N* = 325)	8 (14)	4 (12)	5 (8)	12 (8)	1 (7)	3 (6)	7 (6)	9 (5)	22
London, UK 1970–1982 (*N* = 301)	3 (13)	8 (12)	14 (11)	1 (10)	6 (6)	7 (5)	4 (5)	9 (4)	25
Glasgow, UK 1982–1985 (*N* = 410)	3 (12)	14 (11)	8 (9)	6 (9)	1 (8)	4 (8)	7 (6)	19 (5)	28
Children									
Chicago, IL 1967–1976 (*N* = 305)	14 (17)	6 (16)	19 (11)	23 (10)	18 (9)	9 (8)	4 (5)	1 (4)	29
Birmingham, AL 1979–1984 (*N* = 216)	14 (25)	6 (20)	18 (11)	23 (10)	19 (7)	1 (5)	9 (5)	4 (4)	23

[a] Pneumococcal disease includes pneumonia with bacteremia, meningitis, septicemia, and joint and abdominal cavity infections.

the serious infections in children, and these types account for about 85 percent of all infections.[23,29] The pattern of infecting types was nearly identical for the two cities Chicago and Birmingham.

These data were considered when the revised formulation of the 23-valent pneumococcal vaccine was prepared. The new vaccine contains polysaccharide from each of the most prevalent serotypes among adults and children. Thus the vaccine comprises serotypes accounting for about 90 percent of the infections in the community. Surveillance of pneumococcal capsular types causing bacteremic disease needs to be continued not only to monitor the types in the vaccine but also to attempt to identify shifts of predominant types whether because of naturally occurring circumstances or the increasing use of vaccine. At present, no evidence exists for change in the prevalent capsular types because of vaccine use in the community.

PATHOGENESIS AND CLINICAL MANIFESTATIONS

Pneumonia

The pathogenesis of pneumococcal pneumonia is due to rapid multiplication of the organisms in alveolar spaces. The presence of intra-alveolar exudation enhances multiplication. The pathologic progression of this disease before antimicrobial therapy has been well described and includes four steps. However, each step may be represented in a given pathologic specimen, especially if patients have received antimicrobial therapy. The four steps include congestion, red hepatization, gray hepatization, and resolution. Initially, there is local hyperemia, edema, and neutrophil mobilization. By the second to third day of illness, the lung weight increases three- to fourfold because of blood-tinged fluid, congested capillaries, and alveoli filled with bacteria and red cells. The alveoli then become plugged with fibrin and neutrophils. By the fourth to fifth day, the lungs become gray-white, and the alveoli contain neutrophils but no organisms. There is usually diffuse purulent bronchitis and local adenopathy. Resolution is characterized by complete healing with no evidence of tissue necrosis.

The normal host defense mechanisms of the respiratory tract include the following immunologic and nonimmunologic factors: mucus-secreting cells, epiglottis reflex, cilia, cough reflex, lymphatics, phagocytic leukocytes including polymorphonuclear leukocytes and macrophages, and opsonins. Pneumococcal pneumonia usually develops after aspiration of upper respiratory tract secretions containing pneumococci in patients with impaired host defenses. Conditions that impair pulmonary defenses are many, including alcoholism, anesthesia, stupor, and fluid accumulation in alveoli. The latter condition is most commonly associated with congestive heart failure and probably interfers with the functional capabilities of alevolar macrophages. Since pneumonia follows the aspiration of contaminated secretions, the initial lesion usually occurs in either the lower lobe or the right middle lobe. Lobar pneumonia is more likely to occur in adults, whereas in children and the elderly, bronchopneumonia is usually seen. Usually a single lobe is involved, although two lobes may be infected in 10–25 percent of patients and three lobes in fewer than 1 percent. Pneumonia may be preceded by coryza in 75 percent of the patients, thus suggesting an antecedent viral respiratory tract infection. The incubation period of pneumococcal pneumonia is usually 1–3 days, and the clinical manifestations are unrelated to pneumococcal serotype. Before the use of antimicrobial therapy, natural recovery occurred in 5–7 days and usually coincided with the appearance of circulating antibody. Clinically, recovery was characterized by an abrupt fall in temperature, which was often referred to as *crisis*.

The onset of clinical symptoms is usually abrupt, with a severe shaking chill or rigor in 80 percent of patients. A single episode of vomiting may occur in one-third of patients. A sustained fever of 102–105°F follows almost immediately. Repeated shaking chills are uncommon. Cough productive of rusty sputum occurs in three-quarters of patients. Because of the peripheral location of the initial lesion, pleuritic chest pain is relatively common (75 percent). Patients may be dyspneic, lie on the affected side to splint the involved lung, and may have difficulty in expectoration because of chest pain. Malaise, weakness, anorexia, and general prostration are common. Nausea, vomiting, and headache, however, are less frequent.

On physical examination the patient appears acutely ill and toxic with fever, tachycardia, tachypnea, and shallow respirations. Examination of the chest reveals signs of bronchopneumonia or consolidation. Abdominal distension due to gastric dilatation or paralytic ileus may be present. Abdominal pain may be associated with lower lobe pneumonia and should not be mistaken for an acute abdomen. Extrapulmonary sites of infection such as meninges, endocardium, and joints may be present.

Laboratory findings usually reveal a leukocytosis with an increased number of neutrophils and band forms. Leukopenia, however, may occur in overwhelming infections and in elderly patients. A chest roentgenogram should be obtained to confirm the physical findings and to rule out pleural fluid. Anemia and an elevated bilirubin (indirect) level may suggest mild hemolysis with or without liver disease. Arterial blood gases often reveal hypoxia (a decrease in PO_2) and occasionally a decreased PCO_2. Sputum should be examined both by Gram stain and by the quellung reaction (see below).

A clinical response to appropriate antimicrobial therapy is usually seen within 12–36 hours, although it may take as long as 96 hours. A reduction in fever occurs initially and is followed by a decrease in the respiratory rate, cough, and chest pain. Complete radiologic resolution usually takes 2–3 weeks, although it may be delayed in alcoholics and in patients with chronic lung disease. Subsequent fibrosis is exceedingly uncommon in patients with pneumococcal pneumonia. During the immediate recovery period, herpes labialis may appear. Inappropriate secretion of antidiuretic hormone has been reported with pneumococcal pneumonia.

Most patients with pneumococcal pneumonia, especially those over 50 years of age who have underlying diseases, require hospitalization to ensure adequate diagnostic studies, bed rest, fluid and electrolyte replacement, and adequate ventilation. Patient isolation is unnecessary except during an epidemic or outbreak of pneumococcal disease. Narcotics and sedatives should be avoided if at all possible so that the cough reflex is not suppressed. Because they mask the fever curve, antipyretics should only be used if tachycardia compromises cardiac output. Nasal oxygen is given in cyanosis and hypoxemia are present. Sputum expectoration should be encouraged, especially in the elderly patient, to avoid atelectasis. Many patients have serious underlying cardiac, pulmonary, or metabolic diseases, and careful monitoring of these problems is important.

In patients with persistent fever and tachycardia during antimicrobial therapy, various suppurative complications should be ruled out. These include direct extension into the pleural or pericardial cavities, endobronchial obstruction with distal atelectasis or abscess formation, and extrapulmonary localization such as meningitis, endocarditis, or arthritis. If pneumococci have not been recovered from appropriate clinical specimens, the pulmonary infiltrate may be due to a different respiratory pathogen such as *S. aureus, H. influenzae*, or *K. pneumoniae* or to a noninfectious process, for example, pulmonary infarction or malignancy. Other etiologies of persistent fever include drugs and superinfection.

Local Complications. EMPYEMA. Pleural effusion is the most common complication in pneumococcal pneumonia and occurs in 25 percent of the patients. The fluid is characteristic of an exudate, but Gram stain and cultures do not reveal organisms. The amount of fluid is usually small and does not require specific therapy. Diagnostic aspiration of pleural fluid should always be performed, however, to exclude the presence of empyema. Before antimicrobial therapy, this complication developed in 5–8 percent of the patients; it now occurs in only 10 percent of those patients with pleural effusion and in fewer than 1 percent of all patients. Empyema should be suspected in patients who continue to have fever, tachycardia, and leukocytosis despite adequate antimicrobial therapy. Diagnostic thoracentesis reveals fluid characteristic of an exudate. The gross appearance in the early stages, however, may appear as a transudate. If repeated aspiration is unsuccessful, surgical drainage may be necessary to avoid rupture through the skin (empyema necessitans) or into the bronchus (bronchopleural fistula).

PERICARDITIS. Although the most common form of purulent pericarditis before penicillin therapy, pneumococcal pericarditis is rarely seen at the present time. It occurs almost always with pneumococcal pneumonia (93 percent) and empyema (67 percent) and is due to local dissemination.[30] The clinical picture is similar to other forms of purulent pericarditis, which include precordial pain, fever, tachycardia, and a to-and-fro friction rub on physical examination. An absent friction rub, distant heart sounds, and an enlarged cardiac silhouette should suggest significant pericardial fluid, and the patient should be carefully observed for cardiac tamponade. Noninvasive diagnostic techniques include electrocardiography, echocardiography, body scan, and computer tomography. Pericardiocentesis should be performed to establish the diagnosis. Definitive therapy not only includes antimicrobial therapy but also surgical drainage either through a pericardial window or by pericardiectomy. Constrictive pericarditis should be prevented if at all possible.

LUNG ABSCESS. Necrosis of pulmonary tissue is rarely seen in uncomplicated pneumonia except in type 3 infections. Endobronchial obstruction due to either exudative material, tumor, or a foreign body should be considered in every patient with pneumococcal pneumonia and abscess formation. The clinical signs and symptoms consist of persistent fever, tachycardia, and leukocytosis, and therapy is directed toward relief of the obstruction.

Bacteremia. Bacteremia occurs in approximately 25–30 percent of the patients with pneumococcal pneumonia, although the relative frequency varies widely depending on serotype. Organisms probably enter the blood stream via the lymphatics, hilar nodes, and thoracic duct. The mortality in patients with bacteremic pneumonia is twice that in patients without bacteremia, although the incidence also varies widely when based on serotype. A fulminant clinical course may also be seen in patients with pneumococcal bacteremia and asplenia.[31] Disseminated intravascular coagulation (DIC) can occur in these patients.[32–34] The basis for DIC is unclear, although a lack of bacterial clearance by the spleen and a delay in early antibody formation may explain in part the high mortality in these patients.[32] Pneumococci have been visualized in peripheral blood smears taken from these patients.[34]

Pneumococcal Infections of the Upper Respiratory Tract

Otitis Media. About 76–95 percent of infants and children will have at least one episode of otitis media by the age of 6 years.[35] Recurrent attacks reduce hearing acuity and may have a deleterious effect on learning. The pneumococcus causes about one-half of the cases of bacterial otitis media.[36] Recent bacteriologic studies have revealed that pneumococcal types 19, 6, 23, and 3 (in descending order of frequency) are associated with most otitis media illnesses.[37] Capsular types 6, 19, and 23 are most commonly isolated from healthy carriers in the pediatric population, and these types often cause bacteremic infections in children.[23,28] The role of humoral immunity in pneumococcal otitis media is unclear at the present time. A type-specific serum antibody response to capsular polysaccharide may occur in only a small proportion of children.[38] Pneumococcal vaccine induced very poor responses in infants and children, and the efficacy of the vaccine for preventing otitis media seemed poor.[37,39]

Mastoiditis and Sinusitis. Since the advent of antimicrobial therapy, mastoiditis is rarely seen. Sinusitis, however, is not uncommon. The pneumococcus may be one of the pyogenic bacteria associated with infections of the mastoid or sinuses. Before antibiotics, direct extension from these anatomic areas was one source for the development of pneumococcal meningitis and brain abscess.

Extrapulmonary Pneumococcal Infections

Meningitis. Pneumococcal meningitis can result as a complication of bacteremic pneumonia, mastoiditis and sinusitis, skull fracture with communication between the nasopharynx and the subarachnoid space, or endocarditis. One-quarter of patients with pneumococcal meningitis also have pneumonia. The disease is seen in all age groups, and the mortality is highest in infants and the elderly (approaching 80 percent[24]). The clinical symptoms, spinal fluid profile, and neurologic complications are similar to those in other forms of purulent bacterial meningitis. It is most important to search not only for a primary source of infection in these patients but also for metastatic localization since many patients have bacteremia.

Endocarditis. Before antimicrobial therapy, pneumococcal endocarditis accounted for 10 percent of the cases of microbial endocarditis, but in recent years it occurs in fewer than 1 percent of the patients. Usually a complication of pneumonia or meningitis, endocarditis occurs on either normal or previously damaged heart valves. The clinical course is acute, and unlike viridans streptococcal endocarditis, local tissue destruction of heart valves is common. The aortic valve is often affected, and aortic cusp perforation with acute aortic insufficiency or aortic root fistula formation with septal abscess and conduction abnormalities may be seen. Endophthalmitis with a complete loss of vision requiring subsequent enucleation has been associated with both pneumococcal meningitis and endocarditis.

Arthritis. Pneumococcal arthritis is relatively uncommon and occurs principally in the elderly.[40] Before antibiotic therapy, the incidence of pneumonia in these patients was 70 percent. Now pneumonia occurs uncommonly unless other suppurative foci exist such as empyema or meningitis. Patients may have underlying chronic joint disease, which may delay diagnostic aspiration. The clinical manifestations are similar to other forms of hematogenous pyogenic joint infections. Adjacent osteomyelitis may be detected on radiologic examination. In addition to parenteral antimicrobial therapy, repeated aspiration or closed-tube drainage may be necessary. Intra-articular instillation of penicillin is unnecessary since adequate levels in synovial fluid are achieved after parenteral administration.

Peritonitis. Pneumococci infrequently cause spontaneous peritonitis. These patients have ascites due to either postnecrotic cirrhosis or Laennec cirrhosis.[41] The pathogenesis of this form of peritonitis is unclear, although transient pneumococcal bacteremia associated with respiratory infections may be a precipitating factor. Pneumococci, in addition to other bacteria, grow exceedingly well in vitro in the presence of ascitic fluid.

Laboratory Diagnosis

Isolation of the Organism. Appropriate clinical specimens should always be collected before the administration of antimicrobial therapy. Specimens should be processed immediately or stored at 4°C. Care must be taken to ensure that patients expectorate sputum from the lower respiratory tract. The presence of epithelial cells in sputum samples indicates upper respiratory tract secretions. In addition, expectorated sputum may be contaminated by upper airway secretions including normal oral flora or, in the case of hospitalized patients, gram-negative bacilli and *S. aureus*. If adequate sputum specimens from the lower respiratory tract cannot be obtained, percutaneous transtracheal aspiration should be considered.

Clinical specimens should be examined by Gram stain and, if indicated, by the quellung reaction. Pneumococci may occur singly, in pairs, or in chains. Organisms may appear gram-negative since they are easily decolorized by acetone-alcohol. The presence of polymorphonuclear leukocytes suggests that the specimen has originated from the infected area. However, the presence of gram-positive intracellular organisms may not always be indicative of pneumococcal pneumonia. If the Gram stain suggests pneumococci, a quellung reaction should be performed. This method may be diagnostic and has been correlated with subsequent culture results in 95 percent of adults with pneumococcal pneumonia.[42] Its use in children, however, is limited because of inadequate sputum collection.

Specimens should be processed on blood agar as soon as possible. The addition of gentamicin, 5 μg/ml, to the agar to suppress the growth of other streptococci may increase the sensitivity of the culture. Either infusion or thioglycollate broth may be used for blood cultures. Characteristically, pneumococci grow diffusely in liquid medium and produce a greenish discoloration due to α-hemolysis of blood cells.

Antigen Detection

Counterimmunoelectrophoresis (CIE) provides a rapid method for the detection of capsular polysaccharide antigen in clinical specimens including sputum, blood, cerebrospinal fluid, urine, pleural fluid, and peritoneal fluid.[43] CIE is performed by using, as antibody, Pneumococcal Omni-serum (Statens Serum Institute, Copenhagen, Denmark), which contains anticapsular antibody to 83 serotypes. Highly specific and sensitive for detecting antigen in the cerebrospinal fluid, CIE is positive in about 90 percent of cases of pneumococcal meningitis.[43] However, the proportion of patients with antigen in sputum, blood, or urine varies considerably depending upon the individual study.[44,45] Pneumococcal antigenemia occurs in 45–80 percent, and antigenuria occurs in about 50–65 percent of cases of pneumococcal pneumonia. CIE can detect antigen in sputum when cultures are negative in about one-fourth of cases, but it can be negative when pneumococcus is isolated from sputum. Prior antimicrobial therapy does not appear to alter the CIE results. Pneumococcal capsular types 7 and 14 may not be detected by CIE.

Circulating Antibody

No serologic procedure provides the necessary rapidity of diagnosis of pneumococcal infection in view of the importance of promptly establishing this diagnosis. Since the widespread use of pneumococcal polysaccharide vaccine, circulating anticapsular antibody measured by radioimmunoassay (RIA) has been used extensively to measure type-specific responses to the administration of vaccine and the persistence of antibody.[46] Radioimmunoassay is an involved and complicated procedure. Circulating antibody to pneumococcal hemolysin (pneumolysin) can be measured by enzyme-linked immunosorbent assay (ELISA).[47] Twofold rises or high stable levels of antibody can be detected in about 80 percent of cases with bacteremic pneumonia; however, it is not entirely specific.

IMMUNITY

Natural Immunity

Nonimmunologic host defense mechanisms play an important role in protection against pneumococcal pneumonia. These factors act to filter noxious particles such as bacteria before they reach the alevolar spaces. Impairment of these clearance mechanisms predisposes to the retention of aspirated secretions.

Alveolar macrophages and polymorphonuclear leukocytes are the principal phagocytic cells in bacterial pneumonia.[48] Although the role of the alveolar macrophage in pneumonia has not been well defined, it probably removes aspirated bacteria under normal conditions and promotes resolution of the infected area during healing.

Complement activation also plays an important role early in the course of pneumococcal infections. Alternative complement pathway activation promotes phagocytosis and induces chemotaxis of neutrophils, thereby playing a critical role in host defense before the formation of type-specific capsular polysaccharide antibody.[48]

Acquired Immunity

Type-specific anticapsular antibody appears on the fifth or sixth day of illness, at the time when crisis occurs in untreated patients. Recurrent systemic infections with the same serotype are rare except in patients with hypogammaglobulinemia or persistent foci or infections such as bronchiectasis or sinusitis. Despite the presence of circulating antibody, the pneumococcus may be recovered from the upper respiratory tract for days to weeks. Anticapsular antibody is type specific, protective, and long-lasting, although the effect of prompt antimicrobial therapy on antibody response is unknown. The antibody may be detected by any one of several techniques including agglutination, precipitation, RIA, and enzyme immunoassay. The protective effect of type-specific anticapsular antibodies is to promote phagocytosis of the homologous encapsulated organism by neutrophils.[48]

Pneumococcal Infections in Patients with Immunodeficiency States

Splenectomy and Sickle Cell Disease. Pneumococcal infections in patients with splenectomy follow a rapidly fatal clinical course.[31,33] Disseminated intravascular coagulation may occur in these patients, and organisms can be demonstrated in peripheral blood smears.[32] The basis for this clinical picture may be due to both an impaired clearance of pneumococci from blood and a defect in early antibody formation.

Pneumococcal infections are more common in children with sickle cell disease.[49] The pneumococcus is the most common cause of bacteremia and meningitis in children with sickle cell disease. As in patients with splenectomy, a rapidly progressive and often fatal course is seen. Patients with sickle cell disease have both functional asplenia and defective alternative complement pathway function. A deficiency in normal serum protein opsonins unrelated to the complement system may also be present.

Agammaglobulinemia. Infants and children with various hereditary immunodeficiencies are exceedingly susceptible to pyogenic infections including those due to the pneumococcus. Although these patients have normal complement levels, they are unable to respond to an antigenic challenge with various antigens including pneumococcal capsular polysaccharides.

Hematologic Malignancies. Pneumococcal infections are common in patients with multiple myeloma and acute and chronic lymphocytic leukemia.[50,51] These observations are not surprising since these malignancies result from the proliferation of abnormal clones of plasma cells and B lymphocytes. An impaired primary antibody response has been demonstrated in patients with multiple myeloma and chronic lymphatic leukemia.

ANTIMICROBIAL THERAPY

Penicillin G remains the antimicrobial agent of choice in patients with pneumococcal infections. The comparative susceptibility of pneumococcal isolates to the various penicillins and cephalothin is shown in Table 5. Adequate serum levels can be achieved with each of these agents. Uncomplicated pneumococcal pneumonia responds to intramuscular procaine penicillin, 300,000 to 600,000 units twice a day for 7–10 days. Outpatients may be given procaine penicillin, 600,000 units im, followed by oral phenoxymethyl penicillin (pen V), 250 mg four times a day. If patients are hypotensive, or an empyema is apparent, aqueous crystalline penicillin, 5–10 million units/day, should be administered intravenously. In patients with meningitis, endocarditis, and arthritis, 20 million units of intravenous aqueous crystalline penicillin should be given. Patients allergic to penicillin or its congeners may be given cephalothin or erythromycin for pneumonia and chloramphenicol for meningitis. Pneumococci resistant to chloramphenicol have recently been isolated. Tetracycline should not be given unless the isolate is known to be sensitive since 5–15 percent of pneumococci are resistant to this agent. Clindamycin is not recommended for pneumococcal pneumonia. During the past two decades, pneumococci moderately and highly resistant to penicillin alone and pneumococci multiply resistant to various antibiotics have been found throughout the world.[52] Pneumococci susceptible to penicillin show minimum inhibitory concentrations (MICs) of less than 0.6 μg/ml. By contrast, the MICs of pneumococci of intermediate resistance range from 0.1–1.0 μg/ml and those of pneumococci of high resistance, greater than 2.0 μg/ml. The prevalence of relative resistance reported in clinical isolates varies from 1 to 60 percent, although the highest rates of occurrence have been limited to the Union of South Africa.[52] Most of the first penicillin-resistant pneumococci belonged to capsular types 6A and 19A; a number of other types have been detected that possess relative resistance to penicillin. Types 6A, 6B, 14, and 19A that are resistant to penicillin have been isolated from children in the United States. The earliest (1967–1970) isolates of penicillin-resistant pneumococci were detected in Australia and New Guinea; since then such isolates have been reported in many countries including the United States, United Kingdom, Spain, Switzerland, France, Japan, Canada, Poland, and Israel.[52] Usually the contemporary use of oral antibiotics correlates with the appearance of pharyngeal colonization with resistant pneumococci. Relatively high rates of penicillin-resistant pneumococci associated with invasive disease have been reported among persons residing in Oklahoma City.[53] In that study, 12.2 percent of persons had infections with resistant pneumococci; these occurred mainly in the elderly. The capsular types were 14, 19F, and 23F. These data underscore the necessity to test pneumococcal isolates on a routine basis for penicillin susceptibility.

In 1977, an outbreak due to types 6A and 19A (American type 57) pneumococci resistant to multiple antibiotics occurred in South Africa. These antibiotic-resistant pneumococci had at least five resistant patterns, the multiple-resistant isolates being resistant not only to penicillin (MIC, 0.12–4 μg/ml) but also to tetracycline (MIC, 16–64 μg/ml), chloramphenicol (MIC, 16–32 μg/ml), erythromycin (MIC, 32–64 μg/ml), and clindamycin (MIC, 64–128 μg/ml). Many of these strains also became resistant to rifampin (MIC, >4 μg/ml) after the use of this drug for prophylaxis. All pneumococcal isolates were sensitive to vancomycin, and this agent had to be subsequently used to eradicate the nasopharyngeal carriage of pneumococci. Pneumococci with increased resistance to β-lactam antibiotics do not produce β-lactamases. The intrinsic resistance observed in these isolates is associated with sequential and cumulative alterations in the penicillin-sensitive enzymes termed *penicillin-binding proteins*.[54]

An endemic focus of multiply resistant pneumococci of capsular type 19A has been reported in the United States in Brooklyn, New York, during the years 1983–1984.[55] The MICs of these strains for penicillin ranged from 1.0 to 2.0 μg/ml. They were resistant also to other β-lactam antibiotics, tetracycline, chloramphenicol, and trimethoprim-sulfamethoxazole. The increasing occurrence of multiply resistant pneumococci mandates careful reconsideration of the choice of drugs when the course of disease does not respond to therapy. Further, the

TABLE 5. Comparative Susceptibility of Pneumococcal Isolates to the Penicillins and Cephalothin

Drug	*Minimum Inhibitory Concentration (μg/ml)* Range	Median
Penicillin G	0.01–0.10	0.02
Ampicillin	0.01–0.04	0.02
Nafcillin	0.02–0.20	0.02
Oxacillin	0.04–0.80	0.10
Methicillin	0.10–1.60	0.20
Cephalothin	0.20–0.40	0.20

occurrence of drug-resistant pneumococci provides an additional rational for immunizing high-risk persons with pneumococcal vaccine.

Antimicrobial prophylaxis is less a problem in pneumococcal infections since they are not highly contagious and usually respond to antimicrobial therapy. Oral penicillin G or ampicillin are given prophylactically to children with hypogammaglobulinemia and splenectomy because they are susceptible to serve pneumococcal infections. Cyclical use of appropriate antimicrobial agents may benefit adult patients with severe chronic obstructive pulmonary disease in which recurrent bacterial infections (including pneumococcal) may play a role.

IMMUNOPROPHYLAXIS

Pneumococcal vaccine was introduced in the early 1900s as the major thrust of a program for the prevention of pneumococcal pneumonia among South African gold and diamond miners because the disease was widespread in this population and deaths occurred commonly and threatened the economics of mining.[56] The discovery of pneumococcal types came after these first large-scale tests of pneumococcal vaccine, and Maynard[57] and Lister[58] separately prepared and tested pneumococcal vaccines consisting of a few specific capsular types that appeared to be effective in limited studies among miners. More than 75 years later highly immunogenic pneumococcal vaccines effectively reduce morbidity and prevent death from bacteremic pneumococcal pneumonia in selected populations.[59]

During the 1950s, Austrian called attention to the continuing high case fatality rates in bacteremic pneumococcal disease in the face of the ready availability and use of effective antimicrobial treatment regimens.[21] In a comprehensive examination of bacteremic disease among 529 inpatients at the Kings County Hospital in Brooklyn, NY, he pointed out several salient features: (*1*) case fatality rates in uncomplicated and complicated bacteremic pneumococcal pneumonia remained high; (*2*) most of the deaths occurred in the first 5 days of illness despite treatment; (*3*) many different capsular types were associated with bacteremic infections (unlike in the pre-antibiotic era when types 1, 2, and 3 caused more than three-fourth of infections); and (*4*) case fatality rates increased with age, and they were highest in persons over 50 years of age. Since Austrian's report, several other groups of investigators have added similar supporting data among differing populations in other cities in the United States and in other countries.[22–26,28,29] These studies underscored the importance and provided a rational for using pneumococcal vaccine in the immunoprophylaxis of pneumococcal infections.

By the early 1970s the first polyvalent polysaccharide vaccines were tested for antigenicity and later efficacy. These vaccines consisted of highly purified capsular polysaccharides of the most prevalent serotypes in the United States. A collaborative epidemiologic study conducted by investigators from municipal hospitals in 10 metropolitan communities throughout the United States identified the most common capsular types causing bacteremic infections so that polysaccharides of these serotypes could be incorporated into the vaccine.[60] Pneumococcal vaccine proved highly immunogenic among normal healthy adults.[60] In prospective efficacy trials conducted in the mid-1970s in South Africa among young adult native miners whom experience very high attack rates of pneumococcal infection, the vaccine proved highly beneficial.[60,61] Significantly fewer miners who received a pneumococcal vaccine containing 13 capsular polysaccharides developed disease due to the types in the vaccine as compared with the groups of miners who received either placebo vaccine or meningococcal polysaccharide vaccine. The efficacy of this pneumococcal vaccine in preventing bacteremia to the types contained in the vaccine was about 82 percent. Pneumococcal vaccine also proved efficacious in prospective tests among children older than 2 years with sickle cell anemia.[62] However, among children 7–9 months old, antibody responses to pneumococcal vaccine were poor, and the vaccine did not substantially prevent recurrences of otitis media.[39]

In 1978, commercial pneumococcal vaccine was licensed; it contained (in a single 0.5 ml dose) 50 μg of each of 14 different capsular polysaccharides; these 14 serotypes accounted for about 80 percent of the bacteremic infections. The commercial vaccine was revised in 1983 to include (in a single 0.5 ml dose) 25 μg of each of 23 different capsular polysaccharides (that is, Danish [U.S.] nomenclature types: 1[1], 2[2], 3[3], 4[4], 5[5], 6B[26], 7F[51], 8[8], 9N[9], 9V[68], 10A[34], 11A[43], 12F[12], 14[14], 15B[54], 17F[17], 18C[56], 19A[57], 19F[19], 20[20], 22F[22], 23F[23], and 33F[70]. This new formulation reflected more precisely the major prevailing serotypes, including some types common among children, and included the types that account for about 90 percent of bacteremic infections in the United States and in other countries.[63]

Antibody responses to pneumococcal vaccine have been measured in many different groups, including healthy young adults and healthy elderly adults, healthy children, persons with sickle cell disease, immune disorders, and chronic diseases that affect immune systems, persons receiving renal transplants or undergoing chronic renal dialysis, persons who have had their spleen removed, and persons receiving chemotherapy or radiation therapy (Table 6). Solid evidence is lacking on the level of circulating anticapsular antibody that protects against bacteremic infection. If modest levels of anticapsular antibody, about 500 ng antibody nitrogen per milliliter (measured by RIA), are considered sufficient to provide protection, then most persons receiving pneumococcal vaccine develop these levels of anticapsular antibody for most serotypes.[64–67] The groups of healthy young adults developed the highest levels of antibody and showed the highest proportion of responders to all or nearly all capsular antigens in pneumococcal vaccine. Healthy children over 2 years of age and healthy elderly persons responded somewhat less well; children under 2 years of age responded poorly to pneumococcal polysaccharides.[65,68] The existence of immune dysfunction modulates the response to pneumococcal capsular polysaccharide so that a variable proportion of persons with immune disorders or chronic diseases fail to develop high levels of anticapsular antibody to some serotypes or do not react at all, especially to the weak polysaccharide antigens such as types 6B and 19F.[70–72] The instances of "vaccine failure" usu-

TABLE 6. Anticapsular Antibody Responses Induced by Pneumococcal Vaccine in Persons with Diseases Placing Them at High Risk of Pneumococcal Disease

Underlying conditions causing inadequate antibody production
Lymphadenopathy with human immunodeficiency virus infection
Hodgkin's, treated with chemotherapy
Hodgkin's, after splenectomy
Allegenic bone marrow transplant
Sickle cell disease
Sickle cell disease, children under 2 yr
Sickle cell disease, older children
Systemic lupus erythematosus
Multiple myeloma
Renal transplant
Chronic dialysis
Trisomy 21
Underlying conditions in patients who produce adequate antibody levels
Nephrotic syndrome, steroid responsive
Nephrotic syndrome
Cirrhosis
Chronic obstructive pulmonary disease
Leukemia, treated, in children
Hodgkin's, before treatment
Insulin-dependent diabetes mellitus
Uremia
Splenectomized children, adults
Sjögren syndrome
Aged

ally represent the development of very low levels of anticapsular antibody after the administration of vaccine, for example, values lower than 500 mg antibody nitrogen per milliter by RIA.

Controversy about the benefits of immunizing persons in high-risk populations with pneumococcal vaccine emerged in the early 1980s for several reasons: (*1*) the vaccine had not undergone prospective efficacy tests in persons older than 50 years of age, the population at highest risk for serious pneumococcal disease, and it was unlikely that such studies could be attempted because several hundred thousand test subjects would be required for an adequate trial based on the estimated incidence rates of putative and of bacteremic pneumonia; (*2*) the recognition of "failure of the vaccine" to prevent all bacteremic infections among immunized persons, especially persons unable to mount adequate antibody responses because of underlying immune disorders, immunosuppressive therapy, or chronic diseases; and (*3*) novel approaches to the retrospective analyses of vaccine efficacy presented evidence that pneumococcal vaccine was highly effective in reducing bacteremic disease only in vaccinees of low risk but not in the high-risk (persons with immunosuppressive conditions) and moderate-risk (persons with chronic illnesses) populations.[73,74]

These studies did not detract from the idea that the administration of pneumococcal vaccine to healthy immunocompetent elderly adults induced sufficiently high levels of anticapsular antibody to mediate protection. The studies employing retrospective analysis of pneumococcal vaccine efficacy in the elderly showed the benefits of pneumococcal vaccine immunization of persons capable of mounting immune responses to the capsular polysaccharides.[73] Later prospective studies in moderate- and high-risk elderly adults also showed that the efficacy of pneumococcal vaccine was directly related to the immune responsiveness of the test population. Recent new prospective trials of the 23-valent pneumococcal vaccine in elderly adults confirmed the clinical efficacy of pneumococcal vaccine.[74] It seems reasonable to immunize all adults at about 55 years of age to elicit maximal antibody responses.[59]

Anticapsular antibody induced by the injection of a single dose of pneumococcal vaccine wanes gradually starting about 1 year after the administration of vaccine. The rate of decline probably reflects several aspects including host characteristics, capsular serotype, and intercurrent subclinical and clinical infection. Among healthy young adults 5 years after the administration of vaccine, antibody levels had declined to about three-fourths of the peak levels.[64] Ten years after the administration of vaccine, anticapsular antibody levels remained significantly above peak levels for only two of six serotypes tested.[75] These data suggest that booster immunization with pneumococcal vaccine might be necessary to maintain high levels of antibody and that a second dose of vaccine might be given between 5 and 10 years after the initial dose of vaccine in the adult. The Centers for Disease Control now recommends reimmunization with 23-valent vaccine of persons who received 14-valent vaccine or high risk persons immunized with 23-valent vaccine more than 6 years ago. Recent reports encompassing small numbers of vaccinees suggest that reimmunization with pneumococcal vaccine is not associated with worse adverse reactions than occur during the administration of the initial dose of vaccine.[68,77]

At present, pneumococcal vaccine is recommended for (*1*) adults at high risk of serious pneumococcal infection because of splenic dysfunction or anatomic asplenia, especially sickle cell disease and splenectomy, and because of chronic illness, including Hodgkin's disease, conditions associated with immunosuppression, multiple myeloma, alcoholism, cirrhosis, renal failure, and cerebrospinal fluid leaks; (*2*) adults with chronic cardiovascular and pulmonary diseases; (*3*) healthy adults older than 65 years; (*4*) children older than 2 years with chronic illnesses placing them at high risk of serious pneumococcal infection, including sickle cell disease and splenectomy, conditions associated with immunosuppression, cerebrospinal fluid leaks, and nephrotic syndrome; (*5*) adults and children older than 2 years with asymptomatic or symptomatic human immunodeficiency virus infection. It is not recommended for the prevention of otitis media in infants and young children. Many persons for whom pneumococcal vaccine is recommended also meet the recommendations for influenza virus vaccine; the two vaccines can be administered to one person by employing different sites of injection.

Most adults with bacteremic pneumococcal disease usually have been admitted to the hospital in the previous 5 years for treatment of their underlying disease.[78] They can be targeted for pneumococcal vaccine, and the vaccine should be administered to them before they leave the hospital to prevent a later admission because of pneumococcal disease. Pneumococcal vaccine is highly immunogenic, clinically effective, and exceptionally safe, and it should be used widely to reduce the occurrence of serious pneumococcal disease in high-risk persons.

REFERENCES

1. Pneumococcal polysaccharide vaccine. MMWR. 1981;30:410–2, 417–9.
2. Dubos RJ. The Professor, the Institute and DNA. New York: Rockefeller University Press; 1976.
3. MacLeod CH, Hodges RG, Heidelberger M, et al. Prevention of pneumococcal pneumonia by immunization with specific capsular polysaccharides. J Exp Med. 1945;82:445–65.
4. Austrian R. Life with the Pneumococcus. Philadelphia: University of Pennsylvania Press; 1985.
5. Griffith F. The significance of pneumococcal types. J Hyg. 1928;27:113–59.
6. Avery OT, MacLeod CM, McCarty M. Transformation of pneumococcal types induced by a deoxyribonucleic acid fraction isolated from *Pneumococcus* type III. J Exp Med. 1944;79:137–58.
7. Deibel RH, Seeley HW Jr. Family II. Streptococcaceae. In: Buchananan RE, Gibbons NE, eds. Bergey's Manual of Determinative Bacteriology. 8th ed. Baltimore: Williams & Wilkins; 1974.
8. Larm O, Lindberg B. The pneumococcal polysaccharides: A reexamination. Adv Carbohydr Chem Biochem. 1976;33:295–322.
9. Tomasz A. Surface components of *Streptococcus pneumoniae*. Rev Infect Dis. 1981;3:190–211.
10. Kaplan MH, Volankis JE. Interaction of C-reactive protein complexes with the complement system. I. Consumption of human complement associated with the reaction of CRP with pneumococcal C-polysaccharide and with the choline phosphatides, lecithin and sphingomyelin. J Immunol. 1974;112:2135–47.
11. McDonnell M, Ronda-Lain C, Tomasz A. "Diplophage": A bacteriophage of *Diplococcus pneumoniae*. Virology. 1975;63:577–82.
12. Tiraby JG, Tiraby E, Fox MS. Pneumococcal bacteriophages. Virology. 1975;68:566–9.
13. Ronda-Lian C, Lopez R, Tapia A, et al. Role of the pneumococcal autolysin (murein hydrolase) in the release of progeny bacteriophage and in the bacteriophage-induced lysis of host cells. J Virol. 1977;21:366–74.
14. Bernheimer HP. Lysogeny in pneumococci freshly isolated from man. Science. 1977;195:66–8.
15. Lopez R, Garcia E, Ronda C. Bacteriophages of *Streptococcus pneumoniae*. Rev Infect Dis. 1981;3:212–23.
16. Ronda C, Lopez R, Tomasz A, et al. Transfection of *Streptococcus pneumoniae* with bactriophage DNA. J Virol. 1978;26:221–5.
17. Austrian R. Of gold and pneumococci. A history of pneumococcal vaccines in South Africa. Trans Am Clin Climatol Assoc. 1977;89:141–61.
18. Hendley JO, Sande MA, Stewart PM, et al. Spread of *Streptococcus pneumoniae* in families. I. Carriage rates and distribution of types. J Infect Dis. 1975;132:55–61.
19. Gwaltney JM, Sande MA, Austrian R, et al. Spread of *Streptococcus pneumoniae* in families. II. Relation of transfer of *S. pneumoniae* to incidence of colds and serum antibody. J Infect Dis. 1975;132:62–8.
20. Alvarez S, Guarderas J, Shell CG, et al. Nosocomial pneumococcal bacteremia. Arch Intern Med. 1986;146:1509–12.
21. Austrian R, Gold J. Pneumococcal bacteremia with a special reference to bacteremic pneumococcal pneumonia. Ann Intern Med. 1964;60:759–76.
22. Mufson MA, Kruss DM, Wasil RE, et al. Capsular types and outcome of bacteremic pneumococcal disease in the antibiotic era. Arch Intern Med. 1974;134:505–10.
23. Gray BM, Dillon HC. Clinical and epidemiologic studies of pneumococcal infection in children. Pediatr Infect Dis. 1986;5:201–7.
24. Mufson MA, Oley G, Hughey D. Pneumococcal disease in a medium-sized community in the United States. JAMA. 1982;248:1486–89.
25. Gransden WR, Eykyn SJ, Phillips I. Pneumococcal bacteremia: 325 episodes diagnosed at St. Thomas's Hospital. Br Med J. 1985;290:505–8.
26. Kramer MR, Rudensky B, Hadas-Halperin I, et al. Pneumococcal bacteremia–no change in mortality in 30 years: Analysis of 104 cases and review of the literature. Isr J Med Sci. 1987;23:174–80.
27. Tilghman RC, Finland M. Clinical significance of bacteremia in pneumococcal pneumonia. Arch Intern Med. 1937;59:602–19.

28. Smart LE, Dougall AJ, Girdwood RWA. New 23-valent pneumococcal vaccine in relation to pneumococcal serotypes in systemic and non-systemic disease. J Infect. 1987;14:209–5.
29. Jacobs NM, Lerdkachornsuk S, Metzger WI. Pneumococcal bacteremia in infants and children: A ten-year experience at the Cook County Hospital with special reference to the pneumococcal serotypes isolated. Pediatrics. 1979;64:296–300.
30. Kauffman CA, Watanakunakorn C, Phair JP. Purulent pneumococcal pericarditis. A continuing problem in the antibiotic era. Am J Med. 1973;54:743–50.
31. Bisno AL. Hyposplenism and overwhelming pneumococcal infection: A reappraisal. Am J Med Sci. 1971;262:101–7.
32. Bisno AL, Freeman JC. The syndrome of asplenia, pneumococcal sepsis and disseminated intravascular coagulation. Ann Intern Med. 1970;72:389–93.
33. Haque AU, Min-K-W, From P, et al. Postsplenectomy pneumococcemia in adults. Arch Pathol Lab Med. 1980; 104:258–60.
34. Torres J, Bisno AL. Hyposplenism and pneumococcemia. Visualization of *Diplococcus pneumoniae* in the peripheral blood smear. Am J Med. 1973;55:851–5.
35. Howie VM. Natural history of otitis media. Ann Otol Rhinol Laryngol. 1975;84(Suppl 19):67–72.
36. Howie VM, Ploussard JH, Sloyer JL Jr. The "otitis prone" condition. Am J Dis Child. 1975;129:676–8.
37. Sloyer JL Jr, Ploussard JH, Howie VM. Efficacy of pneumococcal polysaccharide vaccine in preventing otitis media in infants in Huntsville, Alabama. Rev Infect Dis. 1981;3(Suppl):119–23.
38. Sloyer JL Jr, Howie VM, Ploussard JH, et al. Immune response to acute otitis media in children. I. Serotypes isolated and serum and middle ear fluid antibody in pneumococcal otitis media. Infect Immun. 1974;9:1028–32.
39. Karma P. Pukander J, Sipila M, et al. Prevention of otitis media in children by pneumococcal vaccination. Am J Otolaryngol. 1985;6:173–84.
40. Kauffman CA, Watanakunakorn C, Phair JP. Pneumococcal arthritis. J Rheumatol. 1976;3:409–19.
41. Conn HO, Fessel JM. Spontaneous bacterial peritonitis in cirrhosis: Variations on a theme. Medicine (Baltimore). 1971;50:161.
42. Merrill CW, Gwaltney JM, Hendley JO, et al. Rapid identification of pneumococci. Gram stain vs. the quellung reaction. N Engl J Med. 1973;288:510–2.
43. Rytel MW. Counterimmunoelectrophoresis in diagnosis of infectious disease. Hosp Pract. 1975;10:75–82.
44. Morgan AD, Rhind GB, Connaughton JJ, et al. Pneumococcal serotyping and antigen detection in pneumococcal pneumonia of adults. J Infect. 1984;9:134–8.
45. Lenthe-Eboa S, Brighouse G, Auckenthaler R, et al. Comparison of immunological methods for diagnosis of pneumococcal pneumonia in biological fluids. Eur J Clin Microbiol. 1987;6:28–34.
46. Schiffman G, Douglas MR, Bonner MJ, et al. A radioimmunoassay for immunologic phenomena in pneumococcal disease and for the antibody response to pneumococcal vaccines. I. Method for the radioimmunoassay of anticapsular antibodies and comparison with other techniques. J Immunol Methods. 1980;33:133–40.
47. Kalin M, Kanclerski K, Granstrom M, et al. Diagnosis of pneumococcal pneumonia by enzyme-linked immunosorbent assay of antibodies to pneumococcal hemolysin (pneumolysin). J Clin Microbiol. 1987;25:226–9.
48. Johnston RB Jr. The host response to invasion by *Streptococcus pneumoniae:* Protection and the pathogenesis of tissue damage. Rev Infect Dis. 1981;3:282–8.
49. Zarkowsky HS, Gallagher MS, Gill FM, et al. Bacteremia in sickle homoglobinopathies. J Pediatr. 1986;109:579–85.
50. Chou M-Y, Brown AE, Blevins A, et al. Severe pneumococcal infection in patients with neoplastic disease. Cancer. 1983;51:1546–50.
51. Chilcote RR, Baehner RL. Septicemia and association with acute lymphoblastic leukemia. J Pediatr. 1979;94:715–8.
52. Applebaum PC: World-wide development of antibiotic resistance in pneumococci. Eur J Clin Microbiol. 1987;6:367–77.
53. Istre GR, Tarpay M, Anderson M, et al. Invasive disease due to *Streptococcus pneumoniae* in an area with a high rate of relative penicillin resistance. J Infect Dis. 1987;156:732–5.
54. Jacobs MR, Koornhof HJ, Robins-Browne RM, et al. Emergence of multiply resistant pneumococci. N Engl J Med. 1978;299:735–40.
55. Simberkoff MS, Lukaszewski M, Cross A, et al. Antibiotic-resistant isolates of *Streptococcus pneumoniae* from clinical specimens: A cluster of serotype 19A organisms in Brooklyn, New York. J Infect Dis. 1986;153:78–82.
56. Wright AE, Morgan P, Colebrook L, et al. Observations on prophylactic inoculation against pneumococcus infections, and on the results which have been achieved by it. Lancet. 1914;1:1–10, 87–95.
57. Maynard GD. An enquiry into the etiology, manifestations and prevention of pneumonia amongst natives on the Rand recruited from tropical areas. Publ S Afr Inst Med Res. 1913;1:1–101.
58. Lister FS. Prophylactic inoculation of man against pneumococcal infections and more particularly against pneumococcal infections. Publ S Afr Inst Med Res. 1917;10:304–22.
59. LaForce FM, Eickhoff TC. Pneumococcal vaccine: An emerging consensus. Ann Intern Med. 1988;108:757–9.
60. Austrian R, Douglas RM, Schiffman G, et al. Prevention of pneumococcal pneumonia by vaccination. Trans Assoc Am Physicians. 1976;89:184–94.
61. Smit P, Oberholzer D, Hayden-Smith S, et al. Protective efficacy of pneumococcal polysaccharide vaccines. JAMA. 1977;238:2613–6.
62. Amman AJ, Addiego J, Wara DW, et al. Polyvalent pneumococcal polysaccharide immunization of patients with sickle-cell anemia and patients with splenectomy. N Engl J Med. 1977;297:897–900.
63. Bolan G, Broome CV, Facklam RR, et al. Pneumococcal vaccine efficacy in selected populations in the United States. Ann Intern Med. 1986;104:1–6.
64. Mufson MA, Krause HE, Schiffman G, et al. Pneumococcal antibody levels one decade after immunization of health adults. Am J Med Sci. 1987;30:279–89.
65. Roghmann KJ, Tabloski PA, Bentley DW, et al. Immune response of elderly adults to pneumococcus: Variation by age, sex, and functional impairment. J Gerontol. 1987;42:265–70.
66. Paton JC, Toogood IR, Cockington RA, et al. Antibody response to pneumococcal vaccine in children aged 5 to 15 years. Am J Dis Child. 1986;140:135–8.
67. Simberkoff MS, Cross AP, Al-Ibrahim M, et al. Efficacy of pneumococcal vaccine in high-risk patients. N Engl J Med. 1986;315:1318–29.
68. Koskela M, Leinonen M, Haiva V, et al. First and second dose antibody responses to pneumococcal polysaccharide vaccine in infants. Pediatr Infect Dis. 1986;5:45–50.
69. Jarrett MP, Schiffman G, Barland P, et al. Impaired response to pneumococcal vaccine in systemic lupus erythematosus. Arthritis Rheum. 1980;23:1287–93.
70. Schmid GP, Smith RP, Baltch A, et al. Antibody response to pneumococcal vaccine in patients with multiple myeloma. J Infect Dis. 1981;143:590–7.
71. Schildt RA, Rubin RR, Schiffman G, et al. Polyvalent pneumococcal immunization of patients with plasma cell dyscrasias. Cancer. 1981;48:1377–80.
72. Silberman H, Overturf GD, Field RJ, et al. Response of renal allograft recipients to pneumococcal vaccine. Ann Surg. 1980;192:199–201.
73. Shapiro ED, Clemens JD. A controlled evaluation of the protective efficacy of pneumococcal vaccine for patients at high risk of serious pneumococcal infections. Ann Intern Med. 1984;101:325–30.
74. Sims RV, Steinmann WC, McConville JH, et al. The clinical effectiveness of pneumococcal vaccine in the elderly. Ann Intern Med. 1988;108:653–7.
75. Mufson MA, Krause HE, Schiffman G, et al. Pneumococcal antibody levels one decade after immunization of health adults. Am J Med Sci. 1987;30:279–89.
76. Pneumococcal polysaccharide vaccine. MMWR. 1989;38:64–8, 73–6.
77. Mufson MA, Krause HE, Schiffman G, et al. Reactivity and antibody responses of volunteers given two or three doses of pneumococcal vaccine. Proc Soc Exptl Biol Med. 1984;177:220–25.
78. Fedson DS. Improving the use of pneumococcal vaccine through a strategy of hospital-based immunization: A review of its rationale and implications. J Am Geriatrics Soc. 1985;33:142–50.

179. ENTEROCOCCUS SPECIES AND GROUP D STREPTOCOCCI

DANIEL M. MUSHER

MICROBIOLOGY AND EPIDEMIOLOGY

The group D streptococci have traditionally been separated into enterococcal and nonenterococcal species. Based on studies of DNA homology and certain other properties, the classification of group D streptococci has recently undergone a major change. Those organisms that formerly were called enterococci have been reclassified as the genus *Enterococcus* (Table 1). Most

TABLE 1. Group D Streptococci

Enterococcal species
E. faecalis
E. faecium
E. durans
Nonenterococcal species
S. bovis
S. equinus

human infections attributable to group D streptococci are caused by *Enterococcus* (formerly *Streptococcus*) *faecalis* and *Streptococcus bovis*. *Enterococcus* (formerly *Streptococcus*) *faecium* occasionally causes human disease. *Enterococus durans* and *Streptococcus equinus* together account for less than 2 percent of all clinical isolates of enterococci, with the former species predominating.

Group D streptococci are identified in clinical laboratories on the basis of their ability to grow in medium that contains 40 percent bile and to cleave esculin, properties that are lacking in other grouped streptococci, although present in 5 percent of viridans streptococci.[1] In the past few years a test for hydrolysis of L-pyrrolidonyl-β-naphthylamide (PYR reaction) has been used to identify enterococci. This test is reliable, and results are available within minutes. Since *Streptococcus pyogens* also gives a positive reaction, bacitracin susceptibility needs to be studied simultaneously.[2] The common names enterococci or fecal streptococci are given to *E. faecalis, E. faecium*, and *E. durans*; these organisms are distinguished from S. bovis and S. equinus by their ability to grow in broth containing 6.5 percent NaCl. Most group D streptococci are nonhemolytic on sheep blood agar although some are α-hemolytic and some *E. faecalis* strains are β-hemolytic on rabbit or horse blood agar.

Enterococcus faecalis is present in the mouth of normal adults, throughout the small intestines in small numbers (e.g., $10–10^3$ colony-forming units (cfu)/g), and in higher concentrations (10^7 cfu/g) in the feces of normal adults from whom this organism can nearly always be isolated.[3,4] Lower concentrations of *E. faecium* are found in the feces of 25 percent of normal adults. No more than 5–10 percent of normal adults are colonized with *S. bovis* or *S. equinus*, although *S. bovis* is found in a higher percentage of adults with colonic cancer.[5]

Recent data show an increasing prevalence of *E. faecium* in clinical isolates. Because many of these are resistant to penicillin, routine speciation of enterococci and testing of antimicrobial susceptibility may become necessary.

CLINICAL INFECTIONS

Enterococcus faecalis causes disease more frequently than do the other group D streptococci, perhaps because it is more commonly a part of human flora and present in greater concentrations; accordingly, this organism is discussed in this section as the prototype, and others are mentioned when indicated. *Enterococcus faecalis* is implicated in the following kinds of infections: endocarditis, urinary tract infection, intra-abdominal abscess (nearly always in association with other bacteria), soft tissue infection (cellulitis, wound infections, abscess, infected decubitus ulcer), meningitis (rarely), pneumonia (rarely, nosocomial only), and bacteremia due to any of the above, associated with intravenous lines or with no apparent focus.

Group D streptococci are responsible for 10–20 percent of cases of bacterial endocarditis whether on previously normal heart valves or on abnormal or prosthetic valves[6]; *E. faecalis* and *S. bovis* are implicated equally commonly, with occasional cases being attributed to other streptococci in this group.[6–9] *Enterococcus faecalis* is also one of the organisms commonly implicated in polymicrobial bacterial endocarditis.[10] *Enterococcus faecalis* adheres to heart valve tissue more avidly than do viridans streptococci or staphylococci and far more avidly than do facultative gram-negative bacilli.[11] The bacteria stimulate endothelial cells to produce fibronectin or other substances that are as yet incompletely defined[12] and that in turn may stimulate the growth of vegetation.

Endocarditis due to group D streptococci usually occurs in elderly people who have underlying diseases or in drug abusers who inject themselves intravenously. Bacteremia secondary to a recognized source, for example, urinary tract or soft tissue infection (including decubitus ulcers and gangrene), or infection at the site of intravenous lines is often responsible.[13] Unrecognized bacteremia related to the presence of a lesion in the colon and/or instrumentation (e.g., colonoscopy) may be responsible for most cases of endocarditis due to *S. bovis*.[5,14] Several large series of cases have emphasized the lack of differences in the clinical picture of endocarditis due to *E. faecalis* or *S. bovis*[7–9]; most cases follow a subacute course, although some cases of *E. faecalis* endocarditis are more acute in onset. In contrast to endocarditis due to *Staphylococcus aureus*, that due to *E. faecalis* occurring in heroin addicts usually does not involve the tricuspid valve and is not associated with septic pulmonary emboli.[15]

Group D streptococci are responsible for about 5 percent all positive blood cultures[16]; if cases of endocarditis are excluded, enterococci are nearly always responsible. One large metropolitan hospital reported 74 instances of enterococcal bacteremia in the absence of clinical findings of endocarditis during a 15-year period.[17] Nearly all the isolates that were speciated were *E. faecalis* with one each of *E. faecium* and *S. durans*. Sources for enterococcal bacteremia are summarized in Table 2. Garrison et al.[18] presented similar results, although no source for bacteremia was found in 40 percent of the cases. Data on intravenous lines were not presented in these studies; in many of these cases infection associated with an indwelling intravenous line may have been responsible. One-quarter of the 74 patients with enterococcal bacteremia had more than one organism isolated from the blood; indeed, *E. faecalis* is the most frequently identified gram-positive organism in polymicrobial bacteremia,[19–21] probably reflecting the association with devitalized soft tissue or infection in the gastrointestinal or genitourinary tracts. Group D streptococci are also implicated as relatively frequent causes of neonatal sepsis; in this situation *E. faecalis* is four times as common as *S. bovis*.[22]

Urinary tract infection in otherwise healthy women who have no identifiable structural abnormality is due to *E. faecalis* is about 2–3 percent of cases; this percentage may be slightly higher during pregnancy[23] and in women who are taking prophylactic antibiotics to which enterococci are resistant such as trimethoprim-sulfamethoxazole. In elderly ambulatory individuals, enterococci are implicated in asymptomatic bacteriuria in <1 percent of women and 4 percent of men.[24] In contrast, when an indwelling urinary catheter is present, enterococci are among the two or three most frequently isolated bacterial species[25–27], perhaps related in part to antibiotic usage.[25] Nevertheless, bacteremia occurs in only a small percentage of all patients who have urinary catheters and in a disproportionately small percentage of those with enterococcal urinary infection[28,29] despite their prevalence in infecting the urine in catheterized subjects.

Documentation of *E. faecalis* infection in patients with chronic and/or complicated urinary tract infections,[30,31] renal

TABLE 2. Sources of Enterococcal Bacteremia

Source	*Number of Patients*	
Urinary tract	17	
Soft tissue[a]	20	
Burns		10
Decubitus ulcers		5
Wounds		2
Other		3
Intra-abdominal	11	
Abscess		7
Other		4
Perinatal	9	
Mothers		4
Infants		5
Miscellaneous[b]	13	
Unknown	6	
Total	76	

[a] Two of these patients also had urinary tract infection.
[b] These were associated with a number of iatrogenic causes including angiography, instrumentation, surgery, and the implantation of prosthetic devices.
(Data from Shlaes et al.[17])

abscess,[32] or urinary infection associated with kidney stones[33,34] is surprisingly uncommon. As shown in Table 2, when *E. faecalis* bacteremia occurs, a urinary tract source can often be identified.[17,35]

Despite the presence of relatively large numbers of enterococci in the colon, it has been difficult to determine, with certainty, the role of these organisms in producing intra-abdominal infection. In the experimental model, *E. faecalis* does not cause sepsis and produces abscesses only when injected together with other organisms such as *B. fragilis*.[36] Despite their nearly uniform presence in human feces, the enterococci are identified in only 10–25 percent of intra-abdominal abscesses[37–40] and appear in the blood stream much less frequently than do *Escherichia coli* or *B. fragilis* in cases of peritonitis or intra-abdominal abscess; for example, only 1 of 28 blood isolates in 134 patients with intra-abdominal sepsis was *E. faecalis*.[39] Similarly, although enterococci are second only to *E. coli* in the frequency of isolation from human bile,[41,42] these organisms are found only infrequently in blood cultures in cases of acute, suppurative cholecystitis, even when they are present in the bile.[42] In large series of cases of enterococcal bacteremia, only 10–15 percent of cases have been attributed to intraabdominal infection.[43] Despite the fact that some prophylactic antibiotic regimens in widespread use for fecal contamination of the peritoneal cavity are ineffective against *E. faecalis*, the presence of this organism in an abscess after elective surgery has been said to be relatively uncommon,[44,45] although other series have implicated enterococci in one-third of abscesses that occurred when a variety of mixed infections were treated surgically and medically by using moxalactam or clindamycin and tobramycin,[44] and "breakthrough" bacteremia has been described in such circumstances.[47]

Enterococcus faecalis is also commonly identified in infection of previously damaged or compromised soft tissues as, for example, in diabetic or decubitus ulcers, in burns or vascular insufficiency, as well as in wounds and soft tissue infections of the abdomen. Thus, enterococci have been identified in 15–50 percent of cases of surgical abdominal wounds, perineal gangrene, decubitus ulcer, and fetid diabetic limbs. Their pathogenicity has been questioned because of the almost invariable presence of other pathogenic organisms as well as the inability to demonstrate that *E. faecalis* by itself is pathogenic in animal models of infection. Lest the mixed nature of the infection raise suspicion that the enterococcus is not playing an important pathogenic role, it should be noted that soft tissue infection has repeatedly been implicated as the most common source for enterococcal bacteremia.[17,18,43] Infection of apparently undamaged tissues, for example, de novo cellulitis, is almost never due to group D streptococci.

Pneumonia due to group D streptococci is rare; a few cases have been described in severely debilitated, elderly patients,[48,49] especially in association with cephalosporin therapy.[49] Although neonatal meningitis is commonly caused by group D streptococci,[22] cases of meningitis after the neonatal period are rare.[50]

ANTIMICROBIAL SUSCEPTIBILITY AND THERAPY

The distinction between enterococcal and nonenterococcal group D streptococci is especially important when antibiotic susceptibility is considered. Virutally all *S. bovis* organisms are inhibited, and 90 percent of isolates are killed by 0.2 μg/ml penicillin or ampicillin.[51] *Streptococcus bovis* is also susceptible in vitro to many other antibiotics including semisynthetic penicillins, cephalothin (but not necessarily other cephalosporins, e.g. cephalexin), and clindamycin.[52] In contrast, *E. faecalis* is inhibited only by substantially higher concentrations of penicillin or ampicillin (the minimal inhibitory concentration [MIC] for 90 percent of strains [MIC_{90}] = 2–4 μg/ml[53] and is resistant to clinically achievable levels of cephalosporms or clindamycin

TABLE 3. Susceptibility of *Enterococcus faecalis* to Commonly Used Antibiotics[a]

Antibiotic	MIC_{50}	MIC_{90}
Penicillin, ampicillin	1–2	2–4
Carbenicillin, ticarcillin	25	50
Piperacillin, mezlocillin	3	3
Oxacillin, cloxacillin	32	64
Nafcillin	8	32
Cephalothin, cefazolin	25	100
Cefoxitin	25	100
Third-generation cephalosporins	50	100
Clindamycin	100	100
Vancomycin	2	4
Imipenem	0.4	0.8
Rifampin	8	32
Ciprofloxacin	1	1

[a] Expressed as μg/ml.

(Table 3). This organism is also resistant to cloxacillin or dicloxacillin, although some isolates are susceptible to clinically achievable levels of nafcillin.[54] Carbenicillin and ticarcillin have a poor antibacterial effect against *E. faecalis*, although inhibition of most isolates may be achieved by doses used to treat *Pseudomonas* infection; the MIC of mezlocillin and piperacillin is substantially lower and approaches that of penicillin.[53] Enterococci are also intrinsically resistant to achievable serum levels of aminoglycosides.[51] Vancomycin, 2.0–4.0 μg/ml, inhibits *E. faecalis*, and the MIC_{50} of rifampin is 8.0 μg/ml (range, 0.25 to 32 μg/ml).[55] *Enterococcus faecalis* is susceptible to imipenem[56] and ciprofloxacin[57] as well as to the as yet unavailable drug deptomycin.[58] Susceptibility to trimethoprim-sulfamethoxazole in vitro appears to be better than had previously been thought,[59] and consideration should perhaps be given to this combination in treating infected patients. Rare isolates of *E. faecalis* produce β-lactamase and show absolute resistance to penicillins.[60] *Enterococcus faecium* tends to be even more resistant to antibiotics than is *E. faecalis*.[61]

Enterococcus faecalis shows an almost unique tolerance to the effect of penicillin or ampicillin; killing of more than 90 percent of the organisms after overnight incubation at 37°C usually does not occur until concentrations exceed 100 μg/ml.[54,61,62] Vancomycin also fails to kill *E. faecalis*.[55,61,62] The addition of an aminoglycoside to which an isolate has demonstrable susceptibility (albeit to concentrations that can not be reached clinically) causes the synergistic effect of killing *E. faecalis* in vitro in the presence of penicillins or vancomycin[62,63] and bringing about clinical cure in vivo.[63–65] The synergistic effect is thought to be due to increased bacterial uptake of the aminoglycoside that results from damage induced by penicillin or vancomycin.[66,67] Most isolates of *E. faecalis* used to be susceptible to 500–2000 μg/ml of all commonly used aminoglycosides. At the present time, most *E. faecalis* isolates are highly resistant to streptomycin (MIC, >2000 μg/ml), and up to one-third show high-grade resistance to gentamicin (MIC, >500 μg/ml)[68]; plasmid-mediated production of enzymes that inactivate aminoglycosides by adenylation, phosphorylation, or acetylation is largely responsible.[69] These strains tend to be nosocomially acquired and are associated with prior antibiotic therapy and surgical procedures.[70] Occasional isolates of *S. bovis* also show this resistance.[71] When this degree of aminoglycoside resistance is present, synergistic antibacterial activity does not occur in vitro or in vivo.[71–73] In those few clinical situations in which a bactericidal effect is required (endocarditis, sepsis in a granulocytopenic host, and perhaps meningitis or osteomyelitis), susceptibility to the aminoglycoside should be documented early in the course of treatment.[74,75] Each agent should be studied separately since an isolate may be resistant to one aminoglycoside yet sensitive to another. The addition of rifampin to vancomycin produces no synergy in vitro.[55] Certain quinolones have been shown to be bactericidal in vitro and to cure enterococcal endocarditis in experimental animals, but these results are not universally accepted.[57] The bactericidal effect of daptomycin in vitro merits further study. Endocarditis caused by *E. faecalis* that is highly resistant to aminoglycosides is difficult to treat. Certain gentamicin-resistant strains may be susceptible to streptomycin. High doses of ampicillin alone (12–18 g/day) for 8–12 weeks have been successful in a few cases. Surgery may be necessary. Vancomycin should be used in penicillin-allergic patients.

REFERENCES

1. Facklam RR, Carey RB. Streptococci and aerococci. In: Lennette EH, Balows A, Hausler WJ Jr, et al. eds. Manual of Clinical Microbiology. 4th ed. Washington, DC: American Society for Microbiology; 1985:154–75.
2. Wellstood SA. Rapid, cost-effective identification of group A streptococci and enterococci by pyrrolidonyl-β-naphthylamide hydrolysis. J Clin Microbiol. 1987;25:1805.
3. Noble CJ. Carriage of group D streptococci in the human bowel. J Clin Pathol. 1978;31:1182.
4. Kager L, Ljungdahl I, Malmorg AS, et al. Antibiotic prophylaxis with cefoxitin in colorectal surgery. Ann Surg. 1981;193:277.
5. Klein RS, Recco RA, Catalano MT: Association of *Steptococcus bovis* with carcinoma of the colon. N Engl J Med. 1977;297:800.
6. Mandell GL. Enterococcal endocarditis. In: Kaye D, ed. Infective Endocarditis. Baltimore: University Park Press; 1976:101–10.
7. Lowes JA, Williams G, Tabaqchali S, et al. 10 years of infective endocarditis at St. Bartholomew's Hospital: Analysis of clinical features and treatment in relation to prognosis and mortality. Lancet. 1980;1:133.
8. Ravreby WD, Bottone EJ, Keusch GT. Group D streptococcal bacteremia with emphasis on the incidence and presentation of infections due to *Streptococcus bovis*. N Eng J Med. 1973;289:1400.
9. Hoppes WL, Learner PI. Nonenterococcal group D streptococcal endocarditis caused by *Streptococcus bovis*. Ann Intern Med. 1974;81:588.
10. Saravolatz LD, Burch KH, Quinn EL, et al. Polymicrobial infective endocarditis: An increasing clinical entity. Am Heart J. 1978;95:163.
11. Gould K, Ramirez-Ronda CH, Holmes RK, et al. Adherence of bacteria to heart valves in vitro. J Clin Invest. 1975;56:1364.
12. Drake TA, Rodgers GM, Sande MA. Tissue factor is a major stimulus for vegetation formation in endocarditis in rabbits. J Clin Invest. 1984;73:1750.
13. Mandell GL, Kaye D, Levison ME, et al. Enterococcal endocarditis: An analysis of 38 patients observed at the New York Hospital-Cornell Medical Center. Arch Intern Med. 1970;125:258.
14. Murray HW, Roberts RB. *Streptococcus bovis* endocarditis and underlying gastrointestinal disease. Arch Intern Med. 1978;138:1097.
15. Reiner NE, Gopalakrishna KV, Lerner PI. Enterococcal endocarditis in heroin addicts. JAMA. 1976;235:1861.
16. Weinstein MP, Reller LB, Murphy JR, et al. The clinical significance of positive blood cultures: A comprehensive analysis of 500 episodes of bacteremia and fungemia in adults. I. Laboratory and epidemiologic observations. Rev Infect Dis. 1983;5:35–53.
17. Shlaes DM, Levy J. Enterococcal bacteremia without endocarditis. Arch Intern Med. 1981;141:578.
18. Garrison RN, Fry DE, Berberich S, et al. Enterococcal bacteremia. Clinical implications and determinants of death. Ann Surg. 1982;196:43.
19. Hermans PE, Washington JA II. Polymicrobial bacteremia. Ann Intern Med. 1970;73:387.
20. Kiani D, Quinn EL, Burch KH, et al. The increasing importance of polymicrobial bacteremia. JAMA. 1979;242:1044.
21. Reuben AG, Musher DM, Broucke I, et al. Polymicrobial bacteremia: Clinical and microbiologic patterns. Rev Infect Dis. 1989;11:161–83.
22. Klein JO, Marcy SM. Bacterial sepsis and meningitis. In: Remington JS, Klein JD, eds. Infectious Diseases of the Fetus and Newborn Infant. Philadelphia: WB Saunders; 1983;679–734.
23. Stamey TA. Pathogenesis and Treatment of Urinary Tract Infections. Baltimore: Williams & Wilkins, 1980.
24. Boscia JA, Kobasa WD, Knight RA, et al. Epidemiology of bacteriuria in an elderly ambulatory population. Am J Med. 1986;80:208.
25. Warren JW, Tenney JH, Hoopes JM. A prospective microbiologic study of bacteriuria in patients with chronic indwelling urethral catheters. J Infect Dis. 1982;146:719.
26. Breitenbucher RB. Bacterial changes in the urine samples of patients with long-term indwelling catheters. Arch Intern Med. 1984;144:1585.
27. Morrison AJ, Wenzel RP. Nosocomial urinary tract infections due to *Enterococcus*. Arch Intern Med. 1986;146:1549.
28. Krieger JN, Kaiser DL, Wenzel RP. Urinary tract etiology of bloodstream infections in hospitalized patients. J Infect Dis. 1983;148:57.
29. Setia U, Serventi I, Lorenz P. Bacteremia in long-term care facility: Spectrum and mortality. Arch Intern Med. 1984;144:1633.
30. Smith JW, Jones SR, Reed WP, et al. Recurrent urinary infections in men. Characteristics and response to therapy. Ann Intern Med. 1979;91:544.
31. Gleckman R, Crowley M, Natsios GA. Therapy of recurrent invasive urinary-tract infections of men. N Engl J Med. 1979;301:878.
32. Malgieri JJ, Kursh ED, Persky L. The changing clinicopathological pattern of abscesses in or adjacent to the kidney. J Urol. 1977;118:230.
33. Harrison LH, Whitehurst AW, Boyce WH. Adjuvant antimicrobial therapy with renal calculus surgery. J Urol. 1977;118:233.
34. Silverman DE, Stamey TA. Management of infection stones: The Stanford experience. Medicine (Baltimore). 1983;62:44.
35. Gross PA, Harkavy LM, Barden GE, et al. The epidemiology of nosocomial enterococcal urinary tract infection. Am J Med Sci. 1976;76:272.
36. Bartlett JG. Experimental aspects of intraabdominal sepsis. Am J Med. 1984;76:91.
37. Altemeier WA, Culbertson WR, Fullen DW, et al. Intra-abdominal abscesses. Am J Surg. 1973;125:70.
38. Lorber B, Swenson RM. The bacteriology of intra-abdominal infections. Surg Clin North Am. 1975;55:1349.
39. Harding GKM, Buckwold FJ, Ronald AR, et al. Prospective, randomized comparative study of clindamycin, chloramphenicol, and ticarcillin, each in combination with gentamicin, in therapy for intraabdominal and female genital tract sepsis. J Infect Dis. 1980;142:384.
40. Tally FP, McGowan K, Kellum JM, et al. A randomized comparison of cefoxitin with or without amikacin and clindamycin plus amikacin in surgical sepsis. Ann Surg. 1981;193:318.
41. England DM, Rosenblatt JE. Anaerobes in human biliary tracts. J Clin Microbiol. 1977;6:494.
42. Shimada K, Noro T, Inamatsu T, et al. Bacteriology of acute suppurative cholangitis of the aged. J Clin Microbiol. 1981;14:522.
43. Malone DA, Wagner RA, Myers JP, et al. Enterococcal bacteremia in two large community teaching hospitals. Am J Med. 1986;81:601.
44. Feathers RS, Lewis AAM, Sagor GR, et al. Prophylactic systemic antibiotics in colorectal surgery. Lancet. 1977;2:4.
45. Kager L, Liljeqvist L, Malmorg AS, et al. Effect of clindamycin prophylaxis on the colonic microflora in patients undergoing colorectal surgery. Antimicrob Agents Chemother. 1981;20:736.
46. Fitzpatrick B, Warren JW, Caplan ES, et al. A randomized trial of moxalactam (Mox) vs clindamycin/tobramycin (C/T) in the therapy of aerobic-anaerobic infections (Abstract). Antimicrob Agents Chemother. 1982;107:84.
47. Dougherty SH, Flohr AB, Simmons RL. 'Break through' enterococcal septicemia in surgical patients. Arch Surg. 1983;118:232.
48. Duma RJ, Weinberg AN, Medrek TF, et al. Streptococcal infections. A bacteriologic and clinical study of streptococcal bacteremia. Medicine (Baltimore). 1969;48:87.
49. Berk SL, Verghese A, Holtsclaw SA. Enterococcal pneumonia. Occurrence in patients receiving broad-spectrum antibiotic regimens and enteric feeding. Am J Med. 1983;74:153.
50. Bayer AS, Seidel JS, Yoshikawa TT, et al. Group D enterococcal meningitis. Clinical and therapeutic considerations with report of three cases and review of the literature. Arch Intern Med. 1976;136:883.
51. Moellering RC Jr, Krogstad DJ. Antibiotic resistance in enterococci. In: Schlessinger D, ed. Microbiology: 1979. Washington, DC: American Society for Microbiology; 1979;293–8.
52. Moellering RC Jr, Watson BK. Kunz LJ. Endocarditis due to group D streptococci. Am J Med. 1974;57:239.
53. Tofte RW, Solliday J, Crossley KB. Susceptibilities of enterococci to twelve antibiotics. Antimicrob Agents Chemother. 1984;25:532.
54. Glew RH, Moellering RC Jr, Wennersten C. Comparative synergistic activity of nafcillin, oxacillin, and methicillin in combination with gentamicin against enterococci. Antimicrob Agents Chemother. 1975;7:828.
55. Watanakunakorn C, Tisone JC. Effects of a vancomycin-rifampin combination on enterococci. Antimicrob Agents Chemother. 1982;22:915.
56. Neu HC, Labthavikul P. Comparative in vitro activity of *N*-formimidoyl thienamycin against gram-positive and gram-negative aerobic and anaerobic species and its beta-lactamase stability. Antimicrob Agents Chemother. 1982;21:180.
57. Fernandez-Guerrero M, Rouse MS, Henry NK, et al. In vitro and in vivo activity of ciprofloxacin against enterococci isolated from patients with infective endocarditis. Antimicrob Agents Chemother. 1986;31:430.
58. Wanger AR, Murray BE. Activity of LY146032 against enterococci with and without high-level aminoglycoside resistance, including two penicillinase-producing strains. Antimicrob Agents Chemother. 1987;31:1779.
59. Crider SR, Colby SD. Susceptibility of enterococci to trimethoprim and trimethoprim-sulfamethoxazole. Antimicrob. Agents Chemother. 1985;27:71.
60. Ingerman M, Pitsakis PG, Rosenberg A, et al. Beta-lactamase production in experimental endocarditis due to aminoglycoside-resistant *Streptococcus faecalis*. J Infect Dis. 1987;155;1226.
61. Moellering RC Jr. Korzeniowski OM, Sande MA, et al. Species-specific resistance to antimicrobial synergism in *Streptococcus faecium* and *Streptococcus faecalis*. J Gen Microbiol. 1979;111:441.
62. Harwick HJ, Halmanson GM, Guze LB. In vitro activity of ampicillin or vancomycin combined with gentamicin or streptomycin against enterococci. Antimicrob Agents Chemother. 1973;4:383.
63. Mandell GL. Enigmatic enterococcal endocarditis. Ann Intern Med. 1984;100:904.
64. Serra P, Brandimarte C, Martino P, et al. Synergistic treatment of enterococcal endocarditis. Arch Intern Med. 1977;137:1562.
65. Westenfelder GO, Paterson PV, Reisberg BE, et al. Vancomycin-streptomycin synergy in enterococcal endocarditis. JAMA. 1973;223:37.
66. Moellering RC Jr, Weinberg AN. Studies on antibiotic synergism against enterococci. II. Effect of various antibiotics on the uptake of C^{14}-labelled streptomycin by enterococci. J Clin Invest. 1971;50:2580.
67. Storch GA, Krogstad DJ. Antibiotic-induced lysis of enterococci. J Clin Invest. 1981;68:639.

68. Mederski-Samoraj BD, Murray BE. High-level resistance to gentamicin in clinical isolates of enterococci. J Infect Dis. 1983;147:751.
69. Zervos MJ, Mikesell TS, Schaberg DR. Heterogeneity of plasmids determining high-level resistance to gentamicin in clinical isolates of *Streptococcus faecalis*. Antimicrob Agents Chemother. 1986;30:78.
70. Zervos MJ, Dembinski S, Mikesell T, et al. High-level resistance to gentamicin in *Streptococcus faecalis*: Risk factors and evidence for exogenous acquisition of infection. J Infect Dis. 1986;153:1075.
71. Enzler MJ, Rouse MS, Henry NK, et al. In vitro and in vivo studies of streptomycin-resistant, penicillin-susceptible streptococci from patients with infective endocarditis. J Infect Dis. 1987;155:954.
72. Gutschik E. Experimental endocarditis in rabbits. 6. Results of long-term combined therapy of *Streptococcus faecalis* endocarditis with penicillin and streptomycin. Acta Pathol Microbiol Immunol Scand. 1982;90:37.
73. Carrizosa J, Kaye D. Antibiotic synergism in enterococcal endocarditis. J Lab Clin Med. 1976;88:132.
74. Zervos MJ, Patterson JE, Edberg S, et al. Single-concentration broth microdilution test for detection of high-level aminoglycoside resistance in enterococci. J Clin Microbiol. 1987;25:2443.
75. Sahm DF, Torres C. High-content aminoglycoside disks for determining aminoglycoside-penicillin synergy against *Enterococcus faecalis*. J Clin Microbiol. 1988;26:257.

180. STREPTOCOCCUS AGALACTIAE (GROUP B STREPTOCOCCUS)

MORVEN S. EDWARDS
CAROL J. BAKER

HISTORICAL PERSPECTIVE

Group B streptococci (*Streptococcus agalactiae*) were first reported as human pathogens in 1935 by Fry, who described three cases of fatal puerperal sepsis.[1] Before Fry, Lancefield and Hare[2] had identified these organisms in vaginal cultures from asymptomatic postpartum women. Human group B streptococcal infection, however, was reported infrequently until the early 1960s when several authors indicated that disease due to these organisms might be more common than was appreciated previously.[3–5] By the early 1970s, the importance of group B *Streptococcus* as a human pathogen could no longer be overlooked since it had become a frequent cause of infection among febrile postpartum women and neonates. While the appearance of group B *Streptococcus* as a significant pathogen in neonates and young infants represents only one of several well-documented shifts in the prevalence of etiologic agents causing neonatal bacterial infection, its emergence was unusual in that it initially did not replace the existing predominant pathogen, *Escherichia coli*. Therefore, the overall incidence of neonatal sepsis (bacteremia) was increased during the 1970s. More recent reports indicate that the incidence of group B streptococcal neonatal infections has remained unchanged during the last 15 years.[6]

DESCRIPTION

Classification and Morphologic Characteristics

Streptococcus agalactiae is the species designation for streptococci belonging to Lancefield group B. The serologic differentiation of hemolytic streptococci by groups was described in 1933. It is based on the capillary precipitin reaction between the group-specific carbohydrate antigen in the cell wall, which is solubilized by acid treatment of the organisms, with hyperimmune antisera that is prepared by immunization of rabbits with formalin-killed whole cells.[7] Group B streptococci are facultative gram-positive diplococci that are grown easily on a variety of bacteriologic media. Isolated colonies are 3–4 mm in diameter and grayish white in color when cultivated on sheep blood agar. The flat, somewhat mucoid colonies are surrounded by a narrow zone of β-hemolysis that, for some strains, is detectable only on lifting a colony from the agar. While 1–2 percent of strains are nonhemolytic, they are rarely α-hemolytic. To enhance the accurate detection of even low numbers of group B streptococci from sites such as the genital or gastrointestinal tract, a number of selective media have been employed. These usually contain Todd-Hewitt broth with or without sheep red blood cells (5 percent) and antimicrobial agents such as nalidixic acid and gentamicin or colistin.[8]

Identification

Definitive identification of group B streptococci is based on detection of the group B specific cell wall antigen common to all strains. A number of methods, each of which uses hyperimmune group-specific antisera, have been developed for the detection of the group B antigen: countercurrent immunoelectrophoresis, enzyme-linked immunosorbent assay (ELISA), indirect immunofluorescence, staphylococcal coagglutination, and latex agglutination. The latter two are the most widely employed due to their commercial availability and simplicity. When the manufacturer's instructions are followed, each of three commercially available products for serogrouping β-hemolytic streptococci (Phadebact Streptococcus Test Kit, Pharmacia Diagnostics; Sero STAT, Scott Laboratories, Inc.; Streptex, Wellcome Research Laboratories) has been shown to accurately identify each of more than 100 pure-culture group B streptococcal isolates when compared with the Lancefield capillary precipitin method.[9] However, occasional cross-reactions have been observed when the Streptex direct mixed-culture procedure is employed. Nonserologic methods that permit the presumptive identification of group B streptococci include resistance to bacitracin or trimethoprim-sulfamethoxazole, positive sodium hippurate hydrolysis, and production of an orange pigment during anaerobic growth on certain media. β-Hemolytic streptococci that hydrolyze sodium hippurate belong to either groups B or D; these may be distinguished on the basis of hydrolysis of bile esculin agar. Among group D strains, 99 percent hydrolyze bile esculin, whereas 99–100 percent of group B strains fail to react.[10] Production of CAMP factor, which is a thermostable extracellular protein that results in synergistic hemolysis on sheep blood agar with the β-lysin of *Staphylococcus aureus*, is observed in 98–100 percent of group B streptococci. A spot CAMP test, available commercially, allows rapid identification of group B streptococci from a single colony of the primary isolation plate.[11] The combination of the CAMP test with bacitracin sensitivity and the bile esculin reaction has been suggested as an adequate method for the presumptive differentiation of group B from other serogroups of β-hemolytic streptococci.[12]

Serologic Classification

Lancefield defined two cell wall carbohydrate antigens for group B streptococci, the group B specific or "C" substance common to all strains of this serogroup and the type-specific or "S" substance that allows classification into four serotypes: Ia, Ib, II, and III (Table 1).[13] The fifth serotype of group B *Streptococcus*, historically designated type Ic, was characterized by Wilkinson and Eagon.[14] These strains possess a capsular polysaccharide antigen, Ia, that is immunochemically identical to that common to all type Ia strains and a surface protein antigen that is common to all type Ib strains, approximately 60 percent of type II strains, and in an occasional type III strain. However, this protein antigen, historically called the Ibc protein antigen, is not found in type Ia strains. A minor antigenic de-

TABLE 1. Antigenic Determinants of Group B Streptococci

Serotype Designation		*Antigens*		
		Major Polysaccharide	*Proteins*	
Present	*Historical*		*Present*	*Historical*
Ia	Ia	Ia	—	—
Ib/c	Ib	Ib	c	Ibc
Ia/c	Ic	Ia	c	Ibc
II	II	II	c[a]	Ibc[a]
III	III	III	—[b]	—[b]
IV	—	IV	—	—

[a] Sixty percent of type II isolates possess the protein antigen c.
[b] Serotype III strains occasionally may possess the protein antigen c or the proteins X or R.

terminant, the type Iabc polysaccharide was demonstrated by Lancefield to be common to many type I strains. The nomenclature of group B streptococci has been revised to designate the capsular polysaccharides as type-specific antigens and the surface proteins as additional antigenic markers.[15] The simplified designation for the protein antigen Ibc is c, so the former type Ic is presently designated type Ia/c (Table 1), and the former type Ib is type Ib/c. A new serotype, type IV, that contains a unique polysaccharide alone or with protein antigens has been defined recently,[16] and several candidate serotypes are being evaluated. Antibodies against the major and minor polysaccharide antigens, with the exception of the type III antigen, were shown by Lancefield to provide passive protection for mice challenged with homologous—but not heterologous—antigen-containing strains.[17] Although mouse virulence for type III strains could not be achieved in the original mouse-protective assay,[17] others subsequently have modified this experimental model so that antibody to the type III capsular polysaccharide antigen also has been shown to protect against challenge with strains containing the homologous but not the heterologous antigens.[18] In contrast, rabbit antibodies with group B specificity do not protect mice from a lethal challenge.[17]

EPIDEMIOLOGY AND TRANSMISSION

Asymptomatic Colonization

Group B streptococci have been isolated from genital and/or lower gastrointestinal tract cultures of pregnant women at a rate ranging from 5–40 percent.[19–20] These variations in the reported prevalence of asymptomatic colonization relate not only to differences in the culture method employed but also to intrinsic differences in the populations studied (Table 2). When the culture method is selected to optimize the sensitivity of detection and when more than one appropriate site such as the lower vagina or the periurethral or anorectal area is cultured on more than one occasion, the rate of colonization detected usually exceeds 20 percent. Group B streptococci may be harbored in the urinary tract during pregnancy in association with asymptomatic bacteriuria.[21] Even when optimal culture methods are used, a significantly lower prevalence of genital colonization occurs among women who are virgins, older than 20 years of age, or of Mexican-American origin.[22] The serotype distribution of isolates from asymptomatically colonized patients, irrespective of age or sex, is divided evenly among the three major serotypes: I, II, and III.

Pregnancy itself and the timing of cultures during pregnancy do not influence the prevalence of colonization with group B *Streptococcus*. Boyer and associates[23] found that the overall predictive value of a positive second-trimester culture of the vagina or rectum for colonization at delivery was 67 percent while a negative prenatal culture had a predictive value of 92 percent. Thus, the findings of this and other longitudinal studies[24–26] illustrate the limitations of a single genital culture obtained during pregnancy as an accurate predictor of colonization status at delivery.

A growing body of compelling but not conclusive evidence supports the concept that the principal reservoir for group B streptococci may be the lower gastrointestinal tract rather than the female genital tract. Studies documenting a rectal-to-vaginal isolation ratio exceeding 1 and the anorectum as the site most accurately predicting persistence of chronicity of carriage support the possibility that genital colonization may reflect contamination from the rectum.[23,27] Further, group B streptococci have been isolated from the proximal part of the small intestine of adults.[28] The prevalence of oropharyngeal colonization is low in pregnant women (approximately 5 percent), but it approaches 20 percent in homosexual men.

Transmission to Neonates

Mucous membrane colonization of newborns results from vertical transmission of the organism from the mother, either in utero by the ascending route or at the time of delivery. The rate of vertical transmission in neonates born to women colonized with group B streptococci at the time of delivery ranges from 29 to 72 percent (mean, 50 percent).[25,29–31] Paired isolates from mothers and their neonates are of concordant serotypes.[29] The only maternal factor that has been shown to significantly influence the likelihood of vertical transmission is the presence of

TABLE 2. Factors Influencing Detection of Group B Streptococcal Colonization

Feature	*Effect on Isolation Rate*		
	Increased	*Decreased*	*None*
Method employed			
Culture medium	Broth media	Agar media	
	Antibiotic-containing media	Nonselective broth media	
Site(s)	Lower vagina	Cervical os	
	Multiple sites	Single site	
Interval	≥2 cultures in 6–8-wk interval	Single sampling time	
Genital carriage in women			
Pregnancy			+
Timing during pregnancy			+
Day of menstrual cycle	First half		
Age	≤20 yr		
Sexual activity	Active	Virgin	
Birth control method	Intrauterine device		Oral contraceptives
Parity	≤3 pregnancies		≥3 pregnancies
Ethnic origin		Mexican-American	
Marital status			+
Frequency of sexual intercourse/total number of partners			+
Vaginal discharge			+
Socioeconomic group	Lower income		

a high genital inoculum at delivery, as detected by semiquantitative culture methods.[23,24,31,32] Infants born to heavily colonized women are more likely to develop invasive early-onset disease,[23] and infants acquiring heavy colonization have significantly increased rates of early- and late-onset disease.[6]

In addition to exposure at birth, horizontally acquired (nosocomial) colonization of the neonate has been found to contribute to the rate of colonization in some nursery settings. Acquisition is more likely when the maternal population has a high endogenous colonization rate (as influenced by such factors as age, parity, ethnic composition, and socioeconomic status) and when crowded conditions in the nursery promote poor handwashing techniques and transmission to infants via hands of personnel. Although nosocomially acquired rates of colonization in excess of 40 percent have been reported,[33] nosocomial transmission is negligible in smaller, less crowded nurseries.[25,34] Noya and associates[35] described a cluster of late-onset infections that by phage typing appeared to result from a single epidemic strain of type Ib/c group B *Streptococcus*. Epidemiologic analysis suggested that infant-to-infant spread via the hands of personnel was the most likely mode by which five very low birth weight infants developed bacteremic infection. A few smaller case clusters have been attributed to nosocomial acquisition of type III strains. "Community" acquisition of group B streptococci in young infants occurs infrequently. Gardner et al.[36] reported that this mode of acquisition occurred in only 4.3 percent of their patients during the first 2 months of life. None of these infants was colonized at the time of hospital discharge.

The importance of defining the modes of transmission by which neonates acquire asymptomatic colonization with group B streptococci is evidenced by the fact that vertical transmission is required for the development of invasive early-onset infection.[29–31] Several factors have been noted that increase the incidence of invasive early-onset infection among neonates born to colonized mothers. They include rupture of membranes for more than 24 hours before delivery, multiple births, premature rupture of membranes, and maternal fever and/or amnionitis.[23,29–31] While it is clear that some infants who develop late-onset infection acquire the organism from nonmaternal sources,[31] the concordance of serotypes between neonatal and maternal genital isolates at the time of diagnosis in one-half to two-thirds of cases suggests that the vertical route of acquisition also is a major determinant of risk for late-onset infections.[6,37]

Incidence and Serotype Distribution of Infection

The reported incidence of early-onset neonatal group B streptococcal infection, defined as the onset of symptoms during the first 5 days of life, ranges from 0.7 to 3.7 per 1000 live births. Although there is some evidence suggesting that the incidence may be declining, the attack rate up to 1988 remains approximately 2.0 per 1000 live births in most hospitals. Attack rates for early-onset group B streptococcal disease are inversely related to birth weight and may exceed 20 per 1000 live births among infants with birth weights less than 1000 grams.[38] However, approximately 60–90 percent of early-onset infections occur in term infants.[6,38–40] The attack rate for late-onset neonatal infection, which is characterized by the onset of symptoms from 6 days to 3 months of age, is approximately 1 per 1000 live births. This is an estimate that corresponds closely to the attack rate ranging from 0.9 to 1.9 per 1000 live births defined in the 6-year prospective study of Dillon et al.[6]

Beyond early infancy, postpartum women are the only group of patients in whom group B streptococcal disease is diagnosed frequently. These organisms have been estimated to cause 15–25 percent of the cases of postpartum febrile morbidity with or without bacteremia, or an estimated 48,000 cases annually.[41–43] In one population with a known high incidence of carriage, puerperal sepsis due to group B streptococci occurred with an attack rate of 2 per 1000 deliveries.[44] Adults with altered immune status due to diabetes mellitus, chronic hepatic dysfunction, human immunodeficiency virus infection,[45] or malignancies requiring immunosuppressive therapy also are susceptible to group B streptococcal infections. However, its incidence in these hosts appears to be low.

For neonates with early-onset infection without meningitis, the serotype distribution of isolates parallels that of asymptomatically colonized mothers or infants and is divided equally among type I, II, and III strains. However, type III strains of group B streptococci have been isolated from most newborns (80 percent) with early-onset infection in whom meningeal involvement occurs. This serotype is responsible for 93 percent of late-onset infections regardless of clinical expression.[46] The explanation for the apparent tropism of type III strains for the meninges of neonates is poorly understood. Although each of the serotypes has been reported to cause disease in immunocompromised adults, type II strains have been isolated from most adults with meningitis; in contrast, they rarely penetrate the meninges of neonates.[47,48] The mechanisms for this "differential tropism" among different serotypes of group B streptococci in distinct populations of patients have not been defined.

PATHOGENESIS

The association between maternal genital tract colonization with group B streptococci at the time of delivery and risk for the development of invasive neonatal early-onset infection is well established.[29–31] Similarly, there is an enhanced risk for invasive infection rather than asymptomatic colonization in neonates when exposure to the organism is *prolonged* by a rupture of membranes for more than 24 hours before delivery or *intensified* by the presence of maternal amnionitis or a high genital inoculum.[6,23,29–31] However, these factors that influence susceptibility in neonates do not explain fully the low incidence of symptomatic infection among newborns born to colonized mothers at delivery, which is estimated at only 1–2 percent.[49,50]

One explanation for the apparent disparity between the incidence of asymptomatic as compared with invasive infection is the considerable increase in the rate of symptomatic infection that is associated with preterm labor. Infants born at less than 37 weeks' gestation have a 15-fold increase in risk for symptomatic infection when compared with infants at term.[31] Ascending infection by the choriodecidual route may be a primary pathogenetic event initiating the preterm rupture of membranes.[51] The association of group B streptococcal asymptomatic bacteriuria in women who rupture their membranes before the onset of labor supports the hypothesis that group B streptococcal infection may predispose to preterm delivery.[52]

Baker and Kasper[53] reported in 1976 that neonates at risk for invasive type III group B streptococcal infection were those with low concentrations of antibody to the capsular antigen of this serotype; this has been substantiated by others.[54,55] Since infants born prematurely acquire proportionately lower levels of maternal IgG than do those born at term, premature infants are less likely to acquire a level of specific maternal IgG sufficient for "protection" against the development of invasive infection. Although the level of specific anticapsular antibody to type III group B *Streptococcus* required for protection has not been defined, levels less than 2 μg/ml, as determined by a radioactive antigen-binding assay,[53] were detected in 79 neonatal sera collected within 48 hours after the onset of symptoms.[56] Women colonized with type III group B streptococci at the time of delivery whose infants remained well during the first 3 months of life had antibody levels in excess of 2 μg/ml significantly more often (73 percent) than did those whose infants developed early-onset disease (17 percent).[56] Among these latter mothers, the presence of antibody in excess of 2 μg/ml occurred either in association with premature delivery or with the definite or presumed diagnosis of maternal peripartum group B streptococcal infection. A low maternal level of antibody to polysaccharide antigens also is a determinant of neonatal susceptibility to infection due to serotypes Ia, Ib/c, and II group B streptococci.[57–59] Antibody to the group B polysaccharide, however, is not protective.[60]

Although a "deficiency" of type-specific antibody is one critical factor in neonatal susceptibility to symptomatic group B streptococcal infection, other host defense factors also are contributory. For example, the incidence of invasive infection in twins is increased even when corrected for birth weight and gestational age.[61,62] In evaluating the requirements for in vitro opsonization of group B streptococci, Shigeoka et al.[63] have shown that the classical complement pathway and heat-stable opsonins are required for maximal opsonic activity by human sera for type I, II, and III strains. The alternative complement pathway participates in opsonophagocytosis of type III strains when specific antibody is present in a sufficient concentration. The opsonophagocytic requirements for type II group strains are complex, modulated in part but not fully by the c protein as well as the type II polysaccharide antigens, and integrity of the classical complement pathway appears essential for effective opsonophagocytosis in vitro.[64,65] For clinical isolates of type Ia group B *Streptococcus*, opsonization and phagocytosis may proceed via the classical complement pathway in an antibody-independent fashion,[66] and C1 activation may be initiated by interactions with surface-bound capsular polysaccharide of type Ia strains.[67] Deficient activity by a portion of neonatal sera for clinical isolates of this serotype correlated significantly with low levels of the classic pathway components C1q and C4.[68] Since complement proteins in the neonate are not maternally derived and since levels of components in both the classical and alternative pathways are only 30–50 percent of those in maternal or adult control sera at term, physiologically low levels of complement components or their receptors on phagocytes may provide a partial explanation for age-related susceptibility to group B streptococcal disease.

The phagocytic and intracellular killing capacity of neonatal neutrophils is comparable to that of adults under "unstressed" conditions, but neutrophil reserves are exhausted rapidly, and the proliferative rate of granulocytic stem cells is nearly maximal in noninfected neonatal animal; thus their response to infection is limited.[69]

Employing a neonatal rat model of group B streptococcal infection, Zeligs et al.[70] have shown that the recovery of older (7-day-old) animals after experimental challenge correlated with the recovery of myeloid storage pools whereas fatal infection in 2-day-old animals was associated with the failure of depleted myeloid storage pools to respond to the bacterial challenge.

In addition to host factors, bacterial virulence factors undoubtedly contribute to the host–parasite interaction that determines the outcome between exposure and the development of asymptomatic or symptomatic group B streptococcal infection. A high quantity of cell-associated sialic acid and its elaboration in supernatant fluid at high concentrations each has been associated with virulence of type III strains.[71–73] The finding of Rubens et al.[74] that a transposon mutant lacking surface expression of the type III but not the group B specific polysaccharide was avirulent in an experimental model supports the importance of elaborated capsular antigen as a virulence factor.[74] The unique capsular structures of types Ia, Ib, II, and III group B streptococci[75] also might enhance the invasiveness of one serotype over another. While each of these four type-specific polysaccharides contain glucose, galactose, glucosamine, and sialic acid, their structural arrangements are distinct. For example, sialic acid, which constitutes the exclusive terminal residue of the type Ia and III—but not type II—group B streptococcal capsular antigen, inhibits activation of the alternative pathway of complement.[75] Inhibition of this mechanism, which provides a defense for the nonimmune host against bacterial infections, might further explain the occurrence of invasive group B streptococcal disease in some infants.

CLINICAL MANIFESTATIONS

Early-Onset Neonatal Infections

As the incidence of neonatal group B streptococcal infections rose during the 1970s, a bimodal distribution of cases by age at onset of symptoms became apparent. Thus, two distinctive clinical syndromes related to age were described by Franciosi et al.[76] (acute and delayed) and by Baker et al.[77] (early and late onset). Early-onset infection, defined as the development of symptoms during the first 5 days of life, has a mean age at onset of 20 hours.[37,49,76] Maternal obstetric complications are observed frequently (60 percent) in association with early-onset disease; premature infants are affected significantly more often than are infants born at term. The three major clinical expressions of early-onset infection observed in approximately equal frequency are bacteremia with no identifiable focus of infection, pneumonia, and meningitis.

The presenting signs and symptoms of early-onset group B streptococcal infection—lethargy, poor feeding, jaundice, abnormal temperature, grunting respirations, pallor, and in approximately 25 percent of cases, hypotension—are not distinguishable from those of neonates with other types of bacterial infection. Regardless of the focus of infection, respiratory distress is observed frequently.[76,77] Infants with meningitis have a clinical presentation including respiratory distress that initially cannot be distinguished from those without meningeal invasion.[78] Thus, a lumbar puncture is required to identify neonates with meningitis for supportive and specific therapy to be appropriate. One-half of patients with meningitis develop seizures within 24 hours of onset; if they persist, a poor outcome is more likely to result.

Among the approximately 40 percent of infants with early-onset infection who have bacteremia with pneumonia, signs of respiratory distress such as apnea, grunting, tachypnea, and cyanosis are virtually always present. Although pulmonary infiltrates on chest x-ray films may suggest the diagnosis, at least one-half of these infants have a radiographic pattern consistent with and indistinguishable from that of hyaline membrane disease.[79] In most (~80 percent) of these infants, symptoms of respiratory distress are present at or within a few hours after birth. At postmortem examination, atypical hyaline membranes containing group B streptococci are found in the lungs of these infants. This finding provides a partial explanation for the difficulties encountered in clinically distinguishing between infectious and noninfectious forms of respiratory tract disease.[80]

Increased awareness of the disease and improvements in supportive therapy have resulted in decreased mortality among infants with early-onset group B streptococcal infection, and present rates range from 13 to 37 percent.[81,82] While mortality is significantly higher in prematures weighing <1500 g at birth (61 percent), larger infants still account for most deaths.[83]

Late-Onset Neonatal Infections

Late-onset group B streptococcal infection, which may occur occasionally among preterm infants but usually affects the term infant from 7 days to 3 months of age, has a mean age of onset of 24 days.[79] Maternal obstetric complications are rare, and the case-fatality ratio is somewhat lower than that of early-onset infection, 10–15 percent.[49,79,84] Bacteremia with concomitant meningitis (85 percent of cases) has been the predominant clinical manifestation of late-onset infection, but bacteremia without a focus may be becoming increasingly frequent.[6] Regardless of the focus of infection, serotype III strains are isolated from approximately 95 percent of patients. Recently, outbreaks of late-onset diseases, transmitted nosocomially, have been described among hospitalized premature infants.[35] In contrast to infants with early-onset infection, the nonspecific initial symptoms of late-onset disease such as lethargy, poor feeding, and irritability generally occur in association with fever (temperature, ≥38°C), a finding that mandates hospitalization, blood and cerebrospinal fluid (CSF) cultures, and empirical antimicrobial therapy pending laboratory results. These infants may present with fulminant infection characterized by progression, within a few hours, from the absence of symptoms to a moribund state with septic shock, seizures, and CSF Gram stains with sheets of organisms. An increased risk for mortality or permanent neurologic sequelae occurs in patients with this fulminant presentation. Additional clinical findings that have been associated with fatal outcome or permanent neurologic sequelae include neutropenia at admission, prolonged seizures, and high concentrations of type III polysaccharide antigen in admission CSF specimens.[24] A significant number (from 25 to 50 percent) of survivors of group B streptococcal meningitis, whether early- or late-onset type, will have permanent neurologic sequelae.[78,85,86] Approximately one-third of patients with these complications manifest them as severe blindness, deafness, and/or global developmental delay; in the remainder of patients, the deficits are more subtle and may be detectable only when language and cognitive function can be tested adequately.

Bacteremia without an apparent focus and bone and joint infections are the other clinical forms of late-onset group B streptococcal disease that occur relatively frequently. The former patients are generally identified as the result of routine evaluation of the young infant with fever; recovery after appropriate treatment is the rule. These infants should be evaluated carefully for the presence of associated foci of infection such as preauricular or submandibular cellulitis and adenitis,[87] otitis media, conjunctivitis, peritonitis, endocarditis, or deep abscesses.[88] Each of these focal types of infections has also occurred in association with early-onset disease.

Group B streptococcal osteomyelitis is characterized by an indolent onset in which the primary symptom of diminished movement of the singly involved extremity has been noted for many days and, in a few cases, since nursery discharge. It has been postulated that group B streptococcal osteomyelitis might represent a delayed expression of asymptomatic early-onset bacteremia. The observed predilection for involvement of the right proximal humerus may result from bacteremic seeding of this site after minor trauma during vaginal delivery.[89] In contrast, septic arthritis is associated with an acute onset of symptoms, and patients usually have bacteremia documented at the time of admission. Both bone and joint infections are associated with minimal inflammatory changes, and fever is reported in only 20 percent of patients. Lower extremity involvement is commonly observed in infants with septic arthritis, while osteomyelitis has a predilection for involvement of the proximal humerus (60 percent of the cases). However, involvement of the femur, tibia, and flat and small bones has also been reported. In contrast to other bacterial causes of neonatal septic arthritis and osteomyelitis, most infants have no permanent functional impairment of the involved extremity.

Infections in Adults

Bacteremic group B streptococcal infection causes substantial morbidity and mortality among adults. In one analysis from 1975 to 1984, the composite attack rate for group B streptococcal bacteremia was 0.2 cases per 1000 hospital admissions, and 53 percent of group B streptococcal blood culture isolates were from adults.[90] Adults with bacteremia unrelated to pregnancy usually are elderly with ages ranging from 59 to 68 years in recent reports.[90–92] One or more conditions predisposing to infection can be identified in most but not all adults with bacteremia (Table 3). Mortality is increased in older patients, in those with polymicrobial infections, and in those with diabetes mellitus, liver disease, or malignancy. Fatality rates ranging from 8 to 70 percent have been reported,[48,90–93] but if postpartum women, who usually have nonfatal infections, are excluded from these series, mortality exceeds 40 percent.[90–92] Of the 29 adults with bacteremia described by Opal and associates,[90] only 34 percent acquired their infections in the community. Others have described rates of nosocomial infection from 38 to 70 percent,[92,94] but case clustering has not been observed.[90–94] The latter suggests but does not prove that chronic respiratory, genitourinary, or gastrointestinal mucosal infection rather than acquisition of group B streptococci in the hospital is the source for these bacteremias. Additional study of the epidemiology of adult bacteremias is warranted.

TABLE 3. Underlying Conditions in 75 Adults with Bacteremic Group B Streptococcal Infections Unrelated to Pregnancy

Condition	*No. Patients (%)*[a]
Diabetes mellitus	23 (31)
Malignancy	18 (24)
Liver failure and/or history of alcohol abuse	18 (24)
Neurologic impairment	12 (16)
Renal failure	11 (15)
Congestive heart failure	7 (9)
Intravenous catheter related-infection	5 (7)
Steroid administration	5 (7)
Functional or surgical splenectomy	3 (4)
Acquired immune deficiency syndrome	2 (3)

[a] Several patients had more than one underlying condition.
(Data from Polsky et al.,[45] Opal et al.,[90] Gallagher et al.,[71] and Verghese et al.[92])

Postpartum bacteremia due to group B streptococci increased during the 1970s, an increase that paralleled that reported for neonatal infections. Recent reports indicate that group B streptococci account for 10–20 percent of blood culture isolates from women admitted to obstetric services.[24,41,95] Faro[41] reported an incidence of group B streptococcal endometritis or endoparametritis of 1.3 per 1000 deliveries; one-third of these patients had concomitant bacteremia. An uncomplicated outcome after appropriate antimicrobial therapy is the rule for these patients, although complications such as meningitis or endocarditis have been described.[42,93]

Most adult group B streptococcal infections occur in association with one of several sources of infection as detailed below.

Infections of the Female Genital Tract. The greatest number of adult infections due to group B *Streptococcus* occur in postpartum women. The source of these infections is the female genital tract. In one study of 55 women with early postpartum endometritis diagnosed clinically, group B streptococci alone or as a component of polymicrobial infection were among the most commonly isolated facultative aerobes.[96] A variety of clinical manifestations may occur, but the most common of these are endometritis and/or wound infection associated with cesarian section.[37] Most women with endometritis develop signs of infection within 48 hours of delivery. A striking association between abdominal delivery and endometritis has been noted.[44] Minkoff et al.[97] found that, among patients who had cesarian sections, the 19 percent who were colonized with group B streptococci had a significantly increased frequency of premature rupture of membranes, postpartum fever, and endometritis when compared with noncolonized women. These symptoms of endometritis are nonspecific and include fever with or without chills, malaise, moderate uterine tenderness, and normal lochia. In the report by Gibbs and Blanco,[42] the initial lack of symptoms referable to the genital area was followed by the subsequent diagnosis of endometritis in 81 percent of patients and chorioamnionitis in 19 percent. The incidence of life-threatening sequelae of endometritis such as pelvic abscess, septic shock, or septic thrombophlebitis is less than 2 percent.[98] Another frequent manifestation of perinatal maternal morbidity is urinary tract infection. Group B streptococcal peripartum bacteriuria may be asymptomatic or may be diagnosed in association with cystitis or, less frequently, pyelonephritis.[44]

Pneumonia. Group B streptococci behave as opportunistic pathogens in patients whose immune function is altered. The specific mechanisms underlying the predilection for this infection have not been delineated. However, these patients have in common the apparent inability to limit spread of the organism from mucous membrane sites of colonization to the blood stream. The most common underlying conditions among patients with group B streptococcal pneumonia are diabetes mellitus and neurologic disease (for example, stroke or dementia). The seven patients described by Verghese et al.[99] were elderly (median age, 78 years), debilitated, and bedridden. All patients were febrile, had a brisk leukocytosis, and were hypoxic in room air. Chest radiographs showed bilateral or lobar infiltrates. Infection frequently was polymicrobic, although group B streptococci were the predominant organism. Pleural empyema has been described in association with pneumonia.[100] Fatality rates range from 30 to 85 percent.

Endocarditis. A major shift in the clinical expression of group B streptococcal endocarditis has been documented by Lerner et al.[48] In contrast to the predominance of acute mitral valve endocarditis in pregnant women during the preantibiotic era, cases reported since 1945 have had no sex predilection, have been both acute and subacute in onset, and have occurred in older patients (mean age, approximately 50 years).[37,48,101] The mitral valve is still the most commonly affected valve (48 percent); infections involving the aortic (29 percent), mitral and aortic (10 percent), and tricuspid valves (5 percent) also have been described. Underlying heart disease is present in more than half of the cases reported since 1962, rheumatic heart disease being the most common.[101] Valvular disease, atherosclerotic heart disease and mitral valve prolapse also have been described as predisposing features.[101,102] Large friable vegetations are a frequent feature of infection, and embolization may occur early in the course.[101] The mortality rate from group B streptococcal endocarditis is approximately 50 percent.[37,48,93,101,103]

Arthritis and Osteomyelitis. Group B streptococcal arthritis generally is monoarticular, most commonly affecting the knee, hip or shoulder joints, although polyarticular disease with a central pattern has been described.[104] Diabetes mellitus is a common predisposing factor, as is osteoarthritis and infection involving a joint prosthesis. Occasionally, arthritis occurs in the absence of underlying conditions. The most common presenting signs are fever and joint pain in the setting of septicemia. With appropriate antimicrobial therapy, repeated joint aspirations, or open drainage and (usually) removal of a prosthesis, if present, complete recovery occurs in one-half of patients. In the remainder, disease is associated with substantial functional residual. Osteomyelitis as a consequence of adjacent arthritis and vertebral osteomyelitis are primary clinical expressions of bony disease in adults.[104,105]

Skin and Soft Tissue Infections. Group B streptococcal soft tissue infections, including cellulitis, abscess, and infection of decubitus ulcers, are common.[106] In one report of 37 patients, the mean age (44 years) of the two-thirds who had serious underlying conditions was significantly greater than that of normal hosts (21 years) who often acquired infection in association with minor trauma. Abscess formation was observed in 46 percent of these infections. Group B *Streptococcus* was the only organism isolated from 71 percent of patients with an abscess. Appropriate drainage and parenteral antimicrobial therapy affected complete recovery in 89 percent of these patients.[106]

Uncommon Manifestations of Infection. Meningitis due to group B streptococci has been reported in 33 adults, most of whom have had the previously mentioned underlying predisposing conditions.[5,47,48,93,107] With appropriate treatment, most adults have survived the infection, although sequelae such as deafness have been reported.[107] Group B streptococci, alone or as a component of mixed infection, have been isolated from a diabetic with peripheral vascular disease and necrotizing fasciitis of the leg[108] and as a complication of an episiotomy in a normal host.[109] Extensive surgical débridement, volume resuscitation, and antibiotics resulted in the survival of both patients. Other unusual infections include endophthalmitis,[110] a breast abscess in a nonlactating woman,[111] and an epiglottic abscess.[112]

DIAGNOSIS

Isolation of group B *Streptococcus* from blood, CSF, and/or a site of focal suppuration is the only means by which the diagnosis of invasive infection can be documented definitively. Recovery of the organism from mucous membrane sites is of no diagnostic significance. The importance of rapidly establishing a diagnosis for neonates and of documenting infection if antimicrobial therapy has been initiated before culture has led to the development of several antigen detection methods that permit a presumptive diagnosis. Each of the methods reported to date—countercurrent immunoelectrophoresis (CIE), latex particle agglutination (LPA), staphylococcal coagglutination, and enzyme immunoassay—uses hyperimmune group B specific antisera to detect group B streptococcal antigen in various body fluids. Previously, a major limitation of these methods has been their lack of commercial availability. However, LPA reagents prepared for the testing of body fluids, such as Wellcogen Strep B (Wellcome Laboratories) and Directigen (Hynson, Westcott and Dunning, Division of Becton Dickinson & Co), have been shown to have sensitivity comparable to that of methods employing laboratory-prepared hyperimmune antisera.[113,114] Antigen was detected in 91 percent of CSF and/or concentrated urine specimens obtained at the time of admission from infants with group B streptococcal bacteremia or meningitis. A minor limitation of these reagents is the uncommon (approximately 5 percent) occurrence of false-positive reactions.

Several laboratory tests have been reported in which positive results might suggest the diagnosis of group B streptococcal infection, although they are not definitive. These nonspecific diagnostic methods include the presence of gram-positive cocci in gastric or tracheal aspirates in neonates with respiratory distress and abnormalities in neutrophil count.[79]

Intrapartum detection of pregnant women colonized with group B *Streptococcus* would allow accurate identification of high-risk patients who might benefit from early or empirical treatment. This approach, favored by many obstetricians, mandates the availability of rapid, sensitive, and specific methods to detect genital colonization. Two recent reports compared results of conventional cultures with Gram stains of vaginal or cervical swabs from high-risk pregnant women, and found good sensitivity (≥90 percent) but only moderate specificity (approximately 67 percent).[115,116] A nitrous acid extraction method that requires approximately 6 hours for processing of vaginal swabs detected 40 percent of colonized patients, but this included 86 percent of those higher-risk patients with heavy colonization.[117] Employing a similar technique, Howe et al.[118] reported a sensitivity of 100 percent and specificity of 92 percent among parturients with known risk factors for the development of invasive group B streptococcal infection in the neonates.

TREATMENT

The antimicrobial regimens recommended for treatment of group B streptococcal infections in infants and adults are shown in Table 4. Group B streptococci are uniformly susceptible to penicillins in vitro, and penicillin G is the drug of choice when the diagnosis is established. These organisms also are susceptible in vitro to ampicillin, vancomycin, and first- and second-generation cephalosporins, excluding cefoxitin. Of the third-generation cephalosporins, ceftriaxone is the most active.[119,120] The new β-lactam antibiotic imipenem also has good in vitro and in vivo activity.[121] Ciprofloxacin has moderate in vitro activity but has not been evaluated for efficacy.[122] The initial use of ampicillin and an aminoglycoside for suspected neonatal bacteremia or meningitis due to group B *Streptococcus* is based on documentation of in vitro and in vivo synergistic killing of the organism[123,124] and on the need for broad antimicrobial coverage until the diagnosis is established with certainty. After the laboratory diagnosis is established and the clinical response is documented, treatment can be completed with penicillin G alone.

The rationale for the high doses of penicillin G recommended for the treatment of group B streptococcal disease is twofold: (*1*) the minimal inhibitory concentration (MIC) of penicillin G for group B streptococci is 4- to 10-fold greater (range, 0.01–0.4 μg/ml) than that for group A streptococcal strains,[4,37,125] and (*2*) the initial inoculum in the CSF of some infants may be 10^7–10^8 organisms per milliliter.[126] Since inoculum size greatly influences the in vitro susceptibility to penicillin G,[126] these high doses may be required to provide bactericidal activity in vivo. For example, if one performs in vitro testing of penicillin G with a 10^7 or 10^8 inoculum, rather than the standard 10^4–10^5 inoculum of group B streptococci per milliliter, the MIC increases to greater than 128 μg/ml.[126]

Parenteral therapy of 10 days' duration is recommended for the treatment of bacteremia, pneumonia, pyelonephritis, and soft tissue infections, while a 14-day minimum duration is recommended for the treatment of meningitis and a 4-week minimum for the treatment of endocarditis or ventriculitis. Relapses of infection have been reported in association with both inadequate dosage or duration of therapy.[88] Recurrent group B streptococcal infection in which penicillin-tolerant strains were detected at the time of the second infection has been reported.[127,128] The role of penicillin tolerance contributing to incomplete resolution of infection remains ill defined, and more data will be required to resolve the debate concerning the therapeutic implications, if any, in patients with infections due to tolerant strains. High-dose penicillin therapy does not reliably eliminate mucous membrane infection with group B streptococci, a source that may explain recurrences. Treatment with rifampin orally *after* completion of penicillin therapy has been shown in noncontrolled studies to successfully eliminate infection at these sites.[129]

PREVENTION

Two basic approaches, chemoprophylaxis and immunoprophylaxis, have been suggested as means by which prevention of group B streptococcal infections might be accomplished. Recently, new insights into the potential feasibility of both approaches have been achieved. Chemoprophylaxis theoretically could be directed toward women during pregnancy, parturients at the time of delivery, or neonates at birth. As already discussed (see "Epidemiology and Transmission" in this chapter), one problem in achieving prevention of neonatal infection by interruption of vertical transmission at delivery (eradication of maternal genital carriage) is the limited accuracy of a single culture obtained during pregnancy to accurately predict the status of maternal colonization at the time of delivery.[49] In addition, failure to eradicate colonization immediately after oral antimicrobial therapy is noted in 20–30 percent of patients[130,131] and by the time of delivery, this rate increases to nearly 70 percent.[130] In contrast, successful interruption of vertical transmission of colonization has been achieved by the administration of intravenous ampicillin during labor.[132] The efficacy of intrapartum administration of ampicillin in high-risk parturients for the prevention of neonatal sepsis and postpartum febrile morbidity has recently been demonstrated by Boyer and Gotoff[133] in a prospective, randomized study. Screening for detection of genital colonization was performed early in the third trimester, and colonized women who subsequently presented in premature labor or with prolonged rupture of membranes >12 hours received intravenous ampicillin during labor or served as untreated controls. Early-onset disease was not documented among infants whose mothers received ampicillin, while 5 of 79 (6.3 percent) infants born to untreated women had early-onset disease ($p < .02$). Difficulties in implementation of this approach to prevention include the problem of accurately identifying carrier women, the theoretic need to treat large numbers of women to prevent a single neonatal infection, and the potential for adverse reactions to penicillin among recipients. When refined and marketed commercially, rapid diagnostic tests that permit the accurate determination of colonization status *at hospital admission* will promote a targeted selection for the administration of intrapartum prophylaxis. Currently, three special circumstances warrant the administration of intravenous ampicillin to women in labor or to infants at birth (Table 5). The first is the unusual situation (approximately 3–5 percent of patients) in which a woman known to have genital colonization with group B streptococci *also* has two or more factors enhancing the risk for neonatal infection. The second is the woman who has previously delivered an infant who developed invasive group B streptococcal disease. In this circumstance, it is our practice to obtain a total of three rectal *and* lower vaginal cultures from 26 to 34 weeks' gestation. If *any* culture reveals colonization with group B streptococci *or* if any risk factor enhancing neonatal risk for infection is observed, ampicillin is administered intravenously at onset of labor or at the rupture of membranes. Treatment vs. observation of the infant must be individualized. The third situation in which empirical therapy

TABLE 4. Treatment of Group B Streptococcal Infections

	Antibiotic (iv Dose)			
Diagnosis	*Neonate & Infant*	*Adult*	*Alternative Dose for Penicillin-Allergic Adults*	*Duration*
Bacteremia, soft tissue infections	Ampicillin (150–200 mg/kg/day) plus an aminoglycoside initially, then penicillin G (200,000 units/kg/day)	Penicillin G (10 million units/day)	Vancomycin	10 days
Meningitis	Ampicillin (300–400 mg/kg/day) plus gentamicin initially, then penicillin G (500,000 units/kg/day)	Penicillin G (20–30 million units/day)	Chloramphenicol or vancomycin	14 days (minimum)
Osteomyelitis	Penicillin G (200,000 units/kg/day)	Penicillin G (10–20 million units/day)	Vancomycin	3–4 wk
Endocarditis (see Chapter 61)	Penicillin G (400,000 units/kg/day)	Penicillin G (20–30 million units/day) with or without an aminoglycoside	Vancomycin with or without an aminoglycoside	4 wk

TABLE 5. Special Circumstances for Chemoprophylaxis to Prevent Infant Group B Streptococcal Disease

Target	*Indication*	*Approach*
Neonates	Asymptomatic twin of infant with GBS sepsis	Evaluation for sepsis and empirical antibiotic therapy
Mother, intrapartum	Previous delivery of infant with GBS systemic infection	Ampicillin[a] iv until delivery; consider empirical infant therapy
GBS-positive women, intrapartum	Two or more maternal risk factors[b]	Ampicillin[a,c] iv until delivery

Abbreviation: GBS: group B streptococcal.
[a] Initially 2 g, then 1 q4h.
[b] Preterm delivery, premature rupture of membranes, chorioamnionitis, rupture of membranes >12 hours, multiple birth, intrapartum temperature ≥100.6°F.
[c] Or suitable alternative to provide broader coverage if chorioamnionitis is suspected.

should be considered is that of a twin of an infant with invasive infection, in which case the risk to the apparently unaffected twin is enhanced 35-fold.[61,62]

The greatest problem associated with attempting to prevent group B streptococcal disease in neonates by the administration of penicillin at birth is that neonates often are born with established infection. In one prospective nonrandomized study, the incidence of early-onset neonatal infection was significantly lower in patients who received a single intramuscular dose of penicillin G than in those patients who received tetracycline ophthalmic ointment at birth for prophylaxis against gonococcal ophthalmitis.[134] However, the patient population was unusual in this study in that infants with group B streptococcal sepsis were usually asymptomatic at birth. Other investigators have reported that nearly one-half of infants with early-onset group B streptococcal disease are symptomatic either at or within 6 hours of birth.[135–137] In addition, no blood cultures were obtained before penicillin administration, thus making impossible the accurate detection of infection in babies developing symptoms. The efficacy of chemoprophylaxis at birth has been evaluated in premature neonates by Pyati et al.[138] These investigators obtained blood cultures from all infants before administering intramuscular ampicillin within 1 hour of birth. No difference was detected between treated and control infants in the incidence of disease or in the mortality rate. Thus, among neonates with the highest risk for invasive early-onset disease (those weighing <2000 g at birth) and for fatal outcome, penicillin prophylaxis was ineffective in preventing bacteremia or in altering the clinical course of infection.

Since the risk for the development of invasive group B streptococcal disease in neonates correlates significantly with the presence of low levels of maternal antibody to the type-specific antigens of these organisms,[53] immunoprophylactic methods for preventing these infections have been proposed. Purified capsular polysaccharide antigens from group B streptococci have been shown to elicit significant increases in antibody levels in most nonimmune adult volunteers.[139–141] When adults with moderate levels of type-specific antibody are immunized, the rate of antibody response approaches 100 percent. Thus, administration of a polyvalent group B streptococcal polysaccharide vaccine to women during the latter one-third of pregnancy theoretically could provide antibody in levels of sufficient quantity to passively prevent the development of invasive infection in neonates. Confirming the feasibility of this approach, a study in which women were immunized during the last trimester of pregnancy with type III polysaccharide vaccine has documented the immunogenicity of vaccine in pregnancy and shown efficient placental transfer of functionally active IgG antibodies to the neonate.[142] In addition to preventing the development of early-onset disease, this approach to prevention, in contrast to chemoprophylaxis, offers a means that might achieve the prevention of late-onset infection. Although the immunogenicity of group B streptococcal polysaccharides has not been tested among the groups of immunocompromised adults at risk for developing these infections, vaccinating these high-risk patients could potentially reduce their susceptibility to developing invasive infection.

Since levels of maternal immunoglobulin G acquired placentally by the fetus increase proportionately during the last trimester of pregnancy, neonates born at less than 33–34 weeks of gestation are likely to be excluded from the protection that may be afforded by maternal immunization. In these infants, passive immunization with immunoglobulins has been suggested as a means by which group B streptococcal infection could be prevented or—if already established—ameliorated. The commercial availability of immunoglobulin preparations modified for iv use provides a potential means by which this mode of prevention can be assessed. Preliminary investigations indicate that the level of specific antibody to group B streptococcal antigens present in currently available preparations is too low to achieve theoretically "protective" levels of antibody in the neonate unless patients are volume overloaded.[143] However, initial studies have documented the safety of these preparations for neonates,[144,145] and in vitro and animal model experiments suggest that preparations hyperimmune for type-specific group B streptococcal antibodies may be more optimal as therapeutic agents.[143] In all probability, studies designed to test the efficacy of passively administered specific antibody to women in labor or to high-risk neonates at birth will have to await the development of these hyperimmune preparations.

REFERENCES

1. Fry RM. Fatal infections by haemolytic streptococcus group B. Lancet. 1938;1:199–201.
2. Lancefield RC, Hare R. The serological differentiation of pathogenic and nonpathogenic strains of hemolytic streptococci from parturient women. J Exp Med. 1935;61:335–49.
3. Hood M, Janney A, Dameron G. Beta hemolytic streptococcus group B associated with problems of perinatal period. Am J Obstet Gynecol. 1961;82:809–18.
4. Eickhoff TC, Klein JO, Daly AL, et al. Neonatal sepsis and other infections due to group B beta-hemolytic streptococci. N Engl J Med. 1964;271:1221–8.
5. Butter MNW, DeMoor CE. *Streptococcus agalactiae* as a cause of meningitis in the newborn, and of bacteremia in adults. Antonie van Leeuwenhoek. 1967;33:439–50.
6. Dillon HC Jr, Khare S, Gray BM. Group B streptococcal carriage and disease: A 6-year prospective study. J Pediatr. 1987;110:31–6.
7. Lancefield RC. A serological differentiation of human and other groups of hemolytic streptococci. J Exp Med. 1933;57:571–95.
8. Baker CJ, Clark DJ, Barrett FF. Selective broth medium for isolation of group B streptococci. Appl Microbiol. 1973;26:884–5.
9. Slifkin M, Pouchet-Melvin GR. Evaluation of three commercially available test products for serogrouping beta-hemolytic streptococci. Infect Immun. 1983;11:249–55.
10. Facklam RR, Padula JR, Thacker LG, et al. Presumptive identification of group A, B, and D streptococci. Appl Microbiol. 1974;27:107–13.
11. Ratner HB, Weeks LS, Stratton CW. Evaluation of Spot-CAMP test for identification of group B streptococci. J Clin Microbiol. 1986;24:296–7.
12. Facklam RR, Padula JR, Wortham EC, et al. Presumptive identification of group A, B and D streptococci on agar plate medium. J Clin Microbiol. 1979;9:665–72.
13. Lancefield RC. A serological differentiation of specific types of bovine hemolytic streptococci (group B). J Exp Med. 1934;59:441–58.
14. Wilkinson HW, Eagon RG. Type-specific antigens of group B type Ic streptococci. Infect Immun. 1971;4:596–604.
15. Henrichsen J, Ferrieri P, Jelinkova J, et al. Nomenclature of antigens of group B streptococci. Int J Syst Bacteriol. 1984;34:500.
16. Perch B, Kjems E, Henrichsen J. New serotypes of group B streptococci isolated from human sources. J Clin Microbiol. 1979;10:109–10.
17. Lancefield RC, McCarty M, Everly WN. Multiple mouse-protective antibodies directed against group B streptococci. Special reference to antibodies effective against protein antigens. J Exp Med. 1975;142:165–79.
18. Baltimore RS, Kasper DL, Vecchitto JS. Mouse protection test for type III strains of group B *Streptococcus*. J Infect Dis. 1979;140:81–8.
19. Gordon JS, Sbarra AJ. Incidence, technique of isolation, and treatment of group B streptococci. Am J Obstet Gynecol. 1976;126:1023–6.
20. Anthony BF, Eisenstadt R, Carter J, et al. Genital and intestinal carriage of group B streptococci during pregnancy. J Infect Dis. 1981;143:761–6.
21. Persson K, Bjerre B, Elfstrom L, et al. A longitudinal study of group B streptococcal carriage during late pregnancy. Scand J Infect Dis. 1987;19:325–9.

22. Baker CJ, Goroff DK, Alpert S, et al. Vaginal colonization with group B *Streptococcus*: A study in college women. J Infect Dis. 1977;135:392–7.
23. Boyer KM, Gadzala CA, Kelly PD, et al. Selective intrapartum chemoprophylaxis of neonatal group B streptococcal early-onset disease. II. Predictive value of prenatal cultures. J Infect Dis. 1983;148:802–9.
24. Anthony BF, Okada DM, Hobel CJ. Epidemiology of group B *Streptococcus*: Longitudinal observations during pregnancy. J Infect Dis. 1978;137:524–30.
25. Yow MD, Leeds LJ, Thompson PK, et al. The natural history of group B streptococcal colonization in the pregnant woman and her offspring. I. Colonization studies. Am J Obstet Gynecol. 1980;137:34–8.
26. Lewin EB, Amstey MS. Natural history of group B streptococcus colonization and its therapy during pregnancy. Am J Obstet Gynecol. 1981;139:512–5.
27. Dillon HC, Gray E, Pass MA, et al. Anorectal and vaginal carriage of group B streptococci during pregnancy. J Infect Dis. 1982;145:794–9.
28. Anthony BF, Carter JA, Eisenstadt R, et al. Isolation of group B streptococci from the proximal small intestine of adults. J Infect Dis. 1983;147:776.
29. Baker CJ, Barrett FF. Transmission of group B streptococci among parturient women and their neonates. J Pediatr. 1973;83:919–25.
30. Ferrieri P, Cleary PP, Seeds AE. Epidemiology of group B streptococcal carriage in pregnant women and newborn infants. J Med Microbiol. 1976;10:103–14.
31. Pass MA, Gray BM, Khare S, et al. Prospective studies of group B streptococcal infections in infants. J Pediatr. 1979;95:437–43.
32. Ancona RJ, Ferrieri P, Williams PP. Maternal factors that enhance the acquisition of group B streptococci by newborn infants. J Med Microbiol. 1980;13:273–80.
33. Paredes A, Wong P, Mason EO Jr, et al. Nosocomial transmission of group B streptococci in a newborn nursery. Pediatrics. 1976;59:679–82.
34. Steere AC, Aber RC, Warford LR, et al. Possible nosocomial transmission of group B streptococci in a newborn nursery. J Pediatr. 1975;87:784–7.
35. Noya FJD, Rench MA, Metzger TG, et al. Unusual occurrence of an epidemic of type Ib/c group B streptococcal sepsis in a neonatal intensive care unit. J Infect Dis. 1987;155:1135–44.
36. Gardner SE, Mason EO Jr, Yow MD. Community acquisition of group B *Streptococcus* by infants of colonized mothers. Pediatrics. 1980;66:873–5.
37. Baker CJ. Group B streptococcal infections. Adv Intern Med. 1980;25:475–501.
38. Boyer KM, Gadzala CA, Burd LI, et al. Selective intrapartum chemoprophylaxis of neonatal group B streptococcal early-onset disease. I. Epidemiologic rationale. J Infect Dis. 1983;148:795–801.
39. Pyati SP, Pildes RS, Jacobs NM, et al. Penicillin in infants weighing two kilograms or less with early-onset group B streptococcal disease. N Engl J Med. 1983;308:1383–9.
40. Cochi SL, Feldman RA. Estimating national incidence of group B streptococcal disease: The effect of adjusting for birth weight. Pediatr Infect Dis. 1983;2:414–5.
41. Faro S. Group B beta-hemolytic streptococci and puerperal infections. Am J Obstet Gynecol. 1981;139:686–9.
42. Gibbs RS, Blanco JD. Streptococcal infections in pregnancy: A study of 48 bacteremias. Am J Obstet Gynecol. 1981;140:405–11.
43. Institute of Medicine, National Academy of Sciences. Appendix P: New vaccine development: Establishing priorities. In: Diseases of Importance in the United States. v. 1. Washington DC: National Academy Press; 1985:242–439.
44. Pass MA, Gray BM, Dillon HC Jr. Puerperal and perinatal infections with group B streptococci. Am J Obstet Gynecol. 1982;243:147–52.
45. Polsky B, Gold JWM, Whimbey E, et al. Bacterial pneumonia in patients with the acquired immunodeficiency syndrome. Ann Intern Med. 1986;104:38–41.
46. Baker CJ, Barrett FF. Group B streptococcal infection in infants: The importance of the various serotypes. JAMA. 1974;230:1158–60.
47. Wilkinson HW. Group B streptococcal infection in humans. Annu Rev. Microbiol. 1978;32:41.
48. Lerner PI, Gopalakrishna KV, Wolinsky E, et al. Group B *Streptococcus* (*S. agalactiae*) bacteremia in adults: Analysis of 32 cases and review of the literature. Medicine (Baltimore). 1977;56:457–73.
49. Anthony BF, Ikada DM. The emergence of group B streptococci in infections of the newborn infant. Annu Rev Med. 1977;28:355–69.
50. Baker CJ. Summary of the workshop on perinatal infections due to group B *Streptococcus*. J Infect Dis. 1977;136:137–52.
51. Evaldson GR, Malmborg A-S, Nord CE. Premature rupture of the membranes and ascending infection. Br J Obstet Gynecol. 1982;89:793–801.
52. Moller M, Thomsen AC, Borch K, et al. Rupture of fetal membranes and premature delivery associated with group B streptococci in urine of pregnant women. Lancet. 1984;2:69–70.
53. Baker CJ, Kasper DL. Correlation of maternal antibody deficiency with susceptibility to neonatal group B streptococcal infection. N Engl J Med. 1976;294:753–6.
54. Hemming VG, Hall RR, Rhodes PG, et al. Assessment of group B streptococcal opsonins in human and rabbit serum by neutrophil chemiluminescence. J Clin Invest. 1976;58:1379–87.
55. Stewardson-Krieger PB, Albrandt K, Nevin T, et al. Perinatal immunity to group B β-hemolytic *Streptococcus* type Ia. J Infect Dis. 1977;136:649–54.
56. Baker CJ, Edwards MS, Kasper DL. Role of antibody to native type III polysaccharide of group B *Streptococcus* in infant infection. Pediatrics. 1981;68:544–9.
57. Boyer KM, Papierniak CK, Gadzala CA, et al. Transplacental passage of antibody to group B streptococcus serotype Ia. J Pediatr. 1984;104:618–20.
58. Gotoff SP, Papierniak CK, Klegerman ME, et al. Quantitation of IgG antibody to the type-specific polysaccharide of group B streptococcus type Ib in pregnant women and infected infants. J Pediatr. 1984;105:628–30.
59. Gray BM, Pritchard DG, Dillon HC Jr. Seroepidemiological studies of group B *Streptococcus* type II. J Infect Dis. 1985;151:1073–80.
60. Anthony BF, Concepcion NF, Concepcion KF. Human antibody to the group-specific polysaccharide of group B *Streptococcus*. J Infect Dis. 1985;151:221–6.
61. Pass MA, Khare S, Dillon HC. Twin pregnancies: Incidence of group B streptococcal colonization and disease. J Pediatr. 1980;97:635–7.
62. Edwards MS, Jackson CV, Baker CJ. Increased risk of group B streptococcal disease in twins. JAMA. 1981;245:2044–6.
63. Shigeoka AO, Hall RT, Hemming VG, et al. Role of antibody and complement in opsonization of group B streptococci. Infect Immun. 1978;21:34–40.
64. Baker CJ, Webb BJ, Kasper DL, et al. The role of complement and antibody in opsonophagocytosis of type II group B streptococci. J Infect Dis. 1986;154:47–54.
65. Payne NR, Kim Y, Ferrieri P. Effect of differences in antibody and complement requirements on phagocytic uptake and intracellular killing of "c" protein-positive and -negative strains of type II group B streptococci. Infect Immun. 1987;55:1243–51.
66. Baker CJ, Edwards MS, Webb BJ, et al. Antibody-independent classical pathway-mediated opsonophagocytosis of type Ia, group B *Streptococcus*. J Clin Invest. 1982;63:394–404.
67. Levy NJ, Kasper DL. Surface-bound capsular polysaccharide of type Ia group B *Streptococcus* mediates C1 binding and activation of the classic complement pathway. J Immunol. 1986;136:4157–62.
68. Edwards MS, Buffone GJ, Fuselier PA, et al. Deficient classical complement activity in newborn sera. Pediatr Res. 1983;17:685–8.
69. Christensen RD, Hill HR, Rothstein G. Granulocytic stem cell (CFUc) proliferation in experimental group B streptococcal sepsis. Pediatr Res. 1983;17:278–80.
70. Zeligs BA, Armstrong CD, Walser JB, et al. Age-dependent susceptibility of neonatal rats to group B streptococcal type III infection: Correlation of severity of infection and response of myeloid pools. Infect Immun. 1982;37:255–63.
71. Durham DL, Straus DC. Extracellular products of type III *Streptococcus agalactiae* and their relationship to virulence. Curr Microbiol. 1983;8:89–94.
72. Yeung MK, Mattingly SJ. Biosynthetic capacity for type-specific antigen synthesis determines the virulence of serotype III strains of group B streptococci. Infect Immun. 1984;44:217–21.
73. Shigeoka AO, Rote NS, Santos JI, et al. Assessment of the virulence factors of group B streptococci. Correlation with sialic acid content. J Infect Dis. 1983;147:857–63.
74. Rubens CE, Wessels MR, Heggen LM, et al. Transposon mutagenesis of group B streptococcal type III capsular polysaccharide: Correlation of capsule expression with virulence. Proc Natl Acad Sci USA. 1987;84:7208–12.
75. Kasper DL, Baker CJ, Edwards MS, et al. The type III group B streptococcal capsular polysaccharide: Structure, immunospecificity, immunogenicity, and relationship to virulence. In: Weinstein L, Fields BN, eds. Seminars in Infectious Disease. v. 4. Bacterial Vaccines. New York: Thieme-Stratton; 1982:275–8.
76. Franciosi RA, Knostman JD, Zimmerman RA. Group B streptococcal neonatal and infant infections. J Pediatr. 1973;82:707–18.
77. Baker CJ, Barrett FF, Gordon RC, et al. Suppurative meningitis due to streptococci of Lancefield group B: A study of 33 infants. J Pediatr. 1973;82:724–9.
78. Chin KC, Fitzhardinge PM. Sequelae of early-onset group B streptococcal neonatal meningitis. J Pediatr. 1985;106:819–22.
79. Baker CJ. Group B streptococcal infections in neonates. Pediatr Rev. 1979;1:5–15.
80. Katzenstein A, Davis C, Braude A. Pulmonary changes in neonatal sepsis due to group B β-hemolytic streptococcus: Relation to hyaline membrane disease. J Infect Dis. 1976;133:430–5.
81. Baker CJ. Unpublished observations.
82. Gilbert GL, Garland SM. Perinatal group B streptococcal infections. Med J Aust. 1983;1:566–71.
83. Pyati SP, Pildes RS, Ramamurthy RS, et al. Decreasing mortality in neonates with early-onset group B streptococcal infection: Reality or artifact. J Pediatr. 1981;98:625–8.
84. Ferrieri P. GBS infections in the newborn infant: Diagnosis and treatment. Antibiot Chemother. 1985;35:211–24.
85. Edwards MS, Rench MA, Haffar AAM, et al. Long-term sequelae of group B streptococcal meningitis in infants. J Pediatr. 1985;106:717–22.
86. Wald ER, Bergman I, Taylor HG, et al. Long-term outcome of group B streptococcal meningitis. Pediatrics. 1986;77:217–21.
87. Baker CJ. Group B streptococcal cellulitis/adenitis in infants. Am J Dis Child. 1982;136:631–3.
88. Baker CJ, Edwards MS. Group B streptococcal infections. In: Remington JS, Klein JO, eds. Infectious Disease of the Fetus and Newborn Infant. 2nd ed. Philadelphia: WB Saunders; 1983:820–81.

89. Edwards MS, Baker CJ, Wagner ML, et al. An etiologic shift in infantile osteomyelitis: The emergence of the group B streptococcus. J Pediatr. 1978;93:578–83.
90. Opal SM, Cross A, Palmo M, et al. Group B streptococcal sepsis in adults and infants. Contrasts and comparisons. Arch Intern Med. 1988;148:641–5.
91. Gallagher PG, Watanakunakorn C. Group B streptococcal bacteremia in a community teaching hospital. Am J Med. 1985;78:795–800.
92. Verghese A, Mireault K, Arbeit RD. Group B streptococcal bacteremia in men. Rev Infect Dis. 1986;8:912–7.
93. Bayer AS, Chow AW, Anthony BF, et al. Serious infections in adults due to group B streptococci. Am J Med. 1976;61:498–503.
94. Roberts FJ. Group A and group B β-hemolytic streptococcal bacteremia. Rev Infect Dis. 1988;10:228–9.
95. Ledger WJ, Norman J, Gee C, et al. Bacteremia on an obstetric-gynecologic service. Am J Obstet Gynecol. 1975;121:205–12.
96. Rosene K, Eschenbach DA, Tompkins LS, et al. Polymicrobial early postpartum endometritis with facultative and anaerobic bacteria, genital mycoplasmas, and *Chlamydia trachomatis*: Treatment with piperacillin or cefoxitin. J Infect Dis. 1986;153:1028–37.
97. Minkoff HL, Sierra MF, Pringle GF, et al. Vaginal colonization with group B beta-hemolytic streptococcus as a risk fact of for post-cesarean section febrile morbidity. Am J Obstet Gynecol. 1982;142:992–5.
98. Duff P. Pathophysiology and management of postcesarean endomyometritis. Obstet Gynecol. 1986;67:269–76.
99. Verghese A, Berk SL, Boelen LJ, et al. Group B streptococcal pneumonia in the elderly. Arch Intern Med. 1982;142:1642–5.
100. George AL Jr, Savage AM. Fatal group B streptococcal empyema in an adult. South Med J. 1987;80:1436–8.
101. Gallagher PG, Watanakunakorn C. Group B streptococcal endocarditis: Report of seven cases and review of the literature, 1962–1985. Rev Infect Dis. 1986;8:175–88.
102. Backes RJ, Wilson WR, Geraci JE. Group B streptococcal infective endocarditis. Arch Intern Med. 1985;145:693–6.
103. Duma RJ, Weinberg AN, Merdrek RF, et al. Streptococcal infections. A bacteriologic and clinical study of streptococcal bacteremia. Medicine (Baltimore). 1969;48:87–127.
104. Small CB, Slater LN, Lowy FD, et al. Group B streptococcal arthritis in adults. Am J Med. 1984;76:367–75.
105. Pischel KD, Weisman MH, Cone RO. Unique features of group B streptococcal arthritis in adults. Arch Intern Med. 1985;145:97–102.
106. McCarty JM, Haber J. Group B streptococcal soft tissue infections beyond the neonatal period. West J Med. 1987;147:558–60.
107. Harburg TD, Leonard HA, Kimbrough RC III, et al. Group B streptococcal meningitis appearing as acute deafness in an adult. Arch Neurol. 1984;41:214–6.
108. Riefler J III, Molavi A, Schwartz D, et al. Necrotizing fasciitis in adults due to group B *Streptococcus*. Arch Intern Med. 1988;148:727–9.
109. Sutton GP, Smirz LR, Clark DH, et al. Group B streptococcal necrotizing fasciitis arising from an episiotomy. Obstet Gynecol. 1985;66:733–6.
110. Farber BP, Weinbaum DL, Dummer JS. Metastatic bacterial endophthalmitis. Arch Intern Med. 1985;145:62–4.
111. Weiss RL, Matsen JM. Group B streptococcal breast abscess. Arch Pathol Lab Med. 1987;111:74–5.
112. Ridgeway NA, Perlman PE, Verghese A. Epiglottic abscess due to group B *Streptococcus*. Ann Otol Rhinol Laryngol 1984;93:277–8.
113. Baker CJ, Rench MA. Commercial latex agglutination for detection of group B streptococcal antigen in body fluids. J Pediatr. 1983;102:393–5.
114. Rench MA, Metzger TG, Baker CJ. Detection of group B streptococcal antigen in body fluids by a latex-coupled monoclonal antibody assay. J Clin Microbiol. 1984;20:852–4.
115. Feld SM, Harrigan JT. Vaginal gram stain as an immediate detector of group B streptococci in selected obstetric patients. Am J Obstet Gynecol. 1987;156:446–8.
116. Holls WM, Thomas J, Troyer V. Cervical gram stain for rapid detection of colonization with β-*Streptococcus*. Obstet Gynecol. 1987;69:354–7.
117. Wald ER, Dashefsky B, Green M, et al. Rapid detection of group B streptococci directly from vaginal swabs. J Clin Microbiol. 1987;25:573–4.
118. Howe RS, Voychehovski TH, Uraizee F, et al. Neonatal group B streptococcal disease. N Engl J Med. 1987;316:1163.
119. Persson KM-S, Forsgren A. Antimicrobial susceptibility of group B streptococci. Eur J Clin Microbiol. 1986;5:165–7.
120. Kim KS. Antimicrobial susceptibility of GBS. Antibiot Chemother. 1985;35:83–9.
121. Kropp H, Gerckens L, Sundelof JG. Antibacterial activity of imipenem: The first thienamycin antibiotic. Rev Infect Dis. 1985;7(Suppl):389–410.
122. Rolston KVI. Susceptibility of group B and group G streptococci to newer antimicrobial agents. Eur J Clin Microbiol. 1986;5:534–6.
123. Schauf V, Deveikis A, Riff L, et al. Antibiotic-killing kinetics of group B streptococci. J Pediatr. 1976;89:194–8.
124. Deveikis A, Schauf V, Mizen M, et al. Antimicrobial therapy of experimental group B streptococcal infection in mice. Antimicrob Agents Chemother. 1977;11:817–20.
125. Baker CN, Thornsberry C, Facklam RR. Synergism killing kinetics, and antimicrobial susceptibility of group A and B streptococci. Antimicrob Agents Chemother. 1981;19:716–25.
126. Feldman WE. Concentrations of bacteria in cerebrospinal fluid of patients with bacterial meningitis. J Pediatr. 1976;88:549–52.
127. Siegel JD, Shannon KM, De Passe BM. Recurrent infection associated with penicillin-tolerant group B streptococci: A report of two cases. J Pediatr. 1981;99:920–3.
128. Broughton DD, Mitchell WG, Grossman M, et al. Recurrence of group B streptococcal infection. J Pediatr. 1976;89:183–4.
129. Millard DD, Bussey ME, Shulman ST, et al. Multiple group B streptococcal infections in a premature infant: Eradication of nasal colonization with rifampin. Am J Dis Child. 1985;139:964–5.
130. Gardner SE, Yow MD, Leeds LJ, et al. Failure of penicillin to eradicate group B streptococcal colonization in the pregnant woman. Am J Obstet Gynecol. 1979;135:1062–5.
131. Hall RT, Barnes W, Krishnan L, et al. Antibiotic treatment of parturient women colonized with group B streptococci. Am J Obstet Gynecol. 1976;124:630–4.
132. Yow MD, Mason EO, Leeds LJ, et al. Ampicillin prevents intrapartum transmission of group B *Streptococcus*. JAMA. 1979;241:1245–7.
133. Boyer KM, Gotoff SP. Prevention of early-onset neonatal group B streptococcal disease with selective intrapartum chemoprophylaxis. N Engl J Med. 1986;314:1665–9.
134. Siegal JD, McCracken GH Jr, Threlkeld N, et al. Single dose penicillin prophylaxis against neonatal group B streptococcal infections. N Engl J Med. 1981;303:769–75.
135. Baker CJ. Early onset group B streptococcal disease. J Pediatr. 1978;93:124–5.
136. Stewardson-Krieger PB, Gotoff SP. Risk factors in early-onset neonatal group B streptococcal infections. Infection. 1978;6:50–3.
137. Gotoff SP, Boyer KM. Penicillin prophylaxis against neonatal streptococcal infections. N Engl J Med. 1981;304:484.
138. Pyati SP, Pildes RS, Jacobs NM, et al. Penicillin in infants weighing two kilograms or less with early-onset group B streptococcal disease. N Engl J Med. 1983;308:1383–9.
139. Baker CJ, Edwards MS, Kasper DL. Immunogenicity of polysaccharides from type III, group B *Streptococcus*. J Clin Invest. 1978;61:1107–10.
140. Eisenstein TK, DeCuenick BJ, Resavy D, et al. Quantitative determination in human sera of vaccine-induced antibody to type-specific polysaccharides of group B streptococci using an enzyme-linked immunosorbent assay. J Infect Dis. 1983;147:847–56.
141. Baker CJ, Kasper DL. Group B streptococcal vaccines. Rev Infect Dis. 1985;4:458–67.
142. Baker CJ, Rench MA, Edwards MS, et al. Immunization of pregnant women with a polysaccharide vaccine. N Engl J Med. 1988;319:1180–5.
143. Givner LB, Edwards MS, Baker CJ. A polyclonal human IgG preparation hyperimmune for type III, group B *Streptococcus*: In vitro opsonophagocytic activity and efficacy in experimental models. J Infect Dis. 1988;158:724–30.
144. Noya FJD, Rench MA, Garcia-Prats JA, et al. Disposition of an immunoglobulin intravenous preparation in very low birth weight infants. J Pediatr. 1988;112:278–83.
145. Fischer GW, Hemming VG, Hunter KW, et al. Intravenous immunoglobulin in the treatment of neonatal sepsis: Therapeutic strategies and laboratory studies. Pediatr Infect Dis. 1986;5(Suppl):171–5.

181. VIRIDANS AND β-HEMOLYTIC (NON-GROUP A, B, AND D) STREPTOCOCCI*

HARRY A. GALLIS

Streptococci other than *Streptococcus pyogenes, Streptococcus agalactiae*, and the enterococcal and nonenterococcal organisms of group D comprise a diversity of species capable of producing many clinical syndromes in humans and animals. Because Lancefield serogroups frequently cross species lines, these organisms must be distinguished definitively by a variety of antigenic, physiologic, and biochemical characteristics. The practice of separating β-hemolytic strains from the viridans group is no longer valid since many species have diverse hemolytic capabilities.[1] Since much of the clinical and microbiologic literature on these organisms describes a diversity of techniques for speciation, it is confusing or inaccurate to report infections due to "viridans streptococci," "group C strepto-

* The author has made extensive use of the excellent chapters by Richard Roberts, M.D., from the second edition of this text.

cocci," "group G streptococci," etc., in the manner one describes infections due to group A or group B streptococci. It is hoped that the reader will appreciate these difficulties in nomenclature and speciation and will interpret the primary literature by taking these factors into account.

Correlation of the viridans and additional β-hemolytic streptococcal species with serogroup, normal habitat, and clinical manifestations is outlined in Table 1. This chapter and the following chapter on the "*Streptococcus intermedius* group" will emphasize the organisms associated with human disease.

VIRIDANS STREPTOCOCCI

The viridans streptococci possess the general characteristics common to all streptococci (see Chapter 175). However, because of the lack of (*1*) uniformity in cultural and biochemical characteristics, (*2*) correlation between physiologic properties and antigen composition, and (*3*) possession of cell wall carbohydrate serogroup antigens A, B, or D (which identify the pyogenic and fecal streptococci), the identification and pathogenic role of these organisms have largely been ignored except for their etiologic role in bacterial endocarditis. In 1972, on the basis of various biochemical and physiologic properties, transformation studies, cell wall analysis, and computer analysis, Colman and Williams[2] identified five species of viridans streptococci that they termed the human oral viridans streptococci (Table 2). In 1977, Facklam recognized 10 physiologic species.[3] Unfortunately the nomenclature and species identification was not identical to that of Colman and Williams, and these differences continue to cause confusion in the terminology of viridans streptococci. The relationship between the two classifications is shown in Table 2. Because most speciation in the United States is based on Facklam's criteria, this text will follow the most recent modification by Facklam.[4] *Streptococcus intermedius* and its closely related species (*S. anginosus, S. constellatus*, and *S. milleri*) will be discussed in Chapter 182. Two species, *S. uberis* and *S. acidominimus*, will not be discussed in detail due to their rarity as human pathogens.

Clinical Microbiology

The viridans streptococci are nutritionally fastidious bacteria that grow best in complex media and may require a carbon dioxide environment for optimal growth. They produce small colonies on agar with a narrow zone of green (α) or no (γ) hemolysis. A few species such as *S. anginosus* (see Chapter 182)

TABLE 1. Viridans and Additional β-Hemolytic Streptococci

			Clinical Infections	
Species	*Serogroup*	*Normal Habitat*	*Humans*	*Animal*
Viridans (α, γ)				
S. mitis } *S. sanguis* II }	NG, A, C, F, G, H, K, M, O	Human—oropharynx, intestinal tract	Endocarditis, caries	—
S. sanguis I	NG, C, F, H, K	Human—teeth surface, intestinal tract	Endocarditis, caries	—
S. intermedius (*S. anginosus, S. constellatus, S. milleri*)	NG, A, C, F, G, K	Human—oropharynx, teeth surface, skin, intestinal tract	Endocarditis, suppurative infections, bacteremia	—
S. salivarius	NG, F, H, K	Human—oropharynx, intestinal tract	Endocarditis	—
S. mutans	NG, E, F, K	Human—teeth surface, intestinal tract	Endocarditis, caries	—
S. morbillorum	NG	Human—intestinal and urogenital tracts	Endocarditis, suppurative infections	—
S. acidominimus	NG, E, F	Bovine—milk, genital and intestinal tracts	Rare	—
S. uberis	NG, E, F, K	Bovine—milk, oropharynx, skin, intestinal tract	Rare	Mastitis
S. pneumoniae	—	Human—upper respiratory tract	Common	—
S. dysgalactiae (see *S. equisimilis*)	C, G, L	Human—upper respiratory tract, skin, vagina; bovine and sheep	—	Mastitis
S. bovis	D	Human—genital and intestinal tracts; bovine and sheep—intestinal tract	Endocarditis, bacteremia	Endocarditis
S. suis	D (R, S, T)	Swine	Rare	Bacteremia, bone and joint infections
S. lactis	N	Human—oropharynx; bovine—milk	Rare	Mastitis
S. cremoris	N	Human—oropharynx; bovine—milk	Rare	Mastitis
β-hemolytic				
Pyogenes-like				
S. equisimilis (see *S. dysgalactiae*)	C	Human—pharynx and skin; many animal species	See the text	Bacteremia
S. equi and subsp. *S. zooepidemicus*	C	Horse—upper respiratory tract; other animal species (cattle, swine)	Rare	Strangles, respiratory; mastitis
S. lentus	E, P, U	Bovine and swine	—	Cervical adenitis, pneumonia, mastitis
S. canis	G	Human and canine—pharynx, intestinal tract; many animal species	See the text	Bacteremia, adenitis, genital tract
—	L	Human, canine, and swine—pharynx	Endocarditis and cellulitis (rare)	Pneumonia, genitourinary
—	M	Human, canine—pharynx	Suppurative infectopms (rare)	—
Minute				
S. intermedius group	A, C, F, G	Human—oropharynx, skin, intestinal and genital tracts	Bacteremia, suppurative infections	—

TABLE 2. Species of Human Viridans Streptococci

Colman and Williams	Facklam	Serogroup
S. mitior	*S. mitis* *S. sanguis* II	Nongroupable,[a] F, G, H, K, M, O
S. sanguis	*S. sanguis* I	Nongroupable,[a] F, H, K
S. milleri	*S. intermedius* *S. anginosus* *S. constellatus*	Nongroupable,[a] A, C,[a] F,[a] G, K
S. salivarius	*S. salivarius*	Nongroupable,[a] F, H, K
S. mutans	*S. mutans*	Nongroupable,[a] E
	S. morbillorum	Nongroupable
	S. acidominimus	Nongroupable,[a] E, F
	S. uberis	Nongroupable,[a] E, K

[a] Most frequent groups.

and *S. mutans* may include strains that are β-hemolytic. While some of these organisms may react with group A, C, or G antisera, they are biochemically distinct from *S. pyogenes, S. equisimilis*, and the large-colony β-hemolytic group G streptococci.[5] Although the mechanism by which viridans streptococci produce α-hemolysis is unknown, the production of hydrogen peroxide (H_2O_2) may in part be related. Since unheated blood contains catalase, other factors in addition to H_2O_2 must play a role. The cell walls of viridans streptococci, like the pyogenic streptococci, possess peptidoglycan, teichoic acid, and membrane-associated lipoteichoic acid. While group carbohydrate antigens may be detected in some strains (Table 2), there is frequently no correlation between serogroups and biochemical speciation. Many clinical isolates within the same biochemical species produce no known group antigen. Likewise, Lancefield serogrouping should not be the only means of identification of atypical isolates (i.e., minute colonies and CO_2-requiring strains). Viridans streptococci do not produce extracellular exotoxins, although the production of proteolytic enzymes has recently been described (see below). The role of these extracellular products in the pathogenicity of viridans streptococci is unknown.

Species Identification

Since most biochemical speciation in the United States is performed under Centers for Disease Control (CDC) guidelines, these criteria and species designations will be used in this chapter (Table 3). The reader is referred to Table 2 to make the associations with the British scheme. Organisms in the *S. intermedius* group are displayed in tables but discussed in Chapter 182.[2–4]

After the isolation of α-, β- or nonhemolytic streptococci on blood agar, a presumptive identification of non-group A, B, or D is made by bacitracin resistance, a negative CAMP or sodium hippurate reaction, negative or weakly reactive bile esculin (or the PYR test [hydrolysis of L-pyrrolodonyl-β-naphthalamide] see Chapter 13), negative pyruvate reaction, and the absence of growth in 6.5% sodium chloride. (It should be recognized that occasional non-group A streptococci are bacitracin sensitive, and depending upon the site of isolation, i.e., nonpharyngeal, a false-positive presumptive group A assignment may be made.) A heavy saline suspension of a pure growth of the isolate should be inoculated onto the substances described. Excellent correlation has been found with several of the test strip systems that are commercially available.[6] Rapid serologic identification can be performed with slide agglutination tests,[7,8] thus eliminating cumbersome extraction procedures.

Streptococcus Mitis and S. Sanguis II. Colman and Williams designate these organisms *S. mitior*.[2] Cell wall carbohydrate antigens vary (F, G, H, K, M, and O, have been detected), but most strains are nongroupable. The cell walls do not contain rhamnose, which is found in *S. sanguis* I. *S. sanguis II* differs from *S. mitis* primarily in the production of extracellular dextran and fementation of raffinose. Many nutritionally variant streptococci (NVS) fall within the *S. mitis* biochemical species.[9,10]

Streptococcus Sanguis I. Most *S. sanguis* I strains are nongroupable; however, about 15 percent may carry group F, H, C, or K. Over 90 percent are α-hemolytic and produce a dextran polymer. A variety of extracellular enzymes are produced that have unknown pathogenetic significance.[11]

Streptococcus Salivarius. This organism may frequently carry the serogroup K antigen (F and H also dctcctcd) and is usually nonhemolytic. An extracellular levan is produced on sucrose agar.

Streptococcus Mutans. Most strains of *S. mutans* are α- or nonhemolytic, but occasional β-hemolysis is observed. Group antigens E, F, and K have been detected rarely. There are seven serogroups. These organisms frequently require CO_2 for optimal growth and almost always produce dextrans. Since *S. mutans* is frequently bile esculin-positive and occasionally reacts with group D antiserum (cell walls contain a glycerol teichoic acid), this species must be distinguised from *S. bovis*, which does not ferment sorbitol but hydrolyzes starch.

Streptococcus Morbillorum. This organism was not included in the taxonomy of Colman and Williams; however, 46 isolates were characterized by Facklam.[3] None of these strains carried group antigens, half were α-hemolytic, and half showed no reactions on blood agar. Over half of these organisms apparently caused serious infections. Biochemically, *S. morbillorum* is a weak fermenter of sucrose and is nonreactive in most fermentation tests (Table 3). It is distinguished from *S. acidominimus* by a negative sodium hippurate reaction. *S. acidominimus* and *S. uberis*, while rare human pathogens,[3] will not be discussed further in this chapter.

Nutritionally Variant Streptococci. Nutritionally variant streptococci are most commonly isolated from patients with bacterial endocarditis, perhaps accounting for a substantial number of "culture-negative" cases. They vary in their ability to grow in common blood culture media.[12] Most frequently they

TABLE 3. Schema for Biochemical Speciation of Viridans Streptococci

									Glucan		Hemolysis (%)		
Organism	Mannitol	Lactose	Inulin	Arginine	Esculin	Raffinose	40% Bile	Litmus Milk	Agar	Broth	α	γ	β
S. mutans	+	+	+	−	+	+	V	+	+	+	59	29	11
S. sanguis I	−	+	+	V	V	V	V	+	+	V	94	6	0
S. salivarius	−	+	+	−	+	+	V	+	V	−	10	90	0
S. intermedius	−	+	−	V	+	V	V	+	V	−	45	55	0
S. sanguis II	−	+	−	V	−	+	V	+	V	V	95	5	0
S. mitis	−	+	−	V	−	−	V	+	V	−	92	8	0
S. anginosus	−	−	−	V	V	−	V	+	−	−	40	60	0[a]
S. morbillorum	−	−	−	−	−	−	−	−	−	−	50	50	0

[a] Many organisms of this species may be β-hemolytic but are not presented in reviews of "viridans" streptococci.

grow marginally after primary inoculation and fail to grow on subculture onto routine blood agar. However, growth may occur as satelliting colonies around other bacteria (e.g., *Staphylococcus* species contaminating broth or agar cultures) or on media containing thiol compounds such as cysteine or the active forms of vitamin B_6 (pyridoxal or pyridoxamine but *not* pyridoxine).[13] It appears that NVS cannot assimilate pyridoxine and that pyridoxine may bind to vitamin B_6 transport systems, thus inhibiting the uptake of other B_6 analogues.[14] Most of these strains are probably similar to *S. mitis* but occasionally can be allocated to *S. salivarius, S. sanguis, S. anginosus*, or *S. morbillorum*.[15] Many of the *S. mitis* strains possess a red chromophore when boiled in 2N HCl.[16] Patients with endocarditis due to these organisms frequently have antibody to a newly described serotype I antigen found in NVS. This test could potentially be of value in the diagnosis of NVS in "culture-negative" endocarditis.[17]

Pathogenicity

It has been considered that viridans streptococci have a low infective potential and that clinical infections occur after injury to areas of normal habitat. The association of these organisms with dental caries formation and infective endocarditis, however, is well established. The cariogenic property of dextran-producing *S. mutans* has been related to its adherence to tooth enamel with multiplication and the subsequent production of lactic and acetic acids from sugar fermentation. These organic acids then participate in tooth destruction.[18] Adherence to tooth enamel may be inhibited by anti-*S. mutans* salivary IgA. The ability of various viridans streptococci (*S. mitior, S. sanguis, S. mutans*) to lodge on damaged heart valves or platelet–fibrin matrixes also correlates with dextran synthesis. Experimental studies have shown that *S. sanguis* exhibits greater surface adherence when grown in sucrose media to facilitate dextran production than when treated with dextranase.[19] Incubation of *S. sanguis* with nonbactericidal concentrations of penicillin and vancomycin also decreases the adherence of bacteria to the fibrin–platelet matrix.[20,21] Lipoteichoic acid may also mediate such adherence since depletion of lipoteichoic acid results in diminished adherence of group A streptococci to epithelial cells,[22] and inhibitors of cell wall synthesis induce the release of cell wall lipoteichoic acid from *S. sanguis*.[23] The role of various proteolytic enzymes produced by *S. sanguis* in the pathogenicity of this species is presently unknown. The propensity for *S. intermedius* to produce abscesses in major visceral organs suggests that this species possesses pathogenic factors[24] unique to the viridans streptococci (see Chapter 182).

Normal Habitat

The viridans streptococcal species outlined in Table 2 have been termed the human oral streptococci because they compose 30–60 percent of the oral bacterial flora.[2] The locations in the oropharynx where each species most commonly resides are as follows: *S. mitis* and *S. sanguis II*: dental surface and pharynx; *S. sanguis I:* dental surface; *S. salivarius:* hard palate, tongue, and pharynx and *S. mutans:* dental surface. The normal habitat of *S. morbillorum* has not been defined. Viridans streptococci have also been associated with infections of the gastrointestinal and urogenital systems which suggests that they reside on the mucus membranes of these organ systems as well (Table 1).

Clinical Manifestations

The distribution of viridans streptococcal species isolated from various human sources has been reported by two reference laboratories.[1,3] Although most commonly associated with endocarditis, viridans streptococci have also been isolated from infections of all organ systems including the central nervous, respiratory, intestinal, urogenital, and musculoskeletal systems and the skin. Different frequencies of isolation of the viridans species are apparent: *S. sanguis I* and *II*, *S. mitis*, and *S. salivarius* are isolated from all sources, but the two former species are most commonly associated with endocarditis, whereas *S. intermedius* is the species most frequently associated with extracardiac suppurative infections (see Chapter 181). *Streptococcus mutans* and *S. morbillorum* on the other hand, are less frequently isolated from clinical specimens than are the other species and when identified, are often associated with endocarditis. As shown in Table 4, similar isolation frequencies of 1391 extrarespiratory isolates have been recorded since 1976 in the diagnostic microbiology laboratory at The New York Hospital. Fewer than 2.0 percent of isolates were unclassified when employing the identification scheme outlined in Table 3, and Facklam, likewise, was unable to speciate only 40 of 1227 strains.[3]

Multiple bacteria may be isolated from purulent lesions, and the pathogenic role of the viridans species in this clinical setting is often difficult to assess. Positive blood cultures for viridans species without a known source may occur in 70–80 percent of patients and represent either transient bacteremia or contamination.[25] Clinically insignificant positive blood cultures may be polymicrobial and positive in only one of many separate cultures. Although each of the viridans species may be associated with insignificant blood cultures, a thorough evaluation for a suppurative focus should be performed in all patients with *S. intermedius* bacteremia (see Chapter 182).

Bacterial Endocarditis. The viridans streptococci presently account for one-half of bacterial endocarditis (Table 5).[9] Viridans streptococcal endocarditis occurs most often in patients with underlying valvular heart disease. The clinical course is usually subacute, and the cure rate exceeds 90 percent. The relative frequency of the viridans species associated with endocarditis at three medical centers[26–28] is shown in Table 5. *Streptococcus sanguis* I and II and *S. mutans* account for approximately two-thirds of the cases, perhaps secondary to the production of extracellular polysaccharides and teichoic acids, which mediate attachment to cardiac endothelium.

Nutritionally variant streptococci account for 6–7 percent of bacterial endocarditis. Since they require thiol compounds or the active forms of vitamin B_6 for growth in routine laboratory media, they could be one explanation for "culture-negative endocarditis." Media must be supplemented with either pyridoxal hydrochloride or pyridoxamine dihydrochloride for isolation, identification, and subsequent susceptibility testing to antimicrobial agents. A recent review of the clinical course of 49 patients with NVS endocarditis at three medical institutions (The New York Hospital, Mayo Clinic, and Hospital of St. Joseph) indicates that mortality (14 vs. 5 percent), complications including congestive heart failure, prosthetic valve insertion, and embolization (63 vs. 33 percent), and clinical and bacteriologic relapse (8 vs. 1 percent) are more common than in patients with other forms of viridans streptococcal endocarditis.[29] These findings as well as data from the results of antimicrobial therapy in experimental endocarditis due to NVS[30] suggest that all patients with NVS endocarditis should be treated with an antimicrobial regimen appropriate for penicillin-resistant streptococci despite in vitro susceptibility results.

Bacteremia. Since viridans streptococci may transiently invade the blood stream from the oral cavity, it may be difficult to determine the clinical significance of a positive blood culture. Persistently positive cultures indicate either endocarditis or seeding from other infections such as pneumonia, meningitis, sinusitis, otitis, or intra-abdominal infections.[31]

Antimicrobial Therapy

Most viridans streptococci are sensitive to penicillin G, that is, a minimum inhibitory concentration (MIC) ≤ 0.1 μg/ml, al-

TABLE 4. Extrarespiratory Isolation of Human Viridans Streptococci—the New York Hospital, 1976–1982

Source of Clinical Isolates	mitior	sanguis	"intermedius *group*"	salivarius	mutans	morbillorum	*Total*
Central nervous system	2	3	10	2	0	0	17
Cervicofacial	12	4	56	10	1	0	83
Cardiovascular	37	24	9	1	5	0	76
Intestinal	67	36	261	37	6	5	412
Urogenital	27	5	339	15	0	4	390
Bone–joint	6	4	9	1	0	2	22
Skin–wound	28	9	120	14	0	0	171
Bacteremia	104	49	34	23	2	8	220
Total	283	134	838	103	14	19	1391

TABLE 5. "Viridans" Streptococcal Species Associated with Infective Endocarditis

Species	*Data from Refs. 26, 27* (%)	*Data from Ref. 28* (%)
S. sanguis I	31	31
S. sanguis II	25	41 (*S. mitior*)
S. mitis	14	
S. intermedius group[a]	10	8
S. mutans[a]	8	10
S. morbillorum	3	1
S. salivarius	0	2
NVS	0	6
Miscellaneous	8	2

[a] Since some members of these species may be β-hemolytic, they may have been excluded from series on "viridans" endocarditis and reported as group A, C, F, or G.

though a high prevalence of penicillin-resistant organisms in oropharyngeal flora may be recovered from patients receiving oral penicillin prophylaxis.[32] In the New York Hospital experience only 8 and 9 percent of bacteremic isolates from patients with endocarditis are relatively resistant to penicillin G (MIC 0.1–0.2 and >0.2 μg/ml, respectively.[9] Despite the widespread use of penicillin, the susceptibility to penicillin G of isolates associated with endocarditis has not increased since 1944.[28] Minor differences in penicillin G susceptibility have been noted among the viridans streptococcal species.[33] Relative resistance (MIC >0.1 μg/ml) has been observed in 12 percent of *S. mitior*, 9 percent of *S. sanguis*, and 5 percent of the other species.[9] Penicillin G resistant *S. mitior* strains have been isolated in both temporal and geographic proximity to South African resistant pneumococci (see Chapter 178). The MIC for penicillin has ranged from 0.5 to 16 μg/ml. These isolates have properties very similar to resistant pneumococci in that they have major alterations in penicillin-binding proteins (PBP), do not produce β-lactamases, and are resistant to other β-lactam antibiotics but sensitive to vancomycin.[34]

Although viridans streptococci are resistant to the aminoglycosides by disk susceptibility testing, synergy (increase in the rate of bacterial killing over time) using combinations of penicillin G and aminoglycosides has been demonstrated both in vitro[35] and in experimental endocarditis.[36] However, high-level streptomycin resistance (MIC ≥2000 μg/ml) has recently been described; synergy between penicillin G and gentamicin but not streptomycin was demonstrated among these isolates.[36] If high-level streptomycin resistance approaches the prevalence seen among enterococcal isolates, gentamicin might be the preferred aminoglycoside in patients with viridans streptococcal endocarditis as well.

Antibiotic tolerance (minimum bactericidal concentration [MBC] exceeds the MIC ≥32-fold) is due to a defect in bacterial murein hydrolases (autolysins) that mediate the bacteriolytic effects of penicillin. Tolerance has been demonstrated in all viridans species except *S. salivarius*[37] and is probably present in most *S. sanguis* isolates.[38] Tolerant strains are eradicated more slowly than nontolerant strains are in penicillin-treated experimental endocarditis,[39] although differences in killing may only be significant when low doses of penicillin are given.[40] The clinical significance of penicillin tolerance in viridans streptococcal endocarditis is unclear. A relapse after 4 weeks of high-dose parenteral penicillin is rare and has not been associated with tolerance to date. If in vitro tolerance to penicillin G is documented, either high-dose intravenous penicillin or combination penicillin–aminoglycoside therapy should be considered. It should be emphasized that certain laboratory techniques must be used to detect penicillin tolerance. Penicillinase is added to the transferred broth culture, especially if relatively large volumes are used (0.1 ml), and subcultures are incubated for 48 hours.[41]

Other less active antimicrobial agents used in patients who cannot receive penicillin include erythromycin, clindamycin, and chloramphenicol for extracardiac infections, and the cephalosporins and vancomycin for endocarditis. These alternative antibiotics may also be used for prophylaxis in penicillin-allergic patients. Newer agents such as teicoplanin and daptomycin (LY 146032) are currently undergoing clinical trials.[42–44] These agents hold promise because they appear to be bactericidal against penicillin- and vancomycin-tolerant strains.

The antimicrobial susceptibility patterns of NVS differ from *S. mitis* and other viridans streptococci.[45,46] In a combined study of 46 bacteremic isolates from endocarditis patients,[29] two-thirds were penicillin sensitive (MIC ≤0.1 μg/ml), 20 percent had MIC of 0.2–0.4 μg/ml, and 13 percent were resistant (MIC ≥0.5 μg/ml). Eleven percent of strains (all with MBC >50 μg/ml) were tolerant, and in two of the five patients, relapses were documented, thus confirming previous reports of penicillin tolerance.[47] All NVS were sensitive to vancomycin (MIC ≤1.6 μg/ml), but 62 percent were tolerant (compared with only 1 percent of non-NVS *S. mitior*). High-level resistance to streptomycin and gentamicin was not detected, and synergy with either aminoglycoside and penicillin or vancomycin was demonstrated against tolerant strains. These in vitro data and the clinical observatioons discussed previously indicate that all patients with NVS endocarditis should receive combination therapy.

ADDITIONAL β HEMOLYTIC STREPTOCOCCI: PYOGENES-LIKE STREPTOCOCCI

Unlike groups A and B, which contain only one important human pathogen, groups C, F, and G may contain multiple, often heterogeneous species.[5,48] Those organisms that produce a larger colony (>0.5 mm) with a relatively large zone of hemolysis (>2 mm), hence resembling group A, have been referred to as "pyogenes-like" streptococci. These strains are to be distinguished from "minute" β-hemoolytic streptococci (colonies <0.5 mm with a <2 mm zone of β-hemolysis at 24 hours) and most group F streptococci, which are now included in the species *S. anginosus* or the "*S. milleri* group" (Chapter 187). This group of organisms as well as the rare "non-pyogenes" group A strains have created great confusion in the microbiologic and clinical literature that has resulted in a heterogenicity of strains in reports dealing with groups C and G streptococcal infections. Nonpharyngitis isolates and fastidious or atypical organisms isolated from the blood or deep tissue sites (especially intracranial, intrathoracic, or intra-abdominal abscesses) should be characterized biochemically regardless of serogroup. This can now be done reliably with a variety of commerically available "strip" tests.[6]

Clinical Microbiology

Groups C and G possess the usual major properties characteristic of streptococci. Unlike group B streptococci, they are CAMP test– and sodium hippuate–negative. They are distinguished from the rare β-hemolytic group D organisms by their inability to grow in 40% bile. In many diagnostic laboratories, bacitracin disk susceptibility is used as a screening test to separate group A streptococci from pyogenes-like organisms. Studies employing the standard 0.04 unit bacitracin disk indicate that only 6–8 percent of groups C and G streptococci are susceptible.[49] Hence, in body sites such as the pharynx where the major pathogen is *S. pyogenes*, the sensitivity and specificity of this test are excellent.

Because of the variabilities of bacitracin resistance when higher concentrations are used and alterations in hemolysis caused by pH, the type of blood used, aerobic or anaerobic incubation, and the presence of abscence of glucose in the medium, definitive identification requires serogrouping and biochemical testing. Rapid serogrouping can now be performed by latex[8] or coagglutination[7] testing for groups A, B, C, D, F, and G. Only rare cross-reactions occur due to the close structural relationships between carbohydrates of groups A and C and those of groups B and G.[50,51]

Both groups produce a variety of extracellular products including hyaluronidase, streptokinase, DNases, and hemolysins. *Streptococcus equisimilis* is the only group C species that produces streptolysin O and streptokinase, while another hemolysin is produced by *S. equi* and *S. zooepidemicus*.[52] The hyaluronidase and streptokinase are antigenically distinct from the enzymes of *S. pyogenes*. Streptokinase used for human thrombolytic therapy is produced from *S. equisimilis*.[53] The streptolysin O produced by *S. equisimilis* and group G streptococci appears identical to that produced by group A streptococci. Therefore, infections due to these organisms may result in elevation of antibody titers (anti-streptolysin [ASO] and Streptozyme) classically used to screen patients for antecedent group A streptococcal infections.[54] Fibronectin binding has been observed with both groups C and G[55] and may mediate the adherence of streptococci to oral epithelial cells.

Species Identification

Group C and G streptococcal species have been newly amended[56] to include only two species, which now encompass all large-colony group C and G streptococci as well as group L. It is proposed that *S. equi* (and subspecies *zooepidemicus*), both group C with a wide zone of hemolysis, be considered a single species. These organisms have guanidine/cytosine ratios of 41–43 mol percent and over 90 percent similarity by DNA homology. In contrast, *S. dysgalactiae* shows homology with *S. equisimilis*, large-colony group G streptococci, and group L streptococci. The latter differ from *S. dysgalactiae* only in that they are hemolytic. Guanidine/cytosine ratios are 38–40, and biochemically they are similar. Thus, this proposal treats this group much as the viridans streptococci in that serogroups and hemolytic reactions may be diverse within the "species." These organisms are clearly distinct from the groups C and G organisms of the *S. intermedius* group by DNA homology as well as by their failure to produce acetoin (acetylmethylcarbinol) from glucose (Voges-Proskauer [V-P] test). One author has proposed the following scheme to separate β-hemolytic, bacitracin-resistant streptococci: (1) Latex agglutination for A, B, C, D, F, and G; (2) size of the colony at 24 hours; and (3) a quick V-P test.[5] Hence, large-colony, large-zone–hemolysis, V-P–negative streptococci are either *S. dysgalactiae* and its β-hemolytic subspecies of groups C and G or *S. equi* (and its variant *S. zooepidemicus*), group C. The organisms of the "*S. intermedius* group" would contain the minute-colony variants, β-hemolytic (small-zone), V-P–positive strains of groups A, C, G, and F as well as all of the nonhemolytic strains identified by biochemical testing (Chapter 182).

Natural Habitat

The pyogenes-like streptococci are common inhabitants of many animal species (Table 1), and human infections may result from exposure to animals or their products. Group C and G streptococci, however, may also colonize the human pharynx, intestinal tract, and vagina, which may also serve as a source for human disease. Pharyngeal colonization is uncommon in both adults (1–2 percent) and children (<1 percent), although the asymptomatic carrier rate of both group C and G organisms in schoolchildren may be prolonged.[57,58] Colonization of the intestinal tract is uncommon although group G organisms have been recovered more frequently than have group C streptococci (8–13 percent) vs. <1 percent, respectively.[59] Isolation of group C and G organisms from the vagina of healthy peripartum women was first reported in 1935[60] and has been observed in nonpregnant women as well.[57] The vaginal carriage rate appears to be relatively low (<1 percent) as compared with group B and D streptococci.[61] Because of the association of group C and G streptococci with wound infections and cellulitis, these organisms are most certainly normal skin inhabitants. Colonization of neonates by both serogroups has recently been described.[62,63] Positive umbilical cultures were not associated with clinical infections in either study. Group G colonization rates of 41–76 percent were observed over an extended period of time from the nose and umbilicus of neonates at discharge. It is of interest that the recovery (1–3 percent) and infection rate of group B streptococci were low during the same period, thus suggesting mutually exclusive colonization and bacterial interference. With all of the aforementioned studies, however, it is unclear how many of these strains represent large-colony/large-zone-of-hemolysis, pyogenes-like organisms vs. strains of *S. anginosus* carrying C or G antigens. Two investigators found that among bacitracin-resistant group C and G strains isolated from the pharynx, approximately 75 and 15 percent, respectively, were of the *S. intermedius* group.[48,64]

Clinical Manifestations

The isolation and recognition of non-group A and D streptococci was first described by Lancefield and Hare in 1935[60] when β-hemolytic group B, C, and G organisms were recovered from vaginal cultures of healthy and infected parturient women. The association of these serogroups with previous epidemics of erysipelas[65] and puerperal fever[66] became apparent, and severe human infections other than in the genital tract were subsequently reported in the 1940s by Rantz and Kirby[67] and Foley.[68] Subsequently, the role of group C and G streptococci in severe infections was further amplified,[31,69] and numerous reports of these organisms in suppurative infections of various organ systems have been recorded. Although not as common pathogens as group A and B streptococci, group C and G streptococcal infections are associated with a significant morbidity and mortality and present certain unique epidemiologic, clinical and therapeutic features that should be appreciated by physicians and microbiologists.

Clinical infections by group C and G streptococci may be exogenous or endogenous since these organisms commonly reside on the skin or mucous membranes. The former source is often from patient contact with various animals and underscored the prevalence of these infections in certain high-risk groups (i.e., farmers and in rural communities). Outbreaks of pharyngitis have been associated with the ingestion of contaminated animal products including eggs[70] and unpasteurized milk.[71–73] In the past, group C human infections were most commonly caused by *S. equisimilis* (''human C'' streptococcus), although speciation was not performed in many of the earlier studies. More recently, *S. zooepidemicus* has been associated not only with outbreaks of poststreptococcal glomerulonephritis[71,72] but with suppurative infections as well including bacteremia,[73] endocarditis,[74] pneumonia,[75] and meningitis.[76]

Group C and G streptococcal infections are often severe and resemble those caused by group A and B streptococci. They are often associated with bacteremia, and the clinical course may be protracted. Surgical intervention is often required to achieve clinical and microbiologic resolution. Endogenous infections often occur in altered hosts due to age (neonate or elderly), alcoholism, intravenous drug addiction, diabetes mellitus, immunosuppressive therapy with steroids or cytotoxic drugs, or underlying cancer.[31,77] The following is a summary of the suppurative infections caused by group C and G streptococci.

Respiratory Tract Infections. Food- and milk-borne epidemics of group G streptococcal pharyngitis have been reported from many sources.[70] Outbreaks of group C streptococcal pharyngitis unrelated to contaminated food consumption may also occur.[78] The clinical symptoms and course are very similar to group A streptococcal pharyngitis and include fever, mild to severe sore throat, pharyngeal exudates, and cervical adenopathy. The attack rate in a U.S. college epidemic was 31 percent and an ASO titer was elevated in 50 percent of patients. However, asymptomatic infection was present in 23 percent (compared with 2 percent for group A pharyngitis epidemics), which suggests that the epidemic strain may be less virulent than group A strains are. These serogroups have also been recovered from patients with nonepidemic pharyngitis documented by a rise in ASO titer.[79] Group C and G streptococci may be recovered in the clinical laboratory from patients with upper respiratory tract infections (approximately 30 and 10 percent, respectively), although the etiologic role of the serogroups in these studies is unclear.[80,81] In a large report involving children and adolescents with sporadic pharyngitis, 17 percent of the β-hemolytic streptococci isolated were non-group A. Of these organisms, less than half were of groups C and G, and in a small number of patients surveyed, acute and convalescent titer rises to group C and G antigens were rarely demonstrated.[54]

Group C streptococcal pneumonia, although uncommon, is associated with a significant morbidity and may resemble group A disease.[82] It is often preceded by a viral upper respiratory tract infection and is associated with a high incidence of complications including bacteremia with metastatic localization, empyema, and cavitation. Elevated serum aspartate aminotransferase (AST) levels have been noted and suggest hepatic involvement due to direct invasion by the organism or by the release of an extracellular toxin. Pneumonia due to the group G streptococcus is rare.

Skin Infections. Group C and G streptococci are normal skin inhabitants and have been associated with various cutaneous infections including erysipelas, cutaneous ulcers, wound infections, impetiginous lesions, pyoderma, and cellulitis.[65,83,84] Unlike group B and D streptococci, they usually are not important pathogens in patients with peripheral vascular disease but have been observed with increasing frequency in cellulitis after vein harvest for coronary artery bypass grafting and conditions associated with abnormal venous or lymphatic drainage.[85] Lymphangitis and bacteremia may accompany such infections, and immediate medical therapy is often necessary to prevent extensive surgery. These serogroups also have been particularly important in cutaneous infections in patients with underlying malignancies.[31,77]

Puerperal Infections. As mentioned previously, group C and G streptococci are common inhabitants of the female genital tract and have been associated with epidemic and nonepidemic puerperal sepsis.[60,70] Endometritis without bacteremia, on the other hand, may be relatively mild and associated with few systemic symptoms.

Neonatal Sepsis. Group G neonatal sepsis has been documented in 7 of 305 septic newborns over a 5-year period at one institution[63] and has been reported by others as well.[86–89] The clinical setting is very similar to that of early-onset group B streptococcal sepsis in that the child is colonized from the mother after vaginal delivery, a high incidence of maternal obstetric complications is present, and the onset of clinical symptoms is usually within the first week of life. Infants may be either premature or full-term, and the clinical presentation is that of neonatal sepsis including hypothermia, irritability, seizures, apnea, bradycardia, and cardiac arrest.

Endocarditis. Bacterial endocarditis due to group C and G streptococci is uncommon[90–98] and accounts for 8.4 percent of β-hemolytic streptococcal endocarditis and fewer than 1 percent of the total cases.[99] Over a 14-year period at The New York Hospital, only 2 of more than 400 patients with endocarditis were due to group G streptococcus. Although relatively uncommon, group C and G streptococcal endocarditis is associated with a high morbidity and mortality (>30 percent). The duration of symptoms is short, and the usual peripheral manifestations observed in subacute disease are not present. The clinical course is usually marked by valve destruction with resultant hemodynamic abnormalities (congestive heart failure) and recurrent systemic embolization. Abscesses of major organs, including the brain, spleen, and kidneys, and panophthalmitis have been described. Despite the absence of underlying heart disease, hemodynamic compromise often necessitates prosthetic valve insertion. The presumed source of these serogroups has been the gastrointestinal tract (enteritis), skin, and genital tract (septic abortion). Because of the acute and destructive nature of this disease, all patients should receive combination therapy with a penicillin and an aminoglycoside (see above).

Meningitis. Bacterial meningitis due to group C and G serogroups is often associated with infective endocarditis.[76,100] The clinical course is often protracted by a slow response to antimicrobial therapy. The mortality is greater than 50 percent. In the absence of endocarditis, a source is usually not identified.

Septic Arthritis. Patients with group G streptococcal arthritis usually have previously damaged or underlying joint disease such as rheumatoid arthritis, trauma, or prosthetic joints.[101,102] The clinical course is protracted and bacteriologic relapse after medical therapy is not uncommon. Adjacent osteomyelitis from direct extension may occur with persistent infection. Optimal therapy has required open surgical drainage in addition to antimicrobial therapy in many patients.

Bacteremia. Bacteremia due to these serogroups is uncommon and accounts for fewer than 1 percent of all streptococcal blood cultures.[31] Furthermore, since these organisms are normal inhabitants of the skin, contamination may occur. Nevertheless, group C and G streptococcal bacteremia may be associated with severe infections including endocarditis, meningitis, pneumonia, and arthritis.[73,96–98,103] Thus, all bacteremic patients must receive a thorough evaluation for both a source and metastatic localization.

Poststreptococcal Glomerulonephritis. Acute poststreptococcal glomerulonephritis (PSGN) is a well-recognized nonsuppurative sequela after group A streptococcal infections. PSGN has also been associated with group C streptococcal pharyngitis.[71,72] In both outbreaks, the epidemiologic features were similar; the infection was acquired by unpasteurized milk consumption from cattle with mastitis, and the species was *S. zooepidemicus*. Since this species does not produce streptolysin O, no ASO response was noted. Endostreptosin (ESS), a cytoplasmic polypeptide antigen that plays a role in the development of post-group A streptococcal glomerulonephritis, was demonstrated in the cytoplasm of infecting group C isolates, and elevated and persistent anti-ESS antibodies were detected in patients' sera. In an epidemic of acute group A PSGN in Trinidad, three group G and one group C strains were isolated.[104] Although the role of group G streptococci in this outbreak is unclear, the isolates possessed a type 12 M-protein antigen identical to the nephritogenic type 12 antigen of group A streptococci.[105]

Antimicrobial Therapy

The following antibiotics are active against both group C and G streptococci: penicillin G (MIC 0.02–0.06 μg/ml), vancomycin (MIC 0.03–0.5 μg/ml), first-generation cephalosporins (MIC 0.03–0.5 μg/ml), erythromycin (MIC 0.03–1.0 μg/ml), azlocillin and piperacillin (MIC 0.03–1.0 μg/ml), and the new β-lactams except for moxalactam.[106] The activity of moxalactam is similar to that for group B streptococci (MIC 4.0–8.0 μg/ml), and this antibiotic is not indicated for infections caused by these bacteria. Penicillin G is the drug of choice for group C and G infections, and in patients allergic to penicillin, vancomycin, cefazolin, or erythromycin may be used depending on the site and severity of disease. Clinical therapeutic failure has been reported in erythromycin-treated group G arthritis, and erythromycin should not be used for serious, life-threatening infections. Because of its excellent activity (MIC 0.025–0.1 μg/ml), adjunct therapy with rifampin may be useful in such infections.[102] Both clindamycin and chloramphenicol have poor bactericidal activity against group G streptococci.

Conflicting results regarding antibiotic tolerance in both serogroups have been reported. Whereas penicillin- and vancomycin-tolerant group C isolates were uncommon in the study of Rolston et al.[106] Portnoy et al.[107] reported 16 of 17 isolates tolerant to penicillin G (MBC 32- to 512-fold greater than the MIC). Synergy using the combination of penicillin plus gentamicin was demonstrated against all isolates. Based on these in vitro data and the significant morbidity and mortality associated with severe group C streptococcal infections (i.e., endocarditis and meningitis), combination therapy should be employed in these patients. Penicillin tolerance in group G streptococci on the other hand has only been demonstrated in the presence of a high inoculum and stationary growth phase of organisms. Since these in vitro conditions mimic endocarditis and the mortality of group G endocarditis exceeds 30 percent, combination therapy should also be used in this clinical setting. Vancomycin tolerance in group G isolates has been reported,[108] although its demonstration may depend on the phase of growth and laboratory media employed.[96] If vancomycin therapy is considered for serious group G infections, careful antimicrobial susceptibility testing should be performed. If tolerance is demonstrated, combination therapy with an aminoglycoside or possibly rifampin should be instituted.

Additional Pyogenes-like Streptococci

In addition to group C and G streptococci, other pyogenes-like β-hemolytic streptococci have been associated (rarely) with human infections. All are common inhabitants and pathogens in various animals and also have been isolated from the upper respiratory tract of humans. Group E streptococci, once termed *S. infrequens*, contain the single species *S. lentus*. Groups P and U are related to this species. These organisms may be recovered from the urogenital tract and have been associated with bacteremia and empyema.[68] The group L streptococcus, occasionally a cause of infections in dogs, pigs, cattle, and sheep, has been demonstrated to be the cause of an outbreak of wound infection, impetigo and paronychia in meat handlers in England.[109] This organism has also been associated with suppurative parotitis, cellulitis, bacteremic pneumonia, and endocarditis.[31] Group M streptococci have been associated (rarely) with endocarditis. All three serogroups are sensitive to penicillin G, which is the drug of choice for these infections. Serogroup antigens L, M, N, and O have also been detected in viridans streptococci that have been associated (rarely) with bacteremia.[110]

REFERENCES

1. Parker MT, Ball LC. Streptococci and serococci associated with systemic infection in man. J Med Microbiol. 1976;9:275.
2. Colman G, Williams REO. Taxonomy of some human viridans streptococci, In: Wannamaker LW, Matsen JM, eds. Streptococci and Streptococcal Diseases: Recognition, Understanding and Management. New York: Academic Press; 1972:281.
3. Facklam RR. Physiological differentiation of viridans streptococci. J Clin Microbiol. 1977;5:184.
4. Facklam RR. The major differences in the American and British *Streptococcus* taxonomy schemes with special reference to *Streptococcus milleri*. Eur J Clin Microbiol. 1984;3:91–3.
5. Bucher C, Graevenitz AV. Differentiation in throat cultures of group C and G streptococci from *Streptococcus milleri* with identical antigens. Eur J Clin Microbiol. 1985;3:44–5.
6. Facklam R, Bosley GS, Rhoden D, et al. Comparative evaluation of the API 20S and automicrobic gram-positive identification systems for non-beta-hemolytic streptococci and aerococci. J Clin Microbiol. 1985;21:535–541.
7. Hahn G, Nyberg I. Identification of streptococcal groups A, B, C and G by slide co-agglutination of antibody-sensitized protein A-containing staphylococci. J Clin Microbiol. 1976;4:99.
8. Facklam RR, Cooksey RC, Wortham EC. Evaluation of commercial latex agglutination reagents for grouping streptococci. J Clin Microbiol. 1979;10:641.
9. Roberts RB, Krieger AG, Schiller NL. Viridans streptococcal endocarditis: The role of various species including pyridoxal-dependent streptococci. Rev Infect Dis. 1979;1:955.
10. van de Rijn I, Bouvet A. Characterization of a pH-dependent chromophore from nutritionally variant streptococci. Infect Immun. 1984;43:28.
11. Straus DC. Protease production by *Streptococcus sanguis* associated with subacute bacterial endocarditis. Infect Immun. 1982;38:1037.
12. Gross KC, Houghton MP, Roberts RB. Evaluation of blood culture media for isolation of pyridoxal-dependent *Streptococcus mitior (mitis)*. J Clin Microbiol. 1981;14:266.
13. Carey RB, Gross KC, Roberts RB. Vitamin B_6-dependent *Streptococcus mitior (mitis)* isolated from patients with systemic infections. J Infect Dis. 1975;131:722.
14. Schiller NL, Roberts RB. Vitamin B_6 requirements of nutritionally variant *Streptococcus mitior*. J Clin Microbiol. 1982;15:740.
15. Cooksey RC, Thompson FS, Facklam RR. Physiological characterization of nutritionally variant streptococci. J Clin Microbiol. 1979;10:326–330.
16. Bouvet A, van de Rijn I, McCarty M. Nutritionally variant streptococci from patients with endocarditis: Growth parameters in a semisynthetic medium and demonstration of a chromophore. J Bacteriol. 1981;146:1075–82.
17. van de Rijn I, George M, Bouvet A, et al. Enzyme-linked immunosorbent assay for the detection of antibodies to nutritionally variant streptococci in patients with endocarditis. J Infect Dis. 1986;153:116–21.
18. Gibbons RJ, Barghart S. Synthesis of extracellular dextran by cariogenic bacteria and its presence in human dental plaque. Arch Oral Biol. 1967;12:11.
19. Scheld WM, Valone JA, Sande MA. Bacterial adherence in the pathogenesis of endocarditis. Interaction of bacterial dextran, platelets and fibrin. J Clin Invest. 1978;61:1394.
20. Bernard JP, Francioli P, Glauser MP. Vancomycin prophylaxis of experimental *Streptococcus sanguis endocarditis*. Inhibition of bacterial adherence rather than bacterial killing. J Clin Invest. 1981;68:1113.
21. Scheld WM, Zak O, Vosbeck K, et al. Bacterial adhesion in the pathogenesis of infective endocarditis. J Clin Invest. 1981;68:1381.
22. Alkan ML, Beachey EH. Excretion of lipoteichoic acid by group A streptococci. Influence of penicillin on excretion and loss of ability to adhere to human and mucosal cells. J Clin Invest. 1978;61:671.
23. Horne D, Tomasz A. Tolerant response of *Streptococcus sanguis* to betalactams and other cell wall inhibitors. Antimicrob Agents Chemother. 1977;11:888.

24. Ball LY, Parker MT. The cultural and biochemical characters of *Streptococcus milleri* strains isolated from human sources. J Hyg Camb. 1979;82:63–78.
25. Swenson FJ, Rubin SJ. Clinical significance of viridans streptococci isolated from blood cultures. J Clin Microbiol. 1982;15:275.
26. Tuazon CU, Gill V, Gill F. Streptococcal endocarditis: Single vs. combination antibiotic therapy and role of various species. Rev Infect Dis. 1986;8:54–60.
27. Sussman JI, Baron EJ, Tenenbaum MJ, et al. Viridans streptococcal endocarditis: Clinical, microbiological and echocardiographic correlations. J Infect Dis. 1986;154:597–603.
28. Roberts RB, Krieger AG, Gross KC. The species of viridans streptococci associated with microbial endocarditis: Incidence and antimicrobial susceptibility. Trans Am Clin Climatol Assoc. 1977;89:36.
29. Roberts RB, Wilson WR, Bouvet A, et al. Nutritionally variant streptococcal (NVS) endocarditis. In: Proceedings of the 22nd Interscience Conference on Antimicrobiol Agents and Chemotherapy. Washington, DC: American Society of Microbiology; 1982:130.
30. Henry NK, Wilson WR, Roberts RB, et al. Antimicrobial therapy of experimental endocarditis caused by nutritionally variant viridans group streptococci. Antimicrob Agents Chemother. 1986;30:465–7.
31. Duma RJ, Weinberg AN, Medrek TF, et al. Streptococcal infections. A bacteriologic and clinical study of streptococcal bacteremia. Medicine (Baltimore). 1969;48:87.
32. de Louvois J, Gortvai P, Hurley R. Bacteriology of abscesses of the central nervous system: A multicentre prospective study. Br Med J. 1977;2:981.
33. Bourgault AM, Wilson WR, Washington JA II. Antimicrobial susceptibilities of species of viridans streptococci. J Infect Dis. 1979;140:316.
34. Farber BF, Eliopoulos GM, Ward JI, et al: Multiple resistant viridans streptococci: Susceptibility to beta lactam antibiotics and comparison of penicillin-binding protein patterns. Antimicrob Agents Chemother. 1983;24:702.
35. Wolfe JC, Johnson WD. Penicillin-sensitive streptococcal endocarditis. In vitro and clinical observations on penicillin-streptomycin therapy. Ann Intern Med. 1974;81:178.
36. Sande MA, Irvin RG. Penicillin-aminoglycoside synergy in experimental Streptococcus viridans endocarditis. J Infect Dis. 1974;129:572.
37. Holloway Y, Dankert J, Hess J. Penicillin tolerance and bacterial endocarditis (Letter). Lancet. 1980;1:598.
38. Horne D, Tomasz A. Lethal effect of a heterologous murein hydrolase on penicillin-treated *Streptococcus sanguis*. Antimicrob Agents Chemother. 1980;17:235.
39. Brennan RO, Durack DT. Therapeutic significant of penicillin tolerance in experimental streptococcal endocarditis. Antimicrob Agents Chemother. 1983:23, 273.
40. Lowy FD, Neuhaus EG, Chang DS, et al. Penicillin therapy of experimental endocarditis induced by tolerant *Streptococcus sanguis* and nontolerant *Streptococcus mitis*. Antimicrob Agents Chemother. 1983;23:67.
41. Dankert J, Holloway Y, Joldersma W, et al. Importance of minimizing carryover effect of subculture in the detection of penicillin-tolerant viridans group streptococci. Antimicrob Agents Chemother. 1983;23:614.
42. Andrew JH, Wale MC, Wale LJ, Greenwood D. The effect of cultural conditions in the activity of LY146032 against staphylococci and streptococci. J Antimicrob Chemother. 1987;20:213–21.
43. Fass RJ, Halsel VL. In vitro activity of LY 146032 against staphylococci, streptococci, and enterococci. Antimicrob Agents Chemother. 1986;30:781–4.
44. Eliopoulos GM, Willey S, Reiszner E, et al. In vitro and in vivo activity of LY146032, a new cyclic lipopeptide antibiotic. Antimicrob Agents Chemother. 1986;30:532–5.
45. Cooksey RC, Swenson JM. In vitro antimocrobial inhibition patterns of nutritionally variant streptococci. Antimicrob Agents Chemother. 1979;16:514.
46. Gephart JF, Washington JA II. Antimicrobial susceptibilities of nutritionally variant streptococci. J Infect Dis. 1982;146:536.
47. Holloway Y, Dankert J. Penicillin tolerance in nutritionally variant streptococci. Antimicrob Agents Chemother. 1982:22:1073.
48. Kipper-Balz R, Williams BL, Lutticken R, et al. Relatedness of *Streptococcus milleri* with *Streptococcus anginosus* and *Streptococcus constellatus*. Syst Appl Microbiol. 1984;5:494–500.
49. Pollock HM, Dahlgren BJ. Distribution of streptococcal groups in clinical specimens with evaluation of bacitracin screening. Appl Bacteriol. 1974;27:141.
50. Krause RM, McCarty M. Studies on the chemical structure of the streptococcal cell wall. II. The composition of group C cell walls and chemical basis for serologic specificity of the carbohydrate moiety. J Exp Med. 1962;115:49.
51. Curtis SN, Krause RM. Antigenic relationships betwen groups B and G streptococci. J Exp Med. 1964;120:629.
52. Hardie JM. Genus *Streptococcus*. In: Sneath PHA, Mair NS, Sharpe ME, et al., eds. Bergey's Manual of Systematic Bacteriology. v. 2. Baltimore: Williams & Wilkins; 1986:1043–71.
53. Marder VJ. The use of thrombolytic agents: Choice of patient, drug administration, laboratory monitoring. Ann Intern Med. 1979;90:802–8.
54. Schwartz RH, Shulman ST. Group C and group G streptococci. In-office isolation from children and adolescents with pharyngitis. Clin Pediatr (Phila). 1986;25:496–502.
55. Myhre EB, Kuusela P. Binding of human fibronectin to group A, C, and G streptococci. Infect Immun. 1983;40:29.
56. Farrow JAE, Collins MD. Taxonomic studies on streptococci of serological groups C, G and L and possibly related taxa. Syst Appl Microbiol. 1984;5:483–493.
57. Hutchinson RI. Pathogenicity of group C (Lancefield) hemolytic streptococcus. Br Med J. 1946;2:575.
58. Nicholas WC, Steele CP, Bismarck BS. Occurrence of groupable beta-hemolytic streptococci. JAMA. 1962;181:197.
59. Allison VD. Section of comparative medicine. Proc R Soc Med. 1942;35:627.
60. Lancefield RC, Hare R. The serologic differentiation of pathogenic and nonpathogenic strains of hemolytic streptococci from parturient women. J Exp Med. 1935;61:335.
61 Christensen KK, Christensen P, Flamhole L, et al. Frequencies of streptococci of groups A, B, C, D and G in urethra and cervix swab specimens from patients with suspected gonococcal infection. Acta Pathol Microbiol Scand. 1974;82:470.
62. Drusin LM, Ribble JC, Topf B. Group C streptococcal colonization in a newborn nursery. Am J Dis Child. 1973;125:820.
63. Dyson AE, Read SE. Group G streptococcal colonization and sepsis in neonates. J Pediat. 1981;99:944.
64. Ruoff KL, Kunz LJ, Ferraro MJ. Occurrence of *Streptococcus milleri* among beta-hemolytic streptococci isolated from clinical specimens. J Clin Microbiol. 1985;22:149–51.
65. Birkhaug KE. Studies on the biology of the *Streptococcus erysipelatis*. Bull Johns Hopkins Hosp. 1925;36:248.
66. Colebrook DC. The source of infection in puerperal fever due to hemolytic streptococci. Special Report Series No. 205, Medical Research Council. London: His Majesty's Stationery Office; 1935.
67. Rantz LA, Kirby WM: Hemolytic streptococcus bacteremia. A report of thireteen cases with special reference to the serologic groups of the etiologic organisms. N Engl J Med. 1942;227:7230.
68. Foley GE. Further observations on the occurrence of streptococci of groups other than A in human infection. N Engl J Med. 1947;237:809.
69. Feingold DS, Stagg NL, Kunz LJ. Extrarespiratory streptococcal infections. Importance of the various serologic groups. N Engl J Med. 1966;275:356.
70. Hill HR, Caldwell GG, Wilson E, et al. Epidemic of pharyngitis due to streptococci of Lancefield group G. Lancet. 1969;2:371.
71. Duca E, Teodorovici G, Radu C, et al. A new nephritogenic streptococcus. J Hyg Camb. 1969:67:691.
72. Barnham M, Thornton TJ, Lange K. Nephritis caused by *Streptococcus zooepidemicus* (Lancefield group C). Lancet. 1983;1:945.
73. Centers for Disease Control. Group C streptococcal infections associated with eating homemade cheese. MMWR. 1983;32:510.
74. Ghoneim A, Cooke EM. Serious infections caused by group C streptococci. J Clin Pathol. 1980;33:188.
75. Rose HD, Allen JR, Witte G. *Streptococcus zooepidemicus* (group C) pneumonia in a human. J Clin Microbiol. 1980;11:76.
76. Mohr DN, Feist DJ, Washington JA II. Meningitis due to group C streptococci in an adult. Mayo Clin Proc. 1978;53:529.
77. Armstrong D, Blevins A, Louria DB. Groups B, C and G streptococcal infections in a cancer hospital. Ann NY Acad Sci. 1970;72:511.
78. Benjamin JT, Perriello VA, Pharyngitis due to group C hemolytic streptococci in children. J Pediatr. 1976;89:254.
79. Commission on Acute Respiratory Diseases. The role of Lancefield groups of beta-hemolytic streptococci in respiratory secretions. N Engl J Med. 1947;236:157.
80. Murray PR, Wold AD, Washington JA II. Recovery of group A and nongroup A beta-hemolytic streptococci from throat swab specimens. Mayo Clin Proc. 1977;52:81.
81. Forrer CB, Ellner PD. Distribution of hemolytic streptococci in respiratory secretions. J Clin Microbiol. 1979;10:69.
82. Stamm AM, Cobbs CG. Group C streptococcal pneumonia: Report of a fatal case and review of the literature. Rev Infect Dis. 1980;2:889.
83. Portnoy B, Reitler R. Cellulitis due to a hemolytic streptococcus type C. Lancet. 1944;2:597.
84. Belcher DW, Afoakwa SN, Osei-Tutu E, et al. Non-group A streptococci in Ghanaian patients with pyoderma. Lancet.1975;2:1032.
85. Baddour LM, Bisno AL: Non-group A beta-hemolytic streptococcal cellulitis. Association with venous and lymphatic compromise. Am J Med. 1985;79:155–8.
86. Stewardson-Krieger P, Gotoff SP. Neonatal meningitis due to group C beta hemolytic streptococcus. J Pediatr. 1977;90:103.
87. Baker CJ. Unusual occurrence of neonatal septicemia due to group G streptococcus. Pediatrics 1974;53:568.
88. Neiburg PI. Fatal group G streptococcal sepsis in a neonate. Scand J Infect Dis. 1979;2:93.
89. Ancona RJ, Thompson TR, Ferrieri P. Group G streptococcal pneumonia and sepsis in a newborn infant. J Clin Microbiol. 1979;10:758.
90. Rosenthal AH, Stone FM. Puerperal infection with vegetative endocarditis. JAMA. 1940;114:840.
91. Sanders V. Bacterial endocarditis due to a group C beta hemolytic streptococcus. Ann Intern Med. 1963;58:858.
92. Lawrence MS, Cobbs CG. Endocarditis due to group C streptococci. South Med J. 1972;65:487.
93. Finnegan P, Fitzgerald XM, Cumming G, et al. Lancefield group C streptococcal endocarditis. Thorax. 1974;29:245.

94. Bouza E, Meyer RD, Busch DF. Group G streptococcal endocarditis. Am J Clin Pathol. 1978;70:108.
95. Tuazan CU. Group G streptococcus. Am J Med Sci. 1980;279:121.
96. Lam K, Bayer AS. Serious infections due to group G streptococci. Am J Med. 1983;75:561.
97. Vartian C, Lerner PI, Shlaes DM, et al. Infections due to Lancefield Group G streptococci. Medicine (Baltimore). 1985;64:75–88.
98. Auckenthaler R, Hermans PE, Washington JA. Group G streptococcal bacteremia: Clinical study and review of the literature. Rev Infect Dis. 1983;5:196.
99. Blair DC, Martin DB. Beta hemolytic streptococcal endocarditis: Predominance of non group A organisms. Am J Med Sci. 1978;276:269.
100. Low DE, Young MR, Harding GK. Group C streptococcal meningitis in an adult. Arch Intern Med. 1980;140:977.
101. Fujita NK, Lam K, Bayer AS. Septic arthritis due to group G streptococcus. JAMA. 1982;247:812.
102. Nakata MM, Silvers JH, George L. Group G streptococcal arthritis. Arch Intern Med. 1983;143:1328.
103. Mohr DN, Feist DJ, Washington JA II, et al. Infections due to group C streptococci in man. Am J Med. 1979;66:540.
104. Simon WS, Potter EV, Siegal AC, et al. Epidemic nephritis in Trinidad. J Lab Clin Med. 1965;6:1022.
105. Maxted WR, Potter EV. The presence of type 12 M-protein antigen in group G streptococci. J Gen Microbiol. 1967;49:119.
106. Rolston KV, Le Frock JL, Schell RF. Activity of nine antimicrobial agents against Lancefield group C and G streptococci. Antimicrob Agents Chemother. 1982;22:930.
107. Portnoy D, Prentis J, Richards GK. Penicillin tolerance of human isolates of group C streptococci. Antimicrob Agents Chemother. 1981;20:235.
108. Noble JT, Tyburski MB, Berman M. Antimicrobial tolerance in group G streptococci. Lancet. 1980;2:982.
109. Barnham M. Neilson DJ. Group L beta-hemolytic streptococcal infection in meat handlers: Another streptococcal zoonosis? Epidemiol Infect. 1987;9:257–264.
110. Broome CV, Moellering RC, Watson BK. Clinical significance of Lancefield groups L–T streptococci isolated from blood and spinal fluid. J Infect Dis. 1976;133:387.

182. STREPTOCOCCUS INTERMEDIUS GROUP (STREPTOCOCCUS ANGINOSUS-MILLERI GROUP)

HARRY A. GALLIS

Streptococcus intermedius and its close relatives (*Streptococcus* MG, *S. anginosus,* and *S. constellatus*) compose a clinically homogeneous but genetically heterogeneous group of organisms referred to by some authors as *S. milleri,* "*S. milleri* group," or *S. anginosus-milleri* group. Currently, taxonomic controversies still exist between the classification systems of Colman and Williams[1] and Facklam[2]. Because *S. milleri* has yet to be accepted as a valid species, the organisms in this chapter will be referred to as the *S. intermedius* group or complex. The major clinical characteristic of these organisms is a propensity for invasive pyogenic disease that separates them from the other viridans streptococci. They are well known to clinicians and microbiologists by their microbiologic characteristics, e.g., microaerophilic or anaerobic preference, tiny colonies that will not subculture, β-hemolytic group F streptococcus from a brain abscess, etc. This chapter will define the various species biochemically, genetically, and antigenically and then take substantial license in discussing the clinical manifestations as if they were due to a single organism. For an excellent overview, the reader is referred to a recent article.[3]

CLINICAL MICROBIOLOGY

Streptococcus intermedius has the usual biochemical properties that define the genus *Streptococcus* as discussed in Chapter 175. In addition, these organisms frequently are microaerophilic and require CO_2 for normal growth. They may be α-, β-, or nonhemolytic and often contain Lancefield antigens A, C, F, or G. Many exhibit small (<0.5 mm) colonies at 24 hours and were initially described as "minute hemolytic streptococci."[4] The individual organisms within these colonies may be one-half to two-thirds the diameter of other β-hemolytic streptococci. They are not closely related to the larger β-hemolytic organisms of their respective Lancefield serogroups, which accounts for considerable confusion in reports that discuss infections solely on the basis of the Lancefield group without biochemical speciation. DNA–DNA homology studies between the species in the *S. intermedius* group have shown close relationships[5,6] frequently overlapping hemolytic reactions.

TAXONOMY

The various species of streptococci that are closely related to *S. intermedius* have been known since the early 1900s. These organisms have been described as *S. anginosus, S.* MG, minute hemolytic streptococci, *S. intermedius, S. constellatus,* and *S. milleri.* Most of the confusion with regard to these "species" relates to their variation in hemolytic reaction (α-, β-, or nonhemolytic), lactose fermentation, and Voges-Proskauer (V-P) reaction (acetoin from glucose); minute colony morphology; and possession of Lancefield antigens A, C, F, G, or none. Various schemes have been suggested for identifying these organisms. First, if one evaluates bacitracin-resistant (0.04 unit disk) β-hemolytic streptococci (which excludes 99 percent of *S. pyogenes* and only 6–8 percent of other species), many such organisms will fall into typical large-colony morphology group C or group G. Approximately one-third of group C and three-quarters of group G organisms exhibit large zones (>2 mm) of β-hemolysis when incubated anaerobically for 24 hours.[7,8] The remainder as well as β-hemolytic group F generally fall into the *S. intermedius* group.[9,10] It has been suggested[8] that, for rapid identification, bacitracin-resistant streptococci be tested for Lancefield antigens by an agglutination technique, measurement of the zone of hemolysis, and the rapid V-P test. A negative V-P test response will separate the true group C and G organisms but not *S. anginosus* group A.[9] While this scheme deals with the β-hemolytic strains, approximately three-fourths of the organisms in this group are not β-hemolytic. These must be separated from viridans streptococci by biochemical testing. Many of the rapid "strip" tests are suitable.[11] The general characteristics of the *S. intermedius* group are as follows: lactose-, esculin-, salicin-, and arginine-positive; V-P–positive; and mannitol, glycerol, hippurate, and sorbital-negative. Most strains grow best under CO_2, and many form minute colonies on agar. While some strains contain Lancefield antigens A, C, F, or G, most have no Lancefield antigen. Likewise, not all of the β-hemolytic strains have Lancefield antigens, and not all strains with Lancefield antigens are β-hemolytic. Most group F organisms are in the *S. intermedius* group.[10] Antiphagocytic proteins are not produced. Guanidine/cytosine ratios range from 37–43 mol percent. The cell walls usually contain *N*-acetyl-galactosamine and rhamose.[1]

Criteria outlined by the Centers for Disease Control[9] suggest that β-hemolytic groups A, C, F, and G and nongroupable strains be classified as *S. anginosus,* nonhemolytic lactose-positive strains are *S. intermedius,* and lactose-negative strains are *S. constellatus.* It is recognized that the use of the term *S. milleri* connotes organisms that cross all of these groups and cause suppuration; hence this may be a clinically useful term even though the species is not officially accepted.[3,12–16]

PATHOGENICITY

While most of the viridans organisms have low invasive potential, the *S. intermedius* group has long been associated with the propensity to form abscesses. While these infections are not common, they are nonetheless dramatic and frequently life-threatening. The most common associations are dental abscess, brain abscess, liver and other intra-abdominal abscesses (especially periappendiceal or postsurgical), empyema and lung abscess, and skin and soft tissue infections. The virulence factors that separate these organisms from other streptococci have yet to be elucidated. A polysaccharide capsule may be associated with abscess formation,[17] but proteolytic enzymes such as those produced by *S. pyogenes* and antiphagocytic proteins (e.g., M protein) are not present. A 90 kD protein that suppresses lymphocyte and fibroblast proliferation has been identified from *S. intermedius,* but its role in virulence is unknown.[18]

NORMAL HABITAT

These streptococcal species are variably found as part of the normal oral flora, primarily in the gingival crevice and occasionally in dental plaque.[3] Since they do not produce extracellular polysaccharides, the mechanism of adherence probably differs from *S. mutans* and *S. sanguis*.[19] They are less commonly found in saliva or on the buccal mucosa or tongue.[1] They are also variably found in throat swabs, but it is unclear whether this represents "wash-down" from the oral cavity. In addition, the true prevalence is unknown since most authors recognize only the β-hemolytic isolates (especially groups C, F, and G).[7]

Studies of normal fecal flora show these organisms to be present in 16–67 percent of normal individuals, with a lesser frequency in children.[20] They have also been isolated from the normal appendix[21] and vaginal swabs. Isolation from urine specimens most likely represents vaginal contamination.[22,23]

CLINICAL MANIFESTATIONS

Dental Caries and Oral Infections

There is no specific evidence that associates the *S. intermedius* group with dental caries or periodondal disease.[19] The original isolate of *S. milleri* was from a dental abscess, and deeper endodontic and periapical infections are not uncommon. These streptococci may be isolated in mixed or pure culture from a variety of dental sites.[24]

Nasopharyngeal Infection

Streptococcus intermedius is occasionally isolated from the middle ear but is more commonly seen as a pathogen in acute and chronic sinusitis.[25] The association of these organisms with pharyngitis is controversial, and care must be taken to separate them from the large-zone β-hemolytic organisms of groups A, C, and G.[7,8]

Central Nervous System Infections

Streptococci have been isolated from up to 80 percent of patients with brain abscess, with up to 75 percent of these organisms belonging to the *S. intermedius* group. The finding of tiny streptococci in pairs or chains on direct observation of pus from brain abscesses is a common clinical occurrence. These organisms usually display the fastidious cultural characteristics of this group of streptococci. The most frequent predisposing factors are congenital heart disease, sinusitis, otitis media, lung or liver disease, and trauma; however, primary infection without an obvious focus may occur.[3,15,26] Subdural empyema occurs less commonly, and meningitis is rare. In all instances *S. intermedius* may be isolated in pure culture or mixed with anaerobes.

Intra-abdominal Infection and Liver Abscess

The most common intra-abdominal infections involve the liver, appendix, and postoperative situations, usually in mixed culture with bacteroides and other anaerobes. *S. intermedius* group organisms have been isolated from up to 80 percent of liver abscesses and 58 percent of appendiceal abscesses,[3] and it has been suggested that appendicitis associated with these organisms is more likely to result in suppurative complications.[21]

Pleuropulmonary Infections

"Microaerophilic" streptococci are frequent isolates from empyema, lung abscess, and aspiration pneumonia, usually in mixed culture as is seen in most other sites.[3]

Endocarditis

Organisms of the *S. intermedius* group account for between 3 and 15 percent of streptococcal isolates from patients with infective endocarditis.[3] Some authors have suggested that abscesses complicate endocarditis more commonly with these species.[14,26]; however, this has not been found by all.[27] The isolates from endocarditis and dental plaque are more frequently α- or nonhemolytic. Since these organisms lack extracellular polysaccharides, virulence factors such as fimbriae, which mediate attachment, have been postulated.

Miscellaneous Infections

While rare, other infections such as pericarditis, myocardial abscess, splenic abscess, pelvic abscess, osteomyelitis, and septic arthritis have been reported. Since there are occasional reviews of infections due to streptococci of groups C and G, it is difficult to discern which of those organisms are actually of the *S. intermedius* group; hence it is hoped that future reporting of infections due to these organisms will be by species and not by Lancefield group.

ANTIMICROBIAL THERAPY

Since sensitivity testing has not been standardized for fastidious CO_2-requiring streptococci, much of the data in the literature may be based on more rapidly growing strains. Most series report penicillin G minimum inhibitory concentrations (MICs) of <0.06 μg/ml, with rare strains resistant to >1.0 μg/ml. These organisms are usually also susceptible to other penicillins (ampicillin, semisynthetic penicillins), first- and second-generation cephalosporins, cefotaxime, erythromycin, clindamycin, chloramphenicol, and vancomycin, with variable sensitivity to tetracyclines.[3] Most strains are resistant to aminoglycosides; however, synergy may occur in vitro. Infections due to these streptococci have responded well to penicillin G and cephalosporins, with vancomycin, erythromycin, and clindamycin being effective in β-lactam–allergic patients. When abscesses are present, surgical or percutaneous tube drainage should be undertaken as adjunctive therapy.

REFERENCES

1. Colman G, Williams REO. Taxonomy of some human viridans streptococci. In: Wannamaker LW, Matsen JM, eds. Streptococci and Streptococcal Diseases: Recognition, Understanding, and Management. New York: Academic Press; 1972:281.
2. Facklam RR. Physiological differentiation of viridans streptococci. J Clin Microbiol. 1977;5:184.

3. Gossling J. Occurrence and pathogenicity of the *Streptococcus milleri* group. Rev Infect Dis. 1988;10:257–85.
4. Long PH, Bliss EA. Studies on minute hemolytic streptococci: Isolation and cultural characteristics of minute beta hemolytic streptococci. J Exp Med. 1934;60:619.
5. Yajko DM, Hadley WK. Support of the single species concept for *Streptococcus milleri* by DNA hybridization data. Eur J Clin Microbiol. 1985;4:355–6.
6. Ezaki T, Facklam R, Takeuchi N, et al. Genetic relatedness between the type strain of *Streptococcus anginosus* and minute-colony–forming beta-hemolytic streptococci carrying different Lancefield grouping antigens. J Syst Bacteriol. 1986;36:345–7.
7. Bucher C, Graevenitz AV. Differentiation in throat cultures of group C and G streptococci from streptococcus milleri with identical antigens. Eur J Microbiol. 1985;3:44–5.
8. Kipper-Balz R, Williams BL, Lutticken R, et al. Relatedness of *Streptococcus milleri* with *Streptococcus anginosus* and *Streptococcus constellatus*. Syst Appl Microbiol. 1984;5:494–500.
9. Facklam RR. The major differences in the American and British *Streptococcus* taxonomy schemes with special reference to *Streptococcus milleri*. Eur J Clin Microbiol 1984;3:91–3.
10. Libertin CR, Hermans PE, Washington II JA. Beta-hemolytic group F streptococcal bacteremia: A study and review of the literature. Rev Infect Dis. 1985;7:498–503.
11. Facklam RR, Bosley GS, Rhoden D, et al. Comparative evaluation of the API 20S and automicrobic gram-positive identification systems for non-beta-hemolytic streptococci and aerococci. J Clin Microbiol. 1985;21:535–41.
12. Ball LY, Parker MT. The cultural and biochemical characters of *Streptococcus milleri* strains isolated from human sources. J Hyg Camb. 1979;82:63–78.
13. Poole PM, Wilson G. Occurrence and cultural features of *Streptococcus milleri* in various body sites. J Clin Pathol. 1979;32:764–8.
14. Murray HW, Gross KC, Masur H, et al. Serious infections caused by *Streptococcus milleri*. Am J Med. 1978;64:759–64.
15. Shlaes DM, Lerner PI, Wolinsky E, et al. Infections due to Lancefield group F and related streptococci (*S. milleri, S. anginosus*). Medicine (Baltimore). 1981;60–197.
16. Van der Auwera P. Clinical significance of *Streptococcus milleri*. Eur J Clin Microbiol. 1985;4:386–90.
17. Brook I, Walker RI. Pathogenicity of anaerobic gram-positive cocci. Infect Immun. 1984;45:320–4.
18. Arala-Chaves MP, Ribeiro AS, Santarem MMG, et al. Strong mitogenic effect for murine B lymphocytes of an immunosuppressor substance released by *Streptococcus intermedius*. Infect Immun. 1986;54:543–8.
19. Gibbons RJ, Barghart S. Synthesis of extracellular dextran by cariogenic bacteria and its presence in human dental plaque. Arch Oral Biol. 1967;12:11.
20. Unsworth PF. The isolation of streptococci from human faeces. J Hyg Camb. 1980;85:153–164.
21. Poole PM, Wilson G. *Streptococcus milleri* in the appendix. J Clin Pathol 1977;30:937.
22. Ruoff KL, Kunz LJ. Identification of viridans streptococci isolated from clinical specimens. J Clin Microbiol. 1982;15:920–5.
23. Ruoff KL, Fishman JA, Calderwood SB, et al. Distribution and incidence of viridans streptococcal species in routine clinical specimens. Am J Clin Pathol. 1983;80:854–8.
24. Lewis MAO, MacFarlane TW, McGowan DA. Quantitative bacteriology of acute dento-alveolar abscesses. J Med Microbiol. 1986;21:101–4.
25. Evans FO Jr, Sydnor JB, Moore WEC, et al. Sinusitis of the maxillary antrum. N Engl J Med. 1975;293:735–9.
26. Parker MT, Ball LC. Streptococci and aerococci associated with systemic infection in man. J Med Microbiol. 1976;9:275.
27. Sussman JI, Baron EJ, Tenenbaum MJ, et al. Viridans streptococcal endocarditis: Clinical, microbiological, and echocardiographic correlations. J Infect Dis. 1986;154:597–603.

GRAM-POSITIVE BACILLI

183. CORYNEBACTERIUM DIPHTHERIAE

ROB ROY MacGREGOR

The name diphtheria was coined by Bretonneau from the Greek root for leather, describing the tough pharyngeal membrane that is the hallmark of the disease. The definition of diphtheria as a unique syndrome, the explanation of its pathogenesis, and its subsequent control parallel the development of the fields of pathology, bacteriology, and immunology. It has gone from a major health problem to a medical curiosity within recent memory, and stands as a shining example of what can be accomplished with vigorous public health control measures, based on the results of solid scientific investigation.

HISTORY

Although clinical descriptions of sore throat, membrane production, and death by suffocation appear in Hippocratic writings, epidemics of "throat distemper" are not described until the 16th century.[1] A major epidemic occurred in New England in the early 1700s, killing an estimated 2.5 percent of the total population, and up to one-third of all children. Thereafter, similar epidemics were reported at approximately 25 year intervals throughout the 18th and 19th centuries. Diphtheria was not clearly differentiated from other upper respiratory illnesses viewed collectively as "croup" or "distemper" until an epidemic in southern France in 1821 when the clinician-pathologist Pierre Bretonneau first described its unique clinical characteristics.

The first major advance occurred in 1883 when Klebs described chaining cocci and bacilli in microscopic sections of diphtheritic membranes. The following year, working in Koch's laboratory in Berlin, Friedrich Loeffler first isolated the diphtheria bacillus in pure culture, aided by a culture medium of his own design that is still used today. He then demonstrated that the organism could reproduce the disease in guinea pigs, thus fulfilling his mentor's postulates for proof that it was the etiologic agent for diphtheria.[2] Utilizing his special culture medium, he demonstrated that healthy individuals could carry the organism asymptomatically in their throats, thus establishing the carrier state as an important phenomenon in the maintenance and spread of the disease. He also noted that the organisms remained in the membrane without invading the tissues of the throat or more distant sites, and theorized that the neurologic and cardiologic manifestations of the disease were caused by a toxic substance elaborated by the organism. In 1888, Roux and Yersin, working at the Pasteur Institute, proved him correct by demonstrating that bacteria-free filtrates of cultures of diphtheria bacilli were able to kill guinea pigs. Two years later, von Behring, also working in Koch's laboratory, demonstrated that antiserum against the toxin was capable of protecting infected animals from death following infection. Then in 1894, after showing that horses were the most efficient animals at producing antitoxin, Roux reported that its administration reduced mortality from diphtheria among foundlings in Paris from 51 to 24 percent.

In 1913, Schick reported that an individual's local reaction to injection of toxin into the skin could be used to predict susceptibility to infection (a negative reaction indicated presence of protective antitoxin antibodies). At the same time, Theobald Smith and von Behring successfully immunized children with a toxin–antitoxin mixture, and in 1923, Ramon, at the Pasteur Institute, found that exposure of toxin to formalin and heat rendered it nontoxic to recipients while retaining the ability to induce an antibody response. The following year, clinical trials showed that injection of this "toxoid" induced a high level of protection among recipients. Problems of antigenic standardization, determining optimal dosage, frequency of administration, needs for boosting, etc. delayed the widespread use of immunization with toxoid, but between 1930 and 1945, most western countries established programs of childhood immunization. During the 1950s, Freeman, Groman, Barksdale, Pappenheimer, and others demonstrated that toxin production by *Corynebacterium diphtheriae* depended upon the presence of a lysogenic β-phage, and during the following decade, the mechanism by which toxin inhibited protein synthesis was elucidated.[3–5]

THE PATHOGEN

Corynebacterium diphtheriae is a nonsporulating, unencapsulated, nonmotile, pleomorphic gram-positive bacillus. Its name is derived from the Greek *korynee,* or club, referring to its clubbed ends, and *diphtheria,* meaning leather hide, for the characteristic leathery pharyngeal membrane that it provokes. When inoculated on the nutritionally inadequate medium devised by Loeffler, consisting of a heat-coagulated mixture of 75% serum and 25% broth, it initially outgrows other throat flora, and so plates should be inspected for growth at 12–18 hours. The characteristic metachromatic granules and "Chinese character" palisading morphology that differentiate it from other corynebacteria are displayed more prominently on smears taken from colonies grown on this medium when compared with direct smears from clinical specimens. Alternatively, selective media containing potassium tellurite inhibit many of the normal throat flora and identify any *C. diphtheriae* present as gray-black colonies containing reduced tellurite. The species is subdivided into three types—*gravis, intermedius,* and *mitis*—based upon differing colonial morphology on tellurite agar, fermentation reactions, and hemolytic potential.

Exotoxin production by *C. diphtheriae* depends on the presence of a lysogenic β-phage, which carries the gene encoding for toxin (tox^+).[3,5] In its lysogenic phase, the phage's circular DNA integrates into the host bacteria's genetic material as a prophage, with the result that the host cell now can express the gene necessary for synthesis of the polypeptide toxin. When induced by stimuli such as ultraviolet light, the phage enters a lytic cycle, destroying the host cell and releasing new β-phage. Strains of *C. diphtheriae* lacking lysogenic phage do not produce toxin, but they can be converted to toxigenicity in the laboratory by infection with the lysogenic tox^+ phage ("lysogenization"). Recent evidence has been found that such conversion also occurs in nature: culturing in Manchester, England, precipitated by discovery of a clinical case, revealed carriers of both toxigenic and nontoxigenic strains of *C. diphtheriae*. Electrophoretic gel patterns of restriction enzyme digests from both types were identical, suggesting that the resident strain of *C. diphtheriae* in the area was becoming converted by the introduction of a tox^+ β-phage. The origin of the phage was thought to be a child recently returned from Nigeria, carrying a lysogenic organism with a different restriction pattern.[6] Thus, even though the frequency of carriage of tox^+ lysogenic *C. diphtheriae* currently is very low in the West, there is an ongoing risk that resident nontoxigenic strains could become lysogenized by introduction of a β-phage-bearing strain from another part of the world. In addition to the tox^+ gene, significant toxin production requires that bacterial growth be slowed by exhaustion of iron in the environment. Toxigenicity of individual *C. diphtheriae* strains can be demonstrated in vitro by the development of an immunoprecipitin band on antitoxin-impregnated filter paper that has been laid over an agar culture of the organism in question (Elek's test).

EPIDEMIOLOGY

Humans are the only known reservoir for *C. diphtheriae*. The primary modes of spread are via airborne respiratory droplets and/or direct contact with either respiratory secretions or exudate from infected skin lesions. Fomites can play a role in transmission, and epidemics have been caused by contaminated milk. Most respiratory tract disease occurs in the colder months in temperate climates, associated with crowded indoor living conditions and hot dry air. Asymptomatic respiratory carriage is important in perpetuating both endemic and epidemic diphtheria, and immunization reduces an individual's likelihood of being a carrier. Current reservoirs for disease are obscure. In endemic conditions, 3–5 percent of healthy individuals may harbor the organism in their throats,[7] but in the West, where the disease has become very uncommon, isolation of the organism from healthy individuals has become extremely rare. Skin infection, once thought to be primarily a problem in tropical environments, has caused several recent epidemics in Europe and North America among alcoholics and other disadvantaged groups.[8,9] Thus skin carriage of *C. diphtheriae* can act as a silent reservoir for the organism, and it has been found that person-to-person spread from infected skin sites is more efficient than from the respiratory tract.[10,11]

The incidence and pattern of diphtheria in the western world has changed dramatically in the last 50–75 years. From 1921 to 1924, it was the leading cause of death among Canadian children aged 2–14. Since then, the incidence has decreased steadily (Fig. 1), to the point where diphtheria is a rare event. For example, 147,991 cases were reported in the United States in 1920 (151 cases/100,000 population), and 5 or less since 1980 (<0.002/100,000). Over the last 25 years, similar decreases have been seen in Europe.[12,13] The World Health Organization reports similar but less dramatic decreases in incidence worldwide, although the disease remains endemic in many parts of the Third World (with small epidemics globally).[14] Seventeen outbreaks of 15 or more cases occurred in the United States between 1959 and 1980, but there have been none since 1980. When it was common, diphtheria primarily affected children under 15 years of age, but recent epidemics have also involved unimmunized or poorly immunized adults, particularly the urban and rural poor. Minority racial groups have had attack rates 5–20 times higher than whites. Cases in the United States have been distributed primarily in the Southern and Pacific Northwest states, but sporadic cases have been reported throughout the country.[15] Although immunized individuals can still develop clinical diphtheria, prior immunization reduces the frequency and severity of disease: between 1959 and 1970 in the United States, two-thirds of reported cases had received no immunization, 13% more had had one to two doses of toxoid, and only 19 percent reported receiving three or more doses and could be considered fully immunized.[15] Disease was considered severe in 25 percent of unimmunized patients, vs. 6.3 percent of those fully immunized. Nineteen percent of unimmunized patients died, compared with 1.3 percent among those fully immunized; even partial immunization reduced morbidity and mortality by more than 50 percent. The relative distribution of biotypes isolated from cases shifted between the decades 1960–1970 and 1970–1980: during the earlier period, *mitis* was the predominant type (53 percent of isolates), with *gravis* next (27 percent); during the 1970s, *intermedius* became the most common type isolated, and *gravis* fell to 7 percent. Incidence of toxin production correlated with biotype: 98.9 percent of *intermedius* were toxigenic, compared with 84 percent of *gravis* and 34.1 percent of *mitis* strains.[15] In general, *mitis* strains cause less severe disease than do either *gravis* or *intermedius*.

The full explanation for the dramatic decrease in diphtheria's incidence is not evident. Rates began to fall well before the general utilization of toxoid, and epidemics have occurred even in highly immunized populations. Nonetheless, immunization programs have had a major impact: for example, a program in Toronto between 1926 and 1929 reduced the rate of clinical diphtheria in immunized children by 75 percent in comparison with unimmunized controls.[12] However, immunization with toxoid is generally thought only to attenuate the local and systemic effects of toxin without preventing local colonization with the organism. If so, carriage would be expected to remain high in the population, and epidemics should be an ongoing occurrence among the sizable proportion believed to be inadequately immunized. However, disease has become rare, and evidence points to an extremely low incidence of carrier state, despite serologic studies during the 1970s showing what are considered

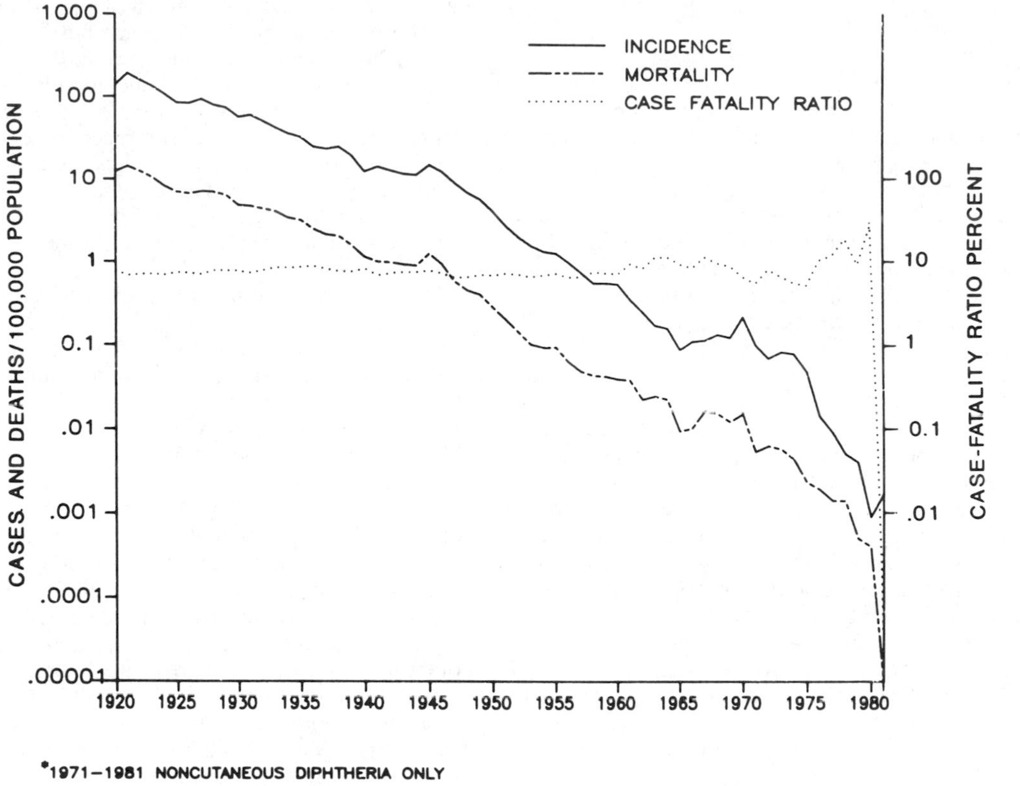

FIG. 1. Diphtheria annual incidence and mortality rates and case–fatality ratios of diphtheria in the United States, 1920–1981.

to be subprotective levels of serum antitoxin in 25 percent of children and 75 percent of adults tested in three cities in the United States.[16] Several factors may contribute to our current good fortune: first, although unproved, historical evidence suggests that diphtheria has occurred in cycles that include gaps of 100 years or more.[1] Second, organisms isolated from immunized individuals are less likely to be toxigenic than are those from unimmunized carriers (64 vs. 94 percent).[16] If toxin production confers no advantage to the organism in an immunized host, its mctabolic cost would put toxigenic organisms at a selective disadvantage, and so loss of this attribute might be predicted.[4] Experience in Rumania supports this hypothesis: 86 percent of surveillence cultures during 1955–1966 were toxigenic, and following an improved immunization program, the percentage dropped to only 7 percent by 1977.[17] Third, some experts believe that the local elaboration of toxin, in the absence of antibody, enhances an organism's ability to colonize. Immunization with toxoid could counteract this selective advantage of toxigenic strians. However, this mechanism cannot be the sole factor in explaining the low frequency of colonization with nontoxigenic strains. Fourth, some virulence factor(s) other than toxin production may exist. For example, in a recent outbreak in Sweden, investigators used genetic probes to demonstrate that all clinical cases were caused by a single strain, although several different toxigenic strains were present in the population.[18] Clearly, additional undefined factors are contributing to the current low rate of *C. diphtheriae* isolation in the United States and elsewhere.

PATHOGENESIS

Corynebacterium diphtheriae is not an invasive organism, ordinarily remaining in the superficial layers of the respiratory mucosa and skin lesions, where it can induce a mild inflammatory reaction in the local tissue. The major virulence of *C. diphtheriae* results from the action of its potent exotoxin, which inhibits protein synthesis in mammalian cells but not in bacteria. The 62,000 dalton polypeptide toxin is comprised of two segments: B, which binds to specific receptors on susceptible cells, and A, the active segment. Following proteolytic cleavage of the bound molecule, segment A enters the cell, where it catalyzes inactivation of the transfer RNA (tRNA) translocase, "elongation factor 2," present in eukaryotic cells but not in bacteria. Loss of this enzyme prevents the interaction of messenger RNA and tRNA stopping further addition of amino acids to developing polypeptide chains[19] (Fig. 2). The toxin affects all cells in the body, but the most prominent effects are on the heart (myocarditis), nerves (demyelination), and kidneys (tubular necrosis). Diphtheria toxin is extremely potent: a single molecule can stop protein synthesis in a cell within several hours, and 0.1 μg/kg will kill susceptible animals.

Within the first few days of respiratory tract infection, toxin elaborated locally induces a dense necrotic coagulum composed of fibrin, leukocytes, erythrocytes, dead respiratory epithelial cells, and organisms (Fig. 3). Removal of this adherent gray-brown "pseudomembrane" reveals a bleeding edematous submucosa. The membrane can be local (tonsillar, pharyngeal, nasal), or extend widely, forming a cast of the pharynx and tracheobronchial tree. The underlying soft tissue edema and cervical adenitis can be intense, and, particularly in the proportionally smaller airways of children, can cause respiratory embarrassment and a "bull neck" appearance. In both adults and children, a common cause of death is suffocation following aspiration of the membrane.

CLINICAL MANIFESTATIONS

Symptoms of infection with *C. diphtheriae* occur locally in the respiratory tract and skin secondary to noninvasive infection

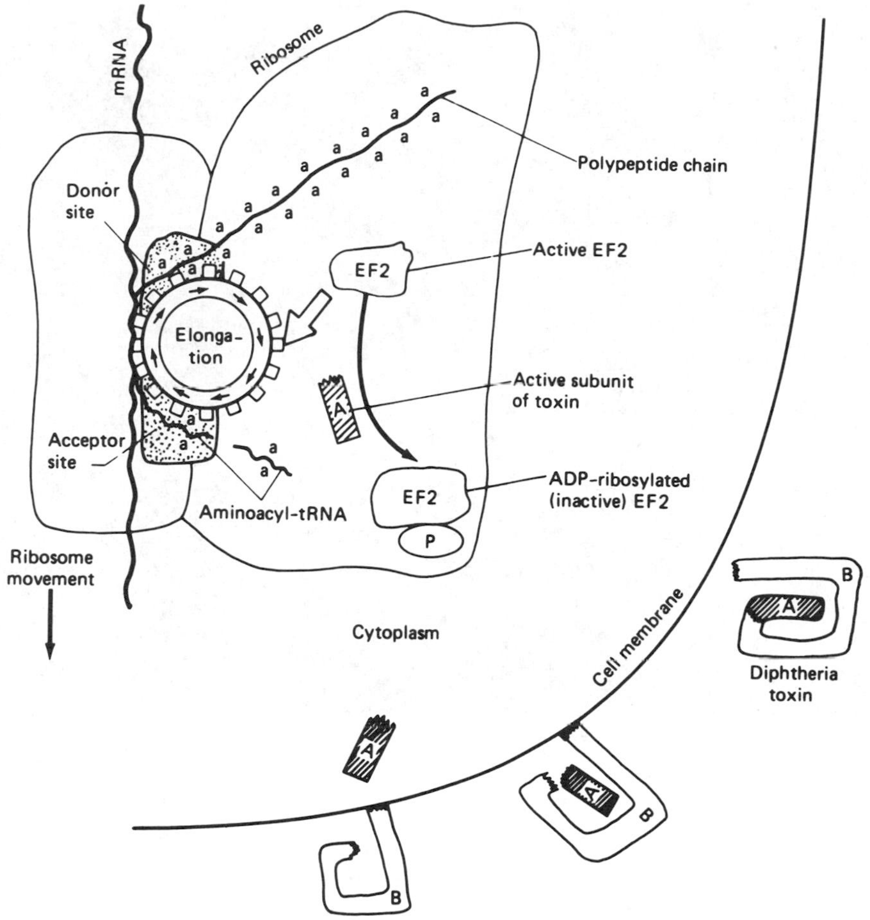

FIG. 2. Action of diphtheria toxin. The toxin-binding (B) portion attaches to the cell membrane, allowing the active (A) portion to dissociate and enter the cell. In the cell, active toxin catalyzes a reaction that ADP-ribosylates and thus inactivates elongation factor 2 (EF2). This factor is essential for ribosomal reactions at the acceptor and donor sites, which transfer triplet code from messenger RNA (mRNA) to amino acid sequences via transfer RNA (tRNA). Inactivation of EF2 stops building of the polypeptide chain.

of these two organs, and at distant sites secondary to absorption and dissemination of diphtheria toxin.

Respiratory Tract Diphtheria

Asymptomatic upper respiratory tract carriage of the organism occurs commonly in areas where diphtheria is endemic and is an important reservoir for maintenance and spread of the organism in a population. However, in the industrial western world, throat colonization has become exceedingly rare except in individuals associated with pockets of infection such as the inner city (homeless people) and rural poverty areas.

Following an incubation period averaging 2–4 days, local signs and symptoms of inflammation can develop at various sites within the respiratory tract.

Anterior Nasal. Infection limited to the anterior nares presents with a serosanguinous or seropurulent nasal discharge often associated with a subtle whitish mucosal membrane, particularly on the septum. The discharge can excite an erosive reaction on the external nares and upper lip, but symptoms generally are quite mild, and signs indicating toxin effects are rare.

Faucial. Including the posterior structures of the mouth and the proximal pharynx, this area is the most common site for clinical diphtheria. Onset is usually abrupt, with low-grade fever (rarely >103°F), malaise, sore throat, mild pharyngeal injection, and development of a membrane typically on one or both tonsils, with extension variously to involve the tonsilar pillars, uvula, soft palate, oropharynx, and nasopharynx (Fig. 4). The membrane initially appears white and glossy, but evolves into a dirty gray color, with patches of green or black necrosis. The extent of the membrane correlates with the severity of symptoms: localized tonsillar disease is often mild, but involvement of the posterior pharynx, soft palate, and periglottal areas is associated with profound malaise, weakness, prostration, cervical adenopathy, and swelling. The latter can distort the normal contour of the submental and cervical area, creating a "bull neck" appearance and causing respiratory stridor.

Laryngeal and Tracheobronchial. Pharyngeal infection may spread downward into the larynx, or occasionally the disease may begin there. Symptoms then include hoarseness, dyspnea, respiratory stridor, and a brassy cough. Edema and membrane involving the trachea and bronchi can embarrass respiration further, and a child so afflicted will appear anxious and cyanotic, use accessory muscles of respiration, and demonstrate inspiratory retractions of intercostal, supraclavicular, and substernal tissues. If this state is not relieved promptly by intubation and mechanical removal of membrane, patients become exhausted and die.

Systemic complications are due to diphtheria toxin, which, although toxic to all tissues, has its most striking effects on the heart and nervous system.

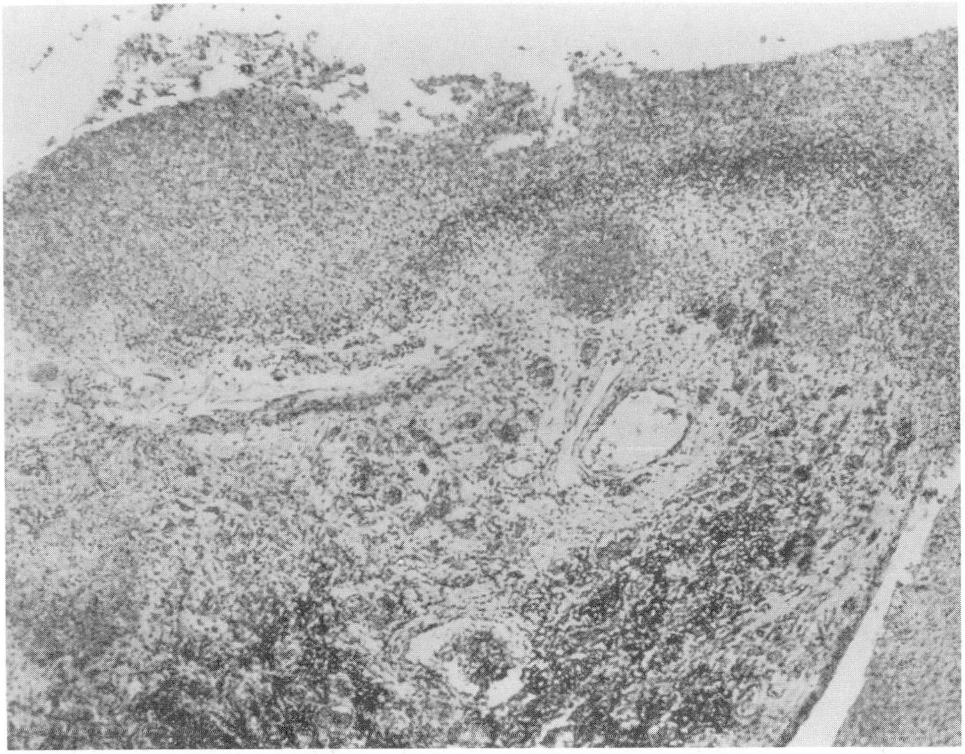

FIG. 3. Diphtheria involving a pharyngeal tonsil. The membrane–tissue junction is clearly marked by intense cellular infiltration. (From Moore,[43] with permission.)

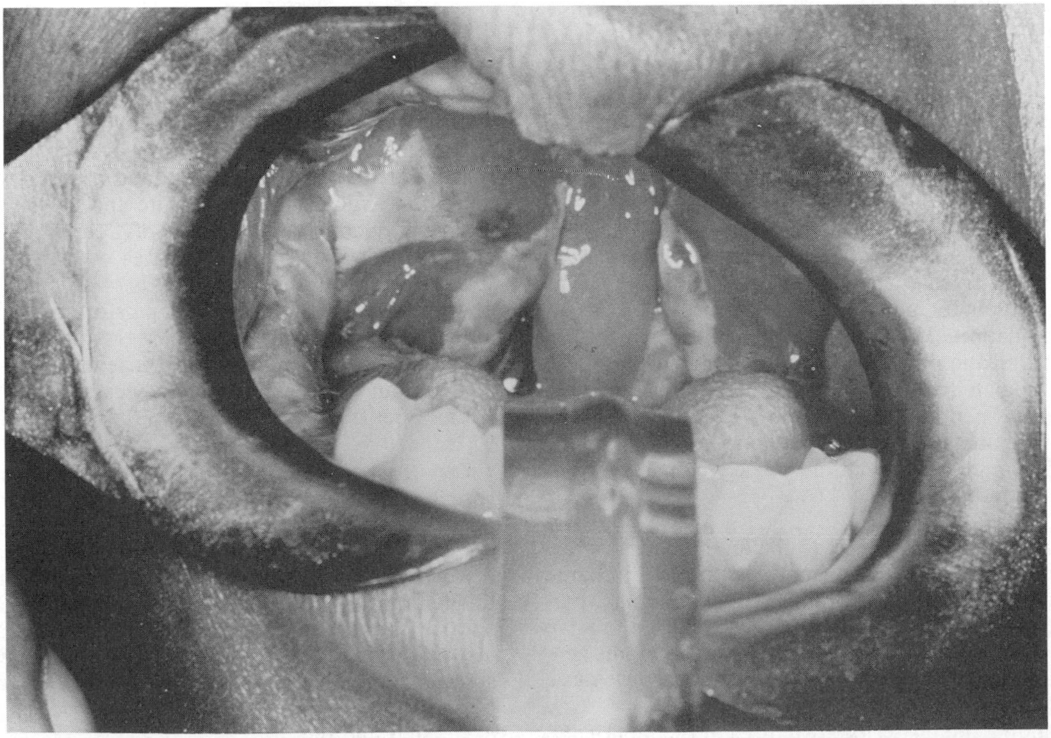

FIG. 4. Pharynx of a 39-year-old woman with bacteriologically confirmed diphtheria. Photograph taken 4 days after the onset of fever, malaise, and sore throat. Hemorrhage due to removal of the membrane by swabbing appears as dark area on the left.

CARDIAC TOXICITY. Subtle evidence of myocarditis can be detected in as many as two-thirds of patients, but 10–25 percent will develop clinical cardiac dysfunction, with the risk to an individual patient correlating directly with the extent and severity of local disease.[20,21] Characteristically, the first evidence of cardiac toxicity occurs after 1–2 weeks of illness, often when the local oropharyngeal disease is improving. Changes in electrocardiograph (ECG) pattern, particularly ST-T wave changes and first-degree heart block, can progress to more severe forms of block, atrioventricular (AV) dissociation, and other arrhythmias, which carry an ominous prognosis. Clinically, myocarditis can present acutely with congestive failure and circulatory collapse, or more insidiously with progressive dyspnea, weakness, diminished heart sounds, cardiac dilatation, and gallop rhythm. Because patients without clinical evidence of myocarditis may have significant electrical changes, it is important to monitor their cardiograms routinely. Elevations of serum AST concentration closely parallel the intensity of myocarditis, and so may be used to monitor its course. From a prognostic standpoint, patients with ECG changes of myocarditis have a mortality rate three to four times higher than those with normal tracings. In particular, AV and left bundle branch blocks carry a mortality rate of 60–90 percent. Patients with prolonged P-R interval and minor T-wave changes generally do well, and these abnormalities ordinarily resolve with time. Patients with bundle–branch blocks and complete AV dissociation have a much higher incidence of death, and survivors may be left with permanent conduction defects.[22]

NEUROLOGIC TOXICITY. This complication is also proportional to the severity of the primary infection: mild disease only occasionally produces neurotoxicity, but up to three-fourths of patients with severe disease can develop neuropathy. Within the first few days of disease, local paralysis of the soft palate and posterior pharyngeal wall occurs commonly, manifested by regurgitation of swallowed fluids through the nose. Thereafter, cranial neuropathies causing oculomotor and ciliary paralysis are also common, and dysfunction of facial, pharyngeal, or laryngeal nerves, although rare, can contribute to the risk of aspiration. Peripheral neuritis develops later, from 10 days to 3 months after the onset of disease in the throat.[23] Principally a motor defect, it begins with proximal muscle groups in the extremities and extends distally, particularly affecting the dorsiflexors of the feet. Dysfunction varies from mild weakness with diminished tendon reflexes to total paralysis. Occasionally motor nerves of the trunk, neck, and upper extremity are involved, as are sensory nerves, resulting in a glove-and-stocking neuropathy. Microscopic examination of affected nerves shows degeneration of myelin sheaths and axon cylinders. Although slow, total resolution of all diphtheritic nerve damage is the rule.

Several excellent clinical descriptions of endemic and epidemic diphtheria in the United States indicate that both the frequency of various symptoms and the severity of disease are inversely proportional to the patient's immunization history.[23–27] Roughly one-half of these reported cases were categorized as mild, often without a membrane. Mortality rates vary from 3.5 to 12 percent, and have not changed in the last 50 years. Rates are highest in the very young and very old. Most deaths occur in the first 3–4 days, from asphyxia or myocarditis; fatal outcome is rare in a fully immunized individual. Sore throat (85–90 percent), fever (50–85 percent), and dysphagia (26–40 percent) are the most common symptoms, and membranes and cervical adenopathy are seen in approximately one-half of the cases. The frequency of complications such as myocarditis and neuritis is directly related to the time between onset of symptoms and administration of antitoxin, and to the extent of membrane formation.

Cutaneous Diphtheria

It has long been recognized that, particularly in the tropics, *C. diphtheriae* can cause clinical skin infections characterized by chronic nonhealing ulcers with a dirty gray membrane and often associated with *Staphylococcus aureus* and group A streptococci. More recently, the significance of this infection in the United States has been emphasized by several outbreaks among alcoholic homeless men and impoverished groups such as native Americans.[9–11] The presentation is indolent and nonprogressive, and is only rarely associated with signs of intoxication. Nonetheless, these infections can induce high antitoxin levels, and thus appear to act as natural immunizing events.[28,29] They also serve as a reservoir for the organism under conditions of both endemic and epidemic respiratory tract diphtheria: cutaneous sites of *C. diphtheriae* have been shown both to contaminate the inanimate environment and to induce throat infections more efficiently than does pharyngeal colonization, and bacterial shedding from cutaneous infections continues longer than from the respiratory tract.[10,11,30] Despite these facts, the clinical significance of isolating the organism from an individual skin lesion is often unclear. Most lesions from which *C. diphtheriae* is isolated are indistinguishable from other chronic dermatologic conditions (eczema, psoriasis, etc.), and only about 15 percent fit the classic description of diphtheritic ulcers given above.[31] Moreover, because *C. diphtheriae* is usually isolated in association with other known skin pathogens, and because the ulcers do not respond to antitoxin therapy, there is debate as to whether or not the isolates are actually causing clinical disease. By 1975, cutaneous diphtheria accounted for 56 percent of total *C. diphtheriae* isolates reported in the United States, and, in 1980, the US Centers for Disease Control (CDC), in an effort to focus attention on respiratory tract diphtheria, removed skin isolates from its yearly diphtheria statistics.

Other Sites

On rare occasions, clinical infection with *C. diphtheriae* can be seen in other sites such as the ear, conjunctivae, or vagina.

DIAGNOSIS

The clinical outcome in diphtheria is improved by the prompt initiation of treatment. Therefore, physicians must act on a presumptive diagnosis, based on several clinical clues: (*1*) mildly painful tonsillitis and/or pharyngitis with associated membrane, especially if the membrane extends to the uvula and soft palate; (*2*) adenopathy and cervical swelling, especially if associated with membranous pharyngitis and signs of systemic toxicity; (*3*) hoarseness and stridor; (*4*) palatal paralysis; (*5*) serosanguinous nasal discharge with associated mucosal membrane; and (*6*) temperature elevation rarely in excess of 103°F. Moderate elevation of white blood cell count and transient proteinuria are common, but nonspecific. In former times when the disease was common, skilled practitioners could often make the diagnosis on examination of methylene blue-stained smears of the membrane or of throat swabs. Currently, rapid diagnosis is sometimes possible with immunofluorescent staining of 4-hour cultures, but definitive identification of *C. diphtheriae* is made on the basis of colonial morphology, microscopic appearance, and fermentation reactions of isolates from bits of membrane or submembrane swabs cultured on Loeffler's or tellurite selective media. Because routine methods of throat culture do not promote the isolation and identification of *C. diphtheriae*, the laboratory must be alerted to use selective media when the disease is suspected. Isolates can be tested for toxin production by inoculation of guinea pigs with and without antitoxin protection, by tissue culture, and by immunodiffusion with agar cultures overlaid with antitoxin-containing strips (Elek plate method).

The differential diagnosis includes faucial mononucleosis, streptococcal or viral pharyngitis and tonsilitis, Vincent's angina, and acute epiglotitis. The membrane of mononucleosis characteristically remains on the tonsils, rarely loses its creamy white appearance, and does not cause bleeding when removed. Streptococcal infection usually produces a more intense local pharyngitis, higher fever, and more pronounced dysphagia. Vincent's angina often involves the gums, and gram stain of the exudate from the necrotic ulcerative pharyngeal lesions shows characteristic fusobacteria and spirochetes. Bacterial epiglotitis secondary to *Haemophilus influenzae* often develops more acutely, and indirect laryngoscopy shows a bright red epiglottis without associated membrane.

TREATMENT

Diphtheria antitoxin (DAT), hyperimmune antiserum produced in horses, has been the cornerstone of therapy for diphtheria since it was first shown to reduce mortality from 7 to 2.5 percent in a controlled trial published in 1898. The antibodies only neutralize toxin before its entry into cells, and so it is critical that DAT be administered as soon as a presumptive diagnosis has been made. The degree of protection is inversely related to the duration of clinical illness preceeding its administration.[24] Although the minimum therapeutic dose has never been determined, traditional (empirical) dosage recommendations assume that the duration of disease and extent of membrane formation roughly indicate the patient's toxin burden. The Committee on Infectious Diseases of the American Academy of Pediatrics recommends 20,000 to 40,000 units of antitoxin for pharyngeal or laryngeal disease of 48 hours' duration; 40,000–60,000 units for nasopharyngeal lesions; and 80,000–100,000 units for extensive disease of 3 or more days' duration and for anyone with brawny swelling of the neck.[32] It recommends administration by intravenous infusion over 60 minutes to inactivate toxin as rapidly as possible, but other experts suggest intramuscular injection of antitoxin for moderate disease, and combined intramuscular/intravenous administration for severe disease. Repeated injections are of no additional benefit. Because up to 10 percent of individuals may show some hypersensitivity to horse protein, even very sick patients must be questioned first concerning known allergy and tested with a 1:10 dilution of DAT instilled onto the conjunctiva or a 1:10–1:100 dilution injected intracutaneously, with epinephrine available for immediate administration. If an immediate reaction occurs, the patient should be desensitized with progressively higher doses of antiserum. The incidence of serum sickness of approximately 10 percent is acceptable in light of the pronounced reduction in mortality effected by antitoxin administration.

Antibiotic therapy, by killing the organism, has three benefits: (*1*) termination of toxin production; (*2*) amelioration of the local infection; and (*3*) prevention of spread of the organism to uninfected contacts. Although several antibiotics, including penicillin, erythromycin, clindamycin, rifampin, and tetracycline, are effective, only penicillin and erythromycin are generally recommended. Intramuscular administration of procaine penicillin G (300,000 units for patients weighing <20 lb., 600,000 units for those over 20 lbs.) at 12-hour intervals is recommended until the patient is able to swallow comfortably, when oral penicillin V (125–250 mg four times a day) or erythromycin estolate or succinate (125–500 mg four times daily) may be substituted for a recommended total treatment period of 14 days. Both drugs are equally effective in resolving fever and local symptoms, and in time to disappearance of membrane. Because erythromycin is marginally superior to penicillin in eradicating the carrier state, some authorities prefer it for initial treatment, despite a significant incidence of thrombophlebitis when it is given intravenously, and of gastrointestinal irritation when given orally. Patients should be maintained in strict isolation throughout therapy and, following therapy, should have three consecutive negative cultures at 24-hour intervals to document eradication of the organism.[32] The carrier state has a slow rate of spontaneous resolution (12 percent after 1 month in one study)[33] and so should be treated to prevent spread of infection. Erythromycin orally for 7 days is the treatment of choice because of several reports demonstrating its greater efficacy in comparison with penicillin.[26,27] However, the issue is clouded by a report showing that 21 percent of cultures taken 2 weeks after completion of erythromycin treatment were again positive for *C. diphtheriae*.[34] Therefore, it is necessary to obtain cultures at least 2 weeks after completing therapy to assure eradication of the organism. A single intramuscular dose of benzathine penicillin G (600,000–1,200,000 units) is prudent when compliance with oral therapy is uncertain.

Supportive care is also important. Bed rest is recommended during the acute phase of illness, but proof of its benefit once the patient feels able to ambulate is lacking. Early in the disease, respiratory and cardiac complications are the biggest threats: airway obstruction can result from aspiration of dislodged pharyngeal membrane, its direct extension into the larynx, or from external compression by enlarged nodes and edema. For this reason, many experts recommend tracheostomy or intubation as an early measure, particularly when the larynx is involved, thereby providing access for mechanical removal of tracheobronchial membranes and avoiding the risk of sudden asphyxia. Vigilance must be maintained to detect the development of primary or secondary bacterial pneumonia. Cardiac complications can be minimized by close electrocardiographic monitoring and the prompt initiation of electrical pacing for conduction disturbances, drugs for arrhythmias, or digitalis for heart failure. Physical therapy should preserve range of motion in paretic extremities while awaiting return of neurologic function. A recent study has shown that treatment of acute diphtheria with prednisone did not reduce the incidence of carditis or neuritis.[35]

PREVENTION

The major manifestations of diphtheria can be prevented in individual patients by immunization with formalin-inactivated toxin. Therefore, recent documentation of inadequate levels of antitoxin in a large proportion of the adult population in North America and Western Europe has caused great concern that a toxigenic strain introduced into these populations could cause a major outbreak of disease. Serum antitoxin levels can be measured by toxin neutralization tests in rabbit skin, in Vero cell culture, or by hemagglutination, with roughly equivalent results. Concentrations of 0.1–0.01 IU (international units) generally are thought to confer protection. For example, data from a recent outbreak showed that 90 percent of clinical cases had antitoxin levels below 0.01 IU/ml, whereas 92 percent of asymptomatic carriers had titers above 0.1 IU/ml.[36] Following immunization, antitoxin levels decline slowly over time so that as many as 50 percent of individuals over age 60 have serum titers below 0.01 IU/ml.[37,38] For this reason, booster doses of toxoid should be administered at 10-year intervals, to maintain antitoxin levels in the protective range.

Recommendations from the Immunization Practices Advisory Committee, published by CDC in 1985[39] are as follows.

For children from 6 weeks to 7 years of age: three 0.5 ml intramuscular injections of diphtheria-pertussis-tetanus (DPT) vaccine should be given at 4–8-week intervals, beginning at 6–8 weeks of age, followed by a fourth dose 6–12 months after the third.

For persons 7 years or more of age: 0.5 ml Td (toxoid—adult) is given twice at a 4–8-week interval, with a third dose 6–12 months later. Because the pertussis component of DPT is responsible for most of its side effects, and the risk of pertussis is much less after age 6, that component of the vaccine is omitted. Moreover, because subjects over age 7 have a higher incidence of local and systemic reactions to the concentration of diphtheria toxoid in pediatric DPT vaccine (7–25 limit flocculation [Lf] units) and because a lower dose of toxoid has been shown to induce protective levels of antitoxin,[40] the Td formulation of vaccine contains a maximum concentration of 2 Lf units of diphtheria toxoid. If the recommended sequence of primary immunizations is interrupted, normal levels of immunity can be achieved simply by administering the remaining doses without need to restart the series.

Booster immunizations: children who have completed their primary immunization before age 4 should receive a booster dose of DPT at the time of school entry. Persons above 7 years of age should receive booster immunization with Td at 10-year intervals. As a help to memory, this should be done at decade or mid-decade intervals (e.g., ages 15, 25, 35, etc., or 20, 30, 40, etc.). It should be noted that, although the recommended booster dose of 1.5–2.0 Lf units will increase antitoxin levels to above 0.01 IU in 90–100 percent of previously immunized individuals,[41,42] some authorities have recommended using 5 Lf units, because antitoxin levels remain above 0.01 IU/ml for a longer period than with 2 Lf units.[41]

Patients should receive toxoid immunization in the convalescent stage of their disease because clinical infection does not always induce adequate levels of antitoxin. Close contacts whose immunization status is incomplete or unclear should promptly receive a dose of toxoid appropriate for their age, and complete the proper series of immunizations. In addition, they should receive prophylactic treatment with erythromycin or penicillin, pending the results of pretreatment cultures. Given these preventive measures, the prophylactic use of antitoxin is considered unwarranted.

REFERENCES

1. English PC. Diphtheria and theories of infectious disease: centennial appreciation of the critical role of diphtheria in the history of medicine. Pediatrics. 1985;76:1–9.
2. Loeffler F. Untersuchugen uber die Bedeutung der Mikroorganismen fur die Entstehung der Diphtherie. Mitt Kaiserlichen Gesundheitsamt. 1884;2:421–99.
3. Groman NB. Conversion by corynephages and its role in the natural history of diphtheria. J Hyg (Camb). 1984;93:405–17.
4. Pappenheimer AM. Diphtheria studies on the biology of an infectious disease. Harvey Lect. 1982;76:45–73.
5. Freeman VJ. Studies on the virulence of bacteriophage-infected strains of *Corynebacterium diphtheriae*. J Bacteriol. 1951;61:675–88.
6. Pappenheimer AM, Murphy JR. Studies on the molecular epidemiology of diphtheria. Lancet. 1983;ii:923–6.
7. Kalapothaki V, Sapounas T, Xirouchaki E, et al. Prevalence of diphtheria carriers in a population with disappearing clinical diphtheria. Infection. 1984;12:387–9.
8. Heath CW, Zusman J. An outbreak of diphtheria among skid-row men. N Engl J Med. 1962;267:809–12.
9. Pedersen AHB, Spearman J, Tronca E, et al. Diphtheria on skid road, Seattle, Washington, 1972–75. Public Health Rep. 1977;92:336–42.
10. Koopman JS, Campbell J. The role of cutaneous diphtheria infections in a diphtheria epidemic. J Infect Dis. 1975;131:239–44.
11. Belsey MA, Sinclair M, Roder MR, et al. *Corynebacterium diphtheriae* skin infections in Alabama and Louisiana. N Engl J Med. 1969;280:135–41.
12. Dixon JMS. Diphtheria in North America. J Hyg (Camb). 1984;93:419–32.
13. Kwantes W. Diphtheria in Europe. J Hyg (Camb). 1984;93:433–7.
14. World Health Organization. Reported Annual Incidence of Diphtheria, Measles, Pertussis, Poliomyelitis, Tetanus and Tuberculosis, 1974–1984. Geneva: World Health Organization; 1986.
15. Brooks GF, Bennett JV, Feldman RA. Diphtheria in the United States, 1959–1970. J Infect Dis. 1974;129:172–8.
16. Chen RT, Broome CV, Weinstein RA, et al. Diphtheria in the United States, 1971–81. Am J Public Health. 1985;75:1393–7.
17. Saragea A, Maximescu P, Meiter E. *Corynebacterium diphtheriae*: microbiological methods used in clinical and epidemiological investigations. Methods Microbiol. 1979;13:62–176.
18. Rappuoli R, Perugini M, Falsen E. Molecular epidemiology of the 1984–86 outbreak of diphtheria in Sweden. N Engl J Med. 1988;318:12–14.
19. Pappenheimer AM. The diphtheria bacillus and its toxin: a model system. J Hyg (Camb). 1984;93:397–440.
20. Boyer NH, Weinstein L. Diphtheritic myocarditis. N Engl J Med. 1948;239:913.
21. Morgan BC. Cardiac complications of diphtheria. Pediatrics. 1963;32:549–57.
22. Ledbetter MK, Cannon AB, Costa AF. The electrocardiogram in diphtheritic myocarditis. Am Heart J. 1964;68:599–611.
23. Dobie RA, Tobey DN. Clinical features of diphtheria in the respiratory tract. JAMA. 1979;242:2197–2201.
24. Naiditch MJ, Bower AG. Diphtheria. A study of 1433 cases observed during a ten year period at the Los Angeles County Hospital. Am J Med. 1954;17:229–45.
25. Kallick CA, Brooks GF, Dover AS, et al. A diphtheria outbreak in Chicago. Illinois Med J. 1970;137:505–12.
26. Zalma VM, Older JJ, Brooks GF. The Austin, Texas, diphtheria outbreak. JAMA. 1970;211:2125–9.
27. McCloskey RV, Eller JJ, Green M, et al. The 1970 epidemic of diphtheria in San Antonio. Ann Intern Med. 1971;75:495–503.
28. Bray JP, Burt EG, Potter EV, et al. Epidemic diphtheria and skin infections in Trinidad. J Infect Dis. 1972;126:34–40.
29. Hewlett EL. Selective primary health care: strategies for control of disease in the developing world. XVIII. Pertussis and diphtheria. Rev Infect Dis. 1985;7:426–33.
30. Belsey MA, LeBlanc DR. Skin infections and the epidemiology of diphtheria: acquisition and persistence of *C. diphtheriae* infections. Am J Epidemiol. 1975;102:179–84.
31. Jellard CH. Diphtheria infection in Northwest Canada, 1969, 1970, and 1971. J Hyg. 1972;70:503–10.
32. Diphtheria. In: Report of the Committee on Infectious Diseases. 19th ed. Evanston: American Academy of Pediatrics; 1982:71–74.
33. Kiselev VI. The use of various antibiotic combinations in the control of diphtheria bacilli carrier statc. Antibiotiki. 1964;9:361–3.
34. Miller LW, Bickham S. Jones WL, et al. Diphtheria carriers and the effect of erythromycin therapy. Antimicrob Agents Chemother. 1974;6:166–9.
35. Thisyakorn USA, Wongvanich J, Kumpeng V. Failure of corticosteroid therapy to prevent diphtheritic myocarditis or neuritis. Pediatr Infect Dis. 1984;3:126–8.
36. Bjorkholm B, Bottiger M, Christenson B, et al. Antitoxin antibody levels and the outcome of illness during an outbreak of diphtheria among alcoholics. Scand J Infect Dis. 1986;18:235–9.
37. Millian SJ, Cherubin CE, Sherwin R, et al. A serologic survey of tetanus and diphtheria immunity in New York City. Arch Environ Health. 1967;15:776–81.
38. Kjeldsen K, Simonsen O, Heron I. Immunity against diphtheria 25–30 years after primary vaccination in childhood. Lancet. 1985;i:900–2.
39. Diphtheria, tetanus, and pertussis: guidelines for vaccine prophylaxis and other preventive measures. JAMA. 1985;254:895–900; 1009–16.
40. Myers MG, Beckman CW, Vosdingh RA, et al. Primary immunization with tetanus and diphtheria toxoids. JAMA. 1982;248:2478–80.
41. Simonsen O, Klaerke M, Klaerke A, et al. Revaccination of adults against diphtheria II: combined diphtheria and tetanus revaccination with different doses of diphtheria toxoid 20 years after primary vaccination. Acta Pathol Microbiol Immunol Scand [C]. 1986;94:219–25.
42. Ruben RL, Nagel J, Fireman P. Antitoxin responses in the elderly to tetanus-diphtheria immunization. Am J Epidemiol. 1978;108:145–9.
43. Moore RA. A Textbook of Pathology. Philadelphia: WB Saunders; 1944.

184. OTHER CORYNEBACTERIA

ARTHUR E. BROWN

In 1896 Lehmann and Neumann proposed that the bacteria morphologically resembling the diphtheria bacillus be incorporated with it into the genus *Corynebacterium*.[1] These nondiphtheria corynebacteria have since been referred to as "diphtheroids" and "coryneforms" and have, in the past, been considered "colonizers" and contaminants. Barksdale referred to the process of lumping these various organisms together on the basis of morphology as "coryneformity."[2] After decades of confusion about their clinical significance, nondiphtheria corynebacteria have begun to emerge as important pathogens. Noteworthy are the increased numbers of opportunistic infections due to nondiphtheria corynebacteria as the survival of severely immunocompromised patients increases. This is contrasted with the decreasing numbers of reported diphtheria cases from 435 in 1970 to 5 in 1981.[3] Because of both increased interest and improved microbiologic techniques, nondiphtheria corynebacteria have been recognized to be the cause of a number of human diseases and are less likely to be dismissed as culture contaminants.

By 1982, four reviews of infections in humans had been published.[4–7] The latter review[7] and a report concerning prosthetic valve endocarditis[8] attempted to determine whether certain species of corynebacteria were associated with specific disease syndromes. Nondiphtheria corynebacteria have been known to cause life-threatening disease. These organisms have caused bacteremia, endocarditis on both prosthetic and native valves, ventriculojugular shunt infection with shunt nephritis, brain abscess, osteomyelitis, empyema, and other serious infections.[4–8] Some species tend to occur with a characteristic clinical syndrome (Table 1).

MICROBIOLOGY

Corynebacteria (from the Greek *koryne*, meaning club, and *bacterion*, little rod) are gram-positive, catalase-positive, aerobic or facultatively anaerobic, asporogenous rods that are usually nonmotile. The cell wall of some species is weaker at the ends, which allows the organism to assume a club shape. During cell division, the daughter cells can remain attached on one side to form L's and V's. The arrangement and cuneiform shape of these cells suggests "Chinese characters." A wide variety of colonial types are found within the genus. Some are small and α-hemolytic and resemble lactobacilli; some are relatively large and white and resemble yeasts. Among the reasons for the difficulty in speciating these organisms are that many require special growth media such as Loeffler or Tinsdale medium or a tellurite plate, most have highly variable biochemical characteristics often requiring supplemental media for detection, and some grow quite slowly. Because of these difficulties and the confusion regarding the taxonomic status of many species that resemble the genus *Corynebacterium*, these organisms have not always been appreciated as pathogens of human disease.[7,9]

SPECIFIC PATHOGENIC CORYNEBACTERIA

Corynebacterium ulcerans

In 1926 Gilbert and Stewart first isolated and named *C. ulcerans* during an investigation of a diphtheria-like illness.[7] Subsequent studies established its pathogenicity and helped to determine the nature of its toxins. Usually a commensal in horses and cattle, *C. ulcerans* causes mastitis in cows and has been isolated from cow's milk. Human infection tends to occur in the summer months among rural populations exposed to domestic livestock, especially cattle. There is no evidence for person-to-person transmission.[7]

Microscopically, the organism is pleomorphic; few metachromatic granules are seen. *Corynebacterium ulcerans* grows well on Loeffler and Tinsdale media and tellurite agar. On blood agar the colonies are somewhat larger and more opaque than are those of *C. diphtheriae* and are generally surrounded by a narrow zone of hemolysis. On Tinsdale medium the brownish black colonies with distinct halos cannot be distinguished from *C. diphtheriae* colonies. *Corynebacterium ulcerans* is urease-positive and nitrate-negative and ferments glucose, maltose, trehalose (slowly), and starch in peptone broth. Liquifaction of gelatin occurs at room temperature.[7,9] Many strains produce the diphtheria toxin.[10] Independent of diphtheria toxin production, some strains produce the dermonecrotic toxin.

Nearly all human isolates of *C. ulcerans* have been cultured from a respiratory site—primarily the throat in asymptomatic persons. However, an exudative pharyngitis and a diphtheria-like disease does occur, including the pseudomembrane formation and cardiac or neurologic manifestations.[11] In presumed toxigenic cases, diphtheria antitoxin should be administered. A presumed case of pneumonia,[12] an ulcer on the hand of a dairy farmer,[9] and a leg ulcer with cellulitis resulting from a puncture wound[13] are also reported to be due to *C. ulcerans*. Although the organism is sensitive to most antibacterial agents in vitro, clinical success with erythromycin would suggest that it is the antibiotic of choice.

Table 1. *Corynebacterium* Species with Characteristic Clinical Manifestations

Species	*Most Common Clinical Presentation*
C. ulcerans	Pharyngitis, diphtheria
C. pseudotuberculosis (C. Ovis)	Suppurative granulomatous lymphadenitis
C. haemolyticum (Arcanobacterium haemolyticum)	Pharyngitis or chronic skin ulcer
C. pseudodiphtheriticum (C. hofmannii)	Prosthetic valve endocarditis
Rhodococcus equi (C. equi)	Necrotizing pneumonia in the immunosuppressed host
C. minutissimum	Erythrasma
C. JK group	Nosocomial skin colonization leading to wound infection or septicemia

Corynebacterium pseudotuberculosis (Corynebacterium ovis)

Called the Preisz-Nocard bacillus in honor of the researchers who first isolated it in the early 1890s from the necrotic kidney of a sheep,[7] *C. pseudotuberculosis* has been the etiologic agent of infections in a variety of other animals including horses, cattle, goats, and deer. The dermonecrotic toxin produced by these organisms was studied by Nicolle and colleagues in 1912 and Hall and Stone in 1916.[7] *Corynebacterium pseudotuberculosis* is known among veterinarians to produce suppurative lymphadenitis, abscesses, and pneumonia in livestock, but the first report of human infection was not until 1966.[14]

Gram stains of direct smears may not show very many diphtheroid bacilli, and the microscopic morphology of in vitro growth may closely resemble that of streptococci, coccobacilli, or pleomorphic bacilli with metachromatic granules. Pinpoint colonies develop after incubation for 24 hours on sheep or horse blood agar. Biochemical reactions vary considerably. A simple test for phospholipase D serves to readily distinguish *C. pseudotuberculosis* and *C. ulcerans* from all other *Corynebacterium* species.[7,9]

Nearly all strains produce a dermonecrotic toxin, and selected isolates produce a diphtheria toxin.[10] There have not been any clinical cases of diphtheria attributed to infection with *C. pseudotuberculosis*.

All 12 reported episodes of human infection with *C. pseudotuberculosis*, except for a veterinary student who developed an eosinophilic pneumonia after exposure in the microbiology laboratory,[15] have been cases of suppurative granulomatous lymphadenitis in patients who had contact with animals or who handled offal and hides or drank raw milk.[16–18] All required a prolonged (several weeks) course of erythromycin or tetracycline and surgery for cure. There is preliminary evidence that contaminated fomites may play a role in the transmission of this disease among animals.[19] A preliminary study suggests that vaccination of lambs may provide these animals with immunologic protection.[20]

Corynebacterium pyogenes (Actinomyces pyogenes)

Corynebacterium pyogenes is a well-recognized animal pathogen that was initially described by Lucet in 1893.[7] This organism is both a commensal and a pathogen among domestic animals and causes a variety of suppurative infections in cattle, sheep, and pigs. Human infection, as rarely as it occurs, most likely represents a zoonosis.

It has been proposed that *C. pyogenes* be transferred to the genus *Actinomyces* as *A. pyogenes*. The organism is an aerotolerant anaerobe that is biochemically very similar to *A. bovis* except that it is hemolytic and actively proteolytic. Gram stains contain both coccal and diphtheroid forms, and on sheep blood agar, *C. pyogenes* produces pinpoint, whitish, β-hemolytic colonies. The hemolytic zone is usually twice the diameter of the colony. *Corynebacterium pyogenes* liquefies gelatin, peptonizes litmus milk, and ferments xylose, while *C. haemolyticum* does not. *Corynebacterium pyogenes* produces a potent soluble hemolysin.[7,9]

There have been a few cases of human infection including cutaneous infections complicated by septicemia, acute ulcerative vulvovaginitis, endocarditis, septic arthritis, osteomyelitis, pneumonia, and empyema reported. However, the specificity of the organism identified in most of these cases could not be distinguished.[6,7,9] Some of these cases may have been due to *C. haemolyticum* because of many shared phenotypic characteristics with *C. pyogenes*.[7] A yearly outbreak of leg ulcers among schoolchildren in rural Thailand is attributed to *C. pyogenes*.[21,22]

Corynebacterium haemolyticum (Arcanobacterium haemolyticum)

Corynebacterium haemolyticum was first isolated from infected American soldiers stationed in the South Pacific during World War II. While this organism closely resembled *C. pyogenes*, the authors felt that it was indeed distinct.[7] It has been accepted as a separate species, and it has now been proposed that *C. haemolyticum* be reclassified in a new genus, *Arcanobacterium*, comprising this single species, *A. haemolyticum*.[23] *Corynebacterium haemolyticum* is only rarely isolated from animals, and its primary epidemiologic reservoir appears to be human since the organism may be found in the pharynx and on the skin of healthy humans.

The microscopic morphology of cells recovered from Loeffler medium is similar to that of *C. diphtheriae*, but growth on tellurite agar is poor. Colonies on sheep blood agar are small with a narrow band of hemolysis. The organism is distinguished from *C. pyogenes* by its failure to hydrolyze gelatin, peptonize litmus milk, and ferment xylose. A dermonecrotic toxin is produced by some strains of *C. haemolyticum*.[7,9]

Infections due to *C. haemolyticum* have most commonly included pharyngitis[24–28] and chronic skin ulcers. The latter is not unlike the epidemic leg ulcers in Thailand that are caused by *C. pyogenes*.[22] Less frequent infections include vertebral osteomyelitis in a diabetic patient, septicemia with an undetermined focus of infection in one patient, brain abscess in two patients,[7] and endocarditis in two patients.[29,30]

While evidence supporting the pathogenic role of *C. haemolyticum* in pharyngitis has been strong,[27,28] this has been challenged by others.[31,32] Because of a lack of exclusion of viral and mycoplasmal pathogens, some of the cases have been questioned.[6,7,31] However, it is possible that *C. haemolyticum* may act opportunistically or synergistically with other infectious agents. The presentation may be similar to that of group A streptococcal infection. When it causes an acute pharyngitis or tonsillitis, with lymphadenitis in about 50 percent of cases, *C. haemolyticum* will be associated initially with a scarlatiniform rash in one-half of cases. The rash involves the trunk and proximal aspects of the extremities and usually will desquamate as the illness progresses. Systemic toxicity such as fever and leukocytosis are usually absent. *Corynebacterium haemolyticum* is sensitive to penicillin, erythromycin, and tetracycline—any of which can be used for therapy.

Corynebacterium pseudodiphtheriticum (Corynebacterium hofmannii)

Corynebacterium pseudodiphtheriticum was most likely first isolated from the throats of humans in 1888 by Von Hoffman. In 1896, Lehmann and Neumann made the detailed description of what was then called *Bacillus pseudodiphtheriticum*. Bergey et al. gave the current name of *C. pseudodiphtheriticum* in 1925.[7] This species of *Corynebacterium* does not produce toxins and is considered part of normal pharyngeal flora in humans.

Differing from other corynebacteria, these organisms generally do not demonstrate pleomorphism, and they take the Gram stain well and evenly. The bacterial cells often lie in parallel rows on smear preparations. *Corynebacterium pseudodiphtheriticum* grows well on all media, and the colonial morphology may closely resemble that of *C. diphtheriae*. While it is inert in carbohydrate fermentation tests, it hydrolyzes urea and reduces nitrates.[7,9]

Human infection had previously been limited to nine cases of endocarditis involving mainly prosthetic valves but rarely natural valves.[4–8,33–35] In 1982, *C. pseudodiphtheriticum* infection was described as the cause of malacoplakia involving the entire urinary tract in a patient with a transplanted kidney.[36] In 1983, *C. pseudodiphtheriticum* was reported as the cause of pneumonia in a man with systemic lupus erythematosus.[37] Since then a case of lung abscess due to *C. pseudodiphtheriticum* has been reported in a patient with the acquired immune deficiency syndrome (AIDS)-related complex.[38] Unfortunately, that patient's human immunodeficiency virus (HIV) serology was not reported. One case each of pneumonia,[39] suppurative lymphadenitis,[40] and a skin graft donor site infection,[41] all due to *C. diphtheriticum* in nonimmunocompromised hosts, have been reported. Antimicrobial sensitivities may vary; therefore, therapy should be guided by susceptibility testing.

Rhodococcus equi (Corynebacterium equi)

Rhodococcus equi (formerly *Corynebacterium equi*) has been recognized as an agent of bronchopneumonia in horses since it was first isolated from infected foals in 1923. Since then it has been found to be a pathogen causing sporadic infections in cattle, sheep, swine, and a cat.[7] Its soil habitat has been confirmed.[42] While *R. equi* is the cause of several important zoonoses, this organism has rarely been isolated from healthy persons. Almost all human infections have occurred in patients with animal exposure histories who have defects in cell-mediated immunity. Infections in both animals and humans are thought to be acquired through the respiratory route.

On Gram stain, the rods vary in length, from cocci to long, curved, clubbed forms. Large, irregular, highly mucoid, pale salmon-pink colonies grow well on ordinary media. *Rhodococcus equi* is differentiated from other pathogenic corynebacteria by its lack of ability to ferment carbohydrates or liquefy gelatin. Some investigators have found the organism to be acid-fast.[7,9]

Of the 17 reported cases of human *R. equi* infection, 16 involve the lung.[7,43–46a] All but the single case of lymphadenitis in a healthy 9-month-old boy[47] occurred in patients with diminished T-cell immunity. Many were receiving corticosteroids. Four were patients with AIDS.[44–46a] The clinical presentation is insidious with fatigue, fever, and a nonproductive cough. Chest radiographs demonstrated cavitary lesions in 11 of these 16 patients. In all instances but one,[46a] an invasive procedure such as bronchoscopy, thoracocentesis, or surgery was required to make the microbiologic diagnosis. The overall mortality was greater than 30 percent. Necrotizing pneumonia due to *R. equi* closely resembles that of tuberculosis or nocardiosis in that nodules and/or cavitation of the upper lobes occurs. Subcutaneous nodular lesions and brain abscess have also been described as in nocardiosis. Furthermore, relapses after short periods of antimicrobial therapy occur. The optimal duration of antimicrobial therapy and the exact role of surgery is uncertain; however, many weeks of antibiotic therapy have been required for cure, and surgical intervention has been applied successfully in most cases. The organism is sensitive to vancomycin, erythromycin, aminoglycosides, and chloramphenicol.

Corynebacterium bovis

This lipolytic coryneform was recovered from cow's milk by Evans in 1916 and called *Bacillus abortus* var. *lipolyticus* and then later named *Bacterium lipolyticus*. Bergey in 1923 used the current name, *Corynebacterium bovis*. Later editions of *Bergey's Manual* have since grouped *B. lipolyticus* with *C. bovis*.[7] These organisms are common commensals in the bovine udder, and their presence in milk causes butterfat to be hydrolyzed, thereby producing rancidity.

Corynebacterium bovis is a nonmotile, slender, gram-positive rod requiring serum, Tween 20 or 80, or egg yolk for growth. Its colonial morphology on nutrient agar is described as whitish, circular, and slightly shiny, whereas it is nonhemolytic on blood agar. *Corynebacterium bovis* is catalse-, urease-, and oxidase-positive but nitrate- and starch-negative.[7,9]

The source of human infection with *C. bovis* is unclear since the organism has not been implicated as a human commensal and since there is rarely an antecedent history of animal exposure. There are seven reported human infections: three cases involving the central nervous system (one each with meningitis,[48] epidural abscess,[48] and a ventriculojugular shunt infection[49]); two cases of prosthetic valve endocarditis[48]; one case of chronic otitis media and mastoiditis[48]; and a case of a chronic leg ulcer that developed in a patient who tripped on a meat bone in a butcher shop.[48] It is noteworthy that three of these seven cases were associated with a prosthetic device and that the shunt infection was associated with "shunt nephritis."[49] Six of these seven cases recovered with antimicrobial therapy; the seventh died of endocarditis. Human isolates of *C. bovis* have been variably sensitive to penicillins; all were sensitive to rifampin. Erythromycin and rifampin may act synergistically and may well be the regimen of choice.

Corynebacterium xerosis

In 1881, an organism with the characteristics of *C. xerosis* was isolated from the conjunctiva of the eye by Raymond. While it was initially considered to be a cause of conjunctivitis, most now believe *C. xerosis* to be a commensal that colonizes the conjunctival sac, nasopharynx, and skin.[7]

Corynebacterium xerosis grows readily on ordinary media and appears on Gram stain as irregularly staining rods. They form small yellow-to-tan colonies and are nonhemolytic. These organisms ferment several carbohydrates, reduce nitrates, and hydrolyze pyrazinamide but do not liquefy gelatin or hydrolyze urea. No toxin production has been reported.[7,9]

Corynebacterium xerosis has been described as the cause of three cases of endocarditis: one in a patient with a prosthetic valve[7] and two in patients with previously normal valves.[50,51] Bacteremia, pneumonia, and surgical wound infection have occurred in five immunocompromised patients.[52] Six additional patients appear to have been colonized with *C. xerosis*.[52] The organism is sensitive to the penicillins, cephalosporins, and vancomycin.

Corynebacterium aquaticum

Initially characterized by Leifson in 1962, *C. aquaticum* is found in both distilled and probably natural fresh water.[7] It is small, coccobacillary, and weakly gram-positive. Slightly yellow colonies that are convex and nonhemolytic appear after overnight incubation on 5% sheep blood agar plates. *Corynebacterium aquaticum* oxidizes glucose and hydrolyzes esculin.[9]

There are six reports of *C. aquaticum* causing human disease. It has been isolated from blood in one patient with endocarditis and another with diabetes.[7] Two cases of relapsing peritonitis have been described in patients undergoing continuous ambulatory peritoneal dialysis (CAPD)[53,54]—one requiring removal of the catheter for cure.[53] One case of *C. aquaticum* meningitis was reported in a 4-week-old infant female born in a hospital where three blood isolates were clustered within the same time frame.[55] A single case of urinary tract infection due to *C. aquaticum* in a neonate 8 days after an uncomplicated vaginal delivery is also described.[55a] *Corynebacterium aquaticum* should be differentiated from *Listeria monocytogenes*, especially in a newborn's cerebrospinal fluid (CSF), urine or in CAPD fluid.

Corynebacterium minutissimum

Although erythrasma has been well described since 1859, its causative agent, *C. minutissimum*, was first described in 1961.[7] Erythrasma is a common superficial infection of the skin that is characterized by pruritic, scaling, reddish brown macular patches occurring in intertriginous areas. This dermatologic condition is usually diagnosed by the typical coral red fluorescence of the skin lesions when examined under Wood's lamp. Gram staining and culture of the pulverized stratum corneum will yield the organism. On special tissue culture medium containing fetal bovine serum, *C. minutissimum* will form colonies of 1 to 2 mm that show the coral red-to-orange fluorescence under long-wave ultraviolet light. *Corynebacterium minutissimum* shares many bacteriologic characteristics with *C. xerosis* but may easily be distinguished from the latter by the fact that *C. minutissimum* does not reduce nitrate. *Corynebacterium minutissimum* produces a porphyrin, hydrolyzes Tween 80, and grows in the presence of hydrogenated castor oil esters.[7,9,56]

There are three reports of human infection with *C. minutissimum* other than erythrasma. One is a case of severe and recurrent breast abscesses in a 42-year-old woman,[56] the second is a case of endocarditis with embolic retinopathy in a patient with mitral valve prolapse,[57] and the third is a case of fatal septicemia in a neutropenic patient with chronic myelogenous leukemia.[58] None of these three patients had clinical evidence of erythrasma; however, all three patients had disruption of the integument.

Corynebacterium striatum

Early reports on *C. striatum* described the organism as a thick diphtheroid with clear-cut bars (striatum) and large irregular granules. *Corynebacterium striatum* is part of the normal flora of the anterior nares and skin, particularly the face and upper part of the torso.[7,9] This organism has been reported as the etiologic agent of a bacteremic pleuropulmonary infection in an elderly man with chronic lymphocytic leukemia.[59] It was also isolated from pulmonary secretions in mixed culture from another patient.[60]

Corynebacterium kutscheri

Corynebacterium kutscheri is a pathogen of experimental rats and mice. Apparently healthy animals can harbor this organism and subsequently develop an active infection when they are stressed. The overt disease is characterized by pseudotuberculous visceral lesions. Infections of rodents in the wild have also been reported.[7,9] There is a single case report of chorioamnionitis in a premature infant.[61]

Group D2

Corynebacterium group D2 is a gram-positive rod described by King in 1972 whose culture and biochemical characteristics resemble those of *Corynebacterium* group JK.[62] During a survey for carriage of antibiotic-resistant diphtheroids, investigators at a cancer center found 6 of 52 isolates to be urease-positive and biochemically less active than were group JK isolates.[63] These six isolates were subsequently found to be group D2.[9] Group D2 organisms do not acidify glucose.[9] *Corynebacterium* D2 isolates are resistant to multiple antibiotics.[62,64]

Group D2 has been isolated from the transtracheal aspirates of an elderly patient with pneumonia[65] and is an etiologic agent involved in alkaline encrusted cystitis, a very severe urinary tract infection that is difficult to treat.[66] Encrusted cystitis is a chronic inflammatory condition of the bladder that was first described by François in 1914 as a localized ulcerative inflammation with deposits of ammonium magnesium phosphate on the surface and on the walls of the ulcer. This disease has been associated with the implantation of urea-splitting microorganisms (mainly *Proteus* spp.) in a bladder that already harbored some form of inflammatory or neoplastic lesion (vesical ground). The urea-splitting activity of D2 plays an important role in its pathogenicity, which is associated with alkaline urine (pH >8.0) and struvite (ammonium magnesium phosphate) stones.[67] Risk factors that relate to infection with *Corynebacterium* group D2 include immunosuppression, previous urinary tract infections with organisms other than group D2, urologic manipulation, and previous urologic disease that created a vesical ground. Because the organism is highly resistant to most antimicrobial agents, vancomycin is recommended until specific antimicrobial sensitivity data become available.[68,69]

Group E

This is a heterogeneous group that includes some organisms that have subsequently been recognized as aerotolerant *Bifidobacterium adolescentis* strains.[9] A single case of pyelonephritis and septicemia in a normal host has been reported.[70]

Group G2

This is a fastidious group of organisms reportedly very similar to *Bacterionema matruchotii* (*C. matruchotii*).[9] Two cases of human infection with group G2 have been reported. The first was a patient who died of endocarditis involving mitral and aortic valve prostheses.[71] The second patient was a male with disseminated intravascular coagulopathy who had large numbers of peripheral blood polymorphonuclear leukocytes each containing as many as 20 bacilli.[72] In these patients, blood cultures did not become positive until after 7 and 10 days of incubation, respectively.

Group JK

Described in 1976,[73] *Corynebacterium* group JK has since been reported to cause sepsis primarily in patients with neoplastic diseases with various risk factors: (*1*) prolonged hospitalization, (*2*) prolonged neutropenia, (*3*) treatment with multiple antibiotics, and (*4*) disruption of the integument.[63,73–76] Most patients are colonized before infection, and most infections are hospital acquired. Group JK corynebacteria appear to exist as part of the skin flora of hospitalized patients, particularly in the inguinal, axillary, and rectal sites, while healthy individuals are generally not colonized with large numbers of these organisms.[75–77] About one-third to one-half of oncology patients admitted to cancer centers are colonized, and this carriage may persist for weeks to months.[75,76,78] Prior broad-spectrum antibiotic therapy in such patients correlates with colonization.[76] Some studies have shown that these organisms are normal flora of the skin that have acquired antibiotic resistance.[79] Outbreaks of infection with group JK have occurred.[80,81]

There is controversy about the transmission of these organisms. One group has found similar plasmids in isolates from different patients, thus suggesting that person-to-person transmission of JK corynebacteria had occurred within the hospital.[82] Other investigators have not been able to demonstrate plasmids.[63,75,80] One group[83] indicated that plasmid profiling was not useful and that restriction endonuclease analysis of chromosomal DNA appears to be the appropriate molecular epidemiologic tool for group JK corynebacteria. This same group found marked heterogeneity among the isolates obtained in their study and suggested that patient-to-patient transmission does not occur.[83]

The alternative suggestion is that antibiotic therapy selects out multiresistant JK strains that are present in low numbers as part of the skin flora.[77,79] A high prevalence of antibiotic-resistant JK colonization in many groups of patients has been demonstrated and is long lasting.[77] Also, there is an inverse relationship between the numbers of antibiotic-susceptible JK and the highly resistant JK, which suggests that the niche vacated by the susceptible JK are then filled by the highly resistant JK.[77]

Gram stain morphology of group JK shows gram-positive coccobacillary or coccal forms that may resemble streptococci. The morphology may often appear in a cuneiform pattern. On sheep blood agar, the colonies are slow growing, small, gray to white, glistening, and usually nonhemolytic. Key biochemical reactions that differentiate JK from other corynebacteria are the inability to produce urease, reduce nitrate, or readily ferment most carbohydrates. No halo is produced on Tinsdale medium. The antibiogram may well be the most distinguishing feature since most isolates are multiply resistant and are frequently only sensitive to vancomycin.[7,9,84] Ultrastructure analysis of these isolates may help in understanding their multidrug resistance patterns.[85]

Infections have occurred most commonly in neutropenic patients or patients with previous cardiac surgery.[7,8,63,73–76] Most of these infections are related to disruption of the integument and present as bacteremia—often associated with indwelling intravenous catheters. Septicemia with *Corynebacterium* group JK occurs most often in patients with lymphoreticular malignancies, often occurring as a terminal event. Among such neutropenic patients with *Corynebacterium* group JK septicemia, skin and soft tissue manifestations were observed in over 25 per cent of cases in one review.[85a] Early prosthetic valve endocarditis due to diphtheroids was found to be due to variably sensitive *Corynebacterium* group JK.[8] At least seven previously reported cases of endocarditis attributed to unspecified diphtheroids were subsequently determined to be due to group JK.[84] Other infections reported include pneumonitis,[86] cavitating pneumonitis,[86a] peritonitis in CAPD,[87] neurosurgical shunt infections,[88] wound infections,[88] infected tibial prosthesis,[89] rash,[86,90] and epicardial abscess related to epicardial catheter placement.[91] Therapy is with vancomycin. Removal of the prosthetic device is required if the infection cannot be controlled medically. This is especially so in cases of endocarditis due to group JK when there is left ventricular failure or paravalvular leak. Prevention of sepsis in high-risk patients is best obtained by controlling the skin colonization of resistant group JK by bathing with an antibacterial soap.[92,93]

REFERENCES

1. Lehmann KB, Neumann R. Atlas und Grundriss der Bakteriologie und Lehrbuch der speciellen bacteriologischen Diagnostik. 1st ed. Munchen: JF Lehmann; 1896.
2. Barksdale L. The genus *Corynebacterium*. In: Starr MP, Stolp H, Truper HG, et al., eds. The Prokaryotes: A Handbook of Habitats, Isolation, and Identification of Bacteria. Berlin: Springer-Verlag; 1981:1827–37.
3. Centers for Disease Control. Fatal diphtheria—Wisconsin 1982. MMWR. 1982;31:553–5.
4. Kaplan K, Weinstein L. Diphtheroid infections of man. Ann Intern Med. 1969;70:919–29.
5. Johnson WD, Kaye D. Serious infections caused by diphtheroids. Ann NY Acad Sci. 1970;174:568–76.
6. Washington JA II. Bacteriology, clinical spectrum of disease, and therapeutic aspects in coryneform bacterial infection. In: Remington JS, Swartz MN, eds. Current Clinical Topics in Infectious Diseases. v. 2. New York: McGraw-Hill; 1981:68–88.
7. Lipsky BA, Goldberger AC, Tompkins LS, et al. Infections caused by nondiphtheria corynebacteria. Rev Infect Dis. 1982:1220–35.
8. Murray BA, Karchmer AW, Moellering RC. Diphtheroid prosthetic valve endocarditis. Am J Med. 1980;69:838–48.
9. Coyle MB, Hollis DG, Groman NB. *Corynebacterium* spp. and other cory-

neform organisms. In: Lennette EH, Ballows A, Hauser WJ Jr, et al., eds. Manual of Clinical Microbiology. Washington, DC: American Society for Microbiology; 1985:193–204.
10. Wong TP, Groman N. Production of diphtheria toxin by selected isolates of *Corynebacterium ulcerans* and *Corynebacterium pseudotuberculosis*. Infect Immun. 1984;43:1114–6.
11. Meers PD. A case of classical diphtheria and other infections due to *Corynebacterium ulcerans*. J Infect. 1979;1:139–42.
12. Siegel SM, Haile CA. *Corynebacterium ulcerans* pneumonia. South Med J. 1985;78:1267.
13. Hadfield TL, Monson MH. *Corynebacterium ulcerans* infection. Clin Microbiol Newsl. 1983;5:104–5.
14. Lopez JF, Wong FM, Quesada J. *Corynebacterium pseudotuberculosis*: First case of human infection. Am J Clin Pathol. 1966;46:562–7.
15. Keslin MH, McCoy EL, McCusker JJ, et al. *Corynebacterium pseudotuberculosis*: A new cause of infectious and eosinophilic pneumonia. Am J Med. 1979;67:228–31.
16. Goldberger AC, Lipsky BA, Plorde JJ. Suppurative granulomatous lymphadenitis caused by *Corynebacterium ovis (pseudotuberculosis)*. Am J Clin Pathol. 1981;76:486–90.
17. Richards M, Hurse A. *Corynebacterium pseudotuberculosis* abscesses in a young butcher. Aust NZ J Med. 1985;15:85–6.
18. House RW, Schousboe M, Allen JP, et al. *Corynebacterium ovis* (pseudotuberculosis) lymphadenitis in a sheep farmer: A new occupational disease in New Zealand. NZ Med J. 1986;99:659–62.
19. Augustine JL, Renshaw HW. Survival of *Corynebacterium pseudotuberculosis* in axenic purulent exudate on common barnyard fomites. Am J Vet Res. 1986;47:713–5.
20. LeaMaster BR, Shen DT, Gorham JR, et al. Efficacy of *Corynebacterium pseudotuberculosis* bacterin for the immunologic protection of sheep against development of caseous lymphadenitis. Am J Vet Res. 1987;48:869–72.
21. Kotrajaras R, Buddhavudhikrai P, Sukroongreung S, et al. Endemic leg ulcers caused by *Corynebacterium pyogenes* in Thailand. Int J Dermatol. 1982; 21:407–9.
22. Kotrajaras R, Tagami H. *Corynebacterium pyogenes*: Its pathogenic mechanism in epidemic leg ulcers in Thailand. Int J Dermatol. 1987;26:45–50.
23. Collins MD, Jones D, Schofield GM. Reclassification of *Corynebacterium haemolyticum* (MacLean, Liebow & Rosenberg) in the genus *Arcanobacterium* gen. nov. as *Arcanobacterium haemolyticum* nom. rev., comb. nov. J Gen Microbiol. 1982;128:1279–81.
24. Green SL, LaPeter KS. Pseudodiphtheritic membranous pharyngitis caused by *Corynebacteriuum hemolyticum*. JAMA. 1981;245:2330–1.
25. Kovatch AL, Schuit KE, Michaels RH. *Corynebacterium hemolyticum* peritonsillar abscess mimicking diphtheria. JAMA. 1983;249:1757–8.
26. Tompkins LS. *Corynebacterium hemolyticum*. Clin Microbiol Newsl. 1983;5:29–30.
27. Miller RA, Brancato F, Holmes KK. *Corynebacterium hemolyticum* as a cause of pharyngitis and scarlatiniform rash in young adults. Ann Intern Med. 1986;105:867–72.
28. Banck G, Nyman M. Tonsillitis and rash associated with *Corynebacterium haemolyticum*. J Infect Dis. 1986;154:1037–40.
29. Worthington MG, Daly BDT, Smith FE. *Corynebacteriuum haemolyticum* endocarditis on a native valve. South Med J. 1985;78:1261–2.
30. Chandrasekar PH, Molinari JA. *Corynebacterium hemolyticum* bacteremia with fatal neurologic complication in an intravenous drug addict. Am J Med. 1987;82:638–40.
31. Greenman JL. *Corynebacteriuum hemolyticum* and pharyngitis. Ann Intern Med. 1987;106:633.
32. Robinson BE, Murray DL. *Corynebacterium hemolyticum* and pharyngitis. Ann Intern Med. 1987;106:778–9.
33. Leonard A, Raij L, Shapiro FL. Bacterial endocarditis in regularly dialyzed patients. Kidney Int. 1973;4:407–22.
34. Rubler S, Harvey L, Avitabile A, et al. Mitral valve obstruction in a case of bacterial endocarditis due *Corynebacterium hofmannii*. NY State J Med. 1982;82:1590–4.
35. Lindner PS, Hardy DJ, Murphy TF. Endocarditis due to *Corynebacterium pseudodiphtheriticum*. NY State J Med. 1986;86:102–4.
36. Nathan AW, Turner DR, Aubrey C, et al. *Corynebacterium hofmannii* infection after renal transplantation. Clin Nephrol. 1982;17:315–8.
37. Donaghy M, Cohen J. Pulmonary infection with *Corynebacterium hofmannii* complicating systemic lupus erythematosus. J Infect Dis. 1983;147:962.
38. Andavolu RH, Jagadha V, Lue Y, et al. Lung abscess involving *Corynebacterium pseudodiphtheriticum* in a patient with AIDS-related complex. NY State J Med. 1986;86:594–6.
39. Miller RA, Rompalo A, Coyle MB. *Corynebacterium pseudodiphtheriticum* pneumonia in an immunologically intact host. Diagn Microbiol Infect Dis. 1986;4:165–71.
40. LaRocco M, Robinson C, Robinson A. *Corynebacterium pseudodiphtheriticum* associated with suppurative lymphadenitis. Eur J Clin Microbiol. 1987;6:79.
41. Lockwood BM, Wilson J. *Corynebacterium pseudodiphtheriticum* isolation. Clin Microbiol Newsl. 1987;9:5–6.
42. Barton MD, Hughes KL. Ecology of *Rhodococcus equi*. Vet Microbiol. 1984;9:65–76.
43. Van Etta LL, Filice GA, Ferguson RM, et al. *Corynebacterium equi*: A review of 12 cases of human infection. Rev Infect Dis. 1983;5:1012–8.
44. Sane DC, Durack DT. Infection with *Rhodococcus equi* in AIDS. N Engl J Med. 1986;314:56–7.
45. Samies JH, Hathaway BN, Echols RM, et al. Lung abscess due to *Corynebacterium equi*. Am J Med. 1986;80:685–8.
46. MacGregor JH, Samuelson WM, Sane DC, et al. Opportunistic lung infection caused by *Rhodococcus (Corynebacterium) equi*. Radiology. 1986;160:83–4.
46a. Weingarter JS, Huang DY, Jackman JD Jr. *Rhodococcus equi* pneumonia—an unusual early manifestation of the acquired immunodeficiency syndrome (AIDS). Chest. 1988;94:195–6.
47. Thomsen VF, Henriques U, Magnusson M. *Corynebacterium equi* Magnusson isolated from a tuberculoid lesion in a child with adenitis coli. Dan Med Bull. 1968;15:135–8.
48. Vale JA, Scott GW. *Corynebacterium bovis* as a cause of human disease. Lancet. 1977;2:682–4.
49. Bolton WK, Sande MA, Normansell DE, et al. Ventriculojugular shunt nephritis with *Corynebacterium bovis*. Am J Med. 1975;59:417–23.
50. Goglio A, Tosi CP, Biroli F. *Corynebacterium xerosis* endocarditis. Clin Microbiol Newsl. 1984;6:83.
51. Eliakim R, Silkoff P, Lugassy G, et al. *Corynebacterium xerosis* endocarditis. Arch Intern Med. 1983;143:1995.
52. Porschen RK, Goodman Z, Rafai B. Isolation of *Corynebacterium xerosis* from clinical specimens. Infection and colonization. Am J Clin Pathol. 1977;68:290–3.
53. Morris AJ, Henderson GK, Bremner DA, et al. Relapsing peritonitis in a patient undergoing continuous ambulatory peritoneal dialysis due to *Corynebacterium aquaticum*. J Infect. 1986;13:151–6.
54. Casella P, Bosoni MA, Tommasi A. Recurrent *Corynebacterium aquaticum* peritonitis in a patient undergoing continuous ambulatory peritoneal dialysis. Clin Microbiol Newsl. 1988;10:62–3.
55. Beckwith DG, Jahre JA, Haggerty S. Isolation of *Corynebacterium aquaticum* from spinal fluid of an infant with meningitis. J Clin Microbiol. 1986;23:375–6.
55a. Tendler C, Bottone EJ. *Corynebacterium aquaticum* urinary tract infection in a neonate, and concepts regarding the role of the organism as a neonatal pathogen. J Clin Microbiol. 1989;27:343–5.
56. Berger SA, Gorea A, Stadler J, et al. Recurrent breast abscesses caused by *Corynebacterium minutissimum*. J Clin Microbiol. 1984;20:1219–20.
57. Herschorn BJ, Brucker AJ. Embolic retinopathy due to *Corynebacterium minutissimum* endocarditis. Br J Ophthalmol. 1985;69:29–31.
58. Guarderas J, Karnad A, Alvarez S, et al. *Corynebacterium minutissimum* bacteremia in a patient with chronic myeloid leukemia in blast crisis. Diagn Microbiol Infect Dis. 1986;5:327–30.
59. Bowstead TT, Santiago SM. Pleuropulmonary infection due to *Corynebacterium striatum*. Br J Dis Chest. 1980;74:198–200.
60. Barr JG, Murphy PG. *Corynebacterium striatum*: An unusual organism isolated in pure culture from sputum. J Infect. 1986;13:297–8.
61. Fitter WF, Se Sa DJ, Richardson R. Chorioamnionitis and funisitis due to *Corynebacterium kutscheri*. Arch Dis Child. 197;55:710–2.
62. Santamaria M, Ponte C, Wilhelmi I, et al. Antimicrobiol susceptibility of *Corynebacterium* group D2. Antimicrob Agents Chemother. 1985;28:845–6.
63. Young VM, Meyers WF, Moody MR, et al. The emergence of coryneform bacteria as a cause of nosocomial infections in compromised hosts. Am J Med. 1981;70:646–50.
64. Roblas RF, Prieto S, Santamaria M, et al. Activity of nine antimicrobial agents against *Corynebacterium* group D2 strains isolated from clinical specimens and skin. Antimicrob Agents Chemother. 1987;31:821–2.
65. Jakobes NF, Perlino CA. "Diphtheroid" pneumonia. South Med J. 1979; 72:475–6.
66. Soriano F, Ponte C, Santamaria M, et al. *Corynebacterium* group D2 as a cause of alkaline-encrusted cystitis: Report of four cases and characterization of the organisms. J Clin Microbiol. 1985;21:788–92.
67. Soriano F, Ponte C, Santamaria M, et al. In vitro and in vivo study of stone formation by *Corynebacterium* group D2 (*Corynebacterium urealyticum*). J Clin Microbiol. 1986;23:691–4.
68. Schoch PA, Ferragamo MA, Cunha BA. *Corynebacterium* group D2 pyelonephritis. Urology. 1987;29:66–7.
69. Aguado JM, Ponte C, Soriano F. Bacteriuria with a multiply resistant species of *Corynebacterium* (*Corynebacterium* group D2): An unnoticed cause of urinary tract infection. J Infect Dis. 1987;156:144–50.
70. Guillard F, Appelbaum PC, Sparrow FB. Pyelonephritis and septicemia due to gram-positive rods similar to *Corynebacterium* Group E (aerotolerant *Bifidobacterium adolescentis*). Ann Intern Med. 1980;92:635–6.
71. Austin GE, Hill EO. Endocarditis due to *Corynebacterium* CDC Group G2. J Infect Dis. 1983;147:1106.
72. Lawrence C, Brown ST, Freundlich LF. Peripheral blood smear bacillemia. Am J Med. 1988;85:111–3.
73. Hande KR, Witebsky FG, Brown MS, et al. Sepsis with a new species of *Corynebacterium*. Ann Intern Med. 1976;85:423–6.
74. Pearson TA, Braine HG, Rathbun HK. *Corynebacterium* sepsis in oncology patients. JAMA. 1977;238:1737–40.
75. Stamm WE, Tompkins LS, Wagner KF, et al. Infection due to *Corynebacterium* species in marrow transplant patients. Ann Intern Med. 1979;91:167–73.
76. Gill VJ, Manning C, Lamson M, et al. Antibiotic-resistant group JK bacteria in hospitals. J Clin Microbiol. 1981;13:472–7.
77. Larson EL, McGinley KJ, Leyden JJ, et al. Skin colonization with antibiotic-

resistant (JK group) and antibiotic-sensitive lipophilic diphtheroids in hospitalized and normal adults. J Infect Dis. 1986;153:701–6.
78. Wichmann S, Wirsing von Koenig CH, Becker-Boost E, et al. Group JK corynebacteria in skin flora of healthy persons and patients. Eur J Clin Microbiol. 1985;4:502–4.
79. McGinley KJ, Labows JN, Zeckman JM, et al. Pathogenic JK group corynebacteria and their similarity to human cutaneous lipophilic diphtheroids. J Infect Dis. 1985;152:801–6.
80. Quinn JP, Arnow PM, Weil D, et al. Outbreak of JK diphtheroid infections associated with environmental contamination. J Clin Microbiol. 1984;19:668–71.
81. Riebel W, Frantz N, Adelstein D, et al. *Corynebacterium* JK: A cause of nosocomial device-related infection. Rev Infect Dis. 1986;8:42–9.
82. Kerry-Williams SM, Noble WC. Plasmids in group JK coryneform bacteria isolated in a single hospital. J Hyg Camb. 1986;97:255–63.
83. Khabbaz RF, Kaper JB, Moody MR, et al. Molecular epidemiology of group JK *Corynebacterium* on a cancer ward: Lack of evidence for patient-to-patient transmission. J Infect Dis. 1986;154:95–9.
84. Riley PS, Hollis DG, Utter GB, et al. Characterization and identification of 95 diphtheroid (group JK) cultures isolated from clinical specimens. J Clin Microbiol. 1979;9:418–24.
85. Blom J, Heltberg O. The ultrastructure of antibiotic-susceptible and multiresistant strains of group JK diphtheroid rods isolated from clinical specimens. Acta Pathol Microbiol Immunol Scand. 1986;94:301–8.
85a. Dan M, Somer I, Knobel B, et al. Cutaneous manifestations of infection with *Corynebacterium* JK. Rev Infect Dis. 1988;10:1204–7.
86. Guarino MJ, Qazi R, Woll JE, et al. Septicemia, rash, and pulmonary infiltrates secondary to *Corynebacterium* group JK infection. Am J Med. 1987;82:132–4.
86a. McNaughton RD, Villaneuva RR, Donnelly R, et al. Cavitating pneumonia caused by *Corynebacterium* goup JK. J Clin Microbiol. 1988;26:2216–7.
87. Pierard D, Lauwers S, Mouton MC, et al. Group JK *Corynebacterium* peritonitis in a patient undergoing continuous ambulatory peritoneal dialysis. J Clin Microbiol. 1983;18:1011–4.
88. Allen KD, Green HT. Infections due to a "group JK" *Corynebacterium*. J Infect. 1986;13:41–4.
89. Claeys G, Vershchraegen G, DeSmet L, et al. *Corynebacterium* JK (Johnson-Kay strain) infection of a Küntscher-nailed tibial fracture. Clin Orthop. 1986;202:227–9.
90. Jerdan MS, Shapiro RS, Smith NB, et al. Cutaneous manifestations of *Corynebacterium* group JK sepsis. J Am Acad Dermatol. 1987;16:444–7.
91. Gronemeyer PS, Weissfeld AS, Sonnenwirth AC. *Corynebacterium* group JK bacterial infection in a patient with an epicardial pacemaker. Am J Clin Pathol. 1980;74:838–42.
92. Brown AE. Neutropenia, fever, and infection. Am J Med. 1984;76:421–8.
93. Blevins A, Lange M, Sobeck K, et al. Prevention and control of *Corynebacterium* CDC JK bacteremia in cancer patients with prolonged neutropenia (Abstract L57). In: Proceedings of the 85th Annual Meeting of the American Society for Microbiology. Las Vegas: American Society for Microbiology; 1985.

185. LISTERIA MONOCYTOGENES

DONALD ARMSTRONG

Listeria monocytogenes is classified among six other species in the genus *Listeria*; none of the others have been implicated in human disease. Taxonomic and chemical studies indicate a similarity to the genus *Brochothrix*, and both genera occupy a position between *Lactobacillus* and *Bacillus*.[1] The organism was first well described as the cause of an epidemic of sepsis in laboratory rabbits and guinea pigs in 1926.[2] An association with a peripheral blood monocytosis was noted, and the name *Bacterium monocytogenes* was applied. The following year an identical organism was isolated from the livers of septic gerbils in South Africa and called *Listerella hepatolytica*.[3] In 1929 it was first identified as an isolate from the blood of a human with an infectious mononucleosis syndrome.[4] Since then, this association has been rare. The first infection during the perinatal period was reported in 1936,[5] and the first case of meningitis in the United States was reported in 1935.[6] There have been a number of summaries of *Listeria* infections over the years, including three international conferences.[7–14] Other names that have appeared in the literature describing organisms that were presumably *L. monocytogenes* are *Corynebacterium infantiseptícum*, *Corynebacterium parvulum*, and *Erysipelothrix monocytogenes*.[7]

MICROBIOLOGY

The organism is a gram-positive, nonspore-forming aerobic rod that is motile at room temperature and hemolytic, characteristics that separte it from similar diphtheroid-like organisms. In Gram stains of clinical specimens, such as cerebrospinal fluid, *L. monocytogenes* may appear coccoid. It can occur in pairs and be mistaken for gram-positive cocci, especially the pneumococci (Fig. 1A). In addition, it may over-decolorize or unevenly stain and be misinterpreted as *Haemophilus influenzae* or some other gram-negative bacillus. Typically the rods resemble diphtheroids (Fig. 1B) and unfortunately may be regarded as "contaminants" and reported as such by the laboratory. A physician should not accept a report stating that a blood or cerebrospinal fluid culture is contaminated. The organism should be identified, and the clinician must decide whether it is a contaminant or a significant isolate. This is particularly important in immunosuppressed patients but should hold true for all patients. The bacterium is catalase-positive and Voges–Proskauer-positive. Esculin is hydrolyzed. Organisms with which it can be confused in the laboratory include *Corynebacterium* species, *Erysipelothrix rhusiopathiae*, beta hemolytic streptococci, or enterococci.[15]

Clinical specimens should be delivered to the laboratory as promptly as possible, and at least 10 ml of spinal fluid should be obtained because the organism may be present in only small numbers. Original isolation has been reported as difficult or slow for uncertain reasons.[15] Once the organism has grown in culture it passes readily. It has been stressed that "The most important single factor likely to result in recovery of *L. monocytogens* from clinical material is a laboratory staff that will carefuly scrutinize diphtheroid-like isolates on the chance that they may not be simple diphtheroids after all."[16] The laboratory may want to use a "cold enrichment" technique for increased sensitivity, particularly on specimens such as stool that may contain mixed flora.[15] This requires refrigerating the specimen from 4 weeks to 6 months so it is an epidemiologic tool rather than an aid to an individual patient's care. An enrichment media and a media for differentiation of *L. monocytogenes* from other common contaminants appear to aid in isolation and identification.[17] The enrichment media was based on Todd–Hewitt broth, with antimicrobials added to inhibit other organisms. The medium allowed recovery of as few as 20 *L. monocytogenes* organisms per gram of feces.

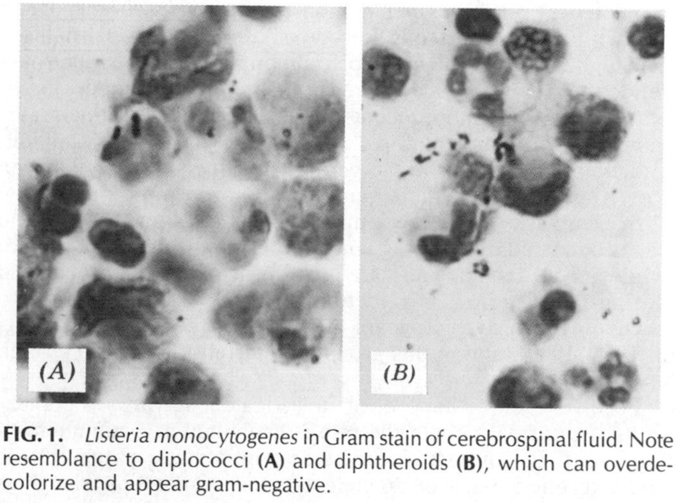

FIG. 1. *Listeria monocytogenes* in Gram stain of cerebrospinal fluid. Note resemblance to diplococci (**A**) and diphtheroids (**B**), which can overdecolorize and appear gram-negative.

A fluorescent antibody technique is available for directly staining clinical specimens such as cerebrospinal fluid, but the results may be difficult to interpret, and the test is not widely used.[15]

Animal inoculation is seldom used for identification now. Rabbits or guinea pigs develop conjunctivitis 1–5 days after inoculation of *L. monocytogenes* into the conjunctival sac (Anton test), and rabbits also develop a monocytosis 3–6 days after intravenous inoculation. Mouse inoculation intraperitoneally has also been used for isolation and identification, as well as for pathogenesis studies. Hepatic abscesses are seen 1–3 days after inoculation.[7,15]

Serologic typing is important for epidemiology. There are at least 11 serotypes, but three cause 90 percent of the clinical infections: types Ia, Ib, and IVb. Clinicians should request that all *L. monocytogenes* isolates be sent by the isolating laboratory to the Centers for Disease Control (CDC) for typing along with acute and convalescent serum specimens from their patients so further epidemiologic information can be accumulated.

Epidemiology

Listeria monocytogenes has been isolated from soil, dust, animal feed, water, sewage, and almost every type of animal cultured,[7,11,18] including asymptomatic humans. Some of the animals from which positive cultures have been obtained are 42 domestic and wild mammalian species, 22 avian species, fish, ticks, a fly, and crustaceans.[7,18] It is evident that the organism is widespread in nature.

The prevalence of symptomatic infection is difficult to estimate. In Denmark there were 2.3 cases per million per year. Similar rates were recorded in Holland, Sweden, and Germany.[18] In the United States reporting was not required, and some states recorded a much higher prevalence than others.[19] During 33 years (1933–1966) there were 731 bacteriologically confirmed cases in the United States; subsequently, in 3 years (1967–1969), 255 cases were reported to the Centers for Disease Control, and these were from only 35 states.[20] It is unlikely that there has been a sharp increase in the incidence, but is more likely that identification is more precise and reporting is more frequent. Increased awareness of listeriosis must be assumed to be due to articles appearing in the medical and microbiology literature more frequently. There are still problems, however, in isolation, recognition, and identification of the organism.

It is thus now evident that the prevalence is higher than the 0.5 cases per million recorded in 1971. In the United States, in 1971, the attack rate was estimated at 0.9/100,000 population at less than 1 year of age, 0.005/100,000 at 5–14 years, and 0.1/100,000 at 55–64 years.[21] From more active CDC surveillance programs in the United States, using discharge summaries from selected hospitals from 1980 to 1982, the incidence rate was projected at 3.6 cases per million per year, which is more in line with those reported in Europe of 2.0–3.0 cases per million. The higher rate of 11.3 cases per million reported in France may reflect a true difference, better reporting, or differences in dietary habits. In a more recent study in 1986, higher attack rates have been found in multiple states surveyed, 6.9 per million, and even higher rates in the perinatal setting (20 per million) in Los Angeles, where there was a cheese-associated outbreak.

In Denmark and in the United States about one-third of the cases occurred during pregnancy or during the neonatal period, while in Sweden and Germany two-thirds of the cases occurred during these periods.[12] Infections in adults are more likely to occur in those over 40 years of age (46 percent of all patients in 1968–1969), and in this group the mortality has been as high as 54 percent.[18,19]

Fecal excretors have been investigated in various populations. In normal people the rate is estimated at a minimum of 1 percent. In contrast, contacts of symptomatic patients have had excretion rates of 26 percent, and workers in slaughter houses have had a rate of 4.8 percent.[12] Where follow-up studies have been done, duration of excretion has been a month or less. The true incidence of carriers and the duration of excretion is probably much higher, since the organism is difficult to isolate from stools.

Although the infection has been regarded among the zoonoses, most cases in the United States occur in urban areas without a history of animal contact. In addition, the incidence is higher in humans in the summer, in contrast to other animals in whom the winter incidence is higher. Contamination of milk due to mastitis in cows and spread to humans in the unpasteurized milk has been well described, as well as infections from ingesting contaminated meat. Contact with infected calves has resulted in skin infections in veterianarians.[7,18,21]

The source of infection in most cases is not clear, except when transplacental transmission occurs. There is increasing evidence of food-borne transmission (see below). There are insufficient instances of serologic documentation of conversions or of significant rises in titer to state that infection represents first contact with the organism or that carriers become symptomatic. In addition, since low level agglutination titers may represent nonspecific or cross reactions with other organisms, results are difficult to interpret.[7,15] Circumstantially, it appears that many people have contact with and may carry the organism, but few develop symptomatic infections. Those who do are immunocompromised in some manner and are selected because of this. The alteration in immune response may be because of pregnancy or may be associated with the neonatal period or with a variety of underlying diseases or types of immunosuppressive therapy.

The distribution of *L. monocytogenes* serotypes has not yet thrown much light on the epidemiology. There have been no definite regional trends, and the most prevalent serotypes have shifted from year to year both in the United States and Europe.[7,9,18,21] One recent study has shown that types Ia and Ib are more common in neonates infected in utero (early neonatal onset), while in those assumed to be infected at or after birth (late neonatal onset) type IVb is more common. Each of the three serotypes, however, occurs in the two syndromes.[22] These interesting findings further stress the need for serotyping all isolates with an aim to elucidate the epidemiology of this infection.

Listeria infections have occurred in clusters in hospitalized patients both in the past and recently.[7,12,23] In one of these reports all the patients were immunosuppressed.[23] There was no ducumented environmental or human focus in these instances. Similarly, clusters in newborn nurseries without an evident source have been described.[12,24]

Food (cole slaw) was implicated as the source of an outbreak of 41 cases of type 4b listeriosis in the Maritime Provinces of Canada in 1981.[25] The cole slaw from which the *L monocytogenes* was isolated was from a farm known to have listeriosis in sheep a year earlier. Their manure was used as fertilizer, and the cabbage wintered over in cold storage sheds before it was sold. Cold enhancement may have played a part. A risk factor for disease was pregnancy, in that 34 of 41 cases were perinatal.

A number of reports implicating vegetables, dairy products, and meats have recently appeared.[26–29] The most recent survey[30] in the United States indicated that as many as 20 percent of cases were food-associated, specifically with raw hot dogs and undercooked chicken.

PATHOGENESIS

Listeria monocytogenes can invade the eye and the skin of humans after direct exposure. This has been observed in laboratory accidents and in veterinarians.[7] It also must cross the placenta during maternal bacteremia and infect the placenta, amniotic fluid, and fetus. In the majority of human cases, however, the portal of entry is not evident. The patients become bacteremic and are considered to be septic due to an unknown source or to have meningitis, presumably from bacteremia. The gastrointestional tract is considered the most likely source[7,12] in these cases, although local lesions are not found. Some patients with systemic listeriosis have had diarrhea, and it has been suggested that the gastrointestinal tract is altered by whatever is causing the diarrhea and allows *L. monocytogenes* to invade. Although the organism has been found in the lungs of patients with disseminated disease, there is no evidence that this a portal of entry. Patients with pleural effusions from which *L. monocytogenes* has been isolated had underlying diseases. These may have been responsible for the effusion, which could have been seeded during bacteremia.[31] Although *L. monocytogenes* has been isolated from urethral exudates, the evidence that it caused urethritis has been weak. The patients either had gonorrhea or a recent history of it, and other causes of urethritis such as *Chlamydia* were not ruled out.[7] The role of *L. monocytogenes* in repeated abortions is also uncertain, but circumstantial evidence is more convincing than that for urethritis.[16]

If the portal of entry is the gastrointestinal tract and more than 1 person in 100 is at least a transient carrier, then why are only certain people affected? It has been observed that many patients with listeriosis are immunosuppressed, either by a basic disease such as a lymphoma or by various agents, usually including adrenocorticosteroids.[16,23,32,33] One report questions this association because, in the series from a general hospital, only 4 of 10 adults with listeriosis were immunosuppressed.[34] Most large series, however, reveal that more than one-half of the cases occur in a clearcut setting of immunodepression.[12,33] From clinical observations of the types of patients infected,[16,23,32,33] and from studies in laboratory animals and in vitro,[35–40] it is apparent that the mononuclear phagocyte is very important in the host response to *L. monocytogenes*. There are both clinical[41] and laboratory[42] studies to suggest that immune globulins are also important. Early studies demonstrated that protective, active immunization could be achieved in mice with sublethal doses of *L. monocytogenes* and that this was not serum dependent.[35] Resistance was subsequently correlated with the development of delayed hypersensitivity skin reactions and with the inactivation of bacilli by macrophages (mononuclear phagocytes).[36] Dependence of lymphocytes was demonstrated by the passage of resistance by injection of immune spleen cells and by the abolition of this activity by treatment of the spleen cells with antilymphocyte serum.[37] Using specific anti-thymus-derived lymphocyte antiserum, the importance of T lymphocytes in host defenses against *L. monocytogenes* was demonstrated in T-cell-depleted mice that failed to develop resistance.[38] Although the importance of the T cell was demonstrated, its exact role still has not been delineated. Both microorganism-specific and -nonspecific activation of mononuclear phagocytes takes place after immunization with *L. monocytogenes*,[39] and it has been demonstrated that delayed hypersensitivity and specific antimicrobial cellular killing are not necessarily correlated in the immunized animal.[40] Antimicrobial macrophage function appeared in mice after immunization with either soluble antigen (via peritoneal diffusion chambers) or live bacteria, both in the presence and absence of measurable delayed hypersensitivity (by the foot pad swelling technique). In addition, studies have shown that macrophages kill *L. monocytogenes* more efficiently in the presence of immune serum than in the presence of normal control serum.[42] It is also apparent that complement is important in opsonization of *L. monocytogenes* by both mouse peritoneal macrophages and polymorphonuclear leukocytes. Chemiluminescence was far greater in the latter compared with the former, yet killing was about the same, suggesting that peritoneal macrophages have an efficient oxygen-independent mechanism of killing or that polymorphonuclear phagocytes have a high level of redundancy in oxygen radical production.[43] It is apparent then, from observations both in experimental animals and humans, that the thymus-derived lymphocyte and mononuclear phagocyte are of prime importance in host defenses against *L. monocytogenes*, and that immune globulins and complement for opsonization are also important.

It is apparent also from clinical observations and laboratory experiments that *L. monocytogenes* can act as a facultative intracellular parasite that sometimes persists in the presence of active immune defenses and effective antibodies.[16] This does not appear to be due to transformation to an L-form, which was once a consideration,[16] and the mechanisms for persistence remain unknown.

In human immunodeficiency virus (HIV)-infected patients or patients with acquired immunodeficiency syndrome (AIDS), there have been relatively few cases of listeriosis recorded since the first report of two bacteremias without meningitis.[44] This raises the possibility that the CD4+ lymphocyte may play a lesser role in host defense of humans than in mice.[45]

A hemolytic and cytolytic toxin called listeriolysin O is a critical factor in the virulence of *L. monocytogenes*.[46] This 52 kD protein is secreted under conditions of low pH and low iron concentration, such as would be present within a phagolysosome. The toxin binds to cholesterol and disrupts membranes, perhaps being the factor that leads to disruption of phagolysosomal membranes and unrestricted growth of *Listeria* within the phagocyte cytoplasm.[47,48] The toxin has physiologic and structural similarities with the hemolysins of *Streptococcus pneumoniae* and *S. pyogenes*: pneumolysin and streptolysin O.[49]

CLINICAL SYNDROMES

The results of an infection with *L. monocytogenes* can be manifest in a number of different syndromes, which I prefer to divide into five categories (Table 1). As noted above, the most common result of contact with the organism appears to be a transient, asymptomatic carrier state. When illness does occur it may be mild and only a brief flu-like syndrome, as seen in some pregnant women.

INFECTIONS IN PREGNANCY

These infections may occur any time during pregnancy, but more often in the third trimester. The patient usually complains of chills and fever and may mention back pain. Physical examination is unrevealing. Although this may suggest a urinary tract infection, the diagnosis is not supported by urine examination or culture, and other laboratory tests are not helpful. The fever and chills may subside with or without therapy, and the only clue to the diagnosis is a positive blood culture. Since these are often not done, some cases may be undetected. There are documented cases in which the gravid woman was not treated and the fetus was not affected by the bacteremia.[12] At other times the infection appears to precipitate labor, and this may result in premature birth of a dead or infected baby.

TABLE 1. Categories of Infections Due to *Listeria monocytogenes*

Category	*Host and Illness*
1. Pregnancy infections	Gravid woman; mild, febrile illness to severe illness
2. Granulomatosis infantiseptica	Neonate, in utero transmission, early grave illness
3. Sepsis[a]	Neonate or adult; moderate to severe illness
4. Meningoencephalitis[a], cerebritis	Neonate or adult, moderate to severe illness
5. Focal infections[b]	Adult or child; localizes from direct contact or bacteremia

[a] Rarely associated with peripheral blood monocytosis.
[b] Includes skin, ocular, lymph node, subacute bacterial endocarditis, osteomyelitis, spinal abscess, peritonitis, cholecystitis.

GRANULOMATOSIS INFANTISEPTICA

Transplacental transmission causes the second category of infection, granulomatosis infantiseptica, which is truly unique for *L. monocytogenes*. The infant has disseminated abscesses and/or granulomas in multiple internal organs, including liver, spleen, lungs, kidney, and brain. This type of infection appears to be limited to in utero infected humans. It resembles most the infections induced in laboratory animals by high-dose inoculation intravenously or intraperitoneally. There may be evidence of amnionitis or meconium-stained amniotic fluid. The infant may be obviously ill or may merely look weak and may develop respiratory or circulatory insufficiency. In these circumstances the meconium and amniotic fluid should be cultured, as well as blood of infant and mother and the maternal vagina and lochia,[12] and the laboratory should be informed of the presumptive or suspected diagnosis. Blood specimens from mother and child should be obtained for serology when the presumptive diagnosis is made, and convalescent specimens should be obtained 2 weeks later. The infant's throat and any skin lesions, which usually appear on the trunk or extremities as papules but may ulcerate, should be cultured. Conjunctivitis may also be present at birth, and the exudate should be smeared and cultured. A lumbar puncture should be done, because the meninges, as well as the brain, may be involved. A Gram stain of any of the specimens mentioned above, such as meconium, skin, or eye lesions, that show gram-positive rods or coccobacillary forms should prompt a presumptive diagnosis of listeriosis and immediate therapy. The child should be treated if the diagnosis is suspected, but not proved, since waiting for culture results could be disastrous. Such a patient would be treated for neonatal sepsis in most institutions, and ampicillin, along with an aminoglycoside, would be included in the treatment regimen (Table 2). The mortality in this syndrome has been close to 100 percent in some series,[12] while in other small series in which the infants have been treated early many have survived.

SEPSIS OF UNKNOWN ORIGIN

The third category includes infections that manifest as sepsis of unknown origin. Patients are adults or neonates with chills and fever. The adults in the majority of cases are immunosuppressed; the neonates become symptomatic after 3 days of age, and it appears that the infection is contracted during or after birth rather than in utero. The mother is almost always asymptomatic. There is nothing to suggest the diagnosis in either adult or neonate except on rare occasions a monocytosis of 8 percent or over may be seen in the peripheral smear. If the patient has an underlying lymphoma, the significance of a monocytosis may be difficult to evaluate.[16] Patients may be hypotensive, and the clinical picture may be the same as that of "gram-negative sepsis." In one series, three of six patients with the sepsis syndrome were hypotensive.[16] A positive blood culture makes the diagnosis. It is probable that during the bacteremia of this type of illness the meninges or brain are seeded, resulting in the fourth category of symptomatic infection—meningoencephalitis or cerebritis.

MENINGOENCEPHALITIS

As with the sepsis syndrome, this occurs in the late neonatal setting (after 3 days of age) and in the immunosuppressed adult. *Listeria monocytogenes* does have a predilection for infecting the central nervous system, especially the meninges. Meningitis is the most common clinical syndrome in many series and is extremely variable in its presentation in both the neonate and adult. As with any neonatal meningitis, failure to thrive, manifested by poor appetite, may be the only warning of the illness. Fever may be low grade or even absent, and bulging fontanelles or stiff neck are not uniformly present. Laboratory examination is not helpful except for cerebrospinal fluid (CSF), which usually contains predominantly neutrophils, but there may be a majority of mononuclear cells. The diphtheroid-like gram-positive bacilli may be absent or may resemble gram-positive cocci and may be mistaken for group B streptococci. Since some *L. monocytogenes* strains are penicillin resistant,[9,16,33] this can be an important distinction.

In the adult, the meningitis may be equally as subtle as in the neonate. In a large series of patients with underlying neoplastic disease, *Listeria* was the most common cause of meningitis,[50] and an increasing number of cases are being reported in patients who have undergone organ transplantation.[23,41] In addition, adults with cirrhosis appear in most series along with normal patients, the latter varying in number from 35 to 60 percent,[12,34] and in one series from a general hospital all patients with central nervous system listeriosis had an underlying disease.[33] Factors in common among the immunosuppressed patients include an

TABLE 2. Differential Diagnosis and Treatment of *Listeria monocytogenes* Infections

Category	Differential Diagnosis	Treatment: First Choice[a]	Treatment: Second Choice[b]
Pregnancy infections	Influenza Pyelonephritis Septic abortion	Ampicillin or penicillin	CTX, erythromycin; ? vancomycin
Granulomatosis infantiseptica	Neonatal sepsis Neonatal meningitis due to enteric bacilli or group B streptococcus	Ampicillin and gentamicin	CTX, erythromycin; ? vancomycin
Sepsis	Sepsis of unknown source due to a large variety of organisms	Ampicillin or penicillin	CTX, erythromycin; ? vancomycin
Meningoencephalitis	Psychiatric illness or metabolic encephalopathy	Ampicillin or penicillin, possibly with gentamicin intrathecally	CTX, erythromycin and/or chloramphenicol; ? vancomycin
	Infection due to *Streptococcus pneumoniae*, *Haemophilus influenzae*, *Neisseria meningitidis*, or *Cryptococcus neoformans* in immunosuppressed patients or to group B streptococci or enteric bacilli in neonates		
Cerebritis	Brain abscess, tumor, stroke	Ampicillin or penicillin	CTX, erythromycin; ? vancomycin
Focal infections	Varies with site	Ampicillin or penicillin	CTX, erythromycin and/or tetracycline; ? vancomycin

Abbreviation: CTX: cotrimoxazole (trimethoprim–sulfamethoxazole) as 20 mg/kg/day of the trimethoprim component in 4 divided doses..
[a] Ampicillin 200 mg/kg/day intravenously in six divided doses; penicillin 300,000 units/kg/day intravenously in six divided doses; gentamicin 6 mg/kg/day intravenously in four divided doses.
[b] Erythromycin 60 mg/kg/day intravenously in four divided doses; tetracycline 15 mg/kg/day intravenously in four divided doses; chloramphenicol 60 mg/kg/day intravenously in four divided doses.

underlying disease or therapy that primarily affects the thymus-derived lymphocyte–mononuclear phagocyte system. Although some patients are neutropenic, most are not. In addition, immunoglobulin levels may be low.[41] The only signs may be low grade fever and personality change. In contrast, fulminant manifestations with coma may be seen, but infrequently. The illness in the adult is more often subacute. Patients with meningitis without demonstrable brain abscess have shown focal neurologic signs. There were 10 such patients found among 78 in a literature review in 1967.[16] Of these patients, nine had cranial nerve signs, two hemiplegia, and one deafness. In 14 cases there was a lymphocytosis or monocytosis of greater than 8 percent. Cerebrospinal fluid counts ranged from 6 to 12,000 cells/mm^3, and differential counts varied from 99 percent polymorphonuclear cells to 98 percent mononuclear cells. Total counts of more than 1000 cells/mm^3 were seen in 32 of 59 patients. Protein concentrations ranged from normal to 735 mg/100 ml, but most were between 100 and 299 mg/100 ml. Glucose levels were not always low; 11 of 28 patients had normal levels. The organism may or may not be seen on Gram stain but will usually grow on culture. On a rare occasion the patient will have a purulent meningitis, negative cerebrospinal fluid cultures, and positive blood cultures for *L. monocytogenes*. This has been described in patients with cerebritis, brain stem infection, or abscess.

Since *L. monocytogenes* is now recognized as one of the organisms to be expected in meningitis of the normal host and is probably the most common cause of meningitis in immunosuppressed patients, it should be included in the differential diagnosis of any patient with meningitis and should be the leading diagnostic possibility in the immunosuppressed patient (Table 2). In the latter situation, in the presence of a normal peripheral leucocyte count the other likely causes are *Cryptococcus neoformans* and *S. pneumoniae*. If the patient has multiple space-occupying lesions, *Toxoplasma gondii* may be responsible, and the CSF findings are not specific. Finding a single space-occupying lesion makes *Nocardia asteroides* the most likely cause. In the presence of neutropenia, Enterobacteriaceae and *Pseudomonas aeruginosa* are more often the cause of meningitis, and a brain abscess may be due to *Aspergillus* species or one of the Mucorales.

CEREBRITIS

Cerebritis is increasingly recognized and reported. The patient may only complain of headache and fever or may present with varying degrees of paralysis resembling a cerebrovascular accident. A computerized tomogram or magnetic resonance imaging scan shows areas of uptake without ring enhancement (Figure 2 illustrates the latter). The cerebrospinal fluid may have no or only a few cells with normal to only slightly abnormal protein and sugar levels. Gram stains and cultures are negative, and the diagnosis is made when the blood culture becomes positive. This entity requires long-term therapy.[51]

FOCAL INFECTIONS

The focal infections caused by *L. monocytogenes* are listed in Table 1. Skin infections are seen in association with granulomatosis infantiseptica and have also been seen in veterinarians as a result of direct contact with infected animals and in laboratory workers as a result of inadvertent direct inoculation. There is nothing distinctive about the ulcerating lesions, and a Gram stain and culture are necessary to establish the diagnosis.[7]

Ocular infections may also be seen as a part of granulomatosis infantiseptica or as a solitary manifestation of a *L. monocytogenes* infection, sometimes after direct inoculation. This takes the form of a purulent conjunctivitis, and the organism can be isolated from the pus. Nonpurulent conjunctivitis has been seen in association with meningitis, but cultures have been negative. Acute anterior uveitis with isolation of the organism from the anterior chamber has been described, and *L. monocytogenes* should be considered in the differential diagnosis of this syndrome.[52]

Lymph node infections have usually involved the cervical lymph nodes, and cases of mixed tuberculous and listerial lymphadenitis have been described.[7,12] Culture of biopsy specimens or purulent drainage are necessary for proof of etiology.

In one report of 12 cases of subacute bacterial endocarditis due to *L. monocytogenes*,[53] there has been nothing distinctive about these cases except that in all, the left side of the heart appeared to be involved and the man to woman ratio was 5:1. The diagnosis must be made by blood cultures in addition to the clinical manifestation.

Other focal infections include arthritis,[16] osteomyelitis,[54] spinal or brain abscess,[7,55] peritonitis,[56] and cholecystitis.[34] Patients with disseminated listeriosis may present with acute hepatitis with serum glutamic-oxaloacetic transaminase levels as high as 9540 and alkaline phosphatase levels as high as 522 IU.[57] There has been nothing distinctive about any of these focal infections except that they tended to occur in immunosuppressed patients.[7,16,55,56]

TREATMENT

There are no controlled studies to establish a drug of choice for the treatment of *L. monocytogenes* infection. Small series and historical comparisons do exist,[58–61] but they do not settle the question. Ampicillin or penicillin appear to be the best drugs. Treatment failures with penicillin have been reported,[9] and in vitro penicillin resistance has been demonstrated to a limited degree.[9,33] Clinical failures do not necessarily indicate antibiotic failure, because in many instances therapy is started late, and particulary in patients with cerebritis or granulomatosis infantiseptica the infection progresses inexorably. Similar treatment failures have been reported with ampicillin.[41] Recent studies have shown that the organisms are sensitive in vitro to levels of both penicillin and ampicillin that are easily achievable in both blood and cerebrospinal fluid. Most isolates are also sensitive to tetracycline, erythromycin, chloramphenicol, trimethoprim-sulfamethoxazole, and cephalothin, and there are case reports documenting responses to each of these antibiotics,[7,8–11,16,20,33,34,58–61] and to combined erythromycin and tetracycline.[16]

There are equally strong advocates of penicillin[34,61] and ampicillin[59,60] and they may be equally effective. Experimental laboratory results show synergism between either ampicillin or penicillin and aminoglycosides against *L. monocytogenes*,[62] and one case report suggests that this can be clinically important.[63] If gentamicin is administered for central nervous system infection, both the intrathecal and systemic routes should be used. Table 2 contains a guide to the therapy for the various syndromes. Trimethoprim–sulfamethoxazole (cotrimoxazole)[64,65] has been successfully used in penicillin-allergic patients with listeriosis. There have been no comparative studies with ampicillin, but cotrimoxazole does seem a reasonable alternative form of therapy at this time. Vancomycin is a possible alternative, but insufficient information is available at present to recommend it.

The appropriate duration of therapy also remains unsettled. Two weeks has proven successful in one series[34] and in a number of case reports, but recurrence has been noted after 2 weeks of therapy in immunosuppressed patients, so 3–6 weeks may be more prudent.[51] This may be particularly true when using bacteriostatic drugs, but the organism tends to persist even in the presence of penicillin treatment in mice.[16]

Mortality varies considerably according to the syndrome and series. Granulomatosis infantiseptica and meningitis in immunosuppressed patients have the highest mortality, ranging in the former from 33 to 100 percent[7,12,21] and in the latter from 12.5 to 43 percent.[16,22,33,50] Survival rates (up to 100 percent) in men-

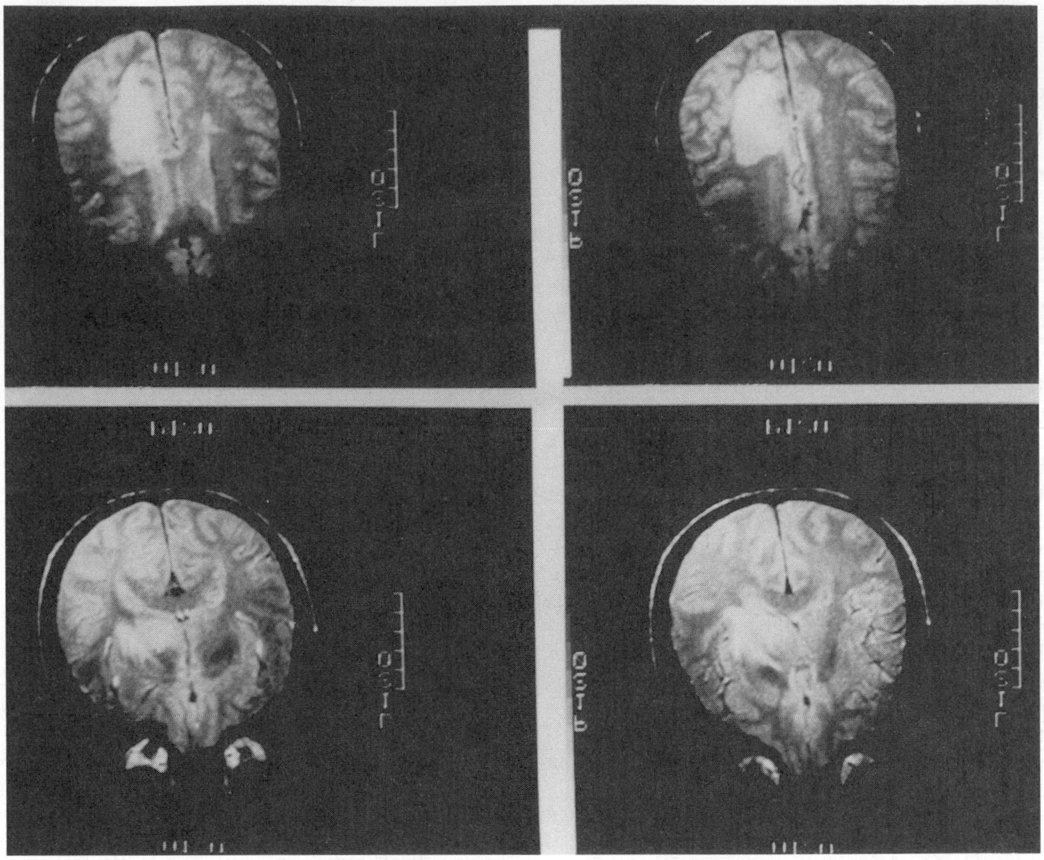

FIG. 2. Magnetic resonance imaging (MRI) scan of the brain of a patient with chronic lymphocytic leukemia, cerebritis, hemiparesis, *L. monocytogenes* in blood cultures, and a negative spinal fluid. Six weeks of ampicillin and gentamicin resulted in a complete recovery.

ingitis have been associated with normal cerebrospinal fluid glucose levels.[16,60] Successful theraphy has repeatedly been associated with early diagnosis and initiation of treatment.

REFERENCES

1. Seeliger HPR, Jones D. Genus *Listeria*. In: Sneath PHA, Mair NS, Sharpe ME, Holt JG, eds. Bergey's Manual of Systematic Bacteriology. Baltimore: Williams & Wilkins; 1986:1235–45.
2. Murray EGD, Webb RA, Swann MBR. A disease of rabbits characterized by a large mononuclear leucocytosis, caused by a hitherto undescribed bacillus. *Bacterium monocytogenes* (in sp). J Pathol Bacteriol. 1926;29:407.
3. Pirie JHH. A new disease of veld rodents "Tiger River Disease." Publ S Afr Inst Med Res. 1927;3:163.
4. Nyfeldt A. Etiologie de la mononucleose infectieuse. Compt Rend Soc Biol. 1929;101:590.
5. Burn CG. Clinical and pathological features of an infection caused by a new pathogen of the genus *Lesterella*. Am J Pathol. 1936;12:341.
6. Burn CG. Characteristics of a new species of the genus *Listerella* obtained from human sources. J Bacteriol. 1935;30:573.
7. Gray ML, Killinger AH. *Listeria monocytogenes* and listeric infections. Bacteriol Rev. 1966;30:309.
8. Hoeprich PD. Infection due to *Listeria monocytogenes*. Medicine (Baltimore) 1958;37:143.
9. Seeliger HPR. Listeriosis. 2nd ed. New York: Hafner; 1961.
10. Gray ML, ed. Second Symposium on Listeric Infections. Bozeman, MT: Artcraft Printers; 1962.
11. Proceedings of the Third International Symposium on Listeriosis, Bilthaven, Netherlands, July 1966.
12. Bejsen-Moller J. Human listeriosis, diagnostic, epidemiological and clinical studies. Acta Pathol Microbiol Scand [Suppl] 1972;229:1–157.
13. Nieman RE, Lorber B. Listeriosis in adults: a changing pattern. Report of eight cases and review of the liteature. 1968–78. Rev Infect Dis. 1980;2:207.
14. Hoff H, Rocourt J, Marget W, eds. *Listeria* and listeriosis. Infection. 1988;16(Suppl 2).
15. Bortolussi R, Schlech WF, Albritton WL. Listeria. In: Lennette EH, Balows WJH, Shadomy HJ, eds. Manual of Clinical Microbiology. 4th ed. Washington, DC: American Society for Microbiology; 1985:205–8.
16. Louria DB, Hensle T, Armstrong D, et al. Listeriosis complicating malignant disease, a new association. Ann Intern Med. 1967;67:261.
17. Mavrothalassitis P. A method for the rapid isolation of *Listeria monocytogenes* from infected material. J Appl Bacteriol. 1977;43:47.
18. Busch LA. Human listeriosis in the United States, 1967–1969. J Infect Dis. 1971;123:328.
19. Ciesielski CA, Hightower AW, Parsons SK, et al. Listeriosis in the United States: 1980–1982. Arch Intern Med. 1988;148:1416–9.
20. Listeriosis Annual Summary, 1969. Dept. of Health, Education and Welfare Publication, Centers for Disease Control, Zoonosis Surveillance, Atlanta, GA, June, 1970.
21. Moore RM, Zehmer RB. Listeriosis in the United States—1971. J Infect Dis. 1973;127:610.
22. Albritton WL, Wiggins GL, Feely JC. Neonatal listeriosis: distribution of serotypes in relation to age at onset of disease. J Pediatr. 1976;88:481.
23. Gantz NM, Myerwitz RL, Medieros AA, et al. Listeriosis in immunosuppressed patients, a cluster of eight cases. Am J Med. 1975;58:637.
24. Levy E, Nassau E. Experience with listeriosis in the newborn. An account of a small epidemic in a nursery ward. Ann Paediatr. 1960;194:321.
25. Schlech WF, Lavigne PM, Bortolussi RA, et al. Epidemic listeriosis—evidence for transmission by food. N Engl J Med. 1983;308:203.
26. Fleming DW, Cochi SL, MacDonald KL, et al. Pasteurized milk as a vehicle of infection in an outbreak of listeriosis. N Engl J Med. 1985;312:404.
27. Ho JL, Shands KN, Griedland G, et al. An outbreak of type 4b *Listeria monocytogenes* infection involving patients from eight Boston hospitals. Arch Intern Med. 1986;146:520.
28. Goulet V, Leonard JL, Celers J. Etude epidemiologique de la listeriose humaine en France en 1984. Rev Epidemiol Sante Publique. 1986;34:191–5.
29. Linnan MJ, Mascola L, Lou XD, et al. Epidemic listeriosis associated with Mexican-style cheese. N Engl J Med. 1988;319:823–8.
30. Schwartz B, Ciesielski CA, Broome CV, et al. Association of sporadic listeriosis with consumption of uncooked hot dogs and undercooked chicken. Lancet. 1988;ii:779–82.
31. Ananthraman A, Israel RH, Magnussen CR. Pleural-pulmonary aspects of *Listeria monocytogenes* infection. Respiration. 1983;44:153.
32. Simpson JF, Leddy JP, Hare JD. Listeriosis complicating lymphoma: report of four cases and interpretive review of pathogenetic factors. Am J Med. 1967;43:39.
33. Buchner LH, Schneierson SS. Clinical and laboratory aspects of *Listeria monocytogenes* infections with a report of ten cases. Am J Med. 1968;45:904.
34. Medoff G, Kunz LJ, Weinberg AN. Listeriosis in humans: an evaluation. J Infect Dis. 1971;123:247.
35. Osebold JW, Sawyer MT. Immunization studies on listeriosis in mice. J Immunol. 1957;78:262.

36. Mackaness GB. Cellular resistance to infection. J Exp Med. 1962;116:381.
37. Mackaness GB, Hill WC. The effect of anti-lymphocyte globulin on cell-mediated resistance to infection. J Exp Med. 1969;129:993.
38. Blanden RV, Langman RE. Cell mediated immunity to bacterial infection in the mouse. Thymus derived cells as effectors of acquired resistance to *Listeria monocytogenes*. Scand J Immunol. 1972;1:379.
39. Krahenbuhl JL, Remington JS. In vitro induction of non-specific resistance in macrophages by specifically sensitized lymphocytes. Infect Immun. 1971;4:337.
40. Osebold JW, Pearson LD, Medin NI. Relationship of antimicrobial cellular immunnity to delayed hypersensitivity in listeriosis. Infect Immun. 1974;9:354.
41. Louria DB, Blevins A, Armstrong D. Listeria infections. Ann NY Acad Sci. 1970;174:545.
42. Njoku-obi AN, Osebold JW. Studies on mechanisms of immunity in listeriosis I. Interaction of peritoneal exudate cells from sheep with *Listeria monocytogenes* in vitro. J Immunol. 1962;89:187.
43. MacGowan AP, Peterson PK, Keane W, et al. Human peritoneal macrophage phagocytic, killing, and chemiluminescent responses to opsonized *Listeria monocytogenes*. Infect Immun. 1983;40:440.
44. Real FX, Gold JW, Krown SE, et al. *Listeria monocytogenes* bacteremia in the acquired immunodeficiency syndrome. Ann Intern Med. 1984;101:883.
45. Kaufmann HE. *Listeria monocytogenes* specific T-cell lines and clones. Infection. 1988;16(Suppl 2):S128–36.
46. Geoffroy C, Gaillard JL, Alouf JE, et al. Purification, characterization, and toxicity of the sulfhydryl-activated hemolysin listeriolysin O from *Listeria monocytogenes*. Infect Immun. 1987;55:1641–6.
47. Kuhn M, Kathariou S, Goebel W. Hemolysin supports survival but not entry of the intracellular bacterium *Listeria monocytogenes*. Infect Immun. 1988;56:79–82.
48. Portnoy DA, Jacks PS, Hinrichs DJ. Role of hemolysin for the intracellular growth of *Listeria monocytogenes*. J Exp Med. 1988;167:1459–71.
49. Mengaud J, Vicente MF, Chenevert J, et al. Expression in *Escherichia coli* and sequence analysis of the listeriolysin O determinant of *Listeria monocytogenes*. Infect Immun. 1988;56:766–72.
50. Chernik NL, Armstrong D, Posner JB. Central nervous system infections in patients with cancer, changing patterns. Cancer. 1977;40:268.
51. Watson GW, Fuller TJ, Elms J, et al. Listeria cerebritis. Arch Intern Med. 1978;138:83.
52. Goodner EK, Okumoto MA. Intraocular listeriosis. Am J Ophthalmol. 1967;64:682.
53. Bassan R. Bacterial endocarditis produced by *Listeria monocytogenes*: case presentation and review of the literature. Am J Clin Pathol. 1975;63:522.
54. Housang ET. Acute *Listeria monocytogenes* osteomyelitis. Infection. 1976;4:113.
55. Spinal abscess due to *Listeria monocytogenes* in a patient with hepatic cirrhosis. J Pathol. 1972;107:9.
56. Clinical pathological conference. N Engl J Med. 1974;291:516.
57. Yu VL, Miller WP, Wing EJ, et al. Disseminated listeriosis presenting as acute hepatitis: case reports and review of hepatic involvement in listeriosis. Am J Med. 1982;73:773.
58. Kalis P, Le Frock JL, Smith W, et al. Listeriosis. Am J Med Sci. 1976;271:159.
59. Gordon RC, Barrett FF, Yow MD. Ampicillin treatment of listeriosis. J Pediatr. 1970;77:1067.
60. Lavetter A, Leedom JM, Mathies AW, et al. Meningitis due to *Listeria monocytogenes*. a review of 25 cases. N Engl J Med. 1971;285:598.
61. Heineman HS. Treatment of *Listeria monocytogenes* meningitis (Letter). N Engl J Med. 1971;285:1026.
62. Gordon RC, Barrett FF, Clark DJ. Influence of several antibiotics, singly and in combination, on the growth of *Listeria monocytogenes*. J Pediatr. 1972;80:667.
63. Shuman RD, Smith CR. Intrathecal gentamicin for refractory gram-positive meningitis. JAMA. 1978;240:469.
64. Scheer MS, Hirschman SZ. Oral and ambulatory therapy of Listeria bacteremia and meningitis with trimethoprim-sulfamethoxazole. Mt Sinai J Med. 1982;49:411.
65. Spitzer PG, Hammer AM, Karchmer AW. Treatment of *Listeria monocytogenes* infection with trimethoprim-sulfamethoxazole: Case report and review of literature. Rev Inf Dis. 1986;8:427–30.

186. BACILLUS ANTHRACIS (ANTHRAX)

F. MARC LaFORCE

Bacillus anthracis is a gram-positive rod that sporulates. The boxcar-shaped organisms seen in tissue smears are characteristic. Bacteria grow well aerobically on blood agar, and colonies are recognized by their stickiness and tendency to stand up in stalagmite fashion when lifted with a bacteriologic loop or an inoculating needle.[1] Organisms are nonmotile, and a specific gamma bacteriophage can be used to help confirm the identity of the organism. Organisms can also be identified in tissue specimens or smears with a direct fluorescent antibody test. All virulent strains are pathogenic for mice. Serologic diagnosis is also possible with a sensitive and specific hemagglutination test.[2]

EPIDEMIOLOGY

Anthrax is primarily a disease of herbivores. Humans become infected as they come into contact with infected animals or their products. Epizootic and enzootic anthrax has long been a problem in Iran, Turkey, Pakistan, and Sudan, and consequently animal products, particularly goat hair, imported from these areas is likely to be contaminated.

Human cases have been divided into two groups: agricultural or industrial. Agricultural cases of human anthrax result from direct contact with animals dying from anthrax. Industrial cases result from contact with anthrax spores that contaminate raw materials such as hides, goat hair, wool, and bones that are used as part of a manufacturing process. Because *B. anthracis* spores can survive for long periods of time, the variety of products that have been linked to human infection is a long and varied one, including such items as shaving brushes, bongo drums, and saddle blankets.

The ultimate reservoir of *B. anthracis* is the soil; however, the cycle of anthrax bacilli in soil is not completely understood. It is clear that simple soil contamination with anthrax spores does not necessarily give rise to cases in animals that graze in such areas. A vegetative phase is necessary whereby anthrax spores multiply to a density sufficient such that grazing animals can become infected. There are a few such anthrax foci in Louisiana, Oklahoma, and Colorado. Multiplication of anthrax in the soil is favored when soil pH is above 6.0 and an early spring rain is followed by a dry spell. Frequently, this is followed by more rain, which is thought to facilitate distribution of new organisms into foraging areas.[3] Local conditions need to be just right, as many epizootics are characterized by a marked degree of focality. On the other hand, if soil conditions are appropriate, it may be possible for spores to persist and multiply regularly for decades. Hundred-year-old descriptions of bad fields with repeated epidemics of anthrax among grazing animals have been reported in Europe. Disease in animals tends to be severe, with high mortality.

Woolsorter's disease, or inhalation anthrax, has a unique epidemiology.[4] Since the disease follows inhalation of anthrax spores, it is never seen as a result of contact with recently infected animals. Rather the disease occurs when aerosols of anthrax spores are generated during the early processing of imported goat hair, a raw product frequently contaminated with anthrax spores. Fortunately the disease was never very common even under conditions guaranteed to cause exposure to aerosolized anthrax spores. On the other hand, sporadic cases have been noted after limited contact with anthrax spores. Inhalation anthrax is very rare, with only two reported United States cases in the last 20 years, the last case occurring in a home craftsman who was weaving a rug using wool that was later shown to have been contaminated with anthrax spores.[4]

In countries where anthrax is enzootic, bones from animals dying of anthrax are frequently used as raw material for the making of bone meal. This material is often used as a fertilizer or as a supplement to animal foods and has accounted for several human cases of cutaneous anthrax.

PATHOGENESIS

Virulence of *B. anthracis* is dependent upon plasmid-mediated production of a three-component exotoxin and an antiphagocytic poly-D-glutamic acid capsule. The toxic proteins, collectively referred to as "anthrax toxin," have been purified and cloned and consist of a protective antigen (PA), an edema factor (EF), and a lethal factor (LF) (see Chapter 1). Anthrax spores inoculated subcutaneously grow rapidly. Growing organisms release toxins that account for marked brawny edema and tissue necrosis. It is generally believed that some degree of immunity develops after cutaneous infection.

Inhaled anthrax spores that are greater than 5 μm pose no problem, as they are physically cleared from the lung by the mucociliary escalator system. Smaller particles are deposited in alveoli or alveolar ducts where they are phagocytized by alveolar macrophages and carried to mediastinal lymph nodes. A hemorrhagic mediastinitis results, followed by bacteremia and intravascular multiplication of organisms. Meningitis often occurs as part of the overwhelming septicemia.

Gastrointestinal anthrax follows ingestion of grossly contaminated undercooked meat. Organisms are transported to mesenteric lymph nodes where they multiply. Hemorrhagic lymphadenitis, ascites, and septicemia follow. Oropharyngeal anthrax has also been reported whereby organisms from contaminated meat are absorbed directly through pharyngeal mucous membranes leading to local swelling, adenopathy, and systemic findings.

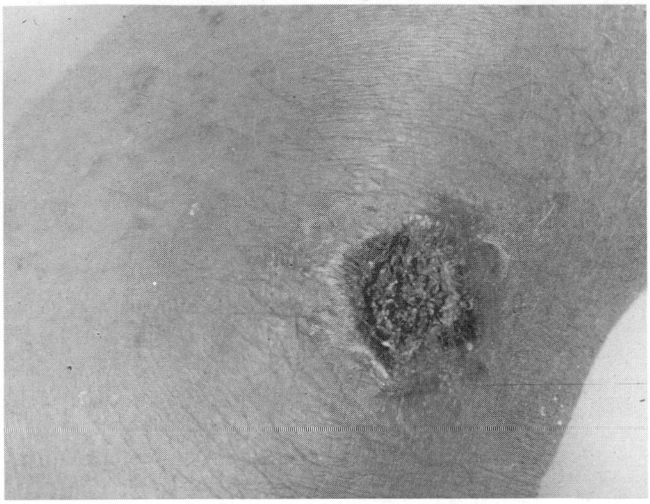

FIG. 2. Cutaneous anthrax of upper forearm on day 14 showing a large necrotic eschar. (Courtesy of Dr. Philip S. Brachman, Atlanta, GA.)

CLINICAL MANIFESTATIONS

Cutaneous anthrax accounts for more than 95 percent of cases (Figs. 1 and 2). The clinical presentation is characteristic, and the diagnosis is not often missed when considered.[5] The infection begins as a small papule that is often pruritic. The papule enlarges and within 24 to 48 hours develops into an ulcer surrounded by vesicles. A black necrotic central eschar develops later and is characteristic. Edema is often striking, particularly with facial lesions. Of diagnostic importance, the lesion is painless. Over 90 percent of cases occur in exposed skin areas such as arms, hands, face, and neck. Anthrax bacilli are easily seen on Gram stain smears and cultures from vesicular fluid. Occasionally massive edema may result in hemoconcentration and hypotension. Lymphangitis and regional lymphadenopathy may occur. Conditions that have been confused with cutaneous anthrax include orf, plague, and tularemia. Untreated cutaneous anthrax is fatal in about 20 percent of cases. Deaths are rare after antimicrobial treatment.

Inhalation anthrax is very difficult to diagnose early. The disease is biphasic, and initial symptoms mimic a severe viral respiratory illness like influenza.[6] This lasts for 2 to 3 days and is followed by a second more acute phase characterized by severe hypoxia and dyspnea. Chest x-ray films consistently show widening of the mediastinum. Patients soon become hypotensive, and about one-half develop meningeal signs. Of 13 well-documented United States cases, 12 have died.

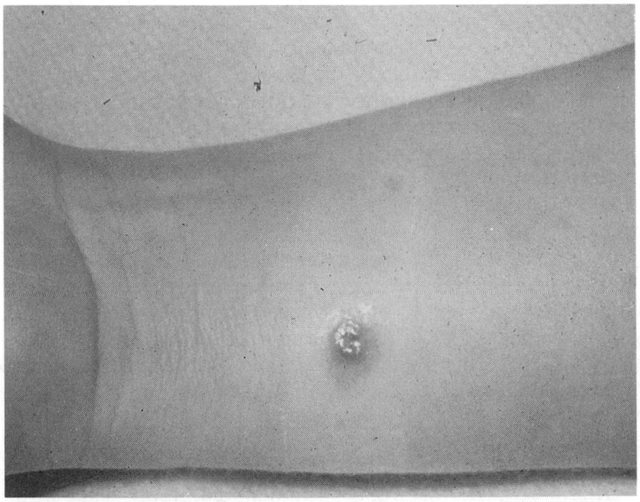

FIG. 1. Cutaneous anthrax of lower forearm on day 4 showing an elevated papule surrounded by a ring of vesicles. (Courtesy of Dr. Philip S. Brachman, Atlanta, GA.)

Gastrointestinal anthrax has never been reported in the United States, but such cases have been reported from developing countries. Presentations may vary and include gastrointestinal pain, bleeding, and rapid development of ascites.

Practitioners in the United States are most likely to see cases of cutaneous anthrax. The surest way not to miss the diagnosis is to consider it in any patient who has a painless ulcer with vesicles and edema and exposure to an animal or animal product.

TREATMENT

Anthrax is effectively treated with penicillin G. In 24 patients with cutaneous anthrax with positive blister cultures who were treated with 2 million units of penicillin, hourly blister cultures yielded negative cultures in all patients 5 hours after the initiation of therapy.[7] Thus, usual recommendations are 2 million units of penicillin G every 6 hours for 2 to 4 days until the edema subsides, at which time oral penicillin therapy can be used. Patients should be treated for 7 to 10 days. Erythromycin, tetracycline, and chloramphenicol are effective alternative drugs in penicillin-sensitive patients. It should be emphasized that antibiotic therapy does not stop the progress of anthrax lesions to an eschar phase, but does decrease systemic manifestations and local edema. Local surgery is contraindicated.

Few good data exist on the treatment of inhalation or gastrointestinal anthrax. High doses of penicillin therapy are recommended (2 million units every 2 hours), although high death rates can be expected. Person-to-person transmission does not occur.

Control of the disease in humans ultimately depends on control of the disease in animals. Animals dying of anthrax should be buried or cremated. Necropsies with spillage of contaminated blood with resultant sporulation of organisms should be avoided. Effective animal vaccines are available, and all cases should be reported to state veterinary authorities.

A human anthrax vaccine consisting of alum-precipitated supernatant material from fermentor cultures of toxigenic, nonencapsulated strains of *B. anthracis* is available from the Michigan Department of Health. The vaccine has been shown to be effective under field conditions, and persons who may be exposed to anthrax should be vaccinated.[8] The ability to prepare purified components of anthrax toxin by recombinant technology has opened the possibility of new anthrax vaccines. For example, immunization with PA toxoid vaccines or PA-producing live vaccines elicits partial or complete protection against anthrax infection.[9]

REFERENCES

1. Doyle RJ, Keller KF, Ezzell JW. Bacillus. In: Lennette EH, Balows A, Hausler WJ, Shadomy HJ, eds. Manual of Clinical Microbiology. 4th ed. Washington, DC: American Society for Microbiology; 1985:211–5.
2. Buchanan TM, Feeley JC, Hayes PS, et al. Anthrax indirect microhemagglutination test. J Immunol. 1971;107:1631–6.
3. Van Ness GB. Ecology of anthrax. Science. 1971;172:1303–7.
4. Brachman PS. Inhalation anthrax. Ann NY Acad Sci. 1980;353:83–93.
5. Gold H. Anthrax. Arch Intern Med. 1955;96:387–96.
6. Plotkin SA, Brachman PS, Utell M, et al. An epidemic of inhalation anthrax, the first in the twentieth century. Am J Med. 160;29:992–01.
7. Ronaghy HA, Azadeh B, Kohout E, et al. Penicillin therapy of human cutaneous anthrax. Curr Ther Res. 1972;14:721–5.
8. Brachman PS, Gold H, Plotkin SA, et al. Field evaluation of human anthrax vaccine. Am J Public Health. 1962;52:632–45.
9. Ivins BE, Welkos SL. Recent advances in the development of an improved human anthrax vaccine. Eur J Epidemiol. 1988;4:12–9.

187. OTHER BACILLUS SPECIES

CARMELITA U. TUAZON

Members of the genus *Bacillus* are aerobic spore-forming rods that can stain as gram-positive or gram-variable and are ubiquitous in nature. *Bacillus* organisms that have been associated with clinical syndromes are listed in Table 1.

Bacillus organisms vary in size from about 3 × 0.4 μm to 9 × 2 μm and appear singly, in a diplobacillary form, or in chains. Most species grow readily on nutrient agar or peptone media. Single colonies are usually 2 to several milliliters in diameter and may have a finely granular, mealy appearance; others are membranous and wrinkled.[1] In broth, a surface scum may be formed with or without turbidity or a heavy flocculent or membranous deposit. Growth is sometimes improved by glucose, but not by blood or serum. *Bacillus subtilis* grows on minimal media containing glucose, citrate, ammonium phosphate, and the usual mineral salts. *Bacillus cereus* requires the addition of certain amino acids. On carbohydrate media most members of the genus form acid only, but a few produce gas, e.g., *B. polymyxa* and *B. licheniformis*. One member of the group *B. megaterium* produces hemolysin like the hemolysin of *Staphylococcus aureus*. *Bacillus cereus* forms oxygen-labile hemolysin resembling streptolysin O.

The optimum temperature for growth varies from 25 to 37°C. In the vegetative form the bacilli are killed in 1 hour by moist heat at a temperature of 55°C. The spores of *B. subtilis* may withstand boiling for hours.[1]

TABLE 1. Clinically Significant *Bacillus* Species

Isolate	*Clinical Syndrome*
B. alvei	Sepsis, meningitis
B. brevis	Corneal ulcer
B. cereus	Bacteremia, pneumonia, ophthalmitis, osteomyelitis, endocarditis
B. circulans	Meningitis
B. coagulans	Corneal abscess
B. laterosporus	Septicemia
B. licheniformis	Bacteremia
B. megaterium or *B. anthracoides*	Meningitis, bacteremia
B. pumilus	Meningitis, bacteremia
B. sphaericus	Peritonitis, pleuritis, pericarditis, pseudotumor of the lung, meningitis, bacteremia
B. subtilis	Meningitis, otitis, mastoiditis, urinary tract infection, bacteremia, pneumonia, endocarditis, ventriculoatrial shunt infection, orbital abscess, panophthalmitis, keratitis, iridocyclitis
B. thuringiensis	Corneal ulcer

EPIDEMIOLOGY

Bacillus organisms are usually found in decaying organic matter, dust, soil, vegetables, and water, and some species are part of the normal human flora. In the hospital setting, the latter site is where the bacteria can readily cause infections in debilitated, immunosuppressed, or traumatized patients. The organism has been implicated as an opportunistic infection in the setting of patients with serious illness who have prolonged survival.

Outbreaks of food poisoning caused by *B. cereus* have been reported from Asia, Australia, Europe, and North America.[2] Other outbreaks of infections related to *Bacillus* organisms include cases of bacteremia related to the contamination of dialysis equipment or wound or burn infections as part of a polymicrobial infection.[3,4]

Epidemiologic studies on the microbiology of street heroin and injection paraphernalia demonstrated *Bacillus* species as the predominant isolates from both specimens.[5,6] Serious infections caused by *Bacillus* species have been reported among drug abusers. Both contaminated heroin and paraphernalia can be implicated as possible sources of the organism.

PATHOGENESIS

The different species of *Bacillus* produce a variety of extracellular products including antimicrobial substances, enzymes, pigments, and toxins in a few species.[2] Enzymes that can be found on culture include amylase, collagenase, hemolysin, lecithinase, phospholipase, protease, and urease. Production of antimicrobial substances before the onset of sporulation is characteristic of the genus and include bacitracin, gramicidin, polymyxin, and tyrocidine.

Two enterotoxins are produced by *B. cereus* during exponential growth, the diarrheal toxin and the emetic toxin. The diarrheal toxin is produced readily on media, e.g., brain–heart infusion broth containing added glucose. The detection of emetic toxin may be difficult initially since ordinary media do not support its production, but growth on a media prepared from rice allows its isolation. The diarrheal toxin causes fluid accumulation in rabbit ileal loops, promotes vascular permeability in rabbits, and is lethal for mice when injected intravenously.

Purulent, pyrogenic, lethal, and necrotic activities are associated with strains of *B. cereus* isolated from patients with severe infections other than those in the gastrointestinal tract. Recent reports have suggested that two lethal toxins may contribute to the virulence of *B. cereus*.[7–9] The two toxins are loop fluid–inducing/skin test/necrotic toxin, which is about 50,000 in molecular weight, and cereolysin, which is a single polypeptide chain with a molecular weight of 55,500. The latter appears to interact with cholesterol as its receptor in the host cell membrane and has vascular permeability activity difficult to distinguish from that of loop fluid–inducing/skin test/necrotic toxin. The strong correlation between the hemolytic activity of a strain and the severity of the clinical infection provides indirect evidence for the putative role of cereolysin as a virulence factor.

Bacillus cereus may have three different forms of enzyme activity related to lecithinase-like activity—phosphatidylcholine hydrolase is the most studied form and is frequently referred to as phospholipase C. This enzyme may have a secondary role in ocular infections by disrupting host cell membrane phospholipids exposed by the action of other toxins.[8]

CLINICAL MANIFESTATIONS

Despite the widespread distribution of *Bacillus* organisms, they are rarely associated with actual infection and are more frequently isolated as a culture contaminant. Isolation of this organism requires careful clinical evaluation to determine the significance of the finding.

Risk factors that have been associated with serious *Bacillus* infections include intravenous drug abuse, sickle cell disease, foreign bodies including intravascular catheters, immunosuppression from malignancy, neutropenia, corticosteroid therapy, or the acquired immune deficiency syndrome.[10]

Clinical manifestations of infections caused by *Bacillus* species include food poisoning, localized infections related to trauma as in ocular infections, deep-seated soft tissue infections, and systemic infections (e.g., meningitis, endocarditis, osteomyelitis, and recurrent bacteremia).[11,11a] Fulminant eye infections are widely recognized complications of non-anthrax *Bacillus* infections.

FOOD POISONING

There are two distinct clinical forms of *B. cereus* food poisoning, emetic and diarrheal.[12] The emetic form is associated with contaminated fried rice and has a short incubation period, usually from 1 to 6 hours, and symptoms are predominantly upper gastrointestinal, manifested by vomiting. It mimics staphylococcal food poisoning. The diarrheal form has a longer incubation period that averages between 10 and 12 hours, and manifestations are related to lower gastrointestinal involvement similar to *Clostridium perfringens* food poisoning. Symptoms usually are abdominal pain, profuse watery diarrhea, tenesmus, and nausea usually lasting no longer than 12–24 hours. Such outbreaks are usually related to the consumption of meat or vegetables, and in one particular outbreak, turkey loaf was implicated.[13] The diarrhea is usually characterized by 3–10 small bowel movements per day, but in some patients it may be voluminous and require the administration of intravenous fluids. In a few patients, the symptoms may last longer, usually for 2–10 days.

The diagnosis of *B. cereus* food poisoning should be suspected in patients who present with upper gastrointestinal symptoms of 1–6 hours' duration after the consumption of fried rice and in those who present with lower intestinal tract illness 6–24 hours after a suspected meal. The diagnosis can be confirmed by the isolation of 10^5 or more *B. cereus* organisms per gram from epidemiologically incriminated food. The isolation of *B. cereus* from stools of patients is not sufficient documentation of the outbreak unless negative stool cultures are obtained from a suitable control group.[12] Serologic typing can be performed for epidemiologic studies, but the antisera are available only in a few centers. No circulating neutralizing antibodies have been detected in symptomatic patients.[13]

Bacillus cereus food poisoning is self-limited and requires no antimicrobial therapy. Treatment is symptomatic, and occasional patients may require fluid replacement if severely dehydrated.

The main preventive measure for *B. cereus* gastroenteritis is proper food handling. The heat-resistant spores of *B. cereus* survive boiling and germinate when boiled rice is left unrefrigerated.[14] Flash frying or brief rewarming of rice before serving is not adequate to destroy the preformed, heat-stable toxin. Prompt refrigeration of boiled rice may help prevent disease.

OCULAR INFECTIONS

Bacillus species have been recognized as ocular pathogens for many years. Dacrocystitis, conjunctivitis, keratitis, iridocyclitis, panophthalmitis, and orbital abscess caused by *B. subtilis* have been described.[15] Previous reports of *B. subtilis* as a causative agent for ocular infections may have been related to faulty speciation. *Bacillus cereus* has been recently recognized as a primary pathogen of ocular infections. In a recent review of post-traumatic *B. cereus* endophthalmitis, *Bacillus* species ranks as the second most common pathogen in five of six series reviewed on post-traumatic endophthalmitis.[16] In post-traumatic ophthalmitis caused by *B. cereus* an intraocular foreign body is often present.[16,17] Such infections have been observed with metal-on-metal projectile injuries. Another setting where *Bacillus* infection occurs is that associated with contamination with soil and dust. Such infection is frequently reported in the setting of a rural or farm environment. The clinical manifestations are characterized by massive destruction of the vitreal and retinal tissue of the eye with resulting visual compromise within the first 12–48 hours after inoculation. The presence of progressive corneal deterioration and ring abscess formation is a complication of panophthalmitis caused by *B. cereus*.[18] Except for infections caused by *Pseudomonas aeruginosa* and *Proteus* species, this finding is almost pathognomonic of *B. cereus*. The ring abscess is usually observed within 48 hours after infection after finding periorbital edema, proptosis, and corneal swelling. Often the vitreal infection spreads to the retina. Patients are frequently systemically ill with fever and leukocytosis.

In the setting of drug abuse, patients present with a rapid fulminant endophthalmitis or panophthalmitis that usually results in a complete loss of vision and enucleation.[5] Initial symptoms include eye pain and decreased vision with chemosis, redness, and proptosis (Fig. 1). Although the exact pathogenesis is unclear, there is indirect evidence that the ophthalmitis is secondary to endogenous infection related to contamination of injection paraphernalia and heroin used by the drug abusers.[6] In one patient, *B. cereus* was isolated from the vitreous aspirate and also from the syringe used by the patient for injecting hydromorphine hydrochloride.[18] In addition to intravenous drugs, e.g., heroin, amphetamine, methylphenidate (Ritalin), cocaine, and hydromorphine hydrochloride, panophthalmitis has been reported after the injection of B vitamin in one patient[19] and in another patient after a blood transfusion.[20]

Early diagnosis is important to achieve successful treatment. One should have a high index of suspicion for *Bacillus* organisms as the pathogen in a patient who presents with ocular infection after trauma or in the setting of drug abuse. Prompt recognition of the infection should allow initiation of appropriate therapy before permanent structural changes occur.[17]

Adequate samples of ocular fluid should be obtained to ensure complete diagnostic evaluation. Because of the serious consequences of panophthalmitis, an aggressive approach with early vitrectomy and vitreal installation of appropriate antibiotics is indicated.[17] Antibiotics administered systemically, intravitreally, topically, and via periocular routes are used in conjunction with surgical intervention. An aminoglycoside, e.g., gentamicin or tobramycin, has been administered locally and systemically but is inadequate to eradicate the infection. Clindamycin or vancomycin is appropriate before the results of culture since *B. cereus* is the most frequent isolate. Clindamycin and gentamicin in combination seem to be favored by the ophthalmologists. Newer drugs, e.g., imipenem and quinolones, appear active, but more experience is needed in their use.[21] In the drug abuse setting both clindamycin and vancomycin have been used as a single agent. The prognosis is poor, and infection usually results in the loss of the eye, but recent experience indicates that with an aggressive approach the eye may be salvaged, although with a loss of vision.[17]

PNEUMONIA

Bacillus cereus is a rare pulmonary pathogen that has been reported to cause pneumonia in the compromised host. A wide

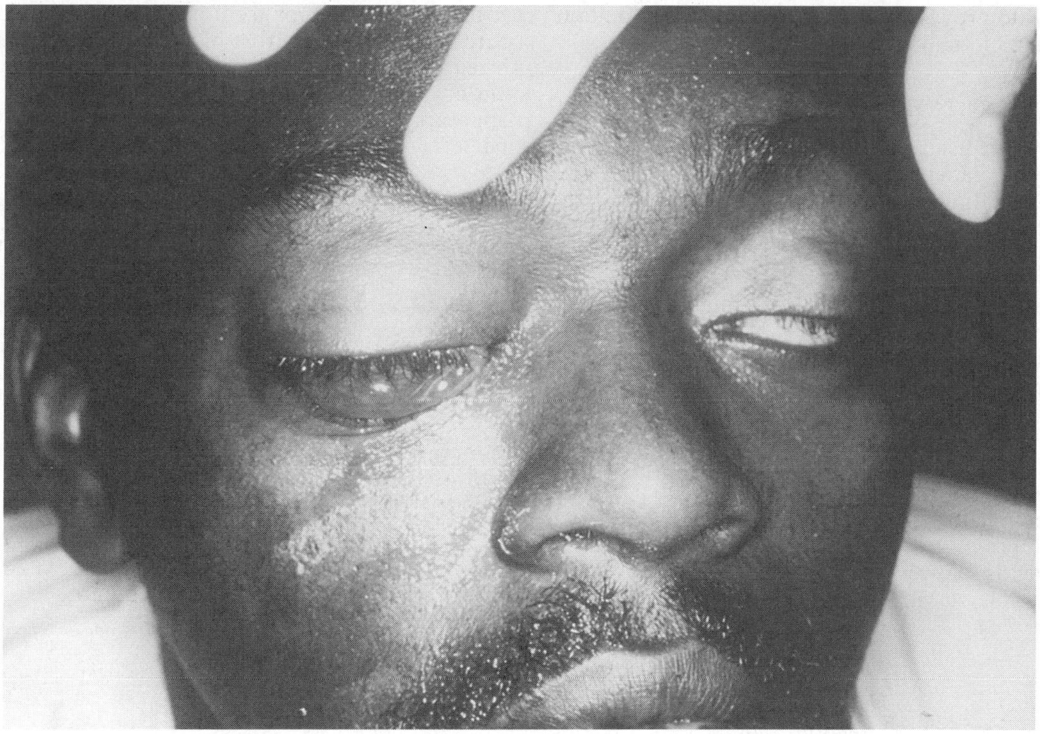

FIG. 1. *Bacillus cereus* endophthalmitis. Note the massive conjunctival edema. (From Shamsuddin et al.,[6] with permission.)

variety of pulmonary presentations have been reported. Cases of necrotizing pneumonitis caused by *B. cereus* have been reported in patients with acute leukemias and hepatic malignancies.[22,23] Very rarely, a cavitating pneumonia may be caused by *B. cereus*.[24] A large pseudotumor of the lung caused by *B. sphaericus* has been reported in a patient with chronic asthma receiving long-term steroid therapy.[25]

The clinical symptoms are indistinguishable from other bacterial pneumonias. The outcome is poor and probably related to the underlying illness. In this setting, early diagnosis is important in preventing death. In immunosuppressed patients consideration should be given to obtaining adequate specimens by transtracheal aspirate or needle aspiration to facilitate establishing the diagnosis.

ENDOCARDITIS

Endocarditis caused by *Bacillus* organisms is rare. In the setting of intravenous drug abuse, endocarditis is a well-recognized complication.[10,11] Similar to ocular infections, the heroin and injection paraphernalia remain the most likely sources of the organism. Most cases are related to drug abuse, but endocarditis has been reported in patients with foreign devices such as a ventricular pacemaker. The clinical presentation and course of endocarditis in the drug abuser is similar to those caused by other pathogens, with a predominance of tricuspid valve involvement and a relatively indolent course.

Infiltrates seen on chest x-ray films among patients with *Bacillus* endocarditis have been attributed to extracellular toxin capable of inducing massive thrombi in pulmonary vessels. In tricuspid endocarditis, however, it may well represent pulmonary septic emboli.

The diagnosis is made by isolation of *Bacillus* species repeatedly from blood cultures plus clinical findings compatible with endocarditis.

Antibiotic therapy with vancomycin or clindamycin has achieved high cure rates in *Bacillus* endocarditis.[10,11] For species other than *B. cereus*, a successful outcome has been reported with use of a cephalosporin.[26] The response to antibiotic therapy is excellent, and surgical intervention is usually not required.

BACTEREMIA AND SEPTICEMIA

Bacteremia with the *Bacillus* species is common, but isolation of the organism from blood cultures does not always indicate infection. In the drug abuser, the spectrum of blood-borne infection can range from transient bacteremia to endocarditis.[27] Again, the drug abuser usually presents with symptoms of fever and positive blood cultures temporally related to heroin injection, findings that implicate heroin injection as the mode of infection. Hemolytic anemia has been reported as a complication of *B. cereus* bacteremia in a drug abuser with hemoglobin SC disease.[28]

Bacillus bacteremia can be a complication among patients with indwelling intravascular catheters. Intravascular devices have played important roles in nosocomial bacteremias including those caused by *Bacillus* species.[29] In half of the cases of *Bacillus* species bacteremia, the device proves to be the source of the bacteremia as evidenced by a positive culture of purulent drainage from a peripheral vein or the recovery of more than 15 colonies from a semiquantitative culture of a catheter tip.[10] In the setting of nosocomial sepsis, isolation of *Bacillus* from blood should suggest an intravascular device as the source.

In patients with positive blood cultures from *Bacillus*, a decision has to be made whether the organism is causing disease. In most cases, especially if the patient is asymptomatic, the bacteremia is self-limited and requires no antimicrobial therapy, which emphasizes the relatively benignity of the process. Appropriate therapy can be readily instituted once a decision has been made that a clinically significant infection is present. Usually infections have an indolent course, and the institution of antimicrobial therapy can await specific sensitivity results. In the setting of *Bacillus* bacteremias occurring in immunosuppressed patients with chronic indwelling intravascular catheters, recent experience suggests that the catheters should be promptly removed to prevent recurrent bacteremia in addition to administering antibiotic therapy.[29]

MUSCULOSKELETAL INFECTIONS

Necrotizing fasciitis caused by *Bacillus* species has been reported in a leukemic patient and in a patient with sickle cell disease.[10,11] In both settings culture from deep tissue specimens grew pure *Bacillus* species. Antibiotic therapy alone is not sufficient, multiple surgical débridement is usually required, and in our patient amputation was necessary.[11] Depending on the species isolated, antibiotic therapy should be tailored accordingly.

Both acute and chronic osteomyelitis are infrequent presentations of *Bacillus* species infection.[10] Acute vertebral osteomyelitis caused by *B. cereus* has been reported in drug abusers and is most likely introduced via the blood stream by injection of contaminated heroin and/or paraphernalia.[11] Chronic osteomyelitis has usually been related to accidental trauma. Cases of vertebral osteomyelitis secondary to *B. cereus* have responded well to prolonged intravenous antibiotic therapy. Chronic osteomyelitis, however, is usually difficult to eradicate, requires multiple surgical procedures, and leads to substantial morbidity.[10]

MENINGITIS

In an earlier review of *Bacillus* infections that included disseminated infection, meningitis was not an uncommon presentation.[15] A wide variety of *Bacillus* species were isolated from cerebrospinal fluid in these patients, including *B. subtilis, B. megaterium* or *B. anthracoides, B. circulans*, and *B. sphaericus*. Most of the patients developed meningitis after spinal anesthesia. The remaining cases were secondary to other infections such as otitis and mastoiditis, urinary tract infection, and infected subdural hematoma. Ventricular shunts may also become infected by *Bacillus* species.[11] Meningitis caused by *Bacillus* species has been associated with a high mortality.[15,30]

Therapy is with intravenous clindamycin, vancomycin, or penicillin, depending on the *Bacillus* species isolated. Removal of any foreign body, such as a ventricular shunt, is necessary to eradicate the infection.[11]

MISCELLANEOUS SYNDROMES

Allergic and respiratory symptoms in workers engaged in the manufacture of laundry detergents containing proteolytic enzymes of *B. subtilis* have been reported.[31]

It is not common for *Bacillus* species to occur in a mixed infection such as surgical wounds, an infected breast prosthesis, and a necrotic tumor. Most patients with such infections are febrile, and the surgical wound or tumor drainage is either purulent, bloody, or serosanguineous.[4]

TREATMENT

Antibiotic susceptibility testing of *Bacillus* species indicates that β-lactam antibiotics are rarely effective in vitro against *B. cereus*, the most common isolate in clinically significant infections.[32] Although there is marked variability among species, non-*B. cereus* strains are susceptible to penicillins, semisynthetic penicillins and cephalosporins. Recent data indicate that imipenem, ciprofloxacin, and gentamicin are highly active.[21] Many strains are also susceptible to tetracycline, chloramphenicol, clindamycin, and erythromycin. The minimum bactericidal concentration (MBC) of the latter drugs may be greater than the minimum inhibitory concentration (MIC), although achievable levels in serum frequently exceed the MBC for these agents.[21] Vancomycin has been found to be bactericidal at or near the same concentration at which it was bacteriostatic.

In immunocompromised patients who have gram-positive aerobic rods isolated from blood cultures, initial coverage with broad-spectrum cephalosporins should be avoided. Vancomycin or clindamycin with or without gentamicin would be most appropriate as initial antibiotic coverage for patients with suspected *Bacillus* infections who are seriously ill.

REFERENCES

1. Wilson G. *Bacillus*: The aerobic spore-bearing bacilli. In: Parker MT, ed. Topley and Wilson's Principles of Bacteriology, Virology and Immunity. Baltimore: Williams & Wilkins; 1983.
2. William RP. *Bacillus anthracis* and other aerobic spore-forming bacilli. In: Braude A, ed. Medical Microbiology and Infectious Diseases. Philadelphia: WB Saunders; 1981.
3. Curtis JR, Wing AJ, Coleman JC. *Bacillus cereus* bacteraemia—a complication of intermittent hemodialysis. Lancet. 1967;1:136–8.
4. Ihde DC, Armstrong D. Clinical spectrum of infection due to *Bacillus* species. Am J Med. 1973;55:839–45.
5. Tuazon CU, Hill R, Sheagren JN. Microbiologic study of street heroin and injection paraphernalia. J Infect Dis. 1974;129:327–9.
6. Shamsuddin D, Tuazon CU, Levy C, et al. *Bacillus cereus* panophthalmitis: Source of the organism. Rev Infect Dis. 1982;4:97–103.
7. Gilbert RJ, Kramer JM. *Bacillus cereus* enterotoxins: Present status. Biochem Soc Trans 1984;12:198–200.
8. Turnbull PCB. *Bacillus cereus* toxins. Pharmacol Ther 1981;13:453–505.
9. Thompson NE, Ketterhagen MJ, Bergdoll MS, et al. Isolation and some properties of an enterotoxin produced by *Bacillus cereus*. Infect Immun. 1984;43:887–94.
10. Sliman R, Rehm S, Shlaes DM. Serious infections caused by *Bacillus* species. Medicine (Baltimore). 1987;66:218–23.
11. Tuazon CU, Murray HW, Levy C, et al. Serious infections from *Bacillus* sp. JAMA. 1979;241:1137–40.

11a. Weber DJ, Rutala WA. Bacillus Species. *Infect Control Hosp Epidemiol.* 1988;9:368–74.

12. Terranova W, Blake PA. *Bacillus cereus* food poisoning. N Engl J Med. 1978;298:143–4.
13. Gianella RA, Brasile L. A hospital food-borne outbreak of diarrhea caused by *Bacillus cereus*: Clinical, epidemiologic and microbiologic studies. J Infect Dis. 1979;139:366–70.
14. Gilbert RJ, Stringer MF, Peace JC. The survival and growth of *Bacillus cereus* in boiled and fried rice in relation to outbreaks of food poisoning. J Hyg Camb. 1974;73:433–44.
15. Farrar WE. Serious infections due to "non-pathogenic" organisms of the genus *Bacillus*: Review of their status as pathogens. Am J Med. 1963;34:134–41.
16. Davey RT Jr, Tauber WB. Post traumatic endophthalmitis: The emerging role of *Bacillus cereus* infection. Rev Infect Dis. 1987;9:110–123.
17. O'Day DM, Smith RS, Gregg CR, et al. The problem of *Bacillus* species infection with special emphasis on the virulence of *Bacillus cereus*. Ophthalmology. 1981;88:833–8.
18. Young EJ, Wallace RJ, Ericsson CD, et al. Panophthalmitis due to *Bacillus cereus*. Arch Intern Med. 1980;140:559–60.
19. Bouza E, Grant S, Jordan MC, et al. *Bacillus cereus* endogenous panophthalmitis. Arch Ophthalmol. 1979;97:498–9.
20. Kerkenezov N. Panophthalmitis after a blood transfusion. Br J Ophthalmol. 1953;37:632–6.
21. Weber DJ, Saviteer SM, Rutala WA, et al. In vitro susceptibility of *Bacillus* spp. to selected antimicrobial agents. Antimicrob Agents Chemother. 1988;32:642–5.
22. Pennington JE, Gibbons ND, Strobeck JE, et al. *Bacillus* species infections in patients with hematologic neoplasia. JAMA. 1976;235:1473–4.
23. Bekemeyer WB, Zimmerman GA. Life threatening complications associated with *Bacillus cereus* pneumonia. Am Rev Respir Dis. 1985;131:466–9.
24. Leff A, Jacobs R, Gooding V, et al. *Bacillus cereus* pneumonia. Survival in a patient with cavitary disease treated with gentamicin. Am Rev Respir Dis. 1977;115:151–4.
25. Isaacson P, Jacobs PH, Mackenzie AMR, et al. Pseudotumor of the lung caused by infection with *Bacillus sphaericus*. J Clin Pathol. 1976;29:806–11.
26. Reller LB. Endocarditis caused by *Bacillus subtilis*. Am J Clin Pathol. 1973;60:714–8.
27. Weller PF, Nicholson A, Braslow N. The spectrum of *Bacillus* bacteremia in heroin addicts. Arch Intern Med. 1979;139:293–4.
28. Rodgers GM, Barrera E Jr, Martin RR. *Bacillus cereus* bacteremia and hemolytic anemia in a patient with hemoglobin SC disease. Arch Intern Med. 1980;140:1103–4.
29. Cotton DJ, Gill VJ, Marshall DJ, et al. Clinical features and therapeutic interventions in 17 cases of *Bacillus* bacteremia in an immunosuppressed patient population. J Clin Microbiol. 1987;25:672–4.
30. Allen BT, Wilkinson HA. A case of meningitis and generalized Shwartzman reaction caused by *Bacillus sphaericus*. Johns Hopkins Med J. 1969;125:8–13.
31. Flindt MLH. Pulmonary disease due to inhalation of derivatives of *Bacillus subtilis* containing proteolytic enzyme. Lancet. 1969;1:1177.

32. Coonrod JD, Leadley PJ, Eickhoff TC. Antibiotic susceptibility of *Bacillus* species. J Infect Dis. 1971;123:102–5.

188. ERYSIPELOTHRIX RHUSIOPATHIAE

J. BRUCE McCLAIN

Erysipelothrix rhusiopathiae (*Erysipelothrix insidiosa*) was first isolated from mice in 1878 by Koch and shortly thereafter by Pasteur and Thuillier from a pig with rouget. Its status as a zoonotic pathogen was established by Loeffler in 1886 and as a human pathogen in 1909 by Rosenbach.[1,2] The terms *sheep joint-ill, swine erysipelas,* and *diamond skin disease* refer to animal illnesses, whereas the terms *erysipeloid, erysipeloid of Rosenbach, whale finger, fish poisoning,* and *seal finger* describe human illness. The term *erysipelas* refers to a rapidly progressive human infection of the soft tissue due to a streptococcus or staphylococcus and should not be used to describe infections with *Erysipelothrix rhusiopathiae*.[2]

Erysipelothrix rhusiopathiae is a gram-positive nonmotile, nonsporulating aerobic or facultatively anaerobic rod. It is pleomorphic, 0.8–2.5 μm in length and 0.3 μm in width. It may exhibit filamentous growth strands that may resemble mycelia but do not branch. On agar it grows as small smooth transparent colonies that may show α-hemolysis on blood agar after 48–72 hours. It ferments glucose, lactose, galactose and fructose and is catalase-, urease-, and oxidase-negative. It can be differentiated from *Listeria monocytogenes* by its lack of motility and its lack of catalase production. It can be differentiated from corynebacteria by its production of H_2S on triple-sugar iron agar slants (TSI).[2] Several serovars have been reported.

EPIDEMIOLOGY

This bacterium is geographically widespread and can be isolated from animals that are not overtly ill as well as from environmental sources in contact with animals. This is not a reportable disease, and no national data on its incidence in humans are available; however, the Centers for Disease Control (CDC) receive an average of one case a year, and a survey of microbiology laboratories in the Washington, D.C., area found no clinical isolates within the last 3 years. Most human cases occur in the summer months. Historically, occupational groups at risk for the illness are slaughterhouse workers, butchers, fishmongers, veterinary workers, food handlers, and trappers. Recent case reports, with few exceptions, are from people in contact with raw seafood or uncooked meat. Since anyone preparing meat or fish is at risk, this disease is an important consideration in the differential diagnosis of infections of the hand.

PATHOGENESIS

Most human cases of the illness result from cutaneous inoculation from some contaminated source; however, 20 percent may have no recognized exposure.[2] There are well-documented cases of endocarditis after the consumption of contaminated food.

Variations in mouse lethality between strains is from 10^1 to $>10^7$ germs, thus demonstrating large strain differences in virulence. Although the factors responsible for this variation are not known, one factor that might determine the degree of virulence is neuraminidase production by the bacterium. This bacterial enzyme can desialate host membranes, thereby making them susceptible to alternative-pathway complement-induced lysis. This property of the organism has been implicated in the arteritis and thrombocytopenia produced in the disseminated form of the rat infection.[3–5]

This infection may be localized, or it may be disseminated. Both forms of the illness have unusual manifestations: (*1*) pain and inflammation in the joints in the regional lymphatic drainage from the site of infection in localized disease, (*2*) a slowly progressive plaquelike skin lesion in the localized disease, and (*3*) a purpuric vasculitic rash in the disseminated form of the illness.

The progressive indurated papular skin lesion may develop central clearing as it resolves. It is characterized histologically by edema of the prickle cells and lymphatic dilatation with perivascular infiltration of neutrophils and basophils. The organism is generally detected in perivascular regions of the dermis.[6]

The purpuric rash is occasionally bullous and is characterized histologically by severe edema in the stratum germinativum and the dermal papillae. There is an intense infiltration of granulocytes in the subpapillary layer and zona reticularis where large collections of germs may be present.[6,7]

CLINICAL MANIFESTATIONS

The incubation period is usually less than 4 days but may be as long as 7. There are two major clinical syndromes: (*1*) localized cutaneous and (*2*) disseminated/endocarditic.[8] There are a number of less common presentations reported as single cases or small series such as chronic arthritis, cerebritis, diffuse cutaneous infection, and osteomyelitis.[1,6,9]

The localized cutaneous form of the illness accounts for 90 percent of preantibiotic reports. It begins after localized inoculation with infectious material. It is characterized by throbbing pain, tingling, itching, and burning, usually with pain or stiffness in the adjacent joint, typically a wrist or finger but occasionally a shoulder or elbow. The skin is indurated in an irregular fashion with distinct borders suggesting an infiltrative process and is accompanied by a violaceous color (Fig. 1).[7] In 10 percent of the cases vesicles that may be hemorrhagic may develop; in 5 percent frank arthritis may develop. Constitutional symptoms such as fever are present in 10 percent of these cases, while 20 percent of the cases will develop proximal spread of the inflammation from the hand to the arm.

Clinical characteristics of erysipeloid that help distinguish its diagnosis from pyogenic cellulitis are the proximal but not distal spread of the skin eruption and the absence of suppuration and

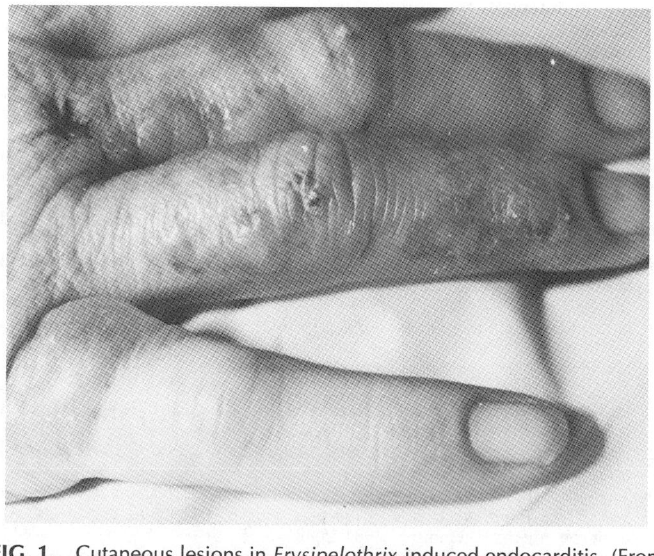

FIG. 1. Cutaneous lesions in *Erysipelothrix*-induced endocarditis. (From Park et al.,[11] with permission.)

pitting edema. The diagnosis is made by culturing the organism from the blood or an infected site. Since *Erysipelothrix* is located deep in the dermis, simple swabbing usually will not detect the pathogen, and biopsy is necessary. There is no available serology.[1,6,9,10]

Most localized cutaneous disease will run a self-limited course averaging 3 weeks. The cutaneous rash will fade by central clearing. One percent of cases will relapse.[1,9,10]

The septicemic form accounts for the majority of recent case reports and is usually associated with endocarditis. Cardinal features of the septicemic form are fever and malaise. Thirty-six percent of cases have a concurrent skin lesion of erysipeloid. Less commonly, a purpuric and petechial rash that is vasculitic in nature occurs and may be accompanied by thrombocytopenia.[1,7,8,11,12]

TREATMENT AND PREVENTION

Erysipelothrix rhusiopathiae is very sensitive to penicillin. All of the 238 strains tested by one investigator were inhibited by less than 0.2 units/ml of penicillin G and less than 0.2 μg/ml of ampicillin, and 95 percent of the strains were susceptible to erythromycin at less than 0.39 μg/ml. Over half of the strains were resistant to oxytetracycline, chloramphenicol, streptomycin, sulfonamides, and kanamycin.[13] Summarized susceptibilities of strains isolated from human endocarditis cases suggests that *Erysipelothrix* is sensitive to cephalothin and clindamycin but is not sensitive to vancomycin.[8,11,13] Since most reported bacteremic cases are associated with endocarditis, presumptive treatment for *Erysipelothrix* endocarditis with daily doses of 12–20 million units of penicillin G should be instituted when bacteremia is encountered. Cephalosporins are an alternative in the penicillin-allergic patients.

There does not appear to be lasting immunity to this germ even in infected individuals. Relapses occur.[1] The development of a veterinary vaccine has been complicated by this lack of immunogenicity. Cross-protection experiments have shown incomplete protection. The current attentuated live vaccine has not been able to consistently protect against infection.[14]

REFERENCES

1. Grieco M, Sheldon C. *Erysipelothrix rhusiopathiae*. Ann NY Acad Sci. 1970;174:523–32.
2. Rosenbach FJ. Experimentelle, morphologische und klinische Studie über die krankheitserregenden Mikroorganismen des Schweinerotlauf, des Erysipeloids und der Mäusesepsis. Z Hyg Infektionskr. 1909;63:343–69.
3. Krasemann C, Muller HE. The virulence of *Erysipelothrix rhusiopathiae* strains and their neuraminidase production. Zentrabl Bakteriol Mikrobiol Hyg [A]. 1975;231:206–13.
4. Nakato H, Shinomiya K, Mikawa H. Possible role of neuraminidase in the pathogenesis of arteritis and thrombocytopenia induced in rats by *Erysipelothrix rhusiopathiae*. Pathol Res Pract. 1986;181:311–9.
5. Nakato H, Shinomiya K, Mikawa H. Adhesion of *Erysipelothrix rhusiopathiae* to cultured rat aortic endothelial cells. The role of bacterial neuraminidase in the induction of arteritis. Pathol Res Pract. 1987;182:255–60.
6. Klauder JV. *Erysipelothrix rhusiopathiae* infection in swine and in human beings. A comparative study of cutaneous lesions. Arch Dermatol Syph. 1944;50:151–9.
7. Erlich JC. *Erysipelothrix rhusiopathiae* infection in man. Arch Intern Med. 1945;78:565–77.
8. Gorby GL, Peacock JE. *Erysipelothrix rhusiopathiae* endocarditis: Microbiologic, epidemiologic and clinical features of an occupational disease. Rev Infect Dis. 1988;10:317–25.
9. Nelson E. Five hundred cases of erysipeloid. Rocky Mtn Med J. 1955;52:40–2.
10. Klauder JV. Erysipeloid as an occupational disease. JAMA. 1938;111:1345–8.
11. Park C, Poretz D, Goldenberg R. *Erysipelothrix* endocarditis with cutaneous lesion. South Med J. 1976;69:1101–3.
12. Procter WI. Subacute bacterial endocarditis due to *Erysipelothrix rhusiopathiae*. Am J Med. 1965;38:820–4.
13. Takahashi T, Sawada T, Ohmae K, et al. Antibiotic resistance of *Erysipelothrix rhusiopathiae* isolated from pigs with chronic swine erysipelas. Antimicrob Agents Chemother. 1984;25:385–6.
14. Takahashi T, Tahagi M, Sawada T. Cross protection in mice and swine immunized with live erysipelas vaccine to challenge exposure with strains of *Erysipelothrix rhusiopathiae* of various serotypes: Am J Vet Res. 1984;45:2115–8.

GRAM-NEGATIVE COCCI

189. NEISSERIA MENINGITIDIS

MICHAEL A. APICELLA

Few infections can cause the civil, medical, and social stress that occurs when serious meningococcal disease enters a community. The rapid onset of disease, the fulminant course of some of the infected, and the mortality and morbidity clearly are reasonable causes for the profound dread of this infection. In addition, the problems of rumor and misinformation frequently add substantially to the woes of medical personnel.

Despite recent advances in understanding the pathogenesis and immunobiology of the meningococcus and the development of effective vaccines against certain meningococcal serotypes, serious infection with this pathogen remains a major worldwide health problem.

Epidemic cerebrospinal fever (meningococcal meningitis) was first described in Geneva by Vieusseaux in 1805.[1] Subsequent reports throughout the nineteenth century confirm its episodic epidemic nature with a propensity for afflicting young children and military recruits assembled in stationary barrack situations.[2] In 1887, Weichselbaum isolated the meningococcus from the cerebrospinal fluid (CSF), and the etiologic relationship between this organism and epidemic meningitis was firmly established.[3] Kiefer in 1896[4] and Albrecht and Ghon in 1901[5] found that healthy persons could become carriers of the meningococcus. Serotypes of the meningococcus were first recognized by Dopter in 1909.[6] This laid the basis for serum therapy in the treatment of meningococcal infection by Flexner in 1913.[7] Glover was the first to note that the carrier rates in military recruitment camps rose with the periods of crowding, and he believed they were associated with an increased incidence of cases.[8] In 1928–1930[9,10] and in 1941[11] significant national and worldwide epidemics occurred. In 1937, sulfonamide therapy radically altered the outcome of meningococcal infection and replaced serum in the treatment.[12] Prophylaxis with sulfonamides eradicated the carrier state[13] and provided a simple and safe method for the prevention of epidemics, particularly in the crowded environments of military barracks. With the advent of antibiotic agents, treatment of meningococcal infection became more effective, and mortality declined. Increasing sulfonamide resistance among meningococci was recognized by Schoenback and Phair[14] in 1941–1943 but did not become a clinically significant problem until the meningococcal epidemics in 1963 in two military bases in California.[15,16] With the subsequent worldwide emergence of resistant strains and with the absence of effective chemoprophylaxis, renewed interest in immunoprevention has occurred and has led to the development of safe and effective vaccines against the groups A, C, Y and W-135 meningococcal serogroups.[17,18]

Many problems still exist in the understanding, prevention, and treatment of meningococcal infection. These include the susceptibilities of certain populations to this infection, its sporadic epidemic nature, the mechanisms responsible for carrier eradication by antibiotics, the reasons for the fulminant nature of the infection, the poor immunogenicity of the group C vaccine in children under the age of 2 years, and the inability of humans to develop antibody to the group B polysaccharide vaccine. Until these and many other questions are answered, meningococcal infections will continue to be a scourge among human populations.

ETIOLOGIC AGENT: MORPHOLOGIC, CULTURAL, AND BIOCHEMICAL CHARACTERISTICS

Neisseria meningitidis is a gram-negative diplococcus (0.6 × 0.8 μm). The adjacent sides are flattened to produce the typical biscuit shape. Because the organism tends to readily undergo autolysis, considerable size and shape variation can be seen in older cultures. The organism produces a polysaccharide capsule, which is the basis of the serogroup typing system. These capsules are not readily visible on Gram stain, but capsules of the serogroup A and C strains can be made to undergo the quellung reaction in the presence of the appropriate serogroup antiserum. The organism is considered fastidious in its growth conditions, thus necessitating the use of appropriate media and growth conditions. These problems in reliable growth may relate as much to nutritional factors as to the presence of substances toxic to the meningococcus in the medium. On solid media, the meningococcus grows as a transparent, nonpigmented, nonhemolytic colony approximately 1–5 mm in diameter. Colonies are convex and, if large amounts of polysaccharide are present, will appear mucoid rather than smooth. Optimal growth conditions are achieved in a moist environment at 35–37°C under an atmosphere of 5–10% carbon dioxide. The organism will grow well on a number of medium bases including blood agar base, trypticase soy agar, supplemented chocolate agar, and Mueller-Hinton agar and will thrive well in cultures grown in Mueller-Hinton agar or trypticase soy broth. Semidefined media such as Frantz medium also provide the necessary nutrients for excellent growth conditions. Confirmation of the presence of this organism in clinical specimens is dependent on a series of carbohydrate fermentations. The meningococcus will ferment glucose and maltose to acid without gas formation and fails to ferment sucrose or lactose. Indole and hydrogen sulfide are not formed. In addition, the organism contains cytochrome oxidase in its cell wall. The enzyme will oxidize the dye tetramethylphenylenediamine (TMPD) from colorless to deep pink. This latter test was initially considered specific for *Neisseria*, but subsequent studies have shown that other genera also exhibit high TMPD-oxidase activities, including *Pseudomonas, Azobacter, Aeromonas,* and *Moraxella*.

Like the gonococcus, the meningococcus has a rapid autolytic rate. Hebeler and Young have demonstrated the presence of an autolysin, an amidase, that acts on the peptidoglycan layer of the gonococcus.[19,20] Whether the mechanism of autolysis is similar in the meningococcus is uncertain. The process appears to be enzymatic since autolysis can be stopped by the addition of potassium cyanide or formalin or by heating cultures to 65°C for 30 minutes.

The importance of iron in the survival of microbes has stimulated interest in the mechanisms *Neisseria* uses in iron acquisition. It has been shown that iron-loaded animals are more susceptible to fatal meningococcal infection.[21] The meningococcus does not produce a soluble siderophore but possess a series of membrane proteins that selectively scavange iron from hemoglobin, transferrin, and lactoferrin.[22,23]

ANTIGENIC STRUCTURE OF THE MENINGOCOCCUS

Capsular Polysaccharides

Shortly after identification of the meningococcus as the etiologic agent in epidemic meningitis and after recognition of healthy nasopharyngeal carriers of the organism, investigations into the application of immunologic methods for the detection and differentiation of meningococci occurred. It became apparent that antigenically diverse meningococci existed, and spurred on by the introduction of serum therapy,[7] English workers identified four antigenically distinct types of meningococci.[24] Because different laboratories were involved, a complex nomenclature evolved that was not resolved until the mid-1950s when serogrouping nomenclature based on capital letters unified all the different systems and simplified the taxonomy. The basis of this specific serogrouping was identified by Scherp and Rake when they isolated the soluble specific polysaccharide responsible for the specificity of the group A meningococcal strains.[25] The relationship between this polysaccharide and the capsule of the meningococcus was established by using the quellung reaction on group A strains.[26] Branham and Carlin, using group C strains, were able to demonstrate that these antigens elicited antibodies that conferred specific protection in mice.[27]

After the introduction of antibiotics, interest in the development of serogroup-specific antigens for use as vaccines diminished greatly, but Watson et al. continued their efforts and identified the specific soluble substance from the group C meningococcus and showed its sialic acid nature.[28]

A major impetus that renewed interest in the immunobiology of the meningococcus was the emergence of sulfonamide-resistant meningococci as a clinical problem. This made antibiotic prophylaxis ineffective, and persistent epidemics of serogroup B and C strains on military recruit reservations during the 1960s prompted reinvestigations into the feasibility of using capsular polysaccharide antigens as vaccine materials.

Meningococci can be segregated by seroagglutination into at least 13 serogroups: A, B, C, D[29,30]; X, Y, Z[31,32]; E, W-135[32]; H, I, K[33]; and L.[34] Capsular polysaccharides responsible for the serogrouping specificity of the groups A, B, C, X, Y, Z, W-135, and L have been purified (Table 1). These polysaccharides have been isolated from the broth supernate of overnight cultures, and a number of effective methods using either detergent precipitation or molecular-sieve and ion-exchange chromatography have been used in their separation.[35–37] Group C polysaccharides can be biochemically divided into neuraminidase-sensitive and neuraminidase-resistant polysaccharides.[38,39] The C strains producing the neuraminidase-sensitive polysaccharide have been designated C-variant strains and have been given the designation C_1.

The role of *O*-acetylation in the specificity of the antigenicity of the groups B and C polysaccharides is not completely known. Evidence now suggests that this substitution is unimportant since both group B- and C-variant strains contain no *O*-acetyl groups[39,40] and, according to Bhattacharjee et al., while *O*-acetyl substitutions are restricted to the C-7 and C-8 atoms of the sialic acid residues, up to 24 percent of the native C_1 polysaccharide is unacetylated.[41] The immunogenicity of the group A and C polysaccharide in humans appears to be a function of their molecular size. Brandt et al. have shown a progressive decrease in the immune response to both the group C and A

TABLE 1. Chemical Composition of Meningococcal Capsular Polysaccharides

Capsular Serogroup Antigen	*Chemical Composition of Capsular Polymer*
A	Partially *O*-acetylated 2-acetamido-2-deoxy-D-mannose-6-phosphate
B	(2 → 8)-linked *N*-acetylneuraminic acid
C_{1+}	*O*-acetylated (2 → 9)-linked *N*-acetylneuraminic acid
C_{1-}	(2 → 9)-linked *N*-acetylneuraminic acid
X	2-acetamido-2-deoxy-D-glucose-4-phosphatate
Y	Partially *O*-acetylated alternating sequence of D-glucose and *N*-acetylneuraminic acid
W-135	Alternating sequence of D-galactose and *N*-acetylneuraminic acid
L	*N*-acetylglucosamine phosphate

polysaccharides in persons immunized with lots of vaccine of decreasing molecular size.[42] In addition, these studies have indicated that the group C vaccine is stable and immunogenic after up to 4 years of storage. The group B polysaccharide has been purified and described immunochemically, but identification of strains that reliably produce polysaccharide and the separation of large quantities of the polysaccharide have been difficult.[40] The polysaccharide may be susceptible to acid accumulation during the stationary growth phase and may undergo degeneration.[43] Increasing the buffering capacity of the medium has been suggested to overcome this problem. The group B polysaccharide has also proved to be a very poor immunogen in humans. At the present time no effective vaccine preparation exists for this serogroup.[44] With the increasing frequency of clinical cases caused by the group Y meningococcus, there has been renewed interest in the capsular polysaccharide strains from this serogroup.[45] The safety and immunogenicity of group Y and W-135 capsular polysaccharides has been demonstrated in humans.[46]

Noncapsular Cell Wall Antigens

The meningococcal outer membrane is similar in structure to other gram negative bacteria. It contains a number of somatic antigens that are important in pathogenesis and immunobiology. The principle antigens that have been studied include the lipooligosaccharide (LOS), which is analogous to the lipopolysaccharide of the enteric gram-negative bacilli, and the outer membrane proteins. The LOS is serologically diverse, with at least 12 different LOS serotypes.[47] The chemical structure of the oligosaccharide portion of the meningococcal LOS from an L3, L7, and L9 serotype has been studied.[48] Interest in the meningococcal outer membrane proteins was stimulated by the work of Gold et al. who showed that a noncapsular typing system could be derived by using bactericidal techniques.[49,50] Using similar methods, Frasch and Chapman succeeded in identifying 11 distinct serotypes of group B meningococci.[51] The antigens responsible for this serotyping system are protein in nature and reside in the outer membrane as part of a lipoprotein–LOS complex. More recently, it has been demonstrated that the serogroup B and C meningococci can be subdivided into at least 15 protein serotypes based on antigenically different outer membrane proteins.[52] The serotype 2 outer membrane protein has been associated with a predilection for disease-causing isolates of the serogroup B meningococcus during epidemics. Recent studies indicate that endemic meningococcal disease appears to be caused by a broad, heterogeneous distribution of serotypes.[53] This is in contrast to epidemics that appear to be caused by a single serotype. Recently, the successful application of molecular biology techniques has resulted in the cloning of a number of important outer membrane protein antigens of the meningococcus, including the H.8 protein[54] and the class 1 outer membrane protein.[55] Recently, Frasch and associates[56] suggested revising the classification system for the somatic antigen serotypes of the meningococcus. These investigators have proposed a new schema based upon the major class 2 (41,000 kD) and class 3 (38,000 kD) outer membrane proteins and the lipooligosaccharides. In their example, a meningococcal strain would be identified by serogroup:protein serotype:lipooligosaccharide serotype. The addition of the class 1 protein (46,000 kD) characteristics could be also used to further define the strain.

By analyzing multilocus enzyme genotypes, Sollander et al. have developed a system for defining the clonal distribution of bacterial isolates.[57] Applying this method the studies of the meningococcus, Olyhoek and coworkers have shown that epidemics caused on a worldwide basis by a strain of serogroup A meningococcus are derived from a single clonotype.[58] Recently, Caugant and coworkers have studied 650 meningococcal strains of different capsular serogroups and have shown that over a period of many years the genetic structure of *N. meningitidis* is basically clonal as a result of low rates of recombination of chromosomal genes.[59]

Meningococci have been shown to have pili.[60] These structures can be maintained under special cultural conditions in vitro, and their role as ligands in attachment to human cells has been studied.[61] Piliated meningococci attach to human nasopharyngeal cells in greater numbers than do meningococci devoid of pili. Trypsin or mechanical shearing causes a loss of pili and decreased attachment. There appears to be wide differences in attachment capability, depending upon the site of isolation of the epithelial cell.[62] Unlike gonococci, piliated meningococci form colonies that are indistinguishable from their nonpiliated isogenic forms.[63]

HUMAN IMMUNOLOGIC RESPONSE TO MENINGOCOCCAL ANTIGENS

Goldschneider et al. have demonstrated that the percentage of people having bactericidal activity in their serum against *Neisseria meningitidis* is inversely proportional to the incidence of meningococcal meningitis during the first 12 years of life.[64,65] At birth, due to maternal transfer of antibodies, approximately 50 percent of the infants have bactericidal antibody titers. The prevalence of bactericidal antibody decreases after birth and reaches its nadir between 6 and 24 months of age. Thereafter, a linear increase in antibody titer occurs until the age of 12. In early adulthood, the prevalence of bactericidal antibody varies with the serogroup but ranges from 67 percent for group A to 86 percent for group B. These same investigators demonstrated the protective nature of bactericidal antibody against homologous serogroups during an epidemic situation. Only 3 of 54 sera from patients contained bactericidal antibody in prebleed specimens against the ultimately infecting serogroup, while 444 of 550 prebleed sera from matched control subjects who did not become infected contained homologous bactericidal antibody. Based on the observations of Goldschneider et al., 38.5 percent of the persons who lacked bactericidal antibody and who acquired the epidemic strain in their nasopharynx in the military recruit environment developed systemic meningococcal disease. Their conclusion was that a deficiency of circulating antimeningococcal antibodies is firmly associated with the establishment of meningococcemia. It appears that bactericidal antibodies are directed against both the capsular polysaccharide and other cell wall antigens that may cross react within the family Neisseriae and with other bacterial genera. Goldschneider et al. demonstrated that the meningococcal carrier state is an immunizing process and that within 2 weeks of colonization production of antibodies to meningococci can be identified.[64,65] Nontypable meningococcal strains, which are seen in carrier studies in children, contain cross-reacting antigens with the encapsulated strains, and bactericidal antibody to these strains develops after nasopharyngeal colonization. Goldschneider et al. also showed that serogroup-specific antibodies arise during the carrier state. The bulk of antimeningococcal antibodies in pooled γ-globulin collected in 1968 were directed against the capsular polysaccharide. In addition, these studies showed that the antibody was primarily directed against the serogroup C meningococcus, which was prevalent in the population at the time of collection. This is in contrast to the low level of antibody directed against the capsular polysaccharide of the group A meningococci, which had not been prevalent in the population for 10–15 years. It would appear that the bulk of protection in the pooled γ-globulin to the C meningococcus is capsular, while protection against group A meningococcus is afforded by cross-reacting antibodies.

Serologic cross-reactions between the meningococcal group A polysaccharide occur with *Bacillus pumilis*, and *Escherichia coli* K1 antigen is immunologically and chemically identical to the group B capsular polysaccharide.[66,67] These unrelated yet immunologically similar antigens may play a very important role in the development of natural immunity to the meningococcus and ultimately in protection against virulent meningococci. Cross-reactivity has now been clearly demonstrated between neonatal tissues and the group B capsular polysaccharide. By using monoclonal antibodies specific for this capsule it has been shown that cross-reactivity exists between central nervous system, cardiac, liver, and renal glycoproteins[68] in the infant rat and the group B polysaccharide. As the animal matures, the cross-reacting antigens persist in the central nervous system. These studies suggest that the poor immunogenicity of this polysaccharide may be due to the fact that it resembles host antigens.

Antibodies to the meningococcus may also enhance susceptibility to infection. By using immunoabsorbent columns to remove serum IgA, Griffiss and Bertram demonstrated that bactericidal activity was deficient in the acute sera of 24 of 28 patients with meningitis or meningococcemia before absorption but was uniformly present after removal of the IgA.[69]

A hypothetic immunoepidemiologic model of epidemic meningococcal disease has been developed that proposes that epidemic susceptibility is acquired by induction of antimeningococcal serum IgA by cross-reacting enteric bacteria. Simultaneous colonization with the appropriate strain of *N. meningitidis* then may result in disseminated disease.[70]

The role of local IgA antibody in protection or modulation of the carrier state is unknown. The meningococcus produces a protease that cleaves the Fc fragment of secretory and serum IgA from the Fab portion of the molecule.[71] The role of this enzyme in the pathogenesis of human disease is unclear. Production of this enzyme among *Neisseria* is confined to the pathogenic members, meningococci, and gonococci.[72]

The Meningococcal Carrier State

The carriage of *Neisseria meningitidis* in the nasopharynx in otherwise healthy humans has been recognized since 1896. Like the carrier states seen with cholera, diphtheria, and typhoid, the dichotomy between the presence of these dread organisms and the absence of the associated disease process seemed a paradox to early investigators. Dopter, before the elucidation of distinct meningococcal serogroups, found organisms in the nasopharynx that had all the characteristics of meningococci but that failed to agglutinate with antimeningococcic serum prepared from strains isolated from spinal fluid. He labeled these parameningococci.[6] Considerable confusion arose, but subsequent investigators demonstrated that all four of the known serotypes, including the parameningococci of Dopter, could cause meningitis.

In 1908, Bruns and Hohn noted a close relationship between the carrier rate in a population and the onset, rise, and decline of an epidemic.[73] Glover noted the same association in the British Army military camps of the First World War and felt that when the carrier rate exceeded 20 percent the community was in danger of an epidemic, usually due to the predominant carrier serotype.[8] Many of Glover's concepts have prevailed until today despite considerable data that fail to support them. Dudley and Brennan showed that high and persistent carrier rates of meningococci, most which were typeable, were not associated with cases of meningococcal meningitis. Hence, to attach any percentage of carrier rates as a bellwether of an epidemic was unsound.[74]

The transmission of the meningococci from carrier to carrier is probably via the respiratory route, but precise data supporting this thesis or on the mechanisms involved are not available. The rate of spread of the carrier state through a population has been the subject of a number of studies. During epidemics in military camps, the rate of new carrier acquisition can be very rapid, while in nonepidemic situations, both military and civilian, the rate of new carrier acquisition can be considerably slower, and the state of carriage can exist for prolonged periods of time. Rake demonstrated that carriers fell into three groups, chronic, intermittent, and transient, and that chronic carriers could be constantly colonized for up to 2 years.[75] He also demonstrated that such factors as coryza unassociated with concomitant rises in other bacterial flora had no effect on the population of meningococci, while streptococcal pharyngitis or any other condition that increases other members of the resident flora of the nasopharynx cause a concomitant decrease in the numbers of meningococci present. Greenfield et al. studied carrier rates in families not exposed to clinically important meningococcal infection during a nonepidemic period. Eighty-eight percent of the strains isolated were groupable, with group B the most common serogroup isolated.[76] During the 32-month observation period, 18 percent of the population were carriers at least once. The median duration of carriage was 9.6 months, and in 38 percent it exceeded 16 months. Adult men had the highest incidence of carriage, ranging from 19 to 33 percent. The adult man introduced the organism into the household 50 percent of the time, and when this occurred, the carrier rate in the children and women in the family increased to levels comparable to those for adult men. The rate of transmission in these circumstances was considered low in comparison with most communicable pathogens, and it was estimated that at this level a susceptible person would have more than a 50 percent chance of escaping carriage even if exposed continually to household carriers for a 5-year period.

Coincident viral infection may affect acquisition of meningococcal nasopharyngeal carriage. It has been noted that, in a study of household contacts, individuals who had a recent history of symptoms of upper respiratory infection had a significantly higher carriage rate when compared with household members without such symptoms.[77]

The carrier state is an immunizing process. Indirect evidence for this phenomenon is the fact that while military recruits have a high frequency of meningococcal carriage and disease seasoned veterans have a much lower carrriage rate and a disease incidence no different from the civilian population. In military recruits, antimeningococcic antibodies have been shown to persist for a minimum of 4–6 months after exposure. These antibodies are of the three major immunoglobulin classes and combine with group-specific and cross-reactive antigens.[64,65] Reller et al. demonstrated the development of bactericidal antibodies to the meningococcus in 38 military recruits who became colonized with nongroupable meningococcal strains. Bactericidal antibody to the homologous strains was present in 39 percent of these men, and in addition, 7–52 percent developed antibodies that were directed against groupable strains.[78] These same investigators found greatly enhanced (10- to 100-fold increase) bactericidal activity to known pathogenic strains of groups A, B, C, and Y after colonization with nongroupable meningococci. This suggests that these organisms may be at least as capable of stimulating cross-reactive antibody as groupable meningococci through either an initial or anamnestic response. An excellent review of the meningococcal carrier state has been recently provided.[79]

Epidemiology of Meningococcal Disease

Meningococcal disease is still a major worldwide health problem. Feldman estimates that during the period 1939–1962 there were almost 600,000 cases in the world and that more than 100,000 of them were fatal.[80] The greatest percentage of these cases was and still is in children.

The case rate during endemic situations varies widely and has almost doubled in the United States over the 6-year period 1975–1981 from 1 to over 2 per 100,000 population. In 1981, there were 3525 cases reported to the Centers for Disease Control as compared with 1478 cases reported in 1978. Infants (816 cases) and children between 1 and 4 years of age (970 cases) accounted for 51 percent of the 1981 patients.[81] Peltola and coworkers have pointed out that shifts in this age distribution of meningococcal disease in a population can forecast an epidemic situation. Relatively more cases arise in the 5- through 19-year-old during epidemic than nonepidemic circumstances.[82,83] Careful surveillance of age distribution patterns may be valuable in recognizing an epidemic during its inception.

The case fatality rate varies depending upon the prevalence of disease, the nature of the infection, and the socioeconomic conditions of the society in which the infections occur. During endemic stiuations in industrialized countries, case fatality can be as low as 7 percent for meningitis and as high as 19 percent for septicemia without meningeal involvement.[84] During epidemic situations, mortality for meningitis can vary from 2 to 10 percent and for septicemia can be as high as 70 percent in some Third World countries.[85,86] In the United States an 8 percent case fatality rate has been reported from major medical centers during endemic periods.[87]

The dramatic effect of antibiotics on the case fatality rate can be seen by comparing two epidemics. Norton and Gordon described an epidemic in Detroit from 1929 to 1931 that involved 1272 patients. The overall case fatality rate was 50 percent, with the highest rate occurring in infants (84 percent) and in adults over the age of 40 (72 percent).[9] During an epidemic in Chile in 1940–1943,[11] the case rate in the province of Valpariso during 1942 was 188.1 per 100,000 population. In Santiago, at the peak of the same epidemic, the case rate in infants was 838.1 per 100,000 population. The meningococcal serotype responsible for this epidemic was group A. Sulfonamides were used in treatment, and the case fatality rate was 16 percent.

Areas of the world that have experienced recent epidemic meningococcal disease are Finland, Mongolia, Alaska, sub-Sahara Africa, and central Canada. Epidemics have occurred in school children in Houston and among skid row populations in Seattle. An excellent review of the epidemic problems in Africa has recently been written by Greenwood.[88]

Clinical Manifestations

The clinical manifestations of meningococcal disease can be quite varied. This can range from transient fever and bacteremia to fulminant disease with death ensuing within hours of the onset of clinical symptoms. Wolfe and Birbara[89] have described four clinical situations.

1. Bacteremia without sepsis. Admission is for an upper respiratory illness or viral exanthem. After recovery and frequently after discharge without specific antimicrobial therapy, the results of blood cultures are reported as positive for *Neisseria meningitidis*. Sullivan and LaScolea recently reported three children with such occult bacteremia who recovered from meningococcal sepsis spontaneously without antibiotics. The level of bacteremia in these children was low, from 22 to 325 organisms/ml.[90]
2. Meningococcemia without meningitis. In these cases the patient is septic, and the signs of leukocytosis, skin rashes, generalized malaise, weakness, headache, and hypotension develop on admission or shortly thereafter.
3. Meningitis with or without meningococcemia. In these patients headache, fever, and meningeal signs are present with a cloudy spinal fluid. The state of the sensorium may vary widely from fully alert to comatose. The deep tendon and other reflexes are normal.
4. The meningoencephalitic presentation. These patients are profoundly obtunded with meningeal signs and septic spinal fluid. The deep tendon reflexes and other reflexes are altered (either absent or rarely hyperactive). Pathologic reflexes are frequently present.

Variations of these manifestations can occur, and the patient can progress from one to the other during the course of disease.

The wide range of clinical expressions requires a high index of suspicion and a careful search for clues of disease, particularly in the endemic situation where a sporadic case is involved. Carpenter and Petersdorf in 53 such cases of meningococcal meningitis reported that headache, confusion, and stiff neck occurred as symptoms in fewer than half the patients.[91] In infants and small children, fever and vomiting are often the only complaints, and children are frequently not brought to the hospital until an insidious impairment in consciousness or convulsions occur.

The signs of meningococcal disease can vary widely. Petechial lesions are a common harbinger of this infection, but occasionally if the patient is not completely undressed when examined or if examination of mucous surfaces such as the palpebral conjunctiva is omitted, important telltale lesions can be missed (Fig. 1). The petechial rash is manifested as discrete lesions 1–2 mm in diameter most frequently on the trunk and lower portions of the body (Figs. 2 and 3). They are commonly seen in clusters under areas where pressure may be applied to the skin by the elastic in underwear or stockings, which demonstrates the importance of completely disrobing the patient for an adequate examination. The petechial lesions can coalesce and form larger lesions that appear ecchymotic. These lesions may actually be secondary to subcutaneous hemorrhage, can occasionally be vesicular, and frequently desquamate as the patients recover. The petechiae correlate with the degree of thrombocytopenia and clinically are important as an indicator in the evolution of bleeding complications secondary to disseminated intravascular coagulopathies (DIC) that ensue. Early in the course of treatment, the progression of petechiae is important to follow both as an index of the effectiveness of therapy and as an index of whether additional therapies should be instituted. One simple way of accomplishing this is to circle areas

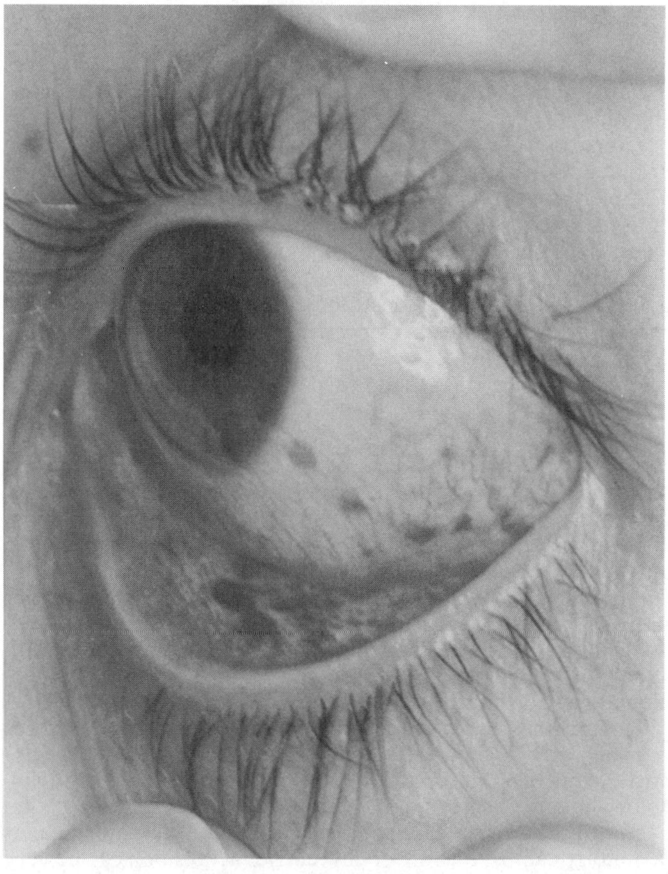

FIG. 1. Palpebral and ocular conjunctival petechiae due to meningococcal sepsis.

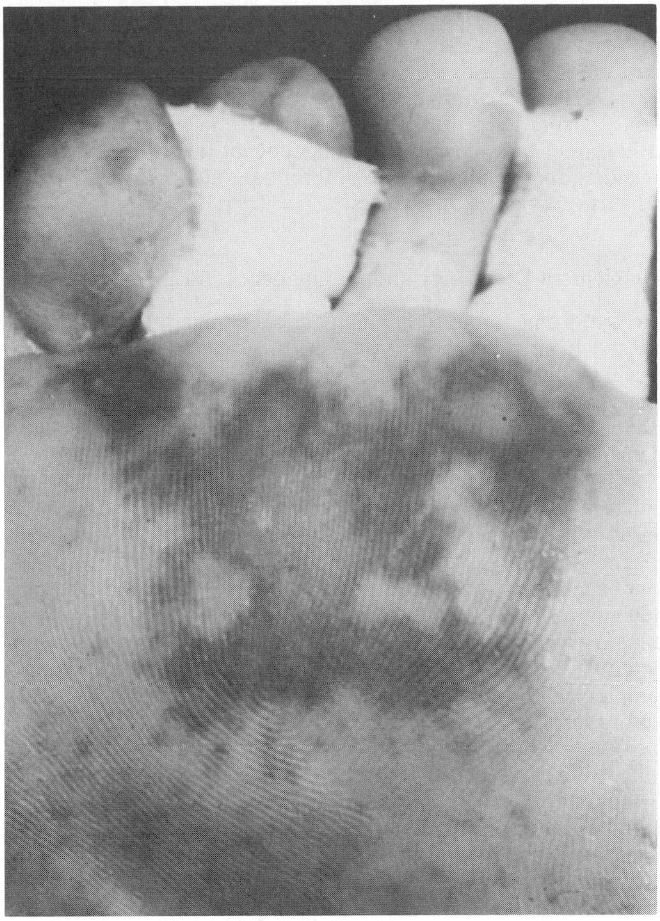

FIG. 2. Subcutaneous ecchymosis on a sole due to meningococcal sepsis.

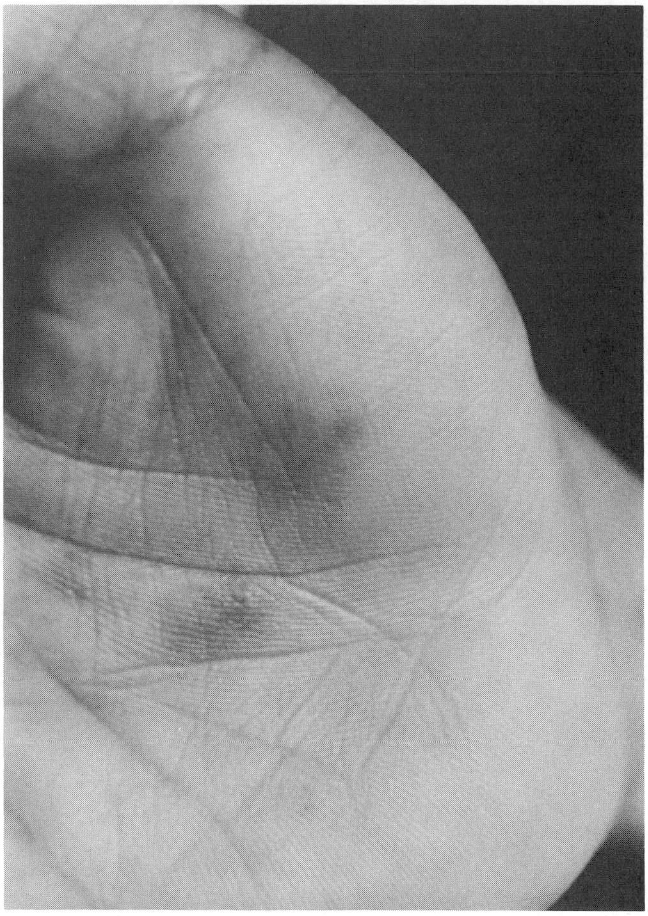

FIG. 3. Embolic lesions on a palm secondary to meningococcal sepsis.

with petechiae, count those within the circle, and document the number of petechial lesions and time of the count on a flow sheet. Counts within each circle should be performed hourly early in the disease or until the patient's condition stabilizes.

A number of authors have described another type of rash associated with meningococcal infection.[80,89] This is a macropapular eruption that can vary somewhat in hue and can be mistaken for a wide variety of viral exanthems, particularly rubella (Fig. 4). This rash is nonpurpuric, nonpruritic, and transient, generally not lasting more than 2 days, and is frequently gone hours after first observation. Generalized muscle tenderness may also be an important differential sign. Occasionally the pain from these myalgias is quite intense and causes considerable discomfort to the patient.

The neurologic problems seen with meningococcal meningitis are somewhat different from those seen with other forms of purulent meningitis. Evidence of meningeal irritation is common except in the very young and old. Feigin and Dodge showed that focal neurologic signs and seizures were less common in meningococcal meningitis than in pneumococcal meningitis or in that due to *Haemophilus* while the levels of unconsciousness were very similar in the three diseases.[92] This correlates with the postmortem findings described by Thomas in which focal cerebral involvement in meningococcal meningitis was rare. The cause of death was related to toxins produced by the agent or by cerebral edema and to the secondary effects on the vital centers in the midbrain region.[93] Ducker and Simmons supported these clinical observations by observing that doses of meningococcal endotoxin, which produced no effect intravenously when introduced into the cerebral ventricular system of dogs, produced massive hemorrhagic pulmonary edema, subendocardial hemorrhages, hemorrhage and edema of both mitral and tricuspid valves, visceral congestion, and adrenal hemorrhage.[94] These lesions are similar to those seen outside the central nervous system in soldiers dying of meningococcal meningitis and bacteremia.[95] The myocardial problems associated with this infection have been stressed by Levin and Painter and by Kanter and associates.[96,97]

Evidence of myocardial failure as manifested by a gallop rhythm, congestive heart failure with pulmonary edema, and high central venous pressures in the face of poor peripheral perfusion has been reported.[96] Treatment of the myocardial failure with cardiac glycosides has resulted in reversing this constellation of problems. Postmortem studies by Hardman[95] and by Gore and Saphir[98] have indicated that myocarditis of varying degrees of severity is present in over half the patients who die of meningococcal disease.

The shock state all too frequently dominates the clinical picture and is an ominous prognostic sign. The patient is poorly responsive, and peripheral vasoconstriction is maximal, with cyanotic, poorly perfused extremities. Arterial blood gas analysis demonstrates evidence of acidosis in the range of pH 7.25–7.3, and depending on the degree of shock, anoxia may be manifested with an arterial PO_2 below 70 mmHg. Probably the most dramatic consequence of this clinical problem is the presence of DIC. Clinical evidence of its occurrence can be obtained by documenting increasing petechiae within prescribed areas, gastric or gingival bleeding, or oozing at the sites of venipuncture or intravenous infusions.

Either concomitant with the initial evaluation of the patient or later in the recovery phase of the illness, a number of unusual complications have been reported. These include arthritis, per-

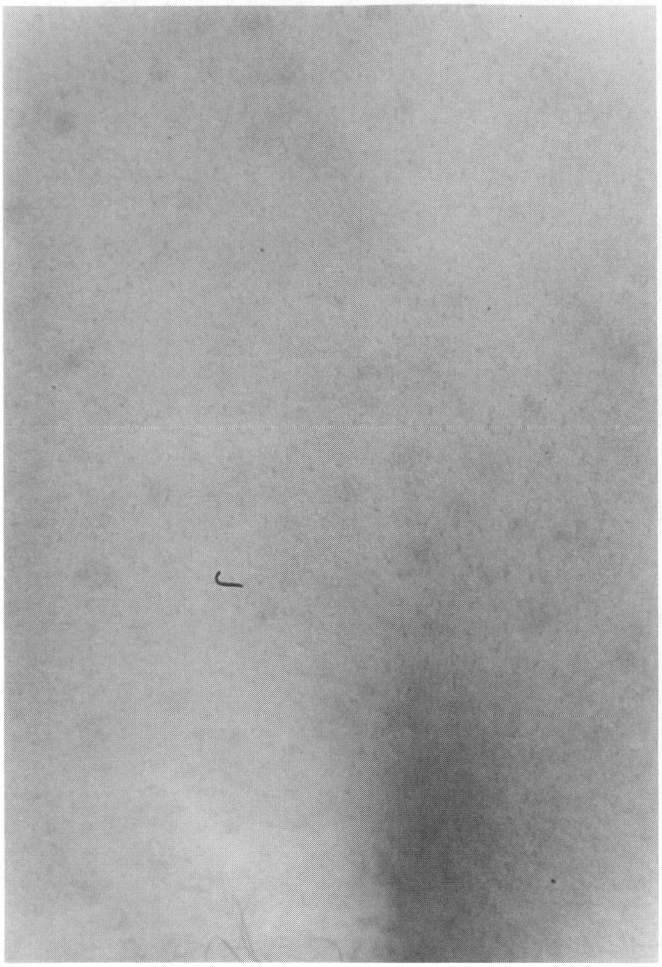

FIG. 4. Rubella-like rash seen early in meningococcal sepsis.

icarditis, conus medullaris syndrome, and cranial nerve dysfunctions, particularly of the sixth, seventh, and eighth cranial nerves.[92,99–103] The pericarditis can cause a massive tamponade. It is of interest that this complication may be unrelated to organism invasion of the pericardium but rather due to an immunologic reaction or toxin. In the report of Pierce and Cooper, the evidence of pericardial involvement occurred after two of the patients were in the recovery phase of their disease.[102] In one of these patients, the first symptoms of pericarditis occurred on the 20th day after the institution of therapy with penicillin. In the other patient, the first symptoms occurred 5 days after therapy began and recurred after pericardiocentesis and prednisone therapy on the 34th hospital day. This patient had a friction rub until the 49th hospital day and was not discharged until almost 3 months after admission. The incidence of this complication, according to Morse and associates, is approximately 19 percent.[101] All the cases of pericarditis seen by these investigators were in the convalescent phase of the disease and in disease caused by the group C meningococcus.[101] A recent report demonstrated a serogroup W-135 in a patient presenting with meningococcal myopericarditis.[104]

Chronic Meningococcemia

Persistent meningococcal bacteremia associated with low-grade fever, rash, and arthritis has been reported.[105,106] The distribution and appearance of the cutaneous lesions are identical to those seen in chronic gonococcemia for which it is mistaken.[80] The frequency of meningococcus in the acute arthritis–dermatitis syndrome appears to be increasing. Rompalo and coworkers compared the isolation of gonococci and meningococci from blood or synovial fluid from 1970–1972 with the period 1980–1983.[107] The ratio of gonococcal to meningococcal isolates changed from 15 to 1 in 1970–1972 to 9 to 5 in 1980–1983. These authors feel that systemic meningococcal infection should be considered more often in the differential diagnosis of the acute arthritis–dermatitis syndrome.

Complement Deficiency and Meningococcemia

The syndrome of chronic meningococcemia must be distinguished from the problem of recurrent episodes of meningococcal meningitis. Studies by Lim and coworkers have recently demonstrated the absence of the sixth complement component in such a patient.[108] In addition, at least one of the patients with recurrent meningococcal disease studied by Alper et al. lacked C3.[109] Studies by Petersen and associates indicated that human deficiency of C8 has been found in some persons with disseminated gonococcal infections and that this complement component is required for serum bactericidal activity against the gonococcus.[110] Ellison and coworkers have evaluated the complement system in 20 patients with first episodes of serious systemic meningococcal infection. Complement deficiency was detected in 6 of 20. Three had deficiencies in a terminal complement protein(s), and three had deficiencies of multiple factors associated with underlying disease states.[111] Densen and coworkers studied a family with properdin deficiency who had a high rate of fatal meningococcal disease.[112] These investigators demonstrated that the bactericidal defect could be corrected by vaccination of this population. Studies by Ross and coworkers suggest that vaccinating individuals deficient in late complement components may shift the burden of host defense from serum bactericidal activity to phagocytosis.[113] These studies would stress the previously unrecognized importance of the complement system in protection against neisserial infections.

Respiratory Infections with the Meningococcus

Meningococcal pneumonia has been a recognized clinical syndrome for over 60 years.[114–117] Because of the nasopharyngeal carriage of the meningococcus, the ability to establish the diagnosis based on the sputum culture alone is hazardous. The incidence of sepsis associated with this type of meningococcal infection appears to be quite low.[115] Therefore, blood cultures may not be of value. Koppes and associates used transtracheal cultures to establish the diagnosis in 68 Air Force recruits with group Y meningococcal pneumonia.[115] In this series, a history of cough, chest pain, chills, and previous upper respiratory infection occurred in over half of the patients. Rales and fever occurred in almost all patients, and evidence of pharyngitis was present in over 80 percent. The disease involved more than one lobe in 40 percent, with the right lower and middle lobe involved most frequently. The prognosis was good—no deaths occurred in the 68 patients with pneumonia. The association of meningococcal infection with preceding viral respiratory infections has been reported. Young and coworkers investigated an outbreak of meningococcal infection in an aged population, most of whom had serologic evidence of influenza.[118] Goldstein and associates have shown that pulmonary clearance of meningococci is diminished in animals previously exposed to an avirulent encephalomyocarditis virus.[119] In a recent study of the etiology of community-acquired pneumonia in Finland, *Neisseria meningitidis* was implicated as the etiologic agent in 6 of 162 cases.[120]

Meningococcal upper respiratory tract infections (pharyngitis) associated with contacts of patients and as a prior symptom and sign in cases of serious meningococcal disease have been described by several authors.[121,122] Suggestions that pharyngeal inflammation is the predecessor to bacteremic dissemination have been made but are unsubstantiated.

Meningococcal Urethritis

Meningococci have been isolated from the urethra and can be the etiologic agent in urethritis.[123,124] An association between orogenital sex and acquisition of the organism has been suggested.[123] In a population of homosexual males, the organism was isolated from the oropharynx (93 percent of isolates), rectum (6 percent of isolates), and urethra (1 percent of isolates).[125]

Laboratory Diagnosis of Meningococcal Infection

The definite diagnosis of serious meningococcal infection has as a prerequisite the bacteriologic isolation of *Neisseria meningitidis* from a usually sterile body fluid such as blood or cerebrospinal, synovial, pleural, or pericardial fluids. The CSF and the blood are the most fruitful sources of positive cultures. In an analysis of 727 cases of meningococcal disease, Hoyne and Brown described the results of 400 blood cultures in which 51.4 percent were positive for meningococci.[126] Spinal fluid examination of 423 patients from the same series indicated that 94 percent were positive for gram-negative diplococci by either smear or culture for the meningococci. Carpenter and Petersdorf indicate that 46 percent of their cases of meningococcal meningitis were positive by CSF culture.[91] In an additional 12 percent of the cases, the diagnosis was made by smear of the spinal fluid and by the clinical manifestations. Levin and Painter studied 28 patients with cultural-proven meningococcal disease, and in 22 of 27 patients tested, the spinal fluid was positive, while 15 of 28 had positive blood cultures.[96] It is of interest that, in 8 of 12 patients considered to have meningococcemia without clinical evidence of meningitis, the spinal fluid cultures were positive. Feldman has quantitated the bacterial counts in CSF with meningococcal meningitis and had a mean of 1.27×10^5 ($150–6 \times 10^7$) organisms per milliliter.[127] The ability to see or to culture the meningococci in the petechial skin and mucosal lesion varies widely. Hoyne and Brown reported identification in 69.8 percent of petechial smears examined.[126] Care should be taken with these specimens because of the difficulty in interpretation. Studies of pericardial fluid have failed to demonstrate the organism by smear or culture.[100,101]

Chemical and cytologic examinations of the spinal fluid in meningococcal infection can yield variable results. Carpenter and Petersdorf examined the spinal fluid of 58 patients with meningococcal meningitis.[91] The median leukocyte count was approximately 1200, with a range from less than 10 to 65,000/μL. Approximately 75 percent had CSF glucose levels below 40 mg/100 ml. Unfortunately, spinal fluid–serum glucose ratios were not given. The CSF protein level ranged from 25 to over 800 mg/100 ml, with the median value approximately 150 mg/100 ml. While not commented on specifically by these authors, the cell type in untreated cases is almost always polymorphonuclear. Partially treated patients may have a pleomorphic spinal fluid.

Studies using counterimmunoelectrophoresis, latex agglutination, and coagglutination have demonstrated the capability of detecting 0.02–0.05 μg of meningococcal antigens per milliliter of spinal fluid of infected patients.[127] The technique offers rapidity in diagnosis, and specificity providing organisms containing cross-reacting antigens are not involved (e.g., *E. coli* K1, which cross reacts with group B meningococcus). False-negative results occur commonly. Feigin, as reported by McCracken, could not detect antigen in the blood and CSF of almost half of his patients with meningococcal meningitis.[122] Feldman has recently shown that this is most probably due to low concentrations of bacteria in certain CSF.[127] McCracken notes that bacterial antigen can be detected longer in the urine than in other body fluids and that concentrated urine specimens in addition to CSF should be studied for antigen.[122] Feign states that there is a direct relationship between poor prognosis of the meningitis and the concentration of antigen in the CSF, while Feldman comments that concentration of bacteria is a more important determinant of prognosis.[128,129] Studies using lactic dehydrogenase or neuraminidase in the CSF as indicators of bacterial infection have recently been reported.[130,131] It is of interest that the levels of both enzymes are substantially elevated in meningococcal meningitis when compared with pneumococcal, *Haemophilus influenzae* type b, or viral central nervous system infections.

Treatment of Meningococcal Infections

The introduction of antibiotics has dramatically altered the prognosis of meningococcal disease. Today, the expected mortality under optimal conditions should not exceed 8–10 percent.[84,87] The random case frequently fares poorer than that in an epidemic because medical personnel are not alerted to the diagnosis and may overlook the early signs and symptoms. The value of early diagnosis in lowering the mortality is exemplified by the results at Fort Dix where an intense surveillance program was established during 1968–1969, and the mortality was less than 5 percent.

In addition to the use of antibiotics, the application of supportive care to treat the problems of DIC, shock, heart failure, prolonged mental obtundation, pericarditis, and pneumonia, which complicate this infection, has had a decided impact on prognosis.

Antibiotic Therapy. The era of chemotherapy for meningococcal infection began with the report of Schwentker et al. in 1937 that demonstrated that sulfonamides could be successfully used in the treatment of meningococcal meningitis and meningococcemia[12] (Table 2). Feldman et al. confirmed these observations. A dramatic change occurred in the prognosis of epidemic meningitis.[135] As new antibiotics were introduced through the 1940s and 1950s, reports appeared that documented the efficacy of several agents used alone and in combination. Early studies of penicillin administered in relatively low doses (120,000 units/day im) indicated that it was not as effective as sulfonamides.[136] Using larger amounts of the drug (360,000 units/day im), Kinsman and D'Alonzo demonstrated that treatment results with penicillin were identical to those with sulfonamides.[137] The efficacy of chloramphenicol as a therapeutic

TABLE 2. Treatment and Prevention of Serious Meningococcal Infection

Problem	*Treatment*
Meningococcal meningitis, meningococcemia, and chronic meningococcemia	Penicillin G—300,000 units/kg/day iv up to 24 million units/day. If penicillin allergic, chloramphenicol, 100 mg/kg/day iv, up to 4 g/day[132]
Antibiotic chemoprophylaxis for household or intimate contacts	Rifampin—adults, 600 mg q12h for 2 days; children, 10 mg/kg q12h for 2 days. *N.B.:* Sulfadiazine (1 g q8h for 3 days) can be used for chemoprophylaxis only if the disease-producing strain is known to be sensitive to 0.1 mg sulfadiazine/100 ml[133]
Immunoprophylaxis	Monovalent A, monovalent C, bivalent A–C, or quadrivalent A, C, Y, and W-135 vaccine is administered once by volume according to the manufacturer. The amount of polysaccharide delivered is usually 50 μg. Vaccination should be considered adjunct to antibiotic chemoprophylaxis for household or intimate contacts of meningococcal disease cases when appropriate serogroups are causing disease[134]

agent was demonstrated by McCrumb and coworkers.[132] In 15 patients treated with this drug, all survived, and only one patient had a complication secondary to the infection, ophthalmoplegia, which cleared subsequently.

The therapeutic efficacy of first-generation cephalosporins was studied in the 1960s. These agents produced variable results, and their use is now contraindicated in treating meningococcal infections.[138,139] Some of the third-generation cephalosporins demonstrate excellent in vitro effectiveness against the meningococcus[140] and probably achieve central nervous system concentrations adequate to treat meningococcal meningeal infection. However, clinical studies are sparse, and the use of these agents should be limited to special circumstances when more conventional therapy cannot be used.

Sulfonamides now have a very limited role in the treatment of meningococcal infections. Studies by Schoenbach and Phair[14] and by Love and Finland[141] revealed small populations of sulfonamide-resistant meningococci. In 1963, an epidemic of group B meningococcal infection occurred at Fort Ord, California, in which the infecting strain was resistant to sulfonamides.[142] Since that time, most isolates, primarily serogroups B and C in this country and group A from worldwide locations, have been resistant to sulfadiazine.[143–145] According to Feldman, strains that fail to grow in the presence of 0.1 mg/100 ml sulfadiazine are sensitive.[144] Those strains with colonies on the 0.1 mg/100 ml but not the 1.0 mg/100 ml plates are "partially resistant," while those that grow at 1.0 mg/100 ml are resistant. This problem has limited the use of sulfonamides only to situations where the strain causing the infection is known to be sulfonamide sensitive before the institution of therapy.

Penicillin therapy for the treatment of meningococcal infections is safe and effective. The drug can be administered intravenously or intramuscularly. The intrathecal route is contraindicated because of the severe neurotoxicity of penicillin in high concentrations in the central nervous system. A goal of antibiotic therapy for meningitis is to establish concentrations of antibiotics in the spinal fluid that approximate 10 times the mean inhibitory concentration (MIC) of the organism for that agent.[146] A dose of 300,000 units/kg/day is recommended, with an upper limit of 24 million units/day as 2 million units q2h.[147] Recent reports of penicillin-insensitive *N. meningitidis* have come from Great Britain and Spain.[148,149] One study has demonstrated that the relative resistance to penicillin is due to a reduced affinity of penicillin binding protein 3 in 11 serogroup B and 4 serogroup C *N. meningitidis* strains isolated from CSF and blood during an epidemic in Spain.[150] Spinal fluid levels of penicillin averaged 0.8 μg/ml on the first day of therapy. This concentration approximated the MIC for penicillin G for the most resistant isolate studied by this group. These strains were also relatively resistant to cefuroxime, but cefotaxime appeared active against these strains. While such resistant meningococcal strains have been infrequently reported to date, clinicians should be alerted to the possibility of their occurrence in unexplained treatment failures or in cases of slowly resolving, documented, meningococcal central nervous system infections. Chloramphenicol is an effective substitute for the penicillin-allergic patient and should be administered intravenously in a dose of 100 mg/kg/day up to a maximum of 4 g/day total dose.[147] Third-generation cephalosporins including cefotaxime, ceftriaxone, and ceftazidime have been used successfully in the treatment of pediatric cases of meningococcal meningitis.[151] The second-generation cephalosporin cefuroxime has also been successfully used in meningococcal meningitis.[152] Relatively small numbers of patients have been treated for meningococcal meningitis with these agents, and their general use should be discouraged at this time. Special circumstances may occur in which they would be the agents of choice, i.e., relatively penicillin-resistant meningococci (care should be taken to choose a sensitive cephalosporin[150]) or drug hypersensitivity reactions, which precludes the use of penicillins and chloramphenicol. The duration of antibiotic therapy will vary somewhat with the presentation and manifestation of the disease and with the response of the patient. At present, when the meningococcus is sensitive to the agents just mentioned, 7–10 days of therapy is usually sufficient (see Chapter 66).

Supportive Care. A common complication of meningococcal disease is vascular collapse and shock. This is primarily due to the effects of meningococcal lipooligosaccharide, which is a potent toxin. Recent studies have indicated that the cytokine tumor necrosis factor α may be a mediator of endotoxic shock since upon injection into animals it induces hypotension, metabolic acidosis, and death.[153–155] Recent data from studies in animals suggest that treatment or pretreatment with polyclonal[154] or monoclonal[156] antibodies against tumor necrosis factor α could be beneficial in purpura fulminans. Girardin and coworkers have demonstrated that serum levels of tumor necrosis factor α, interleukin-1, and γ-interferon correlated with the severity of meningococcemia in children.[157] At the present time, it is not known whether these cytokines play a deleterious or protective role in shock due to meningococcal sepsis. Further studies will be necessary to define this and determine whether intervention to modulate these cytokines would improve the clinical outcome.

In every case of systemic meningococcal infection, the potential for shock must be always considered. Preparations for it and close monitoring of the patients are paramount for effective treatment of vascular collapse. If shock ensues, close hemodynamic monitoring is essential. Central venous pressure, pulmonary artery pressure, pulmonary capillary wedge pressure, blood gases, and cardiac output should be monitored. Calculations of oxygen consumption, systemic vascular resistance, and pulmonary vascular resistance are of considerable value in making decisions about the use of vasoactive drugs for treatment of the shock state. In patients with respiratory distress, the airway should be secured and mechanical ventilation instituted. A flow sheet recording hourly vital signs, physical signs and symptoms, urine output, pertinent laboratory and hemodynamic data, as well as medications is mandatory.

The specific application of therapy in the treatment of shock will vary from patient to patient. The observations by Levin and Painter,[96] Hardeman,[95] and Monsalve and coworkers[158] of the degree of cardiac injury and myocardial depression associated with meningococcal infection is important to note. Volume resuscitation is the first step in the management of decreasing cardiac output. Fluid should be infused until the pulmonary wedge pressure is 8 to 12 mmHg. This will ensure adequate preload in the event vasoactive medications are necessary. If such drugs are necessary for the treatment of shock, dopamine is a frequent first choice in septic shock because of its β-effects on the myocardium. In addition, it has α vasoconstriction effects on the peripheral vasculature and selective dopaminergic effects on the renal and splanchnic vascular beds.[159] In the face of elevated systemic resistance, dobutamine may be preferred because it possesses no peripheral α-effects and does not lead to increased afterload.[160] Epinephrine and norepinephrine should be used in instances of profound shock and myocardial depression where the above agents have failed. Isoproterenol has β_1- and β_2-effects that increase contractility and simultaneously cause vasodilation. In adults, this drug can cause increased myocardial oxygen consumption. When using isoproterenol, further hypotension may take place if adequate fluid replenishment has not occurred before its institution. Cardiac glycosides (digoxin) have been used in the treatment of septic shock.[133] These drugs increase cardiac contractility while reducing cardiac oxygen consumption. If these drugs are used, short-acting agents with close monitoring of potassium levels should be undertaken. Other agents that have limited usefulness in special situations may include sodium nitroprusside, phentolamine, and phenoxybenzamine. Such drugs as nonsteroidal anti-inflammatory agents and naloxone HCl (Narcan) have not to date been shown to be beneficial additions to the management of shock due to meningococcal sepsis. Management of septic shock is discussed further in Chapter 59.

The use of steroids, particularly in patients showing evidence of purpura fulminans and concomitant adrenal hemorrhage (Waterhouse-Fridrichsen syndrome), is still controversial. In the 1950s, several investigators recommended the use of corticosteroid replacement therapy. However, the studies of Belsey and associates were inconclusive in demonstrating a beneficial effect by the application of low-dose steroid in meningococcal infection.[161]

As pointed out earlier, the problem of DIC is ominous. Petechiae are frequent accompaniments of meningococcal sepsis. The development of increasing petechial lesions, confluent ecchymoses, persistently bleeding venipuncture sites, and bleeding gums despite adequate antimicrobial therapy and supportative care is indicative of DIC. The use of heparin in the treatment of this complication of meningococcal disease is controversial.[162,163] If heparin is given, the treatment should be based on a careful study of the clinical situation and laboratory data, particularly that relating to the clotting factors. Interpretation of these observations should be made by one familiar with clotting problems, and therapy should be directed by that person. Physicians experienced in the treatment of the complications of meningococcal disease recognize that as many patients can be harmed by the inappropriate treatment of DIC as by DIC itself. To complicate matters, in severe DIC the problem of plasmin activation with fibrinolysis becomes a clinical reality. This enforces the need for expert direction in the treatment of this complication.

Other major life-threatening complications necessitating therapy include adult respiratory distress syndrome (ARDS), neurologic sequelae ranging from coma to diabetes insipidus, pericarditis, and pneumonia, which is not necessarily meningococcal but may be secondary to aspiration during the obtunded state. This last problem can be insidious and can appear in the convalescent stage of disease. Awareness that it can occur will lead readily to its diagnosis and treatment.

Chemoprophylaxis of the Meningococcal Carrier. Shortly after the clinical use of sulfonamides for the treatment of serious meningococcal disease, it became apparent that short courses of the sulfadiazine resulted in the disappearance of meningococcal carriage for prolonged periods of time.[164,165] As Feldman points out, despite the arguments about the relationships, "if there are no carriers, there are no cases," the use of sulfonamides to reduce carrier rates did decrease the number of cases.[80]

Treatment of the meningococcal carrier state with sulfonamides eradicated carriage quickly and for prolonged periods.[134] The length of time was a function of the initial dose of sulfonamides, and with doses as high as 8 g the carrier rate was reduced from approximately 45 percent to less than 10 percent at 16 weeks. Cheever demonstrated that after two doses of 3 and 2 g of sulfadiazine the carrier rate dropped from 79 to 0 percent in 72 hours.[166] On military bases and in closed environments such as boarding schools, institutions, and family units in which cases arose, this form of chemoprophylaxis was effective in disrupting the spread of meningococcal infections.

With the recognition of widespread sulfonamide-resistant meningococci and the failure of sulfadiazine to impact on the epidemic at Fort Ord,[15,16] these agents have been abandoned for meningococcal chemoprophylaxis except in instances where the meningococcal case strains are known to be sulfa sensitive.

The search for new agents for chemoprophylaxis has been extensive. Penicillin has proved ineffective for several reasons; long-acting mixtures do not eradicate the nasopharyngeal carriage, and while massive doses cause people to become noncarriers, the carrier state recurs promptly after discontinuation of treatment with the drug.[80,167] Two drugs have emerged as candidates for meningococcal prophylaxis. Minocycline and rifampin have been shown to eradicate the carrier state rapidly, and this eradication persists for up to 6–10 weeks after treatment.[168,169] Problems occur with both drugs. Minocycline has been shown to cause vertigo, probably secondary to an effect on the vestibular system.[170] Rifampin treatment can result in the emergence of rifampin-resistant meningococci in 10–27 percent of the patients treated.[171] In addition, rifampin causes red urine in almost all patients, and this can be quite disconcerting unless some forewarning is given.

A number of other agents active against the meningococci in vitro have been tested and have failed to provide prophylaxis. These include erythromycin, trimethoprim, cephalexin, oxytetracycline, and nalidixic acid. Hoeprich has studied a number of these agents and speculates that the primary factor determining effectiveness as a meningococcal prophylactic agent is the ability to achieve bactericidal levels in tears and saliva.[172] Studies by Pugsley and coworkers have demonstrated in 21 persistent meningococcal nasopharyngeal carriers that ciprofloxacin, 500 mg every 12 hours for 5 days, eradicated the meningococcus from the nasopharynx in 100 percent of individuals for up to 13 days after the completion of therapy. An untreated comparative control group had a carriage rate of 85 percent at that time.[173] At the present time, the recommended therapy for meningococcal prophylaxis is rifampin, 600 mg q12h for 2 days for adults and 10 mg/kg q12h for 2 days for children.[174]

The question as to who should receive prophylaxis has concerned public health officials since the advent of effective chemoprophylaxis. Initially with sulfonamides, little discrimination between high-risk and low-risk populations was attempted, and the drug was administered very widely to people without the remotest increased risk of disease. Since the clinical emergence of sulfa resistance and the problem in finding agents that are safe and effective, more attention has been paid to the populations at greatest risk who need chemoprophylaxis. During epidemics and in the endemic situations in civilian populations, household contacts have been shown to be at increased risk of infection.[9,11,87] Analysis by the Centers for Disease Control meningococcal surveillance group showed that the attack rate in this group was 500–800 times greater than that determined for the general population studied.[87] Similar high-risk situations exist in closed populations such as college dormitories, chronic care hospitals, nursery schools,[175] and military barracks. Secondary cases usually occur within 10 days of the primary case, but longer intervals have been described. Close surveillance of this group for at least 10 days would ensure prompt treatment of any secondary cases that might arise in the absence of effective chemoprophylaxis. Hospital personnel are not at increased risk and in general should not receive chemoprophylaxis.[176] Medical staff who have an intimate exposure such as mouth-to-mouth resuscitation should receive prophylaxis.[80,177]

Immunoprophylaxis of Meningococcal Infection

Subsequent to the problem of prevention of epidemic meningococcal disease on military recruit bases after the emergence of sulfa-resistant meningococci, an intense effort was directed at the development of a vaccine for the prevention of meningococcal infections in this high-risk population. The result was the development of two vaccine preparations derived from the capsular polysaccharide of the group A and C meningococci. Artenstein and coworkers demonstrated the effectiveness of the group C vaccine in studies of U.S. Army recruits.[17] Only 1 case of meningococcal disease occurred among 13,763 vaccinees, while 38 bacteriologically proven cases occurred in a control group of 68,072. This was an 87 percent reduction in disease and was proved to be statistically significant. Makela and associates showed that the group A polysaccharide administered to Finnish military recruits significantly lowered the incidence of disease due to this serogroup when compared with an unvaccinated control population.[178] Studies from Finland during a group A epidemic demonstrated the effectiveness of this vaccine in children 3 months to 5 years of age.[18] Recent studies from Africa by Reingold indicate that in this population efficacy 1 year after serogroup A vaccination is less than 30 percent in children below the age of 4 years.[179] The immunologic response of the group C vaccine in children below the age of 2 years is poor, and studies from Brazil indicate that the C vaccine is not protective below the age of 24 months.[180] Studies of the immune response to the A and C vaccine by Gold and coworkers in infants have demonstrated that detectable levels of antibody are generated but that these levels are significantly lower than in older children.[181] In adults, the duration of the group C antibody titer persisted for 2–4 years after vaccination, and in children studied in Egypt who were vaccinated with group A polysaccharide, protection has lasted at least 2 years.[182,183] The vaccine is safe.[184] Reactions appear to be limited to local erythema at the site of injection in approximately 4 percent and some increased irritability in young children in about 6 percent of the vaccine recipients. One series of immunologic hyporesponsiveness to group C antigen was reported in a population of young adult volunteers who had received group A vaccine contaminated with trace amounts of C polysaccharide.[185] It is assumed that this represents an example of low-dose tolerance in humans. Commercial vaccine materials are now carefully tested to ensure that this cross-contamination does not occur. Because the meningococcal vaccines are poorly immunogenic in children below the age of 2 years and because of the lack of a vaccine to the serogroup B meningococcus, chemoprophylaxis is recommended in lieu of vaccine for prevention of secondary cases of meningococcal disease in day care centers.[186]

The use of these vaccines in Third World countries in epidemic areas has become increasingly important. Factors such as underlying parasitic infections, state of nutrition, as well as age of the vaccine recipient play a role in the response to vaccination.[187]

Current commercial vaccines include a quadrivalent product containing polysaccharides of groups A, C, Y, and W-135.[188] There is no vaccine presently available for use in the prevention of group B disease. The group B capsular polysaccharide is not sufficiently immunogenic to produce a reliable antibody response in humans to be effective. Several solutions to this problem are being studied, including the chemical alteration of the capsular B antigen to make it more immunogenic and the search for other cell wall antigens that are capable of eliciting bactericidal antibodies against B meningococci with a minimum of serious side effects.

New vaccines against the meningococcus are under development. These include vaccines developed to somatic antigens such as detoxified lipooligosaccharide and outer membrane proteins and new capsular vaccines comprised of polysaccharide–protein conjugates[189] and those based on anti-idiotype antibodies.[190]

REFERENCES

1. Vieusseaux M. Memoire sur le maladie qui a regne a Geneve au printempts de 1805. J Med Chir Pharmacol. 1805;11:163.
2. Hedrich AW. The movements of epidemic meningitis, 1915–1930. Public Health Rep. 1931;46:2709.
3. Weichselbaum A. Ueber die Aetiologie der akuten Meningitis cerebrospinalis. Fortschr Med. 1887;5:573.
4. Kiefer F. Zur differential Diagnose des Erregers der epidemischen Cerebrospinalmeningitis und der Gonorrhoe. Berl Klin Wochenschr. 1896;33:628.
5. Albrecht H, Ghon A. Uber die Aetiologie und pathologische Anatomie der Meningitis cerebro spinalis epidemica. Wien Klin Wochenschr. 1901;14:984.
6. Dopter C. Etude de quelques germes isoles du rhino-pharynx, voisans du meningocoque (parameningocoques). C R Soc Biol (Paris). 1909;67:74.
7. Flexner S. The results of the serum treatment in thirteen hundred cases of epidemic meningitis. J Exp Med. 1913;17:553.
8. Glover JA. The cerebrospinal fever epidemic of 1917 at "X" depot. J R Army Med Corps. 1918;30:23.
9. Norton JF, Gordon JE. Meningococcus meningitis in Detroit in 1928–1929. I. Epidemiology. J Prev Med. 1930;4:207.
10. French MR. Epidemiological study of 383 cases of meningococcus meningitis in the city of Milwaukee, 1927–1928 and 1929. Am J Public Health. 1931;21:130.
11. Pizzi M. A severe epidemic of meningococcus meningitis in Chile, 1941 and 1942. Am J Public Health. 1944;34:231–8.
12. Schwentker FF, Gelman S, Long PH. The treatment of meningococcic meningitis with sulfonamide. Preliminary report. JAMA. 1937;108:1407.
13. Kuhns DM, Nelson CT, Feldman HA, et al. The prophylactic value of sulfadiazine in the control of meningococcic meningitis. JAMA. 1943;123:335–9.
14. Schoenback EB, Phair JJ. The sensitivity of meningococci to sulfadiazine. Am J Hyg. 1948;47:177–86.
15. Gauld JR, Nitz RE, Hunter DH, et al. Epidemiology of meningococcal meningitis at Ford Ord. Am J Epidemiol. 1965;82:56–72.
16. Bristow MW, Van Peenen PFD, Volk R. Epidemic meningitis in naval recruits. Am J Public Health. 1965;55:1039–45.
17. Artenstein MS, Gold R, Zimmerly JG, et al. Prevention of meningococcal disease by group C polysaccharide vaccine. N Engl J Med. 1970;282:417–20.
18. Piltola H, Makela PH, Kayhty H, et al. Clinical efficacy of meningococcus group A capsular polysaccharide vaccine in children three months to five years of age. N Engl J Med. 1977;297:686–91.
19. Hebeler BH, Young FE. Mechanism of autolysis of *Neisseria gonorrhoeae*. J Bacteriol. 1976;126:1186–93.
20. Hebeler BH, Young FE. Autolysis of *Neisseria gonorrhoeae*. J Bacteriol. 1976;122:385–92.
21. Holbein BE. Enhancement of *Neisseria meningitidis* infection in mice by addition of iron bound to transferrin. Infect Immun. 1981;34:120–5.
22. West WF, Sparling PF. The response of *Neisseria gonorrhoeae* to iron limitation: Alterations in expression of membrane proteins without apparent siderophore production. Infect Immun. 1985;47:388–94.
23. Dyer D, West EP, Sparling PF. Effects of seven carrier proteins on the growth of pathogenic *Neisseria* with heme-bound iron. Infect Immun. 1987;55:1271–5.
24. Gorden MH, Murray EG. Identification of the meningococcus. J R Army Med Corps. 1915;5:411.
25. Scherp HW, Rake GJ. Studies on the meningococcus. VIII. The type I specific substance. J Exp Med. 1935;61:753.
26. Clapp FL, Phillips SW, Stahl HJ. Quantitative use of Neufeld reaction with special reference to titration of type III anti-pneumococcic sera. Proc Soc Exp Biol Med. 1935;33:302.
27. Branham SE, Carlin SA. Comments on a newly recognized group of the meningococcus. Proc Soc Exp Biol Med. 1942;49:141–4.
28. Watson RG, Marinetti GV, Scherp HW. The specific hapten of group C (group II) meningococcus. II. Chemical nature. J Immunol. 1958;81:337–4.
29. Branham SE. Serological relationship among meningococci. Bacteriol Rev. 1953;17:175–88.
30. Branham SE. Reference strains for the serologic groups of meningococcus (*Neisseria meningitidis*). Int Bull Bacteriol Nomen Taxon. 1958;8:1–15.
31. Slaterus K. Serological typing of meningococci by means of microprecipitation. Antonie Van Leeuwenhoek. 1961;27:304–15.
32. Evans JR, Artenstein MS, Hunter DH. Prevalence of meningococcal serogroups and a description of new groups. Am J Epidemiol. 1968;87:643–6.
33. Ding S, Ye R, Zhang H. Three new serogroups of *Neisseria meningitidis*. J Biol Stand. 1981;9:305–15.
34. Ashton FE, Ryan A, Diena B, et al. A new serogroup (L) of *Neisseria meningitidis*. J Clin Microbiol. 1983;17:722–7.
35. Gotschlich EC, Liu TY, Artenstein MS. Preparation and immunochemical properties of the group A, group B, and group C meningococcal polysaccharides. J Exp Med. 1969;129:1349–65.
36. Bundle DR, Jennings JH, Kenny CP. Studies on the group specific polysaccharide of *Neisseria meningitidis* serogroup X and an improved procedure for its isolation. J Biol Chem. 1974;249:4797–801.
37. Robinson JA, Apicella MA. Isolation and characterization of *Neisseria meningitidis* groups A, C, X and Y polysaccharide antigens. Infect Immun. 1970;1:8–14.
38. Apicella MA. Identification of a subgroup antigen on the *Neisseria meningitidis* group C capsular polysaccharide. J Infect Dis. 1974;129:147–53.
39. Apicella MA. Immunological and biochemical studies of meningococcal C polysaccharide isolated by diethylaminoethyl chromatography. Infect Immun. 1976;14:106–113.
40. Liu TY, Gotschlich EC, Dunne FT, et al. Studies on meningococcal polysaccharides. II. Composition and chemical properties of the group B and group C polysaccharide. J Biol Chem. 1971;246:4703–12.
41. Bhattacharjee AK, Jennings HJ, Kenny CP, et al. Structural determination of the sialic acid polysaccharide antigens of *Neisseria meningitidis* serogroup B and C with carbon 13 nuclear magnetic resonance. J Biol Chem. 1975;250:1926–32.
42. Brandt BL, Artenstein MS, Smith CD. Antibody response to meningococcal polysaccharide vaccines. Infect Immun. 1973;8:590–6.
43. Maloney PC, Schneider H, Brandt BL. Production and degrading of serogroup B *Neisseria meningitidis* polysaccharide. Infect Immun. 1972;6:657–61.
44. Wyle FA, Artenstein MS, Brandt BL, et al. Immunologic response of man

to group B meningococcal polysaccharide vaccines. J Infect Dis. 1972;126:514–22.
45. Bhattacharjee AK, Jennings JH, Kenny CP. Characterization of 3-deoxy-D-manno-octulosonic acid as a component of the capsular polysaccharide antigen from *Neisseria meningitidis* serogroup 29E. Biochem Biophys Res Commun. 1974;61:489–93.
46. Griffiss JM, Brandt BL, Broud DO. Human immune response to various doses of group Y and W135 meningococcal polysaccharide vaccines. Infect Immun. 1982;37:205–8.
47. Mandrell RE, Zollinger WD. Lipopolysaccharide serotyping of *Neisseria meningitidis* by hemagglutination inhibition. Infect Immun. 1977;16:471–5.
48. Jennings HL, Johnson KG, Kenne L. The structure of the R-type oligosaccharide core obtained from some lipopolysaccharides of *Neisseria meningitidis*. Carbohydr Res. 1983;121:233–41.
49. Gold R, Wyle FA. New classification of *Neisseria meningitidis* by means of bactericidal reactions. Infect Immun. 1970;1:479–84.
50. Gold R, Winklehake JL, Mars RS, et al. Identification of epidemic strain of group C *Neisseria meningitidis* by bactericidal serotyping. J Infect Dis. 1971;124:593–7.
51. Frasch CE, Chapman SS. Classification of *Neisseria meningitidis* group B into distinct serotypes. III. Application of a new bactericidal-inhibition technique to distribution of serotypes aamong cases and carriers. J Infect Dis. 1973;127:149–54.
52. Frasch CE. Noncapsular surface antigens of *Neisseria meningitidis*. In: Weinstein L, Fields BN, eds. Seminars in Infectious Diseases. New York: Stratton International Medical Book Corp; 1979:304–37.
53. Broud DD, Griffiss JM, Baker CJ. Heterogeneity of serotypes of *Neisseria meningitidis* that cause endemic disease. J Infect Dis. 1979;140:465–70.
54. Kawula TH, Spinola SM, Klapper DG, Cannon JG. Localization of a conserved epitope and an azurin-like domain in the H.8 protein of pathogenic *Neisseria*. Mol Microbiol. 1987;1:179–85.
55. Barlow AK, Heckels JE, Clarke IN. Molecular cloning and expression of *Neisseria meningitidis* class 1 outer membrane protein in *Escherichia coli* K-12. Infect Immun. 1987;55:2734–40.
56. Frasch CE, Zollinger WD, Poolman, JT. Proposed schema for identification of serotypes of *Neisseria meningitidis*. In Schoolnik GK, ed. The Pathogenic *Neisseria*. Washington DC: American Society for Microbiology; 1985:519–24.
57. Selander RK, Caugant DA, Ochman H, et al. Methods of multilocus enzyme electrophoresis for bacterial populations genetics and systematics. Appl Environ Microbiol. 1986;132:2855–61.
58. Olyhoek T, Crowe B, Achtman M. Epidemiological analysis and geographic distribution of *Neisseria meningitidis* group A. In Schoolnik GK, ed. The Pathogenic *Neisseria*. Washington DC: American Society for Microbiology; 1985:530–5.
59. Caugant DA, Mocca IF, Frasch CE, et al. Genetic structure of *Neisseria meningitidis* populations in relation to serogroup, serotype, and outer membrane protein pattern. J Bacteriol. 1987;169:2781–92.
60. DeVoe IW, Gilchrist JE. Piliation and colonial morphology among laboratory strains of meningococci. J Clin Microbiol. 1978;7:379–84.
61. DeVoe IW, Gilchrist JE. Pili on meningococci from primary culture of nasopharyngeal carriers and cerebrospinal fluid of patients with acute disease. J Exp Med. 1975;141:297–305.
62. Stephens DS, McGee ZA. Attachment of *Neisseria meningitidis* to human mucosal surfaces. Influence of pili and type of receptor cell. J Infect Dis. 1981;143:525–32.
63. McGee ZA, Dourmashkin RR, Gross JG, et al. Relationship of pili to colonial morphology. Infect Immun. 1979;24:194–201.
64. Goldschneider I, Gotschlich EC, Artenstein MS. Human immunity to the meningococcus. I. The role of humoral antibody. J Exp Med. 1969;129:1307–26.
65. Goldschneider I, Gotschlich EC, Artenstein MS. Human immunity to the meningococcus. II. Development of natural immunity. J Exp Med. 1969;129:1327–8.
66. Robbins JB, Myerowitz RL, Whesnant JK, et al. Enteric bacteria cross-reactive with *Neisseria meningitidis* groups A and C and *Diplococcus pneumoniae* types I and III. Infect Immun. 1972;6:651–6.
67. Grados O, Ewing WH. Antigenic relationship between *Escherichia coli* and *Neisseria meningitidis*. J Infect Dis. 1970;122:100–3.
68. Finne J, Bitter-Suermann D, Goudis C, et al. An IgG monoclonal antibody to group B meningococci cross reacts with developmentally regulated polysialic acid units of glycoproteins in neural and extraneural tissue. J Immunol. 1987;138:4402–7.
69. Griffiss JM, Bertram MA. Immunoepidemiology of meningococcal disease in military recruits. II. Blocking of serum bactericidal activity by circulating IgA early in the course of invasive disease. J Infect Dis. 1977;136:733–9.
70. Griffiss JM. Epidemic meningococcal disease: Synthesis of a hypothetical immunoepidemiologic model. Rev Infect Dis. 1982;4:159–72.
71. Plaut AG, Gilbert JV, Artenstein MS, et al. *Neisseria gonorrhoeae* and *Neisseria meningitidis*: Extracellular enzyme cleaves human immunoglobulin A. Science. 1975;190:1103–5.
72. Mulks M, Plaut AG. IgA protease production as a characteristic distinguishing pathogenic from harmless Neisseriaceae. N Engl J Med. 1978;299:973–6.
73. Bruns H, Hohn J. Meningokokken im Nasenrachenraum. Klin Jahrb Jena. 1908;285.
74. Dudley SF, Brennan JR. High and persistent carrier rates of *Neisseria meningitidis*, unaccompanied by cases of meningitis. J Hyg (Lond). 1934;34:525.
75. Rake G. Studies on meningococcus infection. VI. The carrier problem. J Exp Med. 1934;59:553.
76. Greenfield S, Sheede PR, Feldman HA. Meningococcal carriage in a population of "normal" families. J Infect Dis. 1971;123:67–73.
77. Olcen P, Kellander J, Danielsson D, et al. Epidemiology of *Neisseria meningitidis* prevalence and symptoms from the upper respiratory tract in family members to patients with meningococcal disease. Scand J Infect Dis. 1981;13:105–9.
78. Reller BL, MacGregor RR, Beaty HN. Bactericidal antibody after colonization with *Neisseria meningitidis*. J Infect Dis. 1973;127:56–62.
79. Broome CV. The carrier state: *Neisseria meningitidis*. J Antimicrob Chemother. 1986;18(Suppl A):25–34.
80. Feldman HA. Meningococcal infections. Adv Intern Med. 1972;18:117–40.
81. Centers for Disease Control. Annual supplement, summary 1975. MMWR 1976;24:30.
82. Peltola H. Meningococcal disease: Still with us. Rev Infect Dis. 1983;5:71–91.
83. Peltola H, Kataja JM, Makela PH. Shift in the age distribution of meningococcal disease as predictor of an epidemic. Lancet. 1982;2:595–7.
84. Andersen BM. Mortality in meningococcal infections. Scand J Infect Dis. 1978;10:277–82.
85. deMorais JS, Munford RS, Risi JB, et al. Epidemic disease due to serogroup C *Neisseria meningitidis* in Sao Paulo, Brazil. J Infect Dis. 1974;129:568–71.
86. Oberli J, Hoi NT, Caravano R, Tan CM, Roux J. Etude d'une epidemie de meningococcie au Viet Nam (provinces du Sud). Bull WHO. 1981;59:585–90.
87. The Meningococcal Disease Surveillance Group. Analysis of endemic meningococcal disease by serogroup and evaluation of chemoprophylaxis. J Infect Dis. 1976;134:201.
88. Greenwood BM. The epidemiology of acute bacterial meningitis in tropical Africa. In: Williams JD, Burnet J, eds. Bacterial Meningitis. New York: Academic Press; 1987:61–92.
89. Wolfe RE, Birbara CA. Meningococcal infections at an army training center. Am J Med. 1968;44:243–55.
90. Sullivan TD, LaScolea LJ. *Neisseria meningitidis* bacteremia in children: Quantitation of bacteremia and spontaneous clinical recovery without antibiotic therapy. Pediatrics. 1987;80:63–87.
91. Carpenter RR, Petersdorf RG. The clinical spectrum of bacterial meningitis. Am J Med. 1962;33:262–75.
92. Feigin RD, Dodge PR. Bacterial meningitis: Newer concepts of pathophysiology and neurologic sequelae. Pediatr Clin North Am. 1976;23:541–56.
93. Thomas HM. Meningococcic meningitis and septicemia. Report of an outbreak in the fourth service command during the winter and spring of 1942–1943. JAMA. 1943;123:264–72.
94. Ducker TB, Simmons RL. The pathogenesis of meningitis. Systemic effects of meningococcal endotoxin within the cerebrospinal fluid. Arch Neurol. 1968;18:123–8.
95. Hardman JM. Fatal meningococcal infections: The changing pathologic picture in the '60's. Milit Med. 1968;133:951–64.
96. Levin S, Painter MB. The treatment of acute meningococcal infection in adults. Ann Intern Med. 1966;64:1049–56.
97. Kanter DM, Mauriello DA, Learner N. Acute meningococcemia with vascular collapse: An analysis of 10 recently treated cases. Am J Med Sci. 1956;232:674–87.
98. Gore I, Saphir Q. Myocarditis, a classification of 1402 cases. Am Heart J. 1947;34:827–31.
99. Gotshall RA. Conus medullaris syndrome after meningococcal meningitis. N Engl J Med. 1972;286:882–3.
100. Herman RA, Rubin HA. Meningococcal pericarditis without meningitis presenting as tamponade. N Engl J Med. 1974;290:143–4.
101. Morse JR, Oretsky MI, Hudson JA. Pericarditis as a complication of meningococcal meningitis. Ann Intern Med. 1971;74:212–7.
102. Pierce I, Cooper E. Meningococcal pericarditis, clinical features and therapy in five patients. Arch Intern Med. 1972;129:918–22.
103. Maron BJ, Macoul KL, Benaron P. Unusual complications of meningococcal meningitidis. Johns Hopkins Med J. 1972;131:64–8.
104. Brasier AR, Macklis JD, Vaughn D, et al. Myopericarditis as an initial presentation of meningococcemia. Unusual manifestations of infection with serotype W135. Am J Med. 1987;82:641–4.
105. Frank ST, Gomez RM. Chronic meningococcemia. Milit Med. 1968;133:918–20.
106. Saslaw S. Chronic meningococcemia: Report of a case. N Engl J Med. 1962;266:605–7.
107. Rompalo AM, Hood EW, Roberts PL, et al. The acute arthritis dermatitis syndrome. The changing importance of *Neisseria gonorrhoeae* and *Neisseria meningitidis*. Arch Intern Med. 1987;147:281–3.
108. Lim D, Gewurz A, Lint TF, et al. Absence of the sixth component of complement in a patient with repeated episodes of meningococcal meningitis. J Pediatr. 1976;89:42.
109. Alper CA, Abramson N, Johnston RB Jr. Increased susceptibility to infection associated with abnormalities of complement-mediated functions and of the third component of complement (C3). N Engl J Med. 1970;282:349–54.
110. Petersen BH, Graham JA, Brooks GF. Human deficiency of the eighth com-

ponent of complement. The requirement of C8 for serum *Neisseria gonorrhoeae* bactericidal activity. J Clin Invest. 1976;57:283–90.
111. Ellison RT, Kohler PF, Curd JG, et al. Prevalence of congenital or acquired complement deficiency in patients with sporadic meningococcal disease. N Engl J Med. 1983;308:913–6.
112. Densen P, Weiler JM, Griffiss JM, et al. Familial properidin deficiency and fatal bacteremia. Correction of the bactericidal defect by vaccination. N Engl J Med. 1987;316:922–6.
113. Ross SC, Rosenthal PJ, Berberich HM, et al. Killing of *Neisseria meningitidis* by human neutrophils: Implications for normal and complement deficient individuals. J Infect Dis. 1987;155:1266–75.
114. Holm MI, Davison WC. Meningococcus pneumonia: I. The occurrence of post-influenzal pneumonia in which *Diplococcus intracellularis meningitidis* was isolated. Bull Johns Hopkins Hosp. 1919;30:324.
115. Koppes GM, Ellenbogen C, Gebhart RJ. Group Y meningococcal disease in United States Air Force recruits. Am J Med. 1977;62:661–6.
116. Putsch RW, Hamilton JD, Wolinsky E. *Neisseria meningitidis*, a respiratory pathogen. J Infect Dis. 1970;121:48–54.
117. Irwin RS, Woelk WK, Coudon WL. Primary meningococcal pneumonia. Ann Intern Med. 1975;82:493–8.
118. Young LS, LaForce FM, Head JJ, et al. A simultaneous outbreak of meningococcal and influenza infections. N Engl J Med. 1972;287:5–9.
119. Goldstein E, Buhlers WC, Akers TC, et al. Murine resistance to inhaled *Neisseria meningitidis* after infection with an encephalomyocarditis virus. Infect Immun. 1972;6:398–402.
120. Kerttula Y, Leinonen M, Koskela M, et al. The etiology of pneumonia, application of bacterial serology and basic laboratory methods. J Infec. 1987;14:21–30.
121. Tobin JL. Complications of meningococcus infection in a series of sixty-three consecutive sporadic cases. Am J Med Sci. 1956;231:241–8.
122. McCracken GH. Rapid identification of specific etiology in meningitis. J Pediatr. 1976;88:706–8.
123. Miller M, Millikin P, Griffin PS, et al. *Neisseria meningitidis* urethritis: A case report. Arch Intern Med. 1979;242:1656–7.
124. Faur YC, Weisburd MH, Wilson ME. Isolation of *Neisseria meningitidis* from the genitourinary tract and anal canal. J Clin Microbiol. 1975;2:178–182.
125. Salet IE, Frasch CE. Seroepidemiologic aspects of *Neisseria meningitidis* in homosexual men. Can Med Assoc J. 1982;126:38–41.
126. Hoyne AL, Brown RH. 727 Meningococcic cases, an analysis. Ann Intern Med. 1948;28:248–59.
127. Feldman WE. Relation of concentrations of bacteria and bacterial antigen in cerebrospinal fluid to prognosis in patients with bacterial meningitis. N Engl J Med. 1977;296:433–5.
128. Feldman WE. Concentrations of bacteria in cerebrospinal fluid of patients with bacterial meningitis. J Pediatr. 1976;88:549–52.
129. Feigin RD, Stechenberg BW, Chang MJ. Prospective evaluation of treatment of *Hemophilus influenzae* meningitis. J Pediatr. 1976;88:542–8.
130. O'Toole RD, Goode L, Howe C. Neuraminidase activity in bacterial meningitis. J Clin Invest. 1971;50:979–85.
131. Beaty HN. Cerebrospinal fluid lactic dehydrogenase and its isoenzymes in infection of the central nervous system. N Engl J Med. 1968;279:1197–202.
132. McCrumb FR, Hall HE, Meridith AM, et al. Chloramphenicol in the treatment of meningococcal meningitis. Am J Med. 1951;10:696–703.
133. Duff P. Pathophysiology and management of septic shock. J Reprod Med. 1980;24:109.
134. Aycock WL, Mueller JH. Meningococcus carrier rates and meningitis incidence. Bacteriol Rev. 1950;14:115–160.
135. Feldman HA, Sweet LA, Dowling HF. Sulfadiazine therapy of purulent meningitis. War Med. 1942;2:995–1007.
136. Mead M, Harris W, Samper BA, et al. Treatment of meningococcal meningitis with penicillin. N Engl J Med. 1944;231:509–17.
137. Kinsman JM, D'Alonzo CA. Meningococcemia: A description of the clinical picture and a comparison of the efficacy of sulfadiazine and penicillin in the treatment of thirty cases. Ann Intern Med. 1946;24:606–17.
138. Mangi RJ, Kundargi RS, Quintiliani R, et al. Development of meningitis during cephalothin therapy. Ann Intern Med. 1973;78:347–51.
139. Brown JD, Mathies AW, Ivler D, et al. Variable results of cephalothin therapy for meningococcal meningitis. In: Hobby G, ed. Antimicrobial Agents and Chemotherapy. Ann Arbor: American Society for Microbiology; 1970:432.
140. Schribner RK, Wedro BC, Weber AH, et al. Activities of eight new beta-lactam and seven antibiotic combinations against *Neisseria meningitidis*. Antimicrob Agents Chemother. 1982;21:678–80.
141. Love BD, Finland M. In vitro susceptibility of meningococcus to 11 antibiotics and sulfadiazine. Am J Med Sci. 1954;228:534–9.
142. Brown JW, Condit PK. Meningococcal infections: Fort Ord and California. Calif Med. 1965;102:171–80.
143. Eickhoff TC, Finland M. Changing susceptibility of meningococci to antimicrobial agents. N Engl J Med. 1965;272:395–8.
144. Feldman HA. Sulfonamide resistant meningococci. Annu Rev Med. 1967;18:495–506.
145. Alexander CE, Sanborn WR, Cherriere G, et al. Sulfadiazine resistant group A *Neisseria meningitidis*. Science. 1968;161:1019.
146. Scheld WM, Sande M. Bactericidal versus bacteriostatic antibiotic therapy of experimental pneumococcal meningitis in rabbits. J Clin Invest. 1983;71:411–9.
147. Berkow R, ed. The Merck Manual of Diagnosis and Therapy. Rahway, NJ: Merck, Sharp & Dohme Laboratories; 1977:1432.
148. Sprott MS, Kearns AM, Field JM. Penicillin insensitive *Neisseria meningitis*. Lancet. 1988;1:1167.
149. Campos J, Mendelman PM, Sako MU, et al. Detection of relatively penicillin G-resistant *Neisseria meningitidis* by disk susceptibility testing. Antimicrob Agents Chemother. 1987;31:1478–82.
150. Mendelman PM, Campos J, Chaffin DO, et al. Relative penicillin G resistance in *Neisseria meningitidis* and reduced affinity of penicillin binding protein 3. Antimicrob Agents Chemother. 1988;32:706–9.
151. Neu HC. Cephalosporins in the treatment of meningitis. Drugs. 1987;34 (Suppl 2):135–53.
152. Shaad UB, Krucko J, Pfenninger J. An extended experience with cefuroxime therapy of childhood bacterial meningitis. Pediatr Infect Dis. 1984;3:410–415.
153. Beutler B, Milsark IW, Cerami AC. Passive immunization against cachectin/tumor necrosis factor protects mice from the lethal effects of endotoxin. Science. 1985;229:869–71.
154. Beutler B, Cerami A. Cachetin: More than a tumor necrosis factor. N Engl J Med. 1987;316:379–85.
155. Tracey KJ, Beutler B, Lowry SF, et al. Shock and tissue injury induced by recombinant human cachetin. Science. 1986;234:470–4.
156. Tracey KJ, Fong Y, Hesse DG, et al. Anti-cachectin/TNF monoclonal antibodies prevent septic shock during lethal bacteremia. Nature. 1987;330:662–4.
157. Girardin E, Grau GE, Dayr J-M, et al. Tumor necrosis factor and interleukin-1 in the serum of children with severe infectious purpura. N Engl J Med. 1988;319:397–400.
158. Monsalve F, Rucabado L, Salvador A, et al. Myocardial depression in septic shock caused by meningococcal infection. Crit Care Med. 1984;12:1021.
159. DeLa Cal MA, Miravelles E, Pascul T, et al. Dose-related hemodynamic and renal effects of dopamine in septic shock. Crit Care Med. 1984;12:22.
160. Fisher CJ, Horowilx BZ, Albertson TE. Cardiorespiratory failure in toxic shock syndrome: Effect of dubutamine. Crit Care Med. 1985;13:160.
161. Belsey MA, Hoffpauir CW, Smith MHD. Dexamethasone in the treatment of acute bacterial meningitis: The effect of study design on the interpretation of results. Pediatrics. 1969;44:503–13.
162. Corrigan JJ Jr, Jordan CM. Heparin therapy in septicemia with disseminated intravascular coagulation. Effect on mortality and on correction of hemostatic defects. N Engl J Med. 1970;283:778–82.
163. Denmark TC, Knight EL. Cardiovascular and coagulation complications of group C meningococcal disease. Arch Intern Med. 1971;127:238.
164. Fairbrother RW. Cerebrospinal meningitis: The use of sulphonamide derivatives in prophylaxis. Br Med J. 1940;2:859–62.
165. Gray FC, Gear J. Sulphapyridine, M and B 693 as a prophylactic against cerebrospinal meningitis. S Afr Med J. 1941;15:139.
166. Cheever FS. The control of meningococcal meningitis by mass chemoprophylaxis with sulfadiazine. Am J Med Sci. 1945;209:74–5.
167. Artenstein MS, Lamson TH, Evans JR. Attempted prophylaxis against meningococcal infection using intramuscular penicillin. Milit Med. 1967;132:1009–11.
168. Guttler RB, Counts GW, Avent CK, et al. Effect of rifampin and minocycline on meningococcal carrier rates. J Infect Dis. 1971;124:199–205.
169. Devine LF, Johnson DP, Rhode SL, et al. Rifampin: Effect of two-day treatment on meningococcal carrier state and the relationship of the levels of drug in sera and saliva. Am J Med Sci. 1971;261:79–83.
170. Jacobson JA, Daniel B. Vestibular reactions associated with minocycline. Antimicrob Agents Chemother. 1975;8:453–6.
171. Weidner CE, Dunkel TB, Pettyjohn FS, et al. Effectiveness of rifampin in eradicating the meningococcal carrier state in a relatively closed population: Emergence of resistant strains. J Infect Dis. 1971;124:172–8.
172. Hoeprich PD. Prediction of antimeningococcic chemoprophylactic efficacy. J Infect Dis. 1971;123:125–33.
173. Pugsley MP, Dworzack DI, Horowitz EA, et al. Efficacy of ciprofloxacin in treatment of nasopharyngeal carriers of *Neisseria meningitidis*. J Infect Dis. 1987;156:211–3.
174. Centers for Disease Control. Vestibular reactions to minocycline. MMWR. 1976;25:31.
175. DeWals P, Herlozhe L, Borlee-Grimee I, et al. Meningococcal disease in Belgium. Secondary attack rate among household day-care nursery and pre-elementary school contacts. J Infect. 1983;1(Suppl 1):53–61.
176. Artenstein MS, Ellis RE. The risk of exposure to a patient with meningococcal meningitis. Milit Med. 1968;133:474–7.
177. Centers for Disease Control. Meningococcal disease–United States. MMWR. 1981;30:113–5.
178. Makela PH, Kayhty H, Weekstrom P, et al. Effect of group A meningococcal vaccine in army recruits in Finland. Lancet. 1975;2:883–6.
179. Reingold AL, Hightower AW, Bolan GA, et al. Age specific differences in duration of clinical protection after vaccination with meningococcal polysaccharide vaccine. Lancet. 1985;2:114–8.
180. Taunay A de E, Galvao PA, de Morais JS, et al. Disease prevention by meningococcal serogroup C polysaccharide vaccine in pre-school: Results after eleven months in San Paulo, Brazil (Abstract). Pediatr Res. 1974;8:429.
181. Gold R, Lepow ML, Goldschneider I, et al. Clinical evaluation of group A and group C meningococcal polysaccharide vaccines in infants. J Clin Invest. 1975;56:1536–47.
182. Wahdan MH, Rizh F, El-Akkad AM, et al. A controlled field trial of a ser-

ogroup A meningococcal polysaccharide vaccine. Bull WHO. 1973;48:667–73.
183. Brandt B, Artenstein MS. Duration of antibody responses after vaccination with group C *Neisseria meningitis* polysaccharide. J Infect Dis. 1975;131:569.
184. Advisory Committee on Immunization Practices. Meningococcal polysaccharide vaccines. Ann Intern Med. 1976;84:179–80.
185. Artenstein MS, Brandt B. Immunologic hyporesponsiveness in man to group C meningococcal polysaccharide. J Immunol. 1975;115:5–7.
186. Broome CV. Use of bacterial vaccines for prevention of penumococcal and meningococcal disease in day care settings. Rev Infect Dis. 1986;8:584–8.
187. Greenwood BM, Bradley AK, Blakebrough IS, et al. The immune response to a meningococcal polysaccharide in an African village. Trans R Soc Trop Med Hyg. 1980;74:340–6.
188. Lepow ML, Beeler J, Randolph M, et al. Reactogenicity and immunogenicity of a quadrivalent combined meningococcal vaccine in children. J Infect Dis. 1986;154:1033–6.
189. Beuvery EC, van Delft RW, Medema F, et al. Immunological evaluation of meningococcal group C polysaccharide–tetanus toxoid conjugate in mice. Infect Immun. 1983;41:609–17.
190. Westerink MAJ, Campagnari AA, Wirth MA, et al. Development and characterization of an anti-idiotype antibody to the capsular polysaccharide of *Neisseria meningitidis* serogroup C. Infect Immun. 1988;56:1120–7.

190. NEISSERIA GONORRHOEAE

H. HUNTER HANDSFIELD

Neisseria gonorrhoeae is the cause of gonorrhea, a common bacterial infection transmitted almost exclusively by sexual contact or perinatally; it predominantly affects the mucous membranes of the lower genitourinary tract and less frequently those of the rectum, oropharynx, and conjunctivae. Ascending genital infection in women leads to the predominant complication, acute salpingitis, one of the most common causes of female infertility in the world. Bacteremic infections, neonatal conjunctivitis, and acute epididymitis are additional important consequences.

Gonorrhea is one of the oldest known human illnesses, and there are references to venereal urethritis in ancient Chinese writings, the biblical Old Testament (Leviticus), and other literatures of antiquity. Galen (AD 130) introduced the term gonorrhea ("flow of seed"), due to confusion of purulent exudate with semen. The causative organism was described by Neisser in 1879 and was first cultivated in 1882 by Leistikow and Loeffler. Although untreated infections were known to heal spontaneously over several weeks or months, reinfections were common; however, in men distinctions often were not made between recurrent gonorrhea and nongonococcal urethritis. Many therapies were tried, but not until the advent of the sulfonamides in the 1930s and of penicillin in 1943 was truly effective therapy available. Growth of fundamental knowledge about the organism and the host response to infection was slow for 80 years, but a remarkable surge of new information began in the early 1970s, and by the late 1980s more was known of the molecular biology of the gonococcus and the pathogenesis of gonorrhea than for the large majority of infectious diseases. Gonorrhea has proved difficult to control in most populations, and it remains a prime example of the influence that social, behavioral, and demographic factors can have on the epidemiology of an infectious disease despite the availability of effective antimicrobial therapy. Several comprehensive reviews have been published recently.[1–3]

THE PATHOGEN

Neisseria gonorrhoeae is a nonmotile, non-spore-forming, gram-negative coccus that characteristically grows in pairs (diplococci) with adjacent sides flattened. It closely resembles the related pathogen, *N. meningitidis*, as well as several species of nonpathogenic *Neisseria*. All *Neisseria* species rapidly oxidize dimethyl- or tetramethylparaphenylene diamine, the basis of the diagnostic oxidase test. Traditionally, gonococci are differentiated from the other *Neisseria* by their ability to grow on selective media, to utilize glucose but not maltose, sucrose, or lactose, to reduce nitrites, and by their inability to grow well at reduced temperature or on simple nutrient agar.[1–3]

Growth and Cultivation

N. gonorrhoeae does not tolerate drying, and clinical specimens should be inoculated immediately onto appropriate agar media. Ideally, plates should be incubated immediately, but inoculated plates may safely be held in candle extinction jars at room temperature for several hours before incubation.[4] The medium must be fresh and moist. Growth is best for most strains at 35–37°C, and many freshly isolated strains have a relative or absolute requirement for added CO_2 (approximately 5 percent) or HCO_3^-. All strains are strictly aerobic. Typical colonies appear in 24–48 hours, and on most media viability is rapidly lost after 48 hours due to autolysis.

Gonococci are inhibited by many fatty acids, and it is therefore necessary to incorporate starch or other substances that absorb fatty acids into most media. All strains have complex growth requirements, including requirements for several vitamins, amino acids, iron, and other factors. For clinical purposes, a satisfactory medium is chocolate agar enriched with glucose and other defined supplements.[5] Isolation of gonococci from sites that normally contain high concentrations of saprophytic microorganisms (pharynx, rectum, and cervix) may be difficult, due to overgrowth of the hardier normal flora. This problem can be largely overcome by use of media containing antimicrobial agents that inhibit most nonpathogenic *Neisseria* and other species but that permit growth of most gonococci (and also meningococci). Chocolate agar that contains vancomycin, colistin, and nystatin (Thayer-Martin medium) has been commonly used for this purpose in the United States.[6] Modified Thayer-Martin medium also contains trimethoprim to inhibit *Proteus* species and is now used extensively.[5] A translucent selective medium called New York City medium, also widely used, contains vancomycin, colistin, trimethoprim, and either nystatin or amphotericin B.[7]

All selective media fail to support the growth of some gonococci, in part because some strains are relatively sensitive to vancomycin. The prevalence of these strains varies geographically, chronologically, and between population groups, and in some settings the use of vancomycin-containing media may significantly impair the diagnosis of gonorrhea.[8,9] Material from sites that usually do not harbor an indigenous flora (e.g., blood, synovial fluid, cerebrospinal fluid) should be cultured on antibiotic-free medium.

For use in situations that preclude immediate inoculation of growth medium, transport systems using media with self-contained CO_2-generating systems are available, but none of these systems can preserve all incubating gonococci. Some non-nutrient transport media (e.g., Amies' modification of Stuart's medium, variations of which are used in many commercial specimen collection kits) can maintain viable gonococci for up to 6 hours before inoculation onto growth media.

Surface Structures

In basic structure, the envelope of *N. gonorrhoeae* is similar to that of other gram-negative bacteria. As the interface between the gonococcus and host, the cell surface has been intensively studied (Fig. 1), and specific surface components have been related to adherence, tissue and cellular penetration, cytotoxicity, and evasion of host defenses both systemically and at the mucosal level.

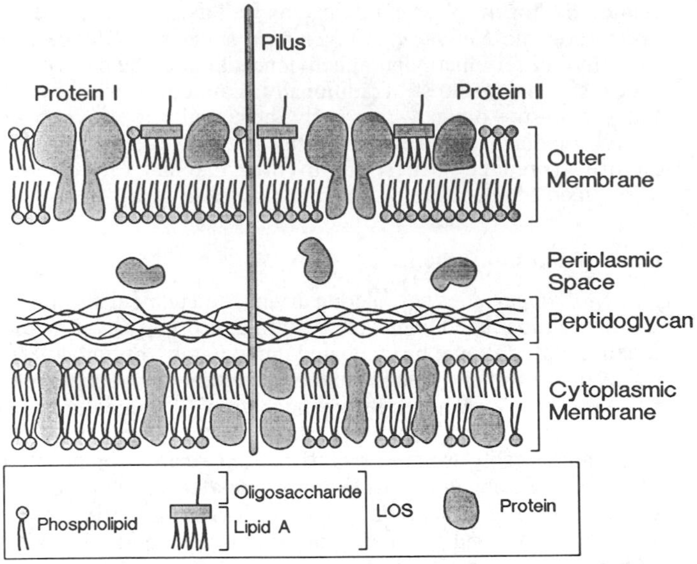

FIG. 1. Schematic representation of the surface structure of *Neisseria gonorrhoeae*, showing the major constituents that contribute to pathogenicity and antimicrobial resistance. (Courtesy of Dr. S. A. Morse, Atlanta, GA.)

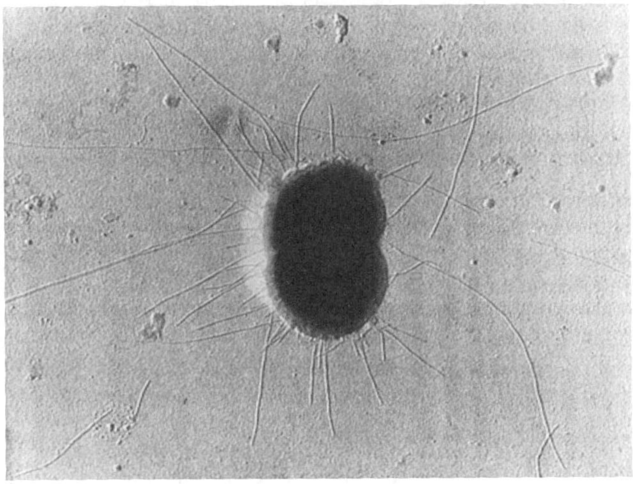

FIG. 2. *Neisseria gonorrhoeae*, with numerous pili extending from the cell surface. (Courtesy of Dr. Gour Biswas, Chapel Hill, NC.)

Pili. Varied colonial forms can be distinguished when *N. gonorrhoeae* is grown on translucent agar.[10] Fresh clinical isolates initially form colony types P^+ and P^{++} (formerly called T1 and T2), and the organisms have numerous pili extending from the cell surface (Fig. 2). After 20–24 hours of growth, P^- (formerly T3 and T4) colonies, in which the cells are nonpiliated, come to predominate. The shift between P^+ or P^{++} and P^- colony types is known as phase variation and is mediated by chromosomal rearrangement.[1–3] Nonpiliated organisms are avirulent in human inoculation experiments.[10] Pili traverse the outer membrane of the gonococcus and are composed of repeating protein subunits (pilin) of molecular weight 19 ± 2.5 kD.[11] Pilin has regions of considerable interstrain antigenic homology, especially near the amino terminus, but there also are areas of extreme antigenic variability near the carboxy terminus.[12,13] In addition, a single strain of *N. gonorrhoeae* can produce pili of varying antigenic composition.[1–3,14] These antigenic variations have compromised the potential utility of pilus-based vaccines against gonorrhea, although research continues on the potential of peptides from the antigenically conserved regions of pilin as the basis for a vaccine.[14]

Piliated gonococci are better able to attach to human mucosal surfaces[13] and are more virulent in several animal models[15] than nonpiliated variants. Pili contribute to resistance to killing by neutrophils,[16,17] although several other surface components also may be involved. In the fallopian tube mucosa model (Fig. 3), pili mediate attachment to nonciliated epithelial cells, which initiates a process of phagocytosis and transport in vacuoles through these cells into intercellular spaces near the basement membrane or directly into the subepithelial space.[15] Concurrently, nearby ciliated mucosal cells lose their cilia and are sloughed.[15] Other factors also mediate attachment, notably protein II, discussed below. Nonpiliated gonococci show attachment and damage to mucosal cells at a lower but measurable rate, and piliated commensal *Neisseria* neither attach nor cause damage in this model.[15]

Outer Membrane. Like all gram-negative bacteria, the gonococcus possesses a cell envelope composed of three distinct layers: an inner cytoplasmic membrane, a middle peptidoglycan cell wall, and an outer membrane. The outer membrane contains lipooligosaccharide (LOS), phosopholipid, and a variety of proteins (Fig. 1).

Protein I has a molecular weight of 32–36 kD and is closely associated in the membrane with LOS. It functions as a porin,[18] providing channels through which aqueous solutes can pass through the otherwise hydrophobic outer membrane, and is believed to play an important role in pathogenesis. Protein I is translocated into the cytoplasmic membrane of erythrocytes with which the gonococcus comes in contact[18]; if this occurs in epithelial cells (which has not yet been demonstrated), it may somehow facilitate endocytosis of the organism (Fig. 3) or otherwise trigger invasion.[14,15,18] Protein I shows stable interstrain antigenic variation and is the basis of the most commonly employed gonococcal serotyping system.[19] Certain protein I serovars are associated with resistance of *N. gonorrhoeae* to the bactericidal effect of normal (nonimmune) human serum and, perhaps as a direct result, with an enhanced propensity to cause bacteremia.[1–3,19] Protein I has been the focus of extensive

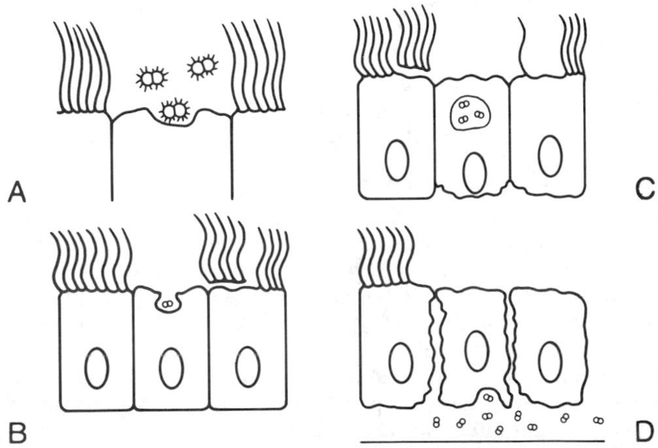

FIG. 3. Schematic representation of the interaction between fallopian tube explant epithelial cells and *N. gonorrhoeae*. **(A)** Attachment of piliated gonococci to surface of nonciliated host cell. **(B)** Endocytosis of gonococci; loss of cilia on adjacent cell, mediated by lipooligosaccharide. **(C)** Transport of gonococci through epithelial cell in endocytotic vacuole, in which the organism may replicate; progression of LOS-associated cytotoxicity. **(D)** Release of organisms into subepithelial space. (From Dalabetta and Hook,[1] with permission.)

investigation directed toward development of a gonococcal vaccine.

Protein II is the designation for several related outer membrane proteins with molecular weights of 20–28 kD.[20] Colonies of *N. gonorrhoeae* that lack protein II appear transparent, whereas those with one or more types of protein II are opaque.[20,21] In contrast to protein I, protein II can vary in amount or be completely absent in a particular gonococcal isolate, and an individual strain of *N. gonorrhoeae* can express up to six protein II variants.[21] Protein II expression in fact varies during natural infection.[22] For example, most mucosal isolates contain protein II, and their colonies are opaque, but most cervical isolates during menstruation and isolates from normally sterile sites, such as fallopian tubes, blood, and synovial fluid, lack protein II and form transparent colonies.[20,23] Colonial opacity has been correlated with virulence in a chick embryo model,[24] adherence to a variety of eukaryotic cell types,[25] attachment to phagocytes,[26] and resistance to nonimmune human serum.[14] Loss of protein II has been associated with resistance to phagocytic killing by neutrophils.[26]

Less is known about protein III, which has a molecular weight of 30–31 kD, is present in all gonococci in close association with protein I and LOS, and has little if any interstrain antigenic variation.[18] Protein III can stimulate blocking antibodies that reduce serum bactericidal activity against *N. gonorrhoeae*.[27]

Several other outer membrane proteins have been identified. These include several proteins (some of which are shared with *N. meningitidis*) that are closely linked with iron utilization and transport and that have molecular weights ranging from 37 kD to >800 kD[28,29]; two proteins of unknown function, both of which carry a common epitope designated H-8[30]; and several poorly characterized growth-related proteins. IgA_1 proteases, present in *N. gonorrhoeae* and *N. meningitidis* but not in nonpathogenic *Neisseria*, are presumed to protect the organism from secretory IgA antibody at mucosal surfaces, but this role has not been proved.[31]

Gonococcal LOS is comprised of lipid A and a core oligosaccharide that, in contrast to the polysaccharide of most gram-negative bacteria, lacks O-antigenic side chains.[32] LOS possesses endotoxic activity, is lethal for experimental animals, and in the fallopian tube explant model (Fig. 3) mediates ciliary loss and the death of adjacent uninfected cells.[15,33] Antigenically variable core oligosaccharide components of LOS are related to the relative resistance of certain strains of *N. gonorrhoeae* to serum bactericidal activity, and perhaps to the clinical manifestations and severity of gonococcal infection.[34,35] These antigenic variations are the basis of an alternative gonococcal serotyping system.[32,35,36]

The peptidoglycan layer may contribute to the inflammatory response in gonococcal infection. For example, gonococcal peptidoglycan fragments are intrinsically toxic in the fallopian tube explant system and cause complement consumption in vitro,[37] and peptidoglycan fragments have been found in apparently sterile synovial fluid of patients with the gonococcal arthritis–dermatitis syndrome.[38] The existence of a polysaccharide capsule surrounding *N. gonorrhoeae* has long been debated, but none has been chemically isolated or characterized. However, gonococci produce a surface polyphosphate that may have capsulelike functions, such as creating a hydrophilic, negatively charged cell surface.[39]

Strain Typing

Studies of the pathogenesis and epidemiology of gonorrhea have been greatly facilitated by the development of reproducible methods for typing *N. gonorrhoeae*. Characterization of gonococcal strains recently has been based on two primary methodologies, auxotyping and serotyping. Auxotyping is based on the requirement of strains for specific nutrients or cofactors, as defined by their ability to grow on chemically defined media that lack these factors.[40] Examples of common auxotypes, among over 30 that have been identified, include prototrophic (Proto), also known as "zero" or "wild-type"; proline-requiring (Pro^-); and strains that require arginine, hypoxanthine, and uracil (AHU^-). The most widely used serotyping system is based on protein I, which may be antigenically classified into two groups, IA and IB.[19] These in turn are divided into serovars based on coagglutination reactions using panels of monoclonal antibodies that react with variable epitopes of protein IA (e.g., serovar IA-4) or IB (e.g., IB-12).[19] In practice, protein I serotyping and auxotyping often are used together to provide enhanced discrimination of strains. This dual system has been instrumental in mapping the geographic and temporal occurrence of gonorrhea in communities, in analyzing the patterns of antibiotic resistance, and in studies of disease transmission.[1,19,41,42]

Gonococci also have been divided into six groups on the basis of LOS typing with polyvalent antisera,[32,35,36] but these types have not yet been related to the epidemiology or clinical manifestations of gonorrhea. In addition, expression of LOS epitopes may vary in vitro or in vivo,[43] perhaps compromising the utility of such typing schemes. Patterns of susceptibility to various antimicrobial agents and analysis of the plasmid content of gonococcal isolates have been used to distinguish gonococcal strains,[42,44] but with less success and reproducibility, as these are not genetically stable characteristics.

Genetics

Plasmids. Many strains of *N. gonorrhoeae* possess a 24.5 MD conjugative plasmid and thereby can conjugally transfer other non-self-transferable plasmids with high efficiency[45]; chromosomal genes are not mobilized. Many gonococci now carry a plasmid (Pc^r) that specifies production of a TEM-1 type of β-lactamase (penicillinase). The two most common Pc^r plasmids have molecular weights of 3.2 or 4.4 MD[46] and are closely related to each other and to similar plasmids found in certain *Haemophilus* species, including *H. ducreyi*.[47] In fact, it is suspected that gonococci first acquired Pc^r plasmids from *H. ducreyi*.[47] Pc^r plasmids are commonly mobilized to other gonococci by the conjugative plasmid.[45] Gonococci with plasmid-mediated high-level resistance to tetracycline (minimum inhibitory concentration [MIC] $\geq$ 16 mg/liter) carry the 24.5 MD conjugative plasmid into which the *tetM* transposon has been inserted.[49] The *tetM* determinant also confers tetracycline resistance to a variety of other bacteria, including some *Streptococcus* and *Mycoplasma* species and various genital organisms, such as *Gardnerella vaginalis* and *Ureaplasma urealyticum*.[49] Owing to its association with the conjugative plasmid, high-level tetracycline resistance is readily transfered to other gonococci. The *tetM* determinant functions by encoding for a protein that protects ribosomes from the effect of tetracycline. Finally, all gonococci contain a small (2.6 MD) cryptic plasmid of unknown function.[49]

Chromosomal Mutations. Chromosomally mediated resistance of *N. gonorrhoeae* to β-lactam antibiotics and the tetracyclines results from a series of individually minor mutations that reduce the permeability of the organism's outer membrane (e.g., the *mtr* and *penB* determinants)[50] or alter penicillin-binding protein-2 to reduce its affinity for penicillin (the *penA* determinant).[50,51] For epidemiologic purposes, such strains are classified as resistant only when the MIC is such that clinical failures are common with the maximum practical therapeutic doses (penicillin G MIC $\geq$ 1.0 mg/liter, tetracycline MIC $\geq$ 2.0 mg/liter).[52] The susceptibility of *N. gonorrhoeae* to cephalosporin antibiotics such as ceftriaxone, which became frequently used in the late 1980s in the United States for treatment of gonorrhea, varies with chromosomally mediated penicillin resistance.[52] To date, however, all isolates have been inhibited by readily attained blood levels of ceftriaxone and are not clinically resistant.

Mutations in biosynthetic and metabolic pathways are common, and may result in dependence on metabolites from the environment for growth. These mutations form the genetic basis for the nutritional requirements that are the basis for auxotyping.[53] Despite these mutations and intrastrain variability in expression of pili, protein II, and LOS, *N. gonorrhoeae* is relatively resistant to external mutagenic stimuli, such as ultraviolet light.[54]

Transformation. The piliated variants of virtually all clinical isolates of *N. gonorrhoeae* are highly competent for the exchange of chromosomal DNA by transformation, but loss of ability to express pili is always accompanied by a dramatic reduction in transformation competence.[55] Uptake of transforming DNA is limited to homologous (gonococcal) DNA, which may reflect recognition of a unique nucleotide sequence on gonococcal DNA by a surface receptor.[56] No bacteriophages have been found in gonococci.

PATHOLOGY

N. gonorrhoeae primarily infects noncornified epithelium. Cornification of the vaginal epithelium, under the influence of estrogen, protects sexually mature women and newborn girls from gonococcal vaginitis, but vaginitis is the predominant manifestation of gonorrhea in prepubertal girls beyond the neonatal period.[57] The histopathology of gonorrhea is not materially different from that of most mucosal pyogenic infections. Attachment to mucosal epithelium, mediated in part by pili and protein II, is followed within 24–48 hours by penetration of the organism between and through epithelial cells to the submucosal tissues.[15,33] A vigorous response by neutrophils ensues, along with sloughing of the epithelium, development of submucosal microabscesses, and exudation of pus. Stained smears usually reveal a large number of gonococci within (or in association with) a few neutrophils, while the majority of cells contain no organisms (Fig. 4). The explanation for this phenomenon remains unclear; some gonococci somehow evade killing mechanisms and continue to multiply intracellularly,[58] but this is unlikely to be the only explanation. In untreated infections, neutrophils are gradually replaced by macrophages and lymphocytes; abnormal lymphocytic and mononuclear infiltration persists in tissues for up to several weeks after *N. gonorrhoeae* can no longer be identified histologically or recovered by culture.

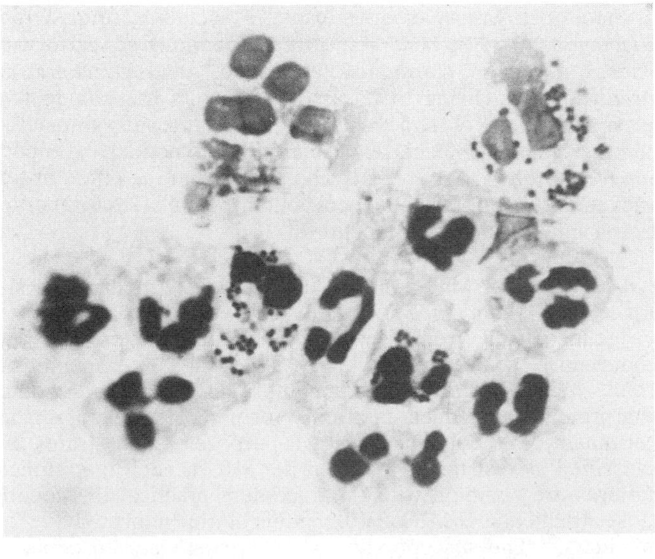

FIG. 4. Gram-stained smear of urethral exudate showing intracellular gram-negative diplococci characteristic of gonorrhea.

EPIDEMIOLOGY

Incidence

Only a few countries possess reporting systems that permit reasonably accurate estimation of the true incidence of gonorrhea. The number of reported cases in the United States (which underestimates the true incidence because of incomplete reporting) rose from about 250,000 cases in the early 1960s to a high of 1.01 million cases in 1978; the peak incidence in modern times, 468 cases per 100,000 population, occurred in 1975[59,60] (Fig. 5). The incidence slowly declined over most of the next decade, then fell by 13 percent in 1987, when 781,000 cases were reported. The incidence nevertheless remained disturbingly high at 324 cases per 100,000 population in 1987. In Sweden, in contrast to the United States, the incidence of gonorrhea fell precipitously and almost continuously after 1970, and the disease had become uncommon by the mid-1980s (Fig. 5); only 2579 cases were reported in 1987, an annual incidence of 31 cases per 100,000 population (Kallings I, unpublished data). The highest incidences of gonorrhea and its complications undoubtedly occur in developing countries, but accurate statistics are not available.

In the United States, the highest attack rates occur in 20–24-year-old women and men[60]; among those who are sexually active, however, the highest risk occurs in 15–19-year-old women.[61,62] Although more cases are reported in men than women, this partly reflects the greater proportion of undiagnosed cases in women than men. The male:female case ratio declined steadily from about 1.5:1 in the 1970s to 1.3:1 in 1987,[60] due in part to dramatically decreasing numbers of cases in homosexually active men, as a result of behavioral changes in response to the epidemic of acquired immune deficiency syndrome.[63] For example, reported cases of gonorrhea in homosexually active men attending public sexually transmitted disease clinics in Seattle fell from 737 cases in 1982 to 29 in 1988 (Handsfield HH, et al., unpublished data). The male:female case ratio has declined among heterosexuals as well.[64] (Handsfield HH, et al., unpublished data), perhaps due to increasingly effective case finding among women.

In the United States, about 286,000 cases of gonorrhea in non-Hispanic whites were reported in 1987, compared with 495,000 cases in all other racial/ethnic groups (Handsfield HH, et al., unpublished data). Owing to differences in the sizes of these populations, the incidence rate is 8–10 times higher in nonwhite populations than in whites, a difference that is only partly explained by greater attendance of nonwhites at public clinics, where case reporting is more complete than in the private health care sector (Rice RJ, et al., unpublished data).[62] During the 1980s, the rate of decline in reported gonorrhea was greater in whites than nonwhites, so that the nonwhite:white incidence ratio rose from 8.2 in 1980 to 10.2 in 1987 (Handsfield HH, et al., unpublished data). In some geographic areas, such as Seattle, cases in blacks rose steadily in the 1980s, cases in whites declined, and cases in other ethnic groups changed little (Handsfield HH, et al., unpublished data). Figure 6 shows the shift in the racial distribution of cases that occurred after a single auxotype/serovar class (Pro^-/IA-4) of β-lactamase-producing *N. gonorrhoeae* was introduced into an urban urea in late 1986.[42] The epidemic strain first appeared in whites but decreased rapidly in that population, while becoming established in blacks. There also was a shift in cases caused by the Pro^-/IA-4 clone from predominantly males to equal numbers of men and women, and the proportion of cases associated with illicit drug use increased steadily from 19 percent in the first quarter of 1987 to 82 percent in the fourth quarter.[42] This study illustrates a pattern of introduction and spread of gonorrhea that

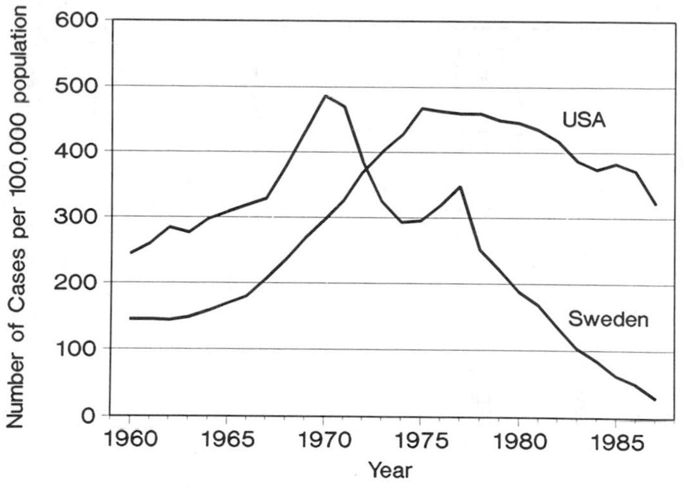

FIG. 5. Incidence of reported gonorrhea in the United States and Sweden, 1960–1987.

probably is common in urban environments in North America, and demonstrates the epidemiologic utility of gonococcal strain typing.

Although nonwhite ethnicity is a marker of gonorrhea risk, it is not in itself a risk factor for gonococcal infection. Other markers associated with increased risk of gonorrhea include lower socioeconomic attainment, lesser education, urban residence, and being unmarried.[61] Gonorrhea appeared to be increasingly associated with illicit drug use in many urban centers in the 1980s, as in the 1987–1988 Seattle outbreak of penicillin-resistant gonorrhea.[42] For unknown reasons, the incidence of gonorrhea in the United States fluctuates seasonally, with consistently more cases reported from July through September and nadirs occurring from January to April.

Transmission

Aside from perinatal transmission, the overriding risk factor for acquiring gonorrhea is sexual intercourse with an infected partner. The risk of transmission of *N. gonorrhoeae* from an infected woman to the urethra of her male partner is approximately 20 percent per episode of vaginal intercourse, rising to 60–80 percent after four or more exposures.[65,66] The risk of male-to-female transmission has been less well studied; it probably approximates 50 percent per contact, rising to ≥90 percent after several exposures.[67] The efficiencies of transmission by other modes of sexual contact are unknown, although rectal intercourse clearly is relatively efficient. Transmission by fellatio is less so, especially from the oropharynx to the urethra,[68,69] and transmission in either direction is rare by cunnilingus.[69] There are conflicting data as to whether women using anovulatory contraceptives are at increased risk for gonorrhea; if so, the magnitude of the effect is small.[70] On the other hand, it appears clear that infected women using anovulatory contraceptives have a reduced risk of acute salpingitis.[71]

Current theory holds that maintenance of gonorrhea in a population or community requires a core group of persons at particularly high risk.[72,73] Epidemiologically, core groups are defined by demographic and social characteristics that directly or indirectly influence sexual behavior, such as young age, urban residence, low educational and socioeconomic levels, nonwhite race, prostitution, and perhaps illicit drug use.[61,72,73] Other determinants may include cultural factors that affect the response to early symptoms, real or perceived reduced access to health care, and similar factors. Many persons with gonorrhea do not belong to the core, but have occasional sexual contact with core group members (e.g., a suburban male who visits an inner city prostitute). However, gonorrhea is not transmitted with 100 percent efficiency, and spontaneous cures are common; in theory, therefore, in the absence of hyperendemic transmission in core group members, the prevalence of infection would decline, perhaps ultimately to zero. Originally developed as a mathematical model,[72,73] the core transmitter hypothesis has been empirically confirmed by several studies,[42,61,74] and a central focus of gonorrhea control is to identify the core group and to target members for case finding, treatment, and educational programs.[73,74] It is probable that the core transmitter concept also is applicable to other sexually transmitted diseases. The differing trends of gonorrhea incidence in various population groups indicate that the gonorrhea epidemic in the United States is "contracting" around an expanding core group. Interestingly, this represents a return to the pattern of gonorrhea and syphilis occurrence in the preantibiotic era, when most cases were associated with prostitution and low socioeconomic attainment.

Gonorrhea most commonly is transmitted by persons who are asymptomatically infected or who have symptoms that they ignore or whose significance is not understood.[75] The behavioral response to symptoms presumably is determined by education and various demographic and sociocultural factors.[61,75] However, except where there is limited access to health care or when persistent sexual activity is an economic necessity (e.g., for some prostitutes), it is probable that most persons with new genital symptoms cease sexual activity and obtain medical attention. It follows that many transmitters are in a subset of infected persons who lack or ignore symptoms and do not spontaneously cease sexual activity and seek treatment. This concept, which applies to all sexually transmitted diseases, underlies the importance of taking active steps to bring the sexual contacts of infected persons to treatment.

Antibiotic-Resistant Neisseria gonorrhoeae

Penicillinase-producing strains of *N. gonorrhoeae* (PPNG), bearing plasmids with the Pc^r determinant, were first documented almost simultaneously in 1975–1976 in the United States, western Europe, the Philippines, and western Africa.[46,76] In retrospect, PPNG strains probably had been contributing for several years to penicillin treatment failures in parts of Asia, the Western Pacific, and Africa. By 1980, PPNG accounted for up to 50 percent of *N. gonorrhoeae* isolates in some arts of the developing world. Figure 7 displays the course of reported PPNG infections in the United States through 1987.[60] For a few years, most isolates in industrialized countries were directly imported from other endemic areas or were detected at the first generation of spread.[76] By 1980, however, sustained transmission was occurring throughout Europe and North America, and indigenous gonococci had acquired Pc^r plasmids.[77] Initially, the predominant Pc^r plasmid in North American gonococci was the 4.4 MD plasmid that was prevalent in Asia and the Philippines, whereas the 3.2 MD plasmid predominated in Europe and Africa.[46,76] By the mid-1980s, however, both of these plasmid types were common throughout the world,[42,78,79] and a few isolates had been identified with at least three other variant plasmids.[80]

The number of PPNG cases in the United States increased rapidly in the mid-1980s (Fig. 7), and by 1988 these strains accounted for over 4 percent of gonorrhea cases and 10–40 percent of gonococcal isolates in several metropolitan areas.[79,81] A few localized outbreaks of single strains of PPNG have been documented[42,77] (Fig. 6), but in most regions a large variety of gonococcal types has been involved.[79,82] For reasons that are unclear, PPNG infection in the United States has been uncommon among homosexually active men with gonorrhea.[78,79] Due to the spread of PPNG and other resistant strains, penicillin no longer is appropriate for routine use in gonorrhea treatment anywhere in the world.

Strains of *N. gonorrhoeae* with plasmid-mediated high-level tetracycline resistance were first documented in the United

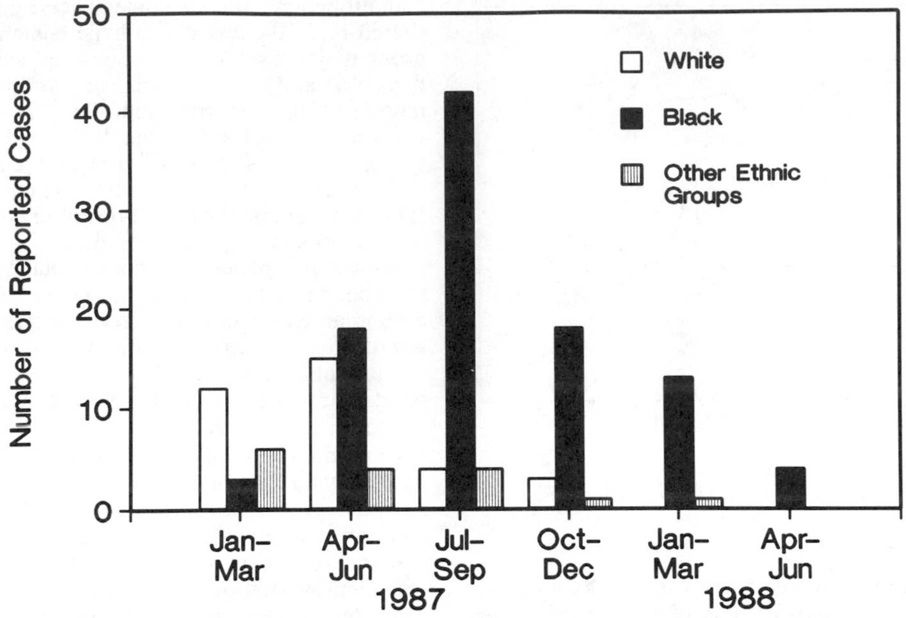

FIG. 6. Ethnic distribution of cases of gonorrhea due to a distinct strain (Pro$^-$/IA-4 auxotype/serovar class) of penicillinase-producing *Neisseria gonorrhoeae* in King County, Washington, July, 1986 to June, 1988. "Other" represents persons of Hispanic origin, ethnic Asians, and Native Americans.

States in 1985.[83] Within 2 years, these strains accounted for several percent of all reported gonorrhea cases in some urban centers and had appeared in small numbers in virtually all areas of the country.[84] Although data are scant on their occurrence outside the United States, plasmid-mediated tetracycline-resistant strains apparently have a worldwide distribution. As for Pc^r plasmids, all strains of *N. gonorrhoeae* probably are competent to acquire and express the *tetM* determinant.[49,50]

The prevalence of gonococcal strains with clinically significant chromosomally mediated resistance to the penicillins and tetracyclines has risen steadily in much of the world, including North America and Europe.[52,85] As of mid-1988, non-PPNG gonococci that had penicillin G MICs ≥ 1.0 mg/liter and/or tetracycline MICs ≥ 2.0 mg/liter accounted for ≥10 percent of all isolates in 20 of 21 sexually transmitted disease clinics that participated in a national program for surveillance of antimicrobial resistance in *N. gonorrhoeae* in the United States; in 10 of the 21 clinics, ≥20 percent of isolates were resistant by these criteria.[81] Although the MICs of ceftriaxone for many such strains are somewhat higher (e.g., 0.015–0.06 mg/liter) than for fully susceptible gonococci (MIC <0.0001–0.008 mg/liter), even these higher levels are greatly exceeded with routinely recommended regimens, and single-dose ceftriaxone therapy is almost always effective.[85,86] A large variety of auxotype/serovar classes is involved, although most strains with chromosomally mediated resistance belong to protein IB serovars.[52] In addition, a circumscribed single-strain outbreak of *N. gonorrhoeae* with relatively high-level chromosomally mediated penicillin resistance (MIC 2–4 mg/liter) has been reported.[87] Relatively resistant strains are especially common in homosexual men,[88] be-

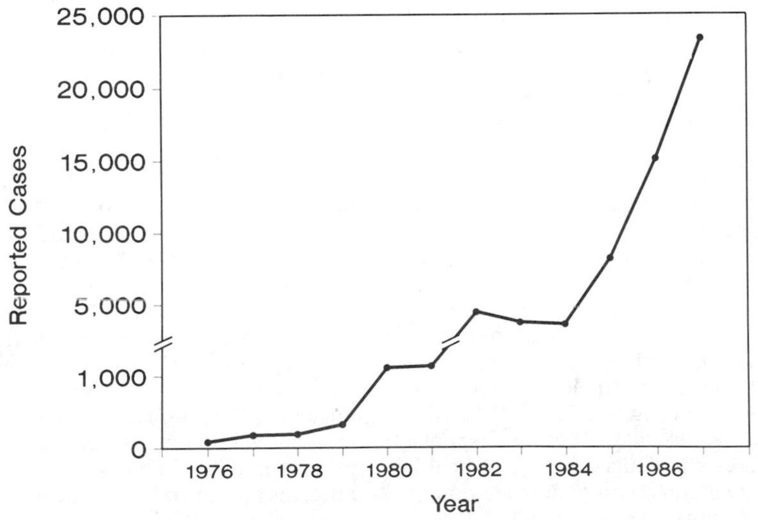

FIG. 7. Reported cases of penicillinase-producing *Neisseria gonorrhoeae* infection in the United States, 1976–1987.

cause a reservoir of rectal infection is required for propagation of gonorrhea in this population, and fecal fatty acids and bile salts select for *mtr* and other genes that result in reduced permeability of the gonococcal outer membrane to antibiotics.[89] The overall prevalence of gonococci with chromosomally mediated resistance is greater than that of PPNG or strains with high-level tetracycline resistance, and in most communities this form of resistance accounts for the majority of treatment failures.[52,85]

CLINICAL MANIFESTATIONS

Genital Infection in Men

Acute urethritis is the predominant manifestation of gonorrhea in men. The incubation period is typically 2–5 days, but ranges from 1 to 10 days or longer[90] (Fig. 8). Urethral discharge and dysuria, usually without urinary frequency or urgency, are the major symptoms. The discharge initially may be scant and mucoid, but within a day or two it becomes overtly purulent. Compared with nongonococcal urethritis, the incubation period is shorter, dysuria usually is more prominent, and the discharge usually is more profuse and more purulent (Fig. 9), but exceptions are common.[91] Most cases of untreated gonococcal urethritis resolve spontaneously over several weeks.

A small proportion of men with urethral gonorrhea remains asymptomatic, and many of these also lack signs of urethritis.[75] However, this depends in part on the infecting organism; some protein IA serovars and the AHU$^-$ auxotype of *N. gonorrhoeae* are more frequently associated with asymptomatic infection in men than other gonococcal types.[19,92,93] The overall incidence of asymptomatic urethral infection is low, but the prevalence may become substantial, because such infections tend to accumulate in the community. The prevalence of asymptomatic urethral infection has approached 50 percent of men with gonorrhea in areas where AHU$^-$ gonococci were prevalent and specific efforts were not made to identify and treat asymptomatic men.[75]

Acute epididymitis is the most commonly recognized complication of urethral gonorrhea, but it is nevertheless uncommon in industrialized countries, accounting for about 10 percent of epididymitis in young men; most cases are due to *Chlamydia trachomatis*.[94] Penile edema, without other overt inflammatory signs, is occasionally seen in gonococcal or nongonococcal urethritis.[95] Penile lymphangitis, periurethral abscess, acute prostatitis, seminal vesiculitis, and infections of Tyson's and Cowper's glands now are rare complications in industrialized countries. Urethral stricture as a result of gonorrhea also is uncommon; it is likely that many strictures in the preantibiotic era resulted from treatment by urethral irrigation with caustic compounds, rather than gonorrhea itself.

Uncomplicated Genital Infection in Women

The primary site of genital infection in women is the endocervix. *Neisseria gonorrhoeae* is also recovered frequently from the urethra or rectum and occasionally from the periurethral (Skene's) glands and the Bartholin's gland ducts, but these rarely are the only infected sites, except in women who have undergone hysterectomy. The natural course of gonorrhea is understood less completely in women than in men, partly because of the frequency of coinfection with other pathogens, such as *C. trachomatis* and *Trichomonas vaginalis*. Most infected women probably develop symptoms,[96] but a substantial minority initially remain asymptomatic or develop only minor symptoms that do not induce them to seek medical care.[97,98] As for men, those with asymptomatic or minimally symptomatic infection accumulate in the population. In settings in which most infections are detected by screening or through case finding efforts among the sexual partners of infected men (e.g., family planning clinics, some sexually transmitted disease clinics), asymptomatic or minimally symptomatic patients may comprise up to 80 percent of women with gonorrhea.[4,97,98] As expected, among women diagnosed in settings that attract symptomatic patients (e.g., emergency departments), the large majority are overtly symptomatic.[96,97]

The incubation period of gonorrhea is more variable and less well defined in women than in men, but most of those who become symptomatic probably do so within 10 days.[96] The dominant symptoms are those of cervicitis and/or urethritis, including increased vaginal discharge, dysuria (usually without urinary urgency or frequency), intermenstrual bleeding (sometimes manifested by postcoital spotting), and menorrhagia.[97,98] These may occur in any combination and they range widely in severity. Abdominal or pelvic pain usually is associated with salpingitis, although this symptom occasionally occurs in infected women in whom laparoscopy shows apparently normal fallopian tubes.[71]

The physical examination typically shows purulent or mucopurulent cervical exudate (Fig. 10) and often other signs of mucopurulent cervicitis, such as edema in a zone of cervical

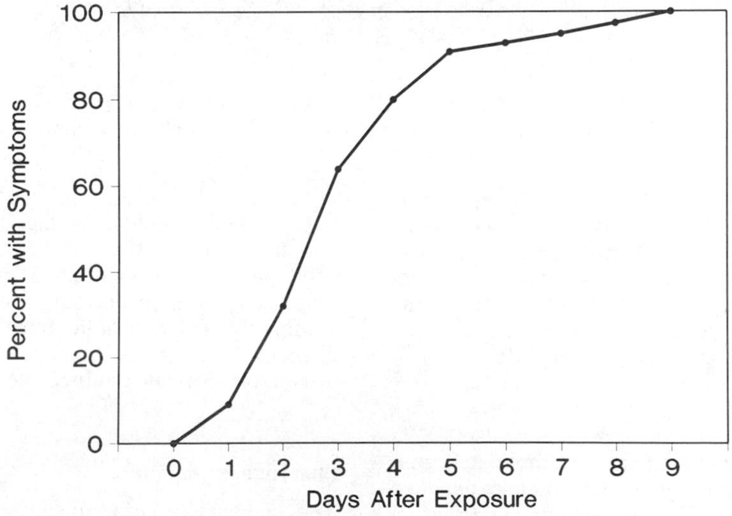

FIG. 8. Incubation period in 44 men with gonococcal urethritis. (Data from Harrison et al.[90])

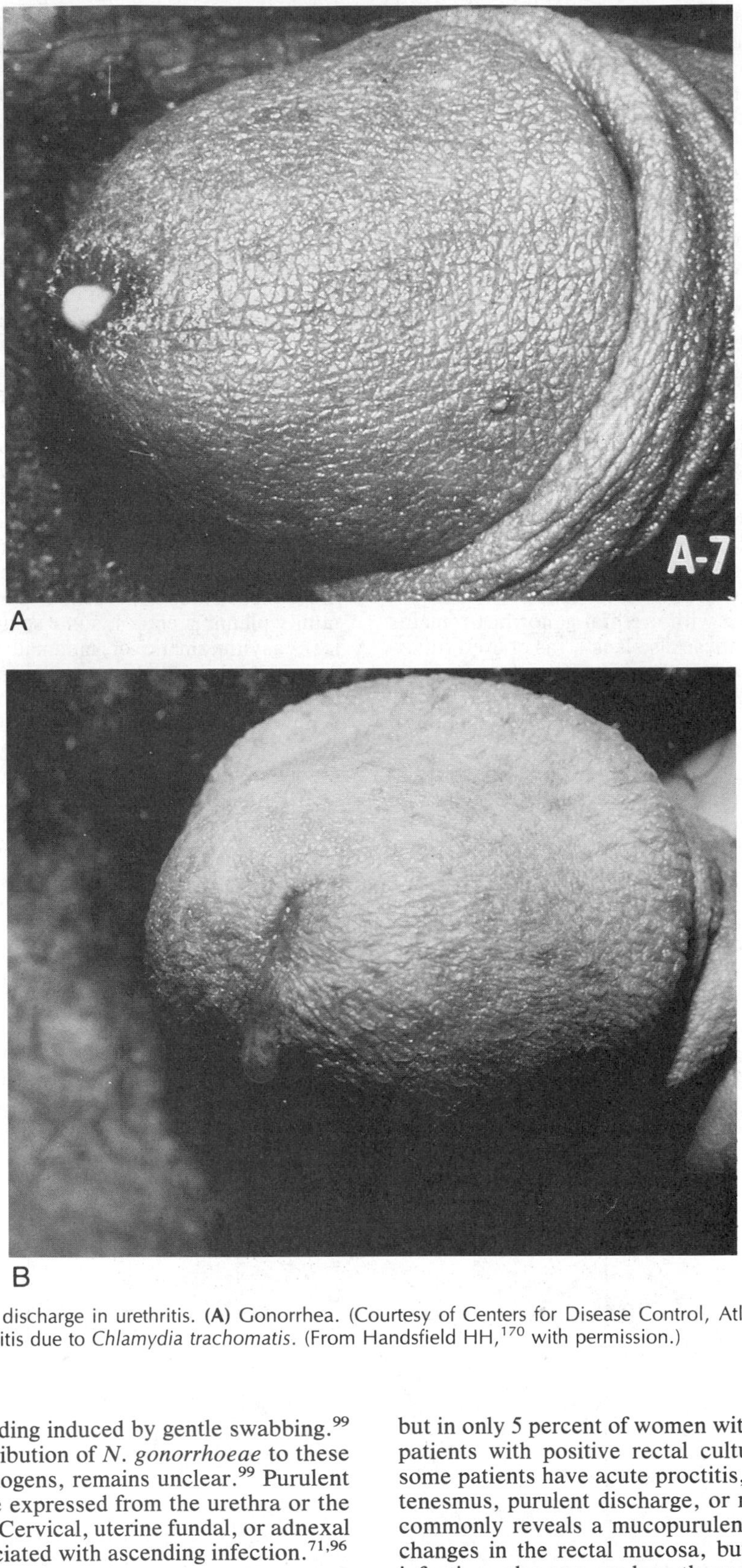

FIG. 9. Urethral discharge in urethritis. **(A)** Gonorrhea. (Courtesy of Centers for Disease Control, Atlanta, GA.) **(B)** Nongonococcal urethritis due to *Chlamydia trachomatis*. (From Handsfield HH,[170] with permission.)

ectopy or endocervical bleeding induced by gentle swabbing.[99] However, the specific contribution of *N. gonorrhoeae* to these signs, vs. that of other pathogens, remains unclear.[99] Purulent discharge sometimes can be expressed from the urethra or the ducts of Bartholin's glands. Cervical, uterine fundal, or adnexal tenderness usually are associated with ascending infection.[71,96]

Anorectral Infection

Approximately 40 percent of women with uncomplicated gonorrhea and a similar proportion of infected homosexual men have positive rectal cultures for *N. gonorrhoeae*. The rectum is the only infected site in about 40 percent of homosexual men but in only 5 percent of women with gonorrhea.[97,98,100,101] Most patients with positive rectal cultures are asymptomatic, but some patients have acute proctitis, manifested by anal pruritis, tenesmus, purulent discharge, or rectal bleeding.[101] Anoscopy commonly reveals a mucopurulent exudate and inflammatory changes in the rectal mucosa, but other sexually transmitted infections also can produce these findings.[100,101]

Pharyngeal Infection

The major risk factor for pharyngeal gonococcal infection is orogenital sexual exposure. Acquired more efficiently by fellatio than cunnilingus,[68,69] pharyngeal infection can be found in 10–20 percent of heterosexual woman with gonorrhea and 10–25 percent of infected homosexual men, but in only 3–7 percent of heterosexual men with gonorrhea.[68,69,88,102] Most pharyngeal infections are asymptomatic, but gonorrhea sometimes causes overt pharyngitis and cervical lymphadenitis.[69] It often is important to document the presence of pharyngeal infection, because the response to some treatments is poor,[68,69,85] and pharyngeal infection may occasionally be the source of continued transmission[68] or systemic dissemination of *N. gonorrhoeae*.[69]

Other Localized Infections

Ocular infection in adults usually results from autoinoculation of the conjunctiva in a person with genital gonorrhea, usually resulting in severe conjunctivitis (Fig. 11); corneal ulceration can supervene rapidly in the absence of prompt antibiotic therapy. However, mild infections occasionally occur, perhaps related to specific strains of *N. gonorrhoeae*.[103] Primary cutaneous infection with *N. gonorrhoeae* is rare, and most cases result from inoculation of a pre-existing lesion or from cutaneous injury at the time of exposure.[104] The usual manifestation is an ulcerative lesion of the genitals, perineum, or finger.[104] *Neisseria gonorrhoeae* has been isolated in cases of acute gingivitis and otherwise unexplained oral ulcerations.

Pelvic Inflammatory Disease

Ascending genital infection occurs in 10–20 percent of women with gonorrhea,[71,97] and is manifested by various combinations of endometritis, salpingitis, tubo-ovarian abscess, pelvic peritonitis, and other local complications.[71] The frequency and considerable morbidity of the acute complications and the long-term sequelae of acute pelvic inflammatory disease (PID) constitute one of the principal reasons to control sexually transmitted diseases in general and gonorrhea and chlamydial infections in particular.[71,105]

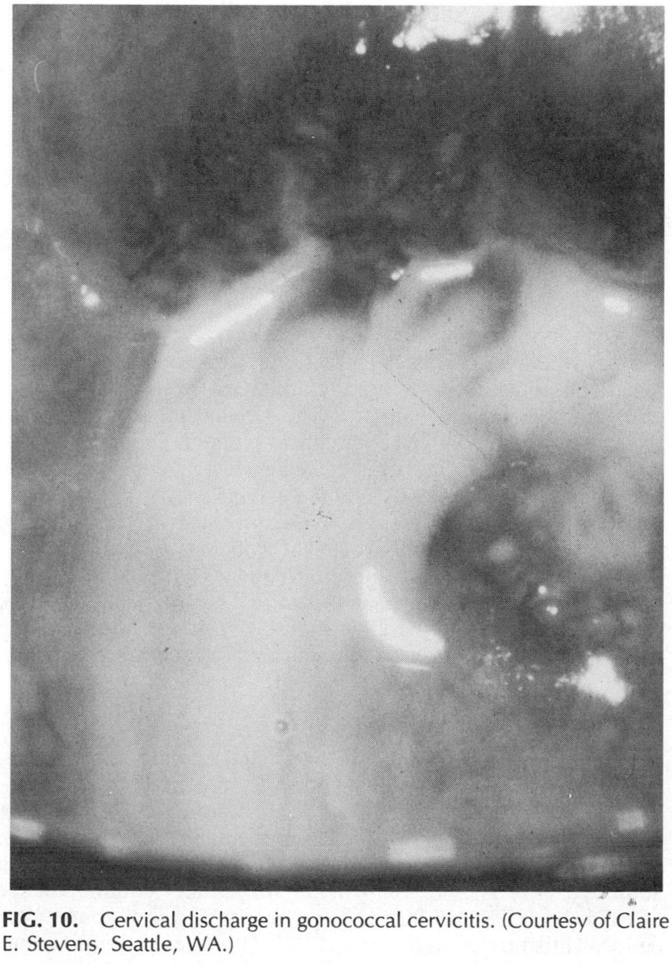

FIG. 10. Cervical discharge in gonococcal cervicitis. (Courtesy of Claire E. Stevens, Seattle, WA.)

The most consistent symptom of PID is low abdominal pain, which is usually but not always bilateral.[73,108] Most women also have symptoms of lower genital tract infection, as described above.[71,106] The onset of gonococcal PID often follows onset of menses by only a few days.[71,96] Some patients have high fever, chills, nausea, and vomiting and appear quite toxic, but all of these features may be absent.[71,96,106] The primary finding on physical examination is pelvic adnexal tenderness, usually but not always bilateral; uterine fundal tenderness, pain elicited on moving the cervix, and one or more tender adnexal masses commonly are present.[71,106] Abdominal examination usually elicits tenderness over the lower quadrants, and signs of peritoneal inflammation are common in severe cases. Findings of mucopurulent cervicitis usually are present, and the majority of women with PID have bacterial vaginosis as well.[106,107] (see Chapters 202 and 95).

Fever, leukocytosis, and an elevated erythrocyte sedimentation rate are common, but all of these are absent in about one-third of laparoscopically documented cases of PID.[71,106] In practice,the clinical diagnosis of PID is imprecise; series using laparoscopy have found that up to one-third of women with clinically diagnosed PID had normal pelvic findings, and several percent of those with other clinical diagnoses in fact had PID.[71,106] In general, gonococcal PID causes more overt clinical inflammatory signs than salpingitis associated only with *C. trachomatis*.[71,106]

In addition to *N. gonorrhoeae*, organisms commonly found in the fallopian tubes or the pelvic peritoneal cavity in PID include *C. trachomatis*, *Mycoplasma hominis*, and various members of the mixed facultative and anaerobic bacterial flora of the vagina[71,106,108] (Fig. 12). The proportion of PID cases associated with gonorrhea has varied from series to series, due to differences in patient selection, improvements in microbiologic diagnosis, and differing background prevalences of gonorrhea, chlamydial infection, and perhaps other predisposing conditions. In the 1980s, roughly 20–40 percent of PID in most urban areas of the United States was associated with gonorrhea,[106] but regional variation is great; in Sweden, where gonorrhea is now uncommon, *N. gonorrhoeae* is a rare cause of PID. The presence of gonococci in the cervix does not prove that the organism is responsible for the salpingitis and does not exclude coinfection with other organisms; moreover, because cervical cultures are relatively insensitive, failure to isolate gonococci or other pathogens does not exclude their contribution to ascending infection.[71,106,108]

Infertility due to fallopian tube obstruction is the most common serious sequela of PID and occurs in 15–20 percent of women following a single episode and 50–80 percent of those with ≥3 episodes of PID.[71,105,106] Infertility may be more common following chlamydial than gonococcal PID, probably because the more acute inflammatory signs associated with gonorrhea bring women to diagnosis and treatment sooner.[105,108] A nationwide epidemic of ectopic pregnancies has followed the epidemic of gonorrhea and chlamydial infections of the 1970s and 1980s, with a lag of several years that corresponds to the difference between the age of maximal risk of sexually transmitted disease and that of desired childbearing.[109] Evidence of prior salpingitis can be found in 50–80 percent of women with ectopic pregnancies.[105] Acute PID predisposes to additional episodes of recurrent PID, particularly with normal vaginal flora, presumably due in part to altered tubal defense mechanisms.[71,106] Use of an intrauterine contraceptive device also pre-

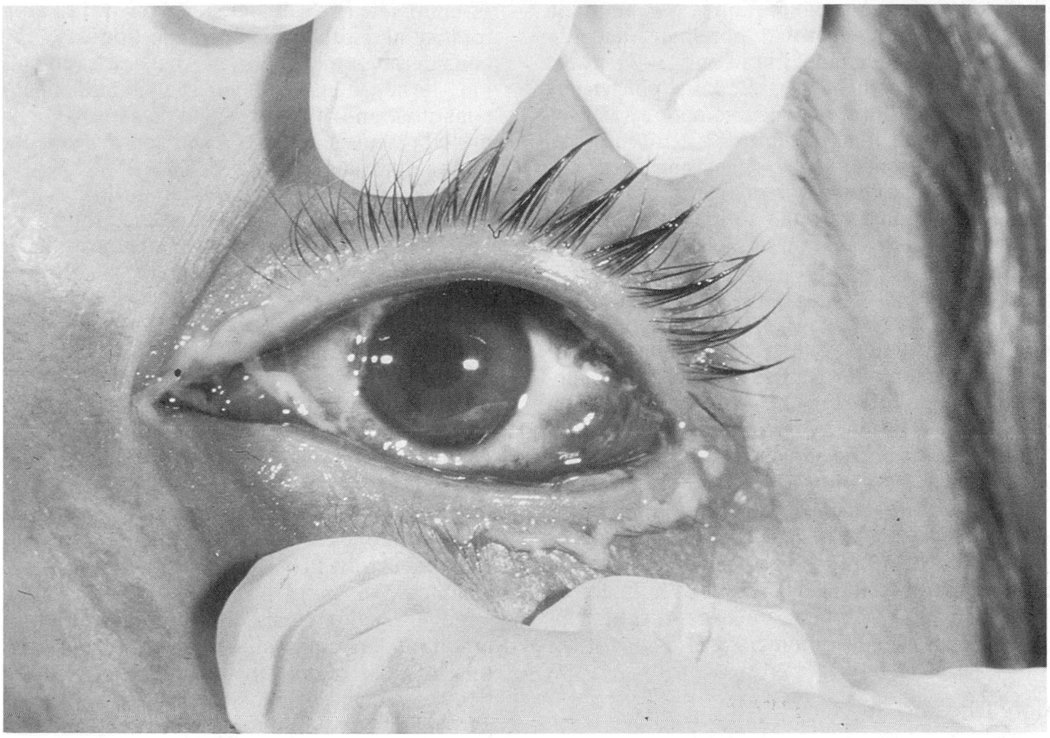

FIG. 11. Acute gonococcal conjunctivitis in an adult. (From Handsfield HH,[170] with permission.)

disposes to recurrent PID.[71,106] Chronic and sometimes disabling pelvic pain is a problem for up to 20 percent of women following PID; it is often difficult to differentiate recurrent PID from chronic pain due to adhesions or other poorly understood mechanisms. True chronic PID is a poorly understood and relatively uncommon condition.

Perihepatitis

Acute perihepatitis (Fitz-Hugh–Curtis syndrome) occurs primarily by spread of *N. gonorrhoeae* or *C. trachomatis* through the peritoneal cavity from the fallopian tube to the liver capsule.[110] However, some cases may result from lymphangitic or bacteremic spread, perhaps explaining rare cases of apparent perihepatitis in men.[110,111] Perihepatitis results in abdominal pain, hepatic tenderness, and right upper quadrant peritoneal inflammatory signs; many cases occur in conjunction with overt PID. Perihepatitis should be considered in the differential diagnosis of right upper quadrant pain in young, sexually active women; it is commonly mistaken for acute cholecystitis or viral hepatitis.[110] If laparoscopy is performed, "violin string" adhesions may be seen between the liver capsule and the parietal peritoneum. The condition responds well to appropriate antimicrobial therapy.

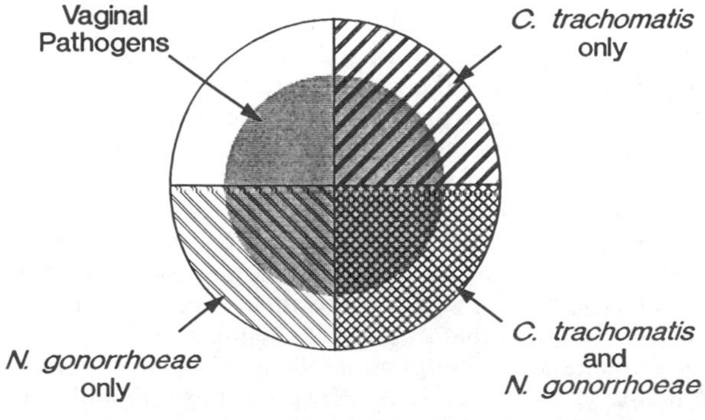

FIG. 12. Schematic representation of the bacteria most commonly involved in the pathogenesis of salpingitis in acute pelvic inflammatory disease. (The overlapping sections are not drawn to proportion.)

Gonorrhea in Pregnancy

Gonorrhea in pregnant women is associated with increased risks of spontaneous abortion, premature labor, early rupture of the fetal membranes, and perinatal infant mortality,[112,113] but it is unclear whether gonococcal infection is directly responsible for these consequences or is merely a marker for high risk due to other pathogenic mechanisms. The clinical manifestations of gonorrhea are unchanged in pregnant women, except that PID is uncommon after the first trimester, when the products of conception completely obstruct the uterine cavity.[112] One study suggests that the prevalence of pharyngeal infection may be higher in pregnant than nonpregnant women with gonorrhea,[114] perhaps due to an increase in the frequency of fellatio as pregnancy progresses. It has been reported that pregnancy is a risk factor for bacteremic dissemination of *N. gonorrhoeae*,[115] but this observation has not been confirmed in recent series.[116,117]

Disseminated Gonococcal Infection

Disseminated gonococcal infection (DGI) results from gonococcal bacteremia and occurs in 0.5–3 percent of infected patients.[115–119] Septic arthritis and a characteristic syndrome of polyarthritis and dermatitis are the predominant manifestations, and DGI is the leading cause of infective arthritis in young adults.[115,116] *Neisseria gonorrhoeae* was a fairly common cause of bacterial endocarditis in the preantibiotic era but gonococcal endocarditis now is uncommon.[115–119] Other rare complications of DGI include meningitis,[120] osteomyelitis,[118] and perhaps pneumonia and the adult respiratory distress syndrome.[121] Overwhelming sepsis accompanied by the Waterhouse-Friderichsen syndrome is said to occur, but no cases have been reported in the past three decades.

Properties of *N. gonorrhoeae* that are associated with dissemination include resistance to the bactericidal action of nonimmune human serum, AHU^- auxotype, specific protein IA serovars, and marked susceptibility to penicillin.[19,122,123] These characteristics also are those associated with asymptomatic gonorrhea in men. Other strains occasionally disseminate, however, and PPNG strains have caused DGI.[124] The best studied host factor that contributes to DGI is homozygous deficiency of complement component C5, C6, C7, or C8, which predisposes to both gonococcal and meningococcal bacteremia.[125] About 5 percent of patients with DGI have such a deficiency, and patients with neisserial bacteremia—especially those with more than one episode—should be screened for these defects using an assay for total hemolytic complement activity. Other host factors that may be associated with an enhanced risk of dissemination include female sex, menstruation, and perhaps pharyngeal gonococcal infection and pregnancy.[69,119]

Women have accounted for up to 80 percent of cases in some series of DGI patients, but this may be due in part to underdiagnosis in men, which in turn is often due to failure to detect asymptomatic urethral infection. In actuality, DGI probably is only modestly more common in women than men.[116,117] In most cases, bacteremia probably begins 7–30 days after infection; in about one-half of affected women, symptoms of DGI begin within 7 days of onset of a menstrual period.[115,116,119] Dissemination may occur from genital, rectal, or pharyngeal infection, and accurate diagnosis requires that all potential sites of primary infection be cultured regardless of the presence or absence of localized symptoms.[115–119]

The most common manifestations of DGI constitute the arthritis–dermatitis syndrome.[119] During the first several days of symptoms, most patients complain of additive and sometimes migratory polyarthralgias that primarily involve the knees, elbows, and more distal joints; axial skeletal involvement is uncommon. Physical examination usually shows objective signs of arthritis or periarticular inflammation (e.g., tenosynovitis) in two or more joints.[115–119] Asymmetrical involvement of only a few joints is an important characteristic that helps to distinguish DGI from polyarthropathy due to most immune complex deposition disorders.[116,119] During this phase, a characteristic dermatitis (Fig. 13) is present in about 75 percent of patients.[115–119] It consists of discrete papules and pustules, often with a hemorrhagic component; other kinds of lesions, such as hemorrhagic bullae and overtly necrotic lesions, occasionally are seen. The lesions usually number 5–40 and occur primarily on the extremities.[115–119] Untreated, the polyarthropathy and dermatitis usually resolve spontaneously, but arthritis often persists and progresses in one or two joints, most commonly the knee, ankle, elbow, or wrist.[115–119] However, any joint, including those of the hands and feet and the sternoclavicular and temporomandibular joints, can be involved. At this stage, the clinical picture is that of septic arthritis. Although this sequence is common, some patients develop septic gonococcal arthritis without prior polyarthritis or dermatitis.[115–119]

The pathogenesis of the clinical manifestation of DGI involves bacteremic inoculation of the skin and the joints or periarticular tissues,[115–119] although immune complexes or other indirect immunologic mechanisms may contribute to some cases.[38,126] Fever and systemic toxicity are common, but usually are mild and often are absent. Polymorphonuclear leukocytosis may or may not be observed. During the polyarthritis–dermatitis stage, gonococci often can be recovered by blood culture, but synovial fluid, if obtained, usually has modest leukocytosis ($<$20,000 leukocytes per mm^3) and is sterile.[115–119] Gonococci often can be seen by immunochemical methods in biopsies of skin lesion, but cultures usually are negative.[127] In the septic joint stage, the synovial fluid is purulent (usually $>$50,000 leukocytes per mm^3), and the culture often is positive, but blood cultures usually are negative.

Overall, only about 50 percent of patients with the arthritis–dermatitis syndrome have positive cultures of the blood or synovial fluid, but *N. gonorrhoeae* can be recovered from a mucosal site in at least 80 percent of patients.[115–119] When DGI is suspected, a minimum of three blood cultures should be obtained; any obtainable synovial fluid should be cultured; all potentially infected mucosal sites (urethra or endocervix, rectum, pharynx) should be cultured, regardless of symptoms or exposure history; and appropriate cultures should be obtained from the sexual partner(s). Although uncommonly positive, gram-stained smears and cultures of pustular skin lesions are simple to perform and should be obtained. The diagnosis of DGI is unequivocal if gonococci are recovered from a systemic site and usually is secure if the organism is isolated from a mucosal site or from the sexual partner of a patient with a typical syndrome that responds to antibiotic therapy.

The differential diagnosis of the gonococcal arthritis–dermatitis syndrome includes meningococcemia,[128] other infective arthritides, and the entire range of inflammatory arthritis. Sexually acquired reactive arthritis (Reiter syndrome and its variants) in particular can be confused with DGI, because these disorders are common in sexually active young adults and are associated with urethritis or cervicitis and with skin lesions that may have a pustular component. Usually, careful clinical and microbiologic assessment readily differentiates these disorders, but a therapeutic antibiotic trial occasionally is required.[116]

Infective endocarditis is an infrequent but serious manifestation of DGI, occurring in an estimated 1–2 percent of patients.[115,116,129] Although usually associated with the arthritis–dermatitis syndrome, gonococcal endocarditis may be the sole manifestation of DGI.[115,129] The aortic valve usually is involved, and the speed of valve destruction and the progression of the clinical course usually are midway between those of "acutte" staphylococcal or pneumococcal endocarditis and "subacute" endocarditis caused by viridans streptococci. Gonococcal meningitis[120] and fulminant septicemia mimicking the Waterhouse–Friedrichsen syndrome are extremely rare manifestations of DGI. One case of adult respiratory distress syndrome and possible pneumonia due to DGI has been reported.[121] Gonococcal osteomyelitis is an uncommon occurrence that usually results from direct extension from untreated septic arthritis.[118]

Neonatal and Pediatric Infections

Infected mothers may transmit *N. gonorrhoeae* to their infants in utero, during delivery, or in the postpartum period.[57] Gonococcal conjunctivitis of the newborn (ophthalmia neonatorum) is the most common clinically recognized manifestation and once was the most common cause of blindness in the United States; it remains a common problem in some developing countries.[130] Prophylaxis by conjunctival instillation of a 1% aqueous solution of silver nitrate is highly effective, although occasional failures occur.[57] Topical application of erythromycin or tetracycline ointment also is effective.[57,131] However, the most important preventive measure is routine screening of pregnant women for gonorrhea and treatment before term. The diagnosis of gonococcal ophthalmia may be suspected clinically when overtly purulent conjunctivitis develops within a week (usually 2–3 days) of delivery, and is confirmed by identification of gonococci in conjunctival secretions by gram-stained smear and culture. Newborns exposed to gonorrhea also can develop septicemia and arthritis,[57,113] but these are uncommon. *Neisseria*

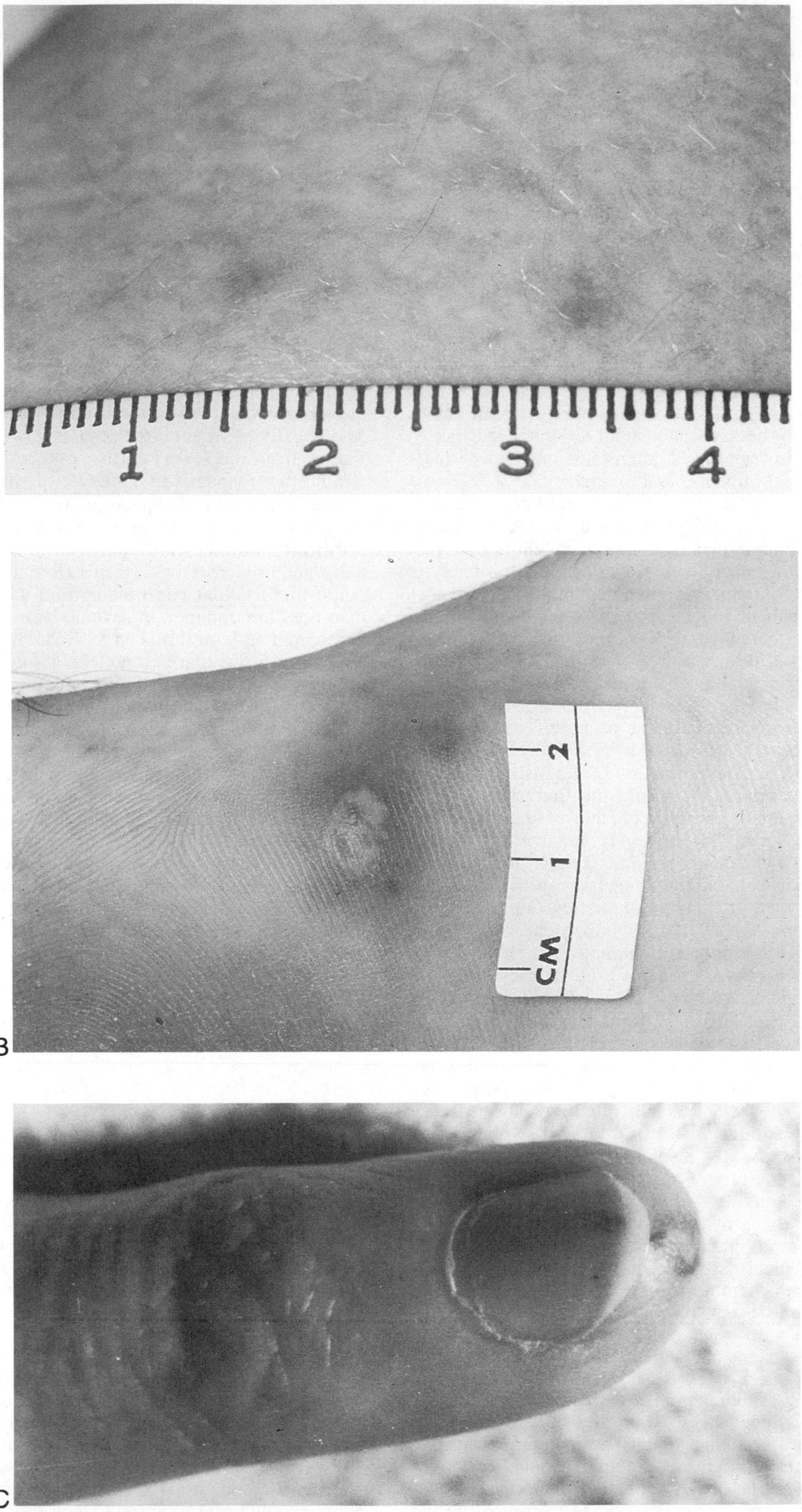

A B C

FIG. 13. Cutaneous lesions in disseminated gonococcal infection. **(A)** Early papular lesions (centimeter rule). **(B)** Hemorrhagic pustular lesion. (From Handsfield HH,[170] with permission.) **(C)** Pustular lesion associated with subungual hemorrhage.

gonorrhoeae often can be recovered from the orogastric aspirates of infants born to infected mothers.[113]

Purulent vaginitis is the primary manifestation of gonorrhea in prepubertal girls[57]; otherwise, beyond the neonatal period the clinical manifestations of gonorrhea in children are not materially different than in adults. After the neonatal period until 1 year of age, most cases in children are said to be acquired nonsexually from an infected parent, usually in a setting of poor hygiene.[57] After 1 year of age, virtually all cases are acquired by sexual abuse, most commonly by an older relative or the mother's nonmarital sexual partner.[132,133]

DIAGNOSIS

The laboratory diagnosis of gonorrhea depends on identification of *N. gonorrhoeae* at an infected site. Isolation by culture is the diagnostic standard and should be used whenever practical, so that the isolate can be screened for antimicrobial resistance.[42,85] In rare instances, however, noncultural diagnostic tests may be useful if isolation is impractical due to lack of access to a laboratory with culture capability or difficulties in transport of specimens. No clinically useful serologic test for gonorrhea has yet been developed.

Culture

A single culture on most selective media has a sensitivity of ≥95 percent for urethral specimens from men with symptomatic urethritis and 80–90 percent for endocervical infection in women, depending on the quality and freshness of the medium and the adequacy of the clinical specimen.[4–7,98,134–136] Dual inoculation of selective and nonselective media may provide the highest yield,[134] but is not logistically practical in many settings. For endocervical culture, inoculation of the selective culture medium with two separate swabs enhances the yield to a degree similar to inoculation of both selective and nonselective media.[134] Although the urethra is commonly infected in women with gonorrhea,[97] culture of urethral specimens does not materially increase the diagnostic yield, except in women who lack cervices due to hysterectomy, and perhaps when purulent exudate is directly expressed from the urethra or Skene's glands. Rectal and pharyngeal specimens should be inoculated onto selective medium only.[134–136] Specimens from other sites (e.g., Bartholin's gland duct) should be collected when indicated by clinical findings. Normally sterile clinical specimens in which competing bacteria are unlikely to be present (e.g., blood, synovial fluid, cerebrospinal fluid) should be inoculated onto nonselective medium, usually enriched chocolate agar, and not selective medium.[116] The yield from synovial fluid is enhanced by inoculating broth medium, as for blood cultures, in addition to agar plates.[116,119]

Male urethral specimens are best obtained by inserting a small swab (e.g., a urethrogenital Calgiswab) 2–3 cm into the urethra,[75] although external discharge is adequate if readily available. When direct collection by swabbing is impractical, the first 10–15 ml of voided urine can be immediately centrifuged and the sediment cultured.[137] Endocervical specimens are collected by first wiping exudate from the exocervix and then placing a swab into the external os and rotating it gently for several seconds, exercising care to avoid contacting the vaginal walls or secretions.[4,5,136] Rectal specimens usually are obtained by passing a swab 2–4 cm into the anal canal, discarding specimens that are heavily contaminated with feces.[100,101] In patients with symptomatic proctitis, the sensitivity of stained smears and perhaps of culture is enhanced by performing anoscopy and collecting purulent secretions or swabbing an area of mucosal inflammation under direct visualization.[101] Pharyngeal specimens are obtained by swabbing the posterior pharynx, including the tonsillar areas and faucial pillars. Whenever practical, swabs should be immediately inoculated onto growth medium at room temperature, which is promptly placed in an enriched CO_2 environment (e.g., a candle extinction jar) and incubated.[4,134,135] However, various non-nutrient transport media (e.g., Amies' modification of Stuart's medium and most commercial transport media) are adequate if the specimen can be transported to the laboratory without refrigeration and inoculated onto growth medium within 6 hours.[135]

The choice of anatomic sites to culture depends on the sites exposed and the clinical syndrome. The urethra usually should be cultured in heterosexual men. Both endocervical and rectal specimens should be collected from women, regardless of whether or not anal intercourse has occurred; most rectal gonococcal infections in women are believed to result from peritoneal contamination with cervicovaginal secretions.[100,138] In most homosexually active men, symptomatic sites plus the rectum should be tested[88,102,136]; the yield from urethral culture in the absence of clinical evidence of urethritis is low in this population,[88] probably because of selection against the antibiotic-sensitive AHU$^-$ gonococci that are most likely to cause asymptomatic urethral infection,[89] as discussed above. Pharyngeal cultures are indicated whenever receptive orogenital exposure has occurred with a potentially infected partner. When examining patients for test of cure after treatment of gonorrhea, all previously infected sites should be cultured. In addition, rectal specimens should be obtained from women, regardless of whether rectal infection was sought or documented before treatment, because up to 70 percent of treatment failures in women are detected only at this site.[139]

Characteristic gonococcal colonies appear on agar medium after 24–48 hours of incubation at 35–37°C.[1–3] Documentation of oxidase-positive gram-negative diplococci confirms a *Neisseria* species, and many laboratories report such isolates from genital sites as presumptive *N. gonorrhoeae*. However, depending on sex and sexual orientation, up to 5 percent of such isolates from the genitals and substantially greater proportions of those from the rectum and pharynx are *N. meningitidis*.[102,140,141] Therefore, sugar utilization reactions or other methods to differentiate these species should be routine for pharyngeal and rectal isolates and are recommended for genital isolates as well.

All gonococcal isolates should be tested for β-lactamase production; the chromogenic cephalosporin, acidometric, iodometric, and paper strip methods all give reliable results in a few minutes.[142] The traditional Kirby–Bauer disc susceptibility test has been difficult to standardize for *N. gonorrhoeae* and is not routinely performed, partly because the organism grows more slowly than most pathogens. In recent years, however, modified disk diffusion assays have been developed to screen gonococci for relative or absolute resistance to tetracycline and penicillin, and the U.S. Public Health Service recommends their routine use for all isolates.[85] Screening for spectinomycin resistance also is indicated in some settings. Determination of the MICs of various antibiotics by the agar dilution method may be indicated for isolates from patients with endocarditis, meningitis, septic arthritis, and other serious complications.

Gram-Stained Smear

Methylene blue and other dyes have been employed to identify gonococci in clinical specimens, but the Gram stain is used almost exclusively in the United States. This test is considered positive when gram-negative diplococci of typical morphology are observed in association with neutrophils (Fig. 4), negative when no such organisms are seen, and equivocal when there are typical morphotypes not associated with neutrophils, or if cell-associated but morphologically atypical organisms are seen. *Neisseria meningitidis* gives identical findings, but nonpathogenic Neisseraceae generally are not associated with neutrophils. Most other apparent gram-negative diplococci actually are bipolar-staining gram-negative rods that are readily differentiated from *Neisseria* species by experienced observers.

Table 1 shows an approximation of the performance of gram-stained smears relative to culture when performed by highly trained personnel. For symptomatic urethritis in men, the performance of the Gram stain is sufficient to make culture confirmation optional,[136,143] except for the desirability of isolating the organism for antimicrobial susceptibility testing. The high specificity of the Gram stain in cervical gonorrhea would theoretically permit reliance on a positive result.[143,144] However, in laboratories that do not test large numbers of women with gonorrhea, the performance of the test often is not as good as shown in Table 1. Nevertheless, the reluctance of many laboratories to perform Gram stains on endocervical specimens is inappropriate; although a negative result means little, a positive smear (Fig. 4) is diagnostically useful. Gram-stained smears should never be used alone for diagnosing infections of the rectum, pharynx, or other sites.

Other Diagnostic Methods

Several tests have been developed in recent years or are under investigation to detect gonococci in infected secretions. These include enzyme immunoassays with polyclonal antigonococcal antibodies[145,146]; fluorescein-conjugated monoclonal antibodies for direct fluorescence microscopy[147]; various genetic probes or DNA–DNA hybridization to detect either plasmid or chromosomal gonococcal DNA[148,149]; and a test based on the observation that amoebocytes from the blood of the horseshoe crab (*Limulus* sp.) form a gel in the presence of endotoxin, including gonococcal lipid A.[150] Potential advantages of these tests over culture include rapid results, utility when specimen transport problems or other issues preclude use of culture, and theoretically improved performance compared with culture, especially in women. However, none of the currently available tests is superior to culture, and most are inferior, especially for endocervical infection; some are no better than the Gram stain. None has yet been adequately studied for rectal and pharyngeal infection. Although genetic or chemical methods to detect PPNG strains are theoretically possible, none is currently available, and no practical methodology currently exists to rapidly identify strains with chromosomally mediated antibiotic resistance.

Tests for complement fixing and anti-pilus antibodies in blood have been developed for investigational use and occasionally have been useful for research, but no serologic test with sufficient sensitivity and specificity for clinical use has yet been developed.[151]

TREATMENT

General Principles

Although the patterns of antimicrobial susceptibility vary from one geographic area or population to another and fluctuate over time, *N. gonorrhoeae* remains susceptible to a wide variety of antibiotics. Failure to cure a case of gonorrhea has public health implications beyond the welfare of the patient, because of the potential for continued transmission and for rapid emergence of antimicrobial resistance. Therefore, whereas 90–95 percent efficacy is considered excellent for many infections, especially in patients who can be closely monitored, acceptable regimens for the treatment of gonorrhea should have efficacies that approach 100 percent, and treatments with efficacies <95 percent should never be used.

A variety of factors in addition to antimicrobial susceptibility influence therapeutic decisions for gonococcal infections, including pharmacokinetic characteristics of the antibiotics, efficacy in complicated vs. uncomplicated infection, differential efficacy at various anatomic sites of infection, toxicity, convenience of administration (for both patient and clinician), and cost. An additional factor, unique to the treatment of gonorrhea and other sexually transmitted infections, is the potential efficacy of treatment for concurrent infections. Historically, this concern focused on syphilis, and this remains an important issue in some countries and for some subpopulations in the industrialized countries (e.g., homosexually active men with multiple partners, inner city drug users). However, by far the most common coexisting infection among heterosexuals with gonorrhea in North America and Europe is genital chlamydial infection. Many studies over two decades have given remarkably consistent results, showing that 15–25 percent of heterosexual men and 35–50 percent of women with gonorrhea also are infected with *C. trachomatis*.[152] These patients are at high risk of postgonococcal urethritis or PID if treatment is not effective for the chlamydial infection.[153] Currently this requires multiple-dose treatment schedules. This fact traditionally has been of great concern, based on the belief that patients with gonorrhea are unreliable and unlikely to adhere to multiple-dose regimens. This concern may be valid for some patients, perhaps especially in less educated populations or those with cultural attitudes affecting compliance, but many persons with gonorrhea probably are no worse than other patients in adherence to multiple-dose regimens of relatively short duration.[154]

Uncomplicated Gonorrhea in Adults

The regimens recommended by the U.S. Public Health Service[85,155] and others[156] in 1987–1988 for treatment of uncomplicated gonorrhea are summarized in Table 2. Ceftriaxone 250 mg intramuscularly (IM) is recommended as initial therapy for all patients in all geographic areas, unless active surveillance of gonococcal antimicrobial susceptibility shows that PPNG strains and those with chromosomally mediated penicillin resistance account for <1 percent and <5 percent, respectively, of *N. gonorrhoeae* isolates in the community.[85] Ceftriaxone has been shown to be effective in single doses of 125 mg IM[86,157,158] and this dose is employed in some sexually transmitted disease clinics.[157] However, 250 mg is the smallest commercially available unit dose and therefore the most convenient in most settings. Ceftriaxone is effective at all potentially infected anatomic sites, including the urethra, cervix, rectum, and pharynx[86,158] and is safe and effective in pregnant women, and preliminary data suggest that it aborts incubating syphilis.[159] The major drawbacks of ceftriaxone therapy are relatively high cost and the necessity for IM rather than oral administration. Although controversy exists concerning the use of cephalosporins in penicillin-allergic patients, cross-reactions appear to be uncommon in persons who receive single doses for gonorrhea.[86]

Spectinomycin 2.0 g IM is highly effective for genital and rectal gonorrhea[85,155] but is ineffective for pharyngeal infection.[157] It is the initial treatment of choice for the rare cases of gonorrhea that persist after ceftriaxone therapy and for patients

TABLE 1. Estimated Performance of Gram Stain Relative to Culture for Detection of Genital and Rectal Gonorrhea

Site	*Percent Sensitivity*	*Percent Specificity*
Male urethra		
Symptomatic	95–100	95–100
Asymptomatic	50–70	95–100
Endocervix	40–60	95–100
Rectum	40–60	90–95[a]

[a] Lower specificity is due to increased prevalence of *N. meningitidis* in the rectum, especially in homosexually active men.[101,141]

TABLE 2. Recommended Treatment of Uncomplicated Gonorrhea in Adults

Initial treatment	
Ceftriaxone 250 mg intramuscularly (IM)[a]	
or	
Spectinomycin 2.0 g IM[b]	
Plus continuing treatment[c] with	
Doxycycline 100 mg orally twice daily for 7 days	
or	
Tetracycline HCl 500 mg orally four times daily for 7 days	
or	
Erythromycin 2.0 g per day orally in divided doses for 7–10 days[d]	

[a] Single doses of 125 mg have proved effective and are used in some clinics, but 250 mg is the smallest commercially available unit dose. Ceftriaxone should be dissolved in 1% lidocaine.
[b] Should be restricted to patients who cannot tolerate ceftriaxone and to those with persistent infection after treatment with ceftriaxone. Not effective for pharyngeal gonococcal infection.
[c] Optional for homosexually active men with gonorrhea; see text.
[d] Should be used only for patients who cannot take doxycycline or tetracycline HCl.
(Modified from Centers for Disease Control.[85,155])

with allergy or intolerance to both the penicillins and cephalosporins. Spectinomycin does not inhibit *Treponema pallidum*, and gonorrhea patients at risk for syphilis who receive this drug should have follow-up serologic tests for syphilis 6–12 weeks later.[85,155]

Amoxicillin 3.0 g orally plus probenecid 1.0 g orally is acceptable as initial treatment for uncomplicated gonorrhea only when active local surveillance shows an absence of resistant gonococci,[85] a situation that is increasingly uncommon.[81] This regimen has reduced efficacy for pharyngeal and perhaps rectal infection, and it should be used only when the physician is convinced the patient will comply with the follow-up doxycycline or tetracycline regimen. Ampicillin 3.5 g may be substituted for amoxicillin, with essentially identical efficacy and tolerance.

Aqueous procaine penicillin G in a dose of 4.8 million units IM, plus probenecid 1.0 g orally, formerly the regimen of choice, is ineffective for infections due to PPNG or strains with high levels of chromosomally mediated penicillin resistance.[87] In addition, procaine penicillin is the least well tolerated and most toxic of the recently recommended regimens, with the potential for acute psychotic reactions due to elevated plasma levels of procaine[160] and for anaphylaxis and other serious allergic reactions.[161] There are few if any legitimate reasons for using procaine penicillin to treat any patient with gonorrhea.

Regardless of the single-dose regimen chosen, heterosexual men and women with gonorrhea should also be treated with doxycycline, 100 mg twice daily, or tetracycline, 500 mg four times daily for 7 days, to eradicate coexisting *C. trachomatis* infection.[85,152,154] Doxycycline is better tolerated than tetracycline, and the twice daily regimen probably enhances compliance.[154] Other tetracycline congeners in equivalent doses also are effective. The tetracyclines should never be used alone for gonorrhea, because problems with compliance, achievable blood levels, and the susceptibility of gonococci in most communities make their use especially conducive to the selection of increasingly resistant strains. Erythromycin, in a divided dose regimen totalling 2.0 g per day, is acceptable in lieu of a tetracycline if the latter is contraindicated or not tolerated.[155] The sulfonamides also should be effective for coexisting chlamydial infection, but they have not been well studied in this setting. Neither erythromycin nor the sulfonamides are effective for gonorrhea when used alone.

Pregnant women with gonorrhea should be treated with ceftriaxone in a single dose of 250 mg; the 125 mg regimen has not been studied. Spectinomycin is effective and probably is safe, but is less acceptable because of the increased likelihood of pharyngeal gonorrhea during pregnancy.[114] The tetracyclines are contraindicated during pregnancy, and most authorities recommend following ceftriaxone with a 7–10 day course of erythromycin.[155]

Because strains of *N. gonorrhoeae* with chromosomally mediated antibiotic resistance are especially common in homosexually active men, ceftriaxone is the sole recommended treatment for uncomplicated gonorrhea in this group,[86,158] regardless of the antimicrobial susceptibility of gonococci in the general population. Follow-up of initial treatment with a tetracycline is optional in this population, because the prevalence of simultaneous chlamydial infection is <10 percent,[152] and serious complications due to *C. trachomatis* are relatively uncommon.

Several other antimicrobial agents have been used effectively or are under investigation for treatment of uncomplicated gonorrhea. Perhaps the most promising regimens employ single doses of the newer quinolone antibiotics, such as ciprofloxacin (500 mg orally), norfloxacin (800 mg orally), and other compounds in various stages of development (e.g., ofloxacin, enoxacin, fleroxacin, and others). These agents are highly active in vitro against *N. gonorrhoeae*, including strains with plasmid-mediated or chromosomally-mediated penicillin or tetracycline resistance, and clinical studies have given promising results.[162,163] Although some quinolones have in vitro activity against *C. trachomatis*, single-dose regimens have not eradicated coexisting chlamydial infections in patients with gonorrhea.[163] These agents are contraindicated in persons <18 years old, pregnant women, and perhaps women not using reliable contraception, groups that collectively comprise up to one-half of all patients with gonorrhea. In addition, some data suggest that widespread use of these drugs may induce clinically significant resistance in *N. gonorrhoeae*.[164]

Regimens employing various cephalosporins, imipenem, aztreonam, combinations of penicillins with the β-lactamase inhibitors sulbactam or clavulanic acid, sulfamethoxazole with trimethoprim, various aminoglycosides, thiamphenicol, and other antibiotics all have been effective in treating uncomplicated gonorrhea, but most of these have no advantages over the recommended regimens. However, single doses of cefuroxime axetil (1.0 g orally) with probenecid (1.0 g orally) have been effective in limited studies[165] and offer an oral β-lactam alternative that is active against antibiotic-resistant gonococci. Single-dose regimens employing new, orally absorbed third-generation cephalosporins (e.g., cefixime, cefpodoxime) may prove useful as well.

Reexamination and repeat cultures for *N. gonorrhoeae* are recommended as a test of cure 4–7 days after completion of treatment, regardless of symptomatic resolution. All initially infected sites, plus the rectal canal in women,[139] should be tested. Most patients with apparently persistent gonorrhea in fact have been reinfected.

Pelvic Inflammatory Disease

Because the specific pathogens responsible for ascending genital infection usually are not known, the recommendations for initial treatment of acute PID are similar regardless of whether the initial lower genital infection is due to *N. gonorrhoeae, C. trachomatis*, or other pathogens.[106,155] Ideally, all women with PID probably should be hospitalized to initiate antibiotic therapy intravenously (IV), as for almost all other intraperitoneal infections, but practical considerations often preclude this option. Definite indications for hospitalization are inability to exclude an acute intra-abdominal emergency such as ectopic pregnancy or appendicitis; certain other diagnostic uncertainties; suspicion of pelvic abscess; marked systemic toxicity; intractable nausea and vomiting; unwillingness or inability of the patient to follow an outpatient regimen or to return for follow-up; and inadequate response to initial outpatient therapy. Pregnant women and prepubertal girls with PID also should be hospitalized.[85,106,155]

The treatment guidelines of the U.S. Public Health Service[85,155] are summarized in Table 3. Few data are available on their relative efficacies. The IV cefoxitin/doxycycline regimen provides excellent coverage for *C. trachomatis, N. gonorrhoeae* (except perhaps for uncommon strains with relatively high levels of chromosomally mediated resistance to cefoxitin),[13] and most but not all of the usual components of the mixed facultative and anaerobic flora that may contribute to PID. This regimen is preferred when gonorrhea or chlamydial infection is suspected. Cefotetan appears to be equivalent to cefoxitin in this setting.[166] The clindamycin/gentamicin regimen has suboptimal activity against *C. trachomatis*, but is active against most strains of *N. gonorrhoeae* and a wide spectrum of vaginal bacteria. This is the preferred regimen when chlamydial and gonococcal infection are unlikely or when a mixed facultative and anaerobic flora are probable, as in recurrent PID and when a pelvic abscess is suspected.[71,106] For both regimens, IV therapy is continued for ≥4 days and for at least 48 hours after definite clinical improvement begins; oral therapy alone (doxycycline or clindamycin) is then continued to complete 10–14 days total treatment.

The treatment of outpatients with PID is the same as for uncomplicated gonorrhea, except that doxycycline is clearly preferable to tetracycline, because of improved compliance and enhanced activity against some anaerobic bacteria. In addition, the treatment period is extended to 10–14 days. For outpatients with severe PID—for example, when hospitalization is indicated but patient refusal or other factors prevent it—some authorities add metronidazole in a dose of 1.0–2.0 g daily in divided doses.[106]

Regardless of the initial treatment, close follow-up is indicated. Clinical progression or failure to improve within 3 days is an indication to reassess the diagnosis, and laparoscopy may be indicated both to confirm the diagnosis of PID and to obtain intra-abdominal culture specimens that may facilitate selection of improved antimicrobial therapy. If an IUD is present, it should be promptly removed; there are no data to suggest that removal need be delayed until antibiotic theray has been initiated. Other adjunctive treatment for PID includes bed rest, analgesia as needed, and sexual abstention for 2–3 weeks, both for comfort and to prevent reinfection.[106]

TABLE 3. Recommended Treatments for Acute Pelvic Inflammatory Disease

Hospitalized patients
Regimen A
Doxycycline 100 mg intravenously (IV) every 12 hours
plus
Cefoxitin 2.0 g IV every 6 hours
Continue both drugs IV for ≥4 days and ≥48 hours after patient improves; then continue doxycycline 100 mg orally twice daily to complete 10–14 days total therapy
OR
Regimen B
Clindamycin 900 mg IV every 8 hours
plus
Gentamicin 2.0 mg/kg IV once, following by 1.5 mg/kg every 8 hours[a]
Continue both drugs IV for ≥4 days and ≥48 hours after patient improves; then continue clindamycin 450 mg orally four times daily to complete 10–14 days total therapy
Outpatients
Ceftriaxone 250 mg intramuscularly (IM)[b]
plus
Doxycycline 100 mg orally twice daily for 10–14 days

[a] Adjust dose if renal function is abnormal or if indicated by serum gentamicin levels.
[b] Cefoxitin 2.0 g IM may be substituted for ceftriaxone in locales where antibiotic-resistant strains of *N. gonorrhoeae* are known to be uncommon.
(Modified from Centers for Disease Control.[85,155])

Acute Epididymitis

Most acute epididymitis in young adults is due to *C. trachomatis*, but *N. gonorrhoeae* accounts for about 10 percent of cases.[94] The majority of cases of gonococcal epididymitis can be managed on an outpatient basis, using the regimen recommended for uncomplicated gonorrhea, but extending doxycycline or tetracycline therapy to 10–14 days.[155] Severe cases should be hospitalized and managed with IM or IV ceftriaxone or an equivalent antibiotic, plus a tetracycline if chlamydial infection cannot be excluded.[94]

Disseminated Gonococcal Infection

Adults with the gonococcal arthritis–dermatitis syndrome should be treated with a 7–10 day course of ceftriaxone, 1.0 g once daily, either IM or IV[85,155]; in some settings, reliable patients without complications may receive this regimen without hospitalization. Therapeutically equivalent doses of other newer third-generation cephalosporins also would be effective. If the infecting organism is documented to be fully susceptible to the penicillins or tetracyclines, many patients who are improving after 3 days can be switched to oral amoxicillin (500 mg 3 times daily), doxycycline, or tetracycline to complete 7–10 days total therapy.[167] Patients with gonococcal endocarditis initially should receive four weeks of parenteral therapy with ceftriaxone or an equivalent third generation cephalosporin.[155] If desired, penicillin could be substituted, depending on the results of antimicrobial susceptibility testing. Meningitis probably should be treated with a 10-day course of ceftriaxone or an equivalent antibiotic.

Gonorrhea in Children

Because there are relatively few cases of gonorrhea in children, treatment has not been as well studied as in adults. Uncomplicated infections normally should be treated with ceftriaxone in a single dose of 125 mg IM; this may be increased to 250 mg in children weighing ≥100 lb (45 kg).[85,155] There are few data on the prevalence of chlamydial infection in pediatric patients with gonorrhea, either perinatally or sexually acquired.[55] The tetracyclines are contraindicated in young children, and erythromycin has not been well studied in this setting; therefore, the usual practice is to obtain microbiologic tests for chlamydial infection and withhold specific treatment unless these are positive. DGI and gonococcal conjunctivitis in children are treated with 7–10 days of ceftriaxone, 25–50 mg/kg body weight per day IM or IV, or with an equivalent regimen of another third-generation cephalosporin. Continuous irrigation of the conjunctivae with physiologic saline solution is often employed in conjunctivitis, but topical antibiotics offer no additional benefit.[85]

Management of Sexual Partners

Management of the sexual partners is an integral part of treating patients with gonorrhea and other sexually transmitted diseases. Failure to ensure that the partner is examined and treated risks reinfection of the patient and continued spread of the infection to others. Depending on local resources and logistic issues, in many industrialized countries health authorities often will assist in the location and notification of the partners of gonorrhea patients; otherwise, the physician and patient should work together to this end. The partners should be examined and treated with one of the recommended antibiotic regimens, regardless of whether or not clinical evidence of gonorrhea is found ("epidemiologic" treatment). Even when presumptive treatment is given, diagnostic tests for *N. gonorrhoeae* should be obtained; failure to document infection, if present, usually precludes active case finding in other sexual partners and distorts statistics on the occurrence of gonorrhea. It is almost never appropriate to treat the sexual partners of patients with gonorrhea or other sexually transmitted diseases without examining them.

PREVENTION AND CONTROL

Condoms, if properly used, provide a high degree of protection from transmission or acquisition of gonorrhea.[168] Other barrier contraceptive methods (diaphragm, cervical cap) and topical spermicides that contain nonoxynol-9 probably are protective, albeit less so than condoms.[168] There is no evidence that such time-honored measures as washing, urinating, or douching after exposure materially reduce the risk of infection.[168] Prophylactic administration of antibiotics immediately before or soon after sexual exposure can reduce the risk of infection, but carries a risk of fostering the spread of resistant gonococci and is not recommended for routine use.[90] Development of a vaccine to prevent gonorrhea is a high research priority,[1–3,61] but to date experimental vaccines containing purified gonococcal pili or recombinant protein I have conferred only partial protection against experimental infection with the homologous strain of *N. gonorrhoeae* and no protection from heterologous challenge.[1,169]

Screening of sexually active persons, especially women, is a mainstay of gonorrhea control and also has the potential to contribute to control of chlamydial infection and other sexually transmitted diseases.[61] Women at risk who are undergoing routine pelvic examination should have specimens collected for culture for *N. gonorrhoeae* and culture or an antigen detection test for *C. trachomatis*. Other key elements in gonorrhea control include conducting appropriate diagnostic testing in persons with compatible clinical syndromes; contact tracing; diagnosis and treatment of the sexual partners of infected persons; use of recommended treatment regimens; and laboratory screening of isolates for antimicrobial resistance.[61] Reporting of cases is important to monitor the gonorrhea epidemic and to facilitate the targeting of control efforts. Finally, public education and personal counseling, in an effort to induce conservative sexual behavior and the use of barrier contraceptives, is central to the control of gonorrhea and all sexually transmitted diseases.[61]

REFERENCES

1. Dallabetta G, Hook EW III. Gonococcal infections. Infect Dis Clin North Am. 1987;1:25–54.
2. Hook EW III, Holmes KK. Gonococcal infections. Ann Intern Med. 1985;102:229–43.
3. Britigan BE, Cohen MS, Sparling PF. Gonococcal infections: a model of molecular pathogenesis. N Engl J Med. 1985;312:1683–94.
4. Pedersen AHB, Bonin P. Screening females for asymptomatic gonorrhea infection. Northwest Med. 1971;70:255–61.
5. Kellogg DS Jr, Holmes KK, Hill GA. Laboratory diagnosis of gonorrhea. *Cumitech 4*. Washington DC: American Society for Microbiology; 1976.
6. Thayer JD, Martin JE Jr. Improved medium selective for the cultivation of *N. gonorrhoeae* and *N. meningititdis*. Public Health Rep. 1966;81:559–62.
7. Faur YC, Weisburd MH, Wilson ME. A new medium for the isolation of pathogenic *Neiseria* (NYC medium): I. Formulations and comparisons with standard media. Health Lab Sci. 1973;10:44–54.
8. Minnett S, Reller LB, Knapp JS. *Neisseria gonorrhoeae* strains inhibited by vancomycin in selective media and correlation with auxotype. J Clin Microbiol. 1981;14:94–9.
9. Windall JJ, Hall MM, Washington JA, et al. Inhibitory effects of vancomycin on *Neisseria gonorrhoeae* in Thayer Martin medium. J Infect Dis. 1980;142:775.
10. Kellogg DS Jr, Peacock WL Sr, Deacon WE, et al. *Neisseria gonorrhoeae*: I. Virulence genetically linked to clonal variation. J Bacteriol. 1963;85:1274–9.
11. Buchanan TM, Chen KCS, Jones RB, et al. Pili and principal outer membrane protein of *Neisseria gonorrhoeae*: immunochemical, structural, and pathogenic aspects. In Brooks GF, et al (eds): Immunobiology of *Neisseria gonorrhoeae*. Washington DC: American Society for Microbiology; 1978:145–54.
12. Segal E, Billyard E, So M, et al. Role of chromosomal rearrangement in *N. gonorrhoeae* pilus phase variation. Cell. 1985;40:293–300.
13. Schoolnik GK, Fernandez R, Tai J-Y, et al. Gonococcal pili: primary structure and receptor binding domain. J Exp Med. 1984;159:1351–70.
14. Heckels JE. Molecular studies on the pathogenesis of gonorrhea. J Med Microbiol. 1984;18:293–307.
15. McGee ZA, Johnson AP, Taylor-Robinson D. Pathogenic mechanisms of *Neisseria gonorrhoeae*: observations on damage to human fallopian tubes in organ culture by gonococci of colony type 1 or type 4. J Infect Dis. 1981;143:413–22.
16. Ofek I, Beachy EH, Bisno AL. Resistance of *Neisseria gonorrhoeae* to phagocytosis: relationship to colonial morphology and surface pili. J Infect Dis. 1974;129:310–6.
17. Dilworth JA, Hendley JO, Mandell GL. Attachment and ingestion of gonococci by neutrophils. Infect Immun. 1975;11:512–6.
18. Blake MS, Gotschlich EC. Gonococcal membrane proteins: speculation on their role in pathogenesis. Prog Allergy. 1983;33:298–313.
19. Knapp JS, Tam MR, Nowinski RC, et al. Serological classification of *Neisseria gonorrhoeae* with use of monoclonal antibodies to gonococcal outer membrane protein I. J Infect Dis. 1984;150:44–8.
20. Swanson J. Colony opacity and protein II compositions of gonococci. Infect Immun. 1982;37:359–68.
21. Black WJ, Schwalbe RS, Nachamkin I, et al. Characterization of *Neisseria gonorrhoeae* protein II phase variation by use of monoclonal antibodies. Infect Immun. 1984;45:453–7.
22. Zak K, Diaz J-L, Jackson D, et al. Antigenic variation during infection with *Neisseria gonorrhoeae*: detection of antibodies to surface proteins in sera of patients with gonorrhea. J Infect Dis. 1984;149:166–74.
23. Draper DL, James JF, Brooks GF, et al. Comparison of virulence markers of peritoneal and fallopian tube isolates with endocervical *Neisseria gon orrhoeae* isolates from women with acute salpingitis. Infect Immun. 1980;27:882–8.
24. Salit IE, Gotschlich EC. Gonococcal color and opacity variants: virulence for chicken embryos. Infect Immun. 1978;22:359–64.
25. Fischer SH, Rest RF. Gonococci possessing only certain P.II outer membrane proteins interact with human neutrophils. Infect Immun. 1988;56:1574–9.
26. Virji M, Heckels JE. The effect of protein II and pili on the interaction of *Neisseria gonorrhoeae* with human polymorphonuclear leucocytes. J Gen Microbiol. 1986;132:503–12.
27. Rice PA, Vayo HE, Tam MR, et al. Immunoglobulin G antibodies directed against protein III block killing of serum-resistant *Neisseria gonorrhoeae* by immune serum. J Exp Med. 1986;164:1735–48.
28. West SE, Sparling PF. Response of *Neisseria gonorrhoeae* to iron limitation: alterations in expression of membrane proteins without apparent siderophore production. Infect Immun. 1985;14:388–94.
29. Morse SA, Mietzner TA, Bolen G, et al. Characterization of the major iron-regulated protein of *Neisseria gonorrhoeae* and *Neisseria meningitidis*. Antonie van Leeuwenhoek. 1987;53:465–9.
30. Cannon JG, Black WJ, Nachamkin I. Monoclonal antibody that recognizes an outer membrane antigen common to the pathogenic *Neisseria* species but not to most nonpathogenic *Neisseria* species. Infect Immun. 1984;43:994–9.
31. Mulks MH, Knapp JS. Immunoglobulin A1 protease types of *Neisseria gonorrhoeae* and their relationship to auxotype and servovar. Infect Immun. 1987;55:931–6.
32. Griffiss JM, Schneider H, Mandrell RE, et al. Lipooligosaccharides: the principal glycolipids of the neisserial outer membrane. Rev Infect Dis. 1988;10:S287–95.
33. Gregg CR, Melly MA, Hellerqvist CG, et al. Toxic activity of purified lipopolysaccharide of *Neisseria gonorrhoeae* for human fallopian tube mucosa. J Infect Dis. 1981;143:432–9.
34. Rice PA, Kasper DL. Characterization of serum resistance of *Neisseria gonorrhoeae* that disseminate: roles of blocking antibody and gonococcal outer membrane proteins. J Clin Invest. 1982;70:157–67.
35. Apicella MA, Westerlink MA, Morse SA, et al. Bactericidal antibody response of normal human serum to the lipooligosaccharide of *Neisseria gonorrhoeae*. J Infect Dis. 1986;153:520–6.
36. Apicella MA, Gagliardi NC. Antigenic heterogeneity of the nonserogroup antigen structure of *Neisseria gonorrhoeae* lipopolysaccharides. Infect Immun. 1979;26:870–4.
37. Rosenthal RS, Folkening WT, Miller DR, et al. Resistance of O-acetylated gonococcal peptidoglycan to human peptidoglycan-degrading enzymes. Infect Immun. 1983;40:903–11.
38. Fleming TJ, Wallsmith DE, Rosenthal RS. Arthropathic properties of gonococcal peptidoglycan fragments: implications for the pathogenesis of disseminated gonococcal disease. Infect Immun. 1986;52:600–8.
39. Noegel A, Gotschlich EC. Isolation of a high molecular weight polyphosphate from *Neisseria gonorrhoeae*. J Exp Med. 1983;157:2049–60.
40. Catlin BW. Nutritional profiles of *Neisseria gonorrhoeae, Neisseria meningitidis*, and *Neisseria lactamica* in chemically defined media and the use

of growth requirements for gonococcal typing. J Infect Dis. 1973;128:178–94.

41. Hook EW III, Judson FN, Handsfield HH. Auxotype/serovar diversity and antimicrobial resistance of *Neisseria gonorrhoeae* in two mid-sized American cities. Sex Transm Dis. 1987;14:141–6.
42. Handsfield HH, Rice RJ, Roberts MC, et al. Localized outbreak of penicillinase-producing *Neisseria gonorrhoeae*: Paradigm for introduction and spread of gonorrhea in a community. JAMA. 1989;261.
43. Demarco de Hormaeche R, Jessop H, Senior K. Gonococcal variants selected by growth *in vivo* or *in vitro* have antigenically different LPS. Microbial Pathogen. 1988;4:289–97.
44. Dillon JR, Bygdeman SM, Sandström EG. Serological ecology of *Neisseria gonorrhoeae* (PPNG and non-PPNG) strains: Canadian perspective. Genitourin Med. 1987;63:160–8.
45. Biswas GD, Blackman EY, Sparling PF. High-frequency conjugal transfer of a gonococcal penicillinase plasmid. J Bacteriol. 1980;143:1318–24.
46. Elwell LP, Roberts M, Mayer LW, et al. Plasmid-mediated beta-lactamase production in *Neisseria gonorrhoeae*. Antimicrob Agents Chemother. 1977;11:528–33.
47. Anderson B, Albritton WL, Biddle J, et al. Common β-lactamase-specifying plasmid in *Haemophilus ducreyi* and *Neisseria gonorrhoeae*. Antimicrob Agents Chemother. 1984;25:296–7.
48. Morse SA, Johnson SR, Biddle JW, et al. High-level tetracycline resistance in *Neisseria gonorrhoeae* is result of acquisition of streptococcal *tetM* determinant. Antimicrob Agents Chemother. 1986;30:664–70.
49. Roberts M, Piot P, Falkow S. The ecology of gonococcal plasmids. J Gen Microbiol. 1979;114:491–4.
50. Cannon JG, Sparling PF. The genetics of the gonococcus. Annu Rev Microbiol. 1984;38:111–33.
51. Spratt BG. Hybrid penicillin-binding proteins in penicillin-resistant strains of *Neisseria gonorrhoeae*. Nature. 1988;332:173–6.
52. Rice RJ, Biddle JW, Jean Louis YA, et al. Chromosomally mediated resistance in *Neisseria gonorrhoeae* in the United States: results of surveillance and reporting, 1983–1984. J Infect Dis. 1986;153:340–5.
53. Shinners EN, Catlin BW. Arginine and pyrimidine biosynthetic defects in *Neisseria gonorrhoeae* strains isolated from patients. J Bacteriol. 1982;151:295–302.
54. Campbell LA, Yasbin RE. Mutagenesis of *Neisseria gonorrhoeae*: absence of error-prone repair. J Bacteriol. 1984;160:288–93.
55. Biswas GD, Sox T, Blackman T, et al. Factors affecting genetic transformation of *Neisseria gonorrhoeae*. J Bacteriol. 1977;129:983–92.
56. Graves JF, Biswas GD, Sparling PF. Sequence-specific DNA uptake in transformation of *Neisseria gonorrhoeae*. J Bacteriol. 1982;152:1071–7.
57. Gutman LT, Wilfert KM. Gonococcal disease in infants and children. In: Holmes KK, et al. Sexually Transmitted Diseases. New York: McGraw-Hill; 1984:238–43.
58. Casey SG, Shafer MW, Spitznagel JK. *Neisseria gonorrhoeae* survive intraleukocytic oxygen-independent antimicrobial capacities of anaerobic and aerobic granulocytes in the presence of pyocin lethal for extracellular gonococci. Infect Immun. 1986;52:384–9.
59. Centers for Disease Control. Summary of notifiable diseases, United States, 1987. MMWR 1987;36:1–59.
60. Centers for Disease Control. Sexually Transmitted Diseases (STD) Statistics, Calendar Year 1987 (No. 136). Atlanta: U.S. Public Health Service; 1988:1–58.
61. Cates W Jr. Epidemiology and control of sexually transmitted diseases: strategic evolution. Infect Dis Clin North Am. 1987;1:1–23.
62. Rice RJ, Aral SO, Blount JH, et al. Gonorrhea in the United States 1975–1984: is the giant only sleeping? Sex Transm Dis. 1987;14:83–7.
63. Handsfield HH. Decreasing incidence of gonorrhea in homosexually active men. West J Med. 1985;143:469–70.
64. Zaidi AA, Aral SO, Reynolds GH, et al. Gonorrhea in the United States, 1967–1979. Sex Transm Dis. 1983;10:72–6.
65. Hooper RR, Reynolds GH, Jones OG, et al. Cohort study of venereal disease: I. The risk of gonorrhea transmission from infected women to men. Am J Epidemiol. 1978;108:136–44.
66. Holmes KK, Johnson DW, Trostle JH. An estimate of the risk of men acquiring gonorrhea by sexual contact with infected females. Am J Epidemiol. 1970;91:170–4.
67. Thin RNT, Williams IA, Nicol CS. Direct and delayed methods of immunofluorescent diagnosis of gonorrhea in women. Br J Vener Dis. 1971;47:27–30.
68. Tice RW, Rodriguez VL. Pharyngeal gonorrhea. JAMA. 1981;246:2717–9.
69. Wiesner PJ, Tronca E, Bonin P, et al. Clinical spectrum of pharyngeal gonococcal infection. N Engl J Med. 1973;288:181–5.
70. McCormack WM, Reynolds GH, Cooperative Study Group. Effect of menstrual cycle and method of contraception on recovery of *Neisseria gonorrhoeae*. JAMA. 1982;247:1292–4.
71. Holmes KK, Eschenbach DA, Knapp JS. Salpingitis: overview of etiology and epidemiology. Am J Obstet Gynecol. 1980;138:893–900.
72. Yorke JA, Hethcote HW, Nold A. Dynamics and control of the transmission of gonorrhea. Sex Transm Dis. 1978;5:51–6.
73. May RM. The transmission and control of gonorrhea. Nature. 1981;291:376.
74. Rothenberg RB. The geography of gonorrhea: empirical demonstration of core group transmission. Am J Epidemiol. 1983;117:688–94.
75. Handsfield HH, Lipman TO, Harnisch JP, et al. Asymptomatic gonorrhea in men: diagnosis, natural course, prevalence and significance. N Engl J Med. 1973;290:117–23.
76. Perine PL, Morton RS, Piot P, et al. Epidemiology and treatment of penicillinase-producing *Neisseria gonorrhoeae*. Sex Transm Dis. 1979;6(Suppl):152–8.
77. Handsfield HH, Sandström EG, Knapp JS, et al. Epidemiology of penicillinase-producing *Neisseria gonorrhoeae* infections: analysis by auxotyping and serogrouping. N Engl J Med. 1982;306:950–4.
78. Centers for Disease Control. Penicillinase-producing *Neisseria gonorrhoeae*—United States, Florida, MMWR. 1986;35:12–4.
79. Centers for Disease Control. Penicillinase-producing *Neisseria gonorrhoeae*—United States, 1986. MMWR. 1987;36:107–8.
80. Dillon JR, Yeung K-H. β-Lactamase plasmids and chromosomally mediated antibiotic resistance in pathogenic *Neisseria* species (Supplement). Clin Microbiol Rev. 1989;2:125–33.
81. Zenilman JM, Schwarcz SK, Knapp JS, et al. National surveillance of antimicrobial resistance in *Neisseria gonorrhoeae* (Abstract 1155). Interscience Conference on Antimicrobial Agents and Chemotherapy, American Society for Microbiology, Los Angeles, October 23–26, 1988.
82. Centers for Disease Control. Multiple strain outbreak of penicillinase-producing *Neisseria gonorrhoeae*—Denver, Colorado, 1986. MMWR. 1987;36:534–43.
83. Centers for Disease Control. Tetracycline-resistant *Neisseria gonorrhoeae*—Georgia, Pennsylvania, New Hampshire, MMWR. 1985;34:563–70.
84. Knapp JS, Zenilman JM, Biddle JW, et al. Frequency and distribution in the United States of strains of *Neisseria gonorrhoeae* with plasmid-mediated, high-level resistance to tetracycline. J Infect Dis. 1987;155:819–22.
85. Centers for Disease Control. Antibiotic-resistant strains of *Neisseria gonorrhoeae*: policy guidelines for detection, management, and control. MMWR. 1987;36(Suppl):1S–18S.
86. Handsfield HH, Hook EW III. Ceftriaxone for treatment of uncomplicated gonorrhea: routine use of a single 125-mg dose in a sexually transmitted disease clinic. Sex Transm Dis. 1987;14:227–30.
87. Faruki H, Kohmescher RN, McKinney WP, et al. A community-based outbreak of infection with penicillin-resistant *Neisseria gonorrhoeae* not producing penicillinase (chromosomally mediated resistance). N Engl J Med. 1985;313:607–11.
88. Handsfield HH, Knapp JS, Diehr PK, et al. Correlation of auxotype and penicillin susceptibility of *Neisseria gonorrhoeae* with sexual preference and clinical manifestations of gonorrhea. Sex Transm Dis. 1980;7:1–5.
89. Morse SA, Lysko OG, McFarland L, et al. Gonococcal strains from homosexual men have outer membranes with reduced permeability to hydrophobic molecules. Infect Immun. 1982;37:432–8.
90. Harrison WO, Hooper RR, Wiesner PJ, et al. A trial of minocycline given after exposure to prevent gonorrhea. N Engl J Med. 1979;300:1074–8.
91. Jacobs NF, Kraus SJ. Gonococcal and nongonococcal urethritis in men: clinical and laboratory differentiation. Ann Intern Med. 1975;82:7–12.
92. Crawford G, Knapp JS, Hale J, et al. Asymptomatic gonorrhea in men: caused by gonococci with unique nutritional requirements. Science. 1977;196:1352–3.
93. Brunham RC, Plummer F, Slaney L, et al. Correlation of auxotype and protein I type with expression of disease due to *Neisseria gonorrhoeae*. J Infect Dis. 1985;152:339–43.
94. Berger RE, Alexander ER, Harnisch JP, et al. Etiology, manifestations and therapy of acute epididymitis: prospective study of 50 cases. J Urol. 1979;121:750–4.
95. Wright RA, Judson FN. Penile venereal edema. JAMA. 1979;241:157–8.
96. Platt R, Rice PA, McCormack WM. Risk of acquiring gonorrhea and prevalence of abnormal adnexal findings among women recently exposed to gonorrhea. JAMA. 1983;250:3205–9.
97. McCormack WM, Stumacher RJ, Johnson K, et al. Clinical spectrum of gonococcal infections in women. Lancet. 1977;1:1182–5.
98. Barlow D, Phillips I. Gonorrhoea in women: diagnostic, clinical and laboratory aspects. Lancet. 1978;1:761–4.
99. Brunham RC, Paavonen J, Stevens CE, et al. Mucopurulent cervicitis—the ignored counterpart in women of urethritis in men. N Engl J Med. 1984;311:1–6.
100. Klein EJ, Fisher CS, Chow AW, et al. Anorectal gonococcal infection. Ann Intern Med. 1977;86:340–6.
101. Quinn TC, Stamm WE, Goodell SE, et al. The polymicrobial origin of intestinal infections in homosexual men. N Engl J Med. 1983;309:576–82.
102. Janda WM, Bohnhoff M, Morello JA, et al. Prevalence and site pathogen studies of *Neisseria meningitidis* and *Neisseria gonorrhoeae* in homosexual men. JAMA. 1980;244:2060–4.
103. Podgore JK, Holmes KK. Ocular gonococcal infection with litle or no inflammatory response. JAMA. 1981;246:242–3.
104. Scott MJ Jr, Scott MJ Sr. Primary cutaneous *Neisseria gonorrhoeae* infection. Arch Dermatol. 1982;118:351–2.
105. Weström L. Incidence, prevalence and trends of acute pelvic inflammatory disease and its consequences in industrialized countries. Am J Obstet Gynecol. 1980;138:880–92.
106. Sweet RL. Pelvic inflammatory disease and infertility in women. Infect Dis Clin North Am. 1987;1:199–215.
107. Spiegel CA. New developments in the etiology and pathogenesis of bacterial vaginosis. Adv Exp Med Biol. 1987;224:127–34.
108. Mårdh P-A. An overview of infectious agents of salpingitis, their biology,

and recent advances in methods of detection. Am J Obstet Gynecol. 1980;138:933–51.
109. Centers for Disease Control. Ectopic pregnancy—United States. MMWR. 1986;35:289–91.
110. Lopez-Zeno JA, Keith LG, Berger GS. The Fitz-Hugh-Curtis syndrome revisited: changing perspectives after half a century. J Reprod Med. 1985;30:567–82.
111. Davidson AC, Hawkins DA. Peuritic pain: Fitz-Hugh-Curtis syndrome in a man. Br J Med. 1982;284:808.
112. Edwards LE, Barrada MMI, Harmann AA, et al. Gonorrhea in pregnancy. Am J Obstet Gynecol. 1978;132:637–41.
113. Handsfield HH, Hodson WA, Holmes KK. Neonatal gonococcal infections: I. Orogastric contamination with *Neisseria gonorrhoeae*. JAMA. 1973;225:697–701.
114. Corman LC, Levison ME, Knight R, et al. The high frequency of pharyngeal gonococcal infection in a prenatal clinic population. JAMA. 1974;230:568–70.
115. Holmes KK, Counts GW, Beaty HN. Disseminated gonococcal infection. Ann Intern Med. 1971;74:979–93.
116. Handsfield HH. Disseminated gonococcal infection. Clin Obstet Gynecol. 1975;18:131–42.
117. O'Brien JA, Goldenberg DL, Rice PA. Disseminated gonococcal infection: a prospective analysis of 49 patients and a review of pathophysiology and immune mechanisms. Medicine. 1983;62:395–406.
118. Masi AT, Eisenstein BI. Dissemianted gonococcal infection (DGI) and gonococcal arthritis (GCA): II. Clinical manifestations, diagnosis, complications, treatment and prevention. Semin Arthritis Rheum. 1981;10:173–97.
119. Holmes KK, Wiesner PJ, Pedersen AHB. The gonococcal arthritis-dermatitis syndrome. Ann Intern Med. 1971;75:470–1.
120. Sayeed ZA, Bhaduri U, Howell E, et al. Gonococcal meningitis: a review. JAMA. 1972;219:1730–1.
121. Walters DG, Goldstein MD. Adult respiratory distress syndrome and gonococcemia. Chest. 1980;77:434–6.
122. Bohnhoff M, Morello JA, Lerner SA. Auxotypes, penicillin susceptibility and serogroups of *Neisseria gonorrhoeae* from disseminated and uncomplicated infections. J Infect Dis. 1986;154:225–30.
123. Knapp JS, Holmes KK. Disseminated gonococcal infection caused by *Neisseria gonorrhoeae* with unique nutritional requirements. J Infect Dis. 1975;132:204–8.
124. Rinaldi RZ, Harrison WO, Fan PT. Penicillin resistant gonococcal arthritis. Ann Intern Med. 1982;97:43–5.
125. Petersen BH, Lee TJ, Snyderman R, et al. *Neisseria meningitidis* and *Neisseria gonorrhoeae* bacteremia associated with C6, C7, or C8 deficiency. Ann Intern Med. 1979;90:917–20.
126. Manicourt DH, Orloff S. Gonococcal arthritis-dermatitis syndrome: study of serum and synovial fluid immune complex levels. Arthritis Rheum. 1982;25:574–8.
127. Tronca E, Handsfield HH, Wiesner PJ, et al. Demonstration of *Neisseria gonorrhoeae* with fluorescent antibody in patients with disseminated gonococcal infection. J Infect Dis. 1974;129:583–6.
128. Rompalo AM, Hook EW III, Roberts PL, et al. The acute arthritis-dermatitis syndrome: the changing importance of *Neisseria gonorrhoeae* and *Neisseria meningitidis*. Arch Intern Med. 1987;147:281–3.
129. Fernandez GC, Chapman AJ Jr, Bolli R, et al. Gonococcal endocarditis: a case series demonstrating modern presentation of an old disease. Am Heart J. 1984;108:1326–34.
130. Laga M, Naaromara W, Brunham RC, et al. Single-dose therapy of gonococcal ophthalmia neonatorum with ceftriaxone. N Engl J Med. 1986;315:1382–5.
131. American Academy of Pediatrics. Prophylaxis and treatment of neonatal gonococcal infections. Pediatrics. 1980;65:1047–8.
132. Folland DS, Burke RE, Hinman AR, et al. Gonorrhesa in pre-adolescent children: an inquiry into the source of infection and mode of transmission. Pediatrics. 1977;60:153–6.
133. Ingram DL, White ST, Durfee MF, et al. Sexual contact in children with gonorrhea. Am J Dis Child. 1982;135:994–6.
134. Bonin P, Tanino TT, Handsfield HH. Isolation of *Neisseria gonorrhoeae* on selective and nonselective media in a sexually transmitted disease clinic. J Clin Microbiol. 1984;19:218–20.
135. Danielsson D, Johanisson G. Culture diagnosis of gonorrhoea: a comparison of the yield with selective and nonselective gonococcal culture media inoculated in the clinic and after transport of specimens. Acta Derm Venereol (Stockh) 1973;53:75–80.
136. Dans PE, Judson F. The establishment of a venereal disease clinic: II. An appraisal of current diagnostic methods in uncomplicated urogenital and rectal gonorrhea. J Am Vener Dis Assoc. 1975;1:107–12.
137. Luciano AA, Grubin L. Gonorrhea screening: comparison of three techniques. JAMA. 1980;243:680–1.
138. Kinghorn GR, Rashid S. Prevalence of rectal and pharyngeal infection in women with gonorrhoea in Sheffield. Br J Vener Dis. 1979;55:408–10.
139. Schroeter AL, Reynolds G. The rectal culture as a test of cure of gonorrhea in the female. J Infect Dis. 1972;125:499–503.
140. Faur YC, Wilson ME, May PS. Isolation of *N. meningitidis* from patients in a gonorrhea screening program: a four-year survey in New York City. Am J Public Health. 1981;71:53–8.
141. Judson FN, Ehret JM, Eickhoff TC. Anogenital infection with *Neisseria meningitidis* in homosexual men. J Infect Dis. 1978;137:458–63.
142. Schoenknecht FD, Sabath LD, Thornsberry C. Susceptibility tests: special tests. In: Lennette EH, et al (eds). Manual of Clinical Microbiology. 4th ed. Washington DC: American Society for Microbiology; 1985:1000–8.
143. Rothenberg RB, Simon R, Chipperfield E, et al. Efficacy of selected diagnostic tests for sexually transmitted diseases. JAMA. 1976;235:49–51.
144. Wald ER. Gonorrhea: diagnosis by Gram stain in the female adolescent. Am J Dis Child. 1977;131:1094–6.
145. Finch CA. Assessment of an enzyme immunoassay for diagnosing gonorrhea. J Reprod Med. 1985;30:250–7.
146. Granato PA, Roefaro M. Comparative evaluation of enzyme immunoassay and culture for the laboratory diagnosis of gonorrhea. Am J Clin Pathol. 1985;83:613–8.
147. Nowinski RC, Tam MR, Goldstein LC, et al. Monoclonal antibodies for diagnosis of infectious diseases in humans. Science. 1983;219:637–44.
148. Jaffe HW, Kraus SJ, Edwards TA, et al. Diagnosis of gonorrhea using a genetic transformation test on mailed clinical specimens. J Infecct Dis. 1982;146:275–9.
149. Totten PA, Holmes KK, Handsfield HH, et al. DNA hybridization technique for the detection of *Neisseria gonorrhoeae* in men with urethritis. J Infect Dis. 1983;148:462–71.
150. Hainer BL, Danylchuk P, Cooper J, et al. Limulus lysate assay in detection of gonorrhea in women from a low incidence population. Am J Obstet Gynecol. 1982;144:67–71.
151. Dans PE, Rothenberg R, Holmes KK. Gonococcal serology: how soon, how useful, and how much? J Infect Dis. 1977;135:330–4.
152. Batteiger BE, Jones RB. Chlamydial infections. Infect Dis Clin North Am. 1987;1:55–81.
153. Stamm WE, Guinan ME, Johnson C, et al. Effect of treatment regimens for *Neisseria gonorrhoeae* on simultaneous infection with *Chlamydia trachomatis*. N Engl J Med. 1984;310:545–9.
154. Jordan WC. Doxycycline vs tetracycline in the treatment of men with gonorrhea: the compliance factor. Sex Transm Dis. 1981;6(Suppl):105–6.
155. Centers for Disease Control. 1985 STD treatment guidelines. MMWR. 1985;34(Suppl):1S–54S.
156. Treatment of sexually transmitted diseases. Med Lett Drugs Therapeut. 1988;30:5–10.
157. Handsfield HH, Murphy VL. Comparative study of ceftriaxone and spectinomycin for the treatment of uncomplicated gonorrhea in men. Lancet. 1983;2:67–70.
158. Judson FN. Treatment of uncomplicated gonorrhea with ceftriaxone: a review. Sex Transm Dis. 1986;13:199–202.
159. Hook EW III, Roddy RE, Handsfield HH. Ceftriaxone therapy for incubating and early syphilis. J Infect Dis. 1988;158:881–4.
160. Downham TF II, Cawley RA, Salley SO, et al. Systemic toxic reactions to procaine penicillin G. Sex Transm Dis. 1978;5:4–9.
161. Jaffe HW, Reynolds GH, Wiesner PJ. National gonorrhea therapy monitoring study: adverse drug reactions. J Am Vener Dis Assoc. 1976;3:29–31.
162. Crider SR, Colby SD, Miller LK, et al. Treatment of penicillin-resistant *Neisseria gonorrhoeae* with oral norfloxacin. N Engl J Med. 1984;311:137–40.
163. Roddy RE, Handsfield HH, Hook EW III. Comparative trial of single-dose ciprofloxacin and ampicillin plus probenecid for treatment of gonococcal urethritis in men. Antimicrob Agents Chemother. 1986;13:169–71.
164. Joyce MP, Aying BB, Vaughan GH, et al. *In vitro* sensitivity of *Neisseria gonorrhoeae* to quinolone antibiotics in the Republic of the Phillippines (Abstract E19). Sixth International Pathogenic *Neisseria* Conference, Pine Mountain, Georgia, October 16–21, 1988.
165. Gottlieb A, Mills J. Cefuroxime axetil for treatment of uncomplicated gonorrhea. Antimicrob Agents Chemother. 1986;30:333–4.
166. Sweet RL, Schachter J, Landers DV, et al. Treatment of hospitalized patients with acute pelvic inflammatory disease: comparison of cefotetan plus doxycycline and cefoxitin plus doxycycline. Am J Obstet Gynecol. 1988;158:736–43.
167. Handsfield HH, Wiesner PJ, Holmes KK. Treatment of the gonococcal arthritis-dermatitis syndrome. Ann Intern Med. 1976;84:661–7.
168. Stone KM, Grimes DA, Magder LS. Personal protection against sexually transmitted diseases. Am J Obstet Gynecol. 1986;155:180–8.
169. Tramont EC, Boslego JW, Chung R, et al. Parenteral gonococcal pilus vaccine. In: Schoolnik GK, Brooks GF, Falkow S, et al, eds. The Pathogenic Neisseriae. Washington, DC: American Society for Microbiology. 1985:316.
170. Handsfield HH. Gonorrhea. In Spittel JA Jr, ed. Clinical Medicine. Philadelphia: Harper & Row; 1984.

191. OTHER GRAM-NEGATIVE COCCI

DIETER H. M. GRÖSCHEL

In addition to the classic pathogens *Neisseria gonorrhoeae* and *Neisseria meningitidis*, other members of the family Neisseriaceae are of clinical importance. These include other *Neisseria* species, and the genera *Moraxella*, including the subgenus *Branhamella*, *Acinetobacter*, and *Kingella*.[1–3] Some of the species closely resemble gonococci and meningococci in Gram-stained smears and, occasionally, on culture media, even selective ones. Thus, identification procedures are needed for the evaluation of clinical isolates that permit the definitive recognition of the classic pathogens and, in addition, allow the clinician to assess the significance of "saprophytes" or unusual gram-negative cocci or coccobacilli in patient specimens. Since *Acinetobacter* differs both bacteriologically and epidemiologically from the other Neisseriaceae, it will be discussed separately in Chapter 198.

NEISSERIA

Neisseria species are identified according to the biochemical and growth characteristics listed in Table 1. *Neisseria meningitidis* and *N. gonorrhoeae* were discussed in previous chapters (189 and 190). The other members of the genus usually grow on nutrient agar at 35°C and on enriched media at 22°C but not on enriched media containing vancomycin, colistin, and trimethoprim except for *N. lactamica* and *N. cinerea*. The classic biochemical identification of *Neisseria* species with cystine-tryptic digest agar media may be difficult; a standard manual of clinical microbiology should be consulted.[4] Novel approaches to identification include rapid carbohydrate degradation tests,[4,5] immunologic tests, and chromogenic enzyme substrate systems.[6,7]

The so-called nonpathogenic neisseriae are common inhabitants of the upper respiratory tract and rarely cause disease. The literature contains numerous reports on infections with these organisms, although their etiologic role is not always clearly established.[8] However, they are occasionally isolated from blood cultures.[9]

Neisseria lactamica

This species resembles *N. meningitidis* by growing on selective media containing vancomycin, colistin, and trimethoprim and producing acid from glucose and maltose. Most strains grow on nutrient agar at 35°C and some on chocolate agar at 22°C. *Neisseria lactamica* can be differentiated from meningococci by its β-galactosidase, which hydrolyzes lactose and the chromogenic substrate o-nitrophenol-β-D-galactopyranoside (OPNG). Spontaneous agglutination and cross-reactions with standard meningococcal typing sera occur[10]; thus biochemical identification is required.

The organism is isolated frequently from the nasopharynx, especially of infants and children, and rarely from the genital tract.[11] The few cases of meningitis or sepsis with *N. lactamica* reported[12–16] responded to penicillin or ampicillin therapy. Asymptomatic carriage of this *Neisseria* species seems to induce cross-reacting antibody to meningococci in infants and children.[10]

Neisseria sicca

A normal inhabitant of the oronasopharynx, the bacterium grows on agar plates in dry, wrinkled colonies that can be emulsified only with difficulty. The rare infections include meningitis,[17,18] endocarditis,[19] prosthetic valve infection,[20] a case of vertebral osteomyelitis with bacteremia,[21] and two cases of pneumonia in immunocompromised women.[22]

Neisseria subflava

This yellow-pigmented species is also a member of the normal pharyngeal flora. It has been isolated from patients with meningitis and sepsis,[18,23] endocarditis,[244–26] and a case of endophthalmitis.[27]

Neisseria mucosa

Growing in large mucoid, often adherent colonies on agar media, this species is differentiated from the others by its ability to reduce nitrate to nitrite and gaseous nitrogen.[4] Case reports and reviews of the literature[8,28–31] describe it as the causative agent of meningitis, endocarditis, pericarditis, empyema,[32] and ocular infection[33,34] as well as visceral botryomycosis[35] and a pulmonary coin lesion,[36] both in patients with chronic granulomatous disease.

Neisseria flavescens

This yellow greenish pigment-producing organism will not acidify the carbohydrates listed in Table 1. The species was first described by Branham[37] after an epidemic of meningitis in Chicago in 1928. Other cases of meningitis[38] and sepsis resembling chronic meningococcemia[39,40] have been reported.

Commensal neisseriae usually are susceptible to penicillin and ampicillin. β-Lactamase–producing *Neisseria perflava* was

TABLE 1. Biochemical and Growth Characteristics of *Neisseria* and *Branhamella*

	Production of Acid from										
Species	Glucose	Maltose	Sucrose	Lactose (ONPG)	Fructose	H_2S[a]	Oxidase	Extra CO_2[b]	Growth at 22°C	Polysaccharide[c]	Pigment[d]
N. gonorrhoeae	+	−	−	−	−	−	+	VI	−	NG	−
N. meningitidis	+	+	−	−	−	−	+	I	−	NG	−
N. lactamica	+	+	−	+	−	+	+	V[e]	V	−	+Y
N. sicca	+	+	+	−	+	+	+	−	+	+	− (sl Y)
N. subflava	+	+	V	−	V	+	+	−	+	V	+Y
N. mucosa	+	+	+	−	+	+	+	−	+	+	− (sl Y)
N. flavescens	−	−	−	−	−	+	+	−	+	+	+Y
N. cinerea	−	−	−	−	−		+	−	V	−	grayish
Branhamella catarrhalis	−	−	−	−	−	+	+	−	V	−	grayish

[a] With lead acetate paper.
[b] VI: very important for growth; I: important for growth.
[c] Synthesis of polysaccharide from 5% sucrose; NG: no growth.
[d] On Loeffler slant; Y: yellow; sl: slightly.
[e] V: variable.

recently isolated from the throat of two healthy people in Belgium.[41] The first reported case of infective endocarditis with *N. flavescens* was caused by a β-lactamase producer.[42] Normal flora must be considered a potential source of β-lactamase transferable to other species, for example, meningococci, in the upper respiratory tract.

Neisseria cinerea

This "nonpathogenic" species may grow on selective (Martin-Lewis) medium.[43] It was recently described as the cause of bacteremia in a child and in an adult alcoholic.[44]

BRANHAMELLA

The genus *Branhamella* was proposed by Catlin[45] in 1970 to separate *Neisseria catarrhalis* from the genus *Neisseria*. It differs from *Neisseria* in its DNA base content and fatty acid composition but is now classified as a subgenus of the genus *Moraxella*.[1]

Branhamella catarrhalis

This saprophytic organism of the upper respiratory tract and, occasionally, of the female genital tract is differentiated from the pathogenic and commensal neisseriae by an inability to produce acid from sugars and polysaccharide from sucrose, a grayish color of the colonies (Table 1), and the ability to hydrolyze deoxyribonucleic acid.[4]

Branhamella catarrhalis has received considerable interest during the past years as a respiratory tract pathogen in immunodeficient and hospitalized patients.[46] It is found on gram-stained sputum smears of patients, frequently phagocytized by polymorphonuclear leukocytes, and reminds the observer of a urethral smear from a patient with gonorrhea. The organism is not very prevalent (7–8 percent) in the oropharyngeal flora in patients and employees of a hospital,[47] but in patients with chronic pulmonary disease, a seasonal relation between the adherence of *Branhamella* to oropharyngeal cells and lower respiratory tract infection was observed.[48] Respiratory tract disease—laryngitis,[49] tracheitis,[50] and pneumonia[51–57]—occurs in infants, children, and adults. Nasopharyngeal cultures from 180 children with cough showed a 66.1 percent isolation rate of *B. catarrhalis*, often in pure culture, in comparison to a 28.3 percent isolation rate in 67 control children.[58] Another study[59] in children with asthma and bronchitis suggested that *B. catarrhalis* may even spread among patients. A study of Belgian miners with anthracosilicosis and exacerbation of chronic bronchitis showed *B. catarrhalis* in the transtracheal aspirate of 15 of 104 patients.[60] In a laboratory study the isolation of more than 10 colonies of *B. catarrhalis* in the primary streak of sputum cultures was associated with clinical respiratory disease in 15 of 16 patients.[61] It plays an important role in otitis media[62–64] and maxillary sinusitis[65] and has been identified as the cause of meningitis,[66] sepsis and endocarditis,[8,52] as well as bacteremia in immunosuppressed[67] and healthy children.[68] There are several reports of ophthalmia neonatorum caused by *Branhamella*[69–72] and single case reports on urinary tract infection in a girl[73] and peritonitis in a 51-year-old woman undergoing chronic continuous ambulatory peritoneal dialysis.[74]

Chapman et al. studied the antibody response in 21 patients (7 pneumonia, 13 chronic bronchitis, 1 sinusitis) and found bactericidal IgG antibody in 18 of 20 convalescent sera.[75] It is of interest that *B. catarrhalis* is an effective B-cell stimulator in vitro.[76,77]

Branhamella catarrhalis, like neisseriae, used to be susceptible to all β-lactam antibiotics, and ampicillin or penicillin was recommended as the drug of choice. In 1977 reports appeared in Europe [78–80] that several β-lactamase–producing isolates had been observed. Only two years later, one of the groups reported that the frequency of β-lactamase producers in routine nasopharyngeal cultures had risen from 4 to 17 percent.[78,81] In the Pacific Northwest all 11 clinically significant isolates of *B. catarrhalis* studied in 1980 produced β-lactamase. This β-lactamase showed more activity to penicillins than to cephalosporins and seemed to differ from the R-plasmid–mediated TEM penicillinase observed in *N. gonorrhoeae*.[80] Plasmids were not detected at that time,[82] but now it is known that there are both plasmid and chromosomally mediated β-lactamases[83] whose detection in the clinical laboratory depends on the assay used[84]; the chromogenic cephalosporin nitrocefin is recommended. The β-lactamase inhibitors clavulanic acid and sulbactam are active against the enzymes produced by *Branhamella*.[83] Although most β-lactamase–producing isolates seem to be responding to achievable concentrations of β-lactam–β-lactamase inhibitor combinations, cephalosporins, and cephamycins, antimicrobial therapy should be guided by in vitro susceptibility tests,[52,82,85] where the inoculum size seems to be important.[86]

MORAXELLA

Known for 90 years as the *Diplobacillus* Morax-Axenfeld, this organism and related gram-negative plump cocci and short rods in pairs are now classified in the genus *Moraxella*.[1,87] Like the previously discussed genera, moraxellae are normal inhabitants of the upper respiratory tract and also can be isolated from the skin and the urogenital tract. Most of the oxidase-positive, strictly aerobic, nonsaccharolytic, and nonmotile bacteria grow on routine media, some also on MacConkey agar. Useful reactions for the identification of *Moraxella* and related bacteria are listed in Table 2. (For a more detailed description of laboratory techniques consult Rubin et al.[88]) Moraxellae are best known as the cause of eye infections[87] but rarely also cause systemic disease.[89] Occasional reports include cases of pericarditis,[90] meningitis,[91] endocarditis,[92] and septicemia.[93] Due to the taxonomic confusion before the 1970s[87] it is difficult to review the older literature for case reports. Until recently, susceptibility to penicillin had been considered a characteristic of the genus. However, β-lactamase–producing strains have been described.[94]

Moraxella lacunata

The classic infection with *M. lacunata* is chronic angular blepharoconjunctivitis.[95] Today *M. lacunata* is the causative agent of only a small percentage of eye infections in the United States.[89,94,96] Occasional epidemics still occur.[97] *Moraxella liquefaciens*, a variant of *M. lacunata*,[87] was implicated in serious invasive disease.[92,93]

The organism requires growth media enriched with serum such as Loeffler medium; some strains will pit the medium surface.

Moraxella nonliquefaciens

This species has been most frequently isolated from human respiratory tract infections[88,96–98] and was recently isolated from an immunosuppressed patient with endophthalmitis.[99] Septicemia was reported in a 75-year-old woman with multiple myeloma after a course of chemotherapy.[100] The organism grows well on blood agar. A penicillin-resistant strain was found among 18 clinical isolates of *M. nonliquefaciens*.[101]

Moraxella osloensis

A common resident of the genital tract, this organism is one of the "*Mimae*" simulating the gonococcus.[102,103] It has been isolated from cases of invasive disease such as septic arthritis[104] and septicemia.[105,106] The bacteria grow well on blood agar and

TABLE 2. Laboratory Procedures Useful for the Identification of *Moraxella*, *Moraxella*-like Organisms, and *Kingella*

Species	Motility	Oxidase	Catalase	OF Glucose	Serum Required	Urease	Indol	Nitrate	Phenylalanine	Gelatin	Assimilation of Acetate	Growth on MacConkey Agar
M. lacunata	−	+	+	−	+	−	−	+	V	V	−	−
M. nonliquefaciens	−	+	+	−	V[a]	−	−	+	−	−	−	−
M. osloensis	−	+	+	−	−	−	−	V	V	−	+	V
M. phenylpyruvica	−	+	+	−	−	+	−	V	+	−	V	V
M. atlantae	−	+	+	−	+	−	−	−	−	−	V	+
M. urethralis	−	+	+	−	−	−	−	−	+	−	V	+
M-5	−	+	+	−	−	−	−	−	V	−	V	V
M-6	−	+	−	−	−	−	−	+	−	−	V	V
K. kingae[b]	−	+	−	F[c]	−	−	−	−	−	−		V
K. indologenes	−	+	−	F	−	−	+	−	−	−		
K. denitrificans	−	+	−	F	−	−	−	+	−	−		−

Key: OF: oxidation or fermentation; −: no reaction.
[a] V: variable.
[b] Most strains hemolytic on blood agar.
[c] May take 3 or more days; some strains require serum supplement.

can be differentiated from other moraxellae by a simple genetic transformation test.[107] This transformation assay has also been used with other moraxellae and is more accurate than biochemical testing is.

Other Moraxellae

Isolates of *Moraxella phenylpyruvica* and *Moraxella urethralis*,[108] formerly M-4, grow well on blood agar and MacConkey agar and are recovered mostly from cultures of the urogenital tract (''*Mima*''). *Moraxella phenylpyruvica*,[87] like *Moraxella atlantae*,[109] formerly M-3, has also been recovered from blood and spinal fluid. *Moraxella*-like bacteria are collected in Centers for Disease Control (CDC) groups M-5 and M-6.[88] M-5 strains have been isolated mainly from dog bite infections and M-6 strains from the respiratory tract. An M-5-like bacterium was isolated from an immunocompromised patient with pneumonia and bacteremia[110] and M-6 from a patient with mitral valve prolapse and endocarditis[111] and from another patient after cardiac catheterization.[112]

KINGELLA

This newly recognized genus[3] contains three species, *Kingella kingae, Kingella indologenes*, and *Kingella denitrificans*.[88] Most strains of *K. kingae* have been obtained from mucous membranes, blood cultures, and bone- or joint-associated sites.[88,113,114]

In most clinical reports the bacterium was isolated from children with septic arthritis[115–117]; one 15-month-old boy had intervertebral disk infection.[118] A review of 12 Swedish and 23 literature cases stressed the link between *K. kingae* and skeletal infections in children.[119] Wolff et al. recently reviewed 20 cases of endocarditis.[120] Petechiae may occur during sepsis,[115] which suggests disseminated gonorrhea.[121] Meningitis in a 21-month-old girl with stomatitis was complicated by bilateral infarcts of the basal ganglia.[122]

Kingella indologenes has been isolated from two cases of eye infections; the first case of endocarditis in a patient with mitral and aortic prosthetic valves was reported recently.[123]

Kingella denitrificans (formerly TM-1) was first recognized on Thayer-Martin medium inoculated with throat swabs during a survey for carriers of meningococci and was also isolated from genitourinary sources. There are several reports on endocarditis caused by this bacterium.[124–127] Antimicrobial therapy, usually with a β-lactam and an aminoglycoside, was successful in all cases.

REFERENCES

1. Krieg NR, Holt JG, eds. Bergey's Manual of Systematic Bacteriology. v 1. Baltimore: Williams & Wilkins; 1984:288,296.
2. Henriksen SD. *Moraxella, Neisseria, Branhamella* and *Acinetobacter*. Annu Rev Microbiol. 1976;30:63.
3. Henriksen SD, Bøvre K. Transfer of *Moraxella kingae*, Henriksen & Bøvre to the genus *Kingella* gen nov in the family Neisseriaceae. Int J Syst Bacteriol. 1976;26:447.
4. Morello JA, Janda WH, Bohnhoff M. *Neisseria* and *Branhamella*. In: Lennette EH, Balows A, Hausler WJ, et al., eds. *Manual of Clinical Microbiology*. ed 4. Washington, DC: American Society for Microbiology; 1985:176.
5. Philip A, Garton GC. Comparative evaluation of five commercial systems for the rapid identification of pathogenic *Neisseria* species. J Clin Microbiol. 1985;22:101.
6. Janda WM, Ulanday MG, Bohnhoff M, et al. Evaluation of the RIM-N, Gonocheck II, and Phadebact systems for the identification of pathogenic *Neisseria* spp and *Branhamella catarrhalis*. J Clin Microbiol. 1985;21:734.
7. Janda WM, Zigler KL, Bradna JJ. API QuadFERM with rapid DNase for identification of *Neisseria* spp and *Branhamella catarrhalis*. J Clin Microbiol. 1987;25:203.
8. Herbert DA, Ruskin J. Are the ''nonpathogenic'' neisseriae pathogenic? Am J Clin Pathol. 1981;75:739.
9. Feder HM, Garibaldi RA. The significance of nongonococcal, nonmeningococcal *Neisseria* isolates from blood cultures. Rev Infect Dis. 1984;6:181.
10. Gold R, Goldschneider I, Lepow ML, et al. Carriage of *Neisseria meningitidis* and *Neisseria lactamica* in infants and children. J Infect Dis. 1978;137:112.
11. Telfer Brunton WA, Young H, Fraser DRK. Isolation of *Neisseria lactamica* from the female genital tract. A case report. Br J Vener Dis. 1980;56:325.
12. Lauer BA, Fisher E. *Neisseria lactamica* meningitis. Am J Dis Child. 1976;130:198.
13. Hansman D. Meningitis caused by *Neisseria lactamica*. N Engl J Med. 1978;299:491.
14. Wilson DH, Overman DL. Septicemia due to *Neisseria lactamica*. J Clin Microbiol. 1976;4:214.
15. Greenberg LW, Kleinerman E. *Neisseria lactamica* meningitis. J Pediatr. 1978;93:1061.
16. Schifman RB, Ryan KJ. *Neisseria lactamica* septicemia in an immunocompromised patient. J Clin Microbiol. 1983;17:934.
17. Bansmer C, Brem J. Acute meningitis caused by *Neisseria sicca*. N Engl J Med. 1948;238:596.
18. Kienitz M, Ritzerfeld W. Meningitis purulenta und Sepsis mit Nachweis von *Neisseria sicca*. Z Med Mikrobiol Immunol. 1966;152:55.
19. Gay RM, Sevier RE. *Neisseria sicca* endocarditis: Report of a case and review of the literature. J Clin Microbiol. 1978;8:729.
20. Ghoneim ATM, Tandon AP. Prosthetic valve endocarditis due to *Neisseria sicca*. A case report. Indian Heart J. 1979;31:246.
21. Doern GV, Blacklow NR, Gantz NM, et al. *Neisseria sicca* osteomyelitis. J Clin Microbiol. 1982;16:595.
22. Gilrane T, Tracy JD, Greenlee RM, et al. *Neisseria sicca* pneumonia. Report of two cases and review of the literature. Am J Med. 1985;78:1038.
23. Demmler GJ, Couch RS, Taber LH. *Neisseria subflava* bacteremia and meningitis in a child: Report of a case and review of the literature. Pediatr Infect Dis. 1985;4:286.
24. Scott RM. Bacterial endocarditis due to *Neisseria flava*. J Pediatr. 1971;78:673.
25. Clark H, Patton RD. Post cardiotomy endocarditis due to *Neisseria perflava* on a prosthetic aortic valve. Ann Intern Med. 1968;68:386.
26. Pollack S, Mogtader A, Lange M. *Neisseria subflava* endocarditis. Case report and review of the literature. Am J Med. 1984;76:752.
27. Stricker RB, Pompilio KJ, Axelrod JL, et al. *Neisseria subflava* endophthalmitis. Am J Ophthalmol. 1982;94:423.
28. Fainstain V, Musher DM, Young EJ. Purulent pericarditis due to *Neisseria mucosa*. Chest. 1978;74:476.
29. Hennessey R, Reinhart JH, McGuckin MB. Endocarditis caused by *Neisseria mucosa* in a patient with a prosthetic heart valve. Am J Med Technol. 1981;47:909.

30. Bricaire F, Frottier J, Bure A, et al. Endocardites à *Neisseria* saprophytes. Sem Hop Paris. 1982;58:263.
31. Davis CL, Towns M, Henrich WL, et al. *Neisseria mucosus* endocarditis following drug abuse. Case report and review of the literature. Arch Intern Med. 1983;143:583.
32. Thorsteinsson SB, Minuth JN, Musher DM. Postpneumonectomy empyema due to *Neisseria mucosa*. Am J Clin Pathol. 1975;64:534.
33. Gini GA. Ocular infection in a newborn caused by *Neisseria mucosa*. J Clin Microbiol. 1987;25:1574.
34. Carter KD, Morgan CM, Otto MH. *Neisseria mucosa* endophthalmitis. Am J Ophthalmol. 1987;104:663.
35. Washburn RG, Bryan CS, DiSalvo AF, et al. Visceral botryomycosis caused by *Neisseria mucosa* in a patient with chronic granulomatous disease. J Infect Dis. 1985;151:563.
36. Claassen JL, Eppes SC, Buckley RH. Pulmonary coin lesion caused by *Neisseria mucosa* in a child with chronic granulomatous disease. Pediatr Infect Dis J. 1987;6:567.
37. Branham SE. A new meningococcus like organism (*Neisseria flavescens* n sp) from epidemic meningitis. Public Health Rep. 1930;45:845.
38. Prentice AW. *Neisseria flavescens* as a cause of meningitis. Lancet. 1957;1:613.
39. Wertlake PT, Williams TW. Septicaemia caused by *Neisseria flavescens*. J Clin Pathol. 1968;21:437.
40. Coovadia YM. *Neisseria flavescens* septicaemia with meningitis. A case report. S Afr Med J. 1984;66:308.
41. Piot P, Roberts M, Ninane G. β-Lactamase production in commensal Neisseriaceae. Lancet. 1979;1:619.
42. Sinave CP, Ratzan KR. Infective endocarditin caused by *Neisseria flavescens*. Am J Med. 1987;82:163.
43. Knapp JS, Totten PA, Mulks MH, et al. Characterization of *Neisseria cinerea*, a nonpathogenic species isolated on Martin-Lewis medium selective for pathogenic *Neisseria* spp. J Clin Microbiol. 1984;19:63.
44. Southern PM, Kutscher AE. Bacteremia due to *Neisseria cinerea*: Report of two cases. Diagn Microbiol Infect Dis. 1987;7:143.
45. Catlin BW. Transfer of organism named *Neisseria catarrhalis* to *Branhamella* gen. nov. Int J Syst Bacteriol. 1970;20:155.
46. Hager H, Verghese A, Alvarez S, et al. *Branhamella catarrhalis* respiratory infections. Rev Infect Dis. 1987;9:1140.
47. Ahmad F, McLeod DT, Power JT, et al. *Branhamella catarrhalis* prevalence in a hospital population. J Hosp Infect. 1985;6:71.
48. Mbaki N, Rikitomi N, Nagatake T, et al. Correlation between *Branhamella catarrhalis* adherence to oropharyngeal cells and seasonal incidence of lower respiratory tract infections. Tohoku J Exp Med. 1987;153:111.
49. Schalén L, Christensen P, Kamme C, et al. High isolation rate of *Branhamella catarrhalis* from the nasopharynx in adults with acute laryngitis. Scand J Infect Dis. 1980;12:277.
50. Ernst TN, Philp M. Bacterial tracheitis caused by *Branhamella catarrhalis*. Pediatr Infect Dis J. 1987;6:574.
51. Berg RA, Bartley DL. Pneumonia associated with *Branhamella catarrhalis* in infants. Pediatr Infect Dis J. 1987;6:569.
52. Doern GV, Miller MJ, Winn RE. *Branhamella (Neisseria) catarrhalis* systemic disease in humans. Arch Intern Med. 1981;141:1690.
53. McNeely DJ, Kitchens CS, Kluge RM. Fatal *Neisseria (Branhamella) catarrhalis* pneumonia in an immunodeficient host. Am Rev Respir Dis. 1978;114:399.
54. Hirota M, Tomonaga A, Komori K, et al. A case of *Branhamella catarrhalis* pneumonia. Kansenshogaku Zasshi. 1978;52:497.
55. Srinivasan G, Raff MJ, Templeton WC, et al. *Branhamella catarrhalis* pneumonia. Am Rev Respir Dis. 1981;123:553.
56. West M, Berk SL, Smith JK. *Branhamella catarrhalis* pneumonia. South Med J. 1982;75:1021.
57. Johnson MA, Drew WL, Roberts M. *Branhamella (Neisseria) catarrhalis*—a lower respiratory tract pathogen? J Clin Microbiol. 1981;13:1066.
58. Brorson J-E, Malmvall B-E. *Branhamella catarrhalis* and other bacteria in the nasopharynx of children with longstanding cough. Scand J Infect Dis. 1981;13:111.
59. Brzin B. *Branhamella catarrhalis* as a human pathogen and a possible hospital infectant. Zentralbl Bakteriol [A]. 1981;249:483.
60. Ninone G, Joly J, Kraytman M. Bronchopulmonary infection due to *Branhamella catarrhalis*: 11 cases assessed by transtracheal puncture. Br Med J. 1978;1:276.
61. von Graevenitz A, Rathbone RR. *Branhamella catarrhalis* in respiratory secretions: Clinical correlation in 16 cases. South Med J. 1981;74:1095.
62. Kamme C. Evaluation of the in vitro sensitivity of *Neisseria catarrhalis* to antibiotics with respect to acute otitis media. Scand J Infect Dis. 1970;2:117.
63. Harrison CJ, Marks MI, Welch DF. Microbiology of recently treated acute otitis media compared with previously untreated acute otitis media. Pediatr Infect Dis. 1985;4:641.
64. VanHare GF, Shurin PA, Marchant CD, et al. Acute otitis media caused by *Branhamella catarrhalis*: Biology and therapy. Rev Infect Dis. 1987;9:16.
65. Brorson J-E, Axelsson A, Holm SE. Studies on *Branhamella catarrhalis* (*Neisseria catarrhalis*) with special reference to maxillary sinusitis. Scand J Infect Dis. 1976;8:151.
66. Cocchi P, Ulivelli A. Meningitis caused by *Neisseria catarrhalis*. Acta Paediatr Scand. 1968;57:451.
67. Bannatyne RM, Kolodej V. *Branhamella catarrhalis* bacteraemia and immunosuppression—part of a larger problem? Diagn Microbiol Infect Dis. 1985;3:65.
68. Baron J, Shapiro ED. Unsuspected bacteremia caused by *Branhamella catarrhalis*. Pediatr Infect Dis. 1985;4:100.
69. Spark RP, Dahlberg DW, LaBelle JW. Pseudogonococcal ophthalmia neonatorum. Am J Clin Pathol. 1979;72:471.
70. Lue YA, Simms DH, Ubriani R, et al. Ophthalmia neonatorum caused by penicillin-resistant *Branhamella catarrhalis*. NY State J Med. 1981;81:1775.
71. Stull TL, Stanford EJ. Pseudogonococcal ophthalmia neonatorum caused by *Branhamella catarrhalis*. Pediatr Infect Dis. 1986;5:104.
72. Romberger JA, Wald ER, Wright PF. *Branhamella catarrhalis* conjunctivitis. South Med J. 1987;80:926.
73. Ahmad F, Calder MA, Croughan MJ, et al. Urinary tract infection caused by *Branhamella catarrhalis*. J Infect. 1985;10:176.
74. Damani NN, Chin ATL. *Branhamella catarrhalis* peritonitis in a continuous ambulatory peritoneal dialysis patient. Nephron. 1987;45:160.
75. Chapman AJ, Musher DM, Jonsson S, et al. Development of bactericidal antibody during *Branhamella catarrhalis* infection. J Infect Dis. 1985; 151:878.
76. Calvert JE, Proctor SJ, Jefferis R. Activation of B chronic lymphocytic leukaemia cells by *Branhamella catarrhalis*. Immunology. 1987;60:45.
77. Forsgren A, Penta A, Schlossman SF, et al. *Branhamella catarrhalis* activates human B lymphocytes following interactions with surface IgD and class I major histocompatibility complex antigens. Cell Immunol. 1988;112:78.
78. Malmvall B-E, Brorson J-E, Johnsson J. In vitro sensitivity to penicillin V and β-lactamase production of *Branhamella catarrhalis*. J Antimicrob Chemother. 1977;3:374.
79. Percival A, Coskill JE, Rowlands J, et al. Pathogenicity of and beta-lactamase production by *Branhamella (Neisseria) catarrhalis*. Lancet. 1977; 2:1175.
80. Van Hoi-Dang AB, Brive–Le Bouguenec C, Barthelemy M, et al. Novel β-lactamase from *Branhamella catarrhalis*. Ann Microbiol (*Paris*). 1978; 129:397.
81. Brorson J-3, Martinell J, Wilkse H. *Branhamella catarrhalis*: Antibiotic susceptibility and β-lactamase production. J Antimicrob Chemother. 1981; 7:208.
82. Doern GV, Siebers KG, Hallick LM, et al. Antibiotic susceptibility of beta-lactamase–producing strains of *Branhamella (Neisseria) catarrhalis*. Antimicrob Agents Chemother. 1980;17:24.
83. O'Grady CE, Nord, eds. Symposium on *Branhamella catarrhalis*. Drugs. 1986;31(Suppl 3):40,64.
84. Doern GV, Tubert TA. Detection of beta-lactamase activity among clinical isolates of *Branhamella catarrhalis* with six different beta-lactamase assays. J Clin Microbiol. 1987;25:1380.
85. Sweeney KG, Verghese A, Needham CA. In vitro susceptibilities of isolates from patients with *Branhamella catarrhalis* pneumonia compared with those of colonizing strains. Antimicrob Agents Chemother. 1985;27:499.
86. Doern GV, Tubert T. Effect of inoculum size on results of macrotube broth dilution susceptibility tests with *Branhamella catarrhalis*. J Clin Microbiol. 1987;25:1576.
87. Henriksen SD. *Moraxella, Acinetobacter* and the *Mimeae*. Bacteriol Rev. 1973;37:522.
88. Rubin SJ, Granato PA, Wasilauskas BL. Glucose-nonfermenting gram-negative bacteria. In: Lennette EH, Balows A, Hausler WJ, et al., eds. Manual of Clinical Microbiology. ed 4. Washington, DC: American Society for Microbiology; 1985:330.
89. Kowalski RP, Harwick JC. Incidence of *Moraxella* conjunctival infection. Am J Ophthalmol. 1986;101:437.
90. Appelbaum A, Giladi A, Borman JBB. *Moraxella* purulent pericarditis. J Cardiovasc Surg. 1974;15:479.
91. Verger P, Laigle JL, Guillard JM, et al. Les méningitis a moraxella chez l'enfant. Bordeaux Med. 1972;5:2189.
92. Silverfarb PM, Lawe JE. Endocarditis due to *Moraxella liquefaciens*. Arch Intern Med. 1968;122:512.
93. Sellers DP, Wise JR, Semer HA. Septicemia due to *Moraxella liquefaciens*. J Maine Med Assoc. 1971;62:73.
94. Rosenthal SL. Clinical role of *Acinetobacter* and *Moraxella*. In: Gilardi GL, ed. Glucose Nonfermenting Gram-Negative Bacteria. West Palm Beach, FL: CRC Press; 1978:105.
95. Fedukowicz HB. External Infections of the Eye. ed 2. New York: Appleton-Century-Crofts; 1978:153.
96. van Bijsterveld OP. The incidence of *Moraxella* on mucous membranes and the skin. Am J Ophthalmol. 1972;74:72.
97. Ringvold A, Vik E, Bevanger LS. *Moraxella lacunata* isolated from epidemic conjunctivitis among teen-aged females. Acta Ophthalmol (Copenh). 1985;63:427.
98. Bøvre K, Henriksen SD. A new *Moraxella* species, *Moraxella osloensis*, and a revised description of *Moraxella nonliquefaciens*. Int J Syst Bacteriol. 1967;17:127.
99. Ebright JR, Lentino JR, Juni E. Endophthalmitis caused by Moraxella nonliquefaciens. Am J Clin Pathol. 1982;77:362.
100. Brorson JE, Falsen E, Nelsson-Ehle H, et al. Septicaemia due to *Moraxella nonliquefaciens* in a patient with multiple myeloma. Scand J Infect Dis. 1983;15:221.
101. Rosenthal SL, Freundlich LF, Gilardi GL, et al. In vitro antibiotic sensitivity of *Moraxella* species. Chemotherapy. 1978;24:360.

102. Svihus RH, Lucero EM, Mikolajczyk MT, et al. Gonorrhea-like syndrome caused by penicillin resistant Mimeae. JAMA. 1961;177:121.
103. Bøvre K, Hagen N, Berdal BP, et al. Oxidase positive rods from cases of suspected gonorrhoea. Acta Pathol Microbiol Scand [B]. 1977;85:27.
104. Feigin RD, San Joaquin V, Middlekamp JN. Septic arthritis due to *Moraxella osloensis*. J Pediatr. 1969;75:116.
105. Butzler JD, Hansen W, Cadranel C, et al. Stomatitis with septicemia due to *Moraxella osloensis*. J Pediatr. 1974;84:721.
106. Lasser AE, Goldman EJ. Moraxella bacteremia. Report of a case resembling gonococcemia with cutaneous manifestations. Cutis. 1978;21:657.
107. Juni E. Simple genetic transformation assay for rapid diagnosis of *Moraxella osloensis*. Appl Microbiol. 1974;27:16.
108. Riley PS, Hollis DG, Weaver RE. Characterization and differentiation of 59 strains of *Moraxella urethralis* from clinical specimens. Appl Microbiol. 1974;28:355.
109. Bøvre K, Fuglesang JE, Hagen N, et al. *Moraxella atlantae* sp nov and its distinction from *Moraxella phenylpyruvica*. Int J Syst Bacteriol. 1976;26:511.
110. Goetz MB, Jones J. Pneumonia and bacteremia caused by a previously undescribed *Moraxella*-like bacterium. J Clin Microbiol. 1982;15:720.
111. Simor AE, Salit IE. Endocarditis caused by M-6. J Clin Microbiol. 1983;17:931.
112. Perez RE. Endocarditis with *Moraxella*-like M-6 after cardiac catheterization. J Clin Microbiol. 1986;24:501.
113. Weaver RE, Hollis DG, Bottone EJ. Gram-negative fermentative bacteria and *Francisella tularensis*. In: Lennette EH, Balows A, Hausler WJ, et al., eds. Manual of Clinical Microbiology, ed 4. Washington, DC: American Society for Microbiology; 1985:309.
114. Ødum L, Fredriksen W. Identification and characterization of *Kingella kingae*. Acta Pathol Microbiol Scand [B]. 1981;89:311.
115. Redfield DC, Overturf GD, Ewing N, et al. Bacteria, arthritis, and skin lesions due to *Kingella kingae*. Arch Dis Child. 1980;55:411.
116. Powell JM, Bass JW. Septic arthritis caused by *Kingella kingae*. Am J Dis Child. 1983;137:974.
117. Raymond J, Bergeret M, Bargy F, et al. Isolation of two strains of *Kingella kingae* associated with septic arthritis. J Clin Microbiol. 1986;24:1100.
118. Woolfrey BF, Lally RT, Faville RJ. Intervertebral diskitis caused by *Kingella kingae*. Am J Clin Pathol. 1986;85:745.
119. Claesson B, Falsen E, Kjellman B. *Kingella kingae* infections: A review and a presentation of data from 10 Swedish cases. Scand J Infect Dis. 1985;17:233.
120. Wolff AH, Ullman RF, Strampfer MJ, et al. *Kingella kingae* endocarditis: Report of a case and review of the literature. Heart Lung. 1987;16:579.
121. Shanson DC, Gazzard BG. *Kingella kingae* septicaemia with a clinical presentation resembling disseminated gonococcal infection. Br Med J. 1984;289:730.
122. Walterspiel JN. *Kingella kingae* meningitis with bilateral infarcts of the basal ganglia. Infection. 1983;11:307.
123. Jenny DB, Letendre PW, Iverson G. Endocarditis caused by *Kingella indologenes*. Rev Infect Dis. 1987;9:787.
124. Goldman IS, Ellner PD, Francke EL, et al. Infective endocarditis due to *Kingella denitrificans*. Am Intern Med. 1980;93:152.
125. Swann RA, Holmes B. Infective endocarditis caused by *Kingella denitrificans*. J Clin Pathol. 1984;37:1384.
126. Khan JA, Sharp S, Mann KR, et al. *Kingella denitrificans* prosthetic endocarditis. Am J Med Sci. 1986;291:187.
127. Brown AM, Rothburn MM, Roberts C, et al. Septicaemia with probable endocarditis caused by *Kingella denitrificans*. J Infect. 1987;15:225.

GRAM-NEGATIVE BACILLI

192. VIBRIO CHOLERAE

WILLIAM B. GREENOUGH III

Illness and death due to dehydrating diarrhea and vomiting can be recognized in the writings of Susruta (Sanskrit), Hippocrates, Galen, and Wang-Shooho. There is still doubt about when cholera in its epidemic form was first described.[1] It is likely that no long-distance spread of cholera took place in Europe and the Americas before the nineteenth century, despite clear descriptions of epidemics on the Indian subcontinent at least from the late fifteenth century, when Portuguese explorers began recounting their experiences in India. Extensions from India to neighboring countries including China seem to have occurred. In 1817 cholera broke out with unusual severity and a high mortality in the area of the Ganges River Delta. Over the next 5 years it spread over much of Asia and the Middle East. A second wave beginning in 1829 reached Europe and America by 1832. New York suffered heavily, and, through the predilection of cholera for the poor, made evident the extent of poverty and lack of sanitation that were closely linked to the epidemic.[2] That Latin America was not spared was emphasized in the recently published novel *Love in the Time of Cholera*.[3] From 1817 to early in the twentieth century six waves of cholera spread across the world. Since then until early in the 1960s the disease contracted in extent across the globe remaining regularly present only in southern Asia.

SPREAD OF EL TOR BIOTYPE

In 1905 Gotschlich isolated six peculiar strains of *Vibrio cholerae* from the dead bodies of returned Mecca pilgrims at the quarantine camp of El Tor.[4] These strains, which produced hemolysins, came from typical cases of cholera and agglutinated in the classical typing serum. However, not until 1961 when the "El Tor" biotype produced an epidemic of major proportions in the Philippines was there general agreement that hemolytic *V. cholerae* could be responsible for severe epidemic human disease.[5] Before 1961 the El Tor variant of *V. cholerae* caused epidemics only in Sulawesi (Celebes). Since then this biotype has spread across Asia,[6] the Middle East, Africa,[7] and more recently parts of Europe. To date the American continent has been spared, although in isolated instances it has been recovered in the United States and Brazil.

There are several characteristics of the El Tor strain that have allowed it to spread across the whole world as previous strains have done. Although fully able to produce the cholera toxin and to cause severe human disease, the ratio of cases to carriers is much less than in cholera due to the "classical" biotype (1:30–100 for "El Tor" versus 1:2–4 for "classical").[8,9] In addition, the duration of carriage following infection and the survival of shed organisms in the environment seem to favor the El Tor biotype. In the heartland of cholera—the Ganges Delta—only since 1969 did the El Tor variant appear, replacing the classical biotype in 1974,[10] thereby completing the displacement of the classical biotype in its heartland.

In 1982 in Bangladesh the classical biotype resurfaced with a new capacity. Not only did it produce more severe illness with higher rates of hospitalization than observed previously, but also it rapidly replaced the El Tor biotype, which had appeared to be well entrenched.[11–13] In the early phase of the 1983 epidemic, although El Tor was still present, the new classical strain predominated. As of this writing no other countries have reported a major reappearance of classical *V. cholerae*, although sporadic isolates have been found.[14]

ENTEROTOXIN

The idea that the clinical manifestations of cholera were due to a toxin really has its roots in the writings of John Snow.[15]

> It would seem that the cholera poison, when reproduced in sufficient quantity, acts as an irritant on the surface of the stomach and intestine, or what is still more probable, it withdraws fluid from the blood circulating in the capillaries, by a power analogous to that by which epithelial cells of the various organs abstract the different secretions of the healthy body.

It is difficult to find a more accurate statement about cholera toxin and its mode of action today. This is not to say that since John Snow's time we have not made great progress; on the contrary, much knowledge has been gathered confirming his brilliant insights. Enterotoxic activity in a cell-free filtrate of *V.*

cholerae cultures was first demonstrated by De in 1953 in the ligated intestine of rabbits[16] and by Dutta and Habbu in 1955 in infant rabbits.[17] Comparative studies of the ability of different strains of *V. cholerae* to produce toxin began with De's studies in 1959.[18] Ten years later methods for the preparation and purification of cholera toxin were established.[19] Simultaneously it was shown that the toxin stimulated active secretion of chloride in the small intestine in a way that exactly simulated and competed with stimuli that increased the level of cyclic AMP in this system.[20] Within a year three laboratories independently demonstrated that cholera toxin did increase levels of cAMP by increasing the activity of adenylate cyclase in intestinal mucosa of rabbits.[21–23] Soon after, this was also shown to be the case in the human intestine during clinical cholera.[24] Since these observations, there has been a rapid proliferation of studies confirming that cholera toxin activates adenylate cyclase in all tissues possessing this enzyme. This effect can be seen in intact tissue and is dependent on a specific receptor, monosialosyl ganglioside (GM_1 ganglioside).[25,26] The toxin has been characterized and contains binding subunits of 11,500 daltons (B), active subunit of 23–24,000 daltons (A_1), and a bridging piece of 5–6000 daltons (A_2) that links A_1 to 5B subunits. The current state of knowledge of the structure and function of this toxin has been well reviewed.[27,28] The importance of this toxin extends well beyond the disease it produces, since it has become a basic tool to assist in elucidating the way in which adenylate cyclase and the cyclic nucleotide system functions. Parallels have also been established between other bacterial toxins and cholera toxin. Once it has entered the cell, the A subunit enzymatically transfers ADP-ribose from cytosolic NAD to a protein (N_s) that regulates the adenylate cyclase system, which is located in the plasma membrane of mammalian cells.[29]

It has also become clear that *Escherichia coli* can produce a toxin that is very similar to the cholera toxin in structure and mode of action.[27,28] Other vibrios that do not agglutinate in the classical Ogawa and Inaba typing sera also produce an enterotoxin similar to that of *V. cholerae*.[30] Other diarrhea-causing bacteria may also produce adenylate cyclase-stimulating substances as in *Salmonella* infections.[31]

The DNA that codes for the adenylate cyclase-activating toxin of *E. coli* (heat-labile toxin) is located in a plasmid that can be transferred to other *E. coli* and perhaps to other enteric bacteria.[32] Close relationships between the *V. cholerae* genetic code for toxin and that of other vibrios or enteric bacteria undoubtedly exist but have not been documented as yet. It has been suggested that the code for toxin in *V. cholerae* is chromosomally linked.[33]

Information on the genetic code for the adenylate cyclase-stimulating cholera toxin and the regulator genes of the structural coding genome[34–36] is now rapidly evolving.

THE PATHOGEN

Classification

Vibrios are one of the most common organisms in surface waters in the world. Their taxonomy is still undergoing rapid changes. This is particularly true with respect to those that may be associated with human diarrheal disease. The two main human pathogens are *V. cholerae* and *V. parahemolyticus*. The way in which these two organisms produce diarrhea is entirely different; *V. parahemolyticus* is an invasive organism affecting primarily the colon, while *V. cholerae* is not invasive, affecting the small intestine through secretion of an exotoxin.

The serotype of *V. cholerae* that causes epidemic human disease, however, has only three determinants, which are of the O or somatic antigens (Table 1). Vibrios of other serogroups can cause sporadic human disease but have not commonly been associated with epidemic human diarrhea. Some of these can produce a cholera-like illness, however[37,38] and do produce a cholera-like enterotoxin.[30] There is considerable importance to understanding the potential relationships between the antigenic markers currently used to identify *V. cholerae*, the cause of epidemic cholera, and other vibrios that seem closely related, which are present the world over.[39]

TABLE 1. Antigenic Determinants of *V. cholerae*

Serotype	*O Antigens*
Ogawa	A,B,
Inaba	A,C
Hikojima	A,B,C

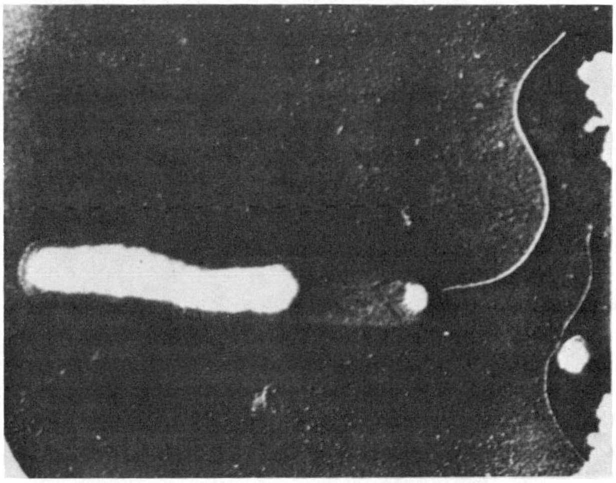

FIG. 1. Electron micrograph of *Vibrio cholerae*. (×50,000)

Relationships to Enterobacteriaceae

Vibrio cholerae is closely related to other members of the Enterobacteriaceae. It differs in that, as isolated from humans with cholera, the organism is a curved rather than a straight rod, is oxidase-positive, grows luxuriantly in alkaline media in the presence of bile salts, and produces a neuraminidase that has the intriguing property of degrading gangliosides to the monosialosyl form, which is the specific receptor for cholera toxin. Antibiotic resistance can be transferred between *V. cholerae* and other members of Enterobacteriaceae. Strains that are resistant to multiple antibiotics have now been observed.[40]

Morphologic Characteristics

The characteristic shape and single polar flagella of *V. cholerae* are seen in Figure 1. The vibrios are short (1.5–3.0 μm by 0.5 μm). They are gram-negative and curved. The characteristic rapid motility is the basis for an immobilization test for their identification.[41] In culture many variants are formed, including spiral forms that had previously resulted in the classification of vibrios as Spirillaceae.

Antigenic Structure

Flagellar (H) antigens are shared by many vibrios, and antisera prepared against them do not distinguish the vibrio causing human epidemic disease from water vibrios.

The somatic (O) antigens do distinguish *V. cholerae* Ogawa, Inaba, and Hikojima, which are responsible for epidemics (Table 1). In most other respects the structure of *V. cholerae* is analogous to other members of the Enterobacteriaceae. Antisera can be raised against vibrios that are not agglutinated by the anti-A, anti-B, or anti-C sera (Table 1). These sera can serve to identify specific strains. A coherent internationally recognized framework for such classification has yet to be worked out, but more than 100 types are currently known. "Endotoxin" is present as in other gram-negative bacteria, and a number of soluble antigens including the enterotoxin are produced. Fewer details are known of the chemical structure of *V. cholerae* lipopolysaccharides than is true in the case of *Salmonella* or *E. coli*, but unique properties have now been described.[42] Variations in the characteristic markers occur both in vivo and in vitro.[43] These changes and their implications are not well understood at present but certainly raise the question of reversion in nature of nonepidemic strains to classical epidemic strains and vice versa.

Genetics

Some of the morphologically distinctive groups of organisms we call vibrios appear to possess close genetic relationships, as seen in DNA compositions and reassociation data.[44,45] Other organisms currently lumped together as vibrios such as *V. parahemolyticus* do not seem closely related to *V. cholerae* nor does their behavior in human disease seem much related except that the gut is attacked. Water vibrios can also be very similar or quite disparate.

Vibrios can experience genetic changes by mutation, transformation, transduction by phage, and conjunction. A number of vibriophages may be used for typing purposes. Knowledge of the genome and plasmids of *V. cholerae* has continued to advance rapidly.[34–36]

Enterotoxin

The enterotoxin that mediates the disease caused by *V. cholerae* has now been completely characterized with respect to its chemical composition, amino acid sequence, and molecular configuration.[27] It is composed of five binding "B" subunits arranged in a circular form; a linking subunit A_2 binds the active adenylate cyclase-stimulating subunit A_1 to the complex. A_1 is bound to A_2 by a disulfide linkage. The molecule has been visualized. The B subunit has been sequenced; the weight has been determined to be 11,500 daltons, and a partial sequence of the A_1 and A_2 units has been published (Fig. 2). Its mode of action is quite well worked out, and interesting similarities exist among the bacterial toxins that interact with NAD.[27]

A newly discovered enterotoxin of *V. cholerae* has been reported in "nontoxigenic" variants and strains from which the gene for the adenylate cyclase-stimulating toxin has been deleted.[47]

DETERMINANTS OF SURVIVAL OF V. CHOLERAE

Although other animals may be experimentally infected with *V. cholerae,* there has been no evidence in nature of a carrier of the organism other than humans. When excreted from the body into water *V. cholerae* survives only for a short time (4–7 days) and in the presence of other competing bacteria even a shorter time. It does not withstand drying or mildly acidic conditions. It will survive more readily in brackish water than in fresh water. Although water seems to be the main source of spread, foods have been implicated on some occasions.[48] There are important differences in survival in the environment between the "classical" and "El Tor" biotypes of *V. cholerae,* the El Tor strain surviving for longer periods both in the host and in nature.[5,48,49]

The new classical strain that appeared in Bangladesh in 1982 has acquired an improved ability to survive for prolonged periods in competition with the existing El Tor strain.[50]

In a recent review attention has been focused on the capacity of *V. cholerae* to undergo reductive division and achieve ultramicro forms that are not recovered by ordinary culture methods. This property, shared with other enteropathogens, may have importance in the latent periods between outbreaks.[51]

Strain Variations

There are several variations that occur in nature with *V. cholerae.* Over a relatively short period of years serotypes shift between Ogawa and Inaba in endemic areas.[52] Similar shifts occur in vitro.[52] Also a transformation to a rough variant is observed in older cultures and also in vivo.[43] The crucial question that remains unanswered is whether there may be a reservoir in nature of *V. cholerae* that is hidden in an as yet undiscovered ecologic niche,[53] and that may become epidemic strains through a genetic change under the right conditions. Over a longer cycle in history there may be changes in biotype. During the last 2 decades we have been the classical biotype displaced by a variant that agglutinates in Ogawa or Inaba sera but that has a different susceptibility pattern for bacteriophages and may hemolyze red cells.[52] Since 1982 a new classical variant that initially displaced the currently entrenched El Tor in Bangladesh now coexists with it.[11–14]

THE DISEASE

Clinical Manifestations

Cholera may be present in an asymptomatic state, as mild diarrhea, or as the typical "full-blown" syndrome, which will be

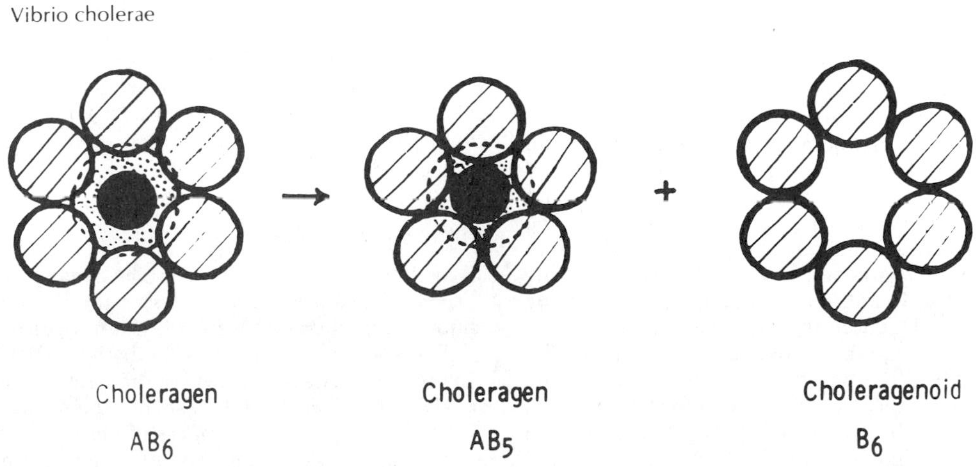

FIG. 2. Postulated model for cholera toxin. (From Lai et al.,[98] with permission.)

TABLE 2. Composition of Cholera Stool[a]

	Concentration (mEq or mmole/liter)			
	Na^+	K^+	Cl^-	HCO_3^-
Adults	135	15	100	45
Children	105	25	90	30

[a] When purging rate is 50 ml/kg/24 hr or more.

discussed in this section. In its extreme manifestation cholera is one of the most rapidly fatal illnesses known. A healthy person may become hypotensive within an hour of the onset of symptoms and may die within 2–3 hours if no treatment is provided. More commonly the disease progresses from the first liquid stool to shock in 4–12 hours with death following in 18 hours to several days. The first symptoms of cholera are an increase in peristalsis, which the patient can sense as a fullness and gurgling in the abdomen. This is followed rapidly by the first loose stool, which is not of the typical "rice water" appearance that is so often referred to in cholera. After several watery movements the stools take on this typical appearance and lose any odor except a mild somewhat fishy smell.

All the symptoms and signs of cholera derive from the depletion of water and salts from the intravascular and extracellular spaces of the body by loss into the gut lumen. The composition of cholera stool varies with its rate of loss from the body, but on the average has the composition shown in Table 2. In the days before successful replacement therapy, the clinical description of cholera included detailed attention to all the stages of hypovolemic shock and dehydration and to the reaction of the body in those surviving prolonged periods of poor circulation and ischemia. If properly treated, only diarrhea will be seen after the acute symptoms and signs of volume loss have been relieved by replacement therapy. Intravenous replacement solutions are listed in Table 3. Vomiting is often present at the early stages of cholera and assumes particular importance with respect to the oral replacement of fluid losses. The clinical appearance of a cholera patient is shown in Figure 3. There is little abdominal pain in cholera, most of the anxiety, muscle cramps, thirst, and faintness being related in their prominence to the rate of fluid loss. On rare occasions ileus may occur at the onset of illness. In such cases there may be profound shock and dehydration without diarrhea. In this situation cholera mimics acute intestinal obstruction. In the older literature this is known as "Cholera Sicca." It can kill particularly rapidly since the physician may lose sight of the amount of fluid that the small and large intestine can sequester.

Initially there is no real difference between cholera and the acute watery diarrheas that are due to enterotoxigenic *E. coli* or "noncholera" vibrios. If cholera is not treated with an antibiotic, however, the diarrhea will continue for a longer time with sustained large volumes lost. A picture of a patient surrounded by the bottles required to treat him is seen in Figure 4. At the most severe extreme of the spectrum of disease it is not unusual for a person to purge 100 percent of his body weight in 4–7 days of diarrhea.[54]

TABLE 3. Intravenous Replacement Solutions

	Concentration (mEq or mmole/liter)				
	Na^+	K^+	Cl^-	HCO_3^-	Glucose
Diarrhea treatment solution (DTS)	118	13	83	48	50
[Dhaka] solution (5/4/1) 5 g NaCl 4 g $NaHCO_3$[a] 1 g KCl	134	13	99	48[a]	0
Ringer's lactate solution (Ringer's)	131	4	109	29	0

[a] Acetate may be substituted for bicarbonated for a more stable solution; sodium acetate anhydrous 3.9 g/liter, or if the triple hydrate is used 6.5 g/liter.

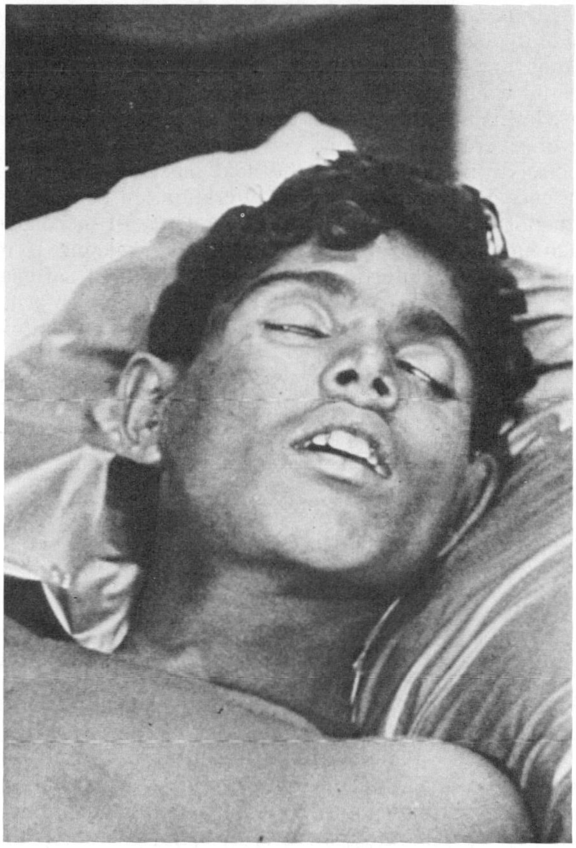

FIG. 3. Severely dehydrated patient with cholera.

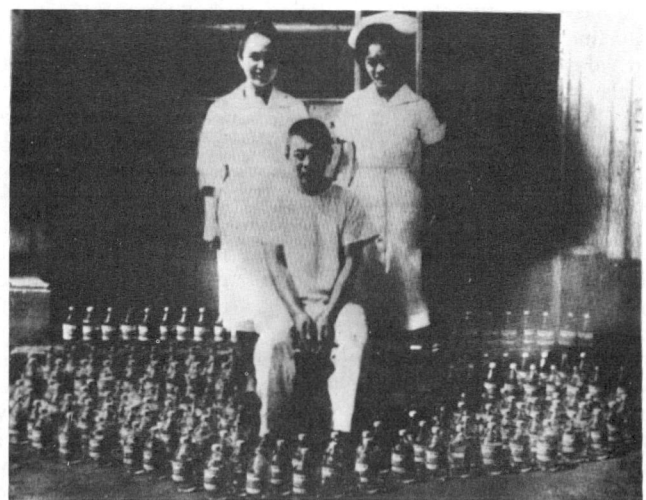

FIG. 4. Recovered cholera patient with bottles of intravenous fluid required to maintain him during his illness.

Complications that occur in cholera can be predicted from the nature of the disease with one exception, which, in the case of children, is most important. Altered consciousness is the rule in cholera, but the mental state is one of being in a somewhat detached state. Cholera patients even without a detectable blood pressure can be aroused and can give lucid and accurate information as to time, place, and person. In children one occasionally sees unconsciousness or convulsions. This may be a sign of hypoglycemia. Since this has obvious therapeutic implications, one must be alert to it. Hypoglycemia can also occur with little change in consciousness. The cause of low blood glucose levels is far from clear and is not related necessarily to states of severe malnutrition.[55]

Electrolyte imbalances are the next most common complication and also may manifest as alterations in consciousness that cannot be accounted for by the severity of the diarrhea. Most common in children in the tropics is hypokalemia. Its manifestations include intestinal ileus, weakness, and cardiac arrhythmias. If inappropriate solutions have been given at home or elsewhere, there may be hypernatremia or water intoxication. Acidosis if not attended to in severe cases can result in a fatal syndrome that is difficult to treat.[56] Renal failure is most often associated with inadequate hydration and the prior administration of a pyrogenic solution or various drugs and stimulants before rehydration. It is usually reversible without dialysis.

The combination of depressed states of consciousness and vomiting leads to a high risk of aspiration with its sequelae. Care must be taken while treating such patients to avoid this risk.

Pathophysiology

Cholera is a topical disease, the organism, *V. cholerae,* never actually entering any tissue of the body. It is swallowed either with water or food. It must survive passage through the stomach to colonize the small intestine even though it is extremely acid sensitive. In the small intestine it must find adequate culture conditions to proliferate. There are several characteristics of pathogenic *V. cholerae* that are important determinants of the colonization process. These include motility, chemotaxis, toxin production, and an as yet unknown colonization adhesion factor(s).[57,58] Once the organism has penetrated the mucous layer and has begun to colonize the lining epithelium of the gut, the intestine begins to secrete an alkaline, bile-rich solution that provides ideal growth medium for the vibrio. The adenylate cyclase-stimulating toxin secreted by the vibrio binds tightly to the GM_1 gangloside receptors of the lining cells and continues to exert its effect for many hours. It is not washed away once attached to its tissue receptor even when there is specific antibody present in the solution.

The mechanism of action of the toxin has been discussed but not its cell specificity in terms of its secretory effect. It is likely that the main source of secretion in the gut is the crypt cells of the small intestine. The villus tip cells are mainly occupied with absorption. The actual mechanism of fluid loss demands a full knowledge of the normal mechanisms of ion traffic in the different cells lining the gut. The new insights gained from studies of cholera have increased this understanding.[59] Probably all levels of the intestine are affected by the cholera toxin. What is seen as cholera stool is the net end-result of nonspecific stimulation of adenylate cyclase in all epithelial cells. The duodenum has the least absorptive capacity, so per unit length the most fluid is lost from this segment.[60,61] The colon has the greatest absorptive capacity and the least secretory capacity and contributes the least to the volume lost in cholera.

In addition to fluid losses it is very likely that the cholera toxin triggers a variety of other phenomena. Since the intestine is a very complex endocrine organ and many hormones are governed by the levels of cyclic nucleotides in the tissues that secrete them, it is likely that cholera toxin disorganizes the delicately integrated humoral systems that coordinate normal intestinal function in ways that have not as yet been defined. The mucous flecks in the stool, which account for the "rice" of the "rice-water," suggest that the discharge of mucus from the intestinal goblet cells is due to cholera toxin. Some data indicate that there is a decrease in the ability to produce gastric acid in cholera patients[62] possibly because the vibrio tends to select persons with low ability to produce acid or because the disease affects the regulation of gastric acid secretion. Thus, although the main features of fluid loss in cholera have been worked out to a considerable degree, there are still many features yet to be described. These are contingent on an improved knowledge of the humoral control mechanisms of the intestine.

Treatment

The treatment of cholera is extraordinarily simple, both in concept and execution. The water and salts lost in the cholera stool must be replaced in comparable amounts and concentrations. The replacement can, except in the most severe cases, be accomplished by mouth. Oral replacement solutions used are listed in Table 4. It cannot be emphasized strongly enough that the earlier replacement can be begun, the less chance there will be for complications secondary to severe volume depletion to occur. Packets of salts and a carrier substance such as glucose of the correct amounts to mix with a given volume of water should be given as soon as it is apparent that the diarrhea is of a sufficient severity to be life threatening. This treatment does not require a physician, nurse, or health worker of any sort. It demands that persons who may be at risk have sufficient knowledge to do the appropriate thing. If a packet of the appropriate mixture of salts is not available, table salt and sugar may be used according to the amounts listed in Table 4. Recently it has been shown that rice can substitute for glucose or sucrose to prepare an effective oral rehydration solution.[63] All except the most severe cases can be managed by oral replacement therapy alone.

Intravenous replacement therapy is needed by an increasing number of patients when the volume of stool output exceeds 100 ml/kg/24 hr or 7 liters/day in a 70-kg person. Intravenous therapy is also needed when appropriate oral rehydration has not been given, and a patient has been allowed to slip into shock.[64] The solutions that may be used are listed in Table 3. When a patient is in shock and has been heavily purging, a true emergency exists. An estimate must be made of the amount of fluid lost, using the guidelines given in Table 5. Initially the deficit must be replaced as rapidly as possible through an 18-gauge needle into a large vein. In this way about 1000 ml can be given in 10–15 minutes, and full initial hydration can be accomplished within an hour in most cases. The initial period is the most critical, and time should not be wasted in trying to do cutdowns. Any vein that can be entered quickly may be used. In our experience in Dhaka the order of preference is as follows: first, peripheral arm veins—if not too constricted; second, external jugular veins (both in adults and children); third, femoral vein; and fourth, in infants, scalp veins. The femoral vein can serve for very rapid infusion of the first 1 or 2 liters until a more stable location is available. Care should be taken to prepare the skin properly since infection can result. Even when a patient appears to have no heartbeat it is worth carrying out a rapid infusion because in near-terminal cholera patients the heart is

TABLE 4. Oral Replacement Solutions

	Weight in Grams of Salts to Add to 1 Liter of Drinking Water	Concentration (mEq or mmole/liter)				
		Na^+	K^+	Cl^-	HCO_3^-	Glucose
WHO solution						
NaCl	3.5	90	20	80	30	111
$NaHCO_3$	2.5					
KCl	1.5					
Glucose	20					
Household solution						
NaCl	5	85		85		111
Glucose[a]	20					

[a] May substitute sucrose 40 g/liter or rice powder 30–80 g/liter.

TABLE 5. Clinical Findings to Estimate Fluid Volume Depletion in Cholera

	Depletion (Percentage of Body Weight)		
Finding	*0–3*	*4–8*	*8–12*
Central pulses (femoral, carotid)	Full	Full	Weak
Peripheral pulses (radial, pedal)	Full	Weak	Absent
Skin turgor	Normal	Decreased	Poor
Eyes	Normal	Slightly sunken	Sunken
Muscles	Normal	Some cramps	Severe cramps
Appearance	Alert; slight thirst	Alert; thirsty	Restless; very thirsty
Urine flow	Normal	Reduced	Absent

inaudible and the pulses virtually absent. During therapy the peripheral and central pulses should be monitored to guide the initial rates of infusion. The blood pressure is of little use because peripheral arteries are constricted while strong central pulses remain. The lung bases should be observed for signs of congestion, particularly in patients who have been neglected and who have had long-standing acidosis.[56] When initial hydration has been successful, then the fluid losses must be matched. In severe cases it is best to leave the intravenous line in place while it is being determined whether the patient is able to keep up with his losses by drinking the oral replacement solution.

Antibodies will shorten the duration of diarrhea and thereby reduce fluid losses in cholera. Tetracycline and its congeners are the drugs of choice in most instances. A dosage of 250 mg every 6 hours for 3–5 days is adequate. In pregnancy cholera tends to lead to abortion, and an effective antibiotic seems indicated although there is no firm evidence that use of antibiotics does reduce the rate of fetal loss. Ampicillin, 250 mg every 6 hours for 5 days, is probably the safest agent in pregnancy. Other effective antimicrobial agents are chloramphenicol, trimethoprim–sulfamethoxazole, furazolidone, and doxycycline. With emergence of multiple antibiotic resistance furazolidone is increasingly useful. There is as yet no information on the oxyquinolones, which should be useful.

The most important life-threatening complication of cholera to recognize early is hypoglycemia. Any alteration in the state of consciousness particularly in a small child or baby must be assumed to be due to this and treated according to the best methods for managing hypoglycemia. This involves the intravenous infusion of 3–4 ml/kg of 25% glucose as a bolus and then adding glucose to the infusion to provide 10 mg/kg/hr. The blood glucose level should be determined and followed if possible in such instances.

Electrolyte imbalances are the next most common problems in the treatment of cholera. They usually present clinically as alterations in the state of consciousness or convulsions especially in the case of a low or high plasma sodium level. In acidosis there may also be, in severe cases, alterations in consciousness, severe hyperventilation, often with symptomatic respiratory distress, and restlessness. In the case of potassium depletion there may be irritability or even some obtundation, ileus that results in marked abdominal distention and an inability to take replacement solutions by mouth, and a marked weakness. For accurate diagnosis and treatment of these complications it is very useful to follow the serum electrolyte levels. Each should be corrected accurately but at a gradual pace to avoid rapid shifts in salts and water across tissues such as the brain to avoid the catastrophic complications associated with cerebral edema. Oral replacement solution is ideally suited to the gradual correction of hypo- or hypernatremia.

Renal failure should be treated conservatively. In most instances there may even have to be early modest potassium replacement in the face of anuria to protect against cardiac arrhythmias. Dialysis is rarely necessary and patients are usually able to eat sufficient calories as carbohydrates to minimize the breakdown of tissue proteins.

Ordinarily cholera has been seen in recent years in parts of the world where atherosclerosis is rare. When this disease has struck populations in Europe such as in Italy or Portugal there is an added risk of infarction of heart, brain, or kidney due to poor perfusion across diseased arteries. In such situations early and effective fluid replacement therapy is even more urgent. This is particularly important since when cholera enters a new nonendemic area the attack rate is similar across all age groups, whereas in an endemic area mostly young children are affected.

Methods of Diagnosis

It is not necessary to make a bacteriologic diagnosis to treat cholera or the related watery diarrheas because the fluids lost from the intestinal tract have approximately the same composition given an equivalent rate of stool output regardless of the etiology. Clinical diagnosis rests on the history of acute onset and the watery stool in the absence of high fever or much abdominal pain. Treatment is based solely on estimating the degree of dehydration by clinical and/or laboratory methods.

The stool when examined microscopically will not show any very distinctive features. Limited numbers of white cells and rarely red cells may be seen, and where there is endemic parasitic disease one may find the prevalent ova and helminths or protozoa. The most effective, rapid way of recognizing cholera specifically is by darkfield or phase microscopy. If cholera stool is viewed under darkfield conditions, vibrios are seen in large numbers with a characteristic motility that gives the appearance of shooting stars. If no antisera are used and one sees the characteristic vibrio and campylobacter motility, it is not possible to distinguish by motility characteristics those vibrios that agglutinate in the Ogawa or Inaba antisera from organisms that do not. If there is an epidemic it is most likely that true *V. cholerae* is what is seen, since the so-called noncholera vibrios do not cause epidemic disease. If the classical antisera for Ogawa and Inaba are available, the rapidly motile vibrio will be totally immobilized by adding the specific homologous antiserum, and an immediate specific diagnosis can be made.[41]

Cultures can be made either directly from stool or from a rectal swab. There are many media on which *V. cholerae* will grow readily, and each has advantages (Table 6). However, it seems best to use a relatively inhibitory medium that will discourage the overgrowth of other microflora and a medium from which colonies can be picked and directly tested by slide agglutination.

When seeking the cause of a nonepidemic clinical case of the disease, it is also desirable to look for noncholera vibrios[37] and enterotoxin-producing *E. coli,* in addition to *V. cholerae*. Unfortunately, neither of these organisms can be readily recognized as a pathogen without resorting to elaborate and controversial serologic reactions or to testing for the ability to produce enterotoxins.

TABLE 6. Media for Culturing *V. cholerae*

	Characteristics		
Agar Medium	*Inhibitory*	*Colony Appearance*	*Direct Slide Agglutination*
Gelatin	No	Clear, hazy ring	Yes
Meat extract	No	Clear-grayish	Yes
MacConkey's	Yes	Clear	No
Monsur	Yes	Black centers	Yes
TCBS	Yes	Yellow	No

HOST DEFENSE

Nonimmune Defenses

For *V. cholerae* to deliver its toxin to the lining cells of the small intestine it must traverse several potentially formidable barriers. The first of these is gastric acid. It has been shown in volunteers who have been fed vibrios that there is a difference of 1 million-fold in the dose required to establish disease in a person with gastric acid as compared with one who has had that acid neutralized.[65] It is likely that, were acid secretion stimulated as by histamine, the stomach would become virtually an absolute barrier to cholera. The importance of acid is further underscored since in situations where sporadic cases are occurring persons who have undergone gastrectomy or who are achlorhydric have higher attack rates.[66]

The next barriers are a complex of propulsive gut motility, the mucous lining layer, and a host of enzymes and bile salts. *Vibrio cholerae* has particular adaptations that permit it to thrive under these conditions, which tend to inhibit the growth of almost all other bacteria. The vibrios' combination of very active motility, a mucinase, chemotaxis directed toward the gut mucosa, and proteases all combine to allow this organism to colonize very successfully in the small intestine.

Those organisms that do not become established in the upper intestine then must compete with other microflora of the lower gut. The conditions in the terminal ileum and colon are unfavorable to vibrio growth. The acidic end products of anaerobic metabolism in the cecum rapidly destroy *V. cholerae*. Thus it is possible to have an infection of this organism in the jejunum and not detect it in the stool. This fact should be remembered when interpreting information on carriers based on data from stool cultures.

Systemic Immune Defenses

After natural infection by *V. cholerae,* circulating antibodies can be detected against several antigens including the toxin. Bacterial agglutinins were first detected in the sera of convalescent cholera patients.[1] Now antibodies to the specific somatic, or O, antigens can be demonstrated in a variety of ways including direct agglutination of heated *V. cholerae,* the agglutination of chicken red blood cells that have been coated with antigens, a vibriocidal test with the end point of vibriolysis, which is complement-dependent, and other complement fixation tests. In addition to the more specific O antigen—antibody reactions, antibodies to the H or flagellar antigens can also be detected after cholera. This antigen, shared with many other enteric organisms, is of no diagnostic value. All these antibodies can also be raised by parenteral injection of antigens as vaccine components.[52]

Vibriocidal antibodies reach a peak 8–10 days after onset of clinical illness and then decrease, returning to baseline 2–7 months later.[67] The vibriocidal response corrfeltes with resistance to infection[68] but as may be seen later may not be the main mediator of protection. The O antigens are determinants of vibriocidal titers and particularly in the case of vaccines may have some type-specific properties.

With the discovery and purification of cholera toxin the measurement of antitoxic immunity became possible. After natural infection patients develop antibodies to toxin. Protection does accrue from circulating antitoxin but probably not at the level induced by natural disease. Protection by circulating immunity to toxin has been shown both by parenteral immunization of animals by toxin or toxoid[69] and by passive transfer of a hyperimmune serum pool to nonimmunized animals. In a natural setting for cholera, however, there is no correlation between antitoxic antibody levels and incidence of the disease.[70]

The early response to somatic antigen after natural infection is in the IgM class. Subsequent challenges by either natural or parenteral vaccine antigens tend to produce an IgG response. Both responses decay after peaking 7–14 days after challenge. The role of circulating antibodies in protection against natural disease is not clear despite the correlation of vibriocidal antibodies with incidence of disease in an endemic area.[68] From experimental work it would seem likely that only IgG would be filtered to any extent across epithelium to the intestinal lumen, and it is only effective if titers are very high.[69] However, both IgG and IgM have been demonstrated in the gut lumen and have been shown to possess activity against cholera antigens.[71] It is likely that the only significance of circulating antibodies except when present in high titers is as epidemiologic markers of an infection or of parenteral immunization.

LOCAL IMMUNE DEFENSES

Since cholera is entirely a topical infection it would seem most likely that topical defenses would be the main determinant of protection against infection by *V. cholerae*. It has been known that recurrent infections are rare in cholera.[72] Also in endemic areas the incidence of disease decreases rapidly with age.[73] Thus there seems no doubt that highly effective immunity does occur in cholera. This has been further documented by volunteer studies in which persons who had previously been challenged with *V. cholerae* and had contracted the classical illness were rechallenged after a period of 3–6 months. Such people proved highly resistant to rechallenge despite rather low circulating antibody titers.[74] Thus it seems clear that there are powerful local immune defenses in the gut that are marshalled against cholera. Early work recognizing local antibody in contrast to serum antibody as a potentially important protective defense against experimental cholera carried out by Burrows has been reviewed.[1] From this awareness has evolved a more detailed knowledge of how local immune mechanisms in the intestines function. Antigens are detected by Peyer's patch lymphocytes. These immature cells then migrate through the lymphatics to the circulation and are "processed" at a site that has not been fully clarified as yet. The "processed" lymphocytes then return to the gut, and perhaps to other tissues, and tend to locate themselves in areas where antigen is present. Their product once back in the gut mucosa is secretory IgA. Studies using cholera toxin as a "probe" have allowed a description of this immunocyte traffic as it pertains to cholera.[75]

The question of how local secretion of IgA or the presence by exudation from the serum of IgG or IgM can mediate destruction of vibrios in an environment where complement does not function has challenged the ingenuity of investigators. There is no such problem with respect to how antitoxic antibodies may work. Clearly, if there is a layer of antibodies adjacent to the epithelium that will bind and deactivate toxin before it attaches to the cells, this will prevent all the disease manifestations. Thus at the surface of the intestine such antibodies may play a very important role in defense against clinical illness if not against infection itself. It is possible that failure by the upper intestine to secrete in response to toxin limits the growth medium available for the multiplication of *V. cholerae* so in fact antitoxic antibodies may at least limit the numbers of vibrios in an important way. Several mechanisms by which the growth of *V. cholerae* can be inhibited are likely. The process by which vibrios attach to gut epithelium is highly specific,[76] and antibodies against whole vibrios interfere with this process. Motility is important in the pathogenesis, and antibodies against whole vibrios or specific O antigen will cause clumping and arrested motion. It is unlikely that phagocytosis or vibriolysis is important in the gut lumen. The importance of antibodies to other specific vibrio traits associated with pathogenicity such as mucinase not yet known.

Measuring antibodies at the mucosal surface of the intestine is very difficult. The mucous layer overlying the epithelium may sequester antibodies within itself and hold them close to the gut surface. The contents of the gut lumen are heterogenous and highly proteolytic. The problem is to measure the antibodies that are present within several microns of the cells of villus tips and crypts. At present satisfactory methods have not been developed to do this. Most of our current knowledge has been derived from observing the traffic of immunocytes[75] and from challenge experiments.[74]

Vaccines

Since natural infection confers quite effective and long-lasting immunity against cholera, it seems reasonable that a vaccine could be made to elicit this protective immunity without disease. Early efforts were directed at preparing vaccines from killed whole vibrios that were injected parenterally. Critical tests of these vaccines did not occur until the early 1960s and showed that some protection could be achieved in populations where cholera was endemic. At best 90 percent protection was seen in the most potent vaccines used. This immunity waned rapidly such that only a trivial residual effect was present after a year.[77] Aluminum-adjuvanted vaccines have extended the duration and quality of protection of whole cell vaccines.[78] Purified polysaccharide fractions of the antigens specific for serotypes have also been used. Inaba polysaccharide and whole cell monospecific Inaba vaccines protected against infection by *V. cholerae,* Inaba El Tor biotype. A monospecific whole cell Ogawa vaccine did not give protection in the same epidemic.[79] In another trial in the Philippines significant protection was conferred by a monovalent Inaba whole cell vaccine against Ogawa infections.[80] Thus it would seem that Ogawa vaccines do not protect against Inaba infection, but Inaba vaccines do cross protect against Ogawa infections. This was in spite of a considerable vibriocidal titer against Inaba that was generated by the Ogawa vaccine, again suggesting that the vibriocidal titer itself is only an accidental correlate of protective immunity.

The addition of adjuvants was initially fraught with difficulties because of a high incidence of local reactions observed when an oil-adjuvant, whole cell vaccine was used in the Philippines. More recently reports of aluminum phosphate-adjuvanted vaccines that were tested both in the Philippines and Calcutta seem promising, with appreciable protection sustained for up to 2 years.[78]

The discovery and isolation of cholera toxin made possible the preparation of toxoid vaccines. To date fairly extensive animal testing has been done with formalinized and gluteraldehyde-dectivated material, and a field trial has been carried out with the gluteraldehyde toxoid.[81] This demonstrated a very low level of protection but seems to have been a poor antigen. A new candidate toxoid vaccine has been prepared recently by Swedish workers without the need of deactivation. This is based on isolated and purified binding (B) subunits that combined with lipopolysaccharide or whole cells would elicit theoretical maximum local immune response. The materials have been given by mouth without side effect to volunteers in Sweden, the United States, and Bangladesh. Local immune responses equal to those seen after natural disease have been observed[82] and protection against challenge documented.[83] Field tests of this oral cholera vaccine have demonstrated substantial protection for more than 1 year.[84]

With the knowledge that the most solid protection against cholera both in volunteers and in nature is conferred by a previous infection and that this protection is evident despite a low level of circulating antibodies, there is a major effort underway to develop a live vaccine strain of *V. cholerae*. The ideal specifications for such a strain would be an organism that possessed all the pathogenicity factors that allowed it to colonize the small intestine (motility, chemotaxis for gut epithelium, mucinase, adhesion factor, and so forth) but that did not produce a complete toxin molecule. It would be desirable for it to produce the binding (''B'' or ''light'') chain of the toxin, since this does not produce diarrhea or damage and would elicit antibodies against itself, thus developing a solid local prevention for binding of the complete toxin molecule. The most rational and effective way to go about preparing such a vaccine strain would be by modern genetic engineering techniques. Previously candidate strains have been sought in nature or by the action of mutagenic agents. Originally, in 1963, Mukerjee isolated four strains of water vibrios from the Middle East and seven strains from Calcutta. The most promising of these strains has been given to humans without causing disease but is known to produce a low level of toxin. It does elicit antitoxic antibodies in infected hosts. Because of this it seems likely that reversion to full toxigenicity might occur in a large-scale trial so this has not been done. The same has been true of a mutant generated by mutagenic agents in the laboratory by Finkelstein more recently. Bhaskaran and Sinha[85] first applied mutagenic methods to generate vaccine strains; however, the strain they chose to test probably lacks a colonizing ability and for this reason has not been pursued. Most recently another strain generated by a mutagen has been reported and has been characterized as a vibrio that produces only B fragments of the toxin.[86] Recombinant live oral cholera vaccines have recently been described that have conferred substantial protection in volunteer studies.[87]

EPIDEMIOLOGY AND PREVENTION

Manner of Spread

There are still many unanswered questions about the spread of cholera. The epidemic disease even in endemic areas is characterized by periods between outbreaks of many months during which there is no evidence of *V. cholerae* in water or food, there are no animals or vectors known, and there are no human carriers in large populations surveyed by rectal swab methods. This is not to say that chronic human carriers do not exist—they do, but they are rare. Where then does *V. cholerae* make its home between outbreaks? One possibility is that the large reservoir of *V. cholerae* not agglutinable by standard typing sera present in surface water throughout the world can, given certain circumstances, undergo genetic change to become a fully virulent epidemic strain. This could occur by a variety of routes, which include plasmid exchanges, transduction by phage, transformation, or mutations. Since mutation is discrete and rare, it is the least likely mechanism, and since ability to detect human carriers is not very good, it is not possible to discriminate between these possibilities. Another possibility supported by some evidence is the existence of *V. cholerae* is a unique ecological niche perhaps with altered growth characteristics.[51,53]

During epidemics there are many persons purging large volumes of vibrio-rich stool, which often contaminates the water that is used for washing, swimming, cooking, or drinking. Early definitive observations on the spread of cholera by water were made by John Snow in England during the epidemic of 1832.[15] In most situations to the present time water seems the principal route of epidemic spread. Food has also been implicated in some epidemics but it is often through the use of contaminated water at some point in the preparation process.[73] Although the El Tor biotype has a longer survival in nature outside of the host than classical strains, it is still fragile and does not last as long as other enteropathogens. It can be said that except in the case of very special conditions in which the water is alkaline (pH 7.5–8.5), cool, shaded, and free of competing bacteria, the life span of *V. cholerae* outside of the human host is usually less than 5 days. Survival in food is even more limited; however, some shellfish if refrigerated can provide a vehicle that is worrisome. These have played a role in outbreaks in the Philippines, Thailand, and more recently in Italy.[88]

As has been pointed out, vibrios that appear identical to *V. cholerae* Inaba or Ogawa but lack the O-specific antigens continuously inhabit surface waters the world over. At present altered forms of *V. cholerae* in specific ecologic associations seem the most plausible reservoir from which epidemic strains could spring.[51,53]

Human carriers do exist and in some instances can shed vibrios for a very long time, even years. Up until 1959 the idea that such carriers played an important role in the spread of disease was not given much credulity.[89] All seem to agree that people with mild illness or in convalescence are important during the epidemic spread of cholera. As has been discussed, however, during a full outbreak there is generally little mystery about how the disease is spreading since there are many cases and a variety of opportunities by which water and food are contaminated. With the advent of the El Tor biotype more importance has been given to human carriers, since this variant persists in man longer and produces more subclinical infection than did classical strains.

There are several important problems about the detection of human carriers. If vibrios are sequestered in the gallbladder or upper intestine, they may not be found in stool since acid conditions in the colon will kill them. Thus a carrier may be silent, detected only if intubation of the upper intestine, or if a purgative is given that is strong enough to result in an alkaline stool. For this reason the number of chronic carriers may be underestimated. Another approach has been to screen the sewerage effluents from populations for *V. cholerae*. During interepidemic periods in Calcutta, positive isolates have been found.[90] There seems no doubt that a role is played by transient human carriers or those with mild cases during epidemic periods. It is possible that the few chronic carriers may explain sequestration in interepidemic periods as well. More attention is needed to this question as well as to the potential for a pool in nature of vibrios that are converted under appropriate conditions from innocuous water vibrios to pathogens capable of epidemic spread.

The pattern of outbreaks has indicated that the greatest risk of disease is among household contacts of symptomatic cholera patients.[91] There is a qualitative difference in attack rates between populations that have continuing experience with cholera and those that do not. In cholera-endemic zones the extent of infection is great,[92] and the highest incidence is in children, sparing the first 2 years of life. In areas not experiencing cholera all age groups are equally attacked. There may be differences in attack rates dependent on which persons in the households are most in contact with soiled clothing, cleaning of stool, and so forth. These may vary according to the cultural settings of the disease. Common source outbreaks do occur and depend on such things as contaminated bottled water (Portugal, 1974) or shellfish (Italy, 1972).[93]

Prevention

It is clear that if there were no opportunities for water or food to be contaminated with cholera vibrios, there would be no spread of the disease. This means that with adequate attention to sanitation and hygiene cholera is not a problem. Much of the world as yet does not have a basic waste disposal system that functions. Even in wealthy countries with excellent technology, examples of raw sewage mingling with surface waters are not rare. Thus few areas of the world are truly inaccessible to the spread of cholera. With the gradual march of the El Tor biotype out of Asia across the Middle East to Africa and Europe over the past decades, it should be apparent that all parts of the world may be affected by the present pandemic and are vulnerable to the new classical strain.

Surveillance of cases of diarrhea or of sewage are perhaps the best early warning methods. If one awaits a cluster of cases of full severity, there will be a rather large community reservoir. In the case of El Tor variants as many as 100 asymptomatic or mild cases exist for each severe illness.[73] When a case is located, if it is an isolated instance, as in importations from affected areas, quarantine procedures may be of help. Most important is to be sure that the disposal of stool is into a system that effectively decontaminates this waste or that vibriocidal agents are used before disposal. In most situations early warning is lacking and the disease is already widespread in the community when discovered. Furthermore the communities attacked are poor, crowded, and characteristically without adequate disposal of human wastes. In such situations few measures have proven effective although many are used and have had claims made for them. It can be said that since the epidemic curve of cholera outbreaks is characteristically abrupt, by the time public health measures are actually applied the epidemic has peaked and is waning. Thus any measure will appear to be highly effective and everyone is satisfied.

Let us look at a few of the measures advocated. Boiling of water for all purposes is an expensive undertaking since it requires a considerable quantity of fuel. When such a program is recommended the authorities should be ready to provide the needed energy source for doing it, otherwise it is usually out of reach economically for the population most at risk—the poor. Clean water sources such as by means of deep tubewells may be provided, but unless these can product sufficient water to supply all needs, there will be little impact. It does no good to provide a safe water source for drinking and cooking if people bathe and wash household articles in contaminated water. Perhaps the simplest and most overlooked measure during an epidemic is effective hand washing which at least may cut down cross contamination within a household where cholera cases are present. Care should be taken when a community is known to harbor cholera that any food products or water that will be used by other communities is not contaminated. Flies may carry *V. cholerae* from contaminated areas but are not a vector of proven importance.

Immunization compaigns with present vaccines are costly and relatively ineffective. They do not reduce the spread of disease only the incidence of clinical cases. New vaccines offer promise but much more work remains before wide application can be realized. One documented benefit is cross protection against diarrhea associated with heat labile toxin producing *E. coli*.

In rural areas of developing countries most of the methods commonly advocated cannot be implemented. Treatment, however, is very simple and highly effective. The major emphasis should be on this. It should never be neglected in favor of control measures that are of doubtful effectiveness.

Role of Treatment

At the present time, since vaccines are not very effective and control measures during outbreaks are also of limited value, the central importance of inexpensive simple and effective treatment seems obvious. With proper management there is no reason for any patient to die from cholera. Although the vast majority of patients will do very well on oral rehydration therapy alone, particularly if started early, there will always be some patients who will require intravenous fluids with the expertise and equipment necessary to give them effectively.

In the affected communities there should be a major effort to teach people how to mix and to give oral rehydrating solution. If no packets of the ideal composition are available, instructions should be provided on how to mix table salt and sugar with an appropriate volume of water. A simple safe prescription is one three-finger pinch of salt and handful scoop of sugar in ½ liter or 1 pint of drinking water. As soon as a mixture that includes bicarbonate and potassium can be provided, this can be readily substituted because the necessity of measuring properly how much water to mix with salts and sugar remains the same for the simple mixture of home ingredients or for a manufactured packet.

A treatment center should be established where seriously fluid-depleted patients can promptly receive intravenous fluids.

This requires 24-hour coverage by trained staff and proper solutions, tubing, and needles. In severe epidemic situations patients can be managed very effectively simply by observing the pulse and appearance without further measurements. Simple but accurate observations on intake and output are possible using cholera cots and buckets (Fig. 5).

Tetracycline or furazolidone should be given to all patients suspected of cholera since they will shorten the diarrhea and will reduce the need for intravenous and oral fluids. In addition, use of an antibiotic will decrease the potential for contaminating the environment. Multiple antibiotic resistance now seems to be an expanding problem,[40,95,96] and tests must be done for this.

Effective sterilization of all stool and vomit is essential before disposal to avoid any chance that the treatment center may be a source of spread of the disease. Despite such measures, in rural areas where patients are brought in small boats, the area around a treatment center will be contaminated, and people in the neighborhood should be protected in all ways possible. It is likely that taking the patient out of his community to a treatment area will reduce the contamination of the home community while somewhat increasing the risk to the area near the hospital.

Anticipation and planning of how to manage epidemic cholera is very important, since the volume of fluids required and the fulminant nature of the disease usually serves to frighten and disorganize even modern facilities. Improvisation is usually needed. Because of the speed with which cholera can kill, and the simplicity and effectiveness of treatment, locating centers near the areas affected is particularly important even if sophisticated facilities are available but are several hours of travel away.[97]

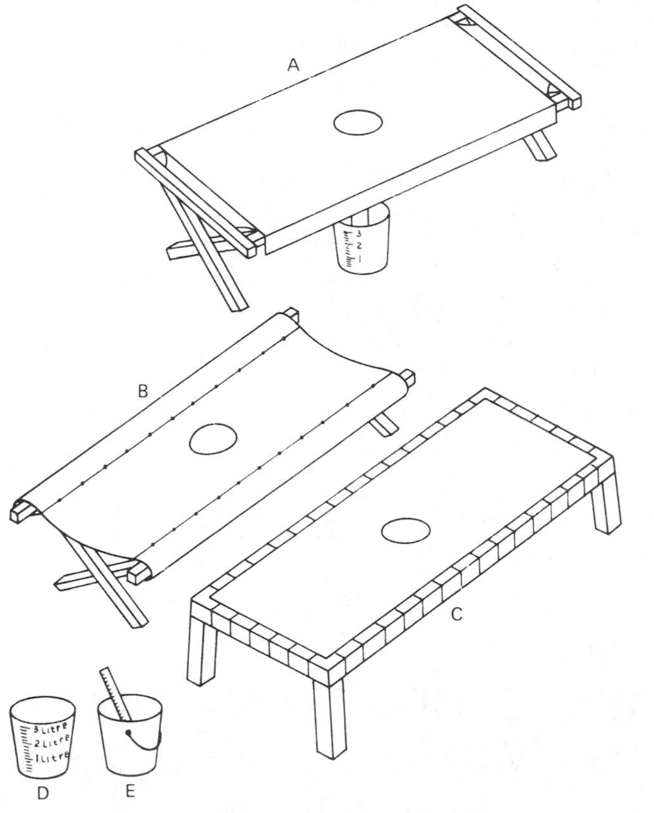

FIG. 5. Several simple cholera cots for patient comfort and ease in measuring stool output during cholera. **(A)** Camp cot with hole on which plastic sheet can be placed; sleeve channels stool to calibrated bucket. **(B)** Camp cot with hole on which plastic sheet can be placed to channel stool to bucket. **(C)** Jute on wood frame bed. **(D)** Calibrated bucket for stool to be placed under cholera cots. **(E)** Bucket with calibrated stick (alternative method). The plastic sheet is desirable but not essential for effective use of these cots. The size of the cots can be adjusted for children or adults.

REFERENCES

1. Pollitzer R. Cholera. Geneva: World Health Organization; 1959.
2. Rosenberg CE. The Cholera Years. Chicago: University of Chicago Press, 1962.
3. Marquez GG. Love in the Time of Cholera. New York: Alfred A. Knopf; 1988.
4. Gotschlich F. Vibrios Choleriques isolés au campement de Tor. Retour du pélerinage de l'annéé, 1905. Report adressé au President du Conseil quarante naine d'Egypt, Alexandria. Quoted in Bull Inst Louis Pasteur. 1905; 3:726.
5. Dizon JJ, Alvero MG, Joseph PR, et al. Studies on El Tor in the Philippines: (1) Characteristics of cholera El Tor in Negros Occidental Province, November 1961 to September 1962. Bull WHO. 1965;33:627.
6. Felsenfeld O. A review of recent trends in cholera research and control. Bull WHO. 1966;34:161.
7. Goodgame RW, Greenough WB III. Cholera in Africa. A message to the West. Ann Intern Med. 1975;82:101.
8. Woodward WE, Mosley WH. The spectrum of cholera in rural Bangladesh 11. Comparison of El Tor, Ogawa and classical Inaba infection. Am J Epidemiol. 1971;96:342.
9. Gerichter CB, Sechter I, Cohan J, et al. A serological survey for cholera antibodies in the population of Jerusalem and surroundings. Isr J Med Sci. 1973;9:980.
10. Bart KJ, Huq Z, Khan M, et al. Seroepidemiologic studies during a simultaneous epidemic of infection with El Tor, Ogawa and classical Inaba *Vibrio cholerae*. J Infect Dis. 1970;12(Suppl):17–24.
11. Samadi AR, Huq MI, Shahid NS, et al. Classical *Vibrio cholerae* biotype displaces El Tor in Bangladesh. Lancet. 1983;1:805–7.
12. Shahid NS, Samadi AR, Khan MK, et al. Classical vs El Tor cholera: a prospective family study of a concurrent outbreak. J Diar Dis Res. 1984;2:73–8.
13. Hugo MI, Sanyal SC, Samadi AR, et al. Comparative behaviour of classical and El Tor biotypes of *Vibrio cholerae* O1 isolated in Bangladesh during 1982. J Diar Dis Res. 1983;1:5–9.
14. Sanyal SC, Sil J, Dutta NK, et al. Present status of classical cholera in India. Indian J Med Res. 1972;60:1564.
15. Snow J. On the Mode of Communication of Cholera. 2nd ed. London: Churchill; 1855. (Reprinted as Snow on Cholera. New York: Hafner; 1965.)
16. De SN, Chaterjee DN. An experimental study of the mechanism of action of *Vibrio cholerae* on the intestinal mucous membrane. J Pathol Bacteriol. 1953;66:559.
17. Dutta NK, Habbu MK. Experimental cholera in infant rabbits. A method for chemotherapeutic investigation. Br J Pharmacol. 1955;10:153.
18. De SE: Enterotoxicity of bacteria free culture filtrates of *Vibrio cholerae*. Nature. 1959;183:1533.
19. Finkelstein RA, Lo Spalluto JJ. Pathogenesis of experimental cholera. Preparation and isolation of choleragen and choleragenoid. J Exp Med. 1969;130:185.
20. Field M, Fromm D, Wallace CK, et al. Stimulation of active chloride secretion in small intestine by cholera exotoxin. J Clin Invest. 1969;48:24a.
21. Schafer DE, Lust WD, Sircar B, et al. Elevated concentration of adenosine 3'5' cyclic monophosphate in intestinal mucosa after treatment with cholera toxin. Proc Natl Acad Sci USA. 1970;67:851.
22. Sharp GWG, Hynie S. Stimulation of intestinal adenylate cyclase by cholera toxin. Nature. 1971;229:266.
23. Kimberg DV, Field M. Johnson J, et al. Stimulation of intestinal mucosal adenylate cyclase by cholera enterotoxin and prostaglandins. J Clin Invest. 1971;50:1218.
24. Chen LC, Rohde JE, Sharp GWG. Properties of adenylate cyclase from human jejunal mucosa during naturally acquired cholera and convalescence. J Clin Invest. 1972;51:892.
25. Van Heyningen WE, Carpenter CCJ, Pierce NF, et al. Deactivation of cholera toxin by ganglioside. J Infect Dis. 1971;124:415.
26. Holmgren J, Lonnroth I, Svennerholm L. Tissue receptor for cholera exotoxin. Postulated structure from studies with GM_1 ganglioside and related glycolipids. Infect Immun. 1973;8:208.
27. Finkelstein RA. Cholera enterotoxin (choleragen): an historical perspective. In: Barua D, Greenough WB III, eds. Topics in Infectious Disease: Cholera. New York: Plenum; 1990.
28. Gill DM, Woolkalis M. Toxins which activate adenylate cyclase. In: Evered D, Whelan J, eds. Microbial Toxins and Diarrhoeal Disease. Ciba Foundation Symposium 112. London: Pittman Publishing; 1985:57–73.
29. Vaughan M. Choleragen, adenylate cyclase, and ADP ribosylation. In: The Harvey Lectures, Series 77. New York: Academic Press; 1983:43–62.
30. Zinnaka Y, Carpenter CCJ Jr. An enterotoxin produced by noncholera vibrios. Johns Hopkins Med J. 1972;131:403.
31. Giannella RA, Gots RE, Charney AN, et al. Pathogenesis of *Salmonella* mediated intestinal fluid secretions. Activation of adenylate cyclase and inhibitions by indomethacin. Gastroenterology. 1975;69:1238.
32. Gyles C, So M, Falkow S. The enterotoxin plasmids of *E. coli*. J Infect Dis. 1974;130:40.
33. Vasil ML, Holmes RK, Finkelstein RA. Conjugal transfer of a chromosomal

gene determining production of enterotoxin in *Vibrio cholerae*. Science. 1975;187:849.
34. Kaper JB, Baldini MM. Genetics. In: Barua D, Greenough WB III, eds. Topics in Infectious Disease: Cholera. New York: Plenum; 1990.
35. Mekalanos JJ, Sublett RD, Romig WR. Genetic mapping of toxin regulatory mutations in *Vibrio cholerae*. J Bacteriol. 1979;139:859.
36. Mekalanos JJ, Moseley SL, Murphy JR, et al. Isolation of enterotoxin structural gene deletion mutations in *Vibrio cholerae* induced by two mutagenic vibriophages. Proc Natl Acad Sci USA. 1982;79:151.
37. McIntyre OR, Feeley JC, Greenough WB III, et al. Diarrhea caused by noncholera vibrios. Am J Trop Med Hyg. 1965;14:412.
38. McIntyre OR, Feeley JC. Characteristics of noncholera vibrios isolated from cases of human diarrhea. Bull WHO. 1965;32:627.
39. Colwell RR, ed. Vibrios in the Environment. New York: John Wiley & Sons; 1984.
40. Glass RI, Huq MI, Lee JV, et al. Plasmid borne multiple drug resistance in *Vibrio cholerae* serogroup 01, biotype El Tor: evidence for a point source outbreak in Bangladesh. J Infect Dis. 1983;147:204–9.
41. Benenson AS, Islam MR, Greenough WB III. Rapid identification of *Vibrio cholerae* by darkfield microscopy. Bull WHO. 1964;30:827.
42. Kabir S. Characterization of the lipopolysaccharide from *Vibrio cholerae* 395 (Ogawa). Infect Immun. 1982;38:1263.
43. Sack RB, Miller CE. Progressive changes in vibrio serotypes in germ-free mice infection with *Vibrio cholerae*. J Bacteriol. 1969;99:688.
44. Colwell RR. Polyphasic taxonomy of the genus *vibrio*. Numerical taxonomy of *Vibrio cholerae, Vibrio parahemolyticus*, and related vibrio species. J Bacteriol. 1970;104:410.
45. Citarella RV, Colwell RR. Polyphasic taxonomy of the genus *vibrio*. Polynucleotide sequence relationships among selected vibrio species. J Bacteriol. 1970;104:434.
46. Kerosky A, Markel OE, Touchstone B, et al. Chemical characterization of cholera toxin and its natural toxoid. J Infect Dis. 1975;133:S14.
47. Sanyal SC, Alam K, Neogi PKB, et al. A new cholera toxin (Letter). Lancet. 1983;1:1337.
48. Felsenfeld O. Notes on food, beverages and fomites with *Vibrio cholerae*. Bull WHO. 1965;33:725.
49. Felsenfeld O. The survival of cholera vibrios. In: Barua D, Burrows W, eds. Cholera. Philadelphia: WB Saunders; 1974:359–66.
50. Huq MI, Sanyal SC, Samadi AR, et al. Comparative behaviour of classical and El Tor biotypes of *Vibrio cholerae* 01 isolated in Bangladesh during 1982. J Diar Dis Res. 1983;1:5–9.
51. Spira WM. The ecology of *Vibrio Cholerae*. In: Barua D, Greenough WB III, eds. Topics in Infectious Disease: Cholera. New York: Plenum; 1990.
52. Barua D. Laboratory diagnosis of cholera, in Barua D, Burrows W (eds): Cholera. Philadelphia, Saunders, 1974, pp 85–126.
53. Huq A, Small EB, West PA, et al. Ecological relationships between *Vibrio cholerae* and planktonic crustacean copepods. Appl Environ Microbiol 45:275, 1983.
54. Hirschhorn N, Kinzie JL, Sachar DB, et al. Decrease in net stool output during intestinal perfusion with glucose-containing solutions. N Engl J Med. 1968;279:176.
55. Hirschhorn N, Lindenbaum J, Greenough WB, et al. Hypoglycemia in children with acute diarrhea. Lancet. 1966;2:128.
56. Greenough WB III, Hirschhorn N, Gordon RS Jr, et al. Pulmonary edema associated with acidosis in patients with cholera. Trop Geogr Med. 1976;28:86.
57. Nelson ET, Clemens JD, Finkelstein RA. *Vibrio cholerae* adherence and colonization in experimental cholera electron microscopic studies. Infect Immun 1976;14:527.
58. Yamamoto T, Yukota T. Electron microscopic study of *Vibrio cholerae* O1 adherence to the mucus coat and villus surface in the human small intestine. Infect Immun. 1988;56:2753–9.
59. Field M. Role of cyclic nucleotides in enterotoxic diarrhea. Adv Cyclic Nucleotide Res. 1980;12:267.
60. Carpenter CCJ, Greenough WB III. Response of the canine duodenum of intraluminal challenge with cholera exotoxin. J Clin Invest. 1968;47:2600.
61. Greenough WB III. Pancreatic and hepatic hypersecretion in cholera. Lancet. 1965;2:991.
62. Sack GH Jr, Pierce NF, Hennessey KN, et al. Gastric acidity in cholera and non cholera diarrhoea. Bull WHO. 1972;47:31.
63. Molla AM, Sarker SA, Hossain M, et al. Rice-powder electrolyte solution as oral therapy in diarrhoea due to *Vibrio cholerae* and *Escherichia coli*. Lancet. 1982;1:1317.
64. Greenough WB III. Cholera. In Conn HF, ed. Current Therapy. Philadelphia: WB Saunders; 1984:13–17.
65. Hornick RB, Music SI, Wenzel R, et al. The Broad Street pump revisited. Response of volunteers to ingested cholera vibrios. Bull NY Acad Med. 1971;47:1192.
66. Gitelson S. Gastrectomy, achlorhydria and cholera. Isr J Med Sci. 1971;7:663.
67. Sack RB, Barua D, Saxena R, et al. Vibriocidal and agglutinating antibody patterns in cholera patients. J Infect Dis. 1966;116:630.
68. Mosley WH. The role of immunity in cholera. A review of epidemiological and serological studies. Tex Rep Biol Med. 1969;27(Suppl. 1):227.
69. Pierce NF, Kaniecki E, Northrup RS. Protection against experimental cholera by antitoxin. J Infect Dis. 1972;126:606.
70. Martin AR, Vernon TB, Mosley WH. Neutralization of the vascular permeability factor of *V. cholerae* in man. Am J Trop Med Hyg. 1969;18:253.
71. Freter R. Coproantibody and bacterial antagonism as protective factors in experimental enteric cholera. J Exp Med. 1956;104:419.
72. Woodward WE. Cholera reinfection in man. J Infect Dis. 1971;123:61.
73. Gangarosa EJ, Mosley WH. Epidemiology and surveillance of cholera. In: Barua D, Burrows W, eds. Cholera. Philadelphia: WB Saunders; 1975:381–403.
74. Levine MM, Black RE, Clements ML, et al. Duration of infection-derived immunity in cholera. J Infect Dis. 1981;143:818.
75. Pierce NF, Gowans JL. Cellular kinetics of the intestinal immune response to cholera-toxoid in rats. J Exp Med. 1975;142:1550.
76. Jones GW, Freter R. Adhesive properties of *Vibrio cholerae*. Nature of the interaction with isolated rabbit brush border membranes and human erythrocytes. Infect Immun. 1976;14:240.
77. Joo I. Cholera vaccines. In: Barua D, Burrows W, eds. Cholera. Philadelphia: WB Saunders; 1975:333–55.
78. Joo I. Aluminum adjuvated vaccines. Forty-third Nobel Symposium; 1979.
79. Mosley WH, Woodward WE, Aziz KMA, et al. The 1968–69 cholera vaccine field trial in rural East Pakistan. Effectiveness of monovalent Ogawa and Inaba vaccines and a purified Inabva antigen with comparative results of serological and animal protection tests. J Infect Dis. 1970;121(Suppl):S1–S9.
80. Watanabe Y. Antibacterial immunity in cholera. In: Barua D, Burrows W, eds. Cholera. Philadelphia: WB Saunders; 1975:283–306.
81. Curlin G. Cholera toxoid field trial. In: Fukumi H, Zinnaka, eds. Twelfth Joint Conference on Cholera. The US–Japan Cooperative Medical Science Program Symposium on Cholera, Sapporo, 1976:276–85.
82. Holmgren J, Svennerholm AM. Cholera and the immune response. In: Hanson LA, Kallos P, Westphal O, eds. Host Parasitic Relationship in Gram-Negative Infections. Basel: S. Karger; 1983:106.
83. Levine MM, Kaper JB, Black RE, et al. New knowledge on pathogenesis of bacterial enteric infections as applied to vaccine development. Microbiol Rev. 1983;47:510–50.
84. Clemens JD, Harris J, Sack DA, et al. Field trial of oral cholera vaccines in Bangladesh: results of one year follow-up. J Infect Dis. 1988;158:60–9.
85. Bhaskaran K, Sinha VB. Attenuation of virulence in *V. cholerae*. J Hyg (Lond). 1967;65:307.
86. Finkelstein RA. Current developments with cholera vaccines: "Where do we go from here?" Prog Clin Biol Res. 1980;47:133.
87. Levine MM, Kaper JB, Herrington D, et al. Safety, immunogenicity and efficacy of recombinant live oral cholera vaccines, CVD 103 and CVD 103-HgR. Lancet. 1988;ii:467–70.
88. de Lorenzo F, Soscia M, Manzillo G, et al. Epidemic of cholera El Tor in Naples 1973. Lancet. 1974;1:669.
89. Dizon JJ. Cholera carriers. In: Barua D, Burrows W, eds. Cholera. Philadelphia: WB Saunders, 1975;367–79.
90. Sinha R, Deb RC, De SP, et al. Cholera carrier studies in Calcutta in 1966–67. Bull WHO. 1967;37:89.
91. Mosley WH, Alvero MG, Joseph PR, et al. Studies of cholera El Tor in the Phillippines. 4. Transmission of infection among neighbourhood and community contracts of cholera patients. Bull WHO. 1965;33:651.
92. McCormack WM, Islam MS, Fahimuddin M, et al. A community study of inapparent cholera infections. Am J Epidemiol. 1969;89:658.
93. Glass RI, Black RE. The epidemiology of cholera. In: Barua D, Greenough WB III, eds. Topics in Infectious Disease: Cholera. New York: Plenum; 1990.
94. Clemens JD, Sack DA, Harris JR, et al. Cross protection by B subunit—whole cell cholera vaccine against diarrhea associated with heat-labile toxin-producing enterotoxigenic *Escherichia coli*: results of a large-scale field trial. J Infect Dis. 1988;158:372–7.
95. Huq MI, Alim ARMA, Mutanda LN, et al. Multiply antibiotic-resistant O group 1 *Vibrio cholerae*—Bangladesh MMWR. 1980;24:109.
96. Glass RI, Huq MI, Alim AR, et al. Emergence of multiply antibiotic resistant *Vibrio cholerae* in Bangladesh. J Infect Dis. 1982;142:939.
97. Baqui AH, Yunus M, Zaman K. Community-operated treatment centres prevented many cholera deaths. J Diar Dis Res. 1984;2:92–8.
98. Lai CY, Mendez E, Chang D. Chemistry of cholera toxin: the subunit structure. J Infect Dis. 1976;133:23–30.

193. OTHER PATHOGENIC VIBRIOS

CHARLES C. J. CARPENTER

In addition to *Vibrio cholerae* 01 and *Campylobacter fetus* (formerly known as *Vibrio fetus*), three additional major groups of vibrios have been clearly associated with human disease. These include the halophilic *V. parahaemolyticus*, of which the epidemiologic and clinical features are reasonably well delineated; other halophilic vibrios including *V. alginolyticus* and *V. vul-*

nificus, which are less common causes of human disease; and the nonhalophilic non-01 *V. cholerae* and *V. mimicus*, which are worldwide in distribution and have frequently been incriminated in human illness.

In the United States, illnesses caused by all of the commonly isolated pathogenic vibrios have a marked seasonal peak in the summer and early fall. This presumably reflects both seasonal changes in recreational water use and the documented increase in numbers of vibrios in both the Chesapeake Bay and the Gulf Coast waters during the warmer months.

VIBRIO PARAHAEMOLYTICUS

Vibrio parahaemolyticus, a halophilic (salt-requiring) vibrio, has long been recognized as the major cause of acute diarrheal disease in Japan.[1] In the past 2 decades, this microorganism has been incriminated in major food poisoning outbreaks along the Atlantic and Gulf Coasts of the United States and on Caribbean cruise ships.[2,3] *Vibrio parahaemolyticus* is a major pathogen in a number of the less-developed countries in which it has been incriminated in up to 20 percent of acute diarrheal illnesses. In the United States, the illness has generally occurred in acute self-limited outbreaks affecting groups of people who have been exposed to common sources of raw or inadequately cooked seafood. In Bangladesh, illness caused by *V. parahaemolyticus* occurs sporadically, with a broad spectrum of clinical manifestations ranging from mild watery diarrhea to a frank dysentery-like syndrome. As suggested by the clinical disease as well as by experimental studies in animals, *V. parahaemolyticus* has the capacity of both producing an enterotoxin and causing an inflammatory reaction in the small bowel mucosa. The enterotoxin, however, seldom causes major degrees of intestinal fluid loss, and the tissue damage caused by this halophilic vibrio is generally less extensive than that observed in shigellosis.

Epidemiology

Because of lack of specificity of the clinical features of the illness, the epidemiologic history usually provides the most important clue to diagnosis. The halophilic *V. parahaemolyticus* is ubiquitous in coastal waters,[1,4,5] and when seafood is inadequately cooked or contaminated by saltwater, the microorganisms can rapidly proliferate to a concentration sufficient to produce disease in humans. In the United States, virtually all confirmed cases have been common-source outbreaks related to the following: (*1*) ingestion of seafood, especially shrimp or crabmeat, that has been inadequately cooked and then allowed to remain at ambient temperatures for several hours; (*2*) ingestion of raw seafood (rarely); or (*3*) contamination of food by seawater (thus, largely limited to shipboard outbreaks). Attack rates are very high in exposed populations; the 51 percent attack rate observed in the very large outbreak after a Louisiana "shrimp boil"[2] is similar to that observed after outbreaks on Caribbean cruise ships.[3]

Secondary spread has not been documented in the Western Hemisphere or in Japan, presumably because of the high level of environmental sanitation and/or the relatively large infective dose.[6] Secondary cases are, however, also rare in areas in which environmental sanitation is less adequate,[5] which suggests that the high infective dose is the most important factor in preventing secondary cases.

Vibrio parahaemolyticus has rarely been cultured from asymptomatic people, and no carrier state has been identified. This microorganism is apparently pathogenic only for humans, and there is no known mammalian reservoir of infection.

Clinical Manifestations

The illness commonly begins with the acute onset of explosive watery diarrhea, often accompanied by mild to moderately severe cramping abdominal pain. In North America and Japan, the onset of illness is generally within 24 hours of ingestion of the contaminated seafood. The median incubation period in the largest documented North American outbreak was 23 hours, with a range of 5–92 hours.[2] The diarrhea is accompanied by low-grade fever, mild chills, and headache in less than one-half of the cases. The electrolyte loss is rarely severe enough to cause decreased skin turgor or postural hypotension. The rare deaths associated with diarrhea caused by *V. parahaemolyticus* have been largely confined to very young children or elderly people with underlying disease.

Laboratory Findings

The diarrheal fluid is characteristically watery, sometimes mucoid, and less often bloody (>15 percent). Microscopic examination of the stool is not of major diagnostic value; in most cases, a few leukocytes are seen (10–20 white blood cells per high-power field), but in some people large numbers of both leukocytes and erythrocytes are observed. Stool culture on appropriate media provides the definitive diagnosis by demonstrating the pleomorphic gram-negative rods, which are facultative anaerobes. *Vibrio parahaemolyticus* grows poorly and is therefore easily overlooked on the standard desoxycholate culture plates. The organism is, however, readily identified on the selective thiosulfate citrate bile salts sucrose (TCBS) agar, on which it appears as a distinct opaque green colony. Final identification is made by standard biochemical tests.[1] Enrichment of fecal culture specimens, especially useful for epidemiologic investigation, can be carried out in hypertonic saline containing 3% sodium chloride in 1% peptone broth, pH 7.4,[6] or in taurocholate-tellurite water.[7] Almost all pathogenic strains of *V. parahaemolyticus* cause β-hemolysis of human erythrocytes (positive Kanagawa reaction), but it is not clear that this property bears any direct relationship to the pathogenicity of the microorganism.[1]

Differential Diagnosis

Since the halophilic *V. parahaemolyticus* is ubiquitous in coastal waters throughout the temperate and tropical zones of the world,[4] this pathogen must be considered in the differential diagnosis of all acute diarrheal illnesses that follow the ingestion of seafood. There are no clinical features that, in the individual case, reliably distinguish diarrhea caused by *V. parahaemolyticus* from that caused by enterotoxigenic *Escherichia coli* or from milder cases of shigellosis or salmonellosis. Vomiting is characteristically less prominent than in disease caused by staphylococcal enterotoxin, and the cramping abdominal pain is generally less severe than that observed in food poisoning caused by *Clostridium perfringens*.

Treatment

No treatment is required by the large majority of patients. The disease is self-limited, and antimicrobial therapy shortens neither the clinical course nor the duration of pathogen excretion. Antiperistaltic agents are of no clear-cut benefit. Occasional patients, usually at the extremes of age, may lose sufficient quantities of fluid to require oral or intravenous electrolyte therapy. In such cases, therapy is guided by the same principles used in the treatment of cholera.

Prevention

Since the illness usually results from the ingestion of raw or inadequately cooked seafood or food that has been rinsed with contaminated seawater, simple means of prevention are available. Most North American outbreaks can be prevented by ensuring that seafoods are prepared at high enough temperatures to kill the microorganisms. *Vibrio parahaemolyticus* can remain viable in shrimp or crabmeat for several minutes at temperatures as high as 80°C, and it is especially important in cooking large quantities of such foods to ensure that all portions of the seafood are exposed to cooking temperatures adequate to kill the microorganism. Of only slightly less importance is the necessity of refrigerating cooked seafood if it is not to be ingested immediately after cooking. Since the generation time of *V. parahaemolyticus*, under the proper circumstances, is less than 15 minutes, a few microorganisms can proliferate to levels sufficient to cause disease in humans if inadequately cooked seafood is left for several hours at ambient temperatures.

Two outbreaks of diarrheal disease due to *V. parahaemolyticus* on Caribbean cruise ships were traced to the use of contaminated seawater, available in the ship's fire system, in one case to wash frozen seafood and in the other to wash the decks of the galley. The contaminated seafood was left at ambient temperatures for several hours before being served. Such outbreaks can obviously be prevented either by avoiding the use of untreated seawater in galleys or by inadequate refrigeration of cooked seafood until it is served.

Prevention of disease due to *V. parahaemolyticus* in Japan remains a problem because of the popularity of uncooked seafood in that nation. Since there is little likelihood either of eradicating the halophilic vibrios from the coastal seawaters or of changing the custom of ingesting raw seafood, *V. parahaemolyticus* will probably remain a major cause of acute diarrheal disease in Japan.

Likewise, in delta areas such as Bangladesh in which people have daily contact with contaminated water, there is little likelihood of altering the incidence of *V. parahaemolyticus* infections in the foreseeable future.

Data are not available to determine whether or not protective immunity is conferred by clinical infection. No effective vaccine is currently available.

OTHER HALOPHILIC NONCHOLERA VIBRIOS

Other halophilic noncholera vibrios that have clearly been implicated in human disease include *V. vulnificus* and *V. alginolyticus*. (*V. fluvialis* and *V. hollisae*, which appear to produce clinical syndromes similar to non-01 *V. cholerae*, and *V. damsela*, which has been implicated in wound infections in a manner similar to *V. vulnificus*, will not be discussed in detail because the role of these seawater-associated vibrios in human disease is less well established.) Like other potentially pathogenic halophilic vibrios, *V. vulnificus* and *V. alginolyticus* are probably part of the normal marine flora and, in the temperate zones, reach sufficient concentrations to cause clinical illness only in the warmer months of the year.

Clinical Manifestations

Unlike *V. parahaemolyticus* and non-01 *V. cholerae*, *V. vulnificus*, and *V. alginolyticus* have not been associated primarily with diarrheal illness but rather with soft tissue infections and/or septicemia. All such illnesses appear to have been associated with the contact of superficial wounds with seawater or with ingestion of seafood.

Vibrio vulnificus (originally described as an L+ or lactose-fermenting vibrio) is the most virulent of the noncholera vibrios and produces two clinical syndromes distinct from those caused by other vibrio species.[8–10] In the compromised host, especially in people with hepatic cirrhosis, *V. vulnificus* has the ability to cross the gut mucosa rapidly and invade the blood stream without causing gastrointestinal symptoms. The clinical picture is one of abrupt onset of chills and fever, often (33 percent) followed by hypotension, usually (75 percent) followed by the development of metastatic cutaneous lesions within 36 hours after onset. The cutaneous lesions begin as erythematous lesions, and rapidly evolve to hemorrhagic bullae or vesicles and then to necrotic ulcers. *Vibrio vulnificus* bacteremia has been fatal in over 50 percent of patients in whom this syndrome has been identified, including all patients in whom hypotension developed. In otherwise healthy people, *V. vulnificus* has been implicated in the rapid development of intense cellulitis, necrotizing vasculitis, and ulcer formation and is often associated with bacteremia after contamination of a superficial wound by warm seawater. The cellulitis generally responds to appropriate antimicrobials, but incision and drainage and/or débidement are often necessary.[10]

V. vulnificus has also, rarely, been associated with acute, self-limited diarrheal illnesses in individuals who were receiving antacid therapy.[11]

Vibrio alginolyticus has been etiologically associated with cellulitis and acute otitis media or otitis externa. These infections have generally occurred in otherwise healthy seawater swimmers or fishermen and have responded well to appropriate antibiotics.[12] *Vibrio alginolyticus* may also occasionally cause life-threatening bacteremia in immunocompromised individuals.

Differential Diagnosis

Vibrio vulnificus should be suspected in any compromised host (especially with underlying cirrhosis) who develops a septicemic illness associated with necrotizing cutaneous lesions within 1–3 days after the ingestion of oysters. Although rare, the clinical syndrome appears to be a distinct one and should suggest this diagnosis.

Similarly, the development of cellulitis on the extremities of people occupationally or recreationally exposed to seawater should suggest *V. vulnificus* (especially in the presence of severe, necrotizing cellulitis) or *V. alginolyticus*.

Vibrio vulnificus and *V. alginolyticus* grow readily on the standard mediums that contain sodium chloride (e.g., MacConkey agar) as well as the selective TCBS medium; final identification is made by standard biochemical tests. It is important to note that *V. vulnificus*, because of its ability to ferment lactose, may be described as "no enteric pathogen" in a routine diagnostic laboratory unless the technician is advised to look specifically for this microorganism.

Treatment

The soft tissue and ear infections caused by *V. vulnificus* and *V. alginolyticus* generally respond well to appropriate antibiotics and, when necessary, surgical drainage. Early administration of antibiotics is critical because the soft tissue infections may spread very rapidly. The response with bacteremic *V. vulnificus* infections in compromised hosts is less predictable. *Vibrio vulnificus* is not uniformly susceptible to the aminoglycosides, which are often used in bacteremia caused by the more common aerobic gram-negative bacilli, and appropriate antimicrobial therapy (a tetracycline is the first choice, with chloramphenicol or a penicillin as an alternative) must be initiated early when the clinical picture suggests infection by this microorganism.[10]

Prevention

Since both *V. vulnificus* and *V. alginolyticus* appear to be part of the normal flora of seawater in warmer climates, there is no sure way of preventing soft tissue infections by occupationally or recreationally exposed people. Because of the high mortality rate of septicemic *V. vulnificus* infection and because of its clear epidemiologic relationship to the ingestion of raw oysters, it would be wise to suggest that immunocompromised people, especially those with hepatic cirrhosis, avoid the ingestion of raw seafoods.

NONHALOPHILIC VIBRIOS: NON-0 GROUP 1 VIBRIO CHOLERAE AND VIBRIO MIMICUS

Vibrio cholerae 0 group 1 has historically been of greatest concern to the medical profession, and other vibrios have often been dismissed as noncholera vibrios (NCVs) or nonagglutinable vibrios (NAGs) because they failed to agglutinate in *V. cholerae* 0 group 1 antiserum. Since vibrios that are biochemically similar to *V. cholerae* but do not agglutinate in *V. cholerae* 0 group 1 antiserum are now toxonomically included in the species *V. cholerae*, they will be referred to as non-01 *V. cholerae* in this discussion. Another nonhalophilic vibrio, *V. mimicus*, closely related to non-0 group 1 *V. cholerae*, has recently been recognized as the cause of sporadic illness over a wide geographic area. These nonhalophilic vibrios require only trace amounts of sodium chloride for growth in culture medium; this growth characteristic distinguishes them from the true halophilic vibrios *V. parahaemolyticus*, *V. vulnificus*, and *V. alginolyticus*, which require larger concentrations of sodium chloride in culture media and have the remarkable ability to grow in 10% sodium chloride.

Clinical Manifestations

Non-01 *V. cholerae* organisms are capable of producing a wide spectrum of diarrheal illnesses ranging from severe watery diarrhea indistinguishable from cholera to the milder traveler's diarrhea of the type commonly associated with enterotoxigenic *E. coli*. Certain clinical isolates of non-01 *V. cholerae* have been shown to produce enterotoxin very similar to if not identical with the *V. cholerae* enterotoxin; other clinical isolates of non-01 cholera strains lack the capacity to produce an identifiable enterotoxin under in vitro conditions.[12] No specific clinical features reliably distinguish the milder diarrheal illnesses caused by non-01 *V. cholerae* from those caused by more commonly recognized enteric pathogens.[13]

V. mimicus has caused sporadic outbreaks of acute diarrheal illness in healthy individuals who have ingested raw seafood, both along the American Gulf Coast[14] and in Bangladesh.[15] The clinical spectrum of this illness is indistinguishable from that caused by *V. parahaemolyticus*. *Vibrio mimicus* may rarely, like *V. alginolyticus*, cause acute otitis in saltwater swimmers.

Laboratory Findings

With intestinal infections caused by both non-01 1 *V. cholerae* and *V. mimicus*, the diarrheal fluid reflects the clinical manifestations and varies from the watery isotonic fluid characteristic of cholera gravis to loose stools in which small numbers of leukocytes and erythrocytes may be seen. The organisms are easily overlooked on standard desoxycholate agar plates but are readily identified on TCBS agar on which they appear as opaque yellow colonies; final speciation is made by type-specific antisera.

Treatment

No treatment is required by the large majority of patients with diarrheal disease, and antimicrobials have not been shown to shorten the clinical course.[13] In occasional patients, especially those in the developing world, the intestinal fluid loss is sufficient to require oral or intravenous electrolyte therapy. In such patients, therapy is guided by the same principles used in the treatment of cholera.

Epidemiology

Non-01 *V. cholerae* are worldwide in distribution and ubiquitous in water sources. Sporadic cases result from the ingestion of very large inocula from contaminated water sources. Likewise, the occasional microepidemics, as have occurred in Czechoslovakia and the Sudan, have apparently resulted from heavy contamination of food and water sources, respectively.[16,17]

In every carefully studied major outbreak of cholera, non-01 vibrios have been isolated from a small proportion of patients (1–5 percent) with illnesses indistinguishable from those caused by *V. cholerae*. There are several possible explanations for this observation, including the loss by certain classic *V. cholerae* of the relevant agglutinating surface antigens, the acquisition by non-01 *V. cholerae* of the gene coding for the production of cholera enterotoxin (unlikely since this gene is chromosomally located in *V. cholerae*), or the acquisition by non-01 *V. cholerae* of the plasmid-mediated gene coding for production of the *E. coli* enterotoxin (possible but never demonstrated either in vitro or in vivo).

Prevention

Since non-01 *V. cholerae* exist in a variety of water sources ranging from freshwater rivers to the oceans, purification of water sources and adequate cooking of fish and other seafoods provide the only certain protection against these occasional pathogens.

REFERENCES

1. Zen-Yoji H, Sakai S, Terayama T, et al. Epidemiology, enteropathogenicity, and classification of *Vibrio parahemolyticus*. J Infect Dis. 1965;115:436.
2. Barker WH, Mackowick PA, Fishbein M, et al. *Vibrio parahemolyticus* gastroenteritis outbreak in Covington, Louisiana, in August 1972. Am J Epidemiol. 1974;100:316.
3. Centers for Disease Control. Gastroenteritis caused by *Vibrio parahaemolyticus* aboard a cruise ship. MMWR. 1978;27:67.
4. Kaneko T, Colwell R, Ecology of *Vibrio parahemolyticus* in Chesapeake Bay. J Bacteriol. 1973;113:24.
5. Bockemuhl J, Amedome A, Triemer A. *Vibrio parahemolyticus* gastroenteritis during the el tor cholera pandemic in Togo (West Africa). Am J Trop Med Hyg. 1975;24:101.
6. Dadisman TA, Nelson R, Molenda JR, et al. *Vibrio parahemolyticus* gastroenteritis in Maryland. I. Clinical and epidemiological aspects. Am J Epidemiol. 1973;96:414.
7. Monsur KA. Bacteriological diagnosis of cholera under field conditions. Bull WHO. 1963;28:387.
8. Bonner JR, Coker AS, Berryman CR, et al. Spectrum of *Vibrio* infections in a Gulf Coast community. Ann Intern Med. 1983;99:464.
9. Pollak SJ, Parris EJ III, Barrett TJ, et al. *Vibrio vulnificus* septicemia. Arch Intern Med. 1983;143:837.
10. Tacket CO, Brenner F, Blake PA. Clinical features and an epidemiologic study of *Vibrio vulnificus* infections. J Infect Dis. 1984;149:558.
11. Johnston JM, Becker SF, McFarland LM. Gastroeneteritis in patients with stool isolates of *Vibrio vulnificus*. Am J Med. 1986;80:336.
12. Blake PA. Disease of humans (other than cholera) caused by vibrios. Annu Rev Microbiol. 1980;34:341.
13. Morris JG, Wilson R, Davis BR, et al. Non-0 group 1 *Vibrio cholerae* gastroenteritis in the United States: Clinical, epidemiologic and laboratory characteristics of sporadic cases. Ann Intern Med. 1982;94:656.
14. Shandera WX, Johnston JJ, David BR, et al. Disease from infection with *Vibrio mimicus*; A newly recognized *Vibrio* species. Ann Intern Med. 1983;99:169.
15. Spira WM, Fedorka-Cray PJ: Purification of enterotoxins from *Vibrio mimicus* that appear to be identical to cholera toxin. Infect Immun. 1984;45:679.
16. Aldova E, Laznickova K, Stepankova E, et al. Isolation of non-agglutinable vibrios from an enteritis outbreak in Czechoslovakia. J Infect Dis. 1968;118:25.
17. World Health Organization. Outbreak of gastroenteritis by non-agglutinable (NAG) vibrios. WHO Weekly Epidemiol Rec. 1969;44:10.

194. CAMPYLOBACTER SPECIES

MARTIN J. BLASER

Campylobacteriosis refers to the group of infections caused by gram-negative bacteria of the genus *Campylobacter*. Among the most common bacterial infections of humans in all parts of the world, campylobacters cause both diarrheal and systemic illnesses and are highly associated with gastritis and peptic ulcer disease. Infection of domesticated animals with campylobacters also is widespread. *Campylobacter* is derived from the greek *Campylo*, meaning curved, and *bacter*, meaning rod, so named to distinguish this genus from identically appearing vibrios.

BACTERIOLOGY

Campylobacters are motile, non-spore-forming, comma-shaped gram-negative rods.[1] Originally isolated from aborted sheep fetuses in 1909, these and similar organisms were called *Vibrio fetus*. However, since these organisms did not ferment carbohydrates and had different Guanine-plus-Cytosine DNA contents from true members of the genus *Vibrio*, a new genus, *Campylobacter*, was created. There are now 14 recognized species within the genus[2]; however, recent taxonomic studies suggest that new species may be named.

Table 1 lists the *Campylobacter* species most commonly associated with human disease and indicates the differentiating characteristics. Certain species such as *C. nitrofigilis* and *C. concisus* have not yet been associated with human illness. In contrast, the "nitrate-negative campylobacters" are associated with diarrheal illnesses, but the appropriate nomenclature for the organisms has not been determined.

Three types of illnesses are associated with *Campylobacter* species—enteric, extraintestinal, and gastric. For each of these illnesses, one *Campylobacter* species predominates while other species are less commonly present. The prototype for enteric infection is *C. jejuni*, for extraintestinal infection it is *C. fetus*, and for gastric infection it is *C. pylori* (Table 2).

Campylobacters grow best in an atmosphere containing 5–10 percent oxygen and are thus considered microaerophilic.[1–3] Although most will not grow under aerobic or anaerobic conditions, *C. jejuni* will grow in candle jars, which permits isolation when the optimal atmosphere can not be achieved. All campylobacters grow at 37°C; however, *C. jejuni* grows best at 42°C. Because *C. jejuni* is the most common enteric pathogen of humans, many laboratories have used incubation at 42°C for optimal isolation; however, the use of this temperature will not allow detection of all species.

Campylobacters multiply more slowly than do the usual enteric flora and therefore cannot be isolated from fecal specimens unless selective techniques are used. The most common isolation methods used in the past include blood-based, antibiotic-containing media. Three such media, Skirrow, Butzler, and Campy-BAP or variations of these have been in wide use.[2,3] The last two media contain cephalothin, which inhibits *C. fetus* and several other *Campylobacter* species but are best suited for isolating *C. jejuni*. Several enrichment broths have been developed, but since ill humans usually excrete 10^6–10^9 *C. jejuni* colony-forming units (cfu)/g stool, enrichment usually is not necessary. Blood-free media also can be used.[4] Due to their small size (0.3–0.6 μm diameter) and motility, campylobacters pass through 0.45 or 0.65 μm filters that retard the usual enteric flora. Filtration methods permit isolation without use of antibiotic-containing media. It is now clear that the use of filtration techniques and nonselective media such as chocolate agar with incubation of plates at 37°C improves stool culture yields of both *C. jejuni* and the "atypical" enteric campylobacters.[5] The development of filtration techniques represents a significant advance over selective media and is now recommended for primary isolation of campylobacters from fecal specimens or swabs.

Visible colonies usually appear on the plating media within 24–48 hours. Occasionally growth takes place after 72–96 hours of incubation, especially for the "atypical" species. The campylobacters can be distinguished from other microorganisms on the basis of several standard criteria and can be distinguished from one another on the basis of biochemical testing.[2,3] Organisms from young cultures have a typical vibrioid appearance (Fig. 1), but after 48 hours of incubation organisms appear coccoid. The ability to hydrolyze hippurate distinguishes *C. jejuni* from most other members of the genus, but hippurate-negative *C. jejuni* isolates also occur. Isolation of campylobacters from sites without a normal flora such as the blood stream is not difficult, although when suspected, incubation of cultures should be extended to 2 weeks. With radiometric detection systems, turbidity of the medium may not be present, and the increase in released radiolabel may be less than usually specified thresholds, which reflects suboptimal conditions for certain of these organisms.[6]

Similar to other bacteria whose ecologic niche is the gastrointestinal tract of mammals, the serotypic diversity of *C. jejuni* is enormous. More than 90 different serotypes based on somatic (0) antigens and 50 different serotypes based on heat-labile (capsular and flagellar) antigens have been identified,[2] and phase variation of flagellar antigens occurs. No group somatic, capsular, or flagellar antigen has been identified; however, the major outer membrane protein and a superficial protein appear to have broad serotypic specificity, factors that may aid in the development of a broadly specific vaccine.

Campylobacter jejuni cannot long withstand drying or freezing temperatures, which are characteristics that limit its transmission.[7] However, *C. jejuni* survives in milk, other foods, or water kept at 4°C for several weeks. Pasteurization effectively destroys the organism, as do the concentrations of chlorine used for water disinfection.

TABLE 1. Differential Characteristics of *Campylobacter* Species as Related to Human Disease

	Growth				H_2S in			Susceptibility to 30 μg disk			
Species	25°	37°	42°	Nitrate Reduction	TSI	Lead Acetate Paper	Hippurate Hydrolysis	Cephalothin	Nalidixic Acid	C-19 Fatty Acid Reduction	Urea Hydrolysis
C. jejuni	−	+	+	+	−	+	+[a]	R	S	+	−
C. coli	−	+	+	+	v	+	−	R	S	+	−
C. laridis	−	+	+	+	−	+	−	R	R	−	−
C. fetus ssp. *fetus*	+	+	v	+	−	v	−	S	R	−	−
C. hyointestinalis	v	+	v	+	+	+	−	S	R	−	−
C. cinaedi	−	+	−	+	−	+	−	S	S	−	−
C. upsaliensis[b]	−	+	+[c]	+	−	+	−	S	S	−	−
C. fennelliae	−	+	−	−	−	+	−	S	S	−	−
C. pylori	−	+	v	−	−	+	−	S	R	+	+

Key: −: does not have the characteristic; +: has the characteristic; v: some strains show the characteristic; R: resistant; S: susceptible.
[a] About 5–10 percent of *C. jejuni* strains are hippurate-negative.
[b] Catalase-negative or weak.
[c] Occasional isolates fail to grow at 42°C.

TABLE 2. Etiologic Agents Associated with Different Clinical Manifestations of *Campylobacter* Infection

	Manifestation		
Pathogen	*Enteric*	*Extraintestinal*	*Gastric*
Major	*C. jejuni*	*C. fetus*	*C. pylori*
Minor	*C. coli* *C. laridis* *C. fetus* *C. fennelliae* *C. cinaedi* *C. upsaliensis* *C. cryaerophila* "Nitrate-negative *Campylobacter*"	*C. jejuni* *C. coli* *C. laridis* *C. fennelliae* *C. cinaedi* *C. sputorum* *C. hyointestinalis*	GCLO-2

EPIDEMIOLOGY

Campylobacteriosis is a worldwide zoonosis. Campylobacters are commonly found as commensals of the gastrointestinal tract of wild or domesticated cattle, sheep, swine, goats, dogs, cats, rodents, and all varieties of fowl.[1,7] *Campylobacter jejuni* has a very varied reservoir, but *C. coli* and *C. hyointestinalis* are most commonly isolated from swine and *C. upsaliensis* from dogs. *Campylobacter fetus* ssp. *fetus* has been isolated from sheep, cattle, and swine,[1] Primary *Campylobacter* infections of animals often occur early in life and may produce morbidity or mortality, but in most infected animals a lifelong carrier state with specific immunity develops. The vast reservoir in animals is probably the ultimate source for most enteric *Campylobacter* infections of humans. Meats originating from infected animals frequently become contaminated with intestinal contents during the slaughtering process.[7] Excreta from infected animals may contaminate soil or water.

Most infections of humans probably result from the consumption of contaminated food and water. Investigations of more than 50 outbreaks indicate that unpasteurized (raw) milk is such a vehicle.[7] Similarly, untreated surface water has been responsible for both endemic and epidemic campylobacteriosis. Backpackers in Wyoming who drank untreated water had *Campylobacter* infections three times as commonly as *Giardia* infections.[8] Several large outbreaks have been traced to defects in municipal water systems.[9] Undercooked meats, especially poultry, have been associated with infection.[10] Other vehicles include raw clams, undercooked beef, and unpasteurized goat's milk and cheeses. Nevertheless, the consumption of undercooked poultry is estimated to be responsible for 50–70 percent of sporadic *Campylobacter* infections in developed countries. Increases in the isolation of *Campylobacter* species represent both improved recognition and increased consumption of poultry in recent years.

Direct contact with infected animals may result in transmission. Household pets, especially young dogs and cats with diarrhea, have been implicated as vectors for campylobacteriosis.[11] Since healthy dogs, cats, rodents, and birds may excrete campylobacters, it is not surprising that human infections associated with these animals also have been reported. Persons with occupational exposure to cattle, sheep, and other farm animals are at increased risk for infection, and laboratory-acquired infections have been reported.

As with other enteric pathogens, fecal–oral person-to-person transmission of *C. jejuni* has been reported. Those in contact with the excreta of infected persons who are not toilet trained (such as infants) are themselves at risk for infection. Infected school-age children may transmit *Campylobacter* infection, but this appears to be much less common. Transmission from infected food handlers who are asymptomatic is at best uncommon. Perinatal transmission from a mother who was not necessarily symptomatic may be due to exposure in utero, during passage through the birth canal, or during the first days of life.[12] Infection has been associated with blood transfusion from an infected patient.[13] Because of a variety of sexual practices in the pre–AIDS era, homosexual men appear to have been at increased risk for *C. cinaedi*, *C. fennelliae*, and other "atypical" campylobacters.[14]

Campylobacter jejuni infections occur year-round in the United States and other developed countries, but with a sharp peak in summer and early fall. *Campylobacter fetus* infections show the same seasonal variation, but the peak is less marked. In tropical countries, the seasonal variation of *C. jejuni* infection is influenced by rainfall. Because of incomplete surveillance, the actual incidence of *Campylobacter* infections in the United States is not known. However, laboratory-based studies in the United States and other developed countries indicate that *C. jejuni* is usually more commonly isolated from fecal specimens from diarrheal patients than is either *Salmonella* or *Shigella*.[15] In England, the number of reported *Campylobacter* infections now exceeds those of *Salmonella* and *Shigella* infections combined, and the incidence continues to increase.

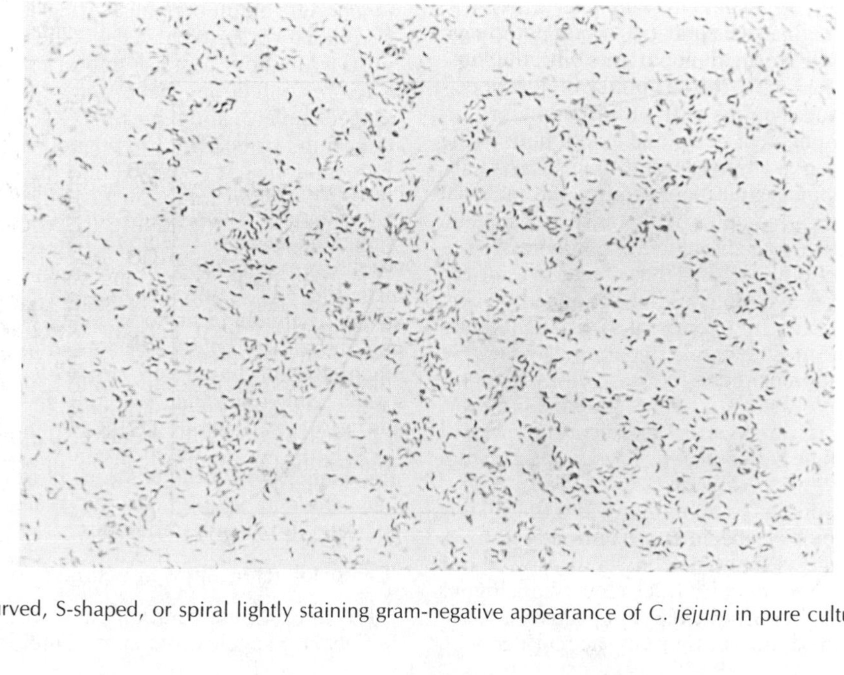

FIG. 1. Fine curved, S-shaped, or spiral lightly staining gram-negative appearance of *C. jejuni* in pure culture. (×1000)

On the basis of estimates of numbers of *Salmonella* infections, there may be more than 2 million *Campylobacter* infections annually in the United States. Population-based studies show a peak incidence in children under 1 year old and in persons 15–29 years old[16]; however, cases have been reported in patients of all ages. The sex ratio appears to be about equal. The prevalence of infection in healthy people is very low (less than 1 percent).

In marked contrast are the results of studies in developing countries. Isolation of *C. jejuni* from healthy persons is much more common and is especially pronounced in the first 5 years of life.[17,18] In these endemic areas, *Campylobacter* infections occurring early in life frequently are symptomatic, whereas later infections are mostly asymptomatic.[18] The substantial age-related difference in the infection-to-illness ratios in the developed and developing countries appears primarily to be due to differences in age- or exposure-related immunity of the populations rather than differences in the isolates.[19] *Campylobacter jejuni* and other campylobacters are important causes of the acute diarrheal illnesses suffered by travelers visiting developing areas.[20]

PATHOGENESIS AND PATHOLOGIC CHARACTERISTICS

Not all *Campylobacter* infections produce illness. Although all factors responsible for this phenomenon are not known, two of the most important appear to be the dose of organisms reaching the small intestine and the specific immunity of the host to the pathogen ingested. Among exposed persons who become ill, the incubation period varies from 1 to 7 days, a characteristic that is probably inversely related to the dose ingested. Most infections occur 2–4 days after exposure. Volunteers have become ill after ingesting as few as 500 organisms, but below a dose of 10^4 organisms, illness was infrequent. *Campylobacter jejuni*, like *Salmonella typhimurium*, is susceptible to hydrochloric acid.[21] Taken together, these data suggest that the infectious dose for *C. jejuni* is similar to that for *Salmonella*. Vehicles such as milk, fatty foods, and water, which favor passage through the gastric acid barrier, probably permit some infections to occur at relatively low doses.

Campylobacter jejuni multiplies in human bile,[21] a characteristic that aids colonization of the bile-rich upper small intestine early in infection. The sites of tissue injury include the jejunum, ileum, and colon, with similar pathologic features in each. Inspection of affected tissues may reveal a diffuse, bloody, edematous, and exudative enteritis,[22] but pathologic examinations are generally performed on patients with the most severe cases. Microscopic examination of rectal biopsy specimens has shown a nonspecific colitis with an inflammatory infiltrate of neutrophils, mononuclear cells, and eosinophils in the lamina propria; degeneration; atrophy; loss of mucus; crypt abscesses in the epithelial glands; and ulceration of the mucosal epithelium.[23,24] Rectal biopsy samples with these nonspecific features have been interpreted as showing acute ulcerative colitis or Crohn's disease. In other cases, the appearance of the rectal biopsy sample has been similar to that produced by *Salmonella* or *Shigella* infections. In a series of 124 patients with *C. jejuni* infection, 18 of the most severely ill patients underwent a sigmoidoscopic examination or rectal biopsy; 17 of these procedures showed colonic involvement.[25] Some patients have terminal ileitis as well as colitis. Host factors are clearly important as well; in volunteers a single strain produced a wide spectrum of clinical manifestation.[26]

The presence of bacteremia in some patients and the finding of cellular infiltration in biopsy specimens from patients with *Campylobacter* colitis suggests that tissue invasion may be one pathogenetic mechanism. No animal model closely analogous to human infection has been reported except in primates. *Campylobacter* outer membranes contain lipopolysaccharides with typical endotoxic activity. Extracellular toxins with cytopathic activities have been found, and classic enterotoxins have also been demonstrated, although generally at low concentrations.[27,28] Two strains lacking detectable enterotoxin production but with low-level in vitro cytotoxin production were fully virulent in volunteers.[26] Infected persons do not develop neutralizing antibodies to these toxins, further casting doubt on their in vivo significance. *Campylobacter jejuni* may adhere to epithelial cells,[29] which favors gut colonization. In vivo passage favors flagellated cells.[30]

Patients in developed countries with *Campylobacter* infection excrete the organism in feces for an average of 2–3 weeks. By 3 months postinfection, convalescent excretion is rare. In developing countries, convalescent excretion is even briefer, probably reflecting high levels of immunity in the population.[19]

Bacteremia sometimes can be detected in patients with *Campylobacter* infections, whether or not they show signs of systemic illness. Most bacteremias reported to the Centers for Disease Control (CDC) have been due to *C. fetus* ssp. *fetus*, whereas *C. jejuni* is by far the more common pathogen. One explanation for the apparently greater tendency for *C. fetus* than *C. jejuni* to cause bacteremia is that the former is usually resistant and the latter susceptible to the bactericidal activity present in normal human serum.[31]

Campylobacter fetus is covered with a surface (S) protein that functions as a capsule.[32] Virtually all human isolates of *C. fetus* possess an S protein that completely disrupts C3b binding to these organisms.[33] The lack of C3b binding explains both serum and phagocytosis resistance. In a mouse model, after oral inoculation strains carrying the S protein develop bacteremia, whereas strains without the S protein do not. The S protein of *C. fetus* appears to be a major virulence factor explaining its extraintestinal spread.

IMMUNITY

Volunteers rechallenged with the homologous *C. jejuni* organism developed infection but were protected from illness.[26] In developing countries where *C. jejuni* infection is hyperendemic, the decreasing case-to-infection ratio with age suggests the acquisition of immunity. Patients infected with campylobacters develop specific IgG, IgM, and IgA antibodies in serum[26,28] and IgA antibodies in intestinal secretions.

In developing countries, specific serum IgA levels rise progressively with age, which reflects recurring exposure to *C. jejuni*. In volunteers, increasing levels of specific serum IgA correlated with increasing specific intestinal levels as well. Supporting the notion that humoral immunity is protective against *C. jejuni* infections have been the numerous reports of prolonged, severe, and recurrent *C. jejuni* infection in patients with congenital or acquired hypogammaglobulinemia.[34,35] In human immunodeficiency virus (HIV)-infected patients as well, a failure of *C. jejuni* infection to respond to antimicrobial therapy correlated with the failure to produce a humoral response to infection.[36]

Despite these exceptions, most patients infected with *C. jejuni* had been previously healthy and recover rapidly from infection. In contrast, patients with *C. fetus* infections much more frequently have evidence of impaired immunity including conditions such as chronic alcoholism, liver disease, old age, diabetes mellitus, and malignancies.[37,38] *Campylobacter fetus* infections may produce diarrheal illnesses in healthy hosts or opportunistic infections in debilitated hosts.[32]

CLINICAL MANIFESTATIONS

Campylobacter jejuni Infections

The clinical manifestations of infections due to all of the *Campylobacter* species that cause enteric illnesses appear identical;

C. jejuni may be regarded as the prototype. Acute enteritis is the most common presentation of *C. jejuni* infection. Symptoms may last from 1 day to 1 week or longer. Often there is a prodrome with fever, headache, myalgia, and malaise 12–24 hours before the onset of intestinal symptoms.[39] In some patients the constitutional symptoms may coincide with the intestinal phase or, less often, may follow it. The most common symptoms are diarrhea, malaise, fever, and abdominal pain.[39–41] Diarrhea may vary from loose stools to massive watery stools or grossly bloody stools. In any patient, the entire spectrum of diarrhea may be seen. For most patients, there are 10 or more bowel movements on the worst day of the illness. Abdominal pain is usually cramping in nature and is improved by defecation; it may be the predominant manifestation of the illness. *Campylobacter* enteritis is frequently self-limiting, with a gradual improvement in symptoms over several days; however, illnesses lasting longer than 1 week occur in about 10–20 percent of patients seeking medical attention, and relapses may be seen in another 5–10 percent of untreated patients.[39]

Infection may also be manifested as an acute colitis, with symptoms of fever, abdominal cramps, and bloody diarrhea persisting for 1 week or longer.[23,42] Fever may be low grade or consist of daily peaks above 40°C. Initially, stools may be watery, but as the illness progresses it may become frankly bloody; tenesmus is a common symptom. In the severest forms, patients appear toxic, and toxic megacolon has been reported.[43] Because of the propensity of *Campylobacter* infection for young adults and this presenting clinical picture, it may be readily confused with ulcerative colitis or Crohn's disease.[23,42] The pathologic findings on rectal biopsy are nonspecific, and the clinical presentation and radiographic findings are also nondiagnostic. Therefore, the clinician should have a high index of suspicion of *Campylobacter* infection when seeing a patient with this symptom complex. Because of the often fastidious nature of these organisms,[44,45] a single negative culture does not rule out infection, especially if the optimal filtration methods are not used for isolation.

Occasionally, acute abdominal pain may be the major or only symptom of infection.[46] Although any quadrant of the abdomen may be affected, it has been right lower quadrant pain that has elicited the most attention. As with *Yersinia enterocolitica* and *Salmonella enteritidis, C. jejuni* may cause pseudoappendicitis.[40] In most cases, the removed appendix has shown minimal or no inflammation. Enlarged mesenteric nodes (mesenteric adenitis) and terminal ileitis[25] also may be responsible for the symptoms. A diagnosis is often made during the postoperative period when diarrhea ensues. *Campylobacter* infection occasionally may present solely as a gastrointestinal hemorrhage.[47] Among neonates, *C. jejuni* infection may present with one or more grossly bloody stools and no other symptoms, with findings suggesting intussusception,[48] or may present with extraintestinal foci.[49]

Fever also may be the sole manifestation of *C. jejuni* infection. Temperature elevation may be so severe and persistent that typhoid fever is the initial diagnosis until *C. jejuni* is isolated from stools. Febrile convulsions in young children before the onset of the enteric phase of illness also may occur.[50]

Bacteremia has been noted in fewer than 1 percent of patients with *C. jejuni* infection. In part, this low frequency reflects the fact that physicians rarely culture the blood of patients with diarrheal illnesses, even when fever is present. Nevertheless, bacteremia appears to be more common during infections of persons at the extremes of life.[7] Meningitis and endocarditis are rare manifestations of *C. jejuni* infections. In general, three patterns of extraintestinal *C. jejuni* infection have been noted.[51] First, there may be a transient bacteremia in a normal host with acute *Campylobacter* enteritis. The bacteremia may be discovered several days after the blood cultures were obtained, by which time the patient usually has completely recovered. The course is benign, and no specific treatment for the positive blood culture is usually indicated. Second, there may be a sustained bacteremia or deep focus of infection in a previously normal host; usually these patients have an acute enteritis as well. The *C. jejuni* isolates are generally relatively or absolutely serum resistant. Bacteremia usually originates from the intestinal tract inflammation and responds to antimicrobial therapy. Third, sustained bacteremia or deep infection may occur in a compromised host; many such patients do not have an acute enteritis. *Campylobacter jejuni* isolates usually are serum sensitive. Antimicrobial therapy, which may need to be prolonged, is required for the elimination or suppression of this infection.

Campylobacter jejuni may cause septic abortion,[52] but sustained bacteremia in a pregnant patient does not necessarily imply fetal infection or a bad outcome. There have been infrequent reports of *C. jejuni* infections being manifested with acute cholecystitis,[53] pancreatitis,[54] and cystitis.[55,56] These are probably reflections of local extension rather than hematogenous (metastatic) foci of infection. A reactive arthritis may occur up to several weeks postinfection in persons with the HLA-B27 histocompatibility antigens,[57] and prolonged rheumatic symptoms also have been reported. Hepatitis, interstitial nephritis, and the hemolytic–uremic syndrome are other reported complications. The Guillain-Barré syndrome (GBS) is an uncommon consequence of *C. jejuni* infection. Nevertheless, from 10 to 30 percent of GBS cases follow *C. jejuni* infections, a finding reflecting in part the high incidence of these infections.[58]

Campylobacter fetus Infections

In contrast to *C. jejuni*, *C. fetus* ssp. *fetus* less frequently causes diarrheal illness. As summarized in Table 3, the clinical, laboratory, and epidemiologic characteristics of *C. jejuni* infections differ significantly from those of *C. fetus* ssp. *fetus*, which often produce systemic manifestations. *Campylobacter fetus* infections may cause intermittent diarrhea or nonspecific abdominal pain without localizing signs. The diarrheal illness may be manifested exactly like *C. jejuni* infection and is more common than was suspected several years ago. Clinical manifestations are similar, and sequelae are uncommon. Nearly all of these patients survive their infections when treated with the appropriate antibiotics and usually do well without antibiotic treatment. *Campylobacter fetus* also may cause a prolonged relapsing illness characterized by fever, chills, and myalgias, without a source of the infection being demonstrated.[37,38,59] Occasionally, secondary seeding to an organ will occur and lead to a more complicated infection[59–61] and sometimes to a fulminant fatal course.

Campylobacter fetus infections appear to have a tropism for vascular sites; vascular necrosis occurs in patients with endocarditis and pericarditis.[62,63] Mycotic aneurysms of the abdominal aorta also occur. Thrombophlebitis may be associated with *C. fetus* bacteremia,[64] but whether it is the primary event or a secondary manifestation of the infection is uncertain. Those patients with a bacteremic illness without localization should be carefully evaluated for the presence of septic thrombophlebitis because when treated with appropriate antibiotics the outcome may be good.

Infections during pregnancy primarily have been manifested by upper respiratory symptoms, pneumonitis, fever, and bacteremia. However, four of five *C. fetus*-infected second-trimester patients delivered dead infants despite antibiotic therapy. One patient was treated with antibiotics and delivered a healthy term infant. All the mothers survived their infection.[65]

Central nervous system (CNS) infections with *C. fetus* occur in neonates and adults. The prognosis is poor for premature infants, but five of six full-term neonates survived infection. Infection is manifested as a meningoencephalitis with a cerebrospinal fluid polymorphonuclear pleocytosis. Subdural effusion may complicate infection. Meningoencephalitis also is the most common CNS manifestation of *C. fetus* infection

TABLE 3. Biologic and Clinical Characteristics of *Campylobacter jejuni, Campylobacter fetus* Subspecies *fetus,* and *Helicobacter pylori*

Feature	Campylobacter jejuni	Campylobacter fetus *ssp.* fetus	Helicobacter pylori
Epidemiologic characteristics			
Reservoir	Avian species, animals	Cattle and sheep	Humans
Affected hosts	Normals, hosts, all ages affected, often in clusters of cases	Opportunist of debilitated hosts, clustering rare, but normal hosts may be affected	Chiefly adults, prevalence of infection increases with age
Laboratory characteristics			
Range of growth temperatures	32–42°C	25–37°C[a]	35–42°C
Usual source of isolation	Feces	Blood stream	Gastric and duodenal biopsy specimens
Clinical characteristics			
As a cause for diarrheal illness	Common	Uncommon	Never
Clinical manifestations	Acute gastroenteritis, colitis	Systemic illness with bacteremia, meningitis, vascular infections, abscesses; gastroenteritis occurs	Gastroduodenal inflammation, ulceration
Outcome of infection	Usually self-limited	May be fatal in debilitated hosts	Persistent, low-grade inflammation

[a] Occasionally grows at 42°C.

in adults.[66] Cerebrovascular accidents, subarachnoid hemorrhages, and brain abscesses also occur. The prognosis is better in adults than in neonates, with approximately 67 percent surviving, although neurologic sequelae are frequent.[59]

Campylobacter fetus has been shown to cause a variety of other types of localized infections, including septic arthritis, spontaneous bacterial peritonitis, salpingitis, lung abscess, empyema, cellulitis, urinary tract infection, vertebral osteomyelitis, and cholecystitis.[59,67,68] Although most patients with these illnesses recovered with appropriate antibiotics and drainage procedures, the courses of their illnesses were frequently prolonged and relapsing. Nevertheless, in other patients, self-limiting bacteremia without any sequelae has been observed.

Other Enteric Campylobacters

The clinical manifestations of infection due to other enteric campylobacters overlap substantially with those of *C. jejuni*.[45,69,70] On average, *C. coli* may produce more mild disease.[19] In homosexual men, *C. cineadi* and *C. fenelliae* infections were more often asymptomatic than were those due to *C. jejuni*.[71] Among immunocompromised patients, especially those with the acquired immunodeficiency syndrome (AIDS), bacteremia by the "atypical" campylobacters appears more common than does *C. jejuni* bacteremia. As with *C. fetus, C. upsaliensis* mostly causes diarrheal diseases in previously normal hosts and bacteremia in compromised hosts; most of the latter strains are serum resistant. *Campylobacter hyointestinalis*, which resembles *C. fetus* in its biochemical characteristics,[72] also may cause bacteremia in compromised hosts. *C. cryaerophila* appears to be associated with acute diarrhea but a firm pathogenic link has not been established.

Campylobacter fetus subsp. *venerealis*, which had never been considered a human pathogen, has now been isolated from stools from two homosexual men in Australia and from two women with bacterial vaginosis. *Campylobacter fetus* subsp. *fetus* has been isolated from two other patients with vaginosis.

Campylobacter sputorum subsp. *sputorum*, which is normal flora in the human mouth and intestine, has been isolated from perianal boils and lung abscesses. *Campylobacter sputorum* subsp. *bubulus*, a commensal of sheep and cattle, has been isolated from boils and skin abscesses from humans.

DIAGNOSIS

A clinical diagnosis of enteric campylobacteriosis may be established by (*1*) demonstration of the organisms in direct microscopy of feces or (*2*) isolation of the organisms. The use of serologic methods for diagnosis is at present a research tool only.

Examination of diarrheal fecal specimens by darkfield or phase-contrast microscopy within 2 hours of passage can permit a rapid presumptive diagnosis of *Campylobacter* enteritis if the characteristic darting motility of the *Campylobacter* species is seen.[41,73] This test is particularly useful in the acute phase of the illness. Similarly, finding vibrio forms on a Gram stain of stools is a very specific means for making a diagnosis, although the sensitivity of this technique is 50–75 percent[74] (Fig. 2). Direct microscopy is also of value for detecting red blood cells and neutrophils, which are present in the feces of 75 percent of patients with *Campylobacter* enteritis.[25,39]

Confirmation of the diagnosis of *C. jejuni* infection is based on a positive stool culture or, occasionally, a positive blood culture. Radiometric blood culture detection systems may be falsely negative for some *Campylobacter* species when using standard procedures.[6] Campylobacters cannot be isolated from fecal specimens unless microaerobic incubation conditions and selective techniques that reduce the growth of competing microorganisms are used.[2] *Campylobacter fetus* is usually isolated from blood cultures 4–14 days after the culture has been obtained.[38] On occasion, *C. fetus* may be isolated from the feces of patients with either diarrheal or systemic infections. If *C. fetus* or other of the atypical species is suspected, incubation at 37°C and the use of media without cephalosporins is necessary. The use of filtration techniques will eliminate this problem. Because of their fastidious nature, failure to isolate campylobacters does not rule out their presence.

THERAPY

Fluid and electrolyte replacement are the cornerstones for treating diarrheal illnesses. Patients with *Campylobacter* infections who are badly dehydrated should undergo rapid volume expansion using intravenous solutions of electrolytes in water. For those with less severe depletion, oral rehydration using glucose and electrolyte solutions is indicated.

Persons infected with *C. jejuni* who are ill enough to seek medical attention and from whom a fecal culture is obtained represent only a subset of all those infected. Nevertheless, even among these patients, fewer than half are candidates for specific antimicrobial therapy.[9] Studies of children with dysentery due to *C. jejuni* showed a clear benefit from early treatment with erythromycin.[75] In contrast, other studies in which the initiation of treatment was delayed for several days until *C. jejuni* was isolated did not show a therapeutic effect.[76] Therefore, rapid presumptive diagnosis of *Campylobacter* infection by means of direct visualization of the organisms in stool is clinically rele-

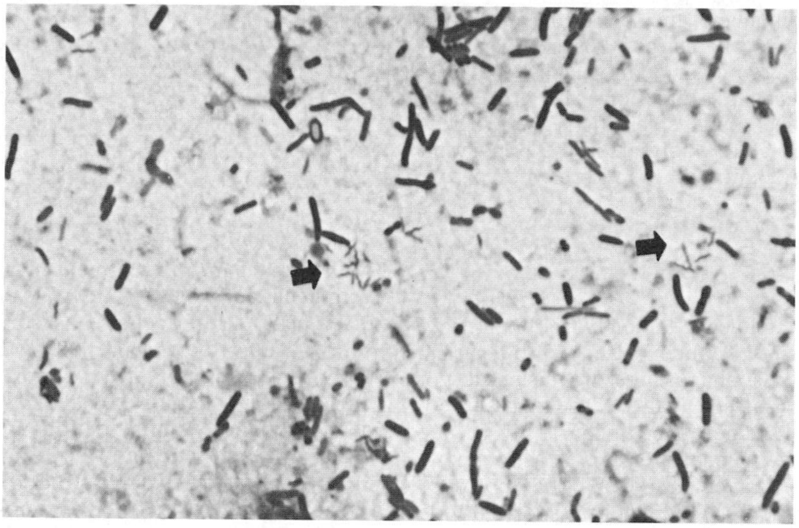

FIG. 2. Gram stain of fecal specimen from a patient with *Campylobacter* enteritis. Arrows point to typical gram-negative fine, small, spiral and *Vibrio*-like organisms. (×1024)

vant. On the basis of anecdotal reports,[23,39,42] wide clinical experience, and the recent controlled trial[75] it is prudent to treat with antibiotics those patients with high fever, bloody diarrhea, or more than eight stools per day; those patients whose symptoms are unimproved or worsening at the time the diagnosis is made; or those in whom symptoms have persisted for more than 1 week.

In vitro, *C. jejuni* is susceptible to a wide variety of antimicrobial agents, including erythromycin, the tetracyclines, the aminoglycosides, chloramphenicol, quinolones, nitrofurans, and clindamycin.[77–679] Because of the ease of administration, a lack of serious toxicity, and its apparent efficacy, erythromycin is the treatment of choice.[41,80,81] The recommended dosage for adults is 250 mg taken orally four times a day for 5–7 days; the recommended dosage for children is 30–50 mg/kg/day in divided doses for the same period. An alternative treatment is ciprofloxacin, 500 mg taken orally twice a day for 5–7 days, which has activity across a broad spectrum of bacteria causing diarrheal illness as well as against campylobacters. Another alternative treatment is tetracycline, except in children under 7 years old; in such patients clindamycin may be used. Most *C. jejuni* isolates are not susceptible to ampicillin or penicillin, and these agents should not be used. However, amoxicillin or ticarcillin plus clavulanic acid may be effective. Susceptibility to sulfonamides and metronidazole is variable. Unlike *Salmonella* infections, treatment with antimicrobial agents does not prolong the carriage of *C. jejuni*; on the contrary, erythromycin eliminates carriage within 72 hours in most patients.[76] *Campylobacter cinaedi* and those *Campylobacter* strains acquired in developing countries, especially *C. coli*, are more likely to be resistant to erythromycin and tetracycline.[82] In such cases when treatment is indicated, until susceptibility is known, alternative agents should be used. The use of antimotility agents appears to prolong the duration of symptoms and has been associated with fatalities.[83] The necessity for treating septic or bacteremic episodes with agents other than erythromycin has not been established. For those patients who are very toxic appearing, treatment with gentamicin, cefotaxime, or chloramphenicol may be indicated, but susceptibility tests should be performed. In hypogammaglobulinemic patients with recurrent *C. jejuni* bacteremias, fresh frozen plasma or intravenous γ-globulin concomitant with appropriate antibiotics may eradicate the infection. Systemic *C. fetus* infections requires parenteral therapy, but erythromycin is not always effective.[84] When isolates have been susceptible, ampicillin treatment has been associated with good results. Patients with endovascular infections due to *C. fetus* require at least 4 weeks of therapy, and gentamicin is probably the agent of choice. Treatment with ampicillin or imipenem/cilastatin are other alternatives. Infections of the CNS should be treated with ampicillin or chloramphenicol for 2–3 weeks. Patients with other serious infections also should be treated with parenteral gentamicin or other aminoglycosides, ampicillin, or chloramphenicol for at least 2 weeks. For patients with diarrheal illness or other less severe infections, treatment need not be as intense or as prolonged.

PROGNOSIS

The vast majority of patients recover fully after *C. jejuni* infections, either spontaneously or after appropriate antimicrobial therapy. The "reactive arthritis" of Reiter syndrome, occurring in HLA-B27–positive persons, closely resembles that seen after *Yersinia*, *Salmonella*, or *Shigella* infections. The Guillain-Barré syndrome is an uncommon sequelum of *Campylobacter* enteritis. Occasional deaths after *C. jejuni* infections have been reported in developed countries[83]; in most cases the victim was an elderly person or a compromised host. However, fatalities in previously healthy young adults may occur, probably as a result of volume depletion. Because in the developing countries most symptomatic *Campylobacter* infections occur in children under 2 years old[18] and frequently produce a dysenteric picture, it is reasonable to conclude that *C. jejuni* infection may play a role in the dehydration and malnutrition that often accompany infantile diarrhea in these areas.

Campylobacter fetus infection may hasten the demise of seriously compromised patients or may be lethal to patients with chronic diseases such as cirrhosis or diabetes mellitus. For compromised hosts with systemic *C. fetus* infections, the prognosis is most dependent on the rapidity with which appropriate antimicrobial therapy is begun. Previously healthy persons infected with *C. fetus* usually survive their illnesses without permanent sequelae.

HELICOBACTER (CAMPYLOBACTER) PYLORI

Epidemiology

Helicobacter pylori (formerly called *C. pylori*) and other related urease-positive organisms are isolated from humans in all parts of the world.[85,86] Although similar organisms have been isolated from other primates and from swine, the role of these animals in human infection is unknown. The largest reservoir appears to be infected humans, and preliminary data suggest that person-to-person transmission occurs. Infection rates are low in persons under 20 in developed countries but then rise progressively until by the age of 60 more than half of the population is infected.[87] In developing countries, infection is more prevalent in all age groups.

Pathogenesis

Helicobacter pylori organisms live in the mucus layer overlaying the antral and fundal gastric epithelium and ectopic gastric tissue in the duodenum and esophagus; the organisms do not appear to invade tissue.[88,89] The survival of these acid-susceptible organisms in the gastric lumen appears largely to be due to the protective effects of the mucus layer as well as to a powerful urease enzyme that generates ammonia.[90] The presence of *H. pylori* overlaying gastric tissue is highly associated with acute infiltrates with neutrophils and other inflammatory cells.[91] Whether or not these organisms cause gastritis or merely colonize the inflamed tissue is not completely resolved at present. However, *H. pylori* infection is specifically associated with the "idiopathic," or "type B," gastritis and not with other forms of gastritis.[92] Furthermore, several lines of evidence including human volunteer studies, antibiotic treatment trials, and animal models suggest that they play a pathogenic role in acute and chronic gastritis.[86] The association of *H. pylori* with gastric metaplasia and duodenitis provides a possible explanation for its consistent association with peptic ulcer disease.[93] Once acquired, these organisms persist for years if not for life,[94] and infected hosts develop long-lasting serologic responses.[87]

Clinical Features

Acute infection with *H. pylori* may be followed immediately by gastritis manifested by epigastric pain, nausea, and vomiting.[95,96] Symptoms usually subside within a few days, but hypochlorhydria may persist for several months.[97] In susceptible individuals, chronic gastritis eventually develops; however, at present the determinants of susceptibility are not known. Chronic gastritis becomes increasingly common among older persons and is usually asymptomatic. The syndrome of non-ulcer dyspepsia is multifactoral in etiology, but *H. pylori* may be responsible for the symptoms in a subset of these patients. Persons with high acid production who are infected with *H. pylori* may be at high risk for the development of duodenal ulcers.

Diagnosis

Helicobacter pylori infection may be diagnosed by isolating these organisms from gastric biopsy specimens with nonselective media such as chocolate agar or a selective medium such as Skirrow's.[98] Plates must be incubated for 2–5 days at 37°C in a moist, microaerobic atmosphere. Comma or S-shaped motile organisms that are oxidase-, catalase-, and urease-positive may be identified as *H. pylori* or as a closely related species.[99] Alternatively, the organisms can be visualized on histologic sections stained with Gram, silver, Giemsa, or acridine orange stains. Assessment of urease activity in biopsy material is another alternative. All of the aforementioned tests require endoscopy and biopsy. The recent development of noninvasive techniques, including the detection of ^{14}C-urea in breath and especially the determination of serum antibodies to *H. pylori* antigens,[87] will greatly facilitate the diagnosis of this infection. Whether *H. pylori* will long remain in the genus *Campylobacter* is uncertain at present.[100,101]

Treatment

Most *H. pylori* organisms are susceptible to a variety of antimicrobial agents including amoxicillin, nitrofurans, metronidazole, and bismuth salts.[102] Treatment with these agents has resulted in the disappearance of the organisms and improvement in gastric histology, but after the termination of therapy, the organisms most often recur, and the histologic appearance of tissues returns to the pretreatment state.[103] No current single-agent therapy has been associated with long-term eradication of the organism.[104] Treatment of patients with duodenal ulcers with agents effective against *H. pylori* prolongs the duration of ulcer healing until relapse as compared with agents directed solely against acid secretion.[105] Evaluation of antimicrobial therapy in patients with inflammatory gastroduodenal lesions must be done in controlled clinical trials before firm antimicrobial treatment recommendations can be made. However, on the basis of the current knowledge, in patients with gastritis who are symptomatic despite appropriate medical therapy, the inclusion of anti-*H. pylori* agents may be warranted.

REFERENCES

1. Smibert RM. Genus *Campylobacter*. In: Krieg NR, Holt HG, eds. Bergey's Manual of Systematic Bacteriology. v. 1. Baltimore: Williams & Wilkins; 1984:111–8.
2. Penner JL. The genus *Campylobacter*: A decade of progress. Clin Microbiol Rev. 1988;1:157–72.
3. Morris GK, Patton CM. *Campylobacter*. In: Lennette E, Balows A, Hausler WJ Jr, et al., eds. Manual of Clinical Microbiology. 4th ed. Washington, DC: American Society for Microbiology; 1985:302–8.
4. Bolton GJ, Hutchinson DN, Coates D. Blood-free selective medium for isolation of *Campylobacter jejuni* from feces. J Clin Microbiol. 1984;19:169–71.
5. Steele TW, McDermott JN. Technical note: The use of membrane filters applied directly to the surface of agar plates for the isolation of *Campylobacter jejuni* from feces. Pathology. 1984;16:263–5.
6. Wang WLL, Blaser MJ. Detection of pathogenic *Campylobacter* species in blood culture systems. J Clin Microbiol. 1986;23:709.
7. Blaser MJ, Taylor DN, Feldman RA. Epidemiology of *Campylobacter jejuni* infections. Epidemiol Rev. 1983;5:157.
8. Taylor DN, McDermott KT, Little JR, et al. *Campylobacter* enteritis associated with drinking untreated water in back-country areas of the Rocky Mountains. Ann Intern Med. 1983;99:38.
9. Mentzing L-O. Waterborne outbreaks of *Campylobacter* enteritis in central Sweden. Lancet. 1981;2:352.
10. Deming MS, Tauxe RV, Blake PA, et al. *Campylobacter* enteritis at a university: Transmission from eating chicken and from cats. Am J Epidemiol. 1987;126:526–34.
11. Skirrow MB. *Campylobacter* enteritis in dogs and cats: A "new" zoonosis. Vet Res Commun. 1981;5:13.
12. Vesikari T, Huttunen L, Maki R. Perinatal *Campylobacter fetus* ss *jejuni* enteritis. Acta Paediatr Scand. 1981;70:261.
13. Pepersack F, Prigogyne T, Butzler JP, et al. *Campylobacter jejuni* post-transfusional septicaemia. Lancet. 1979;2:911.
14. Totten PA, Fennell CL, Tenover FC, et al. *Campylobacter cinaedi* (sp. nov.) and *Campylobacter fennelliae* (sp. nov.): Two new *Campylobacter* species associated with enteric disease in homosexual men. J Infect Dis. 1985; 151:131.
15. Blaser MJ, Wells JG, Feldman RA, et al. *Campylobacter* enteritis in the United States. A multicenter study. Ann Intern Med. 1983;98:360.
16. Riley LW, Finch MJ. Results of the first year of national surveillance of campylobacter infections in the United States. J Infect Dis. 1985;151:956–9.
17. Rajan DP, Mathan VI. Prevalence of *Campylobacter fetus* subsp. *jejuni* in healthy populations in southern India. J Clin Microbiol. 1982;15:749.
18. Glass RI, Stoll BJ, Huq MI, et al. Epidemiologic and clinical features of endemic *Campylobacter jejuni* infection in Bangladesh. J Infect Dis. 1983;148:292.
19. Taylor DN, Echeverria P, Pitarangsi C, et al. The influence of immunity and strain characteristics on the epidemiology of campylobacteriosis. J Clin Microbiol. 1988;26:863.
20. Speelman P, Struelens MJ, Sanyal SC, et al. Detection of *Campylobacter jejuni* and other potential pathogens in travelers' diarrhoea in Bangladesh. Scand J Gastroenterol. 1983;18(Suppl 84):19–23.
21. Blaser MJ, Hardesty HL, Powers B, et al. Survival of *Campylobacter fetus* subsp. *jejuni* in biological milieus. J Clin Microbiol. 1980;11:309.
22. King EO. The laboratory recognition of *Vibrio fetus* and a closely related vibrio isolated from cases of human vibriosis. Ann NY Acad Sci. 1962; 90:700.
23. Lambert ME, Schofield PF, Ironside AG, et al. *Campylobacter* colitis. Br Med J. 1979;1:857.

24. Van Spreeuwel JP, Duursma GC, Meijer CJLM, et al. *Campylobacter* colitis: Histologic, immunohistochemical and ultrastructural findings. Gut. 1985;26:945–51.
25. Blaser MJ, Reller LB, Luechtefeld NW, et al. *Campylobacter* enteritis in Denver. West J Med. 1982;136:287.
26. Black RE, Levine MM, Clements ML, et al. Experimental *Campylobacter jejuni* infection in humans. J Infect Dis. 1988;157:472.
27. Johnson WM, Lior H. Cytotoxic and cytotonic factors produced by *Campylobacter jejuni, Campylobacter coli*, and *Campylobacter laridis*. J Clin Microbiol. 1986;24:275–81.
28. Walker RI, Caldwell MB, Lee EC, et al. Pathophysiology of *Campylobacter* enteritis. Microbiol Rev. 1985;50:81–94.
29. Fauchere JL, Rosenau A, Veron M, et al. Association with HeLa cells of *Campylobacter jejuni* and *Campylobacter coli* isolated from human feces. Infect Immun. 1986;54:283–7.
30. Caldwell MB, Guerry P, Lee EC, et al. Reversible expression of flagella in *Campylobacter jejuni*. Infect Immun. 1985;50:941–3.
31. Blaser MJ, Smith PF, Kohler PA. Susceptibility of *Campylobacter* isolates to the bactericidal activity in human serum. J Infect Dis. 1985;151:227.
32. Blaser MJ, Smith PF, Hopkins JA, et al. Pathogenesis of *Campylobacter fetus* infections. Serum resistance associated with high molecular weight surface proteins. J Infect Dis. 1987;155:696.
33. Blaser MJ, Smith PF, Repine JE, et al. Pathogenesis of *Campylobacter fetus* infections. Failure of C3b to bind explains serum and phagocytosis resistance. J Clin Invest. 1988;81:1434–44.
34. Ahnen DJ, Brown WR. *Campylobacter* enteritis in immune-deficient patients. Ann Intern Med. 1982;96:187.
35. Melamed I, Bujanover Y, Igra YS, et al. *Campylobacter* enteritis in normal and immunodeficient children. Am J Dis Child. 1983;137:752–3.
36. Perlman DM, Ampel NM, Schiffman RB, et al. Persistant *Campylobacter jejuni* infections in patients infected with the human immunodeficiency virus: Association with abnormal serological response to *C. jejuni* and emergence of erythromycin resistance during therapy. Ann Intern Med. 1988;108: 540–6.
37. Fennell CL, Totten PA, Quinn TC, et al. Characterization of *Campylobacter*-like organisms isolated from homosexual men. J Infect Dis. 1984;149:58–66.
38. Bokkenheuser V. *Vibrio fetus* infection in man. I. Ten new cases and some epidemiologic observations. Am J Epidemiol. 1970;91:400.
39. Guerrant RL, Lahita RG, Winn EC Jr, et al. Campylobacteriosis in man: Pathogenic mechanisms and review of 91 bloodstream infections. Am J Med. 1978;65:484.
40. Blaser MJ, Berkowitz ID, LaForce FM, et al. *Campylobacter* enteritis; clinical and epidemiologic features. Ann Intern Med. 1979;91:179.
41. Skirrow MB. *Campylobacter* enteritis: A "new" disease. Br Med J. 1977;2:9.
42. Karmali MA, Fleming PC. *Campylobacter* enteritis in children. J Pediatr. 1979;94:527.
43. McKinley MJ, Taylor M, Sangree MH. Toxic megacolon with campylobacter colitis. Conn Med. 1980;44:496.
44. Tee W, Anderson BN, Ross BC, et al. Atypical campylobacters associated with gastroenteritis. J Clin Microbiol. 1987;25:1248–52.
45. Steele TW, Sangster N, Lanser JA. DNA relatedness and biochemical features of *Campylobacter* spp isolated in Central and South Australia. J Clin Microbiol. 1985;22:71–4.
46. Drake AA, Gilchrist MJR, Washington JA II, et al. Diarrhea due to *Campylobacter fetus* subspecies *jejuni*: A clinical review of 73 cases. Mayo Clin Proc. 1981;56:414.
47. Michalak DM, Perrault J, Gilchrist MJ, et al. *Campylobacter fetus* ss. *jejuni*: A cause of massive lower gastrointestinal hemorrhage. Gastroenterology. 1980;79:742.
48. Anders BJ, Lauer BA, Paisley JW. *Campylobacter* gastroenteritis in neonates. Am J Dis Child. 1981;135:900.
49. Goossens H, Henocque G, Kremp L, et al. Nosocomial outbreak of *Campylobacter jejuni* meningitis in newborn infants. Lancet. 1986;2:146–9.
50. Wright EP, Seager J. Convulsions associated with *Campylobacter* enteritis. Br Med J. 1980;281:454.
51. Blaser MJ, Perez GP, Smith PF, et al. Extraintestinal *Campylobacter jejuni* and *Campylobacter coli* infections: Host factors and strain characteristics. J Infect Dis. 1986;153:552.
52. Gilbert GL, Davoren RA, Cole ME, et al. Midtrimester abortion associated with septicaemia caused by *Campylobacter jejuni*. Med J Aust. 1981;1:585.
53. Mertens A, DeSmet M. *Campylobacter* cholecystitis. Lancet. 1979;1:1092.
54. Gallagher P, Chadwick P, Jones DM, et al. Acute pancreatitis associated with *Campylobacter* infection. Br J Surg. 1981;68:383.
55. Davies JS, Penfold JB. *Campylobacter* urinary infection. Lancet. 1979; 1:1091.
56. Feder HM, Rasoulpour M, Rodriquez AJ. *Campylobacter* urinary tract infection. Value of the urine gram stain. JAMA. 1986;256:2389.
57. Kosunen TU, Kauranen O, Martio J, et al. Reactive arthritis after *Campylobacter jejuni* enteritis in patients with HLA-B27. Lancet. 1980;1:1312.
58. Kaldor J, Speed BR. Guillain-Barré syndrome and *Campylobacter jejuni*: A serological study. Br Med J. 1984;288:1867–70.
59. Franklin B, Ulmer DD. Human infection with *Vibrio fetus*. West J Med. 1974;120:200.
60. Collins HS, Blevins A, Baxter E. Protracted bacteremia and meningitis due to *Vibrio fetus*. Arch Intern Med. 1964;113:361.
61. Park CH, McDonald F, Twohig AM, et al. Septicemia and gastroenteritis due to *Vibrio fetus*. South Med J. 1973;66:531.
62. Loeb H, Bettag JL, Yantz NK, et al. *Vibrio fetus* endocarditis. Am Heart J. 1966;71:381.
63. Killiam HA, Crowder JG, White AC, et al. Pericarditis due to *Vibrio fetus*. Am J Cardiol. 1966;17:723.
64. Vesely D, MacIntyre S, Ratzan KR. Bilateral deep brachial vein thrombophlebitis due to *Vibrio fetus*. Arch Intern Med. 1975;135:994.
65. Eden AH. Perinatal mortality caused by *Vibrio fetus*. Review and analysis. J Pediatr. 1966;68:297.
66. Gunderson CH, Sack GE. Neurology of *Vibrio fetus*. Neurology (NY). 1971;21:307.
67. Kilo C, Hagemann PO, Maryi J. Septic arthritis and bacteremia due to *Vibrio fetus*. Am J Med. 1965;38:962.
68. Lawrence R, Nibbe AF, Levin S. Lung abscess secondary to *Vibrio fetus*, malabsorption syndrome and acquired agammaglobulinemia. Chest. 1971; 60:191.
69. Benjamin JS, Leaper S, Owen RJ, et al. Description of *Campylobacter laridis*, a new species comprising the nalidixic acid resistant thermophilic *Campylobacter* (NARTC group). Curr Microbiol. 1983;8:231–8.
70. Simor AE, Wilcox L. Enteritis associated with *Campylobacter laridis*. J Clin Microbiol. 1987;25:10–2.
71. Quinn TC, Goodell SE, Fennell C, et al. Infections with *Campylobacter jejuni* and *Campylobacter*-like organisms in homosexual men. Ann Intern Med. 1984;101:187–92.
72. Edmonds P, Patton CM, Griffin PM, et al. *Campylobacter hyointestinalis* associated with human gastrointestinal disease in the United States. J Clin Microbiol. 1987;25:685–91.
73. Paisley JW, Mirrett S, Lauer BA, et al. Darkfield microscopy of human feces for the presumptive diagnosis of *Campylobacter* enteritis. J Clin Microbiol. 1982;15:61.
74. Sazie ESM, Titus AE. Rapid diagnosis of *Campylobacter* enteritis. Ann Intern Med. 1982;96:62.
75. Salazar-Lindo E, Sack RB, Chea-Woo E, et al. Early treatment with erythromycin of *Campylobacter jejuni*-associated dysentery in children. J Pediatr. 1986;109:355.
76. Anders BJ, Lauer BA, Paisley JW, et al. Double-blind placebo controlled trial of erythromycin for treatment of *Campylobacter* enteritis. Lancet. 1982;1:131.
77. Vanhoof R, Vanderlinden MP, Dierickx R, et al. Susceptibility of *Campylobacter fetus* subsp. *jejuni* to twenty-nine antimicrobial agents. Antimicrob Agents Chemother. 1978;14:553.
78. Walder M. Susceptibility of *Campylobacter fetus* subsp. *jejuni* to twenty antimicrobial agents. *Antimicrob Agents Chemother*. 1979;16:37.
79. Vanhoof R, Gordts B, Dierickx R, et al. Bacteriostatic and bactericidal activities of 24 antimicrobial agents against *Campylobacter fetus* subsp. *jejuni*. Antimicrob Agents Chemother. 1980;18:118.
80. Blaser MJ, Reller LB. *Campylobacter* enteritis. N Engl J Med. 1981; 305:1444.
81. Skirrow MB. *Campylobacter* enteritis: The first five years. J Hyg. 1982;89:175.
82. Taylor DN, Blaser MJ, Echeverria P, et al. Erythromycin-resistant *Campylobacter* infections in Thailand. Antimicrob Agents Chemother. 1987; 31:438–42.
83. Smith GS, Blaser MJ. Fatalities associated with *Campylobacter jejuni* infections. JAMA. 1985;253:2873.
84. Francioli P, Herzstein, Grob J-P, et al. *Campylobacter fetus* subspecies *fetus* bacteremia. Arch Intern Med. 1985;145:289–92.
85. Blaser MJ, ed. *Campylobacter pylori*, gastritis and peptic ulcer disease. New York: Igaku-Shoin; 1989: In press.
86. Marshall BJ. *Campylobacter pyloridis* and gastritis. J Infect Dis. 1986; 153:650–7.
87. Perez-Perez GI, Dworkin BM, Chodos JE, Blaser MJ. *Campylobacter pylori* antibodies in humans. Ann Intern Med. 1988;109:11–7.
88. Marshall BJ. Unidentified curved bacilli on gastric epithelium in active chronic gastritis. Lancet. 1983;2:1273–5.
89. Price AB, Levi J, Dolby JM, et al. *Campylobacter pyloridis* in peptic ulcer disease: Microbiology, pathology, and scanning electron microscopy. Gut. 1985;26:1183–8.
90. McNulty CAM, Dent JC. Rapid identification of *Campylobacter pylori* (*C. pyloridis*) by preformed enzyme. J Clin Microbiol. 1987;25:1683–6.
91. Blaser MJ. Gastric campylobacter-like organisms, gastritis, and peptic ulcer disease. Gastroenterology. 1987;93:371–83.
92. Drumm B, Sherman P, Cutz E, et al. Association of *Campylobacter pylori* on the gastric mucosa with antral gastritis in children. N Engl J Med. 1987;25:1557–61.
93. Wyatt JI, Rathbone BJ, Dixon MF. *Campylobacter pyloridis* and acid-induced gastric metaplasia in the pathogenesis of duodenitis. J Clin Pathol. 1987;40:841–8.
94. Langenberg WE, Rauws EAJ, Widjojokusomo A, et al. Identification of *Campylobacter pyloridis* isolates by restriction endonuclease DNA analysis. J Clin Microbiol. 1986;24:414–7.
95. Marshall BJ, Armstrong JA, McGechie DB, et al. Attempt to fulfil Koch's postulates for pyloric campylobacter. Med J Aust. 1985;142:436–9.
96. Morris A, Nicholson G. Ingestion of *Campylobacter pyloridis* causes gastritis and raised fasting gastric pH. Am J Gastroenterol. 1987;82:192–9.

97. Ramsey EJ, Carey K, Peterson WL, et al. Epidemic gastritis with hypochlorhydria. Gastroenterology. 1979;76:1449–57.
98. Goodwin CS, Blincow E, Warren JR, et al. Evaluation of cultural techniques for isolating *Campylobacter pyloridis* from endoscopic biopsies of gastric mucosa. J Clin Pathol. 1985;38:1127–31.
99. Kasper G, Dickgiesser N. Isolation from gastric epithelium of *Campylobacter*-like bacteria that are distinct from "*Campylobacter pyloridis*." Lancet. 1985;1:111–2.
100. Goodwin CS, McCulloch RK, Armstrong JA, et al. Unusual cellular fatty acids and distinctive ultrastructure in a new spiral bacterium (*Campylobacter pyloridis*) from the human gastric mucosa. J Med Microbiol. 1985;19:257–67.
101. Romaniuk PJ, Zoltowska B, Trust TJ, et al. *Campylobacter pylori*, the spiral bacterium associated with human gastritis, is not a true *Campylobacter* sp. J Bacteriol. 1987;169:2137–41.
102. Goodwin CS, Blake P, Blincow E. The minimum inhibitory and bactericidal concentrations of antibiotics and anti-ulcer agents against *Campylobacter pyloridis*. J Antimicrob Chemother. 1986;17:309–14.
103. McNulty CAM, Gearty JC, Crump B, et al. *Campylobacter pyloridis* and associated gastritis: Investigator blind, placebo controlled trial if bismuth salicylate and erythromycin ethylsuccinate. Br Med J. 1986;293:645–9.
104. Rauws EAJ, Langenberg W, Houthoff JH, et al. *Campylobacter pyloridis*–associated chronic active gastritis. A prospective study of its prevalence and the effects of antibacterial and anti-ulcer treatment. Gastroenterology. 1988;94:33–40.
105. Coghlan JG, Gilligan D, Humphreys H, et al. *Campylobacter pylori* and recurrence of duodenal ulcers—A 12-month follow-up study. Lancet. 1987;2:1109–11.

TABLE 1. The Tribes and Genera of the Family Enterobacteriaceae That Are Associated with Human Disease

Tribe	Genera
Escherichieae	*Escherichia* *Shigella*
Edwardsielleae	*Edwardsiella*
Salmonelleae	*Salmonella*
Citrobactereae	*Citrobacter*
Klebsielleae	*Klebsiella* *Enterobacter* *Hafnia* *Serratia*
Protease	*Proteus* *Morganella* *Providencia*
Yersinieae	*Yersinia*
Erwinieae	*Erwinia*
Miscellaneous genera (not yet assigned to a tribe)	*Buttiauxella* *Cedecea* *Ewingella* *Kluyvera* *Tatumella* *Rahnella* Various "enteric groups" (not yet assigned to a genus)

195. ENTEROBACTERIACEAE

BARRY I. EISENSTEIN

The large, heterogeneous group of gram-negative bacteria that make up the family Enterobacteriaceae are among the most important medically; a number of genera within the family are major human intestinal pathogens (e.g., *Shigella*, *Salmonella*, *Yersinia*), and several are normal colonizers of the human gastrointestinal tract (e.g., *Escherichia*, *Enterobacter*, *Klebsiella*).[1–4] Because of this colonization tropism, a significant number of member strains are also referred to as "enteric bacteria," a designation that includes other gram-negative bacilli that are commonly found in the gastrointestinal tract such as some species of the families Pseudomonaceae, and Vironaceae. Thus, enteric bacteria and Enterobacteriaceae refer to partially overlapping rather than identical sets of organisms.

Recent taxonomy schemes have employed DNA relatedness data extensively to augment prior phenotype (i.e., biochemical, physiologic, and immunochemical) information.[3] The latest classification by Ewing is presented in Table 1.[4] Certain close relationships are apparent from this scheme (e.g., *Escherichia* and *Shigella*). Typical and distinguishing characteristics of this family are that they are non-spore-forming aerobes capable of anaerobic growth (facultative anaerobes), they reduce nitrates to nitrites (with some exceptions), they do not liquify alginate, they ferment glucose to acid with or without gas, they are oxidase-negative, their growth is not enhanced by NaCl, and they can be either motile (with peritrichous flagella) or nonmotile.[1–4]

Because of their distinctive clinical characteristics and their medical importance, *Yersinia*, *Shigella*, and *Salmonella* are discussed in separate chapters. The remainder of this chapter is divided into two parts: the first summarizes the common traits of the family and how these traits are involved in the pathogenesis of these organisms, and the second focuses on the specific characteristics of the individual pathogenic genera.

GENERAL PROPERTIES

Epidemiology

Members of the family Enterobacteriaceae are widely distributed in the soil and on plants as well as being normal colonizers of the intestinal tracts of humans and animals. It should be recalled, however, that >99 percent of the flora of the human gastrointestinal tract are anaerobes, most of which are members of the genus *Bacteroides*. These organisms are not normally found on body locations outside of the gastrointestinal tract but are an important cause of infections outside of the gastrointestinal tract, particularly the genitourinary system. In individuals with compromise in the normal anatomic barriers to colonization, infection by these bacteria frequently ensues, often leading to pneumonia, septicemia, meningitis, or abscess formation. Hospitalized patients, because of various types of stress, are particularly susceptible to colonization and infection with Enterobacteriaceae such that these organisms are among the leading causes of nosocomial infection.

These bacteria account for approximately 80 percent of significant isolates of gram-negative bacteria in the clinical laboratory and approximately half of all clinically significant isolates.[2] It has been estimated that about half the septicemia isolates, two-thirds the bacterial gastroenteritis isolates, and three-quarters the urinary tract isolates are accounted for by the Enterobacteriaceae.[2]

Because of their important role in hospital outbreaks of infection, it is often necessary to determine whether a given isolate is the same as another recovered from a separate culture site. Such determinations frequently lead to the characterization of the mode of transmission or the point source of transmission, which in turn permits effective control measures. Bacterial spread from one site to another requires growth, DNA duplication, and asexual division. In the absence of major alterations in the genetic content, as with the acquisition of a new plasmid, bacterial offspring are genetically and therefore phenotypically identical to their progenitors. By definition, parent and progeny are "clonal." The evaluation of a number of phenotypic properties, such an antigenic structure and physiologic traits, has been shown to be quite useful in determining clonality and has led to the realization that there are fewer clones extant than would be predicted from all of the theoretic assortments of traits possible. A number of epidemiologic studies have determined that certain clones, identified by unique biochemical signatures, are associated with specific clinical settings (to be discussed below).[5–7]

As an alternative to phenotypic characterization, investigators have recently turned to genetic analyses to obviate the occasional problems with traits that are variably expressed.

Among the simplest has been the use of plasmid analysis to "fingerprint" the isolate, which is useful as long as there has been a minimal amount of selective pressure in the environment, as with antibiotic use, to cause a gain, loss, or change in the plasmid profile.[8–11] Because of this genetic plasticity at the plasmid level, investigators have employed chromosomal analyses for tracking the most stable markers of identity.[12] In this regard the use of restriction fragment length polymorphisms (RFLPs) may be most valuable.

Structure

Enterobacteriaceae share with all bacteria numerous structural features such as a rigid cell envelope surrounding a cytoplasmic membrane, a single chromosome consisting of double-stranded DNA and located throughout the cytoplasm (unlike eukaryotes, there is no nucleus), ribosomes that are smaller and less complicated than eukaryotic ribosomes are, and the absence of mitochondria for oxidative metabolism or an endoplasmic reticulum for protein secretion. As gram-negative bacteria, their cell envelope is characterized by a multilamellar structure. The inner (or cytoplasmic) membrane consists of a phospholipid bilayer with interspersed proteins. The next outer layer consists of a thin (relative to gram-positive bacteria) peptidoglycan along with a periplasmic space. The peptidoglycan is an extensively cross-linked polymer that gives the organism its rigid shape. The complex outer membrane consists of another phospholipid bilayer with extensive intercalation of a number of elements, including lipopolysaccharide (LPS), lipoprotein (which is tethered to the peptidoglycan), multimeric porin proteins (whose membrane-spanning pores facilitate transport), and other outer membrane proteins.[13] Among these proteins are complex, outwardly radiating organelles: flagella, used for locomotion and which arise from a basal structure located in the inner membrane; fimbriae (or common pili), important as adhesins, as discussed in Chapter 2; and sex pili, present in bacteria containing conjugative plasmids and used by the bacteria to mediate conjugative transfer of plasmid DNA.

The Host–Parasite Interaction

Enterobacteriaceae are of great interest to biologists and health care workers not only because several species (especially *Escherichia coli*) are model cells to study general biologic and biochemical processes but because, as a group, these bacteria are important causes of infectious diseases. Extensive clinical investigation has shown that the way in which the parasite interacts with the human host at the cellular and molecular level determines the nature of the disease and the likelihood for recovery. Thus, scientific studies that have made use of *E. coli* and *Salmonella*, in particular, to study fundamental questions of molecular biology have laid an essential foundation for more applied studies aimed at questions of pathogenesis. The use of the tools of molecular genetics, biochemistry, and immunochemistry to study infection is providing insights at the molecular level of pathogenesis heretofore unavailable.

Disease due to bacterial infection typically consists of several sequential but interrelated stages. The initial one involves the entry of the organism into host. Among the Enterobacteriaceae entry is typically through colonization of the gastrointestinal tract, which requires bacterial adherence to mucosal receptors (see Chapter 2). The symptomatic stage of the infection is manifested by a varied assortment of bacterial processes ranging from toxin liberation to invasion and cytologic damage. The springboard for this step is at the initial site of colonization. Finally, the host response, which is directed against individual components of the parasite, typically mediates recovery, although the inflammatory response often contributes to the severity and nature of the disease.

Modern medicine has developed several approaches in dealing with the infectious process. The ability to treat the infection by using antimicrobial agents to kill or inhibit the growth of the organism requires specific targeting of the agents to structures or processes found only in the bacteria. Alternatively, the use of immunologic reagents to prevent, as with prior immunization, or treat an infection generally requires the use of material specific to the pathogen (e.g., an antitoxin). Thus, the vast majority of medical interventions used at the present time to treat or prevent infections are directed at pathogen-specific targets. The topic of pathogen-directed antibiotic therapy is covered extensively in Section E, whereas that of immunization is found in Chapter 295.

Aside from the bacterial targets of antimicrobial therapy, most of the medically relevant components of bacterial pathogens are either secreted (or released) toxins (see Chapter 1) or surface-exposed structures. As mentioned earlier, an important class of surface structures are the fimbriae, which as a group are the major determinants of bacterial adherence to mucosal surfaces (see Chapter 2). These organelles, along with most other surface-exposed structures of gram-negative bacteria, are highly antigenic. This characteristic of bacteria was among the earliest exploited by bacteriologists, who showed the usefulness of antisera raised against different enteric bacteria (e.g., *Salmonella typhi*) in the typing of strains. It was a logical progression to use these sera to probe the antigenic structure of the immunizing bacteria. Therefore, it has been customary for medical microbiologists to view the surface structure of gram-negative bacteria in terms of the classes of antigens found.

Antigenic Structure of the Bacterial Surface

Among the best developed and earliest schemes for the classification of bacterial strains by their antigenic profiles is the use of anti-*Salmonella* sera to classify serotypes of *Salmonella*. Serotyping has been extensively used as well for *E. coli*. The major antigenic groups that react with these antisera are conserved in all species of Enterobacteriaceae.[4] The three classes of antigens are (*1*) the O antigens or somatic antigens, (*2*) the H or flagellar antigens, and (*3*) the K or capsular antigens (the VI antigens of some serotypes of *Salmonella* are subtypes of the capsular antigens).

The O antigens consist of the polysaccharide side chains of the envelope LPS found in all gram-negative bacteria.[14–17] Virulent strains of Enterobacteriaceae (i.e., isolates recovered as the causative agents of infection) typically have smooth LPS. This form of LPS consists of the core part of the LPS, which is linked to lipid A, as well as the repeating polysaccharide. Mutant strains can be recovered, typically after sequential laboratory passage, that no longer synthesize the polysaccharide side chains. Since these strains grow as rough-appearing colonies on laboratory agar, the LPS extracted from these strains has, by convention, been called "rough." These strains have lost their O antigens but may in the process unmask R antigens that are more weakly reactive as a consequence of the small degree of residual antigenicity from the remaining LPS. Gram-negative bacteria cannot survive without at least the core LPS. Unlike the other classes of antigens, the O antigens are absolutely heat stable. The classic reaction to demonstrate the presence of these antigens is agglutination with the type-specific antisera. The O antigenic types are widely shared among all the genera of the Enterobacteriaceae, but in some cases cross-reactivity is particularly pronounced.[4,14] Thus, many of the *E. coli* O serogroups show significant cross-reactivity with members of *Shigella*. Cross-reactivity extends as well to members of *Salmonella*, Citrobacter, and *Klebsiella* and is occasionally seen beyond the Enterobacteriaceae.[18,19] For instance, some *E. coli* O antigens cross react with *Vibrio*, with some human blood groups, and with other cell surface antigens from mammalian tissue.

There is growing recognition that many if not all of these O serogroups represent distinct clones of bacteria. This relationship has been best worked out in *E. coli* where strains within a given serogroup share numerous other biochemical properties as well. Epidemiologic surveys have demonstrated striking associations between certain O serotypes and clinical infections.[5] Although not conclusively proven, it is now generally felt that the O serogroup may act primarily as a marker for a specific clustering of virulence properties needed for a certain infectious process. Thus, certain serogroups possess adhesive factors that are specifically important in urinary tract infection, whereas other serogroups possess colonization factors and toxins that are necessary for gastroenteritis.

H antigens are found on bacterial flagella, which provide many gram-negative bacteria with motility.[4,20] In contrast to the somatic antigens, H antigens are heat labile and consist of protein. In a flagellate organism, the H antigen is dominant to the O antigen so that the reactivity of the O antigen requires prior denaturation of the H antigen, usually accomplished by heat or treatment with acid or alcohol. The agglutination reactions seen with H antigens are more rapid and dramatic than is the agglutination reaction seen with O antigens. A particular property of specific anti-H antibody is that they immobilize flagellate bacteria to which the antibodies are directed. This immunologic reaction is probably important in attenuating the virulence of motile bacteria, particularly in the gastrointestinal and urinary tracts,[21] and was probably responsible for the emergence of flagellar phase variation in *Salmonella*.[22] Phase variation is the property by which a bacterium is capable of alternating the expression of one type of flagellar antigen with an unrelated antigenic type such that the organism can no longer be immobilized by antibody to the first type. It has recently been determined that flagellar phase variation is controlled by an invertible element of DNA that turns on and off the expression of one flagellum type[22] and a repressor gene for the unlinked second flagellar type. The use by bacteria of an invertible element of DNA to drive the genetic expression of a surface organelle is also found in *E. coli* where a similar type of invertible element controls the on and off expression of type 1 fimbriae.[23,24]

The last major class of antigens is the K or capsular antigen.[14,25] K antigens are only partially stable to heat, and although typically composed of polysaccharide-containing capsules, can occasionally be envelope proteins or fimbriae. If the antigen is a capsule, its presence can inhibit the O reaction, which then requires for detection that the capsule be removed or otherwise denatured. Two important examples of K antigens are the VI antigen of *S. typhi*, thought to be important in the virulence of *S. typhi*, and the K1 antigen of *E. coli*, which is associated with neonatal meningitis, bacteremia, and urinary tract infection.[26–30]

Virulence and Virulence Factors

From the perspective of the infectious diseases clinician, virulence of a microorganism can be defined in terms of the nature and severity of the illness that is caused by the infecting agent. From the standpoint of the microbiologist, however, a somewhat different perspective can be taken, a perspective that focuses on the ability of the organism to grow and multiply in a given environmental setting. Pathogenic bacteria both populate a specific niche in the human body and, by definition, produce disease. Thus, a successful pathogen has evolved two classes of host-specific factors: one class promotes survival in the host without harming the host, and the second is specifically involved with disease production. The latter are not associated with nonpathogenic bacteria and can be considered primary virulence factors. The former are sometimes found in nonpathogenic bacteria that occupy the same niche in the host as the pathogenic bacteria (e.g., the gastrointestinal tract), and might be considered secondary, conditional, or auxillary virulence factors; these factors are needed for disease production in that they allow the pathogenic microbe the opportunity to survive in the hostile environment of the host. An example of such a factor is a surface adhesin, which allows the organism to adhere and colonize the mucosal surface. In *E. coli* that are nonpathogenic but are still capable of residing successfully in the human gastrointestinal tract, the presence of adhesins are thought to play an important role in allowing the organism to colonize successfully. In that context, however, these factors are not helping to promote any disease, so they cannot be considered virulence factors. Nevertheless, were the same *E. coli* to also possess an enterotoxin, the organism might be now capable of producing gastroenteritis in the human host, which it could not do in the absence of the adhesin. In this new context, the adhesin can be viewed as a conditional or auxillary virulence factor. In addition to adhesins, the Enterobacteriaceae possess a number of additional auxillary virulence factors. Flagella permit the organism motility, scavenger molecules and receptors such as the siderophore system permit acquisition of limiting nutrients, and capsules block opsonophagocytosis and thereby foil the immunologic machinery of the host.

The primary virulence factors can be further subdivided into those that, by themselves (i.e., in pure isolated form), can replicate at least some part of the illness that the entire organism is capable of producing. The best example of such a factor is a toxin. Nevertheless, most infectious processes are fairly complex, so multiple factors must work together to produce disease. These factors can only play a role in disease production in context of the entire microorganism; while necessary for the disease process, they are insufficient in pure form. An example of these virulence factors are those involved in the intracellular growth of *Salmonella*[31] or the invasive ability of *Yersinia*.[32]

Viewing virulence from the standpoint of the bacterium rather than the host permits a perspective that focuses on the selective pressures operating at the level of the microbe. On some occasions, particularly when the inoculum size of bacteria is relatively high, the selective pressures may be exerted more at the level of the population than at the individual microbe. In this case, heterogeneity in the population, whether genetic or merely phenotypic, would be a benefit to the population undergoing changing environmental pressures. At the individual microbial level, the response of the successful pathogen to a changing environment is the ability to alter expression of important factors that interact with the environment. Since the full spectrum of the infectious process brings the pathogen through many different microenvironments sequentially, many important virulence factors are either genetically regulated or variant so that a flexibility of response to the environment can occur.

Given the fact that the microbe must manifest properties that permit growth within the host while evading its defenses under changing microenvironments, it is evident that the processes of pathogenesis are complex. The successful investigation of these processes therefore requires an assortment of approaches. The very first step in any approach is epidemiologic. At the level of determining what organisms might be responsible for producing disease in a state where one is dealing with a complex flora, correlation studies linking the presence of the microbe with the occurrence of the illness lead to tentative assignments of causality. After the preliminary identification of the microbe, Koch's postulates define the set of experiments needed to be performed to complete the causative linkage. Similarly, at the molecular level of virulence, an initial epidemiologic approach allows assortment of phenotypes with a statistical propensity of disease formation. By analogy, causality at the molecular level can be determined only with molecular purification and characterization of either the candidate gene or gene product. Alternatively, genetic methods can be used to show that a mutation in the candidate virulence gene leads to a loss of virulence.

The approach taken by the student of molecular pathogenesis depends upon the type of virulence factor to be investigated. A primary virulence factor of the subclass that, by itself, is capable of causing damage to the host is usually examined biochemically. Thus, the factor is purified and characterized chemically and in relationship to the effects on host tissue or an animal model. Recently, recombinant methods have been employed to molecularly clone the gene or genes that encode the virulence factor.[33] Then the product can be characterized by sequencing the DNA and thereby providing an inferred amino acid sequence if the factor is a protein or the cloned gene can be used to help in the biochemical purification of the material. Additionally, on some occasions the cloned gene or genes can be shown to enhance the virulence characteristics of an otherwise avirulent microbe.

Primary virulence factors of the type that are necessary but by themselves insufficient for disease production as well as auxillary virulence factors have been most successfully examined by genetic approaches. In this case, the investigator starts with a virulent microbe, mutates a single gene that results in loss of the full infective phenotype of the organism and then characterizes the mutant on the basis of the lost property or properties. Most recently a form of "negative cloning" has been used to isolate mutations in specifically chosen genes.[34] In this approach the investigator first uses the tools of molecular genetics to clone a gene of potential importance in pathogenesis. By then mutating this gene in vitro and reintroducing the mutant allele, a site-specific mutation can be introduced into the otherwise virulent strain.

What follows is a description of a number of virulence factors (Fig. 1) that have been identified in the Enterobacteriaceae along with a discussion, where appropriate, of the approaches used to identify these factors at the molecular level. Mention will be confined to those factors that are essential for or that potentiate the production of infectious disease, keeping in mind that the primary selective pressure for the evolution of these factors is not in the production of disease but rather in the growth promotion of the organism at the site of its propagation.

Adhesins. Virtually all gram-negative bacteria examined ultrastructurally possess surface organelles known as fimbriae or pili.[36–38] As reviewed extensively in Chapter 2, these organelles are indispensable in promoting the adherence of bacteria to mucosal surfaces, which is an essential first step in the colonization of the host by the organism. A typical bacterium has several hundred of these hairlike organelles radiating in a peritrichous fashion from the surface of the cell in all directions, which effectively doubles the radius of the organism. Each individual fimbria consists of about a thousand subunits of an identical protein arranged in a helix. Among these identical subunits and present on each individual fimbriae is a small number of specialized subunits that provide the organelle with its binding specificity.

Fimbriae have been characterized in two different ways, one antigenic, the other functional. Colonization factor antigen (CFA) I and CFA II, defined antigenically, have been found on a number of *E. coli* associated with gastroenteritis. The binding sites on the mucosa to which these fimbriae attach are still unknown, but recent evidence suggests that CFAI binds to a sialoglycoprotein.[39] In contrast, types 1, P, and S fimbriae were initially identified on the basis of their abilities to bind specifically to mannose, digalactose, or sialylgalactoside receptors, respectively. Recently, minor components within types 1,[40,41] and P fimbriae[42,43] have been shown to be responsible for their respective binding abilities and have been characterized genetically and biochemically. These lectinlike subunits are lo-

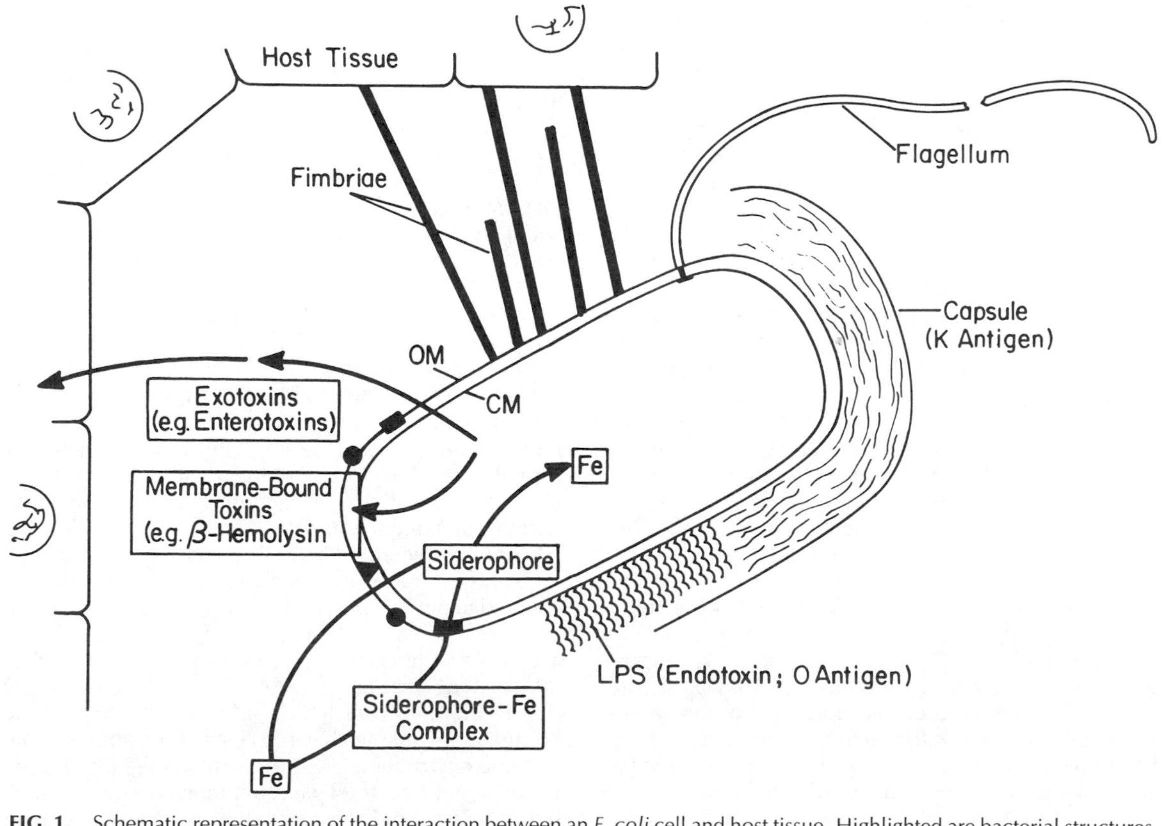

FIG. 1. Schematic representation of the interaction between an *E. coli* cell and host tissue. Highlighted are bacterial structures that are considered important in bacterial pathogenicity. Fe: iron; OM: outer membrane; CM: cytoplasmic membrane; LPS: lipopolysaccharide. (From Eisenstein et al.,[35] with permission.)

cated at the tips of the fimbriae,[44] so the vast part of the organelle is mostly a long extension for the actual ligand.

A number of studies have shown the importance of these adhesins in infection. The plasmid-borne, CFA class of adhesins is extremely important in many forms of *E. coli*-induced gastroenteritis.[45–47] Epidemiologically, P fimbriae are highly associated with *E. coli* strains that are capable of producing urinary tract infection, particularly pyelonephritis,[48–51] and S fimbriae are associated with *E. coli* strains recovered from neonates with sepsis or meningitis.[52] Mutation studies have shown that the specific loss of P fimbriae abrogates the ability of the *E. coli* strain to cause urinary tract infection in the appropriate animal model. The specific epidemiologic linkage of type 1 fimbriae with disease is less clear-cut. *Escherichia coli* found in sites where there is no disease, such as the gastrointestinal tract, and *E. coli* recovered from sites of infection, such as the blood stream and the urinary tract, have been shown to possess type 1 fimbriae in equally high proportion.[53] Nevertheless, recent genetic studies have shown that type 1 fimbriae greatly potentiate the ability of strains of *E. coli* also containing toxin to deliver toxin to susceptible eukaryotic cells.[54] In the same study the type 1 fimbriae were shown to potentiate the ability of the bacteria to extract nutrients by virtue of close adherence from tissue culture cells. Thus, type 1 fimbriae are the type of bacterial factor discussed earlier that potentiates growth hardiness of both pathogenic and nonpathogenic organisms in the human environment and also potentiates the primary virulence factors (i.e., toxins) of pathogenic organisms.

Most bacterial virulence factors that have been studied have been found to be regulated genetically in some way to allow the bacteria to respond flexibly to the environment. A well worked out example by such genetic regulation is discussed below in the context of iron acquisition. A mode of atypical genetic expression is found with type 1 fimbriae in that individual bacteria can oscillate between expressing and not expressing the organelles. Moreover, an individual organism in either state of fimbriation will shift to the alternative phase at a relatively high frequency of once per hundred to thousand divisions. This process of switching back and forth between fimbriate and afimbriate states is quite similar to the flagellar phase variation first described in *Salmonella*. The pathogenic significance of phase variation of flagella in *Salmonella* probably relates to antigenic evasion in that motility can be preserved even under conditions when significant antibody response has been generated against the first phase of flagella.

The role of phase variation in the pathogenic life cycle of *E. coli* is conjectural but may be connected with the fact that type 1 fimbriae not only mediate binding of the bacteria to mucosal surfaces but also to mannose receptors on phagocytic cells. Based on evidence from an animal model of urinary tract infections where *Proteus mirabilis* organisms were inoculated either by the hematogenous or the mucosal route, it has been found that fimbriate organisms are more virulent at the colonization stage of infection whereas afimbriate bacteria are more virulent in the invasive stage of infection.[55] Given the high rate of phase variation, both fimbriate and afimbriate bacteria will be well represented within any given population of *P. mirabilis* or *E. coli*. This population heterogeneity provides survival flexibility under conditions involving rapid changes in the microenvironment, as would occur during an infection. The genetic basis of both fimbrial and flagellar phase variation is the inversion of a small segment of DNA that contains the transcriptional promoter for the respective organelle.[23] Viewed in the broadest context of virulence (i.e., survival of the population in the host), the genetic switch that permits the bacterium to adapt to different environments during an infective process might itself be considered an auxillary virulence factor.[24]

Toxins. Bacterial toxins, reviewed more extensively in Chapter 1, are the most clear-cut examples of virulence factors. Classic biochemical techniques have been used to purify and characterize these molecules.[56] By definition, toxins in pure form interact in some specific way with the host to produce a response as determined by an alteration in the viability or physiology of the target cell system.[57] Cytotoxins and hemolysins destroy cells, whereas many other toxins cause harm to the whole organism in the absence of individual cell death. Some potent toxins are capable of producing the disease caused by the whole pathogen. For instance, tetanus or botulinum toxin, when injected into animals, reproduces the respecive diseases. Likewise, purified endotoxin from gram-negative organisms is capable of reproducing the septic shock picture associated with gram-negative bacteremia. For the most part, however, toxins associated with the Enterobacteriaceae are by themselves insufficient to fully reproduce the infection pathology. Some toxins in fact have unknown roles in the infectious process.

An important piece of epidemiologic evidence that hemolysins are important in some diseases caused by *E. coli* is the finding that over half of *E. coli* organisms isolated in extraintestinal infections possess hemolysin whereas fewer than 10 percent of *E. coli* isolated from the gastrointestinal tract possess hemolysin.[58,59] There seem to be further correlations among virulence factors when one examines the relationship between adhesin production and hemolysin.[52,60] Thus, most uropathogenic *E. coli* contain both the P fimbriae and hemolysin.[53] Experimental studies demonstrating the importance of hemolysin have shown that laboratory-constructed hemolytic strains and nonhemolytic strains mixed with extracted hemolysin are more virulent in animal model studies as compared with strains in which the hemolysin gene has been inactivated.[59,61,62] Other epidemiologic studies show that uropathogenic *E. coli* are also resistant to the bactericidal effect of serum.[63]

A number of molecular varieties of *E. coli* cytotoxins have been described.[64] α-Hemolysins are large molecular weight proteins that can be excreted; β-hemolysins remain cell bound.[59] The cytotoxicity of hemolysins is not limited to red cells but extends to white cells as well and is due to the production of transmembrane pores.[65] There is relative tissue specificity for these toxins; α-hemolysis are more effective cytotoxins of lymphocytes,[66] whereas β-hemolysins are more capable of inhibiting the phagocytosis[67] and chemotaxis[68] of neutrophils. The genetics of hemolysins are probably best worked out for the α variety, which are encoded by both plasmid and chromosomal genes.[59,69] There is little structural homology between the plasmid-encoded and the chromosomally encoded hemolysins, which has led investigators to believe that these hemolysins serve different virulence functions.[70] The regulation of some of these hemolysin genes appears to depend upon iron availability.[71] A different class of cytotoxins are those produced by enteropathogenic *E. coli* (EPEC) and that are very similar to the cytotoxins of *Shigella dysenteriae*.[72–74] EPEC strains, while consisting of a diversity of serogroups, cause virtually identical gastrointestinal disease (see below). The toxins from these different strains are remarkably similar functionally and are uniformally capable of destroying various tissue culture lines, of causing lethality in mice, and of demonstrating gastrointestinal toxicity in suitable animal models.

Unlike the secreted hemolysins, which can act at a long range and whose targets are widespread, the enterotoxins of the enterotoxigenic *E. coli* (ETEC) are cell associated, act at short distances, and exhibit more striking tissue specificity.[56,57] There are two major classes of enterotoxins, the heat-stable toxins (ST) and the heat-labile toxins (LT). The ST is a small molecule that is heavily cross-linked internally with disulfide bonds. It is this cross-linking that provides the stability to heat and enzymatic destruction by proteases (as might be found in the gastrointestinal tract). ST is much more tissue specific than is LT but acts in a similar way in altering the intracellular cyclic nucleotide pools; ST elevates the concentration of cyclic guanine monophosphate (cGMP) which results in altered ion transport and markedly increased fluid excretion by the mucosal cells of the small intestine.[57,75] LT is a much larger molecule and is virtually identical to the cholera toxin of *Vibrio cholerae* in that they display marked serologic cross-reactivity and structural homology.[76] Both are multimeric molecules consisting of a single A polypeptide and a pentameric B polypeptide. The B molecule is the binding part of the toxin and binds to a galactoglycoprotein on the mucosal surface of the small intestinal cells thereby allowing the secondary entry of the A molecule, which is the toxic part of the toxin.[77] Once inside the cell, the A component catalyzes the adenosine diphosphate ribosylation of the guanyl nucleotide-dependent component of adenylate cyclase. The resulting elevated levels of cyclic adenine monophosphate (cAMP) lead to altered electrolyte transport and excessive fluid excretion by the mucosal cells. Tissue cells exhibit an all-or-none susceptibility to LT enterotoxin as a consequence of the tissue binding specificity of the B protomer. Those cells lacking receptors to the B protomer are insensitive to the LT enterotoxin.

Unlike the cytotoxins and enterotoxins whose distribution is restricted to pathogenic strains of the Enterobacteriaceae, endotoxin is ubiquitous in all gram-negative organisms. As discussed earlier, endotoxin consists of the LPS of the outer membrane. Whereas the O antigenic reactivity of the LPS depends upon the auxillary polysaccharide side chains found only in smooth strains, the toxic moiety of LPS resides in the lipid A region found in all strains. Thus all LPS molecules possess endotoxin function, but only some possess O antigenicity. Attempts have been made to raise neutralizing antibodies against the core antigen of LPS, which is conserved in gram-negative bacteria.[78] Some success has occurred with both polyclonal sera[78] and a human monoclonal antibody,[79] which has led to some optimism about the use of these or similar reagents for passive immunotherapy for endotoxic shock. As discussed in Chapter 59, the septic shock response seen in some patients with gram-negative bacteremia can be ascribed almost entirely to the presence of circulating endotoxin. Purified LPS, when administered to animals, causes fever, leukopenia, thrombocytopenia, disseminated intravascular coagulation, and activation of the complement pathways. Other important effects of endotoxin include the release of vasoactive substances and direct cardiovascular function.

Iron Acquisition. The ability to acquire nutrients is an essential attribute of any succcessful organism. As discussed before, the life cycle of a pathogenic microorganism brings it into environments with various degrees of nutritional richness. In the extraintestinal phase of infection by gram-negative bacteria, iron becomes one of the major limiting factors for further growth.[80] This limitation is, in large part, due to the fact that almost all of the iron in the human body is sequestered in either hemeproteins such as hemoglobin and myoglobin or in iron-chelating proteins involved with iron transport such as transferrin and lactoferrin.[80] It is not surprising, then, that the available concentration of iron significantly influences the virulence of *E. coli*.[81] When injected in conjunction with *E. coli*, iron substantially reduces the dose of bacteria needed for lethality.[82] To get around this enormous limitation of iron availability, bacteria have evolved specialized means to acquire iron that involve a high-affinity iron-capturing system capable of competing with the extremely high affinity systems found in the mammalian tissue. Many bacteria are capable of excreting an iron-chelating compound, or siderophore, that the bacteria can then take up again once an extracellular iron siderophore complex has been formed.[80,83] In Enterobacteriaceae the catechol enterobactin is the most commonly occurring siderophore. This compound is excreted by the bacteria when it chelates extracellular iron and is returned back into the bacterial cell where it is then degraded to release the bound iron. *Escherichia coli* strains found specifically in extraintestinal infections have been found to also produce the hydroxymate iron chelator aerobactin, which was initially associated with colicin V plasmids found in many virulent *E. coli* strains.[84,85] More recently it has been found that in some K1 strains of *E. coli* the aerobactin genes are chromosomal.[86]

The evidence that siderophores contribute to virulence is best established for aerobactin. Even though the iron-chelating capacity of aerobactin is significantly less than that of enterobactin and transferrin, aerobactin but not enterobactin has been shown to confer a selective advantage for growth in the body.[87–89] Enterobactin, in contrast, is far more antigenic and elicits an antibody response that inhibits enterobactin's iron uptake efficiency.[90] Both the enterobactin and aerobactin systems are tightly regulated genetically such that, under low iron conditions, expression of both siderophore systems is very high.[80]

An alternative way for the bacterium to acquire iron in the blood stream that may not require any siderophore is hemolysis. Since released hemoglobin contains readily available iron, the action of hemolysin in the blood stream may be equally or more important than is the siderophore systems in providing the bacteria with iron. Contrariwise, the host has evolved mechanisms to decrease its vulnerability to blood-borne bacteria by markedly increasing its sequestration of iron after the onset of pyrexia.[91] The release by the liver of such acute-phase reactants as transferrin is probably an adaptation to the threat of bacteremia.

Capsules. As discussed earlier, the K antigens of *E. coli* consist either of proteinaceous organelles important in colonization of some bacteria usually not associated with human disease (e.g., porcine and bovine gastroenteritis) or consist of polysaccharide capsules. The capsules act in a purely defensive way to promote bacterial virulence by decreasing the ability of antibodies to bind to bacteria and of white cells to phagocytose bacteria. The shieldlike properties depend on two characteristics. First, their polysaccharide composition makes capsules highly hydrophilic, which strongly inhibits phagocytosis by the hydrophobic-surfaced host cells.[92] Second, many capsules are relatively poor immunogens[93] and poor activators of complement.[94] Nevertheless, the antiphagocytic properties of capsules can be overcome by antibodies specifically raised against capsular vaccines, which has been so successful with the pneumococcus, the meningococcus, and *Haemophilus influenzae*. Antibody binding to capsule not only exposes the Fc component of immunoglobulin but also renders the bacterial surface more hydrophobic[92] and allows the activation of the classic pathway of complement.[95]

The best studied capsule found in *E. coli* is the K1 capsular antigen, which is a polymer of *N*-acetyl neuraminic acid. This molecule closely mimics similar compounds found in mammalian tissue and probably is the reason for its poor immunogenicity. In studies with isogenic strains of K1-positive and K1-negative *E. coli*, only the K1-negative mutants were readily killed by complement.[96] Thus, the K1 capsule is unequivocally a virulence factor of the growth-promoting or defensive variety.

Although capsules may be the most important component in allowing gram-negative bacteria to invade the blood stream successfully, other components of the bacterial envelope have been shown to contribute to serum resistance. In some strains of *E. coli* that contain the colicin V plasmid, a particular genetic determinant, *iss*, has been shown to encode resistance to the bactericidal action of serum and complement.[97] Other plasmids, including some R-factors, have also been found to increase the resistance of *E. coli* to serum bactericidal activity.[98] The biochemical basis of non-capsule-mediated serum resistance is not well understood but is believed to be due in some way to the thwarting of the normal deposition of the terminal components of complement.

Plasmids: Drug Resistance and Virulence. Plasmids are self-replicating, nonchromosomal units of DNA that carry their own replication machinery as well as any other genes that might be providing the organism with a phenotype that it would lack if the plasmid were missing. A specialized but extraordinarily important class of plasmids are the R-plasmids, which play a predominant role in antimicrobial resistance among gram-negative bacteria.[99] Most of the individual drug resistance determinants found on R-plasmids come in a self-contained genetic package called a transposon that not only possesses the gene for the drug resistance but also the self-contained ability to relocate itself as a genetic package to other plasmids and even the chromosome.[100] Although such transposition events are relatively infrequent, selection of plasmids containing multiple transposons can be readily selected by exposing the plasmid-containing bacteria to the selective pressure of multiple antimicrobial agents. As a consequence of the enormous use of antimicrobial agents in medicine and in agriculture, most R-plasmids have evolved to the point where they contain multiple transposons and thereby provide a multiple drug resistance phenotype to the bacteria in which they reside.[101–103] As is true with many plasmids, most R-plasmids also possess the machinery for conjugal transfer to other strains and species, thereby further spreading drug resistance.

As has been mentioned in the preceding discussion of individual virulence factors, many, including colonization factors, enterotoxin, and hemolysin, are plasmid borne.[104] Predictably, these virulence factors have been found in plasmids that also contain drug resistance determinants.[105–108] Thus, environmental pressure that selects for further spread of this type of R-plasmid, as would be the case with antimicrobial use, is likely to also promulgate the spread of the linked virulence factors. Even in the absence of the drug resistance determinants, plasmids found in certain strains of virulent bacteria have been found to carry multiple virulence factors. For instance, plasmids found in enterotoxigenic strains of *E. coli* have been shown to carry genes both for enterotoxin production and for the colonization factor antigen found to be important in colonization of the human gastrointestinal tract.[45]

THE SPECIFIC PATHOGENS

Escherichia coli

Escherichia coli is the best-studied free-living organism. Among clinical isolates they can be motile or nonmotile, and most ferment lactose. Other biochemical tests frequently used to identify *E. coli* in the clinical microbiology laboratory are as follows: the methyl red reaction is positive, the Voges-Proskauer (VP) test is negative, urease and phenylalanine deaminase activity is absent, H_2S is not produced, citrate cannot be used as the sole carbon source, and the organism will not grow in the presence of KCN.[4]

Escherichia coli is the most frequent cause of some of the most common bacterial infections, including urinary tract infections, bacteremia, and bacterial-related travelers' diarrhea. It is also a leading cause of neonatal meningitis and can cause a variety of other clinical infections including pneumonia.

Enteric Infections Due to Escherichia coli. *Escherichia coli* was first reported to be an etiologic agent of human infantile diarrhea in the 1920s.[109] In the last decade or so the organism has been recognized as the major cause of bacterial gastroenteritis associated with traveling abroad.[110] Enteric infection caused by *E. coli* can be due to at least four different varieties of bacteria operating through different mechanisms[76]: enterotoxigenic *E. coli* (ETEC) are an important cause of travelers' diarrhea, enteropathogenic *E. coli* (EPEC) are an important cause of childhood diarrhea, enteroinvasive *E. coli* (EIEC) cause a disease that is similar to *Shigella*-like dysentery, and enterohemorrhagic *E. coli* (EHEC) cause hemorrhagic colitis and have been associated with the hemolytic–uremic syndrome in children. These pathogens share the general properties of demonstrating specific interactions with the intestinal mucosa, of elaborating various toxins, and of possessing plasmid-encoded virulence factors.[76]

Travelers' diarrhea is characterized by symptoms of abdominal cramps and frequent explosive bowel movements as a consequence of the copious outpouring of fluid from the gastrointestinal tract.[111] The epidemiology of ETEC disease is typically that of an otherwise healthy individual from an industrialized country visiting tropical or subtropical regions characterized by poor hygienic conditions.[112] ETEC is also an occasional cause of diarrhea in children in the United States.[113,114] A number of epidemiologic studies have been performed on travelers to Mexico. In one large outbreak of gastroenteritis, 72 percent of the ill people and 15 percent of the healthy ones harbored LT-producing ETEC.[111] In that study, the incubation period was 1–2 days, the mean duration of the diarrhea was 3–4 days, and symptoms tended to be mild. An occasional individual presented with more severe illness including fever, chills, and vomiting. Other studies with epidemics due to ST-producing ETEC strains do not differ clinically from the LT-producing strains. Since the organism is passed by the fecal–oral route, contamination most likely occurs through unbottled water and salad vegetables likely to be contaminated with fecal content.

The inoculum of organisms must be high enough to resist the normal defensive barriers of the acid pH of the stomach. Colonization of the small intestine then occurs by virtue of the plasmid-encoded surface fimbriae that enabled the bacteria to adhere to the mucosal surface of the gastrointestinal tract.[45] Typically, the same plasmid encodes the enterotoxin that, as discussed earlier, stimulates massive fluid secretion by the mucosal cells by disrupting intracellular levels of cyclic nucleotides. Human immunity to ETEC gastroenteritis probably depends upon the presence of anti-adhesive factor antibodies that are secreted into the gastrointestinal lumen and block bacterial adherence and colonization.[46,115] Because a number of antigenically diverse fimbriae have been identified with ETEC strains, immunity is likely to be type specific.[47] Presumably the lack of gastroenteritis among adult residents of areas associated with travelers' diarrhea is due to their prior exposure to these colonization antigens and the development of the appropriate humoral immunity. A number of other organisms produce ETEC-like illness in travelers, including various bacteria (e.g., *Shigella*, *Salmonella*, *Campylobacter*), viruses (e.g., rotavirus, Norwalk agent), and parasites (e.g., *Giardia*, *Entamoeba*). Classic cholera caused by strains of *Vibrio cholera* expressing the LT-like cholera toxin produce a disease that is initially similar to that produced by ETEC but then goes on to a much more severe, life-threatening disease. At the present time it is not clearly understood why *V. cholera* has the capacity to cause a disease so much more severe than that produced by ETEC, given the marked similarity in the enterotoxins produced by these two bacteria.

Antimicrobial prophylaxis has been effective for travelers' diarrhea, with protection correlated with the lack of acquisition of the pathogenic bacteria in the stool.[116] But because of increasing drug resistance and the possibilities of side effects, many authorities are recommending that travelers avoid antimicrobial prophylaxis and, instead, use care in their consumption of contaminated food and water. Once disease occurs, antimicrobial agents may be useful in shortening the duration of the disease, but fluid and electrolyte replacement is more important and all that is generally needed.[117] Antimotility drugs may help symptomatology but might also increase the time during which the pathogenic bacteria remain in the gastrointestinal tract.

The mode of pathogenesis of the non-ETEC varieties of gastroenteritis is less well understood at the cellular and molecular level. EPEC strains are an important cause of childhood diarrhea, particularly in underdeveloped countries.[118] They have been incriminated in institutional outbreaks of diarrhea, particularly in nurseries. Based on O antigen identification, there appear to be a limited number of *E. coli* clones associated with this disease, particularly those of serogroups 0608, 025, 026, 0111, 0119, 0125–128, and 0142.[119] These bacteria are capable of disrupting the overlying mucous gel of the host cell.[120] EPEC bacteria have been shown to bind to the membranous cells of Peyer's patches,[121] and "enteroadherence" has been shown to be a mechanism of at least some forms of travelers' diarrhea.[122] Among the classic serotypes of EPEC, the adherence factor is plasmid encoded.[123] Other strains have been shown to produce a Shiga-like toxin. EPEC produces a characteristic lesion in the mucosa with the formation of microcolonies and loss of adjacent microvilli.[124]

The enteroinvasive *E. coli* (EIEC) are capable of cellular invasion and thus are quite different from the typical *E. coli* pathogen, which limits itself to the mucosal surface.[125] As a consequence of cellular invasion, EIEC strains provoke a significant inflammatory response associated with destruction of the intestinal mucosa. Clinically these events result in a picture similar to that of bacterial dysentery, with a high incidence of fever and bloody diarrhea containing inflammatory leukocytes. Fortunately, disease due to EIEC is rare, particularly in the United States. As with ETEC, invasive strains belong to characteristic serogroups, in this case 028, 052, 0112, 0115, 0124, 0136, 0143, 0145, and 0147.[126] The ability to invade is genetically encoded by a large plasmid,[127] and the phenotype can be confirmed with the Sereny test, i.e., the ability to evoke conjunctivitis in guinea pigs.

The enterohemorrhagic *E. coli* belong to the serotype 0157:H7 and were first associated with a multistate outbreak of hemorrhagic colitis in 1982.[128] Unlike classic dysentery, there is no enteroinvasion and inflammation of the mucosa.[129] Typically the patient is afebrile, but in the elderly the disease can be confused with ischemic colitis and can lead to death.[130] These strains have been shown to produce Shiga-like toxins that are cytotoxic for Vero cells.[131,132] At least one Shiga-like toxin is encoded by a lysogenic toxin-converting bacteriophage.[133] Hemolytic–uremic syndrome has been associated with a number of outbreaks with these strains.[134–136]

Urinary Tract Infections. Whereas the major site of normal colonization of the Enterobacteriaceae in the body is the gastrointestinal tract, the most common site for infection is in the urinary tract. Since the urinary tract is normally sterile, any intrusion of bacteria distally (the urethra) to proximally (the kidney) is abnormal. *E. coli* is the most common cause of urinary tract infection and is capable of causing a wide range of illness ranging from uncomplicated urethritis to symptomatic cystitis or pyelonephritis to sepsis.[137] The great majority of uncomplicated infections with *E. coli* (i.e., infections that do not lead to pyelonephritis and sepsis) occur in women by virtue of a shortened urethra and the frequent proximate colonization of the periurethral region with coliform bacteria.[138,139] In contrast, the most important host factor involved in complicated urinary tract infection, whether with *E. coli* or any other bacterium, is the presence of obstruction of normal urinary flow (e.g., prostatic hypertrophy, stones, congenital anomalies) or the presence of a foreign body (e.g., Foley catheter). Whereas specific virulence factors appear to be necessary for uncomplicated infection, relatively nonpathogenic and opportunistic organisms such as *Pseudomonas*, *Proteus*, or *E. coli* lacking virulence factors[140] are capable of causing disease in the presence of a foreign body or obstruction.

A typical patient with uncomplicated cystitis is a sexually active female who was first colonized in the intestine with a uropathogenic strain of *E. coli*. Upon their subsequent colonization of the periurethral region with the help of specific adherence factors, the organisms are propelled into the bladder during sexual intercourse.[141] Postcoital urination may inhibit the subsequent establishment of colonization by these organisms in the bladder and thereby decrease infection. The adherence factor that has been most closely associated with uropathogenic *E. coli* is the P fimbria (or pili associated with pyelonephritis [PAP] pilus).[48–51] The letter designation is derived from the ability of P fimbriae to bind specifically to the P blood group antigen, which contains the disaccharide β-D-Gal 1-4 α-D-Gal.[142] This antigen is present, not only on red cells, but on uroepithelial cells of approximately 99 percent of the population. Well-designed epidemiologic studies have shown that uncomplicated *E. coli* infection is virtually never seen in those individuals lacking the P antigen.[48]

The typical uropathogenic strain of *E. coli* possesses, in addition to P fimbriae, other factors believed needed for the pathogenesis of urinary tract infection. These factors include hemolysin,[143,144] colicin V,[145] and resistance to the complement-dependent bactericidal effect of serum.[146] Most urinary tract infections appear to be due to a small number of O types (04, 06, 075[147]) but these O serogroup strains are also the most prevalent in the gastrointestinal tract.[148] The presence of K antigen is associated with upper urinary tract infections,[149] and antibody to the K antigen has been shown to afford protection against infection in experimental animals.[150] The potential role of hemolysin and resistance to the bactericidal effect of serum on virulence has been discussed previously. It is yet to be shown that the other characteristics of uropathogenic *E. coli* are truly related to their need in virulence or whether they merely reflect a clonal distribution of a handful of strains capable of causing infection.[151]

The use of DNA probe hybridization revealed that uropathogenic *E. coli* possess the genes encoding type 1 fimbriae as well as those for P fimbriae.[53] In contrast to P fimbriae, type 1 fimbriae do not appear to be specific for uropathogenic strains. Type 1 fimbriae may still potentiate colonization of the bladder, perhaps by aggregating masses of bacteria with the mannose-rich Tamm-Horsfall glycoprotein found in the urine.

Respiratory Infections. In contrast to the gastrointestinal and urinary tract infections, which are characterized by *E. coli* exhibiting specific pathogenic features, infections in the respiratory tract appear to be opportunistic.[152,153] Thus, normal hosts become infected with virulent *E. coli* in the gastrointestinal and urinary tracts, but abnormal hosts become infected with nonpathogenic gram-negative organisms elsewhere in the body, particularly the lung. No specific virulence factors have yet been found in *E. coli* that are associated with the respiratory tract disease.

Although one portal of entry of *E. coli* into the lung is hematogenous, the vast majority of gram-negative pneumonias are related to microaspiration of upper airway secretions that have been previously colonized with gram-negative organisms.[154,155] Unlike normal individuals who are infrequently and only transiently colonized by gram-negative organisms, severely ill individuals have an altered physiology that allows such colonization to occur. Recently, some of the molecular details of this association have emerged. Fibronectin is a ubiquitous protein that, among other things, coats the mucosa of the respiratory tract and acts as a specific receptor for many gram-positive bacteria.[156] Severe stress to the body from almost any cause is associated with the presence of a fibronectin-degrading protease in the saliva.[157] With destruction of fibronectin, gram-positive bacteria no longer avidly colonize, which leaves an opening in the ecological niche, and the gram-negative binding receptors underlying the superficial coating of the mucosal tissue become exposed. The result is a markedly enhanced colonization by these gram-negative organisms that, in the context of other inhibitors of normal host response such as foreign bodies in the trachea and a decreased cough reflex, leads to the progression to gram-negative pneumonia.

For these reasons most cases of *E. coli* pneumonia are nosocomial rather than community acquired. Nevertheless, outpatients with severe underlying disease such as diabetes mellitus, alcoholism, and chronic obstructive pulmonary disease are more disposed to gram-negative pneumonias than is the normal population.[152,153] The clinical picture is that of a bronchopneumonia involving the lower lobes, with empyema seen in about a third of the patients and bacteremia in another third of the patients. Among the latter, some of the bacteremias precede the pneumonia and are most frequently secondary to another focus such as the kidneys or the gastrointestinal tract. As expected in a condition that affects primarily debilitated hosts, the death rate is 50 percent or higher. Similar to other gram-negative pneumonias, treatment consists of appropriate antibiotics, drainage of any loculated collections of pus, and respiratory support as required.

Neonatal Meningitis. Infants in their first month of life are particularly predisposed to bacterial meningitis,[158] with *E. coli* and the group B streptococci accounting for the vast majority of cases.[159] In contrast to adult meningitis due to *E. coli*, in neonates there is a strong association between the presence of the K1 capsular antigen and meningitis and, to a lesser extent, with bacteremia.[160,161]

Epidemiologic studies have shown that pregnancy is associated with an increased rate of colonization with K1 strains and that these strains are the ones that are involved in the subsequent neonatal meningitic cases.[162] The pathogenic mechanisms involved with K1 have not yet have been explained, although experiments with neonatal rats show that *E. coli* K1 colonization of the gastrointestinal tract often leads to bacteremia and meningitis.[163] The gastrointestinal tract might be a portal of entry into the blood stream in neonatal humans as well. Fortunately, while such colonization is common, the catastrophic sequelae are rare.

Management of neonatal meningitis requires antibiotic therapy to be initially directed against *E. coli*, the group B streptococci, and the rare *Listeria monocytogenes*. Thus, typical initial therapy should include ampicillin and a third-generation cephalosporin (cefotaxime).

Bacteremia and Miscellaneous Infections Due to Escherichia coli. Although colonization of mucosal surfaces by *E. coli* is frequent, in the gastrointestinal tract, normal, invasive bacteremia is fortunately fairly uncommon. Most strains of *E. coli* are not invasive, particularly in the setting of a normal host with a normal filtering system in the portal circulation (i.e., the liver and spleen). It is much more common to find bacteremia associated with urinary tract infection, particularly when there is obstruction to urinary flow. Given the source of origin, it is not surprising that phenotypic characteristics associated with uropathogenic *E. coli* are also found in bacteremic *E. coli*.[164] Perhaps not unexpectedly, the trait of resistance to the serum bactericidal effect is particularly frequent in the bacteremia isolates. As mentioned previously, a number of biochemical antigenic factors have been shown to correlate with serum resistance, in particular the K1 antigen.

Perhaps the hallmark of gram-negative bacteremia is the systemic reaction to endotoxin or LPS. LPS, ubiquitous in all gram-negative organisms, may be the most toxic component of most bacteremic isolates of *E. coli* and can lead to the life-threatening responses of shock, disseminated intravascular coaggulation, and decomplementation. Passive immunization with antibodies directed against LPS might inhibit many of the toxic effects of endotoxin.[78] Of note, protection has been found when antibodies are limited to those directed against the core antigen shared by all gram-negative bacteria. Most recently, a human monoclonal antibody directed against this core cross-reactive moiety has shown some promise in passive protection studies in animals,[79] which has led to speculation that, in addition to the mainstay of antibiotics and blood pressure control, passive immunotherapy directed against the circulating toxic LPS might prove efficacious for gram-negative bacteria in humans.

Escherichia coli is the leading cause of nosocomial bactermia, with an incidence in 1979 of 2.7 per 10,000 hospital discharges.[165] the primary foci in the hospitalized patient include foreign bodies, in the form of intravenous catheters and endotracheal tubes, and the urogenital, gastrointestinal, and respiratory tracts. As a consequence either of metastatic spread from bacteremia or from contiguous spread, *E. coli* has been found in a wide variety of miscellaneous infections. Contiguous infection is most often found in the distal extremities of individuals with vascular disease, particularly those with diabetes mellitus. In such cases the organism is part of a polymicrobial mixture that includes anaerobic as well as aerobic bacteria. *Escherichia coli* has also been seen in septic arthritis,[166] endophthalmitis,[167] suppurative thyroiditis,[168] intra-abdominal abscess,[169] spontaneous bacterial peritonitis,[170] liver abscess,[171] brain abscess,[172] endocarditis,[173] osteomyelitis, prostatitis,[174] sinusitis, septic thrombophlebitis, and others. As with any bacterial infection, proper management includes the use of antibiotics on the basis of susceptibility patterns of the organism, drainage of pus, and/or surgical débridement when indicated.

TRIBE KLEBSIELLEAE

The four genera *Klebsiella*, *Enterobacter*, *Serratia*, and *Hafnia* belong to the tribe Klebsielleae.[4] Like *E. coli* these organisms are colonizers of the human gastrointestinal tract and are capable of causing a wide variety of clinical syndromes including urinary tract infection, pneumonia, and bacteremia. Unlike the virulent strains of *E. coli* described above, however, this group of organisms is rarely associated with disease in the normal host. Nevertheless, they are a major cause of nosocomial and opportunistic infection.[165]

Klebsiella

The genus *Klebsiella* constitute a group of nonmotile bacteria that have been traditionally speciated into *K. pneumonia*, *K. ozaenae*, and *K. rhinoscleromatis*. This traditional grouping is based on the biochemical reactions of bacteria in the genus. With the introduction of DNA hybridization assays to determine relatedness, the present view is that all these bacteria belong to one species because their DNAs are homologous. But DNA relatedness studies have shown that there is an additional species, *Klebsiella oxytoca*, that is indole-positive.[3] Most clinical laboratories still retain the traditional designations since the distinctions are of some value in epidemiologic investigations. Other important characteristics of these bacteria are that they are unencapsulated, lactose fermenting, H_2S- and indole-negative, and capable of growing in KCN and using citrate as a sole carbon source, and they give a positive VP reaction. A notable characteristic of *Klebsiella* is their large appearance by Gram stain. This property as well as the property of forming large mucoid colonies on agar media is due to a prominent polysaccharide capsule. The large capsule has also made K antigen serotyping more important than O antigen serotyping is for *Klebsiella*. More than 70 types of K antigen have been identified, with some of them showing cross-reactivity with capsules of the pneumococcus and *H. influenzae*. Although the capsule is an important virulence factor in preventing phagocytosis and helping to retard leukocyte migration into infected areas, no capsular type has been found to be associated with greater likelihood of infection. Except for endotoxin, no other constant virulence factor has been found in *Klebsiella* that has been characterized in the molecular detail seen with *E. coli*.[175]

Klebsiella pneumoniae is associated with one important primary infection, lobar pneumonia. Even this classic, community-acquired illness can be reviewed as an opportunistic infection, however, given the subset of individuals who develop this disease. *Klebsiella* lobar pneumonia is virtually limited to people with severe enough underlying problems, particularly alcoholism, diabetes mellitus, and chronic obstructive pulmonary disease, so that their respiratory host defenses are impaired. Typically, the disease produces a severe, acute-onset illness characterized by destructive changes in the lung. Because of the necrotic inflammatory, and hemorrhagic nature of the disease, the sputum is often described as "currant jelly" in quality, and the radiographic appearance is classically that of a swollen infiltrated lobe, which produces the "bowed fissure" radiologic sign. There is a high propensity toward abscess formation, cavitation, empyema, and pleural adhesions. Because of the necrotizing quality of the illness and the debilitated condition of the individuals predisposed to this disease, mortality is high. For this reason treatment has generally been aggressive in the use of multiple antibiotics; a combination of cephalosporin and an aminoglycoside is presently preferred.

Although the most dramatic presentation of *Klebsiella pneumoniae* is as a lobar pneumonia, most cases are more subtle. Most pulmonary disease comes in the form of either bronchopneumonia or bronchitis and is usually hospital acquired. Capsular types 1, 3, 4, and 5 have been particularly associated with respiratory infection, but even among these strains, the predisposition for nosocomial infection outweighs community-acquired disease. Most isolates are found to be associated not with the respiratory tract but with urinary tract infection. In a recent survey, *Klebsiella* was the cause of 9 percent of urinary tract infections and 14 percent of all primary bacteremias in hospitalized patients, the bacteremic rate second by only a slim margin to *E. coli*.[165] *Klebsiella* has been incriminated in 8 percent of all nosocomial bacterial infection. The most common foci for such infections are the urinary tract, lower respiratory tract, biliary tract, and surgical wound sites, in that order.[176] Invasive devices found in hospitalized patients, particularly urinary catheters, endotracheal tubes, and intravenous catheters, markedly increase the disposition to any nosocomial infection, particularly gram-negative rods.[177] Like most gram-negative organisms found in the hospital environment, *Klebsiella* is characteristically resistant to multiple antibiotics. Already naturally resistant to ampicillin and carbenicillin, increasing acquisition of R-plasmids is providing drug resistance to cephalosporins and aminoglycosides with increased frequency.[178,179] The antibiotic treatment of nosocomial *Klebsiella* infections requires susceptibility determinations for optimization. Empirical coverage should be tailored to the drug resistance pattern seen in the local hospital setting.

The other species of *Klebsiella* are less common causes of similar nosocomial infections in hospitalized patients in the United States. *K. ozaenae* and *K. rhinoscleromatis* have been associated with upper respiratory infection, predominantly abroad. Rhinoscleroma, caused by *K. rhinoscleromatis*, is a chronic granulomatous disease involving the mucosa of the upper respiratory system and leads occasionally to bony invasion and airway obstruction.[180] In certain endemic areas in eastern Europe, central Africa, Latin America, and southern Asia, the disease can be quite common,[181] but the disease seems to be generally poorly communicable.[182] The organism is susceptible to a variety of organisms including streptomycin, tetracycline, and trimethoprim-sulfa, and treatment should be prolonged for 6–8 weeks.[183]

The etiologic role of *K. ozaenae* in chronic atrophic rhinitis, called ozaenia, is conjectural. The disease is associated with destruction of the mucosa and a fetid mucopurulent discharge. It is unclear whether antibiotic therapy directed against this organism is of any help in the condition. On the relatively rare occasions when it is found in association with other entities such as pneumonia, it is usually easily treated with a variety of antibiotics, given its high susceptibility. Occasionally the organism is found to be susceptible to ampicillin and carbenicillin, which is in sharp contrast to *K. pneumonae*.[184]

Enterobacter

The genus *Enterobacter* (formerly *Aerobacter*) consists of *E. aerogenes*; *E. cloacae*; *E. agglomerans* (the Herbicola-Lathyri bacteria and formerly called *Erwinia*); two relatively new species, *E. gergoviae* and *E. sakazakii* (formerly called yellow-pigmented *E. cloacae*); and several species not yet associated with human disease.[4] Until the 1960s these organisms were lumped into the classification, *Klebsiella-Aerobacter*, and little distinction was made between them and *Klebsiella*. Unlike *Klebsiella*, *Enterobacter* organisms are motile and tend to be less heavily encapsulated. They do not produce H_2S on triple sugar iron medium, are indole- and methyl red-negative, give a positive VP result, can grow in the presence of KCN, use citrate as a sole carbon source, and can ferment lactose. Simplified tests for decarboxylation of the diamino acids lysine, arginine, and ornithine differentiate *E. cloacae*, *E. aerogenes*, *E. agglomerans*, and *Klebsiella pneumoniae*.[4]

Enterobacter strains are opportunistic pathogens that rarely cause primary human disease. Nevertheless, they are frequent colonizers of hospitalized patients, particularly those treated with antibiotics, and have been associated with burn, wound, respiratory, and urinary infections.[165,185–189] In contrast to most *Klebsiella*, *Enterobacter* organisms are resistant to first-generation cephalosporins and develop antibiotic resistance readily to second-generation cephalosporins.[190]

Enterobacter cloacae accounts for most hospital-acquired infections with this genus and, along with *E. agglomerans*, was associated with a major epidemic of intravenous line contamination that involved 378 patients in 25 hospitals.[191,192] These organisms are capable of horizontal spread in the hospital environment and, like many opportunistic Ennterobacteriaceae, can be spread on the hands of hospital personnel who neglect appropriate aseptic technique, especially hand washing, between patients.

Serratia

Like the genus *Enterobacter*, *Serratia* is an opportunist that has been recognized as a human pathogen only since the 1960s. Before that time, under the assumption the organism was a nonpathogen, the red pigment found in some strains made them attractive as marker organisms to study a number of important questions involving bacterial transmittal. Great controversy arose when it was discovered that the U.S. Army was using these organisms in the 1950s to study population vulnerability to aerosolized bacteria.[193] Although there is no evidence that the aerosolized strain has been specifically involved in subsequent *Serratia* infections, based on the criticism, it is doubtful that any future experiments of this type will ever be publically acknowledged.

Serratia are motile and ferment lactose slowly, if at all. Most strains do not produce lactose or H_2S on triple sugar iron medium but do have a positive VP reaction, use citrate as a sole carbon source, and grow in the presence of KCN. *Serratia* can be differentiated from other Enterobacteriaceae by the production of an extracellular DNase. There are a large number of named species, but only one, *S. marcescens*, has been routinely associated with human disease. There have been rare reports of disease due to *S. liquifaciens* and *S. rubidaea*; these can be distinguished from *S. marcescens* by decarboxylation and fermentation reactions.

The epidemiology of *Serratia* is somewhat different from other Enterobacteriaceae in that *Serratia* appears to be less likely to colonize the gastrointestinal tract but more likely to colonize the respiratory and urinary tracts of hospitalized adults.[193,194] In contrast, among neonates the gastrointestinal tract may be an important resevoir for cross-contamination.[195] Like the other opportunistic bacteria related to *Serratia*, hand-to-hand spread by hospital personnel is the most important factor in horizontal transmission.[193]

Among nosocomial infections, *Serratia* has been found to cause approximately 4 percent of bacteremias and lower respiratory tract infections and 2 percent of urinary tract, surgical wound, and cutaneous infections.[165] In addition to its importance as a hospital-associated opportunist,[193] it has been specifically associated with infections in heroin addicts.[196,197] *Serratia* accounted for 14 percent of addict-associated endocarditis in San Francisco in the early 1970s[196] and has been noted as a cause of osteomyelitis in this population.[197] Most hospital-associated cases are associated with intravenous, intraperitoneal, and urinary catheters[198–201] and instrumentation of the urinary and respiratory tracts.[202,203] *Serratia* organisms, like other members of the Klebsielleae tribe, have also been associated with contaminated intravenous therapy[192] and have been prominent in infections among oncology patients.[204]

In the outpatient setting, *Serratia* is notable for causing septic arthritis among patients receiving intra-articular injections for diagnostic or therapeutic purposes.[205,206] Recently, an epidemic of septic arthritis involving 10 patients was found to be caused by *Serratia* contaminationn of a benzalkonium chloride antiseptic used to soak cotton balls.[207]

Antibiotic treatment of *Serratia* infections is complicated by the high frequency of multiple drug resistance seen in these bacteria. Nevertheless, many if not most strains are susceptible to amikacin,[208,209] with synergy frequently seen with the addition of carbenicillin or ticarcillin.[210] The newer generation β-lactam antibiotics[211–215] as well as the newer quinolones[216,217] may be particularly useful for aminoglycoside-resistant strains.

Hafnia

There remains confusion about the relationship between the genus *Hafnia* and the tribe Klebsielleae. At one time *Hafnia* was considered a member of the genus *Enterobacter* and called *E. hafniae*, but now with the results of DNA relatedness studies as well as biochemical studies, it is defined as a separate genus with one species, *H. alvei*.[2,4] It remains a member of tribe Klebsiella on the basis of the biochemical reactions. The genus is composed of motile bacteria that do not product indole, hydrolyze urea (with rare exceptions), or liquify gelatin. The VP reaction is always positive at 22°C and usually so at 37°C. Lysine and ornithine but rarely arginine are carboxylated.

Hafnia organisms are not frequently involved with infection; when they are, the infections are typically nosocomial.[218,219] Antibiotic susceptibilities appear to be similar to the *Enterobacter* group, so empirical therapy while awaiting antibiotic susceptibilities should be based on patterns for those organisms within the hospital of isolation.

TRIBE PROTEEAE

Proteeae are motile bacteria that deaminate phenylalanine rapidly. Studies employing DNA relatedness have led investigators to conclude that this tribe consists of at least three genera, *Proteus*, *Morganella*, and *Providencia*, and seven species, *Proteus vulgaris*, *Proteus mirabilis*, *Proteus myxofaciens*, *Morganella morganii* (previously *Proteus morganii*), *Providencia alcalifaciens*, *Providencia stuartii*, and *Providencia rettgeri* (previously *Proteus rettgeri*).[1,3,4] The biochemical characteristics of the tribe are that the methyl red reaction is positive, the VP reaction is negative (except for occasional strains of *P. mirabilis*), growth can occur in the presence of KCN, sodium alginate is not used as a sole carbon source, gas production is small, and urea is hydrolyzed rapidly and abundantly by *Proteus*, *Morganella*, and *P. rettgeri* but not by the other *Providencia* spp. Virtually all *Proteus mirabilis* strains are indole-negative, whereas virtually all other strains in the tribe are indole-positive. *Proteus* strains are unique in their ability to swarm on moist agar media. This property is a consequence of their extraordinary motility due to hundreds of flagella per cell.[220]

The swarming *Proteus* species are second only to *E. coli* in the percentage of Enterobacteriaceae encountered in clinical laboratories.[2,165] This high frequency is attributable almost entirely to the propensity of these bacteria to colonize and infect the urinary tract. Several characteristics, one of which is specific for *Proteus*, have been identified that contribute to uropathogenicity. *Proteus*, using the enzyme urease, splits urea into ammonium hydroxide, which raises the urinary pH to levels that promote struvite stone formation.[221–223] These stones act as foreign bodies that obstruct urinary flow and serve as a nidus for persistance of infection, properties that tend to make *Proteus* infections chronic and destructive of renal parenchyma. Urease has also been shown to contribute directly to renal tubular toxicity, in part by alkalyzing the urine. *Proteus*, like most other Enterobacteriaceae, possess fimbriae, important for colonization of the uroepithelium,[224,225] and flagella-dependent motility, important for the spread of infection in the urinary tract.[21] Uropathogenic *Proteus* also synthesize several different hemolysins, which may play a role in virulence.[226–228]

Most *Proteus* infections are due to *P. mirabilis*. Up to 10 percent of all uncomplicated urinary tract infections are caused by this species, which can also cause wound infections, pneumonia, and septicemia in the debilitated. As with many other opportunistic infections, the reservoir for many drug-resistant *Proteus mirabilis* infections in the hospital is in the gastrointestinal tracts of the patients who subsequently become infected.[229] Nevertheless, most nosocomial infections caused by members of the tribe Proteeae are due to the indole-positive species rather than *P. mirabilis*. Recently, it has been shown that the most common organism involved in bacteremia in nursing home patients with chronic indwelling catheters is *Providencia stuartii*.[230,231] Given the enlarging size of this population of patients and the resistance of this organism to multiple antibiotics, it has been suggested that *P. stuartii* may become significantly more important as a nosocomial pathogen in the future.[231] Once established in the hospital setting, the indole-positive Proteeae organisms can cause large outbreaks of nosocomial urinary tract infections.[232,233]

Antibiotic treatment of this group of bacteria can be difficult. Although *P. mirabilis* used to be relatively susceptible to the commonly used antimicrobial agents, many isolates have become more resistant, although not yet as resistant as the indole-positive species. Because of the high frequency of aminoglycoside resistance among the indole-positive isolates, treatment often requires the use of amikacin,[234] the newer β-lactam antibiotics, or the newer quinolones.

OTHER ENTEROBACTERIACEAE

Citrobacter

There are three recognized species in the genus *Citrobacter*, *C. amalonaticus*, *C. diversus*, and *C. freundii*; all have been associated with human disease. While this group was formerly classified within the tribe Salmonelleae on the basis of biochemical similarities, the genus is now placed in the separate tribe Citrobactereae.[4] The genus is composed of motile bacteria with positive methyl red reactions, negative VP reactions, growth on Simmons citrate medium (hence its name), and the ability to hydrolyze urea slowly and weakly by most isolates. Production of H_2S is seen only with *C. freundii*, which may make them mistakenly identified as *Salmonella*. However, in contrast to *Salmonella*, *Citrobacter* usually grows in the presence of KCN. Tests for β-galactosidase with O-nitrophenyl-β-D-galactoside (ONPG) and gas from glucose fermentation are typically positive, whereas tests for DNase, lysine and phenylalanine deamination, and inositol fermentation are negative.[2] Considerable cross-reactivity with the O antigens of other Enterobacteriaceae has been noted.

Although not common, *Citrobacter* has been associated with significant nosocomial infection, particularly involving the urinary and respiratory tracts of debilitated, hospitalized patients.[235,236] But most isolates recovered represent either secondary infection or colonization without apparent clinical significance. In contrast, in neonates *Citrobacter* strains, particularly *C. diversus*, have been found to be an important cause of both meningitis and brain abscess formation.[237,238] Epidemiologic investigations of these cases have shown a high colonization rate in associated but uninfected babies.[239,240] Recently, strains of *C. diversus* recovered from patients with meningitis have been found to be more virulent than are nonmeningitic strains in an animal model and to possess an outer membrane protein not seen in the nonpathologic bacteria.[240] Proof of the molecular association of this protein with disease will require further biochemical and genetic analysis. *Citrobacter* has also been associated with endocarditis[241] and hospital-acquired bacteremias. The latter are often polymicrobial and are accompanied by a high mortality rate, most likely due to the highly debilitated state of the host rather than the intrinsic virulence of the organism.[242]

Treatment requires appropriate antimicrobial susceptibility tests of the infecting organism. Most strains of *C. freundii* and *C. diversus* can be distinguished by their susceptibility patterns; the former are frequently susceptible to carbenicillin but not to cephalothin, whereas the latter are resistant to ampicillin and carbenicillin but sensitive to cephalothin.[236] Most strains are susceptible to the aminoglycoside antibiotics.

Edwardsiella

The organisms of the genus *Edwardsiella* are the only members of the tribe Edwardsielleae and make up three species, *E. tarda*, *E. hoshinae*, and *E. ictaluri*. Only *E. tarda* has been associated with human disease. These bacteria are motile and positive for gas from glucose fermentation, H_2S, indole, lysine decarboxylase, and ornithine decarboxylase.[2] The epithet "tarda" is meant to imply biochemical inactivity since the routine reactions not enumerated above are all negative.[4] Because it does not ferment lactose but does produce H_2S on eneteric media, it can be initially misidentified as *Salmonella*.

Edwardsiella rarely causes disease, but when it does it is most often associated with a *Salmonella*-like gastroenteritis.[243] In a survey of thousands of clinical specimens in Panama, there were 50 human isolates of *Edwardsiella*, of which 10 were associated with an intermittent, watery diarrhea that typically lasted several days and was accompanied by vomiting and low-grade fever; 20 isolates were associated with gastrointestinal carriage only.[244] There are case reports of *E. tarda* causing bacteremia,[245] liver abscess,[243,244] meningitis,[245] and soft tissue infection.[243] Although the organism is susceptible to most commonly used antimicrobial agents,[243] treatment is probably not indicated for uncomplicated gastroenteritis.

Erwinia

The genus *Erwinia* consists of bacteria primarily associated with plants. With the exception of a group known as the Herbicola-Lathyri bacteria, which have been reclassified as *Enterobacter agglomerans*, these bacteria are not associated with human disease. Clinically relevant aspects of *Enterobacter agglomerans* are discussed above under "Tribe Klebsielleae."

Miscellaneous Genera

The Enteric Bacteriology Laboratories of the Centers for Disease Control have, for more than 30 years, received cultures of Enterobacteriaceae from clinical laboratories for identification. Many were atypical strains of known genera, but others have been previously unidentified and assigned to new species or new "enteric groups," pending further classification.[246] Over the last decade identification and classification have been greatly augmented with the use of DNA-DNA hybridization, antimicrobial susceptibility patterns, bacteriophage reactivity, and computer-based algorithms. Thus, whereas in 1972 there were only 11 genera and 26 species in the family, by 1985 there were 22 genera, 69 species, and 29 biogroups, or enteric groups.[246] Over 99 percent of all clinical isolates have already been discussed in this chapter, and 80–95 percent of all isolates recovered in a general hospital setting will be either *Escherichia coli*, *Klebsiella pneumoniae*, or *Proteus mirabilis*.[246] As of 1985 the bacteria recovered from humans belonged to the following rare, mostly newly named genera of Enterobacteriaceae: *Buttiauxella*, *Cedecea*, *Ewingella*,[247] *Kluyvera*, *Rhanella*, and *Tatumella*. In addition the enteric groups 17, 41, 45, 57, 58, 59, 60, and 68 have been isolated from clinical specimens.

REFERENCES

1. Farmer JJ III, Howard BJ, Weissfeld AS. Enterobacteriaceae. In: Howard BJ, Klass J II, Rubin SJ, et al, eds. Clinical and Pathogenic Microbiology. St. Louis: CV Mosby, 1987:289–328.
2. Kelly MT, Brenner DJ, Farmer JJ III. Enterobacteriaceae. In: Lennette EH, Balows A, Hausler WJ Jr, et al, eds. Manual of Clinical Microbiology. 4th ed. Washington, DC: American Society for Microbiology; 1985:263–77.
3. Brenner DJ, Family I. Enterobacteriaceae Rahn 1937. In: Krieg NR, Holt JG, eds. Bergey's Manual of Systematic Bacteriology. Baltimore: Williams & Wilkins; 1984:408–516.
4. Ewing WH. Edwards and Ewing's Identification of Enterobacteriaceae. 4th ed. New York: Elsevier Science Publishing, 1986.
5. Achtman M, Pluschke G. Clonal analysis of descent and virulence among selected *Escherichia coli*. Annu Rev Microbiol. 1986;40:185–210.
6. Hartl DL, Dykhuizen DE. The population genetics of *Escherichia coli*. Annu Rev Genet. 1984;18:31–68.
7. Selander RK, Caugant DA, Whittam TS. Genetic structure and variation in natural populations of *Escherichia coli*. In: Neidhardt FC, Ingraham JL, Low KB, et al, eds. *Escherichia coli* and *Salmonella typhimurium*: Cellular and Molecular Biology. Washington, DC: American Society for Microbiology; 1987:1625–48.
8. Campbell A. Evolutionary significance of accessory DNA elements in bacteria. Annu Rev Microbiol. 1981;35:55–38.
9. Farrar WE Jr. Molecular analysis of plasmids in epidemiologic investigation. J Infect Dis. 1983;148:1–6.
10. Mercer AA, Morelli G, Huezenroeder M, et al. Conservation of plasmids among *Escherichia coli* of diverse origins. Infect Immun. 1984;46:649–57.
11. Waschsmuth K. Genotypic approaches to the diagnosis of bacterial infections: plasmid analyses and gene probes. Infect Control. 1985;6:100–9.
12. Thompkins LS, Troup N, Labigne-Roussel A, et al. Cloned, random chromosomal sequences as probes to identify *Salmonella* species. J Infect Dis. 1986;154:156–62.
13. Nikaido H, Vaara M. Outer membrane. In: Neidhardt FC, Ingraham JL, Low KB, et al, eds. *Escherichia coli* and *Salmonella typhimurium*: Cellular and molecular biology. Washington, DC: American Society for Microbiology; 1987:7–22.
14. Orskov F, Orskov I, Jann B, et al. Serology, chemistry and genetics of O and K antigens of *E. coli*. Bacteriol Rev. 1977;41:667–710.
15. Luderitz I, Staub AM, Westphal O. Immunochemistry of O and R antigens of *Salmonella* and related Enterobacteriaceae. Bacteriol Rev. 1966;30:192.
16. Hitchcock PJ, Leive L, Makela PH, et al. Lipopolysaccharide nomenclature—past, present, and future. J Bacteriol. 1986;166:699–705.
17. Rick PD. Lipopolysaccharide biosynthesis. In: Neidhardt FC, Ingraham JL, Low KB, et al, eds. *Escherichia coli* and *Salmonella typhimurium*: Cellular and molecular biology. Washington, DC: American Society for Microbioloy; 1987:648–62.
18. Drach GW, Reed WP, Williams RC. Antigens common to human and bacterial cells. II. *E. coli* 014 and common Enterobacteriaceae antigen blood groups A and B and *E. coli* 086. J Lab Clin Med. 1972;79:38.
19. Springer GF, Horton RE. Blood group isoantibody. Stimulation in man by feeding blood group–active bacteria. J Clin Invest. 1969;48:1280.
20. MacNab RM. Flagella. In Neidhardt FC, Ingraham JL, Low KB, et al, eds. *Escherichia coli* and *Salmonella typhimurium*: Cellular and molecular biology. Washington, DC: American Society for Microbiology; 1987:70–83.
21. Pazin GJ, Braude AI. Immobilizing antibodies in urine. 2. Prevention of ascending spread of *Proteus mirabilis*. Invest Urol. 1974;12:129–33.
22. Simon M, Zeig J, Silverman M, et al. Phase variation: Evolution of a controlling element. Science. 1980;209:1370.
23. Abraham JM, Freitag CS, Clements JR, et al. An invertible element of DNA controls phase variation of type 1 fimbriae of *Escherichia coli*. Proc Natl Acad Sci USA. 1985;82:5724–7.

24. Eisenstein BI. Pathogenic mechanisms of *Legionella pneumophila* and *Escherichia coli*. ASM News. 1987;53:621–4.
25. Jann K, Jann B. The K antigens of *Escherichia coli*. Prog Allergy. 1982;33:53–79.
26. Wilfert C. *E. coli* menigitis: K_1 antigen and virulence. Annu Rev Med. 1978;29:129–36.
27. Stevens P, Huang SN-Y, Welch WD, et al. Restricted complement activation by *Escherichia coli* with the K-1 capsular serotype: A possible role in pathogenicity. J Immunol. 1978;121:2174–80.
28. Kaisjer B, Jodal U, Hanson LA. Studies in antibody response and tolerance to *E. coli* K antigens in immunized rabbits and in children with urinary tract infection. Int Arch Allerg. 1973;44:260–73.
29. Silver RP, Finn CW, Vann WF, et al. Molecular cloning of the K1 capsular polysaccharide genes of *E. coli*. Nature. 1981;289:696–8.
30. Kaisjer B, Larrson P, Olling S, et al. Protection against acute, ascending pyelonephritis caused by *Escherichia coli* in rats, using isolated capsular antigen conjugated to bovine serum albumin. Infect Immun. 1983;39:142.
31. Fields PI, Swanson RV, Haidaris CG, et al. Mutants of *Salmonella typhimurium* that cannot survive within the macrophage are avirulent. Proc Natl Acad Sci USA. 1986;83:5189–93.
32. Isberg RR, Falkow S. A single genetic locus encoded by *Yersinia pseudotuberculosis* permits invasion of cultured animal cells by *E. coli* K12. Nature. 1985;317:262–4.
33. Eisenstein BI, Engleberg NC. Applied molecular genetics: New tools for the microbiologist and clinician. J Infect Dis. 1986;153:416–30.
34. Ruvkin GB, Ausubel F. A general method for site-directed mutagenesis in procaryotes. Nature. 1981;289:85–8.
35. Eisenstein BI, Jones GW. The spectrum of infectious and pathogenic mechanisms of *Escherichia coli*. Adv Intern Med. 1988;33:231–52.
36. Jones GW, Isaacson RE. Proteinaceous bacterial adhesins and their receptors. CRC Crit Rev Microbiol. 1983;10:229–60.
37. Klemm P. Fimbrial adhesins of *Escherichia coli*. Rev Infect Dis. 1985;7:321–40.
38. Clegg S, Gerlach GF. Enterobacterial fimbriae. J Bacteriol. 1987;169:937–8.
39. Pieroni P, Worobec EA, Paranchych W, et al. Identification of a human erythrocyte receptor for colonization factor antigne I pili expressed by H10407 enterotoxigenic *Escherichia coli*. Infect Immun. 1988;56:1334–40.
40. Maurer L, Orndorff PE. A new locus, *pilE*, required for the binding of type 1 piliated *Escherichia coli* to erythrocytes. FEMS Microbiol Lett. 1985;30:59–66.
41. Minion FC, Abraham SN, Beachey EJ, et al. The genetic determinant of adhesive function in type 1 fimbriae of *Escherichia coli* is distinct from the gene encoding the fimbrial subunit. J Bacteriol. 1986;165:1033–6.
42. Lindberg FP, Lund B, and Normark S. Gene products specifying adhesion of uropathogenic *Escherichia coli* are minor components of pili. Proc Natl Acad Sci USA. 1986;83:1891–5.
43. Uhlin BE, Norgren M, Baba M, et al. Adhesin to human cells by *Escherichia coli* lacking the major subunit of a digalactoside-specific pilus adhesin. Proc Natl Acad Sci USA. 1985;82:1800–4.
44. Lindberg F, Lund B, Johansson L, et al. Localization of the receptor-binding protein adhesin at the tip of the bacterial pilus. Nature. 1987;328:84–7.
45. Evans DJ, Silver RP, Evans DJ Jr. Plasmid controlled colonization factor associated with virulence in *E. coli* enterotoxigenic for humans. Infect Immun. 1975;12:656–67.
46. Levine MM, Kaper JB, Black RE, et al. New knowledge on pathogenesis of bacterial enteric infections as applied to vaccine development. Microbiol Rev. 1983;47:510–50.
47. Mooi FR, de Graaf FK. Molecular biology of fimbriae of enterotoxigenic *Escherichia coli*. Curr Top Microbiol Immunol. 1985;118:119.
48. Lomberg H, Hanson LA, Jacobson B, et al. Correlation of P blood group, vesicoureteral reflux and bacterial attachment in patients with recurrent pyelonephritis. N Engl J Med. 1983;308:1189–92.
49. Kallenius G, Molby R, Svenson S, et al. Occurrence of P-fimbriated *Escherichia coli* in urinary tract infections. Lancet. 1981;2:1369–72.
50. Vaisanen V, Elo J, Tallgren L, et al. Mannose-resistant hemagglutination and P antigen recognition are characteristic of *Escherichia coli* causing primary pyelonephritis. Lancet. 1981;2:1366–9.
51. Svanborg-Eden C, Freter R, Hagberg L, et al. Inhibition of experimental ascending urinary tract infection by an epithelial cell-surface receptor analogue. Nature. 1982;298:560.
52. Korhonen TK, Valtonen MV, Parkkinen J, et al. Serotypes, hemolysin production, and receptor recognition of *Escherichia coli* strains associated with neonatal sepsis and meningitis. Infect Immun. 1985;48:486.
53. O'Hanley P, Low D, Romero I, et al. Gal-Gal binding and hemolysin phenotypes and genotypes associated with uropathogenic *Escherichia coli* N Engl J Med. 1985;313:414.
54. Zafriri D, Oron Y, Eisenstein BI, et al. Growth advantage and enhanced toxicity of *Escherichia coli* adherent to tissue culture cells due to restricted diffusion of products secreted by the cells. J Clin Invest. 1987;79:1210–6.
55. Silverblatt FJ, Ofek I. Influence of pili on the virulence of *Proteus mirabilis* in experimental hematogenous pyelonephritis. J Infect Dis. 1977;138:664–7.
56. Middlebrook J, Dorland RB. Bacterial toxins: Cellular mechanisms of action. Microbiol Rev. 1984;48:199–221.
57. Eidels L, Proia RL, Hart DA. Membrane receptors for bacterial toxins. Microbiol Rev. 1983;47:596–620.
58. Welch RA, Dellinger EP, Minshew B, et al. Haemolysin contributes to virulence of extraintestinal *Escherichia coli* infections. Nature. 1981;294:665–7.
59. Cavalieri SJ, Bohach GA, Snyder IS. *Escherichia coli* alpha-hemolysin: Characteristics and probable role in pathogenicity. Microbiol Rev. 1984;48:326–43.
60. Gadeberg OV, Orskov I. In vitro cytotoxic effect of alpha-hemolytic *Escherichia coli* on human blood granulocytes. Infect Immun. 1984;45:255–60.
61. Waalwijk C, MacLaren DM, de Graaf J. In vivo function of hemolysin in the nephropathogenicity of *Escherichia coli*. Infect Immun. 1983;42:245–9.
62. Waalwijk C, van den Bosch JF, MacLaren DM, et al. Hemolysin plasmid coding for the virulence nephropathogenic *Escherichia coli* strain. Infect Immun. 1982;35:32–7.
63. Hughes C, Hacker J, Roberts A, et al. Hemolysin production as a virulence marker in symptomatic and asymptomatic urinary tract infections caused by *Escherichia coli*. Infect Immun. 1983;39:546–51.
64. Bohach GA, Snyder IS. Chemical and immunological analysis of the complex structure of *Escherichia coli* alpha-hemolysin. J Bacteriol. 1985;164:1071.
65. Bhakdi S, Mackman N, Nicaud JM, et al. *Escherichia coli* hemolysin may damage target cell membranes by generating transmembrane pores. Infect Immun. 1986;52:63–9.
66. Gadeberg OV, Orskov I, Rhodes JM. Cytotoxic effects of an alpha-hemolytic *Escherichia coli* strain on human blood monocytes and granulocytes in vitro. Infect Immun. 1983;41:358–64.
67. Cavalieri SJ, Snyder IS. Effect of *Escherichia coli* alpha-hemolysin on human peripheral leukocyte viability in vitro. Infect Immun. 1982;37:966–74.
68. Pruett TL, Chenoweth DE, Fiegel VD, et al. *Escherichia colii* and human neutrophils: Effect of bacterial supernatant with hemolysin activity upon chemotaxin receptors. Arch Surg. 1985;120:212.
69. Welch RA, Hull R, Falkow S. Molecular cloning and physical characterization of a chromosomal hemolysin from *Escherichia coli*. Infect Immun. 1983;42:178–86.
70. Muller D, Hughes C, Goebel W. Relationship between plasmid and chromosomal hemolysin determinants of *Escherichia coli*. J Bacteriol. 1983;153:846–51.
71. Lebek G, Gruenig HM. Relation between the hemolytic property and iron metabolism in *Escherichia coli*. Infect Immun. 1985;50:682–6.
72. O'Brien AD, LaVeck GD, Thompson MR, et al. Production of *Shigella dysentariae* type 1-like cytotoxin by *Escherichia coli*. J Infect Dis. 1982;146:763–9.
73. O'Brien AD, LaVeck GD. Purification and characterization of a *Shigella dysenteriae* 1-like toxin produced by *Escherichia coli*. Infect Immun. 1983;40:675–83.
74. Strockbine NA, Marques LR, Holmes RK, et al. Characterization of monoclonal antibodies against shiga-like toxin from *Escherichia coli*. Infect Immun. 1985;50:695–700.
75. van Dommelen FS, de Jonge JR. Local changes in fractional saturation of cGMP- and cAMP-receptors in intestinal microvilli in response to cholera toxin and heat-stable *Escherichia coli* toxin. Biochim Biophys Acta. 1986;886:135.
76. Levine MM. *Escherichia coli* that cause diarrhea: Enterotoxigenic, enteropathogenic, enteroinvasive, enterohemorrhagic, and enteroadherent. J Infect Dis. 1987;155:377–89.
77. Holmgren J, Fredman P, Lindblad M, et al. Rabbit intestinal glycoprotein receptor for *Escherichia coli* heat-labile enterotoxin lacking affinity for cholera toxin. Infect Immun. 1982;38:424–33.
78. Ziegler EJ, McCutchan JA, Fierer J, et al. Treatment of gram-negative bacteremia and shock with human antiserum to a mutant *Escherichia coli*. N Engl J Med. 1982;307:1225–30.
79. Teng NNH, Kaplan HS, Hebert JM, et al. Protection against gram-negative bacteremia and endotoxemia with human monoclonal IgM antibodies. Proc Natl Acad Sci USA. 1985;82:1790–4.
80. Bagg A, Neilands JB. Molecular mechanisms of regulation of siderophore-mediated iron assimilation. Microbiol Rev. 1987;51:509–18.
81. Finkelstein RA, Sciortino CV, McIntosh MA. Role of iron in microbe-host interactions. Rev Infect Dis. 1983;5(Suppl):759–77.
82. Griffiths E: Iron and the susceptibility to bacterial infections. In: Beers RF, Bassett EG, eds. Nutritional Factors: Modulating Effects on Metabolic Processes. New York: Raven Press, 1981:463–676.
83. Lankford CE. Bacterial assimilation of iron. Crit Rev Microbiol. 1973;2:273–331.
84. Stuart SJ, Greenwood KT, Luke RK. Hydroxamate-mediated transport of iron controlled by ColV plasmids. J Bacteriol. 1980;143:35–42.
85. Williams PH. Novel iron uptake system specified by ColV plasmids: An important component in the virulence of invasive strains of *Escherichia coli*. Infect Immun. 1979;26:925–32.
86. Valvano MA, Silver RP, Crossa JH. Occurrence of chromosome—or plasmid—mediated aerobactin iron transport systems and hemolysin production among clonal groups of human invasive strains of *Escherichia coli* K1. Infect Immun. 1986;52:192–9.
87. Warner PJ, Williams PH, Bindereif A. ColV plasmid-specified aerobactin synthesis by invasive strains of *Escherichia coli*. Infect Immun. 1981;33:540–5.
88. Williams PH, Carbonetti NH. Iron, siderophores, and the pursuit of virulence: Independence of the aerobactin and enterochelin iron uptake systems in *Escherichia coli*. Infect Immun. 1986;51:942–7.

89. Montgomerie JZ, Kalmanson GM, Guze LB. Enterobactin and virulence of *Escherichia coli* in pyelonephritis. J Infect Dis. 1979;140:1013.
90. Moore DG, Yancey RJ,Lankford CE, et al. Bacteriostatic enterochelin-specific immunoglobulin from normal human serum. Infect Immun. 1980;27:418–23.
91. Kluger MJ, Rothenburg BA. Fever and reduced iron: Their interaction as a host defense response to bacterial infection. Science. 1979;203:374–6.
92. van Oss CJ. Phagocytosis as a surface phenomenon. Annu Rev. Microbiol. 1978;32:19.
93. Robbins JB, Schneerson R, Egan WB, et al. Virulence properties of bacterial capsular polysaccharides—unanswered questions. In: Smith H, Skehel JH, Turner MJ, eds. The Molecular Basis of Microbial Pathogenicity. Weinheim: Verglag Chemie GmbH; 1980:115–32.
94. Stevens P, Huang SN-Y, Welch WD, et al. Restricted complement activation by *Escherichia coli* with the K1 capsular serotype: A possible role in pathogenicity. J Immunol. 1978;121:2174–80.
95. Taylor PW. Bactericidal and bacteriolytic activity of serum against gram-negative bacteria. Microbiol Rev. 1983;47:46–83.
96. Cabello FC. Determinants of pathogenicity of *E. coli* K1. In Timmis KN, Puhler A, eds. Plasmids of Medical, Environmental and Commercial Importance. Amsterdam: North Holland; 1979:155–60.
97. Binns MM, Mayden J, Levine RP. Further characterization of complement resistance conferred on *Escherichia coli* by the plasmid genes *traT* of R100 and *iss* of ColV.I-K94. Infect Immun. 1982;35:654–9.
98. Moll A, Manning PA, Timmis KN. Plasmid-determined resistance to serum bactericidal activity: A major outer membrane protein, the *traT* gene product, is responsible for plasmid-specified serum resistance in *Escherichia coli.* Infect Immun. 1980;28:359–67.
99. Davies J, Smith DI. Plasmid-determined resistance to antimicrobial agents. Annu Rev Microbiol. 1978;32:469–518.
100. Cohen S. Transposable genetic elements and plasmid evolution. Nature. 1976;263:731–8.
101. Falkow S. Infectious Multiple Drug Resistance. London: Pion, 1975.
102. Finland M. Emergence of antibiotic resistance in hospitals, 1935–1975. Rev Infect Dis. 1979;1:4–21.
103. O'Brien TF, Acar JF, Medeiros AA, et al. International comparison of prevalence of resistance to antibiotics. JAMA. 1978;239:1518–23.
104. Elwell LP, Shipley PL. Plasmid-mediated factors associated with virulence of bacteria to animals. Annu Rev Microbiol. 1980;34:465–96.
105. Gowal D, Saxena S, Mago M, et al. Plasmid mediated enterotoxin production and drug resistance amongst *Escherichia coli* from cases of infantile diarrhea. Indian J Pediatr. 1985;52:57–9.
106. Harnet NM, Gules CL. Linkage of genes for heat-stable enterotoxin, drug resistance, K99 antigen, and colicin in bovine and porcine strains of enterotoxigenic *Escherichia coli.* Am J Vet Res. 1985;46:428–33.
107. Murray B, Evans D, Penaranda M, et al. CFA/I-ST plasmids. Comparison of enterotoxigenic *Escherichia coli* (ETEC) of serogroups 025, 063, 078, and 0128 and mobilization from an R factor-containing epidemic (ETEC) isolate. J Bacteriol. 1983;153:566–70.
108. Waalwijk C, Van Den Bosch J, MacLaren D, et al. Hemolysin plasmid coding for the virulence of a nephropathogenic *E. coli* strain. Infect Immun. 1982;35:32–7.
109. Adam A. Biology of colon bacillus dyspepsia and its relation to pathogenesis and to intoxication. Jahrb Kinderberth. 1923;101:295.
110. Ericsson CD, DuPont HL. Traveler's diarrhea: Recent developments. In: Remington JS, Swartz MN, eds. Current Clinical Topics in Infectious Diseases. 6th ed. New York: McGraw-Hill; 1985:66–84.
111. Gorbach SL, Kean BH, Evand DG, et al. Traveler's diarrhea and toxigenic *E. coli.* N Engl J Med. 1975;292:933–6.
112. Steffen R, VanderLinde F, Gyr K, et al. Epidemiology of diarrhea in travelers. JAMA. 1983;249:1176–80.
113. Sack RB, Hirschorn N, Brownlee I, et al. Enterotoxigenic *E. coli*-associated diarrheal disease in Apache children. N Engl J Med. 1975;292:1041–5.
114. Ryder RW, Wachsmuter IK, Buston AE, et al. Infantile diarrhea produced by heat stable enterotoxigenic *E. coli.* N Engl J Med. 1976;295:849–53.
115. Tacket CO, Losonsky G, Link H, et al. Protection by milk immunoglobulin concentrate against oral challenge with enterotoxigenic *Escherichia coli.* N Engl J Med. 1988;318:1240–3.
116. Sack DA, Kaminsky DC, Sack RB, et al. Prophylactic doxycycline for traveler's diarrhea. N Engl J Med. 1978;298:758–63.
117. Ericsson CD, Johnson PC, DuPont HL, et al. Ciprofloxacin or trimethoprim-sulfamethoxazole as initial therapy for traveler's diarrhea. Ann Intern Med. 1987;106:216–20.
118. Ryder RW, Sack DA, Kapikian AZ, et al. Enterotoxigenic *Escherichia coli* and reovirus-like agent in rural Bangladesh. Lancet. 1976;1:659–62.
119. Ewing WH, Tatum HW, Davis BR. The occurrence of *Escherichia coli* serotypes associated with diarrheal disease in the United States. Public Health Lab. 1957;15:118.
120. Ulshen MH, Rollo JR. Pathogenesis of *E. coli* gastroenteritis in man: Another mechanism. N Engl J Med. 1980;302:99–101.
121. Inman LR, Cantey JR. Specific adherence of *Escherichia coli* (strain RDEC-1) to membranous (M) cells of the Peyer's patch in *Escherichia coli* diarrhea in the rabbit. J Clin Invest. 1983;71:1–9.
122. Mathewson JJ, Johnson PC, DuPont HL, et al. A newly recognized cause of travelers' diarrhea: Enteroadherent *Escherichia coli.* J Infect Dis. 1985;151:471–5.
123. Levine MM, Nataro JP, Karch H, et al. The diarrheal response of humans to some classic serotypes of enteropathogenic *Escherichia coli* is dependent on a plasmid encoding an enteroadhesiveness factor. J Infect Dis. 1985;152:550–9.
124. Edelman R, Levine MM. Summary of a workshop on enteropathogenic *Escherichia coli.* J Infect Dis. 1983;147:1108–18.
125. Harris JR, Wachsmuth IK, David BF, et al. High molecular weight plasmid correlates with *Escherichia coli* invasiveness. Infect Immun. 1982;37:1295–8.
126. Sakazaki R, Tamura K, Saito M. Enteropathogenic *E. coli* associated with diarrhea in children and adults. Jpn J Med Sci Biol. 1967;20:387.
127. Small PLC, Falkow S. Identification of regions on a 230-kilobase plasmid from enteroinvasive *Escherichia coli* that are required for entry into HEp-2 cells. Infect Immun. 1988;56:225–9.
128. Riley LW, Remis RS, Helgerson SD, et al. Hemorrhagic colitis associated with rare *Escherichia coli* serotype. N Engl J Med. 1983;308:681–5.
129. Riley LW. The epidemiologic, clinical, and microbiologic features of hemorrhagic colitis. Annu Rev Microbiol. 1987;41:383–407.
130. Ryan CA, Tauxe RX, Hosek GW, et al. *Escherichia coli* 0157:H7 diarrhea in a nursing home: Clinical, epidemiologic, and pathologic findings. J Infect Dis. 1986;154:631–8.
131. Johnson WM, Lior H, Bezanson GS. Cytotoxic *Escherichia coli* 0157:H7 associated with haemorrhagic colitis in Canada. Lancet. 1983;1:76.
132. Padhye VV, Beery JT, Kittell FB, et al. Colonic hemorrhage produced in mice by a unique vero cell cytotoxin from an *Escherichia coli* strain that causes hemorrhagic colitis. J Infect Dis. 1987;155:1249–53.
133. O'Brien AD, Newland JW, Miller SF, et al. Shiga-like toxin-converting phages from *Escherichia coli* strains that cause hemorrhagic colitis or infantile diarrhea. Science. 1984;226:694–6.
134. Karmali MA, Petric M, Steele BT, et al. Sporadic cases of haemolytic–uremic syndrome associated with faecal cytotoxin and cytotoxin-producing *Escherichia coli* in stools. Lancet. 1983;1:619–20.
135. Karmali MA, Petric M, Lim C, et al. The association between idiopathic hemolytic uremic syndrome and infection by verotoxin-producing *Escherichia coli.* J Infect Dis. 1985;151:775–82.
136. Gransden WR, Damm MAS, Anderson JD, et al. Further evidence associating hemolytic uremic syndrome with infection by Verotoxin-producing *Escherichia coli* 0157:H7. J Infect Dis. 1986;154:522–4.
137. Stamm WE, Turck M. Urinary tract infection. Adv Intern Med. 1983;28:141.
138. Fowler JE Jr, Stamey TA. Studies of introital colonization in women with recurrent urinary tract infections: VII. The role of bacterial adherence. J Urol 1977;117:472.
139. Schaeffer AJ, Jones JM, Dunn JK. Association of in vitro *Escherichia coli* adherence to vaginal and buccal epithelial cells with susceptibility of women to recurrent urinary-tract infections. N Engl J Med. 1981;304:1062–6.
140. Johnson JR, Roberts P, Stamm WE. P fimbriae and other virulence factors in *Escherichia coli* urosepsis: Association with patients' characteristics. J Infect Dis. 1987;156:225–9.
141. Buckley RM, McGuckin M, MacGregor RR. Urine bacterial counts following sexual intercourse. N Engl J Med. 1978;298:321.
142. Kallenius G. Structure of carbohydrate part of receptor on human uroepithelial cells for pyelonephritogenic *E. coli*. Lancet. 1981;2:604–6.
143. Minshew BH, Jorgensen J, Counts GW, et al. Association of hemolysin production, hemagglutination of human erythrocytes, and virulence for chicken embryos of extraintestinal *Escherichia coli* isolates. Infect Immun. 1978;20:50–54.
144. Hughes C, Hacker J, Roberts A, et al. Hemolysin production as a virulence marker in symptomatic and asymptomatic urinary tract infections caused by *Escherichia coli.* Infect Immun. 1983;39:546.
145. Davies DL, Falkinere FR, Hardy KG. Colicin V production by clinical isolates of *Escherichia coli.* Infect Immun. 1981;31:574–9.
146. Olling S. Sensitivity of gram negative bacilli to the serum bactericidal activity: A marker of host-parasite relationship in acute and persisting infections. Scand J Infect Dis. 1977;10(Suppl):1–40.
147. Turck M, Petersdorf RG. The epidemiology of nonenteric *E. coli* infections: Prevalence of serological groups. J Clin Invest. 1962;41:1760.
148. Turck M, Ronald AR, Clark H, et al. Studies on the epidemiology of *E. coli* 1960–1968. J Infect Dis. 1969;120:13.
149. Kaijser B. Immunology of *E. coli*: K antigen and its relation to urinary tract infection. J Infect Dis. 1973;127:670.
150. Kaijser B, Ahlstedt S. Protective capacity of antibodies against *E. coli* O and K antigens. Infect Immun. 1977;17:286.
151. Vaisanen-Rhen V, Elo J, Vaisanen E, et al. P-fimbriated clones among uropathogenic *Escherichia coli* strains. Infect Immun. 1984;43:149.
152. Verghese A, Berk SL. Bacterial pneumonia in the elderly. Medicine (Baltimore). 1983;62:271–85.
153. Levison ME, Kaye D. Pneumonia caused by gram-negative bacilli: An overview. Rev Infect Dis. 1985;7(Suppl):656–65.
154. Johanson WG Jr, Woods DE, Chaudhuri T. Association of respiratory tract colonization with adherence of gram-negative bacilli to epithelial cells. J Infect Dis. 1979;139:667–73.
155. Johanson WG Jr, Higuchi JH, Chaudhuri TR, et al. Bacterial adherence to epithelial cells in bacillary colonization of the respiratory tract. Am Rev Respir Dis. 1980;121:55.
156. Abraham SN, Beachey EH, Simpson WA. Adherence of *Streptococcus pyogenes*, *Escherichia coli* and *Pseudomonas aeurginosa* to fibronectin-coated and uncoated epithelial cells. Infect Immun. 1983;41:1261.
157. Woods DE, Strauss DC, Johanson WG Jr, et al. Role of salivary protease

activity in adherence of gram-negative bacilli to mammalian buccal epithelial cells in vivo. J Clin Invest. 1981;68:1435.
158. Haggerty RJ, Ziai M. Acute bacterial menigitis. Adv Pediatr. 1964;13:129.
159. McCracken GH, Sarff ID. Current status and therapy of neonatal *E. coli* menigitis. Hosp Pract. 1974;Oct:57.
160. Robbins JB, McCracken GH, Gotschilch EC, et al. *Escherichia coli* K1 capsular polysaccharide associated with neonatal meningitis. N Engl J Med. 1974;290:1216–20.
161. McCracken GH, Sarff ID, Glode MD, et al. Relation between *Escherichia coli* K1 capsular polysaccharide antigen and clinical outcome in neonatal meningitis. Lancet. 1974;2:246–50.
162. Sarff ID, McCracken GH, Schiffer MS, et al. Epidemiology of *Escherichia coli* K1 in healthy and diseased newborns. Lancet. 1975;1:1099–104.
163. Moxon ER, Glode MP, Sutton A, et al. The infant rat as a model of bacterial meningitis. J Infect Dis. 1977;136(Suppl):186–90.
164. Griffiths E. Candidate virulence markers. In: Sussman M, ed. The virulence of *Escherichia coli*. London: Academic Press; 1985:193–226.
165. Centers for Disease Control. National nosocomial infection study report. Annual summary of 1979, 1982. MMWR.
166. Goldenberg DL, Brandt KD, Catheart ES, et al. Acute arthritis caused by gram-negative bacilli: A clinical characterization. Medicine (Baltimore). 1974;53:197.
167. Faraawi R, Fong IW. *Escherichia coli* emphysematous endophthalmitis and pyelonephritis: Case report and review of the literature. Am J Med. 1988;84:636–9.
168. Saksouk F, Salti I. Acute suppurative thyroiditis caused by *Escherichia coli*. Br Med J. 1977;2:23.
169. Altemeier WA. The bacterial flora of acute perforated appendicitis with periotnitis: A bacteriologic study based upon one hundred cases. Ann Surg. 1938;107:517.
170. Conn HO. Spontaneous peritonitis and bacteremia in Laennec's cirrhosis caused by enteric organisms. Ann Intern Med. 1964;60:568.
171. Rubin RH, Swartz MN, Malt R. Hepatic abscess: Changes in clinical bacteriologic and therapeutic aspects. Am J Med. 1974;57:601.
172. Brewer NS, MacCarty CS, Wellman WE. Brain abscess: A review of recent experience. Ann Intern Med. 1975;83:571.
173. Finland M, Barnes MW. Changing etiology of bacterial endocarditis in the antibacterial era. Ann Intern Med. 1970;72:341.
174. Meares EM. Prostatis: A review. Urol Clin North Am. 1975;2:3.
175. Highsmith AK, Jarvis WR. *Klebsiella pneumoniae* selected virulence factors that contribute to pathogenicity. Infect Control. 1985;6:75.
176. de la Torre MG, Romero-Vivas J, Martinez-Beltran J, et al. *Klebsiella* bacteremia: An analysis of 100 episodes. Rev Infect Dis. 1985;7:143–50.
177. Montgomerie J. Epidemiology of *Klebsiella* and hospital-associated infections. Rev Infect Dis. 1979;1:736–53.
178. Noriega ER, Leibowitz RE, Richmond AS, et al. Nosocomial infection caused by gentamicin resistant, streptomycin sensitive *Klebsiella*. J Infect Dis. 1975;131(Suppl):45.
179. Rennie RP, Duncan IBR. Emergence of gentamicin resistant *Klebsiella* in a general hospital. Antimicrob Agents Chemother. 1978;11:179.
180. Reyes E. Rhinoscleroma. Observations based on a study of two hundred cases. Arch Dermatol Syph. 1946;54:531.
181. Muzyka MM, Gubina KM. Problems of the epidemiology of scleroma. J Hyg Epidemiol Microbiol Immunol. 1971;15:233.
182. Krasilnikov AP, Izraitel NA, Krylou A. Focal incidence of scleroma. J Hyg Epidemiol Microbiol Immunol. 1971;15:243.
183. Altman G, Ostfeld E, Zohar S, et al. Rhinoscleroma. Isr J Med Sci. 1977;13:62.
184. Berger SA, Polloch AA, Richmond AS. Isolation of *Klebsiella ozaenae* and *Klebsiella rhinoscleromatis* in a general hospital. Am J Clin Pathol. 1971;67:499.
185. Mayhall CA, Camb AV, Gayle WE, et al. *Enterobacter cloacae* septicemia in a burn unit center: Epidemiology and control of an outbreak. J Infect Dis. 1979;139:166–71.
186. John JR Jr, Sharbough RJ, Bannister ER. *Enterobacter cloacae*: Bacteremia, epidemiology and antibiotic resistance. Rev Infect Dis. 1982;4:13–28.
187. Steinhauer BW, Eickhoff TC, Kislak JW, et al. The *Klebsiella-Enterobacter-Serratia* division: Clinical and epidemiologic characteristics. Ann Intern Med. 1966;65:1180.
188. Flynn DM, Weinstein RA, Nathan C, et al. Patients' endogenous flora as the source of "nosocomial" *Enterobacter* in cardiac surgery. J Infect Dis. 1987;156:363–8.
189. Burchard KW, Barroll DT, Reed M, et al. *Enterobacter* bacteremia in surgical patients. Surgery. 1986;100:857–61.
190. Olson B, Weinstein RA, Nathan C, et al. Broad-spectrum β-lactam resistance in *Enterobacter*: Emergence during treatment and mechanisms of resistance. J Antimicrob Chemother. 1983;11:299–310.
191. Maki DG, Rhame FS, Mackel DC, et al. Nationwide epidemic of septicemia caused by contaminated intravenous products: Epidemiologic and clinical features. Am J Med. 1976;60:471.
192. Maki DG, Martin WT. Nationwide epidemic of septicemia caused by contaminated infusion products. IV. Growth of microbial pathogens in fluids for intravenous infusion. J Infect Dis. 1975;131:267.
193. Yu VL. *Serratia marcescens*: Historical perspective and clinical review. N Engl J Med. 1979;300:887–93.
194. Farmer JJ, Davis BR, Hickman FW, et al. Detection of *Serratia* outbreaks in hospital. Lancet. 1976;2:455–9.
195. Christensen GD, Koranes SB, Reed L, et al. Epidemic *Serratia marcescens* in a neonatal intensive care unit: Importance of the gastrointestinal tract as a reservoir. Infect Control. 1982;3:127–33.
196. Mills J, Drew E. *Serratia marcescens* endocarditis: A regional illness associated with intravenous drug abuse. Ann Intern Med. 1976;84:29.
197. Ashby ME. Serratia osteomyelitis in heroin users. J Bone Joint Surg [A]. 1976;158:132.
198. Wilfert JN, Barrett FF, Kass EH. Bacteremia due to *Serratia marcescens*. N Engl J Med. 1968;279:286.
199. Stamm WE, Kolff CA, Dones EM, et al. A nursery outbreak caused by *Serratia marcescens*-scalp-vein needles as a portal of entry. J Pediatr. 1976;89:96.
200. Maki DG, Hennekens CG, Phillips CW, et al. Nosocomial urinary tract infection with *Serratia marcescens*: An epidemiologic study. J Infect Dis. 1973;128:579.
201. Schaberg DR, Alford RH, Anderson R, et al. An outbreak of nosocomial infection due to multiply resistant *Serratia marcescens*: Evidence of interhospital spread. J Infect Dis. 1976;134:181–8.
202. Sanders CV, Luby JP, Johanson WG Jr, et al. *Serratia marcescens* infections from inhalation therapy medications: Nosocomial outbreak. Ann Intern Med. 1970;73:15.
203. Webb SF, Vall-Spinosa A. Outbreak of *Serratia marcescens* associated with the flexible fiberbronchoscope. Chest. 1975;68:703.
204. Bodey GP, Rodriguez V, Smith JP. *Serratia* sp. infections in cancer patients. Cancer 1970;25:199.
205. Mayer JW, DeHoratius RJ, Messner RP. *Serratia marcescens*–caused arthritis with negative and positive birefringent crystals. Arch Intern Med. 1976;136:1323.
206. Dorwar BB, Abrutyn E, Schumacher HR. *Serratia* arthritis. JAMA. 1973;225:1642.
207. Nakashima AK, McCarthy A, Martone WJ, et al. Epidemic septic arthritis caused by *Serratia marcescens* and associated with a benzalkonium chloride antiseptic. J Clin Microbiol. 1987;25:1014–8.
208. Weinstein RJ, Young LS, Hewitt WL. Activity of three aminoglycosides and two penicillins against four species of gram-negative bacilli. Antimicrob Agents Chemother. 1975;7:172.
209. Moellering RC Jr, Wennerstein C, Kunz LJ, et al. Resistance to gentamicin, tobramycin and amikacin among clinical isolates of bacteria. Am J Med. 1977;62:873.
210. Weinstein RJ, Young LS, Hewitt WL. Comparison of methods for assessing in vitro antibotic synergism against *Pseudomonas* and *Serratia*. J Lab Clin Med. 1975;86:853.
211. Cone LA, Woodard DR. Aztreonam therapy for serious gram-negative bacillary infections. Rev Infect Dis. 1985;7(Suppl):794–802.
212. Cox CE. Aztreonam therapy for complicated urinary tract infections caused by multidrug-resistant bacteria. Rev Infect Dis. 1985;7(Suppl):767–71.
213. Jones RN. Review of the in vitro spectrum of activity of imipenem. Am J Med. 1985;78:22–32.
214. Thomassen MJ, Demko CA, Doershuk CF, et al. *Pseudomanas cepacia*: Decrease in colonization in patients with cystic fibrosis. Am Rev Respir Dis. 1986;134:669–71.
215. Sutherland R, Beale A, Boon RJ, et al. Antibacterial activity of ticarcillin in the presence of clavulanate potassium. Am J Med. 1985;79:13–24.
216. Bassey CM, Baltch AL, Smith RP. Comparative activity of enoxacin, ciprofloxacin, amifloxacin, norfloxacin, and ofloxacin against 177 bacterial isolates. J Antimicrob Chemother. 1986;17:623–8.
217. Wolfson JS, Hooper DC. The fluoroquinolones: Structures, mechanisms of action and resistance, and spectra of activity in vitro. Antimicrob Agents Chemother. 1985;28:581–6.
218. Washington JA III, Birk RJ, Ritts RE. Bacteriologic and epidemiologic characteristics of *Enterobacter hafniae* and *Enterobacter liquefaciens*. J Infect Dis. 1971;124:379.
219. Berger SA, Edberg SC, Klein RS. *Enterobacter hafniae* infection: Report of two cases and review of the literature. Am J Med Sci. 1977;273:101–4.
220. Kotelko K. *Proteus mirabilis*: Taxonomic position, peculiarities of growth, components of the cell envelope. Curr Top Microbiol Immunol. 1986;129:181–215.
221. MacLaren DM. The significance of urease in *Proteus* pyelonephritis: A historical and biochemical study. J Pathol Bacteriol. 1969;97:43–9.
222. Mosher DM, Griffith DP, Yawn D, et al. Role of urease in pyelonephritis resulting from urinary tract infection with *Proteus*. J Infect Dis. 1975;131:177–81.
223. Braude AI, Siemienski J. Role of bacterial urease in experimental pyelonephritis. J Bacteriol. 1960;80:171–9.
224. Silverblatt FJ. Host–parasite interaction in the rat renal pelvis. A possible role for pili in the pathogensis of pyelonephritis. J Exp Med. 1974;140:1696.
225. Wray SK, Hull SI, Cook RG, et al. Identification and characterization of a uropathogenic isolate of *Proteus mirabilis*. Infect Immun. 1986;54:43–9.
226. Rozalski A, Kotełko K. Hemolytic activity and invasiveness in strains of *Proteus penneri*. J Clin Microbiol. 1987;25:1094–6.
227. Peerbooms PG, Verweij AM, MacLaren D. Vero cell invasiveness of *Proteus mirabilis*. Infect Immun. 1984;43:1068–70.
228. Welch RA. Identification of two different hemolysin determinants in uropathogenic *Proteus* isolates. Infect Immun. 1987;55:2183–90.
229. Chow AW, Taylor PR, Yoshikawa TT, et al. A nosocomial outbreak of infections due to multiply resistant *Proteus mirabilis*: Role of intestinal colonization as a major reservoir. J Infect Dis. 1979;139:621–7.

230. Gaynes RP, Weinstein R, Chamberlin W, et al. Antibiotic-resistant flora in nursing home patients admitted to the hospital. Arch Intern Med. 1985;145:1804–7.
231. Warren JW. *Providencia stuartii*: A common cause of antibiotic-resistant bacteria in patients with long-term indwelling catheters. Rev Infect Dis. 1986;8:61–7.
232. Kaslow RA, Lindsey JO, Bisno AL, et al. Nosocomial infection with highly resistant *Proteus rettgeri*. Am J Epidemiol. 1976;104:278.
233. Iannini PB, Eickhoff TC, LaForce FM. Multidrug resistant *P. rettgeri*: An emerging problem. Ann Intern Med. 1976;55:161.
234. Weinstein RA, Nathan C, Gruensfelder R, et al. Endemic aminoglycoside resistance in gram-negative bacilli. J Infect Dis. 1980;141:338–45.
235. Hodges GR, Degener CE, Barnes WG. Clinical significance of *Citrobacter* isolates. Am J Clin Pathol. 1978;70:37–40.
236. Lipsky BA, Hook ER III, Smith A, et al. *Citrobacter* infections in humans: Experience at the Seattle Veterans Administration Medical Center and a review of the literature. Rev Infect Dis. 1980;2:746–60.
237. Williams WW, Mariano J, Spurrier M, et al. Nosocomial meningitis due to *Citrobacter diversus* in neonates: New aspects of the epidemiology. J Infect Dis. 1984;150:229–55.
238. Kaplan AM, Itabashi HH, Yoshimori R, et al. Cerebral abscesses complicating neonatal *Citrobacter freundii* meningitis. West J Med. 1977;127:418.
239. Ribeiro CD, Davis P, Jones DM. *Citrobacter kozeri* meningitis in a special care baby unit. J Clin Pathol. 1976;29:1094.
240. Kline MW, Mason EO Jr, Kaplan SL. Characterization of *Citrobacter diversus* strains causing neonatal meningitis. J Infect Dis. 1988;157:101–5.
241. MacCulloch D, Menzies R, Cornere BM. Endocarditis due to *Citrobacter diversus* developing resistance to cephalothin. NZ Med J. 1977;85:182.
242. Drelichman V, Band JD. Bacteremias due to *Citrobacter diversus* and *Citrobacter freudii*: Incidence, risk factors, and clinical outcome. Arch Intern Med. 1985;145:1808–10.
243. Jordan GL, Hadley WK. Human infections with *Edwardsiella tarda*. Ann Intern Med. 1969;70:283.
244. Kourvang M, Vesques MA, Saena R. Edwardsiella in man and animals in Panama. Am J Trop Med Hyg. 1977;26:1183.
245. Sonnenwirth AC, Kallus BA. Meningitis due to *Edwardsiella tarda*. Am J Clin Pathol. 1968;49:92.
246. Farmer JJ, Davis BR, Hickman-Brenner FW, et al. Biochemical identification of new species and biogroups of *Enterobacteriaceae* isolated from clinical specimens. J Clin Microbiol. 1985;21:46–76.
247. Pien FD, Bruce AE. Nosocomial *Ewingella americana* bacteremia in an intensive care unit. Arch Intern Med. 1986;146:111–12.

196. PSEUDOMONAS AERUGINOSA

MATTHEW POLLACK

MICROBIOLOGY

Pseudomonas aeruginosa is a gram-negative aerobic rod belonging to the family Pseudomonadaceae. It is rod-shaped, averaging 0.5–0.8 × 1.5–3.0 μm. It occurs singly, in pairs, or in short chains. It is motile, with polar, monotrichous flagella. It produces diffusible fluorescent pigments including pyoverdin and a soluble phenazine pigment called pyocyanin; the latter, produced by somewhat more than one-half of clinical isolates, appears blue or green at neutral or alkaline pH and is the source of the name *aeruginosa*. Some strains also produce dark red or black pigment (pyorubin and pyomelanin, respectively). *Pseudomonas aeruginosa* is nutritionally versatile. Organic growth factors are not required, and it can utilize more than 30 organic compounds for growth. It is an obligate aerobe except in the presence of nitrate. It grows optimally at 37°C and also at 42°C, but not at 4°C. It accomplishes gene transfer by both conjugation and transduction and has G + C content in its DNA of approximately 67 moles percent.[1]

Identification in the clinical microbiology laboratory is relatively simple since *P. aeruginosa* grows readily in a wide variety of media, and the minimal characteristics required for identification are few. It is a gram-negative, straight or slightly curved, motile, nonsporulating rod. It grows aerobically only and does not ferment carbohydrates. It oxidizes sugars such as glucose and xylose, but not maltose. It is indophenol oxidase-, Simmons citrate-, and L-arginine dehydrolase-positive. It produces gas from nitrate and grows in brain–heart infusion broth at 42°C. It is L-lysine decarboxylase- and L-ornithine decarboxylase-negative and produces no hydrogen sulfide or black butt in Kligler's iron agar.

Based on these and other biochemical characteristics, *P. aeruginosa* can be presumptively identified by a number of automated and computer-based gram-negative identification systems. However, these systems cannot always differentiate *P. aeruginosa* from all non-*aeruginosa Pseudomonas* species, which may require differential sugar oxidations, growth at 42°C, and flagella strains. When pyocyanin is present, it is a specific differential characteristic of *P. aeruginosa*. A characteristic sweet grapelike odor in culture may be an equally specific identifying or confirming quality of *P. aeruginosa*.

EPIDEMIOLOGY

Pseudomonas aeruginosa is cosmopolitan in its distribution. It is isolated from soil, water, plants, and animals, including man. It is occasionally pathogenic for plants as well as animals. The minimal nutritional requirements of *Pseudomonas*, as evidenced by its ability to grow in distilled water and its tolerance of a wide variety of physical conditions including temperature, contribute to its ecological success and ultimately to its role as an effective opportunistic pathogen.

The epidemiology of *P. aeruginosa* reflects its predilection for a moist environment. This is apparent in its natural habitat, where its associations with soil and water are closely related, and its identification on plants is a function of humidity. Similarly, human colonization occurs at moist sites such as the perineum, axilla, and ear. Moisture is also a critical factor in hospital reservoirs of *P. aeruginosa* such as respiratory equipment, clean solutions, medicines, disinfectants, sinks, mops, food mixers, vegetables, and so on. Human *Pseudomonas* disease is also associated with water-related reservoirs outside of hospitals including swimming pools, whirlpools, hot tubs, and contact lens solutions.

Pseudomonas aeruginosa is sometimes present as part of the normal microbial flora of man. The prevalence of colonization in healthy persons outside of or upon entry to hospitals is relatively low. Representative site-specific colonization rates are: skin 0–2 percent, nasal mucosa 0–3.3 percent, throat 0–6.6 percent, and stool 2.6–24 percent.[2] In contrast, hospitalization may lead to greatly increased rates of carriage, particularly on the skin in patients with serious burns, in the lower respiratory tract in patients undergoing mechanical ventilation, in the gastrointestinal tract of patients receiving chemotherapy for neoplastic diseases, or at virtually any site in persons treated with antibiotics. In each instance colonization rates may exceed 50 percent, and colonization often presages invasive infection.[3]

Although colonization by *P. aeruginosa* frequently precedes overt infection, the original source of the organism and the precise mode of transmission are often unclear. Potential reservoirs such as uncooked vegetables, hospital sinks, or even flowers in patients' rooms are suspected sources of endemic *P. aeruginosa* strains. Discrete hospital-acquired outbreaks (epidemics) have been more definitively traced to specific reservoirs such as respiratory equipment, endoscopes, transvenous pacemakers, contaminated antistatic mattresses, antiseptics, orthopedic plaster, operating room suction apparatus, contaminated nursery formula, physiotherapy pool, and so on. Patient-to-patient transmission of *Pseudomonas* via the hands of hospital staff or by other fomites is often assumed but difficult to prove.

Because of the prevalence of *P. aeruginosa* in the hospital environment, epidemiologic investigation is facilitated by the use of markers that discriminate among strains.[4] Most frequently used but least discriminatory are antibiograms and biochemical properties as determined by API profiles. In addition, *P. aeruginosa* can be typed on the basis of pyocin (bacteriocin) production or bacteriophage susceptibility patterns. A more specific typing method is by serotyping (or immunotyping) on the basis of immunochemical heterogeneity of outer membrane lipopolysaccharides. Two commonly employed immunotype schemes are the Fisher–Devlin–Gnabasik system, which includes seven types, and the international antigenic typing system (IATS), which embraces a total of 17 different types. Type-specific rabbit antisera may be used in a slide agglutination test to identify different immunotypes. Numerous common-source epidemics have been investigated and reservoirs identified on the basis of immunotyping data. Almost two-thirds of such outbreaks, including those occurring outside as well as within hospitals, have involved IATS serotype 11, which represents only 8 percent of endemic isolates.[5] Perhaps the most sensitive and specific epidemiologic marker identified to date is a DNA probe, which appears to surpass other, conventional typing methods in its discriminatory capacity[6]; this tool is not yet widely available, however.

Pseudomonas aeruginosa is primarily a nosocomial pathogen, and therefore the frequency with which it causes disease can be reliably estimated from annual surveillance data collected by the Centers for Disease Control (CDC) National Nosocomial Infections Study.[7] On the basis of these data, the overall incidence of *P. aeruginosa* infections in U.S. hospitals is 36 per 10,000 discharges. *Pseudomonas aeruginosa* is the fourth most frequently isolated nosocomial pathogen, accounting for 9.9 percent of all hospital-acquired infections. It is the second leading cause of nosocomial pneumonia (13.1 percent of all pneumonias), the third most common cause of urinary tract infections (11.7 percent), and the fourth leading cause of surgical wound infections (7.4 percent). *Pseudomonas aeruginosa* is the fourth most common cause of primary gram-negative bacteremia, and that associated with the highest mortality.[8] Until relatively recently, the incidence and relative frequency of hospital-acquired *P. aeruginosa* infections was on the rise. Whereas *P. aeruginosa* accounted for 6.6 percent of all nosocomial infections documented by the CDC in 1976, this figure increased to 9.9 percent in 1980–1982.[2] Similarly, annual surveillance of hospital-acquired blood stream infections in the state of Virginia reveals that 2.8 percent were caused by *P. aeruginosa* in 1975–1977 compared with 5.9 percent in 1980–1982.[2]

PATHOGENESIS

The pathogenesis of *P. aeruginosa* infections must be understood in the context of its being an opportunistic pathogen. It rarely causes disease in healthy persons, although it is a common human saprophyte. In most cases the disease process begins with some alteration or circumvention of normal host defenses. This may involve a disruption in the integrity of physical barriers to bacterial invasion such as the skin or mucous membranes, or their circumvention as in the case of intravenous lines, urinary catheters, or endotracheal tubes. In other instances, there is an underlying dysfunction of specific immune mechanisms as in neutropenia, hypogammaglobulinemia, complement deficiency, or iatrogenic immunosuppressive states. The ecological resilience of *P. aeruginosa* contributes to its pathogenicity. Its adaptability to a wide variety of physical conditions, minimal nutritional requirements, and relative resistance to antibiotics allow it to survive in large numbers in close proximity to its prospective host.

That the pathogenesis of *Pseudomonas* infections is multifactorial is suggested both by the number of potential virulence factors the organism produces and by the broad spectrum of disease it causes. Multiple pathogenic mechanisms must be assumed in such diverse diseases as *Pseudomonas* septicemia in neutropenic patients, chronic lung infections in persons with cystic fibrosis, endocarditis in heroin addicts, dermatitis in hot tub users, and malignant external otitis in elderly diabetics.

The pathogenesis of *Pseudomonas* infections appears to be complex in that *P. aeruginosa* is both invasive and toxinogenic, a fact that may help explain the variety of diseases and syndromes with which it is identified. *Pseudomonas* infections may be seen as comprising three distinct stages: (*1*) bacterial attachment and colonization; (*2*) local invasion; and (*3*) dissemination and systemic disease. Each stage has as its prerequisite the previous one, but the disease process may stop at any stage. Particular virulence factors of *P. aeruginosa* appear to mediate each of these steps in pathogenesis and to be responsible for characteristic syndromes.

There appears to be a clear relationship between *Pseudomonas* colonization of the respiratory tract and bacterial adherence to epithelial cells.[9] Protein structures on the surface of the bacterium called pili or fimbriae are apparently responsible for adherence to respiratory epithelium, and, by analogy, to other epithelial surfaces as well.[10] Fibronectin ordinarily protects epithelial cells from bacterial attachment, but is apparently lost as the result of illness or other factors involved in hospitalization. The correlation between in vitro adherence of *Pseudomonas* to buccal epithelial cells and in vivo respiratory tract colonization is particularly pronounced in patients with cystic fibrosis and other forms of chronic lung disease. Sputa from these patients contain high levels of protease, which appears to break down the fibronectin coating of epithelial cells leading to enhanced bacterial attachment.[11]

Cellular injury may also play a role in the initial attachment of *Pseudomonas* to epithelial cells. For example, *Pseudomonas* adheres to the desquamating trachael epithelial cells of mice infected with influenza virus but not to normal tracheal epithelium.[12] Epithelial injury from endotracheal intubation can produce the same result. This phenomenon of "opportunistic adherence" may represent an important step in the pathogenesis of *Pseudomonas* keratitis[13] and urinary tract infections,[14] as well as those involving the respiratory tract.

It is clear that *Pseudomonas* pili are attachment organelles or "adhesins," since both purified pili and antibodies to these structures block bacterial attachment to epithelial cells. It is likely that specific molecular sequences on these structures act as ligands that react with complementary sequences (receptors) on host cells. Galactose-binding or mannose-binding lectins of *Pseudomonas* may represent such ligands.[15] The mucoid exopolysaccharide of mucoid *Pseudomonas* strains[16] and the pili of nonmucoid strains represent adhesins for tracheal epithelial cells and for tracheobronchial mucin. The receptors for these adhesins appear to contain *N*-acetylneuraminic acid (sialic acid) and, in the case of tracheobronchial mucin, *N*-acetylglucosamine.[17,18] It has been further proposed that the sialic acid-containing receptor for *Pseudomonas* on tracheal epithelium is a cell surface glycolipid, probably a ganglioside.[19]

Under certain conditions *P. aeruginosa* produces a polysaccharide capsule, referred to as the glycocalyx[20] or mucoid exopolysaccharide.[21] It consists of mannuronic and guluronic acid in a repeating structure termed alginate. This carbohydrate material appears to form a matrix around the bacterium, anchoring it to its environment and to its sister cells and protecting it from host immune factors such as the mucocilliary mechanism of the respiratory tract, phagocytic cells, antibodies, and complement. Mucoid strains of *P. aeruginosa* are often isolated from the sputum of patients with cystic fibrosis.[22] Examination of postmortem lung material from patients with cystic fibrosis provides morphological evidence that *Pseudomonas* forms encapsulated microcolonies in infected alveoli, indicating that formation of the glycocalyx of *Pseudomonas* is an in vivo as well as an in vitro phenomenon.[23] That the mucoid exopolysaccharide or glycocalyx of *Pseudomonas* is a pathogenic factor is further suggested by its antiphagocytic properties[24] and by the greater resistance of mucoid *Pseudomonas* strains to opsonization compared with nonmucoid revertants.[25] Moreover, alginate may inhibit the bactericidal activity of aminoglycoside antibiotics against *P. aeruginosa*.[26]

A number of factors appear to be involved in the ability of *Pseudomonas* to cause invasive disease. While cell-associated surface structures protect the organism from host phagocytes, antibodies, and complement, its extracellular enzymes or toxins break down physical barriers to its penetration, impair host defenses, and render its new milieu more conducive to its physical, nutritional, and reproductive requirements.

Most clinical *P. aeruginosa* isolates produce several extracellular proteases. Two of the best characterized, elastase and alkaline protease,[27] are most clearly associated with virulence. Both are necrotizing in the skin, lung, and cornea, with elastase producing hemorrhage. Elastase has been incriminated in the destructive vascular lesions (ecthyma gangrenosum) associated with septicemic *Pseudomonas* infections and may be responsible for the dissolution of the elastic lamina of blood vessels, which is an important pathologic characteristic of these lesions.[28] The rapidity and degree with which *Pseudomonas* proteases affect local tissue necrosis and disruption of blood vessels underscores their invasive role. Although proteases are not highly cytotoxic, they appear to destroy connections between cells such as the proteoglycan ground substance of the cornea and other supporting structures composed of fibrin and elastin.[29] These enzymes specifically degrade basement membrane-associated laminin,[30] disrupt respiratory cilia,[31] cleave human type III and IV collagen,[32] and solubilize human lung elastin.[33] It has also been suggested[34] that *Pseudomonas* proteases make nutrients available to the bacterium through the breakdown of host tissues at local sites of infection, and, in so doing, aide the proliferative and invasive processes. Finally, *Pseudomonas* proteases may directly alter host defenses through inactivation of complement factors[35] and the cleavage of IgG.[36]

Another toxic protein widely produced by *P. aeruginosa* from clinical sources is the so-called cytotoxin. This 25,000 MW protein, originally called leucocidin because of its cytopathic effects on polymorphonuclear leukocytes,[37] appears to be cytotoxic for most eukaryotic cells. It acts primarily on cell membranes, inhibits polymorphonuclear leukocyte function,[38] and produces pulmonary microvascular injury in at least one experimental model.[39] The apparent pathogenic potential of cytotoxin requires further elucidation.

Pseudomonas aeruginosa produces two hemolysins, one a heat-labile protein called phospholipase c[40] and the other a heat-stable glycolipid.[41] These two substances appear to act synergistically to break down lipids and lecithin. Like *Pseudomonas* proteases, hemolysins can contribute to tissue invasion through their necrotizing effects. It has also been suggested that phospholipase c contributes to the pathogenesis of *Pseudomonas* pneumonia through the degradation of lung surfactants.[42] Phospholipase c production by a high percentage of *Pseudomonas* urinary tract isolates[43] might indicate an as yet undefined role for this enzyme in urinary tract infections as well.

Blood stream invasion and dissemination of *Pseudomonas* from local sites of infection is probably mediated by some of the same cell-associated and extracellular products responsible for more localized disease. In addition to the possible antiphagocytic properties of the mucoid exopolysaccharide, and of lipopolysaccharides contained in the outer cell membrane, *Pseudomonas* blood isolates are usually resistant to the direct bactericidal activity of serum.[44] Although *Pseudomonas* is susceptible to so-called natural antibodies, or IgM, optimal bacterial clearance requires specific IgG antibodies, intact classical and alternative complement pathways, and adequate numbers of functioning polymorphonuclear leukocytes.[45,46] These stringent demands on the host's immune system may be increased by the immunoglobulin-cleaving and complement-inactivating actions of *Pseudomonas* proteases, providing possible mechanisms for the removal of these two important impediments to blood stream invasion.

Although it is not entirely clear how *P. aeruginosa* produces systemic illness, or, in some cases, the death of the infected host, two bacterial products most likely implicated in the systemic toxicity of *Pseudomonas* are its lipopolysaccharide (endotoxin) and exotoxin A.

The lipid A moiety of *Pseudomonas* endotoxin, like that of other bacterial lipopolysaccharides, mediates many of its biological activities. There is considerable indirect evidence implicating endotoxin in the various clinical syndromes associated with gram-negative septicemia. It is likely that circulating endotoxin plays a role in the causation of fever, hypotension, oliguria, leukopenia or leukocytosis, disseminated intravascular coagulation (DIC), and adult respiratory distress syndrome (ARDS). At the cellular and subcellular level, endotoxin activates the clotting, fibrinolytic, kinin, and complement systems. Endotoxin stimulates the production of arachidonic acid metabolites, including prostaglandins and leukotrienes; it promotes the release of β-endorphins; and it induces the production and release of cytokines such as tumor necrosis factor (TNF). All of these factors, TNF in particular,[47,48] appear to mediate endotoxic (septic) shock.

It has been suggested that despite comparable structure, *Pseudomonas* lipopolysaccharides are biologically less potent than those of other gram-negative bacteria. It is more likely, however, that these lipopolysaccharides are roughly comparable in respect to their biological activity.[49] In either case, the various biological assays employed to measure the relative potency of different endotoxins bear an uncertain relationship to naturally occurring endotoxin-mediated disease processes, and the differences measured tend to be small.

The extracellular enzyme, exotoxin A, is produced by a majority of *P. aeruginosa* clinical isolates.[50] It is a potent inhibitor of mammalian protein synthesis by a mechanism identical to that of diphtheria toxin.[51] Both toxins catalyze the transfer of the adenosine diphosphate–ribose moiety of nicotinamide adenine dinucleotide into covalent linkage with elongation factor 2 (EF 2), itself an enzyme that catalyzes the elongation step in polypeptide assembly; this reaction inactivates EF 2, thereby inhibiting protein biosynthesis. Although the enzymatic activities of *Pseudomonas* exotoxin A and diphtheria toxin are similar, the two toxins have distinctive structures and cellular specificities, accounting for their different biological activities and pathogenic roles. The exotoxin A structural gene has been cloned and expressed in *Escherichia coli*.[52] The toxin is a single polypeptide chain of 613 amino acids, and its three-dimensional structure has been elucidated by x-ray crystallography.[53] Three discrete structural domains have been identified with cell recognition, toxin translocation across cell membranes, and enzymatic activity, respectively.[54]

In contrast to *Pseudomonas* proteases, exotoxin A appears to mediate both local and systemic disease processes.[55,56] Its necrotizing activity in locally exposed tissues probably contributes to pathologic lesions at primary and metastatic sites of infection as well as bacterial dissemination. Exotoxin A produces dermonecrosis following intradermal injection in guinea pigs[57] and ocular damage resembling that seen in naturally occurring *Pseudomonas* keratitis after topical application on mouse corneas.[58] Experimental corneal infections produced by toxinogenic *P. aeruginosa* strains are more severe than those produced by nontoxinogenic mutants.[59] Similarly, experimental pulmonary infections caused by a toxin-positive parent strain are accompanied by more parenchymal invasion and inflammatory cell infiltration than those caused by toxinless mutants.[60] These experimental observations support a role for exotoxin A in local tissue damage and in bacterial invasion.

In terms of its possible systemic role, purified exotoxin A is highly lethal for animals, including subhuman primates, and produces shock in dogs and rhesus monkeys.[61] Toxin-producing *Pseudomonas* strains have been associated with greater virulence than nontoxinogenic isolates in bacteremic human infections.[62] In addition, it has been shown that patients with high levels of serum antibodies to exotoxin A at the onset of *Pseudomonas* septicemia have better survival than those with low antibody titers.[63] These data suggest not only a lethal role for exotoxin A in septicemic *Pseudomonas* infections but a protective role for toxin-specific antibodies.

Another potentially pathogenic extracellular enzyme produced by most clinical isolates of *P. aeruginosa* is so-called exoenzyme S.[64] Like exotoxin A, this protein is an adenosine diphosphate ribosyltransferase, although its target protein has not been identified. Purified exoenzyme S is toxic to mice and cytopathic for a variety of tissue culture cell lines.[65] Exoenzyme S-negative *P. aeruginosa* mutants are less virulent then their parent strains in experimental burn[66] and chronic lung infections,[67] apparently on the basis of the enzyme's contribution to bacterial dissemination and lung damage, respectively.

CLINICAL MANIFESTATIONS AND TREATMENT

Endocarditis

Pseudomonas aeruginosa causes infective endocarditis on native heart valves in intravenous (IV) drug users and on prosthetic heart valves. In one study,[68] as much as 58 percent of addict-associated gram-negative bacterial endocarditis was caused by *P. aeruginosa*, although its occurrence is subject to marked regional variation. Conversely, more than 90 percent of all reported *P. aeruginosa* endocarditis is in IV drug users. Most of these patients (87 percent) are young (mean age 29), black males. Although underlying heart disease is relatively uncommon in these patients, some have had previous staphylococcal endocarditis or rheumatic valvular heart disease. The source of the organism is thought to be standing water contaminating drug paraphernalia rather than heroin itself or the addict's skin.[69] In some studies[70,71] there has been a greater association of *Pseudomonas* endocarditis with IV abuse of pentazocine and tripelennamine ("T's and blues") than with heroin. More frequent use of "T's and blues" in shooting galleries, the absence of boiling prior to injection, and the selective survival of *P. aeruginosa* in pentazocine and tripelennamine[72] are factors favoring the association of these drugs with *Pseudomonas* infections. An outbreak of serotype O11 *P. aeruginosa* endocarditis was reported among pentazocine and tripelennamine abusers in Chicago between 1977 and 1980,[71] strongly implying a common source for this epidemic strain.

Although the pathogenesis of infective endocarditis remains controversial, it is thought that the organism establishes itself on the endocardium by direct invasion from the blood stream or via neovascular channels resulting from prior subendothelial injury. In the latter case, foreign materials that are mixed with heroin may cause injury leading to fibrosis of the valve leaflets or mural endocardium. Such fibrosis has been observed in the absence of infection on the heart valves of heroin addicts. The high rate of exposure of the tricuspid valve to both trauma and bacteria in IV drug users probably explains the frequency with which this valve is involved in this group of patients. Finally, *P. aeruginosa* appears to have a particularly high affinity for human endocardium, a characteristic it shares with other more common etiologic agents in endocarditis including *Staphylococcus aureus* and viridans streptococci.[73]

Endocarditis of the tricuspid valve typically presents subacutely, whereas that involving the aortic or mitral valves is usually more acute and fulminant. Fever is almost invariably present initially but may subside with treatment despite persistently positive blood cultures. A cardiac murmur is heard in most patients at the time of hospital admission, and subsequently in virtually all. The tricuspid valve is involved in most cases (70 percent in one large series),[74] but the pulmonic, mitral, and aortic valves, as well as the mural endocardium of either atrium, may also be affected. Biventricular and multiple valve infections are particularly common in *Pseudomonas* endocarditis.[75] Septic pulmonary emboli occur with tricuspid disease and produce cough, sputum, pleuritic chest pain, pulmonary infiltrates (sometimes with abscess), and pleural effusions. Left-sided *Pseudomonas* endocarditis may present with intractable congestive heart failure and large systemic arterial emboli. Brain abscesses, cerebritis, and mycotic aneurysms occur, although meningitis is uncommon except as a terminal event. Splenomegaly is sometimes accompanied by septic infarcts or abscesses. Skin and soft-tissue manifestations such as Janeway lesions, Osler's nodes, and ecthyma gangrenosum are unusual in both right- and left-sided disease.

The diagnosis of *Pseudomonas* endocarditis is made by positive blood cultures in the absence of primary extracardiac sites of infection. Definitive diagnosis is based on culture and histopathologic examination of valvular or endocardial specimens obtained at surgery (or autopsy). In patients with positive blood cultures, an abnormal two-dimensional echocardiography combined with an abnormal chest roentgenogram is highly predictive of *Pseudomonas* endocarditis. Tricuspid involvement with vegetations may be documented by echocardiography or cardiac catheterization and cineangiography, the latter demonstrating valvular insufficiency in 50–70 percent of cases. Repeat echocardiograms may demonstrate vegetations when initial studies are negative.

Aggressive antimicrobial therapy and surgery have improved the prognosis in *Pseudomonas* endocarditis.[76] In tricuspid disease, medical therapy should be initiated with high-dose aminoglycoside (e.g., tobramycin, 8 mg/kg per day) plus an extended spectrum penicillin (e.g., ticarcillin at a dose of 18 g/day). Renal function and aminoglycoside levels must be monitored. If bacteremia persists after 2 weeks of this therapy or the cessation of a 6-week course of antibiotics, tricuspid valvulectomy without valve replacement is indicated. At the time of surgery the pulmonic valve should be closely inspected and if it appears to be involved, it, too, should be removed without replacement. With medical support after tricuspid valvulectomy most patients are hemodynamically stable, although approximately 7 percent may develop right ventricular failure. Patients who are not IV drug users should have the tricuspid valve replaced in a second operation 6–8 months after valvulectomy.[74]

In the case of left-sided *Pseudomonas* endocarditis, combination therapy with an aminoglycoside and extended spectrum penicillin should be instituted in the doses indicated above, and valve replacement accomplished immediately. Computerized axial tomography of the abdomen should be performed prior to surgery, and splenectomy accomplished prior to valve replacement if splenic abscesses are present. As in the case of tricuspid involvement, left-sided disease should be treated with antibiotics for at least 6 weeks. Serum aminoglycoside levels and bactericidal activity should be monitored in order to maintain peak gentamicin or tobramycin levels in the range of 12–20 μg/ml, and at least 10 times the minimum bactericidal concentration (MBC) of the infecting blood isolate, respectively. The higher dose and peak serum concentrations of gentamicin or tobramycin indicated above, compared with those usually recommended for these drugs, have demonstrated efficacy in *Pseudomonas* endocarditis; renal toxicity has been generally mild and reversible.[76]

There is more experience in the treatment of *Pseudomonas* endocarditis with antibiotic combinations that include carbenicillin or ticarcillin than other extended spectrum penicillins. Several treatment failures associated with the emergence of resistant, β-lactamase-producing strains have been reported with aminoglycoside–piperacillin combinations.[77] There has also been limited clinical experience with third-generation cephalosporins, with suboptimal clinical responses documented in several cases of left-sided *Pseudomonas* endocarditis treated with the combination of a third-generation cephalosporin and an aminoglycoside.[70] The efficacy of β-lactam antibiotics, as a group, in *Pseudomonas* endocarditis is limited by several theoretical and practical considerations. The β-lactams may exhibit a slow onset of bactericidal activity, lack the so-called postantibiotic effect, and select for or induce resistant, β-lactamase-producing strains.[78] These shortcomings may be accentuated by the extremely large numbers of organisms present in the vegetations of *Pseudomonas*-infected heart valves, particularly in left-sided endocarditis. The above considerations underlie the need for combination therapy that includes an aminoglycoside, highest possible antibiotic doses consistent with safety, early surgery in the case of left-sided disease, and adequate duration of therapy. Two antibiotics that may have a role in the treatment of *Pseudomonas* endocarditis are imipenem and ciprofloxacin, although to date there is limited clinical experience with either drug. Ciprofloxacin has proven efficacious in animal models of *Pseudomonas* endocarditis, particularly against multiply resistant strains.[79] Its high bactericidal activity in relation to antibiotic concentrations achievable in vegetations, early onset of action, and postantibiotic effect are probably related to its effectiveness.[78,79]

Poor prognostic indicators in *Pseudomonas* endocarditis include delay in initiation of antibiotic therapy, age over 30, presence of left-sided disease, persistent fever on therapy for 2 weeks, mural vegetations, systemic embolization, and mixed infections involving both *P. aeruginosa* and *S. aureus*. The success rate in tricuspid *Pseudomonas* endocarditis with medical therapy, and, if necessary, valvulectomy is about 80 percent. In contrast, the medical cure rate may be as low as 11 percent for left-sided *Pseudomonas* endocarditis.[70] Recent experience suggests, however, that early valve replacement may improve survival dramatically in left-sided disease.[70,80]

Respiratory Infections

Lower respiratory tract infections with *P. aeruginosa* occur almost exclusively in persons with compromised local respiratory or systemic host defense mechanisms. Primary pneumonia occurs in patients with chronic lung disease, congestive heart failure, or both. Exposure to the hospital environment, particularly in an intensive care setting, use of respiratory inhalation equipment, and prior antibiotic therapy increase the likelihood of such infections. Bacteremic *Pseudomonas* pneumonia is seen primarily in patients with malignancies, especially those involving the hematopoietic system, and those who are neutropenic as a result of chemotherapy. Chronic *Pseudomonas* lung infections occur sooner or later in the majority of patients with cystic fibrosis, a genetic disease in which abnormal respiratory secretions impede normal pulmonary toilet; ineffective opsonophagocytic and bactericidal mechanisms may contribute to lower respiratory infections in these patients, especially those due to *P. aeruginosa*.

Primary or nonbacteremic pneumonia[81] results from aspiration of *Pseudomonas* from the pharynx and upper respiratory tract, sites that become colonized during the course of hospitalization, serious illness, and previous antibiotic therapy. Despite rigorous cleaning of ventilator equipment and frequent changes of disposable tubing, direct aerosolization of *Pseudomonas* may still occur in patients receiving respirator therapy. Reservoir nebulizers introduce bacteria directly into the lower respiratory tract. Traditional accounts of *Pseudomonas* pneumonia describe a fulminant, usually fatal infection characterized clinically by chills, fever, severe dyspnea, cough productive of copious purulent sputum, cyanosis, apprehension, mental confusion, and severe systemic toxicity. Chest roentgenograms reveal a diffuse bronchopneumonia, typically bilateral, with distinctive nodular infiltrates, often with small areas of radiolucency. Although this pattern suggests *S. auereus* pneumonia, it is said to be uncommon in other forms of gram-negative pneumonia.[81] Small pleural effusions are common, empyema rare, and a pattern of lobar consolidation only occasionally seen. Pathologically, diffuse bronchopneumonia is marked by microabscess formation, necrosis of alveolar septae, and focal hemorrhages. Bacterial invasion of vessel walls and vascular necrosis are not usually seen in this form of pneumonia.

Bacteremic *Pseudomonas* pneumonia[82–84] occurs primarily, although not exclusively, in neutropenic patients following cancer chemotherapy. The pathogenesis is distinctive in that although the disease often begins, as does the nonbacteremic form, with the introduction of bacteria by the respiratory route, blood stream invasion produces characteristic pulmonary lesions and sometimes metastatic lesions in other viscera as well. Two types of lung lesions have been described.[85] The first consists of poorly defined, hemorrhagic, nodular areas that are frequently subpleural and sometimes surround a small central area of necrosis. Microscopically, these lesions are consistently located around small and medium-sized pulmonary arteries. Intra-alveolar hemorrhages are seen, alveolar necrosis may be present, and inflammatory cell infiltration is largely absent. The second type of lesion is strikingly different from the hemorrhagic lesions. Grossly, they appear as 2–15 mm, firm, yellow-brown or tan, necrotic, umbilicated nodules with a narrow halo of dark red, hemorrhagic parenchyma. Microscopically, some of these lesions are typical abscesses composed of leukocytes and liquifactive necrosis of pulmonary parenchyma. In most cases, however, the lesions demonstrate coagulation necrosis, many bacteria, and necrotic small muscular arteries and veins with bacterial invasion of their walls. These lesions appear to be the pulmonary counterpart of echthyma gangrenosum lesions seen in the skin of patients with bacteremic *Pseudomonas* infections.

Clinically, bacteremic *Pseudomonas* pneumonia is a fulminant disease with death typically occurring 3–4 days after first signs or symptoms of pulmonary or extrapulmonary infection, including those associated with gram-negative sepsis and respiratory failure. Chest roentgenograms obtained early may show pulmonary vascular congestion, interstitial edema, and areas of pulmonary edema. Central venous pressure and pulmonary capillary wedge pressure are typically normal and rule out congestive heart failure as a cause of this roentgenographic picture. Chest roentgenograms obtained 48–72 hours after the initial febrile episode disclose a pattern of parenchymal involvement with a mixture of alveolar and interstitial infiltrates. Cavitation often appears after 48 hours, indicating the necrotizing character of the diffuse bronchopneumonia that has developed by this time. The rapid progression of roentgenogram findings from pulmonary vascular congestion to pulmonary edema, to necrotizing bronchopneumonia, is said to be typical of bacteremic *Pseudomonas* pneumonia.[84]

The treatment of *Pseudomonas* pneumonia includes antibiotics (see treatment of acute exacerbations of lung infections in cystic fibrosis patients, below), maintenance of good pulmonary toilet, respiratory assistance if necessary, and other supportive measures dictated by the presence of septic shock and/or other complications.

Lower respiratory tract colonization with mucoid strains of *P. aeruginosa* is a function of age in patients with cystic fibrosis; few infants under 5 years of age are so colonized, whereas the majority of cystic fibrosis patients over age 18 carry the organism in their respiratory secretions.[86] Although an important pathogenic component of the pulmonary disease in cystic fibrosis probably results from the genetic defect itself, *P. aeruginosa* clearly plays a critical role in the progressive lung lesions and resulting disability observed in most patients with this disease. Although it is not possible, given our present understanding of cystic fibrosis lung disease, to clearly distinguish cause and effect, lower respiratory tract colonization (or infection) with *Pseudomonas* is associated with both acute exacerbations and chronic progression of this disease. In general, more symptomatic patients with more severe and progressive lung disease are more likely to be infected with *Pseudomonas* than those with less serious disease. A direct reflection of this is the greater magnitude of antibody responses to *Pseudomonas*-specific antigens in cystic fibrosis patients with higher Schwachman scores.[87,88]

Respiratory tract colonization with *Pseudomonas* appears to correlate with pathological changes in the bronchial airways in patients with cystic fibrosis.[89] Although it is unclear whether mucus plugging precedes infection or vice versa, airway obstruction begins as bronchiolitis with plugging due to inflammatory exudate; once airway obstruction is established, infections follow. Infection produces more mucus plugging, and this leads to chronic suppuration with resulting bronchiectasis, atelectasis, and ultimately fibrosis. Progressive lung involvement leads to pulmonary insufficiency, and resulting hypoxia is associated with altered cardiopulmonary dynamics, pulmonary hypertension, and cor pulmonale.

The clinical manifestations of *Pseudomonas* pulmonary infections in cystic fibrosis[90] vary widely depending on the duration and severity of underlying lung disease and the acuteness of a particular episode or exacerbation. Initially, patients may have frequent upper respiratory tract infections with a lingering cough after each episode. Other patients may have recurrent bouts of pneumonia with or without a persistent cough between episodes. It is common for some patients to develop lower respiratory tract infection with *Pseudomonas* after previous treatment for persistent staphylococcal colonization or infection. Most patients eventually develop a chronic productive cough of increasing severity, a decrease in appetite, weight loss, and diminished activity, particularly during exacerbations. Other symptoms may include wheezing, tachypnea, and irritability. Low-grade fever often accompanies exacerbations, although high fever is uncommon. Physical signs include evidence of undernutrition, increased anterior–posterior diameter, retractions, cyanosis, inspiratory and expiratory wheezing, rhonchi, localized or generalized moist rales, abdominal distention, and clubbing of fingers and toes. A leukocytosis and left-shift are usually present during acute exacerbations. Blood gases show varying degrees of hypoxemia with or without hypercarbia. Pulmonary function tests reveal an obstructive defect, and, in the presence of chronic fibrosis, a restrictive defect as well. Chest roentgenograms demonstrate overaeration, peribronchial thickening, patchy atelectasis due to mucus plugging of small airways, and patchy pneumonia. In older patients with moderate to more advanced disease, there is severe overaeration, a small heart, depressed diaphragms, and an increased anterior–posterior diameter. Extensive peribronchial infiltration with generalized bronchiectasis may be seen; cyst formation and mucus plugging of dilated bronchi are common findings.

Although there is no cure for *Pseudomonas* pulmonary disease in patients with cystic fibrosis, contemporary therapies have significantly improved survival. Early diagnosis of infection and aggressive treatment are critical to the prevention or postponement of irreversible lung damage. Several years ago, it was established that antibiotics with good in vitro activity against *P. aeruginosa* should be employed, usually in combination, to treat acute exacerbations of *Pseudomonas* lung infection.[91–95] An aminoglycoside like gentamicin, tobramycin, or amikacin, combined with an antipseudomonal penicillin like carbenicillin or ticarcillin, still represents an effective treatment of *Pseudomonas* respiratory infections in patients with cystic fibrosis. However, the introduction of new antipseudomonal penicillins, extended spectrum cephalosporins, carbapenems, monobactams, and quinolones has provided additional therapeutic choices, while stimulating new controversies, in the treatment of these infections. Piperacillin,[96] ceftazidime,[97] imipenem,[98] aztreonam,[99] and ciprofloxacin[100] have all been used, alone or in combination with an aminoglycoside, to effectively treat acute exacerbations of chronic *Pseudomonas* pulmonary infections in patients with cystic fibrosis. However, the use of all of these agents has been associated with the emergence of resistant strains of *P. aeruginosa*. Perhaps the most striking example of this is imipenem, the potent β-lactamase inducer, whose use in cystic fibrosis patients has produced or selected *P. aeruginosa* strains resistant to imipenem as well as other β-lactams including ceftazidime and piperacillin.[101] Yet, all of these agents have produced good clinical responses, in many cases despite the emergence of resistance to them. In fact, one puzzling aspect of therapy for *Pseudomonas* lung infections in patients with cystic fibrosis is the lack of correlation between microbiological and clinical responses. In addition to questions regarding the expanded choice of antimicrobial agents in cystic fibrosis lung infections, controversy has surrounded the use of a single agent (monotherapy) versus antibiotic combinations. While aminoglycoside-containing combinations have been favored for their synergistic activities and prevention of resistance, single drug therapy, most notably with piperacillin[102] or ceftazidime,[103,104] has also proven efficacious.

Since there is now a wide choice of antimicrobial agents effective against lower respiratory tract *Pseudomonas* infections in patients with cystic fibrosis, the selection of particular drugs will depend upon local resistance patterns and prescribing practices. All antibiotics are administered in high doses, by the parenteral route, with the exception of oral quinolones.[105] Altered antibiotic pharmocokinetics in cystic fibrosis patients are due to increased renal tubular secretion, decreased tubular reabsorption, and increased nonrenal clearance.[106] These alterations in antibiotic handling apparently apply to β-lactams as well as aminoglycosides, and may necessitate higher than usual antibiotic doses, greater dosing frequency, and, in the case of aminoglycosides, monitoring of serum drug levels and individualization of dosage regimens. Treatment is usually continued until symptomatic improvement occurs, typically 1–2 weeks. Improvement in both subjective symptoms and objective measures of pulmonary function can be expected.[91,93–95] On the other hand, although *Pseudomonas* may temporarily disappear from the sputum of patients following aggressive antibiotic treatment, it may also persist, develop in vitro resistance to the agent(s) employed in treatment, and (almost inevitably) reappear following discontinuation of therapy.[93,94] Fortunately, clinical improvement is frequently observed despite these less hopeful microbiological events monitored in the sputum.

The role of antibiotic prophylaxis or chronic suppression of *Pseudomonas* lung infections in cystic fibrosis patients is controversial. True prophylaxis, that is, maintenance of patients on an antibiotic with activity against *P. aeruginosa* prior to respiratory tract colonization, has not been adequately studied. Likewise, suppressive therapy, that is, maintenance of patients on an antibiotic once colonization has been established in order to prevent acute exacerbations and arrest chronic progression of *Pseudomonas* lung disease, has been advocated without clear evidence of efficacy. A strategy that shows considerable promise is regular, intermittent therapy of cystic fibrosis patients with chronic *Pseudomonas* lung infections three to four times each year. This aggressive approach, in which patients are treated expectantly rather than in response to acute exacerbations of their chronic infections, may have contributed to recent improvements in mortality observed among Danish cystic fibrosis patients with *Pseudomonas* pulmonary infections.[107,108] Facilitating this approach is the availability of quinolone antibiotics, which were administered to adult cystic fibrosis patients in Denmark.

Another promising treatment is the intermittent aerosolization of antibiotics into the respiratory tracts of cystic fibrosis patients with established *Pseudomonas* lung infections. Among the antibiotics tried have been combinations of an aminoglycoside and antipseudomonas penicillin,[109] ceftazidime alone,[110] and a nebulized aminoglycoside accompanied by an oral quinolone.[111] This approach has reportedly succeeded in reducing patients' symptoms, improving pulmonary function, and decreasing the number of required hospitalizations. Good pulmonary toilet is a critical adjunct to antibiotic therapy in the treatment of chronic lung infections in cystic fibrosis. Inhalation of hydrating and mucolytic agents, postural drainage, and chest physiotherapy are often useful, and bronchial lavage is sometimes employed, to remove respiratory secretions. Whole-lung lavage can be performed using a Carlens tube or segmental lavage accomplished through a bronchoscope.[112] Although the appropriate use of these procedures is not firmly established, segmental lavage should probably be carried out when obstructive secretions or mucus plugs are thought to hamper effective treatment.

Bacteremia

The frequency of *Pseudomonas* bacteremia reflects the invasive potential of *P. aeruginosa* in immunocompromised patients. It tends to occur at the extremes of age, is usually related to nosocomial infections, and is often iatrogenic. Predisposing conditions include hematologic malignancies, immunoglobulin deficiency states, hypocomplementemia, neutropenia, diabetes mellitus, renal transplantation, severe burns, and diffuse dermatidities. Other predisposing factors include cancer chemotherapy resulting in neutropenia or ulceration of the respiratory and gastrointestinal tracts, steroid administration, antibiotic therapy, placement of intravascular lines, urinary tract instrumentation or catheterization, surgery, trauma, and prematurity.

Pseudomonas aeruginosa is the fourth most common cause of primary, hospital-acquired gram-negative bacteremia (behind *E. coli*, *Klebsiella*, and *Enterobacter*)[7] and is probably the third leading cause of all single-organism gram-negative bacteremias (behind *E. coli* and *Klebsiella*).[8,113] Mortality rates vary, but are typically in the 33–38 percent range, at least among cancer patients.[113,114] Some studies indicate a higher mortality among patients with *Pseudomonas* bacteremia compared with other bacteremias (8). It is not clear to what extent this high mortality reflects the more severe underlying illnesses affecting patients subject to *Pseudomonas* bacteremia, and to what extent it is a function of the greater inherent virulence of the organism. The fact that *P. aeruginosa* may cause excess mortality even in patients with less severe underlying diseases[8] underscores its pathogenic potential upon reaching the blood stream.

In general, *Pseudomonas* bacteremia is clinically indistinguishable from other forms of gram-negative sepsis.[115–121] Signs and symptoms are variable and depend on primary site of infection and clinical setting. Common primary sites of infection include the respiratory, gastrointestinal, and urinary tracts, skin and soft tissues, and intravascular foci. Fever is almost always present except in very young or premature infants, and is usually accompanied by tachycardia and tachypnea. Patients apprear toxic, and may manifest apprehension, disorientation, or obtundation. Hypotension is common, and refractory shock may develop as a preterminal event. Respiratory failure occurs in the presence of bacteremic *Pseudomonas* pneumonia or in conjunction with ARDS. Azotemia is common, and renal failure may accompany frank shock. Jaundice appears to occur more often than in other forms of gram-negative sepsis.[116,122] DIC is relatively uncommon.

Skin lesions may be an important distinguishing feature of *Pseudomonas* bacteremia, especially if they represent typical ecthyma gangrenosum.[123–126] These small, round, indurated nodules often begin as vesicles that undergo hemorrhage, necrosis, and ulceration. They are typically surrounded by a rim of erythema and contain little if any pus. Histologically, there is bacterial invasion of small arteries and veins, but little inflammatory infiltrate. *Pseudomonas aeruginosa* can be readily demonstrated in the lesions by Gram stain or culture. Ecthyma lesions usually occur singly or in small numbers on the perineum, buttocks, extremities, or in the axillae, but they may appear anywhere on the body. Ecthyma-like lesions can also be seen on the mucous membranes of the mouth, hard or soft palate, gingiva, or tongue. Although present in a relatively small minority of patients with *Pseudomonas* bacteremia, and rarely associated with other bacterial[127] and fungal[128] etiologies, ecthyma gangrenosum is virtually pathognomonic for *Pseudomonas* disease, especially if microscopic examination reveals typical vascular lesions.

Other types of skin lesions may be seen in conjunction with bacteremic *Pseudomonas* infections.[116] Small painful vesicles occur in clusters on an erythematous base and contain cloudy, bacteria-laden fluid. Flat, sharply demarcated areas of cellulitis may also occur; they tend to enlarge rapidly, becoming hemorrhagic and necrotic. Diffuse maculopapular eruptions, most concentrated on the trunk, have also been described early in *Pseudomonas* sepsis, and metastatic abscesses of the extremities and fingertips are occasionally seen late in the disease.

Antibiotic therapy of *Pseudomonas* bacteremia is frequently instituted prior to a specific etiologic diagnosis. "Empirical" treatment is usually based on a presumptive diagnosis of sepsis suggested by nonspecific signs and symptoms as well as clinical setting. The necessity for beginning treatment immediately once sepsis is suspected, particularly in neutropenic patients, is widely accepted. The number and choice of antibiotics in this setting are controversial, however. The conventional approach to presumptive therapy in the face of neutropenia, or other settings in which *Pseudomonas* is a possible or likely pathogen, is to initiate combination treatment with an aminoglycoside and extended spectrum antipseudomonal penicillin or cephalosporin. The specific choice of agents should be guided by local antibiotic susceptibility patterns and prescribing practices. If a cephalosporin is used, care should be taken to choose an agent like ceftazidime with demonstrated in vitro and in vivo efficacy against *Pseudomonas*; moxalactam and cefotaxime are less satisfactory alternatives in this setting because of their unpredictable activity against *Pseudomonas*. The use of a single antibiotic, so-called monotherapy, in febrile neutropenic patients is the subject of intense debate. Ceftazidime was used successfully as initial therapy in one major study,[129] while another large study reported superior response rates when ceftazidime was combined with a full rather than short course of amikacin.[130] Imipenem monotherapy is currently under investigation in neutropenic cancer patients with suspected sepsis. Some of those advocating monotherapy in this setting also recognize the potential need for modifying the initial antimicrobial treatment when the results of the pretreatment evaluation become available or when the patient remains neutropenic.[129] Despite the continued controversy regarding monotherapy, it is recommended that if *Pseudomonas* sepsis is suspected on the basis of clinical setting or local hospital epidemiology, or if the patient is gravely ill, combination therapy should be instituted with maximum recommended doses of an aminoglycoside and a β-lactam with dependable antipseudomonal activity. Moreover, if *Pseudomonas* bacteremia is documented, similar therapy should be instituted, even if the patient has already responded to a regimen containing a single agent active against *Pseudomonas*. Immunocompromised patients with documented bacteremia due to *Pseudomonas* or other gram-negative bacteria have a higher probability of survival when they receive two antibiotics to which their infecting strains are susceptible, particularly when the two drugs act synergistically.[131,132] The utility of antibiotic synergy is particularly important in persistent, profound neutropenia.[133] In the case of aminoglycoside antibiotics, serum levels should be closely monitored in order to maintain the highest possible levels consistent with safety. The duration of treatment is dictated by the site and severity of the primary infection, promptness of response, and presence or persistence of neutropenia. For example, a nonneutropenic patient with *Pseudomonas* urosepsis who defervesces promptly following removal of a Foley catheter and institution of antibiotics may be managed adequately with 7–10 days of therapy. In contrast, a neutropenic patient with persistent fever and/or other signs of sepsis while on antibiotics may warrant prolonged treatment until the white blood cell count recovers and the fever subsides.

Since no pathophysiologic mechanisms peculiar to *Pseudomonas*-associated septic shock have been adequately elucidated, no specific therapy other than antibiotics is indicated in this condition. Although controversy may still exist over the role of steroid therapy in septic shock,[134] recent studies have not confirmed the efficacy of such treatment.[135,136] Specific immunologic approaches to the therapy of *Pseudomonas* sepsis, such as the passive administration of hyperimmune intravenous immune globulin or *Pseudomonas*-specific monoclonal antibodies, are under active investigation but are not recommended at the present time.

Central Nervous System Infections

Pseudomonas aeruginosa causes meningitis and brain abscess. *Pseudomonas* infections of the central nervous system result from (*1*) extension from a contiguous structure such as ear, mastoid, or paranasal sinus; (*2*) direct inoculation into the subarachnoid space or brain by means of head trauma, surgery, or invasive diagnostic procedures; and (*3*) bacteremic spread from a distant site of infection such as the urinary tract, lung, or endocardium.[137–140] As in other forms of *Pseudomonas* disease, central nervous system infections usually occur in the presence of pre-existing defects in normal host defenses or other predisposing conditions. The latter include recent neurosurgery; penetrating head trauma; tumors of the head and neck; infections of the ear, mastoid, or paranasal sinuses; lumbar punctures; spinal anesthesia; intraventricular shunts or reservoirs; and cerebrospinal fluid (CSF) leaks. In addition, conditions that predispose patients to *Pseudomonas* bacteremia, such as neutropenia and severe burns, increase the risk of metastatic central nervous system infection. In a survey of cancer patients with central nervous system infections,[137] *P. aeruginosa* was the second most common bacterial pathogen isolated in cases of meningitis (after *Listeria monocytogenes*) and the second most frequent cause of brain abscess (*E. coli* was first).

The clinical manifestations of *Pseudomonas* meningitis are like those of other forms of bacterial meningitis and include fever, headache, confusion, and obtundation. The onset of disease may be acute, or even fulminant, particularly when it is associated with bacteremia; septic shock and coma may supervene, and early death is common. In nonbacteremic patients, the onset of clinical disease may be more gradual and insidious, sometimes in the absence of systemic signs and symptoms. This presentation is particularly common in immunosuppressed or cancer patients, and in those whose meningitis is related to neurosurgery or extension from a contiguous site of chronic infection.[141] *Pseudomonas* meningitis is sometimes characterized by a subacute, relapsing course probably due to release of bacteria from loculated areas of infection. Recurrent or chronic *Pseudomonas* meningitis is commonly associated with alteration of normal cranial anatomy secondary to trauma, surgery, and/or malignant disease; indwelling catheters, CSF shunts, or reservoirs; prosthetic materials; active or undrained parameningeal infections; and CSF leaks.

The antibiotic therapy of *Pseudomonas* meningitis is complicated by the in vitro and in vivo resistance of *P. aeruginosa* to many antibiotics and by their poor penetration into the subarachnoid space.[142] Ceftazidime may well be the antimicrobial agent best able to overcome these two limitations. The exquisite susceptibility of most *P. aeruginosa* strains to ceftazidime, coupled with its ability to cross the blood-brain barrier, results in CSF drug levels well in excess of minimum inhibitory concentrations.[143] Although the infrequency of *Pseudomonas* meningitis has precluded large, controlled studies, the efficacy of ceftazidime has been documented by wide clinical experience.[143–145] Successful treatment of *Pseudomonas* meningitis has been reported with ceftazidime employed alone, and in combination with an aminoglycoside administered intravenously or intrathecally. Many documented responses to ceftazidime have followed previously unsuccessful treatment with other agents.[144] While current data suggest that ceftazidime is the antibiotic of choice in *Pseudomonas* meningitis, it is unclear whether it should be used in conjunction with an aminoglycoside. Initial treatment, particularly in desperately ill patients, should probably include both agents administered intravenously at maximal doses consistent with safety. The ability of ceftazidime to enter the CSF in therapeutic concentrations may obviate the need for intrathecal administration of the accompanying aminoglycoside (as previously recommended). However, failure of initial therapy or relapse may necessitate intrathecal therapy, or if there is obstruction of the subarachnoid space or evidence of ventriculitis, direct intraventricular aminoglycoside administration via an intraventricular catheter or reservoir.[146,147] The choice of a particular aminoglycoside should be governed by local susceptibility patterns. Gentamicin, tobramycin, and amikacin have all been administered successfully by both the intrathecal and intraventricular routes; a preservative-free form should be used when available. Extended spectrum cephalosporins other than ceftazidime are probably contraindicated in *Pseudomonas* meningitis on the basis of variable activity against *Pseudomonas*, poor CSF penetration, or both.[142,143,148] Parenteral ciprofloxacin is another very promising antimicrobial agent for use in *Pseudomonas* central nervous system infections on the basis of highly favorable in vitro susceptibility data, good CSF penetration,[149] and equivalent efficacy compared with ceftazidime and tobramycin in experimental *P. aeruginosa* meningitis in rabbits.[150] Adequate clinical experience with ciprofloxacin in *Pseudomonas* meningitis is still lacking, however. The proper duration of antibiotic therapy for *Pseudomonas* meningitis is dictated by the severity and extent of involvement, degree of disruption of normal anatomy, presence or absence of ventriculitis, and by the promptness of response to treatment. A minimum of 2 weeks of therapy should ordinarily be expected, and much longer treatment may be necessary in order to eradicate infection and prevent relapse. Monitoring of lumbar CSF or ventricular fluid by culture, serial cell counts, and determination of antibiotic levels, may help direct therapy and suggest a proper treatment endpoint. Relapses are common and require retreatment.

Pseudomonas brain abscesses should be surgically drained if possible and treated with antibiotics as described above. Intrathecal or intraventricular aminoglycoside administration is not necessary unless persistent meningitis or ventriculitis are present. Abscesses should be monitored during treatment by serial computerized axial tomographic or magnetic resonance scans and antibiotics continued until there is closure or significant diminution in size; 2–6 weeks of therapy may be necessary. Failure of an abscess to diminish in size or progression of symptoms may necessitate reaspiration or surgical exploration and drainage. Cure of *Pseudomonas* central nervous system infections in general may require débridement of necrotic tissue, removal of prosthetic materials, or repair of CSF leaks.

Ear Infections, including "Malignant" External Otitis

Pseudomonas aeruginosa is infrequently found in the normal ear, but often inhabits the external auditory canal in association with injury, maceration, inflammation, or simply wet or humid conditions. It is the predominant bacterial pathogen in cases of external otitis[151] (see Chapter 46) and is presumed to play a contributory if not causal role in this usually benign and self-limited disease. External otitis is clearly associated with swimming ("swimmer's ear") and is said to be more frequent in humid, southern climates.[152] Its clinical manifestations include an itchy or painful, discharging ear, with pain worsened by traction on the pinna, and a tender edematous canal filled with debris. This infection is successfully treated with local measures including topical application of antibiotic- and steroid-containing otic solutions, drying agents, and 2% acetic acid to reduce the growth of *Pseudomonas*. Although external otitis is usually cured by these measures, recurrence is common, particularly in frequent swimmers.

Occasionally, *Pseudomonas* infections of the external auditory canal become locally invasive by penetrating the epithelium and invading underlying soft tissues. This process is usually chronic and indolent, but also destructive and ultimately life-threatening if not promptly and appropriately treated. Invasive, necrotizing, or, more commonly, "malignant external otitis" is a condition found predominantly in elderly diabetics, particularly those with long-standing illness associated with small vessel disease.[152–159] It also occurs occasionally in very young infants suffering from other underlying illnesses,[160,161] and rarely in apparently normal or merely elderly adults.[162]

Tissue invasion by *Pseudomonas* usually begins at the junction between cartilage and bone in the floor of the lateral portion of the external auditory canal, through normal defects in the cartilage called the fissures of Santorini. The invasive process involves soft tissue, cartilage, and ultimately cortical bone and marrow. The necrotizing infection enters the soft tissues of the retromandibular area or parotid space. The infection usually bypasses the tympanic membrane and middle ear, at least early, and enters the mastoid air cells and adjacent temporal bone. Once osteomyelitis of the temporal bone has been established, the infection spreads through the bone at the base of the skull, involving the seventh cranial nerve at the stylomastoid foramen, the ninth, tenth, and eleventh cranial nerves at the jugular foramen, and the twelfth cranial nerve at the hypoglossal canal. Thrombosis of lateral and sigmoid sinuses may occur, and further spread proceeds in sinuses and along other vascular channels with extension throughout the temporal bone all the way to the petrous apex. Extension can then further proceed across the base of the skull, anterior to the foramen magnum, via the basisphenoid and basiocciput or cavernous sinus to the contralateral petrous apex, and from there might involve contralateral cranial nerves. Frank meningitis and brain abscess are relatively uncommon complications.

Presenting symptoms of malignant external otitis include otalgia and otorrhea. A facial nerve palsy may be present initially, whereas involvement of other cranial nerves usually appears later. Some patients report decreased hearing; the pinna may be tender, and the presence of trismus indicates involvement of the temporomandibular area. Systemic symptoms, including fever and weight loss, occur in a small minority of patients. On physical examination, the external auditory canal is abnormal in almost all patients. It usually appears inflamed, swollen, or erythematous, and a purulent discharge is present. In most cases, granulation tissue is seen in the posterior–inferior canal wall or at the junction of the bony and cartilaginous canal. The tympanic membrane is intact in some patients, perforated in others; often it is simply hidden from view by edema, granulation tissue, and debris. Signs of inflammation are often noted in areas outside the ear canal including the pinna, periacuricular and retromandibular areas, and mastoid tip. Local lymphadenopathy and parotid swelling are occasionally present. Bilateral disease is relatively uncommon but does occur.

Leukocytosis is infrequent in malignant external otitis, while CSF pleocytosis and protein elevation are occasionally noted. Although a nonspecific finding, the erythrocyte sedimentation rate (ESR) appears to be strikingly elevated in most cases, with elevations greater than 100 mm/hr sometimes observed.[163] Polytomograms of the mastoid or temporal bone may reveal bony erosions and new bone formation. Computed tomography (CT) scans of the floor of the skull may demonstrate soft tissue densities associated with areas of cellulitis. The anatomic locations of these densities often correspond to specific cranial nerve deficits, e.g., stylomastoid foramen (seventh crainial nerve), jugular foramen (ninth, tenth, and eleventh cranial nerves), or hypoglossal canal (twelfth cranial nerve).[164] Technetium-99 bone scans are more sensitive than roentgenograms in demonstrating early bone involvement, while gallium-67 scans will help discriminate between active inflammation (infection) and conditions such as neoplasms, which simply increase metabolic activity of bone. Magnetic resonance imaging (MRI) may be superior to CT scans in defining the anatomic extent of disease and delineating soft tissue involvement.[165]

Pseudomonas aeruginosa is isolated from cultures of the external auditory canal and specimens obtained at the time of surgery in virtually all patients with malignant external otitis. Although other organisms may be isolated in addition, for practical purposes this may be considered a specific *Pseudomonas* disease.

The treatment of malignant external otitis should be aggressive and persistent, commonly involving both surgery and antibiotics.[152,158] Surgery is aimed at débriding granulation tissue and necrotic material, such as dead bone and cartilage, and draining pus. The nature of the surgery required is determined by sites of involvement and extent of infection. Surgical procedures may include canal débridement, bone or cartilage débridement, mastoidectomy, or facial nerve decompression. Occasionally, a suboccipital approach is used to drain and débride areas of infection in the floor of the skull.[166] In many cases, however, relatively circumscribed surgery may be preferable, in conjunction with aggressive (and effective) antibiotic therapy. Some believe, for example, that facial nerve decompression does not contribute to the recovery of function and should not be routinely performed. Similar opinion holds that the role of surgery in malignant external otitis should generally be limited to local débridement and the excision of accessible foci of infection such as polypectomy or sequestrum removal. This school of thought would reserve more extensive bone resection and drainage of deep-seated cranial abscesses for selected patients whose condition is unresponsive to aggressive medical therapy and more limited surgical débridement.[163]

Appropriate antibiotic therapy of malignant external otitis ordinarily consists of an aminoglycoside in combination with a β-lactam agent with good antipseudomonal activity. Treatment should be continued for a minimum of 4 weeks in the case of relatively limited disease and 6–8 weeks or longer if extensive disease is present, particularly with cranial nerve involvement. Although good data are not available comparing different antibiotic regimens, or single drug vs. combined therapy, some data suggest the greater likelihood of recurrent disease when single rather than combined antibiotics are employed.[158] A retrospective analysis of patients receiving cefsulodin alone compared with those receiving conventional therapy (i.e., an aminoglycoside plus antipseudomonal β-lactam) suggested equivalent efficacy only in patients with "moderate" infections.[167] Although a number of newer agents with potent antipseudomonal activity are available, their use as single agents in this disease is not supported by adequate clinical data. Moreover, the effectiveness of oral therapy with ciprofloxacin and rifampin[168] requires further substantiation. Malignant external otitis is generally so difficult to eradicate, the success or failure of therapy so difficult to assess, and the potential consequences of failed treatment so profound that intensive and prolonged antibiotic therapy, with two agents, is usually indicated. Since there are no precise or universally applicable therapeutic guidelines or end points in this disease, it is preferable to err on the side of over- rather than undertreatment.

It is unclear to what extent earlier recognition and improved treatment of malignant external otitis have improved outcome.[158,163] Overall mortality appears to remain as high as 15–20 percent despite the availability of effective therapy. Patients who present with neurologic deficits have a worse prognosis commensurate with the extent and severity of their infections. It is clear that earlier recognition and institution of appropriate therapy simplifies treatment and improves prognosis. Nonetheless, treatment failures occur and relapses are observed as long as 4–12 months after termination of antibiotic therapy, necessitating careful long-term follow-up. Disease status may be assessed during treatment and post-treatment periods by monitoring pain, ESR, serial technetium-99 scans, and CT or MRI scans.

Otitis media diagnosed during the first 6 weeks of life is frequently caused by gram-negative bacteria, including *Pseudomonas*, and may present atypically.[169] Symptoms include rhinorrhea, irritability, feeding difficulty, cough, and diarrhea. The majority of patients are afebrile. A routine 10-day course of antibiotic treatment may not result in cure, and *Pseudomonas* is often recovered from the ears of treatment failures, whether or not it was the organism initially isolated. An antipseudomonal antibiotic should therefore be included in the initial treatment of children under 6 weeks of age with otitis media, and therapy continued for more than 10 days.

Pseudomonas aeruginosa is the most common bacterial pathogen isolated from the middle and external ear of children and adults with chronic suppurative otitis media. Isolation rates as high as 72 percent have been reported.[170] Although the microbiology of chronic middle ear infections may be complex, *P. aeruginosa* was identified in 67 percent of specimens obtained directly from the middle ear of children with chronic suppurative otitis media and was the only organism grown in 31 percent.[171] Tympanomastoid surgery is considered standard management for chronic suppurative otitis media that is unresponsive to topical and oral antimicrobial therapy. Recent evidence suggests, however, that medical management with parenteral antibiotics and daily aural toilet will result in resolution of most chronic suppurative otitis media, without cholesteatoma, in children, thus, obviating the need for tympanomastoidectomy in the majority of cases.[172] The short- and long-term efficacy of parenteral antibiotic therapy, directed primarily against *Pseudomonas*, requires further confirmation, while the optimal duration of therapy needs to be defined.

Pseudomonas aeruginosa can cause mastoiditis in association with either malignant external otitis or primary acute otitis media.[173] In either case, patients usually have diabetes mellitus or other underlying diseases that adversely affect normal host defenses. In such patients, acute *Pseudomonas* middle ear infections progress to granulomatous mucositis of the mastoid and middle ear, leading to osteomyelitis and bone necrosis. Spontaneous perforation of the tympanic membrane is usual, and seventh cranial nerve palsy is seen in some cases. Treatment consists of local débridement or mastoidectomy and aggressive antibiotic therapy similar to that employed in malignant external otitis. *Pseudomonas* perichondritis of the auricle may follow trauma, burns, or ear surgery.[174] The ear becomes acutely swollen, erythematous, disfigured, and tender, as invading bacteria cause a cellulitis as well as inflammation and necrosis of cartilage. Treatment consists of the insertion of drainage tubes and systemic antipseudomonal antibiotics. Excisional procedures are disfiguring and should be avoided if possible.[174]

Eye Infections

Pseudomonas aeruginosa is a frequent and sometimes devastating pathogen in the human eye. It is one of the most common causes of bacterial corneal ulcer, or keratitis[175] and is also implicated in endophthalmitis.[176] In addition, it has been reported as the etiologic agent in ophthalmia neonatorum,[177] blepharoconjunctivitis,[178] and scleral abscess.[179]

The pathogenesis of *Pseudomonas* eye infections is a function of the peculiar anatomy and physiology of the eye as well as inherent characteristics of the organism itself. The initial attachment of *Pseudomonas* to the ocular epithelium appears to be mediated by sialic acid (*N*-acetylneuraminic acid)-specific receptors,[180] analogous to those responsible for the organisms's attachment to tracheobronchial epithelium. The cornea, aqueous, and vitreous comprise a relatively sequestered and avascular milieu, which, in the normal state, is relatively devoid of humoral and cellular immune elements. When introduced into this locally immunocompromised environment through trauma or hematogenous spread, *Pseudomonas* is capable of rapid proliferation and production of pathogenic extracellular enzymes including elastase, alkaline protease, and exotoxin A. The result can be a rapidly progressive and destructive infection leading to loss of the entire eye. Treatment is complicated by the existence of a blood-eye barrier that impedes access of antibiotics to infected intraocular structures.

Pseudomonas infections of the cornea usually begin with some form of trauma, often minor, which causes an interruption in the epithelial surface and allows bacterial invasion of underlying stroma. *Pseudomonas* keratitis appears to be more common in humid environments, such as the southern United States.[181] It is associated with contact lens use,[182] and the organism appears to adhere to worn, extended-wear soft contact lens.[183] *Pseudomonas* keratitis also has a high incidence in patients with predisposing ocular conditions, particularly those requiring topical steroid therapy, and has been associated with the use of contaminated ocular medications.[184] Also susceptible to *Pseudomonas* keratitis are patients with serious burns, coma, prior ocular irradiation, or exposure to an intensive care environment.[185–187] Pediatric intensive care patients may be particularly susceptible to *Pseudomonas* eye infections associated with tracheostomy, endotracheal intubation, and respiratory care, which apparently result in contamination of unprotected eyes by respiratory secretions.[188] *Pseudomonas* keratitis typically begins as a small central ulcer that spreads concentrically, in some cases to involve the entire cornea and parts of the sclera, and internally to involve deeper portions of the stroma, sometimes leading to corneal perforation.

Clinical signs of *Pseudomonas* keratitis may include a rapidly developing, necrotic, grayish stromal infiltrate in the bed of an epithelial injury, surrounding epithelial edema, severe anterior chamber reaction, and abundant mucopurulent discharge tenaciously adherent to the ulcer surface. The time course of *Pseudomonas* keratitis is variable. Classically, it progresses rapidly over 48 hours or less to involve the entire cornea, in some cases leading to perforation. Alternatively, the infection may evolve subacutely over many days. Fever is either absent or low grade, and other systemic symptoms are unusual. If present, leukocytosis is minimal.

Since a *Pseudomonas* corneal ulcer may lead to the rapid loss of ocular function, it should be approached as a medical emergency. Scrapings are obtained from the floor of the ulcer for Gram stain and culture. The presence of gram-negative rods (or a negative Gram stain) necessitates the immediate initiation of combined topical and subconjunctival (or subtenon) therapy with an aminoglycoside antibiotic such as gentamicin. Topical therapy should consist of an ophthalmic solution rather than ointment, and the optimal aminoglycoside concentration of the preparation is 8 mg/ml or greater (rather than the more dilute 0.3% gentamicin solution commercially available.[189,190] The solution is applied to the affected eye hourly, although continuous lavage has also been advocated.[191] An ophthalmic solution containing a quinolone antibiotic, such as enoxacin, may provide an effective alternative to gentamicin eye drops.[192] Topical therapy alone may be sufficient for relatively small, superficial ulcers,[193] but subconjunctival (or subtenon) administration will ensure higher aminoglycoside concentrations in the corneal stroma, sclera, and aqueous[194]; the latter may be critical if perforation into the anterior chamber is imminent. Once or twice daily subconjunctival injections with 20 mg of gentamicin may be given for the first 3 days of therapy or until negative cultures have been obtained. Ceftazidime may be administered alternatively by the same route. Parenteral therapy should be withheld unless intraocular spread of infection results in endophthalmitis.

Pseudomonas endophthalmitis may result from penetrating injuries, intraocular surgery, posterior perforation of corneal ulcers, or hematogenous spread from other primary sites of infection.[195,196] It is usually a fulminant disease that threatens permanent loss of vision within days or even hours. This rapid progression serves to clinically differentiate *Pseudomonas* endophthalmitis from that caused by less virulent bacteria such as *Staphylococcus epidermidis* and α-hemolytic streptococci, or fungi, which are likely to cause more indolent infections. The most common clinical features are pain, conjuctival hyperemia and chemosis, lid edema, decreased visual acuity, hypopyon, or severe anterior uveitis; involvement of the vitreous and panophthalmitis follow.

Early and aggressive therapy of *Pseudomonas* endophthalmitis can result in the preservation of sight. Aspirated material from the anterior chamber or vitreous cavity should be gram-stained and cultured to establish an etiologic diagnosis. Wound drainage following intraocular surgery may also be cultured, although conjunctival cultures are undependable. Antibiotic therapy normally consists of an aminoglycoside administered by the parenteral, subconjunctival (or subtenon), topical, and intraocular routes, as well as a parenterally and subconjunctivally administered antipseudomonal penicillin. Parenteral, subconjunctival, and intraocular ceftazidime may represent effective alternative therapy.[197,198] although clinical experience is limited. Vitrectomy is frequently indicated to help clear loculated infection and cellular debris, and to facilitate intraocular antibiotic administration. The optimal duration of therapy is not well defined, although antibiotics should probably be continued until there has been marked clinical improvement and intra- and extraocular signs of infection have subsided. Intraocular antibiotic injections may be repeated daily during the first several days of treatment until negative cultures are obtained from the vitreous.

Bone and Joint Infections

Pseudomonas infections of bones and joints result from hematogenous spread from other primary sites or extension from contiguous foci. Blood-borne infections are most commonly seen in IV drug users and in conjunction with urinary tract or pelvic infections. Contiguous infections are usually related to penetrating trauma, surgery, or overlying soft-tissue infections. *Pseudomonas* bone and joint infections occur in children, the elderly, the chronically debilitated, and those with underlying diseases or other predisposing factors. *Pseudomonas* osteochondritis follows puncture wounds of the foot, particularly in children; the sternoclavicular and sacroiliac joints, vertebrae, and symphysis pubis are infected in IV drug users; osteomyelitis occurs in conjunction with vascular insufficiency of the lower extremities in patients with diabetes mellitus; diseased large synovial joints are infected in patients with underlying rheumatoid disease; and infections of the long bones follow open fractures and/or internal fixation procedures.

Blood-borne *Pseudomonas* appear to have a particular predilection for fibrocartilaginous joints of the axial skeleton. These infections often involve joint space, cartilage, synovium, and contiguous bone, such that it is difficult to determine whether arthritis preceded bone involvement, or vice versa. It is likely that these infections often begin in cartilage within the joint space followed by invasion of underlying bone. In addition, the organism may penetrate and damage the epiphyseal plate of growing bone, another cartilaginous structure.

Pseudomonas bone and joint infections are often more indolent than those caused by *S. aureus*, and they tend to be less destructive, or at least less rapidly so. A direct comparison of *P. aeruginosa* and *S. aureus* bone infections in rabbits[199,200] revealed common pathologic features but differences in severity. Compared with staphylococcal osteomyelitis, that caused by *Pseudomonas* was associated with fewer abscesses, less extensive sequestrum formation, less frequent extraosseus extension, and milder roentgenographic changes.

Vertebral osteomyelitis caused by *P. aeruginosa* is occasionally associated with complicated urinary tract infections and genitourinary surgery or instrumentation.[115] This disease often occurs in elderly patients and involves the lumbosacral spine primarily; shared venous drainage between pelvis and spine (Batson's plexus) is the presumed route of infection. Recently reported cases are mainly in IV drug users; the majority of these patients are young males and the cervical spine is more commonly involved (e.g., 27 percent) than in non-drug users (rarely).[201–203] The duration of symptoms is from weeks to months, neck or back pain being most common. Fever and other systemic symptoms are relatively uncommon. Physical signs include local tenderness and decreased range of motion of the spine. Neurologic deficits are found in approximately 15 percent of patients and tend to be mild. When present, temperature elevation is usually low grade. Leukocytosis is variable, and erythrocyte sedimentation rate is almost always elevated. *Pseudomonas* is occasionally isolated from the blood. Plain roentgenograms of the affected spine are sometimes "normal" on admission, but rarely remain so during hospitalization. Tomograms are not usually positive in the face of normal plain films, but are helpful in defining abnormalities when present. These include generalized loss of bone density, a narrowed interspace, destruction of adjacent vertebral endplates, lytic lesions of vertebral bodies, sclerosis, and, particularly late, osteophyte formation. CT or MRI scans may be the most critical means for assessing changes in bone density, soft tissue densities, and anatomic extent of involvement. Technetium bone scans are usually positive, even when roentgenograms are read as "normal," and gallium scans indicate the presence of active infection. Myelograms are occasionally positive due to granulation tissue in the epidural space.

The diagnosis of *Pseudomonas* vertebral osteomyelitis can usually be established by culturing the organism from material obtained by needle biopsy or aspiration. This can sometimes be accomplished under fluoroscopic guidance, but may have to be repeated. Open biopsy may be necessary to make an etiologic diagnosis in as many as one-third of cases. Surgery is usually not required in this disease except when exploration and open biopsy are necessary to establish a diagnosis or decompression is required by a possible epidural or paravertebral abscess (uncommon). Aminoglycoside antibiotics are the primary mode of therapy and should be administered for at least 4 weeks in order to reduce the chance of relapse, which is common with shorter courses of treatment. Although there is no good evidence of increased therapeutic efficacy of antibiotic combinations in this disease, a semisynthetic penicillin with antipseudomonal activity should probably be used in addition to an aminoglycoside. Longer courses of therapy might be considered if there is extensive disease, if the sedimentation rate remains elevated, or if a single antibiotic is employed.

Sternoarticular pyarthrosis due to *Pseudomonas* is another infection found primarily in IV drug users.[204–206] Although sometimes associated with *Pseudomonas* endocarditis, a primary site of infection is usually not discernible, and the pathogenesis of this disease remains obscure. Patients are commonly young males. Joint involvement is usually monoarticular, with the sternoclavicular joint affected more often than sternochondral joints. Major complaints are usually limited to moderate to severe anterior chest discomfort over the affected joint. Painful and restricted movement of the homolateral shoulder is often reported. The duration of symptoms prior to diagnosis is usually months, although more acute presentations sometimes occur. Most patients are persistently febrile, and physical findings include tenderness, swelling, erythema over the affected joint, and limitation of range of motion of the shoulder on the side of involvement. Leukocytosis is sometimes present, and erythrocyte sedimentation rate is always elevated. Arthrocentesis may yield fluid with typical characteristics of pyogenic infection, although smears of the fluid may not reveal bacteria despite subsequent positive culture. Synovial biopsy usually yields the infecting organism, and blood cultures are occasionally positive. Roentgenographic changes include soft-tissue swelling, demineralization of adjacent bone, lytic lesions, and periosteal elevation of the clavicular head, rib, or sternum. Though plain roentgenograms are sometimes read as normal, tomograms usually show abnormalities. Exploratory arthrotomies are usually necessary since contiguous bone involvement is present and requires débridement. In addition, perisynovial or retrosternal abscesses frequently need draining. These infections should be treated for at least 6 weeks with an aminoglycoside antibiotic in combination with an antipseudomonal penicillin. With adequate therapy, full recovery may be expected with minimal functional disability.

Pyogenic infections of the symphysis pubis are associated with prior pelvic surgery and IV drug use, and are usually caused by *P. aeruginosa*.[207,208] The pubic symphysis represents a fibrocartilaginous joint, and, as such, shares with the intervertebral, sternoarticular, and sacroiliac joints a peculiar susceptibility to infection by hematogenously disseminated *Pseudomonas*. Patients with osteomyelitis of the pubis present with hip, groin, thigh, or lower abdominal pain, any of which may be exacerbated by walking. Patients complain of exquisite tenderness over the pubic symphysis and may have fever. The duration of symptoms prior to medical attention ranges from several days to 2 months. Leukocytosis is variable, and erythrocyte sedimentation rate is elevated. Roentgenograms of the pelvis may be normal initially but will eventually show irregularity of the pubic margins and separation at the symphysis pubis. Osteomyelitis of the pubic rami is invariably present and may be extensive. Bone scans are usually positive. The diagnosis is made by needle aspiration or biopsy of the pubic sympysis and culture. This diagnostic procedure is particularly important in order to differentiate pyogenic infection from osteitis pubis. The latter is presumably a noninfectious condition that closely mimics osteomyelitis of the pubis and occurs most commonly after pelvic surgery, childbirth, or trauma.

Most patients with *Pseudomonas* osteomyelitis of the pubis can be cured with antibiotics alone and do not require surgical débridement or drainage. Cures have been documented following aminoglycoside administration alone or in combination with a semisynthetic penicillin. The duration of therapy should be 4 weeks or longer.

Pseudomonas aeruginosa is the most common pathogen implicated in osteochondritis following puncture wounds of the foot.[209–212] Originally described in children, this entity is also found in adults.[213] As the name implies, *Pseudomonas* osteochondritis reflects the peculiar predilection of the organism for cartilage, and involves the small joints and bones of the foot. Typically, a patient experiences early improvement in pain and swelling following a puncture wound of the foot, only to have the symptoms recur or worsen several days later. The average duration of symptoms prior to diagnosis is several weeks, and fever and other systemic signs are usually absent. Examination may reveal a superficial area of cellulitis on the plantar surface of the foot overlying the area of involvement, or merely tenderness to deep palpation. Involvement of the proximal phalanges, metatarsals, metatarsophalangeal joints, tarsal bones, and calcaneus have been reported. Roentgenographic changes are usually present at the time of presentation but sometimes develop later; technetium scans are positive. Aspiration of an affected joint may yield a small amount of purulent fluid with bacteria present on Gram stain or culture.

Appropriate treatment of *Pseudomonas* osteochondritis of the foot includes both surgery and antibiotics. Careful débridement and curettage of necrotic bone appear essential to early cure and minimization of long-term sequelae. Although 2 weeks or less of antibiotic therapy has proven curative in some cases following surgical débridement, a minimum of 4 weeks of treatment with an aminoglycoside antibiotic is preferable. Whether combined therapy with an aminoglycoside and antipseudomonal penicillin is necessary remains controversial. Although delayed treatment sometimes results in residual deformities, and repeated surgical procedures may be required to dispose of devitalized bone or cartilage, functional disability is uncommon, and cure is usually complete.

The term "chronic contiguous osteomyelitis"[214] describes a heterogeneous group of infections that result from direct inoculation of bone or direct extension from overlying or adjacent tissue rather than from a hematogenous source. These infections occur in a variety of clinical settings and are often caused by gram-negative bacteria, among which *P. aeruginosa* is one of the most frequently isolated. A common setting is following a compound fracture, or as a complication of "clean" surgery required in the management of closed fractures of the long bones. In some cases, these infections are acquired following puncture wounds of the foot (see above), or as a complication of peripheral neuropathy with associated pressure necrosis of skin and soft tissue overlying bone. Contiguous *Pseudomonas* bone infection can also result from extension of infection from ischemic ulcers in patients with peripheral vascular disease. Sternal osteomyelitis following heart surgery represents another category of such infections. The heterogeneity of chronic contiguous osteomyelitis in respect to clinical setting, affected host, relative difficulty of therapy, and prognosis complicate interpretation of existing therapeutic literature and establishment of general guidelines for treatment. In one large study, for example, oral ciprofloxacin produced very high cure rates in gram-negative infections associated with nail puncture wounds, pressure necrosis secondary to peripheral neuropathy, and postoperative sternal wounds. The same antibiotic was less effective in post-traumatic or postoperative osteomyelitis of the tibia or femur caused by *Pseudomonas*, and least effective in bone infections associated with underlying peripheral atherosclerotic vascular disease and diabetes mellitus.[214]

In light of the above, general, inclusive therapeutic guidelines are difficult in chronic contiguous *Pseudomonas* osteomyelitis. The immediate goals of antimicrobial therapy are to achieve bactericidal antibiotic levels in blood and bone, and to sustain those levels for the prolonged periods required for the eradication of infection. The combination of an aminoglycoside and antipseudomonal penicillin, both employed in full therapeutic doses for a minimum of 4–6 weeks, is still the standard of therapy. Complicated infections may require longer treatment, as determined by individual circumstances. Surgical débridement, excision of necrotic bone, foreign bodies or sequestra, or removal of prosthetic materials, are often necessary concomitants of therapy. The evaluation of alternative antibiotics for the treatment of *Pseudomonas* bone infections has focused on single agent and oral therapy. Ceftazidime has been used successfully, at an average dose of 4 g per day, to treat both acute and chronic *Pseudomonas* osteomyelitis.[215–217] Treatment failures have been noted, however, including persistence of infection and relapse, in some cases associated with the emergence of resistance. Imipenem has also been employed, with some success, as single agent therapy in chronic *Pseudomonas* bone infections, but clinical experience with this antibiotic is limited.[217] The quinolone antibiotics, ciprofloxacin, ofloxacin, and pefloxacin, have all been evaluated experimentally or clinically for single agent oral therapy of gram-negative osteomyelitis. Following parenteral or oral administration, these antibiotics achieve sustained concentrations in bone and blood well in excess of bactericidal levels for most strains of *P. aeruginosa*. Both ciprofloxacin and ofloxacin have achieved high rates of cure of chronic *Pseudomonas* osteomyelitis in rabbits.[218,219] Moreover, ciprofloxacin[214,220] and pefloxacin[221] have been employed with some success in single agent oral therapy of a variety of acute and chronic *Pseudomonas* bone infections. As in the case of single agent ceftazidime therapy, however, treatment failures, some associated with the emergence of resistance, have been noted. Because of the recalcitrance of *Pseudomonas* osteomyelitis and its association with complicating local or systemic host factors, instances of persistence or relapse requiring retreatment are common and do not necessarily signal the inadequacy of a particular antibiotic.

Urinary Tract Infections

Pseudomonas aeruginosa infections of the urinary tract are usually hospital-acquired and often iatrogenic.[222] They may be related to urinary tract catheterization,[223] instrumentation, or surgery,[224] including renal transplantation.[225,226] Recent data from the Centers for Disease Control National Nosocomial Infections Study indicate that *P. aeruginosa* causes 11.7 percent of all hospital-acquired urinary tract infections.[7] According to this large survey, *Pseudomonas* is the third most common hospital-acquired urinary tract pathogen after *E. coli* and enterococci. Even when not hospital-acquired, *Pseudomonas* urinary tract infections are frequently "complicated" by such factors as obstruction, persistent sites of infection (e.g., chronic prostatitis or stones), previous antibiotic therapy, and recurrent infections. It has been reported that *P. aeruginosa* is the fifth most common cause of recurrent urinary tract infections in school children, and the third most common pathogen when recurrent infections are complicated by obstruction, catheters, or stones.[227] On the other hand, *P. aeruginosa* urinary tract infections are not limited to patients with complicated urinary tract disease but may be seen in outpatient girls and women who do not have sites of persistence or stones.[228] In these cases, *Pseudomonas* may transiently colonize the vaginal introitus, which then serves as a reservoir for subsequent infection.

Pseudomonas aeruginosa appears to be among the most adherent of common urinary pathogens to bladder uroepithelium.[229] It can involve the urinary tract through ascending infection, or by bacteremic spread from another primary site. Conversely, the urinary tract represents one of the most frequent sources of *Pseudomonas* bacteremia (approximately 40 percent of cases in which there was an identifiable single source, in one study).[120]

The clinical manifestations of urinary tract infections caused by *Pseudomonas* are usually indistinguishable from those produced by other bacteria. Rare exceptions occur when ulcerative lesions of the bladder mucosa, ureters, and renal pelvis become necrotic, with sloughing of large pieces of vesical membrane in the urine.[230,231] Another characteristic, if unusual, form of urinary tract involvement by *Pseudomonas* results from bacterial invasion of small and medium-sized blood vessels in the kidneys of bacteremic patients, producing multiple renal infarcts.[232] These lesions apparently represent one of the visceral equivalents of ecthyma gangrenosum.

The appropriate treatment of *Pseudomonas* urinary tract infections depends upon site of involvement, presence or absence of associated sepsis, degree of chronicity, possible sites of persistence (including indwelling Foley catheters), and local patterns of antibiotic susceptibility. Because of these variables, and the paucity of conclusive comparative data regarding specific forms of treatment, it is difficult to make general therapeutic recommendations. Nevertheless, several guidelines are possible. All symptomatic *Pseudomonas* urinary tract infections should be treated. Chronic infections in the presence of a site of persistence, including urinary catheters, are best treated, if feasible, by removing or surgically eliminating the site or source of persistence as well as administering appropriate antibiotics. When a site of persistence such as a catheter cannot be removed, a reasonable approach may be to treat with an antibiotic only for symptomatic episodes or exacerbations, since eradication of infection is unlikely under these circumstances. An alternative approach in this situation, particularly in the presence of frequent, recurrent symptomatic episodes, is an acute "curative" course of an antibiotic followed by chronic suppression. This approach is hampered by the ineffectiveness against *P. aeruginosa* of many oral agents commonly employed to supress urinary tract infections (e.g., trimethoprim–sulfamethoxazole, nitrofurantoin). Although oral fluoroquinolone antibiotics such as norfloxacin[233] and ciprofloxacin[234–236] have been used to treat acute episodes of complicated or chronic *Pseudomonas* urinary tract infections, there is limited experience with these agents employed as chronic suppressive therapy. Another agent with possible suppressive activity against urinary *Pseudomonas* is a methanamine salt administered with an acidifying agent like ascorbic acid.

The aminoglycoside antibiotics are probably still the agents of choice for the parenteral therapy of most urinary tract infections due to *P. aeruginosa*. Gentamicin, tobramycin, amikacin, netilmicin, and sisomicin have all been employed successfully, and are probably equally efficacious. The choice of a specific aminoglycoside should be determined by local susceptibility patterns, availability, and cost. Tobramycin has been advocated in preference to gentamicin in patients with renal dysfunction because of its putatively lower nephrotoxic potential. With the possible exception of bacteremic infections, severe upper tract infections with abscess formation, and infections in neutropenic patients, *Pseudomonas* urinary tract disease can be treated with a single agent. Alternatives to the aminoglycoside antibiotics, particularly in patients with abnormal renal function, are antipseudomonal penicillins, extended spectrum cephalosporins (especially ceftazidime), imipenem, and aztreonam. The oral quinolone antibiotics norfloxacin[233] and ciprofloxacin[234–236] provide a viable alternative to parenteral therapy for *Pseudomonas* urinary tract infections not associated with frank sepsis. Ciprofloxacin is the preferable oral quinolone because of its superior activity against most *P. aeruginosa* isolates and more favorable systemic distribution. Ciprofloxacin has been used successfully to treat a variety of complicated *Pseudomonas* urinary tract infections, often in the presence of a urinary catheter or other structural or functional abnormalities. Initial symptomatic and bacteriologic responses, however, are all too frequently follwed by relapse, in some instances associated with increased resistance to ciprofloxacin. The apparent frequency of relapse is, to some degree, a function of the length of patient follow-up. Although good comparative data are unavailable, the relapse or failure rate in *Pseudomonas* urinary tract infections treated with oral quinolones appears no worse than that observed with parenteral aminoglycoside therapy. In addition, one must recognize that these infections are usually complicated and frequently relapse even in the face of aggressive therapy. On the other hand, the emergence of resistant strains following ciprofloxacin treatment of *Pseudomonas* urinary tract infections is a source of significant practical concern.

The suggested duration of parenteral therapy of *Pseudomonas* urinary tract infections is as follows: 3–5 days for uncomplicated, nonbacteremic infections limited to the bladder; at least 10 days for urosepsis; 2–3 weeks for documented or strongly suspected pyelonephritis, and possibly longer in the case of intrarenal or perinephric abscess. Most parenteral agents suitable for the treatment of *Pseudomonas* disease achieve high urine concentrations, permitting their use in moderate doses, except when the presence of significant renal parenchymal involvement or systemic disease dictate higher doses. Appropriate dosage adjustments should be made for the aminoglycosides in the face of impaired renal function. Optimal dose and duration of oral quinolone treatment of *Pseudomonas* urinary tract infections have not been established and are largely "empirical." Despite the lack of adequate guidance from the literature, it is reasonable to employ ciprofloxacin at a dose of 250–500 mg twice each day for 5–14 days; the higher dose and longer duration of therapy are preferable in complicated infections.

Gastrointestinal Infections

The incidence and potential seriousness of *Pseudomonas* gastointestinal disease is underestimated because it is often clinically inapparent, difficult to separate from that due to other causes, or simply overshadowed by pathologic events outside of the alimentary canal. *Pseudomonas aeruginosa* may produce disease in virtually any portion of the gastrointestinal tract, from the oropharynx to the rectum.[230,237] As in other forms of *Pseudomonas* disease, that involving the gastrointestinal tract occurs primarily in immunocompromised patients. The two most commonly affected groups are young infants[238–244] and those suffering from hematologic malignancies and neutropenia secondary to chemotherapy.[245–248] As well as being a frequent site of *Pseudomonas* infection, the gastrointestinal tract represents an important portal of entry in *Pseudomonas* septicemia. This is perhaps most striking in cancer patients who, following exposure to the hospital environment and broad spectrum antibiotics, develop gastrointestinal colonization with *Pseudomonas*, and upon receiving granulocytopenia-inducing chemotherapy become bacteremic from the large reservoir of *Pseudomonas* in their gut.[3] Although local signs of gastrointestinal involvement by *Pseudomonas* are sometimes overt (e.g., in typhlitis or rectal abscess), these infections are more often clinically inapparent and therefore go unrecognized as a primary focus giving rise to bacteremia.

Although *Pseudomonas* has been associated with relatively mild diarrheal disease in children, its clearest implication as an enteric pathogen is in cases of severe, sometimes fatal necrotizing enterocolitis in young infants.[240,244] A similar disease occurs in neutropenic cancer patients, most commonly with involvement of the distal ileum, cecum, and colon.[245,247,248] In both instances, postmortem examination reveals ulcerating lesions beginning in the bowel mucosa and extending into the submucosa.[240,245] The ulcers are typically hemorrhagic and necrotic and contain many *Pseudomonas*, which can be isolated readily in pure culture. There may be bacterial invasion of blood vessels in the submucosa and extension into the muscularis and serosal layers, sometimes leading to bowel perforation and peritonitis. Although most common in the distal ileum, cecum, and colon, necrotic ulcers may be seen in the oropharynx, esophagus, stomach, and proximal small bowel as well. Bacterial invasion of submucosal blood vessels is occasionally seen in bacteremic patients without demonstrable lesions in the overlying mucosa, probably reflecting its extraintestinal origin. The frequency of vascular involvement and paucity of inflammatory cells characterizing *Pseudomonas*-associated gastrointestinal lesions and ecthyma gangrenosum in the skin underscore their common etiology and pathogenesis.

The clinical syndromes associated with *Pseudomonas* gastrointestinal involvement are not necessarily either distinctive or specific for this pathogen. Young infants with necrotizing enterocolitis typically present with irritability, vomiting, diarrhea, and dehydration, and may have fever, abdominal distention, and signs of peritonitis. Although *Pseudomonas* is clearly implicated as the primary pathogen in many cases of necrotizing enterocolitis, so, too, are *E. coli, Klebsiella pneumoniae*, and other enteric pathogens. Typhlitis, a disease characteristically seen in leukemia patients, involves localized lesions of the cecum associated with necrosis and gangrene, sometimes resulting in perforation and peritonitis.[247] Although *P. aeruginosa* is the most frequently identified pathogen in this disease, other bacteria have been implicated as well. Rectal abscesses represent another localized form of gastrointestinal involvement, usually in neutropenic cancer patients, in which *Pseudomonas* is the most common but not the sole pathogen.[246] These lesions may be associated with few signs of local inflammation and must therefore be suspected and looked for in neutropenic patients with fever; this is particularly true since rectal abscesses can give rise to life-threatening sepsis and must therefore be treated aggressively.

Epidemics of *Pseudomonas*-associated diarrheal disease have been reported in children. The identification of a clear-cut point source in at least one such epidemic subjected to thorough cultural and epidemiologic investigation[239] leaves little doubt as to the primary pathogenic role of *P. aeruginosa*. Clinical manifestations in well-studied epidemics have varied from mild to severe diarrhea with dehydration, vascular collapse, and death. A causal role has also been suggested for *P. aeruginosa* in a syndrome that resembles enteric fever. Sometimes called Shanghai fever, this syndrome is associated variably with diarrhea or constipation, skin rash, and fever lasting 1–2 weeks.[249,250] Although *P. aeruginosa* can be isolated from the stools of patients suffering from this syndrome, its pathogenic role is uncertain. Likewise, the demonstration of *P. aeruginosa* in the stools of patients with choleralike illnesses, and the identification of a putative *Pseudomonas* enterotoxin,[251] does not yet justify the conclusion that *Pseudomonas* is capable of producing toxin-mediated secretory diarrhea.

The therapy of *Pseudomonas* gastrointestinal disease consists of the administration of antibiotics appropriate for the treatment of severe localized or systemic *Pseudomonas* infections, and surgery when bowel necrosis, perforation, obstruction, or undrained pus so dictate.

Skin and Soft-Tissue Infections

Pseudomonas disease of the skin and mucous membranes can result from primary or metastatic foci of infection. As previously indicated (see ''Bacteremia,'' above), *Pseudomonas* bacteremia may produce distinctive skin lesions known as ecthyma gangrenosum.[123,124,252] The salient features of these lesions are hemorrhage, necrosis, surrounding erythema, and the histologic demonstration of vascular invasion by bacteria.[125,126] *Pseudomonas* septicemia may also be associated with subcutaneous nodules,[253–255] deep abscesses, cellulitis,[256] vesicular or pustular lesions,[116,257] and bullae.[255] Metastatic *Pseudomonas* lesions of the skin and mucous membranes can be extensive as well as destructive, sometimes leading to massive necrosis or gangrene involving the face,[258] oropharynx, perineum,[259] or extremeties.[260]

Primary *Pseudomonas* skin and soft-tissue infections may be either localized or diffuse. Common predisposing factors are a breakdown in the integument resulting from burns, trauma, decubitus ulcers, or dermatitis; high moisture conditions such as those found in the perineal area, under the diapers of infants, on the feet of combat troops in the tropics, in the ears of frequent swimmers, or on the skin of whirlpool users; and neutropenia, usually secondary to cancer chemotherapy. The pathogenesis and clinical appearance of primary *Pseudomonas* skin lesions are often similar to metastatic cutaneous foci associated with bacteremia.[261] Common elements are tissue necrosis and hemorrhage. At the microscopic level, locally invasive primary *Pseudomonas* pyoderma may show the same distinctive vascular lesions characteristic of ecthyma gangrenosum associated with septicemic infections. It is not uncommon, in fact, to see a large area of necrotizing *Pseudomonas* pyoderma arising in the perineal area of a neutropenic patient, probably representing a primary infection,[259] and typical metastatic ecthyma lesions elsewhere on the skin of the same patient.[262] Both lesions demonstrate hemorrhage and necrosis, and both are likely to reveal microscopic vascular invasion. The original description of ecthyma gangrenosum was actually based on primary rather than metastatic cutaneous sites of *Pseudomonas* infection.[123]

Pseudomonas wound infections, or pyoderma arising from secondary infection of areas of dermatitis, are often indistinguishable from similar infections caused by other etiologic agents. On occasion, however, these infections may be associated with characteristic blue-green exudate and fruity odor pathognomonic for *Pseudomonas* infection.[257]

Pseudomonas aeruginosa has been implicated as the causative agent in diffuse, pruritic, erythematous, maculopapular, and vesiculopustular rashes occurring in epidemics associated with the use of contaminated whirlpools, hot tubs, spas, and swimming pools.[2,263,264] At least two nosocomial common-source outbreaks have been documented, one traced to a physiotherapy pool[265] and a second in which the hospital water system was implicated.[266] The majority of reported cases of *Pseudomonas* dermatitis have occured as a part of common-source outbreaks associated with IATS serotype 11; other serotypes have also been implicated, however. *Pseudomonas*-associated skin rashes are most evident in areas covered by bathing suits, but can occur more diffusely, sparing only the head and neck. Occasional associated symptoms include headache, dizziness, earache, sore throat, swollen breasts, sore eyes, sore nose, and abdominal cramps. Fever is uncommon and low grade when it occurs. *Pseudomonas* skin rashes are usually self-limited, resolving spontaneously upon discontinuation of exposure. However, in several documented instances associated with a single nosocomial outbreak among immunocompromised patients,[266] *Pseudomonas* folliculitis evolved within 24 hours into severe ecthyma gangrenosum. In most self-limited cases no specific therapy is necessary, although acetic acid compresses have been advocated.[263]

Pseudomonas burn wound sepsis is a dreaded complication of extensive thermal injuries.[267] The extraordinarily high mortality associated with this disease (78 percent in one large 25-year survey) does not appear to have been greatly improved by advances in therapy.[268] *Pseudomonas* burn sepsis results from bacterial colonization of the burn site, destruction of the mechanical barrier to tissue invasion, and multiple, systemic immunologic defects related to serious burns. Although a gram-positive flora predominates at burn sites in the immediate post-burn period, this is soon replaced by gram-negative bacteria, particularly *P. aeruginosa*. *Pseudomonas* rapidly proliferates in the burn eschar, achieving densities of greater than 10^5 bacteria per gram of tissue, followed by invasion of the subeschar space and underlying dermis. Once present in unburned subcutaneous tissue, bacteria spread along fibrous septa, migrate along lymphatics, proliferate in perivascular tissues, and invade blood vessels, resulting in septicemia.

Clinically, *Pseudomonas* burn wound infections are marked by multifocal black, dark brown, or violaceous discoloration of the burn eschar; degeneration of underlying granulation tissue with unexpectedly rapid eschar separation and hemorrhage into subcutaneous tissue; edema and/or hemorrhagic necrosis of previously healthy tissue adjacent to infected burn sites; erythematous nodular lesions in unburned skin; and brown or black neoeschar formation. Systemic manifestations, which may precede bacteremia, include fever or hypothermia, disorientation, obtundation, hypotension, oliguria, ileus, and leukopenia. Metastatic infection may produce ecthyma lesions at sites remote from the infected burn. Pneumonia is common, particularly in the setting of previous inhalation injury.

The appropriate management of *Pseudomonas* burn wound sepsis depends first on early diagnosis based on recognition of local and/or systemic signs and symptoms. If careful daily burn wound inspection reveals any of the wound changes enumerated above, biopsy and quantitative bacterial culture should be undertaken immediately.[267,269] A 500 mg lenticular-shaped tissue sample should include a portion of burn wound and underlying or adjacent unburned tissue. A bacterial density of greater than 10^5 organisms per gram of tissue, or histologic signs such as presence of gram-negative bacilli in unburned tissue, heavy growth of *Pseudomonas* in the subeschar space, vasculitis with perivascular "cuffing," focal hemorrhage, or intense inflammatory reaction at the burn margin indicate burn wound sepsis and the necessity for prompt therapy. An alternative method has been suggested for quantitation of bacteria in burn wounds by means of an absorbent paper disc.[270]

The treatment of *Pseudomonas* burn sepsis includes systemic antibiotic combinations administered in high doses. The choice of agents is governed by local susceptibility patterns that may vary considerably, especially since multiply-resistant *P. aeruginosa* strains are often endemic in burn treatment centers.[271] An aminoglycoside to which the infecting strain is sensitive may be combined with a β-lactam antibiotic active against *Pseudomonas*. There is little role for single agent treatment of *Pseudomonas* burn wound sepsis, since the large populations of bacteria present and problematic antibiotic access to local sites of infection favor the emergence of resistant strains and complicate therapy. Monotherapy with imipenem appears to be specifically contraindicated because of the frequent and rapid development of resistance.[272] In the presence of established burn wound colonization or infection, an absorbable topical agent such as mafenide acetate (Sulfamylon) (silver nitrate and silver sulfadiazine are less well absorbed) should be employed to reduce bacterial populations at the burn site. Subeschar injections of antibiotics, such as carbenicillin, have also been advocated in focal or multifocal infections that do not extend beneath the investing fascia.[273] In addition, silver sulfadiazine and sodium piperacillin appear to act synergistically against some *Pseudomonas* strains, and are active topically in experimental *Pseudomonas* burn sepsis.[274] Surgical removal of infected eschars, débridement of necrotic tissues, or even amputation may be necessary in addition to antibiotic therapy.

Pseudomonas aeruginosa has been implicated in unmanageable exacerbations of acne vulgaris[275] and in other forms of folliculitis.[276] In the first instance, the folliculitis is thought to originate from a *Pseudomonas* otitis externa. Treatment of both the folliculitis and external otitis with acetic acid compresses and topical antibiotics, respectively, apparently results in prompt cure. In the latter case, a self-limited *Pseudomonas* folliculitis has been observed following depilation of the legs, while recurrent papular skin rashes, usually associated with hospitalization, are resistant to treatment and can last from 3 months to 3 years.[276]

Toe web infection, or tropical immersion foot syndrome, is most commonly caused by *P. aeruginosa*.[257,277] Predisposing conditions include high temperature and humidity, physical stress, tight interdigital spaces, and pre-existing tinea-pedis infection. The second, third, and fourth toe webs are commonly involved, with marked scaling and maceration, denudation extending onto the plantar surface, a profuse serous or purulent discharge, and, in some cases, greenish discoloration from elaboration of pyocyanin and greenish-white fluorescence under a Wood's light. Treatment consists of appropriate local measures and a systemic antibiotic with activity against *Pseudomonas* and other gram-negative bacteria.[277]

So-called green nail syndrome describes the appearance of greenish discoloration of the nail plate, usually in association with a *Pseudomonas* paronychia, in persons with a history of frequent submersion of their hands.[257] Although bacterial invasion of the nail plate can occur in some cases, the green discoloration usually results simply from diffusion of pyocyanin pigment from an adjacent paronychia. This discoloration may persist for a number of months after resolution of active infection. Treatment consists of local measures including incision and drainage of the associated paronychia. Not to be confused with green nail syndrome is "green foot," described as greenish discoloration of the toenails and sole of an adolescent's foot associated with documented colonization of rubber-soled basketball shoes by a pigmented strain of *P. aeruginosa*.[278]

REFERENCES

1. Doudoroff M, Palleroni NJ. Genus I. *Pseudomonas*. In: Buchanon RE, Gibbons NE, eds. Bergey's Manual of Determinative Bacteriology. 8th ed. Baltimore; Williams & Wilkins; 1974:217.

2. Morrison AJ, Wenzel RP. Epidemiology of infections due to *Pseudomonas aeruginosa* [Review]. Rev Infect Dis. 1984;6(Suppl):S627.
3. Schimpff SC, Moody M, Young VM. Relationship of colonization with *Pseudomonas aeruginosa* to development of *Pseudomonas* bacteremia in cancer patients. In: Hobby GL, ed. Antimicrobial Agents and Chemotherapy—1970. Washington, DC: American Society for Microbiology;1971:240.
4. Brokopp CD, Farmer JJ. Typing methods for *Pseudomonas aeruginosa*. In: Doggett RG, ed. *Pseudomonas aeruginosa*. New York: Academic Press; 1979:89.
5. Farmer JJ, Weinstein RA, Zierdt CH, et al. Hospital outbreaks caused by *Pseudomonas aeruginosa*: importance of serogroup 011. J Clin Microbiol. 1982;16:266.
6. Ogle JW, Janda JM, Woods DE, et al. Characterization and use of a DNA probe as an epidemiologic marker for *Pseudomonas aeruginosa*. J Infect Dis. 1987;155:119.
7. Centers for Disease Control. Nosocomial infection surveillance, 1980–1982. In: CDC Surveillance Summaries. 1983;32(No. 455):155.
8. Kreger BE, Craven DE, Carling PC, et al. Gram-negative bacteremia III. Reassessment of etiology, epidemiology and ecology in 612 patients. Am J Med 1980;68:332.
9. Higuchi JH, Johanson WG. The relationship between adherence of *Pseudomonas aeruginosa* to upper respiratory cells in vitro and susceptibility to colonization in vivo. J Lab Clin Med. 1980;95:698.
10. Woods DE, Straus DC, Johanson WG, et al. Role of pili in adherence of *Pseudomonas aeruginosa* to mammalian buccal epithelial cells. Infect Immun. 1980;29:1146.
11. Woods DE, Straus DC, Johanson WG, et al. Role of salivary protease activity in adherence of gram-negative bacilli to mammalian buccal epithelial cells in vivo. J Clin Invest. 1981;68:1435.
12. Ramphal R, Small PM, Shands JW, et al. Adherence of *Pseudomonas aeruginosa* to tracheal cells injured by influenza infection or by endotracheal intubation. Infect Immun. 1980;27:614.
13. Ramphal R, McNiece MT, Polack FM. Adherence of *Pseudomonas aeruginosa* to the injured cornea: a step in the pathogenesis of corneal infections. Ann Ophthalmol. 1981;13:421.
14. Sobel JD, Vardi Y. Scanning electron microscopy study of *Pseudomonas aeruginosa* in vivo adherence to rat bladder epithelium. J Urol. 1982;128:414.
15. Gilboa-Garber N, Mizrahi L. Interaction of the mannose-philic lectins of *Pseudomonas aeruginosa* with luminous species of marine enterobacteria. Microbios. 1979;26:31.
16. Ramphal R, Guay C, Pier GB. *Pseudomonas aeurginosa* adhesions for tracheobronchial mucin. Infect Immun. 1987;55:600.
17. Ramphal R, Pyle M. Evidence for mucins and sialic acid as receptors for *Pseudomonas aeruginosa* in the lower respiratory tract. Infect Immun. 1983;41:339.
18. Vishwanath S, Ramphal R. Tracheobronchial mucin receptor for *Pseudomonas aeruginosa*: predominance of amino sugars in binding sites. Infect Immun. 1985;48:331.
19. Ramphal R, Pyle M. Further characterization of the tracheal receptor for *Pseudomonas aeruginosa*. Eur J Clin Microbiol. 1985;4:160.
20. Costerton JW, Brown MRW, Sturgess JM. The cell envelope: its role in infection. In: Doggett RG, ed. *Pseudomonas aeruginosa*. New York: Academic Press; 1979:41.
21. Pier GB. Terminology relating to extracellular polysaccharides produced by *Pseudomonas aeruginosa* (Letter). J Infect Dis. 1985;152:652.
22. Doggett RG, Harrison GM, Carter RG Jr. Mucoid *Pseudomonas aeruginosa* in patients with chronic illnesses. Lancet. 1971;1:236.
23. Lam J, Chan R, Lam K, et al. Production of mucoid microcolonies by *Pseudomonas aeruginosa* within infected lungs in cystic fibrosis. Infect Immun. 1980;28:546.
24. Schwartzmann S, Boring JR III. Antiphagocytic effect of slime from a mucoid strain of *Pseudomonas aeruginosa*. Infect Immun. 1971;3:762.
25. Baltimore RS, Mitchell M. Immunologic investigations of mucoid strains of *Pseudomonas aeruginosa*: comparison of susceptibility to opsonic antibody in mucoid and non-mucoid strains. J Infect Dis. 1980;141:238.
26. Baltimore RS, Cross AS, Dobek AS. The inhibitory effect of sodium alginate on antibiotic activity against mucoid and non-mucoid strains of *Pseudomonas aeruginosa*. J Antimicrob Chemother. 1987;20:815.
27. Morihara K. Production of elastase and proteinase by *Pseudomonas aeruginosa*. J Bacteriol. 1964;88:745.
28. Mull JD, Callahan WS. The role of elastase of *Pseudomonas aeruginosa* in experimental infection. Exp Mol Pathol. 1965;4:567.
29. Kreger AS, Gray LD. Purification of *Pseudomonas aeruginosa* protease and microscopic characterization of pseudomonal protease-induced rabbit corneal damage. Infect Immun. 1978;19:630.
30. Heck LW, Morihara K, Abrahamson DR. Degradation of soluble laminin and depletion of tissue-associated basement membrane laminin by *Pseudomonas aeruginosa* elastase and alkaline protease. Infect Immun. 1986;54:149.
31. Hingley ST, Hastie AT, Kueppers F, et al. Disruption of respiratory cilia by proteases including those of *Pseudomonas aeruginosa*. Infect Immun. 1986;54:379.
32. Heck LW, Morihara K, McRae WB, et al. Specific cleavage of human type III and IV collagens by *Pseudomonas aeruginosa* elastase. Infect Immun. 1986;51:115.
33. Hamdaoui A, Wund-Bisseret F, Bieth JG. Fast solubilization of human lung elastin by *Pseudomonas aeruginosa* elastase. Am Rev Respir Dis. 1987;135:860.
34. Cicmanec JF, Holder IA. Growth of *Pseudomonas aeruginosa* in normal and burned skin extract: role of extracellular proteases. Infect Immun. 1979;25:477.
35. Schultz DR, Miller KD. Elastase of *Pseudomonas aeruginosa*: inactivation of complement components and complement-derived chemotactic and phagocytic factors. Infect Immun. 1974;10:128.
36. Fick RB, Baltimore RS, Gee JBL, et al. Characterization of an IgG protease produced by mucoid and non-mucoid strains of *Pseudomonas aeruginosa*. In: Abstracts of the 1982 Interscience Conference on Antimicrobial Agents and Chemotherapy (Abstract No. 374). Washington, DC: American Society for Microbiology; 1982:132.
37. Scharmann W. Cytotoxic effects of leukocidin from *Pseudomonas aeruginosa* on polymorphonuclear leukocytes from cattle. Infect Immun. 1976;13:836.
38. Bishop MB, Baltch AL, Hill LA, et al. The effect of *Pseudomonas aeruginosa* cytotoxin and toxin A on human polymorphonuclear leukocytes. J Med Microbiol. 1987;24:315.
39. Seeger W, Walmrath D, Neuhof H, et al. Pulmonary microvascular injury induced by *Pseudomonas aeruginosa* cytotoxin in isolated rabbit lungs. Infect Immun. 1986;52:846.
40. Berka RM, Vasil ML. Phospholipase c (heat-labile hemolysin) of *Pseudomonas aeruginosa*: purification and preliminary characterization. J Bacteriol. 1981;152:239.
41. Johnson MK, Boese-Marrazzo D. Production and properties of heat-stable extracellular hemolysin from *Pseudomonas aeruginosa*. Infect Immun. 1980;29:1028.
42. Liu PV. Toxins of *Pseudomonas aeruginosa*. In: Doggett RG, ed. *Pseudomonas aeruginosa*. New York: Academic Press; 1979:63.
43. Berka RM, Gray GL, Vasil ML. Studies of phospholipase c (heat-labile hemolysin) in *Pseudomonas aeruginosa*. Infect Immun. 1981;34:1071.
44. Young LS. Human immunity to *Pseudomonas aeruginosa*. II. Relationship between heat-stable opsonins and type-specific lipopolysaccharides. J Infect Dis. 1972;126:277.
45. Young LS. Human immunity to *Pseudomonas aeruginosa*. I. In vitro interaction of bacteria, polymorphonuclear leukocytes, and serum factors. J Infect Dis. 1972;126:257.
46. Bjornson AB, Michael JG. Biological activities of immunoglobulin M and immunoglobulin G antibodies to *Pseudomonas aeruginosa*. Infect Immun. 1970;2:453.
47. Beutler B, Cerami A. The endogenous mediator of endotoxic shock. Clin Res. 1987;35:192.
48. Mathison JC, Wolfson E, Ulevitch RJ. Participation of tumor necrosis factor in the mediation of gram-negative bacterial lipopolysaccharide-induced injury in rabbits. J Clin Invest. 1988;81:1925.
49. Pollack M. The virulence of *Pseudomonas aeruginosa*. Rev Infect Dis. 1984;6(Suppl):617.
50. Pollack M, Taylor NS. Exotoxin production by clinical isolates of *Pseudomonas aeruginosa*. Infect Immun. 1977;15:776.
51. Iglewski BH, Kabat D. NAD-dependent inhibition of protein synthesis by *Pseudomonas aeruginosa* toxin. Proc Natl Acad Sci USA. 1975;22:2284.
52. Gray GL, Smith OH, Baldridge JS, et al. Cloning, nucleotide sequence and expression in *Escherichia coli* of the exotoxin A structural gene of *Pseudomonas aeruginosa*. Proc Natl Acad Sci USA. 1984;81:2645.
53. Allured VS, Collier RJ, Carroll SF, et al. Structure of exotoxin A of *Pseudomonas aeruginosa* at 3.0 angstrom resolution. Proc Natl Acad Sci USA. 1986;83:1320.
54. Hwang J, Fitzgerald DJ, Adhya S, et al. Functional domains of *Pseudomonas* exotoxin identified by deletion analysis of the gene expressed in *E. coli*. Cell. 1987;48:129.
55. Pollack M. *Pseudomonas aeruginosa* exotoxin A. N Engl J Med. 1980; 302:1360.
56. Pollack M. The role of exotoxin A in *Pseudomonas* disease and immunity. Rev Infect Dis. 1983;5(Suppl):S979.
57. Young LS, Pollack M. Immunologic approaches to the prophylaxis and treatment of *Pseudomonas aeruginosa* infection. In: Sabath LD, ed. *Pseudomonas aeruginosa*: The Organism, Diseases It Causes, and Their Treatment. Bern: Hans Huber Publishers; 1980:119.
58. Hazlett LD, Berk RS, Iglewski BH. Microscopic characterization of ocular damage produced by *Pseudomonas aeruginosa* toxin A. Infect Immun. 1981;34:1025.
59. Ohman DE, Burns RP, Iglewski BH. Corneal infections in mice with toxin A and elastase mutants of *Pseudomonas aeruginosa*. J Infect Dis. 1980;142:547.
60. Woods DE, Cryz SJ, Friedman RL, et al. Contribution of toxin A and elastase to virulence of *Pseudomonas aeruginosa* in chronic lung infections of rats. Infect Immun. 1982;36:1223.
61. Pavlovskis OR, Callahan LT, Pollack M. *Pseudomonas aeruginosa* exotoxin. In: Schlessinger D, ed. Microbiology 1975. Washington, DC: American Society for Microbiology; 1975:252.
62. Cross AS, Sadoff JC, Iglewski BH, et al. Evidence for the role of toxin A in the pathogenesis of infection with *Pseudomonas aeruginosa* in humans. J Infect Dis. 1980;142:538.
63. Pollack M, Young LS. Protective activity of antibodies to exotoxin A and lipopolysaccharide at the onset of *Pseudomonas aeruginosa* septicemia in man. J Clin Invest. 1979;63:276.
64. Iglewski BH, Sadoff JC, Bjorn MJ, et al. *Pseudomonas aeruginosa* exoen-

zyme S: an adenosine diphosphate ribosyltransferase distinct from toxin A. Proc Natl Acad Sci USA. 1978;75:3211.
65. Woods DE, Que JU. Purification of *Pseudomonas aeruginosa* exoenzyme S. Infect Immun. 1987;55:579.
66. Nicas TI, Bradley J, Lochner JE, et al. The role of exoenzyme S in infections with *Pseudomonas aeruginosa*. J Infect Dis. 1985;152:716.
67. Woods DE, Sokol PA. Use of transposon mutants to assess the role of exoenzyme S in chronic pulmonary disease due to *Pseudomonas aeruginosa*. Eur J Clin Microbiol. 1985;4:163.
68. Cohen PS, Maguire JH, Weinstein L. Infective endocarditis caused by gram-negative bacteria: a review of the literature, 1945–1977. Prog Cardiovasc Dis. 1980;22:205.
69. Rajashekaraiah KR, Rice TW, Kallick CA. Recovery of *Pseudomonas aeruginosa* from syringes of drug addicts with endocarditis. J Infect Dis. 1981;144:482.
70. Wieland M, Lederman MM, Kline-King C, et al. Left-sided endocarditis due to *Pseudomonas aeruginosa*. A report of 10 cases and review of the literature. Medicine. 1986;65:180.
71. Shekar R, Rice TW, Zierdt CH, et al. Outbreak of endocarditis caused by *Pseudomonas aeruginosa* serotype O11 among pentazocine and tripelennamine abusers in Chicago. J Infect Dis. 1985;151:203.
72. Botsford KB, Weinstein RA, Nathan CR, et al. Selective survival in pentazocine and tripelennamine of *Pseudomonas aeruginosa* serotype O11 from drug addicts. J Infect Dis. 1985;151:209.
73. Gould K, Ramirez-Ronda CH, Holmes RK, et al. Adherence of bacteria to heart valves *in vitro*. J Clin Invest. 1975;56:1364.
74. Reyes MP, Lerner AM. Current problems in the treatment of infective endocarditis due to *Pseudomonas aeruginosa*. Rev Infect Dis. 1983;5:314.
75. Levine DP, Crane LR, Zervos MJ. Bacteremia in narcotic addicts at the Detroit Medical Center. II. Infectious endocarditis: a prospective comparative study. Rev Infect Dis. 1986;8:374.
76. Reyes MP, Brown WJ, Lerner AM. Treatment of patients with *Pseudomonas* endocarditis with high dose aminoglycoside and carbenicillin therapy. Medicine. 1978;57:57.
77. Jimenez-Lucho VE, Saravolatz LD, Medeiros AA, et al. Failure of therapy in *Pseudomonas* endocarditis: selection of resistant mutants. J Infect Dis. 1986;154:64.
78. Ingerman MJ, Pitsakis PG, Rosenberg AF, et al. The importance of pharmacodynamics in determining the dosing interval in therapy for experimental *Pseudomonas* endocarditis in the rat. J Infect Dis. 1986;153:707.
79. Bayer AS, Blomquist IK, Kim KS. Ciprofloxacin in experimental aortic valve endocarditis due to *Pseudomonas aeruginosa*. J Antimicrob Chemother. 1986;17:641.
80. Myerowitz PD, Gardner R, Campbell C, et al. Earlier operation for left-sided *Pseudomonas* endocarditis in drug addicts. J Thorac Cardiovasc Surg. 1979;77:577.
81. Tillotston JR, Lerner AM. Characteristics of nonbacteremic *Pseudomonas* pneumonia. Ann Intern Med. 1968;68:295.
82. Pennington JE, Reynolds HY, Carbone PP. *Pseudomonas* pneumonia: a retrospective study of 36 cases. Am J Med. 1973;55:155.
83. Rose HD, Heckman MG, Unger JD. *Pseudomonas aeruginosa* pneumonia in adults. Am Rev Respir Dis. 1973;107:416.
84. Iannini PB, Claffey T, Quintiliani R. Bacteremic *Pseudomonas* pneumonia. JAMA. 1974;230:558.
85. Fetzer AE, Werner AS, Hagstrom JWC. Pathologic features of pseudomonal pneumonia. Am Rev Respir Dis. 1967;96:1121.
86. Huang NN, Doggett RG. Antibiotic therapy of *Pseudomonas* infection in patients with cystic fibrosis. In: Doggett RG, ed. *Pseudomonas aeruginosa*. New York: Academic Press; 1979:409.
87. Hoiby N. *Pseudomonas aeruginosa* infection in cystic fibrosis: diagnostic and prognostic significance of *Pseudomonas aeruginosa* precipitins determined by means of crossed immunoelectrophoresis, a survey. Acta Pathol Microbiol Scand [C] 1977;262(Suppl):1.
88. Klinger JD, Strauss DC, Hilton CB, et al. Antibodies to proteases and exotoxin A of *Pseudomonas aeruginosa* in patients with cystic fibrosis: demonstration by radioimmunoassay. J Infect Dis. 1978;138:49.
89. Doggett RG, Harrison GM. Significance of the bacterial flora associated with chronic pulmonary disease in cystic fibrosis. In: Lawson D, ed. Proceedings of the 5th International Cystic Fibrosis Conference. London: Cystic Fibrosis Research Trust; 1967:175.
90. Reynolds HY, Fick RB. *Pseudomonas aeruginosa* pulmonary infections (emphasizing nosocomial pneumonia and respiratory infections in cystic fibrosis). In: Sabath LD, ed. *Pseudomonas aeruginosa*: The Organism, Diseases It Causes, and Their Treatment. Bern: Hans Huber Publishers; 1980:71.
91. Wientzen R, Prestidge CB, Kramer RI, et al. Acute pulmonary exacerbations in cystic fibrosis. A double-blind trial of tobramycin and placebo therapy. Am J Dis Child. 1980;134:1134.
92. Beaudry PH, Marks MI, McDougall D, et al. Is anti-*Pseudomonas* therapy warranted in acute respiratory exacerbations in children with cystic fibrosis? J Pediatr. 1980;97:144.
93. Moller NE, Hoiby N. Antibiotic treatment of chronic *Pseudomonas aeruginosa* infection in cystic fibrosis patients. Scand J Infect Dis. 1981;29(Suppl):87.
94. Hyatt AC, Chipps BE, Kumor KM. A double-blind controlled trial of anti-*Pseudomonas* chemotherapy of acute respiratory exacerbations in patients with cystic fibrosis. J Pediatr. 1981;99:307.
95. Martin AJ, Smally LA, George RH, et al. Gentamicin and tobramycin compared in the treatment of mucoid *Pseudomonas* lung infections in cystic fibrosis. Arch Dis Child. 1980;55:604.
96. Reed MD, Stern RC, Meyers CM, et al. Therapeutic evaluation of piperacillin for acute pulmonary exacerbations in cystic fibrosis. Pediatr Pulmonol. 1987;3:101.
97. Reed MD, Stern RC, O'Brien CA, et al. Randomized double-blind evaluation of ceftazidime dose ranging in hospitalized patients with cystic fibrosis. Antimicrob Agents Chemother. 1987;31:698.
98. Strandvik B, Malmborg AS, Bergan T, et al. Imipenem/cilastatin, an alternative treatment of *Pseudomonas* infection in cystic fibrosis. J Antimicrob Chemother. 1988;21:471.
99. Moss JA, Black PG. Controlled trial of aztreonam vs. tobramycin and azlocillin for acute pulmonary exacerbations of cystic fibrosis. Pediatr Infect Dis J 1988;7:171.
100. Rubio TT, Shapiro C. Ciprofloxacin in the treatment of *Pseudomonas* infection in cystic fibrosis patients. J Antimicrob Chemother. 1986; 18(Suppl):147.
101. Pedersen SS, Pressler T, Jensen T, et al. Combined imipenem/cilastatin and tobramycin therapy of multiresistant *Pseudomonas aeruginosa* in cystic fibrosis. J Antimicrob Chemother. 1987;19:101.
102. Jackson MA, Kusmiesz H, Shelton S, et al. Comparison of piperacillin vs. ticarcillin plus tobramycin in the treatment of acute pulmonary exacerbations of cystic fibrosis. Pediatr Infect Dis J. 1986;5:440.
103. Gold R, Overmeyer A, Knie B, et al. Controlled trial of ceftazidime vs. ticarcillin and tobramycin in the treatment of acute respiratory exacerbations in patients with cystic fibrosis. Pediatr Infect Dis J. 1985;4:172.
104. Bosso JA, Black PG, Matsen JM. Efficacy of aztreonam in pulmonary exacerbations of cystic fibrosis. Pediatr Infect Dis J. 1987;6:393.
105. Hodson ME, Roberts CM, Butland RJ, et al. Oral ciprofloxacin compared with conventional intravenous treatment for *Pseudomonas aeruginosa* infection in adults with cystic fibrosis. Lancet. 1987;1:235.
106. deGroot R, Smith AL. Antibiotic pharmacokinetics in cystic fibrosis. Differences and clinical significance. Clin Pharmacokinet. 1987;13:228.
107. Pedersen SS, Jensen T, Hoiby N, et al. Management of *Pseudomonas aeruginosa* lung infection in Danish cystic fibrosis patients. Acta Paediatr Scand 1987;76:955.
108. Jensen T, Pedersen SS, Nielsen CH, et al. The efficacy and safety of ciprofloxacin and ofloxacin in chronic *Pseudomonas aeruginosa* infection in cystic fibrosis. J Antimicrob Chemother. 1987;20:585.
109. Hodson ME, Penketh RA, Batten JC. Aerosol carbenicillin and gentamicin treatment of *Pseudomonas aeruginosa* infection in patients with cystic fibrosis. Lancet. 1981;2:1137.
110. Stead RJ, Hodson ME, Batten JC. Inhaled ceftazidime compared with gentamicin and carbenicillin in older patients with cystic fibrosis infected with *Pseudomonas aeruginosa*. Br J Dis Chest. 1987;81:272.
111. Carswell F, Ward C, Cook DA, et al. A controlled trial of nebulized aminoglycoside and oral flucloxacillin versus placebo in the outpatient management of children with cystic fibrosis. Br J Dis Chest. 1987;81;356.
112. Ewing CW. Role of the fiberoptic bronchoscope in lung lavage of patients with cystic fibrosis. Chest. 1978;73(Suppl):750.
113. Whimbey EA, Kiehn TE, Brannon P, et al. Bacteremia and fungemia in patients with neoplastic disease. Am J Med. 1987;82:723.
114. Bodey GP, Jadeja L, Elting L. *Pseudomonas* bacteremia: retrospective analysis of 410 episodes. Arch Intern Med. 1985;145:1621.
115. Forkner CE. *Pseudomonas aeruginosa* Infections. New York: Grune & Stratton; 1960:6.
116. Forkner CE, Frei E III, Edgcomb JH, et al. *Pseudomonas* septicemia: observations on twenty-three cases. Am J Med. 1958;25:877.
117. Whitecar JP Jr, Luna M, Bodey GP. *Pseudomonas* bacteremia in patients with malignant diseases. Am J Med Sci. 1970;260:216.
118. Tapper ML, Armstrong D. Bacteremia due to *Pseudomonas aeruginosa* complicating neoplastic disease. J Infect Dis. 1974;130(Suppl):S14.
119. Flick MR, Cluff LE. *Pseudomonas* bacteremia. Am J Med. 1976;60:501.
120. Baltch AL, Griffin PE. *Pseudomonas aeruginosa* bacteremia: a clinical study of 75 patients. Am J Med Sci. 1977;274:119.
121. Jackson MA, Wong KY, Lampkin B. *Pseudomonas aeruginosa* septicemia in childhood cancer patients. Pediatr Infect Dis. 1982;1:239.
122. Vermillion SE, Gregg JA, Baggenstoss AH, et al. Jaundice associated with bacteremia. Arch Intern Med. 1969;124:611.
123. Hitschman F, Kreibich K. Zur pathogenese des Bacillus pyocyaneus und zur Aetiologie des Ekthyma gangrenosum. Wien Klin Wochenschr. 1897; 10:1093.
124. Fraenkel E. Uber die Menschenpathogenitat des Bacillus pyocyaneus. Z Hyg. 1912;72:486.
125. Dorff GJ, Geimer NF, Rosenthal DR, et al. *Pseudomonas* septicemia: illustrated evolution of its skin lesions. Arch Intern Med. 1971;128:591.
126. Teplitz C. Pathogenesis of *Pseudomonas* vasculitis and septic lesions. Arch Pathol. 1965;80:297.
127. Rajan RK. Spontaneous bacterial peritonitis with ecthyma gangrenosum due to *Escherichia coli*. J Clin Gastroenterol. 1982;4:145.
128. Fine JD, Miller JA, Harrist TJ, et al. Cutaneous lesions in disseminated candidiasis mimicking ecthyma gangrenosum. Am J Med. 1981;70:1133.
129. Pizzo PA, Hathorn JW, Hiemenz J, et al. A randomized trial comparing ceftazidime alone with combination antibiotic therapy in cancer patients with fever and neutropenia. N Engl J Med. 1986;315:552.
130. EORTC International Antimicrobial Therapy Cooperative Group. Ceftazi-

dime combined with a short or long course of amikacin for empirical therapy of gram-negative bacteremia in cancer patients with granulocytopenia. N Engl J Med. 1987;317:1692.
131. Klastersky J, Mennier-Carpentier F, Prevost JM. Significance of antimicrobial synergism for the outcome of gram-negative sepsis. Am J Med Sci. 1977;273:157.
132. Love LJ, Schimpff SC, Schriffer CA, et al. Improved prognosis for granulocytopenic patients with gram-negative bacteremia. Am J Med. 1980;68:643.
133. DeJongh CA, Joshi JH, Newman KA, et al. Antibiotic synergism and response in gram-negative bacteremia in granulocytopenic cancer patients. Am J Med. 1986;80(Suppl 5c):96.
134. Sheagren JN. Septic shock and corticosteroids. N Engl J Med. 1981;305:456.
135. Bone RC, Fisher CJ, Clemmer TP, et al. A controlled clinical trial of high-dose methylprednisolone in the treatment of severe sepsis and septic shock. N Engl J Med. 1987;317:653.
136. Veterans Administration Systemic Sepsis Cooperative Study Group. Effect of high-dose glucocorticoid therapy on mortality in patients with clinical signs of systemic sepsis. N Engl J Med. 1987;317:659.
137. Stanley MM. *Bacillus pyocyaneus* infections: a review, report of cases and discussion of newer therapy including streptomycin (concluded). Am J Med. 1947;2:347.
138. Chernik NL, Armstrong D, Posner JB. Central nervous system infections in patients with cancer. Medicine. 1973;52:563.
139. Wise BL, Mathis JL, Jawetz E. Infections of the central nervous system due to *Pseudomonas aeruginosa*. J Neurosurg. 1969;31:432.
140. Bray DA, Calcaterra TC. *Pseudomonas* meningitis complicating head and neck surgery. Laryngoscope. 1976;86:1386.
141. Berk SL, McCabe WR. Meningitis caused by gram-negative bacilli. Ann Intern Med. 1980;93:253.
142. Rahal JJ, Simberkoff MS. Host defense and antimicrobial therapy in gram-negative bacillary meningitis. Ann Intern Med. 1982;96:468.
143. Norrby SR. Role of cephalosporins in the treatment of bacterial meningitis in adults. Overview with special emphasis on ceftazidime. Am J Med. 1985;79(2A):56.
144. Fong IW, Tomkins KB. Review of *Pseudomonas aeruginosa* meningitis with special emphasis on treatment with ceftazidime. Rev Infect Dis. 1985;7:604.
145. Marone P, Concia E, Maserati R, et al. Ceftazidime in the therapy of pseudomonal meningitis. Chemioterapia. 1985;4:289.
146. Wright DF, Kaiser AB, Bowman CM, et al. The pharmacokinetics and efficacy of an aminoglycoside administered into the cerebral ventricles in neonates: implications for further evaluation of this route of therapy in meningitis. J Infect Dis. 1981;143:141.
147. Swartz MN. Intraventricular use of aminoglycosides in the treatment of gram-negative bacillary meningitis: conflicting views. J Infect Dis. 1981;143:293.
148. Modai J, Wolff M, Lebas J, et al. Moxalactam penetration into cerebrospinal fluid in patients with bacterial meningitis. Antimicrob Agents Chemother. 1982;21:551.
149. Norrby SR. 4-Quinolones in the treatment of infections of the central nervous system. Rev Infect Dis. 1988;10(Suppl 1):S253.
150. Hackbarth CJ, Chambers HF, Stella F, et al. Ciprofloxacin in experimental *Pseudomonas aeruginosa* meningitis in rabbits. J Antimicrob Chemother. 1986;18(Suppl D):65.
151. Feinmesser R, Wiesel YM, Argaman M, et al. Otitis externa—bacteriological survey. ORL. 1982;44:121.
152. Chandler JR. Malignant external otitis. Laryngoscope. 1968;78:1257.
153. Dinapoli RP, Thomas JE. Neurologic aspects of malignant external otitis: report of three cases. Mayo Clin Proc. 1971;46:339.
154. Zaky DA, Bentley DW, Lowy K, et al. Malignant external otitis: a severe form of otitis in diabetic patients. Am J Med. 1976;61:298.
155. Damiani JM, Damiani KK, Kinney SE. Malignant external otitis with multiple cranial nerve involvement. Am J Otol. 1979;1:115.
156. Kohut RI, Lindsay JR. Necrotizing ("malignant") external otitis histopathologic processes. Ann Otol Rhinol Laryngol. 1979;88:714.
157. Nadol JB Jr. Histopathology of *Pseudomonas* osteomyelitis of the temporal bone starting as a malignant external otitis. Am J Otolaryngol. 1980;1:359.
158. Doroghazi RM, Nadol JB Jr, Hyslop NE Jr, et al. Invasive external otitis. Report of 21 cases and review of the literature. Am J Med. 1981;71:603.
159. Strauss M, Aber RC, Conner JH, et al. Malignant external otitis: long term (months) antimicrobial therapy. Laryngoscope. 1982;92:397.
160. C'oser PL, Stamm AE, Lobo RC, et al. Malignant external otitis in infants. Laryngoscope. 1980;90:312.
161. Sherman P, Black S, Grossman M. Malignant external otitis due to *Pseudomonas aeruginosa* in childhood. Pediatrics. 1980;66:782.
162. Sutherland GE. Malignant external otitis in a nondiabetic adult. South Med J. 1981;74:516.
163. Rubin J, Yu VL. Malignant external otitis: insights into pathogenesis, clinical manifestations, diagnosis, and therapy. Am J Med. 1988;85:391.
164. Curtin HD, Wolfe P, May M. Malignant external otitis: CT evaluation. Radiology. 1982;145:383.
165. Gherini SG, Brackmann DE, Bradley WG. Magnetic resonance imaging and computerized tomography in malignant external otitis. Laryngoscope. 1986;96:542.
166. Funasaka S, Kumakawa K. Advanced necrotizing external otitis treated by suboccipital craniectomy. Auris Nasus Larynx. 1982;9:9.
167. Meyers BR, Mendelson MH, Parisier SC, et al. Malignant external otitis: comparison of monotherapy vs. combination therapy. Arch Otolaryngol Head Neck Surg. 1987;113:974.
168. Yu VL, Stoehr G, Rubin J, et al. Efficacy of oral ciprofloxacin plus rifampin for therapy of malignant external otitis. In: Program and Abstracts of the Twenty-Seventh Interscience Conference on Antimicrobial Agents and Chemotherapy (Abstract No. 188.) Washington, DC: American Society for Microbiology; 1987:129.
169. Bland RD. Otitis media in the first six weeks of life: diagnosis, bacteriology, and management. Pediatrics 1972;49:18.
170. Brook I, Finegold SM. Bacteriology of chronic otitis media. JAMA. 1979;241:487.
171. Kenna MA, Bluestone CD. Microbiology of chronic suppurative otitis media in children. Pediatr Infect Dis. 1986;5:223.
172. Kenna MA, Bluestone CD, Reilly JS, et al. Medical management of chronic suppurative otitis media without cholesteatoma in children. Laryngoscope. 1986;96:146.
173. Myerhoff WL, Gates GA, Montalbo PJ, et al. *Pseudomonas* mastoiditis. Laryngoscope. 1977;87:483.
174. Bassiouny A. Perichondritis of the auricle. Laryngoscope 1981;91:422.
175. Wilson LA. Bacterial corneal ulcers, In: Duane TD ed. Clinical Ophthalmology. v. 4. New York: Harper & Row; 1978: Ch. 18, 1.
176. Peyman GA, Pague JT, Meisels HI, et al. Postoperative endophthalmitis: a comparison of methods for treatment and prophylaxis with gentamicin. Ophthalmol Surg. 1975;6:45.
177. Armstrong JH, Zacarias F, Rein MF. Ophthalmia neonatorum: a chart review. Pediatrics. 1976;57:884.
178. Rosenoff SH, Wolf ML, Chabuer BA. *Pseudomonas* blepharoconjunctivitis. A complication of combination chemotherapy. Arch Ophthalmol. 1974;91:490.
179. Berler DK, Alper MG. Scleral abscesses and ectasia caused by *Pseudomonas aeruginosa*. Ann Ophthalmol. 1982;14:665.
180. Hazlett LD, Moon M, Berk RS. In vivo identification of sialic acid as the ocular receptor for *Pseudomonas aeruginosa*. Infect Immun. 1986;51:687.
181. Liesegang TJ, Forster RK. Spectrum of microbial keratitis in South Florida. Am J Ophthalmol. 1980;90:38.
182. Alfonso E, Mandelbaum S, Fox MJ, et al. Ulcerative keratitis associated with contact lens wear. Am J Ophthalmol. 1986;101:429.
183. Butrus SI, Klotz SA, Misra RP. The adherence of *Pseudomonas aeruginosa* to soft contact lenses. Ophthalmology 1987;94:1310.
184. Schein OD, Wasson PJ, Boruchoff SA, et al. Microbial keratitis associated with contaminated ocular medications. Am J Ophthalmol. 1988;105:361.
185. Hansen KD, Meyer RF. Amikacin treatment of *Pseudomonas*-caused corneal ulcer. Arch Ophthalmol. 1980;98:1991.
186. Hutton WL, Sexton RS. Atypical *Pseudomonas* corneal ulcers in semicomatose patients. Am J Ophthalmol. 1972;73:37.
187. Tarr KH, Constable IJ. *Pseudomonas* endophthalmitis associated with scleral necrosis. Br J Ophthalmol. 1980;64:676.
188. King S, Devi SP, Mindorff C, et al. Nosocomial *Pseudomonas aeruginosa* conjunctivitis in a pediatric hospital. Infect Control Hosp Epidemiol. 1988;9:77.
189. Leibowitz HM, Kupferman A. Topically administered corticosteroids: effect on antibiotic-treated bacterial keratitis. Arch Ophthalmol. 1980;98:1287.
190. Davis SD, Sarff LD, Hyndfink RA. Relative efficacy of the topical use of amikacin, gentamicin, and tobramycin in experimental *Pseudomonas* keratitis. Can J Ophthalmol. 1980;15:28.
191. Hessburg PC. Treatment of *Pseudomonas* keratitis in humans. Am J Ophthalmol. 1966;61:896.
192. Sugar A, Cohen MA, Bien PA, et al. Treatment of experimental *Pseudomonas* corneal ulcers with enoxacin, a quinolone antibiotic. Arch Ophthalmol. 1986;104:1230.
193. Leibowitz HM, Ryan WJ Jr, Kupferman A. Route of antiobiotic administration in bacterial keratitis. Arch Ophthalmol. 1981;99:1420.
194. Golden B. SubTenon injection of gentamicin for bacterial infections of the eye. J Infect Dis. 1971;124(Suppl):S271.
195. Forster RK. Endophthalmitis. In: Duane TD ed. Clinical Ophthalmology. v. 4. New York: Harper and Row; 1978: Ch. 24, 1.
196. Ayliffe GAJ, Barry DR, Lowbury EJL, et al. Postoperative infection with *Pseudomonas aeruginosa* in an eye hospital. Lancet. 1966;1:1113.
197. Yannis RA, Rissing JP, Buxton TB, et al. Multistrain comparison of three antimicrobial prophylaxis regimens in experimental postoperative *Pseudomonas* endophthalmitis. Am J Ophthalmol. 1985;100:404.
198. Walsted RA, Blika S. Penetration of ceftazidime into the normal rabbit and human eye. Scand J Infect Dis. 1985;(Suppl)44:63.
199. Norden CW, Keleti E. Experimental osteomyelitis caused by *Pseudomonas aeruginosa*. J Infect Dis. 1980;141:71.
200. Norden CW, Myerowitz RL, Keleti E. Experimental osteomyelitis due to *Staphylococcus aureus* or *Pseudomonas aeruginosa*: a radiographic-pathological correlative analysis. Br J Exp Pathol. 1980;61:451.
201. Salahuddin NI, Madhavan T, Fisher EJ, et al. *Pseudomonas* osteomyelitis. Radiologic features. Radiology. 1973;109:41.
202. Wiessman GJ, Wood VE, Kroll LL. *Pseudomonas* vertebral osteomyelitis in heroin addicts. Report of five cases. J Bone Joint Surg. 1973;55:1416.
203. Sapico FL, Montgomerie JZ. Vertebral osteomyelitis in intravenous drug abusers: report of three cases and review of the literature. Rev Infect Dis. 1980;2:196.
204. Tindel JR, Crowder JG. Septic arthritis due to *Pseudomonas aeruginosa*. JAMA. 1971;218:559.

205. Gifford DB, Patzakis M, Ivler D, et al. Septic arthritis due to *Pseudomonas* in heroin addicts. J Bone Joint Surg. 1975;57A:631.
206. Bayer AS, Chow AW, Louie JS, et al. Sternoclavicular pyarthrosis due to gram-negative bacilli. Report of eight cases. Arch Intern Med. 1977;137:1036.
207. Sequeira W, Jones E, Seigel ME, et al. Pyogenic infections of the pubic symphysis. Ann Intern Med. 1982;96:604.
208. del Busto R, Quinn EL, Fisher EJ, et al. Osteomyelitis of the pubis. Report of seven cases. JAMA. 1982;24:1498.
209. Johanson PH. *Pseudomonas* infections of the foot following puncture wounds. JAMA. 1968;204:262.
210. Minnefor AB, Olson MI, Carver DH. *Pseudomonas* osteomyelitis following puncture wounds of the foot. Pediatrics. 1971;47:598.
211. Green NE, Bruno J III. *Pseudomonas* infections of the foot after puncture wounds. South Med J. 1980;73:146.
212. Jacobs RF, Adelman L, Sack CM, et al. Management of *Pseudomonas* osteochondritis complicating puncture wounds of the foot. Pediatrics. 1982;69:432.
213. Siebert WT, Dewan S, Williams TW Jr. Case report. *Pseudomonas* puncture wound osteomyelitis in adults. Am J Med Sci. 1982;283:83.
214. Gilbert DN, Tice AD, Marsh PK, et al. Oral ciprofloxacin therapy for chronic contiguous osteomyelitis cause by aerobic gram-negative bacilli. Am J Med 1987;82(Suppl 4A):254.
215. Gentry LO. Treatment of skin, skin structure, bone, and joint infections with ceftazidime. Am J Med 1985;79(Suppl 2A):67.
216. Bach MC, Cocchetto DM. Ceftazidime as single-agent therapy for gram-negative aerobic bacillary osteomyelitis. Antimicrob Agents Chemother. 1987;31:1605.
217. Gentry LO. Role for newer beta-lactam antibiotics in treatment of osteomyelitis. Am J Med. 1985;78(Suppl 6A):134.
218. Norden CW, Shinners E. Ciprofloxacin as therapy for experimental osteomyelitis caused by *Pseudomonas aeruginosa*. J Infect Dis. 1985;151:291.
219. Norden CW, Niederriter K. Ofloxacin therapy for experimental osteomyelitis caused by *Pseudomonas aeruginosa*. J Infect Dis. 1987;155:823.
220. Greenberg RN, Tice AD, Marsh PK, et al. Randomized trial of ciprofloxacin compared with other antimicrobial therapy in the treatment of osteomyelitis. Am J Med. 1987;82(Suppl 4A):266.
221. Desplaces N, Acar JF. New quinolones in the treatment of joint and bone infections. Rev Infect Dis. 1988;10(Suppl 1):S179.
222. Forkner CE. *Pseudomonas aeruginosa* Infections. New York: Grune & Stratton; 1960:43.
223. Marrie TJ, Major H, Gurwith M, et al. Prolonged outbreak of nosocomial urinary tract infection with a single strain of *Pseudomonas aeruginosa*. Can Med Assoc J. 1978;119:593.
224. Moore B, Forman A. An outbreak of urinary *Pseudomonas aeruginosa* infection acquired during urological operations. Lancet. 1966;2:929.
225. Anderson RJ, Schafer LA, Olin DB, et al. Septicemia in renal transplant recipients. Arch Surg. 1973;106:692.
226. Krieger JN, Brem AS, Kaplan MR. Urinary tract infection in pediatric renal transplantation. Urology. 1980;15:362.
227. Kunin CM. A ten-year-study of bacteriuria in school girls: final report of bacteriologic, urologic and epidemiologic findings. J Infect Dis. 1970; 122:382.
228. Stamey TA. Urinary Infections. Baltimore: Williams & Wilkins; 1972:279.
229. Daifuku R, Stamm WE. Bacterial adherence to bladder uroepithelial cells in catheter-associated urinary tract infection. N Engl J Med. 1986;314:1208.
230. Stanley MM. Bacillus pyocyaneus infections. A review, report of cases and discussion of newer therapy including streptomycin. Am J Med. 1947;2:253.
231. Carrol G, Allen HN, Doubly EK. Study of bacillary infections of the urinary tract. JAMA. 1947;135:683.
232. Fraenkel E. Weitere Untersuchungen uber die Menschenpathogenitat des Bacillus pyocyaneus. Z Hyg Infekt. 1917;84:369.
233. Corrado ML, Grad C, Sabbaj J. Norfloxacin in the treatment of urinary tract infections in men with and without identifiable urologic complications. Am J Med 1987;82(Suppl 6B):70.
234. Leigh DA, Emmanuel FXS, Petch VJ. Ciprofloxacin therapy in complicated urinary tract infections caused by *Pseudomonas aeruginosa* and other resistant bacteria. J Antimicrob Chemother. 1986;18(Suppl D):117.
235. Brown EM, Morris R, Stephenson TP. The efficacy and safety of ciprofloxacin in the treatment of chronic *Pseudomonas aeruginosa* urinary tract infection. J Antimicrob Chemother. 1986;18(Suppl D):123.
236. Malinverni R, Glauser MP. Comparative studies of fluoroquinolones in the treatment of urinary tract infections. Rev Infect Dis. 1988;10(Suppl 1):S153.
237. Barker LF. The clinical symptoms, bacteriologic findings and postmortem appearances in cases of infection of human beings with the bacillus pyocyaneus. JAMA. 1897;29:213.
238. Epstein JW, Grossman AB. Bacillus pyocyaneus in children. Am J Dis Child. 1933;46:132.
239. Ensign PR, Hunter CA. An epidemic of diarrhea in the newborn nursery caused by a milk-borne epidemic in the community. J Pediatr. 1946;29:620.
240. Schaffer AJ, Oppenheimer EH. *Pseudomonas* (pyocyaneus) infections of the gastrointestinal tract in infants and children. South Med J. 1948;41:460.
241. Florman AL, Schifrin N. Observations on a small outbreak of infantile diarrhea associated with *Pseudomonas aeruginosa*. J Pediatr. 1950;36:758.
242. Walker SH. Polymyxin B in *Pseudomonas* and *Proteus* enteritis. J Pediatr. 1952;41:176.
243. Geppert LJ, Baker HJ, Copple BI, et al. *Pseudomonas* infections in infants and children. J Pediatr. 1952;141:555.
244. Stone HH, Kolb LD, Geheber CE. Bacteriologic considerations in perforated necrotizing enterocolitis. South Med J. 1979;72:1540.
245. Amromin GD, Solomon RD. Necrotizing enterpathy: a complication of treated leukemia and lymphoma patients. JAMA. 1962;182:23.
246. Schimpff SC, Wiernik PH, Block JB. Rectal abscesses in cancer patients. Lancet. 1972;2:844.
247. Sherman NJ, Woolley MM. The ileocecal syndrome in acute childhood leukemia. Arch Surg. 1973;107:39.
248. Rodriguez V, Bodey GP. Epidemiology, clinical manifestations, and treatment in cancer patients. In: Doggett RG, ed. *Pseudomonas aeruginosa*. New York: Academic Press; 1979:384.
249. Dold H. On pyocyaneus sepsis and intestinal infections in Shanghai due to *Bacillus pyocyaneus*. Chin Med J. 1918;32:435.
250. Chakravarti DN, Tyagi NN. Pyrexia simulating that of enteric fever caused by *Pseudomonas* pyocyaneus in children. Indian Med Gaz. 1937;72:367.
251. Kubota Y, Liu PV. An enterotoxin of *Pseudomonas aeruginosa*. J Infect Dis. 1971;123:97.
252. Greene SL, Su WP, Muller SA. Ecthyma gangrenosum: report of clinical, histopathologic, and bacteriologic aspects of eight cases. J Am Acad Dermatol. 1984;11:781.
253. Schlossberg D. Multiple erythematous nodules as a manifestation of *Pseudomonas aeruginosa* septicemia. Arch Dermatol. 1980;116:446.
254. Bagel J, Grossman ME. Subcutaneous nodules in *Pseudomonas* sepsis. Am J Med. 1986;80:528.
255. Fleming MG, Milburn PB, Prose NS. *Pseudomonas* septicemia with nodules and bullae. Pediatr Dermatol. 1987;4:18.
256. Roberts R, Tarpay MM, Marks MI, et al. Erysipelas-like lesions and hyperesthesia as manifestations of *Pseudomonas aeruginosa* sepsis. JAMA. 1982;248:2156.
257. Hall JH, Callaway JL, Tindall JP, et al. *Pseudomonas aeruginosa* in dermatology. Arch Dermatol. 1968;97:312.
258. Koopmann CF, Coulthard SW. Infectious facial and nasal cutaneous necrosis: evaluation and diagnosis. Laryngoscope. 1982;92:1130.
259. Berg A, Armitage JO, Burns CP. Fournier's gangrene complicating aggressive therapy for hematologic malignancy. Cancer. 1986;57:2291.
260. Schuster DI. Palatopharyngeal and lower extremity soft tissue loss in an infant secondary to *Pseudomonas* gangrenous cellulitis. Ann Plast Surg. 1981;6:138.
261. Huminer D, Siegman-Ingra Y, Morduchowicz G, et al. Ecthyma gangrenosum without bacteremia. Report of six cases and review of the literature. Arch Intern Med. 1987;147:299.
262. van den Broek PJ, van der Meer JWM, Kunst MW. The pathogenesis of ecthyma gangrenosum. J Infect. 1979;1:263.
263. Washburn J, Jacobson JA, Marston E, et al. *Pseudomonas aeruginosa* rash associated with a whirlpool. JAMA. 1976;235:2205.
264. Thomas P, Moore M, Bell E, et al. *Pseudomonas* dermatitis associated with a swimming pool. JAMA. 1985;253:1156.
265. Schlech WF 3rd, Simonsen N, Sumarah R, et al. Nosocomial outbreak of *Pseudonomas aeruginosa* folliculitis associated with a physiotherapy pool. Can Med Assoc J. 1986;134:909.
266. El Baze P, Thyss A, Caldani C, et al. *Pseudomonas aeruginosa* O-11 folliculitis. Development into ecthyma gangrenosum in immunosuppressed patients. Arch Dermatol. 1985;121:873.
267. Pruitt BA Jr. Infections of burns and other wounds caused by *Pseudomonas aeruginosa*. In: Sabath LD, ed. *Pseudomonas aeruginosa*. The Organism, Diseases It Causes, and Their Treatment. Bern: Hans Huber Publishers; 1980:55.
268. McManus AT, Mason AD Jr, McManus WF, et al. Twenty-five year review of *Pseudomonas aeruginosa* bacteremia in a burn center. Eur J Clin Microbiol. 1985;4:219.
269. Pruitt BA Jr, Foley FD. The use of biopsies in burn patient care. Surgery. 1973;73:887.
270. Williams HB, Breidenbach WC, Callaghan WB, et al. Are burn wound biopsies obsolete? A comparative study of bacterial quantitation in burn patients using the absorbent disc and biopsy techniques. Ann Plast Surg. 1984;13:388.
271. Hansbrough JF, Carroll WB, Zapata-Sirvent RL, et al. Identification and antibiotic susceptibility of bacterial isolates from burned patients. Burns Incl Therm Inj. 1985;11:393.
272. Culbertson GR, McManus AT, Conarro PA, et al. Clinical trial of imipenem/cilastatin in severely burned and infected patients. Surg Gynecol Obstet. 1987;165:25.
273. McManus WF, Goodwin CW Jr, Pruitt BA Jr. Subeschar treatment of burn wound infection. Arch Surg. 1983;118:291.
274. Modak S, Fox CL Jr. Synergistic action of silver sulfadiazine and sodium piperacillin on persistent *Pseudomonas aeruginosa* in vitro and in experimental burn wound infections. J Trauma. 1985;25:27.
275. Leyden JJ, McGinley KJ, Mills OH. *Pseudomonas aeruginosa* gram-negative folliculitis. Arch Dermatol. 1979;115:1203.
276. Alomar A, Ausina V, Vernis J, et al. *Pseudomonas* folliculitis. Cutis. 1982;30:405.
277. Eaglstein NF, Marley WM, Marley NF, et al. Gram-negative bacterial toe web infection: successful treatment with a new third generation cephalosporin. J Am Acad Dermatol. 1983;8:225.
278. LeFeber WP, Golitz LE. Green foot. Pediatr Dermatol. 1984;2:38.

197. PSEUDOMONAS SPECIES (INCLUDING MELIOIDOSIS AND GLANDERS)

JAY P. SANFORD

Members of the genus *Pseudomonas* are motile, gram-negative, strictly aerobic bacteria that are common inhabitants of soil, water, and marine environments.

All are straight or slightly curved bacilli, motile by polar flagella (except *Pseudomonas mallei*), gram-negative, catalase-positive, and usually oxidase-positive and are capable of growth at temperatures of 4–43°C. At least one species (*Pseudomonas mallei*) appears to be a specialized mammalian parasite, while others are occasional animal pathogens.

The current classification in *Bergey's Manual of Systematic Bacteriology* of members of the genus *Pseudomonas* is based on rRNA/DNA homology,[1] which results in five groups (Table 1). Based upon substantial rRNA homology, *Pseudomonas maltophilia* has been assigned to the genus *Xanthomonas*. *Pseudomonas aeruginosa* is discussed in Chapter 196.

Pseudomonas pseudomallei and *P. mallei* are described in this chapter in detail according to the diseases that they can produce, melioidosis and glanders.

Recent reports from a number of cystic fibrosis centers suggest that *Pseudomonas cepacia* is becoming an increasingly frequent and important pulmonary pathogen with instances of fulminant necrotizing pneumonia and bacteremia.[2,3] This concern is heightened by a report of therapeutic failures with ceftazidime, which is highly effective in vitro, in a group of cystic fibrosis patients with severe chronic lung disease.[4]

The remaining pseudomonads can be grouped for consideration. Three broad categories can be defined: those that are opportunistic pathogens (Chapters 286, 287, 291, and 292), those that cause iatrogenic (Chapters 279–281) or egogenic (Chapter 288) infections, and those that present pseudoinfections. In each category the organisms represent environmental microorganisms that have transgressed the usual host defenses.

In most instances the *Pseudomonas* species being considered represent pathogens that have occurred as isolated cases or small outbreaks of nosocomial infection. The clinical manifestations are those of infection itself (e.g., fever) and those that are determined by the site of infection. (See Part II of this text for the major syndromes.) Table 2 is a summary of reported sites of infection. Generalizations about the susceptibility to antimicrobial agents are summarized in Table 3.

TABLE 1. Classification of Pseudomonads That Have Been Isolated from Clinical Specimens

Group/Subgroup	*Genus and Species*
RNA group I	
Fluorescent group	*P. aeruginosa*
	P. fluorescens
	P. putida
Nonfluorescent group	*P. stutzeri*
	P. alcaligenes
	P. pseudoalcaligenes
RNA group II	*P. mallei*
	P. pseudomallei
	P. cepacia
	P. pickettii
RNA group III	*P. acidovorans*
	P. testosteroni
RNA group IV	*P. diminuta*
	P. vesicularis
RNA group V	*Xanthomonas maltophilia*

MELIOIDOSIS

Melioidosis is a glanderslike infectious disease of humans and animals with a protean clinical spectrum first described in its acute fulminant form by Whitmore and Krishnaswami in 1912.[6] Stanton and Fletcher chose the name *melioidosis,* meaning "a resemblance to distemper of asses."[7] Melioidosis bears a striking resemblance to glanders both clinically and pathologically, but it is epidemiologically dissimilar.

Description

Pseudomonas pseudomallei (also known as Whitmore's bacillus) is a small, gram-negative, motile, aerobic bacillus with occasional filamentous chains. When stained with methylene blue, Wayson or Wright stain, marked irregularities with a bipolar "safety pin" pattern are observed. It grows well on standard bacteriologic media.

Epidemiology and Prevalence

Pseudomonas pseudomallei is a natural saprophyte that can be isolated from soil, stagnant streams, ponds, rice paddies, and market produce in the endemic areas. Its ubiquitous nature is illustrated by its isolation as a laboratory contaminant in these areas. *Pseudomonas pseudomallei* is capable of causing disease often in epizootic form among sheep, goats, swine, horses, and seals. Occasional isolates have also been reported from cows, rodents, and cats. Although animals are susceptible to the disease, they apparently do not represent a reservoir for human disease. Attempts to culture *P. pseudomallei* from the urine and feces of a large variety of healthy animals have been unsuccessful. Arthropod-borne infection has never been known to occur naturally, although experimentally transmission has been accomplished in guinea pigs both by the bite of the mosquito (*Aedes aegypti*) and of the rat flea (*Xenopsylla cheopis*). French researchers concluded that humans contract melioidosis by soil contamination of skin abrasions. Ingestion, nasal instillation, or inhalation are other possible methods of spread. Experiments have shown that hamsters can be infected by the respiratory route. In contrast to glanders, infections have been rare in laboratory workers but can occur. Human-to-human transmission of melioidosis has been described only once,[8] that being through venereal transmission from a patient with chronic prostatitis due to *P. pseudomallei* to his wife. The disease is endemic in Southeast Asia, with the greatest concentration of cases reported from Vietnam, Cambodia, Laos, Thailand, Malaysia, and Burma. However, cases in humans or animals have occurred throughout the world between 20 degrees north and south latitudes.[9] Indigenously acquired cases in humans have also been reported from adjacent areas including China, Hong Kong, India, Borneo, the Philippines. Guam, Indonesia, Ceylon, New Guinea, and North Queensland. Cases in humans or animals have been reported from Madagascar, Kenya,[10] central west Africa (Chad, Niger, Upper Volta, Ivory Coast, Gambia[11]), Iran, and Turkey. In 1976 *P. pseudomallei* was isolated from animals in the Paris zoo and from horses in Madrid.[12] Human melioidosis has been described only rarely in the Western hemisphere: Mexico,[13] Panama, Ecuador, Haiti, Brazil, Peru, Guyana, a neonatal case in Hawaii,[14] a case in Georgia,[15] and a possible case in Oklahoma.[16]

Clinically apparent melioidosis remains a relatively rare disease. Prevatt and Hunt were able to find 300 reported cases for their review in 1953.[17] The French Expeditionary Force in Indochina between 1948 and 1954 reported approximately 100 cases among 400,000 troops.[18] As of January, 1973, when all

TABLE 2. Types of Infection by Pseudomonads Other Than Aeruginosa and Pseudomallei

Genus and Species	*Bacteremia*	*Wound Infection*	*Septic Arthritis*	*Empyema/ Pneumonia*	*Abscess*	*Meningitis*	*Endocarditis*	*Urinary Tract*	*Conjunctivitis*	*Otitis Media*
P. fluorescens	X			X	X			X		
P. putida	X	X	X							
P. cepacia	X	X		X			X	X		
P. acidovorans	X									
P. testosteroni	X								X	
P. alcaligenes			X	X					X	
P. stutzeri		X	X						X	X
X. maltophilia	X	X		X	X	X	X	X	X	

(From Gilardi,[5] with permission.)

TABLE 3. Generalizations about Antimicrobial Susceptibilities of Pseudomonads Other Than *P. aeruginosa* and *P. pseudomallei*

Antimicrobial Agent	X. maltophilia	P. cepacia	P. fluorescens	P. putida	P. alcaligenes	P. stutzeri
Chloramphenicol	S	S	—	—	V	S
Polymyxin	S	R	—	—	V	S
Trimethoprim-sulfamethoxazole	S	S	—	—	V	S
Carbenicillin	V	R	R	R	V	S
Piperacillin	V	—	—	—	—	—
Gentamicin	R	R	V	S	S	S
Tobramycin	R	R	—	—	S	—
Amikacin	R	R	S	S	S	S
Cefotaxime	R	S	S	S	S	S
Moxalactam	V	S	S	V	S	S
Cefoperazone	R	S	V	S	S	S
Cefsulodin	V	V	S	S	S	S
Ceftizoxime	R	S	S	S	S	S
Ceftazidime	R	S	S	S	S	S
Aztreonam	R	S	S	S	S	S
Imipenem	R	S	S	S	S	S

Abbreviations: R: resistant (>50 percent of srains resistant); S: susceptible (≥90 percent of strains sensitive); V: variable in susceptibility; —: not reported.

American forces had been withdrawn from Vietnam, there had been 343 reported cases with 36 deaths.[19]

Positive serologic test results were noted in from 0 to about 9 percent of the patients in various fever of unknown origin (FUO) studies in Vietnam.[20,21] In early 1969, a survey done in the III Corps tactical area of the Republic of Vietnam disclosed positive test responses in 5–8 percent of the personnel in tactical units.[22] In later studies done on troops returned to the United States, the prevalence of significant titers was found to be related to the presence and, perhaps, extent of trauma in the patients. Of 200 patients with wounds, 7 had hemagglutinin titers of 1:40 or greater[23] as compared with 18 percent of the patients with open orthopedic wounds and 32 percent of those with burns.[19]

Despite the paucity of recognized cases, serologic surveys indicate that mild or inapparent infection is not uncommon, thus suggesting that contact with the organism occurs frequently. Significant titers have been found in 6–20 percent[24,25] of the indigenous personnel in Vietnam, Thailand, Malaysia, and Northern Australia. Similarly, 2 percent of the Europeans living in Vietnam[26] and 1.1–2 percent[27] of healthy or nonwounded U.S. Army troop personnel returning to the United States after spending 6–12 months in Vietnam had significant hemagglutination titers. On the basis of serologic studies, there are an estimated 225,000 U.S. citizens of the 2,500,000 at risk while serving in Vietnam who have had subclinical infection with *Pseudomonas pseudomallei*.[21] Ten percent of serum specimens from inhabitants of a village in Upper Volta were positive, yet clinical melioidosis has not been recognized in this group.[28] There is adequate documentation that the disease can recur months or years after apparent cure or occur after many years of latency. Intercurrent illness, injury, or stress is an important factor in the latter circumstance.[29,30]

Clinical Manifestations

The clinical manifestations of melioidosis are sufficiently variable to make categorization difficult. Illness can be manifested as an acute, subacute, or chronic process. The incubation period has not been defined; however, based on the development of infection after injury it may be as short as 2 days. After a laboratory accident, an incubation period of 3 days ensued. Clinically inapparent infections may remain latent for a number of years after a person leaves an endemic area and before apparent disease ensues, 26 years being the possible duration of latency in one patient.[31] Males are more often affected than women are, which is thought to represent occupational exposure. Age is also not a determining factor. Melioidosis may be recognized as inapparent infection, asymptomatic pulmonary infiltration, acute localized suppurative infection, acute pulmonary infection, acute septicemic infection, or chronic suppurative infection.

Acute Localized Suppurative Infection. Infection by inoculation of a break in the skin usually results in a nodule with an area of acute lymphangitis and regional lymphadenitis. There is usually fever and generalized malaise. This form of infection may rapidly progress to the acute septicemic form.

Acute Pulmonary Infection. The most common form of the disease has been pulmonary infection, which may represent a primary pneumonitis or hematogenous pneumonitis as a manifestation of the septicemic form.[32] The acute pulmonary infection can vary in severity from a mild bronchitis to overwhelming necrotizing pneumonia. The onset may be abrupt without prodromal symptoms or more gradual with headache, anorexia, and generalized myalgia. Fever occurs in almost all patients, is often in excess of 102°F, and may be associated with rigors. Chest pain, either pleuritic or a dull ache in character, is common. A nonproductive or productive cough with nonspecific sputum or hemoptysis characterizes the illness. Other symptoms may include mild pharyngitis. Tachypnea out of proportion to the fever and findings on physical or x-ray examination may be seen. Chest findings may be minimal but usually consist of rales in the area of pneumonitis. In the absence of dissemination, the spleen and liver are not palpable. Laboratory findings include total leukocyte counts ranging from normal to 20,000/mm^3. Mild normochromic, normocytic anemia may appear during the illness. The pneumonia usually involves the upper lobes with the radiologic appearance of consolidation. Cavitation of the infiltrate frequently occurs. Without specific therapy, the temperature can become normal within a few days; however, the upper lobe cavitation persists and results in a radiologic appearance of tuberculosis. Though uncommon, pleural effusions and pleural masses have been reported.[33] In some instances there is progressive pulmonary spread or hematogenous dissemination with the development of septicemic manifestations.

Acute Septicemic Infections. This is the form originally described by Whitmore primarily among narcotic addicts. Subsequent reports have evidenced less predilection for debilitated patients, although there are reports of patients with diabetes mellitus, steroid-treated lupus erythematosus, and antineoplastic therapy. The onset may be dramatically abrupt, with the dominant symptoms depending on the site of major involvement. In patients with bacteremia complicating pneumonitis, symptoms may include disorientation, extreme dyspnea, severe headache, pharyngitis, diarrhea, and the development of cutaneous pustular lesions on the head, trunk, or extremities. Examination reveals high fever, extreme tachypnea, a flushing of the skin, and cyanosis. Muscle tenderness may be striking. On examination of the chest, signs may be absent, or rales and rhonchi or pleural rubs may be heard. The liver and spleen may be palpable. Signs of arthritis or meningitis may ensue. Patients with the septicemic form usually have a rapidly progressive fatal course, which in some instances may be too fulminant to affect with therapy. The leukocyte count may be normal or slightly increased. Chest x-ray films most commonly show irregular nodular densities, 4–10 mm in diameter, disseminated throughout the lungs. These enlarge, coalesce, and often undergo cavitation as the disease progresses. Other radiologic patterns include unilateral irregular mottled densities with confluence involving one or more lobes.

Chronic Suppurative Infection. In some patients secondary abscesses develop that dominate the clinical picture. Organs involved include the skin, brain, lung, myocardium, liver, spleen, bones including the vertebrae, joints lymph nodes, and even the eye. Such patients may be afebrile.

Diagnosis

Melioidosis should be considered in the differential diagnosis of any febrile illness in a person who has been in an endemic area, especially if the presenting features are those of fulminant respiratory failure, if multiple pustular or necrotic skin or subcutaneous lesions develop, or if there is a radiologic pattern of tuberculosis from which tubercle bacilli cannot be demonstrated.

Microscopic examination of exudate will reveal poorly staining, small, gram-negative bacilli showing the characteristic staining irregularities and "safety pin" bipolar staining with methylene blue or Wright stain. *Pseudomonas pseudomallei* organisms grow on most laboratory media, including eosin-methylene blue agar (EMB) or MacConkey agar, in 24–48 hours. The organisms can be readily differentiated from *P. mallei* and *P. aeruginosa* by standard bacteriologic procedures, which include the hanging drop test for motility. The characteristic wrinkling of the colonies may require 72 hours or longer. The hemagglutination test, agglutination test, and complement fixation test are aids in diagnosis if a fourfold or greater rise in titer is demonstrated in paired sera. Single low titers are difficult to interpret because of nonspecific responses. Differentiation between IgM and IgG antibody responses has not been helpful in distinguishing active from inactive disease.[34] The complement fixation test is said to be specific with titers above 1:8 during the acute illness. Negative serologic test results do not exclude disease. In a recent report, one-third of culture-positive patients had negative serologies at time of diagnosis.[35] The hemagglutination and agglutination tests show more cross-reactions. Titers of 1:160 or more suggest infection.

Treatment

The treatment regimen to be used will vary with the form of the disease. Persons with low-titer positive serologic test responses but without other evidence of infection do not require therapy. The choice of antibiotics in active infection should be based on sensitivity studies, and therapy should be given for a minimum of 30 days. *Pseudomonas pseudomallei* are usually sensitive in vitro to the tetracyclines, chloramphenicol, novobiocin, kanamycin, amoxicillin clavulanate, ticarcillin clavulanate, piperacillin, imipenem,[36] many of the third-generation cephalosporins (cefotaxime, moxalactam, cefoperazone, ceftazidime and ceftriaxone),[37] sulfadiazine or sulfisoxazole, and trimethoprim-sulfamethoxazole and in most instances are resistant to other antibiotics including benzylpenicillin G, erythromycin, ampicillin, streptomycin, colistimethate, ciprofloxacin,[38] aztreonam, ticarcillin, and amdinocillin. In contrast to strains from other areas, fewer than 20 percent of strains from Thailand are sensitive to trimethoprim-sulfamethoxazole.[36] Resistance has developed during therapy.[39] In patients who are not toxic with pneumonitis or chronic suppurative lesions, effective therapy has included tetracycline, 2–3 g/day (40 mg/kg); chloramphenicol, 3 g/day (40 mg/kg); sulfisoxazole, 4 g/day (60 mg/kg); or trimethoprim-sulfamethoxazole (4 mg/kg trimethoprim, 20 mg/kg sulfamethoxazole) for 60–150 days. If the patient is relatively toxic, the use of two of these antimicrobials has been recommended for the initial 30 days, followed by 60–150 days of trimethoprim-sulfamethoxazole alone. In patients with extrapulmonary suppurative lesions, prolonged therapy for 6 months to 1 year should be considered. The potential toxic effects of the therapy must be considered. The usual principles of surgical drainage should be followed. In patients in extremely toxic conditions with severe pneumonitis or the septicemic form of melioidosis, multiple antibiotics should be administered by the parenteral route. Current recommendations for antibiotics in the septicemic form of melioidosis are trimethoprim, 9 mg/kg, and sulfamethoxazole, 45 mg/kg daily, and a third-generation cephalosporin such as ceftazidime (2 g iv q8h). On the basis of in vitro susceptibility, imipenem, 4 g/day (60 mg/kg), should be considered, especially with trimethoprim-sulfamethoxazole–resistant strains. Other alternatives include tetracycline, 4–6 g/day (80 mg/kg); chloramphenicol (80 mg/kg); and one of the following: trimethoprim-sulfamethoxazole (9–45 mg/kg), sulfisoxazole (140 mg/kg), or novobiocin (60 mg/kg). The dosage should be rapidly tapered with clinical improvement.

Prognosis

Before the use of antimicrobials, the mortality of apparent infection was said to be 95 percent. French experience in Indochina indicated that with chloramphenicol therapy the mortality was 20 percent. With better diagnosis and more prolonged appropriate therapy, the mortality in all forms except the septicemic should be low. Even with vigorous appropriate antibiotics and supportive therapy, the mortality in patients with melioidosis septicemia is 50 percent or greater. Very few patients have had long-term follow-up, so the incidence of late relapses cannot be predicted.

Prevention

There is no means of active immunization. If in endemic areas, vigorous cleansing of abrasions and lacerations is recommended.

GLANDERS

Glanders is a serious infectious disease of equine animals that is caused by *Pseudomonas mallei,* which is transmitted occasionally to other domestic animals and to humans.

Description

Pseudomonas mallei is a nonmotile, gram-negative bacillus. When stained with methylene blue, marked irregularities in staining are observed. Organisms grow on most common meat infusion bacteriologic media but require glycerol for optimum growth.

Epidemiology and Prevalence

Glanders is primarily a disease of the horse, mule, or donkey, although goats, sheep, cats, and dogs sometimes naturally contract the disease. Pigs and cattle are said to be absolutely resistant. In horses, the disease may be systemic with prominent pulmonary involvement (glanders) or may be characterized by subcutaneous ulcerative lesions and lymphatic thickening with nodules (farcy). The mode of infection in animals remains controversial; considerations include inhalation, ingestion, or inoculation through breaks in the skin.

Glanders in humans has never been common, but it gains medical importance from the serious nature of the occasional infection. Human disease occurs primarily in persons in close contact with horses, mules, or donkeys, presumably through inoculation of broken skin or the nasal mucosa with the contaminated discharges. A number of instances of infection, presumably of aerosol origin, have been reported in laboratory workers. The degree of potential laboratory hazard is illustrated by a 46 percent incidence of infection in a group of laboratory workers.[43]

With improved sanitation and other control measures, the incidence of glanders has steadily decreased in most countries. There have been no naturally acquired infections reported in the United States since 1938. Sporadic cases still occur in Asia, Africa, and elsewhere in the Americas. As in the instance of melioidosis, age and sex incidence parallel the risk of exposure. Thus, nearly 60 percent of the patients are between the ages of 20 and 40, and reported cases in women are rare.

Clinical Manifestations

Manifestations of the disease in humans are protean and are determined in part by the route of infection. Although categories frequently overlap, manifestations may generally be grouped as acute localized suppurative infection, acute pulmonary infection, acute septicemic infection, and chronic suppurative infection. Infection by way of inoculation of an abrasion or scratch in the skin usually results in a nodule with an area of acute lymphangitis. The period of incubation is usually 1–5 days. Infection of the mucous membranes can result in mucopurulent discharge involving the eye, nose, or lips followed by extensive ulcerating granulomatous lesions, which may or may not be associated with systemic reactions. With systemic invasion, a generalized papular eruption, which may become pustular, is frequent. This septicemic form of disease usually has been fatal in 7–10 days. Infection by inhalation is followed by an incubation period of 10–14 days. The more common symptoms include fever, occasionally associated with rigors, generalized myalgia, fatigue, headache, and pleuritic chest pain. Other symptoms have included photophobia, lacrimation, and diarrhea. Examination findings are usually normal except for fever and occasional lymphadenopathy, especially in the cervical lymph chain, and splenomegaly. Laboratory findings include total leukocyte counts that are usually normal to slightly elevated with 60–80 percent neutrophilic leukocytes. Instances of leukopenia with relative lymphocytosis have been reported. In the acute pulmonary form, chest films characteristically reveal circumscribed densities suggesting early lung abscesses. Other findings can include lobar or bronchopneumonia. In the chronic suppurative form of disease, the most frequent finding is multiple subcutaneous and intramuscular abscesses (83 percent), which most often involve the arms or legs. Approximately one-half of the patients will have lymphatic involvement and nasal discharge or ulceration. Pain at sites other than developing foci and skin eruptions occurs in one-third. Visceral involvement including pulmonary or pleural, ocular, skeletal, hepatic, splenic, and meningeal or intracranial central nervous system involvement occurred in one-quarter or fewer of the 156 patients summarized by Robins.[44]

Diagnosis

Microscopic examination of exudates can reveal small gram-negative bacilli that stain irregularly with methylene blue; however, organisms are generally very scanty, and it is often quite difficult to find them even in acute abscesses. *Pseudomonas mallei* and *P. pseudomallei* cannot be distinguished morphologically. Growth occurs on most meat infusion nutrient media. Blood cultures are usually negative except in the terminal stages of disease. Serologic tests include agglutination titers, which rise rapidly, usually by the second week, to dilutions of 1:640 or greater. Serum from healthy persons has been reported to show agglutination titers in dilutions up to 1:320. The complement fixation test is less sensitive but more specific and is considered positive at dilutions of 1:20 or greater.

Treatment

The limited number of infections in humans has precluded evaluation of most of the antibiotic agents. Sulfadiazine has been found to be an effective agent in experimental animals and in humans.[45] The dosage used has been approximately 100 mg/kg administered in divided doses. In experimental infections, 3 weeks of therapy gave better results than 1 week did. Benzylpenicillin is ineffective in vitro and in experimental infections. Streptomycin is bacteriostatic in vitro but was ineffective in experimental infections in hamsters. More recent antimicrobial agents such as tetracycline, chloramphenicol, the antipseudomonal aminoglycosides, carbenicillin, the polymyxins, and trimethoprim have not been evaluated. In the absence of clinical experience and pending in vitro susceptibility studies, it would seem most reasonable to use the regimens appropriate for patients with various manifestations of melioidosis. In the acute infections, appropriate supportive measures are essential, and in the chronic suppurative infections, the usual principles of surgical drainage should be followed.

Prognosis

The prognosis depends on the type of infection. The acute septicemic form has been uniformly fatal. The localized or chronic forms have a much better prognosis.

Prevention

Next to acquisition from diseased horses, the most common source of natural disease in humans has been contact with human glanders. Isolation is indicated.

REFERENCES

1. Palleroni NJ. Family Pseudomonadaceae. In: Kreig NR, Holt JG, eds. Bergey's Manual of Systematic Bacteriology. v. 1. Baltimore: Williams & Wilkins; 1984:141–219.
2. Goldmann DA, Klinger JD. *Pseudomonas cepacia:* Biology, mechanisms of virulence, epidemiology. J Pediatr. 1986;108:806–12.

3. Isles A, Maclusky I, Corey M, et al. *Pseudomonas cepacia* infection in cystic fibrosis: An emerging problem. J Pediatr. 1984;104:206–10.
4. Gold R, Jin E, Levinson H, et al. Ceftazidime alone and in combination in patients with cystic fibrosis: Lack of efficacy in treatment of severe respiratory infections caused by *Pseudomonas cepacia*. J Antimicrob Chemother. 1983;12(Suppl A):331–6.
5. Gilardi GL. *Pseudomonas*–Identification methods, significance of speciation and pathogenicity for man. In: Lorian V, ed. Significance of Medical Microbiology in the Care of Patients. Baltimore: Williams & Wilkins; 1977:96.
6. Whitmore A, Krishnaswami CS. An account of the discovery of a hitherto undescribed infective disease occurring among the population of Rangoon. Indian Med Gaz. 1912;47:262.
7. Stanton AT, Fletcher W. Trans 4th Congress Far Eastern Assn. Trop Med. 1921;2:196.
8. McCormick JB, Sexton DJ, McMurray JG, et al. Human-to-human transmission of *Pseudomonas pseudomallei*. Ann Intern Med. 1975;83:512.
9. Howe C, Sampath A, Spotnitz M. The pseudomallei group: A review. J Infect Dis. 1971;24:598.
10. Bremmelgaard A, Bygbjerg I, Hoiby N. Microbiological and immunological studies in a case of human melioidosis diagnosed in Denmark. Scand J Infect Dis. 1982;14:271–5.
11. Wall RA, Mabey DCW, Corrah PT, et al. A case of melioidosis in West Africa. J Infect Dis. 1985;152:424–5.
12. Galimand M, Dodin A. Le point sur la melioidose dans le monde. Bull Soc Pathol Exot Filiales. 1982;75:373.
13. Barnes PF, Appleman MD, Cosgrove MM. A case of melioidosis originating in North America. Am Rev Respir Dis. 1986;134:170–1.
14. Osteraas GR, Hardman JM, Bass JW, et al. Neonatal melioidosis. Am J Dis Child. 1971;122:446.
15. Nussbaum JJ, Hull DS, Carter MJ. *Pseudomonas pseudomallei* in an anophthalmic orbit. Arch Ophthalmol. 1980;98:1224.
16. McCormick JB, Weaver RE, Hayes PS, et al. Wound infection by an indigenous *Pseudomonas pseudomallei*-like organism isolated from the soil: Case report and epidemiologic study. J Infect Dis. 1977;135:103.
17. Prevatt AL, Hunt JS. Chronic systemic melioidosis. Am J Med. 1957;23:810.
18. Rubin HL, Alexander AD, Yager RH. Melioidosis: A military medical problem? Milit Med. 1963;128:538.
19. Moore WL Jr. Melioidosis. In: Eickhoff TC, ed. Practice of Medicine. v. 3. Hagerstown, MD: Harper & Row; 1977.
20. Deller JJ, Russell PK. An analysis of fevers of unknown origin in American Soldiers in Vietnam. Ann Intern Med. 1967;66:1129.
21. Clayton AJ, Lisella RS, Martin DG. Melioidosis: A serological survey in military personnel. Milit Med. 1973;138:24.
22. U.S. Army Vietnam Command Health Reports for 1968.
23. Kishimoto RA, Brown GL, Blair EB, et al. Melioidosis: Serologic studies in U.S. Army personnel returning from Southeast Asia. Milit Med. 1971;136:694.
24. Strauss JM, Alexander AD, Rapmund G, et al. Melioidosis in Malaysia. III. Antibodies to *Pseudomonas pseudomallei* in the human population. Am J Trop Med Hyg. 1969;18:703.
25. Ashdown LR, Guard RW. The prevalence of human melioidosis in northern Queensland. Am J Trop Med Hyg. 1984;33:474–8.
26. Brygoo ER. Contribution a l'etude des agglutinine naturelles pour le bacille de Whitmore. Bull Soc Pathol Exot Filiales. 1953;46:347.
27. Sanford JP, Moore WL Jr. Recrudescent melioidosis: A Southeast Asian legacy. Am Rev Respir Dis. 1971;104:452.
28. Dodin A, Terry R. Recherche epidemiologigne du bacille de Whitmore en Afrique. Bull Soc Pathol Exot Filiales. 1974;67:121.
29. Jackson AE, Moore WL Jr, Sanford JP. Recrudescent melioidosis associated with diabetic ketoacidosis: A case report. Arch Intern Med. 1972;130:268.
30. Mackowiak PA, Smith JW. Septicemic melioidosis. Occurrence following acute influenza A six years after exposure in Vietnam. JAMA. 1978;240:764.
31. Mays EE, Rickets EA. Melioidosis: Recrudescence associated with bronchogenic carcinoma twenty-six years following initial geographic exposure. Chest. 1975;68:261.
32. Everett ED, Nelson R. Pulmonary melioidosis: Observations in thirty nine cases. Am Rev Respir Dis. 1975;112:331.
33. Girard DE, Nardone DA, Jones SR. Pleural melioidosis. Am Rev Respir Dis. 1976;114:1175.
34. Ashdown LR. Relationship and significance of specific immunoglobulin M antibody response in clinical and subclinical melioidosis. J Clin Microbiol. 1981;14:361.
35. Guard RW, Khafagi FA, Brigden MC, et al. Melioidosis in far north Queensland. Am J Trop Med Hyg. 1984;33:467–73.
36. Sookpranee T, Sookpranee M, Mellencamp MA, et al. In vitro susceptibility of 199 *Pseudomonas pseudomallei* strains to conventional and new antibiotics (Abstract 544). In: Proceedings of the 28th Interscience Conference on Antimicrobial Agents. Washington, DC: American Society for Microbiology; 1988:204.
37. Ashdown LR, Frettingham RJ. In vitro activity of various cephalosporins against *Pseudomonas pseudomallei*. J Infect Dis. 1984;150:779–80.
38. Gillespie SH, McEniry DW, Felmingham D. In vitro susceptibility of *Pseudomonas pseudomallei* to DNA gyrase inhibitors. J Antimicrob Chemother. 1987;20:612–4.
39. Dance DAB, Wuthiekanum V, White NJ, et al. Antibiotic resistance in *Pseudomonas pseudomallei*. Lancet 1988;1:994–5.
40. DeBuse PJ, Henderson A, White M. Melioidosis in a child in Papua New Guinea. Successful treatment with kanamycin and trimethoprim-sulfamethoxazole. Med J Aust. 1975;2:476.
41. John JF Jr. Trimethoprim-sulfamethoxazole therapy of pulmonary melioidosis. Am Rev Respir Dis. 1976;114:1021.
42. Sanford JP. Melioidosis: Forgotten but not gone. Trans Am Clin Climatol Assoc. 1977;89:201.
43. Howe C, Miller WR. Human glanders: Report of six cases. Ann Intern Med. 1947;26:93.
44. Robins GD. A study of chronic glanders in man with report of a case. In: Studies from Royal Victoria Hospital, Montreal. v. 2. 1906.
45. Miller WR, Pannell L, Ingalls MS. Experimental chemotherapy in glanders and melioidosis. Am J Hyg. 1948;47:205.

198. ACINETOBACTER SPECIES

DAVID M. ALLEN
BARRY J. HARTMAN

Prior to the 1970s, the genus *Acinetobacter* was frequently misidentified because it had few distinctive characteristics. This led to the creation of multiple genera and subsequent taxonomic chaos. Mounting biochemical and genetic evidence confirms its place in the family Neisseriaceae. Realizing the natural prevalence and metabolic versatility of Acinetobacter has permitted a greater appreciation of its role in human disease.

As ubiquitous saprophytes, these gram-negative bacilli of low virulence have been implicated as causes of both community-acquired and nosocomial infections. Advances in immunosuppressive therapy as well as the frequent use of invasive techniques have allowed *Acinetobacter* and other multiply resistant gram-negative opportunists to surpass gram-positive bacteria as the leading causes of nosocomial morbidity.[1]

EPIDEMIOLOGY

Acinetobacter differs from other members of the family Neisseriaceae by the simplicity of its growth requirements.[2] The ability to use a variety of carbon sources via diverse metabolic pathways expands its habitat. This can be demonstrated in nature by the ability of *Acinetobacter* to decompose organic matter in an acidic pH at 30°C.[3]

Related genera (*Moraxella, Neisseria*, and *Kingella*) are parasitic in warm-blooded animals, whereas the free-living *Acinetobacter* organisms can be found on both animate and inanimate objects. Virtually 100 percent of soil and water samples yield *Acinetobacter*, which accounts for 0.001 to ≥50 percent of the organisms present.[4] *Acinetobacter* has been isolated from pasteurized milk, frozen foods,[4] chilled poultry,[5] foundry[6] and hospital air, vaporizer mist, tap water faucets,[7] peritoneal dialysate baths,[8] bedside urinals,[9] washcloths,[10] angiography catheters,[11] ventilators,[12] and plasma protein fractions.[13] Some strains recovered from sink basins have been found to be tolerant of soap.[14]

Acinetobacter has been grown from numerous human sources including sputum, urine, feces, and vaginal secretions.[4] Up to 25 percent of healthy ambulatory adults exhibit cutaneous colonization,[15] and 7 percent have transient pharyngeal colonization.[16] It is the most common gram-negative organism persistently carried on the skin of hospital personnel[17] and was found to colonize 45 percent of inpatient tracheostomy sites.[18] During the Vietnam conflict, it was the most common gram-negative contaminant of traumatic extremity injuries.[19] Of the two subspecies of *Acinetobacter*, var. *lwoffi* has a predilection for the genitourinary (GU) tract, and var. *anitratus* is more frequently isolated from all other sites.[20]

In a review of positive blood cultures in Denver teaching

hospitals from 1975 to 1977, *Acinetobacter* was the cause of 2 percent of all gram-negative bacteremias.[21] The 1984 report of the National Nosocomial Infection Study (NNIS) identified *Acinetobacter* as a pathogen in 0.61 percent of all cases of hospital-acquired infections reported to the Centers for Disease Control (CDC).[22] In a recent series[23] 33 percent of true bacteremias with *Acinetobacter* were polymicrobial. Also noted was a seasonal incidence peaking in late summer. This supported the 1978 NNIS finding that the rate of late summer infections is twice as high as the rate of winter infections.[24]

It is interesting that 40 percent of all infections caused by the genus *Acinetobacter* occur in children under 10 years of age.[25] The reason for this high incidence in pediatrics is unexplained.

HISTORY AND MICROBIOLOGY

Historically, numerous isolates of this ubiquitous organism led to taxonomic confusion. Probably first isolated and described in 1908 as *Diplococcus mucosus,*[26] the bacteria were initially identified by the absence of certain characteristics: no color, no motion, an inability to reduce nitrates, oxidase negativity, and nonfermentation. The lack of distinctive characteristics was used to assist in the nomenclature: *Micrococcus* (small), *Achromobacter* (colorless), *Acinetobacter* (motionless), and *anitratus* (nitrate nonreducing). Later, in an attempt to organize *Neisseria*-like organisms found in urethral smears morphologically, DeBord proposed a new tribe, Mimeae.[27] Two of the three genera of the now obsolete tribe Mimeae later came to be included under the genus *Acinetobacter*. The taxonomic classification listing all oxidase-negative, non-nitrate-reducing, catalase-positive, gram-negative bacteria under the genus *Acinetobacter* was officially recognized in the eighth edition of *Bergey's Manual* (Table 1).

Presently, *Acinetobacter* taxonomy consists of one species: *calcoaceticus* (calcium acetate used as a carbon source). Two recognized subspecies are distinguished by the ability of var. *anitratus* to produce acid from dextrose and var. *lwoffi*'s inability to do so. Further speciation of *A. calcoaceticus* has been delayed until additional distinctive characteristics can be identified. Attempts to organize unique species by using DNA hybridization,[28] bacteriocin typing,[29] and gelatinase and hemolysin production[30] or by differential carbon source utilization[31] have not been practical. Serotyping by agglutination has been unsuccessful due to the inability to readily separate somatic from capsular antibody reactions.[29] In fact, a related lipopolysaccharide (LPS) immunodeterminant found in both *Chlamydia trachomatis* and *Acinetobacter calcoaceticus* var. *anitratus*[32] results in a false-positive response in an enzyme-linked immunosorbent assay (ELISA) when a commercially available assay for chlamydial infections is used in specimens contaminated by *Acinetobacter*.[33]

Acinetobacter organisms are rod shaped during rapid growth and coccoid in the stationary phase. They are generally encapsulated, nonmotile, aerobic Gram-negative organisms that have a tendency to retain crystal violet and be incorrectly identified as gram-positive cocci. Due to a versatility of metabolic requirements, *Acinetobacter* organisms are able to grow in routine laboratory media. Enhanced isolation of *Acinetobacter* from polymicrobial specimens can be accomplished by using media at pH 5.5–6.0 and vigorous aeration at 30°C. Colonies are 1–2 mm, nonpigmented, domed, and mucoid with pitted surfaces. Frequent misidentification of *Acinetobacter* as *Neisseria* on Gram staining is readily clarified by the negative oxidase reaction for *Acinetobacter*. The inability of *Acinetobacter* species to reduce nitrate distinguishes these organisms from Enterobacteriaceae (Table 2).

PATHOGENESIS

The lack of virulence factors for *Acinetobacter* reduces it to the role of an opportunist. Growth in an acidic pH at lower temperatures may enhance its ability to invade devitalized tissue. No known cytotoxins are produced except cell wall LPS. The capsule that surrounds most *Acinetobacter* strains should inhibit phagocytosis and assist in local adhesion; however, this has not been specifically investigated. A selective advantage is suggested by the ability to produce bacteriocins.[29] Overall, without the disruption of normal host defenses, the role of *Acinetobacter* in human infection remains limited.

CLINICAL MANIFESTATIONS

Acinetobacter calcoaceticus has been described as the causative agent of suppurative infections of every organ system.[34] Usually acknowledged to be opportunistic in patients with altered host defenses, *Acinetobacter* infections have been reported to occur in otherwise healthy hosts. The ability to colonize normal and damaged tissue results in frequent isolation but limited clinical significance.[4] Additionally, *Acinetobacter* is often misinterpreted on Gram staining to be other gram-negative organisms more commonly associated with particular clinical conditions (e.g., cerebrospinal fluid: *N. meningitidis*; urethra: *N. gonorrhoeae*; sputum: *Haemophilus influenzae*).

Genitourinary

Isolation of organisms morphologically similar yet biochemically distinct from *Neisseria* led DeBord to formulate the tribe Mimeae.[27] Subsequent studies isolating *Acinetobacter* from pa-

TABLE 1. Chronologic Nomenclature

Acinetobacter calcoaceticus var. *lwoffi* (1968)
- *Achromobacter citroalcaligenes* (1963)
- *Achromobacter hemolyticus* var. *alcaligenes* (1963)
- *Alcaligenes metalcaligenes* (1963)
- *Acinetobacter lwoffi* (1957)
- *Acinetobacter polymorpha* (1957)
- *Achromobacter lwoffi* (1953)
- *Moraxella lwoffi* (1940)
- *Mima polymorpha* (1939)
- *Alcaligenes haemolysis* (1937)

Acinetobacter calcoaceticus var. *anitratus* (1968)
- *Achromobacter hemolyticus* var. *glucidolytica* (1963)
- *Achromobacter conjunctivae* (1963)
- *Acinetobacter anitratum* (1957)
- *Moraxella glucidolytica* (1956)
- *Achromobacter anitratum* (1954)
- *Neisseria winogradsky* (1952)
- B5W (1949)
- *Bacterium anitratum* (1948)
- *Herellea vaginicola* (1942)
- *Micrococcus calco-aceticus* (1911)
- ?*Diplococcus mucosus* (1908)

TABLE 2. Characteristics of the Family Neisseriaceae

Characteristic	Acinetobacter	Neisseria	Moraxella	Kingella
Shape	Paired cocci to medium rods	Paired cocci	Paired cocci to short rods	Paired rods
Oxidase	−	+	+	+
Catalase	+	+	+	−
Reduce nitrates	−	+	±	+
Metabolism	Active, varied	Limited, simple	Limited, simple	Limited, simple
General sensitivity to penicillins	Low	High	High	High
Acid from glucose	+ var. *anitratus* − var. *lwoffi*	−	−	+

(From Henriksen,[2] with permission.)

tients with a penicillin-resistant "gonorrhea-like" urethritis led to the erroneous implication of *Acinetobacter* as a cause of this illness.[35,36] Despite evidence of the colonization of the lower urinary tract with *Acinetobacter*, it is only rarely invasive. However, cases of cystitis and pyelonephritis have been documented in the setting of an indwelling bladder catheter or nephrolithiasis.[34]

Intracranial Infections

Initially described by Cowan in 1938,[26] *Acinetobacter* meningitis occurs infrequently. Although generally found in association with recent neurosurgical procedures,[37] there are reports of *Acinetobacter* meningitis occurring in the healthy host.[38–40] Meningitis can present abruptly or follow a more indolent course.[41] A petechial rash has been noted in up to 30 percent of patients with *Acinetobacter* meningitis.[41] This leads to further confusion with *N. meningitidis* when the Gram stain of the spinal fluid is reviewed. The Waterhouse-Friderichsen syndrome has also been noted in association with *Acinetobacter* meningitis.[38] Intracranial abscesses after neurosurgical procedures have been reported.[42]

Respiratory Tract

Transient colonization of the pharynx has been found in 7 percent of normal healthy persons.[16] Patients with tracheostomies have a much higher rate of colonization. Therefore, it is not surprising that the respiratory system is the most frequent site for *Acinetobacter* infections.[34] Epidemiologically, *Acinetobacter* has been reported to cause community-acquired bronchiolitis and tracheobronchitis in healthy children. It has been speculated that the lack of specific antibodies in the naive host is responsible.[41] Although community-acquired *Acinetobacter* pulmonary infections have been reported in adults, they generally occur in patients with decreased host defenses (alcoholism, tobacco abuse, renal failure, underlying pulmonary disease).[6,43,44] Most pulmonary infections attributed to *Acinetobacter* occur nosocomially, with predisposing factors being endotracheal intubation (or tracheostomy), prior antibiotic therapy, residence in an intensive care unit, recent surgery, and underlying pulmonary disease. Nosocomial spread in the intensive care unit setting has been attributed to ventilatory equipment and to colonized nursing and respiratory therapy personnel.[10,12,45] Nosocomial *Acinetobacter* pneumonias are frequently multilobar. Cavitation, pleural effusion, and bronchopleural fistula formation have been observed. When an *Acinetobacter* pneumonia is undiagnosed or misdiagnosed on Gram stain as *H. influenzae*, ineffective antibiotics may be used and lead to a high mortality rate. Mortality decreases once appropriate antibiotic therapy has been instituted for >3 days.[34] Secondary bacteremia and septic shock are associated with a poor prognosis.

Tracheobronchitis occurs in both children and in compromised adults. The incidence is probably underdiagnosed due to its low mortality. Pulmonary toilet often eradicates the organism without the need for systemic antibiotics.

Soft Tissue

Acinetobacter can cause local cellulitis associated with indwelling venous catheters. Resolution of the catheter-induced cellulitis may occur with catheter removal alone.[46]

Traumatic wounds, burns, and postoperative incisions are often colonized by *Acinetobacter* due to the ability of the organism to thrive on compromised tissue and foreign bodies. Serial observations of traumatic wound colonization and subsequent bacteremia in Vietnam revealed *Acinetobacter* to be present early on wounded extremities and then to produce bacteremia 3–5 days later. Its presence often accompanies other gram-negative bacteria (*Enterobacter, Pseudomonas,* etc.) and gram-positive cocci (*Enterococcus, Staphylococcus*). Synergistic necrotizing fasciitis with *Acinetobacter* and *Streptococcus pyogenes* has been described. Therapeutic intervention may require débridement alone or in combination with systemic antibiotics.[19,34,47,48]

Bacteremia

True *Acinetobacter* bacteremia should be distinguished from pseudobacteremia due to improper blood culturing technique.[7,15] The Nosocomial Infection Surveillance Study of 1984 determined that 0.6 percent of all nosocomial infections involved *Acinetobacter* and that 16.2 percent of these resulted in secondary bacteremia from a primary site.[22] *Acinetobacter* bacteremia is most frequently associated with respiratory infections[13,34] and next by urinary tract, wound, and skin infections. Although descriptions of well-appearing patients with bacteremia are recorded[49] (generally in patients with indwelling catheters), the picture of septic shock is also seen. It is not uncommon to find *Acinetobacter* in polymicrobial bacteremias. Survival in severe trauma (nonburn) patients with bacteremia was found to be higher when the bacteremic organism was of low virulence such as *Acinetobacter* and *Candida*.[47] Mortality of *Acinetobacter* bacteremia has been reported as 22 percent, with a higher mortality in polymicrobial sepsis.[34]

Miscellaneous

Acinetobacter infection can occur at any body site. Reported ocular cases include conjunctivitis,[50] endophthalmitis,[51] corneal ulceration due to soft contact lens contamination, and corneal perforation after misdiagnosis and treatment based on a corneal Gram stain.[52,53] Endocarditis after bacteremia on previously normal valves has been well described, and there is a predilection for the aortic valve.[54,55] Osteomyelitis, septic arthritis, and pancreatic and liver abscesses[4] have also been reported.

THERAPY

Acinetobacter may colonize the pharynx, urethra, skin, conjunctiva, and vagina. Interpretation of culture results must consider colonization and potential contamination from environmental sources. Isolation of *Acinetobacter* from colonized patients requires no specific therapy or precaution.

In patients with clinical presentations suggestive of local cellulitis or phlebitis associated with an intravenous catheter or other foreign body (e.g., stitches), removal of the foreign body with local care will generally be sufficient. The same recommendation can be made for urethritis and cystitis associated with indwelling catheters. Tracheobronchitis related to previous endotracheal intubation may resolve after pulmonary toilet alone. Infections involving the eyes and facial structures often require systemic and local antibiotic therapy. Patients with more extensive tissue involvement with wound dehiscence, fasciitis, and abscesses need débridement, drainage, and intravenous antibiotic therapy. Those with meningitis, endocarditis, osteomyelitis, and bacteremia may require intensive synergistic (combination) intravenous antibiotic therapy. The therapeutic approach to the patient with asymptomatic *Acinetobacter* bacteremia in the setting of an intravenous catheter is not clear beyond the removal of the catheter.

As with many other opportunistic gram-negative organisms, increasing antibiotic resistance has hindered the therapeutic management of active infections.[56] Aminoglycoside-inactivating enzymes, β-lactamases, and plasmid-mediated multiple antibiotic resistance have been identified.[57–59]

In the 1970s, *Acinetobacter* infections were treated with ampicillin, second-generation cephalosporins, minocycline, colistin, carbenicillin, and gentamicin. Most strains are now resistant to ampicillin, carbenicillin, cefotaxime, and chloramphenicol, with some centers reporting up to 84 percent of strains resistant to gentamicin.[57] In 1977, *Acinetobacter* was the most common gentamicin-resistant gram-negative organism isolated at the Massachusetts General Hospital. Tobramycin and amikacin resistance is less common.[60] Strains of *Acinetobacter calcoaceticus* var. *lwoffi* are less resistant than var. *anitratus* is to most antibiotics.[57] In vitro comparative studies of newer agents reveal that the 4-fluoroquinolones, piperacillin, ceftazidime, imipenem, and amikacin retain significant activity against gentamicin-resistant strains of *A. calcoaceticus* var. *anitratus*. Greater activity was noted for these same antibiotics against var. *lwoffi*.[60,61] When in vitro investigation was pursued on var. *anitratus* strains that had been clinically exposed to imipenem over a period of 6 years, imipenem maintained its excellent activity.[62] Bactericidal synergy against *Acinetobacter* has been demonstrated when carbenicillin and an aminoglycoside are combined even in strains where moderate aminoglycoside resistance exists.[63] The clinical relevance is not clear. There is an anecdotal report of successful therapy using the combination of imipenem and 4-fluoroquinolone.[64]

Many mild to moderately severe infections will respond to effective single agents. However, the current approach to treating a serious deep-seated infection involving *Acinetobacter* species should be based on the sensitivities of the specific strain and the use of an effective β-lactam (piperacillin/ticarcillin/ceftazidime) and aminoglycoside combination.

REFERENCES

1. Gardner P, Griffin WB, Swartz MN, et al. Nonfermentative gram-negative bacilli of nosocomial interest. Am J Med. 1970;48:735–49.
2. Henriksen SD. *Moraxella, Neisseria, Branhamella,* and *Acinetobacter*. Annu Rev Microbiol. 1976;30:63–83.
3. Baumann P. Isolation of *Acinetobacter* from soil and water. J Bacteriol. 1968;96:39–42.
4. Henriksen SD. *Moraxella, Acinetobacter* and the Mimeae. Bacteriol Rev. 1973;37:522–61.
5. Thornley MJ. A taxonomic study of *Acinetobacter* and related genera. J Gen Microbiol. 1967;49:211–57.
6. Cordes LG, Brink EW, Checko PJ, et al. A cluster of *Acinetobacter* pneumonia in foundry workers. Ann Intern Med. 1981;95:688–93.
7. Snydman DR, Maloy MF, Brock SM, et al. Pseudobacteremia: False-positive blood cultures from mist tent contamination. Am J Epidemiol. 1977;106:154–9.
8. Abrutyn E, Goodhart GL, Roos K, et al. *Acinetobacter calcoaceticus* outbreak associated with peritoneal dialysis. Am J Epidemiol. 1978;107:328–35.
9. Lowes JA, Smith J, Tabaqchali S, et al. Outbreak of infection in a urological ward. Br Med J. 1980;280:722.
10. Buxton AE, Anderson RL, Werdegar D, et al. Nosocomial respiratory tract infection and colonization with *Acinetobacter calcoaceticus*. Am J Med. 1978;65:507–13.
11. Reyes MP, Ganguly S, Fowler M, et al. Pyrogenic reactions after inadvertent infusion of endotoxin during cardiac catheterizations. Ann Intern Med. 1980;93(Pt I):32–5.
12. Cunha BA, Klimek JJ, Gracewski J, et al. A common source outbreak of *Acinetobacter* pulmonary infections traced to Wright respirometers. Postgrad Med J. 1980;56:169–72.
13. Harvey K, Schuck S. *Acinetobacter* septicaemia following prolonged intravenous therapy. Med J Aust. 1977;2:121–4.
14. Billing E. Studies on a soap tolerant organism: A new variety of *Bacterium anitratum*. J Gen Microbiol. 1955;13:252–60.
15. Al-Khoja MS, Darrell JH. The skin as the source of *Acinetobacter* and *Moraxella* species occurring in blood cultures. J Clin Pathol. 1979;32:497–9.
16. Rosenthal S, Tager IB. Prevalence of gram-negative rods in the normal pharyngeal flora. Ann Intern Med. 1975;83:355–7.
17. Larson EL. Persistent carriage of gram-negative bacteria on hands. Am J Infect Control. 1981;9:112–9.
18. Rosenthal SL. Sources of *Pseudomonas* and *Acinetobacter* species found in human culture materials. Am J Clin Pathol. 1974;62:807–11.
19. Tong MJ. Septic complications of war wounds. JAMA. 1972;219:1044–7.
20. Hoffmann S, Mabeck CE, Vejlsgaard R. Bacteriuria caused by *Acinetobacter calcoaceticus* biovars in a normal population and in general practice. J Clin Microbiol. 1982;16:443–51.
21. Weinstein MP, Reller LB, Murphy JR, et al. The clinical significance of positive blood cultures: A comprehensive analysis of 500 episodes of bacteremia and fungemia in adults. I. laboratory and epidemiologic observations. Rev Infect Dis. 1983;5:35–53.
22. Centers for Disease Control. Nosocomial Infection Surveillance Summary. MMWR. 1987;35:17–29.
23. Smego RA Jr. Endemic nosocomial *Acinetobacter calcoaceticus* bacteremia. Arch Intern Med. 1985;145:2174–9.
24. Retailliau HF, Hightower AW, Dixon RE, et al. *Acinetobacter calcoaceticus*; A nosocomial pathogen with an unusual seasonal pattern. J Infect Dis. 1979;139:371–5.
25. Reynolds RC, Cluff LE. Infection of man with Mimeae. Ann Intern Med. 1963;58:759–67.
26. Cowan ST. Unusual infections following cerebral operations: With a description of *Diplococcus mucosus* (von Lingelsheim). Lancet. 1938;2:1052–4.
27. DeBord GG. Organisms invalidating the diagnosis of gonorrhea by the smear method. Bacteriology. 1939;38:119–20.
28. Bouvet PJ, Grimont PAD. Taxonomy of the genus *Acinetobacter* with the recognition of *Acinetobacter baumannii* sp. nov., *Acinetobacter haemolyticus* sp. nov., *Acinetobacter johnsonii* sp. nov., and *Acinetobacter junii* sp. nov. and emended descriptions of *Acinetobacter calcoaceticus* and *Acinetobacter lwoffii*. Int J Syst Bacteriol. 1986;36:228–40.
29. Andrews HJ. *Acinetobacter* bacteriocin typing. J Hosp Infect. 1986;7:169–75.
30. Gerner-Smidt P. The epidemiology of *Acinetobacter calcoaceticus*: Biotype and resistance-pattern of 328 strains consecutively isolated from clinical specimens. Acta Pathol Microbiol Immunol Scand [B]. 1987;95:5–11.
31. Holt JG, Kreig NR, eds. Bergey's Manual of Determinative Bacteriology. 9th ed. Baltimore: Williams & Wilkins; 1984:288–310.
32. Nurminen M, Wahlstrom E, Kleemola M, et al. Immunologically related ketodeoxyoctonate-containing structures in *Chlamydia trachomatis,* re mutants of *Salmonella species,* and *Acinetobacter calcoaceticus* var. *anitratus*. Infect Immunol. 1984;44:609–13.
33. Saikku P, Puolakkainen M, Leinonen M, et al. Cross-reactivity between Chlamydiazyme and *Acinetobacter* strains. N Engl J Med. 1986;314:922–3.
34. Glew RH, Moellering RC Jr, Kunz LJ. Infections with *Acinetobacter calcoaceticus* (*Herellea vaginicola*): Clinical and laboratory studies. Medicine (Baltimore). 1977;56:79–97.
35. Svihus RH, Lucero EM, Mikolajczyk MT, et al. Gonorrhea-like syndrome caused by penicillin-resistant Mimeae. JAMA. 1961;177:121–4.
36. Kozub WR, Bucolo S, Sami AW, et al. Gonorrhea-like urethritis due to *Mima polymorpha* var. *oxidans*: Patient summary and bacteriological study. Arch Intern Med. 1968;122:514–6.
37. Berk SL, McCabe WR. Meningitis caused by *Acinetobacter calcoaceticus* var *anitratus*: A specific hazard in neurosurgical patients. Arch Neurol. 1981;38:95–8.
38. Townsend FM, Hersey DF, Wilson FW. *Mima polymorpha* as a causative agent in Waterhouse-Friderichsen syndrome. US Armed Forces Med J. 1954;5:673–9.
39. Fred HL, Allen TD, Hessel HL, et al. Meningitis due to *Mima polymorpha*. Arch Intern Med. 1958;102:204–6.
40. Olafsson M, Lee YC, Abernethy TJ. *Mima polymorpha* meningitis: Report of a case and review of the literature. N Engl J Med. 1958;258:465–70.
41. O'Connell CJ, Hamilton R. Gram-negative rod infections. II. *Acinetobacter* infections in general hospital. NY State J Med. 1981;81:750–3.
42. Waage R. *Bacterium anitratum* (B5W) isolated from cerebral abscesses. Acta Pathol Microbiol Scand. 1953;33:268–70.
43. Goodhart GL, Abrutyn E, Watson R, et al. Community-acquired *Acinetobacter calcoaceticus* var *anitratus* pneumonia. JAMA. 1977;238:1516–8.
44. Wands JR, Mann RB, Jackson D, et al. Fatal community-acquired *Herellea* pneumonia in chronic renal disease: Case report. Am Rev Respir Dis. 1973;108:964–7.
45. Stone JW, Das BC. Investigation of an outbreak of infection with *Acinetobacter calcoaceticus* in a special care baby unit. J Hosp Infect. 1985;6:42–8.
46. Gervich DH, Grout CS. An outbreak of nosocomial *Acinetobacter* infections from humidifiers. Am J Infect Control. 1985;13:210–5.
47. Miller RM, Polakavetz SH, Hornick Rb, et al. Analysis of infections acquired by the severely injured patient. Surg Gynecol Obstet. 1973;137:7–10.
48. Amsel MB, Horrilleno E. Synergistic necrotizing fasciitis: A case of polymicrobial infection with *Acinetobacter calcoaceticus*. Curr Surg. 1985;42:370–2.
49. Robinson RG, Garrison RG, Brown RW. Evaluation of the clinical significance of the genus *Herellea*. Ann Intern Med. 1964;60:19–25.
50. Burns RP, Florey MJ. Conjunctivitis caused by Mimae. Am J Ophthalmol. 1963;56:386–91.
51. Peyman GA, Vastine DW, Diamond JG. Vitrectomy and intraocular gentamicin management of *Herellea* endophthalmitis after incomplete phacoemulsification. Am J Ophthalmol. 1975;80:764–5.
52. Wand M, Olive GM, Mangiaracine AB. Corneal perforation and iris prolapse due to *Mima polymorpha*. Arch Ophthalmol. 1975;93:239–41.
53. Herbst RW. *Herellea* corneal ulcer associated with the use of soft contact lenses. Br J Ophthalmol 1972;56:848–50.
54. Altman KA, Sacks F. Bronchopneumonia and endocarditis: Caused by Acinetobacter anitratum (Herellea vaginicola). NY State J Med. 1979;79:1434–5.
55. Thompson WR. *H vaginicola* endocarditis in a heroin addict. JAMA. 1971;215:982.
56. McGowan JE Jr. Antimicrobial resistance in hospital organisms and its relation to antibiotic use. Rev Infect Dis. 1983;5:1033–48.
57. Bergogne-Berezin E, Joly-Guillou ML. An underestimated nosocomial pathogen, *Acinetobacter calcoaceticus*. J Antimicrob Chemother. 1985;16:535–8.
58. Murray BE, Moellering RC Jr. Aminoglycoside-modifying enzymes among clinical isolates of *Acinetobacter calcoaceticus* subsp. *anitratus* (*Herellea*

vaginicola): Explanation for high-level aminoglycoside resistance. Antimicrob Agents Chemother. 1979;15:190–9.
59. Hinchliffe E, Vivian A. Naturally occurring plasmids in *Acinetobacter calcoaceticus*: A P class R factor of restricted host range. J Gen Microbiol. 1980;116:75–80.
60. Stiver HG, Bartlett KH, Chow AW. Comparison of susceptibility of gentamicin-resistant and -susceptible "*Acinetobacter anitratus*" to 15 alternative antibiotics. Antimicrob Agents Chemother. 1986;30:624–5.
61. Rolston KVI, Bodey GP. In vitro susceptibility of *Acinetobacter* species to various antimicrobial agents. Antimicrob Agents Chemother. 1986;30:769–70.
62. Bergogne-Berezin E, Joly-Guillou ML. Comparative activity of imipenem, ceftazidime and cefotaxime against *Acinetobacter calcoaceticus*. J Antimicrob Chemother. 1986;18(Suppl E):35–9.
63. Ramphal R, Kluge RM. *Acinetobacter calcoaceticus* variety *anitratus*: An increasing nosocomial problem. Am J Med Sci. 1979;277:57–66.
64. Ygout J-F, Housset B, Derenne J-P, et al. Hospital-acquired *Acinetobacter baumanii* pneumonitis. Lancet. 1987;1:802.

199. SALMONELLA SPECIES (INCLUDING TYPHOID FEVER)

EDWARD W. HOOK

DESCRIPTION OF THE PATHOGEN

Salmonella are non-spore-forming gram-negative rods of the family Enterobacteriaceae. With the exception of the serotype gallinarum-pullorum, *Salmonella* are motile by peritrichous flagella.

Classification of *Salmonella* is in transition as a result of evidence obtained through DNA hybridization. The *Salmonella–Arizona* group, formerly said to consist of strains belonging to two genera, *Salmonella* and *Arizona*, is now classified on the basis of DNA studies as a single genus, *Salmonella*. The same DNA studies have offered compelling evidence that all *Salmonella* are so closely related in a genetic or evolutionary sense that there is no species differentiation: "there is only one species of *Salmonella*."[1–5] Nevertheless, *Salmonella* strains demonstrate sufficient differences in biochemical reactions, antigenic structure, host adaptations, and geographical distribution to be grouped by DNA hybridization into six distinct subgroups (Table 1), which have been variously designated in proposed taxonomic schemes. Virtually all strains isolated in clinical laboratories and implicated in disease in humans and animals (more than 1800 serotypes, including *S. typhi, S. choleraesuis, S. paratyphi* A, etc.) belong to subgroup I.

Precision in *Salmonella* taxonomy makes for cumbersome, confusing, and unfamiliar clinical and epidemiologic terminology. Therefore, beginning in 1983 it was proposed that the *Salmonella* serotype name be used in reporting.[1] The U.S. Centers for Disease Control advocate this practical approach,[4,5] with cultures reported as shown in Table 2. It was further proposed that designations of *Salmonella* in scientific communications (laboratory reports, surveillance data, and publications) artificially treat the serotypes as species.[4] This system of practical nomenclature is accepted now in much of the world. Thus, in the following pages, serotypes are identified as if they were *Salmonella* species, e.g., *Salmonella typhi*, even though they clearly are not.

Like other enterobacteria, *Salmonella* have somatic (O) antigens, which are lipopolysaccharide components of the cell wall, and flagellar (H) antigens, which are proteins.[6] There are approximately 60 O antigens, which are designated by numbers and letters. The Kauffmann–White scheme categorizes *Salmonella* on the basis of somatic antigens, each group having a major determinant, which is a strongly reacting somatic antigen, and one or more minor somatic antigens.[3] Identification of specific serotypes according to the Kauffmann–White scheme requires definition, too, of flagellar antigens of phases 1 and 2. *Salmonella typhi* also has a capsular or virulence (Vi) antigen composed of a homopolymer of *N*-acetyl galactosaminuronic acid. The presence of Vi antigen on the cell surface may block agglutination by anti-O serum.

Salmonella can be differentiated from other Enterobacteriaceae on the basis of certain biochemical reactions, including fermentation reactions with specific sugars. Most *Salmonella* ferment glucose and mannose to produce acid and gas but do not ferment lactose or sucrose; *S. typhi* does not produce gas. The identification of fermentation variants, i.e., strains with identical antigenic composition but different fermentation characteristics, makes initial screening for *Salmonella* by lactose fermentation somewhat unreliable in endemic areas. For example, a lactose-fermenting *S. typhimurium* easily confused with *Escherichia coli* was endemic in Sao Paulo, Brazil, in the early 1970s.[7] Additionally, a lactose-fermenting *S. typhimurium* initially identified as *Enterobacter aerogenes* was reported to have caused a case of aortic endarteritis and septicemia in the United States.[8]

Plasmid DNAs can serve as markers to identify or "fingerprint" epidemic strains.[9] *Salmonella* isolates can also be characterized according to susceptibility to antibiotics and various bacteriophages.[10] Antibiotic susceptibility patterns, bacteriophage typing, and plasmid fingerprinting are all useful in the epidemiologic study of disease caused by *Salmonella* serotypes of high prevalence.[9,11]

Salmonella organisms grow readily on simple media in aerobic or anaerobic conditions. Cultures of specimens that are normally sterile, such as blood, joint fluid, or cerebrospinal fluid, can be done on ordinary media such as blood agar. Excretions or secretions, such as feces or sputum, which have high concentrations of other microorganisms, are usually grown on selective or differential media, such as bismuth sulfate agar or desoxycholate agar, which contain inhibitors of growth of nonpathogenic organisms of the normal flora. Fecal specimens are also placed in "enrichment media," broths with inhibitors such as selenite or tetrathionate, to increase yield of organisms.

EPIDEMIOLOGY

In the vast majority of cases, human beings acquire *Salmonella* by the ingestion of contaminated food or water. Infection has also resulted from ingestion of contaminated medications or diagnostic agent. Direct fecal–oral spread can occur, particularly in children. Administration of organisms by the intravenous route in platelet transfusions has been documented,[12,13] and transmission of organisms by inadequately sterilized fiber-optic instruments has been reported among patients undergoing upper gastrointestinal endoscopy.[14,15]

Salmonella are primarily pathogens of lower animals. The reservoir of infection in animals constitutes the principal source of nontyphoidal *Salmonella* organisms that infect man, although infection may be transmitted from person to person. *Salmonella* have been isolated from almost all animal species, including poultry (chickens, turkeys, and ducks), cows, pigs, pets (turtles, cats, dogs, mice, guinea pigs, and hamsters), other birds (doves, pigeons, parrots, starlings, sparrows, cowbirds, and so on), sheep, seals, donkeys, lizards, and snakes.[16]

A few *Salmonella* serotypes are highly host-adapted and tend to be virtually "species specific." For example, the only known reservoir for *S. typhi* is man, and infection with this organism strongly implies direct or indirect exposure to a human source. Chimpanzees, mice, and other animals have been infected with *S. typhi* experimentally but are not known to be infected in nature.[17] *Salmonella paratyphi* A, *S. schottmuelleri* (paratyphi B), *S. hirschfeldii* (paratyphi C), and *S. sendai* are thought also

TABLE 1. Properties of Six Subgroups within the Genus *Salmonella* (the *Salmonella–Arizona* Group)

Property or Test	*Results in Salmonella subgroup:* 1	2	3a	3b	4	5
DNA hybridization group of Crosa et al.	1	2	3	4	5	Not studied
Genus according to Ewing	*Salmonella*	*Salmonella*	*Arizona*	*Arizona*	*Salmonella*	*Salmonella*
Salmonella subgenus names formerly used	I	II	III	III	IV	V
Subspecies according to Le Minor et al[1,2]	*choleraesuis*	*salamae*	*arizonae*	*diarizonae*	*houtenae*	*bongori*
Usually monophasic (Mono) or diphasic (Di) flagella	Di	Di	Mono	Di	Mono	Mono
Usually isolated from humans and warm-blooded animals	+	−	−	−	−	−
Usually isolated from cold-blooded animals and the environment	−	+	+	+	+	+
Pathogenic for humans	++++	+	+	+	+	+?
Test[a]						
Dulcitol fermentation	96	90	0	1	0	100
Lactose fermentation	1	1	15	85	0	0
ONPG[b]	2	15	100	100	0	100
Malonate utilization	1	95	95	95	0	0
Growth in KCN medium	1	1	1	1	95	100
Mucate fermentation	90	96	90	30	0	100
Gelatin hydrolysis[c]	−	+	+	+	+	−
D-Galacturonate fermentation[c]	−	+	−	+	+	+
Lysis by O1 bacteriophage[c]	+	+	−	+	−	v

[a] The numbers give the percent positive for the tests after 2 days of incubation at 36°C. The results from the first six tests are based on CDC data. The vast majority of the positive tests occur within 24 hours; reactions positive after 2 days are not considered.
[b] ONPG, o-Nitrophenyl-β-D-galactopyranoside.
[c] Based on the data of Le Minor et al[1,2] 90% or more positive; −, 10% or less positive; v, variable. The rest for gelatin hydrolysis is the rapid film method at 36°C (almost all strains are negative by the tube method at 22°C within 2 days).
(From Farmer et al.,[5] with permission.)

TABLE 2. Some Examples of "Practical Names" for Use in Reporting *Salmonella* Cultures

Reporting by hospital laboratories
Salmonella serogroup C1
Salmonella species
Salmonella species (formerly *Arizona hinshawii*)
Salmonella typhi or *Salmonella* serotype typhi

Reporting by reference laboratories
Salmonella serotype typhimurium[a]
Salmonella serotype typhi,[a] phage type A
Salmonella serotype 50:z_4,z_{24}: (formerly *Arizona hinshawii* 9a,9b:1,3,11)

CDC laboratory report has a place to indicate the *Salmonella* subgroup, which is based on the tests given in Table 2:

		1	2	3a	3b	4	5
Salmonella serotype chameleon[d]	Subgroup	☐	☐	☐	☐	☑	☐

[a] An alternative is to report the serotypes as species, such as *Salmonella typhimurium*, *Salmonella typhi*, and *Salmonella chameleon*.
(From Farmer et al.,[4] with permission.)

to have reservoirs primarily in man, although animal infections are observed occasionally in nature.[18] A few serotypes are also adapted rather specifically to animals. For example, chickens and other birds are the major reservoirs of *S. gallinarum-pullorum*.[18] It should be emphasized, however, that, despite these examples of species adaptation, almost all *Salmonella* serotypes produce disease in both animals and man.

The most accurate information on sources of human salmonellosis is derived from studies of outbreaks. Poultry (chickens, turkeys, ducks) and poultry products (primarily eggs) are the most important sources of human infection and are estimated to be responsible for about one-half of the common-vehicle epidemics.[20] *Salmonella* in feces of infected hens may contaminate the surface of egg shells or penetrate into the interior of the egg through hairline cracks. In hens with ovarian infection, organisms may gain access to the yolk. Large outbreaks of salmonellosis associated with bulk egg products and cracked shell eggs led to the passage of the Egg Products Inspection Act in 1970, which requires pasteurization of all bulk egg products and federally supervised inspection of shell eggs for cracks.[21] Even though this legislation has been associated with a decrease in frequency of egg-associated outbreaks, eggs or foods containing raw or undercooked eggs (homemade eggnog, grilled egg-dipped bread, Caesar salad, pasta made with eggs) continue to be associated with outbreaks.[21]

Meats, especially beef and pork, are quite often implicated, accounting for about 13 percent of the outbreaks, and dairy products, including raw and powdered milk, account for about 4 percent of the epidemics.[22] Pasteurized 2 percent low-fat milk was responsible for a massive outbreak in Illinois in 1985 caused by *S. typhimurium* resistant to ampicillin and other antimicrobials.[23] There were more than 16,000 culture-confirmed cases with epidemiologic data indicating that 150,000–200,000 persons were actually affected. The strain probably came to the processing plant in raw milk from dairy cattle, but the precise method by which previously pasteurized milk was contaminated was not determined.[22]

Pets, especially turtles, are the mode of transmission in 3 percent of the outbreaks.[24] The Food and Drug Administration (FDA) ban on interstate shipment of pet turtles in 1975 was associated with a reduction in frequency but not elimination of turtle-associated salmonellosis.[25] An outbreak of *Salmonella* enterocolitis in 1981 was traced to contact with marijuana, which apparently had been heavily contaminated with animal manure.[26] Food handlers only rarely are identified as sources of outbreaks, and their role as disseminators of infection has been overemphasized.[27,28]

The reservoir of infection among domestic animals is of fundamental importance in the epidemiology of salmonellosis. Animal-to-animal transmission may occur, either directly or indirectly. Animal feeds containing *Salmonella*-contaminated fishmeal or by-products of the meat packing industry, such as bone meal, are major sources of infection among animals. Even though the prevalence of infection may be low among groups of animals, stress and crowding in animal feeding and holding pens before slaughter increase the spread of infection. Processing equipment and the environments of abattoirs and packing plants become contaminated from carcasses of infected animals and contaminate previously uninfected meats passing through the processing line. Thus, raw poultry and raw meat products purchased at retail markets are not infrequently contaminated with *Salmonella*. Meat products contaminated in food-processing plants and shipped to distant sites may lead to infection over wide geographic areas.[29] Contamination of poultry, meat, and other food products probably accounts for the fact that food handlers are more likely to be asymptomatic carriers of *Salmonella* than are members of the general population.[28]

Acquisition of nontyphoidal *Salmonella* organisms from water contaminated with animal or human excreta occurs, but this mode of transmission is more characteristic of *S. typhi* than of nontyphoidal strains.[20,30]

Since humans are the only reservoir of *S. typhi*, direct or indirect contact with a person with typhoid fever or with a chronic carrier is necessary for infection. *Salmonella typhi* is acquired by ingestion of contaminated food or drink. Waterborne typhoid fever, so prevalent in the past, remains a threat where sanitation fails in modern water distribution systems. Breaks in sanitation accounted for a waterborne outbreak of typhoid involving about 230 persons in a camp for migrant farm workers in Dade County, Florida, in 1973.[31] This outbreak of typhoid fever was the largest reported in the United States since 1939. A mentally retarded girl who resided next door to a chronic carrier was probably responsible for contamination of the water supply at a central point in the distribution system. The chlorinator for the water system was defective coincident with the epidemic, and there was demonstrable evidence of coliform contamination of the water. The attack rate of typhoid was 12.6 percent (225/1795) in camp residents, with an increased incidence in those who drank large quantities of camp water. Food, a second major source of *S. typhi*, is usually contaminated by a food handler who is an asymptomatic enteric carrier or by sewage. The outbreak of 507 cases of typhoid fever in Aberdeen, Scotland, in 1964 was traced to canned corned beef from Argentina, which had been cooled in sewage-contaminated river water after canning.[32] In epidemic areas, outbreaks may be related to rainy seasons when sewage-contaminated pools drain downstream.[33] Ingestion of bivalve mollusks such as oysters raised in waters contaminated by sewage was a major source of *S. typhi* in the United States during the early part of the twentieth century; however, sewage treatment and shellfish sanitation programs have eliminated that source almost entirely.[34]

Table 3 lists the 10 *Salmonella* serotypes most frequently isolated from human sources in 1986 and nonhuman sources in 1985 in the United States.[35] These 10 serotypes accounted for about 73 percent of all isolates from humans. A total of 229 different serotypes were identified in the United States in 1986.[35] About 500 different serotypes have been isolated in the United States in the past 10 years. The role of animal reservoirs as a source of human disease is supported by the similarity of serotypes isolated from man and animals, as shown in Table 3. The frequency of isolation of specific serotypes tends to occur in regional patterns, both in the United States and worldwide.[24] Therefore, knowledge of regional patterns of infection may help to localize and to identify sources of infection occurring at distant sites.

Salmonella infections occur with greatest frequency in the United States from July through November (Fig. 1). A seasonal variation is seen worldwide, with peak incidence corresponding to warm weather.

Children under 5 years of age have the highest incidence of salmonellosis. The attack rate is especially high in the first year of life (Fig. 2). About 23 percent of all isolates in 1980 were from infants less than 1 year old, and two-thirds were from persons under 21 years of age. *Salmonella* organisms are isolated from males in the United States slightly more often than from females; the difference in percentage of the total isolates from males and females is slight (for 1980, 50.4 percent of isolates from males, 49.6 percent from females) but has remained consistent for a decade.[35]

The majority of reported isolations of *Salmonella* from humans in the United States comes from "sporadic" cases.[17] However, epidemiologic investigation of such cases reveals in many instances unrecognized outbreaks in families or larger groups. The largest number of outbreaks occurs in the home.[20] If one family member is shown to be infected, approximately one-third of household or family contacts also will be infected.[36] Institutions rank second to the home in frequency of place of occurrence of reported outbreak.[37] Acute care hospitals, pediatric wards, and neonatal nurseries account for about two-thirds of reported institutional outbreaks; nursing homes, psychiatric hospitals, and institutions for the retarded account for the remainder.[37] Banquets, restaurants, food stores, and schools also are not infrequently sources of outbreaks.[20] About 85 percent of all outbreaks are associated with a contaminated common vehicle, usually food or drink, and about 10 percent are spread by cross-infection.

The common vehicles of nosocomial outbreaks include a variety of foods, such as poultry, eggs, meat, dried coconut, protein food supplements, or yeast. Outbreaks also have been related to pharmacologic or diagnostic preparations, especially those of animal origin; pancreatic extract, liver extract, carmine dye, bile salts, pepsin, gelatin, vitamins, thyroid extract, adrenal cortical extract, and pituitary extract have all been implicated as sources of infection.[37]

Cross-infection is especially common in medical institutions,

TABLE 3. The 10 Most Frequently Reported *Salmonella* Serotypes from Human Sources in 1986 and From Nonhuman Sources in 1985

Human Sources 1986			*Nonhuman Sources 1985*		
Serotype	*No. of Isolates*	*% of Total*	*Serotype*	*No. of Isolates*	*% of Total*
1 *S. typhimurium*	10888	25.9	1 *S. typhimurium*	1956	26.4
2 *S. enteritidis*	5967	14.2	2 *S. choleraesuis*	563	7.6
3 *S. heidelberg*	5595	13.3	3 *S. heidelberg*	432	5.8
4 *S. newport*	2431	5.8	4 *S. agona*	259	3.5
5 *S. hadar*	1552	3.7	5 *S. montevideo*	258	3.5
6 *S. infantis*	1104	2.6	6 *S. anatum*	244	3.3
7 *S. agona*	912	2.2	7 *S. saint paul*	220	3.0
8 *S. montevideo*	775	1.8	8 *S. enteritidis*	197	2.7
9 *S. muenchen*	694	1.7	9 *S. san diego*	186	2.5
10 *S. braenderup*	616	1.5	10 *S. newport*	165	2.2
Subtotal	30534	72.7		4480	60.4
Total isolates (all serotypes)	42028	100.0		7417	100.0

(From Centers for Disease Control.[35])

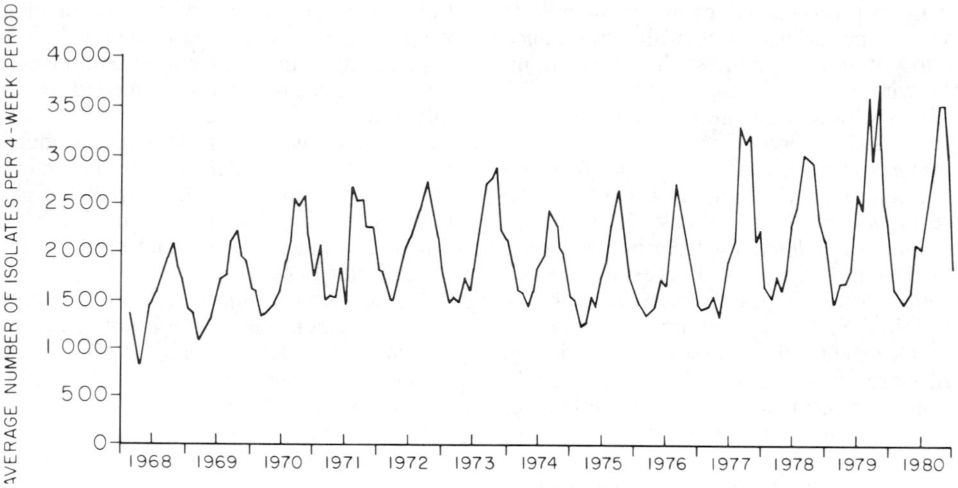

FIG. 1. Seasonal pattern of reported isolations of *Salmonella* in the United States from 1968 through 1980. (From Centers for Disease Control.[35])

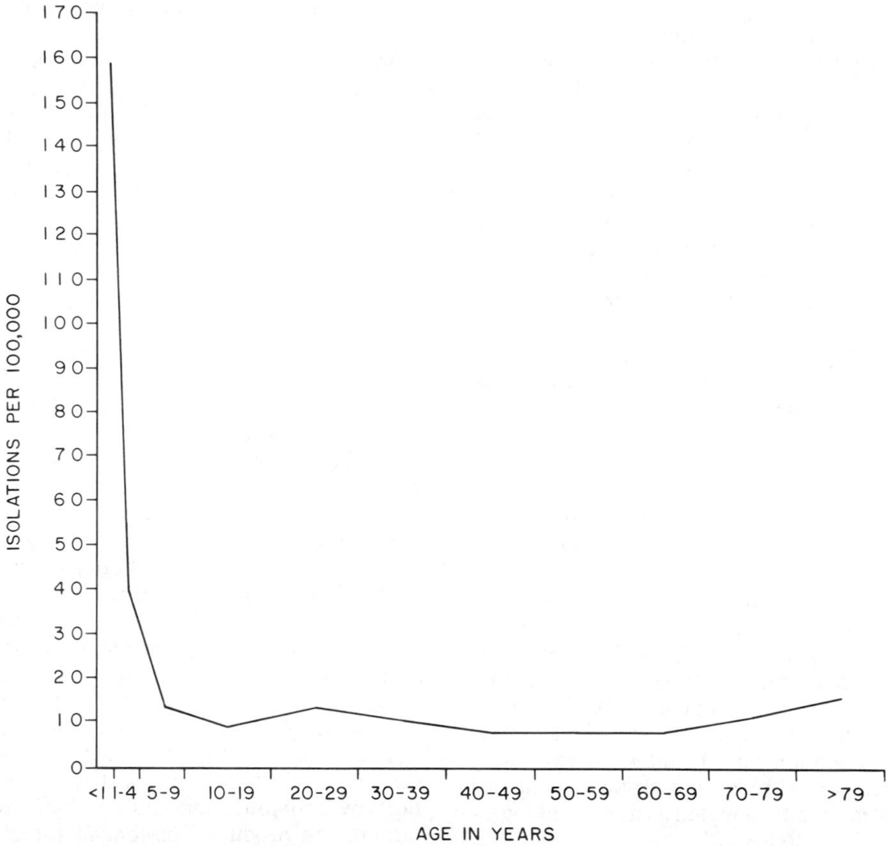

FIG. 2. Isolation rate of *Salmonella* from humans in the United States in 1986 by age group. (From Centers for Disease Control.[35])

accounting for about 60 percent of the nosocomial outbreaks in which the mode of spread is known.[37] Cross-infection with spread by person-to-person contact or by fomites is responsible for virtually all the outbreaks in neonatal nurseries and in pediatric wards and is important in many outbreaks among hospitalized adults.[37,38]

The stage is set for cross-infection when *Salmonella* are introduced into the hospital by admission of, for example, a patient with acute enterocolitis or an asymptomatic carrier with another medical problem or by the introduction of a contaminated common-source vehicle. Hospital personnel then may carry infection on hands or clothing from patient to patient; in some cases, fomites (dust, delivery room suction apparatus, furniture) may be implicated in transmission.[37] Salmonellae have been isolated from vacuum cleaner contents.[39] Diagnostic equipment difficult to sterilize (e.g., fiber-optic endoscopes) has also been implicated in transmission of *Salmonella* infection.[14] Hospital personnel who are excreting *Salmonella* in stools may also occasionally transmit infection to patients.

The vulnerability of hospitalized patients to *Salmonella* infection is related in part to the presence of major underlying diseases and to chemotherapeutic agents that alter resistance to infection. Salmonellosis tends to be unusually severe in institutionalized patients, with an overall case–fatality ratio of 2.3 percent.[37] The case-fatality ratio is highest in nurseries (7.0 percent) and nursing homes (8.7 percent).[37]

There has been a progressive increase in *Salmonella* isolations from humans reported to the Centers for Disease Control during the past 11 years, as shown in Table 4. In 1986, approximately 42,000 isolates of *Salmonella* from humans were reported in the United States.[35] The 1985 figures are skewed upward by the occurrence of the largest *Salmonella* outbreak ever identified in the United States[23]; this outbreak was associated with a low-fat milk product that was widely distributed in Illinois. The overall increase in *Salmonella* infections probably reflects multiple influences, including modern methods of processing foods in bulk and distributing them over wide geographic areas, an increasing number of persons with impaired resistance to infection, wide use of antimicrobials that enhance susceptibility to enteric infection, and better reporting. Nevertheless, *Salmonella* infections are substantially underreported. The number of cases reported in the United States probably represent only 1 to 10 percent of the actual yearly incidence of this infection in the United States.[20,40]

Whereas the incidence of nontyphoidal salmonellosis has actually increased in recent years, there has been an impressive decline in the number of cases of typhoid fever in the United States since 1900.[41,42] The total number of cases of typhoid in the United States currently is less than 500/year or about 0.2 cases per 100,000 per year.[42–44] The decline in incidence of typhoid fever is attributed primarily to improvements in sanitation and, to a smaller extent, to detection and treatment of acute cases and chronic carriers. At least two-thirds of cases of typhoid fever that have occurred in the United States since 1975 can be traced to international travel.[44,45] Tourism in Mexico and India accounts for the majority of the travel-related cases.[42,44,45] In many less well-developed areas of the world, typhoid fever remains endemic, with an annual incidence of 300–500 cases per 100,000 of population in some areas.[44]

PATHOGENESIS

The development of disease after ingestion of *Salmonella* is influenced by the number and virulence of the organisms and by multiple host factors.

A large number of *Salmonella* must be swallowed in most instances to produce disease in healthy human beings. Limited studies with several serotypes, including *S. typhi*, show that, in general, 10^6–10^9 organisms must be ingested to produce symptomatic infection.[18,46,47] However, in the event of infection with unusually virulent organisms or in patients with reduced resistance, symptomatic infection may result from extremely small inocula. In one study, 31 percent of a group of pediatric patients with cystic fibrosis became infected as a result of ingestion of porcine pancreatin, even though less than two organisms were present in each 100 g sample.[48] It is also known that an asymptomatic infection can be established with 10 to 100 times fewer organisms than are needed to produce symptomatic infection.

TABLE 4. *Salmonella* Isolations from Human Sources Reported in the United States from 1976 through 1986

Year	No. of Isolates
1976	23,174
1977	27,071
1978	28,881
1979	31,771
1980	29,338
1981	35,752
1982	37,897
1983	38,886
1984	36,061
1985	56,750
1986	42,028

(From Centers for Disease Control.[35])

Ingested organisms pass from the mouth to the stomach. In the past it was thought that *S. typhi* gained access to the body through the tonsils or pharyngeal lymphatics. However, volunteers gargling large inocula of *S. typhi* (Quailes strain) have failed to acquire disease, and invasion through the pharynx is thought not to occur.[46]

In the stomach *Salmonella* are exposed to gastric acid and low pH, which reduce the number of viable organisms. Most *Salmonella* are killed rapidly at pH 2, which is readily achieved in the normal stomach.[47] Viable bacilli that survive then pass into the small intestine, where the organisms may be further reduced in number or eliminated entirely. The antimicrobial activity observed in the small bowel is related at least in part to the normal microbial flora of the intestine, which elaborate short-chain fatty acids and perhaps other substances capable of killing or inhibiting growth of *Salmonella*. Studies in animals have shown that the increased susceptibility to *Salmonella* infection produced by administration of antibiotics rapidly reverts to normal with reestablishment of the normal intestinal flora.[49,50]

Salmonella that survive the antibacterial mechanisms in the stomach and upper small bowel may multiply in the small intestine. Multiplication of *Salmonella* in the intestinal tract may be asymptomatic, associated only with transient excretion of organisms in stools, or symptomatic, associated with clinical manifestations of either enterocolitis (acute gastroenteritis), enteric fever, or bacteriemia. Blood stream invasion, which occurs with variable frequency, may lead to localization of infection and suppuration at almost any site.

Local factors in the stomach and upper intestinal tract are important determinants of disease. Factors that neutralize the low pH of the stomach or decrease the time the pathogen is exposed to stomach acid diminish local bactericidal action and increase the probability that an infectious inoculum will reach the small intestine. The importance of gastric acidity as a defense mechanism is emphasized by the increased incidence of severe *Salmonella* enterocolitis in persons with achlorhydria, prior gastrectomy, gastroenterostomy, or vagotomy, conditions that reduce acidity or cause faster gastric emptying time.[47,51] The oral administration of buffering compounds also increases susceptibility to intestinal infection.[46,52,53] It has been suggested that ingestion of organisms in food allows for longer exposure to gastric acid, thereby necessitating the presence of a relatively larger inoculum to produce disease, whereas water or other liquids, which have a fast gastric transit time, may be less heavily contaminated and still cause disease.[18]

The small intestine provides other protective mechanisms through motility and normal flora. Alteration of the intestinal flora by antibiotics markedly reduces the size of the inoculum required to produce *Salmonella* infection in animals and humans and prolongs the convalescent carrier state.[46,49,50] Prior antimicrobial therapy also enhances the possibility of infection with antibiotic-resistant *Salmonella* strains.[53,54] Studies of patients with shigellosis suggest that medications that slow intestinal transit time prolong disease, increase the frequency of complications, and extend the convalescent carrier state, but these findings have not yet been extended to patients with *Salmonella* enterocolitis.[55]

Age is an important determinant of disease produced by *Salmonella*. *Salmonella* enterocolitis occurs with highest incidence in children less than 5 years old; newborns and infants less than 1 year of age are especially susceptible. The influence of age on incidence may reflect immaturity of humoral and cellular immune mechanisms, diminished antibacterial action of the normal intestinal flora, a high frequency of fecal–oral contamination, or other factors. In some instances, increasing resistance with age is related to immunity consequent to previous exposure to the organism, even though disease has not been produced.[46] Typhoid fever also occurs with increased frequency in the young in areas of the world such as Mexico, Chile, India, Southeast Asia, and parts of Africa where the disease is endemic. In these areas, adults have acquired substantial resistance through repeated exposure to the organism. However, in more developed areas where enteric fever is not endemic, there is less opportunity for repeated subclinical infections, and the incidence is not age-related.

Patients with impaired cellular and humoral immune mechanisms are at increased risk for development of salmonellosis. Impairments of host defenses caused by malnutrition, malignancy, infection with human immunodeficiency virus or therapeutic measures such as corticosteroid or immunosuppressive therapy also predispose to infection and disease.

In a study of cases admitted to the Johns Hopkins Hospital and the New York Hospital from 1936 to 1958, a major underlying disease was present in 36 percent of 178 patients with *Salmonella* enterocolitis and in 40 percent of 127 patients with *Salmonella* bacteremia, enteric fever, or localized infection.[47] In this study, underlying diseases of the gastrointestinal tract (gastrectomy; achlorhydria; esophageal, gastric, or intestinal malignancies; inflammatory diseases of the bowel) appeared to be common predisposing factors in patients with enterocolitis. The relative importance of changes in intestinal flora, motility, pH, transit time, or other factors in the altered susceptibility is unknown. Patients with enteric fever, bacteremia, or localized infection were more likely to have an underlying disease of the hematopoietic system (sickle hemoglobinopathy, hemolysis, leukemia, or lymphoma) as the associated, predisposing problem. Other studies have confirmed a high percentage of serious underlying disease in patients with *Salmonella* infections.[56,57]

Patients with sickle hemoglobinopathies, malaria, and bartonellosis, all associated with hemolysis, have an increased incidence of *Salmonella* infection. The mechanisms responsible for the alterations in susceptibility in these diverse disease states are multiple and complex. A defect in the alternative complement pathway has been demonstrated in patients with sickle cell anemia and may be causally related to the marked susceptibility of patients with sickle hemoglobinopathies to serious bacteremic infection and osteomyelitis with *Salmonella*.[58] Hemolysis induced experimentally in mice markedly enhances susceptibility to challenge with *S. typhimurium*.[59] Furthermore, in vitro studies have shown that erythrophagocytosis by monocytes impairs the capacity of these cells to phagocytize and kill *Salmonella*.[60] Impairment of host defense may also be related to splenic infarctions leading to autosplenectomy, damage to the immune system resulting in interference with humoral or cellular defenses, or other factors.

Salmonella play a prominent role among the severe systemic infections encountered in patients with acquired immunodeficiency syndrome (AIDS).[61–63] This is not surprising considering the importance of cell-mediated immunity in eradicating *Salmonella* from intracellular sites. Suppression of cellular immunity may account for the tendency of *Salmonella* infections in renal transplant recipients to relapse.[64]

Salmonella serotypes vary in propensity for production of one or the other of the clinical syndromes seen in infected patients. For example, *S. anatum* produces predominantly asymptomatic infection or diarrheal illness and rarely penetrates the intestinal defenses to cause bacteremia.[18] In contrast, certain *Salmonella* serotypes, such as *S. typhi*, regularly penetrate the intestinal mucosa to produce the clinical picture of enteric fever. Other organisms, such as *S. choleraesuis*, regularly invade the blood stream to produce a bacteremic syndrome often associated with localized infection but without the typical manifestations of enteric fever.[65] The particular features of the organism that determine type of disease have not been defined.

Salmonella causing enterocolitis are thought to produce diarrhea by a true infection with mucosal invasion and possibly by elaboration of an enterotoxin that acts on upper intestinal transport. Mucosal invasion alone is not sufficient to account for the intestinal fluid observed in experimental infections.[66] However, *Salmonella* invasion of intestinal mucosa may lead to local production in inflammatory exudates of mediators that stimulate electrolyte secretion and smooth muscle contraction.[67,68] Additional studies are required for definitive characterization of the mechanisms involved in the pathogenesis of *Salmonella* enterocolitis.

The pathogenesis of enteric fever has been extensively studied.[46] The site at which *S. typhi* penetrates the intestinal barrier in man has not been defined with certainty. Jejunal biopsy specimens from infected humans reveal inflammation, suggesting the possibility that the jejunum may be the site of penetration in some patients.[69] However, in the murine typhoid model, penetration probably occurs in the distal ilium where *S. typhimurium* attaches to the microvilli of the brush border; it appears that specific receptors for the organism exist since organisms are attached to less than 5 percent of the microville.[18,70,71] The bacteria apparently invade through Peyer's patches.[72]

Once past the intestinal mucosa, organisms are transported to intestinal lymph follicles where multiplication takes place within mononuclear cells.[46] The pathologic changes in the lymph follicle are characterized by hyperplasia and monocytic inflammatory infiltrates. Poorer phagocytosis by monocytes than by polymorphonuclear leukocytes may account for the progression of organisms to mesenteric lymph nodes and eventually through the thoracic duct to the blood stream; circulating organisms are then removed by reticuloendothelial cells in liver, spleen, and bone marrow.[18] The reticuloendothelial cells undergo hyperplasia. Bloodborne organisms reach the gallbladder, multiply, and secondarily seed the intestine in bile.[73]

Many studies have been directed at the cause of the prolonged fever and toxic symptoms of enteric fever.[45,74,75] For years, circulating endotoxins, lipopolysaccharide components of the bacterial cell wall, were implicated. Injection of an endotoxin into healthy volunteers produces symptoms (headache, fever, abdominal pain, and malaise) and laboratory findings (anemia, leukopenia) remarkably similar to findings in the same volunteers during actual *S. typhi* infection.[46] Furthermore, morphologic lesions similar to those observed in typhoid fever can be produced in rabbits by parenteral administration of endotoxin.[74] Acquired tolerance to the pyrogenic effects of endotoxin has been demonstrated in patients recovering from typhoid fever, suggesting release of endotoxin during the course of infection and a mechanism for resolution of illness. However, other studies argue against circulating endotoxin having a role in the pathogenesis of enteric fever caused by *Salmonella*[76] Volunteers rendered tolerant by repeated parenteral injections of endotoxin developed characteristic signs and symptoms of typhoid fever when experimentally infected with *S. typhi*.[74] In addition, efforts to reproduce a steady febrile state analogous to that seen in typhoid fever by continuous infusion of endotoxin have been unsuccessful because of the rapid development of tolerance. Limulus assay has failed to detect significant circulating endotoxin in symptomatic patients with positive blood cultures for *S. typhi*.[75]

Hornick and Greisman hypothesize that endotoxin contributes to the pathogenesis of enteric fever by enhancing local inflammatory responses at the tissue sites of *S. typhi* multiplication. They suggest that sustained fever is the result of augmented synthesis and release of pyrogen from local inflammatory lesions.[76] Others have suggested that mediators released from mononuclear cells, primarily macrophages, are responsible for the clinical manifestations.[44]

Studies of typhoid fever in volunteers have provided data on the size of inoculum needed to produce disease. Table 5 shows the results with inocula of different sizes of the Quailes strain

TABLE 5. Influence of Inoculum by Oral Route on Incubation Period in Experimental Typhoid Fever in Volunteers

Number of Viable S. typhi	Number with Disease / Number Exposed (Percent)	Incubation Period (Days) Median	Range
10^9	40/42(95)	5	3–32
10^7	16/32(50)	7.5	4–56
10^5	32/116(28)	9	6–33

(From Hornick et al.,[46] with permission.)

of *S. typhi*.[46] The dose required to produce typhoid fever in about 50 percent of healthy volunteers is about 10^7 organisms of this strain given by the oral route. The Quailes strain, like most *S. typhi* and some other *Salmonella* serotypes, has a surface Vi antigen that may inhibit phagocytosis and serum bactericidal activity and that seems to correlate somewhat with the capacity of the organisms to invade the body and to produce disease.[46] In experimental studies, the inoculum required to produce disease is smaller for organisms with Vi antigen than for those without it.[46] In addition, disease associated with Vi-positive strains is characterized by a larger proportion of positive blood and stool cultures than disease caused by the Vi-negative strains.[46] When *Salmonella* lacking Vi antigens are compared, striking variation among serotypes is still encountered in the size of inoculum required to produce disease. Many factors other than Vi antigen obviously are involved in determining the capacity of *Salmonella* to produce disease in the human host.

Localization of *Salmonella* in bone, meninges, heart, lungs, kidneys, spleen, and other organs or tissues can lead to focal abscesses. Abscesses and localized infections are characterized by a polymorphonuclear response; this is true of localized infection even in patients with typhoid fever, where a mononuclear response is observed in typhoidal lesions in the intestines and other tissues. The presence of pre-existing disease resulting in necrotic, scarred, or hyperplastic tissue favors localization of blood-borne organisms. Localized *Salmonella* infections have been seen in many types of benign and malignant tumors, cysts, aneurysms, bone infarctions (as in sickle cell anemia), hematomas, intramuscular injection sites, and effusions into serous cavities.[16] Gallbladder disease, especially stones, seems to favor persistence of *Salmonella* in the biliary tract and predisposes to the chronic enteric carrier state. Involvement of the urinary tract with *Schistosoma hematobium*, with resultant fibrosis and stone formation, leads to an increased incidence of the urinary tract carrier state of *Salmonella* in areas of the world where *S. hematobium* infection is common.[77] Eradication of the urinary carrier state of *Salmonella* can be achieved by treatment of the schistosomiasis. In Brazil, a prolonged bacteremia with *Salmonella* has been described in patients with hepatosplenic schistosomiasis due to *S. mansoni*[78,79] The illness is characterized by prolonged fever, severe anemia, and marked splenomegaly. A somewhat similar syndrome of bacteremia and low-grade fever has been described in patients with *S. hematobium* in Egypt[77,80,81] The same relationship probably exists between *S. japonicum* and *Salmonella*.[82] In these patients, the *Salmonella* apparently have localized in the integument or gut of mature intravascular *Schistosoma* worms, where they are protected from host defenses. Cure of the schistosomasis results in elimination of the *Salmonella* infection.

CLINICAL MANIFESTATIONS

The relative prominence of certain clinical manifestations in persons infected with *Salmonella* forms the basis for the designation of several clinical syndromes: enterocolitis (gastroenteritis), enteric fever, bacteremia, localized infection, and the chronic enteric or urinary carrier state. It should be emphasized that these designations do not delineate well-defined diseases but syndromes or states that may shade one into the other. For example, although gastroenteritis is characteristically a brief illness with diarrhea, fever, positive stool cultures, and negative blood cultures, it may be complicated occasionally by bacteremia or even by localized infection or may be followed by a clinical course characteristic of enteric fever.

Enterocolitis

Acute enterocolitis, also known as gastroenteritis, is the most common clinical expression of *Salmonella* infection. Six to 48 hours after ingestion of contaminated food or water, illness begins in many patients with nausea and vomiting; these symptoms usually resolve within a few hours. Myalgia and headache are common. The cardinal manifestation is diarrhea, which may vary from a few loose stools to fulminant diarrhea.[18,83] In most cases, stools are loose, of moderate volume, and without blood. In exceptional cases, the stools may be watery and of great volume ("choleralike"), or, in other instances, of small volume and associated with tenesmus and gross blood ("dysentery-like"). Temperature elevations to 38–39°C are common, as are chills; both appear in the majority of patients in whom definitive diagnosis is established. Abdominal cramps occur in about two-thirds of the patients and are often localized to the periumbilical region or lower abdominal quadrants.[83] Bowel sounds are increased and abdominal tenderness is present. On microscopic examination, stools show a moderate number of polymorphonuclear leukocytes and, occasionally, red blood cells. Gross blood is unusual but may be seen in severe cases. Peripheral leukocyte count is usually normal, although neutrophilia with a shift toward younger forms may be present.

The duration of fever is less than 2 days in the majority of cases. Diarrhea usually persists less than 7 days, although, rarely, gastrointestinal symptoms may last for several weeks. Prolonged fever and diarrhea suggest a complication or a different diagnosis.

Localization of pain in the right lower quadrant of the abdomen in patients with enterocolitis may lead to a diagnosis of acute appendicitis. At surgery, such patients may have normal appendices or occasionally acute appendicitis, rarely with perforation.

Studies on patients with acute intestinal infection with *Salmonella* have demonstrated that colon involvement is much more common than previously assumed.[84–86] In fact, some studies that have included sigmoidoscopic examination and biopsy of colon mucosa have shown active colitis in most patients with acute intestinal infection caused by *Salmonella*.[84] The colon mucosa shows hyperemia, petechiae, and, in severe cases, a friable mucosa with ulceration. Histologic features include edema, inflammation, erosions, and microabscesses. Because of the frequency of colon involvement, the term "enterocolitis" rather than "gastroenteritis" has been used in this chapter to describe acute intestinal infection with *Salmonella*.

Electrolyte and water depletion may be severe during illness, leading to hypovolemic shock. Toxic dilatation of the colon has been described as a rare complication.[84] The disease is more severe in children, in the elderly, and in patients with achlorhydria, gastrectomy, gastroenterostomy, sickle cell anemia, or other conditions that impair resistance to infection. The frequency of transient bacteremia, estimated to be less than 5 percent in adults, is increased in children and in persons with major underlying diseases. Bacteremia has been shown to occur in 8–16 percent of infants and children 3 years of age or younger who are hospitalized with *Salmonella* enterocolitis and deemed sufficiently ill to require blood culture.[87] In the absence of documented risk factors, the morbidity of infection is the same in enterocolitis patients with or without bacteremia.[87] *Salmonella* intestinal infections tend to be prolonged in children, who continue to excrete organisms in stools for a longer time than adults after clinical manifestations of infection have subsided.

Salmonella enterocolitis can develop in patients who are already hospitalized. The illness may be a nosocomial infection or it may result from activation of pre-existing asymptomatic intestinal infection by antimicrobial therapy, abdominal surgery, or other means.

The differential diagnosis includes viral gastroenteritis, other bacterial enteritides (e.g., those caused by *Shigella, Staphylococcus aureus*, enterotoxin-producing *E. coli, Campylobacter fetus, Vibrio parahaemolyticus, Yersinia enterocolitica*, and *Vibrio cholerae*), pseudomembraneous colitis, inflammatory or granulomatous bowel disease, and certain causes of "surgical abdomen," including acute appendicitis and perforated viscus.

Diagnosis is made by stool culture. Blood cultures are negative in the majority of cases. Agglutination tests are of no value in diagnosis.

One-third to two-thirds of children over 5 years of age and adults continue to have positive stool cultures during the second or third week after onset of illness, even though most patients are totally asymptomatic by that time.[36,88,89] Approximately 5–15 percent of the patients continue to shed organisms in feces for 1–2 months after onset. Almost all adults have negative stool cultures by 6 months after onset; *Salmonella* persist longer in the stools of infants and children than in adults.[89] In the review by Buchwald and Blaser, the median duration of persistence of *Salmonella* in stools was 7 weeks for patients younger than 5 years and 3–4 weeks for older children and adults.[90] Only 40 percent of children younger than 5 years were culture-negative at 20 weeks, whereas 90 percent of older children and adults were negative at that time. Chronic enteric carriers, persons known to excrete *Salmonella* in feces for 1 year or longer, are rare after infections with nontyphoidal *Salmonella* serotypes.

Enteric Fever

Enteric fever is a clinical syndrome produced classically by *S. typhi* and also at times by *S. paratyphi* A, *S. schottmuelleri* (formerly *paratyphi* B), and *S. hirschfeldii* (formerly *paratyphi* C). *Salmonella* serotypes other than those mentioned above can occasionally produce the clinical picture of enteric fever. Enteric fever produced by *S. typhi* is called typhoid fever and that produced by *Salmonella* serotypes other than *S. typhi* is termed paratyphoid fever.

Typhoid fever, the best studied enteric fever, is a severe prolonged disease with a high rate of complications. The clinical features of typhoid and paratyphoid fevers are essentially the same, although paratyphoid tends to be a milder illness than typhoid.[33,46,73,91,92]

The incubation period of typhoid fever is usually 10–14 days but may vary from 7 to 21 days. The incubation period is influenced by the number of organisms ingested. Studies in volunteers ingesting Quailes strain *S. typhi* in milk show an increase in incubation period with decreasing dose of viable organisms (see Table 5).[46] Administration of effective antimicrobials after ingestion of *S. typhi* may prolong the incubation period of typhoid fever.[46]

Manifestations of enterocolitis occasionally occur within hours after the ingestion of food or drink contaminated with *S. typhi* if the dose of organisms is large. In these instances, symptoms of nausea, vomiting, and diarrhea usually resolve completely before the onset of symptoms of typhoid fever.

The onset of typhoid is insidious, in contrast to sepsis produced by most other gram-negative organisms. The initial manifestations are nonspecific and consist of fever, malaise, anorexia, headache, and myalgias. Remittent fever is prominent, with gradually increasing evening temperature elevations from less than 38°C to values in the range of 40°C by the end of the first week of illness. Chills and diaphoreses are seen in about one-third of the patients even in the absence of antimicrobial or antipyretic therapy.[92] Either constipation or diarrhea may occur. Respiratory symptoms, including cough and sore throat, may be prominent. Neuropsychiatric manifestations, including confusion, dizziness, seizures, or acute psychotic behavior, may be predominant in an occasional case.[92,93]

The symptoms of typhoid fever in three large series as tabulated by Hoffman and colleagues are shown in Table 6.[92] Cough, muscle pains, constipation, weakness, and sore thorat were much more common in the Stuart and Pullen series collected in the preantibiotic era than in the other series representative of the antibiotic era.[31,91,92] The factors that account for the differences in the series are not defined, but differences in duration of illness in pre- and postantibiotic eras are probably important.

There is also wide variation in reported frequency of physical signs in typhoid fever, as shown in Table 7.[92] The patient with typhoid fever usually appears acutely ill. Fever is usually prominent, and in many instances the pulse is slow relative to the temperature. Rose spots, 2–4 mm erythematous maculopapular lesions that blanch on pressure, appear characteristically on the upper abdomen in crops of approximately 10 lesions. The lesions are transient and resolve in hours to days.[94] Rose spots are observed in less than 50 percent of the patients. Cervical lymphadenopathy may be present. Examination of the chest may reveal moist rales. The abdomen is tender, especially in the lower quadrants. Abdominal distention is common, and peristalsis is often hypoactive. The sensation of displacing air- and fluid-filled loops of bowel on palpating the abdomen is said to be characteristic.[46] Hepatomegaly is noted in about 25–50 percent of the patients, and a soft, tender spleen can be palpated in about 40–60 percent.[92,95] In about 10 percent of the patients, changes in level of consciousness are present and consist of lethargy, delirium, or coma.[92]

Without antimicrobial therapy, the disease pursues a prolonged course with slow resolution of signs and symptoms

TABLE 6. Symptoms of Typhoid Fever from Three Large Series

Symptoms	*1973 Dade County Outbreak[92] (105 Patients) (Percent)*	*1964 Aberdeen Outbreak[32] (507 Patients) (Percent)*	*1939–1944 Stuart and Pullen Series[91] (360 Patients) (Percent)*
Fever	93	75	100
Headache	59	78	90
Diarrhea	57	37	43
Anorexia	39	NA[a]	91
Abdominal pain	39	35	19
Chills	37	16	37
Vomiting	35	24	54
Cough	28	37	86
Nausea	23	NA	54
Muscle pains	12	25	91
Constipation	10	38	79
Weakness	10	NA	87
Sore throat	6	NA	84
Dizziness	3	NA	25
Seizures	1	0	0

[a] Not available.

TABLE 7. Signs of Typhoid Fever from Three Large Series

Symptoms	*1973 Dade County Outbreak[84] (105 Patients) (Percent)*	*1964 Aberdeen Outbreak[29] (507 Patients) (Percent)*	*1939–1944 Stuart and Pullen Series[83] (360 Patients) (Percent)*
Rose spots	13	46	33
Cervical adenopathy	10	NA[a]	NA
Rales	4	NA	64
Hepatomegaly	52	15	25
Splenomegaly	42	39	64
Neurologic manifestations	5	12	12

[a] Not available.

3–4 weeks after onset if there are no complications. Sustained fever is common during the second and third weeks of disease. Fever decreases slowly by lysis, unlike the resolution by crisis seen in the preantibiotic era in many cases of pneumococcal pneumonia. Headache, confusion, respiratory symptoms, and abdominal pain and distention gradually resolve, and the pulse more characteristically reflects degree of fever. Weakness persists after acute manifestations have subsided. Profound weight loss invariably occurs in the untreated patient. Many of the complications of enteric fever occur during the period of resolution in the third of fourth week after onset.

Therapy with chloramphenicol, amipicillin, or the combination of trimethoprim-sulfamethoxazole shortens the duration of illness. Fever customarily resolves in 3–5 days after initiation of chloramphenicol, but response is influenced by the stage of disease, by complications, and by other factors.

Laboratory findings vary with stage of illness. Anemia develops rather rapidly and reaches a nadir at the end of the third week of illness in the untreated patient, even in the absence of intestinal hemorrhage. Transient leukocytosis may occur during the first 7–10 days of illness, but leukopenia (predominantly neutropenia) subsequently develops and is most severe during the third week of disease. Leukocyte counts ranging from 1200 to 20,000 cells/mm^3 are observed in apparently uncomplicated cases of typhoid.[91] In the Dade County epidemic, the white blood cell count was normal in 74 percent of the patients on admission to the hospital.[92] Despite the presence of rales in some patients, chest roentgenograms are usually normal. The electrocardiogram is normal in most cases, but patients with severe illness may exhibit nonspecific changes in the S-T segment and T waves. Abnormalities of clotting consistent with disseminated intravascular coagulation, including thrombocytopenia, hypofibrinogenemia, or increased levels of circulating fibrinogen-related antigens, have been reported in more than one-half of the patients.[75] There is no correlation of these values with clinical bleeding, and clotting abnormalities resolve with resolution of illness. In the Dade County epidemic, thrombocytopenia or evidence of coagulopathy was detected only occasionally.[92] Transient mild elevations in serum enzyme levels are common during the acute illness. Increased levels of serum glutamic oxaloacetic transaminase (SGOT), alkaline phosphatase, and serum lactic acid dehydrogenase (LDH) occur in one-third or more of patients, and elevations of hydroxybutyric dehydrogenase (HBD) and creatine phosphokinase (CPK) levels are not unusual.[92,93] Jaundice occurs rarely.[93] *Salmonella* antigens of apparently intact bacilli can be demonstrated in hepatic parenchyma of patients with "typhoid hepatitis."[96] A transient mild proteinuria is common during the first week of illness, but abnormalities of creatinine clearance, blood urea nitrogen, and serum creatinine are not seen in uncomplicated cases. Renal biopsy specimens from a few patients with transient proteinuria demonstrated immune complex glomerulitis with Vi antigen in glomerular capillary walls; a later biopsy of one patient showed rapid resolution of glomerulitis.[97] IgA nephropathy with clinical features of gross hematuria, heavy proteinuria, and pathological findings of glomerulonephritis with Vi antigen and IgA in the glomeruli has also been reported in enteric fever.[98]

Definitive diagnosis of typhoid fever is made on the basis of isolation of the organism from the blood. Isolation of the organism from stool, especially in endemic areas, does not establish the diagnosis but does constitute strong presumptive evidence of typhoid in the patient with a typical clinical course. Serologic studies may be helpful, but in many cases of typhoid fever there is no increase in titer of agglutinins during the course of infection, and other illnesses, especially infections with other gram-negative bacilli, may cause nonspecific elevations of agglutinins because of cross-reacting antigens.[99]

In the absence of antimicrobial therapy, blood cultures are positive in over 80 percent of the patients seen in the first week of illness.[91] Twenty to 30 percent of the patients not treated with antimicrobials have positive blood cultures as late as the third week of illness. The majority of isolates of *S. typhi* from blood are obtained as a result of the first blood culture, but a second or third culture should be collected in suspected cases, as these cultures significantly improve the percentage of positives. Culture of bone marrow from the iliac crest, although less practicable than blood culture, yields positive results in about 90 percent of patients with typhoid or paratyphoid fever and is the single most effective method of isolating the causative organism.[44,100,101] Stool cultures, occasionally positive during the incubation period, become positive again in about one-third to two-thirds of the patients during the second through fourth weeks of illness.[46,91]

Antimicrobial therapy diminishes the possibility of recovery of the causative agent from blood, urine, and stool. Prior therapy with antimicrobials is frequent, a result either of self-medication or physicians' treatment of "fever of unknown origin." In patients who have received antimicrobial therapy, cultures of supplementary sites such as bone marrow or even skin snips from rose spots may be a better source of organisms than blood, stool, or urine.[102] The results of bone marrow culture are said not to be influenced by prior chloramphenicol therapy.[100,101] In volunteers infected with *S. typhi* for vaccine studies, culture of a string passed into the duodenum and left there for 12 hours was positive in three of seven cases.[103] The yield of this maneuver in naturally occurring disease is probably no better than cultures of blood and rectal swab.[100]

Serologic studies, although at times helpful, are not reliable in diagnosis. In untreated disease, only about 50 percent of the patients have a fourfold or greater increase in titer of agglutinins (Widal test) against typhoid O antigen at any time during the course of disease. Antimicrobial therapy may also impede immunologic response. In the Dade County epidemic, only 24 percent of patients showed a fourfold or greater increase in antibody titer against O antigen; the titer actually decreased or remained low in 60 percent of patients during therapy.[92] Immunization with typhoid vaccine may produce an impressive increase in titer of anti-O agglutinins, and nonspecific changes in titer may occur during the course of many febrile illnesses. Agglutinins against H antigens, irrespective of change of titer, are not of value in diagnosis. A number of other serodiagnostic methods, e.g., detection of IgM antibody to *S. typhi* lipopolysaccharide antigen by an enzyme-linked immunosorbent assay (ELISA), are being studied and seem promising, but none is ready for routine diagnostic use.[104]

Complications of typhoid fever can be classified as secondary to toxemia (myocarditis, hyperpyrexia, hepatic and bone marrow damage), secondary to local gastrointestinal lesions (hemorrhage and perforation), secondary to prolonged severe illness (suppurative parotitis, decubiti, and pneumonia), secondary to growth and persistence of typhoid bacilli (relapse, localized infection—e.g., meningitis, endocarditis, osteomyelitis, or arthritis—and the chronic carrier state), and secondary to therapy (bone marrow suppression, hypersensitivity reactions, and toxic crisis).[105] In the preantimicrobial era, 12–16 percent of the patients with typhoid fever died, frequently from complications in the third or fourth week of the disease.[91,105] Fatalities still occur occasionally, probably in less than one percent of the patients receiving appropriate antimicrobial and supportive therapy.[44] However, in certain specific geographic areas of Indonesia, India, and Nigeria, case fatality ratios of 9–32 percent have been reported in the past 10–15 years. It is likely that these results are consequent to suboptimal health and medical care rather than an increase in the clinical severity of typhoid fever.[44]

The complications attributed to "toxemia" might well be considered manifestations of severe disease. Toxic myocarditis occurs in severely ill patients, frequently children, and is manifested by tachycardia, weak pulse, muffled heart sounds, and hypotension. The electrocardiogram shows low voltage and T-wave flattening or inversion. Atrial or ventricular arrhythmias may occur. At postmortem, myocardial cells show necrosis, degeneration, and fatty infiltration, although there is some question as to whether these changes reflect a true myocarditis. Profound hyperpyrexia and fulminant hepatic failure are seen rarely. It is usually not possible to say with certainty that hepatic damage is due to typhoid or to an associated condition such as viral hepatitis. Transient bone marrow depression manifested by leukopenia and anemia is common, but persistent bone marrow aplasia rarely, if ever, occurs in the absence of chloramphenicol therapy.

Sequential changes in the lymphoid tissue in the ileocecal area of the intestinal tract occur during typhoid fever and have been classified into four phases: (*1*) hyperplasia, (*2*) necrosis and sloughing, (*3*) ulceration, and (*4*) healing.[73] During the first week of clinical symptoms, hyperplastic changes occur in Peyer's patches in the ileum and in lymphoid follicles in the cecum, causing these tissues to project into the bowel lumen. The hyperplasia regresses after 7–10 days or undergoes necrosis with sloughing of overlying mucosa leading to the formation of characteristic ulcers that parallel the long axis of the ileum. Small punctuate lesions develop in the cecum. Ulcers usually heal completely with little residual scarring, but they may be the sites of hemorrhage or may penetrate to the serosa and lead to bowel perforation. Major intestinal hemorrhage is usually a late complication that occurs during the second or third week of illness. In the preantimicrobial era, gross intestinal hemorrhage occurred in about 5–7 percent of the patients with typhoid, although Stuart and Pullen reported hemorrhage in 21 percent of the patients.[91,105] The incidence of hemorrhage requiring transfusion has been reduced to 1 or 2 percent since the advent of chloramphenicol use.[105] Intestinal hemorrhage rarely causes death. Intestinal perforation usually occurs during the second or third week of illness.[73,105] Perforation is typically single but may be multiple and occurs with the greatest frequency in the terminal ileum where the number of lymphoid aggregates is largest and ulcerations most frequent. In general, perforation has been reported in recent years in 1 percent or less of cases as compared with 2–5 percent in several series collected in the preantibiotic era.[105] Occasional series continue to report high complication rates, e.g., Gupta and colleagues in 1985 reported 125 cases from India in which gut perforations occurred in 9.6 percent of the cases.[106]

Complications of prolonged illness—parotitis, decubitis ulcers, severe wasting—are less severe in antimicrobial-treated patients in whom the duration of the febrile, debilitating illness has been greatly reduced. Pneumonia with patchy or lobar infiltrates can be found in 1–8 percent of the cases and usually occurs late in the illness; the causative bacterium may be the pneumococcus or another microorganism but is seldom *S. typhi*.

Relapse, a recurrence of the manifestations of typhoid after initial clinical response, occurs in about 8–12 percent of the patients who have not received antimicrobial therapy.[46,73,91,105] Antimicrobial therapy may increase the rate of relapse. In several studies, the relapse rate was found to be doubled in patients receiving chloramphenicol therapy for 2 weeks. Ampicillin probably does not affect the rate of relapse. Studies of patients given trimethoprim–sulfamethoxazole indicate that the rate of relapse may be somewhat less than that in patients treated with chloramphenicol.[107–109]

Localization of infection, which may lead to abscess formation, can occur in almost any organ or tissue. Although bacteremia can be assumed to develop in all patients with typhoid, localized infections such as meningitis, endocarditis, osteomyelitis, or thyroiditis occur in less than 1 percent. Pleural effusion occurs in a few patients and may progress to empyema.[110]

The chronic carrier state is defined as documented excretion of *S. typhi* in stool or urine for a year or more. The chronic carrier state usually follows typhoid fever, but as many as one-third of the chronic carriers give no history consistent with this illness. Underlying biliary or urinary tract diseases, especially with stone formation, increase the probability of the chronic enteric or urinary carrier state in patients with typhoid fever. One to 3 percent of the patients with typhoid fever become chronic enteric carriers; however, the incidence is higher in older patients (10.1 percent in the sixth decade) and in women.[111]

Antimicrobial therapy may lead to complications in patients with typhoid fever. The rare idiosyncratic reaction to chloramphenicol characterized by severe aplastic anemia occurs in about 1 of 25,000 persons treated with this antibiotic. Ampicillin and amoxicillin produce rashes and hypersensitivity reactions, and trimethoprim–sulfamethoxazole may cause bone marrow suppression and abnormalities in hepatic function. Toxic crises in patients with typhoid are exacerbations of symptoms of toxemia temporally related to administration of antibiotics. These reactions have been attributed to sudden release of endotoxin and are considered analogous to the Jarisch–Herxheimer reaction seen in patients with syphilis treated with penicillin. The relationship of these "reactions" to antimicrobial therapy is by no means clearly established.[105]

The differential diagnosis of typhoid fever requires consideration of many disease processes characterized by fever and abdominal complaints. Early in the disease the predominance of fever and upper respiratory tract symptoms may suggest influenza or other viral infections. Cough and fever suggest acute bronchitis and, when coupled with rales, raise the question of bacterial pneumonia. Headache, confusion, and fever may prompt consideration of bacterial or aseptic meningitis or meningoencephalitis. Delirium, catatonia, or coma may suggest a diagnosis of psychosis or other neuropsychiatric illness. The abdominal findings may lead to a consideration of acute appendicitis, acute cholecystitis, or intestinal infarction. Bacillary, amebic, or ischemic colitis may enter the differential diagnosis if bloody diarrhea occurs. As fever continues over a period of weeks, other possibilities might include brucellosis, yersinosis, lymphoma, inflammatory bowel disease, Whipple's disease, bacterial endocarditis, miliary tuberculosis, or malaria.

Bacteremia

Salmonella can produce an illness characterized by fever and sustained bacteremia without manifestations of enterocolitis or enteric fever. This syndrome may be caused by any *Salmonella* serotype. Even though blood isolates account for only a small proportion of all *S. typhimurium* isolates from humans, the frequency of infection with this serotype makes it the most common cause of *Salmonella* bacteremia in the United States.[112] *Salmonella choleraesuis* seems to be especially invasive; isolates of this organism are more frequent from blood than from stool.[65,112,113]

The clinical syndrome of *Salmonella* bacteremia is characterized by a hectic febrile course lasting for days or weeks. The organism is isolated from blood, but stool cultures are often negative. Localized suppurative infections develop in about 10 percent of the patients and may become apparent days, months, or even years after the initial bacteremia. Mortality in *S. choleraesuis* infections is higher than in other *Salmonella* infections.

The *Salmonella* bacteremia syndrome is common in patients with AIDS. Organisms are difficult to eradicate from tissue even with prolonged therapy with bactericidal agents, and repeated relapses of infection are common. *Salmonella* bacteremia may be the initial clinical manifestation of AIDS.[61–63,114–116]

Local Infections

Localization of infection may occur at any site after *Salmonella* bacteremia irrespective of the associated clinical syndrome. As might be anticipated, localization at distant sites occurs relatively frequently in patients with the *Salmonella* bacteremia syndrome but rarely in patients with enterocolitis. Localized infection has been reported in the thyroid, meninges, bone, heart, lungs, kidney, adrenals, pancreas, spleen, liver, testes, pericardium, soft tissues, areas of necrosis or infarction, benign or malignant tumors, and cysts.[16,113] The site determines to a large extent the clinical manifestations, although most patients have spiking fever and polymorphonuclear leukocytosis.

Meningitis.[56,113,117–121] Meningitis is a rare complication of *Salmonella* infection and occurs almost exclusively in infants, particularly neonates. Even epidemics of meningitis have been reported during outbreaks of *Salmonella* infection in hospital nurseries. Clinical manifestations are the same as those of any bacterial meningitis in this age group. The clinical course is usually long and marked by relapse. Acute neurologic complications are common and include subdural empyema, cerebral abscesses, and ventriculitis. Acute or chronic hydrocephalus may occur. Mortality is high, probably 40–60 percent, despite appropriate antimicrobial therapy.

Pleuropulmonary Disease.[56,110,113,119,122,123] Saphra and Winter[113] reported 85 cases of respiratory tract involvement with *Salmonella*. Pneumonia or empyema, the predominant types of serious respiratory disease, occur usually in elderly patients or in patients with underlying diseases such as diabetes mellitus, malignancy, cardiovascular disease, or pulmonary disease. Mortality is high. Lung abscesses and infection of malignant pleural effusions also have been reported. *Salmonella* may colonize the upper respiratory tract; thus presence of these organisms in sputum does not necessarily imply lower tract infections.

Endocarditis and Pericarditis.[113,119,124] *Salmonella* endocarditis is very rare. Using strict criteria, Cohen and colleagues found only 42 cases reported since 1939. Seventy-six percent of the patients had pre-existing heart disease, including rheumatic valvular disease, ventricular aneurysm, prosthetic valves, or calcific aortic stenosis. Even with appropriate antibiotic therapy, mortality is extremely high.

Only 10 well-documented cases of purulent pericarditis caused by *Salmonella* have been described in the English literature in the antibiotic era. Prior myocardial infarction, ventricular aneurysm, and gastrectomy seem to be common predisposing conditions.

Arteritis.[56,119,125–127] The literature contains reports of more than 50 cases of *Salmonella* infection with localization in major vessels, including the thoracic and abdominal aortas, coronary arteries, peripheral arteries, arteriovenous fistulae, and aortofemoral bypass grafts. Atherosclerotic infrarenal aortic aneurysms are by far the most common vascular sites of localization. The risk of endothelial infection is high in persons over the age of 50 years who have *Salmonella* bacteremia; more than 90 percent of the reported cases of *Salmonella* arteritis are in patients older than 50 years of age. The distribution of *Salmonella* serotypes associated with this type of vascular infection is similar to that causing salmonellosis in general, except that *S. choleraesuis* is disproportionately represented (over 30 percent), probably because of the high rate of bacteremia associated with this serotype. The mechanism of arterial infection is thought to be direct implantation at a site of endothelial injury in the bacteremia patient or to extension from an adjacent inflammatory lesion such as vertebral osteomyelitis. Mortality is high. Cure of infection will not be achieved by antimicrobial therapy alone. Surgical intervention at an early stage must be considered.

Osteomyelitis and Arthritis.[16,18,56,67,105,113,119,128–130] Before the development of antibiotic therapy for typhoid fever, localization of infection in bone occurred in approximately 1 percent of the cases. Osteomyelitis can develop in normal bone but is especially likely to occur in patients with sickle-cell hemoglobinopathies, systemic lupus erythematosus, hematologic neoplasms, immunosuppressive therapy, bone surgery or trauma, and cirrhosis of the liver. *Salmonella*, not *Staphylococcus*, is the most common cause of osteomyelitis in patients with sickle-cell anemia. Blood-borne *Salmonella* apparently localize in the areas of ischemia and necrosis so common in bone marrow of patients with sickle-cell anemia. *Salmonella* infection of the prosthesis occurs rarely after total hip replacement.[131]

Salmonella infection may be followed about 10 days after onset by a reactive arthritis characterized by migratory polyarthritis without destructive changes. The joints most often involved are knee, ankle, wrist, finger, elbow, shoulder, and sacroiliac. Joint fluid contains polymorphonuclear neutrophils (mean leukocyte count 17,500 mm^3) and is sterile. The vast majority of these patients have HLA-B27 antigen. The arthritis usually lasts several months and responds to anti-inflammatory agents alone. About one-fourth to one-third of the patients have conjunctivitis and/or urethritis, which, with the arthritis, make up the typical triad of Reiter's syndrome.

Salmonella may cause a metastatic suppurative arthritis. Pyogenic arthritis is much less frequent than reactive arthritis.

Splenic Abscess.[119,132–134] Splenic abscess is a rare complication of *Salmonella* infection, but *Salmonella* account for 15 percent of the splenic abscesses reported in the literature. Localization occurs after bacteremia in post-traumatic subcapsular hematomas or splenic cysts. The clinical manifestation is one of left-upper-quadrant tenderness, fever, and leukocytosis. Splenomegaly may be present. With appropriate antimicrobial therapy and surgical drainage, the mortality is less than 10 percent.

Hepatic Abscess.[56,119,135,136] Cohen, Bartlett, and Corey found 10 cases of *Salmonella* pyogenic liver abscesses reported in the English literature in the antibiotic era. Seven of the 10 had pre-existing liver disease including amebic abscesses, echinococcal cysts, and hematomas. Association with biliary tract disease exists in occasional cases. Mortality is high.

Urogenital Tracts.[119] Infection of the urinary and genital tracts with *Salmonella* is rare. *Salmonella* in stools of carriers or persons with acute illness may gain access to the urinary tract to produce cystitis or pyelonephritis. Localization of blood-borne *Salmonella* with abscess formation in the kidneys, testicles, or ovaries is also occasionally reported.

Soft-Tissue Abscesses.[56,113,137] Soft-tissue infections and abscesses occur in 1 percent or less of the patients hospitalized with *Salmonella* infections. The most common sites of infection are adjacent to the gastrointestinal tract. Wound infection after cholecystectomy has been reported, especially in chronic enteric carriers.

Chronic Carrier State

Excretion of organisms in stool after *Salmonella* enterocolitis or enteric fever persists for variable periods of time, usually a few weeks. Persons who continue to excrete organisms for more than a year after disease or after initial discovery of organisms in stool are designated chronic carriers. The incidence of the chronic enteric carrier state after typhoid fever is 1–3 percent.[92,138] Although the chronic carrier state does occur after nontyphoidal salmonellosis, it is quite unusual and is found in far less than 1 percent of the patients.[139] Chronic carriers are asymptomatic.

Incidence of development of the chronic enteric carrier state after typhoid fever increases with age. The average age of the chronic carrier, according to several series, is in the sixth decade.[139–141] Chronic enteric carriers tend to have a much higher incidence of biliary tract disease than the general population, and it has been suggested that the increasing incidence of biliary tract disease with age explains the increased incidence of the carrier state in older patients. The biliary tract is infected in all chronic enteric carriers of *S. typhi*, and 10^6–10^9 viable bacilli are excreted into the duodenum in each milliliter of bile.[142] Chronic enteric carriers excrete large numbers of typhoid bacilli in stools, usually 10^6 or more viable bacilli per gram of feces.[142]

Testing for the presence of antibody to the Vi antigen has been suggested as a mechanism for screening for typhoid carriers. However, only 70 percent of the chronic carriers of *S. typhi* have Vi antibody in titers greater than 1:5.[99]

Patients with *S. hematobium* involvement of the urinary tract have a propensity to become chronic urinary carriers after typhoid fever.[77] Urinary carriers may continue to excrete large numbers of bacilli in urine for months or years.

PREVENTION

The control of *Salmonella* infection transmitted from animals to humans will require control of infection in the animal reservoir, reduction in contamination of foodstuffs prepared from animals, and application of acceptable standards in processing and preparing food in commercial and private kitchens. Adequate refrigeration, caution in preparing foods far in advance of use, and meticulous cleaning of equipment and machines used in food processing are essential preventive practices. However, the widespread infection of animals used as foodstuffs and modern methods of mass production of food make elimination of salmonellosis unlikely in the foreseeable future. Control of *Salmonella* infection transmitted from person to person depends on high standards of personal hygiene; maintenance of a supply of uncontaminated water; proper sewage disposal; and identification, treatment, and follow-up of chronic carriers.[41] Hand washing is of paramount importance in controlling person-to-person spread. Although hands of convalescent carriers are often contaminated after defecation, detectable *Salmonellae* are easily removed by washing the hands with soap and water.[28]

Typhoid vaccine, a saline suspension of acetone- or heat/phenol-killed *S. typhi* enhances the resistance of human beings to infection with *S. typhi* under experimental and natural conditions.[43] Vaccine efficacy ranges from 51 to 67 percent.[143] However, it is known that the degree of resistance produced by presently available vaccines can be overcome easily by increasing the inoculum.[46] Typhoid fever is followed by increased resistance to reinfection, but second attacks of typhoid can occur under conditions associated with heavy exposure to the organism.

Experimental and field studies with a live attenuated oral vaccine prepared from the Ty 21a strain of *S. typhi* have enhanced interest in the possibility of a stable, easily administered oral typhoid vaccine free of the unpleasant side effects of whole cell vaccines.[106,143–146] A recent large-scale field trial in Chile using the live Ty 21a vaccine in enteric coated capsules given in three doses within 1 week demonstrated 67 percent efficacy for at least 3 years.[143] At this stage, the oral live vaccines seem to be about as effective as conventional parenteral whole cell vaccines but with fewer side effects.[147]

There is also renewed interest in testing the capsular polysaccharide of *S. typhi* (Vi antigen) as a parenteral typhoid vaccine. Studies in Nepal have shown efficacy of 75 percent after only one injection of Vi polysaccharide.[148] Although serum antibodies to Vi antigen confer immunity to typhoid fever, it also seems clear that protection against *S. typhi* can occur in the absence of Vi antibody because the protective Ty 21a oral vaccine lacks Vi antigen.[44,148]

Immunization against infection with serotypes other than *S. typhi* has not been shown to be effective in humans, and vaccines containing these serotypes are no longer available in the United States.

Typhoid vaccine should be considered for persons with intimate continuing exposure to a documented typhoid carrier and for persons traveling to areas where there is a recognized appreciable risk of exposure to typhoid. The Public Health Service Advisory Committee on Immunization Practices recommends administration of vaccine to adults and children 10 years and older in doses of 0.5 ml subcutaneously on two occasions separated by 4 or more weeks.[43] Younger children should receive smaller doses. Booster doses every 3 years are recommended under conditions of continued or repeated exposure. Discomfort at the injection site is routine, and febrile reactions to immunization are relatively common.

THERAPY

The type of syndrome produced by *Salmonella* influences the selection and duration of antimicrobial therapy. Antimicrobial therapy is not indicated in transient intestinal carriers or in the vast majority of patients with enterocolitis; however, either chloramphenicol or ampicillin may be life-saving in patients with bacteremia or enteric fever. Trimethoprim–sulfamethoxazole and certain third-generation cephalosporins are also effective in the therapy of enteric fever. Ampicillin, not chloramphenicol, may terminate the chronic carrier state and is preferred in intravascular infections. Although not tested as extensively as ampicillin, amoxicillin can probably be substituted for ampicillin in the therapy of *Salmonella* infection. Despite excellent activity in vitro, a number of antibiotics, including cefamandole, have given very disappointing results in the therapy of *Salmonella* infection.[149] Surgery also plays an important role in the management of localized infections and the chronic enteric carrier state.

Selection of antimicrobials for therapy has been complicated by the emergence of *Salmonella* strains resistant to multiple antimicrobials.[54,150–158] This resistance is generally transferable from organism or organism on plasmids that carry genetic determinants of resistance (R factors); for example, an R factor may confer the ability to produce penicillinase.

The reasons for the emergence of multiple drug resistance in *Salmonella* are incompletely understood but seem related to widespread use of antimicrobials in humans and animals.[156,158–162] Multiply resistant organisms with R factors may be present in the normal gastrointestinal flora. These resistant organisms are selected and grow to high titer in humans receiving antimicrobials to prevent or to cure infection or in animals receiving antimicrobials to improve feed conversion and to promote growth or to prevent or treat infection. If the intestinal tract of humans or animals harbors flora rich in these resistant organisms and is colonized with a strain of a pathogenic bacterium, such as *Salmonella*, which is sensitive to antimicrobials, R factors may be transferred in the gut from the resistant organisms to the previously sensitive pathogenic bacterium.[155] The pathogenic bacterium, now resistant, may spread to produce disease in other animals or man. A number of examples add support to the concept that the use of antimicrobials in animals influences the occurrence of antibiotic-resistant *Salmonella* infections in humans.[156,160] Holmberg and colleagues described a well-studied multistate outbreak of infection with *S. newport* resistant to ampicillin, tetracycline, and other antimicrobials that was spread through hamburger made from beef cattle that had been fed subtherapeutic doses of tetracycline for growth promotion.[156] Illegal use of chloramphenicol in dairies appears to have been associated with an outbreak of hundreds of cases of human infection with *S. newport* resistant to chloramphenicol, ampicillin, and tetracycline in California in 1985. The epidemic strain, spread primarily through hamburger, was isolated from sick cows, the abattoirs where they were slaughtered, and the ground beef prepared from them.[160]

The reported proportion of *Salmonella* strains resistant to antimicrobials varies considerably.[67,54] Geographic differences in circulating *Salmonella* clones and in antimicrobial usage account in part for this variability. The studies of MacDonald and associates, which circumvent some of the biases and problems of earlier studies, examined changes in antimicrobial resistance of *Salmonella* isolated from the same geographic areas in the United States between 1979–1980 and 1984–1985.[54] Resistance to one or more of 13 antimicrobials rose significantly from 16 percent to 24 percent. However, it is of interest that although the overall trend was towards more resistant strains, for some serotypes, for example *S. heidelberg*, the proportion of resistant strains fell significantly between the two periods. The rates of resistance for *Salmonella* isolated during 1984–1985 was tetracycline 13 percent, streptomycin 12 percent, ampicillin 9 percent, sulfamethoxazole 7 percent, nitrofurantoin 4 percent, and chloramphenicol 2 percent. Much higher rates of resistance are reported in certain geographic areas reflecting circulating resistant clones. Often, the acquired resistance involves drugs such as tetracycline, sulfonamides, and streptomycin that are not useful in the treatment of *Salmonella* infections. Of greater clinical importance is the increasing proportion of strains resistant to ampicillin, chloramphenicol, or trimethoprim–sulfamethoxazole, agents useful in the therapy of systemic salmonellosis.[163] With this background of increasing multiple-drug resistance of *Salmonellae*, especially nontyphoidal strains, it has been reassuring to see the development of third-generation cephalosporins and new quinolones that demonstrate impressive bactericidal activity in vitro and in vivo against these organisms, even those resistant to multiple drugs.[120]

Enterocolitis

Most cases of enterocolitis caused by *Salmonella* species resolve quickly and without complications with simple symptomatic therapy. The most important therapeutic consideration is fluid and electrolyte replacement. Parenteral restoration of fluid balance may be required if adequate replacement cannot be achieved by the oral route. Inhibitors of bowel motility are not recommended routinely but may be necessary in patients who must maintain activities during the course of illness. Antimicrobial therapy is not recommended in uncomplicated enterocolitis. Treatment with β-lactam antibiotics, tetracyclines, chloramphenicol, trimethoprim–sulfonamide, and topical aminoglycosides has been shown to have no influence on the duration of fever or diarrhea in these patients.[164] Furthermore, antimicrobials prolong the excretion of organisms in stools; this effect is probably mediated through antimicrobial action on the normal intestinal flora.[88]

It is interesting to speculate that the "lack of effectiveness" of antimicrobials in enterocolitis is related to the brief, self-limited nature of the illness. As judged by observations of patients with enteric fever, response of *Salmonella* infection to antimicrobial therapy is slow, often requiring several days.[46,165] Thus, it is possible that the clinical manifestations of enterocolitis subside before antimicrobials might be anticipated to produce a beneficial effect. The recent reports that ciprofloxacin significantly reduces the duration of diarrhea in patients with *Salmonella* enterocolitis require confirmation.[164]

Although there is little evidence of efficacy of antimicrobials in uncomplicated enterocolitis, antimicrobials should be considered if enterocolitis appears to be evolving into one of the systemic syndromes, that is, enteric fever, chronic bacteremia, or metastatic pyogenic infection. Likewise, antimicrobial therapy should be considered in patients with enterocolitis who have another major disease or condition that impairs host resistance to infection (e.g., neonates and patients with AIDS, sickle hemoglobinopathies, lymphoma, or leukemia).

Antimicrobials may also enhance susceptibility to intestinal infection. A study on the use of a prophylactic antibacterial agent in tourists to endemic areas demonstrated a higher incidence of *Salmonella* infection in those given oxyquinolines to prevent "turista" than in those given no prophylaxis.[166] Activation of asymptomatic *Salmonella* infection by antimicrobial therapy has also been reported.[167]

Enteric Fever

The antimicrobial of choice for enteric fever acquired in most areas of the world is still chloramphenicol in a dosage of 50 mg/kg/day, given orally in four divided doses for at least 2 weeks.[157,158] Response to chloramphenicol is gradual, with temperature returning to normal within 3–5 days in most cases. Ampicillin is also effective in the treatment of enteric fever and should be administered in doses of 100 mg/kg/day in four divided doses by mouth or intravenously for at least 2 weeks.[165] Several studies have demonstrated a slower response rate to ampicillin than to chloramphenicol,[165,168,169] although the latter is associated with more serious potential side effects and perhaps a higher incidence of relapse. Amoxicillin is also effective in the therapy of typhoid fever.[168]

Chloramphenicol-resistant strains have been responsible for outbreaks of typhoid fever in Mexico, Vietnam, India, and Peru, and strains resistant to ampicillin, sulfamethoxazole, and other antimicrobials are reported sporadically.[44,150] In the United States antimicrobial resistance has been a minor problem, with only 2–3 percent of strains of *S. typhi* resistant to chloramphenicol or ampicillin.[44] In a recent study in Britain, where the majority of infections are acquired abroad, especially in India and West Africa, only 11 (0.47 percent) of 2356 strains of *S. typhi* isolated during 1978–1985 were found to be chloramphenicol-resistant.[170] Thus, in general, *S. typhi* has remained remarkably susceptible to antimicrobial agents, especially as compared with the nontyphoidal *Salmonella* and other enteric bacilli.[44]

Ampicillin or amoxicillin is preferred as an alternative to chloramphenicol for therapy of enteric caused by chloramphenicol-resistant organisms. Only occasional strains of *S. typhi* are known to be resistant to both chloramphenicol and ampicillin.[151] Some authorities recommend both chloramphenicol and ampicillin as initial therapy if a drug-resistant strain is suspected; if the organism is found to be resistant to chloramphenicol, ampicillin is continued alone, but, if the organism is sensitive to chloramphenicol, that antibiotic alone is continued.

Trimethoprim–sulfamethoxazole has been used in recent years in the treatment of enteric fever.[171,172] Reports of efficacy have varied from claims of equivalence to chloramphenicol[107,108,173–175] to unsatisfactory bacteriologic response.[176] These variations in results have been attributed to administration of insufficient doses of drug, differences in strains of *S. typhi*, and variation in immunity in different geographic areas. Review of published reports indicates that trimethoprim–sulfamethoxazole is an acceptable alternative to chloramphenicol or ampicillin in the therapy of enteric fever.[109] Recommended dosage of trimethoprim–sulfamethoxazole in adults is 320–640 mg of trimethoprim combined with 1600–3200 mg of sulfamethoxazole per day in two divided oral doses for 2 weeks (4–8 of the 80 mg trimethoprim/400 mg sulfamethoxazole tablets). Side effects include neutropenia and, perhaps, thrombocytopenia. Trimethoprim–sulfamethoxazole is especially useful in *Salmonella* infections caused by organisms resistant to both chloramphenicol and ampicillin. The R factor coding for chloramphenicol resistance also codes for sulfonamide resistance; therefore, only the trimethoprim portion of the drug is active against multiply resistant strains. In fact, successful therapy of enteric fever with trimethoprim alone has been described.[177]

Third-generation cephalosporins, especially cefotaxime, ceftriaxone, and cefoperazone, show excellent in vitro activity against *S. typhi* and nontyphoidal *Salmonella* and are acceptable alternative antimicrobials for treatment of typhoid fever and other systemic *Salmonella* infections including strains resistant to chloramphenicol, ampicillin, or trimethoprim–sulfamethoxazole.[120,178] The literature review by Soe and Overturf indicated a cure rate in typhoid and systemic nontyphoid salmonelloses of about 90 percent.[178] Cefotaxime was the most widely used third-generation cephalosporin for therapy of *Salmonella* infections. Although the results are difficult to compare, cure rates in typhoid fever were higher and relapse rates lower with cefoperazone (97 percent; 0 percent) and ceftriaxone (92 percent; 4 percent) than with cefotaxime (85 percent; 4 percent). In patients with typhoid fever cefoperazone is given in an initial dose of 100 mg/kg intravenously per day (in divided doses at 12-hour intervals) and changed to 50 mg/kg per day when defervescence occurs.[178,179] Therapy is continued for 14 days, although excellent results have been reported with shorter courses of therapy.[178] The dosage of cefotaxime in children is 200 mg/kg per day (maximum 12 gm/day) in four divided doses, and in adults is 2–3 g given three to six times a day. Cefotaxime is administered intravenously over 30 minutes.

Four to five days on the average is required for defervescence. Second-generation cephalosporins have been less effective than third-generation agents in curing typhoid and nontyphoid salmonellosis and should not be used in the therapy of these infections.[149,180]

Ciprofloxacin, a quinoline derivative, is highly active in vitro against *Salmonella* including *S. typhi* and shows promise in the treatment of typhoid fever.[147,181–183] Ramirez, Garcia, and colleagues achieved cure in 36 of 38 patients with typhoid who were treated with 500 mg oral ciprofloxacin every 12 hours for 14 days. The mean duration of fever was 4.2 days.[183,184]

Many antimicrobial agents are active against *S. typhi* and other salmonellae in vitro. However, in general, in vitro response of *Salmonella* serotypes to antibiotics correlates poorly with in vivo response.[185,186]

Supportive therapy for patients with enteric fever includes fluid replacement and maintenance of nutrition. Severely toxemic patients can benefit from a short course of corticosteroids, but, in general, corticosteroids should be reserved for critically ill patients in whom prompt amelioration of the manifestations of toxemia may be life-saving. The duration of corticosteroid therapy should be brief. For some years a 3-day course has been recommended, beginning with 60 mg/day of prednisone or equivalent and rapidly decreasing thereafter to 20 mg/day. Studies reported in 1984 document the beneficial effect of steroids in severe typhoid fever; these studies were carried out using large doses of dexamethasone (an initial dose of 3 mg/kg followed by eight doses of 1 mg/kg every 6 hours) administered intravenously over a 48-hour period.[187] Corticosteroids may increase the relapse rate.[188] Patients with typhoid frequently respond to small doses of salicylates or anti-inflammatory corticosteroids with precipitous falls in temperature to hypothermic levels and transient hypotension. Use of antipyretics should be avoided. Heparin should not be used to treat the subclinical disseminated intravascular coagulation seen in a significant proportion of patients with enteric fever.[75]

The physician must be alert to the development of complications of enteric fever. Intestinal hemorrhage may require blood transfusions. The treatment of intestinal perforation, a condition usually marked by fever, leukocytosis, and findings of abdominal pain and tenderness, is somewhat controversial. Huckstep[73] recommends conservative medical management with antibiotics. However, Archampong[189] has demonstrated that 19 percent of intestinal perforations were multiple or large (some greater than 2.5 cm in diameter) and recommends laparotomy with primary closure or resection and drainage. Archampong showed that mortality was 30 percent when surgery was performed within 5 days of perforation but rose to 76 percent when laparotomy was performed more than 5 days after perforation.

Bacteremia and Localized Infections

Ampicillin, amoxicillin, chloramphenicol, trimethoprim–sulfamethoxazole, or third-generation cephalosporins such as cefotaxime or cefoperazone can be used in the treatment of *Salmonella* bacteremia. However, chloramphenicol should not be used when there is localization of infection at intravascular sites (endocarditis or aneurysmal infection); ampicillin, amoxacillin, or a third-generation cephalosporin is preferred under these circumstances. Bacteremia patients with impaired systemic resistance, for example, patients with AIDS, should also be treated with ampicillin, amoxicillin, or a third-generation cephalosporin.[61–63,114–116] Ciprofloxacin is also reported to be effective in the therapy of recurrent *Salmonella* sepsis.[116] Localized infection with abscess formation usually requires surgical drainage in addition to antimicrobial therapy. In patients with infected aneurysms, best results are obtained with wide excision of the infected site, drainage, and construction of a vascular bypass outside of the infected area.

The duration of therapy is influenced by the site of infection and by the antimicrobial agent. Bacteremia without symptoms of localization should be treated for 10–14 days, whereas localized infections such as osteomyelitis or endocarditis can require therapy for 4–6 weeks or longer. Patients with AIDS should be treated for 3–4 weeks in an effort to prevent relapse; long-term therapy with an oral antimicrobial may be required.

Cefotaxime appears to be the antimicrobial agent of choice in *Salmonella* meningitis.[178] It should be given in doses of 200 mg/kg per day in four divided doses for children and 2–3 g per dose given three to six times a day for adults.

Chronic Carrier State

Ampicillin, 4–5 g/day, combined with probenecid, 2 g/day, both divided into four oral doses, for 6 weeks is the treatment of choice for chronic enteric carriers who have normally functioning gallbladders without evidence of cholelithiasis.[138,141] Amoxicillin, 6 g/day, is as effective as ampicillin.[190] In chronic carriers with gallbladder disease, the rate of failure of ampicillin therapy is about 75 percent, with relapses occurring up to 2 years after discontinuation of therapy.[138,191] However, amoxicillin has been reported to be effective even in patients with gallstones or nonfunctioning gallbladder.[190] The use of a combination of rifampin, trimethoprim, and sulfamethoxazole has been reported to cure 35 of 40 chronic carriers of *S. typhi*, 7 of 19 chronic carriers of *S. paratyphi* B, and 6 of 28 chronic carriers of *S. enteritidis*.[192] Ciprofloxacin has also been reported to be successful in eradication of *S. typhi* in chronic carriers[182,193]; confirmation and long-term follow-up is required. Cholecystectomy is effective in eradicating the chronic carrier state in the majority of cases and should be used in patients who have relapsed after therapy or who cannot tolerate antimicrobial therapy.[139,140]

REFERENCES

1. LeMinor L, Véron M, Popoff M. Taxonomie des *Salmonella*. Ann Microbiol. 1982;133B:223–243.
2. LeMinor L, Véron M, Popoff M. Proposition pour une nomenclature des *Salmonella*. Ann Microbiol. 1982;133B:245–254.
3. LeMinor L. *Salmonella*. In Krieg NR, Holt JG, eds. Bergey's Manual of Systematic Bacteriology. v. 1. Baltimore: Williams and Wilkins; 1984:427–458.
4. Farmer JJ III, McWhorter AC, Brenner DJ, et al. The *Salmonella-Arizona* group of Enterobacteriaceae: nomenclature, classification, and reporting. Clin Microbiol Newsletter. 1984;6:63–66.
5. Farmer JJ III, Davis BR, Hickman-Brenner FW, et al. Biochemical identification of new species and biogroups of Enterobacteriaceae isolated from clinical specimens. J Clin Microbiol. 1985;21:46–76.
6. Davis BD, Dulbecco R, Elsen HN, et al, eds. Microbiology. 3rd ed. New York: Harper & Row; 1980:660–663.
7. Falcão DP, Trabalsi LR, Hickman FW, et al. Unusual Enterobacteriaceae: lactose-positive *Salmonella typhimurium* which is endemic in São Paulo, Brazil. J Clin Microbiol. 1975;2:349.

8. Porschen RK, Hale D, Goodman Z. Misdiagnosed salmonella septicemia and endarteritis due to a lactose-fermenting strain. Bacteriologic and epidemiologic considerations. Am J Clin Pathol. 1977;68:416.
9. O'Brien TR, Hopkins JD, Gilleece ES, et al. Molecular epidemiology of antibiotic resistance in *Salmonella* from animals and human beings in the United States. N Engl J Med. 1982;307:1.
10. Boyd JSK, Parker MT, Maie NS. Symbiotic bacteriophage as a "marker" in the identification of strains of *S. typhimurium*. J Hyg (Camb). 1951;49:442.
11. Gershman M. Single phage-typing set for differentiating salmonellae. J Clin Microbiol. 1977;5:302.
12. Centers for Disease Control. Salmonella Surveillance Summary for 1972. Atlanta: 1972.
13. Rhame FS, Root RK, MacLowry JD, et al. Samonella septicemia from platelet transfusions. Study of an outbreak traced to a hematogenous carrier of *Salmonella choleraesuis*. Ann Intern Med. 1973;76:633.
14. Chmel H, Armstrong D. *Salmonella oslo*: a focal outbreak in a hospital. Am J Med. 1976;60:203.
15. Dean AG. Transmission of *Salmonella typhi* by fiberoptic endocscopy. Lancet. 1977;2:134.
16. Bennett IL Jr, Hook EW. Infectious diseases (some aspects of salmonellosis). Annu Rev Med. 1959;10.1.
17. Edsall G, Gaines S, Landy M, et al. Studies on infection and immunity in experimental typhoid fever. I. Typhoid fever in chimpanzees orally infected with *Salmonella typhosa*. J Exp Med. 1960;112:143.
18. Rubin RH, Weinstein L. Salmonellosis: Microbiologic, Pathologic, and Clinical Features. New York: Stratton Intercontinental Medical Book Corporation; 1977.
19. Buchanan RE, Gibbons NE, eds. Bergey's Manual of Determinative Bacteriology. 8th ed. Baltimore: Williams & Wilkins; 1974.
20. Aserkoff B, Schroeder SA, Brechman PS. Salmonellosis in the United States—A five-year review. Am J Epidemiol. 1970;92:13.
21. Update: *Salmonella enteritidis* infections in the Northeastern United States. JAMA. 1987;257:2408–9.
22. Tacket CO, Dominguez LB, Fisher HJ, et al. An outbreak of multiple-drug-resistant *Salmonella* enteritis from raw milk. JAMA. 1985;253:2058–60.
23. Ryan CA, Nickels MK, Hargrett-Bean NT, et al. Massive outbreak of antimicrobial-resistant salmonellosis traced to pasteurized milk. JAMA. 1987;258:3269–3274.
24. Salmonella Surveillance Summary for 1976. Atlanta: Centers for Disease Control; 1976.
25. Cohen ML, Potter M, Pollard R, et al. Turtle-associated salmonellosis in the United States. JAMA. 1980;243:1247.
26. Taylor DN, Wachsmuth IK, Shangkuan Y, et al: Salmonellosis associated with marijuana. N Engl J Med 306:1249, 1982.
27. Cruickshank JG, Humphrey TJ. The carrier food handler and nontyphoidol salmonellosis. Epidemiol Infect. 1987;98:223–30.
28. Pether JVS, Scott RJD. *Salmonella* carriers; are they dangerous? A study to identify finger contamination with *Salmonellae* by convalescent carriers. J Infect. 1982;5:81–8.
29. Fontaine RE, Arnon S, Martin WT, et al. Raw hamburger: an interstate common source of human salmonellosis. Am J Epidemiol. 1978;107:36.
30. Salmonella Surveillance Report, Annual Summary for 1965. Atlanta: National Communicable Disease Center; 1965.
31. Feldman RE, Baine WB, Nitzkin JL, et al. Epidemiology of *Salmonella typhi* infections in a migrant labor camp in Dade County, Florida. J Infect Dis. 1974;130:334.
32. Walker W. The Aberdeen typhoid outbreak of 1964. Scott Med J. 1965;10:466.
33. Wicks ACB, Holmes GS, Davidson L. Endemic typhoid fever: a diagnostic pitfall. Q J Med. 1971;40:341.
34. Earampamoorthy S, Koff RS. Health hazards of bivalve-mollusk ingestion. Ann Intern Med. 1975;83:107.
35. Salmonella Surveillance Summary for 1986. Atlanta: Centers for Disease Control; 1988.
36. Rosenstein BJ. Salmonellosis in infants and children: epidemiologic and therapeutic considerations. J Pediatr. 1967;70:1.
37. Baine WB, Gangarosa EJ, Bennett JV, et al. Institutional salmonellosis. J Infect Dis. 1973;128:357.
38. Rice PA, Craven PC, Wells JG. *Salmonella heidelberg* enteritis and bacteremia: an epidemic on two pediatric wards. Am J Med. 1976;60:509.
39. Haddock RL. *Salmonella* in vacuum cleaners. Lancet. 1986;1:637.
40. Chalky RB, Blaser MJ. A review of human salmonellosis: III. Magnitude of *Salmonella* infection in the United States. Rev Infect Dis. 1988;10:111–24.
41. Bauer H. The growing problem of salmonellosis in modern society. Medicine. 1973;52:323.
42. Taylor DN, Pollard RA, Blake PA. Typhoid in the United States and the risk to the international traveler. J Infect Dis. 1983;148:599.
43. Public Health Service Advisory Committee on Immunization Practices. Typhoid vaccine. MMWR. 1978;27:231.
44. Edelman R, Levine MM. Summary of an international workshop on typhoid fever. Rev Infect Dis. 1986;8;329–49.
45. Rice PA, Baine WB, Gangarosa EJ. *Salmonella typhi* infections in the United States, 1967–1972: Increasing importance of international travelers. Am J Epidemiol. 1977;106:160.
46. Hornick RB, Greisman SE, Woodward TE, et al. Typhoid fever: pathogenesis and immunologic control. N Engl J Med. 1970;283:686, 739.
47. Hook EW. Salmonellosis: certain factors influencing the interaction of *Salmonella* and the human host. Bull NY Acad Med. 1961;37:499.
48. Lipson A, Meikle H. Porcine pancreatin as a source of *Salmonella* infection in children with cystic fibrosis. Arch Dis Child. 1977;52:569.
49. Miller CP, Bohnhoff M. Changes in the mouse's enteric microflora associated with enhanced susceptibility to salmonella infection following streptomycin treatment. J Infect Dis. 1963;113:59.
50. Bohnhoff M, Miller CP, Martin WR. Resistance of the mouse's intestinal tract to experimental salmonella infection. II. Factors responsible for its loss following streptomycin treatment. J Exp Med. 1964;120:817.
51. Waddell WR, Kunz LJ. Association of *Salmonella* enteritis with operations on the stomach. N Engl J Med. 1956;255:555.
52. Giannella RA, Broitman SA, Zamcheck N. Salmonella enteritis. I. Role of reduced gastric secretion in pathogenesis. Am J Dig Dis. 1971;16:1000.
53. Riley LW, Cohen ML, Seals JE, et al. Importance of host factors in human salmonellosis caused by multiresistant strains of *Salmonella*. J Infect Dis. 1984;149:878–83.
54. MacDonald KL, Cohen ML, Hargrett-Bean NT, et al. Changes in antimicrobial resistance of *Salmonella* isolated from humans in the United States. JAMA. 1987;1496–9.
55. Dupont HL, Hornick RB. Adverse effect of Lomotil therapy in shigellosis. JAMA. 1973;226:1525.
56. Black PH, Kunz LJ, Swartz MN. Salmonellosis—A review of some unusual aspects. N Engl J Med. 1960;262:811,864,921.
57. Wolfe MS, Armstrong D, Louria DB, et al. Salmonellosis in patients with neoplastic disease: a review of 100 episodes at Memorial Cancer Center over a 13-year period. Arch Intern Med. 1971;128:546.
58. Hand WL, King NL. Serum opsonization of *Salmonella* in sickle cell anemia. Am J Med. 1978;64:388.
59. Hook EW, Kaye D, Gill FA. Factors influencing host resistance to *Salmonella* infection. The effects of hemolysis and erythrophagocytosis. Trans Am Clin Climatol Assoc. 1966;78:230.
60. Gill FA, Kaye D, Hook EW. The influence of erythrophagocytosis on the interaction of macrophages and *Salmonella* in vitro. J Exp Med. 1966;124:173.
61. Jacobs JL, Gold JWM, Murray HW, et al. *Salmonella* infections in patients with the acquired immunodeficiency syndrome. Ann Intern Med. 1985;102:186–8.
62. Glaser JB, Morton-Kute L, Berger SR, et al. Recurrent *Salmonella typhimurium* bacteremia associated with the acquired immunodeficiency syndrome. Ann Intern Med. 1985;102:189–93.
63. Smith PD, Macher AM, Bookman MA, et al. *Salmonella typhimurium* enteritis and bacteremia in the acquired immunodeficiency syndrome. Ann Intern Med. 1985;102:207–8.
64. Samra Y, Shaked Y, Maier MK. Nontyphoid salmonellosis in renal transplant recipients: report of five cases and review of this literature. Rev Infect Dis. 1986;8:431–40.
65. Saphra I, Wasserman M. *Salmonella choleraesuis*: a clinical and epidemiological evaluation of 329 infections identified between 1940 and 1954 in the New York Salmonella Center. Am J Med Sci. 1954;228:525.
66. Giannella RA, Rout WR, Formel SB. Effect of indomethacin on intestinal water transport in *Salmonella*-infected Rhesus monkeys. Infect Immun. 1977;17:136.
67. Rubin RH. Human salmonellosis: epidemiology, pathogenesis, and clinical syndromes. Infect Dis Pract. 1982;6:1.
68. Musch MW, Miller RJ, Field M, et al. Stimulation of colonic secretion by lipoxygenase metabolites of arachidonic acid. Science. 1982;217:1255.
69. Sprinz H, Gangarosa EJ, Williams M, et al. Histopathology of the upper small intestines in typhoid fever. Biopsy study of experimental disease in man. Am J Dig Dis. 1966;11:615.
70. Carter PB, Collins FM. The route of enteric infection in normal mice. J Exp Med. 1974;139:1189.
71. Takeuchi A, Sprinz H. Electron-microscope studies of experimental salmonella infection in the preconditioned guinea pig. II. Response of the intestinal mucosa to the invasion by *Salmonella typhimurium*. Am J Pathol. 1967;51:137.
72. Hackett J, Kotlarski I, Mathan V, et al. The colonization of Peyer's patches by a strain of *Salmonella typhimurium* cured of the cryptic plasmid. J Infect Dis. 1986;153:1119–25.
73. Huckstep RL. Typhoid Fever and Other Salmonella Infections. Edinburgh: E & S Livingstone; 1962.
74. Greisman SE, Woodward TE, Hornick RB, et al. Typhoid fever: a study of pathogenesis and physiologic abnormalities. Trans Am Clin Climatol Assoc. 1961;73:146.
75. Butler T, Bell WR, Levin J, et al. Typhoid fever: studies of blood coagulation, bacteremia, and endotoxemia. Arch Intern Med. 1978;138:407.
76. Hornick RB, Greisman S. On the pathogenesis of typhoid fever. Arch Intern Med. 1978;138:357.
77. Farid Z, Bassily S, Kent DC, et al. Chronic urinary salmonella carriers with intermittent bacteraemia. J Trop Med Hyg. 1970;73:153.
78. Neves J, Raso P, Marinko RP. Prolonged septicemic salmonellosis intercurrent with *Schistosomiasis mansoni* infection. J Trop Med Hyg. 1971;74:9.
79. Rocha H, Kirk JW, Heaney CD Jr. Prolonged salmonella bacteremia in patients with *Schistosoma mansoni* infection. Arch Intern Med. 1971;128:254.
80. Hathout S, El-Ghaffer Y, Awny AY. Salmonellosis complicating schistosomiasis in Egypt: a new clinical appreciation. Am J Trop Med Hyg. 1967;16:462.

81. Young SW, Higashi G, Kamel R, et al. Interactions of salmonellae and schistosomes in host-parasitic relations. Trans R Soc Trop Med Hyg. 1973;67:797.
82. Tuazon CU, Nash T, Cheever A, et al. Interaction of *Schistosoma japonicum* with salmonellae and other Gram-negative bacteria. J Infect Dis. 1985;152:722–6.
83. Salmonella enterocolitis—Peru. MMWR. 1977;26:346.
84. Mandal BK, Mani V. Colonic involvement in salmonellosis. Lancet. 1976;1:887.
85. Appelbaum PC, Scragg J, Schonland MM. Colonic involvement in salmonellosis, letter. Lancet. 1976;2:102.
86. Radsel-Medvescek A, Zargi R, Acko M, et al. Colonic involvement in salmonellosis, letter. Lancet. 1977;1:601.
87. Meadow WL, Schneider H, Beem MO. *Salmonella enteritidis* bacteremia in childhood. J Infect Dis. 1985;152:185–9.
88. Aserkoff B, Bennett JV. Effect of antibiotic therapy in acute salmonellosis on the fecal excretion of salmonellae. N Engl J Med. 1969;281:636.
89. Rubenstein AD, Feenster RF, Smith HM. Salmonellosis as a public health problem in wartime. Am J Public Health. 1944;34:841.
90. Buchwald DS, Blaser MJ. A review of human salmonellosis: II. Duration of excretion following infection with nontyphi *Salmonella*. Rev Infect Dis. 1984;6:345–56.
91. Stuart BM, Pullen RL. Typhoid: clinical analysis of three hundred and sixty cases. Arch Intern Med. 1946;78:629.
92. Hoffman TA, Ruiz CJ, Counts GW, et al. Waterborne typhoid fever in Dade County, Florida: clinical and therapeutic evaluations of 105 bacteremic patients. Am J Med. 1975;59:481.
93. Breakey WR, Kala AK. Typhoid catatonia responsive to ECT. Br Med J. 1977;3:357.
94. Litwack KD, Hoke AW, Borchardt KA. Rose spots in typhoid fever. Arch Dermatol. 1972;105:252.
95. Ramachandran S, Godfrey JJ, Perera MVF. Typhoid hepatitis. JAMA. 1974;230:236.
96. Calva JJ, Ruiz-Palacios GM. *Salmonella* hepatitis: detection of salmonella antigens in the liver of patients with typhoid fever. J Infect Dis. 1986;154:373–4.
97. Sitprija V, Pipatanagul V, Boonpucknavig V, et al. Glomerulitis in typhoid fever. Ann Intern Med. 1974;81:210.
98. Indraprasit S, Boonpucknavig V, Boonpucknavig S. IgA nephropathy associated with enteric fever. Nephron. 1985;40:219–22.
99. Typhoid and its serology, editorial. Br Med J. 1978;1:389.
100. Hoffman SL, Punjabi NH, Rockhill RC, et al. Duodenal string-capsule culture compared with bone marrow, blood and rectal-swab cultures for diagnosing typhoid and paratyphoid fever. J Infect Dis. 1984;149:157–61.
101. Guerra-Caceres JG, Gotuzzo-Herencia E, Crosby-Dagnino E, et al. Diagnostic value of bone marrow culture in typhoid fever. Trans R Soc Trop Med Hyg. 1979;73:680–3.
102. Gilman RH, Terminel M, Levine MM, et al. Relative efficacy of blood, urine, rectal swab, bone-marrow and rose-spot cultures for recovery of *Salmonella typhi* in typhoid fever. Lancet. 1975;1:1211.
103. Gilman RH, Hornick RB. Duodenal isolation of *Salmonella typhi* by string capsule in acute typhoid fever. J Clin Microbiol. 1976;3:456.
104. Nardiello S, Pizzella T, Russo M, et al. Serodiagnosis of typhoid fever by enzyme-linked immunosorbent assay determination of anti-*Salmonella typhi* lipopolysaccharide antibodies. J Clin Microbiol. 1984;20:718–21.
105. Rowland HAK. The complications of typhoid fever. J Trop Med Hyg. 1961;64:143.
106. Gupta SP, Gupta MS, Bhardwaj S, et al. Current clinical patterns of typhoid fever: a prospective study. J Trop Med Hyg. 1985;88:377–81.
107. Farid Z, Hassan A, Wahab MFA, et al. Trimethoprim–sulphamethoxazole in enteric fevers. Br Med J. 1970;3:323.
108. Sardesai HV, Karandikar RS, Harshe RG. Comparative trial of co-trimoxazole and chloramphenicol in typhoid fever. Br Med J. 1973;1:82.
109. Butler T, Rumans L, Arnold K. Response of typhoid fever caused by chloramphenicol-susceptible and chloramphenicol-resistant strains of *Salmonella typhi* to treatment with trimethoprim–sulfamethoxazole. Rev Infect Dis. 1982;4:551.
110. Annamalai A, Shreekumar S, Muthukumaran R. Empyema in enteric fever due to *Salmonella paratyphi* B. Dis Chest. 1969;55:72.
111. Typhoid carriers, editorial. Br Med J. 1964;1:1521.
112. Blaser MJ, Feldman RA. Salmonella bacteremia: reports to the Centers for Disease Control, 1968–1979. J Infect Dis. 1981;143:743–6.
113. Saphra I, Winter JW. Clinical manifestations of salmonellosis in man: an evaluation of 7779 human infections identified at the New York Salmonella Center. N Engl J Med. 1957;256:1128.
114. Sperber SJ, Schleupner CJ. Salmonellosis during infection with human immunodeficiency virus. Rev Infect Dis. 1987;9:925–33.
115. Whimbey E, Gold JWM, Polsky B, et al. Bacteremia and fungemia in patients with the acquired immunodeficiency syndrome. Ann Intern Med. 1986;104:511–4.
116. Connolly MJ, Snow MH, Ingham HR. Ciprofloxacin treatment of recurrent *Salmonella* septicaemia in a patient with acquired immune deficiency syndrome. J Antimicrob Chemother. 1986;18:647–8.
117. Kinsella TR, Yogev R, Shulman ST, et al. Treatment of *Salmonella* meningitis and brain abscess with the new cephalosporins: two case reports and a review of the literature. Pediatr Infect Dis J. 1987;6:476–80.
118. West SE, Goodkin R, Kaplan AM. Neonatal Salmonella meningitis complicated by cerebral abscesses. West J Med. 1977;127:142.
119. Cohen JI, Bartlett JA, Corey GR. Extra-intestinal manifestations of salmonella infections. Medicine. 1987;66:349–88.
120. Bryan JP, Rocha H, Scheld WM. Problems in salmonellosis: rationale for clinical trials with newer β-lactam agents and quinolones. Rev Infect Dis. 1986;8:189–207.
121. Rodriguez RE, Valero V, Watanakunakorn C. Salmonella focal intracranial infections: review of the world literature (1984–1984) and report of an unusual case. Rev Infect Dis. 1986;8:31–41.
122. Weiss W, Eisenberg GM, Flippin HF. Salmonella pleuropulmonary disease. Am J Med Sci. 1957;233:487.
123. Barney DP, Fisher R, Schaffner W. Salmonella empyema: a review. South Med J. 1977;70:375.
124. Shanson DC, Brigden W, Weaver EJM. *Salmonella enteritidis* endocarditis. Br Med J. 1977;1:612.
125. Kanwar YS, Malhotra V, Anderson BR, et al. Salmonellosis associated with abdominal aortic aneurysm. Arch Intern Med. 1974;134:1095.
126. Cohen PS, O'Brien TF, Schoenbaum SC, et al. The risk of endothelial infection in adults with salmonella bacteremia. Ann Intern Med. 1978;89:931.
127. Parsons R, Gregory J, Palmer DL. Salmonella infections of the abdominal aorta. Rev Infect Dis. 1983;5:227.
128. Sprecht EE. Hemoglobinopathic *Salmonella* osteomyelitis: orthopedic aspects. Clin Orthop. 1971;71:110.
129. Ortiz-Neu C, Marr JS, Cherubin CE, et al. Bone and joint infections due to *Salmonella*. J Infect Dis. 1978;138:820.
130. Hakansson U, Eitrem R, Low B, et al. HLA-antigen B27 in cases with joint affectations in an outbreak of salmonellosis. Scand J Infect Dis. 1976;8:245–8.
131. Samra Y, Shaked Y, Maier MK. Nontyphoid salmonellosis in patients with total hip replacement: report of four cases and review of the literature. Rev Infect Dis. 1986;8:978–83.
132. Sharr MM. Splenic abscess due to *Salmonella agona*. Br Med J. 1972;1:546.
133. Scott IHK, Thomas HW, Walters RO. Acute splenic abscess due to *Salmonella chester*. Br Med J. 1977;1:688.
134. Chulay JD, Lankerani MR. Splenic abscess: report of 10 cases and review of the literature. Am J Med. 1976;61:513.
135. Poon M, Sanders MG. Hepatic abscess caused by *Salmonella paratyphi* B. Can Med Assoc J. 1972;107:529.
136. Lasch EE. Liver abscess due to salmonellosis: a report on two cases in Upper Volta. Isr J Med Sci. 1966;2:377.
137. Gremillion DH, Geckler R, Ellenbogen C. Salmonella abscess: a potential nosocomial hazard. Arch Surg. 1977;112:843.
138. Kaye D, Merselis JG, Connolly CS, et al. Treatment of chronic carriers of *Salmonella typhosa* with ampicillin. Ann NY Acad Sci. 1967;145:429.
139. Musher DM, Rubenstein AD. Permanent carriers nontyphosal salmonellae. Public Health Rep. 1973;132:869.
140. Freitag JL. Treatment of chronic typhoid carriers by cholecystectomy. Public Health Rep. 1964;79:567.
141. Phillips WE. Treatment of chronic typhoid carriers with ampicillin. JAMA. 1971;217:913.
142. Merselis JG, Kaye D, Connolly CS, et al. Quantitative bacteriology of the typhoid carrier state. Am J Trop Med Hyg. 1964;13:425.
143. Levine MM, Ferreccio C, Black RE, et al. Chilean Typhoid Committee. Large-scale field trial of Ty21a live oral typhoid vaccine in enteric-coated capsule formulation. Lancet. 1987;1:1049–52.
144. Gilman RH, Hornick RB, Woodward TE, et al. Evaluation of a UDP glucose 4 epimerase-less mutant of *Salmonella typhi* as a live oral vaccine. J Infect Dis. 1977;136:717.
145. Wahdan MH, Sérié C, Cerisier Y. A controlled field trial of live *Salmonella typhi* strain TY 21a oral vaccine against typhoid: three-year results. J Infect Dis. 1982;145:292.
146. Woodward TE, Woodward WE. A new oral vaccine against typhoid fever. J Infect Dis. 1982;145:289.
147. Mandal BK. Typhoid fever and other *Salmonellae*. Current Opinion Infect Dis. 1988;1:84–7.
148. Acharya IL, Lowe CU, Thapa R, et al. Prevention of typhoid fever in Nepal with the Vi capsular polysaccharide of *Salmonella typhi*. N Engl J Med. 1987;317:1101–4.
149. DeCarvalho EM, Martinelli R, DeOliveira MMG, et al. Cefamandole treatment of *Salmonella* bacteremia. Antimicrob Agents Chemother. 1982;21:334.
150. Paniker CKJ, Vimala KN. Transferable chloramphenicol resistance in *Salmonella typhi*. Nature, 1972;239:109.
151. McHugh GL, Hopkins CC, Moellering RC, et al. *Salmonella typhimurium* resistant to silver nitrate, chloramphenicol, and ampicillin. Lancet. 1975;1:235.
152. Overturf G, Merton KI, Mathies AW. Antibiotic resistance in typhoid fever. N Engl J Med. 1972;289:463.
152. Lawrence RM, Goldstein E, Hoeprich PD. Typhoid fever caused by chloramphenicol-resistant organisms. JAMA. 1973;224:861.
154. Cherubin CE, Neu HC, Rahal JJ, et al. Emergence of resistance to chloramphenicol in *Salmonella*. J Infect Dis. 1977;135:807.
155. Gangarosa EJ, Bennett JV, Wyatt C, et al. An epidemic-associated episome. J Infect Dis. 1972;126:215.

156. Holmberg SD, Osterhold MT, Senger KA, et al. Drug-resistant *Salmonella* from animals fed antimicrobials. N Engl J Med. 1984;311:617–22.
157. Chin TDY. Therapy of salmonellosis. Ration Drug Ther. 1976;10:1.
158. Anderson ES. Chloramphenicol-resistant *Salmonella typhi*. Lancet. 1973;2:1494.
159. Holmburg SD. Drug-resistant *Salmonella* species from animals fed antimicrobics. Infect Dis Newsletter. 1986;5:25–32.
160. Spika JS, Waterman SH, Soo Hoo GW, et al. Chloramphenicol-resistant *Salmonella newport* traced through hamburger to dairy farms. N Engl J Med. 1987;316:565–70.
161. Cohen ML, Tauxe RV. Drug-resistant *Salmonella* in the United States: an epidemiologic perspective. Science. 1986;234:964–9.
162. DuPont HL, Steele JH. Use of antimicrobial agents in animal feeds: implications for human health. Rev Infect Dis. 1987;9:447–60.
163. Lamb VA, Mayhall CG, Spadora AC, et al. Outbreak of *Salmonella typhimurium* gastroenteritis due to an imported strain resistant to ampicillin, chloramphenicol and trimethoprim–sulfamethoxazole in a nursery. J Clin Microbiol. 1984;20:1076–9.
164. Pichler HET, Diridl G, Sticker K, et al. Clinical efficacy of ciprofloxacin compared with placebo in bacterial diarrhea. Am J Med. 1987;82(Suppl 4A):329–32.
165. Kaye D, Rocha H, Eyckmans L, et al. Comparison of parenteral ampicillin and parenteral chloramphenicol in the treatment of typhoid fever. Ann NY Acad Sci. 1967;145:423.
166. Mentzing LO, Ringertz O. Salmonella infection in tourists. 2. Prophylaxis against salmonellosis. Acta Pathol Microbiol Scand. 1968;74:405.
167. Finger D, Wood WG Jr. Apparent activation of *Salmonella* enteritis by oxytetracycline. Am J Med. 1955;18:389.
168. Pillay N, Adams EB, Coombes DN. Comparative trial of amoxycillin and chloramphenicol in treatment of typhoid fever in adults. Lancet. 1975;2:333.
169. Robertson RP, Wahab MFA, Raasch FO. Evaluation of chloramphenicol and ampicillin in Salmonella enteric fever. N Engl J Med. 1968;278:171.
170. Rowe B, Threlfall EJ, Ward LR. Does chloramphenicol remain the drug of choice for typhoid? Epidemiol Infect. 1987;98:379–89.
171. Trimethorpim–sulfamethoxazole in typhoid. (Editorial). Br Med J. 1970;3:297.
172. Snyder MJ, Perroni J, Gonzalez O, et al. Trimethoprim–sulfamethoxazole in the treatment of typhoid and paratyphoid fevers. J Infect Dis. 1973;128(Suppl):734.
173. Kamat SA. Evaluation of therapeutic efficacy of trimethoprim–sulfamethoxazole and chloramphenicol in enteric fever. Br Med J. 1970;3:320.
174. Franzen C, Lidin-Janson G, Nygren B. Trimethoprim–sulfamethoxazole in enteric infections. Scand J Infect Dis. 1972;4:231.
175. Hassan A, Erian M, Said F, et al. Comparison of co-trimoxazole and chloramphenicol in enteric fever, letter. Br Med J. 1973;3:108.
176. Scragg JN, Rubidge CJ. Trimethoprim and sulfamethoxazole in typhoid fever in children. Br Med J. 1971;3:738.
177. Gargalianos P, Jackson PT, Geddes AM. Trimethoprim in enteric fever. J Antimicrob Chemother. 1986;18:277–9.
178. Soe GB, Overturf GD. Treatment of typhoid fever and other systemic salmonelloses with cefotaxime, ceftriaxone, cefoperazone, and other newer cephalosporins. Rev Infect Dis. 1987;9:719–36.
179. Pape JW, Gerdes H, Orial L, et al. Typhoid fever: successful therapy with cefoperazone. J Infect Dis. 1986;153:272–6.
180. Uwaydah M, Nassar NT, Harakeh H, et al. Treatment of typhoid fever with cefamandole. Antimicrob Agents Chemother. 1984;26:426–7.
181. Mandal B, Flegg P, Dunbar E, et al. Ciprofloxacin in enteric fever. Chemotherapia. 1987;6(Suppl):492–3.
182. Sammalkorpi K, Lahdevirta J, Makela R, et al. Treatment of chronic salmonella carriers with ciprofloxacin (Letter). Lancet. 1987;2:164–5.
183. Ramirez CA, Bran JL, Meja CR, et al. Open, prospective study of the clinical efficacy of ciprofloxacin. Antimicrob Agents Chemother. 1985;28:128–32.
184. Garcia IF, Mejia CR, Ramirez C, et al. Treatment of typhoid fever with ciprofloxacin. A new quinolone antimicrobial. Presented at the International Congress for Infectious Diseases, Cairo, Egypt, April 24, 1985. Reported by BK. Mandal in Bacterial Infections: typhoid fever and other salmonellae. Curr Opinion Gastroenterol. 1986;2:109–12.
185. Kaye D, Merselis JG, Hook EW. Susceptibility of *Salmonella* species to four antibiotics. N Engl J Med. 1963;269:1084.
186. Hook EW. Antimicrobial therapy of *Salmonella* infections. J Egypt Public Health Assoc. 1970;45:206.
187. Hoffman SL, Punjabi NH, Kumala S, et al. Reduction of mortality in chloramphenicol-treated severe typhoid fever by high-dose dexamethasone. N Engl J Med. 1984;310:82.
188. Cooles P. Adjuvant steroids and relapse of typhoid fever. J Trop Med Hyg. 1986;89:229–31.
189. Archampong EG. Operative treatment of typhoid perforation of the bowel. Br Med J. 1969;3:273.
190. Nolan CM, White PC Jr. Treatment of typhoid carriers with amoxicillin. JAMA. 1978;239:2352–4.
191. Johnson WD Jr, Hook EW, Lindsey E, et al. Treatment of chronic typhoid carriers with ampicillin. Antimicrob Agents Chemother. 1973;3:439.
192. Freerksen E, Rosenfield M, Freerksen R, et al. Treatment of chronic *Salmonella* carriers. Chemotherapy. 1977;23:192.
193. Hudson SJ, Ingham HR, Snow MH. Treatment of *Salmonella typhi* carrier state with ciprofloxacin (Letter). Lancet. 1985;1:1047.

200. SHIGELLA SPECIES (BACILLARY DYSENTERY)

HERBERT L. DuPONT

The term *dysentery* was used by Hippocrates to indicate a condition characterized by frequent passage of stools containing blood and mucus accompanied by straining and painful defecation. It was not until the end of the last century, when the causes of amebiasis and bacillary dysentery were determined, that the two great forms of dysentery could be accurately separated. Much of the dysentery in the older historical writings is considered to be of bacillary origin (shigellosis), in view of the absence of liver complications. After the causative agents of the two types of dysentery were determined, the different epidemiologic settings were described. In 1859 in Prague, Lambl, and then later Osler[1] and Councilman and Lafleur,[2] helped to verify the pathogenicity of *Entamoeba histolytica*. In 1898 Shiga[3] conclusively demonstrated that a bacterium was present in the stools of many patients with dysentery and that agglutinins could be demonstrated in the serum of the infected patient. Two years later, Flexner[4] found a similar but serologically different organism in stools of other patients with dysentery acquired in the Philippines. Rogers[5] stated in 1913 that "epidemic dysentery in asylums, jails, or in long-occupied and unsanitary military camps during the war is nearly certain to be bacillary, while sporadic cases in a warm climate are more frequently amebic."

Medical writings since the beginning of recorded history have dealt with the common problems of dysentery in civilian and military populations; perhaps the greatest historical consideration is the influence that bacillary dysentery had on military campaigns. Nearly every long campaign and extended siege has produced epidemics of bacillary dysentery, particularly when sanitary and food sources could not be adequately controlled. In many battles described during the Peloponnesian War, the British campaigns in the eighteenth century, Napoleon's campaigns, the Crimean War, the American Civil War, the Franco-Prussian War, and the Chino-Japanese War, a heavier toll was ascribed to bacillary dysentery than to war-related injuries.[6]

MICROBIOLOGY

Shigella are small gram-negative rods that are members of the family Enterobacteriaceae, tribe Escherichieae, and genus *Shigella*. They are nonmotile and nonencapsulated.

Isolation Techniques

The infecting strain of *Shigella* is generally present in stools in concentrations between 10^3 and 10^9 viable cells per gram of stool, depending on the stage of illness. During the first several days of illness the counts are higher; they drop off to lower levels after several days of clinical disease. During the postconvalescent shedding period, counts fall to 10^2–10^3 viable cells per gram of stool. Recovery of the agent microbiologically is usually not difficult in the early stages of disease due to the higher counts present; it is more difficult during later stages of illness due to lower counts of viable bacteria. Careful selection of material and processing on appropriate media gives a higher yield of organisms. The sooner after passage the specimen is processed, the higher the yield. Stools that stand at room temperature for more than 24 hours have a profound drop in the number of viable cells, and recovery is less likely. A rectal swab obtained and seeded immediately at the bedside is an optimal way to perform a stool culture. In performing bacteriologic identification of *Shigella*, a bit of blood or mucus is seeded onto at least two different media. Generally, stool is plated lightly on a medium with only mild inhibiting factors for gram-negative growth such as MacConkey, xylose-lysine-desoxycholate (XLD) medium, Tergitol-7, or eosin methylene blue (EMB) agar, while a separate specimen is plated heavily on a more inhibitory medium such as *Shigella–Salmonella* (SS) medium. The more plates used, the greater the recovery yield will be. After overnight incubation at 37°C, lactose-negative colonies are picked to triple sugar iron agar (TSI) and lysine iron agar (LIA) slants and reincubated. Those giving a characteristic reaction (alkaline slant, acid butt, and no gas) are tested biochemically and then serologically identified with *Shigella* grouping and typing antisera.

Group and Type Identification

Each of the approximately 40 serotypes of *Shigella* is divided into four groups depending on serologic similarity and fermentation reaction: group A (*S. dysenteriae*), group B (*S. flexneri*), group C (*S. boydii*), and group D (*S. sonnei*). Commercial antiserum is available for determining group- and type-specific antigenicity. *Shigella sonnei* accounts for between 60 and 80 percent of the cases currently reported in the United States.

Invasive Escherichia coli

Certain strains of *E. coli* can cause a clinical illness indistinguishable from shigellosis and should be considered as causative agents of bacillary dysentery. Nearly all the *Shigella*-like *E. coli* have been shown to possess somatic antigens related to *Shigella* serotypes, further demonstrating the similarity of these two groups of organisms. *Escherichia coli* that cause bacillary dysentery have been shown to belong serologically to the following *E. coli* O-groups: 28, 29, 112, 115, 124, 136, 143, 144, 147, 152, 164, and 167. Serotyping may ultimately prove to be useful in detecting these strains. A practical test for determining the virulence of the bacterial isolate (*Shigella* or invasive *E. coli* strain) is the Séreny test.[7] Keratoconjunctivitis develops after 1–7 days in guinea pigs (or rabbits) when an invasive bacterial strain (*E. coli* or *Shigella*) is dropped into the conjunctival sac of the animal (Fig. 1). Recently a different form of bacillary dysentery was shown to be caused by an 0157:H7 strain of *E. coli*.[8] The source of infection characteristically has been contaminated hamburgers obtained at a fast food chain. Serotype 026:H11 *E. coli* has also been implicated as a causative agent of the syndrome. Patients affected acquire dysentery (bloody diarrhea), and a colitis can be documented by endoscopy. The illness differs from that associated with invasive *E. coli* in that high fever is not a feature of this so-called hemorrhagic colitis.

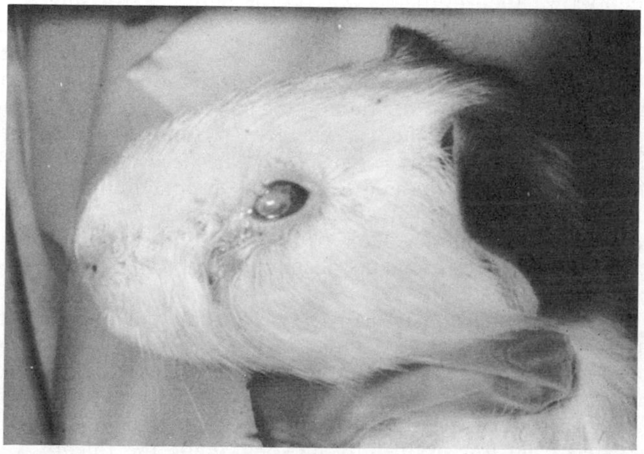

FIG. 1. Guinea pig with keratoconjunctivitis following conjunctival inoculation of invasive *E. coli*. This is a positive Sèreny test.

PATHOGENESIS

Communicability

Bacillary dysentery is the most communicable of the bacterial diarrheas. Volunteer experiments have demonstrated that shigellosis is unique among bacterial enteropathogens in that less than 200 viable cells readily produce the disease in healthy adults.[9] This low dose of organisms probably explains how the illness can be transferred from person to person, why the secondary attack rate is so high when an index case is introduced into a family, and why recurrent bacillary dysentery is an important problem in institutionalized or crowded populations.

Invasiveness

Virulent *Shigella* and other nontoxigenic invasive *E. coli* strains produce disease after invading the intestinal mucosa,[10] with subsequent multiplication and destruction of the mucosa. *Shigella* infection is superficial, and only rarely is there penetration beyond the mucosa. This explains the rarity of obtaining positive blood cultures in shigellosis despite the common occurrence of hyperpyrexia and toxemia. Studies designed to characterize the genetics of virulent *Shigella* strains have shown that the property of invasiveness of *Shigella* and invasive *E. coli* is associated with a mixture of soluble bacterial proteins encoded by a 140-MD plasmid.[11] In some *Shigella* strains a portion of the chromosome also controls invasion of the guinea pig cornea and conjunctiva; it is a locus near the purine E and lactose-galactose regions.[12] Studies using *Shigella-E. coli* hybrids have indicated that the xylose-rhamnose region of the *Shigella* chromosome is also important in determining invasiveness.[13]

Toxigenicity

The Shiga bacillus (*S. dysenteriae* 1) was shown in the early part of this century to produce a neurotoxin that caused paralysis and death in mice and rabbits. It has been suspected since that time that the toxin played an important role in the pathogenesis of clinical illness. Later, an exotoxin in the Shiga bacillus was shown to have enterotoxin activity in the ligated ileal loop model[14] and also to have cytotoxic properties when intestinal mucosa was examined.[15] A possible role for toxin production in the evolution of human shigellosis due to other organisms was further suggested by showing that an *S. flexneri* strain and an *S. sonnei* strain produced a similar toxin, although in decreased amounts, and that sera obtained from patients recently infected with these two species were able to neutralize the activity of Shiga toxin.[16] Undoubtedly, invasiveness is the primary virulence characteristic of *Shigella* strains, but toxin elaboration probably plays a role in the evolution of the local destructive mucosal lesion once the organisms have invaded the colonic mucosa. It is possible that toxin might also help to explain the watery small bowel type of diarrhea that characteristically is seen during the first or second day of illness. Shiga toxin production does appear to be the important virulence property of hemorrhagic colitis *E. coli* (0157:H7).[17]

Anatomic Location of Infection

Volunteer studies have helped to establish the intestinal localization of bacteria in experimental shigellosis. Within 12 hours after swallowing virulent shigellae, the bacteria transiently multiply in the small bowel to concentrations of 10^7–10^9 viable cells/ml of lumenal contents. The counts are higher in the lower portions of the small intestine, although occasionally the infecting strain can be recovered from the stomach for as long as 20 hours after the strain is ingested despite low pH of gastric contents. Abdominal pain and cramping and fever occur while the bacteria are localized in the small bowel. Within a few days, the infecting strain is no longer detectable in small bowel fluid, the patient's temperature becomes lower, and pain and tenderness become more severe and are generally confined to lower abdominal quadrants. Urgency, tenesmus, and bloody mucoid stools (dysentery) often occur in the later stages of infection and correlate with a diffuse colonic localization of the bacteria. The density of intramucosal bacteria is greatest at the lumenal surface and extends in decreasing concentrations to reach the lamina propria and submucosa. Microabscesses form and coalesce to form large abscesses that slough, producing mucosal ulcerations.

EPIDEMIOLOGY

Hippocrates indicated that when a dry winter was followed by a rainy spring, an increase in the number of dysentery cases would follow in the summer. Such an epidemiologic observation has been made by others in more recent years. Tropical environment and poor nutritional standards are associated with an increased prevalence of diarrheal illness in general. However, the relative frequency of specific pathogens appears to be surprisingly similar, irrespective of geographic location. Because of the characteristic clinical picture of bacillary dysentery, this represents one of the most accurately diagnosed and reported classes of infectious diarrhea. The greatest frequency of illness is reported among infants and younger preschool children. Disease rates and also complications and severity follow the degree of malnutrition. Generally bacillary dysentery is a summertime illness. Flies may be important in the transmission of bacillary dysentery,[18–20] especially in tropical climates. Dysentery in warm countries is most prevalent when the fly population is at its highest. Bacteriologic surveys of fly populations have been carried out and indicate that flies can occasionally be shown to be positive for *Shigella* bacteria.[19]

Cyclic Patterns of Disease

Since the description of bacteriologic isolation procedures, cyclic epidemics of bacillary dysentery have been described, each lasting 20–30 years.[21] In Europe during the first 25 years of this century dysentery was generally caused by *S. dysenteriae* 1 (the Shiga bacillus), and mortality was higher than subsequently seen when other serotypes became prevalent. Between 1926 and 1938 *S. flexneri* strains became more important than the Shiga bacillus, and currently *S. sonnei* has replaced other agents as the important cause of bacillary dysentery in European countries and in the United States. A similar trend has occurred in many parts of the world to the point that *S. sonnei* is the most important cause of dysentery in nearly all developed or industrialized countries. It is of interest that in England from the beginning of the seventeenth to the middle of the nineteenth century similar epidemic cycles of bacillary dysentery were described.[6,22] The cyclic pattern of serotypes specific for shigellosis suggests that it takes a certain number of years for herd immunity to reach a critical level in a population before one species of *Shigella* will disappear to be replaced by another. It may be that the disease attacks each generation, rendering the survivors immune and must then wait for the occurrence of nonimmune offspring.[6]

Incidence of Shigellosis by Geography and Host

Bacillary dysentery in Britain is mainly an acute diarrheal disease in school and younger school children. In the United States the highest rate of *Shigella* recovery is in those 1–4 years of age. There has been a change in the seasonal prevalence of bacillary dysentery in the United Kingdom that now correlates with the student enrollment in primary schools. It has been suggested that fecal contamination of lavatory seats in nursery and primary schools occurs from children with diarrhea, and that infection is transmitted to the hands of the younger children.[23] Shigellosis has become an important problem in day care centers for preschool children in the United States. Between 20,000 and 50,000 cases are reported each year in the United Kingdom,[24] and approximately 13,000–19,000 cases each year are reported in the United States. The actual number of cases clearly is far greater than those reported.

In numerous published studies[25–27] an etiologic agent has been identified in 10–40 percent of diarrhea cases, depending on geographic location and severity of illness reported. The major agent identified in these studies was a *Shigella* strain. Bacillary dysentery is primarily a disease of children from 6 months to 10 years of age. Adults often acquire the illness from their children. Children less than 6 months of age do not commonly develop bacillary dysentery. However, in industrialized countries *Shigella* strains may (rarely) cause severe illness in newborns,[28] but in developing countries, where breast feeding is more common, infants are highly resistant to shigellosis,[29] probably due to changes in intestinal flora of breast-fed children or because of the presence of specific antibody in breast milk. *Campylobacter* has been shown to be an important cause of diarrhea in all regions of the world. Its frequency of occurrence often varies inversely with the rate of *Shigella* cases, which is an unexplained observation.

Modes of Spread and Reservoirs in Nature

Most cases of bacillary dysentery are a result of person-to-person transmission. However, in a number of instances widespread epidemics have occurred in military or civilian populations and among persons on board cruise ships due to contaminated food or water. Water and food appear to be particularly important vectors of *Shigella* transmission in developing countries.[30,31] Epidemics of water-borne shigellosis generally appear to be due to wells contaminated with fecal material. Felsen[18] found that dysentery strains could be recovered for up to 6 months from water samples maintained at room temperature. Wells are often located close to cesspools and privies in developing countries where sanitation principles are not followed. In other areas septic tank discharge may empty into lakes, ponds, or other bodies of water close to intakes of camp water supplies or adjacent to bathing beaches. Chlorination of water, if appropriately maintained, will remove the threat of such infections. Food-borne transmission disease is not common compared with direct contact spread, but, when it occurs, it is associated with large outbreaks. During a 5-year period (1964–1968), the Centers for Disease Control in Atlanta reported 21 food-borne or waterborne outbreaks of shigellosis in the United States,[32] indicating the relative rarity of documenting common source epidemics. An epidemiologic observation has been made that when water sanitation improvements are implemented in a community, the incidence of typhoid fever falls, but the prevalence of bacillary dysentery remains unchanged.[18] In contrast to shigellosis, diseases due to *Salmonella, Vibrio cholerae*, and *E. coli* appear epidemiologically to be associated in almost all cases with food- or water-borne transmission. Such a vehicle of transmission is probably necessary with the latter agents because a larger inoculum is necessary to produce illness.[33]

Hand transmission is likely to be a common means of acquiring infection. At a custodial institution, mentally retarded persons were studied for the prevalence of hand transmission of bacteria.[19] Finger and simultaneous fecal cultures were obtained from 268 institutionalized patients. A *Shigella* strain was isolated from the stool of 39 persons, while the fingers were positive in 4 (10 percent of those with a positive stool culture). Additionally, fecal cultures were found to be negative in an additional 229 patients, while a *Shigella* strain was isolated from the hands and fingers of two of these patients with negative stool cultures. *E. coli* was recovered from the fingers of 82 percent of those studied, demonstrating the common occurrence of fecal organisms on the hands among institutionalized persons. These institutionalized patients had adequate washroom and showering facilities and did not show evidence of decreased personal hygiene.

Secondary cases during outbreaks of shigellosis are common. One study demonstrated that 61 percent of the children less than 1 year of age developed bacillary dysentery once an index case occurred in a household.[19] The attack rate was approximately 40 percent for ages 1–4 and 20 percent for all ages once an index case was identified. Secondary attack rates are increased in houses having privies and are reduced in families once sanitary toilet facilities are installed. Transmission rates also correlated with poverty and overcrowding. Following a bout of shigellosis without antimicrobial therapy, fecal excretion of the infecting strain generally lasts 1–4 weeks. Long-term *Shigella* carriage has been well documented in a small percentage of cases and does not appear to correlate with any underlying intestinal dysfunction.[6,34] In contrast to typhoid and cholera carriers, the organisms in dysentery carriage are confined to a colonic site. In the absence of coexistent parasitic infestation of the intestine, these carriers generally will respond to antimicrobial therapy. The long-term carrier may be important to the epidemiology of food- or water-borne illness. The number of organisms excreted by these persons is generally less than is seen with acute dysentery, making them less communicable than active cases.

DIAGNOSIS

History

In any patient with acute diarrheal illness associated with toxemia and systemic symptoms, bacillary dysentery should be considered. This is particularly the case when the illness lasts longer than 48 hours, if there is intrafamily spread with an interval of 1–3 days between cases, if there is fever, and if blood or mucus are seen in stools. The occurrence of hyperpyrexia and seizures in infants and children with shigellosis has lead some to the conclusion that a neurotoxin is important in the pathogenesis of clinical illness, although there is little to support this notion. In patients able to give a careful history, a descending intestinal tract infection is often described. The first symptoms may be fever and abdominal cramping followed by voluminous watery stools (these findings correlate with small bowel site of infection) followed by a decrease in fever and an increase in number of stools with smaller volume ("fractional stools"). In a day or two bloody mucoid stools with fecal urgency and tenesmus may develop. These latter findings reflect a colonic site of infection. It is this evolution of disease symptoms, as the infecting strain descends the intestinal tract, that often leads to a clinical diagnosis of bacillary dysentery and may indicate the need for performing stool culture. Abdominal pain and diarrhea occur in nearly all patients with shigellosis, fever can be documented in approximately one-third of the cases, and mucus is seen in stools of half and gross blood in 40 percent of the cases.[35]

PHYSICAL EXAMINATION

Findings on physical examination are nonspecific and include a variable degree of systemic toxemia, fever (which may be as high as 106°F), abdominal tenderness, especially over the lower abdominal quadrants, and hyperactive bowel sounds. Rectal examination or proctoscopy is generally painful, and an abnormally friable, hyperemic rectal mucosa, increased mucus secretion, and areas of ecchymosis generally are found. Ulcerations of rectal mucosa are seen after several days of illness.

LABORATORY FINDINGS

During the acute illness, the infecting strain is present in large enough numbers that stool cultures generally are positive. In the later stages of the disease it may be necessary to culture material directly from the ulceration through a proctoscope or to incubate fecal material in enrichment broth before plating. In centers where the service is available, direct fluorescent antibody microscopy may be useful in detecting the organism when present in small numbers,[36] but, due to the numerous serotypes potentially responsible for the infection, this procedure does not have widespread application.

The total white blood cell count demonstrates no consistent findings, although leukopenia and brisk leukocytosis are seen on occasion. A "shift to the left" (an increased number of bands compared with segmented neutrophils) when a leukocyte differential count is performed in a patient with diarrhea suggests bacillary dysentery. The single most important laboratory test other than stool culture is the direct microscopic examination of stained fecal smear, which will show prevalent polymorphonuclear leukocytes.[37] A wet-mount preparation is made by adding stool (mucus if it is present) to an equal amount of methylene blue dye. The preparation is then covered with a coverslip and examined microscopically under the high dry objective. Alternately, the specimen can be heat-fixed before staining with dilute methylene blue. The specimen can then be examined under oil after drying. This dry preparation can be stored for later review. Numerous sheets of polymorphonuclear leukocytes are normally found (Fig. 2). Prevalent leukocytes indicate a colitis in which the colonic mucosa is diffusely involved. The leukocyte test when positive indicates a pathologic process, not an etiologic one, and white cells are usually seen also in salmonellosis, *Campylobacter* enteritis, and idiopathic ulcerative colitis.

Serologic evaluation of a patient with bacillary dysentery is generally not helpful in establishing the diagnosis because humoral antibodies do not develop before recovery. Serologic procedures are helpful as an epidemiologic tool in defining the extent of an epidemic in a population known to be infected by a known *Shigella* serotype (especially for the Shiga bacillus). The humoral antibody response correlates with the severity of clinical disease.[35]

TREATMENT AND CLINICAL COURSE

In certain patients with bacillary dysentery (particularly infants and elderly patients), significant dehydration may result from excessive fluid loss through diarrhea and vomiting. The fluid losses can generally be replaced by oral intake since the diarrhea associated with bacillary dysentery is not normally associated with profound fluid and electrolyte depletion. If vomiting or extreme toxemia are prominent features of the illness, especially in the very young or the elderly, intravenous fluid replacement may be necessary.

Antibiotics are useful in the management of shigellosis. In illness due to strains susceptible to antimicrobials, ampicillin or tetracycline will shorten the period of fecal excretion of the infecting strain and will limit the clinical course of illness.[38] Since the infection is normally self-limited, and because antibiotic resistance commonly develops following treatment, some feel that antimicrobial therapy should be reserved for the most severely ill patients.[39] However, since the infection is generally transmitted from person to person, and the infected or colonized person represents the major reservoir of infection, there are public health reasons to treat each patient with a positive stool culture or with known bacillary dysentery. The treatment

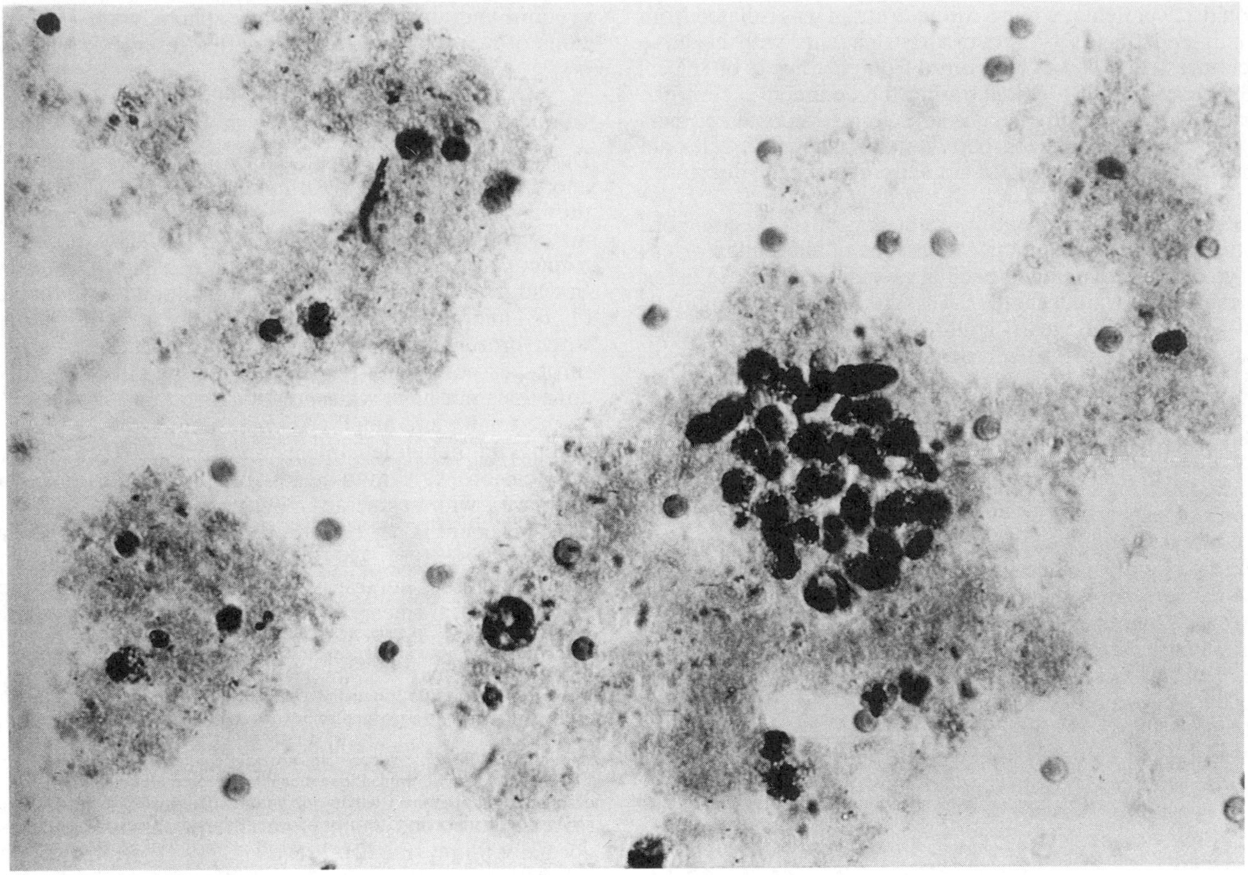

FIG. 2. Methylene blue stain of fecal leukocytes found in colitis. This exudative response may be seen in shigellosis, salmonellosis, *Campylobacter* infection, and colitis due to invasive *E. coli*.

of choice for shigellosis when susceptibility is unknown or when ampicillin/tetracycline-resistant strains are encountered is trimethoprim-sulfamethoxazole.[40,41] The dose is indicated in Table 1. In certain areas of Southeast Asia, Africa, and South America, trimethoprim resistance commonly occurs among prevalent strains of *Shigella*.[42] In these areas, for adult patients with shigellosis or when empiric therapy is aimed at both *Shigella* and *Campylobacter*, ciprofloxacin[43] or norfloxacin[44] will be effective. For children, nalidixic acid can be used in these geographic areas.

Intestinal motility patterns may be important in recovery from infection as well as in preventing the mucosal invasion by a bacterial agent. In such cases, diarrhea might be viewed as a protective mechanism, and its inhibition by motility-active drugs may not be wise. Paregoric has occasionally been shown to worsen clinical salmonellosis,[45] and in occasional patients antidiarrheal drugs such as diphenoxylate (Lomotil) worsen bacillary dysentery and could play a role in the development of toxic dilatation of the colon.[46]

Clinical illness if left untreated generally lasts between 1 day and 1 month, averaging 7 days. Although mortality is unusual in shigellosis except in malnourished children and in the elderly, the clinical illness is more striking and more likely to lead to hospitalization than most other forms of infectious diarrhea. Complications are unusual and generally consist of severe dehydration, febrile seizures, septicemia and/or pneumonia due to coliform organisms (and less commonly the infecting *Shigella* strain), keratoconjunctivitis, and arthritis. Patients with HLA-B27 histocompatability antigen may develop a post-Shigella Reiter syndrome. *Shigella dysenteriae* (the Shiga bacillus) characteristically produces a more serious form of diarrhea, and the mortality of untreated disease during epidemics may be as high as 20 percent. Bacterial strains that produce Shiga toxin (*S. dysenteriae* 1 and *E. coli* in hemorrhagic colitis) often produce the hemolytic uremic syndrome as a complication of illness. A rare fulminating form of bacillary dysentery is seen in children due to massive small intestine invasion by the infecting bacteria, and death early in infection is common (the "Ikari" syndrome).

TABLE 1. Antimicrobial Therapy for Bacillary Dysentery

First Choice		*Alternate*	
Children	*Adults*	*Children (>3 mo)*	*Adults*
TMP 10 mg/kg/day + SMX 50 mg/kg/day in 2 equal doses q12h (po) for 5 days	TMP 160 mg plus SMX 800 mg q12h (po) for 3–5 days	Nalidixic acid 55 mg/kg/day in 4 equally divided doses (po) for 5 days	Ciprofloxacin 500 mg bid (po) for 3–5 days or Norfloxacin 400 mg bid (po) for 3–5 days

Abbreviations: TMP: trimethoprim; SMX: sulfamethoxazole.

CONTROL

Environmental Control

A safe water supply is important for the control of shigellosis and probably represents the single most important factor in areas with substandard sanitation facilities.[47] Chlorination is another factor that is important in decreasing all enteric bacterial infections. Of critical importance to the establishment of a safe water supply system is the general level of sanitation in the area and the establishment of an effective sewage disposal system. Insecticides are useful in decreasing the vector population during peak seasons, and a decrease in the incidence of shigellosis, but not salmonellosis, may be seen after their use.[20] At other times of the year it may be helpful to attack breeding places of insects. Garbage collection and disposal of excreta and sewage may also be useful in controlling the vectors. In many areas it is necessary to examine the techniques of home preparation and storage of food. Important features may be improved such as personal and food hygienic facilities, or refrigeration may be necessary. A major prerequisite in transmission in most cases of bacillary dysentery is the degree of contact and the level of personal hygiene between patients with disease and susceptible persons. Other factors are frequent effective handwashing, voluntary removal of persons with diarrhea from roles as food handlers, and appropriate refrigeration and proper cooking of potentially infected foods. Breast-feeding through the first year of life is an important means of decreasing the incidence of bacillary dysentery in developing countries and in communities with substandard hygienic practices. Also, mothers should be taught how to prepare foods to supplement breast-feeding and to constitute the diet after weaning to improve both sanitation and nutrition. Finally, cases of diarrhea should be adequately diagnosed and isolated, and antimicrobial therapy should be instituted in cases of bacillary dysentery to decrease the reservoir of virulent strains. Degree of symptomatology, personal hygiene, and educability about ways enteric bacteria are spread are important factors that may determine the rate of transmission of the agent, and these factors should influence the decision for antimicrobial therapy.

Immunologic Control

Epidemiologic studies have indicated that a degree of homologous immunity can be demonstrated among those who have recovered from bacillary dysentery.[48–50] These observations have supported the idea that protective vaccine might be developed. It was shown that killed parenteral vaccines failed to protect animals against experimentally produced shigellosis[51] and to protect humans against naturally occurring illness.[52,53] Besredka[53] suggested that immunity against bacillary dysentery conferred by one attack of the disease was due essentially to the sensitization of the intestinal mucosa to dysentery bacilli, and that the antibodies circulating in the serum had a small role or none at all in the protection. After nearly 60 years, Besredka's concept of intestinal immunity still is held as the primary mode through which immunologic control might be feasible. The nature of the intestinal immune response has not been completely characterized. In natural shigellosis, IgA concentrations in stool increase as do anti-*Shigella* secretory IgA antibodies directed to homologous lipopolysaccharide.[54] Also, lymphocytes, monocytes, and granulocytes, in the absence of complement but in the presence of antibody, may serve an anti-*Shigella* function through cell-mediated mechanisms.[55] Formal and coworkers worked with both spontaneously derived avirulent *Shigella* mutants and hybrid strains (*Shigella–E. coli*) in monkeys.[56–58] The most significant work in the area of *Shigella* vaccine development has been carried out by Mel and colleagues, who used streptomycin-dependent mutant strains of *Shigella* as orally administered immunizing agents in Yugoslavian army soldiers and in children living in areas of hyperendemicity.[59,60] These workers demonstrated that immunization with a live attenuated bacterial strain given orally in multiple (at least four) doses would prevent clinical disease but would not alter the carrier status, providing gastric acidity was first decreased by sodium bicarbonate swallowed just before the vaccine. Serotype-specific protection followed vaccination and lasted for at least 6 months, and the immunizing agent remained protective when combined as a bivalent preparation. Volunteer experiments demonstrated that protective immunity imparted by oral immunization approximated that following recovery from disease.[9]

In the future, immunologic control may be possible against a limited number of serotypes of shigellae when attack rates are shown to be particularly high. Further research is being directed toward developing an immunizing strain that multiplies in the intestinal tract so fewer doses may be administered. It may be possible to create such a strain by intergeneric hybridization.[61] Attenuated bacteria can be constructed that are better adapted to host intestinal proliferation and that combine two enteric pathogens in a single vaccine preparation.[62] Also, the importance of exotoxin production by *Shigella* strains must be further studied. It is possible that antitoxic immunity might be important to susceptibility, and that a successful immunizing agent should also include a toxoid component.

REFERENCES

1. Osler W. On the amebae coli in dysentery and in dysentery liver abscess. Johns Hopkins Hosp Bull. 1890;1:736.
2. Councilman WT, Lafleur HA. Amebic dysentery. Johns Hopkins Hosp Rep 1891;2:395.
3. Shiga K. Observations on the epidemiology of dysentery in Japan. Philippine J Sci. 1906;1:485.
4. Flexner S. On the etiology of tropical dysentery. Philadelphia Med J. 1900;6:417.
5. Rogers L. Bacillary dysentery. In: Dysenteries, Their Differentiation and Treatment. London: Oxford University Press: 1913:268.
6. Davison WC. A bacteriological and clinical consideration of bacillary dysentery in adults and children. Medicine. 1922;1:389.
7. Séreny B. Experimental shigella keratoconjunctivitis: a preliminary report. Acta Microbiol Acad Sci Hung. 1955;2:293.
8. Riley LW, Remis RS, Helgerson SD, et al. Hemorrhagic colitis associated with a rare *Escherichia coli* serotype. N Engl J Med. 1983;308:681.
9. DuPont HL, Levine MM, Hornick RB, et al. Inoculum size in shigellosis and implications for expected mode of transmission. J Infect Dis. 1989; In press.
10. LaBrec E, Schneider H, Magnani T, et al. Epithelial cell penetration as an essential step in the pathogenesis of bacillary dysentery. J Bacteriol. 1964;88:1503.
11. Hale TL, Oaks V, Formal SB. Identification and antigenic characterization of virulence-associated, plasmid-coded proteins of *Shigella* spp. and enteroinvasive *Escherichia coli*. Infect Immun. 1985;50:620.
12. Formal SB, Gemski P Jr, Baron LS, et al. Chromosomal locus which controls the ability of *Shigella flexneri* to evoke keratoconjunctivitis. Infect Immun. 1971;3:73.
13. Formal SB, LaBrec EH, Kent TH, et al. Abortive intestinal infection with an *Escherichia coli-Shigella flexneri* hybrid strain. J Bacteriol. 1965;89:1374.
14. Keusch GT, Grady GF, Mata LJ, et al. Pathogenesis of shigella diarrhea. I. Enterotoxin production by *Shigella dysenteriae* 1. J Clin Invest. 1972;51:1212.
15. Keusch GT, Grady GF, Takeuchi A, et al. Pathogenesis of shigella diarrhea. II. Enterotoxin-induced acute enteritis in the rabbit ileum. J Infect Dis. 1972;126:92.
16. Keusch GT, Jacewicz M. The pathogenesis of shigella diarrhea. VI. Toxin and antitoxin in *Shigella flexneri* and *Shigella sonnei* infections in humans. J Infect Dis. 1977;135:552.
17. O'Brien AD, Newland JW, Miller RK, et al. Shiga-like toxin-coverting phages from *Escherichia coli* strains that cause hemorrhagic colitis or infantile diarrhea. Science. 1984;226:694.
18. Felsen J. Bacillary Dysentery Colitis and Enteritis. Philadelphia: WB Saunders; 1945.
19. Hardy A, Watt J. Studies of the acute diarrheal diseases. XVIII. Epidemiology. Public Health Rep. 1948;63:363.
20. Watt J, Lindsay D. Diarrheal disease control studies. I. Effect of fly control in a high morbidity area. Public Health Rep. 1948;63:1319.
21. Kostrzewski J, Stypulkowska-Misiurewicz H. Changes in the epidemiology of dysentery in Poland and the situation in Europe. Arch Immunol Ther Exp. 1968;16:429.

22. Gettings HS. Bacillary dysentery. Trans Soc Trop Med Hyg (Lond). 1915;8:111.
23. Cruickshank R. Diarrheal diseases in the United Kingdom. In: Pemberton J, ed. Epidemiology Reports on Research and Teaching. London: Oxford University Press; 1963:60.
24. Paul H. The Control of Diseases (Social and Communicable). 2nd ed. Baltimore: Williams & Wilkins; 1964:293.
25. Gordon J, Béhar M, Scrimshaw N. Acute diarrheal disease in less developed countries. I. An epidemiological basis for control. In: Control of Gastrointestinal Diseases. Pan Am Health Org, Technical Discussion, Sci Publication 100;1963:26.
26. Ingram V, Rights F, Khan H, et al. Diarrhea in children of West Pakistan: occurrence of bacterial and parasitic agents. Am J Trop Med Hyg. 1966;15:743.
27. Ramos-Alvarez M, Olarte J. Diarrheal diseases of children: the occurrence of enteropathogenic viruses and bacteria. Am J Dis Child. 1964;107:218.
28. Haltalin K. Neonatal shigellosis: report of 16 cases and review of the literature. Am J Dis Child. 1967;114:603.
29. Mata L, Urrutia J, Garcia B, et al. Shigella infection in breast-fed Guatemalan Indian neonates. Am J Dis Child. 1969;117:142.
30. Boyce JM, Hughes JM, Alim ARMA, et al. Patterns of *Shigella* infection in families in rural Bangladesh. Am J Trop Med Hyg. 1982;31:1015.
31. Tjoa WS, DuPont HL, Sullivan P, et al. Location of food consumption and travelers' diarrhea. Am J Epidemiol. 1977;106:61.
32. Donadio J, Gangarosa E. Foodborne shigellosis. J Infect Dis. 1969;119:666.
33. DuPont H, Hornick R. Clinical approach to infectious diarrheas. Medicine. 1973;52:265.
34. Levine M, DuPont H, Khodabandelou M, et al. Long-term shigella-carrier state. N Engl J Med. 1973;288:1169.
35. DuPont H, Hornick R, Dawkins A, et al. The response of man to virulent *Shigella flexneri* 2a. J Infect Dis. 1969;119:396.
36. Thomason B, Cowart G, Cherry W. Current status of immunofluorescence techniques for rapid detection of shigellae in fecal specimens. Appl Microbiol. 1965;13:605.
37. Harris J, DuPont H, Hornick R. Fecal leukocytes in diarrheal illness. Ann Intern Med. 1972;76:697.
38. Haltalin K, Nelson J, Ring R II, et al. Double-blind treatment study of shigellosis comparing ampicillin, sulfadiazone and placebo. J Pediatr. 1967;70:970.
39. Weissman J, Gangarosa E, DuPont H, et al. Changing needs in the antimicrobial therapy of shigellosis. J Infect Dis. 1973;127:611.
40. Nelson JD, Kusmiesz H, Jackson LH, et al. Trimethoprim sulfamethoxazole therapy for shigellosis. JAMA. 1976;235:1239.
41. DuPont HL, Reves RR, Galindo E, et al. Treatment of travelers' diarrhea with trimethoprim/sulfamethoxazole and with trimethoprim alone. N Engl J Med 1982;307:841.
42. Murray BE. Resistance of *Shigella, Salmonella*, and other selected enteric pathogens to antimicrobial agents. Rev Infect Dis. 1986;8:S172.
43. Ericsson CD, Johnson PC, DuPont HL, et al. Ciprofloxacin or trimethoprim/sulfamethoxazole as initial therapy for travelers' diarrhea. A placebo-controlled, randomized trial. Ann Intern Med. 1987;106:216.
44. DuPont HL, Corrado ML, Sabbaj J. Use of norfloxacin in the treatment of acute diarrheal disease. Am J Med. 1987;82(Suppl 6B):79.
45. Sprinz H. Pathogenesis of intestinal infections. Arch Pathol. 1969;87:556.
46. DuPont H, Hornick R. Adverse effects of Lomotil therapy in shigellosis. JAMA. 1973;226:1525.
47. Nyerges V, Eng N. Plan for the control of gastrointestinal diseases. Environmental sanitation, epidemiology, health education and early diagnosis and treatment. In: Control of Gastrointestinal Diseases. Pan Am Health Org, Technical Discussions, Sci Publication 100;1963:36.
48. Cruickshank R. Acquired immunity: bacterial infections. In: Cruickshank R, ed. Modern Trends in Immunology. Washington, DC: Butterworth; 1963:119.
49. DuPont H, Gangarosa E, Reller L, et al. Shigellosis in custodial institutions. Am J Epidemiol. 1970;92:172.
50. Hardy A, Watt J. The acute diarrheal diseases. JAMA. 1944;124:1173.
51. Formal S, Maenza R, Austin S, et al. Failure of parenteral vaccines to protect monkeys against experimental shigellosis. Proc Soc Exp Biol Med. 1967;125:347.
52. Hardy A, DeCapito T, Halbert S. Studies of acute diarrheal diseases. XIX. Immunization in shigellosis. Public Health Rep. 1948;63:685.
53. Besredka A. On the mechanism of dysenteric infection, antidysenteric vaccination per os, and the nature of antidysenteric immunity. Ann Inst Pasteur, Paris. 1919;33:301.
54. Winsor DK Jr, Mathewson JJ, DuPont HL. Comparison of serum and fecal antibody responses of patients with naturally acquired *Shigella sonnei* infection. J Infect Dis. 1988;158:1108.
55. Lowell GH, MacDermott RP, Summers PL, et al. Antibody-dependent cell-mediated antibacterial activity: K lymphocytes, monocytes, and granulocytes are effective against shigella. J Immunol. 1980;125:2778.
56. Formal S, LaBrec E, Palmer A, et al. Protection of monkeys against experimental shigellosis with attenuated vaccines. J Bacteriol. 1965;90:63.
57. Formal S, Kent T, Austin S, et al. Fluorescent-antibody and histological study of vaccinated and control monkeys challenged with *Shigella flexneri*. J Bacteriol. 1966;91:2368.
58. Formal S, Kent T, May H, et al. Protection of monkeys against experimental shigellosis with a living attenuated oral polyvalent dysentery vaccine. J Bacteriol. 1966;92:17.
59. Mel D, Arsic B, Nikolic B, et al. Studies on vaccination against bacillary dysentery. 4. Oral immunization with live monotypic and combined vaccines. Bull WHO. 1968;39:375.
60. Mel D, Gangarosa E, Radovanovic M, et al. Studies on vaccination against bacillary dysentery. 6. Protection of children by oral immunization with streptomycin-dependent Shigella strains. Bull WHO. 1971;45:457.
61. DuPont HL, Hornick RB, Snyder MJ, et al. II. Protection induced by oral live vaccine or primary infection. J Infect Dis. 1972;125:12.
62. Baron LS, Kopecko DJ, Formal SB, et al. Introduction of *Shigella flexneri* 2a type and group antigen genes into oral typhoid vaccine strain *Salmonella typhi* Ty 21A. Infect Immun. 1987;55:2797.

201. HAEMOPHILUS INFLUENZAE

E. RICHARD MOXON

DESCRIPTION OF THE PATHOGEN

Haemophilus influenzae is a small, nonmotile, non-spore-forming bacterium, and a strict parasite of humans found principally in the upper respiratory tract. First reported by Pfeiffer in 1892, the sensational claim that it was the primary agent of epidemic influenza proved fallacious; nonetheless, it has a wide range of pathogenic potential. Its requirement for growth factors, which can be supplied by erythrocytes, accounts for the generic name *Haemophilus* (blood-loving). In microscopic appearance, it is a small (1×0.3 μm) gram-negative bacterium. Stained organisms obtained from clinical specimens vary microscopically from small coccobacilli to long filaments. This variable morphology (pleomorphism) and inconsistent uptake of dyes (e.g., safranin) may result in erroneous interpretations of stained smears.

Aerobic growth of *H. influenzae* requires two supplements known as X factor and V factor, although neither refers to a single substance.[1] X factor can be supplied by heat-stable iron containing pigments that supply protoporphyrins essential for catalases, peroxidases, and cytochromes of the electron-transport chain. The requirement for X factor is used to distinguish *H. influenzae* from *Haemophilus parainfluenzae* (requires only V factor); since X factor is not required for anaerobic growth of *H. influenzae*, confusion may arise if *H. influenzae* is grown anaerobically (e.g., after stab inoculation). The heat-labile V factor, a coenzyme, may be supplied by nicotinamide adenine dinucleotide (NAD), by nicotinamide adenine dinucleotide phosphate (NADP), or by nicotinamide nucleoside. Although present in erythrocytes, V factor must be released from the cell to sustain optimal growth and thus standard blood agar is an unsatisfactory medium. *Haemophilus influenzae* exhibits satellitism around colonies of hemolytic *Staphylococcus aureus* (a source of V factor), and this technique may be used to identify *H. influenzae*. Superior culture results are obtained using media enriched with red cells that have been disrupted by heating (e.g., chocolate agar) or by peptic digestion (Fildes medium). Since excessive heat destroys V factor, commercial media must be quality controlled before use. Although it is not a strict requirement, some *H. influenzae* strains grow best in 5–10 percent carbon dioxide. Viability of *H. influenzae* is lost rapidly, so clinical specimens should be inoculated onto appropriate media without delay. A biotyping scheme[2] devised by Kilian (based on indole production, urease, and ornithine decarboxylase activity) may be used to characterize individual isolates. Biotype III is identical to *Haemophilus aegyptius*, the "Koch-Weeks bacillus."

Colonies of *H. influenzae* are usually granular, transparent (or slightly opaque), circular, and dome-shaped. On chocolate agar most colonies attain a size of about 0.5–0.8 mm during the first 24 hours of growth at 37°C, enlarging to 1.0–1.5 mm by 48 hours. Clinical isolates of *H. influenzae* may be encapsulated, although most do not express this surface antigen. Colonies of encapsulated strains are mucoid (iridescent when grown on transparent media and examined using an indirect source of light) and may attain a size of 3–4 mm. The production of capsule is of major significance to clinicians since it is an important virulence factor. Pittman[3] described six antigenically distinct capsular types, designated a–f.

Using the technique of multilocus enzyme electrophoresis to characterize isolates cultured from carriers and cases of disease obtained over several decades and from all continents, the population structure of *H. influenzae* has been shown to be clonal.[4] These studies also show that most unencapsulated isolates are not capsule-deficient variants of extant capsulate clones; they are genetically distinct and are more heterogeneous in genotype than are clones of capsulate *H. influenzae*.

EPIDEMIOLOGY AND PATHOGENESIS

Haemophilus influenzae is indigenous to humans; no other natural host is known. It is among the bacteria normally found in the pharynx (not the oral cavity) and to a lesser extent also colonizes the mucosae of the conjunctiva and the genital tract. Spread from one individual to another occurs by airborne droplets or by direct contagion with secretions. Exposure to *H. influenzae* begins after birth so that from infancy onwards, carriage of one or more strains for periods of days to months is common, and these organisms are often not eliminated by antibiotic therapy. Surveys have indicated that up to 80 percent of persons are carriers. As a consequence, the presence of *H. influenzae* in cultures obtained from the upper (but not the lower) respiratory tract is a normal finding. Most people are colonized with unencapsulated strains, but in 3–5 percent of people, the isolates have capsules—most commonly serotype b.[5] In general, carriers of *H. influenzae* remain healthy, but occasionally disease occurs. Two contrasting patterns of *H. influenzae* disease can be identified. The first and the most serious in its consequences is invasive infection such as meningitis, septic arthritis, epiglotittis, and cellulitis in which bacteremia is a prominent feature; these infections are usually caused by type b strains and occur in young children. The second category includes less serious but numerically more common infections that occur as a result of contiguous spread of *H. influenzae* within the respiratory tract, e.g., otitis media, sinusitis, conjunctivitis, and bronchopneumonia. These latter infections are usually, but not invariably, caused by unencapsulated strains, and their occurrence is usually conditioned by manifest breakdown of mechanisms that normally act to keep the respiratory tract sterile. These generalizations are not hard and fast; unencapsulated strains are an uncommon but well-recognized cause of neonatal sepsis,[6] including early onset pneumonia and meningitis. They are important in the etiology of invasive lower respiratory tract infections, especially among children living in socially deprived conditions.[7] Unencapsulated strains also cause invasive, bacteremic infections in adults.[8,9] Fifty percent of *H. influenzae* meningitis cases in the older age group are caused by unencapsulated strains and usually occur in persons who have anatomical defects or are otherwise immunocompromised. Obstetric infections such as peritubal abscess are well described.[6] Finally, outbreaks of an apparently new syndrome, Brazilian purpuric Fever, have been described recently in which young children initially presenting with conjunctivitis subsequently develop a serious, potentially fatal form of sepsis mimicking meningococcemia but caused by *H. influenzae* biotype *aegyptius*.[10]

Some key features in the pathogenesis of *H. influenzae* infections are summarized in Figure 1. Factors responsible for colonization are poorly understood. It has been shown experimentally that prior nasopharyngeal infection with influenza and other viruses potentiates bacteremia.[11] Microbial factors include surface adhesins such as filamentous fimbriae (pili), one class of which facilitates attachment to human buccal epithelial cells in vitro and shows specificity for the human blood group antigen Anton.[12] *Haemophilus influenzae* secretes IgAl proteases, the biological significance of which remains speculative.[13] *Haemophilus influenzae* produces at least two factors that inhibit the ciliary activity of human epithelial cells in vitro; one of these has been shown to be lipopolysaccharide and the other factor is of low molecular weight, most likely a heat-stable glycopeptide.[14] Type b strains, which are distinguished by the production of capsular polysaccharide composed of repeating units of ribosyl-ribitol phosphate,[15] account for greater than 95 percent of systemic *H. influenzae* infections in children. The primacy of type b capsule as a crucial virulence factor in the pathogenesis of invasive disease has been well established by the use of genetic techniques and the exploitation of an infant rat model of bacteremia and meningitis.[16] Following intranasal inoculation, *H. influenzae* b invaded the submucosa of the nasopharynx and entered the bloodstream within minutes. Meningitis rarely occured by direct penetration of the central nervous system (CNS) (e.g., via the cribriform plate) but resulted from hematogenous spread. The occurrence of meningitis correlated strikingly with the duration and intensity of bacteremia; experimental manipulations that decreased the efficiency of intravascular clearance (e.g., depletion of complement components or splenectomy) increased the incidence of meningitis.[17] In contrast, prior administration of specific serum antibodies or even priming of the immune response with *Escherichia coli* K100 (which has a capsule that is immunologically cross-reactive with PRP) decreased the severity of bacteremia and the incidence of meningitis.[18]

In many countries, *H. influenzae* b meningitis exceeds cases due to all other bacteria. The Centers for Disease Control surveillance studies of bacterial meningitis estimate that the incidence of *H. influenzae* type b meningitis in the United States is 1.24/100,000 or about 8,000 cases/year.[19] (For comparison, comparable estimated rates for *Neisseria meningitidis* and *Streptococcus pneumoniae* meningitis are 0.72 and 0.30/100,000 population, respectively.) Type b septicemia, meningitis, cellulitis, and septic arthritis mostly affect children aged less than 2 years[20] (peak attack rate 7–14 months) and occur more frequently in males, blacks, and poor families, and in the winter months. Several populations (e.g., Alaskan eskimos,[21] Navajo and Apache Indians)[22] have attack rates significantly higher than the general U.S. population, and the peak incidence of infection is earlier. Epiglottitis tends to occur in older children (aged 2–4 years) and has an estimated incidence of 0.7/100,000. Although epidemics of *H. influenzae* b infection do not occur, outbreaks of systemic infections have been documented among children in day care centers or among persons in closed populations (e.g., a geriatric unit), indicating that type b disease is contagious.[23,24] Among 1147 cases of *H. influenzae* meningitis, 9 associated cases (8 meningitis, 1 epiglottitis) occurred in family members, a 500-fold increase when compared with the general population. The greatest risk (3.4 percent) occurred in contacts aged less than 2 years; no secondary cases occurred in contacts aged 6 years or older.[25]

IMMUNITY

Because of the relative importance of *H. influenzae* b as a cause of meningitis and other systemic infections, careful investigations of the host factors determining susceptibility of humans to strains of this serotype have been made. Fothergill and Wright showed that blood from children aged 3 months to 3 years lacked bactericidal activity against a type b strain, whereas the blood of most neonates, older children, and adults was bactericidal.[26] They proposed that the bactericidal activity

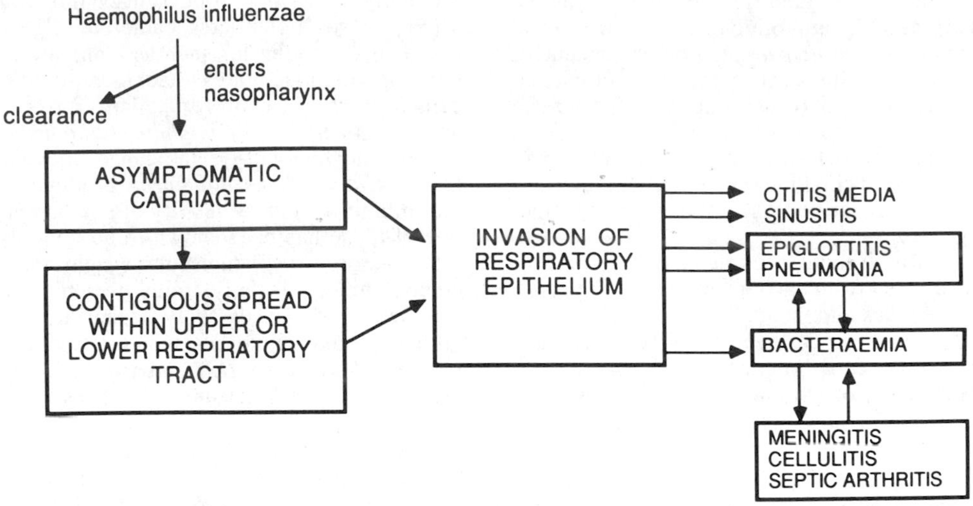

FIG. 1. Some of the diseases and their interrelationships that result from colonization of *Haemophilus influenzae* in the human respiratory tract.

of fresh blood was dependent upon specific antibodies. Alexander observed that when antiserum containing high titers of antibodies to type b capsule was administered as treatment for *H. influenzae* meningitis, a dramatic increase in the phagocytosis of cerebrospinal fluid (CSF) organisms was observed.[27] She suggested that the polyribosyl-ribitol (PRP) capsular polysaccharide was intrinsically antiphagocytic and that efficient ingestion by phagocytes was facilitated by opsonization with type-specific antibodies. This hypothesized role for anti-PRP antibodies as a major determinant in mediating protective immunity has been critically investigated during the last two decades, and its essential validity is established.[28,29] Serum anti-PRP antibodies activate complement-mediated bactericidal[29] and opsonic[30] activity in vitro and mediate protective immunity against systemic infections in humans.[31,32] However, there is an inadequate understanding of the mechanisms determining the age-related, natural acquisition of serum anti-PRP antibodies that occurs in virtually all individuals by ages 3–4 years[33] (Table 1). Indeed, certain data suggest that these antibodies occur in children who have apparently not been colonized with type b organisms.[34] The antigenic stimulus for these antibodies may be exposure to commensals or ingested food possessing cross-reactive epitopes.[35] In support of this, when human volunteers were fed *E. coli* K100, a normal commensal of the gut that has a capsular polysaccharide immunologically similar to

TABLE 1. Titers of Naturally Acquired Antibody to Polyribophosphate of *Haemophilus influenzae* Type b

Age (days)	*No. of Titers*	*Mean $\log_{10}$ Titer ± SD*	*Geometric Mean Titer*[a]
1	29	2.009 ± 0.574[a]	102
2–60	141	1.802 ± 0.569	63.4
61–120	165	1.543 ± 0.494	34.9
121–180	128	1.357 ± 0.377	22.8
181–270	138	1.292 ± 0.348	19.6
271–360	116	1.308 ± 0.463	20.3
361–540	131	1.486 ± 0.513	30.6
541–720	123	1.692 ± 0.611	49.2
721–900	41	1.849 ± 0.577	70.7
901–1080	44	2.061 ± 0.738	115
1081–1440	86	2.178 ± 0.753	151
1441–1800	59	2.383 ± 0.571	242
1801–2160	49	2.385 ± 0.490	243
2161–3600	58	2.248 ± 0.523	177

[a] Titers were measured by a radioactive antigen-binding assay and are expressed in terms of ng of antibody/ml of serum.
(From Anderson et al.,[33] with permission.)

PRP, they responded with increased levels of specific bactericidal and opsonizing antibodies.[36]

The immune response to infection with type b organisms has been investigated in some detail. At the time of infection, serum anti-PRP antibodies are low or absent. In convalescence, levels remain low and responses are poor in children until their age is about 18–24 months.[37] As a consequence, rare instances of second or third episodes of type b infection have been reported. This failure to make serum anti-PRP antibodies, even after generalized infection, is not due to immune tolerance but is typical of a natural delay in the immune response of humans to many polysaccharides and other T-cell-independent antigens, i.e., those that do not activate T-helper cells effectively. Calculations of the minimum serum concentration of anti-PRP antibody associated with protection against *H. influenzae* b disease have been estimated to range from 0.04 to 1.00 μg/ml.[38] These estimates must be interpreted cautiously, taking into account the functional variations (e.g., persistence, avidity of binding) of the different subclasses of anti-PRP antibodies. There is much individual variation in levels of anti-PRP antibodies; many adults lack detectable serum anti-PRP antibody but possess substantial bactericidal and opsonizing activity against type b organisms that cannot be absorbed out with PRP.[29] Thus, despite the deserved attention and proven importance of anti-PRP antibodies, it has been evident for many years that naturally acquired protective immunity to type b disease is mediated by the eclectic activities of antibodies directed against both capsular and somatic antigens. Nonetheless, it is only recently that attempts have been made to define the role and the specificity of serum antibodies to somatic antigens. Natural infection with type b organisms results in antibody responses to somatic antigens (e.g., lipopolysaccharide and outer membrane proteins), and the protective potential of these antibodies has been shown in experimental infections.

The role of local (mucosal) immunity in host defense against *H. influenzae* is poorly understood. A possible role for secretory antibodies, which may act by blocking attachment of *H. influenzae* to respiratory tract mucosa, seems reasonable but is speculative.[39] Conversely, there is some evidence that IgA antibodies, acting either locally at the mucosal level or after entry into the blood stream, may increase susceptibility to infection by blocking the activity of other antibodies.[37]

An important role for complement components in host defense against *H. influenzae* infections was intimated by the initial studies of Fothergill and Wright who found that the bactericidal activity of human serum for *H. influenzae* was abolished by heating to 56°C. *In vitro*, encapsulated and unencapsulated *H. influenzae* are able to activate both the classical and alternative pathways.[40] Additional evidence for a biologically significant role for complement components is suggested by the results of experimental infection and by the increased susceptibility to pyogenic infections of patients with specific congenital deficiencies. Individuals with C2 deficiency (two patients), C3b-inactivator deficiency (two patients), and a single individual with homozygous C3 deficiency have been described in whom increased susceptibility to *H. influenzae* b infections was observed[41] (see Chapter 6).

Killing by cellular ingestion or bactericidal action involves the co-operation of serum components (antibody and complement) and either polymorphonuclear leucocytes (PMN) or cells of the mononuclear–phagocytic system. In vitro, PMN kill *H. influenzae* within minutes when they are incubated in the presence of serum containing type-specific antibodies.[30] However, clearance by cells of the mononuclear–phagocytic system is the major factor mediating blood stream clearance. Individuals without spleens have an increased susceptibility to *H. influenzae* sepsis and meningitis, as do persons with decreased splenic functions, e.g., sickle cell disease.[42] Intensive treatment of individuals with Hodgkin's lymphoma increases susceptibility to *H. influenzae* infections, especially if management includes splenectomy.[43]

Studies of the genetic basis of susceptibility to type b infection has yielded some interesting preliminary results. There are significant differences in both MNS phenotype on erythrocytes and HLA antigen frequencies among individuals with meningitis compared to those with epiglottitis. Furthermore, age-adjusted serum anti-PRP antibody responses following meningitis were lower than for children with epiglottitis.[44] A low responder phenotype has been directly correlated with absence of the G2m(n) allotype.[45] Interestingly, a low incidence of the G2m(n) phenotype is characteristic of blacks and Hispanics, who, in turn, have higher attack rates compared with whites. Furthermore, the G2m(n) allotype is a heavy-chain marker for antibodies of subclass IgG_2, the serum concentration of which is predictive of antibody responses to immunization with polysaccharide antigens. A second marker, Km(1) has been associated with lower antibody responses to PRP and other polysaccharide antigens.[46]

CLINICAL MANIFESTATIONS

Asymptomatic nasopharyngeal colonization with *H. influenzae* is common but occasionally develops into symptomatic disease. Contiguous spread of unencapsulated *H. influenzae* organisms within the upper respiratory tract can result in sinusitis or otitis media. Their spread to the lower respiratory tract is common when there is a breakdown of mechanisms that normally keep it sterile. In chronic pulmonary disease (e.g., cystic fibrosis, bronchiectasis, chronic bronchitis) unencapsulated strains probably play an important role in relation to acute, purulent exacerbations. However, such strains are only rarely associated with systemic infection since they lack determinants necessary for penetration of the mucosal barriers and subsequent survival. However, unencapsulated, type b strains (rarely other serotypes) are invasive; blood stream dissemination leads to metastatic infection (e.g., meningitis, septica arthritis). In the first comprehensive account of systemic *H. influenzae* infections of childhood by Alexander in 1942,[47] three major diseases were described: meningitis, epiglotittis, and pneumonia. The primacy of type b strains and the occurrence of bacteremia were emphasized. More recent reviews[48,49] have appropriately emphasized cellulitis, septic arthritis, and pericarditis, as well as noting the occurrence of other rarer infections caused by type b strains (Table 2).

Increasingly, *H. influenzae* is being recognized as a pathogen

TABLE 2. Carriage and Pathogenicity of *Haemophilus influenzae*

Strains	*Common Upper Respiratory Tract Carriage Rates (%)*	*Principal Manifestations of Pathogenicity*
Nonencapsulated	50–80	Exacerbations of chronic bronchitis, otitis media, sinusitis, conjunctivitis; bacteremic infections rare patients commonly adults
Encapsulated, type b	2–4	Meningitis, epiglottitis, pneumonia and empyema, septic arthritis, cellulitis, osteomyelitis, pericarditis, bacteremia; rarer manifestations include glossitis, tenosynovitis, peritonitis, endocarditis, ventriculitis, associated with infected shunt-tubing
Encapsulated types a, c–f	1–2	Rarely incriminated as pathogens

(From Turk,[49] with permission.)

for adults, particularly those over 50 or with underlying disease. The serotype of isolates obtained from adults with bacteremic pneumonia has been predominantly type b, but nontypeable strains have often been isolated from infections of the meninges[9] or female genital tract.[8]

Meningitis

This is the most common and serious manifestation of systemic infection due to *H. influenzae*. Antecedent symptoms of upper respiratory infection are usual, and an associated or preceding otitis media is also very common. Specific questioning concerning the occurrence of disease in contacts (household, day care centers) is prudent. None of its clinical features distinguish it from other forms of purulent meningitis. It is usually a disease of young infants; adult cases are infrequent and often have a background of recent or remote head trauma, prior neurosurgery, paranasal sinusitis, otitis, or CSF leak. *Haemophilus influenzae* meningitis in neonates is also rare, but such cases can resemble early onset group B streptococcal infection. The most common signs are fever and altered CNS function, but the young child may have few specific signs and nuchal rigidity is often absent. More obvious manifestations, such as seizures or coma, commonly develop as the disease progresses. The disease may be fulminating in onset, with death occurring in a few hours, usually in a child less than 1 year old. However, the more usual pattern consists of several days of mild illness (e.g., upper respiratory tract infection) followed by an ominous deterioration. Insidious development over several weeks, reminiscent of tuberculous meningitis, has also been described, particularly in infants subjected to inadequate antibiotic treatment. Owing to the young age of affected children, subdural effusions are a commonly recognized complication. Clinical suspicion should be greatest when after 2 or 3 days of adequate therapy there is a tense anterior fontanelle, seizures (particularly if focal), hemiparesis, or marked obtundation. In older children, one looks for papilledema and altered mental status. With appropriate management, the overall mortality rate from *H. influenzae* meningitis is less than 5 percent, but apparently permanent sequelae occur in many of the survivors.[50–52] A prospective study of 46 children who had *H. influenzae* meningitis (1975–1977) and adequate follow-up data revealed that hearing or language delay occurred in 35%, mental retardation in 11%, cerebral palsy in 7%, and continuing seizures in 5%. Only 50% were judged to be functioning normally.[53]

Epiglottitis

Acute respiratory obstruction caused by a cellulitis of the supraglottic tissues is a potentially lethal disease with a characteristically fulminating onset. Swelling of the epiglottis and aryepiglotittic folds with complete obliteration of the vallecular and pyriform sinuses is typical. In one study,[54] only 1 of 42 children was correctly diagnosed before admission to the hospital; the message is clear that family physicians and pediatricians need to be familiar with the clinical picture, since it often results in abrupt airway obstruction. Typically, the patient is a child (aged 2–7 years), but occurrence in adults is also well known. The onset is often explosive, initial features being sore throat, fever, and dyspnea progressing rapidly to dysphagia, pooling of oral secretions, and drooling of saliva from the mouth. The child is restless and anxious; he adopts a sitting position, with neck extended and chin protruding in order to reduce airway obstruction. Abrupt deterioration commonly occurs within a few hours, resulting in death in the absence of adequate treatment. Although these abrupt deaths are the result in many instances of airway obstruction, fatal collapse may also result from less well-defined mechanisms associated with the acute toxemia of sepsis. In some cases, the course may be less dramatic, with a prodromal illness of sore throat and hoarseness for 24 hours to 7 days preceding the onset of acute symptoms. The characteristic findings are found above the larynx. The epiglottis is red and swollen and bears a striking resemblance to a bright red cherry obstructing the pharynx at the base of the tongue. This disorder can produce considerable local edema as a result of the loose texture of the submucosa on the lingual aspect of the epiglottis. The trachea appears normal. Examination of the larynx should be done only in a setting in which an airway can be placed, since this examination, if injudiciously performed, may lead to fatal respiratory obstruction.

Pneumonia

The true frequency of primary lung infections due to *H. influenzae* b in children cannot be determined with accuracy but is probably less than 2 percent of all childhood pneumonias.[55] Although acute pneumonitis was apparently common in Alexander's experience 25 years ago, similar cases in the last decade have been rarer. This apparent decrease may reflect the wider use of effective antibiotics, but it is also possible that *H. influenzae* pneumonia occurs more commonly than is recognized. Typically the patient is between 4 months and 4 years old and becomes ill in winter or spring, presenting with a consolidative pneumonia (often with pleural involvement) that is severe enough to require hospitalization. The only clinical feature that tends to distinguish *H. influenzae* pneumonia from bacterial pneumonias due to *S. aureua* or *S. pneumoniae* is a more insidious onset. The development of severe dyspnea, tachycardia, and evidence of cardiovascular failure suggests pericarditis, an uncommon but important complication. Most authors stress the frequency (up to 43 percent) with which primary pneumonia is accompanied by evidence of infection elsewhere (e.g., meningitis, epiglottitis, otitis). *H. influenzae* pneumonia in adults with primary lung disease or alcoholism has been recognized increasingly in recent years (see Chapter 53). The radiologic findings of *H. influenzae* pneumonia, irrespective of age, may be those of a segmented, lobar, bronchopneumonic, or interstitial pattern (listed in descending order of frequency). Cavitation is rare. Pleural effusion has occurred in one-half the cases, but the fluid usually has been sterile.

Cellulitis

This is predominantly seen in young children. The individual presents with fever and a raised, warm, tender area of distinctive reddish-blue hue most often located on one cheek or in the periorbital region. The distinctive color, its location, and age of the child should suggest the etiology. The soft tissue involvement progresses rapidly over a few hours. Some of these children have, or develop, evidence of other septic foci (e.g., meningitis), since an accompanying bacteremia is extremely common.

Bacteremia without Local Disease

Children, particularly those 6–36 months of age, may develop bacteremia without evidence of local disease. Although *S. pneumoniae* is the most common cause of this syndrome, *H. influenzae* is the second most common etiologic agent.[56] Fever, anorexia, and lethargy prompt the visit to a physician; the examination is nondiagnostic. This condition is appreciated most often in those with a temperature greater than 102°F and an increased peripheral neutrophil count. Children with sickle cell disease or with a previous splenectomy are particularly susceptible. Early diagnosis and therapy are critical since these individuals may worsen rapidly and develop septic shock or a localized purulent focus.

Septic Arthritis

Haemophilus influenzae is the most common cause of septic arthritis in children under 2 years of age. Typically, there is involvement of a single large, weight-bearing joint (without osteomyelitis), displaying decreased mobility, pain on movement, and swelling. Positive cultures of blood and joint fluid are usual. However, the signs and symptoms may be more subtle; for example, septic arthritis is an important cause of prolonged fever and irritability (or prolonged antigenemia) during the treatment of other systemic *H. influenzae* diseases (e.g., meningitis). In particular, restrained limbs that are the site of intravenous infusions may be involved. In this context, culture-negative, antigen-positive joint fluid is common. Response to systemic antibiotics is dramatic and often curative, but long-term follow-up is important since residual joint dysfunction occurs in a significant percentage of children.

A review of 29 adults with *H. influenzae* arthritis found that 14 had multiarticular disease and 15 monarticular, 6 being only in the knee.[57] Nineteen had extra-articular infection as well, including meningitis, pneumonia, sinusitis, and cellulitis. Twenty-two had predisposing factors such as ethanolism, trauma, rheumatoid arthritis, systemic lupus erythematosus, diabetes mellitus, splenectomy, multiple myeloma, lymphoma, or common variable hypogammaglobulinemia.

DIAGNOSIS

A provisional diagnosis of meningitis, epiglottitis, facial cellulitis, or septic arthritis will usually be prompted by the history and clinical findings. Confirmation requires microbiologic studies. A positive nasopharyngeal culture for *H. influenzae* is not very helpful because of the high carriage rate among healthy persons. Cultures of blood, CSF, and other normally sterile fluids (e.g., from joints or pleural, subdural, or pericardial spaces) are diagnostic and therefore—under the appropriate circumstances—mandatory. Even if antibiotic therapy has been started, the yield is sufficiently great to recommend that they be taken. Cultures of the inflamed epiglottis are generally positive, but should be taken only when the airway can be guaranteed. Needle aspiration of the middle ear (tympanocentesis), maxillary sinus, the margins of an area of cellulitis, or lung may be helpful in obtaining material for bacterial isolation in selected instances, for example, a very sick patient in whom no diagnosis has been established or in whom complications have developed. Whenever feasible, specimens obtained for culture should also be gram-stained; in about 70 percent of cases of meningitis, CSF smears reveal typical organisms. Detection of capsular antigen in serum,[58] CSF, or concentrated urine using immunoelectrophoresis, latex agglutination, or enzyme-linked immunosorbent assay (ELISA) may be diagnostic and can be found in up to 90 percent of culture-proved cases of meningitis. Despite the widespread distribution of immunologically cross-reactive antigens among bacteria in nature,[36] false-positive reactions are uncommon. Antigen is also often detected in infected pleural, pericardial, or joint fluid and can facilitate diagnosis since it persists after antibiotic therapy. The concentration of PRP in serum or spinal fluid and the duration of antigenemia also provide prognostic information on the clinical outcome and course of the disease.

THERAPY

Without treatment, infection due to *H. influenzae* type b can be rapidly fatal. This is particularly true of meningitis and epiglottitis. Historically, chloramphenicol has produced excellent results in life-threatening infections due to this organism and, in many minds, is still the drug of choice. However, isolates showing resistance to chloramphenicol have been recovered occasionally in the United States and Europe. In a few circumscribed regions, the incidence of resistance has exceeded 50 percent. Routine susceptibility testing is therefore mandatory. Formerly, excellent results were also obtained with ampicillin, but resistant strains were first recognized in the United States in 1973 and are now common. In a recent nationwide study of 757 strains of *H. influenzae* type b, 20 percent had β-lactamase-mediated ampicillin resistance.[59] Ampicillin resistance other than that due to β-lactamase production exists but accounted for only 0.1 percent of the resistant strains in this study. Ampicillin-resistant strains are fully pathogenic and as transmissible as susceptible strains. Because infections with these strains respond poorly to ampicilin, therapy must include other agents until β-lactamase production can be assessed.

There is currently a trend in the United States to use certain parenteral third-generation cephalosporins as initial therapy when life-threatening *H. influenzae* infection is known or suspected in children beyond the neonatal period. A cephalosporin is chosen that is active against *H. influenzae* and that penetrates well into the cerebrospinal fluid; commonly used agents in children include cefotaxime 200 mg/kg/day divided into 6-hourly doses or ceftriaxone 75–100 mg/kg once daily or divided into 12-hourly doses (dose not to exceed 4 g). Despite their superior in vitro activity against the common meningeal pathogens and greater bactericidal activity in CSF, these cephalosporins do not sterilize CSF cultures more rapidly or improve case fatality rates when compared with results of conventional antibiotic regimens.[60]

The American Academy of Pediatrics recommends that initial therapy of known or suspected *H. influenzae* meningitis should be a combination of chloramphenicol and ampicillin.[61] The initial dose of chloramphenicol is 75–100 mg/kg/day divided into 6-hourly doses. Ampicillin is given as 200–300 mg/kg/day divided into 6-hourly doses. If the strain is susceptible to ampicillin, chloramphenicol is discontinued. Treatment should be continued until cultures of blood and CSF are negative and until the patient is afebrile and without clinical or laboratory evidence of infection for 3–5 days. The usual length of therapy is 7–10 days. In an occasional patient with meningitis caused by an ampicillin-susceptible strain, eradication of the infecting strain does not occur, or new signs and symptoms develop shortly after cessation of treatment. Additional therapy with chloramphenicol or an appropriate cephalosporin is indicated. Patients with pericarditis, endocarditis, or osteomyelitis may require courses of up to 3–6 weeks. Chloramphenicol results in dose-related, reversible toxicity to bone marrow. Although this is rarely a clinical problem, special caution must be taken when treating neonates and persons with liver disease in whom serious toxicity may develop. Although idiosyncratic, irreversible bone marrow aplasia due to chloramphenicol is well described, its occurrence is extremely rare.

Oral administration of chloramphenicol is not recommended during the acute stage of meningitis because vomiting, obtundation, and other conditions might interrupt drug therapy. Once acute symptoms have subsided, oral treatment with the same dosage regimen is effective. Hospitalization during this period is advisable to assure compliance.

Antibiotic therapy is only one facet of the management of the child with *H. influenzae* infection, and critical attention must also be given to supportive therapy. For example, in the management of meningitis, optimal ventilation must be insured by maintaining an adequate airway. Fluid administration must be judiciously managed so as to obtain adequate perfusion of tissues, since hypotension and acidosis may accompany severe infection. On the other hand, some degree of cerebral edema and inappropriate secretion of ADH may complicate the course and require fluid restriction. Use of corticosteroid therapy to reduce cerebral edema and its attendant pathophysiology in acute bacterial meningitis has been controversial. Recently, a double-blind, placebo-controlled study of children with acute bacterial meningitis evaluated the effect of dexamethasone 0.15 mg/kg every 6 hours for the first 4 days of therapy, given in conjunction with either cefuroxime or ceftriaxone.[62] Aside from effects on CSF chemistries and antipyretic effects, the significant effect of dexamethasone was on deafness. Of the children with *H. influenzae* meningitis, 11 of 64 receiving placebo and 2 of 73 receiving dexamethasone had moderate or severe hearing loss. Because of the unusually high incidence of deafness in the control group receiving only cefuroxime or ceftriaxone, it remains to be seen whether these results will be broadly applicable.

Seizures may complicate the course of *H. influenzae* disease, and their occurrence should bring to mind the possibility of electrolyte imbalance or subdural effusion. Recurrent generalized or focal seizures require treatment with anticonvulsants.

In the ambulatory setting, ampicillin (50–75 mg/kg/day) or amoxicillin (12–30 mg/kg/day) for 10 days is often satisfactory for the treatment of less severe *H. influenzae* infections (e.g., otitis media). Sinusitis may require prolonged antibiotic therapy with courses of 3 or more weeks being needed. Although poor compliance accounts for many treatment failures in the outpatient setting, ampicillin resistance may also result in an unsatisfactory outcome; several alternatives are available, including erythromycin–sulfisoxazole, cefaclor, trimethoprim–sulfamethoxazole, or amoxicillin–clavulanate.

Cephalosporins are often chosen for treatment of adults with pneumonia when *H. influenzae* is likely or documented. Common parenteral regimens include cefuroxime 0.75–1.5 g every 8 hours, cefotaxime 1.5–2.0 g every 8 hours, or ceftriaxone 1.0–2.0 g every 24 hours. Ambulatory patients for whom oral regimens are appropriate may be given any one of a large variety of regimens, including cefuroxime–axetil, amoxacillin–clavulanate, or trimethoprim–sulfamethoxazole.

PREVENTION

Active Immunization

Several considerations have prompted efforts to develop active immunization against *H. influenzae* type b. The mortality has remained constant at about 5–10 percent for over three decades, and children surviving meningitis sustain an unacceptably high incidence of apparently permanent CNS sequelae. Specific antimicrobial treatment has been complicated by the emergence of strains resistant to preferred antibiotics.

Starting in 1974, a trial of a candidate vaccine consisting of purified type b polysaccharides was undertaken in Finland.[31] This PRP vaccine was given to 49,000 children aged 3 months to 5 years; children who received PRP when aged 24 months or older were protected (estimated efficacy 90 percent). No effect of the vaccine on nasopharyngeal carriage was observed. In 1985 this vaccine was licenced for use in North America and recommended as a routine immunization in susceptible children aged 2 years or older. Subsequently, several million doses of this vaccine have been administered, and adverse effects have been exceptionally rare. However, studies on the efficacy of the vaccine in North America have suggested that the vaccine may be less effective than initially predicted; furthermore, the efficacy data suggested variable results, since no protection was demonstrated in Minnesota, as compared with 44 percent in six areas selected by the Centers for Disease Control, 83 percent in California, and 89 percent in Texas.[63] Since the PRP vaccine was ineffective in preventing type b infections in children less than 18 months (i.e., 70–80 percent of all cases), these potential shortcomings of the PRP vaccine in older children have merely highlighted the potential advantages of the second-generation conjugate vaccines in which the immunogenicity of PRP is enhanced by covalent linkage or complexing of the oligosaccharides to protein. Currently, at least four conjugates are undergoing clinical evaluation. Although differences in the immunogenicity of candidate vaccines have been observed, all elicit significantly enhanced antibody responses when compared with PRP and, in contrast to the latter, are found to prime for a secondary antibody response. One of these conjugates (PRP-D, available in the United States as ProHIBit) has been licensed for use since December, 1987. It is currently recommended for routine use in infants 18 months or older. Clinical studies indicate that all of the conjugate vaccines currently undergoing clinical trials elicit antibodies that are active in complement-mediated bactericidal and opsonic assays and are protective as evidenced by passive immunization of experimentally infected rats. A recently completed efficacy trial of PRP-D has established that it can protect infants against type b disease (efficacy 87 percent: confidence limits 50–96 percent).[32] It can be concluded that effective active immunization strategies for the prevention of type b disease in infants are now a realistic proposition.

Passive Immunization

Individuals with congenital or acquired hypogammaglobulinemia are unduly susceptible to a variety of pathogens, among which infections due to *H. influenzae* are particularly frequent and troublesome. Therapy with intramuscular injections of γ-globulin has been one of the mainstays of management of this form of immunodeficiency. Recently, the availability of intravenous preparations, given as infusions every 3 weeks, has emerged as the preferred way of managing the most severely affected individuals. This has proved particularly beneficial for patients with established, chronic lung disease in which *H. influenzae* infections are often a notorious and intractable problem. Another recent development is the use of a human globulin preparation, bacterial polysaccharide immune globulin (BPIG), prepared from donors actively immunized with PRP vaccine. It contains 10 times the anti-PRP antibodies available in conventional immune globulin. Its pharmacology and protective efficacy have been investigated in Apache Indian infants, who have an exceptionally high incidence of type b infection. Since 40 percent of these infections occur before the age of 6 months, active immunization may not be a feasible proposition. When BPIG was given at 4 monthly intervals (4, 6, and 10 months), significant protection against systemic type b infections was demonstrated.[22]

Chemoprophylaxis

Young children in the same household are at significantly increased risk of secondary invasive infections by *H. influenzae* type b. Estimates of the secondary attack rates in household contacts in the United States are 2–4 percent and in day care centers may be as high as 1.3 percent.[24] It has been suggested that antibiotic treatment of age-susceptible contacts of children with invasive *H. influenzae* could decrease this secondary attack rate. Rifampin (20 mg/kg/dose; maximum dose 600 mg/day) given orally once daily for 4 days is effective in eradicating nasopharyngeal carriage and is currently recommended by the American Academy of Pediatrics for all household contacts (children and adults) where there are children (other than the index case) less than 4 years old. Nursery and day care center contacts should also be considered a household. Nonetheless, several instances of apparent failure of rifampin to prevent secondary cases have been reported, including cases in which the disease isolate was resistant to rifampin.

When a patient with *H. influenzae* meningitis will return from the hospital to a household with a child age 4 years or less, treatment of the patient with rifampin 20 mg/kg (600 mg maximum) once daily for 4 days in recommended prior to discharge in order to eradicate the carrier state and prevent secondary cases.

ACKNOWLEDGMENT

The author wishes to thank Mrs. Sheila Hayes for her expert help in preparing the manuscript.

REFERENCES

1. Evans NM, Smith DD, Wicken AJ. Haemin and nicotinamide adenine dinucleotide requirements of *Haemophilus influenzae* and *Haemophilus parainfluenzae*. J Med Microbiol. 1974;7:359–365.
2. Kilian M. A taxonomic study of the genus *Haemophilus* with the proposal of a new species. J Gen Microbiol. 1976;93:9–62.
3. Pittman M. Variation and type specificity in the bacterial species *Haemophilus influenzae*. J Exp Med. 1931;53:471–492.
4. Musser JM, Granoff DM, Pattison PE, et al. A population genetic framework for the study of invasive diseases caused by serotype b strains of *Haemophilus influenzae*. Proc Natl Acad Sci USA 1985;82:5078–5082.
5. Moxon ER. The carrier state: *Haemophilus influenzae*. J Antimicrob Chemother [Suppl A]. 1986;18:17–24.
6. Wallace RJ, Baker CJ, Quinones FJ, et al. Non-typeable *Haemophilus influenzae* (biotype 4) as a neonatal, maternal and genital pathogen. Rev Infect Dis. 1983;5:123–136.
7. Shann F, Gratten M, Germer S, et al. Aetiology of pneumonia in children in Goroka hospital, Papua, New Guinea. Lancet. 1984;ii:537–541.
8. Wallace RJ, Musher DM, Martin RR. *Haemophilus influenzae* pneumonia in adults. Am J Med. 1978;64:87–93.
9. Spagnuolo PJ, Ellner JJ, Lerner PI, et al. *Haemophilus influenzae* meningitis: the spectrum of disease in adults. Medicine. 1982;61:74–85.
10. Brazilian Purpuric Fever Study Group: Report of a symposium. Ped Infect Dis J. 1989;8:237–49.
11. Michaels RH, Myerowitz RL, Klaw R. Potentiation of experimental meningitis due to *Haemophilus influenzae* by influenza A virus. J Infect Dis. 1977;135:641–645.
12. van Alphen L, van den Berghe N, van den Broek LG. Interaction of *Haemophilus influenzae* with human erythrocytes and oropharyngeal epithelial cells is mediated by a common fimbrial epitope. Infect Immun. 1988;56:1800–1806.
13. Mulks MH, Kornfeld SJ, Plaut AG. Specific proteolytis of human IgA by *Streptococcus pneumoniae* and *Haemophilus influenzae*. J Infect Dis. 1980;141:450–456.
14. Wilson R, Moxon ER. Molecular mechanisms of *Haemophilus influenzae* pathogenicity in the respiratory tract. In: Donachie W, Griffiths E, Stephen J, eds. Bacterial Infections of Respiratory and Gastrointestinal Mucosae. Washington DC: IRL Press. 1988;24:29–38.
15. Crisel RM, Baker RS, Dorman DE. Capsular polymer of *Haemophilus influenzae* type b. I. Structural characterization of the capsular polymer of strain Eagan. J Biol Chem. 1975;250:4926–4930.
16. Moxon ER, Deich RA, Connelly CJ. Cloning of chromosomal DNA from *Haemophilus influenzae:* its use for studying the expression of type b capsule and virulence. J Clin Invest. 1984;73:298–306.
17. Moxon ER, Zwahlen A, Rubin LB. Pathogenesis of *Haemophilus influenzae* meningitis: use of a Rat Model For Studying Microbial Determinants of Virulence. In: Sande M, Smith A, Root R, eds. Bacterial Meningitis. New York: Churchill Livingstone; 1985:23–36.
18. Moxon ER, Anderson P. Meningitis caused by *Haemophilus influenzae* in infant rats: protective immunity and antibody priming by gastrointestinal colonization with *Escherichia coli*. J Infect Dis. 1979;140:47:471–478.
19. Centers for Disease Control. Bacterial meningitis and meningococcemia—United States, 1978. MMWR 1979;28:277–278.
20. Turk D, May JR. *Haemophilus influenzae:* Its Clinical Importance. London: English Universities Press; 1967.
21. Ward JI, Margolis H, Lum M, et al. *Haemophilus influenzae* disease in Alaskan Eskimos: characteristics of a population with an unusual incidence of invasive disease. Lancet. 1981;1:1281–1285.

22. Santosham M, Reid R, Ambrosino DM, et al. Prevention of *Haemophilus influenzae* type b infections in high-risk infants treated with bacterial polysaccharide immune globulin. N Engl J Med. 1988;317:923–929.
23. Glode MP, Daum RA, Goldman DA, et al. *Haemophilus influenzae* type b meningitis: a contagious disease of children. Br Med J. 1980;280:899–901.
24. Marks MI, Dorchester WL. Secondary rates of *Haemophilus influenzae* type b disease among day care contacts. J Pediatr. 1987;111:305–306.
25. Ward JI, Fraser DW, Baraff LI, et al. *Haemophilus influenzae* meningitis: a national study of secondary spread in household contacts. N Engl J Med. 1979;301:122.
26. Fothergill LD, Wright J. Influenzal meningitis: the relation of age incidence to the bactericidal power of blood against causal organism. J Immunol. 1933;24:273–284.
27. Alexander HE, Ellis C, Leidy G. Treatment of type-specific *Haemophilus influenzae* infections in infancy and childhood. J Pediatr. 1942;20:673–698.
28. Robbins JB, Schneerson R, Argaman M, et al. *Haemophilus influenzae* type b: disease and immunity in humans. Ann Intern Med 1973;78:259–269.
29. Anderson P, Johnston R, Smith DH. Human serum activities against *Haemophilus influenzae* type b. J Clin Invest. 1972;51:31–38.
30. Johnston RB, Anderson P, Newman S. Opsonization and phagocytosis of *Haemophilus influenzae* type b. In: Sell SH, Karzon DT, eds. *Haemophilus influenzae*. Nashville: Vanderbilt University Press; 1973:99–112.
31. Peltola H, Kayhty H, Virtanen M, et al. Prevention of *Haemophilus influenzae* type b bacteremic infections with the capsular polysaccharide vaccine. N Engl J Med. 1984;310:1561–1566.
32. Eskola J, Peltola H, Takala AK, et al. Efficacy of *Haemophilus influenzae* type b polysaccharide-diphtheria toxoid conjugate vaccine in infancy. N Engl J Med. 1987;317:717–722.
33. Anderson P, Smith DH, Ingram DL, et al. Antibody to polyribophosphate of *Haemophilus influenzae* type b in infants and children: effect of immunization with polyribophosphate. J Infect Dis. 1977;136:S57–62.
34. Sell SH, Turner DJ, Federspick CF. Natural infections with *Haemophilus influenzae* in childhood. I. Types identified. In: Sell SH, Karzon DL, eds. *Haemophilus influenzae*. Nashville: Vanderbilt University Press; 1973:3–11.
35. Bradshaw MW, Schneerson R, Parke JC, et al. Bacterial antigens cross-reactive with the capsular polysaccharide of *Haemophilus influenzae* type b. Lancet. 1971;1:1095–1096.
36. Schneerson R, Robbins JB. Induction of serum *Haemophilus influenzae* type b capsular antibodies in adult volunteers fed cross-reacting *Escherichia coli* 075.K100:H5. N Engl J Med. 1975;29:1093–1096.
37. Kayhty H, Jousimies-Somer H, Peltola H, et al. Antibody response to capsular polysaccharides of groups A and C *Neisseria meningitidis* and *Haemophilus influenzae* type b during bacteremic disease. J Infect Dis. 1981;143:32–41.
38. Kayhty H, Peltola H, Karanko V, et al. The protective level of serum antibodies to the capsular polysaccharide of *Haemophilus influenzae* type b. J Infect Dis. 1983;147:1100.
39. Pichichero ME, Insel RA. Relationship between naturally occurring human mucosal and serum antibody to the capsular polysaccharide of *Haemophilus influenzae* type b. J Infect Dis. 1983;146:243–248.
40. Quinn PH, Crosson FJ, Winkelstein JA, et al. Activation of the alternative complement pathway by *Haemophilus influenzae* type b. Infect Immun. 1977;16:400–402.
41. Moxon ER, Winkelstein JA. Interaction of *Haemophilus influenzae* with complement. In: Cabello FC, Pruzzo C, eds. *Bacteria, Complement and the Phagocytic Cell*. Berlin: Springer-Verlag; 1988:177–186.
42. Barrett-Connor E. Bacterial infection and sickle-cell anemia: an analysis of 250 infections in 166 patients and review of literature. Medicine. 1971;50:97–112.
43. Weitzman SA, Aisenberg AC, Siber GR, et al. Impaired humoral immunity in treated Hodgkin's disease. N Engl J Med. 1977;297:245–248.
44. Whisnant JK, Rogentine GN, Gralnick MA, et al. Host factors and antibody response in *Haemophilus influenzae* type b meningitis and epiglottitis. J Infect Dis. 1976;133:448–455.
45. Ambrosino DM, Schiffman G, Gotschlich EC, et al. Correlation between G2m(n) immunoglobulin allotype and human antibody response and susceptibility to polysaccharide encapsulated bacteria. J Clin Invest. 1985;75:1935–1942.
46. Granoff DM, Shackleford PG, Pandey JP, et al. Antibody responses to *Haemophilus influenzae* type b polysaccharide vaccine in relation to the K(m)(l) and G2m(23) immunoglobulin allotypes. J Infect Dis. 1986;154:257–264.
47. Alexander HE. *Haemophilus influenzae*. In: Dubos RJ, ed. Bacterial and Mycotic Infections of Man. Philadelphia: JB Lippincott; 1958:470–485.
48. Dajani AS, Asmar BI, Thirmoorthi MC. Systemic *Haemophilus influenzae* disease: an overview. J Pediatr. 1979;94:355–364.
49. Turk DC. Clinical importance of *Haemophilus influenzae*—1981. In: Sell SH, Wright PF, eds. *Haemophilus influenzae*, Epidemiology, Immunology and Prevention of Disease. New York: Elsevier; 1982:3–9.
50. Sell SHW, Webb WW, Pate JE, et al. Psychological sequelae to bacterial meningitis: two controlled studies. Pediatrics. 1972;49:212–217.
51. Sell SH, Merrill RE, Doyne EO, et al. Long-term sequelae of *Haemophilus influenzae* meningitis. Pediatrics. 1972;49:206–211.
52. Feigin RD, Stechenberg BW, Chang MJ. Prospective evaluation of treatment of *Haemophilus influenzae* meningitis. J Pediatr. 1976;88:542–548.
53. Ferry PC, Culbertson JL, Cooper JA, et al. Sequelae of *Haemophilus influenzae* meningitis: preliminary report of a long-term follow-up study. In: Sell SH, Wright PF, eds. *Haemophilus influenzae*, Epidemiology, Immunology and Prevention of Disease. New York; Elsevier; 1982:111–117.
54. Berenberg W, Kevy S. Acute epiglottitis in childhood: A serious emergency readily recognized at the bedside. N Engl J Med. 1958;258:870–874.
55. Ginsburg CM, Howard JB, Nelson JD. Report of 65 cases of *Haemophilus influenzae* pneumonia. Pediatrics. 1979;64:283–286.
56. Marshall R, Teele DW, Klein JO. Unsuspected bacteremia due to *Haemophilus influenzae:* outcome in children not initially admitted to hospital. J Pediatr. 1979;95:690–695.
57. Borenstein DG, Simon GL. *Haemophilus influenzae* septic arthritis in adults. A report of four cases and a review of the literature. Medicine. 1986;65:191–201.
58. Ward JL, Siber GR, Scheifele DW, et al. Rapid diagnosis of *Haemophilus influenzae* type b infection by latex particle agglutination and counterimmunoelectrophoresis. J Pediatr. 1978;93:37–42.
59. Doern GV, Jergensen JH, Thornsberry C, et al. National collaborative study of the prevalence of antimicrobial resistance among clinical isolates of *Haemophilus influenzae*. Antimicrob Agents Chemother. 1988;32:180–5.
60. Committee on Infectious Diseases. Treatment of bacterial meningitis. Pediatrics. 1988;81:904–907.
61. Klein JO, Feigin RD, McCracken GH. Report of the Task Force on Diagnosis and Management of Meningitis. Pediatrics. 1986;78:501–505.
62. Lebel MH, Freij BJ, Syrogiannopoulos GA, et al. Dexamethasone therapy for bacterial meningitis. Results of two double-blind, placebo-controlled trials. N Engl J Med. 1988;319:964–71.
63. Gilsdorf JR. *Haemophilus influenzae* type b vaccine efficacy in the United States. Pediatr Infect Dis J. 1988;7:147–148.

202. HAEMOPHILUS SPECIES

W. LEE HAND

Haemophilus species other than *Haemophilus influenzae* have been considered rare causes of human disease. Because of recent interest in these organisms and refinements in their isolation and identification, it is now apparent that they cause infection more commonly than was previously believed. *Haemophilus* species that have been well documented to produce human illness include *H. parainfluenzae, H. aphrophilus, H. paraphrophilus, H. aegyptius*, (actually a biotype of *H. influenzae*), and *H. ducreyi*. *H. hemolyticus* rarely, if ever, causes clinical disease. Similarly, *H. parahemolyticus* (a species of uncertain validity) is an uncommon pathogen.

Most *Haemophilus* species appear to be normal flora of the mouth and upper respiratory tract. Infections due to these organisms include respiratory tract infection, endocarditis, septicemia, meningitis, brain abscess, and soft tissue infections. *Haemophilus ducreyi* is the etiologic agent of chancroid. *Haemophilus aegyptius* (the Koch-Weeks bacillus) has long been identified as a cause of acute, contagious conjunctivitis. Bacteremic *H. aegyptius* infection is the cause of Brazilian purpuric fever.[1,2] This illness, first recognized in Sao Paulo State, Brazil, in 1984, is a serious systemic illness of children. The disease is preceded by purulent conjunctivitis, which is followed by fever, development of petechial and then purpuric skin lesions, and shock. Since *H. aegyptius* probably should be classified under biotype III of *H. influenzae*,[3,4] this organism and its infections will not be further considered in this chapter.

DESCRIPTION, ISOLATION, AND IDENTIFICATION

Members of the genus *Haemophilus* are small, pleomorphic, gram-negative coccobacilli with fastidious growth requirements.[3] They tend to be slow growing and are strict parasites, needing accessory factors for in vitro growth. Absolute or relative dependence on incubation in carbon dioxide for growth is a characteristic of some species. By definition, these organisms require the presence of X factor (hemin), V factor (nicotinamide adenine dinucleotide, NAD), or both for growth in culture. Both of these factors are found in erythrocytes, but lysis of the red cells is required for release of V factor. This is accomplished by heating erythrocytes in the production of chocolate agar. Requirements for X and V factors and the production of hemolysis on various blood agars are major determinants of separation. Organisms with the "para-" designation require V factor only for growth. The others all require X factor or both X and V factors.

There is considerable uncertainty as to the validity of certain *Haemophilus* species. An extensive study of *Haemophilus* strains by Kilian led him to conclude that *H. aegyptius, H. parahemolyticus*, and *H. paraprohemolyticus* do not deserve specific status.[4] *Haemophilus parahemolyticus* and *H. paraprohemolyticus* were assigned to the *H. parainfluenzae* sp.

Haemophilus aphrophilus was originally described as requiring X factor (hemin) for growth, but there has been subsequent controversy as to the growth requirements for this bacterium (e.g., Refs. 3–6). *Actinobacillus actinomycetemcomitans*, although currently classified in another genus, is similar to *H. aphrophilus*. Growth requirements and some differential characteristics of *Haemophilus* species (excluding *H. influenzae*) are listed in Table 1.

Initial isolation of *Haemophilus* organisms from specimens other than blood should be on chocolate agar incubated in carbon dioxide. In blood culture, the organisms tend to grow as small colonies along the side walls of the bottle or in the red blood cell mass, leaving the broth clear. Routine subculture of blood cultures to chocolate agar with subsequent incubation in carbon dioxide is the most reliable means of isolating the organisms under discussion.[7,8]

In the past, recovery of *H. ducreyi* has presented special problems. However, recent studies indicate that enriched chocolate agar containing Isovitalex and vancomycin (3 μg/ml) is effective for primary isolation of *H. ducreyi* from chancroidal lesions.[9,10] Culture plates should be incubated in a water-saturated atmosphere with 5% CO_2 at a temperature of 33°C.

EPIDEMIOLOGY AND PATHOGENESIS

Haemophilus species are members of the normal flora in the upper respiratory tract (oral cavity and pharynx) and perhaps in the genital area.[4,11–13] *Haemophilus parainfluenzae, H. hemolyticus*, and *H. parahemolyticus* (if considered a separate species) can be recovered from the throat in 10–25 percent of children.[11,13] In one study, *H. aphrophilus* was cultured from gingival scrapings in 35.5 percent of healthy adults.[10] *Haemophilus paraphrophilus* has also been recovered from the mouth and throat of healthy people.[4,14] Obviously, *H. ducreyi* is a pathogen in the genital area, but it should be noted that *H. parainfluenzae* has also been isolated from the urethra and vagina.

Clinical infection due to *Haemophilus* species is the result of local or blood stream invasion from sites of colonization. However, the pathogenicity of these species (*H. parainfluenzae, H. aphrophilus*, and *H. paraphrophilus*) is low as compared with *H. influenzae*.

TABLE 1. Differential Characteristics of Haemophilus Species

Organism	Growth Factor Requirement X	Growth Factor Requirement V	CO_2 Dependence	Hemolysis	Catalase
H. aphrophilus	+	−	+	−	−
H. paraphrophilus	−	+	+	−	±
H. parainfluenzae	−	+	−	−	+
H. hemolyticus	+	+	−	+	+
H. parahemolyticus	−	+	−	+	+
H. ducreyi	+	−	±	±	−

CLINICAL SYNDROMES AND MANIFESTATIONS

Haemophilus species colonizing the mouth and pharynx may cause local (head and/or respiratory tract) infection or systemic disease. Present knowledge indicates that *H. parainfluenzae* is the most frequent pathogen among the *Haemophilus* species. In general, *H. parainfluenzae* infections are clinically similar to those caused by *H. influenzae*. Reported infections caused by this organism include pharyngitis, epiglottitis, otitis media, conjunctivitis, dental abscess, pneumonia, empyema, septicemia, endocarditis, septic arthritis, osteomyelitis, peritonitis, meningitis, brain abscess, and urinary tract and genital (prostatic, urethral) infection.[4,7,8,11,15–28] *Haemophilus aphrophilus* has been noted to be a cause of sinusitis, otitis media, pneumonia and/or empyema, bacteremia, endocarditis, septic arthritis, osteomyelitis, soft-tissue abscesses, wound infections, necrotizing fasciitis, meningitis, and brain abscess.[4–6,12,15,29–32] Cases of laryngitis, epiglottitis, endocarditis, brain abscess, osteomyelitis, and paronychia due to *H. paraphrophilus*, only recently separated from *H. parainfluenzae* as a distinct species, have been documented.[4,14,15,33,34]

Recent evidence indicates that *Haemophilus* species (*H. parainfluenzae, H. aphrophilus*, and *H. paraphrophilus*) can no longer be considered rare causes of endocarditis.[7,8,15,17,29,35–40] *Haemophilus* strains may be the etiologic agents in 5 percent of infective endocarditis cases.[15] The reasons for this apparent recent increase in frequency of *Haemophilus* endocarditis are uncertain. However, improved ability of clinical microbiology laboratories to isolate and to identify these fastidious organisms is probably responsible. It is likely that many of these infections were classified as "culture-negative" endocarditis in the past. *Actinobacillus actinomycetemcomitans*, which is very similar to *H. aphrophilus*, and other small gram-negative rods with fastidious growth requirements may also cause endocarditis.[41,42]

The clinical setting of *Haemophilus* endocarditis is not distinctive. As we might expect from the knowledge that *Haemophilus* colonizes the oral cavity and pharynx, endocarditis may follow dental disease, dental procedures, or other oral trauma. Several cases of polymicrobial endocarditis due to *H. parainfluenzae* plus viridans streptococci have been reported.[16] Other predisposing factors include respiratory tract infections (sinusitis, pneumonia, and possibly otitis media) and intravenous drug abuse.

The onset of *Haemophilus* endocarditis may be relatively abrupt or indolent.[7,8,15–17,29,35–40] A subacute onset, similar to that produced by viridans streptococcal infection, is probably most frequent. Underlying valvular heart disease (including mitral valve prolapse), prosthetic cardiac valves, or intravenous drug abuse are the usual predisposing factors. Most patients are young-to-middle-aged adults. Clinically significant arterial embolization (secondary to large valvular vegetations) is common in *Haemophilus* endocarditis, occurring in 50–60 percent of cases as compared with approximately 25 percent overall in subacute endocarditis. This distinguishing feature of *Haemophilus* endocarditis may in part be due to delayed diagnosis caused by the difficulty in isolating and identifying these organisms from blood cultures. Since *H. paraphrophilus* was rather recently recognized as a distinct species, relatively few cases of endocarditis due to this organism have been reported.[15,34,35] However, some previously reported cases of endocarditis due to *H. parainfluenzae* would now be considered *H. paraphrophilus* infection.

PREVENTION AND TREATMENT

Antibiotic sensitivity studies are often unsatisfactory because of difficulty in growing the organism.[13] In general, tube dilution sensitivities have been more reliable than disk diffusion studies. Serum inhibitory and bactericidal assays, performed in an attempt to monitor the effectiveness of therapy, may also be difficult or impossible to accomplish because of inadequate bacterial growth.

Nearly all tested *Haemophilus* strains have been sensitive to chloramphenicol and aminoglycosides.[5–8,14,16,29,43] The vast majority of strains are also sensitive to trimethoprim-sulfamethoxazole and tetracycline. Most *Haemophilus* organisms are susceptible to ampicillin, but ampicillin resistance, usually associated with β-lactamase production, is recognized with increasing frequency.[22,44–46] *Haemophilus* species are generally sensitive to newer cephalosporins of the "second-generation" (e.g., cefaclor, cefamandole, cefoxitin) and "third-generation" groups (e.g., cefotaxime, ceftriaxone, cefoperazone).[43,44,47,48] Ciprofloxacin, and other new fluoroquinolone antibiotics, have potent activity against *H. influenzae* and other *Haemophilus* species.[49] In contrast, these bacteria are resistant to clindamycin, vancomycin, and usually methicillin.[6,7,16,29]

The usual therapy for *Haemophilus* endocarditis in recent years has been large doses of intravenous ampicillin, often with the addition of an aminoglycoside antibiotic. Ampicillin alone is apparently adequate if the organism is quite sensitive to the antibiotic.[15,35] Obviously, therapy should be based on antibiotic sensitivity studies, but, as noted above, these studies are often difficult to perform. The combination of ampicillin plus an aminoglycoside, a regimen that demonstrates synergy against some *Haemophilus* strains,[8] is often recommended as initial treatment of endocarditis before (and if) satisfactory sensitivity studies can be performed. There is little clinical data on which to base a choice of antibiotic(s) if the organism is resistant to ampicillin. Possible choices would include a second- or third-generation cephalosporin[50] (or possibly trimethoprim-sulfamethoxazole), with or without addition of an aminoglycoside. Preliminary evidence suggests that ceftriaxone may be quite effective in treatment of *Haemophilus* endocarditis.

A high mortality (25–50 percent) has been reported for *Haemophilus* endocarditis.[6,29] However, more recent reports indicate that with appropriate treatment the mortality is probably 10–15 percent. In one study 97 percent (32) of 33 patients with endocarditis due to fastidious gram-negative rods of the HACEK group (*Haemophilus* species [18 patients], *Actinobacillus actinomycetemcomitans* [4], *Cardiobacterium homonis* [6], *Eikenella corrodens* [2], *Kingella kingii* [2]) were successfully treated.[35]

Meningitis or other serious infections due to ampicillin-resistant *Haemophilus* strains should be treated with a third-generation cephalosporin (or perhaps chloramphenicol in patients with meningitis). Less serious infections due to organisms resistant to penicillin G, ampicillin, and first-generation cephalosporins can be treated with trimethoprim-sulfamethoxazole, a newer cephalosporin, or probably ciprofloxacin.

CHANCROID

Chancroid (soft chancre) is a sexually transmitted disease caused by *H. ducreyi*.[51,52] Advances in cultural isolation of the organism have led to improved recognition of chancroid,[9,10] which is a more common cause of ulcerative genital disease than was previously recognized. This infection is worldwide in distribution and is typically associated with low socioeconomic status and poor hygienic conditions. Major outbreaks of infection have recently been reported in Canada and the United States.[53–56] Chancroid is most often seen in nonwhite, uncircumcised men. Only 10 percent of the reported cases are in women, an observation that might be due to a clinically inapparent carrier state, asymptomatic and overlooked lesions, and/or infected prostitutes with large numbers of contacts.[53–57] The latter situation has been especially important in certain outbreaks, both among military and civilian populations.[52–57]

The incubation period for chancroid (from exposure to clinical disease) varies from 1 day to several weeks, with a median of 5–7 days. Lesions are generally confined to the genitalia and perianal areas. Extragenital chancroid (mouth, fingers, or breasts) is rare. Initially the chancroidal lesions usually begin as a tender papule with surrounding erythema, which soon becomes pustular and then erodes to form an ulcer. These ulcers are typically painful, nonindurated, ragged, and undermined with an erythematous halo. The base of the ulcer is composed of granulation tissue, which bleeds easily upon manipulation and may be covered with necrotic exudate. Ulcers may be single or multiple, and up to 10 or more separate ulcerations have been reported.[51–53,55,57–59] Men frequently have single ulcers, whereas women typically are noted to have multiple lesions. Individual ulcers vary from 1 to 20 mm in diameter. Adjacent lesions may merge and form confluent giant or serpiginous ulcerations. Superinfection, especially fusospirochetal, of ulcers may occur and lead to rapid extensive destruction of the external genitalia (phagedenic chancroid). Lesions are most often located on the preputial orifice, internal surface of the prepuce, and frenulum in men and on the fourchette, labia, vestibule, clitoris, cervix, and anus in women.[51–53,55,57,58] Small abrasions appear to facilitate infection.

Tender regional (inguinal) lymphadenopathy is characteristic of chancroid and occurs in approximately half of the patients. This adenopathy is usually unilateral and painful. If untreated the process will progress to suppuration with periadenitis (bubo formation), involving the overlying skin. Spontaneous rupture of the abscess and formation of chronic draining sinuses may follow.

The diagnosis of chancroid on clinical grounds, although commonly attempted, is very difficult and inaccurate, since genital ulcerative disease due to syphilis, *Herpes simplex*, and even lymphogranuloma venereum may be similar. In addition, these infections may be seen in association with chancroid. Culture of material obtained by swab from the purulent ulcer base or by aspiration of a bubo should be performed. As noted above, isolation of *H. ducreyi* is somewhat complicated, but is definitive.[9,10,53,55] Gram stain preparations of exudate material may reveal large numbers of gram-negative coccobacilli, sometimes in "school-of-fish" patterns, but interpretation of these smears is difficult. A positive smear of pus aspirated from a bubo is more reliable for diagnostic purposes. A dot-immunobinding serologic assay for *H. ducreyi* antibody and an immunofluorescence technique to detect organisms in ulcer material have been described, but their value remains to be determined. Biopsy of suspected chancroid ulcers is rarely performed, except to exclude malignancy, but diagnostic histologic findings have been reported by certain investigators.[52,60]

It is essential to exclude syphilis in every case of suspected chancroid, since the two diseases may be confused and since some chancroid patients may have simultaneous primary syphilis.[51,52] Dark-field examinations of exudate material for *Treponema pallidum* and serologic tests for syphilis should be performed. If these studies are negative, some recommend three consecutive monthly serologic tests for syphilis.

Treatment and Prevention

Oral erythromycin (500 mg four times a day) for at least 7 days is well established as an effective therapy for chancroid cases acquired in many areas of the world.[61] Although the clinical data is somewhat limited, a single intramuscular dose of ceftriaxone (250 mg) appears to be as effective as erythromycin in treatment of chancroid.[61–64] The trimethoprim-sulfamethoxazole (or other sulfonamide) combination has been useful in the treatment of chancroid. However, resistance of *H. ducreyi* to sulfonamides has been reported worldwide, and some strains are resistant to trimethoprim.[62,63] Because of this fact, clinical failures with the drug combination have occurred. Nevertheless, oral trimethoprim-sulfamethoxazole (160/800 mg twice a day for 5 or 7 days) continues to be useful in areas where trimethoprim resistance is not common. Single dose trimethoprim-sulfamethoxazole (640/3200 mg) therapy has not provided consistently satisfactory cure rates.[62,63,65]

Many strains of *H. ducreyi* are resistant to tetracycline, which should no longer be used for treatment of chancroid.[66,67] The majority of *H. ducreyi* strains are resistant to ampicillin and amoxicillin, a resistance that is due to plasmid-mediated β-lactamase production.[63,67–69] However, in vitro studies have shown that the organism is susceptible to the amoxicillin/clavulanic acid (a β-lactamase inhibitor) combination product. Limited clinical studies indicate that this drug combination (500 mg/250 mg three times a day) administered for 7 days is effective therapy for chancroid.[63]

Because of the expense and poor patient compliance associated with multiple-dose, multiple-day drug therapies, attempts to identify effective single-dose treatment regimens for chancroid continue. Ceftriaxone in a single dose (see above) is adequate therapy, but the drug must be administrated intramuscularly.[61–64] In one study spectinomycin in a single dose of 2 g given intramuscularly was curative in 94 percent (29) of 31 patients.[70] Ciprofloxacin in a single oral dose of 500 mg was curative in 42 of 44 patients in a single trial. Ciprofloxacin in higher single doses (750 or 1000 mg orally) may prove to be even better therapy, since a 3-day regimen of ciprofloxacin (500 mg twice daily) was effective in all treated patients.[71,72]

In addition to antibiotic therapy, needle aspiration of suppurated (fluctuant) nodes should be accomplished through adjacent uninvolved skin to prevent rupture, sinus formation, and scarring.

It is important to identify all sexual partners of infected individuals, so that these contacts can be treated with an effective antibiotic regimen.[53–57,61,63] Eradication of infection in persons, especially prostitutes, who are the source of multiple cases of infection may be effective in controlling outbreaks of chancroid.[53,54,56] It should be noted that asymptomatic carriage of *H. ducreyi* can occur. Therefore, identification and treatment of sexual partners, whether or not they are symptomatic, is essential. Soap and water cleansing of the genitalia apparently has no prophylactic value after exposure to chancroid, but a properly used condom theoretically may be useful. An additional impetus to the prevention of genital ulcers such as chancroid arises from the observation in African men that these lesions increase the chance of acquiring HIV infection through heterosexual intercourse.[73]

REFERENCES

1. Brazilian Purpuric Fever Study Group. Brazilian purpuric fever: epidemic purpura fulminans associated with antecedent purulent conjunctivitis. Lancet. 1987;2:757–61.
2. Brazilian Purpuric Fever Study Group. *Haemophilus aegyptius* bacteremia in Brazilian purpuric fever. Lancet. 1987;2:761–3.
3. Kilian M. *Haemophilus*. In: Lennette EH, Ballows A, Hausler WJ Jr, Shadomy HJ, eds. Manual of Clinical Microbiology. 4th ed. Washington, DC: American Society for Microbiology; 1985:387–93.
4. Kilian M. A taxonomic study of the genus *Haemophilus* with the proposal of a few species. J Gen Microbiol. 1976;93:9–62.
5. Page MI, King EO. Infection due to *Actinobacillus actinomycetemcomitans* and *Haemophilus aphrophilus*. N Engl J Med. 1966;275:181–8.
6. Sutter VL, Finegold SM. *Haemophilus aphrophilus* infections: clinical and bacteriologic studies. Ann NY Acad Sci. 1970;174:468–87.
7. Dahlgren J, Tally FP, Brothers G, et al. *Haemophilus parainfluenzae* endocarditis. Am J Clin Pathol. 1974;62:607–11.
8. Chunn CJ, Jones SR, McCutchan JA, et al. *Haemophilus parainfluenzae* infective endocarditis. Medicine. 1977;56:99–113.
9. Hammond GW, Lian CJ, Wilt JC, et al. Comparison of specimen collection and laboratory techniques for isolation of *Haemophilus ducreyi*. J Clin Microbiol. 1978;7:39–43.
10. Hannah P, Greenwood JR. Isolation and rapid identification of *Haemophilus ducreyi*. J Clin Microbiol. 1982;16:861–4.
11. Hable KA, Logan BG, Washington JA II. Three *Hemophilus* species. Am J Dis Child. 1971;121:35–7.
12. Kraut MS, Attebery HR, Finegold SM, et al. Detection of *Haemophilus aprophilus* in the human oral flora with a selective medium. J Infect Dis. 1972;126:189–92.
13. Kilian M, Heine-Jensen J, Bulow P. *Haemophilus* in the upper respiratory tract of children. Acta Pathol Microbiol Scand [B]. 1972;80:571–8.
14. Zinnemann K, Rogers KB, Frazer J, et al. A new V-dependent *Haemophilus* species preferring increased CO_2 tension for growth and named *Haemophilus paraphrophilus*, nov. sp. J Pathol Bacteriol. 1968;96:413–9.
15. Geraci JE, Wilkowske CJ, Wilson WR, et al. *Haemophilus* endocarditis: report of 14 patients. Mayo Clin Proc. 1977;52:209–15.
16. Lynn DJ, Kane JG, Parker RH. *Haemophilus parainfluenzae* and *influenzae* endocarditis: a review of forty cases. Medicine. 1977;56:115–28.
17. Treister NW, Sattler FR, Rubenstein DG, et al. Disruption of the aortic valve as a result of *Haemophilus parainfluenzae*. Am Heart J. 1987;114:663–6.
18. Bachman DS. Hemophilus meningitis: Comparison of *H. influenzae* and *H. parainfluenzae*. Pediatrics. 1975;55:526–30.
19. Oill PA, Chow AW, Guze LB. Adult bacteremic *Haemophilus parainfluenzae* infections. Arch Intern Med. 1979;139:985–8.
20. Warman ST, Reinitz E, Klein RS. *Haemophilus parainfluenzae* septic arthritis in an adult. JAMA. 1981;246:868–9.
21. Cooney TG, Harwood BR, Meisner DJ. *Haemophilus parainfluenzae* thoracic empyema. Arch Intern Med. 1981;141:940–1.
22. Rhind GB, Gould GA, Ahmad F, et al. *Haemophilus parainfluenzae* and *H. influenzae* respiratory infections: comparison of clinical features. Br Med J. 1985;291:707–8.
23. Olk DG, Hamill RJ, Proctor RA. *Haemophilus parainfluenzae* vertebral osteomyelitis. Am J Med Sci. 1987;294:114–6.
24. Gallent TE, Malinak LR, Gump DW, et al. *Haemophilus parainfluenzae* peritonitis associated with an intrauterine contraceptive device. Am J Obstet Gynecol. 1977;129:702–3.
25. Blaylock BL, Baber S. Urinary tract infection caused by *Haemophilus parainfluenzae*. Am J Clin Pathol. 1980;71:285–7.
26. Sturm AW. *Haemophilus influenzae* and *Haemophilus parainfluenzae* in nongonococcal urethritis. J Infect Dis. 1986;153:165–7.
27. Clairmont GJ, Zon LI, Groopman JE. *Hemophilus parainfluenzae* prostatitis in a homosexual man with chronic lymphadenopathy syndrome and HTLV-III infection. Am J Med. 1987;82:175–8.
28. Black CT, Kupferschmid JP, West KW, Grosfeld JL. *Haemophilus parainfluenzae* infections in children, with the report of a unique case. Rev Infect Dis. 1988;10:342–6.
29. Elster SK, Mattes LM, Meyers BR, et al. *Haemophilus aphrophilus* endocarditis: review of 23 cases. Am J Cardiol. 1975;35:72–9.
30. Bieger RC, Brewer NS, Washington JA II. *Haemophilus aphrophilus*: a microbiologic and clinical review and report of 42 cases. Medicine. 1978;57:345–55.
31. Petty BG, Burrow CR, Robinson RA, Bulkley GB. *Haemophilus aphrophilus* meningitis followed by vertebral osteomyelitis and suppurative psoas abscess. Am J Med. 1985;78:159–62.
32. Kiddy K, Webberley J. *Haemophilus aphrophilus* as a cause of chronic suppurative pulmonary infection and intraabdominal abscesses. J Infect. 1987;15:161–3.
33. Jones RN, Slepack J, Bigelow J. Ampicillin-resistant *Haemophilus paraphrophilus* laryngo-epiglottitis. J Clin Microbiol. 1976;4:405–7.
34. Bryan JP, Pankey GA. *Haemophilus paraphrophilus* endocarditis. South Med J. 1986;79:480–2.
35. Geraci JE, Wilson WR. Endocarditis due to gram-negative bacteria. Mayo Clin Proc. 1982;57:145–8.
36. Jemsek JG, Greenberg SB, Gentry LO, et al. *Haemophilus parainfluenzae* endocarditis. Am J Med. 1979;66:51–7.
37. Hammond GW, Richardson H, Lian CJ, et al. Two cases of *Haemophilus* endocarditis of prolapsed mitral valve: *Haemophilus paraphrophilus* or *parainfluenzae*? Am J Med. 1978;65:537–41.
38. Blair DC, Weiner LB. Prosthetic valve endocarditis due to *Haemophilus parainfluenzae* biotype II. Am J Dis Child. 1979;133:617–8.
39. Julander I, Lindberg AA, Svanbom M. *Haemophilus parainfluenzae*: an uncommon cause of septicemia and endocarditis. Scand J Infect Dis. 1980;12:85–9.
40. Parker SW, Apicella MA, Fuller CM. *Hemophilus* endocarditis. Two patients with complications. Arch Intern Med. 1983;143:48–51.
41. Geraci JE, Wilson WR, Washington JA II. Infective endocarditis caused by *Actinobacillus actinomycetemcomitans*: report of 4 cases. Mayo Clin Proc. 1980;55:415–9.
42. Wormser GP, Bottone EJ. *Cardiobacterium hominis*: review of microbiologic and clinical features. Rev Infect Dis. 1983;5:680–91.
43. Goldberg R, Washington JA II. The taxonomy and antimicrobial susceptibility of *Haemophilus* species in clinical specimens. Am J Clin Pathol. 1978;70:899–904.
44. Jemsek JG, Martin RR, Greenberg SB, et al. Antimicrobial susceptibility testing of *Haemophilus parainfluenzae* by a kinetic killing-curve method. J Infect Dis. 1980;141:310–6.
45. Scheifele DW, Fussell SJ. Frequency of ampicillin-resistant *Haemophilus parainfluenzae* in children. J Infect Dis. 1981;143:495–8.
46. Scheifele DW, Fussell SJ, Roberts MC. Characterization of ampicillin-resistant *Haemophilus parainfluenzae*. Antimicrob Agents Chemother. 1982; 21:734–9.
47. Watanakunakorn G, Glotzbecker C. Comparative susceptibility of *Haemophilus* species to cefaclor, cefamandole, and five other cephalosporins and ampicillin, chloramphenicol, and tetracycline. Antimicrob Agents Chemother. 1979;15:836–8.
48. Bulger RR, Washington JA II. Effect of inoculum size and beta-lactamase production on in vitro activity of new cephalosporins against *Haemophilus* species. Antimicrob Agents Chemother. 1980;17:393–6.

49. Wollschlager CM, Raoof S, Khan FA. Controlled, comparative study of ciprofloxacin versus ampicillin in treatment of bacterial respiratory tract infections. Am J Med. 1987;82(Suppl 4A):164–8.
50. Calio AJ, Cusumano S, Ullman RF, et al. *Haemophilus parainfluenzae* endocarditis. Heart Lung. 1987;16:222–3.
51. Strakosch EA, Kendell HW, Craig RM, et al. Clinical and laboratory investigation of 370 cases of chancroid. J Invest Dermatol. 1945;6:95–107.
52. Gaisin A, Heaton CL. Chancroid: alias the soft chancre. Int J Dermatol. 1975;14:188–97.
53. Hammond GW, Slutchuk M, Scatiff J, et al. Epidemiologic, clinical, laboratory and therapeutic features of an urban outbreak of chancroid in North America. Rev Infect Dis. 1980;2:867–79.
54. Blackmore CA, Limpakarnjanarat K, Rigau-Perez JG, et al. An outbreak of chancroid in Orange County, California: descriptive epidemiology and disease-control measures. J Infect Dis. 1985;151:840–4.
55. Ronald AR, Plummer FA. Chancroid and *Haemophilus ducreyi*. Ann Intern Med. 1985;102:805–7.
56. Schmid GP, Sanders LL Jr, Blount JH, et al. Chancroid in the United States: reestablishment of an old disease. JAMA. 1987;258:3265–8.
57. Ronald AR. Chancroid: recent advances in treatment and control. Int J Dermatol. 1986;25:31–3.
58. Asin J. Chancroid, a report of 1,402 cases. Am J Syph Gonor Ven Dis. 1952;36:483–7.
59. Kerber RE, Rowe CE, Gilbert KR. Treatment of chancroid. Arch Dermatol. 1969;100:604.
60. Heyman A, Beeson PB, Sheldon WH. Diagnosis of chancroid. JAMA. 1945;129:935–8.
61. Centers for Disease Control. 1985 STD treatment guidelines. MMWR. 1985;34(Suppl 4):765–75.
62. Taylor DN, Pitarangsi C, Echeverria P, et al. Comparative study of ceftriaxone and trimethoprim-sulfamethoxazole for the treatment of chancroid in Thailand. J Infect Dis. 1985;152:1002–6.
63. Schmid GP. The treatment of chancroid. JAMA. 1986;255:1757–62.
64. Bowmer MI, Nsanze H, D'Costa JL, et al. Single-dose ceftriaxone for chancroid. Antimicrob Agents Chemother. 1987;31:67–9.
65. Dylewski J, Nsanze H, D'Costa L, et al. Trimethoprim-sulphamoxole in the treatment of chancroid. Comparison of two single dose treatment regimens with a five day regimen. J Antimicrob Chemother. 1985;16:103–9.
66. Kraus SJ, Kaufman HW, Albritton WL, et al. Chancroid therapy: a review of cases confirmed by culture. Rev Infect Dis. 1982;4(S):S848–56.
67. Bilgeri YR, Ballard RC, Duncan MO, et al. Antimicrobial susceptibility of 103 strains of *Haemophilus ducreyi* isolated in Johannesburg. Antimicrob Agents Chemother. 1982;22:686–8.
68. Handsfield HH, Tolten PA, Fennel CL, et al. Molecular epidemiology of *Haemophilus ducreyi* infections. Ann Intern Med. 1981;95:315–8.
69. Brunton J, Meier M, Ehrman N, et al. Molecular epidemiology of beta-lactamase specifying plasmids of *Haemophilus ducreyi*. Antimicrob Agents Chemother. 1982;21:857–63.
70. Fransen L, Nsanze H, Achola J-N, et al. A comparison of single-dose spectinomycin with five days of trimethroprim-sulfamethoxazole for the treatment of chancroid. Sexually Transmitted Dis. 1987;14:98–101.
71. Naamara W, Plummer FA, Greenblatt RM, et al. Treatment of chancroid with ciprofloxazin: a prospective, randomized clinical trial. Am J Med. 1987;82(Suppl 4A):317–20.
72. Bodhidatta L, Taylor DN, Chitwarakorn A, et al. Evaluation of 500- and 1,000-mg doses of ciprofloxacin for the treatment of chancroid. Antimicrob Agents Chemother. 1988;32:723–5.
73. Simonsen JN, Cameron WD, Garinya MN, et al. Human immunodeficiency virus infection among men with sexually transmitted diseases. N Engl J Med. 1988;319:274–8.

203. GARDNERELLA VAGINALIS

CAROL A. SPIEGEL

HISTORY

In 1953 Leopold described a previously unrecognized *Haemophilus*-like organism associated with prostatitis and cervicitis.[1] Two years later, Gardner and Dukes described *Haemophilus vaginalis* as the etiologic agent of bacterial vaginosis (nonspecific vaginitis).[2] Because it required neither hemin (X factor) nor nicotinamide adenine dinucleotide (V factor), and because it sometimes appeared gram-positive and formed "Chinese letters," it was removed from the genus *Haemophilus* and renamed *Corynebacterium vaginale*.[3] Its taxonomic position remained unclear until studies performed by Greenwood and Pickett[4] and Piot et al.[5] showed a lack of genetic relationship between this organism and other morphologically or physiologically similar genera, at which time it was renamed *Gardnerella vaginalis*.[4]

Improved methods for detection of this organism have changed our understanding of its prevalence in the normal vagina, its association with bacterial vaginosis (BV), and its possible role in urinary tract infection, postpartum sepsis, premature rupture of membranes, and other infections.

THE PATHOGEN

Gardnerella vaginalis[4] is a facultatively anaerobic, oxidase- and catalase-negative, nonsporing, nonencapsulated, nonmotile, pleomorphic, gram-variable rod. It is indole, nitrate, and urease negative. Rare obligate anaerobic strains exist. It requires an enriched medium for growth that must include thiamine, riboflavin, niacin, folinic acid, biotin, and two or more purine and pyrimidine bases. It produces a diffuse β-hemolysis on human but not sheep blood, and acid from some carbohydrates including dextrose, maltose, and starch, but not raffinose. Acetic acid is the major metabolic end product. Starch and hippurate are hydrolyzed.

Electron microscopic studies have described either a gram-positive[6] or gram-negative[7] cell wall or, more recently, a laminated cell wall typical of neither gram-positive nor gram-negative bacteria.[4] The cell wall contains alanine, glutamic acid, glycine, and lysine,[8] and the cell membrane contains predominantly hexadecanoic (16:0), octadecenoic (18:1), and octadecanoic (18:0) acids without hydroxy fatty acids.[9] The amino acid and fatty acid profiles are typical of gram-positive organisms. Endotoxic activity was detected in cell extracts using the *Limulus* amebocyte assay, but lipid A was not present.[4]

Unlike most gram-negative bacteria, *G. vaginalis* is susceptible to penicillin, clindamycin, and vancomycin, and is resistant to colistin and nalidixic acid.[10] The organism is relatively resistant to metronidazole and tinidazole but is susceptible to the hydroxy metabolite of metronidazole.[11]

Because of its unusual cell wall, *G. vaginalis* has not been placed in a family, but it is grouped with gram-negative bacteria in the ninth edition of *Bergey's Manual*.

EPIDEMIOLOGY

The natural habitat for *G. vaginalis* is the human vagina, where it has been found in up to 69 percent of women without signs or symptoms of vaginal infection[12] and in 13.5 percent of girls.[13] The organism is found in nearly 100 percent of women with bacterial vaginosis (BV)[12] and in the urethra of a majority of male partners of women with that diagnosis.[14]

Piot et al. have identified eight biotypes of *G. vaginalis* based on the presence of lipase, hippurate hydrolysis, and β-galactosidase.[15] The same three biotypes predominated in Antwerp, Seattle, and Nairobi. The urethra of men and their partners who had BV were colonized with the same biotype of *G. vaginalis* when the partners were cultured within 24 hours of each other. The distribution of biotypes was the same in women with and without BV. Other biotyping[16] and serotyping[17] schemes have been described, but they have not yet been used to enhance our understanding of the epidemiology of *G. vaginalis* transmission.

PATHOGENESIS

The main syndrome with which *G. vaginalis* is associated is BV. Although *G. vaginalis* is almost universally present in the vagina of women with BV, its role in the pathogenesis of this syndrome is not known. Pili have been seen on *G. vaginalis*,[18] and hemagglutinating activity and adherence to McCoy cells[19] have been demonstrated. The capacity of this organism to adhere to vaginal and urinary epithelial cells may play a role in the pathogenesis of BV and urinary tract infections.[19,20]

In early human studies, either pure cultures of *G. vaginalis*[2,7] or vaginal fluid from a woman with BV[2] was placed in the vagina of women with a normal vaginal exam. Pure cultures were less likely than fresh vaginal fluid to initiate BV, suggesting either that growth on artificial media rendered the *G. vaginalis* nonpathogenic or that other organisms present with *G. vaginalis* in vaginal fluid were required for induction of infection.

Gardnerella vaginalis is not known to produce any toxins, but it has been identified as a member of the vaginal flora with phospholipase A_2 activity.[21] This enzyme initiates labor by converting amniotic phospholipids to free arachidonic acid, which in turn converts long-chain fatty acids in the amnionic and chorionic membranes to prostaglandins. This provides one explanation for the observation that BV is associated with premature rupture of membranes.[22]

Gardnerella vaginalis is serum resistant,[23] a characteristic that may enable this relatively avirulent organism to survive during blood stream invasion that occurs at parturition.

CLINICAL MANIFESTATIONS

Bacterial Vaginosis

Gardnerella vaginalis is almost universally present in the vagina of women with BV, where it is found with a mixed anaerobic flora.[24] BV, probably the most common cause of vaginitis/vaginosis, is associated with an increased vaginal discharge that may have a "fishy" odor, but not with leukorrhea, vulvar burning, or pruritis. It is more common in women who wear an intrauterine contraceptive device.[25] This syndrome is best diagnosed by clinical criteria[26] or Gram stain examination of vaginal fluid[27] rather than culture for *G. vaginalis* (see Chapter 95).

Urinary Tract Infection

Gardnerella vaginalis is a relatively infrequent (0.5 percent) urinary tract isolate. It has been recovered from voided urine from hospitalized patients with symptomatic or asymptomatic bacteriuria; patients with and without pyuria or pyelonephritis; suprapubic aspirates from asymptomatic pregnant women; and, rarely, men.[20,28,29] Because the presence of *G. vaginalis* in midstream urine can represent vaginal contamination, its clinical significance can be difficult to ascertain. However, it does appear to be a pathogen in some patients, predominantly women less than 40 years old (74 percent) and men with compromised renal function. Some cases apparently resolve without appropriate antimicrobial therapy.[28]

Bacteremia

Gardnerella vaginalis causes bacteremia almost exclusively in women and is usually associated with obstetric or gynecologic events[20,30] including postpartum endometritis, postpartum fever, chorioamnionitis, septic abortion, and postcesarian section infection. Neonatal infection has also been reported.[31] The frequency of *G. vaginalis* bacteremia may be underestimated because the organism is susceptible to sodium polyanetholsulfonate (SPS),[32] the anticoagulant contained in most blood culture media. Addition of 1.2 percent gelatin negates the inhibitory effect. *Gardnerella vaginalis* bacteremia may have a relatively benign course and may resolve even in the absence of appropriate antimicrobial therapy.[30]

Other Sources

Gardnerella vaginalis can be recovered from the endometrium and chorioamnion of clinically infected patients in the absence of bacteremia.

DIAGNOSIS, DETECTION, AND IDENTIFICATION

Gardnerella vaginalis produces round, opaque, smooth colonies that are pinpoint in size after 24 hours of incubation and 0.5 mm in diameter at 48 hours. Because the colonies are nondescript on chocolate or Columbia CNA agar, a selective or differential medium is used to improve their detection. Piot and van Dyck have reviewed the available media,[33] which have been made selective by inclusion of antimicrobial agents such as colistin, nalidixic acid, and amphotericin B or differential by inclusion of starch or human blood. β-hemolysis of human blood is a better differential character than starch hydrolysis because the latter is common in members of the vaginal flora. The optimum medium for primary isolation of *G. vaginalis* from a mixed flora is human blood bilayer Tween (HBT),[12] which is composed of Columbia–colistin–nalidixic acid agar (BBL, Cockeysville, Maryland), Proteose Peptone No. 3 (1%; Difco, Detroit, Michigan), amphotericin B (2 mg/liter), and Tween 80 (0.0075%). This medium is poured in two layers, the top one of which is supplemented with 5% outdated human bank blood.

After 24 to 48 hours of incubation in a candle extinction jar, *G. vaginalis* produces colonies with a diffuse zone of β-hemolysis. *Gardnerella vaginalis* is also β-hemolytic when grown on this medium anaerobically, but some anaerobic members of the endogenous and BV-associated flora are β-hemolytic as well.

Gardnerella vaginalis will grow in commercially available blood culture media that are either SPS-free or are supplemented with 1.2% gelatin.[32]

Gardnerella vaginalis can be detected in vaginal fluid by indirect fluorescent antibody methods.[34–36]

There are several identification schemes available for *G. vaginalis*. Thin, gram-negative or gram-variable short rods that are catalase negative and produce a 1–2 mm zone of β-hemolysis with diffuse edges on HBT agar after 48 hours of incubation in CO_2 will be *G. vaginalis* 97.5 percent of the time.[37] This is probably sufficient for identification of vaginal isolates if vaginal cultures are performed.

There are several methods available if more definitive identification is necessary either for research purposes or for identification of extravaginal isolates. The presence of β-hemolysis on human but not sheep blood, negative oxidase and catalase tests, and a positive hippurate test on a small, gram-variable rod represent the minimum criteria for differentiation of *G. vaginalis* from *Haemophilus aphrophilus, Corynebacterium, Bifidobacterium*, and *Lactobacillus*.[38]

Gardnerella vaginalis is positive for α-glucosidase, hippurate hydrolysis, and starch hydrolysis, but negative for β-glucosidase. The sensitivity, specificity, positive predictive value, and negative predictive value of this pattern for identification of *G. vaginalis* are 88, 99, 99, and 91 percent, respectively, when organisms that are β-hemolytic on HBT are tested. The susceptibility of *G. vaginalis* to 50 μg metronidazole, 10% bile, and 150 μg nitrofurantoin, and resistance to 1 mg sulfonamide by disk diffusion using specific media, can also be used.[37]

Susceptibility to sodium polyanetholsulfonate (zone size ≥12 mm) on supplemented *Brucella* blood agar and inhibition by viridans streptococci on chocolate agar have been used to differentiate *G. vaginalis* from members of 13 other genera.[32] Rapid tests for starch and hippurate hydrolysis (both positive) and acid from raffinose (negative) can also be used.[39] An indirect fluorescent antibody test has also been described for identification of clinical isolates.[34]

THERAPY AND SUSCEPTIBILITY

Ninety percent of strains of *Gardnerella vaginalis* are susceptible to penicillin (0.07 mg/liter), ampicillin (0.125 mg/liter), vancomycin (0.5 mg/liter), clindamycin (<0.06 mg/liter), gentamicin (4 mg/liter), metronidazole (4 mg/liter), and its hydroxy metabolite (1 mg/liter).[10,11] It is resistant to cephalexin (64 mg/liter), tetracycline (64 mg/liter), nalidixic acid (>128 mg/liter), colistin (>128 mg/liter), sulfadiazine (>128 mg/liter), and quinolones (>4 mg/liter).[10,40,41] Although erythromycin is active against *G. vaginalis* (0.06 mg/liter), it cannot be used to treat BV adequately, probably due to inactivation by the acid environment of the vagina.[42]

Metronidazole is the drug of choice for treatment of BV.[43] For infections due to *G. vaginalis* alone, such as urinary tract infection or postpartum sepsis, where the anaerobes that accompany it in BV are absent, ampicillin can be used.

PREVENTION

Although *G. vaginalis* biotypes in girls and their mothers have not been compared, horizontal transmission of this organism is possible. Sharing of biotypes by women with BV and their male partners has been shown[15] and implies that sexual transmission from the male to an uncolonized partner is possible. Prevention of BV, however, will probably require control of other members of the vaginosis-associated flora and lactobacilli.

Upper genitourinary tract infection and sepsis in obstetric and gynecologic patients are the most common serious sequelae of vaginal colonization with *G. vaginalis* and, more specifically, with BV. Treatment of BV in the third trimester or before gynecologic procedures is not recommended, as there are no data as to its effectiveness.

REFERENCES

1. Leopold S. Heretofore undescribed organism isolated from the genitourinary system. US Armed Forces Med J. 1953;4:263–6.
2. Gardner HL, Dukes CD. *Hemophilus vaginalis* vaginitis: A newly defined specific infection previously classified "nonspecific" vaginitis. Am J Obstet Gynecol. 1955;69:962–76.
3. Zinneman K, Turner GC. The taxonomic position of "*Haemophilus vaginalis*" (*Corynebacterium vaginale*). J Pathol Bacteriol. 1963;85:213–9.
4. Greenwood JR, Pickett MJ. Transfer of *Haemophilus vaginalis* Gardner and Dukes to a new genus, *Gardnerella: G. vaginalis* (Gardner and Dukes) comb nov. Int J Syst Bacteriol. 1980;30:170–8.
5. Piot P, van Dyck E, Goodfellow M, et al. A taxonomic study of *Gardnerella vaginalis* (*Haemophilus vaginalis*) Gardner and Dukes 1955. J Gen Microbiol. 1980;119:373–96.
6. Reyn A, Birch-Anderson A, Lapage SP. An electron microscope study of thin sections of *Haemophilus vaginalis* (Gardner and Dukes) and some possibly related species. Can J Microbiol. 1966;12:1125–36.
7. Criswell BS, Marston JH, Stenback WA, et al. *Haemophilus vaginalis* 594, a gram-negative organism? Can J Microbiol. 1971;17:865–9.
8. Harper JJ, Davis GHG. Cell wall analysis of *Gardnerella vaginalis* (*Haemophilus vaginalis*). Int J Syst Bacteriol. 1982;32:48–50.
9. Csango PA, Hagen N, Jagars G. Method for isolation of *Gardnerella vaginalis* (*Haemophiluus vaginalis*): Characterization of isolates by gas chromatography. Acta Pathol Microbiol Immunol Scand Sect B. 1982;90:89–93.
10. McCarthy LR, Mickelsen PA, Smith EG. Antibiotic susceptibility of *Haemophilus vaginalis* (*Corynebacterium vaginale*) to 21 antibiotics. Antimicrob Agents Chemother. 1979;16:186–9.
11. Bannatyne RM, Jackowski J, Cheung R, et al. Susceptibility of *Gardnerella vaginalis* to metronidazole, its bioactive metabolites, and tinidazole. Am J Clin Pathol. 1986;87:640–1.
12. Totten PA, Amset R, Hale J, et al. Selective differential human blood bilayer media for isolation of *Gardnerella* (*Haemophilus*) *vaginalis*. J Clin Microbiol. 1982;15:141–7.
13. Hammerschlag MR, Alpert S, Rosner I, et al. Microbiology of the vagina in children: Normal and potentially pathogenic organisms. Pediatrics. 1978; 62:57–62.
14. Pheifer TA, Forsyth PS, Durfee MA, et al. Nonspecific vaginitis: Role of *Haemophilus vaginalis* and treatment with metronidazole. N Engl J Med. 1978;298:1429–34.
15. Piot P, van Dyck E, Peeters M, et al. Biotypes of *Gardnerella vaginalis*. J Clin Microbiol. 1984;20:677–9.
16. Benito R, Vazquez JA, Berron S, et al. A modified scheme for biotyping *Gardnerella vaginalis*. J Med Microbiol. 1986;21:357–9.
17. Ison CA, Harvey DG, Tanna A, et al. Development and evaluation of scheme for serotyping *Gardnerella vaginalis*. Genitourin Med. 1987;63:196–201.
18. Boustouller YL, Johnson AP, Taylor-Robinson D. Pili on *Gardnerella vaginalis* studied by electron microscopy. J Med Microbiol. 1987;23:327–9.
19. Scott TG, Smyth CJ, Keane CT. In vitro adhesiveness and biotype of *Gardnerella vaginalis* strains in relation to the occurrence of clue cells in vaginal discharges. Genitourin Med. 1987;63:47–53.
20. Johnson AP, Boustouller YL. Extra-vaginal infection caused by *Gardnerella vaginalis*. Epidemiol Inf. 1987;98:131–7.
21. Bejar R, Curbelo V, Davis C, et al. Premature labor II. Bacterial sources of phospholipase. Obstet Gynecol. 1981;57:479–82.
22. Gravett MG, Nelson HP, DeRouen T, et al. Independent associations of bacterial vaginosis and *Chlamydia trachomatis* infection with adverse pregnancy outcome. JAMA. 1986;256:1899–1903.
23. Boustouller YL, Johnson AP. Resistance of *Gardnerella vaginalis* to bactericidal activity of human serum. Genitourin Med. 1986;62:380–3.
24. Spiegel CA, Amsel R, Eschenbach D, et al. Anaerobic bacteria in nonspecific vaginitis. N Engl J Med. 1980;303:601–7.
25. Goldacre HJ, Watt B, Loudon N, et al. Vaginal microbial flora in normal young women. Br Med J. 1979;1:1450–3.
26. Amsel R, Totten PA, Spiegel CA, et al. Nonspecific vaginitis: Diagnostic criteria and microbial and epidemiologic associations. Am J Med. 1983;74:14–22.
27. Spiegel CA, Amsel R, Holmes KK. Diagnosis of bacterial vaginosis by direct Gram stain of vaginal fluid. J Clin Microbiol. 1983;18:170–7.
28. Josephson S, Thomason J, Sturino K, et al. *Gardnerella vaginalis* in the urinary tract: Incidence and significance in a hospital population. Obstet Gynecol. 1988;71:245–50.
29. Woolfrey BF, Ireland GK, Lally RT. Significance of *Gardnerella vaginalis* in urine cultures. Am J Clin Pathol. 1985;86:324–9.
30. Reimer LG, Reller LB. *Gardnerella vaginalis* bacteremia:A review of thirty cases. Obstet Gynecol. 1984;64:170–4.
31. Venkataramani TK, Rathbun HK. *Corynebacterium vaginale* (*Haemophilus vaginalis*) bacteremia: Clinical study of 29 cases. Johns Hopkins Med J. 1976;139:93–7.
32. Reimer LG, Reller LB. Effect of sodium polyanetholesulfonate and gelatin on the recovery of *Gardnerella vaginalis* from blood culture media. J Clin Microbiol. 1985;21:686–8.
33. Piot P, van Dyck E. Isolation and identification of *Gardnerella vaginalis*. Scand J Infect Dis. 1983;(Suppl 40):15–8.
34. Svarva PL, Moeland JA. Identification of *Gardnerella vaginalis* by a fluorescent antibody test. Acta Pathol Microbiol Immunol Scand Sect B. 1982;90:453–5.
35. Cano RJ, Beck MA, Grady DV. Detection of *Garderella vaginalis* on vaginal smears by immunofluorescence. Can J Microbiol. 1983;29:27–32.
36. Hansen W, Vray B, Miller K, et al. Detection of *Gardnerella vaginalis* in vaginal specimens by direct immunofluorescence. J Clin Microbiol. 1987;25:1934–7.
37. Piot P, van Dyck E, Totten PA, et al. Identification of *Gardnerella* (*Haemophilus*) *vaginalis*. J Clin Microbiol. 1982;15:19–24.
38. Greenwood JR, Pickett MJ. Salient features of *Haemophilus vaginalis*. J Clin Microbiol. 1979;9:200–4.
39. Yong DCT, Thompson JS. Rapid microbiochemical method for identification of *Gardnerella* (*Hemophilus*) *vaginalis*. J Clin Microbiol. 1982;16:30–3.
40. Jones BM, Kinghorn GR, Geary I. In vitro susceptibility of *Gardnerella vaginalis* and *Bacteroides* organisms, associated with nonspecific vaginitis, to sulfonamide preparations. *Antimicrob Agents Chemother*. 1982;21:870–2.
41. Tjiam KH, Wagenvoort JHT, van Klingeren B, et al. In vitro activity of the two new 4-quinolones A56619 and A56620 against *Neisseria gonorrhoeae, Chlamydia trachomatis, Mycoplasma hominis, Ureaplasma urealyticum* and *Gardnerella vaginalis*. Eur J Clin Microbiol. 1986;5:498–501.
42. Durfee MA, Forsyth PS, Hale JA, et al. Ineffectiveness of erythromycin for treatment of *haemophilus vaginalis*-associated vaginitis: Possible relationship to acidity of vaginal secretions. Antimicrob Agents Chemother. 1979;16: 635–7.
43. Amsel R, Critchlow CW, Spiegel CA, et al. Comparison of metronidazole, ampicillin, and amoxicillin for treatment of bacterial vaginosis (nonspecific vaginitis): Possible explanation for the greater efficacy of metronidazole. In: Finegold SM, ed. U.S. Metronidazole Conference, Proceedings from a Symposium. New York: Biomedical Information Corporation; 1982:225–37.

204. BRUCELLA SPECIES

DENNIS J. MIKOLICH
JOHN M. BOYCE

Brucellosis is an important public health problem that occurs worldwide. It causes significant economic losses among domesticated animals used as sources of meat and dairy products and is frequently transmitted from animals to man in areas where the disease is enzootic.

HISTORY

The first accurate description of brucellosis was published by Marston, who acquired the disease while serving in the British

Army on Malta in 1860. In 1887, Sir David Bruce established the cause of brucellosis by recovering an organism, which he named *Micrococcus melitensis*, from the spleens of several British Army personnel who died of "Malta Fever." In 1905, the organism was first recovered from goats, establishing them as the reservoir of brucellosis on Malta. *Brucella* was first documented as a cause of infectious abortion in cattle by Bang. Subsequent studies revealed that the disease was present in domesticated livestock in most countries where it was sought.

DESCRIPTION OF THE PATHOGEN

Currently, there are six recognized species of brucellae, including *B. abortus* (eight biovars), *B. melitensis*, *B. suis* (four biovars), *B. canis*, *B. ovis*, and *B. neotomae*. All are known human pathogens except *B. ovis* and *B. neotomae*. Brucellae are small, aerobic, gram-negative coccobacilli or short rods. They are nonmotile and non-spore-forming. Many strains of *B. abortus* and *B. ovis* require supplementary CO_2 for growth, particularly for primary isolation, and all species tend to be slow-growing and fastidious; they do not grow well on media commonly used in clinical microbiology laboratories. Growth is optimum on trypticase soy agar, brucella agar, or serum-dextrose agar at 37°C, especially if a biphasic culture system is used.

Brucellae have been shown to have outer membrane proteins that resemble OmpF and OmpA of *Escherichia coli*.[1,2] The lipopolysaccharide complexes present in the cell walls of *B. abortus*, *B. suis*, and *B. melitensis* possess two major surface antigens (A and M), with A predominating in *B. abortus* and M in *B. melitensis*.[1,3] These organisms do not produce exotoxins, but their cell walls contain endotoxin, which differs somewhat in its biologic activity and chemical structure from the endotoxins produced by many enteric bacilli.[4,5] The serologic cross-reactions noted between *Brucella* species and *Yersinia*, *Francisella tularensis*, *Vibrio cholerae*, and salmonellae are due to similarities of the O-specific side chains of the lipopolysaccharide moieties of these organisms.[1,3]

EPIDEMIOLOGY

Brucellosis is primarily a disease of domesticated animals and causes contagious abortion or other reproductive problems in cattle (*B. abortus*), swine (*B. suis*), goats (*B. melitensis*), dogs (*B. canis*), and sheep (*B. ovis*). The organisms can affect the mammary glands and are shed in the milk, especially in cattle, goats, and sheep. *Brucella neotamae* has been recovered from desert wood rats in the western United States. Brucellosis has also been described in camels, hares, feral swine, wild reindeer, and bison.[1]

Brucellosis is transmitted from animals to humans by three routes: direct contact of infected tissues, blood or lymph with conjunctivae or broken skin; ingestion of contaminated meat or dairy products; and inhalation of infectious aerosols.

Brucellosis occurs on all continents and affects about 500,000 individuals annually worldwide. Prior to routine pasteurization of dairy products and implementation of the national bovine brucellosis eradication program, human brucellosis was relatively common in the United States, with more than 5000 cases reported annually. However, immunization of cattle with live, attenuated *B. abortus* strain 19 vaccine, and the state–federal program for testing cattle with subsequent slaughter of infected animals have greatly reduced the incidence of bovine brucellosis. Consequently, the incidence of human brucellosis has decreased dramatically, with 200 or fewer cases being reported annually since 1980 (Fig. 1).

Although brucellosis has been reported from all 50 states, more than one-half of reported cases in recent years occurred in four states (Texas, California, Virginia, and Florida). In contrast to most other states, the number of reported cases in Texas and California has not decreased appreciably during the last 15 years, and as a result, cases from these two states accounted for 37 percent of all cases reported in the United States in the period 1980–1986 (Fig. 1). Onset of illness is more common in the spring and summer months than in the fall and winter.

From 1960 to 1974, swine represented the most common source from which individuals acquired brucellosis in the United States, with cattle being the second most common source.[6,7] In the mid-1970s, there was a resurgence of brucellosis in cattle in the United States, and as a result, cattle were the most common source responsible for human brucellosis in the period 1975–1978.[7,8] Disease associated with exposure to swine or cattle affects mainly individuals employed by the meat-packing industry, livestock producers, and to a lesser extent veterinarians.[6,8,9] Abattoir employees who work in areas where carcasses are disassembled, sawn into pieces, and washed have the highest attack rates.[10,11] Airborne transmission of brucellosis can cause relatively high attack rates among employees who work in other processing areas if air from the "kill floor" flows into adjacent departments.[10]

Direct contact with contaminated tissues of cattle or swine is presumably responsible for a majority of cases among livestock producers, livestock market employees, and veterinarians. Brucellosis acquired by direct contact with animals affects predominantly males between the ages of 20 and 60.[6] This age and sex distribution reflects the importance of abattoir workers and ranchers as the major groups at risk of brucellosis.

From 1965 to 1978, ingestion of unpasteurized dairy products accounted for about 10 percent of cases annually.[6,8] From 1–2 percent of cases each year result from accidental inoculation of veterinarians or livestock producers with *B. abortus* strain 19 vaccine, and another 1–2 percent result from exposure to brucellae in microbiology or research laboratories. Laboratory-acquired disease usually results from accidental spills or airborne transmission.[12,13] Human brucellosis caused by *B. canis* is uncommon, and is usually acquired from dogs or as a result of laboratory accidents.

Interestingly, during the last 5–10 years, the epidemiology of human brucellosis has undergone some changes, especially in Texas and California. In these two states, a majority of recently reported cases have been *B. melitensis* infections associated with ingestion of unpasteurized goat's milk cheese from Mexico.[14] Unlike cases associated with direct exposure to cattle or swine, at least 50 percent of such cases have occurred in persons less than 20 years old, and about 50–60 percent of affected individuals have been females. If bovine and porcine brucellosis continue to come under better control, as they have in recent years,[15] *Brucella* infections associated with unpasteurized dairy products and accidental strain 19 vaccine injections may account for an increasing proportion of cases reported in the United States.

PATHOGENESIS

Brucellae are facultative intracellular bacilli that are capable of evading a number of host defense mechanisms, and can survive inside phagocytic cells for long periods of time.[16–18] *Brucella melitensis* is the most virulent species, followed by *B. suis* and *B. abortus*.[16,17,19]

Brucellae can enter the body via mucous membranes, abraded skin, or inhalation. Polymorphonuclear leukocytes (PMNs) are considered to be the first line of defense against the organism. Both *B. abortus* and *B. melitensis* can be opsonized by normal human serum, which promotes phagocytosis of the organisms by PMNs.[20] PMNs are capable of killing *B. abortus*, but have little ability to destroy intracellular *B. melitenis*.[20] Studies using bovine PMNs suggest that the ability of *Brucella* to remain viable inside PMNs may be due to production of 5′-guanosine monophosphate and adenine, which inhibit degranulation of peroxidase-positive granules in PMNs, thus inhibiting the myeloperoxidase–H_2O_2–halide antibacterial system.[21] Nor-

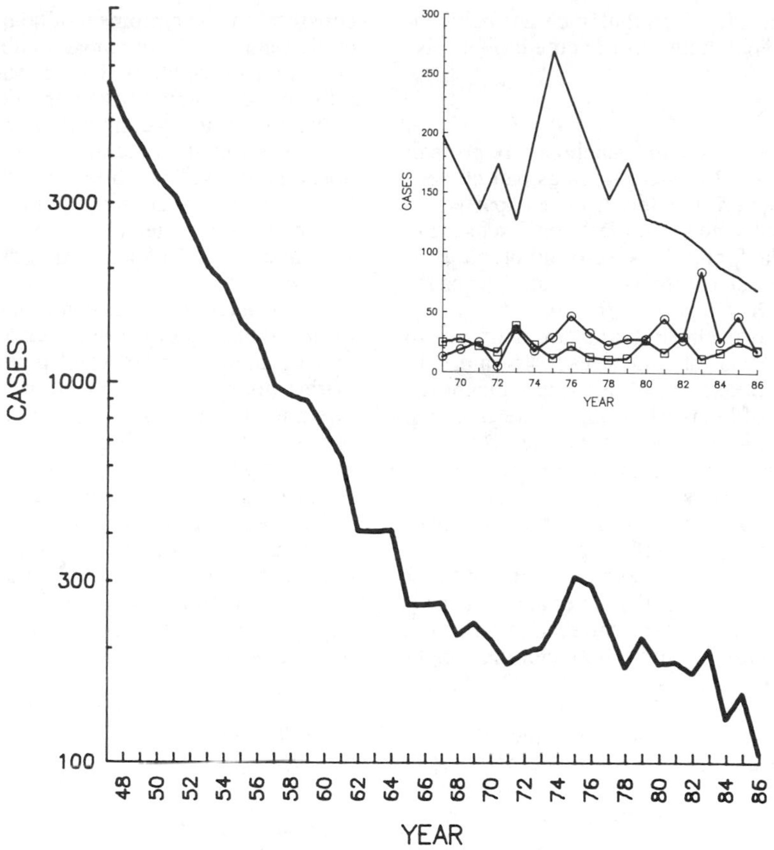

FIG. 1. Reported cases of brucellosis in the United States, 1947–1986. *Inset*: Cases reported in the period 1969–1986. All states except Texas and California (——), Texas (○——○), California (□——□).

mal human serum has good bactericidal activity against *B. abortus*, but not against *B. melitensis*.[20,22] The ability of *B. melitensis* to resist both the bactericidal effect of serum and intracellular killing by PMNs probably accounts for its greater virulence.[20]

Organisms that are not killed by PMNs migrate to regional lymph nodes and then into the blood stream, where they tend to localize in organs of the reticuloendothelial system. Phagocytic cells of the reticuloendothelial system are capable of ingesting brucellae, but some organisms can survive and proliferate intracellularly, especially in the spleen.[16,23] When macrophages become activated, intracellular organisms are apparently killed, with release of endotoxin from the bacterial cell walls. The host response to *Brucella* endotoxin may account for some of the signs and symptoms characteristic of acute brucellosis.[4,16]

The tissue reaction evoked by *Brucella* infection is variable, depending on the animal infected and the species of *Brucella* involved. For instance, when mice are infected with *B. abortus*, they develop grossly visible hepatic granulomas that persist for more than 30 days.[24] In contrast, mice infected with *B. melitensis* develop hepatic microabscesses that disappear within 30 days. In guinea pigs, *B. abortus* causes little tissue reaction, *B. melitensis* causes moderate abscess formation, and *B. suis* causes abscesses in spleen, liver, and testes.[17]

HOST IMMUNITY

Acute brucellosis and live-attenuated vaccines cause both humoral and cell-mediated immune responses.[1,11,25] In experimental animals, specific antibody promotes rapid uptake of brucellae by phagocytic cells, and results in lower numbers of viable organisms in liver and spleen.[23,26,27] However, cell-mediated immunity is considered necessary for eradication of intracellular brucellae. Differences in immune response may depend on the virulence of the infecting strain, inoculum size, age, sex, pregnancy, species, prior antibitoic treatment, and underlying immune state of the host.

In an acute infection in man, IgM rises first and may be the only immunoglobulin detectable for the first week(s).[28] IgM antibody levels begin to drop off about 3 months after onset of illness. IgG antibody levels begin to rise in the second week of the disease, and remain elevated for at least 1 year in untreated patients.[28] In adequately treated patients, IgG *Brucella* antibodies usually disappear or decrease to very low levels by 6 months after onset. Persistent elevation of IgG antibody titers may be due to the presence of viable, intracellular organisms in reticuloendothelial tissue or other foci of infection, but additional studies are needed to confirm this theory. IgA antibody levels become detectable weeks after IgG, but are of no diagnostic value. During reinfection or exacerbation of illness, IgG and possibly IgM brucella antibody titers become elevated.[28] However, the degree to which IgM antibodies become elevated in relapsing brucellosis is controversial, and a recent study found that IgG, but not IgM, antibody levels rose in patients with relapses of brucellosis.[29]

About 7–10 days after infection of experimental animals, lymphokines produced by sensitized T lymphocytes activate macrophages, which subsequently become more efficient at killing intracellular bacteria.[1,30] At about the same time, granulomas form in the liver and spleen, and infected animals develop delayed-type hypersensitivity to *Brucella* antigens.[1,30]

Acute brucellosis is most commonly attributed to infection with the microorganism itself, although immune complex-mediated disease has been described.[31] Gotuzzo et al.[32] detected both rheumatoid factor and antinuclear antibodies in patients with active disease, and have suggested that such autoantibodies may play some role in the pathogenesis of acute brucellosis.

CLINICAL MANIFESTATIONS

The signs and symptoms associated with brucellosis are protean in nature, and no constellation of clinical findings can be considered characteristic. The severity of the disease is partly dependent on the presence or absence of underlying disease, the immune status of the individual, and the species involved. *Brucella melitensis*, and to a lesser extent *B. suis*, tend to cause more severe infections than *B. abortus* or *B. canis*.[33]

The incubation period for brucellosis ranges from 1 week to several months, with an average of 2–3 weeks.[19] Some individuals develop subclinical disease, which is usually diagnosed serologically during surveys of high-risk groups (veterinarians) or during outbreak investigations (abattoir workers).[9] A majority of such patients probably have a mild influenza-like illness, which is seldom followed by sequelae.

About one-third of patients with more symptomatic forms of the illness have acute onset of illness with impressive systemic toxicity, while the remaining two-thirds develop symptoms over 1 or more weeks.[9] Drenching sweats, chills, fever and weakness occur in over 90 percent of cases.[9,19,34] Malaise, headache, and anorexia are also common. Other symptoms including weight loss, myalgias, arthralgias, and back pain are seen in 25–50 percent of patients.[9]

Although an undulating fever pattern was once thought to be characteristic of brucellosis, a majority of affected patients do not exhibit such a response. More commonly, the temperature is normal or slightly elevated in the morning and rises in the afternoon.[19,35] Sustained fever occurs in about 15 percent of cases.[6] Maximum daily temperatures range from 101°F to 104°F.[9]

Lymphadenopathy occurs in 12–21 percent of patients and most commonly affects the cervical and inguinal lymph nodes. Splenomegaly is detected in about 20–30 percent of cases, and may be accompanied by left upper quadrant tenderness.[19]

Recurrent episodes of brucellosis occur in about 5 percent of patients and can be due to relapse or reinfection.[9] Relapses are uncommon in patients who receive appropriate therapy, and usually represent focal suppurative complications such as spondylitis.[16] Although most persons who develop acute brucellosis become immune, reinfections have been documented in individuals with continuing exposure, such as abattoir workers and veterinarians. In general, both relapses and reinfections tend to be milder than the initial episode.[9]

Recurrent exposure to brucellae in seropositive persons may also cause hypersensitivity reactions, which can mimic *Brucella* infection.[36] Such reactions have been reported most frequently in laboratory personnel with frequent contact with *Brucella* antigens and in veterinarians with multiple percutaneous exposures to *B. abortus* strain 19 vaccine.[16,37] Onset of symptoms is usually within minutes to hours of the exposure.

In the 1950s, a good deal was written about "chronic brucellosis," which was usually defined as symptoms lasting more than 1 year after onset.[19,38] A majority of affected patients either had persisting disease caused by inadequate therapy of the initial episode, or had focal suppurative lesions in bone, liver, or spleen.[38] About 20 percent of patients who were diagnosed as having chronic brucellosis complained of persistent fatigue, malaise, and depression that was not accompanied by any clinical, microbiologic, or serologic evidence of active infection.[38,39] This chronic fatigue syndrome was usually seen in patients with pre-existing depressive personality disorders, and has also been seen in patients who are seeking job-related disability payments.[40]

The clinical findings in patients with *B. canis* infection are similar to those seen in other forms of brucellosis.[41–43] The onset is usually insidious, blood cultures are often negative, and constitutional symptoms tend to be milder than with other forms of brucellosis.[41,43] The most notable difference between *B. canis* and other brucellae is that the former seldom causes endocarditis or focal suppurative complications such as spondylitis.

Percutaneous or conjunctival exposure to live, attenuated *B. abortus* strain 19 vaccine is associated with a wide variety of host responses.[36,37,44] Some individuals exposed to strain 19 suffer no local or systemic reactions.[37] More commonly, the exposure causes either (*1*) an immediate local reaction, or (*2*) a systemic illness similar to that caused by natural strains of *B. abortus*.

Local reactions most commonly occur in persons who have a clinical history or serologic evidence of brucellosis in the past, or who have been exposed previously to strain 19 vaccine.[36] Within hours after the injection, patients develop marked pain, swelling, and edema, which sometimes progresses to sloughing of skin at the site of inoculation. Such reactions probably represent an accelerated delayed-type hypersensitivity reaction to *Brucella* antigens (possibly endotoxin).[4,36] Patients who develop a febrile, systemic illness usually have onset a few days to several weeks after exposure. The disease is often milder than that caused by natural strains of *B. abortus*, and seldom causes suppurative complications or endocarditis. Occasionally, patients develop both an immediate local reaction and systemic illness.[37]

COMPLICATIONS

Complications of acute brucellosis have been reported in 1 percent to up to 30 percent of cases. With *B. abortus* or *B. suis*, the complication rate is less than 1 percent in patients who are diagnosed and treated with a few weeks of onset, but the rate increases substantially when infection has been present for more than 60 days before specific antibiotic therapy is started.[9] Complications may affect almost any organ system, as noted below.

Skeletal

Osteoarticular involvement from brucellosis occurs in between 20 and 85 percent of patients in some series, with an increased percentage in those with *B. melitensis*.[35,45–49] Reported findings include arthralgias, arthritis, spondylitis, osteomyelitis, tenosynovitis, bursitis, and sacroiliitis. The type of skeletal involvement seen depends in part on the patient's age and *Brucella* species involved.[47,48] Gotuzzo, et al.[47] reported four syndromes of articular involvement in 103 of 304 patients with brucellosis. The most frequent syndrome was sacroiliitis (46 percent), peripheral arthritis (39 percent), combined sacroiliitis and peripheral arthritis (8 percent), and spondylitis (7 percent).

The onset of arthritis may be acute or insidious, and most commonly involves the hip or knee joint.[48] Synovial fluid cell counts range from 200 to 19,000/mm^3 and reveal a lymphocytic predominance in a majority of cases. Cultures of synovial fluid are often negative, but brucellae have been recovered from synovial fluid in up to 50 percent of cases of *Brucella* arthritis if Ruiz-Castaneda medium is used.[47]

Spondylitis, which is usually seen in elderly patients, often manifests as pain over the involved vertebral bodies, with radiation to the shoulder or flank.[47,49] Ten to 20 percent of patients with spondylitis develop paraspinal abscesses, which may require surgical drainage.[49]

A nondestructive, reactive arthritis that may resolve without antibiotic therapy has been described in patients with brucellosis, and is thought to be due to formation of immune complexes. However, identification of *Brucella* antigen in immune complexes from synovial tissue has not been reported. An association between HLA-B27 alloantigen and spondyloarthritis in chronic brucellosis due to *B. abortus* has been reported, but a subsequent study of patients with *B. melitensis* spondylitis found no such association.[31,50]

About two-thirds of patients with musculoskeletal involvement have positive bone scans demonstrating spinal or extraspinal lesions. Bone scans appear to be more sensitive than bone roentgenograms in detecting spinal lesions due to brucellosis.[51]

Neurologic

Neurologic complications of brucellosis include meningoencephalitis, myelitis, paresis, paresthesias, depression, and psychosis.[19,52] Central nervous system involvement occurs in about 2–5 percent of patients, and usually presents as acute meningoencephalitis.[53] Interestingly, only 33 percent of patients with meningeal involvement have nuchal rigidity.[52] Chronic forms of meningitis have been reported, but are rare.[54] In most cases, the cerebrospinal fluid reveals a lymphocytic pleocytosis with an elevated protein and normal glucose level. Cultures of spinal fluid occasionally yield the organism.[54,55]

An enzyme-linked immunosorbent assay (ELISA) that detects *Brucella*-specific IgG, IgM, and IgA appears to be a sensitive and specific test for rapid diagnosis of neurobrucellosis.[52,56] Computerized tomography may demonstrate basal ganglia calcification, ventricular dilatation, or cerebral edema.[8,53,57]

Genitourinary

Genitourinary involvement has been reported to occur in 2–40 percent of cases, but has affected only about 2–10 percent of patients in recent series.[6,35,58–60] Unilateral epididymo-orchitis is one of the most common genitourinary tract complications. It often causes local pain and swelling, with little or no dysuria. Urinalysis is usually normal, and routine urine cultures are negative.[60] Patients with brucellosis may on rare occasions develop acute interstitial nephritis or pyelonephritis, which cause proteinuria, hematuria, and pyuria.[58,61] Renal involvement may cause caseating granulomas and calcifications similar to those seen in renal tuberculosis.[58] Prostatitis and cystitis due to brucellae have also been reported.[60]

Brucellosis often causes abortions in cattle, swine, goats, and sheep.[1] The high incidence of abortion in these animals is due to localization of brucellae in placental tissue, which contains large amounts of erythritol. Human placental tissue contains very little erythritol, and this fact is presumably responsible for the low incidence of abortions in pregnant women with brucellosis.[19] The role of *Brucella* in causing human abortions has never been evaluated in appropriate case-control studies, so it is not clear if brucellosis causes abortion more frequently than other bacteremic infections that occur in pregnant women. Nonetheless, recovery of brucellae from placental tissue and amniotic fluid in women with abortions provides evidence that pregnant women with acute brucellosis are at some, albeit low, risk of suffering an abortion.[6,54]

Cardiovascular

Endocarditis occurs in less than 2 percent of cases, but is the most common cause of death in patients with brucellosis.[9,19,34,35,58] Brucella endocarditis accounts for less than 1 percent of all cases of infectious endocarditis in most published series, but may account for 8–10 percent of endocarditis cases in some areas where *B. melitensis* infections are endemic.[62,63] A majority of affected patients have been ill for more than 3 months before the diagnosis is made.[63,64] The aortic valve is most commonly involved, with mitral valve or prosthetic valve infection accounting for the remaining cases.[62–65] Echocardiograms often reveal bulky vegetations, and, not surprisingly, embolic phenomena are common.[62,63] Progressive congestive heart failure is the most common cause of death. Valve replacement is warranted in most cases, since few well-documented cases have been successfully treated with antibiotic therapy alone.[62–66] Other cardiovascular complications of brucellosis include myocarditis, pericarditis, and infective aortitis.[66]

Gastrointestinal

Brucellosis often affects the liver in experimentally infected laboratory animals and in humans.[24,67] From 30–60 percent of patients with brucellosis develop abnormal liver function tests, and a smaller percentage develop hepatomegaly.[9] *Brucella abortus* can cause granulomatous hepatitis, with either noncaseating or caseating granulomas.[68] Although *B. melitensis* is also capable of causing granulomatous hepatitis, it may also cause diffuse hepatitis without granuloma formation.[69,70] Hepatic abscesses and cholecystitis have also been described.[67]

In a recent outbreak of brucellosis due to ingestion of goat's milk cheese, about 60 percent of patients gave a history of gastrointestinal complaints such as nausea, vomiting, diarrhea, abdominal discomfort, and anorexia.[14] However, in general, gastrointestinal complaints have been relatively uncommon among patients with brucellosis.[9,35,71]

Spleen

Brucellae frequently localize in the reticuloendothelial system, including lymph nodes, liver, and spleen.[19] This may lead to splenomegaly or abscess formation in the liver or spleen.[19] Splenic calcifications with a radiographic appearance indistinguishable from tuberculosis or histoplasmosis have been reported.[72] Surgical drainage of localized suppurative lesions and splenectomy in chronic brucellosis with secondary hypersplenism and associated thrombocytopenia may be of value if antimicrobial treatment is ineffective.

Pulmonary

Pulmonary involvement in brucellosis may occur following inhalation of infectious aerosols, and possibly via bacteremic spread of the organism to the lungs.[9,73–75] About 15–25 percent of patients with brucellosis develop a cough or other pulmonary symptoms.[9,35,71,73] In some published series, pulmonary symptoms have seldom been accompanied by abnormalities on chest roentgenograms.[9,71] In contrast, Patel et al.[73] found that 16 percent of patients with brucellosis had abnormal chest roentgenograms, which in some cases resembled miliary tuberculosis. Patients in the latter study were ill for an average of 3 months before the diagnosis was made. Hilar adenopathy, perihilar infiltrates, nodular lesions, lung abscess, pleural effusions, and pneumothorax have also been described in patients with brucellosis.[9,73–76]

Hematologic

Anemia, leukopenia, thrombocytopenia, and pancytopenia have been reported more commonly in patients with *B. melitensis* infection than in those infected with other species.[77] The frequency of such abnormalities varies greatly among reported series.[35,77] Hypoprothrombinemia and disseminated intravascular coagulation have been reported in a few cases.

Cutaneous

Cutaneous manifestations of brucellosis occur in about 5 percent of patients.[19] Many transient and often nonspecific skin lesions have been described including erythema nodosum, papules, eczematous rashes, and rubeoliform and scarlatiniform rashes.[78] Petechiae, purpura, and cutaneous granulomatous vasculitis have also been reported.[79]

DIAGNOSIS

Since most patients with brucellosis present with nonspecific signs and symptoms such as fever, chills, arthralgias, and night sweats, questioning patients with findings compatible with brucellosis about potential exposures is of paramount importance. Patients should be questioned about their occupation, ingestion of unpasteurized milk or dairy products such as goat's milk cheese, recent travel to areas where brucellosis is endemic (Mediterranean basin, South America, Mexico), or exposure to livestock or dogs.

When the diagnosis of brucellosis is suspected, the microbiology laboratory should be notified so they can use appropriate media, and take special precautions when handling material that may contain brucellae.[13] A definitive diagnosis of brucellosis is made by recovering the organism from blood, fluid, or tissue specimens. In patients with acute *B. melitensis* infections, cultures of blood and bone marrow will be positive in 70 percent and 90 percent of cases, respectively.[14,80,81] Blood cultures are not positive as often in subacute cases of *B. melitensis* infection or cases caused by other species, but are still recommended. Whenever possible, blood cultures should be processed using the Castaneda technique, which utilizes biphasic medium in a bottle.[82,83] Blood or bone marrow cultures should be incubated for at least 6 weeks. Blood cultures processed in radiometric detection systems may yield positive cultures in less than 10 days.[80] One recent report suggests that lysis centrifugation procedures may yield more positive cultures than standard Castaneda bottles, but this requires confirmation.[84]

In geographic areas where most cases of brucellosis are caused by *B. abortus* or *B. suis*, the diagnosis is often made serologically.[85] Although a number of techniques have been developed for measuring *Brucella* antibodies, the standard tube agglutination test (STA) is probably the most widely used. About 97 percent of culture-proven cases develop a fourfold or greater rise in *Brucella* antibodies as measured by the STA.[85] The antigen used in the STA test is prepared from *B. abortus* and reacts with antibodies directed against *B. abortus*, *B. melitensis*, and *B. suis*, but not *B. canis*.[41] Therefore, if *B. canis* infection is suspected, serology tests specific for *B. canis* must be requested. A *Brucella* STA titer of 1:160 or greater or a fourfold rise in titer is considered presumptive evidence of past or recent infection with brucellae.[85]

The STA test may yield antibody titers of 1:160 or greater for up to 1.5 years after appropriate antibiotic treatment, making it difficult to differentiate persisting, active infection from adequately treated brucellosis.[86] The addition of 2-mercaptoethanol (2-ME) to the STA test inactivates IgM antibodies and permits detection of IgG *Brucella* antibodies. A 2-ME *Brucella* titer of 1:160 or greater obtained more than 1 year after onset of illness is suggestive of ongoing infection with *Brucella*.[86] On the contrary, a 2-ME titer of less than 1:160 is strong evidence against chronic brucellosis if obtained more than 1 year after onset.

False-negative STA tests may occur in patients whose serum contains blocking antibodies.[85] Blocking antibodies result in negative STA titers at low serum dilutions, whereas positive titers are obtained if the patient's serum is diluted sufficiently. If the STA titer is negative in a patient that is suspected of having brucellosis, the laboratory should make a 1:1280 dilution of the serum and repeat the STA test.[85]

The *Brucella* STA test also cross reacts with antibodies from individuals infected with *F. tularensis*, *Yersinia enterocolitica*, or *V. cholerae*, or persons vaccinated against these pathogens.[1,3] However, in persons with tularemia, *Brucella* STA titers are lower than tularemia agglutination titers.

Specific *B. canis* agglutination tests, and an ELISA test using outer membrane proteins of *B. melitensis* have been developed to detect *B. canis* infection.[41,87] The ELISA test measures antibody response in humans to all species of brucellae that are pathogenic.[87] An ELISA using whole-cell and lipopolysaccharide preparations of *B. canis* to detect IgG antibodies to *B. canis*, *B. abortus*, and *B. melitensis*, has also been described.[88]

TREATMENT

Many regimens have been used for treating patients with brucellosis, and there is still considerable debate regarding which regimen, if any, is clearly superior. Patients treated with a single agent such as tetracycline, streptomycin, rifampin, or trimethoprim–sulfamethoxazole have a 10–40 percent chance of suffering a relapse.[9,89] Therefore, many authorities feel that combination therapy is indicated.

In individuals with acute brucellosis that is not accompanied by central nervous system involvement or endocarditis, regimens containing streptomycin have been associated with fewer relapses than single or double drug regimens that do not include streptomycin.[9,35,45,90] Previous World Health Organization treatment guidelines recommended tetracycline 2 g/day for 6 weeks plus streptomycin 1 g/day for 3 weeks.[91] This regimen has been used widely, and is associated with a low rate of relapse. The fact that streptomycin must be given intramuscularly makes this form of therapy difficult to administer in some settings.

Currently, doxycycline 200 mg/day plus rifampin 600–900 mg/day given for 6 weeks is considered the regimen of choice by the World Health Organization.[1] Some investigators favor even longer courses of this regimen if focal suppurative complications are documented. Administration of doxycycline plus rifampin for shorter periods of time (30 days) has been associated with a relapse rate of nearly 40 percent in some studies.[90] Rifampin is considered the drug of choice for treating brucellosis in pregnant women.[1] Trimethoprim–sulfamethoxazole has been used to treat children with acute brucellosis. When therapy is initiated, patients should be observed for evidence of Herxheimer-like reactions.[54,57]

Treatment regimens used for acute, uncomplicated brucellosis may result in relapses in patients with central nervous system involvement because of the low cerebrospinal fluid levels achieved by tetracycline and streptomycin.[35,54] It has been suggested that a combination of rifampin plus a third-generation cephalosporin be used in such patients since both agents achieve good levels in cerebrospinal fluid.[54,92] Alternatively, some authors favor combination therapy with tetracycline or doxycycline plus streptomycin or rifampin, or both.[53] However, there has been very little experience with such regimens, and further studies are needed to determine if such drug combinations will result in fewer relapses in patients with central nervous system complications.

Patients with brucella endocarditis almost always require valve replacement in addition to medical therapy.[62–65] There is no consensus regarding which antibiotic combination is most effective, and the optimal duration of therapy has not been established. Combination therapy with tetracycline, streptomycin, and trimethoprim–sulfamethoxazole for 6 weeks, or rifampin plus trimethoprim–sulfamethoxazole for 6–9 months have been used successfully.[62,63]

In vitro studies have demonstrated that brucellae are usually susceptible to other agents such as imipenem and ciprofloxacin, but insufficient data are available regarding their efficacy in treating patients with brucellosis.[93,94] In animal models of *Brucella* infection, stable plurilamellar vesicle-encapsulated streptomycin has proven to be very effective at eradicating brucellae from affected organs, but such preparations have not been tested in humans.[95]

PREVENTION

Routine vaccination of cattle with *B. abortus* strain 19 vaccine, in conjunction with serologic testing of cattle and slaughter of infected animals, are effective measures for reducing the incidence of bovine brucellosis. In the United States, improved swine husbandry practices and depopulation of infected groups of hogs have lowered the incidence of porcine brucellosis.[15] *Brucella melitensis* Rev 1 and *B. suis* strain 2 vaccines have proven to be very effective in reducing the incidence of caprine and ovine brucellosis.[1,96] Unfortunately, these vaccines are still not used widely in some areas where brucellosis is enzootic in goats.

Control of brucellosis in domesticated livestock is one of the most effective means of preventing human brucellosis. Pasteurization of dairy products, especially in areas where brucellosis is common in cattle, goats, or sheep, is also an important means of preventing human brucellosis. The high incidence of human brucellosis in areas such as the Middle East and Mexico are due to failure to routinely pasteurize milk and dairy products such as cheese.[14,35]

In some countries such as Russia and China, live-attenuated *B. abortus* strain 19-BA or 104M vaccines have been used in individuals at high risk of brucellosis.[1] In France, a phenol-insoluble fraction obtained from *Brucella* has been used to vaccinate high-risk personnel, but the efficacy of this product has not been well established.[1,97] No vaccine is currently available for human use in the United States. Laboratory-acquired brucellosis can be prevented by adherence to biosafety level 3 precautions.[13]

REFERENCES

1. Joint FAO/WHO Expert Committee on Brucellosis. Geneva: World Health Organization; 1986.
2. Winter AJ. Outer membrane proteins of *Brucella*. Ann Inst Pasteur Microbiol. 1987;138:87–9.
3. Bundle DR, Cherwonogrodzky JW, Caroff M, et al. The lipopolysaccharides of *Brucella abortus* and *B. melitensis*. Ann Inst Pasteur Microbiol. 1987;138:92–8.
4. Abernathy RS, Spink WW. Studies with *Brucella* endotoxin in humans: the significance of susceptibility to endotoxin in the pathogenesis of brucellosis. J Clin Invest. 1958;37:219–31.
5. Berman DT, Kurtz RS. Relationship of biological activities to structures of *Brucella abortus* endotoxin and LPS. Ann Inst Pasteur Microbiol. 1987;138:98–101.
6. Fox MD, Kaufmann AF. Brucellosis in the United States, 1965–1974. J Infect Dis. 1977;136:312–6.
7. Centers for Disease Control. Brucellosis Surveillance. Annual Summary, 1975. Atlanta: Centers for Disease Control; 1976.
8. Centers for Disease Control. Brucellosis Surveillance. Annual Survey, 1978. Atlanta: Centers for Disease Control; 1979.
9. Buchanan TM, Faber LC, Feldman RA. Brucellosis in the United States, 1960–1972. An abattoir-associated disease. Part I. Clinical features and therapy. Medicine. 1974;53:403–13.
10. Kaufmann AF, Fox MD, Boyce JM, et al. Airborne spread of brucellosis. Ann NY Acad Sci. 1980;353:105–14.
11. Buchanan TM, Hendricks SL, Patton CM, et al. Brucellosis in the United States, 1960–1972. An abattoir-associated disease. Part III. Epidemiology and evidence for acquired immunity. Medicine. 1974;53:427–39.
12. Pike RM. Laboratory-associated infections: summary and analysis of 3921 cases. Health Lab Sci. 1976;13:105–14.
13. Boyce JM, Kaufmann AF. Transmission of bacterial and rickettsial zoonoses in the laboratory. In: Miller BM, ed. Laboratory Safety: Principles and Practices. Washington, DC: American Society for Microbiology; 1986:90–9.
14. Thapar MK, Young EJ. Urban outbreak of goat cheese brucellosis. Pediatr Infect Dis. 1986;5:640–3.
15. Nelson CJ, Huber JD, Metcalf HE, et al. Status report—1987. Cooperative state–federal brucellosis eradication program. In: Proceedings of the 91st Annual Meeting of the United States Animal Health Association, Salt Lake City, 1987.
16. Spink WW. Host-parasite relationship in brucellosis. Lancet. 1964;2:161–4.
17. Spink WW. Some biologic and clinical problems related to intracellular parasitism in brucellosis. N Engl J Med. 1952;247:603–10.
18. Mackaness GB. The immunological basis of acquired cellular resistance. J Exp Med. 1964;120:105–20.
19. Spink WW. The nature of brucellosis. Minneapolis: University of Minnesota Press; 1956.
20. Young EJ, Borchert M, Kretzer FL, et al. Phagocytosis and killing of *Brucella* by human polymorphonuclear leukocytes. J Infect Dis. 1985;151:682–90.
21. Canning PC, Roth JA, Deyoe BL. Release of 5′-guanosine monophosphate and adenine by *Brucella abortus* and their role in the intracellular survival of the bacteria. J Infect Dis. 1986;154:464–70.
22. Hall WH, Spink WW. Studies of immunity in brucellosis: the bactericidal action of human blood against *Brucella* (Abstract). J Clin Invest. 1947;26:1183.
23. Guerra H, Deter RL, Williams RP. Infection at the subcellular level. II. Distribution and fate of intravenously injected brucellae within phagocytic cells of guinea pigs. Infect Immun. 1973;8:694–9.
24. Young EJ, Gomez CI, Yawn DH, et al. Comparison of *Brucella abortus* and *Brucella melitensis* infections of mice and their effect on acquired cellular resistance. Infect Immun. 1979;26:680–5.
25. Elberg SS. Immunity to brucella infection. Medicine. 1973;53:339–56.
26. Sulitzeanu D. Mechanism of immunity against *Brucella*. Nature. 1965; 205:1086–8.
27. Plommet M, Plommet AM. Immune serum-mediated effects on brucellosis evolution in mice. Infect Immun. 1983;41:97–105.
28. White RG. Immunoglobulin profiles of the chronic antibody response: discussion in relation to *Brucella* infection. Postgrad Med J. 1978;54:595–601.
29. Pellicer T, Ariza J, Foz A. Specific antibodies detected during relapse of human brucellosis. J Infect Dis. 1988;157:918–24.
30. Meyer ME. Brucellosis. In: Samter M, ed. Immunological Diseases. Boston: Little, Brown; 1978:651–9.
31. Hodinka L, Gomor B, Meretey K. HLA-B27-associated spondylarthritis in chronic brucellosis. Lancet. 1978;1:499.
32. Gotuzzo E, Bocanegra TS, Alarcon GS, et al. Humoral immune abnormalities in human brucellosis. Allergol Immunopathol (Madr). 1985;13:417–24.
33. Braude AI. Studies in the pathology and pathogenesis of experimental brucellosis I. A comparison of the pathogenicity of *Brucella abortus*, *Brucella melitensis* and *Brucella suis* for guinea pigs. J Infect Dis. 1951;89:76–82.
34. Dalrymple-Champneys W. Brucella infection and undulant fever in man. London: Oxford University Press; 1960.
35. Lulu AR, Araj GF, Khateeb MI. Human brucellosis in Kuwait: a prospective study of 400 cases. Q J Med. 1988;249:39–54.
36. Spink WW. The significance of bacterial hypersensitivity in human brucellosis: studies on infection due to strain 19 *Brucella abortus*. Ann Intern Med. 1957;47:861–74.
37. Pivnick H, Worton H, Smith DLT, et al. Infection of veterinarians in Ontario by *Brucella abortus* strain 19. Can J Public Health. 1966,57:225–31.
38. Spink WW. What is chronic brucellosis? Ann Intern Med. 1951;35:358–74.
39. Cluff LE, Trever RW, Imboden JB, Canter A. Brucellosis II. Medical aspects of delayed convalescence. Arch Intern Med. 1959;103:398–405.
40. Imboden JB, Canter A, Cluff LE, et al. Brucellosis III. Psychologic aspects of delayed convalescence. Arch Intern Med. 1959;103:106–14.
41. Polt SS, Dismukes WE, Flint A, et al. Human brucellosis caused by *Brucella canis*. Ann Intern Med. 1982;97:717–9.
42. Morisset R, Spink WW. Epidemic canine brucellosis due to a new species, *Brucella canis*. Lancet. 1969;II:1000–2.
43. Blankenship RM, Sanford JP. *Brucella canis*: a cause of undulant fever. Am J Med. 1975;59:424–6.
44. Joffe B, Diamond MT. Brucellosis due to self-inoculation. Ann Intern Med. 1966;65:564–5.
45. Feiz J, Sabbaghian H, Miraldi M. Brucellosis due to *B. melitensis* in children. Clinical and epidemiological observations in 95 patients observed in Central Iran. Clin Pediatr. 1978;17:904–7.
46. Rotes-Querol J. Osteoarticular sites in brucellosis. Ann Rheum Dis. 1957;16:63–8.
47. Gotuzzo E, Alarcon GS, Bocanegra TS, et al. Articular involvement in human brucellosis: a retrospective analysis of 304 cases. Semin Arthritis Rheum. 1982;12:245–55.
48. Mousa ARM, Muhtaseb SA, Almudallal DS, et al. Osteoarticular complications of brucellosis: a study of 169 cases. Rev Infect Dis. 1987;9:531–43.
49. Ariza J, Gudiol F, Valverde J, et al. Brucellar spondylitis: a detailed analysis based on current findings. Rev Infect Dis. 1985;7:656–64.
50. Alarcon GS, Gotuzzo E, Hinostroza SA, et al. HLA studies in brucellar spondylitis. Clin Rheum Dis. 1985;4:312–4.
51. Bahar RH, Al-Suhaili AR, Mousa AM. Brucellosis: appearance on skeletal imaging. Clin Nucl Med. 1988;13:102–6.
52. Mousa ARM, Koshy TS, Araj GF, et al. Brucella meningitis: presentation, diagnosis and treatment—a prospective study of ten cases. Q J Med. 1986;223:873–85.
53. Bouza E, Garcia de la Torre M, Parras F, et al. Brucellar meningitis. Rev Infect Dis. 1987;9:810–22.
54. Young EJ. Human brucellosis. Rev Infect Dis. 1983;5:821–42.
55. Shakir RA, Al-Din ASN, Araj GF, et al. Clinical categories of neurobrucellosis. Brain. 1987;110:213–23.
56. Araj GF, Lulu AR, Saadah MA, et al. Rapid diagnosis of central nervous system brucellosis by ELISA. J. Neuroimmunol. 1986;12:173–82.
57. Shakir AR. Neurobrucellosis. Postgrad Med J. 1986;62:1077–9.
58. Kelalis PP, Greene LF, Weed LA. Brucellosis of the urogenital tract. A mimic of tuberculosis. J Urol. 1962;88:347–53.
59. Ibrahim AIA, Awad R, Shetty SD. Genito-urinary complications of brucellosis. Br J Urol. 1988;61:294–8.
60. Forbes KA, Lowry EC, Gibson TE, et al. Brucellosis of the genitourinary tract; review of the literature and report of a case in a child. Urol Surv. 1954;4:391–412.
61. Dunea G, Kark RM, Lannigan R, et al. Brucella nephritis. Ann Intern Med. 1969;70:783–90.
62. Al-Kasab S, Al-Fagih MR, Al-Yousef S, et al. Brucella infective endocarditis. Successful combined medical and surgical therapy. Thorac Cardiovasc Surg. 1988;95:862–7.

63. Jeroudi MO, Halim MA, Harder EJ, et al. Brucella endocarditis. Br Heart J. 1987;58:279–83.
64. Cohen PS, Maguire JH, Weinstein L. Infective endocarditis caused by gram negative bacteria. A review of the literature; 1945–1977. Prog Cardiovasc Dis. 1980;22:205–39.
65. Fernandez-Guerrero ML, Martinell J, Aguado JM. Prosthetic valve endocarditis caused by *Brucella melitensis*. Arch Intern Med. 1987;147:1141–3.
66. Peery TM, Belter LF. Brucellosis and heart disease II. Fatal brucellosis. A review of the literature and report of new cases. Am J Pathol. 1960;36:673–94.
67. Cervantes F, Carbonell J, Bruguera M, et al. Liver disease in brucellosis. A clinical and pathological study of 40 cases. Postgrad Med J. 1982;58:346–50.
68. Spink WW. Host parasite relationship in human brucellosis with prolonged illness due to suppuration of the liver and spleen. Am J Med Sci. 1964;35:129–36.
69. Young EJ, Suvannoparrat U. Brucellosis outbreak attributed to ingestion of unpasteurized goat cheese. Arch Intern Med. 1975;135:240–3.
70. Young EJ. *Brucella melitensis* hepatitis: the absence of granulomas. Ann Intern Med. 1979;91:414–5.
71. Pfischner WCW, Ishak KG, Neptune EM, et al. Brucellosis in Egypt. A review of experience with 228 patients. Am J Med. 1957;22:915–29.
72. McGarity WC, Serafin D. Brucellosis. Indications for splenectomy. Am J Surg. 1968;115:355–63.
73. Patel PJ, Al-Suhaibani H, Al-Aska AK, et al. The chest radiograph in brucellosis. Clin Radiol. 1988;39:39–41.
74. Harvey WA. Pulmonary brucellosis. Ann Intern Med. 1948;28:768–81.
75. Greer AE. Pulmonary brucellosis. Dis Chest. 1956;29:508–10.
76. Haden RL, Kyger ER. Pulmonary manifestation of brucellosis. Cleve Clin Q. 1946;13:220–7.
77. Crosby E, Llosa L, MiroQuesada M, et al. Hematologic changes in brucellosis. J Infect Dis. 1984;150:419–24.
78. Berger TG, Guill MA, Goette DK. Cutaneous lesions in brucellosis. Arch Dermatol. 1981;117:40–2.
79. Franco Vicario R, Balparda J, Santamaria JM. Cutaneous vasculitis in a patient with acute brucellosis. Dermatologia. 1985;171:126–8.
80. Arnow PM, Smaron M, Ormiste V. Brucellosis in a group of travelers to Spain. JAMA. 1984;251:505–7.
81. Gotuzzo E, Carrillo C, Guerra J, et al. An evaluation of diagnostic methods for brucellosis—the value of bone marrow culture. J Infect Dis. 1986;153:122–5.
82. Castaneda MR. Laboratory diagnosis of brucellosis in man. Bull WHO. 1961;24:73–84.
83. Castaneda MR. A practical method for routine blood cultures in brucellosis. Proc Soc Exp Biol Med. 1947;64:114–5.
84. Etemadi H, Raissadat A, Pickett MJ, et al. Isolation of *Brucella* spp. from clinical specimens. J Clin Microbiol. 1984;20:586.
85. Buchanan TM, Sulzer CR, Frix MK, et al. Brucellosis in the United States, 1960–1972. An abattoir-associated disease. Part II. Diagnostic aspects. Medicine. 1974;53:415–25.
86. Buchanan TM, Faber LC. 2-Mercaptoethanol *Brucella* agglutination test: usefulness for predicting recovery from brucellosis. J Clin Microbiol. 1980;11:691–3.
87. Hunter SB, Bibb WF, Shih CN, et al. Enzyme-linked immunosorbent assay with outer membrane proteins of *Brucella melitensis* to measure immune response to *Brucella* species. J Clin Microbiol. 1986;24:566–72.
88. Devi SJN, Polt SS, Boctor FN, et al. Serological evaluation of brucellosis: importance of species in antigen preparation. J Infect Dis. 1987;156:658–61.
89. Ariza J, Gudiol F, Pallares R, et al. Comparative trial of co-trimoxazole versus tetracycline-streptomycin in treating human brucellosis. J Infect Dis. 1985;152:1358–9.
90. Ariza J, Gudiol F, Pallares R, et al. Comparative trial of rifampin-doxycycline versus tetracycline-streptomycin in the therapy of human brucellosis. Antimicrob Agents Chemother. 1985;28:548–51.
91. Elberg SS. A guide to the diagnosis, treatment and prevention of human brucellosis, WHO document VPH/81.31. Geneva: World Health Organization; 1981.
92. Palenque E, Otero JR, Noriega AR. In vitro susceptibility of *Brucella melitensis* to new cephalosporins crossing the blood-brain barrier. Antimicrob Agents Chemother. 1986;29:182–3.
93. Bosch J, LopezdeGoicoechea MJ, Ariza J, et al. In vitro activity of ciprofloxacin, ceftriaxone, and five other antimicrobial agents against 95 strains of *Brucella melitensis*. J Antimicrob Chemother. 1986;17:459–61.
94. Altes AG, Enciso MD, Garcia PP, et al. In vitro activity of N-formimidoyl thienamycin against 98 clinical isolates of *Brucella melitensis* compared with those of cefoxitin, rifampin, tetracycline, and co-trimoxazole. Antimicrob Agents Chemother. 1982;21:501–3.
95. Fountain MW, Weiss SJ, Fountain AG, et al. Treatment of *Brucella canis* and *Brucella abortus* in vitro and in vivo by stable plurilamellar vesicle-encapsulated aminoglycosides. J Infect Dis. 1985;152:529–35.
96. Kolar J. Control of *Brucella melitensis* brucellosis in developing countries. Ann Inst. Pasteur Microbiol. 1987;138:122–5.
97. Plommet M, Serre A, Fensterbank R. Vaccines, vaccination in brucellosis. Ann Inst. Pasteur Microbiol. 1987;138:117–21.

205. FRANCISELLA TULARENSIS (TULAREMIA)

JOHN M. BOYCE

Francisella tularensis is found primarily in wild mammals and blood-sucking arthropods and in their environment. Infection in humans, usually called tularemia (less commonly rabbit fever or deerfly fever), is characterized by high fever and severe constitutional symptoms that may persist for weeks to several months if not treated appropriately. Although the reported incidence of human tularemia in the United States has declined dramatically in the last 3 decades, the disease is still responsible for appreciable morbidity in some parts of the world and among certain occupational groups.

HISTORY

In 1911, McCoy[1] described a "plague-like disease of rodents" while investigating plague among ground squirrels in California. In 1912, McCoy and Chapin[2] recovered the organism from rodents in Tulare County, California, and named it *Bacterium tularense*. The first bacteriologically confirmed human case was reported by Wherry and Lamb[3] in 1914. Francis,[4] while studying the plaguelike disease in rodents and deerfly fever in Utah in 1919 and 1920, realized that both were manifestations of an illness that was frequently bacteremic, coined the name tularemia, and commented on the role of the deerfly in transmission. In 1924, Parker et al.[5] reported that ticks were naturally infected and were able to transmit the disease. Investigators subsequently discovered tularemia in many other countries.

The organism has previously been called *Bacterium, Baccillus, Brucella,* and *Pasteurella tularensis*. Although the tularemia bacillus and *Pasteurella pestis* (now *Yersinia pestis*) share similarities with respect to pathogenicity, organ pathology, affinity for rodents, and transmission by insects, taxonomists renamed the organism *Francisella* since its small size and growth requirements distinguish if from *Pasteurella*.

DESCRIPTION OF THE PATHOGEN

Francisella tularensis is small, gram-negative, nonmotile coccobacillus that tends to be pleomorphic in culture. It grows poorly or not at all on most ordinary culture media, but growth occurs on glucose cysteine blood agar, glucose blood agar, in thioglycolate broth, and in other media containing sufficient cysteine (or sulfhydryl compounds). On several occasions, it was recovered on buffered charcoal yeast extract (CYE) medium that had been inoculated with specimens from patients with suspected legionellosis.[6] Growth is optimum at 37°C under aerobic conditions, with small, smooth, opaque colonies appearing in 24–48 hours. The organism is usually identified on the basis of its morphologic characteristics, growth requirements, fluorescent staining, and agglutination with specific antisera.

All isolates are serologically homogeneous but may be divided into two categories. Type A (Nearctica) has been recovered from many rodents and from blood-sucking arthropods, is highly virulent in rabbits and humans, uses glycerol, and is citrulline ureidase positive. Type B (Palaearctica) is more commonly recovered from water and aquatic animals, is less virulent in rabbits and humans, does not use glycerol, and is citrulline ureidase negative.

The organism appears to have many antigenic components, including a polysaccharide antigen, a protein antigen that cross reacts with *Brucella*, and an endotoxinlike substance with biologic activity similar to endotoxins produced by other gram-negative bacteria.[7] A majority of strains tested have produced beta-lactamase.

EPIDEMIOLOGY

Francisella tularensis is distributed throughout the northern hemisphere (excluding the United Kingdom) between 30° and 71° north latitude. The organism has been recovered from 100 species of wild mammals (e.g., rabbits, hares, squirrels, voles, muskrats, beavers, deer), at least nine species of domestic animals (e.g., sheep, cattle, cats), birds, some amphibians and fish, many invertebrates (e.g., ticks, deerflies, mosquitoes), mud, and water from streams and wells.[8] In the United States the most important reservoir hosts are rabbits, hares, and ticks. Muskrats have been the source of human infections in both the United States and Canada.

Humans most commonly acquire tularemia after contact with tissues or body fluid of an infected mammal (rabbit) or the bite of an infected arthropod. Less commonly, the disease is transmitted by animal bites (cat, coyote, squirrel), inhalation of infectious aerosols, or ingestion of contaminated water or inadequately cooked meat from an affected animal.[9,10] Most cases are sporadic, but clusters occur among hunters and families, and small epidemics have occurred among muskrat trappers, troops or laborers bitten by ticks or deerflies, and farmers exposed to contaminated dust or water.[10–16]

The incidence of human tularemia in the United States reached a peak in 1939 and has declined steadily to levels of 0.6–1.3/1,000,000 population (Fig. 1). The disease occurs in all 50 states, but the proportion of states reporting large numbers of cases has decreased during the last several decades, and in recent years, nearly 50 percent of reported cases have occurred in Arkansas, Tennessee, Texas, Oklahoma, and Missouri (Fig. 2). The seasonal distribution of cases varies with geographic location. The incidence peaks in the spring and summer months in areas in which tick-borne cases predominate but increases in the winter months in areas in which rabbit-associated cases are prevalent. Since 1950, the proportion of reported cases with onset in the summer months has steadily increased, so that 60% of cases now occur in the months May through September (Fig.

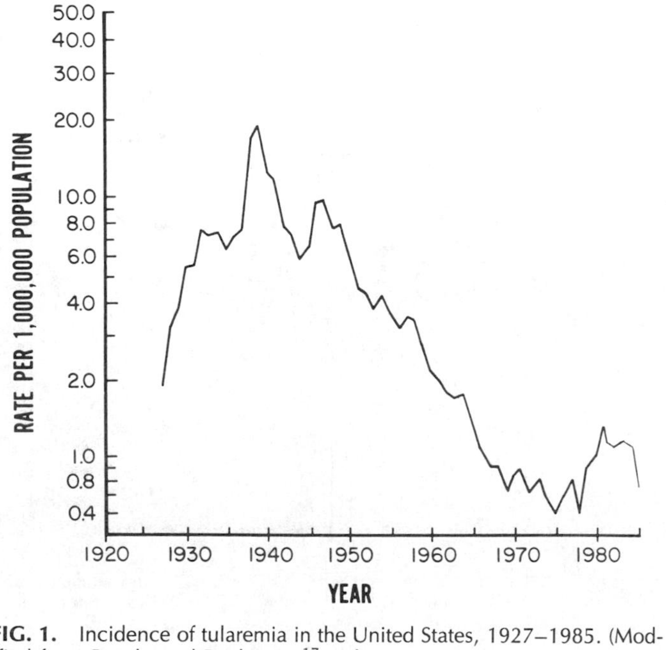

FIG. 1. Incidence of tularemia in the United States, 1927–1985. (Modified from Brooks and Buchanan,[17] with permission.)

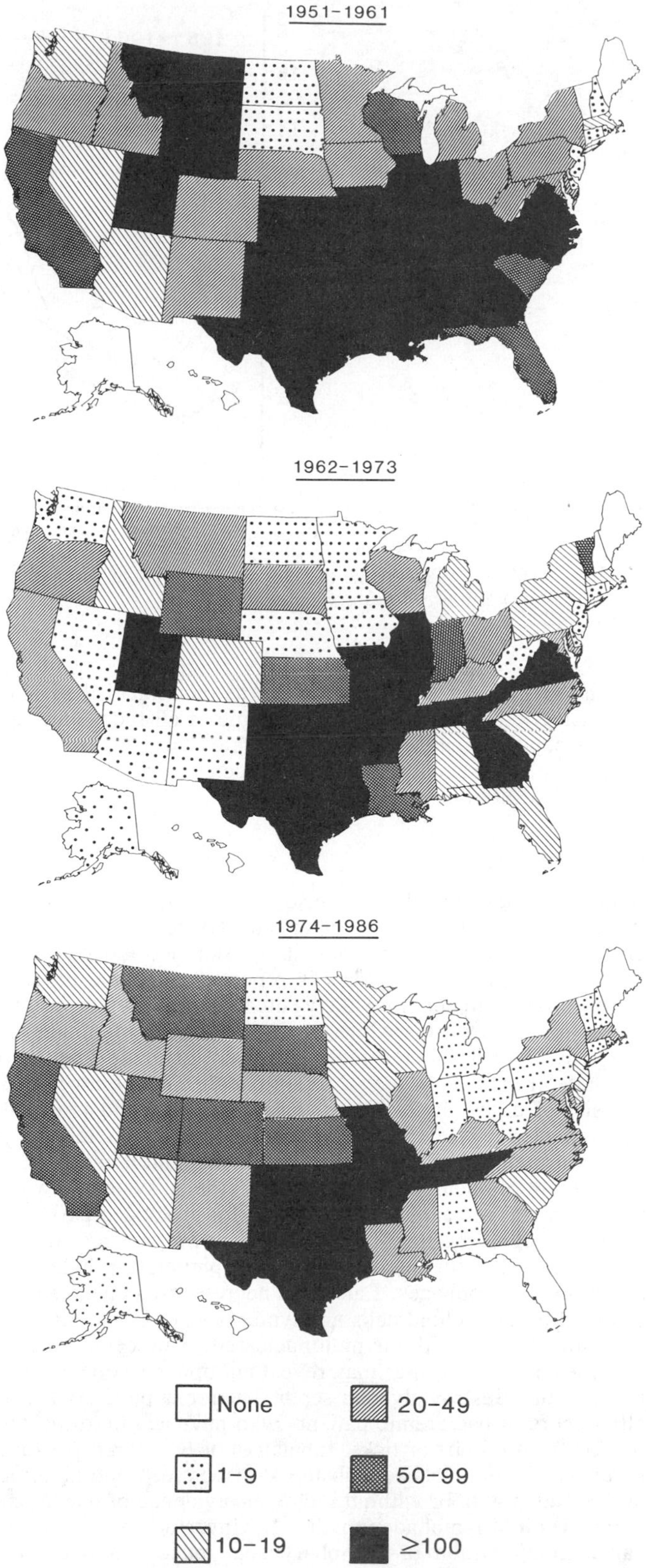

FIG. 2. Reported cases of tularemia, United States, 1951–1986.

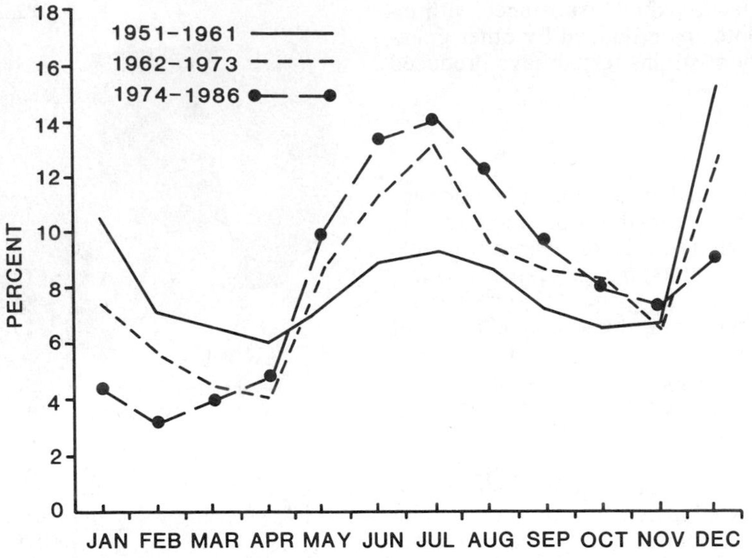

FIG. 3. Percentage of reported cases of tularemia that occurred during each month, United States, 1951–1986. (Modified from Boyce,[18] with permission.)

3). This trend suggests that vector-borne tularemia is becoming increasingly important. Although people of all races and ages are susceptible, age-specific attack rates are highest among adults, with men accounting for 65–75 percent of tick-borne and rabbit-associated cases.

PATHOGENESIS

In humans, 10–50 bacilli will cause disease if inhaled or injected intradermally, whereas 10^8 organisms are required with oral challenge. Portals of entry include the skin and mucous membranes. *Francisella tularensis* is reportedly capable of penetrating intact skin but more likely enters inapparent skin lesions. Ticks inject organisms while feeding or may contaminate the bite wound with infected feces. After an incubation period of 3–5 days (range: 1–14 days), a skin papule usually develops at the site of entry. In 2–4 days, an ulcer forms and is usually accompanied by fever and lymphadenopathy. Bacteremia is common in animals (and probably humans) and is followed by entrapment of bacilli in the reticuloendothelial system in which the organisms are capable of surviving for prolonged periods of time intracellularly. Early lesions in affected organs reveal areas of focal necrosis surrounded by polymorphonuclear leukocytes and a few macrophages. Later, the necrotic areas become surrounded by epithelioid cells and lymphocytes. Caseating granulomata with or without multinucleated giant cells occur in some lesions.[9] The lungs may reveal multiple necrotizing granulomata that destroy alveolar septa. Tularemia pneumonia usually occurs in bacteremic patients who have acquired their infection from rabbits or ticks. Inhalation of *F. tularensis* causes fever, headache, malaise, substernal discomfort, and nonproductive cough with or without radiologic evidence of pneumonia or mediastinal lymphadenopathy.[14,15] Ingestion of bacilli may cause inflammation of the pharyngeal mucosa and cervical lymphadenopathy or a nonspecific febrile illness with no localizing findings.[10]

Inoculation of the conjunctiva or oral mucosa follows contact with a hand or fingers contaminated by tissue fluids from an affected animal or exposure to infectious aerosols.

CLINICAL MANIFESTATIONS

Almost all patients have abrupt onset of fever, chills, malaise, and fatigue and develop one of the following clinical syndromes: ulceroglandular, glandular, typhoidal, oculoglandular, or oropharyngeal tularemia. The ulceroglandular form (75–85 percent of the cases) is characterized by an ulcerated skin lesion and painful regional lymphadenopathy.[9,19,20] Rarely, lymphangitis or nodular sporotrichoid lesions occur proximal to the ulcer. The skin lesion is located on the fingers or hand in over 90 percent of the rabbit-associated cases; in tick-borne cases the ulcer is located on the lower extremities or perineal area (including penis, scrotum, and buttocks) in 50 percent of the cases, on the trunk in 30 percent of the cases, and on the head in 5 to 10 percent of cases. Multiple ulcers may occur in patients who have had contact with many infected animals.[11,20]

About 80–90 percent of the patients with rabbit-associated tularemia have axillary or epitrochlear adenopathy; 60–70 percent of those with tick-borne tularemia have inguinal or femoral adenopathy. Some patients have involvement of several areas (e.g., cervical and axillary adenopathy) (Fig. 4). In glandular tularemia (5–10 percent of the cases) there is fever and tender

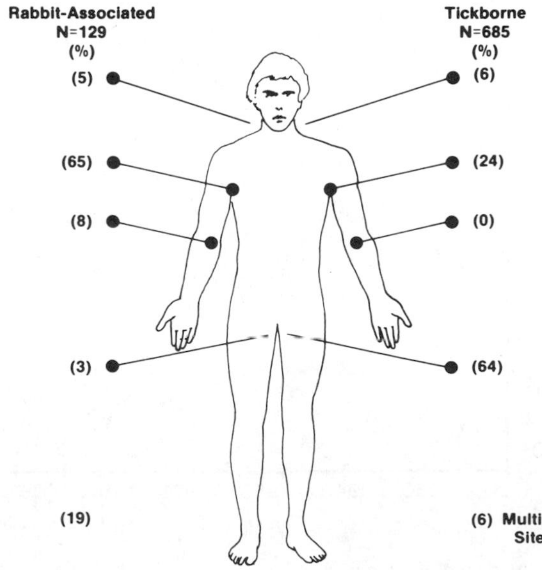

FIG. 4. Distribution of lymphadenopathy in tularemia.

lymphadenopathy but no skin ulcer. In the typhoidal form (5–15 percent of the cases) fever, prostration, and weight loss occur without lymphadenopathy. The protean signs and symptoms and frequent absence of suggestive exposure history make this form of the disease difficult to diagnose. The typhoidal form may occur after intradermal, respiratory, or gastrointestinal challenge.

In the oculoglandular form (1–2 percent of the cases) patients have unilateral, painful, purulent conjunctivitis with preauricular or cervical lymphadenopathy. Chemosis, periorbital edema, and small nodular lesions or ulcerations of the palpebral conjunctiva are noted in some patients. Oropharyngeal tularemia produces an acute exudative or membranous pharyngotonsillitis with cervical lymphadenopathy.[21]

Pleuropulmonary complications are not uncommon in tularemia. Pneumonia, seen in 30–80 percent of the typhoidal cases and in 10–15 percent of the ulceroglandular cases, is characterized by a nonproductive cough, a paucity of findings on physical examination, and patchy ill-defined infiltrates in one or more lobes on chest roentgenograms.[15,16,19,22–24]

Patients may have abnormal chest roentgenograms without respiratory symptoms.[14,20] Some patients develop a lobar pneumonia accompanied by signs of consolidation; lung abscess is rare. Pleural effusions, which are characterized by a predominantly mononuclear cellular response and granulomatous tissue reaction, have occasionally been confused with tuberculous effusions.[12,15] Occasionally, patients have developed adult respiratory distress syndrome (ARDS) as a complication of tularemia.[25]

Rash has been reported in up to 20 percent of the cases in a few series.[4,12] The rash appears several days after the onset of other symptoms and may be macular, maculopapular, pustular, or blotchy. A few cases of tularemia have been accompanied by erythema nodosum or erythema multiforme.[14,20] Some patients develop hepatomegaly and abnormal liver function tests, and a few develop transient renal failure and rhabdomyolysis.[16,26–28] Tularemia pericarditis, peritonitis, meningitis, and osteomyelitis are rare.

Patients with tularemia may present with relatively mild constitutional symptoms, especially when the disease is caused by type B strains of *F. tularensis*.[14,29,30] Tickborne tularemia in children may present as low-grade fever and cervical or occipital lymphadenitis that may resolve spontaneously without specific antimicrobial therapy.[29,30]

Patients with acute onset of fever and painful lymphadenopathy should be carefully questioned about exposure to mammals and ticks. However, failure to elicit a history of animal exposure does not rule out tularemia, since patients with vector-borne, water-borne, or air-borne tularemia are often unaware of their exposure. Glandular or ulceroglandular tularemia may mimic staphylococcal or streptococcal lymphadenitis, infectious mononucleosis, toxoplasmosis, lymphogranuloma venereum, cat-scratch disease, *Pasteurella* infections, plague, or sporotrichosis. Typhoidal tularemia with or without pneumonia may be confused with typhoid fever or with other *Salmonella* infections, brucellosis, malaria, tuberculosis, mycotic infections, Q fever, psittacosis, or legionnaires' disease. The oropharyngeal form mimics streptococcal, viral, or diphtheritic pharyngitis. A history of fever after a tick bite also suggests Rocky Mountain spotted fever, Colorado tick fever, relapsing fever, tick-borne typhus, or Lyme disease.

Francisella tularensis is rarely seen in Gram stains of sputum or exudate from skin ulcers or affected lymph nodes. Cultures of clinical specimens are usually negative since the organism does not grow on most ordinary media. In recent years, a few cases have been diagnosed by radiometric blood culture systems.[28]

Many laboratories are reluctant to attempt isolation of *F. tularensis* because of the risk of creating infectious aerosols in the laboratory. Inoculation of clinical specimens or environmental samples (water) into susceptible laboratory animals is an effective method of recovering the organism but is not generally recommended owing to the risk of infection in laboratory personnel or animal colonies. Therefore, almost all cases are diagnosed serologically. A fourfold rise in the tularemia tube agglutination or microagglutination titer is diagnostic of infection; a single convalescent titer of 1:160 or greater is diagnostic of past or current infection. Agglutination titers are usually negative in the first week of illness and are positive in 50–70 percent of the patients after 2 weeks of illness. Titers reach a maximum in 4–8 weeks and may remain elevated at diagnostic levels for many years after the acute episode. The tularemia skin test becomes positive earlier in the illness and remains positive longer after acute infection than does the agglutination test.[31] Unfortunately, the skin test antigen is not commercially available.

PREVENTION AND THERAPY

To minimize the risk of tularemia, people should avoid skinning or eviscerating rabbits and other wild mammals, especially if the animal appears ill. Wearing gloves while performing such tasks probably reduces the risk of infection. To prevent tickborne disease, tick-infested areas should be avoided when feasible; clothing and the body should be inspected frequently, and ticks should be removed promptly. To remove a tick, grasp near its mouth parts and gradually lift upward; avoid squeezing the body of the tick since its excretions may be infectious. Tick repellents such as diethyltoluamide or dimethyl phthalate may be of value for people whose occupation or avocation results in repeated tick exposures.

Live attenuated tularemia vaccine does not provide complete protection against infection but has been shown to reduce the severity of the disease in vaccinated people who develop overt clinical disease.[32] Laboratory workers (including people handling infected or potentially infected animals) exposed to *F. tularensis* and people whose vocations require repeated contact with wild mammals or vectors in tularemia enzootic areas are candidates for immunization. Inquiries regarding the vaccine should be addressed to the Drug Service, Centers for Disease Control, Atlanta, Georgia.

Streptomycin is still considered the drug of choice for all forms of tularemia.[33,34] Although a number of dosage regimens have been recommended, no one regimen is clearly superior. Streptomycin, 15–20 mg/kg per day intramuscularly in divided doses for 7–14 days, is usually effective. Several reports suggest that gentamicin (3–5 mg/kg per day) is an acceptable alternative to streptomycin.[20,28,35] When the diagnosis of tularemia is in doubt and broader coverage against gram-negative bacteria is desirable, empiric therapy with gentamicin appears reasonable. Additional data are needed to determine whether gentamicin has any advantages over streptomycin for therapy of tularemia. Tetracycline or chloramphenicol may be given, but clinical relapses occur more frequently with these drugs, particularly when administered for less than 14 days.[20,34,36] A loading dose of tetracycline or chloramphenicol, 30 mg/kg orally, is given, followed by 30 mg/kg per day orally in divided doses for 14 days.[37] Relapses are not due to resistant organisms and can be treated with another course of the same drug. Some patients with tularemia have responded to high-dose intravenous erythromycin.[6]

The mortality before the availability of antibiotics was 5–15 percent but has been 1–3 percent in recent years.[20] In typhoidal tularemia the mortality is two to three times higher than in the other forms. Immunity after tularemia is usually lifelong, although a few well-documented reinfections have occurred in laboratory workers. Serum antibodies do not appear to be protective; studies conducted in animals suggest that cell-mediated immunity is important in resisting reinfection.[38]

REFERENCES

1. McCoy GW. A plague-like disease in rodents. Public Health Bull. 1911;43:53–71.
2. McCoy GW, Chapin SW. Further observations on a plague-like disease of rodents with a preliminary note on the causative agent. J Infect Dis. 1912;10:61–72.
3. Wherry WB, Lamb BH. Infection of man with *Bacterium tularense*. J Infect Dis. 1914;15:331–40.
4. Francis E. I. The occurrence of tularemia in nature as a disease of man. Public Health Rep. 1921;36:1731–51.
5. Parker RR, Spencer RR, Francis E. Tularemia infection in ticks of the species *Dermacentor andersoni* Stiles in the Bitterroot Valley, Montana. Public Health Rep. 1924; 39:1057–73.
6. Westerman EL, McDonald J. Tularemia pneumonia mimicking Legionnaire's disease: Isolation of organism on CYE agar and successful treatment with erythromycin. South Med J. 1983;76:1169–70.
7. Finegold MJ, Pulliam JD, Landay ME, et al. Pathological changes in rabbits injected with *Pasteurella tularensis* killed by ionizing radiation. J Infect Dis. 1969;119:635–40.
8. Olsen PF. Tularemia. In: Hubbert WT, McCulloch WF, Schnurrenberger PR, eds. Diseases Transmitted from Animals to Man. Springfield, IL: Charles C Thomas; 1975:191–223.
9. Francis E. A summary of present knowledge of tularemia. Medicine. 1928;7:411–32.
10. Karpoff SP, Antonoff NI. The spread of tularemia through water, as a new factor in its epidemiology. J Bacteriol. 1936;32:243–58.
11. Young LS, Bickness DS, Archer BG, et al. Tularemia epidemic: Vermont, 1968. Forty-seven cases linked to contact with muskrats. N Engl J Med. 1969;280:1253–60.
12. Warring WB, Ruffin JS, Jr. A tick-borne epidemic of tularemia. N Engl J Med. 1946;234:137–40.
13. Klock LE, Olsen PF, Fukushima T. Tularemia epidemic associated with the deerfly. JAMA. 1973;226:149–52.
14. Syrjala H, Kujala P, Myllyla V, et al. Airborne transmission of tularemia in farmers. Scand J Infect Dis. 1985;17:371–5.
15. Teutsch SM, Martone WJ, Brink EW, et al. Pneumonic tularemia on Martha's Vineyard. N Engl J Med. 1979;301:826–8.
16. Martone WJ, Marshall LW, Kaufmann AF, et al. Tularemia pneumonia in Washington, DC. A report of three cases with possible common-source exposures. JAMA. 1979;242:2315–7.
17. Brooks GF, Buchanan TM. Tularemia in the United States: Epidemiologic aspects in the 1960s and follow-up of the outbreak of tularemia in Vermont. J Infect Dis. 1970;121:357–9.
18. Boyce JM. Recent trends in the epidemiology of tularemia in the United States. J Infect Dis. 1975;131:197–9.
19. Sanders CV, Hahn R. Analysis of 106 cases of tularemia. J La State Med Soc. 1968;120:391–3.
20. Evans ME, Gregory DW, Schaffner W, et al. Tularemia: A 30-year experience with 88 cases. Medicine. 1985;64:251–69.
21. Hughes WT Jr, Etteldorf JN. Oropharyngeal tularemia. J Pediatr 1957;51:363–72.
22. Dienst FT Jr. Tularemia. A perusal of 339 cases. J La State Med Soc. 1963;115:114–27.
23. Foshay L. Cause of death in tularemia. Arch Intern Med. 1937;60:22.
24. Miller RP, Bates JH. Pleuropulmonary tularemia. A review of 29 cases. Am Rev Respir Dis. 1969;99:31–41.
25. Sunderrajan EV, Hutton J, Marienfeld D. Adult respiratory distress syndrome secondary to tularemia pneumonia. Arch Intern Med. 1985;145:1435–7.
26. Tilley WS, Garman RW, Stone WJ. Tularemia complicated by acute renal failure. South Med J. 1983;76:273–4.
27. Kaiser AB, Rieves D, Price AH, et al. Tularemia and rhabdomyolysis. JAMA. 1985;253:241–3.
28. Provenza JM, Klotz SA, Penn RL. Isolation of *Francisella tularensis* from blood. J Clin Microbiol. 1986;24:453–5.
29. Schmid GP, Kornblatt AN, Connors CA, et al. Clinically mild tularemia associated with tick-borne *Francisella tularensis*. J Infect Dis. 1983;148:63–7.
30. Markowitz LE, Hynes NA, de la Cruz P, et al. Tick-borne tularemia. An outbreak of lymphadenopathy in children. JAMA. 1985;254:2922–5.
31. Buchanan TM, Brooks GF, Brachman PS. The tularemia skin test. 325 skin tests in 210 persons: Serologic correlation and review of the literature. Ann Intern Med. 1971;74:336–43.
32. Burke DS. Immunization against tularemia: Analysis of the effectiveness of live *Francisella tularensis* vaccine in prevention of laboratory-acquired tularemia. J Infect Dis. 1977;135:55–60.
33. Berson RC, Harwell AB. Streptomycin in the treatment of tularemia. Am J Med Sci. 1948;215:243–9.
34. Corwin WC, Stubbs SP. Further studies on tularemia in the Ozarks. Review of 44 cases during a three-year period. JAMA. 1952; 149:343–5.
35. Mason WL, Eigelsbach HT, Little SF, et al. Treatment of tularemia, including pulmonary tularemia, with gentamicin. Am Rev Respir Dis. 1980;121:39–45.
36. Overholt EL, Tigertt WD, Kadull PJ, et al. An analysis of laboratory-acquired tularemia. Treatment with broad spectrum antibiotics. Am J Med. 1961;30:785–806.
37. Sawyer WD, Dangerfield HG, Hogge AL, et al. Antibiotic prophylaxis and therapy of airborne tularemia. Bacteriol Rev. 1966;30:542–8.
38. Kostiala AAI, McGregor DD, Logie PS. Tularemia in the rat. The cellular basis of host resistance to infection. Immunology. 1975;28:855–69.

206. PASTEURELLA SPECIES

JOHN M. BOYCE

Pasteurellae are primarily animal pathogens but are capable of producing a variety of diseases in humans ranging from focal abscesses to septicemia and endocarditis.

DESCRIPTION OF THE PATHOGEN

Pasteurellae are non-spore-forming, nonmotile, bipolar staining, gram-negative coccobacilli. They are aerobic, facultatively anaerobic, and grow on many ordinary media at 37°C. Recent studies suggest that the genus *Pasteurella* may be divided into 11 different species, but a majority of human *Pasteurella* infections are caused by organisms identified as *P. multocida, P. haemolytica, P. pneumotropica* and *P. ureae*. Most strains of *P. haemolytica* and a few strains of *P. pneumotropica* will grow on media containing bile salts (e.g., MacConkey agar), while other species fail to grow on such media. Primary isolation is facilitated by use of enriched media such as blood or serum agar under increased carbon dioxide tension. Almost all species are oxidase and catalase positive but differ in their biochemical reactions, ability to cause hemolysis on blood agar, and pathogenicity in laboratory animals. *Pasteurella multocida* and *P. haemolytica* both produce lipopolysaccharide endotoxins and possess neuramindase activity.

Several systems for serotyping *P. multocida* and *P. haemolytica* strains have been described. Five serotypes (A, B, D, E, F) of *P. multocida* and 12 serotypes of *P. haemolytica* have been described.[1,2] Serologic cross-reactions occur between some *P. multocida* and *P. pneumotropica* isolates.

EPIDEMIOLOGY

P. multocida is distributed worldwide and has been recovered from the nasopharynx or gastrointestinal tract of many domestic and wild mammals (e.g., cattle, sheep, swine, cats, dogs, rats, opossums, and lions) and birds (e.g., chickens, turkeys, and ducks). The frequency of carriage varies among species: cats (50–70 percent), dogs (12–66 percent), swine (51 percent), and rats (14 percent). The organism causes sporadic and epidemic pneumonia and hemorrhagic septicemia in cattle, sheep, and swine and fowl cholera in chickens, turkeys, and ducks.

Human *P. multocida* infections fall into three broad categories: cases following animal bites, cases associated with nonbite animal exposures, and cases with no known animal exposures. A majority of human infections are related to animal bites.[3] Tindall and Harrison[4] and Lee and Buhr[5] found that 7–17 percent of persons reporting to a hospital for animal bites or scratches developed *P. multocida* infection. The age distribution of cases differs among various series but probably reflects the age of persons sustaining animal bites.[3,6] Although dog bites account for a majority of emergency room visits related to animal bites, 65 percent of bite-associated *P. multocida* infections are caused by cat bites or scratches; dog bites account for the remaining 35 percent. The greater risk of infection associated with cat bites may be related to the higher incidence of *P. multocida* colonization among cats, to the greater degree of virulence exhibited by cat-associated strains, or possibly to differences between the types of wounds inflicted by cats and dogs. Infections have also been reported after the bites of lions, panthers, rabbits, opossums, and rats.

Infections associated with nonbite animal exposures frequently involve the upper respiratory tract, intra-abdominal sites, extremities, or central nervous system of pet owners, livestock handlers, food processors, and other persons who have frequent contact with animals.[7]

Interestingly, 5–15 percent of the patients with *P. multocida* infection have no known animal exposures.[7] In this group, isolates are also predominantly from patients with upper respiratory tract or intra-abdominal disease. Rarely, *P. multocida* has been isolated from the nasopharynx of apparently healthy persons exposed to animals (e.g., veterinary students or animal handlers).[8,9] Hence, it appears that *P. multocida* may exist in humans as part of the normal flora of the upper respiratory tract.

Pasteurella haemolytica is found in the nasopharynx of cattle, sheep, goats, swine, horses, and fowl. The organism also causes epizootics of pneumonia in cattle and sheep, septicemia in lambs, and fowl cholera in chickens and turkeys. Human infections are rare. *P. pneumotropica* has been recovered from the respiratory and gastrointestinal tracts and from the reproductive organs of laboratory animals (e.g., mice and rats) and from dogs and cats and may cause pneumonia, conjunctivitis, peritonitis, abscesses, metritis, and septicemia in these animals. At least 10 human infections have been reported; 5 after dog or cat bites and 5 with little or no known animal exposure.[10–12]

Pasteurella ureae, unlike the other pasteurellae, has only rarely been recovered from animals, and there is no convincing evidence that the organism is transmitted from animals to humans. It has been recovered, often with other potential pathogens, from sputum of patients with chronic respiratory disease and from patients with acute suppurative infections.[13,14]

PATHOGENESIS

After intraperitoneal or parenteral inoculation of *P. multocida* into susceptible animals, organisms multiply rapidly in extracellular spaces, invade the blood stream, reticuloendothelial organs, and lungs within hours, and cause death from overwhelming septicemia. In mice, the LD_{50} of some *P. multocida* isolates from fowl is only 1–2 organisms, while cattle isolates have an LD_{50} of 50–5000 organisms.[1] Virulence is apparently related to the degree of encapsulation of the organism; strains with large capsules are more resistant to phagocytosis in vivo. In mice, the addition of specific antibodies (opsonins) to peritoneal fluid facilitates phagocytosis after intraperitoneal challenge and inhibits the extracellular multiplication of organisms.

Although many strains possess neuraminidase activity, and virulent type B strains recovered from cattle with hemorrhagic septicemia produce hyaluronidase, the importance of these substances as virulence factors is unclear. *Pasteurella haemolytica* strains produce a protein substance that is cytotoxic for bovine alveolar macrophages, peripheral blood monocytes, and polymorphonuclear leukocytes. It appears that this cytotoxin may be important in the pathogenesis of bovine pneumonic pasteurellosis. In general, *P. haemolytica* and *P. pneumotropica* are less virulent than *P. multocida* but cause similar disease in susceptible animals.

Acute localized infections in humans are characterized by edema and infiltration of polymorphonuclear leukocytes, followed by abscess formation in some patients. When organisms invade the blood stream, microabscesses and hemorrhagic lesions may occur in many tissues, such as lung, meninges, or bone.

CLINICAL MANIFESTATIONS

Pasteurella multocida infection in humans usually manifests in one of three ways: focal soft-tissue infection after direct animal contact, chronic respiratory infections, or bacteremia with or without metastatic lesions. Patients with animal bites have acute onset of erythema, pain, and swelling—frequently within hours of the incident (range: few hours to 3 days). Serosanguineous drainage from the lesion is often noted 24 to 48 hours after onset of symptoms. Bite wounds are usually located on the hands and arms, legs, or head–neck area. Regional lymphadenopathy develops in one-third of the cases. Low-grade fever occurs in some patients. Local complications of infected bites, including osteomyelitis, tenosynovitis, and arthritis occur in about 40 percent of cases and are sometimes responsible for prolonged disability of the involved digit or extremity.[15–18] Rarely, children who have sustained bites to the head have developed *P. multocida* brain abscess.

Pasteurella multocida has been recovered in pure culture or with other potential pathogens from patients who have been exposed to animals but who have no history of animal bites. Many of these patients probably had preexisting *P. multocida* nasopharyngeal colonization. Infections in such patients often represent complications of pre-existing chronic respiratory disorders, spread of the organism from the upper respiratory tract to contiguous structures, or complications resulting from *P. multocida* bacteremia (Table 1). Spontaneous peritonitis and septicemia, which occur most often in patients with cirrhosis of the liver, may develop spontaneously or may occur shortly after upper gastrointestinal tract endoscopy.[18,19]

Few human *P. haemolytica* infections have been reported (Table 1). Infections caused by *P. pneumotropica* and *P. ureae* (Table 1) are clinically indistinguishable from diseases caused by *P. multocida* and other more common bacterial pathogens and vary in severity from bite-associated wound infections to septicemia and meningitis.[10–14]

A history of exposure to animals is essential in alerting the physician to the possibility of pasteurellosis. The diagnosis should be strongly considered in patients who develop acute painful cellulitis less than 24 hours after an animal bite (or cat scratch). When the incubation period is longer, the differential diagnosis should include staphylococcal or streptococcal infection, cat-scratch disease, and tularemia. In plague enzootic areas, bubonic plague has been transmitted by cat bite on rare occasions. In patients with no animal contact or with nonbite exposures, the diagnosis depends on demonstration of bipolar staining gram-negative organisms in sputum, pus, or cerebrospinal fluid and isolation of the organism. The bacteriology laboratory should be alerted if a *Pasteurella* infection is suspected since these organisms may initially be confused with *Haemophilus influenzae, Neisseria, Acinetobacter*, or other gram-negative bacilli.

PREVENTION AND THERAPY

Limiting contact with wild and domestic animals is probably the only means of preventing human *Pasteurella* infections. Bite wounds should be promptly cleansed and debrided; surgical closure should be avoided whenever possible. The value of prophylactic administration of antibiotics has not been adequately studied.

Penicillin is considered the drug of choice for *Pasteurella* infections. The optimum dosage, route of administration, and duration of antibiotic therapy have not been adequately evaluated. However, treatment with penicillin V, 500 mg every 6 hours, or tetracycline, 500 mg every 6 hours orally, for 10–14 days should be adequate. Amoxicillin-clavulanic acid has also been

TABLE 1. Types of Infections Associated with Pasteurellae

Organism	Associated Infections
P. multocida	Infected wound, chronic skin ulcers, osteomyelitis, brain abscess, meningitis, otitis, mastoiditis, sinusitis, tonsillitis, pneumonia, empyema, bronchiectasis, bronchitis, epiglottitis, suppurative arthritis, appendiceal abscess, peritonitis, liver abscess, corneal ulcer, panophthalmitis, pyelonephritis, renal abscess, septicemia
P. haemolytica	Infected wound, endocarditis, ?cholecystitis
P. pneumotropica	Infected wound, sinusitis, meningitis, septicemia, ?tonsillitis
P. ureae	Pneumonia, sinusitis, meningitis, septicemia, peritonitis

shown to be effective but is associated with a higher incidence of side effects than penicillin.[20] Ciprofloxacin has good in vitro activity against *P. multocida*, but there is limited experience in using this agent to treat *Pasteurella* infections. Patients with *Pasteurella* septicemia or serious localized infections such as tenosynovitis, arthritis, or osteomyelitis should be hospitalized and treated initially with parenteral penicillin. Alternatives include ampicillin, the parenteral cephalosporins, tetracycline, or chloramphenicol.[18] Appropriate surgical drainage is important in deep-seated infections, and prolonged antibiotic therapy is required in patients with osteomyelitis or endocarditis. Fatal infections rarely occur in the absence of other underlying illnesses.

REFERENCES

1. Carter GR. Pasteurellosis: *Pasteurella multocida* and *Pasteurella hemolytica*. Adv Vet Sci. 1967;11:321.
2. Rimler RB, Rhoades KR. Serogroup F, a new capsule serogroup of *Pasteurella multocida*. J Clin Microbiol. 1987;25:615.
3. Hubbert WT, Rosen MN. I. *Pasteurella multocida* infection due to animal bite. Am J Public Health. 1970;60:1103.
4. Tindall JP, Harrison CM. *Pasteurella multocida* infections following animal injuries, especially cat bites. Arch Dermatol. 1972;105:412.
5. Lee MLH, Buhr AJ. Dog-bites and local infection with *Pasteurella septica*. Br Med J. 1960;1:169.
6. Francis DP, Holmes MA, Brandon G. *Pasteurella multocida* infections after domestic animal bites and scratches. JAMA. 1975;233–42.
7. Hubbert WT, Rosen MN. II. *Pasteurella multocida* infection in man unrelated to animal bite. Am J Public Health. 1970;60:1109.
8. Smith JE. Studies on *Pasteurella septica*. III. Strains from human beings. J Comp Pathol Ther. 1959;69:231.
9. Jones FL Jr, Smull CE. Infections in man due to *Pasteurella multocida*. Pa Med. 1973;76:41.
10. Rogers BT, Anderson JC, Palmer CA, et al. Septicaemia due to *Pasteurella pneumotropica*. J Clin Pathol. 1973;26:396.
11. Cooper A, Martin R, Tibbles JAR. Pasteurella meningitis. Neurology. 1973;23:1097.
12. Medley S. A dog bite wound infected with *Pasteurella pneumotropica*. Med J Aust. 1977;2:224.
13. Starkebaum GA, Plorde JJ. Pasteurella pneumonia: Report of a case and review of the literature. J Clin Microbiol. 1977;5:332.
14. Noble RC, Aarek BJ, Overman SB. Spontaneous bacterical peritonitis caused by *Pasteurella ureae*. J Clin Microbiol. 1987;25:442.
15. Ewing R, Fainstein V, Musher DM, et al. Articular and skeletal infections caused by *Pasteurella multocida*. South Med J. 1980;73:1349.
16. Lucas GL, Bartlett DH. *Pasteurella multocida* infection in the hand. Plast Reconstr Surg. 1981;67:49.
17. Arons MS, Fernando L, Polayes IM, et al. *Pasteurella multocida:* The major cause of hand infections following domestic animal bites. J Hand Surg. 1982;7:47.
18. Weber DJ, Wolfson JS, Swartz MN, et al. *Pasteurella multocida* infections. Report of 34 cases and review of the literature. Medicine. 1984;63:133.
19. Raffi F, Barrier J, Baron D, et al. *Pasteurella multocida* bacteremia: Report of thirteen cases over twelve years and review of the literature. Scand J Infect Dis. 1987;19:385.
20. Goldstein EJ, Reinhardt JF, Murray PM, et al. Outpatient therapy of bite wounds: Demographic data, bacteriology and a prospective, randomized trial of amoxicillin/clavulanic acid versus penicillin ± dicloxacillin. Int J Dermatol. 1987;26:123.

207. YERSINIA SPECIES (INCLUDING PLAGUE)

THOMAS BUTLER

The genus *Yersinia* includes the pathogens *Y. pestis, Y. enterocolitica*, and *Y. pseudotuberculosis*. The yersinioses are zoonotic infections that affect predominantly rodents, pigs, and birds; humans are accidental hosts for infection. *Yersinia pestis* is the cause of plague. The most common clinical form is acute febrile lymphadenitis, called bubonic plague. Less common forms include septicemic, pneumonic, and meningeal plague. Mortality is high in untreated plague, but early antibiotic treatment reduces mortality significantly. *Yersinia enterocolitica* and sometimes *Y. pseudotuberculosis* produce fever, diarrhea, and abdominal pain that mimics acute appendicitis. Common pathologic lesions are acute enteritis and mesenteric lymphadenitis.

YERSINIA PESTIS

History

Plague is a disease of antiquity that has persisted to modern times. Epidemic bubonic plague was vividly described in biblical and medieval times. This disease was estimated to have killed one-fourth of Europe's population in the middle ages. The present pandemic of plague began in China in the 1860s and spread to Hong Kong in the 1890s. The genus is called *Yersinia* because Alexandre Yersin (1863–1943) went to Hong Kong in 1894 and successfully isolated the causative organism in pure culture. This pandemic was subsequently spread by rats transported on ships to California and port cities of South America, Africa, and Asia. Urban plague transmitted by rats was brought under control in most affected cities, but the infection was transferred to sylvatic rodents, which allowed it to become entrenched in rural areas of these countries. In the first half of this century India was severely affected by plague epidemics and suffered more than 10 million deaths. In the 1960s and 1970s, Vietnam became the leading country for plague; during the war it reported more than 10,000 cases a year.[1] Before 1970, *Y. pestis* was called by its earlier name, *Pasteurella pestis*.

Description of the Pathogen

Yersinia pestis is a gram-negative bipolar-staining bacillus that belongs to the bacterial family Enterobacteriaceae. It grows aerobically on most culture media, including blood agar and MacConkey agar. It does not ferment lactose and forms small colonies on MacConkey agar after 24-hour incubation at 35°C. On triple-sugar-iron agar, *Y. pestis* produces an alkaline slant and acid butt. It is nonmotile and negative for citrate utilization, urease, and indole.

Like the other yersiniae, the plague bacillus produces V and W antigens, which confer a requirement for calcium to grow at 37°C.[2] This property, mediated by a 45 megadalton plasmid, is essential for virulence and plays a role in adapting the organism for intracellular survival and growth. Other important virulence factors include the production of lipopolysaccharide endotoxin, a capsular envelope containing the antiphagocytic principle fraction I antigen, the ability to absorb organic iron into the form of hemin, and the presence of the temperature-dependent enzymes coagulase and fibrinolysin.

Epidemiology

Plague occurs worldwide, with most of the human cases reported from developing countries of Asia and Africa (Fig. 1). During 1980–1986, 4522 cases of human plague were reported to the World Health Organization from 17 countries. Of these cases, 431 died. The countries that reported more than 100 cases during 1980–1986 were Tanzania, 927; Vietnam, 895; Brazil, 649; Peru, 512; Uganda, 493; Burma, 335; Madagascar, 270; Bolivia, 175; and the United States, 148. In the United States, all the plague cases occurred in the Southwestern states of New Mexico, Arizona, Colorado, Utah, and California. Most of these occur during the months of May to October, when people are outdoors and come into contact with rodents and their fleas.

Plague is primarily a zoonotic infection. It is transmitted among the natural animal reservoirs, which are predominantly urban and sylvatic rodents, by flea bites, or by ingestion of

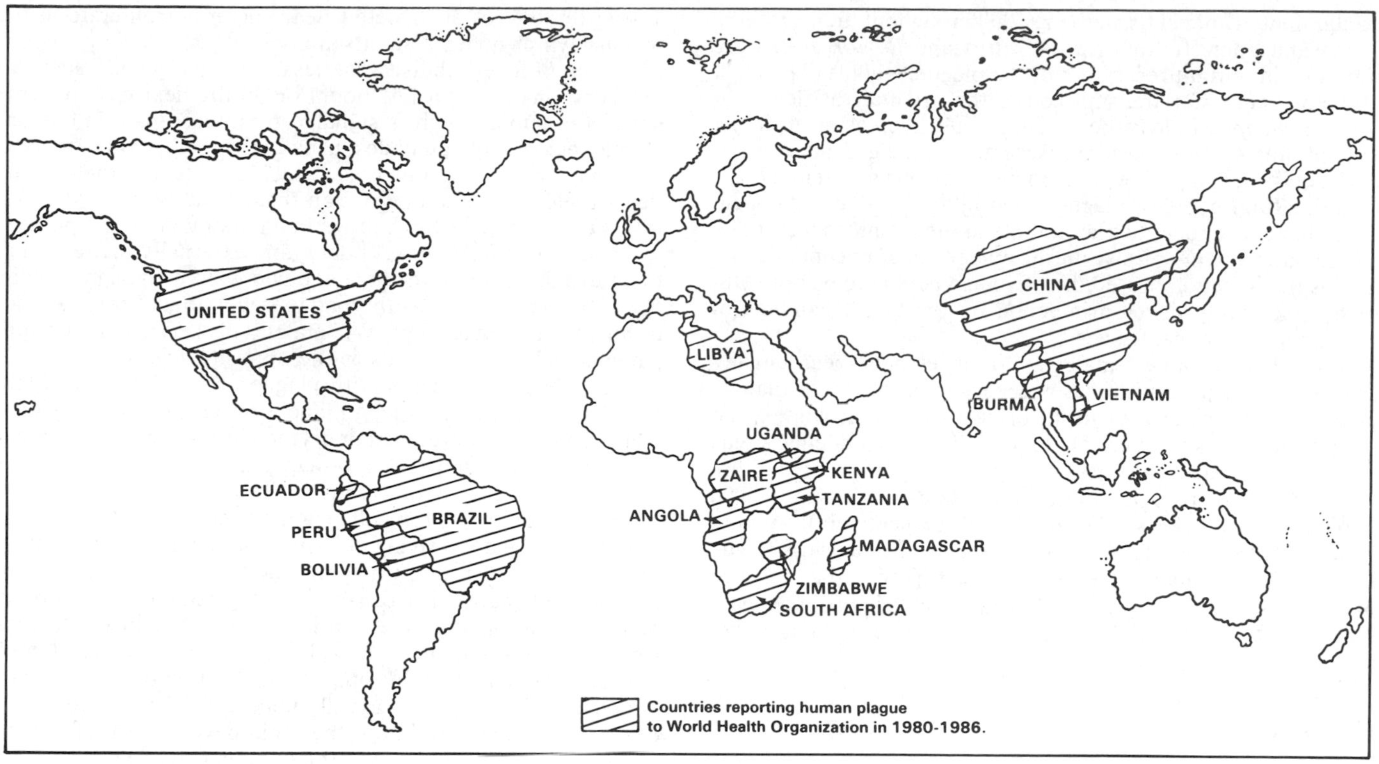

FIG. 1. Countries reporting cases of human plague to the World Health Organization, 1980–1986.

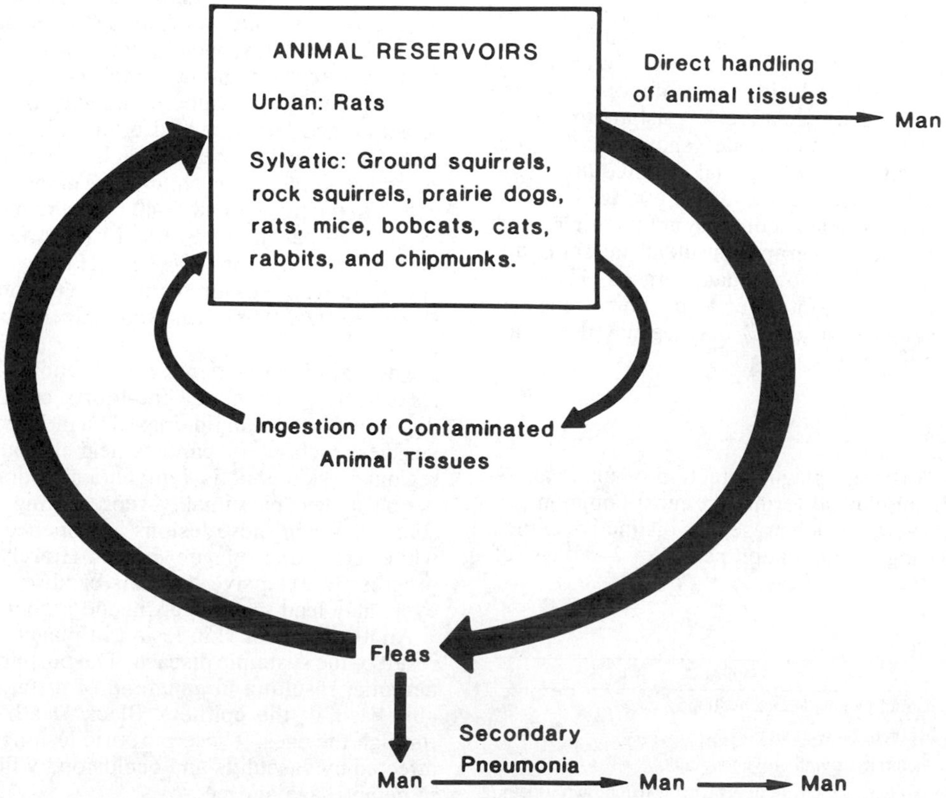

FIG. 2. Transmission of plague. The wide arrows indicate common modes of transmission, the medium arrows indicate occasional transmission, and the thin arrows indicate rare kinds of transmission.

contaminated animal tissues (Fig. 2). Throughout the world, the urban and domestic rats *Rattus rattus* and *R. norvegicus* are the most important reservoirs of the plague bacillus. The most efficient vector for transmission is the oriental rat flea *Xenopsylla cheopis*. In sylvatic foci of plague, such as occur in the United States, the important reservoirs are the ground squirrel, rock squirrel, and prairie dog. Humans become accidental hosts in the natural cycle of plague when bitten by infected rodent fleas; humans appear to play no role in the maintenance of plague in nature. Only rarely, during epidemics of pneumonic plague, is the infection passed directly from person to person. Humans also rarely develop infection by the direct handling of contaminated animal tissues.

In the United States, males and females have been equally affected. Sixty percent of cases occurs in persons less than 20 years old. Although a majority of cases occur in whites, the attack rate among American Indians living in endemic areas such as Arizona, New Mexico, and Utah is 10 times the rate among non-Indians living in the same states (1.4 cases/100,000 population and 0.1/100,000 population, respectively).[3] Within endemic areas, risk factors associated with acquiring plague include direct contact with rodents or carnivores, the presence of harborage and food sources for wild rodents in the immediate vicinity of the home, and possibly failure to control fleas on pet dogs and cats.[4]

Pathogenesis

When a flea ingests a blood meal from a bacteremic animal infected with *Y. pestis*, the coagulase of the organism causes the blood to clot in the foregut, leading to blockage of the flea's swallowing. *Yersinia pestis* multiplies in the clotted blood. During attempts to ingest a blood meal, a blocked flea may regurgitate thousands of organisms into a patient's skin. The inoculated bacteria migrate by cutaneous lymphatics to the regional lymph nodes. The flea-borne bacilli possess a small amount of envelope antigen (fraction 1) and are readily phogocytized by the host's polymorphonuclear leukocytes and mononuclear phagocytes. *Yersinia pestis* resists destruction within mononuclear phagocytes and may multiply intracellularly with elaboration of envelope antigen. If lysis of the mononuclear cell occurs, the bacilli released are relatively resistant to further phagocytosis. The involved lymph nodes show polymorphonuclear leukocytes, destruction of normal architecture, hemorrhagic necrosis, and dense concentrations of extracellular plague bacilli. Transient bacteremia is common in bubonic plague, and in the absence of specific therapy, purulent, necrotic, and hemorrhagic lesions may develop in many organs. Hypotension, oliguria, altered mental status, and subclinical disseminated intravascular coagulation (DIC) may be noted and are attributable to endotoxinemia.[5]

Clinical Manifestations

Bubonic Plague. Although plague infection of man can assume many and protean clinical forms, the most common presentation is bubonic plague, which presents a distinctive clinical picture (Table 1). During an incubation period of 2–8 days following the bite of an infected flea, bacteria proliferate in the regional lymph nodes. Patients are typically affected by the sudden onset of fever, chills, weakness, and headache. Usually at the same time, after a few hours or on the next day, patients notice the bubo, which is signaled by intense pain in one anatomic region of lymph nodes, usually the groin, axilla, or neck. A swelling evolves in this area, which is so tender that the patients typically avoid any motion that would provoke discomfort. For example, if the bubo is in a femoral area, the patients will characteristically flex, abduct, and externally rotate the hip to relieve pressure on the area and will walk with a limp. When the bubo is in an axilla, the patients will abduct the shoulder or hold the arm in a splint. When a bubo is cervical in location, patients will tilt their heads to the opposite side.

TABLE 1. Plague Syndromes

Syndrome	Features
Bubonic	Fever, painful lymphadenopathy (bubo)
Septicemic	Fever, hypotension without bubo
Pneumonic	Cough, hemoptysis with or without bubo
Cutaneous	Pustule, eschar, carbuncle, or ecthyma gangrenosum usually with bubo
Meningitis	Fever, nuchal rigidity usually with bubo

The buboes of patients with plague are oval swellings that vary from 1 to 10 cm in length and elevate the overlying skin, which may appear stretched or erythematous. They may appear either as smooth, uniform, egg-shaped masses or as an irregular cluster of several nodes with intervening and surrounding edema. Palpation will typically elicit extreme tenderness. There is warmth of the overlying skin and an underlying, firm, nonfluctuant mass. Around the lymph nodes there is usually considerable edema, which can be either gelatinous or pitting in nature. Occasionally there is a large area of edema extending from the bubo into the region drained by the affected lymph nodes. Although infections other than plague can produce acute lymphadenitis, plague is virtually unique for the suddenness of onset of the fever and bubo, the rapid development of intense inflammation in the bubo, and the fulminant clinical course that can produce death as quickly as 2–4 days after the onset of symptoms. The bubo of plague is also distinctive for the usual absence of a detectable skin lesion in the anatomic region where it is located as well as for the absence of an ascending lymphangitis near it (Figs. 3 and 4).

The groin is the most common site of the buboes in plague. In clinical reports that have distinguished femoral from inguinal locations, the femoral site was found to be most common. Other common sites are the axillae and cervical region. The reason for a given distribution of buboes is presumed to be the distribution of flea bites, which inoculate the bacteria into the skin to migrate to the regional lymph nodes.

In uncomplicated bubonic plague, the patients are typically prostrate and lethargic and often exhibit restlessness or agitation. Occasionally, they are delirious with high fever, and seizures are common in children. Temperatures are usually elevated, in the range of 38.5–40.0°C, and pulse rates are increased to 110–140 per minute. Blood pressures are characteristically low, in the range of 100/60 mmHg, owing to extreme vasodilation. Lower pressures that are unobtainable may occur if shock ensues. The liver and spleen are often palpable and tender.

The majority of patients with bubonic plague do not have skin lesions; however, about one-fourth of the patients in Vietnam did show varied skin findings. The most common were pustules, vesicles, eschars, or papules near the bubo or in the anatomic region of skin that is lymphatically drained by the affected lymph nodes, presumably representing sites of the flea bites (Fig. 5). When these lesions are opened, they usually contain white cells and plague bacilli. Rarely, these skin lesions progress to extensive cellulitis or abscesses. Ulceration, however, may lead to a larger plague carbuncle.

Another kind of skin lesion in plague is purpura, which is a result of the systemic disease. The purpuric lesions may become necrotic, resulting in gangrene of distal extremities, the probable basis of the epithet "Black Death" attributed to plague through the ages. These purpuric lesions contain blood vessels affected by vasculitis and occlusion by fibrin thrombi, resulting in hemorrhage and necrosis.

Septicemic Plague. A distinctive feature of plague, in ad-

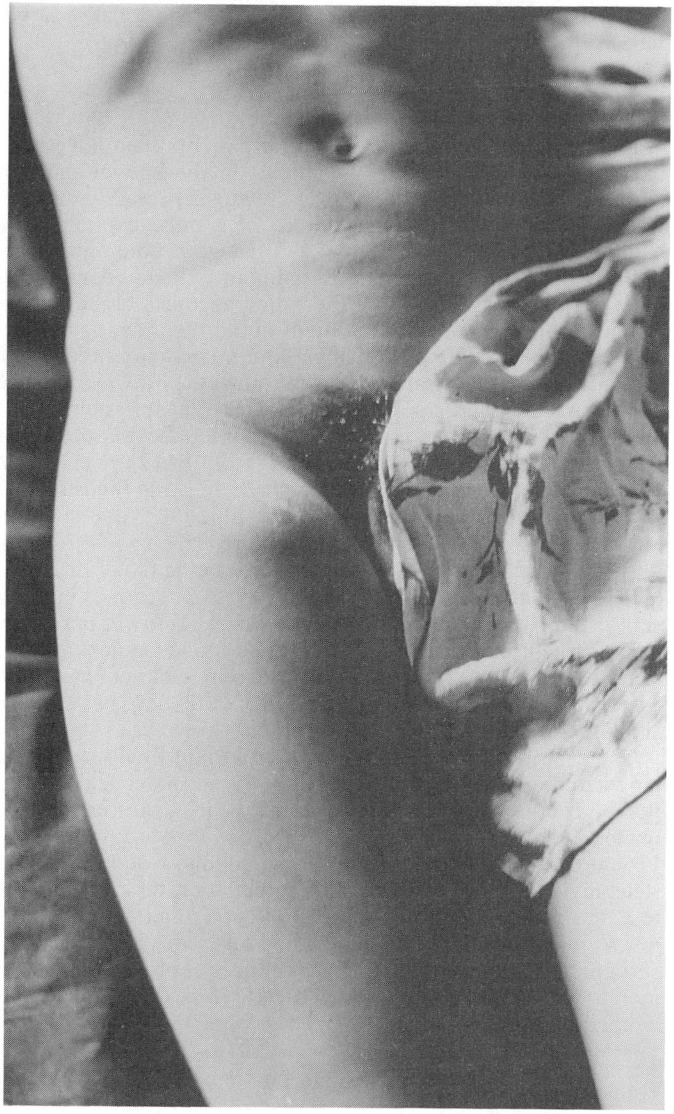

FIG. 3. Right femoral bubo in adult male with plague consists of an enlarged lymph node with desquamation of the overlying skin.

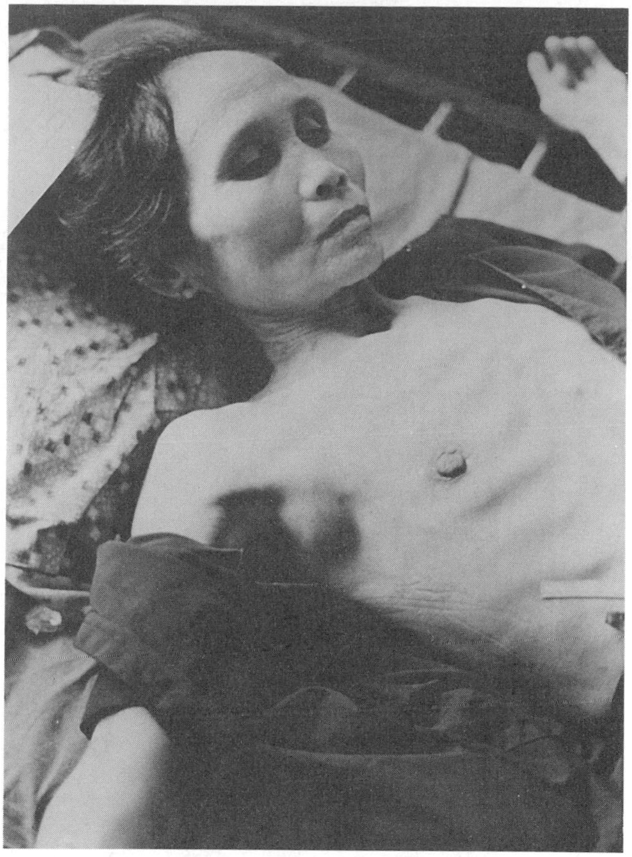

FIG. 4. Right axillary bubo in an adult female who was in septic shock and died the same day.

dition to the bubo, is the propensity of the disease to overwhelm patients with a massive growth of bacteria in the blood. In the early acute states of bubonic plague, all patients probably have intermittent bacteremia. Single blood cultures obtained at the time of hospital admission in Vietnamese patients were positive in 27 percent of cases. A hallmark of moribund patients with plague is high-density bacteremia, so that a blood smear revealing characteristic bacilli has been used as a prognostic indicator in this disease (Fig. 6). Occasionally in the pathogenesis of plague infection, bacteria are inoculated and proliferate in the body without producing a bubo. Patients may become ill with fever and actually die with bacteremia but without detectable lymphadenitis. This syndrome has been termed "septicemic plague" to denote plague without a bubo. In New Mexico 25 percent of plague was septicemic in 1980–1984, and the case fatality rate in these cases (33 percent) was three times higher than in bubonic plague because of delays in diagnosis and treatment.[6,7]

Pneumonic Plague. One of the feared complications of bubonic plague is secondary pneumonia. The infection reaches the lungs by hematogenous spread of bacteria from the bubo. In addition to the high mortality, plague pneumonia is highly contagious by airborne transmission. It presents in the setting of fever and lymphadenopathy as cough, chest pain, and often hemoptysis. Radiographically, there is patchy bronchopneumonia, cavities, or confluent consolidation.[8] The sputum is usually purulent and contains plague bacilli.

Primary inhalation pneumonia is rare now but is a potential threat following exposure to a patient with plague who has a cough. It can be so rapidly fatal that persons reportedly have been exposed, become ill, and died on the same day. Plague pneumonia is invariably fatal when antibiotic therapy is delayed more than 1 day after the onset of illness.

Other Syndromes. Plague meningitis is a rarer complication and typically occurs more than 1 week following inadequately treated bubonic plague. It results from hematogenous spread from a bubo and carries a high mortality rate compared with that of uncomplicated bubonic plague. There appears to be an association between buboes located in the axilla and the development of meningitis. Less commonly, plague meningitis presents as a primary infection of the meninges without antecedent lymphadenitis. Plague meningitis is characterized by fever, headache, meningismus, and pleocytosis with a predominance of polymorphonuclear leukocytes. Bacteria are frequently demonstrable with a Gram stain of spinal fluid sediment, and endotoxin has been demonstrated in spinal fluid with the limulus test.

Plague can produce pharyngitis that may resemble acute tonsillitis. The anterior cervical lymph nodes are usually inflamed, and *Y. pestis* may be recovered from a throat culture or by aspiration of a cervical bubo. This is a rare clinical form of

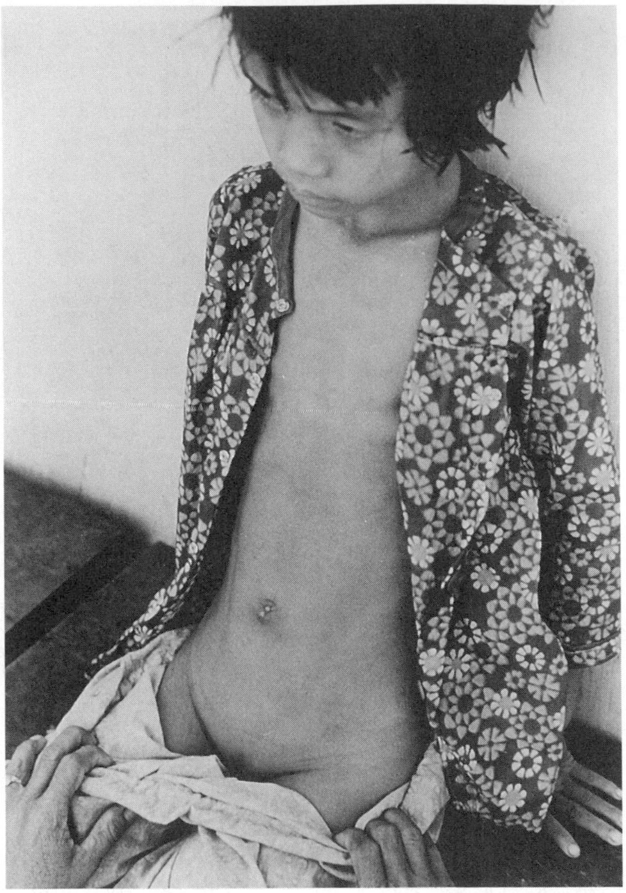

FIG. 5. Pustule on lower rim of umbilicus surrounded by erythema in a young female was the site of the flea bite. She had bilateral enlarged inguinal lymph nodes.

plague that is presumed to follow the inhalation or ingestion of plague bacilli.

Plague presents sometimes with prominent gastrointestinal symptoms of nausea, vomiting, diarrhea, and abdominal pain. These symptoms may precede the bubo or, in septicemic plague, occur without a bubo and commonly result in diagnostic delay.[9]

Laboratory Findings

The white blood cell count is typically elevated in the range of 10,000–20,000 cells per mm^3, with a predominance of immature and mature neutrophils. Severely ill patients tend to have the higher white blood cell counts. Occasionally, some patients, especially children, may develop myelocytic leukemoid reactions with white cell counts as high as 100,000 per mm^3. Examination of the white blood cells in the peripheral blood smear typically reveals cytoplasmic vacuolations, toxic granulations, and Dohle bodies that are characteristic of acute bacterial infections. Blood eosinophils are characteristically diminished or absent in the acute stage of infection but return to normal or elevated levels during convalescence. Blood platelets may be normal or low in the early stages of bubonic plague. Although patients with plague rarely develop a generalized bleeding tendency from profound thrombocytopenia, DIC is common in this infection. Fibrinogen–fibrin degradation products in the sera indicative of DIC were detected in elevated titers in most patients tested in Vietnam. Liver function tests, including serum aminotransferases and bilirubin, are frequently abnormally high. Renal function tests may likewise be abnormal in hypotensive patients.

Diagnosis

Plague should be suspected in febrile patients who have been exposed to rodents or other mammals in the known endemic areas of the world. A bacteriologic diagnosis is readily made in most patients by smear and culture of a bubo aspirate. The aspirate is obtained by inserting a 20 gauge needle on a 10 ml syringe containing 1 ml of sterile saline into the bubo and withdrawing it several times until the saline becomes blood-tinged. Because the bubo does not contain liquid pus, it may be necessary to inject some of the saline and immediately reaspirate it. Drops of the aspirate should be placed onto microscopic slides and air-dried for both Gram and Wayson stains. The Gram stain will reveal polymorphonuclear leukocytes and gram-negative cocobacilli and bacilli ranging from 1 to 2 μm in length. Wayson stain is prepared by mixing 0.2 g of basic fuchsin (90% dye content) with 0.75 g of methylene blue (90% dye content) in 20 ml of 95% ethyl alcohol. This mixture is then poured slowly into 200 ml of 5% phenol. A smear, after being fixed for 2 minutes in absolute methanol, is stained for 10–20 seconds in Wayson's stain, washed with water, and dried. *Yersinia pestis* appears as light blue bacilli with dark blue polar bodies, and the remainder of the slide has a contrasting pink counterstain. Smears of blood, sputum, or spinal fluid can be handled similarly.

The aspirate, blood, and other appropriate fluids should be inoculated onto blood and MacConkey agar plates and into infusion broth. For definitive identification, cultures can be mailed in double containers to the Centers for Disease Control, Plague Branch, P.O. Box 2087, Fort Collins, Colorado, 80522 (telephone: 303-221-6450). At this same laboratory, a serologic test, the passive hemagglutination test utilizing fraction I of *Y. pestis*, can be performed on acute- and convalescent-phase serum. In patients with negative cultures, a 4-fold or greater increase in titer or a single titer of $\geq$1:16 is presumptive evidence for plague infection.

Treatment and Prevention

Antibiotics. Untreated plague has an estimated mortality rate of greater than 50 percent and can evolve into a fulminant illness complicated by septic shock. Therefore, the early institution of effective antibiotic theray is mandatory following appropriate cultures. In 1948, streptomycin was identified as the drug of choice for the treatment of plague by reducing the mortality rate to less than 5 percent. No other drug has been demonstrated to be more efficacious or less toxic. Streptomycin should be administered intramuscularly in two divided doses daily totaling 30 mg per kg of body weight per day for 10 days. Most patients improve rapidly and become afebrile in about 3 days. The 10-day course of streptomycin is recommended to prevent relapses because viable bacteria have been isolated from buboes of patients with plague during convalescence. The risk of vestibular damage and hearing loss due to streptomycin is minimal. This antibiotic should be used cautiously, however, in pregnant women, in older patients who would have trouble adapting to vestibular damage, and in patients with previous hearing difficulty. In such patients, the course of streptomycin can be shortened to 3 days following the disappearance of fever. Renal injury as a result of streptomycin therapy is rare with this regimen; however, renal function should be monitored. If the serum creatinine rises significantly, the dose of streptomycin should be reduced. In mild renal failure, the recommended dose is about 20 mg/kg/day, and in advanced renal failure, it is 8 mg/kg every 3 days.

For patients allergic to streptomycin or in whom an oral drug is strongly preferred, tetracycline is a satisfactory alternative.

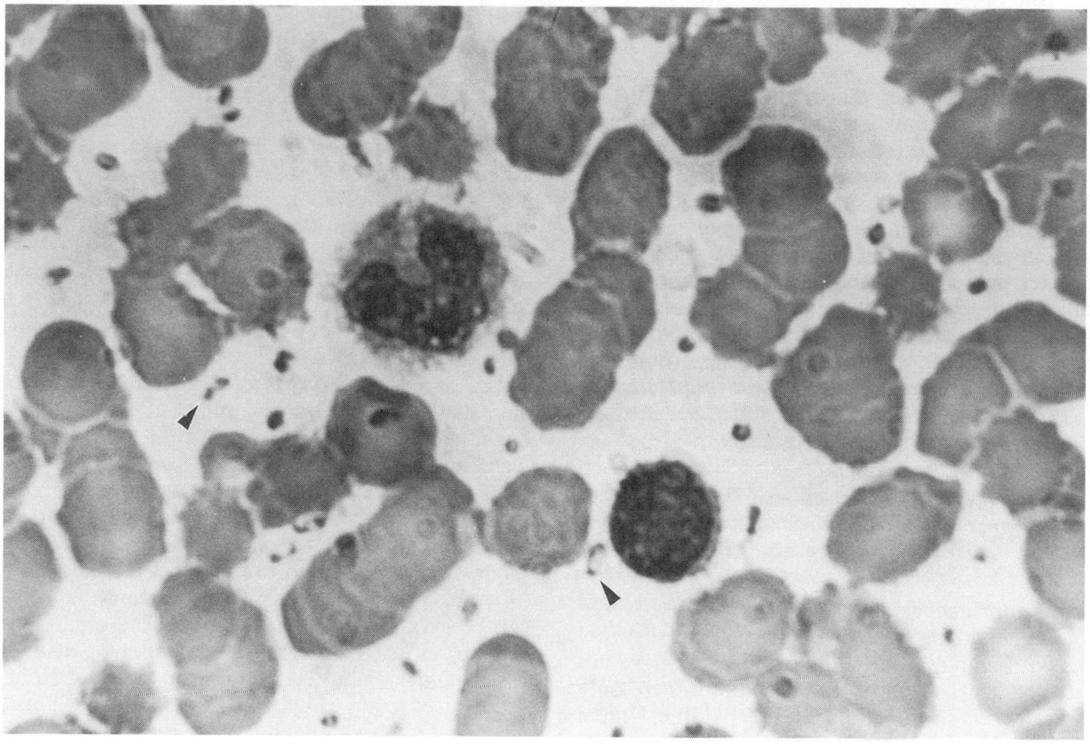

FIG. 6. Fatal plague septicemia with large numbers of bipolar bacilli (arrows) visible on blood smear. Wright stain.

It is administered orally in a dose of 2–4 g/day in four divided doses for 10 days. Tetracycline is contraindicated in children younger than 7 years of age and in pregnant women because it stains developing teeth. It is also contraindicated in renal failure.

For patients with meningitis who require a drug with good penetration into the cerebrospinal fluid and for patients with profound hypotension in whom an intramuscular injection may be poorly absorbed, chloramphenicol should be administered intravenously. This is given as a loading dose of 25 mg/kg of body weight, followed by 60 mg/kg/day in four divided doses. After clinical improvement, chloramphenicol should be continued orally to complete a total course of 10 days. The dosage may be reduced to 30 mg/kg/day to lessen the magnitude of bone marrow suppression, which is reversible after completion of therapy. The irreversible bone marrow aplasia associated with chloramphenicol is so rare (estimated to occur in 1 of 40,000 patients) that its consideration should not deter the use of chloramphenicol in patients seriously ill with plague infection.

Other antimicrobial drugs have been used in plague with varying success. These include sulfonamides, trimethoprim–sulfamethoxazole, kanamycin, and ampicillin. These drugs all appear to be either less effective or more toxic than streptomycin and therefore should not be chosen.

Antibiotic resistance in human isolates of *Y. pestis* has never been reported, nor has resistance emerged during antibiotic therapy. The antibiotics streptomycin, tetracycline, and chloramphenicol given alone are clinically very effective, and relapses are exceedingly rare. Therefore there is no rationale for using multiple antibiotics to treat plague.[10]

Supportive Therapy. Most patients are febrile with constitutional symptoms, including nausea and vomiting. Hypotension and dehydration are common. Therefore intravenous 0.9% saline solution should be given to most patients for the first few days of the illness or until improvement occurs. Patients in shock will require additional quantities of fluid with hemodynamic monitoring and the judicious use of epinephrine or dopamine. There is no evidence that corticosteroids are beneficial in plague. Although DIC is commonly present and purpura occasionally develops in severely ill patients, therapy with heparin has no proven benefit in plague infections.

The buboes usually recede without need of local therapy. Occasionally, however, they may enlarge or become fluctuant during the first week of treatment, requiring incision and drainage. The aspirated fluid should be cultured for evidence of superinfection with other bacteria, but this material is usually sterile.

Precautions. Plague is one of the four internationally quarantinable diseases, along with cholera, smallpox, and yellow fever. Accordingly, all patients with suspected plague should be reported to the Health Department and to the World Health Organization. Patients with uncomplicated infections who are promptly treated present no health hazards to other persons. Those with cough or other signs of pneumonia must be placed in strict respiratory isolation for at least 48 hours after the institution of antibiotic therapy or until the sputum culture is negative. The bubo aspirate and blood must be handled with gloves and with care to avoid aerosolization of these infected fluids. Laboratory workers who process the cultures should be alerted to exercise precautions; however, standard bacteriologic techniques that safeguard against skin contact with and aerosolization of cultures should be adequate.

Vaccine. A formalin-killed vaccine, Plague Vaccine U.S.P. (Cutter Laboratories, Berkeley, CA 94710) is available for travelers to epidemic or hyperendemic areas, for individuals who must live and work in close contact with rodents, and for laboratory workers who must handle live *Y. pestis* cultures. A primary series of two injections is recommended with a 1–3-month interval between them. Booster injections are given every 6 months for as long as exposure continues. In addition to vaccination, persons living in endemic areas should provide themselves with as much personal protection against rodents and fleas as possible, including living in ratproof houses, wearing shoes and garments to cover the legs, and applying insecticide dusts to houses.

Reservoir and Vector Control. The control of plague by health departments requires knowledge of the epidemiology of infected animals, vectors, and the contact of humans with these animals in any particular area. In the United States, the Plague Branch of the Centers for Disease Control in Fort Collins, Colorado has a field team of entomologists, mammalogists, and epidemiologists to investigate cases of plague. A specific approach to each case should be chosen and usually consists of using insecticides around homes, trapping animals, and educating people to avoid contact with certain animals. Urban plague has been successfully controlled in many cities around the world by quarantine, rat control, and the use of insecticides. Sylvatic plague, however, defies definitive control because the wild rodent reservoirs are so widespread and diverse.

YERSINIA ENTEROCOLITICA AND YERSINIA PSEUDOTUBERCULOSIS

History

The agents of the nonplague yersinioses were not discovered by Alexandre Yersin, and because they do not cause widespread epidemics with high mortality like plague they have not attracted as much medical attention. In 1975, there were only 84 cases of *Y. enterocolitica* infection reported in the United States and about 6000 cases in the world literature. During the last decade, however, there occurred an increased interest and recognition of this organism as an important cause of diarrhea and the appendicitislike syndrome. Most of the reported cases were in Scandinavia, other European countries, Canada, and the United States.

Description of the Pathogens

Yersinia enterocolitica and *Y. pseudotuberculosis* are gram-negative, non-lactose-fermenting, urease-positive bacilli that are motile when grown at 25°C but not at 37°C. Both organisms grow on blood, heart infusion, MacConkey, and SS agars at room temperature and at 37°C, and in buffered saline at 4°C. Colonies are often very small after incubation for 24 hours but are readily apparent at 48 hours. More than 50 serotypes and five biotypes of *Y. enterocolitica* have been described.[11] Most strains from patients belong to serotypes O3, O8, and O9 and to biotypes 2, 3, and 4. Six serotypes (I–VI) and four subtypes of *Y. pseudotuberculosis* have been identified, with O-group I accounting for approximately 80 percent of human cases.

The virulence of the yersiniae depends on V and W antigens, which confer dependency on calcium for growth at 37°C. Pathogenic strains are resistant to serum complement, penetrate human epithelial cells (HeLa cells) or guinea pig conjunctivae, are lethal to mice, and demonstrate cytotoxicity.[12–16] Some of these characteristics are mediated by plasmids with weights of 41–82 megadaltons.[17,18] *Yersinia enterocolitica* does not produce a siderophore for iron transport and thus grows better in the presence of other bacteria that produce siderophores and allow the bacteria to transport iron for its growth.[19] Many isolates produce a heat-stable enterotoxin that is similar to the heat-stable enterotoxin produced by *Escherichia coli*.[20] This enterotoxin, which is produced at 22°C but not at 37°C, is probably not important in causing diarrhea during *Yersinia* infection. The organisms produce lipopolysaccharide endotoxin, which has biological properties similar to that of other gram-negative bacteria.

Epidemiology

Yersinia enterocolitica is a relatively infrequent cause of diarrhea and abdominal pain in the United States but is more common in Northern Europe. Infections have been documented in other parts of the world including South America, Africa, and Asia, but *Y. enterocolitica* is rarely a cause of tropical diarrhea.[21] Most isolates from Europe are serotypes O3 and O9, while a majority of the isolates from Canada and the United States are serotypes O3 and O8, respectively. Recently, serotype O3 isolates have been recovered from patients in the New York City area,[22] and serious infections due to serotype O8 have been reported from the Netherlands.[23]

Children and adults and both sexes are susceptible, but children are more often infected than are adults. Transmission of infection occurs by ingestion of contaminated food or water and, less commonly, by direct contact with infected animals or patients.

The natural reservoirs of *Y. enterocolitica* are a variety of animals, including rodents, rabbits, pigs, sheep, cattle, horses, dogs, and cats. Transmission of infection from animals to humans has been suggested through household dogs.[24] In Northern European countries, *Y. enterocolitica* is frequently isolated from pigs' tonsils and tongues at slaughterhouses. Thus, ingestion of incompletely cooked pork and contamination of other foods by pork are important in disease transmission.[25] The ability of this organism to grow at 4°C means that refrigerated meats can be good sources of infection. The organism has been isolated from lakes, streams, and drinking water, but only a few cases have been linked to ingestion of water. Epidemics of food-borne disease have occurred in the United States, including one due to contaminated chocolate milk in New York,[26] one associated with pasteurized milk in Tennessee, and one due to bean sprouts in Pennsylvania. A large outbreak occurred at a Japanese school in 1972 causing 198 pupils to develop fever and abdominal pain. The majority of cases, occur in the winter.

Infection due to *Y. pseudotuberculosis* is the rarest of the yersinioses. It is also a zoonotic infection and has its reservoirs in various rodents, rabbits, deer, farm animals, and birds including turkey, ducks, geese, pigeons, pheasants, and canaries. Although this infection has a worldwide distribution, more cases have been reported from Europe than from other continents. The majority of patients have been children 5–15 years old. Males are affected three times more often than females. Most patients developed their illnesses in the winter. Transmission of this infection is presumed to occur by ingestion of organisms from contact with an infected animal, or common source contamination within a family, such as food or water.

Pathogenesis

The alimentary tract is the portal of entry in most cases. An inoculum of 10^9 organisms may be required to cause infection. After an incubation period of 4–7 days, this infection causes mucosal ulcerations in the terminal ileum (rarely ascending colon), necrotic lesions in Peyer's patches, and enlargement of mesenteric lymph nodes.[27,28] In most cases, the appendix is histologically normal or shows mild inflammation. If septicemia develops, suppurative lesions may occur in various organ systems (e.g., lung, liver, meninges). A reactive polyarthritis, which is more common among patients with histocompatability antigen HLA-B27, is presumably immunologically mediated.

Clinical Manifestations

Entercolitis accounts for two-thirds of all reported cases and is characterized by fever, diarrhea, and abdominal pain lasting 1–3 weeks.[29] In serious cases, rectal bleeding and perforation of the ileum may occur.[30] Fecal excretion of the organism may continue for weeks after symptoms have subsided. Leukocytes and less commonly blood or mucus may be present in the stool. Most patients with this syndrome are less than 5 years of age. Patients with mesenteric adenitis and/or terminal ileitis have fever, right lower quadrant pain, and leukocytosis. This syndrome is most common in older children and adolescents and may be clinically indistinguishable from acute appendicitis.

A reactive polyarthritis, seen in 10–30 percent of adults with *Y. enterocolitica* infection in Scandinavia, begins a few days to a month after onset of acute diarrhea and may involve the knees, ankles, toes, fingers, and wrists.[31] In most cases, two to four joints become inflamed in rapid succession over a period of 2–14 days. Symptoms persist for more than 1 month in two-thirds of cases and for more than 4 months in one-third. After 12 months, most patients are symptomless, but a few will have persisting low back pain, including sacroiliitis, which has been specifically related to the presence of HLA-B27.[32] Ankylosing spondylitis rarely occurs. Synovial fluid examination reveals less than 25,000 white blood cells/mm^3, with 60–95 percent polymorphonuclear leukocytes. Synovial fluid cultures are usually negative. Reiter syndrome with arthritis, urethritis, and conjunctivitis has also been reported. Like arthritis, this complication is much more likely to develop in individuals with the HLA-B27 antigen.[33,34]

Erythema nodosum occurs in up to 30 percent of the Scandinavian cases. Skin lesions appear on the patient's legs and trunk 2–20 days after onset of fever and abdominal pain and resolve spontaneously within a month in most cases. Women outnumber men by 2 to 1.

Recently, exudative pharyngitis has been documented as part of the spectrum of illnesses caused by *Y. enterocolitica*. In one large outbreak in the United States, 8 percent of patients presented with acute pharyngitis and fever, without accompanying diarrhea.[35]

Yersinia enterocolitica septicemia is less common and is most often reported in patients with diabetes mellitus, severe anemia, hemochromatosis, cirrhosis, malignancy, and in elderly patients.[36] Patients with iron overload, such as thalassemic patients who receive frequent transfusions, are at risk for septicemia. The treatment of iron-overloaded patients with desferrioxamine has been particularly associated with *Yersinia* sepsis because this iron chelator enhances the growth of the organism and also appears to inhibit polymorphonuclear leukocyte defense against the infection.[19,37] Septicemic patients may develop hepatic or splenic abscesses, osteomyelitis, wound infections, or meningitis. Endocarditis and mycotic aneurysms due to *Y. enterocolitica* have been reported.[38,39]

By far the most common manifestation of *Y. pseudotuberculosis* infection in humans is mesenteric adenitis, which causes an acute appendicitislike syndrome with fever and right lower quadrant abdominal pain.[29,40] At laparotomy, there is usually a normal appendix and enlarged mesenteric lymph nodes that may be accompanied by inflammation of the terminal ileum. The infection is usually self-limited, and patients who have undergone surgery generally begin to improve promptly after laparotomy. Erythema nodosum and polyarthritis have also been described in patients with *Y. pseudotuberculosis* infection. Less than 30 cases of *Y. pseudotuberculosis*-induced septicemia have been reported in the world literature.[41] About 50 percent of septicemic patients have underlying disease such as cirrhosis, hemochromatosis, or diabetes mellitus.

Diagnosis

Stool, mesenteric lymph node, pharyngeal exudate, peritoneal fluid, or blood cultures may yield *Yersinia*, depending on the clinical syndrome. Recovery of organisms from otherwise uncontaminated material such as blood, cerebrospinal fluid, or mesenteric lymph node tissue is not difficult, but isolation of yersiniae from feces is hampered by their slow growth and by overgrowth of normal fecal flora. Yield of positive stool cultures can be increased by using cold enrichment, alkalai treatment, or selective CIN agar, but these methods are not cost-effective in routine diagnosis because usual enteric culturing methods can detect most clinically significant infections.[42]

Serologic tests are useful in diagnosing *Yersinia* infections provided sera are appropriately absorbed.[11] *Yersinia enterocolitica* and *Y. pseudotuberculosis* cross react with each other and with other organisms such as *Brucella, Vibrio*, and *E. coli. Yersinia pseudotuberculosis* types II and IV cross react with *Salmonella* groups B and D. Agglutinating antibodies appear soon after onset of illness but generally disappear within 2–6 months.

Prevention and Therapy

Public health measures to control *Yersinia* infection should focus on the animal reservoirs in any particular location. The methods of raising and slaughtering pigs can be modified to reduce contamination of meat. For example, workers might prevent contact of meat with the contents of the oral cavity and intestinal tract during slaughter. Meat should not be refrigerated for prolonged periods before consumption.[43] In dairies, care must be taken to prevent contamination of milk after pasteurization.

Yersinia enterocolitica is usually susceptible in vitro to aminoglycosides, chloramphenicol, tetracycline, trimethoprim–sulfamethoxazole, piperacillin, and the third-generation cephalosporins.[44,45] Isolates are usually resistant to penicillin, and resistance to ampicillin, carbenicillin, and first-generation cephalosporins occurs frequently. The value of antimicrobial therapy in cases of enterocolitis and mesenteric adenitis is unclear, since these infections are usually self-limited. Patients with *Y. enterocolitica*-induced septicemia, which has a mortality of 50 percent despite treatment, should receive antibiotic therapy. The drug of choice has not yet been identified, but gentamicin, 5 mg/kg/day intravenously in divided doses or chloramphenicol, 50 mg/kg/day orally or intravenously in divided doses are suggested. Good responses have been reported with trimethoprim–sulfamethoxazole, doxycycline, and ciprofloxacin, whereas failures have occurred with cefuroxime, ceftazidime, cefoperazone, and gentamicin.[45] Laparotomy for suspected appendicitis should be avoided when *Yersinia* infection is a likely diagnosis.

Yersinia pseudotuberculosis is usually sensitive in vitro to ampicillin, tetracycline, chloramphenicol, cephalosporins, and aminoglycosides. Although antibiotic therapy is probably not warranted in most patients with mesenteric adenitis, patients with septicemia should receive ampicillin, 100–200 mg/kg/day intravenously, or streptomycin, 20–30 mg/kg/day intramuscularly, or tetracycline, 20–30 mg/kg/day orally or intravenously in divided doses. The mortality in *Y. pseudotuberculosis* septicemia is 75 percent despite antibiotic therapy.

OTHER YERSINIA SPECIES

Recently, strains that were formerly considered biochemically atypical isolates of *Y. enterocolitica* have been reclassified as *Y. intermedia, Y. frederiksenii*, and *Y. kristensenii. Yersinia intermedia* and *Y. frederiksenii* have seldom been recovered from patients with enterocolitis and have been reported to cause only a small number of soft tissue infections. The pathogenicity of these organisms remains uncertain.

REFERENCES

1. Butler T. Plague and other *Yersinia* Infections. New York: Plenum; 1983.
2. Ferber DM, Brubaker RR. Plasmids in *Yersinia pestis*. Infect Immun. 1981;31:839–41.
3. Kaufmann AF, Boyce JM, Martone WJ. Trends in human plague in the United States. J Infect Dis. 1980;141:522–4.
4. Mann JM, Martone WJ, Boyce JM, et al. Endemic human plague in New Mexico: risk factors associated with infection. J Infect Dis. 1979;140:397–401.
5. Butler T, Levin J, Linh NN, et al. *Yersinia pestis* in Vietnam. II. Quantitative blood cultures and detection of endotoxin in the cerebrospinal fluid of patients with meningitis. J Infect Dis. 1976;133:493–9.

6. Hull HF, Montes JM, Mann JM. Septicemic plague in New Mexico. J Infect Dis. 1987;155:113–8.
7. Leopold JC. Septicemic plague in a 14-month-old child. Pediatr Infect Dis. 1986;5:108–10.
8. Florman AL, Spencer RR, Sheward S. Multiple lung cavities in a 12-year-old girl with bubonic plague, sepsis, and secondary pneumonia. Am J Med. 1986;80:1191–3.
9. Hull HF, Montes JM, Mann JM. Plague masquerading as gastrointestinal illness. West J Med. 1986;145:485–7.
10. Welty TK, Grabman J, Kompare E, et al. Nineteen cases of plague in Arizona. A spectrum including ecthyma gangrenosum due to plague and plague in pregnancy. West J Med. 1985;142:641–6.
11. Wauters G. Antigens of *Yersinia enterocolitica*. In: Bottone EJ, ed. *Yersinia enterocolitica*. Boca Raton, FL: CRC Press; 1981:41–53.
12. Cornelis G, Laroche Y, Balligand G, et al. *Yersinia enterocolitica*, a primary model for bacterial invasiveness. Rev Infect Dis. 1987;9:64–87.
13. Goguen JD, Walker WS, Hatch TP, et al. Plasmid-determined cytotoxicity in *Yersinia pestis* and *Yersinia enterocolitica*. Infect Immun. 1986;51:788–94.
14. Pai CH, DeStephano L. Serum resistance associated with virulence in *Yersinia enterocolitica*. Infect Immun. 1982;35:605–11.
15. Kay BA, Wachsmuth K, Gemski P, et al. Virulence and phenotypic characterization of *Yersinia enterocolitica* isolated from humans in the United States. J Clin Microbiol. 1983;17:128–38.
16. Prpic JK, Davey RB, eds. The genus *Yersinia*: epidemiology, molecular biology and pathogenesis. Basel: Karger; 1987.
17. Portnoy DA, Moseley SL, Falkow S. Characterization of plasmids and plasmid-associated determinants of *Yersinia enterocolitica* pathogenesis. Infect Immun. 1981;31:775–82.
18. Kay BA, Wachsmuth K, Gemski P. New virulence-associated plasmid in *Yersinia enterocolitica*. 1982;15:1161–3.
19. Cantinieaux B, Boelaert J, Hariga C, et al: Impaired neutrophil defense against *Yersinia enterocolitica* in patients with iron overload who are undergoing dialysis. J Lab Clin Med. 1988;111:524–8.
20. Boyce JM, Evans DJ, Evans DG, et al. Production of heat-stable, methanol-soluble enterotoxin by *Yersinia enterocolitica*. Infect Immun. 1979;25:532–7.
21. Carniel E, Butler T, Hossain S, et al. Infrequent detection of *Yersinia enterocolitica* in childhood diarrhea in Bangladesh. Am J Trop Med Hyg. 1986;35:370–1.
22. Bottone EJ. Current trends of *Yersinia enterocolitica* isolates in the New York City area. J Clin Microbiol. 1983;17:63–7.
23. Hoogkamp-Korstanje JAA, de Koning J, Samsom JP. Incidence of human infection with *Yersinia enterocolitica* serotypes O3, O8, and O9 and the use of indirect immunofluorescence in diagnosis. J Infect Dis. 1986;153:138–41.
24. Wilson HD, McCormick JB, Feeley JC. *Yersinia enterocolitica* infection in a 4-month-old infant associated with infection in household dogs. J Pediatr. 1976;89:767–9.
25. Tauxe RV, Vandepitte J, Wauters G, et al. *Yersinia enterocolitica* infections and pork: the missing link. Lancet. 1987;1:1129–32.
26. Black RE, Jackson RJ, Tsai T, et al. Epidemic *Yersinia enterocolitica* infection due to contaminated chocolate milk. N Engl J Med. 1978;298:76–9.
27. Bradford WD, Noce PS, Gutman LT. Pathologic features of enteric infection with *Yersinia enterocolitica*. Arch Pathol. 1974;98:17–22.
28. Ahvonen P. Human yersiniosis in Finland. II. Clinical features. Ann Clin Res. 1972;4:39–48.
29. Marks MI, Pai CH, LaFleur L, et al. *Yersinia enterocolitica* gastroenteritis: a prospective study of clinical, bacteriologic, and epidemiologic features. J Pediatr. 1980;96:26–31.
30. Rabinovitz M, Stremple JF, Wells KE, et al. *Yersinia enterocolitica* infection complicated by intestinal perforation. Arch Intern Med. 1987;147:1662–3.
31. Winblad S. Arthritis associated with *Yersinia enterocolitica* infections. Scand J Infect Dis. 1975;7:191–5.
32. Leirisalo-Repo M. *Yersinia* arthritis. Contrib Microbiol Immunol. 1987;9:145–54.
33. Solem JH, Lassen J. Reiter's disease following *Yersinia enterocolitica* infection. Scand J Infect Dis. 1971;3:83–5.
34. Aho K, Ahvonen P, Lassus A, et al. HL-A antigen and reactive arthritis. Lancet. 1973;2:157.
35. Rose FB, Camp CJ, Antes EJ. Family outbreak of fatal *Yersinia enterocolitica* pharyngitis. Am J Med. 1987;82:636–7.
36. Spira TJ, Kabnis SA. *Yersinia enterocolitica* septicemia with septic arthritis. Arch Intern Med. 1976;136:1305–8.
37. Chiu HY, Flynn DM, Hoffbrand AV, et al. Infection with *Yersinia enterocolitica* in patients with iron overload. Br Med J. 1986;292:97.
38. Appelbaum JS, Wilding G, Morse LJ. *Yersinia enterocolitica* endocarditis. Arch Intern Med. 1983;143:2150–1.
39. Van Noyen R, Peeters P, Van Dessel F, et al. Mycotic aneurysm of the aorta due to *Yersinia enterocolitica*. Contrib Microbiol Immunol. 1987;9:122–6.
40. Weber J, Finlayson NB, Mark JBD. Mesenteric lymphadenitis and terminal ileitis due to *Yersinia pseudotuberculosis*. N Engl J Med. 1970;283:172–4.
41. Yamashiro KM, Goldman RH, Harris D, et al. *Pasteurella pseudotuberculosis*. Acute sepsis with survival. Arch Intern Med. 1971;128:605–8.
42. Kachoris M, Ruoff KL, Welch K, et al. Routine culture of stool specimens for *Yersinia enterocolitica* is not a cost-effective procedure. J Clin Microbiol. 1988;26:582–3.
43. Christiansen SG. The *Yersinia enterocolitica* situation in Denmark. Contrib Microbiol Immunol. 1987;9:93–7.
44. Scribner RK, Marks MI, Weber A, et al. *Yersinia enterocolitica*: comparative in vitro activities of seven new beta-lactam antibiotics. Antimicrob Agents Chemother. 1982;22:140–1.
45. Hoogkamp-Korstanje JAA. Antibiotics in *Yersinia enterocolitica* infections. J Antimicrob Chemother. 1987;20:123–31.

208. BORDETELLA SPECIES

ERIK L. HEWLETT

Descriptions of whooping cough date from 1500, but Baillou, the first modern epidemiologist, is credited with providing the "earliest clear account" of the disease in 1640.[1] The name *pertussis*, meaning violent cough, was first used by Sydenham in 1679.[2] In China the illness is known as "the cough of 100 days." The etiologic organism, initially called *Haemophilus pertussis*, was described by Bordet and Gengou in 1900 and subsequently isolated with the use of a medium that bears their names.[3] A detailed history of pertussis is provided in the classic monograph by Lapin.[2]

DESCRIPTION OF THE PATHOGENS

The genus *Bordetella* now consists of four species—*pertussis, parapertussis, bronchiseptica*, and *avium*. *Bordetella pertussis* and *B. parapertussis* are responsible for disease in humans. *Bordetella bronchiseptica* (or *bronchicanis*) is predominantly an animal pathogen that causes respiratory diseases such as kennel cough in dogs, snuffles in rabbits, and atrophic rhinitis in swine.[4,5] Infrequently, *B. bronchiseptica* is responsible for a whooping cough-like illness in humans and opportunistic infections in compromised hosts.[6,7] *Bordetella avium* is a bronchiseptica-like organism (formerly *Alcaligenes* species) that is an avian pathogen responsible for turkey coryza,[8] but it is not known to infect humans.

The Bordetellae are minute coccobacillary organisms that appear singly or in pairs. The human pathogens (*B. pertussis* and *parapertussis*) are nonmotile; the other two species possess peritrichous flagellae that provide motility.[9] All species are piliated, aerobic, and oxidize amino acids, but do not ferment carbohydrates. The organisms require nicotinamide (or nicotinic acid) for growth at an optimal temperature of 35–37°C. While the starch-blood-agar medium originally described by Bordet and Gengou is still in use, it is clear that the organisms can grow in totally synthetic medium consisting of buffers, minerals, an amino acid energy source, and growth factors such as nicotinamide.[10] Growth is enhanced by, if not dependent upon, compounds such as starch or β-methyl cyclodextrin to absorb and neutralize inhibitory compounds.[11,12] Growth rates and colony sizes differ among the species, with *B. pertussis* requiring 3–6 days for the pinpoint colonies to appear in cultures of clinical specimens. *B. parapertussis* grows slightly faster, produces larger colonies, and in peptone agar or in liquid medium produces a characteristic brownish pigment.

The relatedness of the *Bordetella* species has been addressed in several ways. All *Bordetella* possess DNA with a high G/C (guanosine/cytosine) ratio (66–70 percent).[9] Kloos et al.[13] determined by DNA hybridization that *B. pertussis, B. parapertussis*, and *B. bronchiseptica* are not sufficiently diverse to be classified as distinct species. This conclusion was supported by the work of Musser et al.,[14] who examined genetic diversity of *Bordetella* species by electrophoretic mobility patterns of nonvirulence-related enzymes. In the latter study, *B. parapertussis* was found to be more closely related to *B. bronchiseptica* than to *B. pertussis*.

The *Bordetella* species possess a common O antigen. While

speciation of clinical isolates is accomplished by phenotypic characterization, serotyping is dependent upon heat-labile K agglutinogens.[9] Of the 14 agglutinogens, 6 are specific to *B. pertussis*, with agglutinogen 7 common to the genus. Some of the agglutinogens (factors) have now been identified and characterized biochemically. Factor 1 is a lipooligosaccharide molecule, and factor 2 is fimbrial, consisting of 22-kD subunits.[15,16] There is currently a discrepancy in nomenclature due to slightly different serotyping systems from Eldering in the United States and Preston in Great Britain.[17,18] Typing sera for factors 3 and 6 in the Eldering system and 3 in the Preston system recognize fimbria (21.5 kD subunits.) Eldering factor 3 serum also reacts with a 69-kD surface antigen that may participate in protection.[19,20] In considering the epidemiologic implications of serotype distributions, it is important to note that organisms have the capacity to change serotypes in vitro or in vivo.[21]

Bordetella pertussis produces a number of biologically active substances that are postulated to play a role in disease (reviewed in Refs. 22–24). These include surface components, such as filamentous hemagglutinin (FHA) and the agglutinogens, toxins such as adenylate cyclase toxin, dermonecrotic toxin, pertussis toxin, and tracheal cytotoxin, and a hemolysin.

FHA is a cylindrical protein of 2 × 40–100 nm, with subunits of 220 kD,[25] which derives its name from the ability to agglutinate erythrocytes. It appears to be involved in the attachment of *B. pertussis* to ciliated respiratory epithelia and other types of cells, but has no known toxin activity.[26–28] The structural gene for FHA has been cloned and expressed in *Escherichia coli*, raising the possibility of its production for use in a component vaccine.[29] As mentioned, several of the agglutinogens have been isolated and characterized biochemically. Although the fimbrial nature of agglutinogens 2 and 3/6 suggests a role in attachment to target cells, strains lacking those components do adhere to nonciliated cells and can cause infection.[30] The contribution of these surface proteins to infection remains unresolved.

Adenylate cyclase toxin is an extracytoplasmic enzyme able to interact with and enter mammalian cells.[31,32] Inside the target cell it is activated by endogenous calmodulin to catalyze the production of cyclic AMP from ATP. The resulting accumulation of supraphysiologic levels of cAMP may result in impaired leukocyte functions and even cause cell death.[31–34] The toxin appears to be a single peptide of 216 kD, which may be cleaved to smaller forms during intoxication.[35,36]

Dermonecrotic toxin, also known as mouse lethal toxin or heat-labile toxin, was first discovered by Bordet and Gengou when necrotic lesions developed following intradermal injection of *B. pertussis* into suckling mice.[37] The molecule is predominantly cytoplasmic in location and labile to heating.[38] It has been purified by Endoh et al. and shown to cause vascular smooth muscle contraction, resulting in ischemic necrosis.[39]

A collection of biological responses to the administration of *B. pertussis* organisms in experimental animals is now recognized to be attributable to a single protein toxin, known as pertussis toxin (PT). This molecule elicits lymphocytosis (lymphocytosis-promoting factor, LPF), sensitization to histamine (histamine-sensitizing factor, HSF), and enhancement of insulin secretion (islet-activating protein, IAP). In addition, it is a potent adjuvant. It is a typical A/B toxin, with a binding heterodimer and an active subunit that catalyzes the transfer of ADP-ribose from NAD to certain members of the family of guanine nucleotide binding regulatory (G) proteins in target cells.[40] Regulatory pathways in which pertussis toxin-sensitive G proteins have been demonstrated include: (*1*) inhibition of adenylate cyclase[41]; (*2*) activation of phospholipases[42]; and (*3*) activation of ion channels.[43] The functional consequence of the specific PT-mediated covalent modification is inactivation of the target G protein, resulting in disruption of signal transduction to the affected cell.[41] While many of the effects of pertussis toxin are dependent upon ADP ribosylation, it is clear that the binding oligomer can elicit some responses from the cell surface such as activation of phospholipase C, mobilization of calcium,[44] and production of insulin-like effects.[45] This cell surface interaction (of unknown mechanism) is responsible for the mitogenic action of the toxin demonstrated previously.[46] The pertussis toxin gene has been cloned and sequenced and the subunits expressed in *E. coli*.[47–49] The toxin is produced only by *B. pertussis*, but *B. parapertussis* and *B. bronchiseptica* do contain silent copies of the gene.[50,51]

Tracheal cytotoxin is a component of *Bordetella* species discovered by virtue of its ability to cause ciliostasis, inhibit DNA synthesis, and ultimately to kill tracheal epithelial cells in vitro.[52] The toxin appears to be a tetrapeptide, disaccharide derived from the peptidoglycan and is clearly related to molecules with similar activities from other gram-negative bacteria.[53]

Although *Bordetella* species are hemolytic on blood agar plates, no hemolysin has been isolated or characterized. Avirulent strains are nonhemolytic, and transposon mutants lacking hemolysin are reduced in virulence in a mouse model.[54] The discovery of sequence homology between *E. coli* hemolysin and a portion of the pertussis adenylate cyclase toxin has led to the hypothesis that adenylate cyclase toxin and hemolysin are the same molecule.[55]

When compared with that from other gram-negative organisms, *Bordetella* lipopolysaccharide has several notable features. It is heterogeneous, with two major forms, differing in the phosphate content of the 3-deoxy-2-octulosonic acid portions.[56,57] While the unfractionated material possesses the usual effects of lipopolysaccharide (induction of interleukin-1 production, fever, hypotension, and Schwartzman reaction) the distribution of those activities among the fractions is unusual. Lipid X, but not lipid A, is pyrogenic, and the polysaccharide region is very active as an adjuvant, B-cell mitogen and inducer of resistance to adenovirus in mice.[58,59]

Roles for these multiple factors in the pathophysiology of pertussis can be considered in the context of a generic sequence of events for an infectious disease: entry and attachment to a specific target tissue, production of local damage, and development of systemic disease, all dependent upon an ongoing evasion and disruption of host defense mechanisms.[23] Data from in vitro and in vivo model systems indicate that FHA, some agglutinogens (especially 2 and 3/6), and possibly PT participate in the attachment of *B. pertussis* to the respiratory epithelium.[26–30] Ciliostasis and damage to the epithelium by tracheal cytotoxin disturbs mucociliary clearance, the first line of defense. The inhibition of phagocyte functions (chemotaxis, phagocytosis, oxidative burst, and bactericidal activity) by adenylate cyclase toxin represents an acute, but reversible disruption of immune effector cell function. Pertussis toxin, by covalent modification of proteins, also impairs phagocyte function, but in a more sustained manner.[60] Tracheal cytotoxin, dermonecrotic toxin and/or adenylate cyclase toxin may contribute to local damage to the respiratory mucosa. At present, PT is the leading candidate to account for systemic manifestations of disease.[61] It clearly produces lymphocytosis in experimental animals infected with *B. pertussis*. Pertussis is not, however, a single-toxin disease like tetanus, diphtheria, and botulism. Like *B. pertussis*, *B. parapertussis* can also cause disease, which is generally milder, presumably because it lacks pertussis toxin. Pertussis toxin has been administered intravenously to humans in doses of 0.5–1 μg/kg without causing pertussis or any significant adverse effect.[62] It appears, therefore, that in the context of infection with *B. pertussis*, PT can exacerbate the disease process, but is not solely responsible. This issue is particularly important in the context of component pertussis vaccine design and development.

The production of virulence factors of *B. pertussis* is regulated in several different ways. First, the organisms undergo a genetic event termed *phase variation* by Leslie and Gardiner,[63] resulting in loss of most known virulence factors as well as several other undefined outer membrane proteins. This occurs at a frequency of $1/10^{-4}$–10^{-6} and yields an avirulent strain that exhibits different colony morphology and decreased sensitivity to antibiotics.[64,65] This event appears to result from a DNA frame shift due to insertion of a single nucleotide into the *vir* region of the genome.[66] A similar phenomenon occurs in response to environmental signals such as increased magnesium or nicotinic acid concentration or reduced temperature.[67] This event, termed phenotypic modulation, is reversible upon return to optimal culture conditions. It is not yet clear whether this phenomenon is regulated solely through the *vir* region or at additional sites in the genome.

EPIDEMIOLOGY

Pertussis continues to be a disease of worldwide importance, with an estimated 51,000,000 cases and 600,000 deaths annually.[68] Due to decreased pertussis vaccine usage in several developed nations, there have been dramatic increases in the incidence of disease.[69–71] In most populations, the disease is endemic, with regular epidemic cycles superimposed on the background rate, both at the lower (immunized) rate and the increased rate occurring after a reduction in vaccine use.[69] The epidemics occur in 3–5-year cycles that are attributed to the accumulation of susceptible individuals in the population. Although the actual number of organisms required for infection is not known, *B. pertussis* is clearly very contagious. Attack rates among susceptibles range from 50 to 100 percent, depending upon the nature of exposure.[72] As the organism is localized to the respiratory tract, it is believed that transmission occurs predominantly by aerosol droplet, with highest attack rates for individuals exposed to a coughing patient at a range of ≤5 feet.

Pertussis is novel among childhood infections in that significantly higher attack rates, morbidity, and mortality occur in females. The reason for this feature is unknown. There are no animal reservoirs, and *B. pertussis* is unable to survive for prolonged periods in the environment. Therefore transmission must occur from infected individual to susceptible host. While no prolonged carrier state has been identified,[73–75] asymptomatic culture-positive individuals have been detected during outbreaks.[75,76] These transient "carriers" are unlikely to be a significant source of infection, since they are not coughing.

In the prevaccine era, pertussis was primarily an affliction of children 1–5 years of age, due at least in part to passive protection through maternal antibody. For example, in a study from 1937, 60.2 percent of pertussis patients were 1–5 years of age, with only 19.4 percent less than 1 year of age.[77] In that setting, with most adults having had pertussis as children and being repeatedly exposed in the population, there was a high level of adult immunity. Whole cell pertussis vaccine has clearly been the major cause of overall reduction in the incidence of disease, yet it has probably also affected a shift in the peak age of disease. In 1982–83, 53.1 percent of pertussis cases reported in the United States occurred in children less than 1 year of age.[78] Since vaccine immunity is of limited duration (generally less than 12 years),[72] fully immunized children are well protected, but most adults have little or no immunity for passive transfer to infants. Thus infants, who are at the greatest risk for morbidity and mortality from pertussis, are the least protected. With the limited number of cases in young children, it is clear that adults with atypical, undiagnosed pertussis represent a major source of transmission.[79–81] Even with little attention given to the diagnosis of pertussis in adults, 10–15 percent of reported cases are more than 15 years of age. It is likely, therefore, that at present in the United States adults constitute the majority of patients infected with *B. pertussis*.[81,82]

CLINICAL MANIFESTATIONS

Following an incubation period ranging from less than 1 week to more than 3 weeks, signs and symptoms of the catarrhal phase begin.[2] During the catarrhal phase, the clinical findings, such as rhinorrhea, lacrimation, mild conjunctival infection, malaise, and low-grade fever, are consistent with many different upper respiratory or systemic infectious diseases. Thus, at the onset of symptoms there is no clue to the diagnosis of pertussis except in the setting of known exposure to an active case. Later during this phase, which can be abbreviated to a few days or last as long as 1 week, a dry, nonproductive cough develops. Evolution of the cough to that which is characteristic of the disease heralds onset of the paroxysmal phase.

The cough paroxysm consists of a series of short expiratory bursts, followed by an inspiratory gasp which can result in the typical whoop. Not all children whoop, however, and it is relatively uncommon among infants and adults with pertussis. Paroxysms, which may number more than 30 per 24 hours and be more frequent at night, occur spontaneously or are precipitated by external stimuli such as noises or cold air. They may be sufficiently severe to cause cyanosis and classically end with an episode of vomiting. The cough and vomiting may produce thick mucous plugs and watery secretions. Between paroxysms the patient appears relatively well.

During the late catarrhal and early paroxysmal phases, patients exhibit the typical hematologic feature of the disease, namely leukolymphocytosis. The total white blood cell count, which may sometimes exceed 50,000 cells/mm^3, consists of a relative lymphocytosis with T and B cells and a less striking increase in neutrophils. A slight hyperinsulinemia[83] and reduced glycemic response to epinephrine[84] have been demonstrated during the disease, but neither was associated with hypoglycemia. Pulmonary consolidation is seen on chest radiograph of more than 20 percent of hospital patients.[85] Over this same period of time, the ability to culture *B. pertussis* diminishes progressively.[86] The convalescent phase begins with a decrease in the intensity of the cough and the frequency of paroxysms. After the patient is no longer coughing, an intercurrent respiratory illness such as a cold, can cause recurrence of the paroxysmal cough. This occurs in the absence of detectable *B. pertussis* organisms and does not represent reinfection. Permanent respiratory sequelae of pertussis have not been demonstrated.[87]

The disease, which is generally most severe in infants, may be atypical in that age group and in partially immunized children and adults.[77,78] Infants may present only with apneic spells, and the cough that eventually develops may be paroxysmal but without whoop. In those with partial immunity, the catarrhal phase may be abbreviated or unrecognized and the whoop and leukocytosis absent. Since the adult population represents an increasing proportion of the cases, the disease is frequently not diagnosed until a classical case occurs in a susceptible infant or child.

COMPLICATIONS

The principal complications of pertussis are secondary infections, such as otitis media and pneumonia, and physical sequelae of paroxysmal cough. Pneumonia is a leading cause of death; it can result from aspiration during whooping and vomiting or impaired clearance mechanisms due to the actions of various *B. pertussis* components.[23] Development of these infectious complications is suggested by the onset of fever or a change in the status of the patient between paroxysms.

The increased intrathoracic and intra-abdominal pressures during coughing can result in subconjunctival and scleral hemorrhages, facial and truncal petechiae, epistaxis, hemorrhages in the central nervous system, subcutaneous emphysema, pneumothorax, umbilical and inguinal hernias, and rectal prolapse.

Laceration of the lingual frenulum also occurs with severe cough episodes.

Central nervous system (CNS) abnormalities occur at a relatively high frequency. In children with reported cases of pertussis in the United States, 49 percent were hospitalized, convulsions occurred in 1.9 percent, encephalopathy in 0.3 percent, and death in 0.5 percent.[78] The convulsions may be febrile, in conjunction with secondary infection, or afebrile. There are several mechanisms postulated for these CNS sequelae, such as secondary infection with neurotropic viruses, hypoxia, hypoglycemia, and direct effects of pertussis toxin, but the only one documented pathologically is the parenchymal hemorrhage in the brain due to venous congestion and increased pressure during cough. At the peak of the paroxysmal phase, frequent vomiting can lead, especially in infants and young children in the developing world, to dehydration and nutritional compromise.

DIAGNOSIS

A variety of methods have been developed for detection of *B. pertussis*, its products, or the immune response to them.[89] None, however, is without its limitations in sensitivity, specificity, or practicality. Isolation of *B. pertussis* by culture in the setting of clinical illness is considered the gold standard. The organism can, however, be cultured from asymptomatic contacts who do not develop disease and this isolation by culture is not absolutely specific for the diagnosis of clinical pertussis.[75,76] The starch-based medium developed by Bordet and Gengou (BG medium) is still in use. Supplemented with methicillin or cephalexin to impair growth of normal flora and used at the bedside immediately after preparation, BG medium is equivalent to any medium available.[90] Other media that have been developed have longer shelf life and enable recovery of *B. pertussis* from transported specimens.[89–91] The culture is obtained by calcium alginate nasopharyngeal (NP) swab (cotton inhibits growth of the organism) or aspiration. The cultured specimen must be examined daily for 5–7 days to identify the slow-growing, tiny hemolytic colonies.

The length of time required for culture prompted development of a direct fluorescein-labeled antibody (FA) to detect *B. pertussis* in NP smears.[92] This method, although widely used, is compromised by interobserver variability.[93] The direct FA method is also used to identify *B. pertussis* colonies from culture. Serologic tests for detection of antibodies in serum are useful epidemiologically, but less so during the acute illness.[94] Since the ability to isolate *B. pertussis* by culture decreases progressively during the disease, the use of a combination of culture and an assay for antipertussis antibodies in NP secretions may provide maximal diagnostic sensitivity throughout the course of the illness.[95] Other methods for identification of the organism or its components by DNA hybridization, enzyme assay, or antibodies against its products are promising but still in the developmental stages.[96,97]

In light of the limitations of laboratory procedures for pertussis diagnosis, a clinical case definition was developed to identify individuals with the disease. A cough of 2 weeks' duration was found to be a sensitive and specific marker of pertussis in community outbreaks.[98] Some investigators believe adenovirus can cause a pertussis-like syndrome (see Chapter 122).

PREVENTION

In the prevaccine era, isolation of infected patients was the principal control measure for prevention of pertussis, but because of the nonspecificity of symptoms during the early course of illness, this approach was not successful. Serum from immune individuals was shown to be passively protective during the incubation period, but there is no evidence that presently available pertussis immune globulin is efficacious.[99,100] Antibiotic (erythromycin) prophylaxis is recommended for prevention of disease in contacts of active cases and, although not fully efficacious, has been shown to be a major factor in controlling household transmission and outbreaks.[101–103]

Whole Cell Vaccine

Soon after isolation of *B. pertussis*, work was begun on preparation of a vaccine. Merthiolate-killed, whole cell vaccines were found to be protective, and in the early 1950s the British Medical Research Council trial documented a correlation between protection in a mouse intracerebral potency test and vaccine protection in children.[104] The vaccine currently recommended by the World Health Organization and used throughout most of the world is a killed, whole cell vaccine combined with diphtheria and tetanus (DT) toxoids and aluminum-containing adjuvants (DTP vaccine). The standard immunization schedule includes three primary doses at 2-month intervals beginning at 6–8 weeks of age.[105] Booster doses are given 6–12 months after the third dose and at 4–6 years of age. Because the illness can be severe and life-threatening in infants and newborns, attempts have been made to begin immunization at birth. This approach may, however, compromise the overall response to pertussis vaccine and is not recommended.[106,107]

Whole cell pertussis vaccine is believed to be more than 80 percent efficacious in preventing pertussis, but actual calculation of vaccine efficacy has ranged from 0 to 100 percent, depending upon the preparation used, type of vaccine trial, and case definition.[108] Furthermore, the duration of protection is clearly limited, with attack rates of 95 percent for individuals ≥ 12 years postimmunization.[72] Immunized individuals who do become infected experience less severe disease.[109] A major limitation to whole cell vaccine use has been the associated reactogenicity. When compared with DT, the DTP vaccine has significantly more local and systemic reactions such as pain, swelling, fever, anorexia, fretfulness, and vomiting.[110] Encephalopathy and permanent neurologic sequelae, but not infantile spasms and sudden infant death syndrome, have been associated temporally with pertussis vaccine administration,[111–113] but it appears that few of these are caused by the vaccine.[114] Pertussis vaccine development and use is discussed extensively in a recent review.[114] Consideration of the benefits vs. risks of whole cell vaccine has repeatedly concluded in favor of its continued use.[115] At present, whole cell pertussis vaccine is used in adults only under special circumstances for control of hospital outbreaks. When evaluated in that setting, however, it was found to be less reactogenic in adults than it is reported to be in children.[107,116]

Acellular Vaccine Development

Beginning with the recognition of whole cell vaccine efficacy and reactogenicity, attempts were made to prepare a non-whole cell preparation containing "the protective antigen." Due to concerns about vaccine reactions, several nations such as Sweden, Japan, and Great Britain modified or eliminated whole cell vaccine use.[69–71] Demonstration of the protective effects of pertussis toxin (inactivated) and filamentous hemagglutinin in the mouse potency test led to the development of an acellular vaccine containing principally those two antigens plus agglutinogens and reduced levels of endotoxin compared with whole cell vaccine.[117] This formulation has been used since 1981 in Japan in children 24 months of age and older with apparent efficacy.[118] Pertussis toxoid alone or in combination with filamentous hemagglutinin tested in Swedish children beginning at 6 months of age showed partial protection against infection and good protection against severe disease.[119] These results confirm that pertussis is not a single toxin disease and provide incentive for investigation of other potential vaccine antigens.

TREATMENT

Supportive Care

Infants are at greatest risk of complications with permanent sequelae, and hospitalization should be considered for patients less than 1 year of age. Appropriate measures for such patients with moderate-to-severe disease include close monitoring of vital signs, quantitation of cough paroxysms and associated vomiting cyanosis and apnea, frequent nasotracheal suctioning, and provision of oxygen and parenteral hydration and nutrition.

Specific Therapy

In order to be effective against *B. pertussis*, an antibiotic must penetrate into the respiratory tract. While several antibiotics, including erythromycin, tetracycline, trimethoprim-sulfamethoxazole, and chloramphenicol have been shown to be effective in elimination of *B. pertussis*, erythromycin, especially the estolate ester, appears to be the most reliable, probably due both to its higher serum levels and its ability to enter the respiratory tract.[120] Contrary to previous dogma, erythromycin does appear to reduce severity and duration of disease, even when started during the paroxysmal phase.[121] The recommended dose, 40–50 mg/kg/day (maximum 2 gm/day) in two doses should be given for a full 14 days to prevent bacteriologic relapse, which may occur as a result of inadequate duration of therapy rather than development of drug resistance by the organism.[105] Other antibiotics, such as ampicillin, have activity against *B. pertussis* in vitro but are clinically ineffective and should not be used.

Other therapeutic agents have been evaluated for symptomatic relief during the paroxysmal phase. Several studies indicate that corticosteroids (betamethasone 0.075 mg/kg/day po or hydrocortisone succinate 30 mg/kg/day im) may reduce the number, severity, and duration of cough paroxysms, but at present consideration of use of these agents should be limited to infants with life-threatening pertussis. Salbutamol, a β-adrenergic agonist, has also been proposed for use in clinical pertussis, but there are conflicting data about its efficacy.[122–124] Standard cough suppressants are not effective.

REFERENCES

1. Major RH. A History of Medicine. v. 1. Springfield, IL: Charles C Thomas; 1954:423.
2. Lapin JH. Whooping Cough. Springfield, IL: Charles C Thomas, 1943.
3. Bordet J, Gengou O. Le microbe de la coqueluche. Ann Inst Pasteur. 1906;20:731.
4. Bemis DA, Greisen HA, Appel MJG. Pathogenesis of canine bordetellosis. J Infect Dis. 1977;135:753.
5. Goodnow RA. Biology of *Bordetella bronchiseptica*. Microbiol Rev. 1980;44:722.
6. Ghosh HK, Tranter J. *Bordetella bronchiseptica* infection in man. J Clin Pathol. 1979;32:546.
7. Byrd LH, Anama L, Gutkin M, et al. *Bordetella bronchiseptica* peritonitis associated with continuous ambulatory peritoneal dialysis. J Clin Microbiol. 1981;14:232.
8. Arp LH, Cheville NJ. Tracheal lesions in young turkeys infected with *Bordetella avium*. Am J Vet Rev. 1984;45:2196.
9. Pittman M. Genus *Bordetella*. In: Krieg NR, Holt JG, eds. Bergey's Manual of Systematic Bacteriology. v. 1. Baltimore: Williams & Wilkins, 1984:388–93.
10. Stainer DW. Growth of *Bordetella pertussis*. In: Wardlaw AC, Parton R, eds. Pathogenesis and Immunity in Pertussis. Chichester, England: John Wiley & Sons; 1988:19–37.
11. Parker CD. The genetics and physiology of *Bordetella pertussis*. In: Manclark CR, Hill JC, eds. Third International Symposium on Pertussis. DHEW Publ. No. NIH 79-1830. Washington, DC; 1979:65–9.
12. Imaizumi A, Suzuki Y, Ono S, et al. Heptakis (2,6-0-dimethyl)-cyclodextrin: a novel growth stimulant for *Bordetella pertussis* phase I. J Clin Microbiol. 1983;17:781.
13. Kloos WE, Dobrogosz WJ, Ezzell JW, et al. DNA-DNA hybridization, plasmids, and genetic exchange in the genus *Bordetella*. In: Manclark CR, Hill JC, eds. International Symposium on Pertussis. Washington, DC: US Government Printing Office; 1979:70.
14. Musser JM, Hewlett EL, Peppler MS, et al. Genetic diversity and relationships in populations of *Bordetella* spp. J Bacteriol. 1986;166:230.
15. Zhang JM, Cowell JL, Steven AC, et al. Purification of serotype 2 fimbriae of *Bordetella pertussis* and their identification as a mouse protective antigen. Dev Biol Stand. 1985;61:173.
16. Irons LI, Ashworth LAE, Robinson A. Release and purification of fimbriae from *Bordetella pertussis*. Dev Biol Stand. 1985;61:153.
17. Eldering G, Hornbeck C, Baker J. Serological study of *Bordetella pertussis* and related species. J Bacteriol. 1957;74:133.
18. Preston NW. Type-specific immunity against whooping cough. Br Med J. 1963;2:724.
19. Novotny P, Chubb AP, Cownley K, et al. Bordetella adenylate cyclase: a genus-specific protective antigen and virulence factor. Dev Biol Stand. 1985;61:27.
20. Brennan MJ, Li ZM, Cowell JL, et al. Identification of a 69 kilodalton fimbrial protein as an agglutinogen of *Bordetella pertussis*. Infect Immun. 1988;56:3189.
21. Preston NW, Surapatana N, Carter EJ. A reappraisal of serotype factors 4, 5 and 6 of *Bordetella pertussis*. J Hyg. 1982;88:39.
22. Manclark CJ, Cowell JL. Pertussis. In: Germanier R, ed. Bacterial Vaccines. Orlando, FL: Academic Press; 1984:69.
23. Weiss AA, Hewlett EL. Virulence factors of *Bordetella pertussis*. Annu Rev Microbiol. 1986;40:661.
24. Wardlaw AC, Parton R, eds. Pathogenesis and Immunity in Pertussis. Chicester: John Wiley & Sons; 1988.
25. Sato Y, Cowell JL, Sato H, et al. Separation and purification of the hemagglutinins from *Bordetella pertussis*. Infect Immun. 1983;41:313.
26. Tuomanen E, Weiss A, Rich R, et al. Filamentous hemagglutinin and pertussis toxin promote adherence of *Bordetella pertussis* to cilia. Dev Biol Stand. 1985;61:197.
27. Urisu A, Cowell JL, Manclark CR. Involvement of the filamentous hemagglutinin in the adherence of *Bordetella pertussis* to human WiDr cultures. Dev Biol Stand. 1985;61:205.
28. Gorringe AR, Ashworth LAE, Irons LI, et al. Effect of monoclonal antibodies on the adherence of *Bordetella pertussis* to Vero cells. FEMS Microbiol Lett. 1985;26:5.
29. Brown DR, Parker CD. Cloning of the filamentous hemagglutinin of *Bordetella pertussis* and expression in *Escherichia coli*. Infect Immun. 1987;55:154.
30. Tuomanen E. Bordetella pertussis adhesins. In: Wardlaw AC, Partin R, eds. Pathogenesis and Immunity in Pertussis. Chichester: John Wiley & Sons; 1988:75–91.
31. Confer DL, Eaton JW. Phagocyte impotence caused by an invasive bacterial adenylate cyclase. Science. 1982;217:948.
32. Hewlett EL, Gordon VM. Adenylate cyclase toxin of *Bordetella pertussis*. In: Wardlaw AC, Parton R, eds. Pathogenesis and Immunity in Pertussis. Chichester: John Wiley & Sons; 1988:193–205.
33. Pearson RD, Symes P, Conboy M, et al. Inhibition of monocyte oxidative responses by *Bordetella pertussis* adenylate cyclase toxin. J Immunol. 1987;139:2749.
34. Geber A, Gray MC, Pearson RD, et al. *Bordetella pertussis* adenylate cyclase toxin is lethal for the J774.1A macrophage-like cell line. Clin Res. 1988;36:456A.
35. Hewlett EL, Gordon VM, McCaffrey JD, et al. Purification and characterization of *Bordetella pertussis* adenylate cyclase toxin. Abstracts of the annual meeting of the American Society for Microbiology. 1988;B58.
36. Ladant D, Brezin C, Alonso JM, et al. *Bordetella pertussis* adenylate cyclase: purification, characterization and radioimmunoassay. J Biol Chem. 1988;34:16264.
37. Bordet J, Gengou O. L'endotoxine coquelucheuse. Ann Inst Pasteur. 1909;23:415.
38. Cowell JL, Hewlett EL, Manclark CR. Intracellular localization of the dermonecrotic toxin of *Bordetella pertussis*. Infect Immun. 1979;25:896.
39. Endoh M, Nagai M, Nakase Y. Effect of *Bordetella* heat-labile toxin on perfused lung preparations. Microbiol Immunol. 1986;30:1239.
40. Ui M. The multiple biological activities of pertussis toxin. In: Wardlaw AC, Parton R, eds. Pathogenesis and Immunity in Pertussis. Chichester: John Wiley & Sons; 1988:121–45.
41. Gilman AG. G protein: transducers of receptor generated signals. Annu Rev Biochem. 1987;56:615.
42. Fain JN, Wallace MA, Wojcikiewics RJH. Evidence for involvement of guanine nucleotide-binding regulatory proteins in the activation of phospholipases by hormones. FASEB J. 1988;2:2569.
43. Holz GG IV, Rane SG, Dunlop K. GTP-binding proteins mediate transmitter inhibition of voltage-dependent calcium channels. Nature. 1986;319:670.
44. Rosoff PM, Walker R, Winberry L. Pertussis toxin triggers rapid second messenger production in human T lymphocytes. J Immunol. 1987;139:2419.
45. Tamura M, Nogimori K, Yojima M, et al. A role of the B-oligomer moiety of islet-activating protein, pertussis toxin, in development of biological effects on intact cells. J Biol Chem. 1983;258:6750.
46. Kong AS, Morse JI. The *in vitro* effects of *Bordetella pertussis* lymphocytosis promoting factor in murine lymphocytes. I. Proliferative response. J Exp Med. 1977;145:151.
47. Locht C, Keith JM. Pertussis toxin gene: nucleotide sequence and genetic organisation. Science. 1986;232:1258.
48. Nicosia A, Perugini M, Franzini C, et al. Cloning and sequencing of the

pertussis toxin genes: operon structure and gene duplication. Proc Natl Acad Sci USA. 1986;83:4631.
49. Nicosia A, Bartolini A, Perugini M, et al. Expression and immunological properties of the five subunits of pertussis toxin. Infect Immun. 1987;55:963.
50. Arico B, Rappuoli R. *Bordetella parapertussis* and *Bordetella bronchiseptica* contain transcriptionally silent pertussis toxin genes. J Bacteriol. 1987; 169:2847.
51. Marchitto KS, Smith SG, Locht C, et al. Nucleotide sequence homology to pertussis toxin gene in *B. bronchiseptica* and *B. parapertussis*. Infect Immun. 1987;55:497.
52. Goldman WE, Klapper DG, Baseman JB. Detection, isolation and analysis of a released *Bordetella pertussis* product toxic to cultured tracheal cells. Infect Immun. 1982;36:782.
53. Goldman WE. Tracheal cytotoxin of *Bordetella pertussis*. In: Wardlaw AC, Parton R, eds. Pathogenesis and Immunity in Pertussis. Chichester: John Wiley & Sons; 1988:231–46.
54. Weiss AA, Hewlett EL, Myers GA, et al. Pertussis toxin and extracytoplasmic adenylate cyclase as virulence factors of *Bordetella pertussis*. J Infect Dis. 1984;150:219.
55. Glaser P, Sakamoto H, Bellalou J, et al. Secretion of cyclolysin, the calmodulin-sensitive adenylate cyclase-haemolysin bifunctional protein of *Bordetella pertussis*. EMBO J. 1988;7:3997.
56. Peppler MS. Two physically and serologically distinct lipopolysaccharide profiles in strains of *Bordetella pertussis* and their phenotype variants. Infect Immun. 1984;43:224.
57. Chaby R, Caroff M. Lipopolysaccharides of *Bordetella pertussis* endotoxin. In: Wardlaw AC, Parton R, eds. Pathogenesis and Immunity in Pertussis. Chichester: John Wiley & Sons; 1988:247.
58. Ayme G, Caroff M, Chaby R, et al. Biological activity of fragments derived from *Bordetella pertussis* endotoxin: isolation of a nontoxic, Schwartzman-negative lipid A possessing high adjuvant properties. Infect Immun. 1980;27:739.
59. Winters AL, Baggett DW, Lee JD, et al. Immunomodulation by *Bordetella pertussis*: activiral effects. Dev Biol Stand. 1985;61:233.
60. Becker EL, Kermode JC, Naccachi PH, et al. Pertussis toxin as a probe of neutrophil activation. Fed Proc. 1986;45:2151.
61. Pittman M, Furman BL, Wardlaw AC. *Bordetella pertussis*: respiratory tract infection in the mouse: pathophysiological responses. J Infect Dis. 1980; 142:50.
62. Toyota T, Kai Y,Kakizaki M, et al. Effect of islet-activating protein (IAP) on blood glucose and plasma insulin in healthy volunteers (phase 1 studies). Tohoku J Exp Med. 1980;130:105.
63. Leslie PH, Gardner AD. The phases of Haemophilus pertussis. J Hyg. 1931;31:423.
64. Peppler MS, Schrumpf ME. Isolation and characterization of *Bordetella pertussis* phenotype variants capable of growing on nutrient agar: comparison with phases III and IV. Infect Immun. 1984;43:217.
65. Dobrogosz WJ, Ezzell JW, Kloss WE, et al. Physiology of *Bordetella pertussis*. In: Manclark CR, Hill JC, eds. Third International Symposium on Pertussis. DHEW Publ. No. NIH 79-1830. Washington, DC; 1979:86.
66. Stibitz S, Weiss AA, Falkow S. Regulation of virulence in *Bordetella pertussis*. In: Fahrenbach FJ, ed. Bacterial Protein Toxins. New York: Gustav Fisher; 1988:195.
67. Lacey BW. Antigenic modulation of *Bordetella pertussis*. J Hyg. 1960;58:57.
68. Henderson RH. EPI: "shots" that save lives. World Health. 1987;Jan/Feb:4–7.
69. Kanai K. Japan's experience in pertussis epidemiology and vaccination in the past thirty years. Jpn J Med Sci Biol. 1980;33:107.
70. Cherry JD. The epidemiology of pertussis and pertussis immunization in the United Kingdom and the United States: a comparative study. Curr Probl Pediatr. 1984;14:1.
71. Romanus V, Jonsell R, Bergquist S-O. Pertussis in Sweden after the cessation of general immunization in 1979. Pediatr Infect Dis J. 1987;6:364.
72. Lambert HJ. Epidemiology of a small pertussis outbreak in Kent County, Michigan. Public Health Rep. 1965;80:365.
73. Linnemann CC Jr, Bass JW, Smith MHD. The carrier state in pertussis. Am J Epidemiol. 1968;83:422.
74. Jenkinson D, Pepper JD. A search for subclinical infection during a small outbreak of whooping cough: implications for clinical diagnosis. J R Coll Gen Pract. 1986;36:547.
75. Krantz I, Alestig K, Trollfors B, et al. The carrier state in pertussis. Scand J Infect Dis. 1986;18:121.
76. Broome CV, Preblud SR, Bruner B, et al. Epidemiology of pertussis, Atlanta, 1977. J Pediatr. 1981;98:362.
77. Luttinger P. The epidemiology of pertussis. Am J Dis Child. 1916;12:290.
78. Pertussis—United States, 1982 and 1983. MMWR. 1984;33:573.
79. Linnemann CC Jr, Nasenbeny J. Pertussis in the adult. Annu Rev Med. 1977;28:177.
80. Valenti WM, Pincus PH, Messner MK. Nosocomial pertussis: possible spread by a hospital visitor. Am J Dis Child. 1980;134:520.
81. Maclean DW. Adults with pertussis. J R Coll Gen Pract. 1982;32:298.
82. Biellik RJ, Patriarca PA, Mullen JR, et al. Risk factors for community-and household-acquired pertussis during a large-scale outbreak in central Wisconsin. J Infect Dis. 1988;157:1134.
83. Furman BL, Walker E, Sidey FM, et al. Slight hyperinsulinemia but no hypoglycemia in pertussis patients. J Med Microbiol. 1988;25:183.
84. Badr-El-Din MK, Aref GH, Mazloum H, et al. The beta-adrenergic receptors in pertussis. J Trop Med Hyg. 1976;79:213.
85. Bellamy E, Johnston EDA, Wilson AG. The chest radiograph in whooping cough. Clin Radiol. 1987;38:39.
86. Kwantes W, Joynson DHM, Williams WO. *Bordetella pertussis* isolation in general practice: 1977–79 whooping cough epidemic in West Glamorgen. J Hyg. 1983;90:149.
87. Britten N, Wadsworth J. Long-term respiratory sequelae of whooping cough in a nationally representative sample. Br Med J. 1986;292:441.
88. Huovila R. Clinical symptoms and complications of whooping cough in children and adults. Acta Paediatr Scand [Suppl] 1982;298:13.
89. Onorato IM, Wassilak SGF. Laboratory diagnosis of pertussis: the state of the art. Pediatr Infect Dis J. 1987;6:145.
90. Parker CD, Payne BJ. *Bordetella*. In: Lennette EH, Balows A, et al, eds. Manual of Clinical Microbiology. Washington, DC: American Society for Microbiology; 1985:394.
91. Stauffer LR, Brown DR, Sandstrom RE. Cephalexin-supplemented Jones-Kendrick charcoal agar for selective isolation of *Bordetella pertussis*: comparison with previously described media. J Clin Microbiol. 1983;17:60.
92. Chalvardjian N. The laboratory diagnosis of whooping cough by fluorescent antibody and by culture methods. Can Med Assoc J. 1966;95:263.
93. Broome CV, Fraser DW, English WJ. Pertussis: diagnostic methods and surveillance. In: Manclark CR, Hill JC, eds. Third International Symposium on Pertussis. DHEW Publ. No. NIH 79-1830. Washington, DC. 1979:19.
94. Hakansson S, Sundin CG, Granstrom M, et al. Diagnosis of whooping cough—a comparison of culture, immunofluorescence, and serology with ELISA. Scand J Infect Dis. 1984;16:281.
95. Goodman YE, Wort AJ, Jackson FL. Enzyme-linked immunosorbent assay for detection of pertussis immunoglobulin A in nasopharyngeal secretions as an indicator of recent infection. J Clin Microbiol. 1981;13:286.
96. McLafferty MA, Bromberg K, Harcus DR, et al. Characterization of a DNA probe for identification of *Bordetella pertussis* in clinical specimens. Abstracts of the annual meeting of the American Society for Microbiology. 1987;C322.
97. Confer DL, Eaton JW. *Bordetella* adenylate cyclase: host toxicity and diagnostic utility. Dev Biol Stand. 1985;61:3.
98. Patriarca PA, Biellik RJ, Sanden G, et al. Sensitivity and specificity of clinical case definitions for pertussis. Am J Public Health. 1988;78:833.
99. Bradford WL. Use of convalescent blood in whooping cough. Am J Dis Child. 1935;50:918.
100. Galagtas RC, Nelson KE, Levin S, et al. Treatment of pertussis with pertussis immune globulin. J Pediatr. 1971;79:203.
101. Bass JW. Pertussis: current status of prevention and treatment. Pediatr Inf Dis J. 1985;4:614.
102. Halsey NA, Welling MA, Lehman RD. Nosocomial pertussis: failure of erythromycin treatment and prophylaxis. Am J Dis Child. 1980;134:521.
103. Steketee RW, Wassilack SLF, Adkins WN, et al. Evidence for a high attack rate and efficacy of erythromycin prophylaxis in a pertussis outbreak in a facility for the developmentally disabled. J Infect Dis. 1988;157:434.
104. Medical Research Council. Vaccination against whooping cough. Br Med J. 1959;1:994.
105. Committee on Infectious Diseases, American Academy of Pediatrics. Report of the Committee on Infectious Diseases (Red Book). 21st ed. Elk Grove, IL: American Academy of Pediatrics; 1988:315.
106. Provenzano RW, Wettelow LH, Sullivan CL. Immunization and antibody response in the newborn infant: 1. Pertussis inoculation within twenty-four hours of birth. N Engl J Med. 1965;273:959.
107. Baraff LJ, Leake RD, Burstyn DG, et al. Immunologic response to early and routine DTP immunization in infants. Pediatrics. 1984;73:37.
108. Fine PEM, Clarkson JA. Reflections on the efficacy of pertussis vaccines. Rev Infect Dis. 1987;9:866.
109. Grob PR, Crowder MJ, Robbins JF. Effect of vaccination on severity and dissemination of whooping cough. Br Med J. 1981;282:1925.
110. Cody CL, Baraff LJ, Cherry JD, et al. Nature and rates of adverse reactions associated with DTP and DT immunizations in infants and children. Pediatrics. 1981;68:650.
111. Miller D, Wadsworth J, Diamond J, et al. Pertussis vaccine and whooping cough as risk factors in acute neurological illness and death in young children. Dev Biol Stand. 1985;61:389.
112. Bellman MH, Ross EM, Miller DL. Infantile spasms and pertussis immunisation. Lancet. 1983;1:1031.
113. Hoffman JH, Hinter JC, Damus K, et al. Diphtheria-tetanus-pertussis immunization and sudden infant death: results of the National Institutes of Child Health and Human Development Cooperative Epidemiological Study of Sudden Infant Death Syndrome Risk Factors. Pediatrics. 1987;79:598.
114. Cherry JD, Brunell PA, Golden GS, et al. Report of the task force on pertussis and pertussis immunization—1988. Pediatrics. 1988;81(Suppl):939.
115. Hinman AR, Koplan JP. Pertussis and pertussis vaccine: reanalysis of benefits, risks and costs. JAMA. 1984;251:3109.
116. Linneman CC Jr, Ramundo N, Perlstein PH, et al. Use of pertussis vaccine in an epidemic involving hospital staff. Lancet. 1975;2:1.
117. Sato Y, Kimura M, Fukumi H. Development of a pertussis component vaccine in Japan. Lancet. 1984;1:122.
118. Isomura S. Efficacy and safety of acellular pertussis vaccine in Aichi Prefecture, Japan. Pediatr Infect Dis. 1988;7:258.
119. Ad Hoc Group for the Study of Pertussis Vaccines. Placebo-controlled trial

of two acellular pertussis vaccines in Sweden—protective efficacy and adverse effects. Lancet. 1988;1:955.
120. Bass JW. Pertussis: current status of prevention and treatment. Pediatr Infect Dis J. 1985;4:614.
121. Bergquist S-O, Bernander S, Dahnsjo H, et al. Erythromycin in the treatment of pertussis: a study of bacteriologic and clinical effects. Pediatr Infect Dis J. 1987;6:458.
122. Pavesio D, Ponzone A. Salbutamol and pertussis. Lancet. 1977;1:150.
123. Krantz I, Norrby SR, Trollfors B. Salbutamol vs. placebo for treatment of pertussis. Pediatr Infect Dis J. 1985;4:638.
124. Mertsola J, Viljanen MK, Ruuskamen O. Salbutamol in the treatment of whooping cough. Scand J Infect Dis. 1986;18:593.

209. STREPTOBACILLUS MONILIFORMIS (RAT-BITE FEVER)

RONALD G. WASHBURN

Rat-bite fever is a rare systemic febrile illness typically transmitted by the bite of a rat or other small rodent. The infection has a worldwide distribution and can be caused by either *Streptobacillus moniliformis* or *Spirillum minor*, bacteria commonly found in the oropharyngeal flora of rodents. Streptobacillary disease accounts for the vast majority of cases of rat-bite fever in the United States,[1] while *Spirillum minor* (see Chapter 218) infections occur mainly in Asia.

Illness following rat bites has been known in India for over 2000 years,[2] and the characteristic syndrome of rat-bite fever was recorded in the United States as early as 1839.[3] The causative gram-negative bacillus, initially named *Streptothrix muris ratti*, was recovered from an infected individual in 1916.[4] In 1925, a blood culture isolate from a laboratory worker with fever, rash, and arthritis was called *Streptobacillus moniliformis*, based on its morphologic resemblance to a beaded necklace.[5] In 1926, a similar organism, *Haverhillia multiformis*, was grown from the blood of patients during an epidemic illness resembling rat-bite fever in Haverhill, Massachusetts.[6] Both *H. multiformis* and *Streptothrix muris ratti* were subsequently shown to be identical to *Streptobacillus moniliformis*, the causative agent of streptobacillary rat-bite fever.[2]

BACTERIOLOGY

Streptobacillus moniliformis is a pleomorphic, nonmotile, nonsporing, nonencapsulated gram-negative bacillus measuring 0.3–0.7 μm wide by 1–5 μm long.[7–9] Branching filaments and bead-like chains up to 150 μm long may contain 1–3-μm-wide fusiform swellings. The organism is microaerophilic,[7] requiring a partial pressure of CO_2 between 8 and 10 percent for primary isolation. Trypticase soy agar or broth must be supplemented with 10–20 percent rabbit or horse serum, defibrinated blood, or ascites to support optimal growth. Alternatively, media may be supplemented with a papain digest of ox liver.[10] Sodium polyanethol sulfonate, a substance sometimes added to trypticase soy broth or thioglycollate broth to inhibit the antibacterial activity of human blood, impedes growth of *S. moniliformis* in concentrations of at least 0.0125 percent.[10,11]

On blood agar plates, cotton-like colonies 1.0–2.5 mm in diameter appear following approximately 3 days of incubation at 37°C.[7] In broth media, characteristic flocculent puffballs are seen at the bottom of the tube after 2–6 days. Penicillin-resistant L-phase variants may form either spontaneously or in the presence of penicillin both in vivo and in vitro.[12] These L forms impart a slightly turbid appearance to broth media. Sugar fermentation by *S. moniliformis* is variable but often includes galactose, glucose, maltose, and salicin. Recent evidence suggests that fatty acid profiles on gas liquid chromatographs may hold some promise for rapid identification of *S. moniliformis* isolates.[13,14] In addition, sodium-dodecyl-sulfate (SDS)-polyacrylamide gel electrophoresis patterns of cellular proteins may be useful for epidemiologic studies of Haverhill fever.[15]

EPIDEMIOLOGY

In the United States, persons at risk for percutaneous inoculation with *S. moniliformis* include animal laboratory personnel and individuals (especially children) inhabiting crowded urban dwellings or rural areas infested with wild rats.[1,16–21] Rat-bite fever is typically transmitted by the bite or scratch of wild or laboratory rats or mice, squirrels, or carnivores that prey upon these rodents, including cats, dogs, pigs, ferrets, and weasels.[7,16] A recently reported case followed the bite of a gerbil.[16a] The infection may also be acquired by handling dead rats, with no apparent breach of intact skin.[17] Fifty to one hundred percent of both wild and laboratory rats harbor *S. moniliformis* in their nasopharyngeal flora.[7,17,22,23] Although healthy laboratory mice are generally not colonized with streptobacilli, they do share with rats the susceptibility to epizootic infections characterized by polyarthritis, septicemia, pneumonia, otitis media, and high rates of abortion.[2,7,8,23] *Streptobacillus moniliformis* has also been reported to cause cervical abscesses in guinea pigs and arthritis in turkeys, yielding positive sternal bursa and tendon sheath cultures.[8]

Pathophysiologically, percutaneous inoculation probably produces rat-bite fever when local cutaneous defenses fail and bacteria disseminate. The few available published autopsies describe focal infiltrations of mononuclear cells within tissues invaded by streptobacilli.

Oral ingestion of the organisms spawned several epidemics of Haverhill fever (erythema arthriticum epidemicum), an illness clinically resembling rat-bite fever. Potential sources of such outbreaks include foods such as turkey,[7] or milk or water contaminated with rat excrement.[5,6,17,24–26] Presumably, once ingested, *S. moniliformis* organisms gain access to the peripheral circulation by penetrating the gastrointestinal mucosa.

CLINICAL MANIFESTATIONS

A brief incubation period usually less than 10 days in duration (range 1–22 days) follows the bite of the rat. Abrupt onset of fever, chills, headache, vomiting, and severe migratory arthralgias and myalgias then marks the beginning of the clinical disease. By that time, the wound itself has usually already healed. Indeed, the diagnosis may initially be obscured by the patient's incognizance of a bite that may have occurred during sleep. Regional lymphadenopathy is minimal or absent, in contrast to *S. minor* infection. The peripheral white blood cell count may range as high as 30,000/mm^3 with leftward shift.[7] Up to 25 percent of patients have false-positive serologies for syphilis.

Within 2–4 days following onset of fever, a maculopapular, morbilliform, or petechial rash erupts over the palms, soles, and extremities.[7,9] Skin lesions may become purpuric or confluent[7] or may eventually desquamate.[16] Approximately 50 percent of patients develop asymmetric polyarthritis or true septic arthritis concurrently with the rash or within a few days thereafter.[18,27,28] The knees are most commonly involved, followed by the ankles, elbows, wrists, shoulders, and hips.[24,24a] Typically, the fever subsides spontaneously after 3–5 days without specific antibiotic therapy, and the remaining symptoms gradually resolve within 2 weeks. However, occasionally fever may relapse in an irregular pattern for weeks or months,[12] producing a clinical picture of fever of undetermined origin,[7,8] or arthritis may persist for as long as 2 years. Haverhill fever differs clinically from percutaneously acquired rat-bite fever chiefly in the heightened severity of vomiting and in the high incidence of pharyngitis.[16,25]

Reported complications of *S. moniliformis* infection include endocarditis,[7,8,17,24,29–31] myocarditis,[7,17,22] pericarditis,[2,29] pneumonia,[7,8,17] amnionitis,[32] and anemia.[2,22] Abscesses have been observed in virtually all organs, including brain,[8,33] liver, spleen, and kidney.[7] In infants and young children diarrhea and weight loss may be prominent.[17,21] Mortality of untreated cases overall ranges as high as 13 percent,[7] and endocarditis in the preantibiotic era was uniformly lethal. The majority of these intravascular infections involved valves previously damaged by rheumatic valvulitis or calcification.[8,24]

DIAGNOSIS

In a febrile patient with rash and recent rat exposure, the diagnosis can usually be narrowed to rat-bite fever or leptospirosis. However, the physician caring for a laboratory worker may step into the trap of ascribing a seemingly benign febrile illness to viral infection. Without the clue of an exposure history, the proper diagnosis may grow even more elusive, while such diagnoses as meningococcemia, enteric fever, drug reaction, and viral exanthem enter into consideration. When the rash involves the palms and soles, rat-bite fever may mimic Rocky Mountain spotted fever[34] or secondary syphilis. The presence of oligoarticular or migratory polyarthritis heightens concerns about disseminated gonococcal infection, septic arthritis, infective endocarditis, collagen vascular disease, and acute rheumatic fever.

Direct visualization of pleomorphic branching organisms in Giemsa-, Wayson-, or gram-stained smears of blood, joint fluid, or pus may provide an early clue to the diagnosis. However, laboratory diagnosis rests ultimately on culturing *S. moniliformis* using synthetic media. Specific agglutinins appear within 10 days after onset of illness and reach a maximum within 1–3 months. An initial titer of ≥1:80 or a fourfold rise in titer is considered diagnostic. The highest reported titer is 1:5120.[8] Specific agglutinins usually revert to negative within 5 months to 2 years, but low titers may occasionally persist for as many as 7 years. Experience with serodiagnosis using specific fluorescent antibody and a complement fixation test is limited.

THERAPY AND PREVENTION

Both agents of rat-bite fever, *S. moniliformis* and *S. minor*, are sensitive to penicillin. Procaine penicillin G 600,000 units intramuscularly every 12 hours is effective for either form of the disease, and therapy should continue for at least 10–14 days.[2,16,27] The Jarisch-Herxheimer reaction may complicate initial therapy of *S. minor* infections.[7] Oral tetracycline, 2 g/day, or intramuscular streptomycin, 15 mg/kg/day in two divided doses, are effective alternatives for treatment of penicillin-allergic patients.[2,13] In addition, tetracycline eradicates infections caused by penicillin-resistant L forms of *S. moniliformis*.[19] Experience with erythromycin, chloramphenicol,[34] clindamycin,[17,22] and cephalothin is limited.

Most patients respond promptly to therapy. For individuals who appear well after 5–7 days, therapy can be completed with oral penicillin 2 g/day. Fourteen days of oral penicillin 2 g/day is probably sufficient therapy for patients who present with mild disease.

The recommended treatment for those rare patients with endocarditis is 4.8 million units of procaine penicillin G intramuscularly per day for 4 weeks if the isolate is susceptible to 0.1 μg/ml, or 20 million units of intravenous penicillin G daily for more resistant strains.[30] Streptomycin may be added to improve bactericidal activity or to enhance activity against L forms.[7]

Following a rodent bite, the wound should be thoroughly cleaned, and tetanus prophylaxis should be administered if warranted by the patient's vaccination history. A 3-day course of oral penicillin 2 g/day would seem reasonable, although the prophylactic efficacy of penicillin in this setting is unknown, and the patient should be advised to report subsequent symptoms under any circumstances. Measures to limit the incidence of rat-bite fever include eradication of rats in urban areas, avoidance of nonpasteurized milk and potentially contaminated water, and the use of gloves by laboratory workers when handling rodents.

REFERENCES

1. Anderson LC, Leary SL, Manning PJ. Rat-bite fever in animal research laboratory personnel. Lab Anim Sci. 1983;33:292–4.
2. Roughgarden JW. Antimicrobial therapy of rat-bite fever. Arch Intern Med. 1965;116:39–54.
3. Wilcox W. Violent symptoms from bite of rat. Am J Med Sci. 1839;26:245.
4. Blake FC. Etiology of rat-bite fever. J Exp Med. 1916;23:39.
5. Levaditi C, Nicolau S, Poincloux P. Sur le rôle étiologique de *Streptobacillus moniliformis* (nov.spec.) dans 1-erythème polymorphe aigu septicemique. CR Acad Sci. 1925;180:1188.
6. Parker F Jr, Hudson NP. The etiology of Haverhill fever (erythema arthriticum epidemicum). Am J Pathol. 1926;2:357–79.
7. Gunning JJ. Rat-bite fevers. In: Hunter GW III, Swartzwelder JC, Clyde DF, eds. Tropical medicine. 5th ed. Philadelphia: WB Saunders; 1976:246–7.
8. Rogosa M. *Streptobacillus moniliformis* and *Spirillum minus*. In: Lennette EH, Balows A, Hausler WJ Jr, Shadomy HJ, eds. Manual of Clinical Microbiology. 4th ed. Washington, DC: American Society for Microbiology; 1985:400–4.
9. Joklik WK, Willett HP, Amos DB, eds. Zinsser Microbiology. 18th ed. Norwalk: Appleton-Century-Crofts; 1984:659–60.
10. Shanson DC, Pratt J, Greene P. Comparison of media with and without "panmede" for the isolation of *Streptobacillus moniliformis* from blood cultures and observations on the inhibitory effect of sodium polyanethol sulphonate. J Med Microbiol. 1985;19:181–6.
11. Lambe DW Jr, McPhedran AM, Mertz JA, et al. *Streptobacillus moniliformis* isolated from a case of Haverhill fever: biochemical characterization and inhibitory effect of sodium polyanethol sulfonate. Am J Clin Pathol. 1973;60:854–60.
12. Dolman CE, Kerr DE, Chang H, et al. Two cases of rat-bite fever due to *Streptobacillus moniliformis*. Can J Public Health. 1951;42:228–41.
13. Edwards R, Finch RG. Characterisation and antibiotic susceptibilities of *Streptobacillus moniliformis*. J Med Microbiol. 1986;21:39–42.
14. Rowbotham TJ. Rapid identification of *Streptobacillus moniliformis*. Lancet. 1983;2:567.
15. Costas M, Owen RJ. Numerical analysis of electrophoretic protein patterns of *Streptobacillus moniliformis* strains from human, murine, and avian infections. J Med Microbiol. 1987;23:303–11.
16. Taber LH, Feigin RD. Spirochetal infections. Pediatr Clin North Am. 1979;26:410–11.

16a. Wilkins EGL, Millar JGB, Cockcroft PM, et al. Rat-bite fever in a gerbil breeder. J Infect. 1988;16:177–80.

17. McHugh TP, Bartlett RL, Raymond JI. Rat bite fever: report of a fatal case. Ann Emerg Med. 1985;14:1116–8.
18. Anderson D, Marrie TJ. Septic arthritis due to *Streptobacillus moniliformis*. Arthritis Rheum. 1987;30:229–30.
19. Cole JS, Stoll RW, Bulger RJ. Rat-bite fever: report of three cases. Ann Intern Med. 1969;71:979–81.
20. Collins CH. Laboratory-acquired infections: history, incidence, causes, and prevention. London: Butterworths; 1983:7–13.
21. Raffin BJ, Freemark M. Streptobacillary rat-bite fever: a pediatric problem. Pediatrics. 1979;64:214–7.
22. Taylor AF, Stephenson TG, Giese HA, Pettersen GR, Murray RA. Rat-bite fever in a college student—California. MMWR. 1984;33:318–20.
23. Strangeways WI. Rats as carriers of *Streptobacillus moniliformis*. J Pathol. 1933;37:45–51.
24. McEvoy MB, Noah ND, Pilsworth R. Outbreak of fever caused by *Streptobacillus moniliformis*. Lancet. 1987;2:1361–3.

24a. Holroyd KJ, Reiner AP, Dick JD. *Streptobacillus moniliformis* polyarthritis mimicking rheumatoid arthritis: an urban case of rat bite fever. Am J Med. 1988;85:711–14.

25. Shanson DC, Gazzard BG, Midgley J et al. *Streptobacillus moniliformis* isolated from blood in four cases of Haverhill fever. Lancet. 1983;2:92–4.
26. Place EH, Sutton LE. Infection with *Streptobacillus moniliformis*. Arch Intern Med. 1934;5:659.
27. Mandel DR. Streptobacillary fever: an unusual cause of infectious arthritis. Cleve Clin Q. 1985;52:203–5.
28. Rumley RL, Patrone NA, White L. Rat-bite fever as a cause of septic arthritis: a diagnostic dilemma. Ann Rheum Dis. 1987;46:793–5.
29. Carbeck RB, Murphy JF, Britt EM. Streptobacillary rat-bite fever with massive pericardial effusion. JAMA. 1967;201:703–4.
30. McCormack RC, Kaye D, Hook EW. Endocarditis due to *Streptobacillus moniliformis*: a report of two cases and review of the literature. JAMA. 1967;200:77–9.

31. Simon MW, Wilson D. *Streptobacillus moniliformis* endocarditis: a case report. Clin Pediatr. 1986;25:110–1.
32. Faro S, Walker C, Pierson RL. Amnionitis with intact amniotic membranes involving *Streptobacillus moniliformis*. Obstet Gynecol. 1980;55S:9S–11S.
33. Dijkmans BAC, Thomeer RTWM, Vielvoye GJ, et al. Brain abscess due to *Streptobacillus moniliformis* and *Actinobacterium meyerii*. Infection. 1984;12:34–6.
34. Portnoy BL, Satterwhite TK, Dyckman JD. Rat bite fever misdiagnosed as Rocky Mountain spotted fever. South Med J. 1979;72:607–9.

210. LEGIONELLA PNEUMOPHILA (LEGIONNAIRES' DISEASE)

VICTOR L. YU

In 1976, an outbreak of pneumonia occurred in a hotel at the site of the American Legion convention in Philadelphia.[1] A total of 221 persons contracted pneumonia, and 34 died. Despite intensive investigation, the cause of the outbreak was not found until months later, when Dr. Joseph McDade from the Centers for Disease Control isolated a bacterium from autopsy lung specimens. Following development of a serologic test, high serum antibody titers against this new bacterial isolate were found for most of the outbreak cases.

This bacterium was noted to be different from any other previously described, ultimately leading to creation of a new taxonomic family, the Legionellaceae; a new genus, *Legionella*; and a new species, *pneumophila* (Greek for "lung-loving"). Eleven members of an Odd Fellows' convention also contracted legionnaires' disease at the same Philadelphia hotel in 1974.[2] This outbreak had gone unnoticed until the discovery of *L. pneumophila*.

The first known epidemic of legionnaires' disease occurred in 1965 at a general psychiatric hospital in Washington, DC. Eighty-one patients contracted a respiratory illness, with 15 deaths. Retrospective serologic studies on sera stored for 12 years revealed antibody seroconversion for *L. pneumophila* in 85 percent of the patients.[3]

The first isolation of *L. pneumophila* occurred *in 1947!*[4] An organism had been isolated from a sick guinea pig that had been inoculated with the blood of a patient with a febrile respiratory illness. It was designated as "a rickettsial-like agent," since it failed to grow on various bacteriologic media. Studies performed 30 years later established that this organism was *L. pneumophila*.

The clinical syndromes produced by members of the Legionellaceae family are collectively designated as "legionellosis." "Legionnaires' disease"' is pneumonia caused by *L. pneumophila*, whereas "Pontiac fever" is an acute febrile illness without pneumonia that has been serologically linked to *L. pneumophila* (and other *Legionella* species).

DESCRIPTION OF THE PATHOGEN

There are more than 30 species in the Legionellaceae family, with a total of more than 50 serogroups.[5] *Legionella pneumophila* is responsible for about 90 percent of infections caused by members of the Legionellaceae family. *Legionella pneumophila* contains 14 serogroups, but serogroups 1, 4, and 6 account for the overwhelming majority of strains implicated in human infection.[6]

Separation of *L. pneumophila* from other members of the family can be performed by a number of techniques, including direct fluorescent antibody stains, DNA hybridization reactions, multilocus enzyme electrophoresis, and crossed immunoelectrophoresis.[5,7] The cell walls of all members of the family contain distinctive branched-chain fatty acids with large amounts of ubiquinones, allowing preliminary identification by gas liquid chromatography or cellular ubiquinone analysis.[8]

Morphologic and Physiologic Characteristics

Members of the Legionellaceae family are gram-negative, aerobic, non-spore-forming, unencapsulated bacilli that measure 0.3–0.9 μm in width and 2–20 μm in length. In tissue and clinical specimens, the organisms are coccobacillary measuring 1–2 μm. Elongated filamentous forms may be seen after growth on some culture media.

The organism can be visualized by Gram stain with some difficulty in clinical specimens; basic fuchsin serves as a better counterstain than safranin. The Gimenez stain stains the organism more effectively and is as rapid as the Gram stain. The silver stains, including the Dieterle and Warthin-Starry stains, allow visualization of *Legionella* in paraffin-fixed tissues.

The organism is nutritionally fastidious and does not grow on standard bacteriologic media. Charcoal yeast extract buffered to pH 6.9 is the primary medium used for isolation of these organisms. L-cysteine is a critical ingredient in culture (Fig. 1), while keto-acids and ferric ions together stimulate growth. The active ingredients in yeast extract appear to be purine and pyrimidine derivatives, of which guanine is the most important.[9] The activated charcoal can absorb and detoxify fatty acids and oxygen radicals as well as prevent the oxidation of cysteine.[10] Addition of α-ketoglutaric acid in charcoal yeast extract promotes the growth of *Legionella*, possibly by stimulating production of oxygen-scavenging enzymes.[11]

The media can be made more selective by suppressing other competing microflora using antibacterial agents (cefamandole, polymyxin B, vancomycin), antifungal agents (anisomycin), and inhibitors (glycine).[12] Pretreatment with acid is extremely useful for isolation if selective media are overgrown with other organisms.[13,14] The addition of dyes to the media also enhances

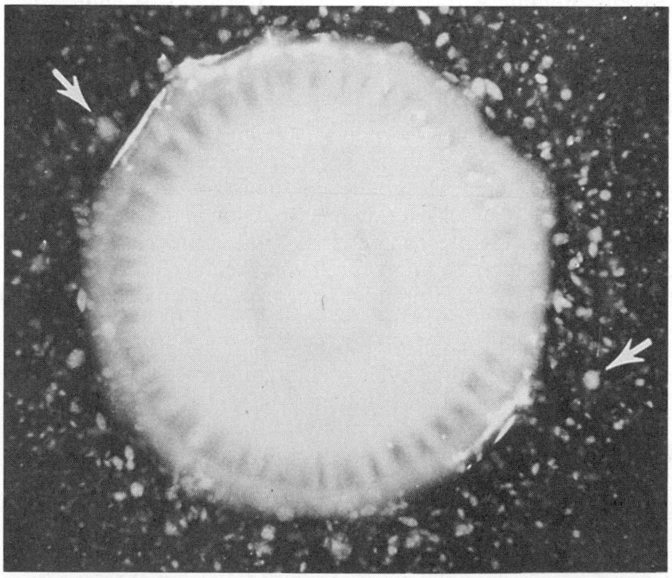

FIG. 1. Demonstration of nutritional symbiosis with environmental microorganisms and *Legionella pneumophila*. The large environmental organism in the center has been plated onto pour plates containing *L. pneumophila* but lacking cysteine (an essential growth ingredient for *L. pneumophila*). The appearance of small, satellite colonies of *L. pneumophila* (arrows) around the peripherry of the environmental organism colony shows that the environmental organism provides cysteine for the *L. pneumophila*. (From Stout et al.,[50] with permission.)

the visibility of the colonies by coloration.[15] The organism grows slowly, requiring 3–5 days for macroscopically visible colonies, and has a typical ground-glass surface, with a distinctive internal appearance when visualized by a stereo microscope. Clinical isolates exhibit optimal growth between 35°C and 37°C.

Legionella pneumophila contains catalase, as do all members of the Legionellaceae family; the reaction is weak, however, when compared with other catalase-positive bacteria. *Legionella pneumophila* is asaccharolytic, oxidase-negative, urease-negative, nitrate-negative, and gelatinase-positive. The organism strongly hydrolyzes hippurate. The organism produces a diffusable, melanin-like, brown pigment on media containing tyrosine and a fluorescent yellow-green pigment on agar medium when exposed to long-wave ultraviolet light lamp.

A single, polar flagella and multiple fimbriae (pili) are present in most strains on primary isolation. Other ultrastructural features typical of gram-negative bacilli include: an inner trilaminar cytoplasmic membrane, a peptidoglycan layer, and an outer trilaminar membrane. A polysaccharide capsule is a variable finding.[16]

The major energy source is derived from amino acids, catabolized via the Krebs cycle.[10,17] Sugars are synthesized by the gluconeogenic enzymes of the pentose cycle and the Embden-Meyerhoff pathway.[10] Carbohydrates are neither fermented nor oxidized.

Extracellular Products

The organism produces a number of enzymes and potential toxins that can be detected in culture supernates or in lysates of intact bacteria including hemolysins, proteases, esterases, phosphatases, aminopeptidases, and endonucleases.[18–23] The exact role of these products in pathogenesis and tissue damage remains uncertain, especially since some of these products are produced by strains avirulent for experimental animals.

Antigenic Characterization

Legionella pneumophila contains a major outer membrane protein[24,25] with a molecular weight of 24,000–29,000. This protein forms ion-permeable channels in contact with lipid membranes, as is characteristic for porins.[26] The lipopolysaccharide of *L. pneumophila* serogroup 1 is tightly bound to this protein.[24] Antibodies detected by indirect immunofluorescence are directed primarily at the lipopolysaccharide.[27]

Heterogeneity in *L. pneumophila* isolates can be demonstrated by a wide variety of methods: monoclonal antibody pattern,[28–30] plasmid analysis,[31,32] immunoprecipitation techniques,[33] agglutination methods,[34] outer membrane protein analysis,[30,35–37] fatty acid profiles,[27] capillary gas liquid chromatography,[38] DNA restriction endonuclease digestion,[39,40] and multilocus enzyme electrophoresis.[41]

EPIDEMIOLOGY

Ecology

The environmental ecology of *L. pneumophila* is particularly pertinent in that legionnaires' disease is one form of pneumonia that theoretically could be prevented with eradication of the organism from its reservoir. The natural habitat for *L. pneumophila* appears to be aquatic bodies, including rivers, lakes, streams, and thermally polluted waters. Although it has been isolated from river banks, mud, and excavations, it has not been isolated from dry soil.

Legionella pneumophila can survive in a wide range of environmental conditions: temperature, 0–63°C; pH, 5.0–8.5; and dissolved oxygen, 0.2–15.0 mg/liter.[42] The organism can survive for years in water samples stored at 2–8°C.

Natural aquatic bodies contain only small numbers of *Legionella*. Since *Legionella* is chlorine-tolerant,[43] the organism survives the water treatment process and passes into the water distribution system, but again only in small numbers.[44,45] Subsequent growth and proliferation occur in man-made habitats, including cooling towers and water distribution systems, which provide favorable water temperatures, physical protection, and nutrients.

The ubiquitous distribution of *L. pneumophila* in man-made aquatic reservoirs is paradoxical considering the difficulties in growth and multiplication under laboratory conditions. Thus some investigators have postulated that *L. pneumophila* is not a free-living aquatic bacterium but one that exists in symbiosis with other microorganisms. Tison et al. found that when *L. pneumophila* was grown in vitro with blue-green algae, it was able to survive and multiply at wider ranges of pH and temperature; *L. pneumophila* was apparently using algae extracellular products as its carbon and energy sources.[46]

Since *L. pneumophila* and amoebae both have a predilection for thermally enriched aquatic habitats, Rowbotham suggested that freshwater amoebae might be natural hosts for *L. pneumophila*.[47] *Legionella pneumophila* can infect and multiply within amoebae and ciliated protozoa.[48,49] When the protozoan host ruptures, large numbers of motile *Legionella* are freed, calling to mind the similar scenario for *Legionella* and human mononuclear cells (see Pathogenesis, below). The intracellular location of the organism may contribute to its survival in otherwise unfavorable environments.

Stout et al. have found that colonization of water distribution systems by *L. pneumophila* is dependent upon a combination of several factors, including water temperature, sediment accumulation, and commensal microflora.[50] Temperature appears to be a particularly critical parameter.[51–54] The organism is most readily found at the bottom of hot water tanks—a relationship that parallels its propensity for colonization in thermally polluted rivers. Environmental bacteria found in hot water storage tanks support the survival of *L. pneumophila* by furnishing essential nutrients (Fig. 1). Interestingly, bacteria populating hot water tanks are more likely to demonstrate a symbiotic relationship with *L. pneumophila* than bacteria populating cold water tanks. The organism is also often found on the surfaces of sediment accumulating in areas of water systems that are prone to stagnation, including distal sites, recirculation lines, and bottoms of storage tanks. Sediment was found to stimulate the growth of commensal microflora in vitro, which in turn stimulated the growth of *L. pneumophila*.[50]

The relevance of these findings was supported in a prospective study of hospital water distribution systems demonstrating that hot water tanks colonized with *L. pneumophila* were significantly more likely to have lower temperatures (< 140°F), have a vertical configuration, be older, and have elevated calcium and magnesium concentrations of water.[54] Vertical tanks would have more diverse temperature strata with thicker sediment accumulation at the bottom of the tank. It should be noted that appearance, degree of cleanliness, and regular preventive maintenance measures of the system were not associated with *Legionella* contamination.

Source of Infection

Cooling towers and evaporative condensers transfer heat to ambient air via direct contact with water. The airstream exits from the cooling tower or evaporative condenser in an aerosol form. It has been presumed that contaminated aerosols are taken into a building by the ventilation-dehumidification system and disseminated to susceptible persons. Pontiac fever has been linked to aerosols from evaporative condensers, cooling towers, air conditioners, and whirlpools.[55–57]

The importance of cooling towers as a disseminator of legionnaires' disease has been questioned.[58] Most of the original epidemiologic investigations implicating cooling towers antedated the discovery that the organism also existed in potable water distribution systems. In addition, it is now known that in many of these outbreaks, cases of legionnaires' disease continued to occur despite disinfection of the cooling towers.

Given the discovery that *L. pneumophila* could colonize water distribution systems,[59,60] subsequent more rigorous investigations have established that water distribution systems are the primary reservoir for dissemination of the organism. Using Evans' applications of Koch's postulates, Best and Johnson established a definitive epidemiologic link of contaminated hospital water distribution systems to nosocomial cases of infection.[61,62] Subsequent studies with molecular fingerprinting techniques (monoclonal antibody subtyping[29,30,63] and plasmid analysis[31,32,64]) have solidified this association. Acquisition of community-acquired legionnaires' disease has now been linked to contamination of residential[65,66] and industrial water supplies.[67]

Mode of Transmission

Surprisingly, the mode of transmission of *L. pneumophila* remains uncertain.[58] Air-borne transmission by aerosolization is the prevailing thesis. The strongest evidence for air-borne spread is Pontiac fever. Pontiac fever was first described in 1968 after an outbreak in a Pontiac, Michigan county health department building. The central air conditioning system may have been contaminated by aerosols from an evaporative condenser. *Legionella pneumophila* was isolated from the lungs of sentinel guinea pigs exposed to the air at the facility. The lung tissue had been frozen and stored for 8 years in anticipation that an unknown organism might someday be discovered.[57]

Since the first environmental isolation of *L. pneumophila* was taken from a showerhead,[68] it has been widely assumed that shower aerosols might be a means for dissemination of the organism. Simulation studies show that only very small numbers of *Legionella* are aerosolized and only for short distances (inches).[69–71] Despite many attempts, an epidemiologic link between showering and acquisition of disease has never been shown.

Humidifiers have been shown to generate aerosols that contain *L. pneumophila* and that cause subclinical infection in guinea pigs exposed to those aerosols.[66,70,72] Inhalation of aerosolized tap water from nebulizers has been linked to hospital-acquired Legionnaires' disease.[73]

Health-care personnel frequently use tap water to rinse respiratory apparatus and tubing for use in mechanical ventilation machines. If tap water was contaminated with *L. pneumophila*, the organism could be directly instilled into the lung.[70,74,75] Patients with legionnaires' disease have been shown to be significantly more likely than patients with other pneumonias to have undergone endotracheal tube placement prior to onset of disease or to have longer duration of incubation.[76,77]

Aspiration of contaminated water or contaminated oropharyngeal secretions has been suggested as a mode of transmission.[78] This hypothesis was supported by a prospective study in which *Legionella* infection was found to be the most common cause of nosocomial pneumonia in a population of oncologic head and neck surgery patients.[62] These patients have a propensity for aspiration as a result of their oral surgery and extensive history of cigarette smoking. Microaspiration was also postulated as the mode for patients with nosocomial legionellosis whose nasogastric tubes were flushed with contaminated water.[79] It should be noted that consumption of water at the implicated hotel during the original 1976 outbreak was significantly associated with acquisition of disease—an association that has been overlooked.[1]

Aerosolization via excavated soil has often been mentioned, but rigorous documenting evidence is absent.

Because pneumonia is the presenting clinical syndrome in more than 95 percent of cases of legionnaires' disease, nonpulmonary portals are not likely. Wound infections have occurred after immersion of the wound in contaminated water or involved hemodialysis fistulas following bacteremic dissemination from pneumonia. Ingestion of the organism followed by bacteremic dissemination from the gastrointestinal tract is an attractive hypothesis, since the organism is now known to be water-borne, and diarrhea is also known to be a prominent symptom of legionnaires' disease. On the other hand, there is little clinical evidence to support this possibility.

Incidence

The incidence of legionnaires' disease is dependent on the degree of contamination of the organism in the aquatic reservoir, the susceptibility of the persons exposed to that water, and the intensity of that exposure. However, it must be kept in mind that the discovery of this infection is also dependent on the availability of specialized laboratory tests and their application to the individual infected patient. Studies have amply documented the presence of unsuspected legionnaires' disease that only surfaced after routine application of these tests.[77,80]

In prospective community-acquired pneumonia studies, the incidence of legionnaires' disease has ranged from 1 to 15 percent,[81–84] while for nosocomial pneumonia the incidence has ranged from 1 to 40 percent.[62,77,85,86]

Cigarette smoking, chronic lung disease, advanced age, and immunosuppression have been consistently implicated as risk factors. Excess alcohol intake has been noted in some studies.[84,87] Surgery is a major predisposing factor in nosocomial infection,[62,85,88,89] with transplant recipients at highest risk.[90–93] Infections in children are rare, although cases have occurred sporadically in immunosuppressed children.

Legionellosis has been classified as "epidemic" and "sporadic," while nosocomial legionellosis has been classified as "endemic" and "hyperendemic." These terms have become less useful with the recognition that they merely designate different prevalences of disease over one spectrum. Thus, while hospitals may be labeled as experiencing "sporadic" disease (implying infrequent cases of nosocomial legionnaires' disease scattered over a long duration), the possibility is that only a proportion of actual cases are diagnosed. These cases surface because of a combination of fortuitous circumstances: clinical suspicion of legionnaires' disease by an individual physician or isolation of the organism from open lung biopsy or postmortem lung culture. Thus situations labeled as "sporadic" or "nonepidemic" may merely represent chance discovery of disease occurring at a low endemic level. Likewise, situations labeled as "epidemic" may merely represent a cyclical peak in a hospital with endemic, but previously undiscovered disease.

PATHOLOGY

Macroscopic examination of lungs taken from patients with legionnaires' disease typically shows a multifocal pneumonia. Lesions are occasionally lobar and difficult to distinguish from pneumococcal pneumonia.

Histologically, the pneumonia is an acute fibrinopurulent pneumonitis characterized by acute alveolitis and bronchiolitis. Proximal bronchioles and bronchi are usually spared. Small focal lesions appear to coalesce to form nodular lesions. Lesions of longer standing also tend to have a nodular appearance and are composed of a central area containing both cell types surrounded by an area of predominantly macrophages.

Destruction of lung architecture has been seen in severe cases, but generally the architecture is well preserved, considering the severity of the inflammatory exudate. Macroscopically visible abscess formation was seen in about 20 percent of autopsy cases in one series.[94] The presence of fibrin-rich exudate in the alveoli, with polymorphonuclear cells and alveolar macrophages, is a prominent finding. A striking lysis of the exudate has been described.[94] Interstitial inflammation, microabscess formation, vasculitis, and pleuritis are common.

Interstitial and intra-alveolar edema with membrane formation is occasionally present, although it may reflect the effects of respiratory therapy rather than infection. Patients who survive appear to suffer few residual lung abnormalities, although pulmonary fibrosis has been described as a sequela.[95]

PATHOGENESIS

Pathogenic microorganisms may potentially enter the lung via aspiration, preceded by oropharyngeal colonization of the organism, direct inhalation, or hematogenous dissemination from another foci of infection. Colonization of the oropharynx has not been demonstrated for *Legionella*, suggesting that subclinical aspiration of contaminated water or direct inhalation are more likely modes of entry. Once organisms enter the upper respiratory tract, clearance is effected by cilia on respiratory epithelial cells. This barrier to entry can be overcome by adherence of the organism to the respiratory epithelial cells. Studies examining the adherence of *L. pneumophila* have not been performed, although the organism does possess pili, which are known to mediate adherence of other organisms to epithelial cells.[96] Symbiosis has also been shown in vitro between oropharyngeal flora and *Legionella*.[97] On the other hand, Baskerville et al. have suggested that *L. pneumophila* has little affinity for respiratory epithelial cells, since little damage is evident on pathologic examination of the airways.[98] *Legionella* organisms are probably cleared by the mucociliary process.[98,99] This hypothesis is supported by the consistent epidemiologic association of increased risk of legionnaires' disease in cigarette smokers, patients with chronic pulmonary diseases, and alcoholics[1,85,89,100]—diseases in which mucociliary clearance is impaired.

After reaching the alveoli, the outcome depends both upon the virulent properties of the organism and the competence of the host in resisting infection. The resident alveolar macrophage is the first phagocytic cell that *Legionella* will encounter. The capability and efficiency of this cell to phagocytose, digest, and kill bacteria makes the alveolar macrophage the critical component in host defense. Alveolar macrophages readily phagocytose *Legionella*, although the process is more avid in the presence of specific opsonizing antibody.[101]

After entry into this mononuclear cell, *L. pneumophila* is enclosed within a specialized, ribosome-lined phagosome (Fig. 2). However, phagosomes containing the organism do not fuse with lysosomes, thus allowing the organism to escape the microbicidal mechanisms of these organelles.[102] The organism then multiplies until the cell ruptures (Fig. 2). Presumably, the liberated bacteria are phagocytosed by newly recruited cells, and the cycle of ingestion, multiplication, and liberation with cell lysis begins anew.

The next line of defense is provided by polymorphonuclear leukocytes and monocytes, recruited from the blood in proportion to the inocula of *Legionella*.[103] Initially, there is an influx of neutrophils, but with the transformation of blood monocytes into macrophages, the inflammatory resposne is composed of roughly equal numbers of neutrophils and mononuclear cells. Although not well studied, these mobile phagocytes are probably attracted by chemotactic factors derived from the alveolar macrophages or the infecting organism. Phagocytosis of *Legionella* is mediated by complement receptors on the monocytes (Fig. 3). *Legionella* fixes complement component C3 to its surface via the alternative pathway; C3 acts as a ligand on the bacterial surface that becomes available for binding to the monocyte receptor.[104] Although blood monocytes can ingest *L. pneumophila* in the absence of specific antibody, its presence as an opsonin improves phagocytosis.[105]

The role of polymorphonuclear leukocytes in host defense against *Legionella* is unclear. Neutropenic patients do not have an undue predilection for legionnaires' disease. Although *L. pneumophila* is susceptible to oxygen-dependent microbicidal systems in vitro,[106] *L. pneumophila* resists killing by polymorphonuclear leukocytes. In vitro *L. pneumophila* is ingested efficiently by neutrophils only in the presence of specific antibody or complement. Unlike monocytes, however, intracellular replication of the organism fails to occur within polymorphonuclear leukocytes.[103,105]

In vitro studies suggest that humoral immunity plays only a secondary role in host defense; for example, antibody does not promote killing of *L. pneumophila* by complement, promotes only modest killing of *L. pneumophila* by phagocytes (polymorphonuclear leukocytes, monocytes, or alveolar macrophages),[105] and does not inhibit intracellular multiplication in monocytes or alveolar macrophages.[101] On the other hand, in patients with legionnaires' disease, type-specific anti-*Legionella* antibody, usually immunoglobulin M initially, followed by immunogobulin G, is measurable within the first several weeks of infection. Moreover, immunized animals develop a specific antibody response with subsequent resistance to *Legionella* challenge.[107,108]

Cell-mediated immunity appears to be the primary host defense against *Legionella*, as is true for other intracellular pathogens (such as *Listeria, Mycobacterium, Toxoplasma*, etc.). Legionnaires' disease is more common and more severe for patients with depressed cell-mediated immunity, including transplant recipients and patients receiving corticosteroids. Legionnaires' disease has occurred simultaneously with cryptococcal meningitis in patients with host defects in cell-mediated immunity[109]; the primary host defense mechanism against cryptococcus is also known to be cell-mediated immunity. Another striking clinical observation is the occurrence of legionnaires' disease in patients with hairy-cell leukemia,[110,110a] a malignancy associated with monocyte deficiency and dysfunction.

Evidence demonstrating the development of cell-mediated immunity includes the appearance of lymphocyte proliferation and cutaneous delayed hypersensitivity to *L. pneumophila* antigens within the first 2 weeks of infection.[108,111–114] In both infected patients and animals, mononuclear cells respond to *L. pneumophila* antigens with proliferation and with the generation of monocyte-activating cytokines, including γ-interferon[115–117] and interleukin-1.[118] The activated macrophages may be nonspecifically armed against *Legionella*.[119,120] Although the activated monocytes and alveolar macrophages inhibit the intracellular multiplication of *L. pneumophila*, killing is not enhanced.[101] Natural killer-like cells triggered by interleukin-2 have been shown to kill mononuclear cells infected by *L. pneumophila*.[121]

Activation of latent infection has been suggested by some workers, although convincing clinical evidence is absent. Furthermore, legionnaires' disease does not occur significantly more frequently in patients with the acquired immunodeficiency syndrome (AIDS) (an illness classically associated with reactivation of pulmonary pathogens) than in other underlying diseases.

Legionella pneumophila strains clearly differ in virulence.[122–124] For example, although multiple strains may colonize water distribution systems, only a few strains are likely to cause disease in patients exposed to the water.[28–31] Agar-passaged strains that lose their virulence are more serum-sensitive, unable to multiply in monocytes or inhibit phagosome–lysosome fusion, and less able to kill guinea pigs.[123–127]

CLINICAL FEATURES

Legionella infection presents in two very different forms: Pontiac fever and pneumonia (legionnaires' disease). It is not known why these two different forms occur, but inocula of the

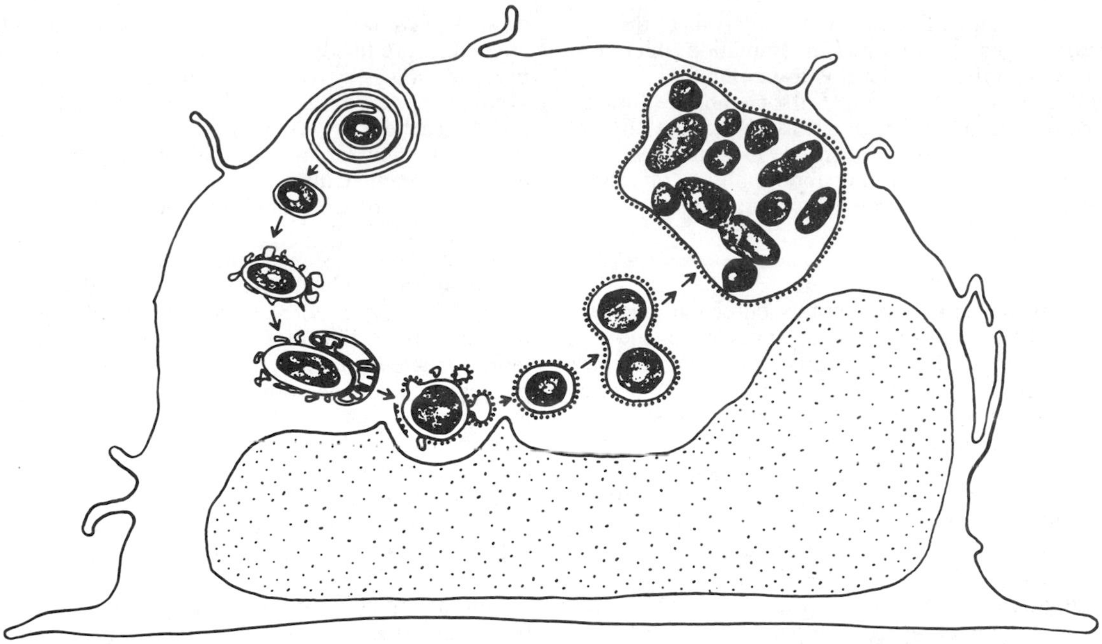

FIG. 2. Replicative cycle of *Legionella pneumophila* within monocytes. *Legionella pneumophila* is phagocytized by a process in which a pseudopod coils around the organism as it is being ingested. A vacuolar phagosome is formed containing *L. pneumophila*: this phagosome is surrounded by smooth vesicles, then mitochondria, and finally ribosomes. The organism multiplies until the phagosome becomes packed and the cell ruptures, thereby liberating the organism. (From Horwitz,[102] with permission.)

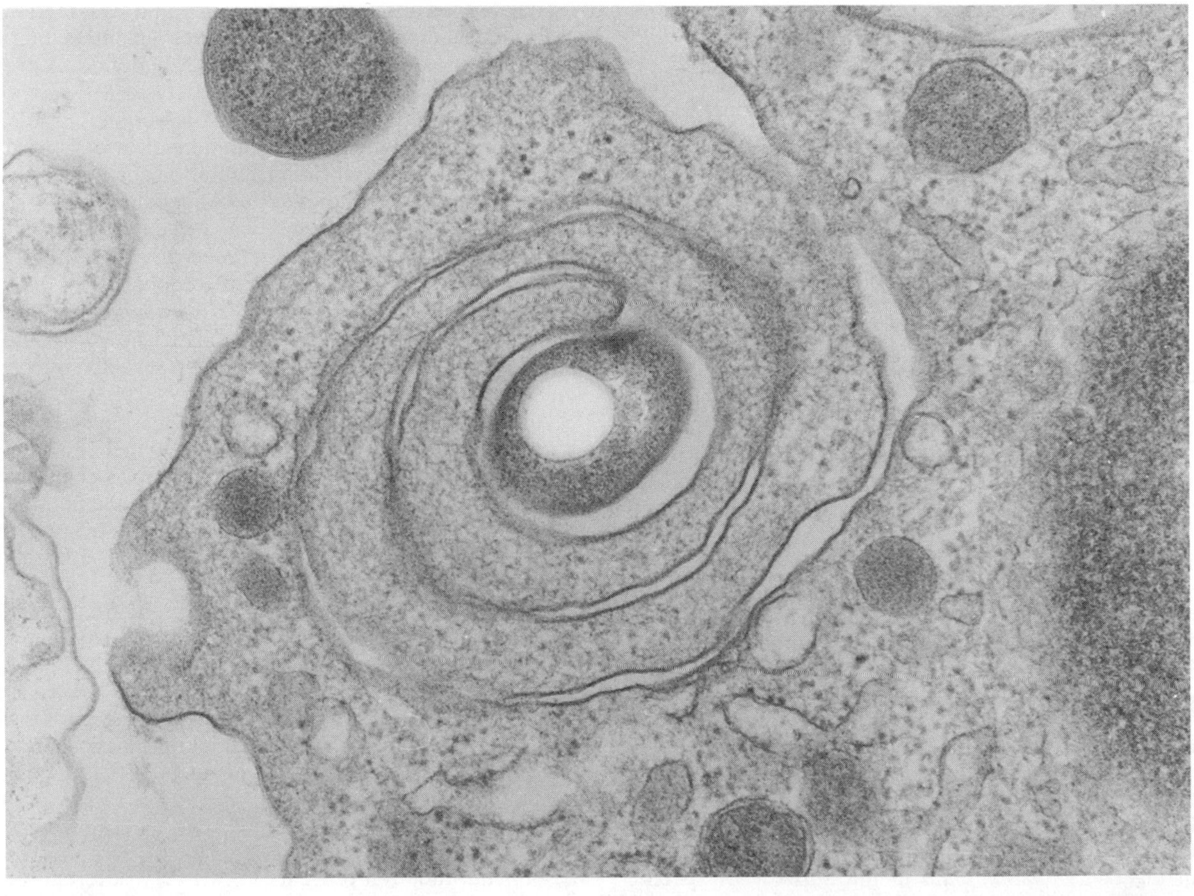

FIG. 3. Human monocyte ingesting *Legionella pneumophila*. A pseudopod of the phagocytic cell coils around the organism (center), which contains a lucent fat vacuole. (electron microscopy, ×28,500) (From Horwitz,[165] with permission.)

organism, differing modes of transmission, and host factors are probably important.

Pontiac Fever

Pontiac fever is an acute, self-limiting, flu-like illness without pneumonia.[57] The incubation period is 24–48 hours, and the attack rate of those exposed is quite high (more than 90 percent). The predominant symptoms are malaise, myalgia, fever, chills, and headache. Nonproductive cough, dizziness, and nausea have also been noted. The chest radiograph remains clear. Only symptomatic therapy is required, and complete recovery within 1 week is the rule.

Legionnaires' Disease

Pneumonia is the predominant clinical finding in legionnaires' disease. The disease encompasses a broad spectrum of illness, ranging from a mild cough and slight fever to coma with widespread pulmonary infiltrates and multisystem failure. The incubation period for legionnaires' disease ranges from 2 to 10 days; the shorter periods are experienced by immunosuppressed patients. In the first 24–48 hours of illness, patients experience nonspecific symptoms including fever, malaise, myalgia, anorexia, and headache.

The cough is initially mild and only slightly productive. Occasionally the sputum may be streaked with blood, but gross hemoptysis is rare. Chest pain, either pleuritic or nonpleuritic, can be a prominent feature for some patients and when coupled with hemoptysis often suggests a diagnosis of pulmonary embolus.

Diarrhea is seen in 25–50 percent of cases, with watery rather than bloody stools. Nausea, vomiting, and abdominal pain are seen in about 10–20 percent of cases. Neurologic symptoms range from headache and lethargy to encephalopathy. Change in mental status is the most common neurologic abnormality,[84,128] although a wide variety of neurologic findings including peripheral neuropathy and cerebellar ataxia have been reported.[129]

Physical examination typically reveals rales early in the course of the disease and findings of consolidation. Bradycardia relative to temperature elevation has been emphasized by some investigators,[100] although we have not found this to be a helpful sign.[84] Hypotension was seen in 17 percent of patients with community-acquired pneumonia.[84] Fever is virtually always present; in one series, 19 percent of patients had temperatures in excess of 40.5°C.[100] Shaking chills are more common in patients in advanced stages of pneumonia.

In a prospective, comparative pneumonia study, clinical manifestations including gastrointestinal and neurologic signs did not occur significantly more frequently in pneumonias caused by *Legionella* than those caused by other organisms.[85] Similarly, laboratory abnormalities including abnormal liver function, hypophosphatemia, hematuria, and hematologic abnormalities, although common, did not occur significantly more frequently in legionnaires' disease than in pneumonias of other etiology. On the other hand, hyponatremia (serum sodium less than 130 mEq/liter) has been found to occur significantly more frequently in legionnaires' disease than in pneumonias of other etiology.[85,100,130]

Although the clinical presentation is nonspecific, the following clues should raise the possibilty of legionnaires' disease in a case of undiagnosed pneumonia: (*1*) a Gram stain of respiratory secretions in which neutrophils are present in large numbers, but few, if any, organisms are visualized; (*2*) hyponatremia (serum sodium less than 130 mEq/ml) (*3*) failure to respond to β-lactam (penicillin or cephalosporin) and aminoglycoside antibiotics; and (*4*) occurrence in a hospital or environment in which the potable water supply is known to be contaminated with *Legionella*.

Extrapulmonary involvement has been documented, including sinusitis, perirectal abscess, pericarditis, pyelonephritis, peritonitis, pancreatitis, and endocarditis. Wound infections could result from dissemination via the blood stream or contamination of the wound by water colonized with *Legionella*.

Legionella prosthetic valve endocarditis has been described in one hospital.[131] Typical symptoms of fever, night sweats, malaise, and symptoms of congestive heart failure were seen. Anemia was a common feature, and its severity correlated with the duration of infection. Unlike endocarditis caused by other organisms, embolic phenomena were not seen, presumably due to the small size of the vegetations.

Many miscellaneous findings have been reported, including disseminated intravascular coagulation, thrombocytopenia, glomerulitis, rhabdomyolysis, various rashes, neuropathics, renal failure, and hepatic failure; they are more likely nonspecific findings related to the severity of the infection, type of underlying disease, and perhaps side effects of drug therapies.

Chest Radiographs

The vast majority of patients have abnormal chest x-ray findings on presentation, and all have abnormalities by the third day.[132] The initial involvement is unilateral for most cases, and there appears to be a modest lower lobe predominance. The initial infiltrate is typically alveolar and may be segmental–lobar or diffuse and patchy. The initial densities may appear as poorly marginated, rounded opacities, which are often pleura-based and may therefore be mistaken for pulmonary infarction. Interstitial infiltrates were described in about 25 percent of the patients in the 1976 Philadelphia outbreak, although such an appearance has not been prominent in subsequent reports. The initial area of infiltration often progresses to more widespread consolidation over the next several days.

The tendency for the radiographic abnormalities to progress after presentation has been widely noted, and several authors suggest that such progression is more frequent in legionnaires' disease than in other pneumonias. Progression of infiltrates has been documented for several days after appropriate and ultimately successful antibiotic therapy.

Pleural effusions are commonplace (24–63 percent of cases) and may occasionally precede the radiographic appearance of the infiltrate.[133] The effusions are typically modest in amount and rarely complicate patient management, although empyema has occurred in individual patients.

Hilar adenopathy and pneumatocoele formation have been reported only rarely. Cavitation and abscess in the immunosuppressed host receiving corticosteroids is not uncommon. Cavitation may occur up to 14 days after presentation, even after appropriate antibiotic therapy and apparent clinical response. Rupture of a cavity into the pleural space, with formation of empyema or bronchopleural fistula, is a rare complication.

The extent of radiographic infiltration does not correlate well with the severity of clinical manifestations or with ultimate outcome. A significant correlation exists between radiographic severity and the presence of *L. pneumophila* in sputum.[133] Presumably increased numbers of organisms in respiratory secretions reflect more extensive disease, as judged radiographically. Radiographic improvement lags behind clinical improvement for several days. The time required to show clearing of infiltrate on a chest radiograph varies, with studies reporting ranges of 1 to 2 months to 3 to 4 months.

LABORATORY DIAGNOSIS

Since legionnaires' disease is not specific in its clinical and radiologic presentation, specialized laboratory tests are necessary to establish the diagnosis[134] (Table 1). Gram stains from normally sterile sites (transtracheal aspirate, lung biopsy, pleural

TABLE 1. Comparison of Specialized Laboratory Tests for Diagnosis of Legionnaires' Disease

Test	Sensitivity (%)	Specificity (%)
Culture		
Sputum	50–70	100[a]
Transtracheal aspirate	90	100[a]
Blood	20	100[a]
Serology	70–96[b]	96–99
Direct fluorescent antibody	25–80	96–99
Urinary antigen[c]	75–90	100
DNA probe	70	95–99

[a] By definition.
[b] IgG and IgM antibody testing in both acute and convalescent sera.
[c] Serogroup 1 only.

fluid) can occasionally suggest the diagnosis; the organisms appear as small, pleomorphic, faintly staining gram-negative rods.

Culture

The definitive method for diagnosis of *Legionella* infection is isolation of the organism from respiratory secretions.[135] Early investigations were hampered by the fact that the causative agent failed to grow on standard bacteriologic media. Buffered charcoal yeast extract agar is now the base medium used for *Legionella* culture. The sensitivity is improved by the addition of antimicrobial agents and dyes[12,15]; the antimicrobial agents prevent the overgrowth of *Legionella* by competing organisms, while the dyes impart a distinctive color to the *Legionella* organisms. A major disadvantage of any culture methodology is the time required for growth, which in the case of *Legionella* can range from 3 to 5 days. The collection of a specimen that truly represents lower respiratory tract secretions is critical for the isolation of the actual pathogenic organism. When dye-containing selective media are used in concert with the buffered charcoal yeast extract agar following acid pretreatment for contaminated specimens, the sensitivity of sputum culture approaches 70 percent.

Transtracheal aspiration specimens are optimal, since contamination by oropharyngeal flora is avoided; for these specimens, the sensitivity may approach 90 percent.[135] The sensitivity of specimens obtained by bronchoscopy is approximately the same as that for sputum; bronchoalveolar lavage gives higher yields than bronchial wash specimens.[136] If there is a pleural effusion, thoracentesis should be performed and the fluid evaluated by direct fluorescent antibody (DFA) stain and culture. *Legionella* has also been isolated from pericardial fluid, rectal abscess, and wounds.

Legionella pneumophila has been isolated from blood using a biphasic medium,[137] a radiometric blood culture system,[131,138] and a lysis–centrifugation blood culture system.[139] In two studies in which *Legionella* bacteremia was found with some frequency,[131,138] blind subculture onto buffered charcoal yeast extract agar from the radiometric culture bottles was required, since growth indices failed to attain the threshold for detection.

Direct Fluorescent Antibody Stain

The first method for detection of *Legionella* in clinical specimens was immunofluorescence. The test can be performed within a few hours, and a positive test is extremely useful. Cross-reactions to non-*Legionella* organisms occur rarely; false-positive DFA tests are usually due to laboratory technique or contaminated reagents rather than cross-reacting bacteria. A major drawback to the DFA stain is the fact that the sensitivity is notably less than that of culture, because positive results depend on the presence of large numbers of organisms in the specimen. A negative test does not rule out disease. The DFA test is more likely to be positive when multilobar infiltrates are present on chest radiograph.[133]

Newer monoclonal antibody reagents are an improvement over the polyclonal reagents. Background staining is improved, and the test is technically easier to perform. DFA reagents for many of the newer species and serogroups are not yet available commercially.

Antibody Detection

Serologic detection of antibodies is the most readily available test for *Legionella*, because sera can easily be sent to referral laboratories. Indirect fluorescent antibody and enzyme-linked immunosorbent assay have been the most popularly used methodologies. Diagnosis is made on a fourfold rise in antibody titer to 1:128; thus both acute and convalescent sera are required, because 4–8 weeks are often required to detect an antibody response. Serology is useful in epidemiologic studies, but it is less helpful to the clinician in making an immediate diagnosis of legionnaires' disease for an individual patient. On the other hand, if the seroprevalence of *L. pneumophila* antibody titers within the community is known to be low, a single elevated titer (1:128 by the indirect fluorescent antibody method) may indicate the presence of acute disease. In the first week of disease, 25–40 percent of patients may have elevated titers.[135,140] False-positive results can occur rarely as a result of antibody cross-reacting to other gram-negative organisms; cystic fibrosis patients with *Pseudomonas aeruginosa* infections, in particular, may have falsely elevated antibody titers.[141,142]

Although the antibody response to legionnaires' disease is polyclonal, IgM antibodies as an individual class are more likely to be elevated than other classes, including IgG antibodies. The use of IgM and IgG assays gives maximal sensitivity (Table 1).

DNA Probe

DNA hybridization tests for *Legionella* ribosomal ribonucleic acid that is genus-specific is commercially available.[143] Results can be available within hours. Sensitivity appears comparable with direct fluorescent antibody methods. False-positive results have been reported, however.[144] The DNA probe cannot replace culture, but it may prove to be a useful adjunct. Prospective pneumonia studies for validation remain to be performed.

Urinary Antigen

Detection of a soluble *L. pneumophila* antigen in urine has been accomplished by radioimmunoassay, enzyme-linked immunoabsorbent assay, and latex agglutination.[145] This test holds unusual promise because it is often easier to obtain urine than adequate sputum in ill patients. The sensitivity is comparable with that of other methodologies, (Table 1) and the test can remain positive for months after the episode of pneumonia.[146] A commercially available test (Dupont, Wilmington, DE) has proven to be the most rapid one available for diagnosis of legionnaires' disease, but it can only be used for serogroup 1 infection. This drawback may be minor, since serogroup 1 accounts for about 70 percent of *L. pneumophila* infection.[6]

TREATMENT

On the basis of in vitro, animal model, and clinical observations, erythromycin remains the treatment of choice for legionellosis. Case fatality rates were lower for patients treated with erythromycin and tetracycline than for those treated with other agents.[1,147] Erythromycin has reduced mortality in both immunocompetent and immunocompromised patients.[148,149]

The recommended dosage for erythromycin is 2–4 g every day, although it should be noted that the 4 g dose can rarely cause ototoxicity, which is reversible upon discontinuation of the drug or decrease in dosage.[150] Although oral erythromycin may be adequate for selected patients, abrupt deterioration can occur in patients with advanced disease who appear stable at the time of diagnosis. Furthermore, the gastrointestinal dysfunction commonly seen in legionnaires' disease may compromise absorption of the oral agent. Thus initiation with the parenteral form seems prudent.

Clinical response, including defervescence and feeling of well-being, usually occurs within 3–5 days. Once a clinical response has been documented, oral therapy with erythromycin, 2 g a day, can replace parenteral therapy (Table 2). Duration of therapy is from 10 to 14 days, although some authorities have recommended longer duration for immunosuppressed patients. Relapse has been reported, although a review of some of these reports suggests that they actually may have been cases of reinfection in patients continually exposed to contaminated water.

In Vitro Susceptibility Studies

The minimal inhibitory concentrations (MIC) of most antibiotics are media-dependent; higher MICs are found in charcoal yeast extract agar media than in Mueller-Hinton broth.[151,152] The organism does produce β-lactamase.[153,154] Susceptibility studies performed in yolk sacs and animals show that erythromycin, tetracycline, and rifampin are the most consistently active agents. The quinolone agents, especially ciprofloxacin and pefloxacin, are highly active in vitro. The excellent penetration of the aforementioned antibiotics into phagocytic cells are presumably the basis for their clinical superiority over β-lactam and aminoglycoside agents.[155,156]

Although controlled studies are not available, we recommend combination erythromycin and oral rifampin therapy as initial therapy for *confirmed* cases of legionnaires' disease. Combination therapy should be strongly considered in patients who have a positive direct fluorescent antibody stain of respiratory tract secretions, since a positive test is an objective marker for advanced pneumonia and is a poor prognostic sign.

We recommend consideration of the immediate addition of erythromycin as the antibiotic of choice for most immunocompetent patients with community-acquired pneumonia if the Gram stain of their sputum shows many neutrophils but a paucity of organisms. Note that such a Gram stain would also suggest the diagnosis of mycoplasma and viral pneumonia and that both mycoplasma and pneumococcal pneumonia would also be covered by erythromycin. Continuation of erythromycin would be based on the results of confirmatory laboratory testing for legionella. The addition of empiric erythromycin should also be considered for any transplant recipient with nosocomial pneumonia if the organism has not been identified. If the water supply of the hospital is known to be contaminated with *L. pneumophila*, this would provide further impetus for using erythromycin pending results of specialized laboratory tests. Gram stain of sputum should be examined, and appropriate respiratory tract cultures should be obtained prior to initiation of empiric therapy.

TABLE 2. Antibiotic Therapy For Legionella Infections

Antimicrobial	*Dose*	*Route*	*Frequency*
Treatment of choice			
Erythromycin[a]	1 g	iv	q6h
	500 mg	po	q6h
Alternative agents[b]			
Rifampin[c]	600 mg	po	q12h
Trimethroprim/	160/800 mg	iv	q8h
sulfamethoxazole[a]	160/800 mg	po	q12h
Doxycycline[a]	100 mg	iv	q12h
Tetracycline[a]	500 mg	iv	q6h
Imipenem	1 gm	iv	q6h
Ciprofloxacin	750 mg	po	q12h

[a] Oral therapy can be implemented following demonstrated improvement on intravenous therapy.
[b] These agents have not undergone controlled evalution for therapy in legionnaires' disease.
[c] Rifampin must be given in combination with another agent.

Tetracyclines (especially doxycycline), trimethoprim-sulfamethoxazole, imipenem/cilastatin, and ciprofloxacin are alternative antibiotic agents that have been used successfully in anecdotal reports[131,157–159] (Table 2).

Prognosis

With appropriate antibiotic therapy, the mortality of legionnaires' disease is low in immunocompetent patients, although in nosocomial infection the mortality may approach 50 percent, especially if antibiotic therapy is started late. Generally the infection responds to erythromycin therapy within 3–5 days. The chest radiograph is not useful for monitoring clinical response.[132] Delay in diagnosis with a consequent delay in initiation of appropriate antibiotic therapy remains the critical factor in outcome determination.

PREVENTION

Since the environmental reservoir for legionnaires' disease has been discovered, prevention of this form of pneumonia is theoretically possible. Because of the prevalence of the organism in aquatic environments, many authorities have advocated culturing of environmental sources only upon the discovery of cases of legionnaires' disease.

On the other hand, recent studies have shown that nosocomial legionellosis could easily exist undiagnosed, especially in hospitals lacking specialized laboratory methods for detecting *Legionella*.[77,86] An important clue to its existence could be the presence of *L. pneumophila* in the hospital water supply. Thus routine environmental culturing in the absence of known cases may be desirable for facilities that house patients at risk for legionnaires' disease, including hospitals and nursing homes. Routine environmental culturing for *Legionella* should certainly be performed in hospitals in which organ and bone marrow transplants are performed, given the high risk for legionnaires' disease in these patients.[88,90–93]

Reservoir Disinfection

Numerous evaluations of various disinfection modalities for man-made water reservoirs have been performed:

Cooling Towers and Evaporative Condensers. Because controlled experiments have not been conducted to demonstrate aerosol dissemination from cooling towers, rational recommendations concerning biocide treatment have been difficult to formulate. Biocides appear to be ineffective in eradicating *L. pneumophila* from cooling towers and only marginally effective in reducing organism numbers.[160] Continuous and shock hyperchlorination have also been ineffective in eradicating *L. pneumophila* from cooling towers. Complicating this issue is the increasing uncertainty on the role that cooling towers play in legionnaires' disease.[58]

Water Distribution Systems. Hyperchlorination was the first disinfection modality applied to water distribution systems. A chlorinator is installed on the incoming water supply and adjusted so that there is a residual concentration of 2–6 ppm. The primary disadvantage is that it is difficult to maintain a stable bacteriostatic residual of chlorine, since chlorine decomposes at the higher temperature found in hot water systems, and *Legionella* are relatively chlorine-tolerant. Other disadvantages include corrosion of the plumbing system[161] and the production of carcinogenic byproducts.

Thermal eradication has emerged as the most widely used method for disinfection of water distribution systems.[61–63] Temperatures of 140°F (60°C) are bactericidal for *L. pneumophila*.[162]

One method consists of raising the hot water temperature to 140–170°F (60–77°C) for several days and then flushing each distal water site with hot water for 30 minutes. Then the temperature of the water is maintained at 150°F (66°C). The major drawback of heat eradication is the logistic difficulties involved in flushing distal sites. The system is also vulnerable to recurrent *L. pneumophila* contamination if the hot water tank temperature drops to lower temperatures. Scalding of patients and health-care personnel is a potential hazard.

Other modalities under investigation include ozonation, instantaneous steam water heaters, ultraviolet light radiation, and generation of metallic ions by electrolysis.[160]

Immunization

The prospects for immunization are promising. A live mutant vaccine has been shown to protect guinea pigs from lethal aerosol doses of *L. pneumophila*.[163] Thus a vaccine for high-risk patients may some day be feasible. The disease is not contagious, so isolation precautions are not needed.[164]

REFERENCES

1. Fraser DW, Tsai T, Orenstein W, et al. Legionnaires' disease: description of an epidemic of pneumonia. N Engl J Med. 1977;297:1186–1196.
2. Terranova W, Cohen ML, Fraser DW. 1974 outbreak of legionnaires' disease diagnosed in 1977. Lancet. 1978;2:122–4.
3. Thacker SB, Bennet JV, Tsai T, et al. An outbreak in 1975 of severe respiratory illness caused by legionnaires' disease bacterium. J Infect Dis. 1978;238:512–9.
4. McDade JE, Brenner DJ, Bozeman FM. Legionnaires' disease bacterium isolated in 1947. Ann Intern Med. 1979;90:659–61.
5. Brenner DJ. Classification of the legionellae. Semin Respir Infect. 1987;2:90–205.
6. Reingold A, Thomason B, Brake B, et al. Legionella pneumonia in the U.S.: the distribution of serogroups and species causing human illness. J Infect Dis. 1984;149:819–24.
7. Collins MT, Bangsborg J, Hoiby N. Antigenic heterogeneity among *Legionella, Fluoribacter*, and *Tatlockia* species analyzed by crossed immunoelectrophoresis. Int J System Bacteriol. 1987;37:351–6.
8. Lambert MA, Moss CW. Cellular fatty acid compositions and isoprenoid quinone contents of 23 *Legionella* species. J Clin Microbiol. 1989;27:465–73.
9. Pine L, Franzus MJ, Malcolm GB. Guanine is a growth factor for *Legionella* species. J Clin Microbiol. 1986;23:163–9.
10. Hoffman P. Bacterial physiology. In: Thornsberry C, et al., eds. *Legionella*—Proceedings of the 2nd International Symposium, Washington, DC. Am Soc Microbiol. 1984;61–7.
11. Pine L, Hoffman PS, Malcolm GB, et al. Role of keto acids and reduced oxygen-scavenging enzymes in the growth of *Legionella* species. J Clin Microbiol. 1986;23:33–42.
12. Vickers RM, Stout JE, Yu VL, et al. Culture methodology for the isolation of *Legionella pneumophila* and other Legionellaceae from clinical and environmental specimens. Semin Respir Infect. 1987;2:274–9.
13. Bopp CA, Sumner JW, Morris GK, et al. Isolation of *Legionella* spp from environmental water samples by low-pH treatment and use of a selective medium. J Clin Microbiol. 1981;13:714–9.
14. Buesching W, Brust R, Ayers L. Enhanced primary isolation of *L. pneumophila* from clinical specimens by low-pH treatment. J Clin Microbiol. 1983;17:1153–5.
15. Vickers RM, Brown A, Garrity GM. Dye containing buffered charcoal yeast extract medium for the differentiation of members of the family Legionellaceae. J Clin Microbiol. 1981;13:380–2.
16. Hebert GA, Callaway C, Ewing EP. Comparison of *L. pneumophila, L. micdadei, L. bozemanii*, and *L. dumoffi* by transmission electron microscopy. J Clin Microbiol. 1984;19:116–21.
17. Tesh MJ, Morse S, Miller RD. Intermediary metabolism in *Legionella pneumophila*: utilization of amino acids and other compounds as energy sources. J Bacteriol. 1981;154:1104–9.
18. Baine WB. Cytolytic and phospholipase C activity in *Legionella* species. J Gen Microbiol. 1985;131:1383–91.
19. Baskerville A, Conlan J, Ashworth L, et al. Pulmonary damage caused by a protease from *L. pneumophila*. Br J Exp Pathol. 1986;67:527–36.
20. Chen GC, Brown A, Lema M. Restriction endonuclease activities in the legionellae. Can J Microbiol. 1986;32:591–3.
21. Friedman RL, Lochner JE, Bigley RH, et al. The effects of *Legionella pneumophila* toxin on oxidative processes and bacterial killing of human polymorphonuclear leukocytes. J Infect Dis. 1982;146:328–34.
22. Thorpe TC, Miller RD. Extracellular enzymes of *L. pneumophila*. Infect Immun. 1981;33:632–8.
23. Lochner TC, Bigley R, Iglewski BH. Defective triggering of polymorphonuclear leukocyte oxidative metabolism by *L. pneumophila* toxin. J Infect Dis. 1985;151:42–6.
24. Hindahl M, Iglewski. Outer membrane proteins from *L. pneumophila* serogroups and other *Legionella* species. Infect Immun. 1986;51:94–101.
25. Nolte FS, Conlin CA. Major outer membrane protein of *L. pneumophila* carries a species-specific epitope. J Clin Microbiol. 1986;12:643–6.
26. Gabay J, Blake M, Niles W, et al. Purification of *Legionella pneumophila* major outer membrane protein and demonstration that it is a porin. J Bacteriol. 1985;162:85–91.
27. Ciesielski CA, Blaser MJ, Wang WLL. Serogroup specificity of *Legionella pneumophila* is related to lipopolysaccharide characteristics. Infect Immun. 1986;51:397–404.
28. Joly JR, McKinney RM, Tobin JO, et al. Development of a standardized subtyping scheme for *L. pneumophila*, serogroup 1, using monoclonal antibodies. J Clin Microbiol. 1986;23:768–71.
29. Dournon E, Bibb WF, Rajagopalan P, et al. Monoclonal antibody reactivity as a virulence marker for *Legionella pneumophila* serogroup 1 strains. J Infect Dis. 1988;157:496–501.
30. Stout J, Joly J, Para P, et al. Comparison of molecular methods for subtyping patient and epidemiologically linked environmental isolates of *Legionella pneumophila*. J Infect Dis. 1988;157:486–95.
31. Plouffe JF, Para MF, Maher WE, et al. Subtypes of *Legionella pneumophila* serogroup 1 associated with different attack rates. Lancet. 1983;2:649–50.
32. Brown A, Lema M, Ciesielski CA, et al. Investigation of a small outbreak of legionnaires' disease by plasmid and peptide analysis of clinical and environmental *Legionella pneumophila*. Infection. 1985;13:163–6.
33. Zanen-Lim OG, van den Broek N, Rietra P. Comparison of strains of *Legionella pneumophila* serogroup 1 isolated in four Amsterdam hospitals from patients and hot water supplies. J Infect Dis. 1984;150:508–12.
34. Thomason BM, Bibb WF. Use of absorbed antisera for demonstration of antigenic variation among strains of *L. pneumophila* serogroup 1. J Clin Microbiol. 1984;19:794–7.
35. Lema M, Brown A. Electrophoretic characterization of soluble protein extracts of *Legionella pneumophila* and other members of the family *Legionellaceae*. J Clin Microbiol. 1983;17:1132–40.
36. Gabay JE, Horwitz MA. Isolation and characterization of the cytoplasmic and outer membranes of legionnaires' disease bacterium (*Legionella pneumophila*). J Exp Med. 1985;161:409–22.
37. Ehret W, Ruckdeschel G. Membrane proteins of Legionellaceae I. Membrane proteins of different stains and serogroups of *Legionella pneumophila*. Zentralbl Bakteriol Mikrobiol Hyg [A]. 1985;259:433–45.
38. Moyer NP, Lange A, Hall N, et al. Application of capillary gas-liquid chromatography for subtyping of *L. pneumophila*. In: Thornsberry C, et al., eds., eds. *Legionella*—Proceedings of the 2nd International Symposium, Washington, DC. Am Soc Microbiol. 1984;274:6.
39. Tompkins LS, Troup N, Wood ST, et al. Molecular epidemiology of *Legionella* species by restriction endonuclease and alloenzyme analysis. J Clin Microbiol. 1987;25:1875–80.
40. Van Ketel R, ter Schegget J, Zanan HC. Molecular epidemiology of *L. pneumophila*, serogroup 1. J Clin Microbiol. 1984;20:362–4.
41. Selander R, McKinney RM, Whittam T, et al. Genetic structure of populations of *L. pneumophila*. J Bacteriol. 1985;163:1021–37.
42. Fliermans CB. Philosophical ecology: *Legionella* in historical perspective. In: Thornsberry C, et al., eds. *Legionella*—Proceedings of the 2nd International Symposium, Washington, DC. Am Soc Microbiol. 1984;285–9.
43. Kuchta JM, States SJ, McNamara AM, et al. Susceptibility of *Legionella pneumophila* to chlorine in tap water. Appl Environ Microbiol. 1983; 46:1134–9.
44. Hsu; SC, Martin R, Wentworth BB. Isolation of *Legionella* species from drinking water. Appl Environ Microbiol. 1984;48:830–2.
45. Witherell LE, Duncan R, Stone K, et al. Investigation of *L. pneumophila* in drinking water. J Am Water Works Assoc. 1988;80:87–93.
46. Tison DL, Pope DH, Cherry WB, et al. Growth of *Legionella pneumophila* in association with blue-green algae (cyanobacteria). Appl Environ Microbiol. 1980;39:346–459.
47. Rowbotham TJ. Isolation of *L. pneumophila* from clinical specimens via amoebae, and the interaction of those and other isolates with amoebae. J Clin Pathol. 1983;36:978–86.
48. Holden EP, Winkler HH, Wood DO, et al. Intracellular growth of *L. pneumophila* within *Acanthamoeba casteanni neff*. Infect Immun. 1984;45:18–24.
49. Fields BS, Shotts EB, Feeley JC, et al. Proliferation of *Legionella pneumophila* as an intracellular parasite of the ciliated protozoan, *Tetrahymena pyriformis*. Appl Environ Microbiol. 1984;47:467–71.
50. Stout JE, Yu VL, Best M. Ecology of *Legionella pneumophila* within water distribution systems. Appl Environ Microbiol. 1985;49:221–8.
51. Peel M, Calwell J, Christopher P, et al. *L. pneumophila* and water temperature in Australian hospitals. Aust NZ J Med. 1985;15:38–41.
52. Lee TC, Stout JE, Yu VL. Factors predisposing to *L. pneumophila* colonization in residential water systems. Arch Environ Health. 1988;43:59–62.
53. Groothuis DG, Veenendaal HR, Dijkstra HL. Influence of temperature on the number of *Legionella pneumophila* in hot water systems. J Appl Bacteriol. 1985;59:529–36.
54. Vickers RM, Stout JE, Yu VL, et al. Culture methodology for the isolation of *Legionella pneumophila* and other Legionellaceae from clinical and environmental specimens. Semin Respir Infect. 1987;2:274–9.

55. Mangione EJ, Remus RS, Tait KA, et al. An outbreak of Pontiac fever related to whirlpool use, Michigan, 1982. JAMA. 1985;77:535–9.
56. Friedman S, Spitalny K, Barbaree J, et al. Pontiac fever outbreak associated with a cooling tower. Am J Public Health. 1987;77:568–72.
57. Kaufmann A, McDade J, Patton C, et al. Pontiac fever: isolation of the etiologic agent (*Legionella pneumophila*) and demonstration of its mode of transmission. Am J Epidemiol. 1981;114:337–47.
58. Muder R, Yu VL, Woo A. Mode of transmission of *L. pneumophila*: a critical review. Arch Intern Med. 1986;146:1607–12.
59. Tobin RS, Ewan P, Walsh K, et al. A survey of *Legionella* pneumophila in water in 12 Canadian cities. Water Res. 1986;20:495–501.
60. Stout JE, Yu VL, Vickers RM, et al. Ubiquitousness of *Legionella pneumophila* in the water supply of a hospital with endemic Legionnaires' disease. N Engl J Med. 1982;306:466–468.
61. Best M, Yu VL, Stout J, et al. Legionellaceae in the hospital water supply—epidemiological link with disease and evaluation of a method of control of nosocomial legionnaires' disease and Pittsburgh pneumonia. Lancet. 1983;2:307–10.
62. Johnson JT, Yu VL, Best M, et al. Nosocomial legionellosis uncovered in surgical patients with head and neck cancer: implications for epidemiologic reservoir and mode of transmission. Lancet. 1985;2:298–300.
63. Meenhorst PL, Reingold AL, Groothuis DG, et al. Water-related nosocomial pneumonia caused by *Legionella pneumophila* serogroups 1 and 20. J Infect Dis. 1985;152:356–64.
64. Nolte FS, Conlin C, Roisin A, et al. Plasmids as epidemiological markers in nosocomial legionnaires' disease. J Infect Dis. 1984;149:251–6.
65. Stout J, Yu VL, Muraca P. Legionnaires' disease acquired from the water supply within the homes of two patients. JAMA. 1987;257:1215–7.
66. Phillips S, Zeff R, Gervich D. Legionnaires' disease. Ann Thorac Surg. 1987;55:56.
67. Muraca PW, Stout JE, Yu VL, et al. Legionnaires' disease in the work environment: implications for environmental health. Am Ind Hyg Assoc J. 1988;584–90.
68. Tobin J, Beare J, Dunnill M, et al. Legionnaires' disease in a transplant unit: isolation of the causative agent from shower baths. Lancet. 1980;2:118–21.
69. Bollin GE, Plouffe JF, Para MF, et al. Aerosols containing *Legionella pneumophila* generated by shower heads and hot water faucets. Appl Environ Microbiol. 1985;50:1128–31.
70. Woo AH, Yu VL, Goetz A. Potential in-hospital mode of transmission for *Legionella pneumophila*: demonstration experiments for dissemination by showers, humidifers, and rinsing of ventilation bag apparatus. Am J Med. 1986;80:567–73.
71. Dennis P, Wright AE, Rutter D, et al. *Legionella pneumophila* in aerosols from shower baths. J Hyg. 1984;93:349–53.
72. Zuravleff JJ, Yu VL, Shonnard J, et al. *Legionella pneumophila* contamination of a hospital humidifier: demonstration of aerosol transmission and subsequent subclincal infection in exposed guinea pigs. Am Rev Respir Dis. 1983;138:657–61.
73. Arnow P, Chou T, Weil D, et al. Nosocomial legionnaires' disease caused by aerosolized tap water from respiratory devices. J Infect Dis. 1982; 146:460–7.
74. Bouvet A, deFenoyl O, Desplaces N. Maladie des legionnaires' due au serogroup 6 de *Legionella pneumophila*—contamination d'un domicile par canule de tracheostomie. Presse Med. 1986;15:35.
75. Kaan J, Simoons-Smit AM, MacLaren D. Another source of aerosol causing nosocomial legionnaires' disease. J Infect. 1985;11:145–8.
76. Markowitz L, Tompkins L, Wilkinson H, et al. Transmission of nosocomial legionnaires' disease in heart transplant patients (Abstract). In: Program and Abstracts of the 24th Interscience 1984 Conference on Antimicrobial Agents and Chemotherapy. Washington, DC: Am Soc Microbiol; 170.
77. Muder RR, Yu VL, McClure J, et al. Nosocomial legionnaires' disease uncovered in a prospective pneumonia study: implications for underdiagnosis. JAMA. 1983;249:3184–92.
78. Yu VL, Stout J, Zuravleff JJ. Aspiration of contaminated water may be a mode of transmission for *Legionella pneumophila* (Abstract). In: Program and Abstracts of 21st Interscience Conference on Antimicrobial Agents and Chemotherapy. Chicago: Am Soc Microbiol; 1981:297.
79. Marrie T, MacDonald S, Clarke K, et al. Nasogastric tubes flushed with contaminated potable water are a risk factor for nosocomial *Legionella pneumophila* (Abstract). In: Program and Abstracts of the 28th Interscience Conference on Antimicrobial Agents and Chemotherapy. Los Angeles: Am Soc Microbiol; 191.
80. Fay D, Baird IM, Aguirre A, et al. Unrecognized legionnaires' disease as a cause of fatal illness. JAMA. 1980;243:2311–3.
81. MacFarlane JT, Finch RG, Ward MJ, et al. Hospital study of adult community-acquired pneumonia. Lancet. 1982;2:255–8.
82. Friss-Moller A, Rechnitzer C, Blak F, et al. Prevalence of legionnaires' disease in pneumonia patients admitted to a Danish department of infectious diseases. Scand J Infect Dis. 1986;18:321–8.
83. Levy M, Dromer F, Brion M, et al. Community-acquired pneumonia—importance of initial noninvasive bacteriologic and radiographic investigation. Chest. 1988;92:43–8.
84. Fang GD, Fine M, Orloff J, et al. Community-acquired pneumonia with emphasis on *Legionella* and TWAR: a prospective multicenter study of 259 cases (Abstract). In: 88th Annual Meeting American Society for Microbiology, Miami Beach, 1988, C44.
85. Yu VL, Kroboth FJ, Shonnard J, et al. Legionnaires' disease: new clinical perspective from a prospective pneumonia study. Am J Med. 1982;73:357–61.
86. Yu VL, Beam TR, Lumish R, et al. Routine culturing for *Legionella* in the hospital environment may be a good idea. Am J Med Sci. 1987;294:97–9.
87. Storch G, Baine W, Fraser DW, et al. Sporadic community-acquired legionnaires' disease in the United States. Ann Intern Med. 1979:596–600.
88. Serota A, Meyer R, Wilson S, et al. Legionnaires' disease in the postoperative patient. J Surg Res. 1980;30:417–27.
89. Korvick J, Yu VL. Legionnaires' disease: an emerging surgical problem. Ann Thorac Surg. 1987;43:341–7.
90. Hofflin JM, Potasman I, Baldwin JC, et al. Infectious complications in heart transplant recipients receiving cyclosporine and corticosteroids. Ann Intern Med. 1987;106:209–16.
91. Kugler JW, Armitage JO, Helms CM, et al. Nosocomial legionnaires' disease. Occurrence in recipients of bone marrow transplants. Am J Med. 1983;74:281–88.
92. Fuller J, Levinson MM, Kline JR, et al. Legionnaires' disease after heart transplantation. Ann Thorac Surg. 1985;39:308–11.
93. Bock B, Edelstein P, Snyder K, et al. Legionnaires' disease in renal transplant recipients. Lancet. 1978;1:410–3.
94. Winn WC, Myerowitz RL. The pathology of the *Legionella* pneumonias: a review of 74 cases and the literature. Hum Pathol. 1981;12:401–22.
95. Chastre J, Raghu G, Soler P, et al. Pulmonary fibrosis following pneumonia due to acute legionnaires' disease. Chest. 1987;91:57–62.
96. Rodgers FG. The role of structure and invasiveness on the pathogenicity of *Legionella*. Zentralbl Bakteriol Microbiol Hyg. 1. Abt [Orig A]. 1983; 255:138–44.
97. Stout JE, Best M, Yu VL, et al. Symbiosis of *Legionella pneumophila* and *Tatlockia micdadei* with human respiratory flora. J Appl Bacteriol. 1986;60:297–9.
98. Baskerville A, Fitzgeorge RB, Broster M, et al. Histopathology of experimental legionnaires' disease in guinea pigs, rhesus monkeys and marmosets. J Pathol. 1983;139:349–62.
99. Davis GS, Winn WC, Gump DW, et al. Legionnaires' pneumonia after aerosol exposure in guinea pigs and rats. Am Rev Respir Dis. 1982;126:1050–7.
100. Kirby BD, Snyder K, Meyer R, et al. Legionnaires' disease: report of 65 nosocomially acquired cases and a review of the literature. Medicine. 1980;59:188–205.
101. Nash TW, Libby D, Horwitz MA. Interaction between the legionnaires' disease bacterium (*L. pneumophila*) and human alveolar macrophages: influence of antibody, lymphokines, and hydrocortisone. J Clin Invest. 1984;74:771–82.
102. Horwitz MA. The Legionnaires' disease bacterium (*Legionella pneumophila*) inhibits phagosome-lysosome fusion in human monocytes. J Exp Med. 1983;158:2108–26.
103. Davis GS, Winn W, Gump DW, et al. The kinetics of early inflammatory events during experimental pneumonia due to *Legionella pneumophila* in guinea pigs. J Infect Dis. 1983;148:823–35.
104. Payne NR, Horwitz MA. Phagocytosis of *Legionella pneumophila* is mediated by human monocyte complement receptors. J Exp Med. 1987; 166:1377–89.
105. Horwitz MA, Silverstein SC. Interaction of the legionnaires' disease bacterium (*Legionella pneumophila*) with human phagocytes I. *L. pneumophila* resists killing by polymorphonuclear leukocytes, antibody, and complement. J Exp Med. 1981;153:386–97.
106. Lochner JE, Friedman RL, Bigley RH, et al. Effect of oxygen-dependent antimicrobiol systems on *Legionella pneumophila*. Infect Immun. 1983; 39:487–9.
107. Rolstad B, Berdal B. Immune defenses against *Legionella pneumophila* in rats. Infect Immun. 1981;32:805–12.
108. Breiman RF, Horwitz MA. Guinea pigs sublethally infected with aerosolized *Legionella pneumophila* develop humoral and cell-mediated immune responses. J Exp Med. 1987;164:799–811.
109. Korvick J, Yu VL. Simultaneous infection with *Cryptococcus neoformans* and *Legionella pneumophila*: in vivo expression of common defects in immunity. Respiration. 1988;53:132–6.
110. Cordonnier C, Farcet JP, Desforges L. Legionnaires' disease and hairy-cell leukemia. Arch Intern Med. 1984;144:2373–5.
110a. Nielson H, Bangsborg J, Rechnitzer C, et al. Defective monocyte function in Legionnaires' disease complicating hairy cell leukemia. Acta Med Scand. 1986;220:381–6.
111. Plouffe JF, Baird IM. Cord blood lymphocyte transformation responses to *L. pneumophila*. J Clin Lab Immunol. 1982;9:119–20.
112. Friedman H, Widen R, Lee I, et al. Cellular immunity to *L. pneumophila* in guinea pigs assessed by direct and indirect migration inhibition; reaction in vitro. Infect Immun. 1983;41:1132–37.
113. Friedman H, Widen R, Klein T, et al. *L. pneumophila*-induced blastogenesis of immune lymphoid cells in vitro. Infect Immun. 1984;43:314–9.
114. Wong KH, McMaster PRB, Feeley JC, et al. Detection of hypersensitivity to *L. pneumophila* in guinea pigs by skin test. Curr Top Microbiol Immunol. 1980;4:105–10.
115. Horwitz MA. Cell-mediated immunity in legionnaires' disease. J Clin Invest. 1983;71:1686–97.
116. Bhardwaj N, Nash T, Horwitz MA. Interferon-gamma-activated human monocytes inhibit the intracellular multiplication of *L. pneumophila*. J Immunol. 1986;137:2662–9.
117. Blanchard DK, Klein TW, Friedman H, et al. Kinetics and characterization

of interferon production by murine spleen cells stimulated with *Legionella pneumophila* antigens. Infect Immun. 1985;49:719–23.
118. Klein TW, Newton CA, Blanchard K, et al. Induction of interleukin 1 by *Legionella pneumophila* antigens in mouse and human mononuclear leukocyte cultures. Zentralbl Bakteriol Mikrobiol Hyg [A]. 1987;265:462–71.
119. Gibson D, Baskerville A, Ashworth L, et al. Non-specific protection against pulmonary *L. pneumophila* infection in guinea pigs immunized and challenged with mycobacteria. Br J Exp Pathol. 1985;66:333–44.
120. Horwitz MA, Lewis W, Cohn ZA. Defective production of monocyte-activating cytokines in lepromatous leprosy. J Exp Med. 1984;159:666–78.
121. Blanchard DK, Stewart WE, Klein TW, et al. Cytolytic activity of human peripheral blood leukocytes against *Legionella pneumophila*-infected monocytes: characterization of the effector. J Immunol. 1987;139:551–6.
122. Winn WC, Chandler FW. Role of virulence factors in *Legionella* infection. Arch Pathol Lab Med. 1982;106:105–11.
123. Klein TW, Friedman H, Widen R. Relative potency of virulent vs. avirulent *L. pneumophila* for induction of cell-mediated immunity. Infect Immun. 1984;44:753–9.
124. Bollin GE, Plouffe JE, Para MF, et al. Difference in virulence of environmental isolates of *Legionella pneumophila*. J Clin Microbiol. 1985;21:674–7.
125. Kishimoto RA, White JD, Chirley F, et al. In vitro response of guinea pig peritoneal macrophages to *L. pneumophila*. Infect Immun. 1981;31:1209–14.
126. Arko R, Wong K, Feeley JC. Immunologic factors affecting the in vivo and in vitro survival of the legionnaires' disease bacterium. Ann Intern Med. 1979;90:680–3.
127. Horwitz MA. Characterization of avirulent *L. pneumophila* that survive, but do not multiply within human monocytes. J Exp Med. 1987;166:1310–28.
128. Johnson JD, Raff M, VanArsdall J. Neurologic manifestations of legionnaires' disease. Medicine. 1984;63:303–10.
129. Weir AI, Bone I, Kennedy D. Neurological involvement in legionellosis. J Neurol Neurosurg Psychiatry. 1982;45:603–8.
130. Miller AC. Hyponatremia in legionnaires' disease. Br Med J. 1982;284:558–9.
131. Tompkins LS, Roessler BJ, Redd SC, et al. *Legionella* prosthetic-valve endocarditis. N Engl J Med. 1988;18:530–5.
132. Muder RR, Yu VL, Parry M. Radiology of *Legionella* pneumonia. Semin Respir Infect. 1987;2:242–54.
133. Kroboth FJ, Yu VL, Reddy S, et al. Clinicoradiographic correlations with the extent of legionnaires' disease. AJR. 1983;141:263–8.
134. Winn WC. *Legionella* and legionnaires' disease; a review with emphasis on environmental studies and laboratory diagnosis. Crit Rev Clin Lab Sci. 1984;21:323–81.
135. Zuravleff JJ, Yu VL, Shonnard J, et al. Diagnosis of legionnaires' disease: an update of laboratory methods with new emphasis on isolation by culture. JAMA. 1983;250:1982–5.
136. Kohorst WR, Schoenfeld SA, Macklin JE, et al. Rapid diagnosis of legionnaires' disease by bronchoalveolar lavage. Chest. 1983;84:186–90.
137. Edelstein PH, Meyer RD, Finegold SM. Isolation of *Legionella pneumophila* from blood. Lancet. 1979;1:750–1.
138. Rihs JD, Yu VL, Zuravleff JJ, et al. Isolation of *Legionella pneumophila* from blood using the BACTEC: a prospective study yielding positive results. J Clin Microbiol. 1985;22:422–4.
139. Reinhardt TJ, Nakahama C, Edelstein P. Comparison of blood culture methods for recovery of *L. pneumophila* from the blood of guinea pigs with experimental infection. J Clin Microbiol. 1987;25:719–21.
140. Harrison TG, Dournon E, Taylor AG. Evaluation of sensitivity of two serological tests for diagnosing pneumonia serogroup 1. J Clin Pathol. 1987;40:77–82.
141. Wang EEL, Manson B, Corey M. False positivity of *Legionella* serology in patients with cystic fibrosis. Pediatr Infect Dis J. 1987;6:256–9.
142. Collins MT, McDonald J, Hoiby N, et al. Agglutinating antibody titers to members of the family Legionellaceae in cystic fibrosis patients as a result of cross-reacting antibodies to cystic fibrosis. J Clin Microbiol. 1984;19:757–62.
143. Wilkinson HW, Sampson J, Plikaytis B. Evaluation of a commercial gene probe for identification of *Legionella* cultures. J Clin Microbiol. 1986;23:217–20.
144. Laussucq S, Schuster D, Alexander WJ, et al. False-positive DNA probe for *Legionella* species associated with a cluster of respiratory illnesses. J Clin Microbiol. 1988;26:1442–4.
145. Kohler RB. Antigen detection for the rapid diagnosis of *Mycoplasma* and *Legionella* pneumonia. Diagn Microbiol Infect Dis. 1986;4(Suppl 3):47.S–59.S.
146. Kohler RB, Winn WC, Wheat LJ. Onset and duration of urinary antigen excretion in legionnaires' disease. J Clin Microbiol. 1984;20:605–7.
147. Beaty HN, Miller AA, Broome CV, et al. Legionnaires' disease in Vermont, May to October, 1977. JAMA. 1978;240:127–31.
148. Brown A, Yu VL, Elder EM, et al. Nosocomial outbreak of legionnaires' disease at the Pittsburgh Veterans Administration Medical Center. Trans Assoc Am Phys. 1980;93:52–9.
149. Keys TF. Therapeutic considerations in the treatment of *Legionella* infection. Semin Respir Infect. 1987;2:770–3.
150. Swanson DJ, Sung RJ, Fine M, et al. A prospective evaluation of erythromycin ototoxicity in patients with pneumonia (Abstract). In: Interscience Conference on Antimicrobial Agents and Chemotherapy 1988. Los Angeles: American Society of Microbiology; 1046.
151. Edelstein PH, Meyer RD. Susceptibility of *L. pneumophila* to 20 antimicrobial agents. Antimicrob Agents Chemother. 1988;18:403–8.
152. Pohlod D, Saravolatz LD. Activity of quinolones against Legionellaceae. J Antimicrob Chemother. 1986;17:540–1.
153. Fu KP, Neu HC. Inactivation of beta-lactam antibiotics by *L. pneumophila*. Antimicrob Agents Chemother. 1979;16:561–4.
154. Weisholtz S, Tomasz A. Response of *L. pneumophila* to beta-lactam antibiotics. Antimicrob Agents Chemother. 1985;27:695–700.
155. Miller MF, Martin J, Johnson P, et al. Erythromycin uptake and accumulation by human polymorphonuclear leukocytes and efficacy of erythromycin in killing of ingested *L. pneumophila*. J Infect Dis. 1984;149:714–8.
156. Vilde J, Dournon E, Rajagopalan P. Inhibition of *L. pneumophila* multiplication within human macrophages by antimicrobial agents. Antimicrob Agents Chemother. 1986;30:743–8.
157. Miller AC. Erythromycin in legionnaires' disease: a reappraisal. J Antimicrob Chemother. 1981;7:217–22.
158. Beasley CRW, Humble M, O'Donnell T. Pilot study: treatment of pneumonia with imipenem/cilastatin. NZ Med J. 1985;98:494–7.
159. Farrell ID, Barker J, Chiodini P, et al. The activity of imipenem on *L. pneumophila* with a note on the treatment of two cases. J Antimicrob Chemother. 1985;16:61–5.
160. Muraca PW, Stout JE, Yu VL. Environmental aspects of legionnaires' disease. J Am Water Works Assoc. 1988;80:78–86.
161. Helms CM, Massanari M, Wenzel RP, et al. Legionnaires' disease associated with a hospital water system (a five year progress report on continuous hyperchlorination). JAMA. 1988;259:2423–7.
162. Stout JE, Best MG, Yu VL. Susceptibility of members of the family Legionellaceae to thermal stress: implications for heat eradication methods in water distribution systems. Appl Environ Microbiol. 1986;52:396–9.
163. Blander SJ, Breiman R, Horwitz MA. A live avirulent *L. pneumophila* induces protective immunity against lethal aerosol challenge (Abstract). Clin Res. 1988;36:578.
164. Yu VL, Zuravleff JJ, Gavlik L, et al. Lack of evidence for person-to-person transmission of legionnaires' disease. J Infect Dis. 1983;147:362.
165. Horwitz MA. Phagocytosis of the Legionnaires' disease bacterium (*Legionella pneumophila*) occurs by a novel mechanism: engulfment within a pseudopod coil. Cell. 1984;36:28.

211. OTHER LEGIONELLA SPECIES

GUO-DONG FANG
VICTOR L. YU

Following the discovery of *Legionella pneumophila* in 1977, other newly discovered organisms (originally termed ALLO for "atypical *Legionella*-like organisms") were isolated on the same culture media used for *L. pneumophila* and were found to share similar biochemical and metabolic features.[1] Almost 30 such species have now been classified into the new family, Legionellaceae.[2]

Eighteen of these species have been implicated in human pneumonia, with 13 isolated by culture from clinical specimens and 5 implicated indirectly by serologic evidence (Table 1). About 85 percent of *Legionella* infections are due to *L. pneumophila* and 15 percent to these other species.[3] More than 10 other species have been isolated from natural aquatic environments but have not yet been implicated in human disease.

In 1977 workers from the University of Pittsburgh and the University of Virginia visualized gram-negative, weakly acid-fast organisms from lung tissue of immunosuppressed patients with acute pneumonitis.[4,5] Almost all of the patients were receiving steroids or cytotoxic chemotherapy; renal transplant recipients were a prominent group. Although organisms could be seen on biopsy and autopsy lung specimens by various stains, they could not be grown on standard bacteriologic culture media. A *Legionella*-like organism was isolated after the clinical specimens were inoculated into guinea pigs and embryonated eggs. Sera from these patients were demonstrated to

TABLE 1. Members of the Legionellaceae Family Implicated in Pneumonia

Legionella pneumophila
Legionella (Tatlockia) micdadei[a]
L. bozemanii
L. dumoffii
L. longbeachae
L. jordanis
L. gormanii
L. feelei
L. hackeliae
L. maceachernii
L. wadsworthii
L. birminghamensis
L. cincinnatiensis
L. oakridgensis[b]
L. anisa[c]
L. cherrii[c]
L. rubrilucens[c]
L. sainthelensi[c]

[a] Pittsburgh pneumonia agent.
[b] Diagnosed by DFA and serology only.
[c] Implicated by serology only.

contain high titers of antibodies against this organism, confirming its etiologic role in pneumonia.

This new organism, originally termed Pittsburgh pneumonia agent (PPA), was found to be serologically and genetically distinct from *L. pneumophila*, although it phenotypically resembled *L. pneumophila* in growth requirements and the presence of branched-chain fatty acids in the cell wall. The organism had been previously isolated in 1943 (named TATLOCK) from the blood of a febrile soldier and in 1959 (named HEBA) from the blood of a patient with a rash;[6,7] both isolations were accomplished via guinea pig inoculation. Following the discovery of PPA, subsequent isolations of other *Legionella*-like organisms were made from infected patients (Table 2).

Investigators from the Centers for Disease Control proposed the name of *Legionella micdadei* for the Pittsburgh pneumonia agent in honor of Joseph McDade, who first isolated *L. pneumophila*.[8] Investigators from the Pittsburgh VA Medical Center proposed that the organism be placed in a separate genus because of significant differences between PPA and *L. pneumophila* in DNA sequence homology and DNA guanine and cytosine content; Garrity et al. proposed the name *Tatlockia micdadei* in honor of Hugh Tatlock, who first isolated the organism in 1943.[9] Garrity et al. also proposed a third genus, *Fluoribacter* (fluorescent rod), for those organisms that showed blue-white autofluorescence on media when illuminated under long-wave ultraviolet light, but were less than 70 percent interrelated to the DNA of *L. pneumophila* and PPA; the species proposed were *Fluoribacter bozemanae*, *Fluoribacter dumoffii*, and *Fluoribacter gormanii*.[9] Brenner argued against the concept of multiple genera within the Legionellaceae family by noting that the methods for isolation and cultivation, the clinical syndrome of pneumonia, and the recommended antibiotic therapy were essentially the same for all species.[2] Reasoned arguments both for and against the concept of additional genera can be reviewed elsewhere.[10–15]

DESCRIPTION OF THE PATHOGENS

The members of the Legionellaceae family have a number of common microbiologic features, including growth on buffered charcoal yeast extract media, failure to grow on blood agar, growth requirement for cysteine, and gram-negative bacillary forms on gram stain.

Legionella (*Tatlockia*) *micdadei* can appear as weakly or partially acid-fast in clinical specimens, although the acid-fast property is not present in organisms grown from culture. Interestingly, patients with Pittsburgh pneumonia have been empirically treated with antituberculosis agents because of false-positive acid-fast smears.[5,16–18]

All species produce a water-soluble, extracellular fluorescent compound when grown on buffered yeast extract agar. When the media is exposed to long-wave ultraviolet light, the organisms and surrounding medium fluoresce yellow-green. Some species also exhibit a blue-white or red intracellular fluorescence within the colony when viewed under ultraviolet light (Table 3). Most species produce a water-soluble or diffusible melaninlike brown pigment as seen on charcoal-free media supplemented with tyrosine (Table 3).

TABLE 2. Historical Overview of the Legionellaceae Implicated in Pneumonia

Strain	Source	Location	Isolated by	Year Isolated	Reference
L. micdadei	Blood, human	Fort Bragg, NC	H. Tatlock	1943	6,8
L. bozemanii	Lung tissue	Key West, FL	F.M. Bozeman	1959	1,63
L. dumoffii	Water, cooling tower	New York, NY	G.W. Gorman	1978	63,64
L. longbeachae	Transtracheal aspirate	Long Beach, CA	R. Porschen	1980	65
L. jordanis	Water, river	Bloomington, IL	G.W. Gorman	1978	66,67
L. gormanii	Soil, creek	Atlanta, GA	G.W. Gorman	1978	68,69
L. feeleii	Water	Windsor, Canada	G.W. Gorman	1981	33,70
L. hackeliae	Bronchial biopsy	Ann Arbor, MI	M. Hackel	1981	58,71
L. maceachernii	Water, home evaporator	Phoenix, AZ	G.W. Gorman	1979	71,72
L. wadsworthii	Sputum	Los Angeles, CA	P.H. Edelstein	1981	73
L. birminghamensis	Lung tissue	Birmingham, AL	S. S. Polt E. Brookings J. Kirklin	1986	49
L. cincinnatiensis	Lung tissue	Cincinnati, OH	J.L. Staneck S.R. Vincent	1982	50
L. oakridgensis	Water, cooling tower	Pennsylvania Minnesota	R.L. Tyndall, C.B. Duncan E.L. Dominque	1981	57,74
L. anisa	Water, sink	Los Angeles, CA	G.W. Gorman	1981	71
L. cherrii	Water, thermal enriched	Minnesota	R.K. Tyndall C.B. Duncan	1982	71
L. rubrilucens	Water, potable	Los Angeles, CA	G.W. Gorman	1980	71,75
L. sainthelensi	Water, spring	Mount Saint Helens, WA	J. Campbell S. Eng	1981	71

The routine clinical biochemical tests are not helpful in distinguishing one species from another. Oxidase reactions are variable (Table 3). Urease, nitrate, and fermentation tests are uniformly negative. All species have catalase activity.

There exist some unique features that can be used for identifying individual species (Table 3). Only *L. pneumophila* and *L. feeleii* hydrolyze hippurate; *L. micdadei, L. feeleii*, and *L. maceachernii* do not produce β-lactamase; *L. micdadei, L. wadsworthii*, and *L. birminghamensis* do not produce brown pigment on tyrosine-containing yeast extract agar; only *L. oakridgensis* is nonmotile. *Legionella micdadei* and *L. maceachernii* also produce blue colonies on media containing bromocresol purple and bromothymol blue dyes, while the other species produce yellow-green to apple-green colonies.[10,19]

The ultrastructures of the *Legionella* species are similar. As seen with scanning electron microscopy, *L. pneumophila, L. bozemanii, L. dumoffii*, and *L. micdadei* possess cytoplasmic vacuoles, trilaminar membranes separated by a periplasic space, a dense peptidoglycanlike layer, a polysaccharide capsule, and a single subpolar flagellum.[20] *Legionella micdadei* is unique in that an extra layer of lucent material exists between the outer membrane and capsule.

Fatty acid profiles and ubiquinone composition are sufficiently unique to allow for confirmation of a *Legionella* species by gas liquid chromatography.[21]

Direct fluorescent antibody testing also allows identification of individual species. Polyclonal and polyvalent reagents are commercially available; one reagent tests for *L. pneumophila*, serogroups 1–6, and another reagent tests for 22 species of the family. A commercially available fluorescent reagent is supposedly capable of detection of 21 species and 33 serogroups of *Legionella*. Individual polyclonal monovalent reagents are available for *L. micdadei, L. bozemanii, L. dumoffii, L. gormanii, L. longbeachae, L. jordanis*, and *L. pneumophila*.

A nucleic acid hybridization probe reactive to *Legionella* ribosomal RNA can determine the presence of a species in a specimen within hours using a single reagent.[22] The commercially available probe cannot, however, differentiate between the various species and serogroups. Outer membrane proteins for the *Legionella* species contain genus-specific and/or species-specific portions that can be used for immunologic and gene probes.[23,24]

Epidemiology

Most *Legionella* species have been recognized as inhabitants of natural aquatic bodies. For six species (*L. dumoffii, L. jordanis, L. gormanii, L. feeleii, L. maceachernii*, and *L. oakridgensis*), discovery of the organism in water preceded its discovery in humans (Table 2). Environmental isolation has not yet been obtained for *L. wadsworthii, L. hackeliae, L. birminghamensis*, and *L. cincinnatiensis* although they have been isolated from clinical specimens in patients with pneumonia.

Like *L. pneumophila*, some of these species (*L. micdadei, L. bozemanii, L. dumoffii*, and *L. feeleii*) have been found to colonize water distribution systems,[25–28] but recovery of these other *Legionella* species is less frequent and technically more difficult. Commensal microflora and sediment known to promote *L. pneumophila* survival in water distribution systems were ineffective in stimulating the growth of *L. micdadei*.[29] Thus the growth kinetics of *L. micdadei* may explain its infrequent presence and low concentration in the water supply, such that only patients with prolonged hospitalization or immunosuppression are susceptible.

Of the other *Legionella* species, *L. micdadei* is the most frequently implicated in infection, accounting for approximately 60 percent of cases of pneumonias caused by species other than *L. pneumophila. Legionella bozemanii* (15 percent), *L. dumoffii* (10 percent), *L. longbeachae* (5 percent), and the other 14 species together (10 percent) account for the remainder.[10,30]

Most patients infected by these *Legionella* species are immunosuppressed, with malignancies and renal transplants constituting the largest portion of such patients. Corticosteroid therapy appears to be a major risk factor for Pittsburgh pneumonia. Patients with nosocomial Pittsburgh pneumonia were significantly more likely to be immunosuppressed than patients with community-acquired Pittsburgh pneumonia.[31]

Seventy-five percent and 60 percent of the reported cases of

TABLE 3. Microbiologic Characteristics of the Legionellaceae

Strain	*Tyrosine YEA browning*[a]	*Gelatin liquefaction*	*Hippurate hydrolysis*	*Oxidase*	*β-Lactamase*	*BCP spot test*[b]	*Colony color on dye medium*[c]	*Autofluorescence*
L. pneumophila	+	+	+	+/−[d]	+	−	Green	−
L. micdadei[e]	−	−	−	+	−	+[f]	Blue	−
L. bozemanii	+	+	−	+/−	+/−	−	Green	+BW[g]
L. dumoffii	+[h]	+	−	−	+	−	Green	+BW[g]
L. longbeachae	+	+	−	+	+/−	−	Green	−
L. jordanis	+	+	−	+	+	−	Green	−
L. gormanii	+	+	−	−	+	−	Green	+BW
L. feeleii	+	−	+/−	−	−	−	Green	−
L. hackeliae	+	+	−	+	+	−	Green	−
L. maceachernii	+	+	−	+	−	+	Blue	−
L. wadsworthii	−	+	−	−	+	−	Green	−
L. birminghamensis	−	+	−	+/−	+	−	Green	−
L. cincinnatiensis	+	+	−	−	+	−	Green	−
L. oakridgensis	+	+	−	−	+(w)[i]	−	Green	−
L. anisa	+	+	−	+	+	−	Green	+BW
L. cherrii	+	+	−	−	+	−	Green	+BW
L. rubrilucens	+	+	−	+	+	−	Green	+R[j]
L. sainthelensi	+	+	−	+	+	−	Green	−

[a] YEA = yeast extract agar.
[b] Bromocresol purple spot test.[9,10]
[c] Buffered charcoal yeast extract agar supplemented with bromocresol purple and bromothymol blue dyes.[19]
[d] +/− = also reported as negative.
[e] Pittsburgh pneumonia agent, *T. micdadei*.
[f] Organism and dye complex fluoresce red when viewed under long-wave ultraviolet light.[10]
[g] BW = blue-white autofluorescence when viewed under long-wave ultraviolet light.
[h] One strain reported negative for browning.[76]
[i] Weakly positive reaction.
[j] R = red.
(Modified from Fang et al.,[10] with permission.)

Pittsburgh pneumonia and *L. dumoffii* were hospital-acquired, while virtually all cases due to the remaining species were sporadic, community-acquired pneumonias.[10]

An outbreak of nosocomial pneumonia caused by *L. dumoffii* was linked to contaminated distilled water. *Legionella dumoffii* was presumably transmitted to susceptible patients by respiratory therapy equipment or room humidifiers.[27] An outbreak of nosocomial pneumonia caused by *L. bozemanii* was linked to the presence of the organism in the hospital water distribution.[26] The outbreak was terminated after the water supply was disinfected using chlorination and heat sterilization.

The mode of transmission of these organisms from the water to the susceptible patient is uncertain. For *L. pneumophila* there is circumstantial evidence involving aerosolization via cooling towers and evaporative condensors, although the importance of these devices in disseminating *Legionella* has been questioned.[32] Interestingly, in pneumonic disease due to the other species, cooling towers and evaporative condensors have not been implicated.

Legionella feeleii was implicated in an outbreak of Pontiac fever in an automobile plant by antibody seroconversion in workers with symptoms of headaches, myalgias, high fever, and fatigue.[33] The organism was isolated from a water-based coolant, which may have been aerosolized, since the attack rate was highest for those workers nearest the coolant source.

Aspiration of contaminated water or oropharyngeal secretions may be a mode of transmission.[34] A patient with cranial nerve paresis and dysphagia with regurgitation developed aspiration pneumonia with lung abscesses after steroid administration.[35] *Legionella micdadei* was isolated from the pleural fluid, and high titers of antibody to *L. micdadei* were subsequently demonstrated. We have observed a case of aspiration pneumonia following a grand mal seizure in which *L. micdadei* was later isolated from sputum. Pittsburgh pneumonia in transplant recipients and surgical patients also tends to occur in the postoperative period, suggesting that postoperative aspiration associated with manipulation of the respiratory tract may be a precipitating factor. Finally, two separate cases of *L. bozemanii* pneumonia occurred following episodes of near drowning.[36,37]

Simultaneous infection with the other *Legionella* species and *L. pneumophila* has been reported, suggesting that the mode of transmission and environmental reservoir of the other *Legionella* species is identical to that of *L. pneumophila*.[10,38–41]

These organisms appear to be less virulent than *L. pneumophila*. Infection tends to occur more often in susceptible immunosuppressed hosts, the course is more benign, and pneumonia responds more readily to antibiotics than in infections by *L. pneumophila*.

The pathology of pneumonia caused by the *Legionella* species is similar to that caused by *L. pneumophila*.[42]

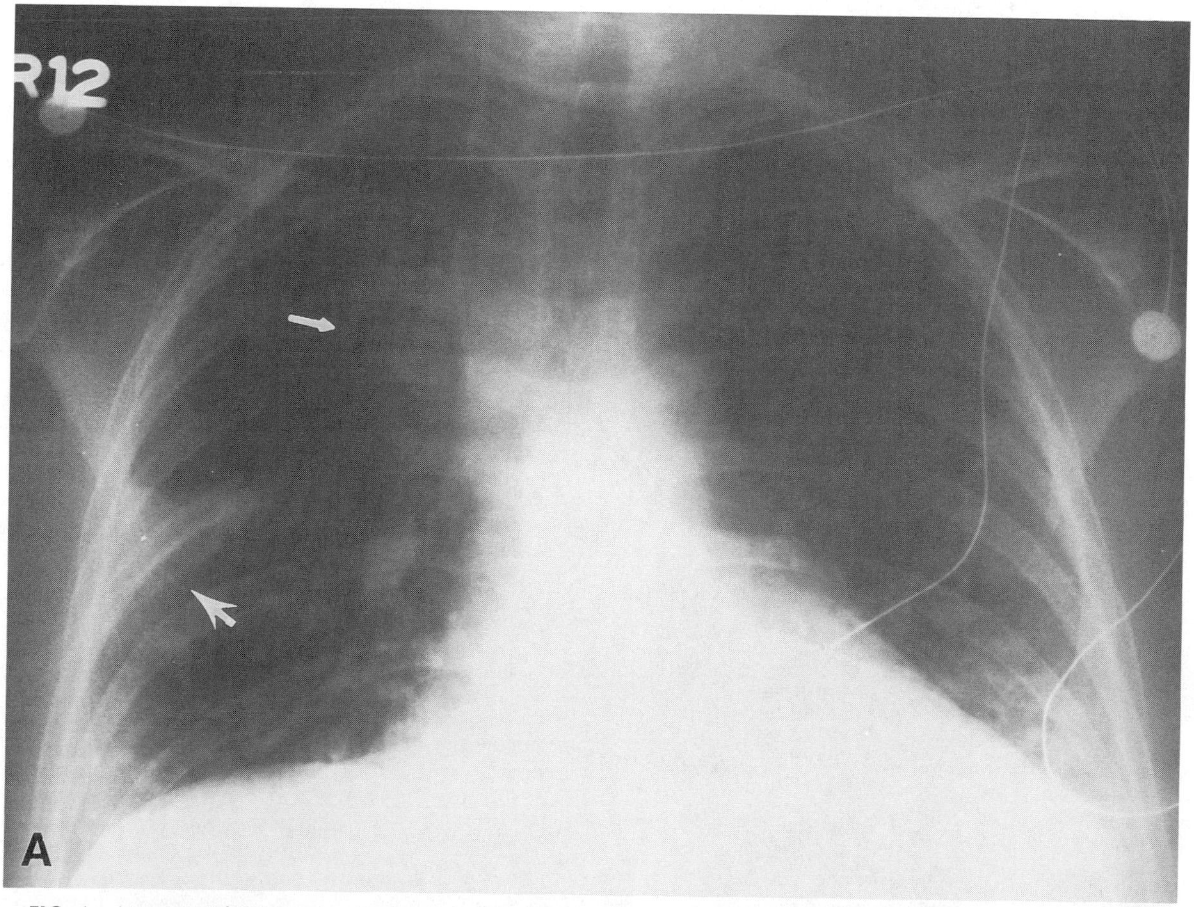

FIG. 1. Nosocomial Pittsburgh pneumonia in a young female receiving steroids for lupus erythematous. On day 3, she experienced abrupt onset of fever, dyspnea, and pleuritic chest pain. **(A)** Poorly marginated densities (small arrow) and a wedge-shaped density (large arrow) were seen on chest x-ray films, suggesting pulmonary embolus, although pulmonary angiography was nonconfirmatory. Direct fluorescent antibody stain and culture of sputum yielded *L. micdadei*. Cavitation in the right upper lobe was seen on day 7 **(B)** and day 10 **(C)**. Computed tomography shows the cavity (arrow, **D**). A residual thin wall cavity was still visible on day 15 **(E)**. The patient ultimately made a full recovery. (From Muder et al.,[51] with permission.) (Figure continues.)

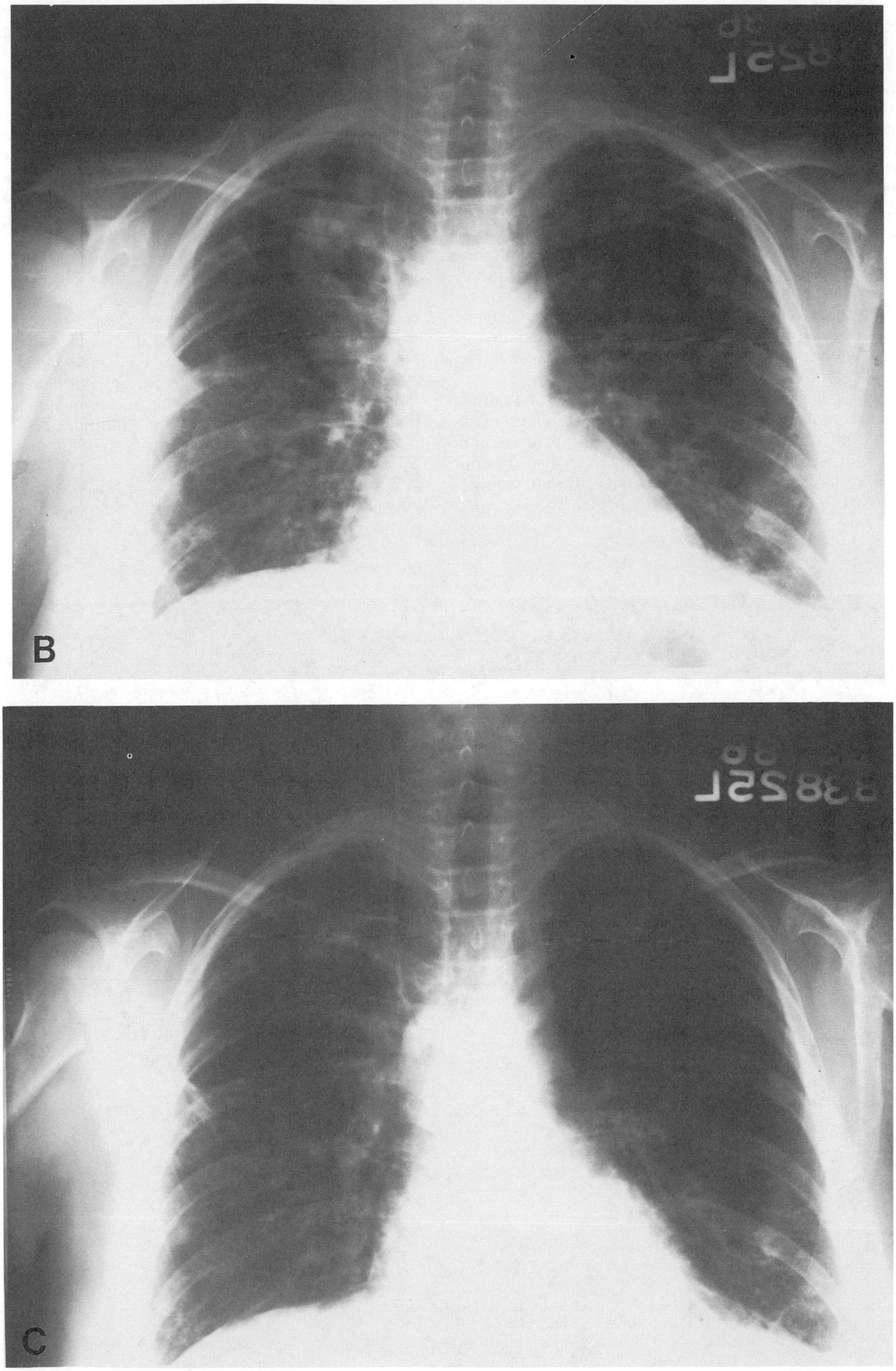

Fig. 1 (*Continued*).

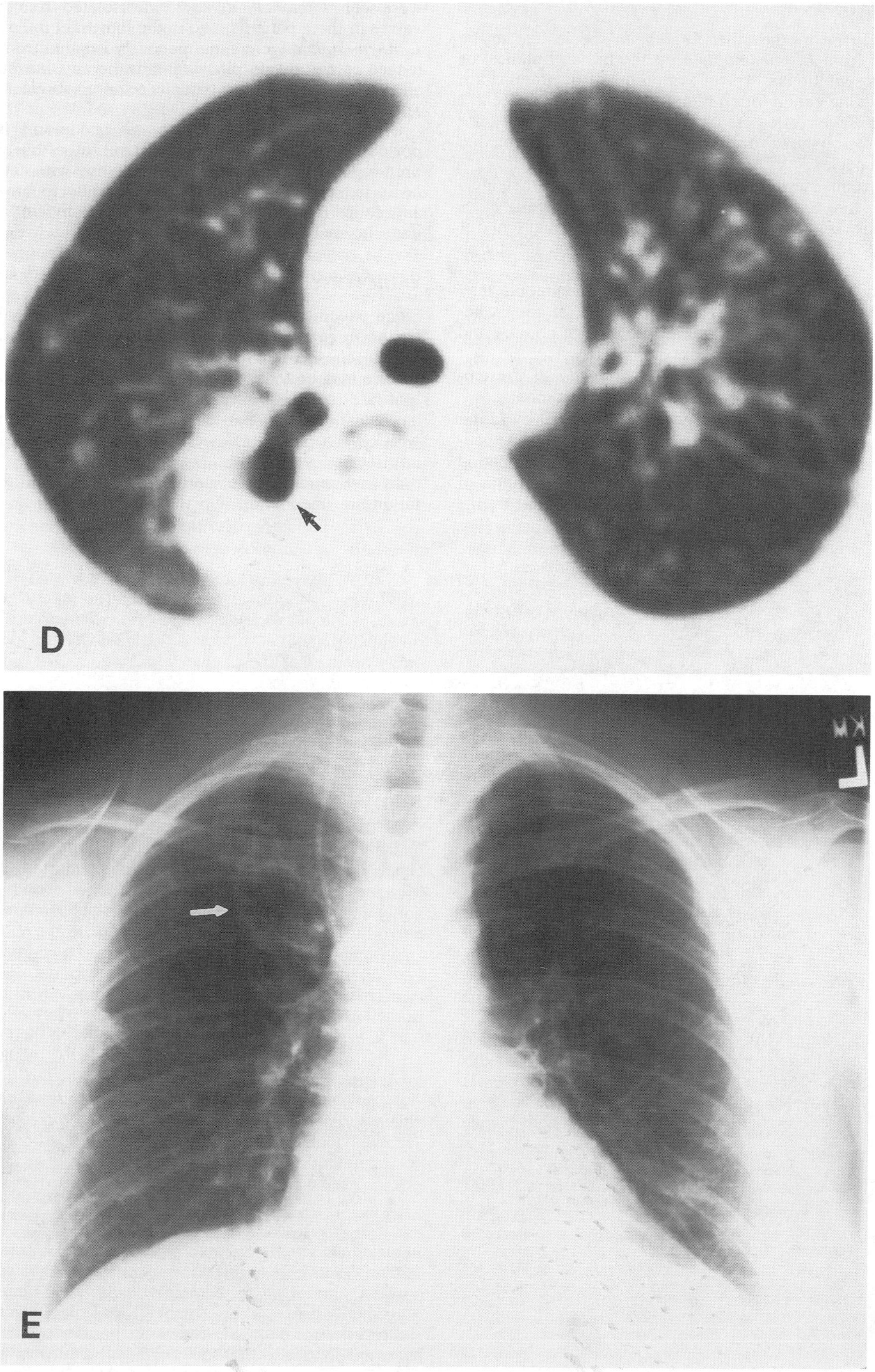

Fig. 1 (*Continued*).

CLINICAL FEATURES

Pneumonia caused by the other *Legionella* species cannot be distinguished from *L. pneumophila* on the basis of clinical or radiologic presentations. Typical symptoms of pneumonia are present, including cough (often nonproductive), pleuritic chest pain, and high fever (often greater than 40°C). Diarrhea , a notable sign in legionnaires' disease, also occurs in infection due to the other species.[10,43]

Hyponatremia (serum sodium less or equal to 130 meq/liter) has been reported to occur significantly more frequently in legionnaires' disease than in any other types of pneumonia; it was seen in 32.4 percent of the patients with Pittsburgh pneumonia.[31]

In immunosuppressed patients, Pittsburgh pneumonia may mimic pulmonary embolism, given the presence of cough, hemoptysis, pleuritic chest pain, and appearance of nodular and pleural-based densities on chest x-ray films (Fig. 1).

Cutaneous abscess has been caused by *L. micdadei*, presumably from bacteremic seeding of a subclinical pneumonia.[44]

Four cases of prosthetic valve endocarditis caused by *L. dumoffii* have been reported from one hospital.[41] All of the pneumonias were hospital-acquired during the perioperative period following valve insertion. The patients had a chronic course of fever, night sweats, weight loss, and anemia; no embolic events were seen. *Legionella dumoffii* was isolated from the prosthetic valves of three patients, and in the fourth, both *L. dumoffii* and *L. pneumophila* were simultaneously isolated from blood. Prolonged erythromycin plus rifampin therapy was successful for all cases, although three patients required surgical replacement of the infected prosthetic valve.

One pediatric case of Pittsburgh pneumonia has been reported in a retrospective serologic survey of hospitalized children.[45] The patient was a 13-year-old boy with acute lymphoblastic leukemia, who responded clinically to broad spectrum antibiotics (which did not include erythromycin) and concomitant increase in his neutrophil count.

RADIOLOGY

Since pneumonia is the most common clinical presentation of all the *Legionella* species, virtually all patients will have abnormal chest x-ray findings at presentation. The initial x-ray picture may be that of a patchy bronchopneumonia, segmental infiltrate, or circumscribed nodular infiltrate. No predilection has been noted for a particular lobe. A few cases have presented with only a pleural effusion without evidence for a clear-cut infiltrate.

In immunocompetent patients, nodular infiltrates and cavitation are uncommon. On the other hand, in an immunosup-

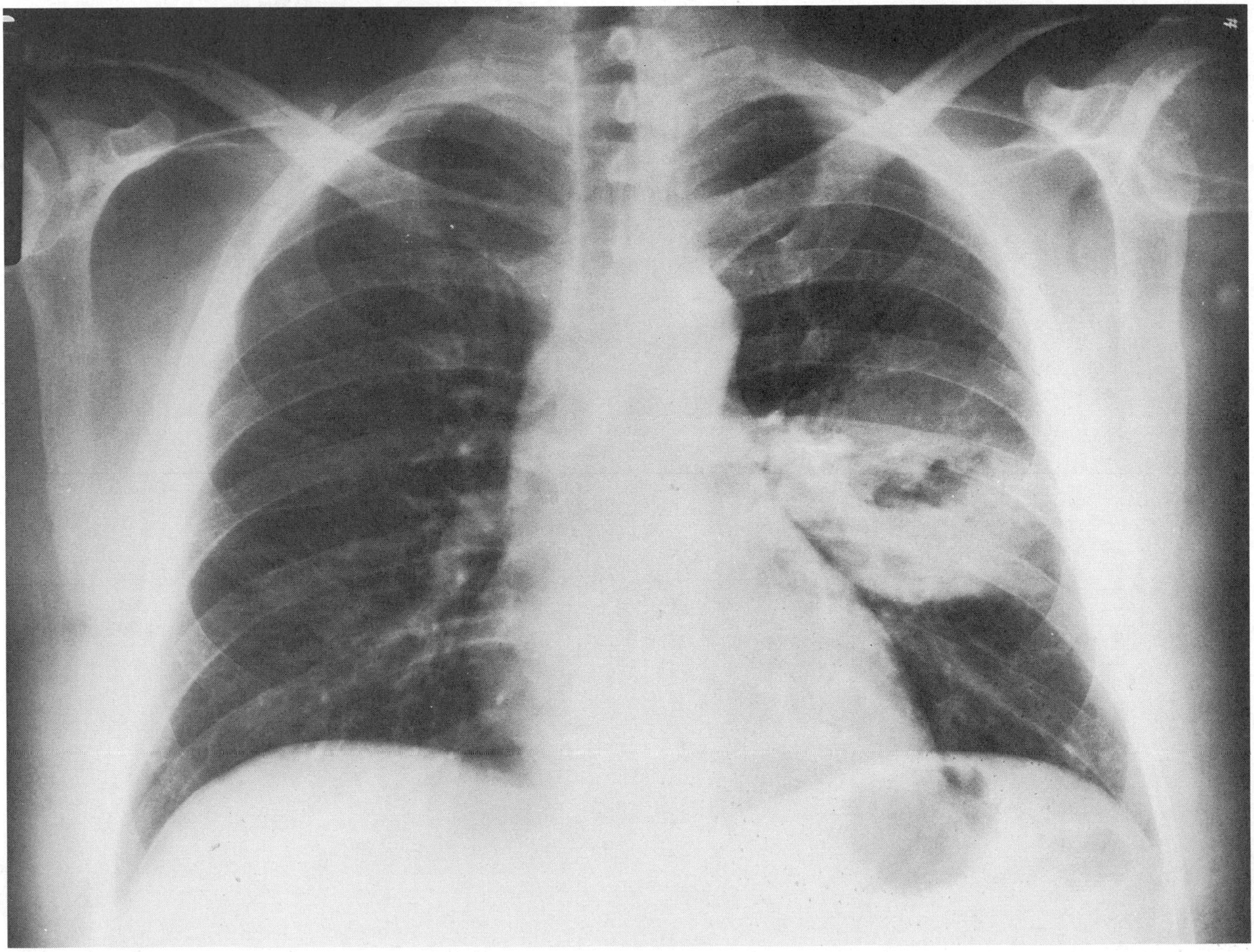

FIG. 2. Nosocomial *L. bozemanii* pneumonia in an immunosuppressed patient. Although the patient responded to erythromycin and rifampin, cavitation occurred within the left lower lobe infiltrate. The infiltrate decreased by month 3 and resolved by month 6.

pressed patient, rapid progression of a patchy alveolar infiltrate to a diffuse multilobe infiltrate is typical. An expanding pulmonary nodule has been a dramatic x-ray finding in some patients.[46] About 10 percent of patients with pneumonia caused by these other *Legionella* species showed evidence of cavitation on chest x-ray film (Figs. 1 and 2;[10] progression of cavitation has occurred despite initiation of appropriate antibiotic therapy.[47,48]

Interestingly, the single reported cases of *L. birminghamensis* and *L. cincinnatiensis* were asymptomatic individuals in which a nodular density was noted incidentally on chest x-ray film.[49,50]

Pleural effusions, usually of small volume, have been found in about 25 percent of patients with Pittsburgh pneumonia,[51,52] although recurrent hemorrhagic pleural effusion has also been described.[47]

Radiologic improvement is quite slow, despite prompt clinical improvement after appropriate antibiotics have been instituted; most patients require more than 3 months of follow-up before resolution can be documented.[26,51]

DIAGNOSIS

The diagnosis of the other *Legionella* species is best established by isolation of the organism from culture using selective media. Direct fluorescent antibody stains and detection of antibodies in sera are available for a limited number of species., The commercially available DNA probe can detect the presence, but not identify the species. It should be noted that unlike *L. pneumophila*, the sensitivity and specificity of the specialized tests for the other *Legionella* species have not been determined. In particular, antibody seroconversion for the other *Legionella* species has not been validated. For example, we suspect that seroconversion to *L. micdadei* may occasionally represent nonspecific cross-reactions to infection by other gram-negative rods; thus cases implicated solely by serology must be evaluated with caution.

TREATMENT

Therapy is similar to that for *L. pneumophila*. Erythromycin appears to be the drug of choice for the other *Legionella* species, based on susceptibility tests conducted in animal models and eggs. Although controlled clinical trials have not been done, erythromycin appears to be more effective for Pittsburgh pneumonia than β-lactam agents and aminoglycosides.[15] Erythromycin combined with rifampin has been quite successful in anecdotal case reports.[26,53] Unlike *L. pneumophila*, many of these organisms do not produce β-lactamases (Table 3), and, indeed, there are numerous anecdotal reports of clinical response to β-lactam agents.[35,44,45,54–58] Trimethoprim–sulfamethoxazole has been effective in immunosuppressed patients with Pittsburgh pneumonia who have failed erythromycin therapy.[47,59,60]

Prevention of nosocomial infection has been accomplished by disinfecting the hospital water supply using heat,[25,26,61] chlorine,[26] and ultraviolet light.[62]

REFERENCES

1. Cordes LG, Gorman GW, Wilkinson HW, et al. Atypical *Legionella*-like organisms: fastidious water-associated bacteria pathogenic for man. Lancet. 1979;2:927–30.
2. Brenner DJ. Classification of legionellae. Semin Respir Infect. 1987;4:190–205.
3. Reingold A, Thomason B, Brake B, et al. *Legionella* pneumonia in the U.S.: the distribution of serogroups and species causing human illness. J Infect Dis. 1984;819–24.
4. Pasculle A, Myerowitz R, Rinaldo C. New bacterial agent of pneumonia isolated from renal transplant recipients. Lancet. 1979;2:58–61.
5. Rogers BH, Donowitz GR, Walker GK, et al. A clinicopathological study of five cases caused by an unidentified acid-fast bacterium. N Engl J Med. 1979;301:959–61.
6. Tatlock H. Studies on a virus from a patient with Fort Bragg fever (pretibial fever). Rev Infect Dis. 1982;4:147–56.
7. Hebert G, Moss CW, McDougal L, et al. The rickettsia-like organisms TATLOCK (1943) and HEBA (1959): bacteria phenotypically similar to but genetically distinct from *L. pneumophila* and the WIGA bacterium. Ann Intern Med. 1980;92:45–52.
8. Hebert GA, Steigerwalt AG, Brenner DJ. *Legionella micdadei* species nova: classification of a third species of legionella associated with human pneumonia. Curr Microbiol. 1980;3:255–7.
9. Garrity GM, Brown A, Vickers RM. *Tatlockia* and *Fluoribacter*: two new genera of organisms resembling *Legionella pneumophila*. Int J Syst Bacteriol. 1980;30:609–14.
10. Fang GD, Yu VL, Vickers RM. Disease due to the Legionellaceae (other than *Legionella pneumophila*): historical, microbiological, clinical and epidemiological review. Medicine. 1989;68:116–32.
11. Joly JR, Kenny GE. Antigenic analysis of *Legionella pneumophila* and *Tatlockia micdadei* (*Legionella micdadei*) by two-dimensional (crossed) immunoelectrophoresis. Infect Immun. 1982;35:721–9.
12. Collins MT, Bangsborg J, Hoiby N. Antigenic heterogeneity among *Legionella, Fluoribacter*, and *Tatlockia* species analyzed by crossed-immunoelectrophoresis. Int J Syst Bacteriol. 1987;37:351–6.
13. Ludwig W, Stackebrandt E. A phylogenetic analysis of *Legionella*. Arch Microbial. 1983;135:45–50.
14. Vickers RM, Yu VL. Clinical laboratory differentiation of Legionellaeae family members with pigment production and fluorescence on media supplemented with aromatic substrates. J Clin Microbiol. 1984;19:583–7.
15. Muder RR, Yu VL, Zuravleff JJ. Pneumonia due to the Pittsburgh pneumonia agent: new clinical perspective with a review of the literature. Medicine. 1983;62:120–8.
16. Yu VL, Zuravleff JJ, Elder E, et al. Pittsburgh pneumonia agent may be a common cause of nosocomial pneumonia—seroepidemiologic evidence. Ann Intern Med. 1982;97:724–5.
17. Myerowitz RL, Pasculle AW, Dowling JN, et al. Opportunistic lung infection due to "Pittsburgh pneumonia agent." N Engl J Med. 1979;301:953–8.
18. Hilton E, Freedman RA, Clintron F, et al. Acid-fast bacilli in sputum: a case of *Legionella micdadei* pneumonia. J Clin Microbiol. 1986;24:1102–3.
19. Vickers RM, Brown A, Garrity GM. Dye containing buffered charcoal yeast extract medium for the differentiation of members of the family *Legionellaceae*. J Clin Microbiol. 1981;13:380–2.
20. Hebert GA, Callaway CS, Ewing EP. Comparison of *Legionella pneumophila, L. micdadei, L. bozemanii*, and *L. dumoffii* by transmission electron microscopy. J Clin Microbiol. 1984;19:116–21.
21. Moss CW, Bibb W, Karr D, et al. Chemical analysis of the genus *Legionella*: fatty acids and isoprenoid quinones. Inserm. 1983;114:375–81.
22. Wilkinson H, Sampson J, Plikaytis B. Evaluation of a commercial gene probe for identification of *Legionella* cultures. J Clin Microbiol. 1986;23:217–20.
23. Butler C, Street E, Hatch T, et al. Disulfide-bonded outer membrane proteins in the genus *Legionella*. Infect Immun. 1985;48:14–8.
24. Sampson J, Plikaytis B, Wilkinson H. Immunologic response of patients with legionellosis against major protein-containing antigens of *L. pneumophila* serogroup 1 as shown by immunoblot analysis. J Clin Microbiol. 1986;23:92–9.
25. Best M, Yu VL, Stout J, et al. Legionellaceae in the hospital water supply—epidemiological link with disease and evaluation of a method of control of nosocomial legionnaries' disease and Pittsburgh pneumonia. Lancet. 1983;2:307–10.
26. Parry MF, Stampleman L, Hutchinson J, et al. Waterborne *Legionella bozemanii* and nosocomial pneumonia in immunosuppressed patients. Ann Intern Med. 1985;103:205–10.
27. Joly JR, Dery P, Gauvneau L, et al. Legionnaires' disease caused by *Legionella dumoffii* in distilled water. Can Med Assoc J. 1986;135:1274–7.
28. Palutke WA, Crane LR, Wentworth BB, et al. *Legionella feeleii*-associated pneumonia in humans. Am J Clin Pathol. 1986;86:348–51.
29. Best MG, Stout J, Yu VL, et al. *Tatlockia micdadei* growth kinetics may explain its infrequent isolation from water and the low prevalence of Pittsburgh pneumonia. Appl Environ Microbiol. 1985;49:1521–2.
30. Kallings I, Kallings LO. Epidemiologic patterns in legionellosis in Sweden. Zentralbl Bakteriol Hyg. 1983;A255–71, 75.
31. Fang GD, Yu VL, Vickers RM. Infections caused by the Pittsburgh pneumonia agent. Semin Respir Infect. 1987;2:262–66.
32. Muder RR, Yu VL, Woo AH. Mode of transmission of *Legionella pneumophila*: a critical review. Arch Intern Med. 1986;81:249–54.
33. Herwaldt LA, Gorman GW, McGrath J, et al. A new *Legionella* species, *Legionella feelii* species nova, causes Pontiac Fever in an automobile plant. Ann Intern Med. 1984;100:333–8.
34. Yu VL, Stout J, Zuravleff J, et al. Aspiration of contaminated water may be mode of transmission for *L. pneumophila*. Intersci Conf Antimicrob Agents Chemother. 1981;297.
35. Donegan EA, Deal MM, Melanephy MC, et al. Primary isolation of a new strain of the TATLOCK/Pittsburgh pneumonia agent (*Legionella micdadei*). West J Med. 1981;134:384–9.
36. Bozeman FM, Humphries JW, Campbell JM. A new group of *Rickettsia*-like agents recovered from guinea pigs. Acta Virol. 1968;12:87–93.
37. Thomason BM, Harris PP, Hicklin MD, et al. A *Legionella*-like bacterium related to WIGA in a fatal case of pneumonia. Ann Intern Med. 1979;91: 673–6.
38. Muder RR, Yu VL, Vickers R, et al. Simultaneous infection with *Legionella pneumophila* and Pittsburgh pneumonia agent—clinical features and epidemiologic implications. Am J Med. 1983;74:609–14.
39. Fumarola D, Miragliotta C, Logroscino G, et al. Simultaneous infection with

Legionella pneumophila and *Legionella micdadei* in an immunologically intact host. A case report. Boll 1st Sieroter Milan. 1984;63:165–6.
40. Tompkins LS, Troup NJ, Woods T, et al. Molecular epidemiology of *Legionella* species by restriction endonuclease and alloenzyme analysis. J Clin Microbiol. 1987;25:1875–80.
41. Tompkins LD, Roessler BJ, Redd SC, et al. *Legionella* prosthetic-valve endocarditis. N Engl J Med. 1988;318:530–5.
42. Wienn WC, Myerowitz RL. The pathology of the legionella pneumonias: a review of 74 cases and the literature. Hum Pathol. 1981;12:401–22.
43. Foltzer MA, Reese RE. Massive diarrhea in *Legionella micdadei* pneumonia. J Clin Gastroenterol. 1985;7:525–7.
44. Ampel NM, Ruben FL, Norden CW. Cutaneous abscess caused by *Legionella micdadei* in an immunosuppressed patient. Ann Intern Med. 1985;102:630–2.
45. Kovatch AL, Jardine DS, Dowling JN, et al. Legionellosis in children with leukemia in relapse. Pediatrics. 1984;73:811–5.
46. Ellis AR, Mayers DL, Martone WJ, et al. Rapid expanding pulmonary nodule caused by Pittsburgh pneumonia agent. JAMA. 1981;245:1558–9.
47. Mehta P, Patel JD, Milder JE. *Legionella micdadei* (Pittsburgh pneumonia agent): two infections with unusual clinical features. JAMA. 1983;249: 1620–3.
48. Wing EJ, Schafer FJ, Pasculle AW. The use of tracheal and pulmonary aspiration to diagnose *Legionella micdadei* pneumonia. Chest. 1982;82:705–7.
49. Wilkinson HW, Thacker WL, Benson RF, et al. *Legionella birminghamensis* sp. nov. isolated from cardiac transplant recipient. J Clin Microbiol. 1987;25:2120–2.
50. Thacker WL, Benson RF, Staneck JL, et al. *Legionella cincinnatiensis* sp. nov. isolated from a patient with pneumonia. J Clin Microbiol. 1988;26:418–20.
51. Muder RR, Yu VL, Parry MF. The radiologic manifestations of *Legionella* pneumonia. Semin Respir Infec. 1987;2:242–54.
52. Muder R, Reddy S, Yu VL, et al. Pneumonia caused by Pittsburgh pneumonia agent: radiologic manifestations. Radiology. 1984;150:633–7.
53. Tang PW, Sandu T, Moss CW, et al. *Legionella bozemanii* serogroup 2: a new etiological agent. J Clin Microbiol. 1984;19:30–33.
54. Ackley A. Community-acquired *Legionella micdadei* pneumonia (Letter). Lancet. 1981;1:221.
55. Boldur I, Brill S, Lahav M, et al. Legionnaires' disease: new etiologic agents. Isr J Med Sci. 1985;21:617–20.
56. Brettman LR, DeHertogh D, Rank EL, et al. *Legionella bozemanii* and empyema (Letter). Ann Intern Med. 1986;105:146–7.
57. Tang PW, Toma S, MacMillan LG. *Legionella oakridgensis*: laboratory diagnosis of a human infection. J Clin Microbiol. 1985;21:462–3.
58. Wilkinson HW, Thacker WL, Steigerwalt AG, et al. Second serogroup of *Legionella hackeliae* isolated from a patient with pneumonia. J Clin Microbiol. 1985;22:488–9.
59. Rudin JE, Evans TL, Wing EJ. Failure of erythromycin in treatment of *Legionella micdadei* pneumonia. Am J Med. 1984;76:318–20.
60. Pope TL, Armstrong P, Thompson R, et al. Pittsburgh pneumonia agent: chest film manifestations. AJR. 1982;138:237–41.
61. Rudin J, Wing E. Prospective study of pneumonia: unexpected incidence of legionellosis. South Med J. 1986;79:417–9.
62. Farr BM, Gratz J, Tartaglino J, et al. Evaluation of ultraviolet light for disinfection of hospital water contaminated with *Legionella*. Lancet. 1988;2:669–72.
63. Brenner DJ, Steigerwalt A, Gorman GW. *Legionella bozemanii*, sp nov and *Legionella dumoffi* sp nov: classification of two additional species of *Legionella* associated with human pneumonia. Curr Microbiol. 1980;4:111–6.
64. Lewallen KS, McKinney RM, Brenner DJ, et al. A newly identified bacterium phenotypically resembling, not genetically distinct from. *Legionella pneumophila*: an isolate in a case of pneumonia. Ann Intern Med. 1979;91: 831–4.
65. McKinney RM, Porschen RK, Edelstein PH, et al. *Legionella longbeachae* species nova, another etiologic agent of human pneumonia. Ann Intern Med. 1981;94:739–43.
66. Cherry WB, Gorman GW, Orrison LH, et al. *Legionella jordanis*: a new species of *Legionella* isolated from water and sewage. J Clin Microbiol. 1982;15:290–7.
67. Thacker WL, Wilkinson HW, Benson RF, et al. *Legionella jordanis* isolated from a patient with fatal pneumonia. J Clin Microbiol. 1988;28:1400–1.
68. Morris GK, Steigerwalt A, Feeley JC, et al. *Legionella gormanii* sp nov. J Clin Microbiol. 1980;12:718–21.
69. Griffith ME, Lindquist DS, Benson RF, et al. First isolation of *Legionella gormanii* from human disease. J Clin Microbiol. 1988;26:380–1.
70. Thacker WL, Wilkinson HW, Plikaytis BB, et al. Second serogroup of *Legionella feelii* strains isolated from humans. J Clin Microbiol. 1985;22:1–4.
71. Brenner DJ, Steigerwalt AG, Gorman GW, et al. Ten new species of *Legionella*. Int J Syst Bacteriol. 1985;35:50–9.
72. Wilkinson HW, Thacker WL, Brenner DJ, et al. Fatal *Legionella maceachernii* pneumonia. J Clin Microbiol. 1985;22:1055.
73. Edelstein PH, Brenner DJ, Moss CW, et al. *Legionella wadsworthii* species nova: a cause of human pneumonia. Ann Intern Med. 1982;97:809–13.
74. Orrison LH, Cherry WB, Tyndall RL, et al. *Legionella oakridgensis*. Unusual new species isolated from cooling tower water. Appl Environ Microbiol. 1983;45:536–45.
75. Wilkinson HW, Reingold AL, Brake BJ, et al. Reactivity of serum from patients with suspected legionellosis against 29 antigens of Legionellaceae and *Legionella*-like organisms by indirect immunofluorescence. J Infect Dis. 1983;147:23–31.
76. Edelstein PH, Pryor EP. A new biotype of *Legionella dumoffii*. J Clin Microbiol. 1985;21:641–2.

212. OTHER GRAM-NEGATIVE BACILLI

JOHN E. McGOWAN, JR.
CARLOS DEL RIO

On occasion, a physician is confronted with infection due to a gram-negative bacillus that does not belong to the groups most frequently encountered (described in previous chapters). A large number of additional gram-negative aerobic bacilli have been reported to cause human infection. However, most of these are rare sources of human disease. Therefore, this chapter will consider selected gram-negative organisms that are included because they are more frequently encountered, because they are of importance in certain clinical or epidemiologic circumstances (nosocomial infection, etc.), or because they present special problems of diagnosis or therapy. Clinical laboratories may identify some of these organisms by group or general description (e.g., "gram-negative nonfermenter," "pseudomonas-like organism") rather than by the level of genus and species. As a result, microbiologic classification and information about some agents considered here is imprecise and subject to refinement as more is learned about organism characteristics.

The initial suspicion of a particular organism from the group considered here often arises from preliminary laboratory data (Gram stain, etc.) implicating a gram-negative rod or from recovery of a gram-negative bacillus that is not a member of Enterobacteriaceae or *Pseudomonas aeruginosa*. The clinical site of infection and the ability of the organism to metabolize carbohydrates fermentatively (in the absence of air) allows an initial assessment of the likely etiology, as shown in Table 1. From such an assessment, the most effective way to provide definitive identification and to test susceptibility of the agent can be selected, inasmuch as some of these organisms require special procedures for antimicrobial susceptibility testing.[1,2] The organisms will be considered in the order in which they are listed in Table 1.

GLUCOSE FERMENTERS

Actinobacillus

The major pathogen of humans in this genus is *Actinobacillus actinomycetemcomitans*. Recent information has led to the proposal that the organism be reclassified as a species of *Haemophilus*.[3] However, common usage has continued to refer to the organism as *Actinobacillus*. Other strains of *Actinobacillus* (*lignieresii, equuli, suis, hominis*, and *capsulatis*) have been recovered from humans on occasion but primarily infect animals.[1]

Actinobacillus actinomycetemcomitans has been described as a human pathogen since 1912, but its role in earlier reports was unclear since it usually was one of polymicrobial isolates from a given site. By the early 1960s, however, recovery of this organism in pure culture from blood and other normally sterile body fluids was reported widely.[4] The name derives from an association with *Actinomyces israeli*, and there is a suggestion that the bacterium may make it possible for lesions typical of actinomycosis to persist even after *A. israeli* is no longer present.[5] Capsular material from this organism inhibits DNA

TABLE 1. Classification of Selected Gram-Negative Aerobic Bacilli by Likely Site of Infection and Biochemical Characteristics

	Most Likely Site of Infection				
Biochemical Group and Organism	*Blood Stream*	*Intestine*	*Soft Tissue*	*Bites*	*Urine*
Glucose fermenters					
Actinobacillus	X				
Aeromonas		X			
Capnocytophaga	X				
Cardiobacterium	X				
Chromobacterium			X		
CDC group DF-2	X				
CDC group DF-3		X			
CDC group EF-4				X	
Plesiomonas shigelloides		X			
Glucose nonfermenters (or weak fermenters)					
Achromobacter	X				
Agrobacterium	X				
Alcaligines	X				
CDC group IVc-2	X				
CDC group IVe (Oligella)					X
CDC group Vd	X				
Eikenella				X	
Flavobacterium[a]	X				
Sphingobacterium[a]	X			X	
Weeksella					X

[a] Weak fermenter.

and collagen synthesis, and the capsule may play an active role in tissue destruction associated with periodontal disease.[6] A bacteriocin ("actinobacillin") produced by the organism is inhibitory to other organisms often present in the mouth.[7] Ultrastructure and surface proteins of the organism vary, depending on whether the organism was cultured aerobically or anaerobically.[8] The organism shares an "enterobacterial common antigen" with Enterobacteriaceae and *Plesiomonas*.[9]

The organism is part of endogenous flora of the mouth and is recovered in patients with periodontal diseases, especially in juvenile periodontitis, a particularly severe localized and destructive form most common in adolescents.[10] *Actinobacillus actinomycetemcomitans* is one of the so-called HACEK organisms, along with *Haemophilus* species, *Cardiobacterium hominis, Eikenella corrodens*, and *Kingella kingii*, which have in common the need for incubation in an atmosphere enhanced with carbon dioxide for recovery in culture and a predilection for infecting the heart valve when causing human disease.[10a] Endocarditis (especially on damaged or prosthetic valves) and wound infection have remained the most frequent sites of *A. actinomycetemcomitans* infection outside the mouth, but pure culture of the organism in meningitis, deep abscess, osteomyelitis, urinary tract infection, and pericarditis have been reported.[11,12] The onset of endocarditis may be insidious, and the course may be protracted.[13] Many but not all patients with endocarditis also have periodontal disease.

Diagnosis of *A. actinomycetemcomitans* is not possible from direct smear, and serologic testing is still experimental[14,15]; therefore culture is the only readily available means, and the fastidious, slow-growing nature of the organism makes this difficult. Soft tissue lesions should be inoculated on blood and chocolate agar because the organism grows poorly on MacConkey agar. The cultures *must* be incubated in an enhanced (5–10 percent) CO_2 atmosphere. By 18–24 hours a few colonies (punctate, nonhemolytic) may be apparent, but the organism grows slowly, and incubation for at least 48 hours is needed. After colonies are seen, the organism continues to grow slowly, sometimes forming a star structure as part of the center of the mature colony. Selective culture media have been developed to enhance growth of the organism.[16] Similarly, the organism may not be apparent in conventional broth or blood culture for the first few days of incubation[17]; on occasion growth has been noted only after 25 days of incubation.[13] In tubes, the organism sometimes will grow only in small "granules" adherent to the sides, and the fluid will remain clear. In automated bacteremia detection systems the organism has been detected within 2–3 days.[13] The Gram stain appearance is coccoid to coccobacillary, similar to the *Haemophilus* strains with which classification is now proposed. Biochemical reactions distinguish *A. actinomycetemcomitans* from similar organisms (Table 2).

Actinobacillus actinomycetemcomitans usually is susceptible in laboratory testing to newer cephalosporins, rifampin, trimethoprim-sulfamethoxazole, aminoglycosides, ciprofloxacin, tetracycline, and chloramphenicol.[17,18] Testing of clinically important strains is required because susceptibility varies from strain to strain. The organism usually tests susceptible or relatively resistant to penicillins in the laboratory, but test result does not necessarily correlate with patient outcome.[11,14,18] Penicillin combined with an aminoglycoside has been the usual treatment for endocarditis due to this organism,[10a] although cephalosporins have been used with success in endocarditis and in one case of pericarditis where pericardiectomy was performed.[11,19] Vancomycin treatment, and prophylaxis with vancomycin and erythromycin have failed in at least one case of endocarditis, and the organism often is resistant to vancomycin and erythromycin.[17]

Recommendations for antimicrobial prophylaxis against endocarditis for patients with damaged heart values who undergo dental procedures apply to this organism as well as to other components of mouth flora.

Aeromonas

Aeromonads are members of the family Vibrionaceae, which are ubiquitous inhabitants of water where they cause disease in amphibians, reptiles, and fish. Four species are recognized: (1) *A. salmonicida*, not associated with disease in humans; (2) *A. hydrophila*; (3) *A. sobria*; and (4) *A caviae*. Three additional species recently have been proposed: *A. media, A. veronii,* and *A. schubertii*.[19a,19b] *A. hydrophila* was first isolated from human feces in 1937 by Miles and Halnan.[20] *Aeromonas* species have been reported as opportunistic pathogens in the immunocompromised host since 1968.[21] In 1981 the organism was first implicated in cases of severe gastroenteritis in Colombia. Since then, a number of reports have associated *Aeromonas* with gastroenteritis in humans[22–24]; however, some controversy about this role exists, partly because the mechanism that causes diarrhea is not clear and *Aeromonas* organisms are not easily isolated on routine enteric media.

The natural habitat of these organisms is water and soil,[25]

TABLE 2. Biochemical Reactions Distinguishing *Actinobacillus actinomycetemcomitans, Haemophilus aphrophilus, Capnocytophaga spp., Cardiobacterium hominis,* DF-2, and *Eikenella corrodens*

Test	A. actinomycetemcomitans	Haemophilus aphrophilus	Cardiobacterium hominis	Eikenella corrodens	Capnocytophaga	*DF-2*
Catalase	Positive	Negative	Negative	Negative	Negative	Positive
Oxidase	Varies	Varies	Positive	Positive	Negative	Positive
Indole	Negative	Negative	Positive	Negative	Negative	Negative
Nitrate reduction	Positive	Positive	Negative	Positive	Varies	Negative

which makes injury with direct exposure to contaminated water a common epidemiologic association in cases of *Aeromonas* infections such as cellulitis, osteomyelitis, and other soft tissue infections. In earlier literature *Aeromonas* was considered an opportunistic pathogen,[21,25] but more recent data indicate that *Aeromonas* can cause a variety of extraintestinal infections, not only in the immunocompromised but also in the healthy host.[26–28,28a]

In humans, four clinical syndromes can be described as part of the spectrum of *Aeromonas* infections: (1) acute diarrhea[22,29]; (2) cellulitis or wound infection,[27,30] usually associated with exposure to water or soil; (3) septicemia, often in immunocompromised patients, especially those with leukemia[31,32]; and (4) a variety of less frequent infections including intra-abdominal abscess,[33,34] hepatobiliary infections,[35] spontaneous bacterial peritonitis in patients with cirrhosis,[36] meningitis,[37] endocarditis,[25] osteomyelitis,[38] urinary tract infections,[34] aspiration pneumonia,[39] tonsillitis, and otitis media.[34] Surgical wound infections due to *Aeromonas hydrophilia* have complicated the use of leeches for wound debridement.[39a]

Acute Diarrhea. The most commonly associated clinical manifestation of *Aeromonas* infection has been diarrhea; studies from several countries, including the United States, show that *Aeromonas* can be recovered from stools of persons with diarrhea significantly more frequently than from asymptomatic controls.[22–24] Ingestion of contaminated water is likely to be the vehicle that permits access of *Aeromonas* to the intestinal tract. The prevalence of asymptomatic fecal carriage of *Aeromonas* varies from 0 percent[23] to approximately 25 percent; highest prevalence was found in Thailand,[24] which suggests that fecal carriage is related to the economic development of the country. *Aeromonas*-associated diarrhea is more frequent during the summer months.[23,40] The disease can present as a self-limited watery diarrhea of short duration, which may be severe enough in children to require hospitalization, or as a more chronic illness that can last more than 2 weeks. This latter presentation is more common in patients over the age of 12. Occasionally, the diarrhea may be so severe as to mimic cholera. Stool smears have not shown fecal leukocytes.[22] The exact mechanism for the diarrhea has not been worked out. A variety of virulence factors have been described including a cytotoxin that has DNA homology and immunologic cross-reactivity with cholera toxin,[41] heat-labile and heat-stable enterotoxins, hemagglutinins, and hemolysis. However, no correlation has been found between toxin production by *Aeromonas* spp. and gastroenteritis.[42]

Cellulitis. Injury with direct exposure to contaminated water is a common epidemiologic association in cases of wound infection, cellulitis, osteomyelitis, and myonecrosis (which can be associated with gas formation).[28] In the setting of a rapidly progressive cellulitis after an injury related to water exposure, *Aeromonas* spp. and *Vibrio vulnificus* infections should be considered in the differential diagnosis.

Sepsis in the Immunocompromised. The source of infection in these patients is a matter for debate because evidence exists in the literature for an endogenous source (i.e., gastrointestinal tract carriage with subsequent blood stream invasion) and exogenous sources such as percutaneous inoculation or nosocomial infection. It is thought that defective hepatic filtration in cirrhosis favors bacteremia with this intestinal inhabitant. *Aeromonas* invasion appears to be especially pathogenic to muscle; both necrotizing myositis and skin lesions of ecthyma gangrenosum have been seen in immunocompromised patients with *Aeromonas* sepsis.[43] *Aeromonas caviae* bacteremia has been described as part of polymicrobial sepsis in the immunocompromised host.[44]

Aeromonas organisms are gram-negative, nonsporulating facultative anaerobic rods that usually are β-hemolytic on blood agar and ferment carbohydrates with acid and gas production. Selective techniques often are necessary for the isolation of *Aeromonas* from mixed cultures. The organism grows well on MacConkey agar (some strains are lactose fermenters, and some are not), but growth on thiosulfate citrate bile salts sucrose (TCBS) medium is variable. In sterile fluid cultures aeromonads grow on standard media and are identified as would be any other gram-negative bacillus. In stool cultures their recognition is more difficult since enteric media is frequently inhibitory for some *Aeromonas* species. Trypticase soy agar supplemented with sheep blood and ampicillin (either 10 or 30 μg/ml) can be used as a selective medium.[29] Growth of colonies on plates usually occurs within 24 hours. *Aeromonas* species are oxidase-positive, and this test is key in separating these organisms from the oxidase-negative Enterobacteriaceae. However, the oxidase reaction may be falsely negative if done on growth from enteric differential media and should preferably be performed on growth from a blood agar plate. A positive oxidase test with a negative spot indole test should make one suspect *Aeromonas*. *Aeromonas hydrophila* is catalase-positive and motile, converts nitrate to nitrite, and is urease negative.[45]

Aeromonas hydrophila is resistant to ampicillin and other penicillins including the ureidopenicillins.[46,47] Sensitivity to tetracyclines is variable; susceptibility to third-generation cephalosporins is more likely than to the earlier cephalosporins. The organism is consistently sensitive to chloramphenicol, trimethoprim-sulfamethoxazole, the newer quinolones, aztreonam, and aminoglycosides except streptomycin.[48] Isolates of *A. sobria* have been shown to be more susceptible to cephalosporins and also are usually susceptible to gentamicin, tobramycin, trimethoprim-sulfamethoxazole, and the newer quinolones but vary in their susceptibility to chloramphenicol, tetracycline, ampicillin, carbenicillin, and amikacin.[48] Motyl et al. have suggested that susceptibility to cephalothin could be used as a potential marker for *A. sobria*.[49] Involvement of plasmids in the antibiotic resistance of *Aeromonas hydrophila* from humans has not been reported, but plasmid transfer exists in isolates from fish.[50] One *A. sobria* isolate has been found to contain a conjugative plasmid that confers multiple antibiotic resistance.[51] β-lactam resistance in *Aeromonas* spp. can be mediated by inducible β-lactamases.[51a]

Capnocytophaga

Capnocytophaga ("eater of carbon dioxide"), previously known as *Bacteroides ochraceus* and DF-1 ("dysgonic fermenter" or a fermenting organism that has difficulty growing in routine media) is a fusiform, gram-negative bacillus that is commonly isolated from the gingival sulcus in people with or without periodontal disease and from periodontal lesions in patients with idiopathic juvenile periodontitis. Recently the importance of this pathogen has been recognized in the granulocytopenic patient with oral mucosal ulcerations.[52,53,53a]

During the 1960s, the Centers for Disease Control (CDC) differentiated a group of thin, gram-negative, saccharolytic rods that were designated as group DF-1. By colony morphology, biochemical features, and DNA homology, *Bacteroides ochraceus*, DF-1, and a group of organisms designated *Capnocytophaga* were demonstrated to be synonymous.[54,55] It was suggested that the latter should be the preferred name.[54] The genus consists of three species, *C. ochracea, C. sputigena*, and *C. gingivalis*.

The mouth appears to be the major habitat of this bacterium[56], where it is important in the etiology of periodontal infections.[57] Indeed, the location of clinical infections suggests the oral cavity or the upper respiratory tract as the site of origin.

Several series suggest that *Capnocytophaga* septicemia is more common in children than in adults.[52,53,58] Whether granulocytopenic children are more likely than are adults to develop oral mucosal defects is unclear. Several virulence factors have been described. Shurin et al. described morphologic and functional abnormalities in neutrophils obtained from two patients with *Capnocytophaga* infections.[59] Sonicates and culture medium of *Capnocytophaga* contained a dialyzable substance that could induce similar changes in neutrophils obtained from normal donors. Wilson et al. have found that isolates of *Capnocytophaga* from blood show considerable serum resistance when compared with isolates from human subgingival plaque.[60] A change in liposaccharide structure was thought responsible for increased serum resistance of blood isolates. β-Lactamase production has been demonstrated in *C. ochracea*.[61]

Capnocytophaga is a cause of serious, life-threatening infections in immunocompromised patients, especially granulocytopenic patients with oral ulcerations. However, infections due to this organism, including bacteremia and endocarditis, have been described in nonimmunocompromised hosts as well.[53a,62–65] The organism also is associated with juvenile periodontitis.

Capnocytophaga are facultatively anaerobic or microaerophilic, capnophilic, fusiform, and dysgonically fermenting gram-negative rods. Their gliding motility on the surface of certain agar media is similar in appearance to *Proteus* spp. but unique in that *Capnocytophaga* organisms do not have flagellae. Organism recovery is most certain from blood or chocolate agar under anaerobic conditions or in the presence of 5–10% CO_2. It may take 2–3 days of incubation before colonies (yellow, nonhemolytic) are apparent. The organisms do not grow on MacConkey agar, and selective media may enhance recovery.[66] Catalase, oxidase, urease, citrate, and indole reactions are all negative. Differentiating characteristics from similar organisms are shown in Table 2. An important differential diagnosis from the laboratory standpoint is the more commonly isolated *Fusobacterium nucleatum*. Strains of *Capnocytophaga* differ from *F. nucleatum* by their ability to ferment carbohydrates, ability to produce succinic and acetic acid, and lack of ability to produce indole.

Special supplementation of the test medium is needed to assess antimicrobial susceptibility. Testing to date suggests that clindamycin, penicillin, ampicillin, antipseudomonal penicillins, imipenem, erythromycin, tetracycline, chloramphenicol, newer quinolones, newer cephalosporins, and metronidazole all may be effective agents.[67,68] Susceptibility results vary for aztreonam, vancomycin, and older cephalosporins, but the organisms usually are resistant to trimethoprim and aminoglycosides.[69,70]

Cardiobacterium

Cardiobacterium hominis is one of the so-called HACEK organisms along with *Haemophilus aphrophilus, Actinobacillus actinomycetemcomitans, Eikenella corrodens*, and *Kingella kingii*, which have in common the need for incubation in an atmosphere enhanced with carbon dioxide for recovery in culture and a predilection for the heart valve when causing human disease.[10a] *Cardiobacterium hominis*, the only species in the genus, originally was called group IID and described as a *Pasturella*-like organism. It is a part of the endogenous flora in the nose, mouth, and throat, has been found occasionally on other mucous membranes, and may be present in the gastrointestinal tract as well.[71] Why the organism is so prone to settle in on heart valves, given its relatively low virulence for infecting other sites, is unclear. Large vegetations and large vessel emboli are characteristic.

Virtually all clinical isolates come from blood, although associated meningitis has been noted as well.[72] Most infected patients have had underlying anatomic defects of the heart valve (rheumatic heart disease, ventricular septal defect, congenital bicuspid valve, etc.); prosthetic cardiac valves have been involved in about 10 percent of reported cases.[73] Many of the patients have had severe periodontitis, often including prior dental procedures without antimicrobial prophylaxis. A subacute presentation with insidious onset (mean of 2–5 months before diagnosis) and the absence of fever at the time of diagnosis is likely.[74] Some of the patients have splenomegaly, anemia, and hematuria, which is consistent with a long period between infection and diagnosis.

The organism is gram-negative but has a pleomorphic appearance, sometimes has swelling of one or both ends, and may be hard to decolorize during the Gram stain procedure.[1] Under the microscope the organisms sometimes form rosettes, but short chains, teardrops, pairs, and clusters are common as well. Supplementation of the medium with yeast extract results in loss of the pleomorphism, and most organisms will become "sticklike" gram-negative rods with rounded ends.[71] Incubation in high humidity and increased (3–5%) carbon dioxide tension maximize recovery of the organism. In such conditions, *Cardiobacterium hominis* grows well on sheep blood agar, chocolate agar, Mueller-Hinton agar, or trypticase soy agar without blood, but grows poorly on MacConkey agar or similar selective media. Colonies of 1–2 mm in diameter form on sheep blood agar, usually by 48–72 hours after incubation at 37°C under increased CO_2 pressure. However, incubation of 5–7 days before growth can be confirmed is not unusual, and cultures should be held for this period if *Cardiobacterium hominis* is suspected.[75] The colonies produce slight α-hemolysis, glisten, and develop a rough appearance, with a serpentine pattern of growth from the edge to adjacent colonies.[71] Identification is made by biochemical testing, as in Table 2; the organism is oxidase-positive, produces indole (although it may take testing of a colony at least 48 hours old for this to be apparent), and is catalase-negative.[1] Serologic testing (fluorescent antibody method) is not standardized and has not become widely available[71]

Susceptibility tests are difficult to perform because of the slow-growing nature of the organism and its growth requirements. When tested, the organism usually is susceptible to β-lactam drugs, chloramphenicol, and tetracycline. Susceptibility to vancomycin, aminoglycosides, erythromycin, and clindamycin has been variable. Penicillin G, with or without the addition of an aminoglycoside, has been the regimen most often employed for therapy. Although microbiologic cure has been achieved frequently, complications have arisen during the course of therapy quite often; systemic embolization, mycotic aneurysm, or progressive cardiac failure have necessitated replacement of the damaged valve in a number of cases.

Chromobacterium

Chromobacterium violaceum is a well-known organism in the southeastern United States where it occasionally is involved in human infection. The organism is a soil and water inhabitant, especially in tropical areas; cases have been reported as well from the northeastern United States, Southeast Asia, and South America.[76] Some strains produce proteases that may be involved in the pathogenesis of human illness. *C. violaceum* now is the only important species causing human disease; *Chromobacterium typhiflavium* now has been reclassified as a Ve-1 strain of *Pseudomonas*, and other species are not known to be pathogenic for humans. Most strains of this organism produce violacein, a pigment insoluble in water (as opposed to the water-soluble pyocyanin of *Pseudomonas*) that imparts a violet-black color to the colonies on solid media. The color may be lost on subculture or after therapy is begun. The organisms produce extracellular products that enhance the activity of β-lactam inhibitors against gram-negative organisms.[77]

Infected patients usually acquire the organism as a result of trauma leading to contamination with soil or water or by ingesting contaminated water. Resulting infection involves urinary tract, gut, or blood stream invasion, with or without an obvious primary focus. An underlying defect of host defenses, especially of the neutrophils, seems to predispose to infection, but a number of cases are described in patients with no known host factor dysfunction. Patients with chronic granulomatous disease appear susceptible, regardless of geographic location.[78] A deficiency of polymorphonuclear leukocyte glucose-6-phosphate dehydrogenase and neutrophil dysfunction also were present in a 3-year-old patient who died with *Chromobacterium violaceum* sepsis.[79] Fever is often high, and spread through the blood stream often leads to secondary sites of infection such as osteomyelitis and abscess in the lung, liver, or abdomen. Reported skin findings include pustular dermatitis, cellulitis, or ulceration.[80,81]

Diagnosis is made by culture of blood, abscess fluid, or skin exudate; serologic tests are not available. Gram stain appearance of the organisms is that of gram-negative long bacilli; occasionally, the organisms will have a slight curve, which makes confusion with vibrios possible. The organisms are facultatively anaerobic and grow readily in 18–24 hours on media containing tryptophan, which include common laboratory media such as sheep blood agar, chocolate agar, Mueller-Hinton agar, trypticase soy broth, and MacConkey agar. Incubation at 30–35°C usually is effective, although growth is enhanced if incubation occurs at 25°C. The organism produces colonies with a violet pigment (hence the species name). The organisms produce hydrogen cyanide, so a faint cyanide smell may be present; the urease and citrate reactions are variable. The oxidase reaction is usually positive but hard to detect in pigmented strains—sometimes demonstrating oxidase can be enhanced by incubating the culture anaerobically, which inhibits pigment formation.[76] Indole reactions are weak and catalase reactions usually are negative.[1] A few strains do not produce pigment, so they may be confused with *Plesiomonas* or *Aeromonas* unless results of indole production are assessed.

Chromobacterium violaceum strains usually are susceptible in the laboratory to chloramphenicol, tetracycline, trimethoprim-sulfamethoxazole, and gentamicin. They are variably susceptible to penicillins and the other aminoglycosides but resistant to most cephalosporins.[76,80] Erythromycin appears ineffective regardless of the susceptibility testing results.[80] Relapse has occurred more than 2 weeks after completion of therapy and apparent cure.[76] Despite therapy, more than half of the reported patients have died, which may reflect the underlying defects in host defenses in most of the victims or late recognition of the etiology.

CDC Group DF-2

DF-2 is the name given to a group of slow-growing gram-negative rod-shaped organisms that have been collected by the CDC. The initials DF stand for "dysgonic fermenter," indicating that these fermentative organisms have difficulty growing in routine media. The first group of dysgonic fermentative organisms (DF-1) contained bacterial strains now recognized as species of *Capnocytophaga*. On the basis of cellular fatty acid composition, DF-2 and IIj may well be additional species of *Flavobacterium*.[82]

The exact reservoir of DF-2 in nature is not known; however, most patients have a history of exposure to oral secretions of a dog, and about half of the cases have followed a dog bite,[83] which suggests that the infection is likely zoonotic.[84] Martone et al. were successful in isolating the organism from the mouth of a patient's dog,[85] and one survey showed DF-2 present in the gingival crevices of 21 percent of dogs and 18 percent of cats.[86] It should be noted, however, that cases of DF-2 infection have occurred without a history of close animal contact.[87]

Although DF-2 is clearly a pathogen, its apparently low virulence is reflected by the rarity of infection in normal hosts. Butler et al.[88] used an experimental rabbit model of endocarditis to show that prior treatment with methylprednisone increased the incidence of bacteremia as well as the number of bacteria per gram of vegetation. Hicklin et al.[83] found that a clinical isolate was serum sensitive; if this applied to the entire genus, it may partly explain the low virulence of the isolates in general. These organisms have been documented to cause fulminating disease, particularly in asplenic persons, alcoholics, and patients receiving corticosteroids.[83,87,89] However, cases also have been reported in people in apparently good health.[90] Splenectomized patients are at risk for developing overwhelming infections with encapsulated bacteria; however, it is not clear why they are also at risk for severe DF-2 infection. Hinrichs and Dunkelberg[91] studied the immune response in a splenectomized patient with DF-2 sepsis. They suggested that a lack of an IgM response was in part responsible for the severity of illness.

Two distinct clinical patterns of illness with DF-2 organisms can be seen. The first is seen primarily in splenectomized patients or patients with cirrhosis and is characterized by shock and disseminated intravascular coagulation.[92] The second pattern of illness is seen more often in individuals with intact spleen and is generally a milder presentation. Cases of meningitis, endocarditis, pneumonia, cellulitis, corneal perforation, and septic arthritis with these organisms have been described.

The organisms can be recovered from blood agar and usually produce punctate colonies after 24 hours of incubation at 35°C in enhanced CO_2 (although in some cases colonies are not detected until the fifth day of incubation). Later they become larger, convex, and smooth, often with a narrow flat edge at the margin of confluent growth and with a bluish-purple hue on blood agar. They do not grow on MacConkey agar but are readily recovered from most blood culture media. Cellular morphology varies with the medium in which the organism is grown; the Gram stain appearance may resemble *Fusobacterium*. There have been some difficulties in subculturing DF-2 from blood culture media, so heart infusion agar (HIA) with 5% rabbit blood incubated for at least 5 days in an environment with enhanced CO_2 is felt to be the best way to subculture the organism.[75,93] However, adequate growth often occurs upon subculture onto sheep blood agar or chocolate agar. In order to show their fermentative characteristics, the organisms need to be grown in carbohydrate broths supplemented with 1.5–3% serum.[93] Biochemically, these organisms are oxidase-positive (although the reaction is often weak), catalase-positive, and *O*-nitrophenyl-β-D-galactosidase (ONPG)-positive. They ferment lactose and maltose. Distinguishing characteristics from similar organisms are shown in Table 2. Examination of the buffy coat by Gram stain is useful in DF-2 infections, especially when the victim has been splenectomized.[94]

Special supplementation of the test medium is needed to assess antimicrobial susceptibility. Isolates of the organism have been shown to be susceptible to penicillins, cephalosporins, imipenem, vancomycin, clindamycin, rifampin, chloramphenicol, ciprofloxacin, and erythromycin; results for trimethoprim-sulfa are variable, and the organisms have tested resistant to aztreonam.[83,95] Resistance to the aminoglycosides is frequent when testing is done by disk diffusion or agar dilution assays, but the same organism may be susceptible when tested by broth dilution.[95] Penicillin is a usual drug for the treatment of a dog bite because both DF-2 and *Pasturella multocida* are susceptible and both may be involved in bites.

It has been suggested that prophylactic penicillin may be warranted for asplenic persons after a dog bite.[83] Further suggested prevention is that splenectomized individuals not keep cats or dogs.[87]

CDC Group DF-3

The organism known as DF-3 (third group of dysgonic fermenters) is distinguished from DF-2 (see above) by negative catalase and oxidase reactions, production of indole by most strains, and fermentation of sucrose and xylose.[96] The organism appears small and coccobacillary and is gram-negative on smear. It produces grey-white colonies with a sweetish odor on blood agar after 1–3 days of incubation. It was detected by the use of cefoperazone-vancomycin agar, a selective medium, for a stool culture of *Campylobacter*. It does not grow on routine enteric media.

DF-3 has been isolated repeatedly from the stools of a patient with common variable hypogammaglobulinemia and chronic diarrhea.[96] The organism was susceptible to carbenicillin, chloramphenicol, tetracycline, clindamycin, and trimethoprim-sulfamethoxazole; it was resistant to most β-lactam drugs, ciprofloxacin, metronidazole, vancomycin, and erythromycin. After therapy with tetracycline, the organism was eradicated, and the patient's symptoms resolved. A second patient in the same report with the same diseases also had a positive stool culture and improved after treatment with tetracycline. A similar organism was isolated from blood of a neutropenic patient.[96a] Although the organism has been recovered from a variety of human sources, these are the only cases suggesting a role in infection.

CDC Group EF-4

Another group of gram-negative bacilli not yet known by genus and species also are defined by the CDC system of letters and numbers defining their microbiologic characteristics. Organisms of group EF-4 belong to the "eugonic fermenters" (organisms that grow well through fermentation of carbohydrates) and were the fourth group so described. Human infection most frequently is associated with human wound infection after dog or cat bites. Bacteremia is rare after such infection but has been reported in a patients with hepatic carcinoma who denied a bite by a dog or cat.[97]

EF-4 bacteria usually appears as short rods on Gram stain, but small coccal forms or long chains of cells also may be present. The organisms grow well on blood agar plates, on which colonies usually form within 24 hours, but grow poorly or not at all on MacConkey and similar agars. The colonies are small and may be slightly yellow-orange in color and smooth; some describe a "popcornlike odor" to the plates after colonies are present.[1] The organisms are oxidase-positive and catalase-positive and reduce nitrate; they are urease-negative and indole-negative. Most of these organisms do not ferment any other sugars besides glucose (defined as group EF-4a); a group of organisms closely related in morphology and growth characteristics do not ferment glucose or any other carbohydrate (group EF-4b). Whether this biochemical distinction has any clinical import is not clear because the latter organisms also have been recovered primarily from wound infections after a cat or dog bite.

A patient with EF-4 bacteremia who was treated with cefazolin and tobramycin remained ill, and the organism was isolated again from blood after therapy was discontinued. The organisms have been tested susceptible to β-lactam drugs, chloramphenicol, tetracycline, and some aminoglycosides in the laboratory, but standardized testing methods and clinical relevance of laboratory testing have not yet been defined.[97]

Plesiomonas shigelloides

This organism, a member of the family Vibrionaceae, has emerged as an enteric pathogen as well as the etiologic agent of various extraintestinal infections.[98,99] The organism was originally isolated in 1947, given the name C27, and designated a member of thc paracolon group of the family Enterobacteriaceae. Later, it was placed in the genus *Plesiomonas*. However, recent studies suggest a common phylogenetic relation between the plesiomonads and the family Enterobacteriaceae, and a proposal has been made to reassign *Plesiomonas* to the tribe Proteaceae.[100] There is only one species in the genus, *Plesiomonas shigelloides*; this organism has been referred to in the literature as C27, *Pseudomonas shigelloides, Aeromonas shigelloides*, or *Vibrio shigelloides*.

P. shigelloides is a water- and soil-associated organism that replicates at temperatures above 8°C. It is found primarily in freshwater or estuary environments within temperate and tropical climates, but it may also be isolated from seawater during the warm-weather months. The usual vehicles of transmission of plesiomonads to humans are food,[99] water, and a variety of animals who may be colonized with the organism. Thus, ingestion of contaminated water or food (such as oysters,[101] shrimp, or chicken[102]), exposure to animals[103] or contaminated waters, and foreign travel[99] could result in transmission of these bacteria. *Plesiomonas shigelloides* usually is considered part of the normal intestinal flora of humans, but up to 3 percent of stool specimens from persons without gastrointestinal disease will grow this organism. The organism produces a cholera-like toxin of unclear importance.[104]

The organism is associated with gastroenteritis[99]; however, failure so far to identify an enteropathogenic mechanism and unsuccessful studies to induce disease in volunteers[105] make it impossible to firmly establish a causal relationship of diarrhea and *Plesiomonas shigelloides*. *P. shigelloides*-associated gastroenteritis is probably underrecognized. Its clinical presentation varies from a mild-self-limited illness to mucoid, bloody diarrhea with polymorphonuclear leukocytes found on fecal smears. The organism is also an infrequent cause of extraintestinal disease, with bacteremia, osteomyelitis,[106] septic arthritis,[107] meningitis,[108] endophthalmitis, cholecystitis, and cellulitis having been reported. Disease produced by this organism seems to be more severe in immunosuppressed patients, who more often develop systemic infection.[109,110]

Plesiomonas shigelloides is a motile, facultatively anaerobic, gram-negative, oxidase-positive bacillus. It is readily isolated from some enteric agars such as MacConkey agar but does not grow well on TCBS medium. Selective techniques may be necessary for isolation of the organism from mixed cultures such as the use of bile peptone broth or trypticase soy broth with ampicillin.[111] The organism grows well at 35°C and produces visible colonies (nonhemolytic) within 24 hours. The organism does not ferment lactose on most enteric agars.

Plesiomonas shigelloides is susceptible to chloramphenicol, tetracycline, trimethoprim-sulfamethoxazole, the aminoglycosides, newer quinolones, imipenem, and third-generation cephalosporins.[45,112,113] Each clinical isolate must be tested because there is great variation from strain to strain. There is increasing resistance to penicillins, which may be due to an inducible β-lactamase similar to that produced by *Aeromonas*.[114]

GLUCOSE NONFERMENTERS (OR WEAK FERMENTERS)

Achromobacter

The genus *Achromobacter* is an enigma to many classification systems; the main species of clinical importance, *Achromobacter xylosoxidans*, now is known in some taxonomic circles as *Alcaligines denitrificans* biotype *xylosoxidans* and in others as *Alcaligenes xylosoxidans* subspecies *xylosoxidans*[115] and appears under *Alcaligines* in *Index Medicus*. However, the name *Achromobacter xylosoxidans* still appears in the clinical literature up to the time this chapter was written, and tests to implement identification by the newer taxonomic criteria are infrequently available in clinical laboratories.[2] Thus, the term *Achromobacter xylosoxidans* will be used in this section. Another organism formerly considered part of the *Achromobacter* genus, the organism known as CDC group Vd, also is not classified consistently in current systems and will be considered separately below.

Achromobacter strains probably are part of the endogenous flora of the ear and gastrointestinal tract and are common contaminants of fluids.[115,116] The organisms resist several commonly employed antimicrobials and disinfectants, qualities aiding their increasing role as a nosocomial pathogen. They produce several types of β-lactamases that hydrolyze a number of the penicillins and older cephalosporins; these enzymes can be plasmid mediated.[117]

Clinical illness due to *Achromobacter* has involved isolates from blood, peritoneal and pleural fluids, urine, respiratory secretions, and wound exudates. Biliary tract sepsis, meningitis (sometimes with lymphocytic predominance in cerebrospinal fluid), pneumonia, peritonitis, urinary tract infection, and bacteremia (including endocarditis on prosthetic valves) have been reported.[115,118,118a] The organism has been implicated in outbreaks of nosocomial infection associated with contaminated fluids (intravenous fluids, hemodialysis fluid, irrigation fluids, mouthwash, etc.), with incubators and humidifiers, and with contaminated soaps and disinfectants.[118,119] Contamination of well water used by the patient was documented in one case of bacteremia.[115] Patients who have been infected often have compromised host defenses, but this is not always the case, especially in nosocomial outbreaks. The organism has been recovered from the eye, ear, and pharynx, but its pathogenic potential in these sites is unproved.

The organism appears as a gram-negative rod on Gram stain. Strains of *Achromobacter xylosoxidans* grow well on blood agar plates; produce flat, spreading, and rough colonies; and have peritrichous flagellae, features that help distinguish it from *Pseudomonas*. The organisms are oxidase-positive, catalase-positive, citrate-positive, and urease-negative, use acetate as the only source of carbon, and oxidize glucose to produce acid. While they may not ferment glucose, they (as the species name indicates) oxidize xylose readily.[119] An isolate of *Achromobacter* can easily be mistaken for a non-*aeruginosa* strain of *Pseudomonas* unless the unusual susceptibility pattern suggests the correct identity.

Usually strains of *Achromobacter xylosoxidans* are susceptible in laboratory testing to a few β-lactam drugs (carbenicillin, piperacillin, some third-generation cephalosporins, imipenem, ticarcillin combined with clavulanic acid) and trimethoprim-sulfamethoxazole.[120] Generally they are resistant to ampicillin, first- and second-generation cephalosporins, the aminoglycosides, and newer fluoroquinolones and vary in response to chloramphenicol, erythromycin, rifampin, and tetracycline.[2,45,113] Similar resistance patterns can be demonstrated by a variety of unrelated strains.[117]

Agrobacterium

Organisms of the genus *Agrobacterium* are well known as plant pathogens, but their role in human disease has become clear only recently. The organisms are present in soil and plants, and the mode by which humans are infected is unclear. Many species are known; *Agrobacterium radiobacter* and organisms of the *Agrobacterium* "yellow group" are the only strains implicated in human disease. An interesting feature of this species is the production of exogenous products typical of the monobactam group of antibiotics.[121]

Prosthetic valve endocarditis, urinary tract infection, septicemia, and peritonitis are among the clinical entities due to *Agrobacterium*.[121–123] The organism was repeatedly recovered from the blood of an elderly patient in France; the patient had been hospitalized for 2 months before the episode of sepsis and had received netilmicin, fosfomycin, amikacin, and mezlocillin before the positive blood cultures. The patient had no known site of trauma leading to inoculation. One patient with urinary tract infection, one with cranial wound infection, and four with peritonitis also are described; in some of these cases the clinical histories raise the possibility of nosocomial infection.[123]

The organism readily grows on blood agar and MacConkey media when incubated aerobically. Colony appearance varies for the different species. Flagellar stains show peritrichous distribution, and strains are catalase-positive and nitrate-positive and oxidize glucose and xylose. Oxidase tests results vary from strain to strain. Rapid hydrolysis of urea, slower hydrolysis of esculin, and oxidation of lactose are key features that help to distinguish this organism from *Achromobacter* spp. and *Pseudomonas* spp., which it otherwise closely resembles. Production of 3-ketolactose is characteristic of the genus, but at least one clinical isolate lacked this ability. In doubtful circumstances, assimilation tests can aid definitive identification, and antibody against the recovered organism has been demonstrated after bacteremia.[122]

Susceptibility of *Agrobacterium radiobacter* has been tested in only a few instances. Isolates from clinical infections have been susceptible to trimethoprim-sulfamethoxazole and chloramphenicol, variably susceptible to β-lactams and aminoglycosides, and resistant to most other tested drugs; septicemia resolved in one case after therapy with cefotaxime, and a strain from a urinary tract infection was susceptible to most penicillins and first- and second-generation cephalosporins but resistant to ceftazidime and aztreonam.[121,122] Bacteremia has persisted during therapy with mezlocillin and amikacin. Newer quinolones have been active against *Agrobacter* spp. in laboratory testing.[113] The "yellow group" organisms have generally shown a more resistant pattern; four tested strains were susceptible to ticarcillin and sulfa and resistant to other tested drugs.[123]

Alcaligenes

Organisms of the *Alcaligenes* genus are another group of nonfermenting gram-negative bacilli found in soil and water, they can also be recovered from the human respiratory tract and gastrointestinal tract in hospitalized patients. Infection results when they are introduced into wounds or colonize those with compromised host defenses. Many of the strains produce β-lactamases, which makes therapy more difficult.[124] In addition, resistance to antimicrobials is enhanced by the extremely small size of diffusion pores in the organism.[125]

The nomenclature of *Alcaligenes* is as confused as any in current clinical taxonomy and changes frequently. Four clinically relevant species are described: *A. denitrificans* (some consider *Achromobacter xylosoxidans* to be a subspecies of this organism), *A. odorans*, *A. piechaudii*, and *A. faecalis*. The last of these is most commonly isolated in clinical microbiology laboratories and can be recovered in a variety of clinical settings. Most isolates of *Alcaligenes faecalis* from blood or respiratory secretions are related to contamination of hospital equipment or fluids with the organism, with resulting human invasion. The organism is seldom a pathogen in urine, and its recovery often serves as a marker for fecal contamination of the urine specimen. It has been described as a part of endogenous skin flora as well. *Alcaligenes odorans* has been found in ear discharges, wounds, sputum, and feces.[2] It is rarely recovered in pure culture from any of these sites. *A. piechaudii* has been recovered from ear discharge.[125a] By contrast, *A. denitrificans* has been recovered as a single pathogen from blood, cerebrospinal fluid, and other normally sterile body fluids as well as in mixed culture from sites usually containing normal flora. Few recent publications have addressed the pathogenic role of these organisms.

Identification of *Alcaligenes* is made by recovery of oxidase-positive, catalase-positive, indole-negative, and urease-negative organisms with flat, spreading edges on blood agar plates. Aerobic incubation is crucial for recovery in culture, and the organisms grow well at 35°C. The organism will also grow on MacConkey agar, unlike the usual strain of *Flavobacterium* or *Eikenella*. One of the species (*A. odorans*) produces a distinctive sweet odor resembling apple cider or strawberries.[2] Distinguishing the organisms and/or confirming identification is made difficult by their lack of reactivity in many biochemical or assimilation tests.[126]

Laboratory testing often shows *Alcaligenes* susceptible to trimethoprim-sulfamethoxazole, with results varying for aminoglycosides and β-lactam drugs; newer fluoroquinolones are variable in their effects but organisms are generally resistant.[113] Nosocomial strains are resistant more often to commonly used drugs.

CDC Group IVc-2

This extremely rare, unusual gram-negative nonfermentative bacillus has been reported to have caused septicemia in two patients during the past few years.[127,128] One of the patients, reported from Israel, had newly diagnosed plasma cell leukemia. In a second case, from the United States, a nosocomial onset of bacteremia developed after arteriography and thrombolectomy in a patient who had no recognized abnormality of host defenses. The reservoir of the organism is assumed to be water and fluids, and bacteremia seemed to arise from wound infection in at least one case.[127]

Organisms of CDC group IVc2 grow well on sheep and horse blood agar as well as on MacConkey agar at 37°C. Short gram-negative rods, oocasionally in chains, are seen on Gram stain. The organisms are motile; have peritrichous flagella; and are oxidase-, citrate-, and urease-positive and negative for nitrate reduction.

Clinical isolates are resistant to ampicillin, cephalothin, cefamandole, aminoglycosides, and chloramphenicol but susceptible to most of the newer β-lactams including ureidopenicillins, third-generation cephalosporins, and imipenem.[127,128] Susceptibility to trimethoprim-sulfamethoxazole has varied in the reported cases.

CDC Group IVe (Oligella)

It now is proposed that these gram-negative bacilli, which were formerly known as CDC group IVe, be called *Oligella ureolytica* because they are able to hydrolyze urea easily.

The likely setting for *Oligella* infection is a patient with a chronic indwelling urinary catheter or other drainage system. The organism's ability to hydrolyze urea may be related to a propensity for the patient to develop urinary stones, perhaps after alkalinization of the urine and precipitation of phosphates. Most clinical isolates come from urine or from secondary blood stream invasion after obstruction of the urinary tract develops. Isolates may be associated with symptomatic urinary tract infection, but many also are recovered from patients with asymptomatic bacteriuria.

Recognition of *Oligella ureolytica* is aided by appearance on Gram stain of pleomorphic gram-negative coccobacilli, with filamentous structures also seen in some cases. Most strains will grow on blood or MacConkey agar but require extended incubation (2–4 days) before growth can be detected. The rapidity of the urease reaction (within 5 minutes on a Christensen urea agar slant) is a distinctive feature. The organism has positive oxidase, motility, and catalase reactions and reduces nitrates to N_2. Most other biochemical reactions are negative.

Aminoglycosides and cephalosporins are agents to which group IVe organisms most often are susceptible.[129] The organisms resist usual serum concentrations of ampicillin, chloramphenicol, erythromycin, penicillin G, tetracycline, and trimethoprim-sulfamethoxazole.

CDC Group Vd

CDC Group Vd is considered part of the *Achromobacter* group in some classifications; those who have reassigned *Achromobacter xylosoxidans* to the genus *Alcaligenes* leave Vd as a free-standing category without genus or species designation. These organisms are similar to *Alcaligenes* and *Pseudomonas* species in their distribution in water, soil, and gastrointestinal tract.[130]

The organisms are generally similar to *Achromobacter xylosoxidans* in biochemical characteristics but hydrolyze urea and grow poorly on cetrimide agar.[2] Two colony morphotypes are seen; one is a small watery translucent colony, with mucoid areas of confluent growth after 48 hours of incubation, while the second, less-common type is pinpoint in size after 24 hours, with a grayish appearance after another 24 hours of incubation.[2,119] The organism grows easily on MacConkey agar, with a large, sticky cell mass on the surface. The organisms oxidize glucose and xylose, but 72 hours or more of incubation may be required before this is apparent. As is true for *A. xylosoxidans*, the organisms have positive catalase and oxidase reactions.[130a]

While the organism has been isolated from a number of human specimen sources including blood, urine, wound, stool, throat, and vagina, it is implicated as the etiologic agent in few; pancreatic abscess, bacteremia in patients with compromised host defenses, nosocomial urinary tract infection, and osteochondritis associated with a nail puncture wound of the foot are described, the first three in patients with compromised host defenses.[130,130a,131] The organisms usually are susceptible to trimethoprim-sulfamethoxazole and imipenem; they differ from *Achromobacter xylosoxidans* in that they sometimes are susceptible to gentamicin (but variably susceptible to other aminoglycosides). One strain tested against norfloxacin was susceptible in vitro, but the patient did not respond to therapy with this drug.[130a]

Eikenella

Eikenella corrodens is a fastidious facultative anaerobic gram-negative bacillus that is part of the normal human oral flora. Henriksen in 1948 identified a gram-negative anaerobic organism that had the peculiar characteristic of creating a depression in the growth medium and referred to this organism as the "corroding bacillus." In 1958, Eiken described and characterized a gram-negative obligate or facultative anaerobic organism for which he proposed the name *Bacteroides corrodens*. Subsequently, the strictly anaerobic organisms continued to be classified as *B. corrodens*, while the facultative anaerobes were reclassified in the new genus *Eikenella*.[132]

Eikenella corrodens is present as endogenous flora in the mouth and upper respiratory tract as well as on other mucous surfaces of the body.[133] Although it is recovered most often in association with other organisms as one component of mixed infection,[134] it has been recovered from sterile sites and in pure culture, which removes doubts about its potential to produce disease.[135,136] Characteristic of *Eikenella* infection is an indolent course, generally taking greater than 1 week from the time of injury to clinical manifestation of disease.[137] Thus, the organism should be considered an opportunistic one capable of causing disease in normal hosts given the appropriate circumstances (such as trauma).

Because *Eikenella* is a member of the endogenous oral flora, it is not surprising that the most common clinical sources of this organism are human bite wounds,[138] head and neck infections,[139] and respiratory tract infections.[134] Gynecologic infections have been described, often in association with an intrauterine contraceptive device.[140] The organism has been isolated from skin infections in drug abusers.[137] *Eikenella* has also been recovered in pure culture from synovial fluid, osteomyelitis exudate, brain, subdural and visceral abscesses, cerebrospinal fluid, and blood.[134,141–143] *Eikenella corrodens* is another of the so-called HACEK organisms, along with *Haemophilus species, Actinobacillus actinomycetemcomitans*, *Cardiobacterium hominis*, and *Kingella kingii*, which have in common the need for incubation in an atmosphere enhanced with carbon dioxide for recovery in culture and a predilection for heart valves when causing human disease.[10a]

Eikenella corrodens is a gram-negative, small straight rod that can be pleomorphic. It grows in either aerobic or anaerobic environments. It is nonmotile and non-spore-forming and does not have a capsule. On blood or chocolate agar and in the presence of 5–10% carbon dioxide, the organism will grow slowly, and it often requires more than 24 hours to recognize the typical pitting of the agar for the 45 percent of isolates that produce this pitting.[2] Colonies are small and grayish, produce a slight greenish discoloration on the blood agar, and elaborate an odor resembling bleach. Strains are oxidase-positive and reduce nitrates to nitrites. Lysine- and ornithine-decarboxylase activity is present in most strains. Many clinical laboratories rely on Gram stain, colony characteristics, production of oxidase, and failure to produce catalase or acid from glucose to identify *Eikenella*.[133] Other characteristics are shown in Table 2.

Susceptibility testing of *E. corrodens* is best done by agar or broth dilution methods using enriched media because the organism is fastidious.[2] Ampicillin, penicillin, second- and third-generation cephalosporins, and tetracyclines have been reported effective in clinical cure.[144,145] However, the organism is uniformly resistant to clindamycin and metronidazole. Recently, a β-lactamase-producing strain of *E. corrodens* has been reported.[146]

Flavobacterium and Weeksella

Flavobacteria are included for this discussion in the group of nonfermenters, although the organisms actually can ferment glucose very slowly. The group name comes from the observation that most members produce a yellow pigment when grown on solid media.

Flavobacteria are commonly inhabitants of soil and water and also are found in food. They are considered by some as endogenous flora of the oropharynx and can live in municipal water supplies despite adequate chlorination. In the hospital, vials, sink traps, tube feedings, and other fluid products can become a reservoir for flavobacteria. Strains produce proteases and gelatinase, which may contribute to virulence; these are responsible for the greenish discoloration around the colonies on blood agar.

Most of the known species of *Flavobacterium* have been isolated only rarely from humans. The most frequent human pathogen is *F. meningosepticum*, which is the only encapsulated strain and, unfortunately, often has colonies that are not pigmented or only weakly pigmented.

Two groups formerly included in *Flavobacterium* now are proposed to form a new genus, *Weeksella*, in part because these organisms vary from other flavobacteria in being susceptible to penicillin. The organisms known as group IIj in the CDC classification scheme[147] now would be named *Weeksella zoohelcum* because most of the infections it produces result from bites or scratches by dogs or cats. A second group, *Flavobacterium* IIf, would become *Weeksella virosa* because it is often associated with urinary tract infection.[147a] The taxonomic position of these and other members of this genus is unsettled.[2,148,148a]

Cases of meningitis, bacteremia, endocarditis (including prosthetic valve), wound infection, and respiratory infection are described for almost all of the species. Most of the cases described have been nosocomial, associated with use of fluids in the hospital (flush solutions for arterial catheters, contaminated syringes in ice chests, respirators, contaminated disinfectants, contaminated anaesthetics, etc.)[149] *Flavobacterium meningosepticum* is the most prominent clinical pathogen, most often appears in outbreaks of meningitis and bacteremia in newborns and premature babies, and results in high case fatality ratios and severe sequelae. More than age must be involved because many other infants develop asymptomatic colonization during the course of a nursery epidemic.[149] Adults developing infection with these organisms frequently have altered host response to infection, but cutaneous infection has been reported in absence of underlying diseases.[149a] *Flavobacterium* IIb has been associated with respiratory tract colonization as well as bacteremia.

Organisms may be long, thin, slightly curved, and occasionally filamentous on Gram stain. They typically form a yellow pigment in culture, grow well to form colonies within 24 hours on blood or chocolate agar, and grow at a much slower rate if at all on MacConkey agar. They produce positive catalase and oxidase reactions, and results are variable in most of the other biochemical reactions commonly employed.[148]

Results of susceptibility testing vary widely when different methods are used; agar disk diffusion methods are less reliable than are dilution methods, and the latter should be employed if at all possible.[150] Most flavobacteria produce β-lactamases and are resistant to penicillin G and other β-lactam drugs.[151] The addition of clavulanic acid produces some lowering of the minimum inhibitory concentration (MIC),[152] while clinical cure has been reported with ciprofloxacin.[153] Many strains are susceptible to erythromycin and tetracycline, but *F. meningosepticum* is more resistant, generally resisting erythromycin, tetracycline, and aminoglycosides as well. Clindamycin, trimethoprim-sulfamethoxazole, imipenem, and rifampin are active in laboratory testing of most strains,[154,155] and rifampin has been employed as part of combination therapy to clear persisting infection.[156] Vancomycin has been successful in the treatment of meningitis in infants[149]; this is the only gram-negative bacillus for which vancomycin has been clinically effective.

Sphingobacterium

Groups IIk-2 and IIk-3 of *Flavobacterium* now have been reclassified as *Sphingobacterium* species because they contain large amounts of sphingophospholipid compounds in the cell membrane, which are not present in the cell walls of flavobacteria.[147] The most prominent human pathogen in the genus is *S. multivorum*, formerly *Flavobacterium multivorum*. This organism has been recovered from culture often, although its causal role has been demonstrated infrequently. Peritonitis, septicemia in a dialysis patient, and bacteremia without dialysis involvement in a patient with lymphoma on induction chemotherapy all are described.[157,158] All cases had a nosocomial onset or were associated with procedures, but the natural habitat of the organism is not well defined; it is assumed to be similar to the flavobacteria.

Sphingobacterium multivorum grows on blood agar, with pinpoint colonies seen after 24 hours and pale yellow or nonpigmented colonies within another 1–2 days of incubation.[2] Growth on MacConkey medium occurs, but more slowly. The organisms are positive for oxidase and catalase, hydrolyze esculin and urease, and produce urease.

The organisms of this group resemble the flavobacteria by demonstrating a natural resistance to many commonly employed drugs and by their ability to grow in antiseptics and disinfectants. Ampicillin has been effective in treating bacteremia,[157] and the combination of trimethoprim-sulfamethoxazole and perfloxacin produced a cure in another bacteremic patient.[158] In vitro susceptibilities have produced conflicting results; in one case, the patient was cured with ampicillin despite resistance in laboratory testing.[157]

Thermophilic Nonfermenters

A report from the CDC in 1985 raised the question of thermophilic (bacteria that survive heating) gram-negative bacteria as a source for some human infections.[159] Isolates with the ability to grow at 50°C were submitted to the CDC over a 22-year period; all were gram-negative, nonfermentative rods or coccobacilli. All were oxidase-positive, grew on heart infusion agar plates but not MacConkey agar, and did not ferment glucose. Cellular fatty acid composition resembled that of *Pseudomonas* species and other glucose-nonfermenting bacteria.

Clinical information was available in 15 cases, including 6 isolates in pure culture from infection at normally sterile body sites (meningitis, 2; bacteremia, 2; endocarditis, 2). Cases occurred in children or adults with compromised host defenses.

The thermophiles had four different forms and were divided into four phenotypes (nonpigmented and slender, coccobacilli, thin rods, pigmented) on this basis. All were susceptible to penicillins and cephalosporins.

"Pink-Pigmented" Gram-Negative Bacilli

Two papers have highlighted hitherto undescribed gram-negative bacilli with pink-pigmented colonies.[159a,159b] The strains have been isolated from blood, cerebrospinal fluid, ascitic fluid, skin lesions, and respiratory tract secretions. Source patients had an underlying chronic disease. The organisms presumably represent a new group of opportunistic pathogens, and deserve further characterization.[159b]

REFERENCES:

1. Weaver RE, Hollis DG, Bottone EJ. Gram-negative fermentative bacteria and *Francisella tularensis*. In: Lennette EH, Balows A, Hausler WJ Jr, et al., eds. Manual of Clinical Microbiology. 4th ed. Washington, DC: American Society for Microbiology; 1985:309–29.
2. Rubin SJ, Granato PA, Wasilauskas BL. Glucose-nonfermenting gram-negative bacteria. In: Lennette EH, Balows A, Hausler WJ Jr, et al., eds. Manual of Clinical Microbiology. 4th ed. Washington, DC: American Society for Microbiology; 1985:330–49.
3. Potts TV, Zaobon JJ, Genco RJ. Reassignment of *Actinobacillus actinomycetemcomitans* to the genus *Haemophilus* as *Haemophilus actinomycetemcomitans* comb. nov. Int J Syst Bacteriol. 1985;35:337–41.
4. Page MI, King EO. Infection due to *Actinobacillus actinomycetemcomitans* and *Haemophilus aphrophilus*. N Engl J Med. 1966;275:181–88.
5. Holm P. Studies on the aetiology of human actinomycosis. II. Do the "other microbes" of actinomycosis possess virulence? Acta Pathol Microbiol Scand. 1951;28:391–406.
6. Kamin S, Harvey W, Wilson M, et al. Inhibition of fibroblast proliferation and collagen synthesis by capsular material from *Actinobacillus actinomycetemcomitans*. J Med Microbiol. 1986;22:245–9.
7. Hammond BF, Lillard SE, Stevens RH. A bacteriocin of *Actinobacillus actinomycetemcomitans*. Infect Immun. 1987;55:686–91.
8. Scannapieco FA, Millar SJ, Reynolds HS, et al. Effect of anaerobiosis on the surface ultrastructure and surface proteins of *Actinobacillus actinomycetemcomitans* (*Haemophilus actinomycetemcomitians*). Infect Immun. 1987;55:2320–3.
9. Bottger EC, Jurs M, Barrett T, et al. Qualitative and quantitative determination of enterobacterial common antigen (ECA) with monoclonal antibodies: Expression of ECA by two *Actinobacillus* species. J Clin Microbiol. 1987;25:377–82.
10. Asikainen S, Jousimies-Somer H, Kanervo A, et al. Certain bacterial species and morphotypes in localized juvenile periodontitis and in matched controls. J Periodontol. 1987;58:224–30.

10a. Meyer DJ, Gerding DN. Favorable prognosis of patients with prosthetic-valve endocarditis caused by gram-negative bacilli of the HACEK group. Am J Med. 1988;85:104–7.

10b. Grace CJ, Levitz RE, Katz-Pollack H, et al. *Actinobacillus actinomycetemcomitans* prosthetic valve endocarditis. Rev Infect Dis. 1988;10:922–9.

11. Horowitz EA, Pugsley MP, Turbes PG, et al. Pericarditis caused by *Actinobacillus actinomycetemcomitans* J Infect Dis. 1987;155:152–3.
12. Ellner JJ, Rosenthal MS, Lerner PI, et al. Infective endocarditis caused by slow-growing, fastidious, gram-negative bacteria. Medicine (Baltimore). 1979;58:145–58.
13. Kristinsson KG, Thorgiersson G, Holbrook WP. *Actinobacillus actinomycetemcomitans* and endocarditis. J Infect Dis. 1988;157:599.
14. Pierce CS, Bartholomew WR, Amsterdam D, et al. Endocarditis due to *Actinobacillus actinomycetemcomitans* serotype c and patient immune response. J Infect Dis. 1984;149:479.
15. Okuda K, Kato T, Naito Y, et al. Precipitating antibody against lipopolysaccharide of *Haemophilus actinomycetemcomitans* in human serum. J Clin Microbiol 1986;24:846–8.
16. Holm A, Rabe P, Kalfas, S, et al. Improved selective culture media for *Actinobacillus actinomycetemcomitans* and *Haemophilus aphrophilus*. J Clin Microbiol. 1987;25:1985–8.
17. Eng RHK, Smith SM, Goldstein EJC, et al. Failure of vancomycin prophylaxis and treatment for *Actinobacillus actinomycetemcomitans* endocarditis. Antimicrob Agents Chemother. 1986;29:699–700.
18. Yogev R, Shulman D, Shulman ST, et al. In vitro activity of antibiotics alone and in combination against *Actinobacillus actinomycetemcomitans*. Antimicrob Agents Chemother. 1986;29:179–81.
19. Watanakunakorn C. The use of beta-lactam antibiotics in the treatment of septicaemia and endocarditis. Scand J Infect Dis. 1984;42(Suppl):110–6.

19a. Kuijper EJ, Steigerwalt AG, Schoenmakers BS, et al. Phenotypic characterization and DNA relatedness in human fecal isolates of *Aeromonas* spp. J Clin Microbiol. 1989;27:132–8.

19b. Hickman-Brenner FW, Fanning GR, Arduino MJ, et al. *Aeromonas schubertii*, a new mannitol-negative species found in human clinical specimens. J Clin Microbiol. 1988;26:1561–4.

20. Miles AA, Halnan ET. A new species of microorganisms (*Proteus melanovogenes*) causing black rot in eggs. J Hyg (Camb). 1937;37:79–97.
21. VonGraevenitz A, Mersh A. The genus *Aeromonas* in human bacteriology: Report of 30 cases and review of the literature. N Engl J Med. 1968;278:587–91.
22. Holmberg SD, Schell WL, Fanning GR, et al. *Aeromonas* intestinal infections in the United States. Ann Intern Med. 1986;105:683–9.
23. Agger WA, McCormick JD, Gurwith MJ. Clinical and microbiological features of *Aeromonas hydrophila*-associated diarrhea. J Clin Microbiol. 1985;21:909–13.
24. Pitarangsi C, Echeverria P, Whitmire R, et al. Enteropathogenicity of *Aeromonas hydrophila* and *Plesiomonas shigelloides*—prevalence among individuals with and without diarrhea in Thailand. Infect Immun. 1982;35:666–73.
25. Davis WA, Kane JG, Garagusi VF. Human *Aeromonas* infections: A review of the literature and a case report of endocarditis. Medicine (Baltimore). 1978;57:267–77.
26. Scott EG, Russell CM, Noell KT, et al. *Aeromonas hydrophila* sepsis in a previously healthy man. JAMA. 1978;239:1742.
27. Lynch JM, Tilson WR, Hodges GR, et al. Nosocomial *Aeromonas hydrophila* cellulitis and bacteremia in a nonimmunocompromised patient. South Med J. 1981;74:901–2.
28. Heckerling PS, Stine TM, Pottage JC, et al. *Aeromonas hydrophila* myonecrosis and gas gangrene in a nonimmunocompromised host. Arch Intern Med. 1983;143:2005–7.

28a. Janda JM, Duffey PS. Mesophilic aeromonads in human disease: Current taxonomy, laboratory identification, and infectious disease spectrum. Rev Infect Dis. 1988;10:980–96.

29. George WL. *Aeromonas*-associated-diarrhea. Clin Microbiol Newsletter 1987;9:121–2.
30. Fulghum DD, Linton WR, Taplin D. Fatal *Aeromonas hydrophila* infection of the skin. South Med J. 1978;71:739–41.
31. Harris RL, Fainstein V, Elting L, et al. Bacteremia caused by *Aeromonas hydrophila* in hospitalized cancer patients. Rev Infect Dis. 1985;7:314–20.
32. Wolff RL, Wiseman SL, Kitchens CS. *Aeromonas hydrophila* bacteremia in ambulatory immunocompromised hosts. Am J Med. 1980;68:238–42.
33. Smith JA. *Aeromonas hydrophila*: Analysis of 11 cases. Can Med Assoc J 1980;122:1270–2.
34. Washington JA. *Aeromonas hydrophila* in clinical bacteriologic specimens. Ann Intern Med. 1972;76:611–14.
35. DeFronzo RA, Murray GF, Maddrey WC. *Aeromonas* septicemia from hepatobiliary disease. Am J Dig Dis. 1973;18:323–31.
36. Conn HO, Fessel M. Spontaneous bacterial peritonitis in cirrhosis: Variations on a theme. Medicine (Baltimore). 1971;50:161–7.
37. Ellison RT, Mostow SR. Pyogenic meningitis manifesting during therapy for *Aeromonas hydrophila* sepsis. Arch Intern Med. 1984;144:2078–9.
38. Karam GH, Ackley AM, Dismukes WE. Posttraumatic *Aeromonas hydrophila* osteomyelitis. Arch Intern Med. 1983;143:2073–4.
39. Baddour LM, Baselski VS. Pneumonia due to *Aeromonas hydrophila*-complex: Epidemiologic, clinical, and microbiologic features. South Med J. 1988;81:461–3.

39a. Abrutyn E. Hospital-associated infection from leeches. Ann Intern Med. 1988;109:356–8.

40. Kuijper EJ, Zanen HC, Peeters MF. *Aeromonas* associated diarrhea in the Netherlands. Ann Intern Med. 1987;106:640–1.
41. Shultz AJ, McCardell BA. DNA homology and immunological cross-reac-

tivity between *Aeromonas hydrophila* cytotonic toxin and cholera toxin. J Clin Microbiol. 1988;26:57–61.
42. Kindschuh M, Pickering LK, Cleary TG, et al. Clinical and biochemical significance of toxin production by *Aeromonas hydrophila*. J Clin Microbiol. 1987;25:916–21.
43. Ketover BP, Young LS, Armstrong D. Septicemia due to *Aeromonas hydrophila*: Clinical and immunological aspects. J Infect Dis. 1973;127:284–90.
44. Janda JM, Brenden R. Importance of *Aeromonas sobria* in *Aeromonas* bacteremia. J Infect Dis. 1987;155:589–90.
45. vonGraevenitz A. *Aeromonas* and *Plesiomonas*. In: Howard BJ, ed. Clinical and Pathogenic Microbiology. St. Louis: CV Mosby; 1987:367–70.
46. Fainstein V, Weaver S, Bodey GP. In vitro susceptibilities of *Aeromonas hydrophila* against new antibiotics. Antimicrob Agents Chemother. 1982;22:513–4.
47. Fass RJ, Barnishan J. In vitro susceptibilities of *Aeromonas hydrophila* to 32 antimicrobial agents. Antimicrobial Agents Chemother. 1981;19:357–8.
48. San Joaquin VH, Scribner RK, Pickett DA, et al. Antimicrobial susceptibility of *Aeromonas species* isolated from patients with diarrhea. Antimicrob Agents Chemother. 1986;30:794–5.
49. Motyl MR. McKinley G, Janda JM. In vitro susceptibilities of *Aeromonas hydrophila*, *Aeromonas sobria*, and *Aeromonas caviae* to 22 antimicrobial agents. Antimicrob Agents Chemother. 1985;28:151–3.
50. McNicol LA, Aziz KM, Huq I, et al. Isolation of drug-resistant *Aeromonas hydrophila* from aquatic environments. Antimicrob Agents Chemother. 1980;17;477–83.
51. Chang BJ, Bolton SM. Plasmids and resistence to antimicrobial agents in *Aeromonas sobria* and *Aeromonas hydrophila* clinical isolates. Antimicrob Agents Chemother. 1987;31:1281–2.
51a. Bakken JS, Saunders CC, Clark RB, et al. Beta-lactam resistance in *Aeromonas* spp. caused by inducible beta-lactamases active against penicillins, cephalosporins, and carbapenems. Antimicrob Agents Chemother. 1988;32:1314–9.
52. Warren JS, Allen SD. Clinical, pathogenic, and laboratory features of *Capnocytophaga* infections. Am J Clin Pathol 1986;86:513–8.
53. Forlenza SW, Newman MG, Lipsey AI, et al. *Capnocytophaga* sepsis: A newly recognized clinical entity in granulocytopenic patients. Lancet. 1980;1:567–8.
53a. Sinnott JT IV, Cullison JP, Juarez-Blanco P. Topics in clinical microbiology–capnocytophaga. Infect Control Hosp Epidemiol. 1988;9:170–3.
54. Newman MG, Sutter VL, Pickett MJ, et al. Detection, identification, and comparison of *Capnocytophaga, Bacteroides ochraceus*, and DF-1. J Clin Microbiol. 1979;10:557–62.
55. Williams BL, Hollis D, Holdeman LV. Synonymy of strains of Centers for Disease Control group DF-1 with species of *Capnocytophaga*. J Clin Microbiol. 1979;10:550–6.
56. Fung JC, Berman M, Fiorentino T. *Capnocytophaga*: A review of the literature. Am J Med Technol. 1983;49:589–91.
57. Newman MG, Socransky SS, Savitt ED, et al. Studies of the microbiology of periodonitis. J Periodontol. 1976;47:373–79.
58. Appelbaum PC, Ballard JO, Eyster ME. Septicemia due to *Capnocytophaga* (*Bacteroides ochraceus*) in Hodgkin's disease (Letter). Ann Intern Med. 1979;90:716–7.
59. Shurin SB, Socransky SS, Sweeney E, et al. A neutrophil disorder induced by *Capnocytophaga*: A dental micro-organism. N Engl J Med. 1979;301:849–54.
60. Wilson ME, Jonak-Urbanczyk JT, Bronson PM, et al. *Capnocytophaga* species: Increased resistance of clinical isolates to serum bactericidal action. J Infect Dis. 1987;156:99–106.
61. Arlet G, Sanson-LePors S, Castaigne S, et al. Isolation of a strain of beta-lactamase-producing *Capnocytophaga ochracea*. J Infect Dis. 1987;155:1346.
62. Parenti DM, Snydman DE. *Capnocytophaga* species: Infections in nonimmunocompromised and immunocompromised hosts. J Infect Dis. 1985;151:140–47.
63. Matlow A, Vellend H. *Capnocytophaga*: A pathogen in imunocompetent hosts. J Infect Dis. 1985;152:233–4.
64. Mosher CB, Corp R. Mediastinal abscess with *Capnocytophaga* spp. in a competent host. J Clin Microbiol. 1986;24:161–2.
65. Buu-Hoi AY, Joundy S, Acar JF. Endocarditis caused by *Capnocytophaga ochracea*. J Clin Microbiol. 1988;26:1061–2.
66. Rummens J, Fossepre J, DeGruyter M, et al. Isolation of *Capnocytophaga* species with a new selective medium. J Clin Microbiol. 1985;22:375–8.
67. Forlenza SW, Newman MG, Horikoshi AL, et al. Antimicrobial susceptibility of *Capnocytophaga*. Antimicrob Agents Chemother. 1981;19:144–6.
68. Sutter VL, Pyeatt D, Kwok YY. In vitro susceptibility of *Capnocytophaga* strains to 18 antimicrobial agents. Antimicrob Agents Chemother. 1981;20:270–1.
69. Rummens J, Gordts B, VanLanduyt HW. In vitro susceptibility of *Capnocytophaga* to 29 antimicrobial agents. Antimicrob Agents Chemother. 1986;30:739–42.
70. Hawkey PM, Smith SD, Haynes J, et al. In vitro susceptibility of *Capnocytophaga* species to antimicrobial agents. Antimicrob Agents Chemother. 1987;31:331–2.
71. Wormser GP, Bottone EJ. *Cardiobacterium hominis*: Review of microbiologic and clinical features. Rev Infect Dis. 1983;5:680–91.
72. Francioli PB, Roussianos D, Glauser MP. *Cardiobacterium hominis* endocarditis manifesting as bacterial meningitis. Arch Intern Med. 1983;143:1483–4.
73. Jolie A, Gnann JW Jr. *Cardiobacterium hominis* causing late prosthetic valve endocarditis. South Med J. 1986;79:1461–2.
74. Robison WJ, Vitelli AS. Infectious endocarditis caused by *Cardiobacterium hominis*. South Med J. 1985;78:1020–1.
75. Weissfeld AS, Howard BJ, Almazan RD, et al. Miscellaneous pathogenic organisms. In: Howard BJ, ed. Clinical and Pathogenic Microbiology. St Louis: CV Mosby; 1987:455–78.
76. Kaufman SC, Ceraso D, Schugurensky A. First case report from Argentina of fatal septicemia caused by *Chromobacterium violaceum*. J Clin Microbiol. 1986;23:956–8.
77. Cooper R, Wells JS, Sykes RB. Novel potentiators of beta-lactam antibiotics. Isolation of SQ28,504 and SQ28,546 from *Chromobacterium violaceum*. J Antibiot (Tokyo) 1985;38:449–54.
78. Sorensen RU, Jacobs MR, Shurin SB. *Chromobacterium violaceum* adenitis acquired in the northern United States as a complication of chronic granulomatous disease. Pediatr Infect Dis. 1985;4:701–2.
79. Mamlok RJ, Mamlok V, Mills GC, et al. Glucose-6-phosphate dehydrogenase deficiency, neutrophil dysfunction, and *Chromobacterium violaceum* sepsis. J Pediatr. 1987,111.852–4.
80. Suarez AE, Wenokur B, Johnson JM. et al. Nonfatal chromobacterial sepsis. South Med J. 1986;79:1146–48.
81. Simo F, Reuman PD, Martinez FJ, et al. *Chromobacterium violaceum* as a cause of periorbital cellulitis. Pediatr Infect Dis. 1984;3:561–3.
82. Dees SB, Powell J, Moss CW, et al. Cellular fatty acid composition of organisms frequently associated with human infections resulting from dog bites: *Pasteurella multocida* and groups EF-4, IIj, M-5, and DF-2. J Clin Microbiol. 1981;14:612–6.
83. Hicklin H, Verghese A, Alvarez S. Dysgonic fermenter 2 septicemia. Rev Infect Dis. 1987;9:884–90.
84. Elliot DL, Tolle SW, Glodberg L, et al. Pet-associated illness. N Engl J Med. 1985;313:985–95.
85. Martone WJ, Zuhl RW, Mison GE, et al. Postsplenectomy sepsis with DF-2: Report of a case with isolation of the organism from the patient's dog. Ann Intern Med. 1980;93:457–9.
86. Westwell AJ, Spencer MB, Kerr KG. DF-2 bacteremia following cat bites. Am J Med. 1987;83:1170.
87. Butler T, Weaver RE, Ramani TKV, et al. Unidentified gram-negative rod infection: A new disease of man. Ann Intern Med. 1977;86:1–5.
88. Butler T, Johnston KH, Gutierrez Y, et al. Enhancement of experimental bacteremia and endocarditis caused by dysgonic fermenter (DF-2) bacterium after treatment with methylprednisolone and after splenectomy. Infect Immun. 1985;47:294–300.
89. Kerr KG. Dysgonic fermenter organisms and post-splenectomy risks. Lancet. 1987;2:1473.
90. Pers C, Kristiansen JE, Scheibel JH, et al. Fatal septicemia caused by DF-2 in a previously healthy man. Scand J Infect Dis. 1986;18:265–7.
91. Hinrichs JH, Dunkelberg WE. DF-2 septicemia after splenectomy: Epidemiology and immunologic response. South Med J. 1980;73:1638–40.
92. Chaudhuri AK, Hartley RB, Maddocks AC. Waterhouse Friderichsen syndrome caused by a DF-2 bacterium in a splenectomised host. J Clin Pathol. 1981;34:172–3.
93. Weaver RE. DF-2 Septicemia. ASCP Check Sample 85-8. Chicago: American Society for Clinical Pathology, 1985.
94. Case records of the Massachusetts General Hospital (case 29-1986). N Engl J Med. 1986;315:241–9.
95. Verghese A, Hamati F, Berk S, et al. Susceptibility of dysgonic fermenter 2 to antimicrobial agents in vitro. Antimicrob Agents Chemother. 1988;32:78–80.
96. Wagner DK, Wright JJ, Ansher AF, et al. Dysgonic fermenter 3-associated gastrointestinal disease in a patient with common variable hypogammaglobulinemia. Am J Med 1988;84:315–18.
96a. Aronsen NE, Zbick CJ. Dysgonic fermenter 3 bacteremia in a neutropenic patient with acute lymphocytic leukemia. J Clin Microbiol. 1988;26:2213–5.
97. Dul MJ, Shlaes DM, Lerner PI. EF-4 bacteremia in a patient with hepatic carcinoid. J Clin Microbiol. 1983;18:1260–1.
98. Brenden RA, Miller MA, Janda JM. Clinical disease spectrum and pathogenic factors associated with *Plesiomonas shigelloides* infections in humans. Rev Infect Dis. 1988;10:303–16.
99. Holmberg SD, Wachsmuth K, Hickman-Brenner FW, et al. *Plesiomonas* enteric infections in the United States. Ann Intern Med. 1986;105:690–94.
100. MacDonell MT, Colwell RR. Phylogeny of the Vibrionaceae, and recommendation for two new genera, *Listonella* and *Shewanella* Syst Appl Microbiol. 1985;6:171–82.
101. Martin DL, Gustafson TL. Plesiomonas gastroenteritis in Texas. JAMA. 1985;254:2063.
102. Newsom R, Gallois C. Diarrheal disease caused by *Plesiomonas shigelloides*. Clin Microbiol Newsletter. 1982;4:158–9.
103. Davis WA, Chretien JH, Garagusi VF, et al. Snake-to-human transmission of *Aeromonas* (PI) *shigelloides* resulting in gastroenteritis. South Med J. 1978;71:474–6.
104. Gardner SE, Fowlston SE, George WL. In vitro production of cholera toxin-like activity by *Plesiomonas shigelloides*. J Infect Dis. 1987;156:720–2.
105. Herrington DA, Tzipori S, Robins-Browne RM, et al. In vitro and in vivo pathogenicity of *Plesiomonas shigelloides*. Infect Immun. 1987;55:979–85.
106. Ingram CW, Morrison AJ, Levitz RE. Gastroenteritis, sepsis, and osteo-

myelitis caused by *Plesiomonas shigelloides* in an immunocompetent host: Case report and review of the literature. J Clin Microbiol. 1987;25:1791–3.
107. Gordon DL, Philpot CR, McGuire C. *Plesiomonas shigelloides* septic arthritis complicating rheumatoid arthritis. Aust NZ J Med. 1983;13:275–6.
108. Pathak A, Custer JR, Levy J. Neonatal septicemia and meningitis due to *Plesiomonas shigelloides*. Pediatrics. 1983;71:389–91.
109. Nolte FS, Poole RM, Murphy GW, et al. Proctitis and fatal septicemia caused by *Plesiomonas shigelloides* in a bisexual man. J Clin Microbiol. 1988;26:388–91.
110. Curti AJ, Lin JH, Szabo K. Overwhelming post-splenectomy infection with *Plesiomonas shigelloides* in a patient cured of Hodgkin's disease: A case report. Am J Clin Pathol. 1983;83:522–4.
111. Rahim Z, Kay BA. Enrichment for *Plesiomonas shigelloides* from stools. J Clin Microbiol. 1988:26:789–90.
112. Reinhardt JF, George WL. Comparative in vitro activities of selected antimicrobial agents against *Aeromonas* species and *Plesiomonas shigelloides*. Antimicrob Agents Chemother. 1983;11:311–8.
113. Auckenthaler R, Michea-Hamzehpour M, Pechere JC. In-vitro activity of newer quinolones against aerobic bacteria. J Antimicrob Chemother. 1986;17(Suppl B):29–39.
114. Miller MA, Finan M, Yousuf M. In-vitro antagonism by *N*-formimidoyl thienamycin and cefoxitin of second and third generation cephalosporins in *Aeromonas hydrophila* and *Serratia marcescens*. J Antimicrob Chemother. 1983;11:311–8.
115. Spear JB, Fuhrer J, Kirby BD. *Achromobacter xylosoxidans* (*Alkaligenes xylosoxidans* subsp. *xylosoxidans*) bacteremia associated with a well-water source: Case report and review of the literature. J Clin Microbiol. 1988;26;598–9.
116. Mandell WF, Garvey GJ, Neu HC. *Achromobacter xylosoxidans* bacteremia. Rev Infect Dis. 1987;9:1001–5.
117. Arroyo JC, Jordan W, Lema MW, et al. Diversity of plasmids in *Achromobacter xylosoxidans* isolates responsible for a seemingly common-source nosocomial outbreak. J Clin Microbiol. 1987;25:1952–5.
118. Sepkowitz DV, Bostic DE, Maslow MJ. *Achromobacter xylosoxidans* meningitis: Case report and review of the literature. Clin Pediatr (Phila). 1987;26:483–5.
118a. D'Amato RF, Salemi M, Mathews A, et al. *Achromobacter xylosoxidans (Alcalignines xylosoxidens* subsp. *xylosoxidans)* meningitis associated with a gunshot wound. J Clin Microbiol. 1988;26:2425–6.
119. Schoch PE, Cunha BA. Nosocomial *Achromobacter xylosoxidans* infections. Infect Control Hosp Epidemiol. 1988;9:84–7.
120. Glupczynski Y, Hansen W, Freney J, et al. In vitro susceptibility of *Alcaligines denitrificans* subsp. *xylosoxidans* to 24 antimicrobial agents. Antimicrob Agents Chemother. 1988;32:276–8.
121. Alos JI, deRafael L, Gonzalez-Palacios R, et al. Urinary tract infection probably caused by *Agrobacterium radiobacter*. Eur J Clin Microbiol. 1985;4:596–7.
122. Freney J, Gruer LD, Bornstein N, et al. Septicemia caused by *Agrobacterium* sp. J Clin Microbiol. 1985;22:683–5.
123. Swann RA, Foulkes SJ, Holmes B, et al. "Agrobacterium yellow group" and *Pseudomonas paucimobilis* causing peritonitis in patients receiving continuous ambulatory peritoneal dialysis. J Clin Pathol. 1985;38:1293–9.
124. Fujii T, Sato K, Inoue M, et al. Purification and properties of inducible penicillin beta-lactamase isolated from *Alcaligenes faecalis*. Antimicrob Agents Chemother. 1985;27:608–11.
125. Ishii J, Nakae T. Size of diffusion pore of *Alcaligenes faecalis*. Antimicrob Agents Chemother. 1988;32:378–84.
125a. Peel MM, Hibberd AJ, King BM, et al. *Alcaligenes piechaudii* from chronic ear discharge. J Clin Microbiol. 1988;26:1580–1.
126. Pickett MJ, Greenwood JR. Identification of oxidase-positive, glucose-negative motile species of nonfermentative bacilli. J Clin Microbiol. 1986;23:920–3.
127. Crowe HM, Brecher SM. Nosocomial septicemia with CDC group IVc-2, an unusual gram-negative bacillus. J Clin Microbiol. 1987;25:2225–6.
128. Dan M, Berger SA, Aderka D, et al. Septicemia caused by the gram-negative bacterium CDC IV c-2 in an immunocompromised human. J Clin Microbiol. 1986;23:803.
129. Welch WD, Porschen RK, Luttrell B. Minimal inhibitory concentrations of 19 antimicrobial agents for 96 clinical isolates of group IVe bacteria. Antimicrob Agents Chemother. 1983;24:432–3.
130. Barson WJ, Cromer BA, Marcon MJ. Puncture wound osteochondritis of the foot caused by CDC group Vd. J Clin Microbiol. 1987;25:2014–6.
130a. Van Horn KG, Gedris C, Ahmed A, et al. Bacteremia and urinary tract infection associated with CDC group Vd biorar 2. J Clin Microbiol. 1989;27:201–2.
131. Kish MA, Buggy BP, Forbes BA. Bacteremia caused by *Achromobacter* species in an immunocompromised host. J Clin Microbiol. 1984;19:947–8.
132. Jackson FL, Goodman YE, Bel FR. Taxonomic status of the facultatively anaerobic organism *Bacteroides corrodens* Eiken to a new genus, *Eikenella*. Int J Syst Bacteriol. 1972;22:73–77.
133. Deker MD. *Eikenella corrodens*. Infect Control. 1986;7:36–41.
134. Suwanagool S, Rothkopf MM, Smith SM, et al. Pathogenicity of *Eikenella corrodens* in humans. Arch Intern Med. 1983;143:2265–8.
135. Javaheri S, Smith RM, Witse D. Intrathoracic infections due to *Eikenella corrodens*. Thorax. 1987;42:700–1.
136. Deker MD, Graham BS, Hunter EB, et al. Endocarditis and infections of intravascular devices due to *Eikenella corrodens*. Am J Med Sci. 1986;292:209–12.
137. Brooks GF, O'Donoghue JM, Rissing JP. *Eikenella corrodens*: A recently recognized pathogen: Infections in medical-surgical patients and in association with methylphenidate abuse. Medicine (Baltimore). 1974;53:325–42.
138. Stoloff AL, Gillies ML. Infections with *Eikenella corrodens* in a general hospital: A report of 33 cases. Rev Infect Dis. 1986;8:50–3.
139. Tveteras K, Kristensten S, Bach V, et al. *Eikenella corrodens*: A recently recognized pathogen in head and neck infections. J Laryngol Otol. 1987;101:592–4.
140. Drouet F, De Montclos H, Boude M, et al. *Eikenella corrodens* and intrauterine contraceptive device. Lancet. 1987;2:1089.
141. Seidel JS, Yamauchi T, Fong C. Arthritis due to *Eikenella corrodens*. J Pediatr. 1975;87:491.
142. Porphyris H. Central nervous system infections due to *Eikenella corrodens*. Surg Neurol. 1983;19:150–3.
143. Raffensperger JG. *Eikenella corrodens* infections in children. J Pediatr Surg. 1986;21:644–6.
144. Goldstein EJ, Citron DM, Vagvolgyi AE, et al. Susceptibility of *Eikenella corrodens* to newer and older quinolones. Antimicrob Agents Chemother. 1986;30:172–3.
145. Goldstein EJ, Gombert ME, Agyare EO. Susceptibility of *Eikenella corrodens* to newer beta-lactamase antibiotics. Antimicrob Agents Chemother. 1980;18:832–33.
146. Trallero EP, Garcia JM, Eguiluz GC, et al. β-Lactamase-producing *Eikenella corrodens* in an intraabdominal abscess. J Infect Dis. 1986;153:379–80.
147. Dees SB, Moss CW, Hollis DG, et al. Chemical characterization of *Flavobacterium odoratum, Flavobacterium breve*, and *Flavobacterium*-like groups IIe, IIh, and IIf. J Clin Microbiol. 1986;23:267–73.
147a. Holmes B, Steigerwalt AG, Weaver RE, et al. *Weeksella virosa* gen. nov. sp. nov. (formerly group IIf), found in human clinical specimens. System Appl Microbiol. 1986;8:185–90.
148. Oberhofer TR, Howard BJ. Nonfermentative gram-negative bacteria. In: Howard BJ, ed. Clinical and Pathogenic Microbiology. St Louis: CV Mosby; 1987:329–358.
148a. Mardy C, Holmes B. Incidence of vaginal *Weeksella virosa* (formerly group IIf). J Clin Pathol. 1988;41:211–4.
149. Ratner H. *Flavobacterium meningosepticum*. Infect Control. 1984;5:237–9.
149a. Bolivar R, Abramovitz W. Cutaneous infection caused by *Flavobacterium meningosepticum*. J Infect Dis. 1989;159:150–1.
150. Harrington SP, Perlino CA. *Flavobacterium meningosepticum* sepsis: Disease due to bacteria with unusual antibiotic susceptibility. South Med J. 1981;74:764–6.
151. Bruun B. Antimicrobial susceptibility of *Flavobacterium meningosepticum* strains identified by DNA-DNA hybridization. Acta Pathol Microbiol Immunol Scand [B] 1987;95:95–101.
152. Raimondi A, Moosdeen F, Williams JD. Antibiotic resistance pattern of *Flavobacterium meningosepticum*. Eur J Clin Microbiol. 1986;5:461–3.
153. Scully BE, Neu HC. Oral ciprofloxacin therapy of infection caused by multiply resistant bacteria other than *Pseudomonas aeruginosa*. J Antimicrob Chemother. 1986;18(Suppl D):179–85.
154. Overturf GD. Use of trimethoprim-sulfamethoxazole in pediatric infections: Relative merits of intravenous administration. Rev Infect Dis. 1987;9(Suppl 2):S168–76.
155. Speciale A, Caccamo F, Pellegrino MB, et al. In vitro activity of imipenem towards gram-negative bacilli. Chemioterapia. 1986;5:291–6.
156. Hirsh BE, Wong B, Kiehn TE, et al.. *Flavobacterium meningosepticum* bacteremia in an adult with acute leukemia. Use of rifampin to clear persistent infection. Diagn Microbiol Infect Dis. 1986;4:65–9.
157. Potvliege C, Dejaegher-Bauduin C, Hansen W, et al. *Flavobacterium multivorum* septicemia in a hemodialyzed patient. J Clin Microbiol. 1984;19:568–9.
158. Freney J, Hansen W, Ploton C, et al. Septicemia caused by *Sphingobacterium multivorum*. J Clin Microbiol. 1987;25:1126–8.
159. Rabkin CS, Galaid EI, Hollis DG, et al. Thermophilic bacteria: A new cause of human disease. J Clin Microbiol. 1985;21:553–7.
159a. Gilardi GL, Faur YC. *Pseudomonas mesophilica* and an untamed taxon, clinical isolates of pink-pigmented oxidative bacteria. J Clin Microbiol. 1984;20:626–9.
159b. Odugbemi T, Nwofor C, Joiner KT. Isolation of an unidentified pink-pigmented bacterium in a clinical specimen. J Clin Microbiol. 1988;26:1072–3.

SPIROCHETES

213. TREPONEMA PALLIDUM (SYPHILIS)

EDMUND C. TRAMONT

Syphilis is a complex systemic illness with protean clinical manifestations caused by the spirochete *Treponema pallidum*. It holds a special place in the history of medicine as the "great imitator" or the "great imposter." It is most often transmitted by sexual contact, and unlike most other infectious diseases, it is rarely diagnosed by isolation and characterization of the causative organism. Instead, less precise methods of diagnosis are used: direct darkfield microscopy and epidemiologic, serologic, and clinical findings. Its natural course is arbitrarily divided into the following phases: (*1*) an incubation period lasting about 3 weeks; (*2*) a primary stage characterized by a nonpainful skin lesion (chancre) associated with regional lymphadenopathy and early bacteremia; (*3*) a secondary bacteremic or disseminated stage accompanied by generalized mucocutaneous lesions and lymphadenopathy; (*4*) a period of subclinical infection (latent syphilis) detected only by serologic tests; and (*5*) in a small number of patients a late or tertiary stage characterized by progressive disease involving principally the ascending aorta and/or the central nervous system, but virtually any organ in the body can be involved.

ETIOLOGY

The causal agent of syphilis is *T. pallidum*, which belongs to the family Spirochaetaceae. Other members of the genus *Treponema* that can infect humans are *T. pertenue* (yaws) and *T. carateum* (pinta). A number of nonpathogenic treponemes have also been isolated, particularly from the oral cavity. Other pathogenic organisms of the family Spirochaetaceae belong to the genera *Borrelia* and *Leptospira*.

The organisms are slender, tightly coiled, unicellular, helical cells 5–15 μm (average, 10–13 μm) long and 0.09–0.18 μm (average, 0.1–0.15 μm) wide. The cytoplasm is surrounded by a trilaminar cytoplasmic membrane, a peptidoglycan layer, a delicate inner mucopeptide layer known as the periplast, an outer lipoprotein membrane containing lipopolysaccharide and an amphorous outer layer detected by ruthenium red staining.[1,2] The ends of the cells are tapered, and three fibrils are inserted into each end. It moves with a drifting rotary motion and usually has a characteristic flexuous or undulating movement about the center of the organism.

Unlike many nonpathogenic treponemes, the virulent treponemes, including *T. pallidum*, cannot be cultivated in vitro.[3] However, they have remained motile in highly enriched and specifically defined media up to 7 days at 35°C and up to 48 hours at 37°C. Carbon dioxide aids survival. They can be maintained viable in liquid nitrogen, less so at −70°C, and in many mammals. Rabbits are the laboratory animals most commonly used for maintaining virulent organisms.[3]

Thus far no metabolic or structural immunologic or virulent marker differences between the pathogenic treponemes have been found, and the speciation between them rests primarily with the associated clinical illness.

The views of the author do not purport to reflect the position of the Department of the Army or the Department of Defense (para 4-3, AR 360-5).

HISTORY

The historical aspects of syphilis make for fascinating reading, and its impact on folklore appears destined to continue.[4,5] Few modern clinicians are aware of the extent of syphilis at the turn of the twentieth century, the individuals of notoriety infected, or the pervasiveness that this disease had on medical practice.[6]

The arguments about the origins of syphilis basically come down to whether syphilis was imported into the "Old World" from the "New World" by the shipmates of Christopher Columbus or whether it was an old disease that spread throughout Europe as a consequence of urbanization. The two theories cannot be reconciled. A pandemic known as the Great Pox (as distinguished from the small pox) ravaged Europe and Asia at the time of the return of Columbus from America and during mass movements of armies and populations in Europe. It cannot be proved with certainty that *T. pallidum* was indeed the cause of this scourge. Nevertheless, the first clear descriptions of this illness were recorded at this time, and the sexual mode of transmission was recognized soon thereafter. As noted in the *Breviary of Helthe*, 1547:[7]

> . . . In englyshe Morbus Gallicus (syphilis) is named the french pockes, whan that I was yonge they were named the spanyshe pockes the which be of many kyndes of the pockes, some be moyst, some be waterashe, some be drye, and some be skorvie, some be lyke skabbes, some be lyke ring wormes, some be fistuled, some be festered, some be cankarus, some be lyke wennes, some be lyke biles, some be lyke knobbles or burres, and some be ulcerous havyinge a lytle drye skabbe in the middle of the ulcerous skabbe, some hath ache in the jioyntes and no singe of the pockes and yet it may be the pockes . . . The cause of these impediments or infyrmytes doth come many wayes, it maye come by lyenge in the shetes or bedde there where a pocky person hath the night before lyenin, it maye come with lyenge with a pocky person, it maye come by syttenge on a draught or sege where as a pocky person did lately syt, it may come by drynkynge oft with a pocky person, but specially it is taken when one pocky person doth synne in lechery the one with another.

The secondary stage of the illness during this period of time was often accompanied by high morbidity and mortality, which attests to the extraordinary virulent nature of the causative organism. It is not known whether the relatively mild nature of present-day syphilis reflects a change in the virulence of the organism, an adaptation of the human host, or the loss of a concomitantly occurring but unknown illness. The proponents of the "New World" or "Columbian Theory" rest their case on the absence of syphilitic bone lesions in old skeletons despite the fact that the pathologic distinction between old bone lesions of leprosy and syphilis is not precise.

One of the difficulties in sorting through older writings is that the distinction between syphilis, gonorrhea, and other "venereal diseases" did not emerge until the late nineteenth century. John Hunter's unfortunate self-inoculation with urethral pus containing both *Neisseria gonorrhoeae* and *T. palldium* only served to prolong misconceptions. However, by the early twentieth century, the etiology, epidemiology, and the clinical manifestations of syphilis were well known as evidenced by the following anonymous poem, which can be dated from the 1920s:

> There was a young man from Back Bay
> Who thought syphilis just went away
> He believed that a chancre
> Was only a canker
> That healed in a week and a day.
>
> But now he has "acne vulgaris"—
> (Or whatever they call it in Paris);
> On his skin it has spread
> From his feet to his head,
> And his friends want to know where his hair is.
>
> There's more to his terrible plight:
> His pupils won't close in the light
> His heart is cavorting,

His wife is aborting,
And he squints through his gun-barrel sight.

Arthralgia cuts into his slumber;
His aorta is in need of a plumber;
But now he has tabes,
And saber-shinned babies,
While of gummas he has quite a number.

He's been treated in every known way,
But his spirochetes grow day by day;
He's developed paresis,
Has long talks with Jesus,
And thinks he's the Queen of the May.

The nickname "lues" came from the Latin *lues venereum*, which means "disease," "sickness,' or "pestilence" and originally was loosely applied to any venereal disease. It became a synonym for syphilis at the turn of the century.

Metchnikoff successfully transferred the disease to chimpanzees in 1903. Two years later, the organism was described in the primary lesion and adjacent lymph nodes of syphilitic patients. Soon thereafter, Wassermann described the complement fixation test for the diagnosis of syphilis by using fetal calf livers laden with *T. pallidum* and, later, extracts of uninfected beef livers and hearts (the forerunner of the present-day nontreponemal tests).

At the same time Ehrlich introduced an arsenic derivative, arsphenamine or Salvarsan, as therapy. Mercury and bismuth preparations were added later. Induced fever therapy (malaria, heat box, hot baths) was quite efficacious, and its benefits were known for more than 300 years. In fact, Dr. Julius Wagner von Jauregg was awarded the Nobel Prize in 1927 for describing the use of malaria injections to treat "paralytica dementia" (neurosyphilis). But these primarily palliative therapies were quickly forgotten; no other disease was as dramatically affected by the discovery of penicillin as syphilis was.

EPIDEMIOLOGY

Syphilis can be acquired by sexual contact, by passage through the placenta (congenital syphilis), by kissing, by transfusion of fresh human blood, or by accidental direct inoculation.[8,9] The overwhelming majority of cases of syphilis are transmitted by sexual intercourse. A patient is most infectious early in the disease (especially when a chancre, mucous patch, and/or condyloma lata are present) and gradually becomes less so over time. For all practical purposes, the patient cannot spread syphilis by sexual contact 4 years after acquiring the illness.

Syphilis can be spread by kissing or touching a person who has active lesions on the lips, oral cavity, breasts, or genitals. Conversely, an infected patient may inoculate syphilis to that area on the body which is kissed. (Wet nurses often spread the disease to infants, especially those from upper-class European families for whom the use of a wet nurse was a socially recognized status symbol.)

Congenital syphilis occurs most frequently when the fetus becomes infected in utero, although it is possible for the neonate to acquire the infection as it passes through the birth canal.

The acquisition of syphilis through transfused blood or blood products is now very rare because of the low incidence of disease, because the requirement that all blood donors have a nonreactive nontreponemal blood test before their blood can be used, and because *T. pallidum* cannot suvive longer than 24–48 hours under the conditions of blood bank storage.[10]

Accidental direct inoculation can occur by a needle prick or when handling infected clinical material. Indeed, syphilis of the fingers is most common in medical personnel.

The number of reported new cases of syphilis in the United States has waxed and waned over the past four decades. It reached its peak during World War II, its nadir in the mid-1950s, rose dramatically in 1960, and then remained relatively stable until 1986 (Fig. 1). A disproportionate number of cases occurred in homosexual men until the mid-1980s when the incidence of

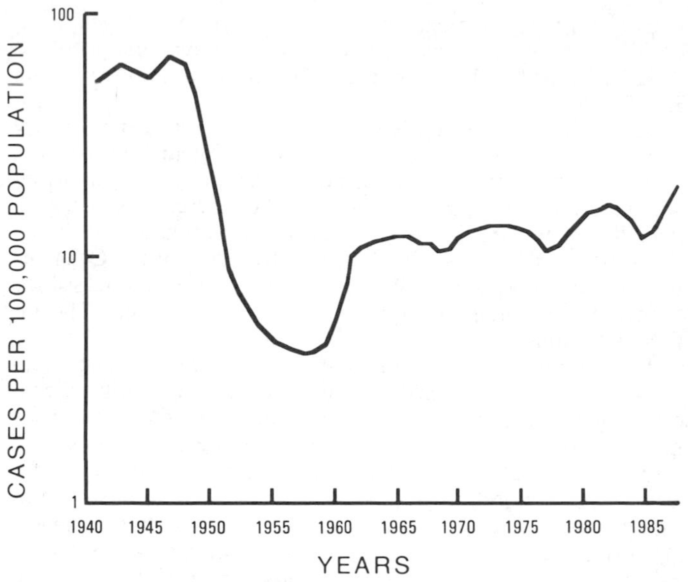

FIG. 1. Primary and secondary syphilis: rate per 100,000 population in the United States, 1941–1987.

new cases among this cohort began to decrease coincident with the adaption of safer sex practices by this group because of the acquired immunodeficiency syndrome (AIDS) epidemic. This was replaced, however, by a rapid increase in new cases occurring primarily among heterosexuals as reflected by a dramatic increase of syphilis in women and neonates (congenital syphilis). Explanations for this resurgence may include (*1*) an increased pool of persons with infectious lesions because of the more virulent nature of syphilis and the difficulty in treating patients with syphilis who had a concomitant human immunodeficiency virus (HIV) infection (see below), (*2*) the redistribution of public health assets to meet other health threats, i.e., AIDS, (*3*) the development of a new highly promiscuous life-style or subculture in which the exchange of sexual favors for drugs, especially in so-called "crack houses," are common, and (*4*) the ineffectiveness of spectinomycin as primary treatment for penicillinase-producing *N. gonorrhoeae* to cure incubating syphilis. Ceftriaxone, which is now recommended as therapy for all antibiotic-resistant strains of *N. gonorrhoeae*, appears to be effective against incubating syphilis.

The vast majority of cases occur in the most sexually active age group (15–30 years old). Since some of these contacts will be "incubating" syphilis and will have no evidence of active disease, aggressive contact tracing and "epidemiologic treatment" of all recently exposed persons are important aspects of syphilis control (i.e., all contacts should be sought and treated unless follow-up examinations can be guaranteed).

PATHOGENESIS

Within hours to days after *T. pallidum* penetrates the intact mucous membrane or gains access through abraded skin, it enters the lymphatics and/or blood stream and disseminates throughout the body. This occurs soon after contact, as evidenced by the fact that patients who have received blood transfusions from syphilitic donors in the seronegative incubation period have become infected.[8,9] Virtually any organ in the body can be invaded, including the central nervous system.[11] The infectious dose will vary from patient to patient, but in rabbits an inoculum containing as few as four spirochetes can establish an infection.[12] The organism divides every 30–33 hours.[13] Clinical lesions appear when a concentration is reached of approximately 10^7 organisms per gram of tissue, and the incubation period is directly proportional to the size of the inoculum.[13]

Clinically, syphilis can be divided into various stages: incubating, primary, secondary, latent, and late syphilis.

The median incubation period is 3 weeks but may vary from 3 to 90 days.

The primary stage refers to the development of the primary lesion, known as a chancre, which occurs at the site of inoculation. It does not develop in every case or may be so inconspicuous as to go unnoticed. Multiple chancres can occur especially in persons infected with HIV. Spirochetes are easily demonstrated in the lesions, especially early ones. Chancres usually heal spontaneously in 2–8 weeks, but often persist for longer periods in immunocompromised hosts, e.g., HIV infected persons.

The secondary or disseminated stage becomes evident in 2–12 weeks (mean, 6 weeks) after contact. This generalized condition with parenchymal, constitutional, and mucocutaneous manifestations occurs at the time when the greatest number of treponemes (high antigen load) are present in the body, particularly in the blood stream. They can also be demonstrated in many other tissues, especially in the skin and lymph nodes. Abnormalities and/or treponemes can be detected in the central nervous system, including the aqueous humor of the eye, in up to 35 percent of these patients.[8,9,11] The immunologic response of the host at this time becomes quite brisk, and an immune-complex glomerulonephritis may occur.[14]

After the secondary stage subsides, the patient enters a latent period in which the diagnosis can only be made by obtaining a positive serologic test response for syphilis. Because relapses of secondary syphilis can occur up to 4 years after contact, this period is divided into early latent (relapses possible) and late latent (relapses very unlikely) stages. Seventy-five percent of relapses occur within the first year, and are a consequence of an immunologic dysfunction in cellular immunity, e.g., last trisemester of pregnancy.

Late syphilis refers to the clinically apparent or inapparent tertiary disease that develops in up to one-third of untreated patients. Most of these lesions involve the vaso vasorum of the aorta and/or the arteries of the central nervous system; the rest consists principally of gummas. The skin, liver, bones, and spleen are the most common sites for gummas to develop.

PATHOLOGIC CHARACTERISTICS

Obliterative endarteritis consisting of concentric endothelial and fibroblastic proliferative thickening is highly suggestive of syphilis (Fig. 2)[9]. These pathologic changes are found in all stages of syphilis. In the primary chancre, polymorphonuclear leukocytes and macrophages can also be seen ingesting treponemes. Hyperkeratosis is frequently found in the skin lesions of secondary syphilis and is especially marked in condylomata.

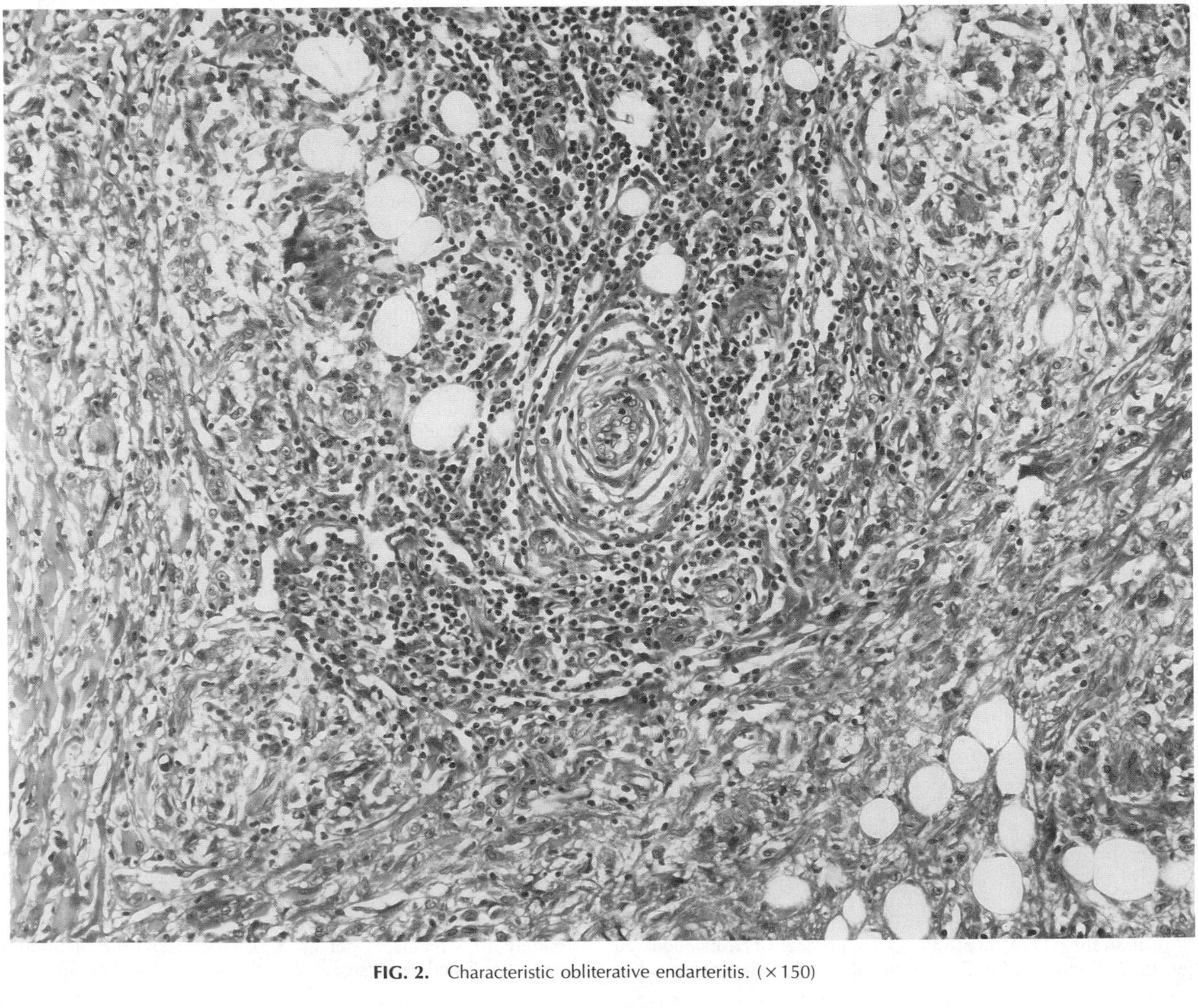

FIG. 2. Characteristic obliterative endarteritis. (×150)

Treponemal antigen, immunoglobulin, and complement deposition in the glomeruli typical of immune-complex glomerulonephritis can be demonstrated in patients who develop a nephrotic syndrome.[14] The obliterative endarteritis of the vaso vasorum and small blood vessels is the principal histopathologic finding in cardiovascular syphilis and meningovascular neurosyphilis. Appropriate staining (i.e., direct fluorescent or silver stains) can be used to demonstrate *T. pallidum*. The gumma is an agranulomatous lesion consisting of a necrotic, coagulated center and small-vessel obliterative endarteritis. It can occur anywhere in the body.

THE NATURAL COURSE OF UNTREATED SYPHILIS

The natural course of untreated syphilis has been studied in a retrospective fashion in 1404 patients who were diagnosed clinically as having early syphilis (the Oslo study, 1891–1951).[15] There are many shortcomings with this study, the most glaring being the lack of laboratory confirmation of syphilis and the method of patient selection. (The darkfield and Wassermann tests were not available at the time this study was initiated). However, since a similar study is unlikely to be ever done again, a brief review is warranted.

From 1890 to 1910, Professor Boeck of the University of Oslo, Norway, hospitalized patients diagnosed as having primary or secondary syphilis. Because he felt that the mercury-containing compounds used at that time were more harmful to the patient than the disease itself was, all of his patients were simply observed. Twenty-four percent of these untreated patients developed relapsing secondary lesions within 4 years (thus the arbitrary designation of early and late syphilis). Twenty-eight percent eventually developed clinical complications of late syphilis; 10 percent developed cardiovascular syphilis, but only those who acquired syphilis after 15 years of age; 6.5 percent developed symptomatic neurosyphilis; and 16 percent developed the late benign syphilis or gummas. Many of the patients had one or more late complications. Of those who went to autopsy, 35 percent of the men and 22 percent of the women had evidence of cardiovascular involvement, especially aortitis. Syphilis was considered the primary cause of death in 15 percent of the men and 8 percent of the women.

A prospective study involving 431 black men with seropositive latent syphilis of 3 or more years' duration was undertaken in 1932 (the Tuskeegee study, 1932–1962).[16] This study showed that hypertension in syphilitic black men 25–50 years of age was 17 percent more common than in nonsyphilitics. Cardiovascular complications including hypertension were more common than neurologic complications were, and both were increased over control populations. Anatomic evidence of aortitis was found to be 25–35 percent more common in autopsied syphilitics, while evidence of central nervous system syphilis was found in 4 percent of the patients. Other studies found higher rates of neurosyphilis.[8]

A third large study involving 382 autopsies of adults revealed similar overall results (the Rosahn study, 1917–1941).[17] Late syphilis was reported in 39 percent, and about 20 percent were felt to have died because of these late complications. Late anatomic lesions at autopsy were as follows: cardiovascular, 83 percent; neurologic, 8 percent; and gummas, 9 percent.

As a result of these studies, the variable waxing and waning course and unpredictable progression to late syphilis was documented. There was an increased overall mortality in syphilitic as compared with nonsyphilitic populations. The development of late complications was shown to occur about twice as often in men than in women, and a racial difference was suggested: blacks were more likely to develop cardiovascular syphilis, whereas whites were more likely to develop neurosyphilis.

CLINICAL MANIFESTATIONS

It was once an adage of medicine that "he who knew syphilis knew medicine." Penicillin therapy changed all that, but one of its legacies is the frequency of delayed and/or erroneous diagnoses that occurs today.[18]

Primary Syphilis

The classic primary chancre beings at the site of inoculation as a single painless papule. It appears after an average 21-day incubation period (3- to 90-day range), quickly erodes, and becomes indurated (Figs. 3 and 4). The base is usually smooth, and the borders are raised and firm and have a characteristic cartilaginous consistency. Unless secondarily infected, the ulcer has a clean appearance and no exudate. The lesion is painless although slightly tender to touch, and there is little pain or bleeding when the ulcer is scraped as for a darkfield examination. Multiple chancres, however, do occur[19], especially in persons infected with HIV. Atypical lesions or the absence of a primary skin lesion are also common. The variations in presentation are dependent upon the number of treponemes inoculated, the immune status of the patient, intercurrent antibiotic therapy, and whether the lesion becomes secondarily infected. In human volunteers with no evidence of a previous infection, a small inoculum produces only a papular lesion, whereas a large inoculum will produce an ulcerative lesion (chancre) in which treponemes can be easily identified. Persons with a history of a previous syphilitic infection will fail to develop any lesions or develop a small darkfield-negative papule, depending on how long their natural infection went untreated.[13] Thus, any genital lesion should raise the suspicion of syphilis, and appropriate studies to establish the diagnosis should be undertaken. The chancre will be located wherever the inoculation took place. The external genitalia are obviously the most frequently involved sites. Other common sites include the cervix, mouth, perianal area, and anal canal in the female and the perianal area, anal canal, and mouth of the male homosexual. A secondary infection of the primary lesion is more common with oral and anal lesions.

Regional lymphadenopathy consisting of moderately enlarged, firm, nonsuppurative, painless lymph nodes or satellite buboes accompany the primary lesion.

The chancre either heals within 3–6 weeks (range, 1–12 weeks) without a trace or leaves a thin atrophic scar. However, the lymphadenopathy usually persists for a longer period of time. The manifestations of secondary syphilis often develop while the chancre is still present.[8,9]

Pathologically, the chancre is characterized by an intense infiltration of plasma cells and scattered histiocytes, a concentric endothelial and fibroplastic proliferative thickening of small blood vessels, and eventually the omnipresent and nearly diagnostic obliterative endarteritis.[9] Spirochetes can be identified by silver, immunofluorescent, or other specific antibody-staining methods (see below).

Primary syphilis must be differentiated prinicpally from herpesvirus infections, chancroid, and traumatic suprainfected genital lesions. Primary genital herpes usually begins as a painful erythematous rash that develops into clusters of vesicles accompanied by regional lymphadenopathy and systemic symptoms. It runs a 10- to 14-day course. Recurrent genital herpes is less florid and is characterized by mild to moderately painful vesicles and no adenopathy. A syphilitic rash is never vesicular except in congenital syphilis. Chancroid is characterized by one or more painful, exudative, indurated ulcers associated with tender lymphadenopathy that eventually suppurate if untreated. The ulcer has overhanging edges and bleeds easily (e.g., when scrapings are collected for a darkfield examination.) Early venereal warts, granuloma inguinale, lymphogranuloma venereum, tuberculosis, atypical mycobacterial infections, tularemia, sporotrichosis, anthrax, rat-bite fever, or any genital ulcer may resemble early primary syphilis.

Secondary Syphilis

Secondary, or disseminated, syphilis is the term used to describe the most clinically florid stage of the infection that results

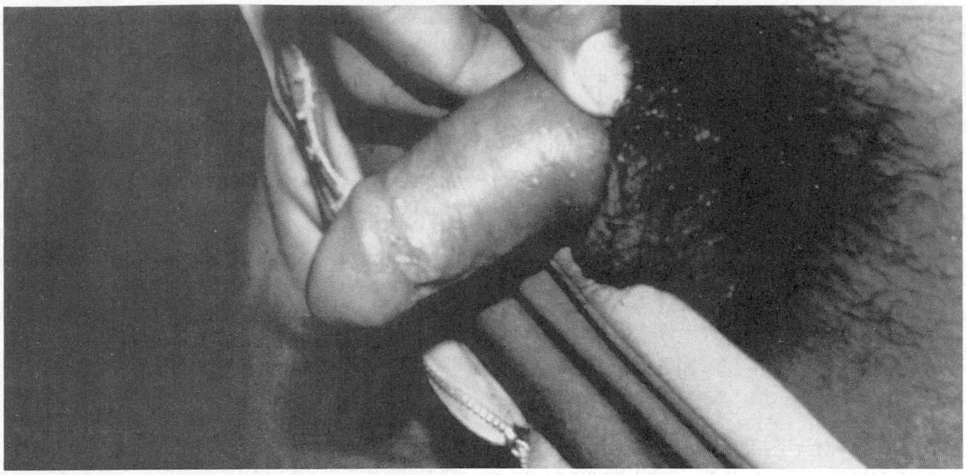

FIG. 3. Primary and syphilitic chancre of the penis.

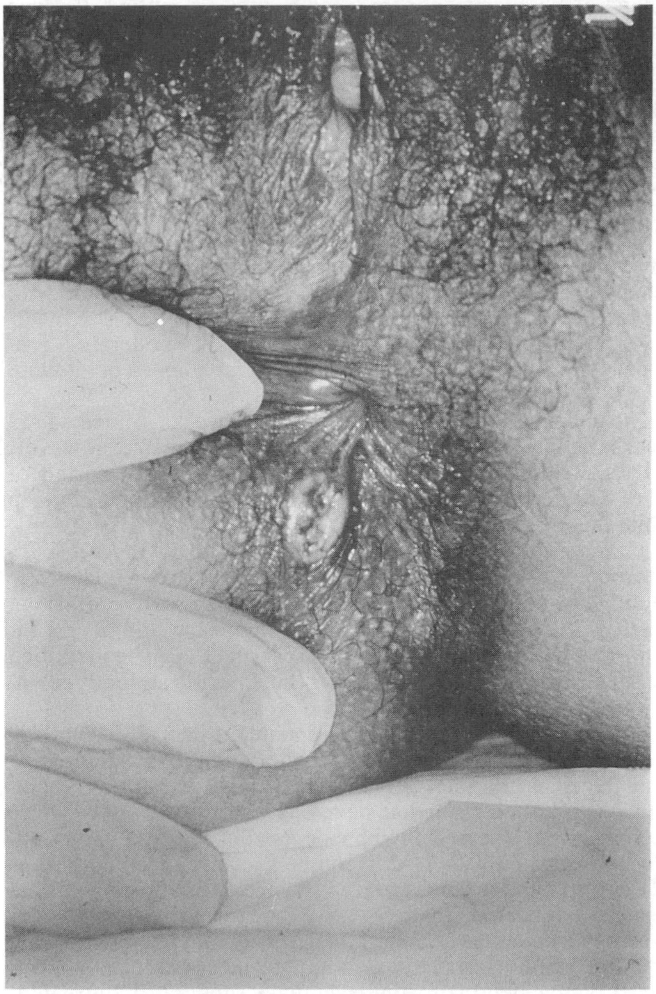

FIG. 4. Primary syphilitic chancre of the perineum.

from multiplication and dissemination of the spirochete and lasts until an immune response develops that exerts some control over the spirochete. It begins 2–8 weeks after the appearance of a chancre, but the time is quite variable. The primary chancre may still be present.[8,9] It is remarkable that, at a time when the host's local immune process appears to be bringing the primary lesions under control, the spirochete disseminates widely and achieves its greatest numbers.

The manifestations of secondary syphilis are widespread and protean (Table 1). The classic and most commonly recognized lesions occur in the skin. Macular, maculopapular, papular, and/or pustular lesions and variations thereof all occur.[8,9,20] Vesicular lesions are conspicuously absent. These lesions usually begin on the trunk and proximal extremities as bilateral pink-to-red discrete mascular lesions 3–10 mm in diameter. Any surface area of the body can become involved. These lesions usually persist from a few days to 8 weeks and often evolve from macules into red papules (hence, maculopapular) and in a few patients finally progress into pustular lesions (pustular syphilids). The degree of endarteritis and perivascular mononuclear infiltration progresses in the same manner. All of the different rashes may be present at one time and become widely distributed to involve the entire body, especially on the palms and soles, locations that strongly suggest the diagnosis (Fig. 5).

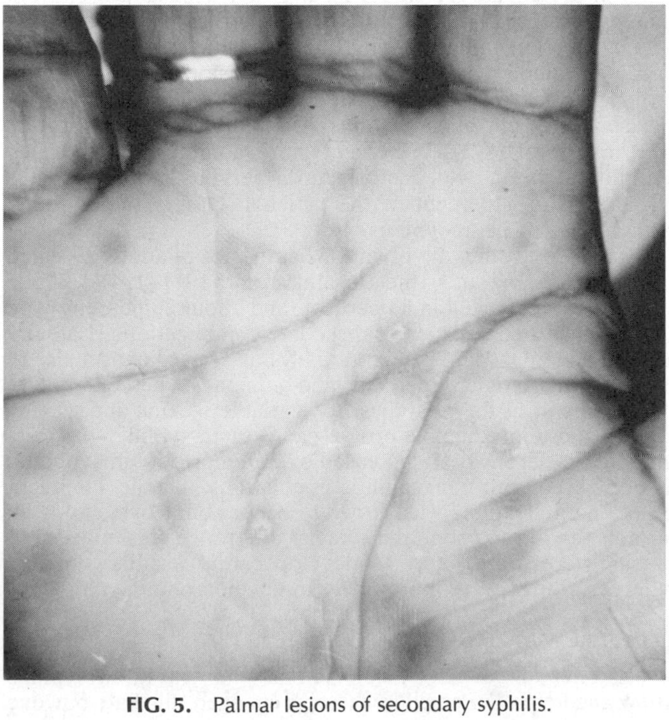

FIG. 5. Palmar lesions of secondary syphilis.

TABLE 1. The Clinical Manifestations of Secondary Syphilis

Manifestation	*Percentage of Cases*
Skin	90
Rash	
Macular	
Maculopapular	
Papular	
Pustular	
Condyloma lata	
Generalized lymphadenopathy	
Pruritus	
Mouth and throat	35
Mucous patches	
Erosions	
Ulcer (aphthous)	
Genital lesions	20
Chancre	
Condyloma lata	
Mucous patch	
Constitutional symptoms	70
Fever of unknown origin	
Malaise	
Pharyngitis, laryngitis	
Anorexia, weight loss	
Arthralgias	
Central nervous system	
Asymptomatic	8–40
Symptomatic	1–2
Headache	
Meningismus	
Meningitis	
Ocular	
Diplopia	
Decreased vision	
Otitic	
Tinnitus	
Vertigo	
Cranial nerve involvement (II–VIII)	
Renal	Unusual
Glomerulonephritis	
Nephrotic syndrome	
Gastrointestinal	Unusual
Hepatitis	Unusual
Intestinal wall invasion	
Arthritis, osteitis, and periostitis	Unusual

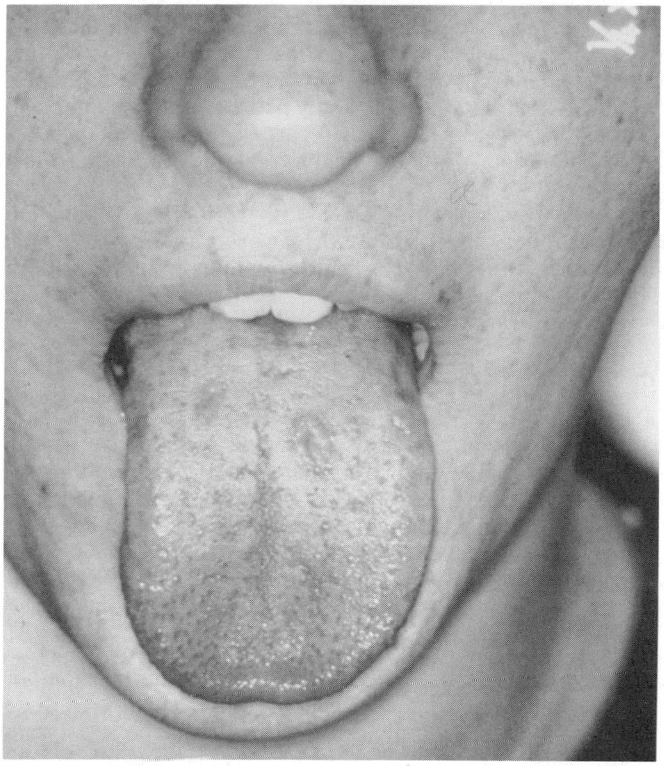

FIG. 6. Mucous patch lesion of secondary syphilis.

When the hair follicles are involved (follicular syphilids), temporary patchy alopecia[8,20] or thinning and a loss of eyebrows and beard may develop. Sometimes a superficial scaling develops (papulosquamous syphilids). In warm, moist intertriginous areas (perianal area, vulva, scrotum, inner aspects of the thighs, the skin under pendulous breasts, nasolabial folds, cleft of the chin, axillary and antecubital folds, webs of the fingers and toes) the papules enlarge, coalesce, and erode to produce painless, broad, moist, gray-white to erythematous highly infectious plaques called condyloma lata. Highly infectious lesions teeming with spirochetes may also develop on mucous membranes (lips, mouth, pharynx, tonsils, vulva, vagina, glans penis, inner prepuce cervix, anal canal). These lesions, referred to as mucous patches, are typically a silvery gray superficial erosion surrounded by a red periphery (Fig. 6). None of these lesions are painful unless secondarily infected.

During relapses of secondary syphilis, the skin lesions tend to be less florid, asymmetrically distributed, and more infiltrated, which suggests a more effective host immune response. Condyloma lata, however, are quite common.

Constitutional symptomatology is also commonly manifested in secondary syphilis. They include low-grade fever, malaise pharyngitis, laryngitis, anorexia, weight loss, arthralgias, and generalized painless lymphadenopathy. Enlargement of the epitrochlear lymph nodes is a unique finding that should always suggest the diagnosis.

The central nervous system will become involved in up to 40 percent of patients[11] as the result of seeding during the inevitable spirochetemia. Headache and meningismus are common, increased cerebrospinal fluid (CSF) protein levels and lymphocyte counts are found in 8–40 percent of the patients,[20a] and acute aseptic meningitis develops in 1–2 percent of the patients. Spirochetes have also been isolated from the CSF of patients with no CSF abnormalities.[11,21] Individual cranial nerves, especially II–VIII, can be involved.[22]

Virtually any organ in the body can be involved. Renal involvement may be in the form of an immune-complex glomerulonephritis (subepithelial electron-dense deposits). Proteinuria is common, an acute nephrotic syndrome may develop, and rarely, hemorrhagic glomerulonephritis occurs.[14]

Syphilitic hepatitis is characterized by an unusually high serum alkaline phosphatase level, a normal or moderately elevated serum bilirubin content, and a histologic picture that includes moderate inflammation with polymorphonuclear cells and lymphocytes, some hepatocellular damage, but no cholestasis.[23] It occurs most often in conjunction with syphilitic proctitis and is seen most frequently in homosexual men. The gastrointestinal tract may also become extensiveley infiltrated and/or ulcerated and can be misdiagnosed as a lymphoma or other cancer.[18,24] Anterior uveitis, usually mild and asymptomatic, occurs in 5–10 percent of the patients with secondary syphilis, and the diagnosis is suggested whenever the uveitis is made worse by steroid treatment.[25,26]

Synovitis, osteitis and periosteitis can also occur.[27,28] These cases are often characterized by nocturnal pain that is increased by heat.[29]

The differential diagnosis of secondary syphilis is extensive, and the appellation "The Great Imitator" is appropriate.

Latent Syphilis

Latent syphilis is by definition that stage of the disease in which a specific treponemal antibody test (fluorescent treponemal antibody absorption [FTA-abs], *Treponema pallidium* hemagglutination [TPHA], microhemagglutination for *T. pallidum* [MHA-TP], *T. pallidum* immobilization [TPI]) is positive but in which there are no clinical manifestations of syphilis, normal cerebrospinal findings, and a normal chest x-ray film. It does not imply a lack of progression of disease. A history compatible with primary or secondary syphilis, exposure to a syphilitic person or delivery of an infant with congenital syphilis may be obtained. Early latent syphilis distinguishes that period of time (first 4 years) during which a relapse may occur (and, therefore, the patient is "infectious"). Ninety percent of the relapses will occur in the first year, and each recurring episode becomes less florid over time. Mucocutaneous relapses are the most common.

Late latent syphilis is associated with resistance to reinfection as well as to infectious relapse.[13] However, a pregnant woman with late latent syphilis can infect her fetus in utero, and an infection can be transmitted via transfused contaminated blood. These patients are treated as if they have late syphilis.

Late Syphilis

Late syphilis (tertiary syphilis) is a slowly progressive inflammatory disease that can affect any organ in the body and can produce clinical illness years after the initial infection. It is generally referred to as neurosyphilis, cardiovascular syphilis, or gummatous syphilis.

Neurosyphilis

Neurosyphilis usually refers to a late stage of the illness rather than to the frequent (up to 40 percent) invasion of the CNS that occurs during the early stages of the disease and that may or may not lead to acute meningeal neurosyphilis (Fig. 7). Late neurosyphilis is usually divided into asymptomatic and symptomatic phases (Table 2).[30] Although this classification recognizes the existence of distinctive forms of neurosyphilis, there is almost always overlap with combinations of meningovascular and parenchymatous features. This is not surprising since neurosyphilis is fundamentally a chronic meningitis involving every portion of the CNS.

The diagnosis of asymptomatic neurosyphilis is given to patients who have no clinical manifestation of neurosyphilis but who have one or more CSF abnormalities. These include pleocytosis, an elevated protein level, a decreased glucose concentration, or a positive Venereal Disease Research Laboratory (VDRL) test response. Local CNS production of treponema antibodies is highly suggestive of an active case of neurosyphilis.[31–34]

The incidence of asymptomatic neurosyphilis in untreated patients ranges from 8 to 40 percent.[35,36] How many of these cases progress to symptomatic neurosyphilis is problematic. With the exception of an Argyll Robertson pupil and tabes dorsalis, the symptoms and signs of neurosyphilis are nonspecific (Table 3), and there is evidence to suggest that symptomatic neurosyphilis can be present in as many as 4 percent of the patients with normal spinal fluid findings.[36] Since lumbar puncture is necessary to make the diagnosis of asymptomatic neurosyphilis and since asymptomatic neurosyphilis occurs in at least 40 percent[11] of the patients, a lumbar puncture should be performed in the follow-up of anyone who may not have been adequately treated, which includes anyone treated with benzathine penicillin (see below).

Late symptomatic neurosyphilis is divided into two major clinical categories that have been correlated with pathologic findings: meningovascular neurosyphilis and parenchymatous neurosyphilis (Table 3). However, a great deal of overlap occurs. (Syphilitic meningitis resembling "aseptic" meningitis may occur during the secondary stage.) Meningovascular neurosyphilis refers to the development of typical endarteritis obliterans, which affects the small blood vessels of the meninges, brain, and spinal cord and leads to multiple small areas of infarction. Parenchymatous neurosyphilis refers to the actual destruction of nerve cells, principally in the cerebral cortex. Thus, the former represents an inflammatory process and the latter a degenerative one, but a mixture of the two pathologic processes is always present. Vascular involvement may lead to a wide spectrum of diseases ranging from hemiplegia to progressive neurologic deficits that are the result of the gradual destruction of nerve tissue by small-vessel endarteritis. Hemiparesis, aphasia, and either focal or generalized seizures may occur and are more frequent now than previously.[36a]

Parenchymatous neurosyphilis includes general paresis and tabes dorsalis, is the result of widespread parenchymal damage, and is a combination of psychiatric manifestations and neurologic findings. Abnormalities correspond to the pneumonic "paresis": Personality (emotional lability, paranoia), Affect (carelessness in appearance), Reflexes (hyperactive), Eye (Argyll

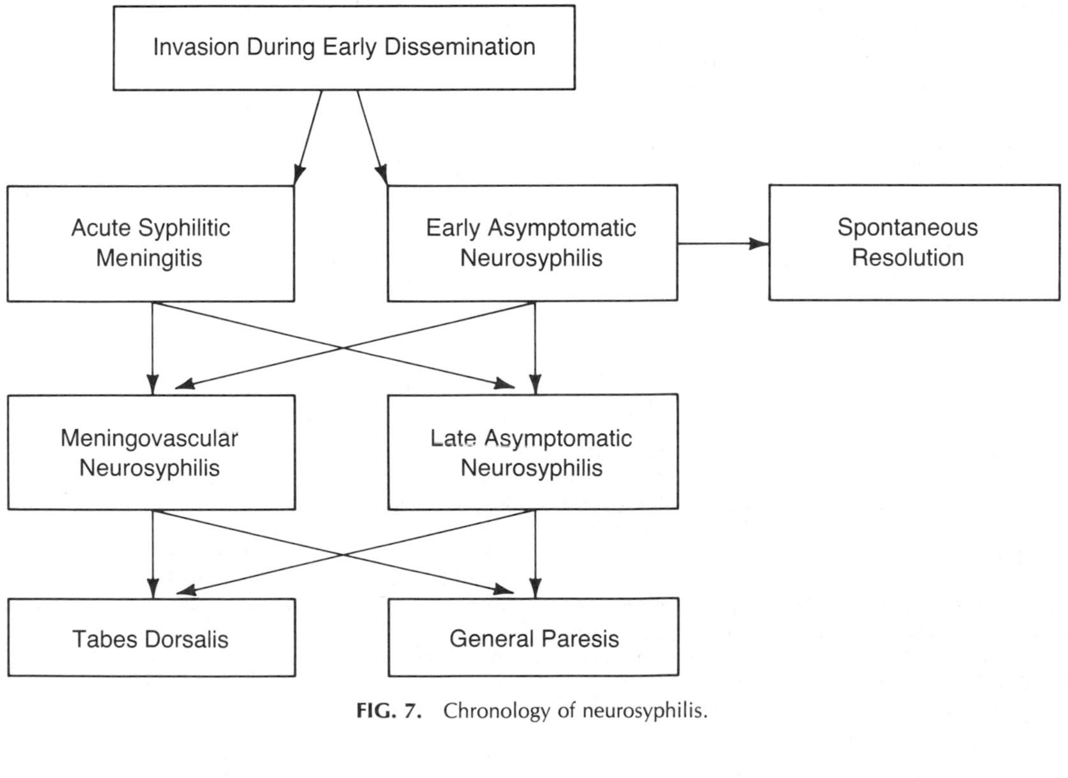

FIG. 7. Chronology of neurosyphilis.

TABLE 2. Classification of Neurosyphilis

Manifestation	*Cases (%) (N = 676)*
Syphilitis meningitis as a complication of secondary syphilis	
Asymptomatic	8–40
Symptomatic	1–2
Asymptomatic late neurosyphilis	31
Symptomatic late neurosyphilis	69
Meningovascular	
Cerebromeningeal	6
Diffuse	
Focal	
Cerebrovascular	10
Spinal	3
Parenchymatous	
Tabetic	30
Paretic	12
Taboparetic	3
Ocular	3
Miscellaneous	2

(Modified from Merritt et al.,[30] with permission.)

TABLE 3. Clinical Manifestations of Neurosyphilis

- Meningovascular
  - Hemiplegia or hemiparesis
  - Seizures
    - Generalized
    - Focal
  - Aphasia
- Parenchymatous
  - General paresis
    - Changes in personality, affect, sensorium, intellect, insight, and judgment
    - Hyperactive reflexes
    - Speech disturbances (slurring)
    - Pupillary disturbances (Argyll Robertson pupils)
    - Optic atrophy tremors (face, tongue, hands, legs)
  - Tabes dorsalis
    - Shooting or lightning pains
    - Ataxia
    - Pupillary disturbances (Argyll Robertson pupils)
    - Impotence
    - Bladder disturbances
    - Fecal incontinence
    - Peripheral neuropathy
    - Romberg sign
    - Cranial nerve involvement (II–VII)

Robertson pupils), Sensorium (illusions, delusions, especially megalomania, hallucinations), Intellect (decreased recent memory, judgment, insight), and Speech (slurred). Spinal cord damage (tabes dorsalis) involves prinicipally demyelinzation of the posterior column, dorsal roots, and dorsal root ganglia that eventually results in the development of an ataxic wide-based gait and footslap, paresthesias, "shooting" or "lightning" pains (sudden onset, rapid radiation, and disappearance), bladder disturbances, fecal incontinence, impotence, loss of position and vibratory sense, absent ankle and knee jerks, and loss of deep pain and temperature sensation. The Romberg sign, the inability to stand with feet together and eyes closed without falling over, is classically present in tabes dorsalis. Trophic degenerative joint disease (Charcot's joints) and traumatic ulcers or sores on the lower extremities and feet as a result of the loss of sensation were prominently featured in old textbooks of physical diagnosis but are seldom seen today.

Ocular disturbances are common. The Argyll Robertson pupil refers to a small irregular pupil that accommodates to near vision but does not react to light or painful stimuli. Optic atrophy may occur usually over a period of months to years. The nerve degeneration usually begins peripherally and proceeds to the center of the nerve, producing progressive concentric constriction of the visual fields (gun barrel sight) with retention of normal vision.

While any cranial nerve can be affected, the most frequent are the 7th and 8th cranial nerves (40 percent), which results in the gradual development of a loss of facial expression; tremors of the lips, tongue, and facial muscles; and difficulty enunciating words, e.g., "methodist–episcopal."

The 2nd, 3rd, and 4th cranial nerves are the next most common (25 percent) nerves affected. Meningovascular syphilis usually occurs 5–10 years after the onset of disease, general paresis 15–20 years after, and tabes dorsalis 25–30 years after.

Two other special forms of neurosyphilis need to be emphasized: syphilitic otitis (asymmetric deafness, tinnitus)[37] and syphilitic eye disease (optic atrophy, asymptomatic progressive visual loss leading to blindness, ptosis).[38] The ear and the eye may be involved during any stage of the disease, including congenital syphilis. They may be the only clinically apparent presentations and usually represent diagnostic dilemmas.[26,38] In early stages they are curable;[39] if untreated they cause irreversible damage.

A positive treponemal antibody test, e.g., TPHA test is found in approximately 7 percent of patients with otherwise unexplained sensorineural hearing loss and in 7 percent of patients with cochleovestibular dysfunction (Menière's disease).[38] Congenital otic syphilis is usually bilateral and more severe than acquired syphilis is. Specialized diagnostic procedures have been developed.[38] Any patient with unexplained hearing loss or vestibular abnormalities, and a positive treponemal antibody test should be treated for syphilitic otitis.[22,37]

Any inflammatory disease of the eye can be mimicked by syphilitic involvement. Uveitis, diffuse chorioretinitis, and vasculitis are the most common disorders and may accompany acute syphilitic meningitis or be an isolated manifestation of secondary syphilis.[20a] Uveitis appears prone to develop after treatment with corticosteroids.[25,26] The differential diagnosis of other systemic diseases includes tuberculosis, rheumatoid arthritis, sarcoidosis, and ocular *Toxocara canis* infections.

The conditions from which neurosyphilis must be differentiated are numerous. They include any degenerative neurologic process, disorders that cause chronic inflammation (e.g., tuberculosis, fungal or sarcoid meningitis, tumors, subdural hematoma, Alzheimer's disease, multiple sclerosis, chronic alcoholism), or any disorder affecting the vasculature of the CNS. The axiom that syphilis can mimic any disease is particularly apropos with regard to the CNS.

Given the vagaries of neurosyphilis, the diagnosis can be very difficult to make. In modern medicine, one is loath to label a patient with a specific etiologic infectious diagnosis without isolation of the infecting organism from the patient (culture, antigen capture, pathologic demonstration). But because *T. pallidum* cannot be cultured in vitro, serologic or antibody tests alone are relied upon to diagnose and follow these patients. However, the demonstration of specific treponemal IgG and IgM antibody production in the CNS is very helpful.[31–34]

The aim of treatment has been to develop a rational and safe therapeutic approach so that the patient has a reasonable expectation that his/her disease will be cured or will not progress to a severe neurologic disability.

However, despite these difficulties, the following points must be remembered: (*1*) A spirochetemia always develops in patients with syphilis before invasion of the CNS. Thus, the diagnosis of neurosyphilis cannot be made without a positive serum treponemal antibody response (e.g., TPHA). (*2*) A positive CSF-VDRL always indicates active neurosyphilis. (*3*) Any CSF abnormality in the appropriate clinical setting strongly suggests active neurosyphilis. (*4*) Local CNS production of antitreponemal antibody is highly suggestive of neurosyphilis. Therefore, any patient with a positive specific serum treponemal antibody test, a positive CSF-VDRL, and/or evidence of local CNS antibody production with or without otherwise explained neurologic findings warrants therapy or close follow-up for neurosyphilis (see below).

Cardiovascular Syphilis

The underlying pathologic lesion of cardiovascular syphilis is the omnipresent endarteritis obliterans, in this case involving the vasa vasorum of the aorta. This results in a medial necrosis with destruction of elastic tissue and subsequent aortitis with a saccular or, occasionally, a fusiform aneurysm. There is a predilection to involve the ascending aorta which leads to weakness of the aortic valve ring and distortion of the cups, and results in aortic regurgitation and coronary artery stenosis. The transverse segment of the aortic arch is the next most frequently involved area, while the aorta below the renal arteries is seldom involved.[8,9] Symptomatic syphilitic aortitis occurs in approximately 10 percent of untreated cases, but the pathologic lesions can be demonstrated on postmortem examination in up to 83 percent of cases of untreated neurosyphilis.[17] A symptomatic syphilitic aortitis should be suspected whenever linear calcifications are noted on chest x-ray films of the ascending aorta, a finding seldom seen in arteriosclerotic disease. Syphilitic aneurysms rarely dissect. Neurologic involvement is common in patients with syphilitic aortitis. Other large arteries such as the temporal artery may also be involved.[40] Because of the success of antibiotic treatment, cardiovascular syphilis is now a medical curiosity in the United States.

Late Benign Syphilis (Gumma)

The gumma is a nonspecific granulomatous-like lesion occurring in late syphilis[8,9] that is rarely seen today. These indolent lesions are most commonly found in the skeletal system, skin, and mucocutaneous tissues but can develop in any organ. They may occur singly or multiply and vary in size from microscopic defects to large tumor-like masses. They are of clinical importance principally as a cause of local destruction. The cutaneous manifestations range from superficial nodules to deep granulomatous lesions, which may break down to form punched-out ulcers. Involution is followed by the development of a thin, atrophic, noncontractile scar arranged in arciform patterns.[8,9] Gummatous hepatitis may cause low-grade fever, epigastric pain and tenderness, and eventual cirrhosis (hepar lobatum). Gummas of the bone may result in fractures or joint destruction, whereas those in the upper respiratory tract can lead to perforation of the nasal system or palate. Trauma may predispose to involvement of a specific site. They must be distinguished from other granulomatous lesions such as tuberculosis, sarcoidosis, and other granulomatous lesions such as tuberculosis, sarcoidosis, and deep fungal infections and from neoplasms. The spirochetes in these lesions are difficult to visualize on microscopic examination. A therapeutic trial of penicillin results in a rapid and dramatic response. Gummas were the most frequent (approximately 15 percent) late complication seen in the Oslo study.

Congenital Syphilis

The incidence of congenital syphilis rose in the mid 1980s coincident with the rise of syphilis in the heterosexual population. Infection of the fetus in utero can occur in any untreated mother but is most likely to occur during the early stages of the infection. The risk of fetal infection decreases progressively thereafter. Infection of the fetus before the fourth month of gestation is rare, thus, early abortion due to syphilis is not seen. Treatment of the mother during the first 4 months of pregnancy usually ensures that the fetus will not be infected. Depending on the severity of the infection, late abortion, stillbirth, neonatal death, neonatal disease, or latent infection may be seen.[8,9]

The clinical pattern is quite variable, but most often there are no abnormal physical findings (Table 4).[8,9,41] In the perinatal period (infantile form) the most striking lesions affect the mucocutaneous tissues and bones. The earliest sign of congenital syphilis is usually a rhinitis (snuffles), which is soon followed by a diffuse maculopapular desquamative rash with extensive sloughing of the epithelium, particularly on the palms, soles, and about the mouth and anus. In contrast to acquired syphilis, a vesicular rash and bullae may develop. These lesions are teeming with spirochetes and have the characteristic obliterative endarteritis and perivascular mononuclear cuffing on microscopic examination that are found in other syphilitic lesions.

TABLE 4. Clinical Signs of Congenital Syphilis

Early	
Osteochondritis	55[a]
Snuffles	40
Rash	40
Anemia	30
Hepatosplenomegaly	20
Jaundice	20
Neurologic signs	20
Lymphadenopathy	5
Mucous patches	5
Late	
Frontal bosses	
Short maxillas	
Saddle nose	
Protruding mandible	
Interstitial keratitis	
Eighth nerve deafness	
High palatal arch	
Hutchinson's incisors	
Mulberry molars	
Sternoclavicular thickening (Higoménakis sign)	
Clutton's joints (bilateral painless swelling of knees)	
Saber shins	
Flaring scapulas	

[a] Percentage of cases.
(Data from Kampmeier[8] and Stokes et al.[9])

There may be a generalized osteochondritis and perichondritis that may affect the architecture of all bones of the skeletal system, most prominently the nose (saddle nose) and the metaphyses of the lower extremities (anterior bowing or "saber shin"). The liver is often heavily infected and is associated with splenomegaly, anemia, thrombocytopenia, and jaundice. The generalized spirochetemia may lead to diffuse inflammatory changes of virtually any organ of the body. Neonatal death is usually due to liver failure, severe pneumonia, or pulmonary hemorrhage. Renal involvement with an immune-complex glomerulonephritis may develop and usually occurs about the fourth month of life.[14] Neonatal congenital syphilis must be differentiated from other generalized congenital infections such as rubella, cytomegalovirus infection, and toxoplasmosis.

If the untreated child survives the first 6–12 months of life, he enters, with a few notable exceptions, a latent period. The late development of cardiovascular syphilis is rare, but interstitial keratitis is quite common. Photophobia, pain, circumcorneal inflammation, and superficial and deep vascularization of the cornea may occur any time between the ages of 5 and 30 years. Asymptomatic or symptomatic neurosyphilis is also common in these patients and resembles the disease in adults. Eighth nerve deafness is particularly common.[42] Necrotizing funisitis, an inflammatory process involving the matrix of the umbilical cord and characterized by perivascular inflammation and obliterative endarteritis, is for all practical purposes pathogonomonic of congenital syphilis. It should be suspected clinically whenever the umbilical cord is swollen and discolored red, white, and blue to resemble a barber's pole.[42a]

Other characteristic stigmata include recurrent arthropathy and bilateral knee effusions (Clutton's joints); centrally notched, widely spread, peg-shaped upper central incisors (Hutchinson's teeth); frontal bossing; and poorly developed maxillas.[9]

Since at least one-third of the mothers who give birth to syphilitic children will not have had prenatal care and about half will have had a nonreactive serologic test during the first trimester of pregnancy, serologic testing is warranted at the time of delivery, especially in high-risk patients.[8,41,43] Because giving penicillin to the neonate is virtually risk free, treatment of all neonates born to syphilitic mothers is warranted.

Atypical Presentations of Syphilis

As noted earlier, the clinical presentations and course of syphilis are quite varied, and the diagnosis can sometimes elude the clinician even under the best of circumstances. Because some patients may have been treated with antibiotics that are suboptimal, i.e., oral penicillin, or inadequate, i.e., spectinomycin, and because of a larger pool of immunocompromised patients (see below) and the relative inexperience of today's clinician with syphilitic patients, there is a sense that unusual patterns and atypical presentations have become more common. However, protean manifestations are the hallmark of syphilis. Older clinicians were never surprised by "unusual findings," and today's clinician should not be either.

LABORATORY DIAGNOSIS

Darkfield Examination Technique

In primary, secondary, and early congenital syphilis, the darkfield examination is the quickest and most direct laboratory method of establishing the diagnosis.[8,9] Examination of a serous transudate from moist lesions such as a primary chancre, condyloma lata, or a mucous patch is the most productive since these lesions will have the largest numbers of treponemes. However, *T. pallidum* can be demonstrated at times from dry skin lesions and lymph nodes by saline aspiration (the saline must be free of bactericidal additives). The surface of the suspected lesion should be cleaned with saline and gently abraded with dry gauze so as not to produce gross bleeding. The serous exudate can then be squeezed onto a glass slide, covered with a coverslip, and examined with darkfield or phase-contrast microscopy. A drop of nonbactericidal saline may be added if the preparation is too thick. *Treponema pallidum* will have a corkscrew appearance and will move in a spiraling (Fig. 8) motion with a characteristic undulation about its midpoint. A lesion should be considered nonsyphilitic only after three negative examinations have been made. Specimens from mouth lesions are worthless since *T. pallidum* cannot be distinguished from nonpathogenic treponemes. A scattering of a few red blood cells will indicate that the specimen is adequate. Cleaning of the lesion with a topical antiseptic or bactericidal saline obscures the diagnosis since dead and nonmotile organisms are difficult to identify. However, if this is inadvertently done, direct or indirect immunofluorescent or immunoperoxidase staining can be used to establish the presence of *T. pallidum*.[44]

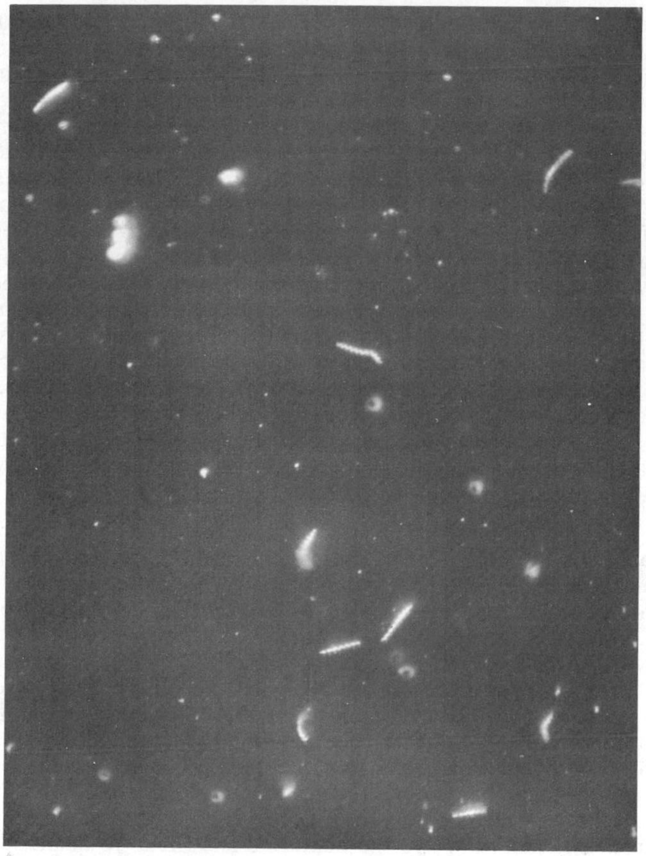

FIG. 8. Darkfield examination. The morphologic characteristics of the spirochetes and the characteristic flexous motion about its center can be appreciated.

Biopsy Specimen

The spirochete can sometimes be demonstrated in biopsy materials. A silver stain is most commonly used, but confusion with elastic tissues can occur. Specific immunofluorescent or immunoperoxidase staining of nonfrozen pathologic specimens are now preferable to silver staining.[45,46]

TABLE 5. Percentage of Patients with Positive Responses to Commonly Used Serologic Tests

	Stage		
Test	*1°*	*2°*	*Late*
Nontreponemal (reaginic tests)			
Veneral Disease Research Laboratory (reaginic) test (VDRL)	70[a]	99[a]	1[b]
Rapid plasma reagin card test (RPR)	80	99	0
Automated reagin test (ART)			
Specific treponemal tests			
Fluorescent antibody absorbed test (FTA-abs)	85	100	98
T. pallidum hemagglutination assay (TPHA, MHA-TP)	65	100	95
Treponemal immobilization test (TPI)	50	97	95

[a] Percentage of patients with positive serologic tests in treated or untreated primary or secondary syphilis.
[b] Treated late syphilis.

Serologic Tests

Confusion surrounds interpretation of the serologic tests for syphilis. This is principally because of the two different types of antibodies measured: the *nonspecific* nontreponemal reaginic antibody and the *specific* antitreponemal antibody. The former is inexpensive, rapid, and convenient for screening large numbers of sera and is also quite helpful as an indication of disease activity. Specific antibody tests establish the high likelihood of a treponemal infection, either at the present time or at sometime in the past (Table 5).

Nontreponemal Reaginic Tests. Much of the confusion about these tests arises from the term *reagin*. This is the result of an unfortunate quirk in the evolution of medical terminology since it has nothing to do with the reagin IgE immunoglobulin involved in allergic reactions. "Syphilis reaginic" antibodies are IgG and IgM immunoglobulins directed against a lipoidal antigen that is the result of the interaction of host tissues with *T. pallidum* and/or from *T. pallidum* itself. The earliest cardiolipin antigens used to measure reaginic antibody were crude extracts made from beef livers or beef hearts. False-positive reactions were quite common. The cardiolipin-cholesterol-lecithin used today is a much purer preparation and gives fewer false-positive reactions. The relationship of these tests with *T. pallidum* infection is fortuitous.

The standard nontreponemal test is the VDRL slide test in which heated serum (56°C) is tested for its ability to flocculate a suspension of a cardiolipin-cholesterol-lecithin antigen. It is now most often used to follow a patient's response to therapy. Most laboratories and blood banks have adapted one of two modifications for routine screening for syphilis: the rapid plasma reagin (RPR) card test or the automated reagin test (ART).

One of the more difficult situations to interpret is the persistent positive VDRL test ("chronic persister") after apparently adequate therapy. This may be a biologically false reaction, or more likely it may indicate persistent active infection or reinfection, especially when the titer is greater than 1:4.

The quantitative RPR test should become nonreactive in primary syphilis 1 year after successful therapy and 2 years after successful therapy in secondary syphilis.[47,48] Most patients with late syphilis should be nonreactive by the fifth year after treatment.[49] The length of time required for the test to become negative correlates with the interval of time between contact and when therapy was instituted and the severity of illness, especially with the type of skin lesions manifested in the secondary stage (i.e., a patient with a macular rash reverts to a negative titer sooner than does a patient with a papular rash).[50] Therefore, a positive RPR response after 1 year in a patient treated for primary syphilis and 2 years for secondary syphilis suggests (*1*) persistent infection, (*2*) reinfection, or (*3*) a biologically false-positive reaction. A patient with late syphilis should have a negative response after 5 years.[47–50]

Specific Treponemal Tests. The principal specific antitreponemal antibody tests done today are the FTA-abs, TPHA, and MHA-TP. The FTA-abs is a standard indirect immunofluorescent antibody test that uses *T. pallidum* harvested from rabbit testes as the antigen. The patient's serum is first absorbed with nonpathogenic treponemal antigen (sorbent) to remove "natural" cross-reacting antibody that may have been raised against saprophytic treponemes of the oral cavity or genital tract. The test has the disadvantage of being standardized at one serum dilution (1:5), and like most other immunofluorescent tests, its interpretation can be quite subjective. Therefore, it requires a great attention to detail, is difficult to standardize from one laboratory to the next, and is difficult to quantitate. Its use as a screening test would be expensive, and when applied to a low-risk population, the number of false-positive reactions would proportionately increase. Thus, its principal use is to verify a positive nontreponemal reaginic test result. Once positive, it remains positive for life.[40,50] Attempts to make the test more predictive of active disease by testing for IgM antibody have not proved useful.[54]

The *T. pallidum* hemagglutination assay (TPHA) is also used to measure specific treponemal antibody. It has the advantage of being easier to peform than the FTA-abs. It uses a "sorbent" to increase specificity, and although it is as specific as the FTA-abs, it is less sensitive in early disease.[50] For practical purposes it is interchangeable with the FTA-abs test. The MHA-TP test is an adaptive of the TPHA utilizing a microtiter plate.

The *T. pallidum* immobilization (TPI) test is rarely used today but was the standard against which all specific treponemal tests were compared. It determines the ability of antibody plus complement to immobilize live *T. pallidum* as visualized under a darkfield microscope (i.e., it is a bactericidal test). It requires the maintenance of replicating *T. pallidum* in rabbits; thus, it is expensive, time-consuming, and difficult to perform. Its utility in today's setting has been questioned.[51] Only a few research laboratories have maintained the capability to perform the TPI test. Recent elucidation of the antigenic structure of the treponeme should lead to simpler tests, especially as increasing incidence results in a greater economic impetus to develop such a test.[52]

The comparative reactivities of the most widely used tests are shown in Table 5. When the diagnosis of syphilis is being seriously considered in an individual patient, the TPHA or FTA-abs test should be done. Once they have become positive and the diagnosis established, their usefulness is limited. A nontreponemal antibody test is very helpful for following the efficacy of therapy. The failure to become negative suggests a persistent infection, reinfection, or a false-positive test response.

The results of the FTA-abs (IgM) test on cord blood to diagnose congenital syphilis has been disappointing,[53] and the best way to follow these infants is with serial quantitative nontreponemal tests performed over a period of several months. As with all serial serologic determinations, the most credible results are those performed simultaneously on appropriately stored serum samples.

Tests for Neurosyphilis. Recent studies have focused on the production of local antitreponemal antibodies in the CNS as a discriminator for CNS invasion.[31–34] This is done by measuring the CSF antitreponemal IgM titer directly[32,34] and by the TPHA-TP–IgG titer in the serum and CSF and correcting for leakage of serum proteins across the blood-brain barrier as follows:

$$\frac{\text{TPHA-IgG titer per mg total IgG (CSF)}}{\text{TPHA-IgG titer per mg total IgG (serum)}} = \text{TPHA-IgG index}^{33}$$

or

$$\frac{\text{CSF-TPHA titer}}{\text{CSF albumin (mg/dl)} \times 10^3 \text{ per serum albumin (mg/dl)}} = \text{TPHA index}^{32}$$

When the former ratio (TPHA-IgG index) is used, the normal range is between 0.5 and 2.0, while patients who are actively producing local CNS antitreponemal antibodies have ratios of 3.0 or greater.[31,33] In the latter test a TPHA index of >100 indicates local antitreponemal antibody production.[32] Leakage of serum proteins into the CSF can be calculated directly by calculating the ratio of serum albumin to CSF albumin or vice versa.[32,33] Oligoclonal antibodies have also been demonstrated.[34a]

The findings of more than five mononuclear cells per cubic millimeter of CSF is also suggestive of active neurosyphilis. A negative CSF-FTA unabsorbed or CSF–TPHA, in essence, rules out neurosyphilis in patients with late disease but not in patients with early disease.[11]

False-Positive Serologic Test for Syphilis. The percentage of false-positive reactions depends on the population being studied. Acute or transient false-positive nontreponemal reaginic test reactions may occur whenever there is a strong immunologic stimulus (acute bacterial or viral infections, vaccination, etc.) Positive reactions persisting for months occur with drug addiction; with autoimmune or connective tissue diseases, especially systemic lupus erythematosus; with aging (up to 10 percent of the persons over the age of 70 years); or in hypergammaglobulinemic states (Table 6). A false-positive nontreponemal reaginic test in this setting tends to be associated with other serum factors frequently associated with autoimmune diseases such as antinuclear, antithyroid, or antimitochondrial antibodies, rheumatoid factor, and cryoglobulins.

A false-positive nontreponemal reaginic test can usually be verified and syphilis excluded by obtaining a negative, specific treponemal antibody test (FTA-abs, TPHA). Unfortunately, sometimes the same illnesses that will result in a false-positive nontreponemal reaginic test (e.g., systemic lupus erythematosus) may also give a positive or borderline positive FTA-abs test reaction. Also, the FTA-abs may be positive when the VDRL is negative.[54] This false reaction can often be distinguished by noting a beaded pattern of immunofluorescence on

TABLE 6. Causes of False-Positive Serologic Test Reactions for Syphilis

Infectious diseases	*Mycoplasma* pneumonia
Lyme disease[a]	Measles
Leptospirosis	Chickenpox
Relapsing fever	Lymphogranuloma venereum
Rat-bite fever (*Spirillum minor*)	Hepatitis
Leprosy	Infectious mononucleosis
Tuberculosis	Early HIV infection
Pneumonococcal pneumonia	Noninfectious diseases
Subacute bacterial endocarditis	Drug addiction
Chancroid	Any connective disease disorder
Scarlet fever	Rheumatoid heart disease
Rickettsial disease	Blood transfusions (multiple)
Malaria	Pregnancy
Trypanosomiasis	"Old age"
Vaccinia (vaccination)	Chronic liver disease

[a] VDRL (RPR)-negative.

the treponemes, but the only definitive way to make the distinction is to obtain the functional TPI test. Other spirochetal illnesses such as relapsing fever (*Borrelia* sp) or yaws, pinta, leptospirosis, rat-bite fever (*Spirillum minor*) will also give positive nontreponemal and treponemal tests, *Borrelia burgdorferi* (Lyme disease) gives a positive FTA-abs but not a positive nontreponemal reaginic reaction (VDRL).

In summary, the reaginic antibody (RPR, VDRL, ART) tests are used for screening large numbers of sera, the specific treponemal tests (TPHA, FTA-abs) for confirming the diagnosis, and the quantitative nontreponemal antibody tests (RPR, VDRL) for assessing the adequacy of therapy.

Isolation of Treponema pallidum

Because *T. pallidum* cannot be cultivated on artificial media, inoculation of laboratory animals (higher primates, rabbit testes) is the only means presently available for isolating the organism.[3,55] The most experience has been with isolation in rabbits. The number of organisms that must be obtained from a human lesion to ensure a positive transfer to the laboratory animals is not known.

The lower portion of the rabbit testis is inoculated with 0.5–3.0 ml of the test material. The rabbits should be kept in a cool (65°F, 17°C) room, and they must be serologically screened ahead of time to exclude concurrent or previous infection with *T. cuniculi* and must be fed antibiotic-free chow. The rabbit testes and/or regional lymph nodes may be harvested after 3 weeks by mincing the testes or lymph nodes and then shaking them in a suitable buffer in a 5–10% CO_2 atmosphere for 30 minutes. This material can be examined by darkfield or fluorescent antibody examination for treponemes, but if negative, it should be injected into another set of test rabbits through at least two passages. Syphilitic infection in the rabbits can also be verified by serologic testing of the rabbit sera.

There has been limited success maintaining *T. pallidum* in tissue culture.[3]

TREATMENT

Although the efficacy of penicillin in the treatment of syphilis is well known, there has never been a well-controlled, carefully planned prospective study to determine the optimal dose or duration of therapy.[56,57] Thus, the following recommendations must be tempered by this knowledge, and it should not be surprising that there are patients who have a persistent infection despite having received "adequate therapy."[11] Nevertheless, by extrapolation from the pharmacokinetics of penicillin therapy, the effect of the drug on *T. pallidum* in experimental conditions, and available clinical data, the current recommendations for the treatment of syphilis are adequate for the overwhelming majority of immunocompetent patients (Table 7). For example, it has been shown in experimental infections (*1*) that *T. pallidum* will regenerate if penicillin blood levels are allowed to fall to subinhibitory levels after 18–24 hours,[58] and from a variety of clinical and experimental data, (*2*) that a level greater than that of 0.03 μg/ml of penicillin is needed to ensure killing of *T. pallidum*[56]; (*3*) that an effective blood level for at least 7 days is necessary to cure early syphilis[56]; and (*4*) that increasing the dose above 0.6 mg/kg over a period of 9 hours does not clear treponemes from primary chancres at an increased rate.[56] Therefore, it can be implied that the most effective antibiotic treatment would be to ensure an adequate blood level over a prolonged period of time. For many years it has been felt that the most convenient way to achieve this goal was to treat with benzathine penicillin, but an awareness of the potential inadequacies of this treatment for CNS invasion[11,21,31] must be maintained. *Treponema pallidum* has been isolated from the CSF of patients with only a chancre,[11] which reflects the spirochetemia that always occurs. Therefore, to reliably cure this readily curable disease, one has to adequately treat treponemes in the CNS (neurosyphilis) even in patients with primary or secondary infections. But benzathine penicillin does not reliably achieve treponemicidal levels in the CSF,[60] numerous treatment failures have been recorded,[11,21,61–63] and the recommendation that benzathine penicillin be considered the treatment of choice was made despite the fact that retreatment was required in as many as 1 of 10 cases.[64,65] On the other hand, there is much clinical experience that suggests that when an early diagnosis is made in an *immunocompetent* host, fewer treponemes exist and the likelihood of completely curing the patient with relatively low doses of penicillin is increased.[56,57] Thus, it seems imprudent to totally abandon 2.4 million units of benzathine penicillin given in two or three doses,[11] which at least gives one some solace in that the patient has circulating penicillin, albeit at low levels, for at least 21 days. Therefore, an increasing number of clinicians now treat syphilis with combination or prolonged therapy to ensure that the most devastating sequela of syphilis, neurosyphilis, does not occur. This is especially true when there is evidence to suggest that the host may be immunocompromised (see below).

Early incubating syphilis is probably aborted when gonorrhea is treated with the currently recommended regimens,[66] spectinomycin excepted.

Because of the high risk of infection, preventive or "epidemiologic" treatment should be given to anyone who was exposed to infectious syphilis within the preceding 3 months. Serologic studies must be done to establish the diagnosis and to follow the adequacy of the response to therapy. These patients should be treated as if they have early syphilis.

Pregnant patients should receive penicillin in dosage schedules appropriate for the stage of syphilis as recommended for nonpregnant patients. Doxycycline should not be used. If the patient has a well-documented penicillin allergy, the choice is more difficult because the efficacy of such treatment for the fetus is not well established. Penicillin desensitization is recommended (see Chapter 21).[67] The patient is given gradually increasing doses of oral or intravenous penicillin over a period of 3–4 hours until full tolerance is achieved.[68] Erythromycin has been used in the past but because of unacceptable failure rates should be used only as a last recourse. Although not yet studied in a prospective fashion, ceftriaxone crosses the placenta and is highly likely to be effective.[59] Tetracycline, erythromycin estolate, and chloramphenicol are *not* recomended because of potential adverse effects on the mother and fetus. The mother should be followed closely during and after the pregnancy, and if an increase in a nontreponemal reagin titer occurs, she must be re-treated.

The risk of infection for the infant is minimal if the mother has received adequate penicillin treatment during pregnancy. However, the child must be examined monthly after delivery and until the nontreponemal reaginic antibody test becomes negative. Because of the small risk of giving penicillin to a newborn, treatment should never be withheld at the expense of "proving the diagnosis," and any child should be promptly treated who is born of a mother who has received inadequate pencillin therapy or treatment with antibiotics other than penicillin and whose treatment status is not well documented or if the infant would be difficult to follow. If neurosyphilis cannot be excluded (which is usually the case), then treatment for asymptomatic neurosyphilis is recommended.[69]

There is no evidence that the efficacy of penicillin treatment of syphilis has diminished over 35 years.[56] However, there is evidence that *T. pallidum* can accept resistant plasmids,[70] and the possibility exists that penicillin treatment may become inadequate in the future.

Tetracycline, chloramphenicol, ceftriaxone, and other cephalosporins have all been shown to be effective alternative antibiotics for treating early syphilis.

Patients also infected with HIV (see HIV below), as with any other immunosuppressed group (see "Immunity," below), present special problems. An intact cellular immune system is an important determinant of the severity of syphilitic disease.

TABLE 7. Recommended Therapy for Syphilis[a]

Stage	*Patients Not Allergic to Penicillin*	*Patients Allergic to Penicillin*[a]
Early syphilis (primary, secondary)	Procaine PCN, 2.4 M units im daily, *plus* Probenecid, 1.0 g po qd × 10 days, *or* Doxycycline, 200 mg po bid × 21 days, *or* Amoxicillin, 3.0 g po bid, *plus* Probenecid, 1.0 g po qd × 14 days, *or* Ceftriaxone,[c] 250 mg im qd or iv × 5 days or 1 gm im qd × 14 days, *or* Benzathine pencillin G,[d] 2.4 million units im weekly for 2 or 3 doses alone or with any of the above oral regimens	Doxycycline, 200 mg po bid × 15 days, *or* Tetracycline hydrochloride, 500 mg po qid × 15 days, *or* Erythromycin (stearate, ethylsuccinate or base), 500 mg qid po × 15 days[b]
Late syphilis (tertiary), neurosyphilis, or HIV infection, especially late-stage IV disease	Aqueous crystalline penicillin G, 2.0–4.0 million units by iv injection q4h × 10 days, *or* Procaine penicillin G, 2.4 million units im, *plus* 1 gm Probenecid, 1 g po daily × 10 days, *or* Amoxicillin, 3 g, + 0.5 g probenicid po bid × 15 days, *or* Doxycycline, 200 mg po bid × 21 days, *or* Ceftriaxone[c] 1 g im or iv × 14 days	Chloramphenicol,[a] 2 gm iv or 500 mg q6h po for 30 days
Pregnancy	Same regimen as for nonpregnant; only penicillin therapy reliably treats the infant	
Congenital syphilis	Aqueous crystalline penicillin G, 50,000 units/kg iv daily in 2 divided doses for a minimum of 10 days, *or* Procaine penicillin G, 50,000 units/kg im daily for a minimum of 10 days	

[a] Therapeutic regimens other than penicillin have not been well studied, especially in patients with syphilis of longer than 1 year's duration; therefore, careful follow-up is mandatory.
[b] Erythromycin is effective in immunocompetent hosts only. Not recommended for pregnant patients.
[c] Ceftriaxone should be diluted in 1% lidocaine solution (1 g/3.6 ml) for im injection.
[d] Treatment failures with benzathine penicillin have been reported. Therefore, the addition of another drug i.e., doxycycline is prudent. Patients treated with benzathine penicillin must be reevaluated at 6-month intervals for neurosyphilis (see the text).
[e] Chloramphenicol is theoretically beneficial treatment for neurosyphilis.

Therefore, these patients should be considered for treatment as if they have neurosyphilis irrespective of their clinical findings, especially when they are in the later stages of their HIV infection.

Late Syphilis, Asymptomatic and Symptomatic Neurosyphilis

Since the central nervous system is invaded during the spirochetemia in at least 40% of patients[11] and since spirochetemia occurs soon after the infection is contracted, all patients with syphilis should be considered to have neurosyphilis, and therefore, a CSF examination is advised. The finding of an elevated mononuclear cell count in the CSF, a positive reactive nontreponemal antibody test (VDRL, RPR), and/or the production of local CNS antitreponemal antibody establishes the diagnosis.[31–34a]

Since benzathine penicillin G seldom produces detectable levels of penicillin in the CSF, this form of penicillin cannot be relied upon as treatment of neurosyphilis[11,12,60,71,72] and, if used, makes it incumbent on the clinician to closely follow the patient with repeated CSF examinations for at least 5 years. To ensure adequate antibiotic levels in the CNS, 12–24 million units of aqueous penicillin G should be given iv for 8–10 days, or 3.0 g amoxicillin bid plus 1.0 g probenecid po for 14 days,[73] or 2.4 million units procaine benzyl penicillin im plus 1 g probenecid po daily for 10 days,[74] or 200 mg doxycycline po bid daily for 21 days,[75] or 1 g ceftriaxone im daily for 14 days,[76] or 2 g chloramphenicol daily for 30 days can be given. Chloramphenicol and cephalothin also reach adequate levels in the aqueous humor of the eye. Follow-up CSF examinations should be done every 3–6 months for at least 3 years or until serum nontreponemal antibodies disappear, local CNS treponemal antibodies disappear, or CSF oligoclonal bands disappear.

Malignancy of the CNS has been associated with a false-positive CSF-FTA, but this has almost always been associated with a negative serum TPHA or FTA-abs reaction.

Treatment of Syphilitic Otitis

Although the evidence is not incontrovertible, patients with possible syphilitic hearing loss should be treated.[37] Treatment should be prolonged (6 weeks to 3 months) and, unless contraindicated, should include prednisone 30–60 mg every day or every other day.[77] Treatment for neurosyphilis would be an alternative choice to parenteral penicillin.

Persistent Infection

The question of persistent infection despite adequate therapy has been a controversial subject ever since the first reports by Collart and associates[78] in 1962 of the isolation of spirochetes after "appropriate therapy." Although the efficacy of treating *T. pallidum* with penicillin is unquestioned, there are some patients in whom the spirochetes become sequestered in areas where adequate levels of penicillin are not easily achieved, for example, the anterior chamber of the eye,[79] the CNS,[11,21] and the labryrinth of the inner ear.[80] Whether these persistent organisms can cause a clinically evident illness at some later date remains speculative. However, there are a number of reports of unusual neurologic, optic, and otic findings in which there is little or no explanation for the pathogenesis except a positive serologic test for syphilis. In the past, attempts at isolation of these persistent organisms have met with variable success, and their validity has been questioned.[81] However, there is now little doubt that *T. pallidum* may persist after treatment, particularly in the CNS, and that these organisms can be isolated by inoculation of appropriate human materials into laboratory animals.[11,21] The challenge facing clinicians is to identify and treat these unfortunate few. Thus, I feel that anyone who has or has had syphilis deserves a CSF examination, and if there are any abnormalities (see above) and/or unexplained neurologic signs or symptoms, the patient should be treated for neurosyphilis.

Follow-up and Re-treatment

All patients with early syphilis and congenital syphilis should have repeat quantitative nontreponemal tests at 3, 6, and 12 months (see above). All patients with secondary syphilis or syphilis of more than 1 year's duration should also have a repeat nontreponemal serologic test 24 months after treatment. Examination of the CSF is also warranted in all patients, especially if they were treated with benzathine penicillin. All patients with documented neurosyphilis must be carefully followed with serologic testing and CSF examinations for at least 5 years unless all abnormal parameters including local CNS production of antibodies normalize.

Re-treatment should be considered whenever (*1*) clinical signs and symptoms of syphilis persist or recur, (*2*) there is a sustained level or an increase in the titer of a nontreponemal test,[47] and (*3*) whenever a positive RPR reaction test persists beyond 12 months in primary syphilis, 24 months in secondary or latent syphilis, and 5 years in late syphilis.

Jarisch-Herxheimer Reaction

The Jarisch-Herxheimer reaction is a systemic reaction occurring 1–2 hours after the initial treatment of syphilis with effective antibiotics, especially penicillin. It consists of the abrupt onset of fever, chills, myalgias, headache, tachycardia, hyperventilation, vasodilatation with flushing, and mild hypotension. It is particularly common when secondary syphilis is treated (70–90 percent) but can occur in any stage (10–25 percent). It lasts 12–24 hours and has been well correlated with the release from the spirochetes of heat-stable pyrogen.[82] Patients should be warned of the reaction before treatment. Varying degrees of severity occur. It is self-limited and can be treated with aspirin every 4 hours over a period of 24–48 hours. Prednisone can also abort the reaction and is warranted as adjunctive therapy when cardiovascular and symptomatic neurosyphilis are being treated since the reaction may have catastrophic consequences.

Immunity

Magnuson and associates[13] were able to demonstrate in human volunteers that immunity developed to reinfection. However, this immunity appeared not to be absolute but became more solid the longer the infection remained untreated. Humoral antibodies are only partially protective since experimental infection in humans and rabbits can be produced when they are present.[14] On the other hand, the granulomatous lesion (gumma), a presumed correlate of cell-mediated immunity, is produced at a time when syphilitic reinfection is resisted. HIV-infected persons who have progressive dysregulation and diminution of their cellular immune status have a propensity to develop more severe disease. Likewise, malnourished individuals who also have a deficit of cellular immune function are prone to develop more severe syphilitic disease.[83]

Furthermore, resistance to infection has been transferred by thymus-dependent lymphocytes in rabbits. Thus, cell-mediated immunity plays a key role in immunity.[83–86] However, cellular immunity may also play an important role in the pathogenesis of syphilis, and there is evidence to suggest that the late complications of the disease are a result of the host's immune response.[83,86]

The likelihood of a susceptible person who is exposed to a patient with infectious syphilis developing syphilis is about 50 percent. However, in controlled volunteer experiments, all volunteers without a history of serologic evidence of previous contact with *T. pallidum* developed syphilis. Obviously, the relative importance of variations in sexual and hygienic practices, immune status, inoculum size, and other factors play an important role in the transmissibility of *T. pallidum*. Congenital syphilis does not convey immunity to syphilis.[87]

SYPHILIS IN HIV-INFECTED PERSONS

Concomitant HIV and syphilis infections are common. Syphilis in HIV-infected patients presents a number of unique problems.[88] A more protracted and malignant course,[89] greater constitutional symptoms, organ involvement, atypical and florid skin rashes, and neurosyphilis especially uveitis[89a,89b,89c] are more likely because of the deleterious impact of HIV on the host's cellular immune system.[90,91] Thus, a more vigorous and/or prolonged course of antibiotics sufficient to cure neurosyphilis appears prudent (Table 7).[88] There is the high possibility that bacteriostatic drugs such as doxycycline or erythromycin may be inadequate because of the immune impairment.[91a]

HIV-infected patients may develop aberrant serologic responses.[89,92] They may develop false-positive or increasing reaginic titers despite adequate therapy, especially during the earlier phases of HIV infection when polyclonal B-cell stimulation is most prevalent. Also, they may fail to develop a response because of an overwhelming antigen load and/or severe immunodysfunction that occurs late in the disease. Finally, antibodies against major histocompatibility complex antigens are capable of binding to *T. pallidum*[93] and, therefore, may result in a false serologic test if an autoimmune component develops as a consequence of the HIV disease process (see Chapter 107). Thus, a high index of suspicion and extraordinary means to establish the diagnosis such as special stains of biopsy specimens may be required.[89]

REFERENCES

1. Hovind-Hougen K. Morphology. In: Shell RF, Muscher DM, eds. Pathogenesis and Immunology of Treponemal Infection. New York: Marcel Dekker; 1983.
2. Johnson C. Composition. In: Shell CF, Muscher DM, eds. Pathogenesis and Immunology of Treponemal Infection. New York: Marcel Dekker; 1983.
3. Jenkin HW, Sandok PL. In vitro cultivation of *Treponema pallidum*. In: Schell RF, Muscher DM, eds. Pathogenesis and Immunology of Treponemal Infection. New York: Marcel Dekker; 1983.
4. Denhie CC. A History of Syphilis. Springfield, IL: Charles C Thomas; 1962.
5. Hall V, Waisbren BA. Syphilis as a major theme of James Joyce's Ulysses. Arch Intern Med. 1980;140:963–965.
6. Parran T. Shadow on the Land, Syphilis. New York: Reynal & Hitchcock; 1937.
7. Waugh MA. Venereal disease in sixteenth-century England. Med Hist. 1973;17:152.
8. Kampmeier RH. Essentials of Syphilology. 3rd ed. Philadelphia: JB Lippincott; 1943.
9. Stokes JH, Beerman H, Ingraham NR. Modern Clinical Syphilology, Diagnosis, Treatment. Case Study. ed 3. Philadelphia: WB Saunders; 1945.
10. Wilcox RR, Guthe T. *Treponema pallidum*. A bibliographical review of the morphology, culture and survival of *T. pallidum* and associated organisms. Bull WHO. 1966;35(Suppl):1.
11. Lukehart S, Hook EW, Baker-Zander SH, et al. Invasion of the Central Nervous System by *Treponema pallidum*. Implications for Diagnosis and Therapy. Ann Intern Med. 1988;109:855–62.
12. Cumberland MC, Turner TB. Rate of multiplication of *Treponema pallidum* in normal and immune rabbits. Am J Syph. 1949;33:201.
13. Magnuson HJ, Thomas EW, Olansky S, et al. Inoculation syphilis in human volunteers. Medicine (Baltimore). 1956;35:33.
14. O'Regan S, Fong JSC, de Chadarevian JP, et al. Treponemal antigens in congenital and acquired syphilic nephritis. Ann Intern Med. 1976;85:325.
15. Clark EG, Danbolt N. The Oslo study of the natural course of untreated syphilis. Med Clin North Am. 1964;48:613.
16. Rockwell DH, Yobs AR, Moore MB. The Tuskeegee study of untreated syphilis; the 30th year of observation. Arch Intern Med. 1964;114:792.
17. Rosahn PD. Autopsy Studies in Syphilis. Journal of Venereal Disease 649 Information Supplement #21. Washington, DC: U.S. Public Health Service Venereal Disease Division; 1947.
18. Drusin LM, Topf-Olstein B, Levy-Zombeck E. Epidemiology of infectious syphilis at a tertiary hospital. Arch Intern Med. 1979;135:901.
19. Chapel TA. The variability of syphilitic chancres. Sex Transm Dis. 1978;5:68.
20. Chapel TA. The signs and symptoms of secondary syphilis. Sex Transm Dis. 1980;7:161.

20a. Merritt HH, Moore M. Acute neurosyphilitic meningitis. Med 1935;14:119.

21. Tramont EC. Persistence of *Treponema pallidum* following penicillin G therapy. JAMA. 1976;236:2206.
22. Saltiel P, Melmed CA, Portnoy D. Sensoneural deafness in early acquired syphilis. Can J Neurol Sci. 1988;10:114–6.
23. Keisler DS, Starke W, Looney DJ, et al. Early syphilis with liver involvement. JAMA. 1982;247:1999.
24. Sachar DB, Klein RS, Swerdlow F. Erosive syphilitic gastritis: Dark-field and immunofluorescent diagnosis from biopsy specimens. Ann Intern Med. 1974;80:512.
25. Ross WH, Sutton HF. Acquired syphilitic uveitis. Arch Ophthalmol. 1980;98:496.
26. Shin DLT, Kass MA, Kolkow AE. Positive FTA-abs tests in subjects with corticosteroid-induced uveitis. Am J Ophthalmol. 1976;86:259.
27. Hansen K, Hvid-Jacobsen H, Lindewald PS, et al. Bone lesions in early syphilis detected by bone scintography. Br J Vener Dis. 1984;60:265–8.
28. Reginato AJ, Schumacher HR, Jiminez S, et al. Synovitis in secondary syphilis. Arch Rheumatol. 1979;22:170.
29. Tight RR, Wagner JF. Skeletal involvement in secondary syphilis detected by bone scanning. JAMA. 1976;235:2326.
30. Merritt HH, Adams RD, Solomon HC. Neurosyphilis. New York: Oxford University Press, 1946.
31. VanEijk RVW, Wolters EC, Tutuarima JA, et al. Effect of early and late

syphilis on central nervous system: Cerebrospinal fluid changes and neurologic deficit. Genitourin Med. 1987;63:77–82.
32. Lugar A, Schmidt BL, Steyer K, et al. Diagnosis of neurosyphilis by examination of the cerebrospinal fluid. Br J Vener Dis. 1981;57:232–7.
33. Muller F, Moskophidis M. Estimation of the local production of antibodies to *Treponema pallidum* in the central nervous system of patients with neurosyphilis. Br J Vener Dis. 1983;59:80–84.
34. Lee JB, Farshy CE, Hunter EF, et al. Detection of immunoglobulin M in cerebrospinal fluid from syphilis patients by enzyme-linked immunosorbent assay. J Clin Microbiol. 1986;24:736–40.
34a. Vartal F, Vandik B, Michaelsen TF. Synthesis of oligoclonal antibodies to *Treponema pallidum*. Ann Neurol 1982;11:35.
35. Chesney AM, Kemp I. Incidence of *Spirochetea pallida* in cerebrospinal fluid during early stages of syphilis. JAMA. 1924;83:1725.
36. Cooperative Clinical Group. Cooperative clinical studies in the treatment of syphilis: Asymptomatic neurosyphilis. Vener Dis Inform. 1937;18:45.
36a. Hotson JR. Modern Neurosyphilis: A partially treated chronic meningitis. West J Med. 1981;135:191.
37. Rothenberg R. Syphilitic hearing loss. South Med J. 1979;72:118.
38. Wilson WR, Zoller M. Electrony-stagmography in congenital and acquired syphilis otitis. Ann Otol. 1981;90:21.
39. Balkany TJ, Dans PE. Reversible sudden deafness in early acquired syphilis. Arch Otolaryngol. 1978;104:60.
40. Smith JL, Isreal CW, Harner RE. Syphilitic temporal arteritis. Arch Ophthalmol. 1967;78:284.
41. Kaufman RE, Jones OG, Bloant JH, et al. Questionnaire survey of reported early congenital syphilis. Am J Sex Transm Dis. 1977;4:135.
42. Kerr AG, Smyth GDL, Cinnamond MJ. Congenital syphilitic deafness. J Laryngol Otol. 1973;86:1.
42a. Fojaco RM, Hensley GT, Moskowitz L. Congenital syphilis and necrotizing funisitis. JAMA. 1989;261:788.
43. Al-Salihi FL, Curran JP, Shetein OA. Occurrence of fetal syphilis after a nonreactive early gestational serologic test. J Pediatr. 1971;78:121.
44. Al-Samarrai HT, Henderson WG. Immunofluorescent staining of *Treponema pallidum* and *Treponema-pertenue* in tissues fixed by formalin and embedded in paraffin wax. Br J Vener Dis. 1977;53:1.
45. Romanowski B, Forsey E, Praad E, et al. Detection of *Treponema pallidum* by fluorescent monoclonal antibody test. Sex Trans Dis. 1987;14:156–9.
46. Beckett JH, Bigbee MA. Immunoperoxidase localization of *Treponema pallidum*. Arch Pathol Lab Med. 1979;103:135.
47. Brown ST, Akbar Z, Larsen SA, et al. Serological response to syphilis treatment. JAMA. 1985;253:1296–9.
48. Fiumara NJ. Treatment of primary and secondary syphilis. Serological response. JAMA. 1980;243:2500.
49. Fiumara NJ. Serologic responses to treatment of 128 patients with late latent syphilis. Sex Transm Dis. 1979;6:243.
50. Fiumara NJ. Reinfection primary, secondary, and latent syphilis. Sex Transm Dis. 1980;7:111.
51. Rein MF, Banks CW, Logan LC, et al. Failure of *Treponema pallidum* immobilization test to provide additional diagnostic information about contemporary problem sera. Sex Transm Dis. 1980;7:101.
52. Alderete JF, Shade-Freeman L, Baseman JB. Immunodiagnostic test for detection of serum antibody to *Treponema pallidum* (syphilis): Fibronectin is a capture vehicle for treponemal adhesions. J Immunol Methods. 1985; 84:365–73.
53. Kaufman RE, Olansky DC, Weisner PJ. The FTA-ABS (IgM) test for neonatal congenital syphilis: A critical review. Sex Transm Dis. 1974;1:79.
54. Tuffanelli DL, Wuepper KO, Bradford LL. Fluorescent treponemal antibody absorption tests. Studies of false-positive reactions to tests for syphilis. N Engl J Med. 1967;276:258.
55. Miller JN. Spirochetes in Body Fluids & Tissues. Springfield, IL: Charles C Thomas, 1971.
56. Idsoe O, Guthe T, Wilcox RR. Penicillin in the treatment of syphilis. The experience of three decades. Bull WHO. 1972;47(Suppl):1.
57. Syphotherapy, 1976. Sex Transm Dis. 1976;3:98.
58. Eagle H. Therapeutic significance of penicillin blood levels. Ann Intern Med. 1948;28:260.
59. Moorthy TT, Lee C, Lim K, et al. Ceftriaxone for treatment of primary syphillis in men: A preliminary study. Sex Transm Dis. 1987;14:116–8.
60. Mohr JA, Griffiths W, Jackson R, et al. Neurosyphilis and penicillin levels in cerebrospinal fluid. JAMA. 1976;236:2208.
61. Green BM, Miller NR, Bynum TE. Failure of penicillin G benzathine in the treatment of neurosyphilis. Arch Intern Med. 1980;140:1117–8.
62. Moskovitz BL, Klimek JJ, Goldman RL, et al. Meningovascular syphilis after 'appropriate' treatment of primary syphilis. Arch Intern Med. 1982;142:139–41.
63. Markovitz PM, Bentner KR, Maggio RP, et al. Failure of recommended treatment for secondary syphilis. JAMA. 1986;255:1767–8.
64. Short DH, Knox JM, Glicksman J. Neurosyphilis: The search for adequate treatment. Ann Dermatol. 1966;93:87–91.
65. Brown S. Update on recommendations for the treatment of syphilis. Rev Infect Dis. 1982;4(Suppl):837–41.
66. Tucker HA, Robinson RCV. Disappearance time of *Treponema pallidum* from lesions of early syphilis following administration of crystalline penicillin. G. Bull Johns Hopkins Hosp. 1947;80:169.
67. Ziaya PR, Hankins GD, Gilstrap LC, et al. Intravenous penicillin desensitization and treatment during pregnancy. JAMA. 1986;256:2561–2.
68. Wendel GD Jr, Stark BJ, Jamison RB, et al. Penicillin allergy and desensitization in serious infections during pregnancy. N Eng J Med. 1985;312:1229–32.
69. McCracken GH, Ginsburg C, Crane DF, et al. Clinical phenomenology of penicillin in newborn infants. J Pediatr. 1973;82:692.
70. Norgand MV, Miller JN. Plasmid DNA in *Treponema pallidum* (Nichols): Potential for antibiotic resistance by syphilis bacteria. Science. 1981;213:553.
71. Speer ME, Taber LH, Clark DB, et al. Cerebrospinal fluid levels of benzathine penicillin G in the neonate. J Pediatr. 1977;91:996.
72. Giles AJH. Tabes dorsalis progressing to general paresis after 20 years despite routine penicillin therapy. Br J Vener Dis. 1980;56:368.
73. Morrison E, Harrison S, Tramont EC. Oral amoxicillin, an alternative treatment of neurosyphilis. Genitourin Med. 1985;61:359–62.
74. Dunlap EM, Al-Egaily, Houang ET. Production of treponemicidal concentration of penicillin in cerebrospinal fluid. Br Med J. 1981;283:646.
75. Yim CW, Flynn NM, Fitzgerald FT. Penetration of oral doxycycline into the cerebrospinal fluid of patients with latent or neurosyphilis. Antimicrob Agents Chemother. 1985;28:347–8.
76. Hook EW III, Baker-Zander S, Moskovitz, et al. Ceftriaxone therapy for asymptomatic neurosyphilis. Sex Transm Dis. 1986;13:185–7.
77. Zoller M, Wilson WR, Nodal JB. Treatment of syphilitic hearing loss. Ann Otol. 1979;88:160.
78. Collart P, Borel L, Darel P. Etude de l'action de la penicilline dans la syphilis tardive: Persistence du treponeme pale après traitement (Primiere Partie, la syphilis tardive experimentale)). Ann Inst Pasteur. 1962;102:596.
79. Smith JL. Spirochetes in Late Seronegative Syphilis. Penicillin Notwithstanding. Springfield, IL: Charles C Thomas; 1969.
80. Mack LW, Smith JL, Walter ER, et al. Temporal bone treponemes. Arch Otolarngol. 1969;90:11.
81. Turner TB, Hardy P, Newman B. Infectivity tests in syphilis. Br J Vener Dis. 1969;45:183.
82. Young EJ, Weingarten NM, Baughn RE, et al. Studies on the pathogenesis of the Jarisch-Herxheimer reaction. J Infect Dis. 1982;146:606.
83. Schell R, Marker D, eds. Pathogenesis and Immunology of Treponemal Infection. New York: Marcel Dekker; 1983.
84. Muscher DM, Baughn RE. Syphilis. In: Samter M, ed. Immunological Diseases. 3rd ed. Boston: Little, Brown; 1978.
85. Baseman JE, Hayes EC. Molecular characterization of receptor binding proteins and immunogens of virulent *Treponema pallidum*. J Exp Med. 1980;151:573.
86. Freidman PS, Turk JL. The role of cell-mediated immune mechanisms in syphilis in Ethiopia. Clin Exp Immunol. 1978;31:59.
87. Fiumara NJ. Acquired syphilis in three patients with congenital syphilis. N Engl J Med. 1974;290:1119.
88. Tramont EC, Syphilis in the AIDS era. N Engl J Med. 1987;316:1600–1.
89. Hicks CB, Benson PM, Lupton GP, et al. Seronegative secondary syphilis in a patient infected with the human immunodeficiency virus (HIV) with Kaposi sarcoma. Ann Intern Med. 1987;107:492–5.
89a. Passo MS, Rosenbaum JT. Ocular syphilis in patients with human immunodeficiency virus infection. Am J Opthal. 1988;106:1.
89b. Zaidman GW. Neurosyphilis and retrobulbar neuritis in a patient with AIDS. Ann Opthalmol. 1986;18:260.
89c. Kamling RT, Villalobos R, Latina M. Recurrent syphilitic uveitis. N Eng J Med. 1989;320:62.
90. Berry CD, Hooton TM, Collier AC, et al. Neurologic relapse after benzathine penicillin therapy for secondary syphilis in a patient with HIV infection. N Engl J Med. 1987;316:1587–9.
91. Johns DR, Tierney M, Felsenstein D. Alternation in the natural history of neurosyphilis by concurrent infections with human immunodeficiency virus. N Engl J Med. 1987;316:1569–72.
91a. Duncan WC. Failure of erythromycin to cure secondary syphilis in a patient infected with the human immunodeficiency virus. Arch Dermatol. 1989;125:82.
92. Radolf JD, Kaplan RP. Unusual manifestations of secondary syphilis and abnormal humoral response to *Treponema pallidum* antigens in a homosexual man with asymptomatic human immunodeficiency virus infection. J Am Acad Dermatol Dis. 1988;18:423–7.
93. Marchitto KS, Kindt TJ, Norgard MV. Monoclonal antibodies directed against major histocompatibility complex antigens bind to the surface of *Treponema pallidum* isolated from infected rabbits and humans. Cell Immunol. 1986;101:633–42.

214. TREPONEMA SPECIES (YAWS, PINTA, BEJEL)

JEFFREY D. CHULAY

The nonvenereal treponematoses are a group of contagious diseases endemic among rural populations in tropical and subtropical countries. All are caused by bacteria that are transmitted primarily by direct contact among children living in unhygienic conditions. The causative organisms are morphologically identical and have only subtle antigenic differences,[1] but differences in clinical manifestations allow the separation of three distinct entities (Table 1). Pinta is characterized by skin lesions only; yaws, by skin and bone lesions; and bejel (endemic syphilis), by mucous membrane as well as by osseous and cutaneous involvement. As with venereal syphilis, all three are characterized by self-limited primary and secondary lesions, a latent period without clinically detectable disease, and late lesions that are frequently destructive. Congenital infection is rarely seen, presumably because primary infection usually occurs before the childbearing years. All three diseases result in host serologic responses indistinguishable from one another and from venereal syphilis. Some degree of protective immunity mediated by both antibody[2] and immune T cells[3] develops with prolonged infection. In animal models[4,5] and human challenge studies[6,7] this protection extends to heterologous treponemal species. This may explain the increasing incidence of venereal syphillis in some regions where yaws has been reduced to very low levels.[8] Although the transmission of the endemic treponematoses can be diminished by improvements in personal hygiene and general living standards, the introduction of penicillin, to which all of these organisms are exquisitely sensitive, has had a dramatic influence on reducing the incidence of these diseases.

DESCRIPTION OF THE PATHOGENS

The genus *Treponema* consists of at least 13 species, among which *T. pallidum* (3 subspecies) and *T. carateum* cause disease in humans.[9] These human pathogens are morphologically indistinguishable and appear as motile tightly coiled helical rods under the darkfield microscope. Their average diameter is 0.13–0.15 μm, and their average length is 10–13 μm.

Because the treponemes that infect humans cannot be continuously cultivated in vitro, their classification rests on differences in host species susceptibility and in the disease manifestations produced in these hosts. *T. p. pallidum,* the most virulent human pathogen, causes venereal syphilis in humans (see Chapter 213) and produces indurated cutaneous and testicular lesions without periorchitis in rabbits. *T. carateum,* the etiologic agent of pinta, is able to infect only humans and chimpanzees. *T. p. pertenue* causes human yaws and produces periorchitis with nonindurated testicular and cutaneous lesions in rabbits. *T. p. endemicum* produces disease in rabbits that is intermediate between that of the syphilis and yaws treponemes. Complicating the classification of these organisms is the fact that with serial passage in rabbits or hamsters there may be a change in the pattern of disease produced.[4,10]

YAWS

History

There is evidence that yaws has probably existed in Africa since prehistoric times where environmental conditions favored its evolution from pinta.[11] It was introduced into the Western Hemisphere by African slaves in the 16th century. Synonyms of the disease include pian, bouba, and frambesia (from the raspberry-like appearance of papillomatous lesions). Castellani identified *T. p. pertenue* in yaws lesions shortly after Schaudinn and Hoffman's discovery of *T. p. pallidum* in 1905. The advent of long-acting penicillin therapy made possible the WHO-sponsored mass treatment campaigns that have dramatically reduced the prevalence of this disease.

Epidemiology and Pathogenesis

Yaws occurs among primitive, rural populations in warm, humid tropical areas of Africa, South America, Southeast Asia, and Oceania (Fig. 1). The number of persons infected, estimated at 50–100 million in the 1950s, was reduced by mass treatment campaigns to fewer than 2 million in the mid-1970s.[12] In the Western Hemisphere, yaws now occurs only sporadically in small regions of Colombia, Guyana, Suriname, and French Guiana, with fewer than 500 cases reported annually in the 1980s.[13] However, there has been a resurgence of yaws in West Africa, with remote communities in Ghana, Togo, and Benin having prevalences approaching those during the 1950s.[14]

Transmission occurs when traumatized skin comes in contact with infectious exudate from active yaws lesions. New cases occur more frequently during the rainy season, and primary infection is usually acquired before puberty. Blood stream invasion shortly after the initial infection leads to subsequent involvement of bone, lymph nodes, and distant skin sites. Histopathologic changes in skin lesions consist of granulomatous inflammation indistinguishable from that seen in pinta or syphilis,[15] with endarteritis common in late lesions. Treponemes, numerous in early skin lesions, are rarely found in bone or late skin lesions.

Clinical Manifestations

After an incubation period of 3–5 weeks, early lesions usually appear on the extremities, especially the legs. These are characterized by papules that enlarge and become papillomatous with superficial erosion (Fig. 2) and then heal spontaneously within 6 months.[16] Weeks to months later a generalized eruption of similar lesions occurs (Fig. 3), although macular and squamous lesions may also be seen. Multiple relapses of these secondary lesions may occur during the first 5 years and are often associated with lymphadenopathy. Osteitis and periostitis can occur during the secondary stage and may involve the fingers

TABLE 1. Differentiation of the Treponematoses

Characteristic	*Venereal syphilis*	*Yaws*	*Pinta*	*Bejel*
Causative organism	*T. pallidum* subsp. *pallidum*	*T. pallidum,* subsp. *pertenue*	*T. carateum*	*T. pallidum,* subsp. *endemicum*
Usual mode of transmission	Sexual; congenital	Skin-to-skin	Skin-to-skin	Mouth-to-mouth; via utensils
Geographic distribution	Cosmpolitan	Warm, humid tropics	Warm, arid tropical Americas	Arid subtropical or temperate zones
Usual age of onset	Adolescent-adult	Childhood	Childhood	Childhood
Primary lesions	Genital chancre	Papillomatous skin lesions	Papulosquamous skin lesions	Oral mucous lesions (rarely seen)
Secondary lesions	Maculopapular skin lesions; condylomata lata; mucous patches	Papillomatous skin lesions; periostitis	Dyschromic papulosquamous skin lesions	Mucous patches; split papules; condylomata lata
Late lesions	Aortitis; neurosyphilis; gummas of skin, bone, and viscera	Destructive skin lesions, hyperkeratoses; gummas of bone and skin	Achromic macular skin lesions	Gummas of bone and skin

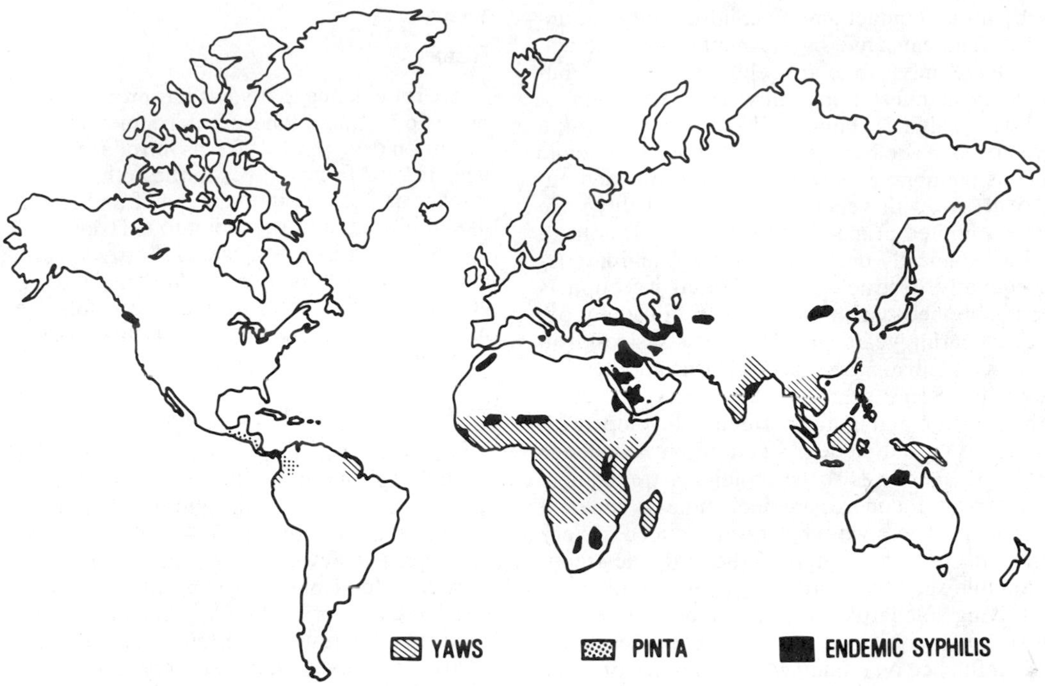

FIG. 1. Geographic distribution of the nonvenereal treponematoses.

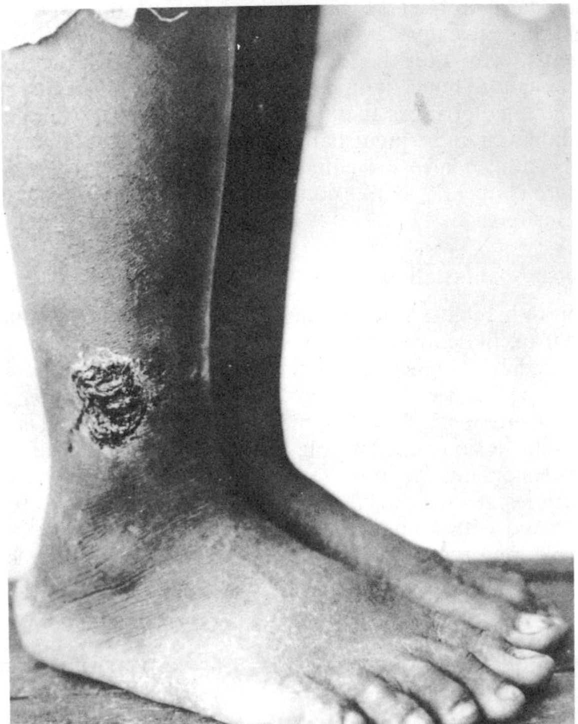

FIG. 2. Primary lesion of yaws (AFIP 39207). (Courtesy of Dr. D. H. Connor, Armed Forces Institute of Pathology, Washington, D.C.)

(polydactylitis), long bones (saber tibia), or paranasal maxillae (goundou). Early lesions do not ulcerate unless they become secondarily infected. In some areas yaws appears to have become attenuated, with primary and secondary lesions characterized by dry papillomas and scaling macules.[17]

The late stage of yaws is characterized by cutaneous plaques, nodules and ulcers, hyperkeratoses of the palms and soles, and gummatous lesions involving the skull, sternum, tibia, or other bones. Ulceration of the skin overlying bone lesions is common, and gummatous erosion of nasopharyngeal structures (gangosa) similar to that seen with venereal syphilis occurs occasionally.

Diagnosis

Yaws should be suspected in persons with chronic skin or bone lesions who have resided in tropical areas where transmission of *T. p. pertenue* occurs (Fig. 1). The diagnosis of yaws can be confirmed by darkfield microscopic examination or fluorescent antibody staining of exudates from cutaneous lesions.[18] In latent yaws, or when treponemes cannot be found, a presumptive diagnosis can be made if cardiolipin (VDRL, rapid plasma reagin [RPR]) or treponemal (fluorescent treponemal antibody absorption [FTA-ABS], microhemagglutination test for *T. pallidum* [MHA-TP]) antibodies are present (see Chapter 213). Depending on their stage and appearance, the lesions of yaws must be differentiated from pyoderma, tropical ulcer, sickle cell anemia, cutaneous leishmaniasis, blastomycosis, leprosy, and tuberculosis[19] as well as from the other treponematoses.

Prevention and Treatment

Yaws responds rapidly to treatment with a single injection of benzathine penicillin G in doses of 1.2 million units for persons aged 10 years and over and 600,000 units for younger children.[20] Although hyperkeratoses may require several months to heal, early lesions usually heal within 1–2 weeks, and relapse is rare. In patients unable to receive penicillin, tetracycline or chloramphenicol at a dose of 25 mg/kg/day for 10–14 days has also been effective.[21] As with syphilis, conversion of seroreactivity occurs most often in patients treated in the early stages of disease. Transmission of the disease can be interrupted by treating contacts and latent cases with penicillin at the dose recommended above.[20]

PINTA

History

Pinta (Sp. blemish), also known as mal de pinto (Sp. to paint) or carate, is probably the oldest human treponematosis.[11] Al-

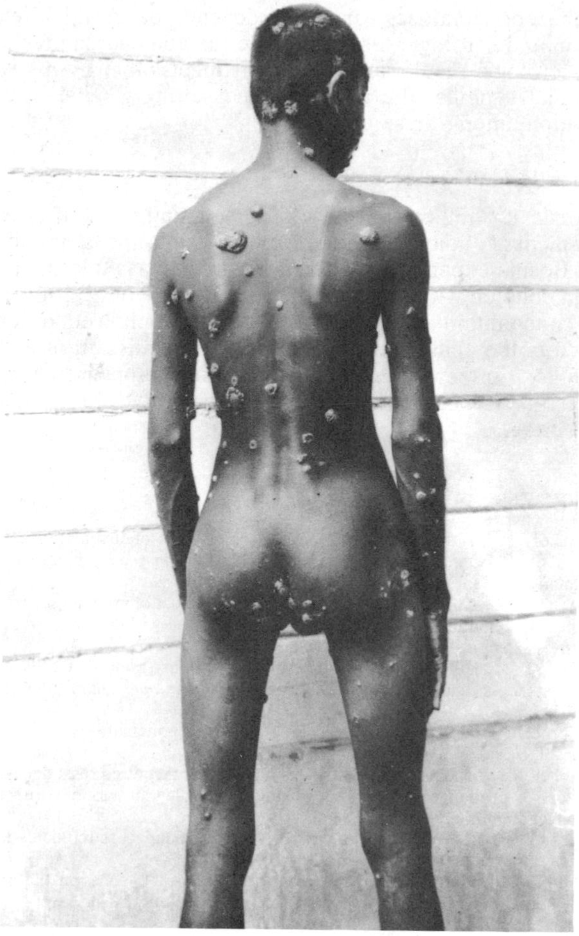

FIG. 3. Disseminated papillomatous nodules in secondary yaws (AFIP 39205). (Courtesy of Dr. D. H. Connor, Armed Forces Institute of Pathology, Washington, D.C.)

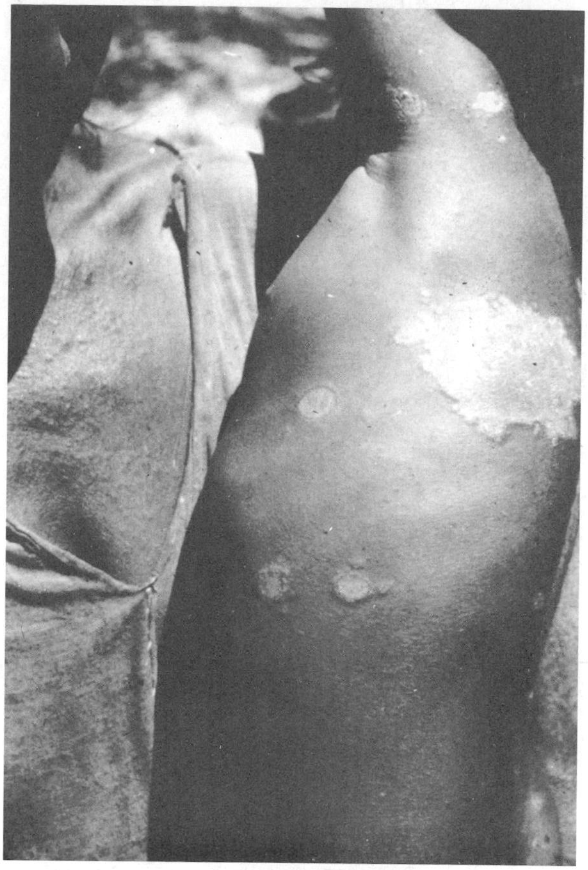

FIG. 4. Large primary and smaller secondary lesions of pinta (AFIP 75-5536-2). (Courtesy of Dr. D. H. Connor, Armed Forces Institute of Pathology, Washington, D.C.)

though it was recognized as early as 1926 that most patients with pinta had Wassermann antibodies, it was not until the identification in 1938 of *T. carateum* from pinta lesions that its treponemal etiology was firmly established.

Epidemiology and Pathogenesis

Pinta occurs only in remote rural areas of southern Mexico, Central America, and Colombia, most commonly in arid inland regions (Fig. 1). Only a few hundred cases have been reported in each of the past several years, a marked reduction from the estimate of 750,000 made 20 years ago.[12] Transmission appears to occur only through contact of broken skin with infectious lesions,[7] after which the organisms multiply locally and spread via the blood stream and lymphatics.

Clinical Manifestations

After an average incubation period of 7–21 days,[7] the initial lesions begin as small, erythematous, pruritic papules on the extremities, face, neck, chest, or abdomen.[22] These enlarge, become slightly squamous, and coalesce with surrounding lesions. Primary lesions may persist for several years before healing with residual hypopigmentation. Disseminated lesions (pintids) appear 3–12 months after the initial lesions, usually as small scaly papules involving the same sites as the primary lesions (Fig. 4). These secondary lesions, and occasionally primary lesions, may develop into dyschromic brown, gray, or blue lesions, especially when located on the face. Pintids may recur up to 10 years into the course of the disease, often in patients with late lesions. The late stage of pinta is characterized by depigmented (achromic) lesions, frequently involving the wrists, elbows, and ankles (Fig. 5). Although pinta does not impair general health or affect longevity, the cosmetic disfigurement frequently results in social ostracism.

Diagnosis

Pinta should be suspected in persons with papulosquamous or abnormally pigmented skin lesions who have resided in remote areas of tropical Latin America (Fig. 1). Except for late achromic lesions, treponemes can usually be demonstrated by darkfield microscopy of fluid from the lesions. Serologic tests (VDRL, FTA-ABS) do not become positive until after the appearance of secondary lesions,[7] which usually persist for life. Differential diagnosis includes neurodermatitis, tinea versicolor, chloasma, and vitiligo.

Prevention and Treatment

A single 1.2 million unit dose of long-acting penicillin G is the treatment of choice.[23] Response to treatment varies depending on the stage of disease. Primary and early secondary lesions heal in 4–6 months, while late secondary lesions require 6–12 months to heal. Leukodermic patches remain at the site of dyschromic and hypochromic lesions, and achromic lesions usually show no improvement. Tetracycline or chloramphenicol in doses as for yaws may be used to treat patients allergic to penicillin. Treatment of latent as well as active cases is important to prevent further transmission of the disease.

BEJEL (ENDEMIC SYPHILIS)

History

It has been known for centuries that a syphilis-like disease could be spread by nonvenereal means. Sibbens in Scotland and ra-

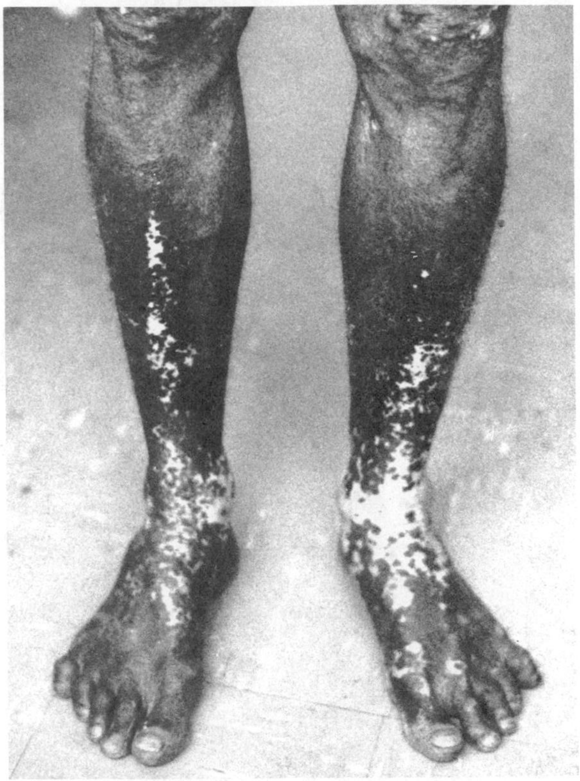

FIG. 5. Achromic lesions of late pinta.

desyge in Norway are of historic interest, while dichuchwa in South Africa, njovera in Rhodesia, skerljevo in Bosnia, and bejel in Syria are local names for more recent examples of this endemic form of syphilis.

Epidemiology and Pathogenesis

Bejel has a focal distribution in Africa, western Asia, and Australia (Fig. 1). The disease affects primarily children and, as with pinta and yaws, occurs only among rural populations with poor standards of living and personal hygiene.[24] In addition to person-to-person spread, transmission is frequently effected via common drinking and eating utensils, with mucosal inoculation felt to be the most common route of infection. The causative organism is *T. pallidum endemicum*.

Clinical Manifestations

The primary lesion is rarely observed, probably because of the small size and oral location of the usual infecting inoculum.[25] Secondary lesions consist of oropharyngeal mucous patches, split papules at the corners of the mouth, condylomata lata, periostitis, and regional lymphadenopathy. Late manifestations, which are clinically apparent more often than are early lesions, include gummatous lesions of the skin, nasopharynx, and bones. Gummas of the breast may be seen in mothers nursing infected infants. Cardiovascular and neurologic lesions are uncommon. As with the other nonvenereal treponematoses, the rarity of congenital disease is probably due to the childhood onset of primary infection in virtually all cases, so blood stream infection does not occur during pregnancy.

Diagnosis

Bejel should be suspected in persons with chronic skin or bone lesions who have lived in endemic areas (Fig. 1). As with the other treponematoses, diagnosis depends on darkfield examination and serologic tests. Because the clinical manifestations and serologic results are often indistinguishable from yaws or venereal syphilis, the epidemiologic setting is vital in differentiation among these diseases.

Prevention and Treatment

A single 1.2 million unit dose of long-acting penicillin G is the treatment of choice for both infected patients and their contacts. The Bosnia experience, where a vigorous mass treatment campaign coupled with the development of efficient health services and concomitant improvements in socioeconomic conditions resulted in the complete interruption of transmission of endemic syphilis,[26] offers hope that with a similar approach the nonvenereal treponematoses may eventually be eradicated elsewhere.

REFERENCES

1. Baker-Zander SA, Lukehart SA. Molecular basis of immunological cross-reactivity between *Treponema pallidum* and *Treponema pertenue*. Infect Immun. 1983;42:634.
2. Azadegan AA, Schell RF, Steiner BM, et al. Effect of immune serum and its immunoglobulin fractions on hamsters challenged with *Treponema pallidum* ssp. *pertenue*. J Infect Dis. 1986;153:1007.
3. Chan JK, Schell RF, LeFrock JL. Ability of enriched immune T cells to confer resistance in hamsters to infection with *Treponema pertenue*. Infect Immun. 1979;26:448.
4. Turner TB, Hollander DW. Biology of the Treponematoses. WHO Monograph Series No. 35, 1957.
5. Schell RF, Azadegan AA, Nitskansky SG, et al. Acquired resistance of hamsters to challenge with homologous and heterologous virulent treponemes. Infect Immun. 1982;37:617.
6. Turner TB. The resistance of yaws and syphilis patients to reinoculation with yaws spirochetes. Am J Hyg. 1936;23:431.
7. Leon Blanco F. Experimental pinta. In: Recent Advances in the Study of Venereal Diseases. A Symposium. Raleigh, NC: Venereal Diseases Education Institute; 1948:275.
8. Willcox RR. Changing patterns of treponemal disease. Br J Vener Dis. 1974;50:169.
9. Smibert RM. Genus *Treponema schaudinn* 1905, 1728. In: Krieg NR, Holt JG, eds. Bergey's Manual of Systematic Bacteriology. Baltimore: Williams & Wilkins; 1984:49.
10. Treponematosis Research. Report of a WHO Scientific Group, WHO Technical Report Series No. 455, 1970.
11. Hackett CJ. On the origin of the human treponematoses. Bull WHO. 1963;29:7.
12. Hopkins DR. After smallpox eradication: Yaws? Am J Trop Med Hyg. 1976;25:860.
13. St. John RK. Yaws in the Americas. Rev Infect Dis. 1985;7(Suppl 2):266.
14. Antal GM, Causse G. The control of endemic treponematoses. Rev Infect Dis. 1985;7(Suppl 2):220.
15. Dooley JR, Binford CH. Treponematoses. In: Binford CH, Connor DH, eds. Pathology of Tropical and Extraordinary Diseases. v. 1. Washington, DC: Armed Forces Institute of Pathology; 1976:110.
16. Hackett CJ: An International Nomenclature of Yaws Lesions. WHO Monogrograph Series No. 36, 1957.
17. Vorst FA. Clinical diagnosis and changing manifestations of treponemal infection. Rev Infect Dis. 1985;7(Suppl 2):327.
18. Perine PL, Nelson JW, Lewis JO, et al. New technologies for use in the surveillance and control of yaws. Rev Infect Dis. 1985;7(Suppl 2):295.
19. Hackett CJ, Loewenthal LJA: Differential Diagnosis of Yaws. WHO Monograph Series No. 45, 1960.
20. Treponemial Infections. Report of a WHO Scientific Group, WHO Technical Report Series No. 674, 1982.
21. Brown ST. Therapy for nonvenereal treponematoses: Review of the efficacy of penicillin and consideration of alternatives. Rev Infect Dis. 1985;7(Suppl 2):318.
22. Marquez F, Rein CR, Arias O. Mal de pinto in Mexico. Bull WHO. 1955;13:299.
23. Rein CR, Kitchen DK, Marquez F, et al. Repository penicillin therapy of pinta in the Mexican peasant. J Invest Dermatol 1953;18:137.
24. Csonka G, Pace J. Endemic nonvenereal treponematosis (bejel) in Saudi Arabia. Rev Infect Dis. 1985;7(Suppl 2):260.
25. Grin EI. Epidemiology and Control of Endemic Syphilis. Report on a Mass-treatment Campaign in Bosnia. WHO Monograph Series No. 11, 1953.
26. Grin EI, Guthe T. Evaluation of a previous mass campaign against endemic syphilis in Bosnia and Herzogovina. Br J Vener Dis. 1973;49:1.

215. LEPTOSPIRA SPECIES (LEPTOSPIROSIS)

W. EDMUND FARRAR

Leptospirosis is an acute generalized infectious disease, characterized by extensive vasculitis, caused by spirochetes of the genus *Leptospira*. It is primarily a disease of wild and domestic mammals; humans are infected only occasionally through direct or indirect contact with animals.

The clinical illness was described by Weil in 1886. The causative organism was first seen by Stimson in 1907, in sections of kidney tissue from a patient dying during a yellow fever epidemic, and was successfully cultivated in 1915 by Inada. In the United States, the incidence of reported cases of leptospirosis increased steadily during the first few decades of the twentieth century, but for the past 20 years about 50–100 cases have been reported annually. Until about 1960 it was generally believed that different serotypes of *Leptospira* produce distinct clinical syndromes. For example, Weil's disease was thought to be caused by *L. icterohaemorrhagiae* and "Fort Bragg fever" (a febrile illness associated with pretibial rash) by *L. autumnalis*. Although there is some correlation between severity of illness and serotype (e.g., jaundice occurs in 83 percent of *icterohaemorrhagiae* infections and in only 13 percent of cases due to *pomona*), the clinical syndromes are not specifically related to serotype, and it is better to refer to the illness caused by all types of *Leptospira* simply as "leptospirosis." Human leptospirosis has been thoroughly reviewed by Feigin and Anderson.[1]

CAUSATIVE MICROORGANISM

Leptospires are finely coiled, motile spirochetes, approximately 0.1 μm in width by 6–20 μm in length, with bent or hooked ends. Unlike other pathogenic spirochetes, they are readily cultivated in artificial media. Approximately 170 serotypes of pathogenic leptospires are recognized. Before 1967 the serotypes were considered as separate species; since that time the antigenically distinct types have been classified as serovars of a single species, *L. interrogans*. For example, an organism referred to as *L. canicola* in the older literature would now be called *L. interrogans* serovar *canicola*. Free-living saprophytic leptospires found in water are often referred to as *L. biflexa*.[2]

EPIDEMIOLOGY

Leptospirosis is a zoonosis of worldwide distribution, affecting many species of wild and domestic mammals. The epidemiology of human infection, in a particular time and place, is determined by the nature of man's contact, both direct and indirect, with infected animals. Man is usually a dead-end host; person-to-person transmission is extremely rare.

Most cases occur in young adult men, and the peak incidence is in summer and early fall. Indirect contact with infected animals, via water or soil contaminated with infected urine, is a more common cause of human infection than direct animal contact. Occupational exposure (farmers, veterinarians, abattoir workers) and recreational exposure (campers, swimmers) are common. Worldwide, rats are the most common source of human infection. In the United States the most important sources of infection, in descending order, are dogs, livestock, rodents, wild mammals, and cats. The serotypes found most commonly in human infection include *canicola, icterohaemorrhagiae, pomona, autumnalis, grippotyphosa, hebdomidis, ballum,* and *australis*.[3,4]

At least two epidemiologic features of leptospirosis make effective control of the disease extremely difficult. (*1*) Leptospires can establish a symbiotic relationship with many animal hosts, persisting for long periods in the renal tubules (with excretion in the urine) without producing disease or pathologic changes in the kidney.[1] Even immunized dogs can excrete infectious leptospires in the urine for long periods of time.[5] (*2*) Wild animals represent an important reservoir for continually reinfecting populations of domestic animals.

PATHOGENESIS AND PATHOLOGIC FINDINGS

After penetrating intact mucous membranes or abraded skin, leptospires enter the blood stream and are rapidly carried to all parts of the body, including the cerebrospinal fluid (CSF) and eye. Hyaluronidase and/or burrowing motility of the organisms have been suggested as mechanisms by which leptospires reach these normally protected sites. Fatally infected animals exhibited many changes suggestive of endotoxemia, but classical endotoxins have never been convincingly demonstrated in these organisms.[1]

Jaundice, which occurs in severe cases, is due primarily to hepatocellular dysfunction, usually without necrosis.[6,7] Hepatic damage is apparently subcellular, and leptospires are rarely seen in the liver. Renal functional abnormalities may be profound and out of proportion to histologic changes seen in the kidney. Renal failure is primarily a result of tubular damage,[7,8] and leptospires are commonly seen in the tubular lumen. The chief cause of the tubular lesion appears to be either hypoxemia or some direct toxic effect of the leptospires. Inflammatory changes in the kidney may be seen in the later stages of development of the renal lesion, and in at least one instance these were associated with circulating immune complexes and deposition of complement components and electron-dense bodies in glomeruli, suggesting immune-complex glomerulonephritis.[9] Hypovolemia and hypotension, caused by loss of intravascular volume as a result of endothelial injury, may contribute to development of renal failure.[8]

During the first week of infection, leptospires may be readily found in the CSF but meningeal signs are absent. Later, when serum antibody appears, meningitis may develop, but leptospires can no longer be found in the CSF. This has led to the suggestion that the meningitis may be due to an antigen–antibody reaction.[6]

Leptospires may persist for months in the aqueous humor, occasionally causing chronic or recurrent uveitis.[10]

Although myalgia may be prominent, early, and severe, histologic changes in muscle are often unimpressive. Early changes include cytoplasmic vacuoles in the myofibrils. Mild infiltration of muscle by polymorphonuclear leukocytes is a late finding in some cases.

Hemorrhagic diathesis due to vasculitis with capillary injury, hemolysis (possibly due to a hemolysin elaborated by some, but not all, serotypes), and focal hemorrhagic myocarditis are seen rarely.

CLINICAL MANIFESTATIONS

Subclinical leptospirosis occurs commonly among persons who are exposed to infected animals. Serologic evidence of infection is found in approximately 15 percent of abattoir and packing house workers and veterinarians. Among patients ill with leptospirosis, 90 percent have the milder anicteric form of the disease, and 5–10 percent have severe leptospirosis with jaundice (Weil's disease).

Leptospirosis may follow a biphasic course (Fig. 1). After an incubation period of 7–12 days (extreme range 2–20 days), the initial "septicemic" phase begins and usually lasts 4–7 days. During this nonspecific "flulike" phase of the illness, leptospires can be isolated from blood, CSF, and most tissues. Defervescence then occurs, and the patient is usually afebrile for

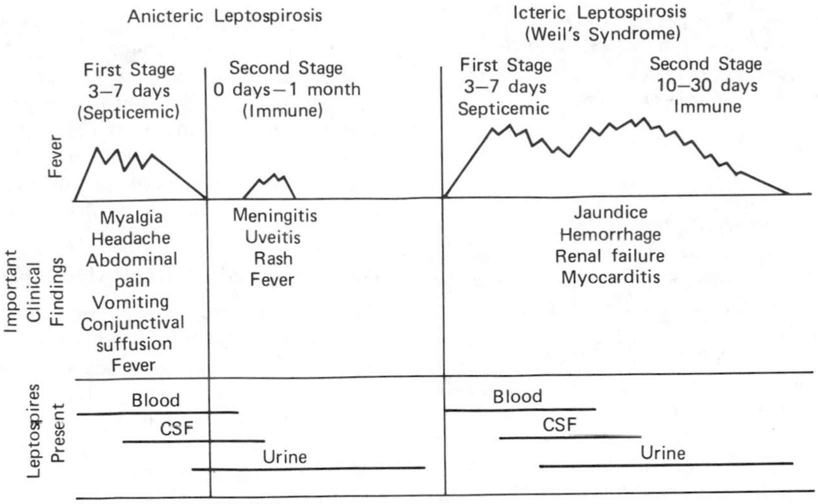

FIG. 1. Stages of anicteric and icteric leptospirosis. Correlation between clinical findings and presence of leptospires in body fluids. (From Feigin et al.,[1] with permission.)

a day or 2. Then the second, "immune" phase of the illness, lasting 4–30 days (occasionally longer), ensues. Early in this stage leptospires disappear from blood and CSF but can still be found in kidney, urine, and aqueous humor. This phase is characterized by the presence of circulating antibody and development of meningitis, uveitis, rash, and (in severe cases) hepatic and renal involvement. In icteric cases leptospires can sometimes be isolated from the blood for 24–48 hours after the appearance of jaundice.

Anicteric Leptospirosis

This common, milder form of leptospirosis is characterized by abrupt onset with fever, headache, severe muscle aches, malaise, prostration, and, in rare cases, circulatory collapse.[1,3,6,11] High remittent fever, chills, persistent headache, severe myalgias, abdominal pain, and nausea and vomiting persist for 4–7 days. Death almost never occurs during this stage. In anicteric infections the second stage may not occur.

In the second or *immune* stage of anicteric leptospirosis fever is usually not present or is low grade and lasts for only 1–3 days. Headache is characteristically intense, unremitting, often throbbing, and poorly controlled with analgesics. It is usually frontal or bitemporal and may be associated with retrobulbar pain. Occurrence of headache in the second phase of illness usually heralds the onset of clinical meningitis. Mild delirium is common, but more severe mental changes, such as hallucinations, are rare. Myalgia most commonly involves muscles of the calf, paraspinal region, abdomen, and neck and may be very severe. Nausea, vomiting, and abdominal pain occur in some combination in up to 95 percent of the patients. Hepatomegaly is uncommon in anicteric leptospirosis, but splenomegaly is found in 15–25 percent of the cases.

The most common physical findings during the second phase are muscle tenderness, conjunctival suffusion, adenopathy, hepatosplenomegaly, and rashes. Most patients have tachycardia, but bradycardia occurs occasionally. Ocular manifestations, including suffusion of the bulbar conjunctiva, photophobia, ocular pain, and conjunctival hemorrhage are relatively common and may suggest the diagnosis. Pulmonary involvement (with infiltrates, cough, and blood-stained sputum), rash, pharyngitis, and cervical and generalized adenopathy are found infrequently. Rather characteristic pretibial slightly raised 1–5 cm erythematous lesions are common in *autumnalis* infections and are part of the syndrome called Fort Bragg fever.[12] The total WBC count is normal or slightly elevated, but most cases exhibit neutrophilia. The erythrocyte sedimentation rate is increased.

The most important clinical syndrome observed in the immune stage of anicteric leptospirosis is aseptic meningitis.[1,6] Although leptospires can be readily found in the CSF during the first stage of illness, they disappear during the second week with the appearance of serum antibody. Eighty to 90 percent of anicteric patients will have CSF pleocytosis during the second week of illness, and 50 percent of these will exhibit clinical signs of meningitis. The aseptic meningitis is nonspecific in its manifestations, and, unless the patient exhibits a distinct biphasic illness or gives a history of exposure to animals, it may be misdiagnosed as viral in nature. Studies at the Centers for Disease Control have demonstrated serologic evidence of *Leptospira* infection in approximately 10 percent of cases of previously unexplained meningitis or encephalitis.[4] The meningitis usually lasts only a few days (rarely 2–3 weeks) and is never fatal in anicteric cases. CSF pressure is often normal, but lumbar puncture may provide dramatic relief of headache. Seventy-five percent of the patients have less than 500 cells/mm^3 of CSF. Polymorphonuclear leukocytes may outnumber mononuclear cells at the onset of meningitis, but mononuclear cells characteristically predominant. CSF protein may be normal or elevated up to 300 mg/100 ml. Glucose concentration is normal. Focal neurologic signs and evidence of encephalitis are uncommon.

Uveitis occurs in approximately 2 percent of the patients, with onset usually several months after the acute illness, and may run a prolonged chronic or recurrent course.[10]

Clinical manifestations in a series of 150 patients with predominantly anicteric leptospirosis are shown in Table 1.[11]

Icteric Leptospirosis (Weil Syndrome)

This severe form of leptospirosis was originally described in infections due to *icterohaemorrhagiae* but can be seen with virtually any serotype of *Leptospira*.[1,6,7] It is characterized by impaired renal and hepatic function, hemorrhage, vascular collapse, severe alterations in consciousness, and a high mortality (5–10 percent now, formerly much higher). The jaundice is usually not associated with hepatocellular necrosis, and after recovery there is no residual hepatic dysfunction.[6,7,13] Death in Weil's disease is rarely due to liver failure. The serum bilirubin level (predominantly direct) is usually below 20 mg/100 ml. The alkaline phosphatase level is moderately elevated, and SGOT and SGPT levels rarely exceed 100–200 units. The combination

TABLE 1. Percentage Frequencies of Symptoms and Signs in 150 Patients with Leptospirosis in South Vietnam

Symptom or Sign	*Percentage*
Headache	98
Fever	97
Myalgia	79
Chills	78
Nausea	41
Diarrhea	29
Abdominal pain	28
Cough	20
Conjunctivitis	42
Splenomegaly	22
Lymphadenopathy	21
Pharyngitis	17
Hepatomegaly	15
Nuchal rigidity	12
Rash	7
Jaundice	1.5

(From Berman et al.,[11] with permission.)

of marked elevation in serum creatine phosphokinase with only modest elevations in transaminases in an acutely jaundiced patient may help differentiate leptospirosis from other forms of acute hepatitis.[14] Hepatomegaly occurs in approximately 25 percent of the cases. A rare complication of severe *autumnalis* infection is acute cholecystitis, which requires surgery.[1]

Severely jaundiced patients are the ones most likely to exhibit renal failure, hemorrhage, and cardiovascular collapse. The severity of the various components of Weil syndrome probably reflects the severity of the underlying vasculitis. Urinalysis is usually abnormal during the leptospiremic phase, with proteinuria, hematuria, and casts commonly found. Azotemia usually appears during the second week. BUN level rarely exceeds 100 mg/100 ml and the serum creatinine, 8 mg/100 ml. The sharp fall in renal blood flow sometimes results in frank acute tubular necrosis, but in most cases renal function is eventually restored to normal. Thrombocytopenia, unaccompanied by other manifestations of disseminated intravascular coagulation,[15] occurs in up to 50 percent of patients with leptospirosis and is closely correlated with the presence of renal failure.[16]

Electrocardiographic abnormalities are common during the leptospiremic phase, and in severe cases congestive heart failure and cardiogenic shock may occur. In one series of 26 fatal cases hemorrhagic myocarditis was found at autopsy in 50 percent.

LABORATORY DIAGNOSIS

The definitive diagnosis of leptospirosis depends on laboratory findings. Criteria for definite diagnosis are either isolation of the organism from any clinical specimen or seroconversion or fourfold or greater rise in antibody titer in the presence of a compatible clinical illness. Presumptive diagnosis of leptospirosis may be based on finding either a microscopic agglutination titer of $\geq 1:100$ or a positive slide agglutination test in the presence of a compatible clinical illness. Since many laboratories have little experience in the diagnosis of leptospirosis, it is desirable to have the studies carried out or at least confirmed in a laboratory thoroughly familiar with the necessary techniques.

Isolation of leptospires from body fluids or tissues requires special laboratory techniques and media but is otherwise not difficult.[17–19] Organisms can be isolated from blood or CSF only during the first 10 days of the illness. They usually appear in the urine during the second week, and biopsy specimens of various tissues have also sometimes yielded the organism. Fletcher's medium and the newer EMJH and Tween 80-albumin media are semisolid media useful in primary isolation of leptospires. Tween 80-albumin medium is now commercially available and may be the best.[19] One to three drops of the specimen to be cultured should be added to 3–5 ml of culture medium. Cultures are incubated for 5–6 weeks at 28 – 30°C in the dark. In semisolid media leptospires grow in a concentrated ring 0.5–1 cm below the surface of the medium, usually appearing 6–14 days after inoculation. Multiple cultures should be done—the type of material cultured depending on the stage of illness. Leptospires remain viable in anticoagulated blood for up to 11 days, so specimens can be mailed to a reference laboratory for culture. Citrate should not be used as anticoagulant because it is toxic to leptospires. Addition of antibacterial agents (neomycin, vancomycin, bacitracin, 5-FU, sulfonamides, cycloheximide) to culture media, or intraperitoneal inoculation of clinical material into hamsters, sometimes facilitates isolation of leptospires from urine or other potentially contaminated specimens. A radiometric method for the rapid detection of *Leptospira* organisms utilizing the BACTEC 460 system (Johnston Laboratories) has recently been described.[20] With this system, leptospiral organisms were detected in human blood after only 2–5 days' incubation.

Leptospires can be seen by darkfield examination, but it requires some expertise to differentiate them from fibrin filaments and other extraneous material. The number of organisms in body fluids is usually small, and except in the case of CSF the method is not likely to be diagnostically helpful. Leptospires can be identified in tissues by silver impregnation techniques.

The laboratory diagnosis of leptospirosis is usually made by means of *serologic tests*.[17,18] The macroscopic slide agglutination test uses killed antigen and is the most useful for screening. The microscopic agglutination test, using live antigen, is more specific. It is utilized for determination of antibody titer and tentative identification of serotype. In both tests antigen pools containing representatives of the most common serogroups are used. In many laboratories an indirect hemagglutination test[21] has replaced the conventional macroscopic agglutination test. Most recently, highly specific and sensitive enzyme-linked immunosorbent assay (ELISA) and Dot-ELISA techniques for detection of leptospiral IgM antibodies have been developed.[22–24] The Dot-ELISA test is inexpensive, simple to perform, utilizes minute amounts of killed antigen, and is easily adapted for use in the field.

Agglutinins appear on the sixth to twelfth day of illness, and the maximum titer is reached in the third or fourth week. Antibiotic therapy may suppress or may delay the development of the antibody response, which is highly variable among individual patients anyway. If the convalescent titer (at least 2 weeks after onset of illness) is negative, another test should be performed 2 weeks later. Low titers may persist for many years after the acute illness. Some patients remain seronegative, primarily because the infecting serotype was not represented in the antigen pools. Cross reactions occur frequently, and serologic tests cannot accurately identify the infecting serotype.

Although isolation of leptospires from patients is rarely attempted, the effort should be made more often because only when the organism is isolated can the infecting serotype be accurately identified. Identification of the serotype is important to find out which ones are frequent causes of human and animal infections in a given locality and also to detect an epidemiologic connection among infections acquired through exposure to a common source.

TREATMENT AND PREVENTION

Since leptospirosis is usually a nonfatal disease with a highly variable clinical course, it has been difficult to assess accurately the effectiveness of antimicrobial therapy, and some controversy about this question remains.[25] Earlier studies suggested that either penicillin G (2.4–3.6 million units/day intravenously) or tetracycline (2 g/day in divided doses by mouth) might shorten the duration of fever and reduce the incidence of renal, hepatic, meningeal, and hemorrhagic complications, but only if therapy was started by the fourth day of illness. Two recent studies indicate that antibiotic therapy may be effective in severe leptospirosis even when treatment is delayed until relatively late in the course of the illness. In a carefully designed study of fatal leptospirosis in the hamster, Alexander and Rule[26] demonstrated that ampicillin, bacampicillin, cyclacillin, piperacillin, mezlocillin, doxycycline, chlorotetracycline, cefotaxime, and moxalactam prevented death of the animals, whereas cephalexin, cefadroxil, cefamandole, and cefoperazone were ineffective. Leptospiruria was eliminated by ampicillin and some of the other β-lactam agents, but not by tetracyclines or certain other β-lactam antibiotics. Earlier studies had suggested that tetracycline, but not penicillin G, can eliminate leptospires from the kidney. Watt et al.,[27] in a placebo-controlled, double-blind study of 42 patients with severe or moderately severe leptospirosis, found that penicillin G (1.5 million units intravenously every 6 hours) reduced the duration of fever, hospitalization, hepatic tenderness, and elevation of the serum creatinine. Leptospiruria was markedly diminished by therapy with penicillin. Seventy-six percent of these patients had renal or hepatic dysfunction, and all but one had been ill for 5 or more days before initiation of therapy.

Recent controlled studies in U.S. soldiers training in Panama have indicated that doxycycline administered in a dose of 200 mg once a week and at the end of training prevented infection.[28] In addition, when doxycycline was administered to patients in a dosage of 100 mg twice daily for 7 days and begun within the first 3 days of onset of disease, severity and duration of symptoms were significantly reduced.[29] Thus doxycycline appears to have both prophylactic and therapeutic value in leptospirosis. Oral ampicillin and amoxicillin have also been reported to be effective.[30] Chloramphenicol is not effective in either experimental animals or human infections.

Taking both experimental animal and clinical studies into account, the following recommendations for treatment of severe or moderately severe leptospirosis seem appropriate. In severely ill patients, treatment with either penicillin G (1.5 million units every 6 hours) or ampicillin (500–1,000 mg every 6 hours), should be initiated by the intravenous route, even if the patient has been ill for several days. In less severe cases, when the patient can tolerate oral therapy, doxycycline (100 mg twice daily), ampicillin, (500–750 mg every 6 hours), or amoxicillin (500 mg every 6 hours) may be employed. Treatment should be continued for 5–7 days.

Careful clinical observation and general supportive therapy are especially important in the management of severe leptospirosis to detect and to deal with such life-threatening complications as renal failure, hypotension, and major hemorrhage. Hemodialysis may be necessary in cases of prolonged and severe renal failure.[31]

Prevention of human leptospirosis is very difficult because of the impossibility of eliminating the large animal reservoir of infection.[32] Vaccination of domestic livestock and pets is widely practiced in the United States[33] and has greatly reduced the incidence of infection in some species. Renal infection can still occur in vaccinated dogs, and humans have become infected from dogs that had been adequately immunized.[5] In specific localities effective rat control, disinfection of contaminated work areas, and prohibition of swimming in contaminated waters have effectively reduced the incidence of disease.

REFERENCES

1. Feigin RD, Anderson DC. Human leptospirosis. CRC Crit Rev Clin Lab Sci. 1975;5:413.
2. Turner LH: Classification of spirochaetes in general and of the genus *Leptospira* in particular. In: Johnson RC, ed. The Biology of Parasitic Spirochetes. New York: Academic Press; 1976:95.
3. Heath CW, Jr, Alexander AD, Galton MM. Leptospirosis in the United States. Analysis of 483 cases in man, 1949–1961. N Engl J Med. 1965;273:857.
4. Kaufman AF. Epidemiologic trends of leptospirosis in the United States, 1965–1974. In: Johnson RC, ed. The Biology of Parasitic Spirochetes. New York: Academic Press; 1976:177.
5. Feigin RD, Lobes LA, Jr, Anderson D, et al. Human leptospirosis from immunized dogs. Ann Intern Med. 1973;79:777.
6. Edwards GA, Domm BM. Human leptospirosis. Medicine 1960;39:117.
7. Arean VM. The pathologic anatomy and pathogenesis of fatal human leptospirosis (Weil's disease). Am J Pathol. 1962;40:393.
8. Sitprija V. Renal involvement in human leptospirosis. Br Med J. 1968;2:656.
9. Lal KN, Aarons I, Woodroffe AJ, et al. Renal lesions in leptospirosis. Aust NZ J Med. 1982;12:276.
10. Alexander A, Baer A, Fair JR, et al. Leptospiral uveitis: report of bacteriologically verified case. AMA Arch Ophthalmol. 1952;48:292.
11. Berman SJ, Tsai C, Holmes K, et al. Sporadic anicteric leptospirosis in South Vietnam. A study in 150 patients. Ann Intern Med. 1973;79:167.
12. Gochenour WS, Jr, Smadel JE, Jackson EB, et al. Leptospiral etiology of Fort Bragg fever. Public Health Rep. 1952;67:811.
13. Ramos-Morales F, Diaz-Rivera RS, Cintrón-Rivera AA, et al. The pathogenesis of leptospiral jaundice. Ann Intern Med. 1959;51:861.
14. Johnson WD, Silva IC, Rocha H. Serum creatine phosphokinase in leptospirosis. JAMA. 1975;233:981.
15. Edwards CN, Nicholson GD, Hassell TA, et al. Thrombocytopenia in leptospirosis: the absence of evidence for disseminated intravascular coagulation. Am J Trop Med Hyg. 1986;35:352–4.
16. Edwards CN, Nicholson DG, Everard COR. Thrombocytopenia in leptospirosis. Am J Trop Med Hyg. 1982;31:827.
17. Alexander AD. Leptospira. In: Lennette EH, Spaulding EH, Truant JP, eds. Manual of Clinical Microbiology. 2nd ed. Washington, DC: American Society for Microbiology; 1974:347.
18. Shotts EB, Jr. Laboratory diagnosis of leptospirosis. In: Johnson RC ed. The Biology of Parasitic Spirochetes. New York: Academic Press; 1976:209.
19. Ellinghausen HC, Jr. Nutrition of leptospires in bovine albumin polysorbate medium. In: Johnson RC, ed. The Biology of Parasitic Spirochetes. New York: Academic Press; 1976:65.
20. Manca N, Verardi R, Colombrita D, et al. Radiometric method for the rapid detection of leptospira organisms. J Clin Microbiol. 1986;23:401–3.
21. Sulzer CR, Jones WL. Evaluation of a hemagglutination test for human leptospirosis. Appl Microbiol. 1973;26:655.
22. Adler B, Murphy AM, Locarnini SA, et al. Detection of specific and anti-leptospiral immunoglobulins M and G in human serum by solid-phase enzyme-linked immunosorbent assay. J Clin Microbiol 1980;11:452.
23. Pappas MG, Ballou WR, Gray MR, et al. Rapid serodiagnosis of leptospirosis using the IGM-specific dot-ELISA: comparison with the microscopic agglutination test. Am J Trop Med Hyg. 1985;34:346–54.
24. Watt G, Alquiza LM, Padre LP, et al. The rapid diagnosis of leptospirosis: a prospective comparison of the dot enzyme-linked immunosorbent assay and the genus-specific microscopic agglutination test at different stages of illness. J Infect Dis. 1988;157:840–2.
25. Stoenner HG. Treatment and control of leptospirosis. In: Johnson RC, ed. The Biology of Parasitic Spirochetes. New York: Academic Press; 1976:375.
26. Alexander AD, Rule PL. Penicillins, cephalosporins, and tetracyclines in treatment of hamsters with fatal leptospirosis. Antimicrob Agents Chemother. 1986;30:835–9.
27. Watt G, Tuazon ML, Santiago E, et al. Placebo-controlled trial of intravenous penicillin for severe and late leptospirosis. Lancet. 1988;1:433–5.
28. Takafuji ET, Kirkpatrick JW, Miller RN, et al. An efficacy trial of doxycycline chemoprophylaxis against leptospirosis. New Engl J Med. 1984;310:497.
29. McClain JBL, Ballou WR, Harrison SM, et al. Doxycycline therapy for leptospirosis. Ann Intern Med. 1984;100:696–8.
30. Münnich D, Lakatos M. Treatment of human leptospira infections with Semicillin (ampicillin) or with Amoxil (amoxycillin). Chemotherapy. 1976;22:372.
31. Kennedy ND, Pusey CD, Rainford DJ, et al. Leptospirosis and acute renal failure—clinical experiences and a review of the literature. Postgrad Med J. 1979;55:176.
32. Faine S, ed. Guidelines for the control of leptospirosis. Geneva: World Health Organization; 1982.
33. Alexander AD. Immunity of leptospirosis. In: Johnson RC, ed. The Biology of Parasitic Spirochetes. New York: Academic Press; 1976:339.

216. BORRELIA SPECIES (RELAPSING FEVER)

WARREN D. JOHNSON, JR.

Relapsing fever is caused by arthropod-borne spirochetes of the genus *Borrelia* and is clinically characterized by recurrent episodes of fever and spirochetemia.[1–4] The human body louse transmits *B. recurrentis*, which causes epidemic relapsing fever, and ticks of the genus *Ornithodoros* transmit the many species of *Borrelia* that cause endemic relapsing fever.

ETIOLOGY

The genus *Borrelia* belongs to the family Treponemataceae, which contains all spirochetal pathogens, including the genera *Treponema* and *Leptospira*.[3] Borrelia are helical, 8–30 μm long and 0.2–0.5 μm wide, have 3–10 loose spirals, are actively motile, and divide by transverse fission.[1,5] They are readily stained with aniline or acid dyes, but strains cannot be distinguished by morphologic characteristics. Borreliae have an outer slime-like layer, a cell wall and cytoplasmic membrane, and numerous internal fibrils.[6] They are promptly killed by desiccation and ultraviolet rays but survive and retain their virulence when frozen at −73°C for many months.[1]

Kelly[7,8] has successfully cultivated several *Borrelia* strains in artificial media with generation times ranging from 18 hours (*B. hermsii*) to 26 hours (*B. recurrentis*). Rodents (rats, hamsters, guinea pigs) injected with some strains develop latent brain infections.[1] Tick-borne borreliae remain viable in their natural tick vectors for up to 12 years, and this represents the optimal method for maintaining organisms.[5] There is tick-spirochete specificity, and this has been used to identify *Borrelia* species.[9,10]

EPIDEMIOLOGY AND TRANSMISSION

Relapsing fever occurs throughout the world, with the exception of a few areas in the Southwest Pacific.[9,10] The distribution and occurrence of epidemic relapsing fever is largely determined by socioeconomic and ecologic factors, whereas the distribution of endemic tick-borne disease is governed by the biology of the tick.

Louse-borne relapsing fever is caused only by *B. recurrentis* and is transmitted from person to person by the human body louse (*Pediculus humanus*).[2] After the louse ingests infective human blood, the spirochetes penetrate the midgut and multiply in the hemolymph. Tissues of the louse are not invaded by spirochetes, so disease cannot be transmitted to man by louse saliva or excrement, nor transovarially to the progeny of the louse. Epidemic relapsing fever therefore results from crushing lice, with the release of infective organisms capable of penetrating intact skin or mucous membranes.[10] Lice are infective for their lifetime (10–60 days). Humans are the only hosts for this organism. Louse-borne relapsing fever usually occurs in epidemics that are associated with catastrophic events, such as war or famine, which result in overcrowding and dissemination of body lice. The last great epidemic was during World War II in North Africa and Europe and caused an estimated 50,000 deaths.[1,2] Louse-borne relapsing fever remains endemic in the highlands of Central and East Africa (Ethiopia, Sudan, Somalia, Chad) and the South American Andes (Bolivia, Peru).[11]

Tick-borne relapsing fever is caused by at least 15 *Borrelia* species and is transmitted to man by soft ticks of the genus *Ornithodoros*. Many rodents and small animals serve as natural reservoirs for these borreliae (chipmunks, squirrels, rabbits, rats, mice, owls, lizards).[9,10] Borreliae contained in the blood meal of the tick rapidly multiply and within hours invade all tissues, including salivary glands, excretory organs, and the genital system. Infection of humans occurs when saliva, or excrement is released by the tick while feeding. Transovarial passage of borreliae to the tick progeny is an important mechanism for perpetuation of the spirochete, since ticks can survive for up to 15 years without feeding.[10] *Ornithodoros* ticks prefer warm, humid environments and altitudes of 1500–6000 feet. They are worldwide is distribution. They inhabit caves, decaying wood, rodent burrows, and animal shelters. Their range of movement is limited (less than 50 yards), but they may be passively carried into human dwellings by rodents. Their presence may pass unnoticed because they are typically night feeders, lack a painful bite, and complete their blood feeding in 5–20 minutes.[10,11] The intrusion of man into their environment creates the opportunity for disease transmission. The largest outbreak of tick-borne relapsing fever in the Western Hemisphere was in 62 campers residing in log cabins (Arizona, 1973).[12] The magnitude of this outbreak may have been related to concurrent epizootic plague that killed many of the natural rodent hosts of the tick.[10]

PATHOPHYSIOLOGY

Borreliae are present in blood during the febrile illness, disappearing before afebrile periods and returning to the blood stream during the subsequent febrile episodes. Spirochetemia in louse-borne disease may reach 100,000 organisms/mm^3 of blood.[2] Borreliae are sequestered in internal organs during the afebrile periods and reemerge antigenically modified.[13] This cyclical process of antigenic variation followed by specific antibody production is responsible for the relapsing course of this disease. With successive relapses, borreliae revert to antigenic types similar to those present in earlier relapses. The ultimate termination of clinical disease has been attributed primarily to the development of specific borreliacidal antibody rather than the activity of phagocytic cells.[1,14]

At autopsy hepatitis and hepatic necrosis, miliary splenic abscesses, central nervous system lesions (hemorrhages, perivascular infiltrates, degenerative lesions), myocarditis, and hemorrhagic, gastrointestinal and renal lesions have been described.[2,3]

CLINICAL MANIFESTATIONS

The clinical manifestations of louse-borne and tick-borne relapsing fever are quite similar.[1–4] The variations that occur may be related to differences in spirochete strains, inoculating dose, host immunity, and general condition of the patients. The clinical features of relapsing fever are summarized in Table 1.

The incubation period of both forms of relapsing fever may be difficult to establish, since louse exposure is often chronic, and the tick bite may not be recognized. Generally, louse-borne disease has a longer incubation period, longer febrile periods and afebrile intervals, but fewer relapses than tick-borne disease. Characteristically, both types of relapsing fever have an acute onset of high fever with rigors, severe headache, myalgias, arthralgias, lethargy, photophobia, and cough. Prodromal symptoms are rare. Initial physical findings often include conjunctival suffusion, petechiae, and diffuse abdominal tenderness with hepatomegaly and splenomegaly. Less common findings include nuchal rigidity, pulmonary rales and rhonchi, lymphadenopathy, and jaundice. During the course of the illness the fever is remittent and accompanied by tachycardia and tachypnea. Hemorrhage is common but rarely severe (pete-

TABLE 1. Summary of Clinical Features of Relapsing Fever

	Mean Value or Incidence	
Manifestation	*Louse-Borne Disease*	*Tick-Borne Disease*
Case fatality rate	4–40%	2–5%
Incubation period	8 days (4–18 days)[a]	7 days (4–18 days)[a]
Duration of first febrile attack	5.5 days	3 days
Duration of afebrile interval	9 days	7 days
Duration of relapses	2 days	2–3 days
Number of relapses	1–2 (1–5)[a]	3 (0–13)[a]
Maximum temperature	101–102°F	105°F
Splenomegaly	77%	41%
Hepatomegaly	66%	17%
Jaundice	36%	7%
Rash	8%	28%
Respiratory symptoms	34% (cough)	16%
CNS involvement	30%	9%

[a] Range.
(From Southern et al.,[3] with permission.)

chiae, epistaxis, hemoptysis, hematuria, hematemesis). Iritis and iridocyclitis may result in permanent impairment of vision. Pneumonia, bronchitis, and otitis media may occur. A truncal skin rash of 1–2 days' duration is common at the end of the primary febrile episode.[3] The rash can be petechial, macular, or papular. Neurologic findings are reported in up to 30 percent of patients and include coma, cranial nerve palsies, hemiplegia, meningitis, and seizures.[3] Myocarditis with associated arrhythmias, cerebral hemorrhage and hepatic failure are the most common causes of death.

The primary febrile episode characteristically terminates abruptly in 3–6 days. This crisis may be associated with fatal hypotension and shock. After 7–10 days, fever and symptoms suddenly recur. The duration and the intensity of the symptoms progressively decrease with each relapse. Louse-borne relapsing fever is usually associated with a single relapse, whereas multiple relapses are the rule in tick-borne disease.

DIAGNOSIS

The definitive diagnosis of relapsing fever is established by the demonstration of borreliae in the peripheral blood of febrile patients (Fig. 1). Spirochetes are found in 70 percent of cases when wet blood smears are examined by darkfield microscopy or in Giemsa- or Wright-stained thick and thin smears.[3,15] Organisms are rarely found during afebrile periods. The diagnostic yield can be increased by the examination of acridine-orange stained smears by fluorescence microscopy.[16]

Agglutinating, complement fixing, borreliacidal, and immobilizing antibodies are detectable in serum. However, these tests are not generally available and, if performed, are of limited diagnostic value due to antigenic variation of strains and the complexity of the relapse phenomenon.[14,15] *Proteus* OXK agglutinin titers are elevated in relapsing fever with the highest titers in patients with louse-borne disease (1:80 or greater). Antibodies to OX19 and OX2 are rare. The serologic tests for syphilis are positive in 5–10 percent of cases. Leukocytosis (to 25,000 cells/mm^3) and an increased erythrocyte sedimentation rate (to 110 mm/hr) are common. The cerebral spinal fluid (CSF) pressure is usually elevated in patients with central nervous system involvement and is associated with a pleocytosis (15–2200 cells/mm^3) and with an elevated protein concentration (to 160 mg/100 ml).[3] Spinal fluid glucose is normal. Spirochetes have been detected in CSF by smear or by animal inoculation in up to 12 percent of the patients with central nervous system signs.

An early clinical diagnosis of louse-borne relapsing fever is not difficult during epidemics unless there is coexisting epidemic typhus, a disease also transmitted by the body louse. During the initial febrile episode of an isolated case of relapsing fever, the differential diagnosis can include malaria, typhoid fever, hepatitis, leptospirosis, rat-bite fever, Colorado tick fever, and dengue.[17] Epidemiologic considerations, the occurrence of relapses, and the demonstration of spirochetemia will exclude these diagnoses.

TREATMENT AND PREVENTION

Relapsing fever has been successfully treated with tetracycline, chloramphenicol, penicillin, and erythromycin.[18–21] Tetracycline in a single oral dose (0.5 g) is the preferred therapy in louse-borne relapsing fever except in pregnant women and children less than 8 years (teeth and bone staining).[21] Erythromycin 0.5 g in a single oral dose is an equally effective alternative therapy.[20] Tick-borne relapsing fever is often treated with either tetracycline or erythromycin 0.5 g every 6 hours for 5–10 days because of the higher rate of treatment failures and relapses in these patients.[3,18,19] The mortality of treated relapsing fever is less than 5 percent.[3] Untreated epidemic louse-borne disease has a mortality of up to 40 percent.[1,2]

Antibiotic treatment typically induces a Jarisch-Herxheimer reaction with severe rigors, leukopenia, increase in temperature, and decrease in blood pressure. The onset of the reaction occurs within 2 hours of initiating therapy and coincides with clearing of the spirochetemia. The reaction appears to be an exaggeration of the crisis observed in untreated patients and is most severe in louse-borne disease. Spirochetal endotoxemia with activation of kinins and fibrinolytic and complement factors may have a major role in both the acute illness and the development of this reaction.[22,23] The Jarisch-Herxheimer reaction is not prevented by the prior administration of hydrocortisone.[18,21]

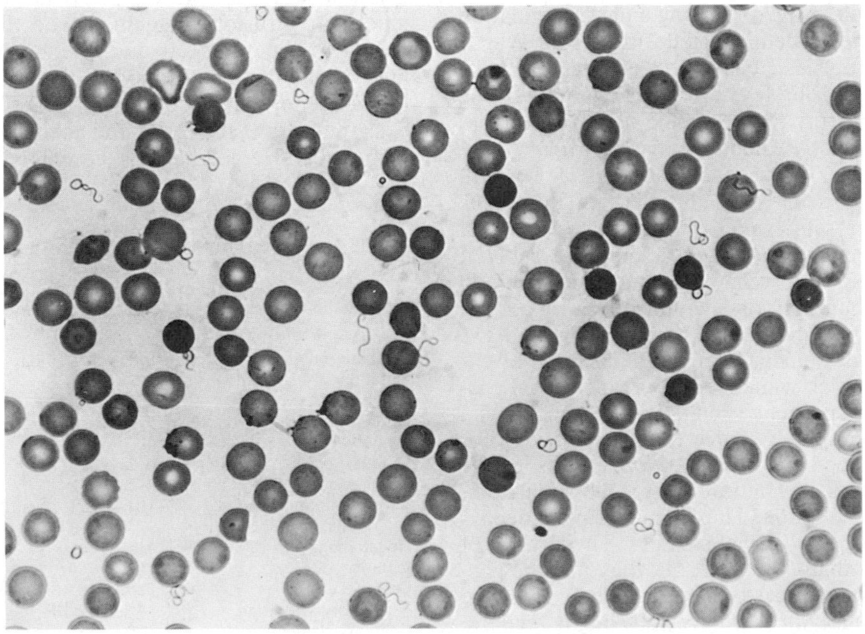

FIG. 1. Peripheral blood smear stained with Wright stain. The *Borrelia* spirochetes can be seen readily. (Original magnification, ×1000) (Courtesy of Dr. Thomas Butler, San Antonio, TX.)

Prevention of relapsing fever requires avoidance or elimination of the arthropod vectors. The varied habitats and the vast geographic areas populated by *Ornithodoros* ticks make their eradication impossible. Insecticides can be used in dwellings and surrounding areas, and insect repellents applied to clothing and persons may further decrease exposure opportunities. Prevention of louse-borne disease is accomplished by good personal hygiene and, if necessary, delousing procedures. DDT-resistant louse strains have developed since World War II, and other insecticides may be required, for example, dimethyl dithiophosphate (malathion).[18]

REFERENCES

1. Felsenfeld O. Borrelia: Strains, Vectors, Human and Animal Borreliosis. St. Louis: Warren H. Green; 1971:180.
2. Bryceson ADM, Parry EHO, Perine PL, et al. Louse-borne relapsing fever. A clinical and laboratory study of 62 cases in Ethiopia and a reconsideration of the literature. Q J Med. 1970;39:129–70.
3. Southern PM Jr, Sanford JP. Relapsing fever: a clinical and microbiological review. Medicine. 1969;48:129–49.
4. Moulton FR, ed. A Symposium on Relapsing Fever in the Americas. Publication No. 18. Washington, DC: American Association for the Advancement of Science; 1942:130.
5. Felsenfeld O. Borreliae, human relapsing fever, and parasite-vector-host relationsips. Bacteriol Rev. 1965;29:46.
6. Hovind-Hougen K. *Treponema* and *Borrelia* morphology. In: Johnson RC, ed. The Biology of Parasitic Spirochetes. New York: Academic Press; 1976:7.
7. Kelly RT. Cultivation and physiology of relapsing fever borreliae. In: Johnson RC, ed. The Biology of Parasitic Spirochetes. New York: Academic Press; 1976:87.
8. Kelly R. Cultivation of *Borrelia hermsii*. Science. 1971;173:443–4.
9. Burgdorfer W. The enlarging spectrum of tick-borne spirochetoses: R.R. Parker Memorial Address. Rev Infect Dis. 1986;8:932–40.
10. Burgdorfer W. The epidemiology of relapsing fevers. In: Johnson RC, ed. The Biology of Parasitic Spirochetes. New York: Academic Press; 1976:191.
11. Felsenfeld O. The problem of relapsing fever in the Americas. Ind Med. 1973;42:7.
12. Center for Disease Control. Relapsing fever. 1973;22:242–6.
13. Stoenner HG, Dodd T, Larsen C. Antigenic variation of *Borrelia hermsii*. J Exp Med. 1982;156:1297.
14. Felsenfeld O. Immunity in relapsing fever. In: Johnson RC, ed. The Biology of Parasitic Spirochetes. New York: Academic Press; 1976:351–8.
15. Burgdorfer W. The diagnosis of relapsing fever. In: Johnson RC, ed. The Biology of Parasitic Spirochetes. New York: Academic Press; 1976:225.
16. Sciotto CG, Lauer BA, White WL, et al. Detection of *Borrelia* in acridine orange-stained blood smears by fluorescence microscopy. Arch Pathol Lab Med. 1983;107:384–6.
17. Le CT. Tick-borne relapsing fever in children. Pediatrics. 1980;66:963–6.
18. Sanford JP. Relapsing fever—treatment and control. In: Johnson RC, ed. The Biology of Parasitic Spirochetes. New York: Academic Press;1976:389–94.
19. Horton JM, Blaser MJ. The spectrum of relapsing fever in the Rocky Mountains. Arch Intern Med. 1985;145:871–5.
20. Perine PL, Teklu B. Antibiotic treatment of louse-borne relapsing fever in Ethiopia: a report of 377 cases. Am J Trop Med Hyg. 1983;32:1096–1100.
21. Bulter T, Jones PK, Wallace CK. *Borrelia recurrentis* infection: clinical trials of antibiotics and management of the Jarisch-Herxheimer-like reaction. J Infect Dis. 1978;137:573–7.
22. Bryceson ADM, Cooper KE, Warrel DA, et al. Studies on the mechanism of the Jarisch-Herxeimer reaction in louse-borne relapsing fever: evidence for the presence of circulating *Borrelia* endotoxin. Clin Sci. 1972;43:343–54.
23. Galloway RE, Levin J, Butler T, et al. Activation of protein mediators of inflammation and evidence for endotoxemia in *Borrelia recurrentis* infection. Am J Med. 1977;63:933–8.

217. BORRELIA BURGDORFERI (LYME DISEASE, LYME BORRELIOSIS)

ALLEN C. STEERE

Lyme disease, originally called Lyme arthritis, was recognized in 1975 because of a close geographic clustering of affected children in Lyme, Connecticut, who were thought to have juvenile rheumatoid arthritis.[1] The illness, which is now known to be caused by a tick-transmitted spirochete, *Borrelia burgdorferi*,[2–4] usually begins in summer with a characteristic skin lesion, erythema chronicum migrans (ECM), accompanied by flulike or meningitis-like symptoms (stage 1).[5,6] Weeks to months later (stage 2), some patients develop cardiac or neurologic abnormalities, musculoskeletal symptoms, or intermittent attacks of arthritis.[5,7–9] Months to years later (stage 3), patients may develop chronic skin, nervous system, or joint abnormalities.[10–14] Serologic testing is the most practical laboratory aid in diagnosis.[3,15–17] All stages of the disorder are usually curable by appropriate antibiotic therapy.[18–20]

Parts of the illness were recognized previously in Europe and were given different names, including erythema chronicum migrans, Bannwarth's syndrome, or acrodermatitis chronica atrophicans.[10,21,22] There are regional differences both in the causative spirochete and in the clinical symptoms of the disease. For example, arthritis is more common in the United States, and neurologic involvement is more frequent in Europe. However, the basic outlines of the disease seem to be similar worldwide, and the entire disease complex is often referred to as Lyme borreliosis. The known geographic distribution of the illness includes at least 33 states of the United States, Europe, Scandinavia, the Soviet Union, China, Japan, and Australia.[23–28]

CAUSATIVE ORGANISM

Borrelia burgdorferi, which grows in Barbour-Stoenner-Kelly (BSK) medium,[29] was first recovered from *Ixodes dammini* ticks in 1982.[2] Although isolation of the spirochete from patients has been difficult, it has now been cultured in several instances each from blood, skin, spinal fluid, and joint fluid samples.[3,4,30] In contrast, recovery of the organism seems as easy from ixodid ticks as it is difficult from patients.[3] *Borrelia burgdorferi* is 11–39 μm long, they have 7–11 flagellae,[31] and their cytosine/guanine ratio is 27.3–30.5 percent (Fig. 1).[32] In one study, the spirochete was found to contain lipopolysaccharide (endotoxin) similar to gram-negative rough-form polysaccharide[33]; in another study, the organism lacked polysaccharide.[34] All isolates of *B. burgdorferi* examined to date have had from four to seven plasmids including supercoiled circular plasmids and linear plasmids.[35] One of these linear plasmids carries the gene that encodes for two of the organism's major outermembrane proteins, the 31 kD Osp A protein and the 34 kD Osp B protein.[36] This gene is variably expressed. Certain plasmids may be lost in culture,[37] which may explain why the organism typically loses pathogenicity in culture. Although isolates of *B. burgdorferi* have shown some heterogeneity (more so in Europe) regarding morphology, DNA homology, plasmids, and outermembrane proteins, there is currently no accepted scheme for subclassification of this organism.

VECTOR OF TRANSMISSION

The vectors of Lyme borreliosis are several closely related ixodid ticks.[38–40] In the northeastern and midwestern United States. *I. dammini* is the vector, and *I. pacificus* is the vector in the West. Other ticks including *I. scapularis, Amblyomma americanum*, and *Rhipicephalus sanguineus* may occasionally be responsible for disease transmission.[41,42] In Europe, *I. ricinus* is the primary vector,[40] and *I. persulcatus* seems to be so in Asia.[25–27] In field studies in Connecticut, the spirochetal pathogen has been found in 10–35 percent of these ticks[2,43]; and on Shelter Island, New York, more than 50 percent of them have been infected with this organism.[44] In *I. pacificus*, the frequency seems to be less[45]; in a survey in California and Oregon, the organism was found in only 2 percent of these ticks.

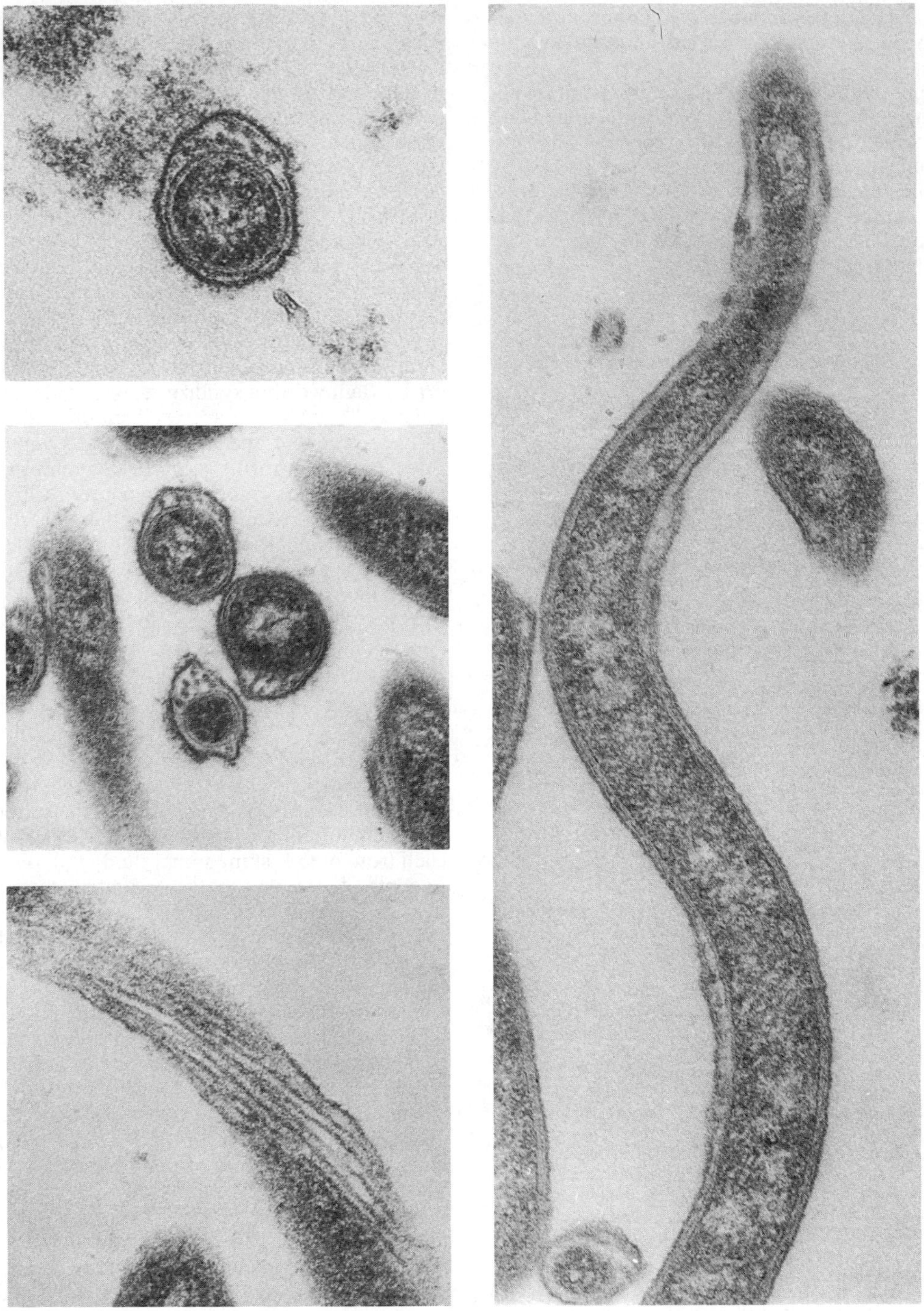

FIG. 1. Electron micrographs of *B. burgdorferi*. The spirochetes have a transverse diameter of about 0.2 μm and 7–11 flagella, which are shown (left panal) in cross section in the upper and middle pictures and in tangential section in the lower picture. In longitudinal section (right panel) the organism has an apparent slime layer, an outer membrane, a flagella, a cell wall, and cytoplasmic constituents; its length is 11–39 μm. (×40,000, except upper left, ×60,000) (From Steere et al,[3] with permission.)

The peak questing periods for adult *I. dammini* are spring and fall; for nymphs, May through July; and for larvae, August and September.[46] The nymphal stage is primarily responsible for transmission of the disease, but all stages of these ticks feed on humans. *Borrelia burgdorferi* seems to be transmitted by regurgitation of midgut contents or by injection of tick saliva during feeding. In studies of experimental transmission in rodents, tick attachment for 24 hours or more was necessary before significant transmission of the spirochete occurred.[47]

ANIMAL HOSTS

Immature *I. dammini* (larvae and nymphs) feed primarily on rodents, particularly on white-footed mice (*Peromyscus leucopus*), and adults usually feed on larger mammals, especially deer (*Odocoileus virginianus*).[48] Infection with *B. burgdorferi* in nature is maintained by horizontal transmission of the organism from infected nymphal *I. dammini* to *Peromyscus leucopus* to larval *I. dammini*, which then molt to infected nymphs to complete the cycle.[49] Deer seem to be quite important for the life cycle of *I. dammini*, and deer are abundant in areas of New England where Lyme disease is endemic.[50]

The tick has been found on and cultured from many other wild and domestic animals[51–53] including birds,[54] which may be responsible for spread of the tick over wide areas. Clinical Lyme disease also affects a wide variety of animal species. Arthritis occurs in dogs, horses, and cattle[55–57]; experimental Lyme arthritis has been produced in LEW/N rats,[58] and ECM has been induced in rabbits.[59] Syrian hamsters inoculated with *B. burgdorferi* develop spirochetemia, and the organisms can be cultured from most of their organs, but they have no signs of illness or significant lesions.[60] Because immature *I. dammini* are aggressive and infect many animal species, the potential for growth and spread of the organism seems large.

EPIDEMIOLOGY

The earliest cases of Lyme disease that have been identified in the United States occurred on Cape Cod in 1962 and in Lyme, Connecticut, in 1965.[61] The illness has now been recognized in at least 33 states. Currently, the disorder occurs primarily in three distinct foci in the United States: in the Northeast from Massachusetts to Maryland, in the Midwest in Wisconsin and Minnesota, and in the West in California and Oregon.[62] Sporadic cases have been recognized along the southeastern coast and in central states as far south as Texas. Lyme borreliosis also occurs throughout Europe and Scandinavia[23] and in Australia.[28] It has recently been recognized in China,[26] Japan,[27] and the Soviet Union where it is found in areas from the western Baltic republics to the maritime region on the Pacific Ocean.[25]

The ages of patients range from 2 to 88 years (median, 28 years), and the sex ratio is nearly 1:1.[6] Age-adjusted attack rates show that the risk of acquiring the illness is similar in all age groups. The onset of the illness is generally between May 1 and November 30; most onsets occur in June and July.[6,38] From 1984 through 1987, the Centers for Disease Control had reports of about 1500 new cases each summer in the United States, but the actual number of cases is likely to be much higher. Asymptomatic infection has been documented with *B. burgdorferi*. In two epidemiologic studies in hyperendemic areas, from 5 to 8 percent of residents tested had subclinical infection, and the estimated ratio of apparent-to-inapparent infection was 1:1.[61,63]

PATHOGENESIS

After injection of *B. burgdorferi* by the tick, the organism migrates outward in the skin (ECM), is spread in lymph (regional adenopathy), or is disseminated in blood to organs, other skin sites, or musculoskeletal tissues. *Borrelia burgdorferi* has been cultured from blood and skin specimens early in the illness,[3,4] from spinal fluid and joint fluid samples after months of illness,[3,30] and from lesions of acrodermatitis as much as 10 years after disease onset.[10] The organism has also been seen in patient specimens of skin, synovium, myocardium, retina, muscle, bone, spleen, brain, and liver.[64–72] These findings and the response of all stages of the disease to antibiotic therapy suggest that the organism may invade and persist, latently or symptomatically, in affected tissues for years.

Initially, the immune response in Lyme disease seems to be suppressed. The mononuclear cells of patients respond minimally to *B. burgdorferi* antigens and less than normal to mitogens.[73,74] Suppressor cell activity is greater than normal. After the first several weeks of infection, mononuclear cells generally have heightened responsiveness to *B. burgdorferi* antigens and to mitogens, less suppressor cell activity than normal, and evidence of B-cell hyperactivity—elevated total serum IgM levels, cryoprecipitates, and circulating immune complexes.[75,76] The specific antibody response to the spirochete develops gradually over months to years to an increasing array of spirochetal polypeptides.[77] Immune antibodies are required for serum-mediated killing of the organism via the classic complement pathway.[78] Both polymorphonuclear leukocytes and monocytes readily phagocytose the spirochete in vitro,[79] but it is not known whether the organism can survive intracellularly. Later in the illness when arthritis is present, antigen-reactive mononuclear cells are concentrated in joint fluid,[74] and in patients with meningitis, such cells are concentrated in spinal fluid.[80] B-cell hyperactivity is usually not found systemically late in the illness.

CLINICAL CHARACTERISTICS

As with other spirochetal infections, Lyme borreliosis generally occurs in stages, with remissions and exacerbations and different clinical manifestations at each stage. The illness usually begins with ECM and associated symptoms (stage 1). It may be followed weeks to months later by neurologic or cardiac abnormalities, musculoskeletal symptoms, or intermittent attacks of arthritis (stage 2) and months to years later by chronic skin, nervous system, or joint involvement (stage 3). However, in an individual patient, the infection is highly variable. At the mild end of the spectrum, some patients have brief involvement in only one system or subclinical infection.[61,63] At the severe end, other patients have abnormalities of the skin, nerves, heart, and joints at the same time. It seems that the disease may begin in any system, and involvement in any system may be transient, recurrent, or chronic. Erythema migrans typically lasts for several weeks but may recur.[5,6] Years later, certain patients develop acrodermatitis chronica atrophicans.[10] The spectrum of neurologic abnormalities ranges from subjective paresthesias to meningopolyneuritis of several months' duration to chronic encephalomyelitis.[8,9,11,12] Joint symptoms also range from subjective arthralgias to intermittent attacks of arthritis to chronic erosive synovitis.[13] Although the skin, nerves, and joints are most commonly affected, almost any system may be involved, including the eyes, heart, lungs, and liver.[7,67,69,71]

SYSTEMS AFFECTED

Skin

Erythema chronicum migrans, which occurs at the site of the tick bite, usually begins as a red macule or papule (Fig. 2, Table 1).[5,6] Of 314 patients in the author's study, 31 percent recalled a tick bite at the skin site where ECM developed 3–32 days later.[6] As the area of redness around the center expands (final median diameter, 15 cm; range, 3–68 cm), most lesions continue to have bright red outer borders (usually flat, but occasionally raised) and partial central clearing (Fig. 2B). The centers of early lesions sometimes become intensely erythematous and indurated, vesicular, or necrotic. In some instances, migrating lesions remain an even intense red, several red rings are found within the outside one, or the central area turns blue before it clears. Although the lesion can be located anywhere, the thigh, groin, and axilla are particularly common sites. If ECM is on the head, only a linear streak might be seen to emerge from the hairline. The lesion is hot to touch, but often not painful.

Within several days after onset of the initial skin lesion (ECM), almost half of the patients in the United States develop multiple annular secondary lesions (Fig. 2, Table 1).[6] Although their appearance is similar to the initial lesions, they are generally smaller, migrate less, and lack indurated centers; they are not associated with previous tick bites. Individual lesions sometimes appear and fade at different times, and their borders sometimes merge. During this period, some patients develop malar rash, conjunctivitis, or rarely, diffuse urticaria. Erythema chronicum migrans and secondary lesions usually fade within 3–4 weeks (range, 1 day to 14 months). However, during or soon after their resolution patients may develop new evanescent lesions (small [2–3 cm] red circles or blotches) for several more

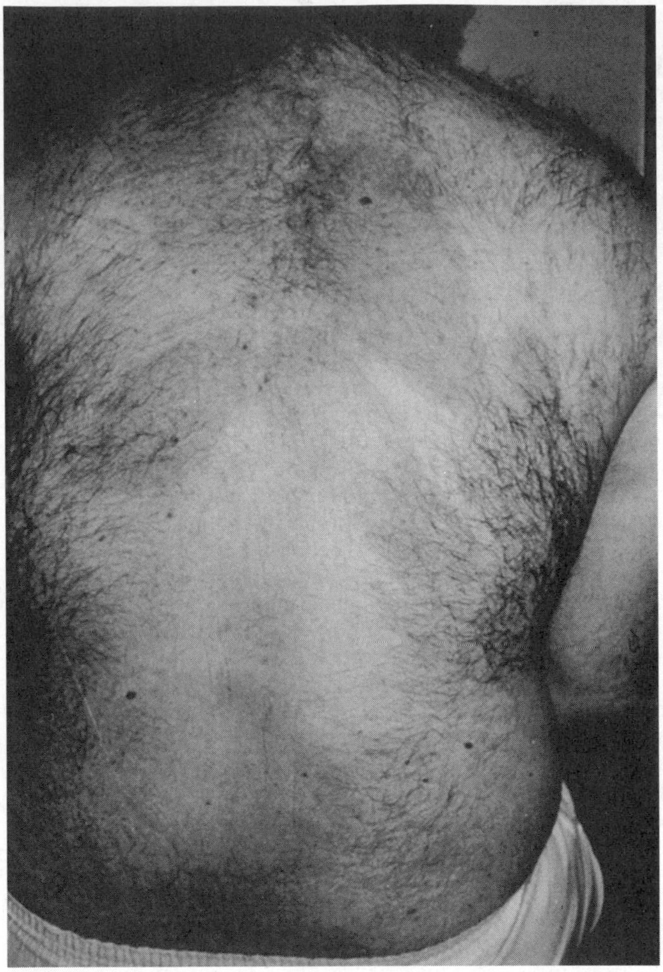

FIG. 2. Four days after the onset of erythema chronicum migrans, secondary lesions have appeared, and several of their borders have merged. (From Steere et al.,[6] with permission.)

TABLE 1. Early Signs of Lyme Disease

Sign	*No. of Patients* N = *314(%)*
Erythema chronicum migrans	314(100)[a]
Multiple annular lesions	150(48)
Lymphadenopathy	
Regional	128(41)
Generalized	63(20)
Pain on neck flexion	52(17)
Malar rash	41(13)
Erythematous throat	38(12)
Conjunctivitis	35(11)
Right upper quadrant tenderness	24(8)
Splenomegaly	18(6)
Hepatomegaly	16(5)
Muscle tenderness	12(4)
Periorbital edema	10(3)
Evanescent skin lesions	8(3)
Abdominal tenderness	6(2)
Testicular swelling	2(1)

[a] Erythema chronicum migrans was required for inclusion in this study.
(From Steere et al.,[6] with permission.)

weeks. On a given day, these lesions appear at different sites, but individual lesions do not migrate. Any of the dermatologic manifestations of the illness may recur.

Erythema chronicum migrans is often accompanied by malaise and fatigue, headache, fever and chills, generalized achiness, and regional lymphadenopathy (Tables 1 and 2).[6] In addition, patients sometimes have evidence of meningeal irritation, mild encephalopathy, migratory musculoskeletal pain, hepatitis, generalized lymphadenopathy or splenomegaly, sore throat, nonproductive cough, or testicular swelling. Except for fatigue and lethargy, which are often constant, the early signs and symptoms are typically intermittent and changing. For example, a patient might experience predominantly headache and a stiff neck for several days. After a few days of improvement, musculoskeletal pain might begin. Associated symptoms may occur several days before ECM and, conversely, may last for months (particularly fatigue and lethargy) after the skin lesions have disappeared.

TABLE 2. Early Symptoms of Lyme Disease

Symptom	*No. of Patients* N = *314(%)*
Malaise, fatigue, and lethargy	251(80)
Headache	200(64)
Fever and chills	185(59)
Stiff neck	151(48)
Arthralgias	150(48)
Myalgias	135(43)
Backache	81(26)
Anorexia	73(23)
Sore throat	53(17)
Nausea	53(17)
Dysesthesia	35(11)
Vomiting	32(10)
Abdominal pain	24(8)
Photophobia	19(6)
Hand stiffness	16(5)
Dizziness	15(5)
Cough	15(5)
Chest pain	12(4)
Ear pain	12(4)
Diarrhea	6(2)

(From Steere et al.,[6] with permission.)

Acrodermatitis chronica atrophicans, which sometimes follows years after erythema migrans, begins with red violacious lesions that become sclerotic or atrophic.[10] These lesions, which may be the presenting manifestation of the disease, may last for many years, and *B. burgdorferi* has been cultured from such lesions as much as 10 years after their onset. Sclerotic lesions may look like localized scleroderma. Patients may also have subluxations of small joints underlying the skin lesions, sometimes accompanied by periosteal thickening.

Musculoskeletal

Within a few weeks to 2 years after the onset of illness, about 80 percent of patients in the United States develop joint symptoms ranging from subjective joint pain to intermittent attacks of arthritis to chronic erosive synovitis.[13] In addition, a few patients have been described with osteomyelitis,[70] myositis,[68] or panniculitis.[81] If musculoskeletal symptoms occur early in the illness, the typical pattern is one of migratory pain in joints, tendons, bursae, muscles, or bones, often without joint swelling. The pain tends to affect only one or two sites at a time and usually lasts a few hours to several days in a given location.

Frank arthritis with marked joint swelling usually does not begin until months after the onset of the illness[5,13] At that time, about 50 percent of patients begin to experience intermittent attacks of joint swelling and pain, primarily in large joints, especially the knee, usually one or two joints at a time. Affected knees are commonly more swollen than painful and are often hot but rarely red. Baker cysts may form and rupture early. However, both large and small joints may be affected, and a few patients have had symmetric polyarthritis. Attacks of arthritis generally last from a few weeks to months separated by periods of complete remission. However, episodes of arthralgia or periarticular involvement—tendinitis, bursitis, or enthesopathy—are commonly interspersed between attacks of arthritis.

The total number of patients who continue to have recurrent attacks decreases by about 10–20 percent each year, but patients have been known to have recurrences for as long as 8 years.

In about 10 percent of patients with arthritis, after a period of intermittent attacks, involvement in large joints becomes chronic, sometimes with erosion of cartilage and bone or permanent joint disability.[13,14] In the author's study of 80 patients with Lyme arthritis, those with chronic involvement had an increased frequency of DR4 and, to a lesser degree, DR3.[82] The relative risk of developing chronic arthritis in patients with both DR4 and DR3 was 46.

As with the other chronic inflammatory arthritides, synovial lesions in Lyme disease show villous hypertrophy, lining cell hyperplasia, fibrin deposition, and mononuclear cell infiltration in the subsynovial lining area.[65,83] T cells, predominantly of the helper/inducer subset, are distributed diffusely in the sublining areas, often with nodular aggregates of tightly intermixed T and B cells.[65] Outside the aggregates, many plasma cells, high endothelial venules, and scattered macrophages are found. HLA-DR and -DQ expression is intense throughout the lesion. When using monoclonal antibodies to outermembrane proteins, a few spirochetes and globular antigen deposits may sometimes be seen in and around synovial blood vessels in areas of lymphocytic infiltration.[65] *Borrelia burgdorferi* is a potent stimulator of interleukin-1, which has been found in the joint fluid of Lyme disease patients.[84] Joint fluid white cell counts range from 500 to 110,000 cells/mm^3 and consist of predominantly polymorphonuclear leukocytes.

Neurologic

Symptoms suggestive of meningeal irritation may occur at the beginning of the illness when ECM is present.[6] Such individuals often have episodic attacks of excruciating headache and neck pain, stiffness, or pressure, typically lasting hours. During the first days of illness, such symptoms are not associated with a spinal fluid pleocytosis or objective neurologic deficit. However, after several weeks to months, about 15 percent of patients in the United States develop frank neurologic abnormalities including meningitis, encephalitis, chorea, cranial neuritis (including bilateral facial palsy), motor and sensory radiculoneuritis, mononeuritis multiplex, or myelitis, alone or in various combinations.[8,9] The usual pattern is fluctuating symptoms of meningitis with superimposed cranial (particularly facial palsy) or peripheral radiculoneuropathy. On examination, such patients usually have neck stiffness only on extreme flexion; Kernig and Brudzinski signs are not present. Facial palsy, or Bell's palsy, frequently occurs alone, and it may be the presenting manifestation of the disease.[85] Most patients with objective neurologic deficits have a lymphocytic pleocytosis in cerebrospinal fluid (CSF) (about 100 cells/mm^3), often with elevated protein levels, but those with facial palsy alone may have normal CSF analyses. Neurologic abnormalities typically last for months but may recur or become chronic.

In Europe, neurologic involvement seems to be associated with the infection more frequently. There, the most common presentation is Bannwarth syndrome, which includes neuritic pain, lymphocytic pleocytosis without headache, and sometimes cranial neuritis.[22] This syndrome has also been called tick-borne meningopolyneuritis (Garin-Bujadoux, Bannwarth)[86], lymphocytic meningoradiculitis, or chronic lymphocytic meningitis.[87] Spinal fluid analyses typically show intrathecal synthesis of IgM or IgG antibody to *B. burgdorferi* and sometimes oligoclonal bands.[88] In one study of such patients who had sural nerve biopsies, the lesions were predominantly axonal, with perivascular infiltration of lymphocytes and plasmacytes around endoneurial, perineurial, or epineurial vessels affecting both myelinated and unmyelinated nerve fibers.[89]

It has recently been recognized that Lyme borreliosis may be associated with chronic neurologic abnormalities that begin months to years after disease onset. The spectrum of such abnormalities is only now being worked out. At the mild end of the spectrum, patients may have intermittent tingling paresthesias of their extremities for years without demonstrable neurologic deficit detected on physical examination.[90] Neurophysiologic testing in such patients often shows abnormal nerve conduction in affected nerves, but spinal fluid analyses generally have normal results. In severe cases, *B. burgdorferi* may invade the central nervous system causing slowly progressive encephalomyelitis, organic brain syndromes, spastic parapareses, transverse myelitis, or dementia.[11,12,91,92] In Minnesota, a young woman developed focal encephalitis with aphasia 6 years after Lyme meningitis.[93] In Sweden, a child experienced progressively destructive Lyme meningoencephalitis for 15 years that was accompanied by tetraplegia, dementia, and sensorineural hearing loss.[94] The results of standard neurologic tests in these patients have been variable. Spinal fluid analyses have generally shown only a minimal or an absent inflammatory response. Magnetic resonance imaging (MRI) scans may show areas of increased density that are consistent with demyelination.[12] Although such patients often have selective concentrations of specific antibody to *B. burgdorferi* in the CSF (particularly in Europe), a test is currently lacking that uniformly indicates active infection in the CNS with this organism.

Cardiac

Within several weeks after the onset of illness, about 8 percent of patients develop cardiac involvement.[7] The most common abnormality is fluctuating atrioventricular block (first-degree, Wenckebach, or complete heart block). However, some patients have evidence of more diffuse cardiac involvement including electrocardiographic changes or a gallium scan[95] compatible with acute myopericarditis, radionuclide evidence of mild left ventricular dysfunction, or rarely, cardiomegaly. None have had heart murmurs. The duration of cardiac involvement is usually brief (3 days to 6 weeks), but it may recur. One patient is known to have died of cardiac involvement of Lyme disease.[66] At autopsy, that patient had a lymphoplasmacellular infiltrate in the epicardium, myocardium, and endocardium, and a few spirochetes were seen in the myocardium. Spirochetes have also been demonstrated in the myocardium in vivo by endomyocardial biopsy.[96]

Other Systems

In addition to conjunctivitis, which is the most common eye abnormality in Lyme disease,[6] patients may develop involvement of deeper tissues in the eye. One patient developed iritis followed by panophthalmitis, which resulted in blindness.[67] Spirochetes were seen in the vitreous debris. Another patient had ischemic optic neuropathy.[97] About 20 percent of patients have evidence of mild hepatitis early in the illness.[6] One patient developed recurrent hepatitis with marked elevations of transaminase levels.[71] A few Dieterle silver-staining spirochetes were found within hepatic sinusoids and parenchyma. Finally, a recent patient was reported with cough, fever, generalized maculopapular rash, myositis, and markedly abnormal liver function test findings.[69] She died of adult respiratory distress syndrome, which was believed to be secondary to Lyme disease.

Congenital Infection

Maternal–fetal transmission of *B. burgdorferi* may cause congenital infection. In one instance, a woman developed Lyme disease during the first trimester of pregnancy and did not receive antibiotic therapy. Her infant, born at 35 weeks' gestational age, died of congenital heart disease during the first week of life.[98] Histologic examination of autopsy material showed *B. burgdorferi* in the spleen, kidneys, and bone marrow. In a later study, 19 cases of Lyme disease were identified in pregnant women.[99] Of the 19 pregnancies, 5 had adverse outcomes including syndactyly, cortical blindness, intrauterine fetal death, prematurity, and rash in the newborn. Finally, during the first trimester of pregnancy, a woman developed ECM, which was treated successfully with oral penicillin.[72] Although she was delivered of a normal-appearing infant at term, the child died suddenly 23 hours after birth. *Borrelia burgdorferi* was demonstrated in the brain and liver of the infant.

LABORATORY DIAGNOSIS

Culture of *B. burgdorferi* from patients permits a definitive diagnosis but is currently a low-yield procedure.[3] Similarly, it is often difficult to find spirochetes in histologic sections. Thus, determination of antibody titers is currently the most practical diagnostic test. In patients, specific IgM antibody titers against *B. burgdorferi* usually reach a peak between the third and sixth week after disease onset; specific IgG antibody titers rise slowly and are generally highest months or years lager (Fig. 3).[3] The initial IgM response is usually directed against the 41 kD flagellar antigen of the spirochete, and a new IgM response may sometimes develop late in the illness to the 34 kD outer-membrane component of the organism. The IgG response appears in a sequential pattern to an increasing array of spirochetal polypeptides over a period of months to years.[77]

Although indirect immunofluorescence was first used to evaluate the antibody response in Lyme disease, enzyme-linked immunsorbent assays (ELISA) were subsequently shown to be more sensitive and specific.[15] Serodiagnosis of early infection, however, has been a problem with either method. In one prospective study using indirect ELISA, only 34 percent of patients had elevated antibody titers acutely, and only 50 percent had them by convalescence.[100] More recently, immunoblotting or IgM-capture ELISA were found to be superior to indirect ELISA for diagnosing early Lyme disease.[16,17] After the first several weeks of infection, patients generally have high antibody titers to *B. burgdorferi*, and testing of one sample is usually adequate for a diagnosis. Antibody to *B. burgdorferi* cross reacts with other spirochetes, including *Treponema pallidum*, but patients with Lyme disease do not have positive VDRL test reactions.

The most common nonspecific laboratory abnormalities, particularly early in the illness, are a high erythrocyte sedimentation rate, an elevated serum IgM level, or an increased serum glutamic oxaloacetic transaminase (SGOT) level (Table 3).[6] Most patients with elevated SGOT levels also have increased levels of serum glutamic pyruvic transaminase (SGPT) and lactate dehydrogenase (LDH). The enzyme levels generally return to normal within several weeks. Patients may be mildly anemic early in the illness and occasionally have elevated white cell counts with shifts to the left in the differential count. A few patients have had microscopic hematuria, sometimes with mild proteinuria (dipstick); values for creatinine and blood urea nitrogen (BUN) have been normal. Throughout the illness, C3 and C4 levels are generally normal or elevated. Tests for rheumatoid factor or antinuclear antibodies are usually negative.

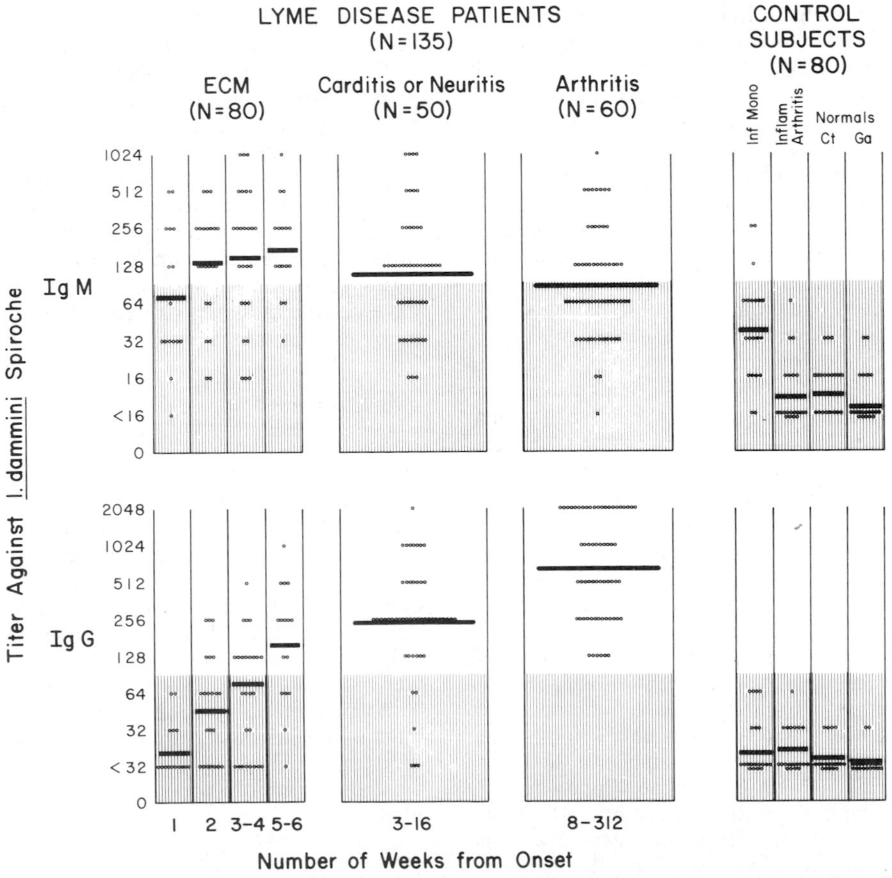

FIG. 3. Indirect immunofluorescent antibody titers against the *I. dammini* spirochete *B. burgdorferi* in serum samples from 135 patients with different clinical manifestations of Lyme disease, from 40 control patients with infectious mononucleosis or inflammatory arthritis, and from 40 healthy control subjects. The heavy bar shows the geometric mean titer for each group; the shaded areas indicate the range of titers generally observed in control subjects. (From Steere et al.,[3] with permission.)

TABLE 3. Laboratory Findings

Finding	*No. of Patients with Abnormal Values, N = 314(%)*	*Median (and Range) of Abnormal Values*
Hematology		
Hematocrit	37(12)	35(36–31)
Leukocytes >10 cells × $10^3/mm^3$	24(8)	12(11–18)
ESR >20 mm/hr	166(53)	35(21–68)
Immunoglobulins		
IgM >250 mg/dl	104(33)	310(252–930)
IgG >1500 mg/dl	10(3)	15880(1520–1760)
IgA >400 mg/dl	12(4)	440(410–580)
Liver function		
SGOT >35 U/ml	59(19)	71(36–251)
SGPT >32 U/ml[a]	47(15)	125(42–491)
LDH >600 U/ml[a]	49(16)	775(608–1080)
Renal function		
Microscopic hematuria (red cells/hpf)	18(6)	15(10–25)

Abbreviations: ESR: erythrocyte sedimentation rate; hpf: high-power field.
(From Steere et al.,[6] with permission.)
[a] Tested only in the 55 patients with abnormal SGOT; creatine phosphokinase levels were normal in all of these patients.

TREATMENT

During 1980 and 1981, we compared phenoxymethyl penicillin, erythromycin, and tetracycline in the treatment of early Lyme disease.[18] ECM and its associated symptoms resolved significantly faster in penicillin- or tetracycline-treated patients than in those given erythromycin (mean duration, 5.4 and 5.7 vs. 9.2 days). More important, 0 of the 39 patients given tetracycline developed major late complications (myocarditis, meningoencephalitis, or recurrent attacks of arthritis) as compared with 3 of 40 penicillin-treated patients (8 percent) and 4 of 29 given erythromycin (14 percent) (p = .07). In 1982, all 49 adult patients were given tetracycline; again none of them developed major complications. Approximately 15 percent of patients experienced a Jarisch-Herxheimer–like reaction (higher fever, redder rash, or greater pain) during the first 24 hours after the start of therapy. In vitro antibiotic sensitivities show that erythromycin, ampicillin, tetracycline, and ceftriaxone are highly active against *B. burgdorferi*; penicillin G, oxacillin, and chloramphenicol are moderately active; and the aminoglycosides and rifampin have no activity.[101,102] However, erythromycin does not seem to be as effective in vivo as in vitro sensitivities would suggest.

For patients early in the illness, I prefer tetracycline, 250 mg or 500 mg four times a day for at least 10 days or for 20 or 30 days if symptoms persist or recur. Doxycycline and amoxicillin may be as effective, but these antibiotics have not yet been tested systematically in early Lyme disease. Phenoxymethyl penicillin, 500 mg four times a day, and erythromycin, 250 mg four times a day, in each instance for at least 10 days, are second- and third-choice alternatives. In children, aged 12 years or under we recommend amoxicillin or phenoxymethyl penicillin, 50 mg/kg/day (not less than 1 g/day or more than 2 g/day) in divided doses for the same duration, or in case of penicillin allergy, erythromycin, 30 mg/kg/day, in divided doses for 15 or 20 days. Early treatment may diminish or abort entirely the subsequent antibody response. Such patients may become reinfected in subsequent summers.[103]

Regardless of the antibiotic agent given, nearly half of patients still experience minor late complications—recurrent episodes of headache or pain in joints, tendons, bursae, or muscles often accompanied by lethargy.[18] However, their physical examinations are usually normal. Symptoms are often reminiscent of those experienced at the beginning of the illness but are generally briefer and less severe. They correlate significantly with the initial severity of the illness. In a given attack, pain usually occurs in one or two sites and lasts from hours to days. With frequent attacks, the pain is often migratory. Patients may continue to have such attacks for several years. The pathogenesis of these symptoms is unclear. We do not know whether they result from a severely depleted number of live spirochetes or from immune-mediated phenomena that do not require the persistence of an intact organism.

In patients who develop frank meningitis, spinal fluid pleocytosis, and cranial or peripheral neuropathies, intravenous penicillin G, 20 million units per day in divided doses for 10 days, is often effective therapy.[19] Headache, stiff neck, and radicular pain usually begin to subside by the second day of therapy and are often gone by 7–10 days, but motor deficits frequently require 7–8 weeks for complete recovery. Ceftriaxone, 2 g per day for 14 days, has also been used successfully in patients with neurologic disease and has the marked advantage of once-a-day dosing.[104] For patients allergic to these medications, tetracycline may be an acceptable alternative.[105]

In patients with high-degree atrioventricular block or a first-degree block of greater than 0.3 seconds, intravenous penicillin, 10 to 20 million units per day or ceftriaxone, 2 g per day, for at least 10 days, and cardiac minitoring is recommended. In patients with complete heart block or deteriorating myocardial function, corticosteroids may be of benefit if the patient does not respond to antibiotic therapy alone within 24 hours.

Established Lyme arthritis can usually be treated successfully with 30-day courses of doxycycline, 100 mg twice a day, or with amoxicillin and probenecid, 500 mg of each four times a day.[106] However, the response to therapy is typically slow, and some patients have required retreatment with oral antibiotics, with intravenous penicillin G, 20 million U per day in divided doses (20), or with ceftriaxone, 2 g per day for 14 days.[104] Synovectomy has been used successfully in patients refractory to antibiotic therapy.

REFERENCES

1. Steere AC, Malawista SE, Snydman DR, et al. Lyme arthritis: An epidemic of oligoarticular arthritis in children and adults in three Connecticut communities. Arthritis Rheum. 1977;20:7.
2. Burgdorfer W, Barbour AG, Hayes SF, et al. Lyme disease—a tick-borne spirochetosis? Science. 1982;216:1317.
3. Steere AC, Grodzicki RL, Kornblatt AN, et al. The spirochetal etiology of Lyme disease. N Engl J Med. 1983;308:733.
4. Benach JL, Bosler EM, Hanrahan JP, et al. Spirochetes isolated from the blood of two patients with Lyme disease. N Engl J Med. 1983;308:740.
5. Steere AC, Malawista SE, Hardin JA, et al. Erythema chronicum migrans and Lyme arthritis: The enlarging clinical spectrum. Ann Intern Med. 1977;86:685.
6. Steere AC, Bartenhagen NH, Craft JE, et al. The early clinical manifestations of Lyme disease. Ann Intern Med. 1983;99:76.
7. Steere AC, Batsford WP, Weinberg M, et al. Lyme carditis: Cardiac abnormalities of Lyme disease. Ann Intern Med. 1980;93:8.
8. Reik L, Steere AC, Bartenhagen NH, et al. Neurologic abnormalities of Lyme disease. Medicine (Baltimore). 1979;58:281.
9. Pachner AR, Steere AC. The triad of neurologic manifestations of Lyme disease: Meningitis, cranial neuritis, and radiculoneuritis. Neurology (NY). 1985;35:47.
10. Asbrink E, Brehmer-Andersson E, Hovmark A. Acrodermatitis chronica atrophicans—a spirochetosis: Clinical and histopathologic picture based on 32 patients; course and relationship to erythema chronicum migrans Afzelius. Am J Dermatopathol. 1986;8:209.
11. Ackermann R, Gollmer E, Rehse-Kupper B. Progressive Borrelien—Enzephalomyelitis. Chronische Manifestation der Erythema-chronicum-migrans. Krankheit am Nervensystem. Dtsch Med Wochenschr. 1985;110:1039.
12. Pachner AR, Steere AC. Central nervous system manifestations of Lyme disease. Arch Neurol. 1989: In press.
13. Steere AC, Schoen RT, Taylor E. The clinical evolution of Lyme arthritis. Ann Intern Med. 1987;107:725.
14. Steere AC, Gibofsky A, Patarroyo ME, et al. Chronic Lyme arthritis: Clinical and immunogenetic differentiation from rheumatoid arthritis. Ann Intern Med. 1979;90:286.
15. Craft JE, Grodzicki RL, Steere AC. The antibody response in Lyme disease: Evaluation of diagnostic tests. J Infect Dis. 1984;149:789.
16. Grodzicki RL, Steere AC. Comparison of immunoblotting with indirect en-

zyme-linked immunosorbent asay using different antigen preparations for diagnosing early Lyme disease. J Infect Dis. 1988;157:790.
17. Berardi VE, Weeks KE, Steere AC. Serodiagnosis of early Lyme disease: Evaluation of IgM and IgG antibody responses by antibody capture enzyme immunoassay. J Infect Dis. 1988;158:754.
18. Steere AC, Hutchinson GJ, Rahn DW, et al. Treatment of the early manifestations of Lyme disease. Ann Intern Med. 1983;99:22.
19. Steere AC, Pachner AR, Malawista SE. Neurologic abnormalities of Lyme disease: Successful treatment with high-dose intravenous penicillin. Ann Intern Med. 1983;99:767.
20. Steere AC, Green J, Schoen RT, et al. Successful parenteral penicillin therapy of established Lyme arthritis. N Engl J Med. 1985;312:869.
21. Afzelius A. Report to Verhandlungen der dermatologischen Gesellschaft zu Stockholm on December 16, 1909. Arch Dermatol Syph. 1910;101:405.
22. Bannwarth A. Chronische lymphocytare Meningitis, entzundliche Polyneuritis und "Rheumatismus." Arch Psychiatr Nervenkr. 1941;113:284.
23. Schmid GP. The global distribution of Lyme disease. Rev Infect Dis. 1985;7:41.
24. Centers for Disease Control. Update: Lyme disease—United States. MMWR. 1984;33:268.
25. Dekonenko EJ, Steere AC, Berardi VP, et al. Lyme borreliosis in the Soviet Union: A cooperative US-USSR report. J Infect Dis. 1988;158:748.
26. Ai C, Wen Y, Zhang Y, et al. Clinical manifestations and epidemiological characteristics of Lyme disease in Hailin County Heilongjiang Province, China. Ann NY Acad Sci. 1988;539:302.
27. Kawabata M, Baba S, Iguchi K, et al. Lyme disease in Japan and its possible incriminated tick vector, *Ixodes persulcatus*. J Infect Dis. 1987;156:854.
28. Steward A, Glass J, Patel A, et al. Lyme arthritis in Hunter Valley. Med J Aust. 1982;1:139.
29. Barbour AG. Isolation and cultivation of Lyme disease spirochetes. Yale J Biol Med. 1984;57:521.
30. Snydman DR, Schenkein DP, Berardi VP, et al. *Borrelia burgdorferi* in joint fluid in chronic Lyme arthritis. Ann Intern Med. 1986;104:798.
31. Hovind-Hougen K, Asbrink E, Stiernstedt G, et al. Ultrastructural differences among spirochetes isolated from patients with Lyme disease and related disorders, and from *Ixodes ricinus*. Zentralbl Bakteriol Hyg. 1986;263:103.
32. Schmid GP, Steigerwalt AG, Johnson SE, et al. DNA characterization of the Lyme spirochete. J Clin Microbiol. 1984;20:155.
33. Beck G, Habicht GS, Benach JL, et al. Chemical and biologic characterization of a lipopolysaccharide extracted from the Lyme disease spirochete (*Borrelia burgdorferi*). J Infect Dis. 1985;152:108.
34. Takayama K, Rothenberg RJ, Barbour AG. Absence of lipopolysaccharide in the Lyme disease spirochete, *Borrelia burgdorferi*. Infect Immun. 1987;55:2311.
35. Barbour AG. Plasmid analysis of *Borrelia burgdorferi*, the Lyme borreliosis agent. J Clin Microbiol. 1988;26:475.
36. Barbour AG, Garon CF. Linear plasmids of the bacterium *Borrelia burgdorferi* have covalently closed ends. Science. 1987;237:409.
37. Schwan TG, Burgdorfer W. Antigenic changes of *Borrelia burgdorferi* as a result of in vitro cultivation. J Infect Dis. 1987;156:852.
38. Steere AC, Broderick TE, Malawista SE. Erythema chronicum migrans and Lyme arthritis: Epidemiologic evidence for a tick vector. Am J Epidemiol. 1978;108:312.
39. Wallis RC, Brown SE, Kloter KO, et al. Erythema chronicum migrans and Lyme arthritis: Field study of ticks. Am J Epidemiol. 1978;108:322.
40. Burgdorfer W, Kierans JE. Ticks and Lyme disease in the United States. Ann Intern Med. 1983;99:121.
41. Schulze TL, Bowen GS, Bosler EM, et al. *Amblyomma americanum:* A potential vector of Lyme disease in New Jersey. Science. 1984;224:601.
42. Rawlings JA. Lyme disease in Texas. Zentralbl Bakteriol Hyg. 1986;263:483.
43. Magnarelli LA, Anderson JF, Apperson CS, et al. Spirochetes in ticks and antibodies to *Borrelia burgdorferi* in white-tailed deer from Connecticut, New York State, and North Carolina. J Wildl Dis. 1976;22:178.
44. Bosler EM, Coleman JL, Benach JL, et al. Natural distribution of the *Ixodes dammini* spirochetes. Science. 1983;220:321.
45. Burgdorfer W, Lane RS, Barbour AG, et al. The western black-legged tick, *Ixodes pacificus:* A vector of *Borrelia burgdorferi*. Am J Trop Med Hyg. 1985;34:925.
46. Wilson ML, Spielman A. Seasonal activity of immature *Ixodes dammini* (Acari: Ixodidae). J Med Entomol. 1985;22:408.
47. Piesman J, Mather TN, Sinsky RJ. Duration of tick attachment and *Borrelia burgdorferi* transmission. J Clin Microbiol. 1987;25:557.
48. Spielman A, Levine JF, Wilson ML. Vectorial capacity of North American *Ixodes* ticks. Yale J Biol Med. 1984;57:507.
49. Levine JF, Wilson ML, Spielman A. Mice as reservoirs of the Lyme disease spirochete. Am J Trop Med Hyg. 1985;34:355.
50. Wilson ML, Adler GH, Spielman A. Correlation between abundance of deer and that of the deer tick, *Ixodes dammini* (Acari: Ixodidae). Ann Entomol Soc Am. 1985;78:172.
51. Anderson JF, Magnarelli LA, Burgdorfer W, et al. Spirochetes in *Ixodes dammini* and mammals from Connecticut. Am J Trop Med Hyg. 1983;32:818.
52. Magnarelli LA, Anderson JF, Burgdorfer W, et al. Parisitism by *Ixodes dammini* (Acari: Ixodidae) and antibodies to spirochetes in mammals at Lyme disease foci in Connecticut, USA. J Med Entomol. 1984;21:52.
53. Anderson JF, Johnson RC, Magnarelli LA, et al. Identification of endemic foci of Lyme disease: Isolation of *Borrelia burgdorferi* from feral rodents and ticks (*Dermacentor variabilis*). J Clin Microbiol. 1985;22:36.
54. Anderson JF, Johnson RC, Magnarelli LA, et al. Involvement of birds in the epidemiology of the Lyme disease agent *Borrelia burgdorferi*. Infect Immun. 1986;51:394.
55. Kornblatt AN, Urband PH, Steere AC. Arthritis caused by *Borrelia burgdorferi* in dogs. J Am Vet Med Assoc. 1985;186:960.
56. Burgess EC, Gillette D, Pickett JP. Arthritis and panuveitis as manifestations of *Borrelia burgdorferi* infection in a Wisconsin pony. J Am Vet Med Assoc. 1986;189:1340.
57. Burgess EC. *Borrelia burgdorferi* infection in Wisconsin horses and cows. Ann NY Acad Sci. 1988;539:235.
58. Barthold SW, Moody KD, Terwilleger GA, et al. Experimental Lyme arthritis in rats infected with *Borrelia burgdorferi*. J Infect Dis. 1988;157:842.
59. Kornblatt AN, Steere AC, Brownstein DG. Experimental Lyme disease in rabbits. Spirochetes found in erythema migrans and blood. Infect Immun. 1984;46:220.
60. Duray PH, Johnson RC. The histopathology of experimentally infected hamsters with the Lyme disease spirochete, *Borrelia burgdorferi*. Proc Soc Exp Biol Med. 1986;181:263.
61. Steere AC, Taylor E, Wilson ML, et al. Longitudinal assessment of the clinical and epidemiologic features of Lyme disease in a defined population. J Infect Dis. 1986;154:295.
62. Steere AC, Malawista SE. Cases of Lyme disease in the United States: Locations correlated with distribution of *Ixodes dammini*. Ann Intern Med. 1979;91:730.
63. Hanrahan JP, Benach JL, Coleman JL, et al. Incidence and cumulative frequency of endemic Lyme disease in a community. J Infect Dis. 1984;150:489.
64. Berger BW, Kaplan MH, Rothenberg IR, et al. Isolation and characterization of the Lyme disease spirochete from the skin of patients with erythema chronicum migrans. J Am Acad Dermatol. 1985;13:444.
65. Steere AC, Duray PH, Butcher EC. Spirochetal antigens and lymphoid cell surface markers in Lyme synovitis: Comparison with rheumatoid synovium and tonsillar lymphoid tissue. Arthritis Rheum. 1988;31:487.
66. Marcus LC, Steere AC, Duray PH, et al. Fatal pancarditis in a patient with coexistent Lyme disease and babesiosis: Demonstration of spirochetes in the heart. Ann Intern Med. 1985;103:374.
67. Steere AC, Duray PH, Kauffmann DJH, et al. Unilateral blindness caused by infection with the Lyme disease spirochete, *Borrelia burgdorferi*. Ann Intern Med. 1985;103:382.
68. Atlas E, Novack SN, Duray PH, et al. Lyme myositis: Muscle invasion by *Borrelia burgdorferi* in a patient with Lyme disease. Ann Intern Med. 1988;109:245.
69. Kirsch M, Ruben FL, Steere AC, et al. Fatal adult respiratory distress syndrome in a patient with Lyme disease. JAMA. 1988;259:2737.
70. Jacobs JC, Stevens M, Duray PH. Lyme disease simulating septic arthritis (Letter). JAMA. 1986;256:1138.
71. Goellner MH, Agger WA, Burgess JH, et al. Hepatitis due to recurrent Lyme disease. Ann Intern Med. 1988;108:707.
72. Weber K, Bratzke HJ, Neubert U, et al. *Borrelia burgdorferi* in a newborn despite oral penicillin for Lyme borreliosis during pregnancy. Pediatr Infect Dis J. 1988;7:286.
73. Moffat CM, Sigal LH, Steere AC, et al. Cellular immune findings in Lyme disease: Correlation with serum IgM and disease activity. Am J Med. 1984;77:625.
74. Sigal LH, Steere AC, Freeman DH, et al. Proliferative responses of mononuclear cells in Lyme disease: Reactivity to *Borrelia burgdorferi* antigens is greater in joint fluid than in blood. Arthritis Rheum. 1986;29:761.
75. Steere AC, Hardin JA, Ruddy S, et al. Lyme arthritis: Correlation of serum and cryoglobulin IgM with activity and serum IgG with remission. Arthritis Rheum. 1979;22:471.
76. Hardin JA, Steere AC, Malawista SE. Immune complexes and the evolution of Lyme arthritis: Dissemination and localization of abnormal Clq binding activity. N Engl J Med. 1979;301:1358.
77. Craft JE, Fischer DK, Shimamoto GT, et al. Antigens of *Borrelia burgdorferi* recognized during Lyme disease: Appearance of a new IgM response and expansion of the IgG response late in the illness. J Clin Invest. 1986;78:934.
78. Kochi SK, Johnson RC. Role of immunoglobulin G in killing of *Borrelia burgdorferi* in the classical complement pathway. Infect Immun. 1988;56:314.
79. Benach JL, Fleit HB, Habicht GS, et al. Interactions of phagocytes with the Lyme disease spirochete: Role of the FC receptor. J Infect Dis. 1984;150:497.
80. Pachner AR, Steere AC, Sigal LH, et al. Antigen-specific proliferation of CFS lymphocytes in Lyme disease. Neurology (NY). 1985;35:1642.
81. Kramer N, Rickert RR, Brodkin RH, et al. Septal panniculitis as a manifestation of Lyme disease. Am J Med. 1986;81:149.
82. Steere AC, Feld J, Winchester RJ. Association of chronic Lyme arthritis with increased frequencies of DR4 and 3 (Abstract). Arthritis Rheum. 1988;31(Suppl):98.
83. Johnston YE, Duray PH, Steere AC, et al. Lyme arthritis: Spirochetes found in synovial microangiopathic lesions. Am J Pathol. 1985;118:26.
84. Habicht GS, Beck G, Benach JL, et al. Lyme disease: Spirochetes induce human and murine interleukin 1 production. J Immunol. 1985;134:3147.
85. Clark JR, Carlson RD, Sasaki CT, et al. Facial paralysis in Lyme disease. Laryngoscope. 1985;95:1341.

86. Horstrup P, Ackermann R. Durch zecken ubertragene Meningopolyneuritis (Garin-Bujadoux, Bannwarth). Fortschr Neurol Psychiatr. 1973;41:583.
87. Skoldenberg BG, Stiernstedt A, Garde G. Chronic meningitis caused by a penicillin-sensitive microorganism? Lancet. 1983;11:75.
88. Wilske B, Schierz G, Preac-Mursic V, et al. Intrathecal production of specific antibodies against *Borrelia burgdorferi* in patients with lymphocytic meningoradiculitis (Bannwarth's syndrome). J Infect Dis. 1984;153:304.
89. Vallat JM, Leboutet MJ, Loubet A, et al. Tick bite neuropathy: An analysis of nerve biopsies from seven cases. Neurology (NY). 1984;34(Suppl):180.
90. Halperin JJ, Little BW, Coyle PK, et al. Lyme disease: Cause of treatable peripheral neuropathy. Neurology (NY). 1987;37:1700.
91. Wokke JHJ, van Gijn J, Elderson A, et al. Chronic forms of *Borrelia burgorferi* infection of the nervous system. Neurology (NY). 1987;37:1031.
92. Reik L Jr, Burgdorfer W, Donaldson JO. Neurologic abnormalities in Lyme disease without erythema chronicum migrans. Am J Med. 1986;81:73.
93. Broderick JP, Sandok BA, Mertz LE. Focal encephalitis in a young woman 6 years after the onset of Lyme disease: Tertiary Lyme disease? Mayo Clin Proc. 1987;62:313.
94. Bensch J, Olcen P, Hagberg L. Destructive chronic *Borrelia* meningoencephalitis in a child untreated for 15 years. Scand J Infect Dis. 1987;19:697.
95. Alpert LI, Welch P, Fisher N. Gallium-positive Lyme disease myocarditis. Clin Nucl Med. 1985;10:617.
96. Reznick JW, Braunstein DB, Walsch RL, et al. Lyme carditis. Electrophysiologic and histopathologic study. Am J Med. 1986;81:923.
97. Schechter SL. Lyme disease associated with optic neuropathy. Am J Med. 1986;81:143.
98. Schlesinger PA, Duray PH, Burke BA, et al. Maternal–fetal transmission of the Lyme disease spirochete, *Borrelia burgdorferi*. Ann Intern Med. 1985;103:67.
99. Markowitz LE, Steere AC, Benach JL, et al. Lyme disease in pregnancy. JAMA. 1986;256:3394.
100. Shrestha M, Grodzicki RL, Steere AC. Diagnosing early Lyme disease. Am J Med. 1985;78:235.
101. Johnson RC, Kodner C, Russell M. In vitro and in vivo susceptibility of the Lyme disease spirochete, *Borrelia burgdorferi*, to four antimicrobial agents. Antimicrob Agents Chemother. 1987;31:164.
102. Preac-Mursic V, Wilske B, Schierz G. European *Borrelia burgdorferi* isolated from humans and ticks: Culture conditions and antibiotic sensitivities. Zentralbl Bakteriol Hyg. 1986;263:112.
103. Pfister HW, Neubert V, Wilske B, et al. Reinfection with *Borrelia burgdorferi*. Lancet. 1986;11:984.
104. Dattwyler RJ, Halperin JJ, Volkman DJ, Luft BJ. Treatment of late Lyme borreliosis — randomized comparison of ceftriaxone and penicillin. Lancet. 1988;1:1191.
105. Ackley A Jr, Lupovici M. Lyme-disease meningitis treated with tetracycline (Letter). Ann Intern Med. 1986;105:630.
106. Liu N, Dinerman H, Levin RE, et al. Randomized trial of doxycycline vs. amoxicillin/probenecid for the treatment of Lyme arthritis: Treatment of non-responders with IV penicillin or ceftriaxone. Arthritis Rheum. (Abstract) In press.

218. SPIRILLUM MINOR (RAT-BITE FEVER)

RONALD G. WASHBURN

Spirillum minor is one of the two etiologic agents of rat-bite fever. The other causative bacterium, *Streptobacillus moniliformis*, is discussed in Chapter 209. *Spirillum minor* causes a significant portion of the cases of rat-bite fever in Asia, but rarely produces infection in the United States.[1,2] In Japan, the infection is called *sodoku* (*so*: rat; *doku*: poison).

In the early years of this century, specimens from patients with *sodoku* were shown to contain spirochetes capable of infecting guinea pigs. These bacteria were initially called *Spirocheta morsus muris* or *Sporozoa muris*.[3] The organism was renamed *Spirillum minus* in 1924[4] and is currently called *Spirillum minor*.[5]

BACTERIOLOGY

Spirillum minor is a short, thick, gram-negative, tightly coiled spiral rod measuring 0.2–0.5 μm by 3–5 μm.[5,6] The organism has two to six regular helical turns.[7] Terminal polytrichous flagella confer darting motility, which can be demonstrated with dark-field examination. *Spirillum minor* cannot be cultured on artificial media.

EPIDEMIOLOGY, PATHOGENESIS, AND PATHOLOGY

The epidemiology of *S. minor* infections is similar to that of streptobacillary rat-bite fever, with the exception that oral ingestion has not been shown to cause spirillary disease. The major route of transmission is through rat bites. Approximately 25 percent of tested rats are positive for *S. minor* in conjunctival and nasopharyngeal secretions, pulmonary lesions, and blood.[6,8] Human-to-human transmission has not been documented.

Relapses of spirillary rat-bite fever have been postulated to be due to seeding of blood and distant foci during periodic reactivation of the primary bite lesion.[6] The few available recorded autopsies show granulomatous inflammation at the original site of inoculation, with epithelial necrosis and mononuclear infiltration of the dermis.[5] Regional lymph nodes are hyperplastic.[6] Deep tissue specimens from distant areas of skin rash contain dilated blood vessels and round cell infiltrates. Liver, spleen, renal tubules, myocardium, and meninges may be hemorrhagic, with areas of necrosis in liver and kidney.

CLINICAL MANIFESTATIONS

The initial bite wound heals promptly but then becomes painful, swollen, and purple approximately 1–4 weeks later, associated with regional lymphangitis and lymphadenitis.[5,6] This local inflammatory lesion ushers in a systemic illness characterized by fever, chills, headache, and malaise. Myalgias and arthritis are rare in this infection, contrasted with streptobacillary rat-bite fever. Leukocytosis with peripheral white blood cell counts in the range of 10,000–20,000/mm^3 may be observed, and up to 50 percent of patients have false-positive syphilis serologies.[6,7] Next, the bite wound commonly progresses to chancrelike ulceration and induration with eschar formation. During the first week of fever, a blotchy violaceous or reddish-brown macular rash erupts over the extremities, face, scalp, and trunk, and then fades during subsequent afebrile intervals. Occasionally, the rash may be urticarial.[9]

Without specific antibiotic therapy, fevers lasting 3–4 days recur at regular intervals between afebrile periods of 3–9 days. Spontaneous cure usually occurs within 1–2 months, but in selected instances fevers have relapsed for years.[9]

The most serious complication of untreated spirillary rat-bite fever is endocarditis. Most of these rare intravascular infections have been observed in patients with pre-existing valvular disease, but one reported case occurred on a normal aortic valve.[10] The spectrum of reported complications also includes myocarditis, pleural effusions, hepatitis, splenomegaly, meningitis, epididymitis, conjunctivitis, and anemia.[3,6,9,11] Overall mortality of untreated *S. minor* infections in the preantibiotic era was 6–10 percent.

DIAGNOSIS

In the absence of a history of rat bite or typical clinical features, other diagnoses that might enter into the differential diagnosis of relapsing fever would include *Borrelia*, malaria, and lymphoma. Since *S. minor* cannot be grown on synthetic media, initial diagnosis relies on direct visualization of characteristic spirochetes in blood, exudate, or lymph node tissue using Giemsa or Wright's stain or dark-field microscopy. Organisms can also be recovered from mice or guinea pigs 1–3 weeks after intraperitoneal inoculation,[3,9] with the precaution that the animals must be prescreened to rule out the presence of pre-existing spirochete infections. No specific serologic test is available for *S. minor* infection.

THERAPY

The usual treatment is procaine penicillin 600,000 units intramuscularly every 12 hours for 10–14 days. Further details are given in Chapter 209.

REFERENCES

1. Anderson LC, Leary SL, Manning PJ. Rat-bite fever in animal research laboratory personnel. Lab Anim Sci. 1983;33:292–4.
2. Cole JS, Stoll RW, Bulger RJ. Rat-bite fever: report of three cases. Ann Intern Med. 1969;71:979–81.
3. Roughgarden JW. Antimicrobial therapy of ratbite fever. Arch Intern Med. 1965;116:39–54.
4. Robertson A. Causal organism of rat-bite fever in man. Ann Trop Med. 1924;18:157.
5. Joklik WK, Willett HP, Amos DB, eds. Zinsser Microbiology. 18th ed. Norwalk: Appleton-Century-Crofts; 1984:741–2.
6. Gunning JJ. Rat-bite fevers. In: Hunter GW III, Swartzwelder JC, Clyde DF, eds. Tropical Medicine. 5th ed. Philadelphia: WB Saunders; 1976:245–6.
7. Rogosa M. *Streptobacillus moniliformis* and *Spirillum minus*. In: Lennette EH, Balows A, Hausler WJ Jr, Shadomy HJ, eds. Manual of Clinical Microbiology. 4th ed. Washington, DC: American Society for Microbiology; 1985:400–4.
8. McHugh TP, Bartlett RL, Raymond JI. Rat bite fever: report of a fatal case. Ann Emerg Med. 1985;14:1116–8.
9. Taber LH, Feigin RD. Spirochetal infections. Pediatr Clin North Am. 1979;26:410–1.
10. McIntosh CS, Vickers PJ, Isaacs AJ. Spirillum endocarditis. Postgrad Med J. 1975;51:645–8.
11. Raffin BJ, Freemark M. Streptobacillary rat-bite fever: a pediatric problem. Pediatrics. 1979;64:214–7.

ANAEROBIC BACTERIA

219. ANAEROBIC BACTERIA: GENERAL CONCEPTS

JOHN G. BARTLETT

Anaerobic bacteria are the numerically dominant components of the normal bacterial flora and they are now recognized as relatively common causes of infections at virtually all anatomic sites.

DEFINITION

There is no universally accepted definition of anaerobic bacteria, but a common requirement is that these bacteria require a reduced oxygen tension for growth and fail to grow on surface media when incubated in air or 10 percent CO_2.[1] Most bacteria will replicate in the absence of oxygen, but those that also grow in air are referred to as "facultative anaerobes," "nonanaerobes," or "aerobes." Anaerobes have substantial differences in oxygen sensitivity.[2] Some anaerobes, especially those that are found in the normal flora and rarely at infected sites, are considered extremely oxygen-sensitive since they will die within several minutes after contact with air. Other anaerobes are considered relatively aerotolerant since they will survive for hours or even days in air, although anaerobic conditions are required for replication. Virtually all anaerobes considered clinically significant are aerotolerant.[3]

The physiologic basis for oxygen sensitivity is poorly understood. Some have suggested that the critical factor is the oxidation-reduction potential (Eh) of the environment. However, studies of *Bacteroides fragilis* in a chemostat indicate that increases in the Eh by chemical manipulation has no effect on growth providing oxygen is not introduced.[4] Growth stops abruptly when oxygen is introduced into the chemostat, indicating that oxygen per se has a direct toxic effect. Superoxide dismutase (SOD) is an enzyme that reduces toxic superoxide radicals and consequently protects microorganisms from their lethal effects. Aerotolerant strains of anaerobic bacteria possess this enzyme, there is a correlation between the concentration of SOD and oxygen tolerance, and the enzyme appears to be inducible with exposure to oxygen.[5] The implication is that SOD favors survival in aerobic conditions and thus serves as a virulence factor.

HISTORICAL PERSPECTIVE

Louis Pasteur is credited with discovering the first obligate anaerobe, *Clostridium butyricum*, in 1861.[1] Numerous papers appeared around the turn of the century in the French and German literature describing the recovery of anaerobic bacteria from a variety of anatomical sites.[6] Among the landmark papers of the time was the publication by Schottmuller,[7] who noted that anaerobic streptococci, rather than group A β-hemolytic streptococci, were actually the most frequent pathogens in puerpural sepsis; he postulated that the infection was endogenously acquired from the normal genital flora, a relatively profound thesis for that time.

Smith noted that the organisms seen in the walls of lung abscess from autopsies resembled the organisms seen in the gingival crevice.[8,9] He postulated aspiration as the mechanism of this infection, and subsequently supported this thesis by reproducing aspiration pneumonia with progression to lung abscess using an intratracheal inoculation of pyorrhea pus in experimental animals. In a tedious series of experiments he isolated 17 organisms from the inoculum and then challenged the animals with each component alone and in various combinations. He found that four organisms (anaerobic streptococci, an anaerobic spirochete, an anaerobic "vibrio," and the fusiform bacillus) were required. This is one of the first studies of synergy, the demonstration that two or more organisms produced an infection that could not be reproduced with a more simplified inoculum.

Altemeier isolated anaerobic bacteria from 96 of 100 cases of appendicitis, most frequently as components of a complex flora.[10] He noted that putrid discharge was the exclusive province of anaerobic bacteria. Infections that were associated with this characteristic odor invariably yielded anaerobes on culture, and the only organisms that reproduced this odor during in vitro growth were anaerobes.[11]

Interest in anaerobes declined with the advent of antibiotics, but was regenerated in the 1960s, probably reflecting three simultaneous developments. First, simplified techniques such as the GasPak jar became available, so that clinical laboratories could cope with oxygen-sensitive forms. Second, organisms that had a long and complicated history of confusing nomenclature were finally categorized into what has become a well-accepted taxonomic classification, thereby facilitating communication. Finally, the frequent isolation of anaerobes by research laboratories, accompanied by the possible therapeutic implications, mandated more widespread use of anaerobic microbiology techniques. Sydney Finegold is credited with spearheading many of these developments.

During the 1960s and 1970s numerous studies redefined the incidence of anaerobic bacteria in various types of infections and bacteriologic patterns at different anatomic sites. Martin reviewed the Mayo Clinic experience showing that 49 percent of 14,839 clinical specimens yielded anaerobic bacteria.[12] Clindamycin evolved as the "gold standard" antimicrobial agent for anaerobic infections in the United States, but the drug received a temporary setback with the report of "clindamycin colitis'' by Tedesdo et al., who found pseudomembranous colitis in 10 percent of 200 clindamycin recipitents at Barnes Hospital in 1973.[13] Subsequently, this was shown to be an epidemic of *Clostridium difficile*-induced disease, so the experience could not be generalized. In England and much of the rest of the world, metronidazole became the ''gold standard,'' at least in part reflecting the fact that it was produced by a British company, that it showed extraordinary in vitro activity against nearly all anaerobes, and that clinical trials showed good in vivo activity as well (although no better than clindamycin). The pathogenic role of anaerobic bacteria was hotly debated, especially in terms of therapeutic implications. One view was that these organisms exist at infected sites due to the concurrent presence of aerobic bacteria, which produced the environmental conditions that permit survival of anaerobes; a logical extension of this thesis is that treatment directed exclusively against the aerobic component of the infection should be adequate.[14] The counter argument was that anaerobes contributed to the pathologic events and required treatment. In fact, some authorities advocated antimicrobials directed against only the anaerobic component of mixed infections,[15] although most took the more conservative view that treatment should be directed against both the aerobic and anaerobic potential pathogens at infected sites.

Arguments favoring the pathogenic role of anaerobes that were commonly quoted at the time include the following:

1. Anaerobic bacteria, especially *B. fragilis*, was a relatively common blood culture isolate, being second only to *Escherichia coli* as a cause of gram-negative bacteremia at the Mayo Clinic.[16]
2. Although the frequency with which aerobic bacteria were concurrently isolated from the infected site was commonly cited as evidence that anaerobes existed only at their discretion, most studies indicated that at least one-third to one-half of infections involving anaerobes yielded an exclusively anaerobic flora.
3. Virulence factors, such as the capsular polysaccharide of *B. fragilis*, provided scientific credibility to the thesis that anaerobes were legitimate pathogens.[17]
4. Experimental animal studies provided testimony to the important role of anaerobic bacteria.[18]
5. Perhaps the most persuasive studies concerned therapeutic trials. One of the most important was a study of penetrating abdominal trauma conducted at Cook County Hospital in the late 1960s in which patients were randomized to receive cephalothin plus kanamycin versus clindamycin plus kanamycin; the major difference between these regimens is the presence or absence of activity vs. *B. fragilis* by clindamycin or cephalothin, respectively.[19] There was a statistically significant difference in outcome favoring the use of the anti-anaerobic drug. A similar study comparing clindamycin–gentamicin and penicillin–gentamicin in 200 patients with postgynecologic surgery infections also demonstrated the need to treat anaerobes.[20]

At the present time, anaerobic bacteria are recognized as relatively frequent pathogens at diverse anatomic sites. Clinicians vary in their interest in pursuing laboratory isolation, since many treat these infections empirically, although most agree that identification of organisms with traditional Gram stains and cultures is preferred when easily accomplished. Nevertheless, this empiric approach is sometimes justifed by the relative difficulty in getting appropriate specimens, the prolonged time sometimes required to recover and identify anaerobic bacteria, the uncertain place of in vitro sensitivity testing of anaerobic bacteria, the fact that many laboratories are still relatively inept at recovering anaerobes, and the observation that empiric treatment generally works.

There continues to be considerable controversy concerning numerous facets of anaerobic infections. These include the role of in vitro sensitivity tests, the relative merits of various antimicrobial agents, and the interactions of various bacteria at infected sites. Nevertheless, these organisms are now generally accepted pathogens. The impact these observations have had on clinical care is evident from antimicrobial usage patterns in hospitals, which generally show that drugs whose existence is justified primarily on the basis of their activity vs. anaerobes, such as clindamycin and cefoxitin, are near the top of the list for antibiotic expenditures in most hospitals.

NORMAL FLORA

Most mucocutaneous surfaces of humans harbor a rich indigenous flora comprised of aerobic and anaerobic bacteria, which varies at different anatomic sites in terms of concentrations and microbial species (Table 1).

The upper airways, including the oral cavity, nasal passages, oropharynx, and nasopharynx, harbor a complex flora that varies at different sites known as ecologic niches.[1,21] This means that the flora of the buccal mucosa is distinctive compared with the flora of the tooth, gum surface, gingival crevice, tongue, or saliva, despite anatomic continuity or juxtaposition. The concentrations of bacteria in saliva are approximately 10^8/ml, of which approximately one-half are anaerobic bacteria and a predominant form is *Veillonella*. In the gingival crevice, the Eh is similar to that of the colon (−300 mv), the concentrations of bacteria reach 10^{12}/ml (the geometric limits with which bacteria occupy space), and anaerobic bacteria account for over 99 percent of the cultivable organisms.[21] The sinuses, eustachian tubes, and respiratory pathogens below the level of the glottis are also generally sterile. Nevertheless, transtracheal aspirations in healthy volunteers show that approximately 20 percent of healthy persons without chronic lung disease harbor small numbers of primarily aerobic bacteria in the lower airways. The most important potential anaerobic pathogens in the upper respiratory tract are *Peptostreptococcus* species (anaerobic streptococci), *Fusobacterium* species (primarily *F. nucleatum*), and *Bacteroides* species (*B. melaninogenicus* group, *B. oralis* group, *B. ruminicola, B. urealyticus*, and *B. disiens*).[21]

The gastrointestinal tract shows marked variations in the concentrations and bacteriologic patterns at different levels.[22–25] The stomach, protected by gastric acidity, contains salivary bacteria that are primarily gram-positive with variable concentrations of anaerobes. In the small bowel, the major mechanism of population control is intestinal motility, so that most of the organisms found are simply passing through. Interruption of flow or a stagnant segment (as with stricture, obstruction, small bowel diverticula, or surgically created blind loops) may result in large concentrations of bacteria with a predominance of anaerobes similar to those found in the colon.[22] This bacterial overgrowth pattern may be responsible for a malabsorption syndrome.

The largest concentrations of anaerobic bacteria are found in

TABLE 1. Bacteriology of the Normal Flora

Anatomic Site	*Total Bacteria (per/ml or g)*	*Ratio Anaerobes:Aerobes*
Upper airway		
Nasal washings	10^3–10^4	3–5:1
Saliva	10^8–10^9	1:1
Tooth surface	10^{10}–10^{11}	1:1
Gingival crevice	10^{11}–10^{12}	1000–1
Gastrointestinal tract		
Stomach	10^2–10^5	1:1
Small bowel	10^2–10^4	1:1
Ileum	10^4–10^7	1:1
Colon	10^{11}–10^{12}	1000:1
Female genital tract		
Endocervix	10^8–10^9	3–5:1
Vagina	10^8–10^9	3–5:1

the relatively stagnant terminal ileum and colon, where concentrations reach 10^{12}/g, and anaerobic bacteria account for 99.9 percent.[23,24] This includes estimates of 400 microbial species including *Peptostreptococcus* species, *Bacteroides* species, *Fusobacterium* species, clostridia, and a diverse array of non-spore-forming gram-positive bacilli (*Bifidobacterium, Eubacterium*, and *Lactobacillus*). The intestinal flora varies not only in its distribution longitudinally, but also in the cross-sectional distribution of bacteria. Organisms that colonize these sites are usually in intimate association with the mucosal surface and the mucous sheath. The colonic flora becomes established after weaning and is thought to remain relatively stable throughout life unless disrupted with intercurrent disease or antibiotic treatment.

The bacteriology of the female genital tract is far less stable than the flora of the gastrointestinal tract. The concentration of bacteria in the vagina and cervix shows a mean of approximately 10^8/ml.[26] However, there is substantial variation, ranging from 10^5 to 10^{11}/ml, simultaneous cultures of the cervix and vagina show unique bacteriologic patterns in an individual, and sequential cultures also show considerable shifts during various stages of the menstrual cycle that may be hormonally influenced.[26,27] Most of the organisms are anaerobic bacteria, although again there is considerable variation, and approximately 20 percent of women have no detectable anaerobes or at least very low concentrations. The dominant anaerobes are *Lactobacillus, Peptostreptococcus*, and *Bacteroides* species; *B. fragilis* is found in only 2–10 percent.[26,27] It should be noted that these comments regarding concentrations and bacterial species apply to healthy nonhospitalized menstruating women; quantitative studies have not been done on premenarche or postmenapausal women, although qualitive cultures in these settings show major differences, with a particularly high yield of coliforms.[28] Other factors that influence bacteriologic patterns include pregnancy, gynecologic surgery, and antibiotic therapy.[29–31]

The skin flora contains large numbers of anaerobic bacteria, the dominant species being *Propionibacterium acnes*, which quantitatively accounts for about one-half of the cultivable flora at most anatomic sites.[32] The skin flora of the perineum and to some extent the lower extremities generally contains components of the colonic flora. The urethra of both sexes contains skin flora as well as *Bacteroides* and *Fusobacterium* species.

PATHOPHYSIOLOGY

Anaerobic infections are usually endogenous, indicating that they originate from the host's own flora. The only important exceptions to this are some of the histotoxic clostridial syndromes such as botulism, *Clostridium perfringens* food poisoning, some cases of gas gangrene in which the organism is acquired from environmental sources, and some cases of *C. difficile*-induced diarrhea or colitis in which this organism may be responsible for endemic or epidemic infections within nursing homes and hospitals. The usual pathophysiologic mechanism for anaerobic infection is a breech in the mucocutaneous barrier, resulting in displacement of the normal flora. This rather simplistic mechanism applies to the great majority of anaerobic infections encountered in clinical practice. The phagocytic, complement-mediated, cell-mediated, and humoral defense mechanisms have all played a definite role in vitro studies and even experimental animal studies of anaerobic infections. However, there seems to be a remarkable paucity of clinical observations to support a pivotal role for these defense mechanisms in a fashion analogous to other organisms. Specifically, patients with neutropenia, defective complement systems, prior splenectomy, congenital or acquired defects in humoral immunity, defective cell-mediated immunity, cancer chemotherapy, or corticosteroid administration infrequently acquire infections involving anaerobic bacteria unless the underlying disease is associated with more commonly recognized predisposing factors such as compromised consciousness with aspiration, carcinoma with obstruction, carcinoma with perforation, mucositis, or perirectal lesions.

Virulence Factors

Anaerobic bacteria include a diverse array of microorganisms that may cause disease by a variety of processes, but the most important virulence factors described are the traditional factors found in aerobic bacteria as well. These include polysaccharide capsules of *B. fragilis* and *B. melaninogenicus*, biologically active endotoxin of fusobacteria, and the production of protein toxins by numerous organisms, (best represented by the histotoxic clostridia.

Virulence factors found in anaerobic gram-negative bacilli are summarized in Table 2.[17,18,33–50] The most extensively studied organism in this group is *B. fragilis*, which, like many other microbes, has a number of potentially important virulence factors. The factor that has received the greatest attention is the capsular polysaccharide which has been studied biochemically, immunologically, and in experimental animals.[17,18,33] The capsule appears to promote abscess formation, possibly by resistance to opsonophagocytosis.[34] The capsular polysaccharide also serves as an appropriate immunogen that confers protection with rechallenge in experimental animals. Protection can be transferred with splenic T cells rather than serum, implicating cell-mediated immunity rather than immunoglobulin, as might be expected.[35,36] The lipopolysaccharide of the cell wall plays a contributing role to "abscessogenic potential" as well.[37] *Bacteroides fragilis*, like many other anaerobes, also produces succinic acid both in vitro and in vivo. This short chain fatty acid appears to inhibit phagocytic killing at the low pH values seen in many infections including abscesses.[38] This is the possible mechanism by which *B. fragilis* and *B. melaninogenicus* appear to confer protection to *Proteus mirabilis* and *E. coli* in vitro.[39,40] *Bacteroides fragilis* also appears to affect the alternative complement pathway.[41,42]

Numerous anaerobes produce a variety of enzymes that may contribute to tissue necrosis or spread through contiguous structures.[43] *Bacteroides fragilis* and *B. melaninogenicus*, like all gram-negative bacteria, contain endotoxin. However, the endotoxin is chemically different from that of coliforms in that

TABLE 2. Virulence Factors of Anaerobic Gram-Negative Bacilli[a]

Virulence Property	*Comment*
Adherence to peritoneal epithelium cells	Found in *B. fragilis* and presumably favors intraperitoneal infection
Capsular polysaccharide	Found in *B. fragilis* and *B. melaninogenicus*; promotes abscess formation, possibly by resistance to opsonophagocytosis
Endotoxin	Fusobacteria have biologically active endotoxin by in vivo assays (Swartzman reaction and chick embryo death test); *Bacteroides* species have endotoxin, but strains tested do not have biologically active endotoxin
Succinic acid	Inhibits phagocytosis and intracellular killing of self and other microbes in the environment at acid pH
Superoxide dismutase production	Produced by clinically significant anaerobes, is inducible with oxygen exposure, and favors aerotolerance
Peroxidase	Favors survival
Hyaluronidase, collagenase, fibrinolysin, neuramidase, chrondrotin sulfatase	Enzymes that may cause tissue destruction and/or promote spread.

[a] See Refs. 17, 18, 33–50.

it lacks KDO and β-hydroxymuristic acid, and, more importantly, it lacks biologic activity in the chick embryo death test, the Schwartzman reaction, and with intravenous inoculation into primates.[45,46] This does not necessarily apply to other anaerobes since *Fusobacterium*, for example, has biologically active endotoxin.

Adjuvants

Anaerobic infections often have additional factors that predispose to infection beyond disruption of normal barriers, which simply accounts for the inoculum. Other contributing factors felt to be important include tissue injury associated with trauma or surgery, impaired blood supply, obstruction of a hollow viscus (respiratory tract, gastrointestinal tract, biliary tract, etc.), or the presence of a foreign body. A common interpretation of these concurrent conditions is that they are important in producing the appropriate environmental milieux that will permit anaerobic bacteria to thrive. With experimental animals, it is commonly noted that relatively large inocula are required to produce infections at a variety of anatomic sites. Factors that notably potentiate virulence include tissue injury or the use of an adjuvant. Typical adjuvants that have been used by various investigators include hemoglobin, sulfates (such as barium sulfate), suture material, agar, sterilized stool, gastric mucin, gum tragacanth, bile salts or even a piece of potato.

Biphasic Disease

An experimental animal model of intra-abdominal sepsis has been studied extensively to define the role of various bacteria in intra-abdominal sepsis.[17,18,51–53] The inoculum in this model consists of cecal contents combined with barium sulfate as an adjuvant placed intraperitoneally in rats in an effort to simulate the septic complications of colonic perforation. The first phase of disease was characterized by generalized peritonitis with a free-flowing peritoneal exudate, and the second phase was characterized by abscess formation (Fig. 1). There was a 43 percent mortality, and all deaths occurred during the first 4 days after challenge. Abscesses were defined as loculated collections within the abdominal cavity, with the characteristic outer wall of collagen, an interface of polymorphonuclear cells, and a central area of necrotic debris and bacteria. Abscesses were initially detected at 5 days following challenge, and all animals sacrificed 7 days after challenge had typical abscesses.

In translating these observations to the clinical setting, it should be noted that the initial phase of the infection, which was generalized peritonitis in the animal model, is more frequently observed as a localized infection at the site of the inoculum, as with appendicitis, diverticulitis, or infection at the site of previous colonic surgery. The subsequent abscess formation may also be localized, as with a periappendiceal abscess or diverticular abscess; when the inoculum is free-flowing there may be abscesses throughout the abdominal cavity, although the favorite sites are the colonic gutters and pelvis due to gravitational flow and the subphrenic spaces due to the negative pressure created by diaphragmatic movement.

Studies of the animal model were designed to distinguish the role of various bacteria as this infection evolved. Initial work showed that blood cultures during the acute peritonitis stage yielded *E. coli*, and quantitative cultures of peritoneal exudate in the early peritonitis stage showed that *E. coli* was the numerically dominant organism; other organisms that were also uniformly present, but in lower concentrations, were the enterococcus *Fusobacterium varium* and *B. fragilis*. Quantitative cultures in the late stage showed that the same four microbial species were universally present, but now *B. fragilis* was the numerically dominant organism, with mean concentrations of $10^{9.8}$/ml. Additional studies were done with "antimicrobial probes," meaning the use of antibiotics to identify specific roles of bacteria. This work showed that gentamicin, which is active against coliforms such as *E. coli* and not active vs. anaerobic bacteria, reduced mortality rates from approximately 37 percent to 4 percent, although 54 of 55 (98 percent) of surviving animals had abscesses at necropsy. Clindamycin, which has the opposite spectrum, had no appreciable effect on mortality, but the incidence of abscess among surviving animals was only 5 percent. Use of the two drugs in combination showed the salutory advantages of each, e.g., a mortality rate of 8 percent and a 6 percent incidence of abscesses in surviving animals. In the final series of experiments the animals were challenged with the four microbial strains that were found at the infected site in pure culture. This work showed that *E. coli* caused early death with a mortality rate that was directly related to the inoculum size. *Bacteroides fragilis* failed to cause lethality, but it induced abscesses in 19 of 20 recipients; in fact, an inoculum comprised of the capsular polysaccharide of *Bacteroides fragilis* without viable bacteria was sufficient to produce typical intra-abdominal abscesses.[17]

The conclusion of this work is that both coliforms and anaerobic bacteria (especially *B. fragilis*) serve as pathogens in this model, although they appear to produce differing biologic events as the infection evolves through its two characteristic stages. *Escherichia coli* appears to be the major pathogen in the early initial generalized peritonitis associated with bacteremia and death. This conclusion is supported by the high incidence of *E. coli* bacteremia early in the infection when lethality occurred, the effect of gentamicin in reducing mortality rates, and the results of monomicrobial challenge in which *E. coli* was the only organism tested that caused death. By contrast, *B. fragilis* appeared to have its major effect in the second stage of the disease. Evidence to support this postulated role in abscess formation were the results of quantitative cultures showing that it was the numerically dominant organism in abscess pus, that clindamycin protected against abscess formation, and that it was the only organism tested to reproduce abscesses with monomicrobial challenge.

Although the pathophysiologic events could be ascribed to just two microbial species, care must be exercised in an overly simplistic interpretation. First, *E. coli* was the coliform in the inoculum, although it is presumed that any member of the Enterobacteraceae family could produce similar results. With regard to abscess formation, it is of interest to note that vaccination with *B. fragilis* polysaccharide capsular material prevents abscess with monomicrobial challenge using *B. fragilis*, but a challenge with stool still produces abscesses, indicating that there are other contributing factors in the pathogenesis of abscesses.[35] It was also noted that certain

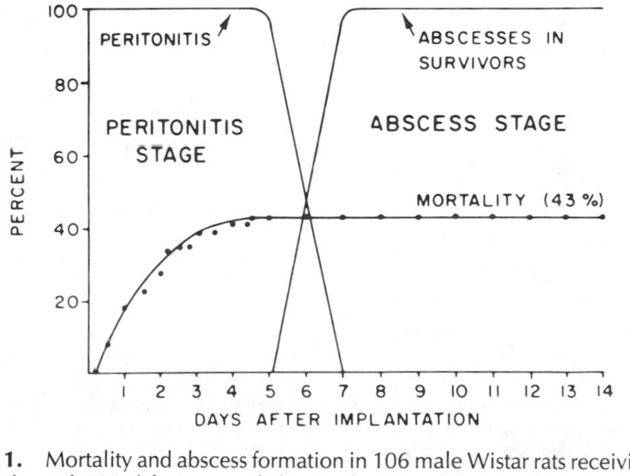

FIG. 1. Mortality and abscess formation in 106 male Wistar rats receiving inoculum obtained from meat-fed animals. Mortality is expressed as cumulative percent.

combinations of bacteria using anaerobes other than *B. fragilis* could produce abscesses in the animal model.[53] Despite these nuances, the animal model has served as a convenient method for interpreting complex events that occur in intra-abdominal sepsis associated with an inoculum of colon contents. A logical conclusion of the observations is that antimicrobial treatment should be directed against coliforms and anaerobes, a thesis that is reasonably well supported in clinical studies.[19,20]

Synergy

A complicating feature of anaerobic infections is their microbiologic complexity. Most studies of anaerobic infections indicate that an average of three to six microbial species are found at the infected site, and these often include aerobic bacteria as well as anaerobes. One problem with this observation is the inherent inability to apply Koch's postulates, since these include the requirement for recovery of a single microbe from an infected site. A second problem is that the polymicrobial nature of the culture results poses great problems in distinguishing commensals, symbionts, and pathogens, which has major implications for treatment, since it is often unrealistic to direct therapy against all components of a polymicrobial infection.

The animal model cited above was studied in an effort to decipher the roles of various bacteria; as noted, two microbial species appeared to be responsible for the pathologic events at two different stages of disease. An additional consideration in these infections is the possibility of synergy, implying that two or more bacteria produce a pathologic process that cannot be produced by a single microbe in pure culture. Because of the complexity of the flora at infected sites, this has always been an attractive thesis to explain the pathophysiology of anaerobic infections. Nevertheless, there are relatively few clear-cut convincing examples of synergy in clinical medicine except for a few studies in experimental models. One example is the study of lung abscess by David Smith noted previously.[8,9] Another example is an indolent destructive skin infection called Meleney's synergistic gangrene, involving *Staphylococcus aureus* and a microaerophilic streptococcus.[54] Inocula of each organism in pure culture into experimental animals fail to produce this lesion, but the combination causes typical necrotic ulcers. It now appears that the *Staphylococcus* produces a hyaluronidase that permits the streptococcus to invade at the inflammatory front.[55]

Another example of synergy concerns the role of *B. melaninogenicus* and a relatively hapless diphtheroid implicated in a necrotizing infection of mucous membranes of the mouth.[56,57] Studies using subcutaneous injections into experimental animals show the combination of organisms produces a more virulent infection in which *B. melaninogenicus* is the actual pathogen and the apparent role for the diphtheroid is simply to provide its obligatory requirement for vitamin K.

There is frequent reference to the assumption that anaerobes exist at infected sites due to the environment milieux produced by a concurrently present aerobic bacteria. Carried to its logical extension, it would appear that elimination of the aerobe would result in death of the anaerobe.[14] There is remarkably little support for this thesis. On the contrary, Ingham et al. have found that succinc acid produced by some anaerobic bacteria interferes with phagocytosis,[40] thus protecting concurrent aerobes so that eradication of the anaerobic component of the infection became the only critical factor for infection control. Altemeier had a more simplistic interpretation of synergy; based on an experimental model of intra-abdominal abscess, he concluded that the total number of bacterial species represented a virulence factor.[58]

Critical review of the medical literature indicates general support for the concept that synergy is an important factor in polymicrobial infection, although careful scrutiny indicates sparse scientific support, except for studies of relatively rare conditions in which specific roles for participating organisms have been defined and more complex animals in which pathogenic mechanisms of synergy are quite elusive.

CLUES TO ANAEROBIC INFECTIONS

There are a number of clinical clues to the presence of anaerobic infections that permit the clinician to make a tentative diagnosis that often becomes the foundation of antimicrobial selection (Table 3).

Infections that occur in continuity to the mucosal surfaces, where anaerobic bacteria comprise the normal flora, frequently involve these microbes. Typical examples include orodental infections, intra-abdominal sepsis, and infections of the female genital tract other than sexually transmitted diseases. In most cases, there is an associated condition that has resulted in a breech in the barrier defense mechanisms.

Infections associated with tissue necrosis and abscess formation are often due to anaerobic bacteria. Anaerobic bacteria have been reported as the dominant bacteria in abscesses at virtually all anatomic sites, including cerebral abscess, peritonsillar abscess, dental abscess, lung abscess, intra-abdominal abscess, tubo-ovarian abscess, and cutaneous abscess. Experimental studies noted above indicate virulence factors, such as the polysaccharide capsule of *B. fragilis* and *B. melaninogenicus*, which appear to be "abscessogenic" and possibly account for this association.

Putrid odor of infections or discharges is considered diagnostic of infection. These organisms produce the same odor with in vitro growth.[11] The characteristic odor tends to be a relatively late feature of most anaerobic infections, and it is generally seen in only about one-third to one-half of patients; nevertheless, when present it is considered diagnostic. The chemical basis for a putrid discharge is not well established, but appears to reflect a combination of metabolic products of anaerobic bacteria that includes short chain volatile fatty acids such as succinic and butyric acid, and methylmercaptan. The short chain volatile fatty acids are produced in vitro as well as in vivo, and their production is used to identify these microbes both with subcultures of isolated strains and with direct analysis of exudate.[59,60] It should be noted that the odor associated with these individual short chain volatile fatty acids, while offensive, is somewhat different than that of exudate-containing anaerobes, so that it must represent some combination that has been elusive to define.

Gas in tissue is another clue to the presence of anaerobic infections, but this is not considered diagnostic since it may be produced by other gas-producing organisms as well.[61] Again, there is a correlation between the clinical observation and in vitro growth of these microbes, since bubbles in broth culture media are an important clue to the recovery of anaerobes. Gas at infected sites may be detected with palpation to detect crepitation, with x-rays, or with scanning techniques. It should be

TABLE 3. Clues to Probability of Anaerobic Bacteria at Infected Sites

Infection adjacent to surfaces that normally harbor anaerobes as normal flora.
Infections, by prior experience, usually involve anaerobic bacteria (Table 4).
Infections characterized by abscess formation or tissue necrosis.
Infections associated with putrid odor.
Infections characterized by gas formation.
Gram stain of exudate showing Polymicrobial flora. Organisms with morphological features of anaerobes.
Failure to cultivate likely pathogens from infected sites that may be ascribed to failure to perform anaerobic cultures, inadequate anaerobic cultures, or prior therapy with antimicrobial agents active vs. anaerobes.
Classic features of toxins produced by histotoxic clostridia: tetanus, botulism, *C. perfringens* food poisoning, gas gangrene, or *C. difficile*-induced diarrhea/colitis.

emphasized that gas at the infected site may represent air introduced during irrigations or other manipulations, the release of CO_2 with hydrogen peroxide, or the rare production of gas by selected aerobic bacteria such as *S. aureus, E. coli* or *Klebsiella* species.

Infections involving a polymicrobial flora are often anaerobic or represent mixtures of aerobic and anaerobic bacteria. This may be readily detected with Gram stains of exudate showing multiple different morphotypes at the infected site. Furthermore, the Gram stain appearance of anaerobic bacteria is often relatively unique. This applies to most anaerobic gram-negative bacilli, such as *Bacteroides* species, which tend to be small, delicate, pale, and pleomorphic. *Fusobacterium nucleatum* shows a typical fusiform shape with pointed ends, and *Fusobacterium necrophorum* shows extreme pleomorphism with round bodies. Anaerobic gram-positive cocci, primarily *Peptostreptococcus*, cannot be distinguished from aerobic or microaerophilic gram-positive cocci on the basis of Gram stain appearance. With regard to gram-positive bacilli, *C. perfringens* usually shows the typical large "box-car" appearance, all clostridia take the Gram stain variably, so that they may appear gram-negative, and strains other than *C. perfringens* or *Clostridium ramosum* often show spores in exudate. Bifidobacteria show typical terminal bifercations and *Actinomyces* has a typical beaded appearance.

The failure to grow likely pathogens in the laboratory is a clue to the presence of relatively fastidious bacteria, such as anaerobes. This may reflect the failure to submit diagnostic specimens that are appropriate for anaerobic culture, the failure of the laboratory to use appropriate microbiologic techniques, or the impact of prior antibiotic treatment. With regard to the latter, it is known that treatment with clindamycin, metronidazole, and possibly other antimicrobial agents as well will rapidly modify the cultivable flora from infected sites so that susceptible strains cannot be easily recovered. Analysis of exudate after therapy also fails to reveal their signature volatile fatty acids.

Additional clues that apply to a relatively small portion of cases include the following: the typical clinical features reflecting toxin activity of the histotoxic clostridia (tetanus, botulism, *C. perfringens* food poisoning, gas gangrene, *C. difficile*-induced diarrhea or colitis); black discoloration or UV light demonstration of red fluorescence, indicating infection involving pigmented *Bacteroides* (the former shows *B. melaninogenicus*); septic thrombophlebitis, suggesting the biologic effect of heparinase produced by *B. fragilis* or other anaerobes; or the woody induration and discharges containing "sulfur granules" and other features characteristic of actinomycosis.

MICROBIOLOGIC METHODS TO ESTABLISH ANAEROBIC INFECTIONS

The clinician and microbiologist must work in concert to provide an optimal recovery rate of anaerobic bacteria. This combined effort is directed toward the proper collection, transport, and processing of specimens.

Specimen Collection

Appropriate specimens must be devoid of contamination by the normal flora. On occasions, the problem of contamination has been obviated with quantitative cultures, but most laboratories do not offer this service so that appropriate specimens are restricted to exudate or tissue obtained directly from the infected site, or the use of normally sterile body fluids (Table 4). In a number of clinical settings these principles are difficult to apply, so that there is simply no opportunity to obtain a meaningful specimen or there is a requirement for specialized collection techniques. As a general rule, liquid or tissue specimens are preferred; swabs should be avoided.

TABLE 4. Specimens Appropriate for Anaerobic Culture

Specimen	*Comment*
Normally sterile body fluids	Includes pleural fluid, peritoneal fluid, bile, cerebrospinal fluid
Abscess contents	Needle aspirates preferred
Wound[a]	Exudate preferrably collected with syringe aspiration using care to decontaminate adjacent areas
Pulmonary	
Pleural fluid	
Transtracheal aspirates[a]	Results with broth cultures only are difficult to interpret
Transthoracic needle aspirates	
Thoracotomy specimens	
Bronchoscopic aspirates[a]	Require double catheter brush with distal occluding plug combined with quantitative culture
Tracheostomy aspirates[a]	Validity not well established, one-third without evidence for infection yield anaerobes, and quantitative cultures may be required
Urinary tract	
Suprapubic aspirates	
Female genital tract	
Culdocentesis	Experience varied
Specimens obtained above pelvic inflection at surgery or laparoscopy	
Transabdominal uterine aspirates	
Intrauterine brush using double catheter device[a]	Requires quantitative cultures; utility in postpartum endometritis is not established
Intra-abdominal	
Aspirates, biopsies	Specimens must be devoid of the gastrointestinal flora
Orodental	
Aspirates of closed spaces	
Paper point specimens	Collected from endodontal canal and preferrably transported in conditions that preserve hydration and anaerobiasis
Sinus aspirates[a]	May require quantitative cultures
Middle ear aspirates	Optimal specimens are obtained with intact tympanic membrane
Soft tissue	
Aspirates of closed spaces, abscesses	
Biopsy using 3 mm dermal punch bx[a]	Sometimes facilitates valid specimen from ulcers subjected to surface contamination (decubitus, diabetic foot, etc.)
Sinuses	
Aspirates using catheter or syringe[a]	Plastic catheter inserted into depths of sinus tract is preferred

[a] Contamination with normal flora is common so that broth cultures are inappropriate and interpretation is facilitated with quantitative or semiquantitative cultures.

Specimen Transport

The optimal method of transporting specimens is immediate delivery so that microbiology processing can begin within 30 minutes ("two fast legs method"). A variety of specialized transport devices permit the maintenance of an oxygen-free environment during transport. Although these are theoretically attractive, there is minimal evidence that they are necessary. A study of the survival of anaerobic bacteria in clinical specimens using quantitative culture techniques of exudate left for various times on the bench showed nearly complete qualitative and quantitative recovery of clinically significant anaerobes with exposure to room air for up to 48–72 hours.[62] Limitations in the study cited include the fact that these were relatively large volumes of exudate retained in a Petri dish representing conditions that do not necessarily apply to all specimens, especially small-volume specimens. Nevertheless, this experiment does suggest that most clinically significant anaerobes survive; as noted above, there is a distinction between the environmental conditions necessary for growth and those necessary for survival, and anaerobes are generally defined by the requirements for replication. Swabs represent a notable exception, although here it appears that drying may be more important than oxygen sensitivity. In this case, the clinician is advised to place the specimen in specially prepared prereduced and anaerobically sterilized (PRAS) semisolid medium such as Cary-Blair medium. The use of other transport devices will depend on the requirements of the individual laboratory, the duration of time between collection and processing, the volume of the specimen (large volumes are preferred), and the idiosyncracies of the people involved.[63]

ANAEROBIC BACTERIA AT INFECTED SITES

Anaerobic bacteria have been reported in infections at virtually all anatomic sites. Nevertheless, a number of recurring studies indicate certain types of infections in which these pathogens are common and other settings in which they are relatively infrequent (Table 5).[64–103]

TABLE 5. Recovery Rates of Anaerobic Bacteria in Infectious Diseases

Disease Catetory (Ref.)	*No. Cases Studied*	*No. with Anaerobes (%)*
Head and neck		
Nontraumatic brain abscess (64)	18	16 (89)
Chronic sinusitis (65)	83	44 (53)
Chronic otitis (66)	68	35 (51)
Perimandibular space infection (67)	31	29 (94)
(68)	21	21 (100)
Peritonsillar abscess (69)		(76)
Dental abscess (70)	10	9 (90)
Chest		
Aspiration pneumonia (71)	70	61 (87)
(72)	47	29 (82)
Lung abscess (73)	57	53 (93)
(74)	26	22 (85)
Empyema (75)	83	63 (76)
(74)	37	23 (62)
Unselected patients (76)	89	29 (33)
(77)	74	16 (22)
Hospital-acquired pneumonia (78)	159	56 (35)
Intra-abdominal sepsis (79)	759	627 (83)
Abscess or peritonitis (80)	72	68 (94)
(81)	64	52 (81)
(82)	40	36 (90)
Appendicial abscess (8)	100	96 (96)
Liver abscess (83)	40	21 (52)
Female genital tract		
Miscellaneous types (84)	33	33 (100)
(85)	91	67 (74)
(86)	50	36 (72)
Pelvic abscess (87)	25	22 (88)
Pelvic inflammatory disease (88)	54	13 (25)
(89)	74	57 (77)
Postpartum endometritis (90)	128	49 (38)
Soft tissue		
Wound infection following elective colon surgery (91)	19	18 (95)
Postappendectomy wounds (92)	65	15 (79)
Cutaneous abscess (93)	135	81 (60)
Diabetic foot ulcer (94)	19	12 (63)
Nonclostridial crepitant cellulitis (95)	12	9 (75)
Pilonidal sinus (96)	45	33 (73)
Breast abscess (97)	41	34 (83)
Necrotizing synergistic cellulitis (98)	57	51 (89)
Paronychia (99)	32	23 (72)
Bite wound infection (100)	34	18 (53)
Bacteremia		
All blood cultures (101)	2,318	209 (9)
Intra-abdominal sepsis (91)	8	7 (88)
Septic abortion (102)	76	48 (63)
Decubitus ulcers (103)		
Endometritis (90)	28	15 (54)

Infections of the Central Nervous System

Focal, purulent intracranial infections that commonly involve anaerobic bacteria include cerebral abscess, subdural empyema, and epidural abscess. Meningitis rarely involves anaerobic bacteria, so that most microbiology laboratories do not even cultivate cerebrospinal fluid anaerobically, and on the rare occasions when anaerobes are recovered this usually reflects either contamination or continuity of the meninges with a parameningeal pyogenic process or brain abscess.

The most carefully studied central nervous system infection that usually involves anaerobes is pyogenic cerebral abscess. Common associated infections include sinusitis, otitis, or mastoiditis, all of which are likely to represent anaerobic infections in which these microbes appear to reach the brain by direct extension or through local vascular spread. Less common concurrent conditions include hematogenous seeding from anaerobic pulmonary infections, intra-abdominal sepsis, or congenital heart disease with right-to-left shunt.

Most of cerebral abscesses are polymicrobial with variations in bacteriologic patterns depending to some extent on the associated condition. The first careful bacteriologic study of nontraumatic brain abscesses in which anaerobic cultures were routinely performed was reported by Heineman and Braude.[64] These investigators recovered anaerobes in 16 of 18 cases, aerobic bacteria were concurrently present in 6, and 2 cases yielded no organisms, possibly reflecting prior antibiotic treatment. *Bacteroides fragilis* is almost invariably present when the associated condition is a middle ear or mastoid infection with local extension to the temporal lobe; coliforms and *Pseudomonas aeruginosa*, various streptococci, and other anaerobic bacteria are often present as well.[104] With sinusitis as the source of the infection, the usual bacteriologic pattern includes a variety of anaerobes other than *B. fragilis* and streptococci including *S. intermedius*. Metastatic abscesses tend to involve a polymicrobial flora similar to that at the site of origin, which is most often a pleuropulmonary infection and less commonly intra-abdominal sepsis. An exception is cerebral abscess occurring in the presence of cynanotic heart disease, in which there is generally a single microbe, usually a streptococcus that may be aerobic, microaerophilic, or anaerobic.

Surgery has generally been considered the most important component of therapy for cerebral abscess, although there is now evidence that many of these patients respond with antimicrobial agents not only early in the cerebritis stage of infection, but also after the abscess wall is well formed.[105] This change in clinical practice is partly ascribed to the recognition and treatment of anaerobic bacteria. With regard to antibiotic selection, the favored drugs have traditionally been those that penetrate the blood-brain barrier and are active against anaerobes; they include metronidazole, penicillin, and chloramphenicol. The role of second- and third-generation cephalosporins is somewhat enigmatic, since none of those that are commonly used for meningeal infections are known to be particularly effective against anaerobic bacteria. Metronidazole has been extensively tested, the clinical experience is good, levels in cerebral abscesses are high, and many now prefer this agent.[104] However, it is not advised as a single agent due to lack of activity against aerobic streptococci (especially *S. intermedius*, gram-negative aerobes, and *Actinomyces* species.

The results of these observations have led to frequent use of combinations of antibiotics for empiric treatment of cerebral abscess under the settings described; such combinations include penicillin G, ampicillin, or a third-generation cephalosporin combined with metronidazole or chloramphenicol. There is little doubt that the mortality rate of cerebral abscess is declining. Most authorities attribute this progress to the important contribution of computerized tomography for both detection of lesions and for following response to therapy, the recognition that anaerobes play an important role in most of these infections, and more appropriate use of antimicrobial agents either with or without aspiration or drainage procedures.[105]

Infections of the Upper Airways

Anaerobic bacteria are involved in a variety of infections of the oral cavity and adjacent structures. Nearly all clinically important dental infections, including pulpitis (endodonic infection),[106] periapical or dental abscess, and perimandibular space infections,[67,68] are likely to involve anaerobes. These three infections often represent a continuum in which the initial lesion is an endodonic infection that progresses to the periapical region and then extends to involve the potential spaces created by fascial insertions along the mandible. Many of the perimandibular spaces are contiguous, but infections are usually localized to specific anatomic sites that are generally adjacent to the portal of entry. The usual presentation is swelling and pain, and the mainstay of treatment is drainage. Special variations that are important to recognize clinically include "Ludwig's angina" (indicating bilateral involvement of the sublingual and submandibular spaces as classically described by Ludwig) and infections involving the posterior compartment of the lateral pharyngeal space as classically described by Lemiere.[107] Lemiere syndrome refers to suppurative thrombophlebitis of the jugular vein with *Fusobacterium* bacteremia and metastatic abscesses, primarily to the lung.

Infections involving the gingival crevice and adjacent gums, including pyorrhea and gingivitis, usually involve anaerobes. An infrequent distinctive form of gingivitis is acute necrotizing ulcerative gingivitis, sometimes known as Vincent's angina or "trench mouth"; this is a relatively fulminant infection associated with severe pain, putrid odor, tissue destruction, and pseudomembrane formation. The bacterial etiology is not well established, although spirochetes have been detected within tissue at the advanced edge of inflammation, and treatment directed against anaerobes is clearly required.[108] A possibly related necrotizing infection of the oral mucous membranes is cancrum oris or "noma," which is characterized by rapid destruction of the bone and face, occurs most frequently in children with malnutrition or systemic disease, and is usually fatal in the absence of antibiotic treatment.

Additional infections adjacent to the upper airways that commonly involve anaerobic bacteria include chronic sinusitis,[65] chronic otitis media,[66] and mastoiditis. Anaerobes are infrequently involved in acute infections at these anatomic sites with a well-characterized repetitive pattern of bacterial pathogens, including *Haemophilus influenzae, Streptococcus pneumoniae, B. catarrhalis* and *Streptococcus pyogenes*. Peritonsillar abscesses are frequently caused by anaerobic bacteria, despite the prevalent impression that they are caused by *S. pyogenes*.[69] Infections of the upper airways and adjacent structures that are infrequently caused by anaerobic bacteria include pharyngitis, parotitis, suppurative adenitis and, as noted, acute sinusitis and acute otitis media.

Microbiologic patterns for the anaerobes tend to follow stereotyped patterns for most of these infections. The dominant anaerobic bacteria involved are *Peptostreptococcus* species, *Fusobacterium* species, and *Bacteroides*- species other than *B. fragilis* including the black-pigmented *Bacteroides* ("*B. melaninogenicus* group"), the *B. oralis* group, the *B. ruminicola* group, *B. disiens*, and the *B. urealyticus* group. Most are sensitive to penicillin, clindamycin, and metronidazole; erythromycin, tetracycline, oral cephalosporins, and antistaphylococcal penicillins are less active.[109] Common aerobes that are concurrently present include *Capnocytophaga* (resistant to oral cephalosporins and metronidazole) and *Eikenella* (resistant to oral cephalosporins, clindamycin, and metronidazole).

Pleuropulmonary Infections

Anaerobic bacteria are relatively frequent and commonly overlooked pathogens in the lower airways. The initial infection is usually aspiration pneumonia, which is commonly followed by suppurative complications including lung abscess or a bronchopleural fistula resulting in an empyema. In general, patients with aspiration pneumonia (pneumonitis) tend to present with typical findings of an acute pneumonia that may not be easily distinguished from other forms of bacterial pneumonia except for the relatively slow tempo of the disease.[110] It should be noted that early in the disease course these patients lack the highly characteristic features that commonly herald the presence of anaerobes such as putrid sputum and necrosis of tissue. The most frequently recognized clues to the bacteriology of anaerobic pulmonary infections are those that are seen relatively late in the course, when there is abscess formation or empyema, the sputum or pleural fluid is putrid (one-half to two-thirds of cases), and there is evidence for chronicity with prolonged symptoms including weight loss and anemia.

Patients with anaerobic pulmonary infections usually have associated conditions that predispose to aspiration such as compromised consciousness (alcoholism, drug addiction, general anesthesia, seizure disorder, stroke, neurologic diseases) or dysphagia. Peridontal disease is often present as well, since this provides the infecting flora.[8] The important anatomic area to note by clinical exam is the gingival crevice, since it is the gingival "pockets" that typically contain large concentrations of the anaerobic bacteria found most frequently in lung abscess. By contrast, saliva has relatively low concentrations of anaerobes, and the dominant organism is *Veillonella*, an anaerobe with little pathogenic clout. Other conditions that predispose to anaerobic infection include bronchiectasis, which was classically described as a debilitating disease associated with putrid discharge. Bronchial obstruction due to foreign body, bronchial stenosis, or a neoplasm also predisposes to anaerobic infection; in a dog model, the insertion of pellets into the lower airways to produce bronchial obstruction is associated with a downstream infection involving anaerobic bacteria from the animal's oral cavity, thus providing experimental support for the role of anaerobes in postobstructive pneumonia.[111]

The clinical presentation of these infections includes the expected features of cough, sputum production, leukocytosis, fever, and dyspnea. Although the list of pulmonary pathogens is legion, anaerobes are on a relative short list of bacterial agents responsible for pulmonary necrosis and chronic pulmonary infections. With regard to anatomic localization, the segments favored by gravitational flow with aspiration in the recumbent position are the superior segments of the lower lobes and the posterior segments of the upper lobes; aspiration that occurs in the upright position favors the lower lobes. The unique features that specifically suggest this infection include the aforementioned putrid sputum or empyema fluid, x-ray evidence of tissue necrosis with cavity formation, the previously noted predisposing conditions, and the chronicity of complaints, which often simulates the clinical features of bronchogenic neoplasms or tuberculosis. The frequent combination of a chronic pulmonary disease characterized by sputum production, dyspnea, fever, weight loss, and cavitation in the upper lobe often suggests pulmonary tuberculosis or a bronchogenic neoplasm.

Bacteriologic patterns in anaerobic pulmonary infections are similar to those described for orodental infections. Most studies were reported in the 1970s, when transtracheal aspiration was in common use, and noted that *B. fragilis* was recovered in 15–20 percent of cases.[71–74,110] This finding was difficult to equate with studies of the oral flora, the presumed source of the inoculum, which consistently showed that virtually no one has upper airway colonization with this microbe. More recent studies suggest that *B. fragilis* was erroneously identified, and other penicillin-resistant *Bacteroides* species presumably account for the discrepancy[110,112] (Table 6). Approximately one-half of these infections involve aerobic bacteria with established or suspected pathogenic potential. Nevertheless, a retrospective analysis of our group of patients, who had pulmonary infections involving an exclusive anaerobic flora, and those with a mixed aerobic–anaerobic flora showed no differences in terms of frequency of putrid discharge or other clinical features typical of anaerobic infections; in fact, response rates were similar when antibiotic treatment was directed exclusively against the anaerobic component.[113] Nevertheless, it should be noted that infections acquired nosocomially, primarily hospital-acquired aspiration pneumonia, tend to involve anaerobes in combination with aerobic gram-negative bacilli and/or *S. aureus*.[78] These latter organisms are regarded as important and potentially devastating pulmonary pathogens in nosocomial pneumonia and should not be ignored in terms of antibiotic selection.

The incidence of anaerobes in pulmonary infections was studied most extensively in the period from 1970 through the early 1980s and showed that anaerobes could be recovered in 60–90 percent of cases of aspiration pneumonia and lung abscess.[71–74] Studies of empyema using appropriate biologic techniques indicate a marked reduction in the incidence of this complication in the antibiotic era, a marked decline in the frequency of pneumococcal empyema since the introduction of penicillin, and a marked increase in the relative frequency of anaerobic empyemas, which now account for 30–50 percent of cases in some series.[75] The frequency of anaerobes in unselected patients with pneumonia has been infrequently studied due to the difficulty of routinely obtaining specimens that are appropriate for anaerobic culture. Nevertheless, one study conducted with transtracheal aspiration in 89 patients showed a yield of 33 percent,[76] and another using bronchoscopy with a specialized protected catheter device for collection of specimens in 74 unselected patients showed a yield of 22 percent.[77]

Therapeutic decisions regarding the selection of drugs for anaerobes involved in pulmonary infections has been the subject of considerable debate. In the 1950s and 1960s penicillins became the drugs of choice based on the extensive studies of William Weiss on patients with putrid lung abscess studied at Philadelphia General Hospital.[114] This choice came under scrutiny in the early 1970s when numerous reports indicated the recovery of penicillin-resistant anaerobes in 15–20 percent of patients. A subsequent comparative study, the only randomized study of treatment conducted up to that time, showed that clindamycin was superior to high-dose intravenous penicillin G in patients with lung abscess.[115] The result of these observations is the evolution of three commonly advocated regimens for anaerobic pulmonary infections:[116] (*1*) Penicillin G given orally or parenterally is preferred by some, who regard it as "the gold standard"; additionally, most patients are not severely ill, so that the clinician often has the opportunity to observe results without serious consequences, the same drug may be used for both oral and parenteral treatment, and there are benefits in terms of side effects and cost. (*2*) Clindamycin is clearly favored for patients who are seriously ill or who have failed to respond to penicillin treatment; some also advocate this drug as the routine first choice for all patients, based on its superiority to penicillin in a clinical trial, the theoretical disadvantage of penicillinase-producing organisms in 15–20 percent of cases, the usual lack of in vitro sensitivity tests to confirm or refute the presence of resistant anaerobes, and the fact that the drug is cost-effective for hospitalized patients since it avoids the delay in response noted with penicillin failures. (*3*) Penicillin combined with metronidazole is occasionally advocated and has limited use in the United States; more extensive use in Europe appears favorable.[110] It should be noted that metronidazole is not advised as a single agent due to the frequent presence and importance of aerobic and microaerophilic streptococci that are resistant to metronidazole. The reported experience with metronidazole as a single agent for anaerobic pulmonary infections shows that approximately one-half were considered therapeutic failures.[110,117] There is minimal information concerning other drugs for anaerobic pulmonary infections, and, although there are probably many that will work reasonably well, relatively few may be used on the basis of published clinical experience in microbiologically confirmed infections.

TABLE 6. Bacteriology of Anaerobic Bacterial Infection of the Lung

	Authors' Experience[110]	*Finegold et al.*[112]
Period reviewed	1968–1975	Early 1980s
Cases	193	196
Total anaerobic isolates	461	656
Average anaerobic isolates/case	2.4	3.3
Bacteroides		
B. fragilis group	38[a]	14
B. melaninogenicus	76[a]	46
B. intermedius	—	60
B. asaccharolyticus	—	6
B. urealyticus	—	18
Other	37	160
Fusobacterium		
F. nucleatum	56	58
F. necrophorium	2	6
Peptosreptococci	87	66
Peptococci	39	—[a]
Gram-positive bacilli		
Clostridium sp.	18	20
Eubacterium sp.	18	46
Actinomyces	5	28
Lactobacillus sp.	8	30
Proprionibacterium sp.	10	12
Bifidobacterium sp.	9	10
Veillonella	23	54

[a] Numbers refer to the number of isolates. Differences in the two series reflect, in part, taxonomic changes and variations in microbiological methods. In the earlier series,[110] the "black-pigmented *Bacteroides* species were reported as *B. melaninogenicus*, whereas the latter series[112] reported these according to their reclassification as *B. melaninogenicus*, *B. intermedius*, and *B. asaccharolyticus*. For gram-positive cocci, the clinically important organisms formerly classified as *Peptococcus* have been reclassified as *Peptostreptococcus*.

Intra-abdominal Sepsis

Infections of the abdominal cavity may be classified as monomicrobial or polymicrobial based on the number of bacterial species at the infected site. Infections that tend to involve a single species include biliary tract infections, pancreatic infections (pancreatic abscess or infected pseudocyst), and primary or "spontaneous" peritonitis. In each instance, the dominant organisms are coliforms, especially *E. coli*, followed by various streptococci; anaerobic bacteria are relatively infrequent. Polymicrobial infections include intra-abdominal abscesses and peritonitis that may be generalized or localized (phlegmon). The dominant bacteria in these cases are combinations of coliforms and anaerobic bacteria, there are an average of four to six microbial species per case, and the dominant isolates in virtually all series are *B. fragilis* (or the "*B. fragilis* group") and *E. coli*[10,79–82] (Table 7).

The pathophysiology of most cases of intra-abdominal sepsis is a breech in the mucosal barrier. Involvement of the colonic flora is especially common, reflecting the frequency of associated diseases at this anatomic segment, including diverticulosis, appendiceal infections, colonic carcinoma, inflammatory bowel disease, and previous colonic surgery. The inoculum of bacteria in such cases presumably involves 400 microbial species that comprise the normal colonic flora; thus the bacteria at the infected site represent a distillate of the inoculum in which organisms presumably survive due to their ability to accommodate to new environmental conditions, such as aerotolerance, and their often poorly understood virulence factors.

The events that follow this type of insult have been studied in the previously noted animal model.[18,118] It should be noted that the "biphasic model" may show considerable variation as

TABLE 7. Bacteriology of Intra-Abdominal Sepsis

Cases studied		759	
Period reviewed		1979–1982	
Bacteriology			
Aerobes only		132 (17%)	
Anaerobes only		7 (1%)	
Anaerobes + aerobes		620 (82%)	
Bacterial isolates			
Aerobes	1256	Anaerobes	1187
E. coli	306	*Bacteroides* sp.	443
P. aeruginosa	121	*B. fragilis*	133
Klebsiella	119	*Clostridium* sp.	256
Proteus sp.	89	*C. perfringens*	50
Enterobacter	46	*Peptostreptococcus*	220
Citrobacter	40	*Fusobacterium*	35
Serratia marcescens	16	*Eubacterium*	60
Gram-negative bacilli (other)	79	Miscellaneous	116
Enterococcus	277		
Staphylococcus aureus	111		
Gram-positive cocci (other)	62		

(Modified from Stone et al.,[79] with permission.)

the lessons are applied to the clinical setting. Rather than generalized peritonitis, the initial inflammatory reaction is often restricted to the site of injury to produce a phlegmon (such as appendicitis or diverticulitis) that subsequently evolves to abscess formation (periappendiceal abscess or diverticular abscess). In other cases, there is more widespread dissemination of bacteria as with free perforation, resulting in generalized peritonitis or subtle leaks; in these cases the second stage of disease is characterized by abscesses that most frequently occur in the pelvis or paracolic gutters due to gravitational flow, or in the subphrenic regions, reflecting upward movement due to the negative pressure created by diaphragmatic movements.

The most important facet of treatment is usually surgical intervention or percutaneous drainage. With regard to antimicrobial therapy, most patients are treated empirically without the benefit of bacteriology results. When cultures are available, results of in vitro sensitivity testing are often useful for drug selection for the coliform component of the infection, although many authorities do not feel that in vitro sensitivity tests are especially useful for the anaerobic component of the infection.[119] The usual treatment is a two-drug regimen with one agent for coliforms (such as an aminoglycoside) and a second agent for anaerobes (such as clindamycin, cefoxitin, or metronidazole). Some of the newer agents, such as imipenem or ticarcillin plus clavulanic acid, have broad activity against both aerobic and anaerobic bacteria involved in intra-abdominal sepsis suggesting that these infections could be treated with a single agent. Numerous comparative clinical trials indicate that multiple regimens are equally effective, with the proviso that the regimen include agents that are likely to be active against both coliforms and anaerobes.[120–124] These studies are difficult to perform and are subject to the following criticisms: most cases involve heterogeneous patient populations in terms of both the host and disease process; the sample size is generally small; surgery often represents the most decisive factor in outcome; the measures used to judge response are often poorly defined or crude, and the reasons for failure are often elusive.[125] Analysis of antibiotic failures in patients with complicated appendiceal infections suggests that contributing factors include the use of regimens with poor activity vs. *B. fragilis* (cefoperazone or cefamandole) or antibiotic-resistant aerobes (especially *P. aeruginosa*).[126] Although treatment directed against *B. fragilis* appears to be important in large clinical trials, analysis of individual cases shows poor correlation between in vitro and in vivo response.[119] Thus the clinician has multiple therapeutic options that appear equally meritorious, with the notation that there are probably subtle differences that have proved elusive to define between drug regimens.

Infections of the Female Genital Tract

Virtually all infections of the female genital tract that are not caused by sexually transmitted pathogens are likely to involve anaerobic bacteria.

The bacteriologic patterns of these infections have undergone considerable redefinition in three periods of study. Early investigators emphasized the role of anaerobic gram-positive cocci, primarily peptostreptococci.[7,87] More recent studies indicate that anaerobic gram-negative bacilli are relatively frequent isolates as well. Workers during the 1970s emphasized the role of *B. fragilis* as well as coliforms, thus drawing analogies with bacteriologic patterns noted in intra-abdominal sepsis.[84–86] These infections were presumably derived from the normal genital tract flora, and a curious discrepancy was the fact that *B. fragilis* is recovered in less than 10 percent of vaginal or cervical cultures. More recent work suggests that *B. fragilis* was probably erroneously identified in these earlier studies, and the true identity of this organism was probably *Bacteroides bivius* and other *Bacteroides* species.[88,89] *Bacteroides bivius* has a sensitivity profile somewhat similar to that of *B. fragilis*, so that the conclusions regarding therapy according to the prior studies were not dramatically altered.

Infections included in this category include a rather diverse group such as Bartholin's gland abscess, adnexal abscess, tubo-ovarian abscess, pyometra, endometritis, pelvic cellulitis, salpingitis, pelvic thrombophlebitis, amnionitis, and wound infections following gynecologic surgery or obstetrical procedures. These infections tend to show the previously noted clinical clues, indicating probable presence of anaerobes such as putrid discharge, gas in soft tissue, and Gram stains showing a polymicrobial flora. Particular problems may be encountered in obtaining appropriate material for valid anaerobic cultures. This has led to the development of specialized techniques such as laparoscopy, culdecentesis or the use of quantitative cultures with telescoping catheters for transcervical sampling of the endometrium.[89,90]

Pelvic inflammatory disease (PID) deserves special comment due to its prevalence, morbidity, and rapidly evolving studies of microbiology. Recent reports utilizing culdocentesis or laparoscopy with fallopian tube sampling implicate a combination of anaerobic and aerobic bacteria (without *Neisseria gonorrhoeae* or *Chlamydia trachomatis*) in 24–95 percent of cases.[89] The isolation rate of *N. gonorrhoeae* from endocervical specimens in these patients ranged from 39 percent to 94 percent. A study of 74 hospitalized women with acute PID showed that anaerobic bacteria were present in 57 (92 percent) of 62 patients with nongonococcal, nonchlamydial infections.[89] The most common organisms in this series were *B. bivius*, anaerobic cocci, *Gardnerella vaginalis*, group B *Streptococcus*, and *E. coli* (Table 8). These studies suggest that PID is often an anaerobic infection even when endocervical cultures yield common sexually transmitted pathogens such as the gonococcus or *C. trachomatis*.

Another common infection involving the female pelvis is "nonspecific vaginitis" which has more recently been referred to as "bacterial vaginosis" or "anaerobic vaginosis."[126–128] Early studies implicated *G. vaginalis* in the etiology of this disease, but more recent work suggests this may be anaerobic infection. Supporting observations include the characteristic putrid discharge, the excellent response to metronidazole, the increased concentrations of succinic acid in the discharge, and quantitative bacterial cultures. A previously unrecognized anaerobe now classified as a new genus, "*Mobiluncus*", has been implicated on the basis of isolation rates and recognition in direct Gram stain.[127,128] An alternative hypothesis is that this represents "dysbiosis," in which there is a secretory response to the aggregate of bacteria in high concentration due to altered pH and the other usual mechanisms of population control.

Antimicrobial agents used in these infections generally follow

TABLE 8. Bacteria Recovered from 74 Patients with Acute Salpingitis[a]

Bacteriology	*No. of Isolates*
Sexually transmitted pathogens	
Neisseria gonorrhoeae	29 (39%)[b]
Chlamydia trachomatis	17 (24%)
Nongonococcal, nonchlamydial isolates	62 (84%)
Anaerobes	57 patients (77%)
Bacteroides bivius	35
Bacteroides sp. (other)	48
Peptostreptococcus sp.	68
Veillonella	19
Aerobes	55 patients (74%)
Gardnerella vaginalis	30
Escherichia coli	18
Group B streptococci	16
Nonhemolytic streptococci	16
Staphylococcus epidermidis	22

[a] Data based on endometrial or fallopian tube cultures in 74 patients hospitalized with acute salpingitis. Sexually transmitted pathogens were recovered from the endocervix.
[b] There were a total of 434 bacterial isolates (7/patient) including 273 anaerobes (4.4/patient) and 161 aerobes (2.6/patient).
(Modified from Sweet,[89] with permission.)

the guidelines noted for intra-abdominal sepsis. For deep and potentially serious infections, the usual recommendation is for a regimen with activity against coliforms and anaerobic bacteria.[129] The role of the enterococcus is often elusive here, as well as with intra-abdominal sepsis, although therapeutic trials have not supported the need for activity against this organism with empirically selected regimens.[86] As with intra-abdominal sepsis, the aerobic gram-negative bacilli are most likely to include relatively resistant organisms in patients who have nosocomial acquisition of infection or recent antibiotic exposure. Important differences compared with intra-abdominal sepsis with regard to bacteriologic patterns include a reduced frequency of coliforms and a predominance of *B. bivius* in place of the "*B. fragilis* group" in infections of the genital tract. These differences presumably reflect variations in the normal flora that represents the inoculum, and they may account for variations in response rates to various antimicrobial regimens.

Soft Tissue Infections

Infections of the skin and soft tissue that commonly involve anaerobic bacteria include cutaneous abscess, infected sebaceous cysts, breast abscesses, infected pilonidal cysts, bite wound infections, paronychia, hidradenitis suppurativa, wound infections associated with surgical procedures involving mucocutaneous surfaces with large populations of anaerobes, synergistic cellulitis, crepitant cellulitis, necrotizing fasciitis, synergistic necrotizing cellulitis, and gas gangrene.

Staphylococcus aureus is traditionally viewed as the most common pathogen in subcutaneous or cutaneous abscesses. However, there is good evidence that anaerobic bacteria account for a major portion.[93] With cutaneous abscesses above the waist, involvement of anaerobic bacteria are less frequent, the most frequent isolates being *S. aureus* or *Peptostreptococcus*; abscesses below the waist are more likely to involve anaerobic bacteria, and the bacteriology of the lesion often reflects the fecal flora, with high recovery rates of *B. fragilis, B. melaninogenicus*, other *Bacteroides* species, and *Peptostreptococcus* species. Similarly, breast abscesses commonly involve *S. aureus*, although anaerobic bacteria account for a substantial portion, and this especially applies to those that are recurrent and subareolar.[97] As expected, pilonidal cyst infections virtually always contain anaerobic bacteria.[96]

Infections associated with bites by humans or animals tend to involve the oral flora of the biter or the skin flora of the recipient.[100] A variation of this theme is the "clinched-fist injury," in which there is a laceration along the knuckles resulting from striking another individual on the teeth. Anaerobic bacteria have been recovered from approximately 50 percent of bite wound injuries, and this applies to dog bites as well as human bites.[100] Other microbiologic considerations in these cases include *Pasteurella multocida* in animal bite infections, *Eikenella corrodens* derived from the normal oral flora, and *S. aureus* derived from the cutaneous flora of the recipient. Another soft tissue infection that involves the oral flora is paronychia. Reported recovery rates for anaerobes range from 30 percent to 75 percent, and are more common in children, presumably due to finger sucking.[99]

Diabetic foot ulcers and decubitus ulcers tend to involve a mixed flora with both anaerobes and coliforms.[94] Perhaps the most convincing studies concern quantitative cultures of deep tissue obtained from amputated extremities.[130] This work shows an average of five microbial species per specimen and quantitative counts of anaerobes that are generally 10–100-fold higher than the counts for aerobes. The dominant anaerobic bacteria in these lesions include the "*B. fragilis* group," other *Bacteroides* species, and *Peptostreptococcus* species. Similar bacteriology findings have been noted with infected decubitus ulcers and diabetic foot ulcers or decubitus ulcer complicated by osteomyelitis or bacteremia.[103]

Deep soft tissue infections involving anaerobic bacteria include necrotizing fasciitis, necrotizing synergistic cellulitis, crepitant cellulitis, and gas gangrene. These are the deep infections involving the fascia causing fasciitis, or within the muscle compartment formed by the enveloping fascia, in which case there is necrosis of the compartment contents. The major pathogens encountered in fasciitis and compartment infections are group A β-hemolytic streptococci, clostridia, and mixtures of aerobic and anaerobic bacteria. The most common is synergistic necrotizing cellulitis, which is a deep soft tissue infection involving both the fascial plane and the muscle compartment.[98] Most of the patients are diabetic and obese, the most frequent sites of involvement are the lower extremities and perianal region, the mortality rate generally ranges from 30 percent to 50 percent (or higher), a characteristic feature is the presence of putrid "dishwater pus" (a thin, grayish discharge), and approximately one-third of patients have an associated bacteremia. There is a relatively high yield of anaerobes in both the "dishwater pus" and blood cultures.[98] Clinical clues in these and other deep soft tissue infections that specifically suggest anaerobic bacteria include putrid discharge, "dishwater pus," and gas in the soft tissue as detected by palpation, x-ray films, or scans. A microbiologically and clinically similar but less common infection is necrotizing fasciitis. The dominant feature here is extension along the fascia with necrosis that may be demonstrated by passing an instrument along the fascial surface. With either fascitis or a compartment infection, the most important facet of treatment is surgery; guidelines for antibiotic regimens for infections involving a mixed aerobic-anaerobic flora are similar to those for intra-abdominal sepsis.

Bacteremia

Anaerobic bacteria account for 5–10 percent of blood culture isolates in patients with clinically significant bacteremia.[101,131,132] This is exclusive of *Propionibacterium*, which almost invariably represents a skin contaminant when recovered from blood cultures. The same applies to some extent to *Clostridium*, since this is often a suspected contaminant as well.[132] Restricting analysis to anaerobes considered clinically significant, most series indicate that the "*B. fragilis* group" accounts for 60–80 percent.[131] A review of the presumed portal of entry for 855 episodes of bacteremia involving anaerobes indicated an intra-abdominal source in 52 percent, the female genital tract in 20 percent, the lower respiratory tract in 6 percent, the upper respiratory tract in 5 percent, and soft tissue infections in 8 percent. Viewed from another vantage point, anaerobic bacteria are commonly found in the majority of patients with bacteremia associated with intra-abdominal sepsis,[91] infections of the female genital tract,[90] decubitus ulcers,[103] and synergistic necrotizing cellulitis.[98] As expected, many of these cases represent polymicrobial bacteremias. The usual clinical features are not particularly distinctive and include fever, chills, and leukocytosis as well as the usual findings at the portal of entry. Hypotension is relatively common, but disseminated intravascular coagulation is rare. The mortality rate is generally reported at 15–35 percent and, as anticipated, is higher when inappropriate antimicrobial agents are used.[133]

TREATMENT

Recommendations for treatment vary according to the clinical presentation, site of infection, and bacteria involved. Drainage of abscesses and debridement of necrotic tissue often represents the most important component of treatment. The expectations of antibiotic therapy show the anticipated differences based on in vitro sensitivity tests, but one of the more important variables that is commonly overlooked concerns time of initiation of treatment with respect to the temporal evolution of the infection. Thus, treatment may be divided into three periods: pretreatment (prophylaxis), treatment in the inflammatory phase ("critical interval"), and treatment in the abscess stage.[134] With prophylaxis, multiple antimicrobial regimens appear to be equally meritorious, including drugs that cannot be recommended for established infections involving anaerobes. An example is the oral administration of neomycin and erythromycin as a bowel prep for patients undergoing elective colon surgery, or the use of ampicillin or cefazolin in gynecologic surgery.[135] A common feature of anaerobic infections is the propensity for abscess formation. Studies in animal models of anaerobic infection indicate that treatment is most effective when delivered early in the course of the inflammatory response; once an abscess has formed, most antibiotics penetrate into it well, but they appear to have little impact on the quantitative counts of bacteria within the abscess.[136] This apparent paradox of bacterial survival in a hostile environment remains unexplained, but may be related to the relatively high concentrations of organisms, lack of bactericidal activity of most antimicrobial agents, or environmental conditions within the abscess that are obviously far different than those used for in vitro susceptibility testing. The clinical experience tends to corroborate these findings in that surgical drainage generally represents a critical determinant in the successful treatment of abscesses. Despite this commonly quoted experience, there are clear exceptions in which abscesses involving anaerobic bacteria resolve with antimicrobial treatment; examples include tubo-ovarian abscesses, liver abscesses, and cerebral abscesses.

With regard to antimicrobial selection, a unique feature of anaerobic infections is that the decision is usually empiric, without the benefit of in vitro susceptibility test results. The reason is the impracticality of meaningful testing and the difficulty in interpreting test results. Most of these infections involve multiple bacteria at the infected site, commonly four to six microbial species or more. This requires considerable time in the microbiology laboratory for separation and identification, many of these organisms are fastidious so that extended incubation periods are required, and there is no good consensus regarding methodology or interpretation of results.[119] For the clinician, the result is that the information is often not available until long after important therapeutic decisions have been required. In addition, there is the virtually impossible job of separating pathogens, symbionts, and commensals in polymicrobial infections, the therapeutic implication being an inherent indecision concerning which microbes require specific treatment.

As a result of the observations noted above, the National Committee for Clinical Laborartory Standards Working Group on Anaerobic Susceptibility Testing[119] has recommended susceptibility testing of anaerobes should not be performed routinely on clinical isolates, but should be restricted to four purposes: (*1*) to determine activity of new antimicrobial agents; (*2*) to monitor susceptibility patterns at various geographic areas to determine changing sensitivity profiles to commonly used agents; (*3*) to monitor sensitivity patterns in local hospitals as a reflection of the influence of antimicrobial pressure; and (*4*) to assist in the management of infections in selected patients.[119] Examples of infections in which routine in vitro susceptibility testing of anaerobic isolates is advocated include cerebral abscess, endocarditis, infections of the bone and joints, infection of prosthetic devices, and refractory or recurrent bacteremia.[119]

Numerous empirically selected regimens are commonly advocated for anaerobic infections that appear to be equally meritorious according to clinical trials, with the major variation being the site of infection. In the past, the common adage was

TABLE 9. In Vitro Activity of Antimicrobial Agents vs. Anaerobes

Agents	*Comments*
Nearly always active	
Metronidazole	Inactive vs. *Proprionibacterium* and *Actinomyces* sp. in vitro; bactericidal vs. most strains
Chloramphenicol	Good activity vs. virtually all clinically significant anaerobes
Imipenem	Resistant to most *Bacteroides* β-lactamases although a novel β-lactamase that inhibits imipenem was found in 2 of 350 *B. fragilis* strains[143]
β-Lactam plus β-lactamase inhibitor	Only carbapenems (imipenem) and cefamycins (cefoxitin) are resistant to hydrolysis by the β-lactams produced by most *B. fragilis*; the addition of a β-lactamase inhibitor dramatically increases in vitro activity[144]
Usually active	
Clindamycin	*B. fragilis* group: 10–20% of strains resistant; some clostridia other than *C. perfringens* are resistant
Cefoxitin	*B. fragilis* group: 10–20% of strains resistant with considerable institutional variation at least partly reflecting usage patterns[138]; poor activity vs. clostridia
Antipseudomonad penicillins	Relatively resistant to β-lactamases of *Bacteroides* sp. and high doses usually employed
Variable activity	
Penicillin	Inactive vs. penicillinase-producing anaerobes; all "*B. fragilis* group" and many strains of *B. melaninogenicus* group, *B. disiens*, *B. bivius*, and some clostridia[139,142]
Cephalosporins (other than cefotetan, cefoxitin, and moxalactam)	Reduced in vitro activity compared with penicillin G vs. most anaerobes and limited published clinical experience to document efficacy
Tetracycline	Inactive vs. many anaerobes and most strains of *B. fragilis*; doxycycline and minocycline are somewhat more active than tetracyclines
Vancomycin	Active against gram-positive anaerobes and inactive vs. gram-negative anaerobes
Erythromycin	Inactive vs. most *Fusobacterium* and many *B. fragilis*
Poor activity	
Aminoglycosides	
Quinolones	
Monobactams	

that infections above the diaphram infrequently involved *B. fragilis*, so that penicillins were commonly regarded as the drug of choice; by contrast, subdiaphragmatic infections were likely to involve *B. fragilis*, making treatment directed against this agent a requirement in the selection of drugs. Recommendations for antimicrobial agents that evolved in the late 1960s and 1970s for anaerobic infections included the use of penicillin for infections above the diaphram and clindamycin, metronidazole, chloramphenicol, or cefoxitin for subdiaphragmatic infections. These drugs emerged as the preferred agents on the basis of in vitro sensitivity tests as well as clinical trials. Subsequently, the issue of drug selection has become complicated by the recognition of increasing resistance, geographic variation in resistant profiles that may reflect drug utilization patterns within hospitals, and a plethora of new drugs.[119,136–139] With infections above the diaphram, the only infection in which *B. fragilis* appears to be a frequent isolate is otogenic cerebral abscess. However, penicilllin-resistant organisms, usually other *Bacteroides* species, are encountered is up to 15–25 percent of infections of the lower respiratory tract.[110,112,111] The result is that alternatives to penicillin are commonly advocated for serious or refractory infections involving anaerobic bacteria at these anatomic sites. With regard to the newer agents, cephalosporins other than cefoxitin play an ill-defined role in anaerobic infections due to vagaries with in vitro sensitivity testing in different laboratories and variable results in comparative clinical trials.

Recommendations for empiric drug selection are made on the basis of in vitro sensitivity tests, studies in animal models, and clinical trials (Table 9).[18,112,119,138–146] Drugs classified as virtually always active include metronidazole, chloramphenicol, imipenem, and the combinations of a β-lactam agent combined with a β-lactamase inhibitor.[119] In vitro resistance of anaerobes to these drugs is sufficiently unusual to be the subject of anecdotal case reports.[143] Other drugs, such as clindamycin or cefoxitin, are less consistently active in vitro against clinically significant anaerobes, but their use is commonly recommended on the basis of an extensive track record with consistently good results. The evolving clinical experience suggests that a single agent may be adequate for polymicrobial infections and that this approach will supplant the traditional dual drug regimens that include an aminoglycoside.[147]

REFERENCES

1. Finegold SM. Anaerobic Bacteria in Human Disease. New York: Academic Press; 1977.
2. Loesche WJ. Oxygen sensitivity of various anaerobic bacteria. Appl Microbiol. 1969;18:723.
3. Tally FP, Steward PR, Sutter VL, et al. Oxygen tolerance of fresh clinical anaerobic bacteria. J Clin Microbiol. 1975;1:161.
4. Onderdonk AB, Johnston J, Mayhew JW, et al. Effect of dissolved oxygen and Eh on *Bacteroides fragilis* during continuous culture. Appl Environ Microbiol. 1976;31:168.
5. Tally FO, Goldin BR, Jacobus NV, et al. Superoxide dismutase in anaerobic bacteria of clinical significance. Infect Immun. 1977;16:20.
6. Veillon A, Zuber A. Sur quelques microbes strictment anaerobies et leur role dans la pathologie humaine. CR Soc Biol (Paris). 1897;49:253.
7. Schottmueller H. Allgemeinen Krankenhaus Hamburg-Eppendorf. Mitt Grenzt Med Chirg. 1910;21:450.
8. Smith DT. Fusospirochetal disease of the lungs, its bacteriology, pathology and experimental reproduction. Am Rev Tuberc. 1927;16:584.
9. Smith DT. Fusospirochetal disease of the lungs, produced with cultures from Vincent's angina. J Infect Dis. 1930;46:303.
10. Altemeier WA. Bacterial flora of acute perforated appendicitis with peritonitis: bacteriologic study based upon 100 cases. Ann Surg. 1938;107:517.
11. Altemeir WA. The cause of the putrid odor of perforated appendicitis with peritonitis. Ann Surg. 1938;107:634.
12. Martin WJ. Isolation and identification of anaerobic bacteria in the clinical laboratory. Mayo Clin Proc. 1974;49:300.
13. Tedesco FJ, Barton RW, Alpers DH. Clindamycin-associated colitis. Ann Intern Med. 1974;81:429.
14. Stone HH, Kolb LD, Geheber CE, et al. Use of aminoglycosides in surgical infections. Ann Surg. 1976;183:660.
15. Gorbach SL, Thadepalli H. Clindamycin in pure and mixed anaerobic infections. Arch Intern Med. 1974;134:87.
16. Wilson WR, Martin WJ, Wilkowske CJ, et al. Anaerobic bacteremia. Mayo Clin Proc. 1972;47:639.
17. Onderdonk AB, Kasper DL, Cisneros RL, et al. The capsular polysaccharide of *Bacteroides fragilis* as a virulence factor: comparison of a pathogenic potential of encapsulated and unencapsulated strains. J Infect Dis. 1977;136:82.
18. Bartlett JG, Onderdonk AB, Louie T, et al. A review: lessons from an animal model of intra-abdominal sepsis. Arch Surg. 1978;113:853.
19. Thadepalli H, Gorbach SL, Broido PW, et al. Abdominal trauma, anaerobes and antibiotics. Surg Gynecol Obstet. 1973;137:270.
20. diZerega GS, Yonekura ML, Roy S, et al. A comparison of clindamycin-gentamicin and penicillin-gentamicin in the treatment of postcesarean endomyometritis. Am J Obstet Gynecol. 1979;134:238.
21. Sutter VL. Anaerobes as normal oral flora. Rev Infect Dis. 1984;6(Suppl 1):S62.
22. Broido PW, Gorbach SL, Condon RE, et al. Upper intestinal microflora control. Arch Surg. 1973;106:90.
23. Finegold SM, Attebery HR, Sutter VL. Effect of diet on human fecal flora. Am J Clin Nutr. 1974;27:1456.
24. Moore WEC, Holdeman LV. Human fecal flora: the normal flora of 20 Japanese-Hawaiians. Appl Microbiol. 1974;27:961.
25. Mackowiak PA. The normal microbial flora. N Engl J Med. 1982;307:83.
26. Bartlett JG, Polk BF. Bacterial flora of the vagina: Quantitative study. Rev Infect Dis. 1984;6(Suppl 1):S67.
27. Sautter RL, Brown WJ. Sequential vaginal cultures from normal young women. J Clin Microbiol. 1980;11:479.
28. Hammerschlag MR, Alpert S, Rosner I, et al. Microbiology of the vagina in children: normal and potentially pathogenic organisms. Pediatrics. 1978;62:57.
29. Goplerud CP, Ohm MJ, Galask RP: Aerobic and anaerobic flora of the cervix during pregnancy and the puerperium. Am J Obstet Gynecol. 1976;126:858.
30. Ohm MJ, Galask RP. Bacterial flora of the cervix from 100 prehysterectomy patients. Am J Obstet Gynecol. 1975;122:683.
31. Ohm MJ, Galask RP. The effect of antibiotic prohylaxis on patients undergoing vaginal operations. Am J Obstet Gynecol. 1975;123:597.
32. Nielsen ML, Raahave D, Stage JG, et al. Anaerobic and aerobic skin bacteria before and after skin-disinfection with chlorhexidine: an experimental study in volunteers. J Clin Pathol. 1975;28:793.
33. Zaleznik DF, Kasper DL. The role of anaerobic bacteria in abscess formation. Annu Rev Med. 1982;33:217.
34. Simon GL, Klempner MS, Kasper DL, et al. Alterations in opsonophagocytic killing by neutrophils of *Bacteroides fragilis* associated with animal and laboratory passage: effect of capsular polysaccharide. J Infect Dis. 1982;145:72.
35. Onderdonk AB, Markham RB, Zaleznik DF, et al. Evidence of T cell-dependent immunity to *Bacteroides fragilis* in an intraabdominal abscess model. J Clin Invest. 1982;69:9.
36. Zaleznik DF, Finberg RW, Shapiro ME, et al. A soluble suppressor T cell factor protects against experimental intraabdominal absceses. J Clin Invest. 1985;75:1023.
37. Zaleznik DF, Zhang Z, Onderdonk AB, et al. Effect of subinhibitory doses of clindamycin on the virulence of *Bacteroides fragilis*: role of lipopolysaccharide. J Infect Dis. 1986;154:40.
38. Rotstein OD, Nasmith PE, Grinstein S. The *Bacteroides* by-product succinic acid inhibits neutrophil respiratory burst by reducing intracellular pH. Infect Immun. 1987;55:864.
39. Ingham HR, Sisson PR, Tharagonnet D, et al. Inhibition of phagocytosis in vitro by obligate anaerobes. Lancet. 1977;2:1252.
40. Ingham HR, Sisson PR, Middleton RL, et al. Phagocytosis and killing of bacteria in aerobic and anaerobic conditions. J Med Microbiol. 1981;14:391.
41. Bjornson AB, Bjornson HS, Ashraf M, et al. Quantitative variability in requirements for opsonization of strains within the *Bacteroides fragilis* group. J Infect Dis. 1983;148:667.
42. Joiner KA, Hawiger A, Gelfand JA. Activation of the alternative complement pathway by blood culture isolates of *Bacteroides fragilis*. Infect Immun. 1981;34:303.
43. Hofstad T. Pathogenicity of anaerobic gram-negative rods: possible mechanisms. Rev Infect Dis. 1984;6:189.
44. Bjornson HS, Hill EO. Bacteroidaceae in thromboembolic disease: effect of cell wall components on blood coagulation in vivo and in vitro. Infect Immun. 1973;8:911.
45. Mansheim BJ, Solstad CA, Kasper DL. Identification of a subspecies-specific capsular antigen from *Bacteroides melaninogenicus* subspecies *asaccharolyticus* by immunofluorescence and electron microscopy. J Infect Dis. 1978;138:736.
46. Mansheim BJ, Onderdonk AB, Kasper DL. Immunochemical and biologic studies of the lipopolysaccharide of *Bacteroides melaninogenicus* subspecies *asaccharolyticus*. J Immunol. 1978;120:72.
47. Fujimura S, Nakamura T. Isolation and characterization of proteases from *Bacteroides melaninogenicus*. Infect Immun. 1981;33:738.
48. Onderdonk AB, Moon NE, Kasper DL, et al. Adherence of *Bacteroides fragilis in vivo*. Infect Immun. 1978;19:1083.
49. Hofstad T, Kalvenes MB. Adhesion of anerobic gram-negative bacteria to mucosal surfaces. Scand J Infect Dis. 1985;46:33.
50. Tally FO, Goldin BR, Jacobus NV, et al. Superoxide dismutase in anaerobic bacteria of clinical significance. Infect Immun. 1977;16:20.
51. Weinstein WM, Onderdonk AB, Bartlett JG. Experimental intra-abdominal abscess in rats: development of an experimental model. Infect Immun. 1974;10:1250.

52. Weinstein WM, Onderdonk AB, Bartlett JG. Antimicrobial therapy of experimental intraabdominal sepsis. J Infect Dis. 1975;132:282.
53. Onderdonk AB, Bartlett JB, Louie T, et al. Microbial synergy in experimental intra-abdominal abscess. Infect Immun. 1976;13:22.
54. Meleney FL. Clinical aspects and treatment of surgical infections. Philadelphia: WB Saunders; 1949.
55. Mergenhagen SE, Thonard JC, Scherp HW. Studies on synergistic infections. I. Experimental infections with anaerobic streptococci. J Infect Dis. 1958;103:33.
56. MacDonald JB, Socransky SS, Gibbons RJ. Aspects of the pathogenesis of mixed anaerobic infections of mucous membranes. J Dent Res. 1963;42:529.
57. MacDonald JB, Sutton RM, Knoll ML. The production of fusospirochetal infections in guinea pigs with recombined pure cultures. J Infect Dis. 1954;95:275.
58. Altemeier WA. The pathogenicity of the bacteria of appendicitis peritonitis. Surgery. 1942;11:374.
59. Gorbach SL, Mayhew JW, Bartlett JG, et al. Rapid diagnosis of anaerobic infections by direct gas-liquid chromatography of clinical specimens. J Clin Invest. 1976;57:478.
60. Spiegel CA, Malangoni MA, Condon RE. Gas-liquid chromatography for rapid diagnosis of intra-abdominal infection. Arch Surg. 1984;119:28.
61. VanBeek A, Zook E, Yaw P, et al. Nonclostridial gas-forming infections. Arch Surg. 1974;108:552.
62. Bartlett JG, Sullivan-Sigler N, Louie TJ, et al. Anaerobes survive in clinical specimens despite delayed processing. J Clin Microbiol. 1976;3:133.
63. Citron DM. Specimen collection and transport, anaerobic culture techniques and identification of anaerobes. Rev Infect Dis. 1984;6:S51.
64. Heineman HS, Braude AL. Anaerobic infection of the brain: observations on eighteen consecutive cases of brain abscess. Am J Med. 1963;35:682.
65. Frederick J, Braude AL. Anaerobic infection of the paranasal sinusitis. N Engl J Med. 1974;290:135.
66. Brook I. The role of anaerobic bacteria in otitis media: microbiology, pathogenesis, and implications on therapy. Am J Otolaryngol. 1987;8:109.
67. Bartlett JG, O'Keefe P. The bacteriology of perimandibular space infections. J Oral Surg. 1979;37:407.
68. Chow AW, Roser SM, Brady FA. Orofacial odontogenic infections. Ann Intern Med. 1978;88:392.
69. Flodstrom A, Hallander HO. Microbiological aspects on peritonsillar abscesses. Scand J Infect Dis. 1976;8:157.
70. Williams BL, McCann GF, Schoenknecht FD. Bacteriology of dental abscesses of endodontic origin. J Clin Microbiol. 1983;18:770.
71. Bartlett JG, Finegold SM. Anaerobic infections of the lung and pleural space. Am Rev Respir Dis. 1974;110:56.
72. Lorber B, Swenson RM. Bacteriology of aspiration pneumonia. A prospective study of community and hospital acquired cases. Ann Intern Med. 1974;81:329.
73. Bartlett JG, Gorbach SL, Tally FP, et al. Bacteriology and treatment of primary lung abscess. Am Rev Respir Dis. 1974;109:510.
74. Beerens H, Tahon-Castel M. Infections Humaines à Bacteries Anaerobies nontoxigenes. Bruxelles: Presses Academiques Europeenes; 1965:91–114.
75. Bartlett JG, Gorbach SL, Thadepalli H, et al. The bacteriology of empyema. Lancet. 1974;1:338.
76. Ries K, Levison ME, Kaye D. Transtracheal aspiration in pulmonary infection. Arch Intern Med. 1974;133:453.
77. Pollack HM, Hawkins EL, Bonner JR, et al. Diagnosis of bacterial pulmonary infections and quantitative protected catheter cultures obtained during bronchoscopy. J Clin Microbiol. 1983;17:255.
78. Bartlett JG, O'Keere P, Tally FP, et al. The bacteriology of hospital-acquired pneumonia. Arch Intern Med. 1986;146:868.
79. Stone HH, Strom PR, Fabian TC, et al. Third-generation cephalosporins for polymicrobial surgical sepsis. Arch Surg. 1983;118:193.
80. Gorbach SL. Management of anaerobic infections: intra-abdominal sepsis. Ann Intern Med. 1975;83:377.
81. Swenson RM, Lorber B, Michaelson TC, et al. The bacteriology of intra-abdominal infections. Arch Surg. 1974;109:398.
82. Moore WEC, Cato EP, Holdeman LV. Anaerobic bacteria of the gastrointestinal flora and their occurrence of clinical infections. J Infect Dis. 1969;119:641.
83. Sabbaj J, Sutter VL, Finegold SM. Anaerobic pyogenic liver abscess. Ann Intern Med. 1972;77:629.
84. Thadepalli H, Gorbach SL, Keith L. Anaerobic infections of the female genital tract: bacteriologic and therapeutic aspects. Am J Obstet Gynecol. 1973;117:1034.
85. Swenson RM, Michaelson TC, Daly MJ, et al. Anaerobic bacterial infections of the female genital tract. Obstet Gynecol. 1973;42:538.
86. Ledger WJ, Gee CL, Pollin P, et al. The use of prereduced media and a portable jar for the collection of anaerobic organisms from clinical sites of infection. Am J Obstet Gynecol. 1976;125:677.
87. Altemeier WA. The anaerobic streptococci in tubo-ovarian abscess. Am J Obstet Gynecol. 1940;39:1038.
88. Eschenbach DA, Buchanan TM, Pollock HM. Polymicrobial etiology of acute pelvic inflammatory disease. N Engl J Med. 1975;193:166.
89. Sweet RL. Pelvic inflammatory disease. Sex Transm Dis. 1986;13:192.
90. Rosene K, Eschenbach DA, Tompkins LS, et al. Polymicrobial early postpartum endometritis with facultative and anaerobic bacteria, genital mycoplasmas, and *Chlamydia trachomatis*: treatment with piperacillin or cefoxitin. J Infect Dis. 1986;153:1028.
91. Bartlett JG, Condon RE, Gorbach SL, et al. Veterans Administration Cooperative study on bowel preparation for elective colon surgery. Ann Surg. 1978;188:126.
92. Sanderson PJ, Wren MWD, Baldwin AWF. Anaerobic organisms in postoperative wounds. J Clin Pathol. 1979;32:143.
93. Meislin HW, Lerner SA, Graves MH, et al. Cutaneous abscesses. Ann Intern Med. 1977;87:145–9.
94. Louie TJ, Bartlett JG, Tally FP, et al. The microbiology of diabetic foot ulcers. Ann Intern Med. 1976;85:461.
95. MacLennan JD. The histotoxic clostridial infections of man. Bacteriol Rev. 1962;26:232.
96. Pearson HE, Smiley DF. *Bacteroides* in pilonidal sinuses. Am J Surg. 1968;115:336.
97. Brook I. Microbiology of non-puerperal breast abscesses. J Infect Dis. 1988;157:377.
98. Stone HH, Martin JD Jr. Synergistic necrotizing cellulitis. Ann Surg. 1972;175:702.
99. Brook I. Bacteriologic study of paronychia in children. Am J Surg. 1981;141:703.
100. Goldstein EJC, Citron DM, Finegold SM. Role of anaerobic bacteria in bite-wound infections. Rev Infect Dis. 1984;6:S177.
101. Chow AW, Guze LB. Bacteroidaceae bacteremia. Medicine. 1974;53:93.
102. Smith JW, Southern PM Jr, Lehmann JD. Bacteremia in septic abortion: complication and treatment. Obstet Gynecol. 1970;35:404.
103. Bryan CS, Dew CE, Reynolds KL. Bacteremia associated with decubitus ulcers. Arch Intern Med. 1983;143:2093.
104. Ingham HR, Selkon JB, Roxby CM. Bacteriological study of otogenic cerebral abscesses: chemotherapeutic role of metronidazole. Br Med J. 1977;2:991.
105. Boom WH, Tuazon CU. Successful treatment of multiple brain abscesses with antibiotics alone. Rev Infect Dis. 1985;7:189.
106. Zavistoski J, Dzink JA, Onderdonk AB, et al. Quantitative bacteriology of endodontic infections. Oral Surg Oral Med Oral Pathol. 1980;1:46.
107. Lemiere A. On certain septicemias. Lancet. 1936;1:701.
108. Loesche WJ, Syed SA, Laughon BE, et al. The bacteriology of acute necrotizing ulcerative gingivitis. J Periodontol. 1982;53:223.
109. Sutter VL, Jones MJ, Ghoneim ATM. Antimicrobial susceptibilities of bacteria associated with periodontal disease. Antimicrob Agents Chemother. 1983;23:483.
110. Bartlett JG. Anaerobic bacterial infections of the lung. Chest. 1987;91:901.
111. Lansing AM, Jamieson WG. Mechanisms of fever in pulmonary atelectasis. Arch Surg. 1963;87:184–9.
112. Finegold SM, George WL, Mulligan ME. Anaerobic infections. Disease-a-Month. 1985;31:8.
113. Bartlett JG. Treatment of anaerobic pleuropulmonary infections. Ann Intern Med. 1975;83:376–7.
114. Weiss W. Oral antibiotic therapy of acute primary lung abscess: comparison of penicillin and tetracycline. Curr Ther Res. 1970;12:154.
115. Levison ME, Mangura CT, Lorber B, et al. Clindamycin compared with penicillin for the treatment of anaerobic lung abscess. Ann Intern Med. 1983;98:466.
116. Drugs for anaerobic infections. Med Lett. 1984;26:87.
117. Sanders CV, Hanna BJ, Lewis AC. Metronidazole in the treatment of anaerobic infections. Am Rev Respir Dis. 1979;120:337.
118. Dunn DL, Simmons RL. The role of anaerobic bacteria in intraabdominal infections. Rev Infect Dis. 1984;6:S139.
119. Finegold SM, et al. Susceptibility testing of anaerobic bacteria. J Clin Microbiol. 1988;26:1253.
120. Nichols RL, Smith JW, Klein DB, et al. Risk of infection after penetrating abdominal trauma. N Engl J Med. 1984;311:1065.
121. Harding GKM, Buckwold FJ, Ronald AR, et al. Prospective, randomized comparative study of clindamycin, chloramphenicol, and ticarcillin, each in combination with gentamicin, in therapy for intra-abdominal and female genital tract sepsis. J Infect Dis. 1980;142:384.
122. Smith JA, Skidmore AG, Forward AD, et al. Prospective, randomized, double-blind comparison of metronidazole and tobramycin with clindamycin and tobramycin in the treatment of intra-abdominal sepsis. Ann Surg. 1980;192:213.
123. Tally FP, McGowan K, Kellum JM, et al. A randomized comparison of cefoxitin with or without amikacin and clindamycin plus amikacin in surgical sepsis. Ann Surg. 1981;193:318.
124. Heseltine PNR, Yellin AE, Appleman MD, et al. Perforated and gangrenous appendicitis: an analysis of antibiotic failures. J Infect Dis. 1983;148:322.
125. Solomkin JS, Meakins JL, Allo MD, et al. Antibiotic trials in intra-abdominal infections. Ann Surg. 1984;200:29.
126. Spiegel CA, Amsel R, Eschenbach D, et al. Anaerobic bacteria in nonspecific vaginitis. N Engl J Med. 1980;303:601.
127. Spiegel CA, Roberts M. *Mobiluncus* gen. nov., *Mobiluncus curtisii* subsp. *curtisii* sp. nov., *Mobiluncus curtisii* subsp. *holmesii* subsp. nov., and *Mobiluncus mulieris* sp. nov., curved rods from human vagina. Int J Syst Bacteriol. 1984;34:177.
128. Spiegel CA, Eschenbach DA, Amsel R, et al. Curved anaerobic bacteria in bacterial (nonspecific) vaginosis and their response to antimicrobial therapy. J Infect Dis. 1983;148:817.
129. Ledger WJ. Selection of antimicrobial agents for treatment of infections of the female genital tract. Rev Infect Dis. 1983;5:S98.

130. Sapico FL, Canawati HN, Witte JL, et al. Quantitative aerobic and anaerobic bacteriology of infected diabetic feet. J Clin Microbiol. 1980;12:413.
131. Finegold SM, George WL, Mulligan ME. Anaerobic infections. Disease-A-Month. 1988;31:4.
132. Gorbach SL, Thadepalli H: Isolation of *Clostridium* in human infections: Evaluation of 114 cases. J Infect Dis. 1975;131:581.
133. Condon RE. *Bacteroides* bacteremia. Arch Surg. 1984;119:897.
134. Bartlett JG, Dezfulian M, Joiner K. Relative efficacy and critical interval of antimicrobial agents in experimental infections involving *Bacteroides fragilis*. Arch Surg. 1983;118:181.
135. Bartlett JG, Condon RE, Gorbach SL, et al. Impact of oral antibiotic regimen on colonic flora, wound irrigation cultures and bacteriology of septic complications. Ann Surg. 1978;188:249.
136. Joiner KA, Lowe BR, Dzink JL, et al. Antibiotic levels in infected and sterile subcutaneous abscesses in mice. J Infect Dis. 1981;143:487.
137. Ohm-Smith MJ, Sweet RL, Hadley WK. Occurrence of clindamycin-resistant anaerobic bacteria isolated from cultures taken following clindamycin therapy. Antimicrob Agents Chemother. 1986;30:11.
138. Tally FP, Cuchural GJ, Jacobus NV, et al. Susceptibility of the *Bacteroides fragilis* group in the United States in 1981. Antimicrob Agents Chemother. 1983;23:536.
139. Murray PR, Rosenblatt JE. Penicillin resistance and penicillinase production in clinical isolates of *Bacteroides melaninogenicus*. Antimicrob Agents Chemother. 1977;11:605.
140. Bawdon RE, Crane LR, Palchaudhuri S. Antibiotic resistance in anaerobic bacteria: molecular biology and clinical aspects. Rev Infect Dis. 1982;4:1075.
141. Wexler HM, Harris B, Carter WT, et al. Six-year retrospective survey of the resistance of *Bacteroides fragilis* group species to clindamycin and cefoxitin. Diagn Microbiol Infect Dis. 1986;4:247.
142. Edson RS, Rosenblatt JE, Lee DT, et al. Recent experience with antimicrobial susceptibility of anaerobic bacteria. Mayo Clin Proc. 1982;57.737.
143. Cuchural GJ, Malamy MH, Tally FP. β-Lactamase-mediated imipenem resistance in *Bacteroides fragilis*. Antimicrobiol Agents Chemother. 1986;30:645.
144. Wexler HM, Finegold SM. In vitro activity of cefoperazone plus sulbactam compared with that of other antimicrobial agents against anaerobic bacteria. Antimicrob Agents Chemother. 1988;32:403.
145. Wexler HM, Finegold SM. *In vitro* activity of cefotetan compared with that of other antimicrobial agents against anaerobic bacteria. Antimicrob Agents Chemother. 1988;32:601.
146. Gorbach SL, Bartlett JG. Anaerobic infections. N Engl J Med. 1974;290:1177.
147. Malangoni MA, Condon RE, Spiegel CA. Treatment of intra-abdominal infections is appropriate with single-agent or combination antibiotic therapy. Surgery. 1985;98:648.

220. CLOSTRIDIUM TETANI (TETANUS)

THOMAS R. CATE

Tetanus (''lockjaw'') is a disease manifested by uncontrolled muscle spasms resulting from the action of the potent neurotoxin tetanospasmin, which is elaborated by *Clostridium tetani*.[1–3] The disease is frequently fatal, especially at the extremes of life, and is preventable by immunization. It occurs predominantly in developing countries among neonates, children, and young adults, but it is still encountered in the United States, especially in unimmunized or inadequately immunized adults over 50 years of age.[4,5]

HISTORY OF TETANUS

Tetanus has been recognized as a clinical entity for many centuries. Understanding of its pathogenesis began in 1884 when Carle and Rattone produced tetanus in rabbits by injecting a suspension from an acne pustule, the site of infection in a fatal human case. In the same year, Nicolaier produced tetanus by inoculation of various small laboratory animals with soil samples. He recognized the presence of long, thin bacilli and was able to perpetuate the organism in mixed culture. Isolation of the organism in pure culture was accomplished in 1889 by Kitasato, who eliminated non-spore-bearing contaminants by means of heat and produced disease in animals by inoculating the isolate. The preparation of toxoid by Behring and Kitasato in 1890 and the production of antitoxin in various animals over the following few years prepared the way for rapid progress in both understanding the pathogenesis of toxigenic diseases and development of prevention and treatment measures.

DESCRIPTION OF THE PATHOGEN

The organism that causes tetanus, *C. tetani,* is a motile, gram-positive, anaerobic, nonencapsulated rod; it can form spores that are characteristically located at one end and give a drumstick or tennis racket appearance.[6] Vegetative forms of the bacillus can be inactivated by heat and disinfectants and are killed by a number of antibiotics. However, the spores are highly resistant to chemical disinfection and can survive in boiling water for a period of several minutes up to an hour. *C. tetani* can be found in human and animal feces, and the widely distributed spores can survive in dry soil for years.

PATHOGENESIS

Clostridium tetani is a noninvasive opportunist that usually depends upon the introduction of its spores into damaged or devitalized tissue along with foreign bodies and/or other bacteria to provide the anaerobic conditions favorable for its growth. On occasion, spores of the bacillus introduced by a prior injury can survive in tissue for months or years and be activated for vegetative growth when minor trauma alters local conditions.[1] Sufficient replication of the organism to produce tetanus can occur in inapparent sites of infection.

The disease tetanus is due to the potent neurotoxin tetanospasmin, which is produced as a protoplasmic protein by vegetative *C. tetani* in a localized site of infection and released predominantly upon lysis of the bacilli.[7] Production of the toxin appears to be plasmid controlled.[8] Tetanospasmin can bind strongly to neural gangliosides, and its most important site of entry to the nervous system is at myoneural junctions of alpha motor neurons.[1,3,9,10] Once the toxin has translocated into the neuron, it is no longer accessible for neutralization. Tetanospasmin is carried by retrograde axonal transport to the neuroaxis where it migrates transynaptically to other neurons, the most important of which are presynaptic inhibitory cells. The toxin binds to presynaptic inhibitory synapses in the neuroaxis and prevents transmitter release. The absence of this inhibition allows lower motor neurons to increase muscle tone and produce rigidity and permits the simultaneous spasms of both agonist and antagonist muscles that characterize tetanus. Tetanospasmin may also promote spontaneous muscle contraction in the absence of an efferent nerve action potential in severe tetanus.

Among factors that determine the clinical course of tetanus in unimmunized individuals are the quantity of toxin produced and the length of the neural pathways that toxin must traverse to reach the neuroaxis.[10] When the quantity of tetanospasmin is sufficient to spread through lymphatics and the blood stream to myoneural junctions throughout the body, those muscles with the shortest neural pathways and, hence, the shortest transport time to the neuroaxis are affected most quickly. Thus, masticatory, facial, and cervical muscles are usually affected first in generalized tetanus and then progressively more distant muscles in a descending fashion. In this type of generalized tetanus, which is the most frequent form of the disease, the release of larger quantities of toxin from a wound into the blood stream will tend to produce both a quicker onset and a more rapid progression of symptoms as well as more severe disease. When the amount of tetanospasmin produced is small and is transported to the neuroaxis only along regional neural pathways, the onset of muscle rigidity will be delayed proportionately to the length of the neural pathway. Muscle involvement may remain localized to the general area of the wound in the latter situation, or ascending tetanus may result if there is sufficient toxin for spread cranially within the spinal cord.

Although spinal inhibitory neurons are most sensitive to the action of tetanospasmin, the toxin can also inhibit acetylcholine release at neuromuscular junctions; such action may explain the facial paralysis that can occur in *cephalic tetanus* (see below). Markedly elevated catecholamine plasma levels and excretion can occur during generalized tetanus and may be due to a loss of inhibition by the intermediolateral cell column of the spinal cord.[3] Other autonomic nervous system functions may also be affected by tetanospasmin. Direct intracerebral injection of tetanospasmin can produce seizures, but the relevance of this finding to human disease is uncertain[3]; the muscle spasms of tetanus are mediated at spinal rather than supraspinal levels of the central nervous system, and the patients can remain fully conscious in the absence of sedatives or dysfunction caused by hypoxia or metabolic derangements. Damage caused by tetanospasmin to the neuromuscular junction, and presumably other synapses, appears to be permanent and require sprouting of new synapses for recovery.

EPIDEMIOLOGY

Clostridium tetani spores are ubiquitous, and essentially any wound or closed, infected area can serve as a nidus for the disease. The incidence of tetanus in any given population varies inversely with the proportion of individuals who have received effective immunization. Tetanus is a major problem in developing countries where compulsory immunization of children is not enforced or required.[4,11] It is often among the 10 most frequent causes of death in such countries, and the number of cases per year worldwide has been estimated at 1 million. Tetanus in developing countries commonly occurs secondary to wounds in school-age boys but also neonatally due to contamination of the umbilical stump, in children from chronic ear infections, postpartum after inexpert attempts to remove a retained placenta, and after procedures such as nonsterile injections, unskilled abortions, earpiercing, scarification rituals, and female circumcision.

In the United States, the incidence of tetanus has stabilized at between 0.03 and 0.04 cases per 100,000 since 1976[5,12] (Fig. 1). Most of the 147 patients reported in the 1985–86 biennium had acute wounds (99, 71 percent) as the source. Chronic wounds or underlying medical conditions such as skin ulcers, abscesses, or gangrene were responsible for most of the remainder (29, 21 percent). Among the latter were three patients (2 percent) with a history of parenteral drug abuse, as has been described previously.[13] Twelve patients (8 percent) had no recognized tetanus-prone wound, and there were no cases of neonatal tetanus. In addition to a much lower overall incidence of tetanus than in developing countries, the United States has also had a markedly different age distribution of cases in recent years (Fig. 2). The disease in the United States occurs predominantly in older adults who are either unimmunized or inadequately immunized.

CLINICAL MANIFESTATIONS

The incubation period of tetanus, the time between an injury and the occurence of first symptoms, is typically within 2 weeks but may range from 2 days to months.[1,10] Shorter incubation periods, particularly those less than a week, tend to be associated with more severe disease. A minority of patients will have no recent injury or apparent site of infection, and this absence should never rule out a diagnosis of tetanus. Among possible explanations is survival of spores for months or years in a site of prior injury and their activation by minor trauma.

Initial symptoms of tetanus may include such complaints as localized or generalized weakness, stiffness or cramping, or difficulty chewing and swallowing food. An early sign is often trismus due to the increase in masseter muscle tone, which gives rise to the complaint of "lockjaw." Increasing muscle rigidity ensues in the generalized disease and progressively involves more muscle groups in a descending or ascending fashion (see above). Reflex spasms usually occur within 1–4 days after the initial symptoms. The interval between initial symptoms and the occurrence of reflex spasms is referred to as the onset period. As with the incubation period, shorter onset periods, particularly those less than 48 hours, tend to be associated with more severe disease.

In generalized tetanus, tonic contractions of various muscle groups may produce findings such as painful opisthotonos, abdominal rigidity, and the characteristic facial expression called risus sardonicus. Laryngospasm and/or involvement of respiratory muscles may prevent adequate ventilation. Difficulty in

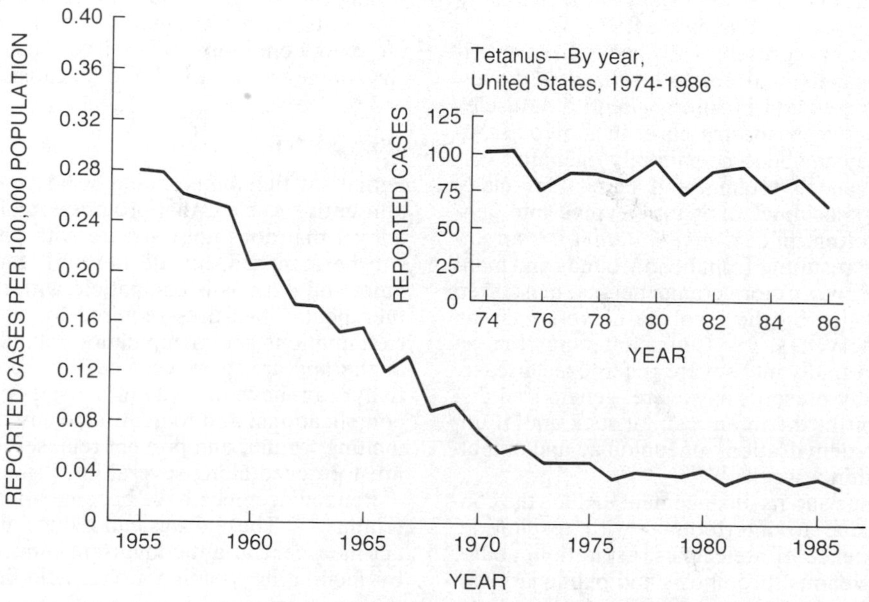

FIG. 1. Tetanus by year, United States, 1955–1986. (From Centers for Disease Control,[12] with permission.)

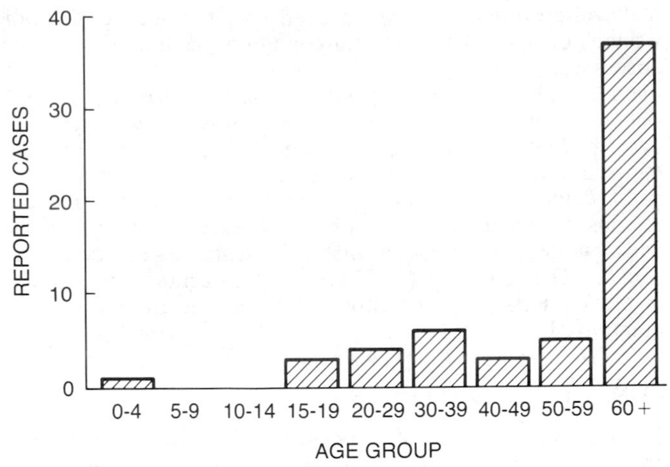

FIG. 2. Tetanus by age group, United States, 1986. (From Centers for Disease Control,[12] with permission.)

swallowing may lead to aspiration. Reflex tetanic spasms lasting several seconds to a few minutes may be precipitated by stimuli such as noise, light, or touch. These sudden spasms of increased muscle contraction cause opisthotonos, flexion, and adduction of the arms with clenched fists over the lower part of the chest and extension of the legs. They are both intensely painful for the fully conscious patient and dangerous; apnea leading to a loss of consciousness, fractures, tendon separations, and rhabdomyolysis may occur.

With neuromuscular blockade, mechanical ventilation, and antibiotics to prevent some of the complications of generalized tetanus, the associated autonomic dysfunction has become a more prominent problem. Its manifestations include "sustained but labile hypertension and tachycardia, irregularities of cardiac rhythm, peripheral vascular constriction, profuse sweating, pyrexia, increased carbon-dioxide output, increased urinary catecholamine excretion, and, in some cases, the late development of hypotension."[14] Otherwise unexplained cardiac arrest presumed to be due to excessive catecholamine output has become one of the major causes of death in severe, generalized tetanus, and the myocarditis observed in such patients resembles that seen in patients with pheochromocytomas.[15] Excessive catecholamine output may also contribute to the markedly negative nitrogen balance seen in this disease.[16]

Most patients with tetanus present with generalized manifestations, but muscle spasms can remain localized to the anatomic area of the inciting wound in some patients.[2,3] Muscles may relax completely between spasms early in the course of *localized tetanus,* but they can become painfully rigid after voluntary movements. Localized tetanus can persist for many weeks before gradually subsiding, or it may evolve into generalized tetanus that is often mild. *Cephalic tetanus* is an unusual form of the disease resulting from head wounds and manifested by dysfunction of one or more cranial nerves, most often VII; musculature innervated by the involved nerve(s) may be paretic until a spasm intervenes.[2,3,17] Cephalic tetanus can remain localized or evolve rapidly into severe generalized disease. *Neonatal tetanus* typically presents as severe, generalized disease within 12 days of birth; the infant cannot suck and, if untreated, usually dies of dehydration, pneumonia, and/or pulmonary hemorrhage within a week.[11,18]

Complications of tetanus and its management include the consequences of hypoxia due to interference with respiration; pneumonia as a consequence of atelectasis, aspiration, and/or mechanical ventilation; venous thrombosis and pulmonary embolus; cardiac arrhythmias, hypertension, and hypotension due to autonomic instability, myocarditis, and/or intravascular volume depletion; fractures of the spine or long bones; infections related to the original wound, decubitus ulcers, and various indwelling catheters (intravascular and bladder); and acute peptic ulcer.[3,14,16,19,20] Mortality varies with the severity of the disease, the age of the patient, and the availability of appropriate medical support. In a series of 82 patients reported from England in 1968,[14] mild tetanus consisting of increased muscle tone and trismus but no major spasms or dysphagia caused no deaths; moderate tetanus with infrequent (less than 12 per 24 hours), mild, short spasms was associated with a case fatality rate of 9 percent, and severe tetanus with more frequent and severe spasms sufficient to interfere with swallowing and ventilation had a case fatality rate of 44 percent. Tetanus tends to be more severe when it occurs at either extreme of life.[21,22] The case fatality rate for neonatal tetanus is about 75 percent.[18,22] Case fatality rates during 1985–86 in the United States were only 5 percent for children and adults less than 50 years old but rose to 42 percent for patients 50 years of age or older.[5] The availability of modern intensive care units has been associated with significant reductions in deaths due to tetanus.[15]

The course of tetanus for patients who survive can be long (1–2 months) and arduous. Spasms may begin to decrease after 10–14 days and disappear after another week or two. Residual weakness, stiffness, and other complaints may persist for a prolonged period,[20,23] but complete recovery can occur from uncomplicated tetanus.

DIAGNOSIS

The diagnosis of tetanus is based primarily on the history and clinical presentation. Only a minority of patients will have sporulated forms of *C. tetani* recognized in Gram stains from a wound or the organism recovered in anaerobic cultures.[1] Moreover, recovery of the organism does not prove a diagnosis of tetanus since it can be part of the flora. A definite history of immunization and/or a serum antitoxin level of 0.01 units/ml or higher makes the diagnosis very unlikely. The differential diagnosis of tetanus includes a number of medical conditions that can simulate one or more of the clinical findings.[3,19,20] Included are such things as meningitis (nuchal rigidity), dental abscess (trismus), peritonitis (abdominal rigidity), rabies (dysphagia), hypocalcemic tetany, epilepsy, decerebrate posturing, and narcotic withdrawal. Dystonic reactions to antipsychotic drugs can be differentiated by a history of ingestion and alleviation of symptoms by benztropine or diphenhydramine. Strychnine poisoning can mimic tetanus in increasing neuronal excitability by interfering with postsynaptic inhibition; emergent treatment of the two conditions is similar, and biochemical studies for strychnine can establish the diagnosis.

TREATMENT

Patients with tetanus should be hospitalized in an intensive care unit until it is clear that progression of disease has stabilized at a level that does not interfere with vital functions and therapy can be managed outside the unit. Surroundings should be as quiet and dark as is compatible with the close observation and therapeutic measures required for management. Unnecessary examinations and manipulations should be avoided. Objectives of therapy are to prevent death, especially from asphyxia initially; to relieve the patient's distress; to minimize and manage complications; and to neutralize any accessible toxin, treat the inciting wound, and prevent relapses and recurrences. Therapy must proceed along several lines simultaneously.

Benzodiazepines have become a mainstay in the therapy for tetanus.[3,24] These drugs can reduce anxiety, produce sedation, act as a central anticonvulsant, and induce muscle relaxation by facilitating γ-aminobutyric acid–inhibitory transmission in the brain stem and spinal cord. Diazepam has been used most frequently, with intravenous doses titrated to the response of muscle rigidity, inhibition of spasms, and sedation. While diazepam may provide adequate relaxation in some patients, others will require neuromuscular blockade with an agent such as pancuronium bromide. The peripheral muscle relaxant dantrolene has also been used successfully in managing tetanus spasms, but prolonged administration of high doses has been associated with hepatotoxicity. If the latter agents are employed, it is important to also provide adequate sedation with a benzodiazepine, barbiturate, and/or narcotic analgesic.

Maintenance of effective ventilation is a primary concern in the management of patients with tetanus. Endotracheal intubation is frequently required to protect the airway and should be given consideration as a prophylactic measure. However, intubation and tracheal suctioning are powerful stimuli for reflex spasms, and adequate sedation and control of muscle spasms must be provided. Tracheostomy can reduce this stimulation and should be performed early when it is apparent that airway protection and/or ventilatory support will be required.

Human tetanus immune globulin (TIG) should be administered intramuscularly as soon as possible to neutralize any tetanospasmin that has not gained entry to the nervous system. Evidence suggests that TIG therapy can cause modest reductions in case fatality rates with tetanus and that 500 units is as effective as the larger doses (3000 units or more) often recommended.[25] No advantage has been shown for injection of TIG into the area of the wound. Intrathecal TIG in a dose of 250 units has been reported to be more effective than is 1000 units given intramuscularly,[26] but the intrathecal route is not officially approved as a mode of administration. Equine antiserum also appears effective in the management of generalized tetanus in doses as low as 10,000 units intramuscularly or intravenously,[27] but it has the disadvantages of occasional anaphylaxis and up to a 25 percent incidence of delayed serum sickness. The administration of antibiotics and wound debridement are potentially important for helping to reduce the toxin load, although arguments can be made for delaying these measures until after the administration of antitoxin since they may transiently increase toxin release. Penicillin is the antibiotic most frequently employed, but a recent report suggests that metronidazole may have greater efficacy.[28] The quantity of tetanospasmin required to produce tetanus is insufficient to induce a protective immune response,[19,29] and patients with this disease require a primary immunization series.

Development of tachyarrhythmias, wildly variable blood pressure, and/or unexplained fever often occurs after the first few days of the management of severe, generalized tetanus. A variety of measures have been employed in an attempt to control these manifestations of autonomic instability. Included have been the β-adrenergic blocker propranolol,[30] the combined α- and β-adrenergic blocker labetalol,[31,32] morphine,[16,33] epidural block,[34] and magnesium sulfate infusions.[35] The efficacy of morphine in this syndrome may relate in part to the replacement of endogenous opiates whose release appears to be inhibited by tetanospasmin.[3] Decreased intravascular volume secondary to dehydration can contribute to the vascular instability. Pulmonary artery catheterization for the measurement of wedge pressure and cardiac output may be necessary for optimal management of this difficult syndrome.

Several general therapeutic measures can be important. Pulmonary emboli have been responsible for the death of tetanus patients, and prophylactic heparinization is recommended. Peptic ulceration with bleeding is not uncommon; prophylaxis with sucralfate may offer an advantage over antacids or histamine type 2 blockers in predisposing less to gastric colonization with bacteria and thus to less nosocomial pneumonia.[36] Decubitus ulcers are a common problem, and the patient should be turned every 4 hours. Patients with tetanus can lose large volumes of fluid through diaphoresis, and they become markedly catabolic. Rhabdomyolysis with myoglobinuria and acute renal failure are also possible complications. The fluids, electrolytes and nutrients required to manage these problems should be given intravenously until the patient is stabilized, the risk of aspiration is reduced, and it is clear that there is no bowel dysfunction such as paralytic ileus. Enteral feedings may then be given via nasogastric tube, although it may be necessary to supplement with intravenous hyperalimentation. Close monitoring for the early detection and treatment of complications is imperative.

PREVENTION

Tetanus is a disease that is preventable by antibody to tetanospasmin.[37] Serum antitoxin levels of 0.01 unit/ml or above are considered protective, although tetanus that is usually mild has occasionally been observed in patients with titers in the range of 0.01–1.0 unit/ml.[1,38] As stated earlier, the quantity of toxin required to produce tetanus is insufficient to induce an immune response that will guarantee protection against recurrent disease.[19,29] Nevertheless, unvaccinated individuals in developing countries are sometimes found to have low serum titers of antitoxin, presumably induced by prolonged release of subclinical amounts of toxin in the intestinal tract.[38,39] For practical purposes, however, tetanus should be considered a disease against which there is no naturally acquired immunity and one that is entirely preventable with appropriate immunization and wound care.[37]

Tetanus toxoid, produced by treatment of tetanospasmin with formaldehyde, is a very good immunogen.[40] Vaccine preparations are standardized according to antigenic potency. The toxoid content of standard tetanus vaccines as measured by flocculation can vary but is usually about 10 "Lf" units. Larger doses (up to 250 Lf) may be desirable in developing countries for single-dose vaccination of adults who are unlikely to return for the completion of a three-dose series.[39] Tetanus toxoid is available as a single-antigen vaccine in an aluminum-adsorbed preparation and in nonadsorbed (fluid) form. The rate of seroconversion is essentially equivalent with either type of vaccine, but adsorbed toxoid is preferred because it induces more persistent antitoxin titers. Tetanus toxoid is frequently administered as one of two or three components in an adsorbed vaccine; it is combined with diphtheria toxoid and pertussis vaccine (DPT) for primary immunization of children younger than 7 years old, with full-dose diphtheria toxoid (DT) for children who are younger than 7 years old and have a contraindication for pertussis vaccination, and with reduced-dose diphtheria toxoid (Td) for immunization of older children and adults. Current recommendations for active immunization via intramuscular injections are given in Table 1. Completion of the primary series will confer humoral immunity to tetanus for at least 10 years in 95 percent or more of vaccinees.[1,38,40] Booster vaccinations are recommended every 10 years to ensure the maintenance of protective antitoxin levels. Reactions to tetanus vaccine are generally minor and local, but the administration of more frequent booster vaccinations increases the risk of both local and sys-

TABLE 1. Schedule of Active Immunization against Tetanus

Dose	*Age/Interval*	*Vaccine*
Age less than 7 yr		
Primary 1	Age 6 wk or older	DPT
Primary 2	4–8 wk after the first dose	DPT
Primary 3	4–8 wk after the second dose	DPT
Primary 4	About 1 yr after the third dose	DPT
Booster	4–6 yr of age	DPT
Additional boosters	Every 10 yr after the last dose	Td
Age 7 and older		
Primary 1	First visit	Td
Primary 2	4–6 wk after the first dose	Td
Primary 3	6 mo–1 yr after the second dose	Td
Boosters	Every 10 yr after the last dose	Td

Abbreviations: DPT: diphtheria and tetanus toxoids and pertussis vaccine adsorbed; Td: tetanus and reduced-dose diphtheria toxoids adsorbed (for adult use).

TABLE 2. Guidelines for the Use of Tetanus Toxoid and Human Tetanus Immune Globulin Following a Wound

Prior Vaccinations with Adsorbed Tetanus Toxoid		Clean, Minor Wounds		All Other Wounds	
Total Number	Years Since Last Dose	Td[a]	TIG	Td	TIG
≥3	<5	No	No	No	No
≥3	5–10	No	No	Yes	No
≥3	>10	Yes	No	Yes	No
≤2, unknown	—	Yes	No	Yes	Yes

[a] Children under 7 years old should receive adsorbed diphtheria and tetanus toxoids combined with pertussis vaccine (DPT), or adsorbed diphtheria and tetanus toxoids (DT) if pertussis vaccine is contraindicated.

Abbreviations: Td: adsorbed tetanus and reduced-dose diphtheria toxoids for adult use; TIG: tetanus immune globulin.

temic reactions.[1,38] Tetanus immunization has been highly successful in reducing the incidence of the disease in the United States (Fig. 1), although older adults are a population segment requiring additional attention (Fig. 2).

Appropriate management of patients presenting with wounds is also very important for preventing tetanus.[1,37,38] Cleansing of the wound, drainage of pus, and meticulous debridement of foreign bodies and necrotic tissue can reduce the likelihood that *C. tetani* will be able to proliferate. Antibiotic therapy for contaminated or infected wounds may also reduce the likelihood of tetanus.[38] Recommendations for specific immunoprophylaxis depend on the patient's prior immunization history and the nature of the wound (Table 2).[40,41] If the patient is known to have received a full immunization series with adsorbed vaccine and the last dose was within the preceding 5 years, no specific immunoprophylaxis is required for any type of wound; however, if the immunization series may have been with fluid toxoid, a booster dose of adsorbed toxoid should be given. Patients who have received a full immunization series with the last dose 5–10 years previously and who have clean, minor wounds need no additional immunoprophylaxis, but those with a tetanus-prone wound should be given a tetanus vaccine booster. Tetanus-prone wounds include those contaminated with dirt, feces, or saliva; puncture wounds; avulsions; and wounds resulting from missles, crushing, burns, and frostbite. Patients who received a full immunization series with the last dose being longer than 10 years previously should be given a booster vaccination with (or without) any type of wound. If the patient is uncertain about prior vaccinations or knows that the full tetanus series has not been received, tetanus vaccine should be given for any type of wound (with arrangements made to complete the series), and additional passive immunization with TIG should be given for tetanus-prone wounds. When vaccine and TIG are given concurrently, separate syringes and separate sites of administration should be used. Also, adsorbed tetanus vaccine should be used to minimize interference by the antitoxin with the active immunization. The dose of TIG recommended for prophylaxis of wounds of average severity is 250 units intramuscularly.[40] Increasing the TIG dose to 500 units[41] and administering 250–500 units to remotely (greater than 10 years) vaccinated patients[38] have been recommended when highly tetanus-prone wounds are present. The latter include wounds that contain devitalized tissue that cannot be debrided, those that have been neglected for 24 hours or longer, and those exposed to very high levels of bacterial contamination such as barnyards, sewers, or colon contents. Special circumstances that call for exceptions to the standard guideline should be carefully noted. Every effort should be made to avoid the treatment errors that still occur in prophylaxis against this eminently preventable disease.[41]

REFERENCES

1. Smith JWG. Tetanus. In: Smith GR, ed. Bacterial Diseases, v. 3. Topley and Wilson's Principles of Bacteriology, Virology and Immunity. 7th ed. Baltimore: Williams & Wilkins; 1983:345–68.
2. Weinstein L. Tetanus. N Engl J Med. 1973;289:1293.
3. Bleck TP. Tetanus: Dealing with the continuing clinical challenge. J Crit Illness. 1987;2:41.
4. Dowell VR Jr. Botulism and tetanus: Selected epidemiologic and microbiologic aspects. Rev Infect Dis. 1984;6(Suppl 1):202.
5. Centers for Disease Control. Tetanus—United States, 1985–1986. MMWR. 1987;36:477.
6. Bytchenko B. Microbiology of tetanus. In: Veronesi R, ed. Tetanus: Important New Concepts. Amsterdam: Excerpta Medica; 1981:28–39.
7. Bizzini B. The chemistry of tetanus toxin. In: Veronesi R, ed. Tetanus: Important New Concepts. Amsterdam: Excerpta Medica; 1981:8–27.
8. Laird WJ, Aaronson W, Silver RP, et al. Plasmid-associated toxigenicity in *Clostridium tetani*. J Infect Dis. 1980;142:623.
9. Mellanby J, Green J. How does tetanus toxin act? Neuroscience. 1981;6:281.
10. Kryzhanovsky GN. Pathophysiology. In: Veronesi R, ed. Tetanus: Important New Concepts. Amsterdam: Excerpta Medica; 1981:109–82.
11. Schofield F. Selective primary health care: Strategies for control of disease in the developing world. XXII. Tetanus: A preventable problem. Rev Infect Dis. 1986;8:144.
12. Centers for Disease Control. Summary of notifiable diseases, United States, 1986. MMWR. 1986;35:39.
13. Cherubin CE. Epidemiology of tetanus in narcotic addicts. NY State J Med. 1970;70:267.
14. Kerr JH, Corbett JL, Prys-Roberts C, et al. Involvement of the sympathetic nervous system in tetanus: Studies on 82 cases. Lancet. 1968;2:236.
15. Trujillo MH, Castillo A, Espana J, et al. Impact of intensive care management on the prognosis of tetanus: Analysis of 641 cases. Chest. 1987;92:63.
16. O'Keefe SJD, Wesley A, Jialal I, et al. The metabolic response and problems with nutritional support in acute tetanus. Metabolism. 1984;33:482.
17. Abde VW, Dekate MP. Cephalic tetanus. J Indian Med Assoc. 1980;74(6):111.
18. Salimpour R. Cause of death in tetanus neonatorium: Study of 233 cases with 54 necropsies. Arch Dis Child. 1977;52:587.
19. Brust JCM, Richter RW. Tetanus in the inner city. NY State J Med. 1974;74:1735.
20. Veronesi R, Focaccia R. The clinical picture. In: Veronesi R, ed. Tetanus: Important New Concepts. Amsterdam: Excerpta Medica; 1981:183–206.
21. Garnier MJ, Marshall FN, Davison KJ, et al. Tetanus in Haiti. Lancet. 1975;1:383.
22. LaForce FM, Young LS, Bennett JV. Tetanus in the United States (1965–1966): Epidemiologic and clinical features. N Engl J Med. 1969;280:569.
23. Illis LS, Taylor FM. Neurological and electroencephalographic sequelae of tetanus. Lancet. 1971;1:826.
24. Olsen KM, Hiller FC. Management of tetanus. Clin Pharm. 1987;6:570.
25. Blake PA, Feldman RA, Buchanon TM, et al. Serologic therapy of tetanus in the United States, 1965–1971. JAMA. 1976;235:42.
26. Gupta PS, Kapoor R, Goyal S, et al. Intrathecal human tetanus immunoglobulin in early tetanus. Lancet. 1980;2:439.
27. Vakil BJ, Tulpule TH, Armitage P, et al. A comparison of the value of 200,000 I.U. of tetanus antitoxin (horse) with 10,000 I.U. in the treatment of tetanus. Clin Pharmacol Ther. 1968;9:465.
28. Ahmadsyah I, Salim A. Treatment of tetanus: An open study to compare the efficacy of procaine penicillin and metronidazole. Br Med J. 1985;291:648.
29. Spenny JG, Lamb RN, Cobbs CG. Recurrent tetanus. South Med J. 1971;64:859.
30. Prys-Roberts C, Kerr JH, Corbett JL, et al. Treatment of sympathetic overactivity in tetanus. Lancet. 1969;1:542.
31. Hanna W, Grell GAC. Oral labetalol in the management of the sympathetic overactivity of severe tetanus. South Med J. 1980;73:653.
32. Domenighetti GM, Savary G, Stricker H. Hyperadrenergic syndrome in severe tetanus: Extreme rise in catecholamines responsive to labetalol. Br Med J. 1984;288:1483.
33. Rie MA, Wilson RS. Morphine therapy controls autonomic hyperactivity in tetanus. Ann Intern Med. 1978;88:653.
34. Lindahl SGE, Dahlgren N, Lundberg D, et al. Adrenergic hyperactivity and epidural block in severe tetanus: A case report. Acta Anaesthesiol Scand. 1985;29:87.
35. Lipman J, James MFM, Erskine J, et al. Autonomic dysfunction in severe tetanus: Magnesium sulfate as an adjunct to deep sedation. Crit Care Med. 1987;15:987.
36. Driks MR, Craven DE, Celli BR, et al. Nosocomial pneumonia in intubated patients given sucralfate as compared with antacids or histamine type 2 blockers: The role of gastric colonization. N Engl J Med. 1987;317:1376.
37. Edsall G. Specific prophylaxis of tetanus. JAMA. 1959;171:471.
38. Veronesi R. Prophylaxis. In: Veronesi R, ed. Tetanus: Important New Concepts. Amsterdam: Excerpta Medica; 1981:238–63.
39. Dastur FD, Awatramani VP, Dixit SK, et al. Response to single dose of tetanus vaccine in subjects with naturally acquired tetanus antitoxin. Lancet. 1981;2:219.
40. Centers for Disease Control. Diphtheria, tetanus and pertussis: Guidelines for vaccine prophylaxis and other preventive measures. Ann Intern Med. 1985;103:896.
41. Brand DA, Acampora D, Gottlieb AD, et al. Adequacy of antitetanus prophylaxis in six hospital emergency rooms. N Engl J Med. 1983;309:636.

221. CLOSTRIDIUM BOTULINUM (BOTULISM)

WILLIAM SCHAFFNER

Botulism is a life-threatening paralytic illness produced by neurotoxins elaborated by *Clostridium botulinum*. The disease occurs under three circumstances: (*1*) *botulism food poisoning* results from eating food that contains preformed toxin; (*2*) *wound botulism* occurs when toxin is produced by *C. botulinum* organisms contaminating traumatic wounds; and (*3*) *infant botulism* is due to toxin production by *C. botulinum* within the gastrointestinal tract of infants.

HISTORY

Because early accounts of botulism frequently incriminated sausages as a source of the illness, the name of the disease was derived from the Latin word for sausage, *botulus*. Outbreaks of "sausage poisoning" were common in southern Germany during the nineteenth century, and Justinius Kerner, a mystic poet and physician, published several monographs on the subject. For a time, botulism was known as "Kerner's disease." Investigating an outbreak in 1895, the Belgian bacteriologist Van Ermengem performed classic experiments in which he isolated the causative anaerobic spore-forming bacillus from an incriminated ham and demonstrated that both the ham and a toxin produced by the organism could induce a paralytic illness in cats.

Botulism occurred only rarely in the United States before World War I. Shortly thereafter, the growth of both commercial and home canning resulted in numerous epidemics. In response to this problem, K. F. Meyer and his associates performed a series of studies that defined the ecology of *C. botulinum*, the circumstances that favored toxin production, and, most important, the conditions under which spores could be destroyed during food processing. This knowledge ensured the safety of commercially canned foods. Although most cases of food-borne botulism today are related to home-canned foods, commercial products and restaurants have been implicated with increasing frequency, and these possibilities must be considered every time botulism occurs.

PATHOGENESIS

Clostridium botulinum is a gram-positive anaerobic bacillus that survives in soil and marine sediment by forming spores that germinate under certain environmental conditions. During growth and autolysis the bacillus releases a potent neurotoxin. Eight immunologically distinct toxin types have been described (types A, B, C_α, C_β, D, E, F, and G). A given bacterial strain produces only a single toxin type. There are marked differences in species susceptibility to the different toxins. Types A, B, and E most commonly produce disease in man; types F and G have only rarely caused human illness. Types C and D are associated with animal botulism, especially in cattle, ducks, and chickens.

On a weight basis, botulinus toxins are the most potent poisons known. While they have not yet been characterized completely, it is known that the toxins are polypeptides with molecular weights approximating 150,000 daltons. The several types differ in their degree of polymerization, their amino acid composition, and their requirement for enzymatic activation.[1] The toxins interfere with neurotransmission at peripheral cholinergic synapses by binding tightly to the presynaptic membrane and preventing the release of the neurotransmitter acetylcholine. Adrenergic fibers are spared. The effect of botulinus toxin on cholinergic pathways in the central nervous system remains in dispute.

The spores of *C. botulinum* are heat resistant; they can withstand 100°C for hours. Fortunately, the toxins are rather heat labile; boiling for 10 minutes or heating at 80°C for 30 minutes will destroy them. Thus, terminal heating of toxin-containing food can prevent illness. Strict anaerobic conditions are not always necessary for toxin production, which procedes best at 30°C but can occur at refrigerator temperatures. Because an environment of low pH is inhospitable to spore germination and toxin production, home-canned acidic foods (such as tomatoes) seem safer than more alkaline varieties, but exceptions occur.

Food items contaminated by toxin of any type may have a completely normal appearance and taste. Types A and B strains (but not type E) also may produce proteolytic enzymes that "spoil" food. Even when only small tastes of such food have dissuaded people from eating further, that nibble has often contained enough toxin to result in full-blown disease.

The toxins are absorbed primarily from the stomach and small bowel. The digestive enzymes do not destroy the toxin molecules. Indeed, pancreatic trypsin seems to enhance the toxicity of type E toxin. Toxin may be absorbed slowly from the colon. In addition, if *C. botulinum* organisms or spores also are ingested and reach the colon, toxin production can occur in the human gastrointestinal tract. Both these mechanisms account for the occasional demonstration of toxin in the blood stream many days after the ingestion of contaminated food.

EPIDEMIOLOGY

The spores of *C. botulinum* are ubiquitous in soil; the distribution of types A and B spores is worldwide. In the United States, type A spores predominate west of the Mississippi River; type B spores are more common in the eastern states. Type E spores are found in the sediments of lakes and the sea, especially in northern latitudes, and have been recovered from the Great Lakes. Although the association is not absolute, toxin types associated with human disease generally follow the geographic distribution of types; type E disease is usually associated with fish products.

The number of cases of food-borne botulism reported annually is increasing. Most cases occur singly or in small clusters and are due to home-canned or prepared foods. This is probably a consequence of a resurgent interest in home canning. Commercially processed foods and foods prepared in restaurants continue to be responsible for occasional outbreaks of botulism.[2] Because commercial foods often have a very wide distribution, patients may be scattered over several states. The physicians attending a single patient may have no clue that an epidemic is in progress. Such episodes constitute a public health emergency and can be detected only if every case is reported immediately to the authorities.

CLINICAL MANIFESTATIONS

Botulism manifests as a neurologic disorder and should be considered in the differential diagnosis of patients complaining of symmetrical descending weakness or paralysis. Symptoms usually begin 12–36 hours (range: 6 hours–8 days) after the ingestion of contaminated food. There may be little in the earliest symptoms that suggests food-borne disease to the physician. Nausea and vomiting are present in only one-third of patients with types A or B disease but are common with type E intoxication.[3] General symptoms of weakness, lassitude, and dizziness appear early. The interruption of cholinergic autonomic transmission results in diminished salivation and extreme dryness of the mouth, tongue, and pharynx, which is unrelieved by drinking fluids. This dryness may be quite painful and cause the patient to complain of "sore throat." Similarly, ileus, constipation, and urinary retention can result.

Neurologic symptoms may occur concurrently, or their onset may be delayed for up to 3 days. The cranial nerves are generally affected first, and ocular symptoms are frequent: diplopia, blurred vision, and photophobia. Bulbar involvement results in dysphonia, dysarthria, and dysphagia. Symmetrical weakness of the extremities occurs, usually in descending fashion and with variable speed. This is accompanied by weakness of the respiratory muscles.

On physical examination, patients are alert, oriented, and *afebrile*. Patients with type B intoxication may be somnolent but can be aroused easily.[4] Postural hypotension often can be demonstrated. Ocular signs may be prominent, with ptosis, extraocular palsies, and dilated, fixed pupils (Fig. 1). Some patients, particularly those with type A disease, may have no obvious ocular involvement.[5] Thus, ocular manifestations provide an important diagnostic clue when they are present, but their absence does not exclude the diagnosis of botulism. The mucous membranes of the mouth are often red, dry, and crusted. Weakness of striated muscle groups, especially of the neck and extremities, ranges from mild impairment to complete paresis. Likewise, deep tendon reflexes may be intact, symmetrically diminished, or absent. Pathologic reflexes cannot be elicited, and sensory examination is always normal. Abdominal distention with absent bowel sounds may be prominent, and urinary retention is common. Respiratory weakness may be evident only by measurement of vital capacity and can progress to respiratory arrest with unexpected suddenness.

After admission to the hospital the intoxication may continue to progress as more muscle groups are involved. Recovery is usually very gradual over weeks to months. Individual patients have been seen months to years after the acute illness with persistent constipation, diminished salivation or lacrimation, intermittent diplopia, and easy fatigue.[6,7]

The clinical diagnosis of botulism is often elusive; many cases are misdiagnosed initially. There are a number of reasons for this: the physician is unlikely to have had previous experience with the disease; if the food is a commercial product, there will be no history of eating home-canned food; the food may have been normal in appearance and taste; the patient may be solitary—not part of a group sharing a meal; and the disease has a natural progression in which different symptoms are prominent at different times in the illness.

A constellation of signs should suggest the diagnosis: (*1*) unexplained postural hypotention; (*2*) dilated, unreactive pupils; (*3*) dry mucous membranes; (*4*) descending paralysis with progressive respiratory weakness; and (*5*) the absence of fever.

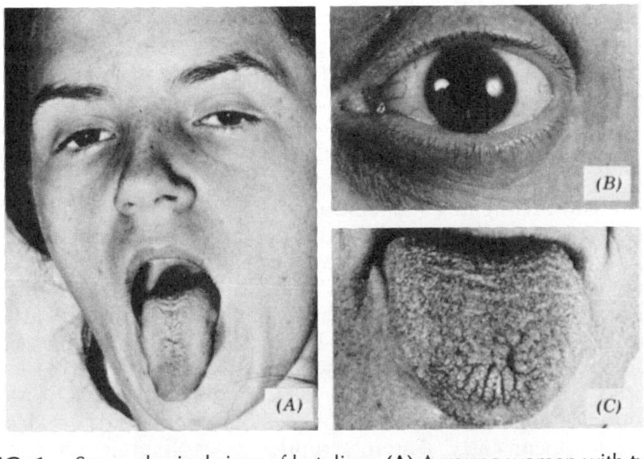

FIG. 1. Some physical signs of botulism. **(A)** A young woman with type B botulism. Bilateral ptosis, dilated pupils, erythematous pharynx, and dry tongue are evident. She also was unable to wrinkle her forehead on request. **(B)** Widely dilated and fixed pupils despite the photographer's bright light in type E disease. **(C)** Extremely dry furrowed tongue in type E botulism.

Early in the illness streptococcal pharyngitis may be diagnosed because of the notable pharyngeal pain and erythema. When nausea, vomiting, abdominal distention, and constipation are prominent and a general ileus pattern is seen on abdominal x-ray films, exploratory laparotomies have been performed in search of intestinal obstruction. Atropine, belladonna, or jimson weed poisoning can produce fixed, dilated pupils and dry mucous membranes but are accompanied by hallucinations and other evidence of central nervous system excitation. The striking weakness and respiratory impairment of botulism have led to confusion with other neuromuscular disorders, most commonly the Guillain-Barré syndrome, especially the C. Miller-Fisher variant with ophthalmoplegia and areflexia. In this disorder the weakness usually begins peripherally and ascends, cranial nerves are usually involved later in the illness, and paresthesias and muscle cramps are common. However, classic cerebrospinal fluid findings (elevation of protein content with no cells and normal pressure) may not be present on initial lumbar puncture. Patients with myasthenia gravis respond dramatically to edrophonium (Tensilon). A few patients with botulism have had modest responses to edrophonium, but not to the degree of patients with myasthenia.[5] Tick paralysis produces an ascending paralysis, is associated with perioral paresthesias, and the offending tick is present. Poliomyelitis is a febrile disease, usually asymmetrical, and produces characteristic changes in the cerebrospinal fluid.

DIAGNOSIS

Routine laboratory studies are of no aid in the diagnosis of botulism. The cerebrospinal fluid examination is normal. The electrocardiogram may reveal nonspecific minor disturbances in T-wave and S-T segment changes and occasional disorders of rhythm.

Electromyography can be useful in documenting electrophysiologic abnormalities consistent with botulism before the results of specialized microbiologic studies are available. It is important that the electromyographer be informed that the diagnosis of botulism is under consideration; a "routine" examination is not likely to be productive. Abnormalities include a decreased amplitude of the evoked muscle action potential to a single supramaximal nerve stimulus as well as enhanced post-tetanic facilitation, muscle fibrillation, and small amplitude polyphasic motor unit potentials of increased number and brief duration.[8]

The diagnosis of botulism can be confirmed by demonstrating: (*1*) botulinus toxin in the blood stream of the patient, (*2*) toxin and/or *C. botulinum* organisms in stool or gastric contents, and (*3*) toxin and/or organisms in the suspect food item. Toxin is detected by bioassay in mice; recovery of *C. botulinum* requires special anaerobic culture techniques. Most hospital laboratories are not equipped to process such specimens optimally; immediate assistance can be obtained from state health departments and the Centers for Disease Control in Atlanta.

TREATMENT

Precipitous respiratory failure is the most ominous threat to the survival of patients with botulism. Close observation and frequent assessments of vital capacity are essential. *Early* elective tracheostomy and the use of ventilatory assistance can be lifesaving. If ileus is profound, nasogastric suction and parenteral nutrition will be necessary. In the absence of ileus, cleansing saline enemas may be administered to remove unabsorbed toxin from the colon. Urinary retention will require indwelling bladder catheterization. The development of fever signifies a complicating nosocomial bacterial infection. Intensive nursing care using meticulous aseptic technique is a major contribution to successful therapy.

The effectiveness of antitoxin therapy is now generally accepted and its use is recommended. In types A and E intoxications its use has produced amelioration of symptoms and has reduced mortality; its efficacy in type B disease is less defined, however.[9] Antitoxin should be administered as soon as possible after specimens for laboratory study are obtained. If a delay has occurred, antitoxin may still be beneficial because botulinus toxin has been demonstrated in the blood of some patients for 30 days. Decisions about the prophylactic use of antitoxin in well persons known to have eaten toxin-containing food must be made on an individual basis.

All preparations of antitoxin are of equine origin; up to 20 percent of the patients have untoward reactions to its administration. Testing for hypersensitivity (with appropriate precautions) should always precede its use. Patients sensitive to horse serum must be desensitized before antitoxin is administered. Polyvalent antitoxin is used because the toxin type is usually unknown at the time antitoxin must be administered and because there is no cross protection between antitoxin types. One vial of antitoxin is administered iv and one, im. This should be repeated again in 2–4 hours if symptoms persist. Trivalent ABE antitoxin is stocked in strategic locations across the United States by the Centers for Disease Control and is available rapidly. The Centers should be contacted at *any hour* about the diagnosis, treatment, and investigation of suspected cases of botulism (phone: days [404] 639-3753; nights, weekends, and holidays [404] 639-2888.

Some physicians administer a course of penicillin therapy with the intent of eradicating bowel carriage of *C. botulinum* and thus forestalling continued toxin elaboration within the gastrointestinal tract. The value of such treatment is uncertain.

Guanidine hydrochloride is a drug that is thought to enhance the release of acetylcholine from terminal nerve fibers. Anecdotal reports suggest that some patients with botulism have reversal of cranial nerve palsies and improvement in respiratory function with use of this drug[10]; approximately half the patients treated have not had demonstrable improvement. Its use should be considered an experimental procedure.

The use of antitoxin and intensive respiratory and supportive therapy have reduced case-fatality ratios from 60 to 25 percent over the last 30 years.

WOUND BOTULISM

Wound botulism is a rare disorder in which toxin is produced by *C. botulinum* infecting a traumatic wound.[11] The patients are usually young males with injuries on the extremities sustained outside the home during work or play. Both types A and B organisms have been implicated, reflecting their presence in soil; type E strains have not yet been associated with wound botulism. The wounds may be thought to be "clean" at the time of initial surgical attention. In the reported cases initial antibiotic therapy did not prevent the development of intoxication. The incubation period between the time of injury and the onset of symptoms ranges from 4 to 14 days. In addition to traumatic wounds, botulism recently was identified as an unusual complication of the wounds caused by iv or nasal drug abuse.[12]

With a few exceptions, the clinical syndrome is entirely like that of food-borne botulism. Fever may be present as a consequence of the wound infection.

Clostridium botulinum has been recovered from wound drainage and from tissue removed in débridement. Toxin can be demonstrated in serum specimens. In addition to wound excision, treatment is as previously indicated. The differential diagnosis includes gas gangrene and tetanus.

INFANT BOTULISM

In 1976 it was first reported that infection with *C. botulinum* could produce the syndrome of the hypotonic ("floppy") infant.[13] This clinical observation has since been amply confirmed, and infant botulism now is recognized as the most common form of botulism in the United States.[14–16]

After a normal gestation and delivery, the affected infants feed and develop appropriately. Most become ill between 3 and 20 weeks of age. Constipation often is the first symptom, but usually is not serious enough to be brought to medical attention. After several days the infant's suck becomes weak, the cry becomes feeble and altered in tone, and oral secretions and food pool in the pharynx. The gag reflex is depressed. Cranial nerve deficits appear, manifested by a flaccid facial expression, ptosis, and ophthalmoplegia. The babies develop generalized muscle weakness, hypotonia, and areflexia. Loss of head control may be striking. Respiratory arrest occurs in almost half the affected children. The infants are afebrile, and cerebrospinal fluid examination is normal. Careful electromyographic examination is exceedingly helpful in establishing the diagnosis. Intensive supportive care will enable the vast majority of infants to recover completely. Antitoxin therapy is not recommended because clinical experience has shown that infants recover completely without it. Furthermore, its use may be associated with an increased risk of anaphylaxis in infants. Concurrent therapy wtih aminoglycoside antibiotics has been associated with potentiation of the neuromuscular paralysis.

Both *C. botulinum* and botulinus toxin have been regularly demonstrated in the stool of these infants. Indeed, both organisms and toxin can be present for prolonged periods (up to 8 weeks) after the infants have recovered completely, often despite antimicrobial therapy. Toxin has been found in the serum of only a few infants.

The evidence indicates that the infant gastrointestinal tract becomes colonized with *C. botulinum* from environmental sources and that toxin production occurs in vivo. Honey contaminated with *C. botulinum* spores is a common source of infection. The mechanism of recovery, despite the continued presence of organisms and toxin in the gut, remains elusive. The mainstay of prevention is to educate mothers and other caregivers not to feed infants honey. Lastly, a provocative study from California postulates that toxin production by *C. botulinum* may account for some cases of the sudden infant death syndrome.[17] Thus, with the recognition of wound botulism and the infant syndromes, the spectrum of disease produced by this microorganism has been expanded dramatically in recent years. In a further curious twist, it should also be noted that preparations of botulinus toxin have been injected therapeutically to ameliorate certain muscle spasm syndromes.[18]

REFERENCES

1. Sakaguchi G. *Clostridium botulinum* toxins. In: Dorner F, Drews J, eds. Pharmacology of Bacterial Toxins, Section 119, International Encyclopedia of Pharmacology and Therapeutics. Oxford: Pergamon Press, 1986:519–48.
2. MacDonald KL, Cohen ML, Blake PA. The changing epidemiology of adult botulism in the United States. Am J Epidemiol. 1986;124:794–9.
3. Koenig MG, Spickard A, Cardella MA, et al. Clinical and laboratory observations on type E botulism in man. Medicine. 1964;43:517–45.
4. Koenig MG, Drutz DJ, Mushlin AI, et al. Type B botulism in man. Am J Med. 1967;42:208–19.
5. Hughes JM, Blumenthal JR, Merson MH, et al. Clinical features of types A and B food-borne botulism. Ann Intern Med. 1981;95:442–5.
6. Mann JM, Martin S, Hoffman R, et al. Patient recovery from type A botulism: morbidity assessment following a large outbreak. Am J Public Health. 1981;71:266–9.
7. Mann J. Prolonged recovery from type A botulism. N Engl J Med. 1983;309:1522.
8. Cherington M, Ginsberg S. Type B botulism: neurophysiologic studies. Neurology. 1971;21:43–6.
9. Tacket CO, Shandera WX, Mann JM, et al. Equine antitoxin use and other factors that predict outcome in type A foodborne botulism. Am J Med. 1984;76:794–8.

10. Cherington M, Ryan DW. Treatment of botulism with guanidine: early neurophysiologic studies. N Engl J Med. 1970;282:195–7.
11. Merson MH, Dowell VR. Epidemiologic, clinical and laboratory aspects of wound botulism. N Engl J Med. 1973;289:1005–10.
12. MacDonald KL, Rutherford GW, Friedman SM, et al. Botulism and botulism-like illness in chronic drug abusers. Ann Intern Med. 1985;102:616–8.
13. Pickett J, Berg B, Chaplin E, et al. Syndrome of botulism in infancy: clinical and electrophysiologic study. N Engl J Med. 1976;295:770–2.
14. Arnon SS, Midura TF, Clay SA, et al. Infant botulism: epidemiological, clinical, and laboratory aspects. JAMA. 1977;237:1946–51.
15. Feldman RA, ed. A seminar on infant botulism. Rev Infect Dis. 1979;1:611–700.
16. Arnon SS. Infant botulism: anticipating the second decade. J Infect Dis. 1986;154:201–6.
17. Arnon SS, Damus K, Chin J. Infant botulism: epidemiology and relation to sudden infant death syndrome. Epidemiol Rev. 1981;3:45–66.
18. Dutton JJ, Buckley EG. Botulinum toxin in the management of blepharospasm. Arch Neurol. 1986;43:380–2.

222. GAS GANGRENE (OTHER CLOSTRIDIUM-ASSOCIATED DISEASES)

JOHN G. BARTLETT

The genus *Clostridium* includes all anaerobic, gram-positive spore-forming bacilli. Most are widely distributed in nature, and many are responsible for diverse clinical syndromes.

MICROBIOLOGY

There are over 60 recognized species of *Clostridium* and many additional isolates that cannot be speciated by currently accepted taxonomic classification.[1] These organisms vary in oxygen tolerance, nutritional requirements, and limiting or optimal temperatures for growth. Some organisms, such as *C. histolyticum* and *C. tertium*, are relatively aerotolerant and may actually replicate, but not sporulate, with aerobic incubation. Other species, such as *C. novyi* type B and *C. haemolyticum*, are strictly anaerobic and will not replicate with oxygen concentrations exceeding 0.05 percent. These variations in aerotolerance are sometimes confusing in distinguishing aerotolerant *Clostridium* from *Bacillus* species. The distinction may usually be made easily by showing that *Bacillus* sp. fail to yield spores when grown anaerobically and that they produce catalase, whereas clostridia rarely produce spores when grown aerobically and infrequently produce catalase.

According to cell wall structure as seen on electron microscopy, clostridia are gram-positive bacteria. However, many strains appear gram-negative or "gram-variable." Loss of gram-negative appearance is most likely in direct stains of clinical material, in cultures after incubation for extended periods, and in species showing terminal spores. The morphology of the species is highly variable—the rods may vary in length and width, and the ends may be rounded, blunt, or tapered (Table 1).

Some clostridial strains such as the two most common clinical isolates, *C. perfringens* and *C. ramosum*, do not readily form spores. Nevertheless, most clostridia will demonstrate spores with incubation at temperatures below those required for optimal growth, usually 30°C. Spore formation is optimally stimulated by heating starch–broth cultures to 70–80°C for 10 minutes or by ethanol shock using an equal volume of 95% ethanol for 45 minutes with subsequent demonstration of survival by incubation at conventional temperatures. Speciation is largely based on morphology, location of spores as terminal or subterminal, biochemical reactions, and gas–liquid chromatography to distinguish products of fermentation.

TABLE 1. *Clostridium* Species: Frequency of Isolation, Gram-Stain Appearance, and Location of Spores

Clostridium spp.	*Frequency*[a]	*Gram-stain appearance*
C. perfringens	89	Large box-car shape with blunt ends, spores rarely seen
C. ramosum	60	Pleomorphic bacilli in chains with bulges, spores rarely seen
C. sporogenes	38	Filamentous with ST spores
C. bifermentans	23	Bacilli with ST spores
C. innocuum	21	Small bacilli with T spores
C. sordellii	16	Bacilli with ST spores
C. paraputrificum	13	Long thin bacilli with T spores
C. subterminale	13	Bacilli often in chains with ST spores
C. cadaveris	12	Pleomorphic bacilli with T spores
C. butyricum	10	Round or blunt ends with large ST spores
C. septicum	9	Pleomorphic with long, thin cells and oval cells, ST spores
C. tertium	9	Large oval T spores

[a] Frequency in clinical specimens from diverse sources.
Abbreviations: T: terminal; ST: subterminal.
(Adapted from Smith,[4] with permission.)

The presence of lecithinase (α-toxin) may be tested using agar plates with egg yolk, in which case there is a zone of opaque precipitate surrounding colonial growth due to lysis of the lecithin in the medium. The reaction may be inhibited by addition of polyvalent gas gangrene antitoxin to the medium (Nagler's test). Nagler's test cannot be used to identify *C. perfringens* definitively, but this is clearly the most common lecithinase-producing *Clostridium* species found in clinical specimens. The egg yolk agar may also be used to demonstrate lipase production. Lipase-producing organisms, such as *C. botulinum*, *C. sporogenes*, and *C. novyi* type A, break down free fats in the egg yolk to liberate free fatty acids, which appear as an oily, iridescent sheen. Other characteristics commonly used for distinguishing species include the ability to ferment various carbohydrates, hydrolyze gelatin, and digest the casein in milk.[1,2] Microbiology laboratories should be able to speciate *C. perfringens* due to its importance in clinical medicine, frequency of recovery, and ease of identification. The need to speciate other clostridia is controversial.

Clostridia are ubiquitous, being found in soil, decaying vegetation, marine sediment, and in the intestinal tract of man, other vertebrates, and insects. They are also commonly recovered from infected sites, but usually as a component of a polymicrobial flora, making it difficult to establish their pathogenic role. The most characteristic and well-documented diseases are the histotoxic clostridial syndromes in which specific clostridial toxins appear to be responsible for the pathophysiology of the disease process (Table 2). The diagnosis in these cases requires the recovery of the putative agent or demonstration of the implicated toxin.

Clostridium perfringens

Clostridium perfringens was first described by Veillon and Zuber in 1898.[3] This is the most frequent clinical isolate of *Clostridium*. It may be found in diverse clinical sources and is responsible for three distinctive histotoxic clostridial syndromes (Table 2). The principle habitats are soil and the intestine of man and animals. Virtually every soil sample ever examined, with the exception of the sands of the Sahara, has been shown to contain *C. perfringens*.[4,5] This organism has also been found in stool specimens from virtually every vertebrate animal investigated, including dogs, cats, lions, tigers, wolves, rats,

TABLE 2. Histotoxic Clostridial Syndromes

Disease	*Agent*	*Toxin*
Enteric diseases		
Food poisoning	*C. perfringens* type A	Enterotoxin
Enteritis necroticans	*C. perfringens* type C	β-Toxin
Antibiotic-associated colitis	*C. difficile*	Toxin A
Neutropenic enterocolitis	*C. septicum* (others)	? β-Toxin
Neurologic syndromes		
Botulism	*C. botulinum*	Botulinal toxins A, B, E, F
Tetanus	*C. tetanus*	Tetanospasm
Soft tissue infection		
Gas gangrene	*C. perfringens* (others)	α-Toxin (others)

TABLE 3. Distribution of Major Toxins Among Types of Clostridia

	Types				
Toxin	*A*	*B*	*C*	*D*	*E*
α	+	+	+	+	+
β	−	+	+	−	−
ε	−	+	−	+	−
ι	−	−	−	−	+

guinea pigs, marmots, elephants, camels, buffaloes, pigs, goats, sheep, horses, cattle, monkeys, chickens, turkeys, sparrows, whales, seals, deer, ducks, antelope, and man.[4–7] Studies of fecal flora by Finegold et al. showed that *C. perfringens* was recovered from 28 of 40 adults subjects in mean concentrations of approximately 10^9/g.[7]

Clostridium perfringens produces 12 toxins, including four major lethal toxins that are used to separate the species into five types classified A to E (Table 3). Only type A strains are found in the microflora of both soil and the gastrointestinal tract. Since these strains are found in the soil as vegetative cells, it is assumed that they are actively replicating and that this is a natural habitat. The addition of types B–E to soil results in their gradual elimination over a period of months, indicating an inability to compete with the native type A strains.[8]

Clostridium perfringens generally has a distinctive box-car appearance on gram stain of clinical material or subcultures. Spores are rarely seen in clinical specimens or in cultures grown in the usual laboratory media.[9] When they do occur, they are oval in shape and subterminal in location. All types produce lecithinase (α-toxin), which can be demonstrated with the Nagler reaction. *Clostridium perfringens* is one of the easiest of all obligate anaerobes to recover. It grows rapidly under anaerobic conditions, with a generation time as short as 8 minutes at 43–45°C. The organism is relatively aerotolerant and shows "stormy fermentation" in milk. On blood agar, the colonies are typically surrounded by a "double zone of hemolysis" with a zone of complete hemolysis and a larger zone of incomplete hemolysis. Virtually all large series indicate that *C. perfringens* is the most common clinical isolate among clostridia, including blood cultures and cultures from infected sites such as intra-abdominal sepsis, genital tract infections, and soft tissue infections.[10–12]

INFECTIONS

Clostridia may be recovered from a diverse array of commonly encountered infections, usually as a component of a polymicrobial flora (Table 4). In most instances, there are no distinctive features, and the role of *Clostridium* as pathogen, symbiont, or commensal is enigmatic. The common denominator of these infections is the fact that they are endogenous, reflecting their normal habitat on mucocutaneous surfaces of the host. Two unique features of clostridial infections that apply to a

TABLE 4. Recovery of Clostridia from Infected Sites

Infected site	*No. Specimens with anaerobes*	*Clostridium perfringens*[a]	*Clostridium sp. (other)*[a]
Blood	175	5	21
Central nervous system	19	0	0
Head and neck	75	0	0
Human bite	25	0	4
Animal bite	33	3	0
Pulmonary	196	5	5
Soft tissue infections			
Above waist	79	4	1
Below waist	135	5	6
Intra-abdominal infections	185	15	44
Perirectal abscess	34	6	59
Foot ulcers	222	2	7
Decubitus ulcers	54	6	39
Osteomyelitis	49	0	2

[a] Results reported for number of isolates per 100 specimens that yielded anaerobes.
(Adapted from Sutter et al.,[154] with permission.)

TABLE 5. Clostridia Isolated from Clinical Specimens

	Blood cultures	*Soft tissue infections*	*Intra-abdominal sepsis*	*Total*
No. isolates	65	87	43	195
C. perfringens	37	20	4	61
C. ramosum	3	15	5	23
C. bifermentans	2	5	4	11
C. sphenoides	2	4	1	7
C. sporogenes	—	3	3	6
C. innocuum	1	3	2	6
C. difficile	1	3	1	5
C. butyricum	—	3	2	5
C. septicum	2	2	—	4
C. tertium	2	1	—	3
C. sordellii	—	3	—	3
C. limosum	2	—	1	3
C. barati	1	1	1	3
Clostridium sp. (other)	3[a]	10[b]	5[c]	18
Clostrium (unclassified)	11	12	13	36

[a] Includes *C. pseudotestanicum* (1), *C. putrificum* (1), and *C. hastiforme* (1).
[b] Includes *C. subterminale* (2), *C. novyi* (2), *C. cadaveris* (1), *C. beijerinckii* (1), *C. fallax* (1), *C. carnis* (1), *C. pseudotetanicum* (1), and *C. ghondi* (1).
[c] Includes *C. fallax* (1), *C. beijerinckii* (1), *C. ghoni* (1), *C. paraputrificum* (1), and *C. carnis*. (1)
(Data from Gorbach and Thadepalli[10] and Gorbach et al.[44])

minority of cases are the penchant for gas formation at the infected site and the histotoxic clostridial syndromes that reflect the activity of specific toxins. Most *Clostridium* species produce large amounts of volatile fatty acids in vitro, presumably accounting for an analogous observation at the infected site in some patients. The result is gas that may be detected by palpation, radiograph, or scans. Examples include crepitant cellulitis,[13] emphysematous cholecystitis,[14,15] emphysematous gastritis,[16] and emphysematous cystitis.[17] In each instance, other pathogens have also been implicated in the pathology of these conditions; many processes may account for the gas formation, but clostridia are the most common.[13] A diverse array of clostridial species is implicated in these infections. About 30 clostridial species have been found at infected sites; *C. perfringens* is the dominant species, accounting for about 20–30 percent of all isolates (Table 1, 4, and 5). The histotoxic clostridial syndromes are discussed below and elsewhere (Table 2).

Bacteremia

Clostridia account for 1–3 percent of all positive blood cultures, and *C. perfringens* is the most common (Tables 1 and 4). In the majority of cases, there is no obvious association between the associated disease process and clostridia bacteremia, leaving the impression that most bacteremias represent either contamination, presumably from the skin, or transient bacteremia of no clinical consequence. One of the earliest studies to note the apparent paradox of bacteremia with a potentially devastating pathogen resulting in no obvious clinical consequence was by Ramsey.[18] This investigator observed 28 women with clostridial bacteremia associated with septic abortion, all of whom had a benign, self-limited course despite the lack of any specific form of antibiotic treatment at the time. An updated report on this thesis was published in 1975 by Gorbach and Thadepalli, who reviewed their experience with positive blood culture of 65 strains of clostridia from 49 patients seen at Cook County Hospital.[10] The authors noted that clostridial bacteremia was usually unrelated to the clinical syndrome and occurred in such settings as pulmonary tuberculosis, aspiration pneumonia, meningococcemia, etc. The interpretation was that the organism either represented a contaminant or simply caused transient bacteremia of no clinical consequence. Other investigators have made similar observations,[18–20] but there are also clinical settings, such as intra-abdominal sepsis, decubitus ulcers, or gynecologic infections, in which clostridial isolates from the blood may be associated with the microbial flora of the infected site without the devastating consequences of clostridial toxins. There is clear-cut clinical relevance in a small minority of conditions, such as infections associated with gas production, clostridial myonecrosis (gas gangrene), and *C. septicum* bacteremia in association with colonic carcinoma or leukemia. The dominant clostridial species isolated from blood cultures regardless of clinical significance is *C. perfringens*, which accounts for 25–50 percent (Tables 4 and 5).[10,11]

Clostridium septicum bacteremia appears to be a unique syndrome associated with specific underlying diseases and a devastating clinical course.[21,31,31a] Toxins produced in vivo by this organism include α-toxin, β-toxin (desoxyribonuclease), and γ-toxin (hyaluronidase). *Clostridium septicum* is a relatively rare cause of gas gangrene and is infrequently encountered in positive blood cultures for clostridia, accounting for only 3 of 360 at the Mayo Clinic during a 15-month review period.[11] When *C. septicum* bacteremia occurs, 70–80 percent of cases are associated with malignancies, most frequently leukemia or colonic carcinoma. There is also an association with neutropenia, especially cyclic neutropenia.[21,26,27,29] Virtually all cases that occur with leukemia do so during relapse.

During World War I, *C. septicum* was second only to *C. perfringens* in causing gas gangrene, and it ranked third in World War II.[32] Unlike the usual cases of gas gangrene, there is no obvious external portal of entry in this more recently recognized syndrome, and the presumed source is the colon. Typical symptoms include sudden onset of fever, abdominal pain, vomiting, and diarrhea and there is commonly rapid progression to shock. The patient may initially appear to have appendicitis, but the fulminant course is clearly atypical. Intravascular hemolysis is rarely encountered. Up to 25 percent of patients have myonecrosis at metastatic sites,[21,31a,33] and others may have unusual presentations such as meningitis,[34] osteomyelitis,[35] septic arthritis,[36] or panophthalmitis.[37] Nearly all patients have evidence of altered integrity of the bowel, such as leukemic infiltrates, neoplasms, or "neutropenic enterocolitis." Neutropenic enterocolitis is seen with congenital neutropenia or neutropenia with cytotoxic chemotherapy. At autopsy or laparotomy, the cecum and adjacent gut show edema, hemorrhage, and necrosis, with typical organisms invading the bowel wall. These lesions presumably represent the portal of entry for organisms comprising the resident colonic flora.

Clostridium septicum is a relatively unusual isolate in normal flora studies; it is recovered in stool in only about 29 percent of cases, although carriage rates in the appendix are reported at 10–63 percent.[38] Rapid institution of antibiotics, preferably penicillin G, will salvage up to one-half of patients, although many patients expire despite aggressive treatment. Patients often need extensive surgery to debride gangrenous lesions of the bowel. Other clostridia that are less commonly implicated include *C. perfringens, C. sphenoides, C. sordelli, C. paraperfringens*, and *C. tertium*.[39–43] Bacteremia with *C. tertium* is the second most frequent blood culture isolate in this setting, but clinically distinctive in the favorable prognosis with antibiotic treatment.[43a]

Intra-abdominal Infections

Clostridia are uniformly present in the colonic flora and are commonly encountered in endogenous infections involving such flora, including intra-abdominal sepsis and wound infections following intestinal surgery. Recovery rates in intra-abdominal sepsis generally range from 30 to 50 percent when appropriate anaerobic culture techniques are used.[44–47] The great majority of these infections are polymicrobial, and the significance of the clostridial isolates is unknown (Tables 4 and 5). An exception is the association of colonic carcinoma with *C. septicum* bacteremia, as reviewed above.

Biliary Tract Infections

Clostridia may be isolated from 10–20 percent of diseased gall bladders at surgery.[48–51] In most instances, the organism can be readily identified by gram stain of bile obtained at surgery. These infections are usually not unique, with two exceptions. First, clostridia in bile are the presumed source for gas gangrene, a rare but devastating complication of biliary tract surgery. The second exception is emphysematous cholecystitis, in which radiographs show gas in the gall bladder lumen, pericholecystic tissue, or biliary radicles.[14,15,52–54] This condition was originally described by Stolz in 1901,[55] and the first report of a preoperative diagnosis based on abdominal radiograph appeared in 1931.[56] At operation the gall bladder is usually tense, there is gas under pressure in the lumen, the mucosa is gangrenous, the mucosa is often separated from the muscularis, pericholecystic abscess formation is common, and the gall bladder lumenal contents are putrid and purulent. Clostridia account for at least half of the cases, and *C. perfringens* is the most common bacterial isolate. Gas from the lumen appears to enter pericholecystic tissue through areas of necrosis in the mucosa and submucosa. Experimental distension of the gall bladder with air causes leakage into the perimuscular layer in the region of duct occlusion, and the submucosal layer is almost entirely elevated before there is rupture into the pericholecystic tissues.[57] This infection is most frequent in diabetics and in men. Complications such as gangrene and abscess formation are sufficiently frequent that the detection of typical findings on radiograph represents a clear indication for early surgical intervention and antimicrobial treatment directed against clostridia.

Female Genital Tract Infections

Clostridia are isolated from 4–20 percent of women with genital tract infections not involving sexually transmitted pathogens.[58–62] The most frequent conditions are tuboovarian and pelvic abscesses. These organisms have been recovered from the normal genital tract flora in approximately 5–10 percent of women, and, when present, the mean concentration was 10^8/ml vaginal secretions.[63,64] Consequently, cultures or stains of exudate that are subject to contamination with this flora cannot be meaningfully interpreted, nor can most clostridia isolated from deep infected sites, or even blood. As reviewed above, Ramsey considered clostridia "benign saprophytes" in blood cultures of women with septic abortion. Similar observations have been noted by others.[10,65–67] Nevertheless, there is the notable exception of uterine gas gangrene, a rare complication that usually occurs in the setting of septic abortion or occasionally in a normal delivery (see below). *Clostridium sordellii* has recently become an organism of special interest in gynecologic infections as a relatively common agent of uterine gas gangrene and as a possible agent of a toxic shock-like syndrome.[68]

Pulmonary Infections

Clostridia may be recovered from 8–10 percent of anaerobic pulmonary infections, with *C. perfringens* accounting for half of the isolates.[69] These organisms have been reported primarily in empyema fluid, but also from transtracheal aspirates.[69] In many cases the clostridia are part of a polymicrobial flora. When the clostridia are recovered as the only isolates, the species is usually *C. perfringens*.[70–77] Aspiration of oropharyngeal flora is considered to be the likely pathophysiologic mechanism in the majority; occasional cases have occurred after penetrating chest injury or thoracotomy with pulmonary resection.[78,79] The clinical features of these infections are not dissimilar to those of anaerobic infections of the lung involving other anaerobic bacteria, although an occasional case is characterized by extensive gas production in the pleural space[72,75] or extensive necrosis of tissue and a rapidly progressive course.[72] The mortality rate for patients with clostridial infections of the lung and pleural space is similar to that for pleuropulmonary infections involving other anaerobic bacteria.[69]

Central Nervous System Infections

Intracranial infections involving *Clostridium* sp. are unusual and often the subject of case reports.[80–85] The great majority represent cerebral abscess, with or without meningeal involvement, in which radiographs typically show focal collections of gas. Most cases involve penetrating trauma, and a characteristic feature is the rapid evolution of symptoms following the traumatic event, often within 24–48 hours. Additional cases are associated with infections of the middle ear. Traumatized muscle associated with hypoxia appears to be the best culture media for clostridia, and the brain would seem relatively unaccommodating. Although these cases are occasionally reported as "gas gangrene of the brain," there is minimal tendency for the spread seen with myonecrosis, and the systemic effects of clostridial toxins are not present. The exception is the occasional case involving the temporal muscle.

Soft Tissue Infections

Clostridia may be isolated from a variety of soft tissue infections including (*1*) common soft tissue infections, in which they represent a component of polymicrobial flora; (*2*) crepitant cellulitis; (*3*) suppurative myositis; and (*4*) gas gangrene.

The first category includes a heterogeneous array of commonly encountered polymicrobial infections such as wound infections following abdominal surgery, perirectal cellulitis, perirectal abscesses, diabetic foot ulcers, decubitus ulcers, infections associated with vascular insufficiency, and stump infections following amputation (Table 4). These infections are not unique compared with similar infections that do not harbor clostridia, so their role in the pathologic events is unclear. Numerous clostridial species may be involved, but the predominant isolates are *C. perfringens* and *C. ramosum* (Table 5). The companion organisms are those that are commonly encountered in intra-abdominal sepsis, and the presumed source is the colonic flora.

Suppurative myositis due to clostridia is similar to "tropical pyomyositis." This occurs most frequently in heroin addicts, usually involving the thigh or forearm and not necessarily in an area of trauma or illicit drug injection.[10] In contrast to tropical pyomyositis, bacteriologic studies fail to yield *Staphylococcus aureus*, but instead yield clostridia either in pure culture or as a component of a polymicrobial flora. This lesion must be distinguished from gas gangrene, which also involves muscle; with myositis, however, there is a suppurative collection without myonecrosis, and there is no evidence of the severe systemic complications associated with gas gangrene. These patients generally respond well to incision and drainage. Operative findings may include abscess formation, localized myositis, and dissecting fasciitis.[10]

Crepitant cellulitis is a soft tissue infection characterized by large amounts of gas formation in the soft tissue.[13,86–89] These infections usually occur in association with trauma, the incubation period from the time of wounding to clinical presentation is usually 3 days or longer, and there is generally minimal systemic toxicity. Findings at the infected site include abundant gas formation, usually far more than in myonecrosis; there is minimal pain, the site shows swelling with little discoloration, and there is a thin, dark discharge, often with the characteristic sweetish or foul odor, that on gram stain shows polymorphonuclear leukocytes and typical bacteria. Clostridia, primarily *C. perfringens*, are the most common cause, although other bacteria such as *Escherichia coli, Klebsiella*, and *S. aureus* may be implicated.[90] Occasionally patients have a more fulminant course, with rapid spread and evidence of clostridial toxemia. In these cases there may be rapid spread through contiguous fascial planes in association with intravascular hemolysis, hypotension, and renal failure.

Gas Gangrene

Clostridial myonecrosis or gas gangrene is a rare but devastating infection characterized by muscle necrosis and systemic toxicity ascribed to toxins elaborated by the putative agent.

Pathogens. The most frequent pathogen is *C. perfringens*, which accounts for approximately 80 percent of cases with positive cultures. Other clostridial species that have been implicated include *C. novyi, C. septicum, C. histolyticum, C. fallax*, and *C. bifermentans*. In some cases there are several species of clostridia isolated from the infected site, and there may also be multiple other species of bacteria at the infected site. The clostridia implicated produce over 20 exotoxins, including 7 that are lethal when injected intraperitoneally into mice (Table 6).

TABLE 6. Toxins Produced by *Clostridium perfringens*

Toxin	*Major strains*	*Biologic activity*[a]
α	A–E	Lethal, necrotizing, hemolytic; lecithinase
β	B, C	Lethal, necrotizing, transmural necrosis with small bowel inoculation
ϵ	B, D	Prototoxin activated by trypsin; lethal, necrotizing; increased vascular permeability, peripheral vasoconstruction
ι	E	Lethal binary toxin dependent on two nonlinked proteins for binding and ADP ribosylation
δ	B, C	Lethal, hemolytic
θ	A–E	Oxygen-labile hemolysin (sulfhydryl group-activated cytolysins), lethal, hemolytic
κ	A, D, E	Collagenase, lethal, necrotizing, gelatinase
λ	B, E	Protease
μ	A, B, D	Hyaluronidase
ν	A–E	Deoxyribonuclease, leukocidin, lethal, hemolytic, necrotizing
Enterotoxin	A	Enterotoxic (ileal loop assays), gut damage, cytotoxic, lethal; binds receptor and induces Ca^{+}-dependent cytotoxicity
Neuraminidase	A–E	Cleaves acetylneuraminic acid residues

[a] Lethality tests performed with systemic administration (intravenous or intraperitoneal), usually in rodent models; "necrotizing" usually refers to dermonecrosis.

The most important toxin is thought to be α-toxin, a phospholipase with a molecular weight of about 30,000 that is responsible for splitting lecithin to phosphoryl choline and diglyceride. Intravenous administration of this toxin in experimental animals produces massive hemolysis, destruction of platelets, and widespread capillary damage. Under appropriate environmental conditions in soft tissue, histotoxic clostridial vegetative forms replicate and produce toxins that promote local spread by diffusion into adjacent soft tissue; systemic absorption of these toxins presumably accounts for the dramatic systemic consequences of gas gangrene. α-Toxin is the most extensively studied of the *C. perfringens* toxins and the role of others, either independently or collectively, is not well established. Kameyama et al. showed that guinea pigs immunized against α-toxin did not develop gas gangrene when challenged with *C. perfringens*, α-toxin, or κ-toxin, although animals immunized with κ-toxin were susceptible to both α-toxin and *C. perfringens*.[91]

Epidemiology. Gas gangrene usually follows wounding associated with trauma or surgery. Routine culturing of traumatic open wounds indicates that 20–80 percent are contaminated by clostridia, although gas gangrene remains a relatively rare infection. In the Western Desert (1940–1942) of World War II, MacLennan reported that 20–30 percent of all battlefield wounds were contaminated by clostridia, but only 0.32 percent of these developed gas gangrene.[92] A review of 187,936 major open wounds of violence by Altemeier and Furste showed that the overall incidence of gas gangrene was 1.7 percent.[93] Furthermore, there was no difference between the flora of wounds that developed gas gangrene and those that did not. These observations emphasize the important contribution of local conditions in promoting replication of vegetative forms with the elaboration of toxins. Factors that promote this process by contributing the tissue hypoxia include the presence of foreign bodies, vascular insufficiency, and concurrent infection with other microbes. Thus the minimum dose required to produce gas gangrene in guinea pigs was reduced 10^3 by injection into devitalized tissue; it was reduced 10^6 by muscle contamination with sterile dirt.[94]

The history of gas gangrene since its discovery in the late 19th century has been closely tied to major wars, due to the high frequency of severe trauma, gross contamination, and delayed surgical intervention characteristic of battlefield conditions. The incidence of gas gangrene in battlefield trauma in World War I was 5 percent, for World War II it was 0.7 percent, for the Korean War it was 0.2 percent, and for the Vietnam conflict it was 0.02 percent (22 cases in 139,000 battle injuries).[87,92,93,95,96] These figures reflect improvements in the management of battlefield trauma with prompt and thorough débridement, especially in the Vietnam conflict, in which rapid evacuation to sites of high-quality trauma surgery was one of the relatively few victories.

During peace time in the United States, approximately half of the cases of gas gangrene follow trauma and half occur postoperatively. The most frequent traumatic injuries are car accidents, followed by crush injuries, industrial accidents, and gunshot wounds. The most frequent antecedent surgical procedures are intestinal surgery, especially colon resection and biliary tract surgery. Occasional cases of gas gangrene are associated with vascular insufficiency to the lower extremities occurring in association with vascular gangrene, diabetic foot ulcers, decubitus ulcers, or as a complication of an amputation. Uterine gas gangrene usually occurs in the setting of a septic abortion, usually a criminal abortion, and less commonly with other gynecologic procedures or following delivery. Spontaneous gas gangrene is a rare form of the infection in which there is no associated traumatic or surgical wounding.

Patients with gas gangrene following trauma are usually male, relatively young, and tend to have extremity involvement. Those with gas gangrene following a surgical procedure are also usually male, but are older, are more likely to have abdominal wall involvement, and carry a worse prognosis. Patients with this condition occurring in association with vascular insufficiency are usually older diabetics; the disease is equally divided between the sexes, and lower extremities are virtually always involved.

The source of the organism has been the subject of some controversy. Clostridia are widely distributed in nature, being found in soil and air samples, including operating room air, dust, food, and clothing.[97,98] Concentrations vary, but any fertile loam contains 10^8/g. The highest concentrations are in the intestinal tract; these strains are also felt to be the most virulent, and an endogenous source is suspected even in cases associated with extensive soil contamination. Person-to-person transmission is rare,[88] although occasional "outbreaks" are reported.[98] In these cases it is sometimes felt that the epidemic strain has exceptional virulence.[98] Relevant studies by Altemeier and Furste showed that *C. perfringens* strains recovered from infected wounds were 10^3–10^6 times more virulent in the minimal dose requirements for infection in guinea pigs compared with soil strains.[94]

Clinical Manifestations. Gas gangrene is usually a fulminant infection characterized by prominent findings at the site of injury and serious systemic toxicity.[87,92,96,99–103] As noted, the usual clinical settings are categorized as (*1*) traumatic injury or penetrating wound; (*2*) surgery, primarily intestinal or biliary tract surgery; (*3*) uterine gas gangrene usually following septic criminal abortion or delivery; (*4*) soft tissue lesions associated with vascular insufficiency; (*5*) intestinal gas gangrene, which is most frequent in compromised hosts; and (*6*) spontaneous gas gangrene.

The usual incubation period from the time of injury to the onset of symptoms ascribed to gas gangrene is 1–4 days (range, 8 hours to 3 weeks). The first symptom noted by the patient is sudden, persistent, and severe pain at the site of the wound. Physical examination at that time typically shows localized tense edema, pallor, and tenderness, although the wound may appear normal in the early stages. Gas may be noted in the soft tissues by palpation, radiograph, or scans. The skin initially appears pale and then progresses to a magenta or bronze discoloration, often followed by the appearance of hemorrhagic bullae (Fig. 1). As the lesion progresses there may be a thin, dirty brown, serosanguineous discharge with a characteristic offensive odor described as sweetish and distinctive compared with the putrid odor of other more common anaerobic infections. Gram stain of the discharge often shows large number of typical gram-positive or gram-variable rods with sparse or no white cells. When *C. perfringens* is involved, the organism shows the typical box-car appearance without spores. The absence of white cells locally is ascribed to the lecithinase, ν-toxin, or other toxins that lyse neutrophils.

The systemic findings that accompany these changes at the wound site may be profound. These include diaphoresis, fever (often low grade), tachycardia, and extreme anxiety on the part of the patient, who often remains exceedingly alert and may sense the severity of the disease process or show apathy. Fever may be deceptively low or absent in the early stages. There is often a disproportionate tachycardia. Late complications include hemolytic anemia, hypotension, and renal failure. Common findings in advanced stages of disease are hemoglobinuria, which may impart the "port wine" discoloration to urine, and hemoglobulinemia. The patient eventually develops coma and the entire body may develop the typical magenta color in the moribund state.

Diagnosis. The diagnosis of gas gangrene is based on the constellation of clinical findings, the demonstration of myonecrosis, and supporting microbiologic data. Clinical clues to this

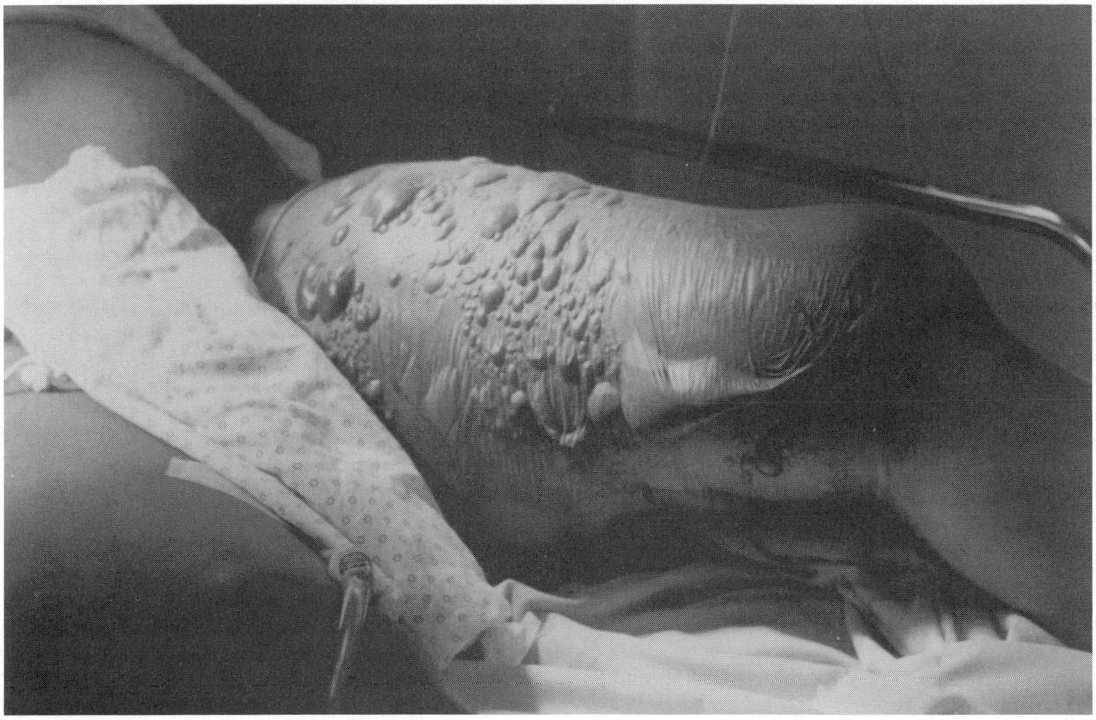

FIG. 1. Thigh lesions in a 61 year old woman with "spontaneous" gas gangrene. She sought physician consultation for a painful bullous lesion on the posterior thigh and was hospitalized 4 hours later when the pain became unbearable. The photograph was taken 4 hours after admission and immediately before a disarticulation procedure that demonstrated myonecrosis with clostridia.

infection include severe systemic toxicity and the occurrence of this infection in the clinical settings noted above, primarily in association with wounding; typical findings at the site of injury, including tense edema, discoloration, and hemorrhagic bullae; evidence of gas in the soft tissues; gram stains of exudate showing typical organisms with sparse white blood cells; the typical discharge with an offensive odor; and computerized tomography showing muscle compartment involvement.

Microbiologic studies may be supportive when clostridia, especially the species implicated in gas gangrene (primarily *C. perfringens*), are identified with direct gram stain of exudate and recovered in cultured of exudate or blood. Nevertheless, most positive cultures for clostridial species, including blood culture isolates, are not associated with the distinctive pathologic features found with the histotoxic clostridial syndromes.[10] *Clostridium perfringens* accounts for approximately 80 percent of cases of gas gangrene. Approximately 15 percent of gas gangrene cases have documented clostridial bacteremia.

The major considerations in the differential diagnosis are other deep and devastating soft tissue infections that share some of the clinical features noted above. The most common among these are crepitant cellulitis, streptococcal fasciitis, necrotizing fasciitis due to a mixed aerobic–anaerobic infection, and synergistic necrotizing cellulitis. The most important diagnostic and therapeutic maneuver in suspected cases is direct visualization of the muscle to confirm myonecrosis, the failure of muscle to respond to electrical stimuli, pale discoloration, and/or failure of the cut surface to bleed. It should be emphasized that many of the characteristic features occur relatively late in the disease course when the patient is already beyond salvage.

Therapy. The most important component of treatment is extensive surgical debridement, with wide excision of involved muscle when the abdominal wall is involved, amputation of an involved extremity, or a hysterectomy with uterine gas gangrene. It is important that all necrotic muscle be debrided, and this often requires reoperation on a daily basis.

Penicillin G is generally regarded as the preferred drug for patients with gas gangrene.[103–105] Recent studies suggest increasing resistance in *C. perfringens*, but such resistance is more striking in some other clostridial species.[105,106] Most authorities continue to regard penicillin as the preferred agent despite these changes, since most strains are still susceptible at levels that are easily achieved. Alternatives for patients who have contraindications to penicillin or when there is concern regarding resistance are chloramphenicol, metronidazole, and imipenem. These drugs are active against virtually all strains of clostridia in vitro, although the published clinical experience is substantially less than that for penicillin G. Other agents with good in vitro activity are erythromycin, rifampin, clindamycin, and tetracycline.[105–107] Cefoxitin is less active than most other cephalosporins versus clostridia in vitro and should be avoided when this diagnosis is suspected. There are also reports of gas gangrene developing during and in spite of surgical prophylaxis with cephalothin.[108]

Despite the nearly universal endorsement of penicillin G, there are disconcerting data not only from in vitro susceptibility studies showing increasing resistance, but also from experimental animal work. Early studies of gas gangrene in guinea pigs by Altemeier showed that tetracycline and chloramphenicol were superior to penicillin.[93,109] More recent studies have been reported by Stevens et al. using a mouse model of gas gangrene. Using a strain of *C. perfringens* that was susceptible to all tested antibiotics and survival as an endpoint, penicillin treatment demonstrated no difference compared with untreated controls.[110] Significantly better outcomes were achieved with clindamycin, metronidazole, rifampin, and tetracycline. The impact that such studies should or will have on antibiotic recommendations is not known.

Other potential forms of treatment include gas gangrene antitoxin and hyperbaric oxygen. The antitoxin was commercially developed as a therapeutic modality in the prepenicillin era as a method of neutralizing circulating toxins. This consisted of horse serum prepared to toxins of five clostridial species implicated in gas gangrene. The clinical experience was variable, but the question of use is now moot since all available supplies are outdated and there appears to be virtually no interest in resuming production.

The use of hyperbaric oxygen is hotly debated by vocal advocates and noted sceptics.[100,101,103,111,112] There is some evidence in experimental animals that mortality rates are reduced, although the hyperbaric oxygen appears less important than surgery or penicillin.[112] The published clinical experience is tarnished by the lack of any properly controlled trials, the frequent inclusion of patients who did not have well-confirmed cases of gas gangrene, and the obvious, unabashed enthusiasm of investigators who often have life-long careers invested in this technique. There does not appear to be a potential benefit in showing demarcation of involved muscle, which may assist the surgeon in defining the extent of resection. In view of the ongoing debate, a common recommendation is to use the procedure if it is readily available. Nevertheless, it would appear inappropriate to delay critical surgery or even risk transport of a critically ill patient for long distances to achieve this therapeutic modality.

Prognosis. The reported mortality rate for gas gangrene encountered in the world wars (prepenicillin era) was 27–31 percent.[32] The reported mortality rate in 116 published studies during the antibiotic era summarizing over 1200 cases was 25 percent.[101] Poor prognostic findings include leukopenia, evidence of intravascular hemolysis, renal failure, elderly age, involvement of the abdominal wall, and "spontaneous gas gangrene."

Enteric Infections

There are four recognized histotoxic clostridial syndromes involving the gut lumen: enteritis necroticans, *C. perfringens* food poisoning, *C. difficile*-induced diarrhea or colitis, and neutropenic enterocolitis (Table 7). In each instance, the enteric pathology is ascribed to the putative agent and/or its toxin from a gastrointestinal source either by microbial invasion (enteritis necroticans and neutropenic enterocolitis) or by the deleterious effects of the toxin on gut epithelium (*C. difficile* colitis and *C. perfringens* food poisoning). The responsible toxin has been described in three of these, and the disease has been reproduced with the postulated toxin in experimental animal studies. The exception is neutropenic enterocolitis, in which *C. septicum* is the usual, but not exclusive, pathogen, and the responsible toxin is not known, although β-toxin is an attractive candidate because of similarities to enteritis necroticans. These conditions show considerable variation in pathophysiologic mechanism, risk factors, clinical presentation, and treatment (Table 7). Neutropenic enterocolitis has been described previously in the section, "Infections," and *C. difficile* colitis is discussed in Chapter 83.

Enteritis Necroticans. Enteritis necroticans is a necrotizing infection of the small bowel caused by the β-toxin of *C. perfringens* type C. This is an important enteric disease of sheep, calves, and piglets in veterinary medicine; its clinical corollary appears to occur only when there is a unique combination of social and nutritional factors in which pig feasts, protein malnutrition, and sweet potatoes all play contributing roles.

HISTORY. The first rigorous study of enteritis necroticans occurred at the end of World War II, when there were hundreds of cases of "Darmbrand" in Germany and Norway involving malnourished individuals.[113] Workers at that time suspected *C. perfringens* type C on the basis of its recovery in stools from afflicted patients and the production of a similar disease by injecting broth cultures of the organism into the small intestine of experimental animals.[114] Subsequent work demonstrated that the pathologic lesion could be ascribed to an exotoxin. Interest in the disease was regenerated in the 1960s when enteritis necroticans, known locally as "pig-bel," was found to be endemic in the highlands of New Guinea. Most of the important studies have been conducted in New Guinea by the team of Lawrence, Murrell, and Walker.[115–120]

PATHOGEN. *Clostridium perfringens* type C is widely distributed in soil and has been found in the stools of many asymptomatic patients as well as animals. Thus exposure is common, and other factors must be invoked in the pathophysiology of the disease. Especially important is the β-toxin, a protein toxin of 30,000–48,000 daltons that is extremely sensitive to proteolytic enzymes.[121] Carrier rates of the putative agent are reportedly 20–70 percent in endemic areas.[116]

EPIDEMIOLOGY. The disease is endemic in the highlands of New Guinea, where surveys in 1964 showed a prevalence of 50 cases per 10,000 population with a mortality rate of 14 per 100,000.[116,119] At the time, it was the most common cause of death in children over 12 months of age in the region; over 86 percent of adults in the area showed circulating antibody to the β-toxin. Sporadic cases have been noted in Southeast Asia, Africa, China, and Western countries. It is commonly thought that the disease is more frequent than generally appreciated, especially in areas where there is extensive malnutrition. This contention is supported by a report of 30 cases in a Khmer refugee camp at the Thai–Kampuchean border in 1985.[122]

The high prevalence of the disease in New Guinea is ascribed to unique cultural habits. Although all people are presumably exposed, it is postulated that the inoculum is especially high during pig feasts, in which there is inadequate heating to eliminate clostridial spores. The organism appears to attach to the small bowel and produce β-toxin, which is protected from proteolytic enzymes by several contributing factors including (*1*) protein malnutrition, resulting in depletion of protease enzymes; (*2*) the dietary staple of sweet potatoes, which contain heat-stable inhibitors of trypsin; and (*3*) a high incidence of colonization with *Ascaris lumbricoides*, which secretes trypsin inhibitors. The high prevalence of the disease in children appears to reflect immunologic naïveté. Experimental support for the proposed mechanism is based on studies showing that inocula of broth cultures or culture filtrates produce typical segmental, transmural necrosis, which can be prevented by combining the filtrate with pancreatin (which destroys toxin B) or by challenge to animals immunized with toxin B vaccine.[120]

CLINICAL AND PATHOLOGIC FEATURES. Enteritis necroticans is a segmental disease of the small intestine. The pathologic spectrum of disease ranges from small necrotic patches with normal intervening mucosa to full thickness necrosis involving large segments.[123,124] With advanced lesions the bowel wall becomes thin and subject to perforation. Microscopic studies show mucosal infarction, with edema, hemorrhage, and a transmural leukocytic infiltrate.

The usual presenting symptoms are abdominal pain, distention, vomiting, and passage of bloody stool.[115–119] The incubation period from the time of exposure to the presumed dietary source is usually about 2 days, but varies from 1 to 7 days. There is considerable variation in the spectrum of clinical features, which range from mild diarrhea simulating common forms of gastroenteritis to acute enteritis and a fulminant course with death in 24 hours.

DIAGNOSIS. The diagnosis in the endemic area is usually established by clinical observations that are sometimes supported by typical pathologic changes in the small bowel noted at surgery or autopsy. The responsible agent may be recognized in bowel contents or stool using fluorescent-stained antibody to the capsular antigen of the putative agent.[122] Cultures are difficult to interpret due to relatively high carrier rates in asymptomatic persons from both the endemic area as well as other

TABLE 7. Comparison of Enteric Diseases Due to Histotoxic Clostridia

	C. perfringens *food poisoning*	*Enteritis necroticans*	C. difficile *induced colitis*	*Neutropenic enterocolitis*
Agent	*C. perfringens* type A	*C. perfringens* type C	*C. difficile*	*C. septicum* (*C. tertium*, *C. perfringens*, others)
Toxin	Enterotoxin	β-toxin	Toxin A	Unclear; β-toxin
MW (daltons)	34–35,000	30–48,000	2400–320,000	?
Trypsin sensitivity	Negative	Positive	Positive	?
Mouse LD_{50} (ng)	80,000	400	50	?
Rabbit ileal loop	Fluid flux, epithelial damage	Segmental transmural necrosis	Mucosal hemorrhage, fluid flux	?
Distribution	Worldwide	New Guinea; other Third World countries	Worldwide	Worldwide
Carrier rate	90–95% for *C. perfringens*; up to 30% for enterotoxin-producing strains	20–70% in endemic areas	3% in healthy adults	2% for *C. septicum* (10–63% in appendix)
Diagnosis	Serology; enterotoxin assay of stools; quantitative culture of food source and stools	Serology; fluorescence-labeled Ab to capsular Ag to demonstrate organism	Tissue culture assay for Toxin B	Blood cultures
Host	Exposure to food-borne source	Malnourished children	Antibiotic exposure, primarily adults	Neutropenia, leukemia (relapse), colon cancer
Clinical findings	Diarrhea, abdominal cramps with minimal systemic toxicity	Bloody diarrhea, vomiting, abdominal pain	Diarrhea ± fecal leukocytes; fever	Septicemia, abdominal pain, vomiting, diarrhea, shock
Pathology	Small bowel epithelial damage, polymorphonuclear infiltrate	Small bowel segmental transmural necrosis	Colitis ± pseudomembranes	Colinic (usually cecal) with hemorrhagic necrosis
Treatment	None (self-limited)	Penicillin ± surgery	Vancomycin or metronidazole orally	Penicillin ± surgery
Mortality	Nil	15–45% (serious cases)	10–20% (serious cases; untreated)	50–100%

geographic regions and the frequent overgrowth of *C. perfringens* type A in stool cultures.[125]

TREATMENT. The preferred antibiotics are chloramphenicol or penicillin G. Supportive measures include intravenous fluids and careful monitoring of serum electrolytes, with special attention to potassium depletion. Intestinal decompression may be required with nasogastric intubation. Indications for surgical intervention include persistent toxicity, persistent intestinal obstruction, suspected perforation, and severe recurrent bleeding. Approximately 50 percent of patients with serious disease require surgery, which generally consists of resecting 50–200 cm of jejunum. Administration of antiserum has no role. Excluding patients with mild disease, the mortality rate is reported at 15–45 percent. More promising is prevention of the disease using β-toxoid vaccine prepared from culture filtrates of the responsible organism.[126,127]

Clostridium perfringens Food Poisoning. Enterotoxin-producing strains of *C. perfringens* type A are responsible for a mild and common form of food poisoning that is found throughout the world and as an occasional cause of sporadic diarrhea that may or may not be associated with antibiotic usage.[128,129]

PATHOGEN. *Clostridium perfringens* type A is responsible for nearly all cases of *C. perfringens* food poisoning, although an identical enterotoxin has been detected in some strains of types C and D.[130] The enterotoxin is a structural component of the spore coat, so that methods of detecting toxigenic potential include ways of enhancing sporulation. The most frequently employed method is the "DS" media described by Duncan and Strong.[131] Yasukawa et al. studied sonicates from 7-hour broth cultures in DS medium with an agar gel double immunodiffusion assay to detect enterotoxin.[132] They found enterotoxin production by 51 of 66 strains from food borne disease cases, compared with 1 of 117 strains recovered from stools of healthy controls. Subsequent work[133] suggested that the frequency of toxigenic potential in this report was low because of a faulty screening process. Heat treatment prior to incubation in DS enhanced toxin production, and reversed passive hemagglutination appeared more sensitive for toxin detection. Using this technique, Uemura showed that 11 of 35 (31 percent) healthy persons harbored toxigenic strains.[133]

The enterotoxin is a polypeptide with a molecular weight of about 35,000 daltons and is susceptible to pronase, but not trypsin, chymotrypsin, or papin.[134–138] Biologic activities of the toxin include the positive rabbit ileal loop assay with fluid accumulation at 90 minutes after challenge; induction of vomiting in cynomolgus monkeys with orogastric challenge; lethality with intravenous challenge to mice (LD_{50} of 80 μg); and cytotoxicity to Vero cells.[139–142] In the small bowel, the enterotoxin binds to a brush border membrane receptor and then induces a calcium ion-dependent breakdown of colloid–osmotic equilibrium, resulting in a size-dependent loss of intracellular material.[141,143,144] This loss alters intracellular metabolic function, including macromolecular synthesis, which is associated with morphologic changes in the cells and eventual cell death. Analogous binding, disrupted equilibrium with loss of intracellular material, and cell death is seen in vitro with Vero cells.[144]

EPIDEMIOLOGY. *Clostridium perfringens* food poisoning follows ingestion of food containing at least 10^8 enterotoxin-producing strains. The most frequent vehicles are cooked meat, poultry, stews, meat pies, and gravies that have become grossly contaminated during long periods of slow cooling and storage at ambient temperature.[145] The spores survive cooking, the heat-activated spores then germinate as the temperature decreases, and optimal growth in meat is achieved at 43–47°C with a generation time of 10–12 minutes.

Clostridium perfringens is a relatively common form of food-borne outbreak. Data from the Centers for Disease Control indicate that *C. perfringens* accounts for approximately 7 percent of such outbreaks in the United States, with an average of 24 victims per outbreak.[145] It is likely that many outbreaks are overlooked due to relatively mild clinical symptoms and the specialized laboratory techniques required for case confirmation.

The initial studies of the diarrhea disease caused by *C. perfringens* concerned food-borne outbreaks. More recently, it has been appreciated that the epidemiologic spectrum of this disease is more extensive. Other settings in which this organism has been implicated include sporadic cases of diarrhea, antibiotic-associated diarrhea, and diarrhea in chronic care facilities.[128,129,146] Patients with these alternative forms appear to have a different clinical presentation in that the diarrhea is more persistent, with an average duration of 11 days.[128]

CLINICAL FEATURES. Most cases occur in the setting of an outbreak due to exposure to a common source, most frequently meat.[145,147] Sporadic cases are presumably common as well, but are unlikely to be investigated. Such exposure is claimed to be an occasional mechanism of antibiotic-associated diarrhea. In outbreaks, the attack rate in exposed persons averages 50–60 percent. One of the largest outbreaks was a banquet in New York City attended by 1800 people, over 900 of whom developed symptomatic disease.[148] The incubation period following exposure is brief, usually 7–15 hours, with a range of 6–24 hours. The usual symptoms are diarrhea in over 90 percent and abdominal cramps in about 80 percent.[145,149] Less frequent symptoms are nausea, (25 percent) vomiting, (9 percent) and fever (24 percent). Nearly all patients have spontaneous resolution of symptoms within 6–24 hours. As noted above, patients with *C. perfringens*-associated diarrhea from nonfood-borne sources have more prolonged illness, which tends to resemble *Campylobacter* infection or salmonellosis.[128]

DIAGNOSIS. *Clostridium perfringens* food poisoning is suspect in any outbreak of diarrhea with abdominal cramps occurring 7–15 hours after ingestion of a common food source. Suggested diagnostic criteria include (*1*) detection of 10^5 *C. perfringens*/g in the common food source; and (*2*) stools obtained within 48 hours of symptoms showing 10^6/g of *C. perfringens* spores.[150] However, mean fecal spore counts of this magnitude may be seen in patients without symptoms.[150] An alternative and generally preferred method is direct analysis of stools for enterotoxin with a reverse passive latex agglutination assay,[151,152] enzyme-linked immunoassay,[153] and a tissue culture assay using Vero cells with neutralizing antibody to inhibit cytopathic effects.[128]

TREATMENT

Clostridial infections represent a heterogeneous group of conditions involving at least 30 different species. Recommendations for treatment vary, although there are some general principles worth reviewing.

The histotoxic clostridial syndromes (Table 2) involve protein toxins with the potential for passive or active immunization. Vaccine is widely endorsed for tetanus, and it is recommended for the prevention of enteritis necroticans in New Guinea, where the disease is endemic. Passive protection with immunoglobulin is advocated for patients with tetanus and for adults with botulism. Antitoxin was previously available for toxins produced by five of the clostridial species responsible for gas gangrene, but efficacy was not well established and the antisera is no longer commercially available. Antitoxin is also available for *C. difficile*, including a *C. sordellii* antitoxin that neutralizes both toxin A and toxin B by antigenic cross-reactivity and monospecific antitoxins to toxin A and toxin B. These preparations have never been tested for potential efficacy by parenteral or enteral administration, which may reflect the nearly uniform therapeutic response to antimicrobial treatment. Thus, with few exceptions, immunotherapy plays a minor role in the treatment of histotoxic clostridial syndromes despite its theoretical attractiveness.

The role of surgery depends on the nature of the infection. Most clostridial infections involve a mixture of aerobic and anaerobic bacteria and obey the usual guidelines for surgery that would apply if clostridia were not present. The clostridial infections that warrant aggressive surgical intervention in terms of timing or extent of resection are emphysematous cholecystitis, neutropenic enterocolitis with *C. septicum* bacteremia, enteritis necroticans, wounds associated with tetanus, some cases of crepitant cellulitis, and all cases of gas gangrene.

With regard to antibiotics, penicillin G is generally considered the drug of choice for clostridial infections. Exceptions are *C. difficile*-induced diarrhea or colitis in which oral vancomycin or metronidazole are the preferred agents, and infant botulism and *C. perfringens* enteritis for which antibiotics are not indicated. Alternative agents that are highly active in vitro versus most clostridial strains are chloramphenicol, imipenem, metronidazole, most expanded spectrum cephalosporins, and combinations of a β-lactamase and β-lactamase inhibitor.[12,105–107] Penicillins other than penicillin G are also highly active, including ampicillin and the antipseudomonad penicillins. The role of cephalosporins and clindamycin is difficult to define. Most cephalosporins other than cefoxitin are quite active in vitro, although it is disturbing that some patients have developed gas gangrene while receiving cephalothin,[108] and the published clinical experience with these agents is limited. Clindamycin is relatively inactive in vitro against some strains other than *C. perfringens*, but this drug shows exceptional in vivo activity in an animal model of gas gangrene.[110]

Despite the nearly universal endorsement of penicillin for clostridial infections, there are a few concerns regarding such a sweeping recommendation, based on in vitro data and experimental animal studies. There appears to be increasing resistance of these organisms to penicillin, although nearly all strains of *C. perfringens* remain susceptible to levels easily achieved with parenteral dosing. β-Lactamase production has been observed with *C. butyricum, C. clostridioforme*, and *C. ramosum*. Decreased affinity of the penicillin-binding proteins has been noted for some strains of *C. perfringens*. Additionally, plasmid-mediated transferrable resistance to tetracycline–chloramphenicol and clindamycin–erythromycin has been observed with *C. perfringens*. These data suggest that resistance is evolving slowly, but most clostridia remain susceptible to a diverse array of antimicrobial agents, with penicillin serving continually as the preferred agent by most authorities. Despite this recommendation, penicillin performs poorly in animal models of gas gangrene, in which survival statistics are significantly better for metronidazole, clindamycin, rifampin, and tetracycline.[93,109,110] The significance of this observation in terms of current recommendations is unknown, but it does suggest that alternative drugs should be considered.

REFERENCES

1. Cato E, George WL, Finegold SM. Genus *Clostridium* Prazmowski. In: Sneath PHA, Mair NS, Sharge ME, Holt JG, eds. 1880 Bergey's Manual of Systematic Bacteriology. v. 2. Baltimore: Williams & Wilkins; 1986:1141–200.
2. Willis AT. Anaerobic Bacteriology: Clinical and Laboratory Practice. 3rd ed. London: Butterworth; 1977:68–172.
3. Veillon A, Zuber A. Recherches sur quelques microbes strictement anaerobies et leur role en pathologie. Arch Med Exp Anat Pathol. 1898;10:517–45.
4. Smith LDS. The Pathogenic Anaerobic Bacteria. 2nd ed. Springfield, IL: Charles C Thomas; 1975:115–324.
5. Smith LDS, Gardner VM. Vegetative cells of *Clostridium perfringens* in soil. J Bacteriol. 1949;58:407–8.
6. Beerens H, Delcourte F. Caractère differential entre *Clostridium perfringens* fécal et tellurique. Ann Inst Pasteur. 1958;95:739–40.
7. Finegold SM, Attebery HR, Sutter VL. Effect of diet on human fecal flora: comparison of Japanese and American diets. Am J Clin Nutr. 1974;27:1456–69.
8. Stringer MF, Watson GN, Gilbert RJ, et al. Fecal carriage of *Clostridium perfringens*. J Hyg. 1985;95:277–88.
9. Kuberski TT. Intraleukocytic spore formation and leukocytic vacuolization during *Clostridium perfringens* septicemia. Am J Clin Pathol. 1977;68:794–6.
10. Gorbach SL, Thadepalli H. Isolation of *Clostridium* in human infections: evaluation of 114 cases. J Infect Dis. 1985;131:S81–S85.
11. Martin WJ. Isolation and identification of anaerobic bacteria in the clinical laboratory. A 2-year experience. Mayo Clin Proc. 1974;49:300.
12. Finegold SM, George WL, Mulligan ME. Anaerobic infections. Dis Mon. 1985;31:10–77.

13. Nichols RL, Smith JW. Gas in the wound: what does it mean? Surg Clin N Am. 1975;55:1289–96.
14. Ram MD, Ghavari MA. Biliary infections and the choice of antibiotics. Am J Gastroenterol. 1974;62:134–8.
15. Mentzer RM Jr, Golden GT, Chandler JG, et al. Emphysematous cholecystitis: an important clinical variant of acute cholecystitis. Rev Surg. 1974;31:454–6.
16. Stephenson SE Jr, Yasrebi H, Rhatigan R, et al. Acute phlegmasia of the stomach. Am Surg. 1970;36:225.
17. Lazurus JA. *Bacillus welchii* infections complicating surgical procedures upon the upper urinary tract. J Urol. 1944;51:315.
18. Ramsay AM. The significance of *Clostridium welchii* in the cervical swab and blood stream in postpartum and postabortum sepsis. J Obstet Gynecol. 1949;56:247.
19. Rathbun HK. Clostridial bacteremia without hemolysis. Arch Intern Med. 1968;122:496.
20. Alpern RJ, Dowell VR Jr. Nonhistotoxic clostridial bacteremia. Am J Clin Pathol. 1971;33:717.
21. Editorial. *Clostridium septicum* and neutropenic enterocolitis. Lancet. 1987;2:608.
22. Alpern RJ, Dowell VR. *Clostridium septicum* infection and malignancy. JAMA. 1969;209:385–8.
23. Koransky JR, Stargel MD, Dowell VR. *Clostridium septicum* bacteremia. Its clinical significance. Am J Med. 1979;66:63–6.
24. Kunkel JM, Rosenthal D. Management of the ileocecal syndrome: neutropenic enterocolitis. Dis Colon Rectum. 1986;29:196–9.
25. Mower WJ, Hawkins JA, Nelson EW. Neutropenic enterocolitis in adults with acute leukemia. Arch Surg. 1986;121:571–3.
26. Rifkin GD. Neutropenic enterocolitis and *Clostridium septicum* infection in patients with agranulocytosis. Arch Intern Med. 1980;140:834–5.
27. Bignold LP, Harvey HPB. Necrotizing enterocolitis associated with invasion by *Clostridium septicum* complicating cyclic neutropenia. Aust NZ J Med. 1979;9:426–9.
28. Boggs DR, Frei E, Thomas LB. Clostridial gas gangrene and septicemia in four patients with leukemia. N Engl J Med. 1958;259:1255.
29. Hopkins DG, Kushner JP. Clostridial species in pathogenesis of necrotizing enterocolitis in patients with neutropenia. Am J Hematol. 1983;14:289–95.
30. Panwalker AP. Unusual infections associated with colorectal cancer. Rev Infect Dis. 1988;10:347–64.
31. Bretzke ML, Bubrick MP, Hitchcock CR. Diffuse spreading *Clostridium septicum* infection, malignant disease and immune suppression. Surg Gynecol Obstet. 1988;166:197–9.
31a. Kornbluth AA, Danzig JB, Bernstein LH. *Clostridium septicum* infection and associated malignancy. Medicine. 1989;68:30–7.
32. MacLennen JD. Anaerobic infections of war wounds in the middle east. Lancet. 1943;2:94.
33. Tikko SK, Distenfield A, Davidson M. *Clostridium septicum* septicemia with identical metastatic myonecrosis in a granulocytopenic patient. Am J Med. 1985;79:256.
34. Gorse GJ, Slater LH, Sobol E, et al. CNS infection and bacteremia due to *Clostridium septicum*. Arch Neurol. 1984;41:882–4.
35. Neimkin RJ, Jupiter JB. Metastatic nontraumatic *Clostridium septicum* osteomyelitis. J Hand Surg. 1985;10:281–4.
36. Macy NJ, Lieber L, Habermann ET. Arthritis caused by *Clostridium septicum*. J Bone Joint Surg. 1986;68:465–6.
37. Insler MS, Karcioglu ZA, Naugle T. *Clostridium septicum* panophthalmitis with systemic complications. Br J Ophthalmol. 1985;69:774–7.
38. George WL, Finegold SM. Clostridia in the human gastrointestinal flora. In: Boriello SP, ed. Clostridia in Gastrointestinal Disease. Boca Raton, FL: CRC Press; 1985:1–37.
39. Felitti VJ. Primary invasion by *Clostridium sphenoides* in a patient with periodic neutropenia. Calif Med. 1973;113:76–8.
40. Gruter H. Gas gangrene following antibiotic-associated enterocolitis in hereditary neutropenia. Arch Anat Cytol Pathol. 1985;33:23–5.
41. Newbold KM, Lord MG, Baglin TP. Role of clostridial organisms in neutropenic enterocolitis. J Clin Pathol. 1987;40:471.
42. Thaler M, Gill V, Pizzo PA. Emergence of *Clostridium tertium* as a pathogen in neutropenic patients. Am J Med. 1986;81:596.
43. Yates P, MacGowan AP, Potter M, et al. Clostridia and neutropenic enterocolitis. Lancet. 1988;1:185.
43a. Speirs G, Warren RE, Rampling A. Clostridium tertium septicemia in patients with neutropenia. J Infect Dis. 1988;158:1336–40.
44. Gorbach SL, Thadepalli H, Norsen J. Anaerobic microorganisms in intraabdominal infections. In: Balows A, DeHann RM, Dowell VR Jr, Guze LB, eds. Anaerobic Bacteria: Role in Disease. Springfield, IL: Charles C Thomas; 1974:399–407.
45. Dunn DL, Simmons RL. The role of anaerobic bacteria in intraabdominal infections. Rev Infect Dis. 1984;6:S139.
46. Moore WEC, Cato EP, Holdeman LV. Anaerobic bacteria of the gastrointestinal flora and their occurrence in clinical infections. J Infect Dis. 1969;119:641.
47. Stone HH, Kolb LD, Geheber CE. Incidence and significance of intraperitoneal anaerobic bacteria. Ann Surg. 1975;181:705–14.
48. Gordon-Taylor G, Whitby LEH. The incidence of anaerobic infections in the gall-bladder. Br J Surg. 1932;19:619.
49. England DM, Rosenblatt JE. Anaerobes in human biliary tracts. J Clin Microbiol. 1977;6:494–8.
50. Lykkegaard Nielsen M, Justesen T. Anaerobic and aerobic bacteriological studies in biliary tract disease. Scand J Gastroenterol. 1976;11:437–46.
51. Shimada K, Inamatsu T, Yamashiro M. Anaerobic bacteria in biliary disease in elderly patients. J Infect Dis. 1977;135:850.
52. Sarmiento RV. Emphysematous cholecystitis: report of four cases and review of the literature. Arch Surg. 1966;93:1009.
53. Edinburgh A, Geffen A. Acute emphysematous cholecystitis. Am J Surg. 1958;96:66.
54. Mentzer RM Jr, Golden GT, Chandler JG, et al. A comparative appraisal of emphysematous cholecystitis. Am J Surg. 1975;129:11.
55. Stolz A. Ueber Gasbildung in den Gallenwegen. Virchows Arch Pathol Anat. 1901;165:90.
56. Hegner CF. Gaseous pericholecystitis with cholecystitis and cholelithiasis. Arch Surg. 1931;22:993.
57. Heifetz CJ, Wyloge EI. Effect of distention of gallbladder with air and its relationship to acute pneumocholecystitis. Ann Surg. 1955;142:283.
58. Thadepalli H, Gorbach SL, Keith L. Anaerobic infections of the female genital tract: bacteriologic and therapeutic aspects. Am J Obstet Gynecol. 1973;117:1034–40.
59. Swenson RM, Michaelson TC, Daly MJ, et al. Anaerobic bacterial infections of the female genital tract. Obstet Gynecol. 1973;42:538–41.
60. DiZerega GS, Yonekura ML, Keegan K, et al. Bacteremia in post-cesarean section endomyometritis: differential response to therapy. Obstet Gynecol. 1980;55:587–90.
61. Sweet RL. Anaerobic infections of the female genital tract. Am J Obstet Gynecol. 1975;122:891.
62. Ledger WJ, Norman M, Gee C, et al. Bacteremia on an obstetric-gynecologic service. Am J Obstet Gynecol. 1975;121:205.
63. Ohm MJ, Galask RP. The effect of antibiotic prophylaxis on patients undergoing vaginal operations. Am J Obstet Gynecol. 1975;123:597.
64. Bartlett JG, Onderdonk AB, Drude E, et al. Quantitative bacteriology of the vaginal flora. J Infect Dis. 1977;136:271.
65. Decker WH, Hall W. Treatment of abortions infected with *Clostridium welchii*. Am J Obstet Gynecol. 1966;95:394.
66. Smith LP, McLean AP, Maughan GB. *Clostridium welchii* septicotoxemia. Am J Obstet Gynecol. 1971;110:135.
67. Pritchard JA, Whalley PJ. Abortion complicated by *Clostridium perfringens* infection. Am J Obstet Gynecol. 1971;111:484.
68. Soper DE. Clostridial myonecrosis arising from an episiotomy. Obstet Gynecol. 1986;68:26S–8S.
69. Bartlett JG. Anaerobic bacterial infections of the lung. Chest. 1987;91:901.
70. Bayer AS, Nelson SC, Galpin JE, et al. Necrotizing pneumonia and empyema due to *Clostridium perfringens*. Am J Med. 1975;59:851.
71. O'Donnell AE. Primary clostridial pneumonia—report of a case. Lancet. 1952;2:367.
72. Sweeting J, Rosenberg L. Primary clostridial pneumonia. Ann Intern Med. 1959;51:805.
73. Jacox R. A case report of an unusual lung abscess due to *Clostridium perfringens* (B. welchii). Ann Intern Med. 1951;34:479.
74. Glaser LF, Glynn R, Ernest HB. Gas bacillus gangrene of lung. JAMA. 1941;116:827.
75. Goldberg NM, Rifkind D. Clostridial empyema. Arch Intern Med. 1965;115:421.
76. Mamborg AS, Rylander M, Selander H. Primary thoracic empyema caused by *Clostridium sporogenes*. Scand J Infect Dis. 1970;2:155.
77. Hardison JE. Primary clostridial pneumonia and empyema. Chest. 1970;57:390–2.
78. Elliot TR, Henry H. Infection of hemothorax by anaerobic gas producing bacilli. Br Med J. 1917;1:413.
79. Lynch JF, Strieder J. Hemothorax complicated by infection with *Clostridium welchii*. N Engl J Med. 1942;226:685.
80. Cairns H, Calvert CA, Daniel P, et al. Complications of head wounds with special reference to infection. Br J Surg [War Surg Suppl]. 1947;1:198.
81. Keogh AJ. Clostridial brain abscess and hyperbaric oxygen. Postgrad Med J. 1973;49:64–6.
82. Russell JA, Taylor JC. Circumscribed gas gangrene abscess of the brain. Case report together with an account of the literature. Br J Surg. 1963;50:434.
83. Colwell FG, Sullivan J, Shuman HH, et al. Acute purulent meningitis due to *Clostridium perfringens*. N Engl J Med. 1960;262:618.
84. Clark PR. Gas gangrene abscess of the brain. J Neurol Neurosurg Psychiatry. 1968;31:391.
85. Gilbert AI, Tolmach RS, Farrell JJ. Gas gangrene of the brain. Am J Surg. 1961;101:366.
86. Qvist G. Anaerobic cellulitis and gas gangrene. Br Med J. 1941;2:4206.
87. MacLennan JD. Anaerobic infections of war wounds in the Middle East. Lancet. 1943;2:94.
88. Wilson TS. The significance of *C. welchii* infections and their relationship to gas gangrene. Can J Surg. 1960;4:35.
89. Filler RM, Griscom NT, Pappas A. Post-traumatic creditation falsely suggesting gas gangrene. N Engl J Med. 1968;278:758–61.
90. VanBeek A, Zook E, Gardner R, et al. Nonclostridial gas-forming infections. Arch Surg. 1974;108:552.
91. Kaneyama S, Sato H, Murata R. The role of alpha toxin of *Clostridium perfringens* in experimental gas gangrene in guinea pigs. Jpn J Med Sci Biol. 1975;25:200.
92. MacLennan JD. The histotoxic clostridial infections of man. Bacteriol Rev. 1962;26:177.

93. Altemeier WA, Furste WL. Gas gangrene. Surg Gynecol Obstet. 1947; 84:507.
94. Altemeier WA, Furste WL. Studies in virulence of *Clostridium welchii*. Surgery. 1949;25:12.
95. Simeone F. Clostridial myositis. In: Symposium on Military Medicine in the Far East Command. Surg Circ Lett Med Section [Suppl]. September, 1951.
96. Brown PW, Kinman PB. Gas gangrene in a metropolitan community. J Bone Joint Surg. 1974;56-A:1445.
97. Lowbury EJL, Lilly HA. The sources of hospital infection of wounds with *Clostridium welchii*. J Hyg. 1958;56:169.
98. Eickhoff TC. An outbreak of surgical wound infections due to *Clostridium perfringens*. Surg Gynecol Obstet. 1962;114:102.
99. Altemeier WA, Fullen WD. Prevention and treatment of gas gangrene. JAMA. 1971;217:806.
100. Caplan ES, Kluge RM. Gas gangrene: review of 34 cases. Arch Intern Med. 1976;136:788.
101. Heimbach RD. Gas gangrene: review and update. HBO Rev. 1980;1:41.
102. Krebs B, Moller BN, Jensen BH. Gas producing infections after lower limb amputatioon because of ischemia. Arch Orthop Trauma Surg. 1986;104:374.
103. Weinstein L, Barza M. Gas gangrene. N Engl J Med. 1973;289:1129.
104. Darke SG, King AM, Slack WK. Gas gangrene and related infection: classification, clinical features and etiology, management and mortality. A report of 88 cases. Br J Surg. 1977;64:104.
105. Schwartzman JD, Reller LB, Wang W-L. Susceptibility of *Clostridium perfringens* isolated from human infections to twenty antibiotics. Antimicrob Agents Chemother. 1977;11:695.
106. Marrie TJ, Haldane EV, Swantee CA, et al. Susceptibility of anaerobic bacteria to nine antimicrobial agents and demonstration of decreased susceptibility of *Clostridium perfringens* to penicillin. Antimicrob Agents Chemother. 1981;19:51–5.
107. Brazier JS, Levett PN, Stannard AL, et al. Antibiotic susceptibility of clinical isolates of *Clostridia*. J Antimicrob Chemother. 1985;15:181.
108. Mohr JA, Griffiths W, Holm R, et al. Clostridial myonecrosis (gas gangrene) during cephalosporin prophylaxis. JAMA. 1978;239:847.
109. Altemeier WA, McMurrin JA, Alt AP. Chloromycetin and aureomycin in experimental gas gangrene. Surgery. 1950;28:621.
110. Stevens DL, Maier KA, Laine BM, et al. Comparison of clindamycin, rifampin, tetracycline, metronidazole, and penicillin for efficacy in prevention of experimental gas gangrene due to *Clostridium perfringens*. J Infect Dis. 1987;155:220.
111. Gibson A, Davis FM. Hyperbaric oxygen therapy in the management of *Clostridium perfringens* infections. NZ Med J. 1986;99:617.
112. Demello FJ, Raglin JJ, Hitchcock CR. Comparative study of experimental *Clostridium perfringens* infection in dogs treated with antibiotics, surgery and hyperbaric oxygen. Surgery. 1971;73:936–41.
113. Zeissler J, Rassfeld-Sternberg L. Enteritis necroticans due to *Clostridium welchii* type F. Br Med J. 1949;11:267.
114. Field HI, Goodwin RFW. The experimental reproduction of enteroxaemia in piglets. J Hyg. 1959;57:81.
115. Murrell TGC, Roth L. Necrotizing jejunitis: a newly discovered disease in the highlands of New Guinea. Med J Aust. 1963;1:61.
116. Lawrence GW, Murrell TGC, Walker PD, eds. Symposium on pig-bel. Papua New Guinea Med J. 1979;22:1–108.
117. Murrell TGC. Some epidemiological features of pig-bel. Papua New Guinea Med J. 1966;9:39–50.
118. Murrell TCG. Pig-bel in Papua New Guinea: an ancient disease discovered. Int J Epidemiol. 1983;12:211.
119. Davis M. A review of pig-bel (necrotizing enteritis) in Papua New Guinea 1961–1984. Papua New Guinea Med J. 1985;2:75.
120. Lawrence G, Cooke R. Experimental pigbel. Br J Exp Pathol. 1980;61:261.
121. Akama K, Otani S, Kameyama S. Purification of β-toxin of *Clostridium perfringens* type C. Jpn J Med Sci Biol. 1968;21:423–6.
122. Karanth S, Coninx R, Dickson C, et al. Enteritis necroticans (pig-bel) on Thai/Kampuchean border? Lancet. 1986;1:1437.
123. Cooke B. The pathology of pigbel. Papua New Guinea Med J. 1979;22:35.
124. Walker PD, Murrell TGC, Nagy LK. Scanning electron microscopy of the jejunum in enteritis necroticans. J Med Microbiol. 1980;13:445–50.
125. Hain E. Origin of *C. welchii* type F in normal stools. Br Med J. 1949;1:271.
126. Rooney J, Shepherd A, Sueby A. *Clostridium welchii* type C antitoxin in the treatment of pig-bel (enteritis necroticans): a controlled trial in Papua, New Guinea. Papua New Guinea Med J. 1979;22:57–9.
127. Lawrence G, Shann F, Freestone DS, et al. Prevention of necrotising enteritis in Papua New Guinea by active immunization. Lancet. 1979;1:227–30.
128. Larson HE, Borriello SP. Infectious diarrhea due to *Clostridium perfringens*. J Infect Dis. 1988;157:390.
129. Luzzi I, Caprioli A, Bisicchia R, et al. A sporadic case of diarrhoea due to enterotoxigenic *Clostridium perfringens*. Microbiol Ecol Health Dis. 1988;1:69–70.
130. Uemura T, Sskjelkvale R. An enterotoxin produced by *Clostridium perfringens* type D. Acta Pathol Microbiol Scand. 1976;84:414–20.
131. Duncan CL, Strong SH. Improved medium for sporulation of *Clostridium perfringens*. Appl Microbiol. 1968;16:82–89.
132. Yasukawa A, Okada Y, Kitase T, et al. Distribution of enterotoxin producing strains of *Clostridium perfringens* type A in human beings, food and soils. J Food Hyg Soc Jpn. 1975;16:313–7.
133. Uemura T. Incidence of enterogenic *Clostridium perfringens* in healthy humans in relation to the enhancement of enterotoxin production by heat treatment. J Appl Bacteriol. 1978;44:411–9.
134. Hauschild AH, Hilscheimer R. Purification and characteristics of the enterotoxin of *Clostridium perfringens* type A. Can J Microbiol. 1971;17:1425–33.
135. Sakaguchi G, Uemura T, Riemann H. A simplified method for purification of *Clostridium perfringens* type A enterotoxin. Appl Microbiol. 1973;27:762–7.
136. Skjelkvale R, Duncal CL. Enterotoxin formation by different toxigenic types of *Clostridium perfringens*. Infect Immun. 1975;11:563–75.
137. Granum PE, Whitaker JR. Improved method for purification of enterotoxin from *Clostridium perfringens* type A. Appl Environ Microbiol. 1980; 39:1120–2.
138. Horiguchi Y, Uemura T, Kamata Y, et al. Production and characterization of monoclonal antibodies to *Clostridium perfringens* enterotoxin. Infect Immun. 1986;52:31–35.
139. Granum PE, Skjelkvale R. Chemical modification and characterization of enterotoxin from *Clostridium perfringens* type A. Acta Pathol Microbiol Scand. 1977;85:89–94.
140. Niilo L. Measurement of biological activities of purified and crude enterotoxin of *Clostridium perfringens*. Infect Immun. 1975;12:440–2.
141. McDonel JL, McClane BA. Binding versus biologic activity of *Clostridium perfringens* enterotoxin in Vero cells. Biochem Biophys Res Commun. 1979;87:497–504.
142. Tolleshang H, Skjelkvale R, Berg T. Quantitation of binding and subcellular distribution of *Clostridium perfringens* enterotoxin in rat liver cells. Infect Immun. 1982;37:486–91.
143. McDonel JL. Binding of *Clostridium perfringens* enterotoxin to rabbit intestinal cells. Biochemistry. 1980;21:4801.
144. McClane BA, McDonel JL. The effects of *Clostridium perfringens* enterotoxin on morphology viability and macromolecular synthesis in Vero cells. J Cell Physiol. 1979;99:191–9.
145. Shandera WX, Tacket CO, Blake PA. Food poisoning due to *Clostridium perfringens* in the United States. J Infect Dis. 1983;147:167.
146. Jackson SG, Yip-Chuck DA, Clark JB, et al. Diagnostic importance of *Clostridium perfringens* enterotoxin analysis in recurring enteritis among elderly, chronic care psychiatric patients. J Clin Microbiol. 1986;23:748.
147. Collee JG, Knowlden JA, Hobbs BC. Studies on the growth, sporulation and carriage of *Clostridium welchii* with special reference to food poisoning strains. J Appl Bacteriol. 1961;24:326.
148. Finegold SM. Anaerobic Bacteria in Human Disease. New York: Academic Press; 1977:511–2.
149. Skjelkvale R, Uemura T. Experimental diarrhoea in human volunteers following oral administration of *Clostridium perfringens* enterotoxin. J Appl Bacteriol. 1977;43:281–6.
150. Birkhead G, Vogt RL, Heum EM, et al. Characterization of an outbreak of *Clostridium perfringens* food poisoning by quantitative fecal culture and fecal enterotoxin measurement. J Clin Microbiol. 1988;26:471.
151. McClane BA, Snyder JT. Development and preliminary evaluation of a slide latex agglutination assay for determination of *Clostridium perfringens* type A enterotoxin. J Immunol Methods. 1987;100:131–6.
152. Harmon SM, Kautter DA. Evaluation of reversed passive latex agglutination test kit for *Clostridium perfringens*. J Food Prot. 1986;49:523–5.
153. McClane BA, Strouse RJ. Rapid detection of *Clostridium perfringens* type A enterotoxin by enzyme-linked immunosorbent assay. J Clin Microbiol. 1984;19:112–5.
154. Sutter V et al, eds. Wadsworth Anaerobic Bacteriology Manual, 3rd ed. St. Louis: CV Mosby; 1980.

223. BACTEROIDES SPECIES

DORI F. ZALEZNIK
DENNIS L. KASPER

Bacteroides species are anaerobic organisms found as constituents of the normal flora of humans in the oral cavity, gastrointestinal tract, and female genital tract. Of this group of organisms, *Bacteroides fragilis* is the single anaerobic species isolated most frequently from infected sites and is a particularly important anaerobic organism. The importance of *Bacteroides* species, in general, derives from the frequency of isolation in infections, virulence factors that appear to influence incidence and types of infections, and antibiotic resistance that alters antibiotic selection when these organisms are suspected. Among the major types of infections caused by these bacteria are abscesses and periodontal disease.

CLASSIFICATION AND BACTERIOLOGY

Clinically, gram-negative anaerobes can be grouped generally using criteria of colonial appearance, morphology under Gram stain, sensitivity to select test antibiotics, and biochemical tests.[1,2] *Bacteroides fragilis* can be distinguished from other *Bacteroides* species and from *Fusobacterium* by growth in the presence of 20% bile (which inhibits most other *Bacteroides* species and *Fusobacterium*), catalase positivity, and resistance to kanamycin, vancomycin, and colistin. Strains also may be indole-positive. *Bacteroides fragilis* grow as 1–3 mm glistening colonies that are nonhemolytic on blood agar plates. By Gram stain, the organism is a pale, gram-negative bacillus that may appear pleomorphic and may stain irregularly; it is aerotolerant. In contrast, members of the *Bacteroides melaninogenicus* group form pigmented, brown to black colonies after approximately 1 week, especially on rabbit blood agar. By ultraviolet light, one may observe a red fluorescence of young colonies that have not yet become pigmented. Organisms of this group are inhibited by bile and are catalase-negative, indole-variable, resistant to kanamycin, and variable to vancomycin and colistin. *Fusobacterium* are longer, slender, gram-negative rods, catalase-negative, indole-positive, and sensitive to kanamycin.

More sophisticated methods for species identification by further biochemical testing include inoculating tubes containing carbohydrates and measuring pH after growth as well as gas-liquid chromatography (GLC) to examine fatty acid end products.[2] Fluorescent antibody reagents also are available for rapid diagnosis, although this has not become a widespread clinical tool.[1] Typing by means of bacteriophages also has been proposed.[3]

With development of newer techniques, DNA homology has provided a means for more precise classification of *Bacteroides* species.[4] Previously termed subspecies of *Bacteroides fragilis*—*B. thetaiotaomicron, B. vulgatus, B. distasonis, B. ovatus,* and *B. uniformis*—as well as *B. fragilis* now are considered separate species based on DNA homology (Table 1). DNA homology has led to the reclassification of the *B. melaninogenicus* group as well into six distinct species including *B. melaninogenicus, B. intermedius, B. gingivalis, B. denticola, B. loescheii,* and *B. corporis*. In addition, other Bacteroides species include members of the *Bacteroides oralis* group—*B. oris, B. buccae, B. capillus*, and *B. pentosaceus*. *Bacteroides bivius* and *B. disiens* are newly recognized *Bacteroides* species and are important in normal vaginal flora.

In recent years an understanding of the genetics of these organisms has begun to emerge, an important area of study well-summarized by Salyers et al.[5] Plasmids containing genes for resistance to clindamycin–erythromycin, including pBF4, pBFTM10, and pBI136, have been identified. Curiously, two of these plasmids also carry a gene for tetracycline resistance that is not expressed in *Bacteroides* species but confers tetracycline resistance on *Escherichia coli* if the organisms are grown under aerobic conditions. Strains of *B. fragilis* also have been identified that appear to carry a clindamycin–erythromycin resistance gene in the chromosome rather than on plasmids. Introduction of new DNA into *Bacteroides* species can be performed by using shuttle vectors for conjugation and by direct transformation. A number of shuttle vectors capable of replication in both *Bacteroides* species and *E. coli* have been studied. Transfer frequencies and expression seem to differ among the organisms. In particular, replication origins for several antibiotic resistance genes from *E. coli* are not expressed in *Bacteroides*. These findings raise questions about transfer of genetic information among colonic colonizing species. Several *Bacteroides* transposons, Tn4351 and Tn4400, have been identified that should facilitate the study of gene mutations. Currently, several cloned genes from *Bacteroides* exist including genes that code for chondroitin lysase II from *B. thetaiotaomicron*, which may play a role in the breakdown of gut endothelial mucopolysaccharides, and a gene that codes for fimbriae or pili of *B. nodosus*, the agent of foot rot in sheep. Introduction of this cloned gene into *E. coli* may facilitate vaccine production.

TABLE 1. Taxonomic Classification of the Major Bacteroides Species

Bacteroides fragilis group	*Bacteroides melaninogenicus* group
B. fragilis	*B. melaninogenicus*
B. thetaiotaomicron	*B. intermedius*
B. vulgatus	*B. gingivalis*
B. distasonis	*B. denticola*
B. ovatus	*B. loescheii*
B. uniformis	*B. corporis*
Bacteroides oralis group	Other *Bacteroides*
B. oris	*B. bivius*
B. buccae	*B. disiens*
B. capillus	
B. pentosaceus	

(Modified from Holdeman et al.,[4] with permission.)

VIRULENCE FACTORS

A number of virulence factors identified in *Bacteroides* species have been postulated to play a role in the pathogenesis of infection. These virulence factors include adherence and invasion properties, enzyme or toxin elaboration, and surface constituents, most notably capsular polysaccharide and lipopolysaccharide of *B. fragilis*.

Adherence and Invasion

Several surface structures of *B. fragilis* and of *Bacteroides* species implicated in periodontal disease, such as *B. gingivalis*, have been studied as attachment factors. Pruzzo et al. demonstrated that strains of *B. fragilis* capable of agglutinating guinea pig and human erythrocytes adhered in vitro to human intestinal and cheek epithelial cell lines.[6] In this experimental system, strains that failed to agglutinate erythrocytes did not adhere to the tissue culture cell lines. The adherent strains were found by electron microscopy to show negative staining characteristics consistent with piliation. Rogemond and Guinet proposed that lectinlike adhesins, which they demonstrated to interact with glycoconjugates, both soluble and membrane-bound, could serve as colonization factors.[7] Onderdonk et al. showed that encapsulated *B. fragilis* adhered well to rat peritoneal mesothelial cells, in contrast to unencapsulated *Bacteroides* species.[8] This adherence could be blocked with capsular polysaccharide.

Fimbriae have been identified as an important attachment factor in *B. gingivalis*. Fimbriae had been postulated to carry both adherence and hemagglutination abilities in this organism, which is an important gingival isolate in human periodontal disease. Yoshimura et al., however, purified fimbriae, which they noted to be a quantitatively important surface structure, but they failed to demonstrated hemagglutinating capacity.[9] Okuda et al. isolated a hemagglutinin from this bacterium to which antibody could be raised.[10] This antibody inhibited the hemagglutinating ability of the organisms and could be demonstrated to bind to the surface of the organisms. Staining the organisms with this antibody outlined vesicular structures by electron microscopy. *Bacteroides melaninogenicus* has been observed to attach to selected gram-positive organisms in vitro, raising the possibility that colonization might be mediated by interaction of resident organisms as well as direct attachment to epithelial surfaces.[11]

Pili and an antipilus vaccine have been demonstrated to play an important protective role in foot rot disease of sheep caused by *B. nodosus*.[12] Protection is specific to the pilus strain of the organism, lending credence to this surface structure as an important attachment factor.

In addition to hemagglutination properties, which may facilitate invasion, investigators have noted that *B. gingivalis* specifically binds and degrades human fibrinogen.[13] Others have speculated that release of phospholipase A by *B. melaninogenicus* and *B. intermedius* may affect the integrity of epithelial cell membranes and thereby lead to cell disruption.[14]

Enzymes and Toxins

Several enzymes have been associated with *Bacteroides* species that may play a role in pathogenesis of disease. In addition to phospholipase A, collagenase has been detected in *B. gingivalis*.[15] Since destruction of collagen has been noted as an important component of the histology of periodontal disease, this enzyme may well play a role.

Enzymes such as collagenase or heparinase may affect the development of specific disease manifestations. Another important enzyme elaborated by *Bacteroides* organisms may facilitate bacterial survival. Many anaerobic species that are encountered frequently in clinical specimens, including *B. fragilis*, display some degree of oxygen tolerance, probably due to the presence of an enzyme, superoxide dismutase. The ability of an anaerobic organism to produce this enzyme and thereby counteract the toxic effect of superoxide radicals may facilitate bacterial survival until a reduced environment hospitable to anaerobes is generated.[16] E. M. Gregory has identified two superoxide dismutases in *B. fragilis*, one that contains iron and one manganese.[17] The enzymes appear to be composed of two subunits of equal size with one combining site for metal and the subunits identical for the two enzymes. The iron-containing superoxide dismutase appeared to be present in the organism, while the manganese-containing enzyme was inducible by growth of the bacterium in the presence of oxygen. This finding led Gregory to speculate that iron stores might either be depleted or highly conserved in the organism under aeration, with the inducible manganese containing enzyme available as a backup system.

Toxins are not a major component of *Bacteroides* species. Myers et al., however, have demonstrated enterotoxinlike activity in a strain of *B. fragilis* that causes diarrheal disease in newborn lambs.[18]

Surface Constituents

The most well-characterized important surface constituents of these organisms have been identified in *B. fragilis* and include a capsular polysaccharide and a lipopolysaccharide. In addition to DNA homology differences between *B. fragilis* and other species of the *B. fragilis* group, *B. fragilis* contain a unique capsular polysaccharide[19] (Fig. 1). No other members of the *Bacteroides* family have been shown to contain an immunologically similar capsular polysaccharide. This capsular polysaccharide has been extracted and purified. Two different prototypic polysaccharides have been identified chemically.[20] One, from the American Type Culture Collection (ATCC), strain 23745, contains nine monosaccharide constituents, including D-galactose, D-glucosamine, L-fucose, L-quinovosamine, D-glucose, L-fucosamine, L-rhamnosamine, galacturonic acid, and 3-amino-3,6-dideoxyhexose. The other polysaccharide, isolated from the National Collection of Type Cultures (NCTC) strain 9343, contains L-fucose, D-galactose, D-glucosamine, D- and L-quinivosamine, and galacturonic acid. Attempts at structural definition of the two capsular polysaccharides have not been successful to date.

Studies using fluorescent antibodies have demonstrated that these two capsule types identify the majority of *B. fragilis* strains and do not react with other *Bacteroides* species.[21,22] A number of studies in animal models of intra-abdominal sepsis have demonstrated the importance of capsular polysaccharide as a virulence factor.[19,23–25]

Bacteroides fragilis also contains a lipopolysaccharide that is chemically and functionally distinct from lipopolysaccharides of aerobic gram-negative bacilli. Chemically, the lipopolysaccharide of *B. fragilis* is composed of four monosaccharides, L-rhamnose, D-galactose, D-glucose, and D-glucosamine.[26] Weintraub et al. characterized the lipopolysaccharide and demonstrated by enzyme-linked immunosorbent assay (ELISA) inhibition studies that this was a shared antigen among *B. fragilis* strains.[26] Absent from this lipopolysaccharide were two critical sugars found in aerobic gram-negative rod lipopolysaccharides, heptose, and 2-keto-3-deoxyoctonate (KDO). The endotoxin moiety of aerobic gram-negative bacilli lipopolysaccharide is lipid A. Hydroxytetradecanoic acid, a major constituent of lipid A, is found in *B. fragilis* lipopolysaccharide but only in small amounts. Wollenweber et al. further determined that branched fatty acids constituted 43 percent of the fatty acid composition of *B. fragilis* lipopolysaccharide and D-3-hydroxy fatty acids 63 percent.[27] β-Hydroxymyristic acid, another constituent of aerobic gram-negative lipopolysaccharide, is not found in *B. fragilis*.

While chemically distinct from aerobic gram-negative rod lipopolysaccharides, it is of greater interest that the lipopolysaccharide of *B. fragilis* is biologically impotent. It induces gelation of limulus lysate at extremely high doses, but this test is the least specific of endotoxin assays.[28] It fails to produce lethality in chick embryos or to induce the Shwartzman reaction.[28] Clinically, *B. fragilis* bacteremia is not commonly associated with disseminated intravascular coagulation (DIC) or purpura, both manifestations of endotoxemia found in aerobic gram-negative rod sepsis. Still, there is experimental evidence that the lipopolysaccharide is a virulence factor.[29]

PATHOGENESIS

The hallmark of infections in which anaerobic organisms play a role is abscess formation. Abscesses are arguably both a host response to infection as well as a unique pathologic process, in which organism and polymorphonuclear leukocytes coexist within a fibrous capsule. Animal models of abscess formation have proved important for the study of the organisms as well as host cellular responses.[30–35]

Two phenotypic suppressor T cells have been implicated in immunity to abscesses caused by *B. fragilis*. Onderdonk et al. demonstrated that immunization of rats with *B. fragilis* capsular polysaccharide protects against abscesses induced by this organism. Passive transfer of hyperimmune globulin from immunized to naive animals did not protect against abscesses, while adoptive transfer of spleen cells and fractionated T cells were protective.[36] Shapiro et al. characterized the responsible T cells as Ly $1^{-}2^{+}3^{+}$, IJ^{+} by selectively depleting immune spleen cell preparations with monoclonal antibodies to T-cell markers.[25,34] Zaleznik et al. identified a small, antigen-specific protein factor (ITF) released from these T cells as critical for protection.[37]

The role of the humoral immune system against *Bacteroides* species has been examined largely in vitro. Bjornson has demonstrated using purified constituents that the alternative complement pathway is crucial for effective opsonization of *B. fragilis* and *B. thetaiotaomicron* in vitro.[38] Antibody from pooled normal human sera facilitated in vitro killing of *B. thetaiotaomicron* but was not required for phagocytic killing of *B. fragilis*. While the work of Onderdonk et al. did not demonstrate a role for hyperimmune globulin (raised by immunization of animals with *B. fragilis* capsular polysaccharide) in prevention of experimental intra-abdominal abscesses, globulin did lead to enhanced blood stream clearance of *B. fragilis*.[36] Joiner et al. proposed a role for the alternative complement pathway in protection against subcutaneous abscesses in mice in studies with cobra venom factor-treated animals.[39] These animals formed larger abscesses than control mice. Table 2 provides a summary of immune mechanisms in response to *B. fragilis*.

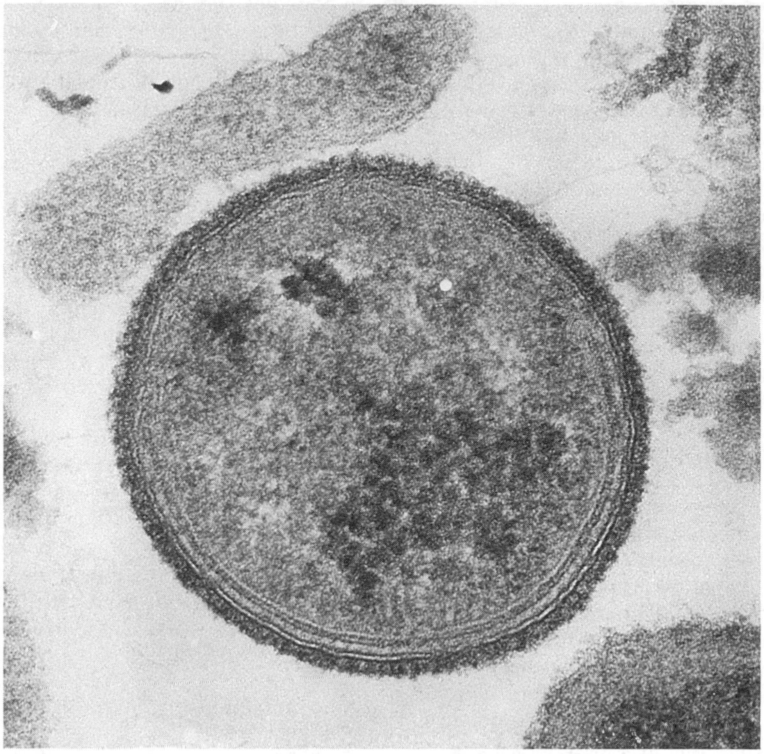

FIG. 1. Electron micrograph of *B. fragilis* strain ATCC 23745, with a thick capsular polysaccharide highlighted by ferritin-labeled antibody. The organisms were incubated first with specific anticapsular antibody followed by ferritin-labeled anti-rabbit IgG. This methodology is more specific for a unique capsular polysaccharide than ruthenium red staining techniques. (×180,000)

TABLE 2. Immunity to *Bacteroides fragilis*

Humoral
Phagocytes are required for in vitro killing.
The alternative complement pathway is activated by *Bacteroides fragilis* in the absence of antibody.
Antibody to capsular polysaccharide enhances killing primarily via the classical complement pathway.[66]
Specific anticapsular antibody does not protect against experimental abscesses but does enhance bacterial blood stream clearance.
Cellular
T cells are required for protection against experimental intra-abdominal abscesses.
Specific protection is induced by the capsular polysaccharide of *Bacteroides fragilis*.
The phenotype of the protective T cells is Ly $1^-2^+3^+$, IJ^+, and protection is not H-2 restricted.
A soluble lymphokine from immune T cells transfers immunity to naive animals, and its activity is antigen-specific.

NORMAL FLORA

The normal flora of humans has been evaluated and varies depending on the location. In the oral cavity, anaerobes including *Bacteroides* species are found in all locations.[40] Fewer anaerobic species are contained in saliva and on the surface of the tongue and teeth, however, than are located in gingival plaque or sulci. In these latter locations members of the *B. melaninogenicus* group figure prominently. The acquisition of anaerobic species in the oral cavity also appears to depend on age, with development of teeth playing a major role.

In the gastrointestinal tract, oral flora at relatively low concentrations are present, with the ligament of Treitz serving as a dividing line. Colonic flora are composed largely of anaerobes in concentrations of 10^{11} compared with 10^8 aerobic organisms per gram of cecal contents.[41] *Bacteroides* species are found commonly. The numerically most prevalent of the *Bacteroides* species are *B. distasonis*, *B. thetaiotaomicron,* and *B. vulgatus*. Although it is the most common anaerobe isolated in clinical infections, *B. fragilis* is notable for its low comparative frequency in the normal colonic flora, only 0.5 percent.[42] This information, as well as the regularity with which a few select anaerobic species are detected in clinical specimens, has led to the prominent focus on virulence factors in the study of these organisms.

Normal vaginal flora also contains *Bacteroides* species, although in lower quantities than gram-positive anaerobes such as *Lactobacillus* or *Peptococcus*. In a study by Bartlett and Polk, 34 percent of 118 samples contained *Bacteroides* other species, which would include *B. bivius* and *B. disiens*, 25 percent *B. melaninogenicus* group, and 14 percent *B. fragilis* group.[43]

CLINICAL PRESENTATIONS

Bacteroides species are encountered frequently in a variety of sites as resident flora and have a propensity for abscess cavities and mixed infections. It is not a surprise, therefore, that these organisms are found in an extensive variety of infections, ranging from brain abscess, sinusitis, and periodontal disease, and intra-abdominal abscesses, to female genital tract abscesses.

Intra-abdominal Infections

Intra-abdominal abscesses, either peritoneal or visceral, are the most prominent manifestation of *Bacteroides* infections and usually involve *B. fragilis*. Infection may arise from a ruptured appendix, diverticulitis with local abscess formation or distant spread, colon tumors, trauma, or surgical manipulation. Visceral sites of abscesses, whether originating from local or hematogenous spread, include liver (most commonly), kidneys, and spleen. Abscesses attached to the visceral peritoneum and omentum as well as subphrenic pockets are observed. Multiple abscesses containing an average of five organisms, two aerobic and three anaerobic, are common as opposed to solitary collections.[44] Gorbach and Bartlett reported isolation of *B. fragilis* in 65 percent of intra-abdominal infections, and anaerobes in as many as 96 percent of cases.[44]

One of the intra-abdominal infections involving anaerobes, is appendicitis with perforation and abscess formation.[45] Diverticulitis involves nonsporulating anaerobes including *Bacteroides* species and can result in perforation followed by generalized peritonitis. More commonly, however, the patient with diverticulitis, even with perforation, will wall off the infection, developing small abscesses that do not require drainage routinely. Abdominal ultrasound, computerized tomography (CT) or gallium scans, or combined liver-spleen and lung scans may facilitate localizing intra-abdominal abscesses. If one diagnostic test is negative, a second may reveal the process.

Among visceral abdominal infections involving *Bacteroides* species, the most common is liver abscess, with nonsporulating anaerobes isolated from approximately 50 percent of liver abscesses.[44] Liver abscess results from both hematogenous spread in association with bacteremia and from contiguous infection, especially within the peritoneal cavity. Infection may spread from the biliary tract or via the portal venous system. Suppurative pyelophlebitis results from direct extension of pelvic or intra-abdominal processes. Symptoms and signs often suggest infection that can be localized readily, but nonspecific symptoms of fever, chills, weight loss, nausea, and vomiting also are observed in many patients. Patients with liver abscesses only have hepatomegaly, right upper quadrant abdominal tenderness, or jaundice in 50 percent of cases.[46] More than 90 percent of patients with liver abscesses will have elevation of the serum alkaline phosphatase, while 77 percent have leukocytosis and 48 percent elevated serum glutamic oxaloacetic transaminase.[46] Fifty percent have associated anemia and elevated serum bilirubin and 33 percent hypoalbuminemia.[46] A basilar pulmonary infiltrate, pleural effusion, or elevated hemidiaphragm may be found on chest x-ray films. In one-third of patients a concomitant bacteremia will be detected.[46] However, some patients, particularly the elderly, may present only with fever and in the course of an evaluation for fever of unknown origin, may have a normal abdominal examination. The diagnosis can be confirmed by ultrasound, CT scan, or radioisotope scanning and occasionally may require multiple studies.

Unlike infections arising from the colon, perforated peptic ulcers, pancreatitis with phlegmon or abscesses, and even acute cholecystitis rarely involve anaerobic species. The exception is gallbladder disease with previous surgery or multiple previous infections in which the anatomy is altered.

Brain Abscess

Bacteroides species, especially oral *Bacteroides* species, are important to consider in brain abscesses, particularly arising from dental sites. A series by Chun et al., isolated anaerobes from 17 (40.4 percent) of 42 specimens from brain abscesses.[47] Of these 17 organisms, three were *Bacteroides* species. When detected in brain abscesses, *Bacteroides* species are most often cultured with other pathogens as part of a mixed process.

Oral Infections

Periodontal disease is extremely common in the adult population in the United States and refers to disease of the support structures for the teeth. In advanced stages, periodontal disease is a major contributor to tooth loss. Infection ranges from gingivitis with spongy gums, easy bleeding, and subgingival plaque to bone destruction. Pockets of pus may develop around teeth, with abscess formation and eventual loosening of teeth as underlying support structures and bone are destroyed.[48] Oral anaerobes, particularly members of the *B. melaninogenicus* group, are felt to play a prominent role in these infections.

Pleuropulmonary Infections

Pleuropulmonary infections, particularly aspiration pneumonia, necrotizing pneumonia, lung abscess, and empyema, frequently involve anaerobes. Usually, multiple species of bacteria, including anaerobic and aerobic organisms, can be isolated from these infections. *Bacteroides fragilis*, while cultured from abscess contents in the lung in as many as 15% of cases, is rarely isolated alone, and therapy has not been directed specifically at this organism.[49] *Bacteroides melaninogenicus* is the most common *Bacteroides* species encountered.[49] In the past, penicillin therapy was felt to be adequate for these mixed, often indolent infections. In recent years a clinical controversy has arisen over this approach, with some advocating initial treatment with clindamycin for lung abscesses.[50] There have been increasing reports of *B. melaninogenicus* resistant to penicillin.[51] However, some clinicians still advocate the treatment of anaerobic infections above the diaphragm with penicillin, reserving other drugs for seriously ill patients and treatment failures.

Pelvic Infections

As discussed above, *Bacteroides* species are important constituents of the normal vaginal flora. These organisms, in turn, figure prominently in infections of the female genital tract. *Bacteroides fragilis*, as is the case with intra-abdominal infections, is a frequent pathogen isolated in as many as two-thirds of pelvic abscesses, while it is not the most common species found in the normal flora.[44] It is important to consider *B. fragilis* in pelvic infections involving abscesses (such as tubo-ovarian) or in postcesarean section or vaginal hysterectomy infections. Salpingitis or endometritis without abscess formation are not as frequently associated with *B. fragilis* as a pathogen.

Bacteremia

Bacteroides fragilis is the second most common gram-negative rod isolated from blood cultures, next to *E. coli*, and is the most common of the *Bacteroides* species to be associated with bacteremia, found in 78% of the cultures reported by Wilson et al.[52] When *B. fragilis* is cultured from the blood, there frequently is an associated localized source of infection, particularly in the abdomen. Wilson et al. reported sources such as peritoneal fluid, surgical wounds, and intra-abdominal collections in 63% of patients with significant anaerobic bacteremia. *Bacteroides fragilis* is a significant pathogen, however, with Chow and Guze reporting 60 percent mortality from *B. fragilis* bacteremia when therapy was not directed at this organism.[53]

Endocarditis

Endocarditis caused by anaerobic organisms is not common, but when it occurs *B. fragilis* is a frequent pathogen, accounting for 11 of 33 infections in a series by Felner and Dowell.[54] In this report, endocarditis with anaerobic organisms was seen more frequently in patients without previous valvular disease than was observed in patients with viridans streptococcal endocarditis.

Skin and Bone Infections

Injury to skin, bone, or soft tissue by trauma, ischemia, or surgery creates a suitable environment for anaerobic infections. These infections are found most frequently when the site is subject to contamination with feces or upper airway secretions.

Common examples include wounds associated with intestinal surgery, decubitus ulcers, or human bites. Anaerobic bacteria can be isolated in cases of crepitant cellulitis, synergistic cellulitis, or gangrene and necrotizing fasciitis. *Bacteroides* species have been isolated from cutaneous abscesses.

While *Bacteroides* species are not common skin flora, these organisms, especially *B. fragilis*, are important pathogens to consider in diabetic foot ulcers. Sapico et al. performed deep tissue cultures of infected feet in 32 diabetic patients.[55] Mixed aerobic and anaerobic specimens were obtained in 25 of these, with *B. fragilis* isolated in 6 and other *Bacteroides* species in an additional 16. Many of these patients seemed predisposed to ulcer formation. Decubitus ulcers also frequently contain *B. fragilis*.

As techniques for culturing anaerobes become more widely applied in clinical laboratories, there are increasing reports of infections involving anaerobes. Osteomyelitis is one such clinical entity and may present as indolent disease.[56] These infections frequently arise in the setting of soft tissue infections in adjacent soft tissues. Hematogenous seeding of bone is uncommon. Nakata and Lewis report that *Bacteroides* species are found in one-third of cases of osteomyelitis in which anaerobes are isolated.[56] Of these species, *B. fragilis* is the most common isolate and may be found in cases of bony infections of the skull as well as other sites where *B. fragilis* would be expected to be a more common contiguous organism. *Bacteroides melaninogenicus* is the next most common *Bacteroides* species detected in osteomyelitis and frequently involves facial bones such as the maxilla and mandible.

TREATMENT

Since most infections with *Bacteroides* species involve collections of pus, one of the mainstays of therapy is drainage of the abscess, if one is present.[45] Choices of antimicrobial agents involve some interesting dilemmas and include both in vitro and therapeutic information. One should not lose sight, however, of the importance of drainage in the appropriate treatment of abscesses. While surgery formerly was required to establish drainage, with the advent of CT scans as well as ultrasound, diagnostic radiologists now are able to perform percutaneous drainage of a number of intra-abdominal sites.[57]

One of the dilemmas in deciding upon antimicrobial therapy for mixed infections always has been determining which organisms were pathogens and which commensals, if any. An important study by Thadepalli et al. examined the necessity to cover for anaerobes in a prospective trial of therapy in penetrating abdominal trauma at Chicago's Cook County Hospital.[58] The regimens compared were cephalothin–kanamycin and clindamycin–kanamycin. By 7 days, there was a dramatic difference in recovery of anaerobes from patients with colonic trauma in the two treatment groups. Twelve of 26 patients (46%) receiving cephalothin–kanamycin were cultured for anaerobes compared with 1 of 25 patients (4%) on clindamycin–kanamycin. This study and others, combined with the experimental data from animal models of intra-abdominal sepsis about *B. fragilis* as a pathogen by itself, suggest that therapy should be directed at this organism if it is a suspected pathogen. As stated above with infections above the diaphragm, the clinical situation is less straightforward, although increasing reports of penicillin-resistant oral *Bacteroides* species raise concerns.

Several classes of antibiotics are of interest in the treatment of *Bacteroides* infections: (*1*) metronidazole, (*2*) clindamycin, (*3*) cephalosporins, especially cefoxitin, (*4*) chloramphenicol, (*5*) broader spectrum penicillins such as ticarcillin and piperacillin, and (*6*) imipenem. Of the newer types of antibiotics marketed today, the quinolones are notable for absence of activity against anaerobes. There is a large reference study from eight widely dispersed U.S. centers on susceptibilities of 1292 isolates from the *B. fragilis* group in 1981 and 1982.[59] In this important study Cuchural et al. documented no resistance among isolates to metronidazole or chloramphenicol. Resistances were highest to tetracycline (a drug of historic interest only, for treatment of anaerobic infections), cefoperazone, and cefotaxime. Cefoxitin resistance was 8 percent in 1981 and 10 percent in 1982. One center (New England Medical Center, Boston), however, showed a rise in resistance to cefoxitin from 14 to 30 percent. Clindamycin resistance in the study was 6 percent in 1981 and 3 percent in 1982. There appeared to be development of some cross-reactive resistance to β-lactam antibiotics in this study, although there were differential sensitivities to a variety of these agents at the beginning of the study. Several other subsequent papers on β-lactam agents against *Bacteroides* species reveal good activity for imipenem, and ticarcillin–clavulanic acid.[60,61] Cefotetan compared favorably with cefoxitin against *B. fragilis* but not against other members of the *B. fragilis* group, for which cefotetan was less active. In general, *B. fragilis* strains are more sensitive to antimicrobials than other member of the *B. fragilis* group (Table 3).

A number of therapeutic trials with small numbers of patients have compared several regimens, including cefoxitin with or without an aminoglycoside, moxalactam, clindamycin plus aminoglycoside, and metronidazole in combination with an aminoglycoside.[62–64] None of these trials have demonstrated superiority of one regimen over another. In patients treated with cefoxitin alone, some treatment failures were observed with facultative gram-negative bacilli resistant to cefoxitin.[62] Centers with resident aerobic flora more resistant to cefoxitin should add an aminoglycoside to the regimen for intra-abdominal sepsis. Small studies of imipenem suggest it will also prove therapeutic against intra-abdominal infections.[61]

While a number of agents provide satisfactory outcomes, information from both in vitro studies and case reports of treatment failures suggests that some regimens may be preferable to others. For example, resistance in *B. fragilis* rarely has been reported with metronidazole, and there was none found in the large Cuchural et al. study.[59] This agent is well tolerated and achieves significant levels both in serum and inside abscesses when administered intravenously or orally. It should be con-

TABLE 3. Antibiotic Susceptibilities of *Bacteroides fragilis* group

Species	*Antibiotic*	*MIC 90% (μg/ml)*	*Range (μg/ml)*
B. fragilis	Metronidazole[a]	1	<0.25–8
	Clindamycin[a]	4	<0.25–>32
	Cefoxitin	16	1–64
	Chloramphenicol[a]	8	0.5–8
	Cefotetan	16	1–64
	Ampicillin/sulbactam	8	0.25–16
	Imipenem	0.125	0.016–8
	Ticarcillin/clavulanic acid	4	0.06–16
B. thetaiotaomicron	Cefoxitin	32	16–64
	Cefotetan	128	32–256
	Ticarcillin/clavulanic acid	4	0.125–8
	Imipenem	0.25	0.125–0.5
B. distasonis	Ceftoxitin	32	4–32
	Cefotetan	64	4–128
	Ticarcillin/clavulanic acid	32	4–32
	Imipenem	0.25	0.016–0.5
B. vulgatus	Ceftoxitin	16	8–16
	Cefotetan	64	8–64
	Ticarcillin/clavulanic acid	16	0.06–32
	Imipenem	0.062	0.062
B. ovatus	Ceftoxitin	64	2–64
	Cefotetan	128	2–256
	Ticarcillin/clavulanic acid	16	0.125–32
	Imipenem	0.25	0.032–0.25

Abbreviation: MIC: minimum inhibitory concentration.
[a] These sensitivities are for the *Bacteroides fragilis* group as a whole rather than for individual species. Sensitivities for the specific species do not vary widely for these antibiotics.
(Data from Refs. 59, 60, 68.)

sidered a first-line therapy against *B. fragilis* infections. The other two widely used antibiotics, clindamycin and cefoxitin, are very useful agents. Despite reports of *B. fragilis* in vitro resistance to one or the other and scattered case reports of clinical failures, there is no compelling evidence against a recommendation of these drugs as first-line agents. Knowledge of local resistance patterns among organisms of the *B. fragilis* group is helpful. In addition, if a specific patient appears not to be responding to one of these antibiotics, consideration should be given to alternative treatment. If the drug in use is cefoxitin, it is wisest not to choose another β-lactam agent in the event cross-resistance has developed.

While the Cuchural et al. study did not demonstrate resistance to chloramphenicol, treatment failures with this antibiotic have been reported increasingly. In animal studies 59 percent of rats developed abscesses while receiving chloramphenicol compared with 5 percent for clindamycin.[65] One theory for this in vivo result is that the anaerobic species may inactivate chloramphenicol. Abscess contents in these rats did contain the inactive derivative of the drug.[65] There are numbers of patients whose infections respond to chloramphenicol, but these data suggest it should not be considered first-line therapy. If the patient receiving chloramphenicol is not responding clinically, the drug should be discontinued in favor of another agent.

Further clinical data are needed to evaluate the role of piperacillin, ticarcillin, ticarcillin plus clavulanate, ampicillin plus sulbactam, or imipenem in anaerobic infections. Third generation cephalosporins generally are not useful even if in vitro sensitivities look promising. Many clinical laboratories still do not routinely perform anaerobic susceptibility testing. One can choose reasonable initial empiric therapy. However, faced with a patient whose infection has been drained and who is on an appropriate agent for the treatment of *Bacteroides* infection but has not responded, a change of antibiotics and attempts to obtain sensitivity information are warranted.

REFERENCES

1. Finegold SM, Martin WJ. Bailey and Scott's diagnostic microbiology. 6th ed. St. Louis: CV Mosby; 1982:309–318.
2. Citron DM. Specimen collection and transport, anaerobic culture techniques, and identification of anaerobes. Rev Infect Dis. 1984;6:S51–8.
3. Booth SJ, Van Tassell RL, Johnson JL et al. Bacteriophages of *Bacteroides*. Rev Infect Dis. 1979;1:325–34.
4. Holdeman LV, Cato EP, Moore WEC. Taxonomy of anaerobes: present state of the art. Rev Infect Dis. 1984;6:S3–10.
5. Salyers AA, Shoemaker NB, Guthrie EP. Recent advances in *Bacteroides* genetics. CRC Crit Rev Microbiol. 1987;14:49–71.
6. Pruzzo C, Dainelli B, Ricchetti M. Piliated *Bacteroides fragilis* strains adhere to epithelial cells and are more sensitive to phagocytosis by human neutrophils than nonpiliated strains. Infect Immun. 1984;43:189–94.
7. Rogemond V, Guinet RMF. Lectinlike adhesins in the *Bacteroides fragilis* group. Infect Immun. 1986;53:99–102.
8. Onderdonk AB, Moon NR, Kasper DL, et al. Adherence of *Bacteroides fragilis* in vivo. Infect Immun. 1978;19:1083–7.
9. Yoshimura F, Takahashi K, Nodasaka Y, et al. Purification and characterization of a novel type of fimbriae from the oral anaerobe *Bacteroides gingivalis*. J Bacteriol. 1984;160:949–57.
10. Okuda K, Yamamoto A, Naito Y, et al. Purification and properties of hemagglutinin from culture supernatant of *Bacteroides gingivalis*. Infect Immun. 1986;54:659–65.
11. Hofstad T. Pathogenicity of anaerobic gram-negative rods: possible mechanisms. Rev Infect Dis. 1984;6:189–99.
12. Lee SW, Alexander B, McGowan B. Purification, characterization, and serologic characteristics of *Bacteroides nodosus* pili and use of a purified pili vaccine in sheep. Am J Vet Res. 1983;44:1676–81.
13. Lantz MS, Rowland RW, Switalski IM, et al. Interactions of *Bacteroides gingivalis* with fibrinogen. Infect Immun. 1986;54:654–8.
14. Bulkacz J, Schuster GS, Baldev S, et al. Phospholipase A activity of extracellular products from *Bacteroides melaninogenicus* on epithelium tissue cultures. J Periodont Res. 1985;20:146–53.
15. McKee AS, McDermid AS, Baskerville A, et al. Effect of hemin on the physiology and virulence of *Bacteroides gingivalis* W50. Infect Immun. 1986;52:349–55.
16. Tally FP, Goldin BR, Jacobus NV, et al. Superoxide dismutase in anaerobic bacteria of clinical significance. Infect Immun. 1977;16:20–5.
17. Gregory EM. Characterization of the O_2-induced manganese-containing superoxide dismutase from *Bacteroides fragilis*. Arch Biochem Biophys. 1985;238:83–9.
18. Myers LL, Firehammer BD, Shoop DS, et al. *Bacteroides fragilis*: a possible cause of acute diarrheal disease in newborn lambs. Infect Immun. 1984;44:241–4.
19. Onderdonk AB, Kasper DL, Cisneros RL, et al. The capsular polysaccharide of *Bacteroides fragilis* as a virulence factor: comparison of the pathogenic potential of encapsulated and unencapsulated strains. J Infect Dis. 1977;136:82–9.
20. Kasper DL, Weintraub A, Lindberg AA, et al. Capsular polysaccharides and lipopolysaccharides from two *Bacteroides fragilis* reference strains: chemical and immunochemical characterization. J Bacteriol. 1983;153:991–7.
21. Weintraub A, Lindberg AA, Kasper DL. Characterization of *Bacteroides fragilis* strains based on antigen-specific immunofluorescence. J Infect Dis. 1983;147:780.
22. Kasper DL, Hayes ME, Reinap BG, et al. Isolation and identification of encapsulated strains of *Bacteroides fragilis*. J Infect Dis. 1977;136:75–81.
23. Weinstein WM, Onderdonk AB, Bartlett JG, et al. Experimental intra-abdominal abscesses in rats: development of an experimental model. Infect Immun. 1974;10:1250–5.
24. Onderdonk AB, Bartlett JG, Louie T, et al. Microbial synergy in experimental intra-abdominal abscess. Infect Immun. 1976;13:22–6.
25. Shapiro ME, Onderdonk AB, Kasper DL, et al. Cellular immunity to *Bacteroides fragilis* capsular polysaccharide. J Exp Med. 1982;154:1188–97.
26. Weintraub A, Larsson BE, Lindberg AA. Chemical and immunochemical analyses of *Bacteroides fragilis* lipopolysaccharides. Infect Immun. 1985;49:197–201.
27. Wollenweber HW, Rietschel ET, Hofstad T, et al. Nature, type of linkage, quantity, and absolute configuration of (3-hydroxy) fatty acids in lipopolysaccharides from *Bacteroides fragilis* NCTC 9343 and related strains. J Bacteriol. 1980;144:898–903.
28. Kasper DL. Chemical and biological characterization of the lipopolysaccharide of *Bacteroides fragilis* subspecies *fragilis*. J Infect Dis. 1976;134:59–66.
29. Zaleznik DF, Zhang Z, Onderdonk AB, et al. Effect of subinhibitory doses of clindamycin on the virulence of *Bacteroides fragilis*: role of lipopolysaccharide. J Infect Dis. 1986;154:40–6.
30. Mayrand D, McBride BC. Ecological relationships of bacteria involved in a simple mixed anaerobic infection. Infect Immun. 1980;27:44–50.
31. Rotstein OD, Pruett TL, Simmons RL. Mechanisms of microbial synergy in polymicrobial surgical infections. Rev Infect Dis. 1985;7:151–70.
32. Ingham HR, Sisson PR, Tharagonnet D, et al. Inhibition of phagocytosis in vitro by obligate anaerobes. Lancet. 1977;2:1252–4.
33. Klempner MS. Interactions of polymorphonuclear leukocytes with anaerobic bacteria. Rev Infect Dis. 1984;6:S41–4.
34. Shapiro ME, Kasper DL, Zaleznik DF, et al. Cellular control of abscess formation: role of T cells in the regulation of abscesses formed in response to *Bacteroides fragilis*. J Immunol. 1986;137:341–6.
35. Nulsen MF, Finlay-Jones JJ, McDonald PJ. T-lymphocyte involvement in abscess formation in nonimmune mice. Infect Immun. 1986;52:633–6.
36. Onderdonk AB, Markham RB, Zaleznik DF, et al. Evidence for T cell-dependent immunity to *Bacteroides fragilis* in an intraabdominal abscess model. J Clin Invest. 1982;69:9–16.
37. Zaleznik DF, Finberg RW, Shapiro ME, et al. A soluble suppressor T cell factor protects against experimental intraabdominal abscesses. J Clin Invest. 1985;75:1023–7.
38. Bjornson AB, Magnafichi PI, Schreiber RD, et al. Opsonization of *Bacteroides* by the alternative complement pathway reconstructed from isolated plasma proteins. J Exp Med. 1987;164:777–98.
39. Joiner KA, Gelfand JA, Onderdonk AB, et al. Host factors in the formation of abscesses. J Infect Dis. 1980;142:40–9.
40. Sutter VL. Anaerobes as normal oral flora. Rev Infect Dis. 1984;6:S62–6.
41. Moore WEC, Cato EP, Holdeman LV. Anaerobic bacteria of the gastrointestinal flora and their occurrence in clinical infections. J Infect Dis. 1969;119:641–9.
42. Moore WEC. Anaerobes as normal flora: gastrointestinal tract. In: Finegold SM, ed. Proc Int Metronidazole Conf Montreal, Quebec, Canada. Princeton, NJ: Excerpta Med; 1977:222–8.
43. Bartlett JG, Polk BF. Bacterial flora of the vagina: quantitative study. Rev Infect Dis. 1984;6:S67–72.
44. Gorbach SL, Bartlett JG. Medical progress: anaerobic infections. N Engl J Med. 1974;290:1177–84, 1237–45, 1289–94.
45. Altemeier WA, Culbertson WR, Fullen WD, et al. Intraabdominal abscesses. Am J Surg. 1973;125:70–9.
46. Rubin RH, Swartz MN, Malt R. Hepatic abscess: changes in clinical, bacteriologic and therapeutic aspects. Am J Med. 1974;57:601–10.
47. Chun CH, Johnson JD, Hofstetter M, et al. Brain abscess: a study of 45 consecutive cases. Medicine. 1986;65:415–31.
48. Newman MG. Anaerobic oral and dental infection. Rev Infect Dis. 1984;6:S107–14.
49. Bartlett JG, Gorbach SL, Tally FP, et al. Bacteriology and treatment of primary lung abscess. Am Rev Respir Dis. 1974;109:510–8.
50. Levison ME, Mangura CT, Lorber B, et al. Clindamycin compared with penicillin for the treatment of anaerobic lung abscess. Ann Intern Med. 1983;98:466–71.
51. Edson RS, Rosenblatt JE, Lee DT, et al. Recent experience with antimicrobial susceptibility of anaerobic bacteria: increasing resistance to penicillin. Mayo Clin Proc. 1982;57:737–41.

52. Wilson WR, Martin WJ, Wilkowske CJ, et al. Anaerobic bacteremia. Mayo Clin Proc. 1972;47:639–46.
53. Chow AW, Guze LB. Bacteroidaceae bacteremia: clinical experience with 112 patients. Medicine. 1974;53:93–126.
54. Felner JM, Dowell VR. Anaerobic bacterial endocarditis. N Engl J Med. 1970;283:1188–92.
55. Sapico FL, Witte JL, Canawati HN, et al. The infected foot of the diabetic patient: quantitative microbiology and analysis of clinical features. Rev Infect Dis. 1984;6:S171–6.
56. Nakata MN, Lewis RP. Anaerobic bacteria in bone and joint infections. Rev Infect Dis. 1984;6:S165–70.
57. Gerzof SG, Robbins AH, Johnson WC, et al. Percutaneous catheter drainage of abdominal abscesses. N Engl J Med. 1981;305:653–7.
58. Thadepalli H, Gorbach SL, Broido PW, et al. Abdominal trauma, anaerobes, and antibiotics. Surg Gynecol Obstet. 1973;137:270–6.
59. Cuchural GJ, Tally FP, Jacobus NV, et al. Antimicrobial susceptibilities of 1,292 isolates of the *Bacteroides fragilis* group in the United States: comparison of 1981 with 1982. Antimicrob Agents Chemother. 1984;26:145–8.
60. O'Keefe JP, Venezio FR, Divincenzo CA, et al. Activity of newer β-lactam agents against clinical isolates of *Bacteroides fragilis* and other *Bacteroides* species. Antimicrob Agents Chemother. 1987;31:2002–4.
61. Tally FP, Gorbach SL. Therapy of mixed anaerobic-aerobic infections. Am J Med. 1985;78:145–53.
62. Drusano GL, Warren JW, Saah AJ, et al. A prospective randomized controlled trial of cefoxitin versus clindamycin-aminoglycoside in mixed anaerobic-aerobic infections. Surg Gynecol Obstet. 1982;154:715–20.
63. Tally FP, Kellum JM, Ho JL, et al. Randomized prospective study comparing moxalactam and cefoxitin with or without tobramycin for the treatment of serious surgical infections. Antimicrob Agents Chemother. 1986;29:244–9.
64. Smith JA, Skidmore AG, Forword AD, et al. Prospective randomized, double-blind comparison of metronidazole and tobramycin with clindamycin and tobramycin in the treatment of intra-abdominal sepsis. Ann Surg. 1981;193:318–23.
65. Onderdonk AB, Kasper DL, Mansheim BJ, et al. Experimental animal models for anaerobic infections. Rev Infect Dis. 1979;1:291–301.
66. Zalcznik DF, Farmer T, Kasper DL. Antibody mediated killing of *Bacteroides fragilis* is strain specific and proceeds via the classical complement pathway. Clin Res. 1988;36:583A.
67. Aldridge KE, Sanders CV, Janney A, et al. Comparison of the activities of penicillin G and new β-lactam antibiotics against clinical isolates of *Bacteroides* species. Antimicrob Agents Chemother. 1984;26:410–3.
68. Wexler HM, Finegold SM. In vitro activity of cefotetan compared with that of other antimicrobial agents against anaerobic bacteria. Antimicrob Agents Chemother. 1988;32:601–4.

224. ANAEROBIC COCCI

JOHN G. BARTLETT

The common and clinically important anaerobic cocci include a diverse group of gram-positive cocci within the genus *Peptostreptococcus*. These organisms are prominent components of the normal flora on human mucocutaneous surfaces, and they are frequent clinical isolates, usually as components of mixed infections involving additional anaerobic bacteria with or without facultative anaerobes.

TAXONOMY

The anaerobic gram-positive cocci include the genera of *Peptostreptococcus, Peptococcus, Ruminococcus, Coprococcus, Gemmiger*, and *Sarcina*. The only organisms in this group that are encountered with any frequency in clinical infections are *Peptostreptococcus* and *Peptococcus*. There has been a recent taxonomic revision in which all of the former species of *Peptococcus* were reclassified in the genus *Peptostreptococcus* with the exception of *Peptococcus niger*.[1] This decision was based on DNA guanine-plus-cytosine content, although there is not universal acceptance of the shift.[2] The most frequent clinical isolates in the revised classification in the genera *Peptostreptococcus* include *P. magnus, P. asaccharolyticus, P. prevotii, P. anaerobius*, and *P. micros*. A new species, *Peptostreptococcus tetradius*, has been proposed to replace the organisms previously classified as "*Gaffkya anaerobia*."[1]

Other relatively recent changes in taxonomic classification include the reclassification of gram positive cocci that produce large quantities of lactic acid with carbohydrate fermentation that were formerly considered anaerobic into the genus *Streptococcus*. These include organisms previously classified as *Peptostreptococcus* or *Peptococcus* that are now classified as *Streptococcus parvulus*, and *Streptococcus morbillorum*. Most strains of these organisms will grow optimally under anaerobic conditions, and some grow in 5–10% CO_2 or air only with several subcultures. Especially important in terms of frequency of isolation and suspected pathogenic potential are organisms formerly classified as *Peptostreptococcus intermedius* which is now collectively referred to as the *Streptococcus intermedius* group.[3]

The anaerobic gram-negative cocci include *Veillonella parvula, V. atypica, V. dispar, Acidaminococcus fermentans*, and *Megasphaera alspenii*. The only organism in this group that is recovered in clinical specimens with any frequency is *V. parvula*, and the pathogenic role of this organism has never been well established.

MICROBIOLOGY

The anaerobic cocci grow well in the nonselective plate and broth media generally recommended for the recovery of anaerobes in clinical specimens. These include the CDC anaerobe blood agar, brain–heart infusion agar, Schaedler agar supplemented with 5% sheep blood, and Brucella agar.[4] Selective media containing vancomycin are generally inhibitory to gram-positive cocci, although these organisms grow well in blood agar plates containing phenylethyl alcohol or neomycin. Growth on both plate media and in broth is often slow, requiring incubation for at least 48 hours or longer. Gram stain performed either directly on specimens or with cultivated organisms fails to show unique features that will distinguish anaerobic, microaerophilic, or facultative gram-positive cocci. Although there is considerable overlap, *P. anaerobius* and *P. productus* are often elongated, appearing in chains or pairs, whereas *P. magnus* is somewhat unique in its large size of 1–2 μm in diameter.

The species of gram-positive cocci are distinguished on the basis of fermentation reactions and products of metabolism as detected by gas–liquid chromatography. These are fastidious organisms that are difficult to cultivate and whose species are laborious to determine. The need for determining species is often questioned since differences in pathogenic potential for the various anaerobic gram-positive cocci are not well defined. Similarly, the utility of in vitro sensitivity tests is controversial, and most authorities do not recommend the procedure owing to the difficulty of the task, the frequent delay in results necessitated by the prolonged incubation period for growth, and the predictability of results. Penicillin G is generally considered the drug of choice, with alternatives being cephalosporins, clindamycin, chloramphenicol, vancomycin, erythromycin, and imipenem. Metronidazole is commonly used for anaerobic infections and is somewhat unpredictable for some anaerobic gram-positive cocci and virtually all aerotolerant strains.

NORMAL FLORA

Anaerobic cocci are found at virtually all mucocutaneous surfaces that harbor a commensal flora. In saliva they account for 30–40 percent of the cultivable flora; approximately half of these organisms are *V. parvula* and the rest include a diverse array of anaerobic gram-positive cocci.[5] Studies of the normal flora of the female genital tract indicate that 60–80 percent of women harbor anaerobic gram-positive cocci in the cervical and vaginal flora in mean concentrations of $10^{8.7}$/g of secretions (mean total concentration of $10^{9.1}$ bacteria/g).[6,7] The dominant organisms found are *P. asaccharolyticus, P. magnus, P. anaerobius*, and *P. prevotii*. *Veillonella* is rarely found at this clinical site. In the fecal flora, anaerobic gram-positive cocci are usually present and found in mean concentrations of approximately 10^{10}/g (total concentration of $10^{11.4}$ bacteria/g of dry weight).[8] One of the most common is *Peptostreptococcus productus*, an infrequent clinical isolate; other species that are found less frequently include *P. magnus, P. prevotii, P. micros, P. parvulus*, and *P. asaccharolyticus*. Other anaerobic cocci that may be found in the fecal flora that are relatively infrequent clinical isolates include *V. parvula, Ruminococcus* species, *A. fermentans*, and *M. elsdenii*. The anaerobic gram-positive cocci also represent normal flora of the skin, urethra, stomach, and small intestine.

RECOVERY IN CLINICAL SPECIMENS

Anaerobic gram-positive cocci are relatively frequent clinical isolates, usually as components of mixed infections involving additional aerobic or anaerobic bacteria. The experience at the Mayo Clinic for three periods of study is summarized in Table 1.[4,9,10] This shows an isolation rate for anaerobic gram-positive cocci of 8.5–31 percent among clinical specimens that yielded any anaerobic bacteria.

The most common clinical isolates are *P. magnus, P. anaerobius, P. micros*, and *P. prevotii* (Table 2).[4] Little is known regarding the relative pathogenic potential and virulence factors of these organisms, although *P. magnus* has been suggested as particularly significant among this group in terms of its frequency of isolation.[10] Data from the Mayo Clinic indicate that this organism accounted for approximately 13 percent of all anaerobic isolates and 51 percent of anaerobic gram-positive cocci in 1983 (Table 2).[4] During this year, anaerobic cocci accounted for 4 percent of anaerobic bacteremias and *P. magnus* was the major blood culture isolate in this group. Although most of the infections were polymicrobial, this organism was recovered in pure culture in approximately 15 percent of the 176 specimens that yielded *P. magnus*. The most frequent types of infections involving *P. magnus* in pure culture were septic arthritis, osteomyelitis (especially infected total hip arthroplasties), and soft tissue infections.

Veillonella species, primarily *V. parvula*, are the most frequently isolated gram-negative anaerobic cocci. These organisms account for 112 of 10,998 (1 percent) anaerobic isolates at the Mayo Clinic during 1971–1972.[9] *Veillonella* represent normal flora, primarily of the upper airways, although the organism is occasionally found in the genital tract and lower gastrointestinal tract as well. In the majority of cases, this represents a contaminant, or it is a component of a polymicrobial flora in which its role as a pathogen is doubtful.

TABLE 1. Frequency of Isolation of *Peptostreptococcus* from Clinical Specimens at the Mayo Clinic during Three Periods of Study

Period Reviewed (Source)	*No. of Specimens Cultivated Anaerobically*	*No. with Anaerobes*	*No. with Anaerobic Gram-Positive Cocci*
1971–1972[9] [a]	27,588	14,839 (54%)	1260 (8.5%)
1974–1978[10] [a]	10,817	2223 (21%)	697 (31%)
1983[4] [b]	Not stated	1340	344 (26%)

[a] Reviews from 1971–1972 and 1974–1978 include some isolates designated as peptostreptococci that have been reclassified as streptococci. Most of these organisms are now classified as *S. intermedius* group (see text).
[b] Analysis is restricted to the "most frequently isolated" anaerobic bacteria excluding *Propionibacterium* sp.

TABLE 2. Anaerobic Bacteria Recovered from Clinical Specimens at the Mayo Clinic in 1983

Organism	*No. of Isolates (%)*
Bacteroides fragilis group	458 (34)
Peptostreptococcus magnus	176 (13)
Bacteroides melaninogenicus group	127 (10)
Clostridium perfringens	97 (7)
Veillonella parvula	55 (4)
Bacteroides ruminicola subsp. *brevis*	49 (4)
Bacteroides oralis	48 (4)
Bacteroides bivius	42 (3)
Clostridium ramosum	41 (3)
Eubacterium lentum	41 (3)
Fusobacterium nucleatum	38 (3)
Peptostreptococcus anaerobius	35 (3)
Peptostreptococcus micros	31 (2)
Peptostreptococcus prevotii	30 (2)

[a] Analysis restricted to "most frequent isolates" excluding *Propionibacterium* sp.
(From Rosenblatt,[4] with permission.)

CLINICAL CONDITIONS

The frequency of peptostreptococci in various anaerobic infections according to the experience at the Wadsworth Veterans Administration Hospital is summarized in Table 3.[11] The data provided indicate that these organisms account for a substantial portion of all anaerobic isolates in clinical specimens, but they also show considerable variation in recovery rates at different anatomic sites. To be emphasized is the observation that the analysis provided uses current taxonomic criteria so that organisms reclassified as aerobic or microaerophilic streptococci are now excluded. This may account for the major differences in isolation rates and the reported bacteriologic results for studies reported prior to the taxonomic change in 1983 or subsequent reports using prior definitions.

Anaerobic Pleuropulmonary Infections

Peptostreptococci account for approximately 10 percent of 656 anaerobic isolates recovered from pulmonary specimens, primarily transtracheal aspirates and pleural fluid.[11,12] Our earlier studies indicated a higher rate with these organisms, accounting for 130 of 461 (28 percent) isolates from similar sources, although these included organisms now classified as *Streptococcus intermedius* and "microaerophilic streptococci." *Veillonella* are sometimes recovered from these specimens as well, but this organism is almost universally present in saliva and its presence may be used as a marker of salivary contamination, so that recovery must be interpreted with caution.

Intra-abdominal Sepsis

Peptostreptococci are components of the normal intestinal flora and may be recovered in 20 percent of specimens from patients with intra-abdominal sepsis.[13,14] In virtually all cases, it represents a component of a polymicrobial infection. The yield of

TABLE 3. Frequency of *Peptostreptococcus* in Anaerobic Infections

Specimen Source	*No. of Specimens with Anaerobes*	*Total No. of Anaerobic Isolates*	*No. of Isolates of Peptostreptococcus/ 100 Specimens*
Baceremia	175	226	7
Central nervous system	19	32	21
Head and neck	75	349	85
Human bite	25	72	48
Animal bite	33	81	21
Pulmonary (TTA, pleural fluid)	196	656	33
Intra-abdominal sepsis	185	203	51
Perirectal abscess	34	158	68
Decubitus ulcer	54	212	107
Foot ulcers	222	645	111
Miscellaneous soft tissue infections (other)	205	578	85
Osteomyelitis	49	139	133

(From Finegold et al.,[11] with permission.)

peptostreptococci is somewhat higher in patients with hepatic abscess.

Female Pelvic Infections

Early studies of the female genital tract focused considerable attention on the role of anaerobic gram-positive cocci in these infections. More recent studies have emphasized an apparently increasing isolation rate of *Bacteroides* species, especially *B. bivus*. Nevertheless, Peptostreptococcus, primarily *P. anaerobius* and *P. provotii*, may be recovered in 25–40 percent of cases, including endometritis, pyometra, pelvic abscess, Bartholin's gland abscess, puerperal sepsis, postgynecologic surgical infections, and polymicrobial pelvic inflammatory disease.[15–20] Bacteremia with *Peptostreptococcus* is especially common in the setting of septic abortion and suppurative thrombophlebitis of the pelvic veins.

Skin and Soft Tissue Infections

Anaerobic bacteria are common isolates in polymicrobial infections of the skin and soft tissue including necrotizing fasciitis, necrotizing synergistic gangrene, infected diabetic foot ulcers, and infected decubiti. In each instance, these are usually polymicrobial infections involving an average of five to eight different anaerobic and aerobic bacterial species. Streptococcal myositis, a condition traditionally and classically ascribed to group A β hemolytic streptococcus, is sometimes caused by other species of streptococci including *Peptostreptococcus*. These organisms may also be found in breast abscesses and infected sebaceous cysts. Care must be exercised in the interpretation of bacterial cultures yielding peptostreptococci from percutaneously collected specimens since these organisms constitute normal skin flora; thus, a pathogenic role is best supported by the observation of typical organisms on direct Gram stain of specimens and their recovery in relatively large concentrations.

Osteomyelitis and Septic Arthritis

Peptostreptococcus is a relatively frequent isolate in infections of bones and joints. As noted above, *P. magnus* appears to play a particularly prominent role.[4] A review of 18 patients with septic arthritis or osteomyelitis involving *P. magnus* showed that all had previously undergone orthopaedic surgery and that 15 had foreign material in place at the time of the infection. The clinical course is characteristically chronic and indolent. These infections obey the usual rules for infected prostheses including the necessity for prolonged courses of antimicrobial therapy combined with removal of the prosthesis.

Bacteremia

Peptostreptococci account for 4–7 percent of blood culture isolates involving anaerobic bacteria at major medical centers.[4,9,10] Intra-abdominal sepsis and gynecologic infections are the most frequent underlying causes. Anaerobic and microaerophilic streptococci account for 5–10 percent of cases of endocarditis, although a relatively small portion of these involve organisms that are currently classified as *Peptostreptococcus*.

TREATMENT

Penicillin G is generally considered the preferred agent for treatment of infections involving *Peptostreptococcus*. Other antibiotics that are also generally active include other penicillins, cephalosporins, clindamycin, chloramphenicol, vancomycin, and imipenem. The activity of tetracycline is unpredictable, and erythromycin is also somewhat variable. Metronidazole is commonly used for anaerobic infections and is somewhat unpredictable in its activity against *Peptostreptococcus*, with at least 10 percent of strains being highly resistant. Occasional strains are also resistant to clindamycin, and this resistance has sometimes been noted with isolates recovered after treatment with clindamycin, although the clinical significance of these findings was not clear since the patients recovered without a change in therapy.[12]

The antimicrobial susceptibility pattern for *Peptostreptococcus* is largely predictable on the basis of the observations noted above. Most authorities recommend that susceptibility testing not be done, with possible exceptions being blood culture isolates (especially from patients with persistent or recurrent bacteremia, endocarditis, and other vascular infection) and isolates from osteomyelitis, septic arthritis, infections of prosthetic devices, and cerebral abscess.[13] The potential utility of the information is obviously magnified in cases in which this organism is isolated in pure culture.

REFERENCES

1. Ezaki T, Yamamoto N, Ninomiya K, et al. Transfer of *Peptococcus indolicus, Peptococcus asaccharolyticus, Peptococcus prevotii*, and *Peptococcus magnus* to the genus *Peptostreptococcus* and proposal of *Peptostreptococcus tetradius* sp. nov. Int J Syst Bacteriol. 1983;33:683–98.
2. Huss VAR, Festl H, Schleifer KH. Nucleic acid hybridization studies and deoxyribonucleic acid base compositions of anaerobic, gram-positive cocci. Int J Syst Bacteriol. 1984;34:95–101.
3. Gossling J. Occurrence and pathogenicity of the *Streptococcus milleri* group. Rev Infect Dis. 1988;10:257–85.
4. Rosenblatt J. Anaerobic Cocci. In: Lennette EH, ed. Manual of Clinical Microbiology. 4th ed. Washington: American Society for Microbiology; 1985:445–9.
5. Socransky SS, Manganiello SD. The oral microbiota of man from birth to senility. J Periodont. 1971;42:485–94.
6. Bartlett JG, Onderdonk AB, Drude E, et al. Quantitative bacteriology of the vaginal flora. J Infect Dis. 1977;136:271–7.
7. Ohm MJ, Galask RP. Bacterial flora of the cervix from 100 prehysterectomy patients. Am J Obstet Gynecol. 1975;122:683–7.
8. Finegold SM, Attebery HR, Sutter VL. Effect of diet on human fecal flora: Comparison of Japanese and American diets. Am J Clin Nutr. 1974;27:1456–69.
9. Martin WJ. Isolation and identification of anaerobic bacteria in the clinical laboratory: A 2-year experience. Mayo Clin Proc. 1974;49:300–8.
10. Bourgault A-M, Rosenblatt JE, Fitzgerald RH. *Peptococcus magnus*: A significant human pathogen. Ann Intern Med. 1980;93:244–8.
11. Finegold SM, George WL, Mulligan ME. Anaerobic Infections. Disease-a-Month. 1985;31:8–77.
12. Ohm-Smith MJ, Sweet RL, Hadley WL. Occurrence of clindamycin-resistant anaerobic bacteria isolated from cultures taken following clindamycin therapy. Antimicrob Agents Chemother. 1986;30:11–4.
13. Finegold SM and the National Committee for Clinical Laboratory Standards Working Group on Anaerobic Susceptibility Testing. Susceptibility testing of anaerobic bacteria. J Clin Microbiol. 1988;26:1253–6.

225. ANAEROBIC GRAM-POSITIVE NONSPORULATING BACILLI

JOHN G. BARTLETT

The genera included here are *Actinomyces, Arachnia, Bifidobacterium, Eubacterium, Lachnospira, Lactobacillus*, and *Propionibacterium*. These are gram-positive or gram-variable rods that are often pleomorphic; some grow in 5–10% CO_2–air incubation despite classification as anaerobic. *Actinomyces* sp. and *Arachnia propionica* cause actinomycosis, which is described elsewhere. The most common clinical isolates of the group are *Propionibacterium acnes* and *Eubacterium lentum*.

NORMAL FLORA

These organisms constitute a major component of the normal flora of mucocutaneous surfaces. *Propionibacterium acnes* is a predominant component of the skin flora and may also be found on mucosal surfaces including the mouth, intestine, urethra, and vagina. Quantitative cultures of stool in 33 healthy persons showed that eubacteria and bifidobacteria accounted for 17 of the 50 isolates recovered in the highest concentrations ($10^{9.8}$–$10^{10.5}$/g of dry weight).[1] Quantitative cultures of vaginal secretions showed that anaerobic gram-positive nonsporulating bacilli were recovered from 35 of 52 specimens in mean concentrations of $10^{8.6}$ gm (mean total concentration of anaerobic bacteria was $10^{9.8}$/g).[2] In the oral cavity, these organisms account for about 5 percent of the salivary flora and 15–25 percent of the gingival flora.[3]

CLINICALLY SIGNIFICANT ISOLATES

Propionibacteria

Propionibacterium acnes is the most common clinical isolate among the anaerobic gram-positive nonsporulating bacilli, accounting for 15–25 percent of anaerobic isolates in some series.[4] They are also common isolates in blood cultures. In the great majority of cases, propionibacteria represent contaminants, so that recovery from normally sterile body fluids is inconsistent and the quantity of organisms is usually small. The major exception is acne. Less frequent exceptions are infections of prosthetic joints, infections of cerebrospinal shunts, osteomyelitis after neurosurgical procedures, and endocarditis.

Eubacteria

The second most frequent clinical isolates from this group are eubacteria, the most common being *E. lentum*. In most instances, this organism is a component of a mixed flora involving multiple other bacteria with better established pathogenic potential. The organism is a major component of the fecal flora and plays a curious role in digitalis toxicity associated with antibiotic use. Approximately 10 percent of patients given digoxin convert a substantial portion of the drug to reduced metabolites that are inactive.[7] *Eubacterium lentum* is the component of the fecal flora considered responsible for this activity. The clinical relevance of the observation concerns the consequences of antibiotic administration to such individuals. Drugs such as erythromycin and tetracycline (and presumably others active against *E. lentum*) may result in serum digoxin concentrations as much as twofold higher.

Bifidobacteria

Bifidobacteria represent a dominant component of the fecal flora of humans, but they are infrequent clinical isolates. When they are recovered, they are usually part of a polymicrobial flora that includes other organisms with better established pathogenic potential. A possible exception is *B. dentium,* formerly classified as *Actinomyces eriksonii*.[8]

REFERENCES

1. Finegold SM, Attebery HR, Sutter VL. Effect of diet on human fecal flora: Comparison of Japanese and American diets. Am J Clin Nutr. 1974;27:1456–69.
2. Bartlett JG, Onderdonk AB, Drude E, et al. Quantitative bacteriology of the vaginal flora. J Infect Dis. 1977;136:271–7.
3. Socransky SS, Manganiello SD. The oral microbiota of man from birth to senility. J Periodontol. 1971;42:485–94.
4. Martin WJ. Isolation and identification of anaerobic bacteria in the clinical laboratory: A 2-year experience. Mayo Clin Proc. 1974;49:300–8.
5. Beeler BA, Crowder JG, Smith JW, et al. *Propionibacterium acnes:* Pathogen in central nervous system shunt infection. Am J Med. 1976;61:935–8.
6. Felner JM, Dowell Vr Jr. Anaerobic bacterial endocarditis. N Engl J Med. 1970;283:1188–92.
7. Lindenbaum J, Rund DG, Butler VP Jr, et al. Inactivation of digoxin by the gut flora: Reversal by antibiotic therapy. N Engl J Med. 1981;305:789–94.
8. Thomas AV, Sodeman TH, Bentz RR. *Bifidobacterium (Actinomyces) eriksonii* infection. Am Rev Respir Dis. 1974;110:663–8.

MISCELLANEOUS BACTERIA

226. BARTONELLA BACILLIFORMIS (BARTONELLOSIS)

NORBERT J. ROBERTS, JR.

The cutaneous manifestations (verrugas) of bartonellosis have been known since the pre-Inca times in Peru. In 1870 the acute form (Oroya fever) was recognized with the occurrence of a severe epidemic of fever and anemia among workmen building the railway between Lima and Oroya. The common bacterial etiology of the two forms was established in 1885 by Daniel Carrión, a Peruvian medical student who developed Oroya fever after having himself inoculated with the blood from a patient's verruga. As a result, bartonellosis has often been designated as Carrión's disease. In 1909 Barton described the circulating causative organism.

DESCRIPTION OF THE PATHOGEN

Bartonella bacilliformis is a small, motile, aerobic pleomorphic bacillus with unipolar flagella that stains reddish purple with Giemsa stain.[1–3] It is gram-negative but counterstains poorly. The organism is often seen in clusters of small bacillary forms, slightly curved, 0.25–0.5 μm in width and 1–3 μm in length, and as coccobacillary forms.[2–4] *B. bacilliformis* grows best at 28–30°C in semisolid nutrient agar containing fresh rabbit serum and rabbit hemoglobin.

EPIDEMIOLOGY

Bartonellosis has a strictly limited regional occurrence that is likely due to the limited habitats of its sandfly vector, *Phlebotomus*.[2,5] *P. verrucarum* and possibly other species of sandfly propagate and transmit this infection in river valleys of the Andes Mountains at altitudes between 2000 and 8000 feet in Peru, Ecuador, and Columbia.[6] In these regions the disease is endemic, with asymptomatic cases and long-term carriers serving as reservoirs of infection.

Both the intrinsic characteristics of the organism and the geographic restriction of the infection distinguish bartonellosis from other hematotropic bacterial infections.[2,3,7,8]

PATHOGENESIS

In nonimmune persons, infection with *Bartonella* via the bite of an infected sandfly results in the manifestations of Oroya fever. Large numbers of bacteria adhere to erythrocytes and invade endothelial cells.[5] When *B. bacilliformis* binds to erythrocytes, it induces deep indentations and deformations of the membrane, with apparent membrane fusion at the neck of the indentation and entry of bacteria within intracellular vacuoles.[9] The bacteria then appear to replicate within the vacuoles without release into the cytoplasm. The infection causes erythrocyte deformation that is only slowly reversible even in the absence of bacterial internalization, which suggests that the internal cytoskeleton has been altered in some way.[9] Cells of the reticuloendothelial system phagocytose and destroy infected erythrocytes and can be shown to contain many organisms.[4,6] In typical patients with acute bartonellosis, the life span of the erythrocytes is thus greatly shortened, and anemia develops, often rapidly and to a severe degree. Coombs test and other tests for agglutinins and hemolysins are negative.[10] Mechanical fragility of the erythrocytes appears to contribute to their destruction, but the fragility does not appear to be related to the intensity of parasitization. Decreased bone marrow erythropoietic response contributes to a rapid development of anemia. In those patients who survive the acute stage, erythropoiesis is markedly enhanced as the infection subsides. Manifestations of complicating infections, especially with *Salmonella* species, most commonly occur in this recovery phase of Oroya fever but may occur in the acute stage of developing anemia.[11]

During recovery, organisms in the blood disappear or decline to a very low level. Resolution of the Oroya fever phase of bartonellosis appears to coincide with the development of immunity that makes second episodes of Oroya fever very unusual.[1,2,6] After a variable latent period, most persons develop a chronic benign form of bartonellosis called *verruga peruana*.[4] Hemangiomatous nodules, which may contain *Bartonella* organisms, develop in the skin and subcutaneous tissue, with minor variations in histologic characteristics and evolution depending on location.[12] These lesions consist of numerous newly formed small vessels with proliferation of endothelial cells. In addition, mast cells as well as lymphocytes and macrophages are present.[12] Old cutaneous verrugas may become quite fibrotic. Uncommonly, lesions have been reported to occur in internal organs and tissues including the central nervous system and bone.

CLINICAL MANIFESTATIONS

Bartonellosis includes two clinical forms of disease, both manifestations of infection by *B. bacilliformis*. The incubation period of bartonellosis is approximately 3 weeks as judged by cases with known times of inoculation.[13,14] However, marked variability is possible, with incubation periods up to 100 days. Apparently healthy persons can be found with blood cultures positive for *B. bacilliformis*.[2]

Oroya Fever

In the nonimmune person, the onset of this form of acute bartonellosis may be either insidious or abrupt. When insidious, the patient may note anorexia, headache, malaise, and a slight fever lasting from 2 to 7 or more days. In these cases, examination of blood smears is frequently negative, and a diagnosis cannot be secured unless blood cultures are obtained. Alternatively, the onset may be sudden, with high fever, severe chills, diaphoresis, headaches, and changes in mentation.[4,14] A sudden marked drop in the number of erythrocytes occurs and gives a peculiar color to the skin that results from slight jaundice combined with pallor due to the severe anemia. The anemia is macrocytic, often hypochromic, with polychromasia, poikilocytosis, Howell-Jolly bodies, basophilic granulations, nucleated erythrocytes, and immature myeloid forms.[4,10] Leukocyte counts are variable, but a shift to the left is usually present regardless of the total leukocyte count.[4] Within several days the erythrocyte count may fall to as low as 500,000/mm^3. The severity of the anemia does not parallel the intensity of the fever. The most rapid diagnosis of Oroya fever may be obtained by eosin/thiazine stain (Diff-Quik, Merz and Dade) of blood smears.[15] Numerous organisms are seen on the blood smear, often adherent to as many as 90 percent of the erythrocytes. IgM antibody may be present not only in patients with Oroya fever but in some healthy individuals as well as those with verrugas.[15]

At this stage, muscle and joint pain and headache may be severe; dyspnea and angina may develop as well as insomnia, delerium, and in terminal cases, coma. Patients often note a feeling of transmission of the cardiac impulse to the head and ears. A generalized nontender lymphadenopathy may develop, but enlargement of the spleen is usually associated with intercurrent infection.[4] Thrombocytopenic purpura may be evident. If the patient survives these changes, a ''critical stage'' then ensues that is characterized by the sudden disappearance of the organism from the erythrocytes. This convalescent phase is marked by a decrease in fever, an increase in the number of erythrocytes, and fewer earlier forms of polymorphonuclear leukocytes. Intercurrent infection[4,6] is most common at this stage and may account for reports of mortality of more than 50 percent.[5] Salmonellosis, amebiasis, malaria, tuberculosis, and invasion by various enteric pathogens are common complications (up to 45 percent of the cases) and adversely affect prognosis, especially during the acute anemic stage. Recurrence of fever or the presence of marked leukocytosis at any time should suggest intercurrent infection.

Verruga Peruana

After resolution of Oroya fever, pain in the bones, joints, and muscles may persist to the stage of verruga development.[4] This cutaneous eruptive form may follow Oroya fever or may develop without prior symptoms, notably in those with previous episodes of bartonellosis. Nodules develop over a period of 1–2 months and may persist for months to years.The verrugas appear most frequently on exposed parts of the body but may also involve mucous membranes and internal organs.[4] Serous membranes may become inflamed, with the organism present in leukocytes of effusions. The cutaneous lesions may vary from red to purple and appear in crops; lesions in stages of growth and regression may be seen in the same patient. The verrugas, may be sessile, miliary, nodular, pedunculated or confluent, with individual lesions reaching 1–2 cm in diameter. They may become secondarily infected and result in a pustular form or may ulcerate or bleed. In the absence of complicating infection, the verrugas are nontender. The diversity of skin lesions, often appearing after subjects leave the endemic area, can pose problems of diagnosis for clinicians and pathologists who encounter either early or late lesions.[12] Joint pains and low-grade fever, often present in the pre-eruptive stage, usually decrease after onset of the eruption. Anemia due to bartonellosis is usually not present at this stage.[4] The organism may be cultured from the cutaneous lesions and occasionally from the blood and bone marrow in this stage.[2,6]

PREVENTION AND TREATMENT

Prevention of infection requires control of the sandfly. For the community, this consists of spraying interiors and exteriors of dwellings with DDT; for the person, protection may be obtained by the use of insect repellents and bed netting. Treatment of acute bartonellosis with chloramphenicol,[5,11] penicillin,[14] and possibly tetracycline and streptomycin[2] produces a dramatic clinical response. Fever often disappears within 24 hours, although organisms may persist longer in the blood.[5] The choice of antibiotic is commonly dictated by the presence of secondary infection. Because of the frequency of complicating *Salmonella* infections,[2] chloramphenicol is often the drug of choice in doses of 2 g or more daily for a minimum of 7 days.[5,11] Blood transfusions may be indicated in cases with severe anemia. Cutaneous verrugal lesions show a variable response to antibiotic therapy; larger and secondarily infected nodules may require surgical excision.

REFERENCES

1. Peters D, Wigand R. Bartonellaceae. Bacteriol Rev. 1955;19:150–9.
2. Weinman D, Kreier JP. *Bartonella* and *Grahamella*. In: Kreier JP, ed. Parasitic Protozoa, v. 4. New York: Academic Press; 1977:197.
3. Kreier JP, Ristic M. The biology of hemotrophic bacteria. Annu Rev Microbiol. 1981;35:325–38.
4. Ricketts WE. Clinical manifestations of Carrión's disease. Arch Intern Med. 1949;84:751–81.
5. Urteaga BO, Payne EH. Treatment of the acute febrile phase of Carrión's disease with chloramphenicol. Am J Trop Med. 1955;4:507–11.
6. Howe C. Carrión's disease. Immunologic studies. Arch Intern Med. 1943;72:147–67.
7. Archer GL, Coleman PH, Cole RM, et al. Human infection from an unidentified erythrocyte-associated bacterium. N Engl J Med. 1979;301:897–900.
8. Dooley JR: Haemotropic bacteria in man. Lancet. 1980;2:1237–9.
9. Benson LA, Kar S, McLaughlin G, et al. Entry of *Bartonella bacilliformis* into erythrocytes. Infect Immun. 1986;54:347–53.
10. Reynafarje C, Ramos J. The hemolytic anemia of human bartonellosis. Blood. 1961;17:562–78.
11. Cuadra M: Salmonellosis complication in human bartonellosis. Tex Rep Biol Med. 1956;14:97–113.
12. Arias-Stella J, Lieberman PH, Erlandson RA, et al. Histology, immunohistochemistry, and ultrastructure of the verruga in Carrión's disease. Am J Surg Pathol. 1986;10:595–610.
13. Ricketts WE. Carrión's disease. A study of the incubation period in thirteen cases. Am J Trop Med. 1947;27:657–9.
14. Schultz MG. Daniel Carrión's experiment. N Engl J Med. 1968;278:1323–6.
15. Knobloch J, Solano L, Alvarez O, et al. Antibodies to *Bartonella bacilliformis* as determined by fluorescence antibody test, indirect haemagglutination and ELISA. Trop Med Parasitol. 1985;36:183–5.

227. CALYMMATOBACTERIUM GRANULOMATIS (DONOVANOSIS, GRANULOMA INGUINALE)

GAVIN HART

Donovanosis has been known by many names, including granuloma contagiosum, granuloma Donovani, granuloma inguinale tropicum, granuloma pudendi tropicum, sclerosing granuloma, and ulcerating granuloma of the pudenda, but the most common synonyms are granuloma inguinale and granuloma venereum.

Donovanosis was probably first described by McLeod in 1882. The causative organism was discovered by Donovan in 1905 and was known as *Donovania granulomatis*. Because of the characteristics of the organism, particularly a prominent capsule, a relationship with *Klebsiella* has often been suggested.[1] However, possibly due to the difficulty in growing *Calymmatobacterium granulomatis* on artificial media, its biochemical and bacteriologic characteristics have not been defined sufficiently to support this classification, and it must currently be regarded as an organism of uncertain affiliation.

DESCRIPTION OF PATHOGEN

The infectious agent is *Calymmatobacterium granulomatis*, a gram-negative bacterium measuring 1.5 μm by 0.7 μm. In tissue smears, the bacteria appear enclosed in vacuolar compartments in large histiocytic cells or occasionally in polymorphonuclear leukocytes or plasma cells.[2] The bacteria reproduce in multiple foci within these cells until the vacuole contains 20–30 organisms, which mature and are then liberated when the infected cell ruptures.

The organisms have a surrounding cell membrane and overlying cell wall and possess a sharply defined capsule when mature. Small filamentous projections, of the size of bacterial fimbriae or pili, extend from the cell wall. Electron microscopy reveals electron-dense granules measuring 35–45 μm in diameter at the periphery of the cell.[1] Culture in the chick embryonic yolk sac has been reported.[3]

EPIDEMIOLOGY

Although fewer than 100 cases are reported annually in the United States, donovanosis is very common in New Guinea, India, central Australia, the Caribbean, and in many other tropical or subtropical environments. In West New Guinea, up to 25 percent of some populations were infected in the 1920s, and 23.5 percent of male patients attending one urban VD clinic in 1972 had donovanosis.[4] A recent epidemic of 20 cases was reported from Texas.[5]

The role of sexual transmission is controversial. Goldberg[6] postulated that the vagina is often infected by autoinoculation from the rectum but clinical disease occurs after sexual or nonsexual trauma of infected sites. Anal intercourse is closely associated with rectal lesions in passive homosexual patients and penile lesions in their active partners.[7] In most cases, lesions cannot be detected in sexual contacts, but a number of studies have detected infection in 12–52 percent of marital or steady sexual partners.[8] The disease is only mildly contagious, and repeated exposure is apparently necessary for the development of most clinical cases. The long incubation period or inconspicuous lesions (such as rectal or vaginal) favor low detection rates in sexual partners.

Zigas[9] screened a New Guinea population and detected lesions in 4.4 percent of the children 1–4 years of age and in 4.9 percent of persons over age 15, whereas no disease was detected in the other age groups. He suggested that the young children were probably infected by sitting on the laps of diseased parents or relatives, whereas adult infection was associated with sexual intercourse.

PATHOLOGY AND CLINICAL MANIFESTATIONS

The primary lesion begins as an indurated nodule that erodes to form a beefy, exuberant, granulomatous, heaped ulcer. This usually progresses slowly, often coalescing with adjacent lesions or forming new lesions by autoinoculation, particularly in the perineal region. Extensive acanthosis and dense dermal infiltrate, mainly plasma cells and histiocytes, occur. Some polymorphonuclear lymphocytes are present in focal collections or scattered throughout the infiltrate, but lymphocytes are rare. The pronounced marginal epithelial proliferation may simulate early epitheliomatous change.[10] Diverse clinical variants may occur that vary from necrotic destructive lesions with profuse exudate to sclerotic forms comprising dry lesions in which scarring is prominent.

The infecting organisms invade mononuclear endothelial cells and, when mature, feature metachromatic bars that stain blue or black with Wright stain. The pathognomonic feature of donovanosis is the large infected mononuclear cell, 25–90 μm in diameter, containing many intracytoplasmic cysts filled with deeply staining Donovan bodies.

Metastatic hematogenous spread to bones, joints, and liver occasionally occurs. Occasionally, the lymphatics are involved, but the frequently seen "suppurating bubo" of the groin is in fact a subcutaneous granuloma (pseudobubo). Secondary infection may occur and aggravate tissue destruction and residual scarring.

SYMPTOMS

The incubation period has been ill defined but is probably 8–80 days. The disease begins as single or multiple subcutaneous nodules that erode through the skin to produce clean granulomatous sharply defined lesions that are usually painless. These lesions, which bleed readily on contact slowly enlarge. Secondary infection may contribute to necrotic debris on an ulcer or at its margin, but surrounding cellulitis rarely occurs. Fibrosis occurs concurrently with extension of the primary lesion, and phimosis or lymphedema of distal tissues is common in the active phase of the disease.

The genitalia are involved in 90 percent of the cases, the inguinal region in 10 percent, the anal region in 5–10 percent, and distant sites in 1–5 percent.[9] Lesions are limited to the genitalia in approximately 80 percent of cases and to the inguinal region in less than 5 percent. Cervical or intravaginal lesions are an uncommon cause of vaginal bleeding.[11] Hematogenous spread of the organism is more common in females,[12] particularly in those with primary lesions on the cervix.

In the man, lesions most commonly occur on the prepuce or glans (Fig. 1), and in the woman lesions on the labia are the most common. The most common distant sites infected are on the head (mouth, lips, throat, face), but involvement of the liver, thorax, and bones[13] has also been reporred.

Systemic disease is associated with severe constitutional toxemia involving a prolonged spiking fever, progressive anemia, and weight loss.[14]

DIAGNOSIS

The clinical manifestation is highly suggestive of the diagnosis in most cases. However, the diagnosis is readily confirmed by a stained crush preparation from the lesion. A piece of clean granulation tissue from a lesion is spread against the slide to be examined. The impression obtained is air-dried and stained with Wright or Giemsa stain.

Donovan bodies appear as clusters of blue- or black-staining organisms with a "safety pin" appearance (from bipolar chromatin condensation) in the cytoplasm of large mononuclear cells.

The crush preparation is designed to facilitate interpretation by minimizing the amount of debris and other organisms that may occur on superficial smears. However identification of Donovan bodies in Papanicolaou smears has been reported.[15,16] The features on a smear from cervical lesions include intact capillaries indicative of epithelial and stromal ulceration, marked inflammatory cell infiltrate consisting predominantly of neutrophils, epithelioid histiocytes representing granuloma formation, and Donovan bodies located in characteristic single or multiple intracytoplasmic vacuoles within large histiocytes.[16] No multinucleated giant cells and very few lymphocytes were observed, thus providing an important distinction from some chronic granulomatous conditions.

Light microscopic examination of formalin-fixed biopsy specimens is a less reliable diagnostic procedure since the pathognomonic Donovan bodies are infrequently seen. However the organisms may be identified by electron microscopy or by light microscopy of sections prepared for electron microscopy by glutaraldehyde fixation and plastic embedding.[2]

Coexisting syphilis and gonorrhea may be detected,[12] and some cases of chancroid may simulate donovanosis.[17]

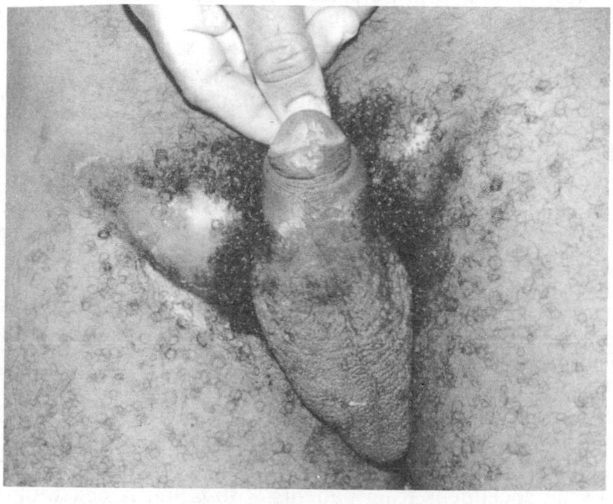

FIG. 1. Lesion of donovanosis on the penis.

PREVENTION AND TREATMENT

Tetracycline (0.5 g every 6 hours orally) is often effective, but failures can occur. Ampicillin is sometimes effective[18] but may require prolonged administration (0.5 g four times a day orally for 12 weeks).[19] Either gentamicin (1 mg/kg twice a day) or chloramphenicol (0.5 g every 8 hours orally) are probably the most effective drugs and cure most lesions within 3 weeks.[20] Erythromycin (0.5 g every 6 hours orally)[21] may be considered in pregnancy, but the results are often disappointing unless it is combined with another antibiotic.[22] Trimethoprim-sulfamethoxazole (two tablets every 12 hours for 10 days) has also proved effective.[23] Penicillin is not effective.[24]

Tetracycline, ampicillin, or trimethoprim-sulfamethoxazole may be used as first-line therapy, and chloramphenicol and gentamicin may be reserved for resistant cases or in communities where failures with the above agents are common. If an antibiotic is effective, the clinical response to treatment, indicated by shrinking and decreasing redness of the lesions, will be evident in 7 days.

Medication should be continued until the lesions have completely healed. If treatment is stopped before this time (after a minimum of 3 weeks of therapy), healing usually continues, but the recurrence rate is greater.

Control measures have never been evaluated, but yearly screening of the total male population aged 15–40 years reduced the prevalence to below 1 percent in one locale.[25]

REFERENCES

1. Kuberski T, Papadimitriou JM, Phillips P. Ultrastructure of *Calymmatobacterium granulomatis* in lesions of granuloma inguinale. J Infect Dis. 1980;142:744.
2. Dodson RF, Fritz GS, Hubler WR, et al. Donovanosis: A morphologic study. J Invest Dermatol. 1974;62:611.
3. Anderson K, Goodpasture EW, DeMonbreun WA. Etiologic consideration of *Donovania granulomatis* cultured in three cases in embryonic yolks. J Exp Med. 1945;8:451.
4. Hart G. Psychological and social aspects of venereal disease in Papua New Guinea. Br J Vener Dis. 1974;50:453.
5. Rosen T, Tschen JA, Ramsdell W, et al. Granuloma inguinale. J Am Acad Dermatol. 1984;11:433.
6. Goldberg J. Studies on granuloma inguinale VII. Some epidemiological considerations of the disease. Br J Vener Dis. 1964;40:140.
7. Marmell M. Donovanosis of the anus in the male. An epidemiologic consideration. Br J Vener Dis. 1958;34:213.
8. Hart G. Chancroid, Donovanosis, Lymphogranuloma venereum. US Department of Health, Education and Welfare, Publication No. (CDC) 75-8302, 1975.
9. Zigas V. Medicine from the past—donovanosis project in Goilala (1951–1954). Papua New Guinea Med J. 1971;14:148.
10. Nayar M, Chandra M, Saxena HMK, et al. Donovanosis—a histopathological study. Indian J Pathol Microbiol. 1981;24:71.
11. Murugan S, Venkatram K, Renganathan PS. Vaginal bleeding in granuloma inguinale. Br J Vener Dis. 1982;58:200.

12. Brigden M, Guard R. Extragenital granuloma inguinale in North Queensland. Med J Aust. 1980;2:565.
13. Kirkpatrick DJ. Donovanosis (granuloma inguinale); a rare cause of osteolytic bone lesions. Clin Radiol. 1970;21:101.
14. Rajam RV, Rangiah PN, Anguli VC. Systemic Donovaniasis. Br J Vener Dis. 1954;30:73.
15. De Boer A, De Boer F, Van der Merwe JV. Cytologic identification of Donovan bodies in granuloma inguinale. Acta Cytol (Baltimore). 1984;28:126.
16. Leiman G, Markowitz S, Margolius KA. Cytologic detection of cervical granuloma inguinale. Diagn Cytopathol. 1986;2:138.
17. Kraus SJ, Werman BS, Biddle JW, et al. Pseudogranuloma inguinale caused by *Haemophilus ducreyi*. Arch Dermatol. 1982;118:494.
18. Breschi LC, Goldman G, Shapiro SR. Granuloma inguinale in Vietnam: Successful therapy with ampicillin and lincomycin. J Am Vener Dis Assoc. 1975;1:118.
19. Thew MA, Swift JT, Heaton CL. Ampicillin in the treatment of granuloma inguinale. JAMA. 1969;210:866.
20. Maddocks I, Anders EM, Dennis E. Donovanosis in Papua New Guinea. Br J Vener Dis. 1976;52:190.
21. Garg BR, Lal S, Bedi BMS, et al. Donovanosis (granuloma inguinale) of the oral cavity. Br J Vener Dis. 1975;51:136.
22. Ashdown LR, Kilvert GT. Granuloma inguinale in Northern Queensland. Med J Aust. 1979;1:146.
23. Garg BR, Lal S, Sivamani S. Efficacy of co-trimoxazole in donovanosis. Br J Vener Dis. 1978;54:348.
24. Robinson HM. The treatment of granuloma inguinale, lymphogranuloma venereum, chancroid and gonorrhea. Arch Dermatol Syph. 1951;64:284.
25. Vogel LC. Een granuloma-venereum (donovanosis)—epidemic in Suid Niew Guinea (1920). Ned T Geneesk. 1965;109:2425.

228. THE AGENT OF CAT SCRATCH DISEASE

GERALD W. FISCHER

Cat scratch disease (CSD) is a common cause of lymphadenopathy in children and adolescents. In addition, many patients have atypical presentations other than regional adenopathy. In 1889, Parinaud described cases of oculoglandular fever associated with conjunctivitis, enlargement of regional lymph nodes, and low-grade fever that persisted for weeks.[1,2] He believed that the disease was contracted from animals and may have described the first cases of CSD. Although tularemia had been associated with Parinaud's oculoglandular syndrome, it became clear that there were other causes as well and that CSD was a common cause of this syndrome.[2] In the early 1930s, Dr. Robert Debré[3] in Paris began to recognize an illness with regional lymphadenopathy that occurred after patients were scratched by cats. Shortly thereafter, Dr. Frank Hanger and Dr. Harry Rose, using aspirated pus from a patient with suppurative CSD adenitis, prepared a skin test antigen that gave positive intradermal reactions in patients with CSD. The first reports on CSD were published in the 1950s,[3,4] and by the early 1980s, CSD had become a well-described entity, with over 700 articles published by investigators around the world.[5]

EPIDEMIOLOGY

CSD occurs worldwide, and in temperate climates the disease is seasonal with approximately 75 percent of cases occurring between September and March.[6] However, cases frequently occur in July and August in warm climates. Over 80 percent of patients are less than 21 years old, and 60 percent are males. About 90 percent of patients have a history of exposure to cats and a cat scratch or bite will have occurred in 75 percent of these individuals. Family outbreaks have been observed in households with cats.[6] Generally, the cases occur within a few weeks of each other, and the animal implicated is usually a kitten. This may suggest that the infectious agent is transmitted from cat to human for only a limited period of time. The mode of transmission is presumably direct contact, since the lymphadenopathy generally follows a scratch, bite, or lick from a young cat. Rarely, a dog, monkey, thorn, or other agent will be implicated in a CSD case. Cats show no evidence of illness and do not react to CSD skin testing. Attempts to isolate the etiologic agent from cats have been unsuccessful.

PATHOLOGY

The lymphatic system is primarily involved, and early in the course of infection, lymph nodes show lymphoid hyperplasia. Later, scattered granulomas appear, and some may contain central areas of necrosis with rare multinucleated giant cells. As the process progresses, stellate areas of necrosis coalesce to form one or more abscesses. Granulomas associated with CSD have also been found in the liver[7] and in osteolytic lesions of bone.[8] If the lymph node capsule ruptures, pus extends into the contiguous tissue and may be surrounded eventually by fibrosis. Since the histopathologic appearance of CSD may resemble that of other infections such as tularemia, lymphogranuloma venereum, and fungal and mycobacterial infections, the histopathology cannot be considered diagnostic for CSD. Warthin-Starry silver stain can be used to demonstrate the small, gram-negative bacillus associated recently with CSD, but these bacteria are generally only found early in the course of infection.

ETIOLOGY

The etiology of CSD has been difficult to identify despite the development of new technologies. However, clinical, epidemiologic, and pathologic studies have implicated an infectious agent. A variety of organisms have been proposed as the cause of CSD, including chlamydia,[9] bacteria,[5,10,11] and viruses.[12,13] A hemagglutinating virus was reported in seven of eight patients with CSD in 1960.[11] The virus was antigenically similar to herpesvirus but differed in its pathogenicity in animals and tissue cultures. The role of viruses in CSD was again raised when herpes-like virus particles were identified in eight of eight randomly selected individuals with a positive CSD skin test.[12] Similar particles were not present in controls. Although intriguing, the role of viruses as etiologic agents in CSD has not been confirmed despite the identification of other lymphadenopathy-associated herpesviruses such as Epstein-Barr virus and cytomegalovirus.

Bacteria have also been proposed as etiologic agents in this disease. In 1961, Boyd and Craig found photochromogenic, acid-fast bacilli in eight patients with CSD.[10] However, no direct association with the disease has been documented. More recently, small, gram-negative bacteria have been suggested as the cause of CSD.[5] Wear and colleagues examined lymph nodes from 39 patients with CSD and found small, pleomorphic, gram-negative bacilli in 34 of 39 lymph nodes.[5] The bacteria were best seen using the Warthin-Starry silver stain, and sera from three convalescent patients reacted with the bacteria in lymph node sections. These bacteria have also been identified in primary skin inoculation lesions, further suggesting an etiologic role.[14] Gerber and colleagues have reported isolating gram-positive bacteria from the lymph node of a patient with CSD.[11] This organism was considered to be of the genus *Rothia* and was proposed to be the same bacterium identified by Wear et al.[5] However, this is unlikely, since the Gram stain and morphologic characteristics are not consistent.

The bacillus identified in 1983 by Wear and colleagues has now been isolated, and three of seven patients with recent CSD had fourfold antibody titer rises against the cultured bacteria.[15] Rabbit antisera to the organism also reacted with the bacterium in tissue specimens from patients with CSD. A cell wall-deficient variant of the bacteria has also been described by these investigators. Further studies to verify its etiologic role in CSD may be forthcoming.[14] Identification of a single pathogen would allow skin test standardization and possibly development of serologic assays to confirm the diagnosis of CSD in patients. In addition, antimicrobial agents could be studied to identify appropriate treatment regimens.

CLINICAL MANIFESTATIONS

Chronic regional lymphadenopathy is the most common clinical feature of CSD and usually develops about 2 weeks after the scratch or contact (Table 1). In spite of having impressive lymphadenopathy, the patient usually appears well. An inoculation site (a scratch, a primary lesion, or both) may be detected in over two-thirds of patients when actively sought. About 3 to 10 days will elapse from the time of the scratch or cat contact until a primary skin papule or pustule forms. Most primary lesions persist for about 1–3 weeks. Low-grade fever lasting for several days occurs in about 30 percent of patients. Malaise or fatigue are noted in about 25 percent, and headache and sore throat in about 10 percent of patients.

Whether or not there is a local cutaneous lesion, lymphadenitis becomes the major manifestation of CSD. The enlarged, tender lymph nodes are most commonly found in the head or neck area. The axillary nodes are frequently involved; less commonly, the epitrochlear, inguinal, femoral, and; rarely, supraclavicular nodes may be enlarged (Fig. 1). Single-node involvement occurs in almost half of the patients, and involvement of multiple nodes in the same site occurs in about 20 percent. About one-third of patients have lymphadenopathy involving several sites. Node enlargement usually persists for 2–4 months but has been known to last for up to 2 years. Suppuration of the involved node occurs in about 10 percent of patients. Transient exanthemata (maculopapular, petechial, or erythema multiforme or nodosum) have been observed in CSD patients, usually lasting for less than 2 weeks.

Atypical manifestations of CSD may also be seen[16,17] (Table 2). The oculoglandular syndrome of Parinaud presents as an ocular granuloma or conjunctivitis with preauricular lymphadenopathy. Most patients are only mildly ill and recover without any residual. Encephalitis or encephalopathy and, rarely, radiculitis are more serious forms of CSD. Children with central nervous system involvement with CSD usually experience sudden onset of neurologic symptoms, often accompanied by fever. This usually occurs within 1–6 weeks of the onset of lymphadenopathy. Severe manifestations with coma may last for several weeks, with gradual complete recovery generally occurring in 1–6 months. The spinal fluid is usually normal, but there may be minimal pleocytosis or elevation of protein. Electroencephalograms show diffuse slowing or focal abnormalities in most patients.

Three previously healthy children, aged 3, 8, and 10 years, were recently described as having hepatic granulomata due to CSD.[7] Illness presented as fever of at least 39°C for more than 3 weeks. Ultrasound or computed tomography showed multiple hepatic nodules, which on biopsy were fibrotic areas containing multiple discrete granulomata. Bacilli consistent morphologically with the putative CSD agent were seen in the liver of two patients and in an axillary lymph node of the third, who had typical CSD in that location. No liver function abnormalities or hepatomegaly was detected. All three patients recovered without sequelae.

Osteitis resembling bacterial osteomyelitis may also occur in children.[8] Biopsy may reveal granulomas, and silver stains may be helpful to identify the small bacilli. An elevated sedimentation rate and a positive bone scan make osteitis due to CSD difficult to differentiate clinically from pyogenic osteomyelitis. A history of cat exposure and scratches is particularly important.

Disseminated angiomatous skin nodules with marked systemic symptoms due to CSD were reported in four patients with the acquired immunodeficiency syndrome (AIDS) or AIDS-related complex.[18] Two also had bone lesions. Some of the skin lesions resembled those of Kaposi's sarcoma.

TABLE 1. Clinical Features of CSD in 908 Patients

Signs and Symptoms	*Percentage*	*Average Duration*	*Range*
Adenopathy	>90	3 M	0.5–12 M
Adenopathy alone	52	3 M	0.5–12 M
Inoculation site	59–93[a]	7 D	7–240 D
Fever (>38.3°C)	32–60[a]	6 D	1–60 D
Malaise, fatigue	29	13 D	1–210 D
Headache	13	4 D	1–7 D
Anorexia, weight loss, emesis	14	5 D	3–30 D
Splenomegaly	12	11 D	7–300 D
Sore throat	9	2 D	1–5 D
Rash	5	9 D	5–14 D
Parotid swelling	2	—	7–28 D
Conjunctivitis	4.5	—	1–11 D

Abbreviations: M: months; D: days.
[a] Includes data from Carithers HA.[17]
(Data from Moriarty and Margileth.[16])

DIAGNOSIS

The diagnosis of CSD is suggested by regional lymphadenopathy that develops slowly over 2–3 weeks in a patient with cat contact and/or scratches. The presence of a primary inoculation papule or pustule at the scratch site strengthens the diagnosis. Other causes of lymphadenopathy must be considered and ruled out. Confirmation of the diagnosis of a typical case requires fulfillment of three of four criteria, whereas all four are necessary in an atypical case, including (*1*) a history of animal (usually a cat or dog) contact, with the presence of a scratch or a primary dermal or eye lesion; (*2*) aspiration of sterile pus from the node (a presumptive diagnostic test) or culture and laboratory data that exclude other etiologic possibilities; (*3*) a positive CSD skin test; and (*4*) a node biopsy revealing histopathology consistent with CSD. Detection of bacteria using Warthin-Starry silver stain or culture may be helpful as more information becomes available concerning the role of gram-negative bacteria.

Tenderness of the node favors CSD or a bacterial adenopathy rather than a neoplasm. Acute lymphadenitis due to bacteria generally develops over 3–4 days. Sonography may be helpful to detect early suppuration of the bubo and to direct needle aspiration when indicated. Early in the disease, a total white blood cell count may show mild leukocytosis and an increased number of polymorphonuclear cells, with eosinophilia in 10–20 percent of patients. The sedimentation rate is usually elevated during the first few weeks.

The cat scratch antigen skin test is positive in 90 percent of patients who are clinically suspected of having CSD and who have had cat contact and/or scratches. However, the skin test only reflects previous exposure to the agent. A negative skin test often occurs if the patient has been ill for less than 3–4 weeks. About 5 percent of patients with typical CSD will have a negative CSD skin test. Since the reaction may persist for years, a positive test may not reflect concurrent disease. Positive reactions have been noted in veterinarians (12–29 percent), healthy persons (4–5 percent) and family contacts of CSD patients. Two negative skin tests at 4-week intervals suggest a disease other than CSD if the patient is not anergic.

The differential diagnosis of CSD includes many known causes of lymphadenopathy.[19] In children and adolescents, lymphogranuloma venereum, syphilis, typical or atypical tuberculosis, other forms of bacterial adenitis, sporotrichosis, tularemia, brucellosis, histoplasmosis, sarcoidosis, toxoplasmosis, infectious mononucleosis, and benign or malignant tumors should be considered. If the patient has an ocular lesion and

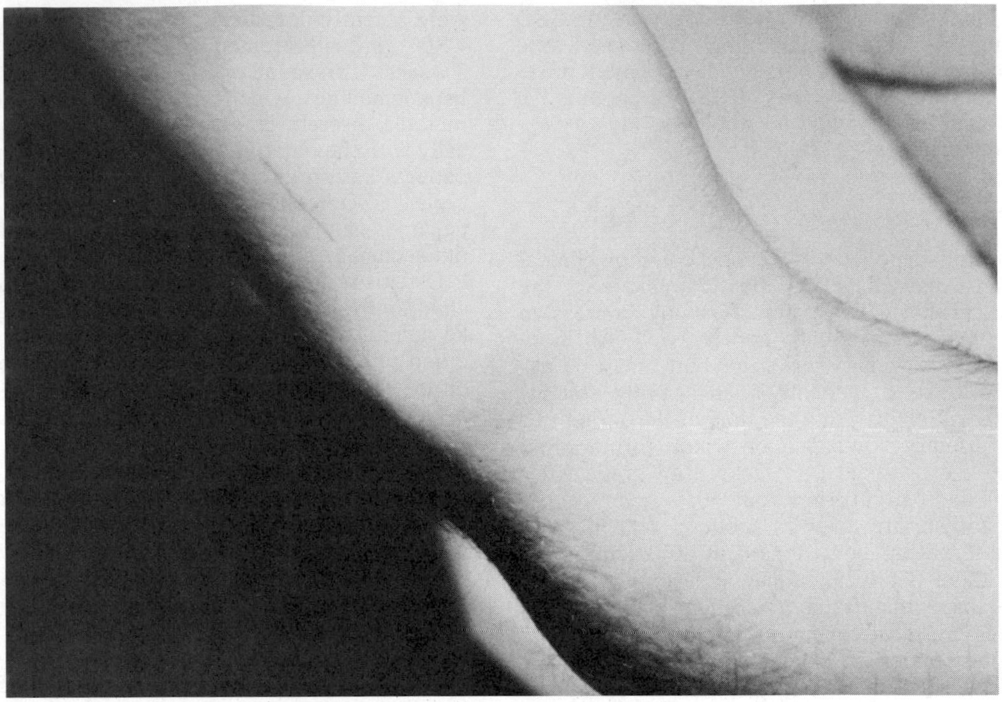

FIG. 1. Epitrochlear lymphadenitis due to CSD.

TABLE 2. Atypical Manifestations of CSD Seen in 1250 Patients

	Percent	*Duration*[a]
Unusual manifestations	11.6	—
Oculoglandular disease	6	3–28 weeks
Encephalopathy	2	7–240 days
Severe, chronic, systemic disease	2	3–21 months
Arthralgias/arthritis	<1	4–84 days
Erythema nodosum	<1	3–42 days

[a] Based on 423 patients from 1984 to 1986.
(Adapted from Moriarty and Margileth,[16] with permission.)

preauricular adenopathy, which would suggest the oculoglandular syndrome of Parinaud, CSD is the most common cause.[20,21]

SKIN TEST

The skin test used today is essentially unchanged from that described by Hanger and Rose. The antigen is made from pus aspirated from the patient's lymph node and is not commercially available. The purulent material is tested for sterility, diluted in saline, heated to 56°C for 72 hours, and then recultured to ensure sterility. A positive test is considered to be at least 5 mm of induration at 48–72 hours. Equivocal reactions can be biopsied to look for subcutaneous granuloma formation. Since there is no current method of assessing biologic activity, skin test antigen potency is difficult to standardize. Clinicians interested in CSD have assessed their preparations by skin testing patients with several antigen lots. Despite several decades of apparent safety, contemporary use of this antigen is of some concern. Potential transmission of infectious agents not killed by mild heating, including human immunodeficiency virus (HIV), hepatitis B, non-A, non-B hepatitis, and Kreutzfeldt-Jakob disease. Potential antigen donors should be generally well and tested serologically for HIV and hepatitis B. This antigen should be used only with all the procedures appropriate for an experimental biologic fluid, including approval by the local institutional review board. Identification of an etiologic agent such as the one described by Wear and colleagues[5] should provide a source of antigen that does not require the use of human material and avoids the potential hazards associated with such biologic substances.

TREATMENT

Specific therapy for CSD is not available. The adenopathy is benign and will subside spontaneously within several months. Careful follow-up examination is important to reassess the size of the bubo and to reassure the patient that the node(s) are slowly receding. If suppuration occurs, aspiration should be considered to relieve the pain and hasten recovery. Needle aspiration is generally preferred to incision and drainage. After washing the skin with an iodophor skin cleanser, aspiration may be accomplished by inserting an 18- or 19-gauge needle tangentially through normal skin at the base of the node. Rarely, reaspiration may be necessary. Characteristically, CSD lymphadenitis is not responsive to antimicrobials, and they are not recommended at this time. However, if the etiology is confirmed to be a bacterium, selected antibiotic therapy based on susceptibility testing may be of value.

Application of moist soaks to the primary skin or eye lesion may effect drainage and shorten the duration of the adenopathy. Excisional biopsy of the ocular granuloma is rarely necessary. Excisional biopsy of the node may be necessary in selected patients, particularly adults, because of persistent pain or for diagnostic purposes.

PROGNOSIS

Complications and sequelae in typical cases are uncommon. One episode appears to confer lifelong immunity. Rarely, a recurrence of sinus track drainage from the nodes originally involved may occur. If the adenopathy is massive (>5 cm), chronic adenopathy may persist for 1–2 years.

PREVENTION

Primary prevention of CSD is not currently feasible because of the large number of household pets (50 million cats in the United

States) and because the suspected cat is invariably well. Since cats probably transmit the agent for only a short period of time, disposal of the cat is not recommended. Up to 10 percent of family members scratched by the same cat may develop CSD. However, the patient with CSD does not require isolation or special precautions since there is no evidence of disease spread from person to person. Declawing of pet cats might be considered.

REFERENCES

1. Parinaud H. Conjonctivite infectieuse transmise par les animaux. Ann Ocul. 1889;101:252–3.
2. Cassady JV, Culbertson CS. Cat-scratch disease and Parinaud's oculoglandular syndrome. Arch Ophthalmol. 1953;50:68–74.
3. Debré R, Lamy M, Jammet M, et al. La maladie des griffes de chat. Bull Mem Soc Med Hop (Paris). 1950;66:76–79.
4. Daniels WB, MacMurray FG. Cat scratch disease, report of one hundred sixty cases. JAMA. 1954;154:1247–51.
5. Wear DJ, Margileth AM, Hadfield TL, et al. Cat scratch disease: A bacterial infection. Science. 1983;221:1403–5.
6. Margileth AM. Cat scratch disease: A therapeutic dilemma. Vet Clin North Am. 1987;155:390–402.
7. Lenoir AA, Storch GA, DeSchryver-Kecskemeti K, et al. granulomatous hepatitis associated with cat scratch disease. Lancet. 1988;1:1132–6.
8. Muszynski MJ, Eppes S, Riley HD. Granulomatous osteolytic lesion of the skull associated with cat-scratch disease. Pediatr Infect Dis. 1987;6:199–201.
9. Chervonskii VI, Terskikh II, Behlehkova AY. Isolation and study of agent of benign lymphoreticulosis (cat scratch fever) in man. Fed Proc. 1964;23(Trans Suppl):T992–4.
10. Boyd GL, Craig G. Etiology of cat-scratch fever. J Pediatr. 1961;59:313–7.
11. Gerber MA, MacAlister TJ, Ballow M, et al. The aetiological agent of cat scratch disease. Lancet. 1985;1:1236–9.
12. Turner W, Bigley NJ, Dodd MC, et al. Hemagglutinating virus isolated from cat scratch disease. J Bacteriol. 1960;80:430–5.
13. Kalter SS, Kim CS, Heberling RL. Herpes-like virus particles associated with cat scratch disease. Nature. 1969;224:190.
14. Margileth AW, Wear DJ, Hadfield TL, et al. Cat-scratch disease, bacteria in skin at the primary inoculation site. JAMA. 1984;252:928–31.
15. English CK, Wear DJ, Margileth AM, et al. Cat-scratch disease, Isolation and culture of the bacterial agent. JAMA. 1988;259:1347–52.
16. Moriarty RA, Margileth AM. Cat scratch disease. Infect Dis Clin North Am. 1987;1:575–90.
17. Carithers HA. Cat-scratch disease: An overview based on a study of 1,200 patients. Am J Dis Child. 1985;139:1124–33.
18. Koehler JE, LeBoit PE, Egbert BM, et al. Cutaneous vascular lesions and disseminated cat-scratch disease in patients with the acquired immunodeficiency syndrome (AIDS) and AIDS-related complex. Ann Intern Med. 1988;109:449–55.
19. Margileth AM. Cervical adenitis. Pediatr Rev. 1985;7:13–24.
20. Margileth AM. Cat scratch disease as a cause of the oculoglandular syndrome of Parinaud. J Pediatr. 1957;20:1000–5.
21. Carithers HA. Oculoglandular disease of Parinaud. Am J Dis Child. 1978;132:1195–1200.

MYCOBACTERIAL DISEASES

229. MYCOBACTERIUM TUBERCULOSIS

ROGER M. DES PREZ
CRAIG R. HEIM

Tuberculosis is an infection, often of lifelong duration, caused by two species of mycobacteria, *Mycobacterium tuberculosis* and *Mycobacterium bovis*. These mycobacteria can cause disease in virtually every organ system in the body, although most prominently the lungs. The disease is characterized histologically by granuloma formation. Tuberculosis is to be distinguished on bacteriologic grounds from disease caused by other superficially similar mycobacterial species.

HISTORY

There is paleopathological evidence of spinal tuberculosis in neolithic and pre-Columbian skeletons and early Egyptian remains. Ancient Greek physicians used the term *phthisis* to indicate its wasting character. However, it did not become a major problem until the crowded urban living conditions of the early industrial revolution created the epidemiologic circumstances favoring its spread. In the seventeenth and eighteenth centuries, tuberculosis caused one-fourth of adult deaths in Europe. The clinical characteristics of phthisis—cough, hemoptysis, prolonged fevers, and wasting—had become well recognized by then, but agreement was lacking as to its cause. In Southern Europe it was believed to be contagious. In northern Europe its occurrence in families led to the belief that it was due to a constitutional predisposition. Virchow thought it was a neoplasm.

Modern concepts of tuberculosis developed in the last half of the nineteenth century as a result of three stellar medical accomplishments. Autopsy studies convinced Laennec that the various forms of pulmonary and extrapulmonary tuberculosis, then regarded as unrelated, were all part of the same disease. In 1865 Francoise Villemin demonstrated that tuberculosis could be transmitted by injection of diseased tissue into guinea pigs. The greatest achievement, however, was Koch's demonstration of the tubercle bacillus and its pathogenicity in 1882.

During the last half of the nineteenth and the first half of the present century the keystone of treatment was rest in the open air, often in specialized hospitals (sanatoria) in locations thought to be salubrious. With the development of diagnostic x-ray films, it became clear that the development of the pulmonary cavity was pivotal in the evolution of disease, and most therapeutic measures were aimed at cavity closure. These included simple bed rest, pneumoperitoneum, therapeutic pneumothorax, and surgical measures to decrease overall lung size such as extraperiosteal plombage and thoracoplasty. Although cases discovered before cavity formation were greatly helped by sanatorium regimens, their impact on advanced disease was much less.

The modern era of tuberculosis treatment began in 1946 with streptomycin (STM).[1] The effect on symptomatic pulmonary disease was dramatic, but more dramatic still was the demonstration that some patients with miliary and meningeal disease, conditions that had been theretofore almost always fatal, recovered with STM therapy. During the STM era, from 1947 to 1952, it became possible for the first time to excise tuberculous tissue without spreading disease; it was established that treatment with at least two drugs (STM and *p*-aminosalicylic acid—PAS) was necessary to avoid drug resistance; and the dose and toxicity of STM were established. In 1952 the much more effective drug isoniazid (INH) became available and tuberculosis became, for the first time, curable in the great majority of patients. In the INH era, from 1952 through 1970 (when rifampin—RMP—came into general use), large-scale cooperative studies established that at least 18 months of treatment were required; that STM added to the effectiveness of INH and PAS in far-advanced but not in less-advanced cases; that resectional pulmonary surgery was rarely if ever necessary; that bed rest and collapse therapy added nothing to prolonged chemotherapy; and that patients under treatment rapidly became noninfectious. With no need for special rest or isolation, the role of specialized sanatoria disappeared and tuberculosis became the province of the general physician and general hospital. The efficacy, low cost, ease of administration, and low toxicity of INH, as then construed, popularized the notion of treating not only active cases but also virtually all people who might, on the basis of a positive tuberculin test, be thought to harbor the infection. It was hoped that the infection in humans could be eradicated thereby, an enthusiasm subsequently tempered by experience.

By 1970, RMP had come to be recognized as equal in efficacy to INH. Since results of 18–24 months of treatment with the then available drugs were so excellent, the role of RMP was not immediately apparent. However, the difficulty of maintaining some patients on therapy for 18–24 months, together with the high cost of long-term supervision, soon led to exploration of shorter courses of therapy. English studies in Africa and the Orient demonstrated that combination regimens containing both RMP and INH could accomplish in 9 months or less what previously had taken 18–24 months to achieve.[1,2] It now is clear that optimal results in drug-sensitive infections can be achieved in 6 months with regimens employing INH, RMP, pyrazinamide (PZA), and either STM or ethambutol (EMB) for 2 months followed by 4 more months of INH and RMP.[3]

MICROBIOLOGY

The term *tubercle bacillus* designates two species of the family Mycobacteriaceae, order Actinomycetales—*M. tuberculosis* and *M. bovis*. They are to be distinguished from many other mycobacterial species of varying pathogenicity and clinical importance that share the staining characteristics referred to as *acid fastness*. Three other species, *M. ulcerans*, *M. microti*, a pathogen for rodents, and *M. africanum*, an organism thought to be intermediate between *M. tuberculosis* and *M. bovis* and a rare cause of human tuberculosis in Africa, are closely related on the basis of bacteriologic features and DNA homology and comprise the other two members of the *M tuberculosis* complex. At present disease due to *M. bovis* is rare, and the terms *tubercle bacillus* and *M. tuberculosis* are, practically speaking, synonymous.[4]

Mycobacterium tuberculosis is an obligate parasite infecting humans, other primates in contact with humans, and other mammalian species in close contact with humans, especially domestic dogs and cats. However, humans are the only reservoir of the organism. It is an aerobic, non-spore-forming, nonmotile bacillus with a large cell wall content of high molecular weight lipids. Growth is slow, the generation time being 15–20 hours, as compared to well under 1 hour for most common bacterial pathogens, and visible colonial growth takes at least 3 and usually 4–6 weeks. The organism tends to grow in parallel groups, leading to the colonial characteristic of serpentine cording.[5]

Through the first half of this century, mycobacteria were speciated by pathogenicity in guinea pigs, rabbits, and fowl. *Mycobacterium tuberculosis* is pathogenic for guinea pigs but not rabbits or fowl; *M. bovis* is pathogenic for both guinea pigs and rabbits but not fowl; and *Mycobacterium avium* is pathogenic only for fowl. (*Mycobacterium avium* is not now regarded as a member of the *M. tuberculosis* complex; although not pathogenic for rabbits or guinea pigs, it is an important pathogen in swine and is closely related to *Mycobacterium intracellulare*.) Pathogenicity in the guinea pig was regarded as a marker of pathogenicity for humans, and isolates not demonstrating this property were regarded as contaminants. This notion was disturbed somewhat by the repeated culture by Feldman of an organism with all of the characteristics of *M. avium* from a pneumoconiotic patient in the 1940s. However, practically speaking, tuberculosis was usually diagnosed by smear and often not even confirmed by guinea pig inoculation.

The advent of chemotherapy engendered more precise mycobacteriology because of the importance of sensitivity testing. It had been noted early that INH-resistant strains differed from INH-sensitive strains in that they were less avid for neutral red dyes, did not produce the enzyme catalase, and were somewhat less pathogenic for guinea pigs. During this period, a number of still more unusual mycobacterial isolates were noted that demonstrated different colonial characteristics, high-grade resistance to both INH and STM, total lack of pathogenicity for the guinea pig, and, in contrast to INH-resistant *M. tuberculosis* strains, a high degree of catalase activity. Early on, there was speculation as to whether they also constituted naturally occurring INH-resistant strains of *M. tuberculosis*. However, study of a large number of these isolates in the laboratory of Ernest Runyon led to a classification of these "anonymous" mycobacteria into four groups on the basis of colonial characteristics. *Mycobacterium tuberculosis* grows slowly (3–6 weeks), and the colonies are buff colored, rough, and friable. Runyon group I is characterized by formation of a yellow or orange pigment only after exposure to light, the photochromogens; group II is characterized by formation of an orange or red pigment in the dark, the scotochromogens; group III is characterized by slow growth, smooth colonies, and a cream color; and group IV, the rapid growers, is characterized by growth in a few days. Although precise speciation has now replaced the Runyon grouping, it is of interest to recount some of the important species that they contained: group I—*M. kansasii*, *M. marinum*, *M. simiae*; group II—*M. scrofulaceum*, *M. xenopi*, *M. gordonae*; group III—*M. avium-intracellulare* complex; group IV—*M. fortuitum-chelonei* complex.[6,7]

The term *acid fast bacilli* (*AFB*) is, practically speaking, synonymous with *mycobacteria*, although some other microbial species, notably *Nocardia*, are variably acid fast. In the Ziehl-Neelsen stain a fixed smear covered with carbol-fuchsin is heated, rinsed, decolorized with acid–alcohol, and counterstained with methylene blue. The Kinyoun stain is modified to make heating unnecessary. The organisms observed with oil immersion are slightly bent rods, 2–4 μm long and 0.2–0.5 μm wide, and appear beaded. In sputum the organisms often lie parallel to one another or two organisms adherent at one end appear as a V shape. It is estimated that 10,000 organisms per milliliter of sputum are required for smear positivity, and a single organism on an entire slide is highly suspicious. Most laboratories now use a fluorochrome stain with phenolic auramine or auramine–rhodamine in the initial staining procedure, a slightly modified acid–alcohol decolorization step, and potassium permanganate counterstaining. The bacteria fluoresce bright orange-yellow against a dark background when viewed with a strong blue light source and can be seen by scanning under low magnification, a less laborious procedure. Sputum or any biologic fluid or material can be examined directly, although thin fluids are often best examined after sedimentation by centrifugation. When sputum digestion and concentration are carried out for culture, a smear of the concentrate is productive. Smears of gastric aspirates are often not done due to the notion that free-living mycobacteria from food or water are so often present as to make a positive finding insignificant. However, studies addressing the point have demonstrated that the majority of such positive smears are due to *M. tuberculosis*.[8] On Gram stain of sputum, *M. tuberculosis* is either weakly gram-positive or appears as colorless rods.

Culture of sputum or tissue requires initial liquefication–decontamination and sedimentation. Historically, this was carried out in 3 or 4 percent sodium hydroxide, although there are now other less inhibitory liquefying–decontaminating materials. Uncontaminated fluids or sterile tissues from deep sources do not need digestion and sterilization. Solid culture media are of two general types, agar based and egg based. Most contain antibacterial additives that are slightly inhibitory for tubercle bacilli as well. Noninhibitory media, on which growth is more rapid, are available. Growth is more rapid in 5–10 percent carbon dioxide. In most laboratories differentiation of *M. tuberculosis* from other mycobacteria can be accomplished by a few simple tests. *Mycobacterium tuberculosis* grows slowly, lacks pigment, produces niacin, reduces nitrates, produces heat-sensitive catalase (inactivated by heating to 68°C at pH 7.0) in relatively small quantity, and is sensitive to INH. INH-resistant strains of *M.*

tuberculosis do not produce catalase. *Mycobacterium bovis* is usually niacin negative and does not reduce nitrates. The other mycobacteria are for the most part niacin negative, do not reduce nitrates, produce heat-stable catalase, usually in large amounts, and are highly resistant to INH. Speciation of mycobacteria other than *M. tuberculosis* can be carried out in most large bacteriologic laboratories or in state reference laboratories.

A radiometric system for culturing mycobacteria is now available. It is positive in 2–6 days, depending on the number of organisms in the specimen (Bactec TB-460 instrument, Johnston Laboratories, Towson, Maryland). Inclusion of a chemical, *p*-nitro-acetylaminohydroxypropio-phenone (NAP), in the incubation mixture will inhibit the growth of *M. tuberculosis* and presumably of *M. bovis*, but not of mycobacteria other than tuberculosis (MOTT). The system does not differentiate between these other species.[9]

Drug sensitivity testing is necessary both as a part of speciation and to design therapy. Most laboratories now provide this as a routine measure. It is performed by comparing growth of appropriately diluted inocula on drug-containing media to growth on drug-free media. Results are reported in terms of the percentage resistant. Generally 6–10 percent resistance or more indicates complete resistance from a clinical point of view. It is probable that rapid sensitivity studies will be made possible by the radiometric system discussed above.[9] Microbial resistance will be discussed in the section on "Treatment of Tuberculosis."

EPIDEMIOLOGY

The two essential factors for rapid spread of tuberculosis are crowded living conditions favoring airborne spread of infection and a population with little native resistance. In the nineteenth century, tuberculosis death rates well over 1000 per 100,000 population accounted for more than 30 percent of all adult deaths in Europe, eliminating those with the least native resistance to the disease. Epidemiologists writing before the chemotherapy era believed that a downward trend had been established at least several decades before reliable mortality and morbidity statistics became available at the turn of the century and that the disease would eventually disappear for the following quantitative epidemiologic reasons.[10,11] It has been stated that 5–15 percent of infected people develop active disease, and half of diseased adults develop pulmonary cavitation and become infectious. (Childhood cases are usually noncavitary and virtually noninfectious, as are extrapulmonary cases and those with noncavitary pulmonary infiltrates.) If 10 percent of those infected develop active disease and 50 percent of those with disease themselves become infectious, it would be necessary for one case to infect 20 people in order to produce another infectious case and maintain the same level of infection in the population. In Holland before World War II one infectious case produced only 13 new infections, and more recent data from Africa indicate 10–14 new infections per source case—rates inadequate to maintain the infection over the long run.[11] At present in developed countries it is estimated that one infectious case produces two to three new cases. (Actually, estimates that 5–15 percent of infected people develop active disease have all been based on heavy exposures such as case contacts and are usually in those who for reasons of age are very susceptible. People infected with small inocula and those infected during disease-resistant periods probably have a much smaller risk.[10,12]

Since the turn of the century, the annual fall in both mortality and morbidity is estimated to have been 4–6 percent in developed countries (Fig. 1). With the widespread application of chemotherapy, this rate has approximately doubled.[11] There is general agreement that the prechemotherapy trend was due to progressively higher natural resistance in the population, since those most susceptible died, and to living conditions less fa-

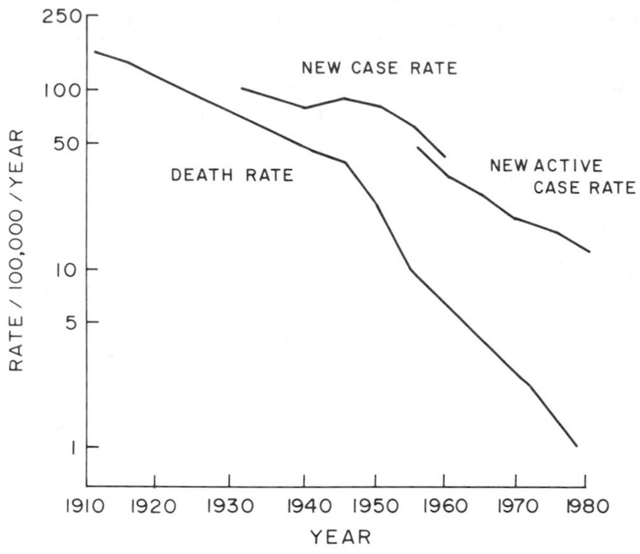

FIG. 1. Tuberculosis death rates, new case rates, and new active case rates, United States, 1910–1980. (From Comstock et al.,[23] with permission.)

vorable to airborne contagion. Epidemic tuberculosis developed in other previously unexposed and therefore still susceptible populations much later, usually when the opportunity for infection coincided with a change in life-style. The disease became rampant in the American Indian population due to exposure to white people and to the change from nomadic to reservation living. In the North American Eskimo population a major epidemic occurred in 1950, with a new-case rate of approximately 2000 per 100,000, infection of 90 percent of the population by age 6, and an enormous death rate. By 1970, due to intense case-finding and treatment efforts, the new-case rate had fallen to 90 per 100,000, achieving in 2 decades what probably would have taken 150 years to achieve without such efforts.[10] Case rates in many areas of the world are presented in Table 1. Worldwide, tuberculosis remains a major health problem, infecting half the world's population and causing an estimated 10 million new cases and 3 million deaths annually, comprising 6 percent of all deaths.

Figure 2 presents tuberculin positivity by age groups in the United States in 1979. These figures are probably representative of other Western developed countries. The annual new-case rate in the United States in 1984 was 9.4 (per 100,000), more in cities over 100,000 in population (20.7) than in smaller cities and rural areas (6.8). The annual death rate was 0.75 overall, but 18.2 in nonwhite males over age 65.[13] In the industrialized West, tuberculosis is increasingly a disease of the urban poor, particularly minorities, often occurring in contact-based microepidemics. A special problem exists in developed countries with large-scale immigration from areas with higher morbidity rates, such as India, Southeast Asia, and Haiti.[14,15] These immigrant groups demonstrate the tuberculosis rates of the country of origin.[16] Special groups, such as drug addicts, patients with end-stage renal disease, residents of institutions for the homeless, to a lesser degree nursing home residents, and patients with the acquired immunodeficiency syndrome (AIDS), demonstrate morbidity rates enormously in excess of those of the general population (Table 2).

Mode of Spread

In the past, infection from ingestion of contaminated milk was commonplace, but now bovine tuberculosis is rare. Skin infection from contamination of a skin abrasion may be seen in pathologists and other laboratory personnel (prosector's wart),

TABLE 1. Tuberculosis Case Rates per 100,000 Population in 1970–1974 for 15 Countries with the Highest, Middle, and Lowest Rates

Highest			*Middle*			*Lowest*		
Country	*Year*	*Rate*	*Country*	*Year*	*Rate*	*Country*	*Year*	*Rate*
Macau	1973	469	St. Lucia	1972	64	Cuba	1972	14
Swaziland	1970	468	Austria	1973	62	United States	1974	14
Bolivia	1972	414	Kenya	1970	61	Martinique	1972	14
Gilbert, Ellice Island	1973	334	Italy	1970	61	Norway	1973	14
Mauritania	1970	332	German Fed Rep	1972	59	Denmark	1973	13
Philippines	1972	328	Angola	1970	58	Australia	1973	12
Wallis, Futuna Island	1973	260	Madagascar	1970	57	Antigua	1973	11
Republic of Korea	1973	249	Iran	1970	56	Trinidad & Tobago	1972	11
South Africa	1973	247	Western Samoa	1973	55	Israel	1973	10
New Hebrides	1973	223	Ghana	1970	55	Virgin Islands, UK	1971	9
Brit Solomon Islands	1973	215	Zaire	1970	54	Cameroon	1970	8
Iraq	1970	214	France	1972	54	Virgin islands, US	1973	6
Brunei	1970	200	Venezuela	1973	54	Grenada	1972	5
Hong Kong	1973	196	Sri Lanka	1972	50	Faeroe Islands	1970	5
Pacific Islands, Trust Territories	1973	175	Ecuador	1973	50	St. Vincent	1972	2

(From Comstock et al.,[23] with permission.)

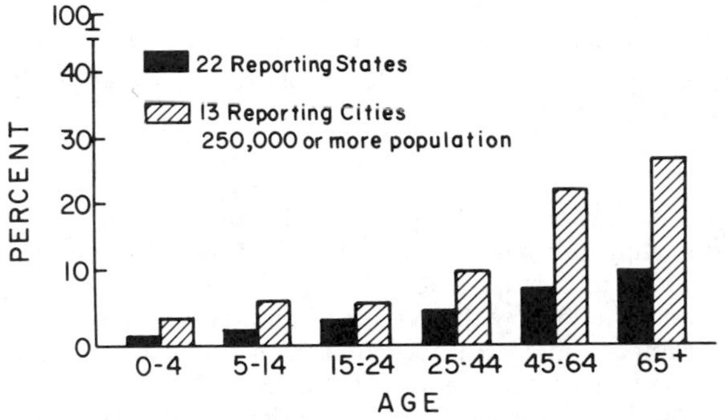

FIG. 2. Percentage of positive tuberculin reactors by age, selected areas, United States, 1979. (From Centers for Disease Control,[212] with permission.)

TABLE 2. Incidence of Active Tuberculosis in Certain Groups

Group	*Incidence per 100,000*	*Reference*
Hostel residents in Glasgow	1,946	
Hostel residents in Boston	317	43
Nursing home residents, tuberculin-positive on admission	2,400	38
Nursing home residents, tuberculin converters	5,900	38
Tuberculin-positive Indochinese refugees		110
All ages, both sexes	926	
Over 65, both sexes	7,160	
Males over 65	14,180	
Dialysis patients, San Francisco	5,800	96
East Indian dialysis patients, London	25,000	114
AIDS patients, New York City	7,000 (approx)	50
Haitian AIDS patients	80,000	48

and venereal transmission has been recorded. However, almost all infections are due to inhalation of *droplet nuclei*, infectious particles of respiratory secretions aerosolized by coughing, sneezing, or talking, which are sufficiently small to dry while airborne, remain suspended for long periods, and reach the terminal air passages, where multiplication is unimpeded and infection begins.[17,18] A cough can produce 3000 infectious droplet nuclei, talking for 5 minutes can produce an equal number, and sneezing can produce many more than that.[10] Accordingly, a room inhabited by a cavitary patient can be infectious even in his or her temporary absence. Although a single infectious unit is thought to be sufficient to infect a tuberculin-negative host, prolonged exposure to an infectious environment is usually required for infection to occur, and brief contact is of little risk. Infection rarely occurs out doors in daylight. In hospital rooms, six air changes per hour largely eliminate environmental infectiousness. Ultraviolet lights positioned so as to avoid patient exposure have been recommended but are rarely used. Large drops of respiratory secretions are of no real concern since they drop to the floor or, if inhaled, are trapped and removed by mucociliary action and coughing. Fomites are not important, and special housekeeping measures for dishes and bed clothes are not necessary. Although data are lacking, it is probable that the practice of having the patient and medical personnel mask for the first week or so of drug treatment has some merit.

Risk of Infection

The most important determinants of contagion are the closeness of contact and the infectiousness of the source, which vary widely among individuals. Cases with positive smears are highly infectious; those positive only on culture are much less so. The degree of sputum positivity and pattern of coughing are important. Compared to some other infections such as measles, one case of which will infect 80 percent of susceptible casual contacts, the infectiousness of tuberculosis is only moderate in most circumstances. Data from Holland in the 1970s indicated that only 50 percent of 0–14-year-old household contacts of smear-positive cases became tuberculin positive and only 5 percent did so when the contact case was culture positive but the smear was negative.[11] The increased risk of infection generally observed in children is probably due to their being more often in the home rather than to any age-related susceptibility to infection per se. It has been estimated that in the United States 27 percent of household contacts of smear-positive cases become infected.[19] However, certain microepidemics in closed environments have demonstrated much higher infection rates.[20] One case of cavitary tuberculosis on the submarine Byrd infected 45 percent of the entire crew; 80 percent of those who slept in the same compartment were infected.[21] In a nursing home epidemic, one case of open tuberculosis infected 31 percent of the susceptible (tuberculin-negative) patients in the home but 79 percent of those on the same wing.[22]

Influence of Chemotherapy on Spread of Infection

People receiving chemotherapy become promptly noninfectious as their cough subsides and the concentration of organisms in the sputum decreases. Just how rapidly treatment reverses infectiousness is not known, but most authorities believe that this occurs within 2 weeks.[10,18] From an epidemiologic point of view, the most important impact of chemotherapy is the virtual elimination of new infections once treatment has been initiated. This striking interruption of the chain of tuberculosis transmission makes case finding and treatment by far the most effective method of tuberculosis control.

Risk of Progression of Infection to Active Disease

It is an accepted approximation that 3.3 percent of people will develop active tuberculosis during the first year after a positive tuberculin test, and a total of 5–15 percent will do so thereafter. The British Medical Research Council vaccine trial provides some precise data concerning the risks of tuberculin conversion in adolescents in a situation of relatively high contagion. A total of 108 (10.4 percent) of 12,876 unvaccinated adolescents developed clinical tuberculosis in circumstances in which the date of their tuberculin conversion was precisely known, 54 percent within 1 year and 78 percent within 2 years.[11] The risk varies with age. As illustrated in Figure 3, it is greatest in the very young, with over 50 percent of those infected under age 6 months in New York City progressing to active, mostly disseminated (miliary-meningeal) disease in one large series. Older children, roughly between ages 3 or 4 and puberty, although as susceptible to infection as younger children, develop disease infrequently, and when it does occur it is most frequently the nonprogressive childhood type of pulmonary tuberculosis.[23] In adolescence and early adulthood, more often in females than in males, the risk of recent infection promptly producing active disease is much greater, and frequently this will be chronic pulmonary tuberculosis of the adult type.[24] Moreover, infection acquired and remaining latent during the relatively disease-resistant period of childhood may become progressive in adolescence or early adulthood due to altered immunologic factors characteristic of this age group, most probably heightened hypersensitivity with an increased tendency to tissue necrosis. Middle-aged adults are less susceptible to progression of infection to disease. However, in old age, a third period of decreased resistance develops, more often in men than women and in nonwhites than whites (Fig. 4). Active disease in the elderly most often represents breakdown of infections acquired earlier in life, but the risk of direct progression of newly acquired infection in this age group is also great.

The likelihood of active disease varies with the intensity and duration of exposure.[25] A number of well-studied microepidemics have illustrated that persons in closest contact with the source case are most at risk not only for infection but also for disease.[21,22,25] The degree of tuberculin positivity has some minor predictive value.[12,23,26] Tall, thin people and black men

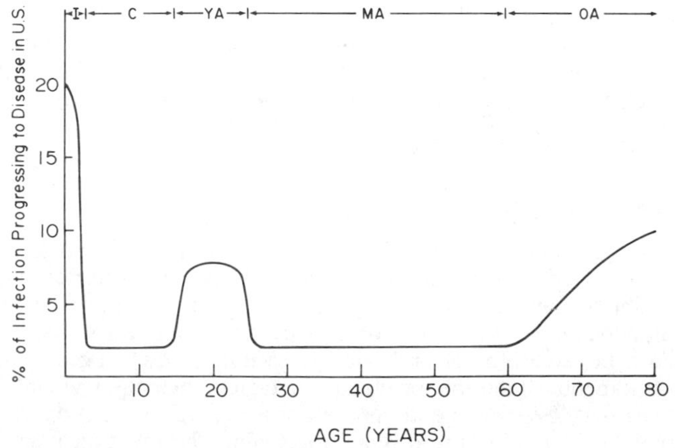

FIG. 3. Estimate of infection progressing to disease in different age groups. I: infancy; C: childhood; Y: young adulthood; MA: midadulthood; OA: old age.

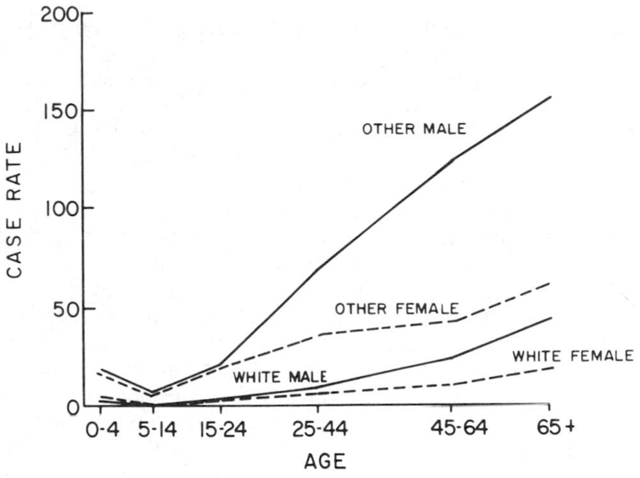

FIG. 4. Tuberculosis case rates for white and other races, males and females by age, United States, 1979. (From Centers for Disease Control,[212] with permission.)

with the histocompatibility type HLA-Bw15 are said to be at increased risk independent of the more important social factors.[15] Malnutrition and intercurrent situations such as alcoholism, homelessness, incarceration, immunosuppression, and AIDS all greatly favor progression of infection to active disease (Table 2).

IMMUNOPATHOLOGIC FEATURES

Tuberculosis is the prototype of infections that require cellular immune responses for their control.[27–29] Infection is associated with a rich antibody response, but no role for this in host defense mechanisms has been demonstrated. Actually it was the demonstration by Merrill Chase in 1945 that cutaneous hypersensitivity to tuberculin could be transferred by cells (adoptive immunity) but not by serum that opened the whole field of cellular immune responses to experimental analysis.

In the first few weeks the host has no defense against the tuberculosis infection. Small inhalational inocula multiply whether free in alveolar spaces or after ingestion by alveolar macrophages. Any bacteriostatic influence of alveolar macrophages on ingested bacilli at this stage must be very slight, a circumstance that has been attributed to interference with phagosome–lysosome fusion by bacterial cell wall lipids. Bacterial multiplication proceeds unimpeded for weeks, both in the initial focus and in lymphohematogenous metastatic foci, until the development of tissue hypersensitivity and cell-mediated immunity supervenes. Tissue hypersensitivity is florid in comparison to other intracellular infections due to the potent immunologic adjuvant activity of mycobacterial lipids.

All people have a native population of lymphocytes capable of recognizing tubercle bacillus antigens, or, more precisely, recognizing antigen processed by macrophages. When such lymphocytes encounter the macrophage–antigen complex, they are activated (transformed) so as to divide, producing a progeny of similarly reactive cells. These in turn replicate and also produce a variety of substances (lymphokines) with the capacity to attract, retain, and stimulate macrophages at the antigen site. Activated macrophages develop high concentrations of lytic enzymes that greatly increase their mycobactericidal capability and also, when released from degenerating cells, cause tissue necrosis. Epithelioid cells, characteristic of the tuberculous granuloma or tubercle, are highly stimulated macrophages. Activated macrophages secrete a fibroblast-stimulating substance, resulting in collagen production and eventual fibrosis. The Langhans giant cell, which consists of fused macrophages oriented around tuberculosis antigen with the multiple nuclei in a peripheral position, represents the most successful type of host tissue response.

When the population of activated lymphocytes reaches a certain size, cutaneous delayed reactivity to tuberculin, or *tissue hypersensitivity*, becomes manifest. The speed with which this occurs varies, but generally it will have developed 6–14 weeks after infection. At the same time, enhanced macrophage microbicidal activity, or *cell-mediated immunity*, appears. It is a matter of dispute whether or not cell-mediated immunity, which connotes resistance to infection, and tissue hypersensitivity, which describes altered cellular reactivity (granuloma formation, tissue necrosis), are endpoints of the same sequence of immunologic and chemical events or are simply parallel and closely associated phenomena depending on different antigens, different lymphocyte populations and/or products, or both. However, in a clinical sense, they seem to be inseparable.

The pathologic features of tuberculosis are the result of the degree of hypersensitivity and the local concentration of antigen.[27,30] Where the antigen load is small and the degree of tissue hypersensitivity high, organization of lymphocytes, macrophages, Langhans giant cells, fibroblasts, and capillaries results in granuloma formation. This hard tubercle is termed a *proliferative or productive* focus and is a very successful tissue reaction with respect to containment of infection, healing with eventual fibrosis, encapsulation, and scar formation. Where both antigen load and degree of hypersensitivity are high, epithelioid cells and giant cells will be sparse or lacking entirely, round cells and granulocytes will be present in a less-organized fashion, and tissue necrosis due to lytic enzymes released from degenerating macrophages may be present, a type of tissue reaction that has been called *exudative*. In the absence of necrosis, exudative lesions may heal completely, but more frequently some degree of tissue necrosis will supervene. Necrosis in tuberculosis tends to be incomplete, resulting in solid or semisolid acellular and amorphous material referred to as *caseous* because of its cheesy consistency. The chemical environment and oxygen tension in caseous material are not favorable to mycobacterial metabolism, and if it inspissates or calcifies, multiplication is largely arrested. However, it is inherently unstable, especially in the lungs, where it demonstrates a tendency to liquefaction and discharge through the bronchial tree, producing a tuberculous cavity and providing conditions in which bacterial populations reach titers five or six logs greater than in noncavitary lesions. Infectious material sloughed from a cavity results in new exudative foci in other parts of the lung (*bronchogenic spread*). The processes of necrosis and healing may occur simultaneously in different areas of the lung. A cross section of a pulmonary cavity demonstrates all of these pathologic reactions, from the least to the most successful in terms of containment of infection, as one progresses from the center outward along a gradient of decreasing antigen concentration. The central cavity, which contains myriad bacilli, is lined by a layer of caseous material with fewer organisms, a more peripheral layer of macrophages and lymphocytes with little organization and still fewer organisms, more peripherally still an area of epithelioid cells and giant cells in which the bacterial content is quite low, and most peripherally a layer of encapsulating fibrosis.

When the degree of hypersensitivity is very low, the tissue reaction may be quite nonspecific, consisting of a few polymorphonuclear leukocytes and mononuclear cells with myriad tubercle bacilli, a condition termed *nonreactive tuberculosis*.[31] The immunologic spectrum from florid hypersensitivity to little or no specific tissue reaction is analogous to the situation in leprosy.

THE TUBERCULIN TEST

Koch's tuberculin was an impure extract of a boiled culture of tubercle bacilli. Koch thought that it was important because of what he perceived to be the therapeutic effect of the reaction of infected individuals to tuberculin, and such was his prestige that this was widely although temporarily accepted. The notion that this reaction might be of diagnostic rather than therapeutic importance has been attributed to Dr. A. Conan Doyle. In 1934 Siebert made a simple protein precipitate of old tuberculin. This purified protein derivative (PPD) quickly became the preferred reagent in most areas of the world. In 1941 a large single lot was adopted as the biologic standard (PPD-S) by which other preparations are standardized. A 5 TU dose of PPD is equivalent to 0.0001 mg of PPD-S protein contained in 0.1 ml of solution. It is slightly stronger than first-strength (1:10,000) old tuberculin (OT). The 250 TU dose is roughly equivalent to second-strength (1:100) OT.[32]

Dosage

The quantitative aspects of tuberculin testing were worked out in careful studies of the response of populations in which the incidence of tuberculosis was accurately known. Trials of different concentrations demonstrated that a dose of tuberculin most nearly equivalent to 5 TU produced the highest proportion of positives in groups of people virtually all of whom were infected, such as sanatorium patients, and the lowest number in groups with a very low incidence of tuberculosis, such as infants from noninfectious environments. Measurement of the size of the induration produced by 5 TU in infected populations demonstrated a unimodal curve with its peak at 16–17 mm, whereas similar studies in mixed (both infected and noninfected) populations produced a bimodal curve with one population demonstrating 0–5 mm induration and the other the larger 16- to 17-mm peak. Subsequently large-scale tuberculin surveys demonstrated that the geographic distribution of people with strong tuberculin reactions (elicited by small doses) and weak tuberculin reactions (requiring large doses) was quite different. Availability of tuberculins prepared from other mycobacterial species made it possible to demonstrate that the geographic distribution of weak tuberculin reactions corresponded to the endemic area of nontuberculous mycobacterial species. Moreover tuberculin surveys using 5 TU in areas in which nontuberculous mycobacteria are not endemic demonstrated a bimodal curve with clear separation between those with no or small reactions (0–5 mm induration) and those with large reactions (12–24 mm induration). In contrast, surveys in areas in which infection with nontuberculous mycobacteria is endemic, such as the southeastern United States, demonstrated many more reactions between 4 and 12 mm induration, a great many of which are now known to be due to cross reactions to PPD-S in people who have had infections with these other mycobacterial agents. The sensitivity (fewest false positives) and specificity (fewest false negatives) of the 5 TU dose was arrived at in part as a result of such surveys, this being the dosage that produced the clearest bimodal curve, and in part based on studies of graded doses in populations with a known high incidence of tuberculosis, as discussed above.[32]

Technical Aspects

Although multiple puncture techniques (*Heaf and Tine tests*) are still used by some for survey work because of their ease of administration, quantitative tuberculin testing requires intracutaneous injection on the volar aspect of the forearm, using a short, beveled No. 26 or 27 needle (*Mantoux test*). Precise intracutaneous injection producing a raised, blanched wheal is necessary. Deeper injections are apt to be washed out by vascular flow, making the dosage uncertain. The reaction is read in 48–72 hours, a positive test usually being defined as greater than 10 mm of induration, not erythema. Induration is determined by viewing the reaction tangentially against a light background. Experienced, careful readers can achieve a precision within 2 mm.

During the 1970s, it was recognized that PPD in solution adheres to glass to the extent that 20 percent of its potency can be lost in 30 minutes and up to 80 percent in 24 hours, and that this can be prevented by the addition of a small amount of the detergent polysorbate 80 (Tween 80). Tween-stabilized tuberculin in solution is light sensitive and, to a lesser degree, temperature sensitive; storage in a refrigerator is necessary.

Interpretation

Ninety percent of persons demonstrating 10 mm of induration in response to a 5 TU tuberculin test and virtually everyone with a 20 mm reaction will be infected. Although the criterion of 10 mm of induration is most useful in surveys and gives most discrimination in populations in which cross-sensitization with other mycobacteria is a problem, indurations of 5–10 mm should be regarded as highly suspicious in areas known to be substantially free of other mycobacterial infections, such as the northeastern United States, and in people such as contacts of active cases in whom tuberculosis is likely to occur.[49]

A tuberculin test cannot sensitize a noninfected person, but it can restimulate or enhance remotely established and subsequently weakened hypersensitivity.[33] This *booster effect* had been known for a long time, but it gained wide attention when the practice of annual testing of hospital personnel was resumed after several years of neglect. The second annual round of testing in these renewed programs resulted in a frequency of tuberculin conversion entirely out of keeping with the local incidence of sputum-positive tuberculosis. It was quickly realized that this was due to the booster effect, which is established within several days of tuberculin injection and persists for over a year. This problem can be circumvented by retesting 1 week later those persons with a very small or negative tuberculin reaction and an uncertain tuberculin history. If the second test is positive, it should be attributed to boosting of a subclinical hypersensitivity state due to old infection rather than to recent conversion with its implication for chemoprophylaxis. This booster phenomenon, which develops within 1 week and may persist for a year or more, is more common in middle-aged and older people. Unfortunately, it may also be observed in persons infected with nontuberculous mycobacteria in areas where these are endemic.[33]

False-positive reactions are all due to infection with nontuberculous mycobacteria. *False-negative reactions*, although uncommon in relatively healthy people, are observed in as many as 20 percent of persons with known active tuberculosis when first tested. Twenty-five percent of those negative to 5 TU will also be nonreactive to 250 TU.[34] Although not all authorities agree, the frequency of both false-positive and false-negative reactions to 250 TU limits the usefulness of this dose.[32] The 1 TU dose may occasionally be useful in very young children who may have a very high degree of tuberculin reactivity. Most false-negative tests in patients with tuberculosis are loosely attributed to general illness and will revert to positive 2 or 3 weeks into treatment when health has been somewhat restored. Protein malnutrition diminishes all cutaneous delayed hypersensitivity reactions. Sarcoidosis is thought to produce a state in which the tuberculin test may be falsely negative, although actually the majority of sarcoidosis patients with tuberculosis will have a positive test, and it is inaccurate to attribute the appearance of tuberculin positivity in sarcoid patients to a decrease in the activity of the sarcoid process.[35] Intercurrent viral infections, reticuloendothelial disease, and therapy with corticosteroids have all been used to explain false-negative tuberculin reactions. It is widespread practice to apply certain ubiquitous antigens (mumps, candida, etc.) in order to diagnose a state of anergy. However, the immunologic reasons for decreased reactivity are multiple, complex, and poorly understood. Efforts to correlate false-negative tuberculin tests with anergy so defined have not been illuminating, and the practice gives little useful information while leading to conclusions that are not always useful or accurate.[34]

Reversion of Tuberculin Reactivity to Negative. The rate of tuberculin positivity in 30-year-old persons in 1930 was over 70 percent. The same age cohort in 1980 demonstrated a rate of under 20 percent, these reactions being true negatives. The most quantitative data on reversion of positive tuberculin tests to negative come from studies by Grzybowski.[36] As illustrated in Table 3, 8.1 percent of known reactors detected in a tuberculin survey had reverted to negative 1 year later. It is probable that the persistence of tuberculin positivity requires the continued presence of living tubercle bacilli in the body, although frequently they will metabolize very slowly. The permanence of the tuberculin test as once construed was probably due to maintenance of hypersensitivity by multiple new aerosol inocula when the opportunity for infection was great, such as is known to be the case in histoplasmosis. Retesting persons with a history of a positive skin test can be done with no risk. A negative result to two tests given a week apart (to exclude the booster effect) should be taken as evidence of true negativity with the same susceptibility to new infection as would have been the case with no history of prior tuberculin positivity.

PATHOGENESIS

As previously discussed, airborne droplet nuclei containing very few or even single infectious units are small enough to avoid entrapment by the bronchial mucociliary apparatus and may reach and multiply in the terminal air spaces. Infection usually begins in the so-called primary infection segments of the lung, the lower division of the lower lobe, the middle lobe, the lingula, and the anterior segment of the upper lobes, in which greater airflow favors deposition of inhaled bacilli. In most cases the initial focus is single, although in one-fourth or more of cases multiple foci will be present, some evolving and some regressing. The bacteria are ingested by alveolar macrophages but multiply nevertheless, eventually destroying the phagocytes. Other macrophages and lymphocytes accumulate in indolent fashion, ingesting bacilli released from degenerating cells, and slowly one or more areas of pneumonitis develop. Infected macrophages spread to regional (hilar, mediastinal, and sometimes supraclavicular or retroperitoneal) lymph nodes, but in the nonimmune host are not retained therein and may spread throughout the body via the blood stream. Distribution of this *occult preallergic lymphohematogenous dissemination* is probably random according to blood flow, but the most important areas are those that favor bacillary growth: the lymph nodes, kidneys, epiphyseal areas of the long bones, vertebral bodies, juxtaependymal meningeal areas adjacent to the subarachnoid space, and, most importantly, the apical-posterior areas of the lungs. Before the development of hypersensitivity (tuberculin reactivity), microbial growth is virtually uninhibited, both in the initial focus and in metastatic foci, thus setting the stage for subsequent evolution of progressive disease in the

TABLE 3. Annual Tuberculin Reversion Rates According to Age Groups, Victoria County, 1959–1962

Age Groups	*Positive Reactors Retested After 1 Year*	*Number of Reversions*	*Reversion Rate*
0–19	99	22	22.2
20–39	200	16	8.0
40–59	525	25	4.8
60 and older	377	34	9.0
Total	1201	97	8.1

(From Grzybowski and Allen.[36])

lung apices and in extrapulmonary sites, either promptly or after latent periods of up to many years in duration.

Evolution of the Primary Infection

Once tuberculin reactivity has developed, the course of the infection depends on the interplay of local factors and the immunologic state. Cellular immunity favors control of infection but tissue hypersensitivity favors either granuloma formation or tissue necrosis, depending in part on whether the local antigen concentration is small or large. In most cases, the ensuing rapid bacterial destruction arrests the whole process, with no remaining evidence that infection had occurred other than a positive skin test. In a few cases, the antigen concentration at the initial pulmonary focus and regional nodes will have reached sufficient size that necrosis and visible calcification ensue, producing the Gohn complex. Much less commonly, pulmonary apical and subapical metastatic foci will also have become large enough that necrosis ensues with the onset of hypersensitivity, producing tiny calcific deposits called *Simon foci* in which latent but viable bacilli often persist.

In children and, uncommonly, in nonwhite young adults[37] and those infected in advanced age,[38] the primary focus may become an area of advancing pneumonia, the so-called progressive primary. Also typically in children, the hilar or mediastinal lymph node component may become very large and may produce bronchial collapse with distal atelectasis.

Several clinical syndromes may be observed at the time of development of tuberculin hypersensitivity or soon thereafter. Again typically in the very young, the initial *preallergic lymphohematogenous dissemination* may blend directly into *hyperacute miliary tuberculosis*, frequently complicated by *tuberculous meningitis* a few weeks later. *Phlyctenular keratoconjunctivitis* is usually unilateral and presents at this time as a severely inflamed eye. *Erythema nodosum* may also occur. When a subpleural metastatic focus has developed due to lymphatic spread from the initial area of pneumonitis, development of hypersensitivity may cause necrosis and rupture of infectious and antigenic material into the pleural space, producing the clinical picture of *serofibrinous pleurisy with effusion*. However, in terms of subsequent disease, the overwhelmingly most important consequence of preallergic lymphohematogenous dissemination is seeding of the apical posterior areas of the lung, where local factors favor both bacterial multiplication and retention. This may progress without interruption or after a latent period of months or years, causing pulmonary tuberculosis of the adult or reinfection type.

Primary (Childhood) and Reinfection (Adult) Tuberculosis

The traditional terms *primary or childhood* and *reinfection or adult pulmonary tuberculosis* came into use as a result of roentgenographic observations made early in this century when infection in childhood was considered to have occurred in everyone.[39] Children's roentgenograms usually revealed large, often massive, mediastinal lymphadenopathy with an often inconspicuous area of pneumonitis in the lower or midlung field. In adolescents and adults the quite different roentgenographic picture of apical or subapical infiltrates, often with cavitation and no hilar adenopathy, was the rule. The inference that in adults this was due to new infection (exogenous reinfection) in a previously sensitized host was based in part on the conviction that infection had always occurred by adolescence and in part on reasoning by analogy to the so-called Koch phenomenon, the observation that a second inoculation in an already infected guinea pig would produce marked local inflammation and necrosis but sharp limitation of the new inoculum. It is now known that this clinical and roentegenographic difference has to do with age-related immunologic factors, at least in large part. In adolescents and young adults, a metastatic focus in the apical-posterior area of the lung may progress in a short time to apical cavitary disease, while the initial focus of infection in the lower lung fields and hilar nodes involutes without clinical or roentgenologic detection.

Chronic Pulmonary Tuberculosis

Apical Localization. In the adult, apical localization of pulmonary tuberculosis has most frequently been attributed to the hyperoxic environment of the apices and the aerobic nature of the tubercle bacillus. However, this theory does not account for several facts: (*1*) other conditions such as histoplasmosis and, most significantly, silicosis also develop most prominently in the posterior subapical areas of the lung; (*2*) tuberculosis is apical-posterior rather than just apical in location; (*3*) in some mountain populations living at ambient oxygen tensions lower than those found in any area of a normal lung at sea level, apical pulmonary tuberculosis is more frequent than in sea-level dwellers of the same country. Another theory, originally proposed by Dock,[40] emphasizes that pulmonary lymph production is deficient at the lung apices, due to hydrostatic factors, and especially at the posterior aspects, where the lung moves very little and lymph flow is minimal. Deficiency in lymph production and drainage would favor retention of bacillary antigen (as well as other substances), resulting in higher antigenic concentrations and tissue necrosis.

The apical localization of pulmonary tuberculosis is characteristic of most adolescents and adults. Stead et al.'s recent study of an epidemic of tuberculosis in a nursing home indicates that infection contracted in the elderly often causes nondescript lower lobe pneumonitis, implying that local progression of the inhaled infection may be as typical in this age group as it is in children.[38]

Endogenous versus Exogenous Reinfection. Principally following the writings of Stead,[39] many have assumed that resistance to exogenous reinfection in the previously infected host is of such a high order that new inocula are destroyed before significant multiplication can occur, and that all or nearly all clinical instances of tuberculosis in the lungs or elsewhere are direct consequences of the initial infection and its hematogenous phase. Although this is probably true in developed countries in which the general level of contagion is small, epidemiologic data make it clear that in areas and times characterized by a high general level of contagion, exogenous reinfection was and probably is the rule.[11,41] A recent contact study in India demonstrated that disease in household contacts of known cases was more commonly observed in the middle-aged and elderly, who on epidemiologic grounds were certain to have been already infected, than in children.[42] In the United States, certain instances have been recorded in which persons known to have been previously infected with drug-sensitive organisms and later exposed to a patient with drug-resistant strains developed new infection with the resistant strain.[43] The practical implication is that tuberculin-positive people exposed to high levels of contagion are at risk of exogenous reinfection, although the risk is certainly much less than in tuberculin-negative people. A recent microepidemic in a shelter for homeless men provided evidence of exogenous reinfection in previously infected individuals. This suggests that in patients with other nonspecific host factors detrimental to containment of infection, tuberculin hypersensitivity might be not only unsuccessful in defending against new inocula but actually harmful by interacting with these new inocula so as to produce tissue necrosis, cavity formation, and progressive disease.[43]

Influence of Age on Tuberculous Infection

Until recently, much of what was taught about clinical patterns of tuberculosis was based on data developed when infection relatively early in life was the rule, and cellular immunity and hypersensitivity were continually being restimulated by frequent inhalation of infectious inocula. While this remains true in situations of high levels of contagion, in the industrialized West clinical manifestations have changed a good deal now that infection is often delayed until later life, and tissue hypersensitivity and cellular immunity may wane and disappear entirely in the absence of restimulation. Once the scourge of the adolescent and young adult, tuberculosis is now most often seen in older people, in whom the clinical manifestations may be different and subtle.

Infection in Infancy. As mentioned, infection in the very young produces disease in a large proportion, 50 percent in those under 6 months of age in one New York study, and when it occurs dissemination (miliary-meningeal disease) is apt to occur.

Infection in Midchildhood. Children past infancy, while quite susceptible to tuberculous infection, are relatively resistant to progressive disease, which when it occurs is most frequently the childhood type of pulmonary tuberculosis. Consolidation and collapse may be observed due to bronchial compression by lymphadenitis. Extrapulmonary tuberculosis in the lymph nodes, the skeleton, and, less commonly, other progressive extrapulmonary foci may develop. However, the usual course of tuberculosis confined to the lung in this age group is involution and healing, and the major danger is subsequent relapse in the more disease-prone period of adolescence.

Infection in Adolescence and Young Adulthood. Initial infection in the adolescent and young adult may demonstrate features (lower lung field pneumonitis, hilar adenitis) noted in children, especially in dark-skinned races.[44] However, more frequently it will appear as chronic upper lobe tuberculosis with no clinical features of childhood disease.[45] Rarely, the roentgenographic picture may be mixed, with features of childhood disease subsiding while those of chronic upper lobe (adult) disease progress. The tendency to apical cavitation early after the initial infection appears soon after puberty and is marked in young adults.[45] Since the majority of young people in industrialized countries are tuberculin negative (Fig. 2), most new cases of pulmonary tuberculosis in adolescents and young adults in these areas are now due to new infections rather than to recrudescence of childhood infections, as was often the case in earlier years. First infections acquired after childhood have much less tendency to cause parenchymal and hilar calcification.

Infection in Midadulthood. The clinical manifestations of tuberculous infection acquired during the middle years are not distinctive, but it has a much better immediate and probably long-term prognosis than infection acquired in the second and third decades, probably because of a reduced tendency to tissue necrosis and progressive disease.[45,46] One small but precisely studied experience documented the progression from tuberculin conversion to cavitary tuberculosis in 23 percent of patients aged 15–19, 13 percent in those aged 20–24, 4 percent in those aged 25–29, and only 2 percent (1 patient out of 42 converters) in those over 30. Progression from tuberculin conversion to cavitary apical disease was prompt, occurring in 3 months in many and within 1 year in most. Elderly individuals were not included in this study.[24]

Infection in Old Age. As mentioned above, tuberculosis is now predominantly a disease of the elderly. Older persons can undergo recrudescence of infection acquired many years earlier as age compromises immune mechanisms, producing the typical apical-posterior disease observed in younger adults. However, studies of tuberculosis in nursing homes by Stead have demonstrated that patients in this age group are often tuberculin negative (70–80 percent), either because they had never been infected or because ancient infections had died entirely with a loss of tuberculin reactivity. Such tuberculin-negative persons may require new infection in the setting of institutionalization and, when this occurs, develop active disease with a frequency approaching that of new infections in adolescents. The disease is usually manifested by nondescript, poorly resolving pneumonitis in the lower, middle, or anterior segments of the upper lobes, sometimes associated with pleural effusion and resembling the primary infection in children, except for much less hilar-mediastinal lymphadenopathy.[38]

Late Hematogenous Tuberculosis

Chronic organ tuberculosis commonly produces abortive episodes of hematogenous spread. However, when aging or other factors compromise cellular immunity and tissue hypersensitivity, such episodes may become progressively frequent and eventually continuous, producing the clinical syndrome of *late hematogenous* or *progressive generalized tuberculosis*. Such cases can be extremely subtle clinically and fatal if not recognized.

Intercurrent Events

General deterioration in health and nutritional status, and factors subsumed under the general category of stress, clearly favor progression of infection. Pregnancy was long regarded as a time of special risk, but it now seems probable that the critical factors are loss of sleep and exhaustion in the postpartum period. Therapy with corticosteroids or oncolytic-immunosuppressive agents compromises host defenses, although exactly how much is not clear; hematopoietic-reticuloendothelial disease, particularly malignancies, often seems to do likewise. The latter are particular problems since disseminated tuberculosis itself can cause hematologic perturbations such as aplastic anemia, thrombocytopenia, leukopenia, and leukemoid reactions sufficiently marked that confusion with leukemia is possible. However, most cases of tuberculosis with hematologic findings suggesting leukemia will be found to consist of both diseases.[47] The postgastrectomy state, jejunal-ileal bypass surgery, and end-stage renal disease are all added risk factors (see the section on "Chemoprophylaxis"). Viral illnesses, particularly in children, predispose to progression of infection (see below). Destructive pulmonary processes such as lung abscess, carcinoma, cavitary histoplasmosis, and pulmonary resection occasionally are followed by activation of previously quiescent or latent pulmonary foci. The relationship of physical injury to the development of bone and joint tuberculosis is well known; tuberculous peritonitis is a recognized uncommon complication of tubal insufflation in infertility clinics; and the development of late generalized hematogenous tuberculosis at times appears to have followed a major trauma such as an automobile accident. All of these associations illustrate that the balance between host and infection can be altered not only by systemic factors but also by local physical disturbance.

Tuberculosis in AIDS. In Haiti, where both diseases are common, the incidence of tuberculosis in AIDS patients has been reported to be as high as 60 percent.[48] In New York City tuberculosis has been observed in 5–11 percent of AIDS patients, ranking it behind *Pneumocystis carinii* and *M. intracellulare* but ahead of all other opportunistic organisms. The disease occurs early in the course of AIDS, often preceding pneumocystis and *M. avium* infection by months or a year or two, suggesting that less severe defects in the immune response suffice for tuberculosis to become progressive. The clinical manifestations are different from those observed in otherwise normal persons, with extrapulmonary disease in up to one-half (compared to 15 percent in healthy persons), and lower-lobe, noncavitary pulmonary tuberculosis is frequent. Substantial efforts to make the diagnosis, including biopsy and culture of tissues such as bone marrow and lymph nodes, are indicated, as the response to chemotherapy will usually be excellent. Treatment should be prolonged, perhaps in this context including indefinite administration of INH after initial multiple-drug therapy. Prophylactic administration of INH in the AIDS patient with a history of active tuberculosis or a positive tuberculin test is indicated, as discussed below.[49,50]

PULMONARY TUBERCULOSIS

Primary Tuberculosis in Childhood

The clinical manifestations of the primary (initial) infection vary depending on the age of the patient. It is most often symptomatic in childhood because of an age-related tendency to extensive regional lymphadenitis and, in the very young, to progressive lymphohematogenous dissemination with miliary-meningeal disease. The initial focus or (in 25 percent or more) foci are most frequently in the lower and midlung zones, but infection in the upper lobe does occur, more often in the anterior segments. At the time of tuberculin conversion fever and lassitude may be briefly present, and rarely, erythema nodosum or phlyctenular keratoconjunctivitis may be seen. Exuberant hilar or mediastinal lymphadenitis may compress central bronchi, causing a brassy cough or even atelectasis of a segment or lobe, or may rupture into a bronchus, seeding infection distally, causing a very symptomatic pneumonia. Uncommonly, local progression of the initial pneumonia with or without caseation and cavity formation occurs, the so-called progressive primary. However, in the majority of those infected in the relatively resistant period of childhood (age 3–15), the process is nonprogressive over the short term; healing, which takes place by involution, encapsulation, and frequently calcification, does not seem to be accelerated by chemotherapy.[45,51] Progression, if any, usually occurs in extrapulmonary metastatic foci or, with the onset of puberty, in the apical posterior aspects of the lung. Treatment of the asymptomatic childhood infection is usually with INH alone for a year except when a drug-resistant infection seems likely. The recommended dose is larger (10–15 mg/kg) than the adult dose, the risk of INH toxicity being negligible in the young. Symptoms associated with bronchial compression will often be benefited by brief corticosteroid treatment (prednisone, 20–40 mg/day). Progressive disease with caseation should be treated with more than one drug for more prolonged periods (see below).

Chronic Pulmonary Tuberculosis

Chronic pulmonary tuberculosis begins as a patch of pneumonitis surrounding a growing bacterial colony in the subapical posterior aspect of an upper lobe, usually appearing just below the clavicle or first rib. A less frequent but still characteristic location is in the apical portion of the lower lobe, where it may be obscured by the heart on chest roentgenogram. Simultaneous progression is uncommon, but foci frequently advance in asynchronous fashion in both upper lobes. The inflammatory response in the sensitized host produces a fibrin-rich alevolar exudate containing a mixture of inflammatory cells. Serial roentgenograms during this phase may demonstrate waxing and waning. If the process accelerates, however, accumulation of large concentrations of antigen in the hypersensitive host will lead to an area of caseous necrosis surrounded by epithelioid cells, granulation tissue, and eventually fibrosis. This process may become arrested by blockage of the bronchocavitary junction, inspissation of the caseous area, and fibrous encapsulation. However, caseation has a marked tendency eventually to liquefy and drain into the bronchial tree, where its bacillary contents are spread by coughing. The cavity, which is the pivotal pathogenic event in the progression of pulmonary tuberculosis, tends to be prevented from collapsing by the rigid peripheral fibrous capsule and the elasticity of the surrounding lung.[30] For reasons usually attributed to the aerobic character of the tubercle bacillus but probably more complicated than that, the pulmonary cavity favors bacillary multiplication to enormous titers, five or six logs greater than found in noncavitary lesions.[52] *The progressive nature of pulmonary tuberculosis in the sensitized host is due to three factors: (1) the tendency of apical caseous foci to liquefy, (2) drainage of this material by the bronchial tree, and (3) the enormous concentrations of organisms in the resulting pulmonary cavities.* The progression from minimal infiltrate to advanced cavitary disease can occur quite rapidly, in a matter of a month or two.

Coughing aerosolizes the material draining from cavities and, on inhalation, distributes it widely throughout the lung (*bronchogenic spread*). Sooner or later new foci develop in susceptible areas, which in turn may undergo caseation, fibrosis, and healing or slough and produce new cavities. The segment or lobe containing the initial cavity is typically involved first with scattered patchy disease, but factors favoring microbial growth in the apices also influence growth of foci spread via the bronchi, and the contralateral apex is often secondarily involved with progressive cavitary disease. New foci of infection may be established in the lower lobe and anterior portions of the upper lobe, but these are usually nonprogressive, healing with solid tubercle formation and fibrosis. Although hematogenous spread can occur when an established pulmonary focus erodes into a vascular channel, usually lymphohematogenous spread is limited by hypersensitivity-induced thrombosis. Regional lymphadenitis, characteristic of the initial infection in children, is not a feature of chronic pulmonary tuberculosis.

The highly infectious secretions from a cavity always cause some degree of endobronchial disease and can often produce extensive areas of inflammation and ulceration in larger draining bronchi. Tuberculous laryngitis may be regarded as an extension of this process, as may local disease throughout the upper airways, mouth, and gastrointestinal tract.

Mechanisms of healing are the same whether they occur spontaneously or under the influence of chemotherapy. In the era before drug therapy, caseous foci surrounded by contracting fibrous tissue might have become inactive. However, viable bacilli almost always persisted in such lesions, which could later become reactivated, either spontaneously or after some physical disturbance due to intercurrent disease or surgery. It is likely that this potential for breakdown of caseous lesions is still the case even in patients treated with maximal chemotherapy. Before drug therapy, open healing of persisting cavities never occurred, although some large, thick-walled cavities in shrunken fibrotic lobes could persist for years with minimal symptoms while remaining highly infectious (*chronic fibroid tuberculosis*). With drug therapy, open healing of cavities does occur with regularity when sputum conversion has been prompt, sometimes with complete reepithelialization. The major risk of cavities persisting after chemotherapy is not relapse of tuberculosis but rather superinfection with organisms of low-grade virulence such as *Aspergillus* or nontuberculous mycobacteria.

Lower Lobe and Endobronchial Tuberculosis. This designation should not be applied to infiltrates and cavities in the apex of the lower lobes, which characterize chronic pulmonary tuberculosis of the ordinary kind, special only in that often the major focus of disease will be obscured by the heart shadow on posterior-anterior roentgenogram. In adults the term *lower lung field tuberculosis* is best reserved for two different but often associated processes, progressive lower lobe pneumonia in recently infected older individuals and endobronchial tuberculosis, often with parenchymal consolidation-collapse. These processes are difficult to diagnose because they are roentgenographically atypical of tuberculosis and have a low bacterial content in comparison to apical disease. They are frequently confused with cancer.

PROGRESSIVE LOWER LOBE DISEASE IN OLDER PERSONS. As mentioned above, studies in nursing homes by Stead have demonstrated that when new tuberculous infection occurs in an older tuberculin-negative individual, the clinical picture is frequently one of nonspecific, unresolving pneumonitis in the lower or middle lobes or anterior segments of the upper lobes similar to primary infection in childhood.[39] Any slowly resolving or nonresolving pneumonitis in an older individual should be considered as possibly due to tuberculosis.

ENDOBRONCHIAL DISEASE. In the older literature, the incidence of endobronchial disease in areas draining apical tuberculous cavities was quite high due to surface contamination by infectious secretions. Now isolated active endobronchial disease is more frequently due to rupture of an adjacent remotely or newly infected node into the bronchial tree or direct spread from parenchymal pneumonic lesions. In one recent series of patients with endobronchial tuberculosis initially seen either because of symptoms of proximal airway obstruction or an unexplained chronic cough, only 25 percent had a history and/or roentgenographic evidence of current or previous pulmonary tuberculosis.[53] The chest roentgenogram showed typical collapse-consolidation in most cases, but in 20 percent it was normal. Sputum smears were usually negative, but the bronchial wash was positive in 85 percent. In 30 percent the observation of bulky, usually white granulation tissue on bronchoscopy led to the erroneous diagnosis of bronchogenic carcinoma. In another recent large series of patients presenting with lower lung field tuberculosis, endobronchial disease was revealed in 32 of 42 who were bronchoscoped.[54] These endobronchial lesions may result in bronchial stenosis in some cases. Cavities are frequently observed but, when present, tend to be large and often associated with an air–fluid level, due presumably to intermittent obstruction and poor drainage.

Tuberculomas. Asymptomatic rounded lesions, single or multiple, may develop either around the parenchymal residua of the initial infection or as a result of fibrous encapsulation of an upper lobe caseous lesion; however, some will cavitate and produce new spread of disease. In some people who have a tendency to excessive fibrogenesis, small caseous or granulomatous residua may become surrounded by concentric layers of fibrous tissue, at times with central or concentric calcification resembling histoplasmomas. Most such lesions are clinically stable and are important only in being confused with cancer.

Symptoms. Early pulmonary tuberculosis causes no symptoms, often being discovered on a chance chest roentgenogram. When the bacillary population has reached a certain size, however, a systemic reaction will cause nonspecific constitutional symptoms such as anorexia, fatigue, weight loss, chilly sensations, afternoon remittent fever, and, when this subsides, night sweats. These symptoms are late rather than early manifestations of disease, gradual in onset, surprisingly well tolerated, and often not recognized at all by the patient until viewed in retrospect after treatment. Symptoms due to local disease are also variable in degree and in time of onset and also indicate the presence of advanced disease. A cough and sputum are usually present due to secretions from the cavity and to bronchial irritation. Coughing to clear cavitary secretions is not severe but may become much more bothersome when bronchial involvement becomes extensive. The mucopurulent sputum is quite nonspecific in character. In chronic bronchitics both the cough and sputum may be ignored. Hemoptysis due to caseous sloughing or to endobronchial erosion is usually minor in degree but connotes advanced disease. Sudden and extensive hemoptysis due to erosion of a pulmonary artery by an advancing cavity (Rasmussen's aneurysm) was a not uncommon terminal event in the predrug era, usually as a result of respiratory insufficiency (drowning) rather than exsanguination.[55] In inactive disease, brisk hemoptysis may be due to aspergillus superinfection of residual cavities (aspergilloma).[56] Chest pain is usually due to extension of inflammation to the parietal pleura. Pleural involvement adjacent to a cavity tends to be associated with visceral-parietal pleural symphysis without effusion (dry pleurisy). Serofibrinous pleurisy with effusion typically occurs early in the course of infection, but also may complicate established chronic pulmonary tuberculosis. Rarely, tuberculous empyema will be discovered. Hemoptysis and chest pain are frightening symptoms and will usually lead to medical attention. Some patients will not seek attention until disease occurs in tissues bathed in the highly infectious pulmonary secretions such as painful pharyngeal ulcers; indolent and nonhealing ulcers of the mouth or tongue; hoarseness and dysphagia due to laryngeal involvement; tuberculous otitis media; gastrointestinal symptoms due to enteric ulceration, perforation, or mass formation; or anal pain due to tuberculous perirectal abscess and fistula formation. Lower lobe tuberculosis due to bronchial lymph node perforation may be associated with or preceded by lithoptysis (stone spitting) and characteristically produces symptoms of severe endobronchial disease such as coughing and often hemoptysis.

Physical Examination. Physical findings are not specific, in general underestimate the extent of the illness, and may be absent in spite of extensive disease. Dullness with decreased fremitus may indicate pleural thickening or fluid. Rales may be appreciated only when the patient breathes in after a short cough (post-tussive rales) but may persist long after healing due to permanent distortion of small bronchioles. With large lesions, signs of consolidation with open bronchi (whispered pectoriloquy, tubular breath sounds) can be heard. Distant hollow breath sounds heard over cavities are called *amphoric* to indicate their similarity to the sound made by blowing across the mouth of a jar (amphora).

Roentgenologic Findings. The chest roentgenogram is central to diagnosis, determination of the extent and character of disease, and evaluation of the response to therapy. Although not specific, certain patterns are highly suggestive of tuberculosis. A patchy or nodular infiltrate in the apical or subapical posterior areas of the upper lobes or the superior segment of a lower lobe is highly suspicious of early chronic tuberculosis. Bilateral upper lobe infiltration with patchy, soft scattered infiltrates, especially with cavitation, is highly suggestive. Cavities may be seen more clearly with apical lordotic films or planigrams. Cavitation in the apical segment of the lower lobe may be obscured by the overlying heart shadow and, in the lateral view, by the dorsal spine, requiring careful scrutiny. Air–fluid levels are uncommon in upper lobe tuberculosis (under 10 percent) but are common in lower lobe cavities. Fresh *bronchogenic spread* from recent spillage of infectious cavity contents will appear as multiple, discrete, soft, fluffy infiltrates either adjacent to a cavity or confluent infiltrate or in more remote parts of the lung. These are seldom progressive and heal by rounding up into more discrete lesions with regular borders.

Both chronicity and certain histopathologic characteristics[57] can be estimated on the chest roentgenogram. Productive lesions (granulomatous) tend to be small and nodular with sharply defined margins indicating few organisms and a good host response. Exudative lesions (pneumonic) tend to have soft, indistinct borders and are more unstable. Fibrotic scars have sharp margins and tend to contrast. Caseation causes increased density. Healing exudative lesions first become smaller and less dense and then, as scarring develops, become more sharply defined. Lower lobe tuberculosis is quite nonspecific roentgenographically. Poorly resolving pneumonia, atelectasis, mass lesions, and large cavities with air–fluid levels have all been observed with some frequency, and initial misdiagnosis is the rule.[57] A pneumonic lesion with enlarged hilar nodes should suggest primary tuberculosis, whether in the upper or lower lung fields and regardless of the age of the patient.

Other Laboratory Findings. A normocytic, normochronic anemia is characteristic of advanced disease, as are lowered serum albumin and elevated globulin. The white blood cell count is usually normal but may be between 10,000 and 15,000 in a minority of patients. Monocytosis, often said to be characteristic of tuberculosis, is actually observed in less than 10 percent of cases. Hematuria or pyuria may indicate coexisting renal tuberculosis. Marked albuminuria is very uncommonly observed and usually indicates amyloidosis. Hyponatremia is present in some advanced cases, with associated findings suggestive of inappropriate secretion of antidiuretic hormone, a syndrome characteristic of tuberculous meningitis but seen with some frequency in pulmonary disease alone. Hyponatremia should also suggest the uncommon association of Addison's disease. Hypercalcemia may be observed in some patients with pulmonary tuberculosis, usually in the first weeks of therapy. It will often appear with vitamin D therapy during early treatment, sharing this characteristic (vitamin D sensitivity) with the hypercalcemia of sarcoidosis. Although usually low grade, it can cause considerable diagnostic confusion if not recognized as attributable to tuberculosis. When prolonged, hypercalcemia can cause renal potassium wasting and hypokalemia. It is suppressible by corticosteroid treatment, although this is seldom required.

Diagnosis. A strong presumptive diagnosis can be made on roentgenographic grounds when the pattern is typical. A positive sputum smear, usual in extensive disease, is almost conclusive in the proper setting. It must be remembered, however, that any destructive process, particularly in the apices, may erode a quiescent focus and cause shedding of acid-fast bacilli. Such excretion of tubercle bacilli is apt to be short-lived, and these necrotizing processes should also be clinically recognizable as other than tuberculosis. The best diagnostic sputum specimen is a good early morning collection. A 24-hour collection is helpful when sputum production is minimal but is often overgrown by mouth organisms. Three daily collections are sufficient for almost all cases; five are certainly so. Aspiration of gastric contents is a time-honored substitute when sputum is not produced. It should be done before the patient gets up, preferably just as he or she wakes up, so that sputum swallowed during sleep is still in the stomach. Smear of gastric contents has been regarded as unreliable because of potential contamination with saprophytic mycobacteria from food or water. In fact, most positive gastric smears containing more than a single organism will be found to be due to tuberculosis.[8] Sputum induction by heated saline aerosols is thought to be more effective than gastric aspiration. A negative tuberculin reaction is not conclusive evidence against tuberculosis even when the dose is 250 TU.[34] Histologic evidence of granuloma formation, even with acid-fast bacilli, is still only strong presumptive evidence of tuberculosis, since similar findings may be produced by mycobacterial other than *M. tuberculosis*. Definitive diagnosis requires culture and speciation of the organism.

FIBEROPTIC BRONCHOSCOPY. Diagnostic fiberoptic bronchoscopy with transbronchial biopsy and bronchial washings is an efficient way to obtain diagnostic materials when sputum does not suffice. However, in the majority of cases, it has been culture of washings rather than histology or acid-fast staining that has provided the diagnosis, and most cases of pulmonary tuberculosis diagnosed by bronchoscopy will later be found to have been positive using specimens obtained in a less invasive manner.[58] Culture of materials obtained at bronchoscopy by rapid radiometric methods (see the section on "Microbiology") has become popular. However, 75 percent of positive mycobacterial cultures from bronchoscopic specimens in one series were mycobacteria other than tuberculosis, and most of these were not causing disease.[9] These authors advise that material obtained at fiberoptic bronchoscopy be submitted for mycobacterial culture only in cases in which tuberculosis is being considered diagnostically on clinical grounds.

Although its usefulness in localized upper lobe infiltrates is not great, fiberoptic bronchoscopy is especially important in lower lobe tuberculosis, in which the number of bacteria is often small and endobronchial involvement is common. Fiberoptic bronchoscopy with transbronchial biopsy is also very important in the early diagnosis of miliary tuberculosis, in which, in contrast to chronic pulmonary tuberculosis, the diagnosis can often be made or at least strongly suspected on histologic grounds alone.[59]

TUBERCULOSIS DIAGNOSED AT AUTOPSY. Reports of undiagnosed tuberculosis as the principal cause of death in autopsy series continue to appear. Usually the patient is old, has other disease processes to which deterioration is attributed, and very frequently is tuberculin negative. Both nonresolving pulmonary processes and extrapulmonary tuberculosis, particularly chronic miliary and meningeal disease, are represented in this group. The usual reason that the diagnosis was missed was failure to test for its presence.[60]

Silicotuberculosis. In older studies the incidence of tuberculosis in silicotics was always far greater, often by an order of magnitude, than in others in the same population, and tuberculosis was an important cause of death.[61] The adjuvant effect of tubercle bacilli does increase the fibrogenetic characteristic of silicosis, but now, when tuberculosis is no longer epidemic in miners, it seems likely that not all cases of conglomerate or progressive massive fibrotic silicosis are due to tuberculosis, as was believed in the past. Nevertheless, there are important peculiarities when these two diseases interact. Silica appears to hamper macrophage bactericidal activity. Cavitation, which can develop in fibrotic masses without infection, will often be considered to be tuberculosis. Diagnosis is sometimes difficult because of a paucity of organisms, often the case in closed fibrotic lesions; the response to therapy is hard to evaluate because roentgenographic lesions do not necessarily change; and the tissue fibrosis seems to favor persistence of infection, making intensive and prolonged treatment advisable.[62]

Tuberculosis and Cancer. Bronchogenic carcinoma and tuberculosis occur together more frequently than would be accounted for by chance. It has been estimated that bronchogenic carcinoma occurs 20 times more frequently in tuberculosis patients than in the general population with the same smoking habits. On the other hand, 1–5 percent of tuberculosis patients admitted to hospitals will also have cancer, the great majority being men who smoke. Several types of interrelationships are important. Tuberculosis is associated with scar carcinoma, and carcinoma developing in quiescent residual tuberculous foci can cause reactivation of infection. Both of these causal sequences imply close anatomic relationship between the cancer and the tuberculous lesion, but in a substantial proportion of patients the two processes may be anatomically separate, implying that people prone to active tuberculosis are also prone to develop cancer, presumably for immunologic reasons. No cell type predominates, as would be expected to be the case if all were scar cancers, the majority of which are adenocarcinomas or alveolar cell carcinomas. It is important to emphasize that many of the cancers are central rather than peripheral.

When tuberculosis and cancer occur together, diagnosis of the latter tends to be obscured. It is good practice to entertain the possibility of cancer in all older smoking men with tuberculosis, at least to the point of obtaining sputum cytologic studies. The diagnosis is not difficult when suspected. There are certain roentgenographic findings that should raise the possibility of cancer complicating tuberculosis, such as progression of one area of shadowing while the remainder of the lesions are regressing, the presence of a large (greater than 3 cm) mass lesion admixed with infiltrative disease, the presence of hilar nodes complicating adult chronic pulmonary tuberculosis, and the development of atelectasis.[63]

Classification of Pulmonary Tuberculosis. The classification of pulmonary tuberculosis dating from the prechemotherapy era emphasized cavitation, as this was critical for prognosis. Although this classification is not presently used, it retains some importance in characterizing cases in which maximum chemotherapy might be elected. *Minimal* disease was defined as an infiltrate no greater in the aggregate than the area from the second chondrocostal junction and the fifth vertebral body to the apex of the lung on one side and containing no cavity and no dense confluent disease. *Moderately advanced* disease was defined as scattered areas of nondense infiltrate greater than *minimal* in extent but less in aggregate area than one lung field; dense confluent infiltrate no greater than one-third of one lung field in extent; or any cavitary disease in which the aggregate diameter of the cavities was less than 4 cm. *Far advanced disease* was defined as anything greater than moderately advanced.

The present classification (American Thoracic Society 1974), based on the concept that proper chemotherapy is curative for any sort of lesion, is as follows: (*O*) no tuberculosis exposure, not infected (no history of exposure, negative tuberculin skin test); (*I*) tuberculosis exposure, no evidence of infection (history of exposure, negative tuberculin skin test); (*II*) tuberculous infection without disease (positive tuberculin skin test, negative bacteriologic studies, no roentgenographic findings compatible with tuberculosis, no symptoms due to tuberculosis); chemotherapy status (preventive therapy), dates, if given; (*III*) tuberculosis: infected, with disease.

The current status of the patient's tuberculosis should be described by the following characteristics: (*1*) location of disease (e.g., pulmonary, pleural, lymphatic); (*2*) bacteriologic status (microscopy and culture with dates); (*3*) chemotherapy status (including dates).

TREATMENT OF TUBERCULOSIS

Prior to the availability of effective drug therapy, approximately half of the patients with active pulmonary tuberculosis died, usually within 2 years, about a quarter recovered, and a quarter become chronic positive cases.[10,11] Sanatorium treatment, while probably effective in noncavitary cases, was much less so in advanced disease. Arrest, when it did occur, carried with it the permanent risk of relapse, observed in 28 percent of one carefully followed series of patients.

During the 1950s and 1960s, it became clear that prolonged chemotherapy could cure almost all patients without traditional measures such as bed rest and collapse therapy, and that isolation was unnecessary since patients on chemotherapy promptly became noninfectious. Although ideally treatment should cure almost all cases, the actual results are often much less successful.[64] A few failures may be due to drug resistance or to improper drug regimens or supervision. The great majority, however, are due to the often carefully concealed failure of the patient to comply with instructions as health returns and the perceived importance of continuing treatment lessens. Accordingly, careful patient education is essential to success. Frequent visits to the physician are important in monitoring drug toxicity and progress but even more vital in reinforcing the seriousness of the treatment enterprise.

Strategies of Treatment Based On Bacterial Characteristics of the Lesion

The bacillary population in pulmonary tuberculosis is thought to consist of organisms in three different physiologic situations: (*1*) rapidly multiplying organisms in the highly favorable, hyperoxic, neutral pH, extracellular environment of the pulmonary cavity; (*2*) much more slowly metabolizing organisms in the somewhat hypoxic and acidic environment of solid caseous material; and (*3*) the acidic (intracellular pH), highly suppressive environment inside the activated macrophage. It has become customary to discuss drugs in terms of their effects on the different populations (Table 4). It should be emphasized, however, that caseation (unabsorbed solid necrosis) favors microbial involution into a metabolically dormant state, protecting trapped organisms from the effects of both antimicrobials and cellular immune mechanisms. Such persisting organisms can be contained only by securing anatomic healing with fibrosis and encapsulation over time.

Antimicrobial Resistance

Populations of tubercle bacilli never exposed to drugs will all contain mutants spontaneously resistant to one or another chemotherapeutic agent at a rate of between 1×10^6 and 1×10^8, a phenomenon termed *genetic resistance*. This is of no practical importance in noncavitary tuberculous lesions in which the bacillary population is small (10^4 or 10^5 per gram of tissue). However, in the enormous populations (10^9 to 10^{11}) characteristic of pulmonary cavities, a relatively large number (10^4 or 10^5) of organisms resistant to one or another drug will be present from the outset, and these, under the selective pressure of single-drug therapy, may promptly multiply and repopulate the lesion.[65] This is one theoretical reason supporting the use of multiple-drug therapy, since the chance of an organism's being spontaneously resistant to two drugs would be extremely small. The presence of a predominantly drug-resistant population in a previously untreated patient is called *primary resistance*. The level of primary resistance in a given population is influenced by the degree of supervision of patients undergoing treatment, since development of drug resistance in treated patients is usually due to improper chemotherapy. Such patients can then spread drug-resistant strains to others. In the United States at large, the level of resistance to a major drug (either INH or STM) has remained at the relatively low level of about 7 percent and seems to have been falling slightly in recent years. However, there are important populations and areas of the country in which the incidence of primary drug resistance is much higher. It is approximately 50 percent in the Oriental wives of servicemen returning from Southeast Asia.[66] Such high levels of resistance are characteristic of societies in which antituberculous medications can be obtained without supervision. Often persons ill with tuberculosis will take the drugs long enough to feel better, discontinue them for economic or other reasons, and then take them again as the illness relapses—ideal conditions for selection and propagation of drug-resistant organisms. There are urban foci of increased resistance in south-

TABLE 4. Actions of Chemotherapeutic Agents

Agent	*Activity*
INH	Bactericidal against both intracellular and extracellular organisms
RMP	Bactericidal against both intracellular and extracellular organisms; maintains activity against very slowly metabolizing bacilli
PZA	Bactericidal only at acidic pH such as within cells; greatest activity in first few months of therapy
STM	Excluded from the intracellular environment; activity only against extracellular organisms
EMB	Bacteriostatic against both intracellular and extracellular organisms

ern California, New York City, and elsewhere, presumably due to the presence of a large number of persons from areas outside of the continental United States characterized by a large incidence of primary drug resistance. In south Texas, one study recorded primary drug resistance in 20 percent of the test population. Importantly, as will be discussed below, primary resistance to RMP was present in approximately 10 percent.[67] A recent increase in primary resistance to RMP has also been noted in a longitudinal study in Brooklyn children.[68] Tuberculosis in homeless individuals living in hostels was found to demonstrate drug resistance in over 60 percent of cases in one study.[43] The country of origin and a history of previous treatment were the two most important predictors of the presence of drug resistance in one study from southern California.[69] The term *secondary resistance* means resistance developing during the course of treatment in a person with an initially drug-sensitive infection. Such cases obviously are major sources of infection of contacts with drug-resistant organisms.

Antituberculous Drugs*

Isoniazid. INH (or H) is the keystone of therapy. It is well absorbed, reaching levels after ingestion equal to those after injection. Its small molecular size allows widespread distribution, and it reaches greater than bactericidal concentrations in all tissues, including caseous foci, the interior of phagocytic cells, and the subarachnoid space. It is metabolized by the liver, both by acetylation and by oxidation via the hepatic p-450 mixed oxidase drug-detoxifying systems. Its major toxicities are two: peripheral neuritis as a result of pyridoxine deficiency and hepatitis. Peripheral neuritis is due to INH-induced depletion of the body's pyridoxine stores by a mechanism or mechanisms that are not understood. It is dose dependent (40 percent at a 20 mg/kg dosage, 20 percent at 10 mg/kg, and 1–2 percent at 5 mg/kg) and more of a problem in certain groups (alcoholics, uremics, malnourished persons, cancer patients, pregnant women) likely to have baseline pyridoxine deficiency. Hepatitis, discussed further below, occurs in 1–2 percent of persons, more often in older individuals, and more often in persons who are slow rather than rapid acetylators, the rate of acetylation of INH being a genetically determined trait.[70] This implies that the toxic moiety is a product of oxidative metabolism rather than of acetylation and provides an explanation for the interaction of INH and RMP, described below. Rarely, INH will cause seizures, usually when ingested in huge doses with suicidal intent.[71]

Rifampin. RMP (or R) is the second major antituberculous agent. Like INH, it reaches therapeutic concentrations in caseous foci and the interior of phagocytic cells, and it penetrates inflamed meninges well. For reasons probably related to its mode of action (inhibition of DNA-dependent RNA polymerase), it is thought to be more effective than INH against organisms that are metabolizing very slowly or only intermittently. Its side effects include gastrointestinal intolerance and, when given on a less than daily schedule at doses larger than 600 mg/day, a number of side effects with what seems to be an immunologic basis, including hemolytic anemia, acute renal failure, and thrombocytopenia. These are rare with daily dosage schedules, however. The most important toxicity by far is hepatitis, discussed further below. RMP may turn urine and other body fluids orange and result in permanent discoloration of soft contact lenses. It is a potent inducer of the hepatic microsomal p-450 mixed oxidase drug-detoxifying system of enzymes. This may result in increased catabolism of some important drugs and hormones, including cortisone, Coumadin, oral contraceptive agents, ketoconazole, phenytoin, and cyclosporine, with important clinical effects such as transplant rejection, adrenal insufficiency, seizures, and unplanned pregnancy.[72]

INH-RMP Hepatotoxicity. The incidence of hepatotoxicity in regimens containing INH but not RMP is approximately 1–2 percent. The incidence is vanishingly small under the age of 20, 0.3 percent between 20 and 35, 1.2 percent between 35 and 49, and 2.3 percent over the age of 50.[73] Recent studies have indicated that the incidence in those over 65 may be as high as 4 percent.[74] Transient, minor elevations of transaminase values occur in 10–20 percent but should not be taken as reason for discontinuation unless the values exceed five times normal. When frank hepatitis develops there is a risk of death, ranging from 6 to 12 percent in three separate studies.[73,75–77] It merits emphasis that most of these fatalities occurred in persons who went on taking the drug in the face of jaundice and associated symptoms of hepatitis. As mentioned, the risk of INH-induced hepatitis is probably greater in slow acetylators, although there is disagreement on this point.[70]

The incidence of hepatotoxicity in regimens containing both INH and RMP is approximately four times that of regimens containing INH alone.[78,79] Moreover there are some important clinical differences. The onset of jaundice with INH alone rarely occurs in the first month and often is delayed for 2 or more months. It is common for INH-RMP-induced jaundice to occur within 1–3 weeks of the onset of treatment and to be rapidly progressive. It is believed, although not established, that INH–RMP hepatotoxicity is due to acceleration of INH oxidation due to the inducing effect of RMP on the heptatic p-450 microsomal mixed oxidase drug-detoxifying system. This conclusion receives some support from the observation that other inducers of this system, notably Dilantin and phenobarbital, have been associated with fulminant hepatic failure in persons receiving INH-RMP.[80] Moreover, in contrast to jaundice complicating INH alone, which is rare in children, the incidence of INH-RMP-induced jaundice in children has been reported to be as high as 25 percent in several series of cases, suggesting an age-related metabolic difference in drug detoxification.[70,81–83]

When hepatitis occurs in patients receiving INH but not RMP, effective regimens based on RMP and a companion drug or drugs can usually be substituted. When hepatitis occurs in patients receiving both INH and RMP, both drugs should be discontinued until the liver function tests return to normal. INH may then be cautiously but usually successfully reintroduced in graduated doses while monitoring liver function tests, and a more prolonged (18–24 months) regimen based on INH and a companion drug or drugs other than RMP can be continued. When patients developing drug-related hepatitis on INH and RMP have demonstrated microbial resistance to INH but not RMP, RMP can usually be gradually reintroduced and a more prolonged (18–24 months) regimen based on RMP and a companion drug or drugs other than INH can be continued. When clinical circumstances dictate that an effort be made to reintroduce both INH and RMP—in the vast majority of instances, this will not be the case—many authorities believe that both drugs can be sequentially reintroduced after a period of time in many patients.[70] Obviously, an attempt to reintroduce drugs that have been associated with hepatitis requires close clinical supervision and close monitoring of liver function tests.

Pyrazinamide. PZA (or Z) has emerged as an essential drug in 6-month regimens, as discussed below. Like INH, it is a nicotinic acid derivative. Studies in the early 1950s suggested that it was so seriously hepatotoxic that it should not be used in first-line treatment regimens. However, this was at a dosage larger and for periods of time longer than are now employed, and PZA as now given is not hepatotoxic and does not add to the hepatotoxicity of INH and RMP.[3,84] One of its metabolites competes with uric acid for secretion at the renal tubular level, resulting in hyperuricemia, fairly frequent mild polyarthralgias

* See Chapter 32 for the dosage and pharmacology.

that are not gout, and, rarely, frank clinical gout.[3] PZA is not active at neutral pH but is active at the more acidic pH found inside phagocytic cells and at the center of caseous lesions. It is regarded, therefore, as having particular effectiveness against intracellular organisms.

Streptomycin. STM (or S), an aminoglycoside, is thought to be excluded from the interior of cells and is active at the neutral pH characteristic of the extracellular space. This has led to the concept that STM and PZA together constitute "one strong drug" and has served as the theoretical basis for initial trials employing INH, RMP, STM, and PZA. Its major toxicity is eighth nerve damage leading to vestibular disturbance and, less frequently, to deafness. This is more of a problem in older persons, and for this reason there is reluctance to administer it to persons much over the age of 50. STM, like all aminoglycosides, is excreted by the kidney, and its dose needs to be reduced in the presence of renal compromise.

Ethambutol. EMB (or E) is a relatively weak component of most multiple-drug regimens and as such is a first-line agent. Its only serious toxicity is optic neuritis, manifested by central scotomata, decreased red-green color vision, decreased visual acuity, and, rarely, concentric contraction of visual fields leading to gun barrel vision. This toxicity is dose dependent, occurring in as many as 3 percent of patients at 25 mg/kg, a dosage often used as a component of four-drug treatment, but is very rare at the more usual dose of 15 mg/kg.[85] Usually optic neuritis develops slowly and reverses when the drug is discontinued, but cases have been reported with a fulminant course leading to blindness over several days.[86] The need to follow visual symptoms closely militates against its use in very young children. EMB can also cause hyperuricemia and, rarely, gout.[87]

Second-Line Agents. *Ethionamide* (*ETH*) is an oral agent with prominent gastrointestinal toxicity, thought to be centrally mediated. *Cycloserine* (*CS*) frequently causes central nervous system disturbances including mood change, psychosis, and seizures. *Kannamycin* and *capreomycin* are aminoglycoside antibiotics with toxicities similar to although somewhat more severe than that of STM. They are probably less effective than STM but do not demonstrate cross-microbial resistance. More than one aminoglycoside cannot be given at the same time. *Para-aminosalicylic* (*PAS*), a weak but formerly frequently used companion drug to INH, now largely replaced by EMB in multiple-drug regimens, is a very disagreeable and difficult to take agent, causing some gastrointestinal upset in most patients as well as frequent hypersensitivity, hepatotoxicity, and, when given as the sodium salt, fluid overload.

Choice of Drug Regimen for Initial Treatment

Before the availability of RMP, excellent results in drug-sensitive infections had been obtained for years with INH and a companion drug, first PAS and subsequently EMB, "reinforced" in extensive disease by administration of STM for 6–12 weeks at the outset of treatment. Repeated observation that shorter courses of treatment led to an unacceptable number of relapses established the necessary duration of treatment as 18–24 months. Results of this then standard treatment were sufficiently good in INH-susceptible infections that when RMP, an agent at least as effective as INH, became available, the only advantages that were readily apparent were treatment of INH-resistant infections and the possibility of decreasing the necessary duration of treatment. Definitive studies in the United States, Great Britain, and elsewhere have now established that treatment of drug-sensitive infections for 9 months with regimens containing INH and RMP provides results just as good (although no better), in terms of reversal of infectiousness and freedom from post-treatment relapse, as those obtained with 18–24 months treatment with non-RMP-containing regimens.[87,88] Other studies sufficiently large to be definitive have demonstrated that 6-month regimens based on an initial 2-month "bactericidal phase" consisting of INH, RMP, STM, and PZA (HRSZ) or EMB rather than STM (HREZ) and a "continuation phase" of INH and RMP for 4 more months also produce results as good as those obtained with longer regimens.[84,87,88] The very real advantages of shorter therapy have led to universal acceptance of 9-month regimens based on INH and RMP as standard therapy and to the increasing use of 6-month regimens. Older regimens excluding RMP have been relegated to infrequent use by both public health authorities and private physicians. Since the only real advantage of 9- or 6-month regimens in drug-sensitive infections is the shorter duration of therapy, a word of caution is perhaps in order. The emergence of drug resistance during therapy is almost always due to careless drug taking on the part of the patient. If this leads to resistance to both major agents, the patient would have highly uncertain prospects for eventual recovery, as was the case in INH-resistant infections before the availability of RMP. This problem has not surfaced often, but experience with these regimens remains short judged in the context of the 30-odd years of drug treatment of pulmonary tuberculosis. As mentioned above, there is no doubt that giving INH and RMP together increases fourfold the incidence of hepatotoxicity compared to that of regimens containing INH but not RMP.[78,79] (PZA does not add to hepatotoxicity in this situation, and the hepatotoxicity of RMP given as a single agent is not well known.) Further, the very bothersome complication of interstitial nephritis seems to be more frequent in patients receiving INH–RMP. Without implying that the problem of toxicity is great, which it is not, it is nevertheless reasonable to consider whether any increased risk is justifiable in the admittedly unusual circumstances of less than extensive disease in which a drug-sensitive infection is highly likely and compliance almost certain. The acceleration of hepatic degradation of many other drugs by RMP, as discussed above,[72] and its poorly understood immunosuppressive effects must also be taken into account. Although to date RMP has proved to be a very safe agent, the more than a decade that intervened between introduction of INH and appreciation of its striking hepatotoxicity illustrates that much time is usually required to understand fully the complexities of any strong drug.

Standard Regimen. The combination of INH (300 mg) plus RMP (600 mg) given once daily by mouth on an empty stomach for 9 months is now an established regimen, advised by many for all forms of tuberculosis, pulmonary and extrapulmonary.[87,88] PZA (25–35 mg/kg) plus either STM (1 g) or EMB (15 or 25 mg/kg) is often added during the early stages of treatment while awaiting sensitivity studies to take into account the possibility of primary drug resistance. This should be done when there is suspicion of a drug-resistant infection on epidemiologic or historical grounds (previous chemotherapy, either as treatment or prophylaxis; contact with a drug-resistant source case; acquisition of infection in places with a known high prevalence of INH resistance such as Asia, Latin America, Africa, and institutions for the homeless).

An intermittent 9-month regimen consisting largely of twice weekly doses has been established as an acceptable alternative on the basis of a now large, well-studied series of cases by one group of investigators. INH and RMP are administered daily as described above for 2 months, and the remainder of the treatment is given twice weekly with the same dose of RMP but a larger (900 mg) dose of INH. Problems with drug resistance have not been reported in this group of cases, and toxicity has been minimal.[87,88]

Six-Month Regimens. Theoretical considerations led to the idea that a combination of STM (effective against extracellular bacilli at neutral pH) and PZA (effective against intracellular bacilli at an acid pH) would constitute one strong drug. This encouraged the notion that addition of this strong drug to INH and RMP would allow still briefer treatment courses. A number of studies have now clearly demonstrated that a 6-month regimen consisting of HRSZ for 2 months followed by 4 months of INH-RMP treatment produces excellent results; and subsequently it has been shown that EMB can be substituted for STM, resulting in an all-oral regimen (HREZ) with no loss of potency.[3,84] The large number of studies that have now been reported allow the following generalizations. (*1*) PZA appears to be the critical additional drug to INH and RMP. Preliminary studies indicate that EMB and STM probably contribute little and are unnecessary in drug-sensitive infections.[3] PZA's highly bactericidal activity is thought to be confined to the first 2 or 3 months of treatment, and it can be discontinued thereafter. Its toxicity is negligible. The dose is 2.0–2.5 g, depending on body size, which is equivalent to 25–35 mg/kg. (*2*) The critical period is the first 2 months of therapy, after which drugs other than RMP and INH can be discontinued. These should be continued throughout the entire 6-month course. (*3*) When the initial bactericidal period of HRSZ or HREZ has been successfully administered, the long-term results of even a very brief (1 or 2 months) continuation phase are surprisingly good. Although such minimal regimens would never be advised as a treatment plan, it seems likely that many recalcitrant patients given four-drug therapy for 2 months will be greatly benefited even when they stop the treatment 1 or 2 months thereafter. Patients whose disease is sufficiently low grade that neither a sputum smear nor a culture is positive will often be cured by the 2-month bactericidal phase of therapy alone. (*4*) Initial resistance to INH, STM, or both does not seem to compromise the results of 6-month treatment employing four drugs in the first 2 months,[89] although most authorities would extend the period of treatment to 9 months in this situation.[88] It should be emphasized that although, as mentioned above, there is some indication that the results using HRZ in the initial 2-month bactericidal phase are as good as those obtained with HRSZ or HREZ in drug-sensitive infections, information regarding the effects of INH or STM resistance in this three-drug treatment plan is not available. For this reason, it seems advisable to continue to use the four drugs in situations in which there is any likelihood of drug resistance. Also, most importantly, *results of 6-month treatment in patients with initial resistance to RMP are very poor*, with unaccepable results being observed in nearly 50 percent.[89] Experience before RMP became available would suggest that RMP-resistant cases should be treated for 18–24 months.

INH-EMB-Based Regimens. An 18- to 24-month course of INH (300 mg) and EMB (15–18 mg/kg for outpatients and 25 mg/kg for inpatients) for moderate or mild drug-sensitive pulmonary tuberculosis, with the addition of STM (1 g) during the first 2 months or until sputum is negative in more advanced or symptomatic disease, is a low-cost, effective, and dependable treatment program with low toxicity.[79] In our opinion, it is the regimen of choice (*1*) in patients with less than extensive disease who can be expected to take drugs reliably and whose supervision consists of no more than monthly clinic or office visits; (*2*) in patients who are likely to be noncompliant but who must nevertheless be treated in a relatively unsupervised fashion; and (*3*) in patients in whom there is more than the usual concern about hepatotoxicity. Although there is no indication that underlying hepatic disease increases the incidence of hepatotoxicity due to antituberculous drugs, its presence certainly complicates the detection of this condition.

An intermittent regimen with these same drugs has also proved highly effective and can be completely supervised. After a 2-month daily course as outlined above, usually in the hospital, a twice-weekly schedule consisting of high-dose INH (15 mg/kg) plus either EMB (50 mg/kg) or STM (25–28 mg/kg) is given under full clinic supervision.

Course of Treatment and Duration of Observation

Usually the diagnosis will have been established before initiation of therapy. In smear-negative cases, five or six sputum specimens and if possible, specimens obtained at bronchoscopy should be submitted before beginning treatment. In severely ill patients treatment should be initiated immediately; a few days of antituberculosis treatment will not interfere with diagnosis. Monthly chest roentgenograms are helpful but not essential in following progress. After 1 month of therapy it is ideal to obtain early morning sputum for culture at 2-week intervals in order to monitor conversion or, if sputum positivity persists, to detect the emergence of drug resistance. It is more practical, however, to obtain several sputum specimens for culture at 2 months of therapy and again at 4 and 6 months. With regimens containing both INH and RMP, conversion by 2 months is the rule, and usually not much longer is required with INH-EMB. In an appreciable minority of patients (20 percent in one study), smears remain positive for periods of time after cultures revert to negative and sporadic positive smears can be seen for long periods, due presumably to breakdown of unstable caseous material containing inactive bacilli.[90] In the uncommon case when sputum cultures continue to be positive after 4 months of treatment, there is a significant threat of emerging drug resistance. In this circumstance, almost never observed when both INH and RMP have been reliably taken in initial therapy, it is important to obtain drug-sensitivity studies for future reference, to raise the question of noncompliance, and to consider seriously the addition of two new drugs to which the organism should be sensitive (on the basis of original sensitivity studies), at least until the result of the new sensitivity studies are known. Addition of only one drug where drug resistance is likely carries the real risk of rapid development of bacterial resistance to the single added drug as well.

Patients receiving INH should be instructed about symptoms suggestive of hepatitis and, when possible, monitored by determination of serum transaminase levels monthly or every 2 months (see the section on "chemoprophylaxis"). This is more important in people receiving both INH and RMP. Patients receiving EMB should be carefully questioned at regular intervals regarding visual symptoms and their visual acuity measured (Snellen chart), and red-green color discimination testing is desirable in those receiving the higher dose of 25 mg/kg. Patients receiving STM should be questioned concerning hearing and vestibular function and tested regularly for high-frequency loss if over 50 years of age.

Relapse after adequate antimicrobial therapy for tuberculosis is so infrequent that prolonged follow-up study is no longer considered necessary.[15,16,18] However, exceptions should be made in the case of unusually extensive disease, slow bacteriologic response to treatment, suspicion of poor compliance on the part of the patient, and high-risk patients by reason of intercurrent disease. Many authorities believe that observation can be discontinued after 9 months of treatment with regimens containing both INH and RMP. It is our present opinion that a total of 2 years of observation is desirable with these regimens as well, with sputum and chest roentgenogram examination every 3–6 months.

Retreatment. Most retreatment patients should be managed by physicians with expertise in tuberculosis treatment. Expert judgment is critical when drug resources are limited. The determination of the susceptibility of the organism to all available drugs is most important.

In infections resistant to INH after initial treatment with INH-EMB or INH-EMB-STM, retreatment with RMP together with two other drugs to which the organism is susceptible under circumstances assuring uninterrupted drug ingestion for at least 24 months is highly effective. Although each case is best handled by individualized therapy, some generalizations are possible. (*1*) A relapse after prompt sputum conversion indicates that drugs have been stopped too soon, usually by the patient. If drugs have been stopped completely, the infection will usually demonstrate the same drug-susceptibility pattern present at the outset and will respond again to the initial drug regimen. (*2*) If drug ingestion and compliance have been irregular, resistant organisms will probably be present. (*3*) A patient with sputum cultures positive for tubercle bacilli after more than 4–6 months of treatment will probably be excreting drug-resistant organisms. (*4*) Under circumstances of suspected or presumed drug resistance, a two- or three-drug combination including at least one unused strong drug (INH, RMP, STM, PZA) and an unused weak drug (EMB, ETH, PAS, CS) may be added to drugs previously given while awaiting drug susceptibility studies. The drugs STM plus PZA are often considered to compose one excellent bactericidal drug. (*5*) The drug CM can replace STM. The drug KM is less effective and more toxic, and its use is limited to last-resort situations. (*6*) Drugs SM, CM, and KM have similar and additive toxicities, and no more than one should be used at the same time. (*7*) In infections resistant to INH, RMP, STM, and PZA, three or four of the weak drugs (ETH, CS, PAS, KM) should be used at the same time and INH also given in high doses (15 mg/kg), since INH retains some suppressive effect even in the presence of high degrees of in vitro resistance.

Other Forms of Treatment. Bed rest, modified rather than absolute, is beneficial during symptomatic disease but has no effect on the overall outcome when effective chemotherapy is given. In treatment failures resistant to all drugs, strict bed rest with continued use of INH may salvage some otherwise hopeless cases and probably is of benefit in retreatment cases resistant to all but the weakest drugs. Surgery is now rarely used in the treatment of pulmonary tuberculosis. It may still have a role in treatment failure cases with resectable cavitary lesions and resistance to all but the weakest chemotherapeutic agents or when lack of patient cooperation compromises the prospects of successful use of limited drug resources.

USE OF CORTICOSTEROIDS. In unusually debilitated patients or those with unusually severe constitutional symptoms, moderate doses of corticosteroids (30–35 mg of prednisone daily) will effect prompt symptomatic improvement, abolish fever, and repair serious anemia and hypoalbuminemia when these are present.[91] The dosage can usually be tapered by 2.5-mg decrements every 3–5 days. When life-threatening hypoxemia (the clinical picture of the adult respiratory distress syndrome) complicates extensive and diffuse pulmonary inflammation in advanced miliary tuberculosis or extensive bronchogenic spread of cavitary tuberculosis, corticosteriods in larger doses (60–80 mg of prednisone daily) may promptly improve arterial oxygenation.[92] When drug fever develops to one or another component of a drug regimen, it is frequently possible to desensitize the patient using a program of decreasing corticosteroids and increasing drug dose over a 4–6-day period.[93] Corticosteroid therapy has no deleterious effect on the course of tuberculosis when chemotherapy is adequate.

Special Treatment Circumstances. CHILDHOOD. Pulmonary tuberculosis in childhood should be treated with INH, 10 mg/kg (maximum of 300 mg daily), and RMP, 15 mg/kg (maximum of 600 mg daily), for a period of 1 year. STM, 20 mg/kg, or EMB, 15 mg/kg, can be added in extensive disease.[87,88] The problem of monitoring visual acuity in very young children limits the safety of EMB in this age group. PZA has not been extensively studied in children, but to date has been found to be safe and is recommended in tuberculous meningitis.[94]

PREGNANCY. Treatment of tuberculosis should not be deferred in pregnancy. In the usual case, INH plus EMB is the regimen of choice. Experience with RMP is less extensive, but the information that exists indicates that it is safe for the fetus and may be used in advanced disease. STM should not be used because of the frequency of eighth nerve toxicity in the fetus, a vulnerability that is not confined to any period of pregnancy. Experience with PZA is too limited to recommend it in pregnancy.[95]

UREMIA AND END-STAGE RENAL DISEASE. INH and RMP can be used in regular doses in uremics, administered after dialysis when this is done. The dosage of EMB should be reduced to 8–10 mg/kg in anephric patients. Recommendations concerning PZA are variable, but it probably can be used at the lower end of the usual recommended dosage, 15–20 mg/kg. STM should not be used except in very unusual circumstances, and then its blood level should be monitored. Pyridoxine supplementation is mandatory in the uremic patient.[96] Biochemical monitoring of hepatotoxicity in uremics may be complicated by the fact that SGOT values are abnormally low in the uremic population.

LIVER DISEASE. Although there is some disagreement on this point, most feel that the selection and dosage of antituberculous agents need not be modified in the presence of alcoholism or liver disease. However, it complicates detection of drug-related liver dysfunction when it does occur; accordingly, clinical and biochemical supervision should be assiduous in this situation.

IMMUNOSUPPRESSED PATIENTS. Tuberculosis appearing during the course of immunosuppressive treatment for intercurrent disease should be treated with the usual drugs and the immunosuppressive therapy continued as indicated for treatment of the underlying process.[97]

CHEMOPROPHYLAXIS

Soon after INH became available, its efficacy and freedom from side effects as then perceived led to its widespread use as a preventive agent. At one time, enthusiasm was such that some suggested treatment of all tuberculin reactors in an attempt to "totally eradicate tuberculosis." This optimism has considerably waned for two reasons. First, it is now realized that the significant hepatotoxicity of INH has to be taken into account. Second, it is now clear that neither INH nor any other drug has much effect on an infection in which microbial multiplication is minimal or absent. Accordingly, the term *prophylaxis* is conceptually misleading; what is actually taking place when it is effective is treatment of a subclinical but active infection.

INH Hepatotoxicity

As mentioned, hepatitis due to INH is rare in people under age 20 and increases with age. A large U.S. Public Health Service (USPHS) study recorded probable hepatitis, defined as a serum SGOT value over 250 Karman units (or elsewhere as five times the upper limit of normal) in 1 per 100,000 people under age 20, 300 between ages 20 and 35, 1200 between ages 35 and 49, 2300 between ages 50 and 64, and 800 over age 64.[73] The lower number in the over-64 age group was felt to be due to a small sample. Recent data indicate an incidence of hepatitis of 4.6 percent (4600 per 100,000) in Arkansas nursing home patients over 65. The incidence in daily drinkers was also high (2650 per 100,000). A large European study reported an incidence of 520 per 100,000; the figure for those under 35 was 280 per 100,000 and for those over 54, 770.[98] Most cases of hepatitis developed within the first 3 months. In the USPHS study, seven (7.6 percent) of the patients with probable hepatitis died.[73] This figure is regarded by many as falsely high, as most deaths were observed in one geographic location (Baltimore) in patients with underlying liver disease. It is generally believed that most deaths occur in persons who persist in taking the drug in spite of symptoms of hepatitis. However, other estimates of the death rate from frank hepatitis in situations in which biochemical monitoring was not carried out include 7.6 percent,[75] 12 percent[76] and 6 percent even when an effort at careful monthly monitoring of symptoms was made.[77] It seems likely that biochemical monitoring will prevent deaths, as the hepatitis is gradually progressive, with a reasonably long subclinical phase. Byrd et al. recorded an incidence of hepatitis of 2300 per 100,000 but no deaths in a biochemically monitored population.[99] It is important to note that many of the patients wih serious biochemical hepatitis in that series were clinically asymptomatic.

Treatment of Contacts of Active Cases

In the large USPHS contact study, the incidence of tuberculosis in nontreated contacts was 1550 per 100,000 compared to 610 in the treated group, a reduction of 61 percent over the 10-year period of observation.[100] In those who were tuberculin negative when first surveyed, the figures (per 100,000) were 510 without and 150 with treatment, a reduction of 59 percent. Estimates of the risk to contacts in other smaller studies are much higher. One small English contact study reported an incidence of 9 percent (9000 per 100,000)[101]; another in New York State reported 2000–3000 per 100,000.[102]

All studies indicate that a year of INH therapy is never 100 percent effective in preventing subsequent disease. Most figures range from 60 to 80 percent, a point insufficiently emphasized. The most important reason for failure is undoubtedly poor compliance. However, there is evidence that INH prophylaxis may not be effective in drug-resistant infections.[103] Whether or not prophylactic monotherapy with INH will result in subsequent INH resistance is not established, but it seems unlikely.[109]

Treatment of many tuberculin-positive contacts is obviously appropriate. The advantage vis-à-vis development of INH hepatitis is clearest among the young, in whom the risk of INH toxicity is least and the likelihood of recent infection is greatest. Usually tuberculin-positive adults who are close or household contacts of active cases should also be treated, but in those over 50 years old or so it may be reasonable to observe rather than treat in view of the greater risk of INH toxicity and the greater possibility that the tuberculin reaction represents ancient infection. The case for treatment of tuberculin-negative contacts of active cases is less secure. Most authorities would advise its use in those under age 5. A period of 3 months of treatment followed by repeat tuberculin testing has been advised. If skin test conversion has taken place, a 12-month course can be completed. If not and if the source of infection has been controlled by treatment, further INH therapy is not necessary. In older tuberculin-negative contacts, the skin test should be repeated in 2 or 3 months and treatment given only if it has become positive.

Treatment of Quiescent, Previously Untreated Pulmonary Tuberculosis

Tuberculin-positive patients with upper lobe fibrotic lesions and patients known to have had active tuberculosis before drugs were available will relapse sufficiently frequently that a year of INH preventive therapy has been widely advised. Representative studies (all figures per 100,000) include a rate of 2450 over 5 years in controls compared to 350 with treatment[105]; 1940 over 7 years in controls compared to 560 with treatment[106]; and 1430 over 5 years in controls compared to 360 with treatment.[98] The risk of relapse decreases in proportion to the length of observation. In the European study, the relapse rate in untreated patients was about 450 per 100,000 in the first year of observation but had fallen to one-third of that by the fifth year, a rate substantially less than the hepatotoxic risk of a year of INH therapy.[98] One analysis has concluded that 6 months of chemoprophylaxis with INH may be enough in this circumstance. However, others have raised the question of whether INH alone is sufficient if these cases actually represent active disease. In a Canadian study, treatment cases were divided into an INH group and an INH-PAS group, both treated for 1 year. Three patients relapsed after INH treatment, two of which demonstrated INH resistance (relapse rate 190 per 100,000); none relapsed after combined drug treatment.[105] Both of these observations, the fall in the rate of development of active disease with longer periods of roentgenographic stability and the greater effectiveness of combined-drug treatment (in one study), suggest that the benefit of chemoprophylaxis in the putatively inactive case is actually confined to those cases which in fact are low-grade active, often with a fairly large bacterial population, for whom single-drug therapy may turn out to have been insufficient. One authority uses maximum therapy (HRSZ) for 3 months and then stops treatment if cultures are negative and the roentgenogram is stable.[107]

Treatment of the Tuberculin Converter

The first 2 years after tuberculin conversion constitute the period of greatest risk with respect to development of active disease. Most authorities would recommend treatment without respect to age in persons with known recent tuberculin conversion.

Treatment of People with Positive Tuberculin Reactions of Uncertain History

All infections in children may be presumed to be recent; in developed countries this is the case in adolescents and young adults as well (Fig. 2). An analysis of the competing risks of tuberculosis and hepatitis by the Centers for Disease Control (CDC) led to the recommendation that tuberculin-positive people under age 35 should receive chemoprophylaxis.[108] Recently issue has been taken with that analysis, leading many to reduce the age under which treatment should be given to 25 or 20, with which position we agree.[75,109] Even in adolescents the actual incidence of active disease in positive reactors is not great, 145 per 100,000 in one experience.[102] However, the risk of INH hepatotoxicity in this age group is so small that treatment is justified.

Treatment of Positive Reactors in Certain Populations with a Known High Incidence of Active Disease

Indochinese refugees demonstrate an astounding prevalence of active tuberculosis, ranging from 491 per 100,000 in the 0–4 age group to 7160 in the 65 and older group. In tuberculin-positive men 65 years and over, a figure of 14,180 per 100,000 (14 percent) has been published.[110] These statistics seem to warrant consideration of treatment in all tuberculin-positive people in this population or at least very careful follow-up studies. In view of the high incidence (50 percent) of drug resistance in Orientals,[66] there is a real question as to whether single-drug chemoprophylaxis should ever be used in this group, a circumstance that considerably complicates the decision to use prophylaxis. Studies on this problem are not yet available. There are other populations—Haitian refugees,[14] possibly Cuban refugees, and certain pockets of high prevalence in urban slum areas[111]—in which widespread prophylactic therapy would be justified, at least in younger people, after ruling out clinically active disease (requiring more than prophylactic regimens) by chest roentgenograms.

Tuberculin-Positive People with Added Risk Factors

Several conditions and situations thought to predispose to activation of tuberculosis have been taken as reasons for preventive chemotherapy in tuberculin-positive people. One study reported that active pulmonary tuberculosis developed in 27 percent (27,000 per 100,000) of patients with roentgenographic evidence suggestive of old, inactive pulmonary tuberculosis after gastrectomy for peptic ulcer disease. Tuberculin-positive, roentgenologically negative post-gastrectomy patients with significant preoperative weight loss developed active pulmonary tuberculosis five times more frequently (1780 per 100,000) than the population from which they came, but there was no such increased incidence in patients with no preoperative weight loss.[112] Prolonged treatment with cortisone in high dosage is thought to predispose to activation of latent tuberculosis, but the actual risk is entirely unknown.[113] Several studies document increased tuberculosis in patients on chronic renal dialysis, figures varying from 1500 to 3300 per 100,000 over 10 years,[96,119] and a somewhat smaller but still significant figure has been reported in renal transplantation patients.[115] The effectiveness and risks of preventive therapy in these patients have not been established, and the pyridoxine-deficient state that regularly occurs in uremia complicates the situation. Preventive therapy with INH has been recommended by some in tuberculin-positive patients with silicosis.[61,62] However, such data as exist indicate that active tuberculosis in silicosis requires prolonged, multiple-drug chemotherapy, and relapse after preventive therapy has been observed. Tuberculin-positive patients with myeloproliferative disorders and hematologic malignancies have also been treated with preventive therapy, especially when corticosteroids were being given, but again with no documentation of risks or benefits. One study has reported that jejunoileal bypass surgery for obesity is associated with an incidence of subsequent tuberculosis 60 times greater than that of the general population (4000 per 100,000). Interestingly, active tuberculosis was most frequently observed when weight had stabilized after the period of rapid loss and was more frequently extrapulmonary than pulmonary.[116] The author recommended chemoprophylaxis in that situation. Chemoprophylaxis is recommended in tuberculin-positive AIDS patients, some advise indefinitely, as approximately 10 percent of AIDS patients in New York City develop active tuberculosis.[49,50] It should be emphasized that with the possible exception of the gastrectomy patient with inactive pulmonary tuberculosis, firm data supporting the usefulness of chemoprophylaxis in all of these situations are lacking.

The Nursing Home Problem

A major analysis by Stead has reported that the risk of men who are tuberculin positive on admission to Arkansas nursing homes subsequently developing tuberculosis was 3.2 percent and the risk in women only slightly less (2.3 percent), and that this could be decreased to 0.3 percent or less with chemoprophylaxis.[74] However, the incidence of toxicity was such (3–4 percent demonstrating hepatic toxicity and an equal percentage demonstrating nonhepatic drug intolerance) that he did not recommend chemoprophylaxis in this group.[117] Others do recommend chemoprophylaxis in tuberculin-positive nursing home patients, however.[118] In Stead's study, the case for chemoprophylaxis in patients who converted to tuberculin positivity after admission, as opposed to those who were reactors on admission, was clear-cut, with an incidence of 11.6 percent active disease in men and 7.6 percent in women and a reduction to 0.2 percent with chemoprophylaxis.[117]

Chemoprophylaxis in Drug-Resistant Infections

Chemoprophylaxis in situations in which the likelihood of drug resistance is high (exposure to hostel populations, Southeast Asians, etc.) has not been systematically worked out. Use of RMP has been advised but has failed in at least one recorded instance, with the development of RMP resistance in the recipient.[103] In this circumstance there is much to recommend treating as if an active drug-resistant infection were present, using a 6-month regimen (HRSZ or HREZ for 2 months and HR for 4 months). This would provide adequate therapy for any infection except one due to RMP-resistant organisms. The rationale underlying this recommendation is that effective chemoprophylaxis is actually treatment of a subclinical but active infection, as discussed above.

Vaccination

Although the data are conflicting, most evidence indicates that Calmette-Guerin bacillus (BCG) vaccination will result in a 60–80 percent decrease in the incidence of tuberculosis in a given population.[119] It is reasonable as a public health measure in situations of quite high prevalence, greater than that existing in the United States and most Western nations at this time. However, its preventive efficacy is almost certainly at least equal to that of chemoprophylaxis. It is applicable only to tuberculin-negative people. Vaccination does not prevent infection but rapidly limits its proliferation, usually to such a degree that clinical disease does not develop.[120] The effectiveness of vaccination in prevention of serious disseminated disease in young children is striking.[111] In the opinion of some authorities, vaccination still makes good sense in the case of certain groups, such as the military and foreign services, that require residence in areas with a serious tuberculosis problem.[111]

EXTRAPULMONARY TUBERCULOSIS

Introduction

It is traditional to divide extrapulmonary tuberculosis into two general groups, each characterized by a different pathogenesis. The first group comprises mucosal infections due to spread of highly infectious respiratory secretions via the respiratory and gastrointestinal tracts (*intracanalicular spread*). Before effective chemotherapy, these infections were frequent complications of uncontrolled cavitary pulmonary disease. However, such lesions are very responsive to chemotherapy and accordingly have become quite rare. The second group comprises those established by *lymphohematogenous spread*, usually at the time of the primary infection and less commonly from established chronic foci. These make up the great majority of cases at present. A third pathogenic mechanism is contiguous spread from a pulmonary or extrapulmonary focus.

The number of cases of pulmonary tuberculosis has continued to decrease yearly in the United States, but the number of extrapulmonary cases has continued at approximately 4000 yearly for a number of years.[121] Accordingly they make up an increasing proportion of the total new case load, at present approximately 15 percent. Extrapulmonary disease is somewhat more common in nonwhites and in women. Figure 5 shows the incidence of various forms of extrapulmonary tuberculosis in the United States in 1979.

General Comments on Treatment of Extrapulmonary Tuberculosis

Although there are essentially no large studies of this problem, experience with cases with coexistent pulmonary and extrapulmonary disease indicates that from an antimicrobial point of view, cavitary pulmonary disease is by far the severest test of chemotherapy and that extrapulmonary manifestations disappear long before the pulmonary disease is arrested. Maximal chemotherapy is indicated in those forms of extrapulmonary disease in which, for anatomic reasons, ongoing inflammation carries an immediate and severe risk, such as in central nervous system disease, spinal tuberculosis, and possibly tuberculous pericarditis. Most other forms of extrapulmonary disease respond rapidly to fairly minimal regimens, especially in situations in which drug-sensitive infections are likely to be present.

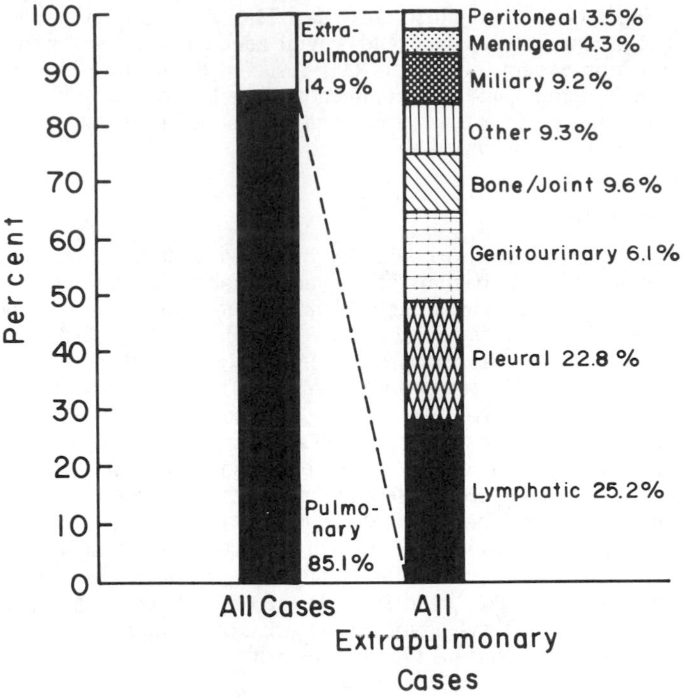

FIG. 5. Percentage distribution of tuberculosis cases by form and site of disease, United States, 1979. (From Centers for Disease Control,[211] with permission.)

In these patients INH-RMP for 9 months or INH-EMB for 18–24 months is appropriate.

Miliary Tuberculosis

The term *miliary tuberculosis* was first used because of the resemblance of the pathologic lesions in acute progressive hematogenous tuberculosis to millet seeds. It has come to be used for all forms of extensive hematogenous disease.[122]

Hematogenous dissemination of tuberculous infection occurs in several different settings. Before development of tuberculin hypersensitivity, blood stream spread probably always occurs to some degree, seeding foci that may later progress to chronic organ tuberculosis. In the vast majority this early lymphohematogenous dissemination stops when tuberculin hypersensitivity develops. In a few, however, it progresses directly to the clinical syndrome of acute miliary tuberculosis. Historically, this was typically a disease of very young children, but at present, when primary infection can occur at any age, this sequence is observed just as frequently in adults.[123–125] Milder, usually nonprogressive lymphohematogenous dissemination also occurs with regularity from chronic foci of organ tuberculosis, as indicated by the frequency with which hepatic granulomata and choroidal tubercles can be found in active pulmonary tuberculosis clinically confined to the lungs. However, seeding from such foci can become recurrent, more and more protracted, and, especially when immune mechanisms are compromised by age or intercurrent illness, eventually progressive, leading to the syndrome of chronic hematogenous tuberculosis (late generalized tuberculosis).[122,126]

Usual Miliary Tuberculosis. The ordinarily transient and mild hematogenous phase of the primary infection may uncommonly be much more extensive and evolve into progressive miliary tuberculosis in the young child. Together with the frequently associated meningitis, this accounts for most tuberculosis deaths in this age group. In children the illness is acute and severe, with high intermittent fevers, night sweats, and occasional rigors. Other manifestations such as pleural effusion, peritonitis, and meningitis occur in as many as two-thirds of the patients. A similar acute illness may occur in adults, although it is usually somewhat more chronic and initially less severe. Table 5 presents selected clinical findings in two recent large series of cases of miliary tuberculosis in adults.[123,124] Both demonstrate the increased frequency in blacks and the importance of underlying conditions such as alcoholism, cirrhosis, neoplasm, and pregnancy. However, the majority of patients have no predisposing conditions. A history of prior tuberculosis is the exception. The usual symptoms of fever, malaise, weight loss, and weakness have little diagnostic specificity. However, headache, when present, will often indicate meningitis, which in the prechemotherapy era supervened in over 50 percent of cases, usually after several weeks of symptoms attributable to miliary disease. Abdominal pain is often due to peritonitis and pleural pain to pleuritis. Physical findings are likewise usually nonspecific, but a careful search should be made for cutaneous rashes, sinus tracts, scrotal masses, and lymphadenopathy, the biopsy specimen of which may be diagnostic. The discovery of a miliary infiltrate on chest roentgenogram is the usual reason that miliary tuberculosis is suspected. It is therefore important to emphasize that people, particularly the elderly, may succumb to miliary tuberculosis before the chest roentgenogram becomes abnormal.[127] Further, as many as one-fourth of patients with proved disease will be tuberculin negative. The white blood cell count is usually normal, and anemia to some degree is the rule. Hyponatremia may be seen in a substantial minority; it is usually associated with meningitis and the laboratory features of inappropriate secretion of antidiuretic hormone.[124] Although some degree of anatomic adrenal involvement is common, frank Addison's disease is rare in the setting of miliary tuberculosis.[128] Elevation of alkaline phosphatase may indicate hepatic involvement. Cultures of sputum and gastric contents will be positive in over one-half of the cases but are usually smear negative and therefore of limited immediate diagnostic help. The urine should also be cultured and will be positive in as many as one-fourth of the cases, and cerebrospinal fluid (CSF) culture should be obtained, as it may be positive when the CSF is otherwise normal and meningeal signs are lacking. Immediate diagnosis is most often made by examination of tissue (lymph nodes or scrotal masses when present, liver biopsy specimens, or bone marrow biopsy specimens). However, transbronchial biopsy is the most direct and productive procedure to obtain tissue and should be performed promptly when the diagnosis is

TABLE 5. Miliary Tuberculosis

	Munt (113)	*Biehl (112)*
Number of cases	69	68
Duration of symptoms	15.7 weeks	2–16 weeks
Longest	30 months	
History of prior TB	6%	4%
Splenomegaly	13%	0.5%
Choroidal tubercles	12%	
Meningitis	19%	17%
Positive tuberculin test	84%	61%
Miliary chest x-ray	97%	93%
Normal white blood count	63%	93%
Significant anemia	29%	
Other foci of TB	23%	32%
Chronic pulmonary	10%	10%
Extrapulmonary	13%	22%
Positive sputum		50%[a]
Positive smear	31%	
Positive culture	63%	
Liver granulomas	66%	
Caseating	33%	
Noncaseating	33%	100%
Marrow granulomas	33%	16%[a]
Caseating with AFB	20%	
Noncaseating	13%	
Mortality	21%	21%

[a] Details of the type of involvement not provided.

suspected. Histology will usually be positive (27 of 34 cases in one recent series[129]), and cultures may be positive when the histology is negative or nonspecifically abnormal. Bronchoalveolar lavage has not yet been systematically evaluated in miliary tuberculosis, but it appears that it will be highly effective. The importance of vigorous diagnostic measures cannot be overemphasized, but treatment should be initiated immediately if a reasonably strong clinical suspicion of miliary tuberculosis exists, as the still appreciable mortality is most often due to delay in diagnosis and treatment. The drug regimen should contain both INH and RMP, but in the pre-RMP era results were excellent with INH-containing regimens.[130] Response may be quite prompt or may require several weeks. Fulminant miliary tuberculosis may be associated with severe refractory hypoxemia (the adult respiratory distress syndrome) and disseminated intravascular coagulation.[131] In such cases adjunctive therapy with corticosteroids (60–80 mg prednisone daily) is indicated. Many advise the use of corticosteroids in debilitated patients with a poor initial response to therapy.

Chronic Hematogenous Tuberculosis. Chronic hematogenous tuberculosis is caused by blood stream spread occurring long after the primary infection.[126] The foci responsible are most often extrapulmonary and most often clinically silent, such as abdominal nodes or small renal or osseous lesions.[122] Such disseminations may lead to acute progressive illness such as that observed in early postprimary miliary disease, but, particularly in older people, it may be low grade and protracted or even episodic, with several waves of illness and interval remission. A cryptic form of hematogenous tuberculosis, often with a histopathologic picture characterized as nonreactive (see below), almost always involves older people, most frequently with underlying illness such as malignancy, uremia, diabetes, alcoholism, or collagen-vascular disease to which the symptoms may be mistakenly attributed. It is usual for the chest roentgenogram to be normal and the tuberculin test negative in chronic hematogenous tuberculosis. The clinical picture frequently consists of fever of unknown origin, but fever itself may be lacking in as many as 20 percent of the cases and the clinical picture may be simple failure to thrive.[132] Diagnosis was made during life in only 15 percent of the largest recent (autopsy) series of such patients but can be made when biopsy specimens are taken of multiple tissues.[125] In that series 90 percent had hepatic involvement.

Nonreactive Tuberculosis and Hematologic Abnormalities. Patients with hematogenous tuberculosis, especially the more chronic sort, may present with a variety of hematologic conditions suggesting primary hematologic disease including pancytopenia, refractory anemia, leukopenia, thrombocytopenia, leukemoid reactions, myelosclerosis, and polycythemia.[47,133] Leukemoid reactions can be sufficiently severe to suggest acute leukemia, although the majority of patients in whom hematogenous tuberculosis coexists with the clinical picture of leukemia will in fact have both diseases. Although these secondary blood dyscrasias can complicate any form of miliary tuberculosis, most occur in cases with the histopathologic picture of nonreactive tuberculosis, which involves areas of necrosis surrounded by normal tissue with little or no specific cellular reaction and very large numbers of bacilli.[31] The clinical picture may be one of acute overwhelming infection, described in the European literature as *Typhobacillosis of Landouzy*,[134] or fever of unknown origin with or without an obscure hematologic illness. Interestingly, meningitis does not complicate cases with this particular tissue reaction, and splenomegaly is the rule.[31,47,133]

Primary Hepatic Tuberculosis. Rarely, miliary tuberculosis may mimic cholangitis with fever and liver function test abnormalities suggestive of intrahepatic or extrahepatic obstructive disease and little evidence of hepatocellular disease. Diagnosis is made by liver biopsy specimens, although in the past patients have been operated on with the presumptive diagnosis of cholelithiasis.[135]

Central Nervous System Tuberculosis

Tuberculous Meningitis. Tuberculous meningitis is usually due to rupture of a subependymal tubercle into the subarachnoid space rather than direct hematogenous seeding of the meninges themselves,[136,137] accounting for the observation that when meningitis complicates miliary disease, it generally develops after several weeks of illness. Meningitis in childhood is usually an early postprimary event; three-fourths of patients have associated pulmonary disease, either miliary tuberculosis, a recent primary pneumonia, or pleural effusion.[138,139] Three-fourths of adults also have evidence of extrameningeal organ tuberculosis, but in a substantial number this is extrapulmonary rather than pulmonary.[137] Whether the critical subependymal tubercle can evolve from foci seeded in an otherwise nonprogressive preallergic hematogenous phase[136] or it is always due to hematogenous spread from an area of extrameningeal chronic organ tuberculosis, although often one that is entirely latent clinically,[137] is a matter of disagreement.

PATHOLOGY. The meningeal involvement is most marked at the base of the brain. In a long-standing case the exudate may become quite thick, gelatinous, and masslike, extending from the pons to the optic nerves, most prominent adjacent to the optic chiasm.[140] The more chronic the process, the more it comes to resemble a fibrous mass, often encroaching on or surrounding the adjacent cranial nerves. Involvement of arteries may lead to localized ischemia or infarction. The middle cerebral artery is most frequently involved, leading to hemiparesis or hemiplegia. Infarction of smaller arteries may cause a variety of symptoms resembling encephalitis. The basilar cisterns and the ventricular foramina may be obstructed by inflammatory exudate or by encroachment of an enlarging tuberculoma, causing hydrocephalus. Less frequently, these same pathologic changes can involve the spinal cord with delayed or absent cerebral symptoms.[141,142]

CLINICAL FINDINGS. The clinical spectrum is very broad, ranging from subtle headache or change in mentation over many weeks to a sudden and severe meningitis. Evidence of concomitant active or inactive extrameningeal tuberculosis will be present in roughly three-fourths of the cases,[138,143,144] miliary shadowing on the chest roentgenogram being the most helpful diagnostic finding. It is important to emphasize, however, that in 25 percent or more of cases there will be no clinical or historical evidence of either active or quiescent tuberculosis; in these cases the source of the hematogenous spread leading to the meningitis is most often a clinically latent focus in a hidden lymph node, a skeletal lesion, or a genitourinary lesion.[137] Tuberculous meningitis can be strongly suspected when meningeal signs are associated with active extrameningeal tuberculosis, but the cornerstone of diagnosis is examination of the CSF. In one recent series,[144] 65 percent of the cases demonstrated between 100 and 500 cells/mm^3, 14 percent contained between 0 and 99, and the remainder between 500 and 1500; the protein was 100–500 mg/100 ml in 65 percent of the cases but under 100 mg/100 ml in 25 percent, and the CSF sugar content, said to be characteristically low, was less than 45 mg/100 ml in only 17 percent of the cases. Lymphocytes were the preponderant cells in 73 percent of the cases, the remainder demonstrating a majority of polymorphonuclear leukocytes, usually early on in the course. Acid-fast bacilli (AFB) were visible on the stained CSF sediment in 37 percent of the cases on initial examination, a figure somewhat higher than in many series. But, importantly, when the fluid from four serial spinal taps was examined, the organisms were seen in 87 percent of the cases. The importance of repeated spinal taps cannot be overemphasized. Initial atypical findings such as a preponderance of polymorphonuclear leukocytes, normal sugar content, or even an entirely negative CSF will almost always evolve to the more typical mononuclear pleocytosis with hypoglycorrhachia over time.

Various neuroradiologic diagnostic modalities such as brain scan, angiography, and air-contrast ventriculography have now been entirely replaced by computer tomography (CT scan) and magnetic resonance imaging.[145] One or more rounded lesions presumed to be tuberculomas in some stage of evolution may be seen in cases that are clinically just meningitis[146] (Fig. 6). CT scanning can also define the presence and extent of basilar arachnoid meningitis, the presence of cerebral infarction, and the presence and course of hydrocephalus—the three pathologic features that are most critical in determining the course of meningitis. One study from a group with extensive experience in treating tuberculous meningitis used CT scan findings for determining the prognosis (patients with an entirely normal scan recovered completely) and for making decisions concerning the use of corticosteroid therapy and surgical shunting procedures for hydrocephalus.[147] Those with a severe degree of basilar exudate did not do well even with shunt surgery.

Fever is usually low grade but may be lacking entirely, the peripheral white blood cell count is normal in most cases, and low-grade anemia is usual. Hyponatremia with the laboratory characteristics of excess antidiuretic hormone has been demonstrated in a substantial minority of patients in one series.[124] Prognosis is influenced by age, the duration of symptoms, and the degree of neurologic deficit. Mortality is greatest under age of 5 and over age 50 (20 and 60 percent, respectively, in the series quoted above), and 80 percent of those who had been ill for more than 2 months died.[144] Clinical staging is based on neurologic status: stage 1—rational with no focal neurologic signs or hydrocephalus; stage 2—confusion or the presence of focal signs such as cranial nerve palsies or hemiparesis; stage 3—stuporous or dense paraplegia or hemiplegia. All 9 patients who were stage 1 at the start of treatment in the above-cited series recovered, 8 without residual neurologic damage. Five out of 11 patients who were stage 3 at the start of treatment died, one recovered with severe neurologic residual damage, and 5 recovered completely.[144] A wide variety of neurologic symptoms such as hemiballismus, decerebrate rigidity, cerebellar symptoms, and hypothalamic–pituitary syndromes may uncommonly be seen.[141] Residual neurologic defects after recovery, observed in about one-fourth of patients, include chronic brain syndrome, hemiparesis, paraplegia, optic atrophy with blindness, oculomotor palsy, deafness, convulsive disorders, and various symptoms of hypothalamic or pituitary dysfunction.[138,148]

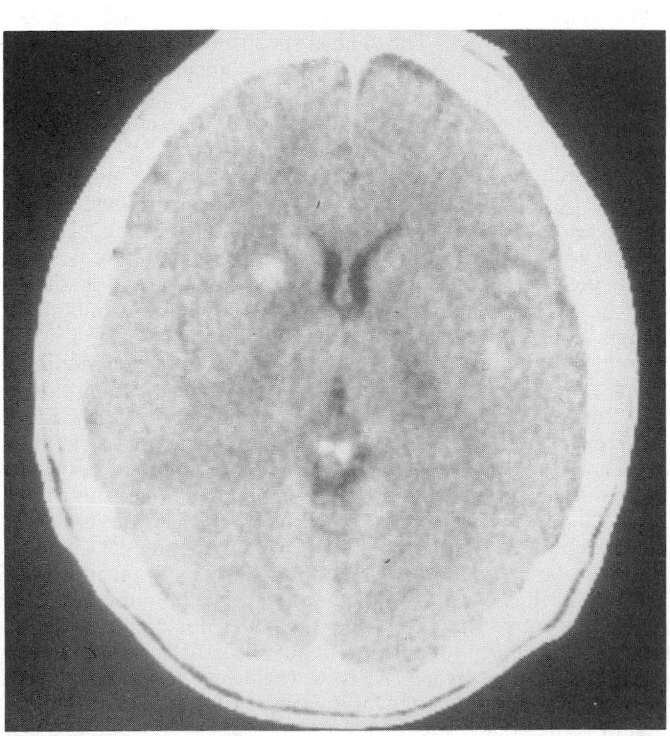

FIG. 6. CT scan showing contrast-enhanced lesions in the cerebral cortex of a patient with tuberculous meningitis. The focal lesions were clinically silent.

TREATMENT. With meningeal inflammation the concentration of INH in the CSF equals that in the blood. Its introduction radically changed the prognosis of tuberculous meningitis.[143] Doses of 10 mg/kg, somewhat higher in children, are advisable until a favorable course has been established, at which point the usual doses suffice. RMP also penetrates the blood-brain barrier fairly well, reaching a concentration on the average half that in blood but well above the minimal inhibitory concentration for *M. tuberculosis* and should also be used (conventional doses).[149] PZA is also recommended in all cases, as it reaches concentrations in the CSF equal to those in serum and significantly adds to the early bactericidal activity of INH plus RMP. ETH and EMB both provide good central nervous system concentrations but are weak drugs, useful only when serious drug resistance is suspected. All of the aminoglycosides penetrate the blood-brain barrier poorly.

Most authorities advise the adjunctive use of corticosteroids in stage 2 and 3 patients in dosages beginning at 60–80 mg prednisone daily. This can often be gradually reduced after 1 or 2 weeks, using the patient's symptoms as a guide to how rapidly to taper. With a favorable response, steroids can be usually discontinued entirely in 4–6 weeks.[150]

TUBERCULOMAS. In the absence of meningitis, tuberculomas act as space-occupying lesions and may present with seizures. CT scanning has revealed that they are more frequently multiple than single, appearing as avascular mass lesions surrounded by edema.[141] Steroid treatment will often reduce edema and decrease symptoms. When the diagnosis is secure, the effects of antimicrobial therapy should be assessed before resorting to surgery, as good resolution is often observed and residual neurologic defects are often less with medical therapy than with surgical excision. When the diagnosis has been made at craniotomy, chemotherapy will prevent the spread of infection. In areas of the world such as India in which tuberculomas are frequent, biopsy performed at craniotomy and assessment of medical therapy without further resection is the approach of choice.[151,152]

TUBERCULOUS SPINAL MENINGITIS. Infrequently, tuberculosis can cause spinal cord disease with little or no intracranial involvement. Advanced spinal meningitis may produce complete encasement of the cord in a gelatinous exudate.[140] An intramedullary tuberculoma or an extradural granulomatous mass can cause symptoms of a cord mass lesion with no meningeal involvement. Also, nerve root compression with pain, lower motor neuron paralysis, upper motor neuron paralysis, bladder or rectal sphincter symptoms, hypesthesia or anesthesia in the distribution of a nerve root, or paresthesias may be seen as a result of spinal involvement. All of these lesions (epidural, meningeal, and intramedullary) can cause subarachnoid block with extremely high CSF protein concentrations, with or without cells.[142,153]

Serofibrinous Pleurisy with Effusion

In the first half of this century, when infection with tuberculosis in childhood or early adulthood was the rule, and probably now in areas of the world where tuberculous infection remains epidemic, serofibrinous pleurisy with effusion, defined as unexplained pleural effusion with a mononuclear pleocytosis and usually some systemic symptoms, was regarded as almost always an early postprimary event due to a large subpleural metastatic focus spread from an ongoing primary infection before the onset of tissue hypersensitivity. With the onset of hypersensitivity (tuberculin reactivity), necrosis of the subpleural focus could cause rupture and delivery of large quantities of infectious antigenic material into the pleural cavity, with consequent exudation of fluid and cells from pleural surfaces.[154] Observations made during thoracotomy demonstrated such major necrotic foci on the visceral pleura together with multiple small tubercles densely distributed over the entire visceral and parietal pleural surfaces.[155] In years past, it was believed that this sequence was rare in established chronic pulmonary tuberculosis, since visceral-parietal pleural symphysis often occurs over chronic lesions, tending to prevent free rupture into the pleural space. However, it is now clear that serofibrinous pleurisy with effusion may in fact be seen in older individuals with chronic pulmonary tuberculosis, as well as in younger people as an early postprimary manifestation. In one recent series, 40 percent of the patients were over 35 years old, 10 percent were over 70, and many had clinically apparent active chronic pulmonary tuberculosis.[156] A minority of cases, perhaps 10 percent, will occur in the setting of progressive hematogenous tuberculosis. These may be associated with other foci of progression in extrapulmonary sites and often with other serous membrane involvement. Cases with coexistent pleural (at times bilateral), peritoneal, and pericardial tuberculosis have been referred to as *tuberculous polyserositis*.

Tuberculous pleurisy itself is usually not progressive, and resolution over several months, with or without treatment, is the rule. However, in the prechemotherapy era, 65 percent of patients with serofibrinous pleurisy with effusion went on to develop progressive chronic organ tuberculosis in the lungs or elsewhere within 5 years, a prognosis strikingly worse than that of primary infections uncomplicated by pleural effusion.[154] Treatment is indicated to interrupt the infection before these more serious manifestations develop.

Clinical Features and Diagnosis. Although at times the clinical picture is low grade and subtle, it is more often abrupt and very symptomatic, easy to confuse with acute bacterial pneumonia.[157] Cough, chest pain, and fever greater than 100°F occur in 85 percent or more of patients, and the fever may be quite high. On the chest roentgenogram, the effusion is usually less than massive and almost always unilateral. Evidence of visible coexistent pulmonary tuberculosis is infrequent, ranging from 5 to 30 percent in different series.

The pleural fluid almost always contains between 500 and 2500 white blood cells, mostly between 1000 and 2000, which in two-thirds of cases will be over 90 percent lymphocytes. In a minority (12 percent in one series) the initial thoracentesis will reveal over 50 percent polymorphonuclear leukocytes, but repeated taps usually show a shift to lymphocytic preponderance. Mesothelial cells, characteristic of neoplastic effusions, are sparse or absent. Serosanguinous effusions are uncommon but do occur in less than 10 percent of cases. The pleural fluid pH is almost always 7.3 or less and may be as low as 7.0. The AFB stain of the fluid sediment is seldom positive, and culture will be positive in 25–33 percent of cases. Pleural needle biopsy will yield granulomatous pleuritis in 75 percent of cases; culture of the biopsy specimen is worthwhile and may be positive even in the 25 percent of cases with nonspecific pleuritis on histologic examination. A small open pleural biopsy will be diagnostic in virtually 100 percent of cases. Cultures of sputum or gastric contents will be positive in 25–33 percent, even in the absence of visible parenchymal involvement. The tuberculin test is positive in the majority of cases (over 90 percent in most series), but a negative reaction cannot be taken as definitive evidence against a tuberculous cause of an effusion. Diagnosis may be not considered at all in older persons with diseases that could explain the effusions, such as cirrhosis or congestive heart failure, until a positive culture is reported weeks later.[158]

Treatment. As mentioned, most often the pleural effusion will resolve in 2–4 months without chemotherapy. Chemotherapy, which does not seem to speed resolution much, is actually directed at prevention of later active disease elsewhere in the body, which, as mentioned, will otherwise evolve in two-thirds of the cases. In that sense it is analogous to treatment of a new tuberculin converter. The use of INH and EMB for 18 months is acceptable therapy, as is INH and RMP for 9 months. Multiple thoracenteses are not necessary once the diagnosis is established and treatment is initiated. A small minority will heal with appreciable pleural fibrosis. Corticosteroid therapy hastens local resolution, but no long-term advantage has been demonstrated.

Tuberculous Empyema and Bronchopleural Fistula

Tuberculous empyema results from a rupture of a major cavitary focus into the pleural space. It is a catastrophic illness usually associated with bronchopleural fistula, and in the era before drug therapy was almost always fatal. The fluid is frankly purulent, as in bacterial empyemas. It is virtually never observed in patients treated with chemotherapy.

Late Complications of Collapse Therapy

Chronic, often calcified pleural shadows that may increase in size and cause pain, bronchopleural fistulas, esophagopleural fistulas, and empyemas, both tuberculous and nontuberculous, can occur many years after remote (prechemotherapeutic) collapse therapy such as extraperiosteal plombage, therapeutic pneumothorax, or thoracoplasty. A CT scan may reveal collections of fluid under a thickened, calcified pleura. The results of prolonged antibiotic therapy, both antituberculous and routine, should be assessed before undertaking surgery. A conservative approach was successful in almost half of the patients in one series, including one with esophagopleural fistula. This is important since surgery is fraught with difficulty in these ancient inflammatory reactions.[159]

Tuberculous Pericarditis

Tuberculous pericarditis is most often due to rupture of an adjacent caseous node into the pericardial sac. Uncommonly, this may occur during chemotherapy,[160] as lymph nodes have a rather unpredictable response to chemotherapy, some involuting promptly and others seeming to progress temporarily under chemotherapy until they rupture or are surgically drained. Less frequently, pericarditis develops as a part of a progressive hematogenous dissemination, often with involvement of other serous sacs.

CLINICAL FEATURES AND DIAGNOSIS. The onset may be subtle, dominated by the cardiovascular consequences of effusion with little to suggest infection, or may be abrupt, with fever and pericardial pain, as observed in 25 percent of the cases in one series.[161] It is probable that all cases have effusion early on, but this may go unrecognized until the clinical picture of chronic constrictive pericarditis supervenes. The anatomic diagnosis of pericarditis with effusion is usually quickly made on the basis of physical findings and laboratory examinations, but etiologic diagnosis is usually difficult. The tuberculin test is usually but not always positive,[161,162] and evidence of extrapericardial tuberculosis is usually lacking. Fever is usual but not invariable, and routine laboratory studies are not helpful. One large series recorded a number of cases of tuberculous pericarditis initially misdiagnosed as idiopathic, uremic, or rheumatoid. Fluid obtained by pericardiocentesis will be similar to the fluid of tuberculous pleurisy, but a positive AFB smear is very uncommon and culture will be positive in only 25–50 percent of cases. In our opinion, diagnostic pericardiocentesis usually should not be done. The risk is substantial and the actual benefit, at least with respect to issues of immediate treatment, is usually limited to excluding pyogenic pericarditis, which often can be done on clinical grounds alone. (Pericardiocentesis to relieve hemodynamic compromise should ideally be performed in a cardiac catheterization laboratory with hemodynamic measurements.) In the absence of associated extrapericardial tuberculosis, diagnosis will often require pericardial tissue. The authors use a subxiphoid approach, which is a small operation, requiring only local anesthesia. This yields a generous specimen. Pericardial fluid is drained at the same time.

TREATMENT. Antibiotic treatment is the same for pericarditis as for pulmonary tuberculosis. However, there are two issues of treatment about which there is no consensus, the role of surgical therapy and the use of adjunctive corticosteroids. Pericardiectomy is obviously indicated for constriction or when effusion causes serious cardiovascular symptoms. How often constriction supervenes is really not known,[163] although some surgeons maintain that this happens in as many as 50 percent of cases treated medically and advocate formal anterior pericardiectomy in the stage of effusion, which is technically easier than after constriction has developed.[164]

Steroid therapy has been advocated to prevent constriction,[162] beginning with 60–80 mg prednisone daily and gradually decreasing the dosage over a period of several weeks as effusion subsides. This is probably effective but should be considered only when the etiologic diagnosis is secure. Obviously it is not necessary when pericardiectomy has been carried out. Whether or not pericardial biopsy by the subxiphoid approach with drainage of fluid will prevent subsequent constriction and therefore obviate the need for further surgery or steroid therapy is not known, but in our limited experience this appears to be the case.

Skeletal Tuberculosis

Pott's Disease (Tuberculous Spondylitis). Half of the cases of skeletal tuberculosis occur in the spine. Infection usually reaches the vertebral bodies via the blood stream, but it may be spread directly from the adjacent lung or by lymphatic spread from parietal pleural disease. The process begins in the anterior part of a vertebral body. The disk space between two involved vertebrae is usually destroyed, producing the characteristic roentgenographic finding of anterior wedging of two adjacent vertebrae with loss of the intervening disk space. (Neoplasm usually spares the intervertebral disk.) The resulting deformity may produce a characteristic posterior prominence or gibbus of the spine. The thoracic spine is involved most frequently, the lumbar spine next, and the cervical and sacral spines least often. Cases of unilateral sacroiliitis due to tuberculosis have been reported.

ABSCESS AND SINUS FORMATION. Pus from a vertebral focus characteristically ruptures anteriorly, enveloping the spine and producing a paraspinal abscess. Since it is confined by tight ligamentous investments, it can develop high pressure, dissect along tissue planes for long distances, and present as a mass in the supraclavicular space, above the posterior iliac crest in Petit's triangle, the groin, the buttock, or even the popliteal fossa.[165] Cases of Pott's abscess perforating into the bowel have been reported, resulting in a gas-filled psoas abscess seen on x-ray film[166]; rupture into the adjacent lung has also been observed.[167] The abscess can also spread infection to other vertebral bodies, sometimes with intervening normal spine.

POTT'S PARAPLEGIA. Paralysis of the lower extremities can develop in several ways. Pressure in a paraspinal abscess can produce ischemic changes in the subjacent cord. In such cases neurologic symptoms are promptly relieved by drainage of the abscess. Caseous or granulating tissue may extrude from the posterior aspect of the vertebral body and impinge on the anterior aspect of the cord. Inflammatory thrombosis of the anterior spinal artery can occur, and rarely, sudden cord transection may result from serious loss of structural integrity.[168]

TREATMENT. Before the availability of chemotherapy, treatment consisted of immobilization, body casting, and often an eventual attempt to stabilize the spine by posterior fusion. Operation in the field of the infection (anterior to the transverse processes) was not possible, as spread of infection would inevitably occur. When it became clear that antibiotic coverage permitted direct operation on diseased tissue, several new orthopedic procedures came into practice, including débridement of the abscess and diseased bone through a posterolateral approach involving resection of one or more transverse processes and the posterior aspects of the ribs (costotransversectomy), actual resection of part of the vertebral body so as to expose the cord and remove material impinging on its anterior aspect (lateral rachotomy), and radical débridement and anterior fusion through an anterior approach. However, a large and carefully studied series of cases by English authors in Africa, in situations in which orthopedic options were limited, have made it clear that in cases without neurologic involvement a strongly favorable response (90 percent) will result from adequate chemotherapy with early ambulation and that casting and surgery add little in the nonadvanced case.[165] Even with paraplegia, 40 percent of patients did well with this conservative approach. These studies give strong support to conservative medical therapy for Pott's disease without neurologic complications, using bed rest only for relief of pain. Large paraspinal abscesses will disappear more rapidly with drainage or débridement, but their presence is not per se an indication for surgical intervention. They should be drained when complicated by paraparesis or paraplegia, although, as mentioned, neurologic improvement can be expected in a substantial minority of cases with drugs alone, and a conservative approach is reasonable as long as the defect is minimal and the initial course favorable. Most feel that prolonged treatment (2 years) with an INH-containing regimen is indicated, and many advise including RMP for 9 months. When drug resistance seems likely, initial treatment with multiple-drug regimens (HRSZ or HREZ) would be advisable. Advanced neurologic defects and severe anatomic instability of the spine require more radical orthopedic approaches.

Peripheral Skeletal Tuberculosis. Tuberculosis of peripheral bones and joints typically is a combination of osteomyelitis and arthritis, monoarticular in 90 percent of cases,[169,170] frequently occurs with no associated evidence of extraskeletal tuberculosis, and often is a consequence of a remote infection. The weight-bearing joints (hip, knee) are involved most often, followed by the ankle, elbow, wrist, and shoulder; but unusual locations (greater trochanter, sternoclavicular joint, ribs, small bones of hands and feet) are also affected. A history of trauma is not uncommon, followed in weeks or months by indolent progressive inflammation. Rarely, multiple lytic lesions in long and flat bones develop, a syndrome called *osteitis cystica tuberculosa multiplex*.

The cause of peripheral skeletal tuberculosis is thought to be a remote and usually long-latent lymphohematogenous focus, often in the epiphyseal region of long bones, which may progress and rupture into the joint space, causing effusion and progressive development of destructive granulation tissue. Small accumulations of fibrin in a joint exudate, termed *rice bodies*, thought to be typical of chronic tuberculous arthritis, are also seen in other granulomatous arthritides.

The earliest clinical manifestation is pain, which may precede both signs of inflammation and x-ray film changes by weeks or even months. X-ray films initially may show only soft tissue swelling, but later they usually reveal some combination of subchondral osteoporosis, para-articular bony destruction, thickening of the overlying periosteum, and eventual cartilage and bone destruction from the proliferating granulation tissue. Cold abscesses and draining sinuses often develop in chronic cases.

In the absence of coexistent active tuberculosis, diagnosis almost always requires a biopsy, which should be done as soon as the suspicion of a tuberculous focus is raised. Histologic findings compatible with tuberculosis constitute sufficient reason to initiate chemotherapy, although a variety of other chronic infections (fungi and nontuberculous mycobacteria) can cause identical clinical and histologic pictures. In early cases treatment with prolonged chemotherapy will result in complete resolution. Casting or other sorts of immobilization are not indicated except for pain control; surgical intervention is necessary only when serious joint instability requires joint fusion, and then only after the results of chemotherapy have been evaluated.

TUBERCULOSIS OF THE CHEST WALL. Rarely but distinctively, tuberculosis may present as single or multiple cold abscesses of the chest wall. Some of these are associated with one or more areas of osteolytic rib tuberculosis. Others are thought to be due to dissection of pus from underlying caseous intercostal nodes.[171,172]

Genitourinary Tuberculosis

Renal Tuberculosis. The majority of cases of pulmonary tuberculosis with no clinical evidence of renal involvement reveal bilateral nonprogressive microscopic renal cortical foci on careful sectioning at postmortem examination.[173] Foci in the cortex have little tendency to progress unless the infection reaches the medulla, where the hypertonic environment is inimical to host defense mechanisms.

Slightly over half of the cases of renal tuberculosis are associated with evidence of extrarenal disease, usually inactive pulmonary lesions, but in less than 10 percent there is associated active extragenitourinary disease. In the remainder, the latent period between prior episodes of tuberculosis and development of renal disease may be several or even many years. Accordingly, it is typically a disease of adults, often middle-aged or older, who are usually not very sick.[174,175]

Even though symptoms are low grade or lacking, the diagnosis can be easily made when considered. Urinary symptoms (dysuria, gross hematuria, and, in late cases, flank pain) were present in 71 percent of patients in one series,[174] but constitutional symptoms were uncommon, and 20 percent of patients were entirely asymptomatic. Continuing tuberculous bacilluria may cause cystitis with urinary frequency and, in late cases, a contracted bladder. Urinary findings are abnormal in 90 percent of cases, consisting of gross or microscopic hematuria or pyuria (albuminuria is uncommon). "Sterile pyuria" is said to be typical of renal tuberculosis, but actually many cases with or without cystitis will also have concomitant infection with ordinary urinary pathogens.[175] The intravenous pyelogram will also be abnormal in 93 percent of cases.[174] Early pyelographic abnormalities are those of any pyelonephritis, consisting of caliceal blunting, at times with reflux of contrast material into the interstitium (caliceal–interstitial reflux). Later changes (papillary cavities similar to those of papillary necrosis, ureteral strictures, "pipe stem" changes, "corkscrewing," "beading," focal calcification, hydronephrosis, gross parenchymal cavitation, and autonephrectomy) have more diagnostic specificity, particularly calcification. Changes may be bilateral and probably always are at the microscopic level, but usually the clinical disease is unilateral. Most patients are tuberculin positive, and culture of three morning urine specimens will reveal the organism in 90 percent of patients. Hypertension is not a feature of renal tuberculosis, and loss of renal function is not observed except in extensive bilateral disease.

Chemotherapy is usually all that is needed for treatment. There is some disagreement as to its duration, British authors favoring shorter (9 month) courses[173] and American authors favoring prolonged (2 years) therapy. All agree on the need for multiple drugs and use INH-RMP-containing regimens. Ureteral cicatrization during healing, producing obstruction, may occur, and the urologic literature recommends pyelograms every 3 months during treatment and yearly for 2 or 3 years thereafter.[176] Indications for surgery include intractable pain, persisting nontuberculous infection due to obstruction, and serious persisting hematuria.[176]

Male Genital Tuberculosis. The majority (80 percent) of cases of male genital tuberculosis are associated with and presumably due to coexistent renal disease.[177] Conversely, the majority of advanced cases of renal disease are associated with some male genital focus. Spread of infection from above involves the prostate, the seminal vesicles, the epididymis, and the testis, in that order. The usual clinical finding is a scrotal mass that may be tender or associated with a draining sinus. Oligospermia is common and may not improve with treatment. Stones may form with treatment of prostatic lesions. Foci of male genital tuberculosis not associated with renal disease are established by lymphohematogenous spread and usually present as an often painful testicular or scrotal mass. Diagnosis is usually established by surgery, and the response to chemotherapy is excellent.

Female Genital Tuberculosis. Female genital tuberculosis begins with a hematogenous focus in the endosalpinx, from which it may spread to the ovary, the endometrium, and rarely the cervix, producing a granuomatous ulcerating mass resembling carcinoma.[178] Symptoms are usually local, consisting of menstrual disorders and abdominal pain, and systemic symptoms are uncommon. It was a major cause of sterility in the past; its treatment by tubal insufflation at times caused tuberculous peritonitis. When pregnancy does occur in the presence of pelvic tuberculosis, an ectopic location is frequent. The presenting symptoms may be those of pelvic inflammatory disease unresponsive to antibiotic therapy. Diagnosis is usually made on the basis of tissue removed at operation (dilatation and curettage, laparotomy, biopsy of the cervix), but the organism can sometimes be cultured from menstrual blood or endometrial scrapings. The response to chemotherapy is excellent, and surgery is needed only for residual large tuboovarian abscesses.

Gastrointestinal Tuberculosis

Before the chemotherapy era, 70 percent of patients with far advanced pulmonary disease developed gastrointestinal tuberculosis due to swallowed infectious secretions, usually symptomatic with diarrhea and abdominal pain. Although it is assumed that present-day cases are also due to swallowed infectious secretions, coexistent evidence of pulmonary tuberculosis is actually present in less than 50 percent of cases and in some series in as little as 25 percent.[179–181] In these cases, the diagnosis is usually an unexpected finding at surgery.

Nonhealing ulcers of the tongue or oropharynx may be due to tuberculosis, and cases have been discovered because of a nonhealing tooth socket after extraction. Esophageal disease is most frequently due to an adjacent caseous node, causing stricture with obstruction, tracheoesophageal fistulae, and, in one reported case, fatal hematemesis from an aortoesophageal fistula.[182] The stomach rarely may be involved with chronic tuberculous ulcerations, and diffuse thickening resembling carcinomatous linitis plastica has been reported. Pyloric obstruction may be caused by spread from adjacent nodes, producing a mass lesion resembling cancer, or by intrinsic hypertrophic changes of the duodenal cap. A variety of small bowel syndromes may be produced, including perforation, obstruction, enteroenteric and enterocutaneous fistulas, massive hemorrhage, and severe malabsorption. Small bowel lesions are frequently multiple. Tuberculosis of the cecum is the most frequent gastrointestinal manifestation, producing symptoms of abdominal pain, anorexia, diarrhea, obstruction, and hemorrhage, which may be massive.[183] The clinical and roentgenographic findings are both suggestive of carcinoma, and often the operative findings are as well. The remainder of the colon can be involved with local hyperplastic changes producing obstruction, ulcerative lesions producing hemorrhage or perforation, or any combination of these manifestations. The colonoscopic finding of transverse ulcerations has been reported to be suggestive, and diagnosis has been made by colonoscopic biopsy.[184] Anal tuberculosis was frequent before the chemotherapy era but still is very important to recognize. Types of involvement include simple ulcer, fistula in ano, fistula associated with a low perirectal abscess, and multiple fistulae associated with complex high perirectal abscesses. The majority of nontuberculous fistulae in ano are in the posterior midline; another location should suggest the possibility of tuberculosis.[185] Pancreatic tuberculosis may present as an abscess or as a mass involving local nodes resembling carcinoma.[186] The biliary tract may be obstructed by tuberculous nodes,[187] and cases of tuberculous ascending cholangitis have been described.[135] Tuberculosis is the most frequent cause of granulomatous hepatitis.[135] Usually this is asymptomatic; less frequently it will cause the chemical picture of disseminated hepatic disease (elevation of alkaline phosphatase out of proportion to bilirubin, normal transaminases), and very rarely, involvement may be massive in the absence of evidence of extrahepatic tuberculosis, which has been called *primary tuberculosis of the liver*.[135]

As mentioned, diagnosis of gastrointestinal tuberculosis is usually made after a surgical procedure. However, the response to chemotherapy is usually excellent, and when the diagnosis is known, surgery should be deferred if possible until the results of chemotherapy have been assessed.

Tuberculous Peritonitis

Tuberculous peritonitis is usually due to rupture of a caseous abdominal lymph node. Less frequently it is spread from a focus in the intestine or fallopian tube, and cases complicating psoas abscess have been recorded.[188] One series from Iran reported evidence of concomitant primary tuberculosis (mediastinal lymphadenopathy, pleural effusion, miliary pulmonary disease) in two-thirds of their cases, mostly in adolescents and young adults.[189] The percentage of cases in which extraperitoneal tuberculosis is clinically evident varies widely in different series. A compilation of 201 cases from four series indicated that the chest x-ray was normal in 34 percent[188,190–192]; in another series it was normal in 44 out of 47 (94 percent) cases.[193] Pleural effusion is the most frequent associated finding. Evidence of other extrapulmonary tuberculosis in bones, nodes, or abdomen may be present. Barium enema studies revealed cecal abnormalities in 2 out of 16 cases in one series.[191]

The clinical picture has been divided into plastic and serous types, the former and less usual being characterized by tender abdominal masses and a doughy abdomen and the latter, and more usual, by ascites and signs of peritonitis. Symptoms of fever, abdominal pain, weight loss, and anorexia are common. One large series emphasized an insidious onset in 94 out of their 100 cases,[192] and in another report the diagnosis was an unsuspected finding in 2 afebrile patients operated on for hernia repair.[190] In contrast, another report emphasized an abrupt onset with chills, fever, ascites, and rebound tenderness resembling acute bacterial peritonitis.[194] Diagnosis has often been made by operation for some combination of tender abdominal mass and acute surgical abdomen, and cases have been mistaken for cholecystitis, appendicitis, and pelvic inflammatory disease.[192] One classic study emphasized the difficulty in diagnosing tuberculous peritonitis in the presence of cirrhosis with ascites.[195] Of 20 patients with both conditions, the diagnosis of tuberculous peritonitis was unsuspected antemortem in 11.

In the absence of recognizable concomitant extraperitoneal tuberculosis, diagnosis most often requires peritoneal biopsy. The tuberculin test is not helpful, the percentage of positive results in various series being 30 percent,[196] 56 percent,[194] 82 percent,[102] and 100 percent.[193] The peritoneal fluid has the biochemical characteristics of an exudate and usually contains between 500 and 2000 cells, mostly lymphocytes. However, as many as 10 percent may initially show a predominance of polymorphonuclear leukocytes.[196] Smear of the fluid is only rarely positive and culture will be positive in approximately 25 percent of cases.[190] Peritoneal biopsy with a Cope needle has resulted in diagnosis in 64 percent of cases and peritoneoscopy plus Cope biopsy in 85 percent in one series.[193] However, bleeding from a peritoneal needle biopsy can become far advanced before it is recognized, and fatalities due to both Cope needle biopsy and peritoneoscopy[197] have been recorded. A small open biopsy will allow all diagnoses to be made safely.

Treatment is conventional chemotherapy, as for pulmonary tuberculosis. One author has advocated the adjunctive use of corticosteroids in order to avoid intestinal obstruction developing during treatment,[193] but this is not generally recommended.

Tuberculous Lymphadenitis

Peripheral Nodes. Tuberculous lymphadenitis usually occurs in otherwise healthy people. Only a minority will have low-grade systemic symptoms. In one large series, the location was cervical or supraclavicular in over 90 percent of cases, in 80 percent only a single node was involved, and evidence of other tuberculosis was present in 18 percent (pulmonary, 7 percent; mediastinal nodes, 9 percent; other, 2 percent).[198] The nodes may be firm and tender during rapid enlargement but later tend to soften, become matted, and may slough and drain. Most cases are tuberculin positive. Diagnosis is made by biopsy. The AFB can be demonstrated on stains in slightly over half of the cases, but nearly all should be culture positive before treatment. The only major diagnostic difficulty is granulomatous lymphadenitis due to mycobacteria other than *M. tuberculosis*, the clinical and histologic pictures of which can be identical, and differentiation is possible only by culture. Treatment is by standard chemotherapy. The response is entirely favorable in about two-thirds of the cases, but in some, persisting pus or large caseous nodes may require surgical resection.

Mediastinal Tuberculous Lymphadenopathy. Mediastinal adenopathy as a part of a primary infection is often visible roentgenologically, especially in children. In dark-skinned races especially, mediastinal adenopathy due to tuberculosis may be seen in young adults as well, which, when not associated with parenchymal disease or fever, may cause confusion with histoplasmosis or other more serious diseases such as lymphoma.[199] Usually involvement is unilateral and is four times more frequent on the right side, but bilateral involvement mimicking sarcoidosis has been recorded. Complications such as bronchoesophageal fistula, bronchial erosion, pericarditis, and superior vena cava syndrome are present in a minority of cases. The response to chemotherapy is excellent.

Mesenteric Tuberculous Lymphadenitis

Rarely, mesenteric lymph nodes will become infected and swollen in the absence of any intrinsic bowel disease or overt peritonitis. These swollen nodes may cause abdominal pain, fever, a palpable mass, or symptoms of partial small bowel obstruction.[181]

Cutaneous Tuberculosis

In the past, a number of cutaneous conditions occurring in the presence of tuberculosis but not containing stainable or culturable organisms have been regarded as allergic reactions to the infection, largely on the basis of histopathology, and grouped under the name *tuberculids*. These include erythema induratum (Bazin's disease), papulonecrotic tuberculids, and others. Recently the validity of this association has been questioned and the lesions have been attributed to other nontuberculous processes such as sarcoidosis.[200] A possible exception to this is erythema nodosum, which in the European literature has been attributed to primary tuberculosis and from which organisms cannot be cultured. This occurs extremely rarely, if at all, in the United States.

A recent reclassification of cutaneous tuberculosis emphasizing the pathogenesis is summarized in Table 6. Skin involvement can be produced by exogenous inoculation (which in the previously nonsensitized host is associated with regional lymphadenitis), by spread from a subjacent focus to the overlying skin (particularly from osteomyelitis, epididymitis, or adenitis), and by hematogenous spread from a distant focus or as a part of a generalized hematogenous dissemination. In all of these conditions, organisms are present in the skin.

Tuberculous Laryngitis

In the prechemotherapy era, laryngeal tuberculosis was observed in over a third of patients dying with pulmonary tuberculosis, often associated with painful ulcers of the epiglottis, pharynx, tonsils, and mouth, as well as middle ear involvement. Laryngeal disease in particular produced a high degree of infectiousness and often terminal widespread bronchogenic dissemination throughout the lungs. The lesions vary from simple erythema to ulceration and exophytic masses resembling carcinoma.[201,202] At present it is estimated that over 50 percent of the cases are due to hematogenous foci rather than surface lesions from highly infectious pulmonary secretions. Symptoms include cough, wheezing, hemoptysis, dysphagia, odynophagia, and otalgia, which can be due to referred pain.

TABLE 6. Classification of Cutaneous Tuberculosis

Proposed Classification of Cutaneous Mycobacteriosis	*Terms Previously Used in Literature*
Inoculation cutaneous mycobacteriosis from an exogenous source	Primary inoculation Tuberculous chancre Tuberculosis primary complex Tuberculosis verrucosa cutis Warty tuberculosis Verruca necrogenica Prosector's wart Tuberculosis cutis verrucosa
Cutaneous mycobacteriosis from local source	
Contiguous spread	Scrofuloderma Tuberculosis colliguativa cutis Orificial tuberculosis
Autoinoculation	Tuberculosis cutis orificialis Tuberculosis ulcerosa cutis et mucosae
Cutaneous mycobacteriosis from hematogenous spread	
Lupus vulgaris	Lupus vulgaris Tuberculosis luposa cutis
Acute hematogenous dissemination	Acute miliary tuberculosis of the skin Tuberculosis cutis miliaris disseminata Tuberculosis cutis acuta generalisata
Nodules or abscesses	Tuberculous gumma Metastatic tuberculous abscess

(From Beyt et al.,[211] with permission.)

Tuberculous Otitis

In prior years tuberculous otitis media was thought to be due to spread of infectious secretions via the eustachian tube and accounted for a significant percentage of chronic suppurative ear conditions. At present the condition is rare, but half of the cases in one large series had no evidence of tuberculosis elsewhere.[203] The classic clinical picture is painless otorrhea with multiple tympanic perforations, exuberant granulations, early severe hearing loss, and mastoid bone necrosis. The diagnosis has been missed for years in the best otolaryngologic hospitals even when tissue has been available. However, in the series quoted above, half of the cases were painful. Tuberculous otitis may be complicated by facial nerve paralysis. The response to drug therapy is excellent, and surgery is not required once the diagnosis is established.[204]

Miscellaneous Forms

Tuberculosis of the thoracic or abdominal aorta with or without aneurysm formation can be established by contiguous spread from tuberculous nodes, pericarditis, spondylitis, paravertebral abscesses, and empyema.[205,206] Dramatic clinical pictures may result, including extensive hematogenous dissemination or rupture into the chest, bronchial tree, or esophagus. Combined medical–surgical therapy is usually required, but only 50 percent or less of recent patients have survived. Uveal tuberculosis can produce a variety of ocular syndromes, including chronic uveitis, iritis, sclerokeratitis, interstitial keratitis, and acute panophthalmitis.[207] Tuberculosis of the breast was observed in 7 out of 10,000 autopsies of tuberculous patients,[208] producing abscesses, sclerosing lesions resembling carcinoma, and multiple nodules. Tuberculosis of the nasopharynx has produced granulomatous and destructive lesions misdiagnosed as Wegener's granulomatosis.[209] Tuberculosis of the adrenal glands may cause adrenal enlargement with or without calcification on abdominal CT scan, as may histoplasmosis. Large glands without calcium may be due to either granuloma or cancer, and granulomatous adrenal destruction can occur without calcification of adrenal enlargement.[210]

REFERENCES

1. D'Esopo ND. Clinical trials in pulmonary tuberculosis. Am Rev Respir Dis. 1982;125(No 3, Pt 2):85–93.
2. Stead WW, Dutt AK. Chemotherapy for tuberculosis today. Am Rev Respir Dis. 1982;125:94–101.
3. Snider DE Jr, Zierski M, Graczyk J, et al. Short-course tuberculosis chemotherapy studies conducted in Poland during the past decade. Eur J Respir Dis. 1986;68:12–18.
4. Wayne LG. Microbiology of tubercle bacilli. Am Rev Respir Dis. 1982;25—No 3, Pt 2):31–41.
5. Youmans AS. The morphology and metabolism of mycobacteria. In: Youmans GP, ed. Tuberculosis. Philadelphia: Saunders; 1979:8.
6. Woods GL, Washington JA II. Mycobacteria other than *Mycobacterium tuberculosis*: Review of microbiologic and clinical aspects. Rev Infect Dis. 1987;9:275–94.
7. O'Brien RJ, Geiter LJ, Snider DE Jr. The epidemiology of nontuberculous mycobacterial diseases in the United States. Results from a national survey. Am Rev Respir Dis. 1987;135:1007–14.
8. Strumph IJ, Tsang AY, Schork MA, et al. The reliability of gastric smears by auramine-rhodamine staining technique for the diagnosis of tuberculosis. Am Rev Respir Dis. 1976;114:971–6.
9. Russell MD, Torrington KG, Tenholder MF. A ten-year experience with fiberoptic bronchoscopy for mycobacterial isolation: Impact of the *Bactec* system. Am Rev Respir Dis. 1986;133:1069–71.
10. Rouillon A, Perdrizet S, Parrot R. Transmission of tubercle bacilli. The effects of chemotherapy. Tubercle. 1976;57:275–99.
11. Styblo K. Recent advances in epidemiological research in tuberculosis. Adv Tuberc Res. 1980;20:1–63.
12. Comstock GW, Edwards LB, Livesay VT. Tuberculosis morbidity in the U.S. Navy: Its distribution and decline. Am Rev Respir Dis. 1974;110:572–80.
13. Centers for Disease Control. Tuberculosis Control Division. Tuberculosis in the United States, 1981–84. Atlanta: Centers for Disease Control; 1986:3.
14. Pitchenik AE, Russell BW, Cleary T, et al. The prevalence of tuberculosis and drug resistance among Haitians. N Engl J Med. 1982;307:162–5.

15. Glassroth J, Robins AG, Snider DE Jr. Tuberculosis in the 1980's. N Engl J Med. 1980;302:1441–50.
16. Sbarbaro JA. Tuberculosis: The new challenge to the practicing clinician. Chest. 1975;68:436–43.
17. Riley RL. Disease transmission and contagion control. Am Rev Respir Dis. 1982;125:16–9.
18. Johnston RF, Wildrick KH. "State of the art" review. The impact of chemotherapy on the care of patients with tuberculosis. Am Rev Respir Dis. 1974;109:636–64.
19. Comstock GW. Epidemiology of tuberculosis. Am Rev Respir Dis. 1982;125(No 3, Pt 2):8–15.
20. Eilertsen E. Epidemics of primary tuberculosis and their significance. Acta Tuberc Scand. 1959;37:203–16.
21. Houk VH, Kent DC, Baker JH, et al. The *Byrd* study. In-depth analysis of a micro-outbreak of tuberculosis in a closed environment. Arch Environ Health. 1968;16:4–6.
22. Stead WW. Tuberculosis among elderly persons: An outbreak in a nursing home. Ann Intern Med. 1981;94:606–10.
23. Comstock GW, Livesay VT, Woolpert SF. The prognosis of a positive tuberculin reaction in childhood and adolescence. Am J Epidemiol. 1974;99:131–8.
24. Gedde-Dahl T. Tuberculous infection in the light of tuberculin matriculation. Am J Hyg. 1952;56:139–214.
25. Davies BH. Infectivity of tuberculosis. Thorax. 1980;35:481–2.
26. Ross HD, Willison JC. The relationship between tuberculin reactions and the later development of tuberculosis: An investigation among Edinburgh school children in 1960–1970. Tubercle. 1971;52:258–65.
27. Rich AR. The Pathogenesis of Tuberculosis, 2nd ed. Springfield, Ill: Charles C Thomas; 1951:1028.
28. Dannenberg AM Jr. Pathogenesis of pulmonary tuberculosis. Am Rev Respir Dis. 1982;125(No 3, Pt 2):25–30.
29. Collins FM. The immunology of tuberculosis. Am Rev Respir Dis. 1982; 125(No 3, Pt 2):42–9.
30. Pratt PC. Pathology of tuberculosis. Semin Roentgenol. 1979;14:196–203.
31. O'Brien JR. Non-reactive tuberculosis. J Clin Pathol. 1954;7:216–25.
32. Snider DE Jr. The tuberculin skin test. Am Rev Respir Dis. 1982;125 (No 3, Pt 2):108–18.
33. Thompson NJ, Glassroth JL, Snider DE Jr, et al. The booster phenomenon in serial tuberculin testing. Am Rev Respir Dis. 1979;119:587–97.
34. Nash DR, Douglass JE. Anergy in active pulmonary tuberculosis. A comparison between positive and negative reactors and an evaluation of 5 TU and 250 TU skin test doses. Chest. 1980;77:32–7.
35. Chusid EL, Shah R, Siltzbach LE. Tuberculin tests during the course of sarcoidosis in 350 patients. Am Rev Respir Dis. 1971;104:13–21.
36. Grzybowski S, Allen EA. The challenge of tuberculosis in decline: A study based on the epidemiology of tuberculosis in Ontario, Canada. Am Rev Respir Dis. 1964;90:707–20.
37. Palmer PE. Pulmonary tuberculosis—usual and unusual radiographic presentations. Semin Roentgenol. 1979;14:204–43.
38. Stead WW, Lofgren JP, Warren E, et al. Tuberculosis as an endemic and nosocomial infection among the elderly in nursing homes. N Engl J Med. 1985;312:1483–7.
39. Stead WW. Pathogenesis of a first episode of chronic pulmonary tuberculosis in man: Recrudescence of residuals of the primary infection or exogenous reinfection? Am Rev Respir Dis. 1967;95:729–45.
40. Goodwin RA, des Prez RM. Apical localization of pulmonary tuberculosis, chronic pulmonary histoplasmosis, and progressive massive fibrosis of the lung. Chest. 1983;83:801–5.
41. Romeyn JA. Exogenous reinfection in tuberculosis. Am Rev Respir Dis. 1970;101:923–7.
42. Kumar RA, Saran M, Verma BL, et al. Pulmonary tuberculosis among contacts of patients with tuberculosis in an urban Indian population. J Epidemiol Community Health. 1984;38:253–8.
43. Nardell E, McInnis B, Thomas B, et al. Exogenous reinfection with tuberculosis in a shelter for the homeless. N Engl J Med. 1986;315:1570–5.
44. Israel S, Long ER. Primary tuberculosis in adolescents and young adults. Am Rev Tuberc. 1941;43:42–55.
45. Dahl RH. First appearance of pulmonary cavity after primary infection with relation to time and age. Acta Tuberc Scand. 1952;27:140–9.
46. Stead WW, Kerby GR, Schlueter DP, et al. The clinical spectrum of primary tuberculosis in adults: Confusion with reinfection in the pathogenesis of chronic tuberculosis. Ann Intern Med. 1968;68:731–45.
47. Cameron SJ. Tuberculosis and the blood: A special relationship. Tubercle. 1974;55:55–72.
48. Pitchenik AE, Cole C, Russel B, et al. Tuberculosis, atypical mycobacteriosis, and the acquired immunodeficiency syndrome among Haitian and non-Haitian patients in south Florida. Ann Intern Med. 1984;101:641–5.
49. American Thoracic Society. Mycobacterioses and the acquired immunodeficiency syndrome. Am Rev Respir Dis. 1987;136:492–6.
50. Louie E, Rice LB, Holzm RS. Tuberculosis in non-Haitian patients with acquired immunodeficiency syndrome. Chest. 1986;90:542–5.
51. Parmar MS. Lower lung field tuberculosis. Am Rev Respir Dis. 1967;96:310–3.
52. Canetti G. Present aspects of bacterial resistance in tuberculosis. Am Rev Respir Dis. 1965;92:687–703.
53. Ip MS, So SY, Lam WK, et al. Endobronchial tuberculosis revisited. Chest. 1986;89:727–30.
54. Chang S, Lee P, Perng P. Lower lung field tuberculosis. Chest. 1987;91:230–2.
55. Plessinger VA, Jolly PN. Rasmussen's aneurysms and fatal hemorrhage in pulmonary tuberculosis. Am Rev Tuberc. 1949;60:589–603.
56. Butz RO, Zvetina JR, Leininger BJ. Ten-year experience with mycetomas in patients with pulmonary tuberculosis. Chest. 1985;87:356–8.
57. Cohen JR, Amorosa JK, Smith PR. The air-fluid level in cavitary pulmonary tuberculosis. Radiology. 1978;127:315–6.
58. Neff TA. Bronchoscopy and Bactec for the diagnosis of tuberculosis: State of the art, or a brief dissertation on the efficient search for the tubercle bacillus? Am Rev Respir Dis. 1986;133:962.
59. Willcox PA, Potgieter PD, Bateman ED, et al. Rapid diagnosis of sputum negative miliary tuberculosis using the flexible fiberoptic bronchoscope. Thorax. 1986;41:681–4.
60. Katz I, Rosenthal T, Michaeli D. Undiagnosed tuberculosis in hospitalized patients. Chest. 1985;87:770–4.
61. Snider DE Jr. The relationship between tuberculosis and silicosis. Am Rev Respir Dis. 1978;118:455–60.
62. Morgan EJ. Silicosis and tuberculosis. Chest. 1979;75:202–3.
63. Mok CK, Nandi P, Ong GB. Co-existent bronchogenic carcinoma and active pulmonary tuberculosis. J Thorac Cardiovasc Surg. 1978;76:469–72.
64. Grzybowski S. The impact of treatment programs on the epidemiology of tuberculosis. Tubercle. 1985;66:69–72.
65. David HL, Newman CM. Some observations on the genetics of isoniazid resistance in the tubercle bacilli. Am Rev Respir Dis. 1971;104:508–15.
66. Byrd RB, Fisk DE, Roethe RA, et al. Tuberculosis in Oriental immigrants: A study in military dependents. Chest. 1979;76:136–9.
67. Carpenter JL, Obnibene AJ, Gorby EW, et al. Antituberculosis drug resistance in South Texas. Am Rev Respir Dis. 1983;128:1055–8.
68. Steiner P, Rao M, Mitchell M, et al. Primary drug-resistant tuberculosis in children. Emergence of primary drug resistance of *M. tuberculosis* to rifampin. Am Rev Respir Dis. 1986;134:446–8.
69. Barnes PF. The influence of epidemiologic factors on drug resistance rates in tuberculosis. Am Rev Respir Dis. 1987;136:325–8.
70. Parthasarathy R, Raghupati G, Sarma B, et al. Hepatic toxicity in South Indian patients during treatment of tuberculosis with short-course regimens containing isoniazid, rifampicin, and pyrazinamide. Tubercle. 1986;67:99–108.
71. Blanchard PD, Yao JD, McAlpine DE, et al. Isoniazid overdose in the Cambodian population of Olmsted County, Minnesota. JAMA. 1986;256:3131–3.
72. Baciewicz AM, Self TH, Bekemeyer WB. Update of rifampin drug interactions. Arch Intern Med. 1987;147:565–8.
73. Kopanoff DE, Snider DE Jr, Caras GJ. Isoniazid-related hepatitis. A U.S. Public Health Service cooperative surveillance study. Am Rev Respir Dis. 1978;117:991–1001.
74. Stead WW, To T. The significance of the tuberculin skin test in elderly persons. Ann Intern Med. 1987;107:837–42.
75. Taylor WC, Aronson MD, Delbanco TL. Should young adults with a positive tuberculin test take isoniazid? Ann Intern Med. 1981;94:808–13.
76. Black M, Mitchell JR, Zimmerman HJ, et al. Isoniazid-associated hepatitis in 114 patients. Gastroenterology. 1975;69:289–302.
77. Dash LA, Comstock GW, Flynn PG. Isoniazid preventive therapy: Retrospect and prospect. Am Rev Respir Dis. 1980;121:1039–44.
78. Tuberculosis Research Centre, Madras, and National Tuberculosis Institute, Bangalore. A controlled clinical trial of 3- and 5-month regimens in the treatment of sputum-positive pulmonary tuberculosis in south India. Am Rev Respir Dis. 1986;134:27–33.
79. Bobrowitz ID. Ethambutol compared to rifampin in original treatment of pulmonary tuberculosis. Lung. 1980;157:117–25.
80. Bartelink AKM, Lenders JWM, Van Herwaarden CLA, et al. Fatal hepatitis after treatment with isoniazid and rifampicin in a patient on anticonvulsant therapy. Tubercle. 1983;64:125–8.
81. Tsagaropoulou-Stinga H, Mataki-Emmanouilidou T, Karida-Kavalioti S, et al. Hepatotoxic reactions in children with severe tuberculosis treated with isoniazid-rifampin. Pediatr Inf Dis. 1985;4:270–3.
82. Rahajoe NN, Rahajoe N, Boediman I, et al. The treatment of tuberculous meningitis in children with a combination of isoniazid, rifampicin, and streptomycin. Preliminary report. Tubercle. 1979;60:245–50.
83. Centers for Disease Control. Adverse drug reactions among children treated for tuberculosis. MMWR. 1980;29:589–91.
84. British Thoracic Society. A controlled trial for 6 months' chemotherapy in pulmonary tuberculosis: Results during the 36 months after the end of chemotherapy and beyond. Br J Dis Chest. 1984;78:330–6.
85. Citron KM. Ethambutol: A review with special reference to ocular toxicity. Tubercle. 1969;50(S):32–6.
86. Chatterjee VKK, Buchanan DR, Friedman AI. Ocular toxicity following ethambutol in standard dosage. Br J Dis Chest. 1986;80:288–91.
87. Medical Section of the American Lung Association. Treatment of tuberculosis and tuberculosis infection in adults and children. Am Rev Respir Dis. 1986;134:355–63.
88. Snider DE Jr, Cohn DL, Davidson PT, et al. Standard therapy for tuberculosis, 1985. Chest. 1985;87:117S–24S.
89. Mitchison DA, Nunn AJ. Influence of initial drug resistance on the response to short-course chemotherapy of pulmonary tuberculosis. Am Rev Respir Dis. 1986;133:423–30.
90. Kim TC, Blackman RS, Heatwole KM, et al. Acid-fast bacilli in sputum

smears of patients with pulmonary tuberculosis: Prevalence and significance of negative smears pretreatment and positive smears posttreatment. Am Rev Respir Dis. 1984;129:264–8.
91. Elsbach P, Edsall JR. ACTH and cortisone as adjuncts in the treatment of advanced pulmonary tuberculosis. Ann Intern Med. 1957;46:332–41.
92. Des Prez RM, Organick A. Corticotropin and corticosteroid therapy in tuberculosis. Arch Intern Med. 1958;101:1129–42.
93. Simpson DG, Hubaytar RT. Hypersensitivity to drugs in the treatment of tuberculosis. Rapid desensitization using cortisone acetate. Am Rev Respir Dis. 1962;86:738–9.
94. Phuapradit P, Vejjajiva A. Treatment of tuberculous meningitis: Role of short-course chemotherapy. Q J Med. 1987;62:249–58.
95. Snider DE Jr, Layde PM, Johnson MW, et al. Treatment of tuberculosis during pregnancy. Am Rev Respir Dis. 1980;122:65–79.
96. Andrew OT, Schoenfeld PY, Hopewell PC, et al. Tuberculosis in patients with end-stage renal disease. Am J Med. 1980;68:59–65.
97. Dantzenberg B, Grosset J, Fechner J, et al. The management of thirty immunocompromised patients with tuberculosis. Am Rev Respir Dis. 1984; 129:494–6.
98. Efficacy of various durations of isoniazid preventive therapy for tuberculosis: Five years of follow-up in the IUAT trial. International Union Against Tuberculosis. Committee on Prophylaxis. Bull WHO. 1982;60:555–64.
99. Byrd RB, Horn BR, Griggs GA, et al. Isoniazid chemoprophylaxis. Association with detection and incidence of liver toxicity. Arch Intern Med. 1970;137:1130–3.
100. Ferebee SH. Controlled chemoprophylaxis trials in tuberculosis. A general review. Bibl Tuberc Med Thorac. 1970;26:28–106.
101. Payne CR. Surveillance of tuberculosis contacts: Experience at Ealing Chest Clinic. Tubercle. 1978;59:179–84.
102. Katz J, Kunofsky S. Logistics of chemoprophylaxis of tuberculosis. Chest. 1971;59:600–5.
103. Fairshter RD, Randazzo GP, Garlin J, et al. Failure of isoniazid prophylaxis after exposure to isoniazid-resistant tuberculosis. Am Rev Respir Dis. 1975;112:37–42.
104. Costello HD, Caras GJ, Snider DE Jr. Drug resistance among previously treated tuberculosis, a brief report. Am Rev Respir Dis. 1980;121:313–6.
105. Grzybowski S, Ashley MJ, McKinnon NE, et al. In Canada: A trial of chemoprophylaxis in inactive tuberculosis. Can Med Assoc J. 1969;101:81–6.
106. Falk A, Fuchs GF. Prophylaxis with isoniazid in inactive tuberculosis. A Veterans Administration cooperative study XII. Chest. 1978;73:44–8.
107. Stead W: Personal communication.
108. Comstock GW, Edwards PQ. The competing risks of tuberculosis and hepatitis for adult tuberculin reactors. Am Rev Respir Dis. 1975;111:573–7.
109. Chemoprophylaxis for tuberculosis. Tubercle. 1981;62:69–72.
110. Special report. Tuberculosis among Indochinese refugees. In: Tuberculosis in the United States. Atlanta: Public Health Centers for Disease Control, Tuberculosis Control Division; 1981:40.
111. Smith DT. Isoniazid prophylaxis and BCG vaccination in the control of tuberculosis. High-risk groups. Arch Environ Health. 1971;23:235–42.
112. Thorn PA, Brookes VS, Waterhouse JA. Peptic ulcer, partial gastrectomy, and pulmonary tuberculosis. Br Med J. 1956;1:603–8.
113. Sahn SA, Lakshminarayan S. Tuberculosis after corticosteroid therapy. Br J Dis Chest. 1976;70:195–205.
114. Cuss FM, Carmichael DJ, Linington A, et al. Tuberculosis in renal failure: A high incidence in patients born in the third world. Clin Nephrol. 1986;25:129–33.
115. Lloveras J, Peterson PK, Simmons RL, et al. Mycobacterial infections in renal transplant recipients. Seven cases and a review of the literature. Arch Intern Med. 1982;142:888–92.
116. Snider DE Jr. Jejunoileal bypass for obesity: A risk factor for tuberculosis. Chest. 1982;81:531–2.
117. Stead WW, To T, Harrison RW, et al. Benefit–risk considerations in preventive treatment of tuberculosis in elderly persons. Ann Intern Med. 1987;107:843–5.
118. Narain JP, Lofgren JP, Warren E, et al. Epidemic tuberculosis in a nursing home: A retrospective cohort study. J Am Geriatr Soc. 1985;33:258–263.
119. Luelmo F. BCG vaccination. Am Rev Respir Dis. 1982;125(No 3, Pt 2): 70–2.
120. Sutherland I, Lindgren I. The protective effect of BCG vaccination as indicated by autopsy studies. Tubercle. 1979;60:225–31.
121. Farer LS, Lowell AM, Meador MP. Extrapulmonary tuberculosis in the United States. Am J Epidemiol. 1979;109:205–17.
122. Auerbach O. Acute generalized miliary tuberculosis. Am J Pathol. 1944;20:121–36.
123. Biehl JP. Miliary tuberculosis. A review of sixty-eight adult patients admitted to a municipal general hospital. Am Rev Tuberc. 1958;77:605–22.
124. Munt PW. Miliary tuberculosis in the chemotherapy era: With a clinical review in 69 American adults. Medicine (Balt) 1972;51:139–55.
125. Chapman CB, Whorton CM. Acute generalized miliary tuberculosis in adults: Clinicopathological study based on 63 cases diagnosed at autopsy. N Engl J Med. 1946;235:239–48.
126. Slavin RE, Walsh TJ, Pollock AD. Late generalized tuberculosis: A clinical pathologic analysis and comparison of 100 cases in the preantibiotic and antibiotic eras. Medicine. 1980;59:352–66.
127. Yu YL, Chow WH, Humphries MJ, et al. Cryptic miliary tuberculosis. Q J Med. 1986;59:421–8.
128. Braidy J, Pothel C, Amra S. Miliary tuberculosis presenting as adrenal failure. Can Med Assoc J. 1981;124:748–9.
129. Willcox PA, Potgieter PD, Bateman ED, et al. Rapid diagnosis of sputum negative miliary tuberculosis using the flexible fiberoptic bronchoscope. Thorax. 1986;41:681–4.
130. Falk A. U.S. Veterans Administration Armed Forces cooperative study on the chemotherapy of tuberculosis: XII. Results of treatment in miliary tuberculosis: A follow-up study of 570 adult patients. Am Rev Respir Dis. 1965;91:6–12.
131. Dyer RA, Chappell WA, Potgeiter PD. Adult respiratory distress syndrome associated with miliary tuberculosis. Crit Care Med. 1985;13:12–5.
132. Proudfoot AT, Akhar AJ, Douglas AC, et al. Miliary tuberculosis in adults. Br Med J. 1969;2:273–6.
133. Oswald NC. Acute tuberculosis and granulocytic disorders. Br Med J. 1963;5371:1489–96.
134. Arends A. Blood disease and so-called generalized non-reactive tuberculosis (typhobacillosis of Landouzy, sepsis tuberculosa acutissima). Acta Med Scandinav. 1950;136:417–29.
135. Harrington PT, Gutierrez JJ, Ramirez-Ronda CH, et al. Granulomatous hepatitis. Rev Infect Dis. 1982;4:638–55.
136. Rich AR, McCordock HA. Pathogenesis of tuberculous meningitis. Bull Johns Hopkins Hosp. 1933;52:5–37.
137. Auerbach O. Tuberculous meningitis: Correlation of therapeutic results with pathogenesis and pathologic changes; general considerations and pathogenesis. Am Rev Tuberc. 1951;64:408–18.
138. Idriss ZH, Sinno AA, Kronfol NM. Tuberculosis meningitis in childhood. Forty-three cases. Am J Dis Child. 1976;130:364–7.
139. Smith AL. Tuberculosis meningitis in childhood. Med J Aust. 1975;1:57–60.
140. Auerbach O. Tuberculous meningitis: Correlation of therapeutic results with pathogenesis and pathologic changes; pathologic changes in untreated and treated cases. Am Rev Tuberc. 1951;64:419–29.
141. Udani PM, Parekh UC, Dastur DK. Neurological and related syndromes in CNS tuberculosis. Clinical features and pathogenesis. J Neurol Sci. 1971;14:341–57.
142. Kocen RS, Parsons M. Neurological complications of tuberculosis: Some unusual manifestations. Q J Med. 1970;39:17–30.
143. Falk A. U.S. Veterans Administration Armed Forces cooperative study on the chemotherapy of tuberculosis: XII. Results of treatment in miliary tuberculosis: A follow-up study of 570 adult patients. Am Rev Respir Dis. 1965;91:6–12.
144. Kennedy DH, Fallon RJ. Tuberculous meningitis. JAMA. 1979;241:264–8.
145. Bullock MR, Welchman JM. Diagnostic and prognostic features of tuberculous meningitis on CT scanning. J Neurol Neurosurg Psychiatry. 1982;45:1098–1101.
146. Stevens DL, Everett ED. Sequential computerized axial tomography in tuberculous meningitis. JAMA. 1978;239:642.
147. Bhargava S, Gupta AK, Tandon PN. Tuberculous meningitis: A CT study. Br J Radiol. 1982;55:189–96.
148. Falk A. U.S. Veterans Administration Armed Forces cooperative study on the chemotherapy of tuberculosis. 13. Tuberculous meningitis in adults, with special reference to survival, neurologic residuals, and work status. Am Rev Respir Dis. 1965;91:823–31.
149. D'Oliveira JJ. Cerebrospinal fluid concentrations of rifampin in meningeal tuberculosis. Am Rev Respir Dis. 1972;106:432–7.
150. O'Toole RD, Thornton GF, Mukherjee MK, et al. Dexamethasone in tuberculous meningitis. Relationship of cerebrospinal fluid effects ot therapeutic efficacy. Ann Intern Med. 1969;70:39–48.
151. Harder E, Al-Kawi MZ, Carney P. Intracranial tuberculoma: Conservative management. Am J Med. 1983;74:570–6.
152. Tandon PN, Bhargava S. Effect of medical treatment on intracranial tuberculoma: A CT study. Tubercle. 1985;66:85–97.
153. Wadia NH, Dastur DK. Spinal meningitides with radiculo-myelopathy. 1. Clinical and radiological features. J Neurol Sci. 1969;8:239–60.
154. Roper WH, Waring JJ. Primary serofibrinous pleural effusion in military personnel. Am Rev Tuberc. 1955;71:616–34.
155. Stead WW, Eichenholz A, Strauss HK. Operative and pathologic findings in twenty-four patients with syndrome of idiopathic pleurisy with effusion, presumably tuberculous. Am Rev Tuberc. 1955;71:472–502.
156. Berger HW, Mejia E. Tuberculous pleurisy. Chest. 1973;63:88–92.
157. Levine H, Szanto PB, Cugell DW. Tuberculous pleurisy. An acute illness. Arch Intern Med. 1968;122:329–32.
158. Epstein DM, Kline LR, Albelda SM, et al. Tuberculous pleural effusions. Chest. 1987;91:106–9.
159. Schmid FG, DeHaller R. Late exudative complications of collapse therapy for pulmonary tuberculosis. Chest. 1986;89:822–7.
160. Hirasing RA, van Bel F. Tuberculous pericarditis developing chemotherapy. Eur J Respir Dis. 1982;63:73–6.
161. Ortbals DW, Avioli LV. Tuberculous pericarditis. Arch Intern Med. 1979; 139:231–4.
162. Rooney JJ, Crocco JA, Lyons HA. Tuberculous pericarditis. Ann Intern Med. 1970;72:72–8.
163. Desai HN. Tuberculous pericarditis. A review of 100 cases. S Afr Med J. 1979;55:877–80.
164. Larrieu AJ, Tyers GF, Williams EH, et al. Recent experience with tuberculous pericarditis. Ann Thorac Surg. 1980;29:464–8.
165. Griffiths DL. Tuberculosis of the spine: A review. Adv Tuberc Res. 1980;20:92–110.

166. Blumenthal DH, Morin ME. Tan A. Intestinal penetration by tuberculous psoas abscess. Am J Roentgenol. 1981;136:995–7.
167. Wardlaw D. Rupture of a paravertebral abscess into the lower lobe of the right lung. J R Coll Surg Edinb. 1977;22:296–9.
168. Hodgson AR, Skinsnes OK, Leong CY. The pathogenesis of Pott's paraplegia. J Bone Joint Surg (Am). 1967;49A:1147–56.
169. Fancourt GJ, Ebden P, Garner P, et al. Bone tuberculosis: Results and experience in Leicestershire. Br J Dis Chest. 1986;80:265–72.
170. Davidson PT, Horowitz I. Skeletal tuberculosis. A review with patient presentations and discussion. Am J Med. 1970;48:77–84.
171. Brown TS. Tuberculosis of the ribs. Clin Radiol. 1980;31:681–4.
172. Rizzoli PB, Passero MA. Tuberculous mediastinal lymphadenitis presenting as chest wall mass. Postgrad Med. 1980;68:97–9.
173. Gow JG. Genito-urinary tuberculosis. A study of the disease in one unit over a period of 24 years. Ann R Coll Surg Engl. 1971;49:50–70.
174. Simon HB, Weinstein AJ, Pasternak MS, et al. Genitourinary tuberculosis. Clinical features in a general hospital population. Am J Med. 1977;63:410–20.
175. Christensen WI. Genitourinary tuberculosis: Review of 102 cases. Medicine. 1974;53:377–90.
176. Cos LR, Cockett AT. Genitourinary tuberculosis revisted. Urology. 1982; 20:111–7.
177. Riehle RA Jr, Jayaraman K. Tuberculosis of the testis. Urology. 1982;20: 43–6.
178. Brown AB, Gilbert CR, TeLinde RW. Pelvic tuberculosis. Obstet Gynecol. 1953;2:476–83.
179. Lambrianides AL, Ackroyd N, Shorey BA. Abdominal tuberculosis. Br J Surg. 1980;67:887–9.
180. Klimach OE, Ormerod LP. Gastrointestinal tuberculosis: A retrospective review of 109 cases in a district general hospital. Q J Med. 1985;56:569–78.
181. Gilinsky NH, Marks IN, Kottler RE, et al. Abdominal tuberculosis. A 10-year review. S Afr Med J. 1983;64:849–57.
182. Dow CJ. Oesophageal tuberculosis: Four cases. Gut. 1981;22:234–6.
183. Verma P, Kapur BM. Massive rectal bleeding due to intestinal tuberculosis. Am J Gastroenterol. 1979;71:217–9.
184. Breiter JR, Hajjar JJ. Segmental tuberculosis of the colon diagnosed by colonoscopy. Am J Gastroenterol. 1981;76:369–73.
185. Whalen TV Jr, Kovalcik PJ, Old WL Jr. Tuberculous anal ulcer. Dis Colon Rectum. 1980;23:54–5.
186. Stambler JB, Klibaner ME, Bliss CM, et al. Tuberculosis abscess of the pancreas. Gastroenterology. 1982;83:922–5.
187. Murphy TF, Gray GF. Biliary tract obstruction due to tuberculous adenitis. Am J Med. 1980;68:452–4.
188. Khoury GA, Payne CR, Harvey DR. Tuberculosis of the peritoneal cavity. Br J Surg. 1978;65:808–11.
189. Borhanmanesh F, Hekmat K. Vaezzadeh K, et al. Tuberculous peritonitis. Prospective study of 32 cases in Iran. Ann Intern Med. 1972;76:567–72.
190. Cromartie RS III. Tuberculous peritonitis. Surg Gynecol Obstet. 1977; 144:876–8.
191. Gonnella JS, Hudson EK. Clinical patterns of tuberculous peritonitis. Arch Intern Med. 1966;117:164–9.
192. Sochocky S. Tuberculous peritonitis. A review of 100 cases. Am Rev Respir Dis. 1967;95:398–401.
193. Singh MM, Bhargava AN, Jain KP. Tuberculous peritonitis. An evaluation of pathogenetic mechanisms, diagnostic procedures and therapeutic measures. N Engl J Med. 1969;281:1091–4.
194. Johnston FF, Sanford JP. Tuberculous peritonitis. Ann Intern Med. 1961;54:1125–33.
195. Burack WR, Hollister RM. Tuberculous peritonitis. A study of forty-seven proved cases encountered by a general medical unit in twenty-five years. Am J Med. 1960;28:510–23.
196. Karney WW, O'Donahue JM, Ostrow JH, et al. The spectrum of tuberculous peritonitis. Chest. 1977;72:310–5.
197. Bastani B, Shariatzadeh MR, Dehdashti F. Tuberculous peritonitis—report of 30 cases and review of the literature. Q J Med. 1985;56:549–57.
198. Summers GD, McNicol MW. Tuberculosis of superficial lymph nodes. Br J Dis Chest. 1980;74:369–73.
199. Bloomberg TJ, Dow CJ. Contemporary mediastinal tuberculosis. Thorax. 1980;35:392–6.
200. Beyt BE Jr, Ortbals DW, Santa Cruz DJ, et al. Cutaneous mycobacteriosis: Analysis of 34 cases with a new classification of the disease. Medicine. 1981;60:95–109.
201. Rohwedder JJ. Upper respiratory tract tuberculosis. Sixteen cases in a general hospital. Ann Intern Med. 1974;80:708–13.
202. Lindell MM Jr, Jing BS, Wallace S. Laryngeal tuberculosis. Am J Roentgenol. 1977;129:677–80.
203. Windle-Taylor PC, Bailey CM. Tuberculous otitis media: A series of 22 patients. Laryngoscope. 1980;90:1039–44.
204. Skolnik PR, Nadol JB Jr, Baker AS. Tuberculosis of the middle ear: Review of the literature with an instructive case report. Rev Infect Dis. 1986;8:403–10.
205. Volini FI, Olfield RC Jr, Thompson JR, et al. Tuberculosis of the aorta. JAMA. 1962;181:78–83.
206. Felson B, Akers PV, Hall GS, et al. Mycotic tuberculous aneurysm of the thoracic aorta. JAMA. 1977;237:1104–8.
207. Ni C, Papale JJ, Robinson NL, et al. Uveal tuberculosis. Int Ophthalmol Clin. 1982;22:103–24.
208. Hamit HF, Ragsdale TH. Mammary tuberculosis. J R Soc Med. 1982;75:764–5.
209. Harrison NK, Knight RK. Tuberculosis of the nasopharynx misdiagnosed as Wegener's granulomatosis. Thorax. 1986;41:219–20.
210. Vita JA, Silverberg SJ, Goland RS, et al. Clinical clues to the cause of Addison's disease. Am J Med. 1985;78:461–6.
211. Beyt BE Jr, Ortbals DW, Santa Cruz DJ, et al. Cutaneous mycobacteriosus: Analysis of 34 cases with a new classification of the disease. Medicine. 1981;60:95.
212. Centers for Disease Control. Tuberculosis Control Division. Tuberculosis in the United States, 1979. Atlanta: Centers for Disease Control; 1981:4–31.

230. MYCOBACTERIUM LEPRAE (LEPROSY)

WARD E. BULLOCK

Leprosy is one of the major unconquered infectious diseases of the world, with the total number of cases exceeding 12 million.[1] Of these, approximately 25 percent bear some form of physical disability as a consequence of the infection.[2] It has been stated with great accuracy that "leprosy is a disease which affects the body of the patient and the mind of the public."[3] Thus, in addition to the medical problems of leprosy, the economic and social consequences are staggering. Until recently, the major burden of the leprosy problem has fallen on the nations with limited resources. However, within the past 20 years, the nations of Western Europe and North America have committed greater support to the study of leprosy, with the result that our understanding of this disease has expanded considerably.

Many physicians in the United States possess limited knowledge of leprosy despite the fact that the number of reported cases in this country is increasing steadily, primarily as the result of increased immigration. In fact, the ratio of native-born to foreign-born cases has shifted from 1:1 during the period 1949–1968 to 1:3.[4] More than 75 percent of 1139 cases reported from 1985 through 1987 occurred in foreign-born persons, with the majority having emigrated from Mexico, the Philippines, Kampuchea, American Somoa, Vietnam, Laos, and India. The number of reported cases is an unknown but probably small fraction of those who actually have leprosy since it is not a reportable disease. Misdiagnosis is common, and when a correct diagnosis is made, many persons insist that the nature of their problem be kept secret. Furthermore, those among the significant population of illegal aliens in the United States who may have a chronic medical problem such as leprosy are not likely to seek medical attention readily. Thus, as our society becomes increasingly cosmopolitan, it behooves all physicians to hone their diagnostic acumen for leprosy to spare patients the ravages of a disease that can only thrive on misdiagnosis or neglect.

MICROBIOLOGIC CHARACTERISTICS OF MYCOBACTERIUM LEPRAE

To date, all attempts to culture *Mycobacterium leprae* in tissue culture or in a synthetic medium have failed. Therefore, information on the microbiology of this organism is extremely limited. When stained by the Ziehl-Neelsen method, it is visualized as an acid-alcohol-fast, slightly curved bacillus, 0.3–0.4 × 4–7 μm, sometimes containing a metachromatic granule near a pole or in the center. The function of these granules is unknown. That the leprosy bacillus is a member of the Mycobacteriaceae is indicated by the fact that it contains mycolic acids characteristic of mycobacteria; these acids are most closely related to the types present in *Mycobacterium tuberculosis* and *M. kan-*

sasii.[5] *Mycobacterium leprae* contains large amounts (2 percent of dry weight) of a specific phenolic glycolipid that contains a particular trisaccharide that apparently is unique to this organism.[6] It also possesses a superficial network of ropelike peptidoglycolipid filaments, the morphologic characteristics and structure of which resemble the surface filaments characteristic of other mycobacteria.[7] Lastly, the leprosy bacillus contains multiple antigens common to other mycobacteria.[8]

The proof that an acid-fast-staining organism that fails to grow in culture truly is *M. leprae* must, of course, be indirect until the cultivation problem is solved. Properties considered to be most specific for *M. leprae* are (*1*) the loss of its acid-fast property by pyridine extraction,[9] although there is debate as to whether this phenomenon is observed exclusively in *M. leprae*. Certainly if a mycobacterial strain fails to lose acid fastness after pyridine extraction, it is probably *not M. leprae*. (*2*) A characteristic growth curve occurs in the footpads of mice with an unusually slow doubling time (11–13 days) in logarithmic phase.[10] Other spp. of mycobacteria either do not multiply in the mouse footpad or grow there more rapidly and produce distinguishable pathology. (*3*) *Mycobacterium leprae* has the ability to oxidize 3,4-dihydroxyphenylalanine (DOPA) enzymatically to pigmented products.[11] Most known spp. of mycobacteria have been found not to contain phenoloxidase activity. Unfortunately, testing for DOPA-oxidase activity is complicated because of a tendency for the substrate to undergo auto-oxidation, which is catalyzed by cations such as copper. (*4*) A characteristic tendency is to infect peripheral nerves of humans or armadillos infected experimentally.[12] No other known *Mycobacterium* possesses this characteristic.

Mycobacterium leprae from either human or armadillo tissue contains large amounts of a unique phenolic glycolipid termed PGL-I. This antigen has a trisaccharide, 3,6-di-o-methyl-β-D-glucopyranosyl-(1 → 4)-2,3-di-o-methyl-α-L-rhamnopyranosyl-(1 → 2)-3-o-methyl-α-L-rhamnopyranose, which elicits a strong antibody response in patients with multibacillary leprosy.[13] Both the natural trisaccharide and synthetic antigens containing the terminal 3,6-di-o-methyl-β-D-glucopyranosyl group have been used for serologic screening, largely using the enzyme-linked immunosorbent assay (ELISA).[13,14] Insensitivity to paucibacillary cases and cross-reactivity with other *Mycobacteria* have limited the use of these tests in diagnosis. Monoclonal antibodies have been prepared that recognize these and other determinants of *M. leprae*.[15,16]

EPIDEMIOLOGY

The epidemiology of leprosy is not well understood, since many years may pass between infection with *M. leprae* and the actual onset of clinical manifestations due to the very slow generation time of this organism. It is generally held that human patients discharging *M. leprae* are the only primary sources of infection. Of interest, however, is the discovery of a naturally occurring, leprosy-like disease among wild armadillos, which suggests that other reservoirs of leprosy may exist in nature.[17]

Many workers have assumed that leprosy is transmitted by direct skin-to-skin contact since a skin lesion is the most frequently recognized early sign and infection rates are highest among children living in close proximity to patients with very bacilliferous forms of the disease (i.e., lepromatous leprosy). Thus, in a typical endemic area, the estimated risk of contracting leprosy is four times higher in household contacts of lepromatous patients than in contacts of tuberculoid cases (paucibacillary) and approximately eight times higher than in noncontacts.[18] Studies on the cell-mediated immune response to *M. leprae* by healthy persons whose job assignments place them in various degrees of contact with leprosy patients indicate that positive responses are higher among those in close contact with the patients.[19]

The role of the skin in the transmission of leprosy has been challenged, since the number of acid-fast bacilli shed from the intact skin of lepromatous patients is very small.[20] On the other hand, the nasal discharge from these persons contains approximately 1×10^8 acid-fast organisms per milliliter,[21] which is equivalent to the number of *M. tuberculosis* in sputum of patients with cavitary pulmonary tuberculosis. This, plus the observation that *M. leprae* may remain viable in dried nasal secretions for several days,[22] suggests that primary infection may be acquired via the respiratory tract. Other potential sources of infection include breast milk, which, in lepromatous patients, contains large numbers of bacilli,[23] and biting insects from which viable acid-fast bacilli have been recovered for at least 72 hours after feeding on lepromatous patients.[24]

Leprosy occurs in all races, although reliable comparisons of relative resistance by race are unavailable. Nevertheless, it is well known that the frequency of the two polar types of leprosy, that is, tuberculoid and lepromatous, varies considerably, both racially and geographically. About 20 percent of the known cases in India are lepromatous, whereas the prevalence is 30–50 percent among whites and among orientals of Japan, China, and Korea. Conversely, tuberculoid cases may constitute up to 90 percent of the total prevalence in endemic areas of Africa.[25] It is likely that genetic factors influence susceptibility to leprosy, although there is as yet no conclusive evidence to support this hypothesis. Concordance of leprosy in monozygotic twins is not sufficiently high to indicate clearly a genetic predisposition, and tests of genetic polymorphic systems have failed to detect significant differences between tuberculoid and lepromatous patients.[26] Studies of human leukocyte antigen (HLA)-phenotype frequencies among leprous patients and controls have yielded inconsistent results.[27,28]

CLINICAL MANIFESTATIONS

The spectrum of disease activity in leprosy is very broad, and it is the position of a person on this spectrum that determines his or her infectivity and long-term prognosis, as well as the likelihood of experiencing damaging nerve reactions or the distressing complication of erythema nodosum. Therefore, it is essential to classify accurately disease activity by careful clinical and histologic evaluation. A widely accepted classification of leprosy is the five-group system of Ridley and Jopling,[29] in which a progression from the most limited form of disease to generalized disease is as follows:

> TT, full tuberculoid → BT, borderline tuberculoid → BB, borderline → BL, borderline lepromatous → LL, full lepromatous.

Persons classified within the borderline zone of the spectrum tend to be clinically unstable and usually move toward the tuberculoid or lepromatous poles, which tend to be regions of greater disease stability.

The Clinical Spectrum

Lesions of TT and BT leprosy typically manifest as large, erythematous plaques with sharply demarcated, raised outer edges. The center usually is flattened, dry, and hairless. *The area is anesthetic*. Sometimes lesions manifest as erythematous or hypopigmented macules; they are few and may be found anywhere except in warmer regions of the body, such as the groin, axilla, and perineum. Damage to peripheral nerves is usually confined to one or two, which may be visibly swollen, as commonly occurs in the greater auricular or superficial peroneal nerves.

In BB leprosy, skin manifestations are more numerous, and satellite lesions may be present near the periphery of larger plaques. The lesions usually are irregularly shaped, erythematous plaques with poorly defined edges and a hypopigmented center, or they may be "target-like" annular lesions formed by a raised erythematous band. The presence of nodules excludes

TT and BT infection. Anesthesia is less marked, and thickened superficial nerves, although more numerous than in TT disease, are less grossly infiltrated.

Patients presenting with BL to LL disease will have extensive skin involvement distributed bilaterally and symmetrically as erythematous macules, papules, or nodules (Figs. 1 and 2). Occasionally in early LL cases, infiltration of the dermis is so diffuse that it imparts a smooth, shiny appearance to the skin, which may appear otherwise normal. As the infection advances, thickening of the facial skin deepens the lines in the forehead and thickens the nose and ears to impart the classic leonine facies. "Succulent" thickening of the ear pinna and lobes is a valuable clinical sign. Eventually there is loss of eyebrows (madarosis) and eyelashes, along with destruction of the nasomaxillary structures. Many patients complain of a chronically "stuffy nose" secondary to atrophic rhinitis. Epistaxis is frequent and later, progressive infection may lead to dacryocystitis, perforation of the nasal septum, destruction of the nasal cartilages, and atrophy of the anterior nasal spine and maxillary aveolar process in the area of the upper incisors.[30] Ophthalmic involvement is also common, (see the section below on "Complications"). Nerve involvement in LL disease is diffuse, although less severe than in tuberculoid cases. Palpable nerve thickening is uncommon, and sensory loss is patchy, typical of mononeuritis multiplex.

Other signs that can provide valuable clues for diagnosis of lepromatous leprosy include (*1*) the presence of a brawny edema involving the feet, lower legs, and dorsal aspects of the hands and digits; swelling of the latter imparts a fusiform, shiny appearance suggestive of scleroderma; (*2*) the presence of erythema nodosum, that is, erythema nodosum leprosum (ENL). Unlike the localized, pretibial erythema nodosum associated with most other conditions, ENL is generally widely disseminated and often involves the face; (*3*) the presence in 10–20 percent of the males of testicular atrophy and gynecomastia as the result of testicular damage by granulomatous pathology.[31]

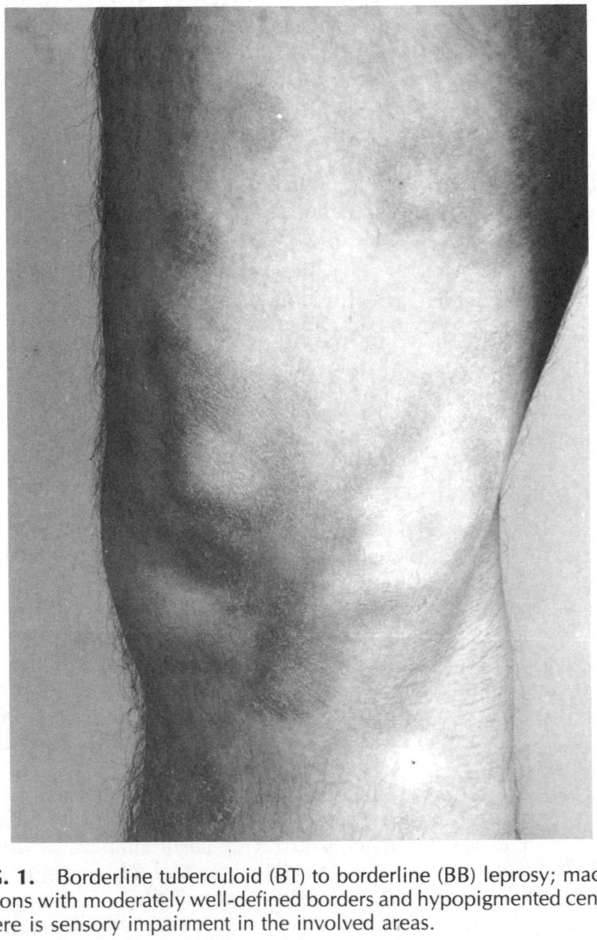

FIG. 1. Borderline tuberculoid (BT) to borderline (BB) leprosy; macular lesions with moderately well-defined borders and hypopigmented centers. There is sensory impairment in the involved areas.

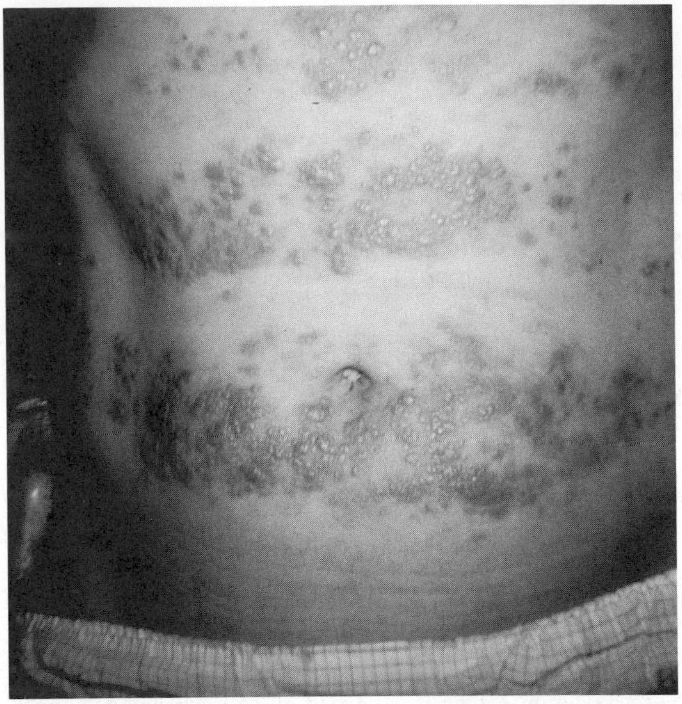

FIG. 2. Lepromatous leprosy (LL); extensive papule formation over abdomen. Minimal or no sensory loss is present in the involved areas.

The Histologic Spectrum

Biopsy specimens of skin lesions from those with TT or BT infection reveal histopathologic changes that are difficult to distinguish from those of sarcoidosis. Within the dermis are foci (often scant) of well-developed epithelioid cells extending into the papillary stroma up to the basal cells of the epidermis. Langhan-type giant cells generally are present, and the granuloma is extensively infiltrated by lymphocytes. A sine qua non for diagnosis is the finding of nerve bundles that are grossly swollen and infiltrated with mononuclear inflammatory cells. Acid-fast bacilli are few or absent. Granulomas have been observed in organs of the reticuloendothelial system; however, the prevalence of these lesions is not established.

As the transition is made through BB and BL to LL forms of leprosy, very distinct changes become evident in the nature of the granulomatous inflammation.[32] The predominant cell type is the macrophage, in which there are typical foamy changes. Langhan-type giant cells are absent, lymphocytes are few, and epithelioid cell formation is poorly developed. Acid-fast bacilli are numerous and in polar cases, 1 g of skin tissue may contain up to 1×10^9 organisms. Characteristically, the granulomatous infiltrate within the dermis remains separated from the basal layer of the epidermis by a thin band of stroma called the *clear zone*. Although there is extensive proliferation of the bacilli within Schwann cells and perineural cells of nerve bundles, structural preservation of axons is better than in tuberculoid disease. A summary of the skin histopathologic changes throughout the spectrum of leprosy is presented in Table 1.

Granulomatous pathologic changes frequently occur in the liver, spleen, and lymph nodes. Within lymph nodes, the paracortical regions are infiltrated by masses of macrophages laden

TABLE 1. Immunologic Manifestations within the Leprosy Spectrum

Manifestation	TT	BT	BB	BL	LL
Lepromin reaction	3+	1+	±	—	—
ENL	—	—	—	±	2+
Bacilli in nose	—	—	—	1+	2+
Bacilli in granuloma	0	1–3+	3–4+	4–5+	5–6+
Epithelioid cells	1+	1+	1+	—	—
Langhan giant cells	1+	2+	—	—	—
Foam cells	—	—	—	1+	3+
Lymphocytes	3+	2+	1+	1+	±
Nerve destruction (skin)	2+	2+	1+	±	—

(Adapted from Ridley,[81] with permission.)

TABLE 2. Abnormal Serologic Activities Associated with Lepromatous Leprosy

Abnormality	Reference No.
False-position VDRL test (>10%)[a]	37
"Autoantibodies"	
To testicular germinal cells[b]	38
To thyroglobulin[b]	39
Antinuclear factors (0–30%)	40
Rheumatoid factor (0–50%)	41
Amyloid-related serum component protein (>50%)	42
Elevated serum C-reactive protein[b] (>50%)	43
Circulating suppressor factor(s)[b]	44, 45
Elevated serum chemotactic factor inactivator[b]	46
Cryoglobulinemia (>30%)	47
Circulating immune complexes[b]	48, 49

[a] Figures in parentheses represent approximate prevalence based on published literature.
[b] Prevalence not established.

with leprae bacilli, which appear to displace large numbers of thymus-derived (T) lymphocytes that normally occupy this area. Germinal centers usually are not involved by the granulomatous pathologic changes and are frequently increased in size and number.[33] Within the spleen, the periarteriolar lymphocyte sheaths of the white pulp frequently are damaged by infiltrates of vacuolated macrophages, and sinusoidal cords of the red pulp are often involved as well.[34]

The Immunologic Spectrum

Persons with tuberculoid disease are capable of manifesting delayed-type hypersensitivity (DTH) to skin tests with antigens of *M. leprae*, and their peripheral blood lymphocytes undergo blast transformation in response to these antigens in vitro. Conversely, the lepromatous patient is profoundly anergic to *M. leprae* by both in vitro and in vivo testing. The most widely available material for skin testing with *M. leprae* antigens is integral lepromin, a crude preparation from the nodules of lepromatous patients. Positive reactions to this lepromin are biphasic in nature, the first phase manifesting as transient erythema and induration, which is maximal at 24–48 hours (the Fernandez reaction). Subsequently, there is progressive nodule formation, which peaks at 3–4 weeks. This phase of the lepromin reaction is considered to be weakly positive when the diameter of nodule formation is between 3 and 5 mm and to be strongly positive when it is greater than 5 mm with ulceration. Histologic examination of a positive reaction reveals a tuberculoid type of inflammation, as described above. The lepromin reaction is not specific since most normal persons produce a positive reaction.

In addition to anergy specific for *M. leprae*, there is also a generalized nonspecific impairment of the DTH response among many patients with lepromatous leprosy. This is reflected by poor skin test reactivity to a variety of microbial antigens and haptens (picryl chloride or dinitrochlorobenzene) as compared with a control population.[35]

Immunoglobulin levels tend to be within normal ranges among tuberculoid patients, whereas polyclonal hypergammaglobulinemia is characteristic of lepromatous leprosy.[36] From 75 to 95 percent of lepromatous sera contain antibodies to *M. leprae* that cross react with other mycobacteria. Furthermore, a number of abnormal serologic activities, which are summarized in Table 2, have been observed in lepromatous patients.

COMPLICATIONS

Erythema Nodosum Leprosum

ENL is a most troublesome complication that occurs only in the more bacilliferous cases at the LL end of the spectrum. The majority of LL patients develop ENL in association with therapy, usually during the first year. Occasionally, however, medical assistance will be sought for the first time because of ENL, which may be triggered by pregnancy, by stress, and by significant alcohol ingestion. Histopathologically, the lesions resemble Arthus-type reactions with localized proliferative vasculitis in which the walls of arteries and veins are invaded by polymorphonuclear cells and eosinophils.[32] Endarteritis and endophlebitis also are common. In severe cases, ENL may persist for months with very high fever, necrosis of the nodules, and leukemoid reactions. Frequently, ENL is associated with polyarthralgia and excruciatingly painful neuritis that can result in sudden loss of peripheral nerve function (e.g., complete foot drop) as the result of increased inflammatory activity within nerve bundles.[50] Red cells and casts are found in the urine of many patients, and biopsy specimens may reveal an immune complex type of glomerulonephritis.[36] Untreated, severe ENL may result in death.

Reversal Reactions

Patients with BL or subpolar forms of lepromatous leprosy who have been maintained on effective therapy for several months may experience reversal reactions. Typically, the leprous skin infiltrates rapidly develop a brawny, raised induration that is erythematous and shiny. In severe cases, the lesions may ulcerate. Associated neuritis is common with nerve swelling, and motor function may be lost in some cases. Histologic examination of lesions in reversal reaction characteristically reveals local diminution in the number of bacilli present, edema formation, and increased numbers of lymphocytes within the inflammatory cell infiltrate. Thus, these reactions appear to represent a localized "upgrading" of the host immune response.

Other Reactions

Nerve abscesses are not uncommon and require surgical drainage. Acute orchitis and tibial periostitis are encountered occasionally and may require corticosteroid therapy, as does an uncommon form of cutaneous vasculitis known as the *Lucio's phenomenon*.[51] This occurs almost exclusively in patients from Latin America who have diffuse lepromatous leprosy.

Deformity

Deformity of the nasomaxillary facial structures results in large measure from primary infection by *M. leprae*, whereas deformity of the hands and feet is secondary to the pathologic changes in the peripheral nerves, with the consequent loss of sensory and motor function. The dysfunctioning and anesthetic hand or foot is extremely susceptible to damage, and if protective and corrective measures are not instituted, repeated trauma and infection will lead to serious deformities as a result of chronic ulceration and resorption of bone in the digits.

Amyloidosis

Secondary amyloidosis is not uncommon in lepromatous patients; however, the prevalence appears to vary somewhat in different geographic areas, ranging from approximately 2 to 31 percent in reported studies.[36] The serum of most LL patients contains elevated levels of a nonimmunoglobulin, amyloid-related serum protein component that is antigenically related to the fibrillar protein found in tissue deposits of secondary amyloid[42]; the role played by this serum component in the formation of amyloid deposits has not been established.

Ophthalmic Complications

Pathologic changes involving the anterior segment of the eye have been observed in 25–30 percent of the patients with LL disease.[52] The lesions frequently detected in these patients are conjunctivitis, superficial punctate keratitis, and leprotic iridocyclitis. The last is insidious, often without pain and, if untreated, may lead to blindness as the result of complicated cataract formation and phthisis bulbi.[52] Secondary damage to the eye often occurs as the result of corneal anesthesia, which in turn is due to granulomatous pathologic changes within the ophthalmic division of the fifth nerve. Thus, trichiasis and repeated rubbing of an anesthetic cornea with the hand or sleeve are major causes of chronic ulceration and eventual blindness.

DIFFERENTIAL DIAGNOSIS

There can be no substitute for alertness to the possibility of leprosy when considering dermatologic, neurologic, or multisystem complaints by persons who are not native to North America or to Western Europe. The same consideration applies to those who have worked or performed military service in endemic areas. Specialists in rheumatology should be especially alert to the possibility of leprosy in patients with peculiar skin manifestations and polyarthralgias or neuritis to avoid misdiagnosis of a collagen disorder. Differentiation of leprosy from lupus erythematosus may be difficult, since in both diseases serum antinuclear factors may be present. Furthermore, immunoglobulin deposits in the basement membrane of skin can be demonstrated in both by immunofluorescence microscopy.[53]

The hypoesthetic or anesthetic skin lesion, with or without associated nerve thickening, must be considered first as leprosy pending the results of a skin biopsy, which is the sine qua non for diagnosis. An adequate biopsy must include both central peripheral areas of a lesion and should be deep enough to remove subcutaneous fatty tissue en bloc. For this reason, an elliptical excisional biopsy, at least 12–15 mm long, is preferred rather than a punch biopsy. In most cases, the diagnosis of BL or LL leprosy can be established fairly easily by examining histologic preparations stained with hematoxylin and eosin and with *special* acid-fast stains. The latter are essential because *M. leprae* in paraffinized tissues frequently is not acid-fast when stained by the Ziehl-Neelsen method. However, the acid-fast property can be restored by clearing the section and impregnating it with an oily substance, such as turpentine or peanut oil, as practiced in the widely used Wade-Fite staining technique.[54] Control sections known to contain acid-fast staining organisms must be prepared simultaneously. Examination of skin biopsy specimens from tuberculoid patients is more difficult, and it may be necessary to search for several hours to find even one or two bacilli. If they are to be found, serial sections of dermal nerves offer the best chance of success. *Mycobacterium leprae* will also take silver stains, and, occasionally, silver-stained organisms will be visible in sections where no acid-fast forms can be seen. Other than the demonstration of acid-fast bacilli in biopsy specimens or in smears of tissue fluid and cells obtained by superficially incising the skin with a scalpel, there is no established laboratory test for leprosy.

THERAPY

Special Problems

The treatment of leprosy, especially the lepromatous form, has proved to be a difficult challenge for several reasons. First, only four major antibacterial drugs are available at present for treatment of leprosy, namely, 4,4′-diaminodiphenylsulfone (i.e., dapsone [DDS]), rifampin, clofazimine (Lamprene), and ethionamide. Second, the inability to grow *M. leprae* in vitro greatly hampers efforts to determine rapidly the minimal inhibitory concentration (MIC) of antibiotics against *M. leprae*, as well as to assess the viability of organisms within infected secretions and tissues. Currently, the only method by which the viability of *M. leprae* can be determined is by means of a rather crude in vivo technique whereby the capacity of the organism to undergo limited multiplication in the mouse footpad is quantitated.[55]

The same method is employed to determine the MIC of *M. leprae*. To do so, several groups of mice are maintained on diets containing different percentages of an antibiotic in order to produce a range of mean serum concentrations equivalent to that attained in the serum of patients during treatment. Suspensions of *M. leprae* are prepared from infected tissues, and 10^3–10^4 organisms are inoculated into the footpads of control mice and mice fed drug-containing diets. After 6–8 months, all mice are killed, homogenates of footpads are prepared, and the number of acid-fast bacilli in each footpad is counted. Yields of $\leq 10^5$ organisms per footpad are accepted as evidence of the inhibition of growth by the test drug at the serum concentration achieved via a given dietary intake. Thus, the MIC is determined. Despite its difficulty, this technique has proved invaluable in developing rational approaches to therapy and in monitoring for the emergence of drug resistance.

The therapy of leprosy is complicated further by the fact that antibiotics necessarily must be given for prolonged periods of time and, in some cases, even for life. Consequently, compliance rates are low since leprosy generally is a quiet disease that does not provide a constant reminder to the patient of the need for long-term treatment.

Of great concern has been the emergence of both primary and secondary resistance to DDS as a consequence of its long-term use as monotherapy. Worldwide, the prevalence of secondary resistance currently ranges from 20 to 190 per 1000 leprosy cases, depending on locale. Primary resistance to DDS of varying prevalence and degree also has been reported worldwide.[56] There is good evidence that DDS-resistant leprosy is fully communicable.[57] Recently, rifampin-resistant strains of *M. leprae* were isolated from multibacillary patients who had relapsed after treatment with rifampin.[58] Because of the need for additional drugs, the encouraging results with ofloxacin in mice warrant further study.[59] Additionally, the use of multidrug regimens has become imperative for treatment of all patients with leprosy.

Finally, the problem of drug resistance by *M. leprae* must be distinguished from that of *persistence,* in which a proportion of drug-sensitive bacilli survive in tissues despite years of therapy. Thus, viable *M. leprae*, still sensitive to low concentrations of DDS, have been isolated from patients even after 10 years of "adequate" therapy, presumably because some bacilli remain metabolically inactive and, therefore, insensitive to the drug. Viable, drug-sensitive *M. leprae* also persist despite prolonged therapy with rifampin, alone or in combination with other drugs.[60] It is unlikely that lepra bacilli remain sequestered from antibiotics, as for example, in nerves, since drug penetration into the peripheral nerves of experimental animals by both DDS and rifampin appears to be good.[61] Concentrations of these respective drugs in the infected skin of leprous patients receiving standard dosages also exceed thhe MIC of *M. leprae*.[62]

Principal Drugs

Dapsone. Outstanding qualities of DDS include its low cost, low toxicity, and the exquisite sensitivity of nonresistant strains of *M. leprae* to its action as a blocker of the *p*-aminobenzoic acid condensation reaction necessary for bacterial folate synthesis. The usual daily dosage is 50–100 mg/day given orally (po). Twenty-four hours after ingestion of 100 mg of DDS, the plasma concentration in a 60-kg person may range from approximately 0.41 to 1.2 μg/ml.[55] This rather wide range is explained by the fact that there are large individual differences in the rates of DDS clearance from the body as the result of genetic polymorphism in the acetylation of DDS. Thus, the half-life ($T_{1/2}$) in plasma varies from approximately 10 to 50 hours, with an average of 28 hours.[55] Regardless of individual acetylator status, however, plasma levels of DDS on daily therapy remain well in excess of the MIC for *M. leprae*, which lies between 0.01 and 0.001 μg/ml.[63] Patients should be checked for glucose-6-phosphate dehydrogenase deficiency before institution of DDS therapy to avoid severe hemolytic episodes. Other toxic effects of DDS that occur uncommonly include agranulocytosis (1 in 10,000 cases), hypoalbuminemia, and an infectious mononucleosis-like syndrome that may be fatal.[64]

Rifampin. The MIC of rifampin against *M. leprae* is less than 1 μg/ml, and it provides a rapid bactericidal effect against organisms in tissues and nasal secretions.[65] As little as a 4-week period of therapy with rifampin prevents multiplication in the mouse footpad of acid-fast bacilli harvested from tissue specimens or nasal secretions of patients with lepromatous leprosy. By contrast, a comparable loss of infectivity cannot be achieved with DDS until 10–12 weeks of treatment.[65]

Institution of rifampin therapy also rapidly reduces the morphologic index (MI) of *M. leprae*; the MI is a measure that expresses the percentage of solidly staining (and, therefore, presumably viable) bacilli within the tissues of patients with multibacillary disease. As depicted in Figure 2, the MI of *M. leprae* in lepromatous patients falls to nearly zero within 4 weeks after starting rifampin therapy, whereas between 3 and 6 months may be required for comparable reduction of the MI after beginning DDS treatment. Although the MI and, therefore, the infectivity of *M. leprae* for mouse footpads decrease rapidly after administration of rifampin, the bacterial index (BI) (i.e., the concentration of morphologically identifiable bacilli in a skin smear or biopsy) declines very slowly in lepromatous patients, often requiring years to reach zero (Fig. 3). Clearly, then, the typical patient with lepromatous leprosy has difficulty not only in disposing of viable *M. leprae* but in clearing nonviable organisms as well. The nature of this dysfunction is unknown but is regarded by many as key to gaining an understanding of the immune deficit(s) that permit the indolent yet inexorable development of the lepromatous state.

Clofazimine. Clofazimine (B663) is a phenazine imino-quinone derivative that is effective in the treatment of leprosy, although its mechanism of action is not well understood. There is some evidence that it may act by inhibiting template formation of the DNA.[66] Clofazimine is highly lipophilic and is deposited within fatty tissues, the skin, and the reticuloendothelial system, where it is taken up by macrophages.[67] Since the compound is a dye, the skin becomes pigmented over time with a coloration varying from a reddish hue to a deep purple. The latter occurs most commonly with high-dosage therapy and is accentuated in the areas of skin infiltrates of patients with lepromatous leprosy.[68] After discontinuation of clofazimine, the pigmentation clears gradually over a period of several months to years. The manner in which the drug is metabolized in the body is poorly understood. It is eliminated very slowly with a $T_{1/2}$ after oral administration that is at least 70 days.[69] Urinary excretion is negligible, whereas approximately 50 percent of an administered dose may be recovered unchanged from the feces, possibly secondary to incomplete absorption from the gut and excretion via the bile, in which high concentrations have been reported.[70] When clofazimine is given in high concentrations (200–300 mg/day) for extended periods of time, it is deposited in the small intestinal wall, thereby causing segmental thickening, which may be associated with midabdominal burning or cramping pain, diarrhea, and, rarely, partial small bowel obstruction.[71]

Ethionamide and Prothionamide. Experience with these drugs in antileprosy therapy is limited. Experiments in mice suggest that they are virtually identical in their activity against *M. leprae* and appear to kill the organism more rapidly than a full dosage of DDS.[56] Both drugs are more expensive than DDS and may induce hepatic toxicity. Hence, they are not regarded

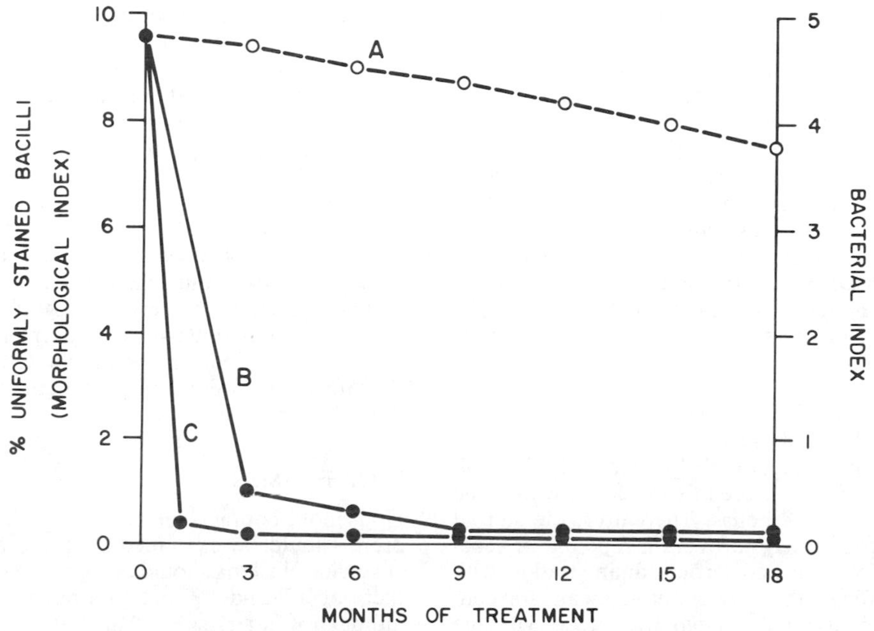

FIG. 3. Effect of treatment on the proportion of uniformly stained bacilli (morphologic index, MI) and bacterial index (BI) in a typical patient with lepromatous leprosy. **(A)** Fall in BI during treatment with dapsone, rifampin, or both drugs; **(B)** fall in MI during dapsone treatment; **(C)** fall in MI during treatment with rifampin or rifampin plus dapsone.

as antibiotics of first choice to be included in multidrug regimens for treatment of lepromatous leprosy.

Current Recommendations for Therapy

In 1982, the World Health Organization (WHO) published new recommendations that multidrug therapy be employed for all forms of leprosy.[56] The principal aim of such therapy is to stem the increase in prevalence of primary and secondary resistance to DDS by *M. leprae* and to reduce the duration of treatment. For treatment of multibacillary forms of leprosy (BB, BL, and LL types), the following triple-drug combination is suggested: (*1*) DDS, 50–100 mg daily, po, self-administered, (*2*) clofazimine, 50 mg daily, po, self-administered, plus a 300-mg dose given once monthly under supervision; and (*3*) rifampin, 600 mg, po, once monthly under supervision. Where clofazimine is totally unacceptable, ethionamide should be considered in a dosage of 250–375 mg daily, po, self-administered.

Combined therapy should be given for a *minimum* of 2 years; if possible, such therapy should be continued until the test results of all skin scrapings and skin biopsies become negative for acid-fast bacilli, a process that may require several years.

The recommendation for intermittent rifampin treatment is made in part because of the heavy, economic burden that the cost of the drug places upon nations with a high prevalence of leprosy. The scientific rationale for this recommendation is based upon limited clinical trials and upon studies of intermittent chemotherapy in the mouse footpad infection model.[65] Despite the early promise of intermittent rifampin therapy and the low incidence of reactions to the drug given in this manner (influenza-like syndrome, thrombocytopenic purpura, and shock), the WHO recommendation is, nevertheless, based upon incomplete data. Therefore, when possible, the author prefers to administer 450 or 600 mg of rifampin daily for a period of 2–3 years.[72]

For treatment of paucibacillary disease (indeterminant, TT, and BT types), the WHO recommends administration of 600 mg rifampin po, once per month under supervision for a 6-month period plus 100 mg DDS po, daily for 6 months, self-administered. If relapse occurs, the treatment regimen is to be repeated. The incidence of relapse depends on the classification and stage of leprosy at the initiation of therapy.[73]

The rationale for this regimen is based on the fact that the number of *M. leprae* in patients with paucibacillary disease rarely exceeds 10^6. Therefore, the risk is quite low of selecting drug-resistant mutants as a result of the drug treatment. In addition, the cell-mediated immune defense mechanisms of these patients are better able to deal with the leprosy bacillus than are those of patients with multibacillary disease.[36] It should be emphasized, however, that the long-term efficacy of intermittent rifampin therapy as recommended by the WHO for paucibacillary disease has not been established. For this reason, some physicians experienced in the treatment of leprosy elect to treat such cases with DDS, 50–100 mg daily, plus rifampin, 450–600 mg daily, for a period of 6 months with continued DDS therapy for a period of 2–5 years.

Treatment of Reactional States

Corticosteroids are the drugs of choice for treatment of severe ENL or reversal reactions. Typically, the patient with ENL will require between 60 and 80 mg of prednisone daily, with some improvement expected after 48 hours. Thereafter, the steroid dosage should be tapered slowly to avoid a rebound of reactional activity. Heretofore, corticosteroid administration with its attendant hazards offered the only effective means for control of ENL. A significant breakthrough was made with the discovery that thalidomide is remarkably effective in treating ENL.[74] Even severe ENL usually is controlled by an oral dosage of 300 mg/day. Generally, this dosage can be tapered over several weeks to 100 mg given at bedtime. The teratogenicity of thalidomide limits its use. However, in situations where pregnancy is not a consideration, prolonged administration has been associated with relatively few side effects. These include drowsiness, eosinophilia, and thrombocytopenia. The mechanism by which thalidomide exerts an anti-inflammatory effect in ENL has not yet been established.

Thalidomide is ineffective against reversal reactions; therefore, high-dose corticosteroid therapy is the mainstay of treatment. Clofazimine in a high dosage of 300 mg, po, per day, exerts an anti-inflammatory effect upon reversal actions and may be employed to augment corticosteroid therapy.[72] After administration of clofazimine in high dosage for 2–4 weeks, it is usually possible to begin tapering both drugs. This must be done carefully, however, as reversal reactions tend to be considerably more persistent and more difficult to treat than ENL.

At no time should specific antileprosy therapy be suspended during the course of treatment for reactional states.

The majority of the patients with leprosy in North America probably can be treated by the general physician with assistance, if need be, from the United States Public Health Service Hospital for Leprosy at Carville, Louisiana, or similar centers in other nations. It is particularly helpful to refer to specialized centers patients who are judged to have possible sulfone-resistant disease, intractable ENL, deformity, and/or marked sensory loss in the hands and feet. Otherwise, patients may be managed in offices, clinics, and hospitals without the necessity of isolation.[75]

Immunotherapy

The problem of drug resistance, microbial persistence, and consequent high rates of relapse in lepromatous leprosy, 1–6 percent per year,[76] clearly indicate the need for immunotherapeutic modalities capable of augmenting the cellular immune response. To date, attempts to improve this response have been rather limited, since the extraordinary complexity of immune defenses against facultative or obligate intracellular pathogens is still poorly understood. Transfer factor therapy has been used in a small number of well-studied patients, and the results suggest that partial correction of the immunologic defect may have been achieved as indicated by accelerated clearing of *M. leprae* from tissues and by histologic evidence for induration of a tuberculoid type of inflammatory response in some lesions with influx of lymphocytes and development of epithelioid and giant cells.[34,77] Clinically, this inflammatory response is recognized by an increase in erythema and edema within lesions, of a type similar to that observed in the more permanent reactions experienced by 10–15 percent of the patients with BL disease *after* the bacterial load has been reduced by treatment for several months.

Currently, clinical trials are underway to assess the therapeutic efficacy of repeated vaccinations with a mixture of heat-killed *M. leprae* and viable Calmette-Guérin bacillus (BCG). Although preliminary results suggest possible benefit from this therapy,[78] well-controlled studies must be conducted before definitive conclusions can be drawn. Other studies are evaluating the effects of administering interleukin-2 or interferon-γ to multibacillary patients.[79]

PROPHYLAXIS

Household contacts of patients with leprosy, especially children, should be examined carefully for signs of leprosy, and suspicious lesions should be biopsied. As a rule, household contacts of TT and BT patients need not be given prophylaxis, although it is advisable that they be examined annually. Children who have had extended household contact with highly bacilliferous persons (i.e., BL or LL) who are shedding organisms in the nasal mucus or from open skin lesions should be considered for DDS prophylaxis, which has been shown to be of value in children under the age of 16 when given according to recommended dosage schedules.[80] Adults appear to be less susceptible to leprosy, and since the efficacy of DDS prophylaxis in this group has not been established, there are no definite recommendations for preventive treatment of older age groups.

Three major trials to determine the preventive role of BCG vaccine against leprosy have yielded different results. Hence, it is not yet possible to recommend BCG as a specific prophylactic measure for prevention of leprosy.[1]

Clinical trials of a vaccine composed of heat-killed *M. leprae* are in progress under the supervision of WHO. However, at least a decade of follow-up will be required before its efficacy can be evaluated.

ACKNOWLEDGMENT

This work was supported by United States Public Health Service Grant NAID 16308.

REFERENCES

1. WHO Expert Committee on Leprosy. Fifth report. Tech Rep Ser. 1977;607.
2. Bechelli LM, Martinez Dominquez V. The leprosy problem in the world. Bull WHO. 1966;34:811.
3. Antia NH. The people we fail to reach. Lepr Rev. 1977;48:155.
4. Enna CD, Jacobson RR, Trautman JR, et al. Leprosy in the United States (1967–1976). Public Health Rep. 1978;93:468.
5. Etemadi AH, Convit J. Mycolic acids for "noncultivable" mycobacteria. Infect Immun. 1974;10:236.
6. Hunter SW, Brennan PJ. A novel phenolic glycolipid from *Mycobacterium leprae* possibly involved in immunogenicity and pathogenicity. J Bacteriol. 1981;147:728.
7. Gordon J, White RG. Surface peptido-glycolipid filaments on *Mycobacterium leprae*. Clin Exp Immunol. 1971;9:539.
8. Navalkar RG, Norlin M, Ouchterlony O. Characterization of leprosy sera with various mycobacterial antigens using double-in-gel analysis, II. Int Arch Allergy. 1965;28:250.
9. Fisher CA, Barksdale L. Cytochemical reactions of human leprosy bacilli and mycobacteria: Ultrastructural implications. J Bacteriol. 1973;113:1389.
10. Shepard CC. The first decade in experimental leprosy. Bull WHO. 1971;44:821.
11. Prabhakaran K, Kirchheimer WF, Harris EB. Oxidation of phenolic compounds by *Mycobacterium leprae* and inhibition of phenolase by substrate analogues and copper chelators. J Bacteriol. 1968;95:2051.
12. Binford CH, Storrs EE, Walsh GP. Disseminated infection in the nine-banded armadillo (*Dasypus novemcinctus*) resulting from inoculation with *M. leprae*: Observations made on 15 animals studied at autopsy. Int J Lepr. 1976;44:80.
13. Chanteau S, Cartel JL, Roux J, et al. Comparison of synthetic antigens for detecting antibodies to phenolic glycolipid I in patients with leprosy and their household contacts. J Infect Dis. 1988;157:770–6.
14. Burgess PJ, Fine PE, Ponnighaus JM, et al. Serological tests in leprosy. The sensitivity, specificity and predictive value of ELISA tests based on phenolic glycolipid antigens, and the implications for their use in epidemiological studies. Epidemiol Infect. 1988;101:159–71.
15. Locniskar M, Zumia A, Mudd DW, et al. Human monoclonal antibodies to phenolic glycolipid-I derived from patients with leprosy, and production of specific anti-idiotypes. Immunology. 1988;64:245–51.
16. Gaylord H, Brennan PJ. Leprosy and the leprosy bacillus; Recent developments in characterization of antigens and immunology of the disease. Ann Rev Microbiol. 1987;41:645.
17. Walsh GP, Storrs EE, Meyers WM, et al. Naturally acquired leprosy-like disease in the nine-banded armadillo (*Dasypus novemcinctus*). Recent epizootiologic findings. J Reticuloendothel Soc. 1977;22:363.
18. Doull JA, Guinto RS, Rodriguez JN, et al. The incidence of leprosy in Cordova and Talisay, Cebu, P.I. Int J Lepr. 1972;10:107.
19. Myrvang B, Negassi K, Lofgren M, et al. Immune responsiveness to *Mycobacterium leprae* of healthy humans. Acta Pathol Microbiol Scand. Sect C. 1975;83:43.
20. Pedley JC: Summary of results of a search of the skin surface for *Mycobacterium leprae*. Lepr Rev. 1970;41:167.
21. Shepard CC. The nasal excretion of *Mycobacterium leprae* in leprosy. Int J Lepr. 1962;30:10.
22. Desikan KV. Viability of *Mycobacterium leprae* outside the human body. Lepr Rev. 1977;48:231.
23. Pedley JC. The presence of *M. leprae* in the lumina of the female mammary gland. Lepr Rev. 1968;39:201.
24. Narayanan E, Shankara Manja K, Bedi BMS, et al. Arthropod feeding experiments in lepromatous leprosy. Lepr Rev. 1972;43:188.
25. Bechelli LM, Martinez Dominguez V. Further information on the leprosy problem in the world. Bull WHO. 1972;46:523.
26. Chakravartti MR, Vogel F. A twin study on leprosy. In: P.E. Becker, W. Lenz, F. Vogel, G. G. Went, eds. Topics in Human Genetics. v. 1. Stuttgart: Thieme; 1973:1–29.
27. Rea TH, Levan NE, Terasaki P. Histocompatibility antigens in patients with leprosy. J Infect Dis. 1976;134:615.
28. Rawlinson WD, Basten A, Britton WJ, et al. Leprosy and immunity: Genetics and immune function in multiple case families. Immunol Cell Biol. 1988;66:9–21.
29. Ridley DS, Jopling WH. Classification of leprosy according to immunity. Int J Lepr. 1966;31:255.
30. Reichart P. Facial and oral manifestations in leprosy. Oral Surg. 1976;41:355.
31. Morley JE, Distiller LA, Sagel J, et al. Hormonal changes associated with testicular atrophy and gynecomastia in patients with leprosy. Clin Endocrinol. 1977;6:299.
32. Ridley DS. Skin biopsy in leprosy. Documenta Geigy. Basel: CIBA-Geigy; 1977.
33. Turk JL, Waters MFR. Immunological significance of changes in lymph nodes across the leprosy spectrum. Clin Exp Immunol. 1971;8:363.
34. Bullock WE. Leprosy: A model of immunological perturbation in chronic infection. J Infect Dis. 1978;137:341.
35. Bullock WE. Studies of immune mechanisms in leprosy: I. Depression of delayed allergic response to skin test antigens. N Engl J Med. 1968;278:298.
36. Bullock WE. Immunobiology of leprosy. In: Good RA, ed. Immunology of Human Infection. New York: Plenum Press; 1981:369.
37. Kent JF, Otero AG, Harrigan RE. Relative specificity of serologic tests for syphilis in *Mycobacterium leprae* infection. Am J Clin Pathol. 1957;27:539.
38. Wall JR, Wright DJM. Antibodies against testicular germinal cells in lepromatous leprosy. Clin Exp Immunol. 1974;17:51.
39. Bonomo L, Dammacco F. Characterization of thyroglobulin antibodies in leprosy: An immunological study of diethylaminoethylcellulose chromatographic fractions. Immunology. 1967;13:565.
40. Bonomo L, Tursi A, Trimigliozzi G, et al. L.E. cells and antinuclear factors in leprosy. Br Med J. 1965;2:689.
41. Cathcart ES, Williams RC Jr, Ross H, et al. The relationship of the latex fixation test to the clinical and serologic manifestations of leprosy. Am J Med. 1961;31:758.
42. Kronvall G, Husby G, Samuel D, et al. Amyloid-related serum component (protein ASC) in leprosy patients. Infect Immun. 1975;11:969.
43. Bush OB Jr. C-reactive protein in leprosy. Int J Lepr. 1958;26:123.
44. Bullock WE, Fasal P. Studies of immune mechanisms in leprosy: III. The role of cellular and humoral factors in impairment of the in vitro immune response. J Immunol. 1971;106:888.
45. Nelson DS, Penrose JM, Waters MFR, et al. Depressive effect of serum from patients with leprosy on mixed lymphocyte reactions: Influence of anti-leprosy treatment. Clin Exp Immunol. 1975;22:385.
46. Ward PA, Goralnick S, Bullock WE. Defective leukotaxis in patients with lepromatous leprosy. J Lab Clin Med. 1976;87:1025.
47. Bonomo L, Dammacco F. Immune complex cryoglobulinaemia in lepromatous leprosy: A pathogenic approach to some clinical features of leprosy. Clin Exp Immunol. 1971;9:175.
48. Gelber RH, Drutz DJ, Epstein WV, et al. Clinical correlates of Clq-precipitating substances in the sera of patients with leprosy. Am J Trop Med Hyg. 1974;23:471.
49. Tung KSK, Kim B, Bjorvatn B, et al. Discrepancy between Clq deviation and Raji cell tests in detection of circulating immune complexes in patients with leprosy. J Infect Dis. 1977;136:216.
50. Pearson JMH, Ross WF. Nerve involvement in leprosy—pathology, differential diagnosis and principles of management. Lepr Rev. 1975;46:199.
51. Rea TH, Levan NE. Lucio's phenomenon and diffuse nonnodular lepromatous leprosy. Arch Dermatol. 1978;114:1023.
52. Choyce DP. The eyes in leprosy. In: Cochrane RG, Davey TF, eds. Leprosy in Theory and Practice. 2nd ed. Baltimore: Williams and Wilkins; 1964:310.
53. Bullock WE, Callerame ML, Panner BJ. Immunohistologic alteration of skin and ultrastructural changes of glomerular basement membranes in leprosy. Am J Trop Med Hyg. 1974;23:78.
54. Wade HW. Demonstration of acid-fast bacilli in tissue sections. Am J Pathol. 1952;28:157.
55. Shepard CC, Ellard GA, Levy L, et al. Experimental chemotherapy of leprosy. Bull WHO. 1976;53:425.
56. WHO Study Group. Chemotherapy of leprosy for control programmes. WHO Tech Rep Ser. 1982;675:7.
57. Jesudasan K, Pannikar V, Christian M. Infectivity of secondary dapsone-resistant cases. Int J Lepr. Other Mycobacteriol Dis. 1988;56:418–21.
58. Guelpa-Lauras CC, Grosset J, Constant-Desportes M, et al. Nine cases of rifampin-resistant leprosy. Int J Lepr. 1984;52:101.
59. Grosset JH, Guelpa-Lauras CC, Perani EG, et al. Activity of ofloxacin against *Mycobacterium leprae* in the mouse. Int J Lepr. Other Mycobacteriol Dis. 1988;56:259–64.
60. Rees RJW, Waters MFR, Pearson JMH, et al. Long-term treatment of dapsone-resistant leprosy with rifampin: Clinical and bacteriological status. Int J Lepr. 1976;44:159.
61. Allen BW, Ellard GA, Gammon TP, et al. The penetration of dapsone, rifampicin, isoniazid and pyrazinamide into peripheral nerves. Br J Pharmacol. 1975;55:151.
62. Peters JH, Murray JF Jr, Gordon GR, et al. Metabolic–bacteriologic relationships in the chemotherapy of lepromatous patients with dapsone or dapsone-rifampin. Int J Lepr. 1978;46:115.

63. Gelber R, Peters JH, Gordon GR, et al. The polymorphic acetylation of dapsone in man. Clin Pharm Ther. 1971;12:225.
64. Frey HM, Gershon AA, Borkowsky W, et al. Fatal dapsone syndrome in a patient treated for lepromatous leprosy. Ann Intern Med. 1981;94:77.
65. Bullock WE. Rifampin in the treatment of leprosy. Rev Infect Dis. 1983;5(Suppl 3):606.
66. Morrison NE, Marley GM. Clofazimine binding studies with deoxyribonucleic acid. Int J Lepr. 1976;44:475.
67. Yawalkar SJ, Vischer W. Lamprene in leprosy. Basle: Ciba Geigy; 1978.
68. Levy L, Randall HP. A study of skin pigmentation by clofazimine. Int J Lepr. 1970;38:404.
69. Levy L. Pharmacologic studies of clofazimine. Am J Trop Med Hyg 1974;23:1097.
70. Mansfield RE. Systemic tissue concentrations of clofazimine (B663). Am J Trop Med Hyg. 1974;23:1116.
71. Mason GH, Ellis-Pegler RB, Arthur JF. Clofazimine and eosinophilic enteritis. Lepr Rev. 1977;48:175.
72. Jacobson RR. The treatment of leprosy (Hansen's disease). Hosp Formulary. 1982;17:1076.
73. Docrrigten G, Ponnighaus JM, Fine PE. Preliminary appraisal of a WHO-recommended multiple drug regimen in paucibacillary leprosy patients in Malawi. Int J Lepr. Other Mycobacteriol Dis. 1988;56:408–17.
74. Iyer CGS, Languillon J, Ramanujam K, et al. WHO coordinated short-term double-bind trial with thalidomide in the treatment of acute lepra reactions in male lepromatous patients. Bull WHO. 1971;45:719.
75. Isolation techniques for use in hospitals. U.S. Public Health Service SDS No. 017-0231-00094-2. Washington, DC: US Government Printing Office; 1975.
76. Noordeen SK. Relapse in lepromatous leprosy. Lepr Rev. 1971;42:43.
77. Hastings RC, Job CJ. Reversal reaction in lepromatous leprosy following transfer factor therapy. Am J Trop Med Hyg. 1978;27:995.
78. Convit J, Aranzazu N, Ulrich M, et al. Immunotherapy with a mixture of *Mycobacterium leprae* and BCG in different forms of leprosy and in Mitsuda-negative contacts. Int J Lepr. 1982;50:415.
79. Nathan CF, Kaplan G, Levis WR, et al. Local and systemic effects of intradermal recombinant interferon-γ in patients with lepromatous leprosy. N Engl J Med. 1986;315:6.
80. Filice GA, Fraser DW. Management of household contacts of leprosy patients. Ann Intern Med. 1978;88:538.
81. Ridley DS. Review of the five-group system for the classification of leprosy according to immunity. Int J Lepr. 1972;40:102.

231. OTHER MYCOBACTERIUM SPECIES

W. Eugene Sanders, Jr.
Edward A. Horowitz

The existence of mycobacteria other than the etiologic agents of tuberculosis and leprosy was recognized over a century ago, shortly after the discovery of the tubercle bacillus by Koch in 1882. Despite the occasional isolation of these organisms from clinical specimens, their presence was for many years considered to be a result of contamination or transient colonization. Diagnosis of tuberculosis was made primarily on the basis of acid-fast smears, and cultures were seldom performed. Early culture techniques also minimized the likelihood of recovery of these other mycobacteria. Hence the role of these other organisms in human disease did not become widely recognized until the 1950s.[1] In the past 3 decades, the relative importance of the other mycobacterial species has progressively increased concurrent with the increasing use of more sophisticated microbiologic methods and the continuing decline in the incidence of tuberculosis.[2,3] In many respects, the study of these microorganisms is still in its infancy. In fact, the pathogenetic role of some species has been recognized only during the past 15 years. As with any new science, the study of these mycobacteria is currently marked by excitement, rapid progress, and occasional controversy.

GENERAL CHARACTERISTICS OF OTHER MYCOBACTERIA

Classification and Nomenclature

In the 1950s, Timpe and Runyon[1] and Runyon[4] provided convincing evidence for the role of other mycobacteria in human disease and proposed a useful method for their classification. The classification scheme was based upon pigment production, rate of growth, and colonial characteristics of the organisms. The four major groups have generally become referred to as photochromogenic, scotochromogenic, nonchromogenic (or nonphotochromogenic), and rapidly growing mycobacteria (Table 1). Throughout the years, a variety of species and subspecies of organisms have been identified within each of Runyon's major groups. The more commonly encountered, medically important species are listed in Table 1. Some species designations have become generally accepted, whereas others remain provisional and, occasionally, the subject of controversy. In the practice of medicine, it may be most useful to refer initially to the other mycobacteria by major grouping as proposed by Runyon and, subsequently, by species when laboratory identification is complete. For example, a presumptive diagnosis might be listed first as "pulmonary infection due to other mycobacteria" and then "pulmonary infection due to photochromogenic mycobacteria" as laboratory evaluation progresses. After complete microbiologic study, the definitive diagnosis may be given, namely, "pulmonary infection due to *Mycobacterium kansasii*."

Microbiology

The species of other mycobacteria are differentiated on the basis of a variety of morphologic, physiologic, and biochemical characteristics (Table 1). Because of the slow growth of some isolates, precise identification can require up to several months to complete. For this reason, tests for susceptibility to antimicrobial agents should be initiated as soon as it is apparent that the organism implicated in disease is likely to grow in pure culture. A variety of serologic tests have been devised that permit characterization of species and often types within species.[2–8,10,11] These serologic tests, although not widely available, are useful investigational and epidemiologic tools. They are seldom of value in the diagnosis or management of individual patients.[2,11,12]

Skin Tests

A variety of skin test reagents have been prepared from various species of other mycobacteria. These include purified protein derivative A (PPD-A), PPD-B, PPD-F, PPD-G, and PPD-Y from *M. avium, M. intracellulare, M. fortuitum, M. scrofulaceum*, and *M. kansasii*, respectively. Cross-reactivity among these reagents[13] due to shared antigens[14] has limited their use primarily to epidemiologic studies. However, Margolith[15] has classified 553 tuberculin-positive children as tuberculous or nontuberculous reactors based on the relative sizes of skin reactions to mycobacterial antigens. This correlated strongly with culture results, especially in cases of adenitis due to *M. avium-intracellulare*. Recently, Vandiviere et al.[16] have demonstrated a correlation of skin test profiles of PPD-S (purified protein derivative from *M. tuberculosis*) and five other mycobacterial antigens with the etiology of pulmonary disease determined subsequently by culture. They also found this method to be useful in selecting therapy for culture-negative patients. The use of multiple simultaneous antigen tests would therefore seem to hold promise as a method of rapid diagnosis in the future.

Epidemiology

Many of the other mycobacterial species are ubiquitous. They have been found in soil,[17,18] water,[19,21] domestic and wild an-

TABLE 1. Distinguishing Characteristics of Medically Important Mycobacteria

Organism	Optimum Temp (°C)	Growth Rate (Days)	Niacin	Nitrate Reduction	Catalase 25°	Catalase 68°	Tween Hydrolysis	Urease	Arylsulfatase	Growth in 5% NaCl	Iron Uptake
M. tuberculosis	37	12–28	+	+	Weak	−	−	+	−	−	−
M. bovis	37	21–40	−	−	Weak	−	−	+	−	−	−
Photochromogens (Runyon group I)											
M. kansasii	37	10–21	−	+	Strong	+	+	+	−	−	−
M. marinum	32	7–14	−	−	Weak	±	+	+	−	−	−
M. simiae	37	7–14	+	−	Strong	+	−	+	−	−	−
Scotochromogens (Runyon group II)											
M. scrofulaceum	37	10–28	−	−	Strong	+	−	+	−	−	−
M. szulgai	37	12–28	−	+	Strong	+	±	+	±	−	−
M. gordonae	37	10–28	−	−	Strong	+	+	−	−	−	−
M. flavescens	37	7–10	−	+	Strong	+	+	+	−	+	−
Nonchromogens (Runyon group III)[a]											
M. avium-intracellulare	37	10–21	−	−	Weak	+	−	−	−	−	−
M. xenopi[b]	42	14–28	−	−	Weak	+	−	−	±	−	−
M. ulcerans	32	28–60	−	−	Strong	+	−	−	−	?	?
M. gastri	37	10–21	−	−	Weak	−	+	+	−	−	−
M. terrae	37	10–21	−	+	Strong	+	+	−	−	−	−
M. triviale	37	10–21	−	+	Strong	+	+	−	±	+	?
Rapid growers (Runyon group IV)											
M. fortuitum	37	3–7	−	+	Strong	+	±	+	+	+	+
M. chelonae sp. *abscessus*	37	3–7	−	−	Strong	+	−	+	+	+	−
M. chelonae sp. *chelonae*	37	3–7	−	−	Strong	+	−	+	+	−	−
M. smegmatis	37	3–7	−	+	Strong	±	+	−	−	+	+

[a] See the text for *M. malmoense* and *M. haemophilum*.
[b] Scotochromogenic. Classified here because of shared antigens.
(Data from References 1–9.)

imals,[2,12] milk,[22,23] and other foodstuffs.[24,25] They may contaminate clinical specimens from the environment or transiently colonize body surfaces or secretions.[2,12,26] Even potentially pathogenic isolates such as *M. avium-intracellulare* may be found as contaminants, colonizers, or etiologic agents of human infection—ranging from subclinical to lethal disseminated disease. The reservoirs of most medically important mycobacteria and their relationship to human disease are shown in Table 2. Despite their widespread distribution in nature, many of the potentially pathogenic mycobacterial species appear to be relatively more common in certain geographic locations. These will be described below in the discussion of specific microorganisms. Depending upon locality, infections due to the other mycobacteria have been reported to account for 0.5–30 percent of all mycobacterial infections.[2,12] In a recent survey of state and territorial public health laboratories by the Centers for Disease Control, organisms other than *M. tuberculosis* were found to account for 35 percent of isolations (not cases) of potentially pathogenic mycobacteria.[27]

Most infections with the other mycobacteria appear to be acquired by aspiration or inoculation of the organisms from a natural reservoir. There is very little evidence to suggest person-to-person transmission of disease.[2,12,18,26] Although there are exceptions, serious infections due to the other mycobacteria tend to occur more commonly in males, in adults of middle age or older, and in individuals with one or more predisposing conditions.[2,12]

Pathology

A variety of careful studies have failed to detect gross or microscopic abnormalities that might permit differentiation of one mycobacterial infection from another. Pulmonary tissues from patients infected with *M. tuberculosis, M. kansasii, M. avium-intracellulare*, and several of the less commonly encountered species may appear identical.[28–31] For example, Corpe and Stergus[29] sent for examination sections of tissue infected with either *M. tuberculosis* or *M. avium-intracellulare* to a group of distinguished pathologists. The panel concluded that it was impossible to differentiate the two conditions on the basis of the histologic morphology. Examination of lymph nodes infected with a variety of mycobacterial species has revealed a broad spectrum of possible inflammatory responses.[12,28,32] Both acute and chronic inflammatory responses have been observed. Acute suppuration, non-necrotic epithelioid tubercles, and caseation have been recorded alone or in combination in the same lymph node and in tissues infected by any one of the many mycobacterial species. In general, the other mycobacterial species are less virulent than *M. tuberculosis* in most laboratory animals. The initiation of experimental infection is usually quite difficult, even when the defenses of the animal have been compromised.[12,33,34]

Diagnostic Considerations

The diagnosis of infection due to the other mycobacterial species occasionally may be suspected by the clinician, radiologist, or pathologist, but only the microbiologist can identify the specific etiologic agent.[2] However, unlike tuberculosis where isolation of a single colony of *M. tuberculosis* is always clinically significant, the other mycobacterial species may colonize body surfaces or secretions for prolonged periods without a relationship to disease. In addition, because of their ubiquity in soil, water, and dust, they are frequent contaminants of clinical specimens. Thus, the differentiation between contamination, colonization, and disease is often quite difficult.

Individual patients often pose unique problems, and they may require more or less time and effort than usual to arrive at a specific etiologic diagnosis of disease. However, there are certain general guidelines that have proved useful in most cases.[35–37] First, the patient should have an illness that is consistent with one or more of the syndromes associated with the other mycobacteria (Table 3). Second, other causes of disease such as *M. tuberculosis* or fungi should be excluded. Third, the species

TABLE 2. Reservoirs of Other Mycobacteria with Relationship to Human Disease and the Environment

Mycobacterium	*Human Pathogen*	*Environmental Contaminant*	*Reservoir*
M. tuberculosis	Yes	No	Humans
M. bovis	Yes	No	Humans, cattle, other mammals
M. kansasii	Yes	Rarely	Water, cattle, swine (rarely)
M. marinum	Yes	Rarely	Fish, water
M. simiae	Yes	No	Primates, possibly water
M. scrofulaceum	Yes	Yes	Soil, water, moist or liquid foodstuffs
M. szulgai	Yes	No	Unknown
M. gordonae	Very rarely	Yes	Water
M. flavescens	Very rarely	Yes	Soil, water
M. avium-intracellulare	Yes	Yes	Soil, water, swine, cattle, birds, fowl
M. xenopi	Yes	Yes	Water
M. ulcerans	Yes	No	Unknown
M. gastri	Very rarely	Yes	Soil, water
M. terrae	Very rarely	Yes	Soil, water
M. triviale	No	Yes	Soil, water
M. fortuitum	Yes	Yes	Soil, water, animals, marine life
M. chelonae	Yes	Yes	Soil, water, animals, marine life
M. smegmatis	Very rarely	Possibly	Moist surfaces, urogenital flora

(Data from References 2, 3, and 11–21.)

TABLE 3. Clinical Syndromes Associated with Other Mycobacterial Species

Syndrome	*Relatively Common Causes*	*Less Frequent Causes*
Chronic bronchopulmonary disease (usually adults)	*M. avium-intracellulare, M. kansasii*	*M. szulgai, M. xenopi, M. simiae, M scrofulaceum, M. fortuitum, M. chelonae, M. malmoense*
Cervical or other local lymphadenitis (especially children)	*M. avium-intracellulare, M. scrofulaceum*	*M. kansasii, M. fortuitum, M. chelonae*
Skin and soft tissue		
Swimming pool granuloma	*M. marinum*	
Sporotrichoid	*M. marinum*	*M. fortuitum, M. chelonae, M. kansasii*
Abscesses, ulcers, sinus tracts	*M. fortuitum, M. chelonae*	*M. haemophilum*
Chronic ulcer (Buruli)	*M. ulcerans*	
Hyperimmune reactions	*M. avium-intracellulare, M. kansasii*	
Skeletal (bone, joint, tendon infection)	*M. kansasii, M. avium-intracellulare, M. fortuitum, M. chelonae*	*M. marinum, M. scrofulaceum*
Disseminated infection	*M. avium-intracellulare, M. kansasii*	*M. fortuitum, M. chelonae, M. scrofulaceum*
Genitourinary disease (relatively rare)	*M. avium-intracellulare*	*M. kansasii*

(Data from References 2, 3, and 12.)

of mycobacterium isolated is crucial. Certain species are rarely if ever associated with human disease, whereas others are seldom environmental contaminants and, therefore, demand further attention (Table 2). Fourth, the site of origin of a positive culture is equally crucial. In the absence of environmental contamination, isolation of a potential pathogen from normally sterile tissues or fluids such as liver or cerebrospinal fluid is clearly significant. Isolations of potential pathogens from secretions such as sputum require confirmation and further study. Fifth, the quantity of growth in cultures from *secretions* is important. In general, disease is associated with relatively heavy growth of the other mycobacterial species, whereas very light or "sparse" growth is usually indicative of colonization or contamination. Exceptions occur; most importantly, very light growth may be found in normally sterile fluids or tissues even in the presence of extensive disease. Finally, in the presence of disease, the organism is usually isolated repeatedly from body secretions. One or two random isolations most often signify environmental contamination of the specimen or one of the laboratory reagents. In light of these observations, the American Thoracic Society has adopted the following requirements for the diagnosis of pulmonary disease caused by the other mycobacterium species:

> A definite diagnosis requires (*1*) evidence, such as a infiltrate visible on a chest roentgenogram, of disease, the cause of which has not been determined by careful clinical and laboratory studies and (*2*) either (*a*) isolation of multiple colonies of the same strain of mycobacteria repeatedly, usually in the absence of other pathogens, or (*b*) isolation of the mycobacteria from a closed lesion from which the specimen has been collected and handled under sterile conditions—for example, an abscess or biopsy tissue.[38]

A description of specific organisms and their diseases follows.

MYCOBACTERIUM KANSASII

Microbiology and Epidemiology

Mycobacterium kansasii is a photochromogenic acid-fast bacillus. In clinical specimens, individual bacilli are relatively long and thick and often appear cross-barred.[2] This somewhat distinctive morphology may provide a clue to etiology; however, definitive diagnosis requires isolation by culture. Strains possess a uniform antigenic structure[2] that most closely resembles *M. tuberculosis*.[39] Infection with *M. kansasii* may confer immunity to subsequent challenge with other mycobacteria,[40] and cross-reactions with other skin test reagents are common.[41] Among the frequently encountered other mycobacterial species, *M. kansasii* is one of the least likely to be recovered from nonhuman sources.[17,42] It has been recovered on rare occasions from water, cattle, and swine (Table 2). Laboratory survival data[43] suggest that water rather than soil might be the natural reservoir.

M. kansasii has been identified as an agent of disease in nearly all parts of the world.[2,12,26] It has been implicated in illness throughout the United States, but the highest incidence occurs in the Southwest and Midwest. Its incidence also appears to be relatively high in England and Wales. The organism infects males more commonly than females in a ratio of 3:1.[12] Most patients are in the fifth decade of life. Infection is relatively rare in children, even in families with cases in adults. The disease occurs more commonly in urban areas[44] and affects patients with a higher income and better standard of living than patients with tuberculosis.[45,46] No ethnic group appears especially prone. However, certain occupational groups are at increased risk such as miners, welders, sandblasters, and painters.[12,47] The pneumoconioses predispose to infection, especially in Europe.[12,44] Chronic obstructive pulmonary disease (COPD) is a very common antecedent to lung infection with *M. kansasii*.[48,49] Up to one-third of patients may give a history of an antecedent spontaneous pneumothorax.[50] Severe infections occur occasionally in otherwise healthy individuals.[2,12,48]

Pulmonary Infection

Mycobacterium kansasii characteristically produces a chronic lung infection that closely resembles pulmonary tuberculosis. Symptoms tend to be somewhat milder than in tuberculosis,[46,51] and they may be totally overshadowed by symptoms of underlying COPD. Most often disease is progressive, but in occasional patients it may remain stable for prolonged periods.[52] Physical findings are minimal, as in tuberculosis. Most routine tests are normal. Elevation of the erythrocyte sedimentation rate (ESR) and a slight leukocytosis are usual. Abnormalities on chest roentgenograms are very difficult to distinguish from those due to tuberculosis.[53,54] A variety of often subtle differences have been reported to be more suggestive of infection due to *M. kansasii*[12,41,55] but cannot be relied upon in most individual cases.[56] A typical roentgenogram with a laminogram is shown in Figure 1. A small percentage of patients will develop a pleural effusion. However, effusion without parenchymal lung disease, as is seen in tuberculosis, is very rarely encountered. The appearance of disseminated disease in the lungs is nearly identical to that due to tuberculosis, fungi, and other causes. Since *M. kansasii* may colonize respiratory secretions without a role in disease,[57] the aforementioned general guidelines for diagnosis should be followed. Cultures should be incubated for prolonged periods because concurrent infection with *M. tuberculosis* may occur.[2,12]

Other Clinical Syndromes

Mycobacterium kansasii may infect extrapulmonary tissues directly, often as a result of inoculation or after hematogenous dissemination. Cervical or other local lymphadenitis has been reported occasionally. Diagnosis and management are identical to that described for *M. scrofulaceum* (see below). Inoculation of the skin has resulted in a syndrome resembling sporotrichosis[58,59] or granulomatous lesions.[60] A variety of manifestations of "hyperimmunity"[12] such as erythema nodosum, multiforme, and induratum as well as macular skin lesions may accompany disseminated infection. Osteomyelitis, soft tissue infection, and tenosynovitis occur occasionally. The clinical presentation, pathology, and roentgenographic appearance are identical to those due to *M. tuberculosis* or the other mycobacterial species. Cellulitis clinically indistinguishable from the usual bacterial cellulitis has been described,[61] as has one case of pericarditis.[62] Genitourinary infection is rare.[2,12] A few cases of granulomatous parenchymal disease have been reported. Involvement of the renal pelvis with obstruction and pyonephrosis is distinctly unusual. Urine cultures may be positive during the course of disseminated infection.[63] Dissemination usually occurs in patients with far advanced disease or in those who are profoundly immunocompromised.[64,65] This syndrome is very rare in children, in contrast with the situation with *M. avium-intracellulare* and *M. tuberculosis*. Anemia and leukopenia or pancytopenia are commonly observed in association with disseminated disease. In some patients these hematologic abnormalities have preceded recognition of the infection. In others, the abnormalities have followed dissemination and appear to have resulted from proliferation of the organisms in the bone marrow.[65] Disseminated disease has been observed in association with the acquired immunodeficiency syndrome (AIDS).[66]

Therapy

Mycobacterium kansasii is among the most predictably sensitive of the mycobacterial species. Treatment of experimental infections in animals reveals a moderately good correlation of

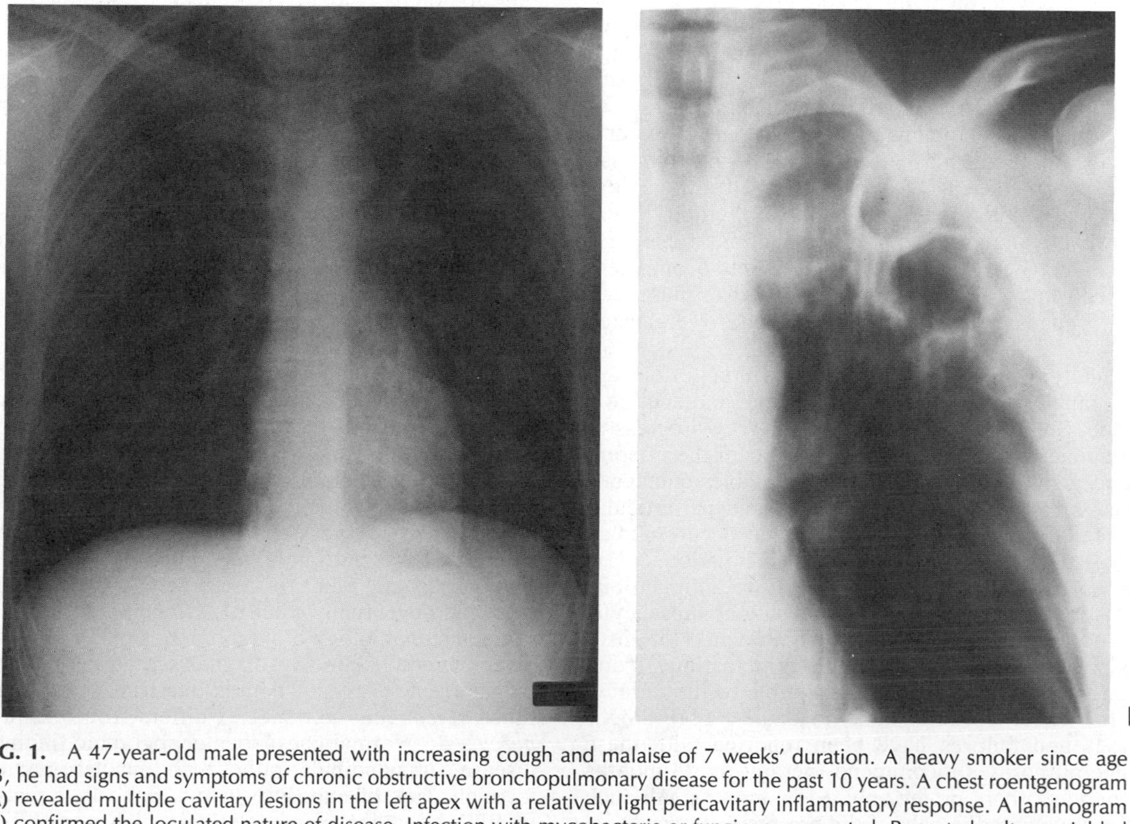

A B

FIG. 1. A 47-year-old male presented with increasing cough and malaise of 7 weeks' duration. A heavy smoker since age 13, he had signs and symptoms of chronic obstructive bronchopulmonary disease for the past 10 years. A chest roentgenogram **(A)** revealed multiple cavitary lesions in the left apex with a relatively light pericavitary inflammatory response. A laminogram **(B)** confirmed the loculated nature of disease. Infection with mycobacteria or fungi was suspected. Repeated cultures yielded heavy growth of *M. kansasii*. His clinical response to chemotherapy with isoniazid, rifampin, and ethambutol was satisfactory.

therapeutic response and in vitro susceptibility. These studies have also demonstrated the importance of using more than one drug to delay or prevent the emergence of resistance during therapy.[12] There have been few carefully controlled clinical studies of treatment in humans, and results of treatment are often difficult to interpret due to the tendency of the disease to improve or remit spontaneously in some (albeit a minority) of infected patients.[52,67] Until recently isoniazid (INH), usually in combination with streptomycin (SM), ethambutol (EMB), or both, has been the mainstay of therapy,[48,50,68] Treatment with these regimens has resulted in conversion of sputum to negative in nearly 90 percent of patients. Unfortunately, relapses have been relatively common (5–15 percent) even when therapy was continued for a year or more after sputum conversion. Recent evidence suggests that multiple-drug regimens containing rifampin (RIF) are superior to combinations lacking this agent.[50,68–70] The role of INH is controversial since *M. kansasii* is usually relatively resistant to this agent in vitro. However, resistance to RIF has developed in patients treated with INH plus RIF and with RIF plus EMB.[71] Therefore, the combination of INH, RIF, and EMB is the current choice for initial treatment. Although a course of 18–24 months has been widely used, preliminary data suggest that 12 months may be adequate in some settings.[72,73] Use of two of the drugs for an additional year may minimize relapse and emergence of resistance. Retreatment regimens should include three drugs not previously used and to which the organism is sensitive. Sulfamethoxazole has recently shown promise as a useful agent in this setting.[71] Surgical resection may be necessary for the management of complications; however, its use does not appear to significantly influence rates of sputum conversion or relapse.[70]

MYCOBACTERIUM MARINUM

Mycobacterium marinum is photochromogenic (Table 1). It grows optimally at approximately 32°C and poorly or not at all at temperatures of 37°C or higher. It shares a variety of antigens with other mycobacteria including *M. tuberculosis*. Infection sensitizes to homologous antigens[74] and to PPD-S.[75,76] Experimental infection confers protection to subsequent challenge with *M. tuberculosis*.[12] *Mycobacterium marinum* inhabits water and marine organisms (Table 2). Infection of humans follows trauma, often minor, in swimming pools, aquariums, or natural bodies of water. Infection may also follow trauma from fish spines or nips by crustaceans. Disease is almost always confined to superficial, cooler body tissues, most often on the extremities. However, one instance of dissemination in this form of the disease has been reported in an immunocompetent child.[77] A spectrum of histopathologic responses has been observed that ranges from frank suppuration to organized granulomas.

Infection usually incubates for 2–8 weeks. Initial lesions appear as small papules that subsequently enlarge and acquire a blue-purple hue. Suppuration then occurs and may progress to ulceration. At times small nodules may appear in the efferent lymphatics and result in a syndrome that resembles cutaneous sporotrichosis. Infections of tendon sheaths and periarticular tissues have been described.[2] Dissemination has occurred in an immunosuppressed patient after renal transplantation.[78] *Mycobacterium marinum* varies in susceptibility to antimicrobial agents. Most strains are resistant to INH, para-aminosalicylic acid (PAS), and SM. RIF and EMB are quite active in vitro. Good results have been obtained with this combination[79,80] and with RIF alone.[81] Some strains are susceptible to the tetracyclines and to trimethoprim-sulfamethoxazole (TMP-SMX). Both successes and failures have been reported with these agents.[82] Some authorities recommend therapy for 18 months or longer, whereas others prefer only a few months. All such reports must be evaluated in light of the presence of occasional spontaneous cures.[83] In general, if the therapeutic response is prompt, it should not be necessary to continue treatment for more than 4–6 weeks after clinical resolution.

MYCOBACTERIUM SIMIAE

Mycobacterium simiae is a photochromogenic acid-fast bacillus. However, in some clinical isolates, pigment production may be slow or scant. If pigment production is poor the organism strongly resembles *M. avium-intracellulare*. Use of the niacin test may promptly differentiate the species. *Mycobacterium simiae* has been isolated from monkeys in captivity and in the wild. It may also be recovered from water. It is a relatively infrequent cause of pulmonary infections.[84,85] Cases have occurred in both monkey handlers and in individuals having no association with these primates. Most patients have given histories of antecedent, nonmycobacterial bronchopulmonary disease. The disease is very difficult to distinguish pathologically and clinically from tuberculosis or other mycobacterial lung infections. Two patients with disseminated infection have been reported.[86] *M. simiae* may also colonize respiratory secretions without a role in disease.[85] In contrast to patients with disease, colonized individuals usually have negative initial acid-fast bacillus smears, fewer positive cultures, and lighter yields of organisms on the few positive cultures. *M. simiae* is resistant to most antimicrobial agents in vitro. Although relatively few patients have been treated, results with multiple-drug regimens have been generally discouraging.[84,85] Whenever possible, selection of drugs should be based upon the results of susceptibility tests. The principles of therapy are the same as those described for infections due to *M. avium-intracellulare* (see below).

MYCOBACTERIUM SCROFULACEUM

Mycobacterium scrofulaceum is a scotochromogenic bacillus that is longer, thicker, and more coarsely beaded than *M. tuberculosis*. Trained microscopists may suspect the presence of this or other mycobacterial species in stained clinical specimens, but precise identification depends upon culture. The vast majority of scotochromogenic mycobacteria are nonpathogenic or very weakly virulent. They are ubiquitous organisms that frequently contaminate specimens, reagents, or standing water. They also readily colonize respiratory secretions of well children and of adult patients with nonmycobacterial disease,[2,12] It is, therefore, important to distinguish *M. scrofulaceum* from these other scotochromogens. *Mycobacterium scrofulaceum* also closely resembles *M. avium-intracellulare* biochemically, antigenically, and in resistance to many chemotherapeutic agents.

M. scrofulaceum is a relatively frequent cause of lymphadenitis and an occasional cause of disease in other tissues. Lymphadenitis due to this organism occurs most commonly in children aged 1–3 years. Secondary cases in households are rare.[87] Lymphadenitis due to *M. scrofulaceum* usually involves a single node or a cluster of nodes in the submandibular area. Other nodes of head, neck, and extremities are involved infrequently. Characteristically, the nodes enlarge slowly over a period of weeks. There are very few local or systemic symptoms. Slight pain may be elicited upon manipulation. Untreated, the infection will usually point to the surface, rupture, form a draining sinus, and eventually calcify. Although minor differences exist in the histopathology of lymph nodes infected with the various mycobacteria, definitive diagnosis requires culture of the etiologic agent.[32] Lymphadenitis due to *M. scrofulaceum* or the other *Mycobacterium* species differs from that due to *M. tuberculosis*. Normal chest roentgenographic findings, unilateral disease, submandibular rather than tonsillar or anterior cervical location, lack of exposure to tuberculosis, negative reactions to PPD in siblings, and relatively high socioeconomic status should suggest infection due to the other mycobacterial species.[2,12,32] Mycobacterial lymphadenitis may resemble that due to cat-scratch disease[32] but may be differentiated by the demonstration of acid-fast bacilli in the tissues. Excision of involved nodes and overlying sinus tract, if present, is almost always curative. Some advocate the use of chemotherapy, but this is seldom necessary with prompt diagnosis and surgery.[2,12,88,89] Relapses are rare.

Infections in other tissues occur occasionally. A very few cases resembling progressive primary tuberculosis have been encountered in children. Rare cases of progressive bronchopulmonary disease in adults have occurred in association with pneumoconioses or extreme debility.[89–91] Occasional infections of bone and soft tissue follow trauma and surgery.[92,93] Disseminated disease is rare. In children, metastatic bone disease may be prominent. Disseminated disease in adults is almost invariably associated with other serious, debilitating illnesses.[2,12] Strains of *M. scrofulaceum* vary in susceptibility to antituberculous and other antibacterial agents such as sulfonamides and erythromycin. There has been little experience with chemotherapy. More often than not the course of the underlying disease appears to have determined the clinical outcome. If possible, therapy should involve the use of three or more drugs that are active in vitro. Initial treatment of serious disease with INH, SM, RIF, and cycloserine (CS) appears reasonable.

MYCOBACTERIUM SZULGAI

First described in 1972,[94] *M. szulgai* is unusual among the scotochromogenic mycobacteria in that clinical isolates have usually been associated with clinical disease. Of the 30 reported cases, 21 involved pulmonary disease similar to that caused by *M. tuberculosis*. Other sites of infection have included skin, olecranon bursa, and cervical lymph nodes. Most of these cases have been recently reviewed.[95,96] One instance of dissemination has been reported, with the organism recovered from sputum, skin lesions, and multiple bone sites.[97] In vitro sensitivity patterns are variable. Very limited in vivo experience suggests that prolonged treatment with three drugs to which the organism is sensitive is rational.

MYCOBACTERIUM AVIUM-INTRACELLULARE

Microbiology and Epidemiology

Microorganisms of the *M. avium* and *M. intracellulare* groups are so similar that they are considered collectively.[2,12] Strains may be differentiated serologically, which may be useful epidemiologically.[2,12,38,98] However, serotyping is not generally available and is seldom helpful in the management of individual patients. *M. avium-intracellulare* has been isolated from soil, water, animals, birds, and foodstuffs.[2,12] It has been shown recently that these organisms can be aerosolized in significant numbers above bodies of water, which suggests that inhalation may be a route for human infection.[99] Humans are frequently colonized, and large segments of certain populations have responded immunologically to these or closely related microorganisms. These organisms are distributed worldwide. Accurate information on their distribution in the United States is not available since there is no mandatory reporting of nontuberculous disease. The best information suggests that immunologic reactivity and symptomatic infection occur throughout the country but are greatest in the Southeast.[2,12,27] The most comprehensive CDC survey[100] of nationwide isolates from October 1981 to September 1983 identified patterns strikingly different from previous surveys. The heavy preponderance of males previously reported was no longer seen, and women actually outnumbered men in the older age groups. Rural cases, previously the majority, were outnumbered by urban cases, although isolates from rural patients were somewhat more likely to represent clinical disease. *M. avium-intracellulare* were the nontuberculous species most frequently isolated from lymph nodes and outnumbered *M. scrofulaceum* by more than five to one. The lungs continue to be the most common site of infection, with pre-existing bronchopulmonary disease a frequent finding. Secondary cases in families have been reported very infrequently[101–103]; however, recent evidence raises the possibility of a genetic predisposition to disease.[104]

Pulmonary Infection

Nearly all cases of symptomatic pulmonary disease occur in adults. Primary pulmonary infections resembling those seen with *M. tuberculosis* are encountered extremely rarely, if at all.[2,12,105] In general, symptoms are quite mild, especially in comparison to tuberculosis and infection due to *M. kansasii*.[106–109] Symptoms of the underlying pulmonary disease, when present, usually predominate. Hemoptysis occurs relatively frequently. Physical examination, routine laboratory tests, and histopathology seldom provide clues to specific etiology. Roentgenographic examination rarely permits differentiation of this infection from tuberculosis, other mycobacterial diseases, or fungal infections (Fig. 2) (see the chest roentgenogram, Fig. 8, in Chapter 56). Subtle differences, somewhat similar to those seen with *M. kansasii*, may raise the suspicion of disease due to these organisms,[54,101–103,110] but confirmation of the diagnosis by culture is necessary. Pulmonary disease due to *M. avium-intracellulare* usually follows an indolent course. However, it may remain relatively stable for prolonged periods, despite persistently positive cultures.[107,109] Rapid progression with or without dissemination appears more likely in patients

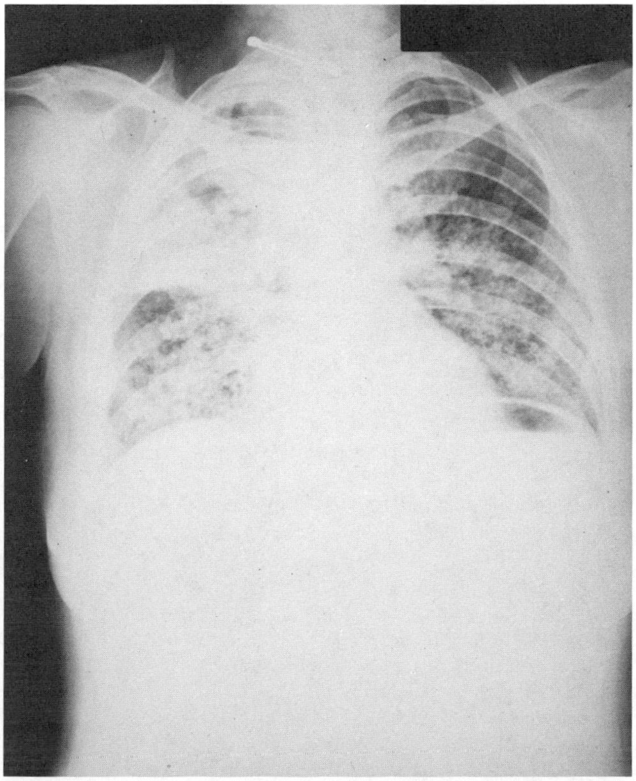

FIG. 2. A 49-year-old woman was admitted with confusion and a low-grade fever. She had a long history of alcohol abuse, liver disease, and gastrointestinal bleeding. Chest roentgenogram after admission revealed extensive bilateral infiltrates consistent with infection due to a variety of possible etiologic agents. Shortly thereafter, the patient developed massive upper gastrointestinal bleeding and hypotension and expired. Postmortem examination revealed disseminated infection with *M. avium-intracellulare* involving the lung, liver, spleen, bone marrow, kidneys, and adrenals.

with severe underlying diseases or extensive infection at time of initial diagnosis.[107,109]

Given the indolent course of most cases and frequent presence of other past or concurrent pulmonary disease, differentiation of active *M. avium-intracellulare* infection from asymptomatic colonization is usually not possible at first encounter. Examination of past radiographs and bacteriologic reports, if available, may be invaluable. In the absence of severe or life-threatening disease, a period of observation while symptoms, radiographs, and sputum cultures are monitored serially is indicated. Repeatedly positive cultures with heavy growth despite a reasonable trial of pulmonary hygiene should be present before a final diagnosis is made.

Other Clinical Syndromes

Mycobacterium avium-intracellulare may cause lymphadenitis indistinguishable from that due to *M. scrofulaceum*.[111] The few instances of lymph node involvement due to true avian strains tend to occur in older children or adults.[112] Treatment is the same as that for *M. scrofulaceum*. Cutaneous manifestations are uncommon. Macronodular lesions may occur during the course of disseminated disease (Fig. 3). Isolated case reports of skin, soft tissue, joint, and bone infections have been summarized by Wolinsky,[2] Chapman,[12] and Namey and Frogameni.[113] Dissemination has occurred in one adult with an infected prosthetic breast implantation[114] and in two children with mastoiditis.[115,116] *Mycobacterium avium-intracellulare* has been isolated from the urine of healthy individuals,[117] patients with disseminated disease and normal genitourinary tracts, and individuals with progressive renal disease similar to that due to *M. tuberculosis*.[12] Patients with disseminated infection have almost always suffered from severe underlying diseases[12,118] although cases in apparently immunocompetent individuals have been reported.[119–121] Osteomyelitis is very common with dissemination, especially in children.[122] It often resembles pyogenic bone infections clinically, although it may progress more slowly.[12] Histopathology of the bone may be consistent with an acute process, with little to suggest a mycobacterial etiology.

Therapy

It is difficult to make definitive recommendations for treatment of *M. avium-intracellulare* infections. Resistance is common, and susceptibilities of individual strains may vary widely.[123–129] No prospective controlled studies to define optimal drug combinations, duration of treatment, or indications for surgical intervention have been performed. Reported retrospective studies[12,50,101,130–139] vary widely in patient populations, extent of disease, therapeutic regimens, and definitions of active disease, relapses, and cures. Such differences make comparisons difficult. The wide resistance of strains of *M. avium-intracellulare* to first-line antimycobacterial agents is presumably a major factor contributing to generally disappointing cure rates. Even so there has been no general agreement on whether or not the use of agents with in vitro activity is related to therapeutic outcome.[2,4] More recently, in a study of 75 patients, responders were shown to have received significantly more drugs to which their isolate was susceptible than did nonresponders.[139] Despite the limited number of patients, potential sam-

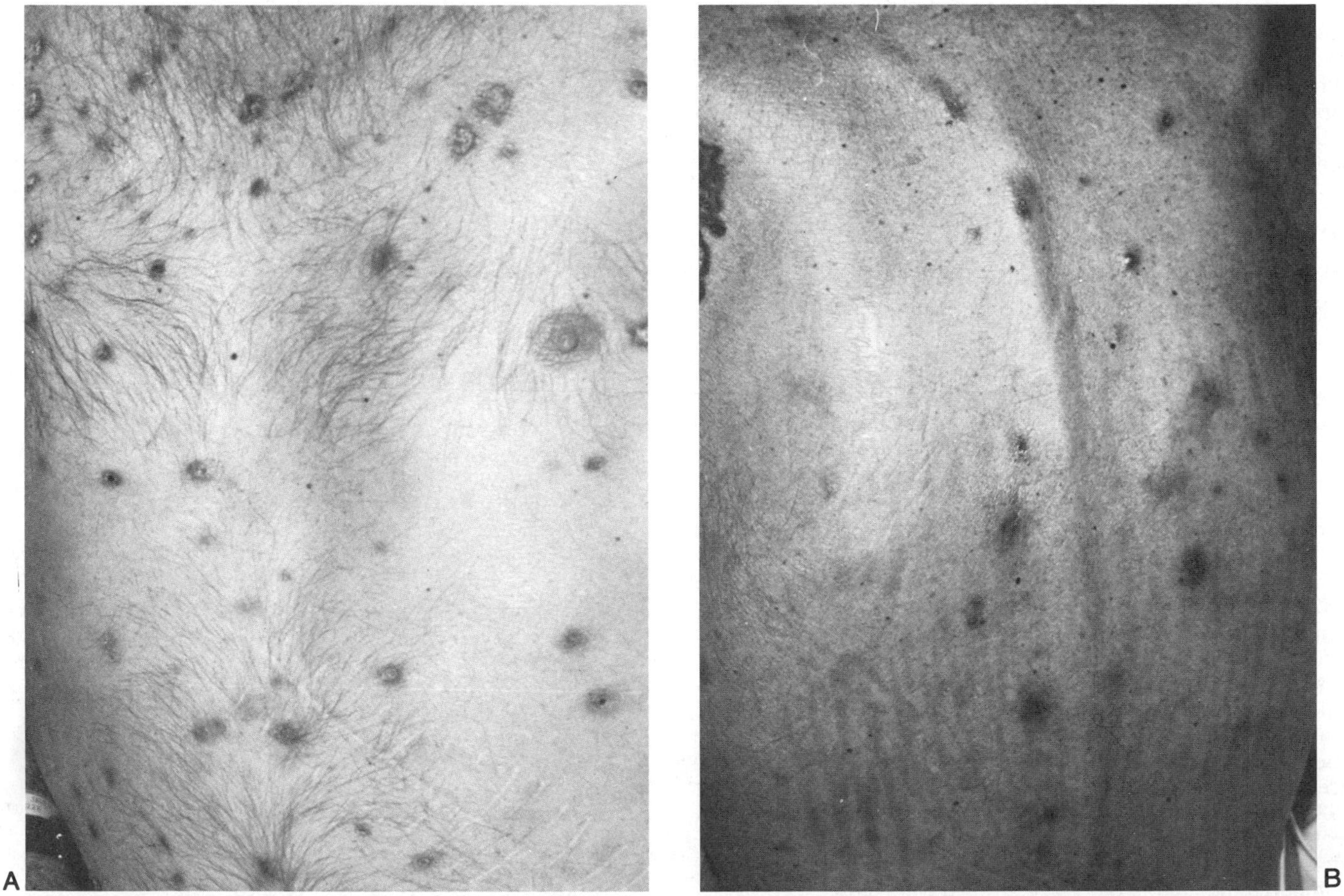

FIG. 3. Maculonodular lesions developed over the chest **(A)** and arms **(B)** of a 59-year-old male with erythroleukemia. Examination of a biopsy specimen of a lesion revealed a poorly organized acute and chronic inflammatory response with large numbers of acid-fast bacilli. Cultures subsequently grew *M. avium-intracellulare*.

pling bias, and imperfect follow-up, the results suggested that it may be prudent to rely on results of susceptibility tests in serious infections until the issue is clarified by further study.

A National Consensus Committee[140] has examined in a thorough and reasoned manner therapeutic issues in light of published data. The consensus recommendations for treatment may be summarized as follows: (1) usual pulmonary infections should be treated with INH, RIF, and EMB for 18–24 months and SM during the first 2–3 months; (2) patients with severe pulmonary disease may benefit from the addition of a fifth or sixth drug (e.g., ethionamide [EM], CS, kanamycin); (3) five- or six-drug regimen, to include rifabutine and clofazimine, is indicated in disseminated disease; (4) resectional surgery combined with chemotherapy may be superior to chemotherapy alone in selected cases; and (5) a solitary pulmonary nodule in an immunologically normal host may be managed with surgical resection alone.

Recently, 46 patients were treated with a uniform four-drug regimen similar to that described above.[137] In 42 (91 percent), sputum cultures converted to negative. Of 10 patients completing 18 months of therapy and followed for 6 months to 4 years, 2 relapsed bacteriologically. Two of 12 patients completing 24 months of therapy reactivated. Interestingly these latter two patients and the four who failed to respond initially had undergone subtotal gastrectomy. Since the two patients who failed on the shorter regimen had not undergone gastrectomy, the investigators concluded that all patients should be treated for 24 months and that gastrectomy should be considered a major risk factor for chemotherapeutic failure.

The Special Problem of Infection in Patients with AIDS

Infection with *M. avium-intracellulare* has become one of the most common complications of AIDS.[141–143] In striking contrast with experience in the pre-AIDS era, most cases present with widespread dissemination. Blood cultures are commonly positive,[144,145] and overwhelming organ involvement is the rule at autopsy.[146] These patients usually have other concurrent opportunistic infections and malignancies, which makes the contribution of this organism to the individual's demise difficult to assess.

Although pulmonary disease similar to that in non-AIDS patients may be seen, most patients present with a gradual onset of fever, night sweats, anorexia, weight loss, and progressive weakness. A gastrointestinal syndrome consisting of abdominal pain, diarrhea, and malabsorption associated with mycobacterial invasion of the intestinal tract has been reported.[147,148] The heavy mycobacterial load combined with the involvement of adjacent lymph nodes has led to the plausible suggestion that the gastrointestinal tract is the organism's portal of entry.[149] Granulomas may be seen in bone marrow and liver biopsy specimens, and their presence in AIDS strongly suggests *M. avium-intracellulare*. However, biopsy material is just as likely to show the presence of acid-fast organisms within foamy macrophages in the absence of well-formed granulomas.

Results of treatment have been generally unsatisfactory, even with the use of agents with a high degree of in vitro activity such as clofazimine and rifabutine.[145,146,150] In fact, with the exception of occasional anecdotal reports of transient clinical improvement or apparent bacteriologic cure,[151] there is little substantive evidence of any predictable or sustained beneficial effect of chemotherapy in the presence of disseminated disease. In vitro data[152] suggest that the poor clinical and bacteriologic response may be related to the lack of mycobactericidal activity of clofazimine and rifabutine at achievable serum levels. As a result, some have replaced rifabutine with RIF, employed amikacin as the aminoglyoside of choice because of its greater bactericidal activity, and selectively added a quinolone to the therapeutic regimen.[153] However, there is at present no evidence that these maneuvers result in improved therapeutic outcome.

The decision whether or not to treat disseminated infection clearly should be individualized.[153] Factors to be considered include severity of infection, the patient's overall state of health, and the potential for drug toxicity or intolerance. In patients in whom the mycobacterial infection appears to be a terminal complication of a far-advanced immunodeficiency state, it may be prudent to withhold chemotherapy. On the other hand, an aggressive trial of therapy may be warranted earlier in the disease when renal and hepatic functions are not severely impaired, the immunodeficiency is less profound, and the patient is informed and likely to be compliant. A five-drug regimen appears rational initially and typically includes amikacin, clofazimine, EMB, RIF or rifabutine, and either INH (only if infection with *M. tuberculosis* is possible), CS, or a quinolone that appears active in vitro. If the patient responds, the aminoglycoside therapy may be discontinued after 4–8 weeks. If the patient fails to respond clinically or microbiologically in 6–8 weeks, it may be appropriate to discontinue antimycobacterial therapy.

Future approaches to chemotherapy for disseminated *M. avium-intracellulare* infections include evaluation of regimens with enhanced mycobactericidal activity or improved penetration into phagocytic cells. Antiviral therapy and the use of immunomodulators offer perhaps the greatest hope for prevention or control of the mycobacterial complications.

MYCOBACTERIUM XENOPI

Mycobacterium xenopi is a scotochromogenic acid-fast bacillus that grows optimally from 42 to 43°C. It is classified with the nonchromogenic organisms because of virulence for birds and antigenic similarities to *M. avium* and *M. intracellulare*. It has been isolated from hot and cold water, including sources in the hospital,[154,155] as well as from other environmental sources.[156] Most infections have resembled pulmonary tuberculosis. Originally thought to be an infrequently encountered and relatively benign disease, recent reviews[156–159] have emphasized an increasing prevalence and the fact that patients may respond unfavorably to chemotherapy or relapse. Patients receiving less than 9 months' treatment in one series[158] invariably had a poor outcome. In vitro sensitivity results were of questionable value. Surgical resection was thought to be beneficial in selected patients not responding to chemotherapy. Empirical therapy should probably include INH, RIF, and either EMB or SM.

Disseminated disease with *M. xenopi* has been reported in a patient with chronic myeloid leukemia treated with busulphan,[160] in two patients with AIDS,[161,162] and in one patient without obvious immune deficiency.[163] The latter patient may have had endocarditis due to *M. xenopi* on a porcine mitral valve.[164]

MYCOBACTERIUM MALMOENSE

This nonphotochromogenic species was first described as a pathogen in 1977 when it was isolated from four patients with pulmonary disease from Malmö, Sweden.[165] Most subsequent reports have been from England, Scotland, and Wales.[166–170] In retrospect, isolates from as far back as 1954 have been recognized.[171] Interestingly, the incidence of disease in the United Kingdom seems to be increasing.[171] To date, five clinical isolates have been reported in the United States.[172,173] At least three of these have represented clinical illness. The organism is microaerophilic and slow growing, sometimes requiring 8–12 weeks for colonies to become visible. It grows at 25 and 37°C, but not at 45°C. Its biochemical profile is similar to that of the *M. avium-intracellulare* complex. It typically but not always hydrolyzes Tween. In the latter case, it may be mistaken for the *M. terrae* complex. In contrast to the broad resistance of the *M. avium-intracellulare* group, most strains of *M. malmoense* are sensitive to EM and CS. This is sometimes the clue leading to the correct identification. Definitive identification is made when the characteristic surface lipid pattern is demonstrated on thin-layer chromatography.

Most infections reported to date have involved the lung. A few cases of adenitis and two instances of disseminated disease[171,174] have been described. Pulmonary disease is clinically and radiographically indistinguishable from tuberculosis. Pre-existing chronic lung disease is frequently present. The organism is usually resistant in vitro to INH, pyrazinamide, and PAS; variably sensitive to RIF and SM; and sensitive to CS and EM. Nevertheless, the best clinical outcomes seem to result from treatment with INH, RIF, and EMB for at least 12 months. Of interest in this regard is a brief report[175] demonstrating that two-drug combinations may lower the minimum inhibitory concentrations (MICs) of each individual drug in vitro.

MYCOBACTERIUM HAEMOPHILUM

This nonchromogenic species was first described in 1978[176] when isolated from skin abscesses of an immunosuppressed patient with Hodgkin's disease. Its unique characteristic is a requirement of hemoglobin or hemin for growth. Optimal growth temperature has variously been reported as 20, 28, and 32°C, but growth is very much retarded at 37°C. Growth may be stimulated by the presence of 10% CO_2. The incubation period is variable, and 8 weeks may be required for colonies to become visible. Fifteen cases of disease with this organism have been reported. Aside from one case of submandibular lymphadenitis in a normal child,[177] these have involved skin and subcutaneous lesions in immunocompromised adults.[176,178–181] Granulomas and numerous acid-fast bacilli may be seen on biopsy specimens. In vitro susceptibilities to antimycobacterial and other antibacterial agents are quite variable and of dubious clinical relevance. All cases so far have responded to combinations of surgery, modification of immunosuppressive drugs, and a variety of antimycobacterial and other agents (doxycycline, TMP-SMX). This limited experience makes it difficult to know which if any of these agents provides optimal treatment or, indeed, if drug treatment is even required for cure.

MYCOBACTERIUM ULCERANS

Mycobacterium ulcerans is an acid-fast bacillus that grows only between 30 and 35°C. It is a cause of chronic, relatively painless, cutaneous (Buruli or Bairnsdale) ulcers. Disease is most prevalent in Australia and Africa; however, cases have been reported in Mexico[182] and in a Nigerian immigrant to the United States.[183] The organism may cause extensive, undermined ulcers, primarily on the extensor surfaces of the extremities. The process begins as a nodule that ulcerates over a period of 4–6 weeks. The centers of the ulcers are necrotic, without caseation, while the organisms are located at the periphery, adjacent to normal tissue.[184] Experience in therapy has been limited and uncontrolled. Success has been reported with local heat,[182] excision and grafting,[182] the combination of SM-INH or diaminodiphenylsulfone (DDS) plus oxytetracycline,[185] and the combination of TMP-SMX, RIF, and minocycline.[186]

RARE PATHOGENS

M. gordonae, M. terrae, M. asiaticum, M. gastri, M. thermoresistibile, M. flavescens, M. smegmatis, and *M. paratuberculosis* are species that are occasionally isolated from clinical specimens and usually regarded as nonpathogenic commensals or environmental contaminants. However, recent reports have shown that all but the last-named can occasionally cause pulmonary and extrapulmonary disease in humans.[187–197a] Therapeutic experience is limited, but chemotherapy has appeared to be efficacious in many of these cases. These organisms can no longer always be ignored, but clinical infection is still a very rare event, and strict diagnostic criteria should be fulfilled before decisions regarding treatment are made.

Preliminary evidence linking an organism similar to *M. paratuberculosis* to Crohn's disease is intriguing.[198,199] However, controversy has been engendered by conflicting data and failure to meet Koch's postulates.

RAPIDLY GROWING MYCOBACTERIA

Microbiology and Epidemiology

The rapidly growing mycobacteria are acid-fast rods that resemble diphtheroids on Gram stain. On primary isolation, they may require from 2 to 30 days for growth. Thereafter, they will usually grow well in 1–3 days. They will flourish on most routine laboratory media as well as those designed for isolation of mycobacteria. *M. fortuitum* and *M. chelonae* (formerly *M. chelonei*) are the major pathogens in this group, although closely related organisms have also been implicated in human disease.[200] Subspecies and serotypes of strains have been described, but precise identification to this level is seldom useful except in epidemiologic investigations. These ubiquitous organisms readily survive nutritional deprivation and extremes of temperature. They may be recovered readily from soil, dust, and water. They have been isolated from tap water, municipal water supplies, moist areas in the hospital, contaminated biologicals, aquariums, domestic animals, and marine life. Most human infections are acquired by inoculation after accidental trauma, surgery, or injection. The source of surgical contamination often has been obscure. The water used to cool cardioplegia solution was suggested as the source for at least some patients in an outbreak of sternal osteomyelitis after open heart surgery.[201] Recently, Safranek et al.[202] traced a series of wound infections to contaminated gentian violet used for skin marking by a plastic surgeon. Incubation periods vary from 1 week to 2 years, but most infections occur within 1 month. Pulmonary infection may be acquired hematogenously or by aspiration. There is no evidence to support person-to-person spread.

Clinical Syndromes

A wide variety of clinical syndromes may be encountered.[200–206] Sporadic infections have involved almost every tissue and organ system, and outbreaks have followed cardiothoracic surgery, peritoneal dialysis, hemodialysis, augmentation mammaplasty, and arthroplasty.[200,206–210] Infections of the skin and soft tissues have been encountered most often. They may resemble pyogenic abscesses with an acute inflammatory reaction and suppuration, or they may progress slowly with chronic inflammation, ulceration, sinus tract formation, and exudates that resemble necrosis of fat. Occasionally, cutaneous infections resemble sporotrichosis. Bronchopulmonary infections usually occur after aspiration, especially of lipoidal material.[203] They are most common in individuals with severe underlying diseases such as cystic fibrosis or in patients receiving immunosuppressive therapy. There are no clinical, radiologic, or histopathologic findings that are diagnostic. Furthermore, these organisms may colonize respiratory secretions without a role in disease. The course of disease is highly variable. In most patients, it is chronic and inexorably progressive. In others it may remain stable for prolonged periods, and rarely, spontaneous recovery may occur. Other clinical syndromes include lymphadenitis, keratitis, suppurative arthritis, osteomyelitis, endocarditis (on natural, prosthetic, or porcine valves), meningitis, peritonitis, and bacteremia related to indwelling intravenous catheters. Dissemination tends to occur very late in the course of disease unless the patient is immunocompromised or profoundly debilitated.

Therapy

The most predictably effective therapy for infections due to the rapidly growing mycobacteria is surgical removal of all involved tissues. Unfortunately, this is often not possible, and chemotherapy must be used. The rapidly growing mycobacteria vary widely in their in vitro susceptibilities to antimicrobial agents.[126,127,211–215] Some have been resistant to all currently available drugs. Amikacin is the most predictably active agent, followed by other aminoglycosides, cefoxitin, doxycycline, and RIF. Occasional isolates may be sensitive to EMB, erythromycin, or sulfonamides. Clinical experience with any of these agents is limited. Although a few patients have responded to therapy with a single drug, combinations appear to be preferable because of a high rate of relapse and emergence of drug resistance.[203,212,214] Selection of agents should be guided by results of in vitro susceptibility tests that employ a relatively large inoculum.[216] Presumptive therapy should probably include amikacin plus one or more of the following: doxycycline, cefoxitin, or RIF.[203,216,217] Treatment should be continued for prolonged periods, probably for no fewer than 4–6 weeks after clinical response.[203,214,217] Imipenem-cilastatin, amoxicillin-clavulanate, and ciprofloxacin are among the newer agents that have shown in vitro activity against some strains of rapid growers and merit consideration in future clinical trials.

THE FUTURE

Diagnosis of disease due to the other mycobacterial species is often delayed because of a lack of familiarity with these organisms.[12,203,205] Tragically, mycobacterial diseases are not considered specifically in the curricula of some U.S. medical schools. Education of students, physicians, and laboratory personnel is needed. The present epidemic of AIDS adds urgency to the problem. Research should concentrate upon defining the pathogenesis of mycobacterial disease and identifying new therapeutic modalities.

REFERENCES

1. Timpe A, Runyon EH. Relationship of "atypical" acid-fast bacilli to human disease: Preliminary report. J Lab Clin Med. 1954;44:202–9.
2. Wolinsky E. Nontuberculous mycobacteria and associated diseases. Am Rev Respir Dis. 1979;119:107–59.
3. Woods GL, Washington JA II. Mycobacteria other than *Mycobacterium tuberculosis:* Review of microbiologic and clinical aspects. Rev Infect. Dis. 1987;9:275–94.
4. Runyon EH. Anonymous mycobacteria in pulmonary disease. Med Clin North Am. 1959;43:273–90.
5. Vestal AL. Procedures for the Isolation and Identification of Mycobacteria. Department of Health, Education and Welfare; CDC publication 76-8230, 1975.
6. Kubica GP. Differential identification of mycobacteria. Am Rev Respir Dis. 1973; 107:9–21.
7. Tsukamura M. A review of the methods of identification and differentiation of mycobacteria. Rev Infect Dis. 1981;3:841–61.
8. Kubica GP, Wayne LG. The Mycobacteria. A Sourcebook. part A. New York: Marcel Dekker; 1984:38–41.
9. Wolinsky E. Mycobacteria: Significance of speciation and sensitivity tests. In: Lorian V, ed. Significance of Medical Microbiology in the Care of Patients. Baltimore: Williams & Wilkins; 1982:103–10.
10. Davidson PT. Introduction (International Conference on Atypical Mycobacteria). Rev Infect Dis. 1981;3:816–8.
11. Brennan PJ. Structures of the typing antigens of atypical mycobacteria: A brief review of present knowledge. Rev Infect Dis. 1981;3:905–13.
12. Chapman JS. The Atypical Mycobacteria and Human Mycobacteriosis. New York: Plenum; 1977:200.
13. Johnston WW, Smith DT. Cross reactions with tuberculin on guinea pigs with single and double experimental infections with mycobacteria. Proc Soc Exp Biol Med. 1964;116:1024–8.
14. Castelnuovo G, Morellini M. The antigens of mycobacteria and their identification by immunoelectrophoretic analysis. Am Rev Respir Dis. 1965;92:29–33.
15. Margileth AM. The use of purified protein derivative mycobacterial skin test antigens in children and adolescents: Purified protein derivative skin test results correlated with mycobacterial isolates. Pediatr Infect Dis. 1983;2:225–31.
16. Vandiviere HM, Dillon M, Melvin IG. Atypical mycobacteria causing pulmonary disease: Rapid diagnosis using skin test profiles. South Med J. 1987;80:5–9.
17. Wolinsky E, Rynearson TK. Mycobacteria in soil and their relation to disease-associated strains. Am Rev Respir Dis. 1968;97:1032–7.
18. Chapman JS. The ecology of the atypical mycobacteria. Arch Environ Health. 1971;22:41–6.
19. Goslee S, Wolinsky E. Water as a source of potentially pathogenic mycobacteria. Am Rev Respir Dis. 1976;113:287–92.
20. Gruft H, Falkinham JO III, Parker BC. Recent experience in the epidemiology of disease caused by atypical mycobacteria. Rev Infect Dis. 1981;3:990–6.
21. Gruft H. Strains of *Mycobacterium kansasii* with weak catalase activity. Am Rev Respir Dis. 1972;106:119–20.
22. Harrington R Jr, Karlson AG. Destruction of various kinds of mycobacteria in milk by pasteurization. Appl Microbiol. 1965;13:494–5.
23. Chapman JS, Speight M. Isolation of atypical mycobacteria from pasteurized milk. Am Rev Respir Dis. 1968;98:1052–4.
24. Stafseth HJ, Buggar RJ, Thompson WH, et al. The cultivation and egg-transmission of the avian tubercle bacillus. J Am Vet Med Assoc. 1934;85:342.
25. Tison F, Devulder B, Roos P, et al. Techniques et resultats de la récherche des mycobactéries dans les viandes. Ann Inst Pasteur (Lille). 1966;17:156–60.
26. Marks J, Jenkins PA. The opportunist mycobacteria—a 20-year retrospect. Postgrad Med J. 1971;47:705–9.
27. Good RC, Snider DE Jr. Isolation of nontuberculous mycobacteria in the United States, 1980. J Infect Dis. 1982;146:829–33.
28. Chapman JS. The Anonymous Mycobacteria in Human Disease. Springfield, IL: Charles C Thomas; 1960:173.
29. Corpe RF, Stergus I. Is histopathology of nonphotochromogenic mycobacterial infection distinguishable from that caused by *Mycobacterium tuberculosis?* Am Rev Respir Dis. 1963;87:289–91.
30. Elston HR, Parrillo OJ, Meiberger M, et al. Pulmonary mycobacteriosis. Report of seven cases. *Arch Intern Med.* 1964;113:365–72.
31. Feldman WH, Auerbach O. Histopathology of granulomatous pulmonary lesions associated with Battey-type mycobacteria. Proceedings of the 22nd Research Conference in Pulmonary Disease. Washington, DC: U.S. Government Printing Office. 1963:239–46.
32. Reid JD, Wolinsky E. Histopathology of lymphadenitis caused by atypical mycobacteria. Am Rev Respir Dis. 1969;99:8–12.
33. Meissner G. The value of animal models for study of infection due to atypical mycobacteria. Rev Infect Dis. 1981;3:953–9.
34. Gangadharam PR, Pratt PF, Davidson PT. Experimental infections with *Mycobacterium intracellulare.* Rev Infect Dis. 1981;3:973–8.
35. Wolinsky E. When is an infection disease? Rev Infect Dis. 1981;3:1025–7.
36. Anonymous. Diagnostic Standards and Classification of Tuberculosis and Other Mycobacterial Diseases. Am Rev Respir Dis. 1981;123:343–58.
37. Ahn CH, McLarty JW, Ahn SS, et al. Diagnostic criteria for pulmonary disease caused by *Mycobacterium kansasii* and *Mycobacterium intracellulare.* Am Rev Respir Dis. 1982;125:388–91.
38. Sommers HM. Disease due to mycobacteria other than *Mycobacterium tuberculosis.* In: Youmans GP, ed. Tuberculosis. Philadelphia: WB Saunders; 1979:386–403.
39. Lind A. Serological studies of mycobacteria by means of diffusion-in-gel techniques (Dissertation). University of Göteburg, 1961.
40. Palmer CE, Long MW. Effects of infection with atypical mycobacteria on BCG vaccination and tuberculins. Am Rev Respir Dis. 1966;94:553–68.
41. Pfuetze KH, Yan Vo L, Reimann AF, et al. Photochromogenic mycobacterial pulmonary disease. Am Rev Respir Dis. 1965;92:470–5.
42. Kubica GP, Bean RE, Palmer JW. The isolation of unclassified (atypical) acid-fast mycobacteria from soil and water samples collected in the state of Georgia. Am Rev Respir Dis. 1963;88:718–20.
43. Joynson DHM. Water: The natural habitat of *Mycobacterium kansasii?* Tubercle. 1979;60:77–81.
44. Marks J. "Opportunist" mycobacteria in England and Wales. Tubercle. 1969;50:78–80.
45. Chapman JS, Dyerly M, Spohn S. Epidemiological notes on *Mycobacterium kansasii* disease. Arch Environ Health. 1968;16:673–8.
46. Lester W, Botkin K, Colton R. Analysis of 49 cases of pulmonary disease caused by photochromogenic mycobacteria. In: Proceedings of the 17th Conference on Chemotherapy of Tuberculosis. Washington, DC: U.S. Government Printing Office. 1958:289–97.
47. Bailey WC, Brown M, Buechner HA, et al. Silicomycobacterial disease in sand-blasters. Am Rev Respir Dis. 1974;110:115–25.
48. Johanson WG Jr, Nicholson DP. Pulmonary disease due to *Mycobacterium kansasii:* An analysis of some factors affecting prognosis. Am Rev Respir Dis. 1969;99:73–85.
49. Ahn CH, Nash DR, Hurst GA. Ventilatory defects in atypical mycobacteriosis. Am Rev Respir Dis. 1976;113:273–9.
50. Davidson PT. The management of disease with atypical mycobacteria. Clin Notes Respir Dis 1979;18:3–13.
51. Zvetina JR. Clinical characteristics of pulmonary infection associated with *M. kansasii.* In: Proceedings of the 25th Research Conference in Pulmonary Disease. Washington, DC: U.S. Government Printing Office. 1966:79–86.
52. Francis PB, Jay SJ, Johanson WG Jr. The course of untreated *M. kansasii* disease. Am Rev Respir Dis. 1975;111:477–87.
53. Shimoide H. Clinical study of atypical mycobacterial infection. III. Disease caused by *Mycobacterium kansasii.* Jap J Tuberc Chest Dis. 1971;30:128–34.
54. Tsai SH, Yue WY, Duthoy EJ. Roentgen aspects of chronic pulmonary mycobacteriosis. An analysis of 18 cases, including one with renal involvement. Radiology. 1968;90:306–10.
55. Christianson LC, Dewlett HJ. Pulmonary disease in adults associated with unclassified mycobacteria. Am J Med. 1960;29:980–91.
56. Woodring JH, Vandiviere HM, Melvin IG, et al. Roentgenographic features

of pulmonary disease caused by atypical mycobacteria. South Med J. 1987;80:1488–97.
57. Atwell RJ, Pratt PC. Unclassified mycobacteria in the gastric contents of health personnel and patients of a tuberculosis hospital. Am Rev Respir Dis. 1960;81:888–92.
58. Owens DW, McBride ME. Sporotrichoid cutaneous infection with *Mycobacterium kansasii*. Arch Dermatol. 1969;100:54–58.
59. Wood LE, Buhler VB, Pollak A. Human infection with the "yellow" acid-fast bacillus. A report of fifteen additional cases. Am Rev Tuberc Pulmonary Dis. 1956;73:917–29.
60. Klinenberg JR, Grimley PM, Seegmiller JE. Destructive polyarthritis due to a photochromogenic mycobacterium. N Engl J Med. 1965;272:190–3.
61. Rosen T. Cutaneous *Mycobacterium kansasii* infection presenting as cellulitis. Cutis. 1983;31:87–9.
62. Palmer JA, Watanakunakorn C. *Mycobacterium kansasii* pericarditis. Thorax. 1984;39:876–7.
63. Phillips S, Larkin JC Jr. Atypical pulmonary tuberculosis caused by unclassified mycobacteria. Ann Intern Med. 1964;60:401–8.
64. Engstrom PF, Dewey GC, Barrett O. Disseminated *Mycobacterium kansasii* infection. Successful treatment of a patient with pancytopenia. Am J Med. 1972;52:533–7.
65. Hagmar B, Kutti J, Lundin P, et al. Disseminated infection caused by *Mycobacterium kansasii*. Report of a case and brief review of the literature. Acta Med Scand. 1969;186:93–9.
66. Sherer R, Sable R, Sonnenberg M, et al. Disseminated infection with *Mycobacterium kansasii* in the acquired immunodeficiency syndrome. Ann Intern Med. 1986;105:710–2.
67. Goldman KP. Treatment of unclassified mycobacterial infection of the lungs. Thorax. 1968;23:94–9.
68. Harris GD, Johanson WG Jr, Nicholson DP. Response to chemotherapy of pulmonary infection due to *Mycobacterium kansasii*. Am Rev Respir Dis. 1975;112:31–6.
69. Ahn CH, Lowell JR, Ahn SS, et al. Chemotherapy for pulmonary disease due to *Mycobacterium kansasii:* Efficacies of some individual drugs. Rev Infect Dis. 1981;3:1028–34.
70. Pezzia W, Raleigh JW, Bailey MC, et al. Treatment of pulmonary disease due to *Mycobacterium kansasii:* Recent experience with rifampin. Rev Infect Dis. 1981;3:1035–9.
71. Ahn CH, Wallace RJ Jr, Steele LC, et al. Sulfonamide-containing regimens for disease caused by rifampin-resistant *Mycobacterium kansasii*. Am Rev Respir Dis. 1987;135:10–6.
72. Ahn CH, Lowell JR, Ahn SS, et al. Short-course chemotherapy for pulmonary disease caused by *Mycobacterium kansasii*. Am Rev Respir Dis. 1983;128:1048–50.
73. Schraufnagel DE, Leech JA, Schraufnagel MN, et al. Short-course chemotherapy for mycobacteriosis *kansasii?* Can Med Assoc J. 1984;130:34–8.
74. Judson FN, Feldman RA. Mycobacterial skin tests in humans 12 years after infection with *Mycobacterium marinum*. Am Rev Respir Dis. 1974;109:544–7.
75. Linell F, Norden A. *Mycobacterium balnei*—a new acid-fast bacillus occurring in swimming pools and capable of producing skin lesions in humans. Acta Tuberc Scand [Suppl] 1954;33:1–84.
76. Philpott JA Jr, Woodburn AR, Philpott OS, et al. Swimming pool granuloma. Arch Dermatol. 1963;88:158–62.
77. King AJ, Fairley JA, Rasmussen JE. Disseminated cutaneous *Mycobacterium marinum* infection. Arch Dermatol. 1983;119:268–70.
78. Gombert ME, Goldstein EJC, Corrado ML, et al. Disseminated *Mycobacterium marinum* infection after renal transplantation. Ann Intern Med. 1981;94:486–7.
79. Van Dyke JJ, Lake KB. Chemotherapy for aquarium granuloma. JAMA. 1975;233:1380–1.
80. Wolinsky E, Gomez F, Zimpfer F. Sporotrichoid *Mycobacterium marinum* infection treated with rifampin-ethambutol. Am Rev Respir Dis. 1972;105:964–7.
81. Donta ST, Smith PW, Levitz RE, et al. Therapy of *Mycobacterium marinum* infections. Arch Intern Med. 1986;146:902–4.
82. Izumi AK, Hanke CW, Higaki M. *M. marinum* infections treated with tetracycline. Arch Dermatol. 1977;113:1067–8.
83. Swift S, Cohen H. Granulomas of the skin due to *Mycobacterium balnei* after abrasions from a fish tank. N Engl J Med. 1962;267:1244–6.
84. Krasnow I, Gross W. *Mycobacterium simiae* infection in the United States: A case report an discussion of the organism. Am Rev Respir Dis. 1975;111:357–60.
85. Bell RC, Higuchi JH, Donovan WN, et al. *Mycobacterium simiae:* Clinical features and follow-up of twenty-four patients. Am Rev Respir Dis. 1983;127:35–8.
86. Rose HD, Dorff GJ, Lauwasser M, et al. Pulmonary and disseminated *Mycobacterium simiae* infection in humans. Am Rev Respir Dis. 1982;126:1110–3.
87. Lincoln EM, Gilbert LA. Disease in children due to mycobacteria other than *M. tuberculosis*. Am Rev Respir Dis. 1972;105:683–714.
88. Abello VB, Riley HD Jr, Rubio T. Atypical mycobacterial infections in children. Scand J Infect Dis. 1971;3:163–7.
89. Wolinsky E. The role of scotochromogenic mycobacteria in human disease. Ann NY Acad Sci. 1963;106:67–71.
90. Gernez-Rieux C, Tacquet A. Les infections humaines a mycobactéries "atypiques" au cours de pneumoconioses. Étude clinique et expérimentale. Bull Int Union Tuberc. 1959;29:330–42.
91. Bhadrakom S, Thasnakorn P, Prijyanonda B, et al. Scotochromogenic acid-fast bacilli isolated from pleural aspirate. J Med Assoc Thailand. 1968;51:33.
92. Cohen MJ, Matz LR, Elphick HR. Infection of the soft tissues of the ankle by a group II mycobacterium (scotochromogen). Med J Aust. 1970;2:679–81.
93. Kelly PJ, Weed LA, Lipscomb PR. Infection of tendon sheaths, bursae, joints and soft tissues by acid-fast bacilli other than tubercle bacilli. J Bone-Joint Surg [Am]. 1963;45:327–36.
94. Marks J, Jenkins PA, Tsukamura M. *Mycobacterium szulgai*—a new pathogen. Tubercle. 1972;53:210–4.
95. Dylewski JS, Zackon HM, Latour AH, et al. *Mycobacterium szulgai:* An unusual pathogen. Rev Infect Dis. 1987;9:578–80.
96. Maloney JM, Gregg CR, Stephens DS, et al. Infections caused by *Mycobacterium szulgai* in humans. Rev Infect Dis. 1987;9:1120–6.
97. Gur H, Porat S, Haas H, et al. Disseminated mycobacterial disease caused by *Mycobacterium szulgai*. Arch Intern Med. 1984;144:1861–3.
98. Schaefer WB. Incidence of serotypes of *Mycobacterium avium* and atypical mycobacteria in human and animal diseases. Am Rev Respir Dis. 1968;97:18–23.
99. Parker BC, Ford MA, Gruft H, et al. Epidemiology of infection by nontuberculous mycobacteria: iv. Preferential aerosolization of *Mycobacterium intracellulare* from natural waters. Am Rev Respir Dis. 1983;128:652–6.
100. O'Brien RJ, Geiter LJ, Snider DE Jr. The epidemiology of nontuberculous mycobacterial diseases: Results from a national survey. Am Rev Respir Dis. 1987;135:1007–14.
101. Yeager H Jr, Raleigh JW. Pulmonary disease due to *Mycobacterium intracellulare*. Am Rev Respir Dis. 1973;108:547–52.
102. Corpe RF. Clinical aspects, medical and surgical, in the management of Battey-type pulmonary disease. Dis Chest. 1964;45:380–2.
103. Lester W. Unclassified mycobacterial disease. Annu Rev Med. 1966;17:351–60.
104. Chakraborty AK, Damle PB, Davidson PT, et al. Disease due to *Mycobacterium intracellulare:* Its possible association with human leukocyte antigens. Rev Infect Dis. 1981;3:1060–3.
105. Prather EC, Bond JO, Hartwig EC, et al. Preliminary report: Epidemiology of infections due to atypical acid-fast bacilli. Dis. Chest. 1961;39:129–39.
106. Kumat SR, Rossiter CE, Gilson JC. A retrospective clinical study of pulmonary disease due to "anonymous mycobacteria" in Wales. Thorax. 1961;16:297–308.
107. Fischer DA, Lester W, Schaefer WB. Infections with atypical mycobacteria. Five years' experience at the National Jewish Hospital. Am Rev Respir Dis. 1968;98:29–34.
108. Ahn CH, Lowell JR, Onstad GD, et al. A demographic study of disease due to *Mycobacterium kansasii* or *M. intracellulare-avium* in Texas. Chest. 1979;75:120–5.
109. Rosenzweig DY, Schlueter DP. Spectrum of clinical disease in pulmonary infection with *Mycobacterium avium-intracellulare*. Rev Infect Dis. 1981;3:1046–51.
110. Tsukamura M, Shimoide H, Segawa I, et al. Clinical features of lung disease due to *Mycobacterium intracellulare*. Kekakku. 1974;49:139–46.
111. Black BG, Chapman JS. Cervical adenitis in children due to human and unclassified mycobacteria. Pediatrics. 1964;33:887–93.
112. Kubin M, Kruml J, Horak Z, et al. Pulmonary and nonpulmonary disease in humans due to avian mycobacteria. I. Clinical and epidemiological analysis of nine cases observed in Czechoslovakia. Am Rev Respir Dis. 1966;94:20–30.
113. Namey TC, Frogameni AD. Coexistent *Mycobacterium intracellulare* arthritis with patellar osteomyelitis in a patient with pulmonary sarcoidosis: A case report and literature review. Orthopedics. 1986;9:425–30.
114. Perry RR, Jaques DP, Lesar MSL, et al. *Mycobacterium avium* infection in a silicone-injected breast. Plast Reconstr Surg. 1985;75:104–6.
115. Wardrop PA, Pillsbury HC. *Mycobacterium avium* acute mastoiditis. Arch Otolaryngol. 1984;110:686–7.
116. Kinsella JP, Grossman M, Black S. Otomastoiditis caused by *Mycobacterium avium-intracellulare*. Pediatr Infect Dis. 1986;5:704–6.
117. Carruthers KJM, Edwards FGB. Atypical mycobacteria in Western Australia. Am Rev Respir Dis. 1965;91:887–95.
118. Koenig MG, Collins RD, Heyssel RM. Disseminated mycobacteriosis caused by Battey-type mycobacteria. Ann Intern Med. 1966;64:145–54.
119. Savage PJ, Dellinger RP. Disseminated tuberculosis caused by *Mycobacterium intracellulare* (Letter). Chest. 1982;82:800–1.
120. Collert S, Petrini B, Wickman K. Osteomyelitis caused by *Mycobacterium avium*. Acta Orthop Scand. 1983;54:449–51.
121. Horsburgh CR Jr, Mason UG, Farhi DC, et al. Disseminated infection with *Mycobacterium avium-intracellulare:* A report of 13 cases and a review of the literature. Medicine (Baltimore). 1985;64:36–48.
122. Saito H, Tasaka H, Osasa S, et al. Disseminated *Mycobacterium intracellulare* infection. Am Rev Respir Dis. 1974;109:572–6.
123. Rynearson TK, Shronts JS, Wolinsky E. Rifampin: In vitro effect on atypical mycobacteria. Am Rev Respir Dis. 1971;104:272–4.
124. Virtanen S. Drug sensitivities of atypical acid-fast organisms. Acta Tuberc Scand. 1961;40:182–9.
125. Guy LR, Chapman JS. Susceptibility in vitro of unclassified mycobacteria to commonly used antimicrobials. Am Rev Respir Dis. 1961;84:746–9.

126. Sanders WE Jr, Hartwig C, Schneider N, et al. Activity of amikacin against mycobacteria in vitro and in murine tuberculosis. Tubercle. 1982;63:201–8.
127. Sanders WE Jr, Schneider N, Hartwig C, et al. Comparative activities of cephalosporins against mycobacteria. In: Nelson JD, Grassi C, eds. Current Chemotherapy and Infectious Disease, v. 2. Washington, DC: American Society for Microbiology; 1980:1075–7.
128. Zimmer BL, DeYoung DR, Roberts GD. In vitro synergistic activity of ethambutol, isoniazid, kanamycin, rifampin, and streptomycin against *Mycobacterium avium-intracellulare* complex. Antimicrob Agents Chemother. 1982;22:148–50.
129. Heifets LB. Synergistic effect of rifampin, streptomycin, ethionamide, and ethambutol on *Mycobacterium intracellulare*. Am Rev Respir Dis. 1982; 125:43–8.
130. Rosenzweig DY. Pulmonary mycobacterial infections due to *Mycobacterium intracellulare-avium* complex. Clinical features and course in 100 consecutive cases. Chest. 1979;75:115–9.
131. Dutt AK, Stead WW. Long-term results of medical treatment in *Mycobacterium intracellulare* infection. Am J Med. 1979;67:449–53.
132. Lester W, Moulding T, Fraser RI, et al. Quintuple drug regimens in the treatment of Battey-type infections. In: Proceedings of the 28th VA–Armed Forces Pulmonary Disease Research Conference. Washington, DC: U.S. Government Printing Office. 1969:83.
133. Davidson PT, Khanijo V, Goble M, et al. Treatment of disease due to *Mycobacterium intracellulare*. Rev Infect Dis. 1981;3:1052–9.
134. Corpe RF. Surgical management of pulmonary disease due to *Mycobacterium avium-intracellulare*. Rev Infect Dis. 1981;3:1064–7.
135. Law SW. Surgical treatment of atypical mycobacterial disease. Dis Chest. 1965;47:296–303.
136. Rosenzweig DY. Course and long-term follow-up of 100 cases of pulmonary infection due to *M. avium-intracellulare* complex. Am Rev Respir Dis. 1976;113:55.
137. Ahn CH, Ahn SS, Anderson RA, et al. A four-drug regimen for initial treatment of cavitary disease caused by *Mycobacterium avium* complex. Am Rev Respir Dis. 1986;134:438–41.
138. Etzkorn ET, Aldarondo S, McAllister CK, et al. Medical therapy of *Mycobacterium avium-intracellulare* pulmonary disease. Am Rev Respir Dis. 1986;134:442–5.
139. Horsburgh CR Jr, Mason UG, Heifets LB, et al. Response to therapy of pulmonary *Mycobacterium avium-intracellulare* infection correlates with results of in vitro susceptibility testing. Am Rev Respir Dis. 1987;135:418–21.
140. Iseman MD, Corpe RF, O'Brien RJ, et al. Disease due to *Mycobacterium avium-intracellulare*. Chest. 1985;87(Suppl):139–49.
141. Greene JB, Sidhu GS, Lewin S, et al. *Mycobacterium avium-intracellulare:* A cause of disseminated life-threatening infection in homosexuals and drug abusers. Ann Intern Med 1982;97:539–45.
142. Fainstein V, Bolivar R, Mavligit G, et al. Disseminated infection due to *Mycobacterium avium-intracellulare* in a homosexual man with Kaposi's sarcoma. J Infect Dis. 1982;145:586.
143. Zakowski P, Fligiel S, Berlin GW, et al. Disseminated *Mycobacterium avium-intracellulare* infection in homosexual men dying of acquired immunodeficiency. JAMA. 1982;248:2980–2.
144. Wong B, Edwards FF, Kiehn TE, et al. Continuous high-grade *Mycobacterium avium-intracellulare* bacteremia in patients with the acquired immune deficiency syndrome. Am J Med. 1985;78:35–40.
145. Young LS, Inderlied CB, Berlin OG, et al. Mycobacterial infections in AIDS patients, with an emphasis on the *Mycobacterium avium* complex. Rev Infect Dis. 1986;8:1024–33.
146. Hawkins CC, Gold JWM, Whimbey E, et al. *Mycobacterium avium* complex infections in patients with the acquired immunodeficiency syndrome. Ann Intern Med. 1986;105:184–8.
147. Gillin JS, Urmacher C, West R, et al. Disseminated *Mycobacterium avium-intracellulare* infection in acquired immunodeficiency syndrome mimicking Whipple's disease. Gastroenterology. 1983;85:1187–91.
148. Wolke A, Meyers S, Adelsberg BR, et al. *Mycobacterium avium-intracellulare*–associated colitis in a patient with the acquired immunodeficiency syndrome. J Clin Gastroenterol. 1984;6:225–9.
149. Damsker B, Bottone EJ. *Mycobacterium avium–Mycobacterium intracellulare* from the intestinal tracts of patients with the acquired immunodeficiency syndrome: Concepts regarding acquisition and pathogenesis. J Infect Dis. 1985;151:179–81.
150. Masur H, Tuazon C, Gill V, et al. Effect of combined clofazimine and ansamycin therapy on *Mycobacterium avium–Mycobacterium intracellulare* bacteremia in patients with AIDS. J Infect Dis. 1987;155:127–9.
151. Pedersen C, Nielsen JD. *Mycobacterium avium* complex and the acquired immunodeficiency syndrome (Letter). Ann Intern Med. 1987;106:165–6.
152. Yajko DM, Nassos PS, Hadley WK. Therapeutic implications of inhibition versus killing of *Mycobacterium avium* complex by antimicrobial agents. Antimicrob Agents Chemother. 1987;31:117–20.
153. Young LS. *Mycobacterium avium* complex infection. J Infect Dis. 1988;157:863–7.
154. Gross W, Hawkins JE, Murphy DB. *Mycobacterium xenopi* in clinical specimens. Am Rev Respir Dis. 1976;113:78.
155. Bullin CH, Tanner EI, Collins CH. Isolation of *Mycobacterium xenopei* from water taps. J Hyg (Lond). 1970;68:97–100.
156. Smith MJ, Citron KM. Clinical review of pulmonary disease caused by *Mycobacterium xenopi*. Thorax. 1983;38:373–7.
157. Costrini AM, Mahler DA, Gross WM, et al. Clinical and roentgenographic features of nosocomial pulmonary disease due to *Mycobacterium xenopi*. Am Rev Respir Dis. 1981;123:104–9.
158. Banks J, Hunter AM, Campbell IA, et al. Pulmonary infection with *Mycobacterium xenopi:* Review of treatment and response. Thorax. 1984;39:376–82.
159. Contreras MA, Cheung OT, Sanders DE, et al. Pulmonary infection with nontuberculous mycobacteria. Am Rev Respir Dis. 1988;137:149–52.
160. Damsker B, Bottone EJ, Deligdisch L. *Mycobacterium xenopi:* Infection in an immunocompromised host. Hum Pathol. 1982;13:866–70.
161. Tecson-Tumang FT, Bright JL. *Mycobacterium xenopi* and the acquired immunodeficiency syndrome (Letter). Ann Intern Med. 1984;100:461–2.
162. Eng RHK, Forrester C, Smith SM, et al. *Mycobacterium xenopi* infection in a patient with acquired immunodeficiency syndrome. Chest. 1984;86:145–7.
163. Weinberg JR, Gertner D, Dootson G, et al. Disseminated *Mycobacterium xenopi* infection. Lancet. 1985;1:1033–4.
164. Price AB, Owen R, Sowter G, et al. Disseminated *Mycobacterium xenopi* infection (Letter). Lancet. 1985;2:383.
165. Schröder KH, Juhlin I. *Mycobacterium malmoense* sp. nov. Int J Syst Bacteriol. 1977;27:241–6.
166. Jenkins PA, Tsukamura M. Infections with *Mycobacterium malmoense* in England and Wales. Tubercle. 1979;60:71–6.
167. Banks J, Jenkins PA, Smith AP. Pulmonary infection with *Mycobacterium malmoense*—a review of treatment and response. Tubercle. 1985;66:197–203.
168. Roberts C, Clague H, Jenkins PA. Pulmonary infection with *Mycobacterium malmoense:* A report of 4 cases. Tubercle. 1985;66:205–9.
169. Connolly MJ, Magee JG, Hendrick DJ. *Mycobacterium malmoense* in the north-east of England. Tubercle. 1985;66:211–7.
170. France AJ, McLeod DT, Calder MA, et al. *Mycobacterium malmoense* infections in Scotland: An increasing problem. Thorax. 1987;42:593–5.
171. Jenkins PA. *Mycobacterium malmoense*. Tubercle. 1985;66:193–5.
172. Warren NG, Body BA, Silcox VA, et al. Pulmonary disease due to *Mycobacterium malmoense*. J Clin Microbiol. 1984;20:245–7.
173. Alberts WM, Chandler KW, Solomon DA, et al. Pulmonary disease caused by *Mycobacterium malmoense*. Am Rev Respir Dis. 1987;135:1375–8.
174. Crellin AM, Owen JR. Disseminated *Mycobacterium malmoense* infection. Br Med J. 1984;289:734.
175. Banks J, Jenkins PA. The effect of combined versus single anti-tuberculosis drugs on in vitro sensitivity patterns of *M. malmoense* and *M. xenopi*. Thorax. 1985;40:697–8.
176. Sompolinsky D, Lagziel A, Naveh D, et al. *Mycobacterium haemophilum* sp., a new pathogen of humans. Int J Syst Bacteriol. 1978;28:67–75.
177. Dawson DJ, Blacklock ZM, Kane DW. *Mycobacterium haemophilum* causing lymphadenitis in an otherwise healthy child. Med J Aust. 1981;2:289–90.
178. Rogers PL, Walker RE, Lane HC, et al. Disseminated *Mycobacterium haemophilum* infection in two patients with the acquired immunodeficiency syndrome. Am J Med. 1988;84:640–2.
179. Moulsdale MT, Harper JM, Thatcher GN, et al. Infection by *Mycobacterium haemophilum*, a metabolically fastidious acid-fast bacillus. Tubercle. 1983;64:29–36.
180. Ryan CG, Dwyer BW. New characteristics of *Mycobacterium haemophilum*. J Clin Microbiol. 1983;18:976–7.
181. Branger B, Gouby A, Oulès R, et al. *Mycobacterium haemophilum* and *Mycobacterium xenopi* associated infection in a renal transplant patient. Clin Nephrol. 1985;23:46–9.
182. Reid IS. *Mycobacterium ulcerans* infection: A report of 13 cases at the Port Moresby General Hospital. Med J Aust. 1967;1:427–31.
183. Lindo SD, Daniels F Jr. Buruli ulcer in New York City. JAMA. 1974;228:1138–9.
184. Dodge OG. Mycobacterial skin ulcers in Uganda: Histopathological and experimental aspects. J Pathol Bacteriol. 1964;88:169–84.
185. Clancey JK, Dodge OG, Lunn HF, et al. Mycobacterial skin ulcers in Uganda. Lancet. 1961;2:951–4.
186. Song M, Vincke G, Vanachter H, et al. Treatment of cutaneous infection due to *Mycobacterium ulcerans*. Dermatologica. 1985;171:197–9.
187. Douglas JG, Calder MA, Choo-Kang YFJ, et al. *Mycobacterium gordonae:* A new pathogen? Thorax. 1986;41:152–3.
188. McIntyre P, Blacklock Z, McCormack JG. Cutaneous infection with *Mycobacterium gordonae*. J Infect. 1987;14:71–8.
189. DeChairo DC, Kittredge D, Meyers A, et al. Septic arthritis due to *Mycobacterium triviale*. Am Rev Respir Dis. 1973;108:1224–6.
190. Edwards MS, Huber TW, Baker CJ. *Mycobacterium terrae* synovitis and osteomyelitis. Am Rev Respir Dis. 1978;117:161–3.
191. Halla JT, Gould JS, Hardin JG. Chronic tenosynovial hand infection from *Mycobacterium terrae*. Arthritis Rheum. 1979;22:1386–90.
192. Kuze F, Mitsuoka A, Chiba W, et al. Chronic pulmonary infection caused by *Mycobacterium terrae* complex: A resected case. Am Rev Respir Dis. 1983;128:561–5.
193. May DC, Kutz JE, Howell RS, et al. *Mycobacterium terrae* tenosynovitis: Chronic infection in a previously healthy individual. South Med J. 1983;76:1445–7.
194. Blacklock ZM, Dawson DJ, Kane DW, et al. *Mycobacterium asiaticum* as a potential pathogen for humans. Am Rev Respir Dis. 1983;127:241–4.
195. Linton IM, Leahy SI, Thomas GW. *Mycobacterium gastri* peritonitis in a

patient undergoing continuous ambulatory peritoneal dialysis. Aust NZ J Med. 1986;16:224–5.
196. Weitzman I, Osadczyi D, Corrado ML, et al. *Mycobacterium thermoresistibile:* A new pathogen for humans. J Clin Microbiol. 1981;14:593–5.
197. Casimir MT, Fainstein V, Papadopolous N. Cavitary lung infection caused by *Mycobacterium flavescens*. South Med J. 1982;75:253–4.
197a. Wallace RJ Jr, Nash DR, Tsukamura M, et al. Human disease due to *Mycobacterium smegmatis*. J Infect Dis. 1988;158:52–9.
198. Van Kruiningen HJ, Chiodini RJ, Thayer WR, et al. Experimental disease in infant goats induced by a mycobacterium isolated from a patient with Crohn's disease. A preliminary report. Dig Dis Sci. 1986;31:1351–60.
199. McFadden JJ, Butcher PD, Chiodini R, et al. Crohn's disease-isolated mycobacteria are identical to *Mycobacterium paratuberculosis,* as determined by DNA probes that distinguish between mycobacterial species. J Clin Microbiol. 1987;25:796–801.
200. Band JD, Ward JI, Fraser DW, et al. Peritonitis due to a *Mycobacterium chelonei*-like organism associated with intermittent chronic peritoneal dialysis. J Infect Dis. 1981;145:9–17.
201. Kuritsky JN, Bullen MG, Broome CV, et al. Sternal wound infections and endocarditis due to organisms of the *Mycobacterium fortuitum* complex. Ann Intern Med. 1983;98:938–9.
202. Safranek TJ, Jarris WR, Carson LA, et al. *Mycobacterium chelonae* wound infections after plastic surgery employing contaminated gentian violet skin-marking solution. N Engl J Med. 1987;317:197–201.
203. Sanders WE Jr. Lung infection caused by rapidly growing mycobacteria. *J Respir Dis* 1982;3:30–8.
204. Hand WL, Sanford JP: *Mycobacterium fortuitum*—a human pathogen. Ann Intern Med. 1970;73:971–7.
205. Dalovisio JR, Pankey GA. Problems in diagnosis and therapy of *Mycobacterium fortuitum* infections. Am Rev Respir Dis. 1978;117:625–30.
206. Wallace RJ Jr, Swenson JM, Silcox VA, et al. Spectrum of disease due to rapidly growing mycobacteria. Rev Infect Dis. 1983;5:657–79.
207. Robicsek F, Daugherty HK, Cook JW, et al. *Mycobacterium fortuitum* epidemics after open heart surgery. J Thorac Cardiovasc Surg. 1978;75:91–6.
208. Repath F, Seabury JH, Sanders CV, et al. Prosthetic valve endocarditis due to *Mycobacterium chelonei*. South Med J. 1976;69:1244–6.
209. Clegg HW, Foster MT, Sanders WE Jr, et al. Infection due to organisms of the *Mycobacterium fortuitum* complex after augmentation mammaplasty: Clinical and epidemiological features. J Infect Dis. 1983;147;427–33.
210. Hoffman PC, Fraser DW, Robicsek F, et al. Two outbreaks of sternal wound infections due to organisms of the *Mycobacterium fortuitum* complex. J Infect Dis. 1981;143:533–42.
211. Sanders WE Jr, Hartwig EC, Schneider NJ, et al. Susceptibility of organisms in the *Mycobacterium fortuitum* complex to antituberculous and other antimicrobial agents. Antimicrob Agents Chemother. 1977;12:295–7.
212. Tice AD, Solomon RJ. Disseminated *Mycobacterium chelonei* infection: Response to sulfonamides. Am Rev Respir Dis. 1979;120:197–201.
213. Dalovisio JR, Pankey GA. In vitro susceptibility of *Mycobacterium fortuitum* and *Mycobacterium chelonei* to amikacin. J Infect Dis. 1978;137:318–21.
214. Dalovisio JR, Pankey GA, Wallace RJ, et al. Clinical usefulness of amikacin and doxycycline in the treatment of infection due to *Mycobacterium fortuitum* and *Mycobacterium chelonei*. Rev Infect Dis. 1981;3:1068–74.
215. Swenson JA, Wallace RJ Jr, Silcox VA, et al. Antimicrobial susceptibility of five subgroups of *Mycobacterium fortuitum* and *Mycobacterium chelonae*. Antimicrob Agents Chemother. 1985;28:807–11.
216. Preheim LC, Bittner MJ, Giger DR, et al. *Mycobacterium fortuitum* sternotomy infections treated with amikacin, cefoxitin, and rifampin: Serum static and killing titers (Abstract 564). In: Proceedings of the 22nd Interscience Conference on Antimicrobial Agents and Chemotherapy. Washington, DC: American Society for Microbiology; 1982.
217. Wallace RJ Jr, Swanson JM, Silcox VA, et al. Treatment of nonpulmonary infections due to *Mycobacterium fortuitum* and *Mycobacterium chelonei* on the basis of in vitro susceptibilities. J Infect Dis. 1985;152:500–14.

DISEASES DUE TO HIGHER BACTERIA

232. NOCARDIA SPECIES

PHILLIP I. LERNER

Nocardiosis is a localized or disseminated infection caused by a soil-borne aerobic actinomycete, usually introduced through the respiratory tract, first described in humans by Eppinger (1890) after Nocard (1888) noted an aerobic actinomycete in *farcin du boeuf* (bovine farcy), an emaciating disease of cattle characterized by pulmonary lesions, multiple cutaneous abscesses, and draining sinuses.[1] The pulmonary event may be transient or subclinical, or may provoke an acute or chronic process mimicking tuberculous or mycotic infections, or malignancy. Hematogenous dissemination spreads particularly to the nervous system and the soft tissues. Uncertain classification in the past linked nocardiosis to the mycoses and to actinomycosis as "aerobic actinomycosis," an error of diagnostic and therapeutic significance.[1]

ETIOLOGY

Classification of Pathogenic Nocardia

Members of the family Nocardiaceae, aerobic actinomycetes, reproduce by fragmenting into bacillary and coccoid elements but are distinguished by filamentous growth with true branching. An array of laboratory features now firmly establish the actinomycetes as bacteria (see Chapter 233). Fragmenting filaments, both vegetative and aerial, are seen, but not conidia.

Nocardia asteroides is the predominant human pathogen. Other pathogenic human spp. include *N. brasiliensis*[2] and *N. caviae*. *Nocardia farcinica,* the agent of bovine nocardiosis, has arguably been implicated in human infection; the validity of that separate designation is not clear.[3,4] They are not commensals in human or animals but natural soil saprophytes often found in decaying organic matter. Other mammals (cats, dogs, guinea pigs) can be infected.

Microbiology and Identification of Pathogenic Nocardia

Nocardia spp. grow readily over a wide temperature range on simple media (e.g., Sabouraud's glucose agar, blood agar); added CO_2 (10%) promotes more rapid growth. Colonies may be smooth and moist, or rugate with a velvety surface, due to a rudimentary aerial mycelium (Fig. 1). Most primary isolates are light orange; pigment variations include cream, yellow, pink, coral, orange, and brick red. *Nocardia* spp. grow poorly on many inhibitory media commonly used for isolation of the pathogenic fungi. The laboratory should be alerted, and specimens must be sent when the patient is not receiving antibiotics. Colonies in pure culture will grow after 48 hours of incubation, but in mixed cultures from clinical material, for example, respiratory secretions, rapidly growing bacteria may obscure small *Nocardia* colonies, and colonial characteristics sufficient to arouse suspicion often take 2–4 weeks to develop, rather than the 4–10 days cited in most textbooks. Multiple specimens must be studied, since simultaneous positive smears and cultures occur only in one-third of cases. The organism may be elusive unless pus from a discharging fistula or an abscess is studied.[5]

The observation of delicate, weakly gram-positive, irregularly stained or beaded branching filaments is extremely important in the recognition of *Nocardia* spp. (Fig. 2). Blood agar is a satisfactory primary isolation medium, but growth in liquid media produces a dry, waxy surface pellicle similar to that of *Mycobacterium* spp. and may aid in visualizing branching filaments. Fragmentation into nondescript coccobacillary forms occurs.[6]

Many *Nocardia* spp. are acid-fast, but compared to *Mycobacteria* spp., they retain fuchsin less tenaciously. Acid fastness is characteristic of organisms in tissue or initial colonial isolates but is quickly lost on subculture; not all pathogenic *Nocardia* strains are acid-fast.[7] A modified Ziehl-Neelsen stain that decolorizes with 1% sulfuric acid instead of acid alcohol is best for demonstrating acid-fast *Nocardia* in clinical specimens.

Nocardia spp. are widely distributed in nature, so the sig-

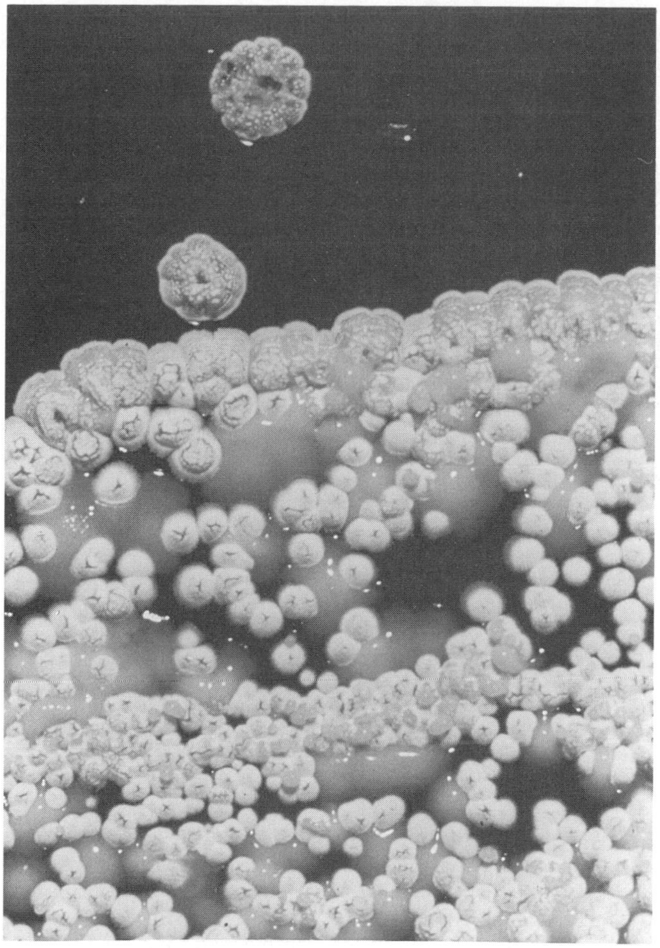

FIG. 1. Rugate colonies of *Nocardia asteroides* on a blood agar plate.

nificance of random sputum isolates has been questioned.[5] Casual false-positive single isolations have been reported from mycobacterial and fungal reference laboratories. Sputum digestion procedures used to isolate mycobacteria render some *Nocardia*-positive sputum specimens falsely negative.[8] *Nocardia* spp. are occasionally skin contaminants or respiratory tract saprophytes.[9–11] Some cultures yielding *Nocardia* may represent milder clinical infections, such as pharyngitis, bronchitis, or otitis media. Young et al. described seven patients with fever or upper respiratory tract symptoms, all with sputum *Nocardia* isolates "of uncertain significance."[5] Four patients had underlying disease, and three did not; none were on steroids. In some, multiple cultures were positive while symptoms continued; therapy was withheld, and all recovered. Respiratory tract colonization (single isolates) occurs in patients with malignancy, tuberculosis, cystic fibrosis, asthma, bronchitis, and allergic aspergillosis.[9] Bronchial obstruction or decreased bronchociliary clearance predisposes to colonization, but infection seldom occurs unless steroids are also part of the picture.[9] The weight of current evidence, from the literature and personal experience, favors the concept that *Nocardia* spp. can indeed at times be respiratory saprophytes in humans. In compromised individuals, it is difficult to withhold therapy when cultures are repeatedly positive.

Precise speciation within the genus *Nocardia* is difficult and is often pursued only in reference laboratories.[7] *Nocardia brasiliensis,* responsible for mycetoma in Mexico and South America, can produce disseminated disease and has been an opportunistic pathogen in this country.[2] Pulmonary and systemic infection with *N. caviae* has been documented in both normal and compromised hosts.[12] The genus *Actinomadura* now designates *Nocardia* spp. of the madurae type, with a different cell wall composition.[7] The species *Actinomadura madurae, A. pelletieri,* and *A. dassonvillei* all cause mycetoma (maduramycosis or madura foot), a chronic, deep subcutaneous tissue and bone infection, usually of the lower limbs (see Chapter 239).

PATHOGENESIS

Nocardia asteroides most commonly infects humans through the respiratory tract.[6] Occasionally the alimentary canal is penetrated, especially the appendix,[13] or, rarely, after dental injury. Traumatic introduction of *Nocardia* spp. from soil may produce, in addition to the classic mycetoma, wound infections (e.g., of compound fractures) or cellulitis, pustules, or pyoderma; these occasionally disseminate.[6,14,15] *Nocardia brasiliensis* may participate in this sequence or occur as an opportunistic organism in a compromised host.[2] Even isolated osteomyelitis occasionally develops in this fashion.[16] A lymphocutaneous sporotrichoid syndrome, often seen with *N. brasiliensis* infection, may be mimicked by *N. asteroides* as well; chancriform lesions have been recorded.[14,17] Post-traumatic keratitis and endophthalmitis have been described.[18,19] A tick bite can introduce the organism,[20] and blood-borne pulmonary infection in a heroin addict has been observed.[21]

A world literature review in 1961 (179 cases) first suggested an increasing incidence and a changing spectrum of infection.[22] Formerly most often a primary infection, nocardiosis now emerges chiefly from an array of debilitating diseases, particularly lymphoreticular neoplasms, chronic pulmonary disorders, notably alveolar proteinosis, and almost any condition requiring long-term corticosteroid usage.[9,11] Other underlying conditions are pemphigus vulgaris, lupus, asthma, glomerulonephritis, Whipple's disease, Goodpasture syndrome, vasculitis, Cushing's disease, cirrhosis, hemochromatosis, ulcerative colitis, bronchiectasis, bronchopulmonary sequestration, tuberculosis, anthracosilicosis, sarcoidosis, and Paget's disease of bone.[1,5,22] Patients with dysgammaglobulinemia and chronic granulomatous disease of childhood are at risk.[23–25] Renal and cardiac transplant recipients are notably prone to nocardiosis,[26,27] the latter being also at risk for subsequent nontuberculous mycobacterosis.[28] Pulmonary or disseminated nocardiosis has also been described in alcoholics.[29] Acquired immunodeficiency syndrome (AIDS) patients are at risk.[30–33] Many antecedent conditions are particularly associated with dysfunction of cellular immunity, but immunoglobulin and leukocyte defects may also be preconditions. Rarely, *Nocardia* spp. invade lung cavities and produce a "fungus ball".

Infections caused by *N. asteroides* result from the organism's ability to evade bactericidal mechanisms of the host, a multifaceted response consisting of early neutrophil mobilization, which inhibits but does not kill *Nocardia* organisms, limiting the spread of infection until the appearance of cell-mediated immunity (CMI), triggered by "activated macrophages" and induction of a T-cell population capable of direct lymphocyte-mediated toxicity to *N. asteroides*[34,35]; both of these cells kill nocardiae in vitro.

Immune T cells are important in clearing *Nocardia* from the lung and in preventing dissemination beyond the lung.[35] Neutrophils predominate in the lesions of nocardiosis, but infections progress unless antimicrobial agents are given or CMI takes over. In the event of an inadequate CMI response, neutrophils may explain the characteristic indolence of human nocardiosis.[35] In chronic granulomatous disease, neutrophils and macrophages are unable to generate a burst of oxidative metabolism during phagocytosis, which impairs intracellular killing of catalase-positive bacteria, such as *Nocardia*.[24] However, *Nocardia* may also be relatively resistant to the metabolites of even a normal oxidative burst.[34]

Filamentous log-phase cells of *Nocardia* are more toxic to

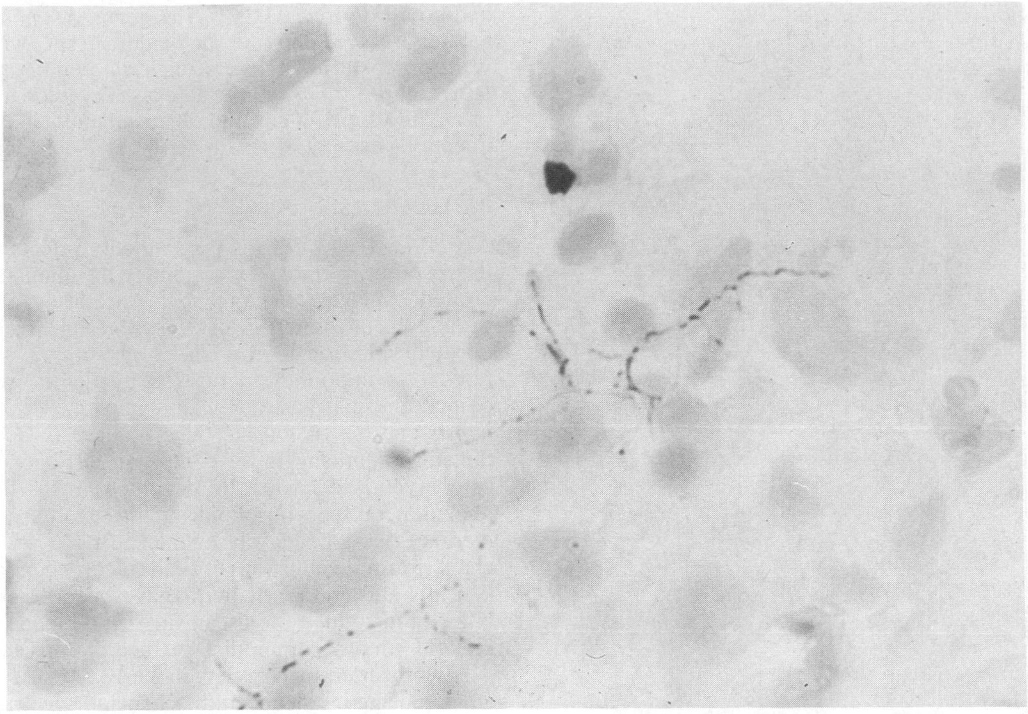

FIG. 2. Gram stain of *Nocardia* sp. demonstrating delicate, beaded, branching filaments. (×900)

mouse macrophages and more virulent for mice than are the easily phagocytized coccoid stationary-phase organisms,[34,36] apparently because they resist phagocytosis more effectively.[35] Enhanced virulence of log-phase cells correlates with the degree of inhibition of macrophage phagosome–lysosome fusion by blocking phagosomal acidification[37] and may relate to the presence of specific cell wall mycolic acids detected only in log-phase cells[38]; these acids may also influence the ability of nocardiae to localize in certain tissues (e.g., brain) and to grow in the host. Lysosomal acid phosphatase is an effective marker of the ability of macrophages to inhibit growth of and kill *N. asteroides*; macrophages isolated from different anatomic sites differ functionally from each other with respect to nocardicidal and acid phosphatase activities.[37] Catalase and superoxide dismutase may represent two additional important virulence factors for *Nocardia*.[39]

There is no evidence for animal-to-person or person-to-person transmission, although rare case clusters suggest the latter possibility.[40,41] Nosocomial cases, not clustered, have been described.[6,9,42] An outbreak in a renal transplant unit discovered the "epidemic strain" of *N. asteroides* (type III antigen) within the dust and air of the unit, suggesting the possibility of respiratory isolation for some immunocompromised patients.[41,43] Plasmid analysis is useful in epidemiologic evaluation of outbreaks,[41] or in recurrences in an individual case.[24]

PATHOLOGY

Nocardiosis produces suppurative necrosis and abscess formation typical of pyogenic infection. Tuberculoid granulomas and Langhan giant cells have been reported, but the typical lesion seldom resembles a granuloma. Tuberculosis and nocardiosis may coexist in the same patient.[1,44]

Pulmonary lesions are often abscesses, generally multiple and confluent; solitary "coin" lesions and miliary patterns are described. Indolent progressive fibrosis resembling fibronodular tuberculosis may be seen. In contrast to the pronounced tissue fibrosis in actinomycosis, nocardiosis seldom provokes more than an occasional partial wall of loose granulation tissue. Rarely, bands of fibrous tissue incompletely encircle the lesions. Daughter abscesses are common; peribronchial lymphadentitis may be present. Confluent abscess formation with little evidence of encapsulation is characteristic of all organs invaded by *Nocardia* spp., unless influenced by prior therapies (Fig. 3), and probably accounts for the ready dissemination of organisms from the initial pulmonary focus.

Extension to the pleura or chest wall may produce empyema, subcutaneous abscess or sinus tracts, or bone involvement resembling to some extent the picture of actinomycosis; this pattern may be associated with fibrosis. Sulfur granules are absent in visceral nocardiosis but appear in infections of the skin or subcutaneous tissues, as in mycetoma and lymphocutaneous syndromes.[14,45]

Nocardia asteroides in tissue sections or pus appears as a beaded, branching filament (Fig. 2) when stained by the Gram method or the Brown-Brenn modification. *Nocardia* spp. are not visible in hematoxylin and eosin preparations or in sections

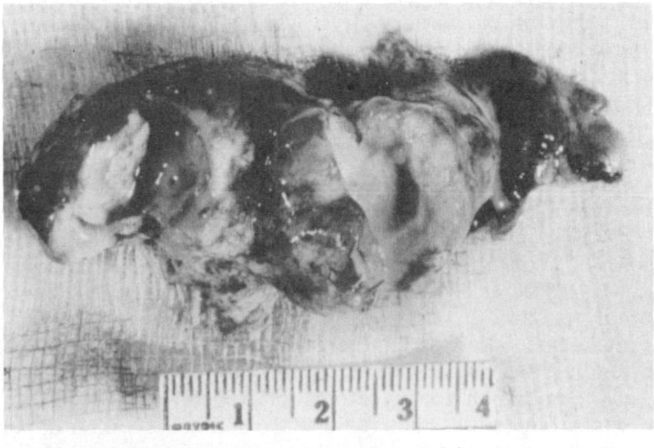

FIG. 3. Multiloculated, thick-walled nocardial brain abscess resected after 3 months of therapy with sulfonamides only.

stained with periodic acid–Schiff (PAS) for fungi. Methenamine-silver preparations stain tissue organisms in the hands of some, but not all, investigators. Overstaining with silver enhances visualization.

SYMPTOMATOLOGY AND DIAGNOSIS

Nocardiosis is an acute, subacute, or chronic suppurative infection with a pronounced tendency to remissions and exacerbations. Men are affected three times as commonly as women. Infection has occurred as early as 4 weeks of age.[46] The most common initial diagnosis, other than pneumonia, is tuberculosis, carcinoma, or lung abscess. In high-risk patients, the diagnosis should be suspected when soft tissue swellings or abscesses and/or central nervous system manifestations, particularly signs of a brain tumor or abscess, develop in conjunction with a current or recent chronic or subacute pulmonary infection.

There is no pathognomonic x-ray picture. Confluent bronchopneumonia may progress to complete consolidation; cavitation (in areas of consolidation or nodules) and pleural involvement are common; empyema is seen in up to 25 percent of cases. X-ray findings include fluffy infiltrates or irregular densities, subpleural plaques, single or scattered nodules or masses, single or multiple abscesses, and alveolar or interstitial reticular infiltrates[47] (Fig. 4) (see also Fig. 4 of Chapter 56). Wegener's granulomatosis can be a mistaken diagnosis in cavitating pulmonary lesions.[48] Calcification is rare. Miliary lesions have been recorded, as have thick-walled cavities and endobronchial lesions,[47,49] yet another feature to confuse with malignancy. The adult respiratory distress syndrome has been described.[50]

Clinical manifestations are not specific: anorexia, weight loss, productive cough, pleural pain, dyspnea, and occasionally hemoptysis, particularly from large cavities.[51] Untreated pulmonary nocardiosis usually runs a chronic course, much like that of tuberculosis, except that lower lobe involvement is more common, but it may also clear spontaneously, obscuring the source of subsequent metastatic infection. Acute pneumonic forms of a few weeks' duration are not rare, however, particularly in the compromised host.

Clinical manifestations also include tracheitis, bronchitis, pleuropulmonary fistula, peritonitis, epididymo-orchitis, iliopsoas abscess, ischiorectal abscess, perirectal abscess, keratoconjunctivitis, hematogenous endophthalmitis, sinusitis, pericarditis, endocarditis (natural and prosthetic valves), aortitis, mediastinitis with superior vena cava obstruction, septic arthritis, peritonitis in chronic peritoneal dialysis, osteomyelitis, and a disseminated miliary picture with diffuse organ abscesses.[16,19,29,33,51–60] Subcutaneous abscesses, single or multiple and generally more firm than fluctuant, lack the induration and fistulous tendency of actinomycosis. *Nocardia* spp. infection in childhood may present as a cervicofacial syndrome and cause cervical adenitis.[61] Dissemination, via blood or possibly lymphatic channels, may occur even from small, inconspicuous pulmonary lesions.[6] Recovery of *N. asteroides* from blood cultures, while not common, does occur, especially in patients receiving immunosuppressive therapy.[11] Unfortunately, many cases are first discovered at autopsy. *Nocardia* spp. have been involved in paratracheal and anterior cervical infections complicating transtracheal aspiration.[62] Peritonsillar abscess has been reported after needle aspiration of tonsillar abscesses.[63]

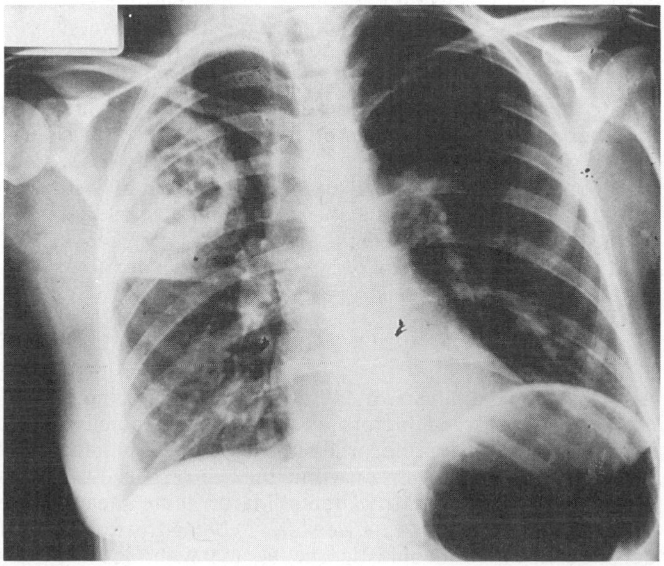

FIG. 4. Cavitary right upper lobe pneumonia due to *Nocardia asteroides*.

The central nervous system is infected in about one-third of all cases and may dominate the clinical picture alone, although this occurs more often in the course of a widespread disseminated infection. Brain abscesses, especially multiloculated lesions, are common; meningitis has been reported,[64–66] as has ventriculitis associated with a ventriculoperitoneal shunt.[46,64] Whereas needle biopsy of a cerebral mass is normally not indicated in patients with confirmed pulmonary nocardiosis,[64] in AIDS patients the potential for multiple organism infection (or infection plus tumor, especially lymphoma) challenges that dictum,[30,31] even though toxoplasmosis is identified nearly 10 times as often as all other causes of intracranial contrast-enhancing rings or nodules in the AIDS population. Epidural spinal cord compression from vertebral osteomyelitis has been observed.[60]

Tests for humoral antibodies or for the demonstration of delayed cutaneous hypersensitivity are not clinically useful, since there are many cross-reactions among *Nocardia* spp. and also between *Mycobacterium* spp. and *Streptomyces* spp.[6] Hemagglutinating and precipitin antibodies to *Nocardia* spp. have been demonstrated in animals; experiences to date in human infections have been limited and inconclusive.[67] Complement-fixing antibody tests are sensitive, but false-positive reactions occur in leprosy and tuberculosis.[68] A recently isolated 55-kilodalton (kD) protein has apparent specificity for *N. asteroides*, and preliminary results with an enzyme immunoassay suggest that antibody titers $\geq$1:256 are sensitive and specific and "not plagued by broad cross-reactivity to sera from patients infected with *M. tuberculosis*."[69] This protein is also present in *N. brasiliensis* and *N. caviae*.[70] There are no skin tests for demonstrating delayed cutaneous hypersensitivity.

While no single clinical feature separates nocardiosis from any other subacute or chronic pulmonary or extrapulmonary infectious process, an appropriate index of suspicion in high-risk patients plus a Gram and a modified acid-fast stain of pus or sputum can often establish the diagnosis in a matter of minutes, since the organism, when seen, is quite characteristic (Fig. 2).

Therapy

Before the advent of sulfonamides, therapy was essentially supportive. Spontaneous remissions were unknown, and surgery alone was seldom of lasting benefit. In 1944 sulfonamides demonstrated beneficial effects, and high-dose therapy administered over a prolonged period of weeks to months soon led to many cures. Sulfonamides were generally recognized as the drugs of choice in nocardiosis, in conjunction with appropriate surgery directed toward drainage of abscesses and empyemas.[1] Animal protection studies in 1951 emphasized poor correlation between in vitro antibiotic susceptibility testing and protection in experimentally infected mice.[71,72] Chlortetracycline, chloramphenicol, and streptomycin exhibited considerable in vitro inhibitory activity but protected experimentally infected mice incompletely or erratically. Sulfadiazine, on the other hand, provided almost complete protection in vivo despite poor in vitro activity. Peabody and Seabury, in a classic review, recommended that sulfadiazine (4–6 g/day; up to 8–9 g/day in severely ill patients) be given along with 2 g/day of an antibiotic, such as chloramphenicol, chlortetracycline, or streptomycin.[1] Since that empirical recommendation, the value of and need for combined therapy have never been tested. There are several reasons for this. (*1*) No one medical center encounters sufficient clinical material to examine therapeutic combinations in a proper study. (*2*) The variable and chronic course of nocardiosis precludes sharp therapeutic endpoints, as metastatic lesions can appear even during or after an apparently effective course of sulfonamide therapy and despite maintenance of the recommended 8–16 mg/100 ml plasma sulfonamide level. (*3*) Surgical therapy frequently influences the ultimate outcome, although brain abscesses may respond to antimicrobial treatment without surgery.[73,74] Sulfisoxazole and triple-sulfonamide combinations are probably as effective as sulfadiazine, although most reported experiences cite the latter preparation. Unfortunately, intravenous preparations of sulfisoxazole and sulfadiazine are no longer available in the United States.

Reliable in vitro antimicrobial susceptibility studies can select alternative therapies when sulfonamide fails or cannot be given because of allergy or patient intolerance. Sulfonamide resistance acquired in vivo has been documented in one case by the author. In vitro assay systems employing homogeneous nocardial suspensions and standardized inocula on agar dilution plates now overcome most of the technical difficulties that beset past studies,[75–77] although uniform growth and homogeneous suspensions cannot be achieved for all isolates.[76–78] Disc diffusion testing is not practical for most antibiotics,[75] but trimethoprim-sulfamethoxazole (TMP-SMX) disc testing readily separates sensitive from resistant strains.[79] Media composition and inoculum effect influence the in vitro susceptibility patterns of *Nocardia*. Pronounced strain-to-strain variability makes in vitro testing important. Sulfonamides demonstrate in vitro inhibitory activity primarily when dilute inocula are used.[75,77,78] Ampicillin exhibits impressive in vitro activity for many strains, while ampicillin-resistant strains produce β-lactamases and, therefore, are often susceptible to amoxicillin-clavulanic acid.[80] Minimal inhibitory concentrations (MICs) of various penicillins are reduced an average of 16-fold in the presence of clavulanic acid.[80] Synergy has been demonstrated with erythromycin-ampicillin, sulfonamide-ampicillin, and ampicillin-cloxacillin.[81–83] Clinical experience with these combinations is currently meager.

Minocycline, with excellent in vitro activity for many strains, continues to accumulate published support for its use as an alternative agent in the treatment of pulmonary nocardiosis,[75–78, 82,84–86] and occasionally even in cerebral infection,[87] even though it does not eradicate tissue organisms in murine experimental cerebral nocardiosis.[88] Antituberculous drugs and antifungal agents, such as amphotericin B and nystatin, have no demonstrable in vitro activity against *Nocardia* spp.

TMP-SMX has received considerable attention in recent years, supplanting sulfonamide as the drug of choice in the minds of many investigators.[79,89] Synergistic action can be demonstrated only for two-thirds of *Nocardia* strains.[75,90] However, treatment failure and late relapses have been recorded[13,91,92]; too little trimethoprim may be present in the commercial fixed-dose combination for optimal activity[93]; thymidine-free media may be necessary to demonstrate synergy, which also depends on the strain tested, inoculum size, length of incubation, and the ratio of the two drugs. The toxicity of the combination is greater than that of sulfonamides alone, especially in patients receiving myelosuppressive therapy.[79] Sulfonamide therapy alone remains an effective therapy even in compromised patients.[26,94] Toxicity may preclude prolonged oral sulfonamide therapy in AIDS patients.[32]

Cycloserine (15 mg/kg of body weight per day in four divided doses) is frequently recommended as a substitute for or an adjunct to sulfonamide therapy.[95] Since the dextro-isomer of alanine, present in all conventional assay media, antagonizes the in vitro activity of cycloserine, alanine-free media are necessary to conduct cycloserine assays. However, in alanine-free assay media augmented with biotin, thiamine, and glucose to permit adequate growth, cycloserine still does not demonstrate impressive in vitro inhibitory activity against *Nocardia* spp.[77,78]

Among the newer antimicrobial agents, amikacin displays impressive in vitro activity against almost 100 percent of tested strains[96,97]; clinical experience, particularly in compromised patients, has been encouraging.[13,98,99] It has also reduced mortality convincingly in a murine intraperitoneal infection model.[94] Imipenem is also consistently active in vitro,[97,100] and a favorable clinical outcome with this combination has been reported in a case of prosthetic aortic valve endocarditis.[55] The combinations of amikacin and imipenem with cefotaxime and TMP-SMX display synergy (fourfold or greater reduction in the MICs of both drugs) for most strains; imipenem-cefotaxime displays synergy in 92 percent of tests, amikacin–TMP-SMX in 83 percent, and imipenem–TMP-SMX in 80 percent, while imipenem-amikacin is predominantly additive.[100] Imipenem and amikacin effectively reduced tissue organism counts in the brains of mice with cerebral nocardiosis.[88] Ceftriaxone, cefuroxime, and cefotaxime also display important in vitro activity[78,96,97]; the last exhibited significant in vivo activity in a murine model of pulmonary nocardiosis.[101] Other antibiotic combinations acting synergistically against susceptible strains of *Nocardia* are amikacin-cefuroxime and amikacin plus amoxicillin-clavulanic acid.[99]

In vitro antimicrobial susceptibility patterns may differ among *Nocardia* spp. In one study, *N. brasiliensis* was notably more sensitive to erythromycin and gentamicin but distinctly more resistant to viomycin and capreomycin than was *N. asteroides*.[77] Other reports also suggest in vitro drug susceptibility differences among *Nocardia* spp.[12,102] Amoxicillin-clavulanic acid is the first promising oral β-lactam antibiotic for treating infections due to *N. brasiliensis*, a rather consistent β-lactamase producer.[103]

Optimal duration of therapy is uncertain. Although a minimum of 6 weeks is usually recommended, sulfonamide therapy is often continued for many months after apparent cure because of the tendency for relapse or the appearance of metastatic abscesses.[92,104] In one study of TMP-SMX efficacy, relapses occurred only rarely when patients were treated for longer than 3 months.[79] The late appearance of a metastatic abscess, even during effective therapy, usually represents the evolution of a previously seeded metastasis, which can progress despite adequate therapy until surgical drainage is achieved.[11] Since multiple opportunistic pathogens often simultaneously or sequentially infect the compromised patient, poor response or the development of a new pulmonary or extrapulmonary lesion may herald the presence of a second pathogen, such as cytomegalovirus, *Pneumocystis carinii*, *Aspergillus*,[23] *Cryptococcus*,[105] or *Mycobacterium tuberculosis*,[32] rather than indicate resistant or progressive nocardiosis.

PROGNOSIS

A retrospective analysis of 147 collected cases of nocardiosis (1945–1968) analyzed factors associated with increased mortality.[106] Disseminated nocardiosis was defined as infection in two noncontiguous organs or within the central nervous system. Mortality was increased in patients (*1*) with acute infection (i.e., symptomatic for less than 3 weeks), (*2*) being treated with corticosteroids or antineoplastic agents, (*3*) with Cushing's disease, and (*4*) with disseminated disease involving two or more noncontiguous organs. Death was always due to sepsis, brain abscess, or overwhelming pneumonia and never to untreated underlying disease. Otherwise healthy patients with pulmonary nocardiosis had a mortality of only 15 percent. Even in patients with serious underlying disease who were receiving no corticosteroids or antineoplastic agents, mortality in pulmonary nocardiosis was only 20 percent. Corticosteroid therapy appeared to be a significant factor in mortality. Dissemination occurred as frequently in previously healthy patients as in other patient categories; corticosteroids did not influence the incidence of dissemination. Antinocardial therapy did not influence the appearance of extrapulmonary lesions.

REFERENCES

1. Peabody JW, Seabury JH. Actinomycosis and nocardiosis. Am J Med. 1960;28:99–115.
2. Smego RA Jr, Gallis HA. The clinical spectrum of *Nocardia brasiliensis* infection in the United States. Rev Infect Dis. 1984;6:164–80.
3. Holm P. Seven cases of human nocardiosis caused by *Nocardia farcinica*. Sabouraudia. 1975;13:161–9.
4. Tsukamura M. Nocardiae that recently caused lung infection in Japan—*Nocardia asteroides* and *Nocardia farcinica*. Microbiol Immunol. 1982;26:341–5.
5. Young LS, Armstrong D, Blevins A, et al. *Nocardia asteroides* infection complicating neoplastic disease. Am J Med. 1971;50:356–67.
6. Palmer DL, Harvey RL, Wheeler JK. Diagnostic and therapeutic considerations in *Nocardia asteroides* infection. Medicine. 1974;53:391–401.
7. Berd D. Laboratory identification of clinically important aerobic actinomycetes. Appl Microbiol. 1973;25:665–81.
8. Murray PR, Heeren RL, Niles AC. Effect of decontamination procedures on recovery of *Nocardia* sp. J Clin Microbiol. 1987;25:2010–1.
9. Rosett W, Hodges GR. Recent experiences with nocardial infections. Am J Med Sci. 1978;276:279–85.
10. Stropnik Z. Isolation of *Nocardia asteroides* from human skin. Sabouraudia. 1965;4:41–4.
11. Frazier AR, Rosenow EC III, Roberts GD. Nocardiosis: A review of 25 cases occurring during 24 months. Mayo Clin Proc. 1975;50:657–63.
12. Arroyo JC, Nichols S, Carroll GF. Disseminated *Nocardia caviae* infection. Am J Med. 1977;62:409–12.
13. Cockerill FR, Edson RS, Roberts GD, et al. Trimethoprim/sulfamethoxazole-resistant *Nocardia asteroides* causing multiple hepatic abscesses. Am J Med. 1984;77:558–60.
14. Kalb RE, Kaplan MH, Grossman ME. Cutaneous nocardiosis. J Am Acad Dermatol. 1985;13:125–33.
15. Kahn FW, Gornick CC, Tofte RW. Primary cutaneous *Nocardia asteroides* infection with dissemination. Am J Med. 1981;70:859–63.
16. De Luca J, Walsh B, Robbins W, et al. *Nocardia asteroides* osteomyelitis. Postgrad Med J. 1986;62:673–4.
17. Tsuboi R, Takamori K, Ogawa H, et al. Lymphocutaneous nocardiosis caused by *Nocardia asteroides*. Arch Dermatol. 1986;122:1183–5.
18. Lass JH, Thoft RA, Bellows AR, et al. Exogenous *Nocardia asteroides* endophthalmitis associated with malignant glaucoma. Ann Ophthalmol. 1981;13:317–21.
19. Chen CJ. *Nocardia asteroides* endophthalmitis. Ophthalmic Surg. 1983;14:502–5.
20. Leggiadro RJ, Miller RB. Cutaneous nocardiosis presenting as a tick-borne infection. Pediatr Infect Dis J. 1987;6:421–2.
21. Vanderstigel M, Leclercq R, Brun-Buisson C, et al. Blood-borne pulmonary infection with *Nocardia asteroides* in a heroin addict. J Clin Microbiol. 1986;23:175–6.
22. Murray JF, Finegold SM, Froman S, et al. The changing spectrum of nocardiosis. Am Rev Respir Dis. 1961;83:315–30.
23. Casale TB, Macher AM, Fauci AS. Concomitant pulmonary aspergillosis and nocardiosis in a patient with chronic granulomatous disease of childhood. South Med J. 1984;77:274–5.
24. Jonsson S, Wallace RJ Jr, Hull SI, et al. Recurrent *Nocardia* pneumonia in an adult with chronic granulomatous disease. Am Rev Respir Dis. 1986;133:932–4.
25. Idriss ZH, Cunningham RJ, Wilfert CM. Nocardiosis in children. Pediatrics. 1975;55:479–84.
26. Simpson GL, Stinson EB, Egger MJ, et al. Nocardial infections in the immunocompromised host: A detailed study in a defined population. Rev Infect Dis. 1981;3:492–507.
27. Gallis HA, Berman RA, Cate TR, et al. Fungal infection following renal transplantation. Arch Intern Med. 1975;135:1163–72.
28. Simpson GL, Raffin TA, Remington JS. Association of prior nocardiosis and subsequent occurrence of nontuberculous mycobacteriosis in a defined, immunosuppressed population. J Infect Dis. 1982;146:211–9.
29. Petersen JM, Awad I, Ahmad M, et al. *Nocardia* osteomyelitis and epidural abscess in the nonimmunosuppressed host. Cleve Clin Q. 1983;50:453–9.
30. Holtz HH, Lavery DP, Kapila R. Actinomycetales infection in the acquired immunodeficiency syndrome. Ann Intern Med. 1985;102:203–205.
31. Adair JC, Beck AC, Apfelbaum RI, et al. Nocardial cerebral abscess in the acquired immunodeficiency syndrome. Arch Neurol. 1987;44:548–50.
32. Rodriguez JL, Barrio JL, Pitchenik AE. Pulmonary nocardiosis in the acquired immunodeficiency syndrome. Chest. 1986;90:912–4.
33. Masters DL, Lentino JR. Cervical osteomyelitis related to *Nocardia asteroides*. J Infect Dis. 1984;149:824–5.
34. Filice GA, Beaman BL, Krick JA, et al. Defense against *Nocardia asteroides* in man. In: Ortiz-Ortiz, L, Bojalil LF, Yakoleff V. eds. Biological, Biochemical, and Biomedical Aspects of Actinomycetes. Orlando, Fla.: Academic Press, 1984:107–18.
35. Filice GA, Niewoehner DE. Contribution of neutrophils and cell-mediated immunity to control of *Nocardia asteroides* in murine lungs. J Infect Dis. 1987;156:113–21.
36. Beaman BL, Maslan S. Virulence of *Nocardia asteroides* during its growth cycle. Infect Immun. 1978;20:290–5.
37. Black CM, Paliescheskey M, Beaman BL, et al. Acidification of phagosomes in murine macrophages: Blockage by *Nocardia asteroides*. J Infect Dis. 1986;154:952–8.
38. Beaman BL, Moring SE. Relationship among cell wall composition, stage of growth, and virulence of *Nocardia asteroides* GUH-2. Infect Immun. 1988;56:557–63.
39. Beaman BL, Black CM, Doughty F, et al. Role of superoxide dismutase and catalase as determinants of pathogenicity of *Nocardia asteroides*: Importance in resistance to microbicidal activities of human polymorphonuclear neutrophils. Infect Immun. 1985;47:125–41.
40. Cox F, Hughes WT. Contagious and other aspects of nocardiosis in the compromised host. Pediatrics. 1975;55:135–8.
41. Stevens DA, Pier AC, Beaman BL, et al. Laboratory evaluation of an outbreak of nocardiosis in immunocompromised hosts. Am J Med. 1981;71:928–34.
42. Baddour LM, Baselski VS, Herr MJ, et al. Nocardiosis in recipients of renal transplants: Evidence for nosocomial acquisition. Am J Infect Control. 1986;14:214–9.
43. Houang ET, Lovett IS, Thompson FD, et al. *Nocardia asteroides* infection—A transmissible disease. J Hosp Infect. 1980;1:31–40.
44. Brown RB, Sands M, Ryczak M. Community-acquired pneumonia caused by mixed aerobic bacteria. Chest. 1986;90:810–4.
45. Dufresne RG Jr, Latour DL, Fields JP. Sulfur granules in lymphocutaneous nocardiosis. J Am Acad Dermatol. 1986;14:847.
46. Law BJ, Marks MI. Pediatric nocardiosis. Pediatrics. 1982;70:560–5.
47. Feigin DS. Nocardiosis of the lung: Chest radiographic findings in 21 cases. Thorac Radiol. 1986;159:9–14.
48. Gibb W, Williams A. Nocardiosis mimicking Wegener's granulomatosis. Scand J Infect Dis. 1986;18:583–5.
49. Henkle JQ, Nair SV. Endobronchial pulmonary nocardiosis. JAMA. 1986;256:1331–2.
50. Schulman LL, Enson Y. *Nocardia* pneumonitis and the adult respiratory distress syndrome. Am J Med Sci. 1987;293:315–9.
51. Curry WA. Human nocardiosis. A clinical review with selected case reports. Arch Intern Med. 1980;140:818–26.
52. Allevato PA, Eisses JF, Mezger E, et al. *Nocardia asteroides* aortitis with perforation of the aorta. Hum Pathol. 1985;16:743–6.
53. Bullock JD. Endogenous ocular nocardiosis; a clinical and experimental study. Trans Am Ophthalmol Soc. 1983;81:451–531.
54. Cons P, Trevino A, Lavalle C. Septic arthritis due to *Nocardia brasiliensis*. J Rheumatol. 1985;12:1019–21.
55. Ertl GM, Schaal KP, Kochsiek K. Nocardial endocarditis of an aortic valve prosthesis. Br Heart J. 1987;57:384–6.
56. Katz P, Fauci AS. *Nocardia asteroides* sinusitis. JAMA. 1977;238:2397–8.
57. Wheeler JS Jr, Culkin DJ, O'Connell J, et al. *Nocardia* epididymo-orchitis in an immunosuppressed patient. J Urol. 1986;136:1314–5.
58. Schwartz JG, Tio FO. Nocardial osteomyelitis: A case report and review of the literature. Diagn Microbiol Infect Dis. 1987;8:37–46.
59. McHenry MC, Duchesneau PM, Keys TF, et al. Vertebral osteomyelitis presenting as spinal compression fracture. Arch Intern Med. 1988;148:417–23.
60. Awad I, Bay JW, Petersen JM. Nocardial osteomyelitis of the spine with epidural spinal cord compression—a case report. Neurosurgery. 1984;15:254–6.
61. Lampe RM, Baker CJ, Septimus EJ, et al. Cervicofacial nocardiosis in children. J Pediatr. 1981;99:593–5.
62. Goldman AL, Light L. Anterior cervical infections: Complications of transtracheal aspirations. Am Rev Respir Dis. 1975;111:707–8.
63. Adair JC, Amber IJ, Johnston JM. Peritonsillar abscess caused by *Nocardia asteroides*. J Clin Microbiol. 1987;25:2214–5.
64. Byrne E, Brophy BP, Pettett LV. *Nocardia* cerebral abscess: New concepts in diagnosis, management, and prognosis. J Neurol Neurosurg Psychiatry. 1979;42:1038–45.
65. Smith PW, Steinkraus GE, Henricks BW, et al. CNS nocardiosis. Response to sulfamethoxazole-trimethoprim. Arch Neurol. 1980;37:729–30.
66. Buggy BP. *Nocardia asteroides* meningitis without brain abscess (Letter). Rev Infect Dis. 1987;9:228–31.
67. Blumer SO, Kaufman L. Microimmunodiffusion test for nocardiosis. J Clin Microbiol. 1979;10:308–12.
68. Shainhouse JZ, Pier AC, Stevens DA. Complement fixation antibody test for human nocardiosis. J Clin Microbiol. 1978;8:516–9.

69. Angeles AM, Sugar AM. Rapid diagnosis of nocardiosis with an enzyme immunoassay. J Infect Dis. 1987;155:292–6.
70. Angeles AM, Sugar AM. Identification of a common immunodominant protein in culture filtrates of three *Nocardia* species and use in etiologic diagnosis of mycetoma. J Clin Microbiol. 1987;25:2278–80.
71. Runyon EH. *Nocardia asteroides*. Studies of its pathogenicity and drug sensitivities. J Lab Clin Med. 1951;37:713–20.
72. Strauss RE, Kligman AM, Pillsbury DM. Chemotherapy of actinomycosis and nocardiosis. Am Rev Tuberc. 1951;63:441–8.
73. Norden CW, Ruben FL, Selker R. Nonsurgical treatment of cerebral nocardiosis. Arch Neurol. 1983;40:594–5.
74. Hall WA, Martinez AJ, Dummer JS, et al. Nocardial brain abscess: Diagnostic and therapeutic use of stereotactic aspiration. Surg Neurol. 1987;28:114–8.
75. Wallace RJ, Septimus EJ, Musher DM, et al. Disk diffusion susceptibility testing of *Nocardia* species. J Infect Dis. 1977;135:568–76.
76. Bach MC, Sabath LD, Finland M. Susceptibility of *Nocardia asteroides* to 45 antimicrobial agents in vitro. Antimicrob Agents Chemother. 1973;3:1–8.
77. Lerner PI, Baum GL. Antimicrobial susceptibility of *Nocardia* species. Antimicrob Agents Chemother. 1973;4:85–93.
78. Dewsnup DH, Wright DN. In vitro susceptibility of *Nocardia asteroides* to 25 antimicrobial agents. Antimicrob Agents Chemother. 1984;25:165–7.
79. Wallace RJ, Septimus EJ, Williams TW, et al. Use of trimethoprim-sulfamethoxazole for treatment of infections due to *Nocardia*. Rev Infect Dis. 1982;4:315–25.
80. Kitzis MD, Gutmann L, Acar JF. In-vitro susceptibility of *Nocardia asteroides* to 21 β-lactam antibiotics, in combination with three β-lactamase inhibitors, and its relationship to the β-lactamase content. J Antimicrob Chemother. 1985;15:23–30.
81. Finland M, Bach MC, Garner C, et al. Synergistic action of ampicillin and erythromycin against *Nocardia asteroides*: Effect of time of incubation. Antimicrob Agents Chemother. 1974;5:344–53.
82. Bach MC, Monaco AP, Finland M. Pulmonary nocardiosis. Therapy with minocycline and with erythromycin plus ampicillin. JAMA. 1973;224:1378–81.
83. Orfanakis MG, Wilcox HG, Smith CB. In vitro studies of the combined effect of ampicillin and sulfonamides on *Nocardia asteroides* and results of therapy in four patients. Antimicrob Agents Chemother. 1972;1:215–20.
84. Bach MC, Gold O, Finland M. Activity of minocycline against *Nocardia asteroides*: Comparison with tetracycline in agar dilution and standard disc-diffusion tests and with sulfadiazine in an experimental infection of mice. J Lab Clin Med. 1973;81:787–93.
85. Petersen EA, Nash ML, Mammana RB, et al. Minocycline treatment of pulmonary nocardiosis. JAMA. 1983;250:930–2.
86. Ochiai T, Amemiya H, Watanabe K, et al. Successful treatment of *Nocardia asteroides* infection with minocycline in kidney transplant patients. Jpn J Surg. 1978;8:138–44.
87. Wren MV, Savage AM, Alford RH. Apparent cure of intracranial *Nocardia asteroides* infection with minocycline. Arch Intern Med. 1979;139:249–50.
88. Gombert ME, Aulicino TM, DuBouchet L, et al. Therapy of experimental cerebral nocardiosis with imipenem, amikacin, trimethoprim-sulfamethoxazole, and minocycline. Antimicrob Agents Chemother 1986;30:270–3.
89. Smego RA, Moeller MB, Gallis HA. Trimethoprim-sulfamethoxazole therapy for *Nocardia* infections. Arch Intern Med. 1983;143:711–8.
90. Adams HG, Beeler BA, Wann LS, et al. Synergistic action of trimethoprim and sulfamethoxazole for *Nocardia asteroides*: Efficacious therapy in five patients. Am J Med Sci. 1984;287:8–12.
91. Stamm AM, McFall DW, Dismukes WE. Failure of sulfonamides and trimethoprim in the treatment of nocardiosis. Arch Intern Med. 1983;143:383–5.
92. Geiseler PJ, Check F, Lamothe F, et al. Failure of trimethoprim-sulfamethoxazole in invasive *Nocardia asteroides* infection. Arch Intern Med. 1979;139:355–6.
93. Bennett JE, Jennings AE. Factors influencing susceptibility of *Nocardia* species to trimethoprim-sulfamethoxazole. Antimicrob Agents Chemother. 1978;13:624–7.
94. Wallace RJ, Septimus E, Musher DM, et al. Treatment of experimental nocardiosis in mice: Comparison of amikacin and sulfonamide. J Infect Dis. 1979;140:244–8.
95. Rhodes ER, Riley HD, Muchmore HG. Cycloserine in the treatment of human nocardiosis. In: Sylvester J, ed. Antimicrobial Agents and Chemotherapy—1961. Ann Arbor, Mich.: American Society for Microbiology; 1962:352–8.
96. Gutmann L, Goldstein FW, Kitzis MD, et al. Susceptibility of *Nocardia asteroides* to 46 antibiotics, including 22 β-lactams. Antimicrob Agents Chemother. 1983;23:248–51.
97. Gombert ME. Susceptibility of *Nocardia asteroides* to various antibiotics, including newer β-lactams, trimethoprim-sulfamethoxazole, amikacin, and *N*-formimidoyl thienamycin. Antimicrob Agents Chemother. 1982;21:1011–2.
98. Meier B, Metzger U, Müller F, et al. Successful treatment of a pancreatic *Nocardia asteroides* abscess with amikacin and surgical drainage. Antimicrob Agents Chemother. 1986;29:150–1.
99. Goldstein FW, Hautefort B, Acar JF. Amikacin-containing regimens for treatment of nocardiosis in immunocompromised patients. Eur J Clin Microbiol. 1987;6:198–200.
100. Gombert ME, Aulicino TM. Synergism of imipenem and amikacin in combination with other antibiotics against *Nocardia asteroides*. Antimicrob Agents Chemother. 1983;24:810–1.
101. Sugar AM, Chahal RS, Stevens DA. A cephalosporin active in vivo against *Nocardia*: Efficacy of cefotaxime in murine model of acute pulmonary nocardiosis. J Hyg (Camb). 1983;91:421–7.
102. Wallace RJ, Wiss K, Curvey R, et al. Differences among *Nocardia* spp. in susceptibility to aminoglycosides and β-lactam antibiotics and their potential use in taxonomy. Antimicrob Agents Chemother. 1983;23:19–21.
103. Wallace RJ, Nash DR, Johnson WK, et al. β-Lactam resistance in *Nocardia brasiliensis* is mediated by β-lactamase and reversed in the presence of clavulanic acid. J Infect Dis. 1987;156:959–66.
104. Stropes L, Bartlett M, White A. Case report: Multiple recurrences of nocardial pneumonia. Am J Med Sci. 1980;280:119–22.
105. Schreiner DT, de Castro P, Jorizzo JL, et al. Disseminated *Nocardia brasiliensis* infection following cryptococcal disease. Arch Dermatol. 1986;122:1186–90.
106. Present CA, Wiernik PH, Serpick AA. Factors affecting survival in nocardiosis. Am Rev Respir Dis. 1973;108:1444–8.

233. ACTINOMYCES AND ARACHNIA SPECIES

PHILLIP I. LERNER

Actinomycosis, a chronic suppurative infection noted for forming external sinuses that discharge characteristic *sulfur granules*, spreads unimpeded by traditional anatomic barriers when endogenous oral commensals invade tissues of the face and neck, lungs, and ileocecal regions. Any tissue may be invaded directly or via metastatic infection. Microbiologists have long had difficulty classifying the pathogens, and early diagnosis continues to elude the clinician.[1]

Actinomyces, slow-growing, filamentous, gram-positive bacteria, exhibit true branching while forming mycelial-type colonies. Although the diseases they produce mimic those of true fungi, they are indisputably prokaryotic bacteria (Schizomycetes) lacking the nuclear membrane of the eukaryotic fungi and the chitin or glucans of fungal cell walls. The narrower filaments (1 μm in diameter) can fragment into bacillary forms, not a property of the tubular hyphae of molds. Reproduction is by bacterial fission, never by spores or budding. Growth is inhibited by many antibiotics but not by polyenes such as amphotericin B. They constitute the order Actinomycetales, with the following families of pathogens: (*1*) Mycobacteriaceae (genus: *Mycobacterium*), (*2*) Actinomycetaceae (genera: *Actinomyces*, *Arachnia*), and (*3*) Nocardiaceae (genus: *Nocardia*).[2] The family Actinomycetaceae remains a heterogeneous, partly ill-defined, and partly unrelated collection of microorganisms despite improved classification of the faultatively anaerobic, filamentous bacteria.[3]

Although Lebert reported antinomycosis in humans in 1857, Bollinger (1877) first described *Actinomyces bovis* ("ray fungus of the cow") in granules from sarcoma-like masses in cattle with "lumpy jaw."[2] Actinomycosis derives from two Greek words, *aktino*, referring to the radiating appearance of the organism in the sulfur granule, and *-mykes*, mistakenly labeling it a fungal infection; thus, actinomycosis refers to infection due to the "ray fungus." Israel (1878) saw similar granules in human autopsy material and described actinomycosis in humans in 1885.[2] The small, hard, yellow granules resembled the elemental sulfur particles then used in pharmaceutical preparations. In 1891, Israel and Wolff grew an anaerobic, filamentous organism from human clinical material, named in 1898 *A. israelii*, but for many years *A. bovis* designated the etiologic agent of both human and bovine disease, since it had priority. In 1940, Erikson proved that they were distinct species.[4] *Actinomyces bovis*, as currently classified, has never been isolated from humans, but *A. israelii* has been isolated from bovine infections.[5] Species designation before 1960 is often uncertain. The history of this infection has been thoroughly reviewed.[2]

Actinomycosis originally designated infection with any pathogenic actinomycete, including aerobic strains. In 1943, Waksman and Henrici separated the pathogenic Actinomycetaceae.[6] The genus *Actinomyces* included microaerophilic and anaerobic pathogens responsible for true actinomycosis. The aerobic nocardioform actinomycetes that they placed in the genus *Nocardia* now constitute a separate family, Nocardiaceae.

ETIOLOGY

Classification of Human Agents of Actinomycosis

Human actinomycosis is caused mainly by *A. israelii*. Three other species and an organism in a related genus, *Arachnia*, all oral commensals, can provoke lesions consistent with classic actinomycosis.[5] In order of importance they are *Arachnia propionica, A. naeslundii, A. viscosus*, and *A. odontolyticus*; all are facultative or anaerobic, gram-positive pathogens. *Actinomyces meyeri* has now been added to this list.[7,8] *Bifidobacterium adolescentis* (formerly *A. eriksonii*) can also produce an actinomycotic infection.[2] Except for *A. viscosus*, they grow best under anaerobic conditions at 37°C. Morphologically, they are usually filamentous or diphtheroidal, the latter feature mimicking the ubiquitous and catalase-positive propionibacteria (*diphtheroids*). Bacilliary and coccoid forms also occur. Characteristic branching (V or Y) can at times be difficult to demonstrate.

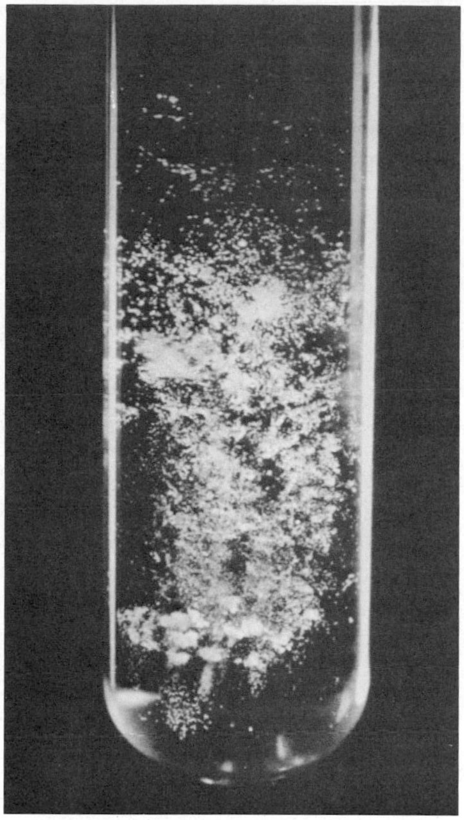

FIG. 1. Discrete bread crumb-like colonies of *A. israelii* (thioglycollate broth).

Microbiologic Characteristics

Actinomyces israelii grows best anaerobically; many strains are microaerophilic, and some even grow aerobically with prolonged incubation in CO_2. Early (overnight) microcolonies are delicately branched filaments radiating from an ill-defined center, the "spider" colony. Mature colonies (5–10 days) are larger, white and opaque, rough-appearing, and heaped up or lobulated ("molar tooth"); smooth variants do occur. In thioglycollate broth, discrete "breadcrumb" colonies form (Fig. 1). Saliva, dental surfaces and calculus, and gingival and tonsillar crypts yield *A. israelii* isolates in 30–50 percent of properly cultured specimens. In early or acute infections, the organisms may appear as free gram-positive filaments (Fig. 2), but in advanced lesions, characteristic granules are usually found (Fig. 3).

Arachnia propionica, morphologically and biochemically similar to *A. israelii*, was originally called *Actinomyces propionicus*. The serologically distinct genus *Arachnia*, created in 1969, produces propionic acid and has diaminopimelic acid in its cell walls.[5] It produces infections similar to those caused by *A. israelii*,[9–11] but macrocolonies are smoother, not molar tooth.

Actinomyces naeslundii has been isolated from blood, brain and other abscesses, cervicofacial infection, gallbladder empyema, suppurative thyroiditis, pleural empyema, pelvic infection in the presence of an intrauterine device (IUD), and a mycotic aneurysm of the splenic artery.[12–15] Granules form less readily, with more free filaments in the tissues.[5] The bacterium grows well in either aerobic or anaerobic conditions but is considered facultative only in the presence of CO_2. Biochemically and antigenically, *A. naeslundii* is quite similar to *A. israelii*.[12]

Odontomyces viscosus, isolated from hamsters with periodontal disease (1963), was catalase positive and grew well aerobically with or without added CO_2. It was reclassified as *A. viscosus* when the genus was modified to include catalase-positive organisms.[5] The most common organism in dental plaque, it is probably etiologic in periodontal disease. Reported infections include various pulmonary and cervicofacial syndromes

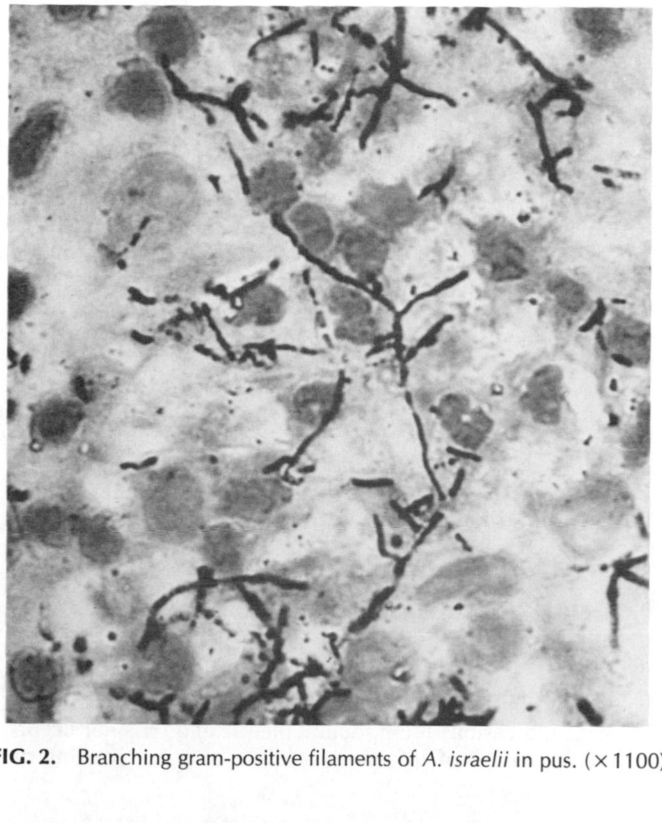

FIG. 2. Branching gram-positive filaments of *A. israelii* in pus. (×1100)

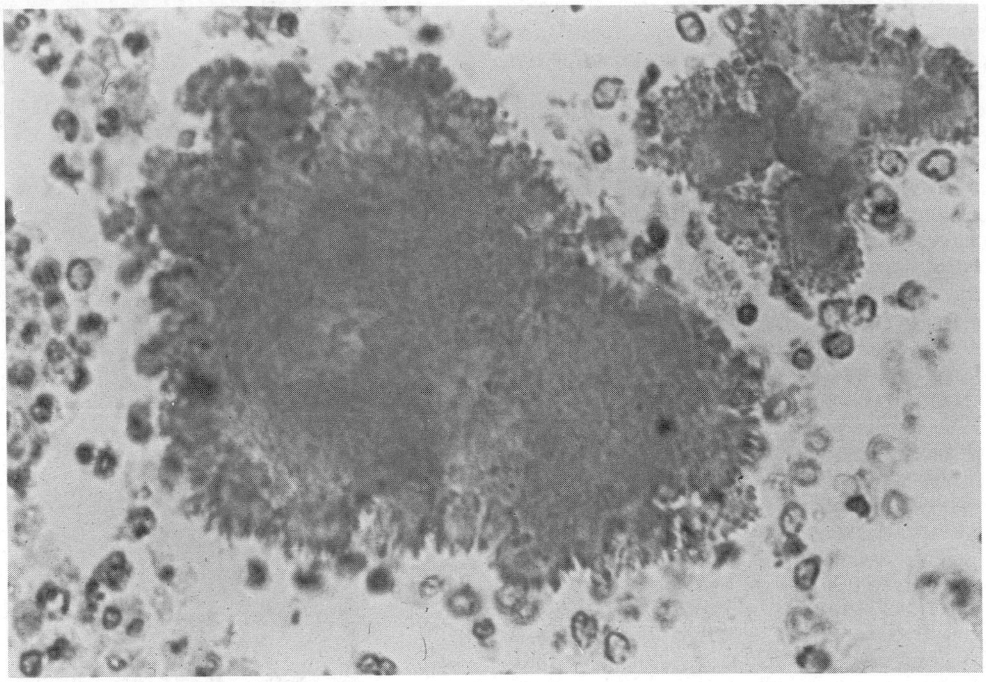

FIG. 3. Sulfur granule revealing an amorphous, amphophilic center surrounded by a rosette of clubbed filaments. (H&E, ×100) (From Lerner,[110] with permission.)

plus bacteremia and endocarditis.[16] It will not grow in a simple medium (e.g., Sabouraud's dextrose agar), produces no aerial filaments, and ferments a variety of carbohydrates, thus avoiding confusion with *Nocardia* spp.

Actinomyces odontolyticus has been associated with all major forms of actinomycosis, including septicemia and disseminated liver abscesses.[17–19] The organism may be present in distinct granules or may be free in the exudate. It is morphologically and physiologically similar to other *Actinomyces* spp.[5]

Actinomyces and *Arachnia* spp. require extended anaerobic or microaerophilic incubation. Specimens should not be taken from patients receiving antibiotics. As Peabody and Seabury note, ". . . by the time the need for special cultural techniques is appreciated, if indeed it is considered at all, the rather ready susceptibility of *A.* [*israelii*] to most available antibiotics has so suppressed its growth that cultures, even when properly sown, are likely to be negative."[20]

The cellular antigens of *A. israelii* are not well defined. Agglutinins and complement-fixing antibodies appear in the sera of some patients, but serologic methods remain impractical, since cross-precipitating antibodies form in other diseases, particularly tuberculosis.[21,22] Immunoelectrophoresis, using monospecific antigen–antibody systems, may yet yield a specific serodiagnostic method.[23,24]

Fluorescein isothiocyanate species-specific antiserum provides rapid and specific identification by direct staining of clinical material, allowing species determination within granules, even in formalin-fixed tissues, and permitting recognition of mixed species in a granule.[25] Conjugates have been prepared for each of the four species of *Actinomyces* and for *Ar. propionica*.[26]

PATHOGENESIS AND PATHOLOGIC CHARACTERISTICS

Actinomyces and *Arachnia* spp. are not highly virulent pathogens, but simply endogenous oral saprophytes—in periodontal pockets and carious teeth, dental plaque and tonsillar crypts—taking advantage of infection, trauma, or a surgical injury to penetrate normally intact mucosal barriers and invade adjacent tissues.[27] Cervicofacial infections follow dental infections and manipulations. Thoracic infection follows apiration of infected oral debris in patients with lingual or gingivodental infection but does not commonly follow cervicofacial infection. Rarely, thoracic infection derives from a penetrating abdominal infection, a retroperitoneal infection, or a mucosal lesion of the esophagus. Abdominal infection often originates in the appendix. Actinomyces are only rarely opportunists in patients on steroids or with leukemia, renal failure, metastatic carcinoma, or acquired immunodeficiency syndrome (AIDS).[1,28] *Primary* actinomycosis, reported in isolated organs or unusual locations and lacking an obvious mucosal point of entry, represents instances where the original source of infection has healed.

Lesions, and even sulfur granules, characteristically contain other bacteria. Holm found *associates* in all closed lesions[29]; others did not,[30,31] but polymicrobic infections are characteristic.[1] Associates may be subcultured as commensals along with supposedly pure cultures. *Actinobacillus actinomycetemcomitans, Haemophilus* spp., fusobacteria, anaerobic and other streptococci, micrococci, staphylococci, *Eikenella corrodens*, and oral bacteroides accompany cervicofacial, nervous system, and thoracic infections; coliforms and intestinal anaerobes are abdominal associates.[1,29–31] Infection can be induced in mice by various *Actinomyces* spp. alone,[5,32] but mixed infections in mice provide evidence of mutualism between different pathogens in the lesions,[33] supporting Holm's conclusion in 1950 that actinomycosis results from a synergistic interaction between *Actinomyces* spp. and a variety of gram-negative associates, the latter augmenting the comparatively weak invasive capacities of the former.[29] Mechanisms of host resistance and immunity to *Actinomyces* spp. are largely unknown, but comparative histopathology of actinomycotic lesions in mice suggests important differences in the host immune response to *A. israelli, A. naeslundii*, and *A. viscosus*.[32] T lymphocytes are not involved either in clearing *A. israelii* from the mouse lung or in preventing disseminated infection, but they may have a role in localized cervicofacial infection.[34]

Antecedent disease and surgery predisposed to infection in

81 of 181 subjects reviewed by Brown[30]; in 100 cases no antecedent event was recorded, although minor dental trauma could not be excluded. Actinomyces granules are commonly found in tonsillar crypts,[5] but they usually provoke little, if any, local tissue reaction and actinomycosis rarely follows tonsillitis or complicates tonsillectomy.[20,30] All age groups are affected, including infants and children.[35] In Brown's series, patients ranged between 10 and 90 years of age, with two-thirds of them between the ages of 30 and 60; males outnumbered females by 4:1.[30] The male prevalence is 3:1 in other series.[1] In childhood, both sexes appear to be infected equally,[35] often with puzzling clinical presentations.[15,36–38]

Gross lesions are single or multiple indurated masses with hard, fibrous walls and soft, central loculations containing pus. Sinus tracts extend to the skin or mucous membrane surfaces or into organs. Chronic infections may remain localized, but the longer the course, the more likely the development of sinuses and/or distant spread. Lesions of the pelvis and abdomen display the highest incidence of sinus development.[30] Histopathology reveals suppuration surrounded by fibrosing, acutely or chronically inflamed granulation tissue.[2] Foamy macrophages account for the yellow color seen grossly. Eosinophils and giant cells are uncommon; plasma cells are scarce acutely but increase with chronicity. Fibrosis may not be prominent in the lung or may be ill-defined, limited, or absent in any early infection. In chronic infection, one typically finds healing by intense, even avascular fibrosis in one area, with acute suppuration nearby.

Sulfur granules are distinctive conglomerate masses of organisms, but aggregates of other organisms, including fungi, nocardia, streptomyces, and staphylococci (botryomycosis) may resemble them; imitators usually lack the characteristic clubbed peripheral fringe.[30] Grossly, the granules are hard, gritty, yellow or dull white by reflected light, and light brown, translucent, or refractile by transmitted light,[31] averaging 2 mm in diameter (Fig. 4). Histologically, they are round or oval, basophilic or amphophilic masses with a radiating rosette or fringe of eosinophilic clubs on the surface.[30] The centers are granular or fibrillar, and a narrow, granular, basophilic band may be present in the outer portion (Fig. 3). The largest ones are very loosely aggregated. Granules may be few and hard to find, and multiple sections of the abscess wall or sinus tract must be meticulously studied.[30] Granules in early lesions may be loosely aggregated, may have poorly developed clubs, and may not be surrounded by chronic inflammatory cells. Not all *Actinomyces* spp. provoke granule formation in tissues as readily as *A. israelii*. The granule represents a mineralized mycelial mass cemented by host calcium phosphate consequent to phosphatase activity from tissue inflammation. Surface *clubs* (Fig. 3) are filaments encased in the same polysaccharide–protein complex.[39] Sulfur granules do not form in vitro. Club-shaped fringes are rare in tonsillar crypt granules, as there is usually little tissue reaction.[25] The true granule reveals masses of gram-positive branching filaments (Fig. 2) when crushed and Gram-stained, a useful diagnostic maneuver.[31,39]

A single filament of *A. israelii* resembles a single filament of *Nocardia asteroides*, but in actinomycotic abscesses, free filaments outside granules are less common, whereas in pyogenic nocardia infiltrates they are numerous. Granules are absent in visceral nocardial lesions and are seen only in mycetoma due to *Nocardia* spp.[40] The presence of acid-fast organisms (by the Putt modification of the Ziehl-Neelsen stain) in actinomycotic sulfur granules suggests that both *A. israelii* and *N. asteroides* could be acid-fast under certain conditions,[40] but the Putt modification produces a positive reaction with many unrelated organisms.[25]

CLINICAL MANIFESTATIONS AND DIAGNOSIS

Cervicofacial Actinomycosis

Actinomycosis should be considered in any cutaneous or soft tissue swelling of the head, face, or neck. A variety of acute, subacute, or chronic lesions from a simple phlegmon to a draining sinus, or an abscess in the cheek, at the angle of the jaw or in the submental area may occur. Cervicofacial actinomycosis evolves in one of two distinct patterns, although the clinical course is variable and patients can display any combination of

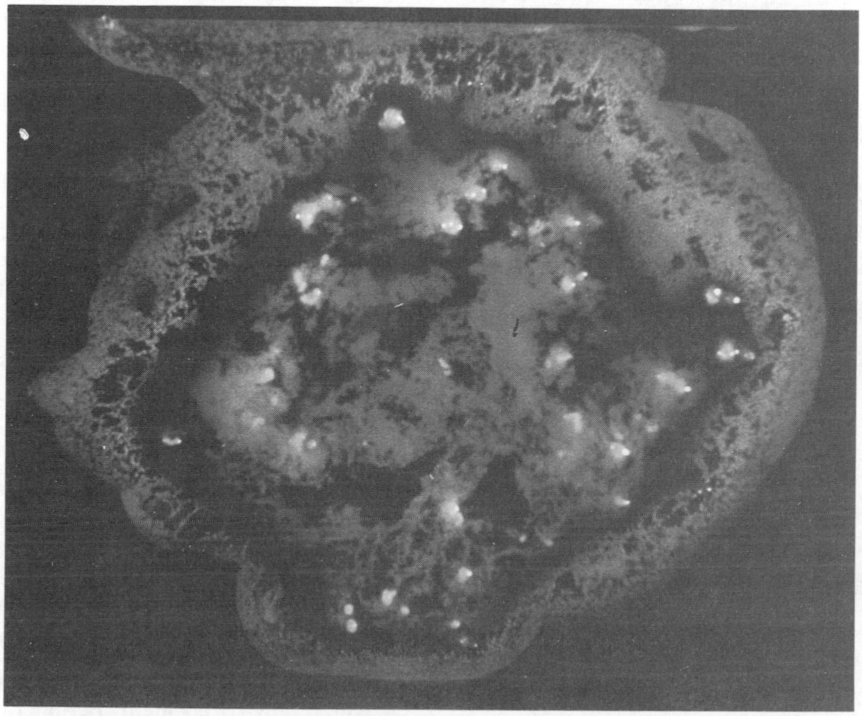

FIG. 4. Macroscopic sulfur granules on a glass slide.

features between the two extremes.[2] The first, a painless lesion, is a slowly enlarging, fluctuant, bluish swelling located at the crossing of the lower border of the mandible by the facial vessels. The second form, more painful and widespread, simulates an acute pyogenic infection in the submandibular (Fig. 5) or paramandibular (Fig. 6) area, at the angle of the mandible, in the parotid region, or in the neck.[41,42] In any area, a pseudotumor (cold abscess) may develop, especially in early cases. Primary infection also may occur in the scalp, palate, lacrimal gland, orbit, tongue, hypopharynx, larynx, trachea, salivary glands, middle ear, mastoid, and paranasal sinuses.[1,2,41–44] Rare maxillary involvement begins as a localized, radiolucent, periapical or periodontal abscess; cutaneous fistulas and hard facial swellings are unusual, but intraoral mucosal drainage occurs more frequently.

A dental portal of entry can usually be implicated, and many, but not all, patients have neglected dental care and display poor oral hygiene, dental decay, periodontal disease, and gingivitis.[30,41] Infection may follow any surgical or traumatic injury to the oral mucous membrane, even a nonpenetrating blow from the outside or the simple eruption of a tooth, particularly a molar.

Infection spreads without regard for facial tissue planes. Adenopathy is not a feature unless contiguous nodes are involved directly. The slowly progressive form manifests primarily as a chronic tissue induration with trismus, ultimately developing draining cutaneous, fistulous tracts. In the acute, rapidly progressive form, with suppuration and abscess formation beneath the skin, trismus and edema of the surrounding tissues are out of proportion to the amount of inflammation (Fig. 6). Antibiotics have modified the natural course of the acutely progressive form, since spontaneous rupture of these masses is currently an uncommon event. Bone changes vary from minor subperiosteal reactions to lytic destruction, without new bone formation but occasionally with definite thickening and sclerosis. The jaw is the most common site of actinomycotic bone involvement.[45] Among 317 patients treated at the Department of Dental Surgery of the University of Cologne (1952–1975), the distribution of lesions was as follows: mandible, 53.6 percent; cheek, 16.4 percent; chin, 13.3 percent; submaxillary ramus and angle, 10.7 percent; upper jaw, 5.7 percent; and mandibular joint, 0.3 percent.[46] Direct bone invasion was rare, but periostitis and post-traumatic osteomyelitis occurred in 11.7 percent of these cases.[46] Primary infection of the thyroid gland,[47] postoperative infection in a thyroidectomy incision, and infection as a complication of transtracheal aspiration have been reported.[48] Actinomycosis of the tongue represents approximately 3 percent of all actinomycotic infections, invading sublingual tissues secondarily.[49] Infection inside the oral cavity can present as an acute abscess, a subacute inflammatory nodule, an infiltrating mass, or a pseudotumor. Infection in tooth extraction sites is common (especially at the third molar) but also occurs in dentigerous cysts with no apparent anatomic connection to the oral cavity.[2]

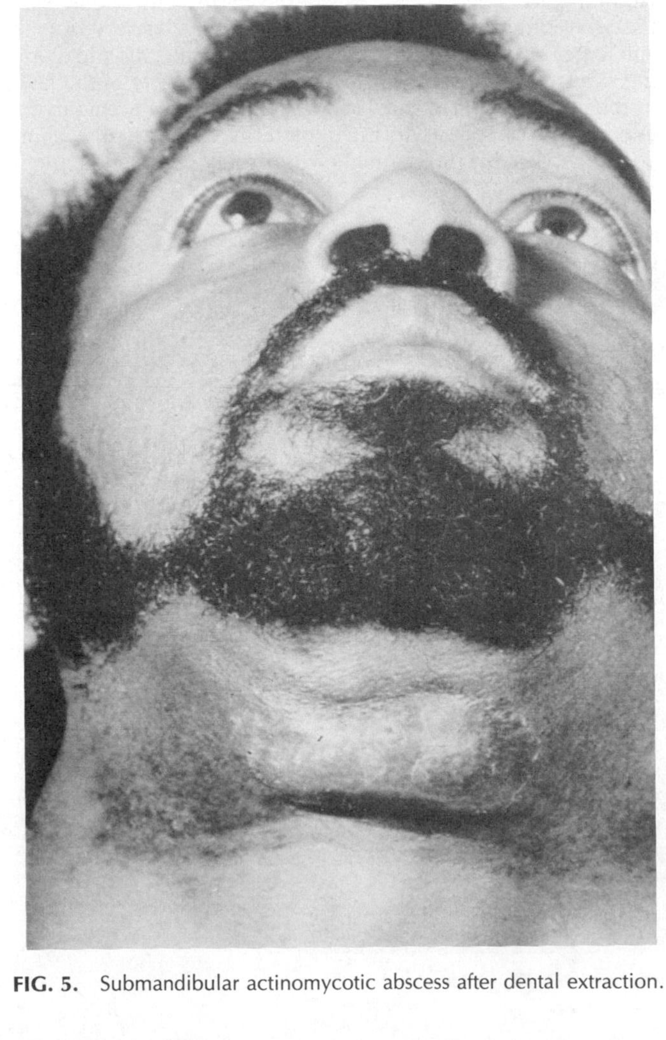

FIG. 5. Submandibular actinomycotic abscess after dental extraction.

Primary bone infection is rare; osseous involvement derives from adjacent soft tissue infection, provoking a periostitis that stimulates new bone formation, often the only x-ray finding. When bone is actively invaded, localized areas of bone destruction are surrounded by increased bone density; bony foci may be interconnected by sinus tracts. Thus, the x-ray appearance can range from a minor subperiosteal reaction and minimal rarefaction to classic osteomyelitis with total lytic destruction or thickening and sclerosis resembling a bone tumor; the mandible is more commonly involved (4:1) than the maxilla.[45] In osteoradionecrosis of the jaws, a serious complication of head-neck radiation therapy, chronic actinomycotic infection may be overlooked for extended periods of time.[50]

Thoracic and Disseminated Actinomycosis

Thoracic infection may involve the lungs, pleura, mediastinum, or chest wall. With no telltale draining sinus (Fig. 7), the correct diagnosis is often long delayed. Infection follows oropharyngeal aspiration, esophageal penetration, direct extension into the mediastinum from the neck, or retroperitoneal or transdiaphragmatic spread from the abdomen. Severe dental disease, abscess, or periodontitis is often the presumed site of primary infection; some patients are edentulous.[51] Bronchitis, emphysema, chronic pneumonitis, or bronchiectasis may be a background feature.[30] Infection mimics tuberculosis or malignancy, particularly when a dense hilar lesion extends into the parenchyma (Fig. 8), and is often discovered when these two diagnoses are being pursued.[51] Constitutional symptoms are nonspecific: weight loss, cough, chest pain, fever, and hemoptysis. Often the expected signs of systemic infection (acute or chronic) may be lacking: Fever may be absent, the white blood cell count may be normal, and anemia need not be present. Hemoptysis is unusual but can occur in a patient with a lung abscess.

Routine cultures seldom yield the pathogen, so cases go unrecognized until empyema or a chest wall fistula leads to the proper studies.[1] Such delays explain Cope's observation of increased hematogenous dissemination in thoracic actinomycosis,[49] If one considers all sites, hematogenous dissemination is not very common in actinomycosis, occurring in 10 percent of cases in Brown's review.[30] Recently, more such cases are being reported.[52] A miliary picture has followed a pelvic infection.[53] Peripheral lesions (skin, subcutaneous tissues, muscle) (Fig. 9) may herald the infection, with pulmonary lesions discovered only by accident. Peripheral skin lesions may suggest a vasculitis on biopsy unless organisms are recognized or cul-

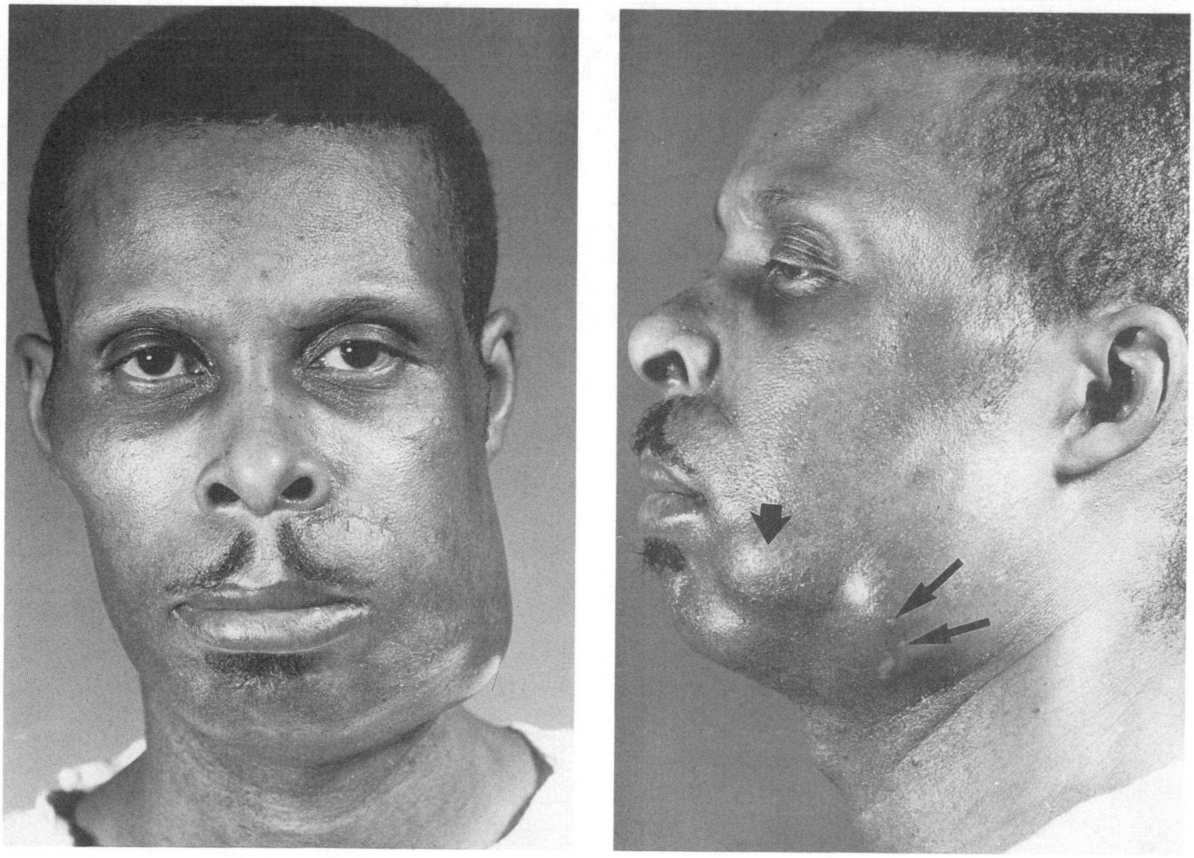

FIG. 6. **(A)** Acute paramandibular actinomycosis (frontal view). **(B)** Acute paramandibular actinomycosis (lateral view). Note two sinus openings (thin arrows) and secondary anterior swelling (large arrow). (Courtesy of Dr. C. Babbush. From Lerner,[110] with permission.)

tured.[54,55] Secondary lesions also harbor associates.[56] Rarely, the organism disseminates in the presence of widespread malignancy.[1]

The classic chronic chest wall sinus discharging granules (Fig. 7) is uncommon today because antibiotics tend to limit infection to the lung. Trapping of granules is enhanced by placing gauze over the fistulous opening. When drainage is copious, one should examine the wall of a tilted tube filled with pus.[57] Pleuropulmonary involvement occurs in less than 2 percent of cases, although small effusions or pleural thickenings were common x-ray findings in one review.[58] Massive empyema is rare[51] but does occur.[59] *Actinomyces* spp. can be one of several participants in a mixed anaerobic empyema, where its primacy can be questioned in the absence of characteristic histopathology.[59]

X-ray findings are nonspecific (see Figs. 2 and 3 of Chapter 56), but some are highly suggestive[58]: (*1*) pulmonary lesions extending through the chest wall; (*2*) wavy periostitis or frank destruction of the ribs, sternum, or shoulder girdle adjacent to a chronic pulmonary process; (*3*) involvement of adjacent lobes by extension (transgression) through an interlobar fissure; and (*4*) characteristic vertebral destruction, extending from mediastinal or retroperitoneal involvement, with erosion of both the body and processes of the affected vertebra, as well as the adjacent ribs. Destruction, combined with new bone formation, produces a mottled effect and, unlike tuberculosis, vertebral collapse and intervertebral disk narrowing are not common, as the disk space is usually spared.[45] Rib periostitis, as a specific x-ray finding, has become uncommon, and the condition most frequently simulated now is a primary bronchogenic carcinoma. Rib abnormalities or destruction can even be due to a combination of carcinoma and actinomycosis.[58] One or more small cavities are found in half the cases; large cavities are rare.[58]

Pulmonary involvement can also resemble a mass, a chronic fibrocavitary process with striking volume contraction resembling tuberculosis, or simply a chronic alveolar infiltrate. Ero-

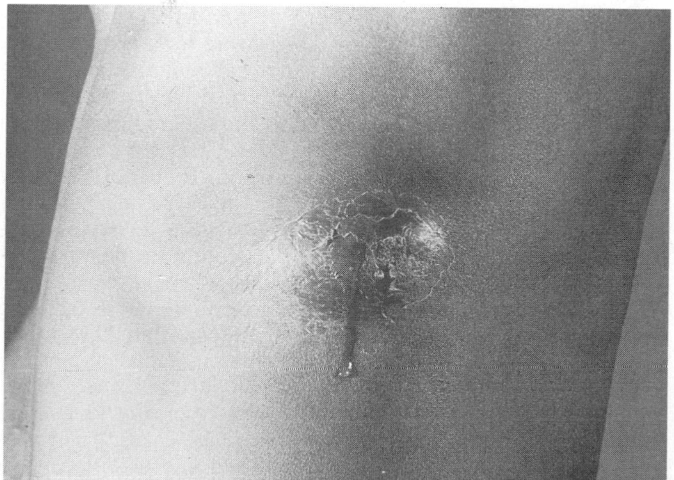

FIG. 7. Spontaneously draining chest wall sinus caused by *A. israelii* in a young man with an asymptomatic pulmonary infiltrate and sulfur granules in sputum cytology.

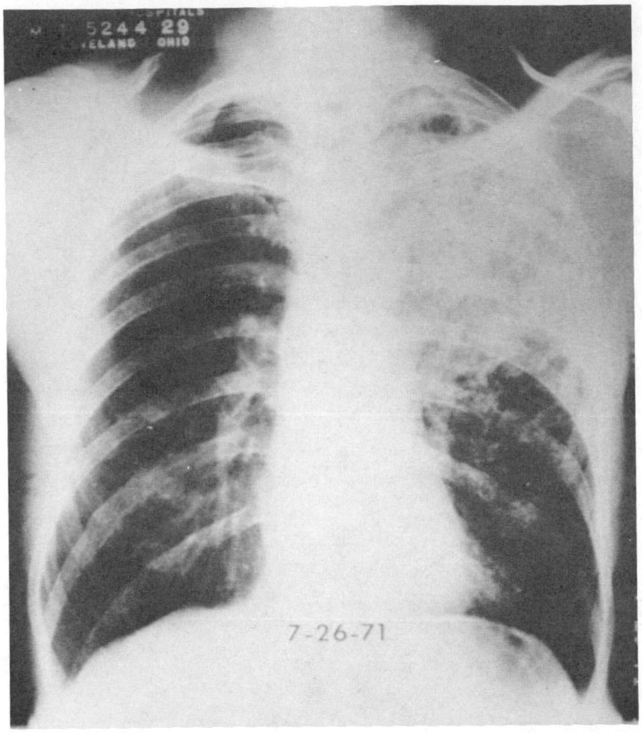

FIG. 8. Cavitating left upper lobe actinomycotic pneumonia treated mistakenly as tuberculosis. See also Figure 2, Chapter 56.

sion into a blood vessel may produce a disseminated miliary picture.[53] Less common are mediastinal involvement, sometimes with superior vena cava obstruction, tracheoesophageal fistula, systemic-to-pulmonary artery fistula, or secondary involvement descending from above (cervicofacial) or ascending from below through the liver and the diaphragm into the right lung base. Sulfur granules in sputum cytologic specimens[60] occasionally resolve the engima of an asymptomatic pulmonary mass, although in most instances the diagnosis is first confirmed after surgical resection for presumptive carcinoma. Pseudotumor may occur without cavitation or obvious bronchial communication, although a normal bronchus entering the lesion (the *open bronchus* sign) usually, but not invariably, excludes neoplasm,[61,62] since an actinomycotic mass can compress, constrict, enter, or distort a bronchus.[63] *Actinomyces* spp. can colonize devitalized tissue, so they can grow in tumors undergoing necrosis. Therefore, the infection not only mimics carcinoma of the lung but may also complicate it; a positive sputum culture alone is not diagnostic. Actinomycosis and tuberculosis also can coexist.[64]

The signficance of *Actinomyces* spp. in bronchopulmonary secretions remains controversial. Kay, in 1948,[65] grew actinomyces from sputum in 65 of 240 patients with a variety of bronchopulmonary infections, but Garrod[31] found no positive cultures in 23 patients with bronchiectasis when he washed the specimens to eliminate salivary contamination. Examining sputa in duplicate, Garrod grew actinomyces from 25 of 49 unwashed specimens but none from washed inocula.

The heart, involved in less than 2 percent of all cases of actinomycosis, usually in young adult men, typically follows intrathoracic disease in over 75 percent of the cases.[66] The pericardium is the most commonly involved site at autopsy (79 percent), with the epicardium, myocardium (50 percent), and endocardium (35 percent) involved in decreasing frequency. Endocarditis (mitral or aortic), usually due to direct extension from the pericardium, occasionally is primary. Friction rub is uncommon, and isolated clinical pericarditis is rare.[67]

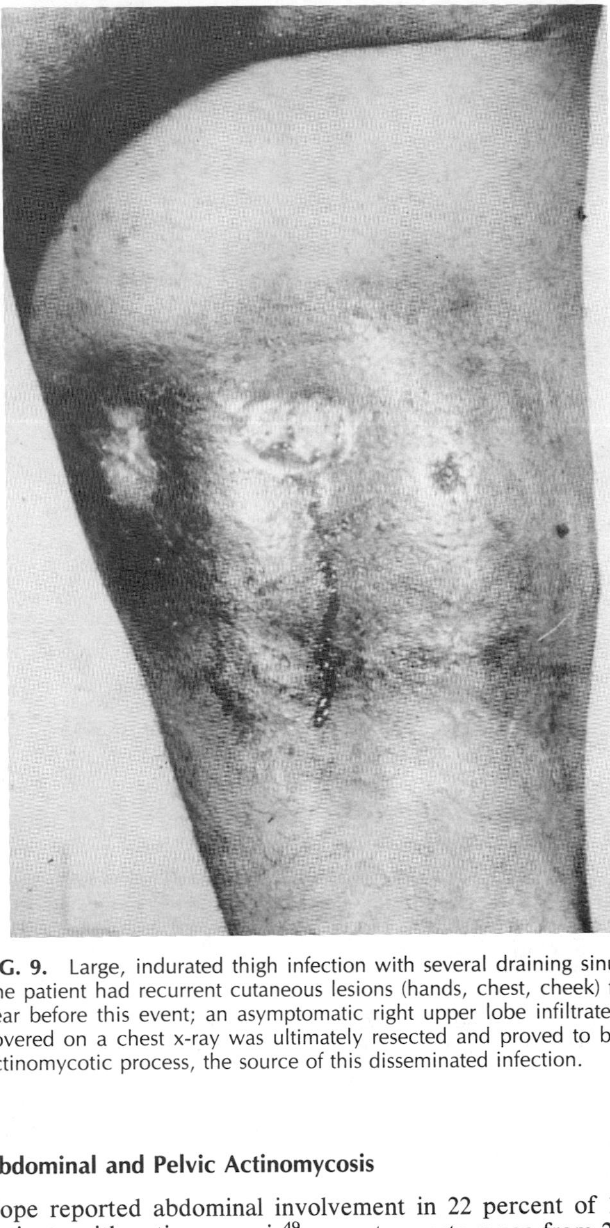

FIG. 9. Large, indurated thigh infection with several draining sinuses. The patient had recurrent cutaneous lesions (hands, chest, cheek) for 1 year before this event; an asymptomatic right upper lobe infiltrate discovered on a chest x-ray was ultimately resected and proved to be an actinomycotic process, the source of this disseminated infection.

Abdominal and Pelvic Actinomycosis

Cope reported abdominal involvement in 22 percent of 1330 patients with actinomycosis[49]; recent reports range from 23 to 53 percent.[1,68] The majority of patients have had prior surgery for an inflammatory bowel condition, most commonly acute appendicitis, or another abdominal emergency.[69] Other antecedents include perforated colonic diverticula and duodenal ulcer, gunshot wound, cholecystectomy, and perforating foreign bodies, such as fish bones.[30] Rarely, nonpenetrating trauma (e.g., a severe blow to the body) antedates the infection.

All forms of actinomycosis are characterized by delayed diagnosis, but the abdominal form heads the list. Latent periods of many months between the inciting event and the recognition of infection are common; a latent period of up to 7 years has been recorded.[69] Diagnosis is also more difficult because of variable pathologic changes, including microabscesses, chronic sinuses and fistulas or abscesses with overwhelming secondary infection, and the avascular "woody" phlegmon (actinomycoma) often excised mistakenly as a colon carcinoma. Correct preoperative diagnosis is made in less than 10 percent of the cases.[70]

Abdominal actinomycosis occurs most frequently in the ileocecal region, being mistaken for Crohn's disease, a cecal carcinoma, tuberculosis, amebiasis, or, if the appendix is intact, a chronic appendicitis.[71] Although ileocecal Crohn's disease offers a favorable antecedent condition, only rarely has actinomycosis been reported to complicate that process.[72] Infection may localize or spread by contiguity, often directed away from the bowel and peritoneal cavity and favoring the subperitoneal or subcutaneous connective tissues to the abdominal wall, paracecally to the subphrenic space, or to the pelvic or perirectal tissues, including the pouch of Douglas.[69] Retroperitoneal infection may simulate tumor or tuberculosis, with extension to the spine.[73] Spread usually occurs by contiguous involvement or vascular channels, rarely by lymphatics. Muscles are often infiltrated, with resultant destruction and fibrosis; bone is infrequently attacked, although vertebral involvement is reported.[10,45,74]

Sinus tracts are not uncommon, but true fistulas from the bowel lumen are surprisingly uncommon, even when the bowel was obviously the source.[68,69] Intermittent episodes of intestinal obstruction occur, however, if the bowel adheres to the inflammatory mass. An antecedent lesion or event may not be evident.[75] Isolated renal, omental, pancreatic, and urachal remnant infections have been reported.[1,76,77]

Infection extending into the pelvic or perianal region can lead to recurrent draining sinuses and fistulas in ano or can manifest simply as a rectal structure.[78] Perianal sinuses of long duration (up to 11 years) may go undiagnosed and may be correctly identified only when characteristic woody induration, sulfur granules, or telltale involvement appears elsewhere in the abdomen. Anorectal disease can also begin primarily in an anal crypt, as a local perianal or ischiorectal abscess, and then spread posteriorly and laterally via the sacrosciatic foramen to the gluteal region.[71]

Gastric actinomycosis mimics ulcer disease or carcinoma. Intramural gastric actinomycosis alone is exceedingly rare; the more common perigastric form declares as an inflammatory mass or abscess adjacent to the stomach or duodenum, usually after perforation of, or surgery for, a peptic ulcer or perforation of the rare solitary intramural gastric actinomycotic focus.[79] Splenic infection may follow gastric perforation.

Hepatic involvement occurs in 15 percent of cases of abdominal actinomycosis and usually arrives via the portal vein from a focus in the bowel, by direct extension from contiguous viscera, or, rarely, via the hepatic artery during disseminated infection.[69] Hepatic lesions may penetrate the abdominal wall, the diaphragm, adjacent viscera, or retroperitoneal tissues.[30] Jaundice is rare, the liver function tests may be normal or abnormal. Reported patterns of hepatic involvement include a solitary intrahepatic mass mimicking neoplasm,[80] multiple liver abscesses,[81] and a disseminated miliary pattern.[18,82,83] Gallbladder and common duct involvement, exceedingly rare, can also occur as isolated events.

Only a small percentage of abdominal cases involve the female pelvic organs, but most cases of pelvic actinomycosis, excluding those associated with IUDs, originate from endogenous intestinal sources. Patients have vague complaints indistinguishable from other insidious malignant or inflammatory pelvic disorders, and the diagnosis is usually made at surgery, unfortunately sometimes after several surgical procedures. Rarely acute, the most common pattern follows a subacute or chronic course lasting for many months or years. Right adnexal involvement is found in 80 percent of the cases; in half of these, involvement is bilateral. When infection derives from intestinal sources, the ovary is the most common organ affected[84]; next in frequency are the tubes and ovaries together, the uterus, the vulva, the cervix, and finally the tubes alone, but endometrial involvement is uncommon unless the organism is introduced directly, as in criminal abortion, with IUDs, infected pessaries, or retained surgical sutures.

Schiffer et al. reported 10 cases of pelvic infection associated with IUDs in a 2-year period, none spreading beyond the genital tract.[85] Presentations of pelvic actinomycosis associated with IUDs range from simple vaginal discharge, to pelvic inflammatory disease with tuboovarian abscess or ureteral obstruction, and, unfortunately, to a "frozen pelvis" mimicking malignancy.[86,87]

When IUD usage was initially recognized as a cause of pelvic actinomycosis, it was believed that the presence of actinomyces-like organisms (ALOs) on Papanicolaou smears of IUD users represented a pathologic state, was predictive of future difficulties, and was an indication for removal of the device. We now appreciate that some 5 percent of healthy women without IUDs harbor ALOs,[88] that the incidence is not higher in IUD users, that not all ALOs seen on Papanicolaou smears represent true actinomyces,[89,90] and that even more precise immunofluorescent staining techniques (limited currently by the absence of commercially available reagents) do not identify high-risk IUD users.[91] Serologic (precipitin) testing might identify IUD users at high risk for developing genital actinomycosis.[92] The overall risk for developing actinomycosis with IUD use seems minuscule given the total number of patient years of IUD use, but prolonged IUD use associated with a stubborn or recurrent pelvic inflammatory condition, especially when tumor is a consideration, should alert gynecologists to the possibility of pelvic actinomycosis and consideration of prolonged antibiotic administration after removal of the IUD.[93]

Urinary tract actinomycosis is rare, as is male genitourinary system infection.[1] The kidneys or bladder can be involved by extension from an intestinal focus, although isolated kidney, bladder, and prostate involvement have all been reported; rarely, sulfur granules in the urine herald this event, but patients may present with a pubic mass, abdominal or rectal pain, or a fistula (ileovesical, appendicovesical or vesicocutaneous).[94–96]

Actinomycosis of the Nervous System

Primary actinomycosis of the central nervous system (CNS) is rare, and, unfortunately, many early reports also include examples of nocardia infection.[97,98] CNS involvement, by direct extension or via metastatic infection, occurs in about 10 percent of cases.[68]

Infection may extend superiorly (sometimes over a period of years) to the base of the skull directly from a cervicofacial focus along connective tissue planes or through foramina at the base of the skull (rarely through bone) and thence into brain (focal CNS infection) or meninges (diffuse basilar meningitis). Perineural spread (from the pharynx via the foramen ovale) to the trigeminal ganglion and from a dental root abscess to the gasserian ganglion represent unusually localized spread, producing tumor-like masses.[98] Direct extension may occur slowly, over a period of years, but Bolton and Ashenhurst[97] concluded that most CNS cases derive from hematogenous spread (teeth or lungs), most commonly producing a single, multiloculated cerebral hemisphere abscess. Smego recently confirmed those findings in a comprehensive tabulation of 70 reported cases of CNS actinomycotic infection.[98] Lesions included brain abscesses (67 percent), which were generally singular, although 9 patients had multiple abscesses with a predilection for the temporal and frontal lobes; meningitis or meningoencephalitis (13 percent); actinomycomas (7 percent) simulating tumors in the cerebral cortices, posterior fossa, or ventricles; subdural empyema (6 percent); and epidural abscess (6 percent). Most infections developed from hematogenous seeding from a distant primary site, most commonly the lungs, mouth, abdomen, or pelvis, including uterine infection secondary to an IUD. Extension of actinomycosis to the vertebral canal and spinal cord may occur by way of intervertebral foramina from a cervical, pulmonary, or abdominal focus,[74,99] and although the dura generally resists penetration, granulation tissue may cause epidural abscess and compression.[98] Brachial plexus involvement has been recorded in thoracic actinomycosis.[100] Draining sinuses were not described in this review of CNS infections, and unlike nocardiosis, where relapse in CNS infection is not uncommon, CNS actinomycosis recurred late in only 1 of 70 instances.[98]

MUSCULOSKELETAL ACTINOMYCOSIS

Secondary involvement of an extremity may result from local spread of cervical, thoracic, or abdominal infection or via hematogenous dissemination (Fig. 9). Because the etiologic agent(s) are exclusively endogenous commensals, primary infection of an extremity is uncommon, and in a recent review of the problem, trauma (including a human bite) preceded infection in 60 percent of the cases.[101] Because of the many clinical and pathologic similarities between isolated actinomycoma of the extremity and mycetoma caused by aerobic actinomycetes, proper identification of the etiologic agent is essential. Osteomyelitis of the long bones of the extremities is exceedingly rare. Before 1950, vertebral actinomycosis was the most common form of osseous actinomycosis reported; the antibiotic era has witnessed a decreased occurrence of widespread actinomycosis with vertebral involvement and increased recognition of bone involvement (jaw) after cervicofacial infection.[45]

THERAPY

Before 1941, death or persistent infection was the end result of all but the most localized disease. With the introduction of penicillin, cure became the rule rather than the exception. Principles for managing actinomycosis remain unchanged since 1960, when Peabody and Seabury[20] emphasized the use of intense, prolonged antibiotic therapy coupled with a sound surgical approach to drainage of abscesses or radical excision of sinus tracts.[71] Penicillin in large doses, given over a period of weeks to months, is the drug of choice, since high concentration are necessary to penetrate areas of fibrosis and suppuration and possibly the granules themselves.[102,103] Occasionally, extensive disease responds to intravenous penicillin alone and may not require surgery.[51,100,104] Cervicofacial infection carries an excellent prognosis for the response to antibiotics alone when recognized early and treated appropriately; tetracycline(s) are as effective as penicillin. Intravenous penicillin G, 10–20 million units/day for 2–6 weeks, followed by oral penicillin (e.g., phenoxymethyl penicillin, 2–4 g/day, to patient tolerance) for 3–12 additional months, is an approximate therapeutic goal for the most deep-seated infections. Specifics in a given case, such as dissemination, critical location (e.g., nervous system, cardiac system) or inability to perform definitive surgery, may alter or extend this formula.[71]

Occasional failures follow the use of penicillin alone. Peabody and Seabury reviewed in vitro and clinical data up to 1960 on sulfadiazine, streptomycin, erythromycin, chloramphenicol, and the tetracyclines.[20] Cures had been achieved with each drug alone or in combinations; in vitro data suggested that actinomyces were inhibited by chloramphenicol (0.005–0.01 μg/ml), by erythromycin (0.005–0.1 μg/ml), and by several tetracyclines. Even streptomycin, considerably less active in vitro, produced excellent clinical results in some cases. Associates may explain such unexpected results.[102] Cures with isoniazid and stilbamidine have been reported.[20] Rifampin therapy for suspected tuberculosis can mask undiagnosed pulmonary actinomycosis.[105]

More recent in vitro testing of 74 strains (seven species) revealed penicillin G minimal inhibitory concentrations (MICs) of 0.03–0.5 μg/ml for all strains of *A. israelii* and 0.06–0.5 μg/ml for all other actinomyces except one strain of *A. naeslundii* and three strains of four *A. bovis* (MIC 1.0 μg/ml).[106] Erythromycin was the most active antimicrobial (MIC 0.12 μg/ml or less). Minocycline and clindamycin were very active in vitro (MICs 0.03–1.0 μg/ml); for a few strains other than *A. israelii*, MICs for clindamycin were 2.0–8.0 μg/ml. MICs for cephalothin, ampicillin, lincomycin, tetracycline, doxycycline, and chloramphenicol were within a therapeutic range for all strains of *A. israelii* and most other species. Metronidazole was conspicuously unimpressive in vitro, as were the aminoglycosides.[106] Similar in vitro results have been reported from Sweden.[107]

Since there are no major species variations in antimicrobial susceptibility among the first-line drugs (penicillin, tetracyclines, erythromycin, clindamycin), infection with strains other than *A. israelii* should also respond to adequate courses of treatment with penicillin G or with any of the penicillin alternatives.[106] Some strains of *A. israelii* are inhibited by sulfonamide concentrations attainable in serum (4.0–8.0 mg/100 ml). Therefore, proven cases of actinomycosis, not mistaken instances of nocardiosis, might on occasion respond to sulfonamides.[106] Cephalosporins (first generation) and clindamycin can now be added to the list of alternative parenteral drugs endorsed by Peabody and Seabury.[20,22] Oral cephalexin and the semisynthetic penicillins, oxacillin and dicloxacillin, are considerably less active in vitro and are best avoided.[106]

Garrod[103] claimed that unsuccessful penicillin treatment may be accompanied by increased in vitro resistance; MICs for two strains of *A. israelii* increased from 0.03 U/ml to 0.2 and >0.5 U/ml, respectively. Boand and Novak found that strains of *A. bovis* (probably *A. israelii*) did not readily adapt to penicillin with serial passage in subinhibitory concentrations of the drug, although four of six strains developed two- to fourfold resistance.[108] The development of in vivo acquired antimicrobial resistance by *Actinomyces* spp., particularly to penicillin G, has not been confirmed. When the response to penicillin is poor, one should search for an undrained abscess, although the possibility of a resistant bacterial associate cannot be entirely dismissed. In fact, some experienced European investigators favor the use of ampicillin (or amoxicillin) for initial therapy because of these concomitant bacterial spp., which are less susceptible in vitro to penicillin G, and even employ metronidazole or clindamycin as secondary agents when *Bacteroides* (*B. fragilis, B. thetaiotomicron*) are present.[46] Imipenem produced an impressive response in an extensive, complicated, and relapsing abdominothoracic infection that had failed to be cured with several earlier surgical procedures and trials of penicillin G.[109]

REFERENCES

1. Weese WC, Smith JM. A study of 57 cases of actinomycosis over a 36-year period. Arch Intern Med. 1975;135:1562–8.
2. Richtsmeier WJ, Johns ME. Actinomycosis of the head and neck. CRC Crit Rev Clin. 1979;11:175–302.
3. Schaal KP, Schofield GM. Classification and identification of clinically significant actinomycetaceae. In: Ortiz-Ortiz L, Bojalil LF, Yakoleff V, eds. Biological, Biochemical and Biomedical Aspects of Actinomycetes. Orlando, Fla.: Academic Press; 1984:505–20.
4. Erikson D. Pathogenic anaerobic organisms of the Actinomyces group. Br Med Res Council. Special Report Series. 1940;No. 240:1–63.
5. Georg LK. The agents of human actinomycosis. In: Balows A, ed. Anaerobic Bacteria Role in Disease. Springfield, Ill: Charles C Thomas; 1974:237–56.
6. Waksman SA, Henrici AT. The nomenclature and classification of the Actinomycetes. J Bacteriol. 1943;46;337–41.
7. Lentino JR, Allen JE, Stachowski M. Hematogenous dissemination of thoracic actinomycosis due to *Actinomyces meyeri*. Pediatr Infect Dis. 1985;4:698–9.
8. Allworth AM, Ghosh HK, Saltos N. A case of *Actinomyces meyeri* pneumonia in a child. Med J Aust. 1986;145:33.
9. Brock DW, Georg LK, Brown JM, et al. Actinomycosis caused by *Arachnia propionica*. Report of 11 cases. Am J Clin Pathol. 1973;59:66–77.
10. Conrad SE, Breivis J, Fried MA. Vertebral osteomyelitis caused by *Arachnia propionica* and resembling actinomycosis. J Bone Joint Surg. 1978;60-A:549–53.
11. Miglets AW. Branson D. *Arachnia propionica* (*Actinomyces propionicus*) as an unusual agent in tympanomastoiditis. Arch Otolaryngol. 1983;109:410–2.
12. Coleman RM, Georg LK, Rozzell AR. *Actinomyces naeslundii* as an agent in human actinomycosis. Appl Microbiol. 1969;18:420–6.
13. Bonnez W, Lattimer G, Mohanraj NA, et al. *Actinomyces naeslundii* as an agent of pelvic actinomycosis in the presence of an intrauterine device. J Clin Microbiol. 1985;21:273–5.
14. Kakkasseril J, Cabanas V, Saba K. Ruptured actinomycotic aneurysm of the splenic artery: A case report of successful resection. Surgery. 1983;93:595–7.
15. Dobson SRM, Edwards MS. Extensive *Actinomyces naeslundii* infection in a child. J Clin Microbiol. 1987;25:1327–9.
16. Eng RHK, Corrado ML, Cleri D, et al. Infections caused by *Actinomyces viscosus*. Am J Clin Pathol. 1981;75:113–6.

17. Hutton RM, Behrens RH. *Actinomyces odontolyticus* as a cause of brain abscess. J Infect. 1979;1:195–7.
18. Ruutu P, Pentikainen PJ, Larinkari U, et al. Hepatic actinomycosis presenting as repeated cholestatic reactions. Scand J Infect Dis. 1982;14:235–8.
19. Peloux Y, Raoult D, Chardon H, et al. *Actinomyces odontolyticus* infections: Review of six patients. J Infect. 1985;11:125–9.
20. Peabody JW, Seabury JH. Actinomycosis and nocardiosis. Am J Med. 1960;28:99–115.
21. Georg LK, Coleman RM, Brown JM. Evaluation of an agar gel precipitin test for serodiagnosis of actinomycosis. J Immunol. 1968;100:1288–92.
22. Lerner PI. Serologic screening for actinomycosis. In: Balows A, ed. Anaerobic Bacteria Role in Disease. Springfield, Ill: Charles C Thomas; 1974:571–84.
23. Holmberg K, Nord CF, Wadstrom T. Serological studies of *Actinomyces israelii* by crossed immunoelectrophoresis: Taxonomic and diagnostic applications. Infect Immun. 1975;12:398–403.
24. Holmberg K. Immunodiagnosis of human actinomycosis. Zentralbl Bakteriol Mikrobiol Hyg. 1981;11(Suppl):259–61.
25. Hotchi M, Schwartz J. Characterization of actinomycotic granules by architecture and staining methods. Arch Pathol. 1972;93:392–400.
26. Happonen RP, Viander M. Comparison of fluorescent antibody technique and conventional staining methods in diagnosis of cervico-facial actinomycosis. J Oral Pathol. 1982;11:417–25.
27. Bowden GHW. Pathogenesis of *Actinomyces israelii* infections. In: Ortiz-Ortiz L, Bojalil LF, Yakoleff V, eds. Biological, Biochemical, and Biomedical Aspects of Actinomycetes. Orlando, Fla: Academic Press; 1984:1–12.
28. Yeager BH, Hoxie J, Weisman RA, et al. Actinomycosis in the acquired immunodeficiency syndrome-related complex. Arch Otolaryngol Head Neck Surg. 1986;112:1293–5.
29. Holm P. Studies on the aetiology of human actinomycosis. 1. The "other microbes" of actinomycosis and their importance. Acta Pathol Microbiol Scand. 1950;27:736–51.
30. Brown JR. Human actinomycosis. A study of 181 subjects. Hum Pathol. 1973;4:319–30.
31. Garrod LP. Actinomycosis of the lung. Aetiology, diagnosis and chemotherapy. Tubercle. 1952;33:258–66.
32. Behbehani MJ, Heeley JD, Jordan HV. Comparative histopathology of lesions produced by *Actinomyces israelii*, *Actinomyces naeslundii*, and *Actinomyces viscosus* in mice. Am J Pathol. 1983;110:267–74.
33. Jordan HV, Kelly DM, Heeley JD. Enhancement of experimental actinomycosis in mice by *Eikenella corrodens*. Infect Immun. 1984;46:367–71.
34. Beaman BL, Gershwin ME, Maslan S. Infectious agents in immunodeficient murine models. Pathogenicity of *Actinomyces israelii* serotype I in congenitally athymic (nude) mice. Infect Immun. 1979;24:583–5.
35. Drake DP, Holt RJ, Childhood actinomycosis. Report of 3 recent cases. Arch Dis Child. 1976;51:979–81.
36. Spinola SM, Bell RA, Henderson FW. Actinomycosis. A cause of pulmonary and mediastinal mass lesions in children. Am J Dis Child. 1981;135:336–9.
37. Stanley IV. Deep actinomycosis in childhood. Acta Paediatr Scand. 1980;69:173–6.
38. Golden N, Cohen H, Weissbrot J, et al. Thoracic actinomycosis in childhood. Clin Pediatr. 1984;24:646–50.
39. Pine L, Overman JR. Determination of the structure and composition of the "sulphur granules" of *Actinomyces bovis*. J Gen Microbiol. 1963;32:209–23.
40. Robboy SJ, Vickery AL. Tinctorial and morphologic properties distinguishing actinomycosis and nocardiosis. N Engl J Med. 1970;282:593–6.
41. Bennhoff DF. Actinomycosis: Diagnostic and therapeutic considerations and a review of 32 cases. Laryngoscope. 1984;94:1198–1217.
42. Hensher R, Bowerman J. Actinomycosis of the parotid gland. Br J Oral Maxillofac Surg. 1985;23:128–34.
43. Shaheen SO, Ellis FG. Actinomycosis of the larynx. J R Soc Med. 1983;76:226–8.
44. Shelton C, Brackmann DE. Actinomycosis otitis media. Arch Otolaryngol Head Neck Surg. 1988;114:88–9.
45. Lewis RP, Sutter VL, Finegold SM. Bone infections involving anaerobic bacteria. Medicine. 1978;57:279–305.
46. Schaal KP, Beaman BL. Clinical significance of actinomycetes. In: Goodfellow M, Mordarski M, Williams ST, eds. The Biology of the Actinomycetes. New York: Acadmic Press; 1983:389–424.
47. Dan M, Garcia A, von Westarp C. Primary actinomycosis of the thyroid mimicking carcinoma. J Otolaryngol. 1984;13:109–12.
48. Rothman NI, Kamholz SL, Pinsker KL. Actinomycotic cervical abscess: A complication of transtracheal aspiration. Chest. 1979;76:228–30.
49. Cope Z. Actinomycosis. London: Oxford University Press; 1938.
50. Happonen RP, Viander M, Pelliniemi L, et al. *Actinomyces israelii* in osteoradionecrosis of the jaws. Oral Surg. 1983;55:580–8.
51. McQuarrie DG, Hall WH. Actinomycosis of the lung and chest wall. Surgery. 1968;64:905–11.
52. Legum LI, Greer KE, Glessner SF. Disseminated actinomycosis. South Med J. 1978;71:463–5.
53. Fisher MS. "Miliary" actinomycosis. J Can Assoc Radiol. 1980;31:149–50.
54. Smith LR, Heaton CL. Actinomycosis presenting as Wegener's granulomatosis. JAMA. 1978;240:247–8.
55. Webb AK, Howell R, Hickman JA. Thoracic actinomycosis presenting with peripheral skin lesions. Thorax. 1978;33:818–9.
56. Butas CA, Read SE, Coleman RE, et al. Disseminated actinomycosis. Can Med Assoc J. 1970;103:1069–71.
57. Varkey B. Sulfur granules. JAMA. 1982;248:3025.
58. Flynn MW, Felson B. The roentgen manifestations of thoracic actinomycosis. Am J Roentgenol Radium Ther Nucl Med. 1970;110:707–16.
59. Harrison RN, Thomas DJB. Acute actinomycotic empyema. Thorax. 1979;34:406–7.
60. Lazzari G, Vineis C, Cugini A. Cytologic diagnosis of primary pulmonary actinomycosis: Report of two cases. Acta Cytol (Balt). 1981;25:299–301.
61. Balikian JP, Cheng TH, Costello P, et al. Pulmonary actinomycosis. Radiology. 1978;128:613–6.
62. Lee M, Berger HW, Fernandez NA, et al. Endobronchial actinomycosis. Mt Sinai J Med. 1982;49:136–9.
63. Broquetas J, Aran X, Moreno A. Pulmonary actinomycosis with endobronchial involvement. Eur J Clin Microbiol. 1985;4:508.
64. Stein CA, Ernst J, Stern M, et al. Thoracic actinomycosis in a recent tuberculin converter. Pediatric Infect Dis. 1983;2:52–5.
65. Kay EB. Actinomyces in chronic bronchopulmonary infections. Am Rev Tuberc. 1948;57:322–9.
66. Dutton WP, Inclan AP. Cardiac actinomycosis. Dis Chest. 1968;54:65–7.
67. Cole FH, Jarrett CL. Primary actinomycosis of the pericardium. South Med J. 1982;75:1028–9.
68. Harvey JC, Cantrell JR, Fisher AM. Actinomycosis: Its recognition and treatment. Ann Intern Med. 1957;46:868–85.
69. Berardi RS. Abdominal actinomycosis. Surg Gynecol Obstet. 1979;149:257–66.
70. Deshmukh N, Heaney SJ. Actinomycosis at multiple colonic sites. Am J Gastroenterol. 1986;81:1212–4.
71. Eastridge CE, Prather R, Hughes FA Jr, et al. Actinomycosis: A 24-year experience. South Med J. 1972;65:839–43.
72. Manley PN, Dhru R. Actinomycosis complicating Crohn's disease. Gastroenterology. 1980;79:934–7.
73. Palmer TE, Venable DD. Retroperitoneal actinomycosis. South Med J. 1986;79:1301–3.
74. Kannangara DW, Tanaka T, Thadepalli H. Spinal epidural abscess due to *Actinomyces israelii*. Neurology. 1981;31:202–4.
75. Lau WY, Boey J, Fan ST, et al. Primary actinomycosis of the abdominal wall. Aust NZ J Surg. 1986;56:873–5.
76. Halevy A, Blenkhard JI, Christodoloupolous J, et al. Actinomycosis of the pancreas. Br J Surg. 1987;74:150.
77. Patel BJ, Moskowitz H, Hashmat A. Unilateral renal actinomycosis. Urology. 1983;21:172–4.
78. Ratliff DA, Carr N, Cochrane JPS. Rectal stricture due to actinomycosis. Br J Surg. 1986;73:589–90.
79. Brink PR, de Ruiter K. Abdominal actinomycosis—a late complication of gastrectomy. Neth J Surg. 1984;36:80–2.
80. Cedermark B, Sundblad R, Willems JS. Suspected neoplasm of the liver with pulmonary metastases cured by surgery and penicillin. Disseminated actinomycosis revisited. Am J Surg. 1981;141:384–6.
81. Mongiardo M, De Rienzo B, Zanchetta G, et al. Primary hepatic actinomycosis. J Infect. 1986;12:65–9.
82. Meade RH. Primary hepatic actinomycosis. Gastroenterology. 1980;78:355–9.
83. Hennrikus EF, Pederson L. Disseminated actinomycosis. West J Med. 1987;147:201–4.
84. Surer F. Actinomycosis of female genital tract. NY State J Med. 1974;74:408–11.
85. Schiffer MA, Elguezabal A, Sultana M, et al. Actinomycosis infections associated with intrauterine contraceptive devices. Obstet Gynecol. 1975;45:67–72.
86. Burkman R, Schlesselman S, McCaffrey L, et al. The relationship of genital tract actinomycetes and the development of pelvic inflammatory disease. Am J Obstet Gynecol. 1982;143:585–9.
87. Spagnuolo PJ, Fransiolli M. Intrauterine device-associated actinomycosis simulating pelvic malignancy. Am J Gastroenterol. 1981;75:144–6.
88. Persson E, Holmberg K, Dahlgren S, et al. *Actinomyces israelii* in the genital tract of women with and without intra-uterine contraceptive devices. Acta Obstet Gynecol Scand. 1983;62:563–8.
89. Gupta PK. Intrauterine contraceptive devices. Vaginal cytology, pathologic changes and clinical implications. Acta Cytol. 1982;26:571–613.
90. O'Brien P, Roth-Moyo L, Davis B. Pseudo-sulfur granules associated with intrauterine contraceptive devices. Am J Clin Pathol. 1981;75:822–5.
91. Pine L, Curtis EM, Brown JM. Actinomyces and the intrauterine contraceptive device: Aspects of the fluorescent antibody stain. Am J Obstet Gynecol. 1985;152:287–90.
92. Persson E, Holmberg K. Clinical evaluation of precipitin tests for genital actinomycosis. J Clin Microbiol. 1984;20:917–22.
93. Persson E. Genital actinomycosis and *Actinomyces israelii* in the female genital tract. Adv Contracept. 1987;3:115–23.
94. Ellis LR, Kenny GM, Nellans RE. Urogenital aspects of actinomycosis. J Urol. 1979;122:132–3.
95. Wajszczuk CP, Logan TF, Pasculle AW, et al. Intra-abdominal actinomycosis presenting with sulfur granules in the urine. Am J Med. 1984;77:1126–8.
96. deSouza E, Katz DA, Dworzack DL, et al. Actinomycosis of the prostate. J Urol. 1985;133:290–1.

97. Bolton CF, Ashenhurst EM. Actinomycosis of the brain. Can Med Assoc J. 1964;90:922–8.
98. Smego RA Jr. Actinomycosis of the central nervous system. Ref Infect Dis. 1987;9:855–65.
99. Deshpande RB, Rao AA. Cervicofacial actinomycosis with upper cervical vertebral involvement and fatal meningitis. J Postgrad Med. 1985;31:223–5.
100. Stanley SL, Lusk RH. Thoracic actinomycosis presenting as a brachial plexus syndrome. Thorax. 1985;40:74–5.
101. Reiner SL, Harrelson JM, Miller Se, et al. Primary actinomycosis of an extremity: A case report and review. Rev Infect Dis. 1987;9:581–9.
102. Holm P. Some investigations into the penicillin sensitivity of human-pathogenic actinomycetes and some comments on penicillin treatment of actinomycosis. Acta Pathol Microbiol Scand. 1948;23:376–404.
103. Garrod LP. The sensitivity of *Actinomyces israelii* to antibiotics. Br Med J. 1952;1:1263–4.
104. Schlech WF III, Gelfand M, Alper B, et al. Medical management of visceral actinomycosis. South Med J. 1983;76:921–2.
105. King JW, White MC. Pulmonary actinomycosis. Rapid improvement with isoniazid and rifampin. Arch Intern Med. 1981;141:1234–5.
106. Lerner PI. Susceptibility of pathogenic Actinomycetes to antimicrobial compounds. Antimicrob Agents Chemother. 1974;5:302–9.
107. Holmberg K, Nord C, Dornbusch K. Antimicrobial in vitro susceptibility of *Actinomyces israelii* and *Arachnia propionica*. Scand J Infect Dis. 1977;9:40–5.
108. Boand A, Novak M. Sensitivity changes of *Actinomyces bovis* to penicillin and stretpomycin. J Bacteriol. 1949;57:501–8.
109. Edelmann M, Cullmann W, Nowak KH, et al. Treatment of abdominothoracic actinomycosis with imipenem. Eur J Clin Microbiol. 1987;6:194–5.
110. Lerner PI: The Lumpy Jaw: Cervicofacial Actinomycosis. Infect Dis Clinic N Amer. 1988;2:203–20.

SECTION F. MYCOSES

234. INTRODUCTION

JOHN E. BENNETT

An understanding of some general properties of fungi and an introduction to some of the specialized terminology will assist the reader in reading the other chapters of this section.

MYCOLOGY

Fungi can be divided into yeasts and molds. Yeastlike fungi are typically round or oval and reproduce by budding. Molds are composed of tubular structures called hyphae that grow by branching and longitudinal extension. Not all pathogenic fungi can be categorized neatly as yeasts or molds. *Coccidioides immitis* and *Rhinosporidium seeberi* are round in tissue but do not bud. Instead, the cytoplasm divides up to form numerous internal spores that, on rupture of the "mother" cell, are released to form new spherical structures. Some fungi can grow either yeastlike or as a mold. In candidiasis and tinea versicolor, the fungus is often seen in both tubular and rounded forms. The so-called dimorphic fungi grow in the host as yeastlike forms but grow at room temperature in vitro as molds. These fungi include the agents of histoplasmosis, blastomycosis, sporotrichosis, coccidioidomycosis, paracoccidioidomycosis, and chromomycosis.

Virtually all fungi reproduce by forming spores through mitosis, a process in which the chromosome number remains the same. No mating precedes this sporulation. A fungal colony with only this asexual spore formation, or with no spore formation, is said to be in the imperfect (asexual) state. Several decades ago, most fungi pathogenic for humans were found only in the imperfect state. Many have subsequently been induced to form sexual spores and have been given new names. These names show the similarity to other fungi in their perfect state. The older name for the fungus is still appropriate for use when the fungus is in the imperfect state. Diagnostic laboratories do not use the specialized procedures necessary to cause sexual spore production in many fungi. Therefore, the microbiology laboratory and the clinician can retain the older name appropriately, for example, *Cryptococcus neoformans,* not *Filobasidiella neoformans*.

Sexual spores arise as a result of mating. Mating only takes place in certain fungi when they are allowed to grow in juxtaposition to a colony of the opposite mating type. Such fungi are called heterothallic and include the agents of histoplasmosis, blastomycosis, and cryptococcosis, as well as some fungi causing ringworm and mucormycosis. Certain other fungi are self-fertile (homothallic). *Pseudallescheria boydii,* for example, forms sexual spores without contact with another colony. Among fungi pathogenic for humans, the sexual spore is formed in a distinctive structure. The fungus transiently becomes diploid and then returns to its usual haploid condition by production of spores through meiosis. The distinctive appearance of the spore-bearing structure and the spores themselves are very helpful in classifying fungi.

Cells of fungi pathogenic for humans are nonmotile and have a rigid cell wall, usually containing chitin and polysaccharides. All fungal cell walls are stained by Gomori methenamine silver and, while the fungus remains viable, the periodic acid–Schiff reagent will also stain the cell wall. Most fungi, except *Candida,* are too weakly gram positive to be seen well on Gram stain. A polysaccharide capsule around the cell wall is characteristic of only one pathogen for humans, *Cryptococcus neoformans,* but occasionally *Sporothrix schenckii* within viscera such as brain or eye has been encapsulated. Inside the fungal cell wall is the sterol-containing cytoplasmic membrane that is the site of action of the polyene macrolide antibiotics, amphotericin B and nystatin. Fungi are not known with surety to have important endotoxins, although intravenous injections of several fungi have been pyrogenic in animals. Exotoxins such as aflatoxin have been produced by certain fungi in vitro, but none yet are known to be produced in vivo.

Fungi can often be identified in tissue even in the absence of culture by taking into account the clinical condition, tissue, inflammatory response, and appearance of the fungus (Table 1). Culture diagnosis is potentially more accurate than histologic features, but many smaller laboratories encounter difficulties in isolating and identifying fungi. The histologic features of a biopsy specimen can be more rapidly diagnostic than culture when mycoses are caused by slow-growing fungi. Biopsy slides are more readily mailed to consultants than cultures, which may arrive nonviable or contaminated. Last, biopsy may provide proof that the fungus is invading tissue and is not just a contaminant or saprophyte growing on debris in a lung cavity or skin ulcer. Ideally, both histologic examination and culture should be done together.

TABLE 1. Typical Appearance of Fungi in Tissue

Yeastlike fungi	
Histoplasma capsulatum	2–3 × 3–4-μm oval, budding uninucleate cells; often intracellular; granulomatous inflammation
Candida glabrata	2.5–3 × 4–5-μm oval budding cells; scanty, nongranulomatous inflammation; necrosis
Candida albicans	3 × 5-μm oval, budding cells usually accomplished by tubular structures (pseudohyphae) with constrictions at septae and branching only at septations
Cryptococcus neoformans	4–6-μm round uninucleate cell with large surrounding capsule; narrow pore between mother and daughter cell; daughter cell detached while small
Sporothrix schenckii	1–3 × 3–10-μm cigar-shaped cell or 2–10-μm round budding cell; pyogenic and granulomatous inflammation
Blastomyces dermatitidis	8–15-μm round multinucleate cell with large pore between mother and daughter cell; daughter cell remains attached until nearly size of mother cell; pyogenic and granulomatous inflammation
Paracoccidioides brasiliensis	2–30-μm multiple, budding, round cells with tiny pore between mother and daughter cell; daughter cell released when small
Coccidioides immitis	5–60-μm thick-walled, nonbudding, round cells that may contain endospores
Agents of chromomycosis	4–12-μm round or oval, brown, thick-walled cells, often in clumps; hyphal forms may be seen in superficial crusts
Molds	
Aspergillus species	2–5-μm wide hyphae, frequently septate, even diameter, Y-shaped branching; vascular invasion; necrosis
Agents of mucormycosis	4–15-μm wide hyphae, rarely septate, uneven diameter, often branch at broad angles; vascular invasion; necrosis

EPIDEMIOLOGY

With rare exceptions, mycoses are not transmissible from patient to patient. Gown, glove, or mask isolation of hospitalized patients with mycoses is not indicated. Ringworm of the scalp in children is transmissible to other children, meaning that caps and combs should not be shared between infected children and playmates. Bandages or casts that become contaminated with draining pus from patients with coccidioidomycosis require care to see that the fungus does not grow several days on the formite. At room temperature the fungus will grow as the spore-bearing mold form, which is infectious.

The diagnostic laboratory should be alerted when specimens from suspected coccidioidomycosis or histoplasmosis cases are sent for culture. Once these cultures grow in the mold form, they can be hazardous to laboratory personnel.

BIBLIOGRAPHY

Al-Doory Y. The Epidemiology of Human Mycotic Diseases. Springfield, IL: Charles C Thomas; 1975.

Al-Doory Y. Laboratory Medical Mycology. Philadelphia: Lea & Febiger; 1980.

Binford CH, Connor DH, eds. Pathology of Tropical and Extraordinary Diseases. Washington, DC.; Armed Forces Institute of Pathology; 1976.

Emmons CW, Binford CH, Utz JP. Medical Mycology. Philadelphia: Lea & Febiger; 1977.

Howard DH, ed. Fungi Pathogenic for Humans and Animals. New York: Marcel Dekker; 1983.

Rippon JW. Medical Mycology. 3rd ed. Philadelphia: WB Saunders; 1988.

235. CANDIDA SPECIES

JOHN E. EDWARDS, JR.

Written descriptions of oral lesions that were probably thrush date to the time of Hippocrates and Galen. Langenbeck, in 1839,[1] found fungi in oral lesions of a patient. By 1841, Berg established the fungal etiology of thrush by inoculating healthy babies with aphthous "membrane material." In 1843, Robin attached to the organism the name *Oidium albicans*. There have been more than 100 synonyms for *Candida albicans*; the two that have persisted are *Monilia albicans*, originated by Zopf in 1890, and *C. albicans*, used by Berkhout in 1923.[2]

In 1861, Zenker described the first well-documented case of deep-seated *Candida*. The first case of *Candida*-induced endocarditis was described in 1940.[3] The most interesting period in the history of *Candida* infections began in the 1940s, when antibiotics were introduced into clinical use. Since then, previously undocumented manifestations of *Candida* infections have appeared, and the incidence of practically all forms of *Candida* infections has risen abruptly. Excellent comprehensive reviews detailing the emergence of *Candida* as a common pathogen are now available.[2,4,5] These emerging infections have included arthritis, osteomyelitis, endophthalmitis, myocarditis, meningitis, peritonitis, myositis, and others that will be elaborated upon in detail in their respective sections of this chapter. In addition to the widespread use of antibiotics, other therapeutic modalities for advanced life support, and surgical procedures such as organ transplants and cardiac valve prostheses, have been important in the expanding incidence of *Candida* infections.

THE PATHOGEN

Candida organisms are yeasts, that is, fungi that exist predominantly in a unicellular form. Both sexual and asexual forms exist. They are small (4–6 μm), thin-walled, ovoid cells that reproduce by budding. They grow well in vented routine blood culture bottles and on agar plates and do not require special fungal media for cultivation. However, biphasic blood culture bottles and lysis centrifugation facilitate recovery.[6] Yeast forms, pseudohyphae, and hyphae may be found in clinical specimens; identification of the hyphae and pseudohyphae is facilitated with 10% potassium hydroxide, which clears the epithelial cells. The organism stains gram-positive.

Candida organisms form smooth, creamy white, glistening colonies that may resemble staphylococcal colonies. A rapid, presumptive identification of *C. albicans* can be made by placing the organism in serum and observing the formation of germ tubes, small projections from the cell surface that appear within 90 minutes.[7] The remainder of the identification and speciation procedures are based primarily on physiologic parameters rather than on morphologic characteristics. Metabolic tests include carbohydrate assimilation and fermentation reactions, nitrate use, and urease production. Chlamydospore formation is also used to identify *C. albicans*. Because of variation in species pathogenicity, speciation is desirable. There are more than 150 species of *Candida*, but only 10 are regarded as important pathogens for humans. They are *C. albicans, C. guilliermondii, C. krusei, C. parapsilosis, C. stellatoidea* (now included within *C. albicans*), *C. tropicalis, C. pseudotropicalis, C. lusitaniae, C.*

rugosa, and *C. glabrata* (now classified as *Torulopsis glabrata*). Technical advances have made definitive speciation within two days possible.[8]

EPIDEMIOLOGY AND ECOLOGY

Candida albicans organisms have been recovered from soil, hospital environments, inanimate objects, and food. However, contamination from humans or animals is probable.[9] Other spp. may live in nonanimal environments, such as soil. Only rarely are *Candida* spp. laboratory contaminants.[10] That principle has not been generally appreciated, and interpretation of positive cultures as laboratory or skin contaminants has led to important errors in patient management.

The organisms are normal commensals of humans and are commonly found on diseased skin, throughout the entire gastrointestinal (GI) tract, expectorated sputum, the female genital tract, and urine of patients with indwelling Foley catheters.[4]

Although the vast majority of *Candida* infections are of endogenous origin, human-to-human transmission is possible. Examples are thrush of the newborn, which may be acquired from the maternal vagina, and balanitis in the uncircumcised man, which may be acquired through contact with a partner who has *Candida* vaginitis. There is also evidence that *Candida* infection can be acquired from the hospital environment.[11,12]

PATHOGENESIS AND PATHOLOGIC FINDINGS

The defense mechanism of intact integument is of importance in maintaining resistance to cutaneous candidiasis; any process causing skin maceration leaves the involved site susceptible to *Candida* invasion, even in healthy individuals. Once the organism invades the dermis[13] or enters the blood stream, polymorphonuclear leukocytes play a role in defense since they have the capacity to damage pseudohyphae[14–16] and to phagocytize and kill blastospores.[17] Of interest is that in many instances the phagocytic vacuoles around *Candida* remain unsealed.[18] In addition to neutrophils, monocytes and eosinophils also ingest and kill *Candida*.[19,20] Monocyte killing in vitro is more efficient than polymorphonuclear killing. The role of platelets in anti-*Candida* defense remains to be elucidated. A platelet-derived factor stimulates germ tube production, and *Candida* cell wall fractions agglutinate platetets.[21] Serum and plasma, even though they contain antibodies and complement components, are incapable of killing *Candida* alone.

Neutrophils and monocytes lacking myeloperoxidase or the capacity to generate hydrogen peroxide and superoxide anion fail to kill *C. albicans* effectively.[19,20] This observation and additional studies suggest that the myeloperoxidase, hydrogen peroxide, and/or superoxide anion system is a major mechanism responsible for intracellular killing of *C. albicans*. Additionally, recent studies have identified a ferrous ion, hydrogen peroxide, iodide system that may be operative in intracellular killing.[22] A further intracellular killing mechanism for phagocytes involves chymotrypsin-like cationic proteins.[23–25] These proteins probably act by increasing membrane permeability.

The role of macrophages and sessile reticuloendothelial cells has also been investigated. Rabbit and mouse alveolar and peritoneal and human lung macrophages have *Candida*-killing capacity.[26,27] Of interest is a study of Taschdjian et al. that showed, by immunofluorescent techniques, organisms within tissue macrophages and sessile reticuloendothelial cells throughout the body in patients with disseminated candidiasis.[28] This observation suggests a defense role for these tissue macrophages.

The role of lymphocytes in defense against *Candida* and the development of *Candida*-induced cell-mediated immunity is an exceptionally complex subject that has recently been reviewed extensively[29] and can be only superficially summarized here. The importance of the defensive role of the lymphocyte can be gleaned from three clinical observations: (*1*) Patients with chronic mucocutaneous candidiasis are infected as a result of dysfunction of their lymphocyte system. (*2*) Delayed-type hypersensitivity reactions to *Candida* antigens are present in approximately 70–80 percent of the healthy population.[30] (*3*) Acquired immunodeficiency syndrome (AIDS) patients are highly susceptible to mucocutaneous candidiasis. However, it should be noted that there is experimental evidence that congenitally athymic (nude) mice have more resistance to *Candida* challenge than controls with normal T lymphocytes.[31,32] Experimental evidence indicates that mannan is the important antigen influencing the lymphocyte responses.[33] Of interest also has been the identification of natural killer cells.[34] Further evidence for the importance of the lymphocyte in defense against *Candida* is the occurrence of the disease in AIDS patients.[35] Despite extensive experimental studies, there is no vaccine commercially available for prevention of either mucocutaneous or systemic candidiasis.

Several observations have substantiated the importance of humoral factors in *Candida* immune defense. The rate of ingestion of *C. albicans* by neutrophils is increased by both heat-labile and heat-stable serum opsonins.[36] IgG and other serum constituents effectively opsonize *C. albicans,* and patients with disseminated candidiasis frequently have a high-titer antibody response. However, the exact role that these antibodies play is open to question, especially in light of evidence showing that antibody is not required for the killing of partially ingested yeast cells.[37,38] Serum iron-binding proteins have been shown to inhibit the growth of *Candida*, presumably by binding iron, which is a *Candida* growth factor.[39] Finally, there are humoral substances that induce *C. albicans* to form pseudohyphae and to clump the organisms in vitro,[40] as well as numerous other humoral substances that have inhibitory effects on *Candida* growth. The significance of these clumping factors and of other inhibitory substances remains to be fully elucidated.

The precise role of complement in anti-*Candida* defense requires further definition. Complement is necessary for optimal opsonization[41] in vitro, and animals deficient in alternate pathway activation are more susceptible to *Candida* challenge.[42] Furthermore, C3b has been found to bind to *Candida* blastospores.[43] Also, evidence for an important role of complement is the finding of complement components deposited in the basement membrane of cutaneous lesions in patients with chronic mucocutaneous candidiasis.[44] Both the classical and alternate pathways are activated by *Candida*. The weight of the evidence suggests that the alternate pathway is the more important. However, the relative roles of the two pathways remain to be determined. Also, a finding of interest that awaits clarification regarding significance is that of *Candida* surface molecules resembling human complement receptors CR2 and CR3.[45–48]

In recent years, adherence capabilities of *Candida* to vaginal and oral epithelial cells, fibronectin, platelet fibrin clots, acrylic, endothelium, and plastics have all been demonstrated, and the topic has been reviewed thoroughly.[49,50] The precise role of adherence in the pathogenesis of *Candida* remains to be defined. Based on investigation in bacterial systems, it is likely to be highly important.

For this usually normal human commensal to become a pathogen, interruption of these normal defense mechanisms is necessary. The factors responsible for this immunocompromise fall into two categories, naturally occurring and iatrogenic. Included in the first category is diabetes mellitus, which predisposes to cutaneous but not disseminated candidiasis.

The most important predisposing factors to *Candida* infection, and especially to disseminated candidiasis, are iatrogenic. The introduction of newer therapeutic modalities for advanced life support into clinical medicine has been primarily responsible for the dramatic change in the incidence of this disease. Of these factors, probably the most important has been the introduction of antibiotics. They suppress normal bacterial flora and allow *Candida* organisms to proliferate, especially in the GI tract. Of interest is that sulfonamides decrease neutrophil *Candida* intracellular killing,[51] and tetracycline, doxycycline, and aminoglycosides have been shown to decrease neutrophil phagocytosis.[52,53]

Factors that may provide a route for *Candida* to enter the vascular system of susceptible patients from the environment include the use of heroin,[54] hyperalimentation fluids, polyethylene catheters,[55] and pressure monitoring devices. The implantation of prosthetic materials, especially cardiac valves and the artificial heart, also is associated with an increased incidence of *Candida* infection. Clinical situations associated with general immune suppression may be further complicated by the use of antibiotics, hyperalimentation fluid, and the other therapeutic modalities mentioned above, usually in the setting of multiple abdominal surgeries, renal transplantation, neoplastic diseases, the use of steroids, and severe burns.

The pathogenic mechanisms by which these clinical conditions and devices increase the incidence of disseminated and mucocutaneous candidiasis are not fully known. For instance, it is not clear whether hyperalimentation fluids simply provide an intravascular hyperglycemic environment that is favorable for the growth of the yeasts or whether they provide a mechanical means (conduit) for their entry into the blood stream. Also, the hyperalimentation catheter tip serves as a nidus for the proliferation of *Candida*, either as a cardiac mural endocarditis or within a deep vein as a fungus-filled fibrin sleeve. The same mechanism may occur in postoperative *Candida*-induced endocarditis, where the damaged endocardium and prosthetic materials localize small numbers of circulating organisms. When burn patients, patients with neoplasia, and postsurgical patients with complications are given multiple antibiotics, there is proliferation of *Candida* organisms in their GI tract, which is presumably a source for dissemination.

Two observations support the hypothesis that the GI tract is a likely source for entrance of *Candida* into the blood stream. Krause et al.[56] reported drinking a suspension containing a massive amount of *Candida*. Despite no recognizable GI disease, the investigator became candidemic and candiduric. Stone et al. have shown that yeasts can cross the GI tract of animals.[57] One would expect patients who have had abdominal surgery and therapy with multiple antibiotics to be at double risk for dissemination from the GI source by having both overgrowth of *Candida* in the GI tract and interruptions of the normal GI tract mucosal integrity. GI tract surgery is now a well-recognized predisposing factor to disseminated candidiasis.[58,59] It is possible that loss of integrity of the GI tract due to either the disease or cytoxic chemotherapy creates a portal by which *Candida* passes from the GI lumen into the blood stream. Alternatively, the growing body of literature regarding *Candida* as a cause of septic thrombophletibis from intraveous catheters suggests that in many cases the catheter entry site in the skin, rather than the GI tract, is the most likely portal of entry.[60]

When the organism invades visceral tissue, microabscesses are formed, generally with normal parenchyma between the microabscesses. When the organism invades tissue, both yeast forms and hyphal forms are present. Whether the formation of filamentous forms of *Candida* is a factor associated with virulence is one of the major unresolved controversies in the field.[61] The initial cellular reaction is polymorphonuclear. Histiocytes, giant cells, and epithelioid cells appear early, and the reaction may take the form of a granulomatous response. Although organisms may be seen on hematoxylin-eosin stains, optimal staining is accomplished with periodic acid–Schiff or methenamine silver. In the severely immunocompromised patient, the inflammatory reaction may be minimal or almost nonexistent, leaving the abscess composed of *Candida* and necrotic tissue.

In superficial candidiasis, the histopathologic change is a chornic dermatitis with the yeast confined to the stratum corneum. However, *Candida* granuloma (see the following section on "Clinical Manifestations") is characterized by invasion into both the epidermis and dermis, as well as by marked hyperkeratosis and acanthosis.

CLINICAL MANIFESTATIONS

As the incidence of diseases due to *Candida* has increased in frequency over the past 30 years, a relatively large number of manifestations, which were previously either not recognized or extremely infrequent, have become well documented. The discussion of these clinical manifestations is facilitated by their subdivision into mucocutaneous and deep organ involvement.

Mucous Membrane Infections

Thrush. Oral *Candida* infection is common and has been extensively reviewed.[62,63] The term *thrush* is applied to a specific form of oral candidiasis characterized by creamy white, curdlike patches on the tongue (Fig. 1) and on other oral mucosal surfaces, which are removable by scraping and leave a raw, bleeding, and painful surface. The patches are actually a pseudomembrane consisting of *Candida*, desquamated epithelial cells, leukocytes, bacteria, keratin, necrotic tissue, and food debris.[64] The diagnosis can be made by the clinical appearance of the lesion and by scraping, using either a potassium hydroxide smear or Gram stain to show masses of hyphae, pseudohyphae, and yeast forms. Simple culturing does not solidify the diagnosis, as *Candida* will grow easily from normal mouths. The classic lesions have been classified by Lehner[64] and include (*1*) acute atrophic candidiasis, a nonspecific atrophy of the tongue that is thought to be a sequela of acute pseudomembranous candidiasis, (*2*) chronic atrophic candidiasis or "denture sore mouth," which is a chronic inflammatory reaction and epithelial thinning under the dental plates, (*3*) angular cheilitis, an inflammatory reaction at the corners of the mouth (not due exclusively to *Candida*), (*4*) *Candida* leukoplakia, firm, white plaques involving the cheek, lips, and tongue that have a protracted course (and, in rare instances, may be precancerous).[65]

Since the introduction of inhaled steroids for the treatment

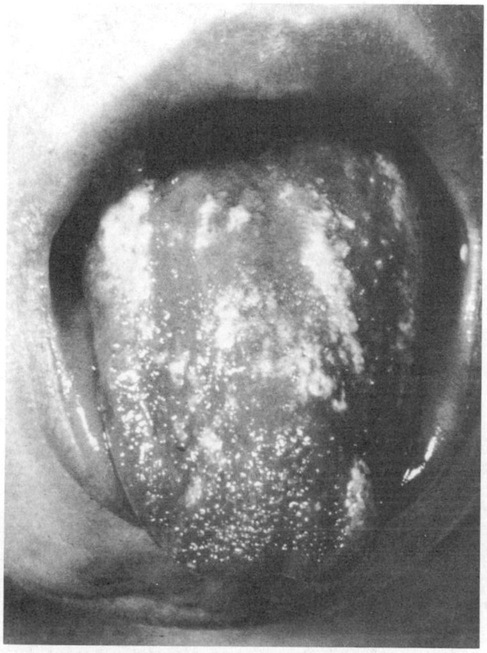

FIG. 1. Typical oral thrush with curd-like white patches over the tongue. (Courtesy of Dr. Arnold Gurevitch, Los Angeles, CA.)

of asthma, especially in children, oral thrush has been reported extensively in patients treated with these agents. The incidence has ranged from 0 to 77 percent.[66] Thrush developing in patients who use inhaled steroids usually resolves spontaneously, without a change in the dose of the agent, or is successfully managed with topical nystatin or clotrimazole.

Other patients with a high incidence of thrush are cancer patients and those with AIDS. Patients with thrush for no obvious reason should be evaluated for AIDS.[67]

Candida Esophagitis. Although there has been a small number of reports of *Candida* esophagitis occurring in patients with no known underlying illness, it is more commonly associated with treatment of malignancy of the hematopoietic or lymphatic systems (Fig. 2) and with AIDS patients. Esophageal disease was believed to occur by direct spread from oral disease (thrush), but reviews have shown that approximately 30 percent of the patients with *Candida* esophagitis have no associated thrush.[68] The most common symptoms of *Candida* esophagitis include painful swallowing, a feeling of obstruction on swallowing, and substernal chest pain. Nausea and vomiting may also occur. The diagnosis is made definitively by biopsy during endoscopy[69,70] (Fig. 3) or by brushing. However, the appropriate clinical setting, associated with the endoscopic appearance of white patches resembling thrush that show masses of hyphae and pseudohyphae upon scraping, is enough evidence to initiate therapy without a histopathologic demonstration of the organisms invading the mucosa. It is important to recognize that *Candida* esophagitis can occur simultaneously with herpes simplex virus esophagitis in severely immunocompromised patients. X-ray examination may be helpful in making a clinical diagnosis; irregularity of the esophageal mucosa as a result of ulcerations may be seen, as well as shoulder defects, diverticulas, fistulas, and dilatation of the esophagus from denervation. Endoscopy is the preferred procedure for diagnosis, however.[70] The pseudomembrane that forms may become so extensive that it causes intraluminal protrusions and partial esophageal obstruction. Perforation of the esophagus due to eosophageal candidiasis is rare. Generally, if perforation occurs, it is in the lower two-thirds of the esophagus. Some patients have had extensive esophageal disease and have been almost asymptomatic, probably as a result of denervation of the esophagus from the disease.[71] Other complications include bleeding and, presumably, dissemination.

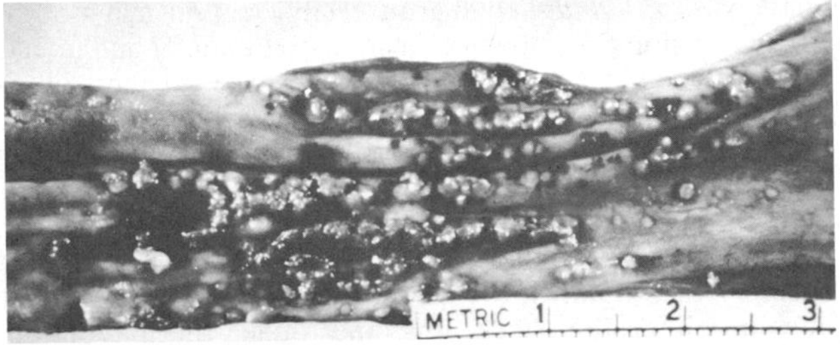

FIG. 2. Severe *Candida* esophagitis at autopsy (Courtesy of Dr. Stephen Targon, Los Angeles, CA.).

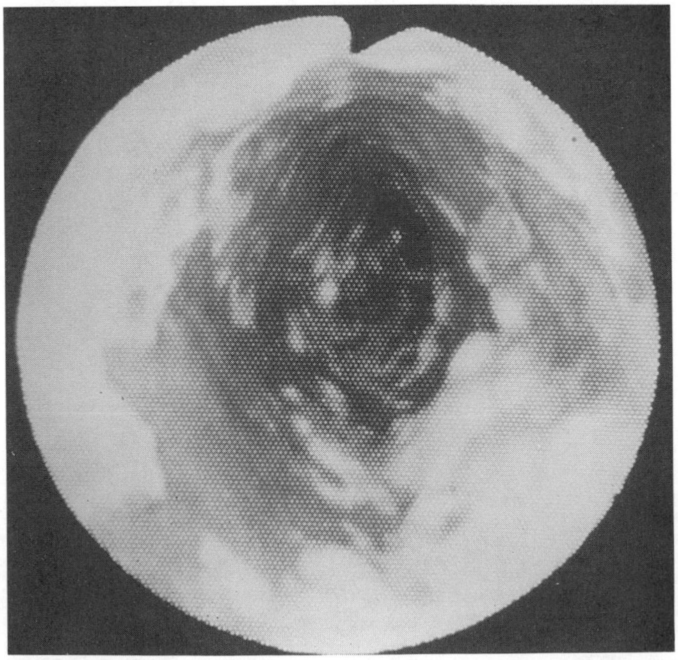

FIG. 3. Numerous *Candida* plaques seen at endoscopy. (Courtesy of Dr. Wilfred Weinstein, Los Angeles, CA.)

Nonesophageal Mucous Membrane Gastrointestinal Candidiasis. The most common setting for GI candidiasis is in patients with neoplastic disease. Eras et al.[72] reviewed their autopsy experience with candidiasis in a cancer hospital and found that involvement of the stomach was by far the next most common site, second only to esophageal candidiasis. The most frequent lesions were single or multiple ulcerations containing *Candida* deep in the ulcer beds. In addition, but with less frequency, chronic gastric ulcer, gastric perforation, and malignant gastric ulcer with concomitant *Candida* infection were seen. The small bowel was third in frequency of involvement (20 percent). Ulceration was the most common lesion. Pseudomembrane formation and ulceration in association with tumor were also noted. Similar to other mucous membrane *Candida* infections, white plaques may be seen on endoscopy of the duodenum, and there may be thickening of mucosal folds in the duodenum and jejunum.[73,74] Equal in frequency to the small bowel was involvement of the large bowel, which again was characterized by ulceraton, superficial erosions, pseudomembrane formation, penetrating ulcers, and perforation. Fifteen percent of the patients had disseminated candidiasis. A topic receiving considerably attention in recent years is gastric candidiasis, which takes two forms: diffuse mucosal involvement (rare) and focal invasion of benign gastric ulcers.[75,76] Whether cimetidine or other H_2-blocking agents play a role in the pathogenesis remains controversial.

Candida Vaginitis. This common infection is seen most frequently in the setting of diabetes mellitus, antibiotic therapy, and pregnancy.[77,78] In addition, use of birth control pills may be a predisposing factor, although this association is controversial. In recent years, *Candida* has assumed the role of the most common cause of vaginitis, with higher frequency rates than *Trichomonas* or nonspecific vaginitis. The introduction of the widespread use of antibiotic therapy may be the most important factor responsible for the emergence of *Candida*-induced vaginitis.

Although *Candida*-induced vaginitis is usually accompanied by a thick, curdlike discharge, occasionally a scanty discharge may characterize the infection. Intense pruritus of the vulva is almost always present. The thick discharge consists of epithelial cells and masses of hyphae and pseudohyphae; a polymorphonuclear leukocyte response is not a component of the inflammatory reaction. The vagina and labia are usually erythematous, and extension onto the vulva and perineum can occur (Fig. 4). In addition, endometritis due to *Candida* has been reported, and the urethra may become secondarily infected.

Cutaneous Candidiasis Syndromes. GENERALIZED CUTANEOUS CANDIDIASIS. This condition is an unusual form of cutaneous candidiasis and is characterized by widespread eruption over

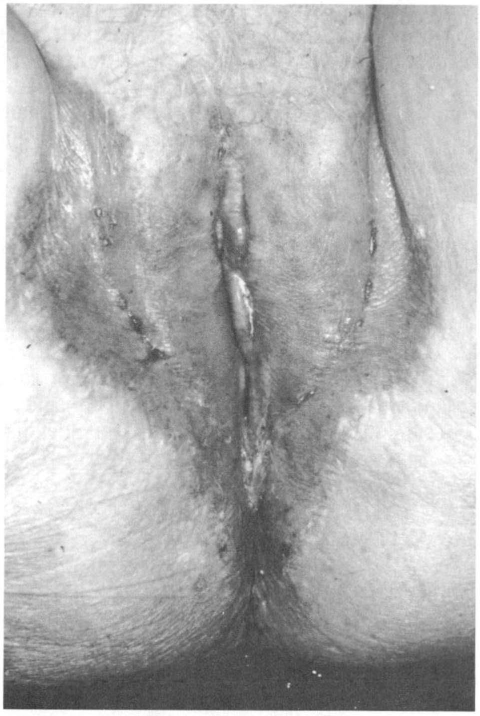

FIG. 4. Extension of *Candida* vaginitis onto the perineum. (Courtesy of Dr. Victor Newcomer, Los Angeles, CA.)

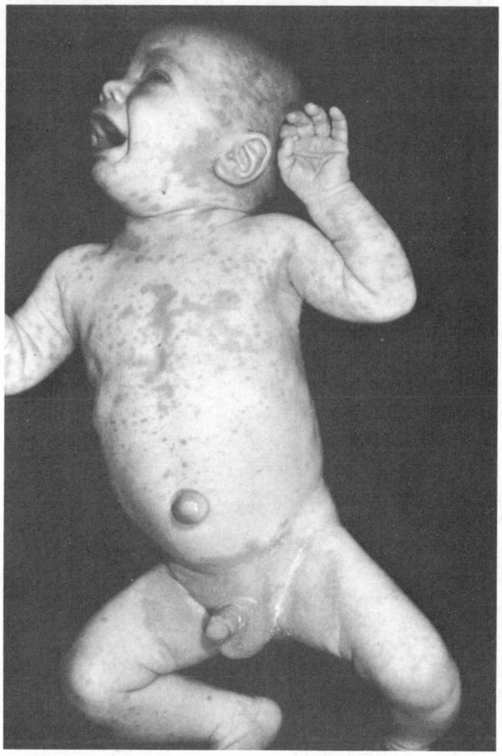

FIG. 5. Generalized candidiasis. (Courtesy of Dr. Victor Newcomer, Los Angeles, CA.)

the trunk, thorax, and extremities, with increased severity in the genitocrural folds, anal region, axillae, hands, and feet (Fig. 5). The process begins as individual vesicles that spread into large, confluent areas. It occurs in both adults and children.[79,80]

Erosio Interdigitalis Blastomycetica. This term applies to *Candida* infection occurring between the fingers or toes (Fig. 6). It has a red base, may extend onto the sides of the digits, is painful, and is predisposed to by maceration.[79]

Candida Folliculitis. Infection at the hair follicles with *Candida* can occur[81,,82] (Fig. 7). Rarely, the condition may become extensive.

Candida Balanitis. This process begins as vesicles on the penis that develop into patches resembling thrush and are accompanied by severe itching and burning. It may spread to the thighs, gluteal folds, buttocks, and scrotum. It can be acquired rarely through sexual intercourse with a partner who has vaginal candidiasis.[83]

Cutaneous Lesions of Disseminated Candidiasis. Three distinct types of lesions have been described in association with disseminated candidiasis. The macronodular lesions (Fig. 8) are 0.5–1.0 cm in diameter, pink to red in color, and may be either single or occur widely distributed over the entire body.[84,85] The most accurate method of making a specific diagnosis is by punch biopsy and demonstration of organisms on histologic section. Most patients who have acquired these lesions have had persistent candidemia. Their presence indicates hematogenous dissemination. In addition, lesions resembling ecthyma gangrenosum have been caused by *Candida* in association with disseminated candidiasis,[86] and purpura fulminans lesions have contained *Candida* on biopsy.[87]

Intertrigo. This common skin condition affects any site where skin surfaces are in close proximity, providing a warm, moist environment. It begins as vesicopustules, which enlarge

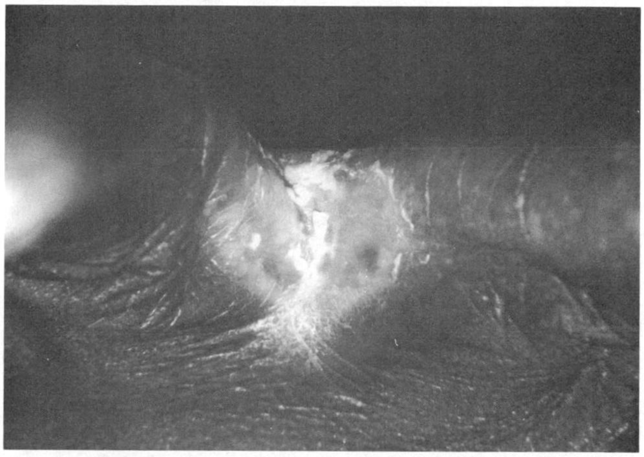

FIG. 6. Erosio interdigitalis blastomycetica. (Courtesy of Dr. Arnold Gurevitch, Los Angeles, CA.)

and rupture, causing maceration and fissuring. The area of involvement has a scalloped border with a white rim consisting of necrotic epidermis, which surrounds an erythematous, macerated base. Frequently, satellite lesions are found that may coalesce and extend the involved area. A variant form of cutaneous candidiasis in the intertriginous region has a miliary appearance resembling miliaria rubra with erythematous macules or vesicopustules.[88]

Paronychia and Onychomycosis. *Candida* is one of the most common causes of paronychia, although its role in the reaction is not entirely clear since many skin bacteria, as well as *Candida*, can usually be recovered by culture of the infected area. The appearance of the reaction is that of a relatively well-localized area of inflammation that becomes warm, glistening, and tense and may extend extensively under the nail (Fig. 9). Unless

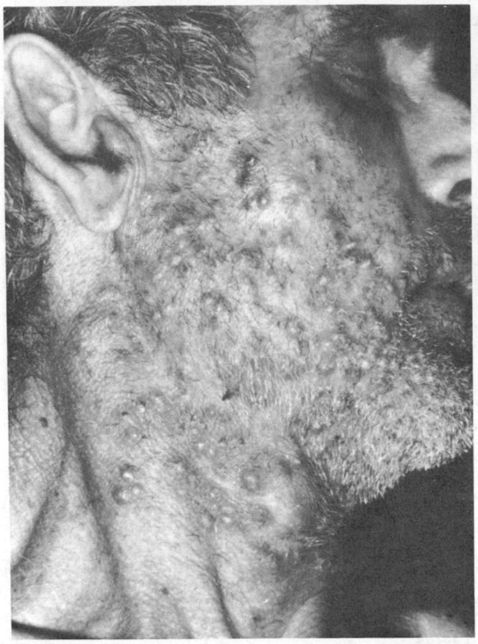

FIG. 7. Severe *Candida* folliculitis in beard distribution. (Courtesy of Dr. Victor Newcomer, Los Angeles, CA.)

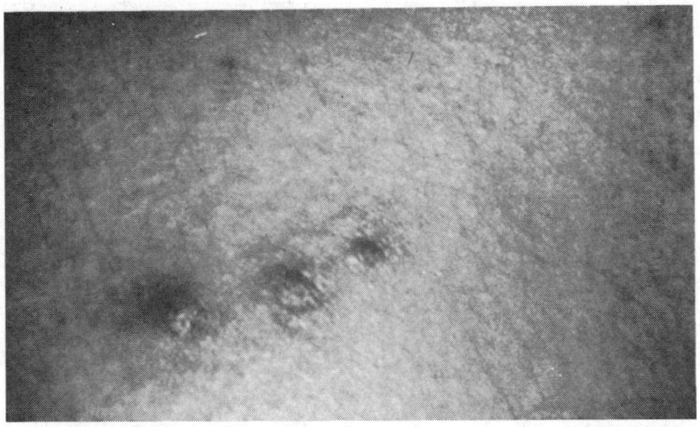

FIG. 8. Macronodular lesions of disseminated candidiasis. (Courtesy of Dr. Richard Meyer, Los Angeles, CA.)

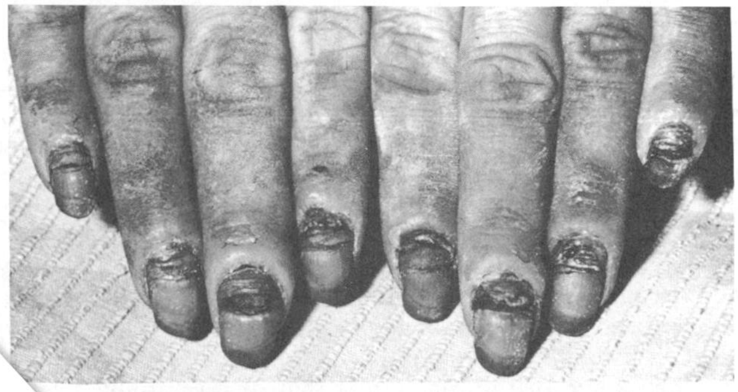

Candida paronychia and onychomycois. (Courtesy of Dr. Victor
r, Los Angeles, CA.)

the disease process is stopped, secondary thickening, ridging, and discoloration occur, and nail loss may result.

Candida paronychia occurs in association with frequent emersion of the hands in water. People who may contract paronychia include diswashers, laundry workers, and young mothers. There is also a higher incidence of paronychia among diabetics than in the nondiabetic population. Specific diagnosis is made by Gram stain or potassium hydroxide preparation and culture showing predominantly *Candida* organisms.

In addition to paronychia, *Candida* may produce infection in the nail itself and is a cause of onychomycosis.[89]

Diaper Rash. *Candida* is a common cause of diaper rash in infants. The condition generally starts in the perianal area and spreads over the perineum in the region of diaper contact (Fig. 10). The process is facilitated by maceration caused by wet diapers. The probable origin is the GI tract. Diagnosis is made by scraping the area and demonstrating the organisms on potassium hydroxide preparation.[90]

Perianal Candidiasis. Although numerous organisms and combinations of organisms have been associated with pruritus ani, either alone or in combination, *Candida* is a frequent cause. The perianal skin develops marked erythema and progresses to maceration (Fig. 11). Intense pruritus results. Complications include involvement of the anal canal and extensive spread over the perineum.

Chronic Mucocutaneous Candidiasis (CMC). This term is used to describe a heterogeneous group of *Candida* infections of the skin, mucous membranes, hair, and nails that have a protracted and persistent course despite what is usually adequate therapy. *Candida* esophagitis can occur and, over the years, cause esophageal stenosis. The major problem, however, is disfiguring lesions of the face, scalp, and hands. Alopecia in areas of infection is common and may be permanent. These infections have been associated with definable, relatively specific, immunlogic abnormalities, which may be responsible for their persistant nature.[91–93]

The major immune defect associated with CMC is failure of T-cell lymphocytes (thymus-derived) to respond to stimulation with *Candida* antigen in vitro by either lymphocyte transformation or synthesis of macrphage inhibition factor (MIF).[92] An in vivo manifestation of this abnormality is reflected in the cu-

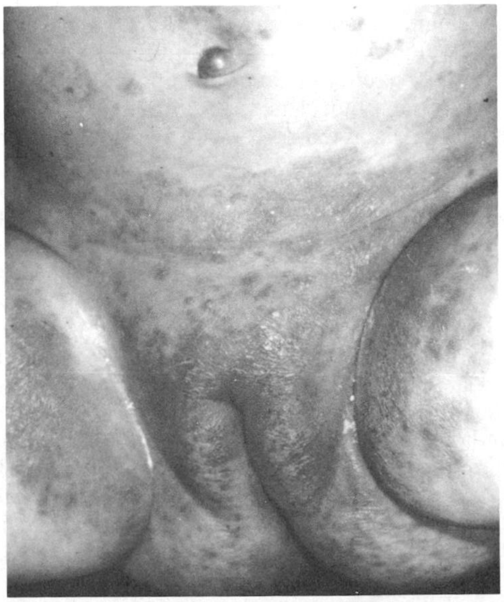

FIG. 10. Severe *Candida* diaper rash. (Courtesy of Dr. Victor Newcomer, Los Angeles, CA.)

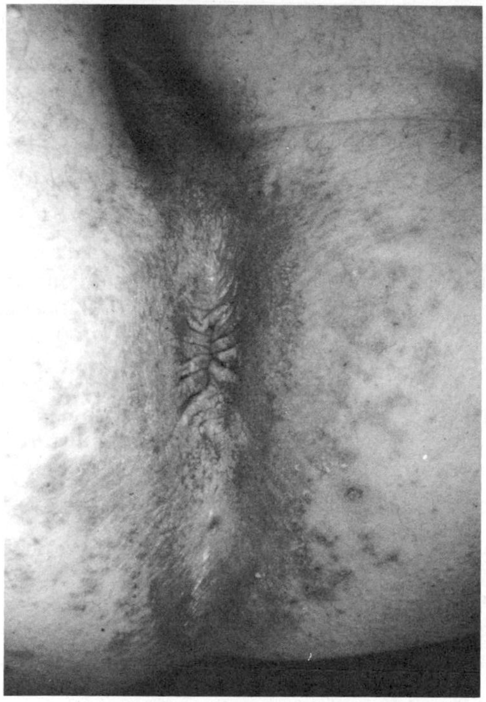

FIG. 11. Perianal candidiasis. (Courtesy of Dr. Victor Newcomer, Los Angeles, CA.)

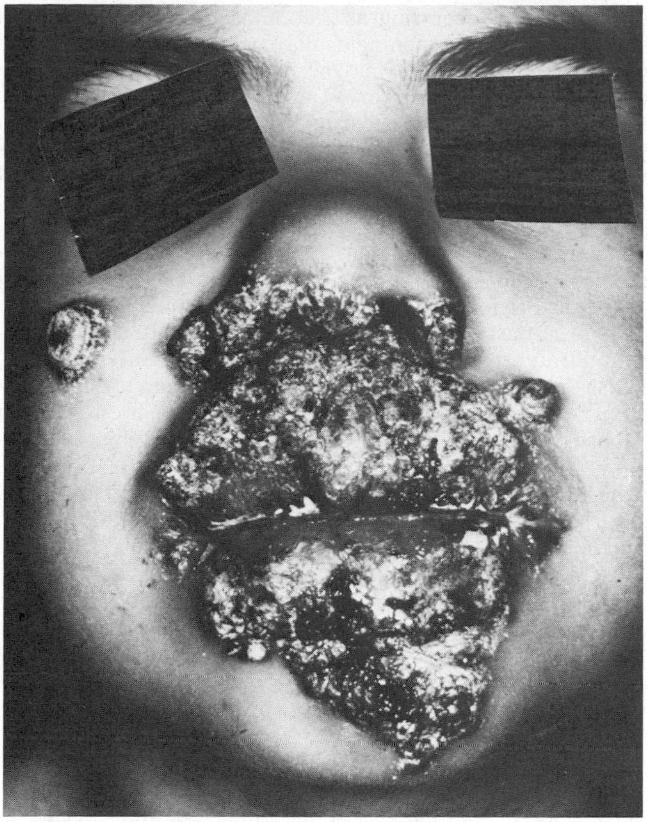

FIG. 12. *Candida* granuloma. (Courtesy of Dr. Victor Newcomer, Los Angeles, CA.)

taneous anergy found in approximately one-half of the patients.[92] Various combinations of the T-cell function abnormalities exist. Some patients' lymphocytes transform in vitro when stimulated by *Candida* antigen, but their skin tests remain negative to the antigen. Certain patients with positive transformations do not synthesize MIF; virtually all patients with negative transformations lack MIF production. Despite these abnormalities of T-cell function (T-cell numbers, lymphocyte proliferative responses to nonspecific mitogens, such as phytohemagglutinins [PHA] and allogenic cells), B-cell lymphocyte numbers and serum immunoglobulins are usually normal. However, some patients have other immune abnormalities, such as cutaneous anergy to such antigens as streptokinase-streptodornase, mumps and tetanus toxoid, defective lymphocyte transformations to nonspecific mitogens (e.g., PHA), defective monocyte chemotaxis, lack of anti-*Candida* antibody in salivary IgA immunoglobulins, plasma inhibitors to *Candida*-stimulated lymphocyte transformations, suppressor lymphocytes, and various degrees of thymic aplasia. Not all patients have these identifiable immune abnormalities.

Most forms of CMC begin in infancy or within the first two decades; rarely, the onset may be after age 30 years. The first manifestation is usually oral thrush, followed by nail infections and then skin involvement. There is a broad spectrum of severity, ranging from chronic involvement of an isolated nail to a severely disfiguring form (*Candida* granuloma) (Fig. 12). An additional facet of CMC is the association of several endocrine disorders in approximately one-half of the patients. Endocrinopathy tends to follow, not precede, CMC, often after an interval of several years. The most common endocrinopathies are hypoparathyroidism and Addison's disease. Hypothyroidism and diabetes mellitus also occur. Autoimmune antibodies to adrenal, thyroid, and gastric tissues are present in approximately one-half of the cases. Thymoma,[94] chronic dermatophytosis, and dental dysplasia have also been associated with CMC. Associations have also been made with vitiligo, polyglandular autoimmune disease, and autoantibodies to melanin-producing cells.[95]

Although most patients with CMC survive for a prolonged period with their disease, if the cutaneous condition and immunodeficiencies are severe enough, they may succumb. Disseminated candidiasis has been a rare complication of this disease; the most common cause of death is bacterial sepsis.

Deep Organ Involvement

Central Nervous System Candidiasis. *Candida* infects both parenchymal brain tissue and the meninges, usually as a complication of disseminated candidiasis. Approximately 50 percent of patients with *Candida* meningitis have had disseminated disease.[96] *Candida* has emerged as the dominant cerebral mycosis in autopsied patients.[97] When infection occurs in brain parenchyma, it generally forms multiple micro- and small macroabscesses scattered throughout the tissue. Rarely, larger abscesses have occurred and may be visualized by computed tomography (CT) scan.[98,99]

Virtually all patients with *Candida* meningitis have had cerebrospinal fluid pleocytosis. Fifty percent have had a lymphocyte pleocytosis with an average count of 600 cells/mm^3. Sixty percent have had hypoglycorrhachia and elevated protein; organisms have been present on wet mount or Gram stain in approximately forty percent.[96] *Candida albicans* has been the responsible pathogen in 90 percent of cases. Occasional cases due to *C. tropicalis* are appearing. Use of hypertonic media was felt to improve recovery of the organism in one case,[100] but this finding has never been confirmed.

The clinical manifestations of central nervous system involvement with diffuse microabscesses may be variable. If the patient is comatose or noncommunicative, detection of abnormalities may be exceptionally difficult. When meningitis is present, the signs of meningeal irritation, typical of any meningeal infection, are frequently present (headache, stiff neck, irritability). In the newborn, diagnosis is often difficult and delayed, leading to permanent neurologic sequelae.

In addition to occurring as a complication of disseminated candidiasis, *Candida* meningitis may result from infection of a ventricular shunt[101,102] or may be introduced by lumbar puncture, trauma, or neurosurgery. Untreated, the mortality rate is very high; it is reduced substantially with antifungal therapy. Hydrocephalus is a reasonably frequently occurring complication of the infection. An increase in the number of cases of *Candida* meningitis reported in neonates is occurring.[103]

Respiratory Tract Candidiasis. In general, *Candida* pneumonia occurs in two forms: (*1*) either local or diffuse bronchopneumonia originating from endobronchial inoculation of the lung[104] or (*2*) as a hematogenously seeded, finely nodular, diffuse infiltrate, which in its early stages may be difficult to distinguish from congestive heart failure or pneumocystis pneumonia.[104,105] Other forms of *Candida* pneumonia are rare, such as those that have been described as necrotizing pneumonia,[105,106] *Candida* pulmonary mycetoma,[107] and transient infiltrates due to *Candida*.[108] X-ray findings are nonspecific, and definitive diagnosis depends on biopsy-proven fungal invasion of pulmonary tissue.[109] Because of a relatively high prevalence of yeasts colonizing the respiratory tract, especially in ill patients, a diagnosis of *Candida* pneumonia cannot be made on the basis of x-ray findings and recovery of yeasts from sputum alone. *Candida* has also caused bronchial infection,[110] laryngeal infection,[111] epiglottitis,[112] and infection of laryngeal prostheses.[113]

Cardiac Candidiasis. MYOCARDITIS AND PERICARDITIS. In addition to causing endocarditis, *Candida* infects both the pericardium and myocardium.[114–120] *Candida* myocarditis occurs as diffuse microabscesses scattered throughout the myocardium with normal intervening myocardial tissue. The relatively high incidence of myocarditis has been stressed by Franklin et al.,[119] who found that 62 percent of their 50 patients with disseminated candidiasis had myocardial involvement. Other retrospective autopsy studies have shown a range from 8.4 to 93 percent. Franklin et al. found the following nonspecific electrocardiographic (ECG) changes in some of their patients: (*1*) supraventricular arrhythmias, (*2*) QRS changes mimicking infarction, and (*3*) pronounced T-wave changes. Five patients had hypotension and shock, which could not be explained by coexistent bacteremia or blood loss. The results of this study and observations in other autopsy series of disseminated candidiasis reveal a surprisingly high incidence of myocarditis (without associated valvular involvement) and point to the importance of thorough cardiac evaluation in patients who may have disseminated candidiasis. Of interest has been the emergence of *Candida* organisms as a cause of pericarditis. A review of purulent pericarditis spanning the years 1960 to 1974 revealed that *Candida* organisms were either the single cause, or were combined with *Aspergillus* in 15 percent of the 26 cases.[120]

The association of *Candida* pericarditis with either cardiac surgery or burns has been emphasized.[114]

Candida Endocarditis. This manifestation of *Candida* was once a distinctly rare phenomenon, but its true incidence has increased simultaneously with the generalized increase in *Candida* infections. Of all the forms of fungal endocarditis, *Candida* is by far the most common. In the last four decades there have been well over 214 reported cases.[121–123] In a detailed review of 319 cases of fungal endocarditis, *Candida* accounted for 67 percent.[122]

Candida endocarditis occurs in association with six clinical factors: (*1*) underlying valvular heart disease, (*2*) heroin addiction, (*3*) cancer chemotherapy, (*4*) implantation of prosthetic valves, (*5*) prolonged use of intravenous catheters (endocarditis, right atrial fungal masses, and infection of atrial myxomas have all been described), and (*6*) superimposed upon pre-existing bacterial endocarditis. Of these associations, by far the most frequent is postoperative cardiac surgery, accounting for approximately 50 percent of the cases. Of interest is the frequency of species other than *C. albicans* that have caused endocarditis; a minimum of 41 percent of the cases have been due to organisms of other species. In heroin addicts, *C. parapsilosis* has been the most common causative organism.[124]

The pathogenic mechanisms for fungal endocarditis are not fully understood, but patients who undergo cardiac surgery are at risk for candidemia by being exposed to multiple antibiotics, prolonged intravenous fluid administration, and intravenous plastic catheters. Both the damaged endocardium and prosthetic material apparently serve as foci for the localization of *Candida* organisms. In addition, contamination of suture material has been implicated in cases reported with concentration along the suture line. Contamination of homografts and heterografts has also been documented.[122] Experimental evidence for a role in the pathogenesis of adherence of *Candida* to platelet fibrin complexes and/or fibronectin is accumulating.[125,126] The mechanisms for adherence and the potential for blocking the adherence are under investigation.[125,126]

The most common valves involved in *Candida* endocarditis have been the aortic and mitral valves. In postoperative *Candida* endocarditis, the type of surgery has not been as important as the length of the postoperative course and complications during the postoperative period. *Candida* infection has been seen in simple valvulotomies and in prosthetic material placement, heterografts, and homografts.[127]

The physical findings and usual symptoms of *Candida* endocarditis are not significantly different from those of bacterial endocarditis, with the exception of the occurrence of large emboli to major vessels. Osler's nodes, Janeway lesions, splinter hemorrhages, hepatosplenomegaly, hematuria, proteinuria, pyuria, and casts all can occur. In addition, although the lesions of hematogenous *Candida* endophthalmitis have been described much more frequently in the setting of disseminated candidiasis without endocarditis, they may also be seen with endocarditis.

The complications of *Candida* endocarditis are very similar to those of bacterial endocarditis and include valve perforation, myocarditis, congestive heart failure, and major emboli. Although the majority of cases of *Candida* endocarditis occur in the 2 postoperative months, some have occurred later, and some patients who have been treated have had recurrent active disease after 2 years,[128] and perhaps as long as 8 years later. Therefore, in following patients treated for postoperative endocarditis, careful follow-up must be extended over a prolonged period.

The majority of patients with *Candida* endocarditis have positive blood cultures. Seelig et al.,[127] in their analysis of 91 cases of *Candida*-induced endocarditis after cardiac surgery, noted that 24 patients (26 percent) had negative blood cultures. Echocardiography is becoming progressively more helpful, and large vegetations may be detected with this technique. Serologic tests for *Candida* antibodies (precipitins) may be of value. However, there is a high incidence of false-negative results with this test, and for reasons that are not understood, there is a high incidence of false-positive results in patients after cardiac surgery.[121,129] An antigen detection method has been successful in rabbits with *Candida*-induced endocarditis,[130] but one study in human patients has been disappointing.[131]

The therapy for *Candida* endocarditis will be discussed in detail in the section below on "Treatment and Prophylaxis." Before the introduction of surgical procedures for the management of *Candida*-induced endocarditis, the mortality rate from this disease was approximately 90 percent. With combined surgical and medical therapy, this mortality rate has dropped to approximately 45 percent.

Candida endocarditis has been seen in association with bacterial endocarditis. Most commonly, staphylococci have been the associated bacteria.

Urinary Tract Candidiasis. Urethral candidiasis can occur in both men and women.[132] In men, the condition results from sexual contact with women who have *Candida* vaginitis. *Candida* prostatic infection has also been reported. In women, it is generally thought to be acquired from extension of *Candida* vaginitis. A history of previous antibiotic use has been found in most patients.

The presence of *Candida* in the urine is common[133–135] and does not necessarily indicate renal tract infection. Antibiotics and Foley catheters have been associated with acquisition of candiduria. Visualization (cystoscopy) and/ or biopsy proof of either fungus balls or tissue invasion is requisite for linking candiduria to infection. While the use of colony counting in urine has been attempted to separate colonization from infection, its usefulness is questionable. However, finding casts in the urine may be helpful in diagnosing renal tissue invasion of the upper renal tract.[136] Most patients with iatrogenic candiduria have spontaneous resolution; however, long-term persistence and fungus ball formation may be complications.[137]

Candida cystitis[138] is most commonly a complication of an indwelling Foley catheter. In the absence of bladder instrumentation, *Candida* cystitis has been associated most often with diabetes mellitus. Symptoms may be absent or may be essentially identical to those of bacterial cystitis. The cytoscopic appearance of the condition is that of a chronic, nonspecific cystitis. A typical thrush membrane has been observed; it resembles deposits of coagulated milk and bleeds upon removal.

Candida infection of the upper urinary tract has been classified into two distinct forms: primary, presumably from an ascending route, and secondary, from hematogenous spread. Papillary necrosis,[139] caliceal invasion, fungus ball formation, and perinephric abscess can result from ascending infection, particularly in the presence of urinary tract obstruction, renal stones, or diabetes mellitus.[140–143] The hematogenous form of disease is by far the most common. The pathologic changes are those of multiple microabsesses, especially in the cortical areas. Of interest is one case of emphysematous pyelonephritis in a diabetic drug addict[144] (and a case of cystitis emphysematosa[145]). The kidney is one of the organs most frequently involved in disseminated disease.

Candida Arthritis, Osteomyelitis, Costochondritis, and Myositis. These manifestations of *Candida* infections were once extremely rare; however, their incidence has increased appreciably in recent years.[146] Sites of localization for hematogenous *Candida*-caused osteomyelitis include the spine (vertebrae and intervertebral disks [Fig. 13]), wrist, femur, cervical spine, costochondral junctions of the ribs, scapula, and proximal humerus.[146,147] Blood cultures usually have been negative, and diagnosis has been made by percutaneous needle aspiration of the involved area. In children, the long bones are generally affected, whereas in adults the axial skeleton predominates.[147] Spinal involvement may be accompanied by disk infection.[148,149] Bone infection may require surgery.[150] X-ray examination findings are nonspecific.

Osteomyelitis as a result of contiguous spread from the skin has also been documented, and there is one reported case of extension of thrush of the mouth into the mandibular bone.

Candida arthritis occurs most frequently as a complication of disseminated candidiasis. It can also occur from trauma, surgery, intra-articular injections of steroids, and as a complication of heroin injection.[151–154] In *Candida* arthritis unassociated with disseminated candidiasis, non-*albicans* species have been the most common. Although the majority of cases of *Candida* arthritis have been acute, chronic *Candida* arthritis has been reported, especialy in leukemic patients.[155] Generally *Candida* arthritis has begun as a suppurative synovitis, and a high percentage of cases have extended to form osteomyelitis. *Candida* costochondritis can occur from hematogenous seeding or as a complication of median sternotomy wound infection.

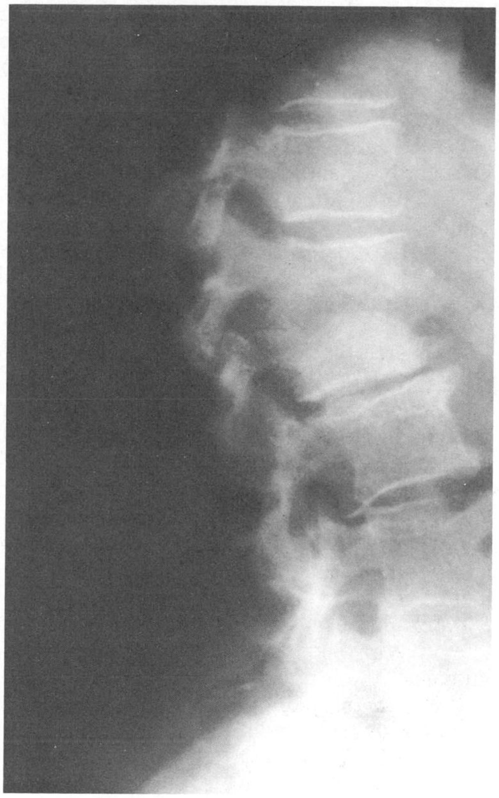

FIG. 13. *Candida* spinal osteomyelitis. Note the involvement of the intervertebral disk and adjacent vertebrae. (From Edwards et al.,[219] with permission.)

Candida infection of muscle has been described in recent years. The majority of patients have been neutropenic and have had pain in the involved muscle.[156] The organisms may be seen on biopsy of the involved muscle.

Candida Infection of Peritoneum, Liver, Spleen, and Gallbladder. A striking increase in the incidence of reported *Candida*-caused peritonitis has occurred in recent years; this infection is a complication of peritoneal dialysis, GI surgery, and perforation of an abdominal viscus.[157–160] Prior antibiotic administration has been an important predisposing factor. For reasons not completely understood, the peritoneal process usually remains localized to the abdomen; the incidence of dissemination is approximately 25 percent in patients acquiring the disease from GI tract perforation. In patients with peritonitis caused by chronic ambulatory peritoneal dialysis, dissemination is distinctly uncommon. Infants disseminate more frequently than adults.

Other GI organs infected with *Candida* that have been reported in recent years include the gallbladder,[161,162] liver,[163,164] spleen,[165,166] and pancreas.[167] Hepatosplenic candidiasis has emerged as an important clinical problem in immunocompromised hosts and is particularly difficult to treat successfully. Most of these infections have occurred in severely immunocompromised patients. CT scans or ultrasound may visualize liver or splenic abscesses. Fungus balls may form in the gallbladder and bile ducts.[161,162,168]

Candida Infection of Vasculature. The incidence of *Candida* intravascular infection has increased significantly in recent years, probably due to the increased number of susceptible patients and the widespread use of indwelling intravascular devices for advanced life support. Both peripheral and deep vascular structures have been involved, as well as both the venous and arterial sides of the circulation[169–176] and implanted prosthetic vascular materials.[177,178] Although the exact pathogenesis is not known, presumably the damaged endothelium becomes susceptible to *Candida* invasion. *Candida* adherence to catheters may also play a role.[179] Complications have included superior cava obstruction, mural endocarditis of the right atrium, tricuspid endocarditis, and pulmonary venous thrombosis. Of importance is that in patients with peripheral septic thrombophlebitis, there may be minimal symptoms and the extent of the disease may be greater than is apparent on initial clinical assessment. These patients require aggressive surgical exploration to determine the extent of the disease process.

Ocular Candidiasis. *Candida* can infect the eye either by hematogenous spread or by direct inoculation, especially during eye surgery. *Candida* can infect virtually any eye structure, including the conjunctiva, cornea, lens, ciliary body, vitreous humor, and the entire uveal tract. Once endophthalmitis occurs, therapy is difficult, and the incidence of permanent intraocular damage is high.

Throughout the 1970s, there has been increased reporting of hematogenous *Candida* endophthalmitis and an actual increase in the incidence of this complication of candidemia.[180,181] The lesions are important because they can cause permanent blindness, and they may provide an indicator of underlying disseminated candidiasis. The lesions are white, cotton ball-like, chorioretinal in origin, and rapidly progress to involve the vitreous humor (Fig. 14). Use of the indirect ophthalmoscope facilitates visualization of their three-dimensional characteristic. Experimental evidence indicates that *C. albicans* may have a much higher frequency of localization to the eye than the other species. Neutropenia inhibits visualization of ocular lesions in the experimental animal[182] and may be associated with lack of formation of easily seen lesions in some neutropenic patients. Diagnosis can be made by the characteristic fundoscopic picture plus, in half the cases, an episode of known candidemia. Aspiration of the anterior chamber is rarely diagnostic. However, elective vitrectomy may be helpful both diagnostically and therapeutically.[183] Symptoms include visual blurring, floating scotomata, and pain.

Syndrome of Disseminated Candidiasis and Candidemia. The problems of management of candidemia and detection of underlying disseminated candidiasis present major enigmas for clinicians dealing with patients who are predisposed to the disseminated form of this disease. The problem is compounded by the absence of positive blood cultures in leukopenic patients with disseminated disease (approximately 80 percent). The interpretation of the significance of recovery of increased numbers of *Candida* from sites such as sputum, urine, feces, and skin is difficult, since the organisms can be recovered frequently from these sites without causing infection.

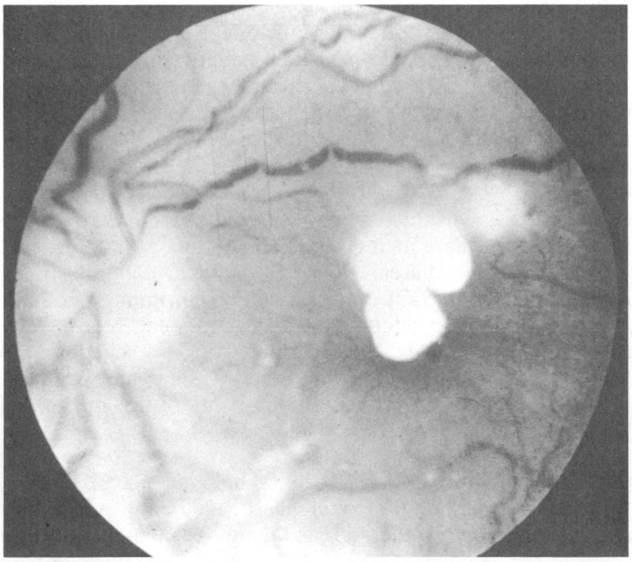

FIG. 14. Advanced hematogenous *Candida* endophthalmitis. (From Fishman et al.,[220] with permission.)

The clinical setting associated with disseminated candidiasis has been previously described. As expected, the populations of patients most commonly affected are those with neoplastic disease, patients who have had complicated postoperative courses, and burn patients.[58,184–187] Of the neoplastic group, the most common association has been with the acute leukemic population.[186,187] Of the postoperative group, the patients who have had organ transplants, heart surgery, or GI tract surgery are at greatest risk.

When *Candida* disseminates, multiple organs are usually involved, with the kidney, brain, myocardium, and eye being the most common. In cancer patients receiving extensive immunosuppressive therapy, recognition of liver and spleen involvement has increased substantially. Other organs less frequently infected include lungs, GI tract, skin, and endocrine glands. The hallmarks of the pathologic changes are diffuse microabscesses with a combined acute suppurative and granulomatous reaction and small macroabscesses. Macroabscesses may also form, especially in liver and spleen.

The rate of premortem diagnosis of disseminated candidiasis has been very low; only approximately 15–40 percent of patients have been diagnosed early enough for appropriate therapy. As an aid to earlier diagnosis, considerable attention has been focused on the detection of serum antibodies to *Candida* and *Candida* antigen.[188] Despite the appearance of more than 100 publications on the serologic diagnosis of disseminated candidiasis, controversies exist regarding the value of various serodiagnostic procedures. Problems with the diagnostic tests have recently been reviewed in detail.[188]

The following conclusions can be drawn from available data: (*1*) The incidence of false-negative test results for antibody has been unacceptably high in most series (probably due to severe immunocompromise) and (*2*) techniques for antigen detection have also been associated with a high incidence of false-negative results (suggesting that antigen may not circulate or circulates in a nondetectable form).

A generalization regarding application of these experimental serodiagnostic tests, which is an amplification of a similar statement made 12 years ago,[189] is still appropriate: A positive serodiagnostic test in a patient likely to have disseminated candidiasis increases the likelihood of the presence of disseminated disease, but a decision on the treatment of a suspect patient cannot be made on the basis of serodiagnostic testing alone and must be based on a comprehensive, multifactorial, repetitive evaluation of the clinical circumstances.

The premortem diagnosis of disseminated candidiasis, therefore, remains a clinical diagnosis. Definitive diagnosis is made by histopathologic demonstration of the organism invading tissues. Of greatest importance in facilitating the diagnosis is awareness of, and persistent evaluation for, the variety of manifestations of disseminated candidiasis that serve as diagnostic clues.

Management of candidemia poses particularly difficult problems. Unquestionably, some patients who have candidemia, especially associated with an indwelling catheter or with administration of intravenous fluids and competent immune status, have spontaneous resolution simultaneous with the removal of the catheter. Among severely immunosuppressed patients, almost all of those with candidemia have disseminated disease.[190] Assuming that a positive blood culture for *Candida* represents "benign" candidemia may be extremely dangerous, and an extensive evaluation of such a patient should be undertaken to disprove the presence of disseminated disease. This evaluation should consist of repeated cultures and careful physical examinations for such manifestations as ocular involvement, osteomyelitis, cutaneous manifestations, and the other complications of disseminated disease that may be recognizable on physical examination. In the immunocompetent patient, the catheter, if present, should be removed, and further blood cultures, as well as evaluation of peripheral smears (Fig. 15), should be performed. Interpretation of the ensuing resolution of the candidemia should be made with the recognition that 50 percent of patients with disseminated candidiasis have not had positive blood cultures, and if the patient is also bacteremic, concomitant fungi may not grow in culture.[191] If candidemia resolves, the patient improves, and repeated examinations disclose no evidence of dissemination, many clinicians withhold treatment. However, most clinical mycologists now recomend amphotericin B treatment in all patients with candidemia and severe neutropenia. Of growing concern is the number of patients who had had complications of candidemia, particularly arthritis, endophthalmitis, endocarditis,[192] and osteomyelitis.[146] The incidence of these complications is undefined, but there are a number of examples in the literature. Whether all patients with candidemia deserve antifungal chemotherapy is unknown at present, and it is not standard practice to treat all candidemic patients. However, if the candidemic patient is inexplicably worsening, amphotericin B should be given.

Miscellaneous Candida Infections. *Candida* infections that have been described but are beyond the scope of this discussion include ear infections, nasal ulcers, lymphadenitis (in leukemics), laryngeal infection, diarrhea, and the ''drunken disease'' syndrome described in Japan thought to be due to *Candida* fermentation of carbohydrate in the GI tract). In addition, *Candida* infections of numerous types have been reported with increasing frequency in antenates,[193] neonates,[194] and older children.[195] The emergence of *C. tropicalis* as a progressively more frequent pathogen in a variety of *Candida* infections, including disseminated candidiasis,[196] should be noted.

TREATMENT AND PROPHYLAXIS

Nystatin has been the primary agent used for mucous membrane and cutaneous candidiasis, and most mild to moderate infections of these sites are treatable with it. Clotrimazole and miconazole have been efficacious for these mucocutaneous syndromes and are topical alternatives to nystatin, especially for vaginal infections. Oral clotrimazole has approximately the same efficacy as oral nystatin for thrush, but it is much more

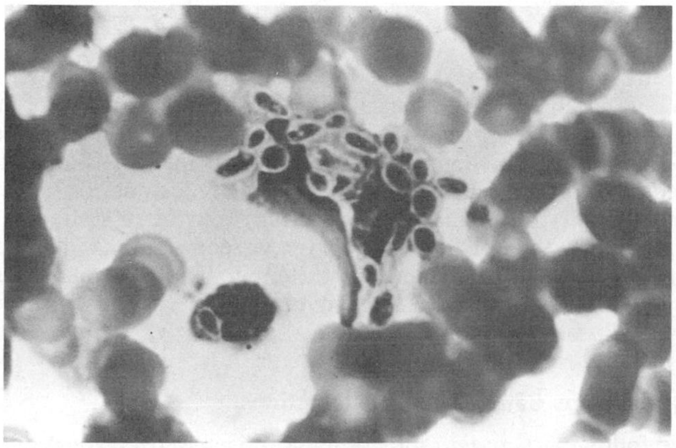

FIG. 15. *Candida* seen on peripheral smear. (Courtesy of Dr. Jack Remington, Palo Alto, CA.)

palatable. Ketoconazole has been effective for mucocutaneous *Candida*, especially chronic mucocutaneous candidiasis syndrome and in patients with esophagitis. Amphotericin B remains the cornerstone of therapy for disseminated and deep organ *Candida* infection. Until more data become available, systemic therapy with miconazole or ketoconazole should rarely be used in treating potentially lethal deep organ *Candida* infections. Insufficient data are available for newer drugs about to enter clinical trials, such as LY121019 and fluconazole. Granulocyte transfusions have been given for *Candida* infection, but they are not used on a wide basis, and their efficacy has not been established from the limited experience to date. Similarly, the role of human granulocytic colony-stimulating factor has not been sufficiently evaluated.

Regarding the prophylaxis of *Candida* infection, the use of oral nystatin or ketoconazole has not been associated with an appreciable decrease in systemic candidiasis in leukemic patients.[197–199] However, there has been one successfu trial in critically ill surgical patients.[200] The most important facet of prophylaxis of *Candida* infections is minimizing the factors that predispose to *Candida* infections.

The total amount of amphotericin B needed to treat any form of *Candida* infection is not known. Derivation of a specific figure is complicated, since some forms of *Candida* infection resolve spontaneously (often correlated with improvement of the immune status of the host). Because the manifestations of *Candida* infections are so varied, their therapy will be discussed individually.

Disseminated Candidiasis

The decision to treat candidemia has been discussed previously in this chapter. Once the decision to treat a patient for presumptive candidiasis has been made, therapy should be initiated with amphotericin B (see Chapter 33). If the patient's course is rapidly worsening, then 5-fluorocytosine (5-FC) can be added to the regimen to provide rapid attainment of therapeutic blood levels.[201] However, bone marrow suppression or diarrhea may be complications of simultaneous use of these agents. Because of a significant incidence of primary resistance to 5-FC[202] and the emergence of resistance during therapy, this drug should not be used alone for management of disseminated disease. Treatment with either amphotericin B or combination therapy is continued until obvious clinical improvement is seen. Unfortunately, there are no controlled studies giving guidelines for the total dose of amphotericin B or 5-FC needed. Serum levels of 5-FC should be monitored.[203]

Candida Endocarditis

The mortality rate is lowest with combined medical and surgical therapy, compared with either medical or surgical treatment alone. McLeod and Remington have summarized these data.[122] Once the diagnosis of *Candida*-caused valvulitis is made, the procedure of choice is to initiate amphotericin B therapy and to perform surgery as soon as possible. After surgery, amphotericin B should be given for 6–10 weeks because of the significant incidence of relapse.[128] At the time of removal of the valve and surrounding vegetations, the area can be washed with an amphotericin-B-containing solution.[204] Some patients with cardiac valvular candidiasis have had relapses years after surgery. Patients with *Candida* endocarditis should be monitored for a minimum of 2 years postoperatively.

Central Nervous System Candida Infection

Based on analysis of current literature, combined amphotericin B and 5-FC, without intrathecal instillation, is the most rational treatment for both meningitis and diffuse parenchymal infection.[98,205] If a shunt is in place, it should be removed, if possible.[101] In exceptionally severe cases, intrathecal antifungals should be used. Indications for surgery of *Candida*-caused brain abscesses remain unclear.

Candida Peritonitis, Gallbladder Infection, and Intra-Abdominal Abscesses

Candida peritonitis due to peritoneal dialysis of adults, if there is no evidence of spread to other organs, may respond to instillation of local amphotericin B at a concentration of 2–4 μg/ml in dialysate fluid.[157] Only limited experiences with intraperitoneal 5-FC and micronazole have been reported. Removal of the catheter is helpful but may not be necessary.[206,207]

Candida coming from an abdominal drain placed at the time of GI surgery should not ordinarily prompt antifungal therapy. Discovery of *Candida* in ascites from an undrained abdomen usually means that intravenous amphotericin B is required. Hematogenous dissemination is uncommon in adults but usual in neonates with peritonitis.[208]

For abscesses in the liver, spleen, or pancreas, intravenous amphotericin B should be given. The failure rate for cure of hepatosplenic candidiasis has been high with amphotericin B, both alone and in combination with 5-FC, unless very long courses of therapy have been given. Reports of cures with liposomal amphotericin have appeared and are promising.[209,210] Surgery, especially splenectomy, and removal of fungus balls from the gallbladder or bile ducts[211] may be indicated when lesions are large or the response to therapy is inadequate. *Candida*-caused cholecystitis may respond to intravenous amphotericin B therapy alone.[211] Further data are necessary for substantiation, however. Failure with ketoconazole has been reported.[212] A *Candida* pancreatic abscess has been successfully drained with CT-guided percutaneous aspiration.[213]

Urinary Candidiasis

Postcatheterization persistent candiduria usually resolves without specific antifungal therapy. If it persists but is asymptomatic, there are two types of patients in whom it should be treated: renal transplant patients and in neutropenic patients. Local amphotericin instillation is a desirable approach. If true cystitis is present, local irrigation with amphotericin B should be undertaken.[135] Usually a solution of 50 mg of amphotericin B in 1 liter of sterile water is infused at a rate of 40 ml/hr. Selected patients may require irrigation through nephrostomy incisions directly into the collecting systems. If fungus balls form, they require surgical removal. For renal parenchymal involvement, intravenous amphotericin B is indicated.

An alternative to amphotericin B for urinary tract infection is 5-FC. This agent is excreted into the urine unchanged in high concentrations. Successful management of urinary tract candidiasis has been documented with this agent. However, the problems of emerging resistance and primary resistance of *Candida* organisms to this agent exist.[202] The role of miconazole and ketoconazole[214] in urinary candidiasis remains conjectural. At least one case of emergence of resistance to miconazole has been reported.[215] Neither ketoconazole nor miconazole is excreted in urine as a biologically active agent. However, fluconazole is excreted in urine.

Thrush

Oral thrush is usually managed successfully with suspensions of nystatin, which are manufactured at a concentration of 100,000 units/ml. The usual adult dose is 4–6 ml of the fluid qid. Nystatin vaginal tablets and clotrimazole troches are also available. These can be sucked four to five times a day. Clotrimazole is approximately as effective as nystatin but is generally much better tolerated. Gentian violet causes staining but is an effective topical agent. Usually 7–10 days of therapy is sufficient; the patient should be treated for 48 hours after becoming asymptomatic. Therapy for denture sore mouth is the same as that for thrush, with the addition of meticulous cleaning of the dentures and correction of ill-fitting plates. Angular cheilitis, which is frequently associated with denture sore mouth, should be treated with either topical nystatin or 3% amphotericin B cream. Management of *Candida*-caused leukoplakia consists of long-term nystatin therapy and surgical resection in persistent cases. *Candida* esophagitis is sometimes manageable with oral nystatin. However, patients with severe disease are unable to swallow the orally administered medicine or simply fail to respond. This circumstance is best managed with low-dose (10–20 mg/day) intravenous amphotericin B[216] or oral ketoconazole. *Candida* intertrigo is most successfully managed by decreasing the moisture of the involved area and by applying amphotericin B lotion or nystatin cream several times a day.

Management of *Candida* diaper rash has been successful with nystatin powder or cream in combination with a corticosteroid, such as Mycolog cream. Amphotericin cream or lotion may also be used. The same agents used for diaper rash are generally successful for pruritus ani. *Candida* vaginitis has been treated with clotrimazole or nystatin suppositories or with miconazole or clotrimazole cream. Mycolog cream can be applied to the vulva. Oral ketoconazole can be used in refractory cases, provided that pregnancy is excluded. The role of itraconazole in mucocutaneous *Candida* infection awaits more extensive evaluation. Promising studies have been performed.[217] *Candida*-caused paronychia is best managed by preventing immersion of the hands in water as much as possible and then by applying amphotericin B lotion. Surgical drainage of the area may become an important addition to the therapeutic maneuvers.

Chronic Mucocutaneous Candidiasis

Topical therapy of skin and mucous membranes achieves only slight improvement in this disease. Intravenous amphotericin B has been effective, but nearly all patients relapse. There have been several attempts to augment therapy through the use of immunostimulating procedures. The most widely used immunostimulating factor has been transfer factor, the cell-free leukocyte extract that can transfer delayed hypersensitivity reactions to previously anergic persons. Other immunostimulants that have undergone even less extensive trials than transfer factor and would still be considered experimental are levamisole, thymosin fraction 5, which is a soluble product extracted from calf thymus, lymphocyte transfusions, thymus transplant, and cimetidine. Oral 5-FC has not been effective. The most important advance in the therapy of this disease is ketoconazole.[218] Numerous reports illustrate successful treatment. Therapy for months or years may be necessary. The side effects of ketoconazole used for extended periods of time require definition.

Ocular Candidiasis

Treatment of intraocular *Candida* infections necessitates the use of parenteral antifungal agents, especially amphotericin B.[180,181] Because of the data demonstrating a synergistic effect of amphotericin B and 5-FC, combination therapy should be used in refractory cases, rapidly developing lesions, or lesions in the vicinity of the macula. Vitrectomy may be of some value in patients with large abscesses in the vitreous and may provide confirmation of the diagnosis.[183] Hematogenous *Candida* endophthalmitis, not extensively involving the vitreous, has occasionally healed spontaneously.

Micellaneous Candida-Caused Infections

The following *Candida* infections not discussed above require systemic amphotericin B: pneumonia,[104] osteomyelitis,[146] and arthritis.[151] Vascular infections require removal of the infected site, followed by systemic therapy. Intra-articular amphotericin B can be used in refractory infections of large joints.

REFERENCES

1. Langenbeck B. Auffingung von Pilzen aus der Schleimhaut der Speiserohre einer Typhus-Leiche. Neue Not Geb Natur Heilk (Froriep). 1839;12:145–7.
2. Rippon JW. Candidiasis and the pathogenic yeasts. In: Medical Mycology. The Pathogenic Fungi and the Pathogenic Actinomycetes. 3rd ed. Philadelphia: WB Saunders; 1988:532–81.
3. Joachim H, Polayes S. Subacute endocarditis and systemic mycosis (monilia). JAMA. 1940;115:205–8.
4. Odds FC. *Candida* and Candidosis. A Review and Bibliography. 2nd ed. London: Bailliere Tindall; 1988.
5. Bodey GP, Fainstein V, eds. Candidiasis. New York: Raven Press; 1985.
6. Body BA, Pfaller MA, Durrer J, et al. Comparison of the lysis centrifugation and radiometric blood culture system for recovery of yeast. Eur J Clin Microbiol Infect Dis. 1988;7:417–20.
7. Reyolds R, Braude AI. The filament-inducing property of blood for *Candida albicans*: Its nature and significance. Clin Res Proc. 1956;4:40.
8. Huppert M, Harper G, Sun SH, et al. Rapid methods for identification of yeasts. J Clin Microbiol. 1975;2:21–34.
9. Ahearn DG. Identification and ecology of yeasts of medical importance. In: Prier JE, Friedman H, eds. Opportunistic Pathogens. Baltimore: University Park Press; 1974:129–46.
10. Hurley R. Pathogenicity of the genus *Candida*. In: Winner HI, Hurley R, eds. Symposium on *Candida* Infections. Edinburgh: Churchill Livingstone; 1966:13.
11. Burnie JP, Odds FC, Lee W, et al. Outbreak of systemic candidiasis in an intensive care unit caused by cross infection. Br Med J. 1985;290:746–8.
12. Burnie JP, Mathews RC, Lee W, et al. Control of an outbreak of systemic *Candida albicans*. Br Med J. 1985;291:1092.
13. Wilson BW, Sohnle PG. Participation of neutrophils and delayed hypersensitivity in the clearance of experimental cutaneous candidiasis. Am J Pathol. 1986;123:241–9.
14. Diamond RD, Krzesicki R, Wellington J. Damage to pseudohyphal forms of *Candida albicans* by neutrophils in the absence of serum in vitro. J Clin Invest. 1978;61:349–59.
15. Levitz SM, Lyman CA, Murata T, et al. Cytosolic calcium changes in individual neutrophils stimulated by opsonized and unopsonized *Candida albicans* hyphae. Infect Immun. 1987;55:2783–8.
16. Diamond RD, Clark RA, Haudenchild CC. Damage to *Candida albicans* hyphae and pseudohyphae by the myeloperoxidase system and oxidative products of neutrophil metabolism in vivo. J Clin Invest. 1980;66:908–17.
17. Fleischmann J, Lehrer RI. Phagocytic mechanism in host response. In: Howard DH, ed. Fungi Pathogenic for Humans and Animals. Part B2. New York: Marcel Dekker; 1985:123–49.
18. Cech P, Lehrer RI. Heterogeneity of human neutrophil phagolysosomes: Functional consequences for candidacidal activity. Blood. 1984;64:147–51.
19. Lehrer RI. The fungicidal mechanisms of human monocytes: 1. Evidence for myeloperoxidase-linked and myeloperoxidase-independent candidacidal mechanisms. J Clin Invest. 1975;55:338–46.
20. Lehrer RI. Measurement of candidacidal activity of specific leukocyte types in mixed cell populations: II. Normal and chronic granulomatous disease eosinophils. Infect Immun. 1971;3:800–2.
21. Skerl KG, Calderone RA, Sveevalsan T. Platelet interactions with *Candida albicans*. Infect Immun. 1981;34:938–43.
22. Levitz SM, Diamond RD. Killing of *Aspergillus fumigatus* spores and *Candida albicans* yeast phase by the iron-hydrogen peroxide-iodide cytotoxic system: Comparison with the myeloperoxidase-hydrogen peroxide-halide system. Infect Immun. 1984;43:1100–2.
23. Selsted ME, Harwig SSL. Purification, primary structure, and antimicrobial activities of a guinea pig neutrophil defensin. Infect Immun. 1987;55:2281–6.
24. Ganz T, Selsted ME, Lehrer RI. Antimicrobial activities of phagocyte granule proteins. In: Hoidal JR, ed. Seminars in Respiratory Infection. V. 1. Orlando, FL: Grune & Stratton; 1986:107–17.
25. Selsted ME, Szklarek D, Ganz T, et al. Activity of rabbit leukocyte peptides against *Candida albicans*. Infect Immun. 1985;49:202–6.
26. Patterson-Delafield J, Martinez RJ, Lehrer RI. Microbicidal cationic proteins in rabbit alveolar macrophages: A potential host defense mechanism. Infect Immun. 1980;30:180–92.
27. Lehrer RI. Host defense mechanisms against disseminated candidiasis. In: UCLA Conference: Severe candidal infections: Clinical perspective, immune defense mechanisms, and current concept of therapy. Edwards JE Jr, mod. Ann Intern Med. 1978;89:91–106.
28. Taschdjian CL, Toni EF, Hsu KC, et al. Immunofluorescence studies of *Candida* in human reticuloendothelial phagocytes: Implications for immunogenesis and pathogenesis of systemic candidiasis. Am J Clin Pathol. 1971;56:50–8.
29. Odds FC. Pathogenesis of candidosis. In: *Candida* and Candidosis. A Review and Biblioigraphy. 2nd ed. London: Bailliere Tindall; 1988:236–78.
30. Furguson AC, Kershnar HE, Collin WK, et al. Correlation of cutaneous hypersensitivity with lymphocytic response to *Candida albicans*. Am J Clin Pathol. 1977;68:499–504.
31. Cutler JE. Acute systemic candidiasis in normal and congenitally thymic-deficient (nude) mice. J Reticuloendothel Soc. 1976;19:121–4.
32. Lee KW, Balish E. Systemic candidiasis in germ free, flora-defined and conventional nude and thymus-bearing mice. J Reticuloendothel Soc. 1981;29:71–7.
33. Domer JE, Stashap PW, Elkins K, et al. Separation of immunomodulary effects of mannan from *Candida albicans* into stimulatory and suppressive components. Cell Immunol. 1986;101:403–14.
34. Scarlingi L, Tissi L, Boccanera M, et al. Modulation of immune reactivity by inactivated *Candida albicans* in mice. Int J Immunother. 1985;1:235–43.
35. Holmberg K, Meyer RD. Fungal infections in patients with AIDS and AIDS related complex. Scand J Infect Dis. 1986;18:179–92.
36. Solomkin JS, Mills EL, Giebink GS, et al. Phagocytosis of *Candida albicans* by human leukocytes: Opsonic requirements. J Infect Dis. 1978;137:30–7.
37. La Force FM, Mills DM, Iverson K, et al. Inhibition of leukocyte candidacidal activity by serum from patients with disseminated candidiasis. J Lab Clin Med. 1975;86:657–66.
38. Chilgren RA, Oh MK, Hong R, et al. Inhibition of PMN leukocyte killing of *Candida albicans* (Abstract). Fed Proc. 1969;28(No 1136):498.
39. Kirkpatrick CH, Rich RR, Bennett JE. Chronic mucocutaneous candidiasis: Model building in cellular immunity. Ann Intern Med. 1971;74:955–78.
40. Louria DB, Smith JK, Brayton RG, et al. Anti-*Candida* factors in serum and their inhibitors: I. Clinical and laboratory observations. J Infect Dis. 1972;125:102–14.
41. Thong YH, Ferrante A. Alternative pathway of complement activation by *Candida albicans*. Aust NZ J Med. 1978;8:620–2.
42. Gelfand JA, Hurley DL, Fauci AS, et al. Role of complement in host defense against experimental disseminated candidiasis. J Infect Dis. 1978;138:9–16.
43. Kozel TR, Brown RR, Pfrommer GS. Activation and binding of C3 by *Candida albicans*. Infect Immun. 1987;55:1890–4.
44. Sohnle PG, Frank MM, Kirkpatrick CH. Deposition of complement components in the cutaneous lesions of chronic mucocutaneous candidiasis. Clin Immunol Immunopathol. 1976;5:340–50.
45. Heidenreich F, Dierich MP. *Candida albicans* and *Candida stellatoidea*, in contrast to other *Candida* species, bind iC3b and C3d but not C3b. Infect Immun. 1985;50:598–600.
46. Edwards JE Jr, Gaither TA, O'Shea JJ, et al. Expression of specific binding sites on *Candida* with functional and antigenic characteristics of human complement receptors. J Immunol. 1986;137:3577–83.
47. Calderone RA, Linehan L, Wadsworth E, et al. Identification of C3d receptors on *Candida albicans*. Infect Immun. 1988;56:252–8.
48. Gilmore BJ, Retsinas EM, Lorenz JS, et al. An iC3b receptor on *Candida albicans*: Structure, function, and correlates for pathogenicity. J Infect Dis. 1988;157:38–46.
49. Rotrosen D, Calderone RA, Edwards JE Jr. Adherence of *Candida* species to host tissues and plastic surfaces. Rev Infect Dis. 1986;8:73–85.
50. Douglas LJ. Adhesion to surfaces. In: Rose AH, Harrison JS, eds. The Yeasts. v. 2. 2nd ed. London: Academic Press; 1987:239–80.
51. Lehrer RI. Inhibition by sulfonamides of the candidacidal activity of human neutrophils. J Clin Invest. 1971;50:2498–2505.
52. Forsgren A, Schmeling D, Quie PG. Effect of tetracycline on the phagocytic function of human leukocytes J Infect Dis. 1974;130:412–5.
53. Ferrari FA, Pagani A, Marconi M, et al. Inhibition of candidacidal activity of human neutrophil leukocytes by aminoglycoside antibiotics. Antimicrob Agents Chemother. 1980;7:87–8.
54. Brandstetter RD, Brause BP. *Candida parapsilosis* endocarditis. Recovery of the causative organism from an addict's own syringes. JAMA. 1980;243:1073.
55. Bozzetti F, Terno G, Bonfantig G, et al. Blood culture as a guide for the diagnosis of central venous catheter spesis. J Parenteral Enteral Nutr. 1984;8:396–8.
56. Krause W, Matheis H, Wulf K. Fungemia and funguria after oral administration of *Candida albicans*. Lancet. 1969;1:598–9.
57. Stone HH, Kolb LD, Currie CA, et al. *Candida* sepsis: Pathogenesis and principles of treatment. Ann Surg. 1974;697–711.
58. Rutledge R, Mandel SR, Wild RE. *Candida* species. Insignificant contaminant or pathogenic species. Am J Surg. 1986;52:299–302.
59. Dehozier JB III, Stratton CW, Potts JR III. Rapid diagnosis of *Candida* species in surgical patients. Am J Surg. 1987;53:600–2.
60. Hauser CJ, Bosco P, Davenport M, et al. Surgical management of fungal peripheral thrombophlebitis. Surgery. 1989;105:510–14.
61. Odds FC. Morphogenesis in *Candida*, with special reference to *C. albicans*. In: *Candida* and Candidosis. A Review and Bibliography. 2nd ed. London: Bailliere Tindall; 1988:42–59.
62. Dreizen S. Oral candidiasis. Am J Med. 1984;30:28–33.
63. Epstein JB, Truelove EL, Izutau KT. Oral candidiasis, pathogenesis and host defense. Rev Infect Dis. 1984;6:96–106.
64. Lehner T. Classification and clinico-pathological features of *Candida* infections in the mouth. In: Winner HI, Hurley R, eds. Symposium on *Candida* Infections. Edinburgh: Churchill Livingstone; 1966:119–37.
65. Jolly M. Premalignant lesions of the oral mucosa. Aust Dent J. 1976;414–22.
66. Vogt FC. The incidence of oral candidiasis with use of inhaled corticosteroids. Ann Allergy. 1979;43:205–10.
67. Syrjanen S, Valle SL, Antonen J, et al. Oral candidal infection as a sign of HIV infection in homosexual men. Oral Surg. 1988;55:36–40.
68. Grieve NWT. Case reports, *Monilia* oesophagitis. Br J Radiol. 1964;37:551–4.
69. Wheeler RR, Peecock JE Jr, Cruz JM, et al. Esophagitis in the immuno-

compromised host: Role of esophagoscopy in the diagnosis. Rev Infect Dis. 1987;9:88–96.
70. Young JA, Elias E. Gastro-oesophageal candidiasis: Diagnosis by brush cytology. J Clin Pathol. 1985;38:293–6.
71. Jones JM. Necrotizing *Candida* esophagitis. Failure of symptoms and roentgenographic findings to reflect severity. JAMA. 1980;244:2190–1.
72. Eras P, Goldstein MJ, Sherlock P. *Candida* infection of the gastrointestinal tract. Medicine. 1972;51:367–79.
73. Joshi SN, Garvin PJ, Sinwoo YC. Candidiasis of the duodenum and jejunum. Gastroenterology. 1981;80:829–33.
74. Minoli G, Terruzzi V, Rossini A. Gastroduodenal candidiasis occurring without underlying diseases (primary gastroduodenal candidiasis). Report on two cases. Endoscopy. 1979;11:18–22.
75. Trier JS, Bjorkman DJ. Esophageal, gastric, and intestinal candidiasis. Am J Med. 1984;30:39–43.
76. Minolig G, Terruzzi V, Ferrara A, et al. A prospective study of relationships between benign gastric ulcer, *Candida*, and medical treatment. Am J Gastroenterol. 1984;79:95–7.
77. Kaufman RH, ed. Vulvovaginal candidiasis. A symposium. J Reprod Med. 1986;31:639–72.
78. Sobel JD. Recurrent vulvovaginal candidiasis. A prospective study of the efficacy of maintenance ketoconazole therapy. N Engl J Med. 1986;315:1455–9.
79. Domonkos AN, Arnold HL Jr, Odom RB, eds. Diseases due to fungi. In Andrews' Diseases of the Skin. Clinical Dermatology. Philadelphia: WB Saunders; 1982:341–403.
80. Alteras I, Feverman EJ, David M, et al. Widely disseminated cutaneous candidosis in adults. Sabouraudia. 1979;17:383–8.
81. Dupont B, Drouhet E. Cutaneous, ocular, and osteoarticular candidiasis in heroin addicts: New clinical and therapeutic aspects in 38 patients. J Infect Dis. 1985;152:577–91.
82. Klotz SA, Drutz DJ, Huppert M, et al. Pityrosporum folliculitis. Its potential for confusion with skin lesions of systemic candidiasis. Arch Intern Med. 1982;142:2126–9.
83. Kozinn PJ, Taschdjian CL. Candidiasis. In Demis DJ, Dobson RL, McGuire J, eds. Clinical Dermatology. v. 3. Hagerstown, Md.: Harper and Row; 1973:unit 17–16.
84. Darcis JM, Etienne M, Demonty J, et al. *Candida albicans* septicemia in heroin addicts. Am J Dermatopathol. 1986;8:501–4.
85. Bodey GP, Luna M. Skin lesions associated with disseminated candidiasis. JAMA. 1974;229:1466–8.
86. Suster S, Rosen LB. Intradermal bullous dermatitis due to candidiasis in an immunocompromised patient. JAMA. 1987;258:2106–7.
87. Silverman RA, Rhodes AR, Dennehy PH. Disseminated intravascular coagulation and purpura fulminans in a patient with *Candida* sepsis. Biopsy of purpura fulminans as an aid to diagnosis of systemic *Candida* infection. Am J Med. 1986;80:679–84.
88. Brophy MC, Dunagin WB. Intertriginous dermatoses. Common puzzling problems. Postgrad Med. 1985;78(7):105–15.
89. Hay RJ, Baran R, More MK, et al. *Candida* onychomycosis—an evaluation of the role of *Candida* species in male disease. Br J Dermatol. 1988;118:47–58.
90. Rasmusson JE. Classification of diaper dermatitis: An overview. Pediatrician. 1987;14(Suppl 1):6––10.
91. Jorizzo JL. Chronic mucocutaneous candidosis. An update. Arch Dermatol. 1982;118:963–5.
92. Stiehm ER. Chronic cutaneous candidiasis, clinical aspects. In: UCLA Conference: Severe Candidal Infections: Clinical Perspective, Immune Defense Mechanisms, and Current concepts of therapy. Edwards JE Jr, mod. Ann Intern Med. 1978;89:91–106.
93. Cleary TG. Chronic mucocutaneous candidiasis. In: Bodey GP, Fainstein V, eds. Candidiasis. New York: Raven Press; 1985:241–52.
94. Kirkpatrick CE, Windhorst DB. Mucocutaneous candidiasis and thymoma. Am J Med. 1979;66:939–45.
95. Howanitz N, Nordlund JL, Lerner AB, et al. Autoantibodies to melanocytes: Occurrence in patients with vitiligo and chronic mucocutaneous candidiasis. Arch Dermatol. 1981;117:705–8.
96. Lipton SA, Hickey WF, Morris JH, et al. Candidal infection in the central nervous system. Am J Med. 1984;76:101–8.
97. Parker JC Jr, McCloskey JJ, Lee RS. The emergence of candidosis, the dominant postmortem cerebral mycosis. Am J Clin Pathol. 1978;70:31–6.
98. Salaki JS, Louria DB, Chmel H. Fungal and yeast infections of the central nervous system. A clinical review. Medicine. 1984;63:108–32.
99. Wietholter H, Thron A, Scholz E, et al. Systemic *Candida albicans* infection with cerebral abscess and granulomas. Clin Neuropathol. 1984;3:37–41.
100. Igra-Siegman Y, Armstrong D, Louria DB. Culture-negative meningitis: Isolation of organisms in hypertonic medium. Isr J Med Sci. 1981;17:383–4.
101. Sugarman B, Massanari M. *Candida* meningitis in patients with CSF shunts. Arch Neurol. 1980;37:180–1.
102. Ehlers RE, Jarrett PB, Kaplan AM. Mixed bacterial and fungal meningitis in a neonate. Dev Med Child Neurol. 1979;21:643–7.
103. Buchs J. *Candida meningitis*: A growing threat to premature and full-term infants. Pediatr Infect Dis. 1985;4:122–4.
104. Armstrong D. *Candida* species. In: Sarosi GA, Davies SF, eds. Fungal Diseases of the Lung. Orlando, Fla.: Grune and Stratton; 1986:Chap. 10:167–73.
105. Cairns MR, Durack DT. Fungal pneumonia in the immunocompromised host. In: Hoidal JR, ed. Seminars in Respiratory Infection. V. 1. Orlando, FL: Grune & Stratton; 1986:166–85.
106. Patriquin H, Lebowitz R, Perreault G, et al. Neonatal candidiasis: Renal and pulmonary manifestations. AJR. 1980;135:1205–10.
107. Watanakunakorn C. Acute pulmonary mycetoma due to *Candida albicans* with complete resolution. J Infect Dis. 1983;148:1131.
108. Wengrower D, Or R, Segal E, et al. Bronchopulmonary candidiasis exacerbating asthma. Case report and review of the literature. Respiration. 1985;47:209–13.
109. Buff SJ, McLeiland R, Gallis HA, et al. *Candida albicans* pneumonia. Radiographic appearance. AJR. 1982;138:645–8.
110. Wengrower D, Or R, Segal E, et al. Bronchopulmonary candidiasis exacerbating asthma. Respiration. 1985;47:209–13.
111. Tashjian LS, Peacock JE Jr. Laryngeal candidiasis. Arch Otolaryngol. 1984;110:806–9.
112. Walsh TJ, Gray WC. *Candida* epiglottis in immunocompromised patients. Chest. 1987;91:482–85.
113. Mahieu HF, van Saene HKF, Rosingh HJ, et al. *Candida* vegetations on silicone voice prostheses. Arch Otolaryngol. 1986;112:321–5.
114. Eng RHK, Sen P, Browne K, et al. *Candida* pericarditis. Am J Med. 1981;70:867–9.
115. Walsh TJ, Hutchins GM. Postoperative *Candida* infections of the heart in children. Clinicopathologic study of a continuing problem of diagnosis and therapy. J Pediatr Surg. 1980;15:325–31.
116. Geisler C, Ernst P, Voglsgaard R. *Candida* pericarditis in a patient with leukemia. Scand J Haematol. 1981;27:75–8.
117. Parker JC Jr. The potentially lethal problem of cardiac candidosis. Am J Clin Pathol. 1980;73:356–61.
118. Ihde DC, Roberts WC, Marr KC, et al. Cardiac candidiasis in cancer patients. Cancer. 1978;41:2364–71.
119. Franklin WG, Simon AB, Sodeman TM. *Candida* myocarditis without valvulitis. Am J Cardiol. 1976;38:924–8.
120. Rubin RH, Moellering RC. Clinical microbiologic and therapeutic aspects of purulent pericarditis. Am J Med. 1975;59:68–78.
121. McLeod R, Remington JS. Postoperative fungal endocarditis. In: Duma RJ, ed. Infections of Prosthetic Heart Valves and Vascular Grafts. Prevention, Diagnosis and Treatment. Baltimore: University Park Press; 1977:163–236.
122. Reyes MP, Lerner AM. Endocarditis caused by *Candida* species. In: Bodeg GP, Fainstein V, eds. Candidiasis. New York: Raven Press; 1985:203–9.
123. McLeod R, Remington JS. Fungal endocarditis. In: Rahimtoola SH, ed. Infective Endocarditis. New York: Grune and Stratton; 1979:211–90.
124. Odds FC. Candida endocarditis, myocarditis, and other cardiovascular Candida infections. In: *Candida* and Candidosis. A Review and Bibliography. 2nd ed. London: Bailliere Tindall; 1988:175–80.
125. Scheld WM, Calderone RA, Alliegro GM, et al. Yeast adherence in the pathogenesis of *Candida* endocarditis. Proc Soc Exp Biol Med. 1981;168:208–13.
126. Calderone RA, Scheld WM. Role of fibronectin in the pathogenesis of candidal infections. Rev Infect Dis. 1987;9(Suppl 4):S400–S403.
127. Seelig MS, Speth CP, Kozinn PJ, et al. Patterns of *Candida* endocarditis following cardiac surgery. Importance of early diagnosis and therapy (an analysis of 91 cases) Prog Cardiovasc Dis. 1974;27:125–60.
128. Galgiani JN, Stevens DA. Fungal endocarditis: Need for guidelines in evaluating therapy. J Thorac Cardiovasc Surg. 1977;73:293–6.
129. Murray IG, Buckley HR, Turner GC. Serological evidence of *Candida* infection after open-heart surgery. J Med Microbiol. 1969;2:463–9.
130. Scheld WM, Brown RS Jr, Harding SA, et al. Detection of circulating antigen in experimental *Candida albicans* endocarditis by an enzyme-linked immunosorbent assay. J Clin Microbiol. 1980;12:679–83.
131. Ryhanen P, Puhakka K, Kujala P, et al. *Candida* immunity in patients undergoing surgical treatment for heart valve disease. J Cardiovasc Surg. 1986;27:72–9.
132. Fernandes M. Monilial urethritis. Mod Treat. 1970;1011–4.
133. Roy JB, Gejer JR, Ohr JA. Urinary tract candidiasis. An update. Urology. 1984;23:533–7.
134. Frangos DN, Nyberg LM Jr. Genitourinary fungal infections. South Med J. 1986;79:455–9.
135. Drutz DJ, Fetchick R. Fungal infections of the kidney and urinary tract. In: Schrier RW, Gottschalk CW, eds. Diseases of the Kidney. v. 1. 4th ed. Boston: Little, Brown; 1988:1015–47.
136. Gregory MC, Schumann GB, Schumann JL, et al. The clinical significance of *Candida* casts. Am J Kidney Dis. 1984;4:179–84.
137. Fisher J, Mayhall G, Duma R, et al. Fungus balls of the urinary tract. South Med J. 1979;72:1281–4.
138. Rohner TJ Jr, Tuliszewski RM. Fungal cystitis. Awareness, diagnosis and treatment. J Urol. 1980;124:142–4.
139. Tomashefski JF Jr, Abramosky CR. *Candida*-associated renal papillary necrosis. Am J Clin Pathol. 1981;75:190–4.
140. Eckstein CW, Kass EJ. Anuria in a newborn secondary to bilateral ureteropelvic fungus balls. J Urol. 1982;127:109–10.
141. Leiter E, Whitehead ED, Desai SB. Fungus balls in renal pelvis. NY State J Med. 1982;82:64–6.
142. Biggers R, Edwards J. Anuria secondary to bilateral ureteropelvic fungus balls. Urology. 1980;15:161–3.
143. Tennant FS, Remmers AR, Perry JE. Primary renal candidiasis associated perinephric abscess and passage of fungus ball in the urine. Arch Intern Med. 1968;122:435–40.

144. Seidenfeld SM, Lemaistre CF, Setiawan H, et al. Emphymatous pyelonephritis caused by *Candida tropicalis*. J Infect Dis. 1982;146:569.
145. Singh CR, Lytle WF. Cystitis emphysematosa caused by *Candida tropicalis*. J Urol. 1983;130:1171–3.
146. Gathe JC Jr, Harris RL, Garland B, et al. *Candida* osteomyelitis. Report of five cases and review of the literature. Am J Med. 1987;82:927–37.
147. Simnpson MB Jr, Merz WG, Kurlinski JP, et al. Opportunistic mycotic osteomyelitis: Bone infections due to *Aspergillus* and *Candida* species. Medicine. 1977;56:475–82.
148. Shaikh BS, Appelbaum PC, Aber RC. Vertebral disc space infection and osteomyelitis due to *Candida albicans* in a patient with acute myelomonocytic leukemia. Cancer. 1980;45:1025–8.
149. Diament MJ, Weller M, Bernstein R. *Candida* infection in a premature infant presenting as discitis. Pediatr Radiol. 1982;12:96–8.
150. Yap S, Ravitch MM, Pataki KI. En bloc chest wall resection for candidal costochondritis in a drug addict. Ann Thorac Surg. 1981;31:182–7.
151. Bayer AS, Guze LB. Fungal arthritis: I. *Candida* arthritis. Diagnostic and prognostic implications and therapeutic considerations. Semin Arthritis Rheum. 1978;8:142–50.
152. Fainstein V, Gilmore C, Hopfer RI, et al. Septic arthritis due to *Candida* species in patients with cancer: Report of five cases and review of the literature. Rev Infect Dis. 1982;4:78–85.
153. Pope TL Jr. Pediatric *Candida albicans* arthritis: Case report of hip involvement with a review of the literature. Prog Pediatr Surg. 1982;15:271–83.
154. Levine M, Rhehm SJ, Wilde AH. Infection with *Candida albicans* of a total knee arthroplasty. Case report and review of the literature. Clin Orthop. 1988;226:235–9.
155. Glauser MP, Gerster JC, Delacretaz F. Chronic *Candida* arthritis in leukemic patients. Rev Infect Dis. 1982;4:1071.
156. Arena FP, Perlin M, Brahman H. Fever, rash, and myalgias of disseminated candidiasis during antifungal therapy. Arch Intern Med. 1981;14:1233.
157. Bayer AS, Blumenkrantz MJ, Montgomerie JZ, et al. *Candida* peritonitis. Report of 22 cases and review of the English literature. Am J Med. 1976;61:832–40.
158. Solomkin JS, Flohr AB, Quie PG, et al. The role of *Candida* in intraperitoneal infections. Surgery. 1980;88:524–30.
159. Eisenberg ES, Leviton I, Sociro R. Fungal peritonitis in patients receiving peritoneal dialysis: Experience with 11 patients and review of the literature. Rev Infect Dis. 1986;309–21.
160. Peoples JB. *Candida* and perforated peptic ulcers. Surgery. 1986;100:758–64.
161. Uflacker R, Wholey MH, Amaral NM, et al. Parasitic and mycotic causes of biliary obstruction. Gastrointest Radiol. 1982;7:173–9.
162. Magnussen CR, Olson JP, Ona FV, et al. *Candida* fungus balls in the common bile duct. Unusual manifestation of disseminated candidiasis. Arch Intern Med. 1979;139:821–2.
163. Thales M, Tastakia B, Shawker TH, et al. Hepatic candidiasis in cancer patients: The evolving picture of the syndrome. Ann Intern Med. 1988;108:88–100.
164. Francis IR, Glazer GM, Amendola MA, et al. Hepatic abscesses in the immunocompromised patient: Role of GT in detection, diagnosis, management, and follow-up. Gastrointest Radiol. 1986;11:257–62.
165. Vasquez TE, Evans DG, Schiffman H, et al. Fungal splenic abscesses in the immunosuppressed patient. Correlation of imaging modalities. Clin Nucl Med. 1987;12:30–8.
166. Helton WS, Carrico CJ, Zaveruha PA, et al. Diagnosis and treatment of splenic fungal abscesses in the immune-suppressed patient. Arch Surg. 1986;121:580–6.
167. Fitzgerald EJ, Lyons K. *Candida* abscess of the pancreas: Diagnosis and treatment by computed tomography-guided percutaneous drainage. Br J Radiol. 1986;59:1121–3.
168. Irani M, Truong LD. Candidiasis of the extrahepatic biliary tract. Arch Pathol Lab Med. 1986;110:1087–90.
169. Torres-Rojas JR, Stratton CW, Sanders CV, et al. *Candida* suppurative peripheral thrombophlebitis. Ann Intern Med. 1982;96:431–5.
170. Walsh TJ, Bustamente CI, Vlahov D, et al. Candidal suppurative peripheral thrombophlebitis: Recognition, prevention, and management. Infect Contr. 1986;7:16–22.
171. Pasternak BM, Samson R, Karp MP. Fungal infection of a vascular prosthesis. Surgery. 1979;85:586–8.
172. Strinden WD, Helgerson RB, Maki DB. *Candida* septic thrombosis of the great vein associated with central catheters. Ann Surg. 1985;202:653–8.
173. Deitch EA, Marini JJ, Huseby JS. Suppurative *Candida* phlebitis of a peripheral vein. J Trauma. 1980;20:618–20.
174. Johnson DE, Bass JL, Thompson TR, et al. *Candida* septicemia and right atrial mass secondary to umbilical vein catheterization. Am J Dis Child. 1981;135:275–7.
175. Knox WF, Hooton VN, Barson AJ. Pulmonary vascular candidiasis and use of central venous catheters in neonates. J Clin Pathol. 1987;40:559–65.
176. Vo NM, Russel JC, Becker DR. Mycotic emboli of the peripheral vessels: Analysis of forty-four cases. Surgery. 1981;90:541–5.
177. Ward RA, Wellhausen SR, Dobbins JJ, et al. Thromboembolic and infectious complications of total artificial heart implantation. Ann NY Acad Sci. 1987;516:638–50.
178. Doscher W, Krishnasastry KV, Deckoff SL. Fungal graft infections: Case report and review of the literature. J Vasc Surg. 1987;6:398–402.
179. Rotrosen D, Gibson TR, Edwards JE. Adherence of *Candida* species to intravenous catheters. J Infect Dis. 1983;147:594.
180. Edwards JE Jr. *Candida* endophthalmitis. In: Bodey GP, Fainstein V, eds. Candidiasis. New York: Raven Press; 1985:211–25.
181. Jones DB. Chemotherapy of experimental endogenous *Candida albicans* endophthalmitis. Trans Am Ophthalmol Soc. 1980;78:846–95.
182. Henderson DK, Hockey LB, Vukalcic LJ, et al. Effect of immunosuppression on the development of experimental hematogenous *Candida* endophthalmitis. Infect Immun. 1980;27:628–31.
183. Barrie T. The place of elective vitrectomy in the management of patients with *Candida* endophthalmitis. Graefes Arch Clin Exp Ophthalmol. 1987;225:107–13.
184. Spebar MJ, Pruitt BA. Candidiasis in the burned patient. J Trauma. 1981;21:237–9.
185. Meunier-Carpentier F, Kiehn TE, Armstrong D. Fungemia in the immunocompromised host. Changing patterns, antigenemia, high mortality. Am J Med. 1981;71:363–70.
186. Hawkins C, Armstrong D. Fungal infections in immunocompromised hosts. Clin Hematol. 1984;13:599–630.
187. Edwards JE Jr, Drutz DJ, Bennett JE, et al. Disseminated Candidiasis. A Major Problem in Cancer and Postoperative Patients. Part I. New York: Academy Professional Information Services; 1986.
188. Bennett JE. Rapid diagnosis of candidiasis and aspergilloses. Rev Infect Dis. 1987;9:398–402.
189. Krick JA, Remington JS. Opportunistic invasive fungal infections in patients with leukemia and lymphoma. Clin Hematol. 1976;5:249–310.
190. Young RC, Bennett JE, Geelhoed GW, et al. Fungemia with compromised host resistance. A study of 70 cases. Ann Intern Med. 1974;80:605–12.
191. Hockey LJ, Fujita NK, Gibson TR, et al. Detection of fungemia obscured by concomitant bacteremia: In vitro and in vivo studies. J Clin Microbiol. 1982;16:1080–5.
192. Beutler SM, Young LS, Lindquist LB, et al. Delayed complications of candidemia. In: Program and Abstracts, 22nd Interscience Conference on Antimicrobial Agents and Chemotherapy. Miami, Fla; 1982:No. 496.
193. Whyte RK, Hussain Z, de Sa D. Antenatal infections with *Candida* species. Arch Dis Child. 1982;57:528–35.
194. Henneberry L. *Candida* sepsis in very low birthweight infant. Neonatal Netw. 1987;5:39–45.
195. Hughes WT. Systemic candidiasis: A study of 109 fatal cases. Pediatr Infect Dis. 1982;1:11–8.
196. Wingard JR, Merz WG, Saral R. *Candida tropicalis*: A major pathogen in immunocompromised patients. Ann Intern Med. 1979;91:539–43.
197. De Gregorio MW, Lee WMF, Ries CA. *Candida* infections in patients with acute leukemia: Ineffectiveness of nystatin prophylaxis and relationship between oropharyngeal and systemic candidiasis. Cancer. 1982;50:2780–4.
198. Hansen RM, Reinerio N, Sohnle PG, et al. Ketoconazole in the prevention of candidiasis in patients with cancer. A prospective, randomized, controlled, double-blind study. Arch Intern Med. 1987;147:710–2.
199. Meunier F. Prevention of mycosis in immunocompromised patients. Rev Infect Dis. 1987;9:408–16.
200. Slotman GJ, Burchard KW. Ketoconazole prevents *Candida* sepsis in critically ill surgical patients. 1987;122:147–51.
201. Polak A. 5-Fluorocytosine and combinations. Ann Biol Clin (Paris). 1987;45:669–72.
202. Stiller RL, Bennett JE, Scholer HJ, et al. Susceptibility to 5-fluorocytosine and prevalence of serotype in 402 *Candida albicans* isolates from the United States. Antimicrob Agents Chemother. 1982;22:482–7.
203. Drutz DJ. In vitro antifungal susceptibility testing and measurement of levels of antifungal agents in body fluids. Rev Infect Dis. 1987;9:392–7.
204. Turnier E, Kay JH, Bernstein S, et al. Surgical treatment of *Candida* endocarditis. Chest. 1975;67:262–8.
205. Smego RA, Perfect JR, Durack DT. Combined therapy with amphotericin B and 5-fluorocytosine for *Candida* meningitis. Rev Infect Dis. 1984;6:791–801.
206. Rodriguez-Perez JC. Fungal peritonitis in CAPD—which treatment is best? Contrib Nephrol. 1987;57:114–21.
207. Struijk DG, Krediet RT, Boeschoten EW, et al. Antifungal treatment of *Candida* peritonitis in continuous ambulatory peritoneal dialysis patients. Am J Kidney Dis. 1987;9:66–70.
208. Johnson DE, Conroy MM, Foker JE, et al. *Candida* peritonitis in the newborn infants. J Pediatr. 1980;97:298–300.
209. Lopez-Berestin G, Bodeg GP, Frankel LS, et al. Treatment of hepatosplenic candidiasis with liposomal amphotericin B. J Clin Oncol. 1987;5:310–7.
210. Shirkhoda B, Lopez-Berestein G, Hlbert JM, et al. Hepatosplenic fungal infection: CT and pathologic evaluation after treatment with liposomal amphotericin B. Radiology. 1986;159:349–53.
211. Schreiber M, Black L, Noah Z, et al. Gallbladder candidiasis in a leukemic child. Am J Dis Child. 1982;136:462–3.
212. Brooks BJ Jr, Williams WL, Sanders CV, et al. Apparent ketoconazole failure in candidal cholecystis. Arch Intern Med. 1982;142:1934–5.
213. Fitzgerald EJ, Lyons K. *Candida* abscess of the pancreas: Diagnosis and treatment by computed tomography-guided percutaneous drainage. Br J Radiol. 1986;59:1121–3.
214. Graybill JR, Galgiani JN, Jorgensen JH, et al. Ketoconazole therapy for fungal urinary tract infections. J Urol. 1983;129:68–70.
215. Holt RJ, Azmi A. The emergence of *Candida albicans* resistant to micon-

azole during the treatment of urinary tract candidosis. Infection. 1978;6:198–9.
216. Medoff G. Controversial areas in antifungal chemotherapy: Short-course and combination therapy with amphotericin B. Rev Infect Dis. 1987;9:403–7.
217. Hay, RJ, Dupont B, Graybill JR, eds. First International Symposium on Itraconazole. Rev Infect Dis. 1987;9(Suppl 1):Jan–Feb.
218. Rosenblatt HM, Stiehm ER. Therapy of chronic mucutaneous candidiasis. In: Graybill JR, ed. Proceedings of a Symposium on New Developments in Therapy for the Mycoses. Am J Med. 1983;74(1B, Jan Suppl):20–2.
219. Edwards JE Jr, Turkel SB, Elden HA, et al. Hematogenous *Candida* osteomyelitis: Report of three cases and review of the literature. Am J Med. 1975;59:89.
220. Fishman LS, Griffin JR, Sapico FL, et al. Hematogenous *Candida* endophthalmitis: A complication of candidemia. N Engl J Med. 1972;286:675.

236. ASPERGILLUS SPECIES

JOHN E. BENNETT

DESCRIPTION OF THE PATHOGEN

Aspergillus is an ubiquitous mold. Disease can be produced by several species and in several ways. "Aspergillosis" has been used to describe illness attributed to allergy, colonization, or tissue invasion by *Aspergillus*.

Aspergillus fumigatus is the usual cause of aspergillosis. *Aspergillus flavus* is the second most important species, particularly in invasive disease of immunosuppressed patients[1] and in lesions beginning in the nose or paranasal sinus.[1–3] *Aspergillus niger*,[1] *A. sydowi*,[4] *A. terreus*,[5] *A. ustus*,[6] *A. versicolor*,[7] *A. amstelodami*,[8] *A. oryzae*,[9] *A. restrictus*,[10] *A. candidus*,[11] and *A. nidulans*[12] have also been reported to cause invasive disease. *Aspergillus* species are identified by appearance of the colony and by microscopic examination of the spore-bearing structures and spores. Mycologic characteristics of the genus *Aspergillus* are the subject of an excellent text.[13]

Aspergillus species produce a variety of toxins in vitro, including aflatoxins, ochratoxins, kojic acid, and clavacin.[14] None of these are known to be produced in the infected host.

EPIDEMIOLOGY

Aspergillus species are ubiquitous in the environment in most countries of the world.[15] The fungus grows well on a variety of substrates, including stored hay or grain, decaying vegetation, soil, and dung. *Aspergillus fumigatus* grows well at 45°C or even higher, making it one of the most common microorganisms found in compost piles.[13] Hospital air has often been found to contain *A. fumigatus*,[16] *A flavus, A. niger*, and other *Aspergillus* species. Unpublished studies in the author's institution found *Aspergillus* present in the air of oncology wards year-round. In various months, the mean number of *A. fumigatus* and *A. flavus* spores taken together ranged from 6 to 14/100 ft^3. One cancer hospital believed their woodpulp-based fireproofing material to be seeding hospital air with *A. flavus*.[17] Determination of *Aspergillus* colony counts in hospital air serves no useful purpose because guidelines for interpreting the results currently do not exist.

Aspergillosis is usually acquired by inhalation of airborne spores. These spores (conidia) are small enough (2.5–3.0 μm for *A. fumigatus*) to reach alveoli or to gain entrance to paranasal sinuses. Conidia in operating room air may enter the implantation site of prosthetic cardiac valves or the eye during cataract surgery. Trauma to the cornea or, in severely immunosuppressed patients, skin trauma may be a nidus for aspergillosis.

Exposure to *Aspergillus* must be nearly universal, but disease is uncommon. Host factors must be of paramount importance. Prevention out of necessity must be restricted to situations of short-term high risk. High-efficiency filters remove *Aspergillus* from the air of operating rooms and laminar flow rooms. Use of laminar flow rooms for seriously immunosuppressed patients is an expensive undertaking that makes medical care more difficult, but aspergillosis has not been observed in patients in laminar flow rooms[18] despite the frequent occurrence of the infection in other parts of the hospital.[19] There is no reason to think that reverse isolation in an ordinary hospital room would be protective. Moving immunosuppressed patients away from dusty hospital renovation[20] and construction[21,22] appears useful, as does keeping potted plants out of their hospital rooms.[23] Hospital air conditioner filters may become heavily contaminated with *Aspergillus*,[22] requiring routine cleaning.

PATHOGENESIS AND PATHOLOGIC CHARACTERISTICS

Host defense primarily relies on the professional phagocytes (neutrophils, monocytes, and macrophages), not upon antibodies or lymphocytes. Complement facilitates neutrophil damage to hyphae and monocyte killing of conidia, as well as providing a source of chemotactic factor.[24,25] However, complement is not necessary for attachment or ingestion of conidia by human or murine alveolar macrophages.[26] A central role for oxidative killing can be assumed from the frequency of aspergillosis in chronic granulomatous disease and from the importance of neutrophils in susceptibility to and recovery from aspergillosis.

Allergic reactions to *Aspergillus* may contribute in some way to the pathology encountered in patients with allergic bronchopulmonary aspergillosis as well as in certain patients with *Aspergillus* either in their paranasal sinus or in ectatic bronchi. Etiology of hemoptysis and pleural fibrosis in fungus ball of the lung is completely unclear. The fungus does not invade lung tissue but remains confined to the cavity and the lumen of ectatic bronchi.

The pathology of invasive aspergillosis depends upon the host. In immunosuppressed patients, vascular invasion is paramount, leading to infarction, necrosis, edema, and hemorrhage in distal tissues. Hyphae are abundant, even forming radially branching clusters in tissue. In contrast, vascular invasion is not seen, and hyphae are sparse in tissue from patients with chronic granulomatous disease.

Hyphae of *Aspergillus* are 2–4 μm wide, frequently septate, and dichotomously branched. In rapidly progressing infections the hyphae tend to be of even diameter. In sites of indolent disease, hyphae may have bulbous widened areas. Sporulation is rarely observed in tissue except for air-containing areas such as lung or paranasal sinus. Cross sections of hyphae or bulbous areas of hyphae are sometimes mistaken for spores. In the absence of sporulation, hyphae cannot be readily distinguished from a large number of pathogenic molds.

CLINICAL MANIFESTATIONS

Ear and Sinus

Otomycosis is the name given to the growth of fungus, usually *Aspergillus*, in the ear canal. Rarely, this represents invasive disease and is potentially lethal.[27] Most often, the fungus is growing on desquamated debris and cerumen and contributes little or nothing to the pathology. Treatment is directed at the underlying chronic otitis externa, not at the fungus. In the paranasal sinus, *Aspergillus* is associated with a variety of different conditions. In the severely neutropenic patient, mucosal invasion beginning in the nose or sinus can spread rapidly to contiguous structures, causing vascular invasion and necrosis.[28] Rarely, previously well patients will have invasive aspergillosis of the sinus, but the disease is indolent and granulomatous. Head or sinus pain, proptosis, and monocular blindness are the most common presenting manifestations.[29] *A. flavus* is particularly common in isolates from invasive aspergillosis of the nose and paranasal sinus. In patients with a history of allergic rhinitis, chronic nasal congestion, and recurrent sinusitis, *Aspergillus* or other molds can be found in sinus mucus, along with eosinophils, neutrophils, and Charcot Leyden crystals. The natural course of the disease, which has been called allergic fungal sinusitis, is poorly defined. In other patients, *Aspergillus* can form a hyphal ball within the sinus. In these noninvasive cases, good surgical drainage is important and often sufficient therapy.

Eye

Minor trauma to the cornea can be followed by deep stromal invasion with *Aspergillus*. Endophthalmitis due to *Aspergillus* can be a late complication of cataract extraction or can be hematogenous. In the latter instance, the patient is usually immunosuppressed,[30,31] has endocarditis,[32] or is a drug addict. For further details see Chapter 99 or the text *Oculomycoses*.[33]

Lung

Allergic bronchopulmonary aspergillosis refers to patients with pre-existing asthma who have eosinophilia, fleeting pulmonary infiltrates due to bronchial plugging, and an immediate type skin test response to *Aspergillus* antigen.[34,35] Total serum IgE and anti-*Aspergillus* IgG are elevated.[35,36] Episodic bronchial plugging seems to lead to central areas of saccular bronchiectasis, which may be perceived as rings or bands on chest x-ray films.[37] IgG antibody to *Aspergillus* is often detected by double diffusion in agar gel.[36] Patients may give a history of expectorating plugs. Hyphae can be seen microscopically in the plugs. The sputum culture intermittently contains *Aspergillus*. Prognosis is variable.[34,38] Some patients experience no permanent loss of pulmonary function despite recurrent exacerbations. Others may develop steroid-dependent asthma or irreversible obstructive lung disease.

Patients with tuberculosis, sarcoidosis, histoplasmosis, asthma, chronic bronchitis, bronchiectasis, and many other chronic pulmonary disorders may acquire colonies of *Aspergillus* growing on secretions in ectatic bronchi, cysts, and cavities (Fig. 1). Masses of hyphae may be seen on chest x-ray films, overlain by a crescent of air (Fig. 2). These are called

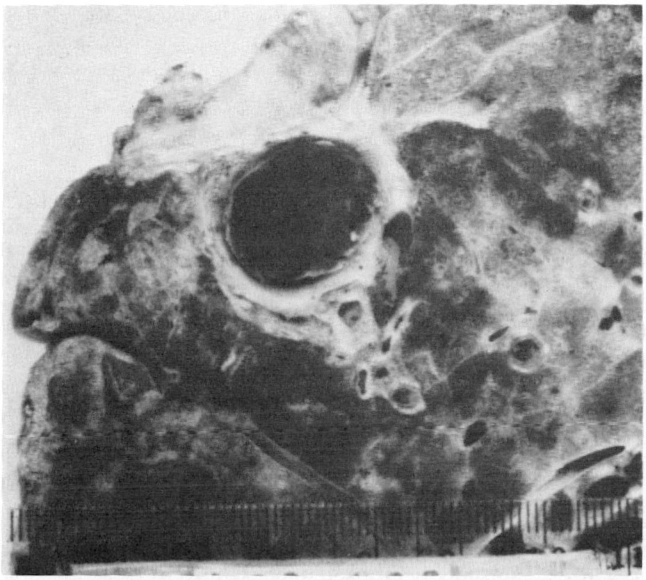

FIG. 1. Aspergilloma in apex of lung at autopsy. Contiguous pleura is thickened.

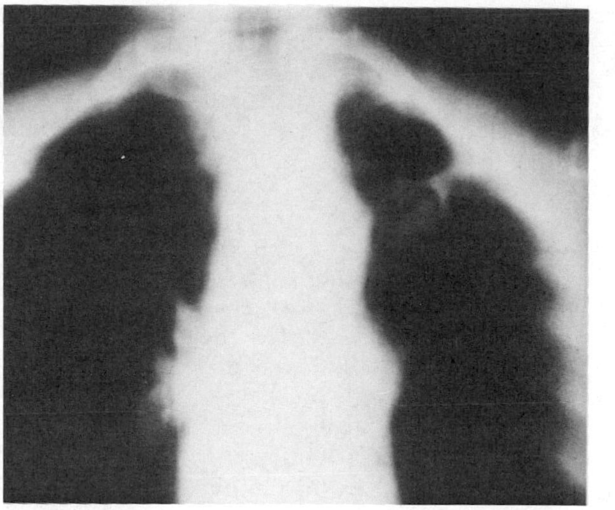

FIG. 2. Aspergilloma on chest x-ray film.

aspergillomas or fungus balls of the lung. Sputum cultures and smears contain *Aspergillus* intermittently. When a fungus ball is visible radiologically, IgG antibody to *Aspergillus* can be demonstrated readily in all patients by a variety of tests.[39] The symptoms and prognosis of this condition are essentially those of the underlying disease. Many patients have hemoptysis, ranging from scant to fatal.[40] Approximately 10 percent of the aspergillomata disappeared spontaneously in one study of 37 patients.[41] Complications of this condition include the spread of *Aspergillus* to the pleura either spontaneously or by surgery, bronchopleural fistula, or bacterial lung abscess.[42] Rarely, spread from the pleura to thoracic vertebral bodies occurs. Use of silk sutures to close bronchial stumps during lung resections on these patients can be followed by *Aspergillus* colonization of the stump and hemoptysis.[43]

Massive inhalation of *Aspergillus* spores by normal children may be followed within 24 hours by fever, dyspnea, and a miliary infiltrate on chest x-ray films. Improvement often begins spontaneously in 2–4 weeks, leading to cure. Occasionally the children have expired from extensive lung lesions[44] or have shown spread to skin[45] or bone.[12] Some of the progressive cases in children have been found to have chronic granulomatous disease, since that condition predisposes to progressive invasive aspergillosis.[46]

Patients with prolonged and profound granulocytopenia are predisposed to acute, rapidly progressive *Aspergillus* pneumonia.[19] Infection begins with high fever, followed in a few days by one or more areas of dense pulmonary consolidation on chest x-ray (Fig. 3).[47] Increase in size of the lesion and spread toward the lung periphery occurs relentlessly. If bone marrow function begins to return, cavitation of the pneumonia is commonly observed, particularly if computerized tomography is done.[48] While cavitation is not diagnostic,[49] this occurrence supports the diagnosis[50] and may be accompanied by expectoration of necrotic lung containing the fungus. Fatal hemoptysis can occur at time of cavitation, particularly if the lesion is close to the hilum. In the absence of bone marrow recovery, dissemination to other parts of the lung, as well as brain, heart, liver, thyroid, and other viscera is common. Survival beyond 2 or 3 weeks is uncommon in profoundly neutropenic patients. Invasive pulmonary aspergillosis is most common in patients with acute leukemia but also occurs in organ transplant recipients and patients receiving high doses of adrenal corticosteroids and cytotoxic therapy.[51–53] Rarely, this infection occurs in neonates,[54,55] cirrhotics,[56] alcoholics,[57] and previously healthy patients.[58]

Invasive pulmonary aspergillosis is different in children and

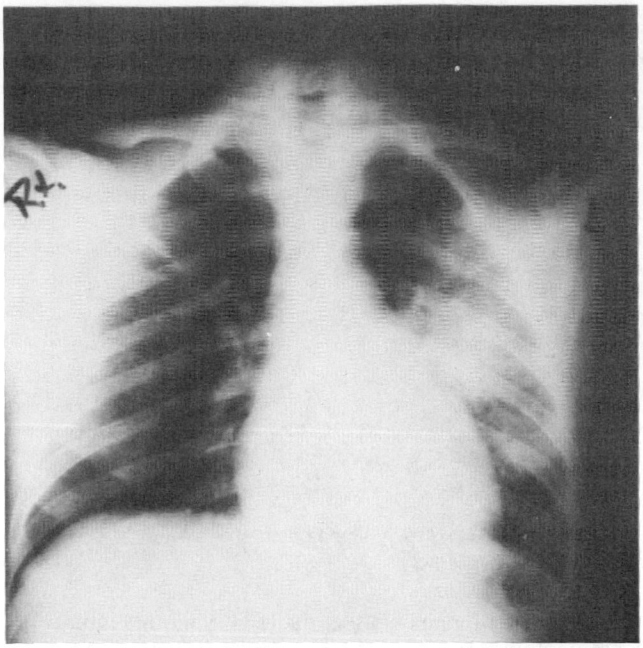

FIG. 3. Fatal invasive pulmonary aspergillosis with acute leukemia.

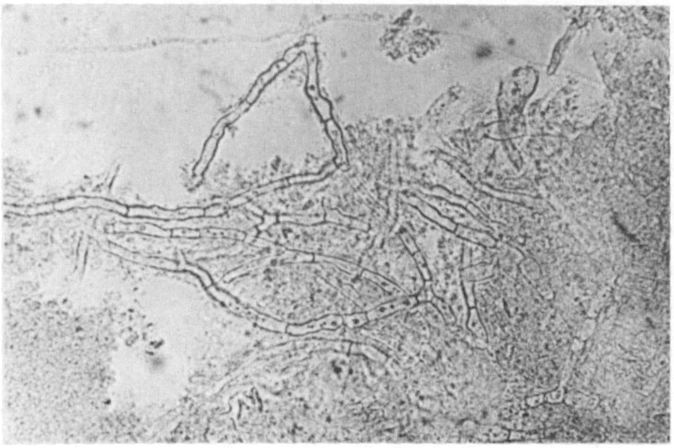

FIG. 4. *Aspergillus flavus* in wet smear from invasive palate lesion of leukemic child. (Original magnification ×900)

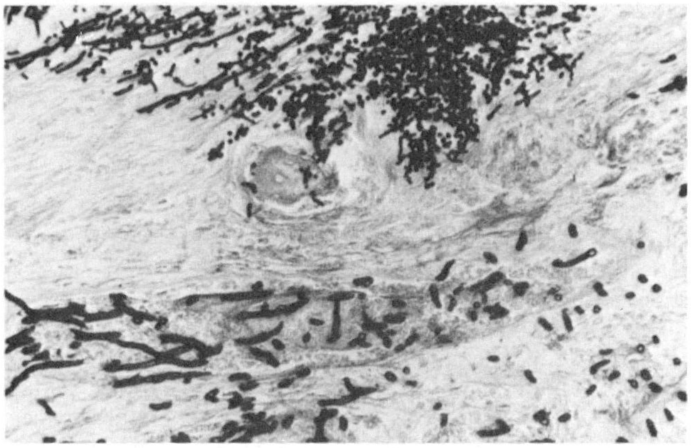

FIG. 5. Aspergillosis in blood vessel and contiguous tissue of gastroesophageal junction. *Candida* pseudohyphae and yeastlike cells in contiguous lesion (methenamine silver, original magnification ×375). (Photomicrograph courtesy of Nathaniel Young.)

young adults with chronic granulomatous disease. Insidious onset of fever, elevated sedimentation rate, and pneumonia are initial manifestations. Chest x-ray films may show one area of pneumonia or numerous small nodular infiltrates. Extension to the thoracic vertebra is common and may lead to compression of the spinal cord.[59] Spread to the pleura, rib, brain, or skin can also occur.

Central Nervous System

Several distinct clinical entities may occur. Immunosuppressed patients may have cerebral vessels occluded by *Aspergillus*, causing cerebral infarction.[19] Rarely, previously normal persons will have a similar event, although histologic examination shows granulation tissue as well as vasculitis.[11] More commonly, the nonimmunosuppressed patient has signs and symptoms of a brain abscess, which, on surgery, is an area of necrosis with numerous hyphae surrounded by dense granulation tissue.[7] Meningitis due to *Aspergillus* is rare but has occurred after drug abuse or transsphenoidal surgery.[60]

Other Sites

Aspergillus may infect a normal, a damaged, or a prosthetic cardiac valve.[61] *Aspergillus*-induced endocarditis resembles bacterial endocarditis in many ways, but *Aspergillus* has rarely been isolated from blood culture. Esophageal or gastrointestinal ulcerations due to *Aspergillus* may occur in the immunosuppressed host.[19] Fatal perforation of the viscus may occur. Immunosuppressed patients may also acquire necrotizing skin ulcers, typically covered by a black eschar, usually on the extremities.[19,62,63] Bone lesions have arisen by direct extension to rib or vertebral body,[46,59,64–66] by hematogenous spread to the vertebra of an immunosuppressed patient,[67–70] or as a complication of removing a herniated lumbar invertebral disc.[71] Infection of the disc space and formation of an epidural abscess have seemed relatively frequent in these few reported cases.

DIAGNOSIS

Demonstration of *Aspergillus* by both culture and microscopic examination of tissue (Figs. 4 and 5) provides the most firm diagnosis. The appearance of hyphae in a smear or a biopsy specimen can be very suggestive but is not diagnostic of aspergillosis when used alone. *Aspergillus* may be isolated in culture due to contamination or, in air-containing tissues such as lung or sinus, may be colonizing and not invading tissue. Isolation of *Aspergillus* from sputum, urine, stool, cornea, or wound, in and of itself, has no diagnostic significance, although the clinical situation must be taken into account. A positive sputum culture from a patient with profound neutropenia and acute leukemia is strongly suggestive of the diagnosis, particularly in a child.[72] A nose culture positive for *Aspergillus* or negative for any organism was found predictive of aspergillosis in one cancer center.[73] Sterility of nasal cultures was attributed to prolonged antimicrobial therapy given for recurrent bacterial infections. Blood, cerebrospinal fluid, and bone marrow specimens from patients with aspergillosis are rarely positive. Serologic tests for aspergillosis have been of interest in allergic bronchopulmonary aspergillosis and aspergilloma,[36,39] but their usefulness in invasive aspergillosis is not established. Attempts to detect circulating *Aspergillus* antigen are being made.[74]

TREATMENT

Surgical excision has been used successfully to treat invasive aspergillosis of the brain[7,75] and paranasal sinus,[2,3] as well as noninvasive sinus colonization.[29] Surgical removal of an infected prosthetic cardiac valve seems to aid response to chemotherapy,[6,61] although the prognosis in *Aspergillus* endocarditis remains dreadful. Surgical excision of an aspergilloma is sometimes indicated for massive hemoptysis, provided the lobe producing hemoptysis is known. Ordinarily, conservative management of aspergilloma lesions is advised.[76] Pleural aspergillosis often responds well to surgical drainage alone.

Intravenous amphotericin B is the drug of choice for invasive aspergillosis. The drug is ineffective in *Aspergillus* residing as a saprophyte in air spaces of the lung and paranasal sinus. Efficacy of the drug is best when diagnosis is made early, immunosuppression is not massive, and amphotericin B doses are advanced rapidly to therapeutic levels.[1,51,52,77,78] A common maintenance dose would be 0.5–0.6 mg/kg/day. Determination of the minimum inhibitory concentration of an *Aspergillus* isolate to amphotericin B has no ready interpretation. The result is dependent on methodology. Using any one technique, very little difference between isolates has been seen.

The combination of flucytosine with amphotericin B has been used in patients with invasive aspergillosis, particularly those with chronic granulomatous disease, but it remains unclear whether flucytosine adds to the effect of amphotericin B. Occasionally, rifampin has been added to amphotericin B, but clinical experience with this combination has not been encouraging. An oral triazole, itraconazole, has had some therapeutic benefit in a few patients with invasive aspergillosis, particularly those with lesser degrees of immunocompromise.[79]

REFERENCES

1. Young RC, Jennings A, Bennett JE. Species identification of invasive aspergillosis in man. Am Clin Pathol. 1972;58:554.
2. Green WR, Font RL, Zimmerman LE. Aspergillosis of the orbit. Report of ten cases and review of the literature. Arch Ophthalmol. 1969;82:302.
3. Sandison AT, Gentles JC, Davidson CA, et al. Aspergilloma of paranasal sinuses and orbit in northern sudanese. Sabouraudia. 1967;6:57.
4. Clinicopathological Conference. A case of fungal endocarditis. Br Med J 1969;3:765.
5. Mershon JC, Samuelson DR, Layman TE. Left ventricular "fibrosis body" aneurysm caused by *Aspergillus* endocarditis. Am J Cardiol. 1968;22:281.
6. Carrizosa J, Levison ME, Lawrence T, et al. Cure of *Aspergillus ustus* endocarditis. Arch Intern Med. 1974;133:486.
7. Venugopal PV, Venugopal TV, Thiruneelakantan D, et al. Cerebral aspergillosis. Report of two cases. Sabouraudia. 1977;15:225.
8. David M, Charlin M, Naudascher M. Infiltration mycosique á *Aspergillus amstelodami* du lobe temporal simulant un abćes encapsulé. Ablation en masse. Guérison. Operatoire. Rev Neurol (Paris). 1951;85:121.
9. Ziskind J, Pizzolato P, Buff EE. Aspergillosis of the brain. Am J Clin Pathol. 1958;29:554.
10. Marsalek E, Zizka Z, Riha V, et al. Plicni aspergilloza S. generalizaci vyvolana druhen *Aspergillus restrictus*. Čas Lék Čes. 1960;99:1285.
11. McCormick WF, Schochet SS, Weaver PR, et al. Disseminated aspergillosis. Arch Pathol. 1975;100:353.
12. Redmond A, Carré IJ, Biggart JD, et al. Aspergillus (*Aspergillus nidulans*) involving bone. J Pathol Bacteriol. 1965;89:391.
13. Raper KB, Fennell DI: The Genus *Aspergillus*. Baltimore: Williams & Wilkins; 1965.
14. Ciegler A, Burmeister HR, Vesonder RF. Poisonous fungi: mycotoxins and mycotoxicoses. In: Howard DH, ed. Fungi Pathogenic for Humans and Animals. v. 3, part B. New York: Marcel Dekker; 1983:413.
15. Sinski JT: The epidemiology of aspergillosis. In: The Epidemiology of Human Mycotic Disease. Springfield, IL: Charles C Thomas; 1975:210–26.
16. Mullins J, Harvey R, Seaton A. Sources and incidence of airborne *Aspergillus fumigatus* (Fres). Clin Allerg. 1976;6:209.
17. Aisner J, Schimpff SC, Bennett JE, et al. *Aspergillus* infection in cancer patients. Association with fireproofing materials in a new hospital. JAMA. 1976;235:411.
18. Levine AS, Siegel SE, Schreiber AD, et al. Protected environments and prophylactic antibiotics. N Engl J Med. 1973;288:477.
19. Young RC, Bennett JE, Vogel CL, et al. Aspergillosis. The spectrum of the disease in 98 patients. Medicine. 1970;49:147.
20. Arnow PM, Andersen RL, Mainoues PD, et al. Pulmonary aspergillosis during hospital renovation. Am Rev Respir Dis. 1978;118:49.
21. Sarubbi FA, Kopf HB, Wilson MB, et al. Increased recovery of *Aspergillus flavus* from respiratory specimens during hospital construction. Am Rev Respir Dis. 1982;125:33.
22. Lentino JR, Rosenkranz MA, Michaels JA, et al. Nosocomial aspergillosis: a retrospective review of airborne disease secondary to road construction and contaminated air conditioners. Am J Epidemiol. 1982;116:430.
23. Muckelmann R, Kunkel G, Staib R, et al. Respirationsallergien verursacht durch Aspergillus-Arten aus der Topferde von Zimmerpflanzen. Prax Pneumol. 1981;8:343.
24. Washburn RG, Gallin JI, Bennett JE. Oxidative killing of *Aspergillus* proceeds by parallel myeloperoxidase-dependent and -independent pathways. Infect Immun. 1987;55:2088–92.
25. Bennett JE. Role of the phagocyte in host defense against aspergillosis. In: vanden Bossche H, Mackenzie DWR, Cauwenbergh G, eds. *Aspergillus* and Aspergillosis. New York: Plenum Press; 1988:115.
26. Kan VL, Bennett JE. Lectin-like attachment sites on murine pulmonary alveolar macrophages bind *Aspergillus fumigatus* conidia. J Infect Dis. 1988;158:407–14.
27. Cunningham M, Yu VL, Tuner J, et al. Necrotizing otitis externa due to *Aspergillus* in an immunocompetent host. Arch Otolaryngol Neck Surg. 1988;114:554–6.
28. Morgan MA, Wilson WR, Neel H, et al. Fungal sinusitis in healthy and immunocompromised individuals. Am J Clin Pathol. 1984;82:597–601.
29. Washburn RG, Kennedy DW, Begley MG, et al. Chronic fungal sinusitis in apparently normal hosts. Medicine. 1988;67:231–47.
30. Naidoff MA, Green WR. Endogenous *Aspergillus* endophthalmitis occurring after kidney transplant. Am J Ophthalmol. 1975;79:502.
31. Darrell RW. Endogenous *Aspergillus* uveitis following heart surgery. Arch Ophthalmol. 1967;78:354.
32. Roney P, Barr C. Chun CH, et al. Endogenous *Aspergillus* endophthalmitis. Rev Infect Dis. 1986;8:955–8.
33. François J, Rysselaere M. Oculomycoses. Springfield, IL: Charles C Thomas; 1972.
34. Malo JL, Hawkins R, Pepys J. Studies in chronic allergic bronchopulmonary aspergillosis. I. Clinical and physiological findings. Thorax. 1977;32:254.
35. Patterson R, Greenberger PA, Radin RC, et al. Allergic bronchopulmonary aspergillosis: staging as an aid to management. Ann Intern Med. 1982;96:286.
36. Malo JL, Longbottom J, Mitchell J, et al. Studies in chronic allergic bronchopulmonary aspergillosis. 3. Immunologic findings. Thorax. 1977;32:269.
37. Malo JL, Pepys J, Simon G. Studies in chronic allergic bronchopulmonary aspergillosis. 2. Radiologic findings. Thorax. 1977;32:262.
38. Nichols D, Dopico GA, Braun S, et al. Acute and chronic pulmonary function changes in allergic bronchopulmonary aspergillosis. Am J Med. 1979;67:631.
39. Kurup VP, Fink JR. Evaluation of methods to detect antibodies against *Aspergillus fumigatus*. Am J Clin Pathol. 1978;69:414.
40. Peña CE. Aspergillosis. In: Baker RD, ed. Human Infection with Fungi, Actinomycetes, and Algae. New York: Springer Verlag; 1971:762–831.
41. Hammerman KJ, Christianson CS, Huntington I, et al. Spontaneous lysis of aspergillomata. Chest 1973;64:697.
42. Colp CR, Cook WA. Successful treatment of pleural aspergillosis and bronchopleural fistula. Chest 1975;68:96.
43. Sawasaki H, Yamada M, Tajima G, et al. Bronchial stump aspergillosis. J Thorac Cardiovasc Surg. 1969;58:198.
44. Strelling MK, Rhaney K, Simmons DAR, et al. Fatal acute pulmonary aspergillosis in two children of one family. Arch Dis Child. 1966;41:34.
45. Vedder JS, Schorr WF. Primary disseminated pulmonary aspergillosis with metastatic skin nodules. JAMA. 1969;209:1191.
46. Altman AR. Thoracic wall invasion secondary to pulmonary aspergillosis. Am J Roentgenol. 1977;129:140.
47. Meyer RD, Young LS, Armstrong D, et al. Aspergillosis complicating neoplastic disease. Am J Med. 1973;54:6.
48. Hruban RH, Meziane MA, Zerhouni EA, et al. Radiologicopathologic correlation of the CT halo sign in invasive pulmonary aspergillosis. J Comput Assist Tomogr. 1987;11:534–6.
49. Gefter WB, Albelda SM, Talbot GH. Invasive pulmonary aspergillosis and acute leukemia. Limitations in the diagnostic utility of the air crescent sign. Radiology. 1985;157:605–10.
50. Kulhman JE, Fishman EK, Siegelman SS. Invasive pulmonary aspergillosis in acute leukemia: characteristic findings on CT, the CT halo sign and the role of CT in early diagnosis. Radiology 1985;157:611–4.
51. Burton JR, Zachery JB, Bessin R, et al. Aspergillosis in four renal transplants. Diagnosis and effective treatment with amphotericin B. Ann Intern Med. 1972;77:383.
52. Gurwith MJ, Stenson EB, Remington JS. Aspergillus infection complicating cardiac transplantation. Arch Intern Med. 1971;128:541.
53. Gustafson TL, Schaffner W, Lavely GB, et al. Invasive aspergillosis in renal transplant recipients: correlation with corticosteroid therapy. J Infect Dis. 1983;148:230.
54. Mangurten HH, Fernandez B. Neonatal aspergillosis accompanying fulminant necrotising enterocolitis. Arch Dis Child. 1979;54:559.
55. Gonzalez-Crussi F, Mirkin LD, Wyllie RM, et al. Acute disseminated aspergillosis during the neonatal period. Clin Pediatr. 1979;18:137.
56. Brown E, Freedman S, Arbeit R, et al. Invasive pulmonary aspergillosis in an apparently nonimmunocompromised host. Am J Med. 1980;69:624.
57. Blum J, Reed JC, Pizzo SV, et al. Miliary aspergillosis associated with alcoholism. Am J Roentgenol. 1978;131:707.
58. Karam GH, Griffin FM. Invasive pulmonary aspergillosis in nonimmunocompromised nonneutropenic hosts. Rev Infect Dis. 1986;8:357–63.
59. Ferris B, Jones J. Paraplegia due to aspergillosis. J Bone Joint Surg. 1985;67B:800–3.
60. Feely M, Steinberg M. *Aspergillus infection* complicating transsphenoidal yttrium-90 pituitary implant. J Neurosurg. 1977;46:530.
61. Barst RJ, Prince AS, Neu H. *Aspergillus* endocarditis in children: case report and review of the literature. Pediatrics. 1981;68:73.

62. Allo MA, Miller J, Townsend T, et al. Primary cutaneous aspergillosis associated with Hickman intravenous catheters. N Engl J Med. 1987;317:1105–8.
63. Carlile JR, Millet RE, Cho CT, et al. Primary cutaneous aspergillosis in a leukemic child. Arch Dermatol. 1978;114:78.
64. Caligiuri P, MacMahon H, Courtney J, et al. Opportunistic pulmonary aspergillosis with chest wall invasion. Arch Intern Med. 1983;143:2323.
65. Glotzbach RE. *Aspergillus terreus* infection of pseudoaneurysm of aortofemoral vascular graft with contiguous vertebral osteomyelitis. Am J Clin Pathol. 1982;77:224.
66. Seres JL, Ono H, Benner EJ. Aspergillosis presenting as spinal cord compression. J Neurosurg. 1972;36:221.
67. Seligsohn R, Rippon JW, Lerner SA. *Aspergillus terreus* osteomyelitis. Arch Intern Med. 1977;137:918.
68. Grossman M. Aspergillosis of bone. Br J Radiol. 1975;48:57.
69. Byrd BF, Weiner MH, McGee ZA. *Aspergillus* spinal epidural abscess. JAMA. 1982;248:3138.
70. Roselle GA, Baird IM. *Aspergillus flavipes* group osteomyelitis. Arch Intern Med. 1979;139, 590.
71. Mawk JR, Erickson DL, Chou SN, et al. *Aspergillus* infections of the lumbar disc spaces. J Neurosurg. 1983;58:270.
72. Yu VL, Muder RR, Poorsattar A. Significance of isolation of *Aspergillus* from the respiratory tract in diagnosis of invasive pulmonary aspergillosis. Am J Med. 1986;81:249–54.
73. Aisner J, Murillo J, Schimpff SC, et al. Invasive aspergillosis in acute leukemia: correlation with nose cultures and antibiotic use. Ann Intern Med. 1979;90:4.
74. Bennett JE. Rapid diagnosis of candidiasis and aspergillosis. Rev Infect Dis. 1987;9:398–402.
75. Henze G, Aldenhoff P, Stephani U, et al. Successful treatment of pulmonary and cerebral aspergillosis in an immunosuppressed child. Eur J Pediatr. 1982;138:263.
76. Faulkner SC, Vernon R, Brown PP, et al. Hemoptysis and pulmonary aspergilloma: operative versus nonoperative treatment. Ann Thorac Surg. 1978;25:389.
77. Aisner J, Schimpff SC, Wiernik PH. Treatment of invasive aspergillosis: relation of early diagnosis and treatment to response. Ann Intern Med. 1977;86:539.
78. Pennington JE. Successful treatment of *Aspergillus* pneumonia in hematologic neoplasia. N Engl J Med. 1976;295:426.
79. De Beule K, De Doncker P, Cauwenbergh G, et al. The treatment of aspergillosis and aspergilloma with itraconazole, clinical results of an open international study (1982–1987). Mykoses. 1988;31:476–85.

TABLE 1. Classification of the Agents of Mucormycosis and Related Diseases

I. Zygomycotina
  A. Zygomycetes
    a. Mucorales
      1. Mucoraceae
        i. *Absidia*
          (a) *A. corymbifera*
          (b) *A. ramosa*
        ii. *Mucor*
          (a) *M circinelloides*
        iii. *Rhizomucor*
          (a) *R. pusillus*
        iv. *Rhizopus*
          (a) *R. oryzae*
          (b) *R. arrhizus*
          (c) *R. rhizopodiformis*
      2. Cunninghamellacaeae
        i. *Cunninghamella*
          (a) *C. bertholletiae*
      3. Mortierellaceae
        i. *Mortierella*
          (a) *M. wolfii*
      4. Saksenaeaceae
        i. *Saksenaea*
          (a) *S. vasiformis*
      5. Syncephalastraceae
        i. *Syncephalastrum*
      6. Apophysomyceae
        i. *Apophysomyces*
          (a) *A. elegans*
      7. Thamnidiaceae
        i. *Cokeromyces*
          (a) *C. recurvatus*
    b. Entomophthorales
        i. *Conidiobolus*
          (a) *C. coronatus* (*Entomophthora coronata*)[a]
          (b) *C. incongruans*
        ii. *Basidiobolus*
          (a) *B. haptosporus* (*B. meristosporus; B. ranarum*)[a]

[a] Obsolete synonyms.
(Data from Howard.[136])

237. AGENTS OF MUCORMYCOSIS AND RELATED SPECIES

ALAN M. SUGAR

Mucormycosis is the common name given to several different diseases caused by fungi of the order Mucorales. Many different species have been implicated as etiologic agents of similar clinical syndromes. The taxonomy of this group is complicated not only by the numerous examples of pathogenic members, but also because of changes in the names of individual species that are made as new advances in classification are accepted. Table 1 summarizes the taxonomic relationships of those Zygomycetes known to be pathogenic. The details of the mycology of the Zygomycetes and problems in taxonomy are beyond the scope of this chapter but can be found elsewhere.[1]

Throughout the years, this group of diseases has been known by other names. For example, references can be found to *phycomycosis* and *zygomycosis*. The former is an allusion to an earlier and more imprecise classification scheme that is no longer used, and the latter reflects the class name of these fungi. As detailed below, not all of the Zygomycetes cause the same type of disease, so that the term *zygomycosis* is too vague and does not accurately convey useful information to the physician. Furthermore, the designation *mucormycosis* is well ingrained in the medical literature and evokes certain useful associations, so that it is best to continue to refer to the mycoses produced by the organisms in the order Mucorales by this name. This convention will be followed in this chapter.

In addition to the Mucorales, the fungi responsible for mucormycosis, the class Zygomycetes contains the Entomophthorales. The fungi in this order also cause distinctive clinical syndromes, but these are clearly separable from those produced by the agents causing mucormycosis. *Entomophthoromycosis* is the currently accepted general term used to describe disease due to these fungi. Diseases caused by the Entomophthorales are extremely rare in North America; they are usually found in Africa, southeast Asia, Indonesia, and South America. Since the clinical and pathologic manifestations of the diseases caused by this group of fungi are different from those produced by the agents of mucormycosis, they will be discussed separately following a discussion of the more common mucormycosis.

MUCORMYCOSIS

The Pathogens

All of the Zygomycetes grow in the environment and in tissue as hyphae and are therefore molds. The taxonomy of the Zygomycetes is based upon a morphologic analysis of the fungus, which will be reviewed below. In addition to morphology, other taxonomically relevant features include carbohydrate assimilation and maximal temperature compatible with growth. These organisms typically grow in 2–5 days on most media. However, cycloheximide inhibits the growth of these fungi, and media that contain this compound, such as Mycosel and Mycobiotic agar, should not be used.

Rhizopus species are the most commonly isolated agents of

mucormycosis, followed by *Rhizomucor*. Differentiation between these genera is accomplished by microscopic examination for the presence and location of rhizoids, the presence of apophyses, and the morphology of the columellae[1,2] (Fig. 1). The capability to identify these strains to this level satisfactorily should be within the grasp of most tertiary care hospital laboratories. Speciation of these organisms is desirable for many reasons, including monitoring the progress of therapy (especially to document the eradication of the original fungus and to determine that a fungus growing from a subsequent clinical specimen is or is not a different contaminating organism) and elucidating any species-specific responses to different antifungal drugs, an important consideration with the current emphasis on development of new classes of antifungal drugs. Disease due to *Cunninghamella*,[3,4] *Saksenaea*,[5,6] and *Apophysomyces*[7,8] is indistinguishable from that caused by the more common Mucorales. Laboratory confirmation of the identity of the organism is the only way to differentiate among the fungi.

Epidemiology

The Mucoraceae are ubiquitous fungi and are common inhabitants of decaying matter. For example, *Rhizopus* species frequently can be recovered from moldy bread. Because of their rapid growth and prolific spore-forming capacity, inhalation of conidia must be a daily experience. The presence of Mucorales spores on nonsterile adhesive tape has been shown to be the source of primary cutaneous mucormycosis.[9–13] Even though these fungi grow in many ecologic niches, the infrequency of disease due to these organisms attests to their low virulence potential in the human host. In contrast to the widespread distribution of these fungi, disease in humans is limited, in most cases, to people with severe immunocompromise, diabetes mellitus, or trauma. Even so, mucormycosis is a rather rare development in any of these patient groups.

Pathogenesis

Most commonly, the fungus gains entry to the body through the respiratory tract. The spores are presumably deposited in the nasal turbinates and may be inhaled into the pulmonary alveoli. In the case of primary cutaneous mucormycosis, spores are introduced directly into abraded skin. They then proliferate and can invade more widely from that initial cutaneous-subcutaneous location.

In order to cause disease, spores must overcome the host's natural immunity and specific humoral and cell-mediated immune mechanisms. Most of our understanding of the pathogenesis of mucormycosis is derived from mouse and rabbit models of infection. Normal animals inoculated with *Rhizopus* do not become ill.[14] However, inhalation of Mucorales spores by animals with diabetes mellitus or those receiving corticosteroids results in death secondary to rapidly progressive pulmonary mucormycosis, often with hematogenous dissemination beyond the lungs.[15–17]

The initial event in fungal cell proliferation is spore germination. In the normal lung, *Rhizopus oryzae* spores are unable to germinate.[15,16,18] Bronchoalveolar macrophages harvested from normal mice readily ingest *Rhizopus* spores and inhibit their germination.[15,19] However, the spores remain viable and can grow if removed from the phagolysosomes. In the lungs of mice with streptozotocin-induced diabetes and in steroid-treated mice, spore germination readily occurs.[15,19] Bronchoalveolar macrophages recovered from these mice do not possess the normal ability to inhibit spore germination.

Neutrophils are prominent components of the host response to the Mucorales. Recruitment of neutrophils into areas of infection is accomplished by fungus-derived and serum-derived chemotactic factors.[20,21] Activation of the alternative complement pathway is the source of the serum-induced chemotaxis.

The mechanisms responsible for the increased susceptibility to mucormycosis in different patient groups are not clear. Oxidative metabolites generated by the phagocyte respiratory burst (e.g., O_2^-, hydrogen peroxide, hypochlorous acid) have been shown to be fungicidal to *R. oryzae* hyphae.[22] How diabetes and steroids interfere with the ability of this fungus to elicit these toxic phagocyte products or the activity of the oxidative metabolites is unknown. Defensins, cationic proteins obtained from mammalian phagocytic cells,[23] also have significant ability to kill *R. oryzae* spores and hyphae.[24] The relative importance of oxidative and nonoxidative fungicidal mechanisms in the normal state and in situations of immunosuppression or diabetes still remains a mystery.

Hyperglycemia or acidosis per se is not sufficient to permit fungal replication within the alveolar macrophage,[12,25] although acidosis without hyperglycemia has been associated with in-

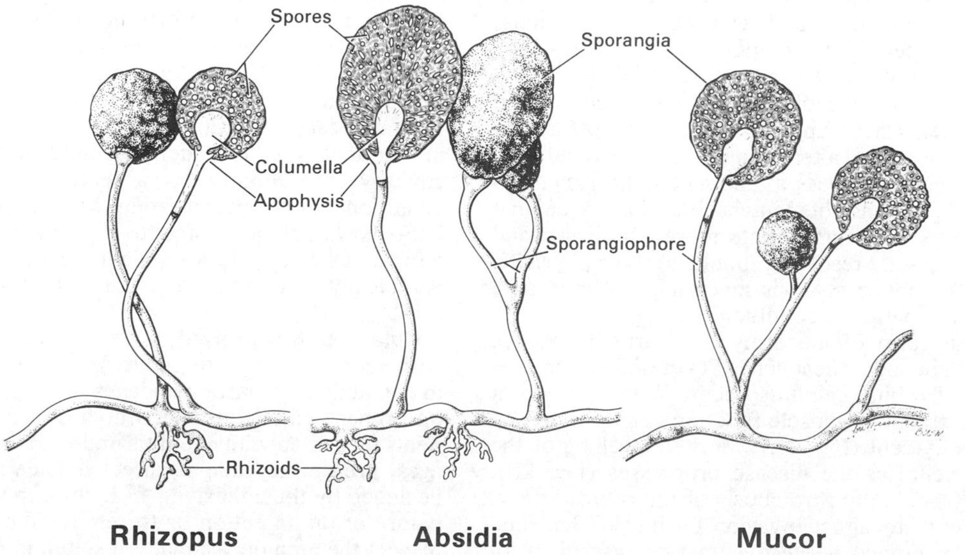

FIG. 1. Diagram of major differentiating morphologic features of three of the most common Mucorales isolated from patients. Note the presence and location of rhizoids, the columella, and the shape of the sporangia. The infectious spores reside within the sporangia. (Illustration by Lori Messenger.)

vasive mucormycosis of humans on occasion.[26,27] Normal human serum can inhibit the growth of *Rhizopus*.[20] In contrast, serum obtained from patients with diabetic ketoacidosis is not inhibitory and may actually enhance fungal growth.[28,29] While neither antibody nor complement is responsible for inhibition of growth of the Mucorales, interactions between transferrin and iron molecules and fungal spores have been described and may be important in determining the rate of fungal cell replication.[30,31] Analysis of the pertinent data does not yet permit the development of a unifying concept of the pathogenesis of mucormycosis. It is clear, however, that undefined defects of macrophages and neutrophils, present in diabetic and steroid-treated animals, are important in allowing the replication of the Mucorales. Moreover, immunologically healthy people can suppress the growth of the Mucorales and clear them from the lung with great efficiency. Finally, the relative paucity of cases of mucormycosis in patients with the acquired immunodeficiency syndrome (AIDS) attests to the relative importance of the neutrophil.

Once the fungus begins to grow, the hyphae invade tissue and have a special affinity for blood vessels. Direct penetration and growth through the blood vessel wall explains the propensity for thrombosis and tissue necrosis, two major hallmarks of the histopathology of mucormycosis. Why blood vessels are a prime target for fungal growth remains unknown.

Clinical Manifestations

The manifestations of mucormycosis can be arbitrarily divided into at least six separate entities, based on clinical presentation and involvement of a particular body site: (*1*) rhinocerebral, (*2*) pulmonary, (*3*) cutaneous, (*4*) gastrointestinal, (*5*) central nervous system, and (*6*) miscellaneous.[32–35] In general, the predilection for one of these types of presentations differs for each of the underlying or predisposing conditions. For example, patients with diabetes most often develop rhinocerebral mucormycosis, neutropenic leukemic patients develop rhinocerebral or pulmonary mucormycosis,[36] and those with protein-calorie malnutrition most often will present with gastrointestinal disease. Disseminated disease, resulting from progression from one of the primary anatomic locations, is particularly troublesome in patients with severe immunologic deficits, such as those with bone marrow transplants or acute leukemia.[37–39]

Rhinocerebral Mucormycosis. This form of mucormycosis is most often found in patients with diabetes mellitus, particularly in the presence of acidosis, and in patients with leukemia, who have been neutropenic for long periods of time and who have been receiving broad-spectrum antibacterial drugs.[40–46] Occasional reports of this form of mucormycosis occurring in renal transplant patients have appeared.[47] Patients presenting with diabetic ketoacidosis and altered mental status should have an improvement in consciousness as the metabolic abnormalities are corrected. Persistence of mental status changes beyond the usual 24–48 hours once appropriate therapy is begun and metabolic abnormalities are resolving should alert the physician to the possibility that mucormycosis involving the brain may be responsible for the patient's condition.

Patients with this form of mucormycosis virtually always complain of facial pain and/or headache. Fever and varying degrees of evidence of orbital cellulitis occur. With invasion of the orbit, loss of extraocular muscle function can develop and proptosis becomes evident (Fig. 2A). Marked swelling of the conjunctiva also occurs as the disease progresses (Fig. 2B). Loss of vision may be due to thrombosis of the retinal artery, presumably secondary to direct invasion by fungal elements. The development of cranial nerve dysfunction, especially of nerves V and VII, occurs with progression of the disease, is manifested by ptosis and pupillary dilatation, and represents a serious prognostic event. Cerebral abscess as a complication of mucormycosis involving the nose and eye can also occur.[48,49] Cavernous sinus and internal carotid artery thrombosis[50] are additional complications that reflect the vascular tropism of the fungus. In the terminal stages of the disease, the underlying predisposing condition continues unabated, and patients may lose consciousness. The end result of such progression is death.

Laboratory studies are nonspecific, but suggestive evidence of the presence of disease can be found on x-ray films of the sinuses. Plain roentgenograms of the sinuses and orbits can reveal sinusoidal mucosal thickening, with or without air–fluid levels.[51] Erosion of bone through the walls of the sinuses or into the orbit can be found as the disease progresses (Fig. 3). Destruction of bone in this region is often dramatically revealed by computed tomography (CT). Abnormalities in soft tissues involved in the disease process can also be visualized by CT scans[52] and thus guide areas of potential surgical intervention.

Recently, there have been several reports of an apparent association between rhinocerebral mucormycosis and the administration of deferoxamine.[53–55] All eight of these patients had been receiving hemodialysis, and all of them died. The mechanisms responsible for this association are unclear and require further study. An additional association with iron metabolism is found in a case of rhinocerebral mucormycosis caused by *Cunninghamella* in a patient with hemochromatosis.[56]

Finally, chronic presentations or late sequelae following apparently successful therapy can be observed.[57,58] Thus, all survivors of acute infection should be monitored for signs of indolent residual infection.

Pulmonary Mucormycosis. Most of the patients with this form of mucormycosis are seriously immunocompromised by virtue of an absolute lack of circulating neutrophils secondary to chemotherapy for malignancy, usually leukemia, and have been receiving broad-spectrum antibiotics for unremitting fever. Other than fever and perhaps dyspnea, there usually are no other symptoms. With continued tissue necrosis, hemoptysis may develop; should a major blood vessel be eroded, fatal pulmonary hemorrhage can result.[59,60] A chest x-ray film will show evidence of infiltration or cavity formation, usually involving one anatomic segment but typically progressing to involve multiple contiguous areas in the same lung.[49] The disease most often begins with unilateral lung involvement but can disseminate more widely as the patient is dying. Patients in intensive care units for prolonged periods are often immunosuppressed as a result of malnutrition and drug use (including corticosteroids), and may be hyperglycemic as a result of parenteral hyperalimentation or glucose intolerance. Thus it is not surprising to read of nosocomial mucormycosis pneumonia in such patients.[61]

Scattered reports can be found of pulmonary mucormycosis with atypical presentations: as a solitary nodule in a diabetic[62]; in a patient with no underlying predisposing condition[63]; as a cavitary pneumonia in a patient without predisposing conditions[64]; or even in a patient with a normal chest x-ray film.[65] Patients with diabetes mellitus can also develop pulmonary mucormycosis with a less fulminant, more subacute course than is typically seen in patients with neutropenia.[66]

Cutaneous Mucormycosis. Sporadic cases of cutaneous mucormycosis continue to occur, but a nationwide epidemic due to contaminated elastic bandages in the 1970s focused attention on primary cutaneous mucormycosis as a distinct entity. Patients presented with cellulitis under areas covered by the bandages, presumably due to direct inoculation of fungi into skin occluded by the adhesive.[9–13] Failure to recognize the mycotic nature of the infection or to remove the bandages in order to inspect the area occasionally resulted in penetration of hyphae into areas below the skin, with subsequent infection of muscle, liver, or other viscera. Use of sterilized bandages and dressings should eliminate this form of mucormycosis. Rarely, intramus-

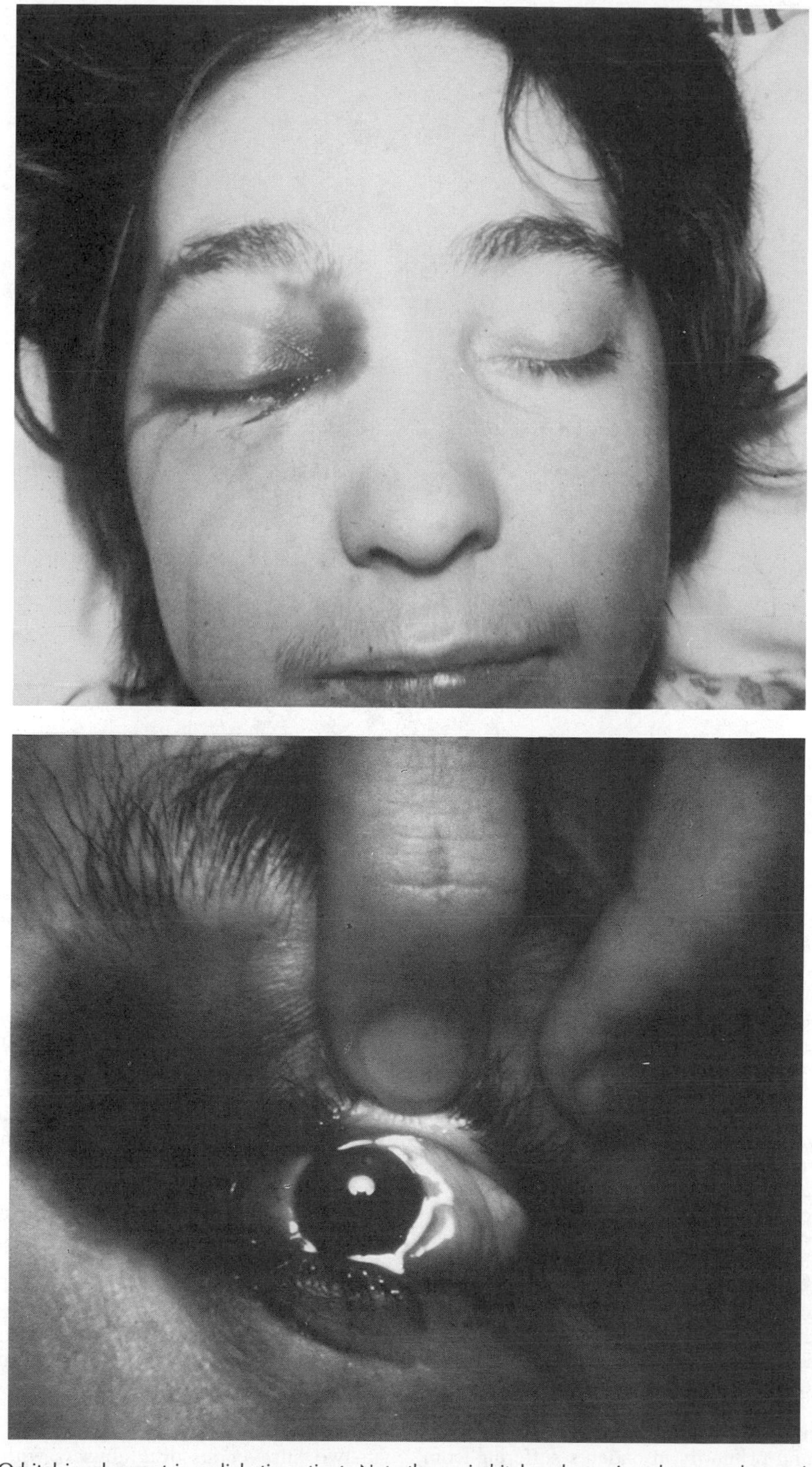

A

B

FIG. 2. (A) Orbital involvement in a diabetic patient. Note the periorbital ecchymosis, edema, and sanguinous discharge from the eye. **(B)** Marked chemosis and proptosis secondary to retro-orbital invasion in rhinocerebral mucormycosis. (Courtesy of Prof. Bertrand Dupont, Paris, France.)

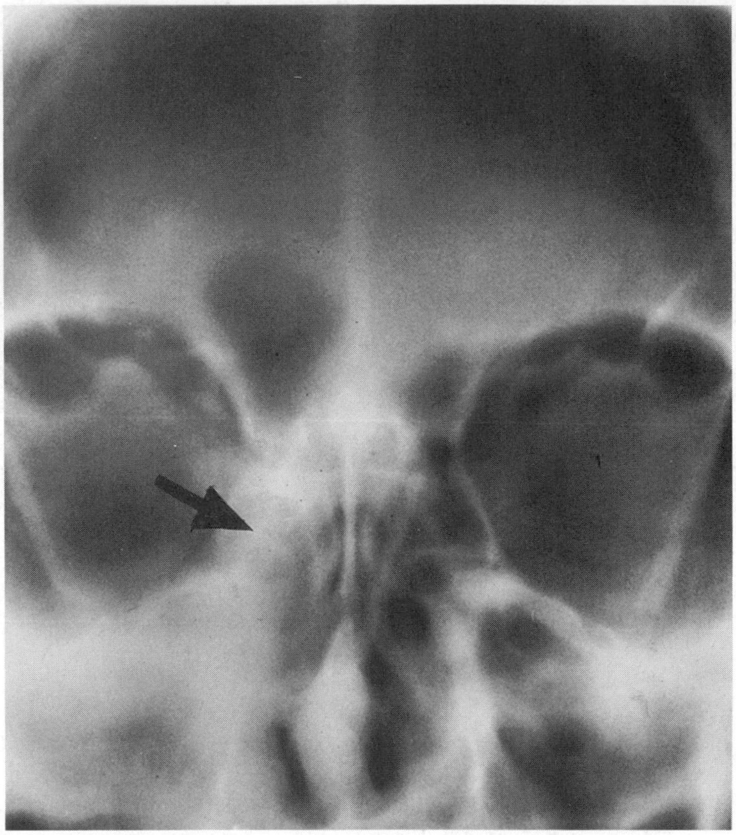

FIG. 3. Tomogram of the head in a patient with rhinocerebral mucormycosis. Note the presence of clouding in the maxillary and ethmoid (arrow) sinuses. (Courtesy of Dr. David A. Stevens, San Jose, CA.)

cular injections have been reported to precede the development of this form of mycormycosis.[67] Cases of cutaneous mucormycosis have been described following minor trauma[8,68–70]; diabetes mellitus is the usual predisposing factor in these patients. Contamination of devitalized tissue during major traumatic accidents also can result in the appearance of this form of mucormycosis.[71] Extensive involvement of burn wounds can result in dissemination of the fungus throughout the body and the death of the patient.[72]

Cutaneous mucormycosis predominantly involves the epidermis and dermis, and necrosis develops secondary to vascular invasion. Cultures have yielded *R. oryzae* or *Rhizopus rhizopodiformis* in most cases.

Patients with pulmonary or other forms of mucormycosis can develop skin lesions distant from the site of primary pathology. This secondary cutaneous involvement of the skin is a result of fungemia, which is almost never documented by positive blood cultures and thus reflects the presence of widely disseminated disease.[38] The involved area is erythematous and painful, with varying degrees of central necrosis.

Gastrointestinal Mucormycosis. Mucormycosis of the gastrointestinal tract is found primarily in patients suffering from extreme malnutrition and is thought to arise from fungi entering the body with food. All portions of the gastrointestinal tract are susceptible to infection, with the stomach, ileum, and colon being the most common sites.[73] As this disease is acute and rapidly fatal, most of the reported cases were diagnosed after the patient died. The initial manifestations of gastrointestinal mucormycosis are abdominal pain and distension associated with nausea and vomiting. Fever and hematochezia may also be found. If the diagnosis is made premortem, the patient is often thought to have an intra-abdominal abscess. Definitive diagnosis can be made only at surgery with appropriate examination of tissue (see below).

Central Nervous System Mucormycosis. This rare manifestation of mucormycosis occurs in severaly debilitated patients. Most often, extension of the fungus from its initial site of invasion in the nose or paranasal sinuses through adjacent bones into the brain is the mode of entry into the central nervous system.[48,74] This complication is recognizable by decreasing consciousness and development of multiple focal neurologic findings of cranial nerves and motor neurons to the rest of the body.

Occasionally, cerebral mucormycosis may occur after open head trauma, presumably as a result of direct implantation of the fungus at the time of injury,[75] or after intravenous injection of illicit drugs.[76–78] The appearance of a black discharge from the wound heralds necrosis of the underlying dura and brain and should suggest the diagnosis of mucormycosis. Occasional reports of isolated cerebral mucormycosis in patients with leukemia[79] or with no predisposing condition[80] have been published.

Isolated mucormycosis of the brain has also been described in two intravenous drug abusers with AIDS.[81] However, the Mucorales seem to be much less commonly found in patients with AIDS than other fungi, such as *Candida* and *Cryptococcus*, and the appearance of mucormycosis in these patients may reflect the occurrence of cerebral mucormycosis in drug addicts.[76–78]

Miscellaneous Forms. Sporadic reports can be found of mucormycosis involving other areas: heart (including endocarditis),[82–85] bones,[8,86–90] kidney,[7] bladder,[91] arterial catheter site with extension to surrounding tissue,[92] mediastinium,[93,94] and trachea.[95] Other conditions involving mucormycosis are osteomyelitis of the clivus resulting in chronic meningitis due to parameningeal irritation,[96] superior vena cava syndrome,[97] and possibly bone marrow necrosis in a patient with a *Mucor*-infected renal cyst.[98]

Diagnosis

The hallmarks of disease caused by the Mucorales are vascular invasion and tissue necrosis; black eschars and discharges should be aggressively sought. The presence of a black nasal discharge should not be dismissed as merely dried blood. It may reflect tissue necrosis and may be an important sign of deep infection. Similarly, black necrotic lesions of the nasal mucosa or hard palate may reflect invasive mucormycosis. Diagnosis is dependent on demonstrating the organism in the tissue of a biopsy specimen. Swabs of discharge or abnormal tissue are not appropriate and often result in erroneous information. Fungal hyphae can be seen on potassium hydroxide preparations of touch slides prepared from the biopsy specimen. Fixed tissue can be stained with hematoxylin and eosin, and fungal hyphae can be seen with this routine histologic stain (Fig. 4). Grocott methenamine silver or periodic acid—Schiff (PAS) staining will also adequately demarcate fungal elements in tissue in most cases (Fig. 5).

Typically, the fungi appear as broad (10–20 μm in diameter), nonseptate hyphae with branches occurring at right angles. Rarely, occasional septae can be visualized. The appearance of Mucorales hyphae in tissue is different from that of *Aspergillus* or *Pseudallescheria*, in that the latter two genera appear as thinner, more regularly shaped fungal elements with more frequent acute angle branching. The hyphae of these genera are also septate. Identification of the genus and species will require culture of tissue and assessment of the morphology of the fungal growth. For unclear reasons, agents of mucormycosis are difficult to isolate from infected tissue and rarely appear in blood culture.

Involved tissue is infiltrated with neutrophils. An inflammatory vasculitis involving both arteries and veins is the rule. Tissue necrosis as a result of blood vessel invasion is prominent. Thrombosis and hemorrhage are also commonly found. In more chronic cases, mononuclear cell infiltration is observed and occasional giant cells may be seen if the infection is present for a sufficient period of time.

Work has begun on the identification of antigens that might be useful as reagents for use in serologic tests.[99–102] However, serodiagnosis of mucormycosis remains investigational and cannot yet be recommended for routine clinical use.

Differential Diagnosis

There are several other infectious diseases that produce manifestations of tissue necrosis and infarction secondary to direct invasion of the vasculature. Infection with *Aspergillus* is most likely to be confused with the rhinocerebral or pulmonary forms of mucormycosis. The only definitive method of differentiating between these two possibilities is by examination of tissue or the results of cultures of a biopsy specimen. Certain aggressive orbital tumors can produce some of the findings of rhinocerebral mucormycosis, but the rapid pace of mucormycosis, the presence of fever, and the development of evidence of necrosis all favor a fungal etiology. Cavernous sinus thrombosis due to extension of staphylococcal lesions of the face can resemble rhinocerebral mucormycosis, but there are no lesions in the nosc or paranasal sinuses. Pulmonary mucormycosis can be mistaken for bland pulmonary embolism, though the progressive extension of the fungal lesion distinguishes the two. On rare occasions, patients with acute leukemia have developed skin lesions identical to those of ecthyma gangrenosa, which more commonly is due to *Pseudomonas aeruginosa*. Blood cultures are usually positive in the latter entity.

Therapy and Prevention

As with any opportunistic infection, the first therapeutic maneuver should be to correct the underlying disease. Aggressive

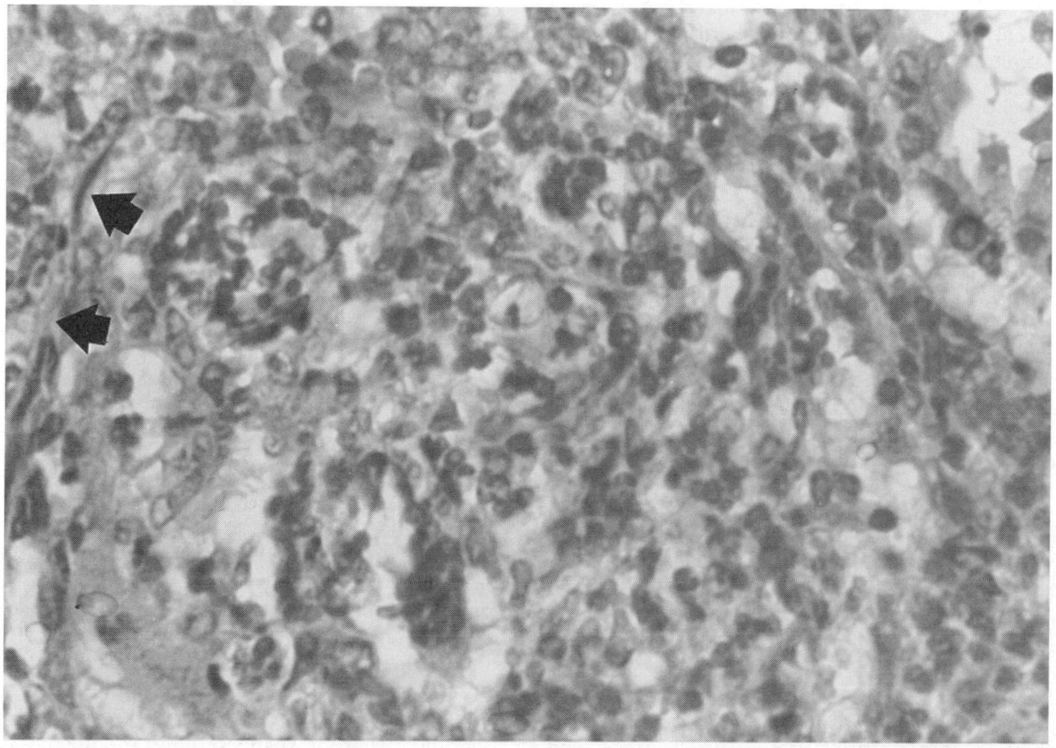

FIG. 4. Photomicrograph of the lung demonstrating a mixed polymorphonuclear/mononuclear cellular infiltrate. The arrow points to a hyphal fragment. (H&E, ×200) (Courtesy of Dr. Alayn Waldorf, Oakland, CA.)

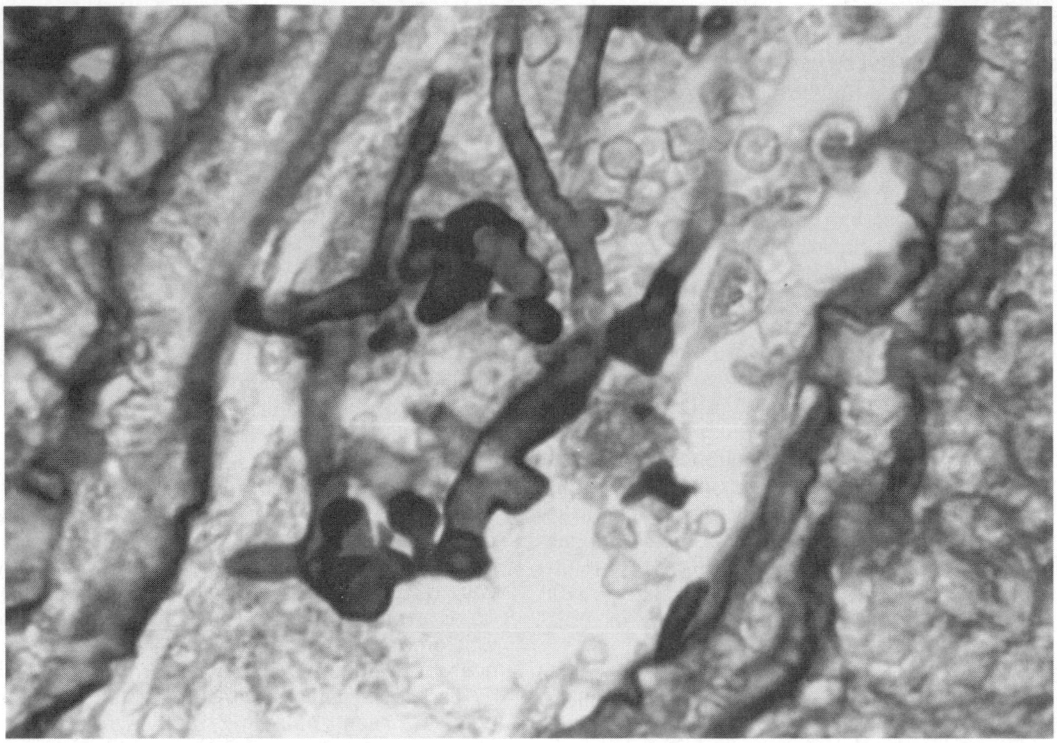

FIG. 5. Photomicrograph of lung demonstrating typical broad, irregularly shaped hyphae with right angle branching, characteristic of the Mucorales. (PAS, ×250) (Courtesy of Dr. Alayn Waldorf, Oakland, CA.)

correction of hyperglycemia and acidemia should be pursued. If possible, doses of immunosuppressive drugs, including steroids, should be decreased and the drugs stopped. The ultimate outcome of mucormycosis depends, in large part, on the prognosis of the underlying disease.

The standard therapy for invasive mucormycosis is treatment with amphotericin B. Since the fungus is relatively refractory to medical treatment, higher than usual doses of amphotericin B have been recommended. Doses typically range from 1.0 to 1.5 mg/kg/day in most patients. Once the patient has been stabilized, alternate-day amphotericin B can be considered. Mucormycosis is one fungal disease that has not been affected by the advent of newer, orally administered azole derivatives. Of the azoles currently approved or under clinical investigation (ketoconazole, itraconazole, or fluconazole), none appears to be active against any of the agents of mucormycosis, save for a single case report of a cure of rhinocerebral mucormycosis achieved with ketoconazole.[103] Thus, amphotericin B remains the only proven effective therapy. The addition of other agents such as rifampin[104] to amphotericin B in an attempt to obtain synergistic antifungal activity is controversial and cannot be recommended as standard therapy. Likewise, the interpretation of in vitro susceptibility tests of single drugs[105] is problematic and adds little to the formulation of treatment plans in individual patients.

While reports have appeared in the literature of patients with mucormycosis recovering with antifungal therapy alone,[106–108] these are clearly the exception and aggressive surgical débridement of necrotic tissue is advisable.[92,109–115] Occasional patients may recover with minimally disfiguring surgery.[35,43,109–111,116] These patients are probably in the minority, and a well-coordinated medical–surgical approach will maximize success. Repeated operations may be required for satisfactory removal of continuously appearing necrotic tissue. Should the patient survive the acute episode, major reconstructive surgery may also be necessary[117] (Fig. 6). Adjunctive oxygen therapy has been considered beneficial in a small number of patients.[117a,117b] Because of the uncontrolled nature of the observations, this form of therapy cannot be recommended at present.

In patients with primary cutaneous involvement, local débridement and topical administration of amphotericin B are satisfactory. However, with any evidence of progression of the disease beyond the skin into the subcutaneous tissue and muscle, or the development of signs and symptoms distant to the focus of infection, systemically administered amphotericin B is advised. The duration of antifungal therapy depends on the response of the infection to treatment and the success in resolving the underlying predisposing conditions.

It is almost impossible to determine accurately the effectiveness of any therapeutic approach to mucormycosis. The disease is too rare to warrant appropriately controlled comparative studies, and cases appear in the literature only if therapy is effective. This reporting bias makes generalization of findings in the published literature difficult when attempting to provide the best possible therapy for a given patient. One way of reconciling differences in approach is to assess the extent of infection at the time of diagnosis; early detection can mean less invasion and tissue destruction, and therefore less need for extensive removal of devitalized tissue because there are fewer fungi in the tissue. Overall, the earlier the diagnosis of mucormycosis is made, the better the outcome. At present, no one approach is preferred over another, and treatment should be individualized.

It is apparent that two factors determine the outcome in all patients: early diagnosis and resolution of predisposing problems. Overall mortality has been about 50 percent, although more recent studies have claimed that up to 85 percent of patients can be successfully treated.[42] Results of treating pulmonary mucormycosis have been quite poor, probably because diagnosis of this form of mucormycosis is so difficult. By the time the disease is suspected and the diagnosis is made, extensive tissue destruction has occurred, the pace of the disease is so rapid, and the general condition of the patient is so poor that

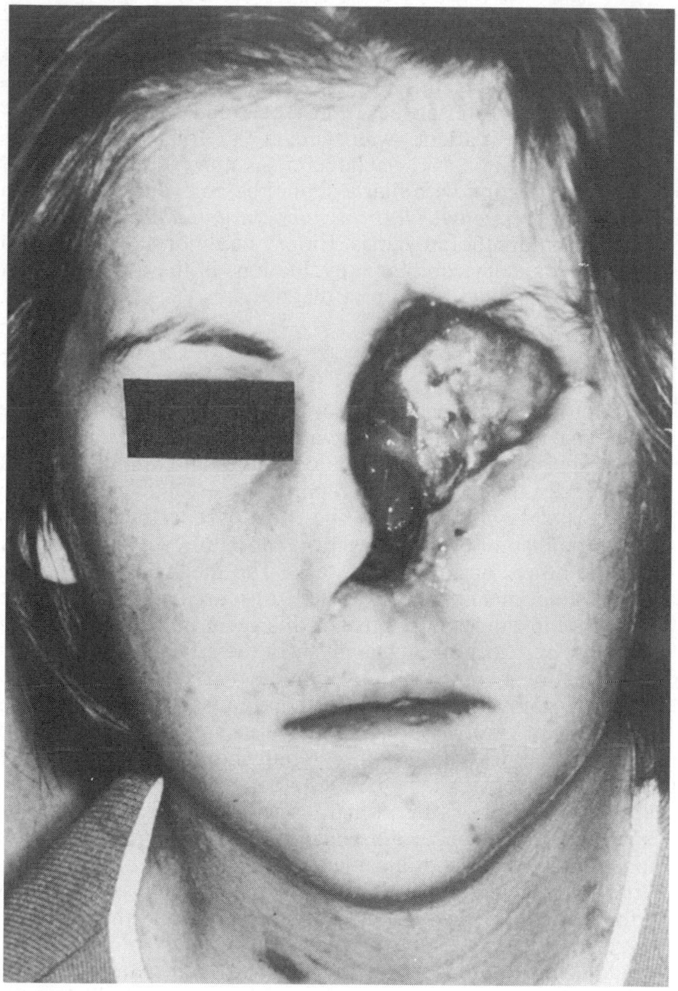

FIG. 6. Photograph of a patient who recovered from rhinocerebral mucormycosis. The residual facial defect following aggressive surgical therapy can be treated with additional reconstructive surgery. (Courtesy of Dr. John E. Edwards, Jr., Los Angeles, CA.)

medical therapy has minimal effect and surgical options are not possible. Occasionally, surgery has appeared helpful.[118]

There is no recognized method for preventing systemic infection with the Mucorales. In patients with severe neutropenia, such as those with bone marrow transplants or leukemia, provision of care in rooms equipped with high-efficiency particulate air filters (HEPA) has been shown to reduce the risks of aspergillosis and mucormycosis.[106] However, due to the high cost of this approach and a lack of effect on the eventual outcome, most centers do not use such filters in the routine care of these patients.

ENTOMOPHTHORAMYCOSIS

The Pathogens

Two genera of the Entomophthorales are responsible for human disease: *Conidiobolus* and *Basidiobolus* (Table 1). Entomophthoramycosis has been arbitrarily subdivided into entomophthoramycosis conidiobolae and entomophthoramycosis basidiobolae on the basis of anatomic localization of the disease and the genus responsible for the pathology at the involved site. The former occurs in the head and face and the latter elsewhere in the body, usually the trunk and arms. This nosology is, however, clearly artificial, since reports of disseminated infection due to *Conidiobolus* have been published.[119,120]

As new information about these organisms is discovered, we can expect to see additional species recovered from human infections and changes in the currently accepted names used for each species. A more widespread geographic distribution of cases also is most likely. Recent reports of disease due to these agents have appeared from the United States[121,122] and Central America.[123]

Epidemiology

These fungi are normal inhabitants of soil throughout the world, including the United States.[124] *Basidiobolus* species have also been isolated from the gut of amphibians and reptiles, including those found in Florida and other areas of the United States.[125] However, most reported cases are from Africa,[126] with cases also occurring in India and other parts of Asia.

Pathogenesis

These organisms are ubiquitous in the environment, even in regions where disease caused by the Entomophthorales is almost never found. Entrance into the body via inhalation or direct inoculation has been postulated,[126,127] but proof for this hypothesis is lacking. Likewise, the mechanisms for host resistance to invasive disease are unknown; however, innate immunity must be fairly high, given the low incidence of disease in most areas of the world.

Echetebu and Ononogbu have described lipase and proteinase activity in supernatants from *Basidiobolus haptosporus*.[128] They postulate that the liberation of lysolecithin from phosphatidylcholine by phospholipase A and a proteinase that can degrade serum proteins may be responsible for the invasive potential of the fungus. Lysolecithin is toxic to mammalian cell membranes, and this may enhance the invasive potential of the organism. However, the ability of the Entomophthorales to produce pathogenetically significant enzymes in vivo is unknown. Moreover, the rarity of disease caused by these agents attests to their low potential for virulence and indicates that some specific abnormality, as yet unknown, must be important in facilitating the initiation and maintenance of infection.

Clinical Manifestations

Entomophthoramycosis conidiobolae is characterized by swelling of the nose, perinasal tissues, and mouth. This is accompanied by symptoms of nasal stuffiness, drainage, and sinus pain. The infection begins as swelling of the inferior nasal turbinates, with subsequent extension into surrounding structures. Nodular subcutaneous masses can be palpated through intact skin. As the disease progresses, generalized facial swelling occurs and the eyes may be unable to be opened as a result (Fig. 7). Systemic symptoms and signs are conspicuously absent. A particularly lucid and instructive summary of this disease has been published by Martinson.[126]

Entomophthoramycosis basidiobolae also begins as nodular subcutaneous lesions. The lesions are typically firm and are not painful. Most frequently, they are located on the trunk, arms, legs, or buttocks.[129] Deeper invasion of muscle underlying involved subcutaneous disease has been described,[130] as has gastrointestinal involvement.[131] While the disease may resolve spontaneously, most cases are slowly progressive until appropriate therapy is administered.

Occasionally, disseminated infection occurs. In one case, the patient presented with low-grade fever, weight loss, cough, and a breast mass.[119] This patient subsequently died of massive pulmonary hemorrhage. Autopsy findings disclosed fungal involvement throughout the body associated with a conspicuous fibrotic reaction.

Biopsy of the submucosal or subcutaneous masses of either form of entomophthoramycosis reveals similar histologic fea-

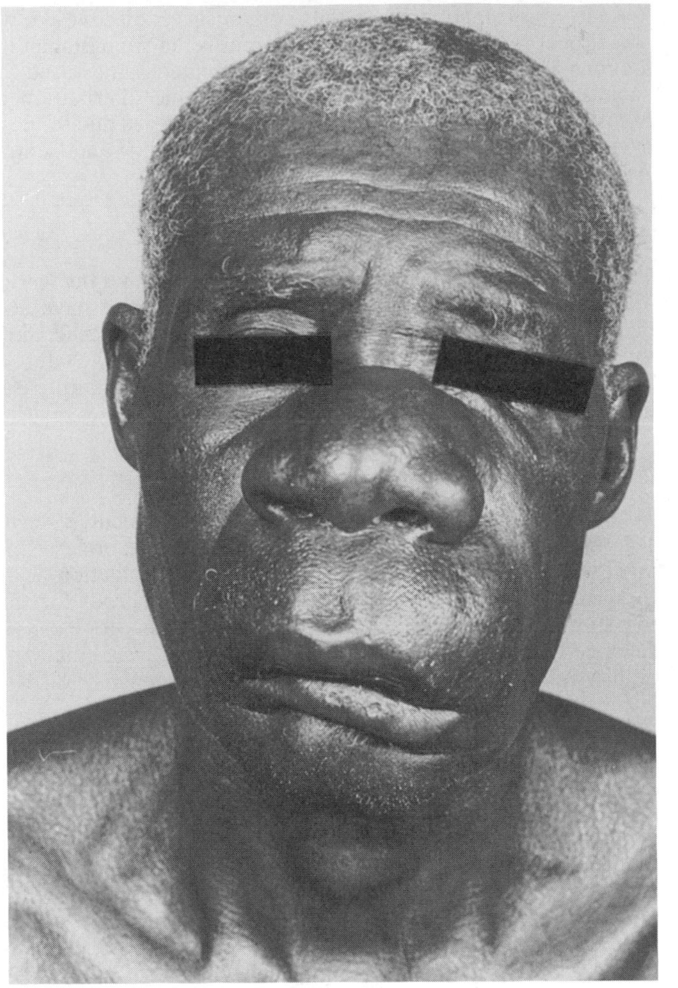

FIG. 7. Photograph of a patient infected with *Conidiobolus* species. Note the marked swelling of the nose and perinasal tissues extending to the periorbital region. (Courtesy of Dr. B. C. Okafor, Enugu, Nigeria.)

tures. Acute and/or chronic inflammatory cells are found in the vicinity of the typical nonseptate, broad, thin-walled hyphae. Occasional hyphal septations can be observed. The hyphae are readily visible on routine hematoxylin and eosin staining but, in contrast to most other fungal pathogens, are not as well demonstrated by PAS or silver staining. Characteristically, the hyphae are surrounded by eosinophilic material, which can appear in a stellate formation or a simple sheath surrounding the hyphae. This has been termed the *Splendore-Hoeppli phenomenon* and is an important histopathologic concomitant of this disease. However, similar perihyphal deposition of eosinophilic material can occur with other fungi or parasites. In contrast to mucormycosis, the Entomophthorales do not invade blood vessels; tissue infarction and necrosis are not found in this disease.

Diagnosis

In areas where entomophthoramycosis is relatively common, the diagnosis can be suspected from the clinical appearance of the patient and the lesions. Definitive diagnosis depends on biopsy of the involved site, with microscopic documentation of tissue invasion and the presence of typical hyphae of either genus.[122] Culture of the fungus is the only way to identify correctly the species present in tissue.

Differential Diagnosis

In tropical areas, a variety of diseases can present with submucosal or subcutaneous nodular lesions associated with swelling. Malignancy and abscess must be ruled out. The presentation in one patient was similar to that of Burkitt's lymphoma.[132] Similarly, onchocerciasis and elephantiasis secondary to infection with filaria should be considered. Infection with *Sporothrix schenckii* or *Mycobacterium ulcerans* also can mimic entomophthoramycosis. Biopsy of abnormal tissue, with pathologic and microbiologic evaluation, is the most efficient method for making the correct diagnosis.

Therapy and Prevention

Therapeutic recommendations for this disease can be made only on the basis of empiric observations. Potassium iodide, trimethoprim/sulfamethoxazole, miconazole, and amphotericin B have all been used. Anecdotal reports suggest that each of these remedies may work; however, the effect of reporting bias makes the determination of which agent is more efficacious and safer than the others an impossible task. The mechanism of action of trimethoprim/sulfamethoxazole is obscure and would be one of the rare instances of the use of this agent in treating mycotic disease. Complicating such analysis of the efficacy of individual treatment regimens is the observation that some cases of entomophthoromycosis, especially those caused by *Basidiobolus* species, may resolve spontaneously. In patients with chronic infection and without life-threatening complications, any of these antimicrobial agents could be considered for use.[133] Susceptibility testing of these fungi, as with other fungi, is not reliable and has an uncertain place in guiding therapeutic decisions. The role of the oral azole antifungals (ketoconazole, itraconazole, and fluconazole) also is not clear, but in consideration of their broad spectrum of antifungal activity and their relative lack of toxicity vis-à-vis the other agents, the use of these drugs should also be evaluated.[134] Indeed, one such patient infected with *Conidiobolus coronatus* was apparently cured after receiving ketoconazole, 600 mg/day.[135]

In addition to medical therapy, a surgical approach to this disease includes removal of accessible nodules and reconstructive surgery to restore a more normal appearance to tissues grossly swollen and deformed by the chronic inflammatory response to the fungus.

Currently, there are no means of preventing this infection or even of identifying those at risk for developing this disease. Thus, there is no role for the use of prophylactic antifungal agents. Early detection of newly acquired infection seems to be the best hope of reducing the serious morbidity associated with long-standing disease.

REFERENCES

1. Rippon JW. Medical Mycology. The Pathogenic Fungi and the Pathogenic Actinomycetes. Philadelphia: WB Saunders; 1988;681–713.
2. Lehrer RI, Howard DH, Sypherd PS, et al. Mucormycosis. Ann Intern Med. 1980;93:93–108.
3. Kwon-Chung KJ, Young RC, Orlando M. Pulmonary mucormycosis caused by *Cunninghamella elegans* in a patient with chronic myelogenous leukemia. Am J Clin Pathol. 1975;64:544–8.
4. Kolbeck PC, Makhoul RG, Bollinger RR, et al. Widely disseminated *Cunninghamella* mucormycosis in an adult renal transplant patient: Case report and review of the literature. Am J Clin Pathol. 1985;83:747–53.
5. Torell H, Cooper BH, Helgeson NGP. Disseminated *Saksenaea vasiformis* infection. Am J Clin Pathol. 1981;76:116–21.
6. Hay RJ, Campbell CK, Marshall WM, et al. Disseminated zygomycosis (mucormycosis) caused by *Saksenaea vasiformis*. J Infect. 1983;7:162–5.
7. Lawrence RM, Snodgrass WT, Reichel GW, et al. Systemic zygomycosis caused by *Apophysomyces elegans*. J Med Vet Mycol. 1986;24:57–65.
8. Wieden MA, Steinbronn KK, Padhye AA, et al. Zygomycosis caused by *Apophysomyces elegans*. J Clin Microbiol. 1985;22:522–6.
9. Gartenberg G, Bottone EJ, Keusch GT, et al. Hospital-acquired mucormycosis (*Rhizopus rhizopodiformis*) of skin and subcutaneous tissue. Epidemiology, mycology and treatment. N Engl J Med. 1978;299:1115–7.

10. Dennis JE, Rhodes KH, Cooney DR, et al. Nosocomial *Rhizopus* infection (zygomycosis) in children. J Pediatr. 1980;96:824–8.
11. Patterson JE, Barden GE, Bia FJ. Hospital-acquired gangrenous mucormycosis. Yale J Biol Med. 1986;59:453–9.
12. Sheldon WJ, Bauer H. The development of the acute inflammatory response to experimental cutaneous mucormycosis in normal and diabetic rabbits. J Exp Med. 1959;110:845.
13. Mead JH, Lupton GP, Dillavou CL, et al. Cutaneous *Rhizopus* infection. Occurrence as a postoperative complication associated with an elasticized adhesive dressing. JAMA. 1979;242:272–4.
14. Waldorf AR, Halde C, Vedros NA. Murine model of pulmonary mucormycosis in cortisone-treated mice. Sabouraudia. 1982;20:217–24.
15. Waldorf AR, Ruderman N, Diamond RD. Specific susceptibility to mucormycosis in murine diabetes and bronchoalveolar macrophage defense against *Rhizopus*. J Clin Invest. 1984;74:150–60.
16. Waldorf AR, Peter L, Polak A. Mucormycotic infection in mice following prolonged incubation of spores in vivo and the role of spore agglutinating antibodies on spore germination. Sabouraudia. 1984;22:101–8.
17. Reinhardt DJ, Licata I, Kaplan W, et al. Experimental cerebral zygomycosis in alloxan-diabetic rabbits: Variation in virulence among zygomycetes. Sabouraudia. 1981;19:245–55.
18. Schaffner A, Davis CE, Schaffner T, et al. In vitro susceptibility of fungi to killing by neutrophil granulocytes discriminates between primary pathogenicity and opportunism. J Clin Invest. 1986;78:511–24.
19. Waldorf AR, Levitz SM, Diamond RD. In vivo bronchoalveolar macrophage defense against *Rhizopus oryzae* and *Aspergillus fumigatus*. J Infect Dis. 1984;150:752–60.
20. Chinn RYW, Diamond RD. Generation of chemotactic factors by *Rhizopus oryzae* in the presence and absence of serum: Relationship to hyphal damage mediated by human neutrophils and effects of hyperglycemia and keotacidosis. Infect Immun. 1982;38:1123–9.
21. Marx RS, Forsyth KR, Hentz ZK. Mucorales species activation of a serum leukotactic factor. Infect Immun. 1982;38:1217–22.
22. Diamond RD, Haudenschild CC, Erickson NF III. Monocyte-mediated damage to *Rhizopus oryzae* hyphae in vitro. Infect Immun. 1982;38:292–7.
23. Ganz T, Selsted ME, Szklarek D, et al. Defensins. Natural peptide antibiotics of human neutrophils. J Clin Invest. 1985;76:1427–35.
24. Levitz SM, Selsted ME, Ganz T, et al. In vitro killing of spores and hyphae of *Aspergillus fumigatus* and *Rhizopus oryzae* by rabbit neutrophil cationic peptides and bronchoalveolar macrophages. J Infect Dis. 1986;154:483–9.
25. Waldorf AR. Host–parasite relationship in opportunistic mycoses. CRC Crit Rev Microbiol. 1985;13:133–72.
26. Espinoza CG, Halkias DG. Pulmonary mucormycosis as a complication of chronic salicylate poisoning. Am J Clin Pathol. 1983;80:508–11.
27. Wong KL, Tai YT, Loke SL, et al. Disseminated zygomycosis masquerading as cerebral lupus erythematosus. Am J Clin Pathol. 1986;86:546–9.
28. Gale GR, Welch A. Studies of opportunistic fungi. I. Inhibition of *R. oryzae* by human sera. Am J Med Sci. 1961;45:604–12.
29. Owens AW, Hacklette MS, Baker RD. An antifungal factor in human serum. I. Studies of *Rhizopus rhizopodiformis*. Sabouraudia. 1965;4:179.
30. Artis WM, Fountain JA, Delcher HK, et al. A mechanism of susceptibility to mucormycosis in diabetic ketoacidosis: Transferrin and iron availability. Diabetes. 1982;31:1109–14.
31. Artis WM, Patrusky E, Rastinejad F, et al. Fungistatic mechanism of human transferrin for *R. oryzae* and *Trichophyton mentagrophytes*: Alternative to simple iron deprivation. Infect Immun. 1983;41:1269–78.
32. Straatsma BR, Zimmerman LE, Gass JDM. Phycomycosis. A clinicopathologic study of fifty-one cases. Lab Invest. 1962;11:963–85.
33. Neame P, Rayner D. Mucormycosis. Arch Pathol. 1960;70:143–50.
34. Meyer RD, Armstrong D. Mucormycosis-changing status. Crit Rev Clin Lab Sci. 1973;4:421–51.
35. Parfrey NA. Improved diagnosis and prognosis of mucormycosis. A clinicopathologic study of 33 cases. Medicine. 1986;65:113–23.
36. Meyer RD, Rosen P, Armstrong D. Phycomycosis complicating leukemia and lymphoma. Ann Intern Med. 1972;77:871–9.
37. Myskowski PL, Brown AE, Dinsmore R, et al. Mucormycosis following bone marrow transplantation. J Am Acad Dermatol. 1983;9:111–5.
38. Meyer RD, Kaplan MH, Ong M, et al. Cutaneous lesions in disseminated mucormycosis. JAMA. 1973;225:737–8.
39. Meyer RD, Rosen P, Armstrong D. Phycomycosis complicating leukemia and lymphoma. Ann Intern Med. 1972;77:871–9.
40. Abramson E, Wilson D, Arky RA. Rhinocerebral phycomycosis in association with diabetic ketoacidosis. Report of two cases and a review of clinical and experimental experience with amphotericin B therapy. Ann Intern Med. 1967;66:735–42.
41. Yanagisawa E, Friedman S, Kundargi RS, et al. Rhinocerebral phycomycosis. Laryngoscope. 1977;87:1319–35.
42. Pillsbury JC, Fischer ND. Rhinocerebral mucormycosis. Arch Otolaryngol. 1977;103:600–4.
43. Meyers BR, Wormser G, Hirschman SZ, et al. Rhinocerebral mucormycosis. Premortem diagnosis and therapy. Arch Intern Med. 1979;139:557–60.
44. England AC III, Weinstein M, Ellner JJ, et al. Two cases of rhinocerebral zygomycosis (mucormycosis) with common epidemiologic and environmental features. Am Rev Respir Dis. 1981;124:497–8.
45. Maniglia AJ, Mintz DH, Novak S. Cephalic phycomycosis: A report of eight cases. Laryngoscope. 1982;92:755–60.
46. Abedi E, Sismanis A, Choi K, et al. Twenty-five years' experience treating cerebro-rhino-orbital mucormycosis. Laryngoscope. 1984;94:1060–2.
47. Morduchowicz G, Shmueli D, Shapira Z, et al. Rhinocerebral mucormycosis in renal transplant recipients: Report of three cases and review of the literature. Rev Infect Dis. 1986;8:441–6.
48. Berthier M, Palmieri O, Lylyk P, et al. Rhino-orbital phycomycosis complicated by cerebral abscess. Neuroradiology. 1982;22:221–4.
49. Price DL, Wolpow ER, Richardson EP Jr. Intracranial phycomycosis: A clinicopathological and radiological study. J Neurol Sci. 1971;14:359–75.
50. Lowe JT Jr, Hudson WR. Rhinocerebral phycomycosis and internal carotid artery thrombosis. Arch Otolaryngol. 1975;101:100–3.
51. Lazo A, Wilner HI, Metes JJ. Craniofacial mucormycosis: Computed tomographic and angiographic findings in two cases. Radiology. 1981;139:623–6.
52. Greenberg MR, Lippman SM, Grinnell VS, et al. Computed tomographic findings in orbital Mucor. West J Med. 1985;143:102–3.
53. Boelaert JR, Vergauwe PL, Vandepitte JM. Mucormycosis infection in dialysis patients. Ann Intern Med. 1987;107:782–3.
54. Windus DW, Stokes TJ, Julian BA, et al. Fatal *Rhizopus* infections in hemodialysis patients receiving deferoxamine. Ann Intern Med. 1987;107:678–80.
55. Goodill JJ, Abuelo JG. Mucormycosis—A new risk of deferoxamine therapy in dialysis patients with aluminum or iron overload? N Engl J Med. 1987;317:34.
56. Brennan RO, Crain BJ, Proctor AM, et al. *Cunninghamella*: A newly recognized cause of rhinocerebral mucormycosis. Am J Clin Pathol. 1983;80:98–102.
57. Finn DG, Farmer JC Jr. Chronic mucormycosis. Laryngoscope. 1982;92:761–3.
58. Ferstenfeld JE, Cohen SH, Rose HD, et al. Chronic rhinocerebral phycomycosis in association with diabetes. Postgrad Med J. 1977;53:337–42.
59. Murray HW. Pulmonary mucormycosis with massive fatal hemoptysis. Chest. 1975;68:65–8.
60. Watts WJ. Bronchopleural fistula followed by massive fatal hemoptysis in a patient with pulmonary mucormycosis: A case report. Arch Intern Med. 1983;143:1029–30.
61. Agger WA, Maki DG. Mucormycosis. A complication of critical care. Arch Intern Med. 1978;138:925–7.
62. Gale AM, Kleitsch WP. Solitary pulmonary nodule due to phycomycosis (mucormycosis). Chest. 1972;62:752–5.
63. Matsushima T, Soejima R, Nakashima T. Solitary pulmonary nodule caused by phycomycosis in a patient without obvious predisposing factors. Thorax. 1980;35:877–8.
64. Record NB Jr, Ginder DR. Pulmonary phycomycosis without obvious predisposing factors. JAMA. 1976;235:1256–7.
65. Aderka A, Sidi Y, Garfinkel D, et al. Roentgenologically invisible mucormycosis pneumonia. Respiration. 1983;44:158–60.
66. Rothstein RD, Simon GL. Subacute pulmonary mucormycosis. J Med Vet Mycol. 1986;24:391–4.
67. Jain JK, Markowitz A, Khilanani PV, et al. Case report: Localized mucormycosis following intramuscular corticosteroid. Case report and review of the literature. Am J Med Sci. 1978;275:209–16.
68. Rothburn MM, Chambers DK, Roberts C, et al. Cutaneous mucormycosis: A rare cause of leg ulceration. J Infect. 1986;13:175–8.
69. Wilson CB, Siber GR, O'Brien TF, et al. Phycomycotic gangrenous cellulitis. A report of two cases and a review of the literature. Arch Surg. 1976;111:532–8.
70. Tomford JW, Whittlesey D, Ellner JJ, et al. Invasive primary cutaneous phycomycosis in diabetic leg ulcers. Arch Surg. 1980;115:770–1.
71. Vainrub B, Macareno H, Mandel S, et al. Wound zygomycosis (mucormycosis) in otherwise healthy adults. Am J Med. 1988;84:546–8.
72. Rabin ER, Lundberg GD, Mitchell ET. Mucormycosis in severely burned patients. Report of two cases with extensive destruction of the face and nasal cavity. N Engl J Med. 1961;264:1286–9.
73. Lyon DT, Schubert TT, Mantia AG, et al. Phycomycosis of the gastrointestinal tract. Am J Gastroenterol. 1979;72:379–94.
74. Gregory JE, Golden A, Haymaker W. Mucormycosis of the central nervous system. A report of three cases. Bull Johns Hopkins Hosp. 1943;73:405–19.
75. Ignelzi RJ, VanderArk GD. Cerebral mucormycosis following open head trauma. Case report. J Neurosurg. 1975;42:593–6.
76. Hameroff SB, Eckholdt JW, Lindenberg R. Cerebral phycomycosis in a heroin addict. Neurology. 1970;20:261–5.
77. Pierce PF Jr, Soloman SL, Kaufman L, et al. Zygomycetes brain abscesses in narcotic addicts with serological diagnosis. JAMA. 1982;248:2881–2.
78. Woods KF, Hanna BJ. Brain stem mucormycosis in a narcotic addict with eventual recovery. Am J Med. 1986;80:126–8.
79. Bachor R, Baczako K, Kern W. Isolated cerebral mucormycosis in a patient with leukemia. Mykosen. 1986;29:497–501.
80. Watson DF, Stern BJ, Levin ML, et al. Isolated cerebral phycomycosis presenting as focal encephalitis. Arch Neurol. 1985;42:922–3.
81. Cuadrado LM, Guerrero A, Lopez Garcia Asenjo JA, et al. Cerebral mucormycosis in two cases of acquired immunodeficiency syndrome. Arch Neurol. 1988;45:109–11.
82. Virmani R, Connor DH, McAllister HA. A report of five patients and review of 14 previously reported cases. Am J Clin Pathol. 1982;78:42–7.
83. Merchant RK, Louria B, Geisler PH, et al. Fungal endocarditis: Review of the literature and report of three cases. Ann Intern Med. 1958;48:242–66.

84. Khica GJ, Berroya RB, Escano FB, et al. Mucormycosis in a mitral prosthesis. J Thorac Cardiovasc Surg. 1972;63:903–5.
85. Tuder RM. Mycoardial infarct in disseminated mucormycosis: Case report with special emphasis on the pathogenic mechanisms. Mycopathologia. 1985;89:81–8.
86. Echols RM, Selinger DS, Hallowell C, et al. *Rhizopus* osteomyelitis. A case report and review. Am J Med. 1979;66:141–5.
87. Gussen R, Canalis RF. Mucormycosis of the temporal bone. Ann Otol Rhinol Laryngol. 1982;91:27–32.
88. Maliwan N, Reyes CV, Rippon JW. Osteomyelitis secondary to cutaneous mucormycosis. Report of a case and a review of the literature. Am J Dermatopathol. 1984;6:479–81.
89. Brown OE, Finn R. Mucormycosis of the mandible. J Oral Maxillofac Surg. 1986;44:132–6.
90. Pierce PF, Wood MB, Roberts GD Jr, et al. *Saksenaea vasiformis* osteomyelitis. J Clin Microbiol. 1987;25:933–5.
91. Axelrod P, Kwon-Chung KJ, Frawley P, et al. Chronic cystitis due to *Cokeromyces recurvatus*: A case report. J Infect Dis. 1987;155:1062–4.
92. Oberle AD, Penn RL. Nosocomial invasive *Saksenaea vasiformis* infection. Am J Clin Pathol. 1983;80:885–8.
93. Leong ASY. Granulomatous mediastinitis due to *Rhizopus* species. Am J Clin Pathol. 1978;70:103–7.
94. Connor BA, Anderson RJ, Smith JW. Mucor mediastinitis. Chest. 1979;75:524–6.
95. Schwartz JRL, Nagle MG, Elkins RC, et al. Mucormycosis of the trachea. An unusual cause of acute upper airway obstruction. Chest. 1982;81:653–4.
96. Jones PG, Gilman RM, Medeiros AA, et al. Focal intracranial mucormycosis presenting as chronic meningitis. JAMA. 1981;246:2063–4.
97. Helenglass G, Elliott JA, Lucie NP. An unusual presentation of opportunistic mucormycosis. Br Med J. 1981;282:108–9.
98. Caraveo J, Trowbridge AA, Amaral BW, et al. Bone marrow necrosis associated with a mucor infection. Am J Med. 1977;62:404–8.
99. Yankey R, Abraham AA. Serological studies of a case of fatal craniofacial mucormycosis. Mycopathologia. 1983;82:105–9.
100. Hessian PA, Smith JMB. Antigenic characterization of some potentially pathogenic mucoraceous fungi. Sabouraudia. 1982;20:209–16.
101. Levy SA, Schmitt KW, Kaufman L. Systemic zygomycosis diagnosed by fine needle aspiration and confirmed with enzyme immunoassay. Chest. 1986;89:146–8.
102. Wysong DR, Waldorf AR. Electrophoretic and immunoblot analyses of *Rhizopus arrhizus* antigens. J Clin Microbiol. 1987;25:358–63.
103. Barnert J, Behr W, Reich H. An amphotericin B-resistant case of rhinocerebral mucormycosis. Infection. 1985;13:134–6.
104. Christenson JC, Shalit I, Welch DF, et al. Synergistic action of amphotericin B and rifampin against *Rhizopus* species. Antimicrob Agents Chemother. 1987;31:1775–8.
105. Eng RHK, Person A, Mangura C, et al. Susceptibility of zygomycetes to amphotericin B, miconazole, and ketoconazole. Antimicrob Agents Chemother. 1981;20:688–90.
106. Bogard BN. Pulmonary mucormycosis. N Engl J Med. 1972;286:606.
107. Hauch TW. Pulmonary mucormycosis: Another cure. Chest. 1977;72:92–3.
108. Brown JF Jr, Gottlieb LS, McCormick RA. Pulmonary and rhinocerebral mucormycosis. Successful outcome with amphotericin B and griseofulvin therapy. Arch Intern Med. 1977;137:936–8.
109. Henriquez M, Levy R, Raja RM, et al. Mucormycosis in a renal transplant recipient with successful outcome. JAMA. 1979;242:1397–9.
110. Rosenberger RS, West BC, King JW. Case report: Survival from sino-orbital mucormycosis due to *Rhizopus rhizopodiformis*. Am J Med Sci. 1983;286:25–30.
111. Smith JL, Stevens DA. Survival in cerebro-rhino-orbital zygomycosis and cavernous sinus thrombosis with combined therapy. South Med J. 1986;79:501–4.
112. West BC, Kwon-Chung KJ, King JW, et al. Inguinal abscess caused by *Rhizopus rhizopodiformis*: Successful treatment with surgery and amphotericin B. J Clin Microbiol. 1983;18:1384–7.
113. Hamill R, Oney LA, Crane LR. Successful therapy for rhinocerebral mucormycosis with associated bilateral brain abscesses. Arch Intern Med. 1983;143:581–3.
114. Breiman A, Sadowsky D, Friedman J. Mucormycosis. Discussion and report of a case involving the maxillary sinus. Oral Surg Oral Med Oral Pathol. 1981;52:375–8.
115. Rakover Y, Vered I, Garzuzi H, et al. Rhinocerebral phycomycosis; combined approach therapy: Case report. J Laryngol Otol. 1985;99:1279–80.
116. Kohn R, Hepler R. Management of limited rhino-orbital mucormycosis without exenteration. Ophthalmology. 1985;92:1440–4.
117. Kaplan AL, Huerta AR, Chiou SJ. Rhinocerebral mucormycosis. West J Med. 1981;135:326–9.
117a. Couch L, Theiler F, Mader T. Rhinocerebral mucormycosis with cerebral extension successfully treated with adjunctive hyperbaric oxygen therapy. Arch Otolaryngol Head Neck Surg. 1988;114:791–4.
117b. Ferguson BJ, Mitchell TG, Moon R, et al. Adjunctive hyperbaric oxygen for treatment of rhinocerebral mucormycosis. Rev Infect Dis. 1988;10:551–9.
118. Bribetz AR, Chuang MT, Burrows L, et al. *Rhizopus* lung abscess in renal transplant patient successfully treated by lobectomy. Chest. 1980;77:102–4.
119. Busapakum R, Youngchaiyud U, Sriumpai S, et al. Disseminated infection with *Conidiobolus incongruus*. Sabouraudia. 1983;21:323–30.
120. Eckert HL, Khoury GH, Pore RS, et al. Deep *Entomophthora* phycomycotic infection reported for the first time in the United States. Chest. 1972;61:392–4.
121. Nathan MD Jr, Keller AR, Lerner CJ, et al. Entomophthorales infection of the maxillofacial region. Laryngoscope. 1982;92:767–9.
122. Dworzack DL, Pollock AS, Hodges GR, et al. Zygomycosis of the maxillary sinus and palate caused by *Basidiobolus haptosporus*. Arch Intern Med. 1978;138:1274–6.
123. Segura JJ, Gonzalez K, Berrocal J, et al. Rhinoentomophthoromycosis: Report of the first two cases observed in Costa Rica (Central America), and review of the literature. Am J Trop Med Hyg. 1981;30:1078–84.
124. Greer DL, Friedman L. Studies on the genus *Basidiobolus* with reclassification on the species pathogenic for man. Sabouraudia. 1966;4:231–41.
125. Okafor JI, Testrake D, Mushinsky HR, et al. A *Basidiobolus* sp. and its association with reptiles and amphibians in Southern Florida. Sabouraudia. 1984;22:47–51.
126. Martinson FD. Clinical epidemiological and therapeutic aspects of entomophthoromycosis. Ann Soc Belg Med Trop. 1972;52:329–42.
127. Herstoff JK, Bogaars H, McDonald CJ. Rhinophycomycosis entomophthorae. Arch Dermatol. 1978;114:1674–8.
128. Echetebu CO, Ononogbu IC. Extracellular lipase and proteinase of *Basidiobolus haptosporus*: Possible role in subcutaneous mycosis. Mycopathologia. 1982;80:171–7.
129. Antonelli M, Vignetti P, Dahir M, et al. Entomophthoromycosis due to *Basidiobolus* in Somalia. Trans R Soc Trop Med Hyg. 1987;81:186–7.
130. Kamalam A, Thambiah AS. Muscle invasion by *Basidiobolus haptosporus*. Sabouraudia. 1984;22:273–7.
131. Schmidt JR, Howard RJ, Chen JL, et al. First culture-proven gastrointestinal enteromophthoromycosis in the United States: A case report and review of the literature. Mycopathologia. 1986;95:101–4.
132. Bittencourt AL, Serra G, Sadigursky M, et al. Subcutaneous zygomycosis caused by *Basidiobolus haptosporus*: Presentation of a case mimicking Burkitt's lymphoma. Am J Trop Med Hyg. 1982;31:370–3.
133. Taylor GD, Sekhon AS, Tyrrell DLJ, et al. Rhinofacial zygomycosis caused by *Conidiobolus coronatus*: A case report including in vitro sensitivity to antimycotic agents. Am J Trop Med Hyg. 1987;36:398–401.
134. Yangco BG, Okafor JI, TeStrake D. In vitro susceptibilities of human and wild-type isolates of *Basidiobolus* and *Conidiobolus* species. Antimicrob Agents Chemother. 1984;25:413–6.
135. Chauvin JL, Drouhet E, Dupont B. Nouveau cas de rhino-entomophtoromycose. Guerison par le ketoconazole. Ann Otolaryngol (Paris). 1982;99:563–8.
136. Howard DH. An introduction to the taxonomy and nomenclature of zoopathogenic fungi. In: Howard DH, ed. Fungi Pathogenic for Humans and Animals (in three parts); Part A, Biology. New York: Marcel Dekker; 1983:3–7.

238. SPOROTHRIX SCHENCKII

JOHN E. BENNETT

Sporotrichosis is the infection caused by the fungus *Sporothrix schenckii* (*Sporotrichum schenckii*). The most common manifestation is a chronic subcutaneous nodular granuloma arising at the site of minor trauma and spreading proximally along lymphatic channels.

MYCOLOGY

Sporothrix schenckii is a dimorphic fungus. Yeastlike cells are formed in the infected host and on enriched culture medium, such as blood cysteine glucose, at 37°C. It grows at room temperature on simple culture media, such as Sabouraud agar, as a white mold that turns brownish black with further incubation. The fungus is identified by the microscopic examination of a sporulating mold culture plus conversion of the mold to yeastlike cells. Identification by histopathologic section is less precise because of variability in the shape and size of yeastlike cells. These cells may be round, oval, or cigar shaped, often 4–6 μm wide.

EPIDEMIOLOGY

Sporothrix schenckii has been isolated most often from soil, living plants, or plant debris.[1] It does not appear to infect plants but occasionally infects animals as well as humans. Disease most often arises as a result of contact with thorny plants, such as roses or sphagnum moss, that implant the fungus in the subcutaneous tissue of the host. Outbreaks have occurred among miners, nursery workers, and other groups handling contaminated timbers, mulch, moss, hay, or other plant materials.[1,2] Most patients with cutaneous sporotrichosis are previously healthy adults less than 30 years old. The number of females and males are approximately equal. In contrast, there is a 6:1 male predominance in patients with extracutaneous sporotrichosis. Such patients are usually more than 30 years old and do not have an obvious cutaneous portal of entry. Many have a history of outdoor occupations in which exposure to plant products would be likely, such as farming. Immunosuppression is uncommon. About one-third of patients with pulmonary sporotrichosis have a history of alcoholism.

CLINICAL MANIFESTATIONS

Sporotrichosis can be divided into two categories that differ in both prognosis and management: cutaneous and extracutaneous infection.

Cutaneous Sporotrichosis

The majority of cases begin at the site of inoculation, usually on an extremity or, particularly in children, on the face. After an incubation period of 1–12 weeks, a small, red, painless papule arises, enlarges slowly, becomes violaceous, and intermittently discharges a small amount of serosanguineous exudate (Fig. 1). Ulceration is common. A lesion remaining confined to a single skin site has been called plaque sporotrichosis. Most often, new lesions appear proximally along paths of lymphatic channels. Although this entity is called *lymphocutaneous sporotrichosis*, lymph nodes are not often infected. Isolation of *S. schenckii* from inguinal or axillary nodes is quite uncommon. Hematogenous dissemination of infection in a patient with lymphocutaneous sporotrichosis is extraordinarily rare, even though a progressive appearance of lesions in proximal sites would suggest a serious outcome in the untreated patient. Fortunately, infection remains confined to subcutaneous tissue, the individual lesions waxing and waning over the months and years. Spontaneous cure has been reported in plaque sporotrichosis[3] but has not been clearly documented in lymphocutaneous disease.

Lesions closely resembling lymphocutaneous sporotrichosis may occur with *Leishmania brasiliensis, Mycobacterium marinum, M. kansasii* and *Nocardia brasiliensis*. Plaque sporotrichosis may be confused with a foreign body granuloma when the lesion is small and nodular. Larger plaque lesions may resemble blastomycosis, chromoblastomycosis, lobomycosis, tuberculosis verrucosa cutis, verruca vulgaris, and Majocchi's granuloma. Isolation of *S. schenckii* on culture of cutaneous exudate is diagnostic. Culture and histology of punch biopsy from skin lesions is usually diagnostic, though more than one attempt may be required. The fungus is often sparse in the lesion. The inflammatory response may be composed of typical granulomas with giant cells and epithelioid cells in the mid and upper dermis; or, a suppurative granulomatous response may be found, with clusters of neutrophils. The epidermis typically shows pseudoepitheliomatous hyperplasia. Fungal cells are confined to the dermis and may be surrounded by a large, periodic acid–Schiff-staining body, forming the so-called asteroid. These are frequent in some series[4] but not in others. Occasionally the fungus can be seen in microscopic examination of exudate from a lesion.

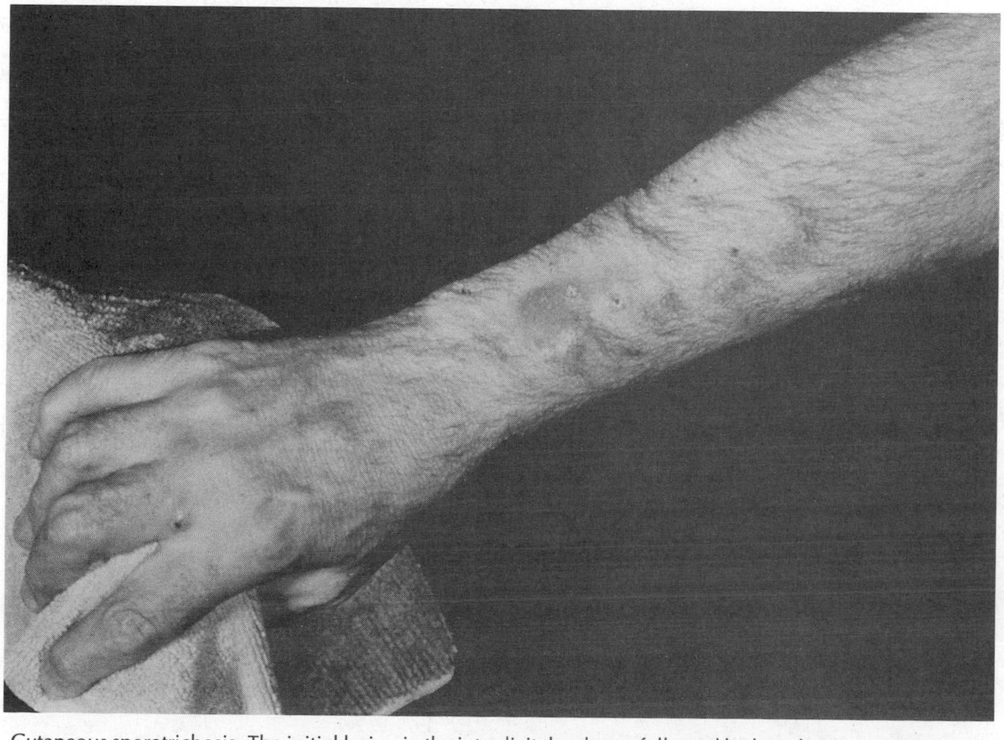

FIG. 1. Cutaneous sporotrichosis. The initial lesion in the interdigital web was followed by lymphangitic spread up the dorsum of the forearm.

Extracutaneous Sporotrichosis

Traumatic inoculation of the conjunctiva or cornea may cause ocular sporotrichosis. Other forms of extracutaneous sporotrichosis are rarely traceable to inoculation.

Osteoarticular sporotrichosis comprises about 80 percent of all extracutaneous cases.[5,6] Infection primarily involves the joint and bone but may also involve the tendon sheath or bursa. The clinical manifestation is that of an extremely indolent arthritis. The knee, ankle, wrist, and elbow are the sites of involvement. The hips, shoulders, and spine are spared. In this disease, signs of cutaneous or other organ involvement are usually absent. Articular signs and symptoms include pain, decreased mobility, effusion, and edema. Systemic symptoms are often minimal. Failure to consider fungal infection as an etiology has led to delay in making the definitive diagnosis for an average of 25 months.[7] This delay results in significant morbidity of the affected joint. *Pulmonary sporotrichosis* is rare. Only 58 cases were found in a recent review.[8] Most are older men with indolent cavitary pneumonitis in one upper lobe (Fig. 2). Productive cough is usual. Many patients have weight loss, anorexia, fatigue, and variable low-grade fever. Hemoptysis or dyspnea may occur. Pleural effusion, hilar adenopathy, or spread beyond the lung is uncommon. The differential diagnosis includes histoplasmosis, coccidioidomycosis, tuberculosis, and infection caused by other mycobacteria.

Most cases of ocular sporotrichosis involve the lids, conjunctiva, or lacrimal apparatus. The pathogenesis is similar to that of cutaneous sporotrichosis. Approximately 15 percent of these infections will involve the orbit. Endophthalmitis has been reported without evidence of pre-existing sporotrichosis.[9]

Central nervous system disease is extremely rare.[10] Neurologic symptoms may be focal or diffuse, but headache and confusion are usually present. There may not be nuchal rigidity. Cerebrospinal fluid shows an elevated leukocyte count composed predominantly of lymphocytes, elevated protein content, and hypoglycorrhachia.

Multifocal cutaneous sporotrichosis: Skin infection beyond a single extremity is probably due to hematogenous spread. Skin lesions resulting from hematogeneous dissemination do not show lymphatic spread.

The inflammatory response in extracutaneous sporotrichosis is usually granulomatous; neutrophils are not prominent. Fungal cells are frequent enough so that they are readily found in methenamine silver-stained sections.

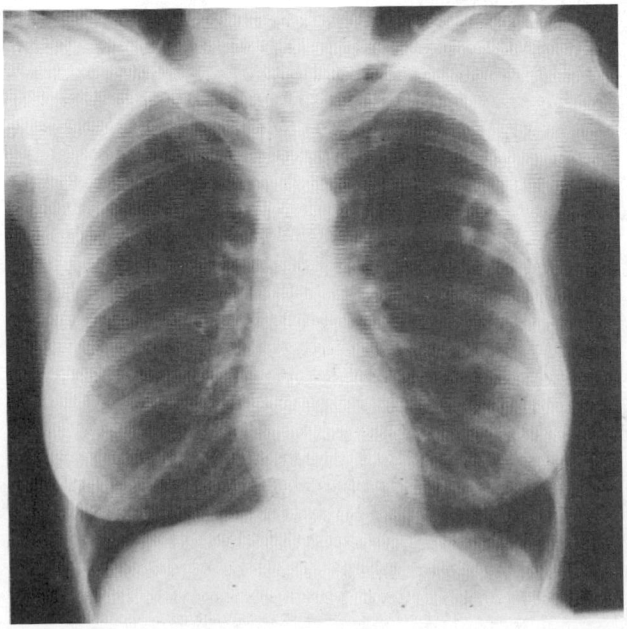

FIG. 2. Chest roentgenogram showing thin-walled left upper lobe cavity resulting from sporotrichosis.

DIAGNOSIS

Diagnosis is best accomplished by culture of the infected tissue, such as skin, joint fluid, bursal fluid, or draining exudate. Cultures of blood, bone marrow, or urine are rarely positive. Although *S. schenckii* was considered to be harmless saprophyte in the sputum of one patient,[11] isolation of this fungus from any body fluid is ordinarily diagnostic.

Antibody to the rhamnomannans and galactomannans of *S. schenckii* may be found in serum of patients with sporotrichosis, but antibody is present in some healthy people.[12] Experimental skin test antigens have provided evidence of exposure in certain populations but are not helpful in clinical situations.

TREATMENT

Cutaneous sporotrichosis is treated with iodides. Therapy is begun with a saturated solution of potassium iodide at a dose of 5 drops tid in milk or juice and increased 3–5 drops/day until a total of 120 drops/day is reached or signs of toxicity occur. If the patient experiences toxicity in the form of increased lacrimation, increased salivation, swelling of the salivary glands, or gastrointestinal symptoms, the therapy should be stopped and reinstituted in several days at a lower dose. A pustular acneiform rash over the cape area of the trunk is frequent and is not an indication for discontinuance of iodides. Rarely, cutaneous disease does not respond to iodide, or serious iodide allergy may preclude continuation of iodide therapy. Heat applied to the lesions is often helpful.[13] Ketoconazole has not been a very effective drug for sporotrichosis, but preliminary reports indicate that itraconazole, 100 mg/day, may be an alternative to iodides in cutaneous infection.[14] Iodides have occasionally been successful in pulmonary sporotrichosis but are rarely useful in osteoarticular infection.

Intravenous amphotericin B is the drug of choice for extracutaneous sporotrichosis. Approximately 2.0–2.5 g are given as 0.5 mg/kg daily. Roughly two-thirds of the osteoarticular patients are cured with a single course of amphotericin B. Residual joint damage is usual. Patients who relapse may respond to a more prolonged course of therapy. Only one-third of the pulmonary patients are cured with amphotericin B. In patients with sporotrichosis confined to one lobe of the lung, lobectomy with or without perioperative amphotericin B is preferred to chemotherapy alone. Meningeal sporotrichosis has proved very difficult to cure with amphotericin B alone. The combination of amphotericin B plus flucytosine may warrant trial in such cases.

PROGNOSIS

Cutaneous sporotrichosis responds well to therapy, and the prognosis is good. Extracutaneous sporotrichosis is more difficult to eradicate, necessitates the use of potentially harmful antifungal medication, and may have marked morbidity and mortality; thus, the prognosis is guarded.

REFERENCES

1. Travassos LR, Lloyd KO. Sporothrix schenckii and related species of ceratocystis. Microbiol Rev. 1980;44:683.
2. Powell KE, Taylor A, Phillips BJ, et al. Cutaneous sporotrichosis in forestry workers. Epidemic due to contaminated sphagnum moss. JAMA. 1978;240:232.
3. Bargman HB. Sporotrichosis of the nose with spontaneous cure. Can Med Assoc J. 1981;124:1027.
4. Bullpitt P, Weedon D. Sporotrichosis: A review of 39 cases. Pathology. 1978;10:249.
5. Wilson DE, Mann, JJ, Bennett JE, et al. Clinical features of extracutaneous sporotrichosis. Medicine. 1967;46:265.

6. Lynch PJ, Voorhees JJ, Harrell ER. Systemic sporotrichosis. Ann Intern Med. 1970;73:23.
7. Crout JE, Brewer NS, Tompkins RB. Sporotrichosis arthritis: Clinical features in seven patients. Ann Intern Med. 1977;86:294.
8. Plus JL, Opal SM. Pulmonary sporotrichosis: review of treatment and outcome. Medicine. 1986;65:143–53.
9. Font RL, Jakobiec FA. Granulomatous necrotizing retinochoroiditis caused by *Sporotrichum schenckii*. Arch Ophthalmol. 1976;94:1513.
10. Ewing GE, Bosl GJ, Peterson PK. Sporotrichosis schenckii meningitis in a farmer with Hodgkin's disease. Am J Med. 1980;68:455.
11. Lowenstein M, Markowitz SM, Nottebart HC, et al. Existence of Sporothrix schenckii as a pulmonary saprophyte. Chest. 1978;73:419.
12. Blumer SO, Kaufman L, Kaplan W, et al. Comparative evaluation of five serologic methods for the diagnosis of sporotrichosis. Appl Microbiol. 1973;26:4.
13. Galiana J, Conti-Diaz IA. Healing effects of heat and rubefacient on nine cases of sporotrichosis. Sabouraudia. 1963;3:64.
14. Restrepo A, Robledo J, Gomez I, et al. Itraconazole therapy in lymphangitis and cutaneous sporotrichosis. Arch Dermatol. 1986;122:413–7.

239. AGENTS OF CHROMOMYCOSIS

KENNETH F. WAGNER

Chromomycosis (also called chromoblastomycosis) is a chronic cutaneous and subcutaneous fungal infection. The disease has been encountered on every continent and in all climates. Most cases occur in tropical and subtropical regions. Specimens from the verrucous, cauliflower-like lesions demonstrate the fungus as sclerotic bodies, singly or in clusters. These sclerotic bodies separate chromomycosis from other related fungal diseases such as phaeohyphomycosis. Histologically, hyperkeratotic pseudoepitheliomatous hyperplasia with keratolytic microabscess formation in the epidermis is seen. Satisfactory treatment of chromomycosis has yet to be developed.

ETIOLOGY AND MYCOLOGY

There is considerable confusion in the literature concerning the terminology of the fungi that cause chromomycosis. I prefer the nomenclature and inclusion of fungi as suggested by McGinnis, with common synonyms in parentheses: *Fonsecaea pedrosoi* (*Hormodendrum pedrosoi, Phialophora pedrosoi, Rhinocladiella pedrosoi*); *Fonsecaea compacta* (*Hormodendrum compactum, Phialophora compacta, Rhinocladiella compacta*); *Phialophora verrucosa*; *Cladosporium carrionii* (*Cladophialophora ajelloi*); and *Rhinocladiella aquaspersa* (*Acrotheca aquaspersa*).[1]

In tissue and exudate, all species produce the same type of dark brown cells, which are septate (sclerotic bodies) and occur singly or in small clusters. On culture, all species form heaped-up dark colonies with short aerial hyphae producing a gray to green or brown to black velvety surface. Because most of the commonly isolated agents of chromomycosis grow slowly, cultures should be held at least 4–6 weeks. Specific identification of the various causal agents requires an experienced mycologist.

EPIDEMIOLOGY

Chromomycosis occurs worldwide and without racial predisposition but is most common in tropical and subtropical areas among barefooted agricultural workers.[2] These cosmopolitan opportunistic pathogens are among the more common fungi found in soil, rotting wood, and decaying vegetation. Traumatic inoculation of fungi into the skin is the main mode of infection. Handling lumber and sitting on wooden planks in Finnish sauna baths have also been implicated as point sources of infection with *F. pedrosoi*.[3] The lower extremities are the most frequently infected sites, with lesions occurring less frequently on the shoulders, chest, trunk, and face. In some areas like Japan and Venezuela upper body sites predominate.[4,5] There is an overwhelming predominance of infection in males. This has been attributed to males having a greater opportunity for soil contact and predisposition to injury while working.[4] Contrary to this observation is a male-to-female ratio of 1/1.1 in 296 cases of chromomycosis in Japan.[5]

F. pedrosoi is the most commonly isolated agent of chromomycosis throughout the world. *C. carrionii* is the major pathogen in Australia, Venezuela, and South Africa. There are only a few cases attributed to *F. compacta* in the literature. Transmission has not been documented to occur from human to human or from animals to humans.

CLINICAL MANIFESTATIONS

The typical verrucous form of chromomycosis appears at a site where traumatic implantation of the fungus has occurred. However, the trauma may have been so long ago that a history of injury is lacking. The primary lesion begins as a small pink scaly papule that may be pruritic. In time (often months to years) a new crop of lesions appears in the same or adjacent areas that are warty, purplish, scaly nodules or can be smooth firm tumors. Peripheral spread can occur with healing in the center as seen in cutaneous blastomycosis (Fig. 1). However, the lesions usually tend to enlarge and become grouped. The older and more distant lesions look like cauliflowers. On the warty surface are small ulcerations or "black dots" of hemopurulent material (Fig. 2). These lesions can be pruritic and rarely are painful. Satellite lesions may develop through scratching and via the lymphatics and may coalesce, resulting in a large verrucous mass.

A second type of lesion is the annular, flattened, papular type with a raised active border (Fig. 3). Through healing the center becomes scarred. Sometimes there is extensive keloid formation in the healing lesions. In advanced cases extensive fibrosis can cause lymphostasis and marked edema of the involved extremity.

The clinical history will usually reveal that the disease had been present for many years with minimal discomfort to the patient. Medical attention is usually sought because of secondary infection, cosmetic reasons, or lymphedema, which can result in elephantiasis. There is usually no fistula formation as seen in mycetomas or invasion of muscle or bone. In rare cases hematogenous spread to the brain, lymph nodes, liver, lungs, and other organs has been reported.[5]

The differential diagnosis of chromomycosis includes lobomycosis, blastomycosis, yaws, tertiary syphilis, tuberculosis verrucosa cutis, leishmaniasis, mycetoma, sporotrichosis, *Mycobacterium marinum*, herpes vulgaris, leprosy, and bromide drug eruption.

PATHOLOGIC FINDINGS

The tissue response in chromomycosis is not specific. It is similar to the responses that can be seen in other mycoses like blastomycosis, coccidioidomycosis, and sporotrichosis.[1] However, the histologic picture of cutaneous chromomycosis is that of a foreign body granuloma interspersed with microabscesses.[4] Numerous neutrophils cluster in the centers of the granuloma. Foreign body giant cells, lymphocytes, eosinophils, and plasma cells are also present. The nonulcerated lesion that is not secondarily infected shows a very high degree of pseudoepitheliomatous hyperplasia.[4] The hyperplasia is not as extreme as in cutaneous blastomycosis or coccidioidal granuloma, but it is considerable and would be termed extreme acanthosis.[4] In early

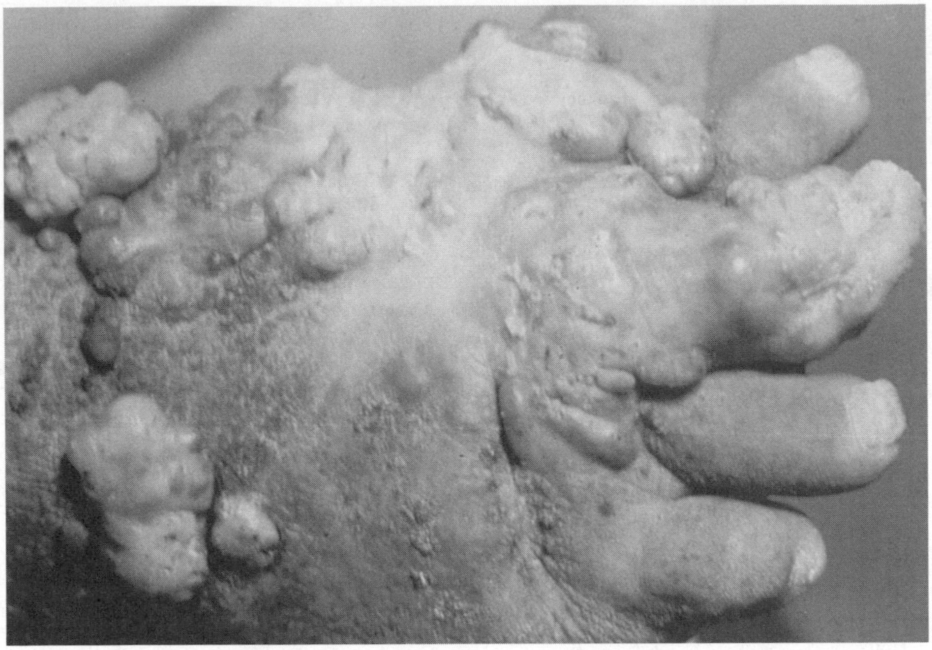

FIG. 1. Verrucous lesions of chromomycosis demonstrate central healing on the foot of a patient in Panama.

lesions in which the organism is found, mostly in the epidermis, including the stratum corneum, hyphal strands are seen more commonly than are sclerotic cells. In older lesions and between nodular lesions changes consistent with chronic fibrosis can be visualized. The process of transepithelial elimination, where blood, foreign matter, and sclerotic bodies are expelled through the epidermis, results in "black dots" found on the lesion's surface (Fig. 2).[1,5a] The fungus is visable in stained and unstained sections. The sclerotic bodies, referred to as medlar bodies, copper pennies, chromobodies, chlamydospores, and sclerotia, are 5–15 μm in diameter, with thick, planate, septal walls, and are often grouped or in chains. These pigmented organisms are easily seen in macrophages, giant cells, or extracellularly on hematoxylin- and eosin-stained material.

DIAGNOSIS

In tissue and exudate, all types of chromomycosis produce the characteristic sclerotic bodies. These are usually more abundant in specimens from verrucous lesions than in material from annular, flat lesions. On examination of the verrucous type of lesions one can usually see "black dot" areas. Scrapings from these areas examined in 10–20% KOH on a microscopic slide will demonstrate the "copper pennies" which appear as pigmented sclerotic bodies. In crusts, pus, and exudate the fungus may appear in the form of long, septate, branched, hyphal strands. Because of frequent contamination with bacteria and other fungi, direct examination of specimens should be confirmed by culture on Sabouraud glucose agar containing chloramphenicol and cycloheximide and kept at 25–30°C for 4–6 weeks.[1] Skin testing and serologic evaluation are not helpful in making the diagnosis.

TREATMENT

In the early stages of the disease when the lesions are small and few in number, wide and deep surgical excision is the treatment of choice. However, most cases seen in clinical practice are advanced and require medical therapy. In general, medical therapy for chromomycosis has been disappointing. Drugs or procedures including topical antifungals, potassium iodide, amphotericin B, thiabendazole, vitamin D_2, 5-fluorocytosine (5-FC), ketoconazole, itraconazole, cryosurgery, and local heat have all been reported to have varying degrees of success. At a daily oral dose of 100–200 mg/kg/day at 6-hour intervals for periods of up to 1 year, 5-FC has been successful in causing the rapid regression of lesions, symptoms, and organisms.[6] However, relapse, resistance, and partial cure are common with 5-FC. Lesions that recur after 5-FC therapy may grow rapidly and show resistance to this agent. Combination therapy with 5-FC and ketoconazole, 200–400 mg/day orally, was successful in a case where ketoconazole alone failed.[7] Apparent cure was achieved in 8 of 9 cases of chromomycosis due to *C. carrionii* and in 2 of 5 cases due to *F. pedrosoi* with itraconazole in doses of 100–400 mg/day orally for 4–8 months.[8] Relapses also occurred after itraconazole. Marked improvement was reported when 5-FC and thermotherapy were used in combination with itraconozole in 3 patients.[8] Thiabendazole in doses of up to 2 g/day orally and amphotericin B intralesionally have been used with limited success.[9,10] Despite successful reports of intravenous amphotericin B plus 5-FC, this author does not recommend its use because minimal inhibitory concentrations of amphotericin B are very high for these fungi. Local thermal treatment by battery-driven pocket warmers may be useful as adjunctive therapy.[11]

REFERENCES

1. McGinnis MR. Chromoblastomycosis and phaeohyphomycosis: New concepts, diagnosis and mycology. J Am Acad Dermatol. 1983;8:1–16.
2. Carrion A. Chromoblastomycosis. Ann NY Acad Sci. 1950;50:1255–1281.
3. Sonck CE. Chromomycosis in Finland. Dermatologia. 1975;19:189–193.
4. Rippon JW. Medical Mycology: The Pathogenic Fungi and the Pathogenic Actinomycetes. 2nd ed. Philadelphia: WB Saunders; 1982:249–76.
5. Fukushiro R. Chromomycosis in Japan. Int J Dermatol. 1983;22:221–9.
5a. Fader RC, McGinnis MR. Infections caused by dematiaceous fungi: Chromoblastomycosis and phaeohyphomycosis. In: Infectious Disease Clinics of North America. 2:4. Philadelphia: WB Saunders; 1988:925–38.
6. Lopes CF, Alvarenga RJ, Cisalpeno EO, et al. Six years experience in treatment of chromomycosis with 5-fluorocytosine. Int J Dermatol. 1978;17:414–8.
7. Silber JG, Gombert ME, Green K, et al. Treatment of chromomycosis with ketoconazole and 5-fluorocytosine. J Am Acad Dermatol. 1983;8:236–38.
8. Borelli D. A clinical trial of itraconazole in the treatment of deep mycosis and leishmaniasis. Rev Infect. Dis. 1987;9(Suppl):57–63.

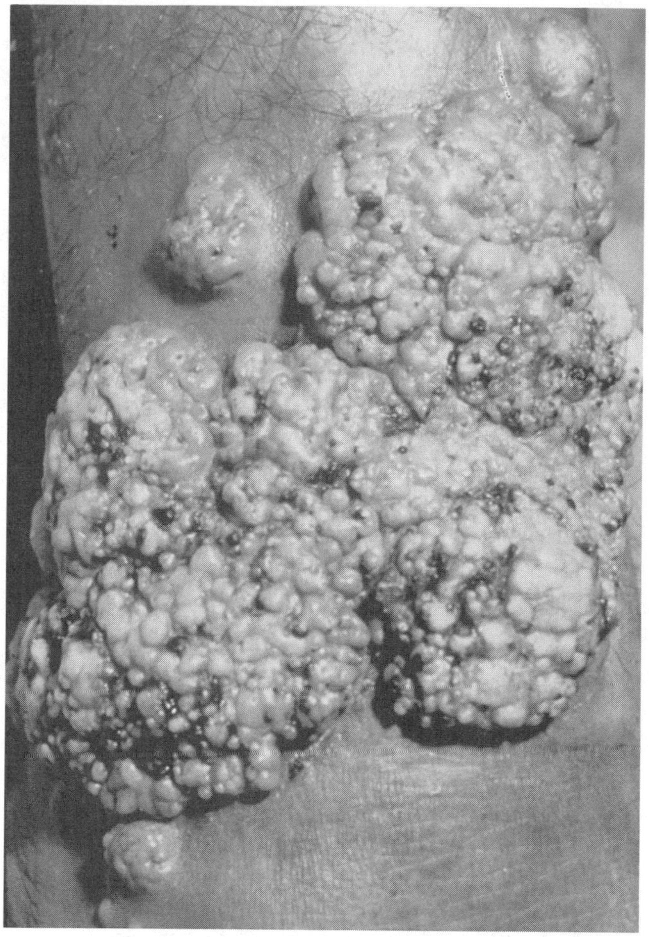

FIG. 2. Pedunculated cauliflower-like chromomycosis lesions showing "black dots" at the apices of microabscesses on the leg of a Panamanian patient.

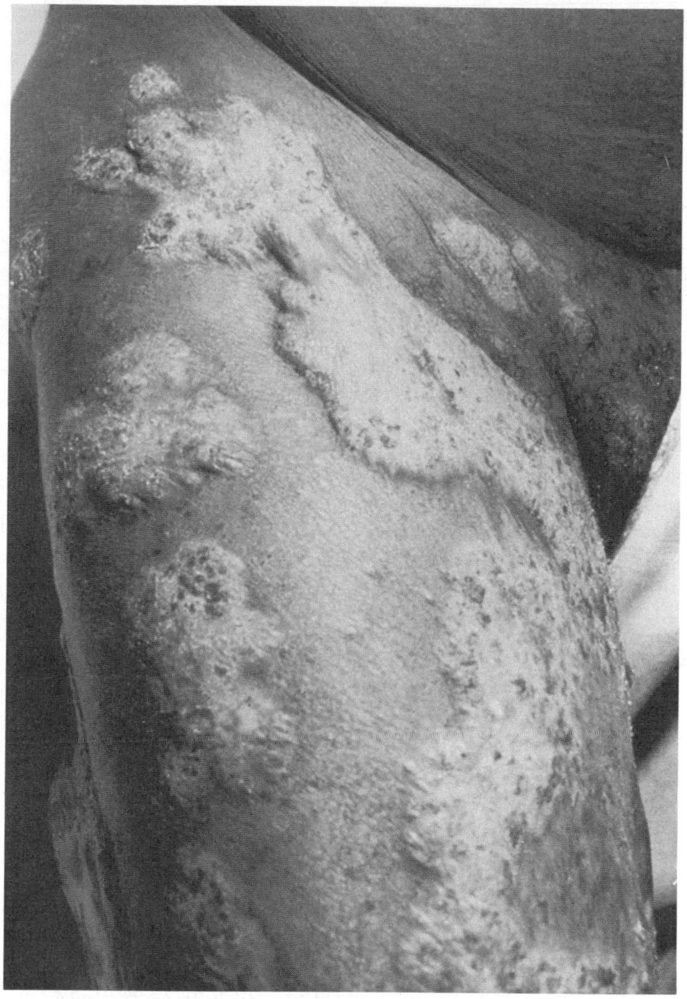

FIG. 3. Annular, flattened papular type of chromomycosis with raised active borders on the leg of a Panamanian patient.

9. Bayles MAH. Chromomycosis: Treatment with thiabendazole. Arch Dermatol. 1971;104:476–85.
10. Whiting DA. Treatment of chromoblastomycosis with high local concentrations of amphotericin B. Br J Dermatol. 1967;79:345.
11. Kinbara T, Fukushiro R, Eryu Y. Chromomycosis—report of two cases successfully treated with local heat therapy. Mykosen. 1982;25:689–94.

240. AGENTS OF MYCETOMA

EL SHEIKH MAHGOUB

Mycetoma (Madura foot) is a local chronic progressive destructive infection of the skin, subcutaneous tissues, fascia, bone, and muscle. After implantation of the organism, the infection, usually on a foot or hand or any site that is subject to trauma, produces a localized swelling containing suppurative granulomas and multiple sinus tracts that extrude grains (granules) of various colors.[1,2] The grains are actual colonies of the causal organism.

ETIOLOGY

Mycetoma caused by true fungi (Eumycetes) is referred to as eumycetoma. The causal fungi described so far include *Pseudallescheria boydii, Madurella mycetomatis, Madurella grisea, Phialophora jeanselmei, Pyrenochaeta romeroi, Leptosphaeria senegaliensis, Neotestudina rosatii, Aspergillus nidulans* or *flavus*, and species of *Fusarium* and *Acremonium*. Actinomycetoma refers to infection caused by aerobic actinomycetes including *Actinomadura madurae, Actinomadura pelletieri, Streptomyces somaliensis, Nocardia brasiliensis, Nocardia asteroides*, and *Nocardia otitidiscaviarum* (*N. caviae*).[3] Several species of dermatophytes also cause a mycetoma-like infection of the scalp and neck,[4,5] but dermatophytes are not considered agents of mycetoma because they do not invade bone.

EPIDEMIOLOGY

In 1842, Gill described the disease for the first time in India in a dispensary in Madur District,[6] hence the derivation of Madura foot, maduromycetoma, *Madurella*, and *Actinomadura madurae*. Both Bidie in 1862 and Carter in 1874[7,8] quite independently from one another have given a full account of the disease and its incidence in India. Today, mycetoma is found worldwide between the Tropics of Cancer and Capricorn. The infection is seen most often in India, Mexico, Niger, Senegal, Somalia, Sudan, Venezuela, Yemen, and Zaire but is not limited to these areas.

The most frequent cause of the disease in the United States is *Pseudallescheria* boydii, which has been isolated frequently from soil in the United States and Canada.[9] *Madurella mycetomatis* and *S. somaliensis* predominate in tropical areas of Africa and India, and *Nocardia brasiliensis* and *A. madurae* are the most common cause of mycetoma in Mexico and Central and South America.[10] *Nocardia asteroides* is reported to predominate in Japan.

PATHOGENESIS AND PATHOLOGIC FINDINGS

Saprophytic soil fungi enter the tissues of the bare foot or hand after local trauma most commonly by a thorn prick. The chest wall and back are infected by sacks contaminated with soil carried over the shoulders. The carrying of wood bundles on the head and shoulders leads to head and neck mycetoma.

The infection begins in the skin and subcutaneous tissues. Mycetoma tends to follow fascial planes in its proximal, lateral, and deep spread as it progressively involves and destroys connective tissue and bone.

Involved tissue reveals a suppurative granuloma. Grains are seen embedded in an abscess composed of neutrophils accompanied by an outer epithelioid cell, plasma cell, and multinucleated giant cell reaction intermingled with areas of fibrosis. Within these suppurative foci the grains are surrounded by an amorphous eosinophilic, homogeneous hyaline-like material termed the *Splendore-Hoeppli phenomenon*. Ultrastructural studies have revealed that this part of the grain matrix is host derived.[11]

The involved area is characterized by tumefaction, multiple sinus formation, and fistulous tracts that communicate with each other, with deep abscesses, and with ulcerated areas of the skin. The progressive proliferation of granulation and scar tissue leads to enlargement and disfigurement of the affected part.

CLINICAL MANIFESTATIONS

Mycetoma is seen most frequently in men between the ages of 20 and 40. A true male-to-female ratio is 5:1. It occurs most often in farmers and other laborers in rural areas who are frequently exposed to penetrating wounds by thorns and splinters. The most common site of infection is the foot, particularly on the dorsum of the fore part. A painless massively swollen indurated foot riddled with sinuses is the most common presentation (Fig. 1). Constitutional complaints are rare, and pyrexia implies secondary bacteria infection. Extrapedal cases appear on other parts of the body in contact with soil during work, sitting, or lying; thus the hand, leg, torso, arm, head, thigh (Fig. 2), and buttocks may also be infected. When the scalp is involved, it usually starts in the back of the head and neck or the frontal part.

The earliest manifestation is a small painless papule or nodule on the sole or dorsum of the foot that progressively increases in size. Such development in usually quicker in actinomycetoma than eumycetoma. The skin lesions swell and rupture with sinus tract formation. As the infection spreads, similar lesions appear on adjacent parts. Old sinuses heal and close up, but new ones open at other sites. Thus, an old mycetoma is characterized by healed scars in addition to sinuses. Months or years later, destruction of deeper tissues, including bone, is manifested as generalized swelling that remains painless except in about 15 percent of patients who report to the hospital primarily because of pain.

The course is progressive as local tissue undergoes a recurring cycle of swelling, suppuration, and scarring. Ultimately, an infected site becomes a swollen deformed mass of destroyed tissue with many fistulas through which grains are discharged. The infection never spreads hematogenously, but regional lymphadenopathy may occur.[12] Involved tissue may become secondarily infected by bacteria.

In the bone, the cortex is invaded, and masses of grains gradually replace osseous tissue and marrow. Radiographs reveal

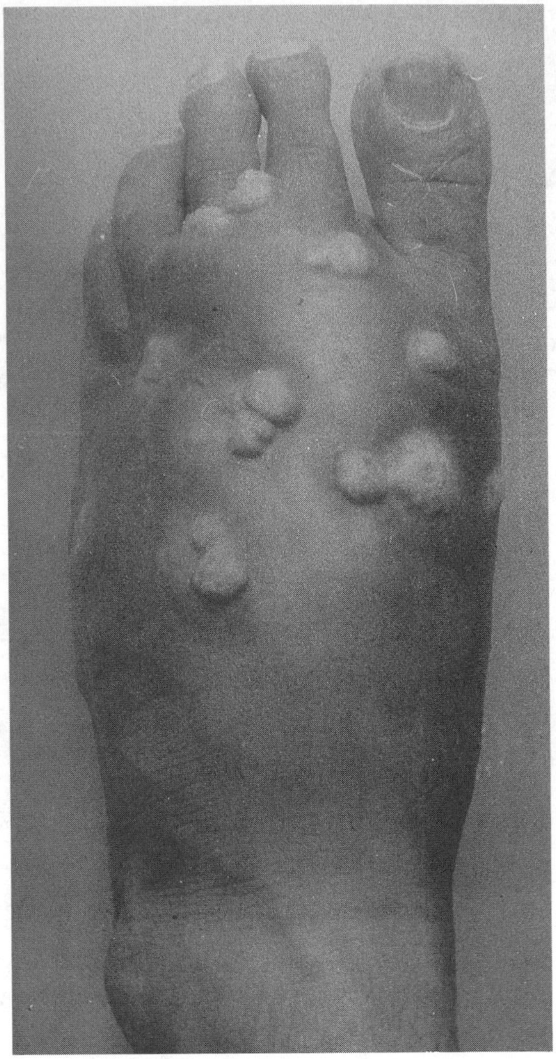

FIG. 1. Actinomycetoma pedis due to *Actinomadura madurae*.

osteolytic lesions called cavities (Fig. 3) and periosteal new bone formation.

Mycetomas of the skull show diffuse thickening of bones due to dense bone formation and a loss of the trabecular pattern, but in a few areas there may be small osteolytic areas as well.[13] Pure osteolytic changes are not seen.

DIAGNOSIS

The triad of signs, indurated swelling, multiple sinus tracts draining grain-filled pus, and the usual localization on a foot characterize a well-developed mycetoma.[14] Characteristic grains in draining sinuses are 0.2–3.0 mm in diameter and may be black, white, yellow, pink, or red depending on the causal organism. Grains may be difficult to locate in histopathologic sections and require multiple cuts through the paraffin-embedded tissue. Hematoxylin-eosin (H&E) stain is adequate to detect the grains (Fig. 4). Tissue Gram staining will detect fine branching hyphae within the actinomycetoma grain, and Gomori methenamine sliver or periodic acid–Schiff (PAS), particularly in the case of pale grains, will detect the larger hyphae of eumycetoma. Species of the agent can often be guessed by the color, size, compaction, and hematoxylin-staining character of the grain.[1]

A more exact species diagnosis is dependent on culture of the grain and isolation of the organism. The grain obtained for

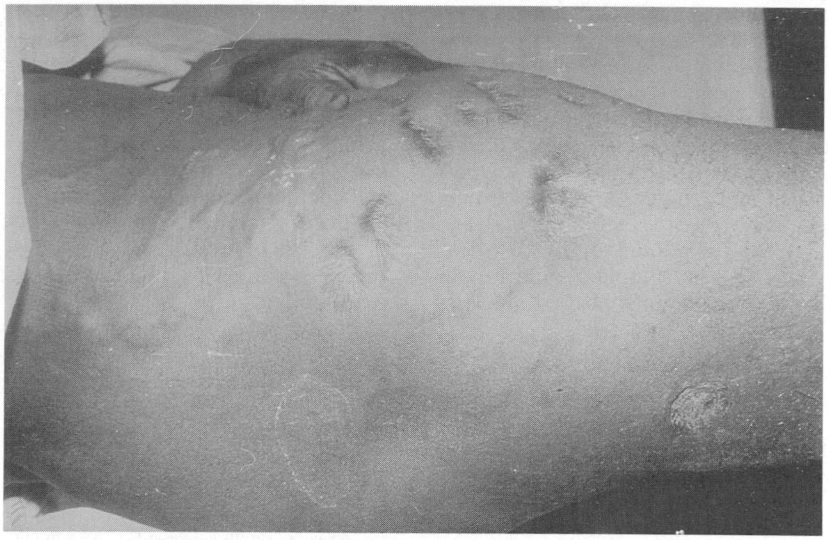

FIG. 2. Mycetoma of the thigh caused by *Streptomyces somaliensis*.

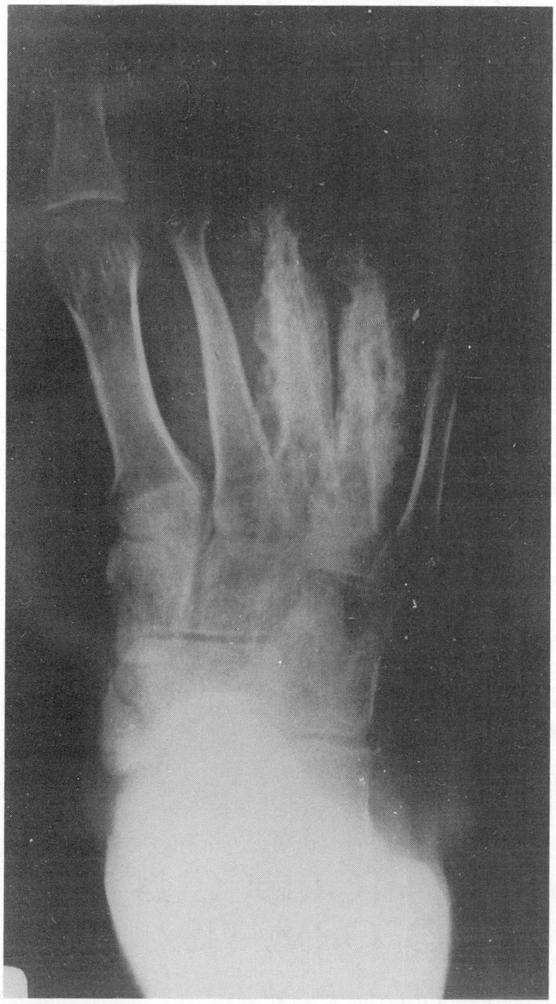

FIG. 3. Radiograph showing small multiple cavities caused by *S. somaliensis*.

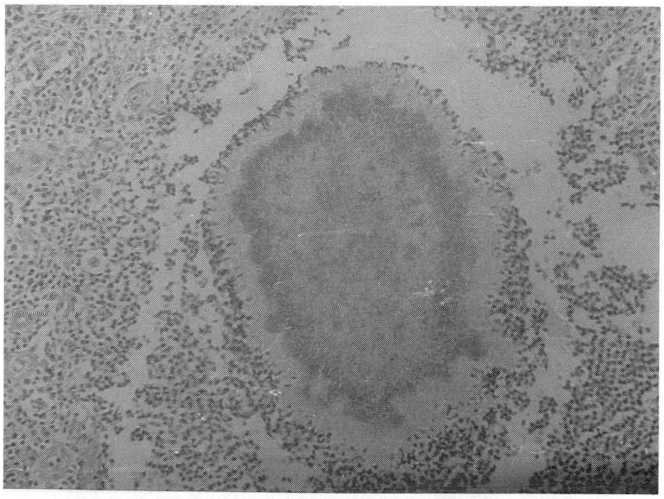

FIG. 4. A young grain of *A. madurae* in the middle of an abscess composed mainly of polymorphonuclear leukocytes. Note the dark coloured basophilic center and pale eosinophilic border. (H&E, ×200)

culture must be as free as possible from bacterial and fungal contamination. A wedge-shaped, deep-seated biopsy provides a good specimen for both histologic and cultural diagnosis. Before being inoculated onto culture media, the grains should be rinsed quickly in 70% alcohol and washed several times in sterile saline. Biopsy specimens are preferred over grains discharged through sinuses because the grains may be contaminated with surface organisms. For primary isolation actinomycetoma grains are grown on Löwenstein-Jensen medium and fungal grains on blood agar. Sabouraud agar without antibacterial antibiotics is a satisfactory culture medium for subcultures.

Serologic diagnosis is at present routinely used in a few centers. Determination of antibodies by means of immunodiffusion (ID) or counterimmunoelectrophoresis (CIE) is used for both serologic diagnosis and follow-up during medical treatment.[15]

DIFFERENTIAL DIAGNOSIS

In endemic areas, a painless, firm, subcutaneous swelling should be regarded as a mycetoma until proved otherwise even in the absence of sinuses. Once mycetoma has invaded bone, the entity is readily confused with chronic bacterial ostoemyelitis. Botryomycosis is a chronic bacterial infection that presents as an indurated fibrotic subcutaneous mass and draining sinuses resembling a mycetoma; grains (colonies of bacteria) are found in the purulent exudate and in tissue sections. Although botryomycosis is most commonly a disease of the skin and subcutaneous tissues, unlike mycetoma, it may also involve viscera. The etiologic agents of botryomycosis include a number of gram-positive cocci (staphylococci, streptococci) and gram-negative bacilli (*Escherichia coli, Pseudomonas, Proteus* species). In the absence of sinuses, mycetoma should be differentiated from benign or malignant tumors, a cold abscess, or a thorn granuloma.[16]

TREATMENT AND PROGNOSIS

Through health education, patients are encouraged to report early to hospitals. However, mycetoma at all stages could be amenable to medical treatment alone or in combination with limited surgery. The latter is sometimes described as bulk-reduction surgery, but amputation or disarticulation should be avoided. The success of treatment depends not only on the differentiation between actinomycetoma and eumycetoma but also on a definitive identification of the causal organism.

In all cases of actinomycetoma, a combination of two drugs is used.[17] One of these is always in streptomycin sulphate in a dose of 14 mg/kg daily for the first month and on alternate days thereafter. In patients with *A. madurae,* dapsone is given orally at 1.5 mg/kg in the morning and evening. Similarly, *S. somaliensis* mycetoma is treated by dapsone first, but if no response

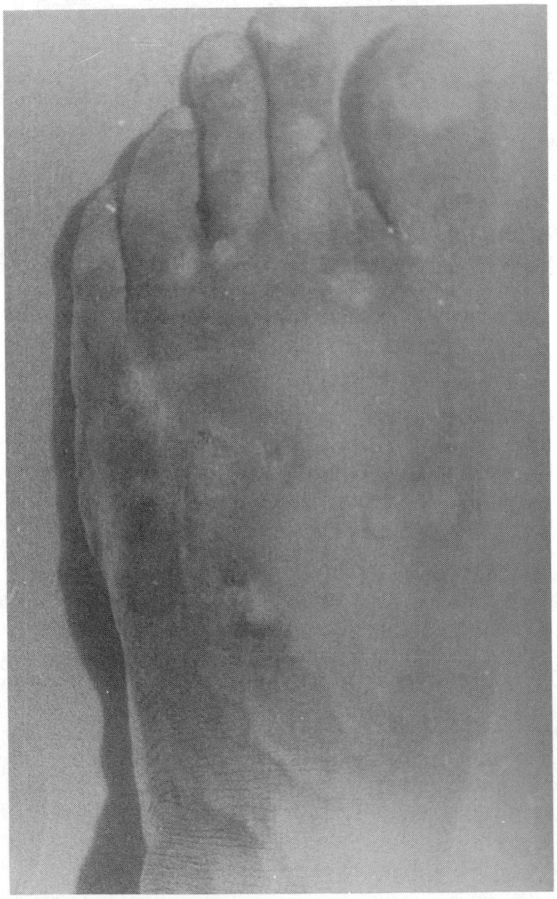

FIG. 5. The same patient with *A. madurae* as in Figure 1 after the end of treatment.

appears after 1 month, treatment is changed to trimethoprim-sulfamethoxazole tablets at 23 mg/kg/day of sulfamethoxazole and 4.6 mg/kg/day of trimethoprim (in two divided doses). *Actinomadura pelletierii* mycetoma responds better to streptomycin and trimethoprim-sulfamethoxazole, which was also our experience with *N. brasiliensis* in Sudan. However, such mycetoma due to *Nocardia* in the Americas is treated with trimethaprim-sulfamethoxazole and dapsone[18] or trimethaprim-sulfamethoxazole and amikacin.[19]

Successful medical treatment in eumycetoma has been thus far recorded in mycetoma caused by *M. mycetomatis.*[20] A cure can be obtained by giving ketoconazole in a dose of 200 mg twice daily.

In all cases of medical management, treatment is given for at least 10 months (Fig. 5). Although side effects are few, patients are regularly followed up by assessing hematologic, kidney, or liver functions, depending on the drug used.

REFERENCES

1. Mahgoub ES, Murray IG. Mycetoma. London: Heinemann; 1973:1–97.
2. Zaias N, Taplin D, Rebell G. Mycetoma. Arch Dermatol. 1969;99:215–25.
3. Tight RR, Bartlett MS. Actinomycetoma in the United States. Rev Infect Dis. 1981;3:1139–50.
4. West BC, Kwon-Chung KJ. Mycetoma caused by *Microsporum audouinii.* First reported case. Am J Clin Pathol. 1980;73:447–55.
5. West BC. Five year follow up of a man with subcutaneous mycetomas caused by *Microsporum audouinii.* Am J Clin Pathol. 1982;77:767.
6. Gill. India Army Medical Reports. London: Churchill. 1874.
7. Bidie G. Notes on Morbus Pedis Entophyticus. Madras Q J Med Sci. 1862;4:222–7.
8. Carter HV. On Mycetoma or the Fungus Disease of India. London: Churchill; 1874.
9. Green WO, Adams TE. Mycetoma in the United States. Am J Clin Pathol. 1964;42:75–91.
10. Lavalle P. Micetomas: La experiencia mexicana. Problemas actuales. In: Libro de resumens II Simposio internacional de micetomas. Taxco, Mexico, 1987.
11. Wethered DB, Markey MA, Hay RJ, et al. Ultrastructural and immunogenic changes in the formation of mycetoma grains. J Med Vet Mycol. 1986;25:39–46.
12. El Hassan AM, Mahgoub ES. Lymph node involvement in mycetoma. Trans R Soc Trop Med Hyg. 1972;66:165–9.
13. Gumaa SA, Mahgoub ES, El Sid MA. Mycetoma of the head and neck. Am J Trop Med Hyg. 1986;35:594–600.
14. Vanbreuseghem R. The early diagnosis of mycetoma. Dermatol Int. 1967;6:123–40.
15. Gumaa SA, Mahgoub ES. Counterimmunoelectrophoresis in the diagnosis of mycetoma and its sensitivity as compared to immunodiffusion. Sabouraudia 1975;13:309–15.
16. Davies AGM. The bone changes of madura foot, observations on Uganda Africans. Radiology. 1958;70:841–47.
17. Mahgoub ES. Medical management of mycetoma. WHO Bull. 1976;54:303–10.
18. Caire P., Arenas R, Suchil P, et al. Tratamiento de micetomas por Nocardia, Experiencia en 50 pacientes. In Libro de Resumenes II Simposio Internacional de Micetomas. Taxco, Mexico; 1987:49.
19. Welsh O, Sauceda E, Gonzalez J. Amikacin y trimetoprim sulphametoxazole. el tratamiento de micetomas actinomicosicos. In: Libro de resumenes II Simposio Internacional de micetomas. Taxco, Mexico; 1987:48.
20. Mahgoub ES, Gumaa SA. Ketoconazole in the treatment of eumycetoma due to *Madurella mycetomatis.* Trans R Soc Trop Med Hyg. 1984;78:376–9.

241. CRYPTOCOCCUS NEOFORMANS

RICHARD D. DIAMOND

Cryptococcosis is a systemic infection caused by the yeastlike fungus *Cryptococcus neoformans*. There are reports that other species of *Cryptococcus* have caused infection, but, to date, none are well documented. Older names for this disease include

European blastomycosis and *torulosis*. The latter name derives from *Torula histolytica*, an old and poorly chosen name for *C. neoformans*.

MYCOLOGY

Cryptococcus neoformans is an encapsulated, yeastlike fungus that reproduces by budding. The cell is round or oval, usually 4–6 μm in diameter, though rarely, larger yeast or pseudomycelia forms may develop. The surrounding capsule may vary greatly in size, depending on growth conditions such as carbon dioxide concentration.[1] At least in experimental studies in mice, the size of the capsule does not appear to be related to virulence,[2] although virulence may be reduced in totally unencapsulated mutants.[3] In any case, the capsule confers several properties on the organism that affect the host response to infection (see the section on "Pathophysiology" below).

IDENTIFICATION

On solid culture media, colonies of *C. neoformans* are smooth, convex, and yellow or tan. Differentiation from other yeastlike fungi involves several procedures. *C. neoformans* grows at 37°C, whereas most nonpathogenic species of *Cryptococcus* do not. In addition, *C. neoformans* does not produce pseudomycelia on cornmeal or rice-Tween agar and hydrolyzes urea during growth on Christensen's agar. For the latter, results of presumptive screening tests may be available in as few as 15 minutes.[4] Glucose is not fermented but is assimilated by the fungus. Dulcitol, inositol, maltose, and sucrose are assimilated, but lactose and nitrate are not.[5] Many strains of *C. neoformans* can use creatinine as a nitrogen source, which may partially explain growth of the organism in creatinine-rich avian feces. Mouse pathogenicity has also been used as a specific procedure for identification of *C. neoformans*. Another useful procedure is based upon the property of *C. neoformans* (but not nonpathogenic yeasts) to produce the brown pigment melanin. The fungal enzyme phenol oxidase acts on certain substrates, such as caffeic acid and dihydroxyphenylalanine, rather than tyrosine, in contrast to melanin synthesis in humans. Indeed, melanin production appears to be related to virulence of cryptococcosis in experimental murine infections,[6] although the mechanism of this effect remains to be established. Originally, agar medium made with glucose, creatinine, and an extract of *Guizotia abyssinica*, a common canary seed (so-called birdseed agar), was used to detect pigment production.[5] Newer modifications of this medium consist of chemically defined substrates, such as caffeic acid in cornmeal agar or paper strips saturated with a solution of L-β-3-dihydroxyphenylalanine-ferric citrate placed on standard agar plates.[7] Use of such media for primary isolation enables immediate separation and presumptive identification of *C. neoformans*, even if colonies of other fungi are present.

Serotypes and Perfect States

Based on antigenic specificity of the capsular polysaccharide, there are four different serotypes of *C. neoformans*—A, B, C, and D[8]—though some strains react with antisera to serotypes A and D. Serotyping may be performed using agglutination or immunofluorescence procedures.[9] Suitable strains of serotypes A and D, which include the large majority of clinical isolates of *C. neoformans*, can be mated to produce the perfect (sexual) state, now termed *Filobasidiella neoformans* var *neoformans*, originally described by Kwon-Chung in 1975.[10] Serotypes B and C are classified as *C. neoformans* var *gattii* because of several characteristics that distinguish them from serotype A and D isolates. First, strains with serotypes B and C form a distinct perfect state,[11] now termed *Filobasidiella neoformans* var *bacillispora*, although a few strains of serotypes A and D have been shown to be able to mate with B and C organisms, albeit with a low survival rate. It has also been noted that serotypes A and D vs. B and C have different geographic distributions and different frequencies of isolation from pigeon droppings.[12,13] Furthermore, biochemical differences between the serotypes of *C. neoformans* are apparent. Most serotype B and C isolates assimilate l-malic, fumaric, and succinic acids produce green pigment on selective (Guizotia seed) media, and can assimilate glycine as a sole carbon source, whereas serotypes A and D isolates generally do not.[14,15] Improved media have been developed for distinguishing serotype B and C from A and D isolates, including blueing of the agar around colonies of B and C but not A and D strains using an agar medium containing L-canavanine, glycine, and bromthymol blue,[15] or inhibition of urease activity by 100 μM ethylenediaminetetraacetic acid (EDTA) in serotype B and C but not A and D strains.[16] Based upon analysis of DNA base composition and sequence homology studies, there are genetic differences between serotype A and D vs. B and C strains as well.[17]

ECOLOGY AND EPIDEMIOLOGY

Relation of Site in Nature to Acquisition of Infections

C. neoformans is a saprobe in nature, with a worldwide distribution rather than any defined endemic area. Since the time of Emmons' original work, the fungus has been found frequently throughout the world in aged pigeon droppings as well as in nesting places such as window ledges and barns.[18] Although *C. neoformans* grows to high concentrations in pigeon feces, the birds are not infected.[18] Soil may also contain the fungus, especially if it is contaminated with bird droppings. Survival of *C. neoformans* in soil may be affected by a variety of biotic factors, as soil bacteria, amoebae, mites, or sow bugs are capable of inhibiting or killing the fungi.[19] Much less commonly, *C. neoformans* has also been isolated from fruits and a variety of other sources in nature. Naturally acquired cryptococcosis occurs in animals as well as in humans, but animal-to-person transmission has not been documented.[18] This is true even after heavy exposure from drinking nonpasteurized milk produced by cattle with cryptococcal mastitis. Rather, circumstantial evidence suggests that disease occurs after the organism is aerosolized and inhaled. In favor of this, viable particles of *C. neoformans* with a size compatible with alveolar deposition (<2 μm) have been isolated in nature from pigeon excreta and soil.[20] Furthermore, healthy persons with a history of heavy exposure to pigeons have a much higher rate of positive delayed skin tests to cryptococcal antigen, or cryptococcin.[21] However, unlike other aerosol-borne mycoses, cases of cryptococcosis rarely occur in clusters, there is no occupational predisposition, histories of exposure to pigeons or dust are not helpful, and there is usually neither historical nor roentgenographic evidence of respiratory infection at the time of diagnosis. Person-to-person transmission has not been documented by the pulmonary route, although a unique case report suggests that a case of cryptococcal endophthalmitis originated from a corneal transplant obtained from a donor who had active cryptococcosis.[22] Furthermore, laboratory workers frequently are exposed to aerosols of the organism, as indicated by a high incidence of positive cryptococcin skin tests,[23] yet laboratory-acquired pulmonary or disseminated cryptocococcosis has never been described. Likewise, rare instances of documented accidental cutaneous inoculation with *C. neoformans* have resulted in localized cutaneous lesions without dissemination.[24] Similarly, recent work on serotypes of *C. neoformans* casts further doubt on the central role of the pigeon in the epidemiology of all cases of cryptococcosis. Though most cases of cryptococcosis are caused by serotype A or D strains, serotypes B and C are responsible for a significant number of infections in tropical and subtropical areas of the world. However, no serotype B or C isolates have been found in pigeon droppings or soil. The ecologic site of these B and C serotype organisms in nature is unknown.

Factors Predisposing to Infection

Because the organism is ubiquitous, it is presumed that exposure to *C. neoformans* is common. Skin test surveys of normal subjects provide some support for this assumption.[21,23] Nevertheless, there must be high natural resistance to infection because new cases were relatively rare, prior to the advent of the acquired immunodeficiency syndrome (AIDS). Review of a large series of cases of cryptococcosis indicates a threefold preponderance of males over females and an excess of white over highly pigmented people.[18] However, this may relate either to differences in host susceptibility or to the likelihood of exposure. There is also an increased incidence of cryptococcosis in patients who are receiving therapeutic doses of corticosteroids, patients with lymphoreticular malignancies (especially Hodgkin's disease), and those with sarcoidosis (even in the absence of corticosteroid therapy).[25] Diabetes mellitus has also been cited as predisposing to cryptococcosis,[18] but the association is less clear-cut than with the above-mentioned factors.[25] Cryptococcosis has been diagnosed frequently after renal transplantation, but corticosteroid therapy appears to be the major factor involved in most cases.[26] Though cyclosporin A suppresses cellular host defense mechanisms, it also appears to inhibit the growth of *C. neoformans* both in vitro and in vivo.[27] A recent large increase in cryptococcosis has occurred in association with AIDS. *C. neoformans* has emerged as the fourth most common cause of life-threatening infections after *Pneumocystis carinii*, cytomegalovirus, and mycobacteria.[28–30] Excluding this latter group of patients, more than half the patients with cryptococcosis have no apparent predisposing factors.[25] The existence of a genetic predisposition to cryptococcosis in humans has not been established, although a single, recent, brief report documented the onset of cryptococcosis 10 years apart in two previously healthy siblings,[31] and genetic factors have been described that increase susceptibility to experimental murine cryptococcosis.[32]

PATHOPHYSIOLOGY

Pathology

C. neoformans elaborates no known exotoxins, so tissue is only displaced by multiplying organisms, with little necrosis and organ dysfunction until late in the course of most infections or earlier with heavy infections. Hemorrhage, infarction, calcification, and extensive fibrosis are extremely rare. The inflammatory response to infection is variable, ranging from minimal to strong. Outside the central nervous system, and to a lesser extent in the meninges, macrophages and giant cells are seen with ingested or adjacent cryptococci together with plasma cells and lymphocytes, but well-formed granulomas are generally not present. Some inflammatory infiltrates are of mixed cell types or contain predominantly neutrophils. The characteristic lesion within the brain, also sometimes seen in other tissues as well, consists of cystic clusters of fungi with no inflammatory response (Fig. 1). These lesions are spread diffusely and prominently throughout the brain, so the disease would be more properly termed a *meningoencephalitis*, rather than a *meningitis*. Typically, the basal ganglia and cortical gray matter are most heavily involved. Large focal collections of organisms with some inflammatory response may occur in the brain (cryptococcoma, cryptococcal granuloma), but these are rare exceptions to the usual diffuse pattern of infection. In severe infections, the brain becomes swollen and soft from the generalized infection. Leptomeninges are often thickened, with distension of the subarachnoid by a white, gelatinous material (largely attributable to the cryptococcal capsular polysaccharide.[33]

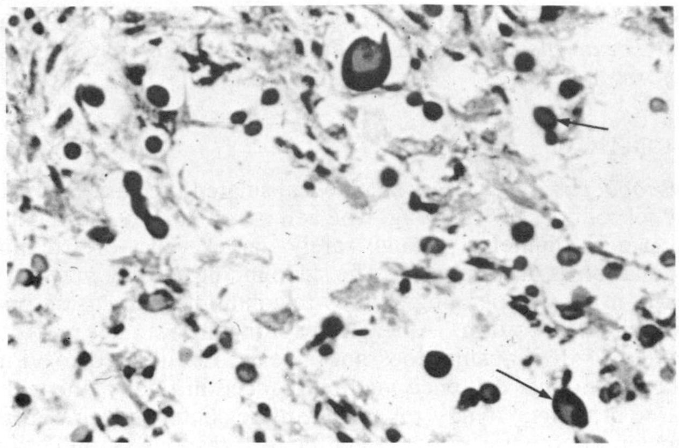

FIG. 1. Cryptococci in brain, delineated by thin, dark-staining cell walls (periodic acid-Schiff). Some cells have characteristic narrow-based buds (arrows). An artifactual halo is visible around organisms as a consequence of shrinkage of the capsule around the cell wall during fixation, rather than tissue necrosis. No inflammatory cells are visible. (×800)

Cellular Host Defense Mechanisms

The mechanisms responsible for the strong, natural host resistance to cryptococcosis have been clarified by a number of experimental studies. It is known from experimental pulmonary infections in mice that neutrophils initially clear most of the cryptococci; then monocytes predominate in the later inflammatory infiltrates.[34] Human neutrophils and monocytes can ingest and kill cryptococci in vitro, using the myeloperoxidase-peroxide-halide mechanism[35] and perhaps neutrophil cationic proteins as well.[36]

Activation of neutrophils with supernatants from stimulated lymphocytes enhances their ability to ingest (and therefore kill) cryptococci with large capsules.[37] Activation of macrophages from the lung[38] or elsewhere[39] by interferon or other factors[40] renders them fungistatic (and perhaps fungicidal) for cryptococci in vitro. This process appears to parallel (but is not directly attributable to) macrophage production of nitrite by an arginase-dependent mechanism.[41] Encapsulated *C. neoformans* organisms may be sufficiently large to preclude phagocytosis, but they can still be surrounded and killed by "rings" of macrophages.[42] Presumably, immunity and macrophage activation require functioning, sensitized T cells.[42,43] In addition to macrophages, natural killer cells can inhibit the growth of cryptococci in vitro by nonphagocytic mechanisms, thereby contributing to clearance of experimental cryptococcosis in vivo.[44,45] However, the significance of the latter activity as a major component of clearance of respiratory-acquired infections has been questioned.[46] Products of natural killer cells also may have an important immunoregulatory role. Anticryptococcal antibodies enhance the inhibitory effects of natural killer cells,[47] and various other effector cells can mediate antibody-dependent, cell-mediated killing of cryptococci.[48] T cells themselves can also be fungistatic for cryptococci.[49]

While the above-mentioned cellular fungicidal mechanisms may be important in clearing cryptococci from sites of infection, defects in these mechanisms do not seem to correlate with susceptibility to cryptococcosis in individual patients. In contrast, patients with cryptococcosis who have no known predisposing factors often have a variety of defects in parameters of cell-mediated immunity. In patients with active disease, or even in those cured and tested several years after treatment, there often are persistent abnormalities in a variety of parameters. These include delayed skin test and in vitro cellular immune responses, such as lymphocyte transformation or production of migration inhibitory factors in response to cryptococcal antigens and, sometimes, to other antigens or to mitogens.[50] Antigen-specific suppression of cell-mediated responses may contribute to such defects. In vitro, whole *C. neoformans* cells stimulate proliferation and interleukin 2 production by T cells from cryptococcosis patients and even from those of healthy persons previously primed with cryptococci; this is followed by an early increase in the number of T8 cells.[51] In experimental murine cryptococcosis, cryptococcal mannoprotein antigens[51] induce and adsorb specifically to a Lyt-1$^+$ IJ$^+$ first-order suppressor T-cell population; these cells not only inhibit the L3T4$^+$ Lyt-2$^-$ cells responsible for initiation of delayed hypersensitivity but also induce second-order suppressor cells, which, in turn, induce third-order Thy-1$^+$ L3T4$^-$ Lyt-2$^+$ IJ$^+$ cells capable of suppressing efferent responses.[52–54] In addition, macrophage-suppressive lymphokines are produced,[55] which might contribute to the observed depression of chemotaxis and the accompanying cutaneous anergy observed in patients with cryptococcosis.[56] In addition, data from experimental studies in guinea pigs suggest that the outcome of most of those experimental infections may be determined by the quantity of the inflammatory response in infectious foci, rather than by the ability of individual leukocytes to kill cryptococci.[57] The cryptococcal cell wall can activate the alternative complement pathway to generate C5a, which is chemotactic for human neutrophils and monocytes,[58,59] a process that may be impaired in some patients with cryptococcosis.[59] In any case, although defects of cellular function occur in association with cryptococcosis in humans, it is not clear whether these defects represent a product of the infection or a preexisting factor that predisposes to the infection.

Cryptococcal Polysaccharide

Within the tissues of the host, *C. neoformans* has a large, distinctive capsule. The major constituent of the capsule appears to be a relatively unbranched chain of α1-3 linked mannose units, substituted with xylosyl or β-glucuronyl groups. Serotype specificity appears to be determined by small structural differences in this glucuronoxylomannan, including the number of xylose residues and the degree of O-acetylation of hydroxyl groups. A galactoxylomannan also is present as a minor capsular constituent.[60,61] Cryptococcal polysaccharide may be immunosuppressive. In humans, long after being cured of cryptococcosis, patients often exhibit prolonged, specific, immunologic unresponsiveness to cryptococcal polysaccharide both in vitro and in vivo, but responses to type III pneumococcal polysaccharide are not depressed compared with responses to challenge in immune, healthy persons.[62] Cryptococcal polysaccharide also inhibits phagocytosis, presumably by binding to the yeast surface and blocking recognition by phagocytes, rather than by changing the surface charge or creating a hydrophobic exterior. The polysaccharide may impair leukocyte migration as well.[63,64] The whole organism and the soluble capsular polysaccharide also activate the alternative complement pathway in serum,[65] although this appears to occur only in the presence of high polysaccharide concentrations.[59] However, some patients have had polysaccharide antigenemia documented within such high ranges.[28–30] This has important implications for the generation of factors that are chemotactic for inflammatory cells, as well as those factors that serve as opsonins for phagocytosis. In a few patients with severe cryptococcosis and fungemia, serum complement and opsonins may be depleted, presumably because of direct activation of the alternative complement pathway by the heavy load of organisms.[66] In any case, the documented, prolonged persistence of cryptococcal polysaccharide in tissues of infected animals for prolonged periods of time[67] creates the possibility for mediation of long-term immunologic effects.

Humoral Host Defense

In addition to cellular anticryptococcal mechanisms, several soluble anticryptococcal factors have been described. Anticryptococcal antibody and complement do not directly damage the organism, but antibody and complement are critical components of some of the cellular host defense mechanisms described above.[47,48,58,59,63,68,69] Despite the observation that B-cell-deficient mice do not appear to have increased susceptibility to cryptococcosis,[70] anticapsular IgG opsonizes *C. neoformans* for phagocytosis by macrophages[68] and, when administered intraperitoneally, can protect against an intravenous cryptococcal challenge.[71] In immunized mice, an intact complement system is required for protection against challenge with *C. neoformans* preopsonized with anticryptococcal globulin.[72] Complement activation by *C. neoformans* results largely in deposition on yeast surfaces of C3bi,[69] which can act as an effective opsonin even in the absence of specific anticryptococcal antibodies in the non-immune host.[73] In addition, C5a contributes to chemoattraction of phagocytic cells.[58,59] An anticryptococcal factor, possibly a globulin, is present in normal serum,[74–76] whereas saliva contains a different fungicidal substance.[76]

Localization to the Central Nervous System

Understanding of potential host defense mechanisms against cryptococcosis provides some important insights into why the disease may localize in the central nervous system (CNS). First, soluble anticryptococcal factors, which are present in normal serum, are absent in cerebrospinal fluid (CSF), which is actually a good growth medium for *C. neoformans*.[76] Second, the inflammatory response to cryptococci in the brain is commonly absent in human disease and is delayed in experimental animals.[57,77] Although cryptococci activate the alternative complement pathway in serum, no significant complement activity is detectable in CSF of patients or healthy persons.[66] Presumably, this could lead to a local deficiency of chemotactic and opsonic factors, which would allow lesions to progress in the brain, while large inflammatory reactions cleared infectious foci outside the CNS. In addition, it has been suggested that high levels of dopamine within the CNS might serve as a substrate for cryptococcal melanin production, thereby favoring local proliferation of more virulent yeasts.[6]

CLINICAL MANIFESTATIONS

Central Nervous System

The onset of CNS cryptococcosis is usually insidious, although the manifestations may be more acute, especially in patients who are receiving corticosteroid therapy or who are being treated for lymphoreticular malignancies. Symptoms are usually present for weeks or months. However, the typical waxing and waning course of the disease, often with completely asymptomatic periods, can be misleading. Complaints may be referable to the CNS, although they may be mild and nonspecific, such as headache, nausea, dizziness, irritability, somnolence, and clumsiness. Careful questioning of the patient and family often uncovers examples of impaired memory and judgment, as well as behavior changes that affect relationships with others. If cranial nerves are involved, the patient may notice decreased visual acuity, diplopia, and facial numbness or weakness. If present, seizures usually occur only late in the course of infections. Like the history, physical findings do not provide specific clues to the diagnosis. Patients are often afebrile or have a mildly elevated temperature peaking at approximately 39°C, exaggerating the normal diurnal pattern. Most patients have minimal or no nuchal rigidity. Papilledema is noted in about one-third of the cases and cranial nerve palsies in about one-fifth. In some patients, hyperreflexia, ankle clonus, or extensor plantar responses can be elicited. Choreoathetoid movements or myoclonic jerks may occur. Except for cranial nerve abnormalities, focal sensory or motor lesions are rare until late in the course of the disease. Large focal granulomas may produce focal neurologic findings but are rare.[18,78] Whether an individual patient has an indolent or a rapidly progressing course seems to correlate with the presence or absence of corticosteroid therapy and/or hematologic malignancy. Dementia may develop because of direct involvement of the brain by the infection. However, late recrudescence of symptoms may indicate the presence of hydrocephalus.

Respiratory System

Pulmonary cryptococcosis may be asymptomatic or may cause production of only scant, sometimes blood-streaked, sputum. The patient may complain of a dull ache in the chest. More specific findings suggesting pulmonary pathologic changes, such as rales or pleural friction rub, are rare. Pulmonary cryptococcosis may progress or regress spontaneously or may remain stable for long periods of time. In most cases of CNS cryptococcosis, pulmonary involvement is not apparent. Conversely, involvement of the respiratory tree often occurs alone, although it may also coexist with extrapulmonary cryptococcosis inside and outside the CNS.

Other Sites

Besides the respiratory system, cryptococcosis may involve several other sites outside the CNS.[18,78] Single or multiple skin lesions may be found in as many as 10 percent of the patients, most commonly as painless lesions of the face or scalp. These nonspecific lesions are often ignored, although they are often the first signs of infection. Lesions may appear as small papules, pustules, or soft subcutaneous masses or as larger ulcers with rolled, slightly undermined edges surrounding a base of granulation tissue (Fig. 2). Umbilicated papules in AIDS patients may resemble molluscum contagiosum. Bleeding into lesions may occur in patients with thrombocytopenia, resulting in palpable purpura. Cellulitis with necrotizing vasculitis has been observed in transplant recipients.[79] Regional lymph nodes are not involved. Bone lesions, which resemble cold abscesses like those seen with tuberculosis, may occur in as many as 5–10 percent of the patients,[78] but joint involvement is unusual. Such lesions may be mistaken clinically for neoplasms. In post-transplant patients, cryptococcal pyelonephritis has been reported as a cause of renal allograft rejection.[80] Other, less common forms of cryptococcosis include chorioretinitis, adrenal involvement, myocarditis, endocarditis, pericarditis, esophagitis, hepatitis, peritonitis, arthritis, bursitis, myositis, renal abscess, and prostatis.[18,78]

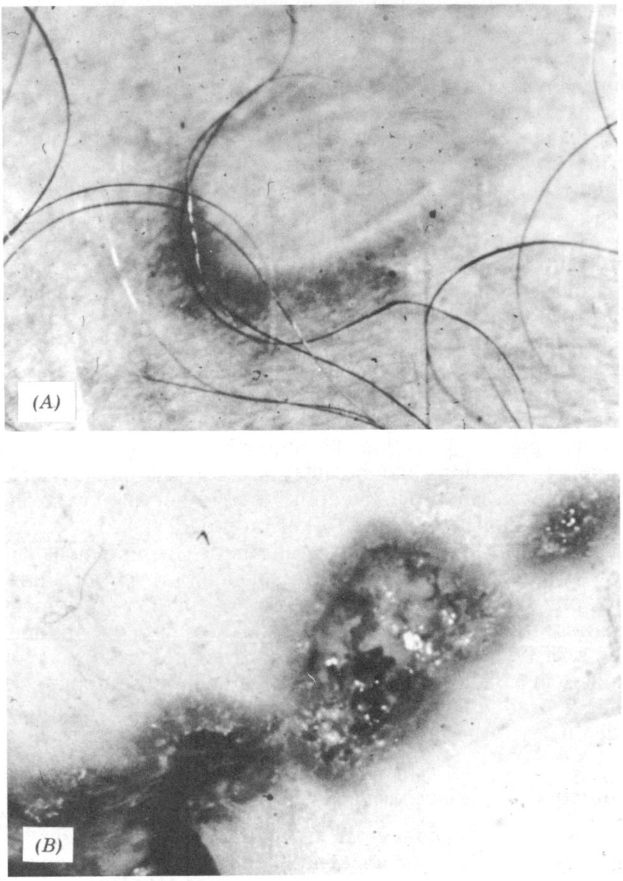

FIG. 2. Nonspecific small lesion of cutaneous cryptococcosis. **(A)** Unusual, extensive ulcerated lesion of the lower face from a different patient **(B)** Papules and other small lesions can sometimes progress to such large lesions.

DIAGNOSIS

Cerebrospinal Fluid Findings

Even with widespread cryptococcosis, there are usually no abnormalities in such routine laboratory test results as hematocrit, peripheral blood leukocyte count, and sedimentation rate, which are often abnormal in other infections. Except for infections in patients with AIDS, CNS involvement is almost always indicated by abnormalities in CSF. Opening pressure is often elevated, glucose is depressed in half the cases, protein concentration is almost always increased, and 40–400 leukocytes/mm^3 are characteristic, with lymphocytes generally outnumbering neutrophils. An eosinophilic pleocytosis may occur rarely. Typically in AIDS patients and occasionally in others, there are minimal or no abnormalities of CSF, but cryptococci grow in cultures. Besides those who have AIDS, this is seen most often in patients with early, asymptomatic CNS disease when lumbar punctures are performed because of cryptococcosis at other sites or in patients who are immunosuppressed and have severe hematologic malignancies complicated by acute, rapidly progressing cryptococcosis. In the latter, the heavy infection may be reflected by the ease of finding the organism in India ink smears of CSF. Although patients often have an indolent waxing and waning course with asymptomatic periods, abnormalities in CSF persist, indicating continued activity of the disease.

Smear and Culture

Detection of the organism by culture is necessary for diagnosis. Although they cannot be used to establish definitely the presence of *C. neoformans*, smears using India ink to define the organism can be valuable in supporting a presumptive diagnosis that guides the direction of further diagnostic efforts. A drop of the sediment of 3–5 ml or more of CSF is mixed on a slide with an equal volume of India ink, and a coverslip is set in place. If correctly made, one should be able to barely read newsprint through the preparation. Since few cryptococci may be present, the entire slide should be examined. When the test is performed in this manner, cryptococci are seen in 50 percent of the patients with cryptococcal meningitis. Strict criteria for identification of organisms should be used, especially for distinctness of the outline of the cell wall and capsule, because artifacts are often mistaken for cryptococci when details of cell structure are ignored (Fig. 3). Some laboratories prefer nigrosin to India ink to reduce the likelihood of confusion of cryptococci with artifacts. Cryptococcosis also has been diagnosed using routine cytologic stains, although false-positive readings have occurred using this technique as well. Similarly, the appearance of cryptococci may vary considerably on Gram-stained smears of pu-

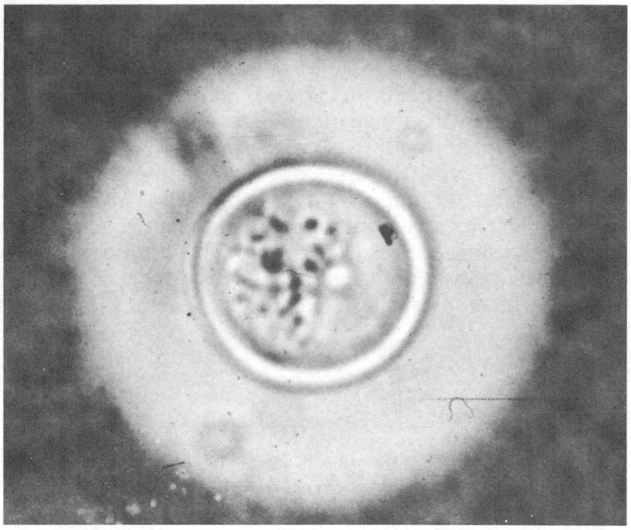

FIG. 3. India ink preparation showing *C. neoformans* in CSF. Although this organism is not budding, it can be differentiated from artifacts by its double refractile cell wall, distinctly outlined capsule, and refractile inclusions in the cytoplasm. (×3600)

rulent specimens, so these may prove to be especially misleading for diagnostic use. Moreover, solutions used in the above procedures may become contaminated with nonpathogenic cryptococci or other fungi. For these reasons, a positive smear must always be confirmed by culture. Centrifuged sediments from 5–10 ml or more of CSF should be cultured on three or more different occasions. Negative cultures do not absolutely rule out cryptococcosis, because often only small numbers of organisms are present in CSF and may be missed. Therefore, large specimens of CSF occasionally are required for diagnosis. In addition, to minimize desiccation of media over a 4- to 6-week incubation period and to increase the culture yield in some difficult cases, it may be helpful to place large volumes of unsedimented CSF on large surfaces of Sabouraud agar on the bottom of Erlenmeyer flasks. Besides repeated sampling of CSF, cultures should be made from suspicious skin and deeper lesions, if present. Urine and sputum should also be cultured, even if there is no clinical or laboratory evidence to suggest involvement of the genitourinary or respiratory systems. In fact, sputum cultures may be positive when there is no roentgenographic evidence of pulmonary infection.[25] Similarly, urine cultures are commonly positive, although renal parenchymal involvement is rare. When sputum cultures are not obtainable, stool cultures may yield the organism.[25] Positive blood cultures occur most often in association with rapid increases in corticosteroid doses, neutropenia, or AIDS, and most often are ominous indicators for patients who have very extensive infections,[25] although some such patients with cryptococcosis can be cured,[81] and blood cultures may rarely become positive after urinary tract instrumentation in localized lesions of the genitourinary tract. Whenever cryptococcosis is documented at any site, this mandates a careful search for lesions elsewhere, both inside and outside the CNS. Isolation of *C. neoformans* should be performed on media without cycloheximide (Actidione). Many media used for the general isolation of fungi contain cycloheximide because it inhibits the growth of nonpathogens, but it inhibits growth of cryptococci as well. *C. neoformans* grows at 37°C but grows more rapidly at lower temperatures (e.g., 30°C), so the latter should be used for primary isolation. The lysis-centrifugation method of blood culture is most rapid and sensitive. Radiometric detection techniques appear to be less sensitive than standard procedures for isolating *C. neoformans* from blood. When *Cryptococcus* is sought, negative radiometric bottles should be subcultured before being discarded.

Histopathology

When tissue specimens are obtained, cryptococcosis may be diagnosed from the histologic sections. The organism is almost colorless and difficult to see with routine hematoxylin and eosin stains. Methenamine silver or periodic acid-Schiff (PAS) stains clearly demarcate the organism and permit recognition of its characteristic size and shape, identifying it as a yeastlike organism that reproduces by formation of narrow-based buds (Fig. 1). *C. neoformans* can then be distinguished from other yeastlike fungi, as well as from artifacts, by Mayer's mucicarmine stain, which colors the cryptococcal capsule rose red but does not stain other fungi that have similar morphologic characteristics.[78] The Masson-Fontana silver stain for melanin also can be used as a specific stain for histologic diagnosis of cryptococcosis.[82]

Serologic Tests

Several serologic tests for cryptococcosis have been described. However, detection of the cryptococcal polysaccharide capsular antigen[83] is the only procedure that is useful clinically on a routine basis. A latex agglutination procedure for detection of antigen is commercially available. Because the antibody-coated latex particles are also agglutinated by rheumatoid factor, controls for rheumatoid factor should be performed on all samples.[84] Use of reducing agents, such as dithiothreitol or mercaptoethanol,[85] or digestion with pronase[86] may also make it possible to test specimens that contain rheumatoid factor by eliminating it without affecting the ability to detect cryptococcal polysaccharide. Both serum and CSF should be tested for antigen. Latex agglutination detects antigen in CSF or serum (or both) from 90 percent or more of the patients with cryptococcal meningitis,[84] but a much lower percentage of serum samples is positive in extraneural cryptococcosis. With controls to exclude the presence of rheumatoid factor, false-positive latex agglutination tests should be unusual. False-positive results may occur due to detection of a cross-reactive antigen in disseminated infections with *Trichosporon beigelii*,[87] due to nonspecific causes in titers up to 1:8, or with some batches of commercial kits in even higher titers. Lack of standardization among manufacturers means that titers cannot be compared without regard to which kit was used. In a recent disturbing national survey of laboratory proficiency, cryptococcal latex agglutination results obtained with four different commercial kits were discarded because neither participating laboratories nor referees could agree on whether the standard test sample was positive or negative.[88] Because of this, positive tests must be confirmed by cultures before a definite diagnosis of cryptococcosis can be made. Anticryptococcal antibodies are detectable in one-third of the patients with cryptococcal meningitis but are also found in a significant percentage of healthy people. Therefore, the presence of antibody is not useful for diagnosis but may have slight clinical value as a prognostic factor signaling a high likelihood for a favorable outcome in cryptococcal meningitis.[25] Several workers have made different preparations of cryptococcin for delayed skin testing,[22,24] but these are useful primarily in epidemiologic and immunologic studies and not at all in diagnosis.

Hydrocephalus

CNS cryptococcosis may be complicated by hydrocephalus. This may be signaled by early or late clinical deterioration, with late development of increased intracranial pressure, or by a recrudescence of abnormalities after initial improvement. When hydrocephalus is suspected, computed tomography (CT) or magnetic resonance imaging is the preferred method for defining the ventricular system and confirming the diagnosis.

Differential Diagnosis

The differential diagnosis of cryptococcosis and other causes of chronic meningitis has been reviewed thoroughly by Ellner and Bennett.[89] Early CNS cryptococcosis may resemble closely other mycoses and tuberculosis, as well as viral meningoencephalitis or meningeal metastases. Cryptococcosis may resemble chronic meningitis due to treatable infections other than tuberculosis (e.g., coccidioidomycosis, histoplasmosis, other mycoses, brucellosis, syphilis) or due to noninfectious causes (e.g., sarcoidosis, chronic benign lymphocytic meningitis).[89] The absence of definite localizing neurologic signs outside the distribution of cranial nerves reduces the likelihood of the diagnosis of intracranial neoplasm. With the increased use of CT scans in the diagnosis of CNS lesions, it has become apparent that even clinically asymptomatic cryptococcosis may produce focal homogenous or doughnut-shaped, contrast-enhanced areas with or without surrounding circumferential areas of decreased density.[90] These must be distinguished from other causes of such intracranial mass lesions, including pyogenic, nocardial or *Aspergillus* abscesses, tuberculosis, hemorrhages, or neoplasms. Immunocompromised patients, particularly those with AIDS, may be completely asymptomatic.[28–30]

When pulmonary cryptococcosis occurs in patients without AIDS, the most common roentgenographic picture resembles tumor: single or multiple circumscribed masses or nodules, more often in the upper lobes, without hilar involvement[91] (Fig. 4). Various other patterns are seen less often, including segmental pneumonia, thick-walled single cavities, lymphadenopathy, pleural effusion, and generalized miliary disease. Patients with AIDS usually manifest fever, cough, and dyspnea, often with pleuritic chest pain, sometimes with x-ray findings of lymphadenopathy or pleural effusions,[92] and most often with diffuse mixed interstitial and intra-alveolar infiltrates.[93] The clinical findings in such patients often are indistinguishable from those of patients with acute pneumonia due to other organisms, such as *Pneumocystis carinii*. Results of bronchoscopy with washings and brushings usually are diagnostic, though biopsy may be necessary to obtain positive specimens. In patients without AIDS, the differential diagnosis is complicated by the fact that patients with pulmonary neoplasms or chronic lung disease may have repeated positive cultures of *C. neoformans* in sputum specimens, apparently due to saprophytic colonization rather than to tissue invasion by the organisms in the lungs or elsewhere.[94,95] Conversely, sputum cultures may be negative with invasive parenchymal cryptococcosis.[25] Therefore, demonstration of tissue invasion by cryptococci is usually necessary for the diagnosis of pulmonary cryptococcis,[96] and surgery may be required to achieve this.

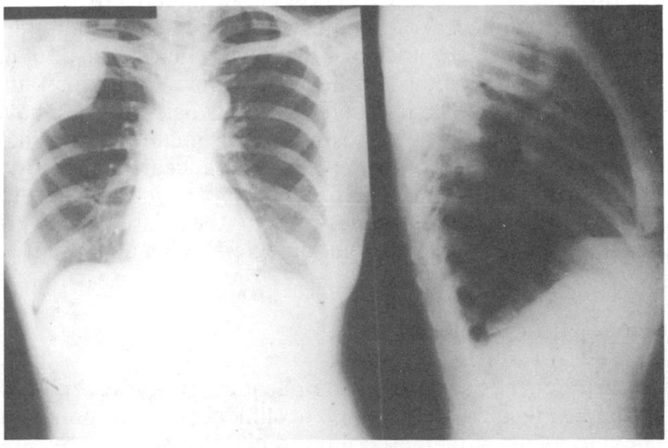

FIG. 4. Chest x-ray film from a patient with pulmonary cryptococcosis that presented as a right upper lobe mass, simulating tumor.

Cutaneous lesions of cryptococcosis are nonspecific and may be mistaken for a wide range of lesions, including those of comedo, lipoma, syphilis, tuberculosis, sarcoidosis, or basal cell carcinoma. However, these lesions are readily accessible for biopsy and offer the opportunity for rapid diagnosis because cryptococci are present in large numbers and are easily identified. Bone lesions are usually round and lytic, without sclerosis at the margins, and resemble bone lesions caused by other fungi and by tuberculosis, especially if a cold abscess is present.

THERAPY

Combination Therapy

Recent evidence indicates that a combination of amphotericin B and flucytosine is at least as effective as amphotericin B alone and should be the treatment of choice for cryptococcal meningitis.[97] Compared with 0.4 mg/kg/day of amphotericin B given alone for 10 weeks, the combination therapy cured more patients, produced fewer failures or relapses, sterilized CSF more rapidly, and resulted in decreased nephrotoxicity during therapy, although the same number of deaths occurred with both the single- and dual-drug treatment regimens.[97] The recommended combination is amphotericin B, 0.3 mg/kg body weight per day intravenously, and flucytosine, 37.5 mg/kg body weight every 6 hours by mouth for 6 weeks. This combination permits the use of a lower than usual dose of amphotericin B. However, azotemia may still occur, causing flucytosine levels to rise. Therefore, renal function should be closely monitored, along with blood flucytosine levels, if possible, and flucytosine levels should be regulated accordingly. This should help to avoid potentially severe reactions to the drug, especially diarrhea and depression of the leukocyte or platelet count, which may be severe enough to necessitate discontinuation of flucytosine. Use of higher doses of amphotericin B greater increases the frequency of toxic reactions to flucytosine. Early occurrence of flucytosine toxicity often precludes the use of combination therapy in patients with AIDS. In general, relapses after 6 weeks of combination therapy appear to be more common in chronically immunosuppressed patients, so that more prolonged treatment may be indicated. Some patients who have no predisposing factors and very mild cryptococcal meningitis may be treated successfully with only 4 weeks of combination therapy,[98] but some so treated will relapse. Thus the advantages of an abbreviated regimen must be weighed against the added difficulties inherent in managing adverse drug effects during retreatment. It should not be overlooked that studies employing 4 or 6 weeks of therapy restricted this recommendation to patients whose cultures were negative by the end of the second week. These studies employed weekly cultures of several milliliters of CSF, done in laboratories experienced in the techniques for recovery of cryptococci.

Amphotericin B

If the combination cannot be given to a particular patient, intravenous amphotericin B alone is effective therapy[25] in doses of 0.4–0.6 mg/kg body weight per day (or double the dose on alternate days). There is no significant development of resistance to amphotericin B during therapy for cryptococcosis. Early toxicity to amphotericin B is manageable by adjusting the dosage and by administering low doses of corticosteroids. It should not be necessary to stop amphotericin B therapy completely because of severe fever, nausea, or early rapid progression of azotemia.[25] Weekly cultures are made of CSF, as well as of specimens from any other sites that were positive before therapy.Therapy is continued for at least 6 weeks, until weekly cultures are negative for 1 month during therapy. Positive India ink smears but negative cultures of CSF do not necessarily indicate continued active disease, but amphotericin B is usually continued to a total dose of 2.5–3.0 g when smears remain positive after cultures have converted to negative. At the end of therapy in most patients, CSF glucose should be normal, and the India ink smear should be negative. However, protein abnormalities (while improving) may be present for years and should not dictate prolongation of therapy. Despite the therapeutic effectiveness of intravenous amphotericin B in most cases of cryptococcal meningitis, measurable levels of the drug in CSF are not achieved during therapy. In only a few selected patients with CNS cryptococcosis, addition of intrathecal injections of amphotericin B, especially by the intraventricular route, may prove useful and even curative.[25,99,100] When it is anticipated that a patient may need intraventricular therapy, careful management of hydrocephalus is necessary, with avoidance of ventricular drainage prostheses whenever possible, because shunts may divert amphotericin B out of CSF during therapy. Because of the effectiveness of intravenous therapy in cryptococcosis, coupled with the risks of intrathecal therapy, intrathecal therapy generally should be reserved for patients who relapse or fail to respond to the usual courses of intravenous amphotericin B or for cases in which nephrotoxicity precludes the use of an adequate intravenous dose of amphotericin B,[99] though this therapy has been advocated for some patients who have a poor prognosis.[100] Patients with AIDS may maintain positive cultures despite the use of any or all of the above treatment regimens, whether used separately or in combination. In those AIDS patients whose cultures are negative at the conclusion of a standard therapeutic regimen, some form of maintenance therapy (amphotericin B, 40–100 mg/day intravenously one to three times weekly) usually is given because of the high likelihood of relapse.[100a]

Flucytosine

Flucytosine, when used alone, can cure some cases of cryptococcal meningitis, but its usefulness is limited by the development of drug resistance during therapy.[101]

Azoles

Ketoconazole has seldom been used in cryptococcosis and achieves only minimal levels in the CNS unless administered in high, toxic doses tolerated by only a minority of patients. A newer, potentially more effective and less toxic triazole derivative, itraconazole, likewise penetrates CSF poorly, whether or not the meninges are inflamed, though it has been used successfully to prolong life in experimental murine cryptococcosis. Unlike other antifungal azoles, another new derivative, fluconazole, is metabolically stable (half-life 22–29 hours), water soluble, and only minimally bound to serum proteins, so that its concentrations in CSF approach those in serum after once-daily oral administration. In the overall management of patients with AIDS, it is particularly desirable to use relatively nontoxic agents without side effects overlapping those of other necessary drugs and to treat in an outpatient setting whenever possible. Therefore, it would be potentially valuable to have an effective, orally administered agent not only for initiation of therapy but for long-term maintenance as well, since the majority of AIDS patients with cryptococcosis appear to relapse even after initially responding to standard treatment regimens. Thus far, uncontrolled trials have been sufficiently promising to warrant studies of anticryptococcal therapy comparing 200–400 mg/day oral fluconazole with standard regimens.[102,102a,102b]

Treatment of Extraneural, Nonrespiratory Lesions

Presumably, therapy for cryptococcosis outside the respiratory and central nervous systems is analogous to that for meningitis, but series are too small to establish this for certain. Some isolated skin lesions appear to become inactive without therapy. However, most cryptococcal lesions of skin, bone, or other organs should be treated with combination therapy or with a total adult dose of 2–3 g of amphotericin B intravenously. Surgical therapy is probably not helpful for most lesions.

Special Considerations in Pulmonary Cryptococcosis

Considerations in the treatment of pulmonary cryptococcosis are different from those in meningeal or nonmeningeal nonpulmonary infection. While the latter require systemic drug treatment, the majority of cases of pulmonary cryptococcosis resolve without antifungal therapy.[99,103] Because sputum cultures are often negative and may be falsely positive, diagnosis must often be made by surgical biopsy. The risk of meningitis as a postoperative complication is low.[103] Total excision may be curative but is not necessary if antifungal therapy is required. Antifungal therapy probably can be postponed during close observation for 2–3 months, as long as CSF is normal and culture is negative, urine cultures are negative, the lesion is small and stable or decreasing in size, and the patient has no predisposing factors (corticosteroid therapy, lymphoreticular malignancy, or AIDS).[103] In general, the natural history of pulmonary cryptococcosis in abnormal hosts appears most often to consist of the development of disseminated infections in the absence of antifungal therapy, in contrast to normal hosts, where self-limited disease requiring no specific therapy most often occurs.[104]

General Considerations in Therapy

Patients with cryptococcosis involving any site should be evaluated every few months for at least 1 year after therapy, even if asymptomatic. Cultural relapses usually occur in the first year after therapy, rarely later. Clinically apparent relapses become obvious much later, usually after significant organ damage has occurred. CSF should be monitored even if the original site of infection was outside the CNS. Conversely, cryptococcosis which originally involved the CNS may relapse with positive cultures in urine or sputum, in addition to CSF.[25] The increased use of CT scans of brains has revealed mass lesions in many patients with CNS cryptococcosis, even in the absence of signs or symptoms of increased intracranial pressure.[90] These masses regress very slowly with treatment. However, there is no evidence to indicate that such patients require either surgery or more prolonged courses of antifungal therapy.

PROGNOSIS

Except in patients with concomitant AIDS, in whom infections only rarely are cured completely, the mortality rate of treated cryptococcal meningitis is probably approximately 25–30 percent. After initial cure, at least with amphotericin B therapy, up to 20–25 percent of the patients relapse. Of those who are cured, 40 percent have significant residual neurologic deficits, including visual loss, cranial nerve palsies, significant motor impairment, or personality change and decreased mental function due to chronic brain syndrome or hydrocephalus. Hydrocephalus can cause late complications or death even when the infection is cured.[25] When severe enough to require shunting, hydrocephalus has a bleak prognosis. Of 10 such patients cited in one study, 6 died, and only 1 remained neurologically normal.[25] In a large series of patients treated with amphotericin B, 55 percent died when predisposing factors (lymphoreticular malignancy or corticosteroid therapy) were present, as opposed to 25 percent in the absence of apparent predisposing factors. However, the worsened outcome was apparently eliminated when corticosteroids were tapered and stopped or when patients were switched to an alternate-day regimen before the end of antifungal therapy. In addition to the above-mentioned factors, failure of anti-fungal therapy was more likely with CSF abnormalities, including an elevated opening pressure, a low glucose level, fewer than 20 leukocytes/mm^3, and a positive India ink preparation. Not surprisingly, indications of extensive infection, such as culture of cryptococci from extraneural sites (especially blood) and high titers of cryptococcal antigen in blood and/or CSF, also signaled a poor outcome. However, prolonged positive cultures during therapy or a positive India ink smear with negative cultures after therapy were not necessarily bad prognostic signs.[25]

Poor prognostic features following combined amphotericin–flucytosine therapy appear similar to those with amphotericin B alone but also include the absence of headache and the presence of abnormal mental status on admission.[98] Some subgroups of patients may require more prolonged courses of treatment than the standard 6-week regimen. For example, based upon small numbers of patients evaluated, renal transplant recipients receiving continuing doses of azathioprine and prednisone have a high risk of treatment failure or relapse of cryptococcosis after completion of anti-fungal therapy. However, experience with assorted individual cases indicates that successful treatment of at least some such patients is possible and that repeated rounds of immunosuppression and even successful retransplantation of kidneys appear feasible without relapse after cure of cryptococcosis. Such renal transplant patients, as well as other groups of patients who are either immuno-compromised or have slow responses to antifungal therapy, often require courses of therapy beyond 6 weeks. Clinical judgment and periodic examinations of the CSF are required to determine whether treatment of such patients should deviate from the standard regimen. Since cryptococcosis in association with AIDS only rarely is cured completely, objectives of therapy are directed toward defining a well-tolerated regimen that is capable of suppressing recrudescence without interfering with treatment of concomitant problems and that is amenable to use in outpatients.

REFERENCES

1. Granger DL, Perfect JR, Durack DT. Virulence of *Cryptococcus neoformans*. Regulation of capsule synthesis by carbon dioxide. J Clin Invest. 1985;76:508–16.
2. Dykstra MA, Friedman L, Murphy JW. Capsule size of *Cryptococcus neoformans*: Control and relationship to virulence. Infect Immun. 1977;16:129–35.
3. Bulmer GS, Sans MD, Gunn CM. *Cryptococcus neoformans*: I. Nonencapsulated mutants. J Bacteriol. 1967;94:1475–9.
4. Zimmer BL, Roberts GD. Rapid selection urease test for presumptive identification of *Cryptococcus neoformans*. J Clin Microbiol. 1979;10:380–1.
5. Jennings A, Bennett JE, Young V. Identification of *Cryptococcus neoformans* in a routine clinical laboratory. Mycopathol Mycol Appl. 1968;35:256–64.
6. Kwon-Chung KJ, Rhodes JC. Encapsulation and melanin formation as indicators of virulence in *Cryptococcus neoformans* Infect Immun. 1986;51:218–23.
7. Kaufmann CS, Merz WG. Two rapid pigmentation tests for identification of *Cryptococcus neoformans*. J Clin Microbiol. 1982;15:339–41.
8. Wilson DE, Bennett JE, Bailey JW. Serologic grouping of *Cryptococcus neoformans*. Proc Soc Exp Biol Med. 1968;127:820–3.
9. Kaplan W, Bragg SL, Cune S, et al. Serotyping *Cryptococcus neoformans* by immunofluorescence. J Clin Microbiol. 1981;14:313–7.
10. Kwon-Chung KJ. A new genus, *Filobasidiella*, the perfect state of *Cryptococcus neoformans*. Mycologia. 1975;67:1197–2000.
11. Kwon-Chung KJ. A new species of *Filobasidiella*, the sexual of *Cryptococcus neoformans* B and C serotypes. Mycologia. 1976;68:942–6.
12. Kwon-Chung KJ, Bennett JE. Epidemiologic differences between the two varieties of *Cryptcoccocus neoformans*. Am J Epidemiol. 1984;120:123–30.
13. Shimizu RY, Howard DH, Clancy MN. The variety of *Cryptococcus neoformans* in patients with AIDS. J Infect Dis. 1986;154:1042.
14. Bennett JE, Kwon-Chung KJ, Theodore TS. Biochemical differences between serotypes of *Cryptococcus neoformans*. Sabouraudia. 1978;16:167–74.
15. Min KH, Kwon-Chung KJ. The biochemical basis for the distribution between the two *Cryptococcus neoformans* varieties with CGB medium. Zentralbl Bakteriol. 1986;261:471–80.
16. Kwon-Chung KJ, Wickes BL, Booth JL, et al. Urease inhibition by EDTA in the two varieties of *Cryptococcus neoformans*. Infect Immun. 1987;55:1751–4.
17. Aulakh HS, Straus SE, Kwon-Chung KJ. Genetic relatedness of *Filobasidiella neoformans* (*Cryptococcus neoformans*) and *Filobasidiella bacillispora* (*Cryptococcus bacillispora*) as determined by deoxyribonucleic acid base composition and sequence homology studies. J System Bacteriol. 1981;31:97–103.
18. Littman ML, Walter JE. Cryptococcosis: Current status. Am J Med. 1968;45:922–32.
19. Ruiz A, Neilson JB, Bulmer GS. Control of *Cryptococcus neoformans* in nature by biotic factors. Sabouraudia. 1982;20:21–9.
20. Neilson JB, Fromtling RA, Bulmer GS. *Cryptococcus neoformans*: Size range of infectious particles from aerosolized soil. Infect Immun. 1977;17:634–8.
21. Newberry WM, Walter JE, Chandler JW, et al. Epidemiologic study of *Cryptococcus neoformans*. Ann Intern Med. 1967;67:724–32.
22. Beyt BE Jr, Waltman SR. Cryptococcal endophthalmitis after corneal transplantation. N Engl J Med. 1978;298:825–6.
23. Atkinson AJ Jr, Bennett JE. Experience with a new skin test antigen prepared from *Cryptococcus neoformans*. Am Rev Respir Dis. 1968;97:637–43.
24. Glaser JB, Garden A. Inoculation of cryptococcosis without transmission of the acquired immunodeficiency syndrome. N Engl J Med. 1985;313:266.
25. Diamond RD, Bennett JE. Prognostic factors in cryptococcal meningitis. A study of 111 cases. Ann Intern Med. 1974;80:176–81.
26. Gallis HA, Berman RA, Cate TR, et al. Fungal infection following renal transplantation. Arch Intern Med. 1975;135:1163–72.
27. Mody CH, Toews GB, Lipscomb MF. Cyclosporin A inhibits the growth of *Cryptococcus neoformans* in a murine mode. Infect Immun. 1988;56:7–12.
28. Kovacs JA, Kovacs AA, Polis M, et al. Cryptococcosis in the acquired immunodeficiency syndrome. Ann Intern Med. 1985;103:533–8.
29. Eng RHK, Bishburg E, Smith SM, et al. Cryptococcal infections in patients with acquired immune deficiency syndrome. Am J Med. 1986;81:19–23.
30. Zuger A, Louie E, Holzman RS, et al. Cryptococcal disease in patients with the acquired immunodeficiency syndrome. Diagnostic features and outcome of treatment. Ann Intern Med. 1986;104:234–40.
31. Krick JA. Familial cryptococcal meningitis. J Infect Dis. 1981;143:133.
32. Marquis G, Montplaisir S, Pelletier M, et al. Genetic resistance to murien cryptococcosis: Increased susceptibility in the CBA/N XID mutant strain of mice. Infect Immun. 1985;47:282–7.
33. Fetter BF, Klintworth GK, Hendry WS. Mycoses of the Central Nervous System. Baltimore: Williams & Wilkins; 1976:100.
34. Gadebusch HH. Mechanisms of native and acquired resistance to infection with *Cryptococcus neoformans*. CRC Crit Rev Microbiol. 1972;1:311–20.
35. Diamond RD, Root RK, Bennett JE. Factors influencing killing of *Cryptococcus neoformans* by human leukocytes in vitro. J Infect Dis. 1972;125:367–76.
36. Ganz T, Selsted ME, Szklarek D, et al. Defensins. Natural peptide antibiotics of human neutrophils. J Clin Invest. 1985;76:1427–35.
37. Kozel TR, Pfrommer GST, Redelman D. Activated neutrophils exhibit enhanced phagocytosis of *Cryptococcus neoformans* opsonized with normal human serum. Clin Exp Immunol. 1987;70:238–46.
38. Weinberg PB, Becker S, Granger DL, et al. Growth inhibition of *Cryptococcus neoformans* by human alveolar macrophages. Am Rev Respir Dis. 1987;136:1242–7.
39. Granger DL, Perfect JR, Durack DT. Macrophage-mediated fungistasis: Requirement for a macromolecular component in serum. J Immunol. 1986;137:693–701.
40. Perfect JR, Granger DL, Durack DT. Effects of antifungal agents and gamma-interferon on macrophage cytotoxicity for fungi and tumor cells. J Infect Dis. 1987;156:316–23.
41. Granger DL, Hibbs JB Jr, Perfect JR, et al. Specific amino acid (L-arginine) requirement for the microbiostatic activity of murine macrophages. J Clin Invest. 1988;81:1129–36.
42. Kalina M, Kletter Y, Aronson M. The interaction of phagocytes and the large-sized parasite, *Cryptococcus neoformans*: Cytochemical and ultrastructural study. Cell Tissue Res. 1974;152:165–74.
43. Graybill JR, Mitchell L, Drutz DJ. Host defense in cryptococcosis: III. Protection of nude mice by thymus transplantation. J Infect Dis. 1979;140:546–52.
44. Hidore MR, Murphy JW. Correlation of natural killer cell activity and clearance of *Cryptococcus neoformans* from mice after adoptive transfer of splenic nylon wool-nonadherent cells. Infect Immun. 1986;51:547–55.
45. Hidore MR, Murphy JW. Natural cellular resistance of beige mice against *Cryptococcus neoformans*. J Immunol. 1986;137:3624–31.
46. Lipscomb MF, Alvarellos T, Toews GB, et al. Role of natural killer cells in resistance to *Cryptococcus neoformans* infections in mice. Amer J Pathol. 1987;128:354–61.
47. Nabavi N, Murphy JW. Antibody-dependent natural killer cell-mediated growth inhibition of *Cryptococcus neoformans*. Infect Immun. 1986;51:556–62.
48. Diamond RD, Allison AC. Nature of the effector cells responsible for antibody-dependent cell-mediated killing of *Cryptococcus neoformans*. Infect Immun. 1976;14:716–20.
49. Fung PYS, Murphy JW. In vitro interactions of immune lymphocytes and *Cryptococcus neoformans*. Infect Immun. 1982;36:1128–38.
50. Schimpff SC, Bennett JE. Abnormalities in cell-mediated immunity in patients with *Cryptococcus neoformans* infection. J Allergy Clin Immunol. 1975;43:430–41.
51. Miller GPG, Puck J. In vitro human lymphocyte responses to *Cryptococcus*

neoformans. Evidence for primary and secondary responses in normals and infected subjects. J Immunol. 1984;133:166–72.
52. Murphy JW, Mosley RL, Cherniak R, et al. Serological, electrophoretic, and biological properties of *Cryptococcus neoformans* antigens. Infect Immun. 1988;56:424–31.
53. Mosley RL, Murphy JW, Cox RA. Immunoadsorption of *Cryptococcus*-specific suppressor T-cell factors. Infect Immun. 1986;51:844–50.
54. Khakpour FR, Murphy JW. Characterization of a third-order suppressor T cell (Ts3) induced by cryptococcal antigen(s). Infect Immun. 1987;55:1657–62.
55. Blackstock R, McCormack JM, Hall NK. Induction of a macrophage-suppressive lymphokine by soluble cryptococcal antigens and its association with models of immunologic tolerance. Infect Immun. 1987;55:233–9.
56. Wilson WR, Ritts RE Jr, Hermans PE. Abnormal chemotaxis in patients with cutaneous anergy. Mayo Clin Proc. 1977;52:196–201.
57. Diamond RD. Effects of stimulation and suppression of cell-mediated immunity on cryptococcosis. Infect Immun. 1977;17:187–94.
58. Laxalt KA, Kozel TR. Chemotaxigenesis and activation of the alternative complement pathway by encapsulated and nonencapsulated *Cryptococcus neoformans*. Infect Immun. 1979;26:435–40.
59. Diamond RD, Erickson NF III. Chemotaxis of human neutrophils and monocytes induced by *Cryptococcus neoformans*. Infect Immun. 1982;38:380–2.
60. Bhattacharjee AK, Bennett JE, Glaudemans CPJ. Capsular polysaccharides of *Cryptococcus neoformans*. Rev Infect Dis. 1984;6:619–24.
61. Cherniak R, Jones RG. Structure determination of *Cryptococcus neoformans* serotype A-variant glucuronoxylomannan by 13-C-N.M.R. spectroscopy. Carbohydrate Res. 1988;172:113–38.
62. Henderson DK, Kan VL, Bennett JE. Tolerance to cryptococcal polysaccharide in cured cryptococcosis patients: Failure of antibody secretion in vitro. Clin Exp Immunol. 1986;65:639–46.
63. Kozel TR, Hermerath CA. Binding of cryptococcal polysaccharide to *Cryptococcus neoformans*. Infect Immun. 1984;43:879–86.
64. Drouhet E, Segretain G. Inhibition de la migration leucocytaire in vitro par un polyoside capsulaire de *Torulopsis* (*Cryptococcus*) *neoformans*. Ann Inst Pasteur. 1951;81:674–6.
65. Diamond RD, May JE, Kane MA, et al. The role of the classical and alternate complement pathways in host defenses against *Cryptococcus neoformans* infection. J Immunol. 1974;112:2260–70.
66. Macher A, Bennett J, Gadek J, et al. Complement depletion in cryptococcal sepsis. J Immunol. 1978;120:1686–90.
67. Muchmore HJ, Scott EN, Felton FG, et al. Cryptococcal capsular polysaccharide clearance in non-immune mice. Mycopathologia. 1982;78:41–5.
68. Eckert TF, Kozel TR. Production and characterization of monoclonal antibodies specific for *Cryptococcus neoformans* capsular polysaccharide. Infect Immun. 1987;55:1895–9.
69. Kozel TR, Pfrommer GST. Activation of the complement system by *Cryptococcus neoformans* leads to binding of iC3b to the yeast. Infect Immun. 1986;52:1–5.
70. Monga DP, Kumur R, Mohapatra LN, et al. Experimental cryptococcosis in normal and B cell deficient mice. Infect Immun. 1979;26:1–3.
71. Dromer F, Charreire J, Contrepois A, et al. Protection of mice against experimental cryptococcosis by anti-*Cryptococcus neoformans* monoclonal antibody. Infect Immun. 1987;55:749–52.
72. Rhodes JC, Wicker LS, Urba WJ. Genetic control of susceptibility to *Cryptococcus neoformans* in mice. Infect Immun. 1980;29:494–9.
73. Kozel TR, Highison B, Stratton CJ. Localization on encapsulated *Cryptococcus neoformans* of serum components opsonic for phagocytosis by macrophages and neutrophils. Infect Immun. 1984;43:574–9.
74. Reiss F, Szilagyi G, Mayer E. Immunological studies of the anticryptococcal factor of normal human serum. Mycopathologia. 1975;55:175–8.
75. Tacker JR, Farhi F, Bulmer GS. Intracellular fate of *Cryptococcus neoformans*. Infect Immun. 1972;6:162–7.
76. Igel JH, Bolande RP. Humoral defense mechanisms in cryptococcosis: Substances in normal human serum, saliva and cerebrospinal fluid affecting the growth of *Cryptococcus neoformans*. J Infect Dis. 1966;116:75–83.
77. Grosse G, Mishra SK, Staib F. Selective involvement of the brain in experimental murine cryptococcosis. II. Histopathological observations. Zentralbl Bakteriol. 1975;233:106–22.
78. Littman ML, Zimmerman LE. Cryptococcosis. New York: Grune & Stratton, 1956.
79. Shrader SK, Watts JC, Dancik JA, et al. Disseminated cryptococcosis presenting as cellulitis with necrotizing vasculitis. J Clin Microbiol. 1986;24:860–2.
80. Hellman RN, Hinrichs J, Sicard G, et al. Cryptococcal pyelonephritis and disseminated cryptococcosis in a renal transplant recipient. Arch Intern Med. 1981;141:128–30.
81. Perfect JR, Durack DT, Gallis HA. Cryptococcemia. Medicine. 1983;62:98–109.
82. Kwon-Chung KJ, Hill WB, Bennett JE. New, special stain for histopathological diagnosis of cryptococcosis. J Clin Microbiol. 1981;13:383–7.
83. Bloomfield N, Gordon MA, Elmendorf DF Jr. Detection of *Cryptococcus neoformans* antigen in body fluids by latex particle agglutination. Proc Soc Exp Biol Med. 1963;114:64–7.
84. Bennett JE, Bailey JW. Control for rheumatoid factor in the latex test for cryptococcosis. Am J Clin Pathol. 1971;56:360–5.
85. Gordon MA, Lapa EW. Elimination of rheumatoid factor in the latex test for cryptococcosis. Am J Clin Pathol. 1974;61:488–94.
86. Stockman L, Roberts GD. Corrected version. Specificity of the latex test for cryptococcal antigen: A rapid, simple method for eliminating interference factors. J Clin Microbiol. 1983;17:945–7.
87. McManus EJ, Jones JM. Detection of a *Trichosporon beigelii* antigen cross-reactive with *Cryptococcus neoformans* capsular polysaccharide in serum from a patient with disseminated *Trichosporon* infection. J Clin Microbiol. 1985;21:681–5.
88. Microbiology Resource Committee, College of American Pathologists. Memorandum to CAP Mycology Survey Participants re 1987 Survey Set F-B. Traverse City, Michigan, 1987.
89. Ellner JJ, Bennett JE. Chronic meningitis. Medicine. 1976;53:341–69.
90. Fujita NK, Reynard M, Sapico FL, et al. Cryptococcal intracerebral mass lesions—The role of computerized tomography and non-surgical management. Ann Intern Med. 1981;94:382–8.
91. Gordonson J, Birnbaum W, Jacobson G, et al. Pulmonary cryptococcosis. Radiology. 1974;112:557–61.
92. Wasser L, Talavera W. Pulmonary cryptococcosis in AIDS. Chest. 1987;92:692–5.
93. Gal AA, Koss MN, Hawkins J, et al. The pathology of pulmonary cryptococcal infections in the acquired immunodeficiency syndrome. Arch Pathol Lab Med. 1986;110:502–7.
94. Duperval R, Hermans PE, Brewer NS, et al. Cryptococcosis, with emphasis on the significance of isolation of *Cryptococcus neoformans* from the respiratory tract. Chest. 1977;72:13–9.
95. Tynes B, Mason KN, Jennings AE, et al. Varient forms of pulmonary cryptococcosis. Ann Intern Med. 1968;69:1117–25.
96. McDonnell JM, Hutchins GM. Pulmonary cryptococcosis. Hum Pathol. 1985;16:121–8.
97. Bennett JE, Dismukes WE, Duma RJ, et al. A comparison of amphotericin B alone and combined with flucytosine in the treatment of cryptococcal meningitis. N Engl J Med. 1979;301:126–31.
98. Dismukes WE, Cloud G, Gallis HA, et al. Treatment of cryptococcal meningitis with combination amphotericin B and flucytosine for four as compared with six weeks. N Engl J Med. 1987;317:334–41.
99. Diamond RD, Bennett JE. A subcutaneous reservoir for intrathecal therapy of fungal meningitis. N Engl J Med. 1973;288:186–8.
100. Polsky B, Depman MR, Gold JWM, et al. Intraventricular therapy of cryptococcal meningitis via a subcutaneous reservoir. Am J Med. 1986;81:24–8.
100a. Zuger A, Schuster M, Simberkoff MS, et al. Maintenance amphotericin B for cryptococcal meningitis in the acquired immunodeficiency syndrome (AIDS) Ann Intern Med. 1988;109:592–3.
101. Bennett JE. Flucytosine. Ann Intern Med. 1977;86:319–22.
102. Saag MS, Dismukes WE. Azole antifungal agents: Emphasis on new triazoles. Antimicrob Agents Chemother. 1988;32:1–8.
102a. Stern JJ, Hartman BJ, Sharkey P, et al. Oral fluconazole therapy for patients with acquired immunodeficiency syndrome and cryptococcosis: experience with 22 patients. Am J Med. 1988;85:477–480.
102b. Sugar AM, Saunders C. Oral fluconazole as suppressive therapy of disseminated cryptococcosis in patients with acquired immunodeficiency syndrome. Am J Med. 1988;85:481–489.
103. Hammerman KJ, Powell KE, Christianson CS, et al. Pulmonary cryptococcosis: Clinical forms and treatment. Am Rev Respir Dis. 1973;108:1116–23.
104. Kerkering TM, Duma RJ, Shadomy S. The evolution of pulmonary cryptococcosis: Clinical implications from a study of 41 patients with and without compromising host factors. Ann Intern Med. 1981;94:611–16.

242. HISTOPLASMA CAPSULATUM

JAMES E. LOYD
ROGER M. DES PREZ
ROBERT A. GOODWIN, JR.

The yeast form of *Histoplasma capsulatum* (derived from inhaled spores) readily parasitizes nonimmune mammalian macrophages, including those of humans. Human infection, histoplasmosis, is the most common and most extensively studied systemic fungus infection in the United States. In heavily endemic areas, virtually the entire population is infected and probably repeatedly reinfected. These encounters are asymptomatic and of no clinical consequence in the vast majority of cases.

Although the organism does not elaborate toxins, its products are highly antigenic and occasionally stimulate vigorous or excessive host reactions. Unusually heavy inhalation inocula cause symptomatic illness, sometimes severe (symptomatic acute pulmonary histoplasmosis). During the acute infection there may be markedly enlarged and inflamed mediastinal lymph nodes, which infrequently cause vascular or bronchial obstruction, acute pericarditis, and other complications. In the late stages of healing, persisting organisms and antigen in caseous nodes rarely may stimulate continuing and destructive encapsulating fibrosis (mediastinal fibrosis), often with fatal results.

This fungus, an organism of generally low human virulence, also may function as an "opportunistic" agent when host immune distrubances allow persisting parasitization of macrophages (disseminated histoplasmosis) or when abnormal pulmonary spaces due to centrilobular or bullous emphysema allow colonization of these spaces and its consequences (chronic pulmonary histoplasmosis).

HISTORICAL SYNOPSIS

Darling, in 1905 in Panama, discovered at an autopsy a new organism that he found in histiocytes of the patient. He named the new agent *Histoplasma capsulatum,* believing it to be an encapsulated plasmodium.[1] During the next 40 years other cases of what was regarded as a rare fatal infection and is now known as disseminated histoplasmosis were reported in the medical literature.[2] In 1934, DeMonbreun[3] recovered the organism from a fatal case and proved that it was a dimorphic fungus rather than a protozoan.

In 1945, Christie and Peterson[4,5] demonstrated that histoplasmosis was a common benign infection that accounted for many cases of pulmonary calcifications previously thought to be due to tuberculosis. In the next few years Palmer, Furcolow, Emmons, and other investigators, mainly from the United States Public Health Service, confirmed these findings[6,7]; demonstrated that soil was the natural habitat of the fungus,[8] which was almost exclusively found in areas where avian and bat excrement collected[9,10]; showed that at such sites (point sources) heavy inhalation of fungal spores caused an acute febrile illness (symptomatic acute pulmonary histoplasmosis)[11]; and by using skin testing programs, mapped endemic areas in the United States and, to a lesser extent, throughout the temperate and tropical zones of the world.[7,12] Furcolow and others (1948–1956) also described the more severe aspects of chronic pulmonary histoplasmosis.[13]

Recent studies[14–16] have contributed to a better understanding of the pathogenesis of the many and varied manifestations of histoplasmosis.

MYCOLOGY

H. capsulatum is the imperfect state of a dimorphic fungus belonging to the class Ascomycetes. The perfect state is *Emmonsiella capsulata.*[17] It exists in its native habitat, the soil, in the mycelial phase but converts to a yeast phase at the body temperature (37°C) of mammals.

The mycelial form consists of septate branching hyphae (1–2.5 μm across) that bear spores at lateral or terminal positions. The spores (the infectious agent) range in size from 2 to 6 μm (microconidia) and 8 to 14 μm (macroconidia). Under proper conditions, many of the macroconidia develop fingerlike appendages over their surfaces and are termed tuberculate spores (Fig. 1A). These are characteristic of the species and are the means whereby identification is made. Spores of all sizes are readily airborne and are of such size, particularly the smaller ones, as to reach alveoli or small bronchioles when inhaled.

The yeast form is ovoid, measuring 1.5–2.0 μm by 3.0–3.5 μm. Reproduction takes place by budding. In viable tissue it is found almost entirely within macrophages. Tissue fixatives produce contraction of the cytoplasm, which causes cytoplasmic stains, for example, hematoxylin and eosin (H & E), to show a surrounding clear area erroneously interpreted in the past as indicating the presence of a capsule (Fig. 1B). Methenamine silver stains the cell membrane (Fig. 1C) and is a much more reliable method of demonstrating the organism but fails to demonstrate tissue morphology. A combined H & E and methenamine silver stain accomplishes both ends.

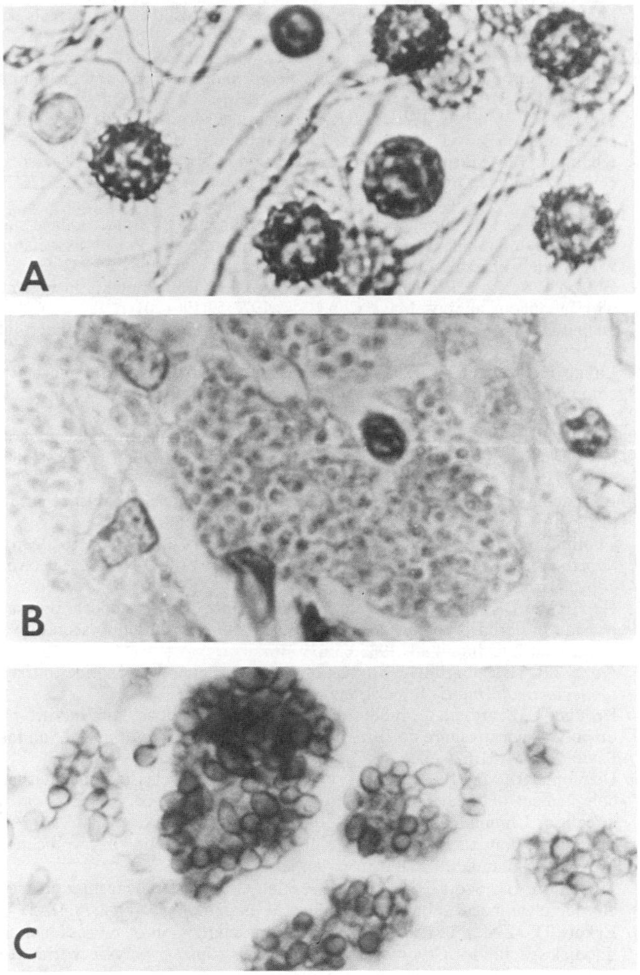

FIG. 1. Mycelial phase, *H. capsulatum.* A microscopic field is picked to show characteristic tuberculated spores (**A**). Macrophages are parasitized by yeast-phase *H. capsulatum* (disseminated histoplasmosis). Fixation has caused cytoplasmic contraction within the organisms, and H & E stain (cytoplasmic stain) erroneously suggests the presence of a capsule (**B**). Methenamine silver stain was used for intracellular yeast forms. The cell wall of the organism stains well, but the stain fails to show tissue morphology (C).

EPIDEMIOLOGY

The general distribution of *H. capsulatum* has been determined by skin testing surveys (Fig. 2), which show a major endemic area in the central United States and spotty areas of infection in tropical, subtropical, and temperate zones of the world.

Cultures of soil specimens have shown that the organism is strikingly more prevalent at sites where heavy accumulations of avian or bat excrement have collected for several years.[9,10] Not all such sites are infested, even in endemic areas, and the involvement of those that are is spotty. This has led to the concept of point sources of microfoci of infection. The more point sources, the more heavily endemic is a given area.

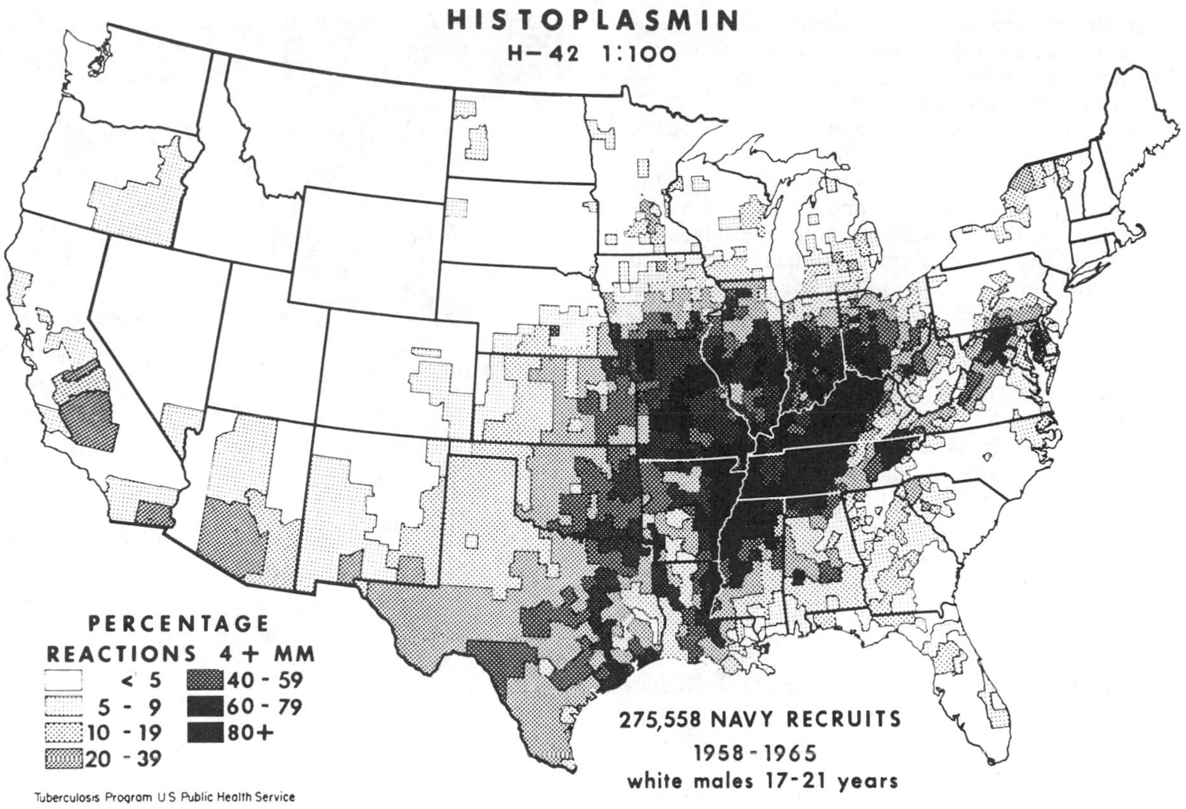

FIG. 2. Positive histoplasmin reactors in naval recruits by county (if lifetime residents). This provides a good indication of relative endemic areas but underestimates the actual number of individuals who have been infected in the past. (From Edwards et al.,[12] with permission.)

Birds are not themselves infected because of high body temperature. Bats (mammals) may be infected, show yeast forms in their feces, and spread the organism to new habitats. The cause of fungus growth stimulation by excrement of either is not well understood. Blackbird roosts, pigeon roosts, chicken houses, chicken manure fertilizer, and sites frequented by bats such as caves, attics, old buildings, and hollow trees in endemic areas are most apt to be point sources. Mechanical disturbances of such sites, dusty circumstances, wind, and enclosed spaces greatly increase the number of airborne spores. Bulldozing an old blackbird roost in dry weather may raise enormous numbers of airborne spores and cause heavy exposures to those nearby but also lesser exposures some distance downwind.

ACUTE PULMONARY HISTOPLASMOSIS

The term *acute pulmonary histoplasmosis* covers the entire range of infection in normal hosts, including rare early and late complications.[14]

Pathogenesis and Pathology

Animal studies[18] show that many inhaled spores reach small bronchioles or alveoli and after 2 or 3 days germinate and release yeast forms of the fungus that are promptly phagocytized by macrophages. In nonimmune hosts the yeasts proliferate within the phagocytes, and more macrophages are recruited to the site, many of which also become infected. These accumulations of infected macrophages and other cells result in a small infiltrate at each infected site. Infected macrophages migrate to the mediastinal lymph nodes and elsewhere in the mononuclear phagocyte system (MPS), especially the spleen and liver. New focal infiltrates develop at these sites and are particularly prominent in the mediastinal lymph nodes.

In the nonimmune animal this process continues for 9–15 days, at which time the onset of acquired immunity causes an intense vasculitis at the site of each infiltrate and results in tissue necrosis and caseation. Macrophages are rendered competent to kill the intracellular parasites, and the lesions heal. The caseous lesions are encapsulated and eventually calcify. Significantly, many yeast forms are trapped in the necrotic tissue and persist even after calcification. It is not known whether they are ever again infectious, although they do act as a source of antigen.

In the immune animal (due to recent infection) the reactions of acquired immunity begin 24–48 hours after the appearance of yeast forms, and therefore, there is but little proliferation of organisms and little reaction. There is every indication that similar changes occur in human infection in both the nonimmune and immune host.

Immunity

Immunity in histoplasmosis is based on cellular immune mechanisms, and it is therefore interesting that the effector cell of that system is also the susceptible tissue in this disease. The natively susceptible macrophage is rendered competent to kill intracellular yeast by the mechanisms of acquired immunity, and in the rare circumstances when this does not occur, persistent disseminated histoplasmosis ensues. Acquired immunity wanes with time, as does skin reactivity. In this it differs from tuberculosis where immunity persists for a much longer period of time.

In the usual infection the number of inhaled spores is small, the number of infiltrates in the lung and mediastinal lymph nodes is small, the encounter is asymptomatic, and at most there are eventually a few small calcifications in the lung, mediastinal lymph nodes, and possibly the liver or spleen.[14] Actually, three-fourths of histoplasmin converters do not demonstrate roentgenologically visible infiltrates or subsequent visible calcifications. In endemic areas calcifications tend to increase during life from repeated infections.

The two most important factors that determine the degree of preimmunity proliferation of organisms and, therefore, the degree of symptoms with the advent of hypersensitivity are the size of the inoculum and the prior immune status of the individual.[14] The quantity of the inoculum roughly determines the number of infiltrates, and the preimmunity incubation period determines the fungus population in each. Moderate inhalation inocula cause symptomatic illness in most nonimmune individuals, with incubation periods of 10–16 days, but are not apt to be symptomatic in fully immune individuals. However, a heavy inhalation exposure will result in symptomatic illness in even the fully immune, although the incubation period is much shorter (3–5 days) and the illness is of shorter duration and less severe. Individuals with waning immunity fall in between the fully immune and the nonimmune with respect to incubation period and severity of illness. The immature native immunity of infants renders them more susceptible to symptomatic illness with mild or heavy exposures.

Symptoms

Symptoms are, in general, nonspecific and rather variable. Fever and headache occur in almost all cases; chills, cough, and chest pain in two-thirds; and less frequently, weakness, weight loss, myalgia, and fatigue.[14] Chest pain varies from vague substernal discomfort to prominent aching substernal pain, usually aggravated by deep breathing. When present, this pain, probably due to enlarged mediastinal nodes, is diagnostically helpful. Gastrointestinal (GI) symptoms, nausea, vomiting, or diarrhea occasionally occur, particularly in children. Coryza, sore throat, or nuchal tension, often misleading symptoms, are sometimes reported. With very heavy inhalation inocula, dyspnea may occur. Rarely it is severe, and death has been reported from acute pulmonary insufficiency. The more symptomatic patients often complain of asthenia persisting after the acute illness for weeks or even months. The duration of illness tends to be related to the severity of symptoms. Mild symptoms (temperature <101°F) may last 1–5 days, and moderate symptoms (temperature of 101–103°F) last an average of 5–7 days. Severe symptoms (temperature of 102–106°F) usually persist for 10 days or so, rarely for 2–3 weeks or longer.

Roentgenographic Findings

The usual infection with a small or modest inhalation inoculum occurs without inducing visible roentgenographic changes in three out of four cases. In the other 25 percent, one, two, or a cluster of small infiltrates or a recognizable enlargement of hilar nodes, or both, may be evident. Eventual calcifications in the lung or hilar lymph nodes occur in only one-fourth of skin test converters. Heavy inhalation inocula result in many small scattered infiltrates (2–5 mm) and usually prominent hilar and mediastinal lymph nodes (Fig. 3). Occasionally the infiltrates may be 10–15 mm across in individuals who develop large fungus populations and greater degrees of hypersensitivity. The larger infiltrates leave caseous nodules that in time calcify and produce rounded calcifications (''buckshot''), their size roughly proportional to the size of the initial infiltrate. Fully immune individuals with short incubation periods show tiny miliary-size infiltrations (1–2 mm), no evident lymphadenopathy, and no subsequent calcifications.[14]

Physical Findings

There is a paucity of physical findings in acute pulmonary histoplasmosis. Occasionally, the liver and spleen are palpable in adults with heavy infections. Hepatosplenomegaly is somewhat more common in infants or young children, and sometimes both organs are impressively enlarged. Erythema nodosum or erythema multiforme may occasionally occur in either symptomatic or asymptomatic infections, more often in symptomatic cases and more commonly in young women. When present, they are often accompanied by arthralgias and, rarely, frank arthritis. Routine laboratory findings are seldom significantly altered.

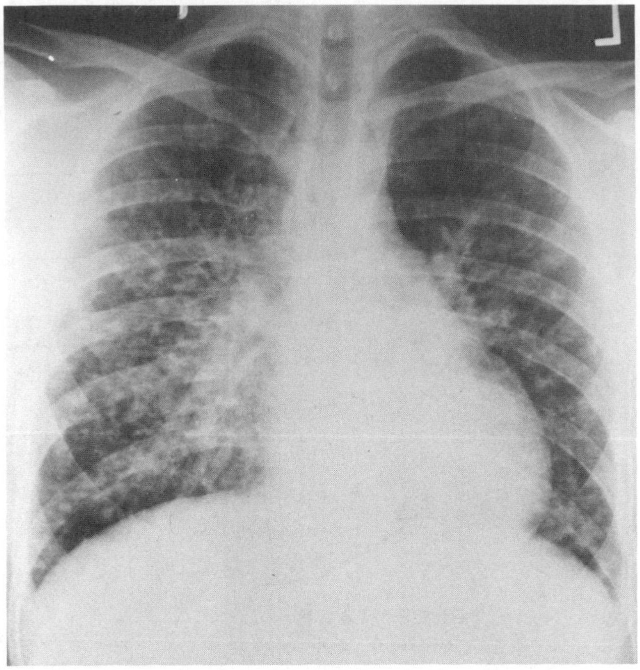

FIG. 3. Acute symptomatic pulmonary histoplasmosis resulting from heavy inhalation exposure to *Histoplasma* spores in a nonimmune individual. The many small infiltrates and the hilar and mediastinal lymphadenopathy are evident.

Diagnosis

The diagnosis begins with thinking of it in the presence of a febrile illness and questioning the possibility of exposure to *Histoplasma* spores. The characteristic roentgenographic findings of small scattered pulmonary infiltrates and hilar adenopathy (Fig. 3) can then provide a strong presumptive clinical diagnosis. A significantly elevated complement fixation (CF) titer would provide strong confirmatory evidence. Cultural or histologic proof is seldom obtained.

Although important in epidemiologic studies, the *histoplasmin skin test* is not often helpful diagnostically and has the disadvantage of occasionally boosting a subsequent complement fixation titer.

Complement fixation is the test that has been most used for the detection of serum antibody to *H. capsulatum*.[19] Complement fixation for yeast-phase antigens is more sensitive than for the mycelial phase, which may be boosted by a prior histoplasmin skin test. A titer of 1:32 or greater or an appropriately timed fourfold increase in titer is evidence of active or recent infection. Background positivity of CF titers in endemic areas may be as high as 30 percent of persons and may reach titers of 1:32. Cross-reactivity to antigens shared with other fungi (especially *Blastomyces*) is a recognized problem.[20] Immunodiffusion (ID) is an agar gel diffusion test that is more specific but less sensitive than CF is. The ID test measures two bands of immunoprecipitation, the M and H bands. The presence of both bands is the most specific serodiagnostic test for histoplasmosis but occurs infrequently. A positive M band alone is fairly specific, more so than positive CF findings; a positive H band alone is rarely seen. Newer and more sensitive tests (radioimmunoassay [RIA]) for the serologic detection of antibody to *H. capsulatum* have been developed, but their higher sensitivity is at the cost of less specificity from more false-positives.[21,22] Detection of *H. capsulatum* antigen in clinical specimens has been reported to be useful in some clinical syndromes (disseminated histoplasmosis).[23]

Treatment

Ordinarily, acute pulmonary histoplasmosis, asymptomatic or symptomatic, requires no specific treatment. Short-course amphotericin B is recommended for unusually prolonged or severe infections and is given to adults in a full dosage of 40–50 mg daily intravenously for 2 or 3 weeks (see the section on disseminated histoplasmosis). Ketoconazole has not been investigated in acute histoplasmosis, but based on its efficacy in other clinical syndromes, it would be an appropriate alternative when given at 400 mg daily for 3 or more months.

Rare Complications

Unusually vigorous host reactions causing greatly enlarged and inflamed mediastinal lymph nodes or excessive encapsulating fibrosis of healing may result in grave damage to structures and organs within the tight confines of the mediastinum in spite of adequate control of the infection.

Tracheal, Bronchial, or Esophageal Obstruction. On rare occasions, marked enlargement of paratracheal lymph nodes has caused serious tracheal obstruction in infants or young children. Enlarged lymph nodes may occasionally obstruct bronchi and cause obstructive pneumonia or bronchiectasis or may compress the esophagus and result in dysphagia. Obstruction of any of these organs, if not critical, usually subsides spontaneously. Surgical excision may be required for serious obstruction. Whether amphotericin B or ketoconazole will significantly accelerate healing is not established, but a trial of either might be considered if circumstances warrant.

Acute Pericarditis. An acutely inflamed caseous lymph node contiguous to the pericardium may induce an acute fibrinous pericarditis without penetration or a granulomatous pericarditis by softening and emptying into the pericardial space.[14] About 40 percent of recognized cases show some degree of tamponade. Most can be controlled by pericardiocentesis, although some thoracic surgeons prefer to perform an immediate anterior pericardiectomy. Spontaneous healing can be expected. Fewer than 15 percent of patients later develop constrictive pericarditis. The presence of mediastinal lymphadenopathy should suggest the diagnosis, and a significantly positive complement fixation test or a fourfold rise in titer will confirm it. Some authorities consider treatment unnecessary, but a good case can be made for the use of a short course of amphotericin B (10–14 days) if given early, with the hope of shortening the course and perhaps diminishing the chance of constriction. Although there is no reported experience, ketoconazole might be tried but is less likely to be promptly effective.

Pleural Effusion. Pleural effusions are not common. Small effusions occur in 50 percent of cases of acute pericarditis and are occasionally seen in ordinary acute infections. When the effusion is massive, it may signify erosion of a lymph node or a parenchymal lesion into the pleural space. In any event, the process is benign and should heal spontaneously.

Mediastinal Granuloma. A group of large caseous lymph nodes, more often in the right paratracheal area, may mat together, break down, and become encapsulated into a single mass. These encapsulated masses are sometimes quite large, measuring up to 10 cm across. It is the thickness of the capsule rather than the size of the mass that determines their clinical significance.[14] A thick (6–10 mm) capsule will invade contiguous tissues, the most common effect being superior vena cava obstruction. If this occurs, an attempt at partial excision or possible evacuation of necrotic contents with or without a venous bypass graft must be weighed against the probability that compensatory changes will eventually relieve the symptoms. Unless symptoms are present, there is no reason to consider surgical intervention and no reason to believe that antifungal agents would be beneficial.

Mediastinal Fibrosis. Even small caseous lymph nodes are often attended by periadenitis and heal with fibrous encapsulation, which becomes adherent to adjacent structures. Rarely, in hypersensitive individuals and with a large antigen load of persistent yeast forms in the caseous center, the stimulus to capsule formation continues, and a fibroma-like massive capsule 1–2 cm in thickness gradually builds up over many years.[24,25] The collagen is laid down in viable adjacent tissues and, depending on the location of the inciting node and the thickness of the capsule, may cause bronchial stenosis, occlusion of pulmonary arteries, veins, or the superior vena cava, or any combination of these, often with fatal results. Common symptoms of mediastinal fibrosis are hemoptysis and dyspnea. Chest radiography findings may be deceptively normal or nearly so, especially if the process is localized to the subcarinal region; computed tomography (CT) may be especially revealing in such circumstances. The symptoms or outcome of mediastinal fibrosis, unlike mediastinal granuloma, are rarely if ever benefited by surgery. The hypothesis that mediastinal granuloma may progress to mediastinal fibrosis was not supported by a recent comprehensive review,[25] so resection of an asymptomatic mediastinal granuloma is not justified by such arguments. There is no reason to believe that amphotericin B would be helpful, but since there is no evidence that it would not and since the consequences are so severe, a trial might be considered.

Broncholithiasis. The vast majority of pulmonary and mediastinal calcifications seen on chest roentgenograms in the United States are due to histoplasmosis. Occasionally, one of the larger calcifications in either the lung or the bronchial lymph nodes may soften and dissect into a bronchus, often causing the expectoration of gritty material or small stones (lithoptysis) with or without hemoptysis or coughing paroxysms.[14] These are benign events and rarely require any specific treatment unless an extruded large stone occludes a bronchus, in which case bronchoscopic removal is indicated.

Esophageal Disturbances. The adhesions of healing periadenitis of adjacent caseous lymph nodes may cause esophageal traction diverticuli or fixation with disturbance of motility.[14] The latter, if severe, requires surgical correction.

Sinuses and Fistulas. Caseous mediastinal lymph nodes, early or late, occasionally soften and dissect into adjacent structures such as the bronchus, pericardium, or esophagus or rarely into two organs to cause a fistula, most commonly bronchoesophageal. The latter usually requires surgical management.

Enlarging Histoplasmoma. The same exuberant fibrotic reaction responsible for the lesion of mediastinal fibrosis is seen more frequently in relation to a caseous nodule in the lung.[26] Slow continuing capsule formation around a 2–4 mm caseous nodule (remnant of a lesion of acute pulmonary histoplasmosis) over 10–15 years results in an enlarging fibroma-like mass up to 3.5 cm in diameter. These can often be recognized by central calcification or laminations of calcification. They are almost always peripheral, do no damage, and can be safely disregarded.

DISSEMINATED HISTOPLASMOSIS

This rare and potentially fatal development is considered to be due to a defect in host immunity and can, therefore, be regarded as an opportunistic infection. Three groups of susceptible hosts are recognized: infants with immature immunity, immunosuppressed individuals, and a group with no known immune defect as measured by present-day methods.

Pathogenesis and Pathology

Persisting infection of a significant number of macrophages implies infection of the entire mononuclear phagocyte system (MPS), often referred to as the reticuloendothelial system. The number of infected macrophages scattered throughout the MPS varies widely, from enormous numbers of heavily parasitized cells to a very few, generally lightly parasitized cells. The degree of involvement of the MPS in a given individual does not progress (from a light to a heavy degree of parasitization) but rather tends to remain constant throughout the course of the illness. The exception to this is in persons treated with corticosteroids or immunosuppressive agents, in whom such treatment may be associated with conversion of a mild and chronic process to an acute and fulminant one.

The major pathologic finding is the diffuse scattering of infected macrophages throughout the MPS and those organs rich in this tissue, notably the visceral lymph nodes, spleen, liver, bone marrow; to a lesser extent the adrenal glands and the submucosa of the intestine; but to some extent any connective tissues in the body.[15] In less extensively involved cases there is a tendency for focal accumulations of infected macrophages to develop in certain organs. These may displace and destroy normal tissue to some extent. Such lesions are found particularly in the adrenals, in the submucosa of the intestine, and most significantly but less commonly, in the adventitia of meningeal or extra-adrenal vessels. Normal host tissue reaction to the presence of parasitized macrophages, whether diffusely scattered or present in focal lesions, is minimal or conspicuously absent. The only reaction is the recruitment of more macrophages, a response known as a histiocytosis. Tuberculoid granulomas, typical of the response in normal hosts, are found only at the mildest and most chronic end of the disease spectrum of disseminated histoplasmosis.

Clinical Manifestations

The disease spectrum parallels the degree of diffuse involvement of the MPS (Fig. 4) and exhibits an equally wide range such that a single clinical description cannot suffice. For convenience, therefore, the spectrum will be divided into three groups, defined as acute, subacute, and chronic.[15]

Acute (Infant-Type) Disseminated Histoplasmosis. In this group there is massive involvement of the MPS that consists of closely packed macrophages engorged with yeast forms. This severe degree of infection is the usual presentation in infants and the occasionally involved young child but is uncommon in adults (Fig. 4). An unrelenting and debilitating fever, with temperatures averaging 101–103°F and often as high as 105°F, is the most conspicuous symptom. GI symptoms are common, particularly nausea, vomiting, and diarrhea. Cough and tachypnea in later stages may indicate the presence of interstitial pneumonia (heavily parasitized macrophages in pulmonary interstitial space). Anemia, leukopenia, or thrombocytopenia, singly or in some combination, are almost always present, often to a serious degree, and frequently cause or contribute to the terminal event. Symptoms of anemia, secondary infection from

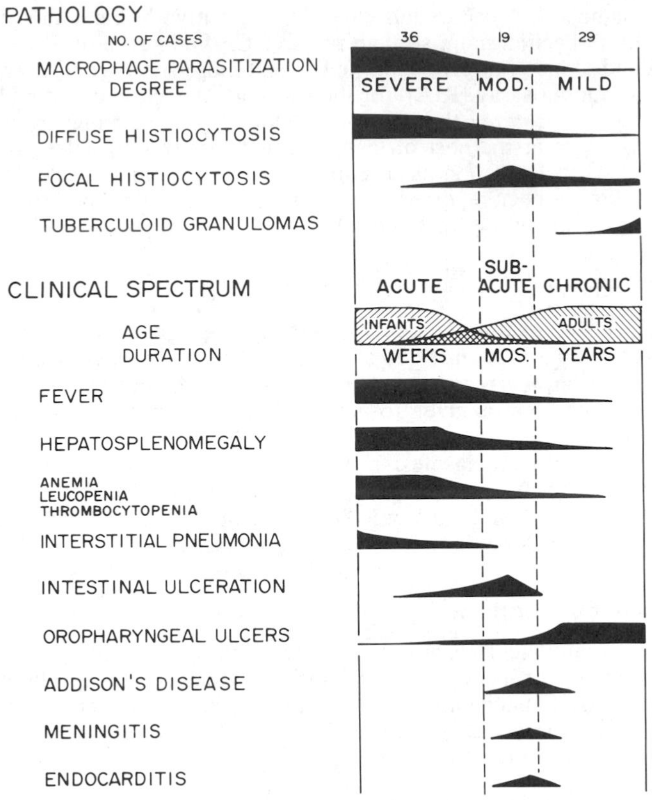

FIG. 4. This schema shows the relationship of the degree of parasitization of macrophages in disseminated histoplasmosis and the corresponding clinical spectrum of acute, subacute, and chronic disease. (From Goodwin et al.,[15] with permission.)

granulocytopenia, or thrombocytopenic bleeding often complicate the late stages of the disease.

The most conspicuous *physical finding* is the always striking enlargement of the liver and spleen, a vivid manifestation of histiocytosis. The visceral lymph nodes are always enlarged, but the peripheral nodes are palpable in only one-third of cases. Occasionally, a superficial and often inconspicuous ulceration may be found in the oropharyngeal mucosa. Ascites and jaundice are occasionally present. Hematologic changes are the most conspicuous *laboratory findings*. The hematocrit is less than 20 in 60 percent of cases, the white blood cell (WBC) count is less than 4000 in 80 percent, and the platelet count is less than 70,000 in 80 percent. Critically low concentrations of one or another cell type are found in at least one-fourth of cases. The chest roentgenogram demonstrates recognizable remnants of the initiating acute pulmonary lesions in at least one-fourth of the patients and clear evidence of diffuse interstitial pneumonia in an equal number. Mild alterations in liver function with no significant change in renal function is the rule.

Untreated, the outcome is invariably fatal, with an average course of 5 weeks.

Subacute (Intermediate-Type) Disseminated Histoplasmosis. A smaller number of patients fall into this intermediate group, which is characterized by a moderate range of parasitization of the MPS (Fig. 4). Two-thirds are adults and one-third, infants. Symptoms are moderate, but there is a notable tendency to develop focal lesions in various organs, some with critical consequences. Fever tends to be moderate, with temperatures in the 100°–101°F range, and is sometimes intermittent. Weight loss and weakness are common due to the greater chronicity of the illness. In about three-fourths of patients some type of focal lesion becomes clinically significant. Intestinal ulceration is common and usually produces GI symptoms. Occasionally, perforation occurs, usually with fatal results. Other focal lesions include complete destruction of the adrenal glands, which causes Addison's disease, endocarditis, severe meningitis, and focal cerebritis. Oropharyngeal ulcers, usually deep and with rolled edges, occur in more than one-fourth of cases and, when present, should lead to the diagnosis.

Hepatosplenomegaly, an important diagnostic finding, is almost always present, although to a lesser degree than in the acute group. Hematologic abnormalities are usual but less marked in degree and seldom clinically important. The chest roentgenogram often shows residuals of the initiating acute pulmonary histoplasmosis but seldom shows interstitial pneumonitis, although mild degrees of the latter are often demonstrable microscopically.

Untreated, the course is fatal in an average of 10–11 months.

Chronic (Adult-Type) Disseminated Histoplasmosis. This group, which is histopathologically characterized by the mildest degree of macrophage parasitization, is made up almost entirely of adults and is characteristic of infection in this age group (Fig. 4). Constitutional symptoms are mild, chronic, and often intermittent. Gradual weight loss, weakness, and fatiguability are the most common symptoms. Fever occurs only in a minority of patients and in these intermittently for short periods. Focal lesions are characteristic of these mild infections. Occasionally Addison's disease, meningitis, or endocarditis may occur. Oropharyngeal ulcers are quite common and, when present, are fortunate diagnostic opportunities in an illness that otherwise is almost impossible to recognize. Papular or plaque-like cutaneous lesions are less common but, when present, provide an easily positive biopsy specimen. Hepatosplenomegaly is either minimal or, more frequently, absent entirely. The liver is more apt to be palpable than is the spleen. Hematologic changes are uncommon and never clinically significant. Unless interrupted by treatment or a fatal focal organ lesion, the course of chronic infection may continue for years, 10–20 years of intermittent illness being not uncommon. Whether these patients ever spontaneously heal is not known.

Details of the focal involvement of organ systems and variations of the clinical manifestations of each are found in a review with a full bibliography.[15] The reader is referred particularly for discussions of the adrenal gland, central nervous system (CNS) involvement, and endocarditis. Patients with underlying disease states thought to involve immunosuppression, such as carcinoma, lymphoma, or serious autoimmune disorders, demonstrate typical clinical manifestations of histoplasmosis when present. Immunosuppressive drugs, particularly corticosteroids, not infrequently appear to have initiated disseminated histoplasmosis or to have converted an established case of mild chronic disease to an acute fulminant form.

Diagnostic Studies

The diagnosis of disseminated histoplasmosis depends on the demonstration of either histologically compatible *intracellular organisms* or a positive culture of blood or viable tissue. There are pitfalls that pathologists and clinicians often fail to take into account. Organisms found in necrotic tissue or even within cells in well-formed tuberculoid granulomas are characteristic residuals of acute pulmonary histoplasmosis and should not be confused with established disseminated disease. Occasionally, a positive culture of blood or urine may be obtained in the more severe but potentially reversible instances of acute pulmonary histoplasmosis. However, the histologic finding of intracellular organisms in viable tissues with no tissue reaction provides firm diagnostic evidence of disseminated histoplasmosis, as does positive blood, bone marrow, urine, or other extrapulmonary tissue cultures when clinical circumstances suggest that the infection has extended well beyond an episode of acute pulmonary histoplasmosis. Improved abdominal imaging techniques (CT and ultrasound) have provided evidence that many patients with disseminated histoplasmosis have bilateral adrenal enlargement; this finding by itself should suggest disseminated histoplasmosis when it is observed in an appropriate clinical setting.[27]

A Wright stain smear or culture of peripheral blood is almost always positive in the severe acute form of disseminated disease, is positive in 50 percent in subacute diseases, and is rarely positive in chronic disease. The use of buffy coat and methenamine silver stain should increase the positive findings, as will bone marrow biopsy with silver stains. New methods for culture of fungi from blood (lysis–centrifugation) appear to be faster and more sensitive.[28] Liver biopsy with methenamine silver stain may be positive in as many as 80 percent of cases, even in chronic disease. Oropharyngeal ulcers due to histoplasmosis are almost always positive on a Giemsa smear of scrapings or culture and always positive on a biopsy specimen with methenamine silver stain. On occasion, histoplasmosis can cause chronic meningitis or mass lesions in the brain after apparent recovery from disseminated histoplasmosis. Assays for antibodies to *H. capsulatum* in cerebrospinal fluid (CSF) may be useful for establishing the diagnosis of chronic meningitis; however, false-positive results have been observed in half the patients with other forms of chronic fungal meningitis.[29]

Treatment

All patients with disseminated histoplasmosis should receive antifungal chemotherapy. Amphotericin B is the drug of choice for severely ill patients, for those with meningitis or endocarditis, or for immunosuppressed patients. The usual total dose is 35 mg/kg.[30] Patients with endocarditis may require more prolonged therapy unless the infection was on a native valve that was removed. The response of meningitis to amphotericin B is slow, but intrathecal therapy is rarely warranted.

Oral ketoconazole has proved to be a useful alternative drug for patients who do not have endocarditis or meningitis and who are not immunosuppressed.[31] For adults, the initial dosage is 400 mg once daily. The duration of therapy is between 6 and 12 months. Ketoconazole can also be used to reduce the chance of relapse in patients with the acquired immunodeficiency syndrome (AIDS) who have just completed a 35 mg/kg course of amphotericin B. Alternatively, weekly amphotericin B can be used for maintenance therapy in AIDS patients after an initial intensive course.

Disseminated Histoplasmosis in AIDS

Disseminated histoplasmosis has been included by the Centers for Disease Control (CDC) as one of the defining infections in AIDS and is the most common defining infection in some endemic areas.[32] Some reports of disseminated histoplasmosis in AIDS have originated from nonendemic areas such as New York in patients long removed from endemic areas, the Caribbean, or South America.[33] Authors recording their experience in endemic areas have emphasized a fulminant course with advanced hematologic abnormalities (thrombocytopenia, leukopenia, anemia), at times producing disseminated intravascular coagulation, respiratory failure, or both. Others recording cases in New York City, a nonendemic area, in persons some years removed from endemic areas have described a prolonged, subacute fever of unknown origin with weight loss and lassitude.[33] This latter experience established with certainty the fact that disseminated histoplasmosis can evolve from a previously subclinical and long dormant focus, a point about which there has been some uncertainty. Especially in these less fulminant cases, pulmonary involvement may be minimal, with chest radiographs demonstrating only sparse interstitial or nodular involvement or entirely normal findings. Diagnosis is usually established by special stains or culture of tissue from bone marrow, skin, liver, or lymph nodes or Wright stain of a buffy coat or marrow smear.

Ketoconazole should not be used alone for initial therapy in immunocompromised patients. Most AIDS patients with disseminated histoplasmosis suffer later relapses, which has led to the recommendation for chronic ketoconazole therapy after a full course of amphotericin B (total of 2 g).

CHRONIC PULMONARY HISTOPLASMOSIS

Occasionally, *H. capsulatum* may play a different opportunistic role. In the face of normal acquired immunity it may take advantage of structural defects of the lung to colonize abnormal pulmonary spaces due to centrilobular and bullous emphysema.[16] This parasitization causes a chronic, destructive disease in the apical areas of the lung that is often mistaken for tuberculosis.

Pathogenesis and Pathology

There are two types of lesions found in chronic pulmonary histoplasmosis, infected air spaces and pneumonic lesions. The infected air spaces are themselves of two types: small rounded fluid-filled spaces, usually in the central lung zones, and larger apical or subapical infected bullous spaces. The nature of the former, infected centrilobular air spaces, is known from histopathologic study of rounded shadows surgically removed on suspicion of carcinoma. In fixed specimens of these, organisms are seen to be sparsely dispersed throughout a bland background, which indicates their fluid nature. The larger apical and subapical "cavities" represent infection of pre-existing bullous air spaces having a caseous lining, with larger numbers of organisms limited almost entirely to its surface. The pneumonic lesions are segmental areas of interstitial pneumonitis that display a marked tendency to develop central or scattered focal areas of coagulation-type necrosis. Histologic evidence favors vasculitis-induced ischemia producing focal or segmental infarcts rather than histolytic products of lymphocyte macrophage interaction (as in tuberculosis) as the cause of this type of tissue necrosis. It is significant that organisms are rarely found in the pneumonic areas unless they enclose an infected air space.[16]

The best explanation of the segmental pneumonic lesions is that they are caused by aspiration of thin, highly antigenic fluid emptied from the small, rounded, infected, and fluid-filled centrilobular emphysematous space or spaces described above. At the time of such an event the few organisms contained in the fluid often infect adjacent bullous spaces, some of which persist as infected cavities.

Clinical Manifestations

Many of the patients have symptoms of pre-existing chronic bronchitis that sometimes mask the symptoms of chronic pulmonary histoplasmosis. In general, symptoms of histoplasmosis are similar to those of tuberculosis but tend to be milder.

The symptoms of the pneumonic lesion differ somewhat from those due to infected "cavities." They often begin abruptly, with mild to moderate degrees of malaise, chilliness, feverishness, fatiguability, or weakness, usually accompanied by a cough productive of mucoid sputum (unless there is pre-existing purulent sputum). Occasionally, night sweats occur. About one-third of patients develop a deep aching chest pain more suggestive of a neoplasm than infection, which may be distressing and is sometimes the major complaint. The cause of this is not clear. At least 20 percent have no symptoms at all during the pneumonic episode. Fever may be recorded in one-half of cases; temperatures are usually less than 101°F but may occasionally go as high as 103–104°F. High fever may continue, gradually diminishing for as long as 2 or 3 weeks, but tends to subside more promptly with rest. Symptoms in general are apt to be prolonged by activity and diminished by rest. With continued activity average symptoms persist for 4 to 5 weeks or longer and may be associated with significant weight loss.

Symptoms of late persistent cavitation are, as a group, milder than those of pneumonic lesions. Mild fatiguability, weakness, and weight loss are the most common constitutional symptoms. Cough and sputum are prominent. In many cases all that is noticed is a gradual increase in symptoms of pre-existing chronic bronchitis. Chronic thick-walled cavities are apt to be attended by purulent sputum and, not uncommonly, blood streaking or frank hemoptysis. Fever and other constitutional symptoms are prominent only in a minority of patients. In most, this form of histoplasmosis aggravates pre-existing or latent symptoms of chronic bronchitis and emphysema and significantly contributes to their progression to eventual pulmonary insufficiency.

Laboratory Findings and Diagnosis

Routine laboratory findings are seldom abnormal. Contrary to what might be expected in a chronic infection, anemia is not usually found unless it is due to another cause. The *histoplasmin skin test* is falsely negative in 20 percent and, if positive, has little or no diagnostic value in endemic areas. The *complement fixation test* also has diagnostic limitations. A single test is negative in 25 percent, only of suggestive titer (less than 1:32) in roughly another 25 percent, and of highly suggestive titer in only one-half of all cases. Also there are cross-reactions to blastomycin that must be taken into account. A high titer in a clinically compatible situation has considerable but not conclusive diagnostic force. *Sputum cultures* are diagnostic if positive, but several may be required in patients with pneumonic lesions or thin-walled cavities in order to establish a positive finding. A single sputum culture will be positive in 70 percent of cases with thick-walled cavities. In experienced hands, a Wright stained *smear* of sputum may be positive (unstained refractile cell wall) in 50–80 percent of patients with positive cultures.

The *diagnosis* is suggested and often strongly supported by the findings on a chest roentgenogram. It is further supported by the demonstration of a significantly positive complement fixation test result and is confirmed by a positive sputum culture or a positive sputum smear.

Roentgenographic Characteristics and Course

The chest roentgenogram is important to the clinician in suggesting the diagnosis and in following the course of chronic pulmonary histoplasmosis. The pneumonic lesion can usually be recognized when seen early, and its behavior on serial studies is quite characteristic (Fig. 5). It is segmental or subsegmental, based on the pleura, usually disposed posterolaterally, and always limited to the apical–posterior zones of the lung. It begins as an interstitial pneumonitis and, if seen early, has a typical interstitial pattern. The pneumonitis usually highlights a few focal radiolucencies of centrilobular emphysema, but in some this is so extensive as to give the interstitial pattern a coarse and interrupted appearance. Soon after onset, focal areas or a large central area of necrosis develops. These can be recognized as dense and sharply marginated areas contained within the pneumonic infiltrate. In a few days or weeks the interstitial pneumonitis subsides. The areas of infarct-like necrosis *contract* over several weeks and in 2 or 3 months resolve entirely to leave only a small fibrotic residuum. Much of the emphysema contained within the involved areas becomes obliterated, thereby contributing further to the loss of lung volume.

Cavities develop as a result of persistent infection of open bullous spaces and mostly appear at the time of a pneumonic episode and particularly when the pneumonitis is disposed im-

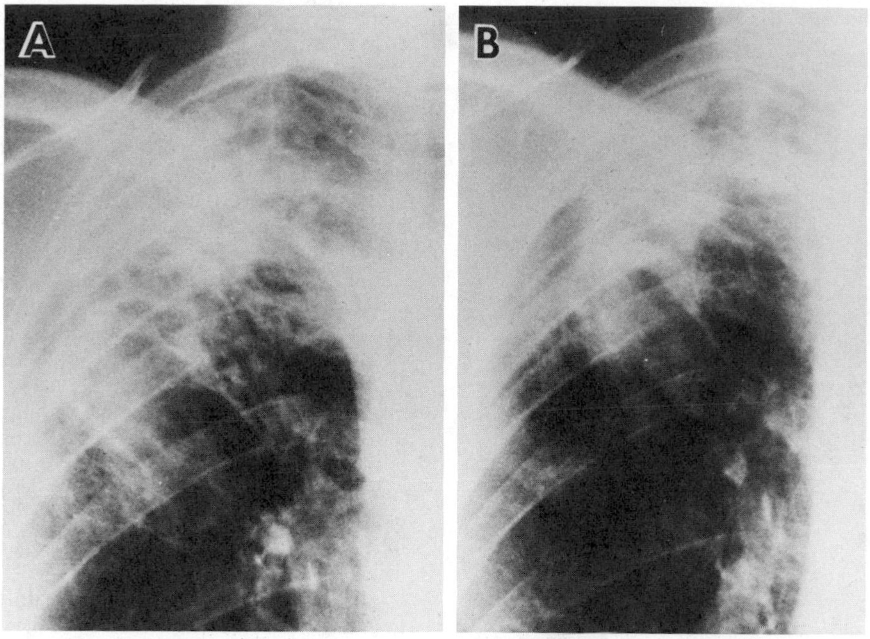

FIG. 5. A typical, fairly early pneumonic lesion of chronic pulmonary histoplasmosis (**A**). Characteristic features are (1) the underlying interstitial pneumonitis seen best in the interspaces is in the lower left area of the photograph. The fine lacy texture is evident. (2) The two large dense areas, one underlying the first anterior rib and clavicle and the other underlying the third anterior rib, are early areas of infarct-like necrosis. (3) The radiolucent areas between the two are areas of centrilobular emphysema. (4) The linear streaks extending into the hilum are characteristic distended peribronchial lymphatics. One month later the interstitial pneumonitis has largely cleared (**B**), and the dense, sharply marginated areas of infarct-like necrosis have *contracted* and pulled together as the emphysematous area has become largely obliterated.

mediately subjacent to apical bullous disease. First the walls of the adjacent bullae are thickened, become roentgenologically visible, and have the appearance of a group of thin-walled cavities. Sometimes the walls thin out further and disappear as the pneumonic infiltrate clears; sometimes the bullae display fluid levels and then gradually become obliterated, presumably because the bronchial communication is obstructed; and sometimes one or more persist as infected thin- or thick-walled cavities. The thickness of the wall has some prognostic significance. Cavities with very thin walls (1 mm) tend to heal spontaneously; those with walls 1–2 mm thick tend to persist with or without mild clinical symptoms; and those with thick walls of 2–4 mm are more symptomatic, have prominent bronchitis-like symptoms, tend to enlarge slowly, and are more often associated with destruction of lung tissue elsewhere. The thick-walled cavities have a larger number of organisms in their necrotic lining. The hypersensitivity response to their products results in slow, continuing necrosis of the inner margin of the fibrous wall, which causes continuous elaboration of new fibrous tissue on the outer wall. This progressive fibrosis destroys adjacent and particularly subjacent lung as the cavity wall slowly advances. This phenomenon has been termed a ''marching cavity'' and is capable of advancing slowly (roughly 1 cm per year) through the entire ipsilateral lung or a large portion of it (Fig. 6).

Thick-walled cavities are also accompanied by increasing fibrosis elsewhere in the lung, particularly in the immediate vicinity of the cavity and at the lung base. These changes are thought to be due to a reaction to aspiration of antigen-rich secretions from the cavity.

Treatment

Rest and *inactivity* are clearly helpful in alleviating symptoms in both pneumonic and cavitary disease. Pneumonic lesions appear to resolve more quickly with rest, but there is little or no benefit of rest in the control of persisting cavities.

The use of *amphotericin B*, 40–50 mg or 0.6 mg/kg body weight daily or three times weekly intravenously for a total of 2.0–2.5 g is recommended for all thick-walled (2–4 mm) cavities, especially if they are enlarging or producing dependent fibrosis. Asymptomatic thin-walled cavities can be watched and treated only if clearly progressive.

Ketoconazole is an appropriate alternative therapy in a dose of 400 mg daily for 6–12 months in patients with persistent cavitation.

PRESUMED OCULAR HISTOPLASMOSIS SYNDROME

As its name suggests, the presumed ocular histoplasmosis syndrome (POHS)[34,35] has not been proved to be caused by histoplasmosis, and the relationship of the ocular syndrome to histoplasmosis remains questionable. *Histoplasma capsulatum* organisms have been demonstrated pathologically in the eyes of patients with two other clinical syndromes, disseminated histoplasmosis and solitary chorioretinal granuloma; however *Histoplasma* organisms have rarely been demonstrated in eyes from patients with POHS.

POHS is a triad of ocular changes that includes scattered yellowish punched-out choroidal lesions, macular subretinal neovascular membranes (with or without hemorrhage), and peripapillary atrophy, all in the absence of inflammatory signs in the vitreous or anterior chamber. The syndrome usually occurs in otherwise healthy young adults who have no signs of active histoplasmosis. The macular neovascular membrane often causes a reduction or loss of visual acuity in one or both eyes.

The association of *Histoplasma capsulatum* with this ocular triad was originally inferred from positive histoplasmin skin testing in the absence of other diseases known to affect the fundus. Skin testing is positive in most patients with ocular

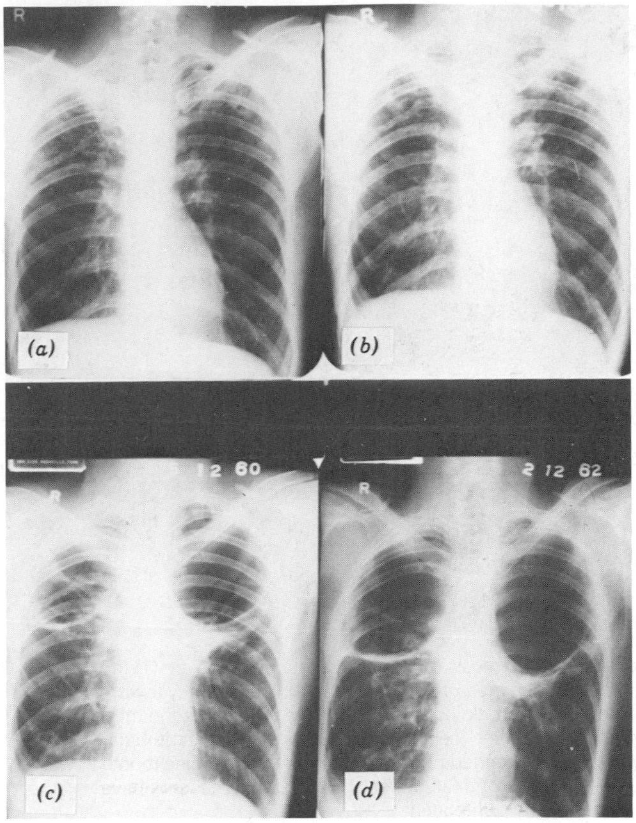

FIG. 6. A composite showing untreated bilateral "marching cavities" of chronic pulmonary histoplasmosis. In 1956, bilateral pneumonic lesions left rather thick-walled (difficult to see) cavities (**A**). Six months later (**B**) there are enlarging thick-walled cavities covering the first anterior interspace bilaterally. The cavities progressively enlarged (**C** and **D**) as the cavity walls have advanced through most of the upper half of both lungs. Fibrotic changes, seen best on the right, cause further destruction. The patient died of pulmonary insufficiency in 1962, having refused treatment throughout because he "didn't feel sick enough."

findings, as it is in the general population in endemic areas, so the diagnostic value of skin testing is negligible in these areas. The failure to meet Koch's postulates does not eliminate the possibility that the retinal syndrome might be a remote manifestation of the initial histoplasmosis infection. However, the best evidence that the syndrome is ever caused by histoplasmosis remains circumstantial—the demonstration of a rough correlation between the regional occurrence of the ocular syndrome and the regional prevalence of histoplasmin skin test positivity.[36]

The typical ocular syndrome can occur clinically in disorders other than histoplasmosis. Although the question is still open about whether POHS is the late result of a remote histoplasmosis infection, it is clearly not an active one, so antifungal therapy is not indicated. In a significant minority, spontaneous improvement of vision occurs. Therapeutic trials of laser photocoagulation have demonstrated at least short-term protection from a loss of visual acuity; corticosteroids or ocular irradiation have also been employed.

HISTOPLASMOSIS DUE TO HISTOPLASMA CAPSULATUM VAR. DUBOISII

H. capsulatum var. *duboisii* is a stable variant found across central Africa that differs morphologically from the parent strain in that the yeast form is considerably larger (7–15 μm). The clinical syndrome associated with human infection with this agent probably has not been fully described. The presently recognized disease entity generally corresponds to the more chronic range of the spectrum of disseminated histoplasmosis. Pathologically, focal lesions are prominent, and these differ in being somewhat more reactive and displaying many parasitized giant cells (multinucleated macrophages) as well as parasitized macrophages. The focal lesions also differ in that they are found predominantly in skin and bone and rarely in the lungs or submucosa of the GI tract including the oropharynx, the lymph nodes, liver, and spleen.[37,38] The clinical spectrum, as might be expected, varies from a single lesion with few or no constitutional symptoms to many lesions of skin and bone that are accompanied by fever, anemia, weight loss, lymphadenopathy, hepatosplenomegaly, and in many, an eventual fatal course.

Almost all cases show cutaneous or subcutaneous lesions.[38] The former usually present as warty, nontender papules a few millimeters across. Some heal spontaneously, whereas others ulcerate and display rolled edges. Less common variations include plaque-like lesions appearing at times eczematoid, psoriasiform, or circinate. Subcutaneous focal lesions are nodular, usually painless, and felt rather than seen, but a few are more inflammatory and tender, and these are apt to break down and form cold abscesses.

The focal lesions of bone are painless at the onset but tend to erode the cortex, at which time they may be tender, and they present as a protruding mass or break down into a cold abscess, which often results in a sinus. Any bone may be involved, but the femur, ribs, and skull are the most common.[37]

The diagnosis is suggested by the character of the skin lesions and by the focal lesions of bone (roentgenologically) and can be confirmed by the finding of large budding yeast forms in smears of cold abscess pus or histologically on biopsy specimens of skin lesions or a culture of either.

In *treatment,* amphotericin B is the drug of choice and is highly effective. It is administered as in disseminated histoplasmosis; patients with more severe disease should receive a total of 2 g, whereas in mild cases a total of 1 g would probably suffice. Sulfamethoxazole (800 mg) plus trimethoprim (160 mg) two or three times daily or ketoconazole 400 mg daily for 1 year have apparently been successful in mild cases, either alone or after a short course of amphotericin B.

REFERENCES

1. Darling ST. A protozoan general infection producing pseudo tubercles in the lungs and focal necrosis in the liver, spleen and lymph nodes. JAMA. 1906;46:1283–85.
2. Parson RJ, Zarafonitis CJD. Histoplasmosis in man: Report of 7 cases and a review of 71 cases. Arch Intern Med. 1945;75:1–23.
3. DeMonbreun WA. The cultivation and cultural characteristics of Darling's *H. capsulatum*. Am J Trop Med. 1934;14:93–125.
4. Christie A, Peterson JC. Pulmonary calcifications in negative reactors to tuberculin. Am J Public Health. 1945;35:1131–47.
5. Christie A, Peterson JC. Histoplasmin sensitivity. J Pediatr. 1946;29:417–32.
6. Palmer CE. Non-tuberculous pulmonary calcification. Public Health Rep. 1945;60:513–20.
7. Palmer CE. Geographic differences in sensitivity to histoplasmin among student nurses. Public Health Rep. 1946;61:475–87.
8. Emmons CW, Morlan HB, Hill EL. Isolation of *Histoplasma capsulatum* from soil. Public Health Rep. 1949;64:892–96.
9. Ajello L. Relationship of *Histoplasma capsulatum* to avian habitats. Public Health Rep. 1964;79:266–70.
10. Emmons CW, Klite PD, Baer GM, et al. Isolation of *Histoplasma capsulatum* from bats in the United States. Am J Epidemiol. 1966;84:103–9.
11. Lehan PH, Furcolow ML. Epidemic histoplasmosis. J Chronic Dis. 1957;5:489–503.
12. Edwards LB, Acquaviva FA, Livesay VT, et al. An atlas of sensitivity to tuberculin, PPD-B, and histoplasmin in the United States. Am Rev Respir Dis. 1969;99(Suppl):1–132.
13. Furcolow ML, Brasher CA. Chronic progressive (cavitary) histoplasmosis as problem in tuberculosis sanatoriums. Am Rev Tuberc. 1956;74:609–19.
14. Goodwin RA, Loyd JE, DesPrez RM. Histoplasmosis in normal hosts. Medicine (Baltimore). 1981;60:231–266.
15. Goodwin RA, Shapiro JL, Thurman GH, et al. Disseminated histoplasmosis. Medicine (Baltimore). 1980;59:1–33.
16. Goodwin RA, Owens FT, Snell JD, et al. Chronic pulmonary histoplasmosis. Medicine (Baltimore). 1976;55:413–452.

17. Kwon-Chung KJ. Sexual stage of *Histoplasma capsulatum*. Science. 1972;177:368–9.
18. Procknow JJ, Connelly AP, Ray CG. Fluorescent antibody technique in histoplasmosis as applied to the pathogenesis of experimental infection in the mouse. Arch Pathol. 1962;73:313–24.
19. Davies SF. Serodiagnosis of histoplasmosis. Semin Respir Infect. 1986;1:9–15.
20. Wheat LJ, French ML, Kamel S, et al. Evaluation of cross-reactions in *Histoplasma capsulatum* serologic tests. J Clin Microbiol. 1986;23:493–9.
21. Wheat LJ, Kohler RB, French ML, et al. Immunoglobulin M and G *Histoplasma* antibody response in histoplasmosis. Am Rev Respir Dis. 1983;126:65–70.
22. Lambert RS, George RB. Evaluation of enzyme immunoassay as a rapid screening test for histoplasmosis and blastomycosis. Am Rev Respir Dis. 1987;136:316–9.
23. Wheat LJ, Kohler RB, Tewari RP. Diagnosis of disseminated histoplasmosis by detection of *Histoplasma capsulatum* antigen in serum and urine specimens. N Engl J Med. 1986;314:83–8.
24. Goodwin RA, Nickell JA, DesPrez RM. Mediastinal fibrosis complicating healed primary histoplasmosis and tuberculosis. Medicine (Baltimore). 1972;51:227–46.
25. Loyd JE, Tillman BF, Atkinson JB, et al. Mediastinal fibrosis complicating histoplasmosis. Medicine (Baltimore). 1988;67:295–310.
26. Goodwin RA, Snell JD. The enlarging histoplasmoma. Concept of tumor-like phenomenon encompassing the tuberculoma and coccidioidoma. Am Rev Respir Dis. 1969;100:1–12.
27. Wilson DA, Nguyen CL, Tytle TL, et al. Sonography of the adrenal glands in chronic disseminated histoplasmosis. J Ultrasound Med. 1986;5:69–73.
28. Paya CV, Roberts GD, Cockerill FR. Laboratory methods for the diagnosis of disseminated histoplasmosis: Clinical importance of the lysis–centrifugation blood culture technique. Mayo Clin Proc. 1987;62:480–5.
29. Wheat LJ, French ML, Batteiger B, et al. Cerebrospinal fluid *Histoplasma* antibodies in central nervous system histoplasmosis. Arch Intern Med. 1985;145:1237–40.
30. Drutz DJ, Spickard A, Rogers DE, et al. Treatment of disseminated mycotic infections. Am J Med. 1968;45:405–18.
31. National Institute of Allergy and Infectious Diseases Mycoses Study Group. Treatment of blastomycosis and histoplasmosis with ketoconazole; results of a prospective randomized clinical trial. Ann Intern Med. 1985;103:861–72.
32. Johnson PC, Khardori N, Najjar AF, et al. Progressive disseminated histoplasmosis in patients with acquired immunodeficiency syndrome. Am J Med. 1988;85:152–8.
33. Salzman SH, Smith RL, Aranda CP. Histoplasmosis in patients at risk for the acquired immunodeficiency syndrome in a nonendemic setting. Chest. 1988;93:917–21.
34. Schlaegel TF. Ocular Histoplasmosis. New York: Grune & Stratton; 1977.
35. Schaegel TF. Update on ocular histoplasmosis. Ophthalmol Clin. 1983;23:1–15.
36. Ellis FD, Schlaegel TF. The geograpic localization of presumed histoplasmic chorioretinitis. Am J Ophth. 1973;75:953–6.
37. Cockshott WP, Lucas AO. Histoplasmosis duboisii. Q J Med. 1964;133:223–38.
38. Lucas AO. Cutaneous manifestations of African histoplasmosis. Br J Dermatol. 1970;82:435–47.

243. BLASTOMYCES DERMATITIDIS

STANLEY W. CHAPMAN

Blastomyces dermatitidis is the dimorphic fungus that causes the systemic pyogranulomatous disease, blastomycosis. Initial infection is through the lungs, usually followed by hematogenous dissemination. Clinical disease most often involves the lungs, skin, bones, and genitourinary system.

HISTORY

The first report of blastomycosis was in 1894 by Gilchrist,[1] who initially speculated that the disease was caused by a protozoan. In collaboration with Stokes, Gilchrist was subsequently able to isolate the organism, to establish that the disease was due to a fungus, and, finally, to infect a dog with the newly isolated fungus.[2–4] Although blastomycosis was originally thought to involve only the skin, a number of cases of systemic disease were soon reported. Analysis of these early cases[5,6] led to the concept that two forms of the disease existed, namely, cutaneous and systemic, and that each represented different portals of entry, skin and lung, respectively. This erroneous concept was not corrected until the work of Schwartz and Baum.[7] By careful clinical and pathologic studies, they established that the primary route of infection was the lungs, and that skin disease or other organ involvement was secondary to dissemination.

THE ORGANISM

Blastomyces dermatitidis is the imperfect (or asexual) stage of *Ajellomyces dermatitidis*. The imperfect stage exhibits dimorphism, growing as a mycelial form at room temperature and as a yeast form at 37°C.[8,9] The mycelial form grows as a white mold that slowly turns light brown. On primary isolation, colonies appear in 1–3 weeks. The branching hyphae are usually 2–3 μm in diameter. Arising at right angles to the hyphae are conidiophores that produce single terminal conidia that vary from 2 to 10 μm in diameter and are of round or oval shape. The conidia are thought to be infectious for humans when the mycelia are disturbed. Conversion of the mycelial form to the yeast form at 37°C is necessary for definitive identification. Yeastlike colonies are wrinkled and cream or tan colored. The yeast cells (Fig. 1) may vary from 5 to 30 μm, but most are 8 to 15 μm in diameter, with a thick cell wall that is highly refractile. The yeast cells are multinucleate, containing 8–12 nuclei, and reproduce by single buds with a broad base between parent and bud. The daughter cell is often nearly as large as the mother cell before detachment. These same yeast cell characteristics in vitro are also noted in tissue or secretions and are used to distinguish *B. dermatitidis* from other fungi.

Two serotypes of *B. dermatitidis* have been identified by exoantigen analysis of yeast organisms.[10] Initial studies indicate that the A-antigen-deficient serotypes are restricted to Africa.[11] The sexual form, *A. dermatitidis*, is heterothallic and requires opposite mating types (+ and −) for fertile cultures.[12,13] Infection occurs with equal frequency with the two mating types.[14] Occasionally, both types are isolated from a single patient.

EPIDEMIOLOGY

A complete understanding of the incidence and epidemiology of blastomycosis has been hindered by the lack of a sensitive,

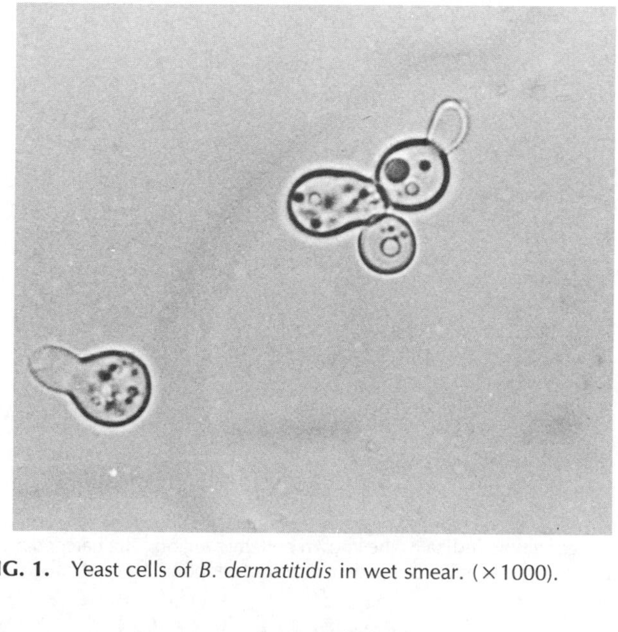

FIG. 1. Yeast cells of *B. dermatitidis* in wet smear. (×1000).

specific skin test reagent and the difficulty in establishing the ecologic niche of *B. dermatitidis* in nature. What we know about blastomycosis is based on the collected studies of sporadic cases in humans and dogs, as well as the studies of nine epidemics or clusters of disease.[15–21] Based on these data, the endemic area in North America (Fig. 2) includes the southeastern and south central states, especially those bordering on the Mississippi and Ohio river basins, the midwestern states and Canadian provinces that border the Great Lakes, and a small area in New York and Canada that follows the St. Lawrence River. Indigenous cases have also been reported in Central and South America, Africa, and perhaps the Middle East.[21]

Initial analysis of sporadic cases indicated that middle-aged men with outdoor occupations that exposed them to soil were at greatest risk for blastomycosis.[15,16] These findings, however, may only reflect the demographics of the rural states from which most of the cases were reported. In contrast, review of the nine case clusters reported to date[22–29] indicates that there is no sex, age, or occupational predilection for blastomycosis. In six of the outbreaks, recreational activities in wooded areas along waterways was the major risk identified. Thus, exposure to soil, whether at work or play, appears to be the common link in reports of sporadic disease and outbreaks.

Attempts to isolate the organism in nature have been difficult and the results inconsistent. Only recently has the organism been isolated in association with human disease. Denton and coworkers reported multiple isolations of *B. dermatitidis* from soil and rotting wood during environmental surveys between 1958 and 1963.[30–32] Yeast phase organisms were said to be recovered from pigeon manure after a single case of blastomycosis, but this report lacks crucial details.[33] Isolation from soil samples of an earthen floor was also reported after a single case of disease in Canada.[34] The recent environmental isolations of *B. dermatitidis* by Klein and coworkers in association with two outbreaks of disease have been important breakthroughs in defining the ecologic niche of the organism.[28,29] In both instances, the organism was isolated from soil containing decayed vegetation or from decomposed wood. Humidity probably played an important role in promoting the growth of the organism because of the proximity to water and recent rainfall in both outbreaks. These studies, in association with other in vitro work,[35] indicate that *B. dermatitidis* exists in nature in warm, moist soil of wooded areas that is also rich in organic debris, such as decaying vegetation or animal manure. The conditions that support the growth of *B. dermatitidis* in these microfoci probably exist for only short periods of time. Thus, when a sporadic outbreak of blastomycosis is recognized, the appropriate local and environmental conditions may no longer exist at the site of exposure, preventing environmental isolation.

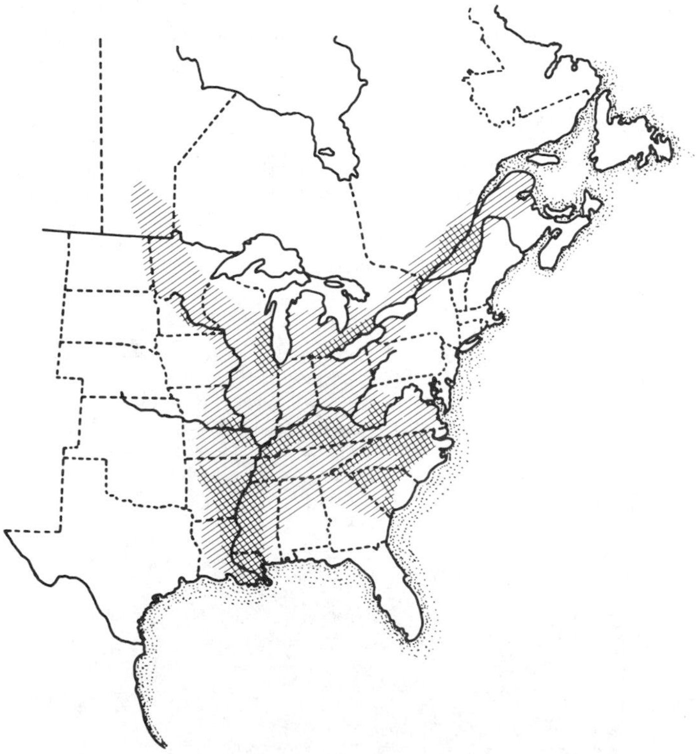

FIG. 2. The incidence and prevalence of blastomycosis in North America. The diagonal line indicates the known endemic region. The hatched areas are those with the highest incidence. (From Rippon,[9] with permission.)

PATHOGENESIS AND PATHOLOGY

The studies of Schwartz and Baum[7] were the first to establish that the portal of entry in humans for blastomycosis appears to be the lung. Thus, the manifestations of disease at other body sites are the result of dissemination from a primary pulmonary infection, even if not clinically recognized. Primary cutaneous blastomycosis has occurred after accidental inoculation in the laboratory or at autopsy[36] and after dog bites.[37] Transmission of disease from person to person by yeast phase organisms has not been documented, except for the rare vaginal infection acquired from a man with genitourinary blastomycosis[38] and a possible case of intrauterine transmission.[39]

Pulmonary infection probably occurs by inhalation of the conidia, which convert to the yeast phase in the lung. The usual inflammatory response consists of clusters of neutrophils, as well as noncaseating granulomas with epithelioid and giant cells. This inflammatory response is simlar to that seen with coccidioidomycosis and sporotrichosis. Although this histopathologic picture recapitulates itself to a variable degree in extrapulmonary sites, the response in cutaneous disease is unique and shows prominent pseudoepitheliomatous hyperplasia with microabscess formation that clinically and histologically may mimic a variety of cutaneous diseases, including squamous cell carcinoma of the skin.[40] The same pseudoepitheliomatous response may also be seen when mucosal surfaces of the mouth, oropharynx, or larynx are involved.

IMMUNITY

The immunologic responses in *B. dermatitidis* infection are not completely defined due to the lack of appropriate antigens. Recent advances in characterizing yeast antigens may overcome this problem in the near future.

Polymorphonuclear Leukocytes

The histopathologic response previously noted implicates both a neutrophil response and a cellular immune response. The polymorphonuclear leukocyte reaction is probably mediated by the release of chemotactic factors from the organism.[41] Human neutrophils have been shown to phagocytize and kill the conidia of *B. dermatitidis* efficiently. However, the phagocytosis and killing of the yeast forms, despite activation of neutrophil metabolic pathways, are poor and may be important in the progression of disease.[42,43] The fungicidal activity of neutrophils can be enhanced in vitro by lymphokine-rich supernatants from immunologically stimulated T lymphocytes and provides a link between cellular immunity and neutrophil function.[44,45]

Cellular Immunity

Delayed hypersensitivity can be induced in mice by subcutaneous injections of live or killed *B. dermatitidis*. Decreased susceptibility to infection parallels the development of the cellular immune response,[46,47] and resistance to infection in mice has been transferred by T lymphocytes.[48] Macrophages harvested from mice with experimental blastomycosis have also been reported to inhibit the replication of *B. dermatitidis*, and interferon-γ treatment, both in vivo and in vitro, has been shown to enhance killing of *B. dermatitidis* by murine alveolar macrophages.[49,50]

The study of cellular immunity in humans has been hindered by the lack of a sensitive, specific antigen for both in vitro studies and skin testing. Recently, the development of specific cellular immunity has been documented in patients with blastomycosis using whole yeast phase organisms and an alkali-soluble, water-soluble yeast extract.[28,51] Macrophages from patients recovering from blastomycosis have also been shown to have enhanced inhibition of intracellular growth of *B. dermatitidis* when compared to controls.[52] Finally, supernatants of antigen-stimulated human lymphocytes have been shown to enhance phagocytosis and intracellular inhibition of the growth of *B. dermatitidis* by both alveolar and monocyte-derived macrophages.[52] Despite these advances, however, an antigen for skin testing is not available. Blastomycin, a culture filtrate of mycelial phase organisms, lacks both specificity and sensitivity. In the Veterans Administration Cooperative Study, only 40 percent of patients with blastomycosis had a positive skin test to blastomycin.[15] Future studies clarifying cellular immunity in human cases of blastomycosis will benefit by the characterization of the fungal antigens.[53,54]

Humoral Immunity

Yeast antigens have been used to evaluate humoral immunity in a variety of serologic tests, each with differing sensitivities and specificities. The complement fixation test has not proved to be useful because of a lack of sensitivity and specificity. Only 50 percent or fewer patients with blastomycosis will develop a positive complement fixation test to blastomycosis.[15] Cross-reactivity with *Histoplasma capsulatum* and to a lesser degree *Coccidioides immitis* has also been a problem.[55]

The immunodiffusion test, which detects precipitin antibodies to the A and B antigen located in the cell wall of the yeast is more specific for blastomycosis. As modified by Kauffman and associates, the presence of antibody to the A antigen has been noted in up to 70–80 percent of patients with blastomycosis.[55–57] However, a recent article reported that patients with localized disease are less likely to have a positive test than those with disseminated disease.[58] It should be noted that the time course for the development of this antibody response, its persistence after infection, and the possible prognostic value of such an antibody response have not been adequately studied. Commercial immunodiffusion test kits are now available.

CLINICAL MANIFESTATIONS

What is known about the clinical manifestations of blastomycosis is derived from careful studies of symptomatic, sporadic cases and the few case clusters reported. It must be emphasized that blastomycosis is a systemic disease with a wide variety of pulmonary and extrapulmonary manifestations. Pulmonary disease may be acute or chronic and mimics infection with pyogenic bacteria, tuberculosis, other fungi, and malignancy. Cutaneous disease, the most common extrapulmonary manifestation, appears similar to disease seen with bromoderma, pyoderma gangrenosum, Majocchi's granuloma, leishmaniasis, *Mycobacterium marinum* infection, and squamous cell carcinoma. *Blastomyces dermatitidis* infection may involve almost every body organ (Table 1), resulting in the diversity of clinical manifestations. Skin, bone, and genitourinary sites of infection are the most common and are most likely to be clinically manifest. Extrapulmonary disease is seen during the chronic form of illness, where approximately two-thirds of patients will have multiple organ involvement.

Although a variety of clinical schema may be used in discussing blastomycosis, that proposed by Sarosi and Davies appears most comprehensive.[65] A modification of this schema is presented in Figure 3. It should be noted that reactivation blastomycosis is controversial, with only few cases being suggestive.[66] Cases attributed to extrapulmonary reactivation may only represent the late clinical manifestations of chronic, subclinical disease that remains active after pulmonary healing. Those factors determining the clinical course after acute infection are not well defined but probably result from a complex interaction of pulmonary anatomy, host defenses, and microbial factors.

Acute Infection

Acute pulmonary infection is often unrecognized unless related to group exposure. Although a wide range of incubation periods have been reported, analysis of point source outbreaks indicates a median incubation time of 30–45 days.[20,21,26,28,29] Symptoms are nonspecific and tend to mimic influenza or bacterial infection with the abrupt onset of myalgias, arthralgias, chills, and fever. Pleuritic pain may be prominent but is usually transient. Cough is initially nonproductive but in many cases becomes productive of purulent sputum. The radiologic findings in the acute stage of disease, whether symptomatic or asymptomatic, are also nonspecific but are usually those of lobar or segmental consolidation, most often in the lower lobes[67,68] (Fig. 4). Pleural effusion is uncommon or, if present, found only in small amounts. Hilar adenopathy is uncommon.

Spontaneous resolution of symptomatic acute pneumonia has been recognized in a few sporadic cases, in case clusters, and after accidental laboratory infection.[69–71] In these cases symptoms usually have resolved in less than 4 weeks, but x-ray film abnormalities have taken longer to clear.

Chronic or Recurrent Infection

Most patients in whom blastomycosis is diagnosed have an indolent onset and progressive disease. The clinical manifestations are diverse, including pulmonary and/or extrapulmonary disease. For the sake of clarity, these will be discussed separately.

Pulmonary Manifestations. The clinical manifestations of pulmonary disease are those of chronic pneumonia, including productive cough, hemoptysis, weight loss, and pleuritic chest pain. Fever, which may not be present, tends to be low grade. The radiologic findings in these patients are variable. Although consolidation may be seen, upper lobe fibronodular infiltrates, with or without cavitation, similar to those of other granulomatous diseases, are more common (Fig. 5).[67,68] Mass lesions that mimic bronchogenic carcinoma are not uncommon[72] (Fig. 6). An occasional patient will have acute deterioration associated with miliary disease due to hematogenous spread[73] (Fig. 7) or diffuse pneumonitis from presumed endobronchial spread.[74] Respiratory failure is common in patients with a miliary pattern, the mortality being 50 percent or greater. Pleural thickening, pleural effusions and pneumothorax may occur. One report noted an unfavorable response to therapy in patients with major pleural disease.[75]

Skin. Skin disease is the most common extrapulmonary manifestation of blastomycosis, occurring in 40–80 percent of cases (Table 1). Although extrapulmonary disease is usually seen in conjunction with active pulmonary disease, skin involvement may occur alone. In some patients with skin disease, asymptomatic pulmonary disease will be found.

Two different types of skin lesions may be seen. The first is the more characteristic verrucous lesions that usually appear on exposed body areas. These often begin as a small papulo-

TABLE 1. Organ Involvement in Blastomycosis on Clinical and Autopsy Findings in Seven Studies

	Study[a]							
Organ System Involved	*Cherniss and Waisbren*[59] *[40]*	*Abernathy*[60] *[35]*	*VA Cooperative Study*[15] *[198]*	*Witorsch and Utz*[61] *[40]*	*Lockwood et al.*[62] *[74]*	*Duttera and Osterhout*[63] *[63]*	*Busey and VA Cooperative Study*[64] *[84]*	*Total*[c]
Lungs	28(70)[b]	27(77)	118(60)	28(70)	59(80)	33(52)	76(90)	369/534(69)
Skin	30(75)	28(80)	118(60)	29(73)	33(45)	36(57)	32(38)	306/534(57)
Bone	19(48)	12(34)	46(23)	11(28)	10(14)	12(19)	6(7)	116/534(22)
Genitourinary	11(28)	5(14)	32(16)	13(33)	13(18)	6(10)	12(14)	92/534(17)
Reticuloendothelial system (liver, spleen, lymph nodes)	5(13)	13(37)	25(13)	7(18)	NS[c]	3(5)	3(4)	56/460(12)
CNS	4(10)	1(3)	9(5)	1(3)	5(7)	4(6)	4(5)	29/534(5)
Mucous membranes	3(8)	2(6)	11(6)	10(25)	NS	NS	NS	26/273(10)
Subcutaneous	25(63)	NS	NS	15(38)	NS	NS	NS	40/80(50)
Other[d]	5(13)	9(26)	18(9)	5(13)	NS	7(11)	2(2)	46/460(10)

[a] Number of cases given in square brackets, [ ]; reference numbers after author.
[b] Number of cases followed by percentage in parentheses.
[c] Total based on studies where stated; NS, not stated.
[d] Other: Thyroid, 10; gastrointestinal, 8; larynx, 8; adrenal, 7; pleura, 6; joints, 5; heart, 2; peritoneum, 1; eye, 1; psoas, 1; retropharynx, 1.

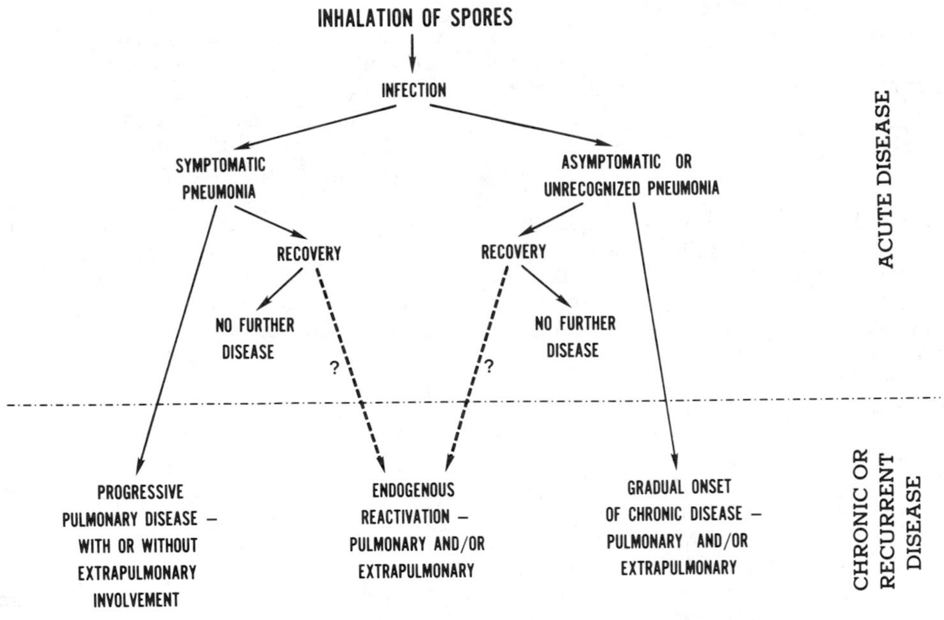

FIG. 3. A clinical classification of blastomycosis. (Adapted from Sarosi and Davies,[65] with permission.)

pustular lesion (Fig. 8) and slowly spread to form a crusted, heaped-up lesion that can vary in color from gray to a violaceous hue (Fig. 9). This lesion is often mistaken for squamous cell carcinoma. Older lesions may show central clearing with scar formation and depigmentation. Microabscess formation tends to occur at the periphery of such lesions, and removal of the eschar peripherally reveals purulent material in which the yeast forms usually are visible on wet preparation.

The second type of lesion is described as ulcerative (Fig. 10), in which the initial pustule spreads as a superficial ulcer or slightly raised lesion, with a bed of red granulation tissue that bleeds easily. Skin lesions of both types may be seen in the same patient. Lesions may also occur on the mucosa of the nose, mouth, and larynx. Skin lesions associated with a pulmonary pathogenesis have little or no regional lymph node involvement or lymphadenitis, in contrast to that seen with inoculation blastomycosis.[36,37]

Subcutaneous Nodules. Although often discussed as a skin manifestation, the clinical syndrome seen in patients with subcutaneous nodules is different from that associated with other skin lesions. Subcutaneous nodules are cold abscesses that are usually seen in conjunction with pulmonary and other extrapulmonary disease. The patient appears acutely ill, systemic manifestations are prominent, and rapid deterioration may result unless prompt therapy is initiated. Lesions sometimes drain spontaneously. Drainage or aspirated pus has abundant numbers of organisms that are readily apparent on microscopic examination.

Bone and Joint. After skin disease, skeletal blastomycosis is next in frequency and is seen in 10–50 percent of cases. The long bones, vertebrae, and ribs are most commonly involved, but almost any bone can be infected.[76,77] A well-circumscribed osteolytic lesion is typical. Patients with bone lesions rarely present with bone pain but rather with contiguous soft tissue abscesses or chronic draining sinuses. Vertebral disease mimics tuberculosis with anterior involvement of the vertebral body, destruction of the interspace, and development of large paraspinous abscesses.

Arthritis usually occurs by extension from a contiguous osteomyelitis. Signs and symptoms may be acute or chronic. Synovial fluid is usually purulent, with organisms readily visible on wet preparation.[78]

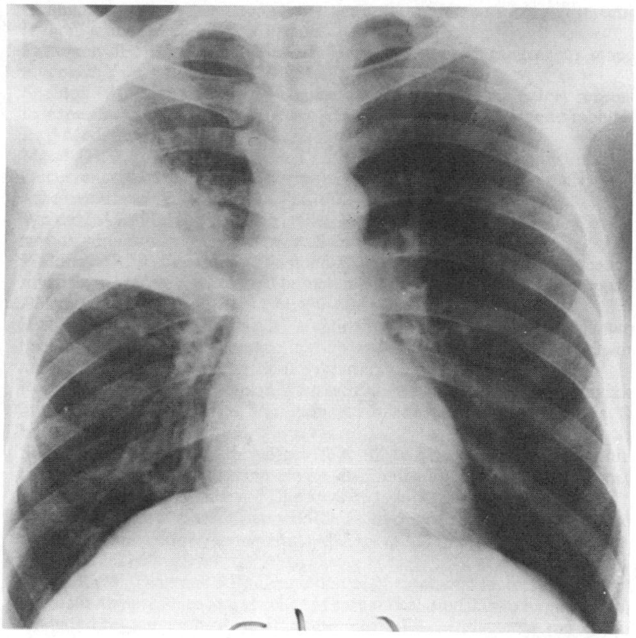

FIG. 4. A confluent infiltrate with a segmental distribution in a patient with blastomycosis.

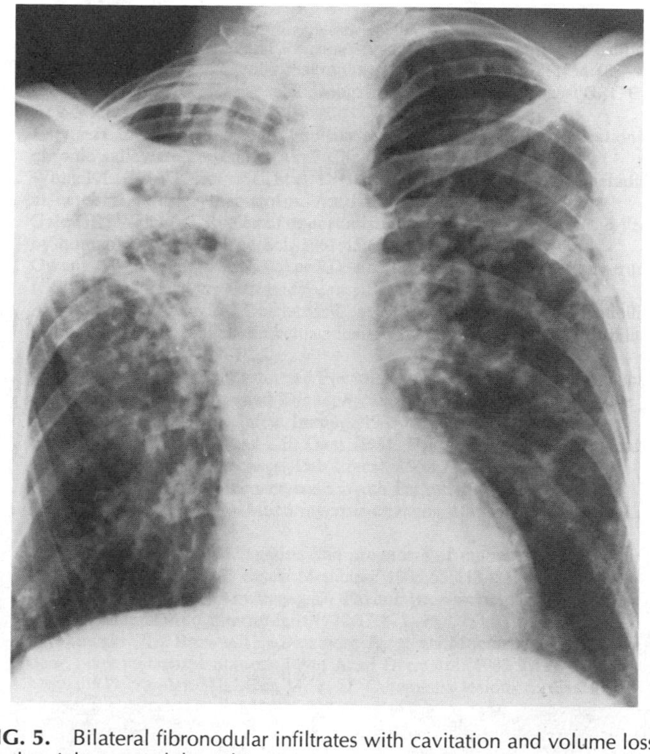

FIG. 5. Bilateral fibronodular infiltrates with cavitation and volume loss in the right upper lobe. This x-ray appearance cannot be distinguished from that of tuberculosis or other granulomatous diseases.

Genitourinary Tract. Up to one-third of the cases in men have been reported to involve the genitourinary tract, primarily the prostate and epididymis.[79] Epididymal disease may spread to the testes. The variable incidence reported may reflect the authors' tenacity to make the diagnosis. Prostatic involvement is most common and is usually manifested by symptoms of obstruction, an enlarged, tender prostate, and pyuria. Cultures of the urine, especially after prostatic massage, are often positive.

Central Nervous System. Disease involving the central nervous system is uncommon. When present, it manifests either as an abscess or as meningitis.[80,81] Abscesses present as mass lesions and may be intracranial or, occasionally, spinal in location. Meningitis is usually a late and fulminant complication of widely disseminated blastomycosis.

Other Sites. Blastomycosis may infrequently involve the liver, spleen, gastrointestinal tract, thyroid, pericardium, adrenal glands, and other sites (Table 1). Most of these represent findings at autopsy in patients with widely disseminated disease. Of note, gastrointestinal disease below the esophagus and overt adrenal insufficiency are rare.

Special Circumstances

Blastomycosis in Children. Although considered rare by some authors, most reviews of blastomycosis note that 2–10 percent of the patients reported are less than 10 years old. A recent common source outbreak of disease involving 46 children noted an attack rate for infection of approximately 50 percent. Of those children infected, about one-half were symptomatic.[28] Pediatric patients manifest the full clinical spectrum of disease as outlined for adults.[82,83]

Blastomycosis in the Compromised Host. Although invasive fungal diseases are common in the immunosuppressed host, only a few reports have indicated that *B. dermatitidis* can act as an opportunistic infection.[84] Blastomycosis in the compromised host is more often disseminated when diagnosed. However, the clinical presentation and the response to therapy are similar to those in the immunocompetent host. This is in contrast to the distinct patterns of disease seen with coccidioidomycosis and histoplasmosis in immunosuppressed patients.

DIAGNOSIS

There is no characteristic clinical syndrome that allows the diagnosis of blastomycosis. Definitive diagnosis requires the growth of the organism from clinical specimens. A presumptive diagnosis may be made by visualization of the characteristic yeast in pus, sputum, secretions, or histopathologic sections. In the appropriate clinical setting, visualization of the fungus can prompt the initiation of antimicrobial therapy.

Direct Examination of Secretions

Sputum or pus is easily examined by wet preparation. A drop of the specimen is placed on the microscope slide, covered with a coverslip, and examined under the high dry objective. Although 10 percent potassium hydroxide has been recommended to aid in finding the organism, it is usually not necessary, as the large, characteristic yeast is easily seen despite cellular debris. Sometimes it is also useful to digest sputum with trypsin and smear the centrifuged sediment. Body fluids such as urine, pleural fluid, or cerebrospinal fluid should be centrifuged and the sediment evaluated in the same way.

When visualized, the yeast cells are easily differentiated from others on the basis of their size, refractile cell wall, and single, broad-based buds (Fig. 1). Occasionally the endospores of *C. immitis* may appear like single yeast cells, but the presence of budding can be used to distinguish *B. dermatitidis*. *Paracoccidioides brasiliensis*, rarely seen in the United States, is distinguished by the presence of multiple, narrow-based buds. Sometimes, *B. dermatitidis* may be as small as *Cryptococcus neoformans*, though the capsule and narrow-based bud of the latter aid in differentiation.

Although bronchoscopy has been recommended as a useful technique for obtaining specimens, it is the experience at the University of Mississippi and Jackson Veterans Administration

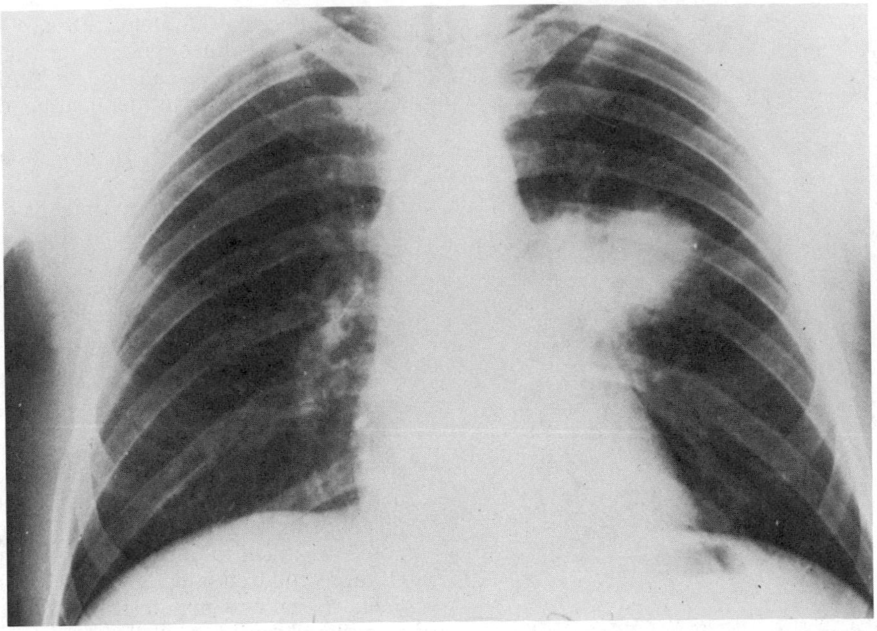

FIG. 6. A perihilar mass lesion in a patient with blastomycosis. This x-ray appearance mimics that of carcinoma of the lung. Patients with this x-ray picture should have bronchoscopy even if wet preparations of sputum reveal the organism in order to rule out a coexisting malignancy.

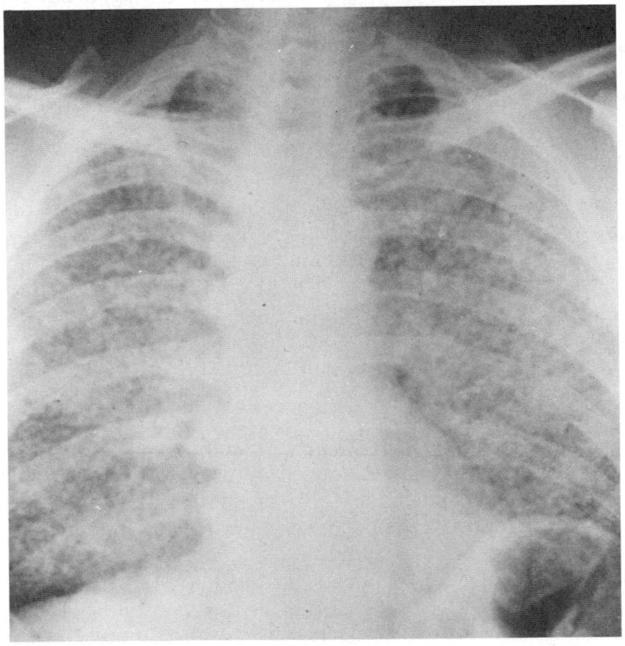

FIG. 7. Miliary blastomycosis in a patient with respiratory failure. (Courtesy of Dr. Guy Campbell, Jackson, MI.)

Medical Centers that bronchoscopy is best reserved for patients not producing sputum or in whom the x-ray film indicates the possibility of malignancy. Bronchial washings and postbronchoscopy sputum samples should be sent for cytology as well as smear and culture, since the organism is often visualized on Papanicolaou preparations.[85]

Histopathologic Examination

The presence of pyogranulomas should alert one to the possibility of blastomycosis. Yeast forms can be difficult to see on

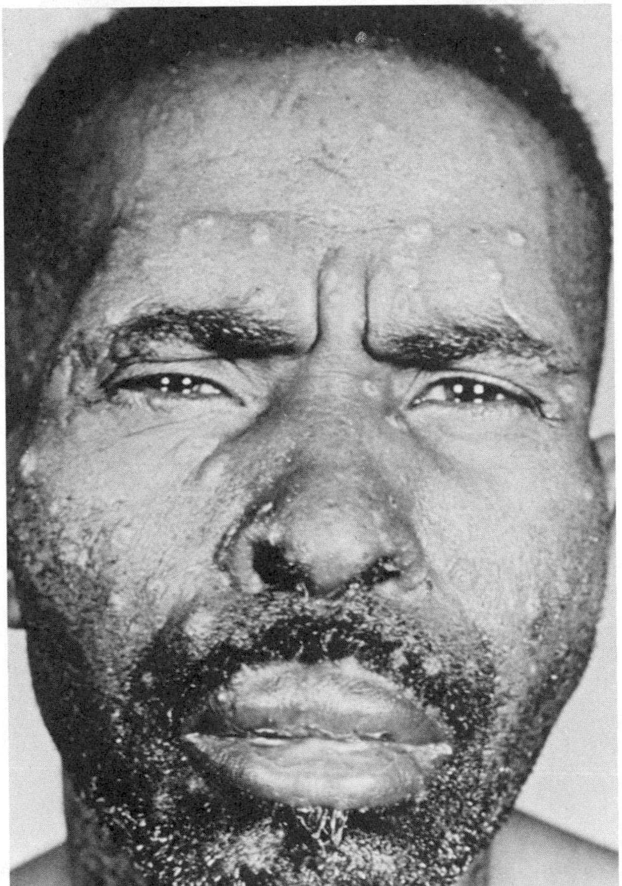

FIG. 8. Multiple papulopustular lesions in a patient with blastomycosis. (Courtesy of Dr. Guy Campbell, Jackson, MI.)

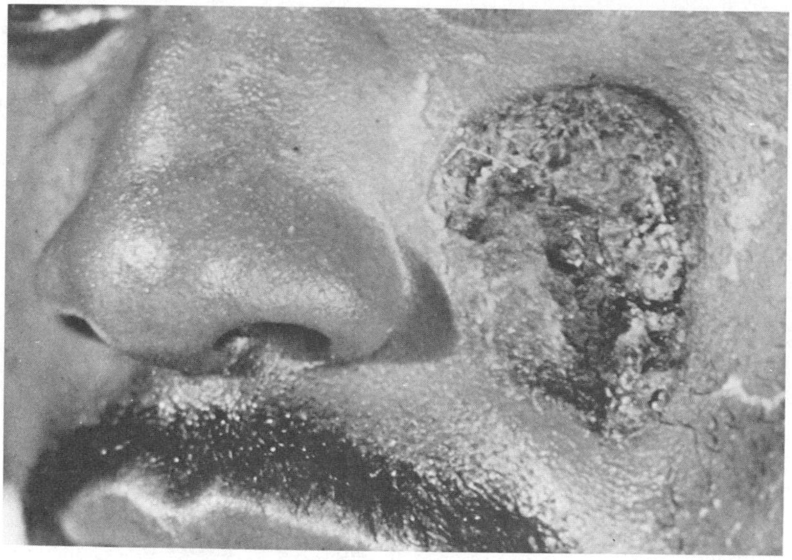

FIG. 9. The typical verrucous skin lesion of blastomycosis. Note the circumscribed edges. (Courtesy of Dr. John F. Busey, Jackson, MI.)

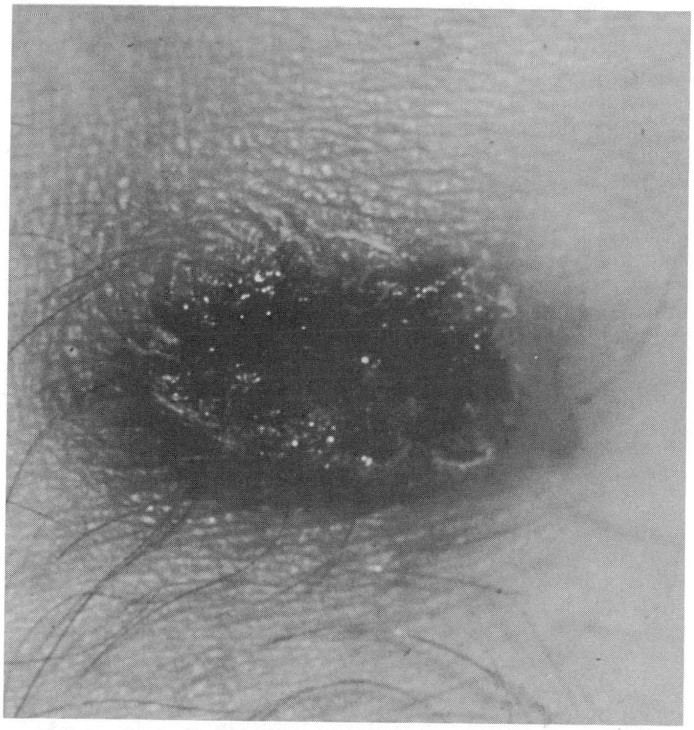

FIG. 10. The ulcerative skin lesion of blastomycosis. These lesions bleed easily.

routine hematoxylin and eosin stains, and special stains should be used to enhance visualization. The Gomori methenamine-silver stain is best used for screening tissue for the presence of fungal elements (Fig. 11). This stain, however, does not allow evaluation of either the fungal morphology or the inflammatory response in the tissue. The periodic acid-Schiff stain, which colors the cell wall pink or red, does allow evaluation of cell morphology and tissue response. Mayer's mucicarmine stains the cell wall of *B. dermatitidis* faintly or not at all. This may be used in differentiating it from *C. neoformans* when necessary.

Culture

Any material obtained should be placed on Sabouraud's or, preferably, more enriched agar (Sabhi, brain heart infusion, Gorman's media, etc.). Initial growth is more dependable at 30°C; thus this temperature is recommended. Specimens contaminated with bacteria should also be cultured on media containing an antibacterial antibiotic such as chloramphenicol. Cycloheximide can be incorporated into the media to inhibit other fungal contaminants. However, this selective media should never be used at 37°C because the yeast phase of *B. dermatitidis* (as well as some opportunistic fungi) is sensitive to cycloheximide, and growth may be inhibited. The mycelial form of *B. dermatitidis* is not diagnostic and requires conversion to the yeast form for confirmation.

Serologic Methods

As mentioned previously, serum complement fixation tests are neither specific nor sensitive. The immunodiffusion test is more sensitive and specific than the complement fixation test.[55–58] Antibody against A antigen has been reported in 52–80 percent of patients with blastomycosis, with almost no cross-reactivity with other fungi.[55] A single report noted that patients with localized disease had a lower rate of positivity (33 percent) when compared to those with disseminated disease (88 percent).[58] Thus, a negative antibody titer, no matter which test is used, should never be used to rule out disease. Neither should a positive titer by itself be an indication for therapy; rather, it should stimulate the clinician to look carefully for the disease.

A radioimmunoassay and an enzyme immunoassay employing commercial antigens have been used by George and coworkers as rapid screening tests for histoplasmosis and blastomycosis.[86,87] Both tests are quite sensitive, but their specificity is no better than that of complement fixation. A sensitive enzyme immunoassay using purified A antigen has been recently reported, but the specificity of this test varies depending on the cut-off titer employed.[88] Using these sensitive tests for initial screening in conjunction with the more specific immunodiffusion test may be useful. However, none of these tests are readily available for clinical use, and their role in the diagnosis of blastomycosis requires further evaluation.

Cellular Immunity Testing

No reagent is currently available for skin testing patients with suspected blastomycosis. Lymphocyte transformation to yeast

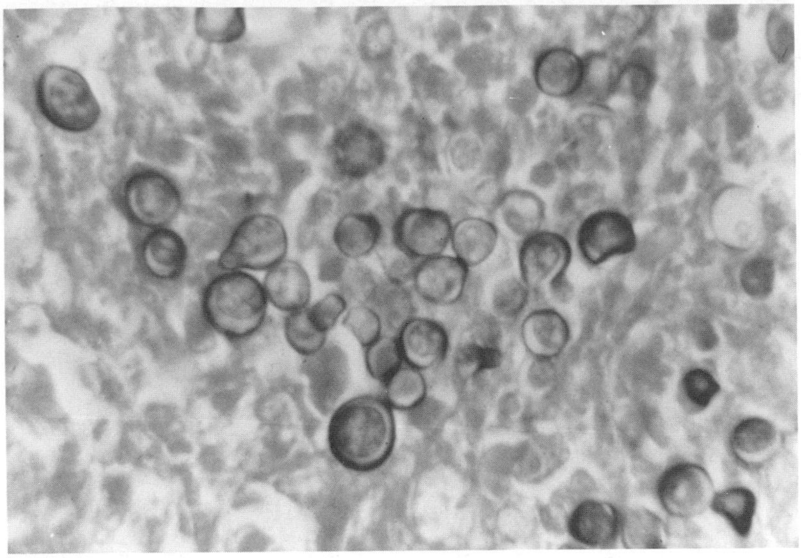

FIG. 11. A Gomori methenamine-silver stain of a laryngeal biopsy specimen in a patient with suspected carcinoma of the larynx. (Courtesy of Dr. James Gorman, Jackson, MI.)

phase organisms and alkali-soluble, water-soluble (ASWS) antigens have been used as an indicator of cell-mediated immunity in patients with blastomycosis. In a recent outbreak, 81 percent of definite and probable cases of blastomycosis had positive lymphocyte transformation tests to the ASWS antigen.[28] This test does not appear to be helpful early in acute disease, as positive tests do not occur for the first 2 weeks of disease. Further, this immunity appears to be long-lived, and a positive test would not necessarily indicate recent infection. Finally, there are only limited data on the specificity of this test. Lymphocyte transformation assays, therefore, are not yet clinically useful and should be considered investigational tests.

TREATMENT

Before the availability of chemotherapy for blastomycosis, the disease as reported had a progressive course with eventual extrapulmonary disease and a mortality exceeding 60 percent. Even though isolated cutaneous disease had a better prognosis, skin lesions were progressive and spontaneous recovery uncommon. Thus, after the introduction of effective antifungal therapy, it was accepted that all patients with blastomycosis should be treated. This concept came under some question after the description of self-limited pulmonary blastomycosis.[69] The decision to withhold therapy for patients with acute pulmonary blastomycosis is difficult and controversial. Although it is true that in some patients blastomycotic pneumonia may resolve without therapy, there is no way of determining which patients will later present with extrapulmonary disease, often with serious sequelae.[66] Further, some patients while under observation may suffer acute exacerbation with miliary disease or endobronchial spread, both associated with high mortality.[73,74] For these reasons, it is the policy at the author's medical center that nearly all patients with active disease are treated. If a cultural diagnosis is made after spontaneous recovery from blastomycotic pneumonia, patients are carefully evaluated for the presence of extrapulmonary disease before deciding not to treat them. If treatment is withheld, patients must be followed carefully for many years for evidence of reactivation or progressive disease.

Amphotericin B was previously considered the treatment of choice for all clinical forms of blastomycosis.[62,64,89] However, recent studies indicate that ketoconazole is an effective alternative in immunocompetent patients with mild to moderate disease.[90–93] Ketoconazole does not cross the blood-brain barrier and should not be used in patients with central nervous system blastomycosis. In a prospective, randomized multicenter trial of patients treated for at least 6 months, there was a 100 percent cure rate in patients treated with 800 mg/day and a 79 percent cure rate in those treated with 400 mg/day.[90] Toxicity was greater with the higher dose. A second study noted a cure rate of 81 percent in 43 patients who completed at least 1 month of therapy with 400 mg/day.[91] Thus, it is recommended to begin ketoconazole as a single daily dose of 400 mg. If the clinical response is not satisfactory, the dose should be increased in 200-mg increments to a maximum of 800 mg/day. Therapy should be continued for at least 6 months.[92,93] Several caveats must be considered when using ketoconazole as therapy. First, gastric acid is necessary for absorption, and ketoconazole blood levels in patients continued on antacid therapy or H-2 blockers may be subtherapeutic.[93,94] Second, both isoniazid and rifampin have been shown to increase hepatic metabolism of ketoconazole and may result in treatment failure.[93,94] Finally, because of its hepatic metabolism, very little ketoconazole is excreted in the urine as active drug. Thus, patients with genitourinary disease may be more resistant to therapy and more likely to relapse after treatment.[90,93–95]

Amphotericin B is now reserved for patients with life-threatening blastomycosis, central nervous system disease, progression of disease on ketoconazole, and those unable to tolerate ketoconazole due to toxicity.[92,93] Although the exact dose and the duration of therapy are uncertain, relapse has been noted to be more common if a total dose of less than 1.5 g is administered. Most authors, therefore, recommend a total dose of 1.5–2.5 g of amphotericin B. In seriously ill patients, 0.3–0.6 mg/kg (not exceeding 50 mg) should be administered daily until objective evidence of improvement is noted. Patients without central nervous system disease have been successfully treated at our medical center by the substitution of ketoconazole in their treatment regimen. For patients who must continue to take amphotericin B, 0.6–0.8 mg/kg (usually 50 mg) may be administered three times per week or every other day on an outpatient basis.[96] Relapse rates of patients treated with amphotericin B are less than 10 percent. Patients with cavitary lung disease appear more likely to relapse than those without cavities.

Hydroxystilbamidine, the first drug available for the treatment of blastomycosis, is now rarely, if ever, used. The drug is administered intravenously in a daily dose of 225 mg until a total dose of 8–12 g has been given. Miconazole, an intravenous imidazole, is infrequently used for blastomycosis.[97] No clinical trials of the treatment of blastomycosis have been published, and, as such, there is no currently defined role for miconazole in this disease. Itraconazole, a new oral imidazole, is currently under active investigation; it appears to be as effective as ketoconazole and may have less toxicity.[98] Future comparative trials will be necessary to define the role of this drug in treating blastomycosis.

Other than for diagnosis, surgery has little role in the treatment of blastomycosis.[99,100] In conjunction with antifungal therapy, surgery appears indicated for the drainage of large abscesses, in the rare patient with large accumulations of empyema fluid or bronchopleural fistula, and the debridement of devitalized bone tissue in patients with osteomyelitis who are responding poorly to therapy. Unless patients have relapses repeatedly in the lung or remain culture positive with appropriate therapy, the surgical resection of large or residual lung cavities is not indicated. Although one paper implies that surgical resection alone may be curative,[101] the likelihood of relapse must be considered. Further, we have seen patients at the author's medical center develop acute, life-threatening disease after surgical resection of lung tissue for diagnostic purposes when blastomycosis was left untreated.[96] Therefore, it is our policy to treat any patient whose resected lung tissue contains *B. dermatitidis* with ketoconazole.

REFERENCES

1. Gilchrist TC. Protozoan dermatitis. J Cutan Gen Dis. 1894;12:496–9.
2. Gilchrist TC. A case of blastomycosis dermatitis in man. Johns Hopkins Hosp Rep. 1896;1:269–83.
3. Gilchrist TC, Stokes WR. The presence of an oidium in the tissues of a case of pseudo-lupus vulgaris. Johns Hopkins Hosp Rep. 1896;7:129–33.
4. Gilchrist TC, Stokes WR. Case of pseudo-lupus vulgaris caused by blastomycosis. J Exp Med. 1898;3:53–78.
5. Martin DS, Smith DT. Blastomycosis I: A review of the literature. Am Rev Tuberc. 1939;39:275–304.
6. Martin DS, Smith DT. Blastomycosis II: A report of thirteen new cases. Am Rev Tuberc. 1939;39:488–515.
7. Schwartz J, Baum GL. Blastomycosis. Am J Clin Pathol. 1951;11:999–1029.
8. Emmons CW, Binford CH, Utz JP, et al. Medical Mycology. 3rd ed. Philadelphia: Lea & Febiger; 1977:342.
9. Rippon JW. Medical Mycology: The Pathogenic Fungi and Pathogenic Actinomycetes. 2nd ed. Philadelphia: WB Saunders; 1982:428.
10. Kaufman L, Standard PG, Weeks RJ, et al. Detection of two *Blastomyces dermatitidis* serotypes by exoantigen analysis. J Clin Microbiol. 1983; 18:110–4.
11. Turner S, Kaufman L. Immunodiagnosis of blastomycosis. Semin Respir Infect. 1986;1:22–8.
12. McDonough ES, Lewis AL. *Blastomyces dermatitidis*: Production of the sexual stage. Science. 1967;156:528–9.
13. McDonough ES, Lewis AL. The ascigerous stage of *Blastomyces dermatitidis*. Mycologia. 1968;60:76–83.
14. McDonough ES, McNamara WJ, Chan DM, et al. Geographic distribution of "+" and "−" isolates of *Blastomyces* (*Ajellomyces*) *dermatitidis* in North America. Am J Epidemiol. 1973;98:63–7.
15. Blastomycosis Cooperative Study of the Veterans Administration. Blastomycosis I: A review of 198 collected cases in Veterans Administration Hospitals. Am Rev Respir Dis. 1964;89:659–72.
16. Menges RE, Doto IL, Weeks RJ. Epidemiologic studies of blastomycosis in Arkansas. Arch Environ Health. 1969;18:956–71.
17. Furcolow ML, Chick EW, Busey JF, et al. Prevalence and incidence studies of human and canine blastomycosis I: Cases in the United States, 1885–1968. Am Rev Respir Dis. 1970;102:60–7.
18. Furcolow ML, Busey JF, Menges RW, et al. Prevalence and incidence studies of human and canine blastomycosis II: Yearly incidence studies in three selected states, 1960–1967. Am J Epidemiol. 1970;92:121–31.
19. Sekshon AS, Borgorus MS, Sims HV. Blastomycosis: Report of three cases from Alberta with a review of Canadian cases. Mycopathologia. 1979;1:53–63.
20. Klein BS, Vergeront JM, Davis JP. Epidemiologic aspects of blastomycosis, the enigmatic systemic mycosis. Semin Respir Infect. 1986;1:29–39.
21. Chick EW. The epidemiology of blastomycosis. In: Al-Dory Y, ed. The Epidemiology of Human Mycotic Disease. Springfield, Ill: Charles C Thomas; 1975:103.
22. Smith JG Jr, Harris JS, Conant NF, et al. An epidemic of North American blastomycosis. JAMA. 1955;158:641–6.
23. Tosh FE, Hammerman KJ, Weeks RJ, et al. A common source epidemic of North American blastomycosis. Am Rev Respir Dis. 1974;109:525–9.
24. United States Department of Health, Education and Welfare, Public Health Service, Centers for Disease Control. Blastomycosis: North Carolina. Morbidity Mortality Weekly Rep. 1976;25:205–6.
25. Kitchen MS, Reiber CD, Eastin GB. An urban epidemic of North American blastomycosis. Am Rev Respir Dis. 1977;115:1063–76.
26. Cockerill FR III, Roberts GD, Rosenblat JE, et al. Epidemic of pulmonary blastomycosis (Nanekagan fever) in Wisconsin canoeists. Chest. 1984; 86:688–92.
27. Armstrong CW, Jenkins SR, Kaufman L, et al. Common source outbreak of blastomycosis in hunters and their dogs. J Infect Dis. 1987;155:568–70.
28. Klein BS, Vergeront JM, Weeks RJ, et al. Isolation of *Blastomyces dermatitidis* in soil associated with a large outbreak of blastomycosis in Wisconsin. N Engl J Med. 1986;314:529–34.
29. Klein BS, Vergeront JM, Disalvo AF, et al. Two outbreaks of blastomycosis along rivers in Wisconsin: Isolation of *Blastomyces dermatitidis* from riverbank soil and evidence of its transmission along waterways. Am Rev Respir Dis. 1987;136:1333–8.
30. Denton JF, McDonough ES, Ajello L, et al. Isolation of *Blastomyces dermatitidis* from soil. Science. 1961;133:1126–7.
31. Denton JF, Disalvo AF. Isolation of *Blastomyces dermatitidis* from natural sites in Augusta, Georgia. Am J Trop Med Hyg. 1964;13:716–22.
32. Denton FJ, Disalvo AF. Additional isolations of *Blastomyces dermatitidis* from natural sites. Am J Trop Med Hyg. 1979;28:697–700.
33. Sarosi GA, Serstock DA. Isolation of *Blastomyces dermatitidis* from pigeon manure. Am Rev Respir Dis. 1976;114:1179–83.
34. Bakerspigel A, Kane J, Schaus D. Isolation of *Blastomyces dermatitidis* from an earthen floor in southwestern Ontario, Canada. J Clin Microbiol. 1986;24:890–1.
35. Dixon DM, Shadomy HJ, Shadomy S. In vitro growth and sporulation of *Blastomyces dermatitidis* on woody plant material. Mycologia. 1977; 69:1193–5.
36. Larson DM, Eckman MR, Alber RL, et al. Primary cutaneous (inoculation) blastomycosis:: An occupational hazard to pathologists. Am J Clin Pathol. 1983;79:253–5.
37. Gnann JW Jr, Bressler GS, Bodet CA, et al. Human blastomycosis after a dog bite. Ann Intern Med. 1983;98:48–9.
38. Craig MW, Davey WN, Green RA. Conjugal blastomycosis. Am Rev Respir Dis. 1970;102:86–90.
39. Watts EA, Gard PD Jr, Tuthill SW. First reported case of intrauterine transmission of blastomycosis. Pediatr Infect Dis. 1983;2:308–10.
40. Daniel WP, Danaar SC, Perry HD. Blastomycosis-like pyoderma. Arch Dermatol. 1979;115:170–3.
41. Sixbey JW, Fields BT, Sun CH, et al. Interactions between human granulocytes and *Blastomyces dermatitidis*. Infect Immun. 1979;23:41–4.
42. Drutz DJ, Frey CL. Intracellular and extracellular defenses against *Blastomyces dermatitidis* conidia and yeasts. J Lab Clin Med. 1985;105:737–50.
43. Schaffner A, Davis CE, Schaffner T, et al. In vitro susceptibility of fungi to killing by neutrophil granulocytes discriminate between primary pathogenicity and opportunism. J Clin Invest. 1986;78:511–24.
44. Brummer E, Sugar AM, Stevens DA. Immunological activation of polymorphonuclear neutrophils for fungal killing: Studies with murine cells and *Blastomycosis dermatitidis* in vitro. J Leukocyte Biol. 1984;36:505–20.
45. Brummer E, Sugar AM, Stevens DA. Enhanced oxidative burst in immunologically activated, but not elicited, polymorphonuclear leukocytes correlates with fungicidal activity. Infect Immun. 1985;49:396–401.
46. Cozad GC, Chang C. T-cell mediated immunoprotection in blastomycosis. Infect Immun. 1980;78:393–403.
47. Morozumi PA, Brummer E, Stevens DA. Protection against pulmonary blastomycosis. Infect Immun. 1982;37:670–8.
48. Brummer E, Morozumi PA, Vo PT, et al. Protection against pulmonary blastomycosis: Adaptive transfer with T lymphocytes, but not serum, from resistant mice. Cell Immunol. 1982;73:349–59.
49. Brummer E, Morozumi A, Philpott DE, et al. Virulence of fungi: Correlation of virulence of *Blastomyces dermatitidis* in vivo with escape from macrophage inhibition of replication in vitro. Infect Immunol. 1981;32:864–71.
50. Brummer E, Hanson LH, Restrepo A, et al. In vivo and in vitro activation of pulmonary macrophages by IFN-γ for enhanced killing of *Paracoccidioides brasiliensis* or *Blastomyces dermatitidis*. J Immunol. 1988;140:2786–9.
51. Bradsher RW. Live *Blastomyces dermatitidis* yeast-induced responses of immune and non-immune human mononuclear cells. Mycopathologia. 1984;87:159–66.
52. Bradsher RW, Balk RA, Jacobs RF. Growth inhibition of *Blastomyces dermatitidis* in alveolar and peripheral macrophages from patients with blastomycosis. Am Rev Respir Dis. 1987;135:412–7.
53. Cox RA, Larsh HW. Isolation of skin test active preparations from yeast phase cell of *Blastomyces dermatitidis*. Infect Immun. 1973;10:42–7.
54. Deighton F, Cox RA, Hall RK, et al. In vivo and in vitro cell mediated immune responses to a cell wall antigen of *Blastomyces dermatitidis*. Infect Immun. 1977;15:429–35.
55. Turner S, Kaufman L. Immunodiagnosis of blastomycosis. Semin Respir Infect. 1986;1:22–8.
56. Kaufman L, McLaughlin DW, Clark MJ, et al. Specific immunodiffusion test for blastomycosis. Appl Microbiol. 1973;26:244–7.
57. Williams JE, Murphy R, Standard PG, et al. Serologic response in blastomycosis: Diagnostic value of double immunodiffusion assay. Am Rev Respir Dis. 1981;123:209–12.

58. Klein BS, Kuritsky WAC, Kaufman L, et al. Comparison of enzyme immunoassay, immunodiffusion and complement fixation tests in detecting antibody in human serum to the A antigen in *B. dermatitidis*. Am Rev Respir Dis. 1986;133:144–8.
59. Cherniss EI, Waisbren BA. North American blastomycosis: A clinical study of 40 cases. Ann Intern Med. 1956;44:105–23.
60. Abernathy RS. Clinical manifestations of pulmonary blastomycosis. Ann Intern Med. 1959;51:707–27.
61. Witorsch P, Utz JP. North American blastomycosis: A study of 40 patients. Medicine. 1968;47:169–200.
62. Lockwood WR, Allison F, Batson BE, et al. The treatment of North American blastomycosis: Ten years experience. Am Rev Respir Dis. 1969; 100:314–20.
63. Duttera MJ, Osterbont S. North American blastomycosis: A survey of 63 cases. South Med J. 1969;62:295–301.
64. Busey JF, Veterans Administrative Cooperative Group. Blastomycosis: III. A comparative study of 2-hydroxystilbamidine and amphotericin B therapy. Am Rev Respir Dis. 1982;105:812–8.
65. Sarosi GA, Davies SF. Blastomycosis. Am Rev Respir Dis. 1979;120:911–38.
66. Laskey W, Sarosi GA. Endogenous activation in blastomycosis. Ann Intern Med. 1978;88:50–2.
67. Halvorsen RA, Duncan JD, Merten DF, et al. Pulmonary blastomycosis: Radiologic manifestations. Radiology. 1984;150:1–5.
68. Rabinowitz JG, Busch J, Buttam WR. Pulmonary manifestations of blastomycosis. Diagn Radiol. 1976;120:25–32.
69. Sarosi GA, Davies SF, Phillips JR. Self-limited blastomycosis: A report of 39 cases. Semin Respir Infect. 1986;1:40–4.
70. Sarosi GA, Hammerman KJ, Tosh FE, et al. Clinical features of acute pulmonary blastomycosis. N Engl J Med. 1974;290:540–3.
71. Baum GL, Lerner PI. Primary pulmonary blastomycosis. A laboratory acquired infection. Ann Intern Med. 1970;73:263–5.
72. Poe RH, Vassallo CL, Plessinger VA, et al. Pulmonary blastomycosis versus carcinoma. A challenging differential. Am J Med Sci. 1972;263:145–55.
73. Griffith JE, Campbell GD. Acute miliary blastomycosis presenting as fulminating respiratory failure. Chest. 1979;75:630–2.
74. Evans ME, Haynes JB, Atkinson JB, et al. *Blastomyces dermatitidis* and the adult respiratory distress syndrome. Am Rev Respir Dis. 1982;126:1099–1102.
75. Kinasewitz GT, Penn RL, George RB. The spectrum and significance of pleural disease in blastomycosis. Chest. 1984;86:580–4.
76. Bassett FH, Tindall JP. Blastomycosis of Bone. South Med J. 1971;65:547–55.
77. Pritchard DJ. Granulomatous infections of bones and joints. Othop Clin North Am. 1975;6:1029–47.
78. Bayer AS, Scott VJ, Guze LB. Fungal arthritis IV. Blastomycotic arthritis. Semin Arthritis Rheum. 1979;9:145–51.
79. Eikenberg HA, Amin M, Lich RJ. Blastomycosis of the genitourinary tract. J Urol. 1975;113:650–2.
80. Gonyea EF. The spectrum of primary blastomycotic meningitis. A review of central nervous system blastomycosis. Ann Neurol. 1978;3:26–39.
81. Roos KL, Bryan JP, Maggio WW, et al. Intracranial blastomycoma. Medicine (Balt). 1987;66:224–35.
82. Laskey WK, Sarosi GA. Blastomycosis in children. Pediatrics. 1980;65:111–4.
83. Steele RW, Abernathy RS. Systemic blastomycosis in children. Pediatr Infect Dis. 1983;2:304–7.
84. Recht AD, Davies SF, Eckman MR. Blastomycosis in immunosuppressed patients. Am Rev Respir Dis. 1982;125:359–62.
85. Trumbull ML, Chesney T McC. The cytological diagnosis of pulmonary blastomycosis. JAMA. 1981;245:836–8.
86. George RB, Lambert RS, Bruce MJ, et al. Radioimmunoassay: A sensitive screening test for histoplasmosis and blastomycosis. Am Rev Respir Dis. 1981;124:407–10.
87. Lambert RS, George RB. Evaluation of enzyme immunoassay as a rapid screening test for histoplasmosis and blastomycosis. Am Rev Respir Dis. 1987;136:316–9.
88. Turner SH, Kaufman L, Jalbert M. Diagnostic assessment of an enzyme-linked immunosorbent assay for human and canine blastomycosis. J Clin Microbiol. 1986;23:294–7.
89. Sarosi GA. Management of fungal disease. Am Rev Respir Dis. 1983;127: 250–3.
90. National Institute of Allergy and Infectious Diseases Study Group. Treatment of blastomycosis and histoplasmosis with ketoconazole: Results of a prospective randomized trial. Ann Intern Med. 1985;103:861–72.
91. Bradsher RW, Rice DC, Abernathy RS. Ketoconazole therapy of endemic blastomycosis. Ann Intern Med. 1985;103:872–9.
92. Sarosi GA, Davies SF, Klein B, et al. Recent developments in blastomycosis. Am Rev Respir Dis. 1986;134:817–8.
93. Sagg MS, Dismukes WE. Treatment of histoplasmosis and blastomycosis. Chest. 1988;93:848–51.
94. Daneshmend TK, Warnock DW. Clinical pharmacokinetics of ketoconazole. Clin Pharmacokinet. 1988;14:13–34.
95. Wise GJ, Goldberg PE, Kozinin PJ. Do the imidazoles have a role in the management of genitourinary fungal infections. J Urol. 1985;133:61–4.
96. Campbell GD, Chapman SW. Blastomycosis. Semin Respir Med. 1987; 9:164–70.
97. Rose HD, Varkey B. Miconazole treatment of relapsed pulmonary blastomycosis. Am Rev Respir Dis. 1978;118:403–8.
98. Dismukes W, Bradsher R, Girard W, et al. Itraconazole therapy for blastomycosis and histoplasmosis. Program and Abstracts of the 26th Interscience Conference on Antimicrobial Agents and Chemotherapy. Washington, DC: American Society for Microbiology; 1986;798A.
99. Hammon JW, Prager RL. Surgical management of fungal diseases of the chest. Surg Clin North Am. 1980;60:897–912.
100. Newson BD, Hardy JD. Pulmonary fungal infections: Survey of 159 cases with surgical implications. J Thorac Cardiovasc Surg. 1982;83:218–26.
101. Edson RS, Keys TF. Treatment of primary pulmonary blastomycosis: Results of long term follow up. Mayo Clin Proc. 1981;56:683–5.

244. COCCIDIOIDES IMMITIS

DAVID A. STEVENS

The initial description of coccidioidomycosis is credited to an intern, Posada, who reported in 1892 a soldier with disseminated disease hospitalized in Buenos Aires.[1] The illness was thought to be mycosis fungoides, but Posada described the etiologic agent in the tissues, thinking it was a protozoan. Four years later Rixford and Gilchrist, reporting a case from San Francisco County Hospital, transmitted the disease via infected tissue to animals and gave the organism its name, *Coccidioides* (resembling the protozoan Coccidia) *immitis* (not mild).[2] In the next decade Ophüls, a Stanford pathologist, identified the organism as a fungus, delineated its life cycle, and identified the lung as the primary portal of entry.[3] By 1929 almost 100 cases had been reported, and the disease was thought to be invariably severe and usually fatal. In that year, Chope, a medical student working in Dickson's laboratory at Stanford, accidentally inhaled a cloud of arthroconidia. Chope was heralded worldwide as a martyr to science, but instead of dying as expected, he developed a severe primary pulmonary infection with erythema nodosum. This was an important clue that eventually led Dr. Myrnie Gifford of the Kern County Health Department and Dickson to realize that the acute self-limited disease seen frequently in Kern County, California, known as San Joaquin Valley fever, was coccidioidomycosis.[4,5] Dickson isolated the fungus from the sputum of such patients. Also in the 1930s, Stewart and Meyer isolated the organism from soil at the site of a small epidemic and postulated widespread natural subclinical immunizing infections.[6] Understanding of the natural history of the infection was thus nearly complete. Gifford and colleagues noted the seasonal variation in incidence and the increased virulence in dark-skinned races and performed epidemiologic skin test studies.[7] Another student of Dickson's, C. E. Smith, refined the skin testing and serologic procedures and used them as tools in extensive epidemiologic and diagnostic studies, made important correlations with the course of the disease, and studied measures to control the organisms in the soil.[8]

MYCOLOGY

The fungus exists in the soil in the mycelial phase.[9] As it matures, alternate cells along a hypha become barrel shaped. The hypha with these structures, termed *arthroconidia*, is easily fragmented, and these spores become airborne and can infect a new site in the soil (saprophytic cycle). They may also be inhaled by an animal host. In the host, the spores swell, become spherical, and develop a thick wall. This new structure, the spherule, reproduces by formation of spherical internal spores, termed endospores (Fig. 1). A single spherule may develop as many as 800 endospores, and when the spherule ruptures, the endospores are released and each in turn can develop into a new spherule (parasitic cycle). If fungus from this phase is re-

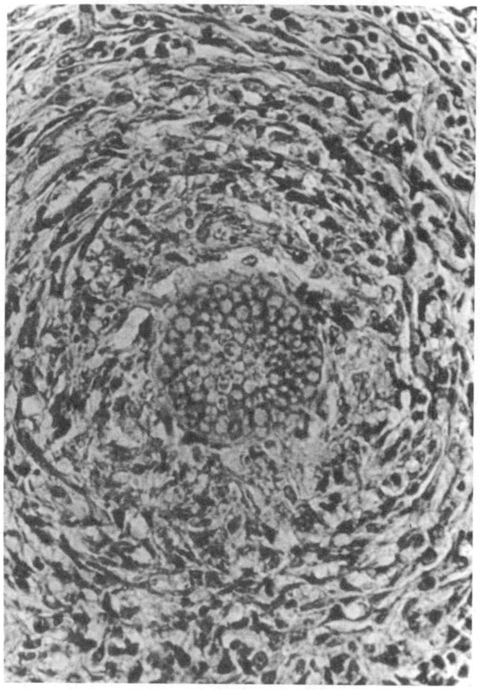

FIG. 1. Mature spherule with endospores, in tissue.

turned to the soil (e.g., via infected body fluids or an animal carcass), the endospore forms an elongated bud, which develops into a hypha. The saprophytic cycle can then begin again.

If infected material is cultured in the laboratory, the fungus also reverts to the mycelial phase. Growth is generally rapid, and flat smooth gray colonies appear in 3–4 days. The optimal temperature is 30°C, but the fungus grows well at 37°C. Hyphae appear in the next few days, and the colonies appear as tufts. Finally, whitish gray cottony annular growth spreads over the plate. Atypical isolates are not infrequent and vary in color, rate of growth, and aerial structures.

In special media the fungus can be induced to remain in the spherule–endospore phase through successive growth cycles.[10]

ECOLOGY AND EPIDEMIOLOGY

Coccidioidomycosis is endemic in certain areas of North, Central, and South America.[11] It is estimated that in the United States alone about 100,000 people are infected annually. Almost all these infections occur in seven southwestern states. It has been shown that the illness in recognized symptomatic cases in otherwise healthy people necessitates an average of 33–35 days missed from work (or school).[12] The estimated cost to the United States is almost 1 million person-days of labor and approximately $6.4 million in medical expenses annually.

Increasingly, cases are being recognized outside the endemic areas. These occur in travelers who have visited an endemic area (in some cases the documented duration of exposure is only a few hours), or as reactivations of infections acquired earlier in former residents of endemic areas, or as infections acquired from fomites from endemic areas (fruit, cotton, landfill are documented sources of infection).[13]

As Maddy demonstrated extensively, the endemic areas coincide generally with the Lower Sonoran Life Zone.[14] This is characterized by arid to semiarid climates, hot summers, few winter freezes, low altitude, alkaline soil, and sparse flora. The creosote bush enjoys the same conditions and has been noted to be coextensive with *C. immitis* soil infection in many areas. In infected soil, positive cultures have been obtained with particular ease in the vicinity of rodent burrows. A variety of animal species has been shown to develop naturally acquired infection.[15]

In recent years, it has been realized that soil infection is present in hitherto unsuspected areas. One of the best sources for these discoveries, unfortunately, is archeology students. Several new foci have been discovered because of digging for Indian artifacts and the resultant miniepidemics of acute coccidioidal infections.[16] Some newly uncovered areas of soil infection do not conform to the ecologic characteristics described above, and it appears that the fungus may be more versatile than previously thought.

The incidence of infection will likely rise, since the endemic areas are in the sunbelt states in which there is a rapidly growing population and because of the increase in mobility and travel.

As can be seen from the above, although this is an infectious disease, it is not a contagious one. The only instances of person-to-person transmission have been in special circumstances such as when attention has not been paid to the potential for the fungus to revert from its tissue phase to its airborne form in contaminated secretions. An example of such transmission is drainage of pus into the interior of a cast, a warm, moist environment where aerial structures can develop, and spores are released into the air when the cast is opened.[17]

PATHOLOGIC FINDINGS

Coccidioidomycosis most resembles tuberculosis in its pathologic manifestations.[18] The predominant tissue reaction is granulomatous. In acute foci purulence may predominate, and in chronic lesions fibrosis may be the main finding. Caseation may occur at any time. The characteristic tissue form of the organism is the spherule, although with careful searching hyphae can be demonstrated in nearly three-fourths of pulmonary cavities in the interior margins and can even be detected in one-third of granulomatous pulmonary lesions.[19] Despite the potential, no person-to-person transmission has been documented from such lesions. A mature endosporulating spherule is pathognomonic (Fig. 1). Many stains have been used to demonstrate this structure, and hematoxylin and eosin often suffice, although in difficult cases (e.g., when caseation is present or organisms are few) I have had the best results with Gomori–methenamine–silver. With this stain, fungi stand out as black against a green background. Some laboratories can use fluorescent antibody techniques to demonstrate spherules in tissue.

Differentiation of *C. immitis* from other organisms is not difficult when mature endosporulating spherules can be located. Sporangia of *Rhinosporidum seeberi* resemble coccidioidal spherules, although the former are much larger and stain with mucicarmine, whereas spherules do not.

At autopsy, positive cultures from tissue have been obtained even after ordinary intravascular formaldehyde embalming.

IMMUNOLOGIC CHARACTERISTICS

After the arthrospore first impacts in the lower airways, the initial host response consists of macrophages and neutrophils.[20] Later, coincident with transformation to the parasitic phase, mononuclear cells are more in evidence. Neutrophils are prominent again when spherules rupture.[21] The fungi apparently activate the complement sequence,[22] generating chemotactic factors.[23] Phagocytosis is attempted by individual cells, although giant cells are required for larger fungal structures. Arthroconidia, endospores, and particularly spherules are quite resistant to killing by neutrophils or products of oxidative metabolism.[24,25,26] A residual hyphal wall layer on arthroconidia and an extracellular matrix surrounding spherules and endospores appear to protect the fungus from phagocytosis and killing.[26] T lymphocytes are stimulated, apparently yielding important interactions with the inflammatory cells, causing their ingress and activating them to facilitate killing.[24,27] Endospores are particularly potent stimuli for lymphocytes.[28] Peripheral blood eosinophilia may be seen in primary infection, particularly in association with erythema nodosum, though peripheral blood and tissue eosinophilia also occurs in progressive disseminated disease.[29]

The correlation among skin tests, serologic tests, and disease status will be discussed in later sections of this chapter. Cellular immunity can be assayed in vitro by techniques such as lymphocyte blastogenesis and lymphokine production. Sometimes in disseminated disease the in vitro tests may be positive when skin tests are negative, suggesting that subtle defects are present. In some instances defects in cellular immunity assays are selective for *C. immitis* antigens, and the patients respond normally to other stimuli.[30,31]

Studies have suggested that the mechanism of cellular unreactivity relates to antigen overload.[32] Recent studies suggest the presence of circulating cells, which can be removed from peripheral blood by nylon wool adherence in vitro, that suppress lymphocyte responses in coccidioidomycosis patients.[33] Others have found plasma factors in such patients that specifically block cell-mediated immune reactions to coccidioidal antigens, probably by acting on abnormal lymphoid receptors.[34,35] Circulating immune complexes, which are present in active disease and correlate with the extent of involvement, are a candidate for this effect,[36] although spherule-produced substances can also be suppressive.[37] Evidence for disordered regulation of immunity in this disease is also demonstrated by elevated serum IgE levels. These levels correlate with the extent of spread of the disease, and the increased IgE is due to both anticoccidioidal antibody and antibody directed to other antigens.[38]

Studies in animals confirm the role of immune response in outcome of disease[20] and suggest that the T lymphocyte is preeminent.[39] Thymectomy[40] or corticosteroid therapy[41] enhances the virulence of the infection.

CLINICAL MANIFESTATIONS

Primary Infection

Sixty percent of those infected have asymptomatic infections or illness indistinguishable from ordinary upper respiratory infections.[42] These people are known to have had a coccidioidal infection only by skin testing. Forty percent develop symptoms of a primary infection 1–3 weeks after exposure. These infections resemble a lower respiratory infection and/or systemic illness with some of the following symptoms: cough, sputum production, chest pain, malaise, fever, chills, night sweats, anorexia, weakness, and arthralgias. Erythema nodosum, 2–10 times more common in women, or an erythema multiforme that involves the upper trunk and extremities may occur. Chest radiographic films show minimal changes, infiltrates or frank pneumonia, or pleural effusion. Hilar nodes may be prominent, suggesting a diagnosis of sarcoidosis. Scalene or supraclavicular nodes may be culture-positive. In most cases, these manifestations resolve spontaneously.

About 5 percent of those infected have pulmonary residua, most commonly a pulmonary nodule or a cavity. The nodules sometimes calcify. The cavity is usually thin walled (Fig. 2). Such patients are often asymptomatic but may have hemoptysis. Coccidioidomycosis is often diagnosed when a nodule is resected to rule out cancer. Pulmonary infection is not resolved in these ways in some patients. Some develop acute progressive pneumonia, often with a fatal outcome; others progress to chronic pulmonary disease.[43]

About 0.5 percent develop disseminated (extrapulmonary) disease, which may involve almost any organ of the body, at one or more sites, although the heart and gastrointestinal tract are rarely involved. Rarely, widespread rapid dissemination may occur with a miliary and usually fatal picture. Major disseminated disease sites are discussed in subsequent sections. It also appears, from evidence of subclinical spontaneously resolving infection in some sites such as the eye and genitourinary tract,[44,45] that hematogenous dissemination without disease or clinical consequences may occur in more patients than the subset with overt dissemination. Development of disease at extrapulmonary sites is uncommon if there have been no such manifestations in the year after quiescence of the initial pulmonary infection, unless host immunity is later impaired, for example, by malignancy or immunsuppressive therapy. Dissemination and fatal disease are far more common in men, pregnant women, immunocompromised hosts, and dark-skinned races.[7,11,46,47] As compared with that in the white race, dissemination is approximately 175 times more common in people in Filipino ancestry, 14 times in blacks, and 2–3 times in people of Mexican ancestry, and there is apparently also increased risk in people of Oriental ancestry.

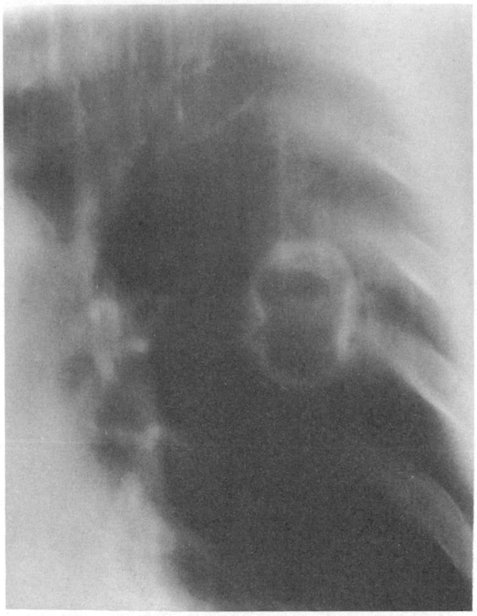

FIG. 2. Thin-walled coccidioidal lung cavity.

Chronic Pulmonary Coccidioidomycosis

In some patients the acute pneumonia does not resolve but progresses to chronic pulmonary disease.[48] Usually cavitary lesions are part of this syndrome (Fig. 3). Diabetics and patients with compromised immunity are disporportionately overrepresented in this group. In these patients the disease may wax and wane over many years. Old granulomatous lesions may break down and new cavities form. Bronchiectasis may be a sequela of chronic or severe acute disease. If a coccidioidal empyema or a bronchopleural fistula develops as a complication of pulmonary disease, it especially contributes to prolonged chronic disease.

Musculoskeletal Coccidioidomycosis

Muscles, tendons, bones, and joints may be involved in disseminated disease, with local pain, swelling, and warmth accompanying the systemic symptoms of infection. Muscle involvement may overlap with subcutaneous foci or with bony involvement, with formation of abscesses or sinus tracts. Over one-third of patients with disseminated disease have bone or joint involvement. Bone lesions are unifocal in 60 percent of

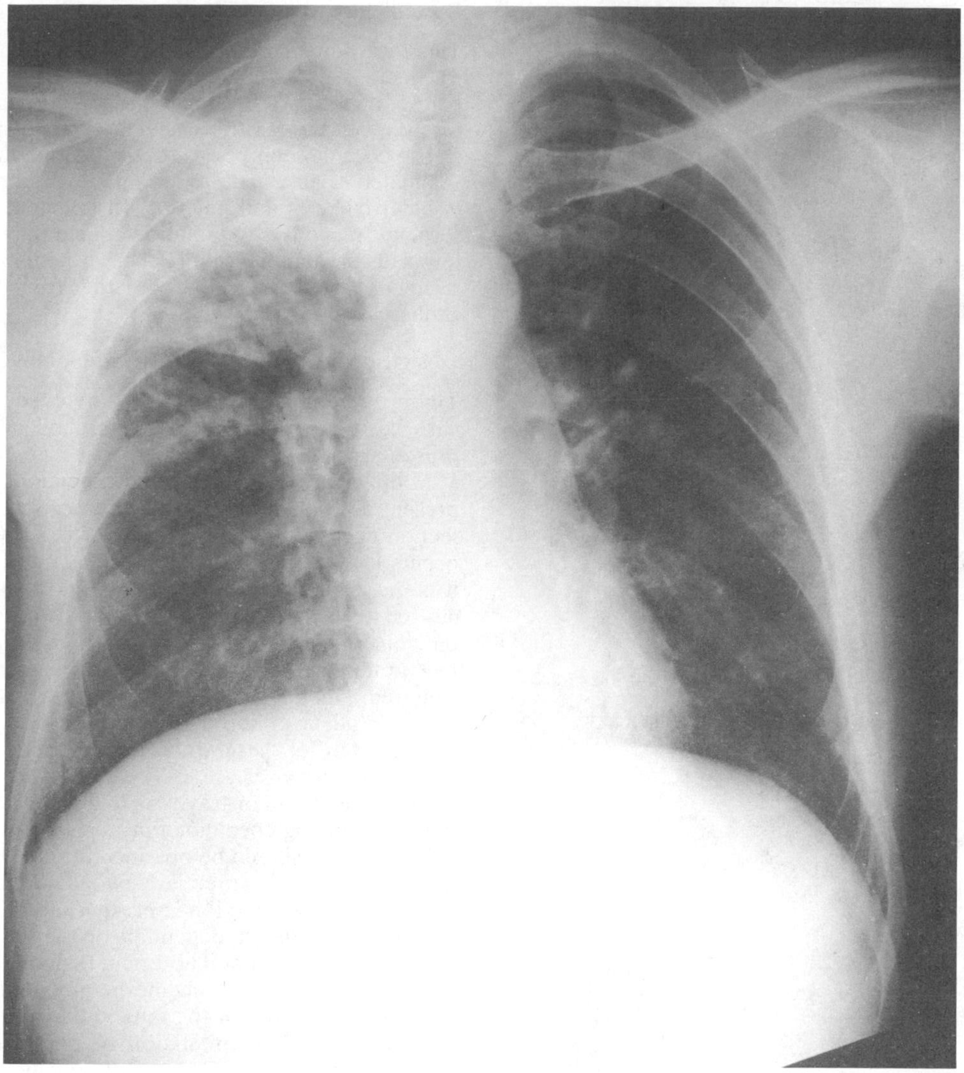

FIG. 3 Chronic progressive coccidioidomycosis with small right upper lobe cavity.

cases.[49] The most commonly involved bones are the skull, metacarpals, metatarsals, spine, and tibia. Lytic lesions are more common than sclerosis (Fig. 4). Bone scans appear more sensitive than radiographic films in detecting foci. Vertebral lesions are most commonly multiple. Unlike in tuberculosis, parts of the arch may be primarily involved, the disk may be relatively spared, and in the thoracic spine the adjacent ribs may be involved. Spread to the meninges is a serious danger.

Joint lesions are unifocal in over 90 percent of patients with joint involvement. The ankle and knee are the sites most commonly involved. Joint disease often occurs adjacent to sites of osteomyelitis. Joint fluid analysis is indistinguishable from bacterial and other fungal arthritis, except that the fungus can usually be seen or cultured. When such culture is unsuccessful, biopsy of the granulomatous synovium frequently is diagnostic.[50]

Meningitis

Meningitis[51,52] usually occurs within 6 months after the primary infection and may appear acutely almost coincident with it. The main areas of involvement are the basilar meninges. Space occupying lesions are rare.

The signs of meningeal irritation common in bacterial meningitis are usually absent. The most common symptom is headache. Fever, weakness, confusion, sluggishness, seizures, abnormal behavior, stiff neck, diplopia, ataxia, vomiting, and focal neurologic defects may occur. In the cerebrospinal fluid (CSF) there is a pleocytosis in which mononuclear cells almost always predominate (eosinophils are sometimes seen), and there are decreased glucose and elevated protein levels. Occasional patients will have only CSF antibody or, more rarely, only a positive culture on presentation. The use of culture and serologic tests will be discussed in subsequent sections. Cisternal or lumbar CSF is a much better indicator of disease activity than is ventricular fluid, the latter commonly having higher glucose and lower protein levels, lower antibody titers, and fewer cells.[53] Patients who relapse after response to therapy usually have pleocytosis or chemical CSF abnormalitieis before CSF antibody recurs.[54]

The diagnosis should be suspected in a patient with a CSF as described above and an appropriate travel or residence history. Supportive evidence includes serum antibody to *C. immitis*, positive coccidioidal skin tests, positive culture from an extraneural site, and exclusion of other causes of chronic meningitis. The diagnosis is confirmed by culture or positive complement fixation test of CSF in the absence of parameningeal disease. Early diagnosis is important, because early treatment

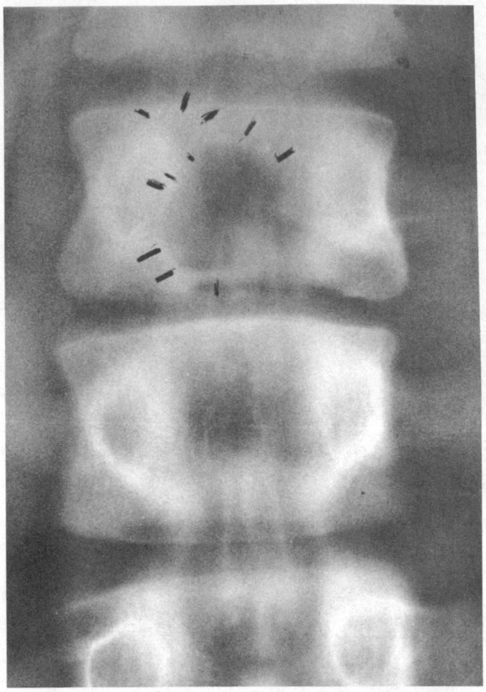

FIG. 4 Osteolytic coccidioidal vertebral lesions (highlighted lesions in vertebral body at top of figure).

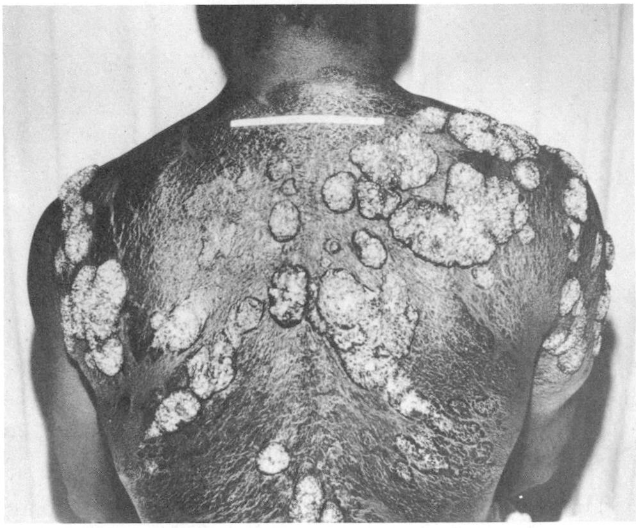

FIG. 5 Severe proliferative verrucous cutaneous coccidioidomycosis.

appears to correlate with successful outcome. Without treatment, about 90 percent of the patients are dead in 1 year.[55]

Cutaneous Coccidioidomycosis

Rashes associated with the primary infection have been discussed above. The skin is a common target organ in disseminated coccidioidomycosis. The appearance is variable, with papules, pustules, plaques, nodules, ulcers, abscesses, or large proliferative lesions (Fig. 5). Probably the most characteristic is a warty appearance. These lesions mimic those due to other fungi, actinomycetes, lues, and tuberculosis.

Rarely (the best documented examples are laboratory accidents) skin lesions result from direct inoculation with contaminated materials.[56] Fortunately, most of these episodes resolve spontaneously without further sequelae.

Coccidioidomycosis in Pediatrics

There are some special considerations in infection in children. The increased risk of dissemination in men appears to be absent before puberty.[11,42] Congenital infection has been reported rarely, even though the placenta is frequently involved in obstetric coccidioidomycosis (described below). Mortality of disseminated disease acquired in infancy is apparently higher than in older children and adults.[57] In infected neonates, the usual serologic responses to infection appear to be blunted. There are few data on amphotericin B use in pediatrics, and doses and regimens are largely extrapolated from the experience in adults.[58]

Obstetric and Gynecologic Coccidioidomycosis

The pelvic organs can be rarely involved in disseminated disease, as occurs in tuberculosis, and with similar clinical presentation.

Although previously resolved coccidioidal infection does not present a problem to women who become pregnant, when infection occurs during pregnancy or is active when conception occurs it may have a dangerous character.[46] In endemic areas it is the leading cause of maternal mortality. Dissemination is 40–100 times more common than in the general population, and only one in eight women survives. The dissemination and mortality rates are higher the later in pregnancy the infection is acquired. Only 60 percent of pregnant patients with active infection produce offspring surviving beyond the neonatal period, and one-third of these are delivered prematurely.

The only defenses are early recognition and early treatment. Pregnant residents or travelers to endemic areas should be suspected of having coccidioidomycosis when a febrile illness develops. Serum should be obtained for a *C. immitis* complement fixation test. If the titer is elevated, a diagnostic work-up is urgent. If active infection is present, abortion or early delivery should be considered, depending on the stage of pregnancy, and the same regimen of amphotericin B should be given as for nonpregnant patients. This chemotherapy appears to enhance survival and to be safe for the fetus if the pregnancy is continued.

Observations of stimulation of parasitic phase *C. immitis* by female sex hormones, and of specific binding proteins for mammalian hormones in the organism, may be relevant to the association of pregnancy with disseminated coccidioidomycosis.[59]

Coccidioidomycosis in the Immunocompromised Host

Coccidioides immitis has an enhanced invasive potential comparable to that of other fungal pathogens in the host whose immunity is impaired by disease (e.g., malignancy, congenital immunodeficiency, acquired immunodeficiency syndrome [AIDS])) or immunosuppressive therapy.[47] It can be an early or late complication of underlying diseases, such as cancer, unlike the opportunistic invaders. Immunosuppressive chemotherapy seems a more important risk factor for dissemination than specific underlying diagnosis or radiotherapy. Lymphocytopenia correlates closely with dissemination. Coccidioidal infection that resolved and became quiescent before the development of an immune impairing condition sometimes can reactivate and disseminate after impairment, but infection acquired after impairment is much more likely to disseminate than that in the normal host. Whereas dissemination is highly lethal in these patients, pulmonary coccidioidomycosis that remains localized to the lung appears not to be necessarily worse than in normal hosts. An unusual feature of disseminated infection in these hosts is concomitant rapidly progressive pulmonary involvement. A combination of diffuse pulmonary disease and widespread dissemination appears the rule in AIDS.[60]

The serologic response in most immunocompromised patients appears to be at least qualitatively intact. The major problem in diagnosis of these patients is lack of suspicion of coccidioidomycosis. This should be considered in patients with a history of a positive skin test, or even of travel or residence in an endemic area, who become immunocompromised. Routine serologic testing of such patients might avert delays in diagnosis of their rapidly fatal infections.

DIAGNOSIS

Mycologic Diagnosis

The organism can be demonstrated by examination and culture with relative ease in pus due to *C. immitis* and, depending on the floridity of the infection, from sputum, joint fluid, aspirates of superficial soft tissue lesions, and resected deep tissues. It is generally more difficult to obtain positive cultures from urine, blood, gastric aspirates, pleural effusions, and peritoneal fluid in cases of coccidioidal involvement. Spinal fluid is culture-positive only about one-third of the time, and visualization of the organism in CSF is extremely rare.

With regard to sputum cultures, selection of purulent parts of the sample, homogenization, or treatment with mucolytic agents followed by centrifugation increases yield.[61] Cytologic preparations appear to be more sensitive than potassium hydroxide preparations.[62] If a satisfactory sputum sample cannot be obtained, transtracheal aspiration, bronchoscopy, or lung biopsy may be indicated, depending on the circumstances.

Enchancement of recovery from samples of fluids obtained in small volumes can be achieved by filtration through sterile bacterial filters and culture and examination of the retentate. This is also especially useful with urine.[45]

Fluids can be examined for the characteristic spherule in the standard potassium hydroxide preparation or in wet mounts using lactophenol cotton blue for contrast. Spherules with endospores must be sought, particularly in respiratory tract samples, because some pollens and some yeasts may cause confusion with immature spherules. Smears stained with a silver stain are particularly helpful.

Cultures of *C. immitis* represent a severe biologic hazard, and suspect isolates should only be handled by experienced laboratories prepared to deal with them, using appropriate safety equipment and procedures.[63]

Several saprophytic fungi resemble *C. immitis* on ordinary media, and if *C. immitis* is suspected, then mycologic media containing cycloheximide can be helpful as an adjunct in either primary isolation or subculture. This drug inhibits many saprophytic fungi.[64] Identification of the organism by its morphologic characteristics in the mycelial phase is difficult, even in the most experienced hands.[9] Further steps are necessary to confirm the mycologic diagnosis. The traditional method has been injection of a suspension of a sporulating culture into rodents and identification of the characteristic spherule phase in them. This can be achieved in a few days to a week or more. More rapid confirmation can be achieved by conversion in special media, either in liquid or on agar, at 40°C and in an increased carbon dioxide atmosphere. Another method with even more rapid confirmation can be performed directly on tissue or fluid materials when structures believed to be spherules are seen. A wet preparation is placed under a sealed coverslip on a microscope slide in an incubator. Periodic examination of the preparation may show the budding development of hyphae. There is a significant biologic hazard risk in handling these.[65,66]

Methods of rapid confirmation involve testing supernatants of liquid media cultures for antigens with reference antisera or immunodiffusion tests with such antisera in agar, detecting extracellular antigens secreted into the agar from cultures growing on it.[67]

Serology and Skin Testing

The mycelial phase antigen, coccidioidin, is most useful in detecting humoral antibody.[68] Serum IgM precipitins can be demonstrated by tube precipitin, latex agglutination, or immunodiffusion methods. These antibodies occur 1–3 weeks after onset of symptoms of primary infection in 75 percent of the cases and disappear within 4 months. Occasionally, precipitins persist when the disease progresses or transiently recur when the disease reactivates. Serum IgG antibodies that fix complement occur later, are present in the more symptomatic primary infections, and may last 6–8 months. This antibody can also be demonstrated by a band in immunodiffusion distinct from the IgM precipitin. The band(s) present in immunodiffusion can be distinguished by demonstration of lines of identity with reference sera that are tube-precipitin-positive, complement-fixing-antibody (CFA) negative, or vice versa. In addition, the antigen in the band corresponding to the CFA test is heat-labile. Occasionally IgG persists longer, at lower levels, even though the infection resolves successfully. By 3 months after onset, 50–90 percent of the patients with symptomatic primary infections have this antibody. At least 90 percent of the patients with primary symptomatic infections show either tube precipitin or CFA.

Elevated CFA titers are the hallmark of disseminated disease. Using the method of Smith and Saito,[69] 95–100 percent of patients without disseminated disease have titers below 1:32 and 99–100 percent have titers below 1:64, whereas 61 percent of the patients with disseminated disease have titers of at least 1:32 and 41 percent have titers at least 1:64. The discriminating titers vary in laboratories that have not standardized the above method, and if such laboratories are used, it would be important to know their data on titers before assessing the significance of an individual result. The exception to the picture described is meningitis, which in serum titers resembles nondisseminated disease unless other disseminated foci are also present. Titration can also be performed with the immunodiffusion test for the band corresponding to CFA. With standardized antigen preparations and conditions, the titers correspond to those in the CFA test. This puts a quantitative specific test in the reach of laboratories not familiar with the CFA test.

The CFA or immunodiffusion titer parallels the course of disease and thus is very helpful. The preceding and current specimens should be run simultaneously for titer comparisons. Rising titers are a bad prognostic sign; falling titers indicate improvement. Overnight binding at 4°C increases the sensitivity of the CFA test. Infection by *Histoplasma capsulatum* may result in low titers to coccidioidin. With some antigen preparations, positive CFA tests have also been reported in other diseases.

A latex agglutination test, available as a commercial kit, appears to be the most sensitive test for precipitin antibodies. However, there is a 6–10 percent rate of false-positive results, and the test is not quantitative. Serum dilution increases the frequency of false-positive tests.[70] Counterimmunoelectrophoresis appears as sensitive and specific as the CFA test and is more rapidly performed. Good results have been reported with radioimmunoassay for antibody. Detection of circulating antigen in sera by radioimmunoassy[71] or enzyme immunoassay[72] is a promising method of rapid diagnosis; acid–heat extraction of specimens appears to reduce interference in the assay.

In meningeal disease, CFA is present in CSF in 70 percent of the patients on initial examination and in almost all patients if the disease progresses. Unless the CSF is concentrated, CFA is absent from CSF in the presence of high serum titers from disease outside the central nervous system. As an exception, CSF may yield a positive CFA in the presence of a parameningeal lesion such as an epidural abscess or an osteomyelitic lesion abutting the dura.[73] The CFA titers in CSF parallel the course of meningeal disease, as described above.

Positive skin tests (>5 mm induration) to coccidioidal antigens are detectable 2–21 days after the first symptoms appear (10–45 days after infection), usually before the first serologic reactions are detectable. Almost every patient with a symptomatic primary infection has a positive skin test by 1 month after onset. Patients with erythema nodosum can develop severe reactions to skin tests and should be tested initially with reagent diluted to 1/100 the usual strength. There is a low degree of cross-reactivity with antigens derived from *Histoplasma capsulatum* and *Blastomyces dermatitidis*. Anergy is common in disseminated coccidioidomycosis. When a negative skin test is obtained in a primary infection, the result suggests that there is latent dissemination or that dissemination will occur later.[8] The mycelial phase antigen, coccidioidin, in dilutions of 1:100 and 1:10, has been the standard in skin testing. However, a parasitic phase antigen, spherulin, may be a more sensitive reagent in detecting dermal-delayed hypersensitivity and is as specific as coccidioidin.[74] Positive skin tests with either reagent do not affect coccidioidal serologic testing, although a positive coccidioidin test may induce antibodies that cross react with histoplasmin.[75] Skin testing is important in diagnosis only in such situations as assessing prior exposure in a patient presenting with a pulmonary nodule, assessing conversion in exposed individuals known to be negative previously, or awaiting serologic results, as an epidemiologic tool or assessing the cellular immunity status in patients with documented coccidioidal disease (prognosis, or assessing response to therapy). Serial testing of negative subjects may, however, produce a positive result.[76]

THERAPY

Chemotherapy

Whereas most patients with symptomatic primary infections recover without therapy, it is generally agreed that a patient with severe primary infection should receive chemotherapy. Because of the possibility of incipient or occult dissemination, patients with high CFA titers (see section on serologic testing) should be treated. Other criteria used to determine the need for treatment are persistent symptoms for over 6 weeks; prostration; extensive, enlarging, or persisting pulmonary involvement; persisting precipitins; negative skin test; infancy; debilitation; pregnancy; concurrent diseases (such as diabetes, asthma, emphysema) likely to be adversely affected by coccidioidal infection; immune impairment; or racial group predisposed to handle the infection poorly. Amphotericin B[77] has been given intravenously to such patients, 1–1.5 mg/kg/day tapering to 1–1.5 mg/kg three times a week to a total dose of 0.5–1.5 g if a clinical response is obtained and more if no response is obtained (using indices such as CFA, skin tests, radiographic films, and other objective clinical measurements). *Coccidioides immitis* appears uniformly susceptible in vitro to amphotericin B.[78]

Once the disease has spread outside the lungs, chemotherapy is almost always indicated. With amphotericin B, courses of 1–2.5 g intravenously are usually used, with more prolonged courses if remission is not achieved.

In addition, local irrigation of sinuses and fistulae, infiltration into lesions, and instillation into abscesses and body cavities with antifungal agents may add to the success of therapy. Intra-articular and intrathecal therapy will be discussed subsequently.

Miconazole is an alternative to amphotericin B therapy.[79] Clinical responses have been reported in series of amphotericin-unresponsive patients with all forms of disseminated or chronic pulmonary disease, given 0.6–1.2 g three times daily. *Coccidioides immitis* isolates are uniformly susceptible in vitro, and development of resistance has not been shown. The drug is less toxic than amphotericin B, but it must be given intravenously or injected locally, thus limiting long-term therapy. Courses have generally been 1–3 months in duration, and the relapse rates have been high (56–78 percent) in those responding to therapy. The place of miconazole in therapy in relation to other drugs has not been determined and requires comparative studies.

The newest addition to our armamentarium is ketoconazole, which is given orally.[80] Like the other two drugs, it is active against *C. immitis* in vitro and in animal models and is the least toxic in clinical studies. Response rates in all forms of the disease (particularly skin and soft tissue), except meningitis, using doses of 200–400 mg/day, are as high as those seen previously with the other drugs. Patients who have not responded to other therapy appear equally responsive. Relapse rates thus far of at least 25 percent, even after at least 12 months of therapy, are disturbing.[81] Doses exceeding 400 mg/day are more toxic and no more effective than lower doses.[82,83]

Itraconazole, an oral triazole currently being investigated in the United States, has produced response rates in nonmeningeal disease during initial trials at least as high as those with ketoconazole.[84] This drug appears to lack side effects possessed by ketoconazole and after further study it may supplant the previous azoles.

Pulmonary Cavity

Surgical removal of cavitary disease is indicated in the presence of persistent, recurrent, or severe hemoptysis; an enlarging cavity despite chemotherapy; or intrapleural rupture. Controversial indications include subpleural location (because of the danger of rupture), a cavity with mycetoma associated with symptoms, persistent *C. immitis* culture-positive sputum, a cavity secondarily infected (because of the possibility of ballooning), and recurrent disease. We must weigh the risks implied in the natural history of these forms when not treated surgically against those associated with a surgical approach.[48] Risks of surgical treatment include bronchopleural fistula, spills occurring at surgery that lead to empyema, and the fact that many patients develop new foci in their remaining lung. Surgery is also indicated for closure of bronchopleural fistulas and where lung expansion is restricted by residua of coccidioidal disease. Preoperative and postoperative chemotherapy is usually considered part of the therapeutic approach when surgery is indicated and particularly when a pneumonic coccidioidal infiltrate, elevated CFA titer, positive sputum cultures, satellite nodule, or lesion that crosses pulmonary fissures is present.

Bone and Joint

A surgical and/or chemotherapeutic approach to bone disease is indicated with active disease is present.[85–87] Surgery contributes to a successful result by resection of infected bone and drainage of adjacent soft tissue purulence. Immobilization is an important part of the regimen. Local chemotherapy via irrigation may have a role. Articular coccidioidomycosis is a chronic, disabling disease, and long-term therapeutic results with a goal of cure have been generally disappointing, except when amputation or arthrodesis plus intravenous amphotericin have been used.[85] Of the less radical therapeutic approaches, allowing joint mobility, a combination of immobilization, synovectomy, systemic amphotericin plus intra-articular amphotericin has produced some long-term successes and at least a functional joint in many cases.[50,86,87] An intra-articular regimen of amphotericin that is commonly used is 15–50 mg (for large joints), depending on tolerance, three times a week for 2 weeks; weekly for 6 weeks; and biweekly for 4 months.[86] Continuous or intermittent irrigation of the drug through tubes has also been used with success.[49] With the availability of oral therapy, it has been commonly used for initial treatment as a substitute for systemic amphotericin, with or without local amphotericin.[80]

Central Nervous System

In coccidioidal meningitis, intrathecal therapy with amphotericin B is the accepted treatment modality. It is common to treat patients who only have coccidioidal meningitis with modest courses (0.5–1.0 g) of systemic amphotericin as well, and this practice is intended at least in part as prophylactic treatment against other occult disseminated foci since intrathecal therapy appears to be the essential part of treatment of every case. This is unlike, for example, the situation with cryptococcal meningitis, in which intravenous amphotericin may be sufficient for many patients.

Intrathecal therapy can be administered by four routes: lumbar, cisternal, ventricular, or cervical. Corticosteroids (e.g., 25 mg of hydrocortisone) are commonly administered simultaneously intrathecally to reduce local reactions. It is advisable to begin therapy with low doses of amphotericin (e.g., 0.01–0.025 mg) if possible and to increase the dose gradually as tolerated. Lumbar delivery is by barbotage or by suspension of the drug in 5-ml hypertonic (10 percent) glucose. With the patient on a table tilted head down, the hypertonic solution reaches the basilar area with minimal dilution.[88] Most experience with lumbar therapy has involved doses of about 0.5 mg, but dose and frequency of treatment may need to be modified according to patient tolerance. Complications of lumbar therapy include local and radicular pain, headaches, paresthesias, nerve palsies (not necessarily corresponding to the level of injection), bladder dystonia, and impotence. The symptoms are usually transient. These problems have largely been attributed to arachnoiditis secondary to amphotericin. However, neurotoxicity (in the form of myelopathy) secondary to the drug has been documented, probably on a vascular basis. Transient symptoms may precede more profound deficits.[89] Cisternal therapy has the advantage of placing the drug closest to the site of maximum infection, the basilar meninges. Doses of 0.01–1.5 mg have been used, usually 0.25 mg or less in 0.5-ml or smaller volumes. Complications of cisternal therapy are rare in experienced hands but include headaches, nausea and vomiting, hypertension, bradycardia, arrhythmias, cranial palsies, dysequilibrium and gait problems, and rarely, upper motor neuron impairment. These complications appear to be due to arachnoiditis, possibly direct neurotoxicity, hemorrhage (with meningismus, compression of brain stem, obstruction of outflow of the fourth ventricle), and/or direct puncture of the brain (usually the medulla, occasionally the cerebellar tonsils or pons, with immediate cough, vomiting, weakness, electric sensations, and respiratory difficulties).[90] Ventricular therapy, such as via an Ommaya reservoir, places the drug distant from the usual principal site of infection but is necessary if ventricular infection is present. Most experience has been with doses beginning at 0.01 mg and gradually increasing to 1.5 mg if tolerated. It is futile in the presence of a ventricular shunt, since the drug is diverted out of the central nervous system. An alternative is placement of the distal end of the tubing in the cisterna magna. Lumbar reservoirs, for lumbar intrathecal delivery, are another variant of reservoir therapy. Bacterial superinfection is a common problem with reservoir therapy.[91] Lateral cervical puncture has had limited use but in experienced hands is reputedly safe and less troublesome than other methods. Delivery by any of the routes suggested may be frustrated by obstruction of flow due to infection and/or fibrosis. Blockage is detected by myelography, radioisotope flow studies, computed tomography, or magnetic resonance imaging (MRI).

An efficacious treatment regimen has yet to be defined by comparative trials. Recommendations for duration of therapy have varied up to treatment for life. Holeman and Johnson,[54] in a large long-term series, have had good results with a regimen of intrathecal treatment three times a week for 3 months or until CSF cells are less than 10/mm^3 (whichever is longer), then one to two times weekly for several months, tapering to once every 1–6 weeks. If CSF cells exceed 10, the frequency is increased until the count falls below this level. If a frank clinical relapse or marked abnormalities in the CSF recur, then the patient is retreated as if a new patient. Therapy is discontinued only after at least 1 year of completely normal CSF on a once every 6 weeks treatment schedule. After cessation of treatment the CSF is examined every 6 weeks for at least 1–2 years. This is important because other studies have indicated that relapse usually occurs in this interval after the end of a course of apparently successful therapy. Winn's regimen.[92] was twice weekly intrathecal therapy until the CSF improved, then once or twice a week until 3 months after the CSF CFA disappeared, with follow-up examinations of the spinal fluid for at least 2 years. Chemical meningitis due to intrathecal drug can be confusing with respect to monitoring CSF indices as a guide to therapy. Both Holeman and Winn reported patients who appear to be cured, with inactive disease without therapy, more than 10 years after onset of meningitis. More aggressive approaches, attempting to reach a dose of 12 mg/month for at least 2 months, have been advocated but without clear evidence of producing more long-term cures.[93] Clinical responses and apparent cures have also been produced, even in amphotericin-unresponsive patients, with intravenous miconazole alone, intrathecal miconazole alone, or a combination of the two routes.[79] Doses of 20 mg intrathecally produce CSF levels that exceed the minimal inhibitory concentrations of *C. immitis* for 24 hours and are well tolerated. Patients with meningeal disease of long duration are less likely to respond. Relapses have occurred after short courses of therapy. Reports suggest that some patients with meningitis may respond to high (≥800 mg/day) doses of oral ketoconazole.[94] A new triazole, fluconazole, which can be given orally, penetrates well into CSF of meningitis patients; preliminary clinical results are encouraging.[95] Responses to itraconazole have also been reported.[84] A drug for meningitis that is effective by the systemic route would represent a significant advance and may be essential for patients with internal obstruction to CSF flow.

An important consideration is awareness of the possibility of hydrocephalus and/or ventricular infection. The former may present as unexplained deterioration in a patient whose CSF shows improvement on therapy or is unchanged, and the latter occurs in a setting of refractoriness to therapy. Computed tomography and MRI have largely replaced earlier methods in the detection of these complications. Shunting of CSF flow may prevent irreversible brain damage. Spread of coccidioidal infection from the distal end of the shunt is a possible risk of such procedure. Use of concomitant intravenous therapy is suggested in such situations while ventricular cultures remain positive.

Immuoprophylaxis and Immunotherapy

The importance of the immune response in control of the infection, as described, has led to approaches directed to manipulation of the host response to prevent disease or to treat it.

Rixford and Gilchrist, in their original studies, showed experimentally infected animals were more resistant to superinfection. The most extensive studies directed to the development of a vaccine have used killed organisms (spherules) rather than attenuated live fungi. A killed vaccine, though protective against challenge in several species,[96] has not been shown to protect humans. Current work is directed to development of purified antigens as more tolerable vaccines that may be protective. If an effective vaccine could be developed for humans, this would be the greatest step forward in the fight against this disease.

Defects in cellular immune reactivity in patients with progressive disease have been described in the section on immunology. Attempts to restore this reactivity as a mode of therapy are therefore logical. Transfer of cellular immunity from an immune donor to an unreactive recipient can be achieved with whole lymphocytes, but this has practical disadvantages (e.g., potential for transmission of other diseases) and theoretical disadvantages (e.g., graft-v.-host reactions). Transfer can also be achieved with subcellular fractions of immune cells, and in coccidioidomycosis efforts have focused on the use of "transfer factor," an extract of disrupted leukocytes with a molecular weight of less than 10,000.[97] Other immunomodulators, including those produced synthetically or by recombinant techniques, show promise in vitro and may represent a future approach to immunotherapy.

REFERENCES

1. Posada A. Un nuevo caso de micosis fungoidea con psorospermias. An Circ Med Argent. 1892;15:585.
2. Rixford E, Gilchrist TC. Two cases of protozoan (coccidioidal) infection of the skin and other organs. Johns Hopkins Hosp Rep. 1896;1:209.
3. Ophüls W, Moffitt HC. A new pathogenic mould (formerly described as a protozoan: *Coccidioides immitis* pyogenes): Preliminary report. Phil Med J. 1900;5:1471.
4. Dickson EC. "Valley fever" of the San Joaquin Valley and fungus *Coccidioides*. Calif West Med. 1937;47:151.
5. Gifford MA. San Joaquin fever. Kern County Health Department Annual Report. 1935–36;22.
6. Stewart RA, Meyer KF. Isolation of *Coccidioides immitis* (Stiles) from the soil. Proc Soc Exp Biol Med. 1932;29:937.
7. Gifford MA, Buss WC, Dowds RJ. Data on *Coccidioides* fungus infection, Kern County, 1901–1936. Kern County Health Department Annual Report. 1936–37;39.
8. Smith CE, Whiting EG, Baker EE, et al. The use of coccidioidin. Am Rev Tuberc. 1948;57:330.
9. Huppert M, Sun SH. Overview of mycology, and the mycology of *Coccidioides immitis*. In: Stevens DA, ed. Coccidioidomycosis: A Text. New York: Plenum Medical; 1980:21.
10. Converse JL. Effect of surface active agents on endosporulation of *Coccidioides immitis* in a chemically defined liquid medium. J Bacteriol. 1957;74:106.
11. Pappagianis D. Epidemiology of coccidioidomycosis. In: Stevens DA, ed. Coccidioidomycosis: A Text. New York: Plenum Medical; 1980:63.
12. Scogins JT. Comparative study of time loss in coccidioidomycosis and other respiratory disease. In: Proceedings of a Symposium on Coccidioidomycosis. US Public Health Service Publication No. 575:1947:132.
13. Rothman PE, Graw RG, Harris JC. Coccidioidomycosis: Possible fomite transmission: A review and report of a case. Am J Dis Child. 1969;118:792.
14. Maddy KT. Observations on *Coccidioides immitis* found growing naturally in soil. Ariz Med. 1965;22:261.
15. Emmons CW. Isolation of *Coccidioides* from soil and rodents. Public Health Rep. 1942;57:109.
16. Werner SB, Pappagianis D, Heindl I, et al. An epidemic of coccidioidomycosis among archeology students in Northern California. New Engl J Med. 1972;286:507.
17. Eckmann BH, Schaefer GL, Huppert M. Bedside interhuman transmission of coccidioidomycosis via growth on fomites: An epidemic involving six persons. Am Rev Respir Dis. 1964;89:175.
18. Huntington RW. Pathology of coccidioidomycosis. In: Stevens DA, ed. Coccidioidomycosis: A Text. New York: Plenum Medical; 1980:113.
19. Puckett TF. Hyphae of *Coccidioides immitis* in tissues of the human host. Am Rev Tuberc. 1954;70:320.
20. Savage DC, Madin SH. Cellular responses in lungs of immunized mice to intranasal infection with *Coccidioides immitis*. Sabouraudia. 1968;6:94.
21. Newcomer VD, Landau JW, Lehman R, et al. The local cellular rsponse in patients with coccidioidomycosis. Arch Dermatol. 1963;88:799.
22. Galgiani JN, Yam P, Petz LD, et al. Complement activation by *Coccidioides immitis*: In vitro and clinical studies. Infect Immun. 1980;28:944.
23. Galgiani JN, Isenberg RA, Stevens DA. Chemotaxigenic activity of extracts from the mycelial and spherule phases of *Coccidioides immitis* for human polymorphonuclear leukocytes. Infect Immun. 1978;21:862.
24. Brummer E, Beaman L, Stevens DA. Killing of endospores, but not arthroconidia, of *Coccidioides immitis* by immunologically activated polymorphonodar neutrophils. In: Einstein HE, Catanzaro A, eds. Coccidioidomycosis: Proceedings of the 4th International Conference on Coccidioidomycosis. Washington, D.C.: National Foundation for Infectious Diseases; 1985:201.
25. Galgiani JN. Inhibition of different phases of *Coccidioides immitis* by human neutrophils or hydrogen peroxide. J Infect Dis. 1986;153:217.
26. Frey CL, Drutz DJ. Influence of fungal surface components on the interaction of *Coccidioides immitis* with polymorphonuclear neutrophils. J Infect Dis. 1986;153:933.
27. Beaman L, Benjamini B, Pappagianis D. Activation of macrophages by lymphokines: Enhancement of phagosome–lysosome fusion and killing of *Coccidioides immitis*. Infect Immun. 1983;39:1201.
28. Deresinski SC, Applegate RJ, Levine HB, et al. Cellular immunity to *Coccidioides immitis*: In vitro lymphocyte response to spherules, arthrospores, and endospores. Cell Immunol. 1977;32:110.
29. Echols RM, Palmer DI, Long GW. Tissue eosinophilia in human coccidioidomycosis. Rev Infect Dis. 1982;4:656.
30. Catanzaro A, Spitler LE, Moser KM. Cellular immune response in coccidioidomycosis. Cell Immunol. 1975;15:360.
31. Cox RA, Vivas JR, Gross R, et al. In vivo and in vitro cell-mediated responses in coccidioidomycosis. Am Rev Respir Dis. 1976;114:937.
32. Bin Ibrahim A, Pappagianis D. Experimental induction of anergy to coccidioidin by antigens of *Coccidioides immitis*. Infect Immun. 1973;7:786.
33. Catanzaro A. Suppressor cells in coccidioidomycosis. Cell Immunol. 1981;64:235.
34. Opelz G, Scheer MI. Cutaneous sensitivity and in vitro responsiveness of lymphocytes in patients with disseminated coccidioidomycosis. J Infect Dis. 1975;132:250.
35. Harvey RP, Stevens DA. In vitro assays of cellular immunity in progressive coccidioidomycosis: Evaluation of suppression with parasitic-phase antigen. Am Rev Respir Dis. 1981;123:665.
36. Cox RA, Pope RM, Stevens DA. Immune complexes in coccidioidomycosis: Correlation with disease involvement. Am Rev Respir Dis. 1982;126:439.
37. Brass C, Levine HB, Stevens DA. Stimulation and suppression of cell-mediated immunity by endosporulation antigens of *Coccidioides immitis*. Infect Immun. 1982;35:431.
38. Cox RA, Baker BS, Stevens DA. Specificity of immunoglobulin E in coccidioidomycosis and correlation with disease involvement. Infect Immun. 1982;37:609.
39. Beaman L, Pappagianis D, Benjamini E. Mechanisms of resistance to infection with *Coccidioides immitis* in mice. Infect Immun. 1979;23:681.
40. Hicks HR, Northey WT. Studies on the response of thymectomized mice to infection with *Coccidioides immitis*. In: Ajello L, ed. Coccidioidomycosis. Tucson: University of Arizona; 1967:183.
41. Newcomer VD, Wright TW, Tarbet JE, et al. The effects of cortisone on experimental coccidioidomycosis. J Invest Dermatol. 1953;20:315.
42. Smith CE, Beard RR, Whiting EG, et al. Varieties of coccidioidal infection in relation to the epidemiology and control of the disease. Am J Public Health. 1946;36:1394.
43. Castellino RA, Blank N. Pulmonary coccidioidomycosis: The wide spectrum of roentgenographic manifestations. Calif Med. 1968;109:41.
44. Rodenbiker HT, Ganley JP, Galgiani JN, et al. Prevalence of chorioretinal scars associated with coccidioidomycosis. Arch Ophthalmol. 1981;99:71.
45. DeFelice R, Weiden MA, Galgiani JN. The incidence and implications of coccidioidouria. Am Rev Respir Dis. 1982;125:49.
46. Harris RE. Coccidioidomycosis complicating pregnancy. Obstet Gynecol. 1966;28:401.
47. Stevens DA. Clinical manifestations and management of coccidioidomycosis in the compromised patient. In: Warnock DW, Richardson MD, eds. Fungal Infection in the Compromised Patient. Chichester, England: John Wiley & Sons; 1982:199.
48. Hyde L. Coccidioidal pulmonary cavitation. Dis Chest. 1968;54(Suppl 1):273.
49. Iger M. Coccidioidal osteomyelitis. In: Ajello L, ed. Coccidioidomycosis, Current Clinical and Diagnostic Status. Miami: Symposia Specialists; 1977:177.
50. Pollock SF, Morris JM, Murray WR. Coccidioidal synovitis of the knee. J Bone Joint Surg. 1967;49A:1397.
51. Kelly PC. Coccidioidal meningitis. In: Stevens DA, ed. Coccidioidomycosis: A Text. New York: Plenum Medical; 1980:163.
52. Bouza E, Dreyer JS, Hewitt WL, et al. Coccidioidal meningitis: An analysis of thirty-one cases and review of the literature. Medicine. 1981;60:139.
53. Goldstein E, Winship MJ, Pappagianis D. Ventricular fluid and the management of coccidioidal meningitis. Ann Intern Med. 1972;77:243.
54. Holeman CW, Johnson P. Long term followup of amphotericin treated coccidioidal meningitis patients. In: Stevens DA, ed. Proceedings of the 21st Annual Meeting of the Coccidioidomycosis Study Group. 1976. (Abstract no 1).
55. Einstein HE, Holeman CW, Sandidge LL, et al. Coccidioidal meningitis: The use of amphotericin B in treatment. Calif Med. 1961;94:339.
56. Wilson JW. The importance of the portal of entry in certain microbial infections: The primary cutaneous "chancriform" syndrome. Dis Chest. 1968;54(Suppl 1):43.
57. Smith CE. Coccidioidomycosis. Pediatr Clin North Am. 1955;2:109.
58. Cherry JD, Lloyd CA, Quilty JF, et al. Amphotericin B therapy in children. J Pediatr. 1969;75:1063.
59. Drutz DJ, Huppert M. Coccidioidomycosis: Factors affecting the host–parasite interaction. J Infect Dis. 1983;147:372.
60. Bronniman DA, Adam RD, Galgiani JN, et al. Coccidioidomycosis in the acquired immunodeficiency syndrome. Ann Intern Med. 1987;106:372.
61. Reed BR, Kaplan W. The use of *N*-acetyl-cysteine and dithiothreitol to process sputa for mycological and fluorescent antibody examinations. Health Lab Sci. 1972;9:118.
62. Warlick MA, Quan SF, Sobonya RE. Rapid diagnosis of pulmonary coccidioidomycosis. Arch Intern Med. 1983;143:723.
63. Johnson JE, Perry JE, Fekety FR, et al. Laboratory-acquired coccidioidomycosis. A report of 210 cases. Ann Intern Med. 1964;60:941.
64. Georg LK, Ajello L, Papageorge C. Use of cycloheximide in the selective isolation of fungi pathogenic to man. J Lab Clin Med. 1954;44:422.
65. Roberts JA, Counts JM, Crecelius HB. Production in vitro of *Coccidioides immitis* spherules and endospores as a diagnostic acid. Am Rev Respir Dis. 1970;102:811.
66. Sun SH, Huppert M, Vukovick KR. Rapid in vitro conversion and identification of *Coccidioides immitis*. J Clin Microbiol. 1976;3:186.
67. Standard PG, Kaufman L. Immunological procedure for the rapid and specific identification of *Coccidioides immitis* cultures. J Clin Microbiol. 1977;5:149.
68. Pappagianis D: Serology and serodiagnosis of coccidioidomycosis. In: Stevens DA, ed. Coccidioidomycosis: A Text. New York: Plenum Medical; 1980:97.
69. Smith CE, Saito MT. Serologic reactions in coccidioidomycosis. J Chronic Dis. 1957;5:571.

70. Pappagianis D, Krasnow I, Beall S. False positive reactions of cerebrospinal fluid and diluted sera with the coccidioidal latex agglutination test. Am J Clin Pathol. 1976;66:916.
71. Weiner MH. Antigenemia detected in human coccidioidomycosis. J Clin Microbiol. 1983;18:136.
72. Galgiani JN, Dugger KO, Ito JI, et al. Antigenemia in primary coccidioidomycosis. Am J Trop Med Hyg. 1984;33:645.
73. Pappagianis D, Saito M, Van Hoosear KH. Antibody in cerebrospinal fluid in non-meningitic coccidioidomycosis. Sabouraudia. 1972;10:173.
74. Stevens DA, Levine HB, Deresinski SC, et al. Epidemiological and clinical skin testing studies with spherulin. In: Ajello L, ed. Coccidioidomycosis, Current Clinical and Diagnostic Status. Miami: Symposia Specialists; 1977:107.
75. Deresinski SC, Levine HB, Kelly PC, et al. Spherulin skin testing and histoplasmal and coccidioidal serology: Lack of effect. Am Rev Respir Dis. 1977;116:1116.
76. Galgiani JN and the Valley Fever Vaccine Group. Development of dermal hypersensitivity to coccidioidal antigens associated with repeated skin testing. Am Rev Resp Dis. 1986;134:1035.
77. Drutz D. Amphotericin B in the treatment of coccidioidomycosis. Drugs 1983;26:337.
78. Collins MS, Pappagianis D. Uniform susceptibility of various strains of *Coccidioides immitis* to amphotericin B. Antimicrob Agents Chemother. 1977;11:1049.
79. Stevens DA. An update on miconazole therapy for coccidioidomycosis. Drugs. 1983;26:347.
80. Galgiani JN. Ketoconazole treatment of coccidioidomycosis. Drugs. 1983;26:355.
81. Stevens DA, Stiller RL, Williams PL, et al. Experience with ketoconazole in three major manifestations of progressive coccidioidomycosis. Am J Med. 1983;74:58.
82. Sugar AM, Alsip SG, Galgiani JN, et al. Pharmacology and toxicity of high-dose ketoconazole. Antimicrob Agents Chemother. 1987;31:1874.
83. Galgiani JN, Stevens DA, Graybill JR, et al. Ketoconazole therapy of progressive coccidioidomycosis: Comparison of 400- and 800-mg doses and observations at higher doses. Am J Med 1988,84.603.
84. Tucker RM, Williams PL, Arathoon EG, et al. Treatment of mycoses with itraconazole. Ann NY Acad Sci. 1988;544:451.
85. Winter WG, Larson RK, Honeggar MM, et al. Coccidioidal arthritis and its treatment: 1975. J Bone Joint Surg 1975;57A:1152.
86. Aidem HP. Intra-articular amphotericin B in the treatment of coccidioidal synovitis of the knee. J Bone Joint Surg. 1968;50A:1663.
87. Greenman R, Becker J, Campbell G, et al. Coccidioidal synovitis of the knee. Arch Intern Med. 1975;135:526.
88. Glynn KP, Alazraki NP, Waltz TA. Coccidioidal meningitis: Intrathecal treatment with hyperbaric amphotericin B. Calif Med. 1973;119:6.
89. Carnevale NT, Galgiani JN, Langston JW, et al. Amphotericin-induced myelopathy. Arch Intern Med. 1980;140:1189.
90. Keane JR. Cisternal puncture complications: Treatment of coccidioidal meningitis with amphotericin B. Calif Med. 1973;119:10.
91. Diamond R, Bennett JE. A subcutaneous reservoir for intrathecal therapy of fungal meningitis. New Engl J Med. 1973;288:186.
92. Winn WA. Coccidioidal meningitis: A follow-up report. In: Ajello L, ed. Coccidioidomycosis. Tucson: University of Arizona; 1965:55.
93. Labadie EL, Hamilton RH. Survival improvement in coccidioidal meningitis by high-dose intrathecal amphotericin B. Arch Intern Med. 1986;146:2013.
94. Graybill JR, Stevens DA, Galgiani JN, et al. Ketoconazole treatment of coccidioidal meningitis. Ann NY Acad Sci. 1988;544:488.
95. Tucker RM, Williams PL, Arathoon EG, et al. Pharmacokinetics of fluconazole in cerebrospinal fluid and serum in human coccidioidal meningitis. Antimicrob Agents Chemother. 1988;32:369.
96. Pappagianis D, Levine HB. The present status of vaccination against coccidioidomycosis in man. Am J Epidemiol. 1975;102:30.
97. Stevens DA. Immunotherapy-transfer factor in coccidioidomycosis. In: Stevens DA, ed. Coccidioidomycosis: A Text. New York: Plenum Medical; 1980:261.

BIBLIOGRAPHY

Drutz DJ, Catanzaro A. Coccidioidomycosis. Am Rev Respir Dis. 1978;117:559.
Stevens DA, ed. Coccidioidomycosis: A Text. New York: Plenum Medical; 1980.

245. DERMATOPHYTOSIS AND OTHER SUPERFICIAL MYCOSES

R. J. HAY

The superficial fungal infections include some of the most common infectious conditions such as ringworm or dermatophytosis and pityriasis versicolor as well as rare disorders including tinea nigra. Their prevalence varies in different parts of the world, but in many tropical countries they are the most common causes of skin disease. Dermatophyte infections and other superficial mycoses are described in this chapter. Superficial candidiasis is discussed in Chapter 234.

DERMATOPHYTOSIS

The dermatophytes are molds that can invade the stratum corneum of the skin or other keratinized tissues derived from epidermis such as hair and nails. They may cause infections, dermatophytoses, at most skin sites, although the feet, groin, scalp, and nails are most commonly affected.[1] The dermatophytes are among the earliest microorganisms that were found to cause infections in humans. *Trichophyton schoenleinii*, the cause of the scalp infection favus, was isolated from a patient and the culture shown to reproduce the typical lesions after inoculation onto human skin as early as 1841. Dermatophyte infections had been described many years before this even though the identity of the cause had not been recognized. The ancient Greek physicians knew about ringworm, and there are descriptions of the manifestations of dermatophytosis in more unlikely sources such as the records of the early Dutch explorers of the sixteenth century who brought back reports of a strange disease of the skin, subsequently known as tinea imbricata caused by *T. concentricum*, in the islanders of the west Pacific.

The Dermatophytes

There are three genera of pathogenic dermatophyte fungi—*Trichophyton, Microsporum*, and *Epidermophyton*. The latter genus is only represented by a single species *E. floccosum*. These keratinophilic organisms probably arose as saprophytic soil fungi, and some dermatophytes, which have only been isolated from soil, have not been shown to cause disease in either animals or humans. Most of the 39 dermatophyte species, however, are parasitic and can cause disease in either humans or animals, often being adapted to a single or narrow range of host species. The dermatophytes are referred to as either zoophilic, anthropophilic or geophilic, depending on whether their primary source is an animal, human, or soil, respectively.

The taxonomy of these fungi is complicated by the fact that most clinical isolates are imperfect fungi, organisms that do not produce sexual structures in culture. However, sexual forms of many of these species are known and have been assigned to one of two genera, *Arthroderma* and *Nannizzia*, which correspond to the imperfect genera *Trichophyton* and *Microsporum*, respectively. The classification of these fungi is difficult, and their exact taxonomic status remains a subject of debate.[2]

The relationships between different dermatophytes are not simply the subject for intellectual dispute. It is important, for instance, to attempt to differentiate strains of the same species in order to understand the spread of infections. Studies of the DNA homology of different species have not proved universally helpful because the fungi are so closely related.[3] Attempts have also been made to classify the dermatophytes acording to their protein composition[4] and production of antibiotics or enzymes such as urease. Both the latter may play a role in determining pathogenicity. For instance, the ability of dermatophytes to produce keratinases will affect their ability to penetrate keratin. The production of elastase has also been proposed as a factor affecting the development of inflammatory responses in ringworm.[5] The significance of the production of antibiotics by dermatophytes is uncertain. The main groups detected have been the penicillins and fusidanes, and these are produced by dermatophytes not only under laboratory culture conditions but also after growth on epidermal sheets in vitro.

Epidemiology

The factors affecting the distribution and transmission of dermatophytosis are largely dependent on the source of the infection[6]—animal, soil, or human—discussed briefly above.

Zoophilic Dermatophyte Infections. The main zoophilic dermatophyte fungi are shown in Table 1. Each organism is primarily an animal pathogen that sometimes causes human infection. In each case there is usually a range of host specificities, from organisms such as *M. nanum*, whose natural host is the pig and which does not infect other animals, to *T. mentagrophytes*, which affects a range of different rodent species as well as cats, dogs, and horses. The host preferences of *T. mentagrophytes* coupled with small clinical and cultural differences has led many mycologists to subdivide this group into different species or subspecies (the *mentagrophytes* complex). Under this classification *T. mentagrophytes quinckeanum* (*T. quinckeanum*) is used to describe the fungus that causes the clinical pattern of favus in mice, an infection associated with the formation of epithelial crusts. In most temperate countries *T. verrucosum*, the cause of cattle ringworm, and *M. canis*, a dermatophyte that causes infections in cats or dogs, are the most common zoophilic dermatophytes that cause human infections. Of all the zoophilic dermatophytes *M. canis* is probably the most prevalent throughout the the world. Its appearance in the tropics is a comparatively recent event, and it is mainly found there as a cause of disease in urban communities.[6] Occasionally the distribution of zoophilic dermatophytes may appear to be difficult to explain, but usually this reflects the distribution of the animal host. For instance *T. erinacei* (*T. mentagrophytes*) is mainly confined to Europe and New Zealand. It is carried by hedgehogs, which were introduced into New Zealand in the nineteenth century from England. *M. persicolor* is a rare cause of human infections in Europe where it has been isolated from the bank vole whose distribution is similarly restricted. *T. simii* is associated with monkeys in India and the Far East, and human infections are only seen in these areas.[7]

Geophilic Dermatophyte Infections. Dermatophytes originating from soil such as *M. gypseum* are infrequent causes of human disease, although they may be seen more commonly in certain parts of the tropics such as the west Pacific and Central America. In other areas they usually cause sporadic infections, although occasionally they may be responsible for outbreaks of human disease in appropriately exposed occupational groups such as gardeners or farm workers.[7]

Anthropophilic Dermatophyte Infections. Dermatophytes that are natural pathogens of humans are the most common cause of human dermatophytosis. They include organisms that mainly cause infections of glabrous skin of the feet or hands as well as a range of pathogens where invasion may involve penetration of the hair shaft. The most common of these organisms in most parts of the world is *T. rubrum*, which causes tinea pedis or tinea cruris in temperate climates and, particularly in the tropics, tinea corporis. Cases of infection due to *T. rubrum* were once rare in the Western Hemisphere, but the infection has spread rapidly during the past 40 years. The ability of this dermatophyte to cause noninflammatory chronic infections of the feet, among other sites, that are easily transmitted is probably an important fctor that has determined its spread in recent years.[6] The large population movements during the Second World War are also thought to have contributed to the spread of the disease. Despite this, a variant with distinct morphologic appearances may be isolated from patients with tinea corporis in remote rural areas of the New and Old World tropics, which suggests that although endemic disease due to this species has been present for a considerable time the key adaptation leading to spread was the appearance of strains capable of causing indolent and noninflammatory infections of peripheral skin sites.[8]

Spread of the organisms that infect glabrous skin is largely through contact with infected desquamated skin scales. Classically this occurs in bathing areas or shower rooms where large numbers of individuals share common facilities, for instance, in military camps or factories.[9] In the U.K. coal mining industry as many as 30–35 percent of coal miners may have dermatophyte infections affecting their feet. In most cases this is due to *T. rubrum*, although *T. interdigitale* (*mentagrophytes*) may also be isolated.[10] Schools and public swimming baths are also sites for infection. By contrast, transmission within the home as a reflection of conjugal or familial cases is not common.[11] *Epidermophyton floccosum* may also cause foot infections, although it is particularly associated with tinea cruris either as a sporadic disease or within institutions such as prisons or military barracks. These infections are not geographically restricted even though there are variations in different countries. In many tropical areas, particularly the Far East, *T. mentagrophytes* is less commonly a cause of interdigital foot disease, and patients are infected by the zoophilic variety of this species on sites other than the feet.[12]

Tinea corporis (tinea imbricata), caused by the anthropophilic dermatophyte *T. concentricum*, has an unusual distribution confined to remote parts of the humid tropics.[13] The main endemic areas are the west Pacific, Malaysia, Assam, and parts of the Amazon basin in Brazil. Infants may be affected shortly after birth, and spontaneous recovery is unusual. Large numbers of viable organisms can be cultured from the houses of infected families. Visitors to endemic areas are rarely infected. Cases have also been described in southern Mexico where the disease appears to fluctuate in severity with the season.

The distribution of some of the other anthropophilic dermatophytes that cause tinea capitis in children as well as other clincal forms of disease such as tinea corporis or onychomycosis may be more restricted. The reasons for this are not entirely clear unless the prevalence of these infections in children, who form a relatively stable population with little opportunity for travel, limits the spread of the disease to certain localities. Whatever the reason, these scalp infections are often found in defined endemic areas (Table 2). The situation is best illustrated by the distribution of *Trichophyton* species causing tinea capitis in West Africa where the endemic areas for *T. soudanense, T. yaoundei*, and *T. gourvilii*, are distinct although there is some overlap.[14] *Trichophyton tonsurans* in the United States and Mexico and *T. violaceum* in India and the Middle East are the predominant causes of scalp infection in some areas. The situation does not always remain stable, and the slow increase in numbers of *T. tonsurans* in the United States after its presumed introduction from Central America illustrates the point.[6] Endemic anthropophilic scalp infections due to *Microsporum* spe-

TABLE 1. Classification of the Main Dermatophytes by Their Primary Reservoir(s)

		Zoophilic	
Anthropophilic	*Geophilic*	*Organism*	*Source(s)*
T. concentricum	*T. ajelloi*	*T. erinacei*[a]	Hedgehogs
T. gourvilii	*T. terrestre*	*T. equinum*	Horses
T. mentagrophytes-interdigitale[a]		*T. mentagrophytes-mentagrophytes*[a]	Rodents
T. megnini	*M. fulvum*	*T. quinckeanum*[a]	Mice
T. rubrum	*M. gypseum*	*T. simii*	Monkeys
T. schoenleinii		*T. verrucosum*	Cattle
T. soudanense		*M. canis*	Cats, dogs
T. tonsurans		*M. gallinae*	Poultry
T. violaceum		*M. nanum*	Pigs
T. yaoundei		*M. persicolor*	Bank voles
M. audouinii			
M. ferrugineum			
E. floccosum			

[a] These organisms are part of the "mentagrophytes" complex and may be classified as a single species.

TABLE 2. Distribution of Dermatophytes Causing Tinea Capitis

Dermatophyte	*Distribution*
T. gourvilii	Central Africa
T. tonsurans	North and central America (Europe—uncommon)
T. soudanense	West and central Africa
T. schoenleinii	North Africa, (United States, Middle East, South Africa, South America—sporadic)
T. verrucosum	Europe
T. violaceum	Indian subcontinent, Middle East, North Africa
T. yaoundei	Central Africa
M. audouinii	Central America, West Africa (Europe—uncommon)
M. canis	Worldwide but uncommon in India and the Far East
M. ferrugineum	Central Africa, Far East

cies are less common. For instance *M. ferrugineum* is found occasionally in the Far East or central Europe. *M. rivalieri* is seen in Africa, Zaire, and Angola. The most widely distributed of this genus is *M. audouinii*. Once common throughout Europe, it is now rare in this area, but it is still an important cause of tinea capitis in West Africa and in parts of the United States and Latin America.

The infection caused by *T. schoenleinii*, favus, has characteristic clinical features. It was once common in Europe but has now largely disappeared from many areas, although there are still pockets of infection in parts of the United States, South America, South Africa (Botswana) and North Africa. One of the features of this disease is the development of crusts or scutula on the scalp. Hairs are invaded, but shedding is delayed because they are not structurally damaged until late in the course of the infection. Although tinea capitis is normally a disease of children; adult women with favus are occasionally seen.

Dermatophytes causing scalp disease may be carried on the skin surface without invading the skin or hair. A small proportion of carriers develop infections within 6 months, others lose the fungus, while the rest remain carriers.[15] The same can also be seen in foot infections where carriage can also occur.

AGE INCIDENCE. Tinea capitis is mainly a disease of childhood, and cases are rare after puberty. Occasionally this infection may occur in elderly women and is associated with scarring alopecia. The reason for the preponderance of the disease in children is thought to be the presence of medium-chain-length fatty (C_8–C_{12}) acids in sebum that inhibit the growth of dermatophytes in postpubertal individuals. By contrast, tinea pedis is usually seen in adolescents or young adults.[16] While foot infections can occasionally occur in young children, in this age group, the nails may be invaded without concomitant skin infection.

Pathogenesis

Transfer of infecting organisms from soil, other animals, or humans is accomplished by means of arthrospores, which are vegetative cells with thickened cell walls formed by dermatophyte hyphae in vitro and vivo. It is likely that these structures are shed by the primary host with shed skin scales or hair. It has been shown that dermatophyte arthrospores can survive for considerable periods outside the host, in some cases for over 15 months. Direct contact between the infected individual and another is not necessary for the development of dermatophytosis. The process of transfer itself is little understood, but invasion of the skin appears to follow adherence of fungal cells to keratinocytes in vitro, a process that is maximal after about 2 or 3 hours. Keratinocytes from different sites do not appear to differ in their binding capacity for arthrospores. Subsequent germination leads to invasion.[17]

Susceptibility to infection is not universal. Studies of mice experimentally infected with *T. quinckeanum* have shown that there is considerable interstrain variation in susceptibility to dermatophytosis.[18] In humans it has been suggested that susceptibility to tinea imbricata is mediated through an autosomal recessive gene, the evidence being based on population studies among tribes of Papua, New Guinea.[19] Similar studies of the more common infections have not been carried out, but familial cases of tinea pedis are not common. The factors determining individual susceptibility to dermatophytosis are not understood, but variations in the composition of inhibitory fatty acids in sebum (see above) offer one explanation. Other skin surface factors thought to be important in determining the outcome of infection include the local carbon dioxide tension and the presence of surface moisture. Sweat and serum also contain inhibitory substances, one of which, transferrin, in its unsaturated state is inhibitory to the growth of dermatophytes.[20]

In experimentally infected mice and guniea pigs the inflammatory response to dermatophytosis is maximal after 9–16 days, and after this stage there is resolution of the infection. The main efferent limb of immunologic resistance is the T lymphocyte. Work in mice with *T. quinckeanum* infections has shown that resistance can be transferred to sublethally irradiated mice with T cells bearing the Thy-1 phenotype (T-helper/inducer cells).[18] Suppressor lymphocyte activity can be detected in cells from the draining lymph nodes at the peak of infection. Immunity cannot be transferred to naive animals with antibody. While it is difficult to extrapolate this data to infected humans, there is evidence that the kinetics of the immune response in humans is similar. For instance, the development of delayed-type hypersensitivity in children with naturally acquired scalp ringworm due to *T. tonsurans* correlates with recovery. Experimentally infected humans develop both delayed-type skin reactions to trichophytin and T-lymphocyte blastogenic responses at the time of recovery.[21] Patients with chronic *T. rubrum* or *T. concentricum* infections have defective T-lymphocyte-mediated responses.[22] These observations suggest that T-lymphocyte activation is critical for recovery in dermatophytosis.

The afferent limb of the immune response is provided by epidermal Langerhans cells, which have been shown to act as antigen-presenting cells in mixed cultures with human lymphocytes. The mechanisms by which T lymphocytes affect recovery are less well understood. Phagocytes, mainly neutrophils and to a lesser extent macrophages, can kill dermatophytes both intracellularly and extracellularly, mainly via oxidative pathways.[18] Dermatophyte antigens have been shown to be chemotactic to human leukocytes and may activate the alternative pathway of complement activation. However, except in inflammatory ringworm, neutrophils are not commonly seen as part of the inflammatory infiltrate in dermatophytosis, and other mechanisms of fungal clearance must be involved. It has been shown that increased epidermal turnover occurs during infection. While this also occurs in heterologous skin grafted onto nu/nu (T-cell-deficient) mice, thus suggesting that an intrinsic response is involved, it is also maximal at the time of development of the maximal immune responses.[23] It is possible that elimination of dermatophytes is also accomplished by increased shedding of the stratum corneum and that the immune system amplifies an endogenous epidermal response to infection.

Different dermatophyte species vary in their ability to elicit an immune response, with some organisms such as *T. rubrum* causing chronic or relapsing infections and others, including *T. verrucosum*, leading to long-term resistance to reinfection.

Clinical Features

The archetypal lesion of dermatophytosis is an annular scaling patch with a raised margin showing a variable degree of inflammation, the center being usually less inflamed than the edge is. This clinical form is sometimes described as tinea circinata. The word *tinea* is used to refer to dermatophyte infections, and it is usually followed by the Latin description of the appropriate site. Hence, tinea pedis is an infection of the feet and tinea capitis, the scalp. The phrase *tinea incognito* is used to describe infections that do not show any of the usual characteristic features of dermatophytosis, often because of inappropriate application of corticosteroid creams.

The clinical appearances of the infection vary with the site, the fungal species involved, and the host's immune response. Zoophilic fungi often cause inflammatory lesions, and in some cases large pustular lesions (kerions) may develop. By contrast, lesions caused by anthropophilic dermatophytes often show little inflammation and may become chronic (see "Pathogenesis").

Dermatophytes cause infections irrespective of the patient's underlying immune status. However, in common with other infections, the clinical appearances alter in immunocompromised individuals. Dermatophyte lesions are usually less inflamed in patients with diseases affecting T-lymphocyte function, but paradoxically, in some patients lesions are pustular as well as extensive. Often there is a marked follicular component to the rash in these individuals.

Tinea Pedis. Tinea pedis is usually caused by infection with either *T. rubrum* or *T. mentagrophytes* (*interdigitale*), less commonly by *E. floccosum*. The infection usually starts in the lateral interdigital spaces of the foot or on the undersurface of the lateral aspects of the toes. The main symptom is itching, although this is very variable. The skin usually cracks and may become severely macerated. In some cases, often where *T. mentagrophytes* is the causative organism, bullae are formed, and there is severe itching. The infection may also spread onto the dorsum of the feet, usually on the lateral side of the foot. Involvement of the sole is common in *T. rubrum* infections, and part or the whole sole becomes erythematous and covered with dry scales. This is most noticeable along the lateral borders of the sole where the appearances are often referred to as "moccasin" or "dry-type" infections. Blisters may also be formed in small clusters on the sole. The course of infection is variable. In noninflammatory forms the interdigital scaling is often chronic or intermittent, whereas if blisters are formed the infection usually resolves but may recur several months later. The main complications of tinea pedis are bacterial cellulitis and fungal invasion of the toenails (onychomycosis) or the skin of the dorsum of the foot and leg.

Tinea pedis is usually seen in young adults or teenage children. It is particularly common in institutions or where common bathing facilities are used. The clinical manifestations of infection are altered in patients with T-lymphocyte abnormalities, including those with the acquired immunodeficiency syndrome (AIDS), where there is often extensive spread of the lesions onto the dorsal surface of the foot.

Scaling between the toes is often referred to as athlete's foot, but similar clinical signs may be produced by a variety of organisms. Erythrasma due to *Corynebacterium minutissimum* may present with scaling and, in particular, maceration between the toe webs. Gram-negative bacteria such as *Pseudomonas* and *Proteus* species may contribute to interdigital disease in patients with closely apposed web spaces or whose work involves immersion in water. These organisms may replace the original dermatophytes in this site, an infection known as dermatophytosis complex.[24] *Staphylococcus aureus* may cause secondary infections of foot eczema, but characteristically this starts on the dorsum of the foot over the first two digits. The mold fungi *Hendersonula toruloidea* and *Scytalidium hyalinum* may cause interdigital scaling as well as nail disease and sole involvement that is indistinguishable from "dry"-type infections caused by dermatophytes.

Tinea Cruris. The most common dermatophytes associated with groin infections are *T. rubrum* and *E. floccosum*. This infection is also called jock itch. The infection starts with scaling and irritation in the groin. The rash usually involves the anterior aspect of the thighs, less commonly the scrotum. The leading edge extending onto the thighs is prominent and may contain follicular papules and pustules. The infection may also spread to the anal cleft. Although tinea cruris is mainly a disease of young adult males, it may affect women, particularly in the tropics, where the infection is often less well delineated and spreads in a band around the waist area.

Tinea cruris is mainly seen in young adult males, and as with tinea pedis, there may be clustering of cases in institutionalized groups such as military camps. The toe webs are also often infected in patients with tinea cruris.

Erythrasma of the groin may also cause a localized rash with itching. However, here the leading edge is less prominent than in tinea cruris, and the rash is covered with fine wrinkles. Erthrasma fluoresces pink under Wood's light. Candidiasis of the groin may also mimic tinea cruris, but an important clue to the presence of *Candida* is the appearance of small satellite pustules beyond the free margin of the rash. Flexural psoriasis causes a vivid red and uniformly scaling rash in the groin, and there is usually at least one other site with typical psoriatic plaques.

Tinea Corporis. Tinea corporis, or ringworm, is one of the most commonly misdiagnosed skin diseases. Cases of this infection are not common in temperate climates, although it is seen more frequently in the tropics. Generally there are a variety of different clinical presentations of this form of dermatophytosis. Most lesions have a prominent edge that may contain pustules or follicular papules, and the center of the lesion is often less inflamed and scaly (Fig. 1). Sites commonly involved are the trunk or legs. Itching is variable, and lesions may

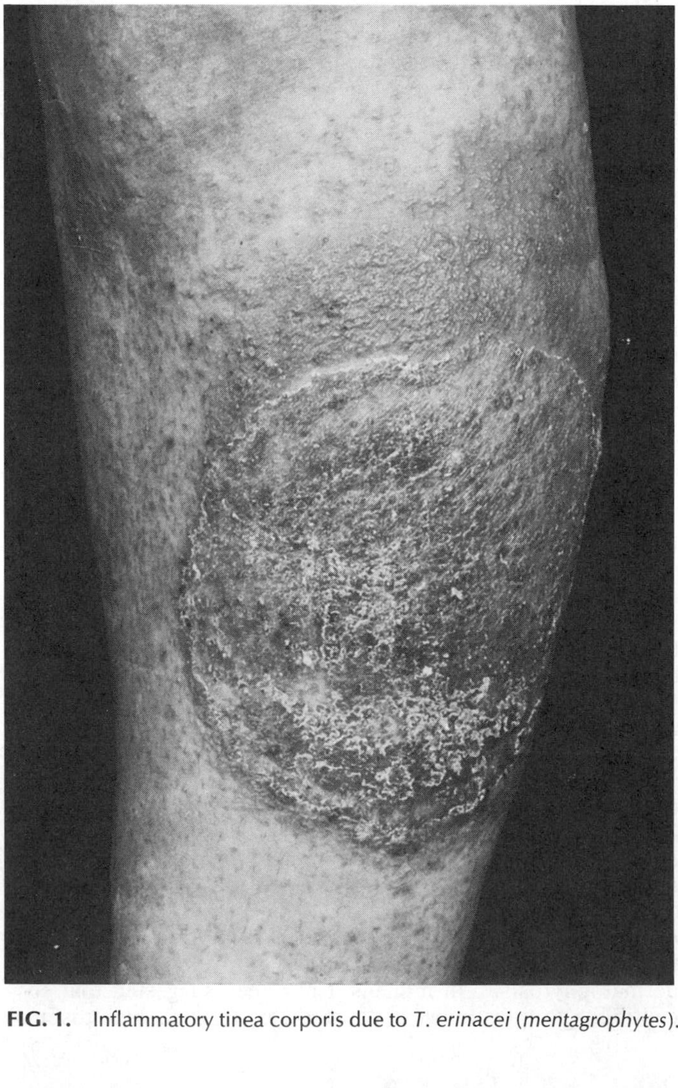

FIG. 1. Inflammatory tinea corporis due to *T. erinacei* (*mentagrophytes*).

be single or multiple. Generally infections due to anthropophilic dermatophytes such as *T. rubrum* are less inflammatory and less clearly demarcated, and in some patients, it is necessary to search for the margin carefully to delineate the rash. Lesions are usually hyperpigmented in pigmented skins. By contrast, zoophilic infections such as those caused by *M. canis* and *T. verrucosum* are more inflammatory, and lesions may become elevated and contain pustules. Infections due to *M. gypseum* are also usually inflammatory and may have a brick red appearance.

These clinical patterns vary with the site of infection. Infections due to *T. rubrum* on the lower parts of the legs may lead to the formation of single or multiple deep nodules that may mimic erythema nodosum.[25] The overlying skin is dry, red, and scaly, which is a useful clue to the correct diagnosis. This form of infection, which is known as nodular folliculitis, follows follicular penetration of the hair follicles of the lower portions of the legs by the fungus. It is mainly seen in women. In patients with defective T-lymphocyte function, scaling is often minimal, and the rash of tinea corporis consists of grouped papules or pustules without significant erythema.

Tinea corporis can occur at any age, although in temperate countries it is most often seen in children and is associated with zoophilic infections.

There are a number of different conditions to be considered in the differential diagnosis of tinea corporis that range from eczema to psoriasis or annular erythema. The important points to look for are the annular scaling margin of lesions and follicular prominence, which are features of dermatophytosis. However, it may be necessary to take scrapings for laboratory culture where there is doubt.

Tinea Imbricata. Tinea imbricata is a variant of tinea corporis that is caused by *T. concentricum*. The geographic distribution of the disease is discussed in Table 2. Patients may be infected at any age, although infants and young children are frequently affected. The main characteristic of the rash is the formation of concentric rings of scales (Fig. 2) over large parts of the body that amalgamate to form waves of scaling.[13] There are other clinical varieties of tinea imbricata, including the diffuse scaling variety where large flakes of skin are prominent. The disease gets it name *imbricata* (Latin, tiled) from this clinical patterns. Other patients may have itchy lichenified lesions on the forearms. The face may be affected as well as the sides of the fingers, but the feet, scalp, axillae, and groin are usually spared. Tinea imbricata is seldom mistaken for other diseases, and the inhabitants of endemic areas easily recognize the appearance of the infection and have specific names for it. In Papua, New Guinea, it is called *sipoma* or *grille*.

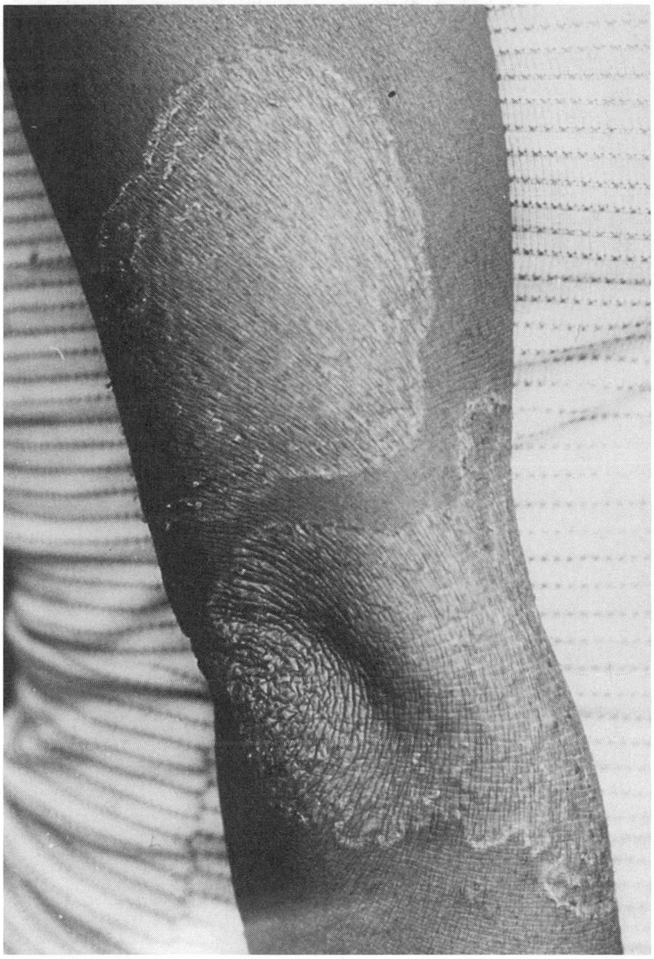

FIG. 2. Early lesions of tinea imbricata showing the first signs of concentric rings.

Dermatophytosis of the Hand (Tinea Manuum). The term *tinea manuum* is used for dermatophyte infections involving the hand. In some patients the dorsum of the hand may be affected, but most commonly the disease occurs on the palmar surface. It is a characteristic of "dry"-type infections at this site to find that only one palm is involved, although in some patients both may be infected. The clinical features are identical to those seen with dry-type infections of the sole. The usual cause is *T. rubrum*, and the feet are often involved in addition to the hands.

Dermatophytosis affecting the palm may be confused with eczema, but the unilateral distribution of the infection and the common accompanying findings of onychomycosis and tinea pedis are helpful clues. Patients with palmar plantar keratoderma (tylosis) are particularly susceptible to superinfection of the palms and soles with dermatophytes.[26] This complication may be difficult to identify, but the skin may blister, and the hand usually itches. In these patients fungi other than *T. rubrum* may be implicated.

Tinea Faciei. Dermatophyte infections of the face are usually caused by the same organisms associated with tinea corporis. Infections due to *T. rubrum* in this site are often particularly difficult to recognize (tinea incognito). The facial skin becomes itchy and red, but the margin of the rash may be difficult to discern (Fig. 3). Some patients report that the facial rash is exacerbated by sun exposure. In other instances lesions are more readily noticeable and affect the ears.

Tinea barbae, infection of the neck and beard area, may be pustular and inflamed because it is often caused by zoophilic organisms such as *T. verrucosum*. It is more localized than sycosis barbae is due to *S. aureus*, a helpful point in distinguishing the two conditions.

Tinea Capitis. Scalp ringworm, or tinea capitis, is a disease of childhood. Its prevalence varies considerably in different parts of the world. The disease is widespread in some urban areas in the United States and Central and South America. Tinea capitis is also common in parts of Africa and India. In northern Europe the disease is sporadic. The main reasons for these differences in the prevalence of infection in different localities are the nature of the infecting organisms and the availability of control measures. Endemic infections affecting large numbers of children are associated with anthropophilic organisms, sporadic disease with zoophilic fungi. Tinea capitis is usually classified by the pattern of hair shaft invasion. Dermatophyte infections where arthrospores are formed on the outside of the hair shaft are known as ectothrix infections, and those where the spores develop within the hair itself, endothrix. In *T. schoenleinii* infections the fungi invade the hair medulla but

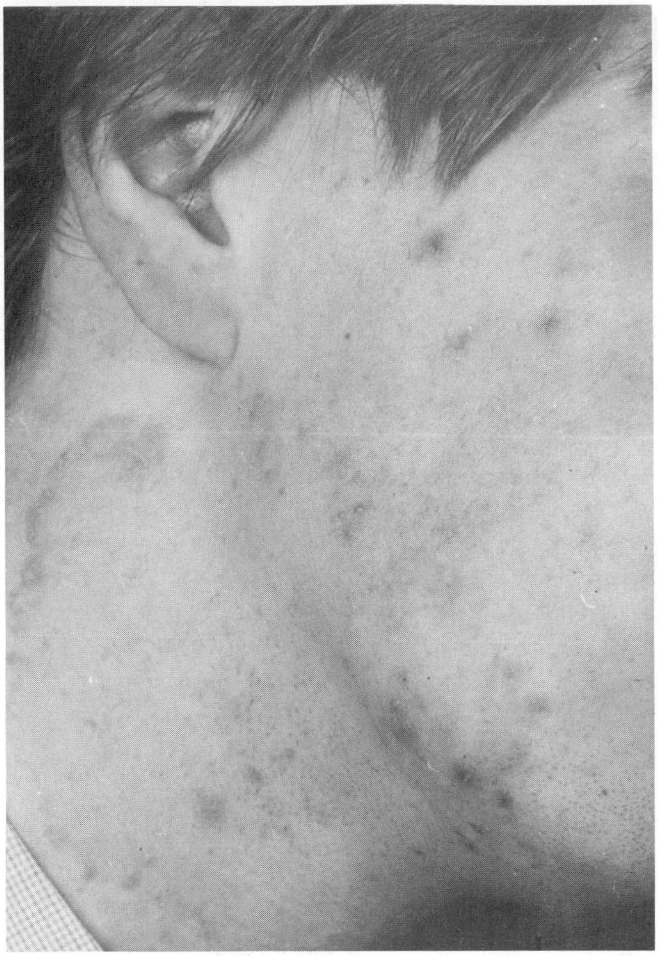

FIG. 3. Tinea faciei due to *T. rubrum*.

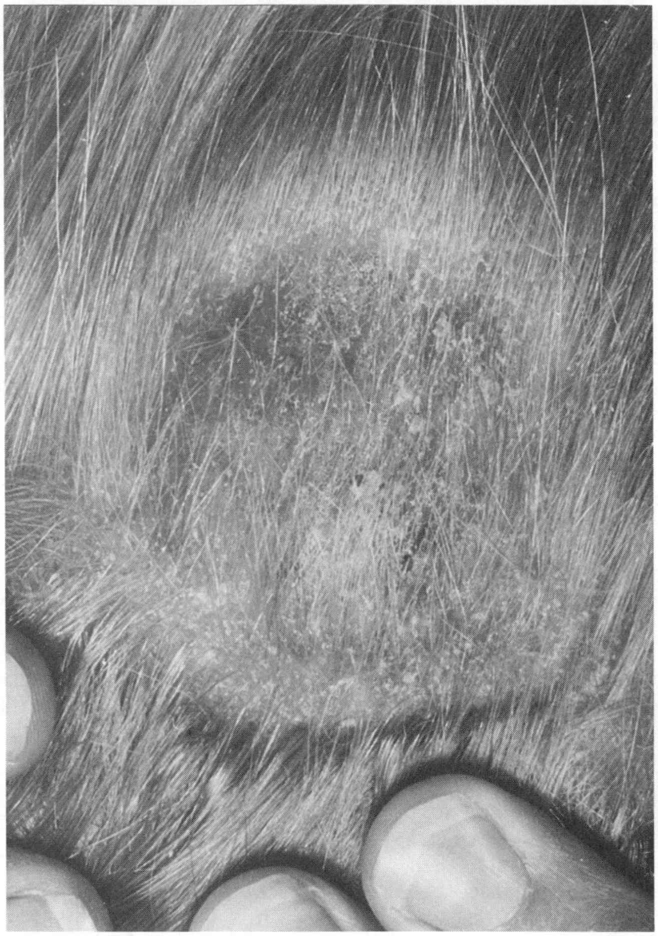

FIG. 4. Scalp ringworm in which an ectothrix infection of the hair is caused by *M. canis*.

then regress and leave tunnels containing air within the hair shaft (the ''favic'' pattern).

The main clinical features of scalp infections due to dermatophytes are the appearance of scaling of the scalp skin that is associated with a variable degree of erythema and inflammation and alopecia. In some cases the infection closely resembles seborrheic dermatitis or dandruff of the scalp. The infection is often accompanied by itching. A pathognomonic feature is hair loss. In ectothrix infections hairs often break a few millimeters or more above the skin surface (Fig. 4). Broken or infected hairs are also slightly swollen and have a dull appearance. In endothrix infections parasitized hairs break at the skin level. In some endothrix infections scattered stumps can be seen within areas of hair loss—black-dot ringworm. In such cases inflammation may be miminal. A further element in tinea capitis is the variable amount of inflammation, but in some cases the whole area becomes pustular and covered with a thick scale or exudative crust. Often one of these elements dominates the clinical pattern. For instance, in some children there is little overt hair loss, the whole infection resembling seborrheic dermatitis. Likewise, in some ectothrix infections a pustular form of dermatophytosis, or kerion, develops. This is less common in endothrix infections. In most kerions the pustules are not a sign of secondary bacterial infection,[27] although this may occur under adherent crusts.

Tinea capitis is rare in adults, although it may occasionally be found in elderly patients and is caused by a variety of fungi such as *T. tonsurans*. It has been associated with scarring alopecia of unknown etiology, pseudopelade, in adults.

In favus the same processes occur, but an important clinical characteristic is the formation of an inflammatory crust, or scutulum, composed of neutrophils and serous exudate around individual hair shafts. With time these amalgamate over the surface of the scalp so that the hair appears to be matted together with a thick crust that is said to have a mousy odor. In many patients the signs are indistinguishable from those seen with other forms of scalp ringworm. Two other characteristics of favus are the late shedding of hairs and the tendency to develop scarring alopecia. The infection may persist into adult life, particular in women.

Untreated scalp ringworm will usually remit spontaneously after puberty. Permanent hair loss is uncommon unless there has been a severe inflammatory response or the patient has favus. A surprising degree of recovery of hair growth occurs, even in children with severe kerions.

Tinea capitis has to be distinguished from seborrheic dermatitis, which usually occurs in older children and does not cause hair loss. Alopecia areata also causes circumscribed areas of hair loss but does not scale, and the exclamation mark hairs seen in this condition, where broken hairs taper from the fractured end toward the skin surface, are pathognomonic.

Onychomycosis Due to Dermatophytes. Onychomycosis, or fungal infection of the nails, usually occurs in individuals with infections of adjacent toe or palmar skin except in the rare cases of childhood nail infection where nail plate invasion may develop without skin involvement. There are several different patterns of nail plate invasion.[28]

The most common clinical pattern of onychomycosis is distal and subungual onychomycosis (DLSO) where the nail plate is invaded from the distal and lateral borders. There is usually associated thickening of the nail, which becomes white, yellow, or brown. The latter color is more common in the rare instances of *T. mentagrophytes* nail disease. In onychomycosis due to endothrix scalp fungi such as *T. soudanense*, the thickening may be minimal, and the nail surface is pitted with small fissures.[29] The most common cause of onychomycosis is *T. rubrum*, which often accompanies long-standing disease, and the infection involves the entire nail plate.

Superficial white onychomycosis (SWO) occurs where the nail plate is invaded from the top surface, which is eventually covered with white crumbly plaques. Other fungi such as *Fusarium* species more commonly cause this pattern of nail invasion. However, in its pure form SWO can be seen with *T. mentagrophytes*, and it may also accompany DLSO in some *T. rubrum* infections.

Rarely invasion appears to originate from the proximal nail plate. This is usually a feature of relapse of treated nails, but rapidly spreading proximal nail plate invasion has also been described in patients with AIDS.[30]

Onychomycosis can occur at any age, although it is more common with increasing age. Males and females are equally affected.

This infection has to be distinguished from onychomycosis due to *Candida* where there is little nail plate thickening but toenail infection is rare. Also *Hendersonula* and *Scytalidium* infections may lead to nail plate invasion. These are difficult to distinguish from infections caused by dermatophytes, but the nail plate is often not grossly thickened and may be severely undermined, and invasion predominantly affects the lateral border of the plate in the early stages of disease. Psoriasis of the nail also causes onycholysis, but the nail plate is typically covered with fine pits.

Deep Dermatophyte Infections. On rare occasions patients known to be immunocompromised or apparently unselected individuals develop dermatophyte infections where the fungi invade subcutaneous tissues via the lymphatics, usually causing clusters of granulomas, lymphedema (Fig. 5) and draining sinuses.[31] Sometimes aggregates of fungal hyphae resembling those found in eumycetomas may be seen in histologic sections. These dermatophyte ''mycetoma'' grains may be surrounded by neutrophil abscesses, but often the fungal hyphae are engulfed by giant cells in tissue sections. Deep dermatophyte infections may extend further to involve draining lymph nodes or other sites including the liver and brain, and they may be fatal.

Dermatophyte Reactions. The immune mechanisms in dermatophytosis may lead to the appearance of secondary rashes called *id reactions*. The most common of these is a type of acute vesicular eczema, or pompholyx that occurs on the hands and feet in patients with inflammatory ringworm of the feet, mainly due to *T. mentagrophytes*. These events are thought to be linked if the original dermatophyte infection becomes inflamed before the appearance of the secondary rash, the latter is maximal on the affected foot, and the patient has a strong delayed-type hyperreactivity (DTH) reaction to intradermal trichophytin. The histology of this id reaction is that of eczema. A second form of id reaction is seen in patients with inflammatory tinea capitis or corporis and is usually caused by zoophilic organisms. It consists of small follicular papules, some of which appear necrotic. This is a form of cutaneous vasculitis that usually subsides spontaneously. Both reactions may be triggered by antifungal therapy. Other less common types of id reaction include annular erythema and erythema nodosum.

Patients with follicular invasion by dermatophytes may develop a residual granuloma in the late stages of the disease called Majocchi's granuloma. It is usually sterile, although sometimes fragments of mycelium can be seen in histologic sections, and resolves slowly with time.

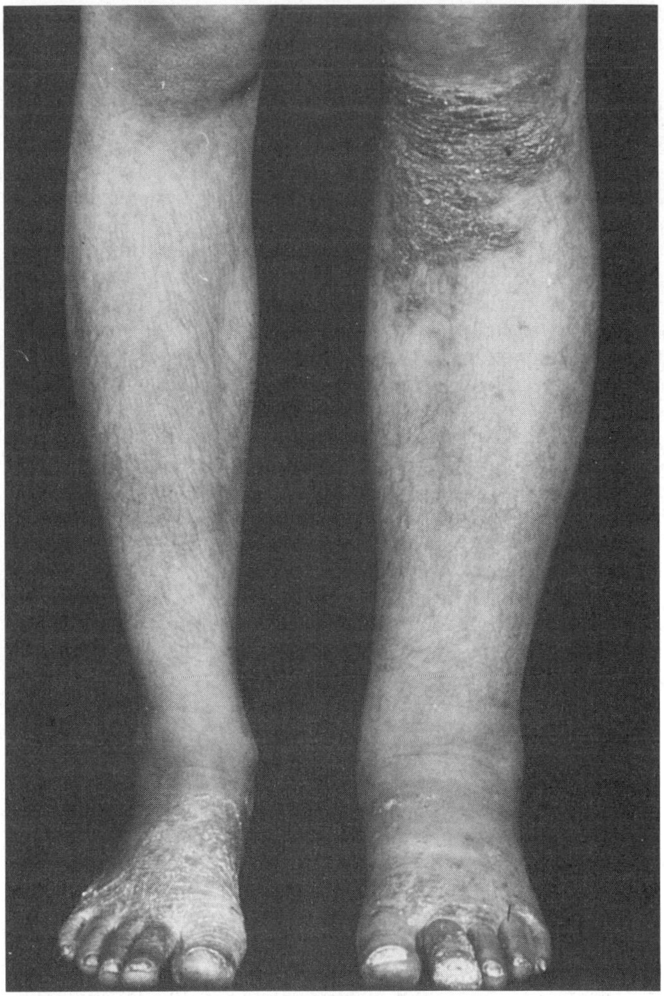

FIG. 5. Deep dermatophytosis in which *T. rubrum* infection is causing unilateral lymphedema after invasion of the lymphatics.

Laboratory Diagnosis

In some cases it is possible to screen patients with scalp infections by using a filtered ultraviolet light source (Wood's light). Infections caused by *Microsporum* species fluoresce green. However *Trichophyton* infections do not fluoresce, apart from favus where the hairs appear yellowish. Fluorescent hairs are infected, and apart from its use as a screening procedure, Woods's light examination may be helpful as a method of selecting hairs for microscopy and culture.

The laboratory diagnosis of dermatophytosis depends on the examination and culture of scrapings or clippings from lesions. It is important to sample the edge of skin lesions and infected nails. In the case of infected hairs broken stubs are best selected and can be removed with forceps without undue trauma. Material should be allowed to soften in 10–20% potassium hydroxide before examining under the microscope. Nails often take up to 2 hours to soften, although the process can be hastened by gentle warming. Fungal hyphae can be seen as chains of arthrospores in cleared scales or clippings.

Dermatophytes infecting hair show characteristic appearances that are helpful in recognition. Some form arthrospores on the outside of the hair shaft, ectothrix infections. The small spores can be seen by focusing the microscope on the edge of the epilated hair shaft. Most of the pathogenic *Microsporum* species that cause tinea capitis have small arthrospores clustered around the outside of hair. By contrast few *Trichophyton* species form ectothrix spores, but those that do, such as *T.*

verrucosum, produce large arthrospores. The majority of *Trichophyton* species causing scalp ringworm form arthrospores within the hair shaft (endothrix infection). With some practice it is possible to make a preliminary identification of the likely genus of invading fungus on the basis of the microscopy of infected hair. *T. schoenleinii* invades hair, but hyphae regress and leave air spaces within the hair shaft.

Scrapings or nail clippings may also be cultured. Primary isolation is carried out at room temperature, usually on Sabouraud agar containing antibiotics (penicillin/streptomycin or choramphenicol) and cycloheximide (Actidione), an antifungal agent that suppresses the growth of environmental contaminant fungi. In the case of nail disease it is important to use some media without cycloheximide because certain fungi such as *Hendersonula* that may infect nails are sensitive to the latter. Most dermatophytes can be identified within 2 weeks, although *T. verrucosum* grows best at 37°C and may only have formed into small and granular colonies at this stage. Identification depends on the gross colonial and microscopic morphology. In some cases other tests involving nutritional requirements and hair penetration in vitro will be necessary to confirm the identification.

Generally the identification of dermatophytes in skin material is simple and worth the effort required to obtain samples. It is particularly helpful in scalp infections where it is important to identify the likely source of infection.

TREATMENT

The usual approach to the management of dermatophyte infections is to treat with topical therapy if possible, but nail and hair infections and widespread dermatophytosis are best treated with oral drugs.[32]

The main topical agents used for dermatophytosis are the keratolytics and compounds with specific antifungal activity. The keratolytic agent used most frequently is Whitfield's ointment (salicylic and benzoic acid compound). This is particularly effective in infections confined to heavily keratinized areas such as the soles or palms. It is inexpensive but messy to use, although a cream formulation of benzoic acid compound is available in some countries.

In the past therapy relied on the use of substances including dyes with weak antifungal activity such as brilliant green and Castellani's paint (magenta and resorcinol). There is now a large group of specific antifungals that may be used in dermatophytosis, although the use of some of these is largely confined to the treatment of tinea pedis. They include drugs such as chlorphenesin, undecylenate, and tolnaftate, which are available in cream or, in some cases, powder form. Few comparative studies have examined their relative merits. Nonetheless, they are effective in uncomplicated cases. More attention has been focused on one particular group of antifungal drugs, the azoles, which include miconazole, clotrimazole, econazole, tioconazole, ketoconazole, oxiconazole, bifonazole, isoconazole, and fenticonazole.[33] These are active against all the common skin fungi, and many can be given once daily. Other potent antifungals used in the treatment of dermatophytosis are cyclopiroxolamine and naftifine. It is difficult to choose between the different groups of these agents on the basis of well-constructed comparative studies.

Generally, topical therapy for tinea pedis has to be continued for at least 2 and possibly 4 weeks; dry-type infections of the sole respond poorly to topical application although the topical medication may be useful to relieve the dryness and scaling. Tinea cruris usually responds within 2 or 3 weeks of the outset of treatment. Some of the azole agents can be used only once daily. Topical treatment for scalp and nail infections are generally ineffective, although cures of nail disease have been claimed for topically applied azoles and cyclopirox olamine. Two new approaches are of potential value in the management of nail disease. The first, a topically applied nail solution containing 28% tioconazole, has been found to produce mycologic and clinical remission on its own or in conjunction with oral griseofulvin. The second such preparation used in nail disease is a combination of 40% urea and bifonazole. Urea is a potent hydrating agent and will soften nails after application under occlusion. The 40% urea paste may be used to remove residual areas of infection after oral therapy for onychomycosis.[34] This combination may also provide useful in addition to oral therapy in nail disease.

The oral agent most often used in dermatophytosis is griseofulvin, which is given in doses of 10 mg/kg daily in either tablet or syrup form.[35] An ultramicrosize formulation is available in some countries in which a lower dose is used. Griseofulvin is generally well tolerated, although it is best taken with food, which also facilitates absorption. It penetrates into the stratum corneum where it reaches concentrations there up to 10 times the plasma levels. Adverse effects include headache, nausea, and abdominal discomfort. Less common reactions are urticaria, diarrhea, and photosensitivity. Griseofulvin may precipitate acute intermittent porphyria and systemic lupus erythemamatosus (SLE) in predisposed subjects. Generally however, the drug is free from serious adverse effects and can be given over a long period. While there are occasional instances of drug resistance, this is not common,[36] most cases of therapeutic failure having other explanations such as poor absorption. Concurrent administration of certain drugs such as phenytoin or phenobarbital may interfere with the absorption of griseofulvin. Oral ketoconazole may also be used for dermatophytosis, although the risk of hepatitis, albeit rare, makes this a second choice for therapy in most instances. However, it is particularly useful in some forms of tinea corporis, in patients unable to tolerate griseofulvin, and in patients who have failed to respond to griseofulvin. Liver function should be monitored regularly through treatment. The new orally active triazole itraconazole is also effective in dermatophyte infections. Preliminary data on the new oral allylamine compound terbinafine indicate that it may also be effective in both dry-type *T. rubrum* infections and onychomycosis. Further experience with these antifungals in a wider range of infections is needed before it will be possible to give more specific recommendations.

Oral therapy is used for scalp ringworm and nail infections. Scalp infections take 6–12 weeks to respond to griseofulvin. Often it is useful to use a topical azole cream in addition and, if crusts are present, to remove these with saline soaks. For the treatment of large numbers of infected children, intermittent therapy with up to 1 g griseofulvin has been suggested, with possible retreatment after 6 weeks. A sustantial percentage of those infected may respond to single-dose therapy.[37] Oral ketoconazole has little place in the treatment of scalp infection, although *T. tonsurans* infections may respond. It is important to attempt to identify the organism causing scalp infection because if the infection is of human origin it can spread to other contacts and it may be necessary to screen classmates or members of the families of children with anthropophilic infections. Zoophilic infections do not usually spread from child to child, although several family members exposed to the same source of infection may develop scalp disease.

Onychomycosis due to dermatophytes is best treated with oral grisefulvin. Fingernail infections will take up to 6 months to respond, and toenail infection may take 1 year or longer. The relapse rate of treated nails is very high, with over 60 percent failing to respond completely or relapsing after initial therapy.[38] For this reason many physicians advise against the treatment of toenail infections unless there is pain or distal sites such as the hands are affected as well.

HENDERSONULA AND SCYTALIDIUM INFECTIONS

Infections caused by the pigmented fungus *Hendersonula toruloidea* closely resemble "dry-type" dermatophytosis due to

T. rubrum. H. toruloidea was originally described as a plant pathogen, but it appears to be a genuine cause of human infection. More recently a similar type of infection has been ascribed to a nonpigmented mold, *Scytalidium hyalinum*. In both cases the affected patients have originated from the tropics.

The precise mechanisms of infection with either organism are unknown. *S. hyalinum* has never been isolated from the environment, and although *H. toruloidea* is a pathogen of certain plants such as fruit trees, patients do not usually give a specific history of exposure. It has been found that healthy individuals in some tropical areas carry these organisms on the feet but do not have overt disease, thus suggesting that asymptomatic carriage may be followed under the appropriate conditions by infection. Infections have been described in immigrants from tropical areas in the United Kingdom, Canada, and France. Patients have also been identified in the southern United States, Trinidad, Colombia, Ecuador, and India, and it is likely that the infection is more widespread. Occasionally it may be seen in patients who have paid short visits to the tropics.

Clinical Features

The clinical signs of skin infection with both *H. toruloidea* and *S. hyalinum* are identical to those associated with dry-type *T. rubrum* infections.[39] There is scaling of the lateral interdigital spaces, over the soles, and on one or both palms. Itching is usually minimal. Onychomycosis may also develop. Often there is early invasion of the lateral border of the nail without significant thickening of the nail plate (Fig. 6), but eventually the whole nail plate may be undermined, and onycholysis may lead to shedding of the complete nail. Hyperpigmented streaks may occur in the nails, although these are not pathognomonic for these infections and can be seen with other forms of inflammatory nail dystrophy.

Diagnosis

Scrapings or nail clippings examined after treatment with potassium hydroxide contain sinuous fungal hyphae. On close inspection the morphology is different from that normally seen with dermatophyte hyphae, but accurate discrimination requires experience. Both organisms grow on Sabouraud's agar but are inhibited if cycloheximide (Actidione) is incorporated into the medium.

Treatment

There is no satisfactory therapy for either infection. Whitfield's ointment may be used to treat *Hendersonula* or *Scytalidium* infections of the sole or the palm. However, none of the specific antifungal drugs currently available produces consistent results.

OTHER FORMS OF ONYCHOMYCOSIS

A number of other fungi may cause onychomycosis. The most common of these is *Scopulariopsis brevicaulis*, which usually causes a nail infection of the great toenails. Some patients with this form of infection have previously abnormal toenails (e.g., onychogryphosis). *Scopulariopsis* infections of the nails have a typical cinnamon color that is caused by the presence of fungal spores seen on direct microscopy of the nail. The fungus is easy to isolate in culture. Treatment may be difficult, but chemical nail removal with 40% urea may be useful.

Superficial white onychomycosis may be caused by *Acremonium* or *Fusarium* species. These infections are similar to those caused by *T. mentagrophytes*, and the identity of the causative organisms should be confirmed by culture.

Occasionally other fungi are isolated from nail material. In many cases they appear to be colonizing the undersurface of dystrophic nail plate. On rare occasions, however, they may contribute to the nail pathology by invasion. This is best established by repeated attempts at culture, and if the organism is isolated on numerous occasions and if hyphae are present in the nail, it is likely that the organism is implicated in the nail disease. Examples of infections caused by a range of different organisms such as *Aspergillus, Fusarium* and *Acremonium* species have been recorded. While there is seldom effective oral therapy for these infections, nail removal with 40% urea is probably the best alternative treatment.

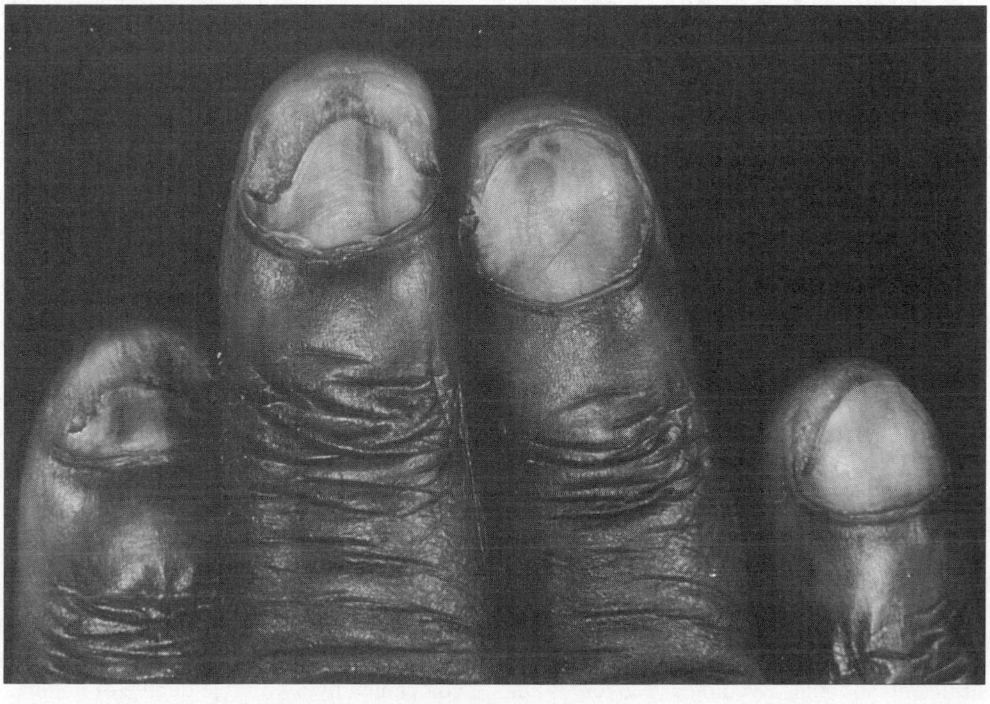

FIG. 6. Onychomycosis due to *H. toruloidea*.

PITYRIASIS VERSICOLOR

Pityriasis or tinea versicolor is a superficial infection caused by *Malassezia furfur*, a lipophilic yeast, which is a normal commensal on the skin surface.[40] The infection is confined to the trunk or proximal aspects of the limbs. Hair and nail plate invasion do not occur.

Organisms

The normal skin is colonized in late childhood and adult life by lipophilic yeasts. Morphologically these are either oval, most common on the scalp, or round, mainly on the trunk, and previously these have been called *Pityrosporum ovale* and *P. orbiculare*, respectively. While both yeast forms are morphologically distinct, they share many similarities both in antigen structure and production of infection in experimental animals. For this reason many workers regard them as members of the same species. Likewise the round, *P. orbiculare* yeasts are identical to those seen in lesions of pityriasis versicolor accompanied by short stubby hyphae, and they are thought to be the same organism in pathogenic phase.

Pathogenesis

The infection is associated with transformation of yeast-phase organisms into hyphal forms, although occasionally patients with pityriasis versicolor will only have oval yeasts present. The stimulus to this phase change is unknown. Infections are more common in the tropics and may appear after sun exposure, which may therefore be a trigger factor. Patients with Cushing syndrome may also develop this infection,[41] but diseases due to T-lymphocyte suppression are not necessarily associated with pityriasis versicolor.

A carboxylic acid called azaleic acid, thought to be produced by the organism in the stratum corneum, is believed to lead to the depigmentation seen in lesions.[42] *Pityrosporum* yeasts grow in the presence of medium-chain-length fatty acids.

Clinical Features

Pityriasis versicolor is usually seen on the trunk or proximal portions of the limbs, although more extensive infections involving the face and waist area are seen in the tropics. Lesions may be hypopigmented or hyperpigmented macules that amalgamate to cover the affected area with scaling plaques. The lesions are usually not itchy. In some patients lesions may remit spontaneously.

The diagnosis can be confirmed by direct microscopy of lesions where the characteristic round yeast forms and short hyphae can be seen. The scrapings can be viewed after clearing with potassium hydroxide but are seen more clearly after staining with a mixture of Parker Quink ink and potassium hydroxide. Lesions fluoresce yellow/green under Wood's light, although this may not be seen on all affected areas. *Pityrosporum* yeasts are difficult to culture unless oil is added to the medium. An overlay of Tween 80 will encourage growth.

Treatment

The most appropriate therapy for pityriasis versicolor is either a topical azole antifungal cream or 2% selenium sulfide lotion or 20% sodium thiosulfate applied daily for 10–14 days.[40] The latter preparations may be irritative. In some cases intermittent applications of 50% propylene glycol in water will prevent a relapse.[43] In severe cases oral ketoconazole or itraconazole will produce remissions. The exact doses of ketoconazole needed to induce a remission are not clear, but 5–10 days (200 mg) of therapy is usually sufficient, although mycologic recovery is not seen for about 30 days because the organisms can still be seen in skin scrapings. In some patients a single dose of 400 mg is effective.

Patients usually have to be warned that the pigmentary changes may only return to normal after many months even after the infection has been successfully treated.

OTHER PITYROSPORUM INFECTIONS

There are two other skin conditions associated with *Pityrosporum* yeasts—*Pityrosporum* folliculitis and seborrheic dermatitis. In addition, this fungus has caused catheter-acquired sepsis (see Chapter 246).

Pityrosporum Folliculitis

There are three main forms of this condition. The first is a folliculitis on the back or upper part of the chest that consists of scattered follicular papules or pustules.[40] These are itchy and often appear after sun exposure. In the second form, which is seen in patients with seborrheic dermatitis, there are numerous small follicular papules over the upper and lower portions of the back and chest. Erythema and greasy perifollicular scales are often seen in these patients. In the third form multiple pustules are seen on the trunk and face in patients with human immunodeficiency (HIV) infection. This type is very similar to the second form, and the patients usually have severe seborrheic dermatitis.

Scrapings or biopsy specimens from lesions show numerous yeasts occluding the mouths of follicles. Treatment with topical azole antifungals may be effective, but often oral therapy with ketoconazole is necessary.

Seborrheic Dermatitis

In the early part of the twentieth century seborrheic dermatitis and dandruff of the scalp were thought to be caused by *Pityrosporum* yeasts because numerous organisms are present in skin scales. This view was subsequently superseded by the belief that the yeasts were secondary to a hyperproliferative state. However, recent evidence suggests that *Pityrosporum* is implicated in the pathogenesis of the condition.[44]

Seborrheic dermatitis responds in most cases to oral ketoconazole or topical azole antifungals. Improvement is associated with disappearance of the organisms, and relapse, with recolonization. Further, the clinical appearances can be mimicked in animals with the application of both live and killed organisms to the skin. Some patients with seborrheic dermatitis have high antibody titers to *Pityrosporum* species.

While it is unlikely that invasion of the epidermis is responsible for the appearance of seborrheic dermatitis, an indirect disease mechanism such as sensitization or toxic damage is possible.

Seborrheic dermatitis can appear in any individual although it is said to be particularly common in patients with neurologic disease such as parkinsonism. Patients with AIDS are also very commonly affected, and the disease causes widespread lesions of the face and trunk.[45] The histology of seborrheic dermatitis is similar in all groups. There is acanthosis and hyperkeratosis with elongation of dermal papillae. An infiltrate of polymorphs in the epidermis above the dermal papillae is also often seen. HIV-positive patients tend to have more plasma cells in the infiltrate. These changes are similar to those seen in some forms of psoriasis.

Clinical Features. The classic features of seborrheic dermatitis comprise a range of different clinical appearances. These include erythema and scaling of the central part of the anterior aspect of the chest and the upper part of the back that are accompanied by a variable degree of itching. On the face there is erythema with greasy scales in the eyebrows, around the alae nasae, behind the ears, and in the external ears. Scaling may also appear in the presternal areas of the chest and on the back. Scaling in the scalp is accompanied by the appearance of pustules in some patients. The clinical appearances are typical, and fungal scrapings are unnecessary.

Other forms of skin disease, including severe erythroderma in infants and an intertriginous rash in adults, have also been called seborrheic dermatitis, but these lesions do not appear to be related to the variety discussed above.

Treatment. The main therapy involves the use of topical azole creams and weak topical corticosteroids such as hydrocortisone, 1%. Relapse is common, but retreatment where necessary is the simplest approach to management.

TINEA NIGRA

Tinea nigra is a superficial form of pheohyphomycosis caused by *Exophiala werneckii*. The infection is confined to the stratum corneum of the palms or soles and is mainly seen in the tropics or subtropics in children or young adults.

The typical lesion of tinea nigra is a superficial scaling macule that is brown or black in color on the palms or soles. The pigmentation is irregularly distributed over larger lesions. Spread of the infection to other sites is very rare, and lesions remain asymptomatic.

The main differential diagnosis is a superficial form of melanoma or a pigmented nevus. The pigmented hyphae can be seen in direct microscopy of skin scrapings treated with potassium hydroxide. The organism can also be cultured from scrapings.

The best therapy is treatment with a keratolytic agent such as Whitfield's ointment or 5–10% salicylic acid ointment.

WHITE PIEDRA

White piedra is an uncommon infection caused by the yeast *Trichosporon beigelii*. It occurs in both the tropics and temperate zones. The infection is a superficial infection of the hair shafts of the scalp, body, or pubic hair. *T. beigelii* may also cause a systemic infection in neutropenic patients.

The organism may be carried on the skin or around the anus. In some patients the infection appears to be sexually transmitted. White piedra is asymptomatic and presents with small yellow concretions on the hair shafts.[46] These are circumscribed, and lesions appear as small nodules, unlike the more diffuse coating of axillary or pubic hair seen in trichomycosis axillaris, which is due to the presence of bacteria on the hair.

The diagnosis may be confirmed by examining an epilated hair mounted in potassium hydroxide. Each nodule contains fungal hyphae, and the organisms can be cultured from infected hairs without difficulty.

Treatment is difficult. Nodules may be removed simply by shaving. Otherwise, coating the hairs with an azole such as econazole or treating the patient with oral ketoconazole may cure the infection. Relapse is common after therapy.

BLACK PIEDRA

Black piedra is another infection of the hair shafts that is caused by a black yeast, *Piedraia hortae*. The disease is rare and mainly confined to parts of the humid tropics. The infection presents with small black nodules on the hairs of the scalp, less commonly elsewhere. These have to be distinguished from pediculosis, but itching is usually absent in black piedra. With direct microscopy these nodules can be shown to be composed of hyphal elements and small ascospores of the causative agent within a dark cement-containing stroma. Treating hairs with a topical salicylic acid, 2% formaldehyde, or an azole cream is usually sufficient, although relapse is common.

REFERENCES

1. Rebell G, Taplin D. Dermatophytes. Their Recognition and Identification. 2nd ed. Miami: University of Miami Press; 1970.
2. De Vroey C. Epidemiology of ringworm (dermatophytosis). Semin Dermatol. 1985;4:185–200.
3. Davison FD, Mackenzie DWR. DNA homology studies in the taxonomy of dermatophytes. J Med Vet Mycol. 1984;22:117–23.
4. Jeffries CD, Reiss E, Ajello L. Analytical isoelectric focusing of secreted dermatophyte proteins applied to taxonomic differentiation of *Microsporum* and *Trichophyton* species (preliminary studies). J Med Vet Mycol. 1984;22:364–79.
5. Rippon JW. Elastase production by ringworm fungi. Science. 1967;157:947.
6. Rippon JW. Epidemiology and emerging patterns of dermatophyte species. In: Current Topics in Medical Mycology I. New York: Springer-Verlag; 1985;208–34.
7. Philpot CM. Geographical distribution of the dermatophytes—a review. J Hyg (Lond). 1978;80:301–13.
8. Smith JMB, Rush-Munro FM. An unusual strain of *Trichophyton rubrum* from Fiji. Sabouraudia 1971;9:153–6.
9. Gentles JC, Evans EGV. Foot infections in swimming baths. Br Med J. 1973;3:260–2.
10. Hope YM, Clayton YM, Hay RJ, et al. Foot infection in coal miners: A reassessment. Br J Dermatol. 1985;112:405–13.
11. Rothman S, Knox G, Windhorst D. Tinea pedis, a source of infection in the family. Arch Dermatol. 1957;75:270–71.
12. Blank H, Taplin D, Zaias N. Cutaneous *Trichophyton mentagrophytes* infections in Vietnam. Arch Dermatol 1969;99:135–44.
13. Hay RJ. Tinea imbricata. In: Current Topics in Medical Mycology 2. New York: Springer-Verlag; 1987;55–72.
14. Verhagen AR. Distribution of dermatophytes causing tinea capitis in Africa. Trop Geogr Med. 1973;26:101–20.
15. Ive FA. The carrier state of tinea capitis in Nigeria. Br J Dermatol. 1966;78:219–21.
16. Blank F, Mann SJ, Peak PA. Distribution of dermatophytosis according to age, ethnic group and sex. Sabouraudia 1974;12:352–61.
17. Zurita J, Hay RJ. The adherence of dermatophyte microconidia and arthroconidia to human keratinocytes in vitro. J Invest Dermatol. 1987;89:529–34.
18. Calderon RA. Immunoregulation of dermatophytosis. Crit Rev Microbiol. 1988. In press.
19. Serjeantson S, Lawrence G. Autosomal recessive inheritance of susceptibility to tinea imbricata. Lancet 1977;1:13–5.
20. King RD, Khan HA, Foye JC, et al. Transferrin, iron and dermatophytes 1. Serum dermatophyte inhibitory component definitely identified as unsaturated transferrin. J Lab Clin Med. 1975;86:204–12.
21. Jones HE, Reinhardt JH, Rinaldi MG. Acquired immunity to dermatophytosis. Arch Dermatol. 1974;109:840–8.
22. Hay RJ, Reid S, Talwet E, et al. Immune responses of patients with tinea imbricata. Br J Dermatol. 1983;108:581–9.
23. Green F, Lee KW, Balish E. Chronic *T. mentagrophytes* dermatophytosis of guinea pig skin grafts on nude mice. J Invest Dermatol. 1982;79:125–31.
24. Leyden JJ, Kligman AM. Interdigita athletes foot, the interaction of dermatophytes and residual bacteria. Arch Dermatol. 1978;114:1466–72.
25. Wilson JW, Plunkett DA. Nodular granulomatous perifolliculitis due to *Trichophyton rubrum*. Arch Dermatol. 1954;64:258–77.
26. Elmros T, Liden S. Hereditary palmo-plantar keratoderma: Incidence of dermatophyte infections and the results of topical treatment with retinoic acid. Acta Derm Venereol (Stockh) 1983;63:254–7.
27. Birt AR, Wilt JC. Mycology, bacteriology and histopathology of suppurative ringworm. Arch Dermatol. 1957;69:441–8.
28. Zaias N. Onychomycosis. Arch Dermatol. 1972;105:263–74.
29. Kalter DC, Hay RJ. Onychomycosis due to *Trichophyton soudanense*. Clin Exp Dermatol. 1988;13:221–227.
30. Weismann K, Knudsen EA, Pedersen C. White nails in AIDS/ARC due to *Trichophyton rubrum* infection. Clin Exp Dermatol. 1988;13:24–7.
31. Allen DE, Snyderman R, Meadows L, et al. Generalised *Microsporum audouinii* infection and depressed cellular immunity associated with a missing plasma factor required for lymphocyte blastogenesis. Am J Med 1977;63:991–1000.
32. Roberts SOB. Treatment of the superficial and subcutaneous mycoses. In: Speller DCE, ed. Antifungal Chemotherapy. Chichester: John Wiley & Sons; 1980;225–84.
33. Hay RJ. Recent advances in the management of fungal disease. Q J Med. 1987;244:631–9.
34. Hay RJ, Roberts D, Richardson M, et al. The evaluation of bifonazole 1% and 40% urea paste in the management of onychomycosis. Clin Exp Dermatol. 1988;13:164–167.
35. Davies RR. Griseofulvin. In: Speller DCE, ed. Antifungal Chemotherapy. Chichester: John Wiley & Sons; 1980:149–82.
36. Artis WM, Odle BM, Jones HE. Griseofluvin-resistant dermatophytosis correlates with in vitro resistance. Arch Dermatol 1981;117:16–9.
37. Beghin D, Van Breuseghem R. Traitement des dermatophyties du cuir chevelu par une dose unique de griseofulvine: Essai d'une dose reduite. Ann Soc Belg Med Trop. 1974;54:477–81.
38. Davies RR, Everall JD, Hamilton E. Mycological and clinical evaluation of griseofulvin for chronic onychomycosis. Br Med J. 1967;3:464–8.
39. Hay RJ, Moore MK. The clinical features of superficial infections caused by

Hendersonula toruloidea and *Scytalidium hyalinum*. Br J Dermatol. 1984;110:677–84.
40. Faergemann J. Lipophilic yeasts in skin disease. Semin Dermatol. 1985;4:173–84.
41. Burke RC. Tinea versicolor: Susceptibility factors and experimental infections in human beings. J Invest Dermatol. 1961;36:389–402.
42. Nazzaro-Porro M, Passi S. Identification of tyrosinase inhibitors in cultures of *Pityrosporum*. J Invest Dermatol. 1978;71:205–8.
43. Faergemann J, Fredriksson T. Propylene glycol in the treatment of pityriasis versicolor. Acta DermVenereol (Stockh). 1980;60:92–3.
44. Shuster S. The aetiology of dandruff and the mode of action of therapeutic agents. Br J Dermatol. 1984;111:235–42.
45. Mathes BM, Douglas MC. Seborrheic dermatitis in patients with acquired immunodeficiency syndrome. J Am Acad Dermatol. 1985;13:947–51.
46. Kalter DCA, Tschen JA, Cernoch PL, et al. Genital white piedra: Epidemiology, microbiology and therapy. J Am Acad Dermatol. 1986;14:982–93.

246. PARACOCCIDIOIDES BRASILIENSIS

ANGELA RESTREPO M.

Paracoccidioidomycosis (South American blastomycosis) is the predominant systemic mycosis in Latin America. It is usually manifested as a chronic, progressive disease of the adult male. Although the lungs are the site of primary infection, dissemination is common, mainly to the mucous membranes, skin, reticuloendothelial system, and adrenals.

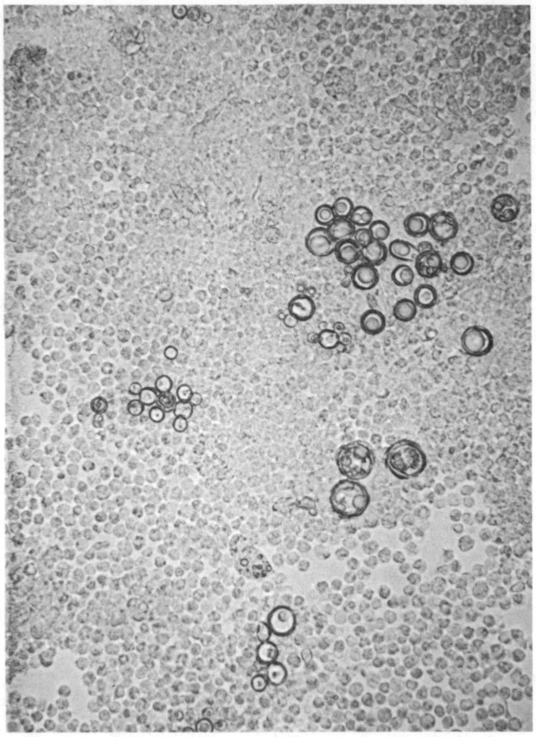

FIG. 1. *Paracoccidioides brasiliensis*: direct KOH preparation from pus. Observe the multiple budding and variation in cell size. (×200).

DESCRIPTION OF THE PATHOGEN

The etiologic agent is a dimorphic fungus, *Paracoccidioides brasiliensis*. Microscopically in cultures at 37°C as well as in tissues and exudates, the fungus appears as an oval-to-round yeast cell, quite variable in size (4–40 μm), that reproduces by multiple budding; the presence of the "pilot wheel" cell is characteristic (Fig. 1). Typically, numerous small (2–4 μm) buds surround the mother cell and are connected to it by means of small cytoplasmic bridges. Colonies produced at 37°C grow in approximately 5–10 days and are soft and cream colored and have a cerebriform aspect.[1,2] When the incubation temperature is lower (19°–28°C), the fungus develops as a mold and produces slow-growing colonies (20–30 days). Initially, they are provided with short tufts of white aerial mycelia, but the colonies become cottony with prolonged incubation; the area beneath is often brownish. Relatively few microscopic structures (chlamydospores, thin septate hyphae) are produced by the mold when grown in the regular mycologic media; when media with reduced carbohydrate content are used, arthroconidia and other types of conidia may be formed. The size of these propagules varies from 4 to 5 μm, and they are infectious.[3,4] This phase probably occurs in nature as well.[5]

ECOLOGY AND EPIDEMIOLOGY

Perhaps the most notable ecologic characteristic of paracoccidioidomycosis is its restricted geographic distribution. It has been reported only in Latin America from Mexico (23 degrees N) to Argentina (34 degrees S); however, some countries within these latitudes are not affected (e.g., the Caribbean Islands, Chile), and the disorder does not afflict persons living in every region of the endemic areas. Endemicity centers in regions with relatively well defined ecologic characteristics, in the tropical and subtropical forests where temperatures are mild and humidity is relatively high and constant throughout the year.[3,5–7] Although cases have been reported in North America, Europe, and Asia,[6,8] patients in those cases had previously been residents in endemic countries. Judging by the number of reported cases (close to 6000), Brazil constitutes the heart of the endemic area, with considerably fewer cases reported from Colombia, Venezuela, and Argentina.[1,2,6,7]

Restricted geographic distribution indicates an equally limited ecologic niche for *P. brasiliensis*, one that has proved elusive. With the exception of two reports on its isolation from soil and one (unconfirmed) from the intestinal contents of bats, attempts to discover the natural habitat have failed.[5,9] Skin test surveys have not offered valuable clues since levels of paracoccidioidin sensitivity have been intermediate, not over 50 percent, in all populations tested.[2,5,6] Nonetheless, most authors agree on the existence of an external habitat and relate the acquisition of infection to contact with an exogenous source of infection. Paracoccidioidomycosis is not contagious from person to person. The route of infection is still a matter of debate. Initially, traumatic implantation was advocated; presently, however, the inhalation theory is accepted by most investigators.[10–14]

The age and sex distribution of clinical cases is peculiar. Paracoccidioidomycosis is rare in children and teenagers, and most patients are 30 or more years of age.[6,7,15,16] Also, males are more commonly afflicted than are females, at a mean ratio of 15:1. This is in contrast with the rate of infection—as determined by a paracoccidioidin skin test—which is alike for both sexes. Of interest, too, is the fact that when the disease occurs in prepubertal patients there is not a sex difference.[16] It has been suggested that the marked sex difference seen in adults could be explained by the inhibitory action displayed by estrogens on the mycelium-to-yeast transition.[17] The occupational distribution reveals a predilection for agricultural workers.[18] Humans are the prevalent hosts for *P. brasiliensis*[5,6]; recently, however, naturally acquired disease has been demonstrated in armadillos.[19]

The disease has long periods of latency, as demonstrated by the nonautochthonous cases reported outside of the endemic area; some of these patients developed overt disease 30 or more years after leaving the endemic regions.[8–18] There is an indication that the fungus can remain dormant in residual lymph node lesions.[20] Dormancy may be the reason why epidemic outbreaks, which could furnish important information on the habitat, have not been reported.[5]

CLINICAL MANIFESTATIONS

It is now accepted that most primary infections are subclinical and occur in persons with a normal immune system. Nonetheless, *P. brasiliensis* has the ability to remain dormant for long periods so that at a later date, if the formerly resistant host becomes immune depressed, the fungus multiplies and the mycosis becomes manifested. The period of latency is usually long, but in young patients it may be brief.[1,12,21] The host's immune defenses are directly related to the clinical form and the severity of the mycosis. Cell-mediated immunity plays a crucial role; it is usually depressed during the peak of infection, partly because of the fungus itself; humoral immunity, on the other hand, is in full function. Upon recovery, the immune balance tends to normalize.[21–24]

Paracoccidioidomycosis is a polymorphic disease, often severe and progressive, although some self-limited cases have been reported.[1,11,13,14,25] In recent years there have been indications of severe manifestations in immunosuppressed patients, including those with the acquired immunodeficiency syndrome (AIDS).[26,27] In younger patients the disorder is subacute and carries a severe prognosis; in adults, the course is chronic and the outcome better.[10–12,16,25] The lungs are the site of the primary infection, but the patient's symptomatology may not reflect this fact. In the juvenile form, for example, the mononuclear phagocyte system is the target organ, and respiratory complaints are minimal. In the adult form, most patients present with respiratory problems either as the sole manifestation of the disease or as contributory pathology to the overall clinical picture.[1,2,11,16,25] Such patients seek medical advice as a result of the following symptoms in order of decreasing frequency: (*1*) mucosal ulcerations occurring mostly in the mouth and nose; (*2*) difficulties in swallowing and changes in voice; (*3*) cutaneous lesions preferentially located on the face; (*4*) enlarged lymph nodes, especially those of the cervical area; and (*5*) respiratory problems such as shortness of breath, persistent cough, purulent or blood-tinged sputum, and chest pain. These symptoms are accompanied by weakness, malaise, fever, and weight loss; usually, more than one lesion is present at the time of the initial consultation.

CHARACTERISTICS OF THE LESIONS

Lungs

The auscultatory findings are minimal in comparison with the radiologic aspects.[28,29] Gallium imaging has indeed revealed the presence of radiologically and clinically unsuspected lesions.[30] Usually, there is some degree of dyspnea.

In the active forms, the x-ray films reveal patchy or confluent nodular infiltrates or condensed lesions, very frequently bilateral and symmetric (Fig. 2). Most changes occur in the central and basal portions of the lungs; the apices usually remain clear. Cavities and hilar adenopathy are not too common. In older cases fibrosis, bullae, and presence of emphysematous areas are the rule. Right ventricular hypertrophy is present in some patients and constitutes the most feared sequela.[1,28–31]

Mucosal Lesions

Infiltrated and ulcerated lesions are observed regularly in the mouth, lips, gums, tongue, palate, and to a lesser extent, the nose, larynx, and pharynx. Such lesions have a granulomatous appearance and may produce edema of the affected area. Ulcerated lesions have a mulberry-like aspect (Fig. 3).

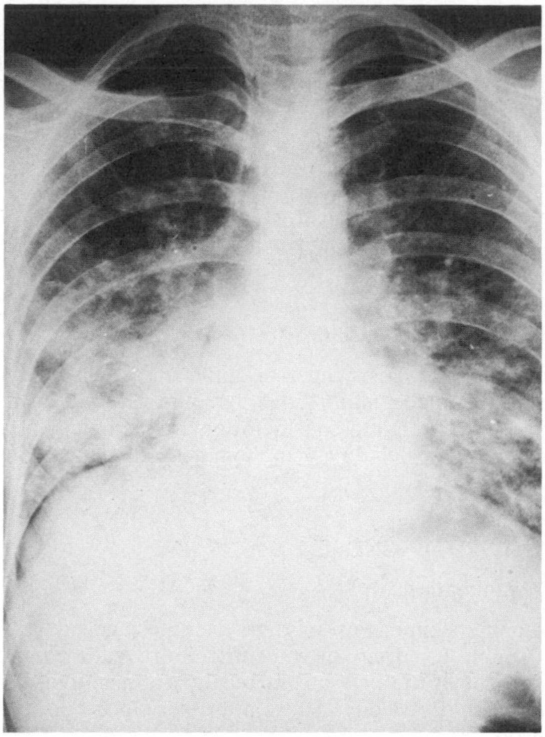

FIG. 2. Paracoccidioidomycosis x-ray film. Infiltrates and nodular lesions are located toward the basal portions of both lungs; the apices appear free.

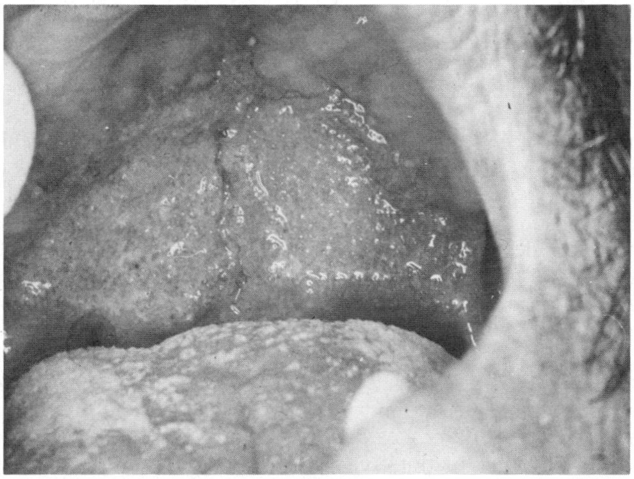

FIG. 3. Paracoccidioidomycosis: lesion of the hard palate.

Skin

Cutaneous lesions are very polymorphic; they tend to appear around the natural orifices. Most commonly, the lesions are warty, ulcerated, and crusted and infiltrate the subcutaneous tissues; they are also granulomatous. Often, skin and mucosal lesions coexist in the same patient.

Lymph Nodes

Cervical, axillary, mesenteric, mediastinal, and other nodes may become enlarged. Draining fistulas may form.

Adrenals

Diminished adrenal function or overt addisonian syndrome may occur. The adrenals are hypertrophied and show nodular lesions.[2,32,33]

Other Lesions

The spleen, liver, gastrointestinal tract, vascular system, bones, central nervous system, and male genitourinary tract are occasionally involved.

DIFFERENTIAL DIAGNOSIS

Paracoccidioidomycosis must be differentiated from tuberculosis, which can coexist in 17–25 percent of the cases.[1,2] Other diseases to be taken into consideration are histoplasmosis, neoplastic disorders including lymphoma, leishmaniasis, leprosy, and syphilis.

LABORATORY DIAGNOSIS

Direct Examination

When such specimens as sputum, exudate, and pus are available, a simple KOH mount will suffice to reveal *P. brasiliensis* in 85 percent of the patients. If results are negative, repeated samples should be collected; sputum should be digested and concentrated. The relative large size of the cells, their refractile walls, and multiple budding make diagnosis simple.

Histologic Studies

Biopsy is often diagnostic. Gomori stain is recommended. If the typical multiple budding cell is not abundant, differentiation from other fungi (*Blastomyces dermatitidis, Histoplasma capsulatum*, and *Cryptococcus neoformans*) should be made. The histologic reaction corresponds to a mixed mycotic granuloma with neutrophils, epithelioid cells, and multinucleate giant cells. Fungi are often found inside the latter cells. A mixed pyogenic, inflammatory reaction is found in ulcerated mucocutaneous lesions and in ruptured lymph nodes. In the subacute progressive form, tissue reactions are diffuse, and phagocytosis is sparse. Lymph nodes have hyperplastic germinal centers and increased numbers of plasmocytes. Skin lesions reveal pseudoepitheliomatous hyperplasia and intraepithelial microabscesses.[34]

Cultures

Culture should be attempted since isolation in culture proves the activity of the process. With contaminated samples, room temperature incubation is preferred; Sabouraud-dextrose or yeast extract agar (in Petri dishes) is recommended for this purpose.

Serologic Tests

Serology is useful not only for the diagnosis but also for the follow-up studies.[2,24] The easiest method, the agar gel immunodiffusion test (ID), demonstrates circulating antibodies in 95 percent of the cases. The test is also specific, and the presence of precipitin bands 1 and 2 practically makes a diagnosis.[24] However, the activity of the process cannot be judged on this basis since these antibodies can be detected years after apparent successful therapy. Another useful test, albeit a cumbersome one, is the complement fixation (CF) test. Its quantitative nature allows a better evaluation of the patient's response to treatment. In contrast with the ID test, cross-reactions with *Histoplasma* antigens are important. Other tests (immunoelectrophoresis, counterimmunoelectrophoresis, and enzyme-linked immunosorbent assay [ELISA]), are also currently used.

Skin Tests

Paracoccidioidin skin testing is not reliable since many active cases (35–50 percent) are nonreactive at the time of diagnosis. However, during the course of treatment, some cases become reactive, and this can be taken as a good prognosis.[23,24] Cross-reactions with histoplasmin are to be expected.[24]

TREATMENT

Paracoccidioidomycosis is the only systemic mycosis amenable to treatment with sulfa drugs (alone or combined with trimethoprim). It can also be treated with amphotericin B and various imidazole derivatives. Because in many cases the diagnosis is not established until late and the patients are usually malnourished, treatment directed merely at suppressing growth of the microorganism is not always successful. Appropriate supportive therapeutic measures (improved diet, rest, correction of anemia, and so forth) are essential.

Sulfonamides

Either sulfadiazine or one of the long-acting compounds (sulfamethoxypyridazine, sulfadimethoxine) can be used. With sulfadiazine, the daily dosage is 4–6 g/day for adults and 60–100 mg/kg/day (in divided doses) for children. This dosage must be continued for several weeks to months, without interruption, until clinical and mycologic improvement is apparent. Then the dosage can be reduced by half. The long-acting compounds require 1–2 g/day for adults during the first 2–3 weeks of treatment; after clinical improvement (approximately 4 weeks), 500 mg/day suffices. Most authors agree that sulfonamide treatment should be continued for 3–5 years to avoid relapses. Periodic clinical, radiologic, and serologic checkups should be conducted. In spite of such a prolonged course of therapy, sulfa drugs are well tolerated; the emergence of resistant strains may pose a problem in some cases. It is imperative to instruct the patient about the necessity of continued therapy since relapses are common if the drug intake is interrupted.[2,35]

Amphotericin B

The dosage and administration pattern of amphotericin B in paracoccidioidomycosis is similar to that recommended for other systemic mycoses. Total dosages have varied from 1200 to 3000 mg; the latter require prolonged periods of hospitalization. Amphotericin B is not curative by itself, and all patients treated with it should also receive maintenance sulfonamide therapy according to the indications previously given. Amphotericin B should be reserved for severe cases and for those unresponsive to other means of therapy.

The two therapeutic measures mentioned are not always successful, and the mortality rate is rather high (17–25 percent); improvement is obtained in 65–70 percent of the cases, while the remainder of cases relapse or fail to improve.[36,37]

Imidazole Compounds

Experience to date has indicated that the orally administered imidazole ketoconazole is of great value in the treatment of paracoccidioidomycosis.[37–39] Improvement has been recorded in 84–95 percent of the cases. A recent follow-up study indicated only a 10% relapse after 5 years.[40] However, a much higher rate has been recorded in a different series of cases.[41] Comparisons between amphotericin B plus sulfonamides and ketoconazole have favored the latter.[42] Ketoconazole should be given at a dose of 200–400 mg/day for a minimum of 6 months and for as long as 12–18 months, depending on the patient's response and the results of mycologic tests. Generally, patients unresponsive to other therapies are also successfully treated with this imidazole.[38,39]

Long-lasting ketoconazole therapy mandates regular check-ups for hepatic dysfunction and gonadal alterations. In general, ketoconazole side effects have been minor in paracoccidioidomycosis.[32,38,39] This fact plus the relatively short periods of therapy that are needed and the facility for oral administration makes ketoconazole an excellent drug for the treatment of this disorder.

Itraconazole, a newer imidazole derivative for oral administration that is presently undergoing clinical trials, appears to be more potent that its predecessor. Administered at a dose of 100 mg/day for periods of 4–12 months, itraconazole produces a prompt remission of all signs and symptoms with the advantage of no toxicity for the liver or interference with steroidogenesis.[43,44] If the relapse rate could also be reduced, this compound would replace ketoconazole as the choice of therapy for paracoccidioidomycosis.

REFERENCES

1. Angulo-Ortega A, Pollak L. Paracoccidioidomycosis. In: Baker RD, ed. The Pathological Anatomy of the Mycoses. Human Infections with Fungi, Actinomycetes and Algae. Berlin: Spring-Verlag; 1971;507–76.
2. Del Negro G, Lacaz CS, Fiorillo AM, eds. *Paracoccidioidomicose* (Blastomycose Sul Americana. Sao Paulo, Brazil: Sarvier Editora; 1982.
3. Bustamante B, McEwen J, Tabares AM, et al. Characteristics of the conidia produced by the mycelial form of *P. brasiliensis*. Sabouraudia. J Med Vet Mycol. 1985;23:407–14.
4. McEwen J, Bedoya V, Patiño MM, et al. Experimental murine paracoccidioidomycosis induced by the inhalation of conidia. J Med Vet Mycol. 1987;25:165–75.
5. Restrepo A. The Ecology of *P. brasiliensis*: A puzzle still unsolved. Sabouraudia. J Med Vet Mycol. 1985;23:323–34.
6. Greer DL, Restrepo A. The epidemiology of paracoccidioidomycosis. In: Al-Doory Y, ed. The Epidemiology of Human Mycotic Diseases. Springfield, IL: Charles C Thomas; 1975:117–41.
7. Marquez SA, Franco MF, Mendes RP, et al. Some epidemiological aspects of paracoccidioidomycosis in Botucatú endemic area, State of Sao Paulo, Brazil. Rev Inst Med Trop Sao Paulo. 1983;25:87–92.
8. Ajello L, Polonelli L. Imported paracoccidioidomycosis: A public health problem in non-endemic areas. Eur J Epidemiol. 1985;1:160–5.
9. Greer DG, Bolaños B. Role of bats in the ecology of *P. brasiliensis*: The survival of *P. brasiliensis* in the intestinal tract of frugivorous bats (*A. literatus*). Sabouraudia. 1977;15:273–82.
10. Giraldo R, Restrepo A, Gutierrez F, et al. Pathogenesis of paracoccidioidomycosis: A model based on the study of 45 patients. Mycopathology. 1976;58:63–70.
11. Londero AT. Paracoccidioidomicose: Patogenia, formas clinicas, manifestacoes pulmonares e diagnóstico. J Pneumol (Brasil). 1986;12:41–60.
12. Franco MF, Montenegro MR, Mendes RP, et al. Paracoccidioidomycosis: A recently proposed classification of its clinical forms. Rev Soc Brasil Med Trop. 1987;20:129–32.
13. Lopez R, Restrepo A. Spontaneous regression of pulmonary paracoccidioidomycosis. Mycopathologia. 1983;82:187–9.
14. Wanke B, Andrade EM, Neto JAL, et al. Paracoccidioidomicose pulmonar assintomatica e regressiva, com posterior diseminacao. Rev Soc Brasil Med Trop. 1983;16:162–67.
15. Ferreira-da-Cruz MF, Wanke B, Galvao-Catro B. Prevalence of paracoccidioidomycosis in hospitalized adults in Rio de Janeiro, Brazil. Mycopathologia. 1987;97:61–4.
16. Londero AT, Melo IS. Paracoccidioidomycosis in childhood. Mycopathologia. 1983;82:49–55.
17. Restrepo A, Salazar ME, Cano LE, et al. Estrogens inhibit mycelium to yeast transformation in the fungus *P. brasiliensis*: Implications for resistance of females to paracoccidioidomycosis. Infect Immun. 1984;46:346–53.
18. Restrepo A, Greer DL. Paracoccidioidomycosis. In: Di Salvo A, ed. Occupational Mycoses. Philadelphia: Lea & Febiger; 1983:43–64.
19. Naiff RD, Ferreira LCL, Barret TV, et al. Enzootic paracoccidioidomycosis in armadillos (*D. novemcinctus* in Pará State, Brasil. Rev Inst Med Trop Sao Paulo. 1986;28:19–27.
20. Restrepo A, de Bedout C, Cano LE, et al. Recovery of *P. brasiliensis* from a partially calcified lymph node lesion by microaerophilic incubation in liquid media. Sabouraudia. 1981;295–300.
21. Franco MF. Host-parasite relationship in paracoccidioidomycosis. J Med Vet Mycol. 1987;25:5–18.
22. Mota NGS, Rezkallah-Iwasso MT, Peracoli MTS, et al. Correlation between cell-mediated immunity and clinical forms of paracoccidioidomycosis. Trans R Soc Trop Med Hyg. 1985;79:765–72.
23. Jimenez BE, Murph JA. Induction of antigen-specific T suppressor cells by soluble *P. brasiliensis* antigen. Infect Immun. 1988;56:734–43.
24. Restrepo A. Immune response to *P. brasiliensis* in human and animal hosts. In: McGinnis MR, ed. Current Topics in Medical Mycology. v. 2. New York: Springer-Verlag; 1987:239–77.
25. Restrepo A, Robledo M, Giraldo R, et al. The gamut of paracoccidioidomycosis. Am J Med. 1976;61:33–42.
26. Sugar AM, Restrepo A, Stevens DA. Paracoccidioidomycosis in the immunosuppressed host. Report of a case and review of the literature. Am Rev Respir Dis. 1984;129:349–2.
27. Londero AT. Paracoccidioidomicose associada a droga imunosupressora en paciente com lupus eritematoso sistémico. J Pneumol (Brasil). 1987;13:224–6.
28. Londero AT, Severo LC. The gamut of progressive pulmonary paracoccidioidomycosis. Mycopathology. 1981;75:65–74.
29. Magalhaes A. Paracoccidioidomycose (Blastomicose Sul Americana). Aspectos radiológicos. Rev Hosp Clin Fac Med Sao Paulo. 1980;35:147–55.
30. Giorgi MCR, Camargo EE, Pinto WP, et al. Gallium-67 imaging in the diagnosis of blastomycosis. Eur J Nucl Med. 1987;13:300–4.
31. Patiño MM, Gomez I, Silva M, et al. El espectro de las manifestaciones radiológicas de la paracoccidioidomicosis. Act Med Colombiana. 1987;12:230–6.
32. Del Negro G, Melo EHL, Rodbard D, et al. Limited adrenal reserve in paracoccidioidomycosis. Clin Endocrinol. 1980;13:553–59.
33. Abad A, Gomez I, Restrepo A. Adrenal function in paracoccidioidomycosis. A prospective study in patients before and after ketoconazole therapy. Infection. 1986;1:22–6.
34. Uribe F, Zuluaga AI, Leon W, et al. Histopathology of cutaneous and mucosal lesions in human paracoccidioidomycosis. Rev Inst Med Trop Sao Paulo. 1987;29:90–6.
35. Del Negro G. Avances terapeuticos em micoses profundas, com enfase a paracoccidioidomicose. Ann Brasil Dermatol. 1987;62:209–12.
36. Campos EP, Sartori JC, Hetch ML, et al. Clinical and serologic features of 47 patients with paracoccidioidomycosis treated by amphotericin B. Rev Inst Med Trop Sao Paulo. 1984;26:212–7.
37. Dillon NL, Sampaio SAP, Habermann MC, et al. Delayed results of treatment of paracoccidioidomycosis with amphotericin B plus sulfonamides versus amphotericin B alone. Rev Inst Med Trop Sao Paulo. 1986;28:263–66.
38. Restrepo A, Gomez I, Cano LE, et al. Treatment of paracoccidioidomycosis with ketoconazole: A 3 year experience. Am J Med. 1983;74(Suppl B):48–52.
39. Negroni R. Estado Actual del empleo del ketoconazol en paracoccidioidomicosis. Rev Argent Micol. 1987;(Suppl):21–6.
40. Robledo MA, Gomez I, Gutierrez F, et al. Evaluación a largo plazo de pacientes con paracoccidioidomycosis tratados con ketoconazol. Acta Med Colombiana. 1985;10:155–60.
41. Marcondes J, Neira DA, Mendes RP, et al. Evaluation of ketoconazole in the treatment of paracoccidioidomycosis. Rev Inst Med Trop Sao Paulo. 1984;26:113–21.
42. Marques SA, Dillon NL, Franco MF, et al. Paracoccidioidomycosis: A comparative study of the evolutionary serologic, clinical and radiologic results for patients treated with ketoconazole or amphotericin B plus sulfonamides. Mycopathology. 1985;89:19–23.
43. Negroni R, Palmieri O, Karen K, et al. Oral treatment of paracoccidioidomycosis and histoplasmosis with itraconazole in humans. Rev Infect Dis. 1987;9(Suppl 1):47–50.
44. Restrepo A, Gomez I, Robledo J, et al. Itraconazole in the treatment of paracoccidioidomycosis. A preliminary report. Rev Infect Dis. 1987;9(Suppl 1):51–6.

247. MISCELLANEOUS FUNGI

JOHN E. BENNETT

PSEUDALLESCHERIA BOYDII

Etiologic Agent

This fungus has been called *Petriellidium boydii* or *Allescheria boydii* when in the perfect state and *Monosporium apiospermum* or *Scedosporium apiospermum* when in the imperfect state. Consequently, the disease induced by the species has been called pseudallescheriasis, petriellidiosis, allescheriasis, or monosporiosis.

Pseudallescheria boydii is a cottony white mold that rapidly turns dark gray with age. The agar under the colony also blackens. The fungus grows well at 30–37°C on a variety of simple culture media, including Sabouraud agar. Microscopically, septate hyphae with oval or club-shaped, pale brown conidia are seen.

Epidemiology, Pathogenesis, and Pathologic Characteristics

Pseudallescheria boydii is a saprophyte that has been isolated from soil, manure, decaying vegetation, and other nature sites in many different countries of the world.[1,2] The fungus enters the body by the airborne route or by penetrating injury. In subcutaneous tissue, the fungus may grow exclusively in grossly visible clumps, called grains. The chronic, suppurative infection resulting from cutaneous inoculation is called mycetoma. This clinical entity is discussed in Chapter 240 and will not be mentioned further here. *Pseudallescheria boydii* infections that do not resemble the clinical entity, mycetoma, are called pseudallescheriasis. This name encompasses a wide variety of clinical conditions. Histopathologically, the fungus may be found as a matted clump of hyphae within but not invading the wall of pulmonary cavities, ectatic bronchi, or paranasal sinuses (Fig. 1). Invasive infection also occurs and is characterized by necrosis and infiltration of the lesion with neutrophils. Hyphae are seen scattered throughout the abscess, not in grains. Vascular invasion by hyphae, so characteristic of aspergillosis and mucormycosis, may also occur in *P. boydii* infections.

Clinical Entities

Pseudallescheriasis often resembles and may be mistaken for aspergillosis, particularly in the ear, paranasal sinus, lung, and eye. *Pseudallescheria boydii* can grow in the cerumen and desquamated debris of the external auditory canal, a condition called otomycosis.[3] Colonization of a poorly draining paranasal sinus may lead to a fungus ball in the sinus[4,5] or, in an immunosuppressed patient, may be followed by progressive invasion and extension to the orbit and meninges.[6,7] Colonization of cysts, cavities, and ectatic bronchi of patients with tuberculosis or other chronic lung diseases possibly contributes to the patient's chronic productive cough or hemoptysis.[3,8–11] A fungus ball may sometimes be detectable radiologically.[3,9] A patient with chronic lung disease has also been reported to develop pleural pseudallescheriasis.[12]

Ocular pseudallescheriasis may result from corneal trauma[13,14] or as a complication of cataract extraction.[15] Hematogenous endophthalmitis from an unknown portal has occurred in an immunosuppressed patient.[16]

Penetrating trauma over the knee has resulted in an indolent arthritis due to *P. boydii*.[16–18] Spinal anesthesia was thought to be the cause of chronic meningitis in one case.[19] In one case known to me, a young drug addict developed chronic *P. boydii* meningitis without a known portal.

The most severe cases of pseudallescheriasis have been reported in patients who were receiving immunosuppressive therapy for organ transplantation,[20] leukemia,[21] lymphoma,[22] systemic lupus erythematosus, or Crohn's disease. In addition to the cases of invasive sinusitis and hematogenous endophthalmitis alluded to above, these patients have had abscesses of lung,[23,24] brain,[22,23,25] or thyroid.[21] A pulmonary portal for the disseminated infection has been assumed but has been infrequently demonstrated. A fishhook penetrating the finger of a renal transplant recipient caused an indolent abscess that dissected into the palm.[26] A patient receiving long-term adrenal corticosteroid therapy developed arthritis surrounded by over 60 ml of pus.[27] Multiple local corticosteroid injections seemed to have predisposed to osteomyelitis of the foot.[28] A subcutaneously implanted pacemaker and prednisone therapy apparently led to tricuspid valve endocarditis.[29] Only an occasional patient with lung,[30] soft tissue, or bone infection[31,32] has no history of trauma or immunosuppression.

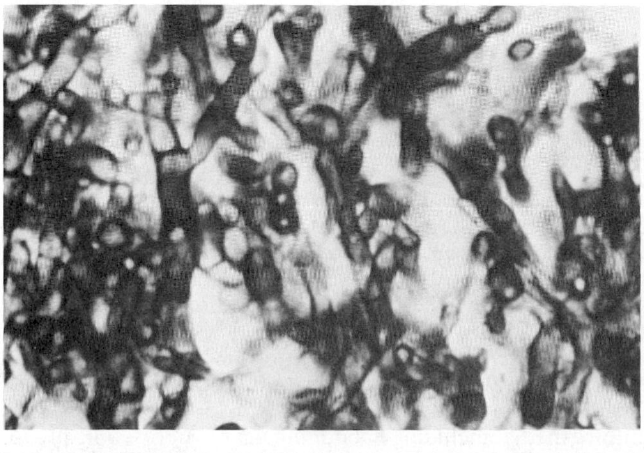

FIG. 1. Clump of *P. boydii* hyphae within maxillary sinus. (Gomori methenamine silver, original magnification ×900)

Diagnosis

Culture is the only reliable means of diagnosis, but histopathologic examination of the lung or sinus lesions is necessary to document invasion. Histopathologic findings alone are not diagnostic, but the presence of septate hyphae in abscesses is compatible with petriellidiosis. Hyphae tend to be 2–7 μm in diameter but may be larger or may show areas of bulbous swelling. Masses of hyphae in air-containing spaces of the lung or paranasal sinus may show conidia[3,6] or clumped groups of hyphae in parallel array, termed a coremium or synnema.[6] These structures more strongly suggest the diagnosis.

One patient with noninvasive pulmonary disease had precipitating antibody to *P. boydii* antigen.[10] The diagnostic value of this test is unknown.

Therapy

Surgical excision or drainage has appeared to assist in the management of fungus ball of the lung,[10,33] sinusitis,[5] pleuritis,[12] endophthalmitis,[16] brain abscess,[34] and in the hand and foot lesions.[26–28] Intravenous amphotericin B in the absence of surgery has not been clearly effective in the few reported cases of invasive[7,16,25,31] and noninvasive[33] pseudallescheriasis. Intravenous amphotericin B plus surgical drainage was successful in treating brain[34] and sinus infection. Favorable results have been noted with amphotericin B eye drops in *P. boydii* keratitis[13] and with intra-articular amphotericin B in *P. boydii* arthritis.[17] In vitro sensitivity testing of molds is difficult to interpret because of technical problems, but the results with *P. boydii* have shown minimum inhibitory concentrations in excess of 250 μg/ml for flucytosine,[16] roughly 2.5–25 μg/ml for amphotericin B,[16,35] and 0.016–0.16 μg/ml for miconazole.[16] Although data about the efficacy of miconazole are not extensive, the drug appears to be beneficial in some cases, particularly when combined with sugrical debridement in the treatment of soft tissue infections.[26,31,36–38] Fragmentary evidence also suggests ketoconazole may be useful.[18,38,39]

PROTOTHECA

Prototheca are unicellular achloric algalike organisms that reproduced by endosporulation. *Prototheca wickerhamii* has been the agent in most human cases except for an occasional case due to *P. zopfi* (also called *P. segbwema*[40]). A review by Pegram et al.[41] contained 29 documented cases. The cases were from broadly dispersed areas of the world, although 12 cases originated in the eastern United States.

Prototheca are ubiquitous in nature and usually enter the body by minor trauma or surgical incisions, causing chronic papulonodular skin lesions. The other major manifestation is olecranon bursitis, with 11 published cases and 1 additional case known to me. Other lesions have included indurated plaques,[42] wound infections,[43] lymphadenitis,[40] and disseminated infection of skin and peritoneum.[44] The infrequency of dissemination in humans contrasts with protothecosis of animals, in which dissemination is usual.

Protothecosis is best diagnosed by biopsy for histologic study and culture. The inflammatory response shows both microabscesses and granulomata with multinucleate giant cells.[45,46] *Prototheca* cells usually range from 8 to 20 μm in diameter, stain well with Gomori methenamine silver or periodic acid–Schiff, and often contain two to eight endospores in each cell or sporangium. White opaque colonies appear in a few days on Sabouraud agar. Identification is by gross and microscopic appearance plus biochemical tests.[47]

Protothecosis has little, if any, tendency to self-healing. Surgical excision of lesions[45,46] and intravenous amphotericin B[42,44,48] have both been used successfully. *Prototheca* species are resistant to flucytosine. One patient responded to ketoconazole, 200 mg/day for 10 weeks.[41]

EMMONSIA CRESCENS

Emmonsia crescens is the causative agent of adiaspiromycosis in humans. Thirteen cases from scattered localities in the world have been reviewed by Emmons and coworkers.[50] At least one additional case exists.[51]

A spore of *E. crescens* inhaled into the lung is capable of growing to a diameter of 200–700 μm. No reproduction occurs in humans, but the huge spore becomes encased in a granuloma with epithelioid cells and multinucleate giant cells. A patient may have one or myriad such granuloma. The infection is usually an incidental autopsy finding, but extensive infection can cause fever, cough, and dyspnea. Diagnosis can be made by culture or by the appearance of the hugh, thick-walled cysts in histopathologic section.

RHINOSPORIDIUM SEEBERI

Rhinosporidiosis is a chronic, usually painless localized infection of the mucous membrane. The lesion increases in size over months or years to form a friable pedunculated mass, typically in the nose or conjunctiva. The etiologic agent, *R. seeberi*, has never been cultured but is thought to be a fungus. *R. seeberi* forms round thick-walled cysts varying from 10 to 200 μm in the submucosa, often visible through the mucosa as white dots. Mature cysts become filled with numerous spores, which on release become new cysts. The infection occurs through the world, although the greatest number of cases has been found in India and Sri Lanka. Lasser and Smith[52] reviewed 28 cases from the United States, 19 in the nose and 9 in the conjunctiva. Twenty-four occurred in men and four in women. No state had an excess of cases. Treatment of choice is surgery.

LOBOA LOBOI

Lobomycosis (Lobo's disease, keloidal blastomycosis) is a chronic skin infection caused by a fungus never isolated in culture but called *Loboa loboi*. More than 100 cases have been reported from Latin America. The disease has not been acquired in the United States except in dolphins off the coast of Florida.[53] The diagnosis is made by finding the typical globose to lemon-shaped cells (about 9 μm in diameter) either singly or in short chains. The fungus remains confined to the skin, progressing slowly over decades. Lesions are nodular, red, hard, and shiny.

DARK-WALLED (DEMATIACEOUS) FUNGI

Phaeohyphomycosis, dematiomycosis, and phaeomycotic cyst are terms referring to infections with dematiaceous fungi (i.e., molds having dark-walled hyphae). Hyphal color is best distinguished on culture in vitro. Hyphae in tissue may be golden brown or colorless, hyphal, or almost yeastlike. Although chromomycosis fits into this definition, it is a discrete entity, described elsewhere. Within the 40 or so species that remain in this category, manifestations of infection are so diverse that terms such as phaeohyphomycosis do not describe a recognizable clinical entity. Nevertheless, there are a few entities and generalizations that can be offered.

Cladosporium trichoides and, rarely, *C. trichoides* var. *chlamydosporum* or *C. bantianum* may produce a brain abscess. Seaworth and coworkers[54] found 22 such cases, including their own case. Most patients with cerebral cladosporiosis have been previously health adults with no obvious portal of entry. Rarely, a lung lesion or history of penetrating trauma has been present. Other dematiaceous fungi have, on rare occasion, caused the same entity.

Nodular and maculopapular skin lesions have been caused by a large number of dark-walled fungi, particularly species of *Exophiala*[55] and *Phialophora*.[56,57] The fungi live as saprophytes in nature, such as on rotted wood, and enter the skin by minor trauma. Phaeomycotic cyst is a variant of this entity, usually caused by *Phialophora* species.[58] The fungus causes a chronic cyst to form at the site of inoculation, usually a leg or hand.

Bipolaris and *Curvularia* are closely rated species with a tendency to cause brain abscess either by spread from the lung or from a contiguous paranasal sinus.[59–61]

Infections with dematiaceous fungi do not respond well to chemotherapy and should be excised when possible. The response to amphotericin B intravenously has been marginal, although the combination of flucytosine and amphotericin B has sometimes appeared beneficial. Intravenous miconazole or oral ketoconazole has appeared to improve lung or skin lesions of some cases.

RARE AGENTS

Trichosporon beigelii (*T. cutaneum*) can be part of the normal human flora and appear in cultures of stool, skin, or urine.[62] Patients with acute leukemia, organ transplantation, prosthetic ardiac valves, or other susceptible states may acquire disseminated trichosporosis.[63,64] Multiple red papular skin lesions may occur during fungemia.[64] An infection of hair shafts, white piedra, is described in Chapter 245.

Fusarium infections, while rare, can present in a wide variety of clinical manifestations.[65] *Paecilomyces varioti* has caused endocarditis in five reported cases.[66]

Malassezia furfur, a lipophilic yeast, colonizes the normal human skin and causes the superficial mycosis, tinea versicolor. The fungus can also cause catheter-acquired sepsis. Almost all the septic cases have been receiving parenteral lipids through a central intravascular catheter such as a Broviac.[67] The majority of patients have been neonates with extended stays in intensive care units, though a few have been adults with malignancy or immunosuppression. Fever has been the most common finding, but bradycardia, apnea, thrombocytopenia, and catheter blockage have been observed in some infants. In one autopsied case, the yeast was observed in lipid-containing areas of pulmonary vascular endothelium. *M. furfur* rarely is detected by conventional culture techniques because the yeast requires fatty acids for growth. Optimum recovery has been culture of blood drawn back through the catheter, using the lysis-centrifugation technique and lipid-enriched agar.[67,68] The fungus adheres to the lumen of the catheter and has not been eradicated by discontinuing lipid infusions or administering miconazole or amphotericin B through the catheter.[69] In vitro, *M. furfur* appears susceptible to both amphotericin B and imidazoles.[70] Cultures of smears[71] or peripheral blood are occasionally positive. The yeast is identified on smear by its size, shape, and the distinctive collarette between mother and daughter cells. Lipid requirement for growth also aids identification. Catheter removal and discontinuing parenteral lipids has been curative.

REFERENCES

1. Ajello L. The isolation of *Allescheria boydii* Shear, an etiologic agent of mycetomas from soil. Am J Trop Med Hyg. 1952;1:227.
2. Mackinnon JE, Conti-Díaz IA, Gezuele E, et al. Datos sobre ecologia de *Allescheria boydii* Shear. Rev Uruguaya Pat Clin Microbiol. 1971;9:37.
3. Milne LJR, McKerrow WS, Paterson WD et al. Pseudallescheriasis in northern Britain. J Med Vet Mycol. 1986;24:377–82.
4. Morgan MA, Wilson WR, Neel HB et al. Fungal sinusitis in healthy and immunocompromised individuals. Am J Clin Pathol. 1984;82:598–601.
5. Winn RE, Ramsey PD, McDonald JC et al. Maxillary sinusitis from Pseudallescheria boydii. Efficacy of surgical therapy. Arch Otolaryngol. 1983;109:123–5.
6. Gluckman SJ, Ries K, Abrutyn E. *Allescheria* (*Petriellidium*) *boydii* sinusitis in a compromised host. J Clin Microbiol. 1977;5:481.
7. Hecht R, Montgomerie JZ. Maxillary sinus infection with *Allescheria boydii* (*Petriellidium boydii*). Johns Hopkins Med J. 1978;142:107.
8. Arnett JC, Hatch HB. Pulmonary allescheriosis. Arch Intern Med. 1975;135:1250.
9. Belitsos NJ, Merz WG, Bowersox DW, et al. *Allescheria boydii* mycetoma complicating pulmonary sarcoid. Johns Hopkins Med J. 1974;135:259.
10. Hainer JW, Ostrow JH, Mackenzie DWR. Pulmonary monosporiosis: Report of a case with precipitating antibody. Chest. 1974;66:601.
11. Rosen P, Adelson HT, Burleigh E. Bronchiectasis complicated by the presence of *Monosporium apiospermum* and *Aspergillus fumigatus*. Am J Clin Pathol. 1969;52:182.
12. Bousley PH. Isolation of *Allescheria boydii* from pleural fluid. J Clin Microbiol. 1977;5:244.
13. Levitt JM, Goldstein J. Keratomycosis due to *Allescheria boydii*. Am J Ophthalmol. 1971;71:1190.
14. Elliott ID, Halde C, Shapiro J. Keratitis and endophthalmitis caused by *Petriellidium boydii*. Am J Ophthalmol. 1977;83:16.
15. Glassman MI, Henkind P, Alture-Werber E. *Monosporium apiospermum* endophthalmitis. Am J Ophthalmol. 1973;76:821.
16. Lutwick LI, Galgiani JN, Johnson RH, et al. Visceral fungal infections due to *Petriellidium boydii* (*Allescheria boydii*). Am J Med. 1976;61:632.
17. Hayden G, Lapp C, Loda F. Arthritis caused by *Monosporium apiospermum* treated with intraarticular amphotericin B. Am J Dis Child. 1977;131:927.
18. Herve F, Douhet E, Dupont B et al. Osteoarthrite mycosique du genou avec destruction articulaire traitee par ketoconazole. Arch Fr Pediatr. 1983;40:309–14.
19. Benham RW, George LK. *Allescheria boydii* causative agent in a case of meningitis. J Invest Dermatol. 1948;10:99.
20. Alsip SG, Cobbs CG. *Pseudallescheria boydii* infection of the central nervous system in a cardiac transplant recipient. South Med J. 1986;79:383–4.
21. Enggano EL, Hughes WT, Kalwinsky DK, et al. *Pseudallescheria boydii* in a patient with acute lymphoblastic leukemia. Arch Pathol Lab Med. 1984;108:619–22.
22. Yoo D, Lee HS, Kwon-Chung KJ. Brain abscesses due to *Pseudallescheria boydii* associated with primary non-Hodgkin's lymphoma of the central nervous system. A case report and literature review. Rev Infect Dis. 1985;78:272–7.
23. Winston DJ, Jordan MC, Rhoses J. *Allescheria boydii* infections in the immunosuppressed host. Am J Med. 1977;63:830.
24. Alture-Werber E, Edberg S, Singer JM. Pulmonary infection with *Allescheria boydii*. Am J Clin Pathol. 1976;66:1019.
25. Gari M, Fruit J, Rousseaux P, et al. *Scedosporium* (*Monosporium*) *apiospermum*: multiple brain abscesses. J Med Vet Mycol. 1985;23:371–6.
26. Lichtman DM, Johnson DC, Mack GR, et al. Maduramycosis (*Allescheria boydii*) infection of the hand. J Bone Joint Surg. 1978;60A:546.
27. Hecke E, Geerts ML, Dooven D. Petriellidiosis of the skin. Mykosen. 1982;26:17.
28. Halpern AA, Nagel DA, Schruman DJ. Allescheria boydii osteomyelitis following multiple steroid injections and surgery. Clin Orthop. 1977;126:232.
29. Davis WA, Isner JM, Bracy AW, et al. Disseminated *Petriellidium boydii* and pacemaker endocarditis. Am J Med. 1980;69:929.
30. Saadah HA, Dixon T. Petriellidium boydii (Allescheria boydii) necrotizing pneumonia in a normal host. JAMA.1981;245:605.
31. Lutwick LI, Rytel MW, Yanez JP, et al. Deep infections from *Petriellidium boydii* treated with miconazole. JAMA. 1979;241:272.
32. Travis LB, Roberts GD, Wilson WR. Clinical significance of *Pseudallescheria boydii*: A review of 10 years' experience. Mayo Clin Proc. 1985;60:531–7.
33. Jung JY, Salas R, Almond CH, et al. The role of surgery in the management of pulmonary monosporiosis: A collective review. J Thorac Cardiovasc Surg. 1977;73:139.
34. Bell WE, Myers MG. *Allescheria* (*Petriellidium*) *boydii* brain abscess in a child with leukemia. Arch Neurol. 1978;35:386.
35. Nielsen HS. Effects of amphotericin B in vitro on perfect and imperfect strains of *Allescheria boydii*. Appl Microbiol. 1967;15:86.
36. Nunery WR, Welsh MG, Sayler R. Pseudallescheria boydii (Petriellidium boydii) infection of the orbit. Ophthal Surg. 1985;16:296–300.
37. Lazarus HS, Myers JP, Brocker RJ. Post-craniotomy wound infection caused by Pseudallescheria boydii. J Neurosurg. 1986;64:153–4.
38. Schiess RJ, Coscia MJ, McClellan GA. Petriellidium boydii pachymeningitis treated with miconazole and ketoconazole. Neurosurgery. 1984;14:220–4.
39. Galgiani JN, Stevens DA, Graybill JR, et al. Pseudallescheria boydii infections treated with ketoconazole. Clinical evaluations of seven patients and in vitro susceptibility results. Chest. 1984;86:219–4.
40. Davies RR, Wilkinson JL. Human protothecosis: Supplementary studies. Ann Trop Med Parasitol. 1967;61:112.
41. Pegram PS, Kerns FT, Wasilauskas BL, et al. Successful ketoconazole treatment of protothecosis with ketoconazole associated hepatotoxicity. Arch Intern Med. 1983;143:1802.
42. Mayhall CG, Miller CW, Eisen AZ, et al. Cutaneous protothecosis. Arch Dermatol. 1976;112:1749.
43. Jones JW, McFadden HW, Chandler FW, et al. Green algal infection in a human. Am J Clin Pathol. 1983;80:102–7.
44. Cox GE, Wilson JD, Brown P. Protothecosis: A case of disseminated algal infection. Lancet. 1974;2:379.
45. Nosanchuk JS, Greenberg RD. Protothecosis of the olecranon bursa caused by achloric algae. Am J Clin Pathol. 1973;59:567.
46. Tindall JP, Fetter BF. Infections caused by achloric algae (protothecosis). Arch Dermatol. 1971;104:490.
47. Sudman MS. Protothecosis. A critical review. Am J Clin Pathol. 1974;61:10.
48. Venezio FR, Lavoo E, Williams JE, et al. Progressive cutaneous protothecosis. Am J Clin Pathol. 1982;77:485.
49. Segal E, Padhye AA, Ajello L. Susceptibility of *Prototheca* species to antifungal agents. Antimicrob Agents Chemother. 1976;10:75.
50. Emmons CW, Binford CH, utz JP, et al. Medical Mycology. 3rd ed. Philadelphia: Lea & Febiger; 1977:493–505.
51. Quilici M, Lebreuil G, Dumon H, et al. A new human case of adiaspiromycosis. Bull Soc Fr Mycol Med. 1976;5:195.
52. Lasser A, Smith HW. Rhinosporidiosis. Arch Otolaryngol. 1976;102:308.
53. Emmons CW, Binford CH, Utz JP, et al. Medical Mycology. 3rd ed. Philadelphia: Lea & Febiger; 1977:379–85.
54. Seaworth BJ, Kwon-Chung KJ, Hamilton JD, et al. Brain abscess caused by a variety of Cladosporium trichoides. Am J Clin Pathol. 1983;79:747.
55. Matsumoto T, Nishimoto K, Kimura K, et al. Phaeohyphomycosis caused by Exophiala moniliae. Sabouraudia. 1984;22:17.
56. Corrado ML, Weitzman I, Stanek A, et al. Subcutaneous infection with *Phialophora richardsiae* and its susceptibility to 5-fluorocytosine, amphotericin B and miconazole. Sabouraudia. 1980;18:97.
57. Meyers WM, Dooley JR, Kwon-Chung KJ. Mycotic granuloma caused by *Phialophora repens*. Am J Clin Pathol. 1975;64:549.
58. Zeifer A, Connor DH. Phaeomycotic cyst. A clinicopathologic study of twenty-five patients. Am J Trop Med Hyg. 1980;29:901.
59. Rohwedder JJ, Simmons JL, Colfer H, et al. Disseminated *Curvularia lunata* infection in a football player. Arch Intern Med. 1979;139:940.
60. Yoshimori RN, Moore RA, Itabashi HH, et al. Phaeohyphomycosis of brain. Granulomatous encephalitis caused by *Drechslera spicifera*. Am J Clin Pathol. 1982;77:363.
61. Washburn RG, Kennedy DW, Begley MG, et al. Chronic fungal sinusitis in apparently normal hosts. Medicine. 1988;67:231–47.
62. Haupt HM, Merz WG, Beschorner WE, et al. Colonization and infection with trichosporon species in the immunosuppressed host. J Infect Dis. 1983;147:199.
63. Hoy J, Hsu KC, Rolston H, et al. Trichosporon beigelii infection: A review. Rev Infect Dis. 1986;8:959–67.
64. Walsh TJ, Newman KR, Moody M, et al. Trichosporonosis in patients with neoplastic disease. Medicine, 1986;65:268–79.
65. Merz WG, Karp JE, Hoagland M, et al. Diagnosis and successful treatment of fusariosis in the compromised host. J Infect Dis. 1988;158:1046–55.
66. Kalish SB, Goldschmidt R, Li C, et al. Infective endocarditis caused by paecilomyces varioti. Am J Clin Pathol. 1982;78:249.
67. Dankner WM, Spector SA, Fierer J, et al. *Malassezia* fungemia in neonates and adults: Complication of hyperalimentation. Rev Infect Dis. 1987;9:743–53.
68. Azimi PH, Levernier K, Lefrak LM, et al. *Malassezia furfur*: A cause of occlusion of percutaneous central venous catheters in infants in the intensive care nursery. Pediatr Infect Dis J. 1988;7:100–3.
69. Powell DA, Marcon MJ. Failure to eradicate *Malassezia furfur* broviac catheter infection with antifungal therapy. Pediatr Infect Dis J. 1987;6:579–88.
70. Marcon MJ, Durrell DE, Powell DA, et al. In vitro activity of systemic antifungal agents against *Malassezia furfur*. Antimicrob Ag Chemother. 1987;31:951–3.
71. Brooks R, Brown L. Systemic infections with *Malassezia furfur* in an adult receiving long-term hyperalimentation therapy. J Infect Dis. 1987;156:410–11.

SECTION G. PROTOZOAL DISEASES

248. INTRODUCTION

JONATHAN I. RAVDIN

The protozoa known to infect humans are a diverse group, as indicated by phylogeny (Table 1), epidemiology (Table 2), clinical manifestations (Table 3), preferred diagnostic studies (Table 4), and chemotherapeutic agents effective in eradicating or arresting infection (Table 5). Protozoa such as *Plasmodium* sp., *Entamoeba histolytica*, *Trypanosoma* sp., and *Leishmania* sp. are major worldwide pathogens and are among the leading causes of disease and mortality in areas of Africa, Asia, and Central and South America. *Giardia lamblia* and *Cryptosporidium* are frequent causes of diarrhea in developing areas and established Western countries. *Pneumocystis carinii* has become of increasing importance due to the worldwide spread of the human immunodeficiency virus (HIV), which after a long latent period induces the onset of the acquired immunodeficiency syndrome (AIDS). *Toxoplasma gondii, Cryptosporidium* sp., and *Sarcocystis* and *Leishmania* sp. all have been noted to cause severe diseases in AIDS patients, and *E. histolytica* remains an important cause of diarrhea in homosexual men with AIDS.

The new or continued importance of protozoan pathogens has stimulated active research in all areas; the most exciting information was recently reviewed and is complete with annotated references.[2] Clinicians are encouraged to familiarize themselves with the material in Tables 2 through 5, which is addressed in depth in the chapters that follow. The key to recognition of protozoan infection is a knowledge of epidemiologic risk factors such as the parasites' geographic distribution (Table 2) and the major modes of clinical presentation (Table 3). The clinical diagnosis of protozoan infection when presenting outside normal areas of high prevalence is usually dependent on physicians considering this possibility in their differential diagnosis. Given present levels of travel, changing immigration patterns, and the immunosuppressive effects of HIV infection, all clinicians need to have a heightened awareness of diseases due to the protozoa. Diagnosis and therapy often require a specialized expertise with use of tests (Table 4) or drugs (Table 5) with which most physicians lack experience. Infectious disease consultants will frequently be called upon to diagnose and manage protozoan in-

TABLE 1. Classification of Protozoa

- Phylum I. Sarocomastigophora (flagella, pseudopodia)
  - Subphylum I. Mastigophora (flagella)
    - Class 2. Zoomastigophorea
      - Order 2. Kinetoplastida
        - Suborder 2. Trypanosomatina
          - *Leishmania, Trypanosoma*
      - Order 5. Diplomonadida
        - Suborder 2. Diplomonadina
          - *Giardia*
      - Order 7. Trichomonadida
        - *Dientamoeba, Trichomonas*
  - Subphylum III. Sarcodina (pseudopodia)
    - Super class 1. Rhizopoda
      - Class 1. Lobosea
        - Subclass 1. Gymnamoebia
          - Order 1. Amoebida
            - Suborder 1. Tubulina
              - *Entamoeba*
            - Suborder 5. Acanthopodina
              - *Acanthamoeba*
          - Order 2. Schizopyrenida
            - *Naegleria*
- Phylum III. Apicomplexa (apical microtuble complex)
  - Class 2. Sporozoea
    - Subclass 2. Coccidia
      - Order 3. Eucoccidia
        - Suborder 2. Eimeriina
          - *Isospora, Toxoplasma*
        - Suborder 3. Haemosporina
          - *Plasmodium*
        - Suborder 3. Piroplasmia
          - Order 1. Piroplasmida
            - *Babesia*
- Phylum VII. Ciliophora (ciliated)
  - Class I. Kinetofragminophorea
    - Subclass 2. Vestibuliferia
      - Order 1. Trichostomatida
        - Suborder 1. Trichostomatina
          - *Balantidium*

(Data from Committee on Systematics and Evolution of the Society of Protozoologists.[1])

TABLE 2. Geographic Distribution and Mechanism of Transmission of Protozoan Infections

Organism	*Geographic Distribution*	*Means of Transmission*
Acanthamoeba sp.	Undefined	Contact lens, ? airborne
Babesia sp.	North America, Europe	Tick-borne, blood transfusions
Balantidium coli	Worldwide	Zoonosis (pigs), water,[a] fecal-oral
Blastocystis hominis	Unknown	Fecal-oral, water
Cryptosporidium sp.	Worldwide	Water, food-borne, fecal-oral, zoonosis
Dientamoeba fragilis	Worldwide	Water, fecal oral
Entamoeba histolytica	Worldwide	Water, fecal-oral, food borne
Giardia lamblia	Worldwide	Water, fecal-oral, food-borne
Isospora sp.	Worldwide	Zoonosis, fecal-oral
Leishmania sp.		
L. tropica	Central Asia, Middle East, North Africa	Sandflies
L. braziliensis and *L. mexicana*	Central and South America	
L. donovani	South America, Central Asia, East Africa	
Naegleria sp.	Worldwide	Freshwater, intranasal exposure
Plasmodium sp.	Africa, Asia, South and Central America, Oceania	Female anopheline mosquitos, inoculation of infected blood
Pneumocystis carinii	Worldwide	Airborne, ? person to person
Sarcocystis sp.	Unknown	Food-borne (meat)
Toxoplasma gondii	Worldwide	Zoonosis (cats), food-borne (meat), congenital
Trichomonas vaginalis	Worldwide	Venereal, during birth, ? nonvenereal
Trypanosoma sp.		
T. cruzi	South and Central America	Reduviid bugs
T. brucei gambiense	West Africa	Tsetse fly
t. brucei rhodesiense	East Africa	Tsetse fly

[a] Ingestion of water contaminated with fecal material.

TABLE 3. Clinical Syndromes Due to Infection by Protozoa

Organism (Disease)	*Major Clinical Syndrome*
Acanthamoeba sp.	Keratitis, granulomatous encephalitis
Babesia sp. (babesiosis)	Fever, malaise, hepatosplenomegaly, and hemolytic anemia, especially in the asplenic
Balantidium coli (balantidiosis)	Colitis
Blastocystis hominis (blastocystis)	Diarrhea, eosinophilia
Cryptosporidium sp. (cryptosporidiosis)	Self-limiting noninflammatory diarrhea; chronic severe diarrhea and cholangitis in AIDS patients
Dientamoeba fragilis	Diarrhea, eosinophilia
Entamoeba histolytica (amebiasis)	Rectocolitis, liver abscess
Giardia lamblia (giardiasis)	Noninflammatory diarrhea with malabsorption
Isospora sp. (isosporiasis)	Diarrhea in AIDS patients
Leishmania sp. (cutaneous, mucocutaneous, and visceral leishmaniasis)	Cutaneous or mucocutaneous ulceration; visceral disease with fever, cachexia, invasive hepatosplenomegaly
Naegleria sp.	Meningoencephalitis
Plasmodium sp. (malaria)	Paroxysmal fever, chills, headache, hepatosplenomegaly
Pneumocystis carinii (pneumocystosis)	Pneumonitis in immunocompromised hosts including AIDS
Sarcocystis sp.	Myositis, fever, eosinophilia
Toxoplasma gondii (toxoplasmosis)	Fever, malaise, lymphadenopathy; chorioretinitis; meningocongenital abnormalities; in immunocompromised host: encephalitis, myocarditis, pneumonitis
Trichomonas vaginalis (trichomoniasis)	Vaginitis, urethritis
Trypanosoma sp. (African sleeping sickness, Chagas disease)	Fever, lymphadenopathy, meningoencephalitis, myocarditis; megaesophagus, congestive cardiopathy

TABLE 4. Diagnostic Tests for Protozoan Diseases

Disease	*Preferred Diagnostic Tests*
Amebiasis	
Intestinal	Stool for ova and parasites, serology
Liver	Ultrasound examination, serology
Amebic keratitis	Corneal scraping for micoscopy and culture
Babesiosis	Thin and thick blood smears
Cryptosporidiosis	Acid-fast and rhodamine staining of fecal samples, serology, small bowel biopsy
Giardiasis	Stool for ova and parasites, stool antigen detection
Granulomatous amebic encephalitis	Brain biopsy
Leishmaniasis	
Cutaneous and mucocutaneous	Biopsy, culture, serology
Visceral	Bone marrow aspiration, culture, serology, lymph node biopsy
Malaria	Wright or Giemsa stain of thin and thick blood smear
Pneumocystosis	Methenamine silver or toluidine blue stain of sputum or bronchoalveolar lavage; if negative, proceed to lung biopsy
Primary amebic meningitis	CSF examination, culture for amebae
Toxoplasmosis	Serology, tissue biopsy, antigen detection
Trichomoniasis	Microscopy of vaginal secretions, culture
Trypanosomiasis	
Chagas disease	Fresh blood or stained smear, blood culture, xenodiagnosis; serology for chronic disease
African sleeping sickness	Blood smear, serology

TABLE 5. Therapeutic Agents Used for Protozoan Infection

Disease	*Agents of First Choice*[a]
Amebiasis	
Intestinal	
Luminal	Diloxanide furoate[b]; paromomycin
Invasive	Metronidazole plus luminal agent
Liver	Metronidazole plus luminal agent
Amebic keratitis	Topical propamidine isethionate or miconazole
Babesiosis	Clindamycin plus quinine
Balantidiasis	Tetracycline or metronidazole
Blastocystis	Iodoquinol or metronidazole
Cryptosporidiosis	None available, can try spiramycin
Dientamoeba infection	Iodoquinol, tetracycline, or paromomycin
Giardiasis	Metronidazole or quinacrine HCl; furazolidone for children
Granulomatous amebic encephalitis	Sulfadiazine
Isosporiasis	Trimethoprim-sulfamethoxazole
Leishmaniasis	
Cutaneous and mucocutaneous	Stibogluconate sodium; amphotericin B for America disease
Visceral	Stibogluconate sodium or pentamidine isethionate
Malaria	Chloroquine phosphate (oral), quinine dihydrochloride (parental)
Chloroquine-resistant *P. falciparum*	Quinine sulfate plus pyrimethamine and sulfadiazine or plus tetracycline
To prevent relapse of *P. vivax* and *P. ovale*	Follow with primaquine phosphate
Pneumocystosis	Trimethoprim-sulfamethoxazole or pentamidine isethionate If adverse reactions, dapsone plus trimethoprim available)
Primary amebic meningitis	Amphotericin B (intravenous and intrathecal)
Toxoplasmosis	Pyrimethamine plus trisulfapyrimidines; spiramycin
Trichomoniasis	Metronidazole
Trypanosomiasis	
Chagas disease	Nifurtimox,[b] benznidazole
African sleeping sickness	
Hemolymphatic stage	Suramin[b] or pentamidine isethionate
CNS involvement	Melarsoprol[b] or tryparsamide plus suramin[b]

[a] Available in the United States, see "Drugs for parasitic infections," Med Lett Drugs Ther. 1988; 30:15–24.
[b] Available from the CDC Drug Service, Centers for Disease Control, Atlanta, GA; telephone, (404) 639-3670 or (404) 639-2888.

fection; this requires maintenance of an updated, in-depth data base as provided by the chapters within this section.

REFERENCES

1. Committee on Systematics and Evolution of the Society of Protozoologists. A newly revised classification of the protozoa. J Protozool. 1980;27:37–58.
2. Petri WA Jr, Ravdin JI. Protozoal Infections. In: Current Opinion in Infectious Diseases. 1988;1:229–237.

249. ENTAMOEBA HISTOLYTICA (AMEBIASIS)

JONATHAN I. RAVDIN
WILLIAM A. PETRI, JR.

Acute and chronic diarrheal illnesses have been of major concern to humans since earliest recorded history.

If there be among you any man that is not clean by reasons of uncleanness that chanceth him by night, then shall he go abroad out of the camp. . . . And thou shalt have a paddle upon thy weapon; and it shall be, when thou wilt ease thyself abroad, thou shalt dig therewith, and shalt turn back and cover that which cometh from thee.

Deuteronomy 23:10 and 23:13

The invasion of Russia by Napoleon was halted by widespread acute diarrheal illness. The atrocities affecting prisoners of war such as at Andersonville during the Civil War and the Bataan Death March in the Philippines during World War II were caused as much by *Entamoeba histolytica* as by prison officials. This protozoan organism is the third leading parasitic cause of death in developing nations[1] and is one of the important health risks to which travelers are exposed. Recently, new information has been acquired on the pathogenesis of invasive amebiasis and the host immune response to the parasite[2–4]; however, it is still unclear why an organism that lives as an intestinal commensal inhabitant in some people causes such severe disease in others. Controversial solutions to this puzzle include the existence of distinct pathogenic and nonpathogenic strains of *E. histolytica* or a single genetic type in which pathogenicity is switched on or off by the influence of bacterial flora and environmental conditions in the gut.[5–9]

Disease caused by *E. histolytica* is expressed most often as ulcerative and inflammatory lesions of the colon that yield a complete spectrum of colonic signs and symptoms. Occasionally, amebae gain access to extraintestinal sites, most commonly the liver, where marked tissue destruction can occur.

Losch, in St. Petersburg, Russia, in 1875, is credited with documenting amebae to be pathogenic by inducing lesions in a dog fed dysenteric stool.[10] Kartulis, in Egypt in 1886, settled the role of amebae as a cause of intestinal and hepatic lesions in patients with diarrhea, and Walker and Sellards dispelled all doubt of the pathogenicity of *E. histolytica* with their detailed studies in the Philippines in 1913. Councilman and Lafleur, pathologists at Johns Hopkins University, provided the information in 1891 to allow a clear distinction between bacillary and amebic dysentery.[11] The history of amebiasis has been highlighted by a number of well-studied epidemics such as that at the Chicago Century of Progress Exposition in 1933[12] and that at the Singer Sewing Machine Plant in Indiana in 1950.[13] But its main impact has been the ability of *E. histolytica* to maintain infection in 20–30 percent of people living in certain areas in the tropics and in up to 5 percent of the people in many temperate climate nations. The most subtle break in personal sanitation allows the organisms to spread and initiate disease.

THE ORGANISM

Entamoeba histolytica belongs to the pseudopod-forming protozoan superclass Rhizopoda within the subphylum Sarcodina.[14] Within their family Entamoebidae, order Amoebida, and class Lobosea are many species that infect humans, including *E. histolytica, E. hartmanni, E. polecki, E. coli*, and *E. gingivalis. E. hartmanni*, previously referred to as "small race" *E. histolytica*, is a distinct species by virtue of morphology, unique antigens, and isoenzyme analysis.[15,16] Most experts agree that the noninvasive *Entamoeba*-like Laredo strain, which grows in culture at a lower temperature (25°C), is a separate species. Classification of *Entamoeba* has been based on morphology, antigenic differences, DNA characterization, isoenzyme analysis, drug susceptibility, host specificity, in vitro growth characteristics, and in vivo virulence.[17]

Currently there is active debate regarding the existence of distinct pathogenic and nonpathogenic strains of *E. histolytica* as defined by the mobility of four isoenzymes (L-malate:NADP$^+$ oxidoreductase, glucose phosphate isomerase, phosphoglucomutase, and hexokinase) on starch gel electrophoresis. This approach to the classification of *E. histolytica* was first described by Reeves and Bischoff[18]; however, Sargeaunt and coworkers[5,9,16] have now studied thousands of clinical isolates and noted greater than 22 distinct isoenzyme patterns (zymodemes). Individual zymodemes have a clear association with the occurrence of asymptomatic infection or symptomatic highly invasive disease.[5,9,16] However, as yet there are no studies defining distinct differences in gene content between such isolates. Mirelman and coworkers[6–8] recently reported that a cloned *E. histolytica* isolate obtained from an asymptomatic patient expressing a "nonpathogenic" zymodeme was induced by coculture in vitro with irradiated viable bacteria to express a "pathogenic" zymodeme with the ability to lyse tissue culture cells and produce liver abscesses in hamsters. Coculture of the ameba with the patient's original bacterial flora resulted in reversion to a "nonpathogenic" zymodeme phenotype. In vivo alteration of zymodeme status has not been adequately studied; at present one should assume that all *E. histolytica* isolates have the capacity to become pathogenic.

E. histolytica trophozoites range in size from 10 to 60 μm, with an average of 25 μm. Trophozoites have a single 3–5 μm nucleus containing fine peripheral chromatin and a central nucleolus; amebae often have ingested erythrocytes (Fig. 1). The cytoplasm consists of a clear ectoplasm and a granular endoplasm that contains numerous vacuoles (Fig. 2). Cysts of *E. histolytica* average 12 μm in diameter (range, 5 to 20 μm) and, depending on their maturity, contain one to four nuclei with morphology identical to trophozoite nuclei. As in other members of the order Amoebida, young *E. histolytica* cysts contain chromatoid bodies with smooth, rounded edges; these are composed of ribosome particles in crystalline arrays.[19] Immature cysts may contain clumps of glycogen that stain with iodine (Fig. 3).

LIFE CYCLE AND EPIDEMIOLOGY

The life cycle of *E. histolytica* is not complex; after encystment of a trophozoite the cyst is excreted and can survive for weeks in a hospitable environment. Ingestion of the cyst results in excystation in the small bowel and trophozoite infection of the colon. The trophozoite undergoes encystment only within the large bowel, possibly associated with conditions that are not ideal for continued activity of the trophozoite. Encystment of xenic cultures of *E. histolytica* can be induced in vitro by hypoosmotic conditions resulting in the appearance of two sialylated glycoproteins and a chitinous cell wall (an *N*-acetyl-D-glucosamine polymer).[20]

Cysts may remain for weeks or months in an appropriately moist environment; outside the body trophozoites degenerate within minutes. In addition, trophozoites are rapidly destroyed by the low gastric pH and enzymes; the encysted stage readily passes this barrier. The cyst, therefore, is the primary reason for the extensive prevalence of the infection throughout the world because it moves from one person to another through fecal contamination of water and vegetables or direct fecal-oral contact.[21]

Knowledge of the epidemiologic risk factors relevant to the acquisition of *E. histolytica* and the occurrence of increased severity of disease (Table 1) is essential for the recognition of patients with amebiasis and an understanding of the importance of this parasite. Epidemiologic surveys for infection with *E. histolytica* are difficult to interpret due to the low number of infected patients who demonstrate the organism on a single stool examination,[23,24] frequent laboratory error in identification,[25] and the variability of detection of serum anti-amebic antibodies after infection. Given these limitations, it is estimated that more than 10 percent of the world's population is infected by *E. histolytica*.[1] Excluding the People's Republic of China, approximately 50 million cases of invasive disease occur in the world each year and result in up to 100,000 deaths.[1] The prevalence of infection is as high as 50 percent in underdeveloped

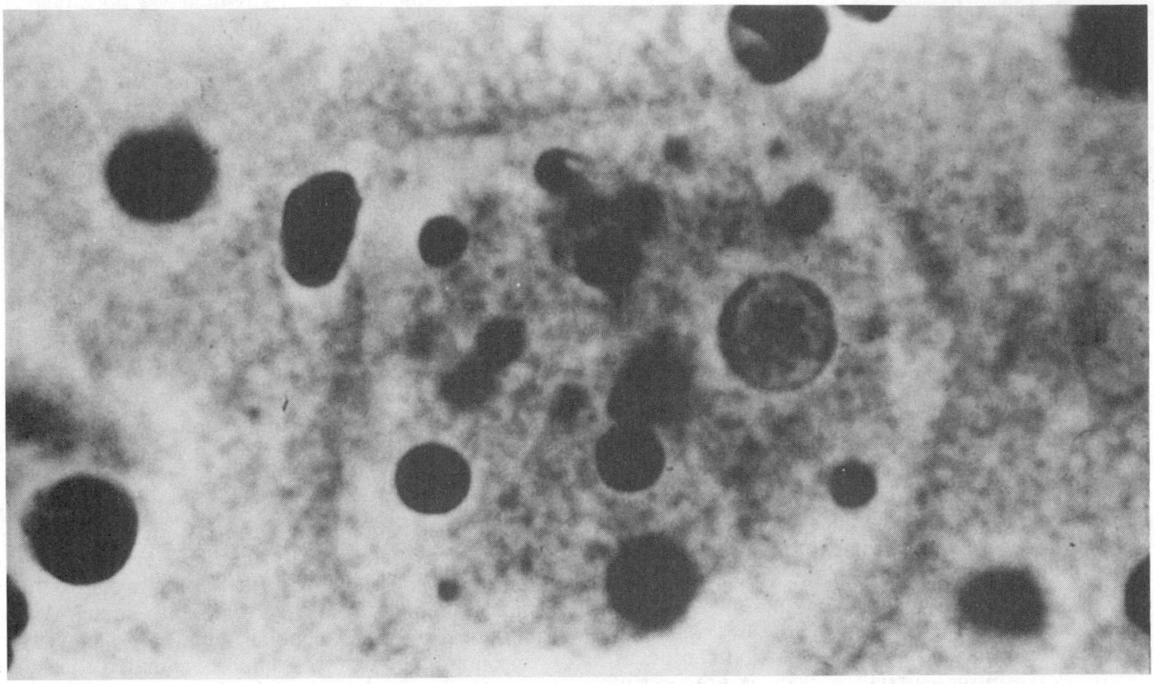

FIG. 1. Trophozoite of *E. histolytica*. A delicate round nucleus with a small central chromatin dot is seen. The trophozoite contains dense ingested red blood cells.

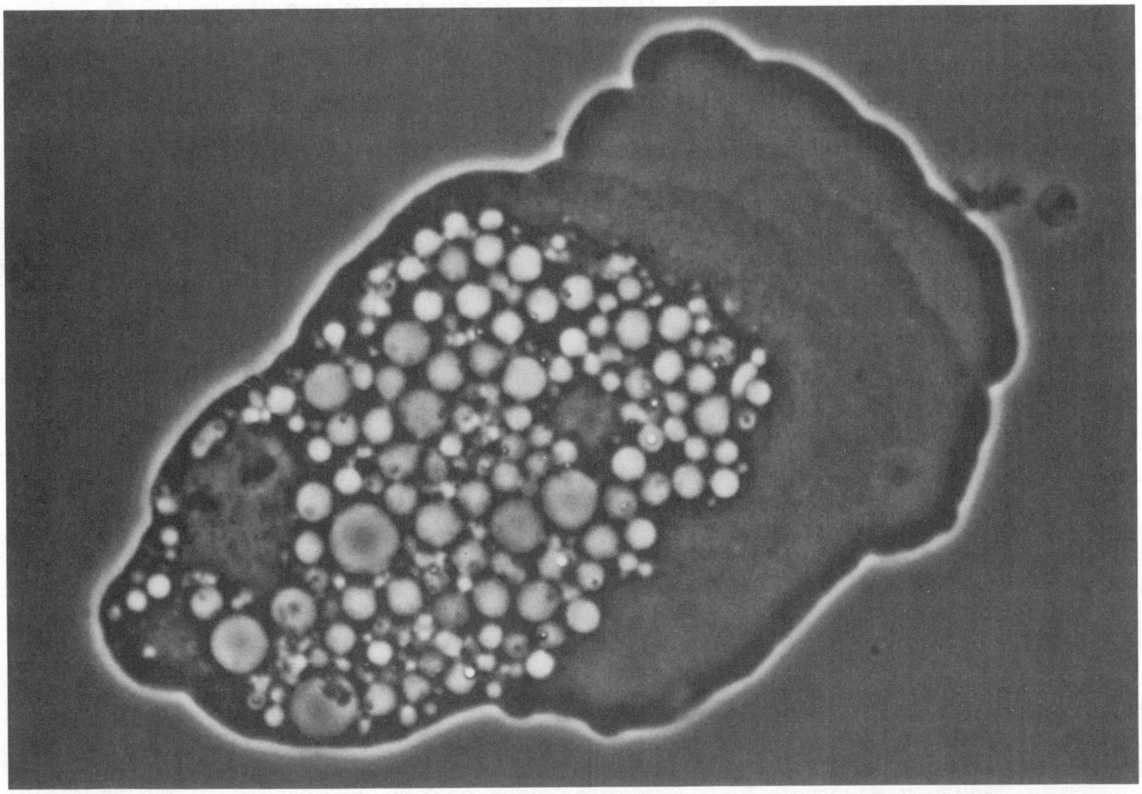

FIG. 2. Phase micrograph of an axenic *E. histolytica* trophozoite strain HM1 : IMSS; note that the cell is oriented with extension of pseudopodia and the highly vesiculated cytoplasm, which is characteristic of virulent axenic strains.

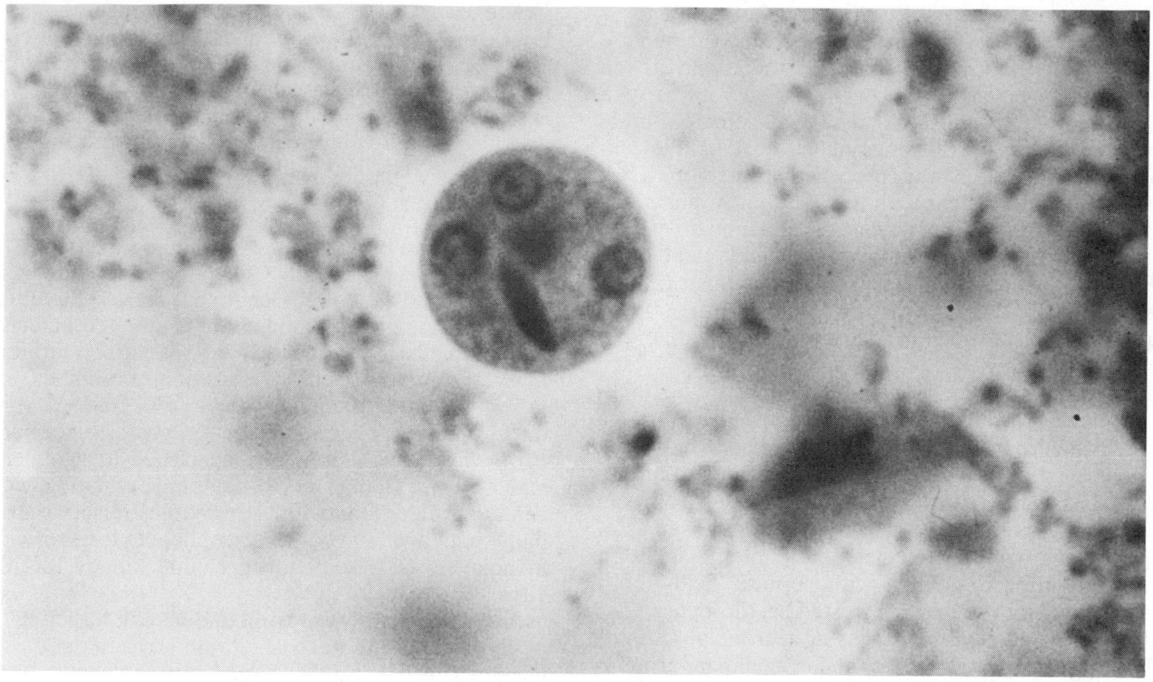

FIG. 3. Mature cyst of *E. histolytica*. Three of the four nuclei are seen in the plane of focus of this photomicrograph.

TABLE 1. Epidemiologic Risk Factors That Apparently Predispose to *E. histolytica* Infection and Increased Severity of Disease

Prevalence	*Increased Severity*
Lower socioeconomic status in an endemic area including	Children, especially neonates
Crowding	Pregnancy and postpartum states
No indoor plumbing	Corticosteroid use
Immigrants from endemic area	Malignancy
Institutionalized population, especially mentally retarded	Malnutrition
Communal living	
Promiscuous male homosexuals	

(From Ravdin,[22] with permission.)

areas,[26,27] and, for example, serologic studies in Mexico City indicate that up to 5 percent of the population experience some form of invasive amebiasis every 2 years.[28] Persistence of a high prevalence of amebic infection depends on cultural habits, sanitation, crowding, and socioeconomic status.[26,28,29] Asymptomatic intestinal infection occurs in 90–99 percent of infected individuals[30–32]; most eliminate the parasite from the gut within 12 months—the mechanisms of such are unknown. In a highly endemic area in Durban, South Africa, a 10 percent prevalence of *E. histolytica* infection resulted in 0.1 percent of the population suffering invasive amebiasis each year.[33,34]

In the United States, the overall prevalence is approximately 4 percent; however, certain high-risk groups have a much higher incidence of infection and disease. Institutionalized populations, especially the mentally retarded, have a very high incidence of *E. histolytica* infection with frequent invasive disease (in up to 73 percent by one serologic survey) and significant mortality.[35–37] Attempts to eradicate amebic infection within individual institutions by the liberal use of anti-amebic drugs or isolation of stool carriers have been unsuccessful.[35,38] Only improved housing and staffing of health care personnel appears to make a substantial impact.[39] There has been a great deal of information regarding the prevalence of amebic infection among sexually promiscuous male homosexuals. In the late 1970s, the prevalence of amebic infection in the gay population of New York City and San Francisco approached 40–50 percent and was one of the many causes of bloody diarrhea in these individuals.[40–44] Although the prevalence of *E. histolytica* infection may be declining with the change in sexual practices due to humen immunodeficiency virus (HIV) infection,[45] recent studies support a continued high prevalence.[46,47] Amebiasis is an important cause of diarrhea in individuals with the acquired immunodeficiency syndrome (AIDS).[48] Additional consequences of coinfection of *E. histolytica* with HIV in the United States or countries such as Haiti[49] or Zaire[50] may result; Petri and Ravdin[51] have suggested that coinfection could stimulate HIV replication. *Entamoeba histolytica* releases a 170 kilodalton (kD) adherence lectin[52] that is a potent T-cell mitogen[53]; stimulation of HIV-infected T-helper cells in vitro with the plant mitogen phytohemagglutinin accelerates HIV expression and T-cell death.[54] Ravdin et al.[55] demonstrated that asymptomatically infected individuals in an endemic area have a substantial prevalence of serum antibody to the purified adherence lectin, thus confirming antigenic exposure.

Many other factors are associated with risk for amebiasis, some unanticipated, such as colonic irrigation without proper sterilization of equipment at a chiropractic clinic in Colorado.[56] Recent immigrants or migrant workers from areas endemic for *E. histolytica* are an important focus of disease in the United States. The overwhelming majority of cases of invasive amebic disease recently reported from academic institutions in the southwestern United States actually occurred in Mexican-Americans.[57–62] Increased risk of amebiasis is associated with foreign travel to any endemic area in the world, especially without taking precautions to avoid enteric infection.[63] The acquisition of *E. histolytica* is usually associated with long-term (greater than 1 month) residence in endemic areas and is usually detected only when symptomatic disease results.[64,65] Additional high-risk groups include children in endemic areas who suffer from fulminant invasive disease with a higher mortality than adults.[66,67]

PATHOLOGY AND PATHOGENESIS

Pathology

Entamoeba histolytica exerts a lytic effect on tissue, a characteristic for which the organism is named. Reports of initial invasion of amebae via mucosal crypts have not been confirmed; amebae appear to invade the colonic epithelium directly.[68,69] Light and electron microscopic studies have been interpreted as showing lysis of mucosal cells on contact with amebae or, alternatively, diffuse mucosal damage before amebic invasion.[69–71] An amorphous, granular, eosinophilic material surrounds trophozoites in tissue, whether in colon, liver, lung, or brain.[68,72,73] Consistent with the fact that trophozoites have the capacity to destroy leukocytes,[74,75] inflammatory cells are found only at the periphery of established amebic lesions.[68,72] Recent in vivo and in vitro studies demonstrate that lysis of host neutrophils by *E. histolytica* results in the release of toxic nonoxidative neutrophil products that contribute to the destruction of host tissues.[76,77]

A spectrum of colonic lesions ranging from nonspecific thickening of the mucosa to the classic flask-shaped ulcer may be associated with amebic infection[70,72] (Fig. 4). In one study only 20 of 53 patients had classic ulcers extending through the mucosa and muscularis mucosa into the submucosa.[72] Amebae can be recognized by a surrounding halo due to fixation artifact, the presence of characteristic nuclear morphology, ingested erythrocytes, and intense staining with periodic acid–Schiff stain or the Gridley stain to detect ingested erythrocytes.[79]

Liver pathology in amebiasis consists of necrotic abscess or periportal fibrosis. The "abscess" contains acellular, proteinaceous debris rather than white cells and is surrounded by a rim of amebic trophozoites invading tissue.[68,73] Amebae establish hepatic infection by ascending the portal venous system rather than the lymphatics.[80,81] Triangular areas of hepatic necrosis, possibly due to ischemia from amebic obstruction of portal vessels, have been observed.[68,80] Amebic liver abscesses probably result from the coalescence of small microabscesses.[80] Liver function abnormalities are frequently present with intestinal amebiasis and are associtaed with periportal inflammation without demonstrable trophozoites.[73,82] Periportal fibrosis has been reported in such patients; whether this reflects past trophozoite invasion or host reaction to amebic antigens or toxins is unclear.

Knowledge of the pathogenic mechanisms of *E. histolytica* has been rapidly expanding[2,4,83]; this has been due in part to the development of an axenic culture medium for the parasite.[84] The pathogenesis of invasive amebiasis requires adherence of *E. histolytica* to the luminal surface of the bowel, amebic cytolytic and proteolytic effects on tissue, and resistance of the parasite to host effector mechanisms. Recent studies have suggested that the associated gut bacterial flora affects amebic invasiveness; in vitro cytopathogenicity can be stimulated by a brief exposure of the trophozoite to certain bacteria.[85,86]

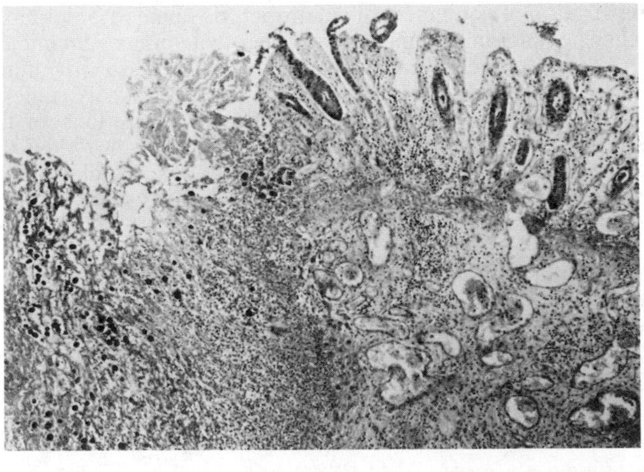

FIG. 4. Light micrograph demonstrating a flask-shaped ulceration in a pathologic specimen from a patient with severe colonic amebiasis. (periodic acid–Schiff stain, ×16) (From Ravdin, et al.,[78] with permission.)

The in vitro adherence of *E. histolytica* trophozoites to Chinese hamster ovary (CHO) cells and human colonic mucins is exclusively mediated by the parasite's galactose (Gal) or *N*-acetyl-D-galactosamine (GalNAc)-inhibitable surface lectin.[52,75,87–89] The Gal/GalNAc adherence lectin participates in the in vitro adherence of *E. histolytica* trophozoites to human leukocytes,[75,90] rat and human colonic mucosa and submucosa,[89] human erythrocytes,[87,91] Chang liver cells,[77] opsonized bacteria or bacteria with Gal/GalNAc-containing lipopolysaccharide,[92] and rat colonic epithelial cells.[88] Ravdin et al.[93] produced monoclonal antibodies that inhibited amebic adherence to CHO cells. By using the lectin's carbohydrate-binding activity and lectin-specific monoclonal antibodies, Petri et al.[52] recently isolated the *E. histolytica* Gal/GalNAc adherence lectin. A chitotriose-inhibitable lectin present in a homogenate of *E. histolytica* was originally described by Kobiler and Mirelman.[94] This 220 kD erythrocyte-agglutinating lectin was recently purified; monoclonal antibodies raised to this lectin partially inhibited amebic erythrophagocytosis or adherence to monolayers of Madin-Darby canine kidney (MDCK) cells in vitro.[95,96]

Axenic *E. histolytica* trophozoites kill target cells only upon direct contact and not via secreted cytotoxins.[87,97] Adherence mediated by the Gal/GalNAc lectin is absolutely required for the in vitro lysis of target cells.[75,87] The death of a target cell may occur up to 20 minutes after amebic adherence; a lethal hit can be delivered within seconds by a trophozoite.[97,98] Amebic cytolytic activity is dependent on parasite microfilament function,[87,97] calcium,[98,99] Ca^{2+}-dependent parasite phospholipase A (PLA) enzyme activity,[99,100] and maintenance of an acid pH in amebic endocytic vesicles.[101] Establishment of adherence by *E. histolytica* trophozoites is followed by a marked sustained elevation of the target cell-free intracellular calcium concentration ($[Ca^{2+}]_i$), which contributes to but may not be totally sufficient for target cell death.[98] The purified *E. histolytica* Gal/GalNAc lectin is a cytotoxin that induces rapid increases in target cell $[Ca^{2+}]_i$.[98] Phorbol esters, tumor-promoting agents, and protein kinase C activators specifically augment parasite cytolytic activity.[102] *E. histolytica* contains an ionophore-like protein of 13–15 kD by sodium dodecyl sulfate–polyacrylamide gel electrophoresis (SDS-PAGE) that induces lipid bilayers or vesicles to leak Na^+, K^+, and to a lesser extent Ca^{2+}.[103,104] This ionophore is packaged within amebae in dense intracellular aggregates, and purified preparations can depolarize erythrocytes.[105,106] Although suggested, there is as yet no evidence that this pore-forming protein directly participates in parasite cytolysis of target cells.

Entamoeba histolytica contains numerous proteolytic enzymes, including a cathepsin B proteinase,[107] an acidic proteinase,[108] a collagenase,[109] and a recently purified major neutral proteinase.[110] Proteinases appear to be involved in dissolution of the extracellular matrix anchoring cells and tissue structure.[110] Amebic glycosidases, such as β-glucosaminidase[111] and a surface membrane-associated neuraminidase[112] may be involved in the degradation of colonic mucins or alteration of target cell surface membrane glycoproteins. *Entamoeba histolytica* sonicate or whole trophozoites can demonstrate enterotoxigenic activity[113–115]; a secretory component may contribute to the diarrheal symptoms observed in intestinal amebiasis.

In vivo models of amebic liver abscess[76] and recent in vitro studies[77] demonstrate that host polymorphonuclear leukocytes constitute the initial host response to *E. histolytica*. Neutrophils demonstrate chemotaxis to amebae,[116] but as mentioned their lysis by *E. histolytica* enhances host tissue destruction. A further understanding of the biochemical and molecular basis for the pathogenicity of *E. histolytica* should aid in the development of a vaccine or pharmacologic strategies to combat this disease.

HOST IMMUNITY

Extensive but anecdotal evidence indicates that cure of amebic colitis or liver abscess is followed by resistance to subsequent invasive amebiasis.[117,118] Serum antibody and coproantibody levels have been demonstrated to increase during invasive disease.[119,120] A protective role for humoral immunity is suggested by the almost universal presence of antibody to the parasite's 170 kD adherence lectin subunit in sera of patients cured of invasive amebiasis.[121] Human immune sera can prevent amebic in vitro adherence[121] despite the parasite's ability to aggregate and shed attached antibodies.[122] In addition to the Gal/GalNAc lectin, the parasite antigens most frequently recognized by human immune sera include 37, 59, and 90 kD glycoproteins[123]; these may be useful for the development of diagnostic tests and vaccines. Production of mucosal anti-amebic IgA antibodies has not been studied. Whether asymptomatic intestinal colonization by *E. histolytica* elicits a protective host immunity response is unknown. Recently, Ravdin et al.[55] demonstrated by immunoblotting anti-amebic antibodies in sera from individuals with asymptomatic infection caused by *E. histolytica* expressing "nonpathogenic" zymodemes. Therefore, as with *Giardia lamblia*,[124] a host antibody response elicited by luminal infection may be responsible for elimination of the parasite and subsequent resistance to reinfection.

Serum from both healthy controls and infected patients (with high antibody titers to *E. histolytica*) are amebicidal to trophozoites through activation of the alternate and classic complement pathways.[125,126] However, amebae isolated from a liver abscess or colonic lesions are resistant to complement-mediated lysis[127]; complement-resistant amebae can be selected in vitro by culture in normal human serum.[128] Complement components are absent from mucosal surfaces; it is unclear, therefore, whether complement plays any role in the prevention of the initial amebic invasion of the colonic mucosa.

Cell-mediated immune defense mechanisms probably have a role in limiting invasive disease and resisting a recurrence after pharmacologic cure. The cell-mediated response consists of antigen-specific lymphocyte blastogenesis with production of lymphokines (including γ-interferon) capable of activating monocyte-derived macrophages to kill *E. histolytica* trophozoites in vitro.[90,129] In addition, in vitro incubation of immune T cells with *E. histolytica* antigen for 5 days elicits cytotoxic T-lymphocyte activity against *E. histolytica* trophozoites.[130] However, in acute disease the T-lymphocyte response to *E. histolytica* may be specifically depressed by a parasite-induced serum factor.[131] The lack of an increased incidence of severe invasive amebiasis in AIDS patients[45] suggests that host resistance to the initial amebic invasion of the colonic mucosa does not involve cell-mediated mechanisms. Clinical correlations of the severity of established invasive disease with cell-mediated immune function include the depression of T-cell numbers and cell-mediated immunity in patients with an amebic liver abscess,[132,133] numerous reports of severe exacerbation of intestinal amebiasis with the occurrence of toxic megacolon during corticosteroid therapy,[134,135] and the fulminant amebic disease in young infants and pregnant women.[66,67,136]

Nonimmune host defenses may be most important in resistance to symptomatic invasive amebiasis. In animal models, mucus trapping of *E. histolytica* trophozoites occurs,[137] and depletion of the colonic mucus blanket is always seen before parasite invasion.[138] Chadee et al. demonstrated that purified rat and human colonic mucins, rich in Gal/GalNAc residues, act as high-affinity receptors for the *E. histolytica* Gal/GalNAc adherence lectin.[88,139] Colonic mucins inhibit amebic adherence to and lysis of colonic epithelial cells in vitro.[88] Therefore, colonic mucin glycoproteins act as an important host defense by binding to the parasite's adherence lectin; however, this interaction probably facilitates intestinal colonization, thus promoting parasitism by *E. histolytica*.

CLINICAL MANIFESTATIONS

The clinical syndromes associated with *E. histolytica* infection are summarized in Table 2; familiarity with these diverse manifestations and epidemiologic risk factors greatly facilitates a rapid, correct diagnosis.

Intestinal Disease

Noninvasive intestinal infection is established by a lack of hematophagous trophozoites, hemoccult-negative stools, and normal mucosa on colonoscopy. Previously, many authorities considered that the presence of serum anti-amebic antibodies signified current or prior invasive amebiasis, but recent studies contradict that assumption.[27,55,140] Patients with noninvasive luminal infection frequently manifest nonspecific gastrointestinal complaints, the etiology of which is difficult to determine.[32] Symptoms such as colicky lower abdominal pain and increased frequency of bowel movements with liquid stools are common and may be intermittent and chronic in nature. We do not have a truly controlled prospective study evaluating the outcome and clinical significance of "noninvasive" amebiasis. In New Delhi, India, a highly endemic area, Nanda et al.[32] studied a selected population of 184 patients who were referred, because of intestinal complaints, to a gastroenterology clinic. Because the total prevalence of symptoms was so high (42 percent with diarrhea), it was not surprising that there was no correlation between a positive stool culture for *E. histolytica* (found in 18.7 percent) and symptoms. Although not statistically significant, 29.4 percent of those infected with *E. histolytica* had an abnormal histology on rectal biopsy as compared with only 9.7 percent in the noninfected group. Both groups had an equal percentage of anti-amebic antibodies detected by standard methods. Fifteen infected patients were followed in the clinic for a mean of 8.6 months, and all spontaneously cleared their infection. However, it is difficult to rule out unknown use of anti-amebic drugs. Banerjee et al.[141] in a study of 167 individuals passing *E. histolytica* cysts found a substantial subsequent incidence of invasive colitis and liver abscess (4 of 69) during a follow-up period of up to 5 years. Jalan and coworkers[147] found that 6 percent of chronic cyst passers had invading trophozoites detected on colonic biopsy. Because most colonized patients studied by Jalan's group have *E. histolytica* antigen, anti-amebic antibodies, or immune complexes in serum, it is debatable whether truly innocuous noninvasive colonization by *E. histolytica* occurs in the highly endemic areas of the developing world.

The presentation of invasive intestinal disease due to *E. histolytica* has been recently reviewed.[22] The signs and symptoms of acute amebic rectocolitis as reported in two large series are summarized in Table 3. Its onset is usually gradual over 1–3

TABLE 2. Clinical Syndromes Associated with *E. histolytica* Infection

Intestinal disease
Asymptomatic infection
Symptomatic noninvasive infection
Acute rectocolitis (dysentery)
Fulminant colitis with perforation
Toxic megacolon
Chronic nondysenteric colitis
Ameboma
Perianal ulceration
Extraintestinal disease
Liver abscess
Liver abscess complicated by:
Peritonitis
Empyema
Pericarditis
Lung abscess
Brain abscess
Genitourinary disease

TABLE 3. Clinical Presentation of Acute Amebic Rectocolitis

Signs and Symptoms	Adams & MacLeod[143] (1958–1972)	Juniper[144] (1957–1962)
Number of cases	3013	55
History <4 weeks	85%	71%
Onset	Gradual	Gradual
Abdominal pain	85%	NA
Diarrhea	100	94
Dysentery	99	94
Weight loss	NA	44
Fever	38	36
Abdominal tenderness	83	12
Heme (+)	All	100
Case fatality	1.9%	9.1% (females, twice that of males)
Uncomplicated	0.5%	NA

Abbreviation: NA: not available.

weeks; in addition to the occurrence of abdominal pain, tenderness, and bloody stools, it is important to note that only one-third of patients are febrile. The liver may be enlarged and exhibit percussion tenderness. When diarrhea is marked, the secondary signs of fluid loss and electrolyte imbalance are observed.[145]

Amebic colitis can affect all age groups and both sexes equally. A key differential point is that virtually all patients have heme-positive stools.[145] Especially in children, colitis can present as rectal bleeding alone without evidence of diarrhea.[146,147] Fecal leukocytes may not be present and are in reduced numbers when compared with patients with shigellosis,[148] presumably due to the ability of amebic trophozoites to lyse human neutrophils.[74,75] Charcot-Leyden crystals are often seen in the stool.

Fulminant colitis is an infrequent presentation of amebic infection that has a very high mortality and a predisposition for occurring in the malnourished,[149] pregnant women,[66] recipients of corticosteroids,[134,135] or the very young.[67,145,150,151] Such patients are severely ill with fever, leukocytosis, profuse bloody mucoid diarrhea, and widespread abdominal pain and are often hypotensive with signs of peritoneal irritation.[66,67,135,147,150,152] Fulminant colitis is often associated with liver abscess; segmental or total necrotic involvement of the colon is frequently present and may necessitate total colectomy and result in a fatal outcome despite anti-amebic and supportive therapy. Single or multiple colonic perforations occur in over 75 percent of cases of fulminant colitis.[150] Intestinal perforation usually presents as a slow leakage rather than an acute event; it is unclear whether surgical intervention is beneficial because attempts to suture such necrotic bowels are usually fruitless.[153]

Toxic megacolon is a well-described complication of acute amebic colitis, occurs in 0.5 percent of cases, and is a definite complication of inappropriate corticosteroid therapy.[154] Recognition is important since these patients do not respond to drug therapy and require colectomy.

Ameboma may be manifested as an annular lesion of the colon that is indistinguishable from colonic carcinoma[150,155] or as a extrahepatic tender palpable mass suggesting a pyogenic abscess. Lesions may be single or multiple and are most common in the cecum and ascending colon. Serum anti-amebic antibodies are usually present in this form of amebiasis; in an endemic area this study should be performed before the surgeon explores the abdomen of such a patient.

Intestinal amebiasis can occur as a chronic nondysenteric syndrome. This was well documented in a series of 159 patients from Pakistan in which most patients had symptoms for more than 1 year (37 percent persisted more than 5 years) that consisted of intermittent diarrhea, mucus, abdominal pain, flatulence, and weight loss.[156] These people have less colonic inflammation and smaller ulcers than do those with inflammatory bowel disease; they have amebae in their stool and serum anti-amebic antibodies, and they respond to anti-amebic drug therapy.[156] Chronic amebic infection may be misdiagnosed as inflammatory bowel disease with potentially disastrous consequences if corticosteroid therapy is begun. Examination of stools and serologic tests for amebic infection should be performed before a diagnosis of idiopathic inflammatory bowel disease is made.[157]

A chronic, irritative bowel syndrome may also follow acute amebic colitis. This illness usually subsides spontaneously. A more serious but similar illness is that referred to as ulcerative postdysenteric colitis.[145] Fortunately, this is not common. It has a pattern similar to ulcerative colitis, with recurrent signs and symptoms of mucus and bloody diarrhea that is unresponsive to anti-amebic therapy, but is associated with high antibody titers against *E. histolytica*. Occasionally this can be manifested as a granulomatous colitis with fistula formation.

Perianal amebiasis may result from extension of severe bowel disease to the skin and results from previous trauma or underlying pathology of the squamous epithelium or is due to fistulous tracts.[158] Lesions can be ulcerative or condylomatous, slowly enlarge over weeks to months, and result in pain and bleeding. Trophozoites are found in the purulent exudate or on biopsy, and these lesions respond well to anti-amebic therapy.

Extraintestinal Amebiasis

An amebic liver abscess can present concurrently with colitis, but more frequently there is no evidence or history of recent intestinal infection by *E. histolytica*,[143] which suggests another risk associated with apparent asymptomatic infection. In a study of 103 residents of Germany with amebic liver abscesses after exposure in endemic areas around the world, 95 percent presented with liver abscesses within 2 to 5 months (median of 3 months) after leaving the endemic area.[159]

Liver abscess can present with an acute onset (less than 10 days) with abdominal pain and fever or subacutely with weight loss prominent and less than half having fever or abdominal pain.[59,143,160–165] Concomitant diarrhea occurs in 30–40 percent of patients; amebae are present in stool even less frequently.[59,143] Abdominal pain is usually localized to the right upper quadrant but can be referred to the shoulder and accompanied by a nonproductive cough.[59,143,162,163] On physical examination there is exquisite point tenderness over the liver,[143] hepatomegaly is present in less than half, dullness and rales at the right lung base are common, and peritoneal signs or jaundice is unusual.[143,160–165] The presence of diffuse peritonitis or a pericardial friction rub indicates extension of the infection beyond the liver and increased mortality.

Laboratory findings include leukocytosis without eosinophilia in 80 percent, mild anemia in more than half, elevated alkaline phosphatase levels in 80 percent, elevated transaminase levels in more aggressive disease, and a high erythrocyte sedimentation rate.[59,143,160–165] Serum cholesterol and albumin concentrations have been noted to be decreased in the majority of patients; hyperbilirubinemia is uncommon and present in the setting of severe disease or peritonitis.[59,143,160–165] Urinalysis frequently has abnormal findings in acute disease with proteinuria common.[59]

Pleuropulmonary amebiasis is the most common complication of amebic liver abscess, usually due to the rupture of a superior right lobe abscess with erosion through the diaphragm to involve the pleural space or lung parenchyma.[143,166] Serous pleural effusion and atelectasis are common accompaniments of liver abscesses and do not indicate extension of disease.[59,143] Patients with pleuropulmonary complications present with cough, pleuritic pain, and dyspnea.[167–169] Empyema due to a rupture of the abscess into the pleural cavity presents with sudden respiratory distress and pain and has a substantial associated mortality (15–35 percent).[167,169] Involvement of lung parenchyma may be by direct or hematogenous extension from the liver. Formation of a hepatobronchial fistula is not uncommon and has been associated with spontaneous cure. The sputum contains large amounts of necrotic material with amebae often demonstrable.[167–169]

Intraperitoneal rupture of liver abscesses occurs in 2–7 percent,[143] with sudden perforation associated with a high mortality.[170] Left lobe abscesses are more likely to progress to rupture due to their later clinical presentation.[143] Such febrile patient with a rigid distended abdomen may suggest an erroneous assumption of a perforated viscus. Pericardial amebiasis is an unusual but serious complication of liver abscesses. Although acute perforation with cardiac tamponade and shock can occur, the usual course is that of fever and abdominal pain progressing to substantial chest pain with signs of congestive heart failure.[143,171] A correct diagnosis is usually dependent on the physician's consideration of the liver as the original source of infection.

Cerebral amebiasis is a rare cause of brain abscess; unfortunately, the onset is abrupt, with rapid progression to death over a period of 12–72 hours without adequate therapy.[172] Amebic brain abscesses must be considered in patients with known amebiasis and alteration of mental states or focal signs; on head computerized tomography (CT scan) the lesions appear irregular without a capsule or surrounding enhancement.[173,174] The diagnosis is made directly by examining tissue for amebic trophozoites; medical therapy with metronidazole and surgical decompression for increased intracranial pressure have improved the outcome of cerebral amebiasis.[172–175]

Genitourinary amebiasis is rare; rectovaginal fistulas in females can result in the spread of *E. histolytica* trophozoites to the genitourinary tract.[176,177] Genital disease presents with painful granulation tissue or ulcers; malignancy is often suspected, and diagnosis is again made by biopsy. Penile amebiasis can result via acquisition from vaginal or anal intercourse.[178,179] Medical therapy without surgery is adequate.[180]

DIAGNOSIS

Intestinal Amebiasis

The diagnosis of intestinal amebiasis is made by identifying *E. histolytica* in the stool. The finding of either trophozoites or cysts confirms the diagnosis of intestinal infection. Substances that interfere with the stool examination should be avoided if possible; these include barium, bismuth, antimicrobials such as tetracycline or erythromycin, antacids, laxatives, and soap or hypertonic enemas.[144] When a laboratory reports either trophozoites or cysts of *E. histolytica*, the physician should carefully review the patient's history, look for potential complications of amebic disease, and then treat the patient accordingly. Laboratories vary tremendously in their ability to diagnose amebiasis.[25] The success of identifying amebas depends on which techniques for identifying trophozoites are used, whether fixed and stained material is examined, whether concentration techniques are used to find cysts, the average specimen load on the laboratory, and the turnover rate of technicians. The best approaches for evaluating stool specimens for amebae are as follows:

1. A specimen obtained during endoscopy should be examined by direct mount in saline of a warm microscope stage for motile, erythrocyte-containing amebae. A small amount of liquid from an area of inflamed bowel is aspirated with a pipette passed through the sigmoidoscope. Liquid stool arriving in the laboratory within 30 minutes after passage can be examined by wet mount in a similar manner. The characteristic motility is that of a directed, linear movement across the microscope stage. Scraping of the ulcer edge or biopsy has a very high yield.
2. Fresh stool specimens should either be smeared and stained with iron hematoxylin or Wheatley trichrome stain or remain fixed in polyvinyl alcohol for later staining (Figs. 1 and 3). This allows the best identification of hematophagous *E. histolytica* trophozoites, the characteristic sign of invasive colonic disease. The nuclear morphology of *E. histolytica*, such as the central position of the nucleolus and the fine peripheral chromatic pattern, is key to differentiate it from commensals such as *Entamoeba coli*.
3. Stool specimens are suspended, after a 6% formalin wash and centrifugation, in formalin–ethyl acetate (9 ml 10% formalin, 3 ml ethyl acetate) to allow concentration of *E. histolytica* cysts at the bottom of the tube after centrifugation.[181] A drop of the sediment is then examined with a drop of dilute iodine solution (1–2% iodine in distilled water) to enhance the morphologic features of the cysts (Fig. 3).
4. Since a single stool examination picks up only one-third of infected patients, at least three specimens should be submitted before excluding the diagnosis of amebiasis.[21,23] A saline-purged specimen may increase the likelihood of diagnosis with less than three specimens. A careful study of whether stool culture for *E. histolytica* would decrease the need for multiple specimens has not been performed, and such cultures are generally not used in clinical practice. Culture media used are not selective for different species of intestinal amebae, and skilled microscopy is still required to determine species identity. Stool culture may be a helpful diagnostic tool in chronic or asymptomatic colonic syndromes with low levels of cyst passage, especially to evaluate the efficacy of cure or the existence of infection when the presence or absence of serum anti-amebic antibodies is not definitive.

Endoscopy with scraping or biopsy is a valuable technique for the diagnostic evaluation of patients with diarrhea and suspected amebiasis[181,182] (Table 4). Amebic colitis is manifested as punctuate hemorrhagic areas or small ulcers (a few millimeters to centimeters in diameter) with exudative centers and hyperemic borders.[182] Rarely, large confluent ulcers are seen. The mucosa may be hyperemic and edematous due to the inflammatory process, and pseudomembranous changes can be present. In the early stage of the disease endoscopy may be normal; therefore, amebiasis should not be excluded on this basis. In addition, disease may be localized to the cecum or ascending colon and be seen only by total colonoscopy.[150,183]

Serologic studies are very helpful in the diagnosis of invasive intestinal amebiasis.[184] Asymptomatic cyst passers usually have negative results by standard serologic methods. Eighty-five percent of the patients with biopsy-proven invasive intestinal amebiasis have serum anti-amebic antibodies as determined by various techniques.[184,185] Indirect hemagglutination (IHA) anti-amebic antibody titers remain elevated ($\geq$1:128) for years after invasive disease. Other studies such as counterimmunoelectrophoresis and gel diffusion precipitation become negative after cure of invasive disease and are helpful in the diagnosis of active amebiasis in an endemic area.[184] It is most important to check an amebic serology in patients with presumed idiopathic inflammatory bowel disease because a false-positive IHA is not seen in this situation.[186]

There is a broad differential diagnosis in patients presenting with a clinical syndrome consistent with intestinal amebiasis. In patients who excrete *E. histolytica* cysts and have nonspecific and episodic abdominal complaints such as bloating,

TABLE 4. Indications for Endoscopy with Biopsy or Scrapings in a Patient with a Clinical Syndrome and Risk Factors Consistent with Amebiasis

Stool exam (−), (+) serology
Stool exam (−), immediate diagnosis required
Stool exam (−), (−) serology, high suspicion
Chronic syndromes or mass lesions

(From Ravdin,[22] with permission.)

cramps, and increased frequency of stools, the differential diagnosis includes giardiasis, viral gastroenteritis, enterotoxigenic *E. coli* infection, *Campylobacter* infection, *Salmonella* infection, cryptosporidiosis, isosporiasis, malabsorption syndromes, and functional bowel disease. Patients with acute amebic rectocolitis need to be differentiated from those with shigellosis, campylobacteriosis, *Salmonella* colitis, or infection with invasive vibrios, *Yersinia enterocolitica*, or invasive *E. coli* strains.[148,151] The most difficult distinction is the differentiation of amebiasis from an acute exacerbation of inflammatory bowel disease.[157] A complete history with attention to epidemiologic risk factors, stool Gram stain (using carbol fuchsin for *Campylobacter*), and examination of stool for amebae are immediately useful. Appropriate culture of stool for bacterial pathogens and obtaining an amebic serology, both of which usually take a few days to obtain results, can be definitive. Immediate endoscopy is recommended if the stool examination is negative and amebic colitis is suspected. A relative contraindication to endoscopy would be patients with fulminant colitis and toxic megacolon in which there is a substantial risk of intestinal perforation during endoscopy. Patients with chronic nondysenteric amebiasis, which can be easily mistaken for inflammatory bowel disease, have serum anti-amebic antibody and amebae present in colonic biopsy specimens.[141,156] Amebiasis must also be differentiated from other localized processes such as carcinoma, lymphoma, tuberculosis, regional enteritis, or *Yersinia* infection. Toxic megacolon is a not infrequent complication of inflammatory bowel disease. Ruling out colitis due to *E. histolytica* is imperative because corticosteroid therapy will exacerbate colonic amebiasis.

Extraintestinal Amebiasis

The diagnosis of amebic liver abscess, pending serologic results, is based on the clinical presentation and recognition of epidemiologic risk factors, a lack of predisposing conditions for pyogenic liver abscess (such as biliary disease, prior appendicitis), and early use of noninvasive imaging studies.

Most important is the performance of an imaging technique to evaluate for the presence of a hepatic lesion. In one study of 75 patients in an endemic area who presented with fever, right upper quadrant pain, nausea, and vomiting, 9 of the 75 had a liver abscess detected by hepatic sonography and hepatobiliary scans, and all were due to *E. histolytica*.[162] These patients were clinically indistinguishable from those with cholecystitis except for their younger age (less than 45 years).[162,163] Imaging techniques available to establish the presence of cystic liver lesions include ultrasound, ^{99m}Tc liver scan, CT scan, magnetic resonance imaging (MRI) scan, and ^{67}Ga scan.[187] None of these methods are absolutely specific in differentiating an amebic liver abscess from a pyogenic abscess or tumor.[188] Sonography is rapid, low in cost, and only slightly less sensitive than is liver or CT scan; simultaneously evaluates the gallbladder; and lacks radiation exposure.[187,188] Liver scans have been used successfully to diagnose amebic liver abscesses in many series[59] but have generally given way to the CT scan in examination of hepatic abnormalities.[189] The CT scan is sensitive but not specific for amebic liver abscess[187–189] (Fig. 5). The use of injected contrast material may help differentiate hepatic abscesses from vascular tumors, an important point if liver aspiration is being contemplated. MRI scans are sensitive in the detection of amebic liver abscess but are no more specific than is older, less costly technology.[190,191] Due to the delay in imaging, gallium scans are not as helpful except if there is uncertainty in regard to pyogenic vs. amebic abscess. Amebic liver abscesses do not contain leukocytes and therefore appear on gallium scans as cold areas, possibly having a "hot" rim. In contrast, a pyogenic abscess presents as an area of increased isotope concentration.[187]

The presence of serum anti-amebic antibodies is often the definitive study in the diagnosis of amebic liver abscess; such antibodies are present in up to 99 percent of patients.[57,59,60,143,165] One pitfall is in patients with an acute presentation of less than 7 days: serologic studies may be negative.[59] If the diagnosis is still in question, a repeat serology 5–7 days later should be positive.

The differential diagnosis for a cystic lesion in the liver that is accompanied by the signs, symptoms, and laboratory abnormalities seen in an amebic liver abscess might also include pyogenic abscess, echinococcal cyst, and hepatoma. Although older studies emphasize that an amebic liver abscess presents as a single large lesion in the right lobe of the liver, recent studies using modern imaging technology demonstrate a high frequency of multiple lesions.[59,187,191] Epidemiologic risk factors, serologic studies, and the presence of calcification will aid in the diagnosis of echinococcal disease. If an amebic or pyogenic etiology cannot be differentiated on clinical grounds and the patient is not stable enough to await serologic studies, liver aspiration with a "skinny needle" under CT or ultrasound guidance should be performed.[192,193] Aspiration of an amebic liver abscess yields a sterile, odorless, brown or yellow liquid with amebae detected on microscopy in the minority of cases. A culture of abscess fluid for *E. histolytica* may be helpful; however, most amebae are in the "wall" of the abscess, and the yield of a culture can be low. Aspiration of a pyogenic abscess is both diagnostic and therapeutic.[160,161] The main risk of aspiration in all cases is peritoneal spillage; amebic peritonitis complicating a liver abscess markedly increases mortality. In addition, aspiration of an echinococcal cyst is to be avoided due to the anaphylactic reaction and seeding with scolices that may accompany leakage into the peritoneum.

Most cases of amebic liver abscess can be diagnosed and treated without aspiration. In some cases antimicrobial therapy directed against enteric gram-negative organisms can be added to metronidazole, pending the results of serologic studies. Therapeutic trials of specific anti-amebic therapy can be helpful diagnostically; most patients will respond within 5 days with decreased pain and fever.[60] The liver abscess cavity usually resolves gradually over months, but persistent cystic lesions are not unusual.[194,195]

TREATMENT

Therapy for amebiasis has been complicated by a number of factors including (*1*) variation of drug effects at the three different sites of amebic replication: the lumen of the bowel, the intestinal submucosa, and extraintestinal sites (Table 5); (*2*) the availability of different drugs in different countries; and (*3*) the development of new drugs and differences of opinion about side effects and efficacy. For example, metronidazole for a 10-day course has been recommended by some as adequate for intestinal disease because the cure rate is 90 percent; others have used these same figures to suggest the use of several drugs because *only* 90 percent are cured.

It is controversial whether asymptomatic, apparently noninvasive *E. histolytica* infection merits therapy. Proponents of the stability of zymodeme analysis suggest that such individuals, especially male homosexuals, are at low risk for invasive disease or the transmission of a pathogenic organism to others and therefore need not be treated.[196,197] This is especially so in an endemic area or subpopulation with a potential high risk for reinfection. However, given the lack of stability of zymodeme expression,[7] the greater than previously appreciated exposure to *E. histolytica* antigens from such infections,[55,140,141] and the potential future occurrence of colitis or liver abscess,[141] we and others[198] presently recommend treatment of asymptomatic *E. histolytica* infection. *E. histolytica* infection should be eradicated in individuals coinfected or at risk for infection with HIV due to the potential stimulation of viral replication by the parasite's mitogenic adherence lectin.[51–53] Additional high-risk

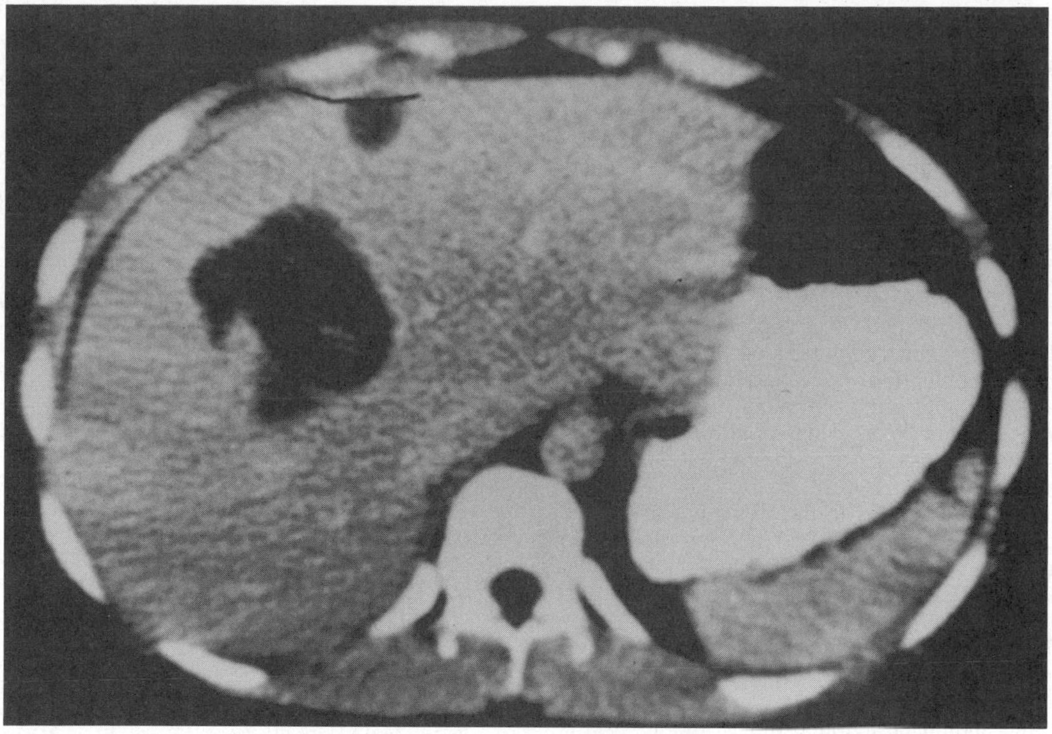

FIG. 5. Abdominal CT scan of a patient with an amebic liver abscess; the irregular multiple defects present in the right lobe of the liver cannot be differentiated from a pyogenic abscess or hepatocellular carcinoma.

TABLE 5. Antimicrobial Agents for Use in Treating Amebiasis

Luminal agents
Diloxanide furoate
Paromomycin
Diiodohydroxyquin
Tissue agents
Bowel wall only
Tetracycline
Erythromycin
Liver only
Chloroquine
All tissues
Metronidazole
Tinidazole
Emetine hydrochloride
2-Dehydroemetine

TABLE 6. Therapeutic Regimens for the Treatment of Amebiasis[a]

Type	*Efficacy (%)*
Cyst passers	
Diloxanide furoate, 500 mg tid for 10 days	87–96
Paromomycin, 30 mg/kg/day in 3 divided doses for 5–10 days	85–90
Tetracycline, 250 mg qid for 10 days, then diiodohydroxyquin, 650 mg tid for 20 days	95
Metronidazole, 750 mg tid for 10 days	90
Invasive rectocolitis	
Metronidazole, 750 mg tid for 5–10 days	>90
Or 2.4 g qd for 2–3 days	>90
Or 50 mg/kg × 1 dose	86
Plus diloxanide furoate or paromomycin	
Tetracycline, 250 mg qid for 15 days, plus chloroquine (base), 600 mg, 300 mg, then 150 mg tid for 14 days	94
Dehydroemetine, 1–1.5 mg/kg/day for 5 days plus diloxanide furoate or paromomycin	90
Liver abscess	
Metronidazole, 750 mg tid for 5–10 days or 2.4 mg qd for 1–2 days plus diloxanide furoate or paromomycin	95
Dehydroemetine, 1–1.5 mg/kg/day for 5 days plus diloxanide furoate or paromomycin	90
Chloroquine (base), 600 mg qd for 2 days, 300 mg base qd for 2–3 weeks (can be added to other regimens)	60

[a] All dosages are for oral administration except dehydroemetine, which is administered intramuscularly; metronidazole can be used intravenously.

groups include nonimmune travelers, malnourished individuals,[149,151] pregnant women,[66] the very young,[67,136,199] and patients being administered corticosteroids.[134,135] In addition, patients cured of luminal amebic infection could be at least partially resistant to reinfection; this has not been adequately studied.

The following recommendations (summarized in Table 6) for treating amebiasis are a synthesis of opinions, with emphasis on the easiest, safest, and most effective combination likely to give maximum cure rates with a single course of therapy. Follow-up stool examination is always necessary because no regimen is completely effective in eradicating intestinal infection. Slightly different treatment regimens in addition to drug toxicities are also summarized in a recent *Medical Letter*.[200]

Intraluminal infection should be treated with diloxanide furoate, 500 mg three times a day for 10 days[201] (this drug is available through the Centers for Disease Control). Paromomycin alone is also an effective treatment of intraluminal infection[202,203] and has the advantage of being a nonabsorbable agent.[204] Diiodohydroxyquin is in limited supply in the United States at present.

Symptomatic amebiasis involving the intestine should be treated with a nitroimidazole (metronidazole or tinidazole [not available in the United States]).[60,143,145,205,206] Metronidazole is administered in a dose of 750 mg three times a day for 5–10 days. This dose of metronidazole causes nausea and abdominal discomfort in a number of patients, but most can successfully complete the course of therapy. Therapy using 2.4 g/day for 2 days has also been reported to be effective in a small number of patients[207]; there is more extensive experience with single-dose therapy using tinidazole.[208] In view of the side effects, which often begin on the second or third day, this short course may be more palatable to the patient. Metronidazole therapy should be followed by an agent known to eradicate the intraluminal encysted organism (Table 6).

Extraintestinal amebiasis should be treated with metronidazole and, to prevent continued intraluminal infection, paromomycin or diloxanide furoate. In patients who are seriously ill due to complications of amebic infection such as peritonitis or a ruptured amebic abscess, many physicians add parenteral emetine for the first few days (a total of two or three doses once a day, 65 mg/dose). This provides the rapid amebicidal action of emetine with a low incidence of cardiotoxicity; however, there is no published evidence of anti-amebic synergy when using these agents in combination. Because of the few cases of incomplete therapy with metronidazole alone, the addition of chloroquine, 600 mg base/day for 2–3 days followed by 300 mg base/day for 2–3 weeks, can be considered but is usually unnecessary.

The role of invasive procedures in the treatment of amebic abscesses has been an area of debate. Needle aspiration of the liver is a safe procedure in experienced hands,[143] but in most patients it is unnecessary for the relief of symptoms.[59,60,192] Approximately 10–15 percent of patients, however, are sufficiently ill to consider reducing the size of the abscess before a full therapeutic response is observed. In these patients, needle aspiration is helpful and indicated.[143,192] Open surgical drainage is not necessary and should be avoided unless the abscess is inaccessible to needle drainage and response to therapy has not occurred in 4 or 5 days. Surgical attempts to correct amebic bowel perforation or peritonitis should be avoided, although some patients may benefit from peritoneal lavage.[209] Once a surgeon has performed a laparotomy on a patient with acute abdominal pain of unknown cause and found the damaged bowel of amebiasis, the temptation is to resect it. This is almost always unsuccessful. The surgeon would be better advised simply to obtain confirmatory specimens for examination and bacterial culture and to rely on anti-protozoal and anti-bacterial agents to control the infection. Maintaining drainage of the peritoneum plus antimicrobial therapy is optimal treatment. Maximum supportive care including meticulous fluid and electrolyte balance is essential in the seriously ill patient.

PREVENTION

Amebic infection is prevented by eradicating fecal contamination of food and water. The most commonly contaminated foods are fresh, ground-grown vegetables such as lettuce. Water is always a prime source of spread of infection. Amebae are not killed by low doses of chlorine or iodine; therefore, simply relying on halide tablets in water as a means of preventing amebic infection is not adequate. Only boiling of water ensures the absence of amebae. Vegetables should be treated with a strong detergent soap and then soaked in acetic acid or vinegar for 10–15 minutes to ensure eradication of the cysts.

In general, in the tropics, unless the boiling of the water and preparation of vegetables has been personally observed, these sources of food and refreshment should be omitted. Even in the finest hotels and restaurants, those preparing the food or placing water in bottles for drinking are often not aware of the potential danger of infection to the nonimmune traveler. Improvement in waste disposal and water purification is the most important factor in reducing the risk of acquiring amebiasis.

Avoiding sexual practices that allow fecal-oral contact can prevent infection in the male homosexual population. At present, there is not a clear means to prevent infection in institutionalized individuals, especially the mentally retarded, although case identification, therapy, improved supervision, and hygiene may be beneficial. Studies of the pathogenesis of amebiasis and host immunity may eventually lead to an immunologic or pharmacologic means to prevent invasive amebic disease.

REFERENCES

1. Walsh JA. Prevalence of *Entamoeba histolytica* infection. In: Ravdin JI, ed. Amebiasis: Human Infection by *Entamoeba histolytica*. New York: Churchill Livingstone; 1988:93–105.
2. Ravdin JI, Pathogenesis of disease with *Entamoeba histolytica*. Studies of adherence toxins and contact-dependent cytolysis. Rev Infect Dis. 1986;8:247–60.
3. Salata RA, Ravdin JI. Review of the human immune mechanisms directed against *Entamoeba histolytica*. Rev Infect Dis. 1986;8:261–72.
4. Petri WA, Ravdin JI. Cytopathogenicity of *Entamoeba histolytica*. Eur J Epidemiol. 1987;3:123–36.
5. Sargeaunt PG, Williams JE, Grene JD. The differentiation of invasive and non-invasive *Entamoeba histolytica* by isoenzyme electrophoresis. Trans R Soc Trop Med Hyg. 1978;72:519–21.
6. Mirelman D, Bracha R, Chayen A, et al. *Entamoeba histolytica*: Effect of growth conditions and bacterial associates on isoenzyme patterns and virulence. Exp Parasitol. 1986;62:142–8.
7. Mirelman D, Bracha R, Wexler A, et al. Changes in isoenzyme patterns of a cloned culture of nonpathogenic *Entamoeba histolytica* during axenization. Infect Immun. 1986;54:827–32.
8. Mirelman D. Effect of culture conditions and bacterial associates on the zymodemes of *Entamoeba histolytica*. Parasitol Today. 1987;3:37–40.
9. Sargeaunt PG. The reliability of *Entamoeba histolytica* zymodemes in clinical diagnosis. Parisitol Today. 1987;3:40–3.
10. Losch FA. Massive development of amebas in the large intestine. Am J Trop Med Hyg. 1875;24:383–92.
11. Kean BY, Mott KE, Russel AJ. Tropical Medicine and Parasitology: Classic Investigations. Ithaca, NY: Cornell University Press; 1978.
12. Select Committee. Amebiasis outbreak in Chicago: Report of a special committee. JAMA. 1934;102:369.
13. LeMaistre CA, Sappenfield R, Culbertson C, et al. Studies of a water-borne outbreak of amebiasis: South Bend, Indiana. Am J Hyg. 1956;64:30–45.
14. Levine ND, Corliss JO, Cox FEG. A newly revised classification of the protozoa. J Protozool. 1980;27:37–58.
15. Miller JH, Swartzwelder JC, Deas JE. An electron microscopic study of *Entamoeba histolytica*. J Parasitol. 1961;47:577.
16. Sargeaunt PG. Zymodemes of *Entamoeba histolytica*. In: Ravdin JI, ed. Amebiasis: Human Infection by *Entamoeba histolytica*. New York: Churchill Livingstone; 1988:370–87.
17. Neal RA. Phylogeny: The relationship of *Entamoeba histolytica* to morphologically similar amebae of the four-nucleate cyst group. In: Ravdin JI, ed. Amebiasis: Human Infection by *Entamoeba histolytica*. New York: Churchill Livingstone; 1988:13–26.
18. Reeves RE, Bischoff JM. Classification of *Entamoeba* species by means of electrophoretic properties of amebal enzymes. J Parasitol. 1968;54:594–600.
19. Barker DC. Differentiation of *Entamoeba*. Patterns of nucleic acids and ribosomes during encystation and excystation. In: Van den Bossche H, ed. Biochemistry of Parasites and Host-Parasite Relationships. Amsterdam: Elsevier Biomedical; 1976:253.
20. Chayen A, Avron B, Nuchamowitz Y, et al. Appearance of sialoglycoproteins in encysting cells of *Entamoeba histolytica*. Infect Immun. 1988;56:673–81.
21. Walsh JA. Transmission of *Entamoeba histolytica* infection. In: Ravdin JI, ed. Amebiasis: Human Infection by *Entamoeba histolytica*. New York: Churchill Livingstone; 1988:106–19.
22. Ravdin JI. Intestinal disease caused by *Entamoeba histolytica*. In: Ravdin JI, ed. Amebiasis: Human Infection by *Entamoeba histolytica*. New York: Churchill Livingstone; 1988:495–510.
23. Healy GR. Diagnostic techniques for stool samples. In: Ravdin JI, ed. Amebiasis: Human Infection by *Entamoeba histolytica*. New York: Churchill Livingstone; 1988:635–49.
24. Mathur TN, Kaur J. The frequency of excretion of cysts of *Entamoeba histolytica* in known cases of non-dysenteric amoebic colitis based on 21 stool examinations. Indian J Med Res. 1973;61:330–4.
25. Krogstad DJ, Spencer HC, Healy GR, et al. Amebiasis: Epidemiologic studies in the United States, 1971–1974. Ann Intern Med. 1978;88:89–97.
26. Bray RS, Harris WG. The epidemiology of infection with *Entamoeba histolytica* in The Gambia, West Africa. Trans R Soc Trop Med Hyg. 1977;71:401–7.
27. Hossain MM, Ljungstrom I, Glass RI, et al. Amoebiasis and giardiasis in Bangladesh: Parasitological and serological studies. Trans R Soc Trop Med Hyg. 1983;77:552–4.
28. Gutierrez G, Ludlow A, Espinos G, et al. National serologic survey II. Search for antibodies against *Entamoeba histolytica* in Mexico. In: Proceedings of the International Conference on Amebiasis. Sepulveda B, Diamond LS, eds. Amebiasis. Mexico City: Instituto Mexicano del Seguro Social; 1976:609–18.
29. Abdel-Hafez MM, el-Kady N, Bolbol AS, et al. Prevalence of intestinal parasitic infections in Riyadh district, Saudi Arabia. Ann Trop Med Parasitol. 1986;80:631–4.
30. Jackson TFHG, Gathiram V, Simjee AE. Seroepidemiological study of an-

tibody responses to the zymodemes of *Entamoeba histolytica*. Lancet. 1985;1:716–9.
31. Jackson TFHG. *Entamoeba histolytica* cyst passers—to treat or not to treat (Editorial)? S Afr Med J. 1987;72:657–8.
32. Nanda R, Baveja U, Anand BS. *Entamoeba histolytica* cyst passers: Clinical features and outcome in untreated subjects. Lancet. 1984;2:301–3.
33. Gathiram V, Jackson TFHG. Frequency distribution of *Entamoeba histolytica* zymodemes in a rural South African population. Lancet. 1985;1:719–21.
34. Gathiram V, Jackson TFHG. A longitudinal study of asymptomatic carriers of pathogenic zymodemes of *Entamoeba histolytica*. S Afr Med J. 1987;72:669–72.
35. Thacker SB, Simpson S, Gordon TJ, et al. Parasitic disease control in a residential facility for the mentally retarded. Am J Public Health. 1979;69:1279–81.
36. Sexton DJ, Krogstad DJ, Spencer HC, et al. Amebiasis in a mental institution: Serologic and epidemiologic studies. Am J Epidemiol. 1974;100:414–23.
37. Petri WA, Ravdin JI. Amebiasis in institutionalized populations. In: Ravdin JI, ed. Amebiasis: Human Infection by *Entamoeba histolytica*. New York: Churchill Livingstone; 1988:576–81.
38. Thacker SB, Kimball AM, Wolfe M, et al. Parasitic disease control in a residential facility for the mentally retarded: Failure of selected isolation procedures. Am J Public Health. 1981;71:303.
39. Brooke MM. Epidemiology and control of amebiasis in institutions for the mentally retarded. Am J Ment Defic. 1963;68:187.
40. Kean BH, William DC, Luminais SK. Epidemic of amoebiasis and giardiasis in a biased population. Br J Vener Dis. 1979;55:375–8.
41. Quinn TC, Corey L, Chaffee RG, et al. The etiology of anorectal infections in homosexual men. Am J Med. 1981;71:395.
42. Phillips SC, Mildvan D, William DC, et al. Sexual transmission of enteric protozoa and helminths in a venereal-disease-clinic population. N Engl J Med. 1981;305:603–6.
43. Markell EK, Havens RF, Kuritsubo RA, et al. Intestinal protozoa in homosexual men of the San Francisco Bay area: Prevalence and correlates of infection. Am J Trop Med Hyg. 1984;33:239–45.
44. Ortega HB, Borchardt KA, Hamilton R, et al. Enteric pathogenic protozoa in homosexual men from San Francisco. Sex Transm Dis. 1983;11:59.
45. Druckman DA, Quinn TC. *Entamoeba histolytica* infection in homosexual men. In: Ravdin JI, ed. Amebiasis: Human Infection by *Entamoeba histolytica*. New York: Churchill Livingstone; 1988:563–75.
46. Peters CS, Sable R, Janda WM, et al. Prevalence of enteric parasites in homosexual patients attending an outpatient clinic. J Clin Microbiol. 1986;24:684–5.
47. Sorvillo FJ, Strassburg MA, Seidel J, et al. Amebic infections in asymptomatic homosexual men, lack of evidence of invasive disease. Am J Public Health. 1986;76:1137–9.
48. Smith PD, Lane HC, Gill VJ, et al. Intestinal infections in patients with the acquired immunodeficiency syndrome (AIDS): Etiology and response to therapy. Ann Intern Med. 1988;108:328–33.
49. Pape JW, Liautaud B, Thomas F, et al. Characteristics of the acquired immunodeficiency syndrome (AIDS) in Haiti. N Engl J Med. 1983;309:945–50.
50. Clumeck N, Sonnet J, Taelman H, et al. Acquired immunodeficiency syndrome in African patients. N Engl J Med. 1984;310:492–7.
51. Petri WA, Ravdin JI. Treatment of homosexual men infected with *Entamoeba histolytica* (Letter). N Engl J Med. 1986;315:393.
52. Petri WA, Smith RD, Schlesinger PH, et al. Isolation of the galactose-binding lectin which mediates the in vitro adherence of *Entamoeba histolytica*. J Clin Invest. 1987;80:1238–44.
53. Salata RA, Ravdin JI. The *N*-acetyl-D-galactosamine–inhibitable adherence lectin of *Entamoeba histolytica*. II. Mitogenicity for human lymphocytes. J Infect Dis. 1985;151:816–22.
54. Zagury D, Bernard J, Leonard R, et al. Long-term cultures of HTLV-III-infected T cells: A model of cytopathogenicity of T cell depletion in AIDS. Science. 1986;231:850–3.
55. Ravdin JI, Simjee AE, Petri WA, et al. Correlation of clinical status and zymodeme analysis with serum Western blot recognition of *Entamoeba histolytica* antigens (Abstract 176). Presented at the 36th Annual Meeting of the American Society of Tropical Medicine and Hygiene, Los Angeles, December 1, 1987.
56. Istre GR, Kriess K, Hopkins RS, et al. An outbreak of amebiasis spread by colonic irrigation at a chiropractic clinic. N Engl J Med. 1982;309:339–42.
57. Shabot JM, Patterson M. Amebic liver abscess: 1966–1976. Dig Dis. 1978;23:110.
58. Abuabara SF, Barrett JA, Hau T, et al. Amebic liver abscess. Arch Surg. 1982;117:239–44.
59. Katzenstein D, Rickerson V, Braude A. New concepts of amebic liver abscess derived from hepatic imaging, serodiagnosis, and hepatic enzymes in 67 consecutive cases in San Diego. Medicine (Baltimore). 1982;61:237–46.
60. Thompson JE Jr, Forlenza S, Verma R. Amebic liver abscess: A therapeutic approach. Rev Infect Dis. 1985;7:171–9.
61. Barnes PF, DeCock KM, Reynolds TN, et al. A comparison of amebic and pyogenic abscess of the liver. Medicine (Baltimore). 1987;66:472–83.
62. Thompson JE Jr, Glasser AJ. Amebic abscess of the liver. Diagnostic features. J Clin Gastroenterol. 1986;8:550–4.
63. Pearson RD, Hewlett EL. Amebiasis in travelers. In: Ravdin JI, ed. Amebiasis: Human Infection by *Entamoeba histolytica*. New York: Churchill Livingstone; 1988:556–62.
64. Pehrson PO. Amoebiasis in a non-endemic country. Scand J Infect Dis. 1983;15:207–14.
65. Merson MH, Morris GK, Sack DA, et al. Traveler's diarrhea in Mexico: A prospective study. N Engl J Med. 1976;294:1299.
66. Lewis EA, Antia AU. Amoebic colitis: Review of 295 cases. Trans R Soc Trop Med Hyg. 1969;63:633–8.
67. Fuchs G, Ruiz-Palacios G, Pickering LK. Amebiasis in the pediatric population. In: Ravdin JI, ed. Amebiasis: Human Infection by *Entamoeba histolytica*. New York: Churchill Livingstone; 1988:594–613.
68. Brandt H, Perez Tamayo R. Pathology of human amebaisis. Hum Pathol. 1970;1:351–85.
69. Griffin JL, Juniper K Jr. Ultrastructure of *Entamoeba histolytica* from human amebic dysentery. Arch Pathol. 1971;91:271–80.
70. Pittman FE, El-Hashimi WK, Pittman JC. Studies of human amebiasis. II. Light and electronmicroscopic observations of colonic mucosa and exudate in acute amebic colitis. Gastroenterology. 1973;65:588–603.
71. Takeuchi A, Phillips BP. Electron microscopic studies of experimental *Entamoeba histolytica* infection in the guinea pig. I. Penetration of the intestinal epithelium by trophozoites. Am J Trop Med Hyg. 1975;24:34–48.
72. Prathap K, Gilman R. The histopathology of acute intestinal amebiasis. Am J Pathol. 1970;60:229–39.
73. Chatgidakis CB. The pathology of hepatic amoebiasis as seen on the Witwatersrand. S Afr J Clin Sci. 1953;4:230.
74. Guerrant RL, Brush J, Ravdin JI, et al. Interaction between *Entamoeba histolytica* and human polymorphonuclear neutrophils. J Infect Dis. 1981;143:83–93.
75. Ravdin JI, Murphy CF, Salata RA, et al. The *N*-acetyl-D-galactosamine–inhibitable adherence lectin of *Entamoeba histolytica*. I. Partial purification and relation to amoebic virulence *in vitro*. J Infect Dis. 1985;151:804–15.
76. Tsutsumi V, Mena-Lopez R, Anaya-Velazquez F, et al. Cellular basis of experimental amebic liver abscess formation. Am J Pathol. 1984;117:81–91.
77. Salata RA, Ravdin JI. The interaction of human neutrophils and *Entamoeba histolytica* increases cytopathogenicity for liver cell monolayers. J Infect Dis. 1986;154:19–26.
78. Ravdin JI, Guerrant RL. A review of the parasite cellular mechanisms involved in the pathogenesis of amebiasis. Rev Infect Dis. 1982;4:1185–207.
79. Joyce MP, Ravdin JI. Pathology of human amebiasis. In: Ravdin JI, ed. Amebiasis: Human Infection by *Entamoeba histolytica*. New York: Churchill Livingstone; 1988:129–46.
80. Aikat BK, Bhusnurmath SR, Pal AK, et al. The pathology and pathogenesis of fatal hepatic amoebiasis: A study based on 79 autopsy cases. Trans R Soc Trop Med Hyg. 1979;73:188–92.
86. Gulati PD, Gupta DN, Chuttani HK. Amoebic liver abscess and disturbances of portal circulation. Am J Med. 1967;45:852–4.
82. Tandon BN, Tandon HD, Puri BK. An electron microscopic study of liver in hepatomegaly presumably caused by amebiasis. Exp Mol Pathol. 1975;22:118.
83. Ravdin JI. Pathogensis of amebiasis: An overview. In: Ravdin JI, ed. Amebiasis: Human Infection by *Entamoeba histolytica*. New York: Churchill Livingstone; 1988:166–75.
84. Diamond LS, Harlow DR, Cunnick CC. A new medium for the axenic cultivation of *Entamoeba histolytica* and other *Entamoeba*. Trans R Soc Trop Med Hyg. 1978;72:431–2.
85. Bracha R, Mirelman D. Virulence of *Entamoeba histolytica* trophozoites. J Exp Med. 1984;160:353–68.
86. Mirelman D. Ameba–bacterial relationship in amebiasis. In: Ravdin JI, ed. Amebiasis: Human Infection by *Entamoeba histolytica*. New York: Churchill Livingstone; 1988:351–69.
87. Ravdin JI, Guerrant RL. Role of adherence in cytopathogenic mechanisms of *Entamoeba histolytica*. J Clin Invest. 1981;68:1305–13.
88. Chadee K, Petri WA, Innes DJ, et al. Rat and human colonic mucins bind to and inhibit the adherence of lectin of *Entamoeba histolytica*. J Clin Invest. 1987;80:1245–54.
89. Ravdin JI, John JE, Johnston LI, et al. Adherence of *Entamoeba histolytica* trophozoites to rat and human colonic mucosa. Infect Immun. 1985;48:292–7.
90. Salata RA, Pearson RD, Ravdin JI. Interaction of human leukocytes with *Entamoeba histolytica*: Killing of virulent amebae by the activated macrophage. J Clin Invest. 1985;76:491–9.
91. Orozco ME, Rodriquez M, Murphy CF, et al. *Entamoeba histolytica*: Cytopathogenicity and lectin activity of avirulent mutants. Exp Parasitol. 1987;63:157–65.
92. Bracha R, Mirelman D. Adherence and ingestion of *Escherichia coli* serotype 055 by trophozoites of *Entamoeba histolytica*. Infect Immun. 1983;40:882–7.
93. Ravdin JI, Petri WA, Murphy CF, et al. Production of mouse monoclonal antibodies which inhibit in vitro adherence of *Entamoeba histolytica* trophozoites. Infect Immun. 1986;53:1–5.
94. Kobiler D, Mirelman D. Adhesion of *Entamoeba histolytica* trophozoites to monolayers of human cells. J Infect Dis. 1981;144:539–46.
95. Rosales-Encina JL, Meza I, Lopez-DeLeon A, et al. Isolation of a 220-kilodalton protein with lectin properties from a virulent strain of *Entamoeba histolytica*. J Infect Dis. 1987;156:790–7.
96. Meza I, Cacares F, Rosales-Encina JL, et al. Use of antibodies to charac-

terize a 220-kilodalton surface protein from *Entamoeba histolytica*. J Infect Dis. 1987;156:798–805.
97. Ravdin JI, Croft BY, Guerrant RL. Cytopathogenic mechanisms of *Entamoeba histolytica*. J Exp Med. 1980;152:377–90.
98. Ravdin JI, Moreau F, Sullivan JA, et al. The relationship of free intracellular calcium ions to the cytolytic activity of *Entamoeba histolytica*. Infect Immun. 1988;56:1505–12.
99. Ravdin JI, Murphy CF, Guerrant RL, et al. Effect of calcium and phospholipase A antagonists on the cytopathogenicity of *Entamoeba histolytica*. J Infect Dis. 1985;152:542–9.
100. Long-Krug SA, Hysmith RM, Fischer KJ, et al. The phospholipase A enzymes of *Entamoeba histolytica*: Description and subcellular localization. J Infect Dis. 1985;152:536–41.
101. Ravdin JI, Schlesinger PH, Murphy CF, et al. Acid intracellular vesicles and the cytolysis of mammalian target cells by *Entamoeba histolytica* trophozoites. J Protozool. 1986;33:478–86.
102. Weikel CS, Murphy CF, Orozco ME, et al. Phorbol esters specifically enhance the cytolytic activity of *Entamoeba histolytica*. Infect Immun. 1988;56:1485–91.
103. Young JE, Young TM, Lu LP, et al. Characterization of a membrane pore-forming protein from *Entamoeba histolytica*. J Exp Med. 1982;156:1677–90.
104. Lynch EC, Rosenberg IM, Gitler C. An ion-channel forming protein produced by *Entamoeba histolytica*. EMBO J. 1982;1:801–4.
105. Rosenberg I, Gitler C. Subcellular fractionation of amoebapore and plasma membrane components of *Entamoeba histolytica* using self-generating Percoll gradients. Mol Biochem Parasitol. 1985;14:231.
106. Young JD-E, Cohn ZA. Molecular mechanisms of cytotoxicity mediated by *Entamoeba histolytica*: Characterization of a pore-forming protein (PFP). J Cell Biochem. 1985;29:299–308.
107. Lushbaugh WB, Hofbauer AF, Kairalla AA, et al. Purification of cathepsin B activity of *Entamoeba histolytica* toxin. Exp Parasitol. 1985;59:328–36.
108. Scholze H, Werries E. A weakly acidic protease has a powerful proteolytic activity in *Entamoeba histolytica*. Mol Biochem Parasitol. 1984;11:293–300.
109. Muñoz MDL, Calderon J, Rojkind M. The collagenase of *Entamoeba histolytica*. J Exp Med. 1982;155:42–51.
110. Keene WE, Petitt MG, Allen S, et al. The major neutral proteinase of *Entamoeba histolytica*. J Exp Med. 1986;163:536–49.
111. Werries E, Nebinger P, Franz A. Degradation of biogene oligosaccharides by Beta-*N*-acetylglucosaminidase secreted by *Entamoeba histolytica*. Mol Biochem Parasitol. 1983;7:127–40.
112. Udezulu IA, Leitch GJ. A membrane-associated neuraminidase in *Entamoeba histolytica* trophozoites. Infect Immun. 1987;55:181–6.
113. Udezulu IA, Leitch GJ, Bailey GB. Use of indomethacin to demonstrate enterotoxic activity in extracts of *Entamoeba histolytica* trophozoites. Infect Immun. 1981;36:795–801.
114. McGowan K, Kane A, Asarkof N, et al. *Entamoeba histolytica* causes intestinal secretion: Role of serotonin. Science. 1983;221:762–4.
115. Feingold C, Bracha R, Wexler A, et al. Isolation, purification, and partial characterization of an enterotoxin from extracts of *Entamoeba histolytica* trophozoites. Infect Immun. 1985;48:211–8.
116. Salata RA, Ahmed P, Ravdin JI. *Entamoeba histolytica* contains a chemoattractant for human polymorphonuclear neutrophils. J Parasitol. 1988. In press.
117. Sepulveda B, Martinez-Palomo A. Immunology of amoebiasis by *Entamoeba histolytica*. In: Cohen S, Warren VS, eds. Immunology of Parasitic Infections, 2nd ed. Oxford: Blackwell Scientific Publications; 1982:170–91.
118. DeLeon A. Prognostico tardio en el absceso hepatico amibiano. Arch Invest Med (Mex). 1970;1(Suppl 1):205–6.
119. Krupp IM, Powell SJ. Comparative study of the antibody response in amebiasis. Am J Trop Med Hyg. 1971;20:421–4.
120. Stamm WP, Ashley MJ, Bell K. The value of amoebic serology in an area of low endemicity. Trans R Soc Trop Med Hyg. 1976;70:49–53.
121. Petri WA, Joyce MP, Broman J, et al. Recognition of the galactose- or *N*-acetylgalactosamine-binding lectin of *Entamoeba histolytica* by human immune sera. Infect Immun. 1987;55:2327–31.
122. Calderon J, Muñoz MDL, Acosta HM. Surface redistribution and release of antibody-induced caps in *Entamoebae*. J Exp Med. 1980;151:184–93.
123. Joyce MP, Ravdin JI. Antigens of *Entamoeba histolytica* recognized by immune sera from liver abscess patients. Am J Trop Med Hyg. 1988;38:74–80.
124. Nash TE, Herrington DA, Losonsky GA, et al. Experimental human infections with *Giardia lamblia*. J Infect Dis. 1987;156:974–84.
125. Huldt G, Davies P, Allison AC, et al. Interactions between *Entamoeba histolytica* and complement. Nature. 1979;277:214–6.
126. Ortiz-Ortiz L, Capin R, Capin NR, et al. Activation of the alternative pathway of complement by *Entamoeba histolytica*. Clin Exp Immunol. 1978;34:10–8.
127. Reed SL, Sargeaunt PG, Braude AI. Resistance to lysis by human serum of pathogenic *Entamoeba histolytica*. Trans R Soc Trop Med Hyg. 1983;77:248–53.
128. Calderon J, Tovar R. Loss of susceptibility to complement lysis in *Entamoeba histolytica* HM1 by treatment with human serum. Immunology. 1986;58:467–71.
129. Salta RA, Murray HW, Rubin BY, et al. The role of gamma interferon in the generation of human macrophages and T lymphocytes cytotoxic for *Entamoeba histolytica*. Am J Trop Med Hyg. 1987;37:72–8.
130. Salata RA, Martinez-Palomo A, Murphy CF, et al. Patients treated for amebic liver abscess develop a cell-mediated immune response effective in vitro against *Entamoeba histolytica*. J Immunol. 1986;136:2633–9.
131. Salata RA, Martinez-Palomo A, Canales L, et al. Immune sera suppresses the antigen specific proliferative response in T-lymphocytes from patients cured of amebic liver abscess. Presented at the 34th Annual Meeting of the American Society of Tropical Medicine and Hygiene, Miami, November 5, 1985.
132. Ganguly NK, Mahajan RC, Gill NJ, et al. Kinetics of lymphocyte subpopulations and their functions in cases of amoebic liver abscess. Trans R Soc Trop Med Hyg. 1981;75:807–10.
133. Ortiz-Ortiz L, Zamacona G, Sepulveda B, et al. Cell-mediated immunity in patients with amebic abscess of the liver. Clin Immunol Immunopathol. 1975;4:127–34.
134. Kanani SR, Knight R. Relapsing amoebic colitis of 12 years' standing exacerbated by corticosteroids. Br Med J. 1969;2:613–4.
135. Balikian JP, Bitar JG, Rishani KK, et al. Fulminant necrotizing amebic colitis in children. Am J Proctol. 1977;28:69.
136. Tucker PC, Webster PD, Kilpatrick ZM. Amebic colitis mistaken for inflammatory bowel disease. Arch Intern Med. 1975;135:681.
137. Leitch GJ, Dickey AD, Udezulu IA, et al. *Entamoeba histolytica* trophozoites in the lumen and mucus blanket of rat colons studied in vivo. Infect Immun. 1985;47:68–73.
138. Chadee K, Meerovitch E. *Entamoeba histolytica*: Early progressive pathology in the cecum of the gerbil (*Meriones unguiculatus*). Am J Trop Med Hyg. 1985;34:283–91.
139. Chadee K, Petri WA, Johnson M, et al. Binding and internalization of purified rat colonic mucins by the Gal/GalNAc adherence lectin of *Entamoeba histolytica*. J Infect Dis. 1988. In press.
140. Bos HM, van den Eijk AA. Enzyme-linked immunosorbent assay (ELISA) in the serodiagnosis of amebiasis. In: Sepulveda B, Diamond L, eds. Amebiasis. Mexico City: Instituto Mexicano del Seguro Social; 1976:721–7.
141. Banerjee RN, Sahani AL, Nag AK, et al. A longitudinal study of intestinal amoebiasis. J Assoc Physicians India. 1976;24:83–8.
142. Jalan KN, Maitra TK. Amebiasis in the developing world. In: Ravdin JI, ed. Amebiasis: Human Infection by *Entamoeba histolytica*. New York: Churchill Livingstone; 1988:535–55.
143. Adams EB, MacLeod IN. Invasive amebiasis. II. Amebic liver abscess and its complications. Medicine (Baltimore). 1977;56:325–34.
144. Juniper K. Parasitic diseases of the intestinal tract. In: Paulson M, ed. Gastroenterologic Medicine. Philadelphia: Lea & Febiger; 1969:172.
145. Adams EB, MacLeod IN. Invasive amebiasis. I. Amebic dysentery and its complications. Medicine (Baltimore). 1977;56:315–23.
146. Jammal MA, Cox K, Ruebner B. Amebiasis presenting as rectal bleeding without diarrhea in childhood. J Pediatr Gastroenterol. Nutr. 1985;4:294–6.
147. Merritt TJ, Coughlin E, Thomas DW, et al. Spectrum of amebiasis in children. Am J Dis Child. 1982;136:785.
148. Speelman P, McGlaughlin R, Kabir I, et al. Differential clinical features and stool findings in shigellosis and amoebic dysentery. Trans R Soc Trop Med Hyg. 1987;81:549–51.
149. Wanke C, Butler T, Islam M. Epidemiologic and clinical features of invasive amebiasis in Bangladesh: A case-control comparison with other diarrheal diseases and postmortem findings. Am J Trop Med Hyg. 1988;38:335–41.
150. Cardoso MJ, Kimura KS, Miguel CLF, et al. Radiology of invasive amebiasis of the colon. J Roentgenol. 1977;128:935.
151. Butler T, Islam I, Azad AK, et al. Causes of death in diarrhoeal diseases after rehydration therapy: An autopsy study of 140 patients in Bangladesh. Bull WHO. 1987;65:317–23.
152. Wopnick S. The recognition of amebiasis in the acute abdomen. Practitioner. 1973;211:71.
153. Monga NK, Sood S, Kaushik SP, et al. Amebic peritonitis. Am J Gastroenterol. 1976;67:366–73.
154. El-Hennawy M, Abd-Rabbo H. Hazards of cortisone therapy in hepatic amoebiasis. J Trop Med Hyg. 1978;81:71–73.
155. Alvarez CR, Zavala RJ, Bautista OJ, et al. Lesiones proliferativas de la pared del colon producidos por *Entamoeba histolytica*. Arch Invest Med (Mex). 1970;1(Suppl 1):227–36.
156. Haider Z, Rasul A. Chronic non-dysenteric intestinal amoebiasis. A review of 159 cases. J Pakistan Med Assoc. 1975;25:75–8.
157. Schleupner CJ, Barritt AS III. Differentiation and occurrence of amebiasis in inflammatory bowel disease. In: Ravdin JI, ed. Amebiasis: Human Infection by *Entamoeba histolytica*. New York: Churchill Livingstone; 1988:582–93.
158. Ruiz-Moreno F. Perianal skin amebiasis. Dis Colon Rectum. 1967;10:65.
159. Knobloch J, Mannweiler E. Development and persistence of antibodies to *Entamoeba histolytica* in patients with amebic liver abscess: Analysis of 216 cases. Am J Trop Med Hyg. 1983;32:727–32.
160. Conter RL, Pitt HA, Tompkins RK, Longmire WP. Differentiation of pyogenic from amebic hepatic abscesses. Surg Gynecol Obstet. 1986;162:114–20.
161. Greenstein AJ, Barth J, Dicker A, et al. Amebic liver abscess: A study of 11 cases compared with a series of 38 patients with pyogenic liver abscess. Am J Gastroenterol. 1985;80:472–8.
162. Schorlemmer RN, Saltzstein EC, Peacock JB, et al. Amebic liver abscess: Differential diagnosis of cholecystitis. Am J Surg. 1983;146:827–9.
163. Boom RA, Fonseca L, Yañez C, et al. Differential diagnosis between amoebic liver abscess and acute cholecystitis. J Med Syst. 1983;7:205–12.
164. Overbosch D, Stuiver PC, van der Kaay HJ. Hepatic amoebiasis: Current

concepts and a report of 25 cases in the Netherlands. Acta Leiden. 1983;51:3–17.
165. Reed SL, Braude AI. Extraintestinal disease: Clinical syndromes, diagnostic profile, and therapy. In: Ravdin JI, ed. Amebiasis: Human Infection by *Entamoeba histolytica*. New York: Churchill Livingstone; 1988:511–32.
166. Rhode FC, Prieto O, Riveros O. Thoracic complications of amoebic liver abscess. Br J Dis Chest. 1979;73:302.
167. Adeyemo AO, Aderounmu A. Intrathoracic complications of amoebic liver abscess. J R Soc Med. 1984;77:17–20.
168. Kubitschek KR, Peters J, Nickeson D, et al. Amebiasis presenting as pleuropulmonary disease. West J Med. 1985;142:203–7.
169. Nwafo DC, Egbue MO. Intrathoracic manifestations of amoebiasis. Ann R Coll Surg Eng. 1981;63:126–8.
170. Eggleston FC, Handa AK, Verghese M. Amebic peritonitis secondary to amebic liver abscess. Surgery. 1982;91:46–48.
171. Wilmot AJ. Clinical Amebiasis. Oxford: Blackwell Scientific Publications; 1962.
172. Orbison JA, Reeves N, Leedham CL, et al. Amebic brain abscess: Review of the literature and report of five additional cases. Medicine (Baltimore). 1951;30:247–82.
173. Becker GL Jr, Knep S, Lance KP, et al. Amebic abscess of the brain. Neurosurgery. 1980;6:192–4.
174. Schmutzhard E, Mayr U, Rumpl E, et al. Secondary cerebral amebiasis due to infection with *Entamoeba histolytica*: A case report with computer tomographic findings. Eur Neurol. 1986;25:161–5.
175. Banerjee AK, Bhatnagar RK, Bhusnurmath SR. Secondary cerebral amebiasis. Trop Geogr Med. 1983;35:333–6.
176. Grigsby WP. Surgical treatment of amebiasis. Surg Gynecol Obstet. 1969;128:609–27.
177. Heinz KPW. Amoebic infection of the female genital tract: A report of three cases. S afr Med J. 1973;47:1795.
178. Mylius RE, Ten Seldam RE. Venereal infection by *Entamoeba histolytica* in a New Guinea native couple. Trop Geogr Med. 1962;14:20.
179. O'Leary RK, Posen J. Amoebiasis of the penis. S Afr Med J. 1984;65:113.
180. Purpon I, Jiminez D, Engelking RL. Amebiasis of the penis. J Urol. 1967;98:372.
181. Young KH, Ballock S, Melvin DM, et al. Ethyl acetate as a substitute for diethylether in the ether-formalin sedimentation technique. J Clin Microbiol. 1979;10:852–3.
182. Blumencranz H, Kasen L, Romeu J, et al. The role of endoscopy in suspected amebiasis. Am J Gastroenterol. 1983;78:15–8.
183. Crowson TD, Hines C Jr. Amebiasis diagnosed by colonoscopy. Gastrointest Endosc. 1978;24:254–5.
184. Patterson M, Healy GR, Shabot JM. Serologic testing for amoebiasis. Gastroenterology. 1980;78:136–41.
185. Kessel JF, Lewis WP, Pasquel CM, et al. Indirect hemagglutination and complement fixation tests in amebiasis. Am J Trop Med Hyg. 1965;14:540–50.
186. Healy GR, Sumner CK. The indirect hemagglutination test for amebiasis in patients with inflammatory bowel disease. Am J Dig Dis. 1972;17:97.
187. Ralls PW, Colletti PM, Halls JM. Imaging in hepatic amebic abscess. In: Ravdin JI, ed. Amebiasis: Human Infection by *Entamoeba histolytica*. New York: Churchill Livingstone; 1988:664–704.
188. Halvorsen RA, Korobkin M, Foster WL, et al. The variable CT appearance of hepatic abscesses. AJR. 1984;142:941–6.
189. Siddiqui HJ, Gharib M, Muscat-Baron J, et al. Liver abscess in Dubai: Analysis of 29 cases and an assessment of the value of CAT scan. Trop Med Parasitol. 1985;79:281–6.
190. Elizondo G, Weissleder R, Stark DD, et al. Amebic liver abscess: Diagnosis and treatment evaluation with MR imaging. Radiology. 1987;165:795–800.
191. Ralls PW, Henley DS, Colletti PM, et al. Amebic liver abscess: MR imaging. Radiology. 1987;165:801–4.
192. Ralls PW, Barnes PF, Johnson MB, et al. Medical treatment of hepatic amebic abscess: Rare need for percutaneous drainage. Radiology. 1987;165:805–7.
193. van Sonnenberg E, Mueller PR, Schiffman RR, et al. Intrahepatic amebic abscesses: Indications for and results of percutaneous catheter drainage. Radiology. 1985;156:631–5.
194. Ralls PW, Quinn MF, Boswell WD, et al. Patterns of resolution in successfully treated hepatic amebic abscess: Sonographic evaluation. Radiology. 1983;149:541–3.
195. Simjee A, Patel A, Gathiram V, et al. Serial ultrasound in amoebic liver abscess. Clin Radiol. 1985;36:61–8.
196. Allason-Jones E, Mindel A, Sargeaunt P, et al. *Entamoeba histolytica* as a commensal intestinal parasite in homosexual men. N Engl J Med. 1986;315:353–6.
197. Goldmeier D, Price AB, Billington O, et al. Is *Entamoeba histolytica* in homosexual men a pathogen? Lancet. 1986;1:641–4.
198. Krogstad DJ. Isoenzyme patterns and pathogenicity in amebic infection. N Engl J Med. 1986;315:390 1.
199. Scragg J. Amoebic liver abscess in African children. Arch Dis Child. 1960;35:171–6.
200. Drugs for parasitic infections. Med Lett. 1988;30:15–24.
201. Wolfe MS. Nondysenteric intestinal amebiasis: Treatment with diloxanide furoate. JAMA. 1973;224:1601–4.
202. Sullam PM, Slutkin G, Gottlieb AB, et al. Paromomycin therapy of endemic amebiasis in homosexual men. Sex Transm Dis. 1986;13:151–5.
203. Courtney KO, Thompson PE, Hodgkinson R, et al. Paromomycin as a therapeutic substance for intestinal amoebiasis and bacterial enteritis. Ann Biochem Exp Med. 1960;20(Suppl):449–56.
204. Norris SM, Ravdin JI. The pharmacology of antiamebic drugs. In: Ravdin JI, ed. Amebiasis: Human Infection by *Entamoeba histolytica*. New York: Churchill Livingstone; 1988:734–40.
205. Powell SJ, Wilmot AJ, Elsdon-Dew R. Further trials of metronidazole in amoebic dysentery and amoebic liver abscess. Ann Trop Med Parasitol. 1967;61:511–4.
206. Simjee AE, Gathiram V, Jackson TFHG, et al. A comparative trial of metronidazole v. tinidazole in the treatment of amoebic liver abscess. S Afr Med J. 1985;68:923–4.
207. Powell SJ. Drug trials in amoebiasis. Bull WHO. 1969;40:956.
208. Lasserre R, Jaroonvesama N, Kurathong S, et al. Single-day drug treatment of amebic liver abscess. Am J Trop Med Hyg. 1983;32:723–6.
209. Kapoor OP, Joshi VR. Multiple amoebic liver abscess. A study of 56 cases. J Trop Med Hyg. 1972;75:4–6.

250. FREE-LIVING AMEBAE

WILLIAM A. PETRI, JR.
JONATHAN I. RAVDIN

HISTORY

Infection of humans with the free-living amebae is fortunately a rare occurrence. Central nervous system (CNS) invasion by *Naegleria* and *Acanthamoeba* has been reported in fewer than 200 patients worldwide, *Acanthamoeba* keratitis in fewer than 100 patients. Distinct from other pathogenic protozoa by nature of their free-living existence, there are no known insect vectors, no human carrier states of epidemiologic importance, and little relationship of poor sanitation to the spread of infection. There are three distinct clinical syndromes caused by the species of free-living amebae that infect humans. Primary amebic meningoencephalitis (PAM) is caused by *Naegleria fowleri*. PAM occurs in healthy children and young adults who usually have been recently swimming in fresh water. The *Naegleria* gain access to the CNS by direct invasion through the nasal mucosa and cribriform plate and cause a rapidly fatal meningoencephalitis. Granulomatous amebic encephalitis (GAE) caused by *Acanthamoeba castellani*, *A. culbertsoni*, and *A. astronyxis* is a subacute opportunistic infection that spreads hematogenously from pulmonary or skin lesions to the CNS, resulting in focal neurologic deficits that progress over days to weeks to a diffuse meningoencephalitis and death. *Acanthamoeba* keratitis is associated with soft contact lens use and minimal ocular trauma and causes a subacute to chronic keratitis.

The history of the free-living amebae begins with Antonie van Leeuwenhoek, the discoverer of the microscope, who in the summer of 1674 described free-living protozoa in a drop of water. Free-living amebae were discovered as contaminants in cultures of monkey kidney tissue cultures by Jahnes et al.[1] in 1957, who observed that the amebae exerted a cytopathic effect on the tissue culture cells. One year later, Culbertson et al.[2] demonstrated that intranasal inoculation of mice with *Acanthamoeba* caused a purulent meningoencephalitis with direct invasion of the CNS via the nasal mucosa. They concluded that "further inquiry into the possible role of the Acanthamoeba in disease processes is desirable."

The first recognized cases of purulent amebic meningoencephalitis in humans were reported in 1965 by Fowler and Carter.[3] Three children and a 28-year-old man, all from the Gulf of St. Vincent area of South Australia, died with fulminant meningoencephalitis. A history of recent swimming in fresh water was not remarked on by the authors. Hemorrhage and necrosis of the olfactory bulbs with inflamed nasal submucosa were seen. Amebae with the distinctive central karyosome of the free-living amebae were seen in the nasal submucosa and olfactory nerves and clustered perivascularly in the brain in the four patients. Cerebrospinal fluid (CSF) examined postmortem in one patient demonstrated free-living amebae. Butt[4] reported an additional three cases from Central Florida, a 10 year old and two 18-year-old boys who had all been swimming in freshwater lakes. Butt named the disease primary amebic meningoencephalitis and demonstrated motile amebae in the CSF of two of the three patients. GAE was later recognized as distinct from PAM,[5] and the first case of *Acanthamoeba* keratitis was diagnosed in the United States in 1973.[6] Infection with free-living amebae is newly recognized but not a new disease: dos Santos[7] reviewed the autopsy records of the Medical College of Virginia and discovered five additional cases of PAM dating back to 1937.

ORGANISMS

Naegleria fowleri was named after the late Malcolm Fowler of Adelaide Children's Hospital of Australia, who with Carter described the initial cases of PAM.[3] *Naegleria fowleri* is the only pathogenic species of *Naegleria* and has also been called *N. aerobia* and *N. invadens*. *Naegleria* have the ability to transform rapidly from the trophozoite to a flagellate form upon transfer to distilled water or a nonnutrient medium.[8,9] The flagellate form spontaneously reverts to the trophozoite, which is the reproductive stage of the protozoan. The trophozoite divides with a unique nuclear mitosis with retention of the nuclear membrane and nucleolus during karyokinesis. The trophozoites are 10–30 μm in diameter and have a clear nucleus with a prominent dense central nucleolus, and pseudopodia (Fig. 1). The granular cytoplasm can contain ingested red blood cells and leukocytes along with cytoplasmic organelles including rough endoplasmic reticulum and mitochondria. The trophozoites feed predominantly on bacteria and have an aerobic metabolism, in contrast to the facultative anaerobic parasite *Entamoeba histolytica*. Encystment of the trophozoite yields an approximately 9-μm-diameter spherical cyst with a central nucleus and a single-layered wall containing an average of two pores. These pores, which are plugged with mucus in the cyst, serve as ports for the emergence of the trophozoite during excystation.[10] *Naegleria fowleri* is thermophilic, with the trophozoite growing well at temperatures as high as 45°C.[11]

Acanthamoeba species pathogenic for humans include *A. castellani, A. polyphaga, A. culbertsoni*, and *A. rhysodes*. These *Acanthamoeba* species were earlier classified as *Hartmanella* species.[9,11] The life cycle of *Acanthamoeba* consists only of the trophozoite and cyst. Trophozoites are 14–40 μm in diameter, contain mitochondria and a single nucleus with a prominent central nucleolus, and have distinctive slender spine-like projections of the plasma membrane (Fig. 2). The cysts have a double-layered wall or envelope, are 12–16 μm in diameter, and also may contain pores in the cyst wall. *Acanthamoeba* have aerobic metabolism and grow best at 25–35°C.

EPIDEMIOLOGY

Naegleria fowleri has been isolated all over the world from soil, river and lake water, and thermally polluted water.[8,9,11] Pathogenic *N. fowleri* proliferate at higher temperatures, with growth occurring at temperatures up to 46°C, compared with pathogenic *Acanthamoeba*, whose growth is inhibited by temperatures above 34–39°C.[12] The presence of *N. fowleri* in fresh water is directly related to water temperature,[13] and *N. fowleri* has been frequently isolated from thermally polluted waters in temperate climates.[14,15] In semitropical locations such as Florida, thermal pollution of the already very warm freshwater lakes in summer and fall is less significant, with at least one *N. fowleri* per 25 ml of water frequently isolated.[13] In the winter as water temperatures drop, *Naegleria* can only be isolated from the lake bottom sediments. *Naegleria* cysts are stable up to 8 months at 4°C.[16] Wellings et al.[13] estimated that there had been a billion exposures of people to *Naegleria*-contaminated fresh water with only seven cases of PAM in Florida over a 14-year period. The factors that protect most individuals from invasive *Naegleria* infection are not understood. The presence of serum agglutinating activity for *N. fowleri* in the majority of young adults tested from the southern United States but not infants indicates that subclinical infection or exposure to *Naegleria* is common.[17] PAM has been reported to have occurred in the central states

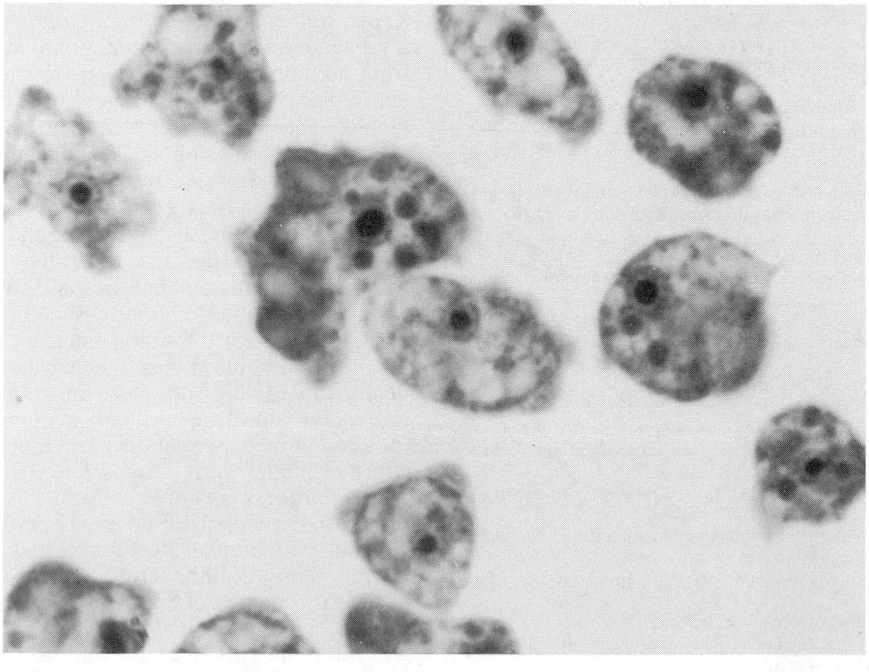

FIG. 1. Trophozoites of *N. fowleri* demonstrating the blunt pseudopodium or lobopodium. The characteristic nucleus contains a centrally placed dense nucleolus. (Iron-hematoxylin, magnification ×800) (From Martinez,[11] with permission.)

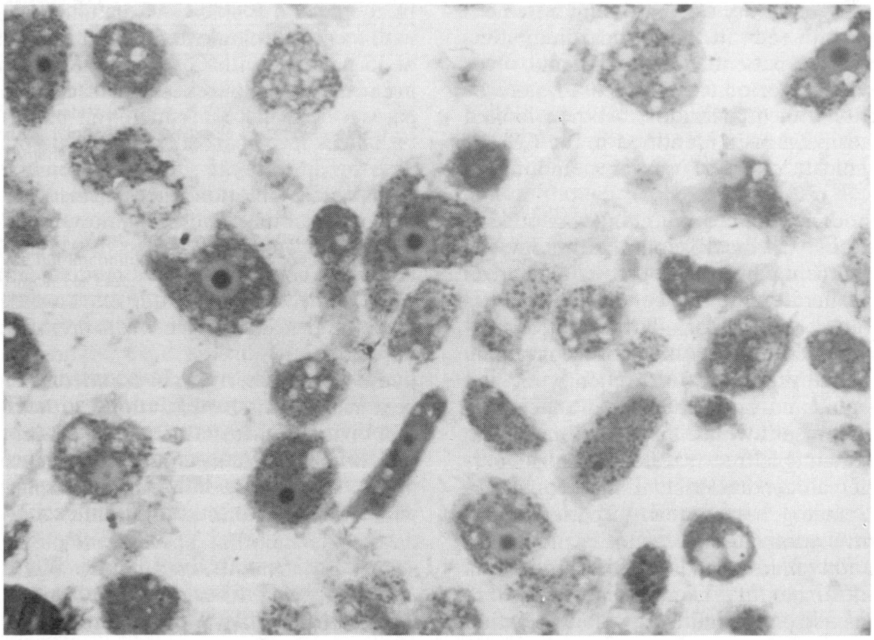

FIG. 2. Trophozoites of *Acanthamoeba glebae* stained with toluidine blue, which demonstrates the round nucleolus surrounded by a nuclear halo and the granular and abundant cytoplasm. (×600) (From Martinez,[11] with permission.)

of the United States, southern Australia, New Zealand, Europe, Africa, and Central America.[9,11] Clusters of cases of PAM with common environmental exposures have occurred.[3,4,9,11]

Acanthamoeba species have also been isolated from soil, water, and air from diverse geographic locations.[9,11] *Acanthamoeba* were cultured from pharyngeal swabs of 38 of 2289 individuals during a study of respiratory viruses in healthy families,[18] and serologic surveys have detected serum antibodies directed against *Acanthamoeba* in healthy people.[19] Despite such evidence of common exposure of the normal population to *Acanthamoeba*, GAE occurs predominantly in debilitated or immunosuppressed individuals.[5,9,11] Underlying illnesses in patients with GAE have included AIDS,[20,21] liver disease, diabetes mellitus, skin ulcers, and renal transplantation. GAE has occurred in patients who are immunocompromised from steroid or chemotherapy treatment.[5,9,11] *Acanthamoeba* keratitis, on the other hand, occurs in healthy people. Of the first 100 cases of amebic keratitis reported to the Centers for Disease Control, 83 percent occurred in people who were contact lens wearers. Corneal infection was associated with the use of homemade saline to clean the lenses and with the wearing of lenses while swimming.[22]

PATHOGENESIS AND PATHOLOGIC FINDINGS

PAM occurs chiefly in healthy children and young adults who have recently swum in warm, freshwater lakes or ponds. Animal models[23] and autopsy studies[3,7–9,11] indicate that CNS invasion by *N. fowleri* occurs after nasal inoculation with the amebae by disruption of the olfactory mucosa. The amebae penetrate the submucosal nervous plexus and the cribriform plate and gain access to the CNS (Fig. 3). *Naegleria fowleri* produces a diffuse meningoencephalitis and purulent leptomeningitis with severest involvement of the cortical grey matter. Cortical hemorrhages and edema with uncal or cerebellar herniation are seen. The olfactory bulbs are hemorrhagic and necrotic. *Naegleria* trophozoites are found in the olfactory nerves and the adventitia and perivascular spaces of small to mid-size arteries and arterioles. No amebic cysts are seen in the brain.[3,7–9,11] A diffuse or focal myocarditis was present in 7 of 16 autopsies of patients

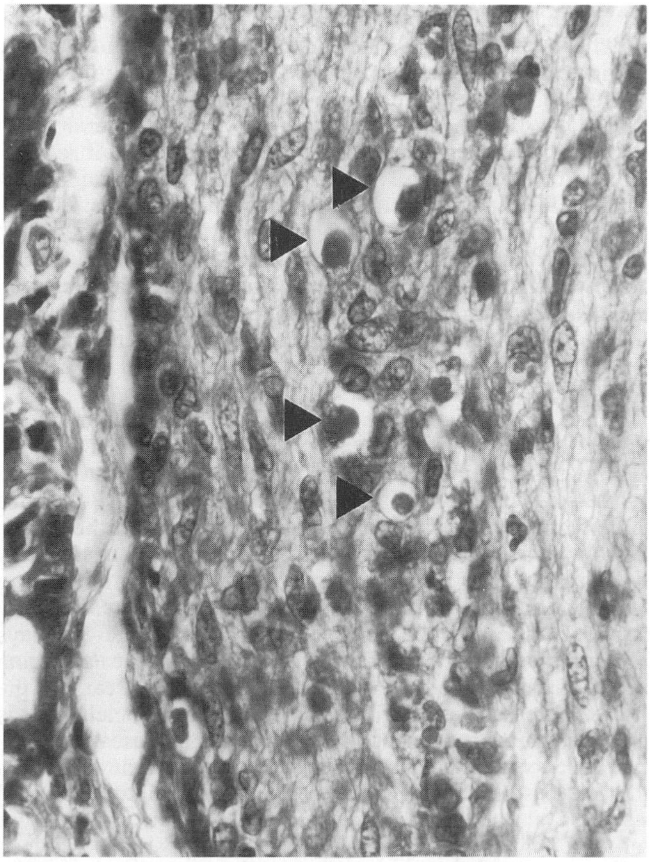

FIG. 3. *Naegleria fowleri* trophozoites (arrowheads) within unmyelinated submucosal olfactory nerve bundles of a 27-year-old man who swam in fresh water 4 days before developing PAM. (H&E, ×500) (From Martinez,[11] with permission.)

with PAM. The inflammatory infiltrate was predominantly neutrophilic, and no amebae were seen in the myocardium. Retrospective chart review of the patients with PAM and myocarditis did not reveal evidence of congestive heart failure or arrhythmias in the patients with myocarditis.[24] When looked for, *Naegleria* trophozoites have been identified in the CSF of all four patients at the Medical College of Virginia[11] and in two of three cases in Florida.[4]

GAE occurs in immunocompromised patients who present with focal neurologic deficits. On macroscopic pathology the leptomeninges are spared except when directly overlying areas of cortical involvement. Moderate to severe cerebral edema occurs, with bilateral uncal or cerebellar tonsillar herniations occasionally seen. Necrotizing granulomatous lesions containing perivascular trophozoites and cysts are most frequently located in the cerebellum, midbrain, and brain stem. Multinucleated giant cells are occasionally present within the granulomas.[5,9,11] The preferential location of amebic trophozoites and cysts perivascularly suggested a hematogenous dissemination of *Acanthamoeba* to the CNS. Hematogenous spread in patients with GAE is supported by identification of *Acanthamoeba* in the skin (Fig. 4), lung, adrenals, and lymph nodes. Amebic skin lesions have been present for weeks to months prior to the development of GAE[21,25]; amebic sinusitis, pneumonitis, or skin infection may be sites of primary human infection that lead to hematogenous dissemination.[5,9,11]

Acanthamoeba keratitis is a corneal infection associated with minor corneal trauma and the use of soft contact lenses in otherwise healthy people. The histologic appearance of corneal infection is similar to *Acanthamoeba* infections of other organs. Both amebic cysts and trophozoites are found within the cornea. There is an acute or mixed inflammatory infiltrate that may contain epithelial and giant cells. However, amebae have also been found in tissue in the absence of an inflammatory infiltrate. Corneal neovascularization occurs to a variable extent.[6,26] Involvement of the posterior chamber of the eye is a rare complication of amebic keratitis but has been observed in enucleation specimens. Sterile inflammation of the posterior segment occurs without isolation or visualization of amebic cysts or trophozoites.[6] The corneal ringlike infiltrate seen with keratitis caused by *Acanthamoeba* and occasionally with gram-negative bacterial, herpes simplex, or fungal etiologies appears to be due to the neutrophil chemoattractant effect of antigen–antibody complexes in the cornea.[6,26]

CLINICAL MANIFESTATIONS

PAM occurs in children and young adults who have previously been in excellent health. Most often the patients with PAM have been swimming in warm, fresh water or have had other exposure to water within the last week. Rarely will there be no history of water exposure: one episode of PAM in an arid region of Nigeria was thought to be due to inhalation of *Naegleria* cysts.[27] The onset of symptoms occurs on average 2–5 days after the last exposure to fresh water, but apparent incubation periods of up to 2 weeks have been reported. Very early in the illness the patient may notice changes in taste or smell. This is followed by an abrupt onset of fever, anorexia, nausea and vomiting, headache, and meningismus in 86–100 percent of patients and mental status changes in two-thirds of patients on initial presentation. Patients rapidly progress to coma, usually without ever developing focal neurologic signs. Most patients are dead within a week after onset of illness.[9,11] Myocarditis has been present in almost half of autopsied patients, but congestive heart failure or arrhythmias are uncommon before death. PAM is a fulminant fatal infection in most patients. There are only two survivors documented—the survival of one child may have been due to early treatment with amphotericin B, miconazole, and rifampin.[28]

GAE is an illness of the immunocompromised and debilitated. In contrast to PAM, GAE has an insidious onset and presents with focal neurologic deficients. Presenting signs and symptoms of 15 patients with GAE included mental status abnormalities in 86 percent; seizures in 66 percent; fever, headache, and hemiparesis in 53 percent; meningismus in 40 percent; visual disturbances in 26 percent; and ataxia in 20 percent.[5] Underlying illnesses in patients with GAE included AIDS, liver disease, renal transplantation, neoplasm, steroid and chemotherapy, diabetes mellitus, and pregnancy.[9] The duration of CNS illness until death was 7 to 120 days (average: 39 days). The incubation period of GAE is difficult to determine as the disease is not associated with freshwater exposure, but *Acanthamoeba* skin ulcers and lesions have been present for months prior to the onset of CNS disease.[5,9,11,25] The skin lesions can be ulcerative,[25] nodular,[20,21] or subcutaneous abscesses[20] and on biopsy demonstrate amebic granulomas. Pneumonitis was present in 2 of 13 patients with GAE.

Acanthamoeba keratitis is frequently misdiagnosed initially as a herpes simplex virus or bacterial or even fungal keratitis, with the average delay to definitive treatment ranging from 11 days to 15 months. The symptoms begin with a foreign body sensation in the affected eye followed by severe pain, photophobia, tearing, blepharospasm, conjunctivitis, and blurred vision. Generally anywhere from several days to several months elapse before the keratitis is at its most advanced, with periods of temporary remission common. These remissions lead to further delays in diagnosis since they are interpreted as responses to antibacterial or antiviral therapy. Signs of amebic keratitis in 36 eyes included iritis in 86 percent, a characteristic corneal ring infiltrate in 78 percent (Figs. 5 and 6), recurrent epithelial breakdown or cataracts in 44 percent, and in the minority hypopyon, elevated intraocular pressure, and anterior nodular scleritis. Most patients will have an anterior uveitis of fluctuating severity.[6] A dendriform epithelial pattern was recently described in three patients as an early sign of *Acanthamoeba* keratitis before stromal involvement (Fig. 7). Recognition of this dendriform pattern enabled early and vision-saving therapy in three patients.[29]

LABORATORY DIAGNOSIS

PAM should be included in the differential diagnosis of children and young adults with meningoencephalitis. Recent exposure to fresh water should raise suspicions of *N. fowleri* infection. The peripheral white cell count is usually elevated, with a predominance of neutrophils. Head computed tomographic (CT) scans in one patient with PAM showed diffuse contrast enhancement of the gray matter and obliterated ambiens, interpeduncular, and quadrigeminal cisterns.[11] The CSF pressure can be elevated, and the CSF is hemorrhagic. White cell counts in the CSF may be low early in disease but later range from 400–26,000 white cells/μl, with neutrophils predominating. Cerebrospinal fluid glucose is low to normal and CSF protein is elevated. In patients with purulent CSF indices and no bacteria demonstrated on Gram stain of CSF sediment, it is very important to examine a wet mount of CSF for amebic trophozoites. These trophozoites are generally destroyed by the fixation procedure for Gram stain and missed if not looked for on a wet mount. Motile trophozoites in the CSF have been seen in 14 of 16 patients with PAM in which a wet mount of CSF was made.[3,4,27,30–34]

GAE in the past has been frequently diagnosed only at autopsy. Brain biopsy is the only way to make the diagnosis during life as *Acanthamoeba* have never been isolated from the CSF of a patient with GAE. Head CT scans in two patients have shown multiple lucent nonenhancing lesions in the cortex.[11,21] Lumbar puncture may be contraindicated in patients with GAE because of the risk of herniation. When it has been performed, the results have been nondiagnostic, with intermediate elevations in white cell count (to 800/μl, lymphocyte predominance)

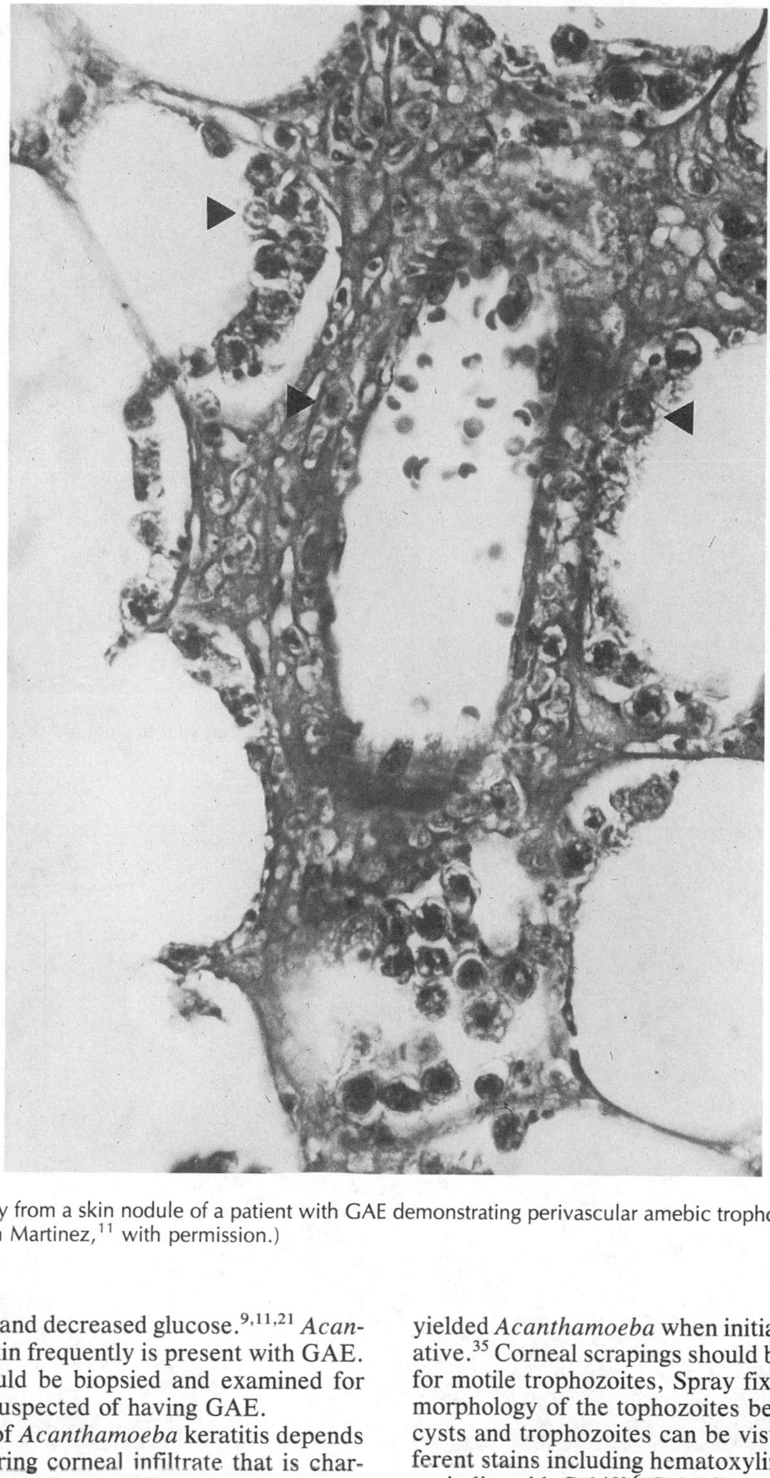

FIG. 4. Skin biopsy from a skin nodule of a patient with GAE demonstrating perivascular amebic trophozoites (arrowheads). (H&E, ×250) (From Martinez,[11] with permission.)

and usually elevated protein and decreased glucose.[9,11,21] *Acanthamoeba* infection of the skin frequently is present with GAE. Skin nodules or ulcers should be biopsied and examined for *Acanthamoeba* in patients suspected of having GAE.

The successful treatment of *Acanthamoeba* keratitis depends on its early diagnosis. The ring corneal infiltrate that is characteristic of this disease is a late sign of stromal involvement. Patchy stromal infiltrates[35] and dendriform epithelial involvement without frank corneal ulcerations[29] can be early signs of amebic keratitis (Figs. 5–7). Diagnosis rests on demonstrating by histopathology or culture *Acanthamoeba* in corneal scrapings or biopsy material. Initial corneal scrapings, Gram stains, and cultures may be misleading because in one-third of cases of amebic keratitis these grew *Staphylococcus epidermidis, Staphylococcus aureus*, α-hemolytic *Streptococcus*, or *Propionibacterium*. A nonnutrient agar overlaid with *Escherichia coli* or *Aerobacter aerogenes* has been used to successfully culture *Acanthamoeba* from 10 of 15 amebic keratitis patients whose previous smear or biopsy had been negative.[6] Culture of the contact lenses and contact lens saline solution has also yielded *Acanthamoeba* when initial corneal scrapings were negative.[35] Corneal scrapings should be examined under wet mount for motile trophozoites, Spray fixatives may best preserve the morphology of the tophozoites before air drying occurs.[36] The cysts and trophozoites can be visualized with a number of different stains including hematoxylin-eosin, Wright, Giemsa, and periodic acid–Schiff.[6] Calcofluor white fluorescently stains the cysts and trophozites in tissue section, facilitating their identification.[37]

TREATMENT

There are two patients known to have survived PAM.[28,38] Both patients received high-dose systemic and intrathecal amphotericin B. Whether other antiamebic agents were given to one patient was not reported[38]; the other successfully treated patient also received systemic and intrathecal miconazole and systemic rifampin and sulfisoxazole.[28] Because of the overall 95 percent mortality of PAM, passive immunotherapy in animal models has been attempted. Intrathecal administration of antinaegleria im-

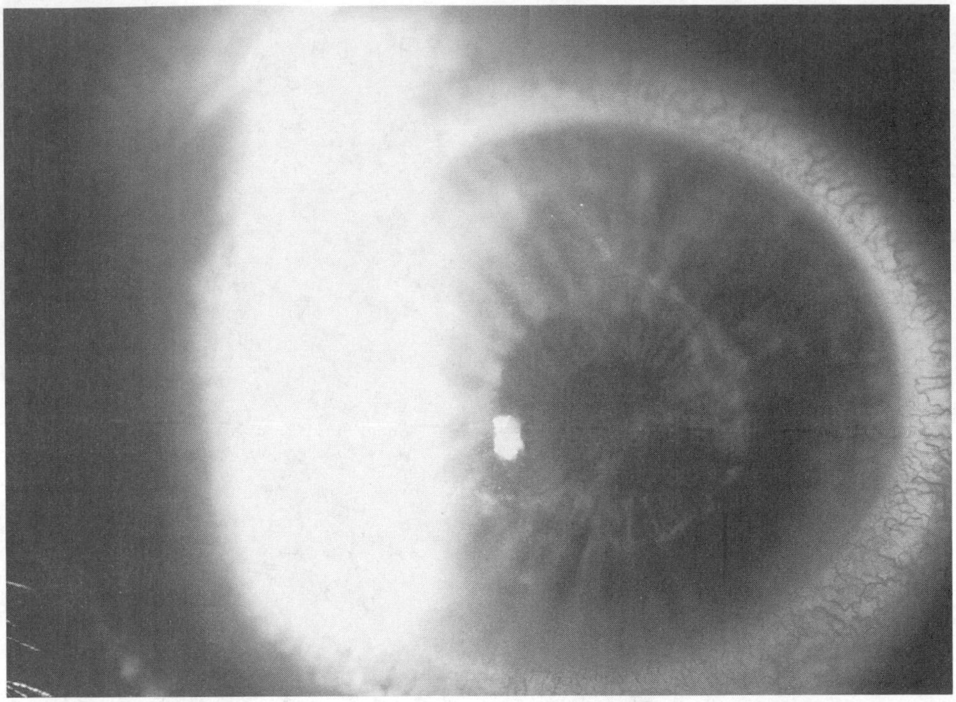

FIG. 5. *Acanthamoeba* keratitis with an early and only partially ring-shaped infiltrate. (From Lindquist et al.,[29] with permission.)

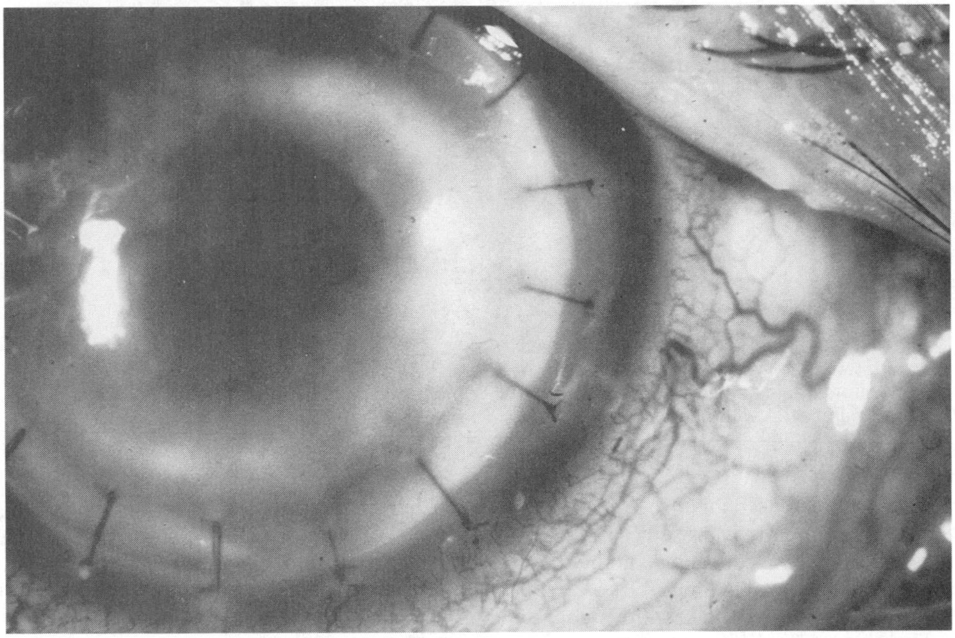

FIG. 6. Progressive ring infiltrate in a corneal graft infected with *Acanthamoeba polyphaga*. (From Cohen et al.,[35] with permission.)

mune serum or an antinaegleria monoclonal antibody prolonged the survival of rabbits inoculated intracisternally with *N. fowleri*.[39] Passive immunotherapy may one day prove to be a useful adjunct to antibiotic treatment of PAM.

Little is known about the treatment of GAE. Most cases have been diagnosed postmortem; premortem diagnosis has generally preceded death by only a few days, making evaluation of therapy difficult. In vitro testing of drug susceptibilities is complicated by interspecies and interstrain differences in antimicrobial sensitivities.[6] Each clinical isolate should be tested for drug sensitivities. In general the diamidine derivatives (propamidine, pentamidine, dibromopropamidine) have the greatest activity against *Acanthamoeba*. Other drugs active in vitro include ketoconazole, miconazole, paramomycin, neomycin, 5-fluorocytosine, and, to a lesser extent, amphotericin B.[6,40,41]

Treatment of *Acanthamoeba* keratitis has been notably more successful than that of GAE or PAM. This relates in large part to the accessibility of the infection to surgical debridement and high concentrations of topical antimicrobial drugs. Successful treatment requires early diagnosis and aggressive surgical and

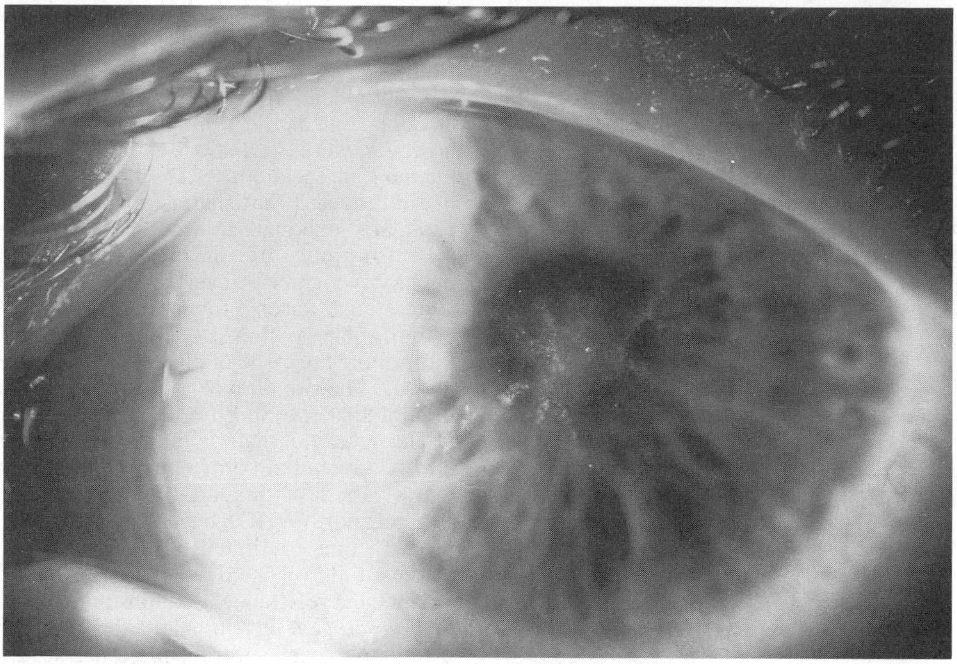

FIG. 7. *Acanthamoeba* keratitis with dendriform epithelial pattern. Radial, linear anterior stromal infiltrates extend nearly to temporal periphery associated with dendriform epithelial irregularity. (From Lindquist et al.,[29] with permission.)

medical management. Recognition of the dendriform pattern on the corneal epithelium, the earliest recognized sign of *Acanthamoeba* keratitis, should be followed immediately with debridement of the abnormal epithelium and institution of antiamebic medical therapy.[6,29,35,42] Medical treatment with topical 1% miconazole nitrate, 0.1% propamidine isethionate, and neosporin should continue for a minimum of 3–4 weeks. Topical propamidine should be administered at least nine times a day, with some authorities recommending it to be administered as often as every 15 to 60 minutes for the first 3 days.[29,43] Early recognition and treatment has eliminated the need in some patients for a late penetrating keratoplasty to restore vision and reduce pain.[6,29,35,42] Propamidine isethionate has caused a reversible epithelial keratopathy after prolonged treatment that can be confused with recurrent amebic keratitis.[44] Crystalline keratopathy caused by viridans streptococci has occurred after topical corticosteroid therapy of *Acanthamoeba* keratitis in two patients, emphasizing both the risks of using topical steroids in this disease and the need for a complete diagnostic reevaluation of patients with amebic keratitis who appear to be failing therapy.[45]

PREVENTION

PAM occurs so rarely that active surveillance for *N. fowleri* in public swimming lakes is probably not justified as a public health measure. However, because of the occurrence of clusters of patients with PAM with common environmental exposures,[3,4,7,33] health officials should consider closing the implicated lake to swimming until corrective actions can be made to limit the growth of *N. fowleri*.

Acanthamoeba keratitis associated with contact lens use is preventable. Contact lenses should be heat disinfected, as hydrogen peroxide disinfection does not kill *Acanthamoeba*. Homemade saline solutions should not be used to clean or store contact lenses, and the lenses should not be worn while swimming in fresh water.[22,35]

REFERENCES

1. Jahnes WG, Fullmer HM, Li CP. Free-living amoebae as contaminants in monkey kidney tissue culture. Proc Soc Exp Biol Med. 1957;96:484.
2. Culbertson CG, Smith JW, Minner JR. *Acanthamoeba*: Observations on animal pathogenicity. Science. 1958;127:1506.
3. Fowler M, Carter RF. Acute pyogenic meningitis probably due to *Acanthamoeba* sp.: A preliminary report. Br Med J. 1965;ii:740.
4. Butt CG. Primary amebic meningoencephalitis. N Engl J Med. 1966;274:1473–6.
5. Martinez AJ. Is *Acanthamoeba* encephalitis an opportunistic infection? Neurology. 1980;30:567–74.
6. Auran JD, Starr MB, Jakobiec FA. *Acanthamoeba* keratitis. A review of the literature. Cornea. 1987;6:2–26.
7. dos Santos JG. Fatal primary amebic meningoencephalitis. A retrospective study in Richmond, Virginia. Am J Clin Pathol. 1970;54:737–42.
8. John DT. Primary amebic meningoencephalitis and the biology of *Naegleria fowleri*. Annu Rev Microbiol. 1982;36:101–23.
9. Sotelo-Avila C. *Naegleria* and *Acanthamoeba*. Free-living amebas pathogenic for man. Perspect Pediatr Pathol. 1987;10:51–85.
10. Schuster FL. Ultrastructure of cysts of *Naegleria* spp: A comparative study. J Protozool. 1975;22:352–9.
11. Martinez AJ. Free-Living Amebas: Natural History, Prevention, Diagnosis, Pathology and Treatment of Disease. Boca Raton, FL: CRC Press; 1985.
12. Griffin JL. Temperature tolerance of pathogenic and nonpathogenic free-living amoebas. Science. 1972;178:869–70.
13. Wellings FM, Amuso PT, Chang SL, et al. Isolation and identification of pathogenic *Naegleria* from Florida lakes. Appl Environ Microbiol. 1977;34:661–7.
14. DeJonckheere J, van de Voorde H. The distribution of *Naegleria fowleri* in man-made thermal waters. Am J Trop Med Hyg. 1977;26:10–5.
15. Sykora JL, Keleti G, Martinez AJ. Occurrence and pathogenicity of *Naegleria fowleri* in artificially heated waters. Appl Environ Microbiol. 1983;45:974–9.
16. Warhurst DC, Carman JA, Mann PG. Survival of *Naegleria fowleri* cysts at 4°C for eight months with retention of virulence. Trans R Soc Trop Med Hyg. 1980;74:832.
17. Marciano-Cabral F, Cline MC, Bradley SG. Specificity of antibodies from human sera for *Naegleria* species. J Clin Microbiol. 1987;25:692–7.
18. Wang SS, Feldman HA. Isolation of *Hartmanella* species from human throats. N Engl J Med. 1967;277:1174–9.
19. Cursons RTM, Brown TJ, Keys EA. Immunity to pathogenic free-living amoeba. Lancet. 1977;2:875–6.
20. Gonzalez MM, Gould E, Dickinson G, et al. Acquired immunodeficiency syndrome associated with *Acanthamoeba* infection and other opportunistic organisms. Arch Pathol Lab Med. 1986;110:749–51.
21. Wiley CA, Safrin RE, Davis CE, et al. *Acanthamoeba* meningoencephalitis in a patient with AIDS. J Infect Dis. 1987;155:130–3.
22. Stehr-Green JK, Bailey TM, Brandt FH, et al. *Acanthamoeba* keratitis in soft contact wearers. A case-control study. JAMA. 1987;258:57–60.
23. Martinez AJ, Duma RJ, Nelson EC, et al. Experimental *Naegleria* meningoencephalitis in mice. Lab Invest. 1973;29:121–33.
24. Markowitz SM, Martinez AJ, Duma RJ, et al. Myocarditis associated with primary amebic (*Naegleria*) meningoencephalitis. Am J Clin Pathol. 1974;62:619–28.

25. Gullett J, Mills J, Hadley K, et al. Disseminated granulomatous *Acanthamoeba* infection presenting as an unusual skin lesion. Am J Med. 1979;67:891–6.
26. Baum J. In: Case records of the Massachusetts General Hospital Case 10-1985. N Engl J Med. 1985;312:634–41.
27. Lawande RV, John I, Dobbs RH, et al. A case or primary amebic meningoencephalitis in Zaria, Nigeria. Am J Clin Pathol. 1979;71:591–4.
28. Siedel JS, Harmatz P, Visvesvara GS, et al. Successful treatment of primary amebic meningoencephalitis. N Engl J Med. 1982;306:346.
29. Lindquist TD, Sher NA, Doughman DJ. Clinical signs and medical therapy of early *Acanthamoeba* keratitis. Arch Ophthalmol. 1988;106:73–7.
30. Butt CG, Baro C, Knorr RW. *Naegleria* (sp) identified in amebic encephalitis. Am J Clin Pathol. 1968;50:568–74.
31. Darby CP, Corradi SE, Holbrook TW, et al. Primary amebic meningoencephalitis. Am J Dis Child. 1979;133:1025–7.
32. Lawande RV, Macfarlane JT, Weir WRC, et al. A case of primary amebic meningoencephalitis in a Nigerian farmer. Am J Trop Med Hyg. 1980;29:21–5.
33. Callicott JH Jr, Nelson EC, Jones MM, et al. Meningoencephalitis due to pathogenic free-living amoebae. Report of two cases. JAMA. 1968;206:579–82.
34. Duma RJ, Rosenblum WI, McGehee RF, et al. Primary amebic meningoencephalitis caused by *Naegleria*. Two new cases, response to amphotericin B and a review. Ann Intern Med. 1971;74:923–32.
35. Cohen EJ, Parlato CJ, Arentsen JJ, et al. Medical and surgical treatment of *Acanthamoeba* keratitis. Am J Ophthalmol. 1987;103:615–25.
36. Wright P, Warhurst D, Jones BR. *Acanthamoeba* keratitis successfully treated medically. Br J Ophthalmol. 1985;69:778–82.
37. Silvany RE, Luckenbach MW, Moore MB. The rapid detection of *Acanthamoeba* in paraffin-embedded sections of corneal tissue with Calcofluor white. Arch Ophthalmol. 1987;105:1366–7.
38. Anderson K, Jamieson A. Primary amoebic meningoencephalitis. Lancet 1972;i:902–3.
39. Lallinger GJ, Reiner SL, Cooke DW, et al. Efficacy of immune therapy in early experimental *Naegleria fowleri* meningitis. Infect Immun. 1987;55:1289–93.
40. Duma RJ, Finley R. In vitro susceptibility of pathogenic *Naegleria* and *Acanthamoeba* species to a variety of therapeutic agents. Antimicrob Agents Chemother. 1976;10:370–6.
41. Nagington J, Richards JE. Chemotherapeutic compounds and *Acanthamoeba* from eye infections. J Clin Pathol. 1976;29:648–51.
42. Holland GN, Donzis PB. Rapid resolution of early *Acanthamoeba* keratitis after epithelial debridement. Am J Ophthalmol. 1987;104:87–9.
43. Moore MB, McCulley JP. Medical and surgical treatment of *Acanthamoeba* keratitis (Letter). Am J Ophthalmol. 1987;104:310–1.
44. Johns KJ, Head WS, O'Day DM. Corneal toxicity of propamidine. Arch Ophthalmol. 1988;106:68–9.
45. Davis RM, Schroeder RP, Rowsey JJ, et al. *Acanthamoeba* keratitis and infectious crystalline keratopathy. Arch Ophthalmol. 1987;105:1524–7.

251. PLASMODIUM SPECIES (MALARIA)

DAVID J. WYLER

Few infectious diseases have had the same impact on the social and economic development of societies as malaria. Although it was not until the seventeenth century that the disease was named by the Italians (*mal'aria,* bad air), the first references to the periodic fevers of malaria can be found in the early Chinese, Chaldean, and Hindu writings. In the fourth century BC, when malaria was endemic in the Mediterranean basin, the Greeks noted an association between exposure to swamps and the subsequent development of periodic fevers and splenomegaly. The recognition of this association led the Greeks, and later the Romans, to drain swamps, a practice that continues to be an important method of controlling the mosquito vector of malaria. In the early seventeenth century, the bark of the quina-quina (cinchona) tree of South America was successfully used in the treatment of intermittent fevers, although it was only in the mid-nineteenth century that quinine was identified as the active alkaloid in the bark. The major breakthrough in understanding the etiology of the disease occurred in 1880 when Charles Louis Alphonse Laveran, a French army surgeon, first saw exflagellated gametocytes in a fresh blood film obtained from a patient with malaria. Five years later, Golgi recognized the multiplication of the asexual blood forms. Only after the development of the Romanowsky polychrome stains in 1891, however, were the distinctive morphologic features of the *Plasmodium* appreciated. At about this time Patrick Manson, who had discovered that filariasis was transmitted by mosquitoes, postulated that malaria was similarly transmitted. Ronald Ross, a British army surgeon in the Indian Medical Service, subsequently recognized developing plasmodia in the mosquito gut, supporting Manson's theory. Through a series of careful studies of bird malaria, Ross conclusively established the major features of the life cycle of plasmodia and received the Nobel Prize in 1902. The site of exoerythrocytic development was not identified until 1948 (Shortt and Garnham).

The history of malaria in this century has been dominated by efforts directed at controlling the vector and at developing potent synthetic antimalarial agents. In 1955, the World Health Organization (WHO) began a worldwide malaria eradication program that continued until 1976, when it was officially declared a failure. The development of resistance to DDT by the vectors and resistance to chloroquine by strains of *Plasmodium falciparum* severely impaired the WHO program and contributed to resurgence of transmission in several areas. Recognizing the limitations of many of the classic approaches to malaria control and the continued impact of the disease on developing nations, scientists have recently begun to direct efforts at seeking newer approaches, such as vaccines, to control malaria.[1]

DESCRIPTION OF THE ORGANISM

Malaria is caused by species of the obligate intracellular protozoa classified in the genus *Plasmodium* within the class Sporozoa (subphylum Apicomplexa), a class that includes certain other human pathogenic protozoa, such as *Toxoplasma gondii* and *Babesia*. In the life cycle of plasmodia, asexual reproduction occurs in humans, and sexual reproduction occurs in the mosquito. Although a large number of *Plasmodium* spp. naturally infect a variety of animals, such as monkeys, rodents, birds, and reptiles, only four species infect humans: *P. falciparum, P. vivax, P. malariae,* and *P. ovale.*[2]* Each sp. has certain morphologic characteristics by which the parasite is identified, as well as biologic and pathogenic features of clinical importance.

Malaria is transmitted by the bites of infected female anopheline mosquitoes or by inoculation of infected blood (e.g., transfusion malaria, congenital malaria). The infective stage, called *sporozoites,* are injected from the mosquito salivary glands into subcutaneous capillaries and circulate to the liver, where they invade hepatic parenchymal cells (Fig. 1). Here the parasites multiply in stages called *exoerythrocytic forms* (or *EE forms*) and become hepatic schizonts. After 1–2 weeks of development, the hepatic schizonts rupture, and each releases thousands of *merozoites,* which enter the circulation and invade erythrocytes. In *P. falciparum* and *P. malariae,* all EE forms rupture more or less at the same time, and none persist chronically in the liver. In contrast, EE forms in *P. vivax* and *P. ovale* exist in two types: the *primary exoerythrocytic forms* that develop and rupture, resulting in an initial wave of parasitemia within weeks after infection, and the *latent exoerythrocytic forms* (also called *hypnozoites*) that may remain in the liver for months or years before they rupture, resulting in relapses of erthrocytic infection. Once the parasites enter the erythrocytic stage, they never reinvade the liver. Therefore, blood-induced

* Humans can be infected experimentally with certain simian malaria species (e.g., *P. knowlesi* and *P. cynomolgi*), and rare cases of naturally acquired human infection with these species have been reported.

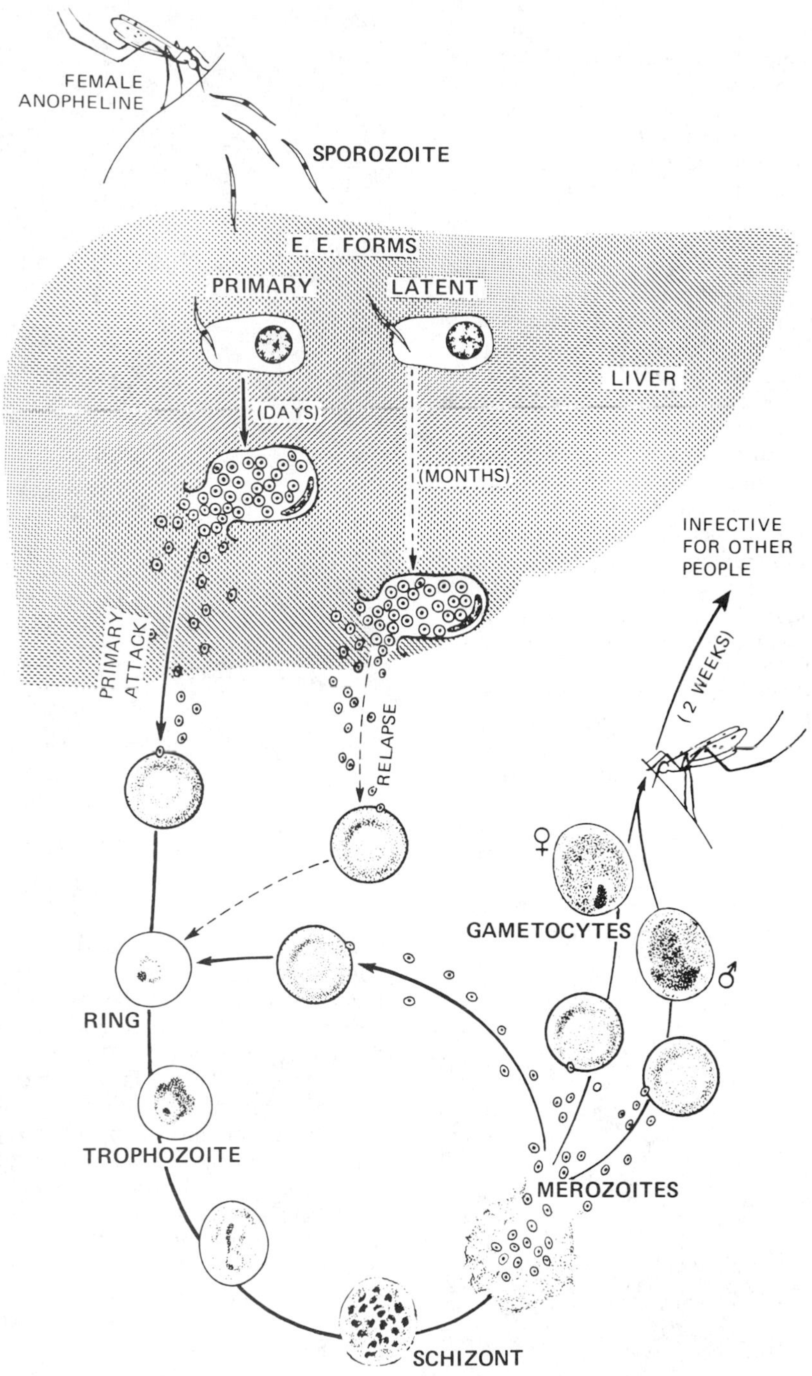

FIG. 1. Life cycle of plasmodia in humans.

infections (e.g., transfusion malaria) never result in development of exoerythrocytic forms.

The invasion of erythrocytes by merozoites entails a highly complex set of events that depend on the interaction between specific surface receptors on merozoites and those on the surface of erythrocytes.[3] Thus, for example, persons whose erythrocytes are Duffy blood-group negative (that is, they lack Duffy a and b determinants) are not susceptible to *P. vivax* infection.[4] In contrast, *P. falciparum* requires determinants on glycophorin (the major surface glycoprotein of erythrocytes) and other sialoproteins for invasion of red cells. Invasion entails movement of a junction that forms between the merozoite and the red cell membrane.[5] Plasmodia develop within a vacuole lined by an erythrocyte plasma membrane that forms during invasion. The age of the erythrocyte is an important determinant of its susceptibility to invasion by different species of the parasite. Only young erythrocytes are infected by *P. vivax* and *P. ovale,* and only mature erythrocytes are susceptible to *P. malariae*. The magnitude of parasitemia is, therefore, limited in malarial infections due to these species. In contrast, *P. falciparum* can develop in erythrocytes of all ages, and parasitemia can reach very high levels. Since the magnitude of parasitemia is an important determinant of mortality in malaria, it is not surprising that infection with *P. falciparum* but not with the other species is frequently fatal if left untreated. Additional erythrocyte characteristics that affect parasite development include hemoglobin composition and enzyme content. The development of *P. falciparum* is suppressed in the presence of fetal hemoglobin, hemoglobin S (HbS), and possibly also in the presence of certain other abnormal hemoglobins.[6] The selective advantage of HbS in innate resistance to falciparum malaria has been well established. Parasites fail to develop in HbS-containing erythrocytes exposed to low oxygen tension, probably because potassium leaks from such infected cells.[7] Although other erythrocyte polymorphisms, for example, glucose-6-phosphate dehydrogenase (G6PD) deficiency, are prevalent in areas of *P. falciparum* endemicity, their protective role in malaria is less certain.[8]

On entering the erythrocyte, merozoites acquire the appearance of signet rings and are called *ring forms*. On Giemsa-stained blood smears, a small purplish nucleus can be seen attached to a fine ring of bluish cytoplasm. As development of the asexual parasite proceeds, the cytoplasm increases in quantity; at this stage the forms are called *trophozoites* (Fig. 2). When nuclear division occurs, the parasites become known as *schizonts* (Fig. 3) and erythrocytes ultimately contain 6–24 individual *merozoites* (the exact number per schizont depends on the species of *Plasmodium*). Rupture of the schizont rapidly ensues, with release of the merozoites into the circulation. Within seconds the merozoites attach to and penetrate new erythrocytes. The process of intracellular maturation leading to development of the schizont, and its ultimate rupture, is called *schizogony*. This process requires approximately 72 hours for *P. malariae* (*quartan* malaria) and 48 hours for the other three species (*tertian* malaria). Among the species of *Plasmodium* that cause human malaria, *P. falciparum* is distinctive in undergoing schizogony while infected erythrocytes are sequestered in capillary and venular beds. Trophozoites and schizonts of *P. falciparum* are generally not present in the peripheral circulation.

The sexual cycle of reproduction begins with the development of *gametocytes* (Fig. 4) from a subpopulation of merozoites. Male and female gametocytes, which can be distinguished from asexual trophozoites and from each other on a morphologic basis, are ingested by susceptible female anopheline mosquitoes during a blood meal. Within the gut of the mosquito, the male gametocyte undergoes a process of *exflagellation,* which results in the release of up to eight *male gametes,* spermlike organisms that fertilize *female gametes* (derived from the female gametocyte). The resulting fertilized *zygotes* invade the gut wall of the mosquito, where they develop into *oöcysts,* each of which contains thousands of sporozoites. This process of *sporogony* requires approximately 10 days and culminates in the rupture of the oöcyst with release of the sporozoites into the hemocoel that surrounds the gut and in sporozoite migration to the salivary glands. When the mosquito subsequently feeds, sporozoites are injected with saliva into the host. In vitro methods are now available for cultivating asexual and sexual blood stages of certain *Plasmodia,* and for studying invasion of host cells by sporozoites and merozoites, and fertilization of gametes.

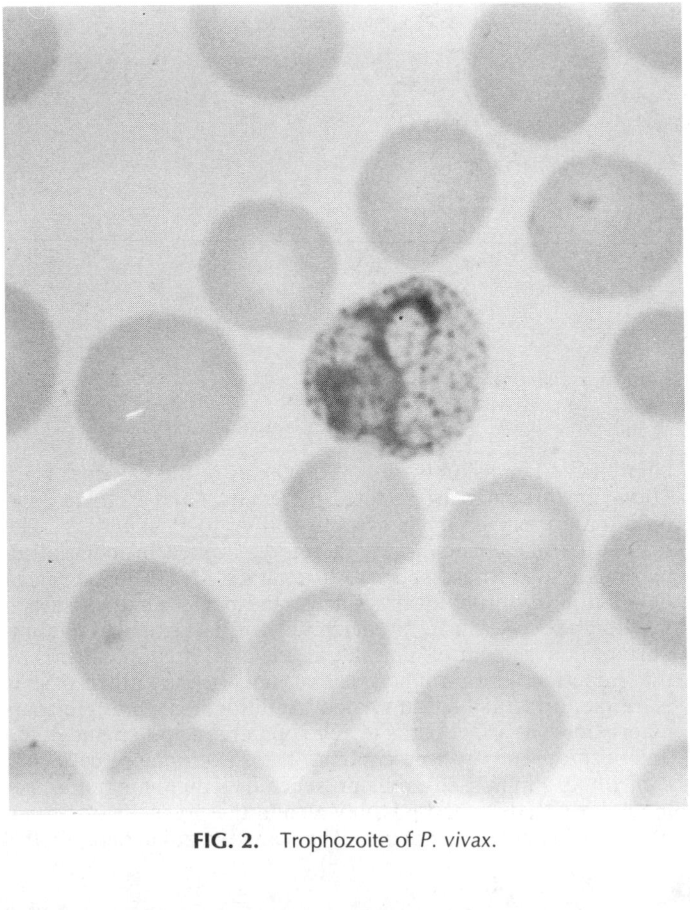

FIG. 2. Trophozoite of *P. vivax*.

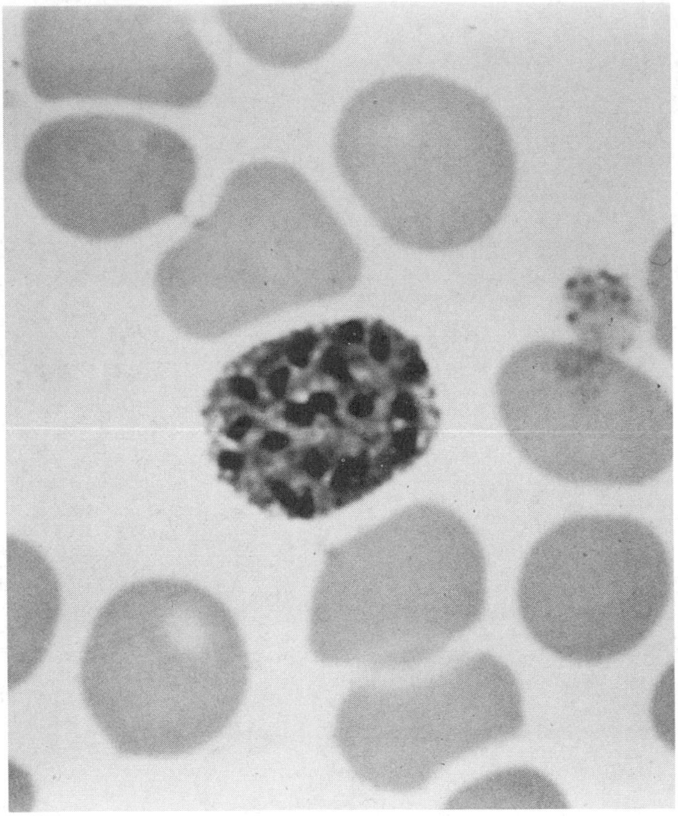

FIG. 3. Schizont of *P. vivax*.

EPIDEMIOLOGY

Malaria is estimated to have a worldwide prevalence of more than 100 million cases associated with approximately 1 million deaths per year in Africa alone and is widely distributed in countries of Africa, Asia, and Latin America. Malaria has been eliminated from the United States, Puerto Rico, Jamaica, the Antilles, Chile, Israel, Lebanon, Japan, Taiwan, North Korea, Australia, and Europe (except for small foci in Greece). Although it is impossible to make precise statements about species distribution, *P. vivax* predominates in India, Pakistan, Bangladesh, Sri Lanka, and Central America, while *P. falciparum* infections occur much less frequently in these countries. *Plasmodium vivax* occurs rarely in Africa because of the resistance to this sp. of most blacks, presumably because they lack the appropriate erythrocyte receptors associated with the Duffy blood group. *Plasmodium falciparum* predominates in Africa, Haiti, and New Guinea. *Plasmodium falciparum* and *P. vivax*

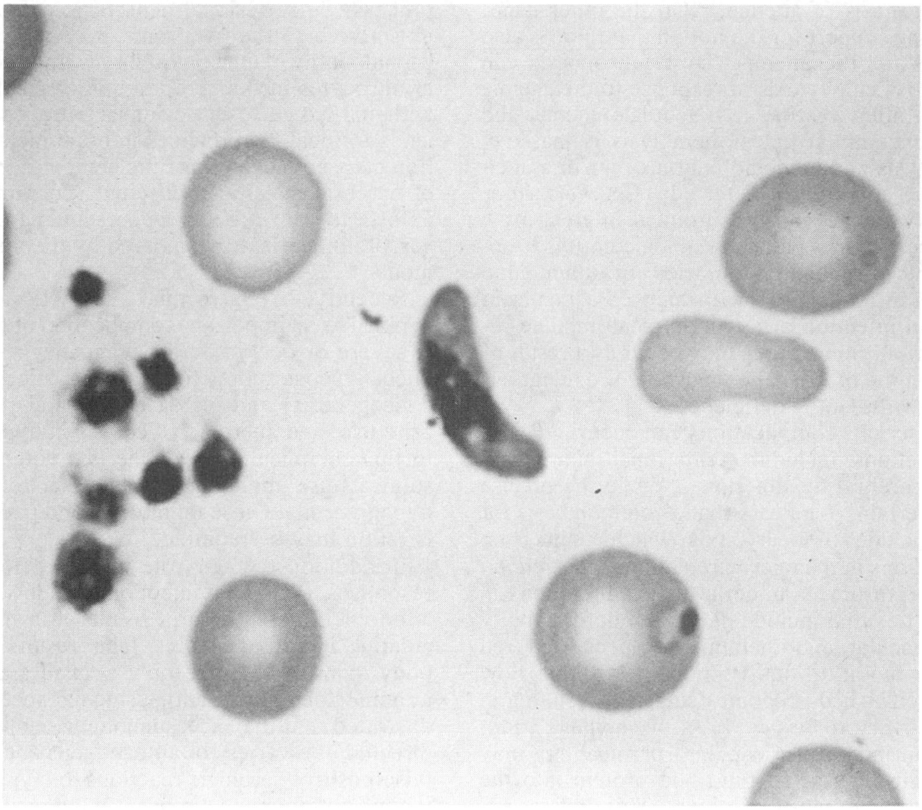

FIG. 4. Gametocyte of *P. falciparum*.

malaria are both prevalent in Southeast Asia, South America, and Oceania. *Plasmodium ovale* occurs primarily in Africa, with rare cases on other continents. The distribution of *P. malariae* is cosmopolitan. In the United States and Europe, malaria is not endemic but occurs as imported or induced (e.g., blood transfusions) cases. Since the anopheline mosquito vectors (*Anopheles quadrimaculatus* and *A. freeborni*) continue to be present in large numbers in the United States, transmission of parasites from imported cases of malaria is a continual risk. In fact, small epidemics due to local transmission of *P. falciparum* and *P. vivax* from imported cases have been recognized in the United States since the 1950s.[9]

The incidence of malaria in the United States has directly paralleled military troop involvement in endemic regions ever since the disease was eradicated from the continental United States in the late 1940s. The close of the Vietnam War era resulted in an initial marked decrease in the total number of cases of malaria in the United States. Travel to endemic areas by American civilians and travel to the United States by citizens from malarious areas are responsible for imported cases. In some imported cases, death (from *P. falciparum*) has resulted from delay in diagnosis or failure to institute appropriate therapy. Congenital and transfusion malaria remain infrequent problems. To minimize the risk of transfusion malaria, the American Association of Blood Banks has recommended that travelers to endemic areas who did not take antimalarial chemoprophylaxis and remained symptom free may donate blood only after a period of 6 months after reentry into the United States. Those persons who took antimalarials, who had malaria, or whose home of origin is an endemic country must wait 3 years before donating blood. Since *P. malariae* can persist in the blood as an asymptomatic infection for more than 50 years, these blood banking rules will not eliminate the risk of transfusion malaria due to this parasite species.[10]

PATHOGENESIS

Neither the presence of sporozoites or exoerythrocytic forms nor gametocytes are directly deleterious to the host, and only the asexual intraerythrocytic parasites cause disease. The pathogenic mechanisms involved in establishing clinical illness can be divided into four basic processes: (*1*) fever and its physiologic consequences, (*2*) anemia, (*3*) tissue hypoxia resulting from anemia and alterations in the microcirculation, and (*4*) initiation of immunopathologic events.

Fever is the hallmark of malaria infection due to all species, and although it has attracted considerable attention for over 2000 years, the basis of malarial fevers remains obscure. The direct temporal association between schizont rupture and the febrile paroxysm has suggested that parasites might liberate a pyrogen, but none has been identified. It has been postulated that endogenous pyrogen is secreted by tissue macrophages, which ingest erythrocyte and parasite debris released at the time of schizont rupture. Tumor necrosis factor/cachectin, an endogenous pyrogen, has been detected in sera of patients with malaria, but its role in the pathogenesis of fever in malaria remains uncertain.[11] Marked vasodilatation results from high fever and causes a decrease in the effective plasma volume, which may result in orthostatic hypotension. As a result, antidiuretic hormone and aldosterone secretion increase. Fluid and electrolyte balance may be further altered by the effects of marked diaphoresis, vomiting, and decreased fluid intake that accompany the paroxysm. Hyponatremia frequently results.[12]

Anemia is a common complication of malaria, and extensive hemolysis may occur in association with very high parasitemias. For the most part, hemolysis results from rupture of infected erythrocytes during schizogony, although the magnitude of hemolysis tends to be greater than can be accounted for by this process alone. Splenic sequestration of erythrocytes in association with the development of splenomegaly probably contributes to the pathogenesis of anemia.[12] On the other hand, there is little compelling support for the notion that there is also an autoimmune basis for the anemia. Dyserythropoesis can occur, and peripheral reticulocytosis in response to the anemia may be delayed even after treatment.[13] Hemoglobinemia and hemoglobinuria are uncommon unless hemolysis is massive. When massive hemolysis and hemoglobinuria occur in association with malaria, the condition is referred to as *blackwater fever*. Although blackwater fever is enshrouded in great mystique, it is not clearly a distinct pathophysiologic entity. It occurs rarely in residents of endemic countries. In nonimmune persons it may occur in association with high parasitemia in cases of *P. falciparum* infection or as an atypical immune response during reinfection. Some cases may occur as a result of hypersensitivity to quinine or after the ingestion of oxidant antimalarials in patients with G6PD deficiency.

A number of other serious complications can occur in *P. falciparum* malarial infections, including acute renal failure, pulmonary edema, and cerebral dysfunction.[14] While the precise mechanisms are not certain, it appears that a common basis for these complications includes tissue hypoxia, which results from the anemia and alterations in the microcirculation. *Plasmodium falciparum*-infected erythrocytes undergo major alterations in their rheologic properties that include decreased deformability and adherence to vascular endothelium via specialized red blood cell membrane modifications ("knobs").[15] Blood flow through the microvascular beds becomes sluggish, resulting in decreased oxygen delivery to tissue. Loss of capillary endothelial integrity and an increase in capillary permeability may occur and can result in leakage of fluid and protein into the interstitial space of certain organs (e.g., lung). This dictates extreme caution in fluid management of patients with complicated falciparum malaria. Microthrombi and putative malarial toxins have been postulated to contribute to the pathogenesis. The histopathologic expression of these processes includes renal cortical changes due to ischemia and acute tubular necrosis.[16] The pulmonary pathologic changes in patients with pulmonary edema as a complication include microvascular congestion with or without thrombus formation, interstitial edema, and hyaline membrane formation.[17] In fatal cases of malaria, the cerebral cortical gray matter may contain congested vessels filled with parasitized erythrocytes, perivascular edema, hemorrhage (ring hemorrhage), and, rarely, glial reaction (malarial granuloma); some of these changes probably represent agonal or postmortem changes.[18,19] Malabsorption and enterocolitis, less common complications of *P. falciparum* malaria, presumably result from similar pathologic processes.[20] Gram-negative sepsis can complicate falciparum malaria. Whether this occurs as a result of a compromise in the integrity of the bowel mucosa, and whether there is defective reticuloendothelial clearance of gram-negative bacteria during malaria, remain to be assessed.

A major role of disseminated intravascular coagulation (DIC) in the pathogenesis of malaria complications has not been established. Some patients develop laboratory evidence of a coagulopathy, with decreased levels of factors V, VII, VIII, X, fibrinogen, and platelets, and prolonged prothrombin and partial thromboplastin times, in addition to having circulating fibrin degradation products. About 5 percent of patients with cerebral malaria develop clinically important bleeding.[21] On the other hand, fatal cases of *P. falciparum* malaria frequently lack pathologic evidence of DIC at postmortem examination. Therefore, neither heparin nor fibrinolytic agents can be justified in treating complications of malaria.

Cerebral malaria is the most common complication of severe malaria (it occurs only in falciparum malaria); death occurs in 20–50 percent of patients. The pathogenesis of cerebral malaria has recently been reassessed by application of modern techniques.[22,23] In contrast to prior notions, it now appears that cerebral edema, reduction in total cerebral blood flow, inflammation, and microthrombus formation are not involved in the process. Since residual neurologic defects are rarely detected in surivivors, the syndrome may represent a metabolic encephalopathy.[14] One possibility is that sequestration of infected erythrocytes in the cerebral microvasculature, in combination with marked glucose use and lactate production by the parasite, leads to local disturbances in brain metabolism. This explanation does not account for the great variability in the prevalence of cerebral malaria in different geographic regions, however. Efforts to gain a better understanding of the pathogenesis of cerebral malaria are hampered by the lack of a suitable animal model.[24]

Recently, hypoglycemia with lactic acidosis has been recognized as an important complication of falciparum malaria that is severe or occurs during pregnancy.[25] It is believed that reduced glucose supply (impaired hepatic glycogenolysis and gluconeogenesis) and increased demand (hyperinsulinemia, parasite use, and anerobic glycolysis in hypoxic tissue) contribute to this complication. Quinine is a potent secretogogue for insulin; its use in antimalarial treatment can aggravate or induce hypoglycemia. Close monitoring and parenteral glucose administration may be required.

In addition to their role in host defense, the immunologic responses to malarial infection include some that may have deleterious effects. Malaria results in a marked increase in circulating immunoglobulins. This results from polyclonal antibody stimulation since only a small amount of the increased immunoglobulin has antiplasmodial specificity. It can be demonstrated that the excess immunoglobulin may have specificity directed at a variety of autoantigens and may result in biologic false-positive serologic reactions for syphilis (VDRL, FTA), although autoimmune disease is not a recognized consequence of malaria.[26] Antibody-mediated splenic sequestration of platelets coated with parasite antigens may contribute to the pathogenesis of thrombocytopenia of malaria.[27] The deposition of immune complexes (composed of plasmodial antigen, IgG, and complement components) in the glomeruli of some children with chronic *P. malariae* infection may result in glomerulonephritis and nephrotic syndrome.[28] This form of immunecomplex glomerulonephritis is unresponsive to antimalarials, corticosteroids, or azothioprine. At present it remains to be determined why this condition only occurs as a complication of malaria due to *P. malariae* and not of malaria due to other species.

The marked reticuloendothelial hyperplasia that results as a response to the sustained intravascular infection not only assists the host in clearing parasites and damaged erythrocytes but also has deleterious effects.[29] Hypersplenism results from the marked splenomegaly and plays a role in the development of anemia, neutropenia, and thrombocytopenia of malaria. In addition, a small number of patients living in endemic regions of Africa, Indonesia, and New Guinea develop massive splenic enlargement and hepatic sinusoidal lymphocytic infiltrates. These patients with so-called tropical splenomegaly syndrome or big spleen disease are often free of detectable circulating plasmodia when diagnosed, although they have high antibody titers to the parasite and respond favorably to chronic antimalarial chemotherapy with a decrease in spleen size and reversal of the pathologic changes in the liver.[30] The etiology of this disease is unknown, but the higher attack rate in kindreds has suggested that these people may represent genetically determined abnormal host responses to chronic malaria. Similarly, the development of Burkitt's lymphoma in Africans living in malaria endemic regions is believed to represent an atypical consequence of Epstein-Barr virus infection in patients with malaria.[31] Although the association of this lymphoproliferative disorder with malaria has not been established with certainty, one possible role that malaria might play as a cofactor in oncogenesis is its effect on the reticuloendothelial system and its ability to induce immunosuppression, thereby compromising host immune surveillance mechanisms directed against tumors. Some clinical observations and more extensive experimental evidence have established that malarial infection prevents the host from mounting certain normal immune responses to a variety of antigens. This immune defect is mediated in part by pigment-laden macrophages and may explain why some patients develop other intercurrent infections.[32]

CLINICAL MANIFESTATIONS

The malarial paroxysm—characterized by high fever, chills, and rigor—is the hallmark of acute malaria. Many patients experience a prodromal period 1 to several days before the onset of the paroxysms and may complain of nonspecific symptoms, such as malaise, headache, myalgia, and fatigue, that are easily mistaken for a viral illness. In addition, patients may complain of more localized symptoms, such as chest pain, abdominal pain, and arthralgias. The ability of malaria to masquerade as other diseases is well known and frequently results in delays in establishing the correct diagnosis.[33] It is particularly important, therefore, that physicians practicing in nonendemic areas maintain a high index of suspicion for malaria in all travelers to endemic countries, intravenous drug addicts, and recipients of blood transfusions. Since symptoms may appear a few days before parasites can be detected by blood smear, it is important to sustain this suspicion and to continue to obtain blood smears for several days before excluding the diagnosis.

The malarial paroxysm has many clinical features in common with those elicited by administering endotoxin to humans, and yet, circulating pyrogens have not been identified during this event. Initially, the patient experiences chills, rigors, and headache. The cold, pale skin with cyanosis of the lips and nail beds and cutis anserina (goose flesh) attest to marked sympathetic discharge. This "cold period" of peripheral vasoconstriction within minutes to 1–2 hours gives way to a "hot phase" in which the temperature not uncommonly rises to 105–106°F, and the patient's skin becomes warm and dry. Tachycardia, tachypnea, cough, severe headache, backache, abdominal pain, nausea, vomiting, and delerium are characteristic of this phase. Orthostatic hypotension resulting from a decrease in effective intravascular volume in the setting of marked peripheral vasodilatation commonly occurs. In 3–6 hours, the patient begins to defervesce and becomes markedly diaphoretic. The temperature may remain elevated between paroxysms in cases of *P. falciparum* malaria. Euphoria and fatigue give way to sleep at this point. Patients may be remarkably asymptomatic between paroxysms, in contrast to many other febrile illnesses. Although these dramatic paroxysms may occur with some regularity, such as every 48 hours in *P. vivax* infections, fever patterns are often irregular. Therefore, it is incorrect to exclude the diagnosis of malaria merely on the basis of irregular fever patterns.

On physical examination, patients frequently are found to have moderate splenomegaly and tender hepatomegaly. Either or both of these signs may be absent when the patient is first examined. The spleen may be extremely delicate due to the sudden stretching of its capsule and is prone to rupture, especially in *P. vivax* malaria. Splenic rupture may also occur spontaneously, even after therapy is instituted. Vigorous palpation of the spleen may be dangerous and should be avoided. Lymphadenopathy does not occur in malaria, and its presence in a patient with malaria should prompt a search for an additional etiology. Other physical findings that have been described in association with malaria but occur with less frequency include jaundice, urticaria, petechial rash, conjunctival suffusion, scleral icterus, retinal vasospasm and hemorrhage, and herpes labialis. Auscultation of the chest may reveal scattered rales in some patients or, rarely, evidence of pulmonary consolidation. Cardiac examination is generally normal except for tachycardia. Fever and anemia may result in flow murmurs and may precipitate congestive heart failure in patients with underlying heart disease. The abdomen may be tender. Despite complaints of myalgia and arthralgia, neither muscle tenderness nor joint effusions are present. Peripheral edema is usually absent. In uncomplicated cases, the neurologic examination is normal, with the exception of delirium and other minor behavioral changes that may result from high fever. Cerebral malaria occurs as a complication of *P. falciparum* infection, although tissue hypoxia resulting from any malaria infection could pose a risk of cerebral ischemia and infarction in patients with cerebrovascular disease. The neurologic abnormalities that have been observed in association with cerebral involvement include (*1*) disturbance of consciousness ranging from somnolence to coma, (*2*) acute organic brain syndromes with altered intellectual function, behavioral changes, or hallucinations, (*3*) major motor seizures, (*4*) meningismus, and, rarely, (*5*) focal neurologic signs. such as Babinski reflexes or hemiparesis, or movement disorders, such as tremors, myoclonus, and choreiform movements. Lumbar puncture is not diagnostic; an increased opening pressure due to cerebral edema and a normal cerebrospinal fluid (CSF) profile may be found. Rarely, an increased CSF protein concentration and lowgrade pleocytosis have been reported, but hypoglycorrhachia does not occur. Although a wide variety of neurologic abnormalities have been described in association with *P. falciparum* infection, other causes occurring concomitantly with malaria have not been excluded in most of the cases reported. Therefore, in patients with cerebral malaria whose neurologic defects are predominantly focal, or in those who have increased erythrocytes or leukocytes in the CSF, evaluation should be undertaken to exclude other pathologic processes. It may be impossible to distinguish febrile convulsions from cerebral malaria in children with *P. falciparum* infection. Worsening cerebral dysfunction in patients with falciparum malaria, even during therapy, may be a sign of hypoglycemia.[25]

Malaria during pregnancy can increase the risk of low birth weight, prematurity, abortion, and stillbirth. *Plasmodium falciparum*-infected pregnant women are at particular risk for developing hypoglycemia. In regions where malaria is endemic, acquired immunity to malaria is commonly lost during pregnancy. The choice of drugs for the prevention and treatment of malaria in pregnancy must consider potential adverse effects on the fetus (see below).

The *diagnosis of malaria* rests on the demonstration of parasites in stained peripheral blood smears (Table 1). Although a higher density of parasites appears in circulation during the paroxysm as schizonts burst and release merozoites, timing in obtaining smears is less important than that smears be obtained several times daily. Symptoms may precede a detectable level of parasitemia by a few days, so smears should be examined at least twice daily until parasites are detected. A diagnosis of malaria can only be excluded by obtaining negative blood smears on several successive days. Efforts to quantitate parasitemia are useful in determining a baseline parasitemia from which the response to therapy can be monitored. Once parasites are detected, thin smears should be examined in an effort to make a species diagnosis (Table 2). Since most physicians are not sufficiently experienced in the morphologic differentiation of plasmodial species, slides should be saved and expert opinion should be sought as soon as possible. Initially, the most important distinction to be made is whether or not the patient has *P. falciparum* malaria. Criteria such as the small size of the rings, the presence of double chromatin knobs (reminiscent of headphones), the tendency for multiple rings to be present in individual erythrocytes, the predominance of rings with few trophozoites and no schizonts in blood smears, and the presence of the characteristic banana-shaped gametocyte, all suggest *P. falciparum*. In any case, if more than 5 percent of the erythrocytes are parasitized, *P. falciparum* malaria should also be suspected. Since the initial therapy for all other species will be the same (chloroquine), immediate determination of the species causing malaria not due to *P. falciparum* is clinically less important. When parasites are not detected on several carefully

TABLE 1. Guide to the Preparation and Examination of Blood Smears in the Diagnosis of Malaria

Thick smear

Thick smears have the advantage of allowing one to examine a larger sample of blood than is possible using thin smears. The principle of the thick smear is that the concentrated erythrocytes are lysed with distilled water, revealing intact parasites. The thick smear should be used only for detecting the presence of parasites and quantitating parasitemia and not for species diagnosis.

1. Place one drop of blood from a finger stick on a thoroughly cleaned glass slide labeled with the patient's name, date, and time.
2. Using the tip of a broken wooden applicator stick or the pointed edge of a glass slide, in a circular motion evenly spread out the blood to a diameter of about ¾ inch (size of a dime).
3. Air dry for at least 30 minutes.
4. Without fixing the smear, stain with Giemsa. Wright stain (used for routine hematologic examinations) may not be optimal for staining plasmodia. Wright-Giemsa stain used in some automatic stainers is suitable. Giemsa stain should be adjusted to pH 7–7.2 to stain Schuffner's dots optimally.

Thin Smear

The thin smear can be used for detecting parasites and should be used for making species diagnosis.

1. Prepare a smear of one drop of blood from a finger stick in a manner used for routine hematologic examinations.
2. Dry the smear and fix it in absolute methanol.
3. Stain with Giemsa.

Quantitation of parasitemia

At low parasite densities, the magnitude of parasitemia can be estimated in terms of the average number of parasitized erythrocytes per oil-emersion field in 5–10 fields. At higher parasite densities, the actual percentage of erythrocytes infected can be determined. An alternative method is to count on thick smears the number of parasites present per 50 white blood cells seen on the smear. By dividing the white blood cell count by 50 and multiplying this number by the number of parasites/50 WBC, the number of parasites/mm^3 can be determined. The goal of quantitating parasitemia is not to achieve great accuracy but rather to determine whether parasitemia is increasing or decreasing during therapy.

examined smears, the presence of granular brownish pigment within monocytes or neutrophils should alert the physician to the presence of malaria. Although serologic tests (IFA and IHA) for malaria are available in the United States through the Centers for Disease Control, Atlanta, Georgia, they should not be relied on to establish a diagnosis of malaria. Serologic tests in malaria are useful in epidemiologic surveys and in identifying infected donors in cases of transfusion malaria.

A variety of abnormalities in routine laboratory tests may be encountered in patients with malaria. In addition to a normochromic, normocytic hemolytic anemia, leukopenia due to a decrease in granulocytes and lymphocytes is often present. However, in the first few days of infection, a transient increase in the percentage of band forms is not unusual. Relative and absolute monocytosis frequently occurs, and monocytes may contain malarial pigment; erythrophagocytosis of normal and parasitized cells may occasionally be recognized. Platelet counts may reach very low levels (less than 50,000/mm^3), but this rarely results in spontaneous hemorrhage and is rapidly reversible with the appropriate antimalarial chemotherapy. Malaria does not cause eosinophilia.

Urinalysis frequently reveals small amounts of protein, probably related to the effects of fever, and is otherwise normal. In the presence of acute tubular necrosis, casts can be seen in the sediment. Children with nephrotic syndrome due to *P. malariae* have marked proteinuria and may also have casts. Elevation in the blood urea nitrogen level may reflect fever and dehydration, but if serum creatinine levels rise disproportionately, renal failure must be considered. Electrolyte balance may be altered by several factors, such as dehydration, vomiting, tissue hypoxia, tachypnea, renal failure, and homeostatic responses to a decrease in effective plasma volume. Repeated serum electrolyte and blood gas determinations are important in assessing the changing status in severely ill patients. Liver function tests may reveal abnormalities, which include elevated transaminase levels and a mild to moderate increase in bilirubin (mostly indirect) but usually normal alkaline phosphatase levels. Marked abnormalities in liver function tests should suggest an associated illness or centrilobular necrosis complicating malaria. Additional tests that may be abnormal include a biologic false-positive VDRL. Hypoglycemia may complicate certain cases of malaria.

THERAPY AND PREVENTION

Treatment of Plasmodium falciparum Malaria

The principles of clinical management of *P. falciparum* malaria include (*1*) early recognition of infection due to *P. falciparum*, (*2*) rapid institution of effective antimalarial chemotherapy by the appropriate route of administration, (*3*) recognition of and therapy for complications, and (*4*) monitoring of the immediate and long-term clinical and parasitologic responses to treatment. Rapid geographic dissemination of multidrug-resistant strains

TABLE 2. Summary of Important Diagnostic and Clinical Features in Human Malaria

	Morphologic Characteristics Useful in Species Diagnosis[a]				
Species	*Infected RBC*	*Trophozoite*	*Schizont*	*Gametocyte*	*Important Clinical Features*
P. falciparum	Normal size; multiply infected RBC more frequent than other species	Small rings with threadlike cytoplasm (blue) and double chromatin dots (red)	Seldom seen in peripheral blood smear	Diagnostic banana-shaped gametocyte	Can achieve very high parasitemia, causing death through complications (severe anemia, renal failure, cerebral dysfunction, pulmonary edema, etc.); pulmonary edema, etc.); A MEDICAL EMERGENCY! Failure to recognize *P. falciparum* and to treat appropriately can lead to death.
P. vivax	Enlarged in size; Schüffner's dots (red) present	Ameboid cytoplasm	Can be seen on smear	Round	Infection limited to younger RBCs; danger of splenic rupture, relapse related to persistence of latent EE forms
P. ovale	Somewhat enlarged, oval in shape, with fringed edges; Schüffner's dots present	Compact cytoplasm	Can be seen on smear	Round	Same as *P. vivax*
P. malariae	Normal size	Compact cytoplasm	Merozoites arranged in rosette around central pigment clump	Round	Limited parasitemia; can be very chronic in subclinical and subpatent forms; can cause nephritis in children
Mixed	Features of each species				

[a] As seen on Giemsa-stained thin smears.

of *P. falciparum* can occur, and serious side effects of some antimalarials may be recognized only with their widespread use. Accordingly, physicians should obtain the most up-to-date information before prescribing antimalarial drugs for therapeutic or prophylactic purposes. Recommendations given in this section are current as of late 1988.

The diagnosis of *P. falciparum* infection should be established without delay since patients, even those who appear clinically stable, may deteriorate rapidly if left untreated. If *P. falciparum* infection can be definitely ruled out, therapy with chloroquine can be instituted on an outpatient basis, since all human malarias not due to *P. falciparum* are sensitive to this agent. Specific species diagnosis can then proceed at a more leisurely pace. On the other hand, if the diagnosis of *P. falciparum* infection is established, cannot be ruled out, or is suspected to exist in a mixed infection (i.e., simultaneous infection with two malarial species), the patient should be hospitalized. Efforts should then be made to determine if the patient has traveled in an area with chloroquine- or Fansidar-resistant *P. falciparum* (Table 3) or has received chloroquine prophylaxis. Suspected chloroquine-resistant falciparum malaria should be treated with a combination of quinine and sulfonamide plus pyrimethamine (most commonly, quinine plus Fansidar) unless the infection was acquired in a region where resistance of *P. falciparum* to the antifolate metabolites is known to occur. Mefloquine (if available) or quinine in combination with a tetracycline is recommended for antifolate (Fansidar)-resistant falciparum malaria.[34] Even after antimalarial therapy begins, patients with *P. falciparum* malaria should be monitored carefully for several days for the appearance of complications, all of which can appear while the patient is being treated. Similarly, blood smears should be examined two or three times a day to determine whether the parasitemia is decreasing, since failure to reduce parasitemia in the first 24–48 hours of chloroquine treatment should raise the possibility of drug failure (Fig. 5E). No parasites should be detectable on smears 4–5 days after completion of a course of chloroquine; persistence of parasites after the fifth day implies treatment failure (Fig. 5F). Since some strains of chloroquine-resistant *P. falciparum* may be suppressed by chloroquine, only to recrudesce days or weeks later, all patients treated with chloroquine should be warned of this possibility (Fig. 5G). Gametocytes may persist in the blood for weeks after asexual forms have been successfully eliminated. Gametocytes do not cause disease in the patient; their presence in the absence of fever and of asexual stage parasites does not dictate the need for treatment.

Chloroquine phosphate can be administered orally according to the regimen outlined in Table 4. Mild gastrointestinal irritation is a common side effect, and pruritus and exacerbation of psoriasis are not uncommon; headache, dizziness, and blurred vision occur infrequently. Since some children vomit the tablets, it is important to observe them for the first hour after each dose. Chloroquine hydrochloride is available for intramuscular administration to patients unable to take oral medication. Potentially fatal adverse reactions (especially in infants and children) have occurred in response to intramuscular chloroquine, so this regimen should be used with great caution. Intramuscular chloroquine was found to be safe in a recent prospective trial carried out in West Africa. Alternatively, chloroquine can be given by nasogastric gavage.

If patients have very high parasitemias (over 5 percent) or are suffering from any of the major complications of *P. falciparum* malaria (severe anemia, renal failure, pulmonary edema, coma, and so forth), quinine dihydrochloride should be given by slow intravenous drip in a large volume of fluid (e.g., 600 mg in 250 ml of 5% glucose in 0.5 normal saline) administered over 8 hours. Some clinicians recommend a loading dose of 20 mg/kg infused over 4h followed by 10 mg/kg in a similar infusion every 8h. Quinine should never be administered by an IV push. The electrocardiogram and vital signs should be monitored for evidence of cardiotoxicity (e.g., widening of the QRS complex, hypotension). Quinine should never be given intramuscularly. As soon as complications have been controlled and the patient

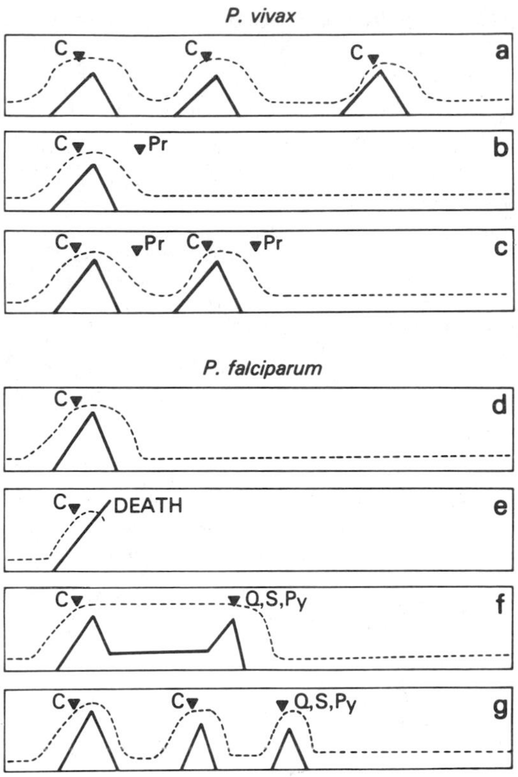

FIG. 5. Representative responses to chemotherapy for *P. vivax* and *P. falciparum* infections. Fever is represented by broken lines; parasitemia is represented by solid lines. C: Chloroquine; Pr: primaquine; S: sulfonamide; Py: pyrimethamine. (**A**) Successful treatment of erythrocytic infection but failure to prevent relapses. (**B**) Relapses prevented with primaquine treatment. (**C**) Initial failure of primaquine to prevent relapses but successful primaquine retreatment after blood forms are eliminated with chloroquine. (**D**) Successful treatment of chloroquine-sensitive *P. falciparum*. (**E–G**) Different patterns of failure of chloroquine against chloroquine-resistant strain of *P. falciparum*. Parasitemia due to chloroquine-resistant strains may (**E**) continue to rise or (**F**) be suppressed to lower but detectable or (**G**) undetectable levels, only to increase at a later time. Although repeated treatment with chloroquine may successfully suppress the infection (**G**) combination chemotherapy may be required to effect a radical cure (**F,G**).

TABLE 3. Geographic Distribution of Chloroquine- and Fansidar-Resistant Strains of *P. falciparum* (as of May 1988)

Chloroquine resistance reported from:
All countries with *P. falciparum* malaria *except:*

AMERICAS	ASIA	AFRICA
Dominican Republic	Middle East	Chad
Haiti		Equatorial Guinea
Central America		Guinea
		Guinea-Bissou
		Liberia
		Senegal
		Sierra Leone

Fansidar resistance reported from:

AMERICAS	ASIA	AFRICA	OCEANEA
Brazil	Thailand[a]	Kenya	Irian Jaya
Panama	Burma[a]	Tanzania	Papua New Guinea
	Kampuchea[a]		Vanuatu
	? Vietnam		

[a] Since Fansidar resistance is widespread only in these countries, therapy against falciparum malaria acquired in these countries should include quinine and tetracycline. Initial therapy against falciparum malaria acquired in the other countries can be with quinine and antifolate drugs, but vigilance should be maintained for the small risk of recrudescence of infection occurring up to 90 days after treatment.

TABLE 4. Recommended Chemotherapy and Prophyiaxis for Malaria

Indication	Drug/Route	Dose: Adult	Dose: Pediatric
Uncomplicated infection with all species except chloroquine-resistant *P. falciparum*	Chloroquine phosphate, po	600 mg base (1 g) followed by 300 mg base (500 mg) in 6 hours then 300 mg base (500 mg)/day for 2 days	10 mg/kg (base) to maximum of 600 mg; half followed by half of this dose in 6 hours and then daily for 2 days
Patient unable to take oral medications	Chloroquine hydrochloride im[a]	200 mg base (250 mg) q6h for maximum of 3 days	5 mg/kg (base) every 12 hours for maximum of 3 days
Severe (complicated) *P. falciparum* infection	Quinine dihydrochloride;[b] see text for iv regimen	600 mg q8h to maximum of 1.8 g/day	25 mg/kg/day; give half dose in 2-hour infusion, followed by second half dose 8 hours later (maximum, 1800 mg/day)
Uncomplicated infection due to chloroquine-resistant *P. falciparum*[c]	Combination of: quinine sulfate (Q), po[d]	650 mg q8h for 7–10 days	Q: 25 mg/kg/day in 3 doses for 10 days
	pyrimethamine (P), po	25 mg bid for 3 days	P: <10 kg: 6.25 mg/day. 10–20 kg: 12.5 mg/day 20–40 kg: 25 mg/day
	sulfadiazine (S) or sulfisoxazole, po	500 mg qid for 5 days	S: 100–200 mg/kg/day in 4 doses (maximum, 2 g/day) for 5 days
Uncomplicated infection due to sulfonamide-pyrimethamine-resistant *P. falciparum*	Combination of quinine sulfate, po tetracycline, po	(see above) 250 mg po qid for 7–10 days	(see above) 6 mg/kg po tid for 7–10 days
Prevention of relapses due to *P. vivax* and *P. ovale*	Primaquine phosphate, po	15 mg base (26.3 mg) day for 14 days	0.3 mg base kg/day for 14 days
Chemoprophylaxis of all species except chloroquinine-resistant *P. falciparum*[e]	Chloroquine phosphate, po	300 mg base (500 mg) once per week. Begin 2 weeks before and continue for 6 weeks after leaving area	< 1 year: 37.5 mg base[f] 1–3 year: 75 mg base 4–6 year: 100 mg base 7–10 years: 150 mg base 11–16 years: 225 mg base
Chemoprophylaxis of chloroquine-resistant *P. falciparum*	See text		

[a] May cause potentially fatal side effects. See text.
[b] Quinine dihydrochloride can be obtained in the United States from the Centers of Disease Control (Drug Service). Monitor vital signs and electrocardiogram. Should be replaced by oral medication as soon as possible. Quinidine can be used as an alternative. See text.
[c] Infection in patients with sulfonamide-pyrimethamine-resistant strains (such as those acquired in Southeast Asia) may recrudesce after this treatment. See text.
[d] In patients who cannot tolerate prolonged treatment with quinine sulfate, this drug may be discontinued after a 3-day course and tetracycline continued; treatment with less than 3 days of quinine sulfate in combination chemotherapy is inadvisable, however.
[e] In addition, patients returning from areas with high transmission rates of *P. vivax* and *P. ovale* should take primaquine phosphate in the doses indicated in the table.
[f] Since children may refuse to take chloroquine tablets because of their bitter taste, it may be necessary to disguise the taste by mixing ground tablets in food. Palatable liquid preparations for pediatric use are readily available in several countries in which malaria transmission occurs.

can take oral medication, a course of chloroquine or one of its alternatives should be started. In the United States, quinine dihydrochloride is available only from the Centers for Disease Control. Since delays in instituting therapy could have disastrous consequences, alternative measures may be necessary to save the patient. Administration of the dextrorotatory diastereoisomer of quinine, quinidine, is at least as effective as quinine in the treatment of falciparum malaria. However, it is more cardiotoxic, with a fourfold greater effect in prolonging the QTc interval.[35] For severe malaria, 15 mg base/kg is infused over a 4-hour period, followed by a similarly slow infusion of 7.5 mg base/kg at 8-hour intervals. Vital signs and the electrocardiogram should be continuously monitored during the infusion. Exchange transfusion can rapidly lower parasitemia and correct severe anemia.

Therapy in chloroquine-resistant *P. falciparum* malaria has been a major concern since 1961, when these strains were first recognized. One problem has been that several of the strains are resistant to the classic individual alternative drugs, such as pyrimethamine and amodiaquine. Presently, the safest and best-studied regimen available is a combination of quinine, a sulfonamide, such as sulfadiazine or sulfisoxazole, and pyrimethamine. Fansidar, a fixed-dose combination of sulfadozine (500 mg/tablet) and pyrimethamine (25 mg/tablet), can be used (three tablets for adults) in place of the individual antifolate drugs. Resistance to antifolates including Fansidar is a problem in Southeast Asia and parts of Brazil; resistant strains have also been encountered elsewhere (Table 3). When drug failure occurs, it is often recognized by an initial response to treatment followed by a subsequent recrudescence days or weeks later (Fig. 5G). Such failures should be treated by a repeated course of combination therapy. Quinine (3–7 days) and tetracycline (1000 mg daily in divided doses for 7–10 days) are efficacious in combination against antifolate-resistant *P. falciparum*,[36] but the antibiotic is not licensed for this use in the United States. Quinine given by mouth may cause cinchonism, a condition characterized by tinnitus, headache, nausea, and altered vision. Given too rapidly by the intravenous route, it may be cardiotoxic. Hypersensitivity to quinine is rare, but when it occurs, it can be manifested by bronchospasm, hemolytic anemia, or thrombocytopenia.

A new antimalarial, mefloquine (Lariam), has emerged from testing of more than 250,000 compounds by the U.S. Army. The drug, a 4-quinoline methanol, is effective in a single dose against chloroquine-resistant *P. falciparum* and the asexual erythrocytic stages of the other three species infective to humans.[34] Mefloquine resistance has emerged in Thailand. Side effects are generally mild, but since mefloquine can cause asymptomatic sinus bradycardia and QT interval prolongation, its use is inadvisable in patients taking certain cardiotropic agents that can alter conduction. Mefloquine is available in Southeast Asia, France, and Switzerland, and may become available in the United States in the future.

In addition to specific antimalarial chemotherapy, patients with *P. falciparum* malaria may require management of the complications. Fluid replacement for dehydration and hypotension should be instituted judiciously for fear of precipitating or aggravating the noncardiogenic pulmonary edema of malaria. Hyponatremia generally represents decreased free water clearance rather than sodium loss and, therefore, should not be treated by sodium loading. Since fluid retention may herald renal failure or pulmonary edema, monitoring of body weight and fluid intake and output is useful. Renal failure or pulmonary edema unresponsive to a therapeutic trial of furosemide requires peritoneal dialysis or hemodialysis. The daily dose of quinine in patients with hepatic or renal failue should be adjusted to one-half to one-third of the regular dose. Serum levels of quinine are not altered by peritoneal dialysis or hemodialysis.

Pulmonary edema may require intubation and assisted ventilation, but usually carries a very poor prognosis regardless of therapy. Although once popular, the administration of corticosteroids to patients with cerebral malaria is inadvisable, since it is ineffective and may be deleterious.[37] Anemia, if severe, may require transfusion of packed red blood cells or of whole blood if hypovolemic shock is also present. Thrombocytopenia in malaria, although severe, generally does not in itself result in significant spontaneous hemorrhage and rarely requires platelet transfusions. The other features of coagulopathy, when present, have been treated with heparin with or without the addition of corticosteroids, low molecular weight dextran, and fresh frozen plasma. These treatment modalities in malaria are controversial, and there is no good evidence that heparin improves patient survival, although it may improve the clotting parameters. In fact, patients with *P. falciparum* malaria have died from hemorrhagic complications of heparin therapy.

Treatment of Malaria Not Due to Plasmodium falciparum

Oral chloroquine phosphate remains the drug of choice in all malarial infections not due to *P. falciparum* since no chloroquine-resistant strains have been encountered. These infections can often be treated on an outpatient basis, provided that contact is maintained with the patient and follow-up visits for obtaining blood smears can be arranged. Patients with chronic diseases that might be aggravated by high fever (e.g., cardiovascular or pulmonary disease, brittle diabetes mellitus) should be hospitalized. No dosage adjustment of chloroquine is necessary for patients with chronic renal failure.

Patients with sporozoite-induced (i.e., mosquito-transmitted) *P. vivax* and *P. ovale* malaria may relapse after chloroquine treatment unless latent exoerythrocytic forms in the liver are eliminated with primaquine, a drug that has no effect on the asexual blood forms (Fig. 5A and B). Primaquine can be given safely after a course of chloroquine and when the patient is afebrile. Since it can induce hemolysis of erythrocytes deficient in G6PD, patients about to receive the drug should first be screened for G6PD deficiency. Patients with the type of deficiency that occurs mainly in blacks can be given the drug, since hemolysis is limited to older erythrocytes; however, hematocrit values should be monitored. Patients with Caucasian-type deficiency should not receive the drug, since severe hemolysis can result. Instead, they should receive chloroquine for the treatment of each relapse (Fig. 5A). Blood-induced infections with *P. vivax* or *P. ovale* do not require primaquine treatment, since no latent EE forms persist to cause relapses.

Monitoring the response of patients treated for malaria not due to *P. falciparum* (fever and blood smears) is important to allow recognition of misdiagnosis (i.e., failure to respond to chloroquine implies that the patient probably has chloroquine-resistant *P. falciparum*). Patients with *P. vivax* who are treated with chloroquine and primaquine may relapse and represent primaquine treatment failures (Fig. 5C). They should receive a second course of chloroquine and primaquine after it has been ascertained that the relapse truly represents *P. vivax* infection and not incorrectly treated chloroquine-resistant *P. falciparum* infection. The rate of primaquine failure (0–30 percent) depends on the locality where the infection is acquired and is the same for each course of therapy given.

Prevention

Attempts to prevent infection should be encouraged in all travelers to areas with the risk of malaria transmission. Malaria risk by country is reported annually in "Health Information for International Travel" (DHHS publication no. (CDC) 88-8280), published by the U.S. Public Health Service and available from the U.S. Government Printing Office, Washington, DC, 20402 (telephone: [202] 783-3238). Updated information regarding prevention of malaria in travelers is available round the clock from the Centers for Disease Control (telephone: [404] 639-1610). Preventive measures include the proper use of mosquito netting at night, clothing that minimizes contact with mosquitoes, and the use of insect repellants. In addition, chemoprophylaxis with chloroquine is used to suppress erythrocytic infection. Chloroquine should be administered 2 weeks before entering, and should be continued for 6 weeks after leaving, a malarious area. One 500-mg tablet (or two 250-mg tablets) of chloroquine phosphate should be taken once a week on the same day of the week (see Table 4 for pediatric doses). The long-term administration of chloroquine at these doses does not cause retinal damage, in contrast to the higher doses. After travelers return from areas with a high risk of *P. vivax* or *P. ovale* infection, primaquine, 15 mg base/day, for 14 days can be administered to patients without G6PD deficiency to prevent relapses.

Prophylaxis of chloroquine-resistant *P. falciparum* malaria is more complicated, and there are differences of opinion regarding the preferable regimen. The prophylactic use of Fansidar is now generally discouraged (other than in exceptional cases) since such use has been associated with serious, potentially fatal complications (erythema multiforme, Stevens-Johnson syndrome, toxic epidermal necrolysis), as well as other complications (serum sickness-like illness, exfoliative dermatitis, urticaria, hepatitis). The prophylactic chloroquine regimen can protect against nonfalciparum malaria and may suppress infection due to *P. falciparum* strains that exhibit relatively low-level resistance. Accordingly, patients traveling to areas with chloroquine-resistant strains should take chloroquine (see Chapter 36) and be given a therapeutic course (three tablets) of Fansidar to take along as a potentially lifesaving *temporary* measure if a febrile illness develops and suitable medical care is unavailable.[38] They should be advised to continue taking prophylactic chloroquine and to seek medical attention even after taking Fansidar. Prophylaxis with the combination of weekly chloroquine and Fansidar (one tablet) can be recommended for the exceptional situation where there will be prolonged exposure in high-transmission areas where the risk of acquiring chloroquine-resistant *P. falciparum* is high and where suitable medical care is unavailable. The traveler should be warned of the side effects and advised to discontinue Fansidar immediately at the first sign of rash or mucosal irritation. Patients with sulfonamide hypersensitivity should not receive Fansidar. Instead, they can be given three doxycycline (100-mg) and three quinine tablets to take along as lifesaving measures for presumptive chloroquine-resistant falciparum malaria. Proguanil, an antifolate drug, is being used in combination with chloroquine in some parts of the world; it is not available in the United States. While proguanil may be effective in Kenya and is not in Thailand and Papua New Guinea, its efficacy elsewhere is uncertain. Amodiaquine is no longer recommended in malaria prophylaxis since it can cause potentially fatal agranulocytosis.

Doxycycline (100 mg) alone, taken once daily (beginning 1–2 days before entering and continuing for 4 weeks after leaving the malarious area) can be recommended for brief visits to forested areas of Thailand, Burma, and Kampuchea where there may be a risk of acquiring chloroquine- and Fansidar-resistant malaria.[39] Tetracyclines should not be taken by children under 8 years of age or by pregnant women. Tetracyclines can cause exaggerated sunburns and candida vaginitis with prolonged use.

Travelers should be advised that no chemoprophylactic regimen is entirely effective and is not a substitute for other preventive modalities. They should realize that any febrile illness—even if it occurs months after leaving an area where malaria is endemic—could be malaria.

Antimalarial Drugs for Pregnant Women

Because of a variety of infectious disease risks, it is generally inadvisable for pregnant women to travel in tropical countries.

On the other hand, when required, chemotherapy and prophylaxis of malaria with chloroquine is generally safe in pregnant women and poses little teratogenic risk. Since antifolate drugs can have teratogenic effects in laboratory animals (although not demonstrated in humans), they should be avoided as prophylactic agents in pregnant women. When it is decided that the risks of inadequately treated chloroquine-resistant falciparum malaria outweigh the theoretical risks of giving pyrimethamine for 3 days, folinic acid should be administered with this antifolate drug. Since clindamycin in combination with quinine has not been demonstrated to be effective against Fansider-resistant *P. falciparum*, there may be no suitable alternative to combination quinine-tetracycline therapy against such infection (unless mefloquine is available). For the treatment of relapsing malaria in pregnant women, primaquine should be avoided, and each relapse should be treated with chloroquine. After delivery, primaquine can be given.

REFERENCES

1. Wyler DJ, Malaria—resurgence, resistance and research. N Engl J Med. 1983;308:875–8, 934–40.
2. Garnham PCC. *Malaria Parasites and Other Hemosporidia*. Oxford: Blackwell Scientific Publications; 1966.
3. Pasvol G, Wilson RJM. Interaction of malaria parasites with red blood cells. Br Med Bull. 1982;38:133–40.
4. Miller LH, Mason SJ, Clyde DF, et al. The resistance factor to *Plasmodium vivax* in blacks: The Duffy blood-group genotype, *FyFy*. N Engl J Med. 1976;295:302–4.
5. Aikawa M, Miller LH, Johnson J, et al. Erythrocyte entry by malarial parasites: A moving junction between erythrocyte and parasite. J Cell Biol. 1978;77:72–82.
6. Friedman MJ. Erythrocytic mechanism of sickle cell resistance to malaria. Proc Natl Acad Sci USA. 1978;75:1994–7.
7. Friedman MJ, Roth EF, Nagel RL, et al. *Plasmodium falciparum:* Physiological interactions with the human sickle cell. Exp Parasitol. 1979;47:73–80.
8. Luzzatto L. Genetics of red cells and susceptibility to malaria. Blood. 1979;54:961–76.
9. Singal M, Shaw PK, Lindsay RC, et al. An outbreak of introduced malaria in California possibly involving secondary transmission. Am J Trop Med Hyg. 1977;26:1–9.
10. American Association of Blood Banks. Standards for Blood Banks and Transfusion Services. 12th ed. Arlington, Va. 1987.
11. Scuderi P, Sterling KE, Lam KS, et al. Raised serum levels of tumour necrosis factor in parasitic infections. Lancet. 1986;2:1364–5.
12. Looaresuwan S, Ho M, Wattanagoon Y, et al. Dynamic alteration in splenic function during acute falciparum malaria. N Engl J Med. 1987;317:675–9.
13. Weatherall DJ, Abdalla S. The anemia of *Plasmodium falciparum* malaria. Br Med Bull. 1982;38:147–51.
14. World Health Organization Malaria Action Programme. Severe and complicated malaria. Trans R Soc Trop Med Hyg. 1986;80(Suppl):1–50.
15. Udeinya I, Schmidt JA, Aikawa M, et al. Falciparum malaria-infected erythrocytes bind to cultured human endothelial cells. Science. 1981;213:555–7.
16. Boonpucknavig V, Sitprija V. Renal disease in acute *Plasmodium falciparum* infection in man. Kidney Int. 1979;16:44–52.
17. Duarte MIS, Corbett CEP, Boulos M, et al. Ultrastructure of the lung in falciparum malaria. Am J Trop Med Hyg. 1985;34:31–5.
18. Spitz S. The pathology of acute falciparum malaria. Milit Surg. 1946;99:555–72.
19. MacPherson GG, Warrell MJ, White NJ, et al. Human cerebral malaria: A quantitative ultrastructure analysis of parasitized erythrocyte sequestration. Am J Pathol. 1985;19:385–401.
20. Olsson RA, Johnston EH. Histopathologic changes and small bowel absorption in falciparum malaria. The importance of anemia in cerebral and uncomplicated falciparum malaria: Role of complications, dyserythropoeisis, and iron sequestration. Am J Trop Med Hyg. 1969;18:355–9.
21. Phillips RE, Looaresuwan S, Warrell DA, et al. Q J Med. 1986;58:305–23.
22. Looaresuwan S, Warrell DA, White NJ, et al. Do patients with cerebral malaria have cerebral edema? A computed tomography study. Lancet. 1983;1:434–7.
23. Warrell DA, Looaresuwan S, Phillips RE, et al. Function of the blood–cerebrospinal fluid barrier in human cerebral malaria: Rejection of the permeability hypothesis. Am J Trop Med Hyg. 1986;35:882–9.
24. Wyler DJ. Steroids are out in the treatment of cerebral malaria: What's next? J Infect Dis. 1988;158:320–4.
25. White NJ, Warrell DA, Chantavanich P, et al. Severe hypoglycemia and hyperinsulinemia in falciparum malaria. N Engl J Med. 1983;309:61–6.
26. Haghighi L, Doust JY, Boroomand K. Biological false positive VDRL test in malaria. Trop Geog Med. 1970;22:482–5.
27. Kelton JG, Keystone J, Moore J, et al. Immune-mediated thrombocytopenia of malaria. J Clin Invest. 1983;71:832–6.
28. Hendrickse RG, Adeniyi A. Quartan malarial nephrotic syndrome in children. Kidney Int. 1979;16:64–74.
29. Wyler DJ, Quinn TC, Chen L-T. Relationship of alterations in splenic clearance function and microcirculation to host defense in acute rodent malaria. J Clin Invest. 1981;67:1400–4.
30. Greenwood BM, Fakunle VM. The tropical splenomegaly syndrome: A review of its pathogenesis. In: The Role of the Spleen in the Immunology of Parasitic Diseases. Basel: Schwabe; 1979:229–44.
31. Morrow RH Jr. Epidemiological evidence for the role of falciparum malaria in the pathogenesis of Burkitt's lymphoma. IARC Sci Pub. 1985;(60):177–86.
32. Wyler DJ. Cellular aspects of immunoregulation in malaria. Bull WHO. 1979;57(Suppl):239–43.
33. Kean BH, Reilly PC. Malaria—the mime: Recent lessons from a group of civilian travellers. Am J Med. 1976;61:159–64.
34. World Health Organization. Development of mefloquine as an antimalarial drug. Bull WHO. 1983;61:169–78.
35. White NJ, Looaresuwan S, Warrell DA, et al. Quinidine in falciparum malaria. Lancet. 1981;2:1069–71.
36. Reacher M, Campbell CC, Freeman J, et al. Drug therapy for *Plasmodium falciparum* malaria resistant to pyrimethamine-sulfadoxine (Fansidar). Lancet. 1981;2:1066–8.
37. Warrell DA, Looaresuwan S, Warrell MJ, et al. Dexamethasone proves deleterious in cerebral malaria. A double-blind trial in 100 comatose patients. N Engl J Med. 1982;306:313–9.
38. Centers for Disease Control. Recommendations for the prevention of malaria in travelers. Morb Mort Weekly Rep. 1988;37:277–84.
39. Pang LW, Boudreau EF, Limsomwong N, et al. Doxycycline prophylaxis for falciparum malaria. Lancet. 1987;1:1161–4.

252. LEISHMANIA SPECIES: VISCERAL (KALA-AZAR), CUTANEOUS, AND MUCOSAL LEISHMANIASIS

RICHARD D. PEARSON
ANASTACIO DE QUEIROZ SOUSA

Leishmaniasis is the general name given to disease caused by any member of the protozoan genus *Leishmania* and can be divided into visceral (kala-azar), cutaneous, and mucosal syndromes. In mammals the *Leishmania* organisms exist as aflagellar amastigotes inside cells of reticuloendothelial origin. They are transmitted by sandflies as flagellated, extracellular, metacyclic promastigotes. The clinical manifestations of leishmaniasis depend on the complex interaction of the parasites' invasiveness, tropism, and pathogenicity and the host's immune responses.[1] Evidence from animal models suggests that susceptibility to *Leishmania* is genetically determined. Cell-mediated immune mechanisms are primarily responsible for controlling infection. The spectrum of human disease ranges from self-healing, localized ulcers to widely disseminated, progressive lesions of the skin and mucous membranes or, in the case of visceral leishmaniasis, the entire reticuloendothelial system. The *Leishmania* species that infect humans, the clinical syndromes that they produce, and their geographic distributions are summarized in Table 1.[2,3]

THE ORGANISMS

In the mammalian host, *Leishmania* are found in cells of reticuloendothelial origin in the amastigote form (Fig. 1), which is 2–3 μm in length and oval or round in shape and lacks an exteriorized flagellum.[3] In Wright- and Giemsa-stained preparations, the cytoplasm appears blue, the nucleus is relatively large and red, and the distinctive kinetoplast is rod shaped and stains intensely red. Multiplication is by binary fission. In the digestive tract of the sandfly vector and in culture, parasites develop through a series of flagellated, intermediate promastigote forms to become infective, metacyclic promastigotes (Fig. 2).[6–8] Promastigotes have a pear- or spindle-shaped body of variable dimensions, the average being 10–15 μm in length and 1.5–3.5 μm in width; the flagella measure 15–28 μm. After inoculation by sandflies, promastigotes are thought to bind to macrophages in the skin. Two parasite surface molecules have been identified that appear to play prominent roles in parasite–phagocyte interactions; an approximate 63 kD glycoprotein (gp63)[9,10] and a lipophosphoglycan.[11,12] Promastigotes activate complement through the alternative pathway and are thereby opsonized. They bind to macrophage receptors for iC3b, mannose/fucose, advanced glycosylation products, and/or fibronectin.[13–21] Promastigotes are phagocytized and convert to intracellular amastigotes within parasitophorous vacuoles.

Although minor ultrastructural differences have been described, it is impossible to differentiate species of *Leishmania* from one another on the basis of morphology in either the amastigote or promastigote stage.[3] Speciation was originally based on a variety of factors such as (*1*) the parasites' behavior in humans, (*2*) epidemiologic differences associated with geographic distribution, (*3*) involvement of specific animal reservoirs, and (*4*) transmission by different species of sandflies. More recently, several biochemical methods of speciation have also been employed: (*5*) isoenzyme determination, (*6*) buoyant density analysis of nuclear and kinetoplast DNA, (*7*) antigenic differences in promastigoate-excreted factors, (*8*) species-specific monoclonal antibodies, (*9*) restriction endonuclease digestion of kinetoplast DNA, and (*10*) species-specific hybridization

TABLE 1. Leishmaniasis[a]

Clinical Syndromes	Leishmania *Species*	*Location*
Visceral leishmaniasis		
Kala-azar: generalized involvement of the reticuloendothelial system (spleen, bone marrow, liver etc.)	*L. donovani donovani*	Indian subcontinent, China
	L. d. infantum	Middle East, Mediterranean littoral, Balkans, western Asiatic area, northwestern Iberia, China, Sub-Saharan Africa
	L. d. archibaldi	Sudan, Kenya, Ethiopia
	L. donovani species	Kenya
	L. d. chagasi	Latin America
	L. mexican amazonensis (?)	Brazil (Bahia State)
	L. tropica (?)	Rare cases reported from Israel and India
Post–kala-azar dermal leishmaniasis	*L. d. donovani*	Indian subcontinent
	L. d. species	Kenya, possibly Ethiopia and Somalia
Old world cutaneous leishmaniasis		
Single or limited number of skin lesions	*L. major*	Middle East, central Asia, Africa, Indian subcontinent
	L. tropica	Mediterranean littoral, Middle East, west Asiatic Area, Indian subcontinent
	L. aethiopica	Ethiopian highlands, Kenya
	L. d. infantum	Occasional cases in Mediterranean basin
	L. d. archibaldi	Sudan, East Africa
	L. donovani species	Kenya
Diffuse cutaneous leishmaniasis	*L. aethiopica*	Ethiopian highlands, Kenya
New world cutaneous leishmaniasis		
Single or limited number of skin lesions	*L. mexicana mexicana* (chiclero ulcer)	Mexico, Central America, Texas (?)
	L. m. amazonensis	Amazon basin and neighboring areas, Brazil, Panama, Venezuela, Trinidad
	L. m. pifanoi	Venezuela
	L. m. garnhami	Venezuela
	L. m. venezuelensis	Venezuela
	L. m. species undetermined	Dominican Republic
	L. braziliensis braziliensis	Brazil, Peru, Ecuador, Boliva, Paraguay, Argentina
	L. b. guyanensis (pian bois, bush yaws)	Guyana, Surinam, northern Amazon basin
	L. b. peruvian (uta)	Peru, western Andes, Argentinian highlands
	L. b. panamensis	Panama and adjacent areas
	L. d. chagasi	Rare cases in Latin America
Diffuse cutaneous leishmaniasis	*L. m. amazonensis*	Amazon basin and neighboring areas
	L. m. pifanoi	Venezuela
	L. m. mexicana	Mexico, Central America (rare)
	Leishmania m. sp	Dominican Republic
Mucosal leishmaniasis	*L. b. braziliensis* (espundia)	Multiple areas in South America
	L. b. panamensis	Panama and adjacent areas

[a] The taxonomy of *Leishmania* species is still in a state of flux. Three "species complexes" have been traditionally identified: the *L. donovani* complex, *L. mexicana* complex, and *L. braziliensis* complex, each having multiple subspecies as indicated above. Lainson and Shaw[2] have recently proposed that the various subspecies be reclassified as distinct species e.g., *L. donovani chagasi* as *L. chagasi*.
(Modified from Lainson et al.,[2] with permission.)

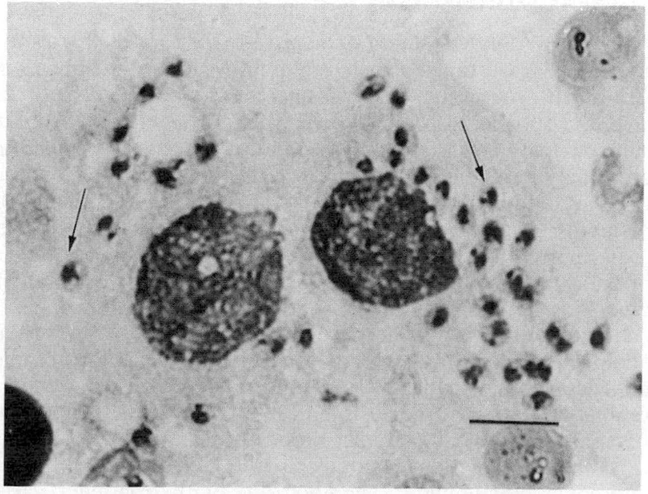

FIG. 1. *Leishmania donovani* amastigotes (arrows) in a touch preparation made from the spleen of an infected hamster. The bar equals 10 μm. (From Pearson et al.,[4] with permission.)

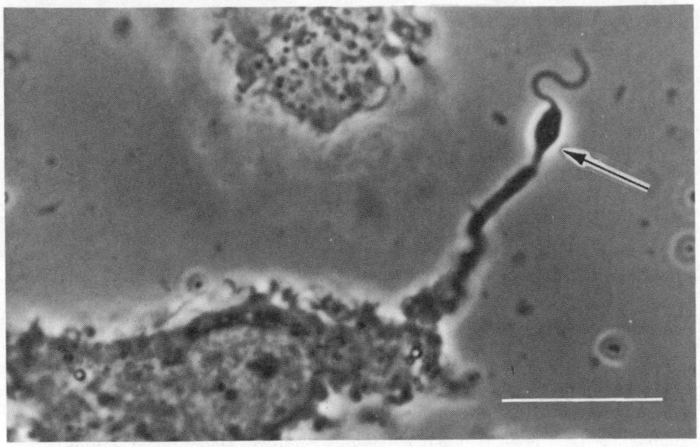

FIG. 2. *Leishmania donovani* promastigote (arrow) attached by its aflagellar pole to a human mononuclear phagocyte in vitro. The bar equals 10 μm. (From Pearson et al.,[5] with permission.)

of kinetoplast DNA.[22–31] Unfortunately, no single method has emerged as a gold standard for speciation, and consensus is still lacking on the taxonomy of *Leishmania*. Lainson and Shaw[2] have recently proposed a revised classification based on all of the above criteria. Clinical isolates are usually identified by species-specific monoclonal antibodies, isoenzyme analysis, or probes for kintoplast DNA. Pulsed-field gradient electrophoresis has been used to separate chromosomes of some *Leishmania* species, and the karyotypes have been found to differ.[32,33]

Sandflies (*Lutzomyia* species and *Psychodopygus* species in the Americas and *Phlebotomus* species elsewhere) are responsible for transmitting *Leishmania*.[3,34] Sandflies breed in cracks in the walls of dwellings, in rubbish, or in rubble piles. They are weak flyers and tend to remain close to the ground near the breeding site. Sandflies ingest amastigotes when they feed on infected mammals. Amastigotes convert to promastigotes in the gut of the sandfly, and parasite replication and development follow. Promastigotes are inoculated into a mammalian host several days later when an infected sandfly attempts to take its next blood meal. Depending on the geographic location and the *Leishmania* species, the major reservoir of infection may be rodents, canine species, other mammals, or humans. With the exception of visceral leishmaniasis in India, the disease is a zoonosis.

VISCERAL LEISHMANIASIS (KALA-AZAR)

Leishmania donovani and *L. chagasi* are responsible for a spectrum of disease ranging from asymptomatic, self-resolving infection to progressive visceral leishmaniasis, which has been termed kala-azar, Dumdum fever, Assam fever, and infantile splenomegaly in various areas of the world. It has become increasingly apparent that most *L. chagasi* or *L. donovani* infections are either asymptomatic or "oligosymptomatic" and self-resolving.[35,36] The ratio of disease to infection has been reported to be approximately 1 to 6.5 in areas with the highest prevalence of kala-azar. Young, malnourished children seem to be at the greatest risk of developing progressive disease. Kala-azar is characterized by a subacute or chronic course with fever, hepatosplenomegaly (often with massive splenic enlargement), anemia, leukopenia, hyperglobulinemia, and progressive emaciation of the affected host. If untreated, the great majority of persons with typical kala-azar proceed to death. In most areas, *L. donovani* infection responds to treatment with pentavalent antimonial compounds. The mortality with treatment varies from an estimated 2–3 percent in South America to 17 percent in one series from East Africa.[37] Multiple factors, including delays in diagnosis and therapy, contribute to mortality.

Epidemiology

Visceral leishmaniasis occurs in widely scattered areas throughout the world. Transmission of the disease depends on three factors: (*1*) an appropriate reservoir of infection, (*2*) a suitable vector, and (*3*) a susceptible population. In South America, the Mediterranean littoral, and China, dogs are thought to be a major reservoir of disease. In Brazil, foxes provide an important wild reservoir that contributes to infection in the domestic reservoir, dogs.[38] In East Africa, rats, gerbils, ground squirrels, other rodents, and small carnivores are important; humans may be an important reservoir during epidemics. In central Asia, wild jackals, foxes, and dogs have been incriminated. Visceral leishmaniasis in India is unique in that no reservoir apart from humans has been identified.

Transmission in India is by a *Phlebotomus* species that is anthropophilic, whereas in other regions it is by sandflies that feed on the appropriate animal host as well as humans. Although rare, *L. donovani* has also been transmitted by blood transfusion[39,40] and after parenteral exposure in the laboratory. Congenital[41,42] and direct person-to-person transmission[43] have also been reported, but are rare.

The characteristics of susceptible human populations are variable and incompletely understood. In East Africa, the disease is most frequent among older children and young adults, probably because they come in contact with infected sandflies during occupational activities. In South America and the Mediterranean littoral, infants and children under 10 years of age are the most commonly infected, although infection in teenagers and young adults does occur. Finally, children and young adults are most commonly affected in India. Except for epidemics of visceral leishmaniasis that have occurred in India and occasionally in East Africa, the disease is sporadic.

Although *L. donovani* is not transmitted in North America or Northern Europe, travelers, military personnel, or immigrants may acquire the disease in endemic areas and, because the incubation period is long, develop clinical illness after returning home. A number of cases have been reported in children and immunocompromised adult travelers who acquired infection in Italy, Greece, Spain, or southern France.[44–48] In general, persons with the acquired immunodeficiency syndrome (AIDS) have had fulminant visceral leishmaniasis and responded poorly to therapy.[49,50]

Pathogenesis

A small granuloma containing amastigote-filled mononuclear cells forms at the site where *L. donovani* is inoculated by the sandfly. The initial lesion is often inapparent, but a small papule may be observed.[51–53] Larger, ulcerative lesions are rare but have been reported in patients with visceral leishmaniasis in East Africa. Amastigotes subsequently disseminate throughout the reticuloendothelial system to the spleen, liver, bone marrow, and lymph nodes. Increased numbers of mononuclear phagocytes in the liver and spleen result in progressive hypertrophy of those organs; the spleen, in particular, may become massively enlarged as splenic lymphoid follicles are replaced by parasitized mononuclear cells. In the liver, there is a marked increase in the number and size of Küpffer cells, many of which are filled with amastigotes. Infected mononuclear phagocytes are also found in the bone marrow, lymph nodes, skin, and other sites.

The outcome of *L. donovani* infection appears to depend on the complex interaction between the parasite's virulence and the immune responses of the host.[1] In the murine model, resistance is determined by a single autosomal gene on chromosome 1, which has been termed *Lsh*.[54] This genetic locus is closely linked to and probably identical with the locus that controls for resistance to *Salmonella typhimurium* and Calmette-Guérin bacillus (BCG).[55] The genetic determinants of human leishmaniasis have not been defined. Epidemiologic evidence indicates that young age and malnutrition both predispose to the development of progressive disease.

The intracellular fate of *L. donovani* and ultimately the course of infection appear to depend on the capacity of T lymphocytes to activate macrophages to kill the parasite.[1] Transfer of T lymphocytes from immune animals to recipient animals confers protection against infection, whereas transfer of immune serum alone does not.[56] Exposure of human monocyte-derived macrophages in vitro to antigen- or mitogen-elicited lymphokines or γ-interferon can effectively activate them to kill amastigotes.[57] Experience with animal models and humans also suggests that the development of potentially effective cell-mediated immune mechanisms may be inhibited during infection.[1] In the murine system[1] there is evidence that both macrophages[58–60] and phenotypic T-helper cell subset(s)[61] may contribute to the progression of disease. Delayed hypersensitivity responses in humans, as assessed by the leishmanin skin test and by in vitro lymphocyte responses to leishmanial antigens,[62,63] are absent during infection but in most instances develop after successful antileishmanial chemotherapy. Paradoxically, antileishmanial antibodies are produced during disease, and there is evidence of polyclonal B lymphocyte activation to account for the observed hypergammaglobulinemia.[64] In person with asymptomatic, self-resolving infection, protective T cells come to predominate, although immune suppression years later can result in the development of symptomatic disease.[65] In kala-azar, protective T cells fail to emerge. In oligosymptomatic disease, there appears to be a standoff between protective T cell populations and disease-enhancing factors. Some cases resolve; others go on to develop classic kala-azar.

Patients with untreated visceral leishmaniasis become progressively cachectic and debilitated. The explanation for their profound weight loss remains uncertain. Cytokines such as tumor necrosis factor/cachectin and interleukin-1 have been postulated to mediate anorexia and wasting.[66,67] Death often is associated with a secondary bacterial or viral infection.

Clinical Manifestations

The clinical features of visceral leishmaniasis are remarkably similar in all parts of the world. The incubation period varies but is usually in the range of 3–8 months[38,47,68] In one case the time that elapsed from arrival in an endemic area to the onset of fever was less than 10 days.[69] Incubation periods as long as 34 months have also been reported.[70] The onset of symptoms may be gradual or sudden. In subacute or chronic cases, victims experience the insidious onset of vague abdominal discomfort, enlargement of the abdomen, fever, weakness, loss of appetite, pallor, cough, and weight loss. Some children have smoldering oligosymptomatic disease with chronic low-grade fever, growth retardation, and organomegaly. A subset of these progresses to full-blown kala-azar.[36] Symptoms often persist for weeks to several months before patients seek medical attention. Fever may be intermittent, remittent with twice-daily temperature spikes, or less commonly, continuous, and it is relatively well tolerated. In acute cases, there may be an abrupt onset of high fever and chills, sometimes with a periodicity that mimics malaria. Sweating with chills, but seldom rigors, accompanies the temperature spikes.

Anemia is almost always present in visceral leishmaniasis and may be severe. It is usually normocytic, normochromic. The anemia appears to be due to a combination of factors, including hemolysis, marrow replacement with *Leishmania* infected mononuclear phagocytes, hemorrhage, splenic sequestration of erythrocytes,[71,72] and hemodilution.[73]

Leukopenia is also prominent with white blood cell counts as low as 1100/mm^3.[32,74,75] It is not known whether the observed neutropenia is due to increased margination, splenic sequestration, an autoimmune process, or a combination of these factors.[75] Severe neutropenia may contribute to secondary bacterial infections. Thrombocytopenia is also observed and contributes to the hemorrhagic tendency. Anemia and leukopenia have not been observed in several cases in which the spleen was previously removed or in patients with visceral leishmaniasis who have undergone splenectomy.[72,76]

Hypergammaglobulinemia, circulating immune complexes, and rheumatoid factors are present in sera of most patients with visceral leishmaniasis.[77,78] The kidneys show evidence of immune complex deposition, and mild glomerulonephritis has been reported in humans[79] as well as in naturally infected dogs. Although mild proteinuria and hematuria are observed in some patients, renal failure is not a feature of the disease.

As time passes, enlargement of the liver and spleen, anemia, and emaciation become more pronounced. The spleen may become enormous. It is usually soft and nontender. The presence of a hard spleen suggests a hematologic disorder or another diagnosis such as schistosomiasis. The liver is enlarged with a sharp edge, soft consistency, and a smooth surface. In rare instances, localized lymphadenopathy has been the only clinical abnormality. Jaundice with mildly elevated liver enzyme levels is occasionally observed and is considered a bad prognostic sign. The skin becomes dry, thin, and scaly, and hair is lost. As the disease progresses, particularly in light-colored patients in India, the skin on the hands, feet, abdomen, and face may become grayish. This discoloration gave rise to the Indian name "kala-azar," which means "black fever." Peripheral edema is occasionally seen late in disease, primarily in children. Hemorrhage may occur from one or multiple sites: epistaxis and gingival bleeding are the most common. Petechiae and ecchymoses may be observed on the extremities. Death in visceral leishmaniasis is often due to bacterial pneumonia, septicemia, concurrent tuberculosis, dysentery, uncontrolled hemorrhage, or severe anemia with its sequelae.

Post–kala-azar dermal leishmaniasis follows the treatment of visceral leishmaniasis in a small percentage of persons in Africa and India. Lesions appear in India up to 2 years after treatment and may persist for as long as 20 years. In contrast, in Africa they usually appear during or shortly after treatment and persist for only a few months.[80,81] These skin lesions vary from depigmented patches to frank nodules and may be confused with leprosy. In a few instances in India, visceral leishmaniasis has recurred in association with post–kala-azar dermal leishmaniasis.

Diagnosis

In an endermic area the constellation of prolonged fever, progressive weight loss, weakness, pronounced splenomegaly, hepatomegaly, anemia, leukopenia, hypergammaglobulinemia, and low albumin levels are highly suggestive of visceral leishmaniasis. A definitive diagnosis depends on the demonstration of amastigotes in tissue or isolation of the organism in culture. Bone marrow aspiration is the safest diagnostic procedure. Amastigotes are seen on Wright- and Giemsa-stained smears in 54–86 percent of cases.[82] Splenic puncture (98 percent positivity)[83] is a more sensitive diagnostic method and has been routinely performed in Kenya. It has been associated with life-threatening hemorrhage in a few cases, particularly in patients with advanced stages of disease who have undergone biopsy at sites other than major medical centers. The morbidity and potential mortality appear to be much less when aspiration is done quickly with a small-bore needle in patients with no laboratory evidence of coagulopathy. Liver biopsy is less likely to yield the diagnosis than splenic puncture is; it too carries the risk of life-threatening hemorrhage. Lymph node aspiration or biopsy may be diagnostic when enlarged nodes are present. In some instances, parasites can be cultured from the buffy coat of blood, and on occasion they can be identified within mononuclear cells in smears of the buffy coat.

Cultures of bone marrow, liver, spleen, lymph node, and particularly in India, blood may reveal the parasite. Specimens are inoculated into Novy-MacNeal-Nicolle (NNN) medium, a biphasic medium, or one of several liquid media that do not contain blood (e.g., Schneider insect medium)[84] and maintained at 22–26°C. Motile promastigotes develop from amastigotes and can be identified in positive cultures in a few days to 4 weeks.

Several tests have been developed to detect specific antileishmanial antibodies. Enzyme-linked immunoabsorbent assays (ELISA),[82,85] which appear to be the most sensitive and specific approach, and indirect immunofluorescent antibody tests have been the most widely used.[86,87] Complement fixation, hemagglutination, and agglutination tests also have their proponents. Each of these tests is to some degree dependent on the *Leishmania* species used as antigen and the method of antigen preparation. Cross-reactions with leprosy, Chagas disease, malaria, schistosomiasis, and cutaneous leishmaniasis can occur. Unfortunately, none of the tests are standardized in commercially available kits, and results of tests for leishmanial antibody provide only suggestive support for the diagnosis.

The leishmanin skin test (Montenegro test) is negative during active visceral leishmaniasis and usually becomes positive only after successful therapy. Although useful in studies of epidemiology, it is of no value in documenting active disease. In post–kala-azar dermal leishmaniasis, the skin test may be positive or negative.

Differential Diagnosis

The clinical picture of visceral leishmaniasis is often indistinguishable from other infectious diseases. Acute presentations may be confused with malaria, typhoid fever, typhus, acute Chagas disease, acute schistosomiasis, miliary tuberculosis, and amebic liver abscess. Subacute or chronic visceral leishmaniasis may be confused with brucellosis, histoplasmosis, infectious mononucleosis, lymphoma, leukemia, agnogenic myeloid metaplasia, hepatosplenic schistosomiasis, and prolonged *Salmonella* bacteremia. In malarious areas, the differential diagnosis includes tropical splenomegaly due to chronic malaria. Post–kala-azar dermal leishmaniasis must be differentiated from leprosy, yaws, and syphilis.

Treatment

Pentavalent antimonial compounds remain the drugs of choice for initial therapy for visceral leishmaniasis.[82,88–91] Two compounds are available: stibogluconate sodium (Pentostam) is used in English-speaking countries including the United States and meglumine antimoniate (Glucantime) in Latin American and Francophile countries. They are chemically similar and appear to have comparable toxicities and therapeutic efficacy in relation to their content of pentavalent antimony (Sb^v).[92] Meglumine antimoniate solution contains approximately 8.5% (85 mg/ml) pentavalent antimony, whereas sodium stibogluconate solutions contain about 10% pentavalent antimony (100 mg/ml). It is recommended that the dosage of drugs be based on the antimony content of the compound administered. Both compounds can be given intramuscularly or intravenously. The dosage recommended for visceral leishmaniasis is 20 mg Sb^v/kg body weight daily to a maximum of 850 mg of Sb^v per day for 20 days.[89] Patients with long-standing disease may require longer therapy. Treatment should be continuous. Primary unresponsiveness, defined as no clinical response to the initial course of Sb^v, ranges from 2 to 8 percent in most areas. Visceral leishmaniasis in Kenya tends to be less responsive. The relapse rate after treatment in Kenya ranges from 5 to 36 percent; elsewhere it is usually less than 10 percent.[91] Patients who do not respond well to an initial course of pentavalent antimony therapy may respond to a second or even a third course. Sb^v can be given at this dose for up to 30 days without additional toxicity. Long-term therapy (120 days) has been reported to be successful in the treatment of post–kala-azar dermal leishmaniasis in India.[93] In some areas, Sb^v, 20 mg/kg body weight, is given to adults without adherence to the 850 mg daily maximum.

The side effects of pentavalent antimonials include anorexia, vomiting, nausea, malaise, myalgia, abdominal pain, arthralgias, weakness, fever, skin rash, cough, headache, and lethargy, but these seldom prevent completion of the treatment course.[88–91] Electrocardiographic changes are dose dependent and include T-wave inversion and a prolonged QT interval. Arrhythmias and sudden death can occur at high doses.[94] Renal dysfunction is a rarely reported toxicity.

Pentamidine (Lomidine) is also active against *L. donovani*, but because of the frequent side effects, which include headache, flushing, faintness, vomiting, abdominal discomfort, hypoglycemia, insulin-dependent diabetes mellitus, and occasionally, vascular collapse, it is reserved for patients who fail to respond to antimonial compounds. Pentamidine isethionate is given intramuscularly in a dose of 2–4 mg/kg body weight per day for up to 15 days. Amphotericin B, 0.5 mg/kg given daily or 1 mg/kg every other day for up to 8 weeks, has also been successfully used for patients who fail to respond to antimony compounds.[95] Allopurinol, allopurinol ribonucleoside, and related pyrazolopyrimidines have been shown to be effective in the treatment of experimental visceral leishmaniasis in rodents, and allopurinol has been used successfully with pentavalent antimonials in some patients who fail to respond to pentavalent antimony alone.[96] Clinical experience, however, is insufficient to justify their use except in controlled experimental trials. Treatment with interferon-γ is theoretically attractive and has appeared promising in animal models[97] and in a small number of patients.

Patients with advanced visceral leishmaniasis should be hospitalized. All patients should receive a high-calorie, high-protein diet with supplemental vitamins. Blood transfusions may be necessary in cases of severe anemia. Associated bacterial infections must be promptly diagnosed and treated with appropriate antibiotics. Splenectomy is not indicated except in the rare instance in which infection does not respond to chemotherapy or in which signs of hypersplenism persist despite apparently adequate chemotherapy.[76]

Unfortunately, there are no tests or rigid criteria to document a cure. The cessation of fever; weight gain; resolution of anemia, leukopenia, and thrombocytopenia; and the disappearance of splenomegaly and hepatomegaly are suggestive. Amastigotes may be seen in bone marrow and splenic aspirates for several weeks after the initiation of successful chemotherapy. Relapses of visceral leishmaniasis usually occur within 6 months after the completion of therapy, but visceral leishmaniasis has been reported in immunosuppressed individuals many years after they have moved from endemic areas. AIDS appears to predispose to the development of severe, progressive disease.[49,50]

Prevention

Despite recent advances in understanding the immunology and molecular biology of leishmania, there is no effective form of immunoprophylaxis or chemoprophylaxis against *L. donovani*. The basic approaches to prevention have been to control the sandfly vectors, to detect and exterminate animal reservoirs, and to treat infected patients.[98] DDT and other residual insecticides have yielded good results in some areas, but spraying is necessary at intervals to maintain vector control. The cessation of DDT spraying for malaria in India, Bangladesh, and southern Iran has been followed by major epidemics of visceral leishmaniasis.[98] In addition, in areas where transmission occurs away from dwellings, residual spraying in houses is of no benefit. Insect repellents and fine mesh netting can provide partial, temporary protection for travelers.

Control of the animal reservoirs of infection is often difficult.

In northeastern Brazil, infected domestic dogs have been identified by mass serologic testing and exterminated, but the risk of *L. donovani* being reintroduced into domestic dogs from infected foxes remains. In epidemics where there is person-to-person transmission as in India and periodically in East Africa, case identification and treatment become major components in control schemes.

CUTANEOUS LEISHMANIASIS OF THE OLD WORLD

The classic form of cutaneous leishmaniasis is the "oriental sore."[2,3,69,99] It has also been termed "bouton d'orient," "bouton de Crete," "bouton d'Alep," "bouton de Biskra," Aleppo evil, Baghdad boil, and Dehli boil in various areas of the world. Cutaneous leishmaniasis occurs throughout tropical and subtropical regions in Asia Minor, China, the Mediterranean littoral, and India and in Africa in Sudan, Ethiopia, and the Congo basin. In general, oriental sores are troublesome and unsightly but not a threat to life.

Epidemiology

Old-world cutaneous leishmaniasis occurs in three major forms, each caused by a different *Leishmania* species. The rural form (*L. major*) is an infection of desert rodents, primarily gerbils, and affects humans in uninhabited areas or in villages on the edge of desert areas in central Asia, North Africa, and the Middle East. Urban cutaneous leishmaniasis (*L. tropica*) infects dogs and humans in such urban areas of the Middle East as Baghdad, Teheran, and Damascus as well as cities in the Mediterranean littoral, India and Pakistan. In cutaneous leishmaniasis (*L. aethiopica*) in Ethiopia, Kenya, and southwest Africa the primary reservoirs are species of hyrax (a small mammal), while rodents constitute secondary reservoirs. In addition to post–kala-azar dermal leishmaniasis, *L. donovani* occasionally causes simple cutaneous leishmaniasis. Old-world cutaneous leishmaniasis is a sporadic disease in endemic areas, but occasionally it occurs in an epidemic pattern, particularly when large groups of susceptible people are exposed during road construction, military maneuvers, or refugee movements.

Pathogenesis and Immunoloy

The promastigote state is inoculated into mammals by the sandfly, and the parasite is subsequently found in its amastigote form in macrophages at the site of inoculation. A granulomatous inflammatory response follows and is characterized by infected and noninfected mononuclear phagocytes, lymphocytes, and plasma cells. A papule forms, enlarges, and eventually ulcerates. Despite evidence of leishmanial antigen-specific lymphocyte responses, cutaneous ulcers often persist for weeks to months. Parasitized mononuclear phagocytes are eventually eliminated from the lesion, lymphocytes become predominant, and epitheloid and giant cells appear. Lesions usually heal slowly and leave a flat, atrophic scar as evidence of disease. Recovery is associated with a high level of resistance to reinfection by the homologous species of *Leishmania*.

Two uncommon variants fall at the extremes of the clinical spectrum of cutaneous leishmaniasis. In leishmaniasis recidivans, a hyperergic variant of cutaneous leishmaniasis, isolated or grouped tubercules appear over or around scars of healed cutaneous ulcers. These lesions often resemble lupus vulgaris. Parasites are present in low number. In diffuse cutaneous leishmaniasis, an anergic variant of cutaneous disease, disease starts as a localized papule that does not ulcerate, and large numbers of organisms progressively disseminate throughout the skin. Both syndromes have a protracted course.

In some respects, the range of immunologic features in cutaneous leishmaniasis parallels that of leprosy. At one end of the spectrum lies diffuse cutaneous leshmaniasis in which there is little evidence of effective cell-mediated immune responses. Heavily parasitized macrophages are abundant throughout the dermis, and few lymphocytes are present. Cutaneous delayed-type hypersensitivity reactions and in vitro lymphocyte responses to leishmanial antigen are absent. Diffuse cutaneous leishmaniasis is somewhat analogous to lepromatous leprosy in which there is massive bacterial infection of macrophages and little evidence of cell-mediated immune responses. At the other extreme lies leishmaniasis recidivans in which parasites are sparse and a mononuclear cell infiltrate predominates. This is somewhat analogous to tuberculoid leprosy in which there is an intense mononuclear infiltrate with few bacteria. However, whereas the character and organization of the granuloma in leprosy are invariably characteristic of the position in the clinical spectrum, this is not so in cutaneous leishmaniasis. When amastigotes are numerous, the cell type is nearly always the macrophage, but when amastigotes are scanty, the character of the granuloma, that is, the composition of the mononuclear response and its organization, is not predictable in contrast to leprosy.[100] Cutaneous ulceration, which pathologically is characterized by focal necrosis of infected macrophages as well as mononuclear cell infiltration,[101] is in all likelihood due to the host's immune response.

The immunology of *L. major* infection has been intensively studied in the murine model. The susceptibility of inbred mice to *L. major* is under genetic control, but the genes involved are distinct from the *Lsh* gene (responsible for resistance to *L. donovani*) and are not involved in the H-2 complex.[102] BALB/c mice, which are susceptible to *L. major*, have progressive local disease followed by widespread dissemination, whereas C57B1 mice, which are considered resistant, can be infected but display localized, self-healing ulcers.[103] At the cellular level, eradication of amastigotes is dependent on T-helper cell activation of macrophages either by the production of cytokines such as interferon-γ[57,104–107] or by direct contact.[108,109] The susceptibility of BALB/c mice to *L. major* seems to be due to a predominance of disease-enhancing rather than protective T cells of phenotypic helper type (Lyt 2−, L3T4+).[110–114] The reason that disease-enhancing T-helper cells predominate in some situations and not others is an area of intense interest.[113] Recent attention has focused on amphipathic surface glycolipids, the lipophosphoglycans (LPGs).[11,12,115] The carbohydrate moiety is anchored in the membrane to lysoalkyl phosphatidylinositol. Immunization of mice with LPG protects them from a parasite challenge, but immunization after hydrolysis with phospholipase C results in disease enhancement.[116] It has been postulated that the manner in which macrophages present LPG or its cleaved carbohydrate moiety in association with Ia antigens may determine which T-cell subsets are activated.[113] Other studies indicate that *Leishmania* amastigotes affect macrophages by decreasing Ia expression and altering lipoxygenase and cyclooxygenase pathways.[60,117] In humans, cutaneous ulcers persist long after antigen-specific T-cell responses develop. Although the explanation for this is not clear, there may be a defect in the influx of protective T cells into the lesion.[118] Alternatively, macrophages might locally suppress the immune response.

The best evidence for immune suppression in human leishmaniasis comes from patients from the Dominican Republic with diffuse cutaneous leishmaniasis.[119,120] Of patients studied extensively, none had delayed cutaneous hypersensitivity reactions or lymphocyte proliferative responses to leishmanial antigens. Decreasing the number of glass-adherent monocytes or the addition of the prostaglandin inhibitor indomethacin permitted expression of lymphocyte responses to leishmanial antigens in vitro, thereby suggesting the presence of a population of suppressor monocytes. In contrast to these patients, patients with localized cutaneous leishmaniasis develop delayed cutaneous hypersensitivity reactions and blastogenic responses to leishmanial antigens during the course of infection.

Clinical Manifestations

The incubation period of old-world cutaneous leishmaniasis varies from 2 weeks to several months and in some cases, has been as long as 3 years.[121] The manifestations of disease are also variable. In the urban or dry form (*L. tropica*), lesions tend to be single, grow slowly, and last for a year or more, whereas in the rural or moist form (*L. major*) lesions may be multiple, mature more rapidly, and tend to heal after several months.

The local lesion starts as a papule at the site where promastigotes are inoculated. The papule gradually increases in size, becomes crusted, and finally ulcerates. The ulcer is usually shallow and circular with well-defined, raised, erythematous borders and a bed of granulation tissue. It gradually increases in size and reaches a diameter of 2 cm or more. Satellite lesions that fuse with the original ulcer may be present. There is frequently a serous or scropurulent discharge, and the center of the granulating base of the ulcer often contains a hard excrescence termed the "Montpellier sign" or rake. A cutaneous horn may also arise. Scrapings of the base in this area are likely to yield parasites. The ulcerative lesion may be accompanied by regional lymphadenopathy. Secondary staphylococcal or streptococcal infection at the site of the ulcer is not uncommon. After a variable period ranging from several months to longer than a year, the ulcer heals and leaves a flat, atrophic, depigmented scar.

Diffuse cutaneous leishmaniasis starts as a localized papule that does not ulcerate. Satellite lesions develop around the initial papule, and organisms subsequently metastasize to distant areas of the skin, often to the face and extremities. The disease progresses slowly and may persist for 20 years or more. The leishmanin skin test is negative.

Leishmaniasis recidivans is the relapsing, tuberculoid form of cutaneous leishmaniasis. It is not uncommon in Iran. The lesions, usually present on the face, spread outward while healing at the center. Mucous membranes may be involved with concomitant nasal destruction. Leishmaniasis recidivans is very chronic and lasts 20–40 years in some cases. The leishmanin skin test is strongly positive, and few if any amastigotes can be identified in the lesion.

Diagnosis

The development of one or more ulcers with the appropriate characteristics in an endemic area is suggestive of leishmaniasis. A definite diagnosis depends on the identification of amastigotes in stained smears of scrapings from the base of the ulcer or from biopsy specimens or aspirates of its border. Material obtained from the surface of the ulcer is often not diagnostic because *Leishmania*-infected macrophages are destroyed in areas of secondary bacterial infection. The diagnosis can also be made by isolating parasites in cultures of aspirates as described for *L. donovani*. Care must be taken to minimize the risk of bacterial and fungal contamination. Although antileishmanial antibodies may be present in the serum, antibody titers are usually low and are not by themselves diagnostic. The leishmanin skin test becomes positive during the course of the disease.

The differential diagnosis of cutaneous leishmaniasis includes cutaneous fungal infections such as blastomycosis, yaws, syphilis, leprosy, cutaneous tuberculosis, atypical mycobacterial infections of the skin, and lupus vulgaris.

Treatment and Prophylaxis

The decision whether or not to treat cutaneous leishmaniasis depends on the location and extent of the lesion. Large or disfiguring lesions are commonly treated with pentavalent antimonial preparations. Although the optimal dosage and duration of therapy are uncertain and may vary from one location to another, 10–20 mg of Sb^{v} per body weight daily for 10–20 days (maximum of 850 mg/day) has been recommended. Therapy can be continued for up to 30 days for lesions that are slow to respond. In persons who fail to respond, a second or even third course of antimony may be successful. *Leishmania aethiopica* infection in East Africa often fails to respond to this dose. In a recent report,[122] a 30-day course of high-dose stibogluconate (20 mg Sb^{v}/kg twice daily) appeared to cure two of three young men with cutaneous *L. aethiopica* infection, but the potential for cardiac toxicity is much greater at doses in excess of 20 mg/kg/day, and deaths have been reported.[94] Secondary bacterial infections should be treated with local care of the ulcer and antibiotics, if necessary. Various forms of cryotherapy or local hyperthermic therapy have been proposed for use alone or in conjunction with systemic drug therapy. Intralesional administration of Sb^{v} has been advocated by some. There have also been reports of cures with several antibiotic and antiprotozoal agents other than pentavalent antimonials, but these have been uncontrolled observations, and interpretation of drug efficacy is difficult since cutaneous leishmaniasis resolves spontaneously. Recently, the topical administration of paromomycin with methylbenzethonium chloride has been reported to be effective in the treatment of *L. major* infections in Isreal. Ketoconazole, 200–400 mg/day for 4–6 weeks, has been reported to be effective in 70 percent of persons with *L. major* lesions[123]; it is not effective against *L. tropica* or *L. aethiopica*.

In the Ethiopian form of diffuse cutaneous leishmaniasis, which responds poorly to antimonials, pentamidine (2–4 mg/kg body weight once or twice a week) has been used successfully.[124] Amphotericin B is an alternative drug for the treatment of antimony failures.

Leishmaniasis recidivans is very resistant to most forms of therapy, although some success has apparently been achieved with locally applied heat or intralesional steroids, with or without concomitant antimonial therapy.

Prophylaxis

Spontaneous resolution of old-world cutaneous leishmaniasis is associated with the development of high-level immunity against the infecting *Leishmania* strain. Historically, mothers living in endemic areas in the Middle East exposed the buttocks of their children to sandflies in order to ensure that infection occurred in an inconspicuous site. People have been immunized in Israel and the Soviet Union with live promastigotes taken from culture. Good results have been obtained with the "Jericho" strain of *L. major*.[125,126] Although this practice has been effective in preventing naturally acquired disease, it has been discontinued in Israel because some of the resulting lesions heal slowly, others become secondarily infected, and parasites may persist at the site of inoculation even after the lesion has healed.[126] Efforts continue toward the development of a defined, component vaccine. Experience in animal models suggests that this is likely to be a successful approach.[1] Sandfly control by the spraying of residual insecticides or elimination of mammalian reservoirs has been effective in limiting disease in some areas. For travelers, insect repellents and fine-mesh netting may reduce sandfly exposure and thereby provide partial protection.

NEW-WORLD CUTANEOUS LEISHMANIASIS

New-world cutaneous leishmaniasis or American cutaneous leishmaniasis is widespread in Latin America where it constitutes a major public health problem (Table 1). The causative agents are subspecies of *L. braziliensis* and *L. mexicana*.[127] On occasion, *L. chagasi* causes simple cutaneous leishmaniasis. Depending on the clinical presentation and geographic location, the disease has been variously called espundia, pian bois (bush yaws), uta, and Chiclero's ear. The spectrum of disease ranges from a single, localized cutaneous ulcer (Fig. 3) to mucocutaneous disease (espundia) (Fig. 4), which is the only form that

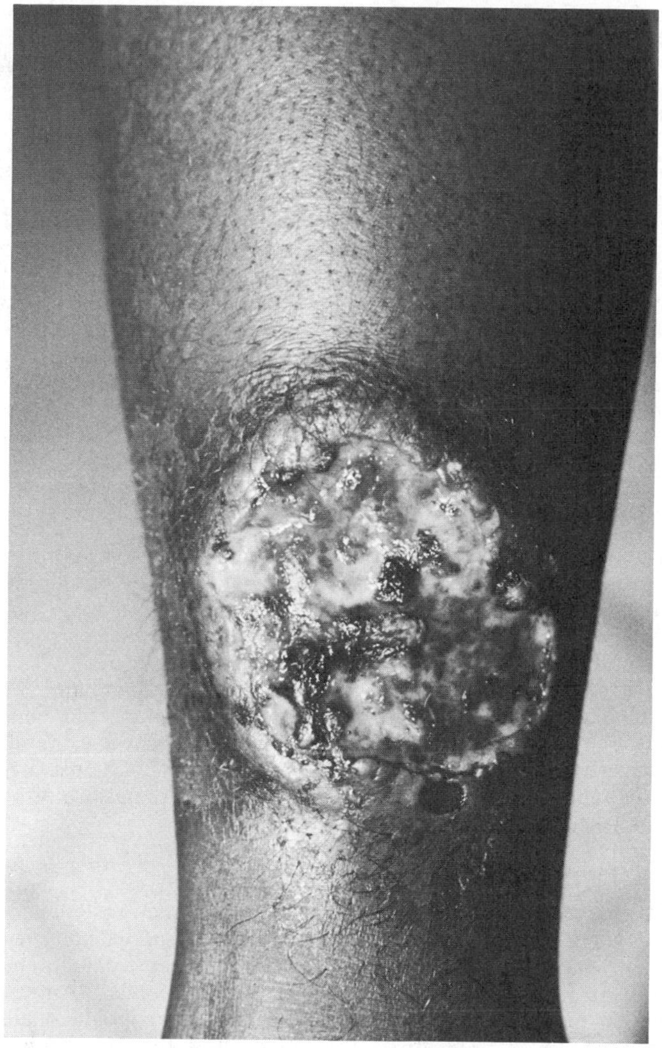

FIG. 3. American cutaneous leishmaniasis. Single, large leg lesion. (Courtesy of Dr. Kurt L. Wiese.)

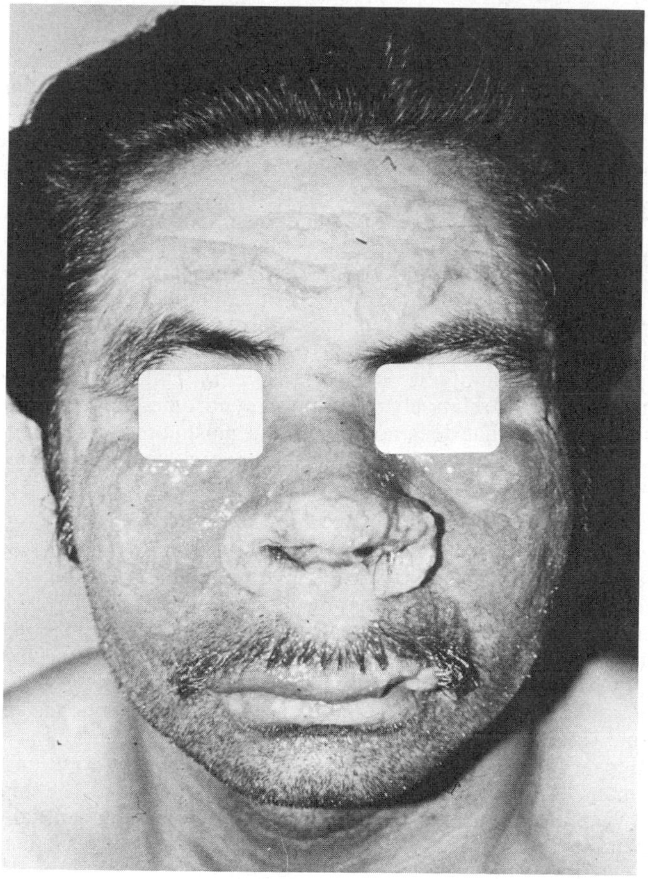

FIG. 4. American mucocutaneous leishmaniasis. There is extensive involvement of the nose and upper lip with destruction of the nasal septum. (From Pearson et al.,[4] with permission.)

carries a significant mortality. In this disorder, involvement of the nose, oral cavity, and pharynx is sometimes so destructive and mutilating that the individual is unable to eat. Prevention of the late sequelae of mucosal leishmaniasis is though to be possible if appropriate therapy is given for cutaneous disease.

Epidemiology

American cutaneous leishmaniasis is endemic in South and Central America.[127] It is found from Texas to northern Argentina. Brazil and Peru are the countries where the disease is most prevalent; Uruguay, Chile, and Canada are the only countries in the Americas where the disease has not been found.[128] Three autochthonous cases have been reported in Texas.[129,130] A focus of diffuse cutaneous leishmaniasis has been identified in the Dominican Republic.[131]

American cutaneous leishmaniasis is a zoonosis. The main reservoirs are small forest rodents, except in the case of *L. peruviana*, where the primary reservoir is the dog.[127] Domestic animals may serve as secondary reservoirs. The vectors are ground-dwelling or arboreal sandflies of the genera *Lutzomyia* and *Psychodopygus*. These sandflies are abundant in the forest, particularly during the hot season or shortly after the summer rains. The disease is most common in persons working at the edge of the forest and in rural settlers. Outbreaks often occur when large areas of forest are being cleared for roads, villages, or farms, as in an outbreak in Brazil among settlers of a new agrarian community.[132]

Pathogenesis

In lesions caused by the *L. braziliensis* complex, amastigotes are often scarce or nondetectable, and the connective tissue reaction is prominent.[133] In a variable percentage of patients,[134] for reasons that are not yet clear, mucous membrane involvement develops months to many years after the cutaneous lesions have healed. Involvement of the nose, oral cavity, and pharynx may be very severe. The disease is characterized by intense mononuclear cell infiltrates with few parasites. Reasons given for the predominance of nasal involvement include a lower skin temperature, which favors parasite growth, failure of cell-mediated immune responses to be effective in cartilage, trauma, or capillary plexus trapping of amastigotes.[51,135] To date, no spontaneous cure of mucosal leishmaniasis has been reported. The lack of an appropriate animal model has hindered research on the immunopathology of mucosal disease.

The pathogenesis and immunology of localized cutaneous leishmaniasis caused by members of the *L. mexicana* complex appear to be similar to that described for *L. major*. Likewise, the syndrome of diffuse cutaneous leishmaniasis observed in Venezuela, Brazil, and the Dominician Republic is similar to that produced by *L. aethiopica* in eastern Africa.

Clinical Manifestations

Cutaneous Leishmaniasis. A wide variety of skin lesions ranging from small, dry, crusted lesions to large, deep, mutilating ulcers are seen in American cutaneous leishmaniasis. There may be a single lesion or multiple ones, usually on an exposed area of the body. Lesions with different characteristics may be seen on the same patient.

In localized cutaneous disease the initial lesion usually appears 2–8 weeks[136] after the sandfly bite as a small, erythematous papule that progresses slowly to form a typical leishmaniotic ulcer: round with raised borders and a granulating base and covered by exudate. The ulcer may persist for months to years. Occasionally, a large vegetation appears that projects above the skin and simulates a neoplasm. Rarely, lesions may assume a keloidal form and give the appearance of lobomycosis.[137] When the primary ulcer is on the hand or foot, lymphatics may be involved, and a chain of nodules may develop along the lymphatics and mimic sporotrichosis.[134,135,138] The characteristics of the cutaneous lesions vary from one geographic area to another, but overlap occurs. Diffuse cutaneous leishmaniasis, a relatively uncommon syndrome, starts as a localized papule that does not ulcerate. Amastigotes disseminate to distant areas of the skin, and the disease runs a protracted course. This is an anergic variant of cutaneous leishmaniasis, and the leishmanin skin test response is negative.

Mucosal Leishmaniasis. *Leishmania braziliensis* can persist after disappearance of the primary cutaneous ulcer and subsequently appear as a mutilating mucosal infection. The percentage of patients who go on to mucosal disease is unknown and probably varies from one location to another. A prospective study in Brazil revealed an annual incidence of cutaneous leishmaniasis of 8.1 per 1000 inhabitants in one hyperendemic region. Most infections occurred in persons 10–30 years of age. Mucosal disease then followed in 2.7 percent of the people with primary lesions after a median duration of 6 years.[139] The time between the primary lesion and mucosal involvement is usually several years, but it may be as soon as 1 month[140] or as late as 24 years.[141] Epistaxis and nasal obstruction are early signs.[142] The process often starts in the septum as a slight swelling and reddening of the mucosa and progresses slowly over time to result in perforation of the septum.[143] When the septum is destroyed, the tip of the nose collapses (tapir nose). Perforation may occur through the skin of the nose or through the soft palate.[136,138] The upper lip is frequently involved as well as the tongue, and then the buccal, pharyngeal, and laryngeal mucosae in that order. Not all of the mucosal involvement is due to direct spread from the nose. Laryngeal leishmaniasis has been misdiagnosed as histoplasmosis and delayed appropriate therapy.[144] Involvement of the trachea[135,138] as well as the genital mucosa may also occur.[138,145] Aspiration pneumonia is a common complication in the late stages of oronasal disease and can result in death.[135]

Diagnosis

The diagnosis of American cutaneous leishmaniasis is based on the identification of amastigotes in tissue, on isolation of the parasite in culture or in hamsters, or on immunologic evidence in the appropriate clinical setting.[146] Aspirates and punch biopsy specimens should be taken from the edge of suspicious skin lesions. Meticulous cleaning of the lesion is necessary to prevent bacterial and fungal contamination. Touch preparations are made, Giemsa stained, and examined for amastigotes. Part of the remainder is used for culture and inoculation of hamsters when possible. A biopsy specimen is fixed for histologic examination. In general, isolates of the *L. mexicana* complex grow well in culture, readily infect hamsters, and produce large lesions that are rich in amastigotes. In contrast, isolates of the *L. braziliensis braziliensis* grow poorly or not at all in culture, they take longer to produce lesions in hamsters, and amastigotes are relatively sparse in infected tissue. The effectiveness of direct diagnosis by identification of the parasite varies with the type and duration of the lesion. The combined overall sensitivity of these methods in leishmanin positive patients is in the range of 50–70 percent.[147] Species-specific monoclonal antibodies and DNA probes have been used successfully to diagnose cutaneous leishmaniasis in tissue samples in experimental studies.[148] They have the advantage of allowing direct diagnosis and speciation, which have relevance in terms of appropriate chemotherapy.

A putative diagnosis of mucosal leishmaniasis is often made on the basis of the clinical findings and a positive leishmanin skin test or the presence of antileishmanial antibodies in serum. The leishmanin test is positive in 86.5[149] to 100 percent of cases[142,150] and the indirect fluorescent antibody test in 62.5 percent when promastigotes are used as the antigen source[151] to 89–96 percent when amastigotes are used.[151,152] Antibody studies may also be useful in evaluating the response to chemotherapy. The indirect fluorescent antibody titer fails after successful chemotherapy,[153] and a subsequent rise in titer suggests a relapse.

The ELISA is positive in 85 percent of those tested during the first 2 years after the primary cutaneous lesion develops.[139]

Differential Diagnosis

Cutaneous leishmaniasis must be differentiated from sporotrichosis, chromomycosis, lobomycosis, cutaneous tuberculosis, atypical mycobacterial infection, syphilis, yaws, leprosy, sarcoidosis, and neoplasms. In mucocutaneous disease, paracoccidioidomycosis, syphilis, tertiary yaws, histoplasmosis, sarcoidosis, basal cell carcinoma, and midline granuloma must be excluded.[136] The nasal polyps that occur in mucocutaneous leishmaniasis may mimic rhinosporidiosis.[154,155] The use of multiple histochemical stains and careful examination of biopsy material, appropriate cultures, and immunologic studies are often necessary to determine the diagnosis.

Treatment

Patients with skin lesions that are disfiguring and those in geographic areas where mucocutaneous disease is prevalent, even if they have only a cutaneous lesion, should be treated. The drugs of first choice are the pentavalent antimonials[51,136] meglumine antimoniate (Glucantime) and sodium stibogluconate (Pentostam).[51,156] The greatest experience in Latin America has been with meglumine antimoniate since sodium stibogluconate is not generally available there.

Various treatment regimens have been used. For uncomplicated cutaneous lesions, the World Health Organization has recommended 10–20 mg Sb^{v}/kg body weight per day (maximum, 850 mg) for 10–20 days. Persons who fail to respond or relapse are given the same dose for twice the duration. Recent data suggest that a daily dose of 20 mg/kg without a limit on the maximum dose is more effective and well tolerated.[157] Most patients with uncomplicated cutaneous disease will respond. Those with mucosal involvement should receive at least 4 weeks of therapy. Many patients require longer courses.[135,136] Up to 100 mg meglumine antimoniate (approximately 28 mg Sb^{v})/kg body weight per day has been given for 20 days of continuous therapy. At these higher dosages 40 percent of patients have suffered side effects.[158] Unfortunately, there are no tests or rigid criteria to document cures. Some have advocated the addition of steroids in persons who develop pronounced inflammation at the site of laryngeal lesions during therapy.

The response of mucosal disease to pentavalent antimonials is often unsatisfactory,[159] and in some regions of South America relapse after apparent cure has been reported to be as high as 50 percent within 1 year of treatment.[158] Patients who do not respond or relapse can be treated with amphotericin B.[159–163] Depending upon the patient's tolerance, 0.5–1.0 mg/kg body weight is given daily or every other day, respectively. A reasonable total adult dose is 1.5–2 g for cutaneous or mucocutaneous disease. Alternatively, pentamidine isethionate, 2–4 mg/kg body weight, can be administered once or twice weekly until the lesions heal. Plastic surgery may be necessary to ameliorate sequelae of mucosal leishmaniasis[164,165] but should not be performed earlier than 1 year after successful chemotherapy because the graft may be lost if a relapse occurs.

Other drugs such as metronidazole, ketoconazole, rifampin, cycloguanil pamoate, allopurinol, nifurtimox, clofazimine, and benznidazole have all been used to treat American cutaneous leishmaniasis, but the experience with them is limited, and they are not recommended for routine treatment. In a recent report immunotherapy with a vaccine consisting of live BCG together with killed leishmania promastigotes was reported to be as effective but less toxic than pentavalent antimony for the treatment of localized cutaneous leishmaniasis in Venezuela.[166]

In areas where there is no mucosal disease and a cutaneous lesion is not disfiguring, the patient can be observed or the lesion treated topically. Some patients with isolated lesions and others with diffuse cutaneous leishmaniasis acquired in the Dominican Republic have been treated successfully with heat applied to the involved areas. Cryosurgery and the application of carbon dioxide snow (dry ice) have also been reported to be effective in some cases.

Prophylaxis

Since American leishmaniasis is a forest zoonosis, little can be done to control the reservoirs or vectors. Care should be taken to avoid establishing settlements at the edge of or within involved forests. Insect repellents can provide limited, partial protection for travelers. In studies in Brazil, a killed promastigote vaccine derived from five *Leishmania* strains reportedly reduced the annual incidence of cutaneous leishmaniasis in military recruits by 86 percent.[167]

REFERENCES

1. Pearson RD, Wilson ME. Host defenses against prototypic intracellular protozoa, the *Leishmania*. In: Walzer PD, Genta RM, eds. Parasitic Infections in the Compromised Host. Immunologic mechanisms and clinical applications. New York: Marcell Deckker; 1988:31–81.
2. Lainson R, Shaw JJ. Evolution classification and geographic distribution. In: Peters W, Killick-Kendrick R, eds. The Leishmaniases in Biology and Medicine. v. 1. London: Academic Press; 1987:2–120.
3. Manson-Bahr PEC, Apted FIC. Manson's Tropical Diseases. 18th ed. London: Bailliere Tindall; 1982:667–73.
4. Pearson RD, Wheeler DA, Harrison LH, et al. The immunobiology of leishmaniasis. Rev Infect Dis. 1983;5:907–27.
5. Pearson RD, Sullivan JA, Roberts D, et al. Interaction of *Leishmania donovani* promastigotes with human phagocytes. Infect Immun. 1983;40:411–6.
6. Giannini MS. Effects of promastigote growth phase, frequency of subculture, and host age on promastigote-initiated infections with *Leishmania donovani* in the golden hamster. J Protozool. 1974;21:521–7.
7. Sacks DL, Perkins PV. Identification of an infective stage of *Leishmania* promastigotes. Science. 1984;223:1417–9.
8. Sacks DL, Hieny S, Sher A. Identification of cell surface carbohydrate and antigenic changes between noninfective and infective developmental stages of *Leishmania major* promastigotes. J Immunol. 1985;135:564–9.
9. Colomer-Gould V, Quintao LG, Keithly J, et al. A common major surface antigen on amastigotes and promastigotes of *Leishmania* species. J Exp Med. 1985;162:902–16.
10. Etges R, Bouvier J, Bordier C. The major surface protein of *Leishmania* promastigotes is a protease. J Biol Chem. 1986;261:9098–101.
11. McConville MJ, Bacic A, Mitchell GF, et al. Lipophosphoglycan of *Leishmania major* that vaccinates against cutaneous leishmaniasis contains an alkylglycerophosphoinositol lipid anchor. Proc Natl Acad Sci USA. 1987;84:8941–5.
12. King DL, Chang Y-D, Turco SJ. Cell surface lipophosphoglycan of *Leishmania donovani*. Mol Biochem Parasitol. 1987;24:47–53.
13. Blackwell JM, Ezekowitz RAB, Roberts MB, et al. Macrophage complement and lectin-like receptors bind *Leishmania* in the absence of serum. J Exp Med. 1985;162:324–31.
14. Wozencraft AO, Sayers G, Blackwell JM. Macrophage type 3 complement receptors mediate serum-independent binding of *Leishmania donovani*. J Exp Med. 1986;164:1332–7.
15. Russell DG, Wilhelm H. The involvement of the major surface glycoprotein (gp63) of *Leishmania* promastigotes in attachment to macrophages. J Immunol. 1986;136:2613–20.
16. Mosser DM, Edelson PJ. Activation of the alternative complement pathway by *Leishmania* promastigotes: Parasite lysis and attachment to macrophages. J Immunol. 1984;132:1501–5.
17. Wilson ME, Pearson RD. Evidence that *Leishmania donovani* utilizes a mannose receptor on human mononuclear phagocytes to establish intracellular parasitism. J Immunol. 1986;136:4681–8.
18. Wilson ME, Pearson RD. Roles of CR3 and mannose receptors in the attachment and ingestion of *Leishmania donovani* by human mononuclear phagocytes. Infect Immun. 1988;56:363–9.
19. Puentes SM, Sacks DL, da Silva RP, et al. Complement binding by two developmental stages of *Leishmania major* promastigotes varying in expression of a surface lipophosphoglycan. J Exp Med. 1988;167:887–902.
20. Mosser DM, Vlassara H, Edelson PJ, et al. *Leishmania* promastigotes are recognized by the macrophage receptor for advanced glycosylation end products. J Exp Med. 1987;165:140–5.
21. Wyler DJ, Sypek JP, McDonald JA. In vitro parasite-monocyte interactions in human leishmaniasis: Possible role of fibronectin in parasite attachment. Infect Immun. 1985;49:305–11.
22. Ebert F. Charakterisierung von *Leishmania donovani*-Stammen mit der Disk-Electrophorese. Z Tropenmed Parasitol. 1973;24:517–24.
23. Gardener PJ, Chance ML, Peters W. Biochemical taxonomy of *Leishmania*. II. Electrophoretic variation of malate dehydrogenase. Ann Trop Med Parasitol. 1974;68:317–25.
24. Brazil RP. Electrophoretic variation of the enzyme phosphoglucomutase in different strains of *Leishmania*. Ann Trop Med Parasitol. 1978;72:289–91.
25. Schnur LF, Chance ML, Ebert F, et al. The biochemical and serological taxonomy of visceralizing *Leishmania*. Ann Trop Med Parasitol. 1981;75:131–44.
26. Rassam MB, Al-Mudhaffar SA, Chance ML. Isoenzyme characterization of *Leishmania* species from Iraq. Ann Trop Med Parasitol. 1979;73:527–34.
27. Decker JE, Schrot JR, Levin GV. Identification of *Leishmania* spp. by radiorespirometry. J Protozool. 1977;24:463–70.
28. Pratt DM, David JR. Monoclonal antibodies that distinguish between New World species of *Leishmania*. Nature. 1981;291:581–3.
29. Arnot DE, Barker DC. Biochemical identification of cutaneous leishmaniasis by analysis of kinetoplast DNA. II. Sequence homologies in *Leishmania* kDNA. Mol Biochem Parasitol. 1981;3:47–56.
30. Wirth DF, Pratt DM. Rapid identification of *Leishmania* species by specific hybridization of kinetoplast DNA in cutaneous lesions. Proc Natl Acad Sci USA. 1982;79:6999–7003.
31. Jackson PR, Wohlhieter JA, Jackson JE, et al. Restriction endonuclease analysis of *Leishmania* kinetoplast DNA characterizes parasites responsible for visceral and cutaneous disease. Am J Trop Med Hyg. 1984;33:808–19.
32. Blackwell J, Pratt DM, Shaw J. Molecular biology of *Leishmania*. Parasitol Today. 1986;2:45–53.
33. Giannini SH, Schittini M, Keithly JS, et al. Karyotype analysis of *Leishmania* species and its use in classification and clinical diagnosis. Science. 1986;232:762–5.
34. Lewis DJ, Ward RD. Transmission and vectors. In: Peters W, Killick-Kendrick R, eds. The Leishmaniases in Biology and Medicine. v. 2. London: Academic Press; 1987:235–62.
35. Badaró R, Jones TC, Lorenco R, et al. A prospective study of visceral leishmaniasis in an endemic area of Brazil. *J Infect Dis*. 1986;154:639–49.
36. Badaro R, Jones TC, Carvalho EM, et al. New perspectives on a subclinical form of visceral leishmaniasis. J Infect Dis. 1986;154:1003–11.
37. Maru M. Clinical and laboratory features and treatment of visceral leishmaniasis in hospitalized patients in northwestern Ethiopia. Am J Trop Med Hyg. 1979;28:15–8.
38. De Alencar JE, Neves J. Leishmaniose visceral (calazar). In: Veronesi R, ed. Doencas Infecciosas e Parasitarias. 7th ed. Rio de Janeiro: Editora Guanabara Koogan SA; 1982:724.
39. Chung HL, Chow HK, Lu JR. The first two cases of transfusion kala-azar. Chin Med J. 1948;66:325.
40. Andre R, Brumpt L, Dreyfuss B, et al. Leishmaniose cutaneeganglionaire et kala-azar transfusionel. Bull Mem Soc Med Hopit. 1957;25–26:584.
41. Low GC, Cooke WE. A congenital case of kala-azar. Lancet. 1926;2:1209–11.
42. Banerji D. Possible congenital infection of kala-azar. J Indian Med Assoc. 1955;24:433–5.
43. Symmers WStC. Leishmaniasis acquired by contagion. A case of marital infection in Britian. Lancet. 1960;1:127–32.
44. Pearson RD, Sousa AQ. Leishmaniasis in travelers. Travel Med. 1985;3:2–8.
45. Steele NP Jr, Foshee WS, Koch F, et al. Visceral leishmaniasis acquired in Greece: Diagnosis and treatment in an American child. South Med J. 1977;70:1481–3.
46. Khot AS, Thompson MH. Visceral leishmaniasis contracted in the Mediterranean area. Arch Dis Child. 1983;58:930–1.
47. Maquire JH, Gantz NM, Moscella S, et al. Leishmanial infections: A consideration in travelers returning from abroad. Am J Med Sci. 1983;285:32–40.
48. Geraci JE, Wilson WR, Thompson JH. Visceral leishmaniasis (kala-azar) as a cause of fever of unknown origin. Mayo Clin Proc. 1980;55:455–8.
49. Clauvel JP, Couderc LJ, Belmin J, et al. Visceral leishmaniasis complicating acquired immunodeficiency syndrome (AIDS) (Letter). Trans R Soc Trop Med Hyg. 1986;80:1010–1.
50. Yebra M, Segovia J, Manzano L, et al. Disseminated-to-skin kala-azar and the acquired immunodeficiency syndrome. Ann Intern Med. 1988;108:490–1.
51. Marsden PD. Current concepts in parasitology: Leishmaniasis. N Engl J Med. 1979;300:350–2.

52. Manson-Bahr PEC. A primary skin lesion in visceral leishmaniasis. Nature. 1955;175:433–4.
53. Manson-Bahr PEC. East African kala-azar with special reference to the pathology, prophylaxis and treatment. Trans R Soc Trop Med Hyg. 1959;53:123–37.
54. Bradley DJ, Taylor BA, Blackwell J, et al. Regulation of *Leishmania* populations within the host: III. Mapping of the locus controlling susceptibility to visceral leishmaniasis in the mouse. Clin Exp Immunol. 1979;37:7–14.
55. Plant JE, Blackwell JM, O'Brien D, et al. Are the *Lsh* and *Ity* disease resistance genes at one locus on mouse chromosome 1? Nature. 1982;297:510–1.
56. Rezai HR, Farrell J, Soulsby EL. Immunological responses of *L. donovani* infection in mice and significance of T cells in resistance to experimental leishmaniasis. Clin Exp Immunol. 1980;40:508–14.
57. Murray HW, Rubin BY, Rothermel CD. Killing of intracellular *Leishmania donovani* by lymphokine-stimulated human mononuclear phagocytes: Evidence that interferon-γ is the activating lymphokine. J Clin Invest. 1983;72:1506–10.
58. Nickol AD, Bonventre PF. Visceral leishmaniasis in congenic mice of susceptible and resistant phenotypes: Immunosuppression by adherent spleen cells. Infect Immun. 1985;50:160–8.
59. Murray HW, Carriero SM, Donelly DM. Presence of a macrophage-mediated suppressor cell mechanism during cell-mediated immune response in experimental visceral leishmaniasis. Infect Immun. 1986;54:487–93.
60. Reiner NE, Malemud CJ. Arachidonic acid metabolism by murine peritoneal macrophages infected with *Leishmania donovani*: in vitro evidence for parasite-induced alterations in cyclooxygenase and lipoxygenase pathways. J Immunol. 1985;134:556–63.
61. Blackwell JM, Ulczak OM. Immunoregulation of genetically controlled acquired responses to *Leishmania donovani* infection in mice: Demonstration and characterization of suppressor T cells in non-cure mice. Infect Immun. 1984;44:97–102.
62. Carvalho EM, Badaró R, Reed SG, et al. Absence of gamma interferon and interleukin 2 production during active visceral leishmaniasis. J Clin Invest. 1985;76:2066–9.
63. Carvalho EM, Teixeira RS, Johnson WD Jr. Cell-mediated immunity in American visceral leishmaniasis: Reversible immunosuppression during acute infection. Infect Immun. 1981;33:498–502.
64. Campos-Neto A, Bunn-Moreno MM. Polyclonal B cell activation in hamsters infected with parasites of the genus *Leishmania*. Infect Immun. 1982;38:871–6.
65. Badaró R, Carvalho EM, Rocha H, et al. *Leishmania donovani*: An opportunistic microbe associated with progressive disease in three immunocompromised patients. Lancet. 1986;1:647–8.
66. Harrison LH, Naidu TG, Drew JS, et al. Reciprocal relationships between undernutrition and the parasitic disease visceral leishmaniasis. Rev Infect Dis. 1986;8:447–53.
67. Cerf BJ, Jones TC, Badaro R, et al. Malnutrition as a risk factor for severe visceral leishmaniasis. J Infect Dis. 1987;156:1030–3.
68. Manson-Bahr PEC, Southgate BA, Harvey AEC. Development of kala-azar in man after inoculation with a leishmania from a Kenya sandfly. Br Med J. 1963;1:1208–10.
69. Manson-Bahr PEC, Apted FIC. Leishmaniasis. In: Manson-Bahr PEC, Apted FIC, eds. Manson's Tropical Diseases, 18th ed. London: Bailliere Tindall; 1982:93–115.
70. Stone HH, Tool CD, Pugsley WS. Kala-azar (visceral leishmaniasis): Report of a case with 34 month incubation period and positive Doan-Wright test. Ann Intern Med. 1952;36:686–93.
71. Knight R, Woodruff AW, Pettitt LE. The mechanism of anaemia in kala-azar: A study of two patients. Trans R Soc Trop Med Hyg. 1967;61:701–5.
72. Woodruff AW, Topley E, Knight R, et al. The anaemia of kala azar. Br J Haematol. 1972;22:319–29.
73. Pippard MJ, Moir D, Weatherall DJ, et al. Mechanism of anaemia in resistant visceral leishmaniasis. Ann Trop Med Parasitol. 1986;80:317–23.
74. Most H, Lavietes PH. Kala-azar in American military personnel. Report of 30 cases. Medicine (Baltimore). 1947;26:221–84.
75. Musumeci S, D'Agata A, Schiliro G, et al. Studies of the neutropenia in kala-azar: Results in two patients. Trans R Soc Trop Med Hyg. 1976;70:500–3.
76. Burchenal JH, Bowers RF, Haedicke TA. Visceral leishmaniasis complicated by severe anemia-improvement following splenectomy. Am J Trop Med Hyg. 1947;27:699–709.
77. Carvalho EM, Andrews BS, Martinelli R, et al. Circulating immune complexes and rheumatoid factor in schistosomiasis and visceral leishmaniasis. Am J Trop Med Hyg. 1983;32:61–69.
78. Pearson RD, Alencar JE, Romito R, et al. Circulating immune complexes and rheumatoid factors in visceral leishmaniasis. J Infect Dis. 1983;147:1102.
79. De Brito T, Hoshino-Shimizu S, Neto VA, et al. Glomerular involvement in human kala-azar. Am J Trop Med Hyg. 1975;24:9–18.
80. Kirk R. Studies in leishmaniasis in the Anglo-Egyptian Sudan: V. Cutaneous and mucocutaneous leishmaniasis. Trans R Soc Trop Med Hyg. 1942;35:257–70.
81. Sen Gupta PC, Bhattacharjee B. Histopathology of post–kala-azar dermal leishmaniasis. J Trop Med Hyg. 1953;56:110–6.
82. Report of the informal meeting on the chemotherapy of visceral leishmaniasis. UNDP/World Bank/WHO Special Programme for Research and Training in Tropical Diseases. Nairobi, Kenya, June 1982.
83. Chulay JD, Bryceson ADM. Quantitation of amastigotes of *Leishmania donovani* in smears of splenic aspirates from patients with visceral leishmaniasis. Am J Trop Med Hyg. 1983;32:475–9.
84. Hockmeyer WT, Kager PA, Rees PH, et al. The culture of *Leishmania donovani* in Schneider's insect medium: Its value in the diagnosis and management of patients with visceral leishmaniasis. Trans R Soc Trop Med Hyg. 1981;75:861–3.
85. Badaró R, Reed SG, Carvalho EM. Immunofluorescent antibody test in American visceral leishmaniasis: Sensitivity and specificity of different morphological forms of two *Leishmania* species. Am J Trop Med Hyg. 1983;32:480–4.
86. Mohammed EAER, Wright EP, Rahman AMA, et al. Serodiagnosis of Sudanese visceral and mucosal leishmaniasis: Comparison of ELISA-immunofluorescence and indirect haemagglutination. Trans R Soc Trop Med Hyg. 1986;80:271–4.
87. Pearson RD, Evans T, Naidu TG, et al. Humoral responses during South American visceral leishmaniasis. Ann Trop Med Parasitol. 1986;80:465–8.
88. Pearson RD, Navin TR, de Sousa AQ, et al. Leishmaniasis. In: Kass EH, Platt R, eds. Current Therapy in Infectious Disease. Burlington, Ontario: BC Becker; 1989. In press.
89. Report of a WHO Expert Committee. The leishmaniasis. Geneva: WHO Technical Report Series 710; 1984.
90. Berman JD. Chemotherapy for leishmaniasis: Biochemical mechanisms, clinical efficacy, and future strategies. Rev Infect Dis. 1988;10:560–86.
91. Information material for physicians—Pentostam (sodium antimony gluconate), HHS, PHS, CDC protocol. Provided by the Centers for Disease Control to physicians administering Pentostam in the United States.
92. Chulay JD, Fleckenstein L, Smith DH. Pharmacokinetics of antimony during treatment of visceral leishmaniasis with sodium stibogluconate or meglumine antimoniate. Trans R Soc Trop Med Hyg. 1988;82:69–72.
93. Thakur CP, Kumar K, Sinha PK, et al. Treatment of post–kala-azar dermal leishmaniasis with sodium stibogluconate. Br Med J. 1987;295:886–7.
94. Thakur CP. Harmful effect of high stibogluconate treatment of kala-azar in India. Trans R Soc Trop Med Hyg. 1986;80:672–3.
95. Prata A. Treatment of kala-azar with amphotericin B. Trans R Soc Trop Med Hyg. 1963;57:266–8.
96. Kager PA, Rees PH, Wellde BT, et al. Allopurinol in the treatment of visceral leishmaniasis. Trans R Soc Trop Med Hyg. 1981;75:556–9.
97. Murray HW, Stern JJ, Welte K, et al. Experimental visceral leishmaniasis: production of interleukin 2 and interferon-γ, tissue immune reaction, and response to treatment with interleukin 2 and interferon-γ. J Immunol. 1987;138:2290–7.
98. Marinkelle CJ. The control of leishmaniasis. Bull WHO. 1980;58:807–18.
99. Ashford RW, Bettini S. Ecology and epidemiology: Old World. In: Peters W, Killick-Kendrick R, eds. The Leishmaniasis in Biology and Medicine. v. 1. London: Academic Press; 1987:365–424.
100. Ridley DS. The pathogenesis of cutaneous leishmaniasis. Trans R Soc Trop Med Hyg. 1979;73:150–60.
101. Ridley MJ, Ridley DS. Cutaneous leishmaniasis: Immune complex formation and necrosis in the acute phase. Br J Exp Pathol. 1984;65:327–36.
102. Mock BA, Fortier AH, Potter M, et al. Genetic control of systemic *Leishmania major* infections; dissociation of intrahepatic amastigote replication from control by the *Lsh* gene. Infect Immun. 1985;50:588–91.
103. Cox FEG. Leishmaniasis and mouse genetics. Nature. 1981;291:111–2.
104. Nacy CA, Meltzer MS, Leonard EJ, et al. Intracellular replication and lymphokine-induced destruction of *Leishmania tropica* in C3H/HeN mouse macrophages. J Immunol. 1981;127:2381–6.
105. Oster CN, Nacy CA. Macrophage activation to kill *Leishmania tropica*: Kinetics of macrophage response to lymphokines that induce antimicrobial activities against amastigotes. J Immunol. 1984;132:1494–500.
106. Hockmeyer WT, Walters D, Gore RW, et al. Intracellular destruction of *Leishmania donovani* and *Leishmania tropica*: Amastigotes by activated macrophages: Dissociation of these microbicidal effector activities in vitro. J Immunol. 1984;132:3120–5.
107. Titus RG, Kelso A, Louis JA. Intracellular destruction of *Leishmania tropica* by macrophages activated with macrophage activating factor/interferon. Clin Exp Immunol. 1984;55:157–65.
108. Sypek JP, Panosian CB, Wyler DJ. Cell contact-mediated macrophage activation for antileishmanial defense. II. Identification of effector cell phenotype and genetic restriction. J Immunol. 1984;133:3351–7.
109. Sypek JP, Panosian CB, Wyler DJ. Antigen recognition by effector T cells in antileishmanial defense. J Infect Dis. 1985;152:1057–63.
110. Howard JG. Immunological regulation and control of experimental leishmaniasis. Int Rev Exp Pathol. 1986;28:79–116.
111. Mitchell GE, Curtis JM, Scollary RG, et al. Resistance and abrogation of resistance to cutaneous leishmaniasis in reconstituted BALB/c nude mice. Aust J Exp Biol Med Sci. 1981;59:539–54.
112. Titus RG, Lima GC, Engers HD, et al. Exacerbation of murine cutaneous leishmaniasis by adoptive transfer of parasite-specific helper T cell populations capable of mediating *Leishmania major*-specific delayed-type hypersensitivity. J Immunol. 1984;133:1594–600.
113. Mitchell GE, Handman E. T-lymphocytes recognize *Leishmania* glycoconjugates. Parasitol Today. 1985;1:61–3.
114. Solbach W, Forberg K, Krammerer E, et al. Suppressive effect of cyclosporin A on the development of *Leishmania tropica*-induced lesions in genetically susceptible BALB/c mice. J Immunol. 1986;137:702–7.
115. Turco SJ, Wilkerson MA, Clawson DR. Expression of an unusual acid glycoconjugate in *Leishmania donovani*. J Biol Chem. 1984;259:3883–9.
116. Handman E. Mitchell GF. Immunization with *Leishmania* receptor for mac-

rophages protects mice against cutaneous leishmaniasis. Proc Natl Acad Sci USA. 1985;82:5910–4.
117. Reiner NE, Ng W, McMaster WR. Parasite-accessory cell interactions in murine leishmaniasis. II. *Leishmania donovani* suppresses macrophage expression for class I and class II major histocompatibility complex gene products. J Immunol. 1987;138:1926–32.
118. McElrath MJ, Kaplan G, Nusrat A, et al. Cutaneous leishmaniasis. The defect in T cell influx in BALB/c mice. J Exp Med. 1987;165:546–59.
119. Petersen EA, Neva FA, Oster CN, et al. Specific inhibition of lymphocyte-proliferation responses by adherent suppressor cells in diffuse cutaneous leishmaniasis. N Engl J Med. 1982;306:387–92.
120. Petersen EA, Neva FA, Barral A, et al. Monocyte suppression of antigen-specific lymphocyte responses in diffuse cutaneous leishmaniasis patients from the Dominican Republic. J Immunol. 1984;132:2603–6.
121. Smith PAJ. Long incubation period in leishmaniasis. Br Med J. 1955;2:1143.
122. Chulay JD, Anzeze EM, Koech DK, et al. High-dose sodium stibogluconate treatment of cutaneous leishmaniasis in Kenya. Trans R Soc Trop Med Hyg. 1983;77:717–21.
123. Weinrauch L, Livshin R, El-On J. Ketoconazole in cutaneous leishmaniasis. Br J Dermatol. 1987;117:666–8.
124. Bryceson ADM. Diffuse cutaneous leishmaniasis in Ethiopia. II. Treatment. Trans R Soc Trop Med Hyg. 1970;64:369–93.
125. Naggan L, Gunders AE, Michaeli D. Follow-up study of a vaccination programme against cutaneous leishmaniasis: II. Vaccination with a recently isolated strain of *L. tropica* from Jericho. Trans R Soc Trop Med Hyg. 1972;66:239–43.
126. Greenblatt CL. The present and future of vaccination for cutaneous leishmaniasis. In: Mizrahi A, Hertman I, Klingberg MA, et al., eds. Progress in Clinical and Biological Research. v. 47. New Developments with Human and Veterinary Vaccines. New York: Alan R Liss; 1980:259–85.
127. Shaw JJ, Lainson R. Ecology and epidemiology: New World. In: Peters W, Killick-Kendrick R, eds. The Leishmaniases in Biology and Medicine. v. 1. London: Academic Press; 1987:291–363.
128. Pessoa SB, Martins AV. Pessôa Parasitologia Medica. 11th ed. Rio de Janeiro: Editora Guanabara Koogan: 1982:78–87.
129. Simpson MH, Mullins JF, Stone OJ. Disseminated anergic cutaneous leishmaniasis. An autochthonous case in Texas and the Mexican states of Tamaulipas and Nuevo Leon. Arch Dermatol. 1968;97:301–3.
130. Shaw PK, Quigg LT, Allain DS, et al. Autochthonous dermal leishmaniasis in Texas. Am J Trop Med Hyg. 1976;25:788–96.
131. Bogaert Diaz H, Rojas RF, de Leon A, et al. Leishmania tegumentaria Americana: Reporte de los primeros tres casos. Rev Dominicana Dermatol. 1975;9:19–33.
132. Da Silva AR, Martins G, Melo JEM, et al. Surto epidemico de leishmaniose tegumentar Americana ocorrido na colonizacao agricola de buriticupu (Estado do Maranhao), Brasil. Rev Inst Med Trop Sao Paulo. 1979;21:43–50.
133. Ridley DS, Marsden PD, Cuba CC, et al. A histological classification of mucocutaneous leishmaniasis in Brazil and its clinical evaluation. Trans R Soc Trop Med Hyg. 1980;74:508–14.
134. Kerdel-Vegas F. American leishmaniasis. Int J Dermatol. 1982;21:291–303.
135. Marsden PD, Sampaio RNR, Rocha R, et al. Mucocutaneous leishmaniasis—an unsolved clinical problem. Trop Doct. 1977;7:7–11.
136. Marsden PD, Nonata RR. Mucocutaneous leishmaniasis—a review of clinical aspects. Rev Soc Bras Med Trop. 1975;9:309–26.
137. Silva D. Leishmaniose tegumentar queloidiana, com lesoes osseas. An Bras Dermatol Sifilolog. 1958;33:3–7.
138. Pupo JA. Estudo clinico da leishmaniose tegumentar Americana—(*Leishmania braziliensis*—Vianna 1911). Rev Hosp Clin Fac Med Sao Paulo. 1946;1:113–64.
139. Jones TC, Johnson WD Jr., Barretto AC, et al. Epidemiology of American cutaneous leishmaniasis due to *Leishmania braziliensis braziliensis*. J Infect Dis. 1987;156:73–83.
140. Villela F, Pestana BR, Pessoa SB. Presenca da *Leishmania brasiliensis* na mucosa nasal sem lesão aparente, em casos recentes de leishmaniose cutanea. O Hospital. 1939;16:953–60.
141. Walton BC, Chinel LV, Eguia OE. Onset of espundia after many years of occult infection with *Leishmania braziliensis*. Am J Trop Med Hyg. 1973;22:696–8.
142. Jaffe L: Further observations on leishmaniasis Americana in the upper respiratory passages in Panama. Arch Dermatol. 1960;72:464–70.
143. Klotz O, Lindenberg H. The pathology of leishmaniosis of the nose. Am J Trop Med. 1923;3:117–41.
144. Zinneman HH, Hall WH, Wallace FG. Leishmaniasis of the larynx. Am J Med. 1961;31:654–8.
145. Aleixo J. Leishmaniose com localizacao genital. An Bras Dermatol Sifilolog. 1945;20:69–71.
146. Furtado T. Criterios para o diagnostico da leishmaniose tegumentar Americana. An Bras Dermatol. 1980;55:81–6.
147. Weigle KA, de Davalos M, Heredia P, et al. Diagnosis of cutaneous and mucocutaneous leishmaniasis in Colombia: A comparison of seven methods. Am J Trop Med Hyg. 1987;36:489–96.
148. Wirth DF, Rogers WO, Barker R Jr, et al. Leishmaniasis and malaria: New tools for epidemiologic analysis. Science. 1986;234:975–9.
149. Montenegro J. Cutaneous reaction in leishmaniasis. Arch Dermatol Syph. 1926;13:187–94.
150. Bonfante-Garrido R, Barreto T. Leishmaniasis tegumentaria Americana en el distrito urdaneta, Venezuela. Bol Of Sanit Panam. 1981;91:30–37.
151. Cuba CAC, Marsden PD, Barreto AC, et al. Parasitologic and immunologic diagnosis of American (mucocutaneous) leishmaniasis. Bull Pan Am Health Organ. 1981;15:249–259.
152. Walton BC, Brooks WH, Arjona J. Serodiagnosis of American leishmaniasis by indirect fluorescent antibody test. Am J Trop Med Hyg. 1972;21:296–99.
153. Walton BC. The indirect fluorescent antibody test for evaluation of effectiveness of chemotherapy in American leishmaniasis (abstract). J Parasitol. 1970;56:480–1.
154. Costa OG. American (mucocutaneous) leishmaniasis. Arch Dermatol Syph. 1944;49:194–6.
155. Jaffe L. Nasal leishmaniasis Americana in Panama. Arch Otolaryngol. 1954;60:601–11.
156. Castro RM. Tratamento de leishmaniose tegumentar Americana. An Bras Dermatol. 1980;55:87–9.
157. Ballou WR, McClain JB, Gordon DM, et al. Safety and efficacy of high-dose sodium stibogluconate therapy of American cutaneous leishmaniasis. Lancet. 1987;2:13–6.
158. Report of the workshop on the chemotherapy of mucocutaneous leishmaniasis. UNDP/World Bank/WHO Special Programme for Research and Training in Tropical Diseases, Brasilia, July 1979.
159. Rocha RAA, Sampaio RN, Guerra M, et al. Apparent glucantime failure in five patients with mucocutaneous leishmaniasis. J Trop Med Hyg. 1980;83:131–9.
160. Furtado TA. Clinical results in the treatment of American leishmaniasis with oral and intravenous amphotericin. In: Welch H, Marti-Ibanez F, ed. Antibiotics Annual 1959–1960. New York: Antibiotica; 1960:631–37.
161. Sampaio SAP, Godoy JT, Paiva L, et al. The treatment of American (mucocutaneous) leishmanias with amphotericin B. Arch Dermatol. 1960;82:627–35.
162. Miranda JL, Lima NDS, Da Cuhna JF. A anfotericina B na terapeutica de leishmaniose tegumentar Americana. O Hospital. 1961;59:31–53.
163. Crofts MAJ. Use of amphotericin B in mucocutaneous leishmaniasis. J Trop Med Hyg. 1976;79:111–3.
164. Farina R. Nose tip collapse through loss of chondro-mucous substance (repair of nasal lining). Plast Reconstr Surg. 1954;13:137–43.
165. Pitanguy I, Ribiero A. Leishmaniasis: Surgical treatment of its sequelae. Plast Reconstr Surg. 1965;30:565–72.
166. Conuit J, Rondon A, Ulrich M, et al. Immunotherapy versus chemotherapy in localized cutaneous leishmaniasis. Lancet. 1987;1:401–5.
167. Mayrink W, Antunes CMF, da Costa CA, et al. Further trails of a vaccine against American cutaneous leishmaniasis (Letter). Trans R Soc Trop Med Hyg. 1986;80:1001.

253. TRYPANOSOMA SPECIES (AMERICAN TRYPANOSOMIASIS, CHAGAS DISEASE): BIOLOGY OF TRYPANOSOMES

LOUIS V. KIRCHHOFF

The genus *Trypanosoma* consists of approximately 20 species of protozoa.[1] Two of these species are pathogenic for humans, and several cause severe and economically important diseases in domestic animals. Broadly defined, the organisms that belong to this genus are protozoan flagellates of the family Trypanosomatidae that pass through different morphologic stages (amastigote, epimastigote, and trypomastigote) in their vertebrate and invertebrate hosts.[2] However, the criterion of three morphologic stages is not fulfilled by each species in the genus. For example, only *Trypanosoma cruzi,* the etiologic agent of American trypanosomiasis, or Chagas disease, and one other species, multiply in the mammalian host as intracellular amastigotes that resemble *Leishmania* and are sometimes referred to as the *leishmanial forms*. In contrast, members of the *Trypanosoma brucei* complex, which cause African sleeping sickness in humans and nagana in animals, do not have an intracellular form and multiply as trypomastigotes that circulate in the mammalian blood stream.

Trypomastigotes are characterized by the presence of one flagellum originating from the kinetoplast, which is an extranuclear and terminally located, DNA-containing giant mitochondrion. The flagellum runs alongside the body of the parasite and is enveloped in an undulating membrane. It extends beyond the body in the form of a free, threadlike structure. The undulating membrane and the free portion of the flagellum confer considerable motility on the organism.

According to the course of their development in the vector, trypanosomes have been classified into two major groups[3]:

1. *Stercoraria:* Multiplication in the mammalian host is discontinuous, typically taking place in the amastigote stage. Development in the vector (Reduviidae, or kissing bug) is completed in the hindgut (posterior station), and contaminative transmission to the vertebrate host takes place. The subgenus *Schizotrypanum* belongs to this group and includes *T. cruzi.*
2. *Salivaria:* Multiplication in the mammalian host is continuous, taking place in the trypomastigote stage. Development in the vector (*Glossina,* or tsetse fly) is completed in the salivary glands (anterior station), and inoculative transmission to the mammalian host occurs. The subgenus *Trypanozoon* belongs to this group and includes, among others, *T. brucei brucei,* which causes disease in animals but is not infective for humans. *Trypanosoma brucei gambiense* and *T. brucei rhodesiense,* the two etiologic agents of African sleeping sickness, or human African trypanosomiasis, are also found in this subgenus. As a group, these three organisms are often referred to as the *T. brucei complex*.

Endemic areas of Chagas disease and African sleeping sickness do not overlap (Fig. 1). Moreover, there are such important differences in the transmission, pathogenesis, and clinical course of the two diseases that they have little in common except the morphologic similarities of the causative agents.

CHAGAS DISEASE

Life Cycle and Transmission

Trypanosoma cruzi, the etiologic agent of American trypanosomiasis, is transmitted by various species of hematophagous triatomine insects, or reduviid bugs[4] (Fig. 2). These vectors are found in large numbers in the wild, where the parasite is transmitted among many mammalian species that constitute the natural reservoir, and in endemic areas they live in the nooks and crannies of substandard dwellings. The insects become infected by sucking blood from animals or humans that have circulating trypomastigotes (Fig. 3). The ingested parasites multiply in the midgut of the insects as epimastigotes, which are flagellates of a distinct morphologic type, and in the hindgut transform into infective metacyclic trypomastigotes that are discharged with the feces at the time of subsequent blood meals. Transmission to a second vertebrate host occurs when mucous membranes, conjunctivas, or breaks in the skin are contaminated with bug feces containing the infective forms. The parasites then enter a variety of host cell types and multiply in the cytoplasm after transformation into amastigotes. When multiplying amastigotes fill the host cell, they differentiate into trypomastigotes, and the cell ruptures. The parasites released invade local tissues or spread hematogenously to distant sites, thus initiating further cycles of multiplication, primarily in muscle cells, and maintaining a parasitemia infective for vectors.

Transmission of *T. cruzi* also occurs through blood transfusion[5,6] and typically takes place in cities when infected but asymptomatic migrants from endemic rural areas donate blood. This mode of transmission constitutes a serious public health problem in several endemic countries. Congenital transmission has been reported as well and is associated with a high fatality rate and severe impairment in surviving infants.[7,8] Finally, numerous laboratory accidents resulting in acute Chagas disease have occurred as a consequence of the facility with which infective forms of the parasite can be produced in the laboratory.[9,10]

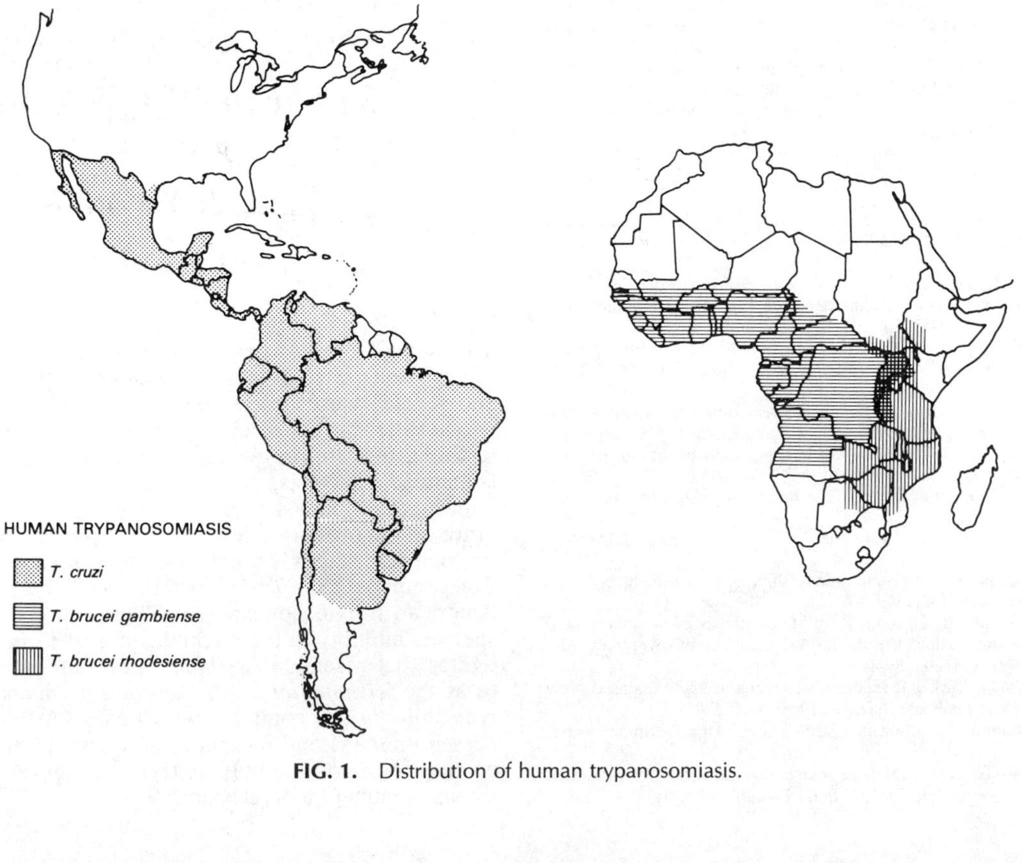

FIG. 1. Distribution of human trypanosomiasis.

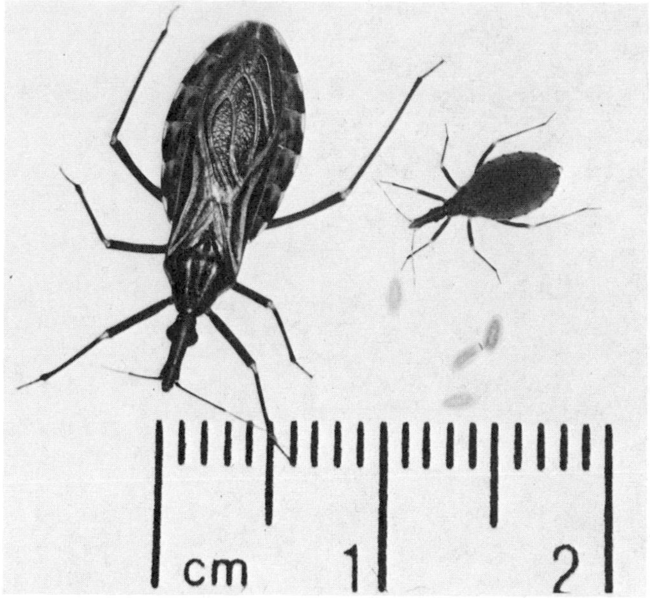

FIG. 2. *Rhodnius prolixus,* a common vector of *T. cruzi.* Eggs, second stage nymph, and adult.

Pathology

In acute Chagas disease, the lesion caused by *T. cruzi* at the site of entry is called a *chagoma* and consists of a local inflammatory response.[11,12] Local histologic changes include intracellular parasitism of muscle and other subcutaneous tissues, interstitial edema, lymphocytic infiltration, and reactive hyperplasia of adjacent lymph nodes. The characteristic pseudocysts seen in sections of infected tissues are intracellular aggregates of amastigotes (Fig. 4). The trypomastigotes that are released when the host cells rupture are readily detected in peripheral blood during the acute phase. Muscles, including the myocardium, are the most heavily parasitized tissues. Myocarditis may develop in association with patchy areas of infected cells and necrosis. A peripheral lymphocytosis accompanies the high parasitemias of the acute illness, and mild elevation of transaminase levels is occasionally seen. In some patients, parasites may be found in the cerebrospinal fluid.[13]

The heart is the organ most commonly affected in chronic Chagas disease. Gross examination of the hearts of chronic chagasic patients who died of intractable heart failure reveals marked bilateral ventricular enlargement, often involving the right side more than the left. Thinning of the ventricular walls is common, as are apical aneurysms and mural thrombi. Widespread lymphocytic infiltration is present, accompanied by diffuse interstitial fibrosis and atrophy of myocardial cells. However, parasites are rarely seen in stained sections of myocardial tissue. The coronary arteries, for the most part, are spared.

Pathologic changes are also common in the conduction system of chronic chagasic hearts and often correlate with premortem rhythm disturbances.[14] Dense fibrosis and chronic inflammatory lesions most frequently involve the right branch and the left anterior branch of the bundle of His, but lesions of this type are found in other parts of the conduction system as well.

The striking features apparent on gross examination of the esophagus or colon of a patient with chronic Chagas disease of the digestive tract (megadisease) are the enormous dilation and muscular hypertrophy of the affected organ. On microscopic examination focal inflammatory lesions with lymphocytic infiltration are seen. A marked reduction in the number of neurons in the myenteric plexus is also apparent, and peri- and intraganglion fibrosis in the presence of Schwann cell proliferation and lymphocytosis is found. In most patients this parasympathetic denervation is confined to the esophagus and/or the colon, but similar lesions have been observed in the biliary tree, the ureters, and other hollow viscera.

The pathogenesis of the cardiac and gastrointestinal lesions of chronic Chagas disease is poorly understood.[15] This subject has been the focus of considerable controversy for several decades, and at present there are basically two schools of thought. Köberle[16] has suggested that the neuronal damage that occurs during acute Chagas disease constitutes the fundamental pathogenic insult that, years later, results in the lesions of the chronic phase. Under this hypothesis, one might expect earlier and more severe symptoms of chronic disease among patients who had comparatively high parasitemias and fulminant courses during the acute phase. To date no studies have been done to establish if this does in fact occur. A second mechanism, pro-

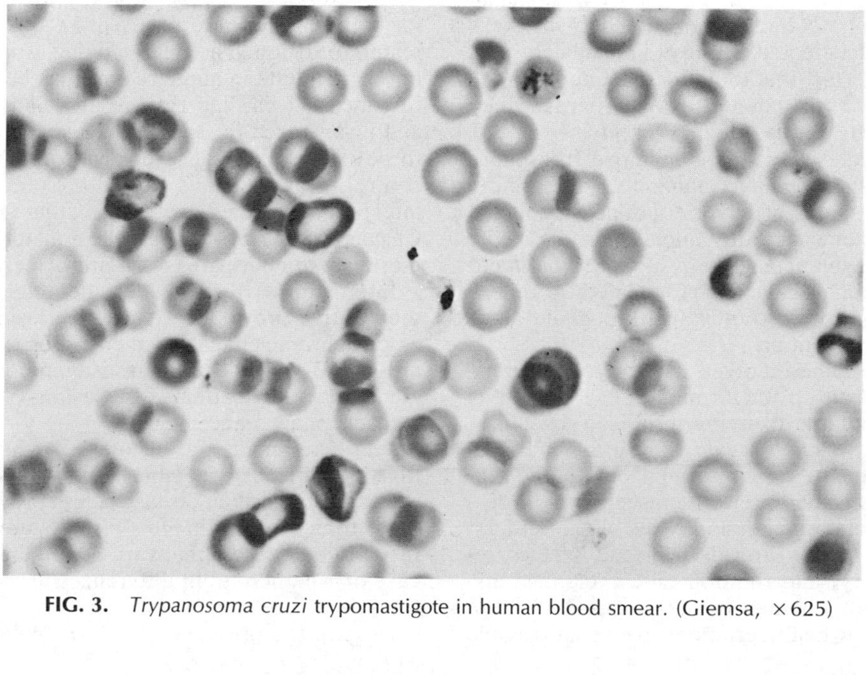

FIG. 3. *Trypanosoma cruzi* trypomastigote in human blood smear. (Giemsa, ×625)

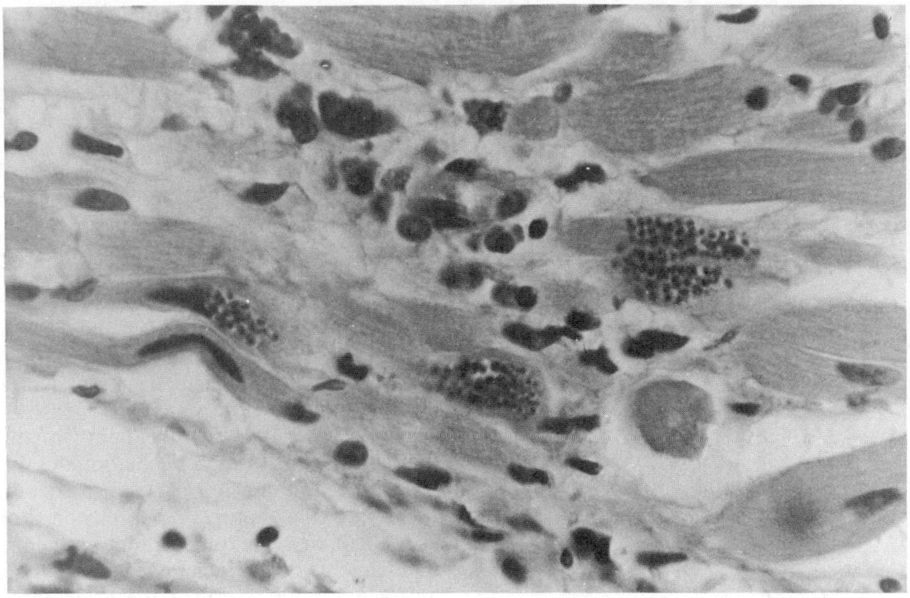

FIG. 4. *Trypanosoma cruzi* pseudocysts of amastigotes in cardiac muscle of a patient with acute Chagas disease. (H&E, ×1560)

posed by Cossio et al.[17] and Santos-Buch and Teixeira,[18] invokes autoimmune mechanisms in the pathogenesis of the lesions of chronic disease. Experimental work done subsequent to these latter studies has failed to resolve the issue[19,20]; thus, the pathogenesis of the lesions of chronic Chagas disease continues to be the subject of debate.[21,22]

Epidemiology

Trypanosoma cruzi infection is a zoonosis, and humans are merely unfortunate hosts whose involvement in the cycle of transmission is not necessary for the perpetuation of the parasite in nature. The reduviid vectors necessary for natural transmission of *T. cruzi* are found in the Americas from the southern half of the United States to southern Argentina.[23,24] Although infected insects have been found throughout this range, their distribution is very uneven. Burrows, hollow trees, palm trees, and other animal shelters are sites where transmission of *T. cruzi* occurs among infected insects and nonhuman mammalian hosts. Vector transmission to humans occurs only in areas where reduviid species that defecate during or immediately after a blood meal are present. This limitation does not apply to the range of the infection in lower mammals, however, because they can acquire the infection by eating infected insects.[25]

Trypanosoma cruzi isolates have been obtained from more than 150 species of wild and domestic mammals.[26] The ability of the parasite to adapt to such a wide variety of hosts, coupled with the long-term parasitemias in the animals, results in the presence of an enormous sylvatic and domestic reservoir in enzootic areas. Infected mammals have been found in the southern United States[27,28] and from there southward throughout all of Latin America to central Argentina.

Historically, humans become involved in the cycle of transmission when land is opened up for farming in enzootic areas where vector species adaptable to living in human dwellings, such as *Rhodnius prolixus, Panstrongylus megistus,* and *Triatoma infestans,* are prevalent. As the natural habitat of the vectors and mammalian hosts is disrupted, the insects take up residence in the thatched roofs, cracks, and holes of the settlers' primitive wood and mud houses. In this way, the infected reduviids become domiciliary, and the domestic cycle of transmission is established. Thus, human trypanosomiasis in Latin America is primarily a public health problem among poor people who live in rural areas. The incidence of new infections is not known because the vast majority go undiagnosed. The mean age of infection in areas of intense transmission is thought to be around 4 years, and in one survey 85 percent of acute cases occurred in children younger than 10 years old.[29] In this study of selected patients, the case fatality rate for acute Chagas disease was 12 percent, but the rate for all new infections is probably less than 1 percent.

Numerous epidemiologic studies of the prevalence of *T. cruzi* infection have been carried out. Currently, it is estimated that 10–12 million people are infected with the parasite, more than half of whom live in Brazil.[30,31] A nationwide study there of more than 1.5 million people from rural areas showed that approximately 10 percent had serologic evidence of infection.[32] Although few prospective data are available, it is generally thought that the majority of seropositive individuals will never develop symptomatic chronic Chagas disease.[33] The mean age of onset of the cardiac and gastrointestinal symptoms of chronic Chagas disease is 35–45 years. However, the age distribution for both types of chronic disease is quite broad and varies from region to region. The relatively high frequency of sudden death in young adults in some regions has been attributed to the disturbances of cardiac rhythm associated with Chagas disease, and in one area in Brazil, chagasic cardiac disease was found to be the leading cause of death in adults.[34] Although vector control measures have altered the prevalence rates of *T. cruzi* infection in selected areas,[31,35,36] there is no doubt that chronic Chagas disease continues to be a major cause of morbidity and mortality in many areas of Latin America.[37]

Interestingly, there is considerable geographic variation in the relative prevalence of cardiac lesions versus megadisease among chronic chagasic patients. For example, in most endemic areas of Brazil, megadisease is common, as is cardiac involvement, and many patients have lesions of both types. In contrast, megaesophagus and megacolon are virtually unknown in Venezuela, Colombia, and Panama. Furthermore, among seropositive individuals in endemic areas of Central America and southern Mexico, cardiac disease is less prevalent than in Brazil and tends to occur later in life. It is not known whether host factors result in this geographic variation in the patterns of clinical disease or whether strain differences in the infecting parasites are the primary determinants.[38]

Despite the presence of *T. cruzi*-infected reduviids in many parts of the southern and western United States, only three autochthonous cases of Chagas disease have been reported: two in Texas and one relatively recent case in California.[39] The rarity of transmission of *T. cruzi* to humans in the United States probably results from the lack of contact between people and infected vectors. Although reduviid bites and associated allergic reactions have been reported,[40] our relatively high housing standards and separate quartering of farm animals discourage the establishment of the domestic cycle of transmission that may result in human infection. In the last 18 years, six confirmed laboratory-acquired infections and nine imported cases of acute Chagas disease have been reported to the Centers for Disease Control (personal communication, D. Juranek). Although the number of autochthonous and imported cases of acute *T. cruzi* infection that go unrecognized may be several times the number reported, the fact remains that acute Chagas disease is rare in the United States.

Since the mid-1970s, enormous numbers of individuals have emigrated to the United States from Central America, a region in which the prevalence of *T. cruzi* infection is quite high.[41] The presence of *T. cruzi* infection in a sizable proportion of these immigrants was established in a recent investigation carried out in the Washington, D.C., area, in which 5 percent of 205 Salvadoran and Nicaraguan immigrants studied were found to be infected.[42] Thus, the epidemiology of chronic *T. cruzi* infection in the United States has been changed markedly by the arrival of these infected immigrants, whose number can be conservatively estimated to be upward of 50,000.

The presence of such a large group of individuals with chronic *T. cruzi* infections raises a number of important public health issues in the United States and in the other industrialized countries to which significant numbers of Central Americans have emigrated. The first of these is the risk of transmission of the parasite by blood transfusion. In a recent prospective study performed in a large blood bank in Los Angeles, 1 of 1022 units examined was found to have been donated by an individual infected with *T. cruzi*.[43] In addition, two instances of transmission of *T. cruzi* by blood transfusion have occurred recently in the United States. In one of these, a bone marrow transplant recipient developed acute Chagas disease and died of chagasic myocarditis after receiving a directed donation from an individual who had emigrated to the United States from an endemic area.[44] In the second instance, an immunosuppressed patient with Hodgkin's disease developed chagasic myocarditis and pericarditis after receiving blood infected with *T. cruzi* from a random donor (I. H. Grant, personal communication). The courses of acute Chagas disease in these two patients were particularly fulminant due to the immunosuppression, and this certainly contributed to the definitive diagnoses. This suggests that other cases of post-transfusion acute Chagas disease may be occurring in immunocompetent patients in whom the infection is not diagnosed because the courses are more benign.

The development of acute Chagas disease in individuals with chronic *T. cruzi* infections living here who undergo immunosuppression should be an additional matter of concern for physicians who care for this immigrant group. Numerous instances of reactivation of acute Chagas disease in *T. cruzi*-infected individuals who are iatrogenically immunosuppressed by treatment for malignancies or after receiving organ transplants have been reported,[45,46] and at least one has occurred in the United States.[47] Additional cases certainly will occur here as the *T. cruzi*-infected immigrants develop diseases that require immunosuppressive therapy. Moreover, acquired immunosuppression also carries with it a risk of reactivation of acute Chagas disease in individuals who harbor the parasite, as evidenced by the recent occurrence of a fatal *T. cruzi* brain abscess in a Salvadoran immigrant infected with the human immunodeficiency virus (D. Gluckstein, personal communication).

Clinical Course

The clinical syndromes of acute *T. cruzi* infection and chronic Chagas disease are quite different. The acute illness results from the first encounter of the host with the parasite, and chronic disease involves late sequelae.

Acute Chagas disease[48] is usually an illness of children, but it can occur at any age. Only a small portion of acute infections caused by *T. cruzi* are recognized as such, due to the mild and nonspecific nature of the symptoms in most patients and to a lack of access to medical care. The first signs of illness occur at least 1 week after invasion by the parasites, but in most cases the incubation period cannot be determined. When the parasite has entered through a break in the skin, a chagoma may be formed, consisting of an indurated area of erythema and swelling accompanied by local lymph node involvement. Romaña's sign (Fig. 5), the classic sign of acute Chagas disease, consists of painless edema of the palpebrae and periocular tissues and may appear when the conjunctiva is the portal of entry. These initial local signs are followed by fever, malaise, anorexia, and edema of the face and lower extremities. Generalized lymphadenopathy and mild hepatosplenomegaly also may appear.

Overt central nervous system signs are not common, but meningoencephalitis develops in some patients and is associated with a very poor prognosis. Severe myocarditis also develops in a small proportion of acute patients, and most deaths are due to the resultant congestive heart failure. Nonspecific electrocardiographic (ECG) changes are seen, but the life-threatening arrhythmias that are frequent in chronic Chagas disease generally do not occur. In untreated patients, symptoms resolve gradually over a period of weeks to months. Areas of local reaction around the eye or other sites of parasite entry can persist for several weeks, as can the lymphadenopathy and splenomegaly. After the spontaneous resolution of the acute illness, the patient enters what is called the *indeterminate phase* of

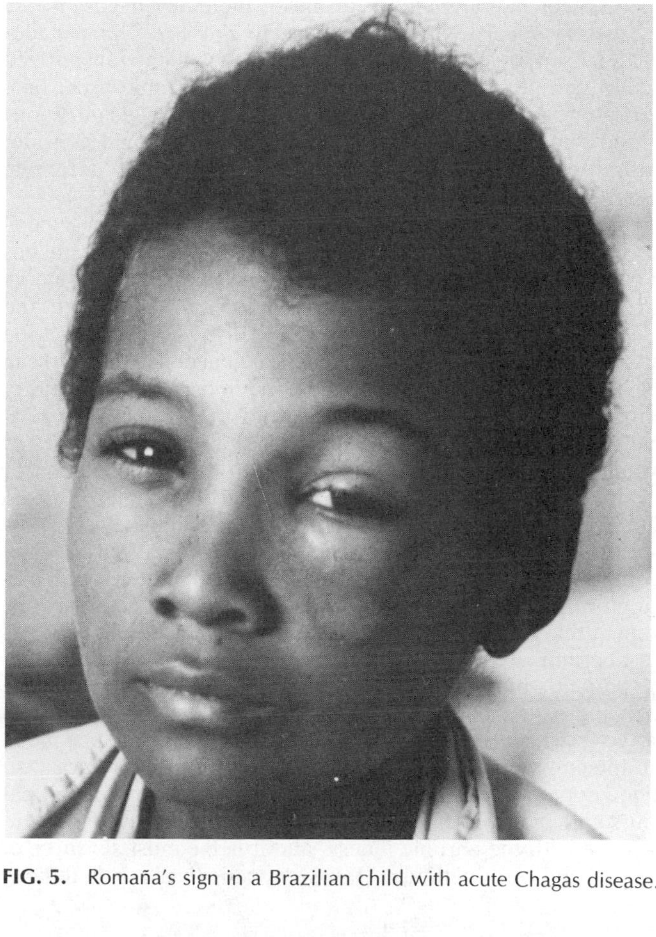

FIG. 5. Romaña's sign in a Brazilian child with acute Chagas disease.

Chagas disease, which is characterized by asymptomatic and subpatent parasitemia and antibodies to a variety of *T. cruzi* antigens.

Chronic Chagas disease becomes apparent years or even decades after the initial infection.[49] The heart is the organ most commonly involved, and symptoms reflect the rhythm disturbances, congestive failure, and thromboembolism that are characteristic of the chronic illness.[50] Dizziness, syncope, and, less commonly, seizures result from a wide variety of arrhythmias. The cardiomyopathy that develops often primarily affects the right ventricle, and the classic signs of right heart failure are frequently present. As in patients with arrhythmias, the progression of symptoms related to the cardiomyopathy may be gradual, but once congestive failure develops, death often occurs in a matter of months. Although some patients have both cardiomyopathy and arrhythmias, most do not.[34] The clinical course is frequently complicated by emboli to the brain or other areas.

In patients with megaesophagus, symptoms are similar to those of idiopathic achalasia and may include dysphagia, odynophagia, chest pain, cough, and regurgitation. Hypersalivation and salivary gland hypertrophy have been observed. Aspiration can occur, especially during sleep, and repeated episodes of aspiration pneumonitis are common. Weight loss and even cachexia in patients with megaesophagus can combine with pulmonary infection to result in death. As in idiopathic achalasia, an increased incidence of cancer of the esophagus has been reported in patients with chagasic esophageal disease.[51]

Patients with chagasic megacolon are plagued by chronic constipation and abdominal pain. Individuals with advanced disease can go for several weeks between bowel movements, and acute obstruction, occasionally with volvulus, can lead to perforation, septicemia, and death.

Diagnosis

The first consideration in the diagnosis of acute Chagas disease is a history consistent with exposure to *T. cruzi*. This includes residence or travel in an environment in which transmission occurs, a recent blood transfusion in an endemic area, or a laboratory accident. The frequency of autochthonous infections in the United States is so low that clinicians should consider naturally acquired acute Chagas disease only as a remote possibility.

The simplest way to make the diagnosis of acute Chagas disease is by direct microscopic examination for motile parasites of fresh anticoagulated blood or of the buffy coat. An alternative but less sensitive method is examination of stained thin and thick blood smears. Concentration of blood by centrifugation after red cell lysis using NH_4Cl (0.083% final concentration) can also be done. The advantage of these methods lies in the rapidity with which they can be performed, but they detect only relatively large numbers of parasites. When repeated attempts to visualize the parasites are unsuccessful, mouse inoculation or culture of the patient's blood on NNN or other suitable media should be tried. These latter techniques are almost always positive in cases of acute Chagas disease, but 7–14 days are usually required before the parasites can be detected in the growth medium or mouse blood. If available, xenodiagnosis might also be done at this point. This technique is carried out by allowing 10–30 laboratory-reared and uninfected reduviid bugs to feed on the patient's blood, either directly or through a thin membrane covering a vial containing blood anticoagulated with preservative-free heparin. Approximately 30 days after the blood meal, the intestinal contents of the bugs are examined for parasites. When done properly, this method is positive in virtually all patients with acute disease as well as in approximately 50 percent of those with the chronic illness, and it is the most sensitive of the parasitologic methods. However, xenodiagnosis is tedious and time-consuming, and the delay involved before the diagnosis can be made is a major disadvantage.

In the diagnosis of acute Chagas disease, serologic testing is of limited usefulness. Immunofluorescence and direct agglutination assays are relatively rapid tests that can detect anti-*T. cruzi* IgM, but seroconversion usually does not occur until 20–40 days after the onset of symptoms.[52]

If chronic Chagas disease is suspected, the first step in making the diagnosis involves determining if antibodies to *T. cruzi* are present. Serologic testing is the method of choice for establishing that an individual is infected and is at risk for developing the symptoms associated with chronic *T. cruzi* infection. Demonstration of the organism is not of primary importance. A number of highly sensitive serologic tests for the detection of anti-*T. cruzi* antibodies are available, such as indirect hemagglutination, complement fixation, immunofluorescence assays, and the enzyme-linked immunosorbent assay (ELISA).[30,53,54] However, a persistent problem with these conventional assays has been the occurrence of false-positive reactions, typically with serum samples from patients with other diseases such as leishmaniasis and syphilis. For this reason, it is generally recommended that three conventional serologic assays be performed on each specimen and that well-characterized positive and negative controls be included in each run. Recently, the use of a highly sensitive and specific procedure for the detection of anti-*T. cruzi* antibodies that employs immunoprecipitation and gel electrophoresis of radiolabeled *T. cruzi* antigens has been described.[55] This assay effectively deals with the problem of false-positive reactions and is available as a confirmatory test in the author's laboratory, but it has not yet been adapted for mass screening.

In a patient who is seropositive for *T. cruzi*, a history of palpitations, dizziness, syncope, or even seizures suggests cerebral hypoperfusion resulting from the rhythm disturbances common in chronic Chagas disease. Right bundle branch block is by far the most common ECG abnormality, but varying degrees of atrioventricular block, left bundle branch block, and premature ventricular contractions, as well as tachyarrhythmias and bradyarrhythmias, are frequently seen.[56] Dyspnea due to arrhythmias or congestive failure may also be a presenting symptom. In the latter case, a chest roentgenogram often shows cardiomegaly, and echocardiography may reveal the chamber enlargement, decreased ventricular wall thickness, apical aneurysm, or reduced ejection fraction that characterize advanced cardiomyopathy.

In seropositive patients who have symptoms of achalasia, radiographic contrast studies using fluoroscopy may demonstrate delayed emptying of the esophagus and, in more advanced cases, varying degrees of esophageal dilation. Endoscopy should also be performed to rule out esophageal cancer and other causes of esophageal dysfunction. Manometry may also be useful in assessing the loss of relaxation of the esophageal sphincter. In general, the symptoms and diagnostic findings in patients with chagasic esophageal disease are indistinguishable from those of idiopathic achalasia.[57]

The diagnosis of chagasic megacolon is suggested by complaints of chronic constipation and abdominal pain, and in patients with advanced disease the colon may be palpable. An air-contrast barium enema is the most effective approach to delineating anatomic changes and functional abnormalities in the colon.

Treatment

Unfortunately, *T. cruzi* is not susceptible to most of the long list of drugs tested for activity over the past several decades, including those effective against African trypanosomes, and thus current therapy is unsatisfactory. There is no drug suitable for general treatment of chagasic patients, although two drugs are being used on an individual basis.[58,59] The first of these, the nitrofuran derivative nifurtimox (Lampit, Bayer 2502), has been in use for two decades, and extensive clinical experience has accumulated. It is the only drug available in the United States for the therapy of Chagas disease. Its precise mechanism of action is not known. In acute Chagas disease, nifurtimox markedly reduces the duration of symptoms and decreases mortality. Likewise, the level and duration of parasitemia are reduced. Despite this efficacy in the treatment of the acute illness, however, nifurtimox achieves a parasitologic cure in only a minority of cases, as indicated by positive xenodiagnoses in many treated patients who are followed for long periods.[60] Geographic variation in the effectiveness of nifurtimox in acute Chagas disease has been observed. Treatment has been found to be most effective in Argentina and Chile, whereas therapy in most of Brazil and in some other countries has been less successful. Therapy with nifurtimox should be initiated as early as possible in cases of acute Chagas disease. Moreover, when laboratory accidents occur in which there is a reasonable likelihood that *T. cruzi* infection will become established, therapy should be initiated without waiting for clinical or parasitologic indications of infection.[9]

The usefulness of nifurtimox in patients with indeterminate phase and chronic Chagas disease has not been established, and post-treatment xenodiagnoses are positive in a large proportion of chronically infected patients given nifurtimox. There is no evidence that patients in the indeterminate phase are less likely to develop symptomatic disease after treatment with the drug; likewise, it has not been shown that it has any effect on symptomatic chronic disease. Thus, there is no indication for treating individuals with chronic *T. cruzi* infections with nifurtimox.

The majority of patients treated with nifurtimox experience adverse side effects. Gastrointestinal complaints include abdominal pain, nausea, vomiting, anorexia, and weight loss. Neurologic symptoms include restlessness, disorientation, insomnia, twitching, paresthesias, polyneuritis, and seizures. These symptoms generally disappear when the dosage is reduced or therapy is discontinued. Nifurtimox is supplied as 30- and 120-mg tablets. The recommended oral dosage for adults is 8–10 mg/kg body weight per day. The dose for adolescents is 12.5–15 mg/kg per day, and for children 1–10 years of age it is 15–20 mg/kg per day. The drug should be given in four divided doses each day, and therapy should be continued for 90–120 days. Nifurtimox can be obtained from the Drug Service of the Centers for Disease Control, Atlanta, Georgia.

Benznidazole (benzonidazole, Radamil, Roche 7-1051), a nitroimidazol derivative, is the second agent that has undergone trials in patients with Chagas disease. The efficacy of this drug is similar to that of nifurtimox in that it is effective in the treatment of acute Chagas disease, but it also has a limited capacity to effect parasitologic cures in patients with acute *T. cruzi* infections, as well as those with chronic Chagas disease. Side effects include peripheral neuropathy, rash, and granulocytopenia. The recommended oral dosage of benznidazole is 5 mg/kg/day for 60 days. Benznidazole is used widely in Latin America, and although it is not presently available in the United States, physicians should be aware of it as an alternative agent for patients who tolerate nifurtimox poorly.

Most patients with acute Chagas disease require no therapy other than nifurtimox, as symptoms are generally self-limited even in the absence of drug treatment. The management of the occasional severely ill acute-phase patient with myocarditis or meningoencephalitis is largely supportive. The treatment of patients with chronic chagasic heart disease is also supportive. Chronically infected individuals should have ECGs done periodically, since pacemakers have been shown to be useful in the management of bradyarrhythmias of chronic Chagas disease.[61] The congestive heart failure of cardiomyopathic Chagas disease is generally treated with measures used in patients with cardiomyopathies due to other causes.

Symptoms associated with the megasyndrome of Chagas disease can usually be managed successfully.[62] The symptoms of megaesophagus, in all but the most severe cases, can be relieved with some success by dietary measures or pneumatic dilation of the esophagogastric junction. A variety of surgical approaches have been tried in patients with advanced disease who do not respond to conservative therapy. Myotomies at the level of the esophageal sphincter, or partial esophageal resections with interposition of a loop of bowel, frequently relieve the symptoms of achalasia, but patients are often plagued by severe reflux esophagitis postoperatively.

Chagasic megacolon in its early stages usually responds to a high-fiber diet, laxatives, and occasional enemas. Patients who no longer respond to these measures develop fecal impaction or, less commonly, colonic volvulus, and require surgery. Various surgical procedures have been used, the most successful of which is a partial resection involving the rectosigmoid and descending colon.

Prevention

Since infection with *T. cruzi* has the potential for causing serious illness in both the acute and chronic phases, and since drug therapy is unsatisfactory, emphasis should be placed on measures to prevent transmission. Programs in some areas involving spraying of households with insecticide have resulted in effective control of vector populations and have broken the domestic cycle of transmission. At present, large-scale application of vector control, along with improvement in housing in the rural areas of endemic regions, appear to offer the best hope for control of Chagas disease. However, their implementation depends on the vagaries of local politics and economic development, and decades may pass before overall control is achieved by this approach. At present, no vaccines are available for the prevention of *T. cruzi* transmission.[63]

In endemic areas, expansion and improvement of programs for screening donated blood for the presence of *T. cruzi* are necessary to reduce transmission by transfusion, which continues to be a major public health problem in many areas of Latin America. Treatment of blood to be transfused with gentian violet effectively inactivates the parasites, but a faster-acting and less colorful agent needs to be developed. In the United States, immigrants from endemic regions should not be allowed to donate blood. The current lack of a commercially available serologic assay to detect *T. cruzi* infection that is rapid, as well as highly sensitive and specific, makes such a policy of donor deferral the best approach at present. Moreover, in view of the possible serious consequences of chronic *T. cruzi* infection, all immigrants from endemic regions should be screened for serologic evidence of infection with the parasite. Identification of infected individuals in this group is important not only to prevent transmission by blood transfusion but also so that physicians who care for these patients become aware of the presence of *T. cruzi* and undertake appropriate diagnostic monitoring and supportive therapy when indicated.

Laboratory personnel should wear gloves and eye protection when working with *T. cruzi*, and suitable containment should be used when dealing with infected insects.[64] Persons traveling in endemic areas should avoid sleeping in dilapidated adobe and wood houses or in dwellings with thatched roofs, since transmission of *T. cruzi* to visitors occasionally occurs under such circumstances.[65] Special precautions for campers, hunters, and others engaging in outdoor activities in the United States are not warranted.

REFERENCES

1. Levine ND, Corliss JO, Cox FEG, et al. A newly revised classification of protozoa. J Protozool. 1980;27:37–58.
2. Hoare CA. The classification of trypanosomes of veterinary and medical importance. Vet Reviews Annotations. 1957;3:1–13.

3. Hoare CA. The Trypanosomes of Mammals: A Zoological Monograph. Oxford: Blackwell; 1972.
4. Brener Z. Biology of *Trypanosoma cruzi.* Ann Rev Microbiol. 1973;27:347–82.
5. Schmuñis GA. Chagas' disease and blood transfusion. In: Dodd RY, Barker LF, eds. Infection, Immunity and Blood Transfusion. New York: Alan R. Liss; 1984:127–45.
6. Bergoglio RM. Enfermedad de Chagas post-transfusional. Experiencia clinica de 48 casos. Prensa Med Argentina. 1984;71:49–52.
7. Bettencourt AL. Congenital Chagas' disease. Am J Dis Child. 1976;130:97–103.
8. Azogue E, La Fuente C, Darras CH. Congenital Chagas' disease in Bolivia: Epidemiological aspects and pathological findings. Trans R Soc Trop Med Hyg. 1985;79:176–80.
9. Brener Z. Laboratory-acquired Chagas' disease: An endemic disease among parasitologists. In: Morel C, ed. Genes and Antigens of Parasites. 2nd ed. Rio de Janeiro: Fundação Oswaldo Cruz; 1984:3–9.
10. Hofflin JM, Sadler RH, Araujo FG, et al. Laboratory-acquired Chagas' disease. Trans R Soc Trop Med Hyg. 1987;81:437–40.
11. Santos-Buch CA. American trypanosomiasis: Chagas' disease. Int Rev Exp Pathol. 1979;19:63–100.
12. Andrade ZA, Andrade SG. Patologia. In: Brener Z, Andrade ZA, eds. *Trypanosoma cruzi* e Doença de Chagas. Rio de Janeiro: Guanabara Koogan; 1979:199–248.
13. Hoff R, Teixeira RS, Carvalho JS, et al. *Trypanosoma cruzi* in the cerebrospinal fluid during the acute stage of Chagas' disease. N Engl J Med. 1978;298:604–6.
14. Andrade ZA, Andrade SG, Oliveira GB, et al. Histopathology of the conducting tissue of the heart in Chagas' myocarditis. Am Heart J. 1978;95:316–24.
15. Andrade ZA. Patogenia da doença de Chagas. Novos aspectos. Arq Bras Cardiol. 1982;38:255–60.
16. Köberle F. Pathogenesis of Chagas' disease. In: Trypanosomiasis and Leishmaniasis with Special Reference to Chagas' Disease. Ciba Foundation Symposium 20 (new series). New York: North-Holland: Elsevier; 1974:137–58.
17. Cossio PM, Diez C, Szarfman A, et al. Chagasic cardiopathy—demonstration of a serum gamma globulin factor which reacts with endocardium and vascular structures. Circulation. 1974;49:13–21.
18. Santos-Buch CA, Teixeira ARL. The immunology of experimental Chagas' disease. III. Rejection of allogeneic heart cells in vitro. J Exp Med. 1974;140:38–53.
19. Khoury EL, Diez C, Cossio PM, et al. Heterophil nature of EVI antibody in *Trypanosoma cruzi* infection. Clin Immunol Immunopathol. 1983;27:283–8.
20. Wood JN, Hudson L, Jessell TM, et al. A monoclonal antibody defining antigenic determinants on subpopulations of mammalian neurones and *Trypanosoma cruzi* parasites. Nature. 1982;296:34–8.
21. Kierszenbaum F. Is there autoimmunity in Chagas' disease? Parasitol Today. 1985;1:4–6.
22. Hudson L. Autoimmune phenomena in chronic chagasic cardiopathy. Parasitol Today. 1985;1:6–9.
23. Brenner RR, de la Merced A, ed. Chagas' Disease Vectors. Boca Raton, Fla.: CRC Press; 1987.
24. Beard CB, Young DG, Butler JF, et al. First isolation of *Trypanosoma cruzi* from a wild caught *Triatoma sanguisuga* (LeConte) (Hemiptera:Triatomae) in Florida, U.S.A. J Parasitol. 1988;74:343–4.
25. Ryckman RE, Olsen LE. Epizootiology of *Trypanosoma cruzi* in Southwestern North America. Part VI. Insectivorous hosts of Triatominae—the perizootiological relationship to *Trypanosoma cruzi*. J Med Entomol. 1965;2:99–106.
26. Goble FC. South American trypanosomes. In: Jackson GJ, Herman R, Singer I, eds. Immunity to Parasitic Diseases in Animals. New York: Appleton-Century-Crofts; 1970:597–689.
27. Kagan IG, Norman L, Allain D. Studies on *Trypanosoma cruzi* isolated in the United States: A review. Rev Biol Trop. 1966;14:55–73.
28. Yaeger RG. The prevalence of *Trypanosoma cruzi* infection in armadillos collected at a site near New Orleans, Louisiana. Am J Trop Med Hyg. 1988;38:323–6.
29. Laranja FS, Dias E, Nobrega G, et al. Chagas' disease—a clinical, epidemiologic, and pathologic study. Circulation. 1956;14:1035–60.
30. Brener Z. Recent developments in the field of Chagas' disease. Bull WHO. 1982;60:463–73.
31. Dias JCP. Control of Chagas' disease in Brazil. Parasitol Today. 1987;3:336–41.
32. Camargo ME, da Silva GR, de Castillo EA, et al. Inquérito sorológico da prevalência da infecção chagásica no Brasil 1975/1980. Rev Inst Med Trop Sao Paulo. 1984;26:192–204.
33. Macedo V. Forma indeterminada da doença de Chagas. J Bras Med. 1980;38:34–40.
34. Amorim D de S. Chagas' disease. Prog Cardiol. 1979;8:235–79.
35. Goldsmith RS, Zarate RJ, Zarate LG, et al. Clinical and epidemiologic studies of Chagas' disease in rural communities in Oaxaca State, and a seven-year follow-up: I. Cerro del Aire. Bull Pan Am Health Organ. 1985;19:120–38.
36. Acquatella H, Catalioti F, Gomez-Mancebo JR, et al. Long-term control of Chagas' disease in Venezuela: Effects on serologic findings, electrocardiographic abnormalities, and clinical outcome. Circulation. 1987;76:556–62.
37. Maguire JH, Hoff R, Sherlock I, et al. Cardiac morbidity and mortality due to Chagas' disease: Prospective electrocardiographic study of a Brazilian community. Circulation. 1987;75:1139–45.
38. Tibayrenc M, Ward P, Moya A, et al. Natural populations of *Trypanosoma cruzi*, the agent of Chagas' disease, have a complex multi-clonal structure. Proc Natl Acad Sci USA. 1986;83:115–9.
39. Schiffler RJ, Mansur GP, Navin TR. Indigenous Chagas' disease (American trypanosomiasis) in California. JAMA. 1984;251:2983–4.
40. Lynch PJ, Pinnas JL. "Kissing bug" bites—*Triatoma* species as an important cause of insect bites in the southwest. Cutis. 1978;22:585–91.
41. Cedillos RA. Chagas' disease in El Salvador. PAHO Bull. 1975;9:135–41.
42. Kirchhoff LV, Gam AA, Gilliam FC. American trypanosomiasis (Chagas' disease) in Central American immigrants. Am J Med. 1987;82:915–20.
43. Kerndt PR, Waskin H, Kirchhoff LV, et al. Prevalence of antibody to *Trypanosoma cruzi* among blood donors in Los Angeles, California. In preparation.
44. Geiseler PJ, Ito JI, Kerndt PR, et al. Fulminant Chagas' disease (CD) in bone marrow transplantation (BMT). Abstracts of the 1987 Interscience Conference on Antimicrobial Agents and Chemotherapy. Washington DC: 169.
45. Barousse AP, Costa JA, Eposto M, et al. Enfermedad de Chagas y inmunosupresión. Medicina (Buenos Aires). 1980;40 (Suppl 1):17–26.
46. Lopez-Blanco OA, Cavalli NH, Jasovich A, et al. Kidney transplantation and Chagas' disease. A two-year follow-up of a patient with parasitemia. Transplantation. 1983;36:211–3.
47. Kohl S, Pickering LK, Frankel LS, et al. Reactivation of Chagas' disease during therapy of acute lymphocytic leukemia. Cancer. 1982;50:827–8.
48. Rassi A. Clinica: Fase aguda. In: Brener Z, Andrade ZA, eds. Trypanosoma Cruzi e Doença de Chagas. Rio de Janeiro: Guanabara Koogan; 1979:247–64.
49. Kirchhoff LV, Neva FA. Chagas' disease in Latin American immigrants. JAMA. 1985;254:3058–60.
50. Cançado JR, Chuster M. Cardiopatia Chagásica. Belo Horizonte, Brazil: Funcação Carlos Chagas; 1985.
51. Camara-Lopes LH. Carcinoma of the eosophagus as a complication of megaesophagus. An analysis of seven cases. Am J Dig Dis. 1961;6:742–56.
52. Schmuñis GA, Szarfman A, Coarasa L, et al. Anti-*Trypanosoma cruzi* agglutinins in acute human Chagas' disease. Am J Trop Med Hyg. 1980;29:170–8.
53. Spencer HC, Allain DS, Sulzer AJ, et al. Evaluation of the micro enzyme-linked immunosorbent assay for antibodies to *Trypanosoma cruzi*. Am J Trop Med Hyg. 1980;29:179–82.
54. Schecter M, Luquetti AO, Rezende JM, et al. Further evaluation of lectin affinity purified glycoprotein (GP90) in the enzyme linked immunosorbent assay (ELISA) for diagnosis of *Trypanosoma cruzi* infection. Trans R Soc Trop Med Hyg. 1985;79:637–40.
55. Kirchhoff LV, Gam AA, Gusmao Rd'A, et al. Increased specificity of serodiagnosis of Chagas' disease by detection of antibody to the 72 and 90 kDa glycoproteins of *Trypanosoma cruzi*. J Infect Dis. 1987;155:561–4.
56. Macedo V, Prata A, da Silva GR, et al. Prevalência de alterações eletrocardiográficas em chagásicos. (Informações preliminares sobre o inquérito eletrocardiográfico nacional). Arq Bras Cardiol. 1982;38:261–4.
57. Raizman RE, Neva FA, Eckert RJ, et al. Chagasic megaesophagus: Similarity to achalasia by manometrics, radiography and response to pneumatic dilitation. Dig Dis. 1975;20:882–8.
58. Brener Z. Present status of chemotherapy and chemoprophylaxis of human trypanosomiasis in the western hemisphere. Pharmacol Ther. 1979;7:71–90.
59. Marr JJ, Docampo R. Chemotherapy for Chagas' disease: A perspective of current therapy and considerations for future research. Rev Infect Dis. 1986;8:884–903.
60. Rassi A, Ferreira HO. Tentativa de tratamento especifico da fase aguda da doença de Chagas com nitrofuranos em esquemas de duração prolongada. Rev Soc Bras Med Trop. 1971;5:235–62.
61. Chuster M. Implante de marcapasso nas bradiarritmias chagásicas. In: Cançado JR, Chuster M, eds. Cardiopatia Chagásica. Belo Horizonte, Brazil: Funcação Carlos Chagas; 1985;289–97.
62. De Rezende JM. Clínica: Manifestações digestivas. In: Brener Z, Andrade AZ, eds. Trypanosoma cruzi e Doença de Chagas. Rio de Janeiro: Guanabara Koogan; 1979:312–62.
63. Brener Z. Why vaccines do not work in Chagas' disease. Parasitol Today. 1986;2:196–8.
64. Hudson L, Grover F, Gutteridge WE, et al. Suggested guidelines for work with live *Trypanosoma cruzi*. Trans R Soc Trop Med Hyg. 1983;77:416–9.
65. Brisseau JM, Cebron JP, Petit T, et al. Chagas' myocarditis imported into France. Lancet. 1988;1:1046.

254. AGENTS OF AFRICAN TRYPANOSOMIASIS (SLEEPING SICKNESS)

LOUIS V. KIRCHHOFF

THE PARASITES AND THEIR TRANSMISSION

The agents of African sleeping sickness are flagellated protozoan parasites that belong to the genus *Trypanosoma*, subgenus *Trypanozoon*.[1,2] A general description of the members of this genus and specific characteristics of the subgenus are presented in the introduction to the previous chapter. Three trypanosome subspecies, *T. brucei brucei, T. brucei rhodesiense*, and *T. brucei gambiense*, will be considered here. They are indistinguishable morphologically, and as a group they are often referred to as the *T. brucei complex*. *Trypanosoma b. brucei* is a parasite of wild and domestic animals that is not infectious for humans. In contrast, *T. b. rhodesiense*, which is primarily a parasite of wild game, can infect humans, and this difference in host specificity forms the basis of the distinction between the two subspecies. *Trypanosoma b. gambiense* primarily infects humans, and infections of wild and domestic animals are of limited importance. For convenience, trinomial designations will be used in this chapter rather than quadripartite names (e.g., *T. b. brucei* rather than *T.* [*T.*] *b. brucei*).

The members of the *T. brucei* complex are transmitted by various species of tsetse flies that belong to the genus *Glossina*.[3] These blood-sucking insects are found only in Africa, where their range covers millions of square kilometers of lowland rain forest and savanna. The parasites undergo a developmental cycle in the insect vectors. Tsetse flies of both sexes become infected with trypanosomes when they ingest blood from infected mammalian hosts that contains trypomastigotes, the form of the parasite that circulates in the blood stream. There are two forms of circulating trypomastigotes: long, slender organisms that are capable of dividing and short, stumpy forms thought to be nondividing parasites that are infective for the insect vectors. Once in the midgut of the tsetse flies, the short blood stream trypomastigotes transform into relatively long, slender procyclic trypomastigotes. After many cycles of multiplication, the procyclic forms migrate to the salivary glands, where they differentiate into epimastigotes and continue to multiply. A final transformation occurs as the epimastigotes become nondividing metacyclic trypomastigotes. Transmission takes place when these infective forms are inoculated during a subsequent blood meal. The cycle is completed when the injected metacyclic forms become blood stream trypomastigotes and begin to multiply in the blood or other extracellular spaces.

The capacity of the African trypanosomes to multiply in the blood stream of their mammalian hosts, where they are continually exposed to humoral defenses, constitutes a fundamental difference between the agents of sleeping sickness and *T. cruzi*, the cause of Chagas disease in the Americas. The African trypanosomes are able to evade immune destruction for long periods because they undergo antigenic variation, a process in which they periodically change the antigenic structure of the coat of glycoproteins that covers the surface of the parasite. The molecular mechanisms that control this complex process have been studied intensively in recent years.[4] When epimastigotes transform into metacyclic trypomastigotes in the salivary glands of the tsetse fly, each parasite synthesizes a surface coat made up of one of about a dozen types of antigenic glycoproteins, called *variant antigen types* (*VATs*). Presumably, this occurs as a preadaptation to the relatively hostile environment of the mammalian host into which the metacyclics must be inoculated if they are to survive. After injection into a mammalian host, the parasites express metacyclic VATs for approximately 5 days, after which they switch to expression of blood stream VATs. Over time the host sequentially mounts specific humoral responses directed against the predominantly expressed VATs. The population of parasites survives because an intrinsic rate of VAT switching provides an apparently endless supply of parasites that have surface glycoprotein coats to which the host has not been exposed previously.

Virtually all transmission of African trypanosomes to both wild and domestic animals, as well as to humans, takes place in the cyclic fashion just described. There is no evidence that these parasites can be transmitted by insects other than tsetse flies, and mechanical transmission by vectors is not important, although it may occur occasionally. Congenital transmission can occur, but in humans it is extremely rare,[5] as is transmission by blood transfusion. A small number of laboratory accidents resulting in infection with African trypanosomes have been reported.[6,7]

PATHOGENESIS AND PATHOLOGY

The pathogenesis of African sleeping sickness is very complex, and many aspects of the process are poorly understood.[8,9] The first sign of infection with African trypanosomes is the acute inflammatory lesion (trypanosomal chancre) that appears a week or so after the bite of an infected tsetse fly and resolves spontaneously over several weeks. Interstitial multiplication of the trypanosomes take place within the chancre, and there is an intense mononuclear cell reaction to the parasites, as well as edema and local tissue destruction.

After this initial local response, the infection evolves over weeks and months into a systemic hemolymphatic illness as the parasites disseminate widely through the lymphatics and the blood stream. Systemic African trypanosomiasis without central nervous system (CNS) involvement is generally referred to as *stage I disease*. The parasites first travel from the site of inoculation to regional lymph nodes, where they proliferate and cause an inflammatory response. They then move through the efferent lymphatics, eventually entering the venous system through the thoracic duct. Multiplication of the parasites continues in the blood stream, and egress of trypanosomes from vessels into interstitial spaces, where multiplication also takes place, is thought to be facilitated by increased vascular permeability.

In stage I of the illness there is widespread lymphadenopathy reflecting marked lymphocytic and histocytic proliferation, which may be followed by fibrosis. Morular cells (Mott cells) are also often present. These cells are plasmacytes with vacuolated cytoplasm and pyknotic nuclei that are thought to play a role in the production of IgM.[10] The spleen may be enlarged, with generalized cellular proliferation, congestion, and focal necrosis. As the disease evolves, an endarteritis with perivascular infiltration of both parasites and lymhocytes may develop in lymph nodes and the spleen.

The heart is frequently involved in this stage of the disease, especially with *T. b. rhodesiense* infections. A pancarditis may develop involving all layers of the heart, including the mural and valvular endocardia.[11] The conducting system may also be affected, and involvement of autonomic innervation of the heart has also been reported.[12] At the cellular level, pathologic changes include intense mononuclear infiltration consisting of lymphocytes, plasmacytes, and morular cells. As the infection progresses, myocytolysis and fibrosis may develop.

A number of hematologic manifestations accompany the development of stage I trypanosomiasis. Normocytic anemia is a regular feature in this phase of the illness and is usually accompanied by a brisk reticulocytosis. Several factors are thought to contribute to the anemia, and immune-mediated hemolysis may be an important mechanism.[10] Platelet counts are often reduced, especially in infections with *T. b. rhodesiense*,[13] and disseminated intravascular coagulation before and during therapy also has been documented.[14] A moderate degree of leukocytosis is usually present, especially in the early months of the infection, and this is accompanied by polyclonal B-cell activation.[15] High titers of immunoglobulins are a striking and constant feature of the illness. They consist primarily of polyclonal IgM that, for the most part, is not directed against specific parasite antigens. A number of other factors, including heterophile antibodies, rheumatoid factor, and anti-DNA antibodies, often are also detected. In addition, high levels of circulating antigen–antibody complexes are uniformly present, and these may play a role in the anemia, tissue damage, and increased vascular permeability that facilitate the dissemination of the parasites.[8] Erythrocyte sedimentation rates are elevated and hypocomplementemia has also been noted.

Stage II of human African trypanosomiasis involves invasion of the CNS. Parasites reach the brain and meninges via the blood stream and cause meningoencephalitis and/or meningomyelitis. In the brain they are found mainly in the frontal lobes, the pons, and the medulla, but other areas may be parasitized as well. Edema and hemorrhages may be evident on gross examination of affected areas at autopsy. Trypanosomes are present in perivascular areas, and nests of organisms can be found without apparent relation to blood vessels. The presence of parasites in the CNS is associated with infiltration of mononuclear cells that are predominantly lymphocytes, plasmacytes, and morular cells. The presence of parasites in the CNS is heralded by abnormal findings in the cerebrospinal fluid (CSF). The CSF may be under increased pressure, and total protein concentration is elevated. The cell count may also be significantly elevated, with mononuclear cells predominating in addition to small numbers of morular cells and eosinophils. Trypanosomes are frequently present in the CSF as well.

EPIDEMIOLOGY

Sleeping sickness was a much greater problem in the past than it is at present.[16] Approximately 50 million individuals are at risk for acquiring the disease, and about 20,000 new cases of human African trypanosomiasis are reported each year.[17] This latter figure is certainly an underestimate, since acquisition of reliable health statistics is difficult in the developing countries where the human trypanosomiases are endemic. West African (gambiense) trypanosomiasis and East African (rhodesiense) trypanosomiasis are epidemiologically distinct diseases. The general geographic distributions of these two illnesses are presented in Figure 1 of the previous chapter, and foci where transmission is known to occur are distributed throughout the indicated areas. Distinguishing epidemiologic and clinical features of the two diseases are presented in Table 1.

TABLE 1. Comparison of West African and East African Trypanosomiasis

	West African (gambiense)	*East African* (rhodesiense)
Organism	*T. b. gambiense*	*T. b. rhodesiense*
Vectors	Tsetse flies (*palpalis* group)	Tsetse flies (*morsitans* group)
Primary reservoir	Humans	Antelope and cattle
Human illness	Chronic (late CNS disease)	Acute (early CNS disease)
Duration of illness	Months to years	<9 months
Lymphadenopathy	Prominent	Minimal
Parasitemia	Low	High
Diagnosis by rodent inoculation	No	Yes
Epidemiology	Rural populations	Tourists in game parks Workers in wild areas Rural populations

West African Trypanosomiasis

West African trypanosomiasis is caused by *T. b. gambiense*, which is transmitted primarily by tsetse flies belonging to the *palpalis* group: *Glossina palpalis*, *G. tachinoides*, and *G. fuscipes*. These vectors inhabit forests and wooded areas along rivers, where favorable conditions of temperature, moisture, and darkness are combined with the availability of mammalian blood. This distribution of the vectors restricts the occurrence of human infection to the tropical rain forests of Central and West Africa. Despite the fact that these tsetse flies adapt to feeding on a variety of mammals, infected humans constitute the only major reservoir of *T. b. gambiense*. The primary determinant of the risk of acquiring the infection is the frequency of contact with the vector. This risk increases during the dry season, when the density of both vectors and humans increases around limited numbers of water holes. Because of this pattern of transmission, West African trypanosomiasis is primarily a problem in rural populations, and tourists rarely become infected with *T. b. gambiense*. The illness caused by *T. b. gambiense* is less severe than that caused by *T. b. rhodesiense*. Thus, a large proportion of infected individuals are asymptomatic for long periods of time and continue to have contact with the vectors. This may be an important element in the persistence of the infection in the reservoir between epidemics.

East African Trypanosomiasis

The etiologic agent of East African trypanosomiasis is *T. b. rhodesiense*. This subspecies is transmitted by tsetse flies of the *morsitans* group, principally *G. morsitans, G. pallidipes*, and *G. swynnertoni*. These vectors are widely distributed in savanna and woodland areas of Central and East Africa. Wild animals are the reservoir of this organism, principally antelope such as the bushbuck and hartebeest. These animals are trypanotolerant and generally do not suffer significant morbidity unless weakened by other illnesses. Cattle are the only domestic animals that can serve as a reservoir of *T. b. rhodesiense*, and infection with the parasite usually causes death if left untreated. Many other wild and domestic animals can be infected with this parasite, but their importance as reservoirs is minimal either because parasitemias are quite low or because they succumb quickly to the infection. The presence of the reservoir of *T. b. rhodesiense* in wild game in vast areas of Africa precludes the opening of these lands for cattle grazing. Humans become infected with *T. b. rhodesiense* only incidentally, since for the most part risk results from contact with tsetse flies that principally feed on wild animals. Thus, the illness is an occupational hazard for individuals, such as game wardens, who work in areas where infected wild animals and vectors are present. In addition, sporadic cases of *T. b. rhodesiense* infection occur among visitors to the game parks of East Africa.

The natural cycle of the African trypanosomes does not exist outside of Africa, and human African trypanosomiasis in the United States is limited to an occasional imported case. During the past 20 years, 15 cases of imported African trypanosomiasis have been reported to the Centers for Disease Control.[18–20] Most of these cases were caused by *T. b. rhodesiense*, and several patients had CNS involvement. Despite the serious nature of the infection, all of the patients were treated effectively.

CLINICAL COURSE

West African Trypanosomiasis

An indurated, painful trypanosomal chancre may develop at the site where parasites were inoculated by an infected tsetse fly. This lesion usually appears 1–2 weeks after the bite of the infected fly and resolves spontaneously over several weeks. The chancre may ulcerate and reach a diameter of several centimeters; regional lymphadenopathy may also develop. However, the trypanosomal chancre is seldom seen in clinical practice. Thus, most patients may develop systemic trypanosomiasis without experiencing the symptoms of localized disease.

The development of stage I (hemolymphatic) disease with dissemination of the parasites is marked by the onset of fever, which may appear weeks or months after acquisition of the infection. The fever is characterized by intermittent bouts of high temperatures lasting for several days, and extended periods may intervene during which the patient is afebrile. As the chronic illness evolves, a wide variety of other signs and symptoms develop. Lymphadenopathy is a fairly constant feature of gambiense trypanosomiasis. The nodes are typically discrete, movable, rubbery, and nontender. With time they frequently become indurated as fibrosis occurs. Supraclavicular and cervical nodes are often visibly discernable, and enlargement of the nodes of the posterior cervical triangle, or Winterbottom's sign, is a classic finding in individuals infected with *T. b. gambiense*. Mild hepatosplenomegaly may be present as well.

Transient edema is a frequent sign during this phase of the illness and can occur in the face as well as in the hands, feet, and other periarticular areas. Pruritis is common, and an irregular circinate rash is often present. The rash is typically located on the trunk, shoulders, buttocks, and thighs and consists of erythematous areas 5–10 cm in diameter with clear centers. Other inconstant findings include malaise, headache, weakness, weight loss, arthralgias, and tachycardia.

Stage II (meningoencephalitic) disease is characterized by the insidious development of protean neurologic manifestations, accompanied by progressive alterations in the composition of the CSF.[21] In gambiense trypanosomiasis CNS findings may develop months or even years after the initiation of the infection. Irritability, personality change, and loss of ability to concentrate may develop before changes in the CSF become evident, and this underscores the arbitrary nature of the distinction between the hemolymphatic and CNS stages of the illness. A picture of progressive indifference develops, associated with daytime somnolence, sometimes alternating with restlessness and insomnia at night. The frequency and progressive nature of the somnolence result in the use of the term *sleeping sickness*. A listless gaze reflects loss of spontaneity, and speech may become indistinct. Extrapyramidal signs often develop and may include choreiform movements of the trunk, neck, and extremities, tremors of the tongue and fingers, and fasciculations of a variety of muscle groups. Ataxia is a frequent sign, and the patient may appear to have Parkinson's disease as a shuffling gait, hypertonia, tremors, and slurred speech develop. The final phase of the CNS disease is one of progressive neurologic impairment ending in coma and death.

Trypanosomiasis in children, which is uncommon because of their relatively limited exposure to the vectors, does not differ greatly from the clinical illness seen in adults. However, the illness tends to run a more acute course, and the distinction between the hemolymphatic and CNS stages is difficult to make.[22] Moreover, due to the protean nature of the symptoms and the lack of pathognomic signs, the diagnosis is often missed in the early stages of the infection and is made only after neurologic impairment has developed.

East African Trypanosomiasis

The most striking general difference between West African and East African trypanosomiases is that the latter illness tends to follow a more acute course, reflecting a relatively less effective adaptation of *T. b. rhodesiense* to humans.[23] The onset of symptoms usually occurs a few days after the patient has been bitten by an infected tsetse fly, but the incubation period may be as long as several weeks. Typically in tourists, systemic signs of infection such as fever, malaise, and headache may appear before the end of the trip or shortly after their return home. As the illness progresses, the pattern of intermittent fever develops and rash is a nearly constant feature of the early weeks of the illness. Lymph node swelling is not prominent is rhodesiense trypanosomiasis, and thus Winterbottom's sign is generally absent. Persistent tachycardia unrelated to the fevers is frequently present early in the course of the illness, and in some patients death may result from arrhythmias and congestive heart failure due to pancarditis even before CNS disease develops. In general, untreated rhodesiense trypanosomiasis usually leads to death in a matter of weeks to months, without a clear distinction between the hemolymphatic and CNS stages.

DIAGNOSIS

Epidemiologic information and clinical findings often combine to suggest the diagnosis of African trypanosomiasis, and a high index of suspicion should be maintained with individuals who have been in endemic areas. However, there are numerous other illnesses common in the tropics that cause symptoms similar to those seen both in the early and late stages of sleeping sickness, and a definitive diagnosis of African trypanosomiasis requires demonstration of the parasite.[24]

If a chancre is present, fluid should be expressed and examined directly under light microscopy for the highly motile trypanosomes. Part of the specimen should be fixed and stained with Giemsa. Aspiration of soft lymph nodes early in the course of the infection can also be used to demonstrate the presence of parasites. This method is more effective in patients with West African trypanosomiasis because of the prominence of lymphadenopathy, but even in such patients, multiple aspirates are sometimes necessary before parasites are found. An enlarged node should be punctured and kneaded gently during aspiration, and the sample obtained should be examined directly and also after staining.

Examination of wet preparations and Giemsa-stained thin and thick smears of peripheral blood is also a sensitive method for detection of infection with African trypanosomes (Fig. 1). This approach is more likely to be successful in the hemolymphatic stage of the illness, and it is much more useful in patients infected with *T. b. rhodesiense* because of the relatively high parasitemias. Since parasitemia levels vary considerably from one day to the next, serial specimens should be examined. If parasites are not seen in blood from a patient whose history and clinical findings point to African trypanosomiasis as the likely diagnosis, efforts should be made to concentrate the organisms. This can be done by examining the buffy coat obtained by centrifuging 10–15 ml of anticoagulated blood. Alternatively, 25–50 ml of anticoagulated blood can be run into a DEAE-cellulose column, and trypanosomes in the eluate can be concentrated by centrifugation.[25] In both of these cases, the specimens obtained should be examined as wet preparations and after Giemsa staining.

Examination of the CSF is mandatory in all patients suspected of having African trypanosomiasis. An increase in the CSF cell count is the first abnormality to be detected. Increased opening pressure of the fluid develops later, as do an elevated IgM level and total protein concentration. Examination of the sediment of centrifuged CSF often reveals trypanosomes in patients with CNS involvement.[26] Any CSF abnormality in a patient in whom trypanosomes have been found in specimens from other sites must be viewed as pathognomonic for CNS involvement, and this has implications for treatment that will be discussed below. CSF IgM levels may remain elevated for long periods after effective therapy.

An additional approach to patients in whom parasites cannot be demonstrated by the above methods is bone marrow aspiration. Trypanosomes may be found by careful examination of

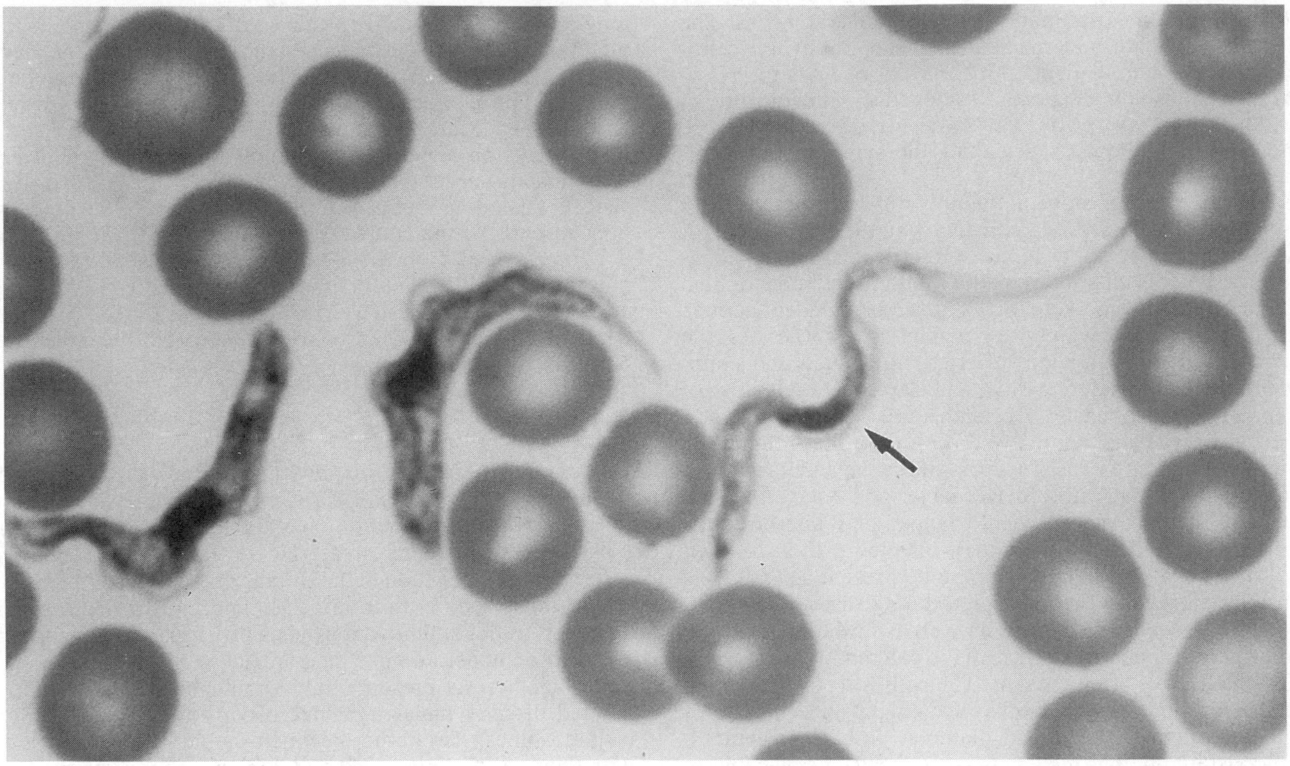

FIG. 1. *Trypanosoma brucei rhodesiense* trypomastigotes in rat blood. The parasite indicated by the arrow is typical of the long, slender forms capable of multiplying in the mammalian host. The other two organisms represent the stumpy, nondividing forms infective for the insect vector. (Giemsa, ×1250) (Courtesy of Dr. G. A. Cook, Iowa City, IA.)

Giemsa-stained specimens. Moreover, material aspirated from the bone marrow can be inoculated into liquid culture medium, as can blood, CSF, or lymph node aspirates obtained from the patient in whom trypanosomiasis is suspected.[27] Finally, the most sensitive method for the detection of infection with *T. b. rhodesiense* is inoculation of small volumes of specimens obtained from the patient into mice or rats. Patent parasitemias will usually develop within a week or two in animals inoculated with specimens from infected individuals. Unfortunately, due to host specificity, *T. b. gambiense* cannot be detected by this method.

A number of serologic assays are available to aid in the diagnosis of African trypanosomiasis, but the variable sensitivity and specificity of these tests mandate that treatment decisions still be based on demonstration of the parasite. Nonetheless, these assays are useful in epidemiologic surveys. Detection of elevated serum IgM levels was used for many years as a screening procedure. More specific methods used currently include the immunofluorescent test[28] and the enzyme-linked immunosorbent assay (ELISA).[29] A simple direct agglutination test for stained trypanosomes performed on cards (CATT)[30] has been developed and is available commercially as a kit.

TREATMENT

The drugs classically used for the therapy of African trypanosomiasis are suramin, pentamidine, and organic arsenicals.[31] More recently, eflornithine has shown promise in the treatment of West African trypanosomiasis. Gambiense and rhodesiense trypanosomiases are treated similarly, and therapy must be individualized based on the presence or absence of CNS disease, side reactions, and occasionally drug resistance of the infecting organisms. Suramin and pentamidine do not penetrate the CNS adequately, and thus the more toxic arsenicals must be used in patients with CNS involvement. Eflornithine gives adequate CNS penetration. In the United States these drugs must be obtained from the Centers for Disease Control, Atlanta, Georgia. Currently recommended treatment protocols are summarized in a recent publication.[32]

The drug of choice for treatment of patients with the hemolymphatic stage of African trypanosomiasis and normal CSF is suramin (Bayer 205, Naphuride, Antrypol). A 100–200 mg test dose should be given. The dosage for adults is 1 g iv on days 1, 3, 7, 14, and 21. The dosage for children is 20 mg/kg iv on days 1, 3, 7, 14, and 21. The drug is administered by slow iv infusion of a freshly prepared 10% aqueous solution. Suramin causes a number of side effects and must be administered under the close supervision of a physician. Approximately 1 patient in 20,000 has an immediate, severe, and potentially fatal reaction to the drug consisting of nausea, vomiting, seizures, and shock. A number of less severe reactions can also occur, including fever, pruritus, photophobia, arthralgias, and skin eruptions. The most important side effect of suramin is renal damage. Transient proteinuria is often seen during treatment. Urinalysis should be done before giving each dose, and if proteinuria increases or casts and red cells appear in the urine sediment, the drug should be discontinued. Suramin should not be used in patients with pre-existing renal insufficiency.

Pentamidine isoethionate (Lomidine) is the alternative drug recommended for patients with hemolymphatic African trypanosomiasis. The drug is effective in treatment of the early stages of gambiense trypanosomiasis, but it has a lower cure rate than suramin. In addition, some *T. b. rhodesiense* infections do not respond to pentamidine. The dosage for both adults and children is 4 mg/kg/day im for 10 days. Frequent, immediate side effects of pentamidine include nausea, vomiting, hypotension, and tachycardia. These reactions are generally transient and do not warrant discontinuation of therapy. Other side effects include nephrotoxicity, abnormal liver function tests, neutropenia, rashes, hypoglycemia, and sterile abscesses.

The drug of choice for therapy of African trypanosomiasis with CNS involvement is the arsenical melarsoprol (Mel B, Arsobal). Melarsoprol will cure both stages of the disease. Thus, it is also indicated for treatment of the hemolymphatic stage in patients in whom suramin and/or pentamidine have failed or could not be tolerated. However, it should never be the first choice for therapy of stage I trypanosomiasis because of its relatively high toxicity. In adults the drug is given in three courses of 3 days each. The recommended dosage is 2–3.6 mg/kg/day iv in three divided doses for 3 days, followed 1 week later by 3.6 mg/kg/day, also in three divided doses for 3 days. This latter course is then repeated 10–21 days later. In debilitated patients, treatment with suramin for 2–4 days before starting melarsoprol and an 18-mg initial dose of the latter drug have been recommended. For pediatric patients, 18–25 mg/kg total should be given over 1 month. An initial dose of 0.36 mg/kg iv should be increased gradually to a maximum of 3.6 mg/kg at 1- to 5-day intervals for a total of 9–10 doses.

Melarsoprol is a highly toxic drug and should be administered with great care. The most important side effects involve the CNS. Reactive encephalopathy is a frequent occurrence, and its incidence has been reported to be as high as 18 percent in some series. It is thought to result from the interaction of the drug with diseased brain tissue and trypanosomes, and it is rare in patients with minimal CNS involvement. It generally occurs during the first course, and its onset may be sudden or insidious. Clinical indications of reactive encephalopathy include high fever, headache, tremor, impaired speech, seizures, and finally coma. The reaction may be fatal, but death rates have been reduced as experience with the drug has accumulated. Melarsoprol should be discontinued at the first sign of encephalopathy. It may be restarted cautiously with small doses a few days after the signs have resolved.

A number of other side effects are associated with melarsoprol therapy. Extravasation of the drug results in intense local reactions and, as with administration of other heavy metals, abdominal pain and vomiting are commonly observed. Jarisch-Herxheimer-type reactions have been reported, as have nephrotoxicity, abnormal liver function tests, and myocardial damage.

The alternative therapeutic approach for patients who cannot tolerate melarsoprol is the combination of the arsenical tryparsamide (Tryparsone, Novatoxyl) and suramin. Tryparsamide is effective against *T. b. gambiense* but not against *T. b. rhodesiense*. It crosses the blood-brain barrier and thus can be used in stage II disease. The dosage of tryparsamide is one injection of 30 mg/kg every 5 days for a total of 12 injections, and that for suramin is 10 mg/kg iv every 5 days, also for a total of 12 injections. The courses of both drugs may be repeated after 1 month. Tryparsamide may also cause encephalopathy; other side effects include fever, abdominal pain, vomiting, rash, tinnitis, and a variety of ocular symptoms.

Recently, experience has been accumulating in the use of eflornithine (difluoromethylornithine, DFMO, Ornidyl) to treat patients with West African trypanosomiasis.[33–35] Initial trials indicate that when given iv, this drug is highly effective in both the hemolymphatic and CNS stages of gambiense trypanosomiasis, and field trials involving larger numbers of patients are underway. This drug produces dramatic reduction of symptoms and rapid clearing of parasites from blood and CSF. The recommended dosage is 400 mg/kg/day iv in 4 divided doses for 14 days, followed by 300 mg/kg/day po, also in 4 divided doses, for 30 days. Frequent side effects include diarrhea and anemia. Thrombocytopenia has been observed, and seizures and hearing loss have been reported rarely. The major advantage of eflornithine is its relative lack of side effects in comparison to melarsoprol. Thus, if its efficacy is confirmed in larger trials, it may have an important role in the treatment of both stage I and stage II *T. b. gambiense* infections. The efficacy of eflornithine in *T. b. rhodesiense* has not been determined. A major disadvantage is the amount of drug that must be given and the duration of therapy; these factors may make widespread use difficult.

PREVENTION

The trypanosomiases constitute complex public health and epizootic problems in many developing countries in Africa. Control programs that focus on eradication of vectors and drug treatment of infected humans and animals have been in operation in some regions for decades. Considerable progress has been made in a number of areas, but at present there is no consensus on the best approach to solving the overall problem of African trypanosomiasis.[3] Individuals can reduce their risk of acquiring infections with trypanosomes by avoiding areas known to harbor infected insects, by wearing clothing that reduces the biting of the flies, and by using insect repellent. Chemoprophylaxis is not recommended because of the high toxicity of the drugs that are active against African trypanosomes, and no vaccine is available to prevent transmission of the parasites.

REFERENCES

1. Hoare CA. The Trypanosomes of Mammals: A Zoological Monograph. Oxford: Blackwell; 1972:401–610.
2. Vickerman K. Developmental cycles and biology of pathogenic trypanosomes. Br Med Bull. 1985;41:105–14.
3. Jordan AM. Trypanosomiasis Control and African Rural Development. London: Longman; 1986:6–24.
4. Donelson JE. Antigenic variation in African trypanosomes. Contrib Microbiol Immunol. 1987;8:138–75.
5. Traub N, Hira PR, Chintu C, et al. Congenital trypanosomiasis: Report of a case due to *Trypanosoma brucei rhodesiense*. E Afr Med J. 1978;55:477–81.
6. Herbert WJ, Parratt D, van Meirvenne N, et al. An accidental laboratory infection with trypanosomes of a defined stock. II. Studies on the serological response of the patient and the identity of the infecting organism. J Infect. 1980;2:113–24.
7. Emeribe AO. Gambiense trypanosomiasis acquired from needle scratch. Lancet. 1988;1:470–1.
8. Greenwood BM, Whittle HC. The pathogenesis of sleeping sickness. Trans R Soc Trop Med Hyg. 1980;74:716–25.
9. Poltera AA. Pathology of human African trypanosomiasis with reference to experimental African trypanosomiasis and infections of the central nervous system. Br Med Bull. 1985;41:169–74.
10. Wery M, Mulumba PM, Lambert PH, et al. Hematologic manifestations, diagnosis, and immunopathology of African trypanosomiasis. Semin Hematol. 1982;19:83–92.
11. Poltera AA, Cox JN, Owor R. Pancarditis involving the conducting system and all valves in human African trypanosomiasis. Br Heart J. 1976;38:827–37.
12. Poltera AA, Owor R, Cox JN. Pathological aspects of human African trypanosomiasis (HAT) in Uganda. A post-mortem survey of fourteen cases. Virchows Arch Pathol Histol. 1977;373:249–65.
13. Robins-Browne RM, Schneider J, Metz J. Thrombocytopenia in trypanosomiasis. Am J Trop Med Hyg. 1975;24:226–31.
14. Barrett-Connor E, Ugoreta RJ, Braude I. Disseminated intravascular coagulation in trypanosomiasis. Arch Intern Med. 1973;131:574–7.
15. Lambert PH, Berney M, Kazyumba GL. Immune complexes in serum and in cerebrospinal fluid in sleeping sickness. Correlation with polyclonal B-cell activation and with intracerebral immunoglobulin synthesis. J Clin Invest. 1981;67:77–85.
16. Duggan AJ. An historical perspective. In: Mulligan HW, ed. The African Trypanosomiases. London: Allen and Unwin; 1970:41–88.
17. Epidemiology and control of African trypanosomiasis. Report of a WHO Expert Committee. WHO Tech Rep Ser. 1986;739:36–58.
18. Bryan RT, Waskin HA, Richards FO, et al. African trypanosomiasis in American travelers: A 20 year review. In: Steffen R, ed. International Travel Medicine. Berlin: Springer-Verlag. In press.
19. Petru AM, Azimi PH, Cummins SK, et al. African sleeping sickness in the United States. Am J Dis Child. 1988;142:224–8.
20. Nieman RE, Kelly JJ, Waskin HA. Severe African trypanosomiasis with spurious hypoglycemia. J Infect Dis. 1989;159:360–2.
21. Haller L, Adams H, Merouze F, et al. Clinical and pathological aspects of human African trypanosomiasis (*T. b. gambiense*) with particular reference to reactive arsenical encephalopathy. Am J Trop Med Hyg. 1986;35:94–9.
22. Buyst H. Sleeping sickness in children. Ann Soc Belg Med Trop. 1977;57:201–12.
23. Gear JHS, Miller B. The clinical manifestations of rhodesiense trypanosomiasis: An account of cases contracted in the Okavango swamps of Botswana. Am J Trop Med Hyg. 1986;35:1146–52.

24. Van Meirvenne N, le Ray D. Diagnosis of African and American trypanosomiases. Br Med Bull. 1985;41:156–61.
25. Lanham SM, Godfrey DG. Isolation of salivarian trypanosomes from man and other animals using DEAE-cellulose. Exp Parasitol. 1970;28:521–34.
26. Cattand P, Miezan BT, de Raadt P. Human African trypanosomiasis: Use of double centrifugation of cerebrospinal fluid to detect trypanosomes. Bull WHO. 1988;66:83–6.
27. Cunningham I. A new culture medium for maintenance of tsetse tissue and growth of trypanosomatids. J Protozool. 1977;24:325–9.
28. Wery M, Wery-Paskoff S, van Wettere P. The diagnosis of human African trypanosomiasis (*T. gambiense*) by the use of fluorescent antibody test. Ann Soc Belg Med Trop. 1970;50:613–34.
29. Ruitenberg EJ, Buys J. Application of the enzyme-linked immunosorbent assay (ELISA) for the diagnosis of human African trypanosomiasis. Am J Trop Med Hyg. 1977;26:31–6.
30. The Testryp CATT (Card Agglutination Test for Trypanosomiasis): A field study on gambiense sleeping sickness in Liberia. Trop Med Parasitol. 1986;37:390–2.
31. Gutteridge WE. Existing chemotherapy and its limitations. Br Med Bull. 1985;41:162–8.
32. Drugs for parasitic infections. Med Lett. 1988;30:15–24.
33. Doua F, Boa FY, Schechter PJ, et al. Treatment of human late stage gambiense trypanosomiasis with α-difluoromethylornithine (eflornithine): Efficacy and tolerance in 14 cases in Côte D'Ivoire. Am J Trop Med Hyg. 1987;37:525–33.
34. Pepin J, Guern C, Milford F, et al. Difluoromethylornithine for arseno-resistant *Trypanosoma brucei gambiense* sleeping sickness. Lancet. 1987;2:1431–3.
35. Taelman H, Schechter PJ, Marcelis L, et al. Difluoromethylornithine, an effective new treatment of Gambian trypanosomiasis. Am J Med. 1987;82:607–14.

255. TOXOPLASMA GONDII

ROBERT E. McCABE
JACK S. REMINGTON

Toxoplasma gondii, an obligate intracellular protozoan that is ubiquitous in nature, is an important cause of infection (*Toxoplasma* infection) and disease (toxoplasmosis) in humans and domestic animals.

Toxoplasma infection may be acute or chronic, symptomatic or asymptomatic. The acute, newly acquired infection is usually asymptomatic in older children and adults; any signs and symptoms (acute toxoplasmosis) are usually of short duration and self-limited. In most cases, the tissue cyst form of the organism persists, but the person has no clinical manifestations (chronic or latent *Toxoplasma* infection). In a few cases, however, *Toxoplasma* is the proven cause of persistent or recrudescent clinical manifestations (chronic toxoplasmosis); chorioretinitis (ocular toxoplasmosis) is an example of the chronic form of the disease.

Acute infection poses the greatest hazard to the immunodeficient patient and to the infant in utero. In immunodeficient patients such as those with the acquired immunodeficiency syndrome (AIDS), the infection may reactivate and produce acute, severe, life-threatening disease such as encephalitis, myocarditis, and/or pneumonitis. The infant infected in utero—with or without signs of the infection at birth—may develop serious untoward sequelae such as impaired vision, neurologic disorders, and sensorineural hearing loss. In addition to personal suffering caused by congenital toxoplasmosis, the cost to society in the United States of caring for such patients is hundreds of millions of dollars each year.[1] Effective measures are available to prevent congenital infection, and chemotherapeutic agents are effective in the treatment of patients with active *Toxoplasma* infection and toxoplasmosis.

ETIOLOGY

Toxoplasma is a sporozoan of the order Coccidia and suborder Eimeria. There is only one species (*T. gondii*), and all strains appear antigenically similar. Forms include trophozoites (formerly termed tachyzoites), tissue cysts, and oocysts.

Trophozoites

Crescent to oval in shape (approximately 4 × 8 μm), trophozoites (Fig. 1) stain well with Wright and Giemsa stains and can invade every mammalian cell type except non-nucleated erythrocytes. The mechanism of cell entry is unknown. Evidence supports cell infection either by active penetration as a result of mechanical and chemical action on the cell membrane or by induction of phagocytosis by the host cell.[2,3] Once within the host cell, the trophozoite resides within a vacuole and multiplies by endodyogeny, a continual process in which two daughter cells form within the mother cell. Continued division results in either cyst formation or host cell lysis. Freezing and thawing, desiccation, and normal gastric secretions (pepsin and hydrochloric acid) are lethal to trophozoites.[1]

Tissue Cysts

A single tissue cyst can vary in size from 10 to 200 μm and may contain as many as 3000 organisms (Fig. 2). The cyst wall is argyrophilic and stains weakly with periodic acid–Schiff (PAS) stain, whereas the organisms within the cyst stain strongly positive with PAS.

Toxoplasma infection is transmitted to carnivores, including humans, by the ingestion of tissue cysts in raw or undercooked meat. Peptic and tryptic digestive enzymes disrupt the cyst wall and release viable organisms that then invade the mucosa of the digestive tract and from there disseminate widely throughout the body. Tissue cysts may be found in any organ but are found most commonly in the brain and in heart and skeletal muscle. They remain viable for the life of the host, are responsible for the chronic (latent) phase of the infection, and possess the potential to reactivate. Freezing (−20°C) and thawing, heating above 60°C, and desiccation destroy tissue cysts.[1]

Oocysts

Oocysts, avoid and 10–12 μm in diameter, are produced only in the intestines of members of the cat family.[4] The oocyst is the form that maintains the life cycle of *Toxoplasma*.

Life Cycle

The definitive hosts of *Toxoplasma* are members of the cat family. After either tissue cysts or oocysts are ingested, viable organisms are released and invade the epithelial cells of the feline intestine where they undergo both an asexual cycle (schizogony) and a sexual cycle (gametogony). Millions of noninfectious, unsporulated oocysts are then shed in cat feces each day for 1–3 weeks.[5] The time of first appearance of oocysts in cat feces depends upon the form of *Toxoplasma* that infected the cat: 3–5 days after ingestion of tissue cysts, 7–10 days after ingestion of trophozoites, and 20–24 days after ingestion of oocysts. After sporulation, oocysts become infectious.[6] Sporulation occurs in 2–3 days at 4°C, 5–8 days at 15°C, and 14–21 days at 11°C. Oocysts do not sporulate below 4°C or above 37°C. Sporulation often depends upon the availability of oxygen and moisture. Oocysts may remain infectious in moist soil for longer than 1 year but can be rendered noninfectious by nearly boiling water or dry heat greater than 66°C. Both cats and incidental hosts may be infected by oocysts; however, only the extraintestinal cycle is observed in incidental hosts.

EPIDEMIOLOGY

Toxoplasma infection is a worldwide zoonosis. The organism infects herbivorous, omnivorous, and carnivorous animals, in-

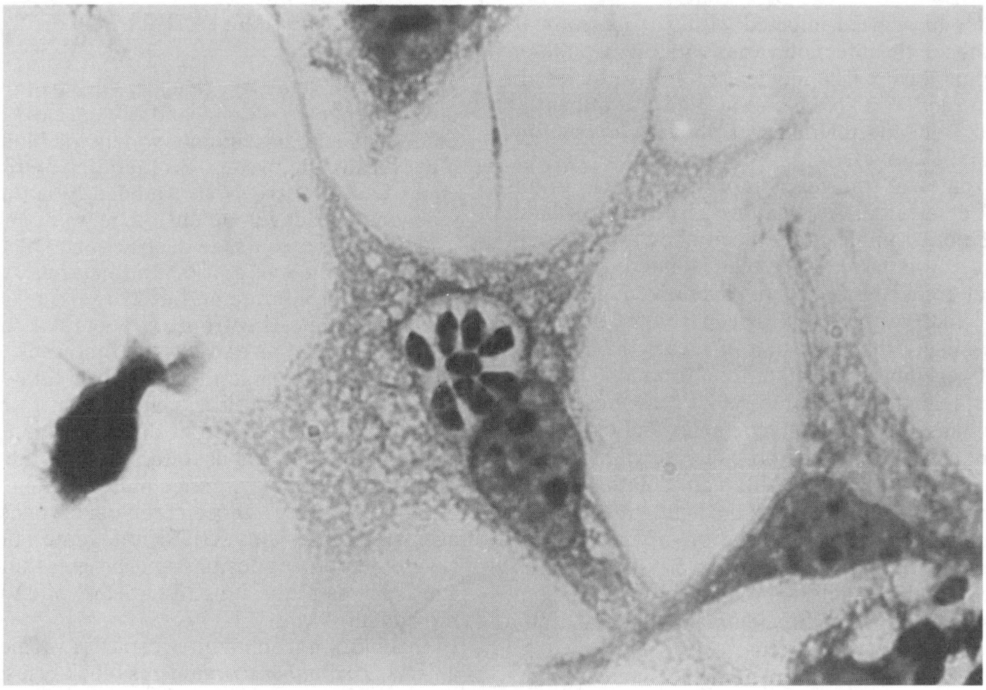

FIG. 1. Eight trophozoites of *T. gondii* are shown in a vacuole of a cultured mouse peritoneal macrophage.

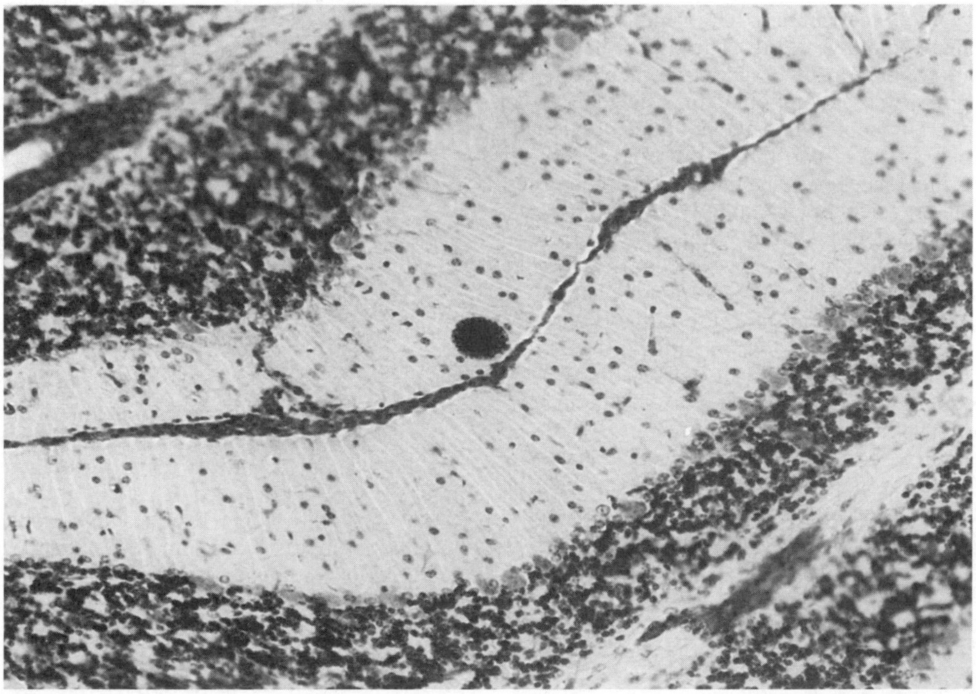

FIG. 2. A single tissue cyst is shown in the cortex of the brain of a mouse infected with *T. gondii*.

cluding all orders of mammals. The prevalence of tissue cysts in meat used for human consumption is high. Excretion of oocysts has been reported in approximately 1 percent of cats in diverse parts of the world. Coprophagous invertebrates such as cockroaches, filth flies, earthworms, snails, and slugs may serve as transport hosts for the oocyst. Although it is possible that *Toxoplasma* infection can be perpetuated in the absence of cats (e.g., via congenital transmission and carnivorism), the presence of cats appears to be of primary importance in transmission of the infection in most areas of the world.[7] However, high prevalences of *Toxoplasma* infection have been found in locales without cats, and low prevalences have been reported in areas with cats.[8]

In humans, the incidence of seropositivity for antibody to *Toxoplasma* increases with increasing age; incidence does not vary significantly between sexes. Slaughterhouse workers may have an increased risk for infection. In many populations such as in El Salvador, Tahiti, and France, the prevalence of seropositivity is more than 90 percent by the fourth decade of life. Serologic surveys indicate that 3–70 percent of healthy adults in the United States have been infected with *Toxoplasma*. In general, the incidence of the infection varies with the population group and geographic locale. The incidence tends to be less in cold regions, in hot and arid areas, and at high elevations, as might be expected from the tolerance of oocysts to environmental conditions (see above).

The two major routes of transmission of *Toxoplasma* to humans are oral and congenital. As many as 25 percent of lamb and 25 percent of pork samples have been shown to contain tissue cysts.[9] Tissue cysts have rarely been isolated from beef. Reports of suspect transmission by unpasteurized goat milk have appeared,[10,11] and *Toxoplasma* has been isolated from eggs as well.[12] It seems likely that ingestion of meats that contain tissue cysts and of vegetables and other food products contaminated with oocysts is the major means of transmission of *Toxoplasma* to humans. Ingestion of vegetables and other food products contaminated with oocysts probably accounts for infection in seropositive vegetarians. Although isolation of trophozoites from secretions of people with the acute infection has been claimed, human-to-human transmission of infection by this route during acute *Toxoplasma* infection has not been established. Outbreaks within families and other groups are common,[13] but there is no evidence of direct human-to-human transmission other than from mother to fetus.

Transmission of the infection from mother to fetus occurs when the mother acquires infection during gestation.[1] (There is only one unequivocal case in which an immunocompetent woman who acquired the acute infection before pregnancy delivered a congenitally infected infant; this woman acquired her infection 2 months before conception [G. Desmonts, Paris, France, 1982, personal communication].) The risk of newly acquired infection in a population of pregnant women depends both on the rate of primary infection in that specific geographic area and on the number of people who have not been previously infected. The interplay of these two intimately related factors may result in similar incidences of congenital infection in areas with widely different prevalences of antibody to *Toxoplasma* in the healthy populations. For example, the prevalences of infection in women of childbearing age in New York City and Paris, France, differ widely (15 and 70 percent, respectively). The incidence of congenital infection in these cities is similar. The reported rates for congenital *Toxoplasma* infection per 1000 live births are 1.3 in New York City, 3 in Paris, 2 in Mexico City, and 6.5 in the Netherlands.[1] More recent data indicate a rate of 0.2 cases per 1000 live births in Birmingham, Alabama; 1 in Basel, Switzerland; 2 in Melbourne, Australia; and 2 in Brussels, Belgium. The seroconversion rate among women of childbearing age in the United States is approximately 0.8 percent per year.[1,14] Thus, approximately 6 of every 1000 women will acquire primary infection with *Toxoplasma* during a 9-month gestation. The population moving from an area of low prevalence of infection to an area of high prevalence of infection (e.g., immigrants to France) at or before the time of childbearing potential may be at increased risk.[15]

Laboratory workers have acquired infection by accidental self-inoculation of organisms.[16] *Toxoplasma* may survive in citrated blood at 4°C for as long as 50 days, and infection has been transmitted by the transfusion of whole blood or white blood cells. Blood and blood products from patients with chronic myelogenous leukemia (e.g., for leukocyte transfusions) may pose a special risk.[17] Transmission of infection by organ transplantation has been documented and may result from transplantation of an organ from a seropositive donor to a seronegative recipient (e.g., heart)[18,19] or reactivation of the chronic infection (e.g., bone marrow transplant recipient). The means of infection may vary among geographic areas, with different sources and mechanisms of transmission operative. Clinically significant reinfection is rarely detected.

PATHOGENESIS AND PATHOLOGIC CHARACTERISTICS

After entering the body (usually via the oral route), trophozoites invade, replicate within, and disrupt host cells, invade contiguous cells, and disseminate widely via blood and lymphatics to other organs and tissues. Proliferation of trophozoites often produces foci of necrosis surrounded by an intense mononuclear reaction. The development of humoral and cellular immunity usually terminates tissue destruction. The barrier to transfer of antibody in the eye and central nervous system may allow organisms to proliferate and destroy tissue at the same time that they are disappearing from extraneural tissues. Tissue cysts can be demonstrated as early as the first week of infection and may be found in any organ. Cysts elicit little or no inflammatory response but persist in a viable latent form and are the likely cause for recrudescence of disease. This form of the infection is asymptomatic and is referred to as chronic (latent) *Toxoplasma* infection.[1] In congenital infection and in immunodeficient patients (e.g., those receiving corticosteroids or cytotoxic agents or those with AIDS), the acute infection may produce severe necrotizing lesions and progress unchecked in vital organs such as brain, lung, and heart, often resulting in death of the patient.

Toxoplasma trophozoites can avoid some host defense mechanisms. *Toxoplasma* organisms block lysosome–phagosome fusion and prevent acidification of the phagosome,[20] thereby escaping killing by macrophages. However, *Toxoplasma* organisms are susceptible to both oxygen-dependent (respiratory burst) and oxygen-independent host cell microbicidal mechanisms.[21] Lymphokines have important roles in the control of *Toxoplasma* infection. γ-Interferon activates macrophages both in vivo and in vitro to kill *Toxoplasma* and confers resistance against *Toxoplasma* in the murine model.[21–23] Human neonatal mononuclear phagocytes generate and respond suboptimally to macrophage-activating factors, e.g., γ-interferon,[24] which may help explain the frequency of signs of infection in neonates in comparison to adults. Parenteral recombinant interleukin-2 protects mice against death due to acute toxoplasmosis.[25] Pregnancy may increase susceptibility to *Toxoplasma*. In a murine model, pregnancy markedly increased mortality after challenge with *Toxoplasma*.[26] The reasons for increased susceptibility during pregnancy in mice have not been elucidated.[27]

Our knowledge of the pathology of infection in humans has come largely from autopsy studies in immunodeficient patients and severely infected infants. Data in immunocompetent adults are limited almost entirely to results obtained from biopsy specimens from lymph nodes.

The histopathologic changes in toxoplasmic lymphadenitis are frequently distinctive and often diagnostic.[28] There is a typical triad of findings: a reactive follicular hyperplasia, irregular clusters of epithelioid histiocytes encroaching on and blurring the margins of the germinal centers, and focal distension of sinuses with monocytoid cells. Langhans giant cells, granulomas, microabscesses, and foci of necrosis are not typically seen. Rarely, trophozoites or tissue cysts are demonstrable.

In the central nervous system there may be an acute focal or diffuse meningoencephalitis with cellular necrosis, microglial nodules, and perivascular mononuclear inflammation that may or may not be associated with intracellular or extracellular organisms.[29] Vascular involvement by trophozoites may produce variable (usually extensive and multiple) necrotic areas of brain parenchyma, often several centimeters in diameter. Lesions may be found in any location. In infants, periaqueductal and periventricular vasculitis and necrosis are distinctive of toxoplasmosis. The necrotic areas may calcify and lead to striking radiographic findings suggestive but not pathognomonic of toxoplasmosis. Hydrocephalus may result from obstruction of the aqueduct of Sylvius or the foramen of Monro. In immunodeficient adults, the major finding is necrotizing encephalitis of gray matter, with multiple, small, and diffusely distributed lesions. Such lesions can be detected by computed axial tomography (CT) and magnetic resonance imaging (MRI). Large single abscesses may also be found, and the patient may present with a mass lesion.[30–33]

Eye infection produces acute chorioretinitis characterized by severe inflammation and necrosis.[34] Granulomatous inflammation of the choroid is secondary to the necrotizing retinitis. There may be exudation into the vitreous or invasion of the vitreous by a budding mass of capillaries. Trophozoites and cysts may be demonstrated in the retina. The pathogenesis of recurrent chorioretinitis is controversial. One school proposes that rupture of tissue cysts releases viable organisms that induce necrosis and inflammation,[35] whereas another school contends that chorioretinitis results from a hypersensitivity reaction triggered by unknown causes.[36]

Organisms have been found in almost all organs and may or may not be accompanied by an intense inflammatory response. Myocardial fibers may contain tissue cysts or large aggregations of organisms without surrounding inflammation, whereas separate areas are infiltrated by mononuclear cells without demonstrable organisms. In immunodeficient patients, areas of necrosis may be widespread.

Skeletal muscle involvement is similar to that of cardiac muscle, and widespread myositis may be evident. Hepatomegaly and mild abnormalities in serum transaminases are common. In the kidney, glomerulonephritis with deposition of *Toxoplasma* antigen and antibody in glomeruli has been reported but appears to be rare.[1]

CLINICAL MANIFESTATIONS

Toxoplasmosis is conveniently considered in four categories: (*1*) acquired in the immunocompetent patient, (*2*) acquired or reactivated in the immunodeficient patient, (*3*) ocular, and (*4*) congenital. In any category, the clinical presentations are not specific for toxoplasmosis, and a wide differential diagnosis must be entertained. Furthermore, methods of diagnosis and their interpretations may differ for each clinical category.

Acute Acquired Toxoplasma Infection in the Immunocompetent Patient

Only 10–20 percent of cases of *Toxoplasma* infection in the adult are symptomatic.[37] Most often, toxoplasmosis presents as asymptomatic cervical lymphadenopathy, but any or all lymph node groups may be enlarged. The nodes are usually discrete and nontender, rarely more than 3 cm in diameter, may vary in firmness, and do not suppurate.[38] However, the nodes may be tender or matted. Fever, malaise, night sweats, myalgias, sore throat, maculopapular rash, hepatosplenomegaly, or small numbers of atypical lymphocytes (<10 percent) may be present.[39] The clinical picture may resemble infectious mononucleosis or cytomegalovirus (CMV) infection, but toxoplasmosis probably causes no more than 1 percent of mononucleosis syndromes.[40] Retroperitoneal or mesenteric lymphadenopathy may produce abdominal pain.[41] Chorioretinitis may occur in cases of acute acquired infection. Although the chorioretinitis is usually unilateral in these cases, it is usually bilateral in cases of congenital toxoplasmosis diagnosed at birth.[42–45]

In the immunocompetent patient, the clinical course is benign and self-limited. Symptoms, if present, usually resolve within a few months and rarely persist beyond 12 months. Lymphadenopathy may wax and wane for months and, in some unusual cases, for 1 year or longer. A form of the disease characterized by chronic lymphadenopathy has been described.[38,46] Rarely an apparently healthy person develops clinically overt, potentially fatal disseminated disease, with myocarditis, pneumonitis, or encephalitis. None of the clinical presentations of acquired toxoplasmosis are distinctive; the differential diagnosis of toxoplasmic lymphadenitis includes lymphoma, infectious mononucleosis, CMV "mononucleosis," cat-scratch disease, sarcoidosis, tuberculosis, tularemia, metastatic carcinoma, and leukemia. Acute acquired toxoplasmosis associated with multiple-organ involvement may mimic other causes of pneumonitis, hepatitis, myocarditis, polymyositis, or fever of unknown origin.[37,41]

The major diagnostic confusion with toxoplasmic lymphadenopathy occurs with Hodgkin's disease and the lymphomas. Toxoplasmic lymphadenopathy is not considered as a diagnostic possibility frequently enough. *Toxoplasma* has been estimated to cause 3–7 percent of clinically significant lymphadenopathy.[38] Serologic test titers diagnostic of acute *Toxoplasma* infection are often obtained after histology of a biopsied node has suggested the possibility of toxoplasmosis.

Acute Toxoplasmosis in the Immunodeficient Host

Toxoplasmic encephalitis, once rare even in immunocompromised patients, it now the most common cause of intracerebral mass lesions in patients with AIDS. It has been estimated that 5–10 percent of AIDS patients in the United States (20,000–40,000 cases by 1991) and approximately 25 percent of AIDS patients in much of western Europe develop toxoplasmic encephalitis.[47–49] Haitian patients may be at a particularly high risk.[50,51] On the basis of serologic studies, toxoplasmic encephalitis is considered to be due to reactivation of the chronic, latent infection.[47,48]

Toxoplasmic encephalitis usually develops in patients already known to have AIDS but occasionally may be the presenting manifestation of AIDS. Disease due to *Toxoplasma* is observed most frequently in the brain but may be seen in the eye,[52] lung,[53] or testes[54] or recovered from tissue culture of blood without a clinically evident seeding focus.[55]

Patients with toxoplasmic encephalitis usually present with a syndrome compatible with multiple mass lesions.[47,48,56–58] Hemiparesis, seizures, visual difficulties, confusion, and lethargy are common; fever and nuchal rigidity have been reported infrequently. The cerebrospinal fluid (CSF) may show no or few white blood cells, low but usually normal glucose concentration, and elevated but occasionally normal protein concentration. Routine analysis of CSF may be completely normal.[47,59,60]

CT scan of the brain is usually abnormal when patients present with symptoms due to toxoplasmic encephalitis.[50,57,60–62] It typically shows multiple intraparenchymal lesions that involve the cerebral hemispheres, thalamus, brain stem, or cerebellum; occasionally only single lesions are found. Contrast-enhanced CT scans demonstrate nodular or ring enhancement in 90 percent of patients, but rarely the focal contrast uptake is not seen. Edema may vary from mild to moderate, and a mass effect may be present. Serial CT scans usually show rapid progression of lesions in the absence of specific therapy. One group[61] has emphasized the importance of a "double dose" of contrast and delayed scans after the administration of contrast for demonstration of lesions. The findings on CT scan are not specific for toxoplasmic encephalitis; similar lesions may be due to tuberculosis, other bacteria, fungi, and lymphoma. Indeed, an AIDS patient may have a single brain abscess with two different organisms or two concurrent abscesses, each caused by different organisms.[50,63] When the CT scan is normal and suspicion is high, MRI scanning may be useful.[50,64]

Serologic tests rarely confirm the diagnosis of toxoplasmic encephalitis in AIDS patients. The test results usually are not consistent with the acute acquired infection (see below) seen in immunocompetent patients, that is, *Toxoplasma*-specific IgM antibody, very high specific IgG antibody titers, serial two-tube rises in titer in acute and convalescent sera, or seroconversion are not usually seen.[48] Attempts to demonstrate specific antibody production in the CSF may be valuable.[47,65] A negative test result for specific IgG antibody diminishes the likelihood of toxoplasmic encephalitis, but approximately 3 percent of patients with toxoplasmic encephalitis do not have *Toxoplasma* antibody in their serum.[48,49]

Although most AIDS patients respond to specific anti-*Toxoplasma* chemotherapy and since such therapy is both toxic and necessary for the remainder of the patient's life,[56] a confirmed diagnosis is highly desirable.[49,50] A brain biopsy with demonstration of *Toxoplasma* organisms is usually necessary for a definitive diagnosis. Interpretation of needle biopsy specimens of the brain is complicated by false-negative results.[49,66] We recognize the reluctance on the part of many neurosurgeons as well as physicians caring for these patients to perform or request open brain biopsy or aspiration. At present empirical chemotherapy appears reasonable in AIDS patients whose brain CT scan is very suggestive of toxoplasmic encephalitis.[51] The patient should respond clinically and radiographically within about 10 days of the start of therapy.[49]

Patients who are being treated with immunosuppressive drugs also are at risk for clinically severe and often fatal toxoplasmosis, although any form of toxoplasmosis may develop in these patients.[30–33] Toxoplasmosis in these patients may be due to either newly acquired or reactivated latent infection. Studies in bone marrow transplant recipients suggest that toxoplasmosis results from reactivation of a latent infection.[67,68] In heart transplant recipients, toxoplasmosis frequently results when a seronegative recipient receives a heart from a seropositive donor.[69,70] Seropositive heart transplant recipients frequently exhibit IgM and IgG serologic antibody titer rises after transplantation without evidence of clinical disease.[69] That toxoplasmosis is markedly underdiagnosed in immunodeficient patients is suggested by the large number of cases diagnosed at some institutions,[71] the large number of autopsy reports,[71,72] and the nonspecific but varied clinical presentation of toxoplasmosis.

Similar to AIDS patients, most other immunodeficient patients who present with toxoplasmosis have disease referable to the central nervous system such as encephalitis, meningoencephalitis, or mass lesions; overt myocarditis or pneumonitis may also be present. As in AIDS patients, the CSF usually reveals mononuclear pleocytosis, an elevated protein concentration, and a normal glucose concentration, although hypoglycorrhachia may occur. Computed axial tomography may detect either multiple diffusely distributed lesions or a single mass lesion and may help direct brain biopsy or aspiration. In the heart transplant recipient, toxoplasmosis may simulate organ rejection. In such cases, toxoplasmosis has been established by endomyocardial biopsy.[69]

Acute infection of the central nervous system by *Toxoplasma* must be differentiated from meningoencephalitis caused by other infectious agents (expecially herpes simplex, fungi, and *Mycobacterium tuberculosis*), brain abscess, cerebral hemorrhage, multifocal leukoencephalopathy, vasculitis such as lupus cerebritis, and tumor. In immunodeficient patients, CSF mononuclear pleocytosis with high protein concentrations in the absence of evidence for bacteria or fungi warrants serious consideration of toxoplasmosis.

Ocular Toxoplasmosis

Toxoplasma infection is an important cause of chorioretinitis in the United States and Europe. The vast majority of cases of *Toxoplasma* chorioretinitis result from congenital infection.[45] Patients are often asymptomatic until later in life, with a peak incidence of symptomatic disease in the second and third decades of life. Clinically apparent reactivation occurs uncommonly after the age of 40 years. The characteristic lesion is a focal necrotizing retinitis that initially appears in the fundus as a yellowish white, elevated cotton patch with indistinct margins, usually on the posterior pole[73] (Fig. 3). The lesions are often in small clusters, and individual lesions in the cluster may be of varying ages. With healing, the lesions pale, atrophy, and develop black pigment. Panuveitis may accompany chorioretinitis, but isolated anterior uveitis has never been proved to occur. Papillitis is usually associated with overt central nervous system disease. Chorioretinitis in those with acquired *Toxoplasma* infection is characteristically unilateral, whereas it is characteristically bilateral in chorioretinitis diagnosed at birth.

Acute chorioretinitis may produce symptoms of blurred vision, scotoma, pain, photophobia, and epiphora. Impairment or a loss of central vision occurs when the macula is involved. As inflammation resolves, vision improves, frequently without complete recovery of visual acuity. Features that suggest toxoplasmosis on ophthalmoscopic examination include bilateral macular involvement, chorioretinal degeneration with a normal-appearing retina surrounding typical punched-out lesions, rapid development of optic nerve atrophy, and clarity of the vitreous and aqueous humor.[73] Relapses of chorioretinitis are frequent (in as many as 13–30 percent of patients after specific chemotherapy),[74,75] but the relapses are rarely accompanied by systemic signs or symptoms.[45] *Toxoplasma* chorioretinitis may resemble the posterior uveitis of tuberculosis, syphilis, leprosy, or presumed ocular histoplasmosis syndrome (POHS).[34,35]

Congenital Toxoplasmosis

Congenital *Toxoplasma* infection or toxoplasmosis results from an acute infection, usually asymptomatic, that is acquired by the mother during gestation. Despite numerous reports to the contrary, only one case of congenital toxoplasmosis is known to have occurred in an immunocompetent woman when she acquired the infection before she conceived (see above).[1,76] Chronically infected women who are immunocompromised (e.g., patients with systemic lupus erythematosus who are being treated with corticosteroids) may transmit the infection to their fetus; the risk of this occurrence is difficult to quantitate but is probably low. The risk to the fetus does not correlate with whether the infection in the mother was symptomatic or asymptomatic during gestation.

To assess the risk of transmission of the organism to the fetus, it is necessary to determine when the pregnant woman acquired the infection with respect to the date of conception. If the pregnant woman was infected before conception, it can be stated *for all practical purposes* that there is no risk of transmission of the organism to the fetus,[1] The data accumulated from prospective studies in France indicate that the incidence and severity of congenital toxoplasmosis vary with the trimester during which infection was acquired.[1,77] Infection acquired in the first trimester by women who were not treated with anti-*Toxoplasma* drugs resulted in congenital infection in 25 percent (an overestimate due to bias for inclusion of infections acquired late in the first trimester). The outcome in these pregnancies may be spontaneous abortion, stillbirth, or severe disease in the newborn. The incidences of fetal infection were 54 and 65 percent for second and third trimester infections, respectively; about 72 and 89 percent of infants infected as the result of second and third trimester infections, respectively, did not have signs of the infection. Treatment of the mother with specific chemotherapy reduces the incidence of congenital infection by about 60 percent.

Clinical manifestations of congenital toxoplasmosis are varied. There may be no sequelae, or sequelae may develop and/or be evident at various times after birth. Most signs and clinical presentations are nonspecific and may mimic disease due to organisms such as herpes simplex, CMV, and rubella. Signs include chorioretinitis, strabismus, blindness, epilepsy, psychomotor or mental retardation, anemia, jaundice, rash, petechiae due to thrombocytopenia, encephalitis, pneumonitis, microcephaly, intracranial calcification, hydrocephalus, diarrhea,

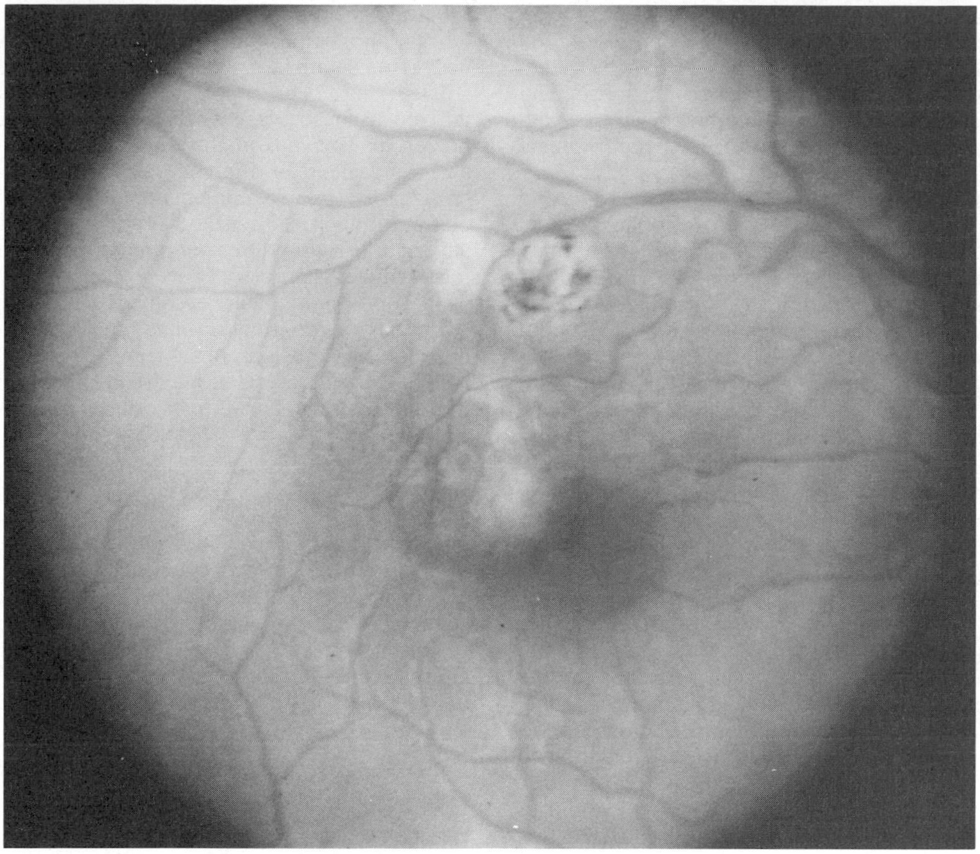

FIG. 3. *Toxoplasma* chorioretinitis.

hypothermia, and nonspecific illness.[1,78] Of note is that *Toxoplasma* infection is not known to cause fetal malformations by affecting host DNA.

A detailed examination may be necessary to detect signs of the infection. In one prospective study,[79] 210 congenitally infected infants were identified: 2 cases (0.9 percent) were fatal, 21 (10.9 percent) had severe disease, 71 (33.8 percent) were mildly afflicted, and 116 (54.4 percent) were without signs of the infection. More intensive examination of the latter 116 infants revealed abnormalities in 39; abnormal CSF was detected in 22 infants, chorioretinitis was seen in 17 infants, and 10 had intracranial calcifications. If clinical signs of infection are evident in the neonate, sequelae are usually severe.[1] Most infants are without obvious signs of disease at birth; delayed-onset disease may be severe or mild. Premature infants often suffer central nervous system disease and ocular disease in the first 3 months of life. Full-term infants frequently develop a milder disease manifested by hepatosplenomegaly and lymphadenopathy that usually appear in the first 2 months of life. In these infants, disease reflecting damage to the central nervous system may occur later, and eye disease may occur months to years after birth.

Recent data collected in follow-up studies suggest that most infants with subclinical infection at birth will subsequently develop signs or symptoms of congenital toxoplasmosis.[80] In one study, clinical evaluation at a mean age of 8.3 years showed that 11 of the 13 infected children who had no signs of the disease after detailed examination in the newborn period suffered sequelae. Some of these children were treated with specific chemotherapy in the newborn period. In each child the initial manifestation was chorioretinitis, which appeared at a mean age of 3.7 years. Three children had unilateral blindness, whereas the other eight children had no loss of visual function. Five children developed neurologic sequelae, including one child with delayed psychomotor development, microcephaly, and seizure disorder and two children with minor cerebellar signs. Sensorineural hearing loss occurred in 3 of 10 children evaluated. A study from The Netherlands[81] reported that five of nine congenitally infected, untreated children followed for up to 14 years developed chhorioretinitis. Information from prospective studies being performed in France suggests that early instigation of specific therapy in those infants with congenital infection but without clinical signs will markedly reduce untoward sequelae.[1,82]

Congenital toxoplasmosis must be differentiated from other members of the TORCH syndrome (i.e., rubella, cytomegalovirus, and herpes simplex), syphilis, *Listeria* and other bacterial infections, other infectious encephalopathies, erythroblastosis fetalis, and sepsis. Herpes simplex, cytomegalovirus, rubella, and syphilis may cause chorioretinitis; both cytomegalovirus and rubella have been associated with hydrocephalus, microcephaly, and cerebral calcification. A markedly elevated CSF protein concentration is a hallmark of congenital toxoplasmosis.[78]

Toxoplasma infection acquired during pregnancy has been implicated in spontaneous abortion, stillbirth, and premature births. *Toxoplasma* organisms have been isolated from the abortuses of women with chronic infection, but the frequency of *Toxoplasma* infection as a cause of abortion is unknown and controversial.[76]

DIAGNOSIS

Since the clinical manifestations of *Toxoplasma* infection may be protean and nonspecific, it must be carefully considered in the differential diagnosis of a large variety of clinical presentations. The right diagnostic test must be performed and appropriately interpreted in light of the patient's clinical situation.

The usefulness of a given diagnostic method may differ considerably with the category of infection, that is, acute acquired *Toxoplasma* infection in the immunocompetent patient, infection in the immunodeficient patient, ocular toxoplasmosis, and congenital toxoplasmosis. Diagnostic methods will be described, followed by a discussion of diagnosis in specific clinical situations.

Acute infection is diagnosed by the isolation of *Toxoplasma* from blood or body fluids; demonstration of trophozoites in histologic sections of tissue or in cytologic preparations of body fluids; demonstration of characteristic lymph node histology or of characteristic test results; or demonstration of *Toxoplasma* tissue cysts in the placenta, fetus, or neonate.[1] Rarely, asymptomatic patients with latent infection will have recurrent parasitemia.[83] Isolation of *Toxoplasma* from the tissues of older children or adults may reflect only the the presence of cysts; one exception to this is that isolation from lymph node tissue in adults may reflect the presence of trophozoites. Finding numerous cysts in tissue secretions suggests but does not prove acute infection.

Isolation of Toxoplasma

Isolation of *Toxoplasma* from blood or body fluids establishes that the infection is acute. In the case of the neonate, isolation of the organism from the placenta is usually diagnostic, and isolation from the fetal tissues is always diagnostic of congenital infection.[1] The organism can be isolated by inoculation of specimens (body fluids; the buffy coat from centrifuged, heparinized blood; or processed tissue) into the peritoneal cavities of mice.[1] Tissue specimens should first be ground in saline with a mortar and pestle or in a tissue homogenizer and then be filtered free of large tissue fragments. Formalin treatment kills the organism. Peritoneal fluid from the mice should be examined 6–10 days after inoculation or earlier if they die. Unlike laboratory strains of *Toxoplasma*, most strains isolated from humans are relatively avirulent for mice. Mice surviving 6 weeks should be tested for antibody to *Toxoplasma*. If antibodies are present, a definitive diagnosis requires demonstration of the organism, usually in cysts, in stained preparations of brain, liver, or spleen from the seropositive mice (e.g., in preparations stained with Wright and Giemsa stains). If cysts are not seen, subinoculation of a suspension of brain, liver, and spleen tissue into fresh mice is necessary. If specimens cannot be processed immediately, they should be stored overnight at 4°C. *Toxoplasma* may be isolated from blood clots stored overnight as well. Tissue cell culture also can be used to isolate *Toxoplasma*: plaques are formed in which the organisms are easily recognized. Tissue cell culture has the advantages of widespread availability (e.g., virology laboratories) and yields results more rapidly than does mouse inoculation. Its sensitivity in comparision to mouse inoculation has not been evaluated carefully.

Histologic Diagnosis

Demonstration of trophozoites in tissue sections or smears of body fluid (e.g., cerebrospinal fluid, amniotic fluid, or bronchoalveolar lavage fluid) establishes the diagnosis of acute *Toxoplasma* infection.[1] Multiple cysts near an inflammatory necrotic lesion probably establishes the diagnosis.[53] It is difficult to demonstrate trophozoites in stained tissue sections. For example, in one report of toxoplasmic encephalitis in AIDS patients,[47] histologic demonstration of *Toxoplasma* was sucessful in only half the specimens obtained from open brain biopsy. Fluorescent antibody staining may be useful, but this method often yields nonspecific results.[84] Recently, the peroxidase–antiperoxidase technique, which uses antisera to *Toxoplasma*, has proved to be both sensitive and specific and has been used successfully in clinical settings to demonstrate the organisms in the central nervous system of patients with AIDS.[48,85,86] Both the fluorescent antibody and peroxidase–antiperoxidase methods are applicable to unfixed or formalin-fixed paraffin-embedded tissue sections.[85] An enzyme-linked immunosorbent assay (ELISA) has been reported to detect *Toxoplasma* antigen in unfixed tissues.[87] Use of fluorescein-labeled monoclonal antibodies to *Toxoplasma* for touch preparations of specimens[88] and rapid electron microscopy[89] have been used successfully to diagnose toxoplasmic encephalitis. A rapid, technically simple, and underused method is the detection of *Toxoplasma* in air-dried, Wright-Giemsa-stained slides of centrifuged (e.g., cytocentrifuge) sediment of cerebrospinal fluid or of brain aspirate or in impression smears of biopsy tissue.

Endomyocardial biopsy has been used successfully to diagnose toxoplasmosis in heart transplant recipients.[69] Characteristic histologic criteria alone are probably sufficient to establish the diagnosis of *Toxoplasma* lymphadenitis in older children and adults.[28]

Skin Tests

Delayed skin hypersensitivity to *Toxoplasma* antigens in cases of acquired infection is often not demonstrable for months or even years after the initial infection. The skin test has been used successfully in population surveys to establish the prevalence of chronic infection and has been proposed as an inexpensive alternative to serologic testing for screening populations (e.g., before pregnancy).[90] False-positive test results are rare.[1]

Antigen-Specific Lymphocyte Transformation and Lymphocyte Typing

Lymphocyte transformation to *Toxoplasma* antigns is a specific and sensitive indicator of previous *Toxoplasma* infection in adults. It has been used successfully to diagnose congenital *Toxoplasma* infection in infants 2 months of age or older.[91]

Recently it has been shown that adult patients with toxoplasmic lymphadenopathy may have abnormal ratios of helper-to-suppressor T lymphocytes in the peripheral blood.[92] A marked increase in suppressor T cells may correlate with the presence of symptoms in acute acquired infection in immunocompetent patients. These abnormalities may persist for months after acquisition of the infection and are not specific for infection with *Toxoplasma*.

Demonstration of Antigen in Body Fluids

The ELISA technique has been adapted to detect antigen in the sera of humans. Antigenemia has been detected in 15 of 23 sera from 22 patients with acute toxoplasmosis.[93] No antigen was detected in the sera of patients either seronegative for antibody to *Toxoplasma* or known to be chronically infected with *Toxoplasma*. These results have been confirmed[94] with the further observation that antigenemia disappeared before IgM antibody disappeared, as detected by the ELISA technique. This suggests that the combination of antigen and antibody testing may be useful in judging the time of acquisition of infection in some cases.

Serologic Tests for Demonstration of Antibody

The use of serologic tests for the demonstration of specific antibody to *Toxoplasma* is the primary method of diagnosis. The problem in serologic diagnosis is the high prevalence of antibody to *Toxoplasma* in most human populations. These antibody titers may persist at high levels (e.g., higher than or equal to 1:512 in the indirect fluorescent antibody [IFA] test) for years in healthy people. A large number of tests has been described, but relatively few are available to the clinician. In the future, more refined tests may become available as specific monoclonal antibodies are developed and specific *Toxoplasma* antigens that may increase the sensitivity or specificity of diagnosis are used.[95,96] Different serologic tests often measure different antibodies that possess unique patterns of rise and fall with time after infection. Many of the tests yield false-positive or false-negative results (or both). The clinician must be familiar with these problems and consult reference laboratories if the need arises. Tests that measure primarily IgG antibody will be described first, followed by tests that measure IgM antibody. The most useful tests for the measurement of IgG antibody are the Sabin-Feldman dye test, the IFA test, and the modified direct agglutination test. In these tests, IgG antibodies appear usually within 1–2 weeks of acquisition of infection, peak within 1–2 months, fall at variable rates, and persist for life.

Sabin-Feldman Dye Test. The Sabin-Feldman dye test is the reference serologic test against which other methods are evaluated.[97] It is a sensitive and specific neutralization test in which the organisms are lysed in the presence of antibody and complement. An international standard reference serum is available from the World Health Organization. The dye test measures primarily IgG antibodies that usually appear 1–2 weeks after initiation of infection, reach peak titers in 6–8 weeks, and then gradually decline over 1–2 years.[1] Low titers probably persist for life. Some patients have persistently high titers (e.g., 1:1000–1:4000) for years. The titer does not correlate with the severity of illness.[98] This test is available in only a few reference laboratories, primarily because live organisms are required.

Indirect Fluorescent Antibody Test. Because the IFA test is easier to perform, safer than the dye test is, and economical, it is used more widely. It appears to measure the same antibodies as the dye test, and its titers tend to parallel dye test titers.[1] The specific reaction between antibody and the antigenic site on the organism is detected by fluorescein-tagged antiserum prepared against serum IgG or whole immunoglobulins. Reliable quantitative titers are frequently difficult to obtain in the IFA test, and only with the dye test can sufficiently accurate quantitative results in IgG antibody determination be obtained for the early diagnosis of congenital infection. False-positive results in the IFA test may occur with sera that contain antinuclear antibodies,[99] and false-negative results may occur in sera with low IgG antibody titers.

Agglutination Test

The agglutination test using formalin-preserved whole trophozoites is available commercially in Europe (Bio-Merieux, Lyon, France) and detects IgG antibody. The test is very sensitive to IgM antibody, and "natural" IgM antibody causes nonspecific agglutination in sera that yield negative results when tested with the dye test and IFA test. This problem is avoided by including 2-mercaptoethanol in the test. The method is accurate, simple to perform, inexpensive, and excellent for screening pregnant women.[100] This method should not be used for the measurement of IgM antibodies. Also available commercially is a kit that uses antigen-coated latex particles to detect agglutination by *Toxoplasma* antibody.[101]

Indirect Hemagglutination Test. The indirect hemagglutination test measures different antibodies than do the dye test and the IFA test and becomes positive days to weeks or months later; titers in the indirect hemagglutination test tend to be higher and remain elevated even longer than do dye test and IFA test titers.[102] There is a wide variation in titers reported by different laboratories. The indirect hemagglutination test should not be used for the diagnosis of congenital infection since it may yield false-negative results in proved cases of infection. It also should not be used for the diagnosis of acute infection in pregnant women since there is a delay in the rise of titers.

Complement Fixation Test. The complement fixation test measures antibodies that appear several weeks later than dye test antibodies do but decline earlier than do dye test antibodies, although complement fixation test results may remain positive for years.[102,103] A positive complement fixation test result does not prove that infection is acute, nor does a negative test result exclude infection.

IgG Enzyme-Linked Immunosorbent Assay. Titers in the IgG-ELISA correlate well with titers in the dye test, indirect hemagglutination test, IFA test, and complement fixation test in some studies but not in others. The usefulness of the IgG-ELISA in the detection of the early antibody response to *Toxoplasma* infection has not been established.

IgM Immunofluorescent Antibody Test. Several assays are available for the measurement of IgM antibody, which appears earlier and declines faster than IgG antibody does. In the IFA test adapted to detect IgM antibody (IgM-IFA), antibody appears within the first week of infection, and titers rise rapidly to levels of 1:80 to 1:1000, then fall to low titers, and usually disappear in a few months. Low titers may persist in some patients for 1 year or longer.[102] Antinuclear antibodies and rheumatoid factor may cause false-positive results.[104] IgG-blocking antibodies can cause false-negative results in this test when the IgG is not removed.[105]

Double-Sandwich IgM Enzyme-Linked Immunosorbent Assay. The double-sandwich IgM-ELISA (DS-IgM-ELISA) is much more sensitive and specific than is either the conventional IgM-ELISA or the IgM-IFA tests.[106,107] False-positive results due to rheumatoid factor and antinuclear antibodies are found in the IgM-IFA test but are not found in the DS-IgM-ELISA.[104] In the conventional IgM-ELISA, false-positive results may occur in sera that contain rheumatoid factor.[106]

IgM Imunosorbent Assay. The IgM immunosorbent assay (IgM-ISAGA; available from Bio-Merieux, Lyon, France), which binds the patient's IgM to a solid surface and uses either formalin-fixed organisms or antigen-coated latex particles to detect IgM antibodies, is both sensitive and specific.[108] The test is simple to perform, does not require the use of enzyme conjugate, and is read in the same manner as the agglutination test. It is more sensitive and specific than is the IgM-IFA test. The presence of rheumatoid factor or antinuclear antibodies does not cause false-positive results in the IgM-ISAGA.

Serologic Diagnosis of Specific Clinical Entities

Acute Acquired Toxoplasma Infection in the Immunocompetent Patient. A negative dye or IFA test titer virtually excludes the diagnosis of acute *Toxoplasma* infection in the immunocompetent person. Acute acquired infection is confirmed by the demonstration of seroconversion from a negative to a positive titer or by the demonstration of a serial two-tube rise from a low to a high titer in sera run in parallel and drawn at 3-week intervals. Although suggestive of acute infection, a single high titer in the dye test, IFA test, or indirect hemagglutination test is not diagnostic. Since the diagnosis of *Toxoplasma* infection is often considered relatively late, serologic test titers may have peaked when the serum was first tested. In such cases, the complement fixation test or the indirect hemagglutination test may be helpful since these tests show positive results later in the course of illness. The agglutination test may be more sensitive than the dye test is for detecting serial two-tube rises in titer.[109] Frequently serial two-tube rises in dye test titers are not detected because the first serum is drawn too late after the acquisition of infection. It is rare in acute *Toxoplasma* infection to have a stable dye or IFA test titer of less than 1:1000.[102,109]

If a high IgM antibody titer is present with a single high IgG antibody titer (e.g., dye or IFA test titer >1:1000), acute infection is probable. A low titer in the DS-IgM-ELISA suggests that infection was acquired 4 months or longer before the serum was drawn,[109] and low titers may persist for longer than a year after infection. In a study of patients with toxoplasmic lymphadenopathy, 50 percent of patients had detectable IgM antibody by the DS-IgM-ELISA test for 7–12 months after the first serum sample was drawn.[109] A negative IgM-IFA test titer does not rule out acute infection. If the patient has received a blood transfusion, serologic tests may measure exogenous rather than endogenous antibody.

Acute Toxoplasma Infection or Toxoplasmosis in the Immunodeficient Patient. The aforementioned criteria for diagnosis in the immunocompetent patient apply to diagnosis of the acute, newly acquired *Toxoplasma* infection in the immunodeficient patient. However, serodiagnosis may be difficult due to a depressed antibody response. For example, among 40 AIDS patients with cerebral toxoplasmosis, only 1 had detectable IgM antibody, and seroconversion or a serial two-tube rise in IgG antibody titer usually was not documented.[48] In another study of toxoplasmic encephalitis in AIDS patients, the modified direct agglutination test frequently showed markedly elevated titers when dye or IFA test titers were low[110] and thus may be useful for diagnosis. French investigators have found a higher incidence of positive IgM test findings and higher IgG titers than have investigators in the United States.[111] For a secure diagnosis in immunodeficient patients, a demonstration of *Toxoplasma* in tissue sections or body fluids is usually needed. The recently developed ELISA technique for detecting *Toxoplasma* antigens in serum and body fluids may prove useful.[93] Demonstration of the intrathecal production of *Toxoplasma*-specific antibody may help to diagnose toxoplasmic encephalitis. In one study, 70 percent of 16 AIDS patients with toxoplasmic encephalitis had intrathecal antibody production as determined by an index of more than 1 and calculated by the formula: index = (CSF dye test titer [reciprocal] × total serum IgG)/(total CSF IgG × serum dye test titer [reciprocal]).[65]

Serologic tests should be performed to identify people who are at risk of acute *Toxoplasma* infection. These include seronegative transplant organ recipients who may acquire the disease from seropositive organ donors,[19,69] seronegative patients who develop an acute acquired infection while immunosuppressed, and seropositive patients who may reactivate their chronic infection during immunosuppression.[67,68,71] Of note is that seropositive recipients of heart transplants frequently exhibit increased titers of IgG and IgM antibody after organ transplantation without clinical evidence of active infection.[69]

Ocular Toxoplasmosis. Low titers of IgG antibody are usual in patients with active *Toxoplasma* chorioretinitis, and IgM antibody usually cannot be detected. *Toxoplasma* chorioretinitis is probably excluded when serologic tests for IgG antibody yield negative results when performed on undiluted serum. When the retinal lesion is characteristic and the serologic titer is positive, most authorities consider that *Toxoplasma* chorioretinitis can be diagnosed with confidence.[34] When the retinal lesion is atypical and the serologic titer is positive, the diagnosis of *Toxoplasma* chorioretinitis is only presumptive since the high prevalence of antibodies in the healthy population precludes the assumption of a causal relationship.

High antibody titers in the aqueous humor (as well as in CSF) may reflect local antibody production, and their presence has proved very useful in diagnosis of active disease. The significance of these titers can be assessed with the following formula, provided the serum dye test titer is less than or equal to 1:1000:

$$C = \left[\frac{\text{Antibody titer in fluid} \times \text{Concentration of } \gamma\text{-globulin in serum}}{\text{Antibody titer in serum} \times \text{Concentration of } \gamma\text{-globulin in body fluid}} \right.$$

If C is greater than or equal to 8, local antibody production is probable and supports the diagnosis of active *Toxoplasma* infection. The method has been used successfully with both dye test and IgM-IFA test titers.[112] A similar approach with an enzyme immunoassay for IgG antibody has been reported for the diagnosis of ocular toxoplasmosis.[113]

Congenital Toxoplasma Infection or Toxoplasmosis. The diagnosis of *Toxoplasma* infection in the neonate is based on finding one (or both) of the following: (*1*) persistent or rising titers in the dye test or IFA test and (*2*) a positive test result for IgM antibody at any titer after birth in the absence of a placental leak.[1]

Since IgG antibody may be transferred passively from the mother to the fetus across the placenta, IgG antibody titers in a newborn may reflect recent or remote infection in the mother. These IgG antibodies have a half-life of approximately 21 days and may persist in the infant for as long as 12 months after birth, depending upon the original antibody titer. Synthesis of IgG antibody by the infant is usually demonstrable by the third month of life if the infant is not treated for toxoplasmosis; antibody synthesis may be delayed until the sixth or ninth month of life if the infant is treated. At the time the infant begins to synthesize IgG antibody, infection can be documented by computing the specific antibody load, that is, the ratio of specific serum antibody titer to the level of serum IgG in the infant. In the absence of infection, the antibody load decreases in the second or third month as the infant produces IgG that does not contain specific antibody to *Toxoplasma*. If the infant is infected with *Toxoplasma*, the antibody load remains the same or increases.[1]

For detection of IgM antibody, the DS-IgM-ELISA is preferred to the IgM-IFA test since the former has greater sensitivity and specificity. The DS-IgM-ELISA detects approximately 75 percent of congenitally infected infants, whereas the IgM-IFA test detects only 25 percent of infected infants. In addition, the IgM-IFA test may yield positive results due to rheumatoid factor made by the fetus and directed against maternal IgG.[114] When maternal IgM has been transferred to the infant via a placental leak, the IgM titer of the infant will fall markedly during the first week of life due to the short half-life (approximately 5 days) of IgM antibody. Even though IgM antibody may not be detected in the infected infant's initial serum specimen, it may be detected later in follow-up sera and thus secure the diagnosis of *Toxoplasma* infection. Use of the Western blot technique has shown that maternal and infant sera may recognize different *Toxoplasma* antigens when the infant is congenitally infected.[96] Thus this technique has promise for the early diagnosis of congenital infection, possibly even in utero.

Toxoplasma Infection in Pregnancy. Acute acquired *Toxoplasma* infection is diagnosed serologically by the same methods used for immunocompetent adults, but special care is directed to a determination of whether infection was acquired before or after conception (see below, "Serologic Screening"). However, this determination is frequently difficult. As noted earlier ("Congenital Toxoplasmosis"), transmission of infection across the placenta to the fetus is relatively unlikely for infections acquired in the first and second trimesters; if abortions are performed routinely for infections acquired in the first trimester, about nine normal fetuses will be aborted for every infected fetus.

Recent data from France show that it is now possible to determine reliably which fetuses are infected, thus allowing more reasoned decisions regarding the aggressiveness of chemotherapy and abortion. A group of 746 pregnant women with acute acquired *Toxoplasma* infection were prospectively identified.[115,116] Fetal blood, amniotic fluid, and fetal ultrasounds to detect ventricular enlargement were obtained at 20–24 weeks of gestation. Fetal blood and amniotic fluid were injected into mice to recover *Toxoplasma*. Of 42 congenitally infected infants, 39 (93 percent) were identified prenatally by at least one of the three tests, but no single test was very sensitive. The mothers who completed their pregnancies were treated aggressively with chemotherapy. Most of the infected infants did not have signs of congenital toxoplasmosis, and the remainder did not have functional deficits. This approach potentially can drastically reduce the ravages of congenital toxoplasmosis. The key to its implementation is a serologic screening program to detect women who acquire the acute infection during gestation and who therefore are candidates for prenatal diagnosis. Prenatal diagnosis of congenital toxoplasmosis can be done reliably only at some referral centers in the United States at present.

TREATMENT

The lack of controlled trials and the variable course of toxoplasmosis have resulted in uncertainty and controversy regarding the specific indications for treatment, the drugs to be used for treatment, and the duration of treatment. A lack of appropriate models of the different types of infection has stalled the development of appropriate treatment regimens. The recent development of models of intracerebral[117] and ocular toxoplasmosis[118] may aid the evaluation of new treatment regimens. The following rccommendations are derived from clinical experience at several medical centers.

Treatment Regimens

Acute Acquired Toxoplasma Infection in the Immunocompetent Patient. Immunocompetent adults with the acquired lymphadenopathic form are usually not treated unless visceral disease is clinically overt or symptoms are unusually severe or persistent. Treatment is usually administered for 2–4 months, followed by reassessment of the patient's condition. Infections acquired by laboratory accident or transfusion of blood products are potentially more severe, and patients with these infections probably should be treated.[16,17]

Acute Toxoplasmosis in the Immunodeficient Patient. Immunodeficient patients should always be treated when the infection is acute. Treatment is given until 4–6 weeks after resolution of all signs and symptoms (often for 6 months or longer). At one medical center, 80 percent of the immunodeficient patients with toxoplasmosis improved with specific therapy.[119] Chronic (latent) asymptomatic infection in the immunodeficient patient is not treated. Patients who have received heart or other organ transplants and who were seropositive for antibody to *Toxoplasma* before receiving the transplant may have rises in serologic test titers and may have IgG or IgM antibodies.[69] These rises in antibody titers may not necessarily reflect active *Toxoplasma* infection.

AIDS has allowed collection of data on the treatment of toxoplasmosis, primarily toxoplasmic encephalitis, in immunodeficient patients. The *Toxoplasma* Encephalitis Study Group retrospectively surveyed 61 AIDS patients with toxoplasmic encephalitis identified up to March 1984 in the United States.[56] Ninety-five percent of the patients were treated initially with pyrimethamine and sulfonamide, with treatment being continued for a median of 43 days. Drug toxicity, observed in 60 percent of the patients, was cited as the most frequent reason for discontinuation of therapy, which was considered necessary in 45 percent of patients. Discontinuation of therapy was frequently associated with relapse of toxoplasmic encephalitis. *Toxoplasma* organisms often were found in brain tissue at autopsy examination, which suggested that therapy did not reliably eradicate *Toxoplasma* from brains of AIDS patients. The overall prognosis of AIDS patients with toxoplasmic encephalitis was poor, with a median survival of 4 months after the start of therapy. The best predictor for a good response was an alert mental status at the start of treatment. The efficacy of corticosteroids could not be determined from this review. French investigators reported similar findings.[111] Complete clinical responses were achieved initially with pyrimethamine and sulfadiazine in 29 percent of the patients, partial improvement in 60 percent, and failure (death) in 11 percent. Of note, 10 episodes of relapse occurred in 6 of 24 evaluable patients. Relapse usually occurred within 6 weeks of discontinuation of therapy; two patients relapsed while receiving pyrimethamine alone at a dose of 25 mg/day. Reinstitution of pyrimethamine and sulfadiazine controlled the relapse in 8 of the 10 episodes. Clinical improvement is usually seen within 1 week[58] of the start of treatment and CT scan improvement within 2–4 weeks.[62]

The high recurrence rate and failure to eradicate *Toxoplasma* from brains suggests a need for prolonged, perhaps lifelong therapy, at least with the presently available agents. However, drug toxicity dramatically compromises the length of therapy and has prompted searches for alternative strategies. Bone marrow suppression and skin rash are particularly frequent with pyrimethamine–sulfa, and bone marrow suppression may be augmented by use of other chemotherapeutic agents such as azidothymidine. In patients with rashes attributed to sulfonamide, investigators have reported successful desensitization to sulfonamide[120,121] or successful use of a different sulfonamide preparation. The sulfonamide has been replaced in some cases by clindamycin (600–1200 mg q6h iv or 600 mg q6h po).[56,122–125] Experience with these strategies is limited at present. Trimethoprim-sulfamethoxazole has proved inferior to pyrimethamine and sulfadiazine in an animal model of toxoplasmosis,[126] and patients have developed toxoplasmic encephalitis while receiving trimethoprim-sulfamethoxazole for suppression of *Pneumocystis carinii*.[56] Thus this combination cannot be recommended for the treatment of toxoplasmic encephalitis. Spiramycin has not prevented toxoplasmic encephalitis in immunosuppressed patients.[127] A new macrolide antibiotic, roxithromycin, provides higher serum levels and has a longer half-life than do presently available macrolides and is effective in a murine model of toxoplasmosis.[128–130] Trimetrexate, a folic acid antagonist that has been used experimentally to treat *Pneumocystis* pneumonia in humans, has been shown effective against *Toxoplasma* in vitro and in vivo.[131]

Ocular Toxoplasmosis. Specific treatment of patients with ocular toxoplasmosis has resulted in the resolution of signs and symptoms. According to one regimen, pyrimethamine and sulfadiazine (or trisulfapyrimidines) are administered for 1 month. Within 10 days, a favorable response can be detected in up to 70 percent of the cases, and lesions are healed, on average, by the 9th or 10th week.[132] The average duration of an untreated attack has been reported to be 4.2 months.[133] If necessary, repeated courses of drugs are administered. Clindamycin (300 mg po q6h for a minimum of 3 weeks) has also been used with favorable clinical results.[74,134,135] Systemic corticosteroids are indicated when lesions involve the macula, optic nerve head, or papillomacular bundle. Photocoagulation has been used both for the treatment of active lesions and for prophylaxis against the spread of lesions since new lesions appear contiguous to old lesions.[136] In some patients, vitrectomy and lentectomy may be necessary.[137]

Acute Acquired Toxoplasma Infection in Pregnant Women. Treatment of the acutely infected pregnant woman does not eliminate but does decrease the incidence of fetal infection. In one study, the incidence of fetal infection was 17 percent in infants born to women who were not treated during pregnancy and 5 percent in infants born to women who were treated during pregnancy[1]; in a second study, the figures were 58 and 23 percent, respectively.[138,139] Two different treatment regimens have proved effective. Spiramycin at 3 g/day given in three or four divided doses can be used throughout gestation.[1] After the first trimester, the combination of pyrimethamine plus sulfadiazine can be used.[134,135] This combination was used with great success in treatment of infected fetuses when the diagnosis was made prenatally as discussed above ("Serologic Diagnosis: *Toxoplasma* Infection in Pregnancy").[115] Other variations of these regimens have been used with apparent success. Because pyrimethamine is teratogenic in laboratory animals, it should not be used during the first 14–16 weeks of pregnancy. There are no data regarding the safety or efficacy of trimethoprim-sulfamethoxazole or clindamycin in this clinical setting, nor are there data on the efficacy of sulfonamides without pyrimethamine.

Congenital Toxoplasmosis. Results of uncontrolled studies in humans and controlled studies in experimental animals suggest that postnatal treatment may prevent the development of untoward sequelae in both symptomatic and asymptomatic infants with congenital *Toxoplasma* infection.[1] The best guidelines for treatment that can be offered at present are shown in Table 1. Healthy-appearing newborns in whom *Toxoplasma* infection is suspected but not confirmed by serologic tests should be treated with pyrimethamine plus sulfadiazine for 21 days, followed by spiramycin or sulfadiazine alone until the diagnosis is established. If the diagnosis is confirmed, treatment should be for a minimum of 6 months in infants born without signs of the infection and for 1 year if there are signs of significant damage.

Drugs

The most effective available therapeutic regimen is the combination of pyrimethamine plus sulfadiazine (or trisulfapyrimidines—sufamerazine, sulfamethazine and sulfadiazine). These agents are active against trophozoites and are synergistic in combination. However, the tissue cyst form of *Toxoplasma* is resistant to presently available antimicrobial agents, including pyrimethamine and sulfadiazine.

Pyrimethamine is lipid soluble, is readily absorbed from the gastrointestinal tract, and has a half-life of 4–5 days. The CSF concentrations have been found to be 10–25 percent of simultaneous plasma concentrations. A study in patients with toxoplasmic encephalitis showed that serum levels varied markedly between patients receiving similar dosages, that toxoplasmacidal levels can be but probably are not always attained in the CSF (especially when pyrimethamine is used without sulfa), and that measurement of serum levels could be useful.[140]

The loading regimen of pyrimethamine for adults is 200 mg/day in two divided doses for 1 day. Sulfa, as described below, is used with pyrimethamine. Regimens after loading doses of pyrimethamine and sulfa depend upon the severity of disease and the immunocompetence of the patient. For immunocompetent patients, pyrimethamine is usually given for 2–4 weeks (or for the second and third trimesters if the patient is pregnant) at 25–50 mg/day, although administration at 2- to 4-day intervals has been suggested in view of pyrimethamine's 4- to 5-day half-life. For immunodeficient patients, pyrimethamine is given for a minimum of 4–6 weeks at 25–50 mg/day. For AIDS patients, 75–100 mg/day is being used for 3–6 weeks, followed by maintenance therapy. For ocular toxoplasmosis, pyrimethamine is used at doses up to 50 mg/day. Pyrimethamine is available only in 25 mg tablets; there is no parenteral form.

TABLE 1. Treatment of the Congenitally Infected Infant[a]

1. Pyrimethamine, 15 mg/m² or 1 mg/kg every 2 days,[b] plus sulfadiazine or trisulfapyrimidines, 100 mg/kg/day in two doses, plus folinic acid, 5 mg every other day. Twice weekly monitor complete blood counts and platelet counts.
2. Spiramycin, 100 mg/kg/day in 2–3 dosages per day; 21-day courses of pyrimethamine plus sulfadiazine may be alternated with 4- to 6-wk courses of spiramycin.
3. Corticosteroids (prednisone 1–2 mg/kg/day) may be added for patients with active chorioretinitis that involves the macula.

[a] The appropriateness of treatment, treatment regimen, and duration of treatment must be considered individually. See the text for additional discussion.
[b] A loading dose is recommended in patients with evidence of severe organ involvement. See the text.

Maintenance therapy is used in AIDS patients because of their high risk of relapse of disease when chemotherapy is stopped. Optimal maintenance therapy for AIDS patients has as yet not been defined. Two regimens are being used at present. One is 50 mg pyrimethamine plus 2 g of sulfa daily; the other is Fansidar at two tablets once weekly. Maintenance pyrimethamine and sulfa at these doses can be tried three times weekly if compliance is not a problem.

Pyrimethamine is a folic acid antagonist, and the most common side effect is dose-related suppression of the bone marrow. A peripheral blood cell and platelet count should be performed twice a week. The risk of these adverse effects may be decreased by concomitant administration of folinic acid (calcium leucovorin). The parenteral form of folinic acid is well absorbed orally, and 5–10 mg of folinic acid (up to 50 mg/day is being used in AIDS patients) may be given orally with orange juice at the same time as the pyrimethamine. Folinic acid does not inhibit the action of pyrimethamine on trophozoites. Less serious side effects of pyrimethamine include gastrointestinal distress, headaches, and a bad taste in the mouth.

Since sulfadiazine, or trisulfapyrimidines, act synergistically with pyrimethamine, one of these drugs is usually given in combination with pyrimethamine. Sulfamethazine and sulfamerazine have activity similar to that of sulfadiazine, whereas all other sulfonamides tested are inferior. The half-life of sulfadiazine is approximately 10–12 hours. A loading dose of 75 mg/kg up to 4 g. is given. Thereafter, 100 mg/kg/day up to 8 g/day is given in two divided doses. The patient must maintain a good urine output to prevent crystalluria and oliguria. Alkalinization of the urine with oral sodium bicarbonate also reduces the chance of crystalluria. The maintenance dose of sulfadiazine for AIDS patients is 500 mg po q6h. Tablets and a liquid oral form of sulfadiazine are available.

Spiramycin, clindamycin, and trimethoprim-sulfamethoxazole are less active than is the combination of pyrimethamine and sulfadiazine. Spiramycin is less toxic than is pyrimethamine plus sulfadiazine, has been used effectively for the treatment of pregnant women, and may be effective in the treatment of infants with congenital infection. This agent is readily available in most countries except the United States. (It can be obtained through the Food and Drug Administration in the United States.) Spiramycin is given orally, 3 g/day for adults, in two to four divided doses. Clindamycin is concentrated in the choroid and has been used in the treatment of ocular disease and also as second-line therapy for toxoplasmic encephalitis in AIDS patients. This drug has not yet proved useful in controlled clinical trials. In studies that report the beneficial effects of trimethoprim-sulfamethoxazole in humans, necessary controls have been omitted; it is therefore unclear whether the effects observed were due to spontaneous resolution or to the sulfonamide component alone. Since sulfamethoxazole is less active than sulfadiazine is, trimethoprim-sulfamethoxazole cannot be recommended at present.

PREVENTION

General Methods

Prevention is most important in seronegative pregnant women and in immunodeficient patients. Prevention is most readily accomplished through education of these patients by their personal physicians. The goal is to avoid ingestion of and contact with cysts or sporulated oocysts. Cysts in meat are made noninfectious by heating the meat to 66°C, by smoking or curing it, or by freezing it to −20°C (which is not attained in most home freezers). Hands should be washed thoroughly after handling raw meat or vegetables, eggs should not be eaten raw, and unpasteurized milk (particularly milk from goats) should be avoided. Vectors such as flies and cockroaches should be controlled.

Cat feces should be avoided altogether. Disposable gloves should be worn while disposing of cat litter material, working in the garden, or cleaning a child's sandbox. Oocysts are killed if the cat litter pan is soaked in nearly boiling water for 5 minutes. If the litter pan is cleaned every day, oocysts will not have a chance to sporulate. Serologic testing of cats is unwarranted since testing will not demonstrate whether the acutely infected cat is excreting oocysts.

Serologic Screening

Acute Toxoplasma Infection or Toxoplasmosis in the Immunodeficient Patient. Transmission of *Toxoplasma* and death due to the infection have resulted from the transfusion of leukocyte-rich blood products and by organ transplantation in immunodeficient patients. Transmission of infection by these routes may occur frequently enough to warrant screening for antibody to *Toxoplasma* in blood product donors and possibly to exclude seropositive people as organ donors to seronegative potential recipients. Prophylactic treatment (pyrimethamine at 25 mg po qd for 6 weeks post-transplantation) has been used with apparent success in seronegative recipients of hearts transplanted from seropositive donors.[141]

Congenital Toxoplasma Infection or Toxoplasmosis. Serologic screening can be used to prevent congenital *Toxoplasma* infection and toxoplasmosis. For a successful screening program and to avoid tragedies, the appropriate tests must be used, the laboratory performing the tests must be competent, and the test results must be interpreted correctly.

The frequency of serologic screening during gestation is an important consideration that is affected by the epidemiology of the infection and the cost of screening, its cost-effectiveness, and its feasibility. In some centers, initially seronegative pregnant women are tested every month during gestation; this schedule is optimal for detecting infection early enough to institute proper medical management. However, based on monetary constraints and epidemiologic considerations in the United States, we have recommended that a serologic test equal in sensitivity, specificity, and reproducibility to the dye test (e.g., IFA test or agglutination test) be performed on all pregnant women as early as possible, at least by 10–12 weeks' gestation, to identify those at risk. Those pregnant women who are seronegative initially should then be tested again, within 20–22 weeks of gestation, to determine whether infection was acquired in the interim. This would allow sufficient time for a decision regarding possible therapeutic abortion to be made or for specific treatment to be started in women with positive results (see the section on treatment, above). A third test would be performed near or at term in seronegative women so that those who acquired infection and their offspring can be identified and appropriately treated. Women identified as possibly having the acute acquired infection can be considered for prenatal diagnosis (see "*Toxoplasma* Infection in Pregnancy"). Appropriate use of prenatal diagnosis can markedly reduce the incidence of clinically significant congenital toxoplasmosis, as has been demonstrated in France.[115,116] However, a systematic screening program as outlined above is necessary to achieve results similar to those in France where systematic, periodic screening is mandated by law.

Women with positive results in the initial test would have a test for IgM antibody performed on the same serum to detect recent infection. In patients with IgG antibodies at any titer, a negative IgM antibody test result in the first trimester, and no clinical signs of acute toxoplasmosis, no further testing would be necessary since the probability of acute acquired infection in these women is very low. Given the same circumstances in the second trimester of pregnancy, a negative DS-IgM-ELISA result rules out, for practical purposes, the acquisition of acute infection before conception. It is for this reason that the DS-IgM-ELISA is preferable.

REFERENCES

1. Remington JS, Desmonts G. Toxoplasmosis. In: Remington JS, Klein JO, eds: Infectious Diseases of the Fetus and Newborn Infant. Philadelphia: WB Saunders; 1983:143.
2. Nichols BA, Chiappino ML, O'Connor GR. Secretion from the rhoptries of *Toxoplasma gondii* during host-cell invasion. J. Ultrastruct Res. 1983;83:85.
3. Schwartzman JD. Inhibition of a penetration-enhancing factor of *Toxoplasma gondii* by monoclonal antibodies specific for rhoptries. Infect Immun. 1986;51:760.
4. Miller NL, Frenkel JK, Dubey JP. Oral infections with *Toxoplasma* cysts and oocysts in felines, other mammals and in birds. J Parasitol. 1970;58:928.
5. Frenkel JK: Toxoplasmosis: Parasite life cycle, pathology, and immunology. In: Hammand DM, ed. The Coccidia. Baltimore: University Park Press; 1973:343.
6. Dubey JP, Miller NL, Frenkel JK. The *Toxoplasma gondii* oocyst from cat feces. J Exp Med. 1970;133:636.
7. Wallace GD. The role of the cat in the natural history of *Toxoplasma gondii*. Am J Trop Med Hyg. 1973;22:313.
8. Wallace GD. Serologic and epidemiologic observations on toxoplasmosis on three Pacific atolls. Am J Epidemiol. 1969;90:103.
9. Dubey JP. A review of toxoplasmosis in pigs. Vet Parasitol. 1986;19:181.
10. Riemann HP, Meyer ME, Theis JH, et al. Toxoplasmosis in an infant fed unpasteurized goat milk. J Pediatr. 1975;87:573.
11. Sacks JJ, Roberto RR, Brooks WF. Toxoplasmosis infection associated with new goat's milk. JAMA. 1982;248:1728.
12. Swartzberg JE, Remington JS. Transmission of *Toxoplasma*. Am J Dis Child. 1975;129:777.
13. Luft BJ, Remington JS. Acute *Toxoplasma* infection among family members of patients with acute lymphadenopathic toxoplasmosis. Arch Intern Med. 1984;144:53.
14. Beach PG. Prevalence of antibodies to *Toxoplasma gondii* in pregnant women in Oregon. J Infect Dis. 1979;140:780.
15. Papoz L, Simondon F, Saurin W, et al. A simple model revelant to toxoplasmosis applied to epidemiologic results in France. Am J Epidemiol. 1986;123:1545.
16. Neu HC. Toxoplasmosis transmitted at autopsy. JAMA. 1967;202:284.
17. Siegel SE, Lunde MN, Gelderman AH, et al. Transmission of toxoplasmosis by leukocyte transfusion. Blood. 1971;37:388.
18. Britt RH, Enzmann DR, Remington JS: Intracranial infection in cardiac transplant recipients. Ann Neurol. 1981;9:107.
19. Ryning FW, McLeod R, Maddox JC, et al. Probable transmission of *Toxoplasma gondii* by organ transplantation. Ann Intern Med. 1979;90:47.
20. Sibley LD, Weidner E, Krahenbuhl JL. Phagosome acidification blocked by intracellular *Toxoplasma gondii*. Nature. 1985;315:416.
21. Murray HW, Rubin BY, Carriero SM, et al. Human mononuclear phagocyte antiprotozoal mechanisms: Oxygen-dependent vs. oxygen-independent activity against intracellular *Toxoplasma gondii*. J Immunol. 1985;134:1982.
22. Suzuki Y, Orellana MA, Schreiber RD, et al. Interferon-gamma: The major mediator of resistance against *Toxoplasma gondii*. Science. 1988;240:516.
23. McCabe RE, Luft BJ, Remington JS. Effect of murine interferon gamma on murine toxoplasmosis. J Infect Dis. 1984;150:961.
24. Wilson CB, Haas JE. Cellular defenses against *Toxoplasma gondii* in newborns. J Clin Invest. 1984;73:1606.
25. Sharma SD, Hofflin JM, Remington JS. In vivo recombinant interleukin 2 administration enhances survival against a lethal challenge with *Toxoplasma gondii*. J Immunol. 1985;135:4160.
26. Luft BJ, Remington JS. Effect of pregnancy on resistance to *Listeria monocytogenes* and *Toxoplasma gondii*. Infections in mice. Infect Immun. 1982;38:1164.
27. Luft BJ, Remington JS. Effect of pregnancy on augmentation of natural killer cell activity by *Corynebacterium parvum* and *Toxoplasma gondii*. J Immunol. 1984;132:2375.
28. Dorfman RF, Remington JS. Value of lymph node biopsy in the diagnosis of acute acquired toxoplasmosis. N Engl J Med. 1973;289:878.
29. Frenkel JK. Pathology and pathogenesis of congenital toxoplasmosis. Bull NY Acad Med. 1974;50:182.
30. Ruskin J, Remington JS. Toxoplasmosis in the compromised host. Ann Intern Med. 1971;74:22.
31. Vietzke WM, Gelderman AH, Grimley PM, et al. Toxoplasmosis complicating malignancy: Experience of the National Cancer Institute. Cancer. 1968;21:816.
32. McLeod R, Berry PF, Marshall WH, et al. Toxoplasmosis presenting as brain abscesses: Diagnosis by computerized tomography and cytology of aspirated purulent material. Am J Med. 1979;67:711.

33. Bobowski SJ, Reed WG. Toxoplasmosis in an adult presenting as a space-occupying cerebral lesion. Arch Pathol. 1958;65:460.
34. O'Connor GR. Manifestations and management of ocular toxoplasmosis. Bull NY Acad Med. 1974;50:192.
35. O'Connor GR. The influence of hypersensitivity on the pathogenesis of ocular toxoplasmosis. Trans Am Ophthalmol Soc. 1970;68:501.
36. Sabates R, Pruett RC, Brockhurst RJ. Fulminant ocular toxoplasmosis. Am J Ophthalmol. 1981;92:497.
37. Remington JS: Toxoplasmosis in the adult. Bull NY Acad Med. 1974;50:211.
38. McCabe RE, Brooks RG, Dorfman RF, et al. Clinical spectrum in 107 cases of toxoplasmic lymphadenopathy. Rev Infect Dis. 1987;9:754.
39. Kean BH. Clinical toxoplasmosis: 50 years. Trans R Soc Trop Med Hyg. 1972;66:549.
40. Remington JS, Barnett CG, Meikel M, et al. Toxoplasmosis and infectious mononucleosis. Arch Intern Med. 1962;110:744.
41. Faruqi AMA, Frank M, Rosvali RV, et al. Acute acquired toxoplasmosis. South Med J. 1976;69:1234.
42. Masur H, Jones TC, Lempert JA, et al. Outbreak of toxoplasmosis in a family and documentation of acquired retinochoroiditis. Am J Med. 1978;66:396.
43. Michaelson JB, Shields JA, McDonald PR, et al. Retinitis secondary to acquired systemic toxoplasmosis with isolation of the parasite. Am J Ophthalmol. 1978;86:548.
44. Gump DW, Holden RA. Acquired chorioretinitis due to toxoplasmosis. Ann Intern Med. 1979;90:58.
45. Perkins FS. Ocular toxoplasmosis. Br J Ophthalmol. 1973;57:1.
46. Sheagren JN, Lunde MN, Simon HB: Chronic lymphadenopathic toxoplasmosis. A case with marked hyperglobulinemia and impaired delayed hypersensitivity responses during active infection. Am J Med. 1976;60:300.
47. Wong B, Gold JM, Brown AE, et al. Central nervous system toxoplasmosis in homosexual men and parenteral drug abusers. Ann Intern Med. 1984;100:36.
48. Luft BJ, Brooks RG, Conley FK, et al. Toxoplasmic encephalitis in patients with acquired immune deficiency syndrome. JAMA. 1984;252:913.
49. Luft BJ, Remington JS. Toxoplasmic encephalitis. J Infect Dis. 1988;157:1.
50. Levy RM, Bredesen DE, Rosenblum ML. Neurological manifestations of the acquired immunodeficiency syndrome (AIDS). Experience at UCSF and review of the literature. J Neurosurg. 1985;62:475.
51. Pitchenik AE, Fischl MA, Walls KW. Evaluation of cerebral-mass lesions in acquired immunodeficiency disease. N Engl J Med. 1983;308:1099.
52. Weiss A, Margo CE, Ledford DK, et al. Toxoplasmic retinochoroiditis as an initial manifestation of the acquired immune deficiency syndrome. Am J Ophthalmol. 1986;101:248.
53. Catterall JR, Hofflin JM, Remington JS. Pulmonary toxoplasmosis. Am Rev Respir Dis. 1986;133:704.
54. Nistol M, Santara A, Paniaqua R, et al. Testicular toxoplasmosis in two men with the acquired immunodeficiency syndrome (AIDS). Arch Pathol Lab Med. 1986;110:744.
55. Hofflin JM, Remington JS. Tissue culture isolation of *Toxoplasma* from blood of a patient with AIDS. Arch Intern Med. 1985;145:925.
56. Haverkos HW. Assessment of therapy for *Toxoplasma* encephalitis. The TE study group. Am J Med. 1987;82:907.
57. Levy RM, Pons VG, Rosenblum ML. Central nervous system mass lesions in the acquired immunodeficiency syndrome (AIDS). J Neurosurg. 1984;61:9.
58. Handler M, Ho V, Whelan M, et al. Intracerebral toxoplasmosis in patients with acquired immune deficiency syndrome. J Neurosurg. 1983;59:994.
59. Horowitz SL, Bentson JAR, Benson DF, et al. CNS toxoplasmosis in acquired immunodeficiency syndrome. Arch Neurol. 1983;40:649.
60. Chan JC, Moskowitz LB, Olivella J, et al. *Toxoplasma* encephalitis in recent Haitian entrants. South Med J. 1983;76:1211.
61. Post MJD, Kursunoglu SJ, Hensley GT, et al. Cranial CT in acquired immunodeficiency syndrome. Spectrum of diseases and optimal contrast enhancement technique. AJR. 1985;145:929.
62. Post MJD, Chan JC, Hensley GT, et al. *Toxoplasma* encephalitis in Haitian adults with acquired immunodeficiency syndrome. A clinical-pathologic-CT correlation. AJR. 1983;140:861.
63. Fischl MA, Pitchenik AE, Spira TJ. Tuberculous brain abscess and *Toxoplasma* encephalitis in a patient with acquired immunodeficiency syndrome. JAMA. 1985;253:3428.
64. Zee CS, Segall HD, Rogers C, et al. MR imaging of cerebral toxoplasmosis. Correlation of computed tomography and pathology. J Comput Assist Tomogr. 1985;9:797.
65. Potasman I, Resnick L, Luft BJ, et al. Intrathecal production of antibodies against *T. gondii* in patients with toxoplasmic encephalitis and AIDS. Ann Intern Med. 1988;108:49.
66. Wanke C, Tuazon CU, Kovacs A, et al. *Toxoplasma* encephalitis in patients with acquired immune deficiency syndrome: Diagnosis and response to therapy. Am J Trop Med Hyg. 1987;36:509.
67. Shepp DH, Hackman RC, Conley FK, et al. *Toxoplasma gondii* reactivation identified by detection of parasitemia in tissue culture. Ann Intern Med. 1985;103:218.
68. John U, Fink M, Gundlach P, et al. Lethal cardiac and cerebral toxoplasmosis in a patient with acute myeloid leukemia after successful allogeneic bone marrow transplantation. Transplantation. 1984;38:430.
69. Luft BJ, Naot Y, Araujo FG, et al. Primary and reactivated *Toxoplasma* infection in patients with cardiac transplants: Clinical spectrum and problems in diagnosis in a defined population. Ann Intern Med. 1983;99:27.
70. McGregor CGA, Fleck DG, Nagington J, et al. Disseminated toxoplasmosis in cardiac transplantation. J Clin Pathol. 1984;37:74.
71. Hakes TB, Armstrong D. Toxoplasmosis. Problems in diagnosis and treatment. Cancer. 1983;52:1535.
72. Gleason TH, Hamlin WB. Disseminated toxoplasmosis in the compromised host. A report of five cases. Arch Intern Med. 1974;134:1059.
73. Koch FLP, Wolf A, Cowen D, et al. Toxoplasmic encephalomyelitis. VII. Significance of ocular lesions in the diagnosis of infantile or congenital toxoplasmosis. Arch Ophthalmol. 1943;29:1.
74. Canamucio CJ, Hallett JW, Leopold IH. Recurrence of treated toxoplasmic uveitis. Am J Ophthalmol. 1963;55:1035.
75. Lakhanpal V, Schocket SS, Nirankeri VS. Clindamycin in the treatment of toxoplasmic retinchoroiditis. Am J Ophthalmol. 1983;95:605.
76. Remington JS: Toxoplasmosis and human abortion. In Meigs JV, Sturgis SH, eds: Progress in Gynecology. V. 4. New York: Grune & Stratton; 1963;303.
77. Desmonts G, Couvreur J. Congenital toxoplasmosis. A prospective study of the offspring of 54 women who acquired toxoplasmosis during pregnancy. Pathophysiology of congenital disease. In: Thalhammer O, Baumgarten K, Pollak A, eds. Perinatal Medicine, Sixth European Congress, Vienna, 1978. Stuttgart: Thieme; 1979.
78. Alford CA, Stagno S, Reynolds DW: Congenital toxoplasmosis: Clinical, laboratory, and therapeutic considerations, with special reference to subclinical disease. Bull NY Acad Med. 1974;50:160.
79. Couvreur J, Desmonts G, Tournier G, et al. Etude d'une serie homogene de 210 cas de toxoplasmose congenitale chez des nourissons ages de 0 a 11 mois et depistes de facon prospective. Ann Pediatr (Paris). 1984;31:815.
80. Wilson CB, Remington JS, Stagno S, et al. Development of adverse sequelae in children born with subclinical congenital *Toxoplasma* infection. Pediatrics. 1980;66:767.
81. de Roever-Bonnet H, Koppe JG, Loewer-Dieger DH: Follow-up of children with congenital *Toxoplasma* infections and children who became serologically negative after 1 year of age, all born in 1964–1965. In: Thalhammer O, Baumgarten K, Pollack A, eds. Perinatal Medicine, Sixth European Congress, Vienna, 1978. Stuttgart: Thieme; 1979:61.
82. Labadie MD, Hazemann JJ. Apport des bilans de sante de l'enfant pour le depistage et l'etude epidemiologique de la toxoplasmose congenitale. Ann Pediatr (Paris). 1984;31:823.
83. Miller MJ, Aronson WJ, Remington JS. Late parasitemia in asymptomatic acquired toxoplasmosis. Ann Intern Med. 1969;71:139.
84. Frenkel JK, Piekarski G. The demonstration of *Toxoplasma* and other organisms by immunofluorescene: A pitfall. J Infect Dis. 1980;141:149.
85. Conley FK, Jenkins HT, Remington JS. *Toxoplasma gondii* infection of the central nervous system. Hum Pathol. 1980;12:690.
86. Moskowitz LB, Hensley GT, Chan JC, et al. The neuropathology of acquired immune deficiency syndrome. Arch Pathol Lab Med. 1984;108:867.
87. van Knapen F, Panggabean SO. Detection of *Toxoplasma* antigen in tissues by means of enzyme-linked immunosorbent assay (ELISA). Am J Clin Pathol. 1982;77:755.
88. Sun T, Greenspan J, Tenenbaum M, et al. Diagnosis of cerebral toxoplasmosis using fluorescein-labeled antitoxoplasma monoclonal antibodies. Am J Surg Pathol. 1986;10:312.
89. Cevezo L, Alvarez M, Price G. Electron microscopic diagnosis of cerebral toxoplasmosis. J Neurosurg. 1985;63:470.
90. Rougier D, Ambroise-Thomas P. Detection of toxoplasmic immunity by multipuncture skin test with excretory-secretory antigen. Lancet. 1985;2:121.
91. Wilson CB, Desmonts G, Couvreur J, et al. Lymphocyte transformation in the diagnosis of congenital *Toxoplasma* infection. N Engl J Med. 1980;302:785.
92. Luft BJ, Pedrotti PW, Engleman EC, et al. Induction of antigen-specific suppressor T cells during acute infection with *Toxoplasma gondii*. J Infect Dis. 1987;155:1033.
93. Araujo FG, Remington JS: Antigenemia in recently acquired acute toxoplasmosis. J Infect Dis. 1980;141:144.
94. Lindenschmidt EG. Enzyme-linked immunosorbent assay for detection of soluble *Toxoplasma gondii* antigen in acute phase toxoplasmosis. Eur J Clin Microbiol. 1985;4:488.
95. Santoro F, Afchain D, Pierce R, et al. Serodiagnosis of toxoplasma infection using a purified parasite protein (P30). Clin Exp Immunol. 1985;62:262.
96. Remington JS, Araujo FG, Desmonts G. Recognition of different *Toxoplasma* antigens by IgM and IgG antibodies in mothers and their congenitally infected newborn. J Infect Dis. 1985;152:1020.
97. Sabin AB, Feldman HA: Dyes as microchemical indicators of a new immunity phenomenon affecting a protozoon parasite (*Toxoplasma*). Science. 1948;108:660.
98. Anderson SE, Remington JS. The diagnosis of toxoplasmosis. South Med J. 1975;68:1433.
99. Araujo FG, Barnett EV, Gentry LO, et al. False-positive anti-*Toxoplasma* fluorescent-antibody tests in patients with antinuclear antibodies. Appl Microbiol. 1971;22:270.
100. Desmonts G, Remington JS. Direct agglutination test for diagnosis of *Toxoplasma* infection: Method for increasing sensitivity and specificity. J Clin Microbiol. 1980;11:562.
101. Walls KW, Remington JS. Evaluation of a commercial latex agglutination method for toxoplasmosis. Diagn Microbiol Infect Dis. 1983;1:265.
102. Welch PC, Masur H, Jones TC, et al. Serologic diagnosis of acute lymphadenopathic toxoplasmosis. J Infect Dis. 1980;142:256.

103. Kean BH, Kimball AC. The complement-fixation test in the diagnosis of congenital toxoplasmosis. Am J Dis Child. 1977;131:21.
104. Naot Y, Barnett EV, Remington JS. Method for avoiding false positive results occurring in immunoglobulin M enzyme-linked immunosorbent assays due to presence of both rheumatoid factor and antinuclear antibodies. J Clin Microbiol. 1981;14:73.
105. Filice GA, Yeager AS, Remington JS. Diagnostic significance of immunoglobulin M antibodies to *Toxoplasma gondii* detected after separation of immunoglobulin M from immunoglobulin G antibodies. J Clin Microbiol. 1980;12:336.
106. Camargo ME, Ferreira AW, Mineo JR, et al. Immunoglobulin G and immunoglobulin M enzyme-linked immunosorbent assays and defined toxoplasmosis serological patterns. Infect Immun. 1978;21:55.
107. Siegel JP, Remington JS. A comparison of methods for quantitating antigen-specific IgM antibody using a reverse enzyme-linked immunosorbent assay. J Clin Microbiol. 1983;18:63.
108. Remington JS, Eimstad WM, Araujo FG. Detection of immunoglobulin M antibodies with antigen-tagged latex particles in an immunosorbent assay. J Clin Microbiol. 1983;17:939.
109. Brooks RG, McCabe RE, Remington JS. Role of serology in the diagnosis of toxoplasmic lymphadenopathy. Rev Infect Dis. 1987;9:1055.
110. McCabe RE, Gibbons D, Brooks RG, et al. Agglutination test for diagnosis of toxoplasmosis in AIDS. Lancet. 1983;2:680.
111. LePort C, Raffi F, Matheron S, et al. Treatment of central nervous system toxoplasmosis with pyrimethamine/sulfadiazine combination in 35 patients with acquired immune deficiency syndrome. Efficacy of long term continuous therapy. Am J Med. 1988;84:94.
112. Desmonts G. Definitive serological diagnosis of ocular toxoplasmosis. Arch Ophthalmol. 1966;76:839.
113. Turanen HJ, Leinikki PO, Jaari KM: Demonstration of intraocular synthesis of immunoglobulin G *Toxoplasma* antibodies for specific diagnosis of toxoplasmic chorioretinitis by enzyme immunoassay. J Clin Microbiol. 1983;17:988.
114. Naot Y, Desmonts G, Remington JS. IgM enzyme-linked immunosorbent assay for the diagnosis of congenital *Toxoplasma* infection. J Pediatr. 1981;98:32.
115. Daffos F, Forestier F, Capella-Pavlovsky M, et al. Prenatal management of 746 pregnancies at risk of congenital toxoplasmosis. N Engl J Med. 1988;318:271.
116. Desmonts G, Daffos F, Forestier F, et al. Prenatal diagnosis of congenital toxoplasmosis. Lancet. 1985;1:500.
117. Hofflin JM, Conley FK, Remington JS. Murine model of intracerebral toxoplasmosis. J Infect Dis. 1987;155:550.
118. Lee WR, Hay J, Hutchison WM, et al. A murine model of congenital toxoplasmic retinochoroiditis. Acta Ophthalmol (Copenh). 1983;61:818.
119. Carey RM, Kimball AC, Armstrong D, et al: *Toxoplasma:* Clinical experiences in a cancer hospital. Am J Med. 1973;54:30.
120. Bell ET, Tapper ML, Pollock AA. Sulphadiazine desensitization in AIDS patients. Lancet. 1985;1:163.
121. Smith RM, Iwamoto GK, Richerson HB, et al. Trimethoprim-sulfamethoxazole desensitization in the acquired immunodeficiency syndrome. Ann Intern Med. 1987;10:335.
122. Rolston KVI, Hoy J. Role of clindamycin in the treatment of central nervous system toxoplasmosis. Am J Med. 1987;83:551.
123. Snow RB, Lavyne MH. CNS toxoplasmosis in a patient with AIDS. Infect Surg. 1983;2:669–79.
124. Araujo FG, Remington JS. Effect of clindamycin on acute and chronic toxoplasmosis in mice. Antimicrob Agents Chemother. 1974;5:647.
125. Danneman BR, Israelski DM, Remington JS. Treatment of toxoplasmic encephalitis with intravenous clindamycin. Arch Intern Med. 1988;148:2477.
126. Grossman PL, Remington JS: The efect of trimethoprim and sulfamethoxazole on *Toxoplasma gondii* in vitro and in vivo. Am J Trop Med Hyg. 1979;28:445.
127. Leport C, Vilde JL, Katlama C, et al. Failure of spiramycin to prevent neurotoxoplasmosis in immunosuppressed patients. JAMA. 1986;255:2290.
128. Chan J, Luft BJ. Activity of roxithromycin (RU 28965), a macrolide, against *Toxoplasma gondii* in mice. Antimicrob Agents Chemother. 1986;30:323.
129. Chang HR, Pechere JCF. Effect of roxithromycin on acute toxoplasmosis in mice. Antimicrob Agents Chemother. 1987;31:1147.
130. Hofflin JM, Remington JS. In vivo synergism of roxithromycin (RU965) and interferon against *Toxoplasma gondii*. Antimicrob Agents Chemother. 1987;31:346.
131. Kovacs JA, Allegra CJ, Chabner BA, et al. Potent effect of trimetrexate, a lipid-soluble antifolate, on *Toxoplasma gondii*. J Infect Dis. 1987;155:1027.
132. Ghosh M, Levy PM, Leopold IH. Therapy of toxoplasmosis uveitis. Am J Ophthalmol. 1965;59:55.
133. Friedman CT, Knox DL. Variations in recurrent active toxoplasmic retinochoroiditis. Arch Ophthalmol. 1969;81:481.
134. Tate GW, Martin RG. Clindamycin in the treatment of human ocular toxoplasmosis. Can J Ophthalmol. 1977;12:188.
135. Tabbara KF, O'Connor GR. Treatment of ocular toxoplasmosis with clindamycin and sulfadiazine. Ophthalmology. 1980;87:129.
136. Ghartey KN, Brockhurst RJ. Photocoagulation of active *Toxoplasma* retinochoroiditis. Am J Ophthalmol. 1980;89:858.
137. Fitzgerald CR. Pars plana vitrectomy for vitreous opacity secondary to presumed toxoplasmosis. Arch Ophthalmol 1980;98:322.
138. Kraubig H. Praventive Behandlung der konnatalen Toxoplasmose. In: Kirchoff H, Kraubig H, eds. Toxoplasmose: Praktische Fragen und Ergebnisse. Stuttgart: Thieme; 1966:104.
139. Kraubig H. Erste praktische Erfahrungen mit der Prophylaxe der konnatalen Toxoplasmose. Med Klin (Munich). 1963;58:1361.
140. Weiss LM, Harris C, Berger M, et al. Pyrimethamine concentrations in serum and cerebrospinal fluid during treatment of acute *Toxoplasma* encephalitis in patients with AIDS. J Infect Dis. 1988;157:580.
141. Hakim M, Esmore D, Wallwork J, et al. Toxoplasmosis in cardiac transplantation. Br Med J. 1986;292:1108.

256. PNEUMOCYSTIS CARINII

PETER D. WALZER

Pneumocystis carinii was discovered in 1909 by Chagas who mistakenly interpreted the organism as a trypanosome. Several years later the Delanöes identified *P. carinii* as a separate genus and species and named the organism in honor of Dr. Carini, another early worker. *Pneumocystis carinii* first came to medical attention when it was implicated as the cause of interstitial plasma cell pneumonia, a disorder of institutionalized debilitated infants of central and eastern Europe after World War II. In the 1960s *P. carinii* became widely appreciated as an important cause of pneumonia in immunocompromised hosts; however, with the development of safe and effective chemotherapy in chemoprophylaxis, interest in the organism waned. The 1980s witnessed a dramatic increase in the incidence of *P. carinii* pneumonia associated with the acquired immunodeficiency syndrome (AIDS). This has presented new clinical challenges and rekindled investigative interest in the organism.

THE PATHOGEN

The taxonomy of *P. carinii* has long been a matter of controversy.[1] Most workers have classified the organism as a protozoan based on morphologic structural properties (e.g., ameboid appearance, presence of filopodia), lack of growth on fungal media, and sensitivity to antiprotozoal drugs. The words used to describe the life cycle stages of the organism have been based on terminology used for protozoa. Investigators favoring a fungal classification of *P. carinii* point to similarities to the ascospore formation in yeasts, the poorly developed organelle system, and the staining with methenamine silver and other reagents that stain fungi. Analysis of ribosomal RNA sequences of microorganisms has recently become an important tool for phylogenetic analysis; when applied to *P. carinii*, data suggest a closer relationship to fungi than to protozoa.[2,3] This has rekindled interest in the fungal characteristics of the organism.

Pneumocystis carinii exists as a saprophyte in the lungs of humans and a variety of animal species in nature. Organisms from these hosts have identical morphologic features, but antigenic as well as animal challenge studies suggest that species or strain differences exist.[4,5] Analysis of the life cycle of *P. carinii* has been based on morphologic studies of human or rat lung sections and, to a lesser extent, on organisms grown in tissue culture.[6,7] Three developmental stages of *P. carinii* have been identified. The *trophozoite* or *trophic form*, the most numerous stage, is small (1–4 μm), pleomorphic, and commonly exists in clusters. This form of the organism is identified on Giemsa stain by its reddish nucleus and blue cytoplasm (Fig. 1A) On electron micrographs there are a nucleus, mitochondria, a few other organelles, and tubular cytoplasmic extensions termed filopodia. The *cyst* is large (5–8 μm), has a thick wall, and contains up to eight daughter forms or intracystic bodies termed sporozoites. The cyst is easily recognizable by stains such as methenamine silver that stain its cell wall (Fig. 1B). The

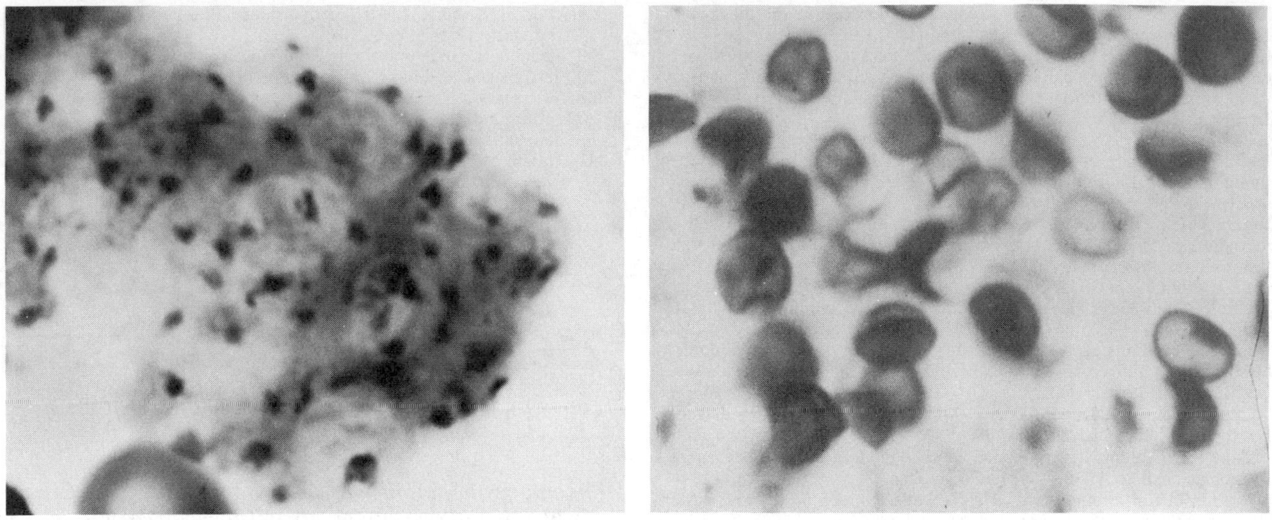

FIG. 1. **(A)** Cluster of *Pneumocystis carinii* trophozoites and cysts. (Diff-Quik, ×2500). **(B)** Cluster of *P. carinii* cysts. (Methenamine silver stain, ×1250).

precyst (4–6 μm) is an intermediate stage, but a definition of its morphologic features has varied among different investigators.

It is generally agreed that trophozoites multiply asexually, perhaps by binary fission. Trophozoites appear to develop into cysts by a sexual cycle, as illustrated by the presence of synaptonemal complexes in precysts. When the cyst reaches maturity, the sporozoites are liberated and then develop into trophozoites. Little is known about the specific factors or conditions that stimulate excystation or encystation of *P. carinii*.

Despite strenuous efforts by many investigators, only limited progress has been achieved with the in vitro cultivation of *P. carinii*.[1] Rat-derived organisms can be propagated on several different cell lines; under optimal conditions, a 10-fold increase in *P. carinii* can be obtained in primary culture and organisms can be serially passaged a few times to naive cultures. Little success has been achieved with human *P. carinii* or with any source of the organism using axenic media. A major impediment to *P. carinii* cultivation has been the lack of reproducibility and standardization among different laboratories. Nevertheless, the available systems have been helpful in studies of *P. carinii* life cycle, of susceptibility to antimicrobial agents, and as a purification step to obtain organisms free from host tissue contaminants.

Within the alveolus *P. carinii* adheres tightly to a specific lining cell, the type 1 pneumocyte,[8] but an intracellular stage in the life cycle has not been found. There is some evidence suggesting that *P. carinii* is covered by alveolar lining fluid and not necessarily in direct contact with inspired air. It seems likely that the organism obtains nutrients from the alveolar fluid constituents or lining cells. Little is known about *P. carinii*'s biochemical pathways; hypotheses have ranged from a metabolism of low-molecular-weight substances (based on the organism's primitive organelle system) to the occurrence of endocytosis. Experimental studies performed on nonreplicating organisms have suggested that *P. carinii* can utilize molecular oxygen and synthesize nucleic acids, proteins, carbohydrates, and phospholipids.[9] Histochemical staining has demonstrated the existence of several dehydrogenase enzymes.[10]

EPIDEMIOLOGY

Studies in immunosuppressed animals have shown that *P. carinii* is communicable and that the airborne route seems to be the major mode of transmission.[11] Questions about the infective form or environmental sources of the organism, vectors, or definitive or intermediate hosts remain unanswered. Person-to-person transmission of *P. carinii* has been suggested by outbreaks and clusters of cases of pneumocystosis in orphanages and hospitals[12] and by the occurrence of the disease in immunosuppressed patients who have prolonged contact with each other. The incubation period is thought to be about 4–8 weeks. There is no evidence that *P. carinii* infection is a zoonosis.

P. carinii has a worldwide distribution. Seroepidemiologic surveys have demonstrated that most healthy children have been exposed to the organism by an early age.[13] Autopsy surveys have revealed subclinical *P. carinii* pulmonary infection in about 5 percent of patients with lymphoreticular neoplasms and rarely in healthy people.[14]

PATHOGENESIS AND PATHOLOGY

Pneumocystis carinii is of such low virulence that inoculation of organisms results in no observable damage to the host. However, such exposure does stimulate an immune response, and recent interest has focused on the use of the immunoblotting technique to delineate the specific antigens involved. A 116-kilodalton (kD) moiety has been found on the surface of *P. carinii* from rats, mice, humans, rabbits, and ferrets.[15,16] Other important rat *P. carinii* antigens are bands of about 45 and 50 kD, while by far the most prominent human *P. carinii* moiety is a broad-based band of about 40 kD.[5] Since these antigens are recognized by a variety of sources of antibody, they possess both shared as well as species-specific determinants. Biochemical data so far suggest that the antigens are composed of protein and carbohydrate constituents.[17]

The attachment of *P. carinii* to the type 1 pneumocyte plays a central role in the host–parasite relationship in this infection.[8] Ultrastructural studies have demonstrated that the surfaces of organism and host cells are closely apposed without fusion of cell membranes or changes in the intramembranous particles, but the specific factors involved in the mechanism of attachment (e.g., receptors, lectins) have not been defined. The surface of *P. carinii* and type 1 cells is rich in carbohydrates, and fluoresceinated lectin probes have revealed that glucose, mannose, and N-acetylglucosamine residues are prominent constituents.[18] Exposure to *P. carinii* does not result in protective immunity, suggesting that the organism possesses evasion mechanisms within the milieu of the alveolar microenvironment.

It is generally considered that impaired cellular immunity is more important than impaired humoral immunity in predisposing to *P. carinii* infection, although the specific host immune defects involved in the process are poorly understood. The patient populations at risk for pneumocystosis include premature, malnourished infants; children with primary immunodeficiency diseases (particularly severe combined immunodeficiency disease); and patients receiving immunosuppressive drugs for the treatment of cancers, organ transplantation, and other disorders.[19] Corticosteroids have been by far the most important form of immunosuppressive therapy; these agents not only lead to the development of pneumocystosis by themselves but also potentiate the effects of chemotherapy protocols involving other cytotoxic drugs. The relationship of corticosteroids to *P. carinii* has also been emphasized by reports of the occurrence of cases of pneumocystosis occurring in patients with Cushing syndrome.[20] The incidence of *P. carinii* pneumonia in different populations of compromised hosts can be directly related to the type and intensity of immunosuppression.[21] This has led to the hypothesis that development of overt disease in these patients represents reactivation of latent infection.

In the 1980s AIDS has become the most common underlying disease predisposing to the development of pneumocystosis.[22] *Pneumocystis carinii* pneumonia occurs in greater than 60 percent and perhaps up to 80–90 percent of AIDS patients in the United States during their lifetime and is the leading cause of mortality. The principal immunologic defect in AIDS is a reduction in number and function of CD4 T helper cells, although impaired function of other cell types also occurs. Blastogenic assays have demonstrated that most healthy adults have good proliferative responses to *P. carinii*, while patients infected with the human immunodeficiency virus (HIV) exhibit a progressive decline in response that parallels severity of this infection.[23] AIDS patients fail to exhibit any proliferative response to *P. carinii* even after recovering from pneumocystosis and receiving zidovudine (AZT) therapy. It is unclear whether the pathogenesis of pneumocystosis in AIDS and other immunodeficiency diseases represents simple reactivation of latent infection or perhaps involves additional exposure to exogenous sources of the organism.

Protein malnutrition is another important risk factor for *P. carinii* infection.[24] Protein malnutrition mainly inhibits cell-mediated immunity and in its most extreme form can induce the development of pneumocystosis under experimental conditions. A more subtle and yet clinically important role for malnutrition is as a complication of the patient's underlying disease or chemotherapy.

Systemic and local antibodies develop in response to *P. carinii* infection and appear to be mainly of the IgG class.[1] Although pneumocystosis has occurred in children whose primary immunodeficiency disease has been characterized mainly by impaired B-cell function, the presence of antibodies has not prevented the development of *P. carinii* pneumonia induced by immunosuppression. Antibodies enhance phagocytosis of *P. carinii* by alveolar macrophages and thereby may function as opsonins.[25] Once engulfed by the macrophage, the organism is immediately digested.

Animal models have been very helpful in studying the pathogenesis, diagnosis, and treatment of pneumocystosis.[26] Rats, mice, rabbits, guinea pigs, and ferrets administered corticosteroids for about 8 weeks spontaneously develop *P. carinii* pneumonia with histologic features identical to those in the human form of the disease. The mechanism here appears to be reactivation of latent infection, since immunosuppressed animals without environmental exposure to *P. carinii* fail to develop the disease.

Sequential studies in the rat model have revealed that *P. carinii* organisms propagate slowly and gradually fill alveolar lumens; at the peak intensity of infection, each lung may contain 10^9–10^{10} organisms. This process is accompanied by the development of the typical foamy alveolar exudate and a series of changes on electron microscopy that culminate in damage to the type 1 cell.[8] There are also alterations in respiratory mechanics and surfactant phospholipids that contribute to this overall picture of diffuse alveolar injury.[27] Host inflammatory changes are inconspicuous and are characterized mainly by hypertrophy and hyperplasia of type 2 pneumocytes (a typical reparative response). Studies of lymphocyte surface markers have revealed a decline in CD4 helper cells in peripheral blood in the lungs but not at other body sites during the development of pneumocystosis in this animal model.[28]

When corticosteroids are withdrawn, the rat regains its weight and mounts a vigorous inflammatory and immune response to clear *P. carinii* from the lung. Alveolar macrophages become very prominent in the phagocytosis of the organism. There also occur a heavy mononuclear cell infiltrate in the lung, the return of T-cell subsets to normal levels, the formation of serum antibodies to *P. carinii*, and the development of pulmonary interstitial fibrosis. Yet, even with the restoration of normal immune function, a few *P. carinii* organisms can be found attached to type 1 cells.

Cases of *P. carinii* pneumonia have occurred spontaneously in a variety of animals with suspected or proved immunodeficiency diseases.[26] Outbreaks of pneumocystosis have been noted in colonies of athymic (nude) and scid mice, providing opportunities to study the pathogenesis of the disease in an immunodeficient animal population under natural conditions.[29] The clinical manifestations of *P. carinii* pneumonia are more severe in older than in younger mice. Once established within an animal colony, the organism may persist for many years. It might seem that these immunodeficient mice would be a good experimental model system, yet attempts to produce pneumonia with exogenous organisms have had conflicting results.

The pathologic features of pneumocystosis in humans reveal densely consolidated lungs with reddish grey cut surfaces. On histologic sections stained with hematoxylin and eosin, the alveoli are filled with pink frothy honeycombed material (Fig. 2); staining with methenamine silver demonstrates masses of organisms. Infants with interstitial plasma cell pneumonia display a prominent plasma cell infiltrate. By contrast, immunosup-

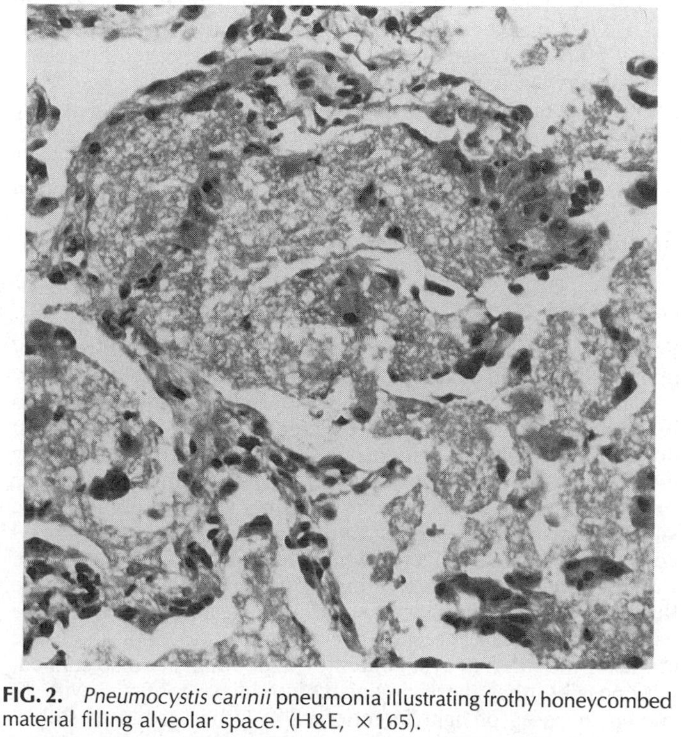

FIG. 2. *Pneumocystis carinii* pneumonia illustrating frothy honeycombed material filling alveolar space. (H&E, ×165).

pressed patients usually only demonstrate interstitial thickening resulting from hyperplasia and hypertrophy of type 2 cells, edema, and a scanty mononuclear cell infiltrate. A variety of atypical histologic features may also be present,[30] but it is not usually possible to determine whether they are due to *P. carinii* or to other conditions that damage the lung.

CLINICAL MANIFESTATIONS

Interstitial plasma cell pneumonia has occurred classically in debilitated infants age 6 weeks to 4 months housed in orphanages or foundling homes under crowded conditions.[31] The disease begins insidiously with symptoms such as poor feeding and progresses gradually to overt respiratory distress and cyanosis. Cases sometimes occurred in explosive outbreaks, giving rise to the term "epidemic" form of *P. carinii* pneumonia. Interstitial plasma cell pneumonia has largely disappeared from industrialized countries but still exists in parts of the world (and in their refugees) where poor socioeconomic conditions abound.[32]

The presenting symptoms of *P. carinii* pneumonia in the compromised host include shortness of breath, fever, and a nonproductive cough.[19] Patients receiving immunosuppressive drugs frequently develop these clinical manifestations after the corticosteroid dose has been tapered and are typically sick for about 1–2 weeks before seeking medical attention. Pneumocystosis in AIDS patients may be a more subtle disease with symptoms lasting from weeks to months.[22,33] On physical examination, tachypnea and tachycardia are frequently present in acutely ill patients. Children may demonstrate cyanosis, flaring of the nasal alae, and intercostal retractions in severe disease. Lung auscultation is usually not helpful, although rales can be heard in about one-third of adults with the disease.

The peripheral blood leukocyte count more likely reflects the patient's underlying disease or immunosuppressive therapy rather than the activity of *P. carinii*. Serum albumin levels may be low if malnutrition is present. The chest roentgenogram classically exhibits bilateral diffuse infiltrates extending from the perihilar region (Fig. 3). In some cases the chest roentgenogram may be completely normal or show such atypical findings as nodules, cavitation, or pneumatocele.[1] There may also be increased lung uptake on gallium scan and enhanced clearance of inhaled technetium 99m diethylenetriamine pentaacetate (tcDPA), a marker for alveolar–capillary membrane permeability.[34,35] Blood gases reveal hypoxemia, increased alveolar–arterial oxygen and gradient, and respiratory alkalosis; in the later stages of *P. carinii* pneumonia, a respiratory acidosis may develop. Pulmonary function abnormalities include impaired vital capacity, total lung capacity, and diffusing incapacity.[36] In general, the changes in blood gases in pulmonary function tests are less severe in AIDS patients than in other immunosuppressed patients.

DIAGNOSIS

Pneumocystosis should be considered in any immunocompromised patient who develops respiratory symptomatology, fever, and an abnormal chest roentgenogram. Since these clinical manifestations may be produced by a long list of infectious and noninfectious agents, diagnosis of *P. carinii* must be made by histopathologic demonstration of the organism.[37] Two basic types of stains have been used. Reagents such as methenamine silver or one of its simpler variants (e.g., toluidine blue O, cresyl echt violet, Gram–Weigert), which selectively stain the wall of *P. carinii* cysts, have been popular among pathologists because they can be used on imprint smears or tissue sections and are easy to interpret. These reagents provide no data about the status of the internal cyst contents; since fungi are also stained, it is possible that these organisms could be confused with *P. carinii* in cases of light infection. The other group of stains, typified by Giemsa or one of its variants (e.g., Diff-Quik, polychrome methylene blue), stain *P. carinii* trophozoites, intracystic bodies, and intermediate forms in imprint smears but cannot be reliably applied to tissue sections. These reagents are rapid and easy to perform, but since they also stain host cells, they require more experience for proper interpretation.

The impact of AIDS has not only increased the proficiency of clinical laboratories in diagnosing *P. carinii* by standard techniques but has also stimulated the development of alternative approaches. Examples include the use of the Gram stain, Wright stain, Papanicolaou smears, and stains such as acridine orange or propidium iodide which are used with fluorescence microscopy. There is increasing attention being devoted to the examination of *P. carinii* in fresh specimens by using phase contrast or Normarski interference contrast microscopy.[38] These techniques provide excellent views of the developmental stages of the organism, and when combined with the use of a vital dye such as erythrosin B, might be very helpful in evaluating organism viability and the effects of chemotherapy. *P. carinii* can be readily detected by immunofluorescent or immunoperoxidase staining (Fig. 4); with the development and commercial availability of monoclonal antibodies, these techniques might gain more widespread clinical application.[39] Now that cloned DNA sequences from the organism are available,[40,41] filter hybridization of clinical specimens can be evaluated as a diagnostic tool.

The collection of specimens that accurately reflect the disease process in the lungs is an essential component of the diagnostic evaluation of patients with suspected pneumocystosis. The infrequent presence of *P. carinii* in sputum or tracheal secretions has severely limited the use of these specimens in non-AIDS patients.[19] However, recent studies have shown that the diagnosis of *P. carinii* can be made in a high proportion of AIDS patients by examination of sputum that has been induced by inhalation of a saline mist.[39] This probably reflects the higher organism burden in patients with AIDS, but quantitative *P. carinii* counts in different patient groups are lacking. It remains to be determined whether reduced sputum will retain its high diagnostic value in routine clinical practice; neverthelesss, it represents a simple, noninvasive, and inexpensive screening procedure.

Fiberoptic bronchoscopy is the most commonly used diagnostic procedure in use in adults today.[42] Bronchoalveolar lavage has generally replaced washings and brushings and causes few serious complications. Transbronchial biopsy may be helpful in some patients but is a more invasive procedure with higher morbidity. The diagnosis of pneumocystosis can usually be established by fiberoptic bronchoscopy in over 90 percent of AIDS patients, although the yield from this procedure in non-AIDS patients is probably not quite as high.

Open lung biopsy, which requires the use of operating room facilities and general anesthesia, has long served as the standard reference procedure for the diagnosis of *P. carinii* because it provides the greatest amount of tissue that can be obtained under direct visualization. Open lung biopsy is performed less frequently than in the past, and there is some controversy over its role in the diagnostic evaluation of lung infiltrates in immunosuppressed patients.[43] I believe that open lung biopsy should be used when bronchoscopy is nondiagnostic or when a patient being treated for *P. carinii* is suspected of having another infection or condition contributing to pulmonary problems. Open lung biopsy has been shown to be superior to transbronchial biopsy when both procedures are performed simultaneously in the same patients[44] and has also been helpful in detecting conditions such as Kaposi's sarcoma of the lungs that have been difficult to diagnose by other techniques.[45]

Needle aspiration or biopsy of the lung was once quite popular but is now usually performed only in children. Enthusiasm for the procedure in adults has waned because of low diagnostic yield and high rate of complications.

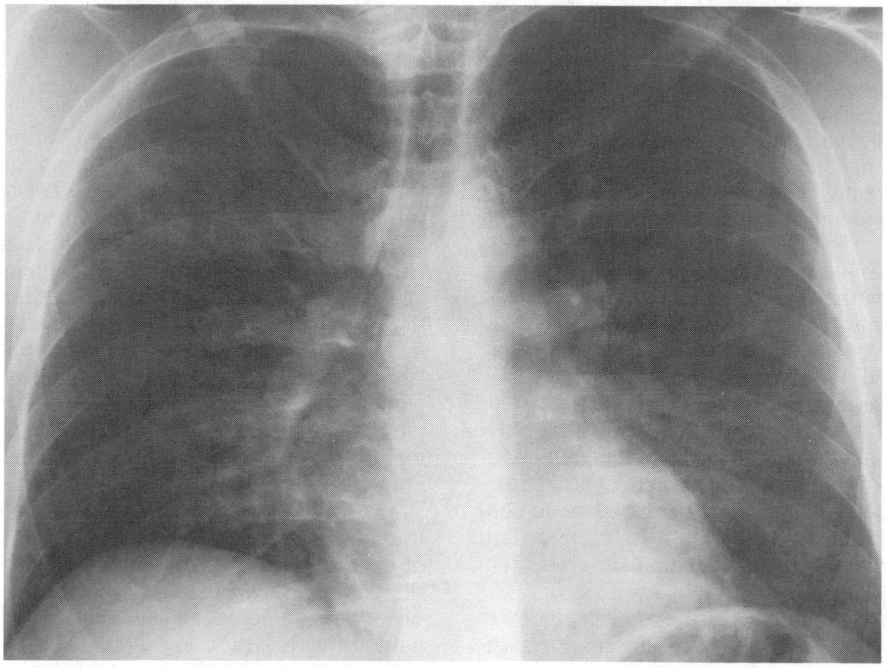

FIG. 3. Chest roentgenogram showing bilateral infiltrates of *P. carinii* pneumonia.

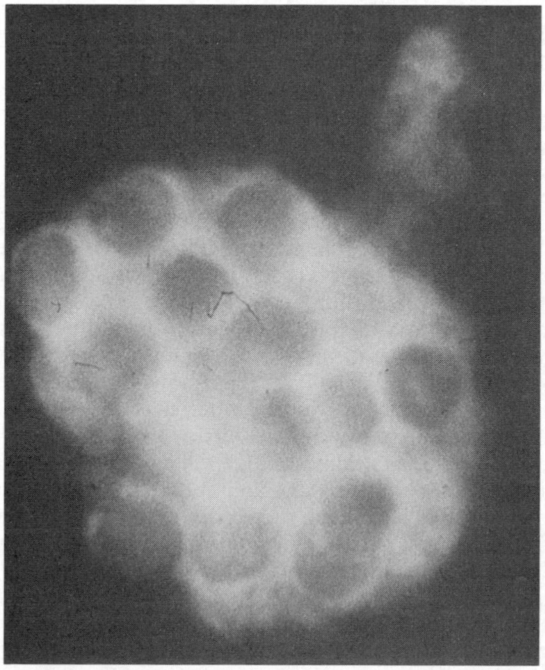

FIG. 4. Clusters of *P. carinii* cysts stained by immunofluorescence. Note peripheral rim pattern of staining. (×1250)

The diagnosis of pneumocystosis should be pursued in an aggressive and systematic manner. Close cooperation is needed among the patient's primary physician, consultants, and clinical laboratories to ensure proper collection and analysis of specimens. Invasive procedures should be performed early in the patient's course to lessen the risk of complications.

Attempts have been made to detect circulating *P. carinii* antigens in serum by counterimmunoelectrophoresis or latex agglutination techniques.[46] Unfortunately, these systems have lacked sufficient sensitivity, specificity, and reproducibility to be of clinical diagnostic value. Serum antibodies to *P. carinii* have been measured by complement fixation, the indirect fluorescent antibody (IFA) technique, and enzyme-linked immunosorbent assay (ELISA) with whole organisms or soluble extracts as the antigen; the high prevalence of serum antibodies to *P. carinii* in the general population has limited the value of these serologic techniques in the diagnosis of pneumocystosis.[13,47] Perhaps measurement of serum antibodies to specific *P. carinii* antigens will be a more fruitful technique.[48]

TREATMENT

Pneumocystis carinii infection in normal hosts is not known to cause symptoms, and thus no treatment is necessary. Untreated pneumocystosis in the form of interstitial plasma cell pneumonia has a mortality rate of about 50 percent, while the disease in the immunocompromised host is almost always fatal. The hospital course is one of progressive hypoxemia and respiratory insufficiency. A variety of factors affect the success of the therapy of *P. carinii* pneumonia including the severity of the disease, prior lung damage, leukocyte or lymphocyte count, the presence of other opportunistic infections, and the status of the patient's underlying medical condition and nutrition.[19,33,49] The need for ventilator support, which is associated with an ominous prognosis, has raised difficult medical and ethical questions for AIDS patients and their physicians about whether to institute such measures.[50]

Dissemination of *P. carinii* beyond the lungs is uncommon but has been well documented (at least 20 cases have been reported in the literature).[51] Recent reports have focused on AIDS patients, although it is unknown whether the extrapulmonary spread of *P. carinii* in this patient population is more frequent than in other immunocompromised hosts. The mechanism of spread of the organism appears to be by hematogenous or lymphatic routes or both. Major sites of extrapulmonary involvement have included lymph nodes, bone marrow, spleen, and liver, but a variety of other locations (e.g., ear, eye, gastrointestinal tract) have also been reported. The presence of *P. carinii* in these locations has usually been suspected by the demonstration of the typical foamy honeycombed material by hematoxylin and eosin stain.

Since the mid-1970s, the major drugs used in the therapy of pneumocystosis have been trimethoprim-sulfamethoxazole (TMP-SMX) and pentamidine isethionate. These drugs are equally effective in patients with AIDS and in other populations of immunocompromised hosts; they have an overall success rate of about 70–80 percent, but even higher rates can be achieved if *P. carinii* pneumonia is mild and therapy is begun promptly.[22,33,52–54]

TMP-SMX exerts its antimicrobial effect on other organisms by inhibiting folic acid synthesis; data obtained so far suggest a similar mechanism of action of *P. carinii*.[55] TMP-SMX is administered orally or intravenously in a dose of 20 mg/kg per day TMP and 100 mg/kg per day SMX in four divided doses. The parenteral route should be used in patients who are very ill or who have gastrointestinal disturbances. The dose of TMP-SMX should be adjusted to achieve optimal serum levels of TMP of 5–8 μg/ml in adults and 3–5 μg/ml in children and levels of SMX of 100–150 μg/ml. The drug is administered for 14 days to non-AIDS patients and is usually well tolerated. Side effects are characterized mainly by gastrointestinal complaints and skin rashes.

Pentamidine isethionate, a diamidine, is an old drug that was first used in the treatment of African trypanosomiasis. Its mechanism of action against *P. carinii* is unknown. Pentamidine isethionate is administered parenterally in a single dose of 4 mg/kg per day for 14 days in non-AIDS patients. The intravenous route has proven to be no more toxic than the intramuscular route[56] and seems to be the preferred method of administration by most clinicians. Pentamidine isethionate is diluted in 50–250 ml of a 5% dextrose solution and infused over at least a period of 1 hour. Pharmacokinetic studies have indicated that serum levels of pentamidine isethionate are quite low even in the presence of moderate renal impairment but may accumulate with repeated dosing; the drug can be found bound to tissues even many months after administration has been stopped.[57,58] Pentamidine isethionate is a toxic drug as evidenced by the fact that side effects occur in about half of non-AIDS patients.[19] These include hypotension, dizziness, cardiac arrhythmias, azotemia, hypocalcemia, hepatic disturbances, and problems at the sites of intramuscular injection. Hypoglycemia may occur and can be followed at a later date by the development of hyperglycemia or frank diabetes mellitus.

Non-AIDS patients respond to the therapeutic effects of TMP-SMX and pentamidine isethionate in a similar manner. Clinical improvement is usually noted after about 4 days of treatment, although there is some variation among individual patients; if there is no response after 5–6 days, it is wise to consider switching to another drug.

The treatment of *P. carinii* pneumonia in patients with AIDS is more complex. These individuals tend to take a longer time before showing a clinical response, and thus it has become customary to administer drugs for 21 days and wait at least 7 days before concluding there is a treatment failure. Even when there has been a clear-cut clinical response, at least half of the AIDS patients will have *P. carinii* present in bronchoalveolar lavage fluid after a course of therapy.[53,59] The specific life cycle stages, viability, and clinical significance of these organisms have not been studied in detail. In contrast to other immunocompromised hosts, patients with AIDS have a high rate of recurrence (about 50 percent) of pneumocystosis that has not been materially altered by drugs (e.g., AZT) that have activity against HIV; it is unclear whether these recurrences represent relapse or true reinfection. Some patients may experience multiple episodes of *P. carinii* pneumonia. It is generally thought that these repeat bouts of the disease are more difficult to treat than the initial episode, but controlled studies are lacking.

A major impediment to *P. carinii* therapy in AIDS is the high frequency of intolerance to antimicrobial drugs.[22,33,53,54] Most patients experience adverse reactions to TMP-SMX that include skin rash, fever, leukopenia, thrombocytopenia, and hepatic dysfunction; these problems usually begin during the second week of therapy and are often of sufficient severity to require discontinuation of the drug. The side effects are generally considered to represent a form of hypersensitivity reaction directed mainly toward the sulfonamide component, but the mechanisms involved are poorly understood. Since substitution of another sulfonamide or sulfone or rechallenge with TMP-SMX has led to widely disparate results in these patients, such actions should only be undertaken with great caution. Adverse reactions to pentamidine isethionate among AIDS patients are generally similar to those among other compromised hosts except that certain side effects are more common (neutropenia) or are particularly troublesome (hypotension, hypoglycemia). Low blood glucose may occur during or after completion of pentamidine isethionate therapy, and clinical manifestations range from an abnormal laboratory finding to life-threatening coma.[60]

The wide experience with TMP-SMX and pentamidine isethionate over the past several years has allowed the formulation of general guidelines for their use. TMP-SMX is the preferred therapy for *P. carinii* pneumonia in non-AIDS patients because of its better tolerance. There is no clear-cut drug of choice in patients with AIDS, but TMP-SMX is probably preferred by most physicians because of its availability in oral and parenteral forms, well-known pharmacokinetics, and broad antibacterial spectrum. Combination therapy with TMP-SMX and pentamidine isethionate is no more effective than either agent used alone and may increase the risk of adverse effects. If one of these drugs has achieved a good clinical anti-*P. carinii* response but has to be discontinued because of toxicity, the other drug is also likely to be effective; however, if one of these drugs has to be withdrawn because of a poor therapeutic response, the second drug is also likely to be ineffective.

A variety of other therapeutic regimens are currently being explored. Rationale for these approaches has come from data obtained in the rat model of pneumocystosis, which has been a reliable predictor of drug activity in humans.[4,61–63] Unfortunately, none of these treatment protocols have been subjected to rigorous controlled clinical trials, and thus conclusions about their value must remain tentative. Most of the attention has focused on inhibitors of folic acid synthesis. Trimetrexate, a lipid-soluble derivative of methotrexate and a potent dihydrofolate reductase (DHFR) inhibitor, has shown promising results in the treatment of pneumocystosis when used alone or in combination with a sulfonamide; bone marrow toxicity can be ameliorated by the administration of high doses of folinic acid.[55,64] Combinations of pyrimethamine and sulfadiazine and trimethoprim and dapsone have been successful in treating small numbers of patients.[65,66] Dapsone has anti-*P. carinii* activity when used alone and may be better tolerated by AIDS patients than are sulfonamides. Since a variety of DHFR inhibitors, sulfonamides, and sulfones are undergoing evaluation, it will be important to determine which compounds offer the greatest value in terms of efficacy and toxicity.

Another interesting therapeutic approach involves the administration of pentamidine isethionate by aerosol, which results in selectively high concentrations of the drug in the lungs.[67] Aerosol pentamidine has mainly been used in patients with mild forms of pneumocystosis and appears to be well tolerated. This form of administration has stimulated interest in determining whether lower parenteral doses of pentamidine isethionate might be used and still be effective.[68] α-Difluoromethlyornithine (DFMO), an inhibitor of polyamine biosynthesis with antitrypanosomal properties, has shown promising results in the treatment of *P. carinii* pneumonia in patients who have failed or could not tolerate standard forms of therapy.[69] Other agents that have shown anti-*P. carinii* activity in animal model or tissue culture systems include diamidines and related compounds (e.g., diminazine, amidocarb, quinapyramine), purine nucleosides (9-deazainosine), and a combination of clindamycin and primaquine.[70–72] Therapy is also discussed in Chapter 110.

General supportive measures such as maintaining adequate oxygen, careful fluid balance, and nutrition are an important part of the management of patients with pneumocystosis. There is controversy over the use of corticosteroids as adjunctive treatment because of the belief that host inflammatory response may be playing a role in the pathogenesis of the pneumonia.[1] In patients who are receiving immunosuppressive drugs for the treatment of cancer or other disorders, it seems prudent to taper steroids and related drugs to the lowest level permitted by the underlying disease. Although some studies have suggested that the administration of corticosteroids is helpful in selected AIDS patients,[73] I believe that the serious side effects of these agents outweigh their empiric use until benefits can be clearly demonstrated from controlled clinical trials.

The long-term follow-up of patients who survive one or more episodes of *P. carinii* pneumonia is beginning to receive attention. Residual pulmonary function abnormalities have been demonstrated in adults but not in children.[74,75] Pulmonary fibrosis can also occur,[76] but since the lung may be subjected to a variety of insults during intensive therapy of pneumocystosis, the precise role of *P. carinii* needs further clarification.

PREVENTION

Recovery from *P. carinii* pneumonia is not accompanied by the development of acquired immunity, and thus the patient is at risk of developing recurrences of the disease as long as the predisposing or immunosuppressive conditions exist. Prospective studies have shown that the administration of TMP-SMX in a dose of 5 mg/kg per day TMP and 25 mg/kg per day SMX administered daily or three times a week can prevent the development of pneumocystosis in immunosuppressed patients.[77] Since the drug does not kill *P. carinii*, it is only effective as a prophylactic agent as long as it is being given.[78,79] Patients usually tolerate the long-term administration of TMP-SMX quite well, but it is still prudent to carefully consider the risks and benefits before starting on such an endeavor. Serious adverse reactions have occurred in renal transplant recipients who were taking other immunosuppressive drugs.[80] Prophylactic TMP-SMX has been shown to be effective in AIDS patients in one prospective but uncontrolled study.[81] However, the toxicity of this and other sulfonamide regimens appears to be quite high.[82] Aerosol pentamidine is a more promising approach,[83] but controlled trials are needed.

Since *P. carinii* may be communicable from person to person, it is prudent in the hospital setting to isolate patients with active disease from direct contact with other susceptible hosts. No official guidelines have been developed, but the most common measures have included use of a private room or respiratory isolation.

REFERENCES

1. Walzer PD, Kim CK, Cushion MT. *Pneumocystis carinii*. In: Walzer PD, Genta RM, eds. Parasitic Infections in the Compromised Host. New York: Marcel Dekker. 1989:83–178.
2. Edman JC, Kovacs JA, Masur H, et al. Ribosomal RNA sequence shows *Pneumocystis carinii* to be a member of the fungi. Nature. 1988;334:519–22.
3. Stringer SL, Stringer JR, Blase MA, et al. *Pneumocystis carinii:* Sequence from ribosomal RNA implies a close relationship with fungi. Exper Parasitol. 1989;68:450–61.
4. Frenkel JK, Good JT, Schultz JA. Latent *Pneumocystis carinii* infection of rats, relapse, and chemotherapy. Lab Invest. 1966;15:1559–77.
5. Walzer PD, Linke MJ. A comparison of the antigenic characteristics of rat and human *Pneumocystis carinii* by immunoblotting. J Immunol. 1987;138:2257–65.
6. Matsumoto Y, Yoshida Y. Sporogony in *Pneumocystis carinii*: Synaptonemal complexes and meiotic nuclear divisions observed in precysts. J Protozool. 1984;31:420–8.
7. Cushion MT, Ruffolo JM, Walzer PD. Characterization of the developmental stages of Pneumocystis by light microscopic techniques. Lab Invest. 1988;58:324–31.
8. Walzer PD. Attachment of microorganisms to host cells: Relevance of *Pneumocystis carinii*. Lab Invest. 1986;54:589–92.
9. Pesanti EL. Phospholipid profile of *Pneumocystis carinii* and its interacting with alveolar type II epithelial cells. Infect Immun. 1987;55:736–41.
10. Mazer MA, Kovacs JA, Swann JC, et al. Histoenzymological study of selected dehydrogenase enzymes in *Pneumocystis carinii*. Infect Immun. 1987;55:727–30.
11. Hughes WT. Natural mode of acquisition for de novo infection with *Pneumocystis carinii*. J Infect Dis. 1982;145:842–8.
12. Singer C, Armstrong D, Rosen PP, et al. *Pneumocystis carinii* pneumonia: A cluster of eleven cases. Ann Intern Med. 1975;82:772–7.
13. Meuwissen JHE, Tauber I, Leewenberg ADEM, et al. Parasitologic and serologic observations of infection with Pneumocystis in humans. J Infect Dis. 1977;136:43–9.
14. Easterly JA. *Pneumocystis carinii* in lungs of adults at autopsy. Am Rev Respir Dis. 1968;94:935–7.
15. Gigliotti F, Stokes C, Cheatham AB, et al. Development of murine monoclonal antibodies to *Pneumocystis carinii*. J Infect Dis. 1986;154:315–22.
16. Graves DC, McNabb SJ, Whorley MA, et al. Analysis of rat *Pneumocystis carinii* antigens recognized using Western immunoblotting. Infect Immun. 1986;54:96–103.
17. Linke MJ, Cushion MT, Walzer PD. Properties of the major rat and human *Pneumocystis carinii* antigens. Infect Immun. 1989;57:1547–55.
18. Cushion MT, DeStefano J, Walzer PD. Surface carbohydrates of *Pneumocystis carinii* detected by fluoresceinated lectin probes. Exp Parasitol. 1988;67:137–47.
19. Walzer PD, Perl DP, Krogstad DJ, et al. *Pneumocystis carinii* pneumonia in the United States: Epidemiologic, clinical and diagnostic features. Ann Intern Med. 1974;80:83–93.
20. Graham BS, Tucker WS. Opportunistic infections in endogenous Cushing's syndrome. Ann Intern Med. 1984;101:334–8.
21. Hughes WT, Feldman S, Aur RJA, et al. Intensity of immunosuppressive therapy and the incidence of *Pneumocystis carinii* pneumonitis. Cancer. 1975;36:2004–9.
22. Mills J. *Pneumocystis carinii* and *Toxoplasma gondii* infections in patients with AIDS. Rev Infect Dis. 1986;8:1001–11.
23. Hagler DN, Deepe GS, Walzer PD. Blastogenic responses to *Pneumocystis carinii* among HIV patients. Clin Exp Immunol. 1988;74:7–13.
24. Hughes WT, Price RA, Sisko F, et al. Protein calorie malnutrition: A host determinant for *Pneumocystis carinii* infection. Am J Dis Child. 1974;128:44–52.
25. Masur H, Jones TC. The interaction in vitro of *Pneumocystis carinii* with macrophages and L cells. J Exp Med. 1978;147:157–70.
26. Walzer PD. Experimental models for *Pneumocystis carinii* infection. In: Young LS, ed. *Pneumocystis carinii* Pneumonia. New York: Marcel Dekker; 1984:7–75.
27. Sheehan PM, Stokes DC, Yeh Y, et al. Surfactant phospholipids and lavage phospholipase A_2 in experimental *Pneumocystis carinii* pneumonia. Am Rev Respir Dis. 1986;134:526–31.
28. Walzer PD, LaBine M, Redington TJ, et al. Lymphocyte changes during chronic administration of and withdrawal from corticosteroids: Relation to *Pneumocystis carinii* pneumonia. J Immunol. 1984;133:2502–8.
29. Walzer PD, Kim CK, Linke MJ, et al. Outbreaks of *Pneumocystis carinii* pneumonia in colonies of immunodeficient mice. Infect Immun. 1989;57:62–70.
30. Weber WR, Askin FB, Dehner LP. Lung biopsy in *Pneumocystis carinii* pneumonia: A study of typical and atypical features. Am J Clin Pathol. 1977;67:11–9.
31. Gajdusek DC. *Pneumocystis carinii*—etiologic agent of interstitial plasma cell pneumonia of premature and young infants. Pediatrics. 1957;19:543–65.
32. Gleason WA, Roden VJ, DeCastro F. *Pneumocystis carinii* in Vietnamese infants. J Pediatr. 1975;87:1001–2.
33. Kovacs JA, Hiemenz JW, Macher AM, et al. *Pneumocystis carinii* pneumonia: A comparison between patients with the acquired immunodeficiency syndrome and patients with other immunodeficiencies. Ann Intern Med. 1984;100:663–71.
34. Coleman DL, Hattner RS, Luce JM, et al. Correlation between gallium lung scans and fiberoptic bronchoscopy in patients with suspected *Pneumocystis carinii* pneumonia and the acquired immune deficiency syndrome. Am Rev Respir Dis. 1984;130:1166–69.
35. Mason GR, Duane GB, Mena I, et al. Accelerated solute clearance in *Pneumocystis carinii* pneumonia. Am Rev Respir Dis. 1987;135:864–8.
36. Coleman DL, Dodek PM, Golden JA, et al. Correlation between serial pulmonary function tests and fiberoptic bronchoscopy in patients with *Pneumocystis carinii* pneumonia and the acquired immune deficiency syndrome. Am Rev Respir Dis. 1984;129:491–3.
37. Walzer PD. Diagnosis of *Pneumocystis carinii* pneumonia. J Infect Dis. 1988;157:629–32.
38. Ruffolo JJ, Cushion MT, Walzer PD. Microscopic techniques for studying *Pneumocystis carinii* in fresh specimens. J Clin Microbiol. 1986;23:17–21.
39. Kovacs JA, Ng VL, Masur H, et al. Diagnosis of *Pneumocystis carinii* pneumonia: Improved detection in sputum with monoclonal antibodies. N Engl J Med. 1988;318:589–93.

40. Wakefield AE, Hopkins JM, Burns J, et al. Cloning of DNA from *Pneumocystis carinii*. J Infect Dis. 1988;158:859–62.
41. Tanabe K, Fuchimoto M, Egawa K, et al. Use of *Pneumocystis carinii* genomic DNA clones for DNA hybridization analysis of infected human lungs. J Infect Dis. 1988;157:593–6.
42. Murray JF, Garay SM, Hopewell PC, et al. Pulmonary complications of the acquired immunodeficiency syndrome: An update. Am Rev Respir Dis. 1987;135:504–9.
43. Robin ED, Burke CM. Lung biopsy in immunosuppressed patients. Chest. 1986;89:276–8.
44. Springmeyer SC, Silverstri RC, Sale GE, et al. The role of transbronchial biopsy for the diagnosis of diffuse pneumonia in immunocompromised marrow transplant recipients. Am Rev Respir Dis. 1982;126:763–5.
45. Ognibene FP, Steis RG, Macher AM. Kaposi's sarcoma causing pulmonary infiltrates and respiratory failure in the acquired immunodeficiency syndrome. Ann Intern Med. 1985;102:471–5.
46. Young LS. Antigen detection in *Pneumocystis carinii* pneumonia. Serodiagnosis Immunother. 1987;1:163–7.
47. Maddison SE, Walls KW, Haverkos HW, et al. Evaluation of serologic tests for *Pneumocystis carinii* antibody and antigenemia in patients with acquired immunodeficiency syndrome. Diagn Microbiol Infect Dis. 1984;2:69.
48. Walzer PD, Stanforth D, Linke MJ, et al. *Pneumocystis carinii*: Immunoblotting and immunofluorescent analysis of serum antibodies during rat infection and recovery. Exp Parasitol. 1987;6:319–28.
49. Brenner M, Ognibene FP, Lack E, et al. Prognostic factors and life expectancy of patients with acquired immunodeficiency syndrome and *Pneumocystis carinii* pneumonia. Am Rev Respir Dis. 1987;136:1199–1206.
50. Wachter RM, Luce JM, Turner J. Intensive care of patients with the acquired immunodeficiency syndrome—outcome and changing patterns of utilization. Am Rev Respir Dis. 1986;134:891–6.
51. Carter TR, Cooper PH, Petri WA, et al. *Pneumocystis carinii* infection of the small intestine in a patient with the acquired immunodeficiency syndrome. Am J Clin Pathol. 1988;89:679–83.
52. Hughes WT, Feldman S, Chaudhary CC, et al. Comparison of pentamidine isethionate and trimethoprim-sulfamethoxazole in treatment of *Pneumocystis carinii* pneumonia. J Pediatr. 1978;92:285–91.
53. Wharton JM, Coleman DL, Wofsy CB, et al. Trimethoprim-sulfamethoxazole or pentamidine for *Pneumocystis carinii* pneumonia in the acquired immunodeficiency syndrome. Ann Intern Med. 1986;105:37–44.
54. Sattler FR, Cowan R, Nielson DM, et al. Trimethoprim-sulfamethoxazole compared with pentamidine for treatment of *Pneumocystis carinii* pneumonia in the acquired immunodeficiency syndrome. Ann Intern Med. 1988;109:280–7.
55. Allegra CJ, Kovacs JA, Drake JC, et al. Activity of antifolates against *Pneumocystis carinii* dihydrofolate reductase and identification of a potent new agent. J Exp Med. 1987;165:926–31.
56. Mallory DL, Parrillo JE, Bailey KR, et al. Cardiovascular effects and safety of intravenous and intramuscular pentamidine isethionate. Crit Care Med. 1987;15:503–5.
57. Conte JE, Upton RA, Lin ET. Pentamidine pharmacokinetics in patients with AIDS with impaired renal function. J Infect Dis. 1987;156:885–90.
58. Donnelly H, Bernard EM, Rothkotter H, et al. Distribution of pentamidine in patients with AIDS. J Infect Dis. 1988;157:985–9.
59. Shelhamer JH, Ognibene FP, Macher AM, et al. Persistence of *Pneumocystis carinii* in lung tissue of acquired immunodeficiency syndrome patients treated for Pneumocystis pneumonia. Am Rev Respir Dis. 1984;130:1161–5.
60. Stahl-Bayliss CM, Kalman CM, Lashkin OL. Pentamidine-induced hypoglycemia in patients with the acquired immune deficiency syndrome. Clin Pharmacol Ther. 1986;39:271–5.
61. Hughes WT, McNabb PC, Markres TD. Efficacy of trimethoprim and sulfamethoxazole in the prevention and treatment of *Pneumocystis carinii* pneumonitis. Antimicrob Agents Chemother. 1974;5:289–93.
62. Kluge RM, Spaulding DM, Spain JA. Combination of pentamidine and trimethoprim-sulfamethoxazole in the therapy of *Pneumocystis carinii* pneumonia in rats. Antimicrob Agents Chemother. 1978;13:975–8.
63. Walzer PD, Kim CK, Foy JM, et al. Inhibitors of folic acid synthesis in the treatment of experimental *Pneumocystis carinii* pneumonia. Antimicrob Agents Chemother. 1988;32:96–103.
64. Allegra CJ, Chabner BA, Tuazon CU, et al. Trimetrexate for the treatment of *Pneumocystis carinii* pneumonia in patients with the acquired immunodeficiency syndrome. N Engl J Med. 1987;317:978–85.
65. Kirby HB, Kenamore B, Guckian JC. *Pneumocystis carinii* pneumonia treated with pyrimethamine and sulfadiazine. Ann Intern Med. 1971;75:505–9.
66. Leoung GS, Mills J, Hopewell PC, et al. Dapsone-trimethoprim for *Pneumocystis carinii* pneumonia in the acquired immunodeficiency syndrome. Ann Intern Med. 1986;105:45–8.
67. Montgomery AB, Debs RJ, Luce JM, et al. Aerosolized pentamidine as sole therapy for *Pneumocystis carinii* pneumonia in patients with acquired immunodeficiency syndrome. Lancet. 1987;2:480–483.
68. Conte JE Jr, Hollander H, Golden JA. Inhaled or reduced-dose intravenous pentamidine for *Pneumocystis carinii* pneumonia. Ann Intern Med. 1987;107:495–8.
69. McCann PP, Bacchi C, Clarkson AB, et al. Inhibition of polyamine biosynthesis by alpha-difluoromethylornithine African trypanosomiasis and *Pneumocystis carinii* as a basis of chemotherapy: Biochemical and clinical aspects. Am J Trop Med Hyg. 1986;35:1153–6.
70. Smith JW, Bartlett MS, Queener SF, et al. *Pneumocystis carinii* pneumonia therapy with 9-deazainosine in rats. Diagn Microbiol Infect Dis. 1987;7:113–8.
71. Walzer PD, Kim CK, Foy JM, et al. Cationic antitrypanosomal and other drugs in the treatment of experimental *Pneumocystis carinii* pneumonia. Antimicrob Agents Chemother. In press.
72. Queener SF, Bartlett MS, Richardson JD, et al. Activity of clindamycin with primaquine against *Pneumocystis carinii* in vitro and in vivo. Antimicrob Ag Chemother. 1988;32:807–13.
73. MacFadden DK, Hyland RH, Inouye T, et al. Corticosteroids as adjunctive therapy in treatment of *Pneumocystis carinii* in patients with acquired immunodeficiency syndrome. Lancet. 1987;1:1477–9.
74. Suffredini AF, Ognibene FP, Lack EE, et al. Nonspecific interstitial pneumonitis: A common cause of pulmonary disease in the acquired immunodeficiency syndrome. Ann Intern Med. 1987;107:7–13.
75. Sanyal SK, Mariencheck WC, Hughes WT, et al. Course of pulmonary dysfunction in children surviving *Pneumocystis carinii* pneumonitis. Am Rev Respir Dis. 1981;124:161–6.
76. Whitcomb ME, Schwarz MI, Charles MA. Interstitial fibrosis after *Pneumocystis carinii*. Ann Intern Med. 1970;73:761–5.
77. Hughes WT, Rivera GK, Schell MJ, et al. Successful intermittent chemoprophylaxis for *Pneumocystis carinii* pneumonitis. N Engl J Med. 1987;316:1627–32.
78. Hughes WT. 1979. Limited effect of trimethoprim-sulfamethoxazole prophylaxis on *Pneumocystic carinii*. Antimicrob Agents Chemother. 1979;16:333–5.
79. Wolff LJ, Baehner RL. Delayed development of pneumocystis pneumonia following administration of short-term high dose trimethoprim-sulfamethoxazole. Am J Dis Child. 1978;132:525–30.
80. Bradley PP, Warden GD, Maxwell JG, et al. Neutropenia and thrombocytopenia in renal allograft patients treated with trimethoprim-sulfamethoxazole. Ann Intern Med. 1980;93:560–2.
81. Fischl MA, Dickinson GM, LaVoie L. Safety and efficacy of sulfamethoxazole and trimethoprim chemoprophylaxis for *Pneumocystis carinii* pneumonia in AIDS. JAMA. 1988;259:1185–9.
82. Pearson RD, Hewlett EL. Use of pyrimethamine-sulfadoxine (Fansidar) in prophylaxis against chloroquine-resistant *Plasmodium falciparum* and *Pneumocystis carinii*. Ann Intern Med. 1987;106:714–8.
83. Golden JA, Hollander H, Chernoff D, et al. Prevention of *Pneumocystis carinii* pneumonia by inhaled pentamidine. Lancet. 1989;i:654–7.

257. GIARDIA LAMBLIA

DAVID R. HILL

Giardia lamblia, a flagellated enteric protozoan, has emerged in recent years as an important cause of endemic and epidemic diarrhea. Its wide distribution throughout the world makes it an important contributor to chronic debilitating diarrheal illnesses and to diarrhea in travelers. In the United States it is the most prevalent enteric parasite and is the leading infectious agent identified in waterborne outbreaks of diarrhea.

DESCRIPTION OF THE PATHOGEN

The genus *Giardia* belongs to the order Diplomonadida and the family Hexamitidae. Separate mammalian hosts were once considered to harbor different *Giardia* species; however, to date only three species have been identified and these primarily by morphologic criteria. They are designated *G. lamblia* (also called *intestinalis* or *duodenalis*), infecting humans and other large mammals, *G. muris*, found in rodents and *G. agilis*, found in frogs.[1] Analysis of *G. lamblia* antigens, isoenzyme patterns, and DNA has allowed a more sophisticated grouping of *Giardia*.[2] These studies, as well as the clinical differences between isolates in experimental human infection, make it clear that both strain and antigenic variation occurs.[3a,3b]

The life cycle of *G. lamblia* comprises two stages: the trophozoite, or freely living stage, and the cyst. The trophozoite is 9–21 μm long and 5–15 μm wide (Fig. 1A) and has a convex dorsal surface and a flat ventral surface containing the disk, which is often referred to as the *sucking* or *adhesive disk*. There are four pairs of posteriorly directed flagellae that appear to be involved in locomotion and perhaps attachment. Their intracytoplasmic projections are termed *axonemes*. The disk cytoskeleton is composed of a clockwise spiral array of microtubules joined by vertical microribbons.[1] The protozoan has two nuclei, each with a prominent central karyosome. On stained preparations these create the characteristic facelike image. Median bodies, tight collections of microtubules, are placed transversely in a clawlike manner in *G. lamblia* and may be helpful in species differentiation.

Of the three morphologic species, only *G. lamblia* has been successfully cultured in vitro.[4] Growth is enhanced by the presence of biliary lipids, intestinal mucous and epithelial cells, thus helping to explain the predilection of *Giardia* to colonize the upper small bowel.[5,6] The trophozoite divides by longitudinal binary fission and has a doubling time in culture of 9–12 hours. It is an aerotolerant anaerobe; metabolizes glucose to ethanol, acetate, and CO_2; lacks mitochondria; and scavenges phospholipids, fatty acids, cholesterol, and pyrimidines from the environment.[7]

Under intestinal influences that are not completely understood, *G. lamblia* trophozoites encyst to form smooth, oval-shaped, thin-walled cysts 8–12 μm long and 7–10 μm wide (Fig. 1B). Encystation may be enhanced by multiple factors, including the presence of secondary bile salts.[8] The major structural component of the cyst wall is chitin.[9] As the cyst matures trophozoite division may occur, forming two daughter trophozoites.

EPIDEMIOLOGY

Giardia lamblia is distributed throughout the world. In the United States *Giardia* was demonstrated in 3.9 percent of more than 300,000 submitted stool specimens, with prevalence rates as high as 16 percent in certain areas, making it the most commonly identified intestinal parasite. In the developing world, *Giardia* is one of the first enteric pathogens to infect infants,[10] with peak prevalence rates of 15–20 percent occurring in children less than 10 years old.[10–12]

Acquisition of the parasite requires oral ingestion of *Giardia* cysts, most often via fecally contaminated water. For the international traveler, this mode of transmission was highlighted by the frequent occurrence of giardiasis in visitors to Leningrad in the early 1970s.[13] In the United States from 1965 to 1984, *G. lamblia* was the most commonly identified pathogen in outbreaks of waterborne diarrheal illness and accounted for 90 outbreaks that affected over 23,500 persons.[14] The first documented outbreak occurred in Aspen, Colorado, in 1965–1966, where it affected at least 123 of 1094 skiers (11 percent).[15] Many subsequent waterborne outbreaks have occurred in the mountainous regions of the northeast, the northwest, and the Rocky Mountain states.[14–18] Common to most of them has been the use of surface water treated by a faulty purification system or by inadequate chlorination and not subjected to flocculation, sedimentation, and filtration.[19,19a] Untreated wilderness water can transmit giardiasis to hikers.[20]

Person-to-person transmission is now the second most commonly identified mode of acquisition and occurs in groups with poor fecal-oral hygiene, such as small children in day care centers, sexually active male homosexuals, and persons in custodial institutions. In children less than 3 years old in day care centers, the prevalence of *Giardia* cyst passage has been as high as 20–50 percent.[21,22] Many of these children are symptomatic and have been shown to spread the disease within their homes and communities.[22] Sexually active gay men have cyst passage rates as high as 20 percent.[23] They may be symptomatic less frequently, but of the many enteric pathogens that this group harbors, one study found that diarrheal symptoms correlated most closely with the presence of *Giardia*.[24] Food occasionally has been documented as a source and may be a more common vehicle for disease transmission than is recognized.[25]

Genetic analysis of *Giardia* isolates from a number of mammalian species,[26] cross-transmission experiments,[27] and the epidemiologic link of at least one waterborne outbreak of giardiasis to beavers implies that many mammalian species serve as reservoirs for *G. lamblia*. This has important implications as efforts are made to protect public water supplies from contamination.

PATHOGENESIS AND IMMUNE RESPONSE

Giardia was once thought to be a harmless commensal, but its association with symptomatic diarrhea,[28] malabsorption in children,[29] disease after waterborne outbreaks, travel, and experimental human infection[3] has clearly established its pathogenicity. The production of diarrhea, and occasionally malabsorption, is most likely the result of a complex interaction of *Giardia* with the host, with the outcome related to the number

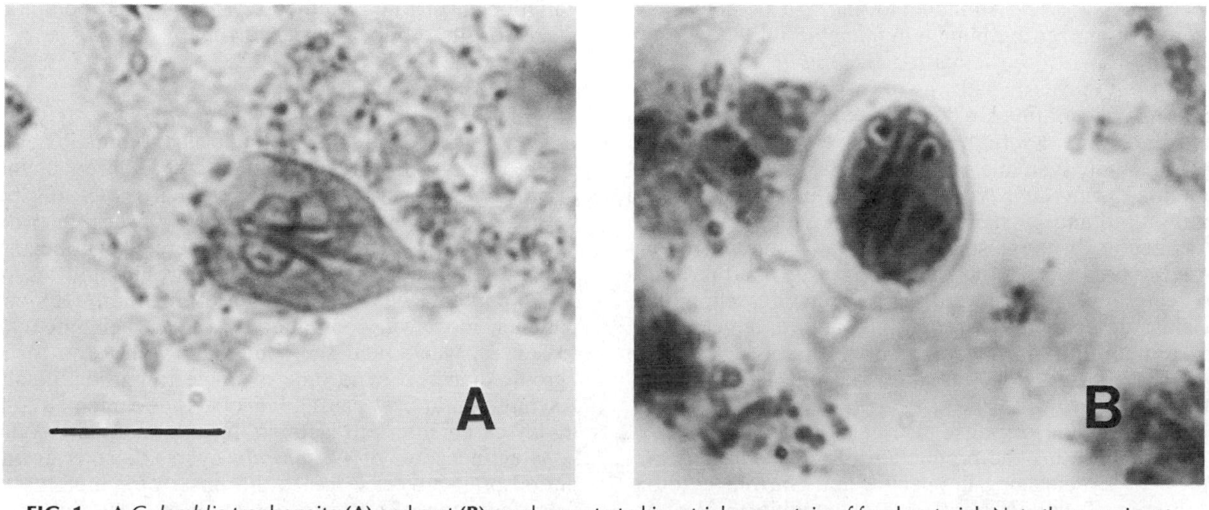

FIG. 1. A *G. lamblia* trophozoite **(A)** and cyst **(B)** are demonstrated in a trichrome stain of fecal material. Note the prominent nuclei in the trophozoite. In the cyst the cytoplasm has separated from the cyst wall; centrally located axonemes, a clawlike median body, and two eccentrically located nuclei can be detected. (Bar equals 10 μm.)

and strain of *Giardia* ingested and the host's immune response to the parasite.

Infection occurs via the oral route usually after ingestion of cysts rather than trophozoites since the latter are readily destroyed by gastric acid. As few as 10–25 cysts may establish infection.[30] After ingestion, under the influence of gastric acid, among other factors, there is excystation of *G. lamblia* trophozoites[31] and subsequent colonization of and multiplication in the upper small bowel. Adherence of *G. lamblia* in the human gut may be via the disk, with attachment at the brush border of enterocytes by either a suction or a clasping mechanism but may also involve specific receptor–ligand interactions.[32,32a]

Several pathogenic mechanisms have been postulated in giardiasis. Electron microscopy has documented disruption of the brush border in some patients[33]; however, the circular disk imprints left on mouse enterocytes by *G. muris*[34] have not been noted in humans. Disaccharidase deficiencies, especially of lactase, are well documented in both humans with *G. lamblia* and animals with *G. muris*.[35,36] In mice infected with *G. muris* there is increased epithelial cell turnover in the crypt region,[36] potentially changing the bowel's absorptive capacity. If the presence of parasites on the epithelial brush border is accounting for diarrhea, a large inoculum of *Giardia* might be expected to enhance the disease, a factor that has been suggested for both humans[30] and mice.[37]

Although some studies have shown invasion of this luminal parasite within the epithelium and submucosa,[38] it is likely that this event is more important in stimulating a host immune response than in the actual production of disease. Simultaneous colonization of the small bowel with *Giardia* and Enterobacteriaceae or yeast may contribute to malabsorption in some patients by the deconjugation of bile salts.[39] There has been no evidence that *Giardia* elaborates an enterotoxin.

The host immune response is the other important component of the host–parasite relationship.[40] Host immunity plays a role in providing protection from disease, in clearance of the parasite, and, in certain instances, in production of disease. Several observations indicate that partially protective immunity may develop to *Giardia*. Prevalence of *Giardia* in areas endemic for the parasite has been higher in younger age groups,[10,41,42] and in an endemic area of the United States, the Colorado Rockies, lower rates of symptomatic disease occurred in long-term residents of the area compared with visitors or short-term residents.[15,43]

The components of host immunity are both humoral and cellular.[40] A systemic antibody response occurs in patients with *Giardia*, and has been useful both diagnostically and in seroprevalence studies.[3,10,44,45] Immunoblotting has detected several antigens recognized by human immune serum.[46,47] Serum has also been shown to be lethal for *G. lamblia* trophozoites via activation of the classic pathway of complement.[48] Because *Giardia* is primarily confined to the lumen of the gastrointestinal tract, gastrointestinal, secretory antibodies may play a more important role than systemic antibodies. Elevation of gut immunoglobulins during *Giardia* infection has been documented by aspirating fluid and by staining intestinal lymphocytes from biopsy specimens. In these studies there is an initial predominence of IgM-staining cells, but elevations of IgG and IgA cells have also been seen.[49–51] In mice, IgA has been the predominant antibody class detected in gut secretions, and its development correlates temporally with clearance of the parasite.[52,53] The absence of specific secretory IgA is associated with failure to resolve the infection.[54,54a]

The cellular immune response also helps to clear parasites, perhaps by coordinating the production of anti-*Giardia* secretory IgA[55,56] or by engaging in specific anti-*Giardia* cytotoxicity.[57] Athymic, T-cell-deficient mice are unable to clear infection with *G. muris* until the mice are reconstituted with lymphoid cells.[58] After reconstitution, these animals develop abnormal intestinal histology that parallels the changes seen in some humans with giardiasis: spruelike lesions with marked flattening of the villi, crypt hypertrophy, and a dense mononuclear cell infiltration of the submucosa.[49,59] The presence of intraepithelial lymphocytes has also been shown to correlate with adverse histologic changes.[36,60] These findings support a role for cellular immunity in the immunopathogenesis of giardiasis. The coordination of this immune response is performed by the T-helper cells.[61] Athymic mice have reduced numbers of T-helper lymphocytes, and depletion of these cells in immunocompetent mice renders them unable to clear infection.[61]

This immune response is likely to be initiated when antigen is taken up by macrophages residing in Peyer's patches.[62] Electron microscopy of the Peyer's patches of *G. muris*-infected mice has demonstrated the ingestion of trophozoites by macrophages with lymphocyte rosetting around them.[63] In vitro, human mononuclear phagocytes and rabbit and mouse peritoneal macrophages are capable of ingesting *Giardia* trophozoites.[64,65] Ingestion is enhanced by anti-*Giardia* antibodies.

Human milk has also been found to be cytotoxic to *Giardia* trophozoites.[66] Cytotoxicity occurs when free fatty acids are released from milk triglycerides by the action of bile-salt-stimulated lipase present in human milk.[67] Both human and animal breast milk has been found to contain anti-*Giardia* antibodies,[65,68,69] and one study has suggested protection of breast-feeding infants from infection.[68]

Predisposition to giardiasis has been documented in patients with common variable immunodeficiency[70] and in children with X-linked agammaglobulinemia.[71] These patients have symptomatic disease with prolonged diarrhea, malabsorption, and marked changes on small bowel biopsy, as described previously, which can include nodular lymphoid hyperplasia. Upon administration of anti-*Giardia* therapy, their symptoms improve and the histologic changes resolve. The finding of nodular lymphoid hyperplasia in giardiasis has also been documented in patients without an underlying immunodeficiency.[72] It remains unclear if selective IgA is a predisposing factor.[50] Children who are chronically malnourished may have associated giardiasis that exacerbates their underlying malnourished state.[73,74] Susceptibility to giardiasis has also been seen in patients with previous gastric surgery and reduced gastric acidity. There does not appear to be an association of giardiasis with blood group specificity.[75] Although patients with AIDS may not have more severe illness with *Giardia*, they do exhibit impaired immune responses to the parasite.[75a,75b]

Small bowel biopsy may demonstrate spruelike lesions or may be normal. One study has correlated the severity of diarrhea with the degree of histologic abnormality on biopsy.[59] The variation in histology indicates the multiple potential mechanisms for the production of diarrhea.

CLINICAL MANIFESTATIONS

Infection with *G. lamblia* includes asymptomatic cyst passage, acute usually self-limited diarrhea, and a chronic syndrome of diarrhea, malabsorption, and weight loss. Of 100 people ingesting *Giardia* cysts, an estimated 5–15 percent will become asymptomatic cyst passers, 25–50 percent will become symptomatic with an acute diarrheal syndrome, and the remaining 35–70 percent will have no trace of infection. Of symptomatic patients, most will spontaneously clear their infection after 1 to several weeks and the remainder will go on to develop a chronic diarrheal syndrome or come to antimicrobial therapy. Asymptomatic cyst passage has been documented for children in day care centers to last as long as 6 months.[21]

After ingestion of *G. lamblia* cysts, there is an incubation period of 1–2 weeks before the onset of symptoms. The time from ingestion of cysts to detection of cysts in the stool may be longer than the incubation period.[3,76] Thus, a stool exam at the time of the onset of symptoms might well be negative.

Symptomatic giardiasis is characterized by the acute onset of diarrhea, abdominal cramps, bloating, and flatulence (Table 1). The patient usually expresses feelings of malaise, nausea, and anorexia and may complain of sulfuric belching. Vomiting, fever, and tenesmus occur less commonly. Initially, stools may be profuse and watery but later are commonly greasy, foul-smelling, and may float. Gross blood, pus, and mucus are usually absent, and, if examined microscopically, the stool is found to be free of polymorphonuclear cells.

One of the most important distinguishing features is the prolonged duration of diarrhea with giardiasis. At the time of presentation, most patients have been symptomatic for more than a week to 10 days. Weight loss of about 10 pounds occurs 50 percent of the time and is another useful clinical feature.[13,15,20,25] Unusually, cases may resolve spontaneously after 3 or 4 days, but most will continue for several weeks. Rarely, a reactive arthritis occurs.[77]

Patients who go on to develop chronic diarrhea have profound malaise, lassitude, occasional headache, and diffuse abdominal and epigastric discomfort often exacerbated by eating. Stools may again be greasy and foul-smelling or frothy, yellowish, occurring in small volume, and frequently passed. Weight loss is usually present. Periods of diarrhea may be interrupted by periods of constipation or normal bowel habits, with the syndrome waxing and waning over months until therapy is given or spontaneous resolution occurs.

Various degrees of malabsorption may be present. Children who present for evaluation for failure to thrive or with a sprue-like illness have been found to have giardiasis.[29] Steatorrhea and malabsorption of vitamins A and B_{12}, protein, and D-xylose have been documented.[73,78,79] The most common disaccharidase deficiency has been that of lactase, occurring in 20–40 percent of cases,[35,59] with post-*Giardia* lactose intolerance sometimes persisting for several weeks after treatment. This is often confused with relapse or reinfection.

The role that chronic infection with *Giardia* plays in the growth and development of children in the developing world has been the subject of much interest.[73,74,80] Some studies point to a deleterious effect on growth,[11,73,74] arguing for the need to treat recurrent disease. Others suggest that reinfection occurs so rapidly in areas of poor sanitation that repeated therapy is impractical.[12,80] These issues are not likely to be resolved until adequate sanitation is provided for persons in the developing world.

DIAGNOSIS

The diagnosis of giardiasis should be considered in all patients with prolonged diarrhea or malabsorption, especially if there is a history of recent travel to an endemic area, the presence of children in the home who attend day care centers, or an active homosexual life-style. The usual method of diagnosis is a stool exam for trophozoites or cysts. A saline wet mount of liquid stool in the acute stage of illness may yield motile trophozoites. More often, however, the stool is semiformed, and trophozoites will not be found. In these cases the stool may again be examined fresh for cysts or after preservation in formalin or polyvinyl alcohol (PVA) and subsequent trichrome or iron hematoxylin staining.[81] Formalin-ether or zinc sulfate flotation concentration techniques may increase the yield. When these techniques are carefully applied, one will identify *Giardia* 50–70 percent of the time after one stool, and some report over 90 percent identification after three stools.[82] Examination of a purged sample does not increase the yield.

Sampling of duodenal contents may be indicated when the stool examination is negative. Three methods have been used: the string test or Entero-Test (Hedeco, Palo Alto, California),[83] duodenal aspiration, and duodenal biopsy. The Enterotest is a gelatin capsule containing a nylon string, the free end of which is secured at the mouth and the capsule swallowed. It dissolves in the stomach and the string continues through the duodenum to the jejunum. After a 4- to 6-hour or overnight incubation while fasting, the string is removed, the bile-stained mucus is squeezed onto a microscope slide, and the specimen is stained or examined fresh for trophozoites. Some studies have reported a significantly increased yield over stool samples by this process.[83] Duodenal aspiration and biopsy are somewhat more cumbersome. Biopsies require touch preparations, Giemsa staining, and a careful search for trophozoites. A biopsy would aid in the identification of histologic pathology not due to giardiasis, and an aspirate could be sampled for small bowel overgrowth.

Testing for systemic anti-*Giardia* antibody, although not widely available, has been useful in seroepidemiologic studies throughout the world.[10,44,45] IgG antibodies remain elevated for long periods of time, making them less helpful diagnostically in areas endemic for giardiasis.[10,84] Serum anti-*Giardia* IgM, however, may be useful in distinguishing current from past giardiasis.[84] Detection of *Giardia* antigens in stool is likely to be useful in the future as a diagnostic test.[85,86] The white blood cell count is usually normal, and eosinophilia is absent. Barium studies are generally nonspecific and may interfere with the examination of stools.

TABLE 1. Symptoms of Giardiasis

	Percent	Range
Diarrhea	89	64–100
Malaise	84	72–97
Flatulence	74	35–97
Foul-smelling, greasy stools	72	57–79
Abdominal cramps	70	44–85
Bloating	69	42–97
Nausea	68	59–79
Anorexia	64	41–82
Weight loss	64	56–73
Vomiting	27	17–36
Fever	13	0–21
Urticaria	9	4–14
Constipation	9	0–17

(Data from Refs. 13, 15, 16, 18, 20, and 25.)

TREATMENT

Routine isolation, culture, and susceptibility testing of *Giardia* have been difficult, with variation in results.[87–89] Most information on drug efficacy, therefore, relies upon clinical experience. Several drugs with excellent efficacy are available for treatment.[90–92] The acridine dye derivative quinacrine is considered by some to be the drug of choice.[92] Given in a dose of 100 mg tid in adults and 6 mg/kg/day in three divided doses in children, for 5–7 days, it has an efficacy of approximately 90 percent; however, it may be poorly tolerated in children,[93] requiring discontinuation. The most common side effects are nausea, vomiting, and abdominal cramping. Yellow discoloration of the skin, urine, and sclerae can occasionally occur, and exfoliative dermatitis and toxic psychosis are rare side effects. Metronidazole, a nitroimidazole, although not approved for use in giardiasis in the United States, is given in a dose of 250 mg tid to adults and 15 mg/kg/day in three divided doses to children for 7 days, with an efficacy of 80–95 percent.[90–92] It is generally better tolerated in the pediatric age group, but concerns about potential mutagenicity make its routine use debatable. Other side effects noted are a metallic taste in the mouth, some nausea, dizziness, and headache, and, rarely, reversible neutropenia. When taken with alcohol, it can give a disulfiram-like effect. High-dose, short-course regimens have lower efficacy rates and may be poorly tolerated. Furazolidone, a nitrofuran, has been advocated as an alternative drug in the pediatric age group because of its availability in liquid suspension form. Given in a dosage of 8 mg/kg/day in three or four divided doses for 10 days it has an efficacy of 80 percent. It may cause gastrointestinal side effects, turn urine brown, and cause mild hemolysis in glucose-6-phosphate dehydrogenase (G6PD)-deficient individuals. In one study it was better tolerated than quinacrine.[93] Although not available in the United States, another nitroimidazole, tinidazole, has shown excellent efficacy (approximately 90 percent) when given in a single 2-g dose.[94] For patients who fail one drug course or infrequently relapse, a second course of the same drug or a switch to a drug from a different class is generally effective.

For pregnant women with giardiasis, there is no consistently recommended therapy because of the theoretical adverse effects of anti-*Giardia* drugs on the fetus. In some women, the disease is mild and therapy may be delayed until after delivery, or at least until after the first trimester. An oral aminoglycoside, paromomycin, has been used with limited experience,[95] but it is attractive because it is not measurably absorbed from the intestine. It is given in a dose of 25–30 mg/kg/day in three divided doses for 5–10 days.[96] More experience with this drug is required before its true efficacy and potential side effects are known.

PREVENTION

The prevention of giardiasis includes the proper handling and treatment of water used for communities and good personal hygiene on an individual basis. Although chlorination alone is sufficient to kill *G. lamblia* cysts, important variables, such as water temperature, clarity, pH, and contact time, alter the efficacy of chlorine, and higher chlorine levels (4–6 mg/liter) may be required.[17,97] Thus, in addition to chlorination, water supplies should also be subjected to flocculation, sedimentation, and filtration.[19] For the traveler to the back country, all water should be considered suspect due to the wide animal reservoir of giardiasis and should be brought to a boil for at least 1 minute, longer at higher elevation. If boiling is impossible, halazone (5 tabs/liter/30 min), a solution of saturated crystalline iodine (12.5 ml/liter/30 min),[98] or other chlorine or iodine preparations may be effective.[97] The traveler should avoid uncooked foods that may have been washed or prepared in contaminated water.

The endemic foci present in day care centers are a major problem. Because of the difficulty of preventing the spread of fecal-oral pathogens and the potential side effects of treatment regimens, some recommend that only symptomatic children be treated.[21] If strict handwashing and treatment of symptomatic children fail to control the diarrhea outbreak, consideration can be given to treating all infected children. Venereal transmission of *Giardia* can be decreased by avoidance of oral-anal and oral-genital sex. At present there is no immuno- or chemoprophylactic strategy for giardiasis.

REFERENCES

1. Feely DE, Erlandsen SI, Chase DG. Structure of the trophozoite and cyst. In: Erlandsen SL, Meyer EA, eds. *Giardia* and Giardiasis. New York: Plenum Press; 1984:3–31.
2. Nash TE, Keister DB. Differences in excretory-secretory products and surface antigens among 19 isolates of *Giardia*. J Infect Dis. 1985;152:1166–71.
3. Nash TE, Herrington DA, Losonsky GA, et al. Experimental human infections with *Giardia lamblia*. J Infect Dis. 1987;156:974–84.

3a. Nash TE, Aggarwal A, Adam RD, et al. Antigenic variation in *Giardia lamblia*. J Immunol. 1988;141:636–41.

3b. Aggarwal A, Nash TE. Antigenic variation of *Giardia lamblia* in vivo. Infect Immun. 1988;56:1420–3.

4. Visvesvara GS. Axenic growth of *Giardia lamblia* in Diamond's TPS-1 medium. Trans R Soc Trop Med Hyg. 1980;74:213–5.
5. Gault MJ, Gillin FD, Zenian AJ. *Giardia lamblia*: Stimulation of growth by human intestinal mucus and epithelial cells in serum-free medium. Exp Parasitol. 1987;64:29–37.
6. Farthing MJG, Keusch GT, Carey MC. Effects of bile and bile salts on growth and membrane lipid uptake by *Giardia lamblia*. Possible implications for the pathogenesis of intestinal disease. J Clin Invest. 1985;76:1727–32.
7. Lindmark DG, Jarroll EL. Metabolism of trophozoites. In: Erlandsen SL, Meyer EA, eds. *Giardia* and Giardiasis. New York: Plenum Press; 1984:65–80.
8. Gillin FD, Reiner DS, Gault MJ, et al. Encystation and expression of cyst antigens by *Giardia lamblia* in vitro. Science. 1987;235:1040–3.
9. Ward HD, Alroy J, Lev BI, et al. Identification of chitin as a structural component of *Giardia* cysts. Infect Immun. 1985;49:629–34.
10. Gilman RH, Brown KH, Visvesvara GS, et al. Epidemiology and serology of *Giardia lamblia* in a developing country: Bangladesh. Trans R Soc Trop Med Hyg. 1985;79:469–73.
11. Farthing MJG, Mata L, Urrutia JJ, et al. Natural history of *Giardia* infection of infants and children in rural Guatemala and its impact on physical growth. Am J Clin Nutr. 1986;43:395–405.
12. Gilman RH, Marquis GS, Miranda E, et al. Rapid reinfection by *Giardia lamblia* after treatment in a hyperendemic third world community. Lancet. 1988;1:343–5.
13. Brodsky RE, Spencer HC, Schultz MG. Giardiasis in American travelers to the Soviet Union. J Infect Dis. 1974;130:319–23.
14. Craun GF. Waterborne giardiasis in the United States 1965–1984. Lancet. 1986;2:513–4.
15. Moore GT, Cross WM, McGuire D, et al. Epidemic giardiasis at a ski resort. N Engl J Med. 1969;281:402–7.
16. Dykes AC, Juranek DD, Lorenz RA, et al. Municipal waterborne giardiasis: An epidemiologic investigation. Beavers implicated as a possible reservoir. Ann Intern Med. 1980;92(Pt 1):165–70.
17. Centers for Disease Control. Waterborne giardiasis—California, Colorado, Oregon, Pennsylvania. Morbid Mortal Week Rep. 1980;29:121–3.
18. Kent GP, Greenspan JR, Herndon JL, et al. Epidemic giardiasis caused by a contaminated public water supply. Am J Public Health. 1988;78:139–43.
19. Jakubowski W. Purple burps and the filtration of drinking water supplies (Editorial). Am J Public Health. 1988;78:123–5.

19a. Porter JD, Ragazzoni HP, Buchanon JD, et al. *Giardia* transmission in a swimming pool. Am J Pub Health. 1988;78:659–62.

20. Barbour AG, Nichols CR, Fukushima T. An outbreak of giardiasis in a group of campers. Am J Trop Med Hyg. 1976;25:384–9.
21. Pickering LK, Woodward WE, DuPont HL, et al. Occurrence of *Giardia lamblia* in children in day care centers. J Pediatr. 1984;104:522–6.
22. Polis MA, Tuazon CU, Alling DW, et al. Transmission of *Giardia lamblia* from a day care center to the community. Am J Public Health. 1986;76:1142–4.
23. Keystone JS, Keystone DL, Proctor EM. Intestinal parasitic infections in homosexual men. Prevalence, symptoms and factors in transmission. Can Med Assoc J. 1980;123:512–4.
24. Quinn TC, Stamm WE, Goodell SE, et al. The polymicrobial origin of intestinal infections in homosexual men. N Engl J Med. 1983;309:576–82.
25. Petersen LR, Cartter ML, Hadler JL. A food-borne outbreak of *Giardia lamblia*. J Infect Dis. 1988;157:846–8.
26. Nash TE, McCutchan T, Keister D, et al. Restriction endonuclease analysis of DNA from 15 *Giardia* isolates obtained from humans and animals. J Infect Dis. 1985;152:64–73.
27. Woo PK. Evidence for animal reservoirs and transmission of *Giardia* infection between animal species. In: Erlandsen SL, Meyer EA, eds. *Giardia* and Giardiasis. New York: Plenum Press; 1984:341–64.
28. Peterson H. Giardiasis (lambliasis). Scand J Gastroenterol. 1972;7(Suppl 14):1–44.
29. Burke JA. Giardiasis in childhood. Am J Dis Child. 1975;129:1304–10.
30. Rendtorff RC. The experimental transmission of human intestinal protozoan parasites: II. *Giardia lamblia* cysts given in capsules. Am J Hyg. 1954;59:209–20.
31. Rice EW, Schaefer FW. Improved in vitro excystation procedure for *Giardia lamblia* cysts. J Clin Microbiol. 1981;14:709–10.
32. Lev B, Ward H, Keusch GT, et al. Lectin activation in *Giardia lamblia* by host protease: A novel host-parasite interaction. Science. 1986;232:71–3.

32a. Inge PMG, Edson CM, Farthing MJG. Attachment of *Giardia lamblia* to rat intestinal epithelial cells. Gut. 1988;29:795–801.

33. Balazs M, Szaltocky E. Electron microscopic examination of the mucosa of the small intestine in infection due to *Giardia lamblia*. Pathol Res Pract. 1978;163:251–60.
34. Owen RL, Nemanic PC, Stevens DP. Ultrastructural observations on giardiasis in a murine model: I. Intestinal distribution, attachment, and relationship to the immune system of *Giardia muris*. Gastroenterology. 1979;76:757–69.
35. Welsh JD, Poley JR, Hensley J, et al. Intestinal disaccharidase and alkaline phosphatase activity in giardiasis. J Pediatr Gastroenterol Nutr. 1984;3:37–40.
36. Gillon J, al Thamery D, Ferguson A. Features of small intestinal pathology (epithelial cell kinetics, intraepithelial lymphocytes, disaccharidases) in a primary *Giardia muris* infection. Gut. 1982;23:498–506.
37. Olveda RK, Andrews JS, Hewlett EL. Murine giardiasis: Localization of trophozoites and small bowel histopathology during the course of infection. Am J Trop Med Hyg. 1982;31:60–6.
38. Saha TK, Gosh TK. Invasion of small intestinal mucosa by *Giardia lamblia* in man. Gastroenterology. 1977;72:402–5.
39. Tandon BN, Tandon RK, Satpathy BK, et al. Mechanism of malabsorption in giardiasis: A study of bacterial flora and bile salt deconjugation in upper jejunum. Gut. 1977;18:176–81.
40. den Hollander N, Riley D, Befus D. Immunology of giardiasis. Parasitol Today. 1988;4:124–31.
41. Oyerinde PO, Ogunbi O, Alonge AA. Age and sex distribution of infections

with *Entamoeba histolytica* and *Giardia intestinalis* in the Lagos population. Int J Epidemiol. 1977;6:231–4.
42. Knight R. Epidemiology and transmission of giardiasis. Trans R Soc Trop Med Hyg. 1980;74:433–6.
43. Istre GP, Dunlop TS, Gaspard GB, et al. Waterborne giardiasis at a mountain resort: Evidence for acquired immunity. Am J Public Health. 1984;74:602–4.
44. Smith PD, Gillin FD, Brown WR, et al. IgG antibody to *Giardia lamblia* detected by enzyme-linked immunosorbent assay. Gastroenterology. 1981;80:1476–80.
45. Miotti PPG, Gilman RH, Santosham M, et al. Age-related rate of seropositivity of antibody to *Giardia lamblia* in four diverse populations. J Clin Microbiol. 1986;24:972–5.
46. Edson CM, Farthing MJG, Thorley-Lawson DA, et al. An 88,000-M_r *Giardia lamblia* surface protein which is immunogenic in humans. Infect Immun. 1986;54:621–5.
47. Taylor GD, Wenman WM. Human immune response to *Giardia lamblia* infection. J Infect Dis. 1987;155:137–40.
48. Hill DR, Burge JJ, Pearson RD. Susceptibility of *Giardia lamblia* trophozoites to the lethal effect of human serum. J Immunol. 1984;132:2046–52.
49. Ridley MJ, Ridley DS. Serum antibodies and jejunal histology in giardiasis. J Clin Pathol. 1976;29:30–4.
50. Jones EG, Brown WR. Serum and intestinal fluid immunoglobulins in patients with giardiasis. Dig Dis. 1974;19:791–6.
51. Thompson A, Rowland R, Hecker R, et al. Immunoglobulin-bearing cells in giardiasis. J Clin Pathol. 1977;30:292–4.
52. Heyworth MF. Antibody response to *Giardia muris* trophozoites in mouse intestine. Infect Immun. 1986;52:568–71.
53. Snider DP, Underdown BJ. Quantitative and temporal analysis of murine antibody response in serum and gut secretions to infection with *Giardia muris*. Infect Immun. 1986;52:271–8.
54. Snider DP, Gordon J, McDermott MR, et al. Chronic *Giardia muris* infection of anti-IgM-treated mice. I. Analysis of immunoglobulin and parasite-specific antibody in normal and immunoglobulin deficient mice. J Immunol. 1985; 134:4153–62.
54a. Snider DP, Skea D, Underdown BJ. Chronic giardiasis in B-cell-deficient mice expressing the *xid* gene. Infect Immun. 1988;56:2838–42.
55. Conley ME, Delacroix DL. Intravascular and mucosal immunoglobulin A: Two separate but related systems of immune defense. Ann Intern Med. 1987;106:892–9.
56. Carlson JR, Heyworth MF, Owen RL. Response of Peyer's patch lymphocyte subsets to *Giardia muris* infection in BALB/c mice. II. B-cell subsets: Enteric antigen exposure is associated with immunoglobulin isotype switching by Peyer's patch B cells. Cell Immunol. 1986;97:51–8.
57. Kanwar SS, Ganguly NK, Walia BNS, et al. Direct and antibody dependent cell mediated cytotoxicity against *Giardia lamblia* by splenic and intestinal lymphoid cells in mice. Gut. 1986;27:73–7.
58. Roberts-Thomson IC, Mitchell GF. Giardiasis in mice: I. Prolonged infections in certain mouse strains and hypothymic (nude) mice. Gastroenterology. 1978;75:42–6.
59. Duncombe VM, Bolin TD, Davis AE, et al. Histopathology in giardiasis: A correlation with diarrhea. Aust NZ J Med. 1978;8:392–6.
60. Wright SG, Tomkins AM. Quantification of the lymphocytic infiltrate in jejunal epithelium in giardiasis. Clin Exp Immunol. 1977;29:408–12.
61. Heyworth MF, Carlson JR, Ermak TH. Clearance of *Giardia muris* infection requires helper/inducer T lymphocytes. J Exp Med. 1987;165:1743–8.
62. Targan SR. The intestine as an immunologic organ. In: Targan SR, moderator. Immunologic mechanisms in intestinal diseases. Ann Intern Med. 1987;106:853–70.
63. Owen RL, Allen CL, Stevens DP. Phagocytosis of *Giardia muris* by macrophages in Peyer's patch epithelium in mice. Infect Immun. 1981;33:591–601.
64. Hill DR, Pearson RD. Ingestion of *Giardia lamblia* trophozoites by human mononuclear phagocytes. Infect Immun. 1987;55:3155–61.
65. Kaplan BS, Uni S, Aikawa M, et al. Effector mechanism of host resistance in murine giardiasis: Specific IgG and IgA cell-mediated toxicity. J Immunol. 1985;134:1975–81.
66. Gillin FD, Reiner DS, Wang CS. Human milk kills parasitic intestinal protozoa. Science. 1983;221:1290–2.
67. Reiner DS, Wang CS, Gillin FD. Human milk kills *Giardia lamblia* by generating toxic lipolytic products. J Infect Dis. 1986;154:825–32.
68. Nayak N, Ganguly NK, Walia BNS, et al. Specific secretory IgA in the milk of *Giardia lamblia*-infected and uninfected women. J Infect Dis. 1987;155:724–7.
69. Islam A, Stoll BJ, Ljungström I, et al. *Giardia lamblia* infections in a cohort of Bangladeshi mothers and infants followed for one year. J Pediatr. 1983;103:996–1000.
70. Ament ME, Rubin CE. Relation of giardiasis to abnormal intestinal structure and function in gastrointestinal immunodeficiency syndromes. Gastroenterology. 1972;62:216–26.
71. LoGalbo PR, Sampson HA, Buckley RH. Symptomatic giardiasis in three patients with X-linked agammaglobulinemia. J Pediatr. 1982;101:78–80.
72. Ward H, Jalan KN, Maitra TK, et al. Small intestinal nodular lymphoid hyperplasia in patients with giardiasis and normal serum immunoglobulins. Gut. 1983;24:120–6.
73. Solomons NW. Giardiasis: Nutritional implications. Rev Infect Dis. 1982; 4:859–69.
74. Gupta MC, Urrutia JJ. Effect of periodic antiascaris and antigiardia treatment on nutritional status of preschool children. Am J Clin Nutr. 1982;36:79–86.
75. Jokipii L, Jokipii AMM. Is predisposition to giardiasis associated with the ABO blood groups? Am J Trop Med Hyg. 1980;29:5–7.
75a. Laughon BE, Druckman DA, Vernon A, et al. Prevalence of enteric pathogens in homosexual men with and without acquired immunodeficiency syndrome. Gastroenterology. 1988;94:984–93.
75b. Janoff EN, Smith PD, Blaser MJ. Acute antibody responses to *Giardia lamblia* are depressed in patients with AIDS. J Infect Dis. 1988;157:798–804.
76. Jokipii AMM, Jokipii L. Prepatency of giardiasis. Lancet. 1977;1:1095–7.
77. Shaw RA, Stevens MA. The reactive arthritis of giardiasis. A case report. JAMA. 1987;258:2734–5.
78. Wright SG. Giardiasis and malabsorption. Trans R Soc Trop Med Hyg. 1980;74:436–7.
79. Sutton DL, Kamath KR. Giardiasis with protein losing enteropathy. J Pediatr Gastroenterol Nutr. 1985;4:56–9.
80. Sullivan PS, DuPont HL, Arafat RR, et al. Illness and reservoirs associated with *Giardia lamblia* infection in rural Egypt: The case against treatment in developing world environments of high endemnicity. Am J Epidemiol. 1988;127:1272–81.
81. Thornton SA, West AH, DuPont HL, et al. Comparison of methods for identification of *Giardia lamblia*. Am J Clin Pathol. 1983;80:858–60.
82. Naik SR, Rau NR, Vinayak VK. A comparative evaluation of three stool samples, jejunal aspirate and jejunal mucosal impression smears in the diagnosis of giardiasis. Ann Trop Med Parasitol. 1978;72:491–2.
83. Rosenthal P, Liebman WM. Comparative study of stool exams, duodenal aspiration, and pediatric Entero-Test for giardiasis in children. J Pediatr. 1980;96:278–9.
84. Goka AKJ, Rolston DDK, Mathan VI, et al. Diagnosis of giardiasis by specific IgM antibody enzyme-linked immunosorbent assay. Lancet. 1986;2:184–6.
85. Nash TE, Herrington DA, Levine MM. Usefulness of an enzyme-linked immunosorbent assay for detection of *Giardia* antigen in feces. J Clin Microbiol. 1987;25:1169–71.
86. Rosoff JD, Stibbs HH. Isolation and identification of a *Giardia lamblia*-specific stool antigen (GSA 65) useful in coprodiagnosis of giardiasis. J Clin Microbiol. 1986;23:905–10.
87. Gordts B, Hemelhof W, Asselman C, et al. In vitro susceptibilities of 25 *Giardia lamblia* isolates of human origin to six commonly used antiprotozoal agents. Antimicrob Agents Chemother. 1985;28:378–80.
88. McIntyre P, Boreham PFL, Phillips RE, et al. Chemotherapy in giardiasis: Clinical responses and in vitro drug sensitivity of human isolates in axenic culture. J Pediatr. 1986;108:1008–10.
89. Inge PMG, Farthing MJG. A radiometric assay for antigiardial drugs. Trans R Soc Trop Med Hyg. 1987;81:345–7.
90. Davidson RA. Issues in clinical parasitology: The treatment of giardiasis. Am J Gastroenterol. 1984;79:256–61.
91. Lerman SJ, Walker RA. Treatment of giardiasis: Literature review and recommendations. Clin Pediatr. 1982;21:409–14.
92. Wolfe MS. Symptomatology, diagnosis, and treatment. In: Erlandsen SL, Meyer EA, eds. *Giardia* and Giardiasis. New York: Plenum Press; 1984:147–61.
93. Craft JC, Murphy T, Nelson JD. Furazolidone and quinacrine. Comparative study of therapy for giardiasis in children. Am J Dis Child. 1981;135:164–6.
94. Speelman P. Single-dose tinidazole for the treatment of giardiasis. Antimicrob Agents Chemother. 1985;27:227–9.
95. Kruetner AK, Del Bene VE, Amstey MS. Giardiasis in pregnancy. Am J Obstet Gynecol. 1981;140:895–901.
96. Rotblatt MD. Giardiasis and amebiasis in pregnancy. Drug Intell Clin Pharmacol. 1983;17:187–8.
97. Jarroll EL, Bingham AK, Meyer EA. *Giardia* cyst destruction: Effectiveness of six small-quantity water disinfection methods. Am J Trop Med Hyg. 1980;29:8–11.
98. Kahn FH, Visscher BR. Water disinfection in the wilderness: A simple, effective method of iodination. West J Med. 1975;122:450–3.

258. TRICHOMONAS VAGINALIS

MICHAEL F. REIN

Trichomonas vaginalis was first described by Donné in 1836.[1] Its acceptance as a primary pathogen was gradual, and the older literature frequently refers to it as a harmless commensal.[2] Closely related organisms are widespread in nature and are important pathogens of cattle, among which they are venereally transmitted, and fowl.[3] Other organisms in the same family also infect humans. *Trichomonas tenax* resides in the anaerobic, periodontal crevices of some patients with pyorrhea and rarely causes respiratory tract infection in patients with underlying pulmonary disease.[4,5] *Pentatrichomonas hominis* can be recovered from the lower gastrointestinal tract, more frequently from patients with symptomatic bowel disease.[4] Trichomonads are highly site specific, and infection has never followed attempts to inoculate one sp. into an anatomic site usually inhabited by another.[4,5]

Infected vaginal discharge contains 10^1–10^5 protozoa/ml, with most women carrying the larger numbers.[6] In fresh preparations, *T. vaginalis* is actively motile and usually pear shaped, with average dimensions of approximately 10×7 μm. The organisms vary somewhat in size and shape and are most easily identified by their characteristic twitching motility. There are four free anterior flagella that appear to arise from a single stalk and a fifth flagellum, which is embedded in the undulating membrane that extends about half way across the organism. *Trichomonas vaginalis* is facultatively anaerobic and can utilize a variety of carbohydrates.[7] All areas of the cell surface are capable of phagocytosis[8] and can ingest bacteria and erythrocytes. The organism generates metabolic energy with unique organelles called *hydrogenosomes*,[9] reproduces by binary fission, and exists only as a vegetative cell, no cyst forms having been described. Recent observations suggest that some isolates contain viral particles.[10,11]

Strains vary with respect to serotype,[4,12] size,[4] surface carbohydrates[13] and proteins,[14–18] hemolytic activity, enzyme complement,[19,20] and experimental virulence.[4,7,21] Trichomonads appear to damage epithelial cells by direct contact[22–26] and cause microulcerations.[27]

Trichomonas vaginalis activates the alternative complement pathway[28] and attracts polymorphonuclear neutrophils (PMN)[29] which can kill the protozoa.[30] Monocytes and macrophages can also kill trichomonads in vitro, but their role in natural infection is uncertain.[31] Humoral and delayed hypersensitivity responses are seen in human infection.[4,7,12,32,33]

EPIDEMIOLOGY

An estimated 3 million American women contract trichomoniasis every year, and the incidence in men is unknown. The venereal nature of trichomoniasis is well established.[4,7] Its incidence is highest among women with multiple sexual partners[34] and in groups with high rates of other sexually transmitted diseases.[7] Thus, patients found to harbor *T. vaginalis* should always be screened for infections with other sexually transmitted pathogens, such as *Neisseria gonorrhoeae, Chlamydia trachomatis*, or human immunodeficiency virus,[7,35,36] which may be clinically silent but of far greater medical consequence than the protozoan infection. The organism is recovered from 66–100 percent of the female partners of infected men[7,33] and 30–80 percent of the male sexual partners of infected women.[7,37] The infection appears to be self-limited in many men,[37] possibly due to the trichomonacidal action of prostatic secretions,[38] including zinc[38] or to the mechanical elimination of urethral protozoa during micturition.

Trichomoniasis is occasionally acquired nonvenereally. The organism will survive for several hours in moist environments, including moist cloths.[7] Thus, the potential for nonvenereal transmission clearly exists, and trichomoniasis is found with high prevalence in some institutionalized populations.

Like the other genital infections, trichomoniasis may be transmitted to neonates during passage through an infected birth canal and is acquired by 2–17 percent of the female offspring of infected women.[7,39] It may not be necessary to treat minimally symptomatic trichomoniasis in the first 3 weeks of life since the infection is often self-limited.[39] Thereafter, trichomoniasis is rare until menarche. The diagnosis of genital trichomoniasis in an older child should raise the question of sexual abuse.[40]

CLINICAL FEATURES

The incubation period in women ranges from about 5 to 28 days.[7,36,41] Symptoms often begin or exacerbate during the menstrual period. Approximately 10–50 percent of infected women attending sexually transmitted disease clinics carry the organism asymptomatically[41]; 50–75 percent of the women developing symptoms complain of discharge,[41] and 25–50 percent note vulvovaginal soreness or irritation.[7,36,41,42] Dysuria, usually mild, or urinary frequency is described by about 30–50 percent of the infected women, and dyspareunia is common. Up to two-thirds of infected women complain of a disagreeable odor, but this symptom may actually be more suggestive of bacterial vaginosis[41,43] (see also Chapters 95 and 202). Abdominal discomfort is described by only 5–12 percent of infected women[7] and should prompt careful evaluation for a second process, such as pelvic inflammatory disease. Unfortunately, none of these symptoms alone or in combination is sufficient to diagnose trichomoniasis reliably since all can accompany other genital infections (see also Chapters 95 and 96).

Examination usually reveals a copious, rather loose discharge that pools in the posterior vaginal fornix. Only about 5–40 percent of the women have a discharge that is clearly yellow or green, but the presence of a yellow vaginal discharge should prompt a careful evaluation for trichomoniasis.[36] Bubbles are observed in the discharge of 10–33 percent of the cases.[7,36,41–43] A yellow discharge may accompany other infections, such as mucopurulent cervicitis.[36,40] Up to half of the infected women have a relatively thick discharge that may be confused with vaginal candidiasis.[42] Symptomatic women usually manifest inflammation of the vaginal walls and exocervix. Punctate hemorrhages, including the so-called strawberry cervix, are observed colposcopically in 45 percent of infected women but in only 2 percent by visual inspection alone.[36,41] Trichomoniasis is a superficial infection, and invasion of the vaginal walls by the parasite has not been observed.[7] Vaginal discharge from 66–91 percent of women with trichomoniasis has a pH level elevated above the normal value of 4.5. An elevated pH level determined with nitrazine paper suggests trichomoniasis or bacterial vaginosis rather than vulvovaginal candidiasis.[43]

Trichomonads can be recovered from the urethra and paraurethral glands in more than 95 percent of the women with trichomoniasis and may explain the association of the infection with urinary frequency.[36] Organisms are rarely isolated from the endocervix.[7] Spread of trichomonads beyond the lower urogenital tract is extremely rare.

Most men carrying trichomonads are completely asymptomatic. Organisms can, however, be isolated from 5–15 percent of patients with nongonococcal urethritis,[37,45] and these men have a syndrome that is not clinically distinguishable from nongonococcal urethritis of other etiologies. Symptomatic men usually have a discharge and dysuria, although the discharge is often so scant that it may be noticed only as a small bead at the meatus upon arising in the morning. Trichomoniasis occasionally causes epididymitis and superficial penile ulcerations, often beneath the prepuce,[37] and involves the prostate gland.[46]

Clinical differentiation of various forms of infectious vaginitis is unreliable,[34,36,41–43,47] and the accurate diagnosis of trichomoniasis in patients of either sex depends on demonstration of the organism in genital specimens. Trichomonads may be identified in vaginal secretions using the wet mount technique (described in Chapter 95), which will detect them in 60–70 percent of the infected women.[7,36,41,48–50] *Trichomonas vaginalis* is most easily recognized by its characteristic movements. The wet mount generally also reveals large numbers of white blood cells,[7,34,36] although asymptomatic women may have very few. In trichomonal infection, epithelial cells appear normal on wet mount, and the bacterial flora consists of either rods or coccobacilli[7] (see also Chapter 95). Endocervical specimens should not be used for the diagnosis of trichomoniasis because the organism is present in the endocervix of only about 13 percent of the women with trichomoniasis.[7] Examination by wet mount of material obtained with a platinum loop from the anterior urethra will reveal the organism in 50–90 percent of the infected men.[7,37,45] Microscopic examination and culture of the urine sediment after prostatic massage is useful in diagnosing trichomoniasis in men, with the culture positive in 95 percent of the cases.[7,37,45] The Gram, Giemsa, Pappenheim, and acridine orange stains are less useful than the wet mount in diagnosing trichomoniasis in patients of either sex.

Unfortunately, a negative wet mount does not rule out trichomoniasis in either group, but trichomonads can be cultured on a number of liquid and semisolid media[36,41,48–50] or in tissue culture,[48] and culture remains the most sensitive (>95 percent) technique for the diagnosis of trichomoniasis. Direct fluorescent antibody staining[49,50] latex agglutination[51] and enzyme linked immunosorbent assay (ELISA) techniques[52,53] are more sensitive than wet mount (80–90 percent) but less sensitive than culture.

Serodiagnosis is plagued by a lack of specificity, particularly in high-risk populations in which antibody may persist from prior infections. Sensitivity is also low. Serologic testing has no current role in the evaluation of the individual patient.[4,7,32]

THERAPY

The development of metronidazole in the early 1960s revolutionized the treatment of trichomoniasis. The drug is activated with reduction of the nitro group by ferredoxin-like proteins possessed only by anaerobic organisms.[54] Short-lived metabolites are felt to act primarily by combining with DNA. Other 5-nitroimidazoles used to treat trichomoniasis outside the United States (e.g., tinidazole, ornidazole) have somewhat different pharmacologic properties but do not vary in effectiveness or toxicity.[54] Systemic therapy eradicates trichomonads from the urinary tract as well as from the vagina, thereby reducing the risk of relapse. Obviously, only systemic therapy is capable of eradicating trichomonads from the male urogenital tract.

Numerous studies have confirmed the efficacy of a single oral 2-g dose of metronidazole in women,[55,56] whereas one recent, large study suggests that this regimen may fail to cure 40 percent of infected men.[45] An alternative regimen consists of 250 mg orally three times daily for 7 days.[55,56]

The advantages of the single-dose regimen include freedom from problems with patient compliance. The lower dose reduces cost and, theoretically, the risk of toxicity. Disadvantages of the single dose are a higher rate of reinfection if sexual partners are not treated simultaneously[57,58] and the possibility of high failure rates in men.[45] In theory, any marginally effective regimen might select for metronidazole-resistant organisms.

The disadvantages of systemic metronidazole are several: Many people taking the drug complain of mild nausea or bad taste, which is more frequent after administration of a large single dose. Metronidazole blocks the metabolism of alcohol, and patients consuming the two concurrently may suffer nausea, vomiting, and flushing.[59] Not merely a narrow spectrum trichomonacide, metronidazole is active against most anaerobic bacteria and will significantly alter normal vaginal flora, occasionally allowing candidal vaginitis to supervene.[60] Metronidazole may increase the anticoagulatory effect of warfarin.

More recently, attention has been called to the capacity of high-dose, long-term metronidazole to induce lung tumors in animals, and it must be regarded as a potential carcinogen. However, data linking clinical use of metronidazole to cancer in humans are weak,[55,62] and its advantages in treating trichomoniasis outweigh its risks. The drug should not be administered indiscriminately, and the doses given should be kept as small as possible.

Metronidazole is contraindicated during the first trimester of pregnancy[63] (see Chapter 25). Although several studies suggest the safety of metronidazole during the last two trimesters,[55,56] it seems prudent to avoid the drug then as well if this is possible. Symptomatic pregnant women might initially be treated with clotrimazole, 100-mg vaginal tablets at bedtime daily for 2 weeks,[55,56] or an allantoin-aminacrine-sulfanilamide preparation. About 20 percent of women are cured by this treatment, and in others symptoms are sufficiently controlled so that definitive therapy may be delayed until later in pregnancy. Women remaining infected should be treated before delivery to prevent transmission to the newborn.[7,39]

As a public health measure, asymptomatically infected women should be treated since they represent an important reservoir of the disease. In addition, about one-third of them will become symptomatic during the following few months. The long-term effects of chronic asymptomatic trichomoniasis are unknown. Initial simultaneous treatment of male sexual partners is particularly important if the single-dose regimen is used.

The number of cases of putative metronidazole treatment failure appears to be increasing. When confronted with a woman who presents with recurrent infection, the clinician should consider the following possibilities. (*1*) Reinfection from an untreated sexual partner remains the most common cause of recurrent disease, especially if the patient received a single-dose regimen.[55,57,58] Nonjudgmental questioning regarding sexual activity may provide necessary information. It is useful to remind women that infected sexual partners are usually completely asymptomatic. (*2*) Noncompliance with multidose regimens may be revealed by careful questioning. (*3*) Very rarely, metronidazole treatment failures have been attributed to increased hepatic inactivation of the drug[63,64] or even, theoretically, to competitive inactivation by bacteria. (*4*) The infecting strain may have decreased sensitivity to metronidazole.[65,66]

Metronidazole Resistance

Metronidazole-resistant *T. vaginalis* has been reported for some years, but its prevalence seems to be increasing.[54,55,66–69] Standard regimens fail to cure infections with some of these resistant strains.[55,66–69] Methods for determining the antimicrobial sensitivity of *T. vaginalis* are not standardized,[67–72] but assays are available at some centers, and suspect organisms should be cultured and tested. Infections with resistant strains might be treated with oral doses of 2 g administered daily along with a 500-mg tablet inserted intravaginally for 7–14 days.[55,68,69] Metronidazole cream is available in some countries, including Canada,[65] but no longer in the United States. Some resistant cases have been cured with high-dose intravenous metronidazole,[73,74] but the minimum effective dose has not been determined.

Because of the frequency of infection in pregnancy, the toxicities of metronidazole, and the apparent development of resistance, therapeutic alternatives to the 5-nitroimidazoles are being actively sought.[72]

REFERENCES

1. Kampmeier RH. Description of *Trichomonas vaginalis* by MA Donne. Sex Trans Dis. 1978;5:119–22.
2. Honigberg BM (ed). Trichomonads Parasitic in Humans. New York: Springer-Verlag. In press.
3. Honigberg BM. Trichomonads of veterinary importance. In: Kreier JP, ed. Parasitic Protozoa, v. 2. New York: Academic Press; 1974;163.
4. Honigberg BM. Trichomonads of importance in human medicine. In: Kreier JP, ed. Parasitic Protozoa, v. 2. New York: Academic Press; 1974:275.
5. Hersh SM. Pulmonary trichomoniasis and *Trichomonas tenax*. J Med Microbiol. 1985;20:1–10.
6. Philip A, Carter-Scott P, Rogers C. An agar culture technique to quantitate *Trichomonas vaginalis* from women. J Infect Dis. 1987;155:304–8.

7. Muller M, Rein MF. *Trichomonas vaginalis*. In: Holmes KK, Mardh P-A, Sparling PF, et al, eds. Sexually Transmitted Diseases. 2nd ed. New York: McGraw-Hill. In press.
8. Francioli P, Shio H, Roberts RB, et al. Phagocytosis and killing of *Neisseria gonorrhoeae* by *Trichomonas vaginalis*. J Infect Dis. 1983;47:87.
9. Muller M. The hydrogenosome. In: Gooday GW, Lloyd D, Trinci APJ, eds. The Eukariotic Microbial Cell. Society for General Microbiology Symposium 30. Cambridge: Cambridge University Press; 1980:127.
10. Wang AL, Wang CC. The double-stranded RNA in *Trichomonas vaginalis* may originate from virus like particles. Proc Natl Acad Sci USA. 1986;83:7956–60.
11. Wang A, Wang CC, Alderete JF. *Trichomonas vaginalis* phenotypic variation occurs only among trichomonads infected with the double stranded RNA viruses. J Exp Med. 1987;166:142–50.
12. Garber GE, Proctor EM, Bowie WR. Immunogenic proteins of *Trichomonas vaginalis* as demonstrated by the immunoblot technique. Infect Immun. 1986;51:250–3.
13. Warton A, Honigberg BM. Analysis of surface saccharides of *Trichomonas vaginalis* strains with various pathogenicity levels by fluorescein-conjugated plant lectins. Z Parasitenkd. 1983;69:149–59.
14. Alderete JF. Identification of immunogenic and antibody binding membrane proteins of pathogenic *Trichomonas vaginalis*. Infect Immun. 1983;80:284.
15. Alderete JF, Suprun-Brown L, Kasmala L. Monoclonal antibody to a major surface glycoprotein immunogen differrentiates isolates and subpopulations of *Trichomonas vaginalis*. Infect Immun. 1986;52:70–5.
16. Krieger JN, Holmes KK, Spence MR, et al. Geographic variation among *Trichomonas vaginalis*: Demonstration of antigenic heterogeneity using monoclonal antibodies and the indirect immunofluorescent technique. J Infect Dis. 1985;5:979–84.
17. Alderete JF, Demes P, Gombosova A, et al. Phenotypes and protein-epitope phenotypic variation among fresh isolates of *Trichomonas vaginalis*. Infect Immun. 1987;55:1037–41.
18. Alderete JF, Kasmala L, Metcalfe E, et al. Phenotypic variation and diversity among *Trichomonas vaginalis* isolates and correlation of phenotype with trichomonal virulence determinants. Infect Immun. 1986;53:285–93.
19. Lockwood BC, North MJ, Scott KI, et al. The use of a highly sensitive electrophoretic method to compare the proteinases of trichomonads. Mol Biochem Parasitol. 1987;24:89–95.
20. Peterson KM, Alderete JF. Acquisition of alpha-1-antitrypsin by a pathogenic strain of *Trichomonas vaginalis*. Infect Immun. 1983;40:640–6.
21. Krieger JN, Poisson MA, Rein MF. Beta-hemolytic activity of *Trichomonas vaginalis* correlates with virulence. Infect Immun. 1983;41:129.
22. Krieger JN, Ravdin JI, Rein MF. Contact-dependent cytopathogenic mechanisms of *Trichomonas vaginalis*. Infect Immun. 1985;50:778–86.
23. Pindak FF, Gardner WA, de Pindak MM. Growth and cytopathogenicity of *Trichomonas vaginalis* in tissue culture. J Clin Microbiol. 1986;23:672–8.
24. Martinotti MG, Martinetto P, Savoia D. Adherence of *Trichomonas vaginalis* to cell culture monolayers. Eur J Clin Microbiol. 1986;5:320–3.
25. Alderete JF, Pearlman E. Pathogenic *Trichomonas vaginalis* cytotoxicity to cell culture monolayers. Br J Vener Dis. 1984;60:99–105.
26. Alderete JF, Garza GE. Specific nature of *Trichomonas vaginalis* parasitism of host cell surfaces. Infect Immun. 1985;50:701–8.
27. Nielsen MH, Nielsen R. Electron microscopy of *Trichomonas vaginalis* Donné: Interaction with vaginal epithelium in human trichomoniasis. Acta Pathol Microbiol Scand (B). 1975;83:305–20.
28. Gillin FD, Sher A. Activation of alternative complement pathway by *Trichomonas vaginalis*. Infect Immun. 1981;34:268.
29. Mason PR, Forman L. In vitro attraction of polymorphonuclear leukocytes by *Trichomonas vaginalis*. J Parasitol. 1980;66:888.
30. Rein MF, Sullivan JA, Mandell GL. Trichomonacidal activity of polymorphonuclear neutrophils: Killing by disruption and fragmentation. J Infect Dis. 1980;142:575.
31. Mantovanic A, Polentaruttic N, Peri G, et al. Cytotoxicity of human peripheral blood monocytes against *Trichomonas vaginalis*. Clin Exp Immunol. 1981;46:391.
32. Mathews HM, Healy GR. Evaluation of two serologic tests for *Trichomonas vaginalis* infection. J Clin Microbiol. 1983;17:840.
33. Mason PR, Patterson BA. Proliferative response of human lymphocytes to secretory and cellular antigens of *Trichomonas vaginalis*. J Parasitol. 1985;71:265–8.
34. McLellan R, Spence MR, Brockman M, et al. The clinical diagnosis of trichomoniasis. Obstet Gynecol. 1982;60:30.
35. Judson FN. The importance of coexisting syphilitic, chlamydial, mycoplasmal and trichomonal infection in the treatment of gonorrhea. Sex Transm Dis. 1979;6:112.
36. Wolner-Hanssen P, Krieger JN, Stevens CE, et al. Clinical manifestations of vaginal trichomoniasis: Implications for strategies for diagnosis and control of the infection. In press.
37. Krieger JN. Urologic aspects of trichomoniasis. Invest Urol. 1981;18:412.
38. Langley JG, Goldsmith JM, Davies N. Venereal trichomoniasis: Role of man. Genitourin Med. 1987;63:264–7.
39. Al-Saliki FL, Curran JP, Wong J-S. Neonatal *Trichomonas vaginalis*: Report of 3 cases and review of the literature. Pediatrics. 1974;53:196.
40. Jones JG, Yamauchi T, Lambert B. Trichomonas vaginalis infestation in sexually abused girls. Am J Dis Child. 1985;139:846–7.
41. Rein MF. Clinical manifestations of urogenital trichomoniasis in women. In Honigberg BM, ed. Trichomonads Parasitic in Humans. New York: Springer-Verlag. In press.
42. Fouts AC, Kraus SJ. *Trichomonas vaginalis*: Reevaluation of its clinical presentation and laboratory diagnosis. J Infect Dis. 1980;141:137.
43. Rein MF, Holmes KK. "Nonspecific vaginitis," vulvovaginal candidiasis, and trichomoniasis: Clinical features, diagnosis, and management. In: Remington JS, Swartz MN, eds. Current Clinical Topics in Infectious Disease. New York: McGraw-Hill; 1983: v. 4, p 281.
44. Chen KCS, Forsyth PS, Buchanan TM, et al. Amine content of vaginal fluid from untreated and treated patients with nonspecific vaginitis. J Clin Invest. 1979;63:828–35.
45. Latif AS, Mason PR, Marowa E. Urethral trichomoniasis in men. Sex Transm Dis. 1987;14:9–11.
46. Gardner WA, Culberson DE, Bennett BD. *Trichomonas vaginalis* in the prostate gland. Arch Pathol Lab Med. 1986;110:430–2.
47. Spence MR, Hollander DH, Smith J, et al. The clinical and laboratory diagnosis of *Trichomonas vaginalis* infection. Sex Transm Dis. 1980;7:168.
48. Smith RF. Detection of *Trichomonas vaginalis* in vaginal specimens by direct immunofluorescence assay. J Clin Microbiol. 1986;24:1107–8.
49. Krieger JN, Tam MR, Stevens CE, et al. Diagnosis of trichomoniasis: Comparison of conventional wet-mount examination with cytologic studies, cultures, and monoclonal antibody staining of direct specimens. JAMA. 1988;259:1223–7.
50. Garber GE, Sibau L, Ma R, et al. Cell culture compared with broth for detection of *Trichomonas vaginalis*. J Clin Microbiol. 1987;25:1275–9.
51. Carney JA, Unadkat P, Yule A, et al. A new rapid agglutination test for the diagnosis of *Trichomonas vaginalis* infection. J Clin Pathol. 1988;41:806–8.
52. Yule A, Gellan MCA, Oriel JD, et al. Detection of *Trichomonas vaginalis* antigen in women by enzymes immunoassay. J Clin Pathol. 1987;40:566–8.
53. Watt RM, Philip A, Wos SM, et al. Rapid assay for immunological detection of *Trichomonas vaginalis*. J Clin Microbiol. 1986;24:551–5.
54. Muller M. Mode of action of metronidazole on anaerobic bacteria and protozoa. Surgery. 1983;93:165.
55. Lossick JG. Treatment of *Trichomonas vaginalis* infection. Rev Infect Dis. 1982;(Suppl):S801.
56. Rein MF. Current therapy of vulvovaginitis. Sex Transm Dis. 1981;8:316.
57. Austin TW, Smith EA, Darwish R, et al. Metronidazole in a single dose for the treatment of trichomoniasis: Failure of a 1-g single dose. Br J Vener Dis. 1982;58:121.
58. Lyng J, Christensen J: A double-blind study of the value of treatment with a single dose tinidazole of partners to females with trichomoniasis. Acta Obstet Gynecol Scand. 1981;60:199.
59. Goodwin DW, Reinhard J. Disulfiramlike effects of trichomonacidal drugs: A review and double blind study. Q J Stud Alcohol. 1972;33:734.
60. Beveridge MM. Vaginal moniliasis after treatment of trichomonal infection with Flagyl. Br J Vener Dis. 1962;38:220.
61. Kazmier FJ. A significant interaction between metronidazole and warfarin. Mayo Clinic Proc. 1976;51:782.
62. Beard CM, Noller KL, O'Fallon WM, et al. Cancer after exposure to metronidazole. Mayo Clin Proc. 1988;63:147–53.
63. Robbie MO, Sweet RL. Metronidazole use in obstetrics and gynecology: A review. Am J Obstet Gynecol. 1983;145:865–81.
64. Robertson DHH, Heyworth R, Harrison C, et al. Treatment failure in *Trichomonass vaginalis* infections in females. I. Concentrations of metronidazole in plasma and vaginal content during normal and high dosage. J Antimicrob Chemother. 1988;21:373–8.
65. Kragden S, Lossick JG, Wilk E. Persistent *Trichomonas vaginalis* infection due to a metronidazole resistant strain. Can Med Assoc J. 1986;134:1373–4.
66. Kulda J, Vojtechovska M, Tachezy J, et al. Metronidazole resistance of *Trichomonas vaginalis* as a cause of treatment failure in trichomoniasis. Br J Vener Dis. 1982;58:394.
67. Muller M, Meingasser JG, Miller WA, et al. Three metronidazole-resistant strains of *Trichomonas vaginalis* from the USA. Am J Obstet Gynecol. 1980;128:808.
68. Lossick JG, Muller M, Gorrell TE. In vitro drug susceptibility and doses of metronidazole required for cure in cases of refractory vaginal trichomoniasis. J Infect Dis. 1986;153:948–55.
69. Muller M, Lossick JG, Gorrell TE. In-vitro susceptibility of *Trichomonas vaginalis* to metronidazole: Treatment outcome in vaginal trichomonas. Sex Transm Dis. 1988;15:17–24.
70. Meingasser JG, Hayworth PG. Sensitivity of *Trichomonas vaginalis* to metronidazole in medium with different concentrations of iron and ascorbate. J Parasitol. 1982;68:1163.
71. Krieger JN, Dickens CS, Rein MF. Susceptibility testing of *Trichomonas vaginalis*: Use of a time kill technique. Antimicrob Agents Chemother. 1985;27:332–6.
72. Sears SD, O'Hare J. In vitro susceptibility of *Trichomonas vaginalis* to 50 antimicrobial agents. Antimicrob Agents Chemother. 1988;32:144–6.
73. Dombrowski MP, Sokol RJ, Brown WJ, et al. Intravenous therapy of metronidazole-resistant *Trichomonas vaginalis*. Obstet Gynecol. 1987;69:524–5.
74. Mattern CFT, Spence MR, Navovitz PC. Properties of metronidazole-resistant *Trichomonas vaginalis*: Possible therapeutic approaches. 21st Interscience Conference on Antimicrobial Agents and Chemotherapy, Chicago, Ill., Paper 766.

259. BABESIA

JEFFREY A. GELFAND

Babesiosis is an infection by malaria-like protozoa (*Babesia*) that parasitize erythrocytes of wild and domestic animals and may cause fever, hemolysis, and hemoglobinuria. Long an economically important disease of cattle, only in the last 30 years has *Babesia* been appreciated to be an occasional pathogen in humans. Typically a mild illness in healthy people, in the asplenic or immunocompromised patient disease may be overwhelming.

The first recorded reference to babesiosis is probably the plague ("murrain") visited upon the cattle of Pharaoh Rameses II (Exodus 9:3).[1] In 1888, during investigations of febrile hemoglobinuria in Rumanian cattle, V. Babes described an intraerythrocytic pathogen that he thought to be a bacterium. In 1893, Theobald Smith and F. L. Kilbourne demonstrated that the organism causing "Texas cattle fever" was a protozoan transmitted by a bloodsucking tick—the first demonstration of an arthropod vector. In 1957, babesiosis was described in Yugoslavia by Skrabalo as a disease of humans.[1] Subsequent early reports involved splenectomized individuals with fulminant disease. In 1969, infection with *Babesia microti* was described in a patient with an intact spleen from the island of Nantucket off the Massachusetts coast. A decade later, a total of 42 clinical ases had been reported from the northeastern section of the United States.

THE PATHOGEN

There are over 70 species worldwide in the genus *Babesia*, and they infect numerous mammals and birds. *B. bovis, B. bigemina, B. divergens*, and *B. major* infect the erythrocytes of cattle; *B. equi*, horses; *B. canis*, dogs; *B. felis*, cats; and *B. microti*, rodents. Originally thought to be host specific, some species can infect a wide range of hosts. Only the rodent strain *B. microti* (in the United States) and the cattle strains *B. divergens* and *B. bovis* (in Europe) have been positively identified as causing disease in humans.[1] Other species of *Babesia* have been implicated in sporadic instances of disease in humans, but these species have not been positively identified.

Babesia species, in the host erythrocyte, vary in size from 1 to 5 μm in length. *B. microti* is 2 by 1.5 μm; *B. divergens*, 4 by 1.5 μm; and *B. bovis*, 2.4 by 1.5 μm. They are pear shaped, oval, or round.[1] Their ring conformation and peripheral location in the erythrocyte frequently leads to their being mistaken for *Plasmodium falciparum*.

The vast majority of cases of human babesiosis have occurred in the northeastern coastal region of the United States, particularly Nantucket Island, Martha's Vineyard, Cape Cod (Massachusetts), eastern Long Island, Shelter Island, and Fire Island (New York). This is likely due to the increasing numbers and close proximity of reservoir, vector, and host. Babesiosis is a zoonotic disease and requires transmission from an animal reservoir to humans via a tick vector. *Ixodes dammini*, the tick vector of Lyme disease, transmits the disease to humans from rodents (primarily the white-footed deer mouse, but also the field mouse, vole, rat, and chipmunk) in the United States[2,3]; the hard-bodied cattle tick *Ixodes ricinus* is thought to transmit bovine babesiosis to humans in Europe.

The tick *Ixodes dammini* has three developmental stages (larva, nymph, adult). In each of these stages, the tick requires a blood meal to mature to the next stage. Blood meals may come from different species. White-tailed deer are the preferred host for the adult tick (but they are not infected with *B. microti*), and it is the reemergence of this host for the tick that appears to be responsible for the spread of *I. dammini*.[4] While obtaining their blood meal on the deer, female ticks are impregnated, with the formation of up to 20,000 eggs. The larval phase requires a blood meal to develop into the next phase, the nymph, which in turn requires another blood meal to become an adult. Rodents, especially the white-footed deer mouse, are the preferred hosts of larval and nymphal phases of the tick.[4]

Babesia microti is enzootic in the white-footed mouse, which acts as the reservoir. The tick larva becomes infected with *B. microti* after feeding on an infected mouse. In endemic areas, rodent infection may be heavy (60 percent on Nantucket Island),[4] and *B. microti* is transmitted from the larval phase of the tick to the nymphal phase (trans-stadial transmission). There is no evidence that *B. microti* can be transmitted transovarially in *I. dammini* (as may occur with *B. bigemina*). The infected nymph then seeks a blood meal and infects another rodent—or a human. Larvae, nymphs, or adult ticks can all feed on humans, but it is the nymph that is the primary vector of *B. microti* to humans. All three stages of tick may feed on the deer, which is not infected by *B. microti*. Thus, the deer appears to be a necessary host for the (adult) tick, while the parasite is maintained in a rodent reservoir. The coming together of all three in large numbers—deer, mouse, and tick—create the conditions for infection in humans.[4]

After passage of the sporozoites from the salivary glands of the tick into the mammalian blood stream, erythrocytes are penetrated and infected. There is evidence that in one babesial species, *B. rodhaini*, penetration of rat erythrocytes requires an intact host alternative complement pathway and an erythrocyte C3b receptor.[5] The parasite activates complement and fixes C3b to its surface, which in turn presumably binds to the rat erythrocyte C3b receptor and infects the cell. Additionally, erythrocytes with C3 on their surface are infected, thus suggesting that complement somehow facilitates the parasite–erythrocyte interaction.[5] There are no data on the involvement of these factors in the interaction between *B. microti* and human erythrocytes.

Upon infection of the host erythrocyte, mature *B. microti* trophozoites undergo asynchronous, asexual budding and divide into two or four merozoites (daughter cells). As parasites exit the erythrocyte, the membrane is damaged, with perforations, protrusions, and inclusions.[6] The actual mechanism of hemolysis is unknown. Because schizogony is asynchronous, massive hemolysis does not occur as it does in *Plasmodium* (with synchronous schizogony).

EPIDEMIOLOGY

There have been over 100 documented human infections with *Babesia*, with additional cases being reported constantly.[7] Babesiosis is still a rarity in Europe, with cases reported from Yugoslavia, France, Russia, Ireland, and Scotland. All occurred in splenectomized individuals and involved bovine *Babesia*.[7] Infection with *B. microti* is no longer a rarity in the coastal areas and islands of Massachusetts, Rhode Island, and New York, and infections with *Babesia* sp. have been reported also in Maryland, Virginia, California, Wisconsin, Minnesota, Georgia, and Mexico.[4,7,8] Restocking of deer populations and curtailment of hunting has increased deer herds in certain areas of the northeast United States, and the proximity of mouse reservoirs to human habitats favors further spread of the disease. The tick vector *I. dammini* now ranges from New Hampshire to Maryland and west to Wisconsin and Minnesota.[4,8]

Most infections with *B. microti* appear to be subclinical. This is borne out by the finding that the seroprevalence (using an immunofluorescent antibody assay) for *B. microti* on Cape Cod was 3.7 percent,[9] while on Shelter Island, in individuals with a high risk of exposure to ticks, it was 4.4 percent in June and reached 6.9 percent by October.[10] Nymphs, the primary vector, feed from May through September, and clinical infection usually occurs 1–3 weeks later.

With asymptomatic infection the rule and a high seroprevalence rate in certain areas, transfusion-associated babesiosis was anticipated—and over a half dozen cases have occurred.[9] Sources of transfusion-associated cases have included platelets and frozen erythrocytes.[9] The incubation period in transfusion-associated disease appears to be longer (6–9 weeks).[9] Finally, transplacental/perinatal transmission of the disease has been described.[10]

CLINICAL MANIFESTATIONS

The clinical manifestations of babesiosis differ markedly between the European and North American cases. All of the European cases have involved splenectomized individuals, and in all nine cases, bovine *Babesia* were involved (*B. bovis, B. divergens*).[7,11] Seven of the nine cases were fatal, and all presented with fulminant, febrile, hemolytic disease.[1,7,11]

In contrast, epidemiologic data from the United States suggest a high incidence of infection of the rodent strain *B. microti* that is either subclinical or mild.[7,9,12] The incubation period after the tick bite is usually 1–3 weeks but occasionally may be as long as 6 weeks.[13] Since the nymph is the primary vector and when engorged is only 2 mm in diameter, most patients do not recall a tick bite.[14] In contradistinction to the European cases, most patients reported in the United States have had intact spleens—only 30 percent have been asplenic, and virtually all of the more than 120 patients with clinical disease have survived (2 have not).[7] The patients with clinical illness and intact spleens are usually 50 years or older—suggesting that age plays a factor in the severity of the clinical response.[14,15] This is similar to the findings in animals. In cattle and horses, babesiosis is mild in younger animals and more severe in older animals.[15] Previously healthy individuals with babesiosis are generally older (mean, >60 years) than are babesiosis patients with antecedent medical problems (mean, 48 years).[14]

Initial symptoms begin gradually and are nonspecific.[15] Malaise, fatigue, anorexia, shaking chills, fever, headache, myalgias, arthralgias, nausea, vomiting, abdominal pain, depression and emotional lability, and dark urine are all common. Photophobia, conjunctival injection, sore throat, and cough have been described as well. Fevers may be sustained or intermittent, and temperatures may reach levels of 40°C.[15] Rash similar to erythema chronicum migrans (ECM) has been described, but this probably represents intercurrent Lyme disease because the same tick is the vector for *Borrelia burgdorferi*; 54 percent of one group of patients with babesiosis had antibodies to the Lyme spirochete.[16] Petechiae, splinter hemorrhages, and ecchymoses have been occasionally noted. Splenomegaly and occasionally hepatomegaly are described in some patients, but lymphadenopathy is absent.

Hemolytic anemia, decreased serum haptoglobin levels, and elevated reticulocyte counts are noted, and the anemia may occasionally be severe.[15] The percentage of erythrocytes parasitized in clinical cases is usually 1–10 percent, but has ranged from less than 1 percent to 85 percent.[16] The total leukocyte count may be normal or mildly decreased, and thrombocytopenia is common. The erythrocyte sedimentation rate may be elevated, and the direct Coombs test may react positively. Urinalysis reveals proteinuria and hemoglobinuria, and blood urea nitrogen (BUN) and serum creatinine levels may be elevated. Mild elevations of the levels of serum bilirubin, alkaline phosphatase, serum aspartate aminotransferase (AST, SGOT), serum alanine aminotransferase (ALT, SGPT), and lactic dehydrogenase (LDH) are usually found. On one occasion, bone marrow examination of a patient with babesiosis revealed macrophages exhibiting hemophagocytosis.

In one series of 17 patients with symptomatic *B. microti* infection, the mean duration of hospitalization was 19.1 days (±2.9), with convalescence lasting 0–18 months.[14] All patients regarded the disease as having been severe. As in other series, patients without pre-existing medical conditions were older.[14]

Thus, *B. microti* produces a high incidence of subclinical infections, but clinical infections are likely in asplenic patients, older individuals, and individuals with pre-existent medical disease (including human immunodeficiency virus [HIV] infection, as recently reported).[17] In patients with clinical disease, symptoms may be severe, but disease is rarely fatal. In contrast, bovine babesiosis, as seen in Europe, occurs in asplenic patients and is always fulminant and usually fatal.

PATHOGENESIS

The critical role of the spleen in the host defense against this disease is emphasized by the higher incidence and greater severity of this disease in asplenic patients and animals. In fact, animals that have recovered from babesiosis can recrudesce after splenectomy, and steroid treatment, which reduces splenic function, can increase infection. Blood percolates through the spleen in intimate contact with splenic endothelium, macrophages, and macrophage products. Erythrocytes must squeeze through intraendothelial spaces. Infected, deformed, and potentially more rigid erythrocytes are more likely to be retained[18] where ingestion by macrophages or the action of macrophage products may serve to control the infection. Complement-sensitized erythrocytes would likely bind under these circumstances. Furthermore, complement activation by *Babesia* could theoretically lead to the generation of tumor necrosis factor (TNF) and interleukin-1 (IL-1).[19] Decreased complement levels, presumably secondary to activation, are frequently found in babesiosis.[20] In addition, increased circulating C1q-binding activity, presumably due to immune complexes, with decreased C4, C3 and CH_{50} levels are seen in patients.[20] The generation of these primarily macrophage-produced mediators (TNF and IL-1) in turn could explain many of the clinical features (fever, anorexia, arthralgias, myalgias) of babesiosis, especially the fulminant shock syndrome of bovine babesiosis. A similar pathogenesis has been proposed for malaria.[21] It is likely that, in the less fulminant situation, TNF functions to enhance killing *Babesia*, as with malaria.[22]

In addition to macrophage factors, other cellular immune functions appear to be important in the host response to *Babesia*. Nude mice and mice with T-lymphocyte hypofunction due to thymectomy, lethal irradiation, or anti-T-lymphocyte serum develop significantly greater parasitemia. The disease itself alters cellular immune function. Patients with acute babesiosis have an increase in T-suppressor/cytotoxic lymphocytes and decreased responses to lymphocyte mitogens with a polyclonal hypergammaglobulinemia.[20]

DIAGNOSIS

Babesiosis is usually diagnosed by microscopic examination of Giemsa- or Wright-stained thin or thick blood smears. The predominant forms seen strongly resemble the ring forms of *Plasmodium falciparum*. They may have a single chromatic dot or two or more chromatic masses. With older stages of *Plasmodium falciparum*, there are brownish pigment deposits (hemozoin).[1] These are absent in Babesiosis. *Babesia* spp. also lack the synchronous stages, shizonts, and gametocytes seen with *Plasmodium* spp. A rare diagnostic feature of *Babesia* is the presence of tetrads of merozoites (Fig. 1). Larger rings may have a central white vacuole that is absent in malaria. Trophozoites may be seen outside erythrocytes with heavier infestation.

An indirect immunofluorescent antibody (IFA) titer for *B. microti* is available through the Centers for Disease Control (Atlanta). Patients with active infection usually have serum titers ≥1024 within a few weeks that fall slowly over months to 1:256 or less. A titer of ≥1:256 is diagnostic for *B. microti*

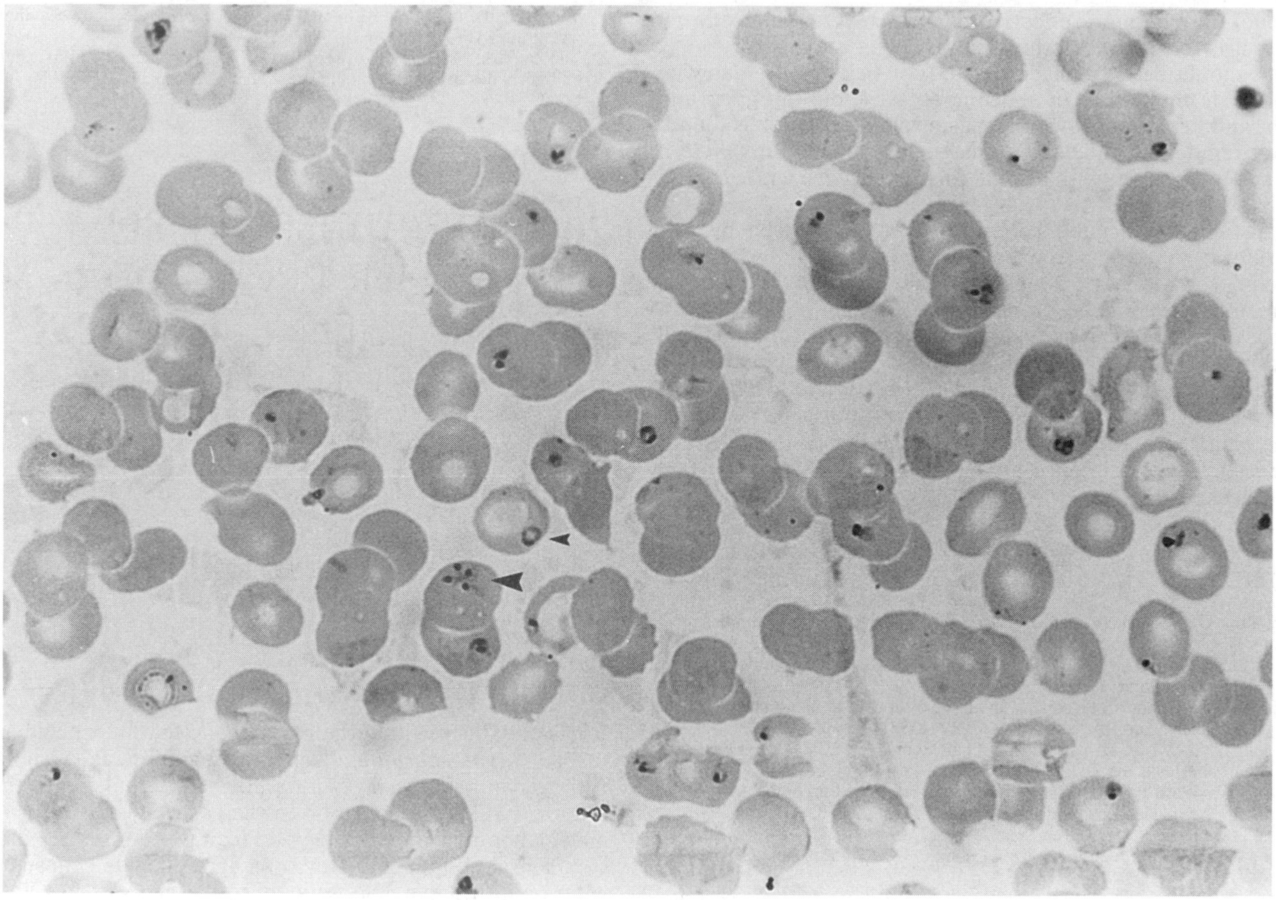

FIG. 1. Human erythrocytes showing heavy infection with *B. microti*. The larger arrows marks a diagnostic but rare tetrad form. The smaller arrow above it marks a ring form with a central pale area (Giemsa stain, ×1,250). (Courtesy of Dr. David Wyler, Boston, MA.)

infection; lower titers may be seen due to cross-reactions between antibodies to *Plasmodium* spp.[23]

Confirmation of suspected *B. microti* infection can be made with intraperitoneal inoculation of 1.0 ml of EDTA–whole blood into the peritoneum of golden hamsters. *B. divergens* replicates readily in gerbils. Within 2–4 weeks, smears will be positive in the infected animals.

TREATMENT

Most patients infected by *B. microti* appear to have a mild illness and recover without specific chemotherapy. Splenectomized patients are more likely to have high level parasitemia and be severely ill, but patients with intact spleens may have severe infection. In patients with serious disease, a combination of clindamycin (20 mg/kg/day in children; in adults, 300–600 mg every 6 hours intravenously or intramuscularly) and oral quinine (25 mg/kg/day in children; in adults, 650 mg every 6–8 hours) taken for 7–10 days appears to be the most effective regimen.[24] Chloroquine, frequently given because of confusion of *B. microti* with *P. falciparum*, is not effective therapy. Other antimalarial and antiprotozoal therapies have likewise been largely unsuccessful, including primaquine, quinacrine, pyrimethamine, pyrimethamine-sulfodoxine, sulfadiazine, tetracycline, minocycline, pentamidine isethionate alone, and trimethoprim-sulfamethoxazole alone.[25] Despite the usual success of the clindamycine-quinine combination, failure of this therapy has been reported.[25] The antitrypanosomal drug diminazene aceturate (Berenil, Hoechst-Roussel Pharmaceuticals, Inc., Somerville, New Jersey) is effective against *B. microti* infections in animals and has been given to one patient who recovered from *B. microti* infection. This patient developed a Guillian-Barré-like disorder.[26] Diminazene was also used unsuccessfully in a fatal case of babesiosis due to *B. divergens*.[11] The combination of pentamidine with trimethoprim-sulfamethoxazole was recently reported to be successful in the treatment of *B. divergens* infection in a splenectomized patient in France.[11] Exchange transfusions are used in profoundly ill patients with high levels of parasitemia and hemolysis. Used concurrently with chemotherapy, exchange transfusion reduces the level of parasitemia and may remove toxic erythrocyte, babesial, or macrophage-produced factors.[27]

PREVENTION

The prevention of babesiosis requires avoidance of areas endemic for *I. dammini* during the period of May through September. This is especially important for splenectomized individuals and others who are immunocompromised. It is quite possible that babesiosis may become a greater problem in the future for patients with the acquired immunodeficiency syndrome (AIDS). In endemic areas, clothing should be worn to cover the lower portion of the body (long pants and socks). Since ticks may crawl up pants legs, tucking pants into boots or socks or cinching the legs at the ankles is helpful. Wearing light-colored clothes enables the ticks to be spotted more easily. Diethyltoluamide (''deet'') and dimethylphthalate insect repellents can be applied to the skin or clothes (especially pants bottoms and socks). It is safer and probably more effective when applied to clothes. A tick repellent with permethrin (Permanone) may be more effective but is not yet available in all states; it is for use on clothing only.

Pets should be carefully inspected for ticks before allowing them inside the home. In endemic areas, avoid tall grass and brush, and keep to well worn roads or paths. If a tick is found, speedy removal is indicated. Grasp below the mouth, where it attaches to the skin, with a small forceps or tweezers, and pull the tick off steadily.

Transfusion-associated babesiosis can be reduced by discouraging blood donors from endemic areas during May through September, by avoiding donors with fevers during the 2 months before intended donation, and by not accepting those with a history of tick bites. It is unlikely that screening of blood will be adopted in the near future, and thus it is anticipated that increases in transfusion-associated babesiosis are likely, given the spread of the tick—and the parasite—into ever-enlarging areas. Clinicians will therefore have to be increasingly alert to the possibility of this once arcane and relatively unimportant disease, babesiosis.

REFERENCES

1. Dammin GJ. Babesiosis. In: Weinstein L, Fields B, eds. Seminars in Infectious Disease. New York: Stratton; 1978:169–99.
2. Healy GR, Spielman A, Gleason N. Human babesiosis: Reservoir of infection on Nantucket Island. Science. 1976;192:479–80.
3. Spielman A, Etkind P, Piesman J, et al. Reservoir hosts of human babesiosis on Nantucket Island. Am J Trop Med Hyg. 1981;30:560–5.
4. Spielman A, Wilson ML, Levine JF, et al. Ecology of *Ixodes dammini*-borne human babesiosis and Lyme disease. Annu Rev Entomol. 1985;30:439–60.
5. Jack RM, Ward PA. *Babesia rodhaini* interactions with complement: Relationship to parasitic entry into red cells. J Immunol. 1980;124:1566–73.
6. Sun T, Tenenbaum MJ, Greenspan J, et al. Morphologic and clinical observations in human infection with *Babesia microti*. J Infect Dis. 1983;148:239–48.
7. Dammin GJ, Spielman A, Benach JL, et al. The rising incidence of clinical *Babesia microti* infection. Hum Pathol. 1981;12:398–400.
8. Steketee RW, Eckman MR, Burgess EC, et al. Babesiosis in Wisconsin: A new focus of disease transmission. JAMA. 1985;253:2675–8.
9. Popovsky MA, Lindberg LE, Syrek AL, et al. Prevalence of *Babesia* antibody in a selected blood donor population. Transfusion. 1988;28:59–61.
10. Esernio-Jenssen D, Scimeca PG, Benach JL, et al. Transplacental/perinatal babesiosis. J Pediatr. 1987;110:570–2.
11. Raoult D, Soulayrol L, Toga B, et al. Babesiosis, pentamidine, and cotrimoxazole. Ann Intern Med. 1987;107:944.
12. Ruebush TK II, Juranek DD, Chisholm ES, et al. Human babesiosis on Nantucket Island: Evidence for self-limited and subclinical infections. N Engl J Med. 1977;297:825–7.
13. Ruebush TK II, Juranek DD, Spielman A, et al. Epidemiology of human babesiosis on Nantucket Island. Am J Trop Med Hyg. 1981;30:937–41.
14. Benach JL, Habicht GS. Clinical characteristics of human babesiosis. J Infect Dis. 1981;144:481.
15. Ruebush TK II, Cassaday PB, March HJ, et al. Human babesiosis on Nantucket Island, clinical features. Ann Intern Med. 1977;86:6–9.
16. Benach JL, Coleman JL, Habicht GS, et al. Serological evidence for simultaneous occurrences of Lyme disease and babesiosis. J Infect Dis. 1985;152:473–7.
17. Benezra D, Brown AE, Polsky B, et al. Babesiosis and infection with human immunodeficiency virus (HIV). Ann Intern Med. 1987;107:944.
18. Looareesuwan S, Ho M, Wattanagoon MB, et al. Dynamic alteration in splenic function during acute falciparum malaria. N Engl J Med. 1987;312:675–9.
19. Okusawa S, Yancey KB, van der Meer JWM, et al. C5a stimulates secretion of tumor necrosis factor from human mononuclear cells in vitro: Comparison with secretion of interleukin-1-beta and interleukin-1-alpha. J Exp Med. 1988;168:443–8.
20. Benach JL, Habicht GS, Hamburger MI. Immunoresponsiveness in acute babesiosis in humans. J Infect Dis. 1982;146:369–80.
21. Clark IA, Virelizier JL, Carswell EA, et al. Possible importance of macrophage-derived mediators in acute malaria. Infect Immun. 1981;32:1058–66.
22. Taverne J, Matthews N, Depledge P, et al. Malarial parasites and tumor cells are killed by the same component of tumor necrosis serum. Clin Exp Immunol. 1984;57:293–300.
23. Ruebush TK II, Chisholm ES, Sulzer AJ, et al. Development and persistence of antibody in persons infected with *Babesia microti*. Am J Trop Med Hyg. 1981;30:291–2.
24. Wittner M, Rowin KS, Tanowitz HB, et al. Successful chemotherapy of transfusion babesiosis. Ann Intern Med. 1982;96:601–4.
25. Clindamycin and quinine treatment for *Babesia microti* infections. MMWR. 1983;32:65–71.
26. Ruebush TK II, Rubin RH, Wolpow ER, et al. Neurologic complications following the treatment of human *Babesia microti* infection with diminazene aceturate. Am J Trop Med. 1979;28:184–9.
27. Jacoby GA, Hunt JV, Kosinski KS, et al. Treatment of transfusion-transmitted babesiosis by exchange transfusion. N Engl J Med. 1980;303:1098–1100.

260. CRYPTOSPORIDIUM AND OTHER PROTOZOA INCLUDING ISOSPORA, SARCOCYSTIS, BALANTIDIUM COLI, AND BLASTOCYSTIS

ROSEMARY SOAVE
CYNTHIA S. WEIKEL

CRYPTOSPORIDIUM

It has only been within the past decade that the coccidian protozoan *Cryptosporidium* gained recognition as a significant pathogen of humans. Tyzzer first described and named the parasite in 1907 when he saw it in the gastric glands of asymptomatic laboratory mice.[1] The protozoan was considered a benign commensal until in 1955 it was recognized as the cause of fatal enteritis in turkeys.[2] Subsequently, the parasite was linked to serious disease in several animal species including calves and lambs, and it is now known to be responsible for major agricultural losses each year.[3–6] Human cryptosporidiosis was first reported in 1976.[7,8] Between 1976 and 1981, a handful of cases were described that primarily involved immunocompromised patients. In 1981–82, *Cryptosporidium* was identified in 47 patients with the acquired immunodeficiency syndrome (AIDS) and was found to be capable of causing severe enteritis.[9] Popularization of stool examination for diagnosis led to reports of cryptosporidiosis in animal handlers[10] and travelers[11,12] and to the realization that the organism parasitizes the immunocompetent host as well.[13] Although the true prevalence of *Cryptosporidium* is not yet known, it has come to be recognized as a common cause of enteritis worldwide.[14–17] However, despite its increased recognition, *Cryptosporidium* remains an elusive and poorly understood pathogen.

The Pathogen

The name *Cryptosporidium* denotes an organism with spores (sporozoites) concealed within an oocyst.[1] Based on having four aflagellar but motile sporozoites with apical complexes, the genus *Cryptosporidium* has been assigned to the phylum Apicomplexa, class Sporozoa.[18] Although taxonomically related to *Toxoplasma, Sarcocystis, Isospora, Eimeria*, and *Plasmodium* species, *Cryptosporidium* has various characteristics that distinguish it from the other coccidia. Twenty species of *Cryptosporidium* have been named for the host in which they were found, including mammals, birds, reptiles, and fish.[14] However, recent cross-transmission experiments indicate an absence of host specificity, thus invalidating many of the named species.[17–20] The exact number of distinct species of *Cryptosporidium* and the nature of differences among various *Cryptosporidium* isolates have not been determined. Based on differences in oocyst size, two species of *Cryptosporidium* affecting mammals have been proposed by Upton and Current:[21] (*1*) the smaller *C. parvum* (2.5 μm diameter oocyst) is thought to be the cause of diarrheal disease in humans and cattle, and (*2*) the larger *C. muris* (5–8 μm diameter oocyst) is known to infect the stomach of mammals. In addition, two species affecting birds, *C. baileyi* and *C. meleagridis*, also appear to be valid.[14]

The *Cryptosporidium* life cycle is basically similar to that of other coccidia in that asexual followed by sexual endogenous stages lead to the production and discharge of oocysts into feces (Fig. 1). Unlike other coccidia, *Cryptosporidium* develops entirely within a single host. Infection is initiated by the ingestion or perhaps inhalation[22,23] of oocysts. Although the infectious dose has not been determined for humans and many animals, 100–150 organisms are known to cause infection in 50 percent of Swiss-Webster mice.[24] The mature (sporulated) *Cryptosporidium* oocyst contains four thin, flat, motile sporozoites (2–4 by 6–8 μm) that exit (excystation) upon dissolution of a single suture on the oocyst wall (Fig. 2). Sporozoites move by gliding and flexing and implant in the host epithelial cell where they round up and develop into trophozoites. Asexual multiplication (merogony) results in the formation of type 1 and type 2 meronts. Type 1 meronts release six to eight merozoites that reinvade the host and reinitiate merogony. The four merozoites released by type 2 meronts initiate the sexual cycle by developing into microgametocyte and macrogametocytes. Aflagellar but motile microgametes fertilize macrogametes, and then they develop into oocysts, thus completing the cycle. Oocysts sporulate in situ and can either reinfect the same host or exit in search of a new host. Some investigators have reported morphologic differences that correlate with oocyst outcome, i.e., thin-walled oocysts reinfect whereas the hardy thick-walled oocysts are expelled into the environment.[25]

Epidemiology

Cryptosporidial infection has been documented in over 30 countries spanning six continents.[14–17,26] Rates of infection range from 0.6 to 20 percent in developed countries and from 4 to 32 percent in underdeveloped nations. Although these studies do not reflect the true prevalence, they do indicate that the parasite is distributed worldwide. The Centers for Disease Control report that in the United States 3–4 percent of patients with AIDS have cryptosporidial enteritis; however, some medical centers are reporting rates of 10–20 percent. In contrast, more than 50 percent of patients with AIDS in Haiti and Africa have cryptosporidiosis. Higher prevalence rates appear to be associated with young age and warm, humid seasons of the year.[26,27] Both sexes are equally affected.[27] Whether breast-feeding protects against the acquisition of *Cryptosporidium* is still controversial.[26,28]

Cryptosporidium may be transmitted from animals to humans, humans to animals, and humans to humans. In addition, fecal contamination of the environment could result in spread via water and possibly food and air.[22,23] Person-to-person spread appears to be responsible for occurrence of infection in (*1*) day care center attendees,[14,26,29–31] (*2*) household contacts of index cases,[6,12,13,27,30,32] and (*3*) hospitalized patients and health care workers.[33–36] Contaminated water has been implicated as the source of infection for travelers[37] and in various outbreaks.[38,39] *Cryptosporidium* oocysts have been found in rivers and other surface water in Arizona, California, Washington, Texas, Colorado, Oregon, and Utah[40,41] as well as in treated and untreated sewage.[42] Contamination of environmental waters is a particularly troublesome problem since chlorination does not kill *Cryptosporidium*. The oocyst is in fact quite hardy and resistant to a number of disinfectants including 3% hypochlorite, iodophors, cresylic acid, benzalkonium chloride, and 5% formaldehyde. Heat (65°C for 30 minutes), prolonged treatment (18 hours) with bleach, or 10% formalin in combination with either bleach or 5% ammonia appear to reduce the infectivity.[6,14] Ongoing studies are aimed at identifying practical and effective ways to destroy cryptosporidial viability and to test and ensure the purity of our water supply.

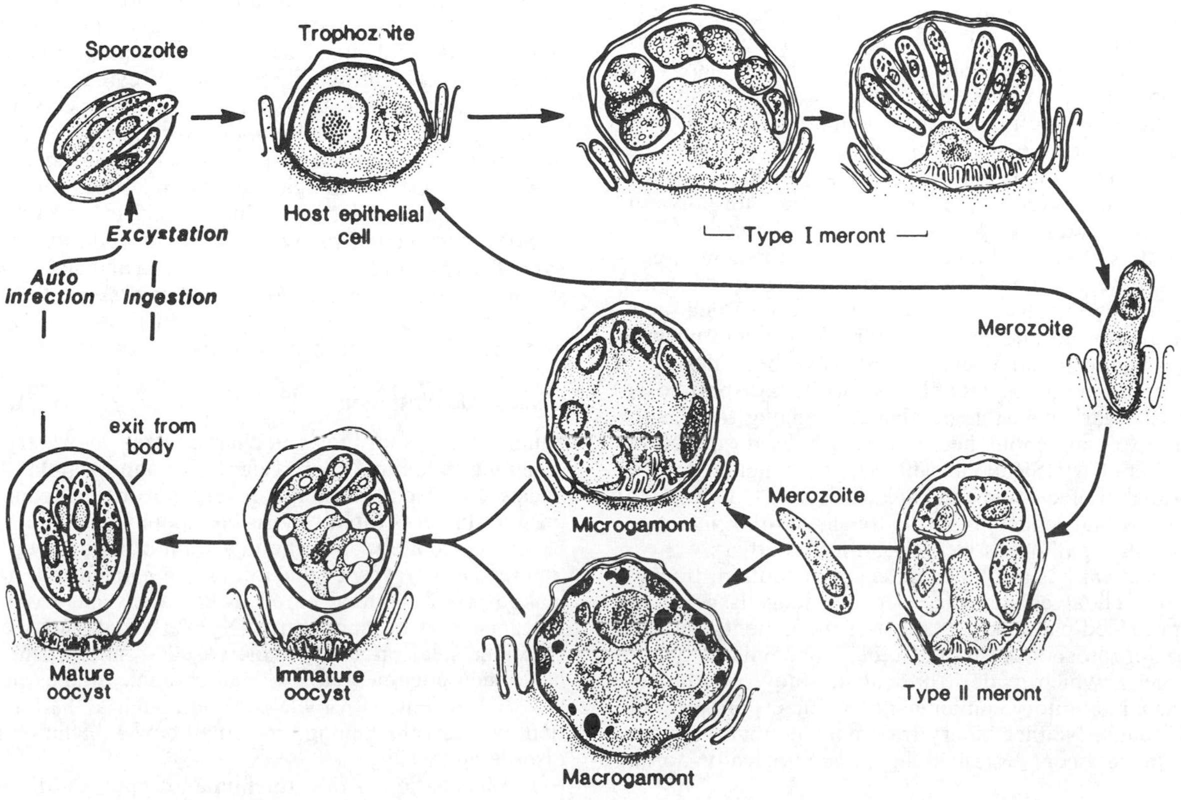

FIG. 1. Diagrammatic representation of the life cycle of *Cryptosporidium*. (From Fayer et al.,[14] with permission.)

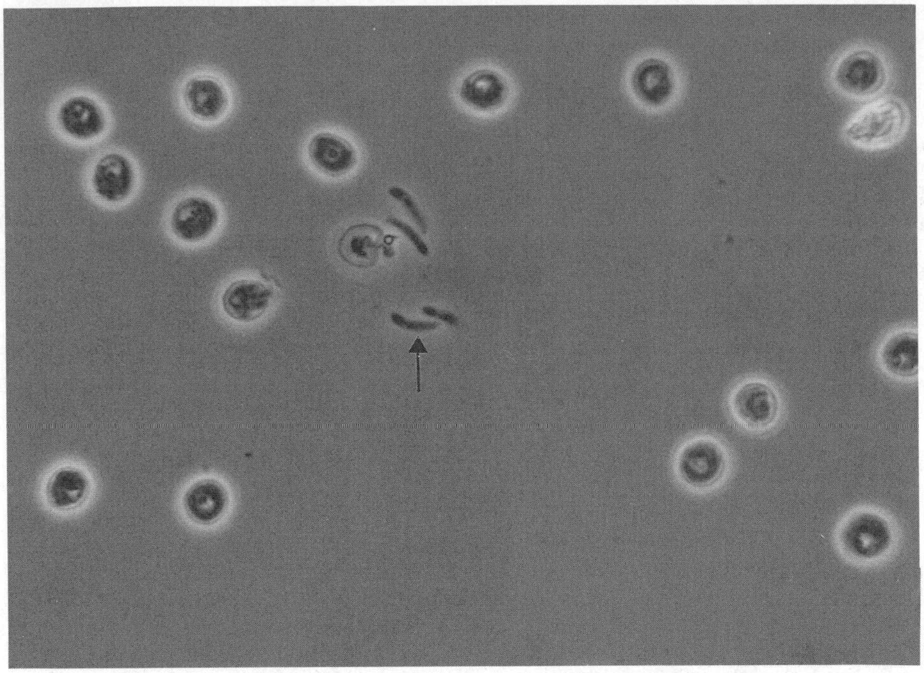

FIG. 2. Excysting *Cryptosporidium* oocyst releasing four sporozoites (arrow). (Phase-contrast, ×630)

Pathology and Pathogenesis

Most of what is known regarding the histopathology of cryptosporidial infection in humans is based on study of biopsied tissue from immunocompromised patients. In these patients, cryptosporidia have been detected throughout the alimentary tract, including the pharynx, esophagus, stomach, duodenum, small intestine, appendix, colon, rectum,[8,14–17,43–47] gallbladder, pancreas, and bile and pancreatic ducts;[44,45,48–51] within colonic submucosal vessels;[52] and in the respiratory tract.[53–56]

Infection is often patchy. The small intestine appears to be the most commonly infected site, but whether this merely reflects the propensity to look there is not known. Histologic changes in the intestine range from minimal to moderate and do not correlate with the degree of infection or clinical symptoms (Fig. 3). They include blunting or a loss of villi, elongation of crypts, and infiltration of the lamina propria with polymorphonuclear leukocytes, lymphocytes, and plasma cells. Ultrastructure studies of infected intestine reveal endogenous stages of the parasite nestled between microvilli and enclosed within a parasitophorous vacuole, i.e., just under the host cell membrane in a unique intracellular yet extracytoplasmic position (Fig. 4). Similar histopathologic findings have been described for only three immunocompetent hosts with cryptosporidiosis.

In contrast, marked histologic changes ranging from acute inflammation to gangrenous necrosis have been described for a small number of AIDS patients who were documented to have cryptosporidial cholecystitis and cholangitis.[44,45,48–51] A few of these patients had concomitant cytomegalovirus infection, whereas no other pathogens were found in the others.

Cryptosporidium has also been detected in sputum, tracheal aspirates, bronchoalveolar lavage, and the lung tissue of immunocompromised patients.[53–56] Most of the patients had gastrointestinal cryptosporidiosis and other concomitant pulmonary pathogens, which made it difficult to know whether the parasite was a respiratory contaminant, colonizer, or true pathogen for humans. Neither biliary tract nor pulmonary cryptosporidiosis have been described in immunologically normal individuals.

In *Cryptosporidium*-infected animals, the degree of pathologic abnormality correlates with the extent of infection. Illness in animals depends on their age and species. Young (neonatal), large (calves, lambs, pigs) mammals develop enterocolitis of variable severity, whereas small mammals such as mice, rats, guinea pigs, and rabbits appear normal.[4–6,14–17,46] Upper respiratory tract infections, often fatal, have been described in wild and domestic birds. Experimental cryptosporidal infection of normal lambs, piglets, and gnotobiotic calves[4–6,57] produced extensive lesions in the small intestine with marked cellular infiltrate into the lamina propria. In recent studies of ileum from spontaneously infected, asymptomatic guinea pigs, *Cryptosporidium* was identified deep within the cytoplasm of M cells.[58] This intracellular location that presumably permits antigenic sampling by the intestinal immune system may be the basis for the lack of symptomatic disease in certain hosts.

Available histopathologic data from humans and animals are confusing and provide few clues to aid in understanding the pathogenic mechanisms by which *Cryptosporidium* causes disease. The cholera-like secretory diarrhea and malabsorption associated with chronic cryptosporidiosis suggest that enterotoxin or hormonally mediated mechanisms as well as physical destruction of the brush border may be operative.

Clinical Manifestations

Human cryptosporidiosis is characterized by watery diarrhea, cramping abdominal pain, weight loss, anorexia, flatulence, and malaise. Nausea, vomiting, fever, and myalgias may also be present. Patients often report that abdominal pain and diarrhea occur immediately after the ingestion of food. Fecal examination reveals cryptosporidial oocysts and mucus but no blood or leukocytes. Peripheral blood leukocytosis and eosinophilia do not appear to be common. D-Xylose and vitamin B_{12} malabsorption, steatorrhea, and increased α_1-antitrypsin clearance have been documented.[43,59] Radiographic studies include features consistent with malabsorption such as barium flocculation, mucosal thickening, and small bowel dilatation as well as disordered motility.

The incubation period for human cryptosporidiosis appears to be between 2 and 14 days. The severity and duration of illness

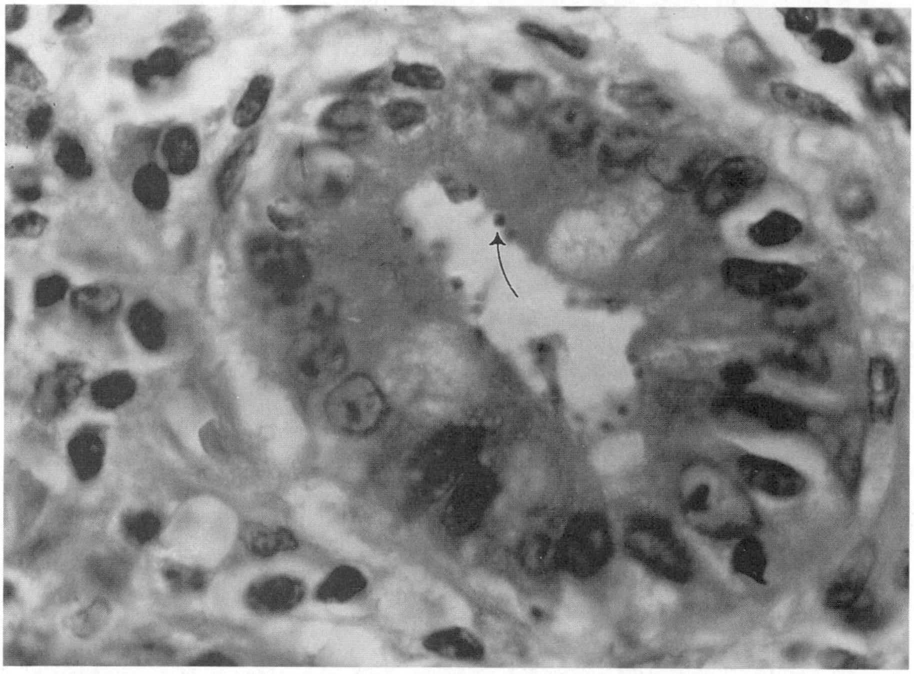

FIG. 3. Cryptosporidia (arrow) on the surface epithelium of the small bowel from a patient with AIDS. (×450)

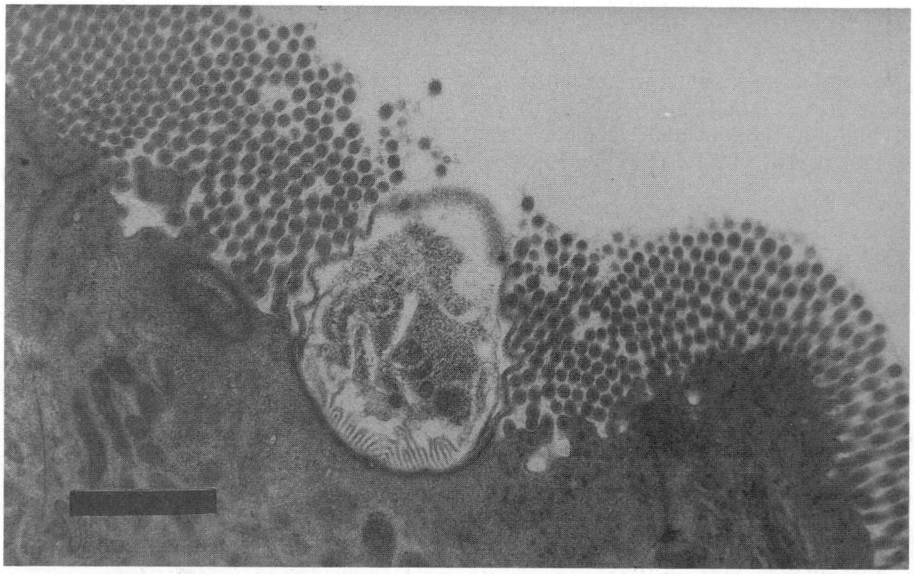

FIG. 4. Electron micrograph of *Cryptosporidium* trophozoite in the brush border of the small intestine of an AIDS patient. (Bar = 2 μm) (From Soave et al.,[15] with permission.)

vary with immunologic competence.[10,13–17,43] For the immunologically intact host, symptoms are often explosive in onset and last an average of 10–14 days but may be prolonged.[13] Fecal clearance of the parasite may lag behind resolution of clinical illness by 1–2 weeks.[60] Illness in these patients is usually severe enough to warrant therapeutic intervention were it available.

In the immunocompromised patient with defects in either cell-mediated or humoral immunity, the course and duration of illness is more variable. Symptoms frequently develop insidiously but increase in severity as immune dysfunction becomes more pronounced. Patients may experience voluminous diarrheal output (1–25 liters daily), profound weight loss (>10 percent of the total body weight), and severe abdominal pain that lasts for months. They often require hospitalization for dehydration, electrolyte imbalance, and severe wasting.

Patients with cryptosporidial cholecystitis have severe abdominal pain localized to the right upper quadrant and epigastric area, nausea, and vomiting in addition to enteritis. Serum levels of alkaline phosphatase and γ-glutamyl transpeptidase are elevated, but serum bilirubin and transaminase levels are normal. Radiographic studies may reveal a dilated gallbladder with thickened walls and dilated bile ducts with luminal irregularities suggestive of sclerosing cholangitis. Patients who underwent cholecystectomy and endoscopic retrograde cholangiopancreatography (ERCP) were found to have cryptosporidia studding the surface epithelium and in the bile (Fig. 5). Transient improvement of symptoms and laboratory abnormalities has been observed after cholecystectomy or endoscopic papillotomy.

Diagnosis

The diagnosis of cryptosporidial enteritis is based on fecal examination.[61–64] Since 1981, various methods for detecting the parasite in fecal smears have been described,[14,65] but their relative merits and comparative sensitivity and specificity have not been fully defined. The use of a modified acid-fast technique allows for differentiation of acid-fast cryptosporidial oocysts from yeast that are similar in size and shape but are not acid-fast (Fig. 6). Infrequently, a minority of oocysts may not take up the acid-fast stain and appear as empty holes in the fecal smear.[66] Variability in oocyst staining characteristics does not seem to hinder diagnosis in experienced hands.

Since the number of negative specimens required to confirm the absence of cryptosporidial infection is not known and oocyst excretion can be intermittent, at least two smears should be obtained.[60] Recently a specific and sensitive direct immunofluorescence antibody (DFA) stain that uses a murine immunoglobulin M monoclonal antibody to the oocyst wall has been developed and marketed.[67] Concentration techniques such as zinc sulfate or Sheather's sucrose flotation are usually not necessary for diagnosis during acute illness but do optimize the detection of oocysts in specimens in which they are rare (e.g., specimens from contacts, environmental samples). Special caution is advised when concentration techniques are used because of the potential for aerosolization of organisms.

Antibodies to cryptosporidia have been detected in the serum of both immunocompetent and immunocompromised hosts by immunofluorescence assay (IFA) and enzyme-linked immunosorbent assay (ELISA).[68–70] When both the IgG and IgM ELISA tests were used, 95 percent of patients with cryptosporidiosis, including patients with AIDS, had antibody when they presented. Although not helpful in the immediate diagnosis of acute illness, the ELISA should prove useful in epidemiologic studies.

Treatment and Prevention

There is currently no known effective therapy for cryptosporidiosis. Fluid and electrolyte replacement is of prime importance in the management of cryptosporidiosis whether or not the infection is self-limited. Illness will resolve in patients receiving corticosteroids or cytotoxic drugs if treatment with them is discontinued. Nonspecific antidiarrheal agents such as kaolin plus pectin (Kaopectate), loperamide (Imodium), diphenoxylate (Lomotil), opiates, or bismuth subsalicylate (Pepto-Bismol) are not consistently efficacious, and their safety in cryptosporidiosis is not known. Limited studies in animals[71,72] and the experimental use of a wide variety of antimicrobial and immunomodulating agents as well as special diets in patients with AIDS have failed to identify effective anticryptosporidial agents.[73] Promising anecdotal reports of success in palliating cryptosporidial diarrhea with the macrolide spiramycin[74] were not confirmed in a recently concluded, placebo-controlled clinical trial. Since poor bioavailability of the oral drug as well as a biliary tract reservoir of infection may have accounted for the disappointing results in many patients, efforts are currently underway to study intravenously administered spiramycin. In addition, novel therapies such as hyperimmune bovine colostrum, cow's milk globulin, and bovine transfer factor are also being investigated.[75–77]

The thick-walled *Cryptosporidium* oocysts are known to be hardy and resistant to numerous disinfectants. Careful hand washing and enteric precautions in the hospital setting are crucial to interrupt person-to-person spread. It is clear that improved techniques for in vitro study of this parasite are badly needed in order to better understanding its unique biologic characteristics and behavior and thus lead to successful control and eradication of *Cryptosporidium*.

SARCOCYSTIS

Coccidian protozoan parasites classified as *Sarcocystis* sp. are worldwide in distribution and cause a zoonotic infection among herbivores, omnivores, and carnivores.[78,79] The parasite has an obligatory two host cycle: sexual reproduction occurs in the intestinal mucosa of the definitive host and results in the shedding of sporocysts in the feces, and asexual multiplication occurs in endothelial cells of the intermediate host preceding the formation of the final asexual stage (sarcocyst) in muscle fibers, usually striated or cardiac.[79] Humans may serve as an incidental, intermediate host when food contaminated with sporocysts

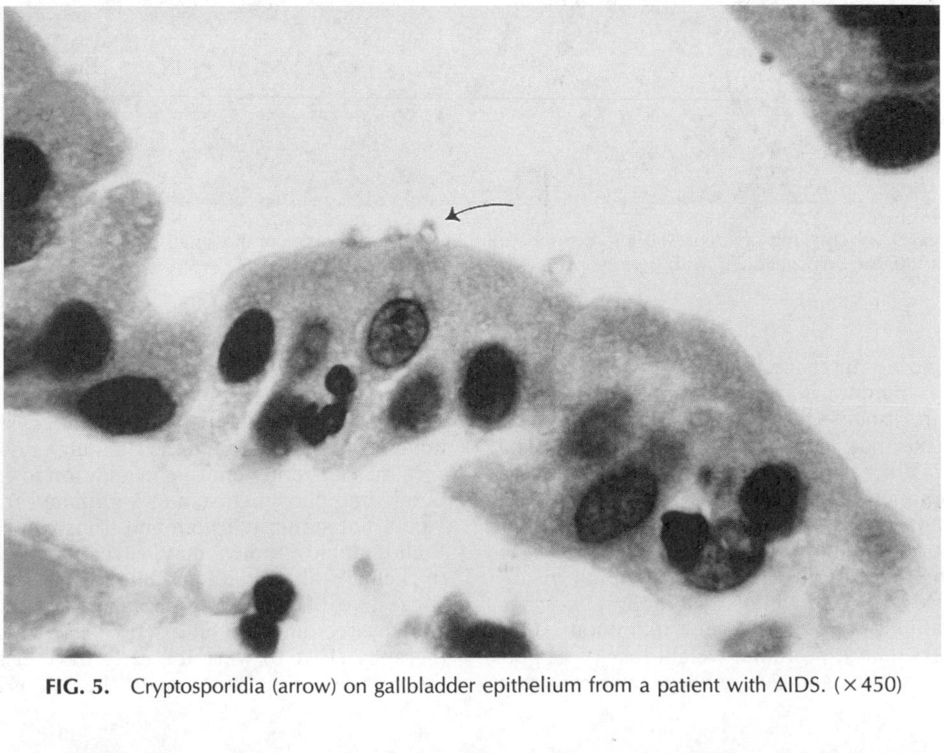

FIG. 5. Cryptosporidia (arrow) on gallbladder epithelium from a patient with AIDS. (×450)

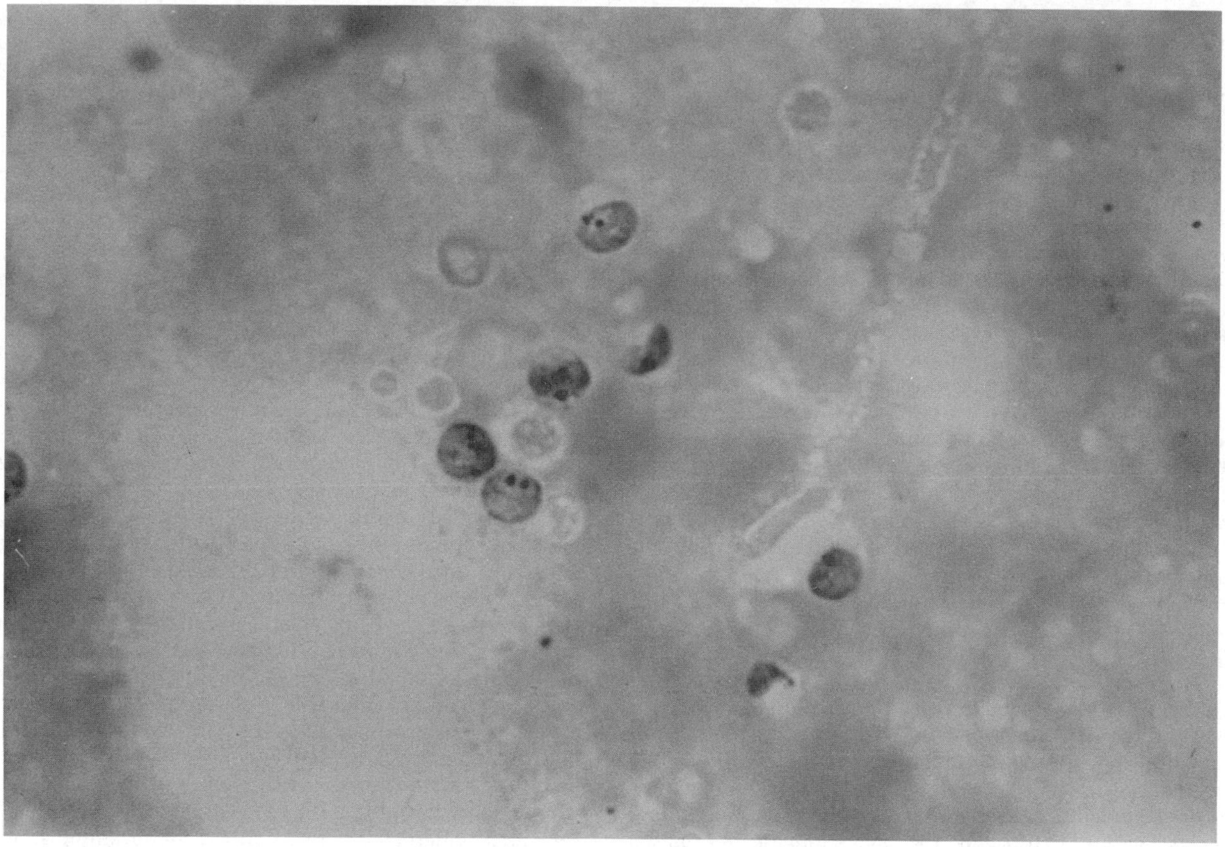

FIG. 6. Cryptosporidia in an acid-fast–stained smear of stool prepared by sucrose flotation. (Courtesy of Dr. Abe Macher, Washington, D.C.)

is accidentally ingested, or for certain species of pig and cattle *Sarcocystis*, humans serve as a definitive host.[79,80] Although *Sarcocystis* is reported to cause significant disease in animals, no clinical manifestations are associated with most human cases of sarcosporidiosis, which are most often encountered as a chance histopathologic finding in muscle.[79,81] Rarely, muscle soreness or swelling has been reported. In muscle, sarcocysts vary greatly in size, with cyst diameters of less than 50 μm to about 300 μm, and cyst lengths up to 5 cm reported.[79,81] Whether humans acting as definitive hosts may suffer any gastrointestinal disturbance is, at present, unclear. Human intestinal mucosa at sites of parasite sexual reproduction has been noted to be intact.[78,80]

BLASTOCYSTIS

Blastocystis hominis, a strict anaerobic protozoan, has been observed by light microscopy in three distinct forms: vacuolated, granular, and ameboid.[82] The vacuolated form of 8–10 μm predominates in fecal specimens. This parasite usually has a single nucleus but occasionally has four or more nuclei and may have a prominent slime capsule. Although infection has been associated with diarrhea in pigs and gnotobiotic guinea pigs and may asymptomatically infect monkey and fowl,[83,84] its importance as a human pathogen has been the subject of considerable debate. Surveys have reported from <1 to 25 percent of stools to be positive, occasionally statistically associated with *Entamoeba histolytica*.[85–91] In limited studies among individuals examined for other enteric pathogens, between 2 and 16 percent have been reported to have only large numbers of *Blastocystis hominis* in their stools; most of these patients reported diarrhea.[86–90]

The clinical syndrome occasionally reported with this infection is not unique. Diarrhea is generally mild to moderate without fecal blood or leukocytes. However, stool outputs of 2–3 liters/day have been reported.[91] Several cases of colitis with fecal leukocytes have been associated with infection with *Blastocystis hominis* but evaluation for other enteric pathogens was limited.[91–94] Colonic biopsy specimens have shown evidence of inflammation, but parasites penetrating the intestinal epithelium in humans have not been reported.[93,94] Diarrhea may be associated with nausea, vomiting, bloating, fatigue, anorexia, abdominal pain, and in a minority of patients, fever.[85,95] Diarrhea has been reported to be prolonged (i.e., greater than 1 month) or intermittent.[85,88–90,92–94,96] Stool eosinophils and mild peripheral eosinophilia have been noted in some patients.[88,92]

Diagnosis is based on stool examination; the presence of five or more organisms per high-powered field (×400) has been suggested to correlate with symptomatic disease.[88,91] However, a clear correlation between numbers of stool parasites and symptoms has not been established. Anecdotically, responses to metronidazole (1.5–2 g/day in divided doses for adults) have been reported.[91,92,95–98] In vitro emetine, metronidazole, and furazolidone have inhibited growth of the parasite more than the other agents tested have.[99] In two cases responses to ketoconazole have been reported.[94]

BALANTIDIUM

Balantidium coli is the largest protozoan and the only ciliate that can produce disease in humans. Its habitat is primarily the colon. There are two forms in the life cycle, just as in *Giardia* and the amoeba: a ciliated trophozoite and an environmentally resistant cyst.[100] The trophozoite is oval and measures about 50–200 μm in length; its membrane is surrounded by hundreds of tiny cilia that provide for its movement through the intestinal wall. Although numerous animal species may harbor *B. coli*, pigs have a particularly high rate of infection and are generally considered the main reservoir for human infection.[100,101] However, balantidiasis has occurred in mental institutions and among Moslems who have no contact with pigs.[100,101]

Humans are usually quite resistant to *B. coli* infection.[101,102] Achlorhydria and poor nutritional status and hygiene decrease resistance.[100] The disease caused by *B. coli* is due to penetration of the organism through the mucosa of the colon with the help of a parasitic hyaluronidase[103] and subsequent replication in the submucosa. Although infection is generally asymptomatic, clinical symptoms range from intermittent watery diarrhea to colitis with stool containing mucus and blood. Severe disease may result in intestinal perforation and peritonitis; rarely, extraintestinal spread occurs, for example, to mesenteric lymph nodes, pleura, or liver.[104–106] Outbreaks of disease have been reported.[101] The differential diagnosis of colitic disease must include amebic and bacillary dysentery. The infection can be diagnosed by finding the rapidly motile trophozoites in fresh stool or in scrapings taken from the periphery of ulcers on sigmoidoscope examinations. Much less commonly, cysts may be observed in human stool.[100,101] Tetracycline is currently considered the treatment of choice, with iodoquinol and metronidazole as alternatives.[107–109]

ISOSPORA

Human isosporiasis is an infection of the gastrointestinal tract that is caused by the coccidian protozoan parasite *Isospora belli*.[110] Although first described in 1915,[111,112] human isosporiasis remains a poorly understood disease. The elliptic *I. belli* oocyst is approximately 22–33 by 10–15 μm in size and contains two sporocysts inside each of which are four sporozoites. Isosporiasis is acquired through the ingestion of sporulated oocysts; the infective dose for humans has not been determined. The parasite invades intestinal epithelium and undergoes the asexual (merogony) and sexual (gametogony) phases of its life cycle in the cytoplasm of the enterocyte. Unsporulated oocysts are excreted in the feces and mature outside the host.

Isospora belli is ubiquitously distributed in the animal kingdom, but its prevalence in humans is not known. It appears to occur more commonly in tropical and subtropical climates. Endemic areas of disease include parts of South America (Santiago, Chile), Africa, and Southeast Asia.[113,114] In the United States, *I. belli* has been implicated in various institutional outbreaks of diarrheal illness and as the cause of enteritis in World War II veterans returning from the Pacific.[113–115] *Isospora* infections have been documented in fewer than 0.2 percent of patients with AIDS in the United States (Centers for Disease Control) and 15 percent of AIDS patients in Haiti.[116] Undoubtedly these figures are underestimates since not all patients are examined for the parasite. Acquisition of *Isospora* from infected animals or humans and contaminated water is suspected but not documented.

Histopathologic study of small intestine biopsy specimens from patients with isosporiasis has revealed atrophic mucosa, shortened villi, hypertrophic crypts, and infiltration of the lamina propria with inflammatory cells, particularly eosinophils.[113,117,118] Organisms have been identified within cytoplasmic vacuoles of enterocytes by using electron microscopy.[119] Extraintestinal involvement of lymph nodes with *Isospora* has been documented in one patient with AIDS[120] and in cats.[121] The pathogenic mechanisms by which *Isospora* causes diarrhea are not known.

The clinical manifestations of isosporiasis include watery diarrhea without blood or inflammatory cells, cramping abdominal pain, and weight loss. Fat malabsorption and peripheral eosinophila (7–15 percent) have been reported in patients with isosporiasis.[113,122] Clinical illness ranges from self-limited enteritis to chronic diarrhea that may persist for months. Chronic or relapsing infection has been described in patients with AIDS[120,122] and in infants and children.[123]

A diagnosis of isosporiasis is established by the identification of *Isospora* oocysts in fecal specimens. Although they are also acid-fast, *Isospora* oocysts they are easily distinguished from cryptosporidia on the basis of size and shape (Fig. 7). *Isospora* may also be detected with a fluorescent auramine stain, but the numerous other techniques described for cryptosporidia have not been evaluated for isosporiasis. Since *Isospora* oocysts may be shed intermittently and in small numbers, concentration methods may be useful in the diagnosis.

Unlike cryptosporidiosis, isosporiasis responds promptly to treatment. A clinical and parasitologic cure may be achieved within 1 week of treatment with oral trimethoprim-sulfamethoxazole (TMP-SMX). Patients with AIDS have a high frequency of recurrence if treatment is stopped, but they will respond favorably to retreatment with TMP-SMX. In order to prevent a recurrence, AIDS patients are often maintained in-

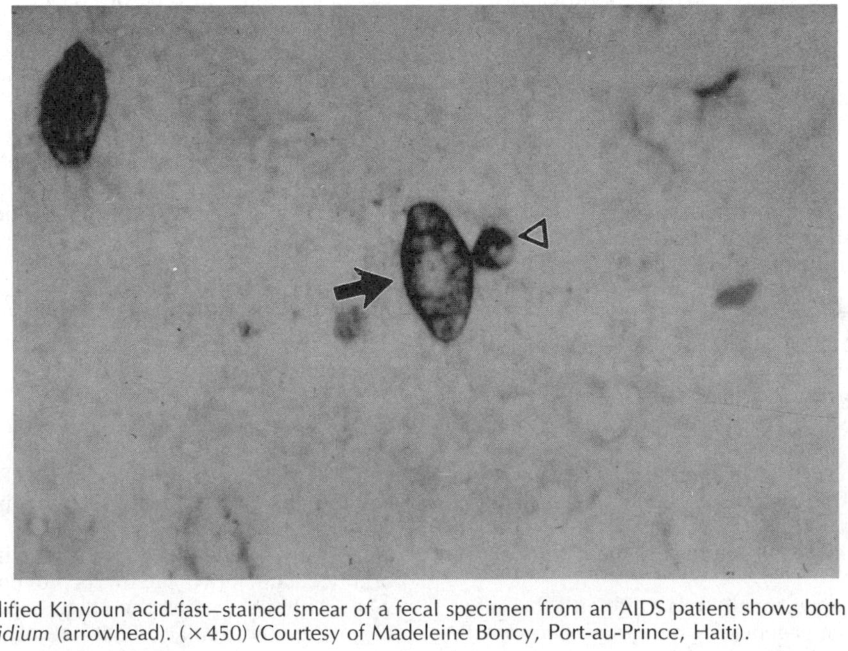

FIG. 7. A modified Kinyoun acid-fast–stained smear of a fecal specimen from an AIDS patient shows both *Isospora* (arrow) and *Cryptosporidium* (arrowhead). (×450) (Courtesy of Madeleine Boncy, Port-au-Prince, Haiti).

definitely on a regimen of suppressive therapy with TMP-SMX at a lower dose or weekly sulfadoxine-pyrimethamine.[124] Unfortunately, however, AIDS patients frequently have adverse reactions to these therapies. Information regarding potentially useful alternate therapy is scanty and often contradictory. There are anecdotal reports of favorable responses to pyrimethamine[125] and roxithromycin,[126] whereas both failure and success have been reorted with the use of metronidazole,[113,117,122] quinacrine,[113,117,127] and nitrofurantoin.[113,117]

REFERENCES

1. Tyzzer EE. A sporozoan found in the peptic glands of the common mouse. Proc Soc Exp Biol Med. 1907–1908;5:12–3.
2. Slavin D. *Cryptosporidium meleagridis* (sp. nov.). J Comp Pathol Ther. 1955;65:262–6.
3. Panciera RJ, Thomassen RW, Garner FM. Cryptosporidial infection in a calf. Vet Pathol. 1971;8:479–84.
4. Anderson BC. Cryptosporidiosis in review. J Am Vet Med Assoc. 1982;180:1455–7.
5. Angus KW. Cryptosporidiosis in man, domestic animals and birds: A review. J R Soc Med. 1983;76:62–70.
6. Tzipori S. Cryptosporidiosis in animals and humans. Microbiol Rev. 1983;47:84–96.
7. Nime FA, Burek JD, Page DL, et al. Acute enterocolitis in a human being infected with the protozoan *Cryptosporidium*. Gastroenterology. 1976;70:592–8.
8. Meisel JL, Perea DR, Meligro C, et al. Overwhelming watery diarrhea associated with a *Cryptosporidium* in an immunosuppressed patient. Gastroenterology. 1976;70:1156–60.
9. Centers for Disease Control. Cryptosporidiosis: Assessment of chemotherapy of males with acquired immune deficiency syndrome (AIDS). MMWR. 1982;31:589–92.
10. Current WL, Reese NC, Ernst JV, et al. Human cryptosporidiosis in immunocompetent and immunodeficient persons: Studies of an outbreak and experimental transmission. N Engl J Med. 1983;308:1252–7.
11. Jokipii L, Pohjola S, Valle SL, et al. Cryptosporidiosis associated with traveling and giardiasis. Gastroenterology. 1985;4:838–42.
12. Soave R, Ma P. Cryptosporidiosis: Traveler's diarrhea in two families. Arch Intern Med. 1985;145:70–2.
13. Wolfson JS, Richter JM, Waldron MA, et al. Cryptosporidiosis in immunocompetent patients. N Engl J Med. 1985;312:1278–82.
14. Fayer R, Ungar BLP. *Cryptosporidium* spp. and cryptosporidiosis. Microbiol Rev. 1986;50:458–83.
15. Soave R, Armstrong D. *Cryptosporidium* and cryptosporidiosis. Rev Infect Dis. 1986;8:1012–23.
16. Janoff EN, Barth Reller L. *Cryptosporidium* species, a protean protozoan. J Clin Microbiol. 1987;25:967–75.
17. Tzipori S. Cryptosporidiosis in perspective. Adv Parasitol. 1988;27:63–129.
18. Levine ND. Some corrections of coccidian (Apicomplexa: Protozoa) nomenclature. J Parasitol. 1980;66:830–4.
19. Tzipori S, Angus KW, Campbell I, et al. *Cryptosporidium*: Evidence for a single-species genus. Infect Immun. 1980;30:884–6.
20. Reese NC, Current WL, Ernst JV, et al. Cryptosporidiosis of man and calf: A case report and results of experimental infections in mice and rats. Am J Trop Med Hyg. 1982;31:226–9.
21. Upton SJ, Current WL. The species of *Cryptosporidium* (Apicomplexa: Cryptosporididae) infeccting mammals. J Parasitol. 1985;71:625–9.
22. Blagburn BL, Current WL. Accidental infection of a researcher with human *Cryptosporidium* (Letter). J Infect Dis. 1983;148:772–3.
23. Hojlyng N, Holten-Andersen W, Jepsen S. Cryptosporidiosis: A case of airborne transmission. Lancet. 1987;2:271–2.
24. Ernest JA, Blagburn BL, Lindsay DS. Infection dynamics of *Cryptosporidium parvum* (Apicomplexa: Cryptosporiididae) in neonatal mice (*Mus musculus*). J Parasitol. 1986;72:796–8.
25. Current WL, Ling PL. Development of human and calf *Cryptosporidium* in chicken embryos. J Infect Dis. 1983;148:1108–13.
26. Navin TR: Cryptosporidiosis in humans: Review of recent epidemiologic studies. Eur J Epidemiol. 1985;1:77–83.
27. Casemore DP, Jackson B. Sporadic cryptosporidiosis in children. Lancet. 1983;2:679.
28. Mata L, Bolanos H, Pizarro D, et al. Cryptosporidiosis in children from some highland Costa Rican rural and urban areas. Am J Trop Med Hyg. 1984;33:24–9.
29. Centers for Disease Control. Cryptosporidiosis among chldren attending day-care centers—Georgia, Pennsylvania, Michigan, California, New Mexico. MMWR. 1984;33:599–601.
30. Heijbel H, Slaine K, Seigel B, et al. Outbreak of diarrhea in a day care center with spread to household members: The role of *Cryptosporidium*. Pediatr Infect Dis J. 1987;6:532–5.
31. Stehr-Green JK, McCaig L, Remsen HM, et al. Shedding of oocysts in immunocompetent individuals infected with *Cryptosporidium*. Am J Trop Med Hyg. 1987;36:338–42.
32. Collier AC, Miller RA, Meyers JD. Cryptosporidiosis after marrow transplantation: Person-to-person transmission and treatment with spiramycin. Ann Intern Med. 1984;101:2056.
33. Dryjanski J, Gold JW, Ritchie MT, et al. Cryptosporidiosis. Case report in a health team worker. Am J Med. 1986;80:751–2.
34. Koch KL, Phillips DJ, Aber RC, et al. Cryptosporidiosis in hospital personnel. Evidence for person-to-person transmission. Ann Intern Med. 1985;102:593–6.
35. Baxby D, Hart CA, Taylor C. Human cryptosporidiosis: A possible cause of hospital cross-infection. Br Med J. 1983;287:1760–1.
36. Martino P, Gentile G, Caprioli A, et al. Hospital acquired cyptosporidiosis in a bone marrow transplantation unit. J Infect Dis. 1988;158:647–9.
37. Ma P, Kaufman DL, Helmick CG, et al. Cryptosporidiosis in tourists returning from the Caribbean. N Engl J Med. 1985;312:647–8.
38. D'Antonio RG, Winn RE, Taylor JP, et al. A waterborne outbreak of cryptosporidiosis in normal hosts. Ann Intern Med. 1985;103:886–8.
39. Gallaher MM, Herndon JL, Nims LJ, et al. Cryptosporidiosis and surface water. Am J Public Health. 1989;79:39–42.
40. Madore MS, Rose JB, Gerba CP, et al. Occurrence of *Cryptosporidium* oocysts in sewage effluents and select surface waters. J Parasitol. 1987;73:702–5.
41. Ongerth JE, Stibbs HH. Identification of *Cryptosporidium* oocysts in river water. Appl Environ Microbiol. 1987;53:672–6.
42. Rose JB, Cifrino A, Madore MS, et al. Detection of *Cryptosporidium* from wastewater and freshwater environments. Water Sci Tech. 1986;18:233–9.
43. Soave R, Danner RL, Honig CL, et al. Cryptosporidiosis in homosexual men. Ann Intern Med. 1984;110:504–11.
44. Guarda LA, Stein SA, Cleary KA, et al. Human cryptosporidiosis in the acquired immune deficiency syndrome. Arch Pathol Lab Med. 1983;107:562–6.
45. Pitlik SD, Fainstein V, Garza D, et al. Human cryptosporidiosis: Spectrum of disease. Report of six cases and review of the literature. Arch Intern Med. 1983;143:2269–76.
46. Navin TR, Juranek DD. Cryptosporidiosis: Clinical, epidemiologic, and parasitologic review. Rev Infect Dis. 1984;6:313–27.
47. Sloper KS, Dourmashkin RR, Bird RB, et al. Chronic malabsorption due to cryptosporidiosis in a child with immunoglobulin deficiency. Gut. 1982;23:80–2.
48. Blumberg RS, Kelsey P, Perrone T, et al. Cryptomegalovirus- and cryptosporidium-associated with acalculous gangrenous cholecystis. Am J Med. 1984;76:118.
49. Margulis SJ, Honig CL, Soave R, et al. Biliary tract obstruction in the acquired immunodeficiency syndrome. Ann Intern Med. 1986;105:207–10.
50. Schneiderman DJ, Cello JP, Laing FC. Papillary stenosis and sclerosing cholangitis in the acquired immunodeficiency syndrome. Ann Intern Med. 1987;106:546–9.
51. Davis JJ, Heyman MB, Ferrell L, et al. Sclerosing cholangitis associated with chronic cryptosporidiosis in a child with a congenital immunodeficiency disorder. Am J Gastroenterol. 1987;82:1196–202.
52. Gentile G, Baldassarri L, Caprioli A, et al. Colonic vascular invasion as a possible route of extraintestinal cryptosporidiosis. Am J Med. 1987;82:574–5.
53. Forgacs P, Tarshis A, Ma P, et al. Intestinal and bronchial cryptosporidiosis in an immunodeficient homosexual man. Ann Intern Med. 1983;99:793.
54. Kocoshis SA, Cibull ML, Davis TE, et al. Intestinal and pulmonary cryptosporidiosis in an infant with severe combined immune deficiency. J Pediatr Gastroenterol Nutr. 1984;3:49.
55. Miller RA, Wasserheit JN, Kirihara J, et al. Detection of *Cryptosporidium* oocysts in sputum during screening for mycobacterium. J Clin Microbiol. 1984;20:1992–3.
56. Manivel C, Filipovich A, Snover DC. Cryptosporidiosis as a cause of diarrhea following bone marrow transplantation. Dis Colon Rectum. 1985;28:741–2.
57. Heine J, Pohlenz JFL, Moon HW, et al. Enteric lesions and diarrhea in gnotobiotic calves monoinfected with *Cryptosporidium* species. J Infect Dis. 1984;150:768–75.
58. Marcial MA, Madara JL. Cryptosporidium: Cellular localization, structural analysis of absorptive cell–parasite membrane–membrane interactions in guinea pigs and suggestion of protozoan transport by M cells. Gastroenterology. 1986;90:583–94.
59. Koch KL, Shankey TV, Weinstein GS, et al. Cryptosporidiosis in a patient with hemophilia, common variable hypogammaglobulinemia, and the acquired immunodeficiency syndrome. Ann Intern Med. 1983;99:337–40.
60. Jokipii L, Jokipii AMM. Timing of symptoms and oocyst excretion in human cryptosporidiosis. N Engl J Med. 1986;315:1643–7.
61. Henricksen SA, Pohlenz JFL. Staining of cryptosporidia by a modified Ziehl-Neelsen technique. Acta Vet Scand. 1981;22:594–6.
62. Tzipori S, Angus KW, Gray EW, et al. Vomiting and diarrhea associated with cryptosporidial infection. N Engl J Med. 1980;303:818.
63. Garcia LS, Bruckner DA, Brewer TC, et al. Techniques for the recovery and identification of *Cryptosporidium* oocysts from stool specimens. J Clin Microbiol. 1983;18:185–90.
64. Ma P, Soave R. Three-step stool examination for cryptosporidiosis in 10 homosexual men with protracted watery diarrhea. J Infect Dis. 1983;147:824–8.
65. Crawford FG, Vermund SH. Human cryptosporidiosis. CRC Crit Rev Microbiol. 1988;16:113–59.

66. Weikel CS, Johnston CI, Auxilia Dora Soursa M, et al. Cryptosporidiosis in Northeastern Brazil: Association with sporadic diarrhea. J Infect Dis. 1985;151:963.
67. Sterling CR, Arrowood MJ. Detection of *Cryptosporidium* and cryptosporidiosis. Rev Infect Dis. 1986;8:1012.
68. Campbell PM, Current WL. Demonstration of serum antibodies to *Cryptosporidium* sp. in normal and immunodeficient humans with confirmed infections. J Clin Microbiol. 1983;18:165–9.
69. Tzipori S, Campbell I. Prevalence of *Cryptosporidium* antibodies in 10 animal species. J Clin Microbiol. 1981;14:455–6.
70. Ungar BL, Soave R, Fayer R, et al. Enzyme immunoassay detection of immunoglobulin M and G antibodies to *Cryptosporidium* in immunocompetent and immunocompromised patients. J Infect Dis. 1986;153:570–8.
71. Tzipori S, Campbell I, Angus KW. The therapeutic effect of 16 antimicrobial agents on *Cryptosporidium* infection in mice. Aust J Exp Biol Med Sci. 1982;60:187–90.
72. Rehg JE, Hancock ML, Woodmansee DB. Characterization of cyclophosphamide-rat model of cryptosporidiosis. Infect Immun. 1987;55:2669.
73. Soave R. Therapy and prevention of coccidiosis. In: Schlessinger D, ed. Microbiology—1984. Washington DC: American Society for Microbiology; 1984:232–6.
74. Portnoy D, Whiteside ME, Buckley E III, et al. Treatment of intestinal cryptosporidiosis with spiramycin. Ann Intern Med. 1984;101:202–4.
75. Tzipori S, Roberton D, Chapman C. Remission of diarrhea due to cryptosporidiosis in an immunodeficient child treated with hyperimmune bovine colostrum. Br Med J 1986;293:1276.
76. Kotler D. Preliminary observations of the effect of cow's milk globulin upon intestinal cryptosporidiosis in AIDS (Abstract). Third International Conference on AIDS. Washington, DC, June 1987.
77. Louie E, Borkowsky W, Klesius PH, et al. Treatment of cryptosporidiosis with oral bovine transfer factor. Clin Immunol Immunopathol. 1987;44:329.
78. Greve E. Sarcosporidiosis—an overlooked zoonosis. Dan Med Bull. 1985;32:228–30.
79. Beaver PC, Gadgil RK, Morera P. Sarcocystis in man: A review and report of five cases. Am J Trop Med Hyg. 1979;28:819–44.
80. Bunyaratvej S, Bunyawongwiroj P, Nitiyanant P. Human intestinal sarcosporidiosis: Report of six cases. Am J Trop Med Hyg. 1982;31:36–41.
81. Jeffrey HC. Sarcosporidiosis in man. Trans R Soc Trop Med Hyg. 1974;68:17–29.
82. Zierdt CH, Rude WS, Bull BS. Protozoan characteristics of *Blastocystis hominis*. Am J Clin Pathol. 1967;48:495–501.
83. Phillips BP, Zierdt CH. *Blastocystis hominis:* Pathogenic potential in human patients and in gnotobiotes. Exp Parasitol. 1976;39:358–64.
84. Yamada M, Yoshikawa H, Tegoshi T, et al. Light microscopical study of *Blastocystis* spp. in monkeys and fowls. Parasitol Res. 1987;73:527–31.
85. Garcia LS, Bruckner DA, Clancy MN. Clinical relevance of *Blastocystis hominis*. Lancet. 1984;1:1233–4.
86. Taylor DN, Blaser MJ, Blacklow N, et al. Polymicrobial aetiology of traveller's diarrhoea. Lancet. 1985;1:381–3.
87. Babcock D, Houston R, Kumaki D, et al. *Blastocystis hominis* in Kathmandu, Nepal. N Engl J Med. 1986;313:1419.
88. Sheehan DJ, Raucher BG, McKitrick JC. Association of *Blastocystis hominis* with signs and symptoms of human disease. J Clin Microbiol. 1986;24:548–50.
89. Markell EK, Udkow MP. *Blastocystis hominis:* Pathogen or fellow traveler? Am J Trop Med Hyg. 1986;35:1023–6.
90. Pikula ZP. *Blastocystis hominis* and human disease. J Clin Microbiol. 1987;25:1581.
91. Diaczok BJ, Rival J. Diarrhea due to *Blastocystis hominis:* An old organism revisited. South Med J. 1987;80:931–2.
92. Vannatta JB, Adamson D, Mullican K. *Blastocystis hominis* infection presenting as recurrent diarrhea. Ann Intern Med. 1985;102:495–6.
93. Russo AR, Stone SL, Taplin ME, et al. Presumptive evidence for *Blastocystis hominis* as a cause of colitis. Arch Intern Med. 1988;148:1064.
94. Cohen AN. Ketoconazole and resistant *Blastocystis hominis* infection. Ann Intern Med. 1985;103:480–1.
95. Gallagher PG, Venglarcik JS III. *Blastocystis hominis* enteritis. Pediatr Infect Dis. 1985;4:556–7.
96. Zierdt CH, Tan HK. Ultrastructure and light microscope appearance of *Blastocystis hominis* in a patient with enteric disease. Z Parasitenkl. 1976;50:277–83.
97. LeBar WD, Larsen EC, Patel K. Afebrile diarrhea and *Blastocystis hominis*. Ann Intern Med. 1985;103:306.
98. Ricci N, Toma P, Furlani M, et al. *Blastocystis hominis:* A neglected cause of diarrhoea? Lancet. 1984;1:966.
99. Zierdt CH, Swan JC, Hosseini J. In vitro response of *Blastocystis hominis* to antiprotozoal drugs. J Protozool. 1983;30:332–4.
100. Arean VM, Koppisch E. Balantidiasis—a review and report of cases. Am J Pathol. 1956;32:1089–108.
101. Walzer PD, Judson FN, Murphy KB, et al. Balantidiasis outbreak in Truk. Am J Trop Med Hyg. 1973;22:33–41.
102. Young MD. Attempts to transmit human *Balantidium coli*. Am J Trop Med. 1950;30:71–2.
103. Tempelis CH, Lysenko MG. The production of hyaluronidase by *Balantidium coli*. Exp Parasitol. 1957;6:31–6.
104. Castro J, Vazquez-Iglesias JL, Arnal-Monreal F. Dysentery caused by *Balantidium coli*—report of two cases. Endoscopy. 1983;15:272–4.
105. Vidan JR, Frauca A, Martinez B, et al. Parasitosis hepatica por *Balantidium coli*. Med Clin (Barc). 1985;85:299–300.
106. Lahiri VL, Elhence BR, Agarwal BM. *Balantidium* peritonitis diagnosed on cytologic material. Acta Cytol (Baltimore). 1977;21:123–4.
107. Drugs for parasitic infections.
108. Zaman V, Natarajan PN. In vitro trials of metronidazole against *Balantidium coli*. Trans R Soc Trop Med Hyg. 1969;63:152.
109. Garcia-Laverde A, De Bonilla L. Clinical trials with metronidazole in human balantidiasis. Am J Trop Med Hyg. 1975;24:781–3.
110. Soave R, Johnson WD Jr. *Cryptosporidium* and *Isospora belli* infections. J Infect Dis. 1988;157:225–9.
111. Woodcock HM. Notes on the protozoan parasites in the excreta. Br Med J. 1915;2:709–11.
112. Wenyon CM. Observations on the common intestinal protozoa of man: Their diagnosis and pathogenicity. Lancet. 1915;2:1173–83.
113. Brandborg LL, Goldberg SB, Briedenbach WC. Human coccidiosis—a possible cause of malabsorption. The life cycle in small-bowel mucosal biopsies as a diagnostic feature. N Engl J Med. 1970;283:1306–13.
114. Faust EC, Giraldo LE, Caicedo G, et al. Human isosporosis in the Western Hemisphere. Am J Med. 1983;10:343.
115. Smitskamp H, Dey-Muller E. Geographical distribution and clinical significance of human coccidiosis. Trop Geogr Med. 1966;18:133–6.
116. DeHovitz JA, Pape JW, Boncy M, et al. Clinical manifestations and therapy of *Isospora belli* infection in patients with acquired immunodeficiency syndrome. N Engl J Med. 1986;315:87.
117. Trier JS, Moxey PC, Schimmel EM, et al. Chronic intestinal coccidiosis in man: Intestinal morphology and response to treatment. Gastroenterology. 1974;66:923–35.
118. Webster BH. Human isosporiasis: A report of three cases with necropsy findings in one case. Am J Trop Med. 1957;6:86–9.
119. Liebman WM, Thaler MM, DeLorimier A, et al. Intractable diarrhea of infancy due to intestinal coccidiosis. Gastroenterology. 1980;78:579.
120. Restrepo C, Macher AM, Radany EH. Disseminated extraintestinal isosporiasis in a patient with acquired immunodeficiency syndrome. Am J Clin Pathol. 1987;87:536.
121. Dubey JP, Frenkel JK. Extra-intestinal stages of *Isospora felis I. rivolta* (Protozoa: Eimeridiae) in cats. J Protozool. 1972;19:89–92.
122. Forthal DN, Guest SS. *Isospora belli* enteritis in three homosexual men. Am J Trop Med Hyg. 1984;33:1060.
123. Faira JA, Brust MB. Human isosporiasis caused by *Isospora belli*, Wenyon 1923. Salvador-Bahia. Rev Inst Med Trop Sao Paulo. 1983;251:47–9.
124. Pape JW, Verdier R, Johnson WD. Treatment and prophylaxis of *Isospora belli* infection in patients with the acquired immunodeficiency syndrome. N Engl J Med. 1989;320:1044–7.
125. Weiss LM, Perlman DC, Sherman J, et al. *Isospora belli* infection: Treatment with pyrimethamine. Ann Inter Med. 1988;109:474–5.
126. Musey KL, Chidiac C, Beaucaire G, et al. Effectiveness of roxithromycin for treating *Isospora belli* infection. J Infect Dis. 1988;158:646.
127. Ma P, Kaufman D, Montana J. *Isospora belli* diarrheal infection in homosexual men. AIDS Res. 1984;1:327.

261. MICROSPORIDIA

RALPH T. BRYAN

The phylum Microspora consists of approximately 80 genera and over 700 species. Organisms belonging to this phylum are referred to collectively as *microsporidia*, and the disease they produce is termed *microsporidiosis*. Microsporidia are obligate intracellular, spore-forming protozoal parasites. They are ubiquitous in nature and have been found in most major animal groups.[1] First identified in 1857, microsporidia have long been recognized as a cause of disease in many nonhuman hosts. Historically, these organisms have caused serious economic problems for the silkworm, honeybee, and commercial fishing industries. They have also been shown to be sources of significant disease in laboratory rodents, rabbits, fur-bearing animals, and primates. Infections in laboratory animals have caused serious problems with interpretation of experimental results.[1–3] Their importance as human pathogens has only recently been recognized.[4–6]

DESCRIPTION OF THE PATHOGEN

Depending on the species, microsporidian spores range in size from 1 to 20 μm. Those species infecting mammals tend to be smaller, with diameters in the 1–2 μm range, and are usually ovoid or piriform in shape. Ultrastructurally, all microsporidian spores possess a characteristic coiled polar filament or tubule (Fig. 1). Upon ingestion by a host, the spore is stimulated by changes in pH and ionic concentrations to evert its coiled tubule. The tubule then penetrates the host cell and injects the infective agent or sporoplasm into the nondisrupted host cell cytoplasm. Thereafter, merogony and sporogony proceed sequentially, resulting in a new generation of sporoblasts. Subsequent maturation and spore organelle synthesis give rise to new spores, which are then capable of further multiplication, dissemination to different cells, and/or passage into the environment via skin, urine, or feces.[1] Spores passed into the environment can, in some species, remain viable for up to 4 months.[7] Transmission is thought to occur primarily via the fecal-oral route, but transplacental and transovarial transmission also occur.[2,8] Direct inoculation may play a role in transmission in some cases.[9,10]

Among the numerous microsporidian genera, only four have been implicated in human disease: *Nosema, Encephalitozoon, Pleistophora,* and *Enterocytozoon. Nosema* and *Pleistophora* are generally considered to be pathogens of insects and fish, respectively, whereas *Encephalitozoon* usually infects nonhuman mammals. Organisms of the genus *Enterocytozoon* have been described only in human patients with the acquired immunodeficiency syndrome (AIDS). Although *Nosema, Pleistophora,* and particularly *Encephalitozoon* are well studied, very little is known about *Enterocytozoon.*

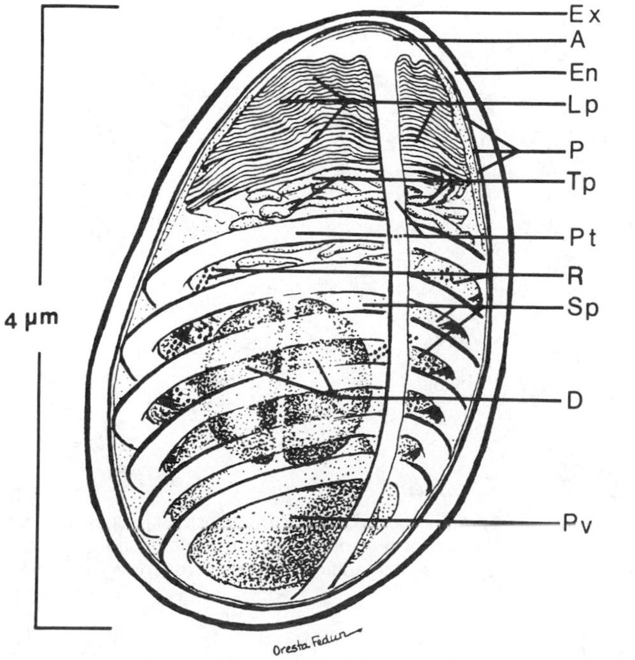

FIG. 1. Diagram of the internal structure of a microsporidian spore. The spore coat has an outer electron-dense exospore and an inner, thicker, electron-lucent endospore. The extrusion apparatus (anchoring disc, polar tubule, lamellar polaroplast, and tubular polaroplast) dominates the spore contents and is diagnostic of microsporidia. The number of polar tubule coils depends on the particular species and can vary from a few to over 30. Ex: exospore; En: endospore; P: unit membrane; A: anchoring disc; Pt: polar tubule; Lp: lamellar polaroplast; Tp: tubular polaroplast; Pv: posterior vacuole; R: ribosomes; Sp: sporoplasm; D: diplokaryon nuclei. (From Cali and Owen,[5] with permission.)

PATHOGENESIS

Of the microsporidian species known to infect mammals, *Encephalitozoon cuniculi* has been the most thoroughly studied. Infection with *E. cuniculi* begins in intestinal epithelial cells. In the mouse, the first extraintestinal site to show signs of infection is the liver. Thereafter, spores are thought to travel via blood, via lymph, or within infected macrophages to distant anatomic locations.[2] As infection progresses, central nervous system vasculitis and severe interstitial nephritis predominate.[1] In contrast, the primary pathologic site in infections with *Enterocytozoon bieneusi* appears to be the small bowel. Corresponding inflammation, however, is minimal or absent. It is unknown whether or not *En. bieneusi* infections are associated with extraintestinal pathologic lesions similar to those seen with *E. cuniculi.*

EPIDEMIOLOGY

Very little is known about the epidemiology of microsporidiosis. Several case reports indicate that immunosuppression or trauma may play a key role in infection.[9–15] Serologic surveys performed with assays for antibodies to *E. cuniculi* suggest that travelers and residents in tropical countries may have increased exposure to this organism, but clinical correlation and definitive epidemiologic findings are lacking.[16–20] Nevertheless, microsporidia are being increasingly implicated as a cause of human disease, particularly in patients with AIDS. Six microsporidial infections in patients without AIDS are documented in the literature (Table 1). Four of the six patients had either traveled to or resided in tropical countries. The fifth patient was an infant with thymic aplasia,[11] and the sixth was a Japanese boy with no known immunodeficiencies or exposure to the tropics.[21]

AIDS-related cases of microsporidiosis are being recognized with increasing frequency. As of this writing, 15 cases have been well documented in patients from Europe, the United States, Haiti, South America, and Uganda (Table 2). Moreover, a series examining small bowel biopsy specimens from 80 AIDS patients from New York City and Washington, D.C., has identified some 20 cases of intestinal infection with *En. bieneusi* (J. Orenstein, personal communication).

CLINICAL MANIFESTATIONS

Although reports of possible cases appeared as early as 1924,[1,13,22] conclusive evidence for human infection with microsporidia was not available until 1959. The definitive case involved a 9-year-old Japanese boy who presented with symptoms of recurrent fever, loss of consciousness, headache, and convulsions. He was not known to be immunocompromised in any way, but was noted to have a negative tuberculin skin test despite having received Calmette-Guérin bacillus vaccine (BCG) 4 months before his admission. Examination of his cerebrospinal fluid (CSF) and urinary sediments revealed organisms consistent with microsporidia.[21]

No further cases were reported until 1973, when the first human case proven by autopsy was published.[11] The patient was a 4-month-old boy with thymic aplasia who presented with severe diarrhea and malabsorption. Autopsy revealed disseminated microsporidia in the lungs, stomach, small and large bowels, kidneys, adrenal glands, myocardium, liver, and diaphragm. The implicated organism was identified by electron microscopy as *Nosema connori.*[23] Also in 1973 and again in 1981, two cases with corneal involvement were documented by biopsy and enucleation.[9,10] Neither patient had any overt evidence of underlying immunodeficiency, but both were residents of the tropics (Sri Lanka and Botswana). The organisms involved appeared to represent unique species, but their generic

TABLE 1. Microsporidiosis: Confirmed Human Cases (Non-AIDS)

Reference	*Clinical History*	*Genus*	*Location*
Matsubayashi et al.[21]	9-year-old boy with seizure disorder	*Encephalitozoon*	Japan
Margileth et al.[11]	4-month-old boy with thymic aplasia and disseminated microsporidia	*Nosema*	Washington, D.C.
Ashton and Wirasinha[9]	11-year-old boy with keratitis	Genus unknown	Sri Lanka
Pinnolis et al.[10]	26-year-old woman with corneal ulceration	Genus unknown	Botswana
Bergquist et al.[19]	2-year-old boy with seizures	*Encephalitozoon*	Columbia (Diagnosis in Sweden)
Davis et al.[24]	45-year-old man with keratitis/iritis	Genus unknown	S. Carolina (travel to Central America)

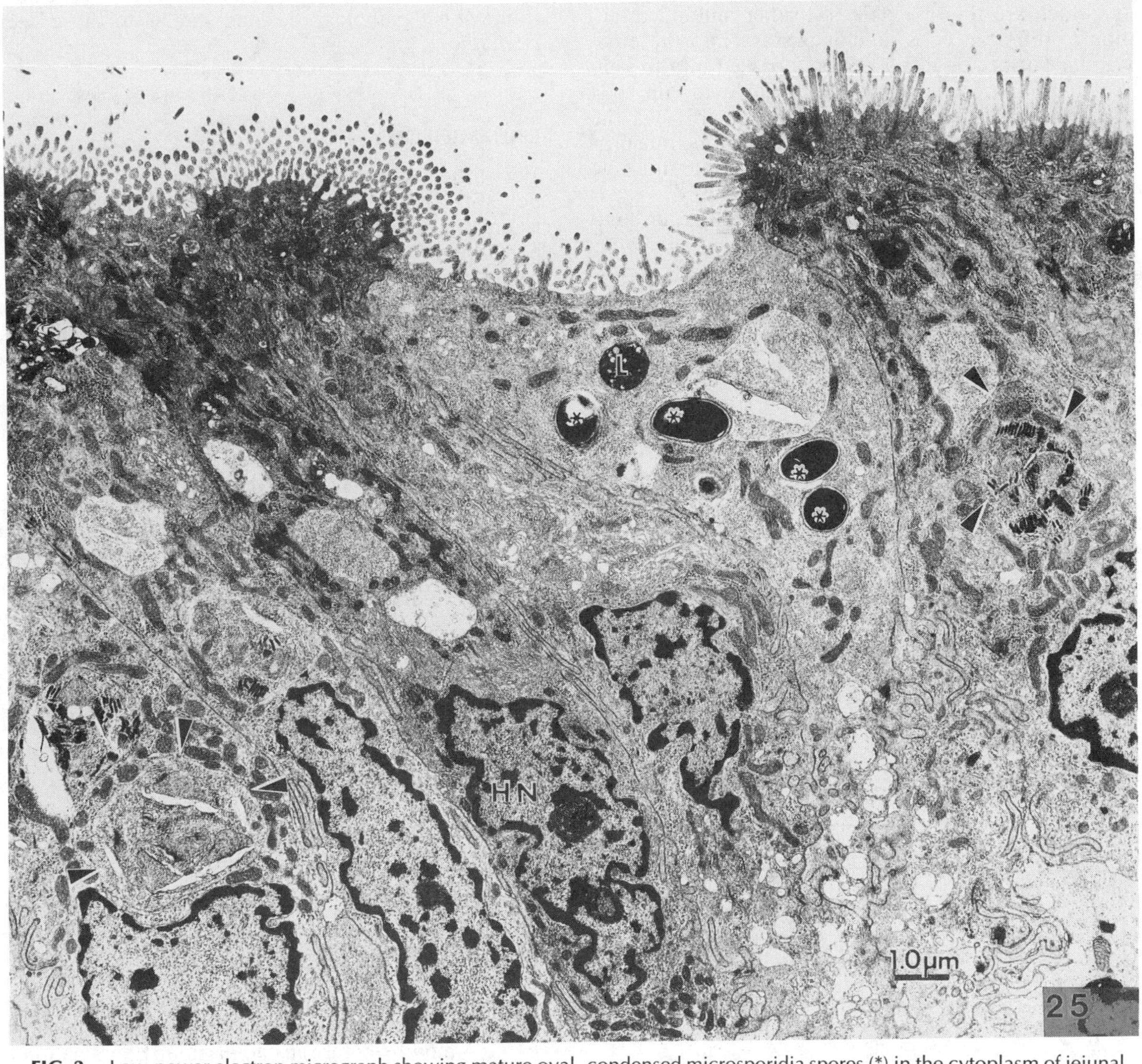

FIG. 2. Low-power electron micrograph showing mature oval, condensed microsporidia spores (*) in the cytoplasm of jejunal enterocytes near the villus tip. Spores can be differentiated from an adjacent multivesicular lysosomal body (L) by their spore coats and oval shape. Dividing sporogonial forms containing spiral polar tubules are present in adjacent enterocytes (arrows). HN: Host nucleus. (From Cali and Owen,[5] with permission.)

classifications were uncertain. Hence, the organisms were classified as members of the "collective group" *Microsporidium*.[1] The next case reported was that of a 3-year-old Columbian boy who had presented in Sweden with seizures and hepatomegaly. A thorough search for immunologic abnormalities revealed normal B-cell counts but low (1.0) T-cell helper/suppressor ratios. Diagnosis was based on the discovery of 1.5 × 2.5 μm gram-positive, oblong organisms in his urinary sediment. Identical organisms were recovered from mice that had been injected with the patient's urine.[17,19] In 1988 another case of microsporidial keratitis was detected in a 45-year-old South Carolina man who had recently traveled to Central America.[25]

Reports of microsporidial infection in patients with AIDS first appeared in 1985 (Table 2). The predominant manifestations of this infection in AIDS patients appear to be chronic diarrhea and weight loss. In the vast majority of cases, *En. bieneusi* is

TABLE 2. Microsporidiosis in Patients with AIDS

Reference	*Patient/Locale/Symptoms*	*Basis of Diagnosis*	*Genus*
Dobbins and Weinstein[25]	42 YO M/Florida/diarrhea, wt. loss	Intestinal Bx	*Enterocytozoon*
Modigliani et al.[12]	29 YO M/Haiti/diarrhea, wt. loss	Intestinal Bx	*Enterocytozoon*
Ledford et al.[13 a]	20 YO M/Florida/wt. Loss, myopathy	Muscle Bx	*Pleisitophora*
Owen[14]	45 YO M/California/diarrhea, wt. loss	Intestinal Bx	*Enterocytozoon*
Terada et al.[15]	35 YO M/Florida/diarrhea, hepatitis	Liver Bx/autopsy	*Encephalitozoon*
Lucas and Wamukota[29]	M/Uganda/slim disease	Intestinal Bx	*Enterocytozoon*
Lucas and Wamukota[29]	M/Uganda/slim disease	Intestinal Bx	*Enterocytozoon*
Rijpstra et al.[27]	40 YO M/Argentina/diarrhea, wt. loss	Intestinal Bx	*Enterocytozoon*
Rijpstra et al.[27]	30 YO M/Netherlands/diarrhea, wt. loss	Intetinal Bx	*Enterocytozoon*
Rijpstra et al.[27]	30 YO M/England/diarrhea, wt. loss	Intestinal Bx	*Enterocytozoon*
Curry et al.[30]	34 YO M/England/diarrhea, wt. loss	Intestinal Bx	Not stated
Canning et al.[31]	M/England/diarrhea	Intestinal Bx	*Enterocytozoon*
Dobbins[b]	35 YO M/Florida/diarrhea, wt. loss	Intestinal Bx	*Enterocytozoon*
Gourley and Swedo[26]	40s YO M/Texas/diarrhea, wt. loss	Intestinal Bx	*Enterocytozoon*
Gourley and Swedo[26]	30s YO M/Texas/diarrhea, wt. loss	Autopsy	*Enterocytozoon*

Abbreviations: YO: year-old; M: male; wt.: weight; Bx: biopsy.
[a] Diagnosis of AIDS in question.[32]
[b] Personal communication.

the implicated organism. Most AIDS patients with microsporidiosis appear to meet diagnostic criteria for human immunodeficiency virus wasting syndrome or, as it is referred to in Africa, *slim disease*.[1,4–6,14]

DIAGNOSIS

Currently, definitive diagnosis of microsporidiosis requires biopsy and electron microscopy (Fig. 2). Although other biopsy sites have resulted in diagnoses (e.g., muscle and liver), the small intestine appears to provide the highest diagnostic yield (R. Owen, personal communication). In biopsy specimens obtained from other gastrointestinal sites (stomach, colon, rectum), organisms either were not found or were rare in comparison to small bowel specimens.[12,25,26] Various developmental forms (spores, sporonts, plasmodia, schizonts) may be seen in biopsy specimens, but their small size, poor staining qualities, and lack of surrounding tissue reaction often make diagnosis difficult. Although many microsporidian spores are gram-positive and contain a periodic acid–Schiff (PAS)-positive anterior granule, most stain poorly with routine tissue stains such as hematoxylin-eosin.[1] For AIDS patients with *En. bieneusi*, however, Giemsa-stained touch preparations[27] and basic fuschin/methylene blue/Azure 2 stained semithin plastic sections of duodenal biopsy specimens may facilitate diagnosis (J. Orenstein, personal communication). Nevertheless, species-specific identification of organisms still depends on electron microscopic description of ultrastructural characteristics.

Serologic tests (carbon immunoassay, indirect fluorescent antibody, and enzyme-linked immunosorbent assay) have been useful in detecting IgG and IgM antibodies to *E. cuniculi* in several species of animals.[1] Similarly, antibodies to *E. cuniculi* have been found in various human populations, but clinical correlation has been somewhat limited. Furthermore, *E. cuniculi* is the only microsporidian species infecting mammals for which serologic assays are available. Microsporidia of the genus *Enterocytozoon* (the genus most frequently found in patients with AIDS) have not been propagated in cell culture or laboratory animals, so serologic assays have yet to be developed. It is not known if antigens of *E. cuniculi* cross react with those of *Enterocytozoon*.

TREATMENT

Although chloroquine phosphate and fumagillin have demonstrated some growth inhibitory effect on *E. cuniculi* grown in cell culture, no effective therapy has been demonstrated in vivo in animals or humans.[7,28] Limited experience in treating infection due to *En. bieneusi* suggests that pyrimethamine,[27] metronidazole,[27] or trimethoprim/sulfamethoxazole[6] may be effective.

REFERENCES

1. Canning EU, Lom J. The Microsporidia of Vertebrates. London: Academic Press; 1986.
2. Gannon J. A survey of *Encephalitozoon cuniculi* in laboratory animal colonies in the United Kingdom. Lab Anim. 1980;14:91–4.
3. Cox JC. Altered immune responsiveness associated *Encephalitozoon cuniculi* infection in rabbits. Infect Immun. 1977;15:392–5.
4. Shadduck JA. Human microsporidiosis and AIDS. Rev Infect Dis. 1989;11:203–7.
5. Cali A, Owen R. Microsporidiosis. In: Balows A, ed. The Laboratory Diagnosis of Infectious Diseases: Principles and Practice. New York: Springer-Verlag; 1988:929–50.
6. Current WL, Owen RL. Cryptosporidiosis and microsporidiosis. In: Farthing MJG, Keusch GT, eds. Enteric infection: Mechanisms, manifestations, and management. London: Chapman and Hall Medical; 1989:223–49.
7. Waller T. Sensitivity of *Encephalitozoon cuniculi* to various temperatures, disinfectants and drugs. Lab Anim. 1979;13:227–30.
8. Zeman DH, Baskin GB. Encephalitozoonosis is squirrel monkeys (*Saimiri sciureus*). Vet Pathol. 1985;22:24–31.
9. Ashton N, Wirasinha PA. Encephalitozoonosis (nosematosis) of the cornea. Br J Ophthalmol. 1973;57:669–74.
10. Pinnolis M, Egbert PR, Font RL, et al. Nosematosis of the cornea. Arch Opthalmol. 1981;99:1044–7.
11. Margileth AM, Strano AJ, Chandra R, et al. Disseminated nosematosis in an immunologically compromised infant. Arch Pathol. 1973;95:145–50.
12. Modigliani R, Bories C, Le Charpentier Y, et al. Diarrhea and malabsorption in acquired immune deficiency syndrome: A study of four cases with special emphasis on opportunistic protozoan infestations. Gut. 1985;26:179–87.
13. Ledford DK, Overman MD, Gonzalvo A, et al. Microsporidiosis myositis in a patient with acquired immunodeficiency syndrome. Ann Intern Med. 1985;102:628–30.
14. Owen RL. Intestinal *Microsporidia* infection in humans: Clinical description and diagnostic approach (Abstract). American Society of Microbiology Annual Meeting. Atlanta, Georgia; March 1987.
15. Terada S, Reddy R, Jeffers LJ, et al. Microsporidian hepatitis in the acquired immunodeficiency syndrome. Ann Intern Med. 1987;107:61–2.
16. Singh M, Kane GJ, Mackinlay L, et al. Detection of antibodies to *Nosema cuniculi* (protozoa: microsporidia) in human and animal sera by the indirect fluorescent antibody technique. Southeast Asia J Trop Med Public Health. 1982;13:110–3.
17. Antibody to *Encephalitozoon cuniculi* in man. WHO Weekly Epidemiol Rec. 1983;58:30–2.
18. Hollister WS, Canning EU. An enzyme-linked immunosorbent assay (ELISA) for detection of antibodies to *E. cuniculi* and its use in determination of infections in man. Parasitology. 1987;94:209–19.

19. Bergquist NR, Stintzing G, Smedman L, et al. Diagnosis of encephalitozoonosis in man by serological tests. Br Med J. 1984;288:902.
20. Bergquist R, Morfeldt-Mansson L, Pehrson PO, et al. Antibody against *Encephalitozoon cuniculi* in Swedish homosexual men. Scand J Infect Dis. 1984;16:389–91.
21. Matsubayashi H, Koike T, Mikata T, et al. A case of *Encephalitozoon*—like body infection in man. Arch Pathol. 1959;67:181–7.
22. Levaditi C, Nicolau S, Schoen R. Nouvelles recherches sur l'*Encephalitozoon cuniculi*. CR Soc. Biol. Paris. 1924a;40:662–6.
23. Strano AJ, Cali A, Neafie RC. Microsporidiosis. In: Binford CH, Connor DH, eds. Pathology of Tropical and Extraordinary Diseases. Washington, DC: Armed Forces Institute of Pathology; 1976:336–9.
24. Davis RM, Font RL, Keisler MS, et al. Corneal microsporidiosis: A case report. Submitted for publication.
25. Dobbins WO III, Weinstein WM. Electron microscopy of the intestine and rectum in acquired immunodeficiency syndrome. Gastroenterology. 1985;88:738–49.
26. Gourley WK, Swedo TL. Intestinal infection by microsporidia *Enterocytozoon bieneusi* of patients with AIDS: An ultrastructural study of the use of human mitochondria by a protozoan (Abstract). Lab Invest. 1988;58:35A.
27. Rijpstra AC, Canning EU, van Ketel RJ, et al. Use of light microscopy to diagnose small-intestinal microsporidiosis in patients with AIDS. J Infect Dis. 1988;157:827–31.
28. Shadduck JA. Effect of fumagillin on in vitro multiplication of *Encephalitozoon cuniculi*. J Protozool. 1980;27:202–8.
29. Lucas SB, Wamukota W. HIV and the local African population. In: Pounder RE, Chiodini PL, eds. Advanced Medicine. v. 23. London: Bailliere Tindall; 1987:102–11.
30. Curry A, McWilliam LJ, Haboubi NY, et al. Microsporidiosis in a British patient with AIDS. J Clin Pathol. 1988;41:477–8.
31. Canning EU, Hollister WS, Caun K, et al. Microsporidian infection due to Enterocytozoon: Relationship with immunosuppression and HIV (Abstract). Trans R Soc Trop Med Hyg. 1988;82:651.
32. Macher AM, Neafie R, Angritt P, et al. Microsporidial myositis and the acquired immunodeficiency syndrome (AIDS): A four-year follow-up (Letter). Ann Intern Med. 1988;109:343.

SECTION H. DISEASES DUE TO HELMINTHS

262. INTRODUCTION

KENNETH S. WARREN

Helminths, or worms, are unique among the infectious agents of humans because of their size, their prevalence, the complexity of their life cycles and migrations within the host, their ability to induce an eosinophilia, and particularly because of their inability to undergo direct replication in the definitive human host.

Whereas bacteria, protozoa, fungi, and viruses must be viewed under light or electron microscopes, all the helminths are visible to the naked eye, ranging in length from 2 to 10,000 mm. Thus, the mathematical ecologists Anderson and May have termed the former organisms *microparasites* and the latter *macroparasites*.[1] Worms may well be the most prevalent of the infectious agents of humans, it having been estimated that there are almost as many helminthiases as people, considering multiple infections.[2] Three of the helminths account for close to 1 billion infections each (*Ascaris*, *Trichuris*, and the hookworms), and two for 0.25 billion each (the schistosomes and filariae). In the United States it was estimated in the 1970s that there were 54 million helminth infections, the majority due to enterobiasis.[3]

The helminths are divided into three groups, as shown in Table 1—the nematodes (round worms) and two groups of flat worms, the trematodes (flukes) and the cestodes (tapeworms). As can be seen in Table 1, the means by which the worms infect humans, by ingestion, by skin penetration, or by injection by insects, bears no particular relation to their group.

The helminth life cycles may be exceedingly simple, such as those of *Enterobius* and *Trichuris*, in which eggs pass out of the gut, embryonate, and, when ingested, develop into egg-producing worms in the gut. Similarly, larvae encysted in meat or on vegetables also pass down into the intestines, where they develop into the tapeworms or the intestinal fluke. A more complex system involves ingestion of eggs or skin penetration by larvae and migration through the lungs to the final habitat in the lumen or blood vessels of the gut (*Ascaris*, hookworms, *Strongyloides*, and schistosomes). Finally, other helminths, which are ingested or injected (by insects), migrate through the tissues to their final habitats: *Trichinella*—muscles; *Clonorchis, Fasciola, Echinococcus*—liver; *Paragonimus, Echinococcus*—lungs; *Onchocerca*—skin; and *Wuchereria*—lymphatics. Outside the body the simplest systems involve eggs alone, increasing in complexity through skin-penetrating larvae, development of infectious larvae in the flesh of other animals or in biting insects, and, finally, alternation of generations in which the digenetic trematodes undergo sexual reproduction in a definitive host and asexual reproduction in snails.

Another characteristic not shared with any other infectious agents is a close association between the helminths and the eosinophil, a white blood cell whose function has remained a mystery. Recent studies, however, suggest that this intriguing cell plays a role in immunity in both schistosomiasis and trichinosis.[4] Those worms most strongly associated with eosinophilia are the filariae, *Strongyloides, Trichinella, Fasciola*, and the schistosomes.

Finally, and most important, is the fact that the majority of helminths do not multiply in the definitive human host. They have been characterized as guerrillas "repeatedly infiltrating host defenses as individuals or in small groups and gradually building up into large forces; warfare is usually by attrition and tends to be prolonged."[5] Important exceptions to this situation are *Strongyloides*, whose larvae may become infectious while in the gut, resulting in overwhelming autoinfection, and *Echinococcus*, the dog tapeworm, humans being the intermediate hosts in which larval multiplication takes place within the so-called hydatid cyst.

The lack of replication in humans by most adult worm species has multiple consequences, the most important being pathogenesis, immunity, and treatment. There is an overdispersed distribution of worms in human populations, with most persons harboring low worm burdens.[6,7] The association of disease with

TABLE 1. Major Helminth Infections of Humans

Organism	Common Name	Means of Infection	Major Disease Manifestation[a]
Nematodes			
Ancylostoma duodenale	Hookworm	Skin	Anemia
Ascaris lumbricoides	Giant roundworm	Oral	Intestinal obstruction
Enterobius vermicularis	Pinworm	Oral	Anal pruritus
Onchocerca volvulus	River blindness	Insect	Blindness
Strongyloides stercoralis	Strongyloidiasis	Skin	Autoinfection
Trichinella spiralis	Trichinosis	Oral	Myositis
Trichuris trichiura	Whipworm	Oral	Rectal prolapse
Wuchereria bancrofti	Filariasis	Insect	Elephantiasis
Trematodes			
Clonorchis sinensis	Liver fluke	Oral	Biliary obstruction
Fasciola hepatica	Liver fluke	Oral	Hepatomegaly
Fasciolopsis buski	Intestinal fluke	Oral	Diarrhea
Paragonimus westermani	Lung fluke	Oral	Cough
Schistosoma haematobium	Blood fluke	Skin	Hydronephrosis
Schistosoma japonicum	Blood fluke	Skin	Hepatosplenomegaly
Schistosoma mansoni	Blood fluke	Skin	Hepatosplenomegaly
Cestodes			
Diphyllobothrium latum	Fish tapeworm	Oral	Anemia
Taenia saginata	Beef tapeworm	Oral	None
Taenia sodium	Pork tapeworm	Oral	Epilepsy from cysticercosis
Echinococcus granulosus	Hydatid cyst	Oral	Cyst

[a] These manifestations are relatively infrequent and tend to be related to the intensity of infection, exceptions being *Strongyloidiasis* and *Echinococcus*.

heavy worm burdens is most clearly illustrated in the case of hookworm infection. Each *Ancylostoma* ingests about 0.15 ml of blood per day. In patients with low worm burdens, blood loss is negligible and anemia does not occur, but those harboring 1000 worms may lose more than 100 ml of blood daily. While it had always been assumed that patients with very low worm burdens were immune and those with high burdens were not, it is possible that the opposite may be true,[6] as few worms may not provide a significant antigenic stimulus for the development of immunity. Finally, treatment of some of the helminth infections requires highly toxic drugs. It may be preferable, therefore, not to treat patients with low worm burdens who have no signs or symptoms of disease; those with many worms may be treated with low, nontoxic doses of drugs to greatly reduce worm burdens rather than with the high, toxic doses of drugs needed to achieve a "cure."

To conclude, it is essential to understand the unique characteristics of the helminths in order to cope adequately with these infectious agents either on an individual or a population basis. The effect of understanding the characteristics of helminth infections on disease control is dramatically illustrated by a recent publication on "targeted mass treatment" of schistosomiasis mansoni.[8] A single treatment of the 30 percent of the population of a Kenyan village with the heaviest infections (using one-half the package insert dose of an antischistosomal drug) resulted in a 97 percent drop in parasite egg output. One year later egg output remained at 10 percent of the pretreatment level, and there was a marked decrease in hepatomegaly, the major clinical manifestation of schistosomal disease.[8]

REFERENCES

1. Anderson RM, May RM. Population biology of infectious diseases: Part I. Nature 1979;280:361–7.
2. Stoll NR. This wormy world. J Parasitol. 1947;33:1–18.
3. Warren KS. Helminthic diseases endemic in the United States. Am J Trop Med Hyg. 1974;23:723–30.
4. Butterworth AE. Cell-mediated damage to helminths. Adv Parasitol. 1984;23:143–235.
5. Warren KS. The guerrilla worm. N Engl J Med. 1970;282:810–1.
6. Warren KS. The control of helminths: Nonreplicating infectious agents of man. Am Rev Publ Health. 1981;2:101–16.
7. Anderson RM, May RM. Helminth infections of humans: Mathematical models, population dynamics, and control. Adv Parasitol. 1985;24:1–101.
8. Mahmoud AAF, Arap Siongok TK, Ouma JH, et al. Effect of targeted mass treatment on intensity of infection and morbidity in schistosomiasis mansoni. Lancet. 1983;1:849–51.

263. INTESTINAL NEMATODES (ROUNDWORMS)

ADEL A. F. MAHMOUD

The phylum Nematoidea, or roundworms, is the second largest phylum in the animal kingdom, encompassing as many as 500,000 species. Members of this phylum are elongated, with bilaterally symmetric bodies containing an intestinal tract and a large body cavity. Many roundworm species are free living, but few are parasites of humans. Infection with intestinal roundworms, however, constitute the largest group of helminthic infections of humans. For example, it is estimated that worldwide there are 1 billion cases of ascariasis and 800 million of trichuriasis. The life cycle of parasitic nematodes is important clinically because some of these infections can be transmitted directly from infected to uninfected people, whereas in others eggs must undergo a process of maturation outside the human host and in a third category the parasites may spend a part of their life cycle in the soil before becoming infective to humans. As with other parasitic infections, definitive diagnosis depends on demonstration of the stage of the life cycle in the host. Serologic methods are of no clinical significance in diagnosis and should not be used as an indication for therapy. Nematodes, like most other worms infectious to humans, do not multiply in the host, an important biologic and clinical feature that means that to increase parasite load in an infected individual, exposure to the infective stage is necessary. The exception to this characteristic of worm infections is strongyloidiasis in the immunosuppressed, where the parasite is capable of increasing its larval stage with the host in the absence of exposure to worms from the environment. The major parasitic nematodes with their mode of infection and final habitat in the host are outlined in Table 1.

TRICHURIASIS

Infection with the nematode *Trichuris trichiura* is among the most prevalent helminthiasis; approximately 800 million cases occur wordwide, most abundantly in warm, moist regions.[1] In the United States it has recently been estimated that 2.2 million people are infected with *T. trichiura*, mainly in the rural south-

TABLE 1. Important Intestinal Roundworm Infections of Humans

Infection	*Mode of Transmission*	*Superfamily*	*Species Infecting Humans*	*Infective Stage*	*Final Habitat*
Trichuriasis	Direct	Trichuroidea	*Trichuris trichiura*	Eggs	Large intestines
Enterobiasis	Direct	Oxyuroidea	*Enterobius vermicularis*	Eggs	Cecum
Ascariasis	Modified direct	Ascaroidea	*Ascaris lumbricoides*	Mature eggs	Small intestines
Hookworm	Skin penetration	Strongyloidea	*Ancylostoma duodenale*	Larvae	Small intestines
			Necator americanus	Larvae	Small intestines
Strongyloidiasis	Skin penetration	Rhabditoidea	*Strongyloides stercoralis*	Larvae	Small intestines

east. Infection rates up to 75 percent were found in young schoolchildren in Puerto Rico.

The normal habitat of *T. trichiura* is in the cecum and ascending colon. The body of the pinkish gray adult worms (mean length 40 mm) is divided into an attenuated whip-like anterior part that is three-fifths its length and a more robust posterior part. The head or anterior part of the worm penetrates and anchors itself to the intestinal mucosa.

Life Cycle

Humans are the principal hosts for *T. trichiura*, and infection is transmitted directly (Fig. 1). The mean expected life span of adult worms is 1 year, and during this period each female worm produces 5000–20,000 eggs/day. The ova (50–54 × 22 μm) are barrel shaped, with a thick shell and translucent polar prominences, and are unsegmented at oviposition. After excretion in the feces, embryonic development takes place under optimal conditions of moisture and shade in 2–4 weeks. When the embryonated egg is ingested by humans, the larva escapes from the shell in the upper small intestine. These larval worms penetrate the intestinal villi, where they lie for 3–10 days before slowly moving downward into the lumen of the cecum, where the anterior three-quarters of the worms remain within the superficial mucosa, and the short posterior end is free in the human. Worms develop to mature ovipositing adults in 1–3 months.

Epidemiology

Trichuriasis has a worldwide prevalence; it is most common, however, in poor rural communities and areas in which sanitary facilities are lacking. The intensity of infection is usually light; children in the 5- to 15-year age group have the highest prevalence and probably have heavier worm loads than adults. Infection results from ingestion of embryonated ova by direct contamination of hands, food, or drink or indirectly through flies and other insects.

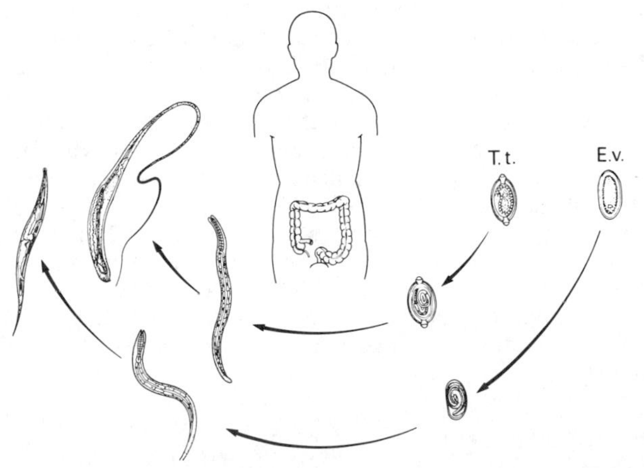

FIG. 1. Life cycle of direct infecting nematodes. Eggs are passed with stools in *T. trichiura* (T.t.) or are deposited at the perianal region in *E. vermicularis* (E.v.). They embryonate in a short time and infection is acquired by ingestion. Eggs hatch in the intestine and larvae migrate to their final habitat in the colon (T.t.) or cecum (E.v.).

Humans are the principal host of *T. trichiura*, but the parasite has also been found in monkeys, lemurs, and hogs. Soil pollution by human or animal feces, therefore, constitutes the major determining factor in the spread of infection.

The morbidity due to trichuriasis in endemic communities is not fully understood. Although most infected people harbor low worm burdens, a small proportion acquire heavy infections. Clinical impressions point to this subpopulation of heavily infected people (mainly children) as most likely to suffer from disease.

Clinical Syndromes

Infection with *T. trichiura* in humans is mainly asymptomatic; however, several clinical features have been described on the basis of uncontrolled morbidity surveys. Adult worms embed their heads in the intestinal mucosa and have been shown to suck approximately 0.005 ml of blood/worm/day.[2] This negligible amount of blood loss does not usually produce significant anemia. Furthermore, it has been demonstrated that healthy children with heavy *Trichuris* infection (mean worm burden 406) lose an amount of blood within an acceptable range. Although a plethora of abdominal signs and symptoms have been associated with *T. trichiura* infections, the underlying mechanisms are unknown. In heavily infected people it appears that infection may manifest itself as mild anemia, bloody diarrhea, growth retardation, and rectal prolapse.[3] Associated conditions such as malnutrition and other parasitic infections seem to play a significant role in the pathogenesis of the above-mentioned symptoms and signs. Although a portion of the worms are embedded in the mucosa of the large bowel, no significant eosinophilia has been reported in trichuriasis.

Diagnosis

Fecal examination by the simple smear technique is sufficient since the level of egg output is so high (about 200 eggs/g of feces per worm pair). Diagnosis is made by finding the characteristic lemon shaped ova. Since light infections are usually asymptomatic, there is no need to use concentration techniques to detect *Trichuris* eggs.

Management

In the past, a light *Trichuris* infection has not been considered to constitute an indication for therapeutic intervention, since the drugs available were either ineffective or toxic. The availability of mebendazol (Vermox), however, has changed the indications for therapy since it is essentially nontoxic and is highly effective, giving a cure rate of 70–90 percent and a reduction in egg output of 90–99 percent.[4] Mebendazole is administered in a dose of 100 mg twice a day for 3 days regardless of body weight. The drug is poorly absorbed from the gastrointestinal tract and has essentially no side effects.

ENTEROBIASIS

Enterobiasis, or pinworm, is also highly prevalent throughout the world, particularly in countries of the temperate zone. In the United States it is the most common of all helminthic infections, with an estimated 42 million cases.[5] Pinworm infection is particularly common among children and is not associated with any specific socioeconomic levels.[6] Enterobiasis is most prevalent in congested districts, in institutionalized groups, and among members of the same family.

Life Cycle

Enterobius vermicularis is a small (1 cm in length) white threadlike worm inhabiting the cecum and adjacent gut (Fig. 1). A gravid female worm contains an average of 11,100 ova and has a life span of 11–35 days. The gravid females migrate at night to the perianal and perineal regions for oviposition; ova are infrequently laid in the intestines. The stimulus for oviposition seems to be a subclinical temperature and an aerobic environment. Ova are laid either in clusters or in a stream but are not widely distributed in the perianal region. *Enterobius* ova are ovoid but flattened on one side and measure approximately 56 × 27 μm. The eggs embryonate within 6 hours and are transferred from the perianal region to night clothes, bedding, and dust and air. The most common mode of transmission, however, is via the hands of the patient, particularly beneath the fingernails, through scratching or handling clothes and bed linen. On ingestion, the embryos hatch in the duodenum, molt twice, and develop into adult worms in 36–53 days.

Epidemiology

The prevalence of pinworm infection is lowest in nurslings and reaches its maximum in schoolchildren 5–14 years old.[7] The absence of an extended extracorporeal development stage favors direct transmission. Eggs are infective within 6 hr of ovideposition and may remain so for 20 days.

Pinworm is primarily a familial or institutional infection, with no predilection to specific socioeconomic conditions. For as yet unknown reasons, enterobiasis is less prevalent in blacks than in whites. Since the life span of the worms is relatively brief, long-standing infections must be due to continuous reinfection. Estimates of worm burdens in infected people have shown an average of 58 worms in the 4- to 10-year-old group, compared with 16 worms in the 11- to 16-year-old group. No data are available, however, on the intensity of infections in adults.

Clinical Syndromes

The clinical presentations in enterobiasis are related largely to perianal and perineal pruritis. Although various classifications of symptoms into local, secondary, and reflex nervous symptoms have been proposed, it is important to realize that a large proportion of pinworm infections are essentially asymptomatic.[8,9] In a hospital based study of children 2–12 years old none of the signs and symptoms largely ascribed to enterobiasis was significantly more common in infected than in uninfected children.[10]

The most common complaints are local itching and restless sleep due to nocturnal anal pruritis. Occasionally the migration of the parasite may produce ectopic disease such as appendicitis, chronic salpingitis, or ulcerative lesions in the small or large bowel. There is no evidence that enterobiasis is associated with significant eosinophilia or elevated serum IgE levels.

Diagnosis

Although pinworms can be seen by the naked eye, they may easily be confused with bits of white thread. Diagnosis is readily made by examination of an adhesive cellophane tape pressed against the perianal region early in the morning. A single examination detects 50 percent of infections, three examinations detect 90 percent, and five examinations detect 99 percent. As the infection usually runs in families, diagnosis in one person necessitates the examination of all members.

Management

Drug therapy is recommended for all infected members of families with symptomatic infections. Mebendazole (Vermox) in a single oral dose of 100 mg results in cure rates of 90–100 percent.[11] Although personal cleanliness is a useful general principle, its role in management of enterobiasis is trivial and tends only to enhance the psychologic trauma and stigmata associated with this infection.

ASCARIASIS

Ascariasis, or roundworm, infection is the most common helminthic infection of humans with an estimated worldwide prevalence of 1 billion. The causative organism, *Ascaris lumbricoides*, is cosmopolitan in distribution, being most abundant in tropical countries. In the United States it has been estimated that 4 million people, mainly in the southeast, have *Ascaris* infection.[5]

The white or reddish yellow adult worms (15–35 cm in length) live in the lumen of the small intestine, most commonly in the jejunum and middle ileum. Infection with *Ascaris* appears to be asymptomatic in the vast majority of cases but may produce serious pulmonary disease or obstruction of biliary or intestinal tracts in a small proportion of infected people.

Life Cycle

Ascaris lumbricoides is a parasite of humans; adult worms inhabit the lumen of the small intestine and have a life span of approximately 10–24 months. Each female worm produces a daily output of 200,000 ova. The fertile ovum is broadly oval, has a thick shell with an outer course mammillated albuminous covering, and measures 45–70 μm in length by 35–50 μm in breadth (Fig. 2). After their passage with feces and under favorable environmental conditions, fully developed infective embryos are formed within the eggs in 5–10 days. When ingested by humans, they hatch in the small intestine; the embryos penetrate its wall and migrate via venous blood to the

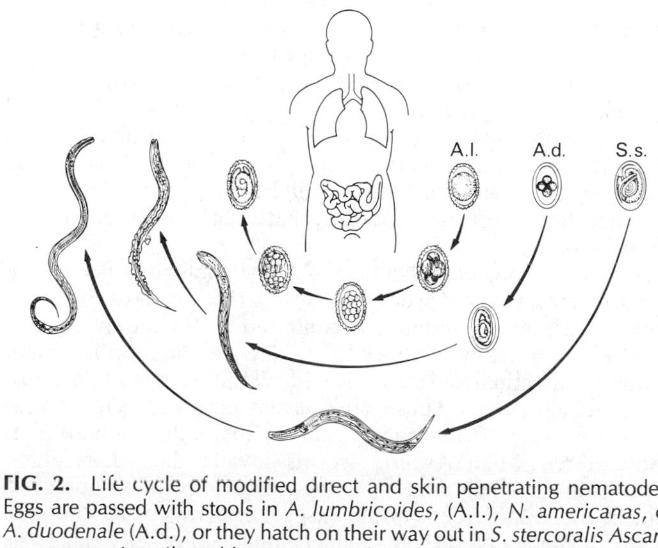

FIG. 2. Life cycle of modified direct and skin penetrating nematodes. Eggs are passed with stools in *A. lumbricoides*, (A.l.), *N. americanas*, or *A. duodenale* (A.d.), or they hatch on their way out in *S. stercoralis Ascaris* eggs mature in soil, and humans are infected on ingestion of these eggs. In hookworm and strongyloidiasis humans are infected by skin penetration by filariform larvae. In all three infections larvae pass through a migratory phase via the lungs before reaching maturity at their final habitat in the small intestine.

heart and lungs, where they break out into the alveoli and pass up through the bronchi and trachea. They are then swallowed to return to the intestines and become mature worms. The time required to produce a gravid female has been estimated to be 2 months.

Epidemiology

Ascaris infection occurs at all ages but is most common in preschool- and young school-age children.[12] Incidence is approximately the same for both sexes, but in blacks of the southeastern United States, it is over three times that in whites. Transmission of *A. lumbricoides* is usually hand to mouth. It is enhanced by the extremely high output of eggs by fecund female worms and the ability of ova to resist unfavorable external environment. *Ascaris* eggs can live for 2 years at 5–10°C, can survive for 3 months in the absence of oxygen, and can resist desiccation for 2–3 weeks at 22°C.[13] In moist, loose, sandy soil ova remain viable up to 6 years and can survive freezing winter temperatures.

In endemic areas, most people have light to moderate worm burdens. For example, a recent survey in Colombia reported that 72 percent of the infected people had less than 1–19 eggs/mg feces and only 5 percent had more than 200 eggs/mg feces.

Clinical Syndromes

The pathologic lesions encountered in ascariasis depend on the intensity of infection and the organs involved. Although overt disease is rare in roundworm infection, the more common problems are pulmonary and nutritional disorders; obstruction of the intestinal or biliary tract; and seasonal pneumonitis. The pulmonary manifestations of ascariasis occur during the stage of larval migration through the lungs and resemble Löffler syndrome.[14,15] Transient respiratory symptoms associated with pulmonary infiltration and peripheral blood eosinophilia are the main features of this syndrome. Considering the endemicity and prevalence of *Ascaris* infections, it is amazing that only a very small proportion of infected people have pulmonary symptoms. In some endemic areas such as Saudi Arabia, where transmission of *Ascaris* is seasonal, the so-called seasonal pneumonitis has frequently been reported.[15]

Children with moderately heavy *Ascaris* infection were shown to have impairment of digestion or absorption of dietary proteins.[16] In a recent study children with an average worm burden of 71 had a 72 percent impairment of dietary nitrogen absorption, and two-thirds had a moderate steatorrhea. Some of these studies were performed in areas in the developing world in which additional nutritional deficiencies cannot be excluded. In contrast, a controlled study performed in the southern United States on the nutritional status of children with *Ascaris* infection revealed no significant difference between uninfected and infected groups.[17]

A more serious complication of *Ascaris* infection is encountered when a mass of worms obstructs the lumen of the small bowel. This acute abdominal condition is commonly seen in children with heavy infections.[18,19] The presentation is similar to acute intestinal obstruction with vomiting, abdominal distension, and cramps. These patients may pass worms in vomitus or in stools during an attack. Another obstructive syndrome is encountered when *Ascaris* worms invade the biliary duct, mostly the common duct.[20] A single ascarid is usually present, and in about 15 percent of the cases the worms were shown to be dead. Clinically, these patients complain of colicky epigastric pain, nausea, and vomiting. Jaundice is rare, since the syndrome is acute and patients usually seek immediate clinical help.[21]

Because of the great prevalence of ascariasis, aberrant ascarids situated at different tissue sites in infected people have been described. Worms were found escaping through umbilical and hernial fistulas, in the fallopian tubes and urinary bladder, and in the lungs and heart. These ectopic locations of ascarids may give rise to difficult diagnostic problems, but fortunately they are very rare.

Diagnosis

Because of the enormous daily output of eggs by gravid ascarids, direct smear examination of stools is sufficient for diagnosis.

Management

The drug of choice for treatment of intestinal infections with *A. lumbricoides* is mebendazole (Vermox). It is given as 100 mg twice daily for 3 days.[22] In cases in which intestinal or biliary obstruction is suspected, piperazine citrate (Antepar) is recommended.[23] It is administered as piperazine syrup by instillation through a nasogastric tube, 150 mg/kg initially, followed by six doses of 65 mg/kg at 12 hour intervals. Piperazine narcotizes the worms and helps relieve the obstruction of the intestinal or biliary tract.

HOOKWORM

Human infection with the two species of hookworm, *Ancylostoma duodenale* and *Necator americanus*, is estimated to affect approximately one-fourth of the world's population. The present geographic distribution of hookworm infections lies in the tropical and subtropical zones between 45°N and 30°S latitude.[24] The remarkable success in controlling hookworm infection in the United States during the early part of this century has not, however, occurred in other parts of the world. Iron deficiency anemia due to hookworms and other nutritional factors looms across most of the developing world. A low degree of prevalence of the infection still exists in the southeastern United States.[5]

Life Cycle

Adult hookworms are small, cylindrical (approximately 1 cm long), grayish white nematodes. Hookworms live chiefly in the upper small intestine, attached to the mucosa by their strong buccal capsules. The average daily blood loss for *N. americanus* worm is about 0.03 ml and for *A. duodenale* is 0.2 ml.[25] Human hookworms have a mean life span of approximately 5 years, although it is probable that the majority of worms disappear within 2 years.

Adult worms lay an average of 7000 eggs daily. The eggs are ovoidal and thin shelled and measure 58 × 36 μm. They pass out with the stools, and under suitable conditions of soil humidity and temperature, the eggs hatch into larvae that molt once to become infective for humans (Fig. 2). Contact with contaminated soil for 5–10 minutes is required for skin penetration. The larvae are carried by the circulation to the lungs, penetrate the alveolar walls, and make their way up the trachea to be swallowed and carried to their final habitat in the small intestines. Gravid females start egg deposition 4–6 weeks after skin penetration.

Epidemiology

The distribution and prevalence of hookworm infections are limited by environmental conditions. Ova fail to develop at temperatures below 13°C. Although larvae require relatively little moisture, drying and direct sunlight are destructive. The superficial position of infective larvae on the topsoil affords easy access for the penetration of human skin. Other major epidemiologic features of hookworm transmission concern methods of disposal of fecal waste and the human habit of walking barefoot.

Clinical Syndromes

Disease manifestations may occur early during the course of infection, with "ground itch," intense pruritis, erythema, and papule vasicular rash at the site of larval penetration.[26] The migration of the larvae through the lungs may produce a Löffler-like syndrome with transitory chest symptoms, diffuse opacities on roentgenograph film, and eosinophilia in sputum and peripheral blood. The major manifestations of hookworm disease, however, are iron deficiency anemia and hypoalbuminemia due to intestinal blood loss. The development of these clinical features depends not only on the worm burden but on the amount of absorbable dietary iron.

Along with the phase of worm attachment to the small intestine mucosa, abdominal pain, diarrhea, and weight loss may be noted.[24] In addition, malabsorption has been reported in children and, less commonly, in adults.

Diagnosis

Direct fecal smear examination is adequate for diagnosis of clinically significant hookworm infections. This technique will identify egg counts of more than 1200 eggs/ml. For quantitative purposes, the modified Stoll method can be used.[24]

Management

Mebendazole (Vermox) is the current drug of choice.[27] It is administered as 100 mg twice a day for 3 days regardless of the patient's body weight. This regimen results in a 95 percent cure rate and a 99.9 percent reduction of egg counts. Anemia should be corrected by iron therapy.

STRONGYLOIDIASIS

Infection with the nematode *Strongyloides stercoralis* is potentially lethal because of its capacity to cause an overwhelming autoinfection, particularly in the immunosuppressed host. Strongloidiasis, although uncommon in comparison with the other major intestinal nematodes, is widely distributed in the tropics. In the United States a prevalence of 0.4–4 percent has been estimated in the southern states.

Strongyloides stercoralis worms can survive and reproduce as parasitic forms in humans or as free-living forms in soil.[28] The parasitic female is a colorless semitransparent nematode 2.2 mm in length, whereas the male is considerably shorter (0.7 mm). Adult worms inhabit the upper small intestine, where the females burrow through the mucosa but usually not through the muscularis mucosa.

Life Cycle

The life cycle of *S. stercoralis* is complex and is not fully understood. Parasitic forms that exist in humans, the principal host, deposit ova as they burrow their way into the intestinal mucosa (Fig. 2). Larvae ordinarily hatch in the mucosa, bore through the epithelium to the intestinal lumen, and are passed in the feces. They can either molt and differentiate into free-living adult males and females or metamorphose into the filariform infectious forms. The free-living adults either continue their life cycles in the soil or produce filariform infective larvae. The usual route of infection in humans is through skin contact with soil contaminated with the infective filariform larvae. Humans may also be infected via the lower gastrointestinal tract or perianal region from larvae that transform into infective organisms during their passage with feces. This "autoinfection" cycle explains the overwhelming larvae invasion seen in strongyloides hyperinfection syndrome. The larvae then pass by way of the blood stream to the lungs, break into the alveolar spaces, and ascend to the glottis, where they are swallowed to their final habitat in the small intestines. Deposition of eggs begins about 28 days after the initial infection.

Epidemiology

Transmission of *S. stercoralis* depends on suitability of the soil, climatic conditions, and sanitation. In temperate zones, incidence is highest in institutions (5–35 percent). Autochthonous cases have been reported in the United States and may be due to autoinfection. Contrary to most other worm infections, the patient's worm burden in strongyloidiasis is dependent not only on the size of larval inoculum but also on the degree of autoinfection. This process may be enhanced in people with compromised immune systems and may lead to a fatal outcome from an overwhelming infection.

Clinical Syndromes

The symptoms of strongyloidiasis correspond to the three stages of infection: invasion of the skin, migration of larvae, and penetration of the intestinal mucosa by adults.[29] Although approximately one-third of the people with strongyloidiasis are asymptomatic, the remainder may have symptoms related to one or more of the stages of parasite migration in the host. The skin and pulmonary symptoms resemble those encountered in hookworm disease: pruritic papular erythematous rash and a Löffler-like syndrome with eosinophilia.

The more characteristic clinical features are, however, seen simultaneously with the intestinal phase of strongyloidiasis. Burning or colicky abdominal pain, often epigastric, occurs and is associated with diarrhea and the passage of mucus. Some patients may complain of nausea, vomiting, and weight loss with evidence of malabsorption or of protein-losing enteropathy.[30] Eosinophilia is a prominent feature of this infection. In addition, 5–22 percent of patients may develop a generalized or localized urticarial rash beginning perianally and extending to the buttocks, abdomen, and thighs.[31]

Massive larval invasion of the lungs and other tissue may occur with autoinfection, particularly in immunocompromised hosts.[32,33] Disseminated strongyloidiasis has been described in patients with lymphomas, leukemias, lepromatous leprosy and in those treated with corticosteroids; more recently it has been reported in association with human immunodeficiency virus (HIV) infection.[34] Severe generalized abdominal pain, diffuse pulmonary infiltrates, ileus, shock, and meningitis or sepsis from gram-negative bacilli may occur. Eosinophilia may be absent.

Diagnosis

Definitive diagnosis depends on the demonstration of *S. stercoralis* larvae in the feces or duodenal fluid. A concentration technique such as the zinc sulfate method should be used for stool examination. Sampling of duodenal contents can easily be accomplished by the use of Enterotest (Hedeco, Palo Alto, Calif.). Repeated examinations may be necessary to exclude the diagnosis.

Management

All people infected with *S. stercoralis* should be treated with the aim of eradicating the infection. Thiabendazole (Mintezol) is the only known effective agent. It is given in a dose of 25 mg/kg twice a day for 2 days. In the hyperinfection syndrome, early diagnosis and treatment for 2–3 weeks may be lifesaving, but the mortality is very high despite treatment.[36] Patients with a past history of exposure to *S. stercoralis* should be thoroughly examined and treated before undergoing any immunosuppressive therapy.

REFERENCES

1. Bundy DAP, Cooper ES. Human trichuris and trichasiasis. Adv Parasitol. 1988. In press.
2. Layrisse M, Aparcedo L, Martinez-Torres C, et al. Blood loss due to infection with *Trichuris trichiura*. Am J Trop Med Hyg. 1967;16:613.
3. Gilman RH, Chong UH, Davis C, et al. The adverse consequences of heavy *Trichuris* infection. Trans R Soc Trop Med Hyg. 1983;77:432–8.
4. Bundy DAP, Cooper ES. Trichuriasis. In: Warren KS, Mahmoud AAF, eds. Tropical and Geographical Medicine. 2d ed. 1989. In press.
5. Warren KS. Helminthic diseases endemic in the United States. Am J Trop Med Hyg. 1974;23:723.
6. Pawlowski, ZS. Enterobiasis. In: Pawlowski ZS, ed. Clinical Tropical Medicine and Communicable Diseases. v. 3. 1988. In press.
7. Aaswell-Elkins M, Elkins DB, et al. The distribution and abundance of *Enterobium vermicularis* in a South Indian fishing community. Parasitiology. 1987;95:339–54.
8. Symmers W, St. C. Pathology of oxyuriasis. Arch Pathol. 1950;50:475.
9. Wagner ED, Eby WC. Pinworm prevalence in California elementary school children and diagnostic methods. Am J Trop Med Hyg. 1983;32:998–1001.
10. Welsh NM: Recent insights into childhood "social diseases" gonorrhea, scabies, pediculosis, pinworms. Clin Pediatr. 1978;17:318–22.
11. Pawlowski ZS. Enterobiasis. In: Warren KS, Mahmoud AAF, eds. Tropical and Geographical Medicine. 2d ed. 1989. In press.
12. Crampton DWT, Nesheim MC, Pawlowski ZS, ed. Ascariasis and Its Public Health Significance. London: Taylor and Francis; 1985.
13. Sinniah B. Daily egg production of *Ascaris lumbricoides*: The distribution of eggs in the feces and the variability of egg counts. Parasitology. 1982;84:167.
14. Spillman RK. Pulmonary ascariasis in tropical communities. Am J Trop Med Hyg. 1975;24:791.
15. Gelpi AP, Mustafa A. *Ascaris* pneumonia. Am J Med. 1968;44:377.
16. Stephenson LS. The contribution of *Ascaris lumbricoides* to malnutrition in children. Parasitology. 1980;81:221–33.
17. Blumenthal DS, Schults MG. Effects of *Ascaris* infection on nutritional status in children. Am J Trop Med Hyg. 1976;25:682.
18. Blumenthal DS, Schultz MG. Incidence of intestinal obstruction in children infected with *Ascaris lumbricoides*. Am J Trop Med Hyg. 1974;24:801.
19. Pinus J. Surgical complications of *Ascaris*. In: Rikham PP, Hecker W Chi, Pievot J, eds, Pediatric Surgery in Tropical Countries. Baltimore-Munich; Urban & Schwarzenberg; 1982:79.
20. Chin-Che C, Cheng-Teh H. Biliary ascariasis in childhood: A clinical analysis of 788 cases. Chin Med J [Engl]. 1966;85:167.
21. Khuroo MS, Zargar SA. Mahagan R, et al. sonographic appearances in biliary ascariasis: Gastroenterology. 1987;83:267–72.
22. World Health Organization. Prevention and control of intestinal parasitic infections: Report of a WHO expert committee. WHO Technical Rep Ser 749, Geneva, World Health Organization, 1987.
23. Swartwelder JC, Miller JH, Sappenfield RW. The use of piperazine for the treatment of human helminthiases. Gastroenterology. 1957;33:87.
24. Schad GA, Banwell JG. Hookworms. In: Warren KS, Mahmoud AAF, eds. Tropical and Geographical Medicine. 2d ed. 1989. In press.
25. Roche M, Layrisse M. The nature and causes of "hookworm anemia." Am J Trop Med Hyg. 1966;15:1030.
26. Miller TA. Hookworm infection in man. Adv Parasitol. 1979;17:315–83.
27. The Medical Letter on Drugs and Therapeutics: Drugs for Parasitic Infections. v. 30. New Rochelle, NY: Medical Letter; 1988:15–24.
28. Chent TC. General Parasitology. New York: Academic Press; 1973:626.
29. Grove DI. Strongyloidiasis. In: Warren KS, Mahmoud AAF eds. Tropical and Geographical Medicine. 2d ed. 1989. In press.
30. Milner PF, Irvine RA, Carton CJ, et al. Intestinal malabsorption in *Strongyloides stercoralis* infestation. Gut. 1965;6:574.
31. Smith JD, Goette DK, Odom RB. Larva currens: Cutaneous strongyloidiasis. Arch Dermatol. 1976;112:1161.
32. Scowden EB, Schaffner W, Stone WJ. Overwhelming strongyloidiasis: An unappreciated opportunistic infection. Medicine. 1978;57:527.
33. Igra-Siegman Y, Kapila R, Sen P, et al. Syndrome of hyperinfection with *Strongyloides stercerolis*. Rev Infect Dis. 1981;3:397–407.
34. Purtilo DT, Meyers WM, Connor DH. Fatal strongyloidiasis in immunosuppressed patients. Am J Med. 1974;56:488.
35. Beal CB, Viens P, Grant RGL, et al. A new technique for sampling duodenal contents: Demonstration of upper small bowel pathogens. Am J Trop Med Hyg. 1970;19:349.
36. Grove DI. Treatment of strongyloidiasis with thiobendazole: An analysis of toxicity and effectiveness. Trans R Soc Trop Med Hyg. 1982;76:114–8.

264. TISSUE NEMATODES (TRICHINOSIS, DRACUNCULIASIS, FILARIASIS)

DAVID I. GROVE

The tissue-dwelling roundworms constitute a major global health problem. They are widely scattered around the world, especially in the tropics, and infect millions of people. Some are parasites of humans only, while others have an animal reservoir. All these parasites have complex life cycles involving arthropod intermediate hosts except for *Trichinella spiralis,* which is transmitted directly from one host to the next by ingestion of infective larvae. Like most helminths, the adult worms do not multiply within the human host; therefore, the worm load and severity of disease depend in large measure on the intensity and frequency of exposure to the infective forms. The relative pathogenicity of the adult worms vs. the larval forms varies according to the species of infecting worm. Definitive diagnosis requires isolation and identification of the parasite, but in some infections this may be difficult. Effective therapy is available for only some of these infections. While some parasites present almost insurmountable control problems, others can be avoided by simple preventive measures. Infections acquired by ingestion of contaminated food or water will be considered first, and then those transmitted by blood-sucking flies will be discussed.

TRICHINOSIS

Trichinosis develops when undercooked flesh contaminated with infective larvae of *Trichinella spiralis* is eaten. Most infections are asymptomatic, but heavy exposure may lead to diarrhea, periorbital edema, myositis, fever, and prostration.[1]

Life Cycle

When raw or inadequately cooked meat containing viable larvae of *T. spiralis* is eaten, the organisms are freed from the cyst walls by acid–pepsin digestion in the stomach and pass into the small intestine. They attach to the mucosa at the bases of the villi and develop into adult worms, the males being about 1.5 × 0.05 mm and the females 3.5 × 0.06 mm in size. Each fertilized female releases about 500 larvae over a period of 2 weeks and then is expelled in the feces. The newborn larvae seed the skeletal muscles via the blood stream. They burrow into individual muscle fibers and then over the next 3 weeks increase 10 times in length, coil, and become capable of infecting a new host. A cyst wall develops around the larva and may eventually calcify. Larvae may remain viable for several years.

Epidemiology

Trichinella spiralis is distributed throughout the world apart from Australia and many of the Pacific islands. It is widely spread in nature among a large number of carnivorous animals, humans being an incidental host. In the United States, it is most prevalent in the northeast and on the west coast. While only 100–200 cases are reported in the United States each year, an autopsy survey in 1968 revealed that 4 percent of the cadavers were infected.[2] Humans usually become infected by eating inadequately processed pork. The vast majority of swine in the United States are fed with grain and are generally uninfected. The small proportion fed with garbage may become infected when given uncooked trichinous scraps, usually pig meat, or when the carcasses of infected wild animals such as rats are eaten. A number of cases in North America have resulted from eating poorly cooked bear meat. Epidemics occur when families or small communities consume trichinous meat from a common source.

Pathologic Characteristics

During the first 2–3 weeks after infection the small intestine shows a mild, partial villous atrophy and an inflammatory infiltrate of polymorphs, eosinophils, lymphocytes, and macrophages in the mucosa and submucosa. Adult worms may be seen in the epithelial layer near the bases of the villi. The most striking changes are in the skeletal muscles. The fibers become edematous, lose their cross-striations, undergo basophilic degeneration, and their nuclei proliferate. The typical coiled worm, the cyst wall derived from the host cell, and the surrounding lymphocytic and eosinophilic infiltrate may be seen within the muscle fiber. In severe cases, focal interstitial myocarditis, meningitis, and encephalitis may be seen.

Clinical Features

Most infections are subclinical. The development of symptoms depends mainly on the size of the inoculum of viable larvae. Consequently, the frequencies of the symptoms and signs of trichinosis vary widely from outbreak to outbreak. Their relative frequencies are shown in Table 1.[3–11] Symptoms attributable to adult worms in the intestines may be found during the first week after infection. Diarrhea is the most common symptom, but patients may also complain of abdominal discomfort and vomiting. Patients with extremely heavy worm burdens may develop a fulminant enteritis. Symptoms associated with systemic invasion by larvae are much more common and usually appear during the second week after infection. Fever is frequently present, although it is of variable intensity and duration. Periorbital edema may be associated with subconjunctival hemorrhages and chemosis. Myositis with pain, swelling, and weakness is also common; it usually develops first in the extraocular muscles and then involves the masseters, neck muscles, limb flexors, and lumbar muscles. Some patients may complain of headache, cough, shortness of breath, hoarseness, and dysphagia. Occasionally a rash that may be macular or petechial is observed. Retinal or subungual splinter hemorrhages are sometimes seen. These systemic symptoms usually peak 2–3 weeks after infection and then slowly subside, although malaise and weakness may persist for weeks. Occasionally a patient dies, usually from a myocarditis but sometimes from encephalitis or pneumonia.

TABLE 1. Frequencies of Symptoms and Signs of Trichinosis Condensed from Nine Reported Outbreaks

Symptom/Sign	*Mean*	*Range*
Fever	91	(71–100)
Myalgia	89	(68–100)
Weakness and malaise	82	(50–94)
Periorbital edema	77	(29–100)
Headache	52	(0–100)
Cutaneous rash	20	(0–67)
Trunk and limb edema	18	(0–75)
Diarrhea	16	(0–48)
Nausea	15	(0–67)
Subconjunctival hemorrhages	9	(0–65)
Subungual splinter hemorrhages	9	(0–60)
Cough	6	(0–40)
Vomiting	3	(0–13)

(Data from references 3–11.)

Diagnosis

Trichinosis should be suspected in a patient who has any of the cardinal features of periorbital edema, myositis, fever, and eosinophilia. If questioning reveals the recent consumption of poorly cooked meat, particularly pork products, the likelihood of the diagnosis is greatly increased. Further confirmation is provided if others who have eaten the same meat have similar symptoms. An eosinophilia is usually found: it begins about the 10th day and may reach very high levels. The erythrocyte sedimentation rate is usually normal. Elevated serum creatine phosphokinase and lactic dehydrogenase levels indicate considerable muscle involvement. Antibodies are not detectable until at least 3 weeks after infection; a bentonite flocculation antibody titer of 1:5 or more or a fourfold rise in titer may help to establish the diagnosis. This test is simple, rapid, and reproducible. Serum may be sent to the Centers for Disease Control (Atlanta). The skin test for *Trichinella* remains positive for years after exposure; therefore, it does not differentiate between past and recent infections. Muscle biopsy is usually unnecessary; if doubt remains, a sample taken from a tender swollen muscle may confirm the diagnosis.

The protean manifestations of trichinosis require differentiation of this infection from a large number of other diseases. The gastrointestinal symptoms may mimic gastroenteritis. Systemic symptoms may cause confusion with influenza, typhoid fever, sinusitis, dermatomyositis, glomerulonephritis, and angioneurotic edema. The rash may resemble that found in measles, scarlet fever, and typhus.

Treatment

There is no satisfactory treatment for trichinosis. In the rare instance when a patient is known to have ingested trichinous meat within 24 hours, thiabendazole should be administered in an oral dose of 25 mg/kg/day for 1 week. This drug has little effect on muscle larvae and has not been shown to alter the course of the disease in established infections. The mainstays of treatment are bed rest and salicylates. Corticosteroids may be used in critically ill patients, but the evidence for benefit is equivocal. It has been claimed that mebendazole was effective when given 5 months after the onset of infection[12]; this uncontrolled, single case report must be viewed with some skepticism.

Prevention

The most effective method of killing *Trichinella* larvae is by proper cooking: the thermal death point is 55°C, so meat should be cooked until there is no trace of pink fluid or flesh. Storage in a home freezer (−15°C) for 3 weeks usually sterilizes meat, but smoking, salting, and drying are unreliable.

DRACUNCULIASIS

Dracunculiasis (dracontiasis, guinea worm infection) develops after drinking water containing crustaceans infected with *Dracunculus medinensis*. It is characterized by a chronic cutaneous ulcer from which the worm protrudes.

Life Cycle

When water containing infected copepods is drunk, larvae are released in the host stomach, pass into the small intestine, penetrate the mucosa, and reach the retroperitoneum where they mature and mate. The female worm (1–2 mm in diameter and up to 1 m long) migrates to the subcutaneous tissue, usually of the legs, about 1 year later. The overlying skin ulcerates, and a portion of the worm protrudes. On contact with water, large numbers of larvae are released from a loop of uterus prolapsed through either the mouth or a rupture in the body wall. These are in turn ingested by crustaceans in which they undergo further development whereby the life cycle is continued.[13]

Epidemiology

Dracunculus medinensis is spread sporadically through the tropics, particularly Africa, the Middle East, and India, and is estimated to afflict about 140 million people. Fur-bearing animals may be infected, but their importance as a disease reservoir is uncertain. Shallow ponds, cisterns, and wells are the usual habitat of the crustacean intermediate hosts. The disease is prevalent in areas where people bathe or wade in water used for drinking purposes. Manifestations in a community are markedly seasonal. This reflects both the developmental cycle of the parasite, which requires an incubation period of about 1 year, and the influence of climate on the types of water sources used. The disability resulting from infection may be of great economic importance if the timing of clinical manifestations coincides with a busy period of the agricultural year.[14]

Clinical Features

There are often no clinical signs until the worm reaches the surface and is ready to discharge larvae. A stinging papule develops at this point, usually on the lower portions of the legs. At this time, some patients may have a generalized reaction with urticaria, nausea, vomiting, diarrhea, and dyspnea. Over the next few days the lesion vesiculates, and then the blister ruptures and forms a painful ulcer within which part of the worm is often visible. If the area is douched with fluid, a milky fluid containing larvae wells up. Discharge continues intermittently, and the worm is slowly absorbed or extruded over the next few weeks, after which the ulcer heals. Multiple ulcers are common, and secondary infection is frequent.[13] Immunity to reinfection does not develop.

Diagnosis

The clinical picture is characteristic. Larvae can be found on microscopic examination of the discharge fluid.

Treatment

Thiabendazole, 25 mg/kg twice daily for 2 days,[15] or metronidazole, 5 mg/kg twice daily for 1 week,[16] have no effect on the worms themselves but produce resolution of inflammation within several days. This permits easy removal of the worm over a week or so by progressively rolling out the emerging worm onto a small stick. Secondary bacterial infection should be treated as necessary.

Prevention

Guinea worm infection can be prevented by boiling or chlorinating drinking water or by sieving it through a cloth. Control on a public health scale requires improved water supplies. The years 1981–1990 have been designated by many international agencies as the International Drinking Water Supply and Sanitation Decade. This led to hopes that dracunculiasis may be eradicated from the globe by the end of the decade. Thus far, there has only been a modest reduction in the incidence of Guinea worm intection.[17]

BANCROFTIAN AND BRUGIAN FILARIASIS

Bancroftian filariasis and brugian (Malayan) filariasis are similar clinical conditions resulting from the transmission of *Wuchereria bancrofti, Brugia malayi,* and *B. timori* to humans by mosquitoes. Symptomatic patients have acute lymphatic inflammation or the effects of chronic lymphatic obstruction such as hydrocele, elephantiasis of the limbs, and chyluria.[18]

Life Cycle

After the bite of an infected mosquito, infective larvae pass into the lymphatics and lymph nodes where they mature over the next few months into white, threadlike adult worms, the males being about 40 × 0.1 mm and the females 100 × 0.25 mm in size. The adults live for many years, and the fertilized females discharge microfilariae approximately 150 × 7 μm in size via the lymphatics into the blood stream. The number of microfilariae found in the peripheral blood varies. There is usually a surge of microfilariae into the blood during the middle of the night, a phenomenon known as nocturnal periodicity. Patients from the South Pacific with *W. bancrofti* infection have a much less pronounced peak that is maximal during the day. *B. malayi* infections produce nocturnal peaks of varying intensity. If microfilariae are ingested by a mosquito during feeding, the organisms develop into infective larvae over the next 2 weeks and are ready to repeat the cycle (Fig. 1).

Epidemiology

Wuchereria bancrofti is distributed widely throughout the tropics and subtropics, while *B. malayi* is restricted to South and Southeast Asia. *B. timori* is restricted to the eastern Indonesian archipelago. It is estimated that 250 million people are infected with these parasites. There is no animal reservoir for *W. bancrofti,* but *B. malayi* has been found in felines and primates. Even in endemic areas, only a small proportion (less than 1 percent) of mosquito bites are infective. It is probable that patent infections are produced only when a susceptible person receives a large number of infective larvae and that obstructive disease develops only when exposure continues for many years.

Pathologic Characteristics

Lymphatics harboring adult worms display endothelial proliferation, fibrin deposition, and a granulomatous inflammatory infiltrate of eosinophils, lymphocytes, and macrophages. Molting and the death of worms probably exacerbate the inflammation, which is succeeded by fibrosis and obstruction to lymph flow.

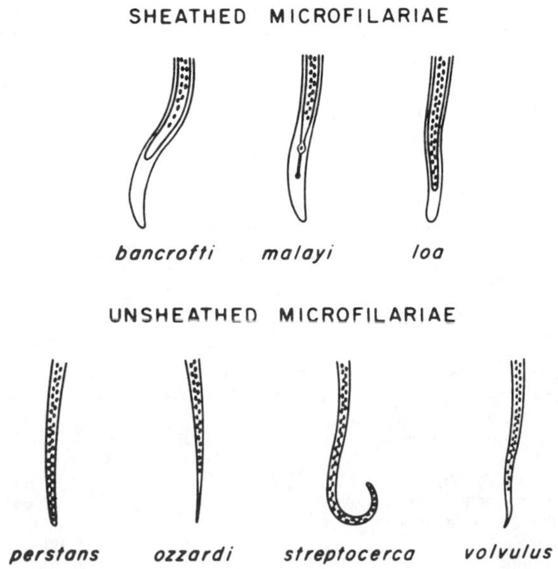

FIG. 1. Comparative features of microfilariae.

Clinical Features

Many patients are asymptomatic despite the presence of a microfilaremia. Clinical manifestations are due either to acute inflammation or to chronic lymphatic obstruction. Attacks of lymphangitis or lymphadenitis with fever, headache, backache, and nausea occasionally occur. Acute funiculitis, epididymitis, or orchitis may be seen. These acute episodes usually subside after a few days to several weeks but may recur. Chronic lymphadenopathy is frequently found and may be the only manifestation of filariasis. In long-standing cases lymphedema may develop. Chronic hydrocele is the most common feature. The lower limbs are involved less frequently; at first there is pitting edema that is most marked pretibially, but eventually nonpitting edema may involve the whole limb. In elephantiasis, the skin of the leg or scrotum becomes thickened, fissured, and warty. Ulceration and secondary infection may occur. Occasionally lymph varices may be seen, especially in the genital region. Chyluria develops when swollen lymphatics burst into the urinary tract.

Diagnosis

The definitive diagnosis of bancroftian filariasis and brugian filariasis depends on demonstration of the parasite. Unfortunately, microfilariae are frequently absent from the blood in both the early and late stages of the disease. A blood sample should be taken around midnight unless the patient is from the South Pacific. The smear is stained and examined for microfilariae: if none are found, a concentration method should be used.[19] Microfilariae may occasionally be found in hydrocele fluid or chylous urine. Eosinophilia is usually absent except during episodes of acute inflammation. Serologic tests for antibody such as bentonite flocculation, indirect hemagglutination, and indirect fluorescent antibody tests may be of some help but do not differentiate among the various forms of filariasis or between past and current infection. Recently, immunoassays to measure filarial antigen in serum have been described.[20–21a] Unfortunately, these tests have been more successful in detecting antigenemia in patients with microfilaremia than in infected, amicrofilaremic individuals. Nevertheless, if they can be improved and become available routinely, they may greatly facilitate the diagnosis of filariasis. Adult worms can sometimes be found in lymph node biopsy specimens, but this procedure is not generally justified. If microfilariae cannot be found, the diagnosis must be made on clinical grounds by the exclusion of other causes.

Treatment

There is no satisfactory treatment for filariasis. Diethylcarbamazine citrate in an oral dose of 3 mg/kg three times daily for 3 weeks reduces the number of microfilariae in the peripheral blood. The effect on adult worms is much less certain; it is probably more effective against adults of *B. malayi* than *W. bancrofti* but may well precipitate acute inflammation around the dead or dying worms. It has been suggested that diethylcarbamazine administered in a much higher total dose and spaced at weekly or monthly intervals may give better long-term therapeutic results.[22] Acute inflammatory reactions should be treated with anti-inflammatory agents. Mild lymphedema may be controlled with elastic stockings. Surgery is useful in the management of hydrocele but has little place in patients with elephantiasis of the legs.

Prevention

The most effective preventive measure is avoidance of mosquitoes by the use of screens, nets, and insect repellents.

LOIASIS

Loiasis is caused by *Loa loa* and is transmitted to humans by tabanid flies. It is characterized by transient subcutaneous swellings. Occasionally the worm is seen migrating through the subconjunctiva.

Life Cycle

The white, threadlike adult worms, measuring 30–70 × 0.3 mm, migrate through the connective tissues. The sheathed microfilariae, 300 × 8 μm, appear in the blood during the day and may be ingested by tabanid (horse) flies in which they develop into infective larvae.

Epidemiology

Loa loa is irregularly distributed in West and central Africa. The vectors are diurnally biting flies (*Chrysops* species) that live in the canopy of the rain forest. They are attracted by people moving through open spaces in the jungle. Monkeys harbor *L. papionis* (transmitted by nocturnally biting *Chrysops*), which is able to hybridize with *L. loa* and produce fertile offspring, but there is no significant interchange of parasites between monkeys and humans.[23]

Clinical Features

Many patients are asymptomatic, although they may have high eosinophil levels in the peripheral blood. Transient swellings of localized subcutaneous edema, called Calabar swellings, may develop. Usually only one swelling occurs at a time. The onset may be preceded by localized pain and itching for several hours. It is nonerythematous, 10–20 cm in diameter, and lasts for several days to weeks. Calabar swellings are commonly seen around joints such as the wrist or the knee and recur irregularly at either the same or different sites. Other patients complain of pruritus or have urticaria. Occasionally a worm may be seen passing through the subconjunctiva where it produces an intense conjunctivitis lasting several days. Infected visitors to endemic areas may have a hyperreactive state characterized by more frequent recurrences of fugitive swellings, greater eosinophilia, increased debilitation, and more complications, particularly the development of renal disease, either before or after treatment with diethylcarbamazine.[24] Other complications that may be seen are endomyocardial fibrosis, retinopathy, encephalopathy, peripheral neuropathy, and arthritis.

Diagnosis

The disease should be suspected in a patient with a typical history who has lived in West or central Africa. The diagnosis is established by finding microfilariae in the daytime blood as described in the section on bancroftian filariasis. Failure to find microfilariae does not rule out the diagnosis. Occasionally the adult can be extracted from the eye.

Treatment

Diethylcarbamazine eliminates microfilariae from the blood and may kill adult worms. It is administered as described in the section on onchocerciasis.

Prevention

Personal protection depends on avoiding places where biting flies are numerous, by wearing protective clothing, and by using insect repellents. Mass treatment of villages will interrupt transmission; diethylcarbamazine is administered in doses of 5 mg/kg/day for 3 consecutive days each month.[23]

ONCHOCERCIASIS

Onchocerciasis (river blindness) is caused by *Onchocerca volvulus* and is transmitted to humans by blackflies. It is characterized by an itchy dermatitis, subcutaneous nodules, and keratitis.[25]

Life Cycle

After the bite of an infected *Simulium* blackfly, larvae penetrate the skin and migrate into the connective tissues. They develop into white filiform adults, the males being 30 × 0.2 mm and the females 400 × 0.3 mm in size. The worms are often found tangled together in nodules of fibrous tissue where they may live for years. Each female produces large numbers of unsheathed microfilariae 200–300 × 6–8 μm in size that migrate through the skin and connective tissues. The life cycle is continued when they are ingested by female blackflies and develop into infective larvae.

Epidemiology

Onchocerca volvulus infects 30 million people in West, central, and East Africa and another 1 million people in scattered foci in Central and South America. There is no known animal reservoir. Onchocerciasis tends to be focal in distribution within its endemic areas. In Africa, the flies breed in fast-flowing streams in both the savannah and rain forest and tend to bite low on the body. In America, the flies breed in small streams on the hillsides and bite more frequently around the head. Heavy parasite loads and severe disease require repeated infection.

Pathologic Characteristics

A granulomatous inflammatory reaction followed by fibrosis develops around the adult worms. The microfilariae in the subcutaneous tissues may produce a low-grade inflammatory reaction, destruction of the elastic fibers, and fibrosis.[26,27]

Clinical Features

Early skin lesions produce an itchy, erythematous, papular rash. In severe infections, cutaneous lymphedema with leathery thickening and depigmentation may be seen. Ultimately, a loss of elasticity with chronic lymphadenopathy may produce pendulous sacs containing inguinal and femoral lymph nodes. Firm, nontender, freely mobile fibrous nodules that may be several millimeters to centimeters in size and may contain the adult worms may be found. They are more commonly located over bony prominences. Impaired visual acuity is the most serious complication. The most common lesion is punctate keratitis followed by pannus formation and corneal fibrosis. Microfilariae can often be seen in the cornea and anterior chamber with a slit lamp. Iridocyclitis, glaucoma, choroiditis, and optic atrophy may develop.[28]

Diagnosis

The diagnosis is made either by demonstrating microfilariae in skin snips or in the cornea or anterior chamber on slit-lamp examination or by finding adult worms in a nodule biopsy specimen. Impalpable nodules can sometimes be demonstrated by ultrasound techniques.[29] Bloodless skin snips are taken without anesthesia by raising small cones of skin about 3 mm in diameter with the tip of a needle and then cutting them off with a razor blade. Snips should be taken from over the scapulas and iliac crests and from the buttocks and thighs. They are allowed to stand for half an hour in a drop of 0.9% saline and then are examined under a microscope for microfilariae. Ultrasound detection of changes in the vitreous humor have been described recently.[29a] Eosinophilia is common. Serologic tests do not differentiate among the various forms of filariasis. If the diagnosis is strongly suspected but parasites cannot be found, a single oral test dose of 50 mg of diethylcarbamazine can be given (Mazzotti reaction). If an exacerbation of the rash occurs within a few hours, the diagnosis is likely.

Treatment

Traditionally, patients with skin disease have been treated with diethylcarbamazine. This drug kills microfilariae but has little effect on the adult worm. Severe reactions such as rash, fever, generalized body pains, keratitis, and iritis may occur, so the dose must be built up gradually as follows: day 1, 50 mg; day 2, 50 mg three times; day 3, 100 mg three times; and days 4–21, 3 mg/kg three times a day. Recent studies have shown that a new agent, ivermectin, is safer and more effective than diethylcarbamazine is.[30–33] This agent is now the drug of choice. Unfortunately, like diethylcarbamazine, ivermectin kills microfilariae but not adult worms. The rates of decrease in numbers of microfilariae in the skin and anterior chamber of the eye and the severity of Mazzotti reactions are less, and the duration of the reduction in microfilarial loads is longer with ivermectin when compared with diethylcarbamazine. Studies reported thus far have used a single oral dose of approximately 150 μg/kg. This drug is likely to become generally available soon. Adult worms can be killed by suramin, but this drug is toxic. In the past it has been recommended that it should only be administered to patients who have recurrent skin disease after several courses of diethylcarbamazine therapy or to patients with eye disease. After a test dose of 100 mg, 1 g is given intravenously each week for 6 weeks. If proteinuria or abundant casts appear in the urine or an exfoliative dermatitis develops, treatment with the drug should be stopped. After the advent of ivermectin, this recommendation needs to be reviewed when sufficient data become available. Surgical removal of nodules should be performed whenever practical. Expert ophthalmologic advice should be sought before the treatment of eye lesions.

Prevention

Personal protection depends on avoiding places where biting flies are numerous and on wearing protective clothing. A major control program is in progress in West Africa. The vector is being attacked by larvicides applied to breeding places; the onchocerciasis-infected population is gradually being replaced by a healthy population.

MANSONELLA INFECTIONS

Mansonella ozzardi, transmitted by blackflies and midges, is found in latin America. Adult worms are found in the visceral fatty tissues. Unsheathed microfilariae that are not periodic may be found in the peripheral blood. Most patients are asymptomatic.

Mansonella perstans, also transmitted by midges, is found in Africa and South America. Adult worms live in the body cavities. Unsheathed microfilariae may be found in the peripheral blood, especially at night. Most patients are asymptomatic.

Mansonella streptocerca is transmitted to humans by biting midges. It is found in central Africa and is characterized by dermatitis. Microfilariae are found in skin snips, and treatment is with diethylcarbamazine.[34]

TROPICAL PULMONARY EOSINOPHILIA

Tropical pulmonary eosinophilia is a disease syndrome caused by microfilariae in the tissues, especially the lungs.[35,36] It is unclear whether the causative organisms of this occult filariasis are parasites of animals or humans, although recent evidence suggests that the latter is more likely.[37] It is scattered throughout the tropics but is most commonly seen in southern Asia. Patients have recurrent episodes of a paroxysmal, dry cough, wheezing, and dyspnea. There is frequently malaise, anorexia, and weight loss. Physical examination often reveals scattered rhonchi and crepitations. Some patients may have hepatomegaly and lymphadenopathy. The symptoms usually fluctuate in severity over many months. The absence of microfilariae from the blood makes a definitive diagnosis difficult. Eosinophilia is almost always present, often at extremely high levels. Chest x-ray films usually reveal scattered reticulonodular opacities. Antibodies to filarial worms are found in the serum. A presumptive clinical diagnosis can usually be made without recourse to lung biopsy, and the diagnosis is established by a successful response to therapy. The administration of diethylcarbamazine orally in a dose of 3 mg/kg three times daily for 2 weeks is an effective treatment. There may be an initial exacerbation of symptoms, but the eosinophil level falls, and the chest x-ray picture clears over a few weeks.

REFERENCES

1. Gould SE, ed. Trichinosis in Man and Animals. Springfield, IL: Charles C Thomas; 1970.
2. Zimmerman WJ, Steele JH, Kagan IG. The changing status of trichiniasis in the United States population. Public Health Rep. 1968;83:957.
3. Corridan JP, Gray JJ. Trichinosis in South west Ireland. Br Med J. 1969;1:727.
4. Doege TC, Thienprasit P, Headington LT, et al. Trichinosis and raw bear meat in Thailand. Lancet. 1969;1:459.
5. Hathaway FH, Blaney L. Trichinosis: Report of an epidemic. Ann Intern Med. 1947;26:250.
6. Khamboonruang C, Nateewatana N. Trichinosis: A recent outbreak in Northern Thailand. Southeast Asian J Trop Med Public Health. 1975;6:74.
7. Kratz F. Die trichinenepidemie zu Hedersleben, 1866. Quoted in: Gould SE, ed. Trichinosis in Man and Animals. Springfield, IL: Charles C Thomas; 1970;274–5.
8. Oppenheim JM, Whims CB, Frisch AW. Trichinosis: Clinical and laboratory observations in a group of 256 cases. Milit Surg. 1947;101:294.
9. Schmitt N, Bowmer EJ, Simon PC, et al. Trichinosis from bear meat and adulterated pork: A major outbreak in British Columbia, 1971. Can Med Assoc J. 1972;107:1087.
10. Shookhoff HB, Birnkrant WB, Greenberg M. An outbreak of trichinosis in New York City, with special reference to the intradermal and precipitin tests. Am J Public Health. 1946;36:1403.
11. Wand M, Lyman D. Trichinosis from bear meat: Clinical and laboratory features. JAMA. 1972;220:245.
12. Levin ML. Treatment of trichinosis with mebendazole. Am J Trop Med Hyg. 1983;32:980.
13. Muller R. *Dracunculus* and dracunculiasis. Adv Parasitol. 1971;9:73.
14. Muller R. Guinea worm disease: Epidemiology, control and treatment. Bull WHO. 1979;57:683.
15. Sastry SC, Jayakumar K, Lakshminarayana V. The treatment of dracontiasis with thiabendazole. J Trop Med Hyg. 1978;81:32.
16. Sharma VP, Rathore HS, Sharma MM. Efficacy of metronidazole in dracunculiasis: A clinical trial. Am J Trop Med Hyg. 1979;28:658.
17. Hopkins DR. Dracunculiasis eradication: A mid-decade status report. Am J Trop Med Hyg. 1987;37:115.
18. Sasa M, ed. Human Filariasis: A Global Survey of Epidemiology and Control. Baltimore: University Park Press; 1976.
19. Methods for the diagnosis of microfilaremia. WHO Tech Rep Ser. 1974;542:50.
20. Huijin Z, Zhenghou T, Reddy MV, et al. Parasite antigens in sera and urine of patients with bancroftian and brugian filariasis. Am J Trop Med Hyg. 1987;36:554.
21. Weil GJ, Jain DC, Malhotra SA, et al. A monoclonal antibody-based enzyme immunoassay for detecting antigenemia in bancroftian filariasis. J Infect Dis. 1987;156:350.

21a. Weil GJ, Sethumadhavan KVS, Santhanam S, et al. Persistence of parasite antigenemia following diethylcarbamazine therapy of bancroftian filariasis. Am J Trop Med Hyg. 1988;38:589.

22. Ottesen EA. Efficacy of diethylcarbamazine in eradicating infection with lymphatic-dwelling filariae in humans. Rev Infect Dis. 1985;7:341.
23. Fain A. Les problemes actuels de la loase. Bull WHO. 1978;56:155.
24. Nutman TB, Miller KD, Mulligan M, et al. *Loa loa* infection in temporary residents of endemic regions: Recognition of a hyperresponsive syndrome with characteristic clinical manifestations. J Infect Dis. 1986;154:10.
25. Nelson GS. Onchocerciasis. Adv Parasitol. 1970;8:173.
26. Mackenzie CD, Williams JF, Sisley BM, et al. Variations in host responses and the pathogenesis of human onchocerciasis. Rev Infect Dis. 1985;7:802.
27. Connor DH, George GH, Gibson DW. Pathologic changes of human onchocerciasis: Implications for future research. Rev Infect Dis. 1985;7:809.
28. Thylefors B. Ocular onchocerciasis. Bull WHO. 1978;56:63.
29. Homeida MA, Mackenzie CD, Williams HF, et al. The detection of onchocercal nodules by ultrasound technique. Trans R Soc Trop Med Hyg. 1986;80:570.

29a. Reyna O, Zea Flores, Nowell de Arevalo AM, et al., Ultrasound detection of changes in the vitreous humor of onchocerciasis patients from Guatemala. Trans R Soc Trop Med Hyg. 1988;82:606.

30. Greene BM, Taylor HR, Cupp EW, et al. Comparison of ivermectin and diethylcarbamazine in the treatment of onchocerciasis. N Engl J Med. 1985;313:133.
31. Lariviere M, Vingtain P, Aziz M, et al. Double-blind study of ivermectin and diethylcarbamazine in African onchocerciasis patients with ocular involvement. Lancet. 1985;2:174.
32. Awadzi K, Dadzie KY, Schulz-Key H, et al. The chemotherapy of onchocerciasis XI. A double-blind comparative study of ivermectin, diethylcarbamazine and placebo in human onchocerciasis in northern Ghana. Ann Trop Med Parasitol. 1986;80:433.
33. Dadzie KY, Bird AC, Awadzi K, et al. Ocular findings in a double-blind study of ivermectin versus diethylcarbamazine versus placebo in the treatment of onchocerciasis. Br J Ophthalmol. 1987;71:78.
34. Meyers WM, Connor DH, Harman LE, et al. Human streptocerciasis. Am J Trop Med Hyg. 1972;21:528.
35. Webb JKG, Job CK, Gault EW. Tropical eosinophilia. Lancet. 1960;1:835.
36. Neva FA, Otteson EA. Current concepts in parasitology: Tropical (filarial) eosinophilia. N Engl J Med. 1978;298:1129.
37. Otteson EA, Neva FA, Paranajape RS, et al. Specific allergic sensitisation to filarial antigens in tropical eosinophilia syndrome. Lancet. 1979;1:1158.

265. TREMATODES (SCHISTOSOMIASIS) AND OTHER FLUKES

ADEL A. F. MAHMOUD

Flukes are parasitic worms of the class Trematoda. The classic shape of a digenetic trematode is that of a thick, oval leaf, although there are many variations in both shape and size. The length of different fluke species varies from less than 1 mm to several centimeters. An oral and, in most species, a ventral sucker are characteristic external features. The principal internal organs are a blind biforcate intestinal tract and prominent reproductive organs, which are arranged in a specific manner in each species.

All species parasitic in humans belong to the digenetic group in which sexual reproduction in the adult worms is followed by asexual multiplication in the larvae stages (alternation of generations). Most flukes infecting humans are hermaphrodites, with the exception of the schistosomes. The more important parasitic trematodes of humans are summarized in Table 1. Since some of these species have a tissue migratory stage in the host, eosinophilia is a prominent clinical sign of trematode infections.

BLOOD FLUKES

Schistosomiasis

The five human blood flukes *Schistosoma mansoni, S. japonicum, S. mekongi, S. haematobium*, and *S. intercalatum* make up the group of major importance in flatworm infections of humans, not only because they currently infect more than 200 million people but also because their prevalence is on the increase.[1] The major areas of agricultural development in Africa, South America, and Asia are endemic; schistosome distribution is expanding with the introduction of more agricultural programs. Schistosomiasis may cause a severe degree of morbidity and pathologic changes that, if left undiagnosed and untreated, may result in major disability or mortality.

In the United States infection with human schistosomes has

TABLE 1. Important Parasitc Trematodes of Humans

Type of Flukes	Disease	Species Infecting Humans	Intermediate Hosts		Final Habitat
			Primary	Secondary	
Blood	Schistosomiasis	*S. haematobium*	Snails	None	Vesical plexus
		S. japonicum	Snails	None	Superior mesenteric veins
		S. mansoni	Snails	None	Inferior mesenteric veins
Liver	Clonorchiasis	*C. sinensis*	Snails	Fish	Bile ducts
	Opisthorchiasis	O. felineus *O. viverrini*	Snails	Fish	Bile ducts
	Fascioliasis	*F. hepatica*	Snails	Watercress	Bile ducts
Intestinal	Fasciolopsiasis	*F. buski*	Snails	Aquatic plants	Small intestines
Lung	Paragonimiasis	*P. westermani*	Snails	Crabs	Lungs

been estimated to exceed 400,000 persons.[2] These are mainly immigrants from endemic areas, particularly Puerto Rico, Brazil, the Middle East, and the Phillippines. Fortunately, the infection cannot be transmitted in this country because of the absence of the appropriate snail intermediate host.

Adult schistosome worms are distinct from most other flukes in that they exist as separate sexes. In *S. japonicum, S. mekongi, S. mansoni*, and *S. intercalatum* infection, mature worms inhabit the portal and mesenteric vessels; in *S. haematobium*, the vesical plexus. The lateral edges of the body of the male worm are folded to enclose a groove where the female usually lies. It has been estimated that each female produces 300 eggs daily in *S. mansoni* and *S. haematobium* and 3000 eggs in *S. japonicum* infections.

Life Cycle. Humans are the principal definitive host for the five schistosome species. Adult worms (1–2 cm in length) living in the venous system of the intestines or the urinary bladder start their sexual reproduction by mating and passing characteristically shaped eggs (145 × 55 μm but slightly smaller in *S. japonicum* and *S. mekongi*) that find their way to the outside via the host excreta (Fig. 1). In fresh water the eggs hatch and release ciliated motile miracidia that soon penetrate into the body of the snail intermediate host. For each species and for each geographic strain of the schistosomes there is a specific snail intermediate host. Therefore, it is believed that the geographic distribution of schistosomiasis depends on the distribution of the specific snails and that it is the absence of these snails in the continental United States that prevents the transmission of the infection in this country. Inside the snail, the miracidia multiply asexually, and in 4–6 weeks hundreds of motile, forked-tail cercariae emerge. These are the infective forms. On encountering human skin, the cercariae penetrate it with the help of their glandular secretions. In the process of invasion of the human host the cercariae lose their tails and change into schistosomulae that migrate to the lungs and the liver; in about 6 weeks they mature to adult worms that mate and descend via the venous system to their final habitat. The life span of the schistosome worms has been the subject of controversy. On the basis of data obtained from persons who left an endemic area and who years later were found to be still passing eggs, a claim has been made that the worms can live up to 30 years. The mean life span of the worms, however, seems to be much shorter. In a study where a group of Yemeni immigrants moved to a nonendemic country, the mean life span of *S. mansoni* worms has been shown to be 5–10 years.[3] In *S. haematobium* infections recent investigations suggest that its life span may even be shorter than that of *S. mansoni*.[4]

Epidemiology. Each of the five species of schistosomes that infect humans has a specific geographic distribution. *Schistosoma mansoni* occurs in Arabia, Africa, South America, and the Caribbean; *S. japonicum*, in Japan, China, and the Philippines; *S. mekongi*, in Southeast Asia; *S. haematobium*, in Africa and the Middle East; and *S. intercalatum*, in West and central Africa. Two major factors are responsible for the endemicity of schistosomiasis in specific geographic areas: the presence of the specific snail intermediate host and the method of disposal of human excreta.

The specificity of the snail intermediate host is remarkable not only in regard to the species of schistosomes but also to the geographic strain of the parasites. The kinetics of snail infections are important; at any one time period the infection rate of snails in an endemic area is very low, and although they shed an enormous number of cercariae, the latter also have extremely low counts in bodies of water.[6] Attempts to measure cercarial density in the field by filtration techniques in most cases have resulted in an extremely low recovery of organisms from large volumes of water. Adding to these findings the diurnal, seasonal, and yearly variations in snail infection rates, it would appear that the rate of exposure of persons in endemic areas to schistosome infections must be low. This is contrary to the old belief that the frequent contact with schistosome-infected water provides an ample opportunity for continual infection. In fact, epidemiologic surveys in endemic areas have shown that there are peaks of intensity and prevalence of infection in the younger members of the population and that both decrease by age.[4] The distribution of the infection in these communities fits a negative binomial curve, with most infected persons harboring low worm burdens and only a small proportion having heavy infections. The implications of these epidemiologic findings are relevant to our understanding of the dynamics of the infection in communities and the role of immunity or ecology in its control.

The prevalence and degree of morbidity in schistosomiasis have been shown to correlate well with the worm burden as estimated by fecal or urinary egg counts.[7,8] In addition, recent information points to a possible link between HLA antigens and the development of hepatosplenomegaly in schistosomiasis mansoni or japonica.[9,10]

Pathogenesis. Three major disease syndromes occur in schistosomiasis. In their chronologic order they are dermatitis, Katayama fever, and the chronic fibro-obstructive sequelae. These syndromes coincide with and are related to the three different stages of development of the parasite within the host: cercariae, mature worms, and eggs. The penetrating cercariae have been associated with a papular pruritic rash called swimmer's itch, or schistosome dermatitis. While this reaction is seen occasionally in infections with human schistosomes, it occurs most often and is most severe when nonhuman (bird) cercariae penetrate the skin.[11] Almost all these organisms die in the dermis, which results in the typical skin rash. Schistosome dermatitis is a sensitization phenomenon since it occurs in previously exposed persons; the papules are delayed in onset, and skin biopsy specimens have revealed edema and massive cellular infiltrate in the dermis and epidermis. Studies in experimental animals have demonstrated both humor and cell-mediated immune responses against the cercarial stage of *S. mansoni* that can be adoptively transferred to unexposed recipients.[12]

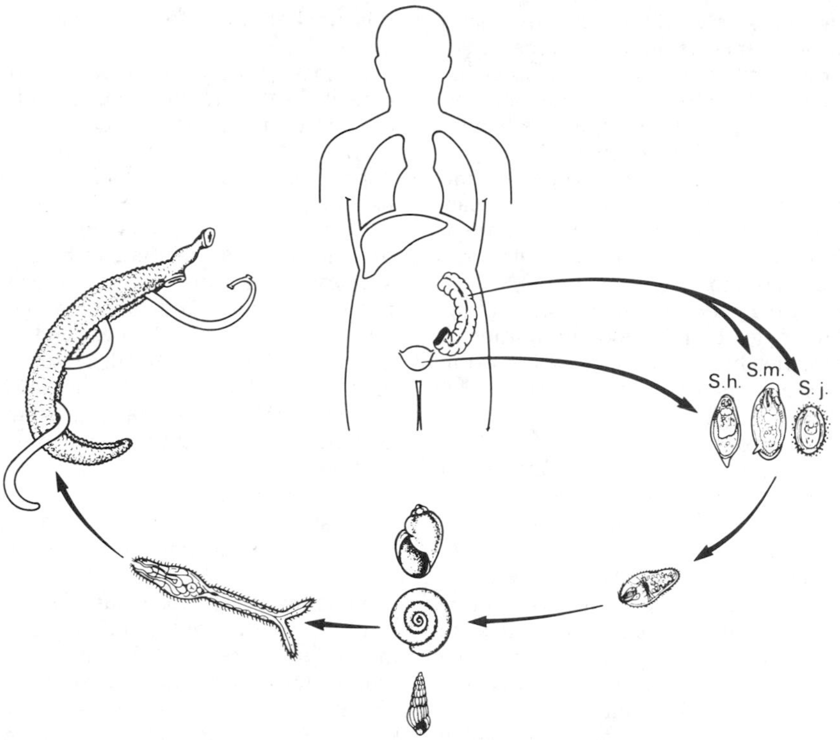

FIG. 1. Life cycle of schistosomes. Eggs are passed with stools in *Schistosoma mansoni* (S.m.) and *Schistosoma japonicum* (S.j.) and with urine in *Schistosoma haematobium* (S.h.). The eggs hatch in fresh water, miracidia invade specific snail intermediate hosts, and in a few weeks forked-tail cercariae are liberated. These infective forms penetrate human skin, pass through a migratory phase in the lung and the liver, and then pass to their final habitat in the portal venous system (s.m. and S.j.) or in the urinary bladder venous plexus (S.h.). Two other species infect humans, although less frequently. *Schistoma intercalatum* produces terminal spined eggs that may be found in feces, while *S. mekongi* produces eggs similar to but smaller than those of *S. japonicum*, which may also be found in stools. Both of these two species of schistosomes have characteristic snail intermediate hosts.

When the worms have matured and egg deposition begins, a condition known as Katayama fever, or acute schistosomiasis, may be noticed. It is a serum sickness-like syndrome that is usually seen in primary heavy infections, particularly those due to *S. japonicum*. It may be due to immune complex formation initiated by the massive antigenic challenge produced by the eggs.[13]

During the chronic stages of the infection, the mature worms constantly produce large numbers of eggs, some of which remain in the body. Since the habitat of *S. mansoni, S. intercalatum, S. japonicum*, and *S. mekongi* worms is the mesenteric blood vessels, the intestines are involved primarily, and egg embolism results in secondary involvement of the liver. In *S. haematobium* infections the main system involved is the urinary tract. The host response to the eggs retained in the tissues results in granuloma formation consisting mainly of lymphocytes, macrophages, and eosinophils.[14] In *S. mansoni* and *S. haematobium* infections the granulomatous response has been shown to be an immunologic reaction of the delayed hypersensitivity type.[15,16] In contrast, *S. japonicum*-induced granulomas seem to have different kinetics, and it has been suggested that they may be due to antigen–antibody complexes.[17]

Tissue injury in chronic schistosomiasis is initiated by the egg-induced granulomas. The inflammatory infiltrate leads to replacement of normal tissue followed by extensive collagen deposition and scarring. The large avascular granulomas and the residual fibrous tissue cause the major pathologic lesions in chronic schistosomiasis: obstruction to portal blood flow in the liver, to pulmonary blood flow in the lungs, and to urine flow through the ureters and bladder. During the early stages of schistosome infection in humans and in experimental animals, the granulomatous response is exuberant but it later modulates.[18] The occurrence of this modulation of granulomatous hypersensitivity is an important factor in protecting the host against its immunopathologic response to schistosome eggs and appears to play a significant role in limiting the progress of disease.[19,20]

Schistomiasis in humans and in experimental animals seems to be associated with a partial degree of resistance to reinfection.[21] While the evidence for immunity in humans is controversial, several mechanisms for immunity against schistosomiasis have been demonstrated in animals. One form of acquired resistance has been shown to depend on antibodies, is mediated by eosinophils, and is directed against the invading immature worms, while other effector mechanisms involving mononuclear phagocytes, neutrophils, and platelets have been described.[22–24]

Clinical Syndromes. ACUTE SCHISTOSOMIASIS. Schistosome dermatitis occurs occasionally within 24 hours after penetration of the cercariae. It is a pruritic papular skin rash known as swimmer's itch. This syndrome appears to be a sensitization phenomenon since it rarely occurs on primary exposure. Swimmer's itch has been demonstrated in infected persons experimentally reexposed to *S. mansoni* and *S. haematobium* cercariae. The more severe forms of schistosome dermatitis follow infection with avian schistosomes and is common in the region of the Great Lakes of the north central United States.

The next clinical phase of schistosomiasis coincides with the beginning of oviposition, 4–8 weeks after infection. Katayama fever was described in Japan where it used to occur and has been known to be most severe after *S. japonicum* infections.[25] A few reports have described a similar syndrome in Puerto Rico and other areas endemic for *S. mansoni*, usually in patients with heavy infections; it is, however, rarely seen in schistosomiasis due to *S. haematobium* or other species infecting humans. Patients with Katayama fever have an acute onset of fever, chills, sweating, headache, and cough. On physical examination, enlargement of the liver, spleen, and lymph nodes is noted. Eosinophilia occurs in most cases and averages about 40 percent of the differential leukocyte count. Most symptoms and signs disappear within a few weeks, but death may occur, particularly in schistosomiasis due to *S. japonicum*. At postmortem examination, massive infection is invariably found, with large numbers of eggs in the intestines and liver.

CHRONIC SCHISTOSOMIASIS. Most persons with schistosomiasis harbor a low to moderate worm load, and a good proportion of these persons are asymptomatic. In patients with heavy worm loads, however, the chronic characteristic sequela of the disease eventually reveals itself.

The patient with chronic schistosomiasis caused by *S. mansoni, S. japonicum*, or *S. mekongi* may conplain of fatigue and abdominal pain with intermittent diarrhea or dysentery. The two most commonly affected sites are the intestines and the liver. Intestinal schistosomiasis results from the chronic granulomatous lesions in the bowel wall.[26] Polyps have been observed, but only in some endemic areas in Egypt.[27] Blood loss from ulcerations may lead to a moderate degree of anemia. In *S. mansoni, S. japonicum*, and *S. mekongi* infections, many eggs remain in the venous portal circulation and are carried into the liver. The eggs with their associated granulomas result in a presinusoidal block to portal blood flow and in the development of portal hypertension and portal-systemic collateral circulation. Hemodynamic studies of hepatic schistosomiasis reveal that both intrasplenic and portal pressures are markedly elevated whereas the wedge hepatic vein pressure is normal.[28] The total volume of hepatic blood remains within normal range by increasing the arterial blood flow. Liver cell perfusion is not reduced; consequently, liver function test results remain normal for a long time. These circulatory and immunologic processes also lead to enlargement of the spleen. Clinically, the earliest sign of chronic schistosomiasis due to *S. mansoni, S. japonicum*, or *S. mekongi* is enlargement of the liver. With progression of liver disease, splenomegaly develops. The spleen may reach massive dimensions and is usually firm. The hepatosplenic stage may be associated with abdominal pain or dragging pain in the left upper quadrant. Sudden episodes of hermatemesis from bleeding esophageal varices may occur, but they are associated with low mortality. Patients may not bleed again for many years, or bleeding may recur at fairly frequent intervals. Persons with compensated liver disease will have relatively normal hepatic function with normal serum albumin and elevated γ-globulin levels. The white blood cell count may show a moderate degree of eosinophilia. Intestinal and eosphageal blood losses and the development of hypersplenism may lead to a moderate degree of anemia in some patients. The terminal stage of hepatosplenic schistosomiasis is heralded by the development of decompensated liver disease. Jaundice, ascites, and liver failure may follow. It is not known, however, whether this is a natural progression of the schistosome disease or whether it is related to additional factors such as nutritional deficiencies or hepatic viral infections.

In *S. haematobium* infections the initial pathologic lesions are located in the ureters and bladder.[29] Exuberant granulomatous reactions to the eggs may lead to obstruction of urinary flow or papillomatous irregularities of the bladder wall. On intravenous pyelography or ultrasonography, obstruction, hydronephrosis, hydroureters, and filling defects in the bladder may be demonstrated. Patients usually complain of terminal hematuria and dysuria. The end stages of schistosomiasis due to *S. haematobium* progress through hydronephrosis, secondary infections, and uremia. In some endemic areas an association has been demonstrated between *S. haematobium* infection and both the *Salmonella* urinary carrier state[30] and bladder cancer.[31]

In some parts of West and central Africa, *S. intercalatum* parasitizes the mesenteric veins of humans; terminal-spine eggs are passed in stools of infected individuals. The clinical syndromes caused by *S. intercalatum* infection in humans are poorly defined. Infected individuals may complain of abdominal pain and bloody diarrhea.[32]

Until recently, *S. japonicum* was considered the only species of schistosomes that infects humans in the Far East. A new species, *S. mekongi*[33] is now considered to be the main human pathogen in mainland Indochina. The parasite differs from *S. japonicum* by its smaller eggs and its specific intermediate snail host. There are no controlled studies yet that describe the specific clinical features of human infection with *S. mekongi*. On the basis of examining a small number of Laotian immigrants with *S. mekongi*, hcpatomegaly was, however, the main clinical finding.[34]

The clinical descriptions given above have concentrated on the major sites affected by the five human schistosomes. Two other syndromes that are occasionally seen will be outlined briefly.

Pulmonary schistosomiasis is manifested by symptoms and signs of cor pulmonale and may occur as a complication of hepatosplenic disease.[35] Patent portosystemic collateral circulation in these patients enables the schistosome eggs to bypass the liver, and they are then trapped in the pulmonary capillaries. This syndrome may also be seen in schistosomiasis due to *S. haematobium* since the eggs can escape from the vesical plexus via the inferior vena cava to the lungs. Obstruction to pulmonary blood flow follows because of arteritis and granuloma formation. Pulmonary hypertension may be demonstrated, but the cardiac output usually remains within normal values.

Central nervous system schistosomiasis is rare but constitutes 3 percent of the complications of *S. japonicum* infections.[25] In these cases the brain is the usual site of disease, which is manifested as a space-occupying lesion or as a generalized encephalopathy. Furthermore, schistosomiasis caused by *S. japonicum* is considered one of the important causes of focal epilepsy in the Far East. In *S. haematobium* and *S. mansoni* infections, granulomatous lesions around ectopic eggs have been described in the spinal cord. These patients have a transverse myelitis-like syndrome, and a diagnosis may be difficult since active intestinal or urinary tract infection may not be easy to demonstrate.[36]

Diagnosis. The geographic distribution of schistosomiasis is well defined. Therefore, an important step in establishing the diagnosis is to inquire about the travel history of the patient. Detailed information should also be obtained about any history of water contact, skin rash, or an acute febrile episode (Katayama fever). A definitive diagnosis can be made only by finding schistosome eggs in feces or urine or in a biopsy specimen, usually from the rectum. Since assessing the intensity of infection in schistosomiasis is an essential part of the clinical evaluation, quantitative techniques for stool and urine examination are strongly recommended.[37] At present, the Kato thick smear is the procedure of choice for the determination of eggs in the feces. A 50 mg sample of feces that has been pressed through 105 mesh stainless steel bolting cloth (W. S. Tyler, Cleveland) is placed on a glass slide and covered with a cellophane coverslip (no. 124PD, Film Department, E.I. DuPont de Nemours, Wilmington, DE) impregnated with 50% glycerine. The slide is inverted and pressed onto a bed of filter paper, turned face up, and left for a period of 24–48 hours, during which time the fecal matter clears. The embryo within the egg also clears, but the characteristic shape of the egg shell can easily be seen.

Urine for the diagnosis of *S. haematobium* infection is best collected between noon and 2 PM. Counts can be made by passing a 10 ml aliquot of the urine sample through a Nuclepore filter (13 mm in diameter with a pore size of 8 μm) held in a PT-103 chamber (Nuclepore Corp., Pleasanton, CA).[37] The filter is removed, placed face down on a microscope slide, and examined immediately at 40× magnification. The terminal-spined eggs are clearly seen with no necessity of staining procedures.

Rectal biopsy can be used to diagnose any of the five species of human schistosomes. An anoscope is introduced, and small pieces of the mucosa are pinched off by a sharp curette. Four tissue samples are usually obtained; each is compressed between two glass slides and examined for eggs at low magnification.

A variety of immunologic diagnostic techniques such as skin or serologic tests have been described but are not of practical use in the diagnosis of schistosomiasis. Crude antigenic extracts of schistosome materials are used in these tests that compromise their specificity and sensitivity, and they provide no quantitative data on the intensity of infection. One practical and useful application of serologic tests, however, is in the case of central nervous system or ectopic schistosomiasis with no demonstrable infection in the feces, urine, or rectal mucosa. A positive serologic test in this instance may provide a useful clinical pointer for diagnosis and therapy.

Management. Drug management of schistosomiasis has changed drastically over the past few years. Safe, effective, and orally administered chemotherapeutic agents are now available for the treatment of major human schistosome infections. Praziquantel is a new broad spectrum anthelmintic agent that is effective against all five human schistosome species.[38] It is administered as a single oral dose of 40 mg/kg body weight for individuals with *S. mansoni* or *S. haematobium* infection. In subjects with schistosomiasis japonica, praziquantel is administered as 20 mg/kg body weight three times for 1 day. Praziquantel has also been found to be effective against *S. mekongi*. The drug results in a remarkable degree of parasitologic cure and reduction of egg counts. Side effects are mild and include abdominal discomfort, fever, and headache.

Several other oral compounds have been proved just as effective but with limited range of parasite specificity. Metrifonate (Bayer, Germany) is effective against *S. haematobium* infection. It is given orally at 7.5 mg/kg body weight, to be repeated twice at 2-week intervals. Oxamniquine (Pfizer) is effective against *S. mansoni* infection. The recommended dose is 15–20 mg/kg body weight. Individuals who were infected in Egypt or East Africa may need higher doses, up to 60 mg/kg body weight given in divided doses.

LIVER FLUKES

The major liver flukes of humans are *Clonorchis sinensis*, the Chinese liver fluke, and various species of *Opisthorchis*, which are largely found in Southeast Asia and Russia. *Fasciola hepatica* is one of the most important diseases of sheep and cattle that, incidentally, infects humans; several hundred cases have been reported in Latin America, Europe, Asia, and North Africa.

Clonorchiasis

The Chinese, or oriental, liver fluke *C. sinensis* is a parasite of fish-eating mammals in the Far East. Although humans are incidental hosts, millions of persons are infected, mainly in China. Hong Kong, Vietnam, and Korea. The adult fluke is a flat, elongated worm (approximately 15 × 3 mm). They inhabit the distal biliary capillaries where they deposit relatively small, yellow operculated eggs (30 × 14 μm) that are fully embryonated when they pass out of the body in feces (Fig. 2). The eggs are then ingested by specific snails, inside which they hatch into miracidia; these organisms multiply enormously, which results in large nubmers of cercariae that pass into the water. On coming into contact with certain freshwater fish, the cercariae penetrate under the scales or into the skin where they encyst as metacercariae, which are the infective forms. Humans acquire clonorchiasis by the ingestion of raw or inadequately cooked fish; the metacercariae excyst in the duodenum and pass through the ampulla of Vater where adult worms mature inside the bile ducts.

Clinical Syndromes. Controlled studies have revealed that most persons with *C. sinensis* infections are asymptomatic.[39] No gross changes can be detected in the liver in mild or early infection, but localized obstruction of bile ducts and thickening of their walls may be seen in heavy infection. Clinically, persons with heavy worm loads may suffer from cholangitis and cholangiohepatitis.[40] An increased incidence of cholangiocarcinoma in the Chinese of Hong Kong has been associated with *C. sinensis* infections. Pathologically, these tumors are adenocarcinomas originating from the hyperplastic epithelial lining of the bile ducts.

Diagnosis and Management. A definitive diagnosis of clonorchiasis depends on demonstration of the characteristic eggs in the feces. To improve the chance of finding eggs, a stool concentration technique such as formol-ether may be necessary. Praziquantel is now the drug of choice for the treatment of clonorchiasis.[38] Surgery to relieve biliary tract obstruction may rarely be needed.

Opisthorchiasis

Human infections with *O. felineus* and *O. viverrini* are clinically similar to clonorchiasis. These two parasites are common liver flukes of cats and dogs that can occasionally be transmitted to humans. Infection with *O. felineus* is endemic in Southeast Asia and eastern Europe, whereas *O. viverrini* infection is commonly found in Thailand. The life cycle and symptoms are similar to those of *C. sinensis* infection.[40] Diagnosis is established by fecal examination. Praziquantel has been found to be effective in treating infected individuals.[38]

Fascioliasis

Infection with the liver fluke *F. hepatica* is a cosmopolitan zoonosis throughout the sheep-raising areas of the world. Human infections have been reproted, particularly from South America, Europe, Africa, China, and Australia. The adult fluke is large, flat, brownish, and leaf shaped and measures approximately 2.5 cm × 1.0 cm. The final habitat of mature worms in their natural hosts (mainly sheep and cattle) or in humans is the biliary system where they deposit their eggs (Fig. 2). The large oval, yellowish brown, operculate ova (140 μm × 75 μm) pass to the intestines, are evacuated in the feces, and complete their development in water. In a few days mature miracidia hatch and must reach their specific snail intermediate host within 8 hours. Inside the lymph spaces of the snail, multiplication takes place, and unforked-tail cercariae emerge, and undergo encystment into metacercariae on aquatic grasses, plants, and sometimes soil. The infective metacercariae when swallowed excyst, and the larvae penetrate the intestinal wall into the peritoneum, whence they usually pass through the liver capsule and tissues to the biliary tract. Approximately 12 weeks are needed from infection to oviposition in humans.

Clinical Syndromes. Unlike clonorchiasis, infection with *F. hepatica* has two distinct clinical phases corresponding to the hepatic migratory phase of its life cycle and to the presence of the worms in their final habitat in the bile ducts.[40] The early phase is characterized by fever and pain in the right upper quadrant that are associated with enlargement of the liver. Marked

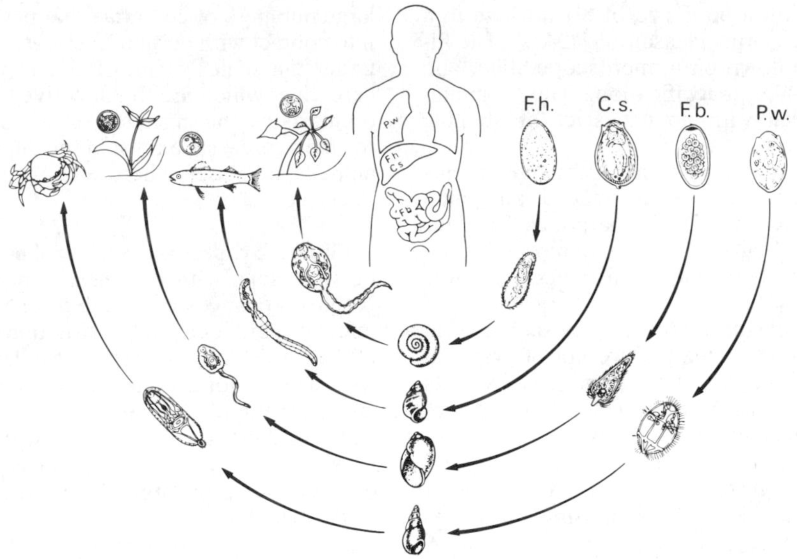

FIG. 2. Life cycle of important parasitic flukes. Eggs are passed with stools in *Fasciola hepatica* (F.h.), *Clonorchis sinensis* (C.s.), and *Fasciolopsis buski* (F.b.) or in sputum in *Paragonimus westermani* (P.w.) infections. The next stage of multiplication occurs in specific snail intermediate hosts, followed by liberation of cercariae, which encyst on the second intermediate hosts (aquatic plants, fish, or crabs). These metacercariae are the infective stage, and humans develop the infection after consumption of the second intermediate hosts. The final habitats of these flukes are the liver (F.h. and C.s.), intestines (F.b.), or lungs (P.w.).

eosinophilia is usually seen. A few weeks after this acute episode and as the worms enter the bile canaliculi, the symptoms may decline or disappear completely. Individual cases with obstruction of bile ducts and biliary cirrhosis have been reported, but they are extremely rare. Most infections are found incidentally during surgery or routine stool examination.

Diagnosis and Management. Laboratory diagnosis is based on finding the characteristic ova in the feces or bile. A concentration method such as formol-ether is necessary to enhance the chance of finding eggs. Praziquantel is currently the drug of choice for treating fascioliasis.[41]

INTESTINAL FLUKES

Fasciolopsiasis

Human infection with the large intestinal fluke *Fasciolopsis buski* is endemic in the Far East and Southeast Asia. Adult worms are thick and fleshy and range in length from 2 to 7.5 cm and in breadth from 0.8 to 2.0 cm. These flukes inhabit the duodenum and jejunum and produce large operculated eggs (135 × 80 μm) (Fig. 2). On reaching fresh water, the eggs develop into miracidia that hatch and must reach a specific snail intermediate host to multiply and to develop into free-living cercariae. These organisms will, in turn, encyst into metacercariae on almost any aquatic plant. The metacercariae, or infective forms, can survive in most environments for periods up to 1 year. When the infected plants are ingested by humans, the metacercariae excyst in the intestines, and the parasites develop into mature worms within 3 months.

Clinical Syndromes. Adult flukes live in the upper portion of the small intestine and are usually attached to its mucosa. Fasciolopsiasis appears to be mostly asymptomatic.[40] Controlled field studies demonstrated no significant difference between infected and control persons as regards their development or intestinal absorption capabilities. In heavy infections, however, the major symptoms relate to the presence of the worms in the intestines. Diarrhea, abdominal pain, and signs of malabsorption in the stools (undigested food) may be encountered.

Diagnosis and Management. A definitive diagnosis depends on demonstration of adult worms or eggs in stools. Adult worms recovered from feces should be examined by an experienced parasitologist. Eggs that resemble those of *F. hepatica* can be demonstrated by fecal smear examination or by the use of a concentration technique such as formol-ether. The treatment of choice of symptomatic fasciolopsiasis is praziquantel. It is administered orally at 25 mg/kg body weight three times per day for 1 day.[41]

Heterophyiasis

Human infection with the minute intestinal fluke *Heterophyes heterophyes* is common in the Nile delta, in the Far East, and in Southeast Asia. These flukes are small, less than 2 mm in length, and they inhabit the small intestines. The life cycle is similar to *F. buski*, but the metacercariae encyst in freshwater or brackish water fish. Infection is acquired by consumption of undercooked or salted fish. Adult worms deposit small operculate eggs (30 × 15 μm) that can be detected in the stools. Clinically, heterophyiasis is manifested as abdominal pain associated with mucous diarrhea. There are no controlled studies to indicate the specificity of these symptoms and the relationship of morbidity to worm loads. Treatment is recommended for symptomatic patients; the drug of choice is praziquantel, as described above for fasciolopsiasis.

LUNG FLUKES

Paragonimiasis

Human infection by the lung flukes *Paragonimus westermani* and several other species is widely distributed over three continents. Endemic foci have been found in West Africa, in almost every country in the Far East and the Indian subcontinent, and in several parts of Central and South America. Adult worms measuring 7–12 mm × 4–7 mm encapsulate within the parenchyma of the lung, usually close to bronchioles. On reaching maturity the worm deposits golden brown operculate eggs (100 × 10 μm) that pass into the bronchioles and are coughed up (Fig. 2). Eggs can be detected in the sputum of infected persons or in their feces if they swallow their sputum. In fresh water, the eggs mature and liberate free-swimming miracidia that infect the specific snail intermediate host. After a rather protracted period of development and reproduction in the snail (3–5 months), stumpy-tailed cercariae emerge. They encyst in the muscles and viscera of crayfish and freshwater crabs. Human infection is initiated by consumption of these freshwater crustaceans, either raw or pickled. Metacercariae excyst in the duodenum, penetrate the intestinal wall, and enter the peritoneal cavity. The next migratory phase takes the metacercariae through the diaphragm to the pleural cavities and then into the lungs where they finally lodge. Egg deposition starts 5–6 weeks after infection.

Clinical Syndromes. Most light and moderate infections are asymptomatic. The important clinical manifestations of paragonimiasis are eosinophilia and chest complaints.[40] Cough productive of brownish sputum with intermittent hemoptysis is the initial manifestation. The condition then evolves to a picture of chronic bronchitis or bronchiectasis with profuse expectoration and pleuritic chest pain. Lung abscesses, pleural effusion, and rarely, masses due to ectopic worms in the abdomen or central nervous system may be encountered. The clinical picture of cerebral paragonimiasis may resemble epilepsy, cerebral tumors, or embolism of the brain.

Diagnosis and Management. Examination of the sputum or feces provides the opportunity for finding the characteristic operculated eggs. In cases of ectopic paragonimiasis, serologic examination (complement fixation test) may be helpful. Once the diagnosis is established, therapy should be initiated. Praziquantel is given orally in a dose of 25 mg/kg body weight three times per day for 1 day.[41]

REFERENCES

1. Mahmoud AAF, Abdel Wahab MF. Schistosomiasis. In: Warren KS, Mahmoud AAF, eds. Tropical and Geographical Medicine. 2nd ed. New York: McGraw-Hill; In press.
2. Warren KS. Helminthic diseases endemic in the United States. Am J Trop Med Hyg. 1974;23:723.
3. Warren KS, Mahmoud AAF, Cummings P, et al. Schistosomiasis mansoni in Yemen in California: Duration of infection, presence of disease, therapeutic management. Am J Trop Med Hyg. 1974;23:902.
4. Anderson RM. Determinants of infection in human schistosomiasis. In: Mahmoud AAF, ed. Clinical Tropical Medicine and Communicable Diseases. London; Bailliere-Tindall; 1987:279–300.
5. World Health Organization. Atlas of the Global Distribution of Schistosomiasis. Parasitic Diseases Programme. Geneva: World Health Organization; 1987.
6. Sturrock RF. Biology and ecology of human schistosomes. In: Mahmoud AAF, ed. Clinical Tropical Medicine and Communicable Diseases. London: Bailliere-Tindall; 1987:249–66.
7. Siongok TKA, Mahmoud AAF, Ouma JH, et al. Morbidity in schistosomiasis mansoni in relation to intensity of infection: Study of a community in Machakos, Kenya. Am J Trop Med Hyg. 1976;25:273.
8. Abdel-Salam E, Abdel-Fattah M. Prevalence and morbidity of *Schistosoma haematobium* in Egyptian children. A controlled study. Am J Trop Med Hyg. 1977;26:463.
9. Abdel Salam E, Abdel Khalik A, Abdel Meguid A, et al. Association of HLA class I antigens (A1, B5, B8 and CW2) with disease manifestations and infection in human schistosomiasis mansoni in Egypt. Tissue Antigens. 1986;23:142–6.
10. Kojima S, Yano A, Sasazuki T, Ohta N. Association between HLA and immune responses in individuals with chronic schistosomiasis japonica. Trans R Soc Trop Med Hyg. 1984;78:325–9.
11. Orris L, Combes FC. Clam digger's dermatitis: Schistosome dermatitis from sea water. AMA Arch Dermatol Syphilol. 1952;66:367.
12. Colley DG, Savage AM, Lewis FA. Host responses induced and elicited by cercariae, schistosomula and cercarial antigenic preparation. Am J Trop Med Hyg. 1977;26(Suppl):88.
13. Hiatt RA, Sotomayor ZR, Sanchez G, et al. Factors in the pathogenesis of acute schistosomiasis mansoni. J Infect Dis. 1979;139:659–66.
14. Moore DL, Grove DI, Warren KS. The *Schistosoma mansoni* egg granuloma: Quantitation of cell populations. J Pathol. 1977;121:41.
15. Warren KS, Domingo EO, Cowan RBT. Granuloma formation around schistosome eggs as a manifestation of delayed hypersensitivity. Am J Pathol. 1967;51:735.
16. Kassis AI, Warren KS, Mahmoud AAF. The *Schistosoma haematobium* egg granuloma. Cell Immunol. 1978;38:310.
17. Olds GR, Mahmoud AAF. Kinetics and mechanisms of pulmonary granuloma formation around *Schistosoma japonicum* eggs injected into mice. Cell Immunol. 1981;60:251.
18. Mahmoud AAF. Regulation of immunopathology in parasitic infections. In: Ogra PL, Jacobs DM, eds. Regulation of the Immune Response. S Karger AG; 1983:267.
19. Warren KS. Determinants of disease in human schistosomiasis. In: Mahmoud AAF, ed. Clinical Tropical Medicine and Communicable Diseases. London: Bailliere-Tindall; 1987:301–31.
20. Colley DG. Dynamics of the human immune response to schistosomes. In: Mahmoud AAF, et al. Clinical Tropical Medicine and Communicable Diseases. London: Bailliere-Tindall; 1987:315–32.
21. Butterworth AE. Potential for vaccines against human schistosomes. In: Mahmoud AAF, ed. Clinical Tropical Medicine and Communicable Diseases. London: Bailliere-Tindall; 1987:465–83.
22. Mahmoud AAF. The ecology of eosinophils in schistosomiasis. J Infect Dis. 1981;145:613–22.
23. Capron A, Dessaint JP, Capron M, et al. Immunity to schistosomes: Progress toward vaccine. Science. 1987;238:1065–72.
24. Ellner JJ, Mahmoud AAF. Phagocytes and worms: David and Goliath, revisited. Rev Infect Dis. 1982;4:698–714.
25. Olveda RM, Domingo EO. Schistosomiasis japonica. In: Mahmoud AAF, ed. Clinical Tropical Medicine and Communicable Diseases. London: Bailliere-Tindall; 1987:397–418.
26. Abdel-Wahab MF, Mahmoud SS. Schistosomiasis mansoni in Egypt. In: Mahmoud AAF, ed. Clinical Tropical Medicine and Communicable Diseases. London: Bailliere-Tindall; 1987:371–98.
27. Lehman JS, Farid Z, Bassily S, et al. Colonic calcification and polyposis in schistosomiasis. Radiology. 1971;98:379.
28. Prata A. Schistosomiasis mansoni in Brazil. In: Mahmoud AAF, ed. Clinical Tropical Medicine and Communicable Diseases. London: Bailliere-Tindall; 1987:349–70.
29. Wilkins A, Gilles H. Schistosomiasis haematobia. In: Mahmoud AAF, ed. Clinical Tropical Medicine and Communicable Diseases. London: Bailliere-Tindall; 1987:333–48.
30. Young SW, Higashi G, Kamel R, et al. Interaction of salmonellae and schistosomes in host parasite relations. Trans R Soc Trop Med Hyg. 1973;67:797.
31. World Health Organization. Progress in assessment of morbidity due to *Schistosoma haematobium* infection: A review of recent literature. Geneva: World Health Organization; 1987.
32. World Health Organization. The Control of Schistosomiasis. Geneva: World Health Organization Technical Report Series 728; 1985:113.
33. Voge M, Bruckner D, Bruce JI. *Schistosoma mekongi* sp. *n.* from man and animals compared with four geographic strains of *Schistosoma japonicum*. J Parisitol. 1978;64:577.
34. Hofstetter M, Nash TE, Cheever AW, et al. Infection with *Schistosoma mekongi* in southeast Asian refugees. J Inf Dis. 1981;144:420.
35. Abdel Wahab MF: Schistosomiasis in Egypt. Boca Raton, FL: CRC; 1982:150.
36. Scrimgeour EM, Gajdusek DC. Involvement of the central nervous system in *Schistosoma mansoni* and *Schistosoma haematobium* infection. A review. Brain. 1985;108:1023–38.
37. Peters PAS, Kazura JW. Update on diagnostic methods for schistosomiasis. In: Mahmoud AAF, ed. Clinical Tropical Medicine and Communicable Diseases. London: Bailliere-Tindall; 1987:419–34.
38. Mahmoud AAF. Praziquantel for the treatment of helminthic infections. In: Stollerman GH, ed. Advances in Internal Medicine. v. 32. Chicago: Year Book Medical Publishers; 1987:193–206.
39. Straus WG. Clinical manifestations of clonorchiasis. A controlled study of 105 cases. Am J Trop Med Hyg. 1962;11:625.
40. Harinasuta T, Bunnag D. Liver, lung and intestinal trematodiasis. In: Warren KS, Mahmoud AAF, et al. Tropical and Geographical Medicine. 2nd ed. New York: McGraw-Hill; In press.
41. Medical Letter. Drugs for parasitic infections. Med Lett. 1988;30:15–24.

266. CESTODES (TAPEWORMS)

THOMAS C. JONES

Segmented worms, or tapeworms, cause illness in humans in either of the two stages of their life cycle: the adult stage, which causes signs and symptoms referable to the gastrointestinal (GI) tract, where the adult tapeworm resides, and the larval stage, which causes signs and symptoms secondary to enlarging larval cysts in various tissues of the mammalian host. These worms have been recognized since the beginning of recorded history beause of the impressive length of the adult (up to 30 feet) and because of the fluid-filled cysts in the larval stage that give meat a "measled" appearance. Four of the more common tapeworms of humans cause primarily GI symptoms because humans are a *definitive* host; these are *Taenia saginata, T. solium, Diphyllobothrium latum*, and *Hymenolepis nana*. The definitive host is the mammal that allows full development of the cestode into an adult segmented worm. *Taenia solium* and *H. nana* also find the human an acceptable *intermediate* host. The intermediate host allows penetration of the intestinal mucosa by the larval stage and survival of this larval form in tissue for varying periods of time. Humans can only support the larval or intermediate stage of *Echinococcus granulosus*, and symptoms due to the large cysts in visceral organs, such as liver and lung, are observed. Since these diseases are quite different from each other, they will be discussed in separate sections after a brief discussion of cestode biology, immunity, and pathogenesis of infection.

BIOLOGY AND LIFE CYCLE

The adult tapeworm is extremely functional, as demonstrated by its two main parts: one, the head, or *scolex*, designed for attachment; the other, the *proglottids*, designed as efficient hermaphroditic egg machines. The *strobila* includes everything except the scolex (e.g., a neck region from which the segments [proglottids] develop). These are at first immature; they then mature and finally become the gravid proglottids at the other end of the worm.

Attachment of the tapeworm to the mucosal surface in the intestinal tract is accomplished by four muscular suction cups on the scolex in *T. saginata*. In *T. solium* a *rostellum* is also present with a group of hooks surrounding it. *Diphyllobothrium latum* has two sucking grooves, which give its head a distinctive appearance.

Tapeworms have, within each proglottid, male and female reproductive organs, a primitive nervous system, a muscular system, and excretory canals. They also have an efficient surface for absorption of nutrients since they lack an alimentary canal.[1] The diet of the host has marked effects on the growth and development of cestodes.[2] The surface of the proglottid demonstrates a pattern of microvilli consistent with an absorptive surface similar to intestinal mucosa of vertebrates.[3]

During development of the proglottids, spermatogenesis and ovarian maturation occur. In compressed stained preparations the vitellaria, ovary, testes, genital atrium, and uterus can be identified. The degree of branching of the uterus and its size relative to the proglottid serve as differential features among organisms (Fig. 1). The fertilized eggs accumulate in large numbers in the gravid uterine horns. These eggs can be released into the host's intestine, or the intact terminal gravid proglottids may separate from the rest of the tapeworm. Both eggs and proglottids can be found in the stool.

Ingestion of these eggs by a susceptible intermediate host provides continuation of the tapeworm life cycle. The eggs develop into larvae (called *oncospheres* or, in the case of *D. latum*, *corocidia*). The oncosphere is capable of penetrating the intestinal mucosa of the intermediate host and migrating in this larval stage.

Development of larvae into the encysted forms differs among the cestodes, and this has led to different terms to describe the encysted stages. The oncospheres of *T. saginata* and *T. solium* each develop into small fluid-filled sacs containing a single head. These are called *cysticerci*, or bladder worms, and are usually less than a few centimeters in diameter. *Cysticercosis* refers to the disease in cattle caused by the intermediate stage larvae of *T. saginata* and the disease caused by the intermediate stage larvae of *T. solium* infection in pigs and humans. In *H. nana* each oncosphere develops into a cystlike larva, but the sac contains no fluid, and it is termed *cystlike* or *cysticercoid*. Similarly, variations in this larval stage in the intermediate hosts of *D. latum* have led to their being termed *procercoid* and *plerocercoid* larvae. An oncosphere that develops a germinal membrane allowing production of many scolices within a single fluid-filled cyst is called a *coenurus*. When membranes can generate other germinal tissue within a cyst (such as brood capsule and daughter cysts) containing numerous scolices, this is termed a *hydatid*. This is the typical cyst of echinococcosis. A slight variation of this kind of larval development is seen in *Echinococcus multilocularis*, in which the germinal membrane is so situated that new cysts develop on the outside of the original cyst. The new scolices do not remain enclosed within the enlarging cyst but instead can spread like a malignant neoplasm into adjacent host tissue.

Ingestion of tissues containing cysts and viable scolices by

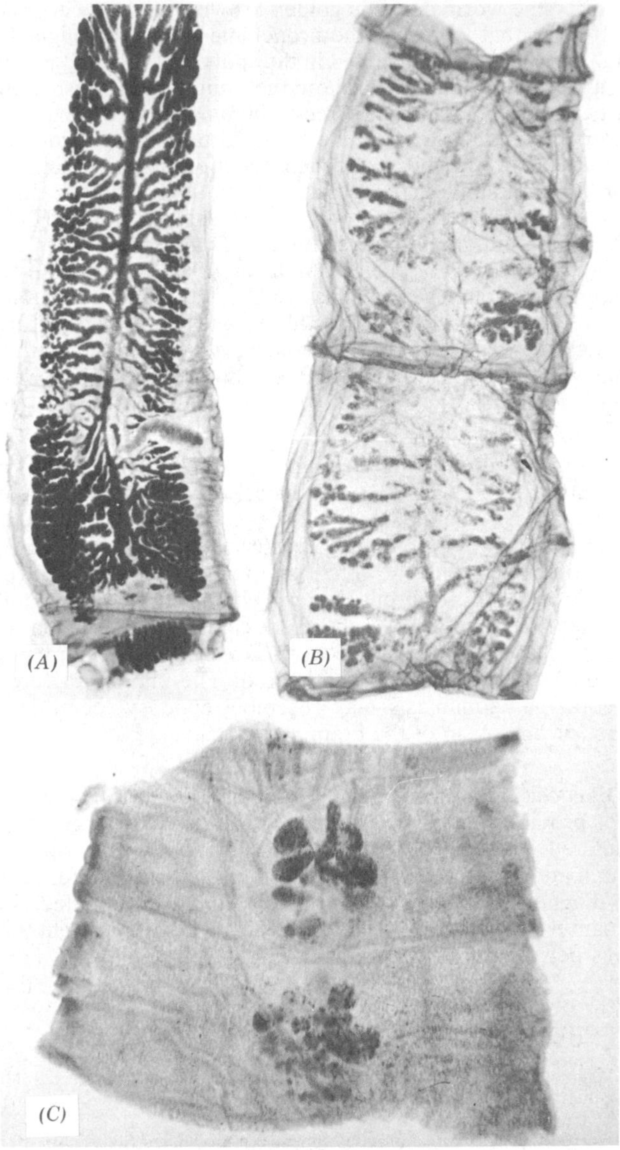

FIG. 1. Stained proglottids of *Taenia saginata* (**A**), *T. solium* (**B**), and *Diphyllobothrium latum* (**C**). Note the different amounts of uterine branching and the relative size of the uterus to the proglottid. (Approx. ×6) (Courtesy of Cornell University Medical College, Department of Internal Medicine, New York, NY.)

the appropriate definitive host allows development of the larval stage into an adult and completion of the life cycle.

PATHOGENESIS AND IMMUNITY

Adult tapeworms within the lumen of the host's intestinal tract usually cause no demonstrable changes in the mucosa or the submucosa. The worm may induce a moderate eosinophilia in some patients. It is possible that some interference with small bowel motility occurs in view of the common intestinal complaints of patients harboring adult worms, but this has not been documented.

Immunity plays only a limited role during adult worm infection, and there is little effect on the duration of infection or the host's susceptibility to reinfection. Immune responses in eradication of *Hymenolepis* infection may be an exception to this general observation.[4] It is possible that immune mechanisms participate in limiting the species specificity of tapeworm infections.[5] In contrast to this limited role for immunologic mechanisms in adult tapeworm infections, immunity during the intermediate stage of larval development is quite important.

The larvae of *T. solium* migrate throughout different tissues of the host, causing varied tissue reactions. The most important site for cysticerci to develop is within the central nervous system. The inflammatory response surrounding the organism begins at the time of larval migration but is markedly intensified as the cyst begins to degenerate. The reaction includes all cellular elements, including neutrophils, fibroblasts, and giant cells. This reaction at the base of the brain causes cysticercic meningitis. In brain substance a localized fluid-filled, space-occupying lesion may increase in size, degenerate, and calcify. In endemic areas, patients with epilepsy may show the numerous calcified lesions on skull x-ray films. Cysticercus may also involve other organs but with much less frequency. Involvement of muscle, skin, eyes, and the heart have all been described.

There is little information on the development of immunity in human cysticercus, and some believe that the presence of cysts in different stages of development is a sign of repeated infections.[6] On the other hand, humoral antibody response and particularly complement-mediated organism lysis,[4] delayed hypersensitivity, and protection of immunized animals has been shown experimentally.[4,7]

The larvae of *E. granulosus* enter the portal circulation, and the majority are trapped in sinusoids of the liver, although some pass through to the lungs, heart, and other sites. An initial inflammatory response may be seen within hours, followed by disintegration of most larvae. If any larvae survive, they can develop into hydatids within 5 days. A barrier of host tissue forms around the developing hydatid, the adventitial membrane, thought to be a combination of compressed host tissue and inflammatory cells. In old cysts this may calcify. The majority of the cysts are found in the right lobe of the liver. Growing cysts can compress and rupture into bile ducts, pleural and peritoneal cavities, bronchi, and the intestinal lumen.

Immunity to *Echinococcus* has been of particular interest because *E. multilocularis* can behave like a malignant tumor. In a series of experiments using *E. multilocularis* in the cotton rat, it has been shown that cell-mediated immunity controls metastatic dissemination during the early phase of infection, and that Calmette-Guérin bacillus suppresses growth and metastases of the hydatid.[8,9] In addition, humoral responses and complement activation occur and have been shown to be effective against protoscolices of *Eichinococcus* spp. in vitro.[4]

During intestinal infection with *H. nana*, in which the cysticercoid stage occurs within villi of the intestinal mucosa, there is usually little evidence of an inflammatory reaction. Only in heavy experimental infections in rats has necrosis and atrophy of the mucosa been described in *H. nana* infections. Immunity may be very important in the control of this infection, since mice given eggs of *H. nana* become resistant to reinfection (i.e., the number of cysticercoids found in the mucosa after challenge is reduced).[10] Treatment of mice with antimouse thymocyte serum completely abolishes this acquired immunity.[11]

TAENIA SAGINATA (THE BEEF TAPEWORM)

The human is the only definitive host for this cestode, and infection occurs when poorly cooked muscle of diseased cattle is ingested. The cysticercus in the muscle of beef resists digestion by gastric juices. The larva is released, in part due to the action of bile salts on the encysted organism, and in approximately 2 months develops into an adult worm. The body of this tapeworm may be more than 30 feet long and can contain more than 1000 proglottids. Eggs produced within the uterus are released into the fecal stream. The embryo of the egg characteristically contains three pairs of hooklets that are useful in identifying *Taenia* species. When these eggs are ingested by cattle, oncospheres penetrate the intestinal wall, and the disease of cattle, *Cysticercus bovis*, results. Buffalo, giraffe, and llama are also recognized as natural hosts.[12]

The infection occurs throughout the world. Its prevalence is determined by the eating (rare meats) and sanitation habits (human fecally contaminated grazing lands) of people. It has been particularly common in Yugoslavia, Moslem countries, Ethiopia, and Kenya. It is common, but less frequent, in Central and South America.

Symptoms due to *T. saginata* infection are minimal and usually consist of mild abdominal cramps and "hunger pains." Weight loss may occur but is most likely secondary to factors other than competition with the worm for the host's intestinal nutrients. Rarely, a bolus of worm has caused intestinal or appendiceal obstruction. The most common complaint is the uncomfortable sensation exerienced by the patient as the motile, muscular proglottids force their way through the anal sphincter. Long strips of worm up to several feet in length can be passed. This frightening experience may be associated with symptoms such as dizziness, headache, weakness, and tingling. The only systemic reaction to the worm is a mild to moderate eosinophilia.

The diagnosis of *T. saginata* is made by examining the stool for proglottids. The uterus has 15–30 lateral branches, a feature distinguishing it from *T. solium* (Fig. 1). It has been stated that the presence of an accessory lobe of the ovary and the absence of a vaginal sphincter muscle are more reliable criteria for identifying *T. saginata*. The eggs of the *Taenia* species are indistinguishable from each other; however, their presence is diagnostic of tapeworm infection and will stimulate a search for proglottids in subsequent specimens. Occasionally a tapeworm is first seen on upper GI and small bowel radiologic studies.

Treatment of *T. saginata* infection of humans has been simplified with the availability of the drug niclosamide. Four tablets (2 g) are chewed thoroughly by the patient after a light meal.[13] This drug has a direct toxic effect on the entire worm, causing it to release from the mucosa and to undergo marked degenerative changes. The drug can occasionally cause abdominal cramps and nausea but is otherwise quite free of side effects. Paromomycin (Humatin), 1 g every 4 hours in four doses, and praziquantel, a single dose of 10 mg/kg, are also effective.[14]

Beef tapeworm infection is prevented when meat is cooked thoroughly. This is particularly important in areas where cysticercosis of cattle is common and where inspection programs are incomplete. Alternatively, prevention of human fecal contamination of grazing lands will break the cycle, as will the careful enforcement of meat inspection procedures.

TAENIA SOLIUM (PORK TAPEWORM)

Adult Stage Taeniasis

As in the case of beef tapeworm, humans are the only definitive hosts of this *Taenia* species. Humans acquire the disease by ingesting measled pork containing the cysticercus. Other vertebrates, such as dogs, cats, and sheep, may serve as intermediate hosts.

The adult *T. solium* may reach a length of 10–20 feet. The eggs produced are morphologically indistinguishable from those of *T. saginata*.

Acquisition of this tapeworm occurs only after the ingestion of measled meat. The infection occurs most commonly in Eastern Europe, Central and South America, Spain, Portugal, and parts of Africa, China, and India.

Clinical manifestations of the intestinal infection are nonexistent or mild. Certain reports have indicated some irritation to the intestinal mucosa, perhaps secondary to embedding of the hooklets in the mucosa. Eosinophilia may also be seen in response to this infection. The diagnosis is made by examining the feces for the eggs and proglottids of *T. solium*. A major technique for distinguishing this organism is identifying in the proglottids a uterus with fewer branches than are seen in *T. saginata* (seven to 12 branches). Seeing the hooklet-lined rostellum of the scolex is the most reliable means of diagnosis of *T. solium*. The absence of an accessory lobe of the ovary and the presence of a vaginal sphincter muscle are also helpful diagnostic features.

Treatment of adult taeniasis due to *T. solium* is the same as outlined for *T. saginata*. Reverse peristalsis and vomiting should be prevented in patients with *T. solium* because of the potential for inadvertently initiating the intermediate stage cycle in humans.

Infection with *T. solium* has been almost completely eliminated in countries where pork is avoided or cooked completely. Control of human fecal contamination of pig feeding areas has also decreased the frequency of infection.

Human Cysticercosis

Cysticercosis in humans is due to infection with eggs of *T. solium* acquired by contact with contaminated human feces. In the intermediate stage it is referred to as *Cysticercus cellulosae*. The routes by which a human may become the intermediate host include contact with food or water contaminated with human feces (the most common source); autoinfection from anus to mouth by a person with the adult tapeworm; and least likely, reverse peristalsis and internal infection. The oncosphere develops rapidly after penetrating the host's intestinal wall. Within 3 weeks the scolex is visible in the cyst, and by 10 weeks it is a fully infective larva. The cyst is usually 0.5–1 cm in diameter and contains the invaginated head (with more than 20 hooklets) and a yellow, viscous fluid. The cyst remains viable for 3–5 years and then degenerates.[6] At this time, cysts evoke an inflammatory reaction and often calcify.

Cysticercosis is most common in Mexico and in certain parts of Africa and South America.

The cysticercus can develop in almost any tissue of the body, and clinical manifestations reflect the organ involved. The most common clinical problem is alteration of central nervous system function. Lesions are most often found within the cerebrum, in the subarachnoid space at the base of the brain (causing the *Cysticercus racemosus* form), and in the ventricles. The cerebellum, brain stem, and spinal cord are less frequently involved. The symptoms and signs include headache, papilledema, hemiparesis, decreased vision, and seizures. Rarely, the disease may manifest as small mass lesions in the eye, heart, muscle, skin, or peritoneal cavity.

Diagnosis is occasionally made by a roentgenogram of the skull or extremities that shows the small calcific densities. The best diagnostic test is computed tomography (CT) of the head, which shows clearly the numerous forms of the space-occupying lesions and hydrocephalus.[15,16] Serologic tests for cysticercus antibodies are of value in confirming the diagnosis. Tests for antibody in serum have recently improved and are now 80–95 percent sensitive and specific.[17] Sensitivity is improved by testing the spinal fluid as well.[15] The best tests available at present are the enzyme-linked immunosorbent assay (ELISA) and the hemagglutination tests using cyst vesicular fluid as antigen.[17] The protein portion, with a molecular weight of 103 kD, appears particularly useful. The diagnosis is sometimes made by identifying the characteristic cysts at surgery.

Until recently, treatment of cysticercosis was usually surgical, either removing the obstructing tissue from the ventricles or inserting ventricular fluid shunts. During the past 5 years, praziquantel has been shown to be effective in killing the larval stage of cysticercosis. Patients with active infection with living organisms have been shown to exhibit marked improvement and even cure of the disease by the use of praziquantel.[15,18] Treatment is with 50 mg/kg/day in three divided doses for 2 weeks.[13] Patients with a long history of seizures, brain calcification and normal cerebrospinal fluid, indicating that the organisms are no longer alive, will not respond to treatment. Praziquantel leads to degeneration of the organism and therefore acute inflammation. This requires the use of corticosteroids in most patients during praziquantel therapy.[15] Symptomatic treatment of seizures is a part of the long-term management of cysticercosis.

Prevention of infection by control of deposition of human excrement is most important. Continued control by meat inspection of human infection with the adult stage of *T. solium* will also decrease the prevalence of cysticercosis.

DIPHYLLOBOTHRIASIS

Humans are but one of the raw-fish-eating mammals that serve as a definitive host for *Diphyllobothrium latum* (the fish tapeworm). Other animals, particularly foxes, dogs, cats, bears, and seals, can also support maturation of the adult tapeworm. Thus, prevention of human fecal contamination of water will not necessarily decrease continued spread of the disease, as it will in *Taenia* infections. The life cycle of *D. latum* is further complicated by the presence of two intermediate stages rather than one.

The adult in the mammalian intestinal tract is the largest tapeworm of humans, reaching 40–50 feet in length. Eggs released from the gravid proglottids are operculated. When they reach fresh water they develop into an embryo over several weeks, releasing a ciliated oncosphere, the *coracidium*. This free-swimming form must be eaten within a few days by a copepod (crustacean). In the copepod the intestinal wall is penetrated by the developing larva, and in the hemocoelom it develops over the next 2 weeks into a *procercoid*. When the copepod is ingested along with other plankton by a fish, the procercoid penetrates the abdominal cavity and changes into a *plerocercoid*, also termed a *sparganum*. If the fish is eaten raw by a mammal, the plerocercoid is released to develop into an adult *D. latum* in 3–4 weeks.

The infection occurs in areas where ingestion of raw fish is common, such as Finland, Sweden, Japan, the Baltic countries, and among Canadian and Alaskan Eskimos. In the United States it is seen among Jewish cooks who sample gelfilte fish during its preparation.

Large numbers of worms can be present in the intestinal tract. In general, symptoms are mild, but complications, such as obstruction, have been recorded, although these are rare. The most important effect of the fish tapeworm on the host is its ability to compete effectively for certain vitamins, such as vitamin B_{12}. This cestode can split the vitamin B_{12}–intrinsic factor complex formed in the lumen of the mammalian intestinal tract. Vitamin B_{12} that is split from the intrinsic factors is not absorbed by the host but may be used by the parasite. Low serum vitamin B_{12} levels result, and in a small percentage of infected persons (2 percent) sufficient decrease in absorption leads to megaloblastic anemia and the associated neurologic symptoms. It has been suggested that a product (lysolecithin) of the tapeworm contributes to the severity of the anemia.[19] Folate absorption by the host may also be diminished in the presence of tapeworm and contribute to this kind of anemia.[6] Decrease in the levels of ascorbic acid, thiamine, and riboflavin has also been described. The typical clinical picture of megaloblastic anemia includes pallor, glossitis, and loss of tongue papillae. Neurologic symptoms and signs include numbness, paresthesias, loss of vibration sense, weakness, and unsteady gait.

Diagnosis of diphyllobothriasis is made by examining stool specimens for the characteristic operculated eggs and proglottids of *D. latum*. The proglottids contain a uterus, which occupies only the middle third of the segment and has relatively few short branches (Fig. 1). This tapeworm may be suspected by its displacement of barium during upper GI radiologic studies. The tapeworm can be confirmed as the cause of anemia by the presence of free gastric acid and of intrinsic factor, and by the correction of vitamin B_{12} deficiency after removal of the worms.

The same drugs used to treat *Taenia* infections are used to treat diphyllobothriasis. A single injection of cyanocobalamin (vitamin B_{12}), 1 mg/ml, and supplemental doses of folic acid and B complex vitamins will reverse the host deficiency of these vitamins. Fish tapeworm infection is prevented by thorough cooking of freshwater fish. Freezing for more than 24 hours may also kill the plerocercoid larvae.

HYMENOLEPIASIS

Hymenolepis nana (the dwarf tapeworm) is the only tapeworm in which the life cycle can be maintained in nature by humans acting as both the definitive and intermediate host. In this situation, humans spread the disease to other humans by fecal contamination of the environment. This infection is found in all parts of the world, particularly in Africa, South America, and Eastern Europe. It is a particularly common problem among children in institutions and in other crowded, unsanitary areas. For instance, at the Willowbrook State School in New York, 8 percent of the children had *H. nana*.[20]

The name of the organism, *nana*, meaning dwarf, is derived from the small size of the adult worm, which measures only 1–2 inches in length. The scolex has suckers and a rostellum with 20–30 hooklets. The eggs produced by gravid proglottids are characteristic because of their clear double membranous shells. When these eggs are ingested the oncospheres are released, penetrate villi in the mucosa of the intestinal tract, and develop into the cysticercoid larvae. After 4 days these larvae rupture from the villus and mature into adult worms in 10–12 days, thus completing the life cycle. This cycle can be repeated within the host's intestinal tract (internal autoinfection), causing gradually increasing numbers of adult worms in an infected child.

The clinical symptoms are related to mucosal irritation by adult and by cysticercoid stages, leading to abdominal cramps and diarrhea. Some children with heavy infections have also had symptoms of dizziness and even seizures, thought to be associated with some neurotoxic product absorbed from these worms.

The diagnosis is established by identifying the double-membrane eggs in the stool. Patients are treated with 2 g/day of niclosamide for 5–7 days. The reason for the longer course of treatment is that recently encysted larvae may keep releasing organisms for 4 days, the duration of cysticercoid development. By treating the patient for more than 5 days, newly developed cysticercoid larvae are released into the intestine and are destroyed during maturation into adult worms. The drug is ineffective against the cysticercoid stage itself. The illness is prevented by interrupting the cycle of fecal contamination. Paromomycin and praziquantel are also effective.

ECHINOCOCCOSIS (HYDATID DISEASE)

The tapeworm *Echinococcus granulosus* persists in nature by infecting dogs, which house the adult worm in their intestinal tract, and sheep or cattle, which become the intermediate hosts by ingesting the contaminated dog feces. The dog ingests beef or lamb containing the larva and completes the cycle. Humans become involved accidentally by contact with contaminated dog feces, as do sheep, and thereby become the hosts for the gradually enlarging cyst, the hydatid. The adult worm in the dog is only a few millimeters in length and has only three proglottids, one immature, one mature, and one gravid. Large numbers of eggs are produced, therefore, not by a worm with growing proglottids but by the large number of scolices within each hydatid capable of developing into hundreds of adult worms. The worm lives for only 6 months. The eggs produced are extremely resistant to environmental changes. When humans ingest these eggs, oncospheres penetrate the mesenteric vessels and are carried to various organs of the body. The liver and lungs are commonly infected and are the sites of development of hydatid cysts.[6]

The small oncosphere undergoes dramatic changes after implantation, increasing in size to 2 or 3 inches in a few months. The embryo develops a central cyst, which has an inner germinal layer containing numerous nuclei. Small masses of these nuclei are at the sites where special germinating cystic structures called *brood capsules* form. These increase in number, become vacuolated, and remain attached to the germinal membrane by a pedicle. The new larvae (scolices) develop in large numbers from the germinal layer within the brood capsule. The hydatid cyst is filled witih fluid, and the developing capsules are filled in turn with cysts and scolices. When a scolex develops from the germinal membrane, there is first a local thickening; then a small bud develops, followed by a complex mature scolex with suckers and hooklets.

The cyst increases in size at the rate of about 1 cm/year. It is this gradually enlarging mass that compresses adjacent host structures leading to the signs of echinococcosis in humans.

Echinococcosis is seen in most sheep- and cattle-raising areas of the world, including Australia, New Zealand, Argentina, Uruguay, Chile, parts of Africa, Eastern Europe, and the Middle East. It is particularly common in Lebanon and Greece.

The most common location of hydatid cysts is the liver (60 percent), usually in the right lobe. Liver tissue adjacent to the cyst shows evidence of cholestasis, congestion, and atrophy. The cyst may rupture into the biliary tract, leading to cholangitis and intermittent ductal obstruction. Cysts may also rupture through the capsule of the liver into the peritoneal cavity or through the diaphragm into the pleural space. Rupture into the peritoneal cavity leads to the formation of new daughter cysts throughout the peritoneum. Cysts growing in the peritoneal cavity can compress and rupture into adjacent abdominal viscera. However, it is most common for the enlarging cyst to remain intact for many years. Splenic, renal, cerebral, ocular, and osseous hydatids have been described. Eosinophilia and the development of antibody to antigens of *Echinococcus* are common. Allergic symptoms, such as urticaria, asthma, and anaphylaxis, are rare.

Hydatid disease is suggested by the presence of a symmetrical tumor mass, detected by palpation, routine roentgenograms of the abdomen or chest, radioactive scans, or sonography. The mass may be outlined by a smooth rim of calcification, a characteristic finding, but one that may not be present in the young growing cysts. Eosinophilia should lead one to obtain a more specific serologic test for echinococcosis. The most reliable test uses partially purified hydatid antigen or antigen 5 in a double designated arc 5 diffusion test (Ref. 21, reviewed in Ref. 4). To facilitate the use of this test, an enzyme immunoassay has been developed to provide a screening step to identify appropriate sera.[22] Complement fixation, hemagglutination, latex agglutination, and bentonite flocculation tests are also available. A skin test using hydatid fluid (Casoni) was relied upon in the past, but because of its low sensitivity and specificity, its use is no longer justifiable.[4] Diagnostic aspiration of intact cysts *should not* be performed because of the danger of rupture and spillage of cyst contacts.

Surgical removal of the intact cyst is the preferred form of therapy. If this is impossible, marsupialization and sterilization of the cyst contents with 2% formalin, hypertonic solutions (such as 30% sodium chloride), and 1% iodine may be effective. Not all cysts need to be removed; however, when they are shown to be enlarging and likely to compromise host organ function, removal is indicated. The use of imidazoles as an adjunct to surgery or in inoperable cases of echinococcosis has been advocated. It is clear that some patients respond well, with decreasing cyst size, control of metastatic foci, or treatment of *E. multilocularis* with mebendazole or albendazole. Albendazole may be superior to mebendazole.[23] It has been used in doses of 10 mg/kg/day for 8 weeks in the treatment of inoperable cases and as preoperative therapy for 4 days. Praziquantel may also have a role in the treatment of echinococcosis. It is very effective in treating the adult worm in the intestinal tract of the dog, and it has been shown to have efficacy in hydatid disease.[24]

The cycle of infection can be broken by keeping dogs free of infection by proper disposal of carcasses and entrails of dead sheep, cattle, and hogs.

Another species of tapeworm causing echinococcosis is *E. multilocularis*. This species has been restricted to the Northern Hemisphere (Canada, Alaska, Northern Europe, USSR). The usual intermediate hosts are small rodents, with foxes and dogs serving as the definitive hosts. Humans acquire this infection by eating fecally contaminated berries and vegetables. The germinal membrane is not confined within a single cyst, and scolices develop in an uncontrolled manner, invading adjacent tissue and spreading to distant sites (metastases). Clincally, it manifests as an infiltrative process of the liver (in 90 percent of the cases). There has been little possibility for surgical resection of this multicystic, invasive process. Imidazoles may be useful in the treatment of this disease.

A new species of *Echinococcus, E. vogeli*, has been identified in South America, and it may be responsible for most human hydatid disease in the region.[25]

OTHER TAPEWORMS OF HUMANS

Humans may become the definitive hosts of two uncommon tapeworms by ingesting larvae present in fleas. These tapeworms usually occur in children because of their close contact witih dogs and cats. The adult of *Dipylidium caninum* measures 5–30 inches in length and resides in the intestinal tracts of dogs, cats, and wild carnivores. Eggs are taken in by fleas or dog lice, in which the cysticercus stage develops. If the infected fleas are ingested by dogs or by humans, the adult form develops. These tapeworms can cause mild GI symptoms, restlessness, and eosinophilia. The diagnosis is established by finding proglottids of the tapeworm in stool. Treatment with niclosamide is the therapy of choice, as in other tapeworm infections for which humans are the definitive hosts.

Humans may also be infected by the rodent tapeworm, *Hymenolepis diminuta*. The disease follows ingestion of a flea that has taken in eggs deposited in rat stool. An adult worm, 5–20 inches in length, develops in the intestinal tract of humans. The most common symptoms are diarrhea and mild abdominal discomfort. *Hymenolepis diminuta* is treated with niclosamide. These tapeworms can be prevented by avoiding contact with fleas, by keeping dogs and cats free of them, and by controlling rodent populations.

Another rare disease acquired from dogs is the tapeworm, *Multiceps multiceps*. The disease, termed *coenurosis*, occurs when humans become the intermediate stage for the larvae developing in a coenurus, a cyst with many scolices but without brood capsules or daughter cysts.[6] The adult tapeworm in dogs or wolves yields eggs that develop into a coenurus in sheep, cattle, horses, antelopes, and other herbivorous mammals. Humans occasionally become infected by also ingesting these eggs. The oncospheres penetrate the intestinal tract, enter the circulation, and reach the central nervous system, where they develop into cysts. The clinical signs are those of intracerebral cystic lesions. This disease may be difficult to distinguish from the more common tapeworm larval infections of humans, cysticercosis and echinococcosis. The most common manifestation is basal arachnoiditis, causing the posterior fossa syndrome. Internal hydrocephalus may be the presenting event. Eye involvement has been described occasionally. Spinal fluid pleocytosis and elevated protein content are common. There is no specific treatment available at this time, although the surgical approaches used in cysticercosis may be helpful in some cases. Drug therapy, such as with imidazoles, should be considered.

REFERENCES

1. Wardle RA, McLeod JA. The Zoology of Tapeworms. Minneapolis: University of Minnesota Press; 1952.
2. Komuniecki R, Roberts LS. Developmental physiology of cestodes: XIV. Roughage and carbohydrate content of host diet for optimal growth and development of *Hymenolepis diminuta*. J Parasitol. 1975;61:427–33.
3. Lumsden RD, Oaks JA, Alworth WL. Cytological studies on the absorptive surfaces of cestodes: IV. Localization and cytochemical properties of membrane-fixed cation binding sites. J Parasitol. 1970;56:737–47.
4. Williams JF. Cestode infections. In: Cohen S, Warren KS, eds. Immunology of Parasitic Infections. 2nd ed. London: Blackwell; 1982:676–714.
5. Isaak DD, Jacobson RH, Reed ND. Thymus dependence of tapeworm (*Hymenolepis diminuta*) elimination from mice. Information Immobiliere. 1975;12:1478–9.
6. Vik R, Tansusat P, Marquez-Monter H, et al. In: Marcial-Rojas RA, ed. Pathology of Protozoal and Helminthic Diseases with Clinical Correlation. Baltimore: Williams and Wilkins; 1971:572–657.
7. Rickard MD, Arundel JH, Adolph AJ. A preliminary field trial to evaluate the use of immunization for the control of naturally acquired *Taenia saginata* infection in cattle. Res Vet Sci. 1981;30:104–8.
8. Baron RW, Tanner CE. The effect of immunosuppression on secondary *Echinococcus multilocularis* infections in mice. Int J Parasitol. 1976;6:37–42.
9. Rau ME, Tanner CE. BCG suppresses growth and metastasis of hydatid infections. Nature. 1975;256:318–9.
10. Ito A, Yamamoto M. The mode of active protection against *Hymenolepis nana* reinfection in mice inoculated with different doses of shell-free eggs. Jpn J Parasitol. 1976;25:247–52.
11. Okamoto K, Zoizumi M. *Hymenolepis nana:* Effect of antithymocyte serum on acquired immunity in mice. Exp Parasitol. 1972;32:56–61.
12. Faust EC, Russell PF, Jung RC. Clinical Parasitology. Philadelphia: Lea and Febiger; 1970:502.
13. Medical Letter editors: Drugs for parasitic infections. Med Lett Drugs Ther. 1986;28:9.
14. Vermund SH, MacLeod S, Goldstein RG. Taeniasis unresponsive to a single dose of niclosamide: Case reprot of persistent infection with *Taenia saginata* and a review of therapy. Rev Infect Dis. 1986;8:423–6.
15. Earnest MP, Reller LB, Filley CM, et al. Neurocysticercosis in the United States: 35 cases and a review. Rev Infect Dis. 1987;9:961–79.
16. Nash TE, Neva FA. Recent advances in the diagnosis and treatment of cerebral cysticercosis. N Engl J Med. 1984;311:1492–6.
17. Larralde C, Laclette JP, Owen CS, et al. Reliable serology of *Taenia solium* cysticercosis withi antigens from cyst vesicular fluid: ELISA and hemagglutination tests. Am J Trop Med Hyg. 1986;35:965–73.
18. Sotelo J, Escobedo F, Rodriguez-Carbajal J, et al. Therapy of parenchymal brain cysticercosis with praziquantel. N Engl J Med. 1984;310:1001–7.
19. Totterman G. On the pathogenesis of pernicious tapeworm anaemia. Ann Clin Res. 1976 (suppl 18);8:1–48.
20. Yoeli M, Most H, Hammond J, et al. Parasitic infections in a closed comunity. Results of a 10-year survey in Willowbrook State School. Trans R Soc Trop Med Hyg. 1972;66:764–76.
21. Coltorti EA, Varela-Diaz VM. Detection of antibodies against *Echinococcus granulosus* arc 5 antigens by double diffusion test. Trans R Soc Trop Med Hyg. 1978;72:226–9.
22. Coltorti EA. Standardization and evaluation of an enzyme immunoassay as a screening test for the seroepidemiology of human hydatidosis. Am J Trop Med Hyg. 1986;35:1000–5.
23. Okelo GBA. Hydatid disease: Research and control in Turkana, Ill. Albendazole in the treatment of inoperable hydatid disease in Kenya—a report of 12 cases. Tran R Soc Trop Med. 1986;80:193–7.
24. Pearson RD, Guenant RL. Praziquantel: A major advance in antihelminthic therapy. Ann Intern Med. 1983;99:195–8.
25. D'Alessandro A, Rausch RL, Cuello C, et al. *Echinococcus vogeli* in man

with a review of polycystic hydatid disease in Colombia and neighboring countries. Am J Trop Med Hyg. 1979;28:303–17.

267. VISCERAL LARVA MIGRANS AND OTHER UNUSUAL HELMINTH INFECTIONS

THEODORE E. NASH

EOSINOPHILIA: CLINICAL SIGNIFICANCE

Eosinophilia is commonly, but not always, associated with invasive helminth infections and, when present, suggests their presence. The degree of eosinophilia can vary dramatically and is influenced by a number of factors. Helminths whose migrations through the tissues are limited, such as infections localized to the skin or intestinal tract, are associated with little or no eosinophilic response. However, helminths that migrate through the internal tissues, either as part of their normal life cycle or ectopically, usually cause eosinophilia. Once the migration is completed and the tissues are no longer exposed to the parasite, eosinophilia wanes. In some helminth infections, the parasites are effectively separated from the host by encystment or a walling off process that limits the eosinophilic response. Acute, as compared with chronic, infections tend to provoke higher responses, as do heavy compared to light infections. Eosinophilia also depends on the ability of the host to respond. Expected responses may not be found in septic patients or in some immunologically impaired patients. Although many helminths may cause eosinophilia, in most instances the possibilities can be narrowed by understanding the possible exposures, life cycle, prepatent and incubation periods, usual disease manifestations, and expected laboratory findings. The diagnostic procedures used to detect infections differ for each parasite, so that a clear idea of the potential causes is essential. The physician must understand the sensitivity of the diagnostic procedures and the abilities of the laboratory personnel performing them. Intestinal ascaris infections are readily detected. On the other hand, some parasitic infections may be difficult to detect, such as the larvae of strongyloides or the ova of intestinal schistosomes, and special stool concentration methods may be needed. Patients may present during the prepatent period before the parasite can be detected, such as in ascariasis or schistosomiasis. Repeated stool examinations eventually diagnose both infections. The usefulness of serologic testing varies, but serology can be very helpful both in suggesting diagnoses and in ruling out infections. Few serologic tests for parasitic infections have been standardized, so the sensitivity and specificity may differ from published values.

Most helminths that infect humans are relatively host-specific to humans, undergo normal migration and development, and are found in typical anatomic locations. However, these helminths may at times undergo abnormal or aborted migrations and cause symptoms or signs because of their unusual or ectopic location. A good example of this is the deposition of schistosome ova and the subsequent granulotomous, inflammatory lesions in the spinal cord or brain in schistosoma infections. Helminths of animals can also infect humans. Some helminths, such as *Echinococcus granulosus* and *Trichinella spiralis,* commonly infect humans, migrate and develop normally, and reside in similar locations, as in the usual host. In contrast, other helminths of animals are unable to develop or migrate normally. Commonly, they undergo prolonged, aberrant migrations or locate abnormally in the tissues as underdeveloped larvae, inciting an eosinophilic inflammation that is responsible for many of the symptoms and signs of these infections. Although a large number of animal parasites may infect humans, most do so rarely. In contrast, some helminths of animals infect humans more commonly and cause distinctive clinical syndromes sometimes associated with characteristic epidemiology, exposure history, and geographic locations (Table 1). More often than not, similar clinical syndromes are caused by a group of related parasites. The diagnosis is suggested on clinical and epidemiologic grounds. Although pathologic examination of tissue can sometimes establish the diagnosis, the detection of larvae is commonly unrewarding. Serologic tests are at times helpful (see below under "Visceral Larva Migrans [Toxocariasis]), but usually are either not fully evaluated, experimental, or unavailable.

Visceral Larva Migrans (Toxocariasis)

Visceral larva migrans (VLM) is a syndrome characterized in its most florid state by eosinophilia, fever, and hepatomegaly. It is caused primarily by infection with *Toxocara canis* but also be *T. cati* and other helminths less frequently.[1–3]

Life Cycle in the Dog

Toxocara canis infects dogs and related mammals by a number of mechanisms.[1] After ingestion of viable eggs, two routes of development occur. In the first, eggs hatch in the small intestine, and the resulting larvae migrate to the liver, lung, and trachea. They are then swallowed and mature in the lumen of the small intestine, where eggs are shed. Other larvae migrate to and remain dormant in the muscles but are capable of development even years after the primary infection, particularly in pregnant bitches. During pregnancy, larvae again develop and infect the pups transplacentally and transmammarily. Not uncommonly, infective larvae are found in the feces of the pups, and the bitch can be reinfected in the process of caring for her pups. Eggs ingested by rodents and other mammals hatch, and the larvae become encapsulated in the muscles for long periods of time. These animals, when eaten, can infect dogs. Eggs are not infectious when passed in the feces and take 3–4 weeks to develop. They are hardy and often remain viable for months. Large numbers of viable eggs contaminate the environment because of the high prevalence of infection in dogs and the ability of eggs to survive relatively harsh environmental conditions.

TABLE 1. Clinical Syndromes Associated with Unusual Helminth Infections in Humans

Clinical Syndrome	*Parasite*	*Usual Host*
Visceral larva migrans	*Toxocara canis* *Toxocara cati*	Dogs Cats
Eosinophilic gastroenteritis	*Anisakis* spp. *Phocanema* spp.	Sea mammals Sea mammals
Cutaneous larva migrans	*Ancylostoma braziliense* *Ancylosloma caninum*	Canines, felines Canines, felines
Eosinophilic meningitis	*Angiostrongylus cantonensis* *Gnathostoma spinigerum*	Rat Felines, other mammals
Pulmonary or cutaneous nodules	*Dirofilaria* spp.	Dog, other mammals
Abdominal angiostrongyliasis	*Angiostrongylus costaricensis*	Cotton rat
Capillariasis	*Capillaria philippinensis*	?
Swimmer's itch	*Trichobilharzia* spp.	Birds

Infection in Humans

Prevalence. Toxocariasis is prevalent wherever dogs are found and *Toxocara* eggs are able to survive. The prevalence of infection or disease in humans is not known, but seroepidemiology studies show wide differences in prevalence depending on the population tested. In the United States, seropositivity ranged from 2.8 percent[4] in an unselected population to 23.1 percent[5] in a kindergarten population in the southern United States to 54 percent[6] in a rural community selected for study because of elevated levels of antibodies noted in a few individuals. None of the seropositive persons had recognizable disease.

Clinical Manifestations. VLM occurs most commonly in children less than 6 years of age.[3,4] Compared to control populations, infected children more commonly have a history of pica and an association with a puppy. Patients are more commonly black and from rural areas. Disease manifestations vary and range from asymptomatic infection to fulminant disease and death, but it is increasingly appreciated that most infections are asymptomatic. Those who come to medical attention most commonly complain of cough, fever, wheezing, and other generalized symptoms.[3–7] The liver is the organ most frequently involved and hepatomegaly is a common finding, although almost any organ can be affected. Splenomegaly occurs in a minority, and lymphadenopathy has been noted. Lung involvement with radiologic findings has been documented in 32–44 percent, but respiratory distress occurs rarely. Skin lesions such as urticaria and nodules have also been described. Seizures have been noted to occur with increased frequency in VLM; however, severe neurologic involvement is infrequent but is associated with increased mortality. Eye involvement in VLM is unusual but has been documented (see below under "Ocular Larva Migrans"). Eosinophilia, usually accompanied by leukocytosis, is the hallmark of VLM. Other laboratory findings include hypergammaglobulinemia and elevated isohemagglutinin titers to A and B blood group antigens, which are due to the host's immune response to cross-reacting antigens on the surface of *T. canis* larvae.

Diagnosis. The diagnosis of VLM is usually suggested clinically by the presence of eosinophilia and/or leukocytosis in a young child accompanied by hepatomegaly or signs and symptoms of other organ involvement. A history of pica and exposure to puppies is common. The diagnosis is definitively confirmed by finding larvae in the affected tissues by histologic examination or by digestion of tissue; however, larvae are frequently not found. The enzyme-linked immunosorbent assay (ELISA) employing extracts or excretory-secretory products of *T. canis* larvae appears specific and useful in confirming the clinical diagnosis.[8] However, toxocara antibody titers in populations without clinically apparent VLM vary dramatically, ranging from 2 percent to over 50 percent. In some populations, elevated titers occur in patients without clinically apparent VLM and are not indicative of an active infection.

Differential Diagnosis. Eosinophilia, fever, and hepatomegaly are caused by other parasitic infections. These include acute schistosomiasis, *Fasciola hepatica* infections, *Ascaris lumbricoides* abscess of the liver, acute liver fluke infections (*Clonorchis sinensis* and *Opisthorchis viverrini*), complications from *Echinococcus* infection of the liver, *Capillaria hepatica,* and other invasive helminths. Diseases not caused by parasitic infections should also be considered. Children with mild disease may only manifest eosinophilia.

Treatment and Management. Most patient recover without specific therapy. Treatment with anti-inflammatory or antihelminthic drugs may be considered with severe complications that are usually due to involvement of the brain, lungs, or heart. There is no proven effective therapy, although thiabendazole, mebendazole, diethylcarbamazine, and other antihelminthics have been used. Indeed, injury to the parasite may provoke a more intense inflammatory response leading to worsening of the clinical picture. Corticosteroids have been used with and without specific antilarval therapy, with some reports of improvement.

Prevention. VLM can be easily prevented by a number of simple but effective measures that prevent *T. canis* eggs from contaminating the environment and children from ingesting eggs. Dogs, particularly puppies, should be periodically tested and treated for *T. canis* and other worms. Pica should be prevented.

OCULAR LARVA MIGRANS

Ocular larval migrans (OLM) is caused by an infection of the eye with *T. canis* larvae.[9] Although a present or past history of clinically recognized VLM has occasionally been noted, almost all patients present with unilateral eye involvement without a past history or present systemic symptoms or signs. Presumably, a larva by chance becomes entrapped in the eye, resulting in an eosinophilic inflammatory mass. Children are most commonly affected and, on the average, are older (mean, 8.6 years in one study) than those diagnosed with VLM. The findings are most commonly those of a posterior or peripheral inflammatory mass. In fact, this entity was first recognized after examination of eyes enucleated for the treatment of presumed retinoblastoma.[9] Eosinophilia, hepatomegaly, and other signs and symptoms of VLM are lacking. The diagnosis is established clinically. Although the serum titers to toxocara larvae are higher than those of a control population,[10] many patients with OLM have low or negative titers. However, elevated vitreous[11] and aqueous fluid titers[12] to toxocara larvae compared to serum levels have been documented and appear to be useful in establishing the diagnosis. There is no specific therapy.

ANISAKIASIS

Anisakiasis is caused by the accidental infection of humans by larvae of marine mammals found in saltwater fish and squid. The clinical syndrome, caused by penetration of larvae into the stomach or small intestine and characterized by upper and/or lower abdominal symptoms, is suggested by a history of ingestion of raw, salted, pickled, smoked, or poorly cooked fish.

Life Cycle in Marine Mammals

Larvae of *Anisakis, Phocanema,* and occasionally other genera can accidentally infect humans.[1,13–15] The adults are found in the stomach of marine mammals. The eggs, passed in the feces, hatch as free-swimming larvae and are ingested by certain crustaceans that, after further development, are infectious for fish and squid. (Infectious larvae can be transferred by ingestion from fish to fish.) In fish the larvae are found in the muscles and/or peritoneal cavity. When ingested by appropriate marine mammals, such as dolphins, seals, and whales, they burrow head first into the stomach, leaving a portion free in the lumen of the host. When consumed by humans, the larvae attempt and many times succeed in burrowing into the stomach or intestine, resulting in typical symptoms.

Clinical Syndrome

Anisakiasis occurs after ingestion of raw or improperly cooked marine fish. The disease, initially recognized in The Netherlands after ingestion of raw herring, is most frequently reported from Japan, where raw fish are commonly eaten. In the United

States, infection is still uncommon but is now more frequently recognized because of increased ingestion of raw fish, particularly salmon. Cod, halibut, pollock, greenling, herring, and mackerel are other implicated fishes.

Clinical manifestations are caused by penetration of worms into the gastrointestinal tract, usually the stomach or lower small intestine, most commonly the ileum.[14–16] Occasionally, throat irritation is followed by coughing up the characteristic worm. Initial invasion is associated with acute symptoms, while the presence of worms for longer periods causes chronic symptoms. The location of the worms and symptoms depends somewhat on the genus, with *Phocanema* more commonly associated with infection of the stomach and *Anisakis* with the intestine. Symptoms usually occur within 48 hours after ingestion, but this pattern is variable. In gastric anisakiasis, patients complain of intense abdominal pain, nausea, and vomiting. Small intestinal involvement results in lower abdominal pain and signs of obstruction mimicking appendicitis. Symptoms may be chronic, sometimes lasting for months and, rarely for years. These symptoms are associated with intestinal masses containing the parasite and are sometimes confused with tumor, regional enteritis, or diverticulitis.

Laboratory Findings. Eosinophilia is usually not present in either gastric or intestinal anisakiasis. Leukocytosis has been noted in almost two-thirds of cases in one series with intestinal involvement.

Diagnosis. Anisakiasis should be considered in anyone with a history of ingestion of raw marine fish and suggestive abdominal symptoms. A definitive diagnosis can be established by endoscopy, radiographic studies, or pathologic examination of tissue. In the upper gastrointestinal tract, worms are found partially embedded in any area of the stomach and may be associated with localized mucosal edema, erosions, or mass lesions.[17,18] Upper gastrointestinal radiographic studies may note the outline of a worm associated with mucosal edema or tumor formation. Removal of the worm during endoscopy definitively establishes the diagnosis and is curative.[16] Intestinal anisakiasis is diagnosed clinically. Varying degrees of thickening of the walls and narrowing of the lumen of the ileum or jejunum are found on radiographic studies.[17,18] Lesions resolve with 2–3 weeks.[17] Occasionally, removal of the intestinal mass is required to establish the diagnosis and effectively treat the patient. Tissues show inflammatory masses, many eosinophils, and the characteristic helminth. Serologic test are not generally available and are of limited usefulness.

Treatment. Symptoms improve spontaneously in most patients without specific therapy, but treatment is hastened by removing worms lodged in the stomach during endoscopy. In one series of intestinal anisakiasis, all 12 patients became asymptomatic by 2 weeks.[17] One Japanese investigator commonly uses antacids after removal of stomach worms.

Prevention. Larvae resist heating up to 50°C, as well as pickling, salting, and some methods of smoking. Infection can be prevented by cooking or freezing fish for 24 hours before ingestion.

CUTANEOUS LARVAL MIGRANS (CREEPING ERUPTION)

Cutaneous larval migrans is characterized as serpiginous, reddened, elevated, pruritic skin lesions usually caused by *Ancylostoma braziliense,* the dog and cat hookworm.[1,19] Other animal hookworms including *A. caninum, Uncinaria stenocephala, Bunostomum phlebotomum,* and others; the human hookworms, *Strongyloides stercoralis* and *Gnathostoma spinigerum;* and, rarely, insect larvae can cause similar findings. Like human hookworms, *A. braziliense* larvae infect dogs and cats by burrowing through the skin. The adults reside in the intestine and shed eggs, which undergo development into infectious larvae outside the body in places protected from desiccation and temperature extremes, such as sandy, shady areas around beaches or under houses. Infections are most common in warmer climates such as the southeastern United States and occur in children more commonly than in adults. Larvae penetrate the skin, causing tingling followed by itching, vesicle formation, and typically raised, reddened, serpiginous tracks that mark the prior route of the parasite.[1,19,20] In severe infections, persons may have hundreds of tracks. Little further development of the parasite occurs. Usually there are few, if any, systemic symptoms, but some reports have documented lung infiltrates and, rarely, severe lung dysfunction and recovery of parasites in the sputum. Eosinophilia has been noted in some infections.[20] The skin lesions are readily recognized, and the diagnosis is made clinically. Biopsy specimens usually show an eosinophilic inflammatory infiltrate, but the migrating parasite is usually not identified. For this reason, biopsies are usually not indicated to establish the diagnosis. Without treatment, skin lesions gradually disappear.[21] Both topical (10% aqueous suspension qid)[22] thiabendazole and oral administration (25 mg/kg bid for 2 days)[21] are effective. In one study, most patients treated with thiabendazole responded within the first week compared to the more than 4 weeks required for comparable improvement in the placebo-treated group.[21]

EOSINOPHILIC MENINGITIS DUE TO HELMINTHS

Infection of humans with larvae of *Angiostrongylus cantonensis,* the rat lung worm, is characterized by invasion of the brain leading to signs and symptoms of meningitis associated with an eosinophilis pleocytosis in the cerebiospinal fluid (CSF) and peripheral eosinophilia.[23] The adults of *A. cantonensis* reside in the lungs of rats.[1] Eggs hatch in the lungs and the larvae are swallowed, expelled in the feces, and seek an appropriate molluscan intermediate host, where the parasite develops into the infective third-stage larva. Infective larvae are found in a number of molluscs including slugs, land snails, and a land planarian, but are also found in a number of unrelated animals including freshwater prawns, land and coconut crabs, and frogs. After ingestion by rats, the infective larvae migrate to the brain and eventually to the lungs. In humans, the migration of the larvae to the brain causes eosinophilic meningitis. Although adult worms do not develop in humans, it is unclear if the larvae remain in the central nervous system or are killed elsewhere.

Epidemics and sporadic infections occur most commonly in the South Pacific,[24] Southeast Asia,[25] and Taiwan.[26] The most commonly recognized sources of human infection are raw or undercooked snails, prawns, or crabs. Contamination of foods such as leafy vegetables by larvae deposited by slugs or snails may also occur. Clinical manifestations vary, and although fatalities occur, particularly in massive infections, most patients have a relatively uncomplicated course.[23–26] In one well-characterized epidemic the incubation period ranged from 1 to 6 days after ingestion of infected snails.[24] Symptoms include headache, stiff neck, fever, rash, pruritus, abdominal pain, constitutional complaints, nausea, and vomiting. Neurologic involvement varies from no complaints to paresthesias and pain, weakness, various focal neurologic findings (sixth and fouth cranial nerve palsies are frequently noted), coma, and death. In general, the patients do not appear to be as ill as in bacterial meningitis. Signs of meningitis are frequent but nonspecific. CSF leukocytosis with more than 10 percent eosinophils is always present. CSF glucose values are usually normal, but depressed values have been noted. A fall followed by a rise in the number of eosinophils in the CSF at 50–90 days has been documented in some patients, although they are usually asymptomatic.

The diagnosis is established clinically, but occasionally a characteristic larva is found in the CSF at the time of lumbar puncture. The diagnosis is suggested by a history of eating raw or partially cooked implicated foods and recent travel to endemic areas. Serologic tests have not been fully evaluated, nor are they readily available.

There is no proven therapy. Repeated CSF lumbar punctures appear to be helpful in treating associated headaches, presumably by decreasing CSF pressure. Recovery usually occurs by 2 months, although prolonged symptoms and signs have occasionally been noted.

Infection with *G. spinigerum* may also cause eosinophilic meningitis.[27,28] Infections occur mostly in Southeast Asia, particularly in Thailand and Japan. The larvae migrate in the tissues and clinically cause intermittent swellings that are most noticeable in the subcutaneous tissues. Occasionally, the larvae find their way into the nervous system and cause a myeloencephalitis. Permanent neurologic deficits and death are more common than with *A. cantonensis,* and red cells are more likely to be found in the CSF. The diagnosis is established clinically, and serologic tests not generally available. Other helminth infections such as cysticercosis and paragonimiasis can result in eosinophilic meningitis. Recently, fatal eosinophilic meningoencephalitis due to infection with the raccoon ascarid, *Bayliscaris procyonis,* has been described. Infection occurs after the accidental ingestion of *B. procyonis* eggs, which are found in raccoon feces.[29]

ABDOMINAL ANGIOSTRONGYLIASIS

Clinical manifestations of human infections of *Angiostrongylus costaricensis* are due to penetration and development of the parasite in the lower small bowel and adjacent colon, and are characterized by abdominal pain, vomiting, and a right lower quadrant mass.[30] In the normal host, the rat, adult parasites reside in the arteries and arterioles of the ileocecal area of the intestine. Eggs deposited in the tissue hatch, and the larvae escape in the feces. They are then ingested by the slug intermediate host and after further development become infectious for rats after ingestion. After maturation in the lymphatics, the larvae penetrate the arterioles and arteries in the ileocecal area of the rat, where they reside as adults. In humans, the parsite follows a similar pattern of migration, except that eggs are retained in the tissues and larvae do not appear in the feces. Adults are found most commonly in the arteries and arterioles around the ileocecum and deposit eggs there. Both the eggs and worms provoke an inflammatory response resulting in occluded vessels and an eosinophilic, granulomatous, edematous mass. Infections of humans, most commonly children, have recently been recognized in Central and South America and, rarely, in Africa. The manner of human infection is not usually known, but it may occur after accidental ingestion of infected slugs or after ingestion of foods contaminated with larvae deposited in the mucous slime trail of slugs. Patients are mild to moderately ill and complain of abdominal pain and tenderness, vomiting and fever, and, in about 50 percent of the cases,[31] a right lower quadrant mass. Surgery reveals that the cecum, ascending colon, ileum, and appendix are involved to varying degrees. The syndrome resembles appendicitis, except for the presence of eosinophilia and leukocytosis. The diagnosis is suspected clinically and confirmed by examination of biopsied or excised areas. X-ray findings are nonspecific and show filling defects and spasticity of the ileum, cecum, or colon. Serologic tests are not generally available. Most patients undergo laparotomy with removal of the inflamed areas; the natural history of infected children is unclear. Some clinically diagnosed children are treated with diethylcarbamazine and thiabendazole (75 mg/kg/day for 3 days) without undergoing surgery. It is not known whether specific antihelminthic therapy is effective. Massive ascaris infections may present with intestinal masses and may be confused with infections due to *A. costaricensis.*

DIROFILARIASIS

Accidental infections in humans with *Dirofilaria* result most commonly in a lung nodule or subcutaneous mass. Two groups of parasites of the genus *Dirofilaria* accidentally infect humans.[1] The clinical presentations are generally different, reflecting the final location of the adults in the usual animal host. The adult worms of *Dirofilaria immitis,* the dog heart worm and the only important parasite in the first group, reside in the right heart and pulmonary vessels and are usually located in the lungs in humans. *Dirofilaria immitis* is transmitted by mosquito to its most common host, the domesticated dog, and other related mammals. After development in the subcutaneous tissues, the parasites migrate as young adults to the right heart and pulmonary vessels. In humans, the immature filariae migrate similarly but do not develop and instead die, causing a local vasculitis leading to pulmonary infarcts. Histologic examination usually reveals a dead worm in an infarct with vasculitis and with granulomatous and sometimes eosinophilic inflammation. Most infections occur in the southeastern United States, where infections and transmission to dogs and accidental transmission to humans are most likely to occur. Persons are asymptomatic in more than half of the infections and show a coin lesion on a routine chest x-ray film.[32,33] Others complain of cough, chest pain, or hemoptysis, most likely due to pulmonary infarction. In some instances, lung infiltrates are noted that resolve into nodules.[34] Eosinophilia occurs in less than 15 percent of cases. The diagnosis can be made with certainty only by biopsy. Although serologic tests are available, their sensitivity and specificity are not adequate to rule out other potential life-threatening conditions such as a tumor.

Adults of the second group of filariae (subgenus *Nochtiella*) reside in the subcutaneous tissue of various mammals and cause inflammatory subcutaneous masses in humans.[35] These parasites include *Dirofilaria tenuis* (raccoon), *D. ursi* (bear), *D. subdermata* (porcupines), and *D. repens* (dog and cat in Europe and Asia). Patients present with inflammatory subcutaneous masses containing increased numbers of eosinophils. As in infections with *D. immitis,* there are few if any systemic symptoms, and eosinophilia is not usually present. The diagnosis is established by biopsy. However, careful inspection of the entire tissue may be needed to find the parasite. In addition, both groups of parasites can be differentiated histologically, with *D. immitis* demonstrating a smooth cuticle compared to the ridged cuticle in the *Nochtiella* group.

Capillariasis

Capillaria philippinensis inhabits the small bowel of humans, causing diarrhea and malabsorption.[36] Infections have been recognized in the Philippines, primarily in northern Luzon, and in Thailand, and one case has been reported from Iran. The life cycle is incompletely understood; however, fresh fish contain larvae infectious for humans and birds.[37] The latter may be an important reservoir host. After raw freshwater fish are eaten, the larvae invade the jejunum and ileum, and the resulting adults produce both eggs and larvae. Unlike almost all helminths that infect humans, with the exception of *S. sterocoralis,* the parasite multiplies in the gut, a process known as *autoinfection,* resulting in an overwhelming infection. In fulminant cases, autopsies reveal a thickened, edematous small bowel with a flattened mucosa containing a mononuclear infiltrate. Numerous adults, larvae, and eggs are present in both the lumen and the mucosa. Almost all the signs and symptoms are related to progressive diarrhea and malabsorption. Patients complain of borborygmi, abdominal pain, vomiting, weight loss, and malaise resulting in wasting, abdominal distension, and edema. Laboratory examinations document the typical findings of protein-losing enteropathy; fat, mineral, and vitamin malabsorption; and electrolyte loss.[36] Fever and eosinophilia are uncommon, although eosinophilia has been noted after therapy. The diagnosis is established by detecting the characteristic *Trichuris trichiuria*-like ova or larvae in the stool. No serologic tests are available. Untreated, mortality rates of up to one-third have been documented, but specific antihelminthic therapy is effective and lifesaving.[38] Therapy in the past included thiabendazole, 25 mg/kg for 30 days, but mebendazole, 200 mg/kg bid po for 20 days, has largely supplanted thiabendazole treatment. Relapses should be treated with prolonged courses of therapy. Infection is prevented by eating properly cooked freshwater fish.

SWIMMER'S ITCH

Cercariae, the infective form of a large number of blood flukes of birds (commonly *Trichobilharzia*), nonhuman mammals, and, less commonly, human schistosomes can cause a characteristic dermatitis in humans associated with penetration of the cercariae into the skin.[1] Unlike human schistosomes, cercariae from animals do not develop further in humans, and their clinical manifestations are almost always limited to the skin. Infections are frequent in many areas of the world but are particularly common in persons exposed to the freshwater lakes of the northern United States. However, infections also occur after exposure to saltwater (clam digger's itch). Although there is variation in the clinical manifestations after the initial exposure, symptoms are typically mild and sometimes go unnoticed.[39,40] The patient complains of itching followed by the appearance of macules at the site of penetration of the cercariae. By 24 hours, the macules have disappeared and begin to be replaced by papules. After repeated exposures, reactions occur earlier than 24 hours after exposure and are more severe. Papules are larger and associated with erythema, itching, and edema. By 4–7 days symptoms subside, but in severe cases they may last for weeks.

Cercariae are produced by various species of molluscs, which are the intermediate hosts of these parasites. Control of infection can be obtained by ridding bathing areas of the molluscan intermediate host or the definitive host or by avoiding infected bodies of water. There is no specific antihelminthic therapy.

REFERENCES

1. Beaver PC, Jung RC, Cupp EW. Clinical Parasitology. Philadelphia: Lea and Febiger; 1984.
2. Beaver PC, Snyder CH, Carrera GM, et al. Chronic eosinophilia due to visceral larva migrans. Report of three cases. Pediatrics. 1952;9:7.
3. Huntley CC, Costas MC, Lyerly BS. Visceral larva migrans syndrome: Clinical characteristics and immunologic studies in 51 patients. Pediatrics. 1965;36:523.
4. Glickman LT, Schantz PM. Epidemiology and pathogenesis of zoonotic toxocariasis. Epidemiol Rev. 1981;3:230.
5. Worley G, Green JA, Frothingham TE, et al. *Toxocara canis* infection: Clinical and epidemiological associations with seropositivity in kindergarten children. J Infect Dis 1984;159:591.
6. Jones WE, Schantz PM, Foreman K, et al. Human toxocarias in a rural community. Am J Dis Child. 1980;134:967.
7. Mok CH. Visceral larva migrans. A discussion based on review of the literature. Clin Pediatr. 1968;7:565.
8. Glickman L, Schantz P, Dombroske R, et al. Evaluation of serodiagnostic tests for visceral larva migrans. Am J Trop Med Hyg. 1978;27:492.
9. Wilder HC. Nematode endophalmitis. Trans Am Acad Ophthalmol Otolaryngol. 1950;55:99.
10. Schantz PM, Meyer D, Glickman LT. Clinical, serologic, and epidemiologic characteristics of ocular toxocariasis. Am J Trop Med Hyg. 1979;28:24.
11. Biglan AW, Glickman LT, Lobes LA. Serum and vitreous *Toxocara* antibody in nematode endophthalmitis. Am J Ophthalmol. 1979;88:898.
12. Felberg NT, Shields JA, Federman JL. Antibody to *Toxcara canis* in the aqueous humor. Arch Ophthalmol. 1981;99:1563.
13. Smith JW, Wootten R. *Anisakis* and anisakiasis. In: Lumsden WHR, Muller R, Baker JR, eds. Advances in Parasitology. v. 16. London: Academic Press; 1978:93–163.
14. Van Thiel PH, Kuipers FC, Roskam RTH. A nematode parasitic to herring, causing acute abdominal syndromes in man. Trop Geogr Med. 1960;2:97.
15. Yokogawa N, Yoshimura H. Clinicopathologic studies of larval anisakiasis in Japan. Am J Trop Med Hyg. 1967;16:723.
16. Sugimachi K, Inokuchi K, Ooiwa T, et al. Acute gastric anisakiasis. Analysis of 178 cases. JAMA. 1985;253:1012.
17. Matsui T, Iida M, Murakami M, et al. Intestinal anisakiasis: Clinical and radiologic features. Radiology. 1985;157:299.
18. Kusuhara T, Watanabe K, Fukuda M. Radiographic study of acute gastric anisakiais. Gastrointest Radiol. 1984;9:305.
19. Kirby-Smith JL, Dove WE, White GF. Some observations on creeping eruption. Am J Trop Med Hyg. 1929;9:179.
20. Hitch JM. Systemic treatment of creeping eruption. Arch Dermatol Syph. 1947;55:664.
21. Katz R, Ziegler J, Blank H. The natural course of creeping eruption and treatment with thiabendazole. Arch Dermatol. 1965;91:420.
22. Davis CM, Israel RM. Treatment of creeping eruption with topical thiabendazole. Arch Dermatol. 1968;97:325.
23. Rosen L, Chappell R, Laqueur GL, et al. Eosinophilic meningoencephalitis caused by a metastrongylid lung-worm of rats. JAMA. 1962;179:620.
24. Kliks MM, Kroenke K, Hardman JM. Eosinophilic radiculomyeloencephalitis: An angiostrongyliasis outbreak in American Samoa related to ingestion of *Achatina fulica* snails. Am J Trop Med Hyg. 1982;31:1114.
25. Punyagupta S, Juttijudata P, Bunnag T. Eosinophilic meningitis in Thailand: Clinical studies of 484 typical cases probably caused by *Angiostrongylus cantonensis*. Am J Trop Med Hyg. 1975;24:921.
26. Yii C-Y. Clinical observations on eosinophilic meningitis and meningoencephalitis caused by *Angiostrongylus cantonensis* on Taiwan. Am J Trop Med Hyg. 1976;25:233.
27. Chitanondh H, Rosen L. Fatal eosinophilic encephalomyelitis caused by the nematode *Gnathostoma spinigerum*. Am J Trop Med Hyg. 1967;16:638.
28. Punyagupta S, Juttijudata P. Two fatal cases of eosinophilic myeloencephalitis, a newly recognized disease caused by *Gnathostoma spinigerum*. Trans R Soc Trop Med Hyg. 1968;62:801.
29. Fox AS, Kazacos KR, Gould NS. Fatal eosinophilic meningoencephalitis and visceral larva migrans caused by the raccoon ascarid *Bayliscaris procyonis*. N Engl J Med. 1985;312:1619.
30. Morera P, Cepedes R. *Angiostrongylus costaricensis* n. sp. (Nematoda: Metastrongyloidea), a new lungworm occurring in man in Costa Rica. Rev Biol Trop. 1971;18:173.
31. Loria-Cortes R, Lobo-Sanahuga JF. Clinical abdominal angiostrongylosis: A study of 116 children with intestinal eosinophilic granuloma caused by *Angiostrongylus costaricensis*. Am J Trop Med Hyg. 1980;29:538.
32. Beaver PC, Orihel TC. Human infection with filariae of animals in the United States. Am J Trop Med Hyg. 1965;14:1010.
33. Cifferri F. Human pulmonary dirofilariasis in the United States: A critical review. Am J Trop Med Hyg. 1982;31:302.
34. Kochar AS. Human pulmonary dirofilariasis: Report of three cases and brief review of the literature. Am J Clin Pathol. 1985;84:19.
35. Beaver PC, Wolfson JS, Waldron MA. *Dirofilaria ursi*-like parasites acquired by humans in the northern United States and Canada: Report of two cases and brief review. Am J Trop Med Hyg. 1987;37:357.
36. Whalen GE, Strickland GT, Cross HJ, et al. Intestinal capillariasis: A new disease in man. Lancet. 1969;1:13.
37. Cross JH, Basaca-Sevilla V. Experimental transmission of *Capillaria philippinensis* to birds. Trans R Soc Trop Med Hyg. 1983;77:511.
38. Whalen GE, Rosenberg EB, Gutman RA. Treatment of intestinal capillariasis with thiabendazole, bithionol, and bephenium. Am J Trop Med Hyg. 1971;20:95.
39. Olivier L. Schistosome dermatitis, a sensitization phenomenon. Am J Hyg. 1949;49:290.
40. MacFarlane MV. Schistosome dermatitis in New Zealand. Part II. Pathology and immunology of cercarial lesions. Am J Hyg. 1949;50:152.

SECTION I. ECTOPARASITES

268. INTRODUCTION

BARBARA BRAUNSTEIN WILSON
PEYTON E. WEARY

An ectoparasite is an organism that lives on or in the skin of its host and derives sustenance from that host. This term can include those organisms that live on the host only long enough to obtain a blood meal as well as those that burrow into the superficial layers of the skin and remain there for weeks to months or even years if left untreated. The burrowing organisms are sometimes grouped separately under the category of "endoparasites"; however, in general as well as in this text, the term *ectoparasites* includes these organisms. Biting or vesicating arthropods that inflict injury on humans but do not parasitize the host are excluded from this category.

Arthropods are classified as either insects (Hexapoda) or arachnids (Arachnida) (Table 1). Insects are six-legged arthropods and include lice, bedbugs, fleas, and flies. The arachnids have eight legs and include mites, ticks, and spiders. Only selected ectoparasites will be discussed in the following chapters.

Although ectoparasitic infestations are no longer a major public health problem in the United States, on a worldwide basis ectoparasitic disease and diseases transmitted by ectoparasites as vectors present very serious health and economic problems. In tropical climates very few natives escape some type of ectoparasitic disease, and the consequences of such disease can be multilating, incapacitating, debilitating, or fatal. Not only do ectoparasites cause enormous economic losses to humans by virtue of human parasitism, they also parasitize domestic animals used for food and contribute greatly to the malnutrition found in underdeveloped countries.

Many bacterial, spirochetal, viral, rickettsial, helminthic, and protozoal diseases can be transmitted to humans by arthropod vectors. Table 2 lists some arthropod-borne diseases.

ERADICATION, CONTROL AND PREVENTION

For most ectoparasites, eradication is not a practical approach because of the substantial reservoir of wild animals that allow perpetuation of the species. Elimination of some species from domestic animals is reasonable in certain climates but is a virtual impossibility in other regions of the world. In many instances improvements in sanitation and improved socioeconomic factors will do more to reduce parasitism for humans than will attempts to eliminate the organisms.

It is sometimes possible, however, to control important diseases in humans and livestock by controlling the arthropod vectors responsible for the transmission of those diseases. Such large-scale programs often require cooperation between governmental agencies at various levels for effective implementa-

TABLE 1. Classification of Selected Important Ectoparasites (Phylum Arthropoda)

Common Name	*Class*	*Order*	*Family*	*Genus*	*Species*
Lice (pediculosis)	Insects (Hexapoda)	Anoplura (sucking lice)	Pediculidae	*Pediculus*	*P. humanus* var. *corporis*—human body louse
					P. humanus var. *capitis*—human head louse
				Phthirus	*Ph. pubis*—pubic or "crab" louse
Bedbugs	Insecta (Hexapoda)	Hemiptera (true bugs)	Cimicidae (bedbugs)	*Cimex*	*C. lectularius*—temperate regions
					C. hemipterus—tropical regions
Fleas	Insecta (Hexapoda)	Siphonaptera (fleas)	Pulicidae	*Pulex*	*P. irritans*—human flea
				Ctenocephalides	*C. canis*—dog flea
					C. felis—cat flea
			Tungidae	*Tunga*	*T. penetrans*—borrowing flea (tungiasis)
Flies (myiasis)	Insecta (Hexapoda)	Diptera (true Flies)	Gasterophilidae	*Gasterophilus*	*G. intestinalis*—creeping eruption
			Oestridae	*Dermatobia*	*D. hominis*—human botfly (myiasis)
			Calliphoridae	*Auchmeromyia*	*A. luteola*—Congo floor maggot (myiasis)
				Cordylobia	*C. anthropophaga*—tumbu fly (myiasis)
				Chrysomyia	*Ch. bezziana*—Old World screw worm fly (myiasis)
				Lucilia	*L. sericata*—green bottle fly (myiasis)
				Phormia	*P. regina*—black bottle fly (myiasis)
				Calliphora	Several species—blue bottle fly (myiasis)
			Sarcophagidae	*Sarcophaga*	Several species—flesh flies (myiasis)
				Wohlfahrtia	Several species—flesh flies (myiasis)
Mites	Arachnida	Acarina	Sarcoptidae	*Sarcoptes*	*S. scabiei* var. *hominis*—itch mites (human scabies)
					S. scabiei var. *canis*—canine scabies
			Trombiculidae	*Eutrombicula*	E. alfreddugési—common chigger
			Pyemotidae	*Pyemotes*	*P. ventricosus*—straw or grain itch
			Dermanyssidae	*Dermanyssus*	*D. gallinae*—fowl mite
				Ornithonyssus	*O. bacoti*—rat mite
Ticks	Arachnida	Acarina	Ixodidae (hard tick)	*Dermacentor*	*D. variabilis*—dog tick
					D. andersoni—wood tick
				Amblyomma	*A. americanum*
					A. cajennense
				Ixodes	*I. holocyclus*
					I. dammini
			Argasidae (soft tick)	*Ornithodoros*	*O. moubata*

TABLE 2. Selected Diseases Transmitted by Arthropods

Infectious Disease	*Vector*
Arboviruses (including yellow fever, dengue fever, and encephalitis)	Mosquitoes and ticks
Babesiosis	Hard ticks
Brugia malayi (*Wuchereria bancrofti*)	Mosquitoes
Endemic relapsing fever (*Borrelia duttoni*)	Soft ticks
Epidemic relapsing fever (*Borrelia recurrentis*)	Human body lice
Epidemic typhus (*Rickettsia prowazekii*)	Human body lice
Filariasis	Mosquitoes
Leishmaniasis (*Leishmania* spp.)	Phlebotomid flies
Lyme disease (*Borrelia burgdorferi*)	Hard ticks
Malaria (*Plasmodium* spp.)	Mosquitoes
Murine typhus (*Rickettsia mooseri*)	Rat fleas, lice
Onchocerciasis (*Onchocerea volvulus*)	Black flies
Plague (*Yersinia pestis*)	Rat fleas
Q fever (*Coxiella burnetii*)	Hard ticks
Rickettsial pox (*Rickettsia akari*)	Mouse mites
Rocky Mountain spotted fever (*Rickettsia rickettsii*)	Hard ticks
Scrub typhus (*Rickettsia tsutsugamushi*)	Mites
Trench fever (*Rickettsia quintana*)	Human body lice
Trypanosomiasis (African)	Tse tse flies
Trypanosomiasis (American; *Trypanosoma cruzi*)	Triatomid drugs
Tularemia (*Francisella tularensis*)	Flies, hard ticks

tion. Methods used to control arthropod vectors include the use of insecticides or environmental manipulations that would limit breeding and spread of the undesirable arthropod species. Unfortunately, the widespread use of insecticides may induce the development of resistance in the arthropods, thereby requiring the development of new and different toxic agents. Extensive use of insecticides may create anxiety and controversy because of the possible hazardous effects they may have on the environment.

Diseases spread by arthropods may be limited not only by controlling the arthropod vector but also by preventing access of the arthropod to its host. When possible, fine screening should be used on windows and doors to prevent entrance of flying arthropods into the dwelling. Insect repellents that are applied to the skin or clothes are also an effective means for protecting humans from arthropods. The active ingredient in most of the insect repellents available in the United States contain either *N,N*-diethyl-*m*-toluamide (deet) or ethyl hexanediol.

There is a great need to more clearly define the factors that are responsible for attracting ectoparasites to the skin of humans, and important work is underway in this area. When we understand these basic epidemiologic facts more precisely, better insect repellents can be produced, which would greatly improve the ability of humans to prevent parasitism. As with other organisms, cycles of increased pathogenicity occur among parasitic organisms, as attested to by epidemics of scabies. Better knowledge of the mechanisms whereby this occurs may also help in controlling these disorders.

BIBLIOGRAPHY

DeOreo GA. Pigeons acting as vector in acariasis caused by *Dermanyssus gallinae* (DeGeer 1778). Arch Dermatol. 1958;77:422.

Fox JG. Outbreak of tropical rat mite dermatitis in laboratory personnel. Arch Dermatol. 1982;118:676.

Hall RD. A case of human myiasis caused by *Phormia regina* (Diptera: Calliphoridae) in Missouri, USA. *J Med Entomol.* 1986;23:578–9.

Hewitt M, Barrow GI, Miller DC, et al. Mites in the personal environment and their role in skin disorders. Br J Dermatol. 1973;89:401.

Honig PJ. Arthropod bites, stings, and infestations: Their prevention and treatment. Pediatr Dermatol. 1986;3:189–97.

James MT. Herm's Medical Entomology. 6th ed. New York: Macmillan; 1969.

Kunkle GA, Greiner EC. Dermatitis in horses and man caused by straw itch mite. J Am Vet Med Assoc. 1982;181:467.

Lane RP, Lovell CR, Griffiths WAD, et al. Human cutaneous myiasis. A review and report of three cases due to *Dermatobia hominus*. Clin Exp Dermatol. 1987;12:40–5.

Moschella SL, Hurley HJ, eds. Dermatology. Philadelphia: WB Saunders; 1985.

269. LICE (PEDICULOSIS)

BARBARA BRAUNSTEIN WILSON
PEYTON E. WEARY

THE ORGANISMS

The order Anoplura contains more than 200 species, of which only members of the family Pediculidae are parasitic for humans. The species of importance are ***Pediculus humanus*** var. ***corporis***, the human body louse, ***Pediculus humanus*** var. ***capitis***, the human head louse, and ***Phthirus pubis***, the pubic or crab louse. (For the complete classification see Table 1, Chapter 266.)

Eggs laid by the fertilized adult female are firmly glued to body hairs or fibers of clothing and appear as small globoid or oval protrusions called nits (Fig. 1). Approximately 7–10 days after deposition small voracious nymphs emerge that must feed within 24 hours to survive. After 2–3 weeks and three successive molts, the mature adults mate. The fertilized females produce 250–300 eggs over the next 20–30 days before death.

The body louse and the head louse are virtually identical—small (2–4 mm), grayish white, flattened, wingless, and elongated parasites with pointed heads. From each segment of the fused triple-segmented thorax a pair of jointed legs protrude that end in clawlike projections (Fig. 2). The pubic louse is distinctively different in shape, being much wider and shorter than its cousins are and resembling a crab, whence its nickname.

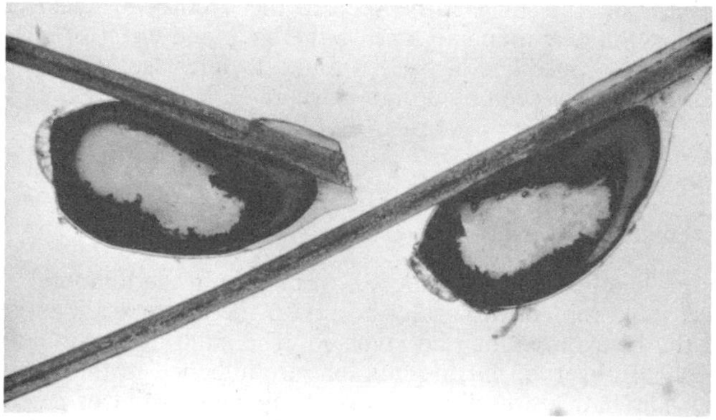

FIG. 1. Nits (ova) of *Pediculus humanus* var. *capitis* attached to scalp hairs.

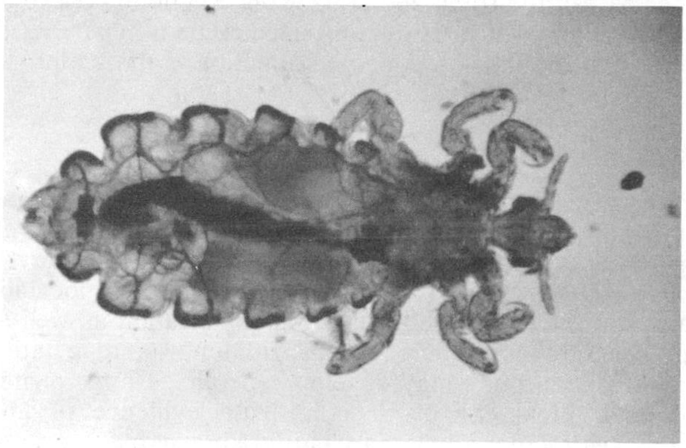

FIG. 2. *Pediculus humanus* var. *capitis.*

EPIDEMIOLOGY

Lice infestations have been observed in virtually every inhabited area of the world. At times of war, overcrowding, or widespread inattention to personal hygiene, major epidemics have occurred.

PEDICULOSIS CAPITIS

Persons from all social and economic backgrounds can become infested with head lice, and infestations can reach epidemic proportions, especially among schoolchildren. The disease is uncommon in blacks and is seen most frequently in young females, presumably because of their longer hair styles. Lice are transferred by close personal contact and the sharing of hats, combs, and brushes.

PEDICULOSIS CORPORIS

Pediculosis corporis (body lice) is seen primarily where there is overcrowding and poor sanitation. The body louse lays its eggs and resides in the seams of the clothing rather than on the skin of its host. The body louse leaves the clothing only to obtain a blood meal from its host. Nits present in the clothing are viable for up to 1 month. Besides causing significant cutaneous disease, the human body louse is a vector for epidemic typhus, trench fever, and louse-borne relapsing fever.

PHTHIRUS PUBIS

Phthirus pubis (pubic lice) infestation is transmitted by sexual or close body contact and less often by the sharing of personal clothing or bedding. The pubic louse resides primarily in the pubic hair but can also be seen in the eyebrows, eyelashes, axillary hair, and coarse hair on the back and chest of males. The pubic louse has also been found to infest scalp hair (unpublished case seen by author Barbara B. Wilson, M.D.).

CLINICAL MANIFESTATIONS

Pediculosis Capitis

Adult head lice and nits localize primarily in the temporal and occipital areas of the scalp; however, the entire scalp as well as the beard area may be involved. The adult lice may be difficult to observe, but the nits that are attached to the base of the hairshaft are easily seen. The major complaint of persons afflicted with head lice is pruritus of the scalp. Scratching leads to excoriations and secondary bacterial infection that is manifested by weeping and crusting of the scalp as well as tender occipital and cervical adenopathy. A pruritic, symmetric, morbilliform eruption may develop on the body, especially on the upper part of the trunk and arms. This eruption is felt to be an "id" reaction, which is hypothesized to be a hypersensitivity reaction to the inflammation and infection in the scalp.

Pediculosis Corporis

Except in cases of very severe infestations, the adult louse is not usually seen on the skin but rather in the seams of the clothing. Patients complain of pruritus and develop small erythematous macules, papules, and excoriations that are located primarily on the trunk. Secondary impetiginization as well as an "id" reaction may occur. Persons with long-standing untreated pediculosis corporis may develop generalized hyperpigmentation and thickening of the skin with evidence of numerous healed excoriations, an entity known as "vagabonds' disease."

Phthirus Pubis

The primary complaint of perons infested with *Phthirus pubis* is marked pruritus of all affected areas, which may include axillary and coarse truncal hairs and eyelashes as well as pubic hair. One may or may not see erythematous macules and papules with excoriations and secondary infection, and if it occurs, it is usually less severe than that seen in pediculosis capitis and corporis. The nits and occasionally the adult pubic lice can be seen attached to the base of the hairs.

Small gray to bluish macules measuring less than 1 cm in diameter may be seen on the trunk, thighs, and upper parts of the arms. These lesions, known as "maculae cerulae," are felt to be caused by an anticoagulant that is injected into the skin by the biting louse. Infestation of the eyelashes by pubic lice can cause crusting of the lid margins. In such cases, the nits are readily seen at the base of the lashes.

THERAPY

Symptomatic treatment of pruritus in all three types of infestation consists of adequate doses of antihistamines such as hydroxyzine, 25 to 50 mg three to four times daily. Medium- to high-potency topical corticosteroids such as triamcinolone or fluocinolone cream should be applied to affected areas two to three times daily. When secondary bacterial infection is present, *Staphylococcus aureus* is a frequent cause, and patients should be treated with a systemic antibiotic such as erythromycin or dicloxacillin, 250 mg four times a day for 10 days.

Pediculosis Capitis

There are several different pediculicides that can be used to effectively treat head lice. These include 1% lindane or gamma benzene hexachloride shampoo (Kwell), pyrethrin liquid with piperonyl butoxide (RID, A-200 pyrinate liquid), 1% permethrin creme rinse (Nix) and 0.5% malathion lotion (Prioderm).

A recent study has shown that, when compared with lindane and the pyrethrins, malathion lotion was most effective and was the only product that showed excellent ovicidal activity.[1] Objections to malathion include an unpleasant odor and a treatment time of 8–10 hours as compared with the 10-minute therapy required by the other agents. Unfortunately, malathion is no longer available in the United States.

All of the other available pediculicides are probably comparable in efficacy. They are all cosmetically acceptable and easy to use, each requiring only a 10-minute application to the scalp. This treatment is repeated in 1 week.

Lindane is the only pediculicide that requires a prescription, but it offers no advantage over the other agents. There have been toxic side effects reported with lindane including seizures and even death; however, toxicity is not a problem when treating pediculosis because of the short periods of skin contact required and therefore minimal systemic absorption of the agent.

Nits should be removed from the hairs by applying a solution of equal parts of vinegar and water and then combing the hair with a fine-toothed comb that has been dipped in vinegar. Combs and brushes should be soaked in the pediculicide for 1 hour. Articles of clothing that have been in contact with an infested individual within the previous 3 days should be laundered in the hot cycle of the washing machine or dry cleaned.

Pediculosis Corporis

Body lice can be eradicated by either discarding the clothing, when practical, or by laundering clothes in the hot cycle and then carefully ironing the seams of clothing. Body lice can also be eliminated by dusting the clothing with either 1% malathion powder or 10% DDT powder.

Phthirus Pubis

As for pediculosis capitis, *Phthirus pubis* may be treated with lindane, permethrin, pyrethrin, or malathion as described above. The pediculicides should be applied to all affected areas except the eyelids. Eyelid infestation can be effectively treated by applying a thick layer of petrolatum to the eyelid margins twice a day for 8 days. Clothes and bedding of an infested individual should be laundered as described for pediculosis capitis.

PREVENTION

The spread of pediculosis capitis can be minimized by improving living conditions and personal hygiene and by avoiding the sharing of hats, combs, and hair brushes. Classroom epidemics are best prevented by frequent examination of the scalps of the students. Body lice are rarely seen in those with good personal hygiene who change their clothes frequently. Pubic lice are best prevented by avoiding sexual or close body contact with infested individuals.

REFERENCE

1. Meinking TL, Taplin D, Kalter DC, et al. Comparative efficacy of treatments for pediculosis capitis infestations. Arch Dermatol. 1986;122:267–71.

BIBLIOGRAPHY

Honig PJ. Arthopod bites, stings and infestations: their prevention and treatment. Ped Dermatol. 1986;3:189–97.
Moschella SL, Hurley JH. eds. Dermatology. Philadelphia: WB Saunders; 1985.

270. SCABIES

BARBARA BRAUNSTEIN WILSON
PEYTON E. WEARY

Scabies is a disease of great antiquity and possibly the cause for the "7-year itch" known to humanity for centuries. Napoleon's troops during the Russian campaign were thought to have had rampant scabies. Periodic epidemics of scabies are thought to occur at approximately 30-year intervals and persist for approximately 15 years.[1]

THE ORGANISMS

The organisms that cause scabies belong to the order Acarina, the family Sarcoptidae, and the genus *Sarcoptes*. Human scabies is caused by the itch mite *Sarcoptes scabiei* var. *hominis*. The scabies mite is one of the cutaneous parasites that burrow into the skin of its host, and therefore, some experts prefer to call it an "endoparasite" rather than an "ectoparasite."

Two to three eggs are laid daily by the fertilized female in burrows several millimeters in length created at the base of the stratum corneum of the epidermis. After 72–84 hours larvae emerge and, after several moults, become adult mites and mate after about 17 days. The males die shortly, but the gravid females proceed to burrow and complete the life cycle.

The full-grown adult female is only about 0.35 mm in length, rounded, with three pairs of short stubby legs. The organisms may be demonstrated in the burrows by an application of mineral oil to the skin overlying a burrow followed by vigorous scraping to the point where minimal bleeding occurs (Fig. 1). Under the microscope the scraped material may demonstrate mites, mite feces, or eggs. It is often difficult to demonstrate the organisms in older lesions or in nodular lesions.

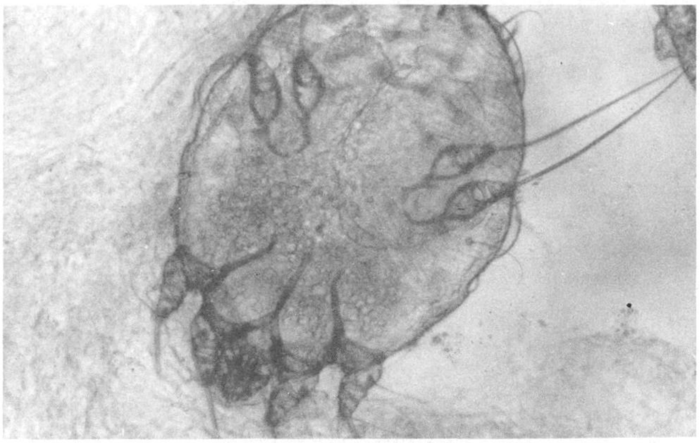

FIG. 1. Organism of scabies in a wet mount preparation.

EPIDEMIOLOGY

The disorder is worldwide in distribution, but the actual prevalence is unknown. There has been a substantial increase in the incidence of scabies in the United States since 1973. Epidemics have been associated with both world wars, so conditions of poverty, poor hygiene, overcrowding, malnutrition, and sexual promiscuity probably are contributory factors. The cyclic pattern may reflect the development of immunologic resistance of certain population groups at risk. Although the scabies mite can cause significant cutaneous disease, it is not a vector for infectious diseases.

Scabies is transmitted by intimate personal contact, often sexual in nature, but casual contact, including that of nursing attendants, may be adequate for transmission, and institutional epidemics can occur. The clinical picture of scabies is usually fairly characteristic but is extremely variable depending on the degree and duration of the infestation. Fastidious individuals who wash frequently may have fewer and more subtle lesions, while those who neglect themselves are more likely to have extensive cutaneous disease.

CLINICAL MANIFESTATIONS

Human Scabies

Most individuals infested with the scabies mite complain of intense itching that is usually more severe at night. Erythematous papules and excoriations are noted in areas of predilection such as the interdigital web spaces, wrists, elbows, anterior axillary folds, periumbilical skin, pelvic girdle, buttocks, penis, knees, and sides of the feet. In infants and small children the palms, soles, face, and scalp may be affected. One should look carefully for classic linear burrows, particularly in the interdigital spaces and on the penis (Fig. 2). Assistance in demonstrating the burrows can be provided by the application of blue or black ink to the skin overlying a suspected burrow. By capillary action the ink will be pulled into the burrow. Removal of the excess external ink with an alcohol swab will leave the ink in the burrow, thus demonstrating its presence. It is the burrow containing the organism and its eggs and feces that will yield a positive scraping. At times, scabies in infants may be vesicular or even bullous, and secondary pyoderma may obscure the underlying disorder. A background eczematous eruption may be present and is probably related to the development of hypersensitivity by the host to the scabies mite. Treatment with topical or systemic corticosteroids may alter the clinical picture such that the disease remains unrecognized, an entity known as "scabies in-

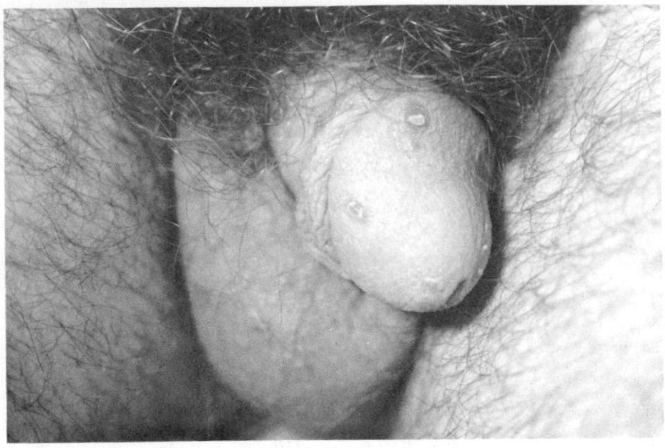

FIG. 2. Typical lesions of scabies on the penis.

cognito." Scabies may even present as an urticarial eruption, and IgE deposits have been demonstrated in cutaneous vessels of scabetic lesions and in high concentrations in the serum of such patients.[2] A small percentage of infested persons have a nodular variant of scabies that presents as scattered pruritic reddish brown nodules, particularly on the penis and scrotum and in the axillae. These lesions are thought to be a manifestation of strong delayed hypersensitivity to retained mite products and may take weeks or months to disappear after adequate therapy.

Norwegian Scabies

A severe variant of scabies known as Norwegian or crusted scabies can occur, usually in institutionalized persons, particularly those with Down syndrome, and in individuals who are debilitated or immunosuppressed.[3,4] Many thousands of mites inhabit the skin and produce widespread scaling and thickening of the skin that may resemble psoriasis. Thickened nails, alopecia, generalized hyperpigmentation, eosinophilia, and pyoderma with lymphadenopathy may also occur.

Animal Scabies

Occasionally dogs with sarcoptic mange caused by *Sarcopte scabeii* var. *canis* can be responsible for minor epidemics of mite bites, usually in members of a family. The lesions are pruritic, papular, or urticarial and are located primarily on the trunk, arms, axillae, and breasts. No burrows are seen since the organisms cannot complete their life cycle on humans. Eradication of the infestation of the animal produces prompt subsidence of the condition.

THERAPY AND PREVENTION

The treatment of scabies remains controversial.[5–7] The most extensively used topical medication, 1% lindane lotion or gamma benzene hexachloride (Kwell), has been faulted for its potential neurotoxicity, particularly in infants. Most cases of toxicity, however, have been caused by improper use of the medication or by its use in premature infants or individuals with underlying cutaneous disorders that allow greater absorption of the agent into the blood stream.[7,8] If the lotion is applied from the neck to the toes and left on for 12 hours in nonpregnant adults and 6 hours in children older than 1 year, it appears to safely exterminate the mites in most cases. A second application of lindane is recommended 1 week after the first.

Lindane should be used with caution, or alternate therapy should be used in persons with widespread dermatitic or scaly skin because their skin may demonstrate increased systemic absorption of topical medications. All patients should be instructed not to apply the lindane more than twice in a 1-month period. It is recommended that alternate therapy be given for pregnant women and young children under 1 year of age. Crotamiton (Eurax) 10% cream or lotion or 5% precipitated sulfur in petrolatum are probably safe to use in children under 1 year old and in pregnant women; however, its safety has not been established in clinical trials.[6] Treatment failure is quite high for these agents. Eurax is applied to the skin and left on for 24 hours. A second application is recommended the next day. Precipitated sulfur is applied daily for 3 days. The scalp should be treated in infants and young children, but this is not necessary in adults in whom the scalp is spared.

One common mistake made by patients that may contribute to the lack of eradication of the mite is the failure to reapply whatever medication is lost after washing the hands during the treatment period. Medication should be reapplied after each washing since the hands are common sites for infestation. The nails should be cut before therapy. Because of the high infestivity rate, other members of the family and intimate friends should be treated simultaneously. Recently worn clothes and bed linens should be laundered by using the hot cycle of the washing machine or dry cleaned.

Although it is not yet available, permethrin 5% dermal cream shows promising results, when compared with lindane, as an effective antiscabetic agent in preliminary trials.[9]

Patients should be treated symptomatically with an oral antihistamine such as hydroxyzine, 25 mg to 50 mg three to four times a day. A soothing topical antipruritic preparation such as Sarna lotion, which contains menthol and phenol, can be applied as needed and may provide some relief from itching. Topical corticosteroids can also be applied two to three times daily to decrease inflammation and pruritus. Patients should be warned that, after adequate therapy, pruritus, probably caused by retained mite parts, may persist for up to 2 weeks.

REFERENCES

1. Cohen HB. Scabies continues. Int J Dermatol. 1982;21:134.
2. Chapel TA, Krugel L, Chapel J, et al. Scabies presenting as urticaria. JAMA. 1981;246:1440.
3. Youshock E, Glazer SD. Norwegian scabies in a renal transplant patient. JAMA. 1981;246:2608.
4. Rav RC, Baird IM. Crusted scabies in a patient with acquired immunodeficiency syndrome. J Am Acad Dermatol. 1986;15:1058–9.
5. Orkin M, Maibach HI. Current views of scabies and pediculosis pubis. Cutis. 1984;33:85–97.
6. Honig PJ. Arthropod bites, stings and infestations: Their prevention and treatment. Pediatr Dermatol. 1986;3:189–97.
7. Rasmussen JE. Lindane—a prudent approach. Arch Dermatol. 1987;123:1008–10.
8. Friedman SJ. Lindane neurotoxic reaction in non-bullous congenital ichthyosiform erythroderma. Arch Dermatol. 1987;123:1056–8.
9. Taplan D, Meinking TL, Porcelain SL, et al. Permethrin 5% cream: A new treatment for scabies. J Am Acad Dermatol. 1986;15:995–1001.

271. MAGGOTS (MYIASIS)

BARBARA BRAUNSTEIN WILSON
PEYTON E. WEARY

Myiasis is the term used for the invasion of living, necrotic, or dead animal or human tissues by the larvae (maggots) of various dipterous (two-winged) flies. For many centuries maggots have been observed to infest necrotic tissue of wounds and dead animals, and their cleansing action on necrotic tissue was once used medically to débride wounds. Animal myiasis can adversely affect the economy of a culture that is dependent on domestic animals.

THE ORGANISMS

Some of the more important dipterous flies capable of producing myiasis belong to the genera *Gasterophilus, Dermatobia, Auchmeromyia, Cordylobia, Chrysomyia, Lucilia, Phormia, Calliphora, Sarcophaga,* and *Wohfartia* (see Table 1 in Chapter 268 for further classification).

The life cycle of the flies varies with the species and method of infestation. In general, the eggs may be deposited on unbroken skin, on wounds, or in dead tissue. The larvae hatch from the eggs and then burrow into the adjacent tissue where they mature into adult flies that emerge to complete the cycle. The larvae are variable in size and shape but often appear as small, white, elongated, soft segmented worms (grubs) (Fig. 1.).

Cattle and many other mammals provide the most common reservoirs for most of these insects.

EPIDEMIOLOGY

While more often observed in tropical areas, human cases of myiasis have been reported from many countries, and animal infestations occur worldwide.[1] Human myiasis is more common where sanitation and personal hygiene are poor.

There are three types of myiasis:

1. Specific—the larvae infest only the living tissue of various organs.
2. Semispecific—the larvae normally infest bodies of dead animals or other dead organic matter, but on occasion the eggs or larvae are deposited in diseased (necrotic) tissue of living hosts from which they may sometimes invade viable tissue.
3. Accidental—the larvae are ingested and find their way into the gastrointestinal or genitourinary tissues. For more details one should consult standard texts on tropical diseases.[2]

CLINICAL MANIFESTATIONS

While maggots are not carriers of infectious agents, the maggots themselves may cause significant disease. The clinical manifestations of myiasis vary greatly depending not only on the species of maggot but also on the localization of the infestation. Myiasis may be a benign, mild, even asymptomatic disease, or it may be severe and catastrophic. Maggots may parasitize the skin, vaginal/urinary tract, gastrointestinal tract, and various cavities of the body such as the nasal pharynx, sinuses, eyes, and auditory canals.[3] Cutaneous disease caused by maggots may present in any of the following ways:

1. Furuncle-like lesions in which rupture of the abscess often results in the release of the maggot.

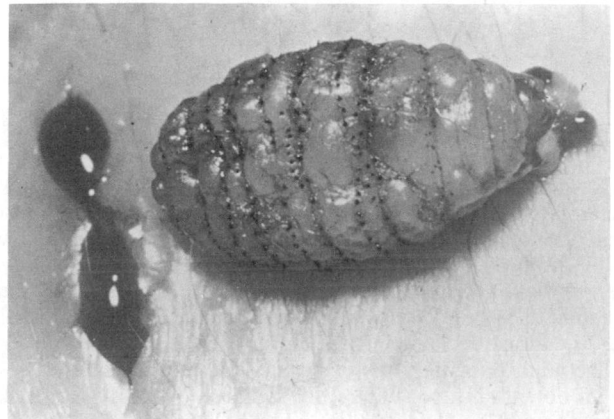

FIG. 1. Organism removed from the skin of a patient with myiasis.

2. A "creeping eruption" in which the larva creates a painful, serpiginous, erythematous line in the wake of its path through the skin. This particular lesion can be distinguished from creeping eruption caused by hookworms (cutaneous larva migrans) because the maggots move more slowly through the skin and are larger and therefore more likely to be seen with the unaided eye.
3. Infestation of open wounds and necrotic tissue, which may lead to purulence and secondary infection.
4. Transient, pruritic or painful, erythematous, cutaneous swellings may occur where the burrowing larva travels slowly through the skin. Eventually an opening may develop in the skin through which one end of the larva may protrude.
5. Larvae of flies can also develop on the external surface of the skin, normally in folds, where they feed on accumulated epidermal debris. This type of infestation is most likely to occur in individuals with an eczematous eruption or poor personal hygiene.

Ophthalmomyiasis refers to invasion of the eye by larvae of dipterous flies. In some instances, the larvae remain external to the globe, and in others either the anterior chamber or posterior segment of the eye may be affected, in which case subretinal tracks can be identified. Orificial involvement of such sites as the ear, nose, urethra, gingiva, or vagina may produce severe and obscure problems. In some cases, migration to various internal organs (e.g., brain) may be incapacitating or life-threatening. The disorder tungiasis, in which the mature flea *Tunga penetrans* invades the skin of humans to enter a gravid state, may resemble myiasis.

SAPROPHYTIC DISEASE

When maggots remain confined to dead tissue, aside from the repulsive nature of the process, they often produce surprisingly little additional damage, although suppuration may be a complication.

TREATMENT

Parasitic and saprophytic myiasis lesions are usually treated surgically, although certain cultures have developed unique and ingenious methods for removal by virtue of promoting migration of the larvae into dead animal tissue strapped to the skin. Débridement of devitalized tissue may prevent saprophytic infestation.

REFERENCES

1. Morgan RJ, Moss HB, Honska WL. Myiasis. Arch Dermatol. 1964;90:180.
2. Binford CH, Connor DH. Pathology of Tropical and Extraordinary Diseases. Washington, DC: Armed Forces Institute of Pathology; 1976.
3. Leclerq M. Entomological Parasitology. 1st ed. Oxford, England: Pergamon Press; 1969.

BIBLIOGRAPHY

Hall RD. A case of human myiasis caused by *Phormia regina* (Diptera: *Calliphoridae*) in Missouri, USA. J Med Entomol. 1986;23:578–79.

Lane RP, Lovell CR, Griffiths WAD, Sonnex TS. Human cutaneous myiasis. A review and report of three cases due to *Dermatobia hominis*. Clin Exp Dermatol. 1987;12:40–45.

Moschella SL, Hurley HJ. eds. Dermatology. Philadelphia: WB Saunders; 1985.

272. MITES (INCLUDING CHIGGERS)

BARBARA BRAUNSTEIN WILSON
PEYTON E. WEARY

THE ORGANISM

Mites belong to the order Acarina, and over 30,000 different species have been described. Mites may be free living or may parasitize plants, insects, animals, or humans.[1] Adult mites have a fused head and thorax and four pairs of legs. The size of the mite varies with the species.

Mites are important medically not only because they can cause significant cutaneous disease in humans, but some species are also known vectors of infectious diseases such as rickettsialpox, scrub typhus, murine typhus, Q fever, tularemia, plague, and tsutsugamushi fever.

The mites that are most likely to affect humans include chiggers (harvest mites), animal mites, food mites, grain mites, and scabies. Except for the mite *Sarcoptes scabeii* var. *humanus* (see Chapter 268), which parasitizes only humans, mites are only occasional predators of humans. Unlike the scabies mites, the occasional predators do not burrow into their hosts' skin, but they may remain attached to the skin surface for minutes to hours while they obtain a blood meal.

CHIGGERS

The common chigger, also known as the harvest mite or red bug, belongs to the family Trombiculidae and is prevalent in the southern United States, especially during the summer and fall months. Chiggers live on grasses and shrubs, and it is the larval form that attaches itself to passing animals or humans. After obtaining a blood meal, the larvae drop off, and within hours, extremely pruritic, erythematous papules appear (Fig. 1). Occasionally the larvae may be seen in the center of the lesions, but these have usually dropped off or have been scratched off by the time the eruption appears. Lesions are most frequent on the legs and are especially likely to occur where clothing is snug against the skin such that it may impede the migration of the larvae. The severity of the eruption depends on the allergic sensitivity of the host to the mite's oral secretions. If the reaction is severe, fever and/or a background eczematous eruption may develop. Erythema multiforme-like eruptions have also occurred.

ANIMAL MITES

Humans may be the occasional host of mites that are the usual parasites of animals. Canine scabies (*Sarcoptes scabeii* var. *canis*) from infested dogs and *Cheyletiella* species infesting the coats of dogs, cats, and rabbits may bite humans. The rat mite (*Ornithonyssus bocoti*), the fowl mite (*Dermanyssus gallinae*), and the mouse mite (*Allodermanyssus sanguineus*) can likewise temporarily infest humans exposed to the infested animals.

FOOD, GRAIN, AND STRAW MITES

Grocerymen and warehouse workers who handle food such as cheese, flour, or vegetables infested with mites and farmers exposed to grain or straw mites may likewise develop pruritic eruptions secondary to mite bites. The clinical appearance for these as well as the animal mite bites consists of pruritic erythematous macules and papules that may show a central red punctum with vesiculation or crusting.

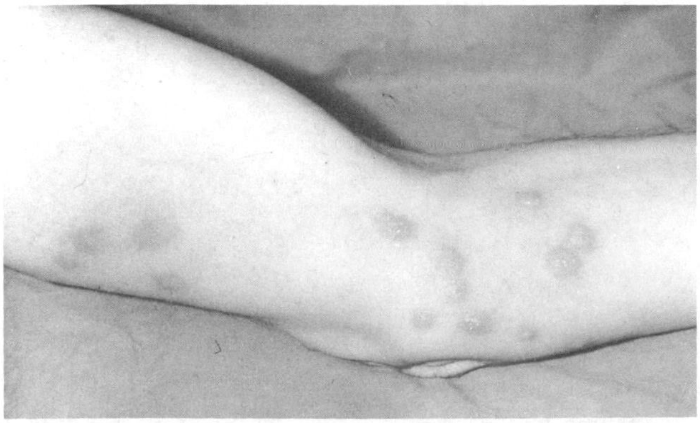

FIG. 1. Intense reaction to chigger bites.

OTHER MITES

Demodex folliculorum, the follicle mite, commonly infests the hair or sebaceous follicles of the face and eyelids of humans and some animals. They are suspected of producing, at times, facial granulomas and eyelid irritation as seen in acne rosacea, but their pathologic role is not clear. An allergy to house dust mites is suspected as a causative factor in some cases of atopic eczema and respiratory allergies.

The house dust mite antigen has also been implicated as a possible etiologic factor in Kawasaki syndrome.[2,3]

TREATMENT AND PREVENTION

Treatment of mite bites is symptomatic. Oral antihistamines such as hydroxyzine, 25 to 50 mg by mouth three to four times daily, and the application of potent topical steroids such as fluocinonide cream twice a day give temporary relief of pruritus. Most lesions resolve spontaneously within a week. Elimination of animal or fomite sources of infestation or spraying an infested area with chemicals may reduce or eliminate human mite infestations. Insect repellents are useful for prevention.

REFERENCES

1. Moschella SL, Hurley JH, eds. Dermatology. Philadelphia: WB Saunders; 1986.
2. Furusho K, Ohba I, Soeda T, et al. Possible role for mite antigen in Kawasaki disease. Lancet. 1981;8239:194.
3. Globe MP, Brogden R, Joffe LS, et al. Kawasaki syndrome and house dust mite exposure. Pediatr Infect Dis. 1986;5:644–8.

BIBLIOGRAPHY

DeOreo GA. Pigeons acting as vector in acariasis caused by *Dermanyssus gallinae* (DeGeer 1978). Arch Dermatol. 1958;77:422.

Fox JG. Outbreak of tropical rat mite dermatitis in laboratory personnel. Arch Dermatol. 1982;118:676.

Hewitt M, Barrow GI, Miller DC, et al. Mites in the personal environment and their role in skin disorders. Br J Dermatol. 1973;89:401.

Kunkle GA, Greiner EC. Dermatitis in horses and man caused by straw itch mite. J Am Med Assoc. 1982;181:467.

273. TICKS (INCLUDING TICK PARALYSIS)

BARBARA BRAUNSTEIN WILSON
PEYTON E. WEARY

Ticks are classified into three families, the Ixodidae (hard ticks), the Argasidae (soft ticks), and the Nuttalliellidae.[1] Ticks of the Ixodidae family are most likely to parasitize humans and will be the primary subject of discussion in this chapter; however, the soft tick, *Ornithodoros moubata*, is an important vector of endemic relapsing fever caused by *Borrelia duttoni* (for further classification see Table 1 in Chapter 266).

The adult hard tick has eight legs and a hard plate (scutum) on its dorsal surface, which distinguishes it from the soft tick (Figs. 1 and 2). There are four stages in the life cycle of the tick: egg, larva, nymph, and adult, all of which except the egg

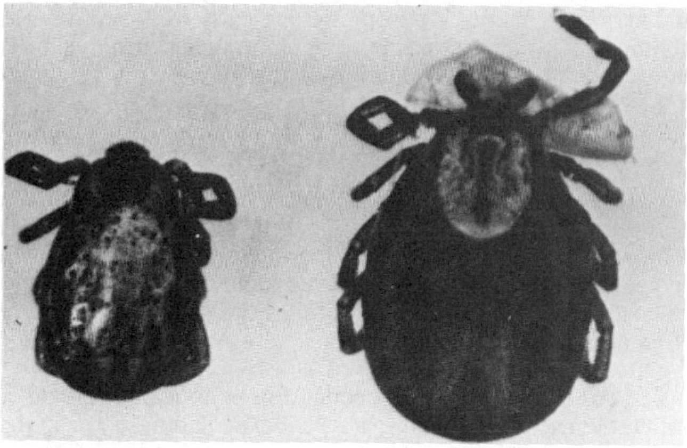

FIG. 1. Nymph and adult ticks (*Dermacentor variabilis*).

stage require blood meals. The life cycle of some species extends over a 2-year period. The tick obtains its blood meal by embedding its head in the skin, a process that usually produces no symptoms. If the tick goes unnoticed, it may remain attached to the skin, engorging itself with its host's blood for days at a time.

EPIDEMIOLOGY

Because of a large animal reservoir, humans are only occasional hosts for ticks. The larvae, nymphs, and adults tend to gravitate to grasses alongside animal trails, from which they attach themselves to passing hosts. Following engorgement, most ticks drop off the host to undergo further maturation, to mate, and to lay eggs.

Ticks are important vectors for the transmission of rickettsial, viral and, bacterial diseases discussed in other chapters (see Table 2, Chapter 266). Ticks of the genus *Dermacentor* (Fig. 1) are known to cause tick paralysis, and are vectors of Rocky Mountain spotted fever and tularemia. Ticks of the genera *Ixodes* and *Amblyomma* are known to transmit Lyme disease. Other human diseases that may be transmitted by hard ticks include arboviruses, Q fever, tick-bite fever and babesiosis.

Tick infestation can cause great economic losses to industries dependent upon domestic animals such as cattle and sheep by causing damaged hides or a decrease in an animal's weight gain. Ticks can also transmit infectious diseases such as babesiosis or rickettsial diseases to domestic animals.

CLINICAL MANIFESTATIONS

Uncomplicated Bites

During the process of attachment and feeding, the tick produces little or no discomfort to the host. Following removal, in uncomplicated bites, a punctum surrounded by erythema may be visible for 1–2 weeks. Rarely, a delayed hypersensitivity reaction with fever, pruritus, and urticaria may develop, with the initial tick bite eliciting little or no response.

Tick Bite Granuloma

Occasionally, following a tick bite, a persistent, firm, pruritic, erythematous papule or nodule may develop. Microscopically, one sees a granulomatous reaction, which is felt to represent a reaction to retained foreign material at the bite site. If the granuloma persists, it may require surgical excision for relief of pruritus.

TICK PARALYSIS

A rare but very alarming reaction may occasionally occur in which prolonged attachment (5–7 days) of certain species of ticks may result in paralysis of its host. The paralysis begins in the lower extremities and ascends symmetrically to involve the trunk, upper extremities, and head within a few hours. A neurotoxin isolated from the tick salivary gland is felt to be responsible for the neurologic symptoms. Ticks most often responsible for causing tick paralysis are *Ixodes holocyclus* in Australia, *Dermacentor andersoni* in western North America, and *Dermacentor variabilis* in eastern North America.[2] In most cases, removal of the tick leads to rapid resolution of symptoms; however, the response may be slow and associated with electromyographic evidence of denervation. Tick paralysis caused by *I. holocyclus* can be especially severe, and the host may die despite removal of the tick. A hyperimmune serum against *I. holocyclus* has been developed and is an effective treatment for

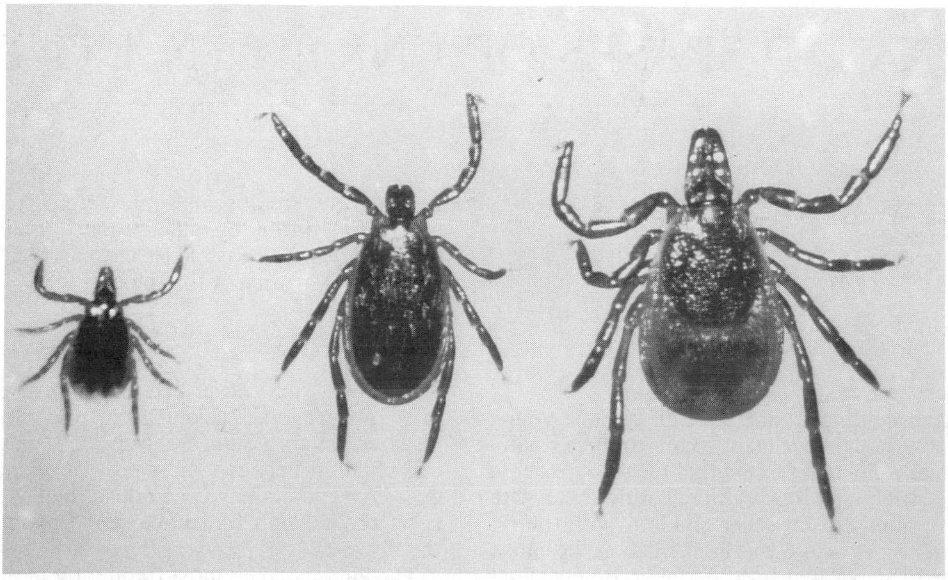

FIG. 2. Nymph, adult male, and adult female ticks (*Ixodes dammini*). (Courtesy of Dr. Willy Burgdorfer, Hamilton, MT.)

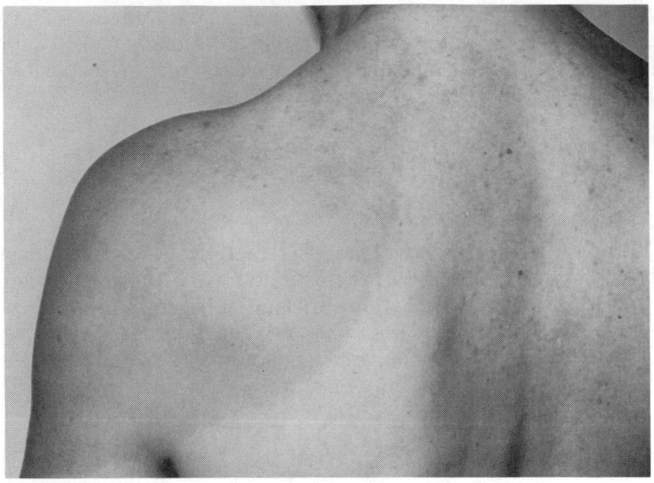

FIG. 3. Expanding erythematous annular lesion of erythema chronicum migrans on the shoulder of a patient with Lyme disease.

tick paralysis caused by this species of tick; however, it is ineffective against other species.

Lyme Disease

The most common tick-borne disease in the United States is Lyme disease, which is covered in detail elsewhere in this book (see Chapter 217). The known vectors of Lyme disease include *Amblyomma americanum* and several species of *Ixodes*, the most well-known of which is *Ixodes dammini* (Fig. 2). Lyme disease is a multisystem disorder caused by the spirochete *Borrelia burgdorferi*. At the site of the tick bite, an erythematous papule may develop and expand into an erythematous annular lesion with central clearing, an eruption known as erythema chronicum migrans[3] (Fig. 3). Secondary annular lesions may also develop weeks to months later at locations distant from the original tick bite. Patients with Lyme disease may also have internal involvement, primarily of the cardiac, rheumatologic, and nervous systems. Appropriate and early treatment with antibiotics such as tetracycline, penicillin, or erythromycin usually results in prompt resolution of the disease.[4]

ERADICATION AND PREVENTION

A well-organized and carefully implemented program can successfully control medically or economically important ticks in a limited geographic area. Such programs include the widespread use of acaricides in domestic animals or the breeding of domestic animals that are resistant to tick infestations. Spraying of an area with appropriate chemicals may temporarily reduce the tick population.

Persons exposed by their occupation or avocation should examine themselves for ticks, and children should be examined periodically by their parents during the tick season (midspring to midsummer). If found, removal can be accomplished in various ways.[5] Some claims are made that application of various irritants (alcohol, nailpolish, a hot match) will cause the tick to let go, but these methods are not uniformly successful. Most ticks can be successfully removed in their entirety by gently grasping the tick's mouthparts where they are imbedded in the skin with a forceps and pulling gently. The tick should not be squeezed during the process, since feces and tissue juices may transmit infection. If necessary, the tick may be removed by performing a small shave excision. Periodic removal of ticks from household pets is important to prevent spread within the household. Insect repellents are useful, and protective clothing is very helpful to prevent tick bites.

REFERENCES

1. Kettle DS. Medical and veterinary entomology. New York: John Wiley & Sons; 1982.
2. Jellison WL, Gregson JD. Tick paralysis in northwestern U.S. and British Columbia. Rocky Mountain Med J. 1950;47:28.
3. Berger BW. Erythema chronicum migrans of Lyme Disease. Arch Dermatol. 1984;120:1017–21.
4. Eichenfield AH. Diagnosis and treatment of Lyme disease. Pediatr Ann. 1986;15:583–4, 587, 591–4.
5. Needham GR. Evaluation of five popular methods for tick removal. Pediatrics. 1985;75:997–1002.

SECTION J. DISEASES OF UNKNOWN ETIOLOGY

274. ROSEOLA (EXANTHEM SUBITUM)

ANNE A. GERSHON

Roseola is an acute febrile illness, largely of infants and young children, that has been thought for many years to have a viral etiology. About 30 years ago it was found that the disease could be produced in susceptible children by inoculating them with bacteria-free serum obtained from other children with the illness.[1] In 1988, human herpesvirus 6 was implicated as the cause of roseola. This virus was isolated from peripheral blood lymphocytes from four 6-month-old infants with clinical roseola. Antibodies were absent from acute serum, but each child seroconverted during convalescence.[2] Should this report be confirmed, it will be possible to learn more about the epidemiology and natural history of this illness.

EPIDEMIOLOGY

Roseola was first described and named by Zahorsky[3] in 1910. It is now recognized as one of the most common exanthematous diseases of very young children.[4] It is most often seen in infants and children between the ages of 6 months and 3 years; only occasional adults have been described as having roseola. There is no predilection for either sex. Immunity appears to follow the disease.[4]

The illness occurs most frequently in the late spring and midautumn. The disease appears to be somewhat contagious, although the secondary attack rate in households is not high. It is also unusual to find a history of contact with the disease before onset, and the attack rate after exposure is low. Rare outbreaks of roseola have been described.[5,6] However, it is controversial whether these were outbreaks of roseola or an infection with a similar clinical picture such as an enterovirus infection or rubella.

The incubation period of roseola after exposure to the disease appears to be about 10–15 days.[4] After injection of serum it was found to be 9 days.[1]

CLINICAL MANIFESTATIONS

A prodromal period is unusual, but if it occurs it is often mild, with fever, slight coryza, minimal reddening of the pharynx and tympanic membranes, and some swelling of the eyelids. The disease itself begins with fever, which may reach 104°F or higher. The fever usually lasts for 3–5 days, but during this time the infant or child usually does not look particularly ill. Often adenopathy in the cervical and posterior auricular regions is noted. Strikingly, as the fever falls a maculopapular rash appears, usually on the trunk or neck. In roseola the rash appears within 48 hours after the fever disappears; this sequence is clinically diagnostic of the illness.[4] The rash may last for a few hours to a few days.[4]

COMPLICATIONS

Complications are uncommon. Convulsions may accompany the illness, but these are almost invariably febrile. Classically, convulsions appear as the temperature is rising.[4] Occasional infants with roseola have been noted to have a bulging fontanel as part of their illness.[7] Rarely encephalopathy has been associated with roseola. Thrombocytopenic purpura has also been described after roseola,[8] but this too is extremely rare. It has been suggested that thrombocytopenia may be secondary to an immune reaction set off by the causative agent.

DIAGNOSIS

Routine laboratory studies reveal an initial leukopenia with neutropenia, followed by a leukocytosis. The cerebrospinal fluid is normal in roseola, even if seizures have occurred. Since the etiologic agent has not been identified, it is impossible to make a specific laboratory diagnosis. Therefore, the diagnosis is usually based on the characteristic clinical picture: a young child with unexplained high fever who looks relatively comfortable and who develops a maculopapular rash as his or her temperature falls.

TREATMENT

There is no specific treatment for roseola; antibiotics are ineffective. Antipyretics should be given as indicated for a temperature above 101°F. Isolation of patients with roseola is unnecessary since the illness is not very communicable.

REFERENCES

1. Kempe CH, Shaw EB, Jackson JR, et al. Studies on the etiology of exanthema subitum (roseola infantum). J Pediatr. 1950;37:561.
2. Yamanishi K, Okuno T, Shiraki K, et al. Identification of human herpesvirus-6 as a causal agent for exanthem subitum. Lancet. 1088;1:1065–7.
3. Zahorsky J. Roseola infantilis. Pediatrics. 22:60, 1910;22:60.
4. Berenberg W, Wright S, Janeway CA. Roseola infantum (exanthem subitum). N Engl J Med. 1949;241:253.
5. Clemens H. Exanthem subitum (roseola infantum): Report of 80 cases. J Pediatr. 1945;26:66.
6. James U, Freier A. Roseola infantum: An outbreak in a maternity hospital. Arch Dis Child. 1949;24:54.
7. Oski F. Roseola infantum. Am J Dis Child. 1961;101:376.
8. Nishimura K, Igarashi M, Ishii A, et al. Thrombocytopenia purpura associated with exanthem subitum. Jpn J Pediatr. 1972;25:809.

275. KAWASAKI SYNDROME (MUCOCUTANEOUS LYMPH NODE SYNDROME)

JACOB A. LOHR

Kawasaki syndrome, originally called mucocutaneous lymph node syndrome, is a diffuse vasculitis of unknown etiology.[1–3] The criteria by which the disorder is diagnosed are noted in Table 1.[4]

Japanese investigators have detailed information on more than 80,000 cases. The Centers for Disease Control have recorded more than 2300 confirmed cases occurring in the United States since July 1976.

The male-to-female ratio is 1.6:1.[5] Eighty percent of the patients are younger than 4 years of age. The syndrome is unusual after the age of 8 years.

Asians, especially of Japanese ancestry, are at greatest risk for acquiring the disease, but the syndrome can affect any ethnic group. Blacks have an intermediate risk, and the risk for whites is the least. Sporadic cases appear to be the rule, but epidemics, with incidences of up to 150 cases per 100,000 children, have occurred in separate geographic areas in the United States.[6,7] No evidence for person-to-person spread or common-source exposure has been documented. Although cases in the United States are most frequent in the winter and spring,[5] the syndrome is not limited by seasonal, geographic, socioeconomic, or environmental barriers.[8] Recurrences and second cases within families are unusual. Recently reported case fatality rates are less than 1 percent.[9]

ETIOLOGY

The etiology of Kawasaki syndrome remains unknown. Toxic, allergic, and immunologic causes have been suspected, but most investigations have centered on identifying an infectious etiology. Streptococcal, staphylococcal, rickettsial, leptospiral, and viral (including a recent focus on retroviral) agents have all been investigated.[9,10] Although patients with documented infectious diseases have fulfilled the criteria for a diagnosis of Kawasaki syndrome, the vast majority of cases in large series and epidemics remain etiologically unexplained.[6,7] Toxic agents such as mercury have been suspected but later dismissed when investigated more extensively. A number of immunologic abnormalities including hyperimmunoglobulinemia, circulating

TABLE 1. Diagnostic Criteria for Kawasaki Syndrome

Fever of 5 or more days' duration
Presence of four of the following five conditions
1. Bilateral conjunctival injection
2. Change(s)[a] in the mucous membranes of the upper respiratory tract such as an injected pharynx; injected lips; dry, fissured lips; strawberry tongue
3. Change(s)[a] of the peripheral extremities such as peripheral edema, peripheral erythema, desquamation, periungual desquamation
4. Rash, primarily truncal; polymorphous but nonvesicular
5. Cervical lymphadenopathy
Illness cannot be explained by other known disease processes

[a] One criterion is sufficient to establish the condition.

immune complexes, and abnormalities of peripheral blood lymphocyte populations have been described,[11–14] but the pathogenetic importance of these changes is not known.

CLINICAL FINDINGS

Kawasaki syndrome is a triphasic illness that progresses from an *initial phase* of approximately 10 days to a *subacute phase* of approximately 25 days and concludes with a *convalescent phase* that terminates between the 6th and 10th week of illness.[15]

Characteristic of the first phase are fever, conjunctival congestion, involvement of lips and oral cavity, reddening and swelling of palms and soles, rash, lymphadenopathy, and behavioral changes.

Fever is usually the initial symptom and is present in all cases.[5] Lasting through most of the acute phase or even well into the subacute phase and associated with a toxic appearance, the fever has a remittent pattern with temperatures ranging from 101°F to 104°F.[3,10] A few days after the fever, the bulbar conjunctivae become congested or hyperemic, without discharge or exudate, in 96 percent of cases.[2,5,10,15] The palpebral conjunctivae are less involved.[3] The conjunctivae usually clear as the fever subsides but may be abnormal for 3–5 weeks.[15] Ninety-nine percent of the patients have dryness, redness, and fissuring of lips; protuberance of the tongue papillae, which is clinically indistinguishable from the "strawberry tongue" of streptococcal disease; or profuse reddening and dryness of the oral and pharyngeal mucosal,[5] These mouth changes appear 1–3 days after the onset of fever.[15] The strawberry tongue and mucosal and lip redness disappear before or with fever; the lip fissures heal 1–2 weeks later. Eighty-eight percent of the patients have red palms and soles, which appear on the third to fifth day of illness and remain for 5–15 days.[2] Seventy-six percent also have indurative edema of the hands and feet.

Ninety-nine percent of the patients experience an erythema multiforme, morbilliform, or scarlatiniform exanthem that appears 1–5 days after the onset of fever and disappears within a week.[2,5] Its distribution is primarily truncal but may include the extremities and face.

Lymphadenopathy is the least frequent of the characteristic findings and is seen in only 50–82 percent of cases.[5,15] The adenopathy appears approximately 3 days into the illness and lasts for up to 3 weeks. Usually there is enlargement in excess of 1.5 cm of a single cervical node. The node is minimally tender, firm, nonsuppurative, often red, and rarely, warm.[15] Behavioral changes, although not part of the diagnostic criteria, are present in most patients during the acute phase. Marked irritability, significant mood changes, and disturbed sleep patterns prevail.

The subacute phase includes desquamation and thrombocytosis.[10] Arthralgias, arthritis, and cardiac dysfunction may also appear in this phase.

The membranous desquamation of the fingertips occurs in 94 percent of the children[2] (Fig. 1). It usually begins in the periungual area and extends over the entire palmar region within a week.[15] The feet are involved in a similar fashion but follow the palmar desquamation by a few days.

Arthralgias and arthritis may be a prominent part of the clinical course in fewer than half of the patients.[2,15] The knees, hips, and elbows are the joints most frequently affected. Resolution may take weeks, but it is complete and without known sequelae.[16]

The most significant finding in Kawasaki syndrome is carditis, which accounts for the fatalities seen with the disease.[2] Clinical evidence of cardiac involvement occurs in approximately 20 percent of patients and includes aneurysms, myocarditis, arrhythmias, mitral insufficiency, myocardial infarction, or sudden death.[10] Routine angiography of 150 unselected patients by Kato and colleagues[17] revealed aneurysms in 17 percent and vascular obstruction in 2 percent of the patients. Yoshikawa et al.[18] have demonstrated that biplanar echocardiography is almost as sensitive as angiography in detecting coronary aneurysms. Follow-up angiography 1–2 years after diagnosis in 16 patients with aneurysms revealed resolution in 8 patients (50 percent).[17]

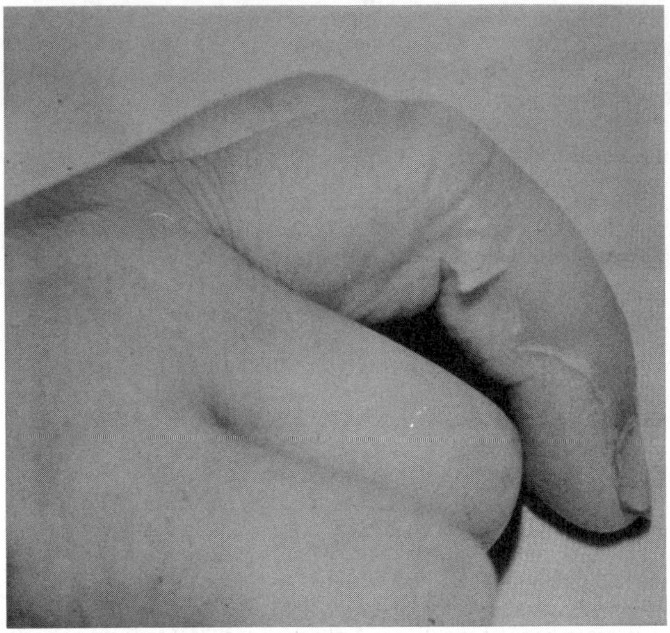

FIG. 1. Hand of a child with Kawasaki syndrome. Desquamation of the skin of finger is occurring.

The convalescent phase begins when clinical symptoms subside and usually quietly ends when the erythrocyte sedimentation rate returns to normal, but serious, even fatal cardiac dysfunction may commence or reappear during this phase.[10] Transverse lines in the fingernails or toenails may also appear during this phase.[2]

Other reported clinical features that may appear during the clinical course of the illness include aseptic meningitis[3]; diarrhea, abdominal pain, and hydrops of the gall bladder[11]; hepatic dysfunction; urethritis and meatal ulcers[3]; otitis media[19]; uveitis[20]; hypertension; cranial nerve palsies; hemolytic–uremic syndrome; aneurysms of the aorta or medium-sized noncoronary arteries[10]; myositis[21]; and necrosis of abdominal organs, testes, or digits of the hands.[22]

Atypical cases not fulfilling classic diagnostic criteria but associated with significant, even fatal coronary artery disease are being recognized with increasing frequency.[23,24] Especially in young infants, the illness may be more severe and more difficult to diagnose.[25]

PATHOLOGIC FINDINGS

Fujiwara and Hamashima[26] reported the pathologic findings from a study of 20 hearts. They demonstrated that the disease begins as a small-vessel and coronary artery angiitis associated with a pancarditis, progresses to coronary artery aneurysm and thrombus formation, and may terminate as scarring and severe stenosis of the coronary arteries. Yutani et al.[27] reported finding round-cell myocarditis and fibrosis in all of 201 unselected patients who underwent endomyocardial biopsy.

LABORATORY STUDIES

Hematologic findings include mild anemia,[2] leukocytosis associated with a minimal to marked shift to the left,[2,3] marked thrombocytosis,[3] and an increased erythrocyte sedimentation rate.[2,3] During the convalescent phase, neutropenia may occur and may last for months.[16]

Pyuria is common, and up to 100 white blood cells per high-power field may be found.[2,3] It generally lasts 2–5 days. The pus cells are apparently of urethral origin.[3] Mild to moderate proteinuria can occur, but microscopic hematuria is rare.[2,3]

The occasional cerebrospinal fluid pleocytosis is mild with white blood cell counts of less than 100 cells/mm^3 and a lymphocyte predominance.[3] Mild increases in serum transaminase levels are seen.[2,3] Significant elevations of bilirubin levels are uncommon, but clinical jaundice has been recorded.[2]

DIFFERENTIAL DIAGNOSIS

The differential diagnosis is extensive and includes scarlet fever, staphylococcal scalded skin syndrome, toxic shock syndrome, Rocky Mountain spotted fever, leptospirosis, measles, rubella, roseola, enteroviral disease, infectious mononucleosis, cervical adenopathy, allergic disease, Stevens-Johnson syndrome, serum sickness, juvenile rheumatoid arthritis, lupus erythematosus, periarteritis nodosa, Reiter syndrome, scleroderma, and acrodynia. These diseases can usually be ruled out by historical data, careful physical examinations, simple laboratory tests, and observation of the course.

THERAPY

Specific therapy is unknown. Antibiotics have not been effective in modifying the course of the disease.[2] Anticoagulants have been suggested,[3] but there are no data to support their use.

Steroids have been tried for their anti-inflammatory effects, but Kato and associates found their use to be associated with an increased likelihood of aneurysm formation when compared with aspirin therapy or no anti-inflammatory therapy.[28]

Aspirin is recommended as a part of the standard therapy because of its therapeutic effects on inflammation or platelet aggregation.[10] A dosage of 80–100 mg/kg/day administered in divided doses will usually provide serum salicylate levels of 15–25 mg/dl, which have been shown to significantly reduce the duration of fever in a majority of patients. Aspirin has a modest benefit for the arthritis or arthralgia that occurs later.[3] Dosage should be reduced to 3–5 mg/kg/day after the fever is controlled and before thrombocytosis occurs in the subacute phase. This dosage is more appropriate for inhibiting platelet aggregation and is continued until the erythrocyte sedimentation rate returns to normal or longer if coronary artery abnormalities have occurred.[10]

A recently introduced and widely accepted mode of therapy is high-dose intravenous γ-globulin (IVGG). In a collaborative study, IVGG, 400 mg/kg/day for 4 days, and aspirin, 100 mg/kg/day for 14 days, were more effective in preventing cardiac abnormalities than was aspirin alone for 14 days.[29] The mechanism for the apparent effectiveness of IVGG is not known.

Surgical approaches including aortocoronary bypass grafting for the child with severe coronary artery disease have been devised, but results are often disappointing, especially if surgery is attempted during the subacute or early convalescent phase.[30,31]

REFERENCES

1. Kawasaki T. MCLS—Clinical observation of 50 cases (in Japanese). Jpn J Allergy 1967;16:178–222.
2. Kawasaki T, Kosaki F, Okawa S, et al. A new infantile acute febrile mucocutaneous lymph node syndrome (MLNS) prevailing in Japan. Pediatrics. 1974;54:271–6.
3. Melish ME, Hicks RM, Larson EJ. Mucocutaneous lymph node syndrome in the United States. Am J Dis Child. 1976;130:599–607.
4. Centers for Disease Control. Kawasaki disease—New York. MMWR 1980;130:29:61–3.
5. Bell DM, Morens DM, Holman RC, et al. Kawasaki syndrome in the United States. Am J Dis Child. 1983;137:211–4.
6. Bell DM, Brink EW, Nitzkin JL, et al. Kawasaki syndrome: Description of two outbreaks in the United States. N Engl J Med. 1981;304:1568–76.
7. Centers for Disease Control. Multiple outbreaks of Kawasaki syndrome—United States. MMWR. 1985;34:33–5.
8. Japan MCLS Research Committee. Diagnostic Guidelines of Infantile Acute Febrile Mucocutaneous Lymph Node Syndrome, ed 2. Tokyo: Japan Red Cross Central Hospital; 1974.
9. Rauch AM. Kawasaki syndrome: Review of new epidemiologic and laboratory developments. Pediatr Infect Dis J. 1987;6:1016–21.
10. Melish ME: Kawasaki syndrome: A new infectious disease? J Infect Dis. 1981;143:317–24.
11. Goldsmith RW, Gribetz D, Strauss L. Mucocutaneous lymph node syndrome (MLNS) in the continental United States. Pediatrics. 1976;57:431–5.
12. Mason WH, Jordon SC, Sakai R, et al. Circulating immune complexes in Kawasaki syndrome. Pediatr Infect Dis J. 1985;4:48–51.
13. Leung DYM, Siegel RL, Grady S, et al. Immunoregulatory abnormalities in mucocutaneous lymph node syndrome. Clin Immunol Immunopathol. 1982;23:100–12.
14. Leung DYM, Chu ET, Wood N, et al. Immunoregulatory T cell abnormalities in mucocutaneous lymph node syndrome. J Immunol. 1983;130:2002–4.
15. Melish ME: Kawasaki syndrome (mucocutaneous lymph node syndrome). Pediatr Rev. 1980;2:107–14.
16. Calabro JJ, Williamson P, Yunus M, et al. Kawasaki disease (KD): A rising pediatric dilemma. Arthritis Rheum. 1981;24(Suppl):88.
17. Kato H, Koike S, Tanaka C, et al. Coronary heart disease in children with Kawasaki disease. Jpn Circ J. 1979;43:469–75.
18. Yoshikawa J, Yanagihara K, Owaki T, et al. Cross-sectional echocardiographic diagnosis of coronary artery aneurysms in patients with the mucocutaneous lymph node syndrome. Circulation. 1979;59:133–9.
19. Brown JS, Billmeier GJ, Cox F, et al. Mucocutaneous lymph node syndrome in the continental United States. J Pediatr. 1976;88:81–3.
20. LaPointe N, Chad Z, Lacroix J, et al. Kawasaki disease: Association with uveitis in seven patients. Pediatrics. 1982;69:376–9.
21. Koutras A. Myositis with Kawasaki's disease. Am J Dis Child. 1982;136:78–9.
22. Mercer S, Carpenter B. Surgical complications of Kawasaki's disease. J Pediatr Surg. 1981;16:444–8.
23. Rowley AH, Gonzalez-Crussi F, Gidding SS, et al. Incomplete Kawasaki disease with coronary artery involvement. J Pediatr. 1987;110:409–13.
24. Cloney DL, Teja K, Lohr JA. Fetal case of atypical Kawasaki syndrome. Pediatr Infect Dis J. 1987;6:297–9.
25. Burns JC, Wiggins JW Jr, Toews WH, et al. Clinical spectrum of Kawasaki disease in infants younger than 6 months of age. J Pediatr. 1986;109:759–63.
26. Fumjiwara H, Hamashima Y. Pathology of the heart in Kawasaki disease. Pediatrics. 1978;61:100–7.
27. Yutani C, Go S, Kamiya T, et al. Cardiac biopsy in Kawasaki's disease. Arch Pathol Lab Med. 1981;105:470–3.
28. Kato H, Kolke S, Yokoyama T. Kawasaki disease: Effect of treatment on coronary artery involvement. Pediatrics. 1979;63:175–9.
29. Newberger JW, Takahashi M, Burns JC, et al. The treatment of Kawasaki syndrome with intravenous gamma globulin. N Engl J Med. 1986;315:341–7.
30. Hirose H, Kawashima Y, Nakano S, et al. Long-term results in surgical treatment of children 4 years old or younger with coronary involvement due to Kawasaki disease. Circulation. 1986;74(Suppl 1):77–81.
31. Kitamura S, Kawachi K, Harima R, et al. Surgery for coronary heart disease due to mucocutaneous lymph node syndrome. Am J Cardiol. 1983;51:444–8.

SPECIAL PROBLEMS

PART IV

SECTION A. NOSOCOMIAL INFECTIONS

276. ORGANIZATION FOR INFECTION CONTROL

RICHARD P. WENZEL

The primary function of a hospital infection control program is to minimize risks to patients, employees, and visitors. Various activities need to be organized (Fig. 1) so that useful data can be obtained for decision making. Important information gleaned by the infection control team will receive high priority for discussion by the members of the infection control committee. If accepted by this committee, their recommendations are forwarded to a committee of clinicians for approval and eventually to an advisory committee formulating hospital policy.

The imperatives for a good infection control program are medical, administrative, economic, legal, social, and ethical. Above all, they are medical and ethical, and these must be the primary interests of the infection control team. In today's health-conscious society, one must be sensitive to all concerns but not subjugate medical and ethical issues to those of legal, administrative, or other areas.

The problems of hospital-acquired, or nosocomial, infections are substantial. At least 5 percent of patients hospitalized in U.S. acute care institutions acquire an infection that was neither present nor incubating on admission.[1] The resulting 2 million or more hospital-acquired infections add a significant morbidity, mortality, and economic burden to the outcomes expected from the underlying diseases alone.[2–11] Estimates of the direct effects of hospital-acquired infections have been 30,000 or more deaths and $5 billion or more in indirect costs related to excess stay. With respect to the 120,000 or more blood stream infections alone, it has been suggested that they carry such high (25 percent) attributable or direct mortality that they represent a leading cause of death.[12]

An important question is how best to structure the activity of the infection control team to meet the needs of the hospital and patients. It is the author's opinion that some type of on-ward surveillance is essential, not only to define high-risk practices and identify higher than optimal rates but also to provide visibility for consultation. The Centers for Disease Control's (CDC) study on the efficacy of nosocomial infection control (SENIC) has determined that hospitals with increasing levels of surveillance activities had progressively lower rates of infection.[13] Although the mechanisms behind such findings are not known, it is likely that visibility, access to the staff, and the staff's perception of the importance of infection control may have been important factors.

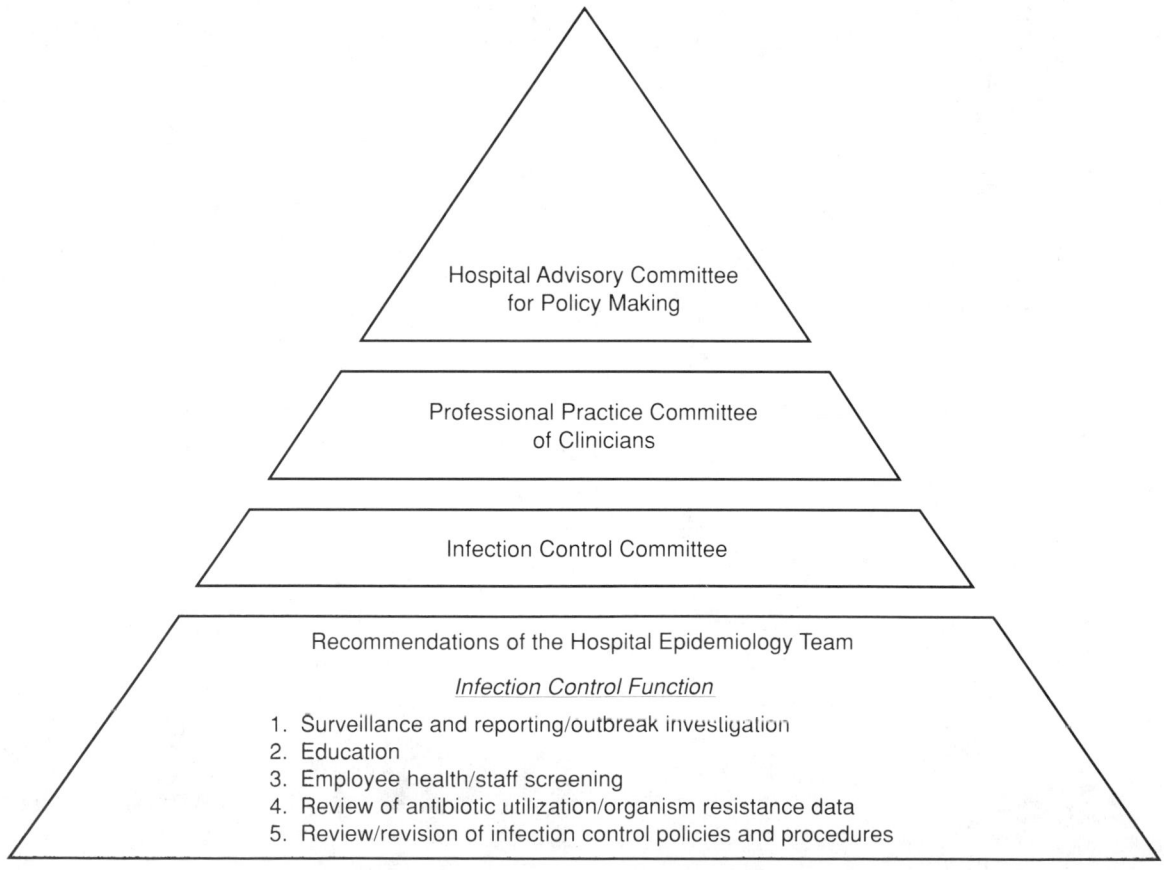

FIG. 1. The purpose of an infection control program is to minimize the risk of infection for hospital patients, employees, and visitors.

HOW MUCH SURVEILLANCE

In hospitals with limited resources, infection control practitioners may not be able to survey the entire hospital. A priority list for surveillance activities must be developed, and it has been suggested that critical care areas be top priority. Although the latter usually comprise 5–10 percent of hospital beds, they are the focus of 33–45 percent of all nosocomial blood stream and pulmonary infections.[14] Furthermore, the critical care units are often the birthplace of antibiotic resistance, the location of most epidemics in the hospital,[15] and the place where many device-related (and thus preventable) infections occur. Additionally, the infection control practitioner will identify more infections per hour of surveillance on critical care units than on general wards in the hospital.[14] Nosocomial blood stream infection should also be a top priority, and all should be detected using laboratory-based surveillance.

A secondary list of priorities would include various operative procedures or device-related infections, and each hospital can choose how many and which ones to survey. Thereafter, if sufficient personnel are available, hospitalwide surveillance could be conducted, at least for a period of time, to determine other priority areas. The details of developing an efficient surveillance system and validating its accuracy have been described.[16]

Recently, a review of surveillance and use of computers in hospital infection control has been published.[17] It is reasonable to assume that the computer will occupy a more important place in future infection control and surveillance activities. For example, as hospitals become totally computerized, it is likely that the infection control practitioners will have easier access to the starting point, that is, screening data such as the Kardex itself or microbiology laboratory reports. They can then identify high-risk patients on a daily basis and immediately perform selective chart reviews. Useful summaries that would be otherwise too tedious will become routine. The procedure might involve scanning the data on the last 1000 or more infections at one site, determining the organisms, locations, and underlying illnesses, and identifying high-risk procedures and locations. It is also very possible that as libraries become computerized, one will be able to compare local hospital rates quickly with those reported in the literature.

With the vast amount of data collected in centralized reporting systems, the computer is essential. Statistical analyses will eventually be built into the reporting system, and potential epidemics, otherwise difficult to recognize, can be identified and flagged for in-depth review.

EDUCATION

There are few studies to show optimal methods of education. Indeed, awareness of the importance of certain procedures, such as handwashing, has not been followed by a high frequency of practice in critical care units.[18] Nevertheless, an inference from the SENIC study is that hospitals performing in-service education particularly related to procedures had lower infection rates than those with no such organized activities. Thus, educational efforts should be encouraged and their outcomes measured. As a routine activity on the wards, it seems reasonable for the infection control practitioner to meet briefly (15 minutes) with the ward team to review the monthly surveillance data, highlighting areas of concern. Similarly, in academic units where the ward team rotates every 4 weeks, it might be reasonable for the practitioner to review isolation policies, specific problems, and infection exposure guidelines with the new group (physicians, and students) monthly.

EMPLOYEE HEALTH AND STAFF SCREENING

One function of the employee health division is to ensure that those taking care of ill patients are themselves healthy and do not transmit disease to patients. The health records of all employees should be examined before their employment, and potential health care workers should be advised of the possible risks of being an employee. Once employed, hospital workers should be instructed in the proper techniques involving asepsis that are important in routine, day-to-day infection control. They should be aware of the potential they have for transmitting disease from themselves to patients or from one patient to another. Vaccinations that are important for maintaining health should be offered, and an annual purified protein derivative skin test should be repeated on those persons who are initially skin test negative. In addition, when an employee with a negative skin test history is exposed to the initially undiagnosed patient with tuberculosis, further skin testing approximately 3 months after exposure should be performed. One can then determine if a conversion occurred as a result of the exposure.

A periodic review of policies related to exposure to patients with viral hepatitis, tuberculosis, meningococcal infections, or the acquired immunodeficiency syndrome (AIDS) may prevent panic when hospital employees later work with such patients. Importantly, the employee health group should be available to discuss infections of special concern to pregnant women, including viral hepatitis, cytomegalovirus, rubella and parvovirus (fifth disease). Certainly there should be clear lines of communication between the employee health and infection control teams.

ANTIBIOTIC USE AND ORGANISM RESISTANCE

Few programs have a formal approach to optimal antibiotic use, and in fact this activity is frequently handled by the pharmacy and therapeutics committee. Nevertheless, it seems reasonable for an institution to examine at least the relationships between drug use and subsequent antibiotic resistance for isolates from specific anatomic sites such as the blood stream. The data examined will generate important information for clinicians who need to initiate empiric therapy for nosocomial blood stream infections pending the identification of the organism and the antibiogram. It is emphasized that the best data are obtained if nosocomial isolates are distinguished from commonly acquired isolates; if only blood stream isolates are tested (true pathogens with high mortality); and if only one isolate per patient is counted in the numerator and the denominator. A second analysis would include a table reporting secular trends for nosocomial blood stream isolates, distinguishing gram-positive from gram-negative (Table 1). Furthermore, total grams of usage by year could be plotted on one axis and the proportion of unique nosocomial blood stream isolates that were resistant to the drug in the following year on the other axis. This would identify the nature of the relationship between antibiotic use and subsequent resistance.

POLICIES AND PROCEDURES

A routine review of policies and procedures should be performed. Usually this occurs just before the visit of the Joint

TABLE 1. Secular Trend Reports for Nosocomial Blood Stream Isolates

Nosocomial Blood Stream Pathogens:	*1988*	*1989*	*1990*	*1991*
Gram-positive isolates				
Resistance to methicillin	(*N* =)	(*N* =)	(*N* =)	(*N* =)
S. aureus	—	—	—	—
Coagulase-negative staphylococci	—	—	—	—
Gram-negative isolates				
Resistance to commonly used antibiotics				
Drug X	—	—	—	—
Drug Y	—	—	—	—
Drug Z	—	—	—	—

Committee for Accreditation of Healthcare Organizations, during which time it may not be most efficient. The orderly annual or every-2-year review seems optimal. However, when a problem arises, such as the management of contacts of a case with pertussis or the proper isolation of a patient with fifth disease, it is useful at that time to review the hospital's policy and make necessary revisions. Similarly, whenever new equipment becomes available or new data accrue regarding a device, that time may be propitious for a review of the procedure.

INFECTION CONTROL COMMITTEE

Every hospital seeking accreditation is required by the Joint Commission on Accreditation of Healthcare Organizations (JCAHO) to have an infection control committee.[19] The purpose of the committee is to use the expertise of members from various departments of the hospital so that the existing policies on infection control can be continually reviewed and nosocomial infection problems can be identified and resolved. The qualifications for membership should include interest, expertise, and, if possible, influence within the hospital. It is likely that administrative changes will be effected more easily if the representatives also possess the desired qualities of tact and charisma.

The chairman of the committee is usually but not always a physician and is usually a clinician. Some hospitals have preferred to have a pathologist as chairman, since the clinical microbiology laboratory is often under his direction. In 40 percent of hospitals surveyed by the CDC in the late 1970s, a pathologist was the head of the infection surveillance and control program.[20] The JCAHO requires an administrator, a nurse, a microbiologist, an internist, and all infection control practitioners to be members of the committee. The latter are the nurses or equivalent persons who perform the day-to-day infection control duties. In general, one-third to one-half of the members are physicians, and approximately one-third are nurses. Although physicians who specialize in infectious diseases are on the committee in many hospitals, the remaining clinicians represent varied departments. Nurses on the committee always include the surveillance personnel, and some hospitals choose to appoint inservice and/or employee health nurses. Administrators, microbiologists, and pharmacists are often asked to serve. Most hospital epidemiologists quickly point out that although there may be up to 15 or more members, most of the work and influence arise from a nucleus of four or five members with a vested interest in infection control.

Committee Meetings

Many hospitals' infection control committees meet monthly, and they are required by the Joint Commission to meet at least bimonthly. The most important aspect of a successful committee is to have an organized plan for each meeting. If a detailed topic is to be discussed, it is advisable that a typewritten summary of the data be presented to the members approximately 48 hours before the meeting, explaining the purpose of the discussion. The committee should convene on a monthly basis, preferably at a regular time, such as the second Wednesday of each month, and a breakfast or luncheon meeting seems beneficial. Most committees spend just a few minutes on old business and a review of the minutes, and then immediately proceed with a summary of the current infection report. In large hospitals it is not reasonable to spend time describing every patient with an infection. Instead, it is necessary to summarize existing infection problems, seeking evidence for a common source and developing potential control measures. Because of the high mortality rate of hospital-acquired blood stream infections, these should be carefully analyzed according to patient location, organism, predisposing illnesses and procedures, and other common preinfection events. Specifically, the antibiograms of blood stream isolates should be updated as a guide to empiric therapy. Questions to be answered include the following: (*1*) What proportion of *Staphylococcus aureus* or important coagulase-negative staphylococcal isolates are resistant to methicillin? (*2*) What proportion of gram-negative rod isolates are resistant to gentamicin, tobramycin, amikacin, or the frequently used new cephalosporins? If infection problems are identified as a result of reporting, they should occupy the next area of business.

When no particular problem has been identified by surveillance, the director of the meeting should have planned a review of one or two policies or procedures by the committee. The agenda might include the management of the human immunodeficiency virus (HIV) serum antibody-positive employee, the indications for administration of the hepatitis B vaccine to employees, tuberculin skin test policies for employees, antibiograms for common nosocomial pathogens, intravenous catheter-associated infections, and others. The hospital's resident expert in the area under discussion should be invited to the meeting for political reasons, as well as for his or her other medical expertise. Before the meeting, it should have been determined what other institutions are doing about the policy or procedure in question, what the CDC is currently recommending, and what data are available in the scientific literature to support various options. The purpose of the committee should not be to discuss members' recall of the literature, but instead to use the data as the starting point for a discussion of reasonable policy alternatives. When a decision is made, the recommendations of the infection control committee should be clearly stated, signed by the administrator, and presented in very short order to the policy committee for immediate action (Fig. 1). It is desirable for an administrator be a member of both the infection control committee and the policy committee to expedite changes.

Occasionally, the committee becomes aware that a particular infection control problem is related to a specific member of the hospital's medical team. When the facts are clear, it is the responsibility of the committee to advise that person of a need to change a policy or procedure—often a delicate matter. In the interest of a good program, it seems reasonable that the infection control practitioner not be the person to present this information. Instead, the chairman of the committee and/or the administrator should personally visit the chairman of that physician's department. The ideal person should, of course, be sensitive, tactful, and genuinely interested in the improvement of medical care at the facility. It is hoped that such a person would not be perceived as a policing member of the committee.

OUTBREAKS

Once an outbreak is identified, the infection control team should investigate immediately. The various steps of investigating an outbreak (Table 2) begin with the proof that an outbreak has occurred (i.e., statistical evidence that the current rate of infection is significantly greater than the known endemic rates). The endemic rates are most easily ascertained by a review of surveillance data, but they may have to be obtained retrospectively by chart reviews. It is important to ascertain if the surveillance definitions or methods have changed in the epidemic and pre-epidemic periods or if microbiologic identification of organisms has changed.

Once a problem has been identified (such as postoperative wound infections after cardiac bypass surgery), a case definition must be clearly outlined. Then the charts of all patients should be reviewed and an epidemic curve plotted so that one can readily ascertain the extent of the problem and its time relationships to prior procedures or admission to the hospital. Line lists (raw data) and lists of graphic materials can then be made relating the problem being investigated to prior procedures, locations, physicians, medications, and so forth, and a hypothesis

TABLE 2. Steps for Investigating an Outbreak

1. Provide a case definition and then prove that the outbreak exists. Show statistically that current rates are significantly higher than prior rates.
2. Plot an epidemic curve with the number of cases on the Y-axis and the calendar date on the X-axis.
3. Review the charts of infected patients, listing the dates of admission, all procedures, medications, medical personnel attending them, and locations.
4. Organize the data on line lists and summarize them to determine if common events occurred in infected patients.
5. Plot the data for all common events. The number of patients should be on the Y-axis, and the X-axis should include the interval between infection (days) and an operation, a suspected medication, a nonoperative procedure, contact with various medical personnel, and so forth.
6. Formulate a hypothesis about likely cause–effect relationships.
7. Compare infected patients with controls who are of the same age, sex, and service. Show whether or not a statistical difference exists in the infected group with respect to exposure to a given physician, meal, operation, procedure, medication, and so forth.
8. Institute temporary infection control measures.
9. If a statistical difference suggests a common source, document the suspected source microbiologically with appropriate cultures.
10. Institute further infection control measures needed.
11. Continue surveillance of the problem. Document actual control by reduction of rates.
12. Write a report of the investigation and place it in the records of the infection control committee.

can be formulated. Once a hypothesis regarding the cause of the event is made, a controlled study may need to be performed to confirm or negate it. Controls should be a random sample of those patients of the same age, sex, and service who had the same procedures but who did not become infected. The committee should look at the statistical difference in terms of exposure to one or more procedures or medications, physicians, nurses, and so forth in the infected group compared to the controls. It is important not to "overmatch" cases and controls initially, since the cause of the problem might not be apparent after application of statistical analysis. For example, if the cause of blood stream infections were related to contaminated arterial monitoring transducers, and if all cases were closely matched to controls who also had transducers, no difference would be apparent in the analysis.

The hospital must fully support the investigation of such outbreaks once they are identified, including laboratory support for culturing of personnel or the environment, when necessary, in unusual circumstances. Furthermore, since many clues can be gleaned from a review of the employee health service data, records of all personnel involved should be reviewed early in the investigation. The primary investigating team should include the hospital epidemiologist, the microbiology laboratory person who will be in charge of the investigation, the employee health director, and infection control practitioners. The infection control practitioners should be employed in the on-ward investigation and chart reviews.

When the possible reservoirs and modes of transmission are identified, temporary infection control measures necessary to contain the disease should be implemented, and the investigation should be continued until hypotheses are confirmed. Ideally, confirmation includes microbiologic documentation, for example, culture of *S. aureus* with the plasmid pattern in the nares of an anesthesiologist, as was found in postoperative wound infections, or finding the same serotype of *Klebsiella pneumoniae* on the hands of a respiratory therapist, as was found in several respiratory medication reservoirs and in patients with respiratory-associated pneumonias. If a common source can be confirmed, final infection control recommendations must be implemented. It is essential that the infection control team follow through with the surveillance once the control measures have been instituted to establish that control has been achieved.

LEGAL ASPECTS

The infection control committee should be clearly aware of the legal aspects of infection control. It is important that the hospital understand what constitutes negligence in general and particularly negligence related to infection control. The four legal criteria for negligence include (*1*) a duty to or standard of care for the patient, (*2*) failure to perform that duty or to meet the standard, (*3*) proof that the plaintiff was injured directly as a result of the failure of the defendant to perform the duty or to meet the standard, and (*4*) damages as a result of the injury.

The role of the hospital with respect to the law is complex, for we are asked to define our policies and procedures, and in some cases we are told what they should be; yet failure by hospitals to follow those policies to the letter has been used by plaintiffs in a court of law. In this regard, some authorities suggest indicating in the policy statement that some judgment is required in performing hospital duties, since hospitals and physicians need a certain degree of flexibility in individual cases and need not be held rigidly bound to a protocol defined in the infection control manual. It also appears that patients are more likely to sue physicians and hospitals when there has been little communication and understanding of possible risks, such as infection after surgery. Therefore, in today's litigious society, physicians may need to inform patients of the risks of infection associated with various hospital procedures and should point out the efforts being made to minimize them.

The standards of care that the plaintiff can use are not only those set by the hospitals themselves but also those set by decisions of prior court suits, by government of other regulatory agencies, and by the CDC. Since 1981, the CDC has issued a number of guidelines on the prevention and control of nosocomial infections. Since it is likely that they will be used in legal decisions, it seems prudent for the hospitals that do not agree and will not comply with the guidelines to document the rationale and alternative policies used. Lawyers in the field of infection control liability often point out that good surveillance data have helped hospitals defend themselves, since a definite risk of infection associated with a certain procedure was clearly documented. Thus, finding an individual infection by itself does not necessarily indicate negligence. Furthermore, surveillance data are tangible documentation of the continual efforts by the hospital to identify (and, by inference, to reduce) the infection problems.

The role of the infection control committee with respect to legal responsibilities is to be sure that the hospital complies with regulatory agencies and follows its own standards assiduously. Regrettably, important policy positions and federal laws that are published in the *Federal Register* are not duplicated in a more widely read document.

JOINT COMMITTEE ON ACCREDITATION OF HEALTHCARE ORGANIZATIONS

The Joint Committee on Accreditation of Healthcare Organizations (JCAHO) is a nongovernmental, nonprofit organization that, among its other duties, accredits hospitals. It is based in Chicago, and its governing body is a 20-member board appointed by the American College of Medicine, American College of Surgeons, Americal Medical Association, and the American Hospital Association. The JCAHO has stated that they not only expect the hospital to have a hospitalwide infection control program and an infection control committee responsible to the medical staff, but also to maintain specific written infection control policies and procedures for all services throughout the hospital. The infection control committee must be aware of the suggestions of this accrediting body: JCAHO requires written definitions of nosocomial infections, a reporting system, a review of all departments within the hospital, and written infection control policies for each department. They demand all necessary laboratory support for infection control, an active employee health program including orientation of all new employees, and a review of antibiotic use. Accreditation is voluntary, and hospitals pay a fee for the 1- to 3-day accreditation review by a team consisting of a physician, nurse, administrator, and, more recently, a laboratory technologist.

HOSPITAL ADMINISTRATION

In recent years with an unsteady economy, the influence of the hospital administrator has increased. Faced with difficult choices, administrators may not view infection control activities as cost effective and may consider reducing support. The problem is compounded by the fact that most hospital administrators in the United States have no formal medical training; only 2.5 percent have a medical degree, and most have no training in nosocomial infection prevention.[21] However, it is likely that current and future economic incentives from national and state welfare organizations and from other third-party payers may modulate the current concerns of administrators if improved infection control activities with reduced infection rates shorten costly hospital stays.

LOCAL AND STATE HEALTH DEPARTMENTS

Because patients admitted to the hospital may have communicable diseases that must be reported to the health department, it is prudent for the infection control team to communicate frequently with both local and state health departments. All state health departments in turn report to the CDC. Communicable diseases of importance are then summarized by the CDC in the *Morbidity and Mortality Weekly Report* and in an annual summary. Common source outbreaks of nosocomial infections are also of interest to local and state health departments and to the CDC and should definitely be reported. Should additional help be needed to investigate an outbreak, these governmental agencies may elect to send help immediately or to suggest alternative means for solution.

REFERENCES

1. Haley RW, Culver DH, White JW, et al. The nationwide infection rate: A new need for vital statistics. Am J Epidemiol. 1985;121:159.
2. Rose R, Hunting KJ, Townsend TR, et al. Morbidity/mortality and economics of hospital-acquired bloodstream infections: A controlled study. South Med J. 1977;70:1267.
3. Townsend TR, Wenzel RP. Nosocomial bloodstream infections in a newborn intensive care unit: A case-matched control study of morbidity, mortality, and risk. Am J Epidemiol. 1981;114:73.
4. Freeman J, McGowan JE Jr. Risk factors for nosocomial infection. J Infect Dis. 1978;138:811.
5. Spengler RF, Greenough WE III. Hospital costs and mortality attributed to nosocomial bacteremias. JAMA. 1978;240:2455.
6. Freeman J, Rosner BA, McGowan JE Jr. Adverse effects of nosocomial infection. J Infect Dis. 1979;140:732.
7. Green JW, Wenzel RP. Endometritis following cesarean section: A controlled study of the increased duration of hospital stay and direct cost of hospitalization. Ann Surg. 1977;185:264.
8. Donowitz LG, Wenzel RP. Endometritis following cesarean section: A controlled study of the increased duration of hospital stay and direct cost of hospitalization. Am J Obstet Gynecol. 1980;137:467.
9. Haley RW, Schaberg DR, von Allmen SD, et al. Estimating the extra charges and prolongation of hospitalization due to nosocomial infections: A comparison of methods. J Infect Dis. 1980;141:248.
10. McGowan JE Jr. Cost and benefit in control of nosocomial infection: Methods for analysis. Rev Infect Dis. 1981;3:790.
11. Dixon RE. Costs of nosocomial infections and benefits of infection control programs. In: Wenzel RP, ed. Prevention and Control of Nosocomial Infections. Baltimore: Williams & Wilkins; 1987:19.
12. Wenzel RP. The mortality of hospital-acquired bloodstream infections: Need for a new vital statistic. Trans Am Clin Climatol Assoc. 1987;98:43–8.
13. Haley RW, Culver DH, White JW, et al. The efficacy of infection surveillance and control programs in preventing nosocomial infections in university hospitals. Am J Epidemiol. 1985;121:182–205.
14. Wenzel RP, Osterman CA, Donowitz LG, et al. Identification of procedure-related nosocomial infections in high-risk patients. Rev Infect Dis. 1981;3:701.
15. Wenzel RP, Thompson RL, Landry SM, et al. Hospital-acquired infections in intensive care unit patients: An overview with emphasis on epidemics. Infect Control. 1983;4:371–5.
16. Wenzel RP, Osterman CA, Husting KJ, et al. Hospital-acquired infections. I: Infection Surveillance in a University Hospital. Am J Epidemiol. 1976; 103:251.
17. Wenzel RP, Streed SA. Surveillance and use of computers in hospital infection control. J Hosp Infect. In press.
18. Albert RK, Condie F. Handwashing patterns in medical intensive care units. N Engl J Med. 1981;304:1465–6.
19. Joint Commission on the Accreditation of Hospitals. Infection control. In: AMH/84 Accreditation Manual for Hospitals. Chicago: Joint Commission on the Accreditation of Hospitals; 1983:69.
20. Haley RW: The "Hospital Epidemiologist" in U.S. hospitals, 1976–1977: A description of the head of the infection surveillance and control program. Infect Control. 1980;1:21.
21. Brachman PS, Haley RW. Nosocomial infection control: Role of the hospital administrator. Rev Infect Dis. 1981;3:783.

BIBLIOGRAPHY

Wenzel RP. Handbook of Hospital Acquired Infections. Boca Raton, Fla: CRC Press; 1981.

Bennett JV, Brachman PS. Hospital Infections. Boston: Little, Brown; 1986.

Wenzel RP. Prevention and Control of Nosocomial Infections. Baltimore: Williams & Wilkins; 1987.

277. ISOLATION

STEPHEN A. STREED
RICHARD P. WENZEL

Patient isolation had its developmental roots in the public health field, where individuals or families with communicable diseases were quarantined in their homes or sent to a facility dedicated to the long-term care of similarly afflicted patients. The quarantine was lifted or the patient was released from the facility only after the perceived danger of the general public had passed. The analogous containment of infectious agents within the health care setting has been achieved by patient isolation. Although the practice of physically separating infected from noninfected patients and other susceptible persons has persisted, efforts to integrate the care of most infected patients were promoted by the Centers for Disease Control (CDC) publication "Isolation Techniques for Use in Hospitals," initially published in 1970[1] and revised in 1983.[2] An essential feature of all of the CDC recommendations is a heightened awareness of potentially infectious patients. A growing number of authors[3] and advisory[4] or regulatory agencies[5] have suggested a more generalized application of barriers specifically designed to prevent acquisition or transport of certain blood- and/or body fluid-borne viral agents, such as the human immunodeficiency virus (HIV) or the hepatitis B virus (HBV). Thus, the implementation of *universal precautions* or *body substance isolation*[4] is being recommended for all patients, without specific knowledge of or special regard for the infectious potential of the patient.

ALTERNATIVE APPROACHES TO PATIENT ISOLATION

Category-Specific Isolation

Both the 1970 and 1983 guidelines recommended the use of seven general categories of isolation or precautions. Under this system, patients with infections are placed in one or more of the categories, based upon the known or suspected infectious agent, its potential mode(s) of transmission, and the site and extent of the infection. Color-coded cards specific to each category are placed outside the patient's room, and all persons entering the room are expected to follow the instructions on the card. Clean supplies (gloves, gowns, masks, etc.) needed to carry out the isolation protocols properly are placed either on a dedicated isolation cart or in an anteroom, depending on the design and resources of the hospital. Protocols for certain agent–infection site combinations call for a private room and/or special air-handling capabilities, and require that appropriate protective attire be worn by persons entering the room. Under this system, however, most agent–infection site combinations are be managed safely without special facilities or room requirements, resulting in minimal disruption of the usual patient care and visitor routines. The use of protective attire is dependent upon the likelihood of the caregiver to come in contact with items contaminated with the agent. Specialized linen and supply handling and room cleaning are indicated only in certain circumstances. Handwashing is indicated for all seven categories before entering and upon leaving the patient's room. The specifications for each category are summarized (Table 1).

Disease-Specific Isolation

Disease-specific isolation, as described by the CDC in 1983,[2] is designed to increase the cost effectiveness of patient care by recommending only those practices needed to interrupt the transmission of the given agent. The unique characteristics of each agent and infection site are considered, and the barriers appropriate to that combination are implemented. This system uses a single, general-purpose specification card that is placed outside the patient's room. The card is a "menu" of all protocols from which the staff member selects precautions appropriate for the disease. A table of infectious diseases and their indicated precautions is provided to assist in the selection process. Handwashing, before and after caring for the patient, continues to be recommended for all patient care circumstances, irrespective of the isolation status of the patient. The disease-specific system may have certain advantages, compared to the category-specific system, in that it promotes a more efficient use of supplies and personnel time by not requiring adherence to general protocols. The tailoring of barrier placement to a specific agent should result in optimal use of resources. Alternatively, since this system depends heavily on knowledge of the specific agent, delays in agent identification may result in confusion and inadequate barrier placement. Furthermore, since greater skill is required to identify the disease and its indicated barriers correctly, there may be correspondingly greater potential for error in protocol assignment.

Universal Precautions

Since it is not possible to obtain complete medical and social histories for all patients, it is now recommended that a system of *universal precautions* be implemented for all patients undergoing medical care.[4] Universal precautions are directed specifically at blood- and/or body-fluid-borne viral agents such as HIV or HBV. This system specifies the following precautions:

1. All health care workers should routinely use appropriate barrier precautions to prevent skin and mucous membrane exposure when contact with blood or other body fluids of any patient is anticipated. Gloves should be worn for touching the blood or body fluids, mucous membranes, or nonintact skin of all patients; for handling items or surfaces soiled with blood or body fluids; and for performing venipuncture or other vascular access procedures. Gloves should be changed after contact with each patient. Masks and protective eyewear or face shields should be worn during procedures that are likely to generate droplets of blood or other body fluids to prevent exposure of mucous membranes of the mouth, nose, and eyes. Gowns or aprons should be worn during procedures that are likely to generate splashes of blood or other body fluids.
2. Hands and other skin surfaces should be washed immediately and thoroughly if contaminated with blood or other body fluids. Hands should be washed immediately after gloves are removed.
3. All health care workers should take precautions to prevent injuries caused by needles, scalpels, and other sharp instruments or devices during procedures; when cleaning used instruments; during disposal of used needles; and when handling sharp instruments after procedures. To prevent needlestick injuries, needles should *not* be recapped, purposely bent or broken by hand, removed from disposable syringes, or otherwise manipulated by hand. After they are used, disposable syringes and needles, scalpel blades, and other sharp items should be placed in puncture-resistant containers for disposal; these containers should be located as close as practical to the area of use. Large-bore reusable needles should be placed in a puncture-resistant container for transport to the reprocessing area.
4. Although saliva has not been implicated in HIV transmission, to minimize the need for emergency mouth-to-mouth resuscitation, mouthpieces, resuscitation bags, or other ventilation devices shouuld be available for use in areas in which the need for resuscitation is predictable.
5. Health care workers who have exudative lesions or weeping dermatitis should refrain from all direct patient care and from handling patient care equipment until the condition resolves.
6. Pregnant health care workers are not known to be at greater risk of contracting HIV infection than health care workers who are not pregnant; however, if a health care worker develops HIV infection during pregnancy, the infant is at risk of developing infection resulting from perinatal transmission. Because of this risk, pregnant health care workers should be especially familiar with and strictly adherent to precautions to minimize the risk of HIV transmission.[4]

TABLE 1. Summary of CDC Category-Specific Isolation Standards

Category	*Private Room*	*Gown*	*Gloves*	*Masks*	*Handwashing*
Strict	+	+	+	+	+
Respiratory	+	–	–	For those in close contact with patient	+
Tuberculosis	+	Only to prevent gross contamination	–	If patient is coughing	+
Contact	+	If soiling is likely	If contact with infective material occurs	For those in close contact with patient	+
Enteric	Only if patient's hygiene is poor	If soiling is likely	If contact with infective material occurs	–	+
Drainage/Secretion	–	If soiling is likely	If contact with infective material occurs	–	+
Blood/body fluids	Only if patient's hygiene is poor	If soiling with blood or body fluids is likely	If contact with blood or body fluids occurs	–	+

Implementation of universal precautions makes the use of blood and body fluid precautions obsolete under the category-specific system, since all of the former protocols are now recommended for use with all patients. Use of additional precautions under the category- or disease-specific systems may be indicated by the infection status of the patient.

Health care facilities are now charged by the Occupational Health and Safety Administration (OSHA) with the responsibility of identifying and classifying workplace tasks that staff members are likely to encounter into the following categories according to the potential risk of exposure to infectious materials:

Category 1. Tasks that involve exposure to blood, body fluids, or tissues.
Category 2. Tasks that involve no exposure to blood, body fluids, or tissues, but employment may require performing unplanned category 1 tasks.
Category 3. Tasks that involve no exposure to blood, body fluids, or tissues, and category 1 tasks are not a condition of employment.

Once the tasks are classified, engineering controls, work practices, and protective equipment appropriate to the task are essential to minimize the probability of HIV or HBV transmission. Hospitals will bear the responsibility for task classification, provision of protective equipment and supplies, and personnel training and education to ensure appropriate use of protective measures.[5]

Body Substance Isolation

A departure from the CDC category- or disease-specific systems has been proposed by Lynch et al.[3] that combines some of the features found in earlier systems with features of the universal precautions guidelines. This system is referred to as *body substance isolation* and is used for all patients. Gloves are recommended for any contact with mucous membranes, nonintact skin, and moist body substances. The role of handwashing is deemphasized somewhat, in large part due to the assumed protective effect of the gloves. Additional measures are used for diseases that are known to include an airborne transmission component, but most other infections are managed without specific precautions. The recommendations are as follows:

1. Gloves are worn for anticipated contact with blood or body fluids. Handwashing is not required unless there is a tear or puncture in the gloves and visible soilage occurs. Gloves are changed between patients.
2. Handwashing after other types of patient contact is indicated and is directed to the removal of transient microbial flora.
3. Gowns, aprons, masks, or goggles should be worn when blood or body fluids are likely to contact the clothing, skin, or face.
4. Disposable and reusable items should be contained securely enough to prevent leakage.
5. Needles should not be recapped, and all sharp instruments should be placed in puncture-resistant containers for disposal.
6. Private rooms may be necessary for some patients with diseases transmitted via the airborne route or for patients who soil the environment with body substances.

Under this system, a "Body Substance Isolation Is for All Patient Care" sign is placed in all patients' rooms. An additional "Stop Sign Alert," with instructions, is placed outside the rooms of patients with airborne infections, and masks are provided for susceptible persons entering the room. No other forms of isolation or precaution are recognized under this system. Gloves are made readily available at the bedside of all patients, and additional supplies are stored on the nursing unit or on a special cart at the bedside as patient care needs dictate. The skill level of the health care worker is considered when assessing the need for protective attire (e.g., the skilled phlebotomist may not need to wear gloves, while less skilled personnel may find glove use desirable). This is in contrast to the universal precautions approach, which requires the use of barriers based upon the exposure potential of the care being provided, irrespective of the skill level of the care provider.

Discussion

There is no system of isolation that is applicable to all hospitals. Selection of the optimal system for a given facility must ultimately depend upon a complex blend of clinical, economic, political, and philosophical considerations and must be workable within the physical and resource structure of the facility. A combination of either category- or disease-specific isolation and universal precautions would appear to be a prudent approach, given the de facto community standard established by the CDC and the need to respond to OSHA specifications pertaining to universal precautions. Body substance isolation may not fully meet these standards and specifications, and thus should be used with caution until specific data are obtained regarding the suitability of this system.

The purpose of an isolation or precaution sign is to identify infectious patients and to instruct visitors and staff members regarding safe practices while in the vicinity of those patients. Since recognition of the hazard potential, both by the system itself and by individuals within the system, is the critical first step in its containment, the isolation method that actively alerts and instructs may ultimately prove to be most effective.

REFERENCES

1. Centers for Disease Control. Isolation Techniques for Use in Hospitals. DHEW Pub. No. (PHS) 70-2054. Washington, DC: U.S. Government Printing Office; 1970.
2. Garner JS, Simmons BP. Guideline for isolation precautions for use in hospitals. Infection Control. 1983;4:245–325.
3. Lynch P, Jackson MM, Cummings MJ, et al. Rethinking the role of isolation practices in the prevention of nosocomial infections. Ann Intern Med. 1987;107:243–6.
4. Recommendations for prevention of HIV transmission in health care settings. MMWR. 1987;(36, No 2S).
5. Joint Advisory Notice. Protection Against Occupational Exposure to Hepatitis B Virus (HBV) and Human Immunodeficiency Virus (HIV). Washington, DC: Department of Labor/Department of Health and Human Services; Oct. 19, 1987.

278. STERILIZATION, DISINFECTION, AND DISPOSAL OF INFECTIOUS WASTE

MICHAEL A. MARTIN
RICHARD P. WENZEL

Medical and surgical devices may serve as vehicles for the transmission of infectious agents to susceptible hosts. Before such devices can be used on a patient without posing a risk of infection, some or all of the microorganisms on its surface must be removed. Likewise, after a device has been used, it must once again be rendered safe for use in a subsequent patient or it must be disposed of. The latter option generates a large amount of potentially infectious waste, which is a cause of concern for persons in the hospital as well as in the community.

DEFINITIONS

Sterilization is the destruction or elimination of all forms of life; it can be accomplished by a physical or a chemical process. *Disinfection* is the elimination of all vegetative microorganisms, but not bacterial or fungal spores, from an inanimate object. Other related terms are commonly used and deserve mention. A *germicide* is an agent that destroys microorganisms, especially pathogens, on either living tissue or inanimate objects. An *antiseptic* is a substance applied to skin or living tissue that prevents or arrests the growth or action of microorganisms either by inhibiting their activity or by destroying them. *Pasteurization* refers to the process of exposing an object to hot (77°C) water for 30 minutes. Its purpose is to destroy all pathogenic microbes except bacterial spores. A *sanitizer* is a substance applied to inanimate objects that reduces the number of bacteria to levels judged safe by public health departments. *Cleaning* is the removal of foreign (especially organic) material from objects. *Decontamination* is the removal of pathogenic microorganisms from objects so that they are safe to handle.[1,2]

STERILIZATION

Sterilization may be accomplished by the use of heat, gases (especially ethylene oxide), glutaraldehyde, irradiation (ionizing, ultraviolet, and microwave), and filtration. The major methods used in hospitals are heat and ethylene oxide.[2–6]

Heat

The oldest and most widely recognized agent for destruction of microorganisms is heat. Both moist and dry heat sterilize, but dry heat kills at a slower rate and requires higher temperatures and longer exposure times. Even boiling water at ambient pressure is not an effective sterilizing agent, because its temperature cannot be raised above 100°C, thereby allowing many spores to survive. Saturated steam under pressure, however, provides an efficient, inexpensive method to sterilize in a relatively short time. Moreover moist heat has the advantage of penetrating many materials. The pressure of the steam per se has no influence on sterilization; increased pressure increases the temperature of the steam inside a chamber of fixed volume.

The desired endpoint of sterilization is the elimination of all microbial life forms. Because bacterial endospores are among the microorganisms most resistant to chemical and physical agents of sterilization, they are used as biologic indicators of the completeness of the process. Heat resistance varies among different microorganisms and depends upon the type of heat. The spores of *Bacillus stearothermophilus* are more resistant to moist heat and are used to monitor sterilization processes using steam. The inactivation of 100,000 of these spores by saturated steam at 121°C requires an exposure time of 12 minutes. At the same temperature, 1 million spores of *B. subtilis* are inactivated in less than 1 minute. However, *B. subtilis* var. *niger* is more resistant to dry heat than is *B. stearothermophilus*. Vegetative bacteria such as *Staphylococcus aureus* do not usually survive exposure to moist heat at 80°C for more than 10 minutes.

The thermal resistance of bacterial spores has been related to structural components such as dipicolonic acid, which is chelated with calcium ions in the spore wall and is absent from vegetative cells. Most viruses are inactivated at 60°C within 20 minutes, although longer exposures and higher temperatures are required for the more resistant small, nonenveloped RNA viruses such as poliovirus.

Steam sterilization is carried out in a variable pressure chamber called an *autoclave*, of which there are several types based on the method by which air in the chamber is removed. In downward displacement autoclaves, steam entering at the top of the chamber forces the more dense chamber air out through a discharge valve at the bottom. These units have been used widely in U.S. hospitals since the early twentieth century and are still used in most hospitals for sterilization of unwrapped or lightly wrapped materials such as laboratory media, water, pharmaceuticals, infectious waste, and nonporous articles. Prevacuumed, high-temperature sterilizers, widely used since the 1960s, remove air from the chamber before steam enters. They are used for porous materials such as towels and surgical gowns. To evaluate the efficacy of air removal in these units, the Bowie-Dick tape test has been employed. Autoclave tape, placed in the center of a stack of surgical towels, undergoes a color change on exposure to steam. A smaller disposable test pack is now available. The recommended exposure times, temperatures, and pressures for saturated steam sterilization are as follows: 15 minutes at 121°C and 103 kPa pressure (250°F, 15 psi); 10 minutes at 126°C and 138 kPa (260°F, 20 psi); and 3 minutes at 134°C and 203 kPa (273°F, 29.4 psi).[7] Although one can monitor cycle times, temperatures, and pressures, the exact conditions within the materials wrapped in packs is not known. Therefore, weekly biologic sterility testing with spores of *B. stearothermophilus* is recommended by the Centers for Disease Control (CDC) and the Joint Commission on Accreditation of Hospitals (JCAH). Test spores of *B. stearothermophilus* are incubated at 55°C. Either spore strips (Fig. 1) or a device that contains the spores in a self-contained incubation system is used. A chemical acid-base dye indicator is added to growth medium contained in small tubes with appropriate spores (Fig. 2). A change in the color of the liquid medium indicates growth and possibly ineffective conditions for sterilization. However, a single positive spore test does not necessarily indicate that objects processed in the same sterilizer are not sterile. It does require that the sterilizer be rechecked for proper temperature, pressure, and use and that the test be repeated. If the sterilizer is found to be defective, a recall of objects should be initiated. Importantly, all implantable objects should be recalled for any load in which the spore test is positive.

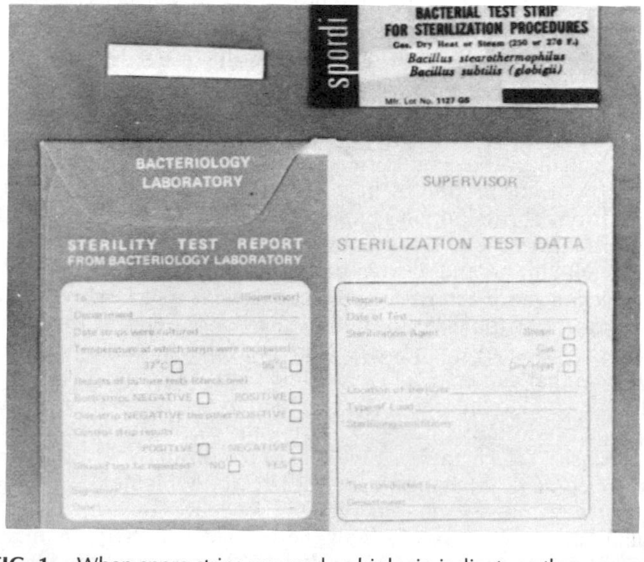

FIG. 1. When spore strips are used as biologic indicators, they are sent to the bacteriology laboratory for incubation and detection of growth. The rectangular spore strip itself is shown in the upper left-hand corner. The manufacturer places the strip inside a cellophane package, which is illustrated in the upper right-hand corner, and the cellophane package is located inside the larger paper envelope (bottom of figure). This type of biologic monitoring could be used for either gas or steam sterilization processing, since both types of spores are included on the paper strip. The central sterile supply personnel complete the data on the right half of the envelope, and the laboratory staff complete the data on the left half after incubation in appropriate media. In the combination strips, incubation for 7 days should be at 55°C if strips were exposed to steam and at 35°C if strips were exposed to gas.

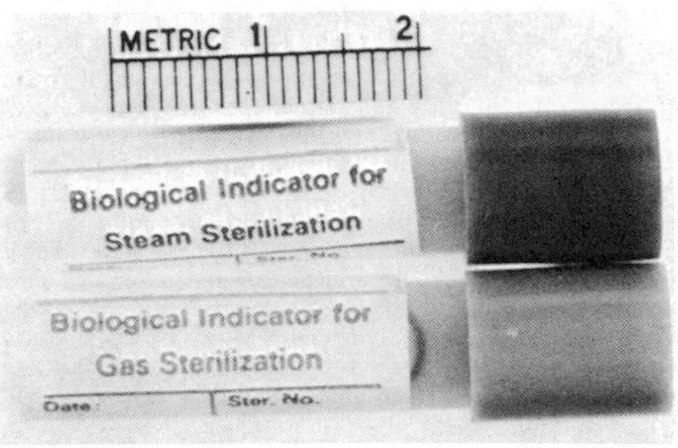

FIG. 2. Biologic indicator tubes containing spores of *Bacillus subtilis* (for gas sterilization) or *B. stearothermophilus* (for steam sterilization), growth media, and a color indicator. The tubes are placed in the cneter of the load about to be sterilized and are crushed 10 minutes after sterilization (when the tube is cool) to allow the spores to contact the growth media. The tubes are made of plastic and have a glass capsule encased within. Crushing the capsule breaks the glass, allowing the culture fluid inside to come in contact with spores located at the top of the tube. Then the tubes are incubated for 7 days. Results of the test can be read by the central sterile supply personnel. A change in color from blue to yellow means that sterilization has not been achieved.

When spore strips are used, they should be inoculated with sterile forceps in trypticase soy or a similar broth; thioglycolate broth is inhibitory and should not be used. Care should be taken that the spore strip cultures are not secondarily infected by unsterile forceps or a contaminated water bath. The alcohol flame technique for ''sterilizing'' forceps should be avoided because alcohol may contain viable spores that resist the flaming process. In addition, there has been at least one report of presumed autoclave failure due to false-positive spore strip tests related to contamination of the broth used as a growth medium. The contaminant, *Bacillus coagulans,* resulted in broth turbidity at 55°C, the optimal incubation temperature for *B. stearothermophilus*.[3] The authors recommended incubating an uninoculated tube of trypticase soy broth for quality control at 55°C in addition to the usual 37°C quality check.

Packaging should be performed in such a way as to ensure effective transmission of heat and steam and protection from oxidation, corrosion, and blunting of sharp instruments. In addition, fabric packs should never exceed the dimensions 30 × 30 × 50 cm, should always be positioned on end, and should not weigh more than 5.5 kg. Empty basins and large trays of instruments should be located at the bottom end of the autoclave to prevent condensate from wetting materials beneath. Objects that can trap cold air should always be positioned with the open end to the side (facing neither up nor down) to facilitate escape of air and condensate during the sterilization process.

''Flash'' sterilization (autoclave sterilization by the unwrapped method, using steam at 132°C for 3 minutes) was originally developed as an emergency procedure for dropped surgical instruments but is now performed routinely in many operating rooms in the United States.[9] The Association for the Advancement of Medical Instrumentation has recommended that it be restricted to unplanned or emergency situations and that implantable devices never be sterilized by this method.[10] Although sterilization failure is rarely a cause of serious bacterial nosocomial infections, episodes have been reported. Two surgical patients developed tetanus due to inadequate sterilization of talc glove powder.[11] Additionally, an outbreak of *Pseudomonas aeruginosa* serotype 011 meningitis and intra-abdominal infections resulted from failure of flash sterilization of extension tubing used for cerebral ventriculoperitoneal shunts.[12]

Ethylene Oxide

Two gases, ethylene oxide and formaldehyde, have been used extensively in the sterilization of medical products. Currently, the most widely used gaseous sterilizing agent in the United States is ethylene oxide (EtO). It is used almost exclusively by hospitals and manufacturers of medical devices to sterilize items that cannot be sterilized by heat or radiation. Such items include those made of plastic, rubber, cotton, wool, and silk, as well as electronic equipment.[2,4,6] EtO, an epoxide with the molecular formula CH_2CH_2O, is a colorless gas (bp 10.4°C at 760 torr) that is water soluble. EtO is an explosive gas even at 3% vapor and air; therefore, it is mixed with either carbon dioxide or fluorinated hydrocarbons to increase its safety for hospital use. Carbon dioxide is less expensive, but because of high vapor pressure it must be contained in expensive steel chambers. In contrast, the fluorinated material is more expensive, but it can be contained in less costly metal containers. Many EtO sterilizers, however, use 100% EtO in chambers kept under significant negative pressure for safety. If they are properly designed and operated, there is no evidence of risk of explosion using 100% EtO in hospitals.

The microbicidal activity of EtO is primarily due to alkylation of nucleic acids by the replacement of a labile hydrogen with a hydroxyethyl group, $-CH_2CH_2OH$. EtO inactivates all microorganisms that contain nucleic acids. Since spores of *B. subtilis* are relatively resistant, this microorganism is the biologic indicator of choice for EtO.[2,4] Spores should be incubated at 35–37°C. The frequency of testing recommended by the CDC is at least once a week, although live bacterial spores should be used with each load of implantable or intravascular items undergoing gas sterilization.[13]

The Occupational Safety and Health Administration (OSHA) has declared that exposure to EtO presents a carcinogenic, mutagenic, neurologic, and sensitization hazard to workers.[14] In 1984, OSHA reduced the time-weighted average permissible exposure limit for EtO from the previous 50 mg/liter (50 ppm) to 1 mg/liter. Determinations of employee exposure from breathing-zone air samples are required. The odor of EtO is detectable at about 700 mg/liter. Exposure to high concentrations of EtO can occur in three situations: (*1*) when the door of the sterilizer is opened in close proximity to the cabinet; (*2*) with unvented sterilizers; and (*3*) with unvented aerators. Hospitals should be aware of these high-risk locations and times and make efforts to minimize exposure.

Some of the unwanted side effects associated with the use of EtO and the fluorohydrocarbon mixtures are marbling, which occurs in some plastics, and fogging of certain types of endoscopic instruments. If the process includes application of heat to 60°C or more, certain lens cements will dissolve, allowing moisture to enter the chamber.

One must be careful to follow the exact specifications of the manufacturer. When EtO is also used commercially to sterilize biologicals such as antibiotics, the pharmaceutical industry must be prepared to show that no toxicity has been imparted and that there has been no loss of biologic activity. In hospitals using a gas sterilizer that incorporates a heating coil, the manufacturers recommend the use of EtO at a concentration of ≥450 mg/liter and at an adequate relative humidity. Sterilization of heat-sensitive objects with ionizing radiation has been suggested as an alternative to the use of toxic gases, but currently the cost is prohibitive.

EtO sterilization is carried out in a pressure chamber with the capacity to evacuate air, to warm and moisturize the product uniformly, to add EtO at a specific temperature, and to remove EtO after a specified time interval. The major factors that affect the inactivation of microorganisms by EtO are gas concentration, temperature, relative humidity, and exposure time. In general, doubling the concentration or vapor pressure will halve the sterilization time. Also, for each increase of 10°C there is a doubling of the activity. Sterilization with EtO is most rapid at a relative humidity of 30% and is increasingly slower above and below this point.

The sterilization process includes the use of two separate chambers: a gas sterilization unit and an aeration cabinet. The latter is used to allow the noxious gas to dissipate rapidly (8–12 hours) from gas-sterilized items. Without a heated aeration cabinet, aeration times up of to 1 week would be necessary to make materials safe for reuse. Two large manufacturers of EtO sterilization systems use 100% EtO and 12% EtO plus 88% freon, respectively.

The major advantage of using EtO is its ability to sterilize heat-sensitive items. Exposure to EtO can be carried out at lower temperatures and pressures to achieve sterilization. EtO is able to penetrate through a mass of materials, and it dissolves in rubber and plastics. The disadvantages of EtO gas sterilization include the long cycle time, exposure, and toxicity.

DISINFECTION

It would be optimal if all medical and surgical devices could be sterilized by steam autoclaving. Since this is not possible, one must often choose from among a number of chemical disinfectants. Spaulding[15] outlined an approach to this problem in which he defined three categories of disinfectants, based on their level of germicidal action (Table 1), and three categories of instruments based on the degree of infection risk involved in their use (Table 2). *High-level disinfectants* are effective against bacterial endospores if the exposure time is long enough. *Intermediate-level* disinfectants are tuberculocidal but not sporicidal. *Low-level disinfectants* will not reliably destroy bacterial endospores, tubercle bacilli, or small, nonlipid RNA viruses (e.g., enteroviruses). Some disinfectants, known as *chemosterilizers,* will produce sterility if the contact time is long enough. Items to be disinfected are categorized as critical, semicritical or noncritical based on their degree of contact with the patient (Table 2). This scheme is an oversimplification, especially with regard to items in the semicritical category, over which there is debate about whether sterilization or high-level disinfection is the appropriate minimum level of treatment. Organic material, such as blood, pus, and feces, absorbs and inactivates germicides, leaving only the excess free chemical to act. Therefore, thorough cleansing and rinsing are essential before disinfection. This is especially important for reprocessing of respiratory therapy equipment. Aqueous glutaraldehyde solutions and pasteurization are frequently used. In a recent study, the authors demonstrated the efficacy of a synergized glutaraldehyde-phenate solution (Sporocidin) in disinfecting respiratory therapy equipment contaminated during patient use.[16]

It should be pointed out that since the summer of 1982, the Environmental Protection Agency (EPA) has discontinued efficacy testing of disinfectants after registration with the agency. Whether this action will have any effect on infection control is unclear. Currently, therefore, testing of efficacy can be performed in clinical microbiology laboratories, commercial laboratories, or state health department laboratories.

Disinfectants that are widely used at present include alcohols, hypochlorites and other chlorine compounds, formaldehyde, glutaraldehyde, hydrogen peroxide, iodophors, phenolics, and quaternary ammonium compounds.

There have been numerous reports of infections due either to failure of disinfectants to kill certain microbes or to contaminated disinfectants. The quaternary ammonium compounds, especially benzalkonium chloride, have been cited most often. Shickman et al.[17] reported an outbreak of *P. aeruginosa* bacteremias manifesting as fever, chills, and hypotension occurring about 1 hour after cardiac catheterization. The catheters were immersed in benzalkonium chloride before the procedure, and *P. aeruginosa* was isolated from benzalkonium aspirated from the lumen of the catheter. In another hospital outbreak of blood stream and other infections due to *Enterobacter cloacae,* the organism was recovered from an aqueous solution of benzalkonium chloride-containing gauze sponges. The authors were able to contaminate the disinfectant experimentally with the epidemic strain of bacteria in the presence, but not in the absence, of sterile cotton gauze.[18] An outbreak of *Pseudomonas cepacia* bacteremia in 1975 was also related to the inactivation of benzalkonium chloride in the presence of organic material (rayon sponges).[19] Furthermore, chlorhexidine[20,21] and phenols[22] have also been incriminated in reports of contaminated disinfectants. *Pseudomonas* spp., especially *P. cepacia* and *P. aeruginosa,* are the isolates most frequently associated with infections related to contaminated disinfectants.[23]

A summary of all the disinfectants in current use is beyond the scope of this chapter and can be found in several excellent reviews.[2,24,25]

TABLE 1. Levels of Disinfection According to Type of Microorganism

	Bacteria				Viruses	
Level	*Vegetative*	*Tubercle Bacillus*	*Spores*	*Fungi*[a]	*Lipid and Medium Size*	*Nonlipid and Small*
High	+[b]	+	+[c]	+	+	+
Intermediate	+	+	±[d]	+	+	±[e]
Low	+	−	−	±	+	−

[a] Includes asexual spores but not necessarily chlamydospores or sexual spores.
[b] A plus sign indicates that a killing effect can be expected when the normal-use concentrations of chemical disinfectants or pasteurization are properly employed; a minus sign indicates little or no killing effect.
[c] Only with extended exposure times are high-level disinfectant chemicals capable of actual sterilization.
[d] Some intermediate-level disinfectants can be expected to exhibit some sporicidal action.
[e] Some intermediate-level disinfectants may have limited virucidal activity.
(From Gainer and Favero,[13] with permission.)

Infectious Waste

It is estimated that acute care hospitals generate about 5–6 kg of solid waste per patient per day and that 5–7 percent of this is infectious waste.[26] The topic of disposal of infectious waste from hospitals is currently an area of controversy, and there are few data upon which to base rational conclusions. Thus, much current practice is based on state and local regulations as well as guidelines from various national agencies. In 1976, Congress enacted the Resource Conservation and Recovery Act (RCRA, P.L. 94-580), which charged the EPA with the responsibility of formulating "cradle-to-grave" regulations for hazardous waste. Hazardous waste is defined in this act as "solid waste . . . [that may] pose a substantial present or potential hazard to human health or the environment when improperly . . . managed" (42 USC 6091 et seq). The EPA, in turn, has defined infectious wastes as "wastes that in all probability contain pathogenic agents that, because of their type, concentration, and quantity, may cause disease in persons exposed to the waste."[27] At the time of this writing, the EPA has not issued any regulations regarding the disposal of infectious waste. However, Congress is considering a bill that would require the EPA to promulgate such regulations. Public awareness of this issue has been heightened by several instances of hospital waste mismanagement that have been widely reported (e.g., plastic tubing and vials washed ashore on Long Island beaches), as well as concern that waste from patients with human immunodeficiency virus (HIV) infection may pose a public health hazard.

There are few studies to support the hypothesis that hospital waste has ever caused infections. A study that quantified the microbial load associated with hospital waste found that it was no more contaminated with microbes than household waste; moreover, common nosocomial pathogens (e.g., *P. aeruginosa, Enterobacter* ssp., *Klebsiella* ssp., and group D streptococci) were detected more often in household waste.[28] Although there

TABLE 2. Guidelines for Cleaning, Disinfecting, and Sterilizing Medical Equipment

Classification	*Definition*	*Example*	*Minimal Level of Disinfection*	*Example of Agents*
Critical	An object introduced directly into the blood stream or into other normally sterile areas of the body	Surgical instruments, cardiac catheters, implants, components of a heart-lung oxygenator	Sterilization	Steam, EtO, chemosterilizers
Semicritical	An object that comes into contact with intact mucous membranes	Flexible fiberoptic endoscope, endotracheal tube, anesthesia breathing circuit	High-level chemical disinfection or wet pasteurization (sterilization is preferable)	Glutaraldehyde, hydrogen peroxide, ethyl alcohol, chlorine
Noncritical	An object that comes into contact with intact skin	Blood pressure cuff, table top, electrocardiographic leads	Cleaning or low-level disinfection	

(From Garner and Favero,[13] with permission.)

are numerous reports of nosocomial transmission of infection related to sharp objects in hospital waste,[29,30] there is only one reported instance of in-hospital transmission of infection not related to sharp objects. This involved a hospital's chute hydropulping waste system that was a reservoir of airborne *Pseudomonas*.[31] Moreover, there is no evidence that hospital waste disposal practices have caused disease in the community.[32] With regard to concern over transmission of HIV related to exposure to hospital waste, a study at the CDC showed that drying HIV caused a 10- to 100-fold reduction in HIV concentration within several hours.[33]

Both the CDC[13] and the EPA[27] have issued guidelines on the management of infectious waste (Table 3). In addition to those shown in the table, the EPA designates items such as contaminated laboratory waste, surgery and autopsy waste, dialysis unit waste, and contaminated equipment as possibly infectious waste, leaving the decision to an authorized person at the hospital.

Recommended methods of treatment of infectious waste include steam sterilization or incineration.[34,35] Disposal can be maintained by one of two methods: incineration or landfilling. Incineration seems preferable and theoretically has many advantages, including its performance on site, thereby eliminating the need to travel any distance from the hospital. It also has the advantage of reducing the waste to only 10 percent of the original volume of material, but it is generally much more expensive than landfilling. Pollution standards for incinerators are strict today, and this is a particularly important consideration because combustion of polyvinyl chloride leads to the production of hydrochloric acid, smoke, and ash.

Collection of materials for incineration should include consideration for protecting housekeeping and waste disposal personnel from injuries from sharp objects. The best method is to use specially designed boxes rather than simple plastic bags. Transportation to a remote site must comply with standards for shipping hazardous waste.

The two phases of incineration involve solid refuse combustion in an ignition chamber and the gaseous phase of combustion, which is the result of a downdraft or a mixing of air in a second chamber. The retention times and operating temperatures in the secondary combustion areas vary from one manufacturer to another but range from 0.2 second at 1315°C to 0.5 second at 815°C. It should be mentioned that poor incineration is not always a design problem but can be a performance problem, since sometimes the least skilled people are given the responsibility of operating these highly expensive (≥$30,000) and sometimes complex machines.

TABLE 3. Types of Solid Waste Designated as Infectious and Recommended Disposal Methods

	CDC		*EPA*	
Source or Type of Solid Waste	*Infectious Waste*	*Disposal/ Treatment Method*	*Infectious Waste*	*Disposal/ Treatment Method*
Microbiological	Yes	S, I	Yes	S, I, TI, C
Blood/blood products	Yes	S, I, Sew	Yes	S, I, Sew, C
Pathologic tissue	Yes	I	Yes	I, SW, CB
Sharp objects	Yes	S, I	Yes	S, I
Waste from patients on communicable disease isolation precautions	?	GIPH	Yes	S, I

Abbreviations: I: incineration; S: steam sterilization; TI: thermal inactivation; C: chemical disinfection (for liquids only); Sew: sanitary sewer (the EPA requires secondary treatment); SW: steam sterilization with incineration or grinding; CB: cremation or burial by a mortician; GIPH: handle according to the current edition of *CDC Guidelines for Isolation Precautions in Hospitals*. (Modified from Rutala and Sarubbi,[26] with permission.)

Biologic waste is not only great in quantity but comes from diverse sources, including physicians' offices, outpatient facilities, and veterinary hospitals. It is obvious that, with the huge amount of material constantly being dumped, there must be some regulation. Currently, there are no data to show that the risk of infection is significantly greater in workers handling solid waste materials. Nevertheless, reasonable precautions should be maintained by these workers. It is essential that no scavenging of any part of hospital waste be permitted.

CURRENT ISSUES IN DISINFECTION, STERILIZATION, AND DISPOSAL OF HOSPITAL WASTE

Human Immunodeficiency Virus

HIV is a 100-nm RNA virus with a lipid envelope.[36] In general, the presence of lipid in a virus is associated with a high degree of susceptibility to all germicides.[37] Using a quantitative bioassay, Martin et al.[38] found that alcohols, hypochlorite, hydrogen peroxide, phenolics, paraformaldehyde, and the detergent NP-40 (but not Tween-20) inactivated HIV at concentrations well below those commonly employed. Spire et al.,[39] using an assay for reverse transcriptase activity, examined the inactivation of HIV by commonly used disinfectants. They suggested that 25% ethanol or 1% glutaraldehyde should be sufficient to disinfect medical instruments, and that 0.2% sodium hypochlorite should be sufficient for cleaning floors and benches. Formalin 0.1% required 48 hours to render reverse transcriptase activity undetectable. Resnick et al.[40] pointed out that assays for reverse transcriptase activity are not reliable alternatives to tests for infectious virus, as the ability to detect reverse transcriptase activity is rapidly lost upon dilution. Using a highly concentrated viral preparation, they found that infectious cell-free virus could be recovered from dried material for 3–7 days. In an aqueous environment, HIV retained its infectivity for more than 2 weeks at room temperature (23–27°C). Sodium hypochlorite 0.5% (a 10% solution of household bleach), alcohol 70%, or NP-40 0.5% completely inactivated HIV after 1 minute of exposure.

Reusable devices should receive high-level disinfection or sterilization by steam or EtO. As a general rule, any contaminated equipment that can withstand heat should be autoclaved. Endoscopes should be sterilized with EtO or receive high-level disinfection with a mycobactericidal agent, such as soaking in 2% glutaraldehyde for 45 minutes.[41]

Disposable items that are visibly contaminated should be

placed in a waterproof bag and disposed of like other infectious waste. Standard dishwashing and laundering procedures will adequately decontaminate eating utensils and linens. Visibly contaminated linens should first be placed in a hot-water-soluble bag and then in a waterproof plastic bag for transport to the laundry.

Patients infected with HIV can undergo hemodialysis and do not require isolation from other patients. The dialyzer is disposable. Recommendations for disinfecting the dialysis fluid pathways of the hemodialysis machine (exposure to 500–750 mg/liter of sodium hypochlorite for 30–40 minutes) were originally aimed at controlling bacterial contamination but are also effective against HIV.[42]

Creutzfeldt-Jakob Disease Agent

Current evidence suggests that Creutzfeldt-Jakob disease (CJD) and several other transmissible neurodegenerative diseases may be caused by infectious agents known as *prions*,[43] a term defined by Prusiner as "a small proteinaceous infectious particle which resists inactivation by procedures that modify nucleic acids." Person-to-person transmission of the agent has been reported in association with corneal transplantation[44] and with silver electrodes used for stereotactic electroencephalographic exploration for excision of epileptic foci.[45] In the latter case, the electrodes had been treated with 70% ethanol and exposure to formaldehyde vapor for 48 hours. Recently, potential occupational transmission of CJD has been described in three histopathologists.[46–46b] Transmission studies have shown that primates can be infected via the percutaneous route. Brain, spinal cord, and cerebrospinal fluid from humans or animals with CJD have regularly transmitted infection when inoculated into animals. Other visceral organs (liver, lung, kidney) transmit infection less predictably. Blood has been found to be infective in studies using guinea pigs. The agent associated with CJD is resistant to many of the standard disinfection and sterilization procedures including boiling, ultraviolet irradiation, ionizing radiation, 70% ethanol plus formaldehyde vapor, glutaraldehyde, and 4% formaldehyde (10% formalin, as used to preserve pathologic specimens).[47] Thus, brain biopsy specimens or other tissue fixed in formalin should be considered infectious.[48] Taylor and McConnell showed that brain tissue from mice with scrapie was infectious even after autoclaving.[48a] Previous recommendations for the handling of material from patients with CJD relied heavily on data from experiments with the prion associated with scrapie.[49] More recent data based on studies using guinea pig and mouse-adapted isolates from patients with CJD show that three techniques will inactivate the agent: (*1*) autoclaving for 1 hour at no less than 121°C and 103 kPa pressure (250°F, 15 psi); (*2*) exposure to 1 N or 0.1 N sodium hydroxide for 1 hour at room temperature; and (*3*) exposure to 0.5% sodium hypochlorite (a 10-fold dilution of household bleach).[50,51] Compared with hypochlorite, 1 N sodium hydroxide was more active against large titers of scrapie agent, less corrosive to fabrics and plastic surfaces, and less irritating to skin. The authors recommended that contaminated skin be disinfected with a 5- to 10-minute exposure to 1 N sodium hydroxide followed by extensive washing with water. At this time, EtO cannot be recommended for sterilizing instruments potentially contaminated with the agent of CJD.[51]

Hepatitis B Virus

Hepatitis B virus (HBV) is a 42-nm DNA virus with a lipid envelope. It has been detected on a wide variety of inanimate environmental surfaces. HBV in human plasma retained its infectivity for a chimpanzee after the virus was dried and stored at 25°C for 7 days.[52] Lack of a method of propagating HBV in the laboratory has hindered the understanding of HBV inactivation by physical and chemical agents. Studies suggest that 500 mg/liter sodium hypochlorite, 70% isopropyl alcohol, 80% ethyl alcohol, and 2% glutaraldehyde are effective.[53,54] Heat is the preferred treatment. Autoclaving at 121°C and 103 kPa for 15 minutes, exposure to dry heat at 160°C for 2 hours, and boiling in water at 100°C for 10 minutes will inactive HBV. Environmental surfaces should be disinfected with sodium hypochlorite (500–5000 mg/liter). For other devices, a high-level disinfectant such as 2% glutaraldehyde is recommended.[55]

Endoscopes

Flexible fiberoptic endoscopes (colonoscopes, bronchoscopes, etc.) pose a number of problems with regard to decontamination. They are expensive, contain narrow channels and valves that are difficult to clean, are unable to withstand heat sterilization, and are often introduced into the next patient within 10 minutes of previous use.[56] Infections after gastrointestinal endoscopy are infrequent.[57] Nonetheless, reports of infection due to inadequately decontaminated endoscopes, especially those used for endoscopic retrograde cholangiopancreatography, illustrate their potential as a source of nosocomial infection. The organisms most often associated with infections due to gastrointestinal endoscopes are *Salmonella* spp.[57–60] and *P. aeruginosa*.[57,61–64] Nosocomial infections from contaminated bronchoscopes have also been reported, including outbreaks of pulmonary infections due to *Serratia marcescens*,[65] and possibly to *Mycobacterium tuberculosis*.[66] In the latter report, a 30-minute exposure to 2% glutaraldehyde failed to disinfect suction valves contaminated with mycobacteria. In many of the reported cases, the disinfectants used on the endoscopes were less active against gram-negative bacteria than glutaraldehyde or povidone-iodine solutions. Both the type of disinfectant and the technique used are important. Like other instruments, the endoscope must be carefully cleaned before disinfection or sterilization to remove any organic material. Ideally, endoscopes should be sterilized with EtO. If this is not possible, several alternatives for soaking in commercial preparations are recommended usually with 30-minute contact times: 8% aqueous formaldehyde, 2% alkalinized glutaraldehyde, or an iodophor with 5000 mg/liter available iodine.[67,68] In a study of automated cleaning and disinfecting machines, Babb et al. found that 2% alkaline glutaraldehyde was the most effective disinfectant, but it caused a hypersensitivity reaction in some of the personnel.[56] The CDC does not recommend the use of quaternary ammonium compounds, phenolics, or alcohols. All accessories of the endoscopes, such as cytology brushes, biopsy probes, and cleaning brushes, should be either disposable or sterilized by autoclaving after each use. After soaking, the unit should be rinsed three times in either sterile distilled water or tap water with 10 mg/liter hypochlorite. The endoscope should then be dried by personnel wearing sterile gloves and using sterile towels, placed in a sterile wrapper, and kept until ready for reuse. The risk of transmission of HBV via endoscopes is probably very low.[69–71] However, one reported case of hepatitis B was almost certainly acquired from a contaminated endoscope,[72] and Morris et al.[73] reported a patient whose serum tested positive for hepatitis B surface antigen after exposure to a contaminated endoscope. Such reports emphasize the need for adequate cleaning and high-level disinfection or even sterilization of endoscopes after procedures.

REFERENCES

1. Block SS. Definition of terms. In: Block SS, ed. Disinfection, Sterilization, and Preservation. 3rd ed. Philadelphia: Lea and Febiger; 1983:877–81.
2. Rutala WA. Disinfection, sterilization, and waste disposal. In: Wenzel RP, ed. Prevention and Control of Nosocomial Infections. Baltimore: Williams and Wilkins; 1987:257–82.
3. Joslyn L. Sterilization by heat. In: Block SS, ed. Disinfection, Sterilization, and Preservation. 3rd ed. Philadelphia: Lea and Febiger; 1983:3–46.
4. Caputo RA, Odlaug TE. Sterilization with ethylene oxide and other gases. In: Block SS, ed. Disinfection, Sterilization, and Preservation. 3rd ed. Philadelphia: Lea and Febiger; 1983:47–64.

5. Alder VG, Simpson RA. Sterilization and disinfection by heat methods. In: Russel AD, Hugo WB, Ayliffe GAJ, eds. Principles and Practice of Disinfection, Preservation, and Sterilization. Oxford: Blackwell; 1982:433–53.
6. Christensen EA, Kristensen H. Gaseous sterilization. In: Russell AD, Hugo WB, Ayliffe GAJ, eds. Principles and Practice of Disinfection, Preservation, and Sterilization. Oxford: Blackwell; 1982:548–68.
7. Ernst RR. Sterilization by heat. In: Block SS, ed. Disinfection, Sterilization and Preservation. 2nd ed. Philadelphia: Lea and Febiger; 1977:481.
8. Gurevich I, Holmes JE, Cunha BA. Presumed autoclave failure due to false-positive spore strip tests. Infect Control. 1982;3:388–92.
9. Kotilainen HR, Gantz NM. An evaluation of three biological indicator systems in flash sterilization. Infect Control. 1987;8:311–6.
10. Maki DG, Hassemer CA. Flash sterilization: Carefully measured haste. Infect Control. 1987;8:307–10.
11. Sevitt S. Source of two hospital-infected cases of tetanus. Lancet. 1949; 2:1075–8.
12. Ho JL, Highsmith AK, Wong ES, et al. Common-source *Pseudomonas aeruginosa* infection in neurosurgery. In: Proceedings and Abstracts of the Annual Meeting of the American Society for Microbiology. Abstract L-10. Washington, DC: American Society for Microbiology; 1981:80.
13. Garner JS, Favero MS. CDC guideline for handwashing and hospital environmental control, 1985. Infect Control. 1986;7:231–43.
14. Federal Register. Occupational exposure to ethylene oxide: Final standard. 29 CRF Part 1910. Washington, DC: Department of Labor, Occupational Safety and Health Administration; June 22, 1984.
15. Spaulding EH. Chemical disinfection of medical and surgical materials. In: Lawrence CA, Block SS, eds. Disinfection, Sterilization, and Preservation. Philadelphia: Lea and Febiger; 1968:517–31.
16. Townsend TR, Wee SB, Koblin B. An efficacy evaluation of a synergized glutaraldehyde-phenate solution in disinfecting respiratory therapy equipment contaminated during patient use. Infect Control. 1982;3:240–4.
17. Shickman MD, Guze LB, Pearce ML. Bacteremia following cardiac catheterization. N Engl J Med. 1959;260:1164–6.
18. Malizia WF, Gangarosa EJ, Goley AF. Benzalkonium chloride as a source of infection. N Engl J Med. 1960;263:800–2.
19. Frank MJ, Schaffner W. Contaminated aqueous benzalkonium chloride—an unnecessary hospital hazard. JAMA. 1976;236:2418–9.
20. Mitchell RG, Hayward AC. Post-operative urinary tract infections caused by contaminated irrigating fluid. Lancet. 1966;1:793–5.
21. Coyle-Gilchrist MM, Crewe P, Roberts G. *Flavobacterium meningosepticum* in the hospital environment. J Clin Pathol. 1976;29:824–6.
22. Newman KA, Tenney JH, Oken HA, et al. Persistent isolation of an unusual *Pseudomonas* species from a phenolic disinfectant system. Infect Control. 1984;5:219–222.
23. Rutala WA, Cole EC. Antiseptics and disinfectants—safe and effective? Infect Control. 1984;5:215–8.
24. Favero MS. Chemical disinfection of medical and surgical materials. In: Block SS, ed. Disinfection, Sterilization and Preservation. 3rd ed. Philadelphia: Lea and Febiger; 1983:469–92.
25. Hugo WB, Russell AD. Types of antimicrobial agents. In: Russell AD, Hugo WB, Ayliffe GAJ, eds. Principles and Practice of Disinfection, Preservation, and Sterilization. Oxford: Blackwell; 1982:8–106.
26. Rutala WA, Sarubbi FA. Management of infectious waste from hospitals. Infect Control. 1983;4:198–204.
27. United States Environmental Protection Agency. EPA Guide for Infectious Waste Management. Pub. No. EPA/530-SW-86-014. Springfield, VA: National Technical Information Service; May 1986.
28. Kalnowski G, Wiegand H, Ruden H. The microbial contamination of hospital Waste. Zentrlbl Bakteriol [B]. 1983;178:364–79.
29. McCormick RD, Maki DG. Epidemiology of needle-stick injuries in hospital personnel. Am J Med. 1981;70:928–32.
30. Jacobson JT, Burke JD, Conti MT. Injuries of hospital employees from needles and sharp objects. Infect Control. 1983;2:100–2.
31. Grieble HG, Bird TJ, Nidea HM, et al. Chute-hydropulping waste disposal system: A reservoir of enteric bacilli and *Pseudomonas* in a modern hospital. J Infect Dis. 1974;130:602–7.
32. Rutala WA. Infectious waste—a growing problem for infection control. Asepsis. 1987;9(4):2–6.
33. Centers for Disease Control. Recommendations for prevention of HIV transmission in health-care settings. MMWR. 1987;36(Suppl 2S):10S.
34. Rutala WA, Stiegel MM, Sarubbi FA. Decontamination of laboratory microbiological waste by steam sterilization. Appl Environ Microbiol. 1982; 43:1311–6.
35. Peterson ML, Statzenberger FJ. Microbiological evaluation of incineration operations. Appl Microbiol. 1969;18:8–13.
36. Ho DD, Pomerantz RJ, Kaplan JC. Pathogenesis of infection with human immunodeficiency virus. N Engl J Med. 1987;317:278–86.
37. Klein M, Deforest A. Principles of viral inactivation. In: Block SS, ed. Disinfection, Sterilization, and Preservation. 3rd ed. Philadelphia: Lea and Febiger; 1983:422–34.
38. Martin LS, McDougal JS, Loskoski SL. Disinfection and inactivation of the human T lymphotropic virus type III/lymphadenopathy-associated virus. J Infect Dis. 1985;152:400–3.
39. Spire B, Barre-Sinoussi F, Montagnier L, et al. Inactivation of lymphadenopathy-associated virus by chemical disinfectants. Lancet. 1984;2:899–901.
40. Resnick L, Veren K, Salahuddin SZ, et al. Stability and inactivation of HTLV-III/LAV under clinical and laboratory environments. JAMA. 1986;255:1887–91.
41. Conte JE Jr. Infection with human immunodeficiency virus in the hospital—epidemiology, infection control, and biosafety considerations. Ann Intern Med. 1986;105:730–6.
42. Centers for Disease Control. Recommendations for providing dialysis treatment to patients infected with human T-lymphotropic virus type III/lymphadenopathy-associated virus. MMWR. 1986;35:376–8, 383.
43. Prusiner SB. Prions and neurodegenerative diseases. N Engl J Med. 1987; 317:1571–81.
44. Duffy P, Wolf J, Collins G, et al. Possible person-to-person transmission of Creutzfeldt-Jakob disease. N Engl J Med. 1974;290:692–3.
45. Bernoulli C, Siegfried J, Baumgartner G, et al. Danger of accidental person-to-person transmission of Creutzfeldt-Jakob disease by surgery. Lancet. 1977;1:478–9.
46. Miller DC. Creutzfeldt-Jakob disease in histopathology technicians. N Engl J Med. 1988;318:853–4.
46a. Sitwell L, Lach B, Atack E, et al. Creutzfeldt-Jakob disease in histopathology technicians. N Engl J Med. 1988;318:854.
46b. Brown P, Cathala F, Raubertas RF, et al. The epidemiology of Creutzfeldt-Jakob disease: Conclusion of a 15 year investigation in France and review of the world literature. Neurology. 1987;37:473–7.
47. Jarvis WR. Precautions for Creutzfeldt-Jakob disease. Infect Control. 1982; 3:238–9.
48. Brown P, Gibbs CJ Jr, Gajdusek DC, et al. Transmission of Creutzfeldt-Jakob disease formalin-fixed, paraffin-embedded human brain tissue. N Engl J Med. 1986;315:1614–5.
48a. Taylor DM, McConnell I. Autoclaving does not decontaminate formalin-fixed scrapie tissues. Lancet. 1988;i:463–4.
49. Gajdusek DC, Gibbs CJ Jr, Asher DM, et al. Precautions in medical care of, and in handling materials from, patients with transmissible virus dementia (Creutzfeldt-Jakob disease). N Engl J Med. 1977;297:1253–8.
50. Brown P, Rohwer RG, Gajdusek CD. Sodium hydroxide decontamination of Creutzfeldt-Jakob disease virus. N Engl J Med. 1984;310:727.
51. Brown P, Gibbs CJ Jr, Amyx HL, et al. Chemical disinfection of Creutzfeldt-Jakob disease virus. N Engl J Med. 1982;306:1279–82.
52. Bond WW, Favero MS, Peterson NJ, et al. Survival of hepatitis B virus after drying and storage for one week. Lancet. 1981;1:550–1.
53. Bond WW, Favero MS, Petersen NS, et al. Inactivation of hepatitis B virus by intermediate-to-high level disinfectant chemicals. J Clin Microbiol. 1983;18:535–8.
54. Kobayashi H, Tsuzuki M, Koshimizu K, et al. Susceptibility of hepatitis B virus to disinfectants or heat. J Clin Microbiol. 1984;20:214–6.
55. Bond WW, Peterson NJ, Favero MS. Viral hepatitis B: Aspects of environmental control. Health Lab Sci. 1977;14:235–52.
56. Babb JR, Bradley CR, Deverill CEA, et al. Recent advances in the cleaning and disinfection of fibrescopes. J Hosp Infect. 1981;2:329–40.
57. Vennes JA. Infectious complications of gastrointestinal endoscopy. Dig Dis Sci. 1981;26(July Suppl):60–4S.
58. Colin-Jones DG, Cockel R, Schiller KFR. Current endoscopic practice in the United Kingdom. Clin Gastroenterol. 1978;7:775–86.
59. Beecham HJ, Mitchell LC, Parkin WE. *Salmonella typhimurium* transmitted by fiberoptic upper gastrointestinal endoscopy. JAMA. 1979;241:1013–5.
60. Noy MF, Harrison L, Holmes GKT, et al. The significance of bacterial contamination of fiberoptic endoscopes. J Hosp Infect. 1980;1:53–61.
61. Earnshaw JJ, Clark AW, Thun BT. Outbreak of *Pseudomonas aeruginosa* following endoscopic retrograde cholangiopancreatography. J Hosp Infect. 1985;6:95–7.
62. Allen JI, Allen MO, Olson MM, et al. *Pseudomonas* infection of the biliary system resulting from use of a contaminated endoscope. Gastroenterology. 1987;92:759–63.
63. Classen DC, Jacobson JA, Burke JP, et al. Serious pseudomonas infections associated with endoscopic retrograde cholangiopancreatography. Am J Med. 1988;84:590–6.
64. Allen JI, O'Conner-Allen M, Olson MM, et al. *Pseudomonas* infection of the biliary system resulting from use of a contaminated endoscope. Gastroenterology. 1987;92:759–63.
65. Webb SF, Vall-Spinosa A. Outbreak of *Serratia marcescens* associated with the flexible fiberbronchoscope. Chest. 1975;68:703–8.
66. Wheeler PW, Kaiser AB. Mycobacterial contamination of bronchoscopy specimens and possible pulmonary infection due to an inability to disinfect the suction valves of bronchoscopes. In: Program and Abstracts of the 27th Interscience Conference on Antimicrobial Agents and Chemotherapy. Abstract 71. New York: American Society for Microbiology; 1987:108.
67. Simmons BP, Hooton TM, Mallison GF. CDC guidelines for the prevention and control of nosocomial infections; guideline for hsopital environmental control. Am J Infect Control. 1983;11:97–120.
68. Ad Hoc Committee on Infection Control in the Handling of Endoscopic Equipment: Guidelines for cleaning and disinfection of flexible fiberoptic endoscopes used in gastrointestinal endoscopy. AORN J. 1978;28:907–10.
69. Moncada RE, Denes AE, Berquist KR, et al. Inadvertent exposure of endoscopy patients to viral hepatitis B. Gastrointest Endosc. 1978;24:231–2.
70. Hoofnagle JH, Blake J, Buskell-Bales J, et al. Lack of transmission of type B hepatitis by fiberoptic upper endoscopy. J Clin Gastroenterol. 1980;2:65–9.
71. Bond WW, Moncada RE. Viral hepatitis B infection risk in flexible fiberoptic endoscopy. Gastrointest Endosc. 1978;24:225–30.

72. Birnie GG, Quigley EM, Clements BG, et al. Endoscopic transmission of hepatitis B virus. Gut. 1983;24:171–4.
73. Morris IM, Cattle DDS, Smits BJ. Endoscopy and transmission of hepatitis B. Lancet. 1975;2:1152.

279. BACTEREMIA DUE TO PERCUTANEOUS INTRAVASCULAR DEVICES

DAVID K. HENDERSON

The relentless progress of medical science and technology has been accompanied by the development of a host of new devices, each with its own complications. Included in the list of devices to be discussed are peripheral and central intravenous catheters, total parenteral nutrition (TPN) catheters, flow-directed balloon-tipped pulmonary artery catheters, arterial lines, and catheters placed to afford long-term central venous access such as Hickman or Broviac catheters.

Maki has suggested that more than 25,000 patients develop device-related bacteremia in the United States each year.[1] Such device-associated infections occur as sporadic cases as well as in case clusters caused by the same organism. Most sporadic nosocomial bacteremias, however, are not device related but occur as a result of distant localized infection that then seeds the blood stream.[2] Primary bacteremias (i.e., those without an obvious infected focus outside the blood stream) account for only one-fourth of sporadic nosocomial bacteremias.

Conversely, more than three-fourths of the nosocomial bacteremias occurring in case clusters are primary bacteremias, and more than 75 percent of these are device associated.[2] Much of what we know about the epidemiology and pathogenesis of device-associated infections has been learned from a careful study of these case clusters of device-associated infection.

Both local and systemic infection may result from contamination of intravascular devices. Local cellulitis, abscess formation, septic thrombophlebitis, device-associated bacteremia, or endocarditis all occur as complications of intravascular therapy and monitoring.

PATHOGENESIS

Bacteria may gain access to an intravascular device at several points (Fig. 1). Each of the potential access sites depicted in Figure 1 has been associated with both sporadic cases and case clusters of nosocomial bacteremia. Whereas the skin entry site has long been thought to be the most important portal of entry for invading microorganisms, the relative importance of the remaining sites is not known. Over the past 5 years, several investigators have focused attention on this problem. Discussion of the current state of these investigations is perhaps most easily accomplished through assessment of each potential portal of entry.

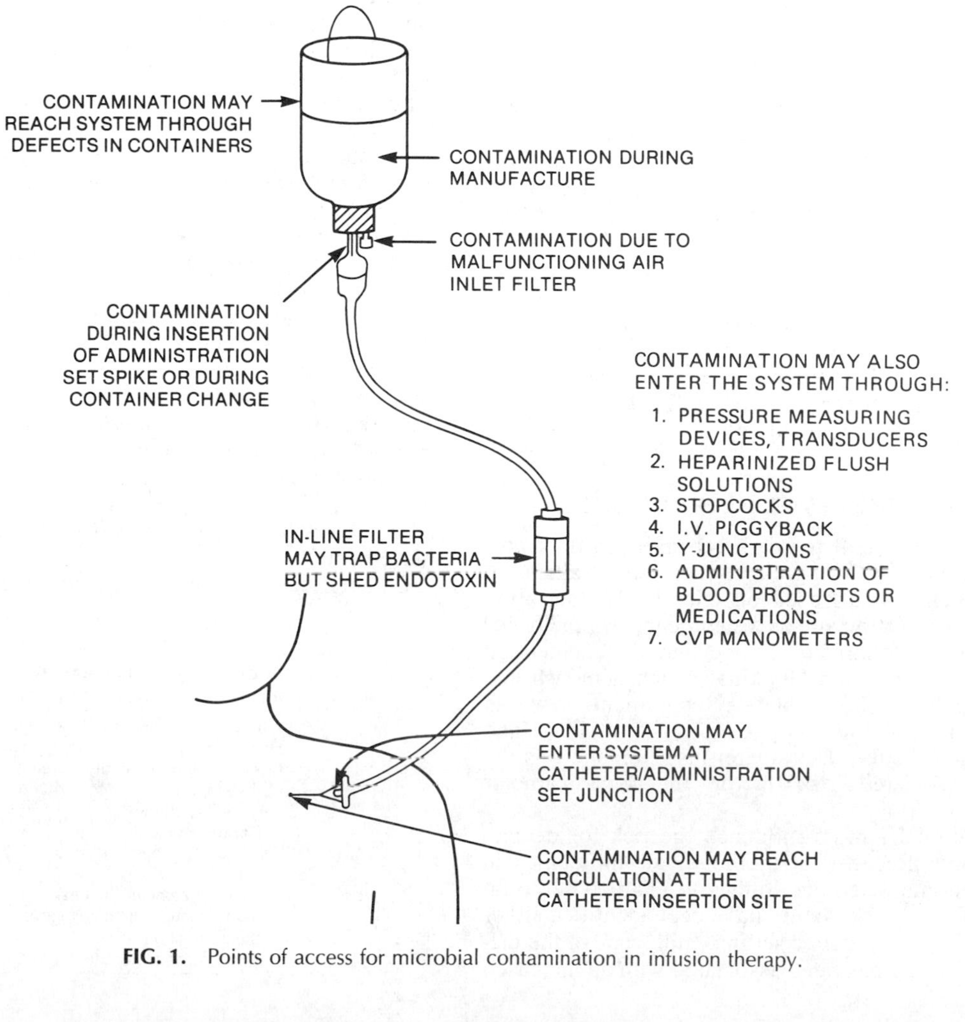
CONTAMINATION MAY REACH SYSTEM THROUGH DEFECTS IN CONTAINERS
CONTAMINATION DURING MANUFACTURE
CONTAMINATION DUE TO MALFUNCTIONING AIR INLET FILTER
CONTAMINATION DURING INSERTION OF ADMINISTRATION SET SPIKE OR DURING CONTAINER CHANGE
CONTAMINATION MAY ALSO ENTER THE SYSTEM THROUGH:
1. PRESSURE MEASURING DEVICES, TRANSDUCERS
2. HEPARINIZED FLUSH SOLUTIONS
3. STOPCOCKS
4. I.V. PIGGYBACK
5. Y-JUNCTIONS
6. ADMINISTRATION OF BLOOD PRODUCTS OR MEDICATIONS
7. CVP MANOMETERS
IN-LINE FILTER MAY TRAP BACTERIA BUT SHED ENDOTOXIN
CONTAMINATION MAY ENTER SYSTEM AT CATHETER/ADMINISTRATION SET JUNCTION
CONTAMINATION MAY REACH CIRCULATION AT THE CATHETER INSERTION SITE

FIG. 1. Points of access for microbial contamination in infusion therapy.

CONTAMINATION OF THE INFUSATE

Infusion-related sepsis has been reviewed in detail,[2,3] and both manufacture-related[4,5] and in-use contamination of infusate[2,6,7] have been documented as causes of device-associated sepsis.

Another factor influencing the pathogenesis of infusate-associated infection is the composition of the fluid. Different infusion fluids support the growth of differing pathogens. The microbiology of outbreaks of infusate-related sepsis is somewhat monotonous; pathogens such as *Enterobacter, Citrobacter*, and *Serratia* predominate.[2] No infusate is entirely free of risk; even distilled water can support the growth of *Pseudomonas cepacia*.[8] Parenteral nutrition solutions are superb substrates for the growth of certain microorganisms.[9] Casein hydrolysate solutions support the growth of many bacteria and fungi.[10] Lipid emulsions support bacterial growth extremely well,[11,12] and their use has also been associated with a risk for fungemia caused by the lipid-dependent yeast *Malassezia furfur*.[13] This latter risk has also been primarily identified in the neonatal intensive care setting but has been less commonly seen in adults.[13]

Parenteral nutrition solutions may also become contaminated during compounding in the hospital pharmacy.[14,15] Two similar outbreaks of *Candida parapsilosis* infections were linked to the backflow of yeasts into TPN solution because a vacuum pump was used improperly.[14,15]

The composition of the infusate also influences the degree of irritation of the vascular intima at the site of infusion. Fluids that are not isotonic, those at nonphysiologic pH, and those containing particulates all may irritate the vascular wall, thus provoking thrombus formation. Such thrombi may be seeded—either hematogenously or by direct extension.

CONTAMINATION AT JUNCTIONS

Contamination of the catheter hub–infusion tubing junction as a significant contributor to device-associated infection has been championed by Sitges-Serra and colleagues.[16–19] These investigators have suggested that endemic coagulase-negative staphylococcal bacteremias often arise as a result of contamination of the catheter hub with these organisms. Other investigators have incriminated the hub–tubing junction (particularly when it does not allow a good fit) in the pathogenesis of epidemics of coagulase-negative staphylococcal infection.[20,21] More recently, Maki and Ringer have found hub contamination to be the second most heavily weighted risk factor for catheter-associated infection in a large, prospective study.[22] In addition, a number of outbreaks of bacteremia have been traced to contaminated medications, either those added directly to the system or those piggybacked into a side port.

CONTAMINATION AT THE DEVICE INSERTION SITE

Many authorities believe that the catheter insertion tract provides the major avenue for the ingress of microbial invaders.[1–3, 20–23] Several studies have focused on microbial colonization around the catheter insertion site as a significant risk factor for catheter-associated infection.[24,25] Supporting this contention are the studies of Cooper and Hopkins, which demonstrated organisms on the exterior surface of catheters rather than within the catheter lumen.[26] In the prospective study of Maki and Ringer, colonization around the catheter insertion site was the most strongly associated risk factor for local catheter infection.[22]

Numerous additional factors influence the risk for device-associated infection. Because of methodologic difficulties in performing appropriate scientific studies to characterize relative risk, many of these risk factors have been identified either retrospectively or in the epidemic setting. Still, each of the factors identified in Table 1 has been associated with an increased risk of device-associated infection.[2] In addition, several other factors have been incriminated as increasing the risk for device-associated infection and bacteremia. Several of these factors are outlined in Table 2. Of these, a few deserve special mention.

TABLE 1. Patient-Related Risk Factors for Device-Associated Bacteremia

Age ≤ 1 year, ≥ 60 years
Granulocytopenia
Immunosuppressive chemotherapy
Loss of skin integrity (e.g., burns, psoriasis)
Severity of underlying illness
Presence of distant infection

Alteration of the patient's skin flora, either as a result of antimicrobial therapy or by colonization with an epidemic strain carried on the hands of hospital personnel, is a common event preceding catheter site infection. In addition, certain therapeutic devices (e.g., semipermeable membrane dressings) may actually increase the cutaneous microbial burden surrounding the catheter insertion site.[27,28]

Failure of hospital personnel to perform appropriate hand washing technique, particularly in the intensive care unit setting, has been well documented.[29,30] Numerous epidemics of device-associated bacteremia have been linked to the carrying of the epidemic strain on the hands of hospital personnel.

A few outbreaks of infection have been linked to the application of contaminated antiseptic ointment or disinfecting solutions onto the skin of patients.[31,32] Even the iodophors have been found to contain viable organisms.[33,34]

Manipulating the system for repositioning, for obtaining a sample, or for any other reason increases the likelihood that the catheter may become contaminated. This point has been best illustrated in studies of infectious complications associated with catheters used for TPN (discussed below).

Several catheter-related characteristics have been suggested to be associated with an increased risk for catheter-associated infection. Catheters that irritate the vascular intima and provoke thrombogenesis and catheters made of materials that are in themselves thrombogenic are likely to be associated with an increased risk for device-associated infection.

Older studies have suggested that stiff catheters were associated with higher infection rates.[35] Such catheters are likely to be more mobile in the insertion tract and are thought to be more thrombogenic. Stillman and colleagues demonstrated a clear association between the thrombogenicity of a catheter and the risk for device-associated infection.[36] Subsequently, Linder and coworkers have confirmed these observations by demonstrating that flexible silicone elastomer and polyurethane catheters are less thrombogenic than polyvinylchloride catheters.[37] Despite differences in thrombogenicity, some authorities believe that all catheters become coated with a fibrin sheath shortly after placement.[38,39]

Catheter composition may influence the risk for infection in

TABLE 2. Additional Factors Associated with Increased Risk for Device-Associated Infection

Alteration in patient's cutaneous microflora
Health care provider hygiene (hand washing)
Contaminated ointment or cream
Catheter composition/construction
Flexibility/stiffness
Thrombogenicity
Microbial adherence properties
Size of catheter
Number of catheter lumens
Distant infection (hematogenous seeding)
Catheter function/use
Catheter management: entry into the system

another way. Sheth and coworkers have shown that certain microorganisms, most notably staphylococci, are able to adhere better to a catheter made from polyvinychloride than to a Teflon catheter.[40] Rotrosen and colleagues demonstrated increased adherence of *Candida* species to polyvinylchloride catheters when compared with Teflon catheters.[41] One might hypothesize that materials that facilitate microbial adherence may be associated with an increased risk for device-associated infection.

The physical size of the catheter (and therefore the size of the defect in the skin's intrinsic host defenses) is also likely to be correlated with increased risk. Similarly, increasing the number of lumens in a catheter has been suggested to increase the risk for catheter-associated infections. Several studies have now suggested that the use of triple-lumen catheters is associated with an increased risk for catheter-associated infection when compared with single-lumen catheters;[42–48] however, not all studies have found this difference.[49,50]

The presence of distant infection resulting in hematogenous seeding of the intravascular device has been incriminated in the pathogenesis of device-associated infection in some series.[24,51,52] Several factors may influence the risk for catheter seeding including catheter composition, local thrombus formation at the catheter insertion site, intensity of bacteremia, the pathogen, duration of catheterization, duration of bacteremia, and the patient's ability to mount an immunologic response to the infection.

Finally, the way the catheter is used may influence risk. For example, risks for infection with flow-directed, balloon-tipped pulmonary artery catheters may be higher because of the way these catheters are used.[53] In critically ill patients these catheters are used intensively; they are frequently repositioned to obtain accurate readings; they are used to obtain samples for the measurement of cardiac output; and they are often used to obtain mixed venous blood to measure oxygen and carbon dioxide tensions. Catheter management—insertion and care—also may influence risk for infection. Several studies have shown that catheters placed by less experienced personnel are at increased risk for infection,[54–56] and a number of studies have suggested that the number of times the system is entered also influences the risk for infection.[57–61] In addition to the factors outlined above, the risk of developing catheter-associated bacteremia is related to the patient and his intrinsic host defense mechanisms as well as to factors related to the patient's hospital environment or therapy (Table 1). Most such patient-related factors cannot be altered by the physician; however, these data can be used when deciding on the necessity for and duration of intravenous therapy.

In addition to patient-related risk factors, several hospital-related risk factors for catheter-acquired bacteremia have been either identified or proposed (Table 3). In contraposition to the patient-related factors, such hospital-related factors can often be altered for patient benefit.

MICROBIOLOGY

Staphylococci continue to predominate as the most frequently encountered pathogens in device-related infections. Although *Staphylococcus aureus* is a frequent cause of device-associated infection, the coagulase-negative staphylococci have become the most common causes of these infections in the past 10 years.

TABLE 3. Hospital-Related Risk Factors for Catheter-Acquired Infection

Type of catheter (plastic > steel)
Location of catheter (central > peripheral[2,62]; femoral > jugular/subclavian)
Type of placement (cutdown > percutaneous[62–64])
Duration of placement (at least 72 hr > less than 72 hr[2,22,62,63])
Emergent placement > elective
Skill of venipuncturist (others > iv team[2])

TABLE 4. Microbiology of Device-Associated Bacteremia

Staphylococcus aureus
Staphylococcus epidermidis
Klebsiella species[a]
Enterobacter species[a]
Serratia marcescens[a]
Candida albicans[b]
Candida species[b]
Pseudomonas aeruginosa[c]
Pseudomonas cepacia[c]
Citrobacter freundii[a]
Corynebacteria (especially JK strains)[d]

[a] Frequently associated with contaminated infusate.
[b] Most often associated with TPN; usually along the catheter path, but occasionally as a result of contaminated infusate.
[c] May arise from a water source (e.g., infusate) or may reflect cutaneous colonization.
[d] JK bacteremia occurs almost exclusively in severely immunosuppressed patients who are or have been receiving broad-spectrum antibiotics and who have indwelling intravascular devices.

Although there are some minor microbiologic differences among the devices or therapies under discussion, as a genus, staphylococci account for one-half to two-thirds of the episodes of bacteremia associated with these devices. Recent studies have suggested that coagulase-negative staphylococci may be able to adhere to plastic catheters more aggressively than can other organisms.[65,66] This property would result in a selective advantage for coagulase-negative staphylococci in causing device-associated infections.

Other commonly encountered isolates are listed in Table 4. The occurrence of some of the more unusual isolates, (e.g., *Enterobacter* sp., *Pseudomonas cepacia, Citrobacter freundii*) as a clear cause of device-associated infection should at least suggest the possibility of a contaminated infusion product[2] or of an aqueous environmental reservoir for these pathogens.[74]

Other organisms may cause such infections (e.g. *Flavobacterium, Acinetobacter* sp.); however, such organisms have been infrequently associated with either infusion-related or cannula-related infections.[6,75]

DIAGNOSIS

Clinical detection of catheter-associated septicemia is sometimes difficult. Signs of local inflammation are present in only about one-half of the cases.[2] Maki has summarized key issues in the diagnosis of device-associated bacteremia.[2] In addition to the presence of one of the indwelling intravascular devices listed above, several other clinical features should alert the physician to the possibility of device-associated bacteremia. Salient features of device-associated sepsis that help distinguish it from other bacteremic syndromes are listed in Table 5.

Although none of these criteria specifically identifies the intravascular device as the source of sepsis, the presence of these clinical findings should at least raise the possibility of device-associated bacteremia.

TABLE 5. Factors Differentiating Device-Associated Bacteremia from Other Septic Syndromes

Local phlebitis and/or inflammation at catheter insertion site
Lack of other source for bacteremia
Sepsis occurring in a patient not otherwise at high risk for bacteremia[2]
Localized embolic disease distal to cannulated artery[67,68]
Hematogenous *Candida* endophthalmitis in patients receiving TPN[69,70]
Presence of ≥15 colonies of bacteria on semiquantitative culture of the catheter tip[67,71–73]
Sepsis apparently refractory to "appropriate" antimicrobial therapy
Resolution of febrile syndrome after device removal
Typical (*S. aureus, S. epidermidis*) or unusual (*P. cepacia, Enterobacter agglomerans, E. cloacae*) microbiology
Clustered infections caused by infusion-related organisms

Cultures of the catheter tip itself have been reported to be of variable value. Before the development of the semiquantitative culturing technique reported by Maki and colleagues,[71,72] most clinical microbiology laboratories used broth culture of catheter tips in an attempt to detect contaminated catheters. This technique yielded results that were highly variable and unreliable.[2,71,72]

Using the semiquantitative culture technique, which defines a positive catheter tip culture as yielding 15 or more colonies,[71,72] in combination with a relatively strict definition of catheter-associated sepsis,[2] Maki and colleagues have reported a specificity ranging between 76 and 96 percent and a predictive value of a positive culture ranging between 16[72] and 31[71] percent in four studies.[67,71–73] Data regarding the sensitivity of the semiquantitative culture technique are not available since the authors have incorporated having a positive culture as part of their definition of both local catheter infection and catheter-acquired bacteremia.[2,67,71–73]

The cutoff point of 15 colonies per catheter was arbitrary. The authors note that most infected catheters yield confluent growth when using the semiquantitative technique.[2]

To culture the catheter, the point at which it enters the skin should be marked, and the catheter should be removed aseptically. Sterile scissors (plastic catheters) or a sterile hemostat (steel needles) should be used to sever the catheter distal to the skin entry site (Fig. 2).

Several investigators have tried to modify Maki's technique to improve the predictability of the procedure. Cleri and coworkers have reported a technique for quantitatively culturing catheters in broth.[76] This system, which is a bit more cumbersome for the laboratory to use, was felt by these authors to have three advantages over the system described by Maki et al. These were (*1*) the ability to detect organisms within the lumen of the insert, (*2*) the ability to evaluate relative numbers of organisms from different catheter segments, and (*3*) the ability to compare relative numbers of organisms present in mixed infections.[76] Although the relative merits of these procedures remain to be delineated, the ease of performing the semiquantitative technique described by Maki and coworkers[71,72] has brought it into widespread clinical use.

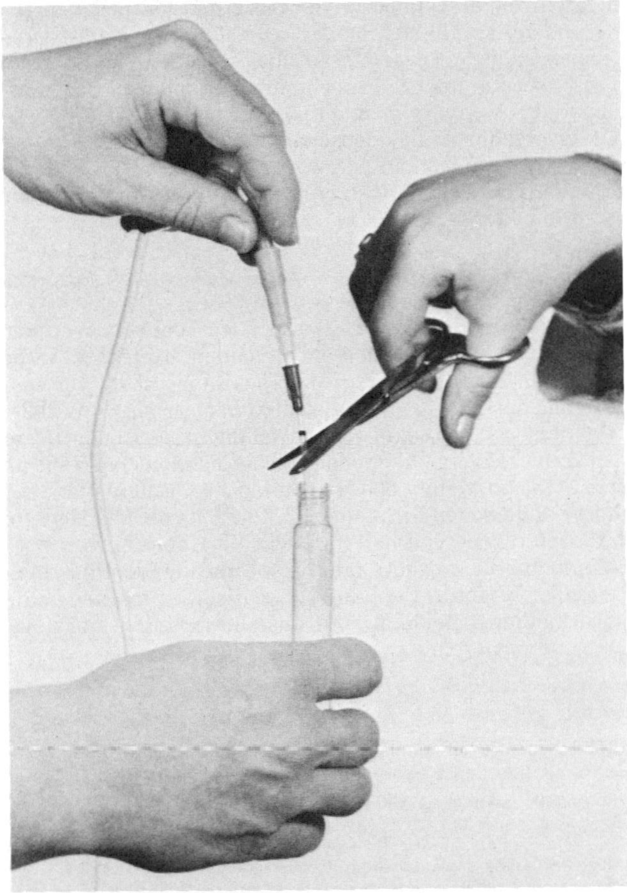

FIG. 2. Procedure for culturing an intravenous catheter when a blood stream infection is thought to result from contamination of the catheter itself. The black band on the catheter above the scissors indicates the former skin surface–catheter interface. Using sterile scissors, cut the catheter as shown and allow the catheter tip to drop into the sterile screw-capped container.

Other investigators have suggested alternative techniques for diagnosing catheter-associated infections.[26,77–80] Cooper and Hopkins evaluated directly Gram staining the catheter segment and found this technique to be more rapid and at least as sensitive and specific as the semiquantitative culture. Collignon and coworkers[77] have advocated Gram staining of "impression smears" from the catheter, while Zuffrey et al. have used acridine orange staining of the catheter.[80] Spencer and Kristinsson reported that the Gram stain technique failed to diagnose infection adequately.[81] Although some experience is being gained with the direct gram stain, none of these newer techniques has been used enough to assess its overall utility. Some authors have recommended a combination of direct and microbiologic techniques.[77]

Finally, Mosca et al. have emphasized the benefits of obtaining blood cultures by using the Isolator system, which allows for a quantitative estimate of microbial burden in the specimen.[82]

On the basis of currently available data, conclusions cannot be drawn regarding the relative merits of various blood culturing techniques in confirming the diagnosis of catheter-acquired sepsis. Wing and colleagues used a comparison of quantitative cultures obtained peripherally and quantitative cultures obtained by drawing blood back through the putatively contaminated catheter to document the occurrence of catheter-acquired sepsis.[83] Tonnesen et al. reported that blood drawn through venous or arterial catheters gave concordant results with cultures obtained by peripheral venipuncture in 92 percent of cases.[84] In 5 percent of cases, results of catheter pull-back cultures were considered to represent false-positives (most were *S. epidermidis*), and in an additional 2 percent, catheter-drawn cultures were reported to be falsely negative.[84] Similar results were reported by Felices et al.,[85] who compared the results of cultures obtained by peripheral venipuncture with cultures obtained through central venous catheters. The incidence of false-positive draw-back cultures may greatly depend on the type of access port used to draw the cultures and the care taken in obtaining the specimen. If the details of the method used to obtain the culture are unknown, it is imprudent to rely entirely on cultures obtained by drawing blood through an indwelling catheter. In unusual circumstances, however, these cultures may provide valuable information.[83]

DEVICE-SPECIFIC ISSUES

Peripheral Intravenous Cannulization

Steel needles have been associated with lower rates of local infections, bacteremic infections, and local phlebitis than have plastic catheters.[62,63] Tully et al., however, demonstrated that steel catheters placed by an intravenous team nurse were associated with significantly less phlebitis but significantly more episodes of infiltration than were Teflon catheters.[86] In this study all catheters were removed in less than 72 hours; infection rates for both catheter types were extremely low, and there were no differences in local or systemic infection rates between the two groups.[86]

The location of catheter placement also may influence subsequent infection rates. Catheters placed in the lower extremities, particularly those placed in the femoral veins, are associated with increased risk for many complications, including infection.[62,63,87,88]

If data are evaluated on the basis of infection per number of catheters placed, central lines are associated with higher infection rates than are peripheral catheters. If, on the other hand, data are assessed on the basis of infections (both local and systemic) per day of catheterization, central lines are associated with a lower sepsis rate than are peripheral catheters.[2] For several reasons, including the increased risks of serious complications such as pneumothorax, hemothorax, puncture of the great arteries, and thrombosis or thrombophlebitis of the great veins, central catheter placement should be reserved for situations in which a peripheral catheter either cannot be placed or cannot be used.

Catheters placed percutaneously are associated with a lower infection rate than are those placed by cutdown.[62–64] Leaving any catheter in place for longer than 72 hours significantly increases the risk of infection[2,22,62,63]; catheters placed emergently are also at higher risk for infection, presumably due to breaks in technique at the time of placement. Several authors have suggested that catheters placed by members of an intravenous therapy team are associated with lower complication rates than are those placed by other health care professionals.

Techniques for the placement and care of indwelling venous cannulae have been reviewed in detail.[62,63] Several aspects of catheter maintenance and care are controversial and await definitive studies to document their efficacy. Issues that are the focus of such controversy are listed in Table 6. Several of these issues deserve further comment.

Although several authorities have recommended the use of an antimicrobial skin ointment to cover the catheter insertion site,[2,62,63,89] no study has documented the efficacy of such substances in preventing catheter-acquired bacteremia. Rhame and colleagues reviewed the composite experience of six different studies that were designed to address this issue.[62] In five of these studies, there were no differences between topical antimicrobial agents and placebo. In the smallest series in this review (a study of 78 catheter insertions) there were 3 infections in the placebo group and 0 in the therapy group.[62] Maki and Band[90] prospectively studied the following three regimens of catheter care: (*1*) application of polymyxin-neomycin-bacitracin ointment at insertion and every 48 hours, (*2*) application of iodophor ointment at insertion and every 48 hours, or (*3*) no ointment. In their study of 827 random catheter insertions there were no differences in either catheter-acquired sepsis (two cases in each group) or local inflammation (38.9 vs. 41.9 vs. 41.7 percent). The only difference noted was in semiquantitative cultures of catheter tips.[90] In the polymyxin-neomycin-bacitracin ointment group there were 6 positive cultures; in the iodophor group, there were 10; and in the control group, there were 18. This difference was greatest in catheters that were left in place for over 4 days.

Thus, information regarding the efficacy of these antimicrobial ointments or creams for intravascular cannulae is contradictory and confusing, and the clinical utility of these compounds remains questionable.

The use of in-line membrane filters has also been advocated as a mechanism for reducing the incidence of catheter-acquired infection.[91] Since, as was pointed out earlier, the major points of entry are the skin insertion site and, perhaps, the catheter hub, one might suspect that such devices would be of limited usefulness in preventing most catheter-acquired septicemias. No study has concluded by recommending the routine inclusion of such filters in all intravenous setups; nor has any study demonstrated conclusive evidence that the routine use of such filters results in a lowering of the infusion-related bacteremia rate.

In isolated situations (e.g., if there is particulate matter in the infusate, if the solution must hang for an extended period of time, or perhaps in a situation in which an infusate such as TPN solution supports the growth of microorganisms extremely well), the addition of these filters to the system is of theoretic value. However, even in cases in which the infusion fluid is contaminated, organisms trapped on the filter may shed endotoxins into the patient's circulation.[92]

In the past, several authorities have recommended placing a sterile dressing over the catheter entry site,[62,63] and others have made recommendations for the routine care (usually on a daily or every-other-day basis) of the entry site. Recently, Maki and Ringer compared the efficacy of a sterile, dry gauze dressing with two semipermeable membrane dressings, one of which was impregnated with an iodophor.[22] No difference was seen among the four groups: (*1*) gauze changed every 48 hours, (*2*) gauze left in place for the life of the catheter, (*3*) transparent membrane left in place for the life of the catheter, and (*4*) iodophor membrane left on for the life of the catheter.[22]

Finally, two studies have demonstrated that routinely changing intravenous administration sets at 48 rather than 24 hours was not associated with a significant increase in the infusion-related bacteremia rate.[93,94] More recently Snydman and coworkers[95] and Maki and colleagues[96] have compared the relative safety of changing administration sets at 72-hour intervals with changing them at 48 hours. Neither study identified an increased risk with the 72-hour interval.

Thus, it now seems safe, in addition to practical and reasonable, to insert a peripheral catheter, dress it, hook up the administration set, and change all three at 72-hour intervals.

TABLE 6. Factors Not Documented to Affect Risk for Catheter-Acquired Infection

Topical antimicrobial ointment
In-line membrane filters
Dressing materials
Frequent changes of administration set

Central Venous Catheters

Since central venous catheters frequently remain in place longer than peripheral intravenous ones do, certain problems either occur with more frequency or are unique to these catheters. In addition, due to the placement of these catheters in the great veins, complications of placement such as infective endocarditis and suppurative thrombophlebitis of the great veins represent life-threatening events.

Michel and colleagues studied 390 catheters placed into the subclavian vein, by identical technique, in an attempt to determine risk factors associated with microbial colonization.[97] In this study, the presence of distant infection, bacteremia, or tracheostomy was associated with an increased risk for catheter colonization.[97] Unfortunately, these authors chose to culture the catheters by using the broth culture technique, which yields notoriously unreliable results.[2,62,63]

The presence of either intraluminal or extraluminal fibrin has been proposed as predisposing to the development of catheter-associated infection.[2,36,39] Stillman and colleagues studied 94 central catheters and found that all of 11 catheters categorized as infected in their study and 30 out of 83 not found to be either infected or colonized had gross visible evidence of either intraluminal or surface thrombin at the time of removal.[36]

Manipulation of the catheter (either for blood drawing, intermittent medication administration, or flushing) may increase the risk of contamination. As with peripheral catheters, the use of antiseptic or antibiotic ointments on central venous catheter insertion sites has been recommended by several authorities;[2,62,63,89] however, proof of the efficacy of these compounds in reducing infection remains to be demonstrated. In a study by Prager and Silva[98] antiseptic cream was of no benefit in preventing either infection or colonization of central catheters. If a traditional central venous pressure (CVP) manometer is being used g. 1), the manometer itself may represent a potential site for bacterial entry into the system.

The issue of whether central catheters should be changed over a guidewire remains controversial. Although the guidewire technique is commonly used, little scientific evidence supports its use if catheter-associated infection is expected. Maher and colleagues used this technique successfully for catheter exchange in situations assessed as "low risk for infection."[99] Use of guidewire obviates the need for a second percutaneous puncture of the great veins and may be preferable for catheter exchanges judged routine or mandated by some reason other than suspected infection.

Exchange over a guidewire may also be associated with lower risks for some complications (e.g., bleeding, pneumothorax). If a guidewire is to be used for catheter exchange, culture of the removed or "old" catheter tip should be performed. In addition, blood cultures should be drawn through the "old" line before removal. If either of these cultures becomes positive, the "new" catheter should be removed and cultured. If central access is still desired, a third catheter should be placed at a new puncture site. In situations in which the catheter is being removed for suspected sepsis, in my opinion, exchange over a guidewire should not be attempted.

The umbilical vein catheter that is commonly used for vascular access in neonates presents some unique problems. Because of the extensive microbiologic flora of the umbilical stump,[100] these catheters are at high risk for both colonization and infection.[101–103] Although high rates of umbilical catheter-associated infection have been reported in several studies,[101–103] not all centers report such high rates.[104–106] One study has reported a much lower incidence of infectious complications when the umbilical artery (rather than the umbilical vein) was cannulated for infusion.[104]

Issues regarding catheter composition and effectiveness of subcutaneous tunneling of catheters and risks associated with electronic monitoring devices will be discussed in the sections below.

Total Parenteral Nutrition

Several aspects of the delivery of TPN separate this mode of intravascular therapy from others. First, the composition of the infusate supports the growth of different microorganisms, most notably certain of the *Candida* species.[9,10] Second, TPN catheters are often required to remain in place much longer than either peripheral or other central venous cannulae. For this reason, problems with catheter contamination become much more of a concern. Third, the hypertonicity of the solution tends to cause thrombosis, which may result in an increased risk of infection. Fourth, because patients who require TPN are frequently severely ill due to neoplasms, trauma, or inflammatory bowel disease, the risk for bacteremia is higher. Therefore, the potential for hematogenous seeding of the catheter is high.

For these and other reasons, the placement, management, and care of catheters used for TPN has received a great deal of attention. Ryan and colleagues, in a prospective study of 200 catheters, documented that the risk of catheter-associated infection increased significantly when the integrity of the delivery system was interrupted.[57] Numerous other studies support this concept.[58–60] More recently Snydman and colleagues found that the occurrence of so-called line violations was highly associated with the development of TPN catheter-associated sepsis.[61] For these reasons the Centers for Disease Control (CDC) have recommended that the administration of TPN be performed by a team[107] (Table 7). In their study, Snydman and colleagues also attempted to correlate the results of twice-weekly 1 ml pour-plate blood cultures with the subsequent development of catheter colonization and sepsis. Similar to the previously cited studies,[84,85] although concordance was high among blood cultures, catheter tip cultures, and peripheral blood cultures, cultures obtained through the TPN catheter demonstrated a reasonably high incidence of false positivity, primarily due to *S. epidermidis* contamination.[61]

TABLE 7. Prevention of Infusion-Related Infection in TPN

Administration of TPN should be under the supervision of a team of health care professionals (usually a nurse, pharmacist, and physician). Both the decision for appropriateness of TPN therapy and protocols for insertion, maintenance, and delivery of TPN should be under the responsibility of this team
TPN solution should be prepared using sterile or aseptic technique when possible in a laminar flow hood. Once prepared, the solution should be infused immediately or stored at 4°C
Placement of the catheter should be performed by using sterile technique including, at a minimum, mask, gloves, drapes, and appropriate skin preparation (preferably with 1% iodine)
Once placed, the catheter should be anchored to avoid movement, which may result in local irritation of the insertion site or transport of organisms along the insertion path
If possible the system should be kept closed, avoiding unnecessary entry for blood drawing and administration of other fluids or blood products via the TPN line
Other aspects of TPN administration are either of empirical or theoretic value or have been demonstrated to be of value in small studies. These techniques or procedures await definitive studies to document their merit; they include the following:
Routine application of antiseptic cream at the site of catheter insertion (either at the time of venipuncture or at routine dressing change)
Routine dressing changes, skin defatting with acetone, and skin preparation with antiseptics
Routine use of semipermeable dressing materials (e.g., OP-SITE)
Routine use of in-line membrane filters
Use of silicone or other less traumatic, nonthrombogenic catheters; use of heparin-bonded catheters; use of low-dose heparin infusions
Tunneling the catheter subcutaneously to increase the anatomic distance between cather insertion site and the point at which the catheter enters the vessel

(Modified from Goldmann et al.[107] with permission.)

Candida infection has been a particular problem in patients receiving TPN.[69,70,108] Curry and Quie reported a 16 percent incidence of candidemia among patients receiving TPN in a prospective study in a hospital that did not have a TPN team.[108] In another prospective study of 131 postoperative patients who were receiving TPN, 13 patients were detected as developing chorioretinal lesions consistent with hematogenous *Candida* endophthalmitis; 7 of the patients had positive blood cultures for *Candida*.[70] Although most of these infections are presumed to arise as a result of yeast contamination at the catheter entry site, occasional outbreaks of *Candida* infection due to a TPN solution that was intrinsically contaminated have been reported.[15,16] Because of the risk of intrinsic as well as in-use contamination of TPN solutions with *Candida* or other microorganisms, some authorities have recommended the routine use of an in-line membrane filter to prevent infusion-related sepsis.[91] Such filters have been implicated as a common cause of catheter dysfunction, and their efficacy in preventing catheter-acquired infection remains to be documented.

Because the TPN catheter frequently must be left in place for an extended period of time and because of the increased thrombogenicity of the TPN fluid, several modifications of the delivery system of the catheter itself have been advocated. Among the suggested mechanisms for decreasing infections in TPN are (*1*) either bonding heparin or a heparin-like substance to the catheter or infusing heparin with the infusate in an attempt to minimize fibrin sheath formation;[109,110] (*2*) constructing the catheter of a more flexible substance, thereby producing less trauma to the vascular endothelium;[111,112] and (*3*) tunneling the catheter under the skin in an attempt to decrease access of pathogens to the circulation.[112,113] In one small study the addition of 1 unit/ml of heparin to the infusate decreased septic complications;[110] however, a subsequent study failed to demonstrate a benefit from adding heparin to the infusate.[110] Several papers have reported lower infectious complication rates with silicone elastomer catheters.[111,112] Two small studies have failed to show any benefit of increasing the distance between the anatomic insertion site and the site at which the catheter enters the vessel.[112,113]

Most of the studies cited above contain only small numbers of patients. Additionally, in all the aforementioned studies, although these newer technologies produced statistically significantly lower infection rates than did the controls, these technologies failed to lower the catheter sepsis rate below rates published by centers with large experiences with TPN.[114,115] For these reasons these data are still at too preliminary a stage for definitive conclusions to be drawn regarding the efficacy of these techniques.

The routine use of antibiotic cream at the insertion site under the dressing may promote colonization of the skin (and ultimately the catheter) with *Candida*.[89] For this reason, many authorities recommend the use of antiseptic ointment (such as an iodophor). No controlled study has demonstrated the efficacy of these ointments in preventing catheter-acquired sepsis. Similarly, several authorities recommend routinely changing the dressing, repreparing the skin, and inspecting the catheter insertion site either daily,[89] every other day,[57] three times weekly,[112] or at longer intervals.[58] Although the use of antimicrobial creams and visualizing the insertion site to look for signs of local infection would seem reasonable, the theoretic possibility exists that the additional manipulations of the line caused by these procedures might actually be detrimental.[116] Topical antimicrobials have also been shown to invalidate cultures of the catheter insertion site.

A final and often difficult issue is deciding when to remove a TPN catheter for suspected sepsis. In the past, most authorities recommended the removal of a TPN line whenever infection was suspected. In separate studies, Ryan et al.[57] and Maher et al.[99] have suggested that nearly 70 percent of catheters removed for suspected sepsis are apparently removed unnecessarily. Thus, the TPN team is often faced with the dilemma of whether or not to remove the catheter from a patient in whom the evidence for infection is equivocal. Such a patient may have many reasons for fever; therefore, the diagnosis of infection may be difficult. Often patients are severely immunosuppressed and/or thrombocytopenic, and the risks associated with catheter replacement may be quite high. Several clinical features may help the physician decide how to manage the catheter.[2,117] The presence of positive blood cultures (particularly due to *Candida* or *S. epidermidis*) in the absence of another source for the infection or in the presence of hemodynamic instability, embolic phenomena, leukocytosis, or profound leukopenia may herald the onset of catheter-associated sepsis. In addition, the development of new glucose intolerance in a TPN patient whose carbohydrate metabolism had been previously well regulated may be an early subtle sign of bacteremia.[117]

Long-Term Central Venous Access

In 1973, Broviac and colleagues reported their initial experience with the use of a chronic indwelling right atrial catheter for the delivery of long-term parenteral nutrition.[118] Since this initial report, modifications of the catheter system have been published, and the situation in which these catheters have been used has broadened considerably. Initial reports suggested that the rate of catheter infection in non-neutropenic patients was approximately one infection per 5.5 patient years.[119] Venous access has long been a problem for patients receiving chemotherapy for malignancy. Hickman and colleagues modified the Broviac catheter for use in patients undergoing bone marrow transplantation.[120] This catheter can be used for the administration of intensive chemotherapy, the administration of other medicines and fluids, transfusion, and phlebotomy. These catheters spare the patient both physical and psychological trauma.

Several centers have reported their experience using these catheters, and many series report remarkably low rates of infection. Press and colleagues summarize 1088 catheter placements from 18 studies in their literature review. In their summary data, these authors report approximately 0.14 infections per 100 catheter days.[121]

Several issues regarding the care and maintenance of these catheters remain unsettled. Among these issues are (*1*) whether or not a dressing should be placed over the exit site (and if so, what dressing materials and how frequently should the dressing be changed), (*2*) whether or not the system should be routinely flushed (and if so, how frequently and with what), (*3*) whether or not blood cultures obtained through the catheter are reliable indicators of catheter contamination, and (*4*) what are the indications for catheter removal, and can either or both local infection and/or bacteremia be treated with the catheter in place?

Although definitive answers to these questions remain elusive, at the Warren G. Magnuson Clinical Center of the National Institutes of Health, a sterile dry gauze dressing or a semipermeable membrane is kept in place over the exit site. These dressings are changed at least twice weekly. We also use an every-other-day heparin flush (5 ml of 100 units/ml) to attempt to keep the catheters open.

The issue of "pull-back" blood cultures has been discussed earlier. Repeated isolation of the same organism from cultures drawn through the catheter indicates a need for therapy. Individual positive cultures and sporadic positive cultures are difficult to interpret in the absence of clinical or laboratory correlates.

The problem of how best to treat an infection in a patient with a long-term venous access catheter in place is a difficult one. Hiemenz and colleagues report success in treating 90 percent of proved bacteremias while leaving the catheter in place.[122] Others have reported similar successes.[122–125] Some organisms (e.g., *Bacillus* sp., *Candida* sp.) may be difficult to eradicate,[126] although Hartman and Shuchat had some success in treating *Candida* infections.[125] Guidelines for managing these infections have been summarized by Hiemenz et al.[126]

There are two additional issues regarding long-term access devices: first, several centers have reported remarkable success—few infections and few other complications as well—with totally implantable access devices.[127–129] In the largest of these studies the rate of infections for each 100 catheter-days was 0.43—comparable to other implantable catheters.[129] Second, use of these catheters has been associated with a new and fortunately rare complication, septic thrombosis of the atrium.[130]

Flow-Directed, Balloon-Tipped Pulmonary Artery Catheters

The use of the indwelling, balloon-tipped pulmonary artery catheter[131] has revolutionized the management of hemodynamically unstable, critically ill patients. The placement of such a catheter in one of the great veins, across the tricuspid and pulmonic valves, and into the pulmonary vasculature is not without complications, however. Michel et al. demonstrated that 29 out of 153 pulmonary artery catheter tips produced microbial growth in thioglycolate broth.[132] Although no patient in this study was felt to develop sepsis secondary to the contaminated catheter, other studies have suggested a reasonably high rate of contamination with occasional episodes of catheter-related sepsis.[133]

Katz and colleagues retrospectively studied complications associated with the placement of 392 balloon-tipped catheters; of these, 17 (4.2 percent) were assessed to be associated with bacteremia.[133] Maki has estimated that 3–5 percent of these catheters in place for more than 72 hours will produce bacteremia.[2] Another problem relatively unique to the flow-directed, balloon-tipped pulmonary artery catheter is that such catheters may traumatize the right-sided heart valves and the right-sided endocardium.

In a study of 102 consecutive autopsies of patients who died in the hospital, 26 (25.5 percent) had had an indwelling intracardiac catheter inserted before death.[134] Six of these patients were excluded from analysis (four patients died 48 hours or less after catheter placement; two patients had permanent transvenous pacemakers in place for many years with the anticipated endocardial fibrosis). Of the remaining 20 patients, 6 had vegetations present, and 88 percent of the patients had some evidence of intracardiac damage.[134] One patient had infective endocarditis on the tricuspid valve. Other studies have reported slightly lower but significant incidences of right-sided heart vegetations among monitored patients coming to autopsy.[135] Green and colleagues noted a 10-fold increase in the incidence of valvular vegetations when they compared a period of time before the introduction of balloon-tipped pulmonary artery catheters with a time in which the catheters were in wide use.[135] Severely burned patients may be at even higher risk for this complication.[136]

No prospective study has addressed risk factors associated with infection of these catheters, nor have studies assessed the efficacy of devices designed to decrease the risk of catheter-associated infection (e.g., leaving the introducer sheath in the vein to protect the catheter).[132] Other aspects of the monitoring equipment (e.g., transducer dome, heparin flush) will be discussed in the section on arterial lines.

Arterial Lines, Transducers, and Transducer Domes

The widespread use of arterial lines for blood pressure monitoring or for obtaining arterial samples for blood gas determinations has yielded yet another source of device-associated infection. In addition, the technical electronic equipment used for hemodynamic monitoring—transducers and their associated paraphernalia—have also been cited as a source of device-associated infection.

Stamm and colleagues reported an outbreak of *Flavobacterium* bacteremia among monitored patients in an intensive care unit.[6] Ultimately, these organisms were cultured from in-use radial artery catheters, from stopcocks, and from ice used to cool syringes for blood gas determinations.[6] Adams et al. reported a series of 147 radial artery cannulations in infants in whom umbilical artery cannulation failed.[68] In this series there were two episodes of catheter-related sepsis. Band and Maki used the semiquantitative catheter tip culture technique to study 130 arterial catheters in 95 patients.[67] In their series 23 catheters were classified as "local infection" (i.e., ≥15 colonies per semiquantitative culture), and there were 5 episodes of sepsis.[67] Factors associated with increased risk for infection were (*1*) duration of catheterization (especially longer than 96 hours), (*2*) placement by cutdown rather than percutaneously, and (*3*) clinical signs of local inflammation.

More recently, Maki and Hassemer reported a prospective study designed to assess the endemic rate of bacteremia associated with arterial monitoring.[137] Transducer chamber fluid was demonstrated to be contaminated in nearly 12 percent of the cases. There were eight cases of bacteremia—four definitely related and four possibly related to the extrinsic contamination.[137]

Several epidemics of infection due to improper sterilization of reusable transducer domes have been reported.[138–140] More recently, however, with the introduction of disposable transducer domes, one might assume that these problems would be overcome. Buxton and colleagues reported an epidemic of *Enterobacter* infections that was associated with the contamination of disposable transducer domes during their initial setup.[140] The chambers and domes were apparently contaminated by the hands of hospital personnel who had handled heavily contaminated transducer heads.[138] West and colleagues also reported

TABLE 8. Prevention of Infection Associated with Hemodynamic Monitoring

Place arterial lines, central venous lines, and flow-directed, balloon-tipped catheters by using sterile technique. Mask and sterile gloves should be worn at a minimum. The skin should be prepared with an effective antiseptic solution (e.g., 1% iodine in alcohol)
Place the catheters percutaneously and anchor well to avoid catheter movement. Dress the insertion site appropriately
Use heparinized saline (not glucose) for continuous flush solutions
Do not reuse transducer domes; sterilize reusable part of transducer setup with either glutaraldehyde or ethylene oxide between patients
Replace chamber domes and continuous flow devices every 48–72 hours[8]; if possible replace arterial lines every 96 hours[24]
Use sterile fluid to fill the chamber dome; use aseptic technique in the assembly
Avoid placing unnecessary junctions or stopcocks into the apparatus; minimize manipulation of the system.

Serratia sepsis due to transducer dome cracks.[141] In this hospital, supposedly disposable transducer domes were being resterilized with resultant cracks or breaks in the dome membrane.[141]

Another potential reservoir for nosocomial bacteremia is the heparin flush solution used to irrigate certain intravascular devices continually. This fluid has been implicated as a reservoir for outbreaks of device-associated bacteremia in more than one case.[142,143]

Several authors have made recommendations regarding the prevention of infection associated with intravascular monitoring devices.[2,67,137,138,143,144] A summary of these recommendations is presented in Table 8.

PREVENTION OF DEVICE-ASSOCIATED BACTEREMIA

Techniques to be used to prevent device-associated bacteremia have been reviewed by Maki[2] and Murphy and Lipman[145] and have been outlined elsewhere in this chapter. Several additional points should be emphasized. First, a systematic approach to this issue including the development of a standard approach is likely to be beneficial.[146] For central catheters the development of a multidisciplinary team has been advantageous.[107,147]

Emphasis should be placed on attention to detail including hand washing,[29,30,148] optimal management of the insertion site, limitations of entry into the system, careful management of the administration set and the catheter itself,[149] and the maintenance of a high index of suspicion for infectious complications.

Finally, new scientific approaches are needed to help establish better techniques for catheter management,[25,27,96,150] and further technological advances such as bonding antimicrobial agents to the intravascular device[151] may also reduce risks for device-associated infection. Increased attention to such details can significantly lower the endemic rate of device-associated infection as well as decrease the number of epidemics of such infections.

REFERENCES

1. Maki DG. Sepsis arising from extrinsic contamination of the infusion and measures for control. In Phillips J, Meers PD, D'Arcy DF, eds. Microbiologic Hazards of Intravenous Therapy. Lancaster, England: MTP Press; 1977:99–143.
2. Maki DG. Epidemic nosocomial bacteremias. In: Wenzel RP, ed. Handbook of Hospital Acquired Infections. Boca Raton, FL. CRC Press; 1981:371–512.
3. Maki DG. Nosocomial bacteremia: An epidemiologic overview. Am J Med. 1981;70:719–32.
4. Maki DG, Rhame FS, Mackel DC, et al. Nationwide epidemic of septicemia caused by contaminated intravenous products: I: Epidemiologic and clinical features. Am J Med. 1976;60:471–85.
5. Felts SK, Schaffner W, Melly MA, et al. Sepsis caused by contaminated intravenous fluids: Epidemiologic, clinical and laboratory investigation of an outbreak in one hospital. Ann Intern Med. 1972;77:881–90.

6. Stamm WE, Collella JJ, Anderson MS, et al. Indwelling arterial catheters as a source of nosocomial bacteremia: An outbreak caused by *Flavobacterium* species. N Engl J Med. 1975;292:1099–102.
7. Holmes CJ, Allwood MC. The microbial contamination of intravenous infusions during clinical use. J Appl Bacteriol. 1979;46:247–57.
8. Carson LA, Favero MS, Bond WW, et al. Morphological biochemical and growth characteristics of *Pseudomonas cepacia* from distilled water. Appl Microbiol. 1973;25:476–83.
9. Goldmann DG, Martin WT, Worthington JW. Growth of bacteria and fungi in total parenteral nutrition solutions. Am J Surg. 1973;126:314–8.
10. Maki DG. Growth properties of microorganisms in infusion fluid and method of detection. In: Phillips I, ed. Microbiologic Hazards of Intravenous Therapy. Lancaster, England: MTP Press; 1977:13–47.
11. Crocker KS, Noga R, Filibeck DG, et al. Microbial growth comparisons of five commercial parenteral lipid emulsions. J Parenter Enteral Nutr. 1984;8:391–5.
12. Jarvis WR, Highsmith AK. Bacterial growth and endotoxin production in lipid emulsion. J Clin Microbiol. 1984;19:17–20.
13. Dankner WM, Spector SA, Fierer J. *Malassezia* fungemia in neonates and adults: Complication of hyperalimentation. Rev Infect Dis. 1987;9:743–837.
14. Plouffe JF, Brown DG, Silva J, et al. Nosocomial outbreak of *Candida parapsilosis* fungemia related to intravenous infusions. Arch Intern Med. 1977;137:1686–9.
15. Solomon SL, Khabbaz RF, Parker RH, et al. An outbreak of *Candida parapsilosis* bloodstream infections in patients receiving parenteral nutrition. J Infect Dis. 1984;149:98–102.
16. Sitges-Serra A, Puig P, Jaurrieta E, et al. Catheter sepsis due to *Staphylococcus epidermidis* during parenteral nutrition. Surg Gynecol Obstet. 1980;151:481–3.
17. Sitges-Serra A, Puig P, Linares J, et al. Hub colonization as the initial step in an outbreak of catheter-related sepsis due to coagulase negative staphylococci during parenteral nutrition. J Parenter Enteral Nutr. 1984;8:668–72.
18. Sitges-Serra A, Linares J, Perez JL, et al. A randomized trial on the effect of tubing changes on hub contamination and catheter sepsis during parenteral nutrition. J Parenter Enteral Nutr. 1985;9:322–5.
19. Linares J, Sitges-Serra A, Garau J, et al. Pathogenesis of catheter sepsis: A prospective study with quantitative and semiquantitative cultures of catheter hub and segments. J Clin Microbiol. 1985;21:357–60.
20. Deitel M, Krajden S, Saldanha CR, et al. An outbreak of *Staphylococcus epidermidis* septicemia. J Parenter Enteral Nutr. 1983;7:569–72.
21. Pemberton LB, Lyman B, Mandal J, et al. Outbreak of *Staphylococcus epidermidis* nosocomial infections in patients receiving total parenteral nutrition. J Parenter Enteral Nutr. 1984;8:325–6.
22. Maki DG, Ringer M. Evaluation of dressing regimens for prevention of infection with peripheral intravenous catheters: Gauze, a transparent polyurethane dressing, and an iodophor-transparent dressing. JAMA. 1987; 258:2396–403.
23. Snydman DR, Murray SA, Kornfield SF et al. Total parenteral nutrition-related infections: Prospective epidemiologic study using semiquantitative methods. Am J Med. 1982;695–9.
24. Bjornson HS, Colley R, Bower RH, et al. Association between microorganism growth at the catheter insertion site and colonization of the catheter in patients receiving total parenteral nutrition. Surgery 1982;92:720–7.
25. Maki DG, McCormack KN. Defatting catheter insertion sites in total parenteral nutrition is of no value as an infection control measure. Am J Med. 1987;83:833–40.
26. Cooper GL, Hopkins CC. Rapid diagnosis of intravascular catheter-associated infection by direct Gram-staining of catheter segments. N Engl J Med. 1985;18:1142–50.
27. Kelsey MC, Gosling M. A comparison of the morbidity associated with occlusive and non-occlusive dressings applied to peripheral intravenous devices. J Hosp Infect. 1984;5:313–21.
28. Craven DE, Lichtenberg A, Kunches LM, et al. A randomized study comparing a transparent polyurethane dressing to a dry gauze dressing for peripheral intravenous catheter sites. Infect Control. 1985;6:361–6.
29. Preston GA, Larson EL, Stamm WE. The effect of private isolation rooms on patient care practices, colonization, and infection in an intensive care unit. Am J Med. 1981;70:641–5.
30. Albert RK, Condie F. Hand-washing patterns in medical intensive care units. N Engl J Med. 1981;304:1465–6.
31. Weinstein RA, Emori TG, Anderson RL, et al. Pressure transducers as a source of bacteremia after open heart surgery: Report of an outbreak and guidelines for prevention. Chest. 1976;69:338–44.
32. Frank MJ, Schaffner W. Contaminated aqueous benzalkonium chloride: An unnecessary hospital infection hazard. JAMA. 1976;236:2418–9.
33. Berkelman RL, Lewin S, Allen JR, et al. Pseudobacteremia attributed to contamination of povidone-iodine with *Pseudomonas cepacia*. Ann Intern Med. 1981;95:32–6.
34. Craven DE, Moody B, Connolly MG, et al. Pseudobacteremia caused by povidone-iodine solution contaminated with *Pseudomonas cepacia*. N Engl J Med. 1981;305:621–3.
35. Welch GW, McKeel DW Jr, Silverstein P, et al. The role of catheter composition in the development of thrombophlebitis. Surg Gynecol Obstet. 1974;138:421–4.
36. Stillman RM, Soliman S, Garcia L, et al. Etiology of catheter-associated sepsis. Arch Surg. 1977;112:1497–9.
37. Linder LE, Curelaru I, Gustavsson B, et al. Material thrombogenicity in central venous catheterization: A comparison between soft, antebrachial catheters of silicone elastomer and polyurethane. J Parenter Enteral Nutr. 1984;8:399–406.
38. Bozzetti F. Central venous catheter sepsis. Surg Gynecol Obstet. 1985; 161:293–301.
39. Peters WR, Bush WH, McIntyre RD, et al. The development of fibrin sheath on indwelling venous catheters. Surg Gynecol Obstet. 1973;137:43–7.
40. Sheth NK, Franson TR, Rose HD, et al. Colonization of bacteria on polyvinyl chloride and Teflon intravascular catheter in hospitalized patients. J Clin Microbiol. 1983;18:1061–3.
41. Rotrosen D, Calderone RA, Edwards JE Jr. Adherence of *Candida* species to host tissues and plastic surfaces. Rev Infect Dis. 1986;8:73–85.
42. Wolfe BM, Ryder MA, Nishikawa RA, et al. Complications of parenteral nutrition. Am J Surg. 1986;152:93–9.
43. Pemberton LB, Lyman B, Lauder V, et al. Sepsis from triple- vs. single-lumen catheters during total parenteral nutrition in surgical or critically ill patients. Arch Surg. 1986;121:591–4.
44. Appelgran KN. Triple-lumen catheters. Technological advance or setback? Arch Surg. 1987;53:113–6.
45. Hilton E, Haslett TM, Borenstein MT, et al. Central catheter infections: Single vs. triple-lumen catheters influence of guidelines on infection rates when used for replacement of catheters. Am J Med. 1988;84:667–72.
46. Vo NM, Waycaster M, Godfrey J. Triple-lumen catheters for parenteral nutrition. South Med J. 1988;81:214–7.
47. Yeung C, May J, Hughes R. Infection rate for single-lumen vs. triple-lumen subclavian catheters. Infect Control Hosp Epidemiol. 1988;9:154–8.
48. Mantese VA, German DS, Kruminski DL, et al. Colonization and sepsis from triple-lumen catheters in critically ill patients. Am J Surg. 1987; 154:597–601.
49. Miller JJ, Venus B, Matthew M. Comparison of the sterility of long-term central catheterization using single-lumen, triple-lumen and pulmonary artery catheters. Crit Care Med. 1984;12:634–7.
50. Kelly CS, Ligas JR, Smith CA, et al. Sepsis due to triple-lumen central venous catheters. Surg Gynecol Obstet. 1986;163:14–6.
51. Kovalevich DS, Faubion WC, Bender JM, et al. Association of parenteral nutrition catheter sepsis with urinary tract infections. J Parenter Enteral Nutr. 1986;10:639–41.
52. Pettigren RA, Lang DSR, Haycock DA, et al. Catheter-related sepsis in patients on intravenous nutrition: A prospective study of quantitative catheter cultures and guideline changes for suspected sepsis. Br J Surg 1985;72:52–5.
53. Hampton AA, Sheretz RJ. Vascular-access infections in hospitalized patients. Surg Clin North Am. 1988;68:57–71.
54. Bernard RW, Stahl WM, Chase RM Jr. Subclavian vein catheterizations: A prospective study. II. Infectious complications. Ann Surg. 1971;173:191–200.
55. Sitzmann JV, Townsend TR, Siler MC, et al. Septic and technical complications of central venous catheterization: A prospective study of 200 consecutive patients. Ann Surg. 1985;202:766–70.
56. Armstrong CW, Mayhall CG, Miller KG, et al. Prospective study of catheter replacement and other risk factors for infection of hyperalimentation catheters. J Infect Dis. 1986;154:808–16.
57. Ryan JA, Abel RM, Abbott WM, et al. Catheter complications in total parenteral nutrition: A prospective study of 200 consecutive patients. N Engl J Med. 1974;290:757–61.
58. Powell-Tuck, J, Lennard-Jones JE, Lowes JA, et al. Intravenous feeding in a gastroenterological unit: A prospective study of infective complications. J Clin Pathol. 1979;32:549–55.
59. Sanderson I, Deitel M. Intravenous hyperalimentation without sepsis. Surg Gynecol Obstet. 1973;136:577–85.
60. Sanders RA, Sheldon GF. Septic complications of total parenteral nutrition. Am J Surg. 1976;132:214–20.
61. Snydman DR, Murray SA, Kornfeld SF, et al. Total parenteral nutrition-related infections: Prospective epidemiologic study using semiquantitative methods. Am J Med. 1982;73:695–9.
62. Rhame FS, Maki DG, Bennett JV. Intravenous cannula-related infections. In Bennett JV, Brachman PS, eds. Hospital Infections. Boston: Little, Brown; 1979:433–42.
63. Maki DG, Goldmann DA, Rhame FS. Infection control in intravenous therapy. Ann Intern Med. 1973;79:867–87.
64. Moran JM, Atwood RP, Rowe MI. A clinical and bacteriologic study of infections associated with venous cutdowns. N Engl J Med. 1965;272:554–60.
65. Christensen GD, Simpson A, Bisno AL, et al. Adherence of slime-producing strains of *Staphylococcus epidermidis* to smooth surfaces. Infect Immun. 1982;37:318–26.
66. Peters G, Locci R, Pulverer G. Adherence and growth of coagulase negative staphylococci on surfaces of intravenous catheters. J Infect Dis. 1982;146:479–82.
67. Band JD, Maki DG. Infections caused by arterial catheters used for hemodynamic monitoring. Am J Med. 1979;67:735–41.
68. Adams JM, Speer ME, Rudolph AJ. Bacterial colonization of radial artery catheters. Pediatrics. 1980;65:94–7.
69. Montgomerie JZ, Edwards JE Jr. Association of infection due to *Candida albicans* with intravenous hyperalimentation. J Infect Dis. 1978;127:197–201.

70. Henderson DK, Edwards JE Jr, Montgomerie JZ. Hematogenous *Candida* endophthalmitis in patients receiving parenteral hyperalimentation fluids. J Infect Dis. 1981;143:655–61.
71. Maki DG, Jarrett F, Sarafin HW. A semiquantitative method for identification of catheter-related infection in the burn patient. J Surg Res. 1977;22:513–20.
72. Maki DG, Weise CE, Sarafin HW. A semiquantitative method for identifying intravenous-catheter-related infection. N Engl J Med. 1977;296:1305–9.
73. Band JD, Maki DG. Steel needles used for intravenous therapy: Morbidity in patients with hematologic malignancy. Arch Intern Med. 1980;140:31–4.
74. Henderson DK, Baptiste RM, Parrillo J, et al. Indolent epidemic of *Pseudomonas cepacia* bacteremia and pseudobacteremia in an intensive care unit traced to a contaminated blood gas analyzer. Am J Med. 1988;84:75–81.
75. Smith PW, Massanari RM. Room humidifiers as the source of *Acinetobacter* infections. JAMA. 1977;237:795–7.
76. Cleri DJ, Corrado ML, Seligman SJ. Quantitative culture of intravenous catheters and other intravascular inserts. J Infect Dis. 1980;141:781–6.
77. Collignon P, Chan R, Munro R. Rapid diagnosis of intravascular catheter-related sepsis. Arch Intern Med. 1987;147:1609–12.
78. McGeer A, Righter J. Improving our ability to diagnose infections associated with central venous catheters: Value of Gram's staining and culture of entry site swabs. Can Med Assoc J. 1987;137:1009–15.
79. Vanhuynegen L, Parmentier P, Porvliege C. In situ bacteriologic diagnosis of total parenteral nutrition catheter infection. Surgery. 1988;103:174–7.
80. Zuffrey J, Rime B, Franciou P, et al. Simple method for rapid diagnosis of catheter-associated infection by direct acridine orange staining of catheter tips. J Clin Microbiol. 1988;26:175–7.
81. Spencer RC, Kristinsson KG. Failure to diagnose intravascular associated infection by direct Gram-staining of catheter segments. J Hosp Infec. 1986;7:305–6.
82. Mosca R, Curtas S, Forbes B, et al. The benefits of isolator cultures in the management of suspected catheter sepsis. Surgery. 1987;102:718–23.
83. Wing EJ, Norden CW, Shadduck RK, et al. Use of quantitative bacteriologic techniques to diagnose catheter-related sepsis. Arch Intern Med. 1979; 139:482–8.
84. Tonnesen A, Peuler M, Lockwood WR. Cultures of blood drawn by catheters vs. venipuncture. JAMA. 1976;235:1877.
85. Felices FJ, Hernandez JL, Ruiz J, et al. Use of the central venous pressure catheter to obtain blood cultures. Crit Care Med. 1979;7:78–9.
86. Tully JL, Friedland GH, Baldini LM, et al. Complications of intravenous therapy with steel needles and Teflon catheters. Am J Med. 1981;70:702–6.
87. Crane C: Venous interruption for septic thrombophlebitis. N Engl J Med. 1962;262:947–51.
88. Munster AM: Septic thrombophlebitis: A surgical disorder. JAMA. 1974;230:1010–1.
89. Jarrard MM, Freeman JB. The effects of antibiotic ointments and antiseptics on the skin flora beneath subclavian catheter dressings during intravenous hyperalimentation. J Surg Res. 1977;22:521–6.
90. Maki DG, Band JD. A comparative study of polyantibiotic and iodophor ointments in prevention of vascular catheter-related infection. Am J Med. 1981;70:739–44.
91. Wilmore DW, Dudrick SJ. An in-line filter for intravenous solutions. Arch Surg. 1969;99:462–3.
92. Rusmin S, DeLuca PP. Effect of antibiotics and osmotic change on the release of endotoxin by bacteria retained on intravenous in-line filters. Am J Hosp Pharm. 1975;32:378–80.
93. Buxton AE, Highsmith AK, Garner JS, et al. Contamination of intravenous infusion fluid: Effects of changing administration sets. Ann Intern Med. 1979;90:764–8.
94. Band JD, Maki DG. Safety of changing intravenous delivery systems at longer than 24-hour intervals. Ann Intern Med. 1979;91:173–8.
95. Snydman DR, Reidy MD, Perry LK, et al. Safety of changing intravenous (IV) administration sets containing burettes at longer than 48 hour intervals. Infect Control. 1987;8:113–6.
96. Maki DG, Boiticelli JT, LeRoy ML, et al. Prospective study of replacing administration sets for intravenous therapy at 48 vs. 72 hour intervals: 72 hours is safe and cost-effective. JAMA. 1987;258:1777–81.
97. Michel L, McMichan JC, Bachy JL. Microbial colonization of indwelling central venous catheters: Statistical evaluation of potential contaminating factors. Am J Surg. 1979;137:745–8.
98. Prager RL, Silva J Jr. Colonization of central venous catheters. South Med J. 1984;77:458–61.
99. Maher MM, Henderson DK, Brennan MF. Central venous catheter exchange in cancer patients during total parenteral nutrition. NITA J. 1982;5:54–60.
100. Fairchild JP, Graber CP, Vogel EN, et al. Flora of the umbilical stump. J Pediatr. 1958;53:538–46.
101. Anagnostakis D, Kamba A, Petrochilou V, et al. Risk of infection associated with umbilical vein catheterization: A prospective study in 75 newborn infants. J Pediatr. 1973;86:759–65.
102. Balagtas RC, Bell CE, Edwards LD, et al. Risk of local and systemic infections associated with umbilical vein catheterization: A prospective study in 86 newborn patients. Pediatrics. 1971;48:359–67.
103. Hall RT, Rhodes PG. Total parenteral alimentation via indwelling umbilical catheters in the newborn period. Arch Dis Child. 1976;51:929–34.
104. Symansky MR, Fox HA. Umbilical vessel catheterization: Indications, management, and evaluation of the technique. J Pediatr. 1972;80:820–6.
105. Powers WF, Tooley WH. Contamination of umbilical vessel catheters: Encouraging information. Pediatrics. 1972;49:470–1.
106. Munson DP, Thompson TR, Johnson DE, et al. Coagulase-negative staphylococcal septicemia: Experience in a newborn intensive care unit. J Pediatr. 1982;101:602–5.
107. Goldmann DA, Maki DG. Infection control in total parenteral nutrition. JAMA. 1973;223:1360–4.
108. Curry CR, Quie PG. Fungal septicemia in patients receiving parenteral hyperalimentation. N Engl J Med. 1971;285:1221–5.
109. Bailey MJ. Reduction of catheter-associated sepsis in parenteral nutrition using low-dose intravenous heparin. Br Med J. 1979;1:1671–73.
110. Ruggiero RP, Aisenstein TJ. Central catheter fibrin sleeve; heparin effect. J Parenter Enteral Nutr. 1983;7:270–3.
111. Bottino J, McCredie KB, Groschel DHM, et al. Long-term intravenous therapy with peripherally inserted silicone elastomer central venous catheters in patients with malignant diseases. Cancer. 1979;43:1937–43.
112. Mitchell A, Atkins S, Royle GT, et al. Reduced catheter sepsis and prolonged catheter life using a tunnelled silicone rubber catheter for total parenteral nutrition. Br J Surg. 1982;69:420–2.
113. Meyenfeldt MMF, Stapert J, deJong PCM, et al. TPN catheter sepsis: Lack of effect of subcutaneous tunnelling of PVC catheters on sepsis rate. J Parenter Enteral Nutr. 1980;4:514–7.
114. Copeland EM, MacFayden BV, McGown C, et al. The use of hyperalimentation in patients with potential sepsis. Surg Gynecol Obstet. 1974;137:377–80.
115. Wilmore DW, Dudrick SJ. Safe long-term venous catheterization. Arch Surg. 1969;98:256–8.
116. Burke JP, Garibaldi RA, Britt MR, et al. Prevention of catheter-associated urinary tract infections: Efficacy of daily meatal care regimens. Am J Med. 1981;70:655–8.
117. Henderson DK, Myers RF, Laniak JM. Catheter-acquired infection in total parenteral nutrition. NITA J. 1982;5:62–8.
118. Broviac JW, Cole JJ, Scribner BH. A silicone rubber atrial catheter for prolonged parenteral alimentation. Surg Gynecol Obstet. 1973;136: 602–6.
119. Blacklock HA, Hill RS, Clarke AG, et al. Use of modified subcutaneous right-atrial catheter for venous access in leukaemic patients. Lancet. 1980;1:993–5.
120. Hickman RO, Buckner CD, Clift RA, et al. A modified right atrial catheter for access to the venous system in marrow transplant recipients. Surg Gynecol Obstet. 1979;148:871–5.
121. Press OW, Ramsey PG, Larson EB, et al. Hickman catheter infections in patients with malignancies., Medicine (Baltimore). 1984;63:189–200.
122. Hiemenz JW, Robichaud KJ, Johnston MR, et al. Bacteremia in patients with indwelling silastic catheters. Proc Am Soc Clin Oncol. 1982;1:57.
123. Prince A, Heller B, Levy J, et al. Management of fever in patients with central vein catheters. Pediatr Infect Dis. 1986;5:20–24.
124. Olson TA, Fischer GW, Lupo MC, et al. Antimicrobial therapy of Broviac catheter infections in pediatric hematology oncology patients. J Pediatr Surg. 1987;22:839–42.
125. Hartman GE, Shuchat ST. Management of septic complications associated with Silastic catheters in childhood malignancies. Pediatr Infect Dis J. 1987;6:1042–7.
126. Hiemenz J, Skelton J, Pizzo PA. Perspective on the management of catheter-related infections in cancer patients. Pediatr Infect Dis. 1987;5:6–11.
127. Strum S, McDermed J, Korn A, et al. Improved methods for venous access: The Port-a-cath, a totally implanted catheter system. J Clin Oncol. 1986;4:596–603.
128. Becton DL, Kletzel M, Golladay ES, et al. An experience with an implanted port system in 66 children with cancer. Cancer. 1988;61:376–8.
129. Brothers TE, VanMoll LK, Niederhuber JE, et al. Ensminger WD. Experience with subcutaneous infusion ports in three hundred patients. Surg Gynecol Obstet. 1988;166:295–301.
130. Haddad W, Idowu J, Georgeson K, et al. Septic atrial thrombosis. A potentially lethal complication of Broviac catheters in infants. Am J Dis Child. 1986;140:778–80.
131. Swan HJC, Ganz W, Forrester J. Catheterization of the heart in man with the use of a flow-directed balloon-tipped catheter. N Engl J Med. 1970;283:447–51.
132. Michel L, Marsh HM, McMichan JC, et al. Infection of pulmonary artery catheters in critically ill patients. JAMA. 1981;245:1032–6.
133. Katz JD, Cronan LH, Barash PG, et al. Pulmonary artery flow-guided catheters in the perioperative period. JAMA. 1977;237:2832–4.
134. Ford SE, Manley PN. Indwelling cardiac catheters. An autopsy study of associated endocardial lesions. Arch Pathol Lab Med. 1982;106:314–7.
135. Greene JF Jr, Fitzwater JE, Clemmer TP. Septic endocarditis and indwelling pulmonary artery catheters. JAMA. 1975;233:891–2.
136. Ehrie M, Morgan AP, Moore FD, et al. Endocarditis with the indwelling balloon-tipped pulmonary artery catheter in burn patients. J Trauma. 1978;18:664–6.
137. Maki DG, Hassemer CA. Endemic rate of fluid contamination and related septicemia in arterial pressure monitoring. Am J Med. 1981;70:733–8.
138. Weinstein RA, Stamm WE, Kramer L, et al. Pressure monitoring devices: Overlooked source of nosocomial infection. JAMA. 1976;236:936–8.
139. Phillips I, Eykyne S, Curtis MA, et al. *Pseudomonas cepacia* (*multivorans*) septicemia in an intensive care unit. Lancet. 1971;1:375–7.
140. Buxton AE, Anderson RL, Klimek J, et al. Failure of disposable domes to

prevent septicemia from contaminated pressure transducers. Chest. 1978;74:508–13.
141. West CM, Wayle B, Touneson A, et al. Nosocomial *Serratia marcescens* bacteremia associated with reuse of disposable monitoring domes (Abstract 429). In: Seventeenth Interscience Conference on Antimicrobial Agents and Chemotherapy. New York. Washington, DC: American Society for Microbiology; 1977.
142. Walton JR, Shapiro BA, Harrison RA. *Serratia* bacteremia from mean arterial pressure monitors. Anesthesiology. 1975;43:113–4.
143. Donowitz LG, Marsik FJ, Hoyt JW, et al. Control of nosocomial *Serratia marcescens* bacteremia traced to contaminated pressure transducers. JAMA. 1979;242:1749–51.
144. Hawley HB. Bacterial infection from intravascular monitoring devices. Infect Control. 1983;4:399–401.
145. Murphy LM, Lipman TD. Central venous catheter care in parenteral nutrition: A review. J Parenter Enteral Nutr. 1987;11:190–201.
146. Wyatt TD, Timoney R. The effect of introducing a policy for catheter care on the catheter infection rate in a small hospital. J Hosp Infect. 1987;9: 230–4.
147. Faubion WC, Wesley JR, Khalidi N, et al. Total parenteral nutrition catheter sepsis: Impact of the team approach. J Parenter Enteral Nutr. 1986;10: 642–5.
148. Steere AC, Mallison GF. Handwashing practices for the prevention of nosocomial infections. Ann Intern Med. 1975;83:683–90.
149. Stotter AT, Ward H, Waterfield AH, et al. Junctional care: The key to prevention of catheter sepsis in intravenous feeding. J Parenter Enteral Nutr. 1987;11:159–62.
150. Gabel KS, Geelhoed GW, Zalkind DL. A comparative study of a new skin preparation method for peripheral intravenous lines. Am J Surg. 1988; 54:307–10.
151. Trooskin SZ, Donetz AP, Harvey RA, et al. Prevention of catheter sepsis by antibiotic bonding. Surgery. 1985;97:547–51.

280. NOSOCOMIAL RESPIRATORY INFECTION

JAMES E. PENNINGTON

The lung currently accounts for 15 percent of all hospital-acquired infections in the United States.[1] Nosocomial pneumonia is associated with mortalities ranging from 20 to 50 percent[2–6] and is the most common fatal nosocomial infection. On the basis of epidemiologic studies,[5] it is estimated that about 15 percent of all hospital-associated deaths are directly related to hospital-acquired pneumonia. Any reduction in the incidence and mortality from this particular infectious complication would have a major impact upon hospital-associated mortality.

INCIDENCE AND MORTALITY

The incidence of hospital-acquired lower respiratory infections in the United States is estimated to be 0.6 percent (6 cases per 1000 discharges),[1] or approximately 300,000 cases per year.[7] The majority of nosocomial pneumonias occur in intensive care unit settings or postsurgical recovery areas, where the incidence may be from 7 percent to as high as 20 percent.[4,8,9]

Mortalities reported for hospital-acquired pneumonia have ranged from 20 percent, in a multihospital survey that included several community hospitals,[2] to 50 percent or higher in university referral hospitals.[3,4] While bacteremia occurs in fewer than 10 percent of nosocomial pneumonias,[1] it is associated with a threefold increase in mortality.[2] Of even greater relevance appears to be the relationship of mortality to etiologic agents (Table 1). It is clear that the prognosis associated with aerobic gram-negative bacillary pneumonias is considerably worse than that with gram-positive or viral agents. In one report,[4] *Pseudomonas aeruginosa* was identified as a gram-negative pulmonary pathogen associated with uniquely high mortality (70 percent), as compared with other gram-negative bacilli (33 percent). Mortalities associated with gram-positive organisms (usually *Staphylococcus aureus*) are lower but not negligible. The mortalities reported for nosocomial legionnaires' disease[10] may be somewhat overstated since a number of fatal cases have been diagnosed retrospectively, without a trial of specific therapy. However, since nosocomial legionnaires' disease occurs predominantly in compromised hosts, death rates higher than those reported for sporadic community-acquired legionnaires' disease might be expected. Whereas viral nosocomial pneumonias are usually not fatal, deaths can occur, particularly in children with congenital heart disease[11] or adults with debilitating diseases.[12,13]

TABLE 1. Relationship between Etiologic Agent and Mortality from Hospital-Acquired Pneumonia

Series (Ref no.)	*Etiologic Agent*	*Mortality (%)*
Graybill (3)	Gram-positive cocci	24
Stevens (4)	Gram-positive cocci	5
Graybill (3)	Gram-negative bacilli	56
Stevens (4)	Gram-negative bacilli	50
Valenti (18)	Virus	7
Kirby (10)	*Legionella pneumophila*	25

The particularly high mortalities associated with gram-negative bacillary nosocomial pneumonia should not be surprising. Several features of that infection make therapy difficult. These include (1) a necrotizing and hemorrhagic lung pathology, rendering local lung defenses less effective and making adequate antibiotic penetration difficult; (2) pathogens that generally require higher dosages of potentially toxic antibiotics; and (3) hosts that generally are among the most debilitated in the hospital.

ETIOLOGIES

The majority of nosocomial pneumonias are caused by gram-negative bacilli (Table 2). The National Nosocomial Infections Study consistently reports that more than 60 percent of nosocomial pneumonias are caused by aerobic gram-negative bacilli.[1] In fact, gram-negative bacilli accounted for six of the top seven etiologic agents identified in the last reported survey (1984). In rank order, these organisms were *Pseudomonas aeruginosa* (16.9 percent); *Staphyloccus aureus* (12.9 percent); *Klebsiella* sp. (11.6 percent); *Enterobacteriaceae* sp. (9.4 percent); *Escherichia coli* (6.4 percent); *Serratia marcescens* (5.8 percent); and *Proteus* sp. (4.2 percent). *Streptococcus pneumoniae* accounted for less than 3 percent of the nosocomial pneumonias. Others have also reported that nosocomial pneumonias are predominantly caused by gram-negative bacilli. This has been noted both in community hospitals,[2] and in university hospitals.[4] It should be pointed out, however, that defining the precise etiology of most hospital-acquired pneumonias is difficult. In one series, using strict criteria for identifying etiologic agents (e.g., correlation of sputum and blood cultures or repetitive isolation of the same organisms from purulent sputum), 44 percent of all nosocomial pneumonias were of uncertain etiology.[3] For example, only by employing molecular epidemiologic methods was *Branhamella catarrhalis* verified as a nosocomial respiratory pathogen.[14]

TABLE 2. Etiologic Agents Causing Hospital-Acquired Pneumonia

Common	*Less Common*
Pseudomonas aeruginosa	Anaerobic mouth flora
Staphylococcus aureus	*Streptococcus pneumoniae*
Klebsiella sp.	Other enteric gram-negative bacilli
Enterobacter sp.	*Branhamella catarrhalis*
	Influenza A virus
Escherichia coli	*Haemophilus influenzae*
Pediatric wards: respiratory syncytial virus	*Legionella* sp.
	Aspergillus

Less frequent etiologies for hospital-acquired pneumonias are also noted in Table 2. Several of these may occur more frequently than generally acknowledged. This potential for underreporting is due to difficulties with the diagnostic techniques necessary for certain etiologic agents. Also, while epidemic viral pneumonia has been recognized in the hospital setting,[15–17] only with prospective monitoring and careful evaluation of specimens by a diagnostic virology lab can the true incidence of endemic viral pneumonias in the hospital setting be determined. One such survey reported that viral agents accounted for 19.7 percent of all nosocomial lower respiratory infections during a 17-month surveillance period in a general hospital.[18] As in other reports, the majority of nosocomial viral pneumonia cases in that study occurred in pediatric wards. In fact, when carefully monitored, viruses are the most common cause of nosocomial respiratory infections in pediatric wards.[15] Although data are less well established for adults, it appears that nosocomial viral respiratory infections are much less common in adult medical and surgical wards.[19]

In recent years, attention has been directed toward two viral pathogens, respiratory syncytial virus (RSV) and influenza A, as important etiologic agents for nosocomial respiratory infection.[12,20,21] In one study, more than 40 percent of hospitalized infant contacts developed RSV infection during hospitalization.[20] In another report,[13] seven hospitalized adults with debilitating disease developed nosocomial influenza A pneumonia after exposure to a single index case. Like these two reports, most studies have emphasized the role of RSV infection among pediatric patients and influenza among adults. However, these viral agents are clearly not limited to these specific settings.[22–24] Nosocomial respiratory infections with other viral agents are less well described. However, occasional outbreaks with such agents as parainfluenza virus (e.g., in neonatal nurseries) have been reported.[15] Since routine bacteriologic cultures of respiratory secretions will not allow for isolation of viral pathogens, clinician awareness that viral agents may cause nosocomial pneumonia must be emphasized, particularly during periods of communitywide epidemic viral illness.

As with viral agents, the diagnosis of Legionnaires' disease requires special serologic and microbiologic techniques. Although it is generally believed that fewer than 10 percent of nosocomial pneumonias are caused by *Legionella* sp.,[25] the true incidence of this infection as a sporadic nosocomial pneumonia is unknown. For example, in hospital settings with contamination of potable water by *Legionella* sp., this pathogen may account for up to 30 percent of all nosocomial pneumonias.[26,27] Other bacterial pathogens that should be mentioned are *Hemophilus influenzae*, which occurs with increased frequency in patients with chronic lung disease,[28] but is otherwise rare,[1] and anaerobic bacteria, which may be associated with large-scale aspirations (e.g., during extubation) but are otherwise not considered to be common in this setting.[1]

While the subject of pneumonia in the immunocompromised host is discussed elsewhere in this text, it should be mentioned that pneumonias caused by *Aspergillus* sp.[29] and, to a lesser extent, *Torulopsis glabrata*[30] may occur in such patients after nosocomial exposures. This should be suspected when these pneumonias begin to occur in frequencies out of proportion to those expected in the hospital setting.

PREDISPOSING FACTORS

A number of factors that increase the risk of pneumonia in the hospital setting have been identified (Table 3). First and foremost is intubation of the respiratory tract. Both short-term intubations for surgery and longer-term intubation for respiratory failure are associated with the highest of reported frequencies (17–20 percent) for nosocomial pneumonia.[4,9] In one report, the incidence of nosocomial pneumonia for intubated patients was four times higher than that for nonintubated patients, and tracheostomy further increased this risk.[31] In a recent prospective study, 21 percent of 233 intubated patients developed nosocomial pneumonia, and associated mortality was 55 percent.[6] The major risk factors associated with pneumonia in the intubated patients were presence of intracranial pressure monitors, fall–winter season, use of cimetidine (see "Pathogenesis" below), and tubing changes every 24 hours instead of 48 hours.[6] A number of other factors likely account for the enhanced risk of pneumonia among intubated patients. Apart from the obvious fact that such patients are often the most critically ill, the presence of an endotracheal tube eliminates the action of the inertial filtration system of the nose and conducting airways and the mucociliary clearance system of the airways. Also, mechanical irritation and injury of respiratory mucosa may predispose to local colonization of airways with potential bacterial pathogens.

TABLE 3. Predisposing Factors for Hospital-Acquired Pneumonia

Intubation
Intensive care unit
Antibiotics
Surgery
Chronic lung disease
Advanced age
Immunosuppression

Respiratory equipment itself may serve as a source of bacteria causing nosocomial pneumonia. In past years, the major risk of infection was associated with contaminated mainstream reservoir nebulizers, designed to deliver aerosols of small particle size suspended in the effluent gas.[32,33] These observations led to the current trends in respiratory therapy to utilize cascade humidifiers, which do not generate microaerosols. Nevertheless, respiratory equipment continues to serve as a source of bacterial contamination. For example, side-arm medication nebulizers may become contaminated with bacteria after a single use.[34] Also, condensate in dependent regions of disposable tubing may become contaminated.[35] Evidence now suggests that less frequent (48 hour) rather than more frequent (24 hour) tubing changes result in a lower risk of pneumonia, presumably due to less frequent manipulation of tubes and possible reflux of condensate into airways.[6,36]

The use of antibiotics in the hospital setting has been associated with increased risk of nosocomial pneumonia.[37–39] These so-called superinfections presumably occur as a consequence of selection for more resistant bacterial pathogens during treatment of a primary infection (see "Pathogenesis," below). In one report, 149 patients treated in the hospital with penicillin or erythromycin for community-acquired bacterial pneumonia experienced a 16 percent incidence of pulmonary superinfections.[39] Etiologic agents were either gram-negative bacilli or *Staph. aureus*. While a concomitant group of non-antibiotic-treated hospitalized patients was not available in this series for comparison, this incidence is several times that reported in the general hospital population.[1]

Postsurgical patients clearly are at increased risk for pneumonia.[9] In one hospital experience, 50 percent of all nosocomial pneumonias occurred in postoperative patients.[40] Others have reported a 17.5 percent incidence of nosocomial pneumonia among patients undergoing elective thoracic or abdominal procedures.[9] Obesity, advanced age, and severity of underlying disease were all associated with increased risk for nosocomial pneumonia in that study. The relative importance of intubation, prophylactic antibiotics, and stress of the surgical procedure in predisposing to pneumonia is not yet well defined in surgical patients, however.

It is often stated that chronic pulmonary diseases are associated with increased risk of nosocomial pneumonia. Whereas several studies suggest that this is the case,[28,37] it is also noteworthy that these particular patients require assisted ventilation more frequently than others. In one report, mortalities from nosocomial pneumonia in intubated patients with or without underlying chronic lung disease were not significantly different.[4] Advanced age has also been associated with an increased risk for nosocomial pneumonia.[4,9] Finally, immunosuppression and myelosuppression clearly are predisposing factors for nosocomial pneumonias.[3,10,29]

PATHOGENESIS

Nosocomial pneumonia can develop either as a result of aspiration of upper airway flora or secondary to bacteremia. Metastatic pneumonias resulting from septic pelvic thrombophlebitis, right-sided endocarditis, "urosepsis," or simply bacteremia in the compromised host are all well described. However, the majority of nosocomial pneumonias appear to result from aspiration of potential pathogens that have colonized the mucosal surfaces of the upper airways.[37,41] In fact, the relative predictive value of positive surveillance cultures of the upper airways in high-risk patients has been determined. In one study,[37] 213 patients admitted to a medical intensive care unit were monitored with frequent cultures of the posterior oropharynx. Ninety-five patients (45 percent) became colonized with aerobic gram-negative bacilli by the end of 1 week in the hospital. Of these 95 colonized patients, subsequent nosocomial pneumonia developed in 22 (23 percent). Pneumonia developed in only 4 of 118 noncolonized patients (3.3 percent). The risk factors for upper airway colonization with gram-negative bacilli appear to be (*1*) more advanced degrees of illness, (*2*) longer duration in the hospital, (*3*) prior or concomitant use of antibiotics, (*4*) intubation, (*5*) azotemia, and (*6*) underlying pulmonary disease.[37,38,42]

The source of organisms colonizing the upper airway has been a controversial subject. Whereas a fecal-to-oral route of contamination has long been suspected for bedridden patients, this could not readily explain the frequency of colonization by such organisms as *P. aeruginosa*, which are distinctly unusual inhabitants of the human gastrointestinal tract. In one study, daily cultures were monitored from rectal, hypopharyngeal, and tracheal sites in 21 patients requiring prolonged intubation.[43] Enterobacteriaceae were commonly cultured from the hypopharynx and rectum before their appearance in tracheal cultures. In contrast, non-Enterobacteriaceae (e.g., *P. aeruginosa, Acinetobacter*), were rarely found in those sites before their appearance in the trachea. This suggested that environmental sources existed primarily for non-Enterobacteriaceae and that colonizing Enterobacteriaceae originated primarily from the patients' endogenous flora. Studies by others suggest that the most important vector for transmission of environmental flora is the hands of health care personnel.[44] Unfortunately, although hand washing and other infection control methods may reduce cross-contamination with certain potential pathogens, it appears that the patient's endogenous flora will continue to provide a source for upper airway colonization. Further, the recent popularity of gastric alkalinization to prevent stress ulcers and bleeding in hospitalized patients is producing larger numbers of patients with extensive bacterial overgrowth in the upper gastrointestinal tract. This, in turn, appears to lead to airway colonization secondary to aspiration of gastric microflora.[45,46] In one recent report, use of cimetidine was a major risk factor for nosocomial pneumonia in the intensive care unit.[6] Furthermore, a recent controlled trial demonstrated a greater frequency of nosocomial pneumonia in patients receiving gastrointestinal bleeding prophylaxis by gastric alkalinization as compared to patients receiving sucralfate, a compound that does not act to raise gastric pH.[47]

Considerable data are now available to describe mechanisms for bacterial colonization of the respiratory epithelium. Both bacterial factors (e.g., pili)[48] and host factors (e.g., epithelial receptors, fibronectin on cell surfaces, and protease content in saliva)[49–51] appear to play roles in the colonization process. In particular, fibronectin appears to play an integral part in modulating oropharyngeal bacterial ecology. Under normal conditions, mucosal cells are coated with fibronectin, which in turn selects for adherence of gram-positive cocci and prevents adherence of gram-negative bacteria to cells.[49,50] Increased protease content of saliva is associated with loss of fibronectin from buccal cell surfaces and increased adherence (in vitro) and colonization (in vivo) of airway mucosa with gram-negative bacilli.[51] One recent study has identified polymorphonuclear leukocytes in airway secretions as the source of this protease.[52] Furthermore, in vitro bacterial adherence assays, utilizing respiratory epithelial cells obtained from high-risk patients, may have some predictive value for subsequent airway colonization.[53] Other factors that have been demonstrated as important for airway colonization are epithelial tissue damage[54] and reduction of the normal microbial flora of the upper airway during antibiotic administration.[55] As these mechanisms become better defined, improved methods for preventing airway colonization may be developed.

DIAGNOSTIC CONSIDERATIONS

In contrast to community-acquired pneumonia, it may be difficult to determine whether or not a pneumonia has developed in a hospitalized patient.[56,57] The classic clinical findings for pneumonia, such as new fever, new pulmonary infiltrate, cough, sputum production, and elevated leukocyte count, may not be present in the hospitalized patient with nosocomial pneumonia. Alternatively, these findings may be present, yet may not be caused by pneumonia. It is not surprising, therefore, that considerable debate generally surrounds the isolation of potential gram-negative (or *Staph. aureus*) bacillary pathogens from cultures of the airways in such patients. Does this represent "colonization" or actual nosocomial "infection"? If infection, is it pneumonia or simply tracheobronchitis? Even the presence or absence of purulent tracheobronchial secretions will not be sufficient to answer the latter question (although it will be helpful in answering the former).

A recent study clearly illustrates the lack of clinical precision in diagnosing nosocomial pneumonia.[56] In that study, histopathologic and clinical diagnoses were correlated for 30 consecutive adult patients who died in association with adult respiratory distress syndrome. Particular attention was given to whether or not premortem clinical diagnoses of pneumonia could be verified by autopsy findings. In some cases, autopsies revealed unsuspected pneumonia, and in other cases, clinically suspected pneumonias were not confirmed by examination of lung tissues. Overall, nosocomial bacterial pneumonia was misdiagnosed in 30 percent of the patients. Obviously, the difficulty in distinguishing between bacterial colonization and infection of the lower respiratory tract will inevitably lead to some errors in management. Such errors may include treatment of colonized patients with broad-spectrum antibiotics or, alternatively, withholding of treatment from infected patients. Clinical experience, coupled with careful physical and microbiologic observations, can be expected to assist the clinician in this difficult setting, however.

The initial evaluation of a patient with suspected nosocomial pneumonia must address several questions: Has there been a change in clinical status, unexplained by other events (e.g., myocardial infarction, pulmonary embolism); and specifically, has there been a sudden increase in lung infiltrate, a drop in arterial Po_2, a change in fever pattern, and, most importantly, an increase in quantity and purulence of respiratory secretions? Although these clinical criteria for nosocomial pneumonia may lack both sensitivity and specificity, they may be the only available parameters for the clinician.

Microbiologic evaluation of the patient with suspected nosocomial pneumonia may or may not be helpful. Sputum or respiratory secretions (obtained by endotracheal aspiration) should be examined microscopically using a Gram stain. Unfortunately, these specimens are often contaminated with upper airway flora. Likewise, cultures of such specimens may or may not reflect the microbiology of infected lung tissues. Isolation of a single organism from blood cultures may help to distinguish between contaminating and infecting bacterial isolates in sputum. Blood cultures are positive in fewer than 10 percent of patients with nosocomial pneumonias, however.[1]

A number of specialized microbiologic methods, and also several invasive methods for obtaining specimens, have been described as potentially useful for improving diagnostic specificity for nosocomial pneumonia.[58] Quantitative sputum cultures, "washed" sputum cultures, and microscopic "screening" of sputa for the presence of upper airway cells suggesting contamination have all been advocated as means for determining the significance of bacterial isolates. These methods may be impractical for widespread use, however, and in fact have met with some controversy regarding their actual usefulness. Transtracheal aspiration (not possible in intubated patients), percutaneous thin-needle lung aspiration (not advised for patients on positive pressure breathing modes), and shielded-tip bronchoscopic sampling of lower airway secretions have all been suggested as methods to prevent upper airway contamination of respiratory specimens. While these methods may, in fact, increase diagnostic specificity in certain patients, they may not be well tolerated by certain critically ill patients with suspected pneumonia. In addition, reports have illustrated a rather high rate of false-positive results for cultures obtained by these procedures.[59,60] One report compared the accuracy of quantitative respiratory secretion cultures obtained by shielded-tip bronchoscopy to that of cultures of lung tissue obtained by open lung biopsy in patients with assisted ventilation.[60] Specimens were collected from intubated patients immediately after they expired. While excellent microbiologic correlation between lung tissues and bronchoscopic specimens with $\geq 10^3$ colony forming units of bacteria per milliliter was noted for patients with histologic evidence of pneumonia, there was a 40 percent incidence of false-positive results among the bronchoscopic specimens obtained from patients without pneumonia. No false-negatives were found. If patients had not received prior antibiotics, however, false-positive results were reduced to 13 percent. More recent studies by the same investigators continue to emphasize the usefulness of shielded-tip bronchoscopy with quantitative cultures for excluding pneumonia.[57] Even more recently, experimental studies in intubated baboons have suggested that quantitative cultures of bronchoalveolar lavage (BAL) specimens also might be useful in the diagnosis of pneumonia in subjects with assisted ventilation.[61] Finally, immunologic methods for diagnostic evaluation of respiratory specimens (e..g., direct fluorescent antibody for *Legionella* sp. or crossed-immunoelectrophoresis for pneumococcal antigens) have been described. Unfortunately, the vast majority of nosocomial pneumonias are caused by pathogens for which no immunologic diagnostic techniques currently exist.

TREATMENT

Once it has been decided that a nosocomial infection of the lower respiratory tract exists, several issues must be considered in selecting therapy. Patient-related considerations are as follows: (*1*) has the patient recently received antibiotics, which could select for more resistant organisms; (*2*) does the patient have underlying chronic bronchitis, which would increase the risk of *H. influenzae,* or cystic fibrosis, which would increase the risk of *P. aeruginosa* and *Staph. aureus;* and (*3*) does the patient's sputum smear reveal a predominant gram-positive or gram-negative flora? Another consideration must be the recent experience with nosocomial pathogens in a given hospital or intensive care unit. Has there, for example, been a particularly high incidence of pneumonias caused by multiantibiotic-resistant *Acinetobacter* or *Serratia* during recent months? Or, is there a known problem with *Legionella* sp. in the patient's hospital? Particularly relevant to pediatric and psychiatric wards are concomitant outbreaks of viral or mycoplasmal respiratory infections in the community. Finally, have prior surveillance cultures of the patient's respiratory secretions revealed potential pathogens with unusual antibiotic sensitivity patterns? All of these factors must be considered when selecting an initial antibiotic regimen for treatment of suspected pneumonia. Of equal importance in making a therapeutic decision is a thorough understanding of which pathogens are most likely to cause nosocomial pneumonia in general (see "Etiologies," above).

Therapy selected for empiric treatment of nosocomial pneumonia, before definitive microbiologic identification of the pathogen, must be broad enough to ensure coverage for aerobic gram-negative bacilli, including such highly resistant organisms as *P. aeruginosa, Serratia marcescens,* and *Acinetobacter,* and also for *Staph. aureus.* On the basis of these considerations, several regimens have been employed for empiric treatment of nosocomial pneumonia. These include a semisynthetic penicillin plus an aminoglycoside; clindamycin plus an aminoglycoside; or a cephalosporin plus an aminoglycoside. In special situations, coverage for other organisms must also be included. These coverages include mouth anaerobes when obvious aspiration has occurred, *H. influenzae* in patients with known chronic lung disease, and *Legionella* sp. in certain hospitals. There is little evidence that two agents with gram-negative activity offer advantages over a single agent for treating gram-negative pneumonias. Nevertheless, the potential for additive or even synergistic therapeutic efficacy of two-drug regimens against gram-negative pathogens has led to popularity of cephalosporin–aminoglycoside combinations in this setting. Considerable interest has developed recently in the use of single-agent ("monodrug") coverage for life-threatening nosocomial infections. Most clinical studies of broad-spectrum β-lactam antibiotics as monodrug coverage for nosocomial sepsis have not been limited to treatment of pneumonia. However, several recent reports have examined this approach specifically for pulmonary indications.[62–66] In general, clinical efficacy of monodrug empiric treatment of nosocomial sepsis has been equivalent to that with combination regimens. However, problems have also been associated with this approach, including emergence of antibiotic-resistant bacteria during therapy.[62,67] In some cases serious bacterial superinfections have occurred.[62]

The duration of treatment for nosocomial pneumonia is often extended. In some cases, treatment is necessary for longer than 1 month. Also, in some cases, it will be impossible to eradicate the original pathogen from sputum despite clinical improvement. The continued presence of an endotracheal tube plus the necrotizing nature of gram-negative pneumonias undoubtedly contribute to this persistence of pathogens in airways and the necessity for protracted periods of therapy. Needless to say, the risk for emergence of resistant microorganisms during such therapy is considerable and has been proposed as an additional reason to utilize two different classes of antibiotics with gram-negative activity.[68]

The role of aminoglycosides in treating gram-negative nosocomial pneumonia deserves further comment. Evidence exists that aminoglycosides are more active than β-lactam antimicrobial agents against certain resistant gram-negative bacilli, such as *P. aeruginosa.*[69,70] Thus, many consider aminoglycosides a critical component of therapy for life-threatening gram-negative infections of the lung. Unfortunately, the therapeutic ratios for aminoglycosides in serum are narrow, and the penetration of aminoglycosides from blood into the infected respiratory tissues may be insufficient to achieve local drug concentrations above the minimal inhibitory concentration necessary for the infecting organism.[71] Accordingly, several approaches have been utilized to improve delivery of aminoglycosides into infected lung tissues. These include computer-assisted individualized dosing,[72] bolus dosing with unconventionally large doses,[73] and direct instillation of aminoglycoside into the respiratory tract via endotracheal or tracheostomy tube.[74] In a prospective randomized study,[74] groups of patients with nosocomial gram-negative pneumonia were treated with systemic antibiotics plus either 25 mg of sisomicin in saline suspension instilled into the respiratory tract every 8 hours or saline–placebo instillations. Significantly, more patients experienced improvement in the group receiving local aminoglycoside treatment. Superinfections with resistant flora were no different among the groups. Further investigation of local aminoglycoside therapy for pneumonia will be necessary before the relative risks and benefits can be defined. However, for selected patients, local aminoglycoside instillation therapy may be warranted.

There is growing interest in immunologic methods of treatment of gram-negative pneumonia.[75] A number of passive immune sera, including the J-5 cross-protective antisera,[76] and hyperimmune *Pseudomonas* globulin[77,78] are potentially valuable agents for treatment of gram-negative pneumonias. Clinical data are insufficient, however, to establish a definitive therapeutic role for passive immune globulins in nosocomial pneumonia at this time.

PREVENTION

The primary objective in preventing nosocomial pneumonia is to reduce the acquisition of potential bacterial pathogens in upper airways and thus to reduce the potential for aspiration of these organisms into the lower respiratory tract. Three general approaches have been utilized to achieve this objective: (*1*) attention to environmental factors (e.g., hand washing, specialized isolation procedures, monitoring of respiratory equipment for bacterial contamination); (*2*) prophylactic antibiotics, and (*3*) immunologic intervention. It is clear that attention to the patient's environment, particularly for those patients in intensive care units, will decrease the risk of nosocomial pneumonia.[33] Guidelines for decontamination of respiratory apparatus, proper suctioning techniques for intubated patients, proper hand washing policies, and handling of inhalation medications in the ICU setting have been published.[79] There is evidence that some of these recommendations, such as changing disposable respiratory equipment every 24 hours, are not correct.[36]

The use of prophylactic antibiotics to prevent colonization of airways with gram-negative bacilli has also been proposed.[80,81] In one study, aerosolized polymyxin B sulfate was utilized for patients admitted to a respiratory ICU.[80,82] While prophylactic topical polymyxin B sulfate led to decreased airway colonization and fewer subsequent pneumonias, there was a distinct increase in antibiotic resistance among respiratory pathogens in this setting. Pneumonia-related mortalities actually began to rise in the latter phase of this study. Experience by others with prophylactic endotracheal gentamicin has also demonstrated reduced rates of airway colonization at the expense of more resistant organisms.[81] Thus, the benefits of topical respiratory antibiotic prophylaxis did not clearly outweigh the attendant risks.

Oropharyngeal or gastrointestinal bacterial flora appear to be an important source of airway colonization in hospitalized patients. Accordingly, several groups in Europe have recently employed topical prophylactic antibiotics for "decontamination" of the oropharynx and gastrointestinal tract in patients at high risk for nosocomial pneumonia. In one study,[83] trauma patients requiring assisted ventilation for more than 5 days received daily polymyxin, tobramycin, and amphotericin B, applied to oropharyngeal mucosa and also instilled via gastric feeding tube. In order to prevent the emergence of resistant bacteria, intravenous cefotaxime was also given. Although this study was not controlled, the incidence of nosocomial pneumonia was less than that during the 2 year period prior to institution of antibiotic prophylaxis. In a separate and controlled study, also conducted in intubated critically ill patients, topical polymyxin, gentamicin, and amphotericin B were applied daily to the oropharynx and nostrils, and polymyxin plus gentamicin was also instilled via gastric feeding tube.[84] Systemic antibiotics were not employed in this study. Pneumonias occurred in 1 of 19 (5 percent) patients receiving the topical prophylaxis, and 9 of 20 (45 percent) controls. There was no difference in mortality between the groups, however. While these observations are encouraging, larger, controlled studies employing this approach will be needed before the impact on morbidity, mortality, and emergence of resistant bacteria can be fully evaluated.

Finally, considerable rationale has been presented for the development of immunologic protection of the respiratory tract against gram-negative bacilli during hospitalization.[2] Unfortunately, an effective mechanism to achieve this goal has not been described. There are several potential approaches to providing immune enhancement of lung defenses. One method would be to provide organism-specific immunization for pathogens known to be associated with particularly high mortalities. This approach has been evaluated for *P. aeruginosa* pneumonia, using prophylactic immunization with a lipopolysaccharide vaccine.[85] Although results from that study suggest that immunization reduced the incidence and mortality of *Pseudomonas* pneumonia, the experience was limited to only 34 vaccinated patients. Furthermore, side effects from lipopolysaccharide *Pseudomonas* vaccines are severe. A number of less toxic *Pseudomonas* vaccines are under investigation and may eventually be useful for immunologic interventions in settings associated with unusually high risk of *Pseudomonas* pneumonia. The usefulness of newly developed preparations for passive *Pseudomonas* immunization has yet to be demonstrated.[77]

An alternative, and perhaps even more rational, immunologic approach would be to confer protection against the wide range of gram-negative bacillary species that serve as potential pathogens for the human respiratory tract. So-called cross-protective vaccines or antisera, such as the J-5 mutant of *E. coli* 0 111, might be candidate immunogens. Clinical studies with J-5 antisera suggest a protective role against gram-negative septicemia;[76,86] however, prophylactic administration of J-5 antisera did not protect against nosocomial pneumonia.[86]

Limited success has been achieved in controlling nosocomial viral respiratory infection. It is thought that respiratory syncytial virus (RSV) is spread primarily by direct inoculation of large droplets or by direct contact (i.e., hands, fomites).[87] Thus, secretion precautions may be useful for known cases. In one study, isolation, cohorting of infected infants, and cohorting of staff to infected infants reduced the spread of RSV among patients but not among hospital personnel.[88] More recently, it has been shown that use of masks, goggles, gloves, and gowns will reduce nosocomial spread of RSV.[89,90] In contrast to RSV, influenza virus is spread by small particle aerosols. Thus, influenza can be spread more rapidly and is generally even more difficult to control. Prophylactic immunization with influenza vaccines, including for hospital workers, would be the most rational approach to control of nosocomial influenza respiratory infection. Remarkably, fewer than 20 percent of high-risk patients are immunized each year,[17] and probably fewer health care workers receive influenza vaccine.[11] Since prophylactic amantadine hydrochloride has also been shown to be effective against influenza A infection, use of this agent should be encouraged for protection of high-risk patients during nosocomial spread of influenza.[91,92]

In summary, it must be emphasized that nosocomial pneumonia is a discouraging problem. Despite our rather extensive understanding of the pathogenesis of this infectious disease, there is little evidence that significant progress is being made in either preventing or better treating nosocomial pneumonias. It can, thus, be argued that nosocomial pneumonia deserves the highest of priorities as a theme for both clinical and basic investigations.

REFERENCES

1. Centers for Disease Control. National Nosocomial Infections Study Report. Annual Summary. 1984. MMWR. 1986;35:17SS–29SS.
2. Stamm WE, Martin SM, Bennett JV. Epidemiology of nosocomial infections due to gram-negative bacilli: Aspects relevant to development and use of vaccines. J Infect Dis. 1977;136:S151–60.
3. Graybill JR, Marshall LW, Charache P, et al. Nosocomial pneumonia. Am Rev Respir Dis. 1973;108:1130–40.
4. Stevens RM, Terex D, Skillman JJ, et al. Pneumonia in an intensive care unit. Arch Intern Med. 1974;134:106–11.
5. Gross PA, Neu HC, Aswapokee P, et al. Deaths from nosocomial infections: Experience in a university hospital and a community hospital. Am J Med. 1980;68:219–23.
6. Craven DE, Kunches LM, Kilinsky V, et al. Risk factors for pneumonia and fatality in patients receiving continuous mechanical ventilation. Am Rev Respir Dis. 1986;133:792–6.
7. Gross PA. Epidemiology of hospital-acquired pneumonia. Semin Respir Infect. 1987;2:2–7.
8. Hemming VG, Overall JC Jr, Britt MR. Nosocomial infections in a newborn intensive care unit. N Engl J Med. 1976;294:1310–16.
9. Garibaldi RA, Britt MR, Coleman ML, et al. Risk factors for postoperative pneumonia. Am J Med. 1981;70:677–80.
10. Kirby BD, Snyder KM, Meyer RD, et al. Legionnaires' disease: Report of sixty-five nosocomially acquired cases and review of the literature. Medicine. 1980;59:188–205.
11. MacDonald NE, Hall CB, Suffin SC, et al. Respiratory syncytial viral infection in infants with congenital heart disease. N Engl J Med. 1982;307:397–409.
12. Blumenfeld HL, Kilbourne ED, Louria DB, Robers DE. Studies on influenza in the pandemic of 1957–1958: I. An epidemiologic, clinical and serologic investigation of an intrahospital epidemic, with a note on vaccination efficacy. J Clin Invest. 1959;38:199–212.
13. Kapila R, Lintz DI, Tecson FT, et al. A nosocomial outbreak of influenza A. Chest. 1977;71:576–9.
14. Patterson TF, Patterson JE, Masecar BL, et al. A nosocomial outbreak of *Branhamella catarrhalis* confirmed by restriction endonuclease analysis. J Infect Dis. 1988;157:996–1001.
15. Hall CB. Nosocomial viral respiratory infections: Perennial weeds on pediatric wards. Am J Med. 1981;70:670–6.
16. Wenzel RP, Deal EC, Hendley JO. Hospital-acquired viral respiratory illness on a pediatric ward. Pediatrics. 1977;60:367–71.
17. Glezen WP. Viral pneumonia as a cause and result of hospitalization. J Infect Dis. 1983;147:765–70.
18. Valenti WM, Hall CB, Douglas RG Jr, et al. Nosocomial viral infections: I. Epidemiology and significance. Infect Control. 1979;1:33–7.
19. Kimball AM, Foy HM, Cooney MK, et al. Isolation of respiratory syncytial and influenza viruses from the sputum of patients hospitalized with pneumonia. J Infect Dis. 1983;147:181–4.
20. Hall CB, Douglas RG Jr, Geiman JM, et al. Nosocomial respiratory syncytial virus infections. N Engl J Med. 1975;293:1343–6.
21. Hoffman PC, Dixon RE. Control of influenza in the hospital. Ann Intern Med. 1977;87:725–8.
22. Hall CB, Douglas RG Jr: Nosocomial influenza infection as a cause of intercurrent fevers in infants. Pediatrics. 1975;55:673–7.
23. Meibalane R, Sedmak GV, Sasidharan P, et al. Outbreak of influenza in a neonatal intensive care unit. J Pediatr. 1977;91:974–6.
24. Mathur U, Bentley DW, Hall CB. Concurrent respiratory syncytial virus and influenza A infections in the institutionalized elderly and chronically ill. Ann Intern Med. 1980;93:49–52.
25. England AC III, Fraser DW. Sporadic and epidemic nosocomial legionellosis in the United States. Am J Med. 1981;70:707–11.
26. Yu VL, Kroboth FJ, Shonnard J, et al. Legionnaires' disease: New clinical perspective from a prospective pneumonia study. Am J Med. 1982;73:357–61.
27. Korvick JA, Yu VL, Fang G. Legionella species as hospital-acquired respiratory pathogens. Semin Respir Infect. 1987;2:34–47.
28. Simon HB, Southwick FS, Moellering RC, et al: *Hemophilus influenzae* in hospitalized adults: Current perspectives. Am J Med. 1980;69:219–26.
29. Aisner J, Schimpff SC, Bennett JE, et al. Aspergillus infections in cancer patients. JAMA. 1976;235:411–2.
30. Aisner J, Schimpff SC, Sutherland JC, et al. *Torulopsis glabrata* infections in patients with cancer. Am J Med. 1976;61:23–8.
31. Cross AS, Roup B. Role of respiratory assistance devices in endemic nosocomial pneumonia. Am J Med. 1981;70:681–5.
32. Reinarz JA, Pierce AK, Mays BB, et al. The potential role of inhalation therapy equipment in nosocomial pulmonary infection. J Clin Invest. 1965;44:831–9.
33. Pierce AK, Sanford JP, Thomas GD, et al. Long-term evaluation of decontamination of inhalation-therapy equipment and the occurrence of necrotizing pneumonia. N Engl J Med. 1970;282:528–31.
34. Craven DE, Lichtenberg DA, Goularte TA, et al. Contaminated medication nebulizers in mechanical ventilator circuits: Source of bacterial aerosols. Am J Med. 1984;77:834–8.
35. Craven DE, Goultarte TA, Make BJ. Contaminated condensate in mechanical ventilator circuits: A risk factor for nosocomial pneumonia? Am Rev Respir Dis. 1984;129:625–8.
36. Craven DE, Connolly MG Jr, Lichtenberg DA, et al: Contamination of mechanical ventilators with tubing changes every 24 or 48 hours. N Eng J Med. 1982;306:1505–9.
37. Johanson WG Jr, Pierce AK, Sanford JP, et al. Nosocomial respiratory infections with gram-negative bacilli. Ann Intern Med. 1972;77:701–6.
38. Louria DB, Kaminski T. The effects of four anti-microbial drug regimens on sputum superinfection in hospitalized patients. Am Rev Respir Dis. 1962;85:649–65.
39. Tillotson JR, Finland M. Bacterial colonization and clinical superinfection of the respiratory tract complicating antibiotic treatment of pneumonia. J Infect Dis. 1969;119:597–624.
40. Eickhoff JC. Pulmonary infections in surgical patients. Surg Clin North Am. 1980;60:175–83.
41. Reynolds HY. Bacterial adherence to respiratory tract mucosa—a dynamic interaction leading to colonization. Semin Respir Infect. 1987;2:8–19.
42. Johanson WG, Pierce AK, Sanford JP. Changing pharyngeal bacterial flora of hospitalized patients. N Engl J Med. 1969;281:1137–40.
43. Schwartz SN, Dowling JN, Benkovic C, et al. Sources of gram-negative bacilli colonizing the tracheae of intubated patients. J Infect Dis. 1978;138:227–31.
44. Maki DG, Alvarado CJ, Hassemer CA, et al. Relation of the inanimate hospital environment to endemic nosocomial infection. N Engl J Med. 1982;25:1562–6.
45. DuMoulin GC, Paterson DG, Hedley-Whyte J, et al. Aspiration of gastric bacteria in antacid-treated patients: A frequent cause of postoperative colonisation of the airway. Lancet. 1982;1:242–5.
46. Pingleton SK, Hinthorn DR, Liu C. Enteral nutrition in patients receiving mechanical ventilation. Am J Med. 1986;80:827–32.
47. Driks MR, Craven DE, Bartolome R, et al. Nosocomial pneumonia in intubated patients given sucralfate as compared with antacids or histamine type 2 blockers. N Engl J Med. 1987;317:1376–82.
48. Woods DE, Straus DC, Johanson WG Jr, et al. Role of pili in adherence of *Pseudomonas aeruginosa* to mammalian buccal epithelial cells. Infect Immun. 1980;29:1146–51.
49. Abraham SN, Beachey EH, Simpson WA. Adherence of *Streptococcus pyogenes, Escherichia coli,* and *Pseudomonas aeruginosa* to fibronectin-coated and uncoated epithelial cells. Infect Immun. 1983;41:1261–8.
50. Woods DE, Straus DC, Johanson WG Jr, et al. Role of fibronectin in the prevention of adherence of *Pseudomonas aeruginosa* to buccal cells. J Infect Dis. 1981;143:784–90.
51. Woods DE, Straus DC, Johanson WG Jr, et al. Role of salivary protease activity in adherence of gram-negative bacilli to mammalian buccal epithelial cells in vivo. J Clin Invest. 1981;68:1435–40.
52. Dal Nogare AR, Toews GB, Pierce AK. Increased salivary elastase precedes gram-negative bacillary colonization in postoperative patients. Am Rev Respir Dis. 1987;135:671–5.
53. Johanson WG Jr, Higuchi JG, Chaudhuri TR, et al. Bacterial adherence to epithelial cells in bacillary colonization of the respiratory tract. Am Rev Respir Dis. 1980;121:55–63.
54. Ramphal R, Small PM, Shands JW Jr, et al. Adherence of *Pseudomonas aeruginosa* to tracheal cells injured by influenza infection or by endotracheal intubation. Infect Immun. 1980;27:614–9.
55. Sprunt K, Redman W. Evidence suggesting importance of role of interbacterial inhibition in maintaining balance of normal flora. Ann Intern Med. 1968;68:579–90.
56. Andrews CP, Coalson JJ, Smith JD, et al. Diagnosis of nosocomial bacterial pneumonia in acute, diffuse lung injury. Chest. 1981;80:254–8.
57. Fagon JY, Chastre J, Hance A, et al. Detection of nosocomial lung infection in ventilated patients. Amer Rev Respir Dis. 1988;138:110–6.
58. Winterbauer RH, Dreis DF. New diagnostic approaches to the hospitalized patient with pneumonia. Semin Respir Infect. 1987;2:57–66.
59. Joshi JH, Wang K-P, De Jongh CA, et al. A comparative evaluation of two fiberoptic bronchoscopy catheters: The plugged telescoping catheter versus the single sheathed nonplugged catheter. Am Rev Respir Dis. 1982;126:860–3.
60. Chastre J, Viau F, Brun P, et al. Prospective evaluation of the protected specimen brush for the diagnosis of pulmonary infections in ventilated patients. Am Rev Respir Dis. 1984;130:924–9.
61. Johanson WG Jr, Seidenfeld JJ, Gomez P, et al. Bacteriologic diagnosis of nosocomial pneumonia following prolonged mechanical ventilation. Am Rev Respir Dis. 1988;137:259–64.
62. Cone LA, Woodard DR, Stoltzman DS, et al. Ceftazidime versus tobramycin–ticarcillin in the treatment of pneumonia and bacteremia. Antimicrob Agents Chemother. 1985;28:33–6.
63. Greenberg RN, Reilly PM, Luppen KL, et al. Aztreonam therapy for gram-negative pneumonia. Am J Med. 1985;78S:31–3.
64. Salata RA, Gebhart RL, Palmer DL et al. Pneumonia treated with imipenem/cilastatin. Am J Med. 1985;78S:104–9.
65. Schentag JJ, Reitberg DP, Cumbo TJ. Cefmenoxime efficacy, safety, and pharmacokinetics in critical care patients with nosocomial pneumonia. Am J Med. 1984;77S:34–42.
66. Trenholme GM, Pottage JC Jr, Karakusis PH. Use of ceftazidime in the treatment of nosocomial lower respiratory infections. Am J Med. 1985;79S:32–6.
67. Winston DJ, McGrattan MA, Busuttil RW. Imipenem therapy of *Pseudomonas aeruginosa* and other serious bacterial infections. Antimicrob Agents Chemother. 1984;26:673–7.

68. Gerber AU, Vastola AP, Brandel J, et al. Selection of aminoglycoside-resistant variants of *Pseudomonas aeruginosa* in an in vivo model. J Infect Dis. 1982;146:691–7.
69. Bundtzen RW, Gerger AU, Cohn DL, et al. Postantibiotic suppression of bacterial growth. Rev. Infect Dis. 1981;3:28–37.
70. Corrado ML, Landesman SH, Cherubin CD. Influence of inoculum size on activity of cefoperazone, cefotaxime, moxalactam, piperacillin, and N-formimidoyl thienamycin (MK 0787) against *Pseudomonas aeruginosa*. Antimicrob Agents Chemother. 1980;18:893–6.
71. Pennington JE. Penetration of antibiotics into respiratory secretions. Rev Infect Dis. 1981;3:67–73.
72. Cipolle RJ, Seifert RD, Zaske DE, et al. Hospital acquired gram-negative pneumonias: Response rate and dosage requirements with individualized tobramycin therapy. Therapeutic Drug Monitoring. 1980;2:359–63.
73. Martin AJ, Smalley CA, George RH, et al. Gentamicin and tobramycin compared in the treatment of mucoid pseudomonas lung infections in cystic fibrosis. Arch Dis Childhood. 1980;55:604–7.
74. Klastersky J, Carpentier-Meunier F, Kahan-Coppens L, et al. Endotracheally administered antibiotics for gram-negative bronchopneumonia. Chest. 1979;75:586–91.
75. Pennington JE. New therapeutic approaches to hospital-acquired pneumonia. Semin Respir Infect. 1987;2:67–73.
76. Ziegler EJ, McCutchan JA, Fierer J, et al. Treatment of gram-negative bacteremia and shock with human antiserum to a mutant *Escherichia coli*. N Engl J Med. 1982;307:1225–30.
77. Collins MS, Roby RE. Protective activity of an intravenous immune globulin (human) enriched in antibody against lipopolysaccharide antigens of *Pseudomonas aeruginosa*. Am J Med. 1984;76:168–74.
78. Class I, Junginger W, Kloss T. *Pseudomonas* immunoglobulin in surgical intensive care patients on mechanical ventilation. Infection. 1987;15S:67–70.
79. Simmons BP, Wong ES. Guidelines for prevention of nosocomial pneumonia. Infect Control. 1982;3:327–33.
80. Greenfield S, Teres D, Bushnell LS, et al. Prevention of gram-negative bacillary pneumonia using aerosol polymyxin as prophylaxis. J Clin Invest. 1973;52:2935–40.
81. Klastersky J, Huysmans E, Weerts D, et al. Endotracheally administered gentamicin for the prevention of infections of the respiratory tract in patients with tracheostomy: A double-blind study. Chest. 1974;65:650–4.
82. Feeley TW, DuMoulin GC, Hedley-Whyte J, et al. Aerosol polymysin and pneumonia in seriously ill patients. N Engl J Med. 1975;293:471–5.
83. Stoutenbeek CP, van Saene HKF, Miranda DR, et al. The effect of selective decontamination of the digestive tract on colonization and infection rate in multiple trauma patients. Intensive Care Med. 1984;10:185–92.
84. Unertl K, Ruckdeschel G, Selbmann HK, et al. Prevention of colonization and respiratory infections in long-term ventilated patients by local antimicrobial prophylaxis. Intensive Care Med. 1987;13:106–13.
85. Polk HC Jr, Borden S, Aldrett JA. Prevention of *Pseudomonas* respiratory infection in a surgical intensive care unit. Ann Surg. 1973;177:607–15.
86. Baumgartner J, McCutchan JA, Van Melle G, et al. Prevention of gram-negative shock and death in surgical patients by antibody to endotoxin core glycolipid. Lancet. 1985;2:59–63.
87. Hall CB, Douglas RG. Modes of transmission of respiratory syncytial virus. J Pediatr. 1981;99:100–3.
88. Hall CB, Geiman JM, Douglas RG Jr. et al. Control of nosocomial respiratory syncytial viral infections. Pediatrics. 1978;67:728–32.
89. Agah R, Cherry JD, Garakian AJ, et al. Respiratory syncytial virus infection rate in personnel caring for children with RSV infections. Am J Dis Child. 1987;141:695–7.
90. Leclair JM, Freeman J, Sullivan BF, et al. Prevention of nosocomial respiratory syncytial virus infections through compliance with glove and gown isolation precautions. N Engl J Med. 1987;317:329–33.
91. Arden NH, Patriarca PA, Fasano MB, et al. The roles of vaccination and amantadine prophylaxis in controlling an outbreak of influenza A (H3N2) in a nursing home. Arch Intern Med. 1988;148:865–8.
92. Atkinson WL, Arden NH, Patriarca PA, et al. Amantadine prophylaxis during an institutional outbreak of type A (H1N1) influenza. Arch Intern Med. 1986;146:1751–6.

281. NOSOCOMIAL URINARY TRACT INFECTIONS

JOHN W. WARREN

Urinary tract infections (UTIs) are the most common infections occurring in hospitals and nursing homes. In hospitals, where the epidemiology has been better investigated, about 80 percent of nosocomial UTIs are associated with the use of urethral catheters.[1–3] Another 5–10 percent occur after other genitourinary manipulations.[1,4] The remainder are not associated with urologic procedures, and although the etiologies of these infections are not well understood, one can speculate that a proportion occur in patients who simply have developed an episode of bacteriuria in the hospital rather than in the community.[5–7] The emphasis of this chapter will be upon catheter-associated bacteriuria, by far the most common type of nosocomial UTI.

CATHETER-ASSOCIATED BACTERIURIA

Each year millions of urinary catheters are placed in patients in acute care hospitals, rehabilitation units, and chronic care facilities.[8] Sequential studies in the same institution over a decade suggest that the use of indwelling urethral catheters is increasing.[9] With the exception of occasional nonbacterial urethritis[10] and mechanical trauma,[11,12] virtually all complications of urinary catheterization are results of consequent bacteriuria. Catheter-associated bacteriuria represents the most common infection acquired in acute care[2] and long-term care[13] facilities.

This prominence is long-standing, for the urinary catheter is among the most venerable of medical devices.[14–16] For centuries, a urethral catheter system was a tube inserted into the bladder that drained urine into an open container. The universal development of bacteriuria from these open catheters elicited in the 1950s a major advance in catheter design, the closed catheter system.[17–21] This system is composed of an indwelling bladder catheter inserted into a collection tube that is fused to a collection bag on its distal end. This arrangement allows drainage through a tube into a receptacle so that the urine is always contained within a lumen protected from the contaminated environment. Universal bacteriuria occurred by 4 days with open catheters[22] but is now more than 30 days in closed catheter systems.[21,23] Although no well-designed controlled trials comparing open with closed catheters have been performed, reports have been sufficiently persuasive that the closed system has become the standard for patients requiring indwelling urethral catheters.[21,23–26]

The closed catheter system has only postponed but has not eliminated catheter-associated bacteriuria. Insertion of the catheter may push or drag urethral organisms into the bladder.[27] Once indwelling, the catheter over time enhances uropathogen colonization of the urethra, particularly in women.[28,29] The lumen and external surfaces of the catheter act as conduits for bacterial entry into the bladder.[28,30–32] The tube offers a niche on its luminal and external surfaces for bacteria to develop a microenvironment within a biofilm layer.[33–36] Uroepithelial cells of catheterized patients may transiently allow greater numbers of bacteria to adhere to their surfaces, a phenomenon that may precede the onset of bacteriuria.[37] As a foreign body, the catheter may cause mechanically or chemically induced inflammation of the urethra and bladder mucosa[10] yet may blunt adequate antibacterial polymorphonuclear leukocyte function.[38,39] The bacteria it eventually hosts may include urease-producing organisms that can elicit struvite and apatite crystallization with resulting catheter obstruction[40,41] and subsequent increased intravesical pressure, transmucosal migration,[42] or vesicoureteral reflux of bacteria.

PATHOGENESIS

The majority of bacteria causing catheter-associated bacteriuria are from the patients own colonic flora[32] and may be native inhabitants or new immigrants, that is, exogenous organisms from the hospital environment.[43–45] Just as with the pathogenesis of UTI in noncatheterized patients, these colonic bacteria may migrate across the perineum to colonize the periurethral area. Additionally, exogenous organisms may directly colonize the periurethral area or catheter equipment.[46–48] Organisms may be transferred to the patient by the hands of health care personnel[46–50] or infrequently by contaminated products[8] or containers.[46]

BACTERIAL

Entry

Once in or on the patient or on the catheter system surface, organisms may enter the bladder through one of three ways: (1) at the time of catheter insertion; (2) through the catheter lumen; or (3) along the catheter–mucosa interface. Furthermore, several reports suggest that there is a risk of bacteriuria in the hours or days after catheter removal.[51–55]

Catheter Insertion. The normal distal urethra is colonized with bacteria, though usually not coliforms. Insertion of a catheter through the urethra into the bladder may carry some of these organisms along. The process of catheter insertion, urine drainage, and immediate removal is associated with rates of bacteriuria ranging from less than 1 percent of healthy people to 20 percent of elderly hospitalized patients.[27] Overall, the incidence of bacteriuria in hospitalized patients undergoing a single "in-and-out" catheterization is about 3 percent.[2] Most prospective studies of indwelling urethral catheters have excluded patients with bacteriuria in specimens obtained within 24 hours after catheter insertion. While some may have had pre-existing bacteriuria, the number of patients is frequently higher than one would expect based on age- and sex-linked prevalences of asymptomatic bacteriuria; a number of these patients likely became bacteriuric at the time of catheter insertion.[32]

Intraluminal. Once in place, the indwelling closed catheter system may be opened at two sites. Although contrary to appropriate hygiene, the junction between the catheter and the collection tube may be disconnected for, say, catheter irrigation or urine collection; bacteriuria may be associated with such interruptions.[25,31] The second site, the drainage tube of the collection bag, is one that must be opened periodically to provide appropriate care.[21,25] If the lumen of the drainage tube is contaminated with bacteria, for example, from an unwashed container previously used to collect urine from a bacteriuric patient,[46] organisms may enter the drainage bag and before the next emptying multiply to high concentrations. Even after the bag is drained, organisms may persist in the urine film coating the inside of the collection bag and multiply as the bag refills with urine. Bacteria in the bag, introduced by contamination of the catheter–collection tube junction or the drainage tube, may ascend the collection tube and catheter through the urine itself[56] or by growth of organisms along the internal surface.[33]

Extraluminal. The success of the closed catheter system is because it has greatly limited intraluminal entry of organisms. However, even with meticulous attention to maintenance of the closed system, the opportunity for bacterial entry exists in the space between the external catheter and the urethral mucosa. Garibaldi et al.[30] demonstrated that periurethral colonization with gram-negative rods or enterococci within 24 hours after catheterization was followed by bacteriuria significantly more frequently than in patients not so colonized. Futhermore, Schaeffer and Chmiel[28] and Kunin and Steele[29] have demonstrated progressive uropathogen colonization of the urethra in catheterized patients, particularly women. Such colonization precedes bacteriuria with the same strain in up to two-thirds of patients,[23,28,32] a sequence that may be related to the density of colonizing bacteria.[28]

After Catheter Removal. Even after removal of a catheter, the patient may remain at increased risk of bacteriuria for an unknown period of time. Hartstein et al.[55] found that 10 of 88 (11 percent) patients developed bacteriuria within 24 hours after catheter removal. This rate was higher than any single daily rate during the 12 days of catheterization itself. Additional studies have identified similar proportions of patients becoming bacteriuric after catheter removal.[51–54] This development may be related to uropathogens in the urethra during catheterization.[32] Most prospective investigations of catheter-associated bacteriuia have not included cultures of urine specimens obtained after catheter removal.[57,58] Such studies are needed to determine the incidence, pathophysiology, and consequences of this phenomenon.

Within the Catheterized Urinary Tract

The catheterized urinary tract appears to be a hospitable environment for bacteria. The majority of bacterial strains that enter are able to multiply to high concentrations within a day or so.[23,59] This is in marked contrast to the noncatheterized urinary tract, where small numbers of organisms introduced in the bladder are eliminated efficiently.[60,61] In the catheterized urinary tract, the bacteria may maintain themselves through interaction with surfaces by way of specific and nonspecific adherence mechanisms. Specific adhesins include fimbria binding to uroepithelial cells or the catheter surface.[37,62,63] Among nonspecific mechanisms, glycocalyx, or biofilm, which covers and secures bacteria against a mucosal or catheter surface, has been demonstrated on drainage bags, catheters, and uroepithelium.[33,34] Organisms contained within the biofilm appear to be well protected from the mechanical flow of urine, possibly other host defense mechanisms, and even antibiotics.[35] The biofilm may allow the contained sessile organisms to establish a microenvironment from which some may move into the urine; these planktonic microbes are those that are voided and enumerated as bacteriuria by the patient's medical care providers.

With time, the presence of bacteria elicits an inflammatory response resulting in acute and chronic cystitis with pyuria[64] and production of antibody.[64–66] These processes occurring in long-term catheterized patients with only bladder bacteriuria diminish the utility of antibody-coated bacteria as an assay for localization of infection to the upper urinary tracts.[65] Organisms may move up the ureter to one or both kidneys where a similar biofilm microenvironment may develop within the pelvis or tubular system. Invasion through the unicellular epithelium there[67] may allow entry of bacteria into the interstitium; the subsequent inflammatory response is recognized pathologically as acute pyelonephritis.[68–70] With continued catheterization and bacteriuria, chronic renal inflammation may develop and, particularly with stone formation, chronic pyelonephritis may follow.[71] While the conventional wisdom is that bacteremia associated with urinary tract infection is from a renal site, the presence of acute and chronic cystitis in long-term catheterized patients suggests that occasional bacteremia may follow invasion of bladder mucosa.

Risk Factors for Bacteriurua

Most studies of risk factors for catheter-associated bacteriruia have been univariate analyses unable to discriminate between independent risk factors and those that are associated but not independent.[1,2,21,25,55] However, several multivariate analyses have clarified risks of catheterization.[6,72,73] Such an analysis by Platt and colleagues[72] was of 1474 catheterizations and revealed nine independent risk factors for bacteriruia:

1. Duration of catheterization
2. Absence of use of a urinemeter
3. Microbial colonization of the drainage bag
4. Diabetes mellitus
5. Absence of antibiotic use
6. Female patient

7. Indications for other than drainage during surgery or output measurement
8. Abnormal serum creatinine
9. Errors in catheter care

Shapiro et al.,[73] in a smaller prospective study using multivariate analysis, revealed many of the same risk factors and additionally showed that patients catheterized relatively late in their hospitalization had an increased rate of bacteriuria compared with those catheterized earlier. They further found that for those patients who were to undergo prolonged catheterization, the risk of bacteriuria was higher in the first few days than that of patients catheterized for only a few days. This suggested to the authors that prolonged catheterization was a marker for patients at higher risk of bacteriuria and that this risk was present even in the early catheterization period.

Interestingly, both these multivariate analyses demonstrated that two prominent risk factors of earlier univariate studies, that is, patient age and medical training of the person inserting the catheter, were confounding and not independent variables in the development of bacteriuria.

Duration of Catheterization

The duration of catheterization is the most important risk factor for the development of catheter-associated bacteriuria.[6,21,25,55,72] It depends on the indications for catheterization, which may be grouped into four main categories: *(1)* urine output measurement; *(2)* surgical operation; *(3)* urine retention; and *(4)* urinary incontinence.

A graph of patients by duration of their catheterization would show a bimodal frequency distribution with peaks at 2–4 days and at 3–6 months or more. The first peak would represent hospitalized patients with transient indications for catheterization; the second would be composed of nursing home patients with perceived permanent indications for urine drainage assistance. Once the urethral catheter is in place, the daily incidence of bacteriuria is 3–10 percent.[21,25,31,55,74] The majority of catheterized patients will be bacteriuric by the end of 30 days,[21,23,66] a convenient dividing line between short-term and long-term catheterization (Table 1).

TABLE 1. Comparison of Short-Term and Long-Term Urethral Catheterization

Characteristic	*Short-Term (less than 30 days)*	*Long-Term (30 days or more)*
Patient		
Type of illness	Acute, surgical	Chronic, neurologic
Location	Hospital	Nursing home
Indications	Output measurement Surgery Urine retention Incontinence	Incontinence Urine retention
Usual catheter duration	2–4 days	Months to years
Bacteriuria		
Incidence	3–10%/day	3–10%/day
Prevalence	15%	90%
Number of species/patient	Single	Polymicrobial
Common species	*E. coli* *K. pneumoniae* *Proteus mirabilis* *Pseudomonas aeruginosa*	*Providencia stuartii* *Proteus mirabilis* *E. coli* *M. morganii*
Proved prevention of bacteriuria	Closed catheter system Systemic antibiotic	None
Complications	Fevers Acute pyelonephritis Bacteremia Death	Fevers Acute pyelonephritis Bacteremia Death Catheter obstruction Urinary stones Chronic renal inflammation Peri-urinary infections Renal failure Bladder cancer
Medical goal	Postpone bacteriuria	Prevent complications of bacteriuria
Options	Diapers and pads External collection devices Intermittent catheterization Suprapubic catheterization	Diapers and pads External collection devices Intermittent catheterization Suprapubic catheterization Urinary diversions Prosthetic bladder sphincters

Short-Term Catheterization. Between 15 and 25 percent of patients in acute care hospitals may have a catheter in place sometime during their stay.[2] Most are in place for only a short time: up to one-third are in place for less than 1 day,[25,74] and both the mean and median durations are between 2 and 4 days.[2,21,25,31,55] Nevertheless, between 10 and 30 percent of these catheterized patients develop bacteriuria,[2,21,25] significantly greater than the 1 percent found among noncatheterized patients.[2] Because of the large number of patients catheterized, catheter-associated bacteriuria is the most common hospital-acquired infection, representing about 40 percent of such infections and constituting the majority of the 900,000 patients with nosocomial bacteriuria in American hospitals each year.[75]

Among short-term catheterized patients, *Escherichia coli* is the most frequent bacteriuric species isolated. Other common organisms are *Pseudomonas aeruginosa, Klebsiella pneumoniae, Proteus mirabilis, Staphylococcus epidermidis,* and enterococci[1,8,21,31,72,76] (Table 2). Particularly when antibiotics are in use, yeasts may be isolated as well.[31,72,77] To establish a diagnosis, many investigators have required organism concentrations of at least 100,000 cfu/ml of urine;[78] others have selected lower concentrations.[79] As noted, most bacteria first identified at low concentrations will over succeeding days reach a density of 100,000 cfu/ml or more.[59] Thus, identifying the onset of bacteriuria even in small numbers is of epidemiologic significance.

COMPLICATIONS. *Symptomatic UTI.* The majority of episodes of short-term catheter-associated bacteriuria are asymptomatic.[2,55,74] However, fevers or other symptoms of UTI occur in 10–30 percent of patients with catheter-associated bacteriuria;[2,55,74] daily cultures of urine indicate that many symptomatic UTIs occur on the first day of bacteriuria.[3,74] Of catheter-associated bacteriuric patients, only 1–5 percent will develop clinical bacteremia.[1,3,69,70,74] Bacteremias from nosocomial UTIs represent 6–15 percent of the total nosocomial bacteremias.[3,69] Men with catheter-associated bacteriuria are at greater risk than women for the development of bacteremia.[3] In some reports, certain bacteriuric organisms, for example, *Serratia marcescens*, may be more likely than others to cause bacteremia.[1,3] The mortality directly attributed to bacteremia from nosocomial bacteriuria is 13 percent; most deaths are in patients with severe underlying diseases.[69] At autopsy, patients with catheter-associated bacteriuria dying in a hospital may have acute pyelonephritis, urinary stones, or perinephric abscesses.[69,70] Even without overt evidence of systemic infection, catheter-associated bacteriuria appears to be related to an increased risk of death.[80]

Long-Term Catheterization. Although the magnitude of long-term urethral catheter use has not been directly measured, extrapolations from several studies[13,81–85] suggest that at any given time more than 100,000 patients in American nursing homes have urethral catheters in place. Many of these patients have been catheterized for months and in some cases years. The two most frequent indications are *(1)* urinary incontinence (mostly women), and *(2)* bladder outlet obstruction (mostly men). Urinary incontinence is by far the more common; women constitute up to 80 percent of long-term catheterized patients.[85] In nursing homes, the prevalence of patients with urinary incontinence ranges up to 50 percent;[83] because continually wet skin may become macerated and lead to decubitus ulcers, the catheter may be used as a preventive or management technique. Of nursing home patients with long-term urethral catheters, 34–69 percent have decubitus ulcers.[82,83,86]

Even with excellent care, all patients become bacteriuric if catheterized long enough. This universal prevalence of bacteriuria in long-term catheterized patients[87,88] is a function of two related phenomena. The first is an incidence of new episodes of bacteriuria similar to that seen in short-term catheterized patients[87] and, over time, caused by a wide variety of gram-negative and gram-positive bacterial species. The second is the ability of some of these strains to persist for weeks and months in the catheterized urinary tract.[87] Two of the more common and persistent species are *E. coli* and *Providencia stuartii*; their persistence is related to specific adherence factors. The adhesin of *E. coli* is type 1 pilus, a well-studied adhesin for uroepithelium and Tamm-Horsfall protein.[62] For *Providencia stuartii*, the adhesin is named MR/K and appears to mediate adhesion to the catheter surface itself.[63] *Providencia stuartii* (as well as other species in the Proteeae tribe) uses the catheter as a niche,[89] a likely reason for its being found frequently in catheterized but rarely in noncatheterized urinary tracts.[90,91]

These phenomena result in polymicrobial bacteriuria in 75–95 percent of urine specimens from long-term catheterized patients. Such specimens commonly have two to four bacterial species, each at concentrations of 10^5 cfu/ml or more;[86–88] some may have up to six to eight species at that concentration.[86] These are not only common uropathogens such as *E. coli, Pseudomonas aeruginosa,* and *Proteus mirabilis*, but also less familiar species such as *Providencia stuartii* and *Morganella morganii*[13,66,86,87,92–94] (Tables 1 and 2). The high prevalence of polymicrobial bacteriuria and of unfamiliar uropathogens at high concentrations is sometimes not recognized or appreciated by clinicians and laboratories.[95] Furthermore, in many patients additional strains are present at low numbers. Many of these strains appear to be unable to multiply to high concentrations,[96] a finding in contrast to the situation in short-term catheterized urinary tracts[59] and possibly related to competition from the established bacterial strains.

COMPLICATIONS. Complications of long-term catheter-associated bacteriuria fall into two categories. The first includes symptomatic UTIs such as seen with short-term catheterization, that is, fever, acute pyelonephritis, and bacteremia; as in short-term catheterized patients, some of these episodes may result in death. The second group encompasses those occurring during long-term catheterization: obstruction, urinary tract stones, chronic renal inflammation, local peri-urinary infections, renal failure, and (with catheterization for years) bladder cancer.

Symptomatic UTI. Although two-thirds of febrile episodes in aged long-term catheterized patients may arise from the urinary tract,[86] the incidence is suprisingly low, about one febrile episode per 100 days of catheterization.[86,97] In women at least, most such episodes are of low-grade fever, last for 1 day or less, and resolve without antibiotic therapy.[86] However, bacteremia may occur during some of these fevers, even by "non-uropathogens" such as *Providencia stuartii* or *M. morganii*.[86,90,91] Bacteremia and death are more frequent during episodes of fever of more than 102°F (38.8°C).[86] Autopsies have revealed acute pyelonephritis in more than one-third of patients dying with long-term catheters in place.[68]

Catheter Obstructions. In long-term catheterized patients a catheter obstruction may be a problem and, in some patients, a recurrent one.[98,99] The complex material that obstructs urinary catheters is composed of bacteria, glycocalyx, Tamm-Horsfall protein, and precipitated crystals.[33,36,40,41,100] *Proteus mirabilis* bacteriuria is associated with catheter obstruction[41] probably because of its potent urease,[101,102] which hydrolyzes urea to ammonia, increasing urine pH and causing crystallization of struvite and apatite in the catheter lumen.[103–105] Electron microscopy has demonstrated the development of these crystals within the bacterial biofilm.[106] Although some catheter obstructions are associated with the onset of fever, the great majority are not,[86] possibly because of early detection and removal of the obstructed catheter.

Urinary Stones. A similar bacterial process may occur in the urinary tract itself, resulting in the crystallization of struvite and apatite in the form of so-called "infection stones," a common problem in long-term catheterized patients.[107] Such stones in the bladder, often crusting around the catheter balloon and tip, are relatively benign.[108] However, renal stones may be more serious, leading to chronic pyelonephritis and renal dysfunction.[71]

Chronic Renal Inflammation. Chronic renal inflammation, common in long-term catheterized persons,[66,71,109–112] is related directly to the duration of catheterization.[66,112] However, chronic pyelonephritis, that is, chronic renal inflammation with the additional components of deformed calyces and overlying parenchymal scarring, is found in only a minority of chronically inflamed kidneys and is often associated with the presence of pelvic or renal stones.[112]

Other Complications. In the past, additional complications were seen in long-term catheterized patients with injured spinal cords, mostly men, now usually managed with intermittent catheterization.[71,113] Such complications included peri-urethral infections such as urethritis, urethral fistulae, epididymitis, scrotal abscesses, prostititis, and prostatic abscesses.[71] Chronic renal failure was often diagnosed in catheterized spinal-injured patients and was frequently associated with intrarenal stones and chronic pyelonephritis.[71,110,111,113–115] In those catheterized for 10 years or longer, bladder metaplasia and cancer were found more frequently than in the noncatheterized population.[116,117]

TABLE 2. Organisms Isolated from Catheter Bacteriuria (% of Total)

Organism	Catheterization: Short-term[72] (Incidence)	Catheterization: Long-Term[87] (Weekly prevalence)
Providencia stuartii	0	384 (24)
Proteus species	8 (6)	232 (15)
Escherichia coli	33 (24)	228 (14)
Pseudomonas aeruginosa	12 (9)	188 (12)
Enterococcus	9 (7)	124 (8)
Morganella morganii	0	118 (7)
Klebsiella species	11 (8)	68 (4)
Coagulase-negative staphylococci	11 (8)	53 (3)
Other gram-negative bacilli	10 (7)	93 (6)
Other gram-positive bacteria	6 (4)	56 (4)
Yeasts	35 (26)	0
Total	136 (100)	1599 (100)

PREVENTION

Prevention can be addressed in three stages: *(1)* prevention of the catheterization itself; *(2)* once the catheter is in place, prevention of bacteriuria; and *(3)* once bacteriuria occurs, prevention of its complications.

Prevention of Urethral Catheterization

Obviously, the most direct method to prevent catheter-associated bacteriuria is to prevent catheterization. The last several decades have seen major advances in understanding complications of catheterization, in weighing its risks and benefits, and in determining appropriate indications for catheter insertion.[8,26,82,118–125] This understanding has prompted the use of alternatives to the urethral catheter. For instance, for incontinent patients, health care providers have encouraged a greater use of patient training, biofeedback, medications, surgery, and special clothes and bedclothes as management techniques.[120] Additionally several devices have been further explored as options to the urethral catheter.

External Collection Devices. For men with urinary incontinence, external collectors applied about the penis that empty through a collection tube into a drainage bag have been widely used. Although these avoid problems of a tube in the urinary tract, urine within the condom catheters may have high concentrations of organisms, the urethra and skin may be colonized with uropathogens, and bladder bacteriuria may develop, particularly in patients who frequently manipulate the condom.[126–128] Careful collection of urine in a new condom by well-trained individuals is necessary to distinguish bladder bacteriuria from skin or condom contamination.[129,130] Although no properly designed controlled trials have been performed, condom catheters appear to be associated with a lower incidence of bacteriuria than indwelling urethral catheters. However, contaminated external devices can be reservoirs for the spread of a nosocomial infection.[126,128,131] Complications include local problems such as skin breakdown, maceration, and ulceration; urethral diverticuli; and ischemic disease including penile gangrene from constriction by the condom's roller ring.[132–135]

For incontinent women, affixation of an external device capable of effectively collecting urine has been a continuing problem. Innovative devices exploiting the technology of ostomy adhesives are presently undergoing trials.[136]

Intermittent Catheterization. For postoperative patients with temporary urine retention, one or more periodic in-and-out catheterizations may be sufficient to drain urine until normal voiding returns. Bacteriuria may follow single catheterizations and is dependent in part on the patient. In general, the younger and healthier the patient, the lower the incidence; for all hospitalized patients the incidence of bacteriuria from a single catheterization is about 3 percent.[2] One group has shown in a randomized trial that instillation of 50 ml of 2% povidone iodine before catheter removal was associated with a lower rate of bacteriuria.[137]

For chronic urine retention, prolonged intermittent catheterization is useful. Many spinal cord-injured patients or others with neurogenic bladders can use their bladders as containers for urine storage yet cannot initiate urination. Insertion of a sterile or clean catheter every 3–6 hours by caregivers or the patient, drainage of urine, and immediate removal of the catheter provide periodic bladder emptying.[138–143] However, bacteriuria develops in 27–100 percent of such patients within the first month.[140,144–148] Incidences of bacteriuria range from 21 to 27 new episodes per 100 patient-weeks.[149–151] These rates in spinal cord-injured patients are less than half that of patients with long-term indwelling catheters.[87] Oral or topical antibiotics and methenamine preparations have been used to postpone bacteriuria for short periods in intermittently catheterized patients.[145,148,151,152] All patients eventually become bacteriuric, and whether such practices would be beneficial over months and years of intermittent catheterization has not been shown. The bacteriuria is usually asymptomatic, and although no well-designed comparisons have been performed, intermittent catheterization may be an improvement over indwelling catheterization in regard to local periurethral infections, febrile episodes, bladder and renal stones, and deterioration of renal function.[139,142,153] Complications may include urethral trauma and, if vesicoureteral reflux is present, renal deterioration.

Suprapubic Catheterization. Short-term suprapubic catheterization has been used in gynecologic, urologic, and other types of surgery. The concept supporting its use is that the lower density of bacteria on the anterior abdominal skin will yield lower rates of bacteriuria than that associated with catheters in the urethra. Another feature is that clamping of the suprapubic catheter allows testing of voiding per urethra, obviously an advantage not shared with the urethral catheter. Although a number of workers have reported their results, many studies are inadequately designed to compare suprapubic with urethral catheterization.[154–161] However, Andersen and colleagues[162] have performed a randomized trial of suprapubic versus indwelling urethral catheterization in patients undergoing gynecologic operations. Clamping to test for return of normal voiding allowed the suprapubic catheters to be removed earlier than the urethral catheters (mean of 3.7 versus 5.0 days). Because the endpoint was bacteriuria at 5 days, not only did the patients with suprapubic catheters have less time at risk, but some may have been able to clear catheter-associated bacteriuria by the time urine specimens were cultured 1 to 2 days after catheter removal. Patients with suprapubic catheters undergoing culposuspension had a lower prevalence of bacteriuria at 5 days than patients with urethral catheters. However, there was no significant difference between the two catheterization methods among patients undergoing vaginal repairs. Although not seen in this study, complications of suprapubic catheterization include cellulitis, leakage, and hematoma at the puncture site and occasional catheter prolapse through the urethra. For comfort and convenience, patients and caregivers usually prefer suprapubic over indwelling catheters.[154,155,157,158,160–162] Suprapubic catheterization appears promising and deserves well-designed trials to evaluate its effectiveness in different patient populations now requiring short-term and long-term urethral catheters.

Urinary Diversions. Occasionally, intractable incontinence in women has been treated by structuring a nonbladder storage unit for urine.[163] These urinary diversions include ileal and colonic conduits requiring collection bags on the abdominal wall as well as diversions that are continent and are emptied by intermittent catheterization through the stoma.[163,164] Bacteriologic investigations of these diversions have shown that bacteriuria is common, perhaps more in ileal than in colonic devices and in those requiring a collection bag than in those not requiring one.[165–167] Acute pyelonephritis, chronic pyelonephritis, and renal dysfunction are complications, particularly in conduits in which ureteral reflux is a consequence.[164]

Prosthetic Bladder Sphincters. For selected incontinent patients prosthetic bladder sphincters are options for management. The implanted prosthesis exerts pressure against the proximal urethra, thus obstructing the flow of urine from the bladder. Some devices are passive and the patient voids by simply overcoming the pressure of the device.[168] More complex devices use hydraulic pressure and an implanted manual pump.[169,170] Complications of all these devices include mechanical failure, erosion of the components into surrounding tissue, and infections. Infections may be acute or indolent and may result in fistula formation; cure may require administration of antimicrobial agents and removal of the prosthesis. The number of such devices in use is small.

Prevention of Bacteriuria

Once a urethral catheter is in place, only two principles are universally recommended for prevention of bacteriuria: (1) maintain the closed catheter system and (2) minimize the duration of catheterization. These and associated catheter hygiene practices have been well described.[119–123]

Maintain Closed System. Urine specimens should be obtained without opening the catheter–collection tube junction.[25,31] Use of a presealed junction diminishes the incidence of bacteriuria, most notably in patients not receiving antibiotics, and diminishes mortality.[171] The system should only be opened at the bag drainage tube; personnel must avoid touching the end of the drainage tube to possibly contaminated containers.[46] Communication of appropriate techniques to caregivers has been a largely successful effort of infection control teams. Longitudinal studies in the same institution suggest that continued attention has resulted in fewer errors of catheter hygiene.[57,74] Perhaps not coincidentally, the incidence of bacteriuria in that institution has fallen to 3 percent/day of catheterization.[74,121]

Minimize Duration. If the catheter can be removed before bacteriuria develops, postponement becomes prevention. Hartstein and colleagues,[55] using a predetermined list of durations appropriate for each indication, found that the duration of catheterization averaged one-third longer than necessary. Importantly, the majority of bacteriurias occurred after the catheter would have been removed had the appropriate catheter durations been observed.[55]

Additional Efforts. Modifications intended to further postpone bacteriuria include (1) second-line defenses for organisms that have entered the closed catheter system; (2) prevention of urethral bypass of the closed system; and (3) systemic antibacterial compounds concentrated in the urine.

ORGANISMS ENTERING THE CLOSED CATHETER SYSTEM. Attempts have been made to kill organisms that have entered the interior of the closed system or at least to prevent their proximal movement. Several methods of irrigation of the catheter with antibacterial solutions have been developed but have not been effective in postponing bacteriuria.[31,172,173] Such practices have required either another catheter junction (for continuous irrigation) or frequent opening of the closed system (for intermittent irrigation); these modifications have offered additional opportunities for entry of bacteria, which are often resistant to the irrigating antibiotic.[31] Likewise, controlled studies of antibacterial compounds in the collection bag have generally demonstrated no effectiveness in curtailing bacteriuria.[174–176] The only one that showed an effectiveness reported a rate of bag contamination which was two to four times higher than that of the other trials.[177] Another strategy directed at the drainage bag includes use of devices that ensure a discontinuous column of urine in the catheter–collection tube, thus presumably obstructing bacterial movement toward the bladder. Certain catheter vents and urinometers might be worth further study in some situations.[178,179]

These second-line defenses would be of value only when the integrity of the closed catheter system is broken. However, with adequate hygiene, bacterial entry into the lumen of the system is minimal and such efforts are superfluous.[122,180] In areas in which catheter systems are opened frequently or in which a particular antibiotic-resistant or known highly virulent organism must be controlled, these techniques may be useful[119,174,177] and should be examined with controlled trials.

PREVENTION OF URETHRAL BYPASS. Numerous antibacterial compounds have been applied at the catheter–urethra interface in attempts to block this most common site of bacterial entry. Most such studies have shown little if any clinical usefulness in postponing bacteriuria.[9,181–184] An intriguing variation of this theme is the use of silver-coated catheters, which, in two recent controlled trials,[23,185] have postponed bacteriuria, in one demonstrably because of a decrease in urethral entry.[23] If economical, this type of device may show promise.

SYSTEMIC ANTIBACTERIAL COMPOUNDS. Antibacterial substances in renal and bladder urine have been examined as a potential third line of defense. Up to 80 percent of catheterized patients, because of underlying diseases or procedures, are administered antibiotics during but not because of catheterization. Comparisons of these patients with those not receiving antibiotics have generally shown that antibiotic use is associated with a lower incidence of bacteriuria.[23,25,30,55,72–74] Furthermore, several trials of antibiotic prophylaxis have found that antibiotic recipients have lower incidences of bacteriuria than controls.[54,66,186–188] Nevertheless, the studies that have observed patients for a sufficient time have revealed that antibiotics are effective in postponement but not prevention of bacteriuria.[23,25,54,55,66,72,73,187] Antibiotics appear to be effective for the first several days of use, and then resistant organisms begin to appear in the urine.[54,66,186,189] Most authorities believe that the use of antibiotics to postpone bacteriuria is not indicated because of side effects, cost, and emergence of antibiotic-resistant bacteria in the patient and the medical unit.[119–121,123,124] Schaeffer[122] does recommend prophylactic antibiotics for patients who are at "high risk" of complications from UTI. A recent trial[186] demonstrated that three doses of intramuscular ampicillin around the time of catheter insertion resulted in lower prevalences than both the control group and a group receiving thrice daily ampicillin for the duration of catheterization. Although the longer-term antibiotic therapy resulted in antibiotic-resistant organisms causing bacteriuria, the peri-insertional antibiotic regimen did not. The potential benefits of this regimen should be examined in further studies.

Although methenamine is an antibacterial agent that is commonly used in catheterized patients, it is not effective even if urine can be made sufficiently acidic.[147,190–193] Its antibacterial action depends on hydrolysis to formaldehyde; at least 60 minutes of exposure to acidic urine is necessary to form a bactericidal concentration of formaldehyde.[194–196] Urine draining through an unobstructed catheter does not accumulate in the bladder for sufficient time for this concentration to form. However, such a concentration develops in the collecting bag, and methenamine may be effective in preventing interpatient spread,[121] a hypothesis that requires testing.

Prevention of Complications of Bacteriuria

Once bacteriuria develops, theoretically one could prevent its complications if several criteria were met:

1. The complication was of sufficient frequency and/or seriousness to justify attempts at prevention.
2. Bacteriuria could be identified in time to prevent the complication.
3. A procedure were effective in prevention.
4. The advantages of the procedure outweighed its disadvantages.

Symptomatic UTI. Symptomatic UTI (fever, urinary symptoms, acute pyelonephritis, and/or bacteremia) is a complication of catheter-associated bacteriuria. A study by Garibaldi et al.[74] is instructive in addressing the value of antibiotic therapy of asymptomatic bacteriuria in the prevention of symptomatic infection. This group studied 608 short-term catheterized patients of whom 76 (13 percent) acquired bacteriuria. Of these, 25 developed symptomatic UTI, two with bacteremia. These 25 represented one-third of the bacteriuric patients but only 4 percent of the total catheterized; the two with bacteremia were only 0.3 percent of the total catheterized patients. Of the 25 with symptomatic UTI, 15 (60 percent) developed symptoms on the first day of bacteriuria as identified by daily cultures of catheter urine. The investigators thought that prevention of symptomatic UTI would be possible in only the 10 bacteriuric patients who developed late symptoms. To detect the onset of bacteriuria, more than 2500 daily urine cultures were required. Assuming that all the late symptomatic UTIs could have been prevented, 250 urine cultures would be necessary to prevent each one. Furthermore, more than 1000 urine cultures would be required to prevent one bacteremia. Other studies tend to confirm these findings. Hartstein et al.[55] and Haley and colleagues[2] found even lower rates of symptomatic UTI and of bacteremia among patients with catheter-associated bacteriuria. Sweet et al.[175] found that a majority of febrile episodes occurred within 24 hours of onset of catheter-associated bacteriuria. These findings do not provide firm support for surveillance or treatment of asymptomatic catheter-associated bacteriuria, even if one assumes that antibiotic administration could prevent most symptomatic UTIs. However, to the extent that this assumption provides support for such practice, the basis is even less sure for there has not been a properly designed trial measuring effectiveness and adverse effects of antibiotic therapy for this indication.

One can make a stronger statement about therapy of the omnipresent and usually asymptomatic bacteriuria of long-term catheterized patients. Because of the continuing incidence of new episodes of bacteriuria, antibiotic therapy of some type would have to be administered much of the time. At least one study of cephalexin administered to long-term catheterized patients whenever a susceptible organism was present revealed that there was no effect on the incidence of new episodes of bacteriuria, the number of bacterial strains per urine specimen, or most importantly, the incidence of febrile episodes.[189] The only change that did ensue was a subsequent marked increase in the prevalence of antibiotic-resistant organisms, a finding of others as well.[197]

In general, clinicians should not treat asymptomatic bacteriuria as long as the catheter remains in place.[55,120–124] However, because of the study by Platt et al.[80] that reported excess mortality related to short-term catheter-associated bacteriuria, often without apparent evidence of systemic infection, this stance may be modified as further data accumulate. Additionally, specific exceptions may pertain if certain bacterial strains in the institution are known to cause a high incidence of bacteremia. For instance, some investigators have reported that *Serratia marcescens* may be such an organism.[1,3] In this regard, it is interesting that Krieger et al.[3] have reported a prolonged period between the onset of bacteriuria by *Serratia marcescens* and the development of bacteremia. This prolonged lag time, with a median of 24 days, may allow antibiotic therapy of *Serratia marcescens* bacteriuria to prevent bacteremia by this species.[3] As noted above, however, no controlled trials of such treatment for this or any other species have been performed.

Some students of UTIs believe that therapy of asymptomatic bacteriuria is appropriate if the catheter is to be soon removed.[120,122,123] With or without antimicrobial therapy, catheter-associated bacteriuria in many patients (but not all) will disappear after catheter removal.[53,55,58,70,198–200] Patients with catheter-associated bacteriuria appear to have an increased incidence of postcatheterization symptomatic UTIs[58,162] and a higher prevalence of bacteriuria at 1 year[162] than those who did not develop bacteriuria during their catheterization. Therefore, obtaining a culture of urine around the time of catheter removal seems reasonable. The timing of the postcatheter culture may be important; several days after catheter removal (e.g., at the time of hospital discharge) might be optimal.[58] Postponing culture until this time might, on the one hand, allow some patients to clear a catheter-associated bacteriuria and, on the other, identify a new bacteriuria occurring just after catheter removal.[55] If organisms are found, oral antibiotic therapy might be administered; alternatively, a second urine culture at the first posthospitalization visit could be obtained[122] and a decision made at that time. These approaches require study.

Catheter Obstructions. Even if a technique were uniformly effective in preventing catheter obstructions, this result would have little impact on febrile episodes. This is because of the relatively low proportion of fevers associated with catheter obstruction[86,97] and, in at least one study in women, the relatively low proportion of obstructions associated with fever.[86] However, certain patients have recurrent obstructions, and for these, particularly if fevers or bacteremias are associated, measures to prevent recurrences might be useful. Unfortunately, the very simple technique of once daily catheter irrigation with normal saline has been demonstrated in a crossover randomized trial to be ineffective in diminishing obstructions or fevers.[201] Methenamine preparations may diminish the incidence of catheter obstruction,[192,193,202] apparently not because of antimicrobial activity but perhaps because of biochemical alteration of salt solubility. Another possibility is the use of the oral urease inhibitor acetohydroxamic acid,[203] but this compound is associated with venous thromboses and pulmonary emboli.[204]

Urinary Stones. Acetohydroxamic acid has been demonstrated to be effective in reducing stone formation in noncatheterized patients with struvite and apatite stones caused by urease-producing organisms.[204] This therapy might be considered in long-term catheterized patients with such stones who have recurrent fevers, bacteremias, acute pyelonephritis, hydronephrosis, chronic pyelonephritis, or renal dysfunction. However, the risks of this therapy should prompt caution in its use.

Prevention of Patient–Patient Transmission

Once bacteriuria has developed, its consequences may extend beyond the individual patient. The periurethral bacterial flora, the surfaces of the catheter system and collection containers,[46,48] the "persistent, huge reservoir of contaminated urine,"[119] as well as the feces[44,45] and skin[7,205] of the patient are sources for contamination of the hands of medical personnel who may carry the bacteria to other patients.[46–48,50] Such patient–patient transmission leads to clusters of nosocomial bacteriurias, particularly with nonfecal isolates such as *Serratia, Pseudomonas,* and *Citrobacter* species, which also tend to be resistant to many antibiotics.[48,49,131,206–208] Schaberg et al.[208] found that 15 percent of nosocomial bacteriurias occurred in such clusters. Patients transferred from one institution to another have been the source of subsequent outbreaks in the second institution.[197,207,209]

Furthermore, plasmids encoding antibiotic resistance can move between bacteria,[45,205,210,211] often in the intestinal flora. In addition, the transfer of such plasmids from one species to another has been a phenomenon suspected clinically to have occurred in the urine of catheterized patients.[205,206,212] Such conjugation has been demonstrated in vitro in urine at room temperature for 4–8 hours;[213] these conditions are those present in the collection bag of the patient with polymicrobial bacteriuria.

Because many clusters or epidemics of catheter-associated bacteriuria are caused by antibiotic-resistant organisms, therapeutic options for each patient are limited, making the control of such outbreaks more critical. Clusters of catheter-associated bacteriuria must be recognized to be controlled; thus, some type of surveillance system should be developed in each institution. Such systems are often targeted at high-risk areas such as intensive care units.[121] The isolation of *Serratia marcescens* or *Pseudomonas aeruginosa* from the catheter urine of even a single patient may be sufficient evidence to initiate control measures.[121] Those developing such surveillance programs should realize that a common effect of culture reports on the patient's chart is to elicit antimicrobial therapy from the physician.[189,197]

Efforts to stop clusters or epidemics of catheter-associated bacteriuria can be divided into three categories: (1) diminishing the number of bacteria in reservoirs; (2) diminishing contact spread; and (3) modifying risk factors.[8,47] To diminish reservoirs, consideration might be given to systemic or bag antibiotics[119,122,174,177] or to systemic methenamine with urine acidification.[121] If intestinal colonization is a factor, oral nonabsorbable antibiotics might be considered.[8,47] For limiting contact spread, the caregiver would do well to view the catheterized urinary tract as an open wound.[47] The most important procedure is hand washing between patients, including after patient contact in which only skin surfaces are touched.[50,205] Others include use of gloves and segregation of catheterized patients,[214] particularly those infected from those uninfected. An approach that apparently appeals more to common sense than to actual practice is the notification to an institution to which the patient is being transferred of the presence of catheter-associated bacteriuria. Many of the risk factors for bacteriuria[72,73] are patient features that cannot be modified. Of those that can be, the two most critical are errors of closed catheter hygiene and prolonged catheterization.

TREATMENT OF COMPLICATIONS

For the patient who develops fever or signs of bacteremia, the clinician should rule out sources outside the urinary tract, catheter obstruction, and especially among men, periurethral infection; cultures of urine and blood should be obtained. Many clinicians would empirically treat such patients with parenteral antibiotics at doses high enough to achieve concentrations in the serum adequate to treat bacteremia from a known or suspected bacteriuric species. The selection of antibiotics should be based on knowledge of organisms common in the medical unit and Gram stain of the patient's urine at the time of the fever. Not surprisingly, survival of patients with bacteremia from nosocomial UTIs is related to the administration of antibiotics active against the bacteremic strain.[69] The catheterized patient with lower abdominal pain, dysuria, and/or urgency and without fever or other evidence of systemic infection may benefit from an oral antibiotic active in vitro in the same doses used for non-catheter-related UTIs. Appropriate durations of parenteral or oral therapies have not been well established. For patients with increasing renal dysfunction or evidence of recalcitrant or recurring bacteremia, a search for urinary stones may be helpful[69] in anticipation of direct intervention.

NOSOCOMIAL BACTERIURIA NOT ASSOCIATED WITH A CATHETER

About 10 percent of nosocomial bacteriurias are associated with urinary procedures other than catheterization. The pathogenesis of the 10–20 percent of nosocomial UTIs not associated with any instrumentation is not well understood. Boscia et al.,[5] studying ambulatory, aged, noncatheterized residents of the community and of nursing homes, found that 30 percent of women were bacteriuric during a 12-month period. However, only 6 percent were persistently bacteriuric with the same species, the other 24 percent having intermittent bacteriuria. A similar phenomenon but of smaller numbers was detected among aged men. These findings may be pertinent to understanding a very large study in American hospitals that revealed that hospital-acquired UTIs occurring in the absence of instrumentation were significantly associated with age, female sex, and history of previous UTIs.[6] These characteristics define a population group, hospitalized or not, that has a relatively high incidence of asymptomatic bacteriuria. Furthermore, rates of bacteriuria are higher in debilitated than in healthy individuals,[5] and hospitalization appears to enhance colonization of the skin with potential pathogens[7]; these findings suggest that hospitalized patients have higher incidences of asymptomatic bacteriuria than nonhospitalized patients.

REFERENCES

1. Stamm WE, Martin SM, Bennett JV. Epidemiology of nosocomial infections due to gram-negative bacilli: Aspects relevant to development and use of vaccines. J Infect Dis. 1977;136S:S151–S160.
2. Haley RW, Hooton TM, Culver DH, et al. Nosocomial infections in U.S. hospitals, 1975–1976: Estimated frequency by selected characteristics of patients. Am J Med. 1981;70:947–59.
3. Krieger JN, Kaiser DL, Wenzel RP. Urinary tract etiology of bloodstream infections in hospitalized patients. J Infect Dis. 1983;148:57–62.
4. Echols RM, Palmer DL, King RM, et al. Multidrug-resistant *Serratia marcescens* bacteriuria related to urologic instrumentation. Southern Med J. 1984;77:173–7.
5. Boscia JA, Kobasa WD, Knight RA, et al. Epidemiology of bacteriuria in an elderly ambulatory population. Am J Med. 1986;80:208–14.
6. Hooton TM, Haley RW, Culver DH, et al. The joint associations of multiple risk factors with the occurrence of nosocomial infection. Am J Med. 1981;70:960–70.
7. Stratford B, Gallus AS, Matthiesson AM, et al. Alteration of superficial bacterial flora in severely ill patients. Lancet. 1968;i:68.
8. Garibaldi RA. Hospital acquired urinary tract infection. In: Wenzel RP, ed. CRC Handbook of Hospital Acquired Infections. Boca Raton, FL: CRC Press; 1981:513–37.
9. Burke J, Jacobson J, Garibaldi R, et al. Evaluation of daily meatal care with poly-antibiotic ointment in prevention of urinary catheter-associated bacteriuria. J Urol. 1983;129:331–4.
10. Syme R. Epidemic of acute urethral stricture after prostate surgery. Lancet. 1982;2:1925.
11. Freed J, Krespi Y. Urologic catheter: Unusual complications. NY State J Med. 1979;79:1892–3.
12. Barnes-Snow E, Luchi R, Doig R. Penile laceration from a Foley catheter. J Am Geriatr Soc. 1985;33:712–4.
13. Garibaldi RA, Brodine S, Matsumiya S. Infections among patients in nursing homes. Policies, prevalence and problems. N Engl J Med. 1981;305:731–5.
14. Clark A: Remarks on catheter fever. Lancet. 1883;1:1075–7.
15. Dukes C. Urinary infections after excision of the rectum: Their cause and prevention. Proc R Soc Med. 1928;22:1–11.
16. Beeson PB. The case against the catheter. Am J Med. 1958;24:1–3.
17. Pyrah LN, Goldie W, Parsons FM, et al. Control of *Pseudomonas pyocyanea* infection in a urological ward. Lancet. 1955;ii:314–7.
18. Gillespie WA. Infection in urological patients. Proc R Soc Med. 1956;49:1045–7.
19. Gillespie WA, Linton KB, Miller A, et al. The diagnosis, epidemiology and control of urinary infection in urology and gynecology. J Clin Pathol. 1960;13:187–94.
20. Gillespie WA, Lennon GG, Linton KB, et al. Prevention of urinary infection in gynecology. Br Med J. 1964;2:423.
21. Kunin CM, McCormack RC. Prevention of catheter-induced urinary-tract infections by sterile closed drainage. N Engl J Med. 1966;274:1155.
22. Kass EH. Asymptomatic infections of the urinary tract. Trans Assoc Am Physicians. 1956;69:56.
23. Schaeffer AJ, Story KO, Johnson SM. Effect of silver oxide/trichloroisocyanuric acid antimicrobial urinary drainage system on catheter-associated bacteriuria. J Urol. 1988;139:69–73.
24. Thornton GF, Andriole VT. Bacteriuria during indwelling catheter drainage. II. Effect of a closed sterile drainage system. JAMA. 1970;214:339–42.
25. Garibaldi RA, Burke JP, Dickman ML, et al. Factors predisposing to bacteriuria during indwelling urethral catheterization. N Engl J Med. 1974;291:215.
26. Stamm WE. Guidelines for prevention of catheter-associated urinary tract infections. Ann Intern Med. 1975;82:386–90.
27. Turck M, Goffe B, Petersdorf RG. The urethral catheter and urinary tract infection. J Urol. 1962;88:834–7.
28. Schaeffer AJ, Chmiel J. Urethral meatal colonization in the pathogenesis of catheter-associated bacteriuria. J Urol. 1983;130:1096–9.
29. Kunin CM, Steele C. Culture of the surface of urinary catheters to sample urethral flora and study the effect of antimicrobial therapy. J Clin Microbiol. 1985;21:902–8.
30. Garibaldi RA, Burke JP, Britt MR, et al. Meatal colonization and catheter-associated bacteriuria. N Engl J Med. 1980;303:316–8.
31. Warren JW, Platt R, Thomas RJ, et al. Antibiotic irrigation and catheter-associated urinary-tract infections. N Engl J Med. 1978;299:570.
32. Daifuku R, Stamm W. Association of rectal and urethral colonization with urinary tract infection in patients with indwelling catheters. JAMA. 1984;252:2028–30.
33. Nickel JC, Grant SK, Costerton JW. Catheter-associated bacteriuria, an experimental study. Urology. 1985;26:369–75.
34. Nickel JC, Gristina P, Costerton JW. Electron microscopic study of an infected Foley catheter. Can J Surg. 1985;28:50–2.
35. Nickel JC, Ruseska I, Wright JB, et al. Tobramycin resistance of *Pseudomonas aeruginosa* cells growing as a biofilm on urinary catheter material. Antimicrob Agents Chemother. 1985;27:619–24.
36. Ladd TI, Schmiel D, Nickel JC, et al. Rapid method for detection of adherent bacteria on Foley urinary catheters. J Clin Microbiol. 1985;21:1004–6.
37. Daifuku R, Stamm W. Bacterial adherence to bladder uroepithelial cells in

catheter-associated urinary tract infection. N Engl J Med. 1986;314:1208–13.
38. Zimmerli W, Lew PD, Walkvogel FA. Pathogenesis of foreign body infection. Evidence for a local granulocyte defect. J Clin Invest. 1984;73:1191–200.
39. Zimmerli W, Waldvogel FA, Vaudaux P, et al. Pathogenesis of foreign body infection: Description and characteristics of an animal model. J Infect Dis. 1982;146:487–97.
40. Hedelin H, Eddeland A, Larsson L, et al. The composition of catheter encrustations, including the effects of allopurinol treatment. Br J Urol. 1984;56:250–4.
41. Mobley HLT, Warren JW. Urease-positive bacteriuria and obstruction of long-term urinary catheters. J Clin Microbiol. 1987;25:2216–7.
42. Mehrotra RML. An experimental study of the vesical circulation during distension and in cystitis. J Pathol Bacteriol. 1953;66:79–89.
43. Shooter RA, Walker KA, Williams VR, et al. Faecal carriage of *Pseudomonas aeruginosa* in hospital patients: Possible spread from patient to patient. Lancet. 1966;2:1331–4.
44. Selden R, Lee S, Wang WLL, et al. Nosocomial Klebsiella infections: Intestinal colonization as a reservoir. Ann Intern Med. 1971;74:657–64.
45. Brun-Buisson C, Philippon A, Ansquer M, et al. Transferable enzymatic resistance to third-generation cephalosporins during nosocomial outbreak of multiresistant *Klebsiella pneumoniae*. Lancet. 1987;2:302–6.
46. Rutala WA, Kennedy VA, Loflin HB, et al. *Serratia marcescens* nosocomial infections of the urinary tract associated with urine measuring containers and urinometers. Am J Med. 1981;70:659–63.
47. Schaberg DR, Weinstein RA, Stamm WE. Epidemics of nosocomial urinary tract infection caused by multiply resistant gram-negative bacilli: Epidemiology and control. J Infect Dis. 1976;133:363–6.
48. Maki DG, Hennekens CG, Phillips CW, et al. Nosocomial urinary tract infection with *Serratia marcescens*: An epidemiologic study. J Infect Dis. 1973;128:579–87.
49. Kaslow RA, Lindsey JO, Bisno AL, et al. Nosocomial infection with highly resistant *Proteus rettgeri*—report of an epidemic. Am J Epidemiol. 1976;104:278–86.
50. Casewell M, Phillips I. Hands as route of transmission for Klebsiella species. Br Med J. 1977;2:1315–7.
51. Marple CD. The frequency and character of urinary tract infections in an unselected group of women. Ann Intern Med. 1941;14:2220.
52. Brehmer B, Madsen PO. Route and prophylaxis of ascending bladder infection in male patients with indwelling catheters. J Urol. 1972;108:719–21.
53. Butler HK, Kunin CM. Evaluation of specific systemic antimicrobial therapy in patients while on closed catheter drainage. J Urol. 1968;100:567.
54. Britt MR, Garibaldi RA, Miller WA, et al. Antimicrobial prophylaxis for catheter-associated bacteriuria. Antimicrob Agents Chemother. 1977;11:240.
55. Hartstein AI, Garber SB, Ward TT, et al. Nosocomial urinary tract infection: A prospective evaluation of 108 catheterized patients. Infect Control. 1981;2:380–6.
56. Weyrauch HM, Bassett JB. Ascending infection in an artificial urinary tract; an experimental study. Stanford Med Bull. 1951;9:25.
57. Burke J, Larsen R, Stevens L. Nosocomial bacteriuria: Estimating the potential for prevention by closed sterile urinary drainage. Infect Control. 1986;7:96–9.
58. Davies A, Shroff K. When should a urine specimen be examined after removal of a urinary catheter? J Hosp Infect. 1983;4:177–80.
59. Stark RP, Maki DG. Bacteriuria in the catheterized patient. What quantitative level of bacteriuria is relevant? N Engl J Med. 1984;311:560–4.
60. Bran JL, Levison ME, Kaye D. Entrance of bacteria into the female urinary bladder. N Engl J Med. 1972;286:626.
61. Buckley RM, McGucken M, MacGregor RR. Urine bacterial counts following sexual intercourse. N Engl J Med. 1978;298:321.
62. Mobley HLT, Chippendale, MG, Tenney JH, et al. Expression of type 1 fimbriae may be required for persistence of *E. coli* in the catheterized urinary tract. J Clin Microbiol. 1987;25:2253–7.
63. Mobley HLT, Chipendale GR, Tenney JH, et al. MR/K hemagglutination of *Providencia stuartii* correlates with catheter adherence and with persistence in catheter-associated bacteriuria. J Infect Dis. 1988;157:264–71.
64. Kostiala AAI, Nyren P, Jokinen EJ, et al. Prospective study on the appearance of antibody-coated bacteria in patients with an indwelling urinary catheter. Nephron. 1981;30:279–85.
65. Hulter H, Borchardt K, Mahood J, et al. Localization of catheter-induced urinary tract infections: Interpretation of bladder washout and antibody-coated bacteria tests. Nephron. 1984;38:48–53.
66. Nyren P, Runeberg L, Kostiala AI, et al. Prophylactic methenamine hippurate or nitrofurantoin in patients with an indwelling urinary catheter. Ann Clin Res. 1981;13:16–21.
67. Warren JW, Mobley HLT, Trifillis AL. Internalization of *Escherichia coli* into human renal tubular epithelial cells. J Infect Dis. 1988;158:221–3.
68. Warren JW, Muncie HL Jr, Hall-Craggs M. Acute pyelonephritis associated with bacteriuria during long-term catheterization: A prospective clinicopathological study. J Infect Dis. 1988;158:1341–6.
69. Bryan C, Reynolds K. Hospital-acquired bacteremic urinary tract infection: Epidemiology and outcome. J Urol. 1984;132:494–8.
70. Gordon D, Bune A, Grime B, et al. Diagnostic criteria and natural history of catheter-associated urinary tract infections after prostatectomy. Lancet. 1983;1:1269–71.
71. Tribe CR, Silver JR. Renal failure in paraplegia. London: Pitman Medical Publishing Co; 1969:35–53.
72. Platt R, Polk BF, Murdock B, et al. Risk factors for nosocomial urinary tract infection. Am J Epidemiol. 1986;124:977–85.
73. Shapiro M, Simchen E, Izraeli S, et al. A multivariate analysis of risk factors for acquiring bacteriuria in patients with indwelling urinary catheters for longer than 24 hours. Infect Control. 1984;5:525–32.
74. Garibaldi RA, Mooney BR, Epstein BJ, et al. An evaluation of daily bacteriologic monitoring to identify preventable episodes of catheter-associated urinary tract infection. Infect Control. 1982;3:466–70.
75. Haley R, Culver D, White J, et al. The nationwide nosocomial infection rate: A new need for vital statistics. Am J Epidem. 1985;121:159–67.
76. Morrison AJ, Wenzel RP. Nosocomial urinary tract infections due to enterococcus. Arch Intern Med. 1986;146:1549–51.
77. Hamory BH, Wenzel RP. Hospital-associated candiduria: Predisposing factors and review of the literature. J Urol. 1978;120:444–8.
78. U.S. Department of Health and Human Services. NNIS Manual: National nosocomial infections surveillance system. Public Health Service, Centers for Disease Control; 1988:XIII-5–XIII-9.
79. Warren JW, Muncie HL Jr, Bergquist EJ, et al. Sequelae and management of urinary infection in the patient requiring chronic catheterization. J Urol. 1981;125:1–8.
80. Platt R, Polk BF, Muyrdock B, et al. Mortality associated with nosocomial urinary tract infection. N Engl J Med. 1982;307:637.
81. Kunin CM, Chin QF, Chambers S. Indwelling urinary catheters in the elderly. Am J Med. 1987;82:405–11.
82. Marron KR, Fillit U, Peskowitz M, et al. The non-use of urethral catheterization in the management of urinary incontinence in the teaching nursing home. J AM Geriatr Soc. 1983;31:278–81.
83. Ouslander JG, Kane RL, Abrass IB. Urinary incontinence in elderly nursing home patients. JAMA. 1982;94:661–6.
84. Ribeiro BJ, Smith SR. Evaluation of urinary catheterization and urinary incontinence in a general nursing home population. J Am Geriatr Soc. 1985;33:479–82.
85. Warren JW, Steinberg L, Hebel JR, et al. The prevalence of urethral catheterization in Maryland nursing homes: Estimates for the United States. Arch Intern Med. In press.
86. Warren JW, Damron D, Tenney JH, et al. Fever, bacteremia, and death as complications of bacteriuria in women with long-term urethral catheters. J Infect Dis. 1987;155:1151–8.
87. Warren JW, Tenney JH, Hoopes JM, et al. A prospective microbiologic study of bacteriuria in patients with chronic indwelling urethral catheters. J Infect Dis. 1982;146:719–23.
88. Steward DK, Wood GL, Cohen RL, et al. Failure of the urinalysis and quantitative urine culture in diagnosing symptomatic urinary tract infections in patients with long-term urinary catheters. Am J Infect Control. 1985;13:154–60.
89. Tenney JH, Warren JW. Bacteriuria in women with long-term catheters: Paired comparison of the indwelling and replacement catheter. J Infect Dis. 1988;157:199–202.
90. Warren JW. *Providencia stuartii*: A common cause of antibiotic-resistant bacteriuria in patients with long-term indwelling catheters. Rev Infect Dis. 1986;8:61–7.
91. McHale PJ, Walker F, Scully B, et al. *Providencia stuartii* infections: A review of 117 cases over an eight year period. J Hosp Infect. 1981;2:155–65.
92. Alling B, Brandberg A, Seeberg S, et al. Aerobic and anaerobic microbial flora in the urinary tract of geriatric patients during long-term care. J Infect Dis. 1973;127:34–9.
93. Hunt TE, Hader WJ. Intensive investigation and treatment of urinary tract infections in paraplegics. Med Serv J Can. 1966;22:548–58.
94. McLeod JW, Glasg MB, Mason JM, et al. Survey of the different urinary infections which develop in the paraplegic and their relative significance. Microbiology. 1965;3:124–43.
95. Damron D, Warren J, Chippendale M, et al. Do clinical microbiology laboratories accurately report bacteriology in urine from patients with long-term urinary catheters? J Clin Microbiol. 1986;24:400–4.
96. Tenney JH, Warren JW. Long-term catheter-associated bacteriuria: Species at low concentration. Urology. 1987;30:444–6.
97. Ouslander JG, Greengold B, Chen S. Complications of chronic indwelling urinary catheters among male nursing home patients: A prospective study. J Urol. 1987;138:1191–5.
98. Kunin CM, Chin QF, Chambers S. Formation of encrustations on indwelling urinary catheters in the elderly: A comparison of different types of catheter materials in "blockers" and "nonblockers." J Urol. 1987;138:899–902.
99. Muncie HL, Warren JW. Fate of long-term urethral catheters in female nursing home patients. Submitted for publication.
100. Bruce AW, Sira SS, Clark AF, et al. The problem of catheter encrustation. Can Med Assoc J. 1974;111:238–9.
101. Jones B, Mobley H. Genetic and biochemical diversity of ureases of *Proteus, Providencia,* and *Morganella* species isolated from urinary tract infection. Infect Immun. 1987;55:2198–2203.
102. Mobley HLT, Jones B, Jerse AE. Cloning of urease gene sequences from *Providencia stuartii.* Infect Immun. 1986;54:161–9.
103. Nemoy NJ, Stamey TA. Surgical, bacteriological, and biochemical management of "infection stones." JAMA. 1971;215:1470.

104. Williams HE. Nephrolithiasis. N Engl J Med. 1974;290:33.
105. Takeuchi H, Takayama H, Konishi T, et al. Scanning electron microscopy detects bacteria within infection stones. J Urol. 1984;132:67–9.
106. McLean R, Nickel JC, Noakes VC, et al. An in vitro ultrastructural study of infectious kidney stone genesis. Infect Immun. 1985;49:805–11.
107. Nikakhtar B, Vaziri ND, Khonsari F, et al. Urolithiasis in patients with spinal cord injury. Paraplegia. 1981;19:363–6.
108. Hardy AG. Complications of the indwelling urethral catheter. Paraplegia. 1968;6:5.
109. Carty M, Brocklehurst J, Carty J. Bacteriuria and its correlates in old age. Gerontology. 1981;27:72–5.
110. Dietrick RB, Russi S. Tabulation and review of autopsy findings in fifty-five paraplegics. JAMA. 1958;166:41.
111. Talbot HS. Renal disease and hypertension in paraplegics and quadriplegics. Med Serv J Can. 1966;22:570.
112. Hall-Craggs M, Hebel JR, Muncie HL, et al. Chronic pyelonephritis and severe mononuclear renal inflammation in long-term catheterized aged nursing home patients. Submitted for publication.
113. Najenson T, Mendelson L, Sabransky H, et al. Upper urinary tract in patients after traumatic spinal cord injury. Paraplegia. 1969;7:85.
114. Donnelly J, Hackler RH, Bunts RC. Present urologic status of the World War II paraplegic: 25-year followup. Comparison with status of the 20-year Korean War paraplegic and 5-year Vietnam paraplegic. J Urol. 1972;108:558.
115. Jousse AT, Wynne-Jones M, Breithaupt DJ. A followup study of life expectancy and mortality in traumatic transverse myelitis. In: Proceedings of the Sixteenth Veterans Administration Spinal Cord Injury Conference; 1967;198–202.
116. Kaufman JM, Fam B, Jacobs S, et al. Bladder cancer and squamous metaplasia in spinal cord injury patients. J Urol. 1977;118:967–71.
117. Locke JR, Hill DE, Walzer Y. Incidence of squamous cell carcinoma in patients with long-term catheter drainage. J Urol. 1985;133:1034–5.
118. Wong ES. Guideline for prevention of catheter-associated urinary tract infections. Am J Infect Control. 1983;11:28–36.
119. Kunin CM. Detection, prevention and management of urinary tract infections. 4th ed. Philadelphia: Lea & Febiger; 1987:245–97.
120. Slade N, Gillespie WA. The urinary tract and the catheter: Infection and other problems. New York: John Wiley & Sons; 1985.
121. Garibaldi RA. Hospital-acquired urinary tract infections: Epidemiology and prevention. In: Wenzel RP, ed. Prevention and Control of Nosocomial Infections. Baltimore: Williams & Wilkins; 1987:335–43.
122. Schaeffer AJ. Catheter-associated bacteriuria. Urol Clin North Am. 1986;13:735–47.
123. Schaberg DR, Zervos MJ. Nosocomial urinary tract infection. Compr Ther. 1986;12:8–11.
124. Warren JW. Catheter-associated urinary tract infections. Infectious Dis Clin North Am. 1987;1:823–54.
125. Nordqvist P, Ekelund P, Edouard L, et al. Catheter-free geriatric care. Routines and consequences for clinical infection, care and economy. J Hosp Infect. 1984;5:298–304.
126. Fierer J, Ekstrom M. An outbreak of *Providencia stuartii* urinary tract infections. Patients with condon catheters are a reservoir of the bacteria. JAMA. 1981;245:1553–5.
127. Hirsh DD, Fainstein V, Musher DM. Do condom catheter collecting systems cause urinary tract infection? JAMA. 1979;242:340–1.
128. Montgomerie JZ, Morrow JW. Pseudomonas colonization in patients with spinal cord injury. Am J Epidemiol. 1978;108:328–36.
129. Ouslander JG, Greengold BA, Silverblatt FJ, et al. An accurate method to obtain urine for culture in men with external catheters. Arch Intern Med. 1987;147:286–8.
130. Nicolle LE, Harding GKM, Kennedy J, et al. Urine specimen collection with external devices for diagnosis of bacteriuria in elderly incontinent men. J Clin Microbiol. 1988;26:1115–9.
131. Shlaes DM, Currie CA. Endemic gentamicin resistance R factors on a spinal cord injury unit. J Clin Microbiol. 1983;18:236–41.
132. Golji H. Complications of external condom drainage. Paraplegia. 1981;19:189–97.
133. Jayachandran S, Mooppan U, Kim H. Complications from external (condom) urinary drainage devices. Urology. 1985;25:31–4.
134. Melekos M, Asbach HW. Complications from urinary condom catheters. Urology. 1986;27:88.
135. Steinhardt G, McRoberts JW. Total distal penile necrosis caused by condom catheter. JAMA. 1980;244:1238–44.
136. Johnson DE, O'Reilly JL, Warren JW. Clinical evaluation of an external urine collection device for non-ambulatory incontinent women. J Urol. 1989;141:535–7.
137. Van Den Broek PJ, Dahha TJ, Mouton RP. Bladder irrigation with povidone-iodine in prevention of urinary-tract infections associated with intermittent urethral catheterization. Lancet. 1985;i:563–5.
138. Guttmann L, Frankel H. The value of intermittent catheterization in the early management of traumatic paraplegia and tetraplegia. Paraplegia. 1966;4:63.
139. Firlit CF, Canning JR, Lloyd FA, et al. Experience with intermittent catheterization in chronic spinal cord injury patients. J Urol. 1975;114:234.
140. Hardy AG. Experiences with intermittent catheterization in acute paraplegia. Med Serv J Can. 1966;22:538.
141. Herr HW. Intermittent catheterization in neurogenic bladder dysfunction. J Urol. 1975;113:477.
142. Pearman JW. Urological follow-up of 99 spinal cord injured patients initially managed by intermittent catheterisation. Br J Urol. 1976;48:297.
143. Perkash I. Intermittent catheterization and bladder rehabilitation in spinal cord injury patients. J Urol. 1975;114:230.
144. Haldorson AM, Keys TF, Maker MD, et al. Nonvalue of neomycin instillation after intermittent urinary catheterization. Antimicrob Agents Chemother. 1978;14:368–70.
145. Kuhlemeier K, Stover S, Lloyd L. Prophylactic antibacterial therapy for preventing urinary tract infections in spinal cord injury patients. J Urol. 1985;134:514–7.
146. Stickler DJ, Wilmot CB, O'Flynn JD. The mode of development of urinary infection in intermittently catheterized male paraplegics. Paraplegia. 1970;8:243–52.
147. Vainrub B, Musher DB. Lack of effect of methenamine in suppression of, or prophylaxis against, chronic urinary infection. Antimicrob Agents Chemother. 1977;12:625.
148. Kevorkian CG, Merritt JL, Ilstrup DM. Methenamine mandelate with acidification: An effective urinary antiseptic in patients with neurogenic bladder. Mayo Clin Proc. 1984;59:523–9.
149. Anderson RU. Prophylaxis of bacteriuria during intermittent catheterization of the acute neurogenic bladder. J Urol. 1980;123:364–6.
150. Donovan WH, Stolov WC, Clowers DE, et al. Bacteriuria during intermittent catheterization following spinal cord injury. Arch Phys Med Rehabil. 1978;59:351–7.
151. Mohler JL, Cowen DL, Flanigan RC. Suppression and treatment of urinary tract infection in patients with an intermittently catheterized neurogenic bladder. J Urol. 1987;138:336–40.
152. Krebs M, Halvorsen R, Fishman I, et al. Prevention of urinary tract infection during intermittent catheterization. J Urol. 1983;131:82–5.
153. Diokno A, Sonda L, Hollander J, et al. Fate of patients started on clean intermittent self-catheterization therapy 10 years ago. J Urol. 1983;129:1120–2.
154. Abrams PH, Gaches CGC, Green NA, et al. Role of suprapubic catheterization in retention of urine. J R Soc Med. 1980;73:845–8.
155. Barham KA. Suprapubic bladder drainage in gynecological surgery. Aust NZ J Surg. 1973;43:32–6.
156. Frymire LJ. Comparison of suprapubic versus Foley drains. Obstet Gynecol. 1971;38:239–44.
157. Hodgkinson CP, Hodari AA. Trocar suprapubic cystostomy for postoperative bladder drainage in the female. Am J Obstet Gynecol. 1966;96:773–83.
158. Hofmeister FJ, Martens WE, Strebel RL. Foley catheter or suprapubic tube? Am J Obstet Gynecol. 1970;107:767–79.
159. Ingram JM. Suprapubic cystotomy by trocar catheter: A preliminary report. Am J Obstet Gynecol. 1972;113:1108–13.
160. Kariher DH, Fernandez IA, Trombetta GC, et al. Use of suction with suprapubic bladder drainage. Obstet Gynecol. 1970;35:401–4.
161. Shapiro J, Hoffmann J, Jersky J. A comparison of suprapubic and transurethral drainage for postoperative urinary retention in general surgical patients. Acta Chir Scand. 1982;148:323–7.
162. Andersen JT, Heisterberg L, Hebjorn S, et al. Suprapubic versus transurethral bladder drainage after colposuspension/vaginal repair. Acta Obstet Gynecol Scand. 1985;64:139–43.
163. Anonymous. Urinary diversion for incontinence. Lancet. 1986;1:363–4.
164. Goldwasser B, Webster G. Continent urinary diversion. J Urol. 1985;134:227–36.
165. Mansson W, Colleen S, Mardh P-A. The microbial flora of the continent cecal urinary reservoir, its stoma and the peristomal skin. J Urol. 1986;135:247–50.
166. Schmidt JD, Hawtrey CE, Flocks RH, et al. Complications, results and problems of ileal conduit diversions. J Urol. 1973;109:210–6.
167. Hill MJ, Hudson MJ, Stewart M. The urinary bacterial flora in patients with three types of urinary tract diversion. J Med Microbiol. 1983;16:221–6.
168. Kaufman JJ, Raz S. Passive urethral compression with a silicone gel prosthesis for the treatment of male urinary incontinence. Mayo Clin Proc. 1976;51:373.
169. Scott FB, Bradley WE, Timm GW. Treatment of urinary incontinence by implantable prosthetic sphincter. Urology. 1973;1:252.
170. Small MP. The Rosen incontinence procedure: A new artificial urinary sphincter for the management of urinary incontinence. J Urol. 1980;123:507.
171. Platt R, Murdock B, Polk BF, et al. Reduction of mortality associated with nosocomial urinary tract infection. Lancet. 1983;1:1893–7.
172. Bastable JRG, Peel RN, Birch DM, et al. Continuous irrigation of the bladder after prostatectomy: Its effect on post-prostatectomy infection. Br J Urol. 1977;49:689–93.
173. Savage, JE, Phillips B, Lifshitz S, et al. Bacteriuria in closed bladder drainage versus continuous irrigation in patients undergoing intracavitary radium for treatment of gynecologic cancer. Gynecol Oncol. 1982;13:26.
174. Gillespie W, Jones J, Teasdale C, et al. Does the addition of disinfectant to urine drainage bags prevent infection in catheterized patients? Lancet. 1983;1:1037–9.
175. Sweet DE, Goodpasture HC, Holl K, et al. Evaluation of H_2O_2 prophylaxis of bacteriuria in patients with long-term indwelling Foley catheters: A randomized controlled study. Infect Control. 1985;6:263–6.
176. Thompson RL, Haley CE, Searcy MA, et al. Catheter-associated bacteriuria. Failure to reduce attack rates using periodic instillations of a disinfectant into urinary drainage systems. JAMA. 1984;251:747–51.
177. Maizels M, Schaeffer AJ. Decreased incidence of bacteriuria associated with

periodic instillations of hydrogen peroxide into the urethral catheter drainage bag. J Urol. 1980;123:841–5.
178. Blenkharn JJ. Prevention of bacteriuria during urinary catheterization of patients in an intensive care unit: Evaluation of the "Ureofix 500" closed drainage system. J Hosp Infect. 1985;6:187–93.
179. Monson TP, Macalalad FV, Hamman JW, et al. Evaluation of a vented drainage system in prevention of bacteriuria. J Urol. 1977;117:216–9.
180. Kunin CM. The drainage bag additive saga. Infect Control. 1985;6:261–2.
181. Burke JP, Garibaldi RA, Britt MR, et al. Prevention of catheter-associated urinary tract infections. Efficacy of daily meatal care regimens. Am J Med. 1981;70:655–8.
182. Butler HK, Kunin CM. Evaluation of polymyxin catheter lubricant and impregnated catheters. J Urol. 1968;100:560–72.
183. Kunin CM, Finkelberg Z. Evaluation of an intraurethral lubricating catheter in prevention of catheter-induced urinary tract infections. J Urol. 1971;106:928–30.
184. Monson T, Kunin CM. Evaluation of a polymer-coated indwelling catheter in prevention of infection. J Urol. 1974;111:220–2.
185. Lundberg T. Prevention of catheter-associated urinary-tract infections by use of silver-impregnated catheters. Lancet. 1986;1:1031.
186. Mountokalakis T, Skounakis M, Tselentis J. Short-term versus prolonged systemic antibiotic prophylaxis in patients treated with indwelling catheters. J Urol. 1985;134:506–8.
187. Polk BF, Tager IB, Shapiro M, et al. Randomized clinical trial of perioperative cefazolin in preventing infection after hysterectomy. Lancet. 1980;1:437–40.
188. Bivens MD, Neufeld J, McCarty WD. The prophylactic use of Keflex and Keflin in vaginal hysterectomy. Am J Obstet Gynecol. 1975;122:169–75.
189. Warren JW, Anthony WC, Hoopes JM, et al. Cephalexin for susceptible bacteriuria in afebrile, long-term catheterized patients. JAMA. 1982;248:454–8.
190. Gerstein AR, Okun R, Gonick HC, et al. The prolonged use of methenamine hippurate in the treatment of chronic urinary tract infection. J Urol. 1968;100:767–71.
191. Norberg B, Norberg A, Parkhede U, et al. Effect of short-term high-dose treatment with methenamine hippurate on urinary infection in geriatric patients with an indwelling catheter. IV. Clinical evaluation. Eur J Clin Pharmacol. 1979;15:347–61.
192. Norrman K, Wibell L. Treatment with methenamine hippurate in the patient with a catheter. J Int Med Res. 1976;4:115–7.
193. Wibell L, Schenynius A, Norrman K. Methenamine-hippurate and bacteriuria in the geriatric patient with a catheter. Acta Med Scand. 1980;207:469–73.
194. Musher DM, Griffith DP, Richie Y. The generation of formaldehyde from methenamine: Effect of urinary flow and residual volume. Invest Urol. 1976;13:380.
195. Musher DM, Griffith DP. Generation of formaldehyde from methenamine: Effect of pH and concentration, and antibacterial effect. Antimicrob Agents Chemother. 1974;6:708.
196. Shohl AT, Deming CL. Hexamethylenamin: Its quantitative factors in therapy. J Urol. 1920;4:419.
197. Bjork DT, Pelletier LL, Tight R. Urinary tract infections with antibiotic resistant organisms in catheterized nursing home patients. Infect Control. 1984;5:173–6.
198. Levin J. The incidence and prevention of infection after urethral catheterization. Ann Intern Med. 1964;60:914–22.
199. Sanford JP. Hospital-acquired urinary-tract infections. Ann Intern Med. 1964;60:903–13.
200. Tyler CW, Oseasohn R. The relationship of in-lying catheterization to persistent bacteriuria in gynecologic patients. Am J Obstet Gynecol. 1963;86:998–1002.
201. Muncie HL, Hoopes JM, Damron DJ, et al. Once-daily irrigation of long-term urethral catheters with normal saline: Lack of benefit. Arch Intern Med. 1989;149:441–3.
202. Norberg A, Norberg B, Parkhede U, et al. Randomized double-blind study of prophylactic methenamine hippurate treatment of patients with indwelling catheters. Eur J Clin Pharmacol. 1980;18:497–500.
203. Burns P, Gauthier J. Prevention of urinary catheter incrustations by acetohydroxamic acid. J Urol. 1984;132:455–6.
204. Williams JJ, Rodman JS, Peterson CM. A randomized double-blind study of acetohydroxamic acid in struvite nephrolithiasis. N Engl J Med. 1984;311:760–3.
205. Casewell MW, Phillips I. Aspects of the plasmid-mediated antibiotic resistance and epidemiology of Klebsiella species. Am J Med. 1981;70:459–62.
206. Shlaes DM, Lehman M-H, Currie-McCumber CA, et al. Prevalence of colonization with antibiotic resistant gram-negative bacilli in a nursing home care unit: The importance of cross-colonization as documented by plasmid analysis. Infect Control. 1986;7:538–45.
207. Penner JL, Hinton NA, Hamilton LJ, et al. Three episodes of nosocomial urinary tract infections caused by one O-serotype of *Providencia stuartii*. J Urol. 1981;125:668–71.
208. Schaberg DR, Haley RW, Highsmith AK, et al. Nosocomial bacteriuria: A prospective study of case clustering and antimicrobial resistance. Ann Intern Med. 1980;93:420–4.
209. Schaberg DR, Alford RH, Anderson R, et al. An outbreak of nosocomial infection due to multiply resistant *Serratia marcescens*: Evidence of inter-hospital spread. J Infect Dis. 1976;134:181–8.
210. Rubens CE, Farrar WE Jr, McGee ZA, et al. Evolution of a plasmid mediating resistance to multiple antimicrobial agents during a prolonged epidemic of nosocomial infections. J Infect Dis. 1981;143:170–81.
211. Schaberg DR, Rubens CE, Alford RH, et al. Evolution of antimicrobial resistance and nosocomial infection: Lessons from the Vanderbilt experience. Am J Med. 1981;70:445–8.
212. Thompkins LS, Plorde JJ, Falkow S. Molecular analysis of R-factors from multiresistant nosocomial isolates. J Infect Dis. 1980;141:625–36.
213. Schaberg DR, Highsmith AK, Wachsmith IK. Resistance plasmid transfer by *Serratia marcescens* in urine. Antimicrob Agents Chemother. 1977;11:449–40.
214. Maki D, Hennekens C, Bennet J: Prevention of catheter-associated urinary tract infection. JAMA. 1972;221:1270–1.

282. NOSOCOMIAL VIRAL HEPATITIS

BRADLEY N. DOEBBELING
RICHARD P. WENZEL

In 1949 Leibowitz et al.[1] focused on the risk of viral heptatitis in hospital personnel by relating the illness in a nurse to the multiple needlesticks she sustained in the course of her duties in the blood bank. The extent of the problem was quantified in 1966 by Bryne, who calculated a mean annual attack rate of 51 cases per 100,000 hospital employees.[2] The relatively high risk to laboratory workers was subsequently shown to be related to their handling of blood, and later control and diagnostic sera used in clinical laboratories were discovered to be contaminated with hepatitis B surface antigen (HBsAg). It is now recognized that high-risk locations are hemodialysis units, emergency and operating rooms, clinical laboratories, organ transplantation wards, and oncology wards. A number of studies have shown that exposure to blood and blood products is the most important risk factor.[3–5] In one series the infection rate among employees with the highest exposure to blood was estimated at 1.05/100 person-years.[4] The frequency of sharps injuries appeared to correlate with the rate of hepatitis B virus (HBV) infection in hospital employees in some studies.[4,5] Other risk factors include country of origin, history of jaundice, male sex, increasing age, and race (possibly confounding the country of origin).[4,5]

OCCUPATIONAL CATEGORIES

In a 1976 report from the Centers for Disease Control,[6] the presence of HBsAg or anti-HBsAb was detected in 14 and 16 percent of dentists and physicians, respectively, compared with 4 percent of first-time blood donors. The prevalences of HBsAg in physicians, dentists, and first-time blood donors were 0.8, 1.7, and 0.3 percent, respectively. The risks sharply increased with age in physicians and dentists, and it was noted that professionals in surgical subspecialties had a seropositivity rate 1.6 times greater than those in nonsurgical subspecialties. The prevalence of HBV markers among personnel at large teaching hospitals and urban medical centers ranges from 10 to 25 percent.[3–5,7] Among community hospitals the mean prevalence of seropositivity throughout the United States prior to 1983 was 8.4 percent, while the seroprevalence at a given institution ranged from 0 to 16.7 percent.[8] The differences in seropositivity among hospitals may partly reflect the national origin of their employees.[9] Importantly, it should be noted that studies of the prevalence of HBV markers appear to overestimate the incidence of infection in most settings.[10]

In 1975 the annual rate of hepatitis in dental professionals was reported to be 6.7 percent compared with 2.4 percent for lawyers with the same age distribution; the prevalence of HBV seropositivity for oral surgeons was 21 percent compared with

5 percent for general dentists.[11] In the same study, fewer than 7 percent of the dentists used gloves all the time despite evidence suggesting that failure to use gloves is associated with a higher prevalence of hepatitis B infection. Recently, a serologic survey of dentists revealed a 0.9 percent chronic carrier rate, a 6.7 percent natural immunity rate, and a 35 percent vaccine acceptance rate.[12]

The World Health Organization (WHO) estimates that the incidence of hepatitis infection in medical and ancillary staff is from three to six times that in those in other professions. The rate of infection of health care workers is directly related to duration of employment.[13] The probability of infection may be as high as between 0.6 and 1.4 percent for each year working in a hospital in an endemic country.[11] The incidence of hepatitis B infection among hospital employees appears to be declining; this decrease is perhaps related to better infection control procedures as well as vaccine availability. A statewide survey of hospital employees in Minnesota revealed a significant decline in the number of cases from 127/100,000 persons in 1975 to 8/100,000 in 1983.[10] A similar decline in clinical disease was noted in hospital staff in Sweden during successive 5 year periods, from 1969–73 (102/100,000 person-years) to 1979–83 (10.4/100,000 person-years).[14] The risk of developing HBV infection is still relatively high for surgical house officers and operating room workers; emergency room and intensive care unit personnel; blood bank, laboratory, and pathology technologists; medical house officers and pathology residents; as well as hemodialysis and intravenous nurses and technologists.[3,15]

HEMODIALYSIS UNITS

The high incidence of viral hepatitis in hemodialysis units was recognized in the mid-1960s by Ringertz and Nystrom.[16] In the early 1970s, the incidences of infection for dialysis staff and patients were reported to be 3.4 and 4.4 cases, respectively, per 100 people at risk per year.[17] By the mid-1970s estimates were that 6.2 percent of the patients and 5.2 percent of the staff contracted hepatitis B infection within 1 year of association with a hemodialysis unit.[18] In the latter study, the finding of particular significance was that dialysis units that separated HBsAg-positive from HBsAg-negative patients had significantly lower rates of infection in patients and staff. From 1976 to 1983, the annual incidence of HBV infection declined significantly among patients from 3 to 0.5 percent and among staff from 2.6 to 0.5 percent in hemodialysis centers.[19] In the same series the incidences of non-A, non-B hepatitis among hemodialysis patients and staff were 1.8 and 0.5 percent, respectively, in 1983.

The cumulative incidences of new HBV infection in Israel, a country with a high endemic rate, in patients and staff are 16 and 15 percent, respectively, at 1 year; at 2 years, they are 31 and 22 percent.[20] Chronic carriers were relatively frequent among patients in the study (7 percent compared with 2 percent of the general population). Similarly, nurses in the study were at particularly high risk to develop new infections.

Hepatitis B surface antigenemia is relatively common among hemodialysis patients. Although HBsAg-positive patients in one series of 101 chronic hemodialysis patients were not significantly different from antigen-negative patients in terms of morbidity, hospital stay, or mortality, this may reflect a type II error.[21] Recent availability of a monoclonal radioimmunoassay appears to improve the detection of HBsAg in hemodialysis patients by 120 percent over conventional polyclonal radioimmunoassays.[22]

Most investigators agree that the reservoir for HBV in hemodialysis units is primarily the patients who are chronic carriers of HBsAg. The major mode of transmission is thought to be contact with blood or serum of such patients, although all cases cannot be explained on the basis of such exposure.[23] Environmental contamination also may be important, since HBsAg may remain viable for up to 7 days on machine control knobs, intravenous infusion poles, marking pens, walls, and surfaces of machines.[24] The risk is obviously high in these areas, and the need for strict aseptic technique is clear.

Non-A, non-B hepatitis is now the most common cause of hepatitis in dialysis centers.[18] While dialysis patients developing hepatitis receive transfusions more frequently than controls, the occurrence of non-A, non-B hepatitis in patients not receiving blood products argues for the importance of the dialysis center in transmitting the infection.[25]

The introduction of infection control strategies for the prevention of HBV infection has had a major impact on the disease's incidence among dialysis patients and staff. By 1983, 86 percent of centers were segregating HBsAg-positive patients by using separate machines and rooms.[19] Similarly, 84 percent of centers screened all patients monthly for HBsAg, an increase from 57 percent in 1976. While essentially all centers use some form of routine cleaning of environmental surfaces, 67 percent used high-level disinfectants. Centers using room and machine separation practices had a 0.5 percent incidence of HBsAg, significantly lower than those using only machine or no segregation practices, 0.9 and 1.1 percent, respectively. New cases continued to occur, however, even at those centers not providing dialysis to HBsAg-positive patients.

Control measures for limiting hepatitis in dialysis units include the following:

I. Area
   A. The dialysis unit itself should be a separate part of the hospital, preferably with limited access.
   B. There should be designated staff toilet facilities separate from those for hospital patients.
   C. HBsAg carriers should be separated from HBsAg-negative dialysis patients by using different rooms and machines for each.

II. Surveillance
   A. There should be surveillance of hospital patients and employees with viral hepatitis to identify changes in incidence rates.
   B. All anti-HBsAb-negative patients and personnel in dialysis centers should have serologic screenings for HBsAg every 1 to 6 months depending on the background incidence.

III. Hygiene practices
   A. Protective clothes, including laboratory coats over scrub suits or gowns and disposable gloves, should be worn in dialysis units. The protective clothing should not be worn outside the area; it should be discarded before eating, drinking, or smoking.
   B. There should be no eating, drinking, or smoking in the dialysis unit.
   C. Scrupulous personal hygiene should be maintained; this includes no scratching of the head or biting of the nails or pencils.
   D. Strict hand washing procedures should be followed with a foot-operated soap dispenser and knee-operated handles, if possible.

IV. Laboratory practices
   A. High-visibility labeling should be used on all blood specimens.
   B. Needles used to draw blood should not be recapped.
   C. In the laboratory, blood specimens should be pipetted and not poured; stoppers should be twisted gently to avoid aerosols. Pipetting should not be done by mouth.
   D. Automated techniques should be used whenever possible, and there should be a special area for testing the samples of HBsAg.

V. Other
  A. All contaminated materials should be autoclaved or incinerated if possible.
  B. All surfaces that become contaminated with blood should be washed in 0.5–1.0% sodium hypochlorite.
  C. Extreme care should be taken in cleaning and in sterilizing nondisposable dialysis equipment such as the venous pressure gauge.
  D. Whenever possible, disposable supplies should be used.

PERSON-TO-PERSON TRANSMISSION

Despite the high-risk of seroconversion of patients and staff in certain hospital settings, there are no current recommendations to screen all patients routinely for HBsAg and anti-HBsAb. Furthermore, there are not sufficient data to recommend removing hospital personnel from routine duties if they are HBsAg-positive. A prospective study of six health care workers who were chronic hepatitis B carriers (including three who were HBeAg-positive) failed to document any hepatitis B transmission, suggesting that the risk is probably less than 1 percent.[26] Obviously, however, any employee with acute viral hepatitis should be restricted from working. While there is clear evidence that transmission of hepatitis B from health care workers to susceptible patients occurs, it happens relatively infrequently.[27] There is currently no evidence that hepatitis B may be transmitted by food.[28]

Hepatitis B infection is an apparent risk of working with institutionalized mentally retarded students. The prevalence of HBV markers among staff at a day school was independently associated with classroom contact with a HBsAg-positive student, duration of employment at the school, and previous work with mentally retarded students.[29] Among teachers with daily classroom contact, the incidence of HBV infection is estimated at 2.6 percent per year.[29] In a prospective study, 2.4 percent of HBsAg-negative employees seroconverted during 539 person-years.[30] Because of the difficulty in determining nonoccupational causes of seroconversions in the institutional setting, all seroconversions are usually labeled as occupationally related.

Several outbreaks among hospital employees have occurred when an apparently healthy patient was attended during the incubation of the disease. Hospital outbreaks have been reported in both England and Australia when trauma victims were taken to the operating rooms, and subsequently to the intensive care units, before acute HBV infections were suspected.[31,32] Both instances underscore the importance of considering all patients' blood as potentially infectious.

The attack rate of hepatitis B in patients exposed to HBsAg-positive dentists has been recently estimated to vary from 1 in 40 to 1 in 400.[33] Nine outbreaks of hepatitis B involving from 3 to 55 clinically infected patients have been linked to oral surgeons or dentists.[33–36] One outbreak of 9 clinically ill patients actually resulted in two deaths, although no other deaths have been reported.[35] Dentists who were thought to have infected patients were HBsAg-positive and HBeAg-positive (if tested).[34,36] Both the length of exposure and degree of trauma involved (i.e., tooth extraction, other surgery) frequently correlated with the likelihood of infection.[33–36] Transmission of infection typically did not occur when dentists and oral surgeons wore gloves but was likely when they did not.

Documented transmission of HBV from other health care providers has also been demonstrated. The first outbreak was reported in 1972, when a nurse in a surgical ward transmitted infection to 11 patients.[37] Subsequently, nosocomial transmission has been linked to a general practitioner,[38,39] two surgeons,[40,41] two gynecologists,[42,43] and two technicians.[40,44] The spread of infection from patient to health care provider to patient was first recognized in 1976 and was subsequently confirmed in a retrospective series.[44,45]

BLOOD TRANSFUSIONS

In 1968 Cohen and Dougherty illustrated the risks of viral hepatitis after transfusion of blood from the Red Cross, from a proprietary bank, and from narcotics addicts to be 1.4, 8.3, and 98 per 1000 units, respectively.[46] Subsequently, Alter et al. estimated that by exclusion of commercial blood donors and donors positive for HBsAg, they could reduce the risk of post-transfusion hepatitis from 20 cases per 1000 units to 3.7 cases per 1000 units (a 0.37 percent risk of hepatitis per unit).[47]

Furthermore, it is possible that the risk of infection with HBsAg-positive blood is low in donors who do not also have HBeAg. This is suggested by the study of hepatitis after needlestick exposure to blood containing HBsAg.[48] When the "donors" had HBeAg and HBsAg, 14 out of 20 recipients acquired hepatitis B. When the donors had HBsAg but no HBeAg, none of the 11 recipients acquired hepatitis. Although we cannot immediately extend the findings to whole blood, future studies of post-transfusion hepatitis may confirm these data.

In a survey of 132 anti-HBsAb-positive recipients of blood transfusions, none acquired hepatitis B, but 16 of 371 (4.3 percent) without anti-HBsAb did acquire hepatitis B.[49] Thus, anti-HBsAb appears to offer protection against infection and illness. Nevertheless, with multiple transfusions, such as are required for open heart surgery, anti-HBsAb may not completely protect against hepatitis B infection.[50] Core antibody (anti-HBc) does not appear to be related either to protection or to recovery from infection.

The implementation of changes in blood component screening policies for HBsAg in July 1972 has dramatically decreased the incidence of post-transfusion hepatitis B. The recent addition of testing for surrogate markers for non-A, non-B hepatitis (alanine aminotransferase [ALT] in the winter of 1986—1987, anti-HBc in the spring of 1987) should further reduce post-transfusion hepatitis due to non-A, non-B. Similarly, changes in the screening of voluntary donors starting in 1983, as well as HIV antibody testing, should reduce the number of hepatitis carriers accepted as donors, thus decreasing the incidence of subsequent hepatitis.[51]

Current data on the incidence of post-transfusion hepatitis are limited. In a series of 1513 recipients of blood from four centers, 156 (10.3 percent) developed non-A, non-B hepatitis as defined by abnormally elevated ALT levels.[52] This method of case definition overestimates the number of clinical cases, although a more specific definition awaits determination of specific viral markers. The incidence of reported clinical cases of non-A, non-B hepatitis in Philadelphia declined from 8–9/10,000 transfusions earlier to 4/10,000 transfusions in 1983.[53] A further reduction of the incidence of non-A, non-B transfusion-related hepatitis by 50 to 60 percent may be possible, depending on the thresholds chosen for a "positive" surrogate marker and the proportion of denied units of blood.[54]

Hepatitis has been associated with a variety of intravenous products other than blood, including fibrinogen; factors II, VII, VIII, IX, X; and contaminated commercially prepared plasma protein products. Heat-treated factor VIII transmitted non-A, non-B hepatitis in up to 84 percent of previously nontransfused hemophiliacs.[55] Outbreaks of infection among surgical patients receiving clotting factor products for bleeding underline the importance of limiting use to persons with known factor deficiencies.[56] Intravenous γ-globulin therapy, particularly in hypogammaglobulinemic patients, has been associated with apparent transmission of non-A, non-B hepatitis and subsequent cirrhosis.[57] Until a test becomes widely available to identify specific causes of non-A, non-B hepatitis, the putative link of intravenous γ-globulin and viral hepatitis remains unconfirmed.

Hepatitis A has occasionally been shown to cause post-transfusion hepatitis. Outbreaks of hepatitis A have also occurred in a neonatal intensive care unit[58] and a bone marrow transplant center through transfusion of contaminated packed red blood cells and platelets, respectively.

Barring commercial contamination, there is thought to be no risk with plasma protein fraction. The authors are unaware of any reports of viral hepatitis related to the intramuscular preparations of γ-globulin. A number of other infections reported to be transmitted by blood include cytomegalovirus, Epstein-Barr virus, syphilis, Colorado tick fever, Rocky Mountain spotted fever, babesiasis, malaria, and the acquired immunodeficiency syndrome (AIDS).

THE DELTA AGENT

The HBsAg-associated δ-antigen represents a marker of a transmissible defective agent distinct from hepatitis B virus yet requiring HBV replication for its synthesis and expression.[59] δ-Infection is endemic in southern Italy, South America, parts of Africa, the Middle East, the South Pacific, and much of the world.[60] In North America, it is limited largely to hemophiliacs, intravenous drug abusers, and occasional male homosexuals. In the hospital setting, patients and employees who are chronic carriers of HBsAg are at risk of developing acute hepatitis and possibly chronic liver disease if they are subsequently exposed to the δ-agent.

Nosocomial transmission has occurred from a parenteral drug abuser undergoing hemodialysis to another asymptomatic carrier of hepatitis B who was regularly dialyzed on the same machine.[61] It would seem reasonable to segregate delta-positive dialysis patients if they were identified from chronic HBsAg carriers who were δ-negative. Other potential exposures include needlestick injuries and blood transfusions and will likely be described in the near future. Fulminant hepatitis was seen in three HBsAg-positive renal transplant patients, with δ-antigen found in the hepatocytes of two of the patients.[62] It was postulated by the authors that the hepatocellular failure seen in the patients was due to δ-superinfection. Preoperative δ-infection has been suggested as a contraindication to liver transplant, although graft reinfection occurred in only four of eight transplanted patients with evidence of preoperative δ-virus infection, one of whom was treated successfully with repeat transplant.[63] Since the δ-agent cannot exist without HBsAg, susceptibile patients and staff should receive the hepatitis B vaccine to prevent both infections.

HEPATITIS A

Hospital-associated outbreaks of hepatitis A virus (HAV) were infrequently reported in the past, presumably because of the lack of a carrier state, the transient viremia, and a decline in viral shedding once the patient becomes symptomatic.[45] Recently, nosocomial outbreaks have been reported with increasing frequency, although this change may be due to better recognition of HAV infection with improved serodiagnostic tools. Most episodes have occurred in the nursery or neonatal intensive care unit and typically have involved a patient hospitalized during the incubation period of HAV for an unrelated problem.[64] The risk of spread to staff is increased if any one of several factors enhancing fecal–oral transmission, including infancy, mental retardation, fecal incontinence, diarrhea, vomiting, and nasogastric drainage, is present.[65] Premature infants are frequently asymptomatic and may be responsible for secondary transmission. Adults also have occasionally been responsible for outbreaks, often with an underlying illness which masked the diagnosis of HAV infection.[64] Outbreaks have been traced to adults from endemic areas,[66] those who were sewage workers,[67] as well as a nurse who had developed infection from eating raw seafood.[68] The ease with which HAV infection is spread in the hospital emphasizes the importance of flawless technique in gowning, gloving, and hand washing when exposure to bodily fluids is anticipated. Eating, drinking, smoking, as well as placing other objects in the mouth while in the work area are all strongly discouraged.

Other mechanisms of transmission include food-borne outbreaks[69] and blood transfusions. Although rare, post-transfusion HAV infection was well documented in a young girl receiving a single unit of packed red blood cells.[70] HAV antigen was demonstrated in the donor's hepatocytes, as well as plasma from the original unit. The ability to test for IgM antibody to HAV has allowed demonstration of several other cases of post-transfusion HAV infection.[71] The infrequent occurrence of post-transfusion HAV infection may be due to the lack of a carrier state, the brief duration of viremia, and possibly the resulting passive immunity when several units are transfused. Transmission by transfusion may subsequently result in secondary spread within the hospital, particularly among infants.

PERINATAL/REPRODUCTIVE TRANSMISSION

Perinatal transmission of HBV infection has serious consequences for the infant, since most become chronic carriers and are at risk for eventual development of cirrhosis and hepatocellular carcinoma.[72,73] Postexposure prophylaxis of infants with either hepatitis B immunoglobulin (HBIg) or hepatitis B vaccine alone has been effective in up to 75 percent of infants born to HBsAg-positive mothers.[74–77] Combination therapy, or passive–active immunization, has been shown to be even more efficacious, reducing the chronic carrier rate to 5 to 10 percent, even among the highest-risk infants born to mothers with both HBeAg and HBsAg.[74,78,79]

The Centers for Disease Control (CDC) currently recommend that infants at risk receive HBIg (0.5 ml intramuscularly) and the initial vaccine dose at separate sites within the first 12 hours of life, with subsequent vaccine doses at 1 and 6 months of age.[28] Although reduced doses of HBIg have been suggested as a cost-saving measure, they cannot be recommended. In a series from Taiwan the lack of a statistically significant difference in HBsAg carrier rates at 1 year (17.7 vs. 40 percent) between infants receiving either 0.5 ml or 0.25 ml HBIg at birth may have been due to the small number of infants in each group.[80]

The CDC recommends routine HBsAg screening only in women in high-risk categories, estimating that up to 90 percent of potentially infected infants will thus be detected.[28] Recently published series from three large inner city hospitals, however, suggest that these criteria would have identified only half of the HBsAg-positive women giving birth at their institutions.[81–83] Universal screening should be considered,[84] particularly at hospitals with a high prevalence of HBsAg-positive carriers, because of the devastating consequences of infection and the ease of prevention. If these measures were implemented throughout the world, they could potentially lead to the virtual elimination of HBV infection within several generations.

While hepatitis B is well recognized as a common cause of sexually transmitted disease, its transmission by artificial insemination was only recently demonstrated.[85] Sperm donors should be routinely screened for HBsAg as part of their initial evaluation.

EMPLOYEE HEALTH

Management of hospital employees exposed to patients with hepatitis or to their blood is often difficult, especially in the presence of a strong emotional reaction and the absence of data. The most difficult areas include personnel with mucous membrane exposure or blood spilled on employees with dermatitis. Both situations should probably be handled as any percutaneous exposure, although few data exist.

Immunoprophylaxis of hepatitis A is typically undertaken

after identification of an index case. Immune serum globulin (ISG) has been shown to prevent infection or lessen severity of clinical disease if administered within 2 weeks of exposure,[86] with an efficacy of 80 to 90 percent. Postexposure prophylaxis with ISG (0.02 ml/kg) is recommended for (*1*) hospital employees with enteric exposure to infected patients, (*2*) day care center staff and attendees if a case is recognized among employees or children, (*3*) residents and staff of custodial care institutions with close contact to a case, (*4*) classroom contacts during an apparent outbreak, (*5*) kitchen contacts of infected food handlers.[87]

Postexposure prophylaxis for hepatitis B is recommended for accidental percutaneous exposures and sexual contacts of HBsAg-positive persons, as well as perinatal exposures.[88] One dose of hepatitis B immune globulin (HBIg), 0.06 ml/kg intramuscularly, followed by the hepatitis B vaccine series is recommended for percutaneous exposure to known HBsAg-positive patients. Percutaneous exposures to patients with unknown serology should lead to initiation of the vaccine, while HBIg administration may await confirmation of positive serology. If the source of the needlestick or mucous membrane exposure is unknown, 5 ml (approximately 0.06 ml/kg) of ISG should be administered for prophylaxis against hepatitis A and possible protection against non-A, non-B hepatitis. Sexual contacts should receive a single dose of HBIg 0.06 μl/kg within 14 days of exposure, with vaccine recommended for homosexual men and regular sexual contacts of HBV carriers.[88]

Both types of globulin should be administered intramuscularly when indicated. Pregnancy is not a contraindication to use of either ISG or HBIg, although a few hypersensitivity reactions have been reported.[89] Administration of ISG and HBIg have not been associated with any known transmission of the human immunodeficiency virus (HIV).

VACCINE PROPHYLAXIS

The plasma-derived, inactivated HBV vaccine (Heptavax-B) was licensed by the Food and Drug Administration in November 1981. Clinical trials have shown that the vaccine is safe and highly antigenic and helps to prevent infection with the hepatitis B virus. The sequelae of HBV should also be prevented by an effective vaccine: immune complex diseases, chronic hepatitis and cirrhosis, δ-agent infections, and hepatocellular carcinoma. The vaccine has been used primarily by health care workers with frequent blood exposure, staff and patients in hemodialysis units, and institutions for the developmentally disabled. Economic considerations ($128 for the series of three injections), as well as unfounded fear about the safety of a vaccine made from pooled plasma specimens, have led to its underutilization. The CDC recommends increased use among high-risk groups for acute HBV infection, especially homosexual males, parenteral drug abusers, and heterosexuals exposed to HBV carriers.[90]

The decision to screen recipients prior to vaccination depends on the prevalence of immunity in a population, as well as the costs of screening and vaccination.[28] The relative cost-effectiveness of any combination of the variables may be estimated; for example, given a seroprevalence of less than 8 percent and screening costs greater than $10 per person, vaccination without screening is cost-effective.[28] For routine purposes, only one antibody test need be used (anti-HBc or anti-HBsAb), if at all. In Italy, a country with a high seroprevalence for HBsAg, screening has been shown to be most cost-effective when done sequentially: i.e., anti-HBc, anti-HBsAb, then HBsAg.[91] Patients were then vaccinated if anti-HBc was absent, anti-HBsAb was found in low concentrations (<10 mIU/ml), or the patient was HBsAg-negative.

Recent release of a HBV vaccine prepared in yeast by recombinant DNA technology (Recombivax-HB) provides another choice in vaccine selection. Reported side effects have been rare, typically soreness at the site of injection or mild systemic symptoms (17 vs. 15 percent, respectively) similar to those associated with the plasma-derived vaccine.[92] When used at equivalent doses (20 μg/dose), the recombinant vaccine is somewhat more immunogenic (significantly so only at 30 days).[93] When used at the currently recommended dose (10 μg), which is half the dose of the plasma-derived vaccine, the recombinant vaccine developed geometric mean antibody titers ranging from 30 to 100 percent of those seen with the previous vaccine.[92] Although no large efficacy trials have been undertaken in adults, the vaccines appear equivalent in neonates.[79] There are no data suggesting greater safety with either vaccine.

Primary vaccination requires a series of three intramuscular injections at 0, 1, and 6 months, preferably in the deltoid. The plasma-derived vaccine should be dosed at 20 μg (1.0 ml) for adults and older children, 10 μg (0.5 ml) for children under 11 years, and 40 μg (2.0 ml) for hemodialysis and immunosuppressed patients.[28] The CDC currently recommends the recombinant vaccine be dosed at 10 μg for adults and older children, and 5 μg for children less than 11 years.[90] A specially formulated preparation of the recombinant vaccine containing 40 μg in a smaller volume with less aluminum hydroxide should be available in the future for the hemodialysis and immunosuppressed population. At the present time, these patients should receive 40 μg doses of the plasma-derived vaccine. Intradermal injections of 2 μg (0.1 ml) of the plasma-derived vaccine were compared to the usual dose injected intramuscularly in 50 patients as a cost-saving measure.[94] No significant difference was seen between the two groups in rate of seroconversion or mean titer of anti-HBs at 1 year, although titers were somewhat lower in the intradermal group. In general, the intradermal injections were better tolerated, but more difficult to administer correctly.

Vaccine should be stored at 2–8°C (36–46°F); however, freezing should be avoided since it destroys the potency of the vaccine.[80] A low rate of seroconversion has been associated with injection in the buttocks and correlates with older age.[95,96] Additionally, failures have been associated with certain batches of vaccine.[96] Only approximately half of a large series of hemodialysis patients seroconverted after primary vaccination (using 40 μg doses), while there was no clear protective effect of vaccination, perhaps because of a low attack rate in the population, as well as the low rate of seroconversion.[97]

Postvaccination antibody testing may be done within 6 months of completing the vaccine series. Revaccination of nonresponders produces adequate anti-HBsAb in approximately one-third of patients who received deltoid injections previously. Revaccination of nonresponders receiving a primary series of vaccinations in the buttocks has been shown to be over 75 percent effective and is recommended.[28]

Vaccinated patients tend to lose demonstrable protective antibody with time. The use of booster doses is controversial, although not recommended currently by the CDC, a position based on the apparent protective effect against viremia and clinical HBV infection seen in homosexual males up to 5 years after vaccination.[98] It is difficult to draw many conclusions from the study, however, in that there was a very high attrition rate (43 percent at 3 years), higher doses of vaccine were used (40 μg), and there was evidence of continued antigenic stimulation in the population suggested by the high rate of HBV infection in nonresponders. Other authors have recommended the use of a booster dose when the level of protective antibody falls below 10 mIU/ml,[87] or sequentially every 4 to 5 years, until better data are available.[99] Hemodialysis patients should receive semiannual testing, with booster doses when anti-HBsAb is less than 10 mIU/ml.

Vaccination is safe and not contraindicated in pregnancy, and it has not been associated with any transmission of HIV. The plasma-derived vaccine undergoes three separate steps to kill any viral particles, including treatment with pepsin, urea, then formalin. There have been no seroconversions to HIV in over 1 million vaccinees at low risk for AIDS.[99]

REFERENCES

1. Leibowitz S, Greenwald L, Cohen I, et al. Serum hepatitis in a blood bank worker. JAMA. 1949;140:1331–3.
2. Byrne EB. Viral hepatitis: An occupational hazard of medical personnel. Experience of the Yale–New Haven Hospital, 1952 to 1965. JAMA. 1966;195:362–4.
3. Dienstag JL, Ryan DM. Occupational exposure to hepatitis B virus in hospital personnel: Infection or immunization? Am J Epidemiol. 1982;115:26–39.
4. Hadler SC, Doto IL, Maynard JE, et al. Occupational risk of hepatitis B infection in hospital workers. Infect Control. 1985;6:24–31.
5. Hicks CG, Hargiss CO, Harris JR. Prevalence survey for hepatitis B in high-risk university hospital employees. Am J Infect Control. 1985;13:1–6.
6. Smith JL, Maynard JE, Berquist KR, et al. Comparative risk of hepatitis B among physicians and dentists. J Infect Dis. 1976;133:705–6.
7. Denes AE, Smith JL, Maynard JE, et al. Hepatitis B infection in physicians: Results of a nationwide seroepidemiologic survey. JAMA. 1978;239:210–2.
8. McLean AA, Monahan GR, Finkelstein DM. Prevalence of hepatitis B serologic markers in community hospital personnel. Am J Public Health. 1987;77:998–9.
9. Kalish SB, Fisher B, Wallemark CB, et al. Prevalence of antibody to hepatitis B virus in foreign-born hospital employees. Am J Med. 1987;83:824–8.
10. Osterholm MT, Garayalde SM. Clinical viral hepatitis B among Minnesota hospital personnel: Results of a ten-year statewide survey. JAMA. 1985;254:3207–12.
11. Feldman RE, Schiff ER. Hepatitis in dental professionals. JAMA. 1975;232:1228–30.
12. Siew C, Gruninger SE, Mitchell EW, et al. Survey of hepatitis B exposure and vaccination in volunteer dentists. J Am Dent Assoc. 1987;114:457–9.
13. Solvas JG, Castillo JL, Vela MCM, et al. The risk of infection with hepatitis B virus in relation to length of hospital employment. J Hosp Infect. 1987;9:43–7.
14. Christenson B. Acute infections with hepatitis B virus in medical personnel during a 15-year follow-up. Am J Epidemiol. 1985;122:411–7.
15. Jovanovich JF, Saravolatz LD, Arking LM. The risk of hepatitis B among select employee groups in an urban hospital. JAMA. 1983;250:1893–4.
16. Ringertz O, Nystrom B. Viral hepatitis in connection with hemodialysis and kidney transplantation. Scand J Urol Nephrol. 1967;1:192–8.
17. Garibaldi RA, Forrest JN, Bryan JA, et al. Hemodialysis-associated hepatitis. JAMA. 1973;225:384–9.
18. Snydman DR, Bergman D, Bryan JA. Hemodialysis-associated with hepatitis in the United States, 1974. J Infect Dis. 1977;135:687–91.
19. Alter MJ, Favero MS, Maynard JE. Impact of infection control strategies on the incidence of dialysis-associated hepatitis in the United States. J Infect Dis. 1986;153:1149–51.
20. Fraser GM, Fraser D, Chazan R, et al. Hepatitis B infections in a chronic hemodialysis unit in a country where hepatitis B is endemic: A prospective study. Am J Epidemiol. 1987;126:500–5.
21. Josselson J, Kyser BA, Weir MR, et al. Hepatitis B surface antigenemia in a chronic hemodialysis program: Lack of influence on morbidity and mortality. Am J Kidney Dis. 1987;9:456–61.
22. Fujita YK, Kamata K, Kameda H, et al. Detection of hepatitis B virus infection in hepatitis B surface antigen-negative hemodialysis patients by monoclonal radioimmunoassays. Gastroenterology. 1986;91:1357–63.
23. Shusterman N, Singer I. Infectious hepatitis in dialysis patients. Am J Kidney Dis. 1987;9:447–55.
24. Bond WW, Favero MS, Petersen NJ, et al. Survival of hepatitis B virus after drying and storage for one week. Lancet. 1981;1:550–1.
25. Seaworth BJ, Garrett LE, Stead WW, et al. Non-A, non-B hepatitis and chronic dialysis—another dilemma. Am J Nephrol. 1984;4:235–9.
26. LaBrecque DR, Muhs JM, Lutwick LI, et al. The risk of hepatitis B transmission from health care workers to patients in a hospital setting—a prospective study. Hepatology. 1986;6:205–8.
27. Galambos JT. Transmission of hepatitis B from providers to patients: How big is the risk? Hepatology. 1986;6:320–5.
28. Centers for Disease Control. Recommendations for protection against viral hepatitis. MMWR. 1985;34(22):313–24, 329–35.
29. Remis RS, Rossignol MA, Kane MA. Hepatitis B infection in a day school for mentally retarded students: Transmission from students to staff. Am J Public Health. 1987;77:1183–6.
30. Lohiya G, Lohiya S, Caires S, et al. Occupational risk of hepatitis B from institutionalized mentally retarded HBsAg carriers: A prospective study. J Infect Dis. 1986;154:990–5.
31. Shanson D. The risks of transmission of the HTLV-III and hepatitis B virus in the hospital. Infect Control. 1986;7(Suppl 2):128–32.
32. Radvan GH, Hewson EG, Berenger S, et al. The Newcastle hepatitis B outbreak: Observations on cause, management and prevention. Med J Aust. 1986;144:461–4.
33. Hadler SC, Sorley DL, Acree KH, et al. An outbreak of hepatitis B in a dental practice. Ann Intern Med. 1981;95:133–8.
34. Kane MA, Lettau LA. Transmission of HBV from dental personnel to patients. J Am Dent Assoc. 1985;110:634–6.
35. Shaw FE Jr, Barrett CL, Hamm R, et al. Lethal outbreak of hepatitis B in a dental practice. JAMA. 1986;255:3260–4.
36. Centers for Disease Control. Outbreak of hepatitis B associated with an oral surgeon—New Hampshire. MMWR. 1987;36:132–3.
37. Garibaldi RA, Rasmussen CM, Holmes AW, et al. Hospital-acquired serum hepatitis: Report of an outbreak. JAMA. 1972;219:1577–80.
38. Grob PJ, Moeschlin P. Risks to contacts of a medical practitioner carrying HBsAg. N Engl J Med. 1975;293:197.
39. Grob PJ, Bischof B, Naeff F. Cluster of hepatitis B transmitted by a physician. Lancet. 1981;2:1218–20.
40. Haerem JW, Siebke JC, Ulstrup J, et al. HBsAg transmission from a cardiac surgeon incubating hepatitis B resulting in chronic antigenemia in four patients. Acta Med Scand. 1981;210:389–92.
41. Coutinho RA, van Lent PA, Stoutjesdijk L, et al. Hepatitis B from doctors. Lancet. 1982;1:345–6.
42. Communicable Disease Surveillance Centre and Epidemiological Research Laboratory. Acute hepatitis B associated with gynecological surgery. Lancet. 1980;1:1–6.
43. Carl M, Blakey DL, Francis DP, et al. Interruption of hepatitis B transmission by modification of a gynecologist's surgical technique. Lancet. 1982;1:731–3.
44. Snydman DR, Hindman SH, Wineland MD, et al. Nosocomial viral hepatitis B: A cluster among staff with subsequent transmission to patients. Ann Intern Med. 1976;85:573–7.
45. Maynard JE. Nosocomial viral hepatitis. Am J Med. 1981;70:439–44.
46. Cohen SN, Dougherty WJ. Transfusion hepatitis arising from addict blood donors. JAMA. 1968;203:427–9.
47. Alter HJ, Holland PV, Purcell RH, et al. Posttransfusion hepatitis after exclusion of commercial and hepatitis B antigen-positive donors. Ann Intern Med. 1972;77:691–9.
48. Alter HJ, Seeff LB, Kaplan PM, et al. Type B hepatitis: The infectivity of blood positive for e antigen and DNA polymerase after accidental needlestick exposure. N Engl J Med. 1976;295:909–13.
49. Melnick JL, Dreesman GR, Hollinger FB. Approaching the control of viral hepatitis type B. J Infect Dis. 1976;133:210–29.
50. Holland PV, Walsh JH, Morrow AG, et al. Failure of Australia antibody to prevent post-transfusion hepatitis. Lancet. 1969;2:553–5.
51. Bove JR. Transfusion-associated hepatitis and AIDS: What is the risk? N Engl J Med. 1987;317:242–5.
52. Aach RD, Szmuness W, Mosley JW, et al. Serum alanine aminotransferase of donors in relation to the risk of non-A, non-B hepatitis in recipients: The transfusion-transmitted virus study. N Engl J Med. 1981;304:989–94.
53. Dahlke MB. Designated blood donations. N Engl J Med. 1984;310:1195.
54. Richard D. The usefulness of surrogate markers anti-HBc and ALT for post-transfusion non-A, non-B hepatitis prevention. J Virol Methods. 1987;17:105–17.
55. Colombo M, Mannucci PM, Carnelli V, et al. Transmission of non-A, non-B hepatitis by heat-treated factor VIII concentrate. Lancet. 1985;2:1–4.
56. Centers for Disease Control. Non-A, non-B hepatitis associated with a factor IX complex infused during cardiovascular surgery—Arizona. MMWR. 1986;35(24):391–9.
57. Webster ADB, Lever AML. Non-A, non-B hepatitis after intravenous gammaglobulin. Lancet. 1986;1:322.
58. Noble RC, Kane MA, Reeves SA, et al. Posttransfusion hepatitis A in a neonatal intensive care unit. JAMA. 1984;252:2711–5.
59. Rizzetto MB, Hoyer B, Canese MG, et al. Delta agent: Association of delta antigen with hepatitis B surface antigen and RNA in the serum of delta-infected chimpanzees. Natl Acad Sci Proc. 1980;77:6124–8.
60. Zanetti AR, Ponzetto A, Forzani B, et al. Worldwide epidemiology and modes of transmission of delta hepatitis. Infection. 1987;15:85–6.
61. Lettau LA, Alfred HJ, Glew RH, et al. Nosocomial transmission of delta hepatitis. Ann Intern Med. 1986;104:631–5.
62. Kharsa G, Degott C, Degos F, et al. Fulminant hepatitis in renal transplant recipients. The role of the delta agent. Transplantation. 1987;44:221–3.
63. Colledan M, Gislon M, Doglia M, et al. Liver transplantation in patients with B viral hepatitis and delta infection. Transplant Proc. 1987;19:4073–6.
64. Baptiste R, Koziol D, Henderson DK. Nosocomial transmission of hepatitis A in an adult population. Infect Control. 1987;8:364–70.
65. Krober MS, Bass JW, Brown JD, et al. Hospital outbreak of hepatitis A: risk factors for spread. Pediatr Infect Dis. 1984;3:296–9.
66. Skidmore SJ, Gully PR, Middleton JD, et al. An outbreak of hepatitis A on a hospital ward. J Med Virol. 1985;17:175–7.
67. Edgar WM, Campbell AD. Nosocomial infection with hepatitis A. J Infect. 1985;10:43–7.
68. Ebisawa I, Kurosu Y, Hatashita T. Nursery-associated hepatitis A traced to a male nurse. J Hyg Camb. 1984;92:251–4.
69. Eisenstein AB, Aach RD, Jacobsohn W, et al. An epidemic of infectious hepatitis in a general hospital: Probable transmission by contaminated orange juice. JAMA. 1963;185:171–4.
70. Hollinger FB, Khan NC, Oefinger PE, et al. Posttransfusion hepatitis type A. JAMA. 1983;250:2313–7.
71. Sherertz RJ, Russell BA, Reuman PD. Transmission of hepatitis A by transfusion of blood products. Arch Intern Med. 1984;144:1579–80.
72. Stevens CE, Beasley RP, Tsui J, et al. Vertical transmission of hepatitis B antigen in Taiwan. N Engl J Med. 1975;292:771–4.
73. Beasley RP, Hwang LY, Lin CC, et al. Hepatocellular carcinoma and hepatitis B virus. A prospective study of 22,707 men in Taiwan. Lancet. 1981;2:1129–33.
74. Beasley RP, Hwang LY, Stevens CE, et al. Efficacy of hepatitis B immune

globulin for prevention of perinatal transmission of the hepatitis B virus carrier state: Final report of a randomized double-blind, placebo-controlled trial. Hepatology. 1983;3:135–41.
75. Beasley RP, Hwang LY, Lee GCY, et al. Prevention of perinatally transmitted hepatitis B virus infections with hepatitis B immune globulin and hepatitis B vaccine. Lancet. 1983;2:1099–102.
76. Wong VCW, Ip HMH, Reesink HW, et al. Prevention of the HBsAg carrier state in newborn infants of mothers who are chronic carriers of HBsAg and HBeAg by administration of hepatitis B vaccine and hepatitis B immunoglobulin. Lancet. 1984;1:921–6.
77. Lo KJ, Tsai YT, Lee SD, et al. Immunoprophylaxis of infection with hepatitis B virus in infants born to hepatitis B surface antigen-positive carrier mothers. J Infect Dis. 1985;152:817–22.
78. Stevens CE, Toy PT, Tong MJ, et al. Perinatal hepatitis B virus transmission in the United States: Prevention by passive–active immunization. JAMA. 1985;253:1740–5.
79. Stevens CE, Taylor PE, Tong MJ, et al. Yeast-recombinant hepatitis B vaccine: Efficacy with hepatitis B immune globulin in prevention of perinatal hepatitis B virus transmission. JAMA. 1987;257:2612–6.
80. Ko TM, Lin KH, Ho MM, et al. Reduced doses of hepatitis B immune globulin in the prevention of perinatal transmission of hepatitis B. J Med Virol. 1987;21:301–9.
81. Kumar ML, Dawson NV, McCullough AJ, et al. Should all pregnant women be screened for hepatitis B? Ann Intern Med. 1987;107:273–7.
82. Jonas MM, Schiff ER, O'Sullivan MJ, et al. Failure of Centers for Disease Control criteria to identify hepatitis B infection in a large municipal obstetrical population. Ann Intern Med. 1987;107:335–7.
83. McQuillan GM, Townsend TR, Johannes CB, et al. Prevention of perinatal transmission of hepatitis B virus: The sensitivity, specificity and predictive value of the recommended screening questions to detect high-risk women in an obstetric population. Am J Epidemiol. 1987;126:484–91.
84. Stevens CE. Perinatal hepatitis B virus infection: Screening of pregnant women and protection of the infant. Ann Intern Med. 1987;107:412–3.
85. Berry WR, Gottesfeld RL, Alter HJ, et al. Transmission of hepatitis B virus by artificial insemination. JAMA. 1987;257:1079–81.
86. Hall WT, Madden DL, Mundon FK, et al. Protective effect of immune serum globulin (ISG) against hepatitis A infection in a natural epidemic. Am J Epidemiol. 1977;106:72–5.
87. Schiff ER, Brooks WS, Fisher R, et al. Immunoprophylaxis of viral hepatitis: A practical guide. Am J Gastroenterol. 1987;82:287–91.
88. Valenti WM. Hepatitis B prevention: 1. A review of ACIP's newest guidelines. Infect Control. 1986;7:74–7.
89. Centers for Disease Control. Immune globulins for protection against viral hepatitis. MMWR. 1977;26(52):425–8, 441–2.
90. Centers for Disease Control. Update on hepatitis B prevention. MMWR. 1987;36:353–66.
91. Corrao G, Zotti C, Tinivella F, et al. HBV pre-vaccination screening in hospital personnel: Cost-effectiveness analysis. Eur J Epidemiol. 1987;3:25–9.
92. Zajac BA, West DJ, McAleer WJ, et al. Overview of clinical studies with hepatitis B vaccine made by recombinant DNA. J Infect. 1986;13(Suppl A):39–45.
93. Zahradnik JM, Couch RB, Gerin JL. Safety and immunogenicity of a purified hepatitis B virus vaccine prepared by using recombinant DNA technology. J Infect Dis. 1987;155:903–8.
94. Redfield RR, Innis BL, Scott RM, et al. Clinical evaluation of low-dose intradermally administered hepatitis B virus vaccine: A cost reduction strategy. JAMA. 1985;254:3203–6.
95. Klotz SA, Normand R, Silberman R. Hepatitis B vaccine in healthy hospital employees. Infect Control. 1986;7:365–9.
96. Weber DJ, Rutala WA, Samsa GP, et al. Obesity as a predictor of poor antibody response to hepatitis B plasma vaccine. JAMA. 1985;254:3187–9.
97. Stevens CE, Alter HJ, Taylor PE, et al. Hepatitis B vaccine in patients receiving hemodialysis: Immunogenicity and efficacy. N Engl J Med. 1984;311:496–501.
98. Hadler SC, Francis DP, Maynard JE, et al. Long-term immunogenicity and efficacy of hepatitis B vaccine in homosexual men. N Engl J Med. 1986;315:209–14.
99. Hollinger FB. Hepatitis B vaccines—to switch or not to switch. JAMA. 1987;257:2634–6.

283. HIV-1 IN THE HEALTH-CARE SETTING

DAVID K. HENDERSON

Shortly after the first descriptions of the acquired immunodeficiency syndrome (AIDS) were published,[1–4] the Centers for Disease Control (CDC) issued the first set of guidelines designed to minimize the risk for transmission of this syndrome.[5] At that time the agent responsible for AIDS had not yet been identified; these early recommendations were based on what, to that point, had been learned about the epidemiology of AIDS. For health-care providers, these early epidemiologic studies were disquieting rather than reassuring. The epidemiology of AIDS in the community appeared to parallel the epidemiology of hepatitis B, and health-care workers were already aware of the significant risks for occupational/nosocomial transmission of this disease.[6–8]

Discovery of the agent responsible for AIDS[9,10] and the subsequent development of serologic tests for antibodies directed against the human immunodeficiency virus, type I (HIV-1) have allowed health-care professionals the opportunity to gain further insight into the relative risks for occupational/nosocomial transmission of HIV-1.

The purpose of this chapter is to summarize the current state of knowledge regarding these risks and to discuss appropriate means for minimizing these risks as well as other issues relevant to the management of HIV-1-infected individuals in the health-care setting.

OCCUPATIONAL/NOSOCOMIAL TRANSMISSION OF HIV-1

Routes of Transmission

In the community, HIV-1 infection is primarily a sexually transmitted disease, but it can also be spread by direct inoculation, such as might occur as a result of sharing needles in the process of intravenous substance use, or through receipt of transfusions of blood or blood products that are contaminated with HIV-1.

In the health-care setting, the major risk for transmission is associated with percutaneous exposure to blood or blood-containing body fluids contaminated with HIV-1.[11–15] Although other types of exposures may be occasionally responsible for occupational/nosocomial infection,[16] the relative risk for transmission by these routes is likely to be significantly smaller than for percutaneous exposure.[13]

Percutaneous Exposures

HIV-1 primarily infects cells bearing the CD4 epitope (primarily T4 lymphocytes and cells of the macrophage–monocyte line). These cells are most commonly found in blood, but are also found (usually in significantly smaller concentrations) in other body fluids. One might hypothesize that percutaneous exposure to large quantities of body fluids containing the highest concentrations of these cells would be most likely to transmit HIV-1 infection. For example, transfusion of a unit of blood known to be contaminated with HIV-1 has been shown to be an extremely efficient mechanism for transmission of HIV-1.[17,18] In the health-care setting, then, the type of exposure that would seem most likely to fulfill these criteria is an accidental injection of blood or a transcutaneous exposure to a sharp object contaminated with blood that contains cells infected with HIV-1.

Eighteen health-care and/or scientific laboratory workers have developed documented HIV-1 antibody seroconversions following an adverse exposure in the health-care setting[13,15,16,19–31a] (summarized in Table 1, sections A and B). Of these 18, 13 reported percutaneous exposures,[13,15,19–26,28,31,31a] 11 reported needlestick injuries,[13,15,19–24,26,28,31,31a] and 2 reported cuts with sharp objects contaminated with material containing HIV-1.[25,26,30]

Of the 8 HIV-1-seropositive health-care workers who are reported as possible occupational infections, but in whom seroconversions were not documented in sequential serum samples, 5 related a history of at least one percutaneous injury.[12,15,19,32,33]

TABLE 1. Health-Care Workers Reported to Have Acquired Occupational HIV Infection

	Authors (Ref.)	Sex	Occupation	Exposure
A.	Documented seroconversion following percutaneous exposures			
	Anonymous[22]	F	Nurse	Needlestick
	Oskenhendler et al.[23]	F	Nurse	Needlestick
	Neisson-Vernant et al.[24]	F	Nurse	Needlestick
	Stricof and Morse[21,a]	F	Nurse	Needlestick
	CDC[20]	F	Nurse	Needlesticks
	CDC[20]	F	Nurse	Needlestick
	Weiss et al.[25]	M	Lab worker	Cut with contaminated sharp object
	Gerberding et al.[13]	F	Nurse	Needlestick
	CDC[15]	F	Nurse	Needlestick, rapid progression to AIDS
	Ramsey et al.[28]	F	Nurse	Needlestick
	Henderson et al.[30]	F	Lab Worker	Cut with contaminated sharp object
	Michelet et al.[31]	F	Nurse	Needlestick
	Wallace and Harrison[31a]	M	Medical Corpsman	Needlestick
B.	Documented seroconversion following other exposures			
	CDC[27]	F	Mother	Multiple cutaneous exposures to blood
	CDC[16]	F	Emergency room worker	Prolonged exposure of nonintact skin to blood
	CDC[16]	F	Phlebotomist	Mucous membrane exposure
	CDC[16]	F	Medical technologist	Blood on nonintact skin
	Gioannini et al.[29]	F	ICU nurse	Large cutaneous/mucous membrane exposure
C.	Health-care workers found seropositive following HIV-related injury/exposure			
	Weiss et al.[12b]	F	Health-care worker	Two needlestick injuries
	Weiss et al.[12b]	F	Health-care worker	Biopsy forceps injury
	Weiss et al.[12b]	M	Health-care worker	Capillary tube injury
	Weiss et al.[23]	M	Lab worker	Frequent opportunity for cutaneous exposure to virus
D.	Health-care workers found seropositive: no documented HIV-1-related exposure, no community risk behavior			
	Weiss et al.[12b]	F	Nurse	N/A (reported anonymously)
	Gilmore et al.[43]	F	Health care administrator	None known
	Klein et al.[32]	M	Dentist	None reported (history of cuts and needlesticks; sources unknown)
	Ponce de Leon et al.[33]	M	Medical technician	None known specifically (history of numerous exposures)

Mucous Membrane Exposures

Of the 17 documented HIV-1 antibody seroconversions among health-care workers, 2 were associated with significant mucous membrane exposures to blood from HIV-1-infected patients[16,29] (Table 1, section B). Both were extensive exposures.

Other Exposures

Two of the seventeen health-care workers who seroconverted following occupational/nosocomial exposures reported getting blood from an HIV-1-infected patient either on an open wound or on nonintact skin.[15,16] One of the seventeen reported extensive cutaneous contact with blood and other body fluids from an HIV-1-infected patient.[27] In each of these instances, transmission is presumed to have occurred as a result of the health-care worker getting contaminated blood or blood-containing body fluids on nonintact skin (i.e., inapparent parenteral transmission).

Occupational/nosocomial transmission of other blood-borne infectious diseases by inapparent parenteral inoculation (e.g., hepatitis B) is well documented. Fewer than 50 percent of health-care professionals who develop hepatitis B recall a specific percutaneous injury.[34] One research laboratory worker acquired infection with the same strain of HIV-1 that was being processed in the laboratory, presumably through contact with concentrated viral preparation on nonintact skin.[15,25,26] I am aware of no evidence that supports transmission of HIV-1 in the health-care setting by any other route of transmission. Both Friedland[18] and Lifson[35] have presented formidable evidence that "casual-contact" transmission, environmental transmission, or aerosol/respiratory transmission is not occurring.

Body Fluids Implicated

HIV-1 has been cultured from blood, semen, tears, saliva, vaginal secretions, breast milk, cerebrospinal fluid, urine, alveolar fluid, and synovial fluid. Furthermore, it seems entirely plausible that careful study of other body fluids will eventually yield HIV-1 in culture. In the community, transmission of HIV-1 has been associated with blood, semen, and vaginal secretions. In the health-care setting, most of the cases of occupational/nosocomial infection with HIV-1 have been associated with exposure to blood.[12,13,15,16,19–22,24,27–31a] Three instances of occupational infection have been associated with something other than blood.[23,25,26] In two of these instances, scientific laboratory workers were exposed to culture fluid containing high titers of HIV-1.[15,25,26] In the third instance a clinical health-care worker sustained a needlestick injury with a needle that had been used to aspirate bloody pleural fluid from a patient who had AIDS.[23]

HIV-1 INFECTION IN HEALTH-CARE WORKERS

AIDS

A few cases of AIDS in health-care workers who deny participation in behaviors known to place individuals at risk for HIV-1 infection have been reported as anecdotes in the literature.[36–39] In addition, as part of routine AIDS surveillance activities, epidemiologists at CDC have asked state and local health authorities to question AIDS patients regarding their past employment histories, specifically requesting that the local authorities ask whether the individual had worked in a health-care or clinical laboratory setting since 1978.[15] Periodic summaries of these data have been reported, initially by Lifson and colleagues[40] and more recently by Chamberland et al.[41] Through May, 1988, 53,010 patients with AIDS whose employment histories were known had been reported to CDC.[41] Of these cases, 2,805 (5.3 percent) occurred in individuals who related a history of working in a health-care or laboratory setting since 1978.[41] This percentage compares favorably to the 5.7 percent of the work force in the United States that is employed in the health-care industry.[15,42]

When compared with all other AIDS patients, health-care workers with AIDS were more likely to relate a history of male homosexuality or bisexuality and less likely to relate a history of intravenous substance abuse (Table 2).[41] Comparing demographic information obtained from health-care workers who

TABLE 2. Characteristics of Health-Care Workers (HCWs) and All Other Patients Reported to CDC with AIDS

Characteristic	*HCW* (N = 2805)	p *Value*	*All Others* (N = 50,205)
Male sex	92%	NS	92%
Mean age (years)	37	NS	37
Caucasian	63%	<0.0001	59%
Black	26%	NS	25%
Hispanic	9%	<0.0001	15%
Male homosexual/bisexual	74%	<0.001	63%
IV drug user (IVDA)	6%	<0.001	19%
Male homosexual/bisexual IVDA	7%	NS	7%
Heterosexual exposure	5%	NS	4%
Transfusion of blood/ blood products	3%	NS	4%
No reported/identified risk	5%	<0.001	3%

(Modified from Chamberland et al.,[41] with permission.)

have AIDS with all other AIDS patients reported to CDC demonstrates minimal differences (Table 2).

Health-care workers were also more likely to report no known risk factors for HIV-1 infection (5.3 percent for the health-care workers vs. 2.8 percent for all other AIDS patients ($p < 0.001$, chi-square test)[41] (Table 2). The reasons that health-care workers are overrepresented in this population are not known, but they may include underreporting of risk behaviors by health-care workers as well as occupational exposure and infection.[15] The percentage of health-care workers classified as having "no identified risk" has remained reasonably stable over time,[41] and the percentage of all of the "no identified risk" cases accounted for by health-workers has remained quite stable over time at approximately 9–10 percent.[41] Health-care workers initially reported to CDC as having AIDS with "no identified risk" were more likely to be female (29 percent for health-care workers vs. 24 percent for all other patients reporting "no identified risk")[41] and were more likely to reside outside of the five states reporting the most cases.[41]

As of May, 1988, 236 cases of AIDS had been reported to CDC as having occurred in health-care workers who reported no known risk for HIV-1 (Table 3).[41] Of the 236, information from the "no identified risk" investigation was incomplete for 112 (21 of these patients either died before a thorough history regarding risk behaviors could be taken or refused to be interviewed regarding participation in risk behaviors; 91 were still being investigated by CDC).[41] For 124 of the 236, secondary interviews or other follow-up information had been obtained by investigators at CDC by May, 1988. Of the 124, 84 (68 percent) had been reclassified into one of the traditional transmission categories, leaving only 40 health-care workers whose investigations had been completed in the "no identified risk" transmission category.[41] These 40 individuals represent less than 0.1 percent of all cases of AIDS reported to CDC at that time and 1.4 percent of all health-care workers with AIDS reported to CDC.[41]

Chamberland and her colleagues have performed a detailed analysis of the 40 health-care workers with AIDS who remained in the "no identified risk" category following further investigation (Table 1, section E).[41] These investigators noted some striking differences when comparisons were made between this group of 40 health-care workers and all health-care workers in the United States.[41] For example, 29 (73 percent) of the 40 are males, although according to the United States Bureau of Labor,[42] 77 percent of U.S. health-care workers are female. When the occupations of these 40 health-care workers were compared with health-care workers who have AIDS associated with an identified risk behavior, the only occupation that was significantly overrepresented among the "no identified risk" cases was maintenance workers (20 percent for "no identified risk" cases vs. 6 percent for those with identifiable risk factors ($p < 0.004$, Fisher's exact test).[41]

TABLE 3. Health Care Workers Who Have AIDS Associated with No Identified Risk

Authors (Ref.)	*Summary*
Chamberland et al.[41]	236 cases initially reported to CDC as having AIDS with "no identified risk"
	84 reclassified into traditional transmission category
	21 on whom further information unobtainable; 91 still under investigation
	40 (29 males, 11 females) completed CDC interview and remained "no identified risk"; includes 8 physicians, 1 dentist, 5 nurses, 11 nurses' aides, 7 service workers, 4 technicians, 1 physical therapist, 1 emergency medical technician, 1 embalmer, and 2 others
	16/40 had at least 1 needlestick in the past 10 years; 24/40 had "no exposure"
	25/40 worked in a hospital, 6 in a nursing home
Barker[39]	Male physician in Baltimore reported percutaneous exposure to blood in 1983; developed AIDS in 1986
Bygbjerg[36]	Female Danish surgeon died of AIDS in 1977 following multiple exposures in Zaire during 1975 and 1976
Belani et al.[37]	Male operating room technician (Baltimore) retrospectively reported needlestick injury after being diagnosed with AIDS; denied risk behaviors
Grint and McEvoy[38]	Female housewife developed AIDS 2½ years after caring for a dying 33-year-old Ghanian man who later was shown to be HIV-infected; "health-care worker" provided care without barriers, had frequent contact with secretions and excreta; during this time, worker had small cuts on hand and also had an acute exacerbation of chronic eczema

[a] Also reported by McCray et al.[19]
[b] Also reported by CDC.[44]

HIV-1 Antibody Seropositivity

Case Reports. The difficulty in obtaining accurate histories regarding participation in behaviors known to place individuals at risk for HIV-1 infection is emphasized by the studies of Lifson et al.[40] and Chamberland and her colleagues.[41] In addition, because of the question of compensation, health-care workers may have an added incentive to mislead interviewers regarding participation in risk behaviors. Nonetheless, several well-documented cases of occupational/nosocomial transmission of HIV-1 have demonstrated that there is a risk for transmission of this virus in the health-care setting.

Three general types of case reports have appeared in the medical literature describing occupational HIV-1 infection: (*1*) reports describing health-care workers identified as being positive for antibody to HIV-1 who deny participation in risk behaviors and do not recall any adverse exposures to blood or body fluids from an HIV-1-infected patient (4 cases) (Table 1, section D)[12,32,33,43]; (*2*) case reports of health-care workers identified as being positive for antibody to HIV-1 following an adverse exposure to blood, body fluids, or culture fluids containing HIV-1, but for whom no serum sample is available from the health-care worker near the time of the adverse exposure to demonstrate that the health-care worker was not infected prior to the exposure (4 cases) (Table 1, section C)[12,25,44]; and (*3*) case reports describing health-care workers who sustained injuries, had blood specimens drawn near the time of their injuries that demonstrated absence of HIV-1 antibody, who were followed prospectively and subsequently found to seroconvert (18 cases) (Table 1, Sections A and B).[13,15,16,19–31a]

Taken together, these reports describe 26 health-care workers who were found to be HIV-1-infected in these studies. In 2 of these cases,[12,44] the infected health-care worker's sexual partner was also found to be infected, and heterosexual transmission of the virus could not be excluded.[44]

Prevalence Studies. Several studies have attempted to address the issue of HIV-1 transmission in the health-care setting by measuring the prevalence of HIV-1 infection in cohorts of health-care workers.[12,19,32,43,45–52] These studies are summarized in Table 4. The very low prevalence of HIV-1 infection among these health-care workers provided the first indirect evidence that the risk for transmission of HIV-1 in the health-care setting was small. When compared with the prevalence of infection in the population at large, health-care workers did not appear to be overrepresented among individuals with documented HIV-1 infection.

More recently, Kelley and coworkers analyzed data from the United States Army's HIV-1 screening program to determine if health-care workers in this branch of the military were overrepresented in the population of individuals determined to

TABLE 4. HIV-1 Seroprevalence Studies in Health Care Workers

Authors (Ref.)	*No. Evaluated*	*No. Reporting HIV-Related Needlestick Exposure*	*No. Reporting Other HIV-Related Exposures*	*No. HIV-1 Seropositive*	*No. of Seropositives Reporting Community Risk*	*No. of Seropositives Reporting No Community Risk*	*Overall Prevalence (%)*	*Prevalence Excluding Seropositives Who Report Community Risk (%)*	*Comment*
Weiss et al.[12]	359	42	NS	8	6	2*	2.2	0.57	One worker entirely anonymous; the second had seropositive sexual partner; heterosexual transmission could not be excluded (44)
Marcus et al.[55]	1054	856	198	4	0	4*	0.38	0.38	One seropositive worker has seropositive sexual partner (also included in series reported by Weiss et al [12]); includes individuals in CDC longitudinal study
Weiss et al.[25]	265	10	35	1	0	1	0.38	0.38	Laboratory worker with frequent opportunities for cutaneous exposures to virus cultures and concentrated virus preparations
Klein et al.[32]	1322	NS	NS	5	4	1	0.38	0.08	One seropositive dentist; no known history of parenteral exposure to HIV; history of multiple needlestick injuries; treats known high-risk patients
Gilmore et al.[43]	1590	NS	NS	2	1	1	0.13	0.06	One female office worker (no patient or specimen contact) found positive
Hirsch et al.[45]	85	30	3	0	0	0	0	0	
Weiss et al.[46]	188	NS	NS	0	0	0	0	0	
Shanson et al.[47]	151	7	NS	1	1	0	0.66	0	
Ebbesen et al.[48]	961	NS	NS	0	0	0	0	0	
Lubick et al.[49]	10	NS	NS	0	0	0	0	0	
Harper et al.[50]	325	NS	NS	0	0	0	0	0	
Boland et al.[51]	45	3	2	0	0	0	0	0	
Gerberding et al.[52]	264	22	NS	0	0	0	0	0	Survey of dental personnel
Total	6619	970	238	21	12	8	0.32	0.12	

have positive HIV-1 serologies.[53] Female medical personnel in the Army were less likely to have HIV-1 antibodies than were female nonmedical personnel. Although male health-care providers did have a higher prevalence of HIV-1 infection, this risk could not be related to level or intensity of blood exposure.[53] In this study, the major adjusted risk factor for HIV-1 infection among male health-care personnel was marital status, with unmarried male medical personnel having a relative risk for infection of 3.2 when compared with married medical personnel.[53]

Prospective/Longitudinal Studies. MAGNITUDE OF RISK ASSOCIATED WITH PERCUTANEOUS EXPOSURE TO BLOOD OR BLOOD-CONTAINING BODY FLUIDS FROM A PATIENT WITH HIV-1 INFECTION. The case reports of occupational/nosocomial transmission of HIV-1 clearly document that there is an occupational risk for HIV-1 transmission; the prevalence studies cited above suggested that the risk for transmission of HIV-1 was apparently small.[54] Neither the anecdotal reports nor the prevalence studies allow estimation of the magnitude of risk for infection. Longitudinal cohort studies of health-care workers involved in the day-to-day care of HIV-1-infected patients and in the handling and processing of specimens from such patients provide the best available evidence regarding the magnitude of risk for transmission of this virus in the health-care setting.

As of August, 1988, I am aware of 10 ongoing prospective studies that are attempting to measure the magnitude of risk for HIV-1 transmission in the health-care setting.[28,30,52,55–61] All 10 studies are following health-care workers who have reported percutaneous exposures to blood or body fluids from a patient known to have HIV-1 infection (Table 5). In these studies 1320 health-care workers have reported a total of 1389 percutaneous exposures to blood or other body fluids from a patient known to harbor HIV-1. Five instances of occupational/nosocomial infection are recorded in these 10 studies, for an overall risk of transmission per injury of 0.36 percent (95 percent confidence interval 0.12–0.84 percent, Poisson). The risk for transmission calculated per participant is 0.38 percent (95 percent confidence interval 0.12–0.88 percent Poisson). Thus the risk for transmission of HIV-1 following a documented percutaneous exposure to blood or blood-containing body fluids from a patient known to have HIV-1 infection is approximately 1 in 250 injuries.

MAGNITUDE OF RISK ASSOCIATED WITH MUCOUS MEMBRANE EXPOSURE TO BLOOD OR BLOOD-CONTAINING BODY FLUIDS FROM A PATIENT WITH HIV-1 INFECTION. Eight studies have evaluated health-care workers who have reported mucous membrane exposures to blood or body fluids from a patient who has HIV-1 infection[28,30,52,55–59] (Table 6). Although anecdotal case reports document that HIV-1 can be transmitted following a mucous membrane exposure in the health-care setting,[16,29] none of the 8 studies have detected a seroconversion following this type of exposure.[28,30,52,55–59] In these studies, 538 health-care workers have reported a total of 921 mucous membrane exposures with no seroconversions. Pooling the results of these studies, the upper boundary of the 95 percent confidence interval for the rate of transmission per mucous membrane exposure is 0.33 percent, with the actual risk likely to be significantly smaller.

MAGNITUDE OF RISK IN THE ABSENCE OF AN ADVERSE EXPOSURE TO BLOOD OR BODY FLUIDS. Three of these studies are also following health care workers who provide care for HIV-1-infected pa-

TABLE 5. Summary of Published Prospective Studies of the Risk for Occupational/Nosocomial Transmission of HIV-1 Following Percutaneous Exposure[a]

Authors (Ref.)	*Health-Care Workers Studied*	*No. of Percutaneous Exposures Reported*	*No. of Seroconversions*	*Seroconversion Rate per Person (%)*	*Seroconversion Rate Per Event (%)*
Marcus et al.[55]	582	582	3	0.52	0.52
Gerberding et al.[52]	180	224	1	0.56	0.45
Henderson et al.[30]	108	126	0	0	0
McEvoy et al.[57]	76	76	0	0	0
Kuhls et al.[56]	45	52	0	0	0
Wormser et al.[58]	48	48	0	0	0
Elmslie et al.[59]	115	115	0	0	0
Ramsey et al.[28]	31	31	1	3.23	0
Hernandez et al.[60]	58	58	0	0	0
Pizzocolo et al.[61]	77	77	0	0	0
Total	1320	1389	5	0.38	0.36

[a] All study participants included in this table have (*1*) sustained a percutaneous exposure to blood or blood-containing body fluids from a patient known to be HIV-1-infected; (*2*) had serum samples obtained within 30 days of exposure to document seronegativity at the time of exposure; and (*3*) been followed for a minimum of 90 days following exposure.

TABLE 6. Summary of Published Prospective Studies of the Risk for Occupational/Nosocomial Transmission of HIV-1 Following Mucous Membrane Exposure[a]

Authors (Ref.)	*Health-Care Workers Studied*	*No. of Mucous Membrane Exposures Reported*	*No. of Seroconversions*	*Seroconversion Rate per Person (%)*	*Seroconversion Rate Per Event (%)*
Marcus et al.[55]	38	38	0	0	0
Gerberding et al.[52]	168	401	0	0	0
Henderson et al.[30]	234	337	0	0	0
McEvoy et al.[57]	24	24	0	0	0
Kuhls et al.[56]	34	81	0	0	0
Wormser et al.[58]	3	3	0	0	0
Elmslie et al.[59]	24	24	0	0	0
Ramsey et al.[28]	13	13	0	0	0
Total	538	921	0	0	0

[a] All study participants included in this table have (*1*) sustained a mucous membrane exposure to blood or blood-containing body fluids from a patient known to be HIV-1-infected; (*2*) had serum samples obtained within 30 days of exposure to document seronegativity at the time of exposure; and (*3*) followed for a minimum of 90 days following exposure.

tients but who do not relate a history of a percutaneous or mucous membrane exposure to blood or other body fluids from these patients[30,52,56] (Table 7). No seroconversions have been documented among study participants in these studies in the absence of an adverse exposure. In addition, the elegant studies of household contacts of HIV-1-infected patients (reviewed in ref. 18) suggest minimal risk associated with this type of exposure. The magnitude of risk for occupational/nosocomial transmission of HIV-1 in the absence of an adverse event is so small as to currently elude estimation. In all likelihood, this risk will continue to be below the limits of detection.

Risk Factors. Although there has been a great deal of speculation about factors associated with an increased risk for occupational/nosocomial transmission of HIV-1, no study has demonstrated that any single risk factor (with the possible exception of the percutaneous route of injury) is associated with an increased risk for transmission of HIV-1 in the health-care setting. Although it seems probable that certain procedures or techniques are likely to be associated with an increased level of risk for occupational/nosocomial infection, none have yet been documented. In addition, a variety of other factors may influence the risk for occupational HIV-1 infection. Factors that have been proposed as possible contributors to this risk are listed in Table 8. These factors may relate to the injury, to the patient (i.e., the source/donor), or to the health-care worker (i.e., recipient). A number of the anecdotal case reports of occupational infection have been associated with deep or severe injuries[15,19–22,25,30]; however, a few have occurred after superficial injuries.[23,24] Donors for 12 of the 17 evaluable seroconversions (one health-care worker became infected following two exposures—one to blood from a patient who had AIDS, the other to a patient who was only HIV-1 seropositive) were patients meeting the CDC criteria for AIDS.[15,19–22,24,28,30–31a] Conversely, 4 of the documented infections occurred following adverse exposures to blood from patients infected with HIV-1 who did not meet the criteria for AIDS. Reason argues that some, if not most, of the factors listed in Table 8 contribute to this risk; however, we all await definitive studies that allow us to define and characterize the relative contribution of these (and presumably other) risk factors.

The prospective studies cited above that are attempting to measure the magnitude of risk for occupational/nosocomial transmission of HIV-1 are all measuring the risk associated with a single event. A number of other factors will obviously affect the cumulative risk for an individual health-care worker. Occupations that are associated with an increased likelihood of adverse exposures are clearly more likely to be associated with an elevated cumulative risk for occupational infection with blood-borne pathogens. Using the hepatitis B virus (HBV) model for comparison, prevalence studies demonstrate that roughly 30 percent of surgeons (in the era prior to the availability of the hepatitis B vaccine) had serologic evidence of exposure to HBV.[62] Other occupations in the health-care setting that are associated with increased risk for adverse exposures have also been associated with an increased risk for HBV infection.[62] Thus, although the "one-hit" risk for infection with HIV-1 following an adverse exposure is relatively small, as yet no data have been generated that address cumulative risk for various health-care occupations. A variety of other factors will probably influence an individual health-care professional's risk, including (but by no means limited to) prevalence of HIV-1 infection in the health-care worker's patient population, level of experience, frequency of performing invasive procedures, types of invasive procedures performed, case load, and frequency of unsafe work practices.

TABLE 7. Summary of Published Prospective Studies of the Risk for Occupational/Nosocomial Transmission of HIV-1 As a Result of Routine Patient Care Activity in the Absence of any Adverse Exposure[a]

Authors (Ref.)	*Health-Care Workers Studied*	*No. of Seroconversions*	*Seroconversion Rate (%)*
Gerberding et al.[52]	120	0	0
Henderson et al.[30]	689	0	0
Kuhls et al.[56]	120	0	0
Total	929	0	0

[a] All study participants included in this table have been followed for at least 6 months.

TABLE 8. Factors Possibly Influencing Risks for Occupational/Nosocomial Transmission of HIV-1

Factors related to the injury
- Route of exposure
- Depth of injury
- Size of defect in integument
- Amount of contamination
- Type of contamination (i.e., body fluid, culture material, etc.)
- Amount of time elapsed since specimen was withdrawn from the source (donor) (i.e., was injury associated with a "hot needle"?)
- Concentration of virus/virus-infected cells in fluid
- Presence of CD4-positive cells at site of exposure

Patient (donor)-related factors
- Donor's stage of HIV-related illness
- Presence/absence of free virus in the circulation (viremia)
- Presence/absence of circulating p24 antigen
- Number and concentration of HIV-1-infected cells in the circulation
- Antiviral chemotherapy

Employee (recipient)-related factors
- Histocompatibility
- Lack of skin integrity
- Poor hygiene (e.g., handwashing)
- Inadequate first aid following exposure
- Concurrent viral infection (e.g., EBV, CMV) resulting in increased CD4 expression
- Chronic inflammation at/around skin entry site
- Immunologic status

Relative Risk in the Health-Care Setting. Although the risk for occupational/nosocomial transmission of HIV-1 infection has been the source of significant anxiety for many health-care professionals during the past 7 years, it is important to keep the relative risk for occupational HIV-1 infection in perspective. For a blood-borne infectious disease, the risk for HIV-1 transmission following an occupational percutaneous exposure is relatively small. For example, as noted above, the risk for transmission of HIV-1 following a percutaneous injury is approximately 0.36 percent. The risk for infection with HBV following a percutaneous exposure to blood from a patient known to be hepatitis B "e" antigen-positive has been estimated to be between 27 and 43 percent[6–8]; the risk for such an exposure to result in clinically significant hepatitis in these studies ranged between 6 and 24 percent.[6–8] Despite the availability of a safe and effective vaccine, CDC has estimated that approximately 12,000 new cases of hepatitis B infection related to occupational exposure occur in health-care workers in the United States annually.[63] The Occupational Safety and Health Administration (OSHA) has estimated that between 167 and 202 health care workers died from occupationally acquired hepatitis B infection in 1987.[64] Perhaps most tragically, OSHA also estimates that only 30–40 percent of the "at risk" health-care worker population have received the hepatitis B vaccine.[65]

Thus, while it is clear that there are definite and definable risks for transmission of HIV-1 in the health-care setting, it is equally clear that the magnitude of risk for occupational/nosocomial infection with this virus compares favorably with risks that health-care workers have been taking (and, unfortunately, have been far too cavalier about) for decades. The health-care setting was not a risk-free environment prior to the advent of AIDS and HIV-1 infection. In addition to the risk for occupational acquisition of hepatitis B infection, a number of other pathogens, such as *Mycobacterium tuberculosis* and rubella virus, have been identified as representing defined occupational risks to health-care workers; risks associated with the management of patients infected with other pathogens, such as the agent responsible for non-A, non-B hepatitis and the human T-lymphotropic virus, type 1, remain to be characterized. Furthermore, it seems likely that additional occupational/nosocomial pathogens will be identified in the future.

In the past, such risks have not precluded the provision of high-quality health-care. When contrasted with the occupational risks all of us have been taking for years, this new risk provided by AIDS/HIV-1 infection does not seem to warrant the attention that it has received. When assessed in the appropriate context, decisions not to provide care to HIV-1-infected individuals seem incongruent.

Management of HIV-1-Infected Health-Care Workers

The risk for staff-to-patient transmission of HIV-1 has also been a topic of some concern. The first clear guidance issued on this subject was published by CDC in October, 1985.[11] Subsequently CDC issued a set of guidelines for the management of HIV-1-infected personnel who perform invasive procedures.[66] These guidelines used hepatitis B infection as a model for HIV-1 transmission, since no data were available that addressed the risk for staff-to-patient transmission of HIV-1. Although patient-to-health-care-worker transmission of hepatitis B is a relatively common event, staff-to-patient transmission is rare.[11] Since HIV-1 appeared to be even less transmissible than HBV in the health-care setting, CDC recommended that HIV-1-infected health-care workers who are otherwise fit for duty and who do not perform invasive procedures be allowed to perform their usual duties.[11] In subsequent guidelines, CDC recommended that HIV-1-infected individuals who perform invasive procedures be evaluated on a case-by-case basis.[66] In August, 1987, CDC revised and consolidated all previous recommendations for preventing the transmission of HIV-1 in the health-care setting.[20] These guidelines state, "The question of whether workers infected with HIV—especially those who perform invasive procedures—can adequately and safely be allowed to perform patient-care duties or whether their work assignments should be changed must be determined on an individual basis. These decisions should be made by the health-care worker's personal physician(s) in conjunction with the medical directors and personnel health service staff at the employing institution or hospital."[20]

These recommendations have been made despite the fact that, as yet, no cases of staff-to-patient transmission of HIV-1 have been reported. Nonetheless, these recommendations seem reasonable in light of the fact that a clear potential (albeit a small one) for transmission of HIV-1 would exist in certain settings. Although several such instances must have arisen over the past 5 years, only one report has attempted to analyze an infected health-care worker's patients for potential staff-to-patient transmission.[67] This study examined the registry of AIDS cases reported to an infected surgeon's home state and cross checked that list for any of the 400 patients who had invasive procedures performed by this surgeon during the preceding 5 years.[67] Although this study has serious limitations,[68] none of the infected surgeon's patients were identified as having been reported with AIDS. The difficulties inherent in performing such a study (confidentiality, medical liability, etc.) are prodigious. Finally, it should be noted that the occurrence of the first case of documented staff-to-patient transmission of HIV-1 will probably precipitate even more conservative or restrictive policies in many institutions.

From a practical standpoint, even the "case-by-case" management of infected health-care workers is fraught with some difficulties. Not all occupations are likely to be at equal risk for staff-to-patient transmission. Furthermore, it seems entirely reasonable to assume that even infected individuals participating in the same occupation would be associated with different levels of risk, depending on a variety of technical factors. For example, during abdominal/pelvic surgery some gynecologic surgeons blindly palpate in the pelvic cavity for the suture-needle tip; others do not. Such a practice is likely to be associated with a higher risk for patient-to-staff transmission of blood-borne pathogens and, ultimately, will probably be associated with an increased risk for staff-to-patient transmission as well. Deciding how to assess each individual in a rational and fair manner will not be easy.

Decisions regarding the management of infected workers will occasionally have to be made on the basis of data that are either subtle or difficult to quantitate. For example, although not all authorities agree, some reports have suggested that subtle signs of HIV-1-associated dementia appear very early in the course of HIV-1 infection.[69] Whether such subtle changes might impair performance remains unclear. In any event, it would seem prudent to assess HIV-1-infected personnel in the same way that personnel who have other illnesses are assessed, rather than attempting to single out those who may be infected with HIV-1 for special testing or assessment.

The question of whether or not an individual infected worker should be reassigned to different duties is also a difficult one. If the infected worker agrees to the reassignment, then things will go smoothly. If not, problems could easily arise. Although to my knowledge this issue has not yet been tested in court, many authorities believe that AIDS (and probably HIV-1 infection) will be viewed by the courts as a handicap.[70] If HIV-1 infection is found by the courts to be a handicap, then the concept of "reasonable accommodation" will govern issues of staff reassignment. If HIV-1 infection is, in fact, found to be a handicap, involuntary termination of employment of an infected health-care worker may well be viewed by the court as discrimination against the employee solely on the basis of his or her handicap.

PREVENTION OF TRANSMISSION

As early as 1982,[5] CDC began issuing recommendations regarding the use of infection control precautions in caring for AIDS patients and handling laboratory specimens from these patients. Since these first recommendations were published, CDC has issued a number of extensions, modifications, and revisions of these initial recommendations.[11,20,66,71–79] In addition to the CDC recommendations, several authorities in the field have made recommendations regarding the management of HIV-1-infected patients in the health-care setting.[13,58,80–88] Although, as might be expected, there are some minor differences in approach, virtually all of these recommendations are designed to minimize the risk for percutaneous, mucous membrane, and cutaneous exposures to blood and blood-containing body fluids.

Universal Precautions

In August, 1987, CDC issued new guidelines designed to minimize the risk for transmission of HIV-1 in the health-care setting.[20] These guidelines have come to be called "universal precautions." The general intent of these precautions is clear—all patients may harbor blood-borne pathogens; therefore, blood and blood-containing body fluids from all patients should be considered a hazard.[20] The major tenets of the universal precautions recommendations are summarized in Table 9. Although these concepts seem both practical and reasonable, acceptance of the new recommendations has been far from universal.

There are several reasons why health-care workers have found implementation of these new recommendations difficult. Perhaps the major reason that acceptance of these recommendations has been less than enthusiastic is the fact that cutaneous exposures to blood and blood-containing body fluids in the

TABLE 9. Summary of Universal Precautions and Recommendations

Handwashing should be performed before and after patient contact, immediately if hands are contaminated with blood or other body fluids, and after removing gloves.
Gloves should be worn when soiling of the hands with blood or body fluids is *likely*.
Gowns are generally not indicated; however, gowns should be worn if soiling of exposed skin or clothing is *likely*.
Masks are generally not indicated; however, masks should be worn when splashing or splattering of blood or other body fluids is *likely*. A mask alone is not sufficient protection but should be worn in combination with protective eyewear.
Protective eyewear is usually not indicated; however, protective eyewear should be worn when splashing or splattering of blood or other body fluids is *likely*. Personal eyewear often offers adequate protection. Eyewear should always be worn with a mask (See above).
A private room is generally not indicated; however, a patient should be placed in a private room if hygienic practices are poor or if the environment is *likely* to be soiled with blood or body fluids.
Patients may receive regular food service on reusable dishes; no special precautions are indicated for meal service.
Reusable, contaminated equipment should be cleaned of visible organic material, placed in an impervious container and returned to central hospital supply for decontamination and reprocessing.
Contaminated needles and other disposable sharp objects should be handled carefully. Used needles should never be bent, clipped, or recapped. Contaminated sharp objects should be discarded immediately after use into a puncture-resistant container designed for this purpose. Needle containers should not be overfilled; containers should be sealed and discarded when two-thirds to three-fourths full.
To minimize the risks for exchange of body fluids, pocket masks or mechanical ventilation devices should be readily available in areas in which resuscitation procedures are *likely* to be needed.
Spills of blood or blood-containing body fluids should be cleaned up by: first, donning gloves (and other barriers if indicated); second, wiping up excess material with disposable towels; third, cleansing with soap and water; and fourth, disinfecting with a dilute solution (1:100 for smooth surfaces; 1:10 for porous surfaces) of household bleach (sodium hypochlorite) and water. Diluted bleach solution should be no more than 24 hours old. Large spills or spills containing broken glass or sharp objects should first be covered with disposable towels; second, saturated with 1:10 bleach solution and allowed to stand for at least 10 minutes; and third, cleaned up as outline above.
Health-care workers who have open lesions, dermatitis, etc. should refrain from direct patient care and from directly handling contaminated equipment. Such employees should be evaluated by employee health services or by a private physician to assess illness for duty.
Compliance with these precautions is the responsibility of the health-care employer. Employers must provide: orientation, training, and continuing education for all health-care workers, along with adequate barriers and supplies. Employers are required to monitor compliance with universal precautions. Employers should develop mechanisms for counseling and retraining of noncompliant employees and should develop appropriate disciplinary action for repeatedly noncompliant employees.

(Modified from Centers for Disease Control.[20])

health-care setting have been extremely common occurrences for years. Such exposures have become "business as usual" for far too many health-care professionals. For example, in one study conducted prior to the implementation of universal precautions, 442 hospital-based health-care workers reported sustaining more than 10,000 cutaneous exposures to blood in a 1-year period.[89] More than 2700 of these exposures were to blood from a patient known to harbor HIV-1 infection—despite the fact that during the study period such patients were placed on a category of isolation called "blood and body fluids precautions," which requires the use of gloves for procedures likely to result in cutaneous contamination with blood or other body fluids.[89]

In general, infection control practices and procedures have not been given the highest priority by health-care providers. Gerberding and her coworkers noted that 56 percent of the participants in their prospective study of health-care workers involved in the care of HIV-1-infected patients reported using infection control precautions judged inadequate by the investigators.[52] The reason that health-care workers have maintained such a cavalier attitude toward infection control is unclear. One reason may be that most of us simply learned about these concepts incorrectly. We were not taught that these exposures represented a serious risk to our health. Thus it has become curiously acceptable to health-care professionals to have 200 of our colleagues die each year of hepatitis B and its complications.[65] Clearly, HIV-1 infection provides us with another opportunity to reassess our health-care practice priorities.

Many health-care professionals feel that infection control procedures are cumbersome to use—that these procedures reduce dexterity, are uncomfortable, or take too much time. Others believe that isolation garb may inhibit the patient-provider relationship. Finally, because most types of occupational infections are reasonably uncommon, many health-care workers have adopted an "it-will-never-happen-to-me" attitude.

Another general problem with implementing universal precautions has been related to the availability of barriers. Since these recommendations were issued by CDC,[20] disposable gloves and other barriers have been in short supply, and some institutions have had a difficult time maintaining adequate stocks. In addition, health-care workers have frequently complained that the quality of available barriers is quite variable. Gloves often leak, and there is apparently no standard or requirement that gloves or other barriers meet defined specifications. Finally, most often because of financial considerations, some institutions have chosen not to make these barriers universally available. In light of the United States Department of Labor Joint Advisory Notice discussed below,[65] this latter stance may be imprudent.

Unfortunately, none of the above reasons obviate the risks for occupational/nosocomial infection. All health-care workers need to reevaluate their approach to infection control. Implementation of, and strict adherence to, universal precautions could have a profound impact on the occurrence of a variety of occupational infections in the health-care setting.

Others have felt that the universal precautions recommendations were not specific enough, arguing (*1*) that since the major risk for HIV-1 transmission was associated with exposure to blood, many, if not most, other body substances should not require such stringent requirements; and (*2*) that the recommendations do not make clear which barriers should be used with which procedures. Additionally, some hospital officials have argued that certain of the universal precaution recommendations are neither practical nor cost-effective for their own institutions. For example, in remote areas of the United States where the prevalence of both HIV-1 and HBV infection is extremely low, it may not be cost-effective to advocate the use of barriers for every patient. Blood banking administrators have also argued that it is impractical to ask phlebotomists in donor areas to wear gloves because these individuals are managing several patients at a time, and the patients have already been screened for bloodborne infections.

CDC responded by issuing a clarification of some of these issues,[79] noting a number of body substances to which the universal precautions do not apply, including feces, nasal secretions, sputum, sweat, tears, urine, and vomitus (when these substances do not contain visible blood).[79] In addition, this clarification (*1*) discusses how to determine which barriers to use for specific procedures; (*2*) discusses in more detail the rationale for wearing gloves for phlebotomy (and allows some flexibility in deciding when gloves should be worn); and (*3*) discusses waste handling practices appropriate for universal precautions.

In hospitals housing large populations of patients who harbor blood-borne infections, excluding some body fluids from consideration for universal precautions may be impractical as well as imprudent. At the Warren G. Magnuson Clinical Center of the National Institutes of Health, the Hospital Infections Committee has chosen to continue recommending the use of universal precautions for handling urine, feces, vomitus, sputum, and oral secretions from all patients, in addition to applying these precautions during the handling of the various body fluids outlined in the revised CDC recommendations.[79]

An issue that is frequently raised regarding the implementation of universal precautions is the question of whether samples from patients known to harbor blood-borne infections should be specially labeled. Handsfield and his coworkers, working in a hospital where such labels are supposed to be routinely used, found that the majority of samples containing either hepatitis B surface antigen or antibody to HIV-1 did not have labels applied.[90] Although cogent and coherent arguments can be made to support either the use or the elimination of such labels,[91] in our hospital we have continued to use special labels for all patients known to harbor any blood-borne pathogen—simply because those patients present a known (and higher level of) risk. Nonetheless, we do advocate the use of universal precautions for all samples. Kelen and colleagues, in an HIV-1 seroprevalence survey of patients admitted to the Johns Hopkins Emergency Room, found a 5.2 percent prevalence of HIV-1 infection in these patients. Among trauma victims in this survey, 13.6 percent of patients had detectable levels of antibody to HIV-1.[92] Only 27 of the 119 seropositive patients in this study presented with known, symptomatic HIV-1 infection. Thus one could conclude from the studies of Handsfield et al. and Kelen et al. that the samples that may not be perceived as representing a risk for transmission of blood-borne infections may clearly be associated with such a risk.

One aspect of the universal precautions recommendations that was decidedly different from prior guidelines issued by CDC was the fact that, for the first time, the universal precautions guidelines discussed the issue of compliance and the responsibility for monitoring compliance, stating, "Employers of health-care workers should ensure that policies exist for . . . monitoring adherence to recommended protective measures. When monitoring reveals a failure to follow recommended precautions, counseling, education, and/or retraining should be provided, and, if necessary, appropriate disciplinary action should be considered."[20] Thus, for the first time the burden of compliance with infection control precautions has been placed on the employer, rather than on the employee.

Shortly after the universal precautions recommendations were published, in October, 1987, the United States Department of Labor and the Department of Health and Human Services issued a joint advisory notice regarding the risk for transmission of HBV and HIV-1.[65] The intent of this joint advisory notice was to provide, and require that health care institutions develop, a systematized method of implementing precautions designed to prevent transmission of blood-borne infectious diseases. Although most of the recommendations are similar in intent to the universal precautions guidelines, there are additional recommendations as well, and the cover letter for the joint advisory notice stated that OSHA was initiating a program of enforcement for the recommendations contained in the advisory notice to ensure that the recommendations were being followed by health-care institutions.[65] Significant details of the OSHA recommendations—especially aspects not included in the CDC recommendations—are outlined in Table 10.[65] The formalization of the universal precautions recommendations into rigid standard operating procedures has been the source of some controversy. Prior recommendations from CDC were intended only as guidelines. In fact, in the past, CDC has often encouraged individual institutions to modify their recommendations to meet specific institutional needs[93]; it remains to be seen whether OSHA will permit such flexibility.

TABLE 10. Summary of OSHA Guidelines

All health-care workplace tasks should be categorized as follows:

- Category I. Procedures involving expected exposures to blood, body fluids or tissues.
- Category II. Procedures involving no routine exposure, but may involve unplanned exposure to blood, body fluids or tissues.
- Category III. Procedures involving no exposures to blood, body fluids or tissues.

Employers should establish standard operating procedures (SOPs) for all category I and II tasks.

Both employees and patients should be educated regarding protective equipment and safe work practices.

Employers are responsible for ensuring that all employees are adequately trained and protected.

No worker should perform a category I task before receiving appropriate training to guarantee that the employee

A. Understands the mechanisms of transmission of HIV-1 and HBV.
B. Identifies and categorizes tasks as category I, II, or III.
C. Understands the types of protective barriers available, their general function, and their rationale for use.
D. Understands appropriate actions to take if an unexpected category I task presents itself.
E. Knows requirements for safe work practices and protective barrier for his/her specific tasks.
F. Knows where barrier supplies are stored and how to use and discard each barrier appropriately; understands the general limitations of each barrier.
G. Knows how to manage spills of blood or body fluids; knows how to manage personal exposures.

Employers should use the safest procedures and equipment that are both available and practical.

Employers should offer hepatitis B vaccine at no cost to all employees whose job entails category I tasks.

Employers should offer, at no cost, serologic monitoring for HIV-1 and HBV following known or suspected parenteral exposures to blood or body fluids. This program should include attention to employee confidentiality and a medical counseling service for all employees identified as seropositive for either infection.

Employers must maintain appropriate records documenting task categorization, SOPs, training records, surveillance/compliance monitoring activities, and investigation of adverse exposures.

(Modified from Department of Labor.[65])

Management of Opportunistic Infections

Some concern has been raised about risks for occupational/nosocomial transmission of certain of the opportunistic pathogens commonly found in patients who have AIDS. The majority of these opportunistic pathogens cause problems only for patients who have severely compromised cellular immunity (e.g., *Pneumocystis carinii, Mycobacterium avium-intracellulare*). Some of the infections are not transmitted from person to person (e.g., toxoplasmosis). Others represent minimal, if any, risk for occupational transmission (e.g., cryptococcosis, histoplasmosis, candidiasis). Only a few of these infections represent moderate occupational risks. Certain of the infections that do represent some risk (e.g., hepatitis B[52,54] and non-A, non-B hepatitis[54]) are transmitted in the health-care setting similarly to HIV-1. Thus precautions that are appropriate for managing HIV-1 infection should afford adequate protection against these pathogens as well.

Of the remaining opportunistic infections associated with some risk for transmission in the health-care setting, tuberculosis,[58] certain diarrheal illnesses,[58] and herpesvirus infections[52,56,58] are most frequently incriminated. Tuberculosis, which occurs primarily among patients in specific HIV-1 transmission categories,[58] can be transmitted in the health-care setting.[58,93] In addition, the diarrheal pathogens salmonella, shigella, and cryptosporidium have been transmitted occupationally.[58] For these reasons, it should be emphasized that implementation of universal precautions does not replace the need to implement additional appropriate categories of isolation (e.g., respiratory/acid-fast bacillus precautions for patients who have documented pulmonary tuberculosis or undiagnosed pulmonary infection consistent with the diagnosis of tuberculosis and/or enteric precautions for patients diagnosed with infectious diarrhea or for patients who have undiagnosed diarrheal syndromes consistent with an infectious etiology).[20,93]

Since dissemination of herpes zoster occurs frequently in

HIV-1-infected patients, such patients should be managed as "immunocompromised" (see Chapter 284). Health-care workers who are susceptible to varicella zoster virus (VZV) are at risk for occupational infection and should not provide care for patients who have active VZV infection (either varicella or dermatomal zoster).

Like other severely immunosuppressed patients, AIDS patients often shed herpes simplex viruses (HSV-I, HSV-II) from oral and genital lesions and in oral secretions. Health-care workers are at risk for cutaneous inoculation with HSV-I and HSV-II (i.e., whitlow) and should use recommended barrier precautions when suctioning, providing oral care, or providing care for open lesions for *any* patient.[20,79,93]

Finally, significant concern has been raised regarding the risks (particularly for pregnant health-care workers) for acquiring occupational/nosocomial cytomegalovirus (CMV) infection. To my knowledge, patient-to-staff transmission of CMV has not been documented (see Chapter 284). In addition, in prospective studies attempting to assess this risk, neither Gerberding and colleagues[52] nor Kuhls et al.[56] found an increased rate of CMV infection among personnel providing care for HIV-1-infected patients. For these reasons, CDC has concluded that pregnant health-care workers need not be restricted from caring for HIV-1-infected patients, while emphasizing that ". . . pregnant health-care workers should be especially familiar with and strictly adhere to precautions. . . ."[20]

Thus the documented or suspected presence of transmissible infectious diseases in *any* patient should trigger the implementation of appropriate isolation precautions.

Whereas the presence of HIV-1 infection in a patient may influence the physician's differential diagnosis, HIV-1 infection, in itself, does not require respiratory, enteric, or strict isolation precautions. Once the physician has established the differential diagnosis, isolation precautions should be chosen based on the most likely possibilities in the physician's differential diagnosis. In this respect, and in many others, AIDS and HIV-1-infected patients are no different from any patient who has compromised host defenses.

Management of Needles and Sharp Objects

Since percutaneous exposure to blood or blood-containing body fluids represents the highest risk to health-care personnel, special attention should be given to the handling and disposal of sharp objects in the hospital. A number of studies have identified inappropriate handling of needles and syringes as the primary risk for the occurrence of percutaneous injuries in the hospital.[19,63,94] Although not all such injuries may be preventable,[19,63] emphasis should be placed on practices that minimize the risk for these injuries. Jagger and colleagues note that poor instrument and device design contributes significantly to the increased risk[63]; nonetheless, some practices, such as recapping sharp objects, should be avoided whenever possible.

The use of impervious needle disposal units has been suggested as a possible method for reducing the frequency of needlestick injuries among health-care workers, and these devices have been shown to decrease the frequency of some types of injuries.[95–97] Since recapping injuries are among the most common presumably preventable injuries, Edmond and coworkers placed impervious needle disposal containers at patients' bedsides to facilitate disposal and to discourage resheathing.[98] Unfortunately, the presence of the bedside container had little impact on employee behavior in this study, and neither the frequency of resheathing nor the frequency of percutaneous injuries decreased during the study period.[98]

Decontamination and Sterilization

Although HIV-1 has been shown to be capable of survival in the environment,[99] there are no reported instances in which the environment has been thought to be a reservoir for HIV-1 transmission. Studies of household contacts of HIV-1-infected individuals (reviewed in Refs. 18 and 36) demonstrate absence of transmission of HIV-1 except to sexual contacts or to children born to mothers infected at the time of delivery. In combination with the longitudinal studies of health-care workers participating in the care of HIV-1-infected patients, such studies provide the best evidence that the risk for environmental transmission of HIV-1 is very small.

Procedures and techniques that have been previously recommended for routine sterilization and disinfection of hospital equipment also destroy HIV-1.[20] Detailed information regarding disinfection and sterilization is reviewed in the universal precautions guidelines.[20] Although a variety of disinfecting solutions have been suggested to have efficacy against HIV-1,[100] CDC continues to recommend the use of sodium hypochlorite (household bleach) for disinfection of contaminated surfaces. The bleach should be diluted 1:100 from the bottle (1 part bleach to 99 parts water) for small spills on smooth surfaces and should be diluted 1:10 (1 part bleach to 9 parts water) for spills on porous surfaces. Once diluted, bleach solutions maintain adequate potency for only 24 hours. Fresh solutions should be prepared daily. The majority of larger spills should be first wiped up (e.g., with disposable paper towels) and then disinfected appropriately.[20] Special recommendations have been published for managing spills of culture fluid containing large amounts of virus.[78]

Support Services and Waste Disposal

Although some confusion has arisen regarding appropriate techniques for the management of support services (i.e., housekeeping and laundry) under universal precautions, the 1987 guidelines[20] and the recent clarification of those guidelines issued by CDC[79] emphasize that universal precautions were not intended to modify previous recommendations for these services. These new recommendations provide a uniform approach to the management of these services in the hospital. For the housekeeping service, the guidelines summarize older recommendations and stress the importance of thorough routine cleaning.[20] For the laundry service, the recommendations note that soiled linen should be handled as little as possible and that all soiled linen should be placed in bags in the location where it has been used. In our hospital, we have chosen to place linen that is visibly contaminated with blood or body fluids in an isolation linen container. CDC recommends that such linen be placed and transported in bags that minimize the risk for leakage.[20]

Recommendations for techniques appropriate for disposal of infective waste were also not significantly changed when the universal precautions guidelines were issued. Although some centers felt that the new guidelines required incineration of all patient-related material, the supplementary recommendations issued by CDC clarified this issue.[79] A summary of these general recommendations regarding the management of hospital-related waste is included in Table 11.

Management of Employees Sustaining Adverse Exposures to Blood or Blood-Containing Body Fluids

Recommendations for the management of health-care workers who sustain adverse exposures to blood or blood-containing body fluids from a patient who has HIV-1 infection have been published by CDC[20] and others.[58,85,101] In my opinion, it is imperative that each institution develop a systematic approach to the management of these exposures that is consonant both with CDC recommendations as well as local laws and regulations. Several issues associated with the management of employees sustaining such exposures are both difficult and controversial. The approach that the Warren G. Magnuson Clinical Center at

TABLE 11. Hospital Waste Disposal Practices and Universal Precautions

No published evidence demonstrates that hospital waste has been associated with disease in the community; no published evidence documents that hospital waste represents more risk than residential waste.

Nonetheless, intuitively, some hospital wastes seem to be more likely to be associated with higher risk; therefore special handling/processing of these wastes as medical pathologic waste (MPW) seems warranted. Included in this category are the following:

A. Waste from the clinical laboratories (e.g., microbiology, clinical chemistry, hematology, blood bank, serology).
B. Waste from the anatomic and surgical pathology areas.
C. Wastes containing large amounts of blood or blood-containing body fluids.

Bulk blood, pleural fluid, suctioned fluids, secretions, and excretions can be poured down the drain (into the sanitary sewer) if such procedures are consonant with local and state regulations regarding waste disposal. The individual discarding these wastes should use appropriate barriers to prevent cutaneous and/or mucous membrane exposures.

Other wastes capable of being ground up and flushed into the sanitary sewer may be discarded in this fashion, if such procedures are consonant with local and state regulations.

If medical pathologic waste is to be placed in a landfill, it should be first be either incinerated or autoclaved.

All waste disposal policies should be based on institutional needs and designed to comply with local and state regulations governing waste management.

the National Institutes of Health has developed to manage such exposures is outlined in Table 12. Several points are worthy of further emphasis. Education is an extremely important part of any prevention program. Employees should be intensively educated regarding the importance of managing these exposures according to institutional policy. Although each injury should be considered individually, institutions should provide guidance to their employee health services regarding which general types of injuries should be further evaluated and which require no further assessment. After administering first aid, the employee should report the injury to his or her supervisor and, as soon as possible, to the employee health service. After obtaining informed consent from the "donor" patient as well as from the "recipient" health-care worker, blood should be drawn for both hepatitis and HIV-1 testing (Table 12). The institution should have knowledgeable counselors available (both for the employee and the patient) to explain the risks attendant on the tests as well as the need for performing the tests. Each institution should develop a policy for the management of exposures in instances in which the "donor" is either unable or refuses to give consent for these tests. An employee would require follow-up if he or she sustains a significant exposure to blood from a patient known to be infected with HIV-1, from a patient known to have indeterminate HIV-1 serologies, or from a patient whose HIV-1 serologies are unavailable. Employees requiring such follow-up should be counseled in detail regarding (*1*) the epidemiology, routes of transmission, and transmissibility of HIV-1; (*2*) the risk for occupational/nosocomial transmission of HIV-1 following such an injury; (*3*) the importance of notifying the employee health service of any acute febrile illness; and (*4*) techniques effective in minimizing the risk for transmission of HIV-1 to sexual partners, family members, and other household contacts. Additional blood samples should be drawn for serologic evaluation at 6 weeks, 12 weeks, 6 months, and 1 year following the exposure. If the employee develops an intercurrent illness consistent with acute HIV-1 infection, additional serologies should be obtained and the employee should be evaluated with more sophisticated tests (if they are available), such as p24 antigen testing or gene amplification.[102]

The follow-up schedule for employees sustaining adverse exposures is somewhat controversial. CDC recommends testing at 6 weeks, 12 weeks, and 6 months following an exposure.[20] Recently, concern has been raised that the period of time that elapses between HIV-1 infection and the production of detectable levels of anti-HIV-1-antibodies (i.e., the "window of infectivity") may be longer than was initially suggested.[103,104] Ranki et al.[103] and Wolinsky et al.[104] have shown that this "window of infectivity" may be as long as 14 months (or longer) for individuals acquiring infection sexually.

The "window of infectivity" is known with reasonable precision for 14 of the 18 health-care workers who have documented occupational HIV-1 infections[13,15,16,18–24,29,30,31a] (Table 1, Sections A and B); all 14 were found to be seropositive within six months of exposure; 8 of the 14 were seropositive within 4 months.[13,15,16,19–24,29,30,31a] Two of the remaining four health-care workers were seronegative at 3 months following exposure, but seropositive 6 months later (i.e., 9 months after exposure). Neither was evaluated between the 3- and 9-month samples.[28]

As yet, no health-care worker has been identified as seroconverting later than 6 months following exposure. It should be noted that many, if not most, of the 1858 health-care workers who have chosen to participate in longitudinal studies and who have sustained adverse exposures (Tables 5 and 6) have been followed for more than 1 year after their exposures. Some have been followed for as long as 6 years.[30]

Use of more sophisticated techniques, such as polymerase chain reaction (PCR) technology, may further clarify this issue. Nonetheless, based on currently available information, it would seem prudent to recommend a minimum of 12 months' serologic follow-up for employees sustaining documented adverse exposures (Table 12).

The issue of whether azidothymidine (AZT) prophylaxis should be offered to a health-care worker who has sustained a significant injury is a difficult one. If the risk for transmission following a documented percutaneous exposure to blood or blood-containing body fluids from a patient known to be infected with HIV-1 is 0.4 percent, proving efficacy of AZT in this setting will be very difficult. Even if one assumes 100 percent efficacy and 100 percent accuracy of enrollee's histories (broad assumptions, at best), in a double-blind, placebo-controlled trial, a sample size of 1500 per group (3000 enrollees total) would be needed for a two-tailed comparison to demonstrate significance at the 5 percent level. If the efficacy is only 90 percent, sample size requirements would increase dramatically.

Conversely, two studies suggest that AZT may have theoretical application in this situation.[105,106] Ruprecht and colleagues demonstrated that AZT was capable of suppressing infection and disease (but not preventing infection) in mice that were treated 4 hours after infection with Rauscher murine leukemia virus.[105] In their study these authors noted that the use of therapeutic doses of AZT led to significant side effects (bone marrow suppression) that accompanied prolonged (i.e., longer than 6 weeks') therapy.[105] It should be noted, however, that in a number of studies, AZT has been well tolerated (with minimal hematologic toxicity) by otherwise healthy individuals when administered for 6 weeks.

Tavares and coworkers evaluated AZT administered at various times following infection of cats with the feline leukemia virus.[106] In the animals that received AZT within 1 hour of infection, no sign of persistent infection could be detected.[106] In this experiment, some of the cats that did not receive AZT until 3 days following infection were apparently cured as well.[106]

Still, for all the reasons cited above, this issue is a difficult one and will be extremely hard to resolve scientifically. Nonetheless, Burroughs-Wellcome, the manufacturer of AZT, has initiated a collaborative study with the National Institute of Allergy and Infectious Diseases in an attempt to address these questions. Studies designed to document factors associated with an increased risk for transmission of HIV-1 (see Table 7) might be able to clarify risk to such an extent that a clinical trial designed to assess efficacy would have a much higher likelihood

TABLE 12. Guidelines for Management of Exposures to Blood and Blood-Containing Body Fluids

Source[a] (Donor) Laboratory Results	Employee Laboratory Studies to Obtain	Employee's Laboratory Results	Treatment	Follow-up
HBsAg-Positive; HBsAg-, anti-HBS-, anti-HIV-1-negative; AST/ALT normal; NANB not suspected	AST/ALT: save serum	HBsAG- or anti-HBS-positive	None	None
		HBsAg-anti-HBS-negative	HBIG 0.06 ml/kg; begin hepatitis B vaccine series[b]	HBsAG, anti-HBS, anti-HBc 6 months following injury
AST/ALT abnormal or normal; NANB hepatitis suspected; anti-HIV-, HBsAg-negative	AST/ALT; save serum	N/A	Optional NANB prophylaxis, 2 ml IG[c]	AST/ALT at 1, 3, and 6 months after exposure; optional NANB prophylaxis, 2 ml IG, 1 month after exposure[c]
HBsAg-negative; anti-HIV-negative; AST/ALT-NANB not suspected	None	None	None	None
Unknown; classified as high risk[d]	HBsAg; Anti-HBs; AST/ALT; save serum	HBsAG- or anti-HBS-positive	Optional NANB prophylaxis, 2 ml IG[c]	AST, ALT at 1, 3, and 6 months; 2 ml IG at 1 month[c]
		HBsAg-, anti-HBs-negative	HBIG 0.06 ml/kg; begin hepatitis B vaccine series[b]; optional for NANB, 2 ml IG[c]	HBsAg, anti-HBS in 6 months; ALT/AST in 1, 3, and 6 months; optional for NANB, 2 ml IG at 1 month[c]
Unknown; classified as low risk[e]	Save serum	N/A	Optional for HBV and NANB, 5 ml IG[f]	None
Unknown; classified as negligible risk	None	None	None	None
Anti-HIV-positive or indeterminate HBsAG-positive; ALT/AST normal or abnormal; NANB not suspected	Anti-HIV[g] HBsAg; Anti-HBs; AST/ALT; Save serum	Anti-HIV negative[h] HBsAg/anti-HBs-positive Anti-HIV-negative[h]; HBsAg-anti-HBs-negative	Optional NANB prophylaxis, 2 ml IG[c] Optional AZT prophylaxis[i] HBIG 0.06 ml/kg; begin hepatitis B vaccine series[c] Optional AZT prophylaxis[i]	Anti-HIV at 6 weeks, 3, 6, and 12 months; continue AZT for 6 weeks; monitor for toxicity weekly Anti-HIV at 6 weeks, 3, 6, and 12 months; HBsAg, anti-HBs; continue AZT 6 weeks; monitor for AZT toxicity weekly[i]
Anti-HIV-positive or indeterminate AST/ALT abnormal or normal; NANB suspected HBsAg-negative	Anti-HIV[g]; AST/ALT; save serum	Anti-HIV-negative[h]	Optional NANB prophylaxis 2 ml IG[c]; optional HIV AZT prophylaxis[i]	Anti-HIV at 6 weeks, 3, 6, and 12 months; AST/ALT at 1, 3, and 6 months; AZT: continue for 6 weeks; monitor AZT toxicity weekly; optional for NANB, 2 ml IG at 1 month[c]
Anti-HIV-positive or indeterminate HBsAg-negative; AST/ALT-NANB not suspected	Anti-HIV[g]; save serum	Anti-HIV-negative[h]	Optional HIV AZT prophylaxis[i]	Anti-HIV in 6 weeks, 3, 6, and 12 months; continue AZT for 6 weeks; monitor AZT toxicity weekly

[a] If the source of the injury is known; obtain written, informed consent, and order: HBsAg, AST/ALT, and anti-HIV.
[b] If the employee refuses hepatitis B vaccine, a second dose of HBIG should be administered in 1 month.
[c] Value of ISG prophylaxis for NANB is not proven; if given, prophylaxis should be administered as soon after the exposure as is possible.
[d] Location of exposure makes it likely that injury may have come from patient infected with one of these blood-borne pathogens, for example, needlestick occurred in hepatitis laboratory.
[e] Location of injury makes it unlikely that needle, etc. was contaminated with blood/body fluids containing HIV, NANB, or HBV.
[f] Prophylaxis for both HBV and NANB; administer as soon after exposure as possible.
[g] Employee should be prospectively followed for possible HIV-1 exposure by Employee Health Service.
[h] If the employee is found to be HIV-1-seropositive on the initial specimen, (i.e., seropositivity is not related to the injury, he/she should nonetheless be notified immediately of the confirmed result, counseled appropriately, and referred for appropriate follow-up.
[i] Value of AZT prophylaxis for HIV-1 exposure is unknown; if given, prophylaxis should be administered as soon after the exposure as is possible. Employees receiving AZT should be counseled about possible toxicity, given written, informed consent, and monitored weekly for signs of hematologic toxicity. Not an approved indication for this drug; nationwide experimental protocol in progress (see text).

Abbreviations: HIV: human immunodeficiency virus; anti-HIV: antibodies directed against HIV; HBsAg: hepatitis B surface antigen; anti-HBs: antibodies directed against HBsAg; AST/ALT: aspartate aminotransferase/alanine aminotransferase; HBIG: hepatitis B immune globulin; ISG: standard immune serum globulin; NANB: non-A, non-B hepatitis.

(Courtesy of Dr. James M. Schmitt, Occupational Medical Service, National Institutes of Health, Bethesda, MD.)

of success. For now, decisions on AZT prophylaxis for health-care workers sustaining exposures to blood or blood-containing body fluids will have to be made on an individual basis in accord with institutional policies and recommendations.

As noted above, the risks for HIV-1 transmission as a result of exposures other than percutaneous exposure to blood are currently too small to be estimated. Management of employees sustaining mucous membrane exposures or cutaneous exposures to blood or blood-containing body fluids from a patient infected with HIV-1 should be based on principles similar to those for the management of percutaneous exposures—modified by what is known about the magnitude of risk of transmission for such exposures. Although HIV-1 transmission has been documented following mucous membrane exposures[16,29] and following blood exposure on nonintact skin,[16,27] these types of exposures occur quite commonly in hospitals providing care for HIV-1-infected patients,[52,54,64,89] and none of the prospective studies assessing risk for HIV-1 transmission in the health-care setting have identified any seroconversions associated with these types of exposures.[19,28,30,52,54–58]

Routine Serologic Surveillance

Although CDC[20] and OSHA[65] have recommended that serologic testing be made available to employees who sustain adverse exposures to blood or blood-containing body fluids, because HIV-1 transmission has been documented to occur rarely in the absence of a percutaneous exposure, both groups stopped short of recommending routine serologic surveillance of health-care workers for HIV-1 infection. For a variety of reasons, instituting a mandatory program of serologic screening for clinical employees is probably not advisable. Nonetheless, many institutions have decided to offer a voluntary program of serologic surveillance of clinical and clinical laboratory personnel. Offering serologic surveillance for hospital employees may help allay anxiety and make provision of high-quality care for HIV-1-infected patients easier. In our own hospital, the Occupational Medical Service offers voluntary confidential HIV-1 testing for health-care workers who have direct patient contact or who process blood or blood-containing body fluids as part of their routine duties. If an institution decides to begin such a program for its clinical employees, several important issues should be considered. Among these are the following: (*1*) employees should give written informed consent before entering the program; (*2*) employees should be given information regarding risk behaviors for HIV-1 infection and risks associated with having the test performed prior to entry into the study; (*3*) participants should be notified that the results from testing will become a part of their official employee health service medical records; (*4*) results from such a program must be held in strict confidentiality by the institution; and (*5*) individuals identified as HIV-1-infected should be counseled regarding the meaning of the test and directed to appropriate institution and community resources. Finally, it should be noted that there are several pitfalls associated with such a program. The ELISA tests that are currently marketed for screening for HIV-1 infection are antibody tests; both false-positive and false-negative tests occur. In low prevalence populations false-positive ELISA tests will occur more frequently than true positives. In our own experience many false-positive ELISA tests may also produce one band in the Western blot test kits (i.e., an indeterminate test). Institutions initiating serologic surveillance programs should anticipate the occurrence of indeterminate results and have a plan for further evaluation of individuals who have such results. Identification of incidental positives (whether related or unrelated to occupational exposures) may result in compensation claims. CDC and NIH have recommended routine medical surveillance (presumably including serologic studies) in "all laboratories that test specimens, do research, or produce reagents involving HIV."[78]

Counseling

The availability of skilled counselors who can provide knowledge, reassurance, and assistance to health-care workers sustaining exposures to blood or blood-containing body fluids from an HIV-1-infected patient is an integral part of a good employee health service. Such a counselor should maintain a state-of-the-art level of knowledge regarding the magnitude of risk for transmission of HIV-1 associated with various types of exposures in the health-care setting and should also be knowledgeable regarding risks for and prevention of transmission to sexual partners, spouses, family members, and other household contacts. Finally, an important part of this counseling service is to provide perspective for the exposed employee.

LEGAL AND ETHICAL ISSUES

The introduction of HIV-1 into the health-care setting has raised a number of difficult questions, many of which will ultimately be resolved in the courts. In addition, HIV-1 infection has presented the health-care professional with a number of moral and ethical dilemmas. Although limitations of space preclude an exhaustive discussion of these issues, several of them relate directly to the management of HIV-1-infected individuals in the health-care setting.

HIV-1 Antibody Testing of Patients

The use of the HIV-1 antibody tests for routine, or in some instances, mandatory testing of patients has been a controversial issue.[11,13,20,107–121] Although CDC has recommended testing of hospitalized patients to determine prevalence,[111] neither CDC nor most other authorities have advocated mandatory routine testing of patients. When the likelihood of adverse exposure to blood is high, some centers have advocated testing.[20] Another argument for testing of patients is that the physicians providing care would alter procedures if they knew the patient was infected with a blood-borne pathogen. For example, some surgeons have argued that, for patients known to be carriers of HIV-1 or hepatitis B, inexperienced personnel should not be permitted in the operating room. In addition, they suggest that hand-to-hand passes of needles and other sharp objects should be forbidden in such cases; no sharp objects should be allowed to lie in the surgical field; retraction of tissues should be performed with instruments rather than hands; no hands other than the surgeon's should be allowed in the wound; use of sharp instruments for cutting or sewing should be minimized; and all operative personnel should wear impervious gowns. Although one might argue that such precautions might be prudent for all surgical procedures, routine use of these procedures would probably result in prolongation of operative times, and would consequently be associated with an increased risk for other operative complications.[20]

If an institution decides to initiate a program of routine preoperative testing of patients, individuals responsible for the program should be certain that it contains several components: (*1*) patients should give informed consent for the test, and the consent should be documented in the patient's medical record before the blood is drawn; (*2*) prior to obtaining the blood and as part of the informed consent process, the physician should explain the rationale for ordering the test as well as the risks to the patient of having this serologic result in his or her medical record; (*3*) as part of the informed consent procedure, the patient should receive counseling about the test and what the result will mean; (*4*) patients identified as seropositive should be notified of their results and counseled on its meaning and on techniques for preventing transmission; (*5*) results from such testing should be maintained with as much confidentiality as is possible; and (*6*) the results of such testing should not be used to deny the patient care or to cause the patient to receive suboptimal care.[20]

Right of Health-Care Workers to Refuse to Give Care

The issue of whether or not a physician can legally refuse to provide care for a patient simply because he or she has HIV-1 infection has yet to be decided in the courts. Although many argue that physicians are morally and ethically bound to provide care for all patients,[114,120–124] others have argued that physicians are not required to evaluate or treat HIV-1-infected patients.[124] The American Medical Association has noted that "a physician may not ethically refuse to treat a patient whose condition is within the physician's current realm of competence, solely because the patient is seropositive."[122] Although these issues are complex, most authorities have agreed with the AMA position.

Confidentiality and the Physician's "Duty to Warn"

Perhaps more than any other illness, AIDS and HIV 1 infection have emphasized the need for maintenance of the confidentiality of a patient's medical record. Numerous personal and professional tragedies associated with the violation of patient confidentiality have been related in the lay press. Although every effort should be made to ensure patient confidentiality, I should emphasize that confidentiality of a patient's records should never be absolutely guaranteed. In many academic institutions, hundreds (sometimes thousands) of individuals have access to patient records. One should never promise something that cannot be delivered.

Although maintenance of patient confidentiality is extremely important, it should not be considered absolute. Although again somewhat controversial, most authorities (citing the case of Tarasoff vs. the Regents of California)[125] have argued that a physician does have a duty to warn (for example) the patient's sexual partner if the patient refuses to notify the partner that he or she is infected with HIV-1.[108,114,122] The AMA has advocated that, if the physician is unable to convince the patient to notify a partner, the physician should report the patient to the local public health authorities. If the authorities fail to notify the partner, the physician should then notify the partner.[122] Clearly, the optimal method of partner notification is to convince the infected individual of the importance of notifying his or her sexual partners. Counseling the individual can often convince the patient of the need for notification.

REFERENCES

1. Centers for Disease Control. *Pneumocystis* pneumonia. MMWR. 1981;30:250–2.
2. Gottlieb MS, Schroff R, Schranker HM, et al. *Pneumocystis carinii* pneumonia and mucosal candidiasis in previously healthy homosexual men: evidence of a new acquired cellular immunodeficiency. N Engl J Med. 1981;305:1425–31.
3. Masur H, Michelis MA, Greene JB, et al. An outbreak of community-acquired *Pneumocystis carinii* pneumonia: initial manifestation of cellular immune dysfunction. N Engl J Med. 1981;305:1431–8.
4. Siegal FP, Lopez C, Hammer G, et al. Severe acquired immunodeficiency in male homosexuals, manifested by chronic perianal ulcerative herpes simplex lesions. N Engl J Med. 1981;305:1439–44.
5. Centers for Disease Control. Acquired immune deficiency syndrome: precautions for clinical and laboratory staffs. MMWR. 1982;31:577–80.
6. Seefe LB, Wright EC, Zimmerman HJ, et al. Type B hepatitis after needlestick exposure: prevention with hepatitis B immune globulin. Final report of the Veterans' Administration Cooperative Study. Ann Intern Med. 1978;88:285–93.
7. Grady GF, Lee VA, Prince AM, et al. Hepatitis B immune globulin for accidental exposures among medical personnel: final report of a multicenter controlled trial. J Infect Dis. 1978;138:625–38.
8. Werner BJ, Grady GF. Accidental hepatitis-B-surface-antigen-positive inoculations: use of "e" antigen to estimate infectivity. Ann Intern Med. 1982;97:367–9.
9. Barré-Sinoussi F, Chermann JC, Rey F, et al. Isolation of a T-lymphotropic retrovirus from a patient at risk for the acquired immunodeficiency syndrome. Science. 1983;220:868–71.
10. Gallo RC, Salahuddin SZ, Popovic M, et al. Frequent detection of cytopathic retroviruses (HTLV-III) from patients with AIDS and at risk for AIDS. Science. 1984;224:500–3.
11. Centers for Disease Control. Summary and recommendations for preventing transmission of infection with human T-lymphotropic virus type III/lymphadenopathy-associated virus in the workplace. MMWR. 1985;34:681–95.
12. Weiss SH, Saxinger WC, Rechtman D, et al. HLTV-III infection among health care workers. Association with needle-stick injuries. JAMA. 1985;254:2089–93.
13. Gerberding JL, Henderson DK. Design of rational infection control policies for human immunodeficiency virus infection. J Infect Dis. 1987;156:861–4.
14. Wormser GP, Joline C, Duncanson F, et al. Needle-stick injuries during the care of patients with AIDS (Letter). N Engl J Med. 1984;310:1461–2.
15. Centers for Disease Control. Update: acquired immunodeficiency syndrome and human immunodeficiency virus infection among health-care workers. MMWR. 1988;37:229–34;239.
16. Centers for Disease Control. Update: human immunodeficiency virus infections in health-care workers exposed to blood of infected patients. MMWR. 1987;36:285–9.
17. Ward JW, Deppe DA, Samson S, et al. Human immunodeficiency virus infection from blood donors who later developed the acquired immunodefiency syndrome. Ann Intern Med. 1987;106:61–2.
18. Friedland GH, Klein RS. Transmission of the human immunodeficiency virus. N Engl J Med. 1987;317:1125–35.
19. McCray E, The Cooperative Needlestick Surveillance Group. Occupational risk of the acquired immunodeficiency syndrome among health care workers. N Engl J Med. 1986;314:1127–32.
20. Centers for Disease Control. Recommendations for prevention of HIV transmission in health-care settings. MMWR. 1987;36(Suppl 2S):1S–19S.
21. Stricof RL, Morse DL. HTLV-III/LAV seroconversion following a deep intramuscular needlestick injury (Letter). N Engl J Med. 1986;314:1115.
22. Anonymous. Needlestick transmission of HTLV-III from a patient infected in Africa. Lancet. 1984;2:1376–7.
23. Oskenhendler E, Harzic M, LeRoux J-M, et al. HIV infection with seroconversion after a superficial needlestick injury to the finger (Letter). N Engl J Med. 1986;315:582.
24. Neisson-Vernant C, Arfi S, Mathez D, et al. Needlestick HIV seroconversion in a nurse (Letter). Lancet. 1986;2:814.
25. Weiss SH, Goedert JJ, Gartner S, et al. Risk of human immunodeficiency virus (HIV-1) infection among laboratory workers. Science. 1988;239:68–71.
26. Centers for Disease Control, Division of Safety, National Institutes of Health. Occupationally acquired human immunodeficiency virus infections in laboratories producing virus concentrates in large quantities: conclusions and recommendations of an expert team convened by the Director of the National Institutes of Health (NIH). MMWR. 1988;37(Suppl 4):19–22.
27. Centers for Disease Control. Apparent transmission of human T-lymphotropic virus type III/lymphadenopathy-associated virus from a child to a mother providing health care. MMWR. 1986;35:75–9.
28. Ramsey KM, Smith EN, Reinarz JA. Prospective evaluation of 44 health care workers exposed to human immunodeficiency virus-1, with one seroconversion (Abstract). Clin Res. 1988;36:22A.
29. Gioananni P, Sinicco A, Cariti G, et al. HIV infection acquired by a nurse. Eur J Epidemiol. 1988;4:119–20.
30. Henderson DK, Fahey BJ, Saah J, et al. Longitudinal assessment of the risk for occupational/nosocomial transmission of human immunodeficiency virus, type I in health care workers (Abstract). Presented at the 28th Interscience Conference on Antimicrobial Agents and Chemotherapy, Los Angeles, October, 1988.
31. Michelet C, Cartier F, Ruffault A, et al. Needlestick HIV infection in a nurse (Abstract). Abstract 9010. Presented at the IV International Conference on AIDS, Stockholm, Sweden, June, 1988.

31a. Wallace MR, Harrison WO. HIV seroconversion with progressive disease in a health care worker after needlestick injury. Lancet. 1988;1:1454.

32. Klein RS, Phelan JA, Freeman K, et al. Low occupational risk of human immunodeficiency virus infection among dental professionals. N Engl J Med. 1988;318:86–90.
33. Ponce de Leon RS, Sanchez-Mejorada G, Zaidi-Jacobsen M. AIDS in a blood-bank technician. Infect Control Hosp Epidemiol. 1988;318:86–90.
34. Hoofnagle J. Acute hepatitis. In: Mandell GL, Douglas RG Jr, Bennett JE, eds. Principles and Practice of Infectious Diseases. 2nd ed. New York: John Wiley & Sons; 1985:1002–29.
35. Lifson AR. Do alternate modes for transmission of human immunodeficiency virus exist? A review. JAMA. 1988;259:1353–6.
36. Bygbjerg JC. AIDS in a Danish Surgeon (Zaire, 1976) (Letter). Lancet. 1984;1:676.
37. Belani A, Dutta D, Rosen S, et al. AIDS in a hospital worker (Letter). Lancet. 1984;1:676.
38. Grint P, McEvoy M. Two associated cases of the acquired immune deficiency syndrome (AIDS). PHLS Commun Dis Rep. 1985;85:4.
39. Barker T. Physician sues Johns Hopkins after contracting AIDS. Am Med Assoc News. 1987;June 19:8.
40. Lifson AR, Castro KG, McCray E, et al. National surveillance of AIDS in health-care workers. JAMA. 1986;256:3231–4.
41. Chamberland M, Conley L, Lifson A, et al. AIDS in health-care workers—a surveillance report. Abstract 9020. Presented at the IV International Conference on AIDS, Stockholm, Sweden, June, 1988.
42. Bureau of Labor Statistics. Employment and Earnings. Washington, DC: U.S. Department of Labor, Bureau of Labor Statistics; 1988;35:12,93,194.
43. Gilmore N, Ballachey M-L, O'Shaughnessy M, et al. HTLV-III/LAV serologic survey of health care workers in a Canadian teaching hospital. Ab-

stract 200. Presented at the 2nd International Conference on AIDS, Paris, France, June, 1986.

44. Centers for Disease Control. Update: evaluation of human T-lymphotropic virus type III/lymphadenopathy-associated virus infection in health-care personnel—United States. MMWR. 1985;34:575–8.
45. Hirsch MS, Wormser GP, Schooley RT, et al. Risk of nosocomial infection with human T-cell lymphotropic virus III (HTLV-III). N Engl J Med. 1985;312:1–4.
46. Weiss SH, Goedert JJ, Sarngadharan MG, et al. Screening test for HTLV-III (AIDS agent) antibodies. Specificity, sensitivity, and applications. JAMA. 1985;253:221–5.
47. Shanson DC, Evans R, Lai L. Incidence and risk of transmission of HTLV-III infection to a staff at a London hospital, 1982–85. J Hosp Infect. 1985;Suppl C:15–22.
48. Ebbesen P, Melbye M, Scheutz F, et al. Lack of antibodies to HTLV-III/LAV in Danish dentists (Letter). JAMA. 1986;256:2199.
49. Lubick HA, Schaeffer LD. Occupational risk of dental personnel survey (Letter). J Am Dent Assoc. 1986;113:10–12.
50. Harper S, Flynn N, VanHorne J, et al. Absence of HIV antibody among dental professionals, surgeons, and household contacts exposed to persons with HIV infection (Abstract). Abstract THP.215. Presented at the 3rd International Conference on AIDS, Washington, D.C., June, 1986.
51. Boland M, Keresztes J, Evans P, et al. HIV seroprevalence among nurses caring for children with AIDS/ARC (Abstract). Abstract THP.212. Presented at the 3rd International Conference on AIDS, Washington, D.C., June, 1986.
52. Gerberding JL, Bryant-LeBlanc CE, Nelson K, et al. Risk of transmitting the human immunodeficiency virus, cytomegalovirus, and hepatitis B virus to health care workers exposed to patients with AIDS and AIDS-related conditions. J Infect Dis. 1987;156:1–8.
53. Kelley P, Brundage J, Burke D, et al. Evidence supporting low risk estimates for HIV transmission in health care settings. Abstract 9004. Presented at the IV International Conference on AIDS, Stockholm, Sweden, June, 1988.
54. Henderson DK, Saah AJ, Zak BJ, et al. Risk of nosocomial infection with human T-cell lymphotropic virus type III/lymphadenopathy-associated virus in a large cohort of intensively exposed health care workers. Ann Intern Med. 1986;104:644–7.
55. Marcus R, The Cooperative Needlestick Surveillance Group. CDC's health-care workers surveillance project: an update. Abstract 9015. Presented at the IV International Conference on AIDS, Stockholm, Sweden, June, 1988.
56. Kuhls TL, Viker S, Parris NB, et al. Occupational risk of HIV, HBV, and HSV-2 infections in health care personnel caring for AIDS patients. Am J Public Health. 1987;7:1306–9.
57. McEvoy M, Porter K, Mortimer P, et al. Prospective study of clinical, laboratory, and ancillary staff with accidental exposures to blood or body fluids from patients infected with HIV. Br Med J. 1987;294:1595–7.
58. Wormser GP, Joline C, Sivak S, et al. Human immunodeficiency virus infections: considerations for health care workers. Bull NY Acad Med. 1988;64:203–15.
59. Elmslie K, O'Shaughnessy JV. National surveillance program on occupational exposure to HIV among health-care workers in Canada. Can Dis Week Rep. 1987;13:163–6.
60. Hernandez E, Gatell JM, Puyuelo T, et al. Risk of transmitting the HIV to health care workers (HCW) exposed to HIV infected body fluids. Abstract 9003. Presented at the IV International Conference on AIDS, Stockholm, Sweden, June, 1988.
61. Pizzocolo G, Stellini R, Cadeo GP, et al. Risk of HIV and HBV infection after accidental needlestick. Abstract 9012. Presented at the IV International Conference on AIDS, Stockholm, Sweden, June, 1988.
62. West DJ. The risk of hepatitis B infection among health professionals in the United States: a review. Am J Med Sci. 1984;287:26–33.
63. Jagger J, Hunt EH, Brand-Elnaggar J, et al. Rates of needle-stick injury caused by various devices in a university hospital. N Engl J Med. 1988;319:284–8.
64. Fahey BJ, Meehan PE, Henderson DK. The risk of HIV-1 transmission in health care workers. Infect Med. 1988;5:224–37.
65. Department of Labor. Joint Advisory Notice: Department of Labor/Department of Health and Human Services. Federal Register. 1987;52:41818–24.
66. Centers for Disease Control. Recommendations for preventing transmission of infection with human T-lymphotropic virus type III/lymphadenopathy-associated virus during invasive procedures. MMWR. 1986;35:221–3.
67. Sacks JJ. AIDS in a surgeon (Letter). N Engl J Med. 1985;313:1017–8.
68. Mascoli R. More on AIDS in a surgeon (Letter). N Engl J Med. 1986;314:1190.
69. Grant I, Atkinson JH, Hesselink JR, et al. Evidence for early central nervous system involvement in the acquired immunodeficiency syndrome (AIDS) and other human immunodeficiency virus (HIV) infections: studies with neurophysiologic testing and magnetic resonance imaging. Ann Intern Med. 1987;107:828–36.
70. Dickens BM. Legal rights and duties in the AIDS epidemic. Science. 1988;239:580–5.
71. Centers for Disease Control. Prevention of acquired immune deficiency syndrome. MMWR. 1983;32:101–3.
72. Centers for Disease Coontrol. Acquired immunodeficiency syndrome (AIDS): precautions for health-care workers and allied professionals. MMWR. 1983;32:450–1.
73. Centers for Disease Control. Recommendations for preventing possible transmission of human T-lymphotropic virus type III/lymphadenopathy-associated virus from tears. MMWR. 1985;34:533–4.
74. Centers for Disease Control. Recommendations for providing dialysis treatment to patients infected with human T-lymphotropic virus type III/lymphadenopathy-associated virus. MMWR. 1986;35:376–83.
75. Favero MS. Recommended precautions for patients undergoing hemodialysis who have AIDS or non-A, non-B hepatitis. Infect Control. 1985;6:301–5.
76. Centers for Disease Control. Recommended infection-control practices for dentistry. MMWR. 1985;35:237–42.
77. Centers for Disease Control. Human T-lymphotropic virus type III/lymphadenopathy-associated virus: agent summary statement. MMWR. 1986;35:540–2;547–9.
78. Centers for Disease Control. Agent summary statement for human immunodeficiency viruses (HIVs), including HTLV-III, LAV, HIV-1, and HIV-2. MMWR. 1988;37(Suppl 4):1–17.
79. Centers for Disease Control. Update: universal precautions for preventions of transmission of human immunodeficiency virus, hepatitis B virus, and other bloodborne pathogens in health-care settings. MMWR. 1988;37:337–82;3878.
80. Conte JE Jr, Hadley WK, Sande M. Infection-control guidelines for patients with the acquired immunodeficiency syndrome. N Engl J Med. 1983;309:740–4.
81. Federico JV, Gershon RRM. AIDS—safety practices for clinical and research laboratories. Infect Control. 1984;5:185–7.
82. LaCamera D. AIDS: precautions for health care personnel. Top Clin Nurs. 1984;6:45–52.
83. Norris SM, Limon L. Recommendations for decontaminating manikins used in cardiopulmonary resuscitation training: 1983 update. Infect Control. 1984;5:399–402.
84. Adams A, Lowy FD. Infection control and the hospitalized AIDS patient. Infect Control. 1985;6:200–201.
85. Conte JE Jr. Infection with human immunodeficiency virus in the hospital. Ann Intern Med. 1986;105:730–6.
86. Advisory Committee on Infection within Hospitals. Management of HTLV-III/LAV infection in the hospital. Chicago: American Hospital Association; 1986.
87. Gerberding JL, The UCSF Task Force on AIDS. Recommended infection control policies for patients with human immunodeficiency virus infection. N Engl J Med. 1986;315:1562–4.
88. Lynch P, Jackson MM, Cummings MJ, et al. Rethinking the role of isolation practices in the prevention of nosocomial infection. Ann Intern Med. 1986;107:243–6.
89. Henderson DK, Fahey BJ, Willy ME. Frequency and intensity of cutaneous exposures to blood and body fluids among health care providers in a referral hospital. Abstract 9017. Presented at the IV International Conference on AIDS, Stockholm, Sweden, June, 1988.
90. Handsfield HH, Cummings J, Swenson PD. Prevalence of antibody to human immunodeficiency virus and hepatitis B surface antigen in blood samples submitted to a hospital laboratory: implications for handling specimens. JAMA. 1987;258:3395–7.
91. Gottfried SE. The labeling of specimens as infectious (Letter). JAMA. 1988;259:1807–8.
92. Kelen GD, Fritz S, Qaqish B, et al. Unrecognized human immunodeficiency virus infection in emergency department patients. N Engl J Med. 1988;318:1645–50.
93. Garner JS, Simmons BP. Guideline for isolation precautions in hospitals. Infect Control. 1983;4(Suppl):245–325.
94. McCormick RD, Maki DG. Epidemiology of needle-stick injuries in hospital personnel. Am J Med. 1981;70:928–32.
95. Krasinski K, LaCouture R, Holzman RS. Effect of changing needle disposal systems on needle puncture injuries. Infect Control. 1987;8:59–62.
96. Ribner BS, Landry MN, Gholson GL, et al. Impact of a rigid, puncture resistant container system upon needlestick injuries. Infect Control. 1987;8:63–6.
97. Schmitt JM, Mc Shalley ED, Henderson DK. Accidental percutaneous injuries in health-care workers: a five year experience (Abstract). Abstract 1140. Presented at the 26th Interscience Conference on Antimicrobial Agents and Chemotherapy, New Orleans, LA, October, 1986.
98. Edmond M, Khakoo R, McTaggart B, et al. Effect of bedside needle disposal units on needle recapping frequency and needlestick injury. Infect Control Hosp Epidemiol. 1988;9:114–5.
99. Resnick L, Veren K, Salahuddin SZ, et al. Stability and inactivation of HTLV-III/LAV under clinical and laboratory environments. JAMA. 1986;255:1887–91.
100. Martin LS, McDougal S, Loskoski SL. Disinfection and inactivation of human T lymphotropic virus type III/lymphadenopathy-associated virus. J Infect Dis. 1985;152:400–3.
101. Kuhls TL, Cherry JD. The management of health-care workers' accidental parenteral exposures to biological specimens of HIV seropositive individuals. Infect Control. 1987;8:211–3.
102. Kwok S, Mack DH, Mullis KB, et al. Identification of human immunodeficiency virus sequences by using in vitro enzymatic amplification and oligomer cleavage detection. J Virol. 1987;61:1690–4.
103. Ranki A, Krohn M, Allain J-P, et al. Long latency period precedes overt seroconversion in sexually transmitted human-immunodeficiency-virus infection. Lancet. 1987;2:589–93.

104. Wolinsky S, Rinaldo C, Farzedegan H, et al. Polymerase chain reaction (PCR) detection of HIV provirus before HIV seroconversion. Abstract 1099. Presented at the IV International Conference on AIDS, Stockholm, Sweden, June, 1988.
105. Ruprecht RM, O'Brien LG, Rossoni LD, et al. Suppression of mouse viraemia and retroviral disease by 3'-azido-3'deoxythymidine. Nature. 1986;323:467–9.
106. Tavares L, Roneker C, Johnston K, et al. 3'-Azido-3'deoxythymidine in feline leukemia virus-infected cats: a model for therapy and prophylaxis of AIDS. Cancer Res. 1987;47:3190–4.
107. Bayer R, Levine C, Wolf SM. HIV antibody screening: an ethical framework for evaluating proposed programs. JAMA. 1986;256:1768–74.
108. Gostin L, Curran WJ. AIDS screening, confidentiality, and the duty to warn. Am J Public Health. 1987;77:361–5.
109. Lenox JL, Redfield RR, Burke DS. HIV antibody screening in a general hospital population (Letter). JAMA. 1987;257:2914.
110. Meyer KB, Pauker SG. Screening for HIV: can we afford the false positive rate? N Engl J Med. 1987;317:238–41.
111. Centers for Disease Control. Public Health Service guidelines for counseling and antibody testing to prevent HIV infection and AIDS. MMWR. 1987;36:509–515.
112. AMA Board of Trustees. Prevention and control of AIDS. Cleve Clin J Med. 1987;54:477–87.
113. Gambino R. Screening for HIV (Letter). N Engl J Med. 1988;318:378–9.
114. Walters L. Ethical issues in the prevention and treatment of HIV infection and AIDS. Science. 1988;239:597–603.
115. Parker JE. Screening for HIV (Letter). N Engl J Med. 1988;318:379.
116. Mortimer PP. Screening for HIV (Letter). N Engl J Med. 1988;318:379.
117. Trueblood HW. Screening for HIV (Letter). N Engl J Med. 1988;318:379–80.
118. Pelroth MG. Screening for HIV (Letter). N Engl J Med. 1988;318:380.
119. Mayer KB, Pauker SG. Screening for HIV (Letter). N Engl J Med. 1988;318:380.
120. Osborne JE. AIDS: politics and science. N Engl J Med. 1988;318:444–7.
121. Hagen MD, Meyer KB, Pauker SG. Routine preoperative screening for HIV. Does the risk to the surgeon outweigh the risk to the patient? JAMA. 1988;259:1357–9.
122. AMA Council on Ethical and Judicial Affairs. Ethical issues involved in the growing AIDS crisis. JAMA. 1988;259:1360–1.
123. Zuger A, Mlles SH. Physicians, AIDS, and occupational risk: historical traditions and ethical obligations. JAMA. 1987;258:1924–8.
124. Kim JH, Perfect JR. To help the sick: an historical and ethical essay concerning the refusal to care for patients with AIDS. Am J Med. 1988;84:135–8.
125. Tarasoff vs. the Regents of the University of California. California Reporter (California Supreme Court). 1976;131:14–42.

284. NOSOCOMIAL HERPESVIRUS INFECTIONS

DAVID K. HENDERSON

Although five herpesviruses commonly infect humans (Table 1), recent evidence has been presented that suggests that a sixth may also be an important pathogen,[1,2] and a seventh, Herpesvirus simiae is a rare cause of human infection. With the exception of the varicella-zoster virus (VZV) the remaining herpesviruses infecting humans apparently require close personal contact for person-to-person spread and are therefore not classified as highly contagious. Three properties shared by some members of this family of viruses are important to emphasize: (*1*) all of these viruses can, after causing a primary infection, persist in a latent state in the body and subsequently cause recrudescent or reactivation infection; (*2*) many if not all of the herpesvirus family produce marked immunomodulating effects on the infected host, and certain of the viruses have been incriminated as being oncogenic; and (*3*) differentiation of recrudescent infection from primary infection is often difficult and makes identification of true nosocomial infections problematic. This distinction is often made on the basis of serologic evidence, the reliability of which may be questionable. Because recrudescent infections are common among immunosuppressed patients, they are discussed in detail in the chapters of this book dealing with each of the different viruses. For that reason, recrudescent infections have been omitted from the discussion that follows.

TABLE 1. Herpes Viruses Infecting Humans

Herpes simplex viruses (HSV-I and HSV-II)
Varicella-zoster virus (VZV)
Cytomegalovirus (CMV)
Epstein-Barr virus (EBV)
Human herpesvirus 6 (HHV-6)
Herpesvirus simiae (herpes B virus) (rare)

These viruses have become important nosocomial pathogens for several reasons, including the presence of some of these agents in blood, blood products, and organ transplants and the high prevalence of these infections in the population at large.

The purpose of this chapter is to discuss the risk of nosocomial transmission of each of these agents and to discuss appropriate techniques to be used to prevent transmission of these agents to patients and personnel in the hospital.

HERPES SIMPLEX VIRUSES

Risk of Nosocomial Transmission

Transmission of herpes simplex virus (HSV-I and HSV-II) from infected patients to staff has been well documented.[3–10] Both HSV-I and HSV-II have been associated with the occurrence of herpetic whitlow.[8–13] Primary HSV-I infection has also been reported after mouth-to-mouth resuscitation.[8] Although a great deal of attention has been focused on the problem of HSV-II infection in obstetric and neonatal intensive care unit (ICU) settings, HSV-I has also been associated with outbreaks of infection in hospital personnel and their families.[9] Once in a nursery or an ICU, for example, an infant with HSV infection may serve as a reservoir for transmission to other infants, although the risk of such transmission appears to be small.[9] Whereas HSV infection occurring as a result of the infant acquiring infection during delivery has been well documented, postpartum acquisition of HSV has been much less common and more difficult to document, and the diagnosis has been made most often on empirical grounds.[14] Transmission of HSV-I from staff to patients has also been reported. Linnemann and colleagues used restriction enzyme analysis to demonstrate that two cases of HSV-I infection in neonates in the same nursery were caused by viruses with identical DNA "fingerprints."[15] More recently Sakadka et al. have reported two clusters of HSV-I infections at two separate hospitals.[16] Both clusters involved three neonates, and in both instances all three infants had HSV-I isolates that produced virtually identical endonuclease cleavage profiles.[16] Although not proved definitively, an environmental reservoir (radiant warmer) was incriminated in one cluster. In the other, three infants born at one hospital approximately 1 year apart were infected with strains of HSV-I that yielded identical restriction endonuclease patterns. The authors postulated that health care workers providing care for these infants developed periodic reactivation of HSV-1 infection that resulted in transmission to the infants.[16] Although never measured, the risk of nosocomial transmission of HSV to susceptible patients, including neonates, appears to be quite small.

Mechanism of Nosocomial Transmission

The frequent occurrence of whitlow in ICU personnel, respiratory care personnel, and dentists argues for a primary role for cutaneous inoculations of HSV-I from oral secretions of infected patients directly into the skin of health care providers. Although many if not most whitlows represent primary infection with HSV, reactivation infection or recrudescence can occur,[10,12,17] and one experimental study has demonstrated the possibility for reinfection.[18]

Oral lesions due to HSV-I contain large quantities of virus and represent a potential reservoir for nosocomial transmission. In one study oral lesions were found to have an average of $>10^8$ plaque-forming units/ml of vesicular fluid.[19] Moreover, high titers of virus remained in lesions of severely immunocompromised patients for 3 weeks or longer.[19] More recently, Turner et al. demonstrated that HSV-I could be cultured from the hands of six of nine adults with oral lesions.[20] In addition, in the same study HSV-I isolates were shown to survive drying on skin, plastic, and cloth for up to 4 hours. Both patients and hospital personnel can harbor inapparent reactivation infections. In one prospective study, 9.6 percent of asymptomatic staff members of an obstetric hospital were found to have HSV in saliva.[21]

HSV-contaminated breast milk has been inferentially incriminated as being responsible for the postpartum transmission of HSV in one instance[22]; however, HSV infection of either mother or child is not a contraindication to breast-feeding.

Prevention of Nosocomial Transmission

Institution of universal precautions[23] should minimize the risk for the transmission of HSV-1. By following universal precautions, health care workers should avoid direct cutaneous exposure to HSV-I lesions. For patients who have extensive oral, genital or cutaneous disease, the use of drainage and secretion precautions is appropriate. All personnel having skin-to-skin contact with an HSV-infected patient should use good hand washing techniques. Personnel performing procedures involving oral or genital secretions (e.g., suctioning, placement of an oral airway, dental work, irrigation of a Foley catheter, dressing changes) should wear gloves. Such patients are a reservoir for whitlow but probably represent minimal risk to other patients, with only the following few exceptions. Patients with disseminated HSV lesions should not be roomed with immunocompromised patients or with patients who have severe atopic histories or defects in skin integrity (burn patients, eczema, etc.). Alternatively, in a nursery, a neonatal ICU, or a burn ward, such patients are optimally managed by using strict isolation or, when possible, cohort nursing.

A special problem arises when the mother of a newborn has active nongenital HSV infection. Kibrick has recommended that the newborn be placed in a private room, that the mother only be allowed to handle or feed the baby after her lesions have crusted over, and that once the mother has had contact with the baby, the baby be placed on drainage and secretion precautions.[24] Management of mothers and babies exposed to mothers with genital infections is also outlined in Table 2. Optimal care of infants born to infected mothers would include placing the infant in a "special" nursery on drainage and secretion precautions during hospitalization (for up to 14 days). Such infants should be evaluated frequently for signs of HSV infection. Infants developing signs or symptoms of active infection should be maintained on drainage and secretion precautions; if more extensive disease develops, strict isolation or cohort nursing in a private room or in an isolation room in the ICU may be more effective. If such a room is not available, the infant should be separated from other infants in the nursery or ICU. Placing the infant in an incubator or isolette may raise the consciousness of the staff regarding the potential for transmission.[24] A similar approach has been recommended by Gibbs.[25]

Mothers with active genital lesions should be allowed to feed or handle their infants. However, before handling her baby, the mother should cover all lesions, carefully wash her hands, and put on clean hospital garb. If an infant is restricted to an ICU or nursery for life support purposes, the mother may visit that area if all lesions are crusted over and covered. Additionally, in the circumstance in which vaginal delivery by a mother known or suspected of having active genital HSV infection is attempted, fetal scalp monitoring should not be performed due to the risk of infection due to inoculation.[26]

Management of Infected or Exposed Personnel

Hospital personnel who have active oral or other cutaneous infection should not be permitted to care for high-risk patients until the lesions are entirely crusted and dry. Examples of such high-risk patients include premature infants, newborns, severely immunocompromised patients, burn patients, and patients with diseases affecting skin integrity. In the event that an infected individual must work to provide adequate care in a high-risk area, all lesions should be covered by dressings (or a mask). When possible, gloves should be worn, and strict hand washing techniques should be used.

In the event of apparent outbreak or cluster of infections caused by HSV-I, restriction enzyme analysis of DNA from viral isolates has proved to be an extremely useful epidemiologic tool.[16,27]

VARICELLA-ZOSTER VIRUS

Risk of Transmission

Of the members of the herpesvirus family, the varicella-zoster virus (VZV) is by far the most contagious. For this reason most adults have been exposed to the virus and have a prior history of chickenpox (varicella). The risk of transmission is highest in pediatric populations. Among adults, patients and staff from rural areas and locales where the incidence of VZV infection

TABLE 2. Recommendations for Peripartum Care of Pregnant Women with Herpes Simplex Infections

Genital Lesions Present at Term	*Primary Genital Lesions*	*Secondary Genital Lesions*	*Status of Membranes*	*Recommended Route of Delivery*	*Isolation of Mother*	*Isolation of Newborn*
Yes	+	–	Intact or ruptured <4–6 hr	Cesarean section	Yes	Yes
	+	–	Ruptured >4–6 hr	Vaginally	Yes	Yes
	+	or +	Baby has been delivered vaginally	—	Yes	Yes
	–	+	Ruptured >4–6 hr	Vaginally	Yes	Yes
	–	+	Intact or ruptured <4–6 hr	Cesarean section	Yes	Yes
No, cervical culture +	–	–	Intact or ruptured <4–6 hr	Cesarean section	Yes	Yes
	–	–	Ruptured >4–6 hr	Vaginally	Yes	Yes
No, + history, inactive	–	–	Intact or ruptured	Vaginally	No	No
No, active nongenital HSV	–	–	Intact or ruptured	Vaginally	Yes	No at birth (yes after maternal contact)
No, history of nongenital HSV, inactive	–	–	Intact or ruptured	Vaginally	No	No

(Modified from Kibrick,[24] with permission.)

is lower (e.g., tropical climates) are at highest risk for acquisition.[28]

The major concern with nosocomial transmission of VZV infection occurs in areas housing potentially susceptible immunosuppressed patients (e.g., pediatric oncology ward). In immunocompetent patients, both primary infections (varicella) and recrudescent VZV infections (herpes zoster) are usually benign, self-limited infections. In patients who are immunosuppressed either by an underlying illness or by therapy for an underlying illness, both primary[29–31] and recrudescent VZV infections[31–33] are associated with increased morbidity and mortality. Patients with certain congenital and acquired immunodeficiency (AIDS) syndromes may also be at high risk for severe or fatal primary infections. Finally, some authors have reported that varicella occurring during pregnancy is associated with increased severity.[34,35] Others have stressed that this increase in severity is typical of varicella in an adult population[36,37] and that complications of VZV infection in pregnancy occur no more frequently than in the entire adult population. Whether immunocompromised patients who have had chickenpox are at risk for exogenous reinfection is a matter of some controversy. Several investigators have suggested that immunocompromised patients may be at risk to acquire exogenous reinfection with VZV in the form of typical dermatomal zoster,[38,39] as a second case of varicella or chickenpox,[40,41] or as atypical generalized zoster,[39] a syndrome reported to resemble disseminated zoster without an antecedent dermatome. One epidemiologic study has suggested such a possibility[40]; however, this study has considerable shortcomings,[42,43] and molecular epidemiologic information regarding this outbreak is not available. Gershon and coworkers have demonstrated reinfection varicella in immunosuppressed patients.[41] Currently, most authorities believe that primary VZV infection generally produces lifetime protection against exogenous reinfection. If cases of exogenous reinfection do occur, they must be quite uncommon.

Mechanisms of Transmission

Nosocomial transmission of VZV infection does occur. Several studies have clearly demonstrated airborne transmission from an index case with varicella to susceptible children.[44–46] Also, a susceptible patient or staff member may acquire primary infection as a result of direct contact with lesions from a patient with dermatomal zoster.[36] Despite some published evidence suggesting that dermatomal zoster may be transmitted from patient to patient,[38,39,47,48] most authorities believe that dermatomal zoster represents recrudescent infection rather than a transmissible illness.[36,49–51] One report suggested that a patient with localized zoster was the index case in a nosocomial outbreak of VZV infection.[52] Since the index case was bedfast and several of the secondary cases were younger than 1 year old (and, therefore, not ambulatory), the authors postulated that the transmission must have occurred either via the airborne route or via the hands of hospital personnel. In any event, such occurrences would appear to be extremely uncommon.

Prevention of Nosocomial Transmission

Because VZV is highly contagious and because VZV infection may be life-threatening in certain patient populations,[29–31] many authorities have made recommendations regarding techniques to be used to prevent nosocomial transmission of VZV infection.[40,53–58] If possible, patients with active VZV infections should not be hospitalized. If patients with active infections must be hospitalized, most authorities recommend that patients with dermatomal zoster be placed on drainage and secretion precautions and that the patient's door be labeled with a sign warning people who have not had chickenpox not to enter the patient's room. Severely immunocompromised patients who develop dermatomal zoster (i.e., those with hematologic or reticuloendothelial malignancies, those with AIDS, and those receiving high-dose corticosteroids or multidrug chemotherapy) should be placed on strict isolation precautions because of the high incidence of dissemination. In such instances, if the primary dermatome begins to heal without signs of dissemination, precautions may be relaxed to drainage and secretion precautions. Patients with varicella or disseminated zoster should be placed on strict isolation precautions. Because of the airborne transmission of VZV,[44,45] Leclair et al. Gustafson and colleagues have recommended that hospitalized patients with varicella be placed downwind from other potentially susceptible patients. Anderson and coworkers documented the absence of VZV transmission over a 1-year period in a pediatrics hospital by using negative-pressure ventilation rooms.[57]

If a susceptible immunocompromised patient is exposed to a patient with VZV infection, transmission of the infection can be prevented by the administration of hyperimmune globulin (varicella-zoster immune globulin [VZIG]). To be effective, VZIG should be administered as soon as possible after exposure. The Centers for Disease Control (CDC) recommend that VZIG be given within 96 hours of exposure.[58] VZV infections are common, and in spite of good infection control procedures, VZV is frequently introduced into the hospital environment in an uncontrolled fashion.[43–48,59–63] Because of the urgency involved in identifying exposed, susceptible, immunosuppressed patients,[48] an organized approach to a potential outbreak is advisable. We have developed an algorithm to manage potential nosocomial outbreaks of VZV infection[49] (Fig. 1). Others have used a similar approach.[64,65]

Description of the Algorithm

Cases of VZV infection are identified by routine ward rounds, by routine surveillance activities, and by referrals from patient care areas. Once a suspected case is identified, the diagnosis is confirmed, either by hospital epidemiology service staff members or by staff of the clinical virology laboratory. If the suspected diagnosis is incorrect, the investigation is aborted. Once the diagnosis is confirmed, the investigation is divided into two separate areas: (*1*) the patient-related epidemiologic investigation and (*2*) the staff-related epidemiologic investigation. Because of the necessity for administering passive immunoglobulin prophylaxis to exposed, susceptible, immunocompromised children within 96 hours of exposure to be effective, the initial focus of the investigation is on patients.

An in-hospital "travel history" is first obtained from the index case. Because in-hospital exposures may take place in any of a number of patient-related areas, several diverse areas must be considered in history taking (Fig. 1). When any of these areas are included in the patient's travel history, the departmental records from that area are examined. Patients documented to be in that area at the same time as the index case are included in the population at risk.

The second component of the patient-related investigation is the direct identification of patients at high risk for severe complications of primary VZV infection (Fig. 1). Three methods are used to identify such patients: (*1*) a computer list of all hospitalized pediatric patients, (*2*) a list of all ambulatory care patients including those children who might be staying outside the hospital but returning daily for chemotherapy and/or blood drawing, and (*3*) questioning the inpatient pediatrics staff.

Once the population at risk has been determined, the immunologic status of all patients on the list is assessed. If the patient is found to be potentially immunosuppressed (i.e., hematologic malignancy receiving chemotherapy, high-dose steroid therapy, congenital or acquired immunodeficiency), the patient and his medical staff are questioned regarding the potential for exposure and for a prior history of chickenpox. If the patient is potentially exposed and has a negative or equivocal history of VZV infection, a baseline serology is drawn, and VZIG is

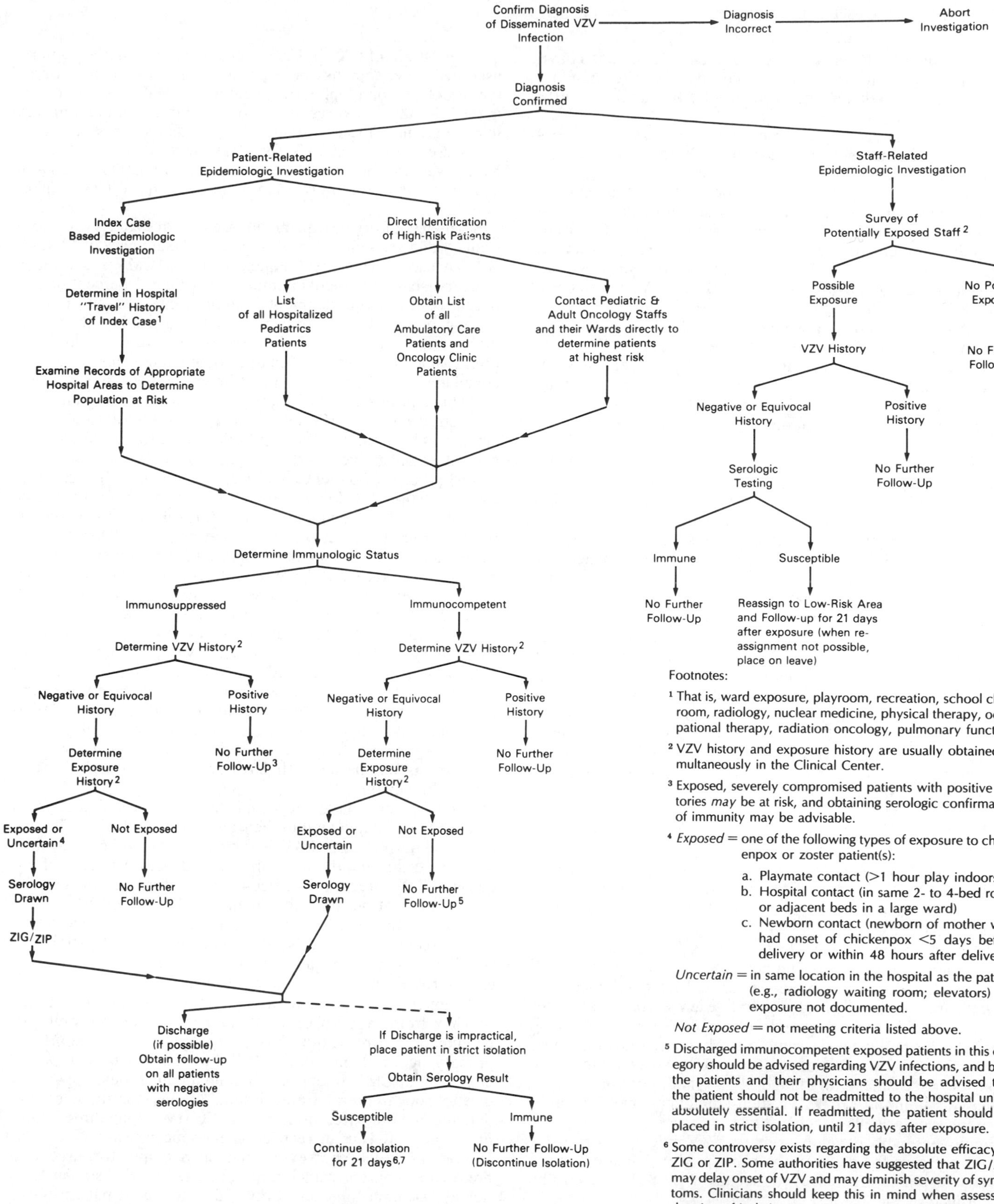

Footnotes:

[1] That is, ward exposure, playroom, recreation, school classroom, radiology, nuclear medicine, physical therapy, occupational therapy, radiation oncology, pulmonary function.

[2] VZV history and exposure history are usually obtained simultaneously in the Clinical Center.

[3] Exposed, severely compromised patients with positive histories *may* be at risk, and obtaining serologic confirmation of immunity may be advisable.

[4] *Exposed* = one of the following types of exposure to chickenpox or zoster patient(s):

a. Playmate contact (>1 hour play indoors)
b. Hospital contact (in same 2- to 4-bed room or adjacent beds in a large ward)
c. Newborn contact (newborn of mother who had onset of chickenpox <5 days before delivery or within 48 hours after delivery).

Uncertain = in same location in the hospital as the patient (e.g., radiology waiting room; elevators) but exposure not documented.

Not Exposed = not meeting criteria listed above.

[5] Discharged immunocompetent exposed patients in this category should be advised regarding VZV infections, and both the patients and their physicians should be advised that the patient should not be readmitted to the hospital unless absolutely essential. If readmitted, the patient should be placed in strict isolation, until 21 days after exposure.

[6] Some controversy exists regarding the absolute efficacy of ZIG or ZIP. Some authorities have suggested that ZIG/ZIP may delay onset of VZV and may diminish severity of symptoms. Clinicians should keep this in mind when assessing duration of isolation.

[7] Usual incubation period for VZV is 9–21 days; hence, the immunocompetent, susceptible, exposed patient should be placed in strict isolation 8 days following exposure. Isolation should be continued until 22 days following exposure. In an immunocompromised patient the incubation period may be shorter. Therefore, an exposed, susceptible, immunocompromised patient who did not receive prophylaxis should be placed in isolation immediately after the patient is identified as being at risk. If the patient did not receive prophylaxis, isolation should be continued for 21 days following exposure.

FIG. 1. Algorithm for the evaluation of a potential nosocomial outbreak of VZV infection.

administered. If VZIG is not available, many blood banks have plasma from patients recovering from zoster (zoster-immune plasma [ZIP]), which contains high-titer antivaricella antibody.[66]

If the patient is determined to have had primary VZV infection or is determined not to have been exposed, no further follow-up is needed.

If patients on the potentially exposed list are found to be immunocompetent, exposure and VZV histories are obtained after a work-up of the immunocompromised patients. Exposed, susceptible immunocompetent patients have serologies drawn and, when possible, are discharged. Those with negative exposure histories or positive histories of prior VZV infection need no further follow-up.

If patients must remain hospitalized, serologic determination of immunity by using a sensitive technique, such as FAMA,[67] immune adherence hemagglutination (IAHA),[68] or enzyme-linked immunosorbent assay (ELISA),[69] may help determine which exposed patients are susceptible. Less sensitive tests such as the complement fixation test are not reliable indicators of immunity.[70]

Exposed, susceptible, immunocompetent patients should be placed in strict isolation from 9 days after the first possible exposure until 21 days after the last possible exposure. Exposed, susceptible, immunosuppressed patients (even those receiving VZIG or ZIP) should be placed in strict isolation at the time the patient is identified as being at risk until at least 21 days after the last possible exposure. Some studies have suggested that the administration of ZIP or earlier preparations of VZIG to exposed, susceptible, immunosuppressed patients may actually lengthen the incubation period for such patients. Although instances of lengthened incubation periods have not been reported with newer preparations of VZIG, physicians responsible for the care of such patients should be mindful of this possibility when planning extended in-hospital care for the patient. Exposed, susceptible, immunosuppressed patients may be candidates for the varicella vaccine.[71,72] Additional studies have suggested a role for transfer factor in the prevention of primary VZV infection in such patients.[73,74]

Management of Infected or Exposed Personnel

The other major aspect of the work-up of a potential nosocomial outbreak of VZV infection is the assessment of potentially exposed staff (Fig. 1). Exposure and VZV histories are taken from all potentially exposed staff. Potentially exposed staff who relate negative or equivocal histories of VZV infection should have serologic assessment of immunity with a sensitive test.[67–69]

Exposed, susceptible employees should be reassigned to a low-risk area or placed on administrative leave from 9 days after the first possible exposure until 21 days after the last possible exposure. If employees desiring to work in an area with a high prevalence of VZV infection are found to be susceptible on the basis of assessment of humoral[67–69] and, possibly, cell-mediated[75] immunity to VZV, such employees may be candidates for the varicella vaccine.[71,72]

Employees who develop primary VZV infection or zoster should not care for or be in the same area with patients until the last lesion is crusted over (usually 7 or 8 days after the appearance of the last lesion).

CYTOMEGALOVIRUS

Risk for Nosocomial Transmission

The nosocomial epidemiology of cytomegalovirus (CMV) infection is incompletely understood. Part of the difficulty in assessing the magnitude of risk for nosocomial transmission lies in the difficulty in discriminating between endogenous reactivation infection and exogenous reinfection (i.e., infection with a second strain of CMV). The term *secondary infection* will be used here to encompass both possibilities. In several settings, the risk of an individual patient acquiring CMV infection, either in the hospital or as a result of iatrogenic intervention, appears to be quite high. Premature infants and infants in newborn nurseries are at increased risk for CMV acquisition.[76–83] Studies have suggested that from 14 to 30 percent of infants residing in a neonatal ICU for more than 1 month acquire CMV infection.[76–78]

Recipients of organ transplants are also at high risk for both primary and secondary CMV infection. A summary of 12 studies that used various techniques to assess CMV infection in renal transplant recipients demonstrated that 53 percent of seronegative transplant recipients acquired infection and that 85 percent of seropositive transplant recipients either shed culturable virus or developed a fourfold rise in anti-CMV antibody titer.[84] Since these results include some studies that used only complement fixation to document infection, these numbers are probably conservative estimates of the risk of a renal transplant recipient acquiring CMV infection. Heart transplant recipients are also at high risk for CMV infection. Post-transplant, 62 percent of seronegative heart transplant patients seroconverted, and 60 percent of patients who were seropositive before heart transplantation developed fourfold rises in antibody titer after transplantation.[85] Recipients of heterologous bone marrow infusions or grafts are also at increased risk for CMV infection. In one study 39 percent of all seronegative patients acquired primary infection, and 61 percent of seropositive bone marrow recipients developed evidence of secondary CMV infection.[86]

Recipients of granulocyte transfusions have also been demonstrated to be at risk for acquiring CMV infection. In the study cited above,[86] 48 percent of seronegative bone marrow recipients who received granulocyte transfusions seroconverted as compared with 33 percent of seronegative recipients who did not receive granulocyte transfusions. In an earlier study, Winston and colleagues demonstrated that 61 percent of patients receiving granulocyte transfusions developed evidence of CMV infection as compared with 26 percent of age- and disease-matched recipients.[87]

Several studies have suggested that the transfusion of fresh whole blood is implicated in the transmission of CMV. The risk for the acquisition of CMV has been shown to be associated with increasing numbers of units transfused. The risk of acquiring CMV infection has been estimated to be between 2.4 and 2.7 percent per unit of transfused whole blood.[88–89]

Although the risk for CMV transmission by parenteral exposure seems clear, the issue of whether hospital patients or hospital personnel are at risk for acquiring CMV by nonparenteral routes of exposure is less clear.

Although apparently uncommon, nonparenteral transmission of CMV from patient to patient has been reasonably well documented.[90–93] Breast milk has been implicated as a source of primary neonatal infection.[83,92,94] Two studies have reported clustering of CMV infections in neonatal nurseries, apparently due to nonparenteral transmission.[90,91] One of these studies documented nonparenteral spread of CMV among three infants in a neonatal ICU using restriction endonuclease analysis.[91] The author concluded, however, that such common-source outbreaks are apparently uncommon. In a study using similar technology, Demmler and coworkers demonstrated patient-to-patient transmission of a single strain of CMV in a busy chronic care pediatrics hospital.[93] The authors isolated CMV from patients' hands, from health care workers' hands, and from hospitalized infants' diapers.[93]

The issue of whether hospital personnel are at risk for acquiring CMV infection is a controversial one. Some investigators have suggested that hospital personnel are at slightly higher risk for seroconversion than are age-matched controls who did not have patient contact.[95] The intensive studies by Ahlfors and colleagues in Sweden, however, found little evidence that nurses were at greater risk for acquiring CMV infection than were other age-matched Swedish women.[96,97] A study using restriction enzyme analysis of CMV DNA demonstrated no correlation between the CMV strain infecting a neonate and the strain of CMV found to be infecting a nurse who cared for the infant.[98] In a second study using similar technology, significant differences were found in DNA from CMV isolates obtained from a physician who became infected while caring for a CMV-infected child and the isolate from the child.[99] In both studies the health care professionals were pregnant, and both elected to have abortions. CMV with identical restriction patterns to the maternal isolates was grown from each of the infected fetuses.[98,99]

Several more recent studies have suggested minimal or negligible risk for patient-to-staff transmission of CMV.[93,100–106] Balfour and Balfour compared CMV infection rates in three groups of nurses—those working in neonatal intensive care units, those working in renal transplant/dialysis units and student nurses—with age-matched blood donors.[100] No association was found between the prevalence of infection among patients and seroconversion, and these authors concluded that nurses were no more likely to develop CMV infection than were the age-matched blood donor controls.[100]

Demmler and colleagues[93] also found no association between CMV seroconversion and occupational exposure to CMV in two pediatric hospitals in Texas. This study also found no correlation between prevalence of infection in patients and seroconversion in health care providers.[93] Adler and coworkers used restriction endonucleases to evaluate CMV isolates from 34 hospitalized newborn infants and from the one seronegative health care worker who developed primary CMV infection during the 3-year study period.[101] No two isolates were identical.

Brady and colleagues demonstrated annual seroconversion rates for CMV-serosusceptible pediatric house staff of 3.8 percent.[102] Although appropriate controls were not available for this study, similar rates have been documented for other medical and nonmedical personnel.[93,97,107]

Hatherly found no seroconversions among obstetrics staff caring for CMV-infected patients,[103] and Blackman and coworkers concluded that the risk of CMV transmission from infected disabled children to educational and health care personnel providing care for these children was low.[104]

Finally, since patients who are infected with the human immunodeficiency virus (HIV) (particularly those who have AIDS) are known to harbor and shed large quantities of herpesviruses, both Gerberding and colleagues[105] and Kuhls et al.[106] have evaluated health care workers providing care for HIV-1-infected patients for serologic evidence of CMV infection. Neither study found an elevated rate of CMV acquisition.

Conversely, other investigators, while failing to demonstrate patient-to-staff transmission of CMV, have postulated that the risk for transmission is likely to be higher for personnel working with patients who have a high prevalence of CMV infection.[108,109] Although such a hypothesis seems plausible, to my knowledge, no direct evidence supports this contention.

At this time there are no instances of patient-to-staff transmission of CMV that are documented by restriction enzyme analysis of CMV isolates. One investigator has, however, used endonuclease analysis to document apparent nonparenteral transmission of CMV from an infected infant to his seronegative mother.[83] Thus, the magnitude of the risk of patient-to-staff transmission of CMV, especially when appropriate isolation procedures are observed, would appear to be small.[107]

Mechanisms of Nosocomial Transmission

In the instances in which primary infection with CMV is documented to have occurred in the hospital setting, the parenteral route of transmission has almost always been implicated.

Most primary infections in the neonatal ICU can be traced to the transfusion of whole blood contaminated with CMV.[76–82] Consumption of breast milk contaminated with CMV has been suggested to be an important nonparenteral mechanism of transmission of CMV to neonates.[83,92,94] The possibility has also been raised, but not to my knowledge documented, that fomites[92] or health care professionals[91–93] may be vectors for nonparenteral transmission of CMV in unusual circumstances.

Renal transplant recipients can acquire primary CMV infection from blood transfusions,[56,84,110,111] from leukocyte infusions, or from the transplanted organ itself.[56,112,113] Recipients of bone marrow allografts can acquire CMV infection through receipt of an infected allograft, through transfused blood or platelets, or perhaps most likely, through infected leukocyte infusions.[91,92] Weller[114] and others have postulated that intimate contact is required for the transmission of CMV infection. If nonparenteral transmission is occurring in the hospital, it must be due to exposure of a susceptible individual (patient or employee) to contaminated excreta or secretions, presumably via the oral or respiratory routes.

Prevention of Nosocomial Transmission

Several precautionary measures can be implemented to minimize the risk of CMV transmission in a high-risk setting in the hospital. Choosing organ seronegative donors for renal transplant recipients who are seronegative is an effective way of minimizing the risk for subsequent CMV infection in this setting. Betts has advocated using the donor serologic status as a major determinant in selecting a donor kidney for a seronegative recipient.[113]

Winston et al. have suggested that seronegative donors be given priority as potential leukocyte donors because of the evidence that CMV is leukocyte associated and that the development of CMV infection in recipients of leukocytes is often a serious problem.[87]

Both Lang et al.[111] and Tolkoff-Rubin et al.[110] have recommended transfusing patients at high risk for CMV infection with either leukocyte-depleted blood or with washed, frozen red cells to minimize the risk of CMV transmission. In addition, several studies have demonstrated a decreased risk for primary CMV infection that is associated with the transfusion of frozen, deglycerolized red blood cells.[110,115–117] Most recently Brady and colleagues have extended their earlier studies to demonstrate that transfusing either blood from CMV-seronegative donors or frozen, deglycerolized red blood cells was associated with significantly lower CMV excretion rates in preterm infants receiving these transfusions than was found in similar infants who received either saline washed red blood cells or conventionally processed whole blood.[117]

Yeager and colleagues[81] and Benson et al.[82] have demonstrated the efficacy of transfusing blood from seronegative donors into seronegative recipients to prevent the transmission of CMV to neonates. In one study, CMV infections were entirely prevented by administering seronegative blood to neonates.[81] One of these approaches would also be advisable if a seronegative transplant recipient who has received an organ from a seronegative donor requires transfusion. Since human milk may also be a reservoir for CMV infection in neonates,[83,92,94] Yeager et al. have also recommended that donors of milk be screened and that a premature infant of a seronegative mother receive milk from the mother or from seronegative donors.[81]

Since most pregnant women secreting CMV in cervical mucus are asymptomatic and, unlike infection with the herpes simplex viruses, since perinatal infection with CMV is not associated with symptomatic illness in the newborn, no precautions are advocated for mothers known to be secreting CMV at delivery.

Placing immunosuppressed patients who are infected with CMV (e.g., patients with AIDS, transplant recipients, or babies with congenital infection) on isolation precautions may be prudent, in part because such patients excrete large quantities of virus in many different body fluids.[56] Appropriate precautions for such patients should include gloves for contact with wounds or lesions or for contact with blood, secretions, or excreta. Also, infected patients in the neonatal ICU should be segregated from noninfected babies. Other precautions advisable in caring for such patients would include handling linens and other reusable patient care items as isolation materials and emphasizing hand washing after each patient contact. In general, strict adherence to universal precautions[23] should further minimize the already small risk for occupational/nosocomial infection.

Management of Infected, Exposed and Potentially Exposed Personnel

The risk for staff-to-patient transmission of CMV has received little attention in the literature. Only one study has attempted to assess this risk. Demmler and colleagues found no evidence of CMV transmission among patients cared for by four CMV-shedding health care workers.[93] These authors concluded that, although a theoretic possibility, the risk for staff-to-patient transmission of CMV was sufficiently small to allow infected health care workers to continue working.[93] Based on currently available evidence regarding the transmission and transmissibility of CMV, such an approach seems entirely reasonable.

The issue of limiting exposure of pregnant health care workers to CMV-infected patients remains somewhat controversial.

Although, as noted above, data documenting CMV transmission from patient to staff are nonexistent, a commonsense approach to the care of infected patients is appropriate. In an earlier edition of this text[118] I recommended the conservative approach previously advocated by Valenti[56] to the management of CMV-infected patients by pregnant health care workers. Several factors have caused our Hospital Infections Committee to reassess this difficult and controversial issue; in a later publication Valenti has modified his recommendations as well.[119]

First, a number of additional manuscripts (see "Risk for Nosocomial Transmission," above) have been published that further document that the risk for occupational/nosocomial infection with CMV is quite small. Because the number of seroconversions in these studies is small, a very large study would be required to measure the magnitude of the small risk of CMV transmission to health care workers precisely. Nonetheless, the expanded, consistent data base is reassuring.

Second, numerous investigators have pointed out that many patients who are excreting CMV (e.g., immunosuppressed patients, AIDS patients, dialysis patients, transplant recipients, pediatric patients) have no signs or symptoms of CMV infection. Such patients are frequently not identified as being infected or infectious during the course of hospitalization. Presumably, most patients shedding CMV who are hospitalized will not be specifically identified as having CMV infection; for this reason a broader approach to our patient population seems prudent.

Third, since the magnitude of the risk to pregnant health care workers is currently below the limits of detection, the administrative problems associated with a more restrictive policy (i.e., if pregnant health care workers are restricted, how should one manage health care workers who "think they might be" or "are trying to become" or "are not trying to prevent becoming" pregnant?) may not be justified.

Fourth, the recent issuance by the CDC (and adoption by our hospital) of universal precautions guidelines[23] should further reduce the already small risk for CMV transmission from patients to health care workers.

A subsequent clarification of the universal precautions policy recently issued by CDC noted that these precautions do not apply to feces, urine, saliva, sweat, sputum, or tears.[120] In this update, the CDC emphasizes that universal precautions are supplementary or baseline precautions and that these new precautions are not designed to replace standard infection control policy. Specifically, this update notes that prior CDC recommendations[121] recommend wearing gloves to prevent gross microbial contamination of hands. This latter recommendation deserves careful consideration when handling urine from any patient. Although universal precautions do not apply to saliva, the prior recommendation for gloving before digital examination of mucous membranes remain in effect.

These new recommendations also allow the health care worker to use judgment in deciding whether or not barriers (such as gloves) are needed. These new guidelines emphasize the importance of hand washing, which, if practiced appropriately, should minimize the risk for occupational CMV infection.

Finally, the issue of routine screening of health care workers for antibody to CMV is also controversial. Several recent papers have addressed this issue[103,119,122–126]; the lack of consensus is apparent. The CDC has not advocated routine screening.[122,123] Conversely, Adler[124] and Plotkin[125] support periodic serologic testing for "potentially pregnant" employees whose jobs entail exposure to CMV-infected patients. Brady[126] argues that, on the basis of the magnitude of risk, serologic testing is not warranted and may in fact cause increased anxiety. Onorato et al. argue that no data indicate that routine testing will have any impact on the risk of congenital CMV infection.[123] Our Hospital Infections Committee and Occupational Medical Service have decided not to offer routine screening of employees. Since the risk for patient-to-staff transmission is as yet unmeasurable and since adherence to universal precautions will further reduce this risk, we do not recommend reassignment of pregnant health care workers. Rather, we have chosen to educate staff aggressively regarding CMV and other occupational risks and to emphasize the importance of good hygiene and universal precautions during pregnancy. For all these reasons, we do not recommend reassignment of pregnant health care workers.

EPSTEIN-BARR VIRUS

Risk for Nosocomial Transmission

The risk of nosocomial transmission of Epstein-Barr virus (EBV) appears to be very small. Only a handful of instances of nosocomial transmission of EBV to patients have been identified.[89–97]

Transmission of EBV from patient to staff or staff to patient has not been described, although Ginsburg and colleagues have described an outbreak of infectious mononucleosis in personnel working in an outpatient clinic,[127] and Chang et al. have described the apparent transmissibility of EBV in a relatively crowded nursery providing domiciliary care.[128]

Mechanisms of Transmission

Patients who have been shown to have acquired nosocomial EBV infection have been recipients of blood or plasma transfusions[129–136] or bone marrow allografts[137] apparently infected with EBV. EBV appears to be one of the least contagious of the herpesviruses, and most authorities believe that intimate contact is required for transmission of the virus.[138]

Prevention of Nosocomial Transmission

Patients known to have EBV in their secretions may be a reservoir for infection if extremely poor hygiene practices are followed by health care workers. In 1975, the CDC recommended that patients with infectious mononucleosis be placed on secretions precautions.[139] In more recent recommendations the CDC states that isolation precautions are not necessary but adds the codicil that oral secretions may be infectious.[121] Adherence to universal precautions, use of appropriate barriers, and attention to hand washing and hygiene practices will further reduce the risk for occupational infection.

Management of Infected or Exposed Personnel

Staff who acquire infection with EBV (e.g., infectious mononucleosis) may secrete virus much longer than symptoms persist,[140] but if good hygienic practices are followed (e.g., hand washing), such personnel probably do not transmit the infection.

HUMAN HERPESVIRUS 6

Risk for Nosocomial Transmission

Recently an additional herpesvirus capable of infecting humans has been identified. First called human B-lymphotropic virus[1] and then human herpesvirus 6 (HHV-6),[2] this agent has recently been postulated as the cause of roseola infantum (exanthem subitum)[141] (see Chapter 274). This childhood exanthem is reasonably contagious and may represent a risk for nosocomial transmission, particularly in pediatric hospitals. This virus is also found (presumably as an opportunist) in the peripheral blood of AIDS patients.[2]

Mechanisms of Transmission

Because of the level of contagiousness this virus may well be transmitted by the respiratory route, perhaps in a fashion similar to varicella-zoster virus (VZV). Data regarding the epidemiology and putative routes of transmission of HHV-6 are at too preliminary a stage for comment.

Prevention of Nosocomial Transmission

Because of the contagiousness of the exanthem and because we are just beginning to learn about the epidemiology of HHV-6, hospitalized patients who have roseola should be treated similarly to patients with VZV infection.

HERPESVIRUS SIMIAE

Herpesvirus simiae, also called herpes B virus, commonly causes infection in Old World monkeys. In rare instances this virus has been found to infect humans, usually causing a severe and often fatal encephalomyelitis.[142,143] Most instances of human infection have occurred in monkey handlers, and most but not all instances of infection have occurred after monkey bites or scratches. One instance of zosterlike apparent reactivation infection has been documented.[142] Person-to-person transmission has not been documented.

An outbreak of four cases of B-virus infection in Pensacola, Florida, in 1987, including two deaths as well as the first documented case of human-to-human transmission, focused national attention on the possibility of occupational transmission of herpes B.[144] Herpes B infection in humans has been considered to be a rare disease. Only 22 cases are reported in the literature.[145,146] Although symptomatic herpes B infection in humans has been thought to be associated with severe illness (20 of the 22 cases had encephalitis, and 15 of the 20 died [145]); 2 of the 4 cases reported in the Pensacola outbreak had mild illnesses.[144] Both these individuals received antiviral therapy. The frequency with which infected individuals develop mild or asymptomatic infectious is unknown.

In response to these four cases the CDC developed a detailed set of guidelines to prevent herpes B infection in animal handlers.[145] Adherence to these guidelines should minimize the risk for symptomatic infection.

If an animal handler is scratched or bitten by a monkey known to be harboring the B virus, experimental studies have suggested that transmission can be prevented by the administration of acyclovir.[144–147] One of the four cases from the Pensacola outbreak recovered after oral acyclovir treatment; the other who recovered received intravenous acyclovir.[144] Employees sustaining significant injuries should be considered for postexposure treatment with acyclovir.[145]

REFERENCES

1. Salahuddin SZ, Ablashi DV, Markham PD, et al. Isolation of a new virus, HBLV in patient with lymphoproliferative. Science. 1986;225:69–72.
2. Lopez C, Pellett P, Stewart J, et al. Characterizations of human herpesvirus-6. J Infect Dis. 1988;157:1271–3.
3. Stern H, Eleck SD, Millar DM, et al. Herpetic whitlow: A form of cross-infection in hospitals. Lancet. 1959;2:871–4.
4. Rosato FE, Rosato EF, Plotkin SA. Herpetic paronychia—an occupational hazard of medical personnel. N Engl J Med. 1964;270:979–82.
5. Hanbrick GW Jr, Cox RP, Senior Jr. Primary herpes infection of the finger in medical personnel. Arch Dermatol. 1962;85:583–9.
6. Bart BJ, Fisher I. Primary herpes simplex infection of the hand: Report of a case. J Am Dent Assoc. 1965;71:74–7.
7. Brooks SL, Rowe NH, Drach JC, et al. Prevalence of herpes simplex virus disease in a professional population. J Am Dent Assoc. 1981;102:31–4.
8. Hendricks AA, Shapiro EP. Primary herpes simplex infection following mouth-to-mouth resuscitation. JAMA. 1980;243:257–9.
9. Adams G, Stover BH, Keenlyside RA, et al. Nosocomial herpetic infections in a pediatric intensive care unit. Am J Epidemiol. 1981;113:126–32.
10. Gill MJ, Arlette J, Buchan K. Herpes simplex virus infections of the hand. A profile of 79 cases. Am J Med. 1988;84:89–93.
11. Nahmias AJ, Roizman B. Infection with herpes-simplex viruses 1 and 2 (first of three parts). N Engl J Med. 1973;289:667–74.
12. Haburchak DR. Recurrent herpetic whitlow due to herpes simplex virus type 2. Arch Intern Med. 1978;138:1418–9.
13. Glogau R, Hanna L, Jawetz E. Herpetic whitlow as part of genital virus infection. J Infect Dis. 1977;136:689–92.
14. Light IJ. Postnatal acquisition of herpes simplex virus by the newborn infant: A review of the literature. Pediatrics. 1979;63:480–2.
15. Linneman CC Jr, Buchman TG, Light IJ, et al. Transmission of herpes simplex virus, type 1 in a nursery for the newborn: Identification of viral isolates by DNA fingerprinting. Lancet. 1978;1:964–6.
16. Sakadka H, Saheki Y, Uzuki K, et al. Two outbreaks of herpes simplex virus, type 1 nosocomial infection among newborns. J Clin Microbiol. 1986;24:36–40.
17. Crane LR, Lerner AM. Herpetic whitlow: A manifestation of primary infection with herpes simplex virus type 1 or type 2. J Infect Dis. 1978;137:855–6.
18. Blank H, Haines HG. Experimental reinfection with herpes simplex virus. J Invest Dermatol. 1973;61:223–5.
19. Daniels CA, LeGoff SG. Shedding of infectious virus/antibody complexes from vesicular lesions of patients with recurrent herpes labialis. Lancet. 1975;2:524–8.
20. Turner R, Shehab Z, Osborne K, et al. Shedding and survival of herpes simplex virus from "fever blisters." Pediatrics. 1982;70:547–9.
21. Hatherly LI, Hayes K, Jack I. Herpes virus in an obstetric hospital: II. Asymptomatic virus excretion in staff members. Med J Aust. 1980;2:273–5.
22. Dunkle LM, Schmidt RR, O'Connor DM. Neonatal herpes simplex infection possibly acquired via maternal breast milk. Pediatrics. 1979;63:250–1.
23. Centers for Disease Control. Recommendation for prevention of HIV transmission in health-care settings. MMWR. 1987;36(Suppl 2):1–18.
24. Kibrick S. Herpes simplex infection at term: What to do with mother, newborn, and nursery personnel. JAMA. 1980;243:157–60.
25. Gibbs RS: Infection control of herpes simplex virus in obstetrics and gynecology. J Reprod Med. 1986;31(Suppl):395–8.
26. Kaye EM, Dooling EC. Neonatal herpes simplex meningoencephalitis associated with fetal scalp monitor electrodes. Neurology (NY). 1981;31:1045–7.
27. Buchman TG, Roizman B, Adams G, et al. Restriction endonuclease fingerprinting of herpes simplex virus DNA: A novel epidemiological tool applied to a nosocomial outbreak. J Infect Dis. 1978;138:488–98.
28. Nassar NT, Touma HC. Brief report: Susceptibility of Filipino nurses to the varicella zoster virus. Infect Control. 1986;7:71–2.
29. Feldman S, Hughes WT, Daniel CB. Varicella in children with cancer: Seventy-seven cases. Pediatrics. 1975;56:388–97.
30. Myers MG: Viremia caused by varicella-zoster virus: Association with malignant progressive varicella. J Infect Dis. 1979;140:229–33.
31. Dolin R, Reichman RC, Mazur MH, et al. Herpes zoster-varicella infections in immunosuppressed patients. Ann Intern Med. 1978;89:375–88.
32. Feldman S, Chaudary S, Ossi M, et al. A viremic phase for herpes zoster in children with cancer. J Pediatr. 1977;91:597–600.
33. Feldman S, Hughes WT, Kim HY. Herpes zoster in children with cancer. Am J Dis Child. 1973;126:178–84.
34. Fish SA. Maternal death due to disseminated varicella. JAMA. 1960;173:978–81.
35. Triebwasser JH, Harris RE, Bryant RE, et al. Varicella pneumonia in adults.

Report of seven cases and a review of the literature. Medicine (Baltimore). 1967;46:409–23.
36. Brunell PA. Varicella zoster virus. In: Mandell GL, Douglas RG, Bennett JE, eds. Principles and Practice of Infectious Diseases. New York: Churchill Livingstone; 1979:1295–1306.
37. Brunell PA. Varicella-zoster infections in pregnancy. JAMA. 1967;199:93–5.
38. Rado JP, Tako J, Geder L, et al. Herpes zoster house epidemic in steroid-treated patients. Arch Intern Med. 1965;116:329–35.
39. Schimpff S, Serpick A, Stoler B, et al. Varicella-zoster infection in patients with cancer. Ann Intern Med. 1972;76:241–54.
40. Morens DM, Bregman DJ, West M, et al. An outbreak of varicella-zoster virus infection among cancer patients. Ann Intern Med. 1980;93:414–9.
41. Gershon AA, Steinberg SP, Gelb L. Clinical reinfection with varicella zoster virus. J Infect Dis. 1984;149:137–42.
42. Henderson DK, Laniak JM, Myers RF, et al. Prevention of nosocomial varicella zoster disease. Ann Intern Med. 1981;95:515–6.
43. Henderson DK, Laniak JM, Myers RF, et al. Varicella-zoster virus infection among cancer patients. Ann Intern Med. 1981;95:655–6.
44. Leclair JM, Zaia JA, Levin MJ, et al. Airborne transmission of chickenpox in a hospital. N Engl J Med. 1980;302:450–3.
45. Gustafson TL, Lavely GB, Brawner ER, et al. An outbreak of airborne nosocomial varicella. Pediatrics. 1982;70:550–6.
46. Krasinski K, Holtzman RS, LaCoufure R, et al. Hospital experience with varicella-zoster virus. Infect Control. 1986;7:312–6.
47. Feinstein A, Trau H, Schewach-Millet M. Herpes zoster in a husband and wife. Int J Dermatol. 1980;19:514–6.
48. Berlin BS, Campbell T. Hospital-acquired herpes zoster following exposure to chickenpox. JAMA. 1970;211:1831–3.
49. Miller LH, Brunell PA. Zoster, reinfection or activation of latent virus? Observations on the antibody response. Am J Med. 1970;49:480–3.
50. Haynes RE. Varicella zoster infections in normal and compromised hosts. In: Galasso GJ, ed. Antiviral Agents and Viral Diseases of Man. New York: Raven Press; 1979:647–79.
51. Weller TH: Varicella-herpes zoster virus. In: Evans A, ed. Viral Infections of Humans—Epidemiology and Control. New York: Plenum Press; 1975:457–80.
52. Asano Y, Iwayama S, Miyata T, et al. Spread of varicella in hospitalized children having no direct contact with an indicator zoster case and its prevention by a live vaccine. Biken J. 1980;23:157–61.
53. Myers MG, Rasley D, Hierholzer WJ. Hospital infection control for varicella zoster virus infection. Pediatrics. 1982;70:199–202.
54. Steele RW, Coleman MA, Fiser M, et al. Varicella zoster in hospital personnel: Skin test reactivity to monitor susceptibility. Pediatrics. 1982;70:604–8.
55. Hayden GF, Meyers JD, Dixon RE. Nosocomial varicella: II. Suggested guidelines for management. West J Med. 1979;130:300–3.
56. Valenti WM, Betts RF, Breese Hall C, et al. Nosocomial viral infections: II. Guidelines for prevention and control of respiratory viruses, herpesviruses, and hepatitis viruses. Infect Control. 1980;1:165–78.
57. Anderson JD, Bonner M, Scheifele DW, et al. Lack of nosocomial spread of varicella in a pediatric hospital with negative pressure ventilated rooms. Infect Control. 1985;6:120–1.
58. Centers for Disease Control. Varicella zoster immune globulin. MMWR. 1981;30:15–6, 21–3.
59. Laniak JM, Myers RF, Henderson DK. Algorithm for the control of nosocomial varicella zoster virus infections (Abstract). In: Proceedings of the 82nd Annual Meeting of the American Society for Microbiology. Washington, DC: American Society for Microbiology; 1982:87.
60. Meyers JD, MacQuarrie MB, Merigan TC, et al. Nosocomial varicella: I. Outbreak in oncology patients at a children's hospital. West J Med. 1979;130:196–8.
61. Weber DJ, Rutala WA, Parnam C. Impact and costs of varicella prevention in a university hospital. Am J Public Health. 1988;78:19–23.
62. Haiduven-Griffiths D, Fecko H. Varicella in hospital personnel: A challenge for the infection control practitioner. Am J Infect Control. 1987;15:207–11.
63. Alter SJ, Hammond JA, McVey CJ, et al. Susceptibility to varicella zoster virus among adults at high-risk for exposure. Infect Control. 1986;7:448–51.
64. Mendelson MH, Legg E, Hirschman SZ. Program for preventing nosocomial varicella-zoster virus infection: Application and implications (Abstract). In: Proceedings of the 26th Interscience Conference on Antimicrobial Agents and Chemotherapy. Washington, DC: American Society for Microbiology; 1986:307.
65. Weitekamp MR, Schan P, Aber RC. An algorithm for the control of nosocomial varicella zoster virus infection. Am J Infect Control. 1985;13:193–8.
66. Balfour HH, Groth KE, McCullough J, et al. Prevention or modification of varicella using zoster immune plasma. Am J Dis Child. 1977;131:693–6.
67. Williams V, Gershon A, Brunell PA. Serologic response to varicella-zoster membrane antigens measured by indirect immunofluorescence. J Infect Dis. 1974;130:669–72.
68. Gershon AA, Kalter ZG, Steinberg S. Detection of antibody to varicella-zoster virus by immune adherence hemagglutination. Proc Soc Exp Biol Med. 1976;151:762.
69. Stanley J, Myers MG, Edmond B, et al. An enzyme-linked immunosorbent assay for detection of antibody to varicella zoster virus. J Clin Microbiol. 1982;15:205–11.
70. Brunell PA, Gershon AA, Uduman SA, et al. Varicella-zoster immunoglobulins during varicella, latency, and zoster. J Infect Dis. 1975;132:49–54.
71. Izawa T, Ihara T, Hattori A, et al. Application of live varicella vaccine in children with acute leukemia or other malignant diseases. Pediatrics. 1977;60:805–9.
72. Brunell PA, Shehab Z, Geiser C, et al. Administration of live varicella vaccine to children with leukaemia. Lancet. 1982;2:1069–72.
73. Steele RW, Myers MG, Vincent MM. Transfer factor for the prevention of varicella-zoster infection in childhood leukemia. N Engl J Med. 1980;303:355–9.
74. Steele RW. Transfer factor and cellular reactivity to varicella zoster antigen in childhood leukemia. Cell Immunol. 1980;50:282–9.
75. Gershon AA, Steinberg S, Smith M. Cell-mediated immunity to varicella zoster virus demonstrated by viral inactivation with human leukocytes. Infect Immun. 1976;13:1549–53.
76. Spector SA, Schmidt W, Ticknor W, et al. Cytomegaloviruria in older infants in intensive care units. J Pediatr. 1979;59:444–6.
77. Ballard RA, Drew L, Hufnagle KG, et al. Acquired cytomegalovirus infection in preterm infants. Am J Dis Child. 1979;133:482–5.
78. Spector SA, Edwards DK, Coen RW. Association of acquired cytomegalovirus infections and bronchopulmonary dysplasia in premature infants. Pediatr Res. 1982;16:309.
79. Yeager AS: Transfusion-acquired cytomegalovirus infection in newborn infants. Am J Dis Child. 1974;128:478–83.
80. Yeager AS, Jacobs H, Clark J. Nursery-acquired cytomegalovirus infection in two preterm infants. J Pediatr. 1972;81:332–5.
81. Yeager AS, Grumet FC, Hufleigh EB, et al. Prevention of transfusion-acquired cytomegalovirus infections in newborn infants. J Pediatr. 1981;98:281–7.
82. Benson JWT, Bodden SJ, Tobin JP. Cytomegalovirus and blood transfusion in neonates. Arch Dis Child. 1979;54:538–41.
83. Spector SA, Spector DH: Molecular epidemiology of cytomegalovirus infection in premature twin infants and their mother. Pediatr Infect Dis. 1982;1:405–9.
84. Glenn J. Cytomegalovirus infections following renal transplantation. Rev Infect Dis. 1981;3:1151–78.
85. Pollard RB, Arvin AM, Gamberg P, et al. Specific cell-mediated immunity and infections with herpes viruses in cardiac transplant recipients. Am J Med. 1982;73:679–87.
86. Hersman J, Meyers JD, Thomas ED, et al. The effect of granulocyte transfusions on the incidence of cytomegalovirus infection after allogeneic marrow transplantation. Ann Intern Med. 1982;96:149–52.
87. Winston DJ, Winston SH, Howell CL, et al. Cytomegalovirus infections associated with leukocyte transfusions. Ann Intern Med. 1980;93:671–5.
88. Prince AM, Szmuness W, Millian SJ, et al. A serologic study of cytomegalovirus infections associated with blood transfusions. N Engl J Med. 1971;284:1125–32.
89. Armstrong JA, Tarr GC, Youngblood LA, et al. Cytomegalovirus infection in children undergoing open heart surgery. Yale J Biol Med. 1976;49:83–91.
90. Gurevich I, Cunha BA. Non-parenteral transmission of cytomegalovirus in a neonatal intensive care unit. Lancet. 1981;2:222–4.
91. Spector S. Transmission of cytomegalovirus among infants in hospital documented by restriction-endonuclease-digestion analyses. Lancet. 1983;1:378–81.
92. Stagno S, Reynolds DW, Pass RF, et al. Breast milk and the risk of cytomegalovirus infection. N Engl J Med. 1980;302:1073–7.
93. Demmler GJ, Yow MD, Spector SA, et al. Nosocomial cytomegalovirus infections within two hospitals caring for infants and children. J Infect Dis. 1987;156:9–16.
94. Hayes K, Danks DM, Gibas H. Brief recordings: Cytomegalovirus in human milk. N Engl J Med. 1972;287:177–8.
95. Yeager AS. Longitudinal, serological study of cytomegalovirus infections in nurses and in personnel without patient contact. J Clin Microbiol. 1975;2:448–52.
96. Ahlfors K. Epidemiological studies of congenital cytomegalovirus infection. Scand J Infect Dis. 1982;34(Suppl):1–36.
97. Ahlfors K, Ivarsson SA, Johnsson T, et al. Risk of cytomegalovirus infection in nurses and congenital infection in their offspring. Acta Paediatr Scand. 1981;70:819–23.
98. Yow MD, Lakeman AD, Stagno S, et al. Use of restriction enzymes to investigate the source of a primary cytomegalovirus infection in a pediatric nurse. Pediatrics. 1982;70:713–6.
99. Wilfert CM, Huang ES, Stagno S. Restriction endonuclease analysis of cytomegalovirus deoxyribonucleic acid as an epidemiologic tool. Pediatrics. 1982;70:717–21.
100. Balfour CL, Balfour HH Jr. Cytomegalovirus is not an occupational risk for nurses in renal transplant and neonatal units. Results of a prospective surveillance study. JAMA. 1986;256:1909–14.
101. Adler SP, Baggett J, Wilson M, et al. Molecular epidemiology of cytomegalovirus in a nursery: Lack of evidence for nosocomial transmission. J Pediatr. 1986;108:117–23.
102. Brady MT, Demmler GJ, Anderson DC. Cytomegalovirus infection in pediatric house officers: Susceptibility to and rates of primary infection. Infect Control. 1987;8:329–32.
103. Hatherley LI. Is primary cytomegalovirus infection an occupational hazard for obstetric nurses? A serologic study. Infect Control. 1986;7:452–5.

104. Blackman JA, Murph JR, Bale JF Jr. Risk of cytomegalovirus infection among educators and health-care personnel serving disabled children. Pediatr Infect Dis J. 1987;6:725–9.
105. Gerberding JL, Bryant-LeBlanc CE, Nelson K, et al. Risk of transmitting the human immunodeficiency virus, cytomegalovirus, and hepatitis B virus to health-care workers exposed to AIDS patients and AIDS-related conditions. J Infect Dis. 1987;156:1–8.
106. Kuhls TL, Viker S, Parris NB, et al. Occupational risk of HIV, HBV and HSV-2 infections in health care personnel caring for AIDS patients. Am J Public Health. 1987;77:1306–9.
107. Dworsky ME, Welch K, Cassady G, et al. Occupational risk for primary cytomegalovirus infection among pediatric health-care workers. N Engl J Med. 1983;309:950–3.
108. Pass R. Epidemiology and transmission of cytomegalovirus. J Infect Dis. 1985;152:243–8.
109. Gurevich I, Tafuro P. Caring for the infectious patient: Risk factors during pregnancy. Infect Control. 1984;5:482–8.
110. Tolkoff-Rubin NE, Rubin RH, Keller EE, et al. Cytomegalovirus infection in dialysis patients and personnel. Ann Intern Med. 1978;89(Part 1):625–8.
111. Lang DJ, Ebert PA, Rodgers BM, et al. Reduction of post-transfusion cytomegalovirus infection following use of leukocyte-depleted blood. Transfusion. 1977;17:391–5.
112. Ho M, Suwausirikul S, Dowling JN, et al. The transplanted kidney as a source of cytomegalovirus infection. N Engl J Med. 1975;293:1109–12.
113. Betts RF. Cytomegalovirus vaccine in renal transplants. Ann Intern Med. 1979;91:780–2.
114. Weller TH. The cytomegaloviruses: Ubiquitous agents with protean clinical manifestations. N Engl J Med. 1971;285:203–14.
115. Betts RF, Cestero RVM, Freeman RB, et al. Epidemiology of cytomegalovirus in end-stage renal disease. J Med Virol. 1979;4:89–96.
116. Brady MT, Milan JD, Anderson DC, et al. Use of deglycerolized red blood cells to prevent post-transfusion infection with cytomegalovirus in neonates. J Infect Dis. 1984;150:334–9.
117. Brady MT, Demmler GJ, Seavy D, et al. Method of blood processing affects cytomegalovirus excretion in newborn nurseries. Am J Infect Control. 1987;15:245–8.
118. Henderson DK. Nosocomial herpesvirus infections. In: Mandell GL, Douglas RG, Bennett JE, eds. Principles and Practice of Infectious Diseases. 2nd ed. New York: Churchill Livingstone; 1985:1630–7.
119. Valenti WM. Infection control and the pregnant health care worker. Am J Infect Control. 1986;14:20–7.
120. Centers for Disease Control. Update: Universal precautions for prevention of transmission of human immunodeficiency virus, hepatitis B virus, and other bloodborne pathogens in health care settings. MMWR. 1988;37:277–82, 287–8.
121. Garner JS, Simmons BP. Guidelines for isolation precautions in hospitals. Infect Control. 1983;4(Suppl):245–325.
122. Williams WW. Guidelines for infection control in hospital personnel. Infect Control 1983;4:(Suppl):326–49.
123. Onorato IM, Morens DM, Martone WJ, et al. Epidemiology of cytomegalovirus infections: Recommendations for prevention and control. Rev Infect Dis. 1985;7:479–97.
124. Adler SP. Nosocomial transmission of cytomegalovirus. Pediatr Infect Dis. 1986;5:239–46.
125. Plotkin SA. Cytomegalovirus in hospitals. Pediatr Infect Dis. 1986;5:177–8.
126. Brady MT. Cytomegalovirus infections: Occupational risk for health professionals. Am J Infect Control. 1986;14:197–203.
127. Ginsburg CM, Henle G, Henle W. An outbreak of infectious mononucleosis among the personnel in an outpatient clinic. Am J Epidemiol. 1976;104:571–5.
128. Chang RS, Rosen L, Kapikian AZ. Epstein-Barr virus infections in a nursery. Am J Epidemiol. 1981;113:22–9.
129. Gerber P, Walsh JH, Rosenblum EN, et al. Association of Epstein-Barr infection with the post-perfusion syndrome. Lancet. 1969;1:593–5.
130. Purtilo DT, Paquin LA, Sakamota K, et al. Persistent transfusion-associated infectious mononucleosis with transient acquired immunodeficiency. Am J Med. 1980;68:437–40.
131. Corey L, Stamm WE, Feorino PM, et al. HBsAg-negative hepatitis in a hemodialysis unit: Relation of Epstein-Barr virus. N Engl J Med. 1975;293:1273–8.
132. Solem JH, Jorgensen W. Accidentally transmitted infectious mononucleosis: Report of a case. Acta Med Scand. 1969;186:433–7.
133. Blacklow NR, Watson BK, Miller G, et al. Mononucleosis with heterophil antibodies: Epstein-Barr virus infection acquisition by an elderly patient in hospital. Am J Med. 1971;51:549–52.
134. Turner AR, MacDonald RM, Cooper BA. Transmission of infectious mononucleosis by transfusion of pre-illness plasma. Ann Intern Med. 1972;77:751–3.
135. Henle W, Henle G, Harrison FS, et al. Antibody responses to the Epstein-Barr virus and cytomegalovirus after open-heart and other surgery. N Engl J Med. 1970;282:1068–74.
136. Virolainen M, Anderson LC, Lalla M, et al. T-lymphocyte proliferation in mononucleosis. Clin Immunol Immunopathol. 1973;2:114–20.
137. Sullivan JL, Wallen WC, Johnson FL. Epstein-Barr virus infection following bone-marrow transplantation. Int J Cancer. 1978;22:132–5.
138. Hoaglund RJ. The transmission of infectious mononucleosis. Am J Med Sci. 1955;229:262–72.
139. Centers for Disease Control. Isolation Techniques for Use in Hospitals. ed 2. U.S. Dept. of Health, Education, and Welfare Publication No. (CDC) 76-8314. Washington, DC: Government Printing Office; 1975.
140. Miller G, Niederman JC, Andrews LL. Prolonged oropharyngeal excretion of Epstein-Barr virus after infectious mononucleosis. N Engl J Med. 1973;288:229–32.
141. Yamanishi K, Shiraki K, Kondo T, et al. Identification of human herpesvirus-6 as a causal agent for Exanthem subitum. Lancet. 1988;1:1065–7.
142. Fierer J, Basely P, Braude AL, et al. Herpes B virus encephalomyelitis presenting as ophthalmic zoster. Ann Intern Med. 1973;79:225–8.
143. Bryan BL, Espana CD, Emmuns RW, et al. Recovery from encephalomyelitis caused by Herpesvirus simiae. Arch Intern Med. 1975;135:368.
144. Centers for Disease Control. B virus infections in humans—Pensacola, Florida. MMWR. 1987;36:289–90, 295–6.
145. Centers for Disease Control. Guidelines for prevention of Herpesvirus simiae (B virus) infections in monkey handlers. MMWR. 1987;36:680–2, 687–9.
146. Palmer AE. B virus, Herpesvirus simiae: Historical perspective. J Med Parasitol. 1987;16:99–130.
147. Boulter EA, Thornton B, Bauer DJ, et al. Successful treatment of experimental B virus (Herpesvirus simiae) infection with acyclovir. Br Med J. 1980;280:681–3.

285. POSTOPERATIVE INFECTIONS AND ANTIMICROBIAL PROPHYLAXIS

ALLEN B. KAISER

In 1862, Louis Pasteur's ingenious experiments into the nature of putrifaction were officially endorsed by the Paris Academy of Science. The endorsement signaled an end to the long-held belief that the exposure of organic material to air brought about the "spontaneous generation" of microorganisms, and the concepts of "sepsis" and "asepsis" became firmly established. A scant three years later, in what must be regarded as a paradigm of applied science, Joseph Lister demonstrated the incredible implications of antisepsis in his practice of orthopedic surgery. For the first time in recorded history, major surgical procedures could be performed with a reasonable expectation of primary wound healing and recovery. Essential enhancements for preventing and controlling wound "sepsis" were provided by the antibiotic revolution of the 1940s, ushering in the highly technical, highly invasive, and highly successful era of modern surgery. As noted by McDermott and Rogers,[1] the greatest impact of the antibiotic revolution may be related, in the long run, to its essential role in supporting the advancements of modern surgery. Indeed, surgery as we know it today would be impossible in an environment in which infection was likely or, once established, untreatable. As a case in point, recent reports have indicated that further advances in the implantation of the artificial heart—the epitome of applied technology in surgery—must await improved methods of infection control.[2]

Despite the fundamental role of antisepsis and antibiotics in the development of modern surgery, implementation of these discoveries in the practice of surgery has not occurred without opposition. As late as 1880, for example, William Halstead was ordered from the operating theater when he challenged a senior surgeon's disregard for antiseptic techniques. The early use of antibiotics for prophylaxis in surgical procedures was also questioned as respected academicians freely voiced their disapproval of antibiotic prophylaxis in clean surgical procedures.[3] For a number of years the value of prophylactic antibiotics in preventing infections of the surgical wound remained in doubt.

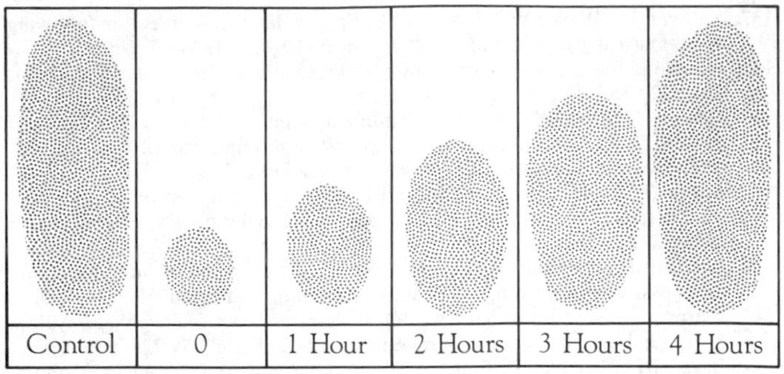

FIG. 1 Relationship between the timing of antimicrobial administration and the effectiveness of prophylaxis as shown by the size of wound infection. Lesion sizes were measured as mean diameter (mm) of induration developing 24 hours after intradermal inoculation of *S. aureus*.

A consensus in favor of their use did not emerge until two concepts of perioperative prophylaxis and infection were established. First, investigators in Cincinnati and Boston demonstrated that, despite the use of standard aseptic techniques, *Staphylococcus aureus* could be regularly isolated from the operative field.[4–6] It became apparent that aseptic technique could decrease but not eliminate bacterial contamination of the surgical field. Therefore, the possibility could be considered that perioperative antibiotics could supplement aseptic techniques in containing the inevitable contamination of the operative wound. The second major finding related to the importance of the timing of the administration of the prophylactic antibiotic. As early as 1946, Howes[7] had noted a correlation between the amelioration of infection and the interval between the contamination of the wounds and the administration of antibiotics. Several years later, Burke,[8] working in a guinea pig model of wound infection, demonstrated the remarkable brevity of the "window" of prophylactic efficacy. Burke noted that antibiotics given shortly before or at the time of bacterial inoculation of the subcutaneous tissue of the guinea pig produced a remarkable diminution in the size of the subsequent wound infection compared with lesions in animals not receiving antibiotic prophylaxis (Fig. 1). By delaying the administration of antibiotics by only 3 or 4 hours, resulting lesions were identical in size to those of animals receiving no antibiotic prophylaxis whatsoever. Thus, "failures" of antimicrobial prophylaxis noted in earlier clinical studies could be traced to the fact that preoperative or intraoperative antibiotics had not been given.[9,10] The efficacy of prophylactic antibiotics has now been verified for hundreds of surgical procedures with a wide variety of antimicrobials when care has been given to provide adequate serum and tissue levels of antibiotics during the surgical procedure. Perioperative antibiotics and aseptic techniques have become routine aspects of care in most major surgical procedures. However, much remains to be learned regarding the pathophysiology and epidemiology of surgical wound infections, the value of increasingly stringent methods of asepsis, and the optimal choice, dose, and duration of perioperative antibiotics.

PRINCIPLES OF PREVENTION AND CONTROL OF SURGICAL WOUND INFECTION

Determinants of Surgical Wound Infection

In reviewing the principles underlying the prevention and control of surgical wound infections, it is axiomatic to appreciate the inevitability of bacterial contamination of the surgical wound. State-of-the-art aseptic technique has been associated with a dramatic drop in, but not the elimination of, this phenomenon. Even under laminar flow operating room environments, bacteria can be predictably isolated from wound surfaces at the close of the surgical procedure.[11] However, given the regularity with which bacteria contaminate wound tissues during surgery, wound infection remains the exception and not the rule. This was the case even in the era when prophylactic antibiotics were not routinely administered. The ability of tissues to contain the contaminating bacteria, thereby avoiding an infecting process, is related to existing local and systemic immune processes. The milieu of the surgical wound may be viewed as a balance of opposing forces. (Fig. 2). As the number and virulence of contaminating bacteria increases, so does the chance for the development of a postoperative infection. The importance of the microbial load in determining whether a wound becomes infected or not has been appreciated for years. On the basis of expected degree of microbial contamination, surgeons and hospital epidemiologists have historically stratified surgical procedures into clean, clean-contaminated, and contaminated (Table 1). However, since perioperative antibiotic prophylaxis has become standard of care for most surgical procedures, such categorization is less meaningful in estimating the risk of infection. With antibiotic prophylaxis, expected infection rates have decreased dramatically for all surgical categories, and other risk factors such as the degree of tissue trauma and the presence of foreign material have assumed a much more important role as determinants of surgical wound infection.

The presence of traumatized or devitalized tissues, hematomas, and foreign material enhances the opportunity for infection. Classic investigations by Elek and Coneh[12] have established the role of "local variables" in the infecting process. Working with *S. aureus* infections of the skin of human volunteers, these researchers conclusively established the role of foreign material in potentiating wound infection. By including

TABLE 1. Classification of Operative Wounds by Level of Bacterial Contamination

	% Infection Rate	
	Preoperative Antibiotics Routinely Administered	
Classification Criteria[65]	*No*[a]	*Yes*[b]
Clean wound A nontraumatic wound in which no inflammation was encountered, no break in technique occurred, and respiratory, alimentary, and genitourinary tracts were not entered.	5.1	0.8
Clean-contaminated wound A nontraumatic wound in which a minor break in technique occurred or in which the gastrointestinal, genitourinary, or respiratory tracts were entered without significant spillage. This category includes transection of the appendix or cystic duct in the absence of acute inflammation and entrance into the biliary or genitourinary tracts in the absence of infected bile or urine.	10.1	1.3
Contaminated wound A fresh, traumatic wound from a relatively clean source or an operative wound in which there is a major break in technique, gross spillage from the gastrointestinal tract, or entrance into the genitourinary or biliary tract in the presence of infected urine or bile. This includes incisions encountering acute nonpurulent inflammation. Also included in this contaminated category are dirty wounds, such as traumatic wounds from a dirty source or with delayed treatment, fecal contamination, foreign bodies, a devitalized viscus, or pus from any source that is encountered.	21.9	10.2

[a] Data obtained from a multicenter study performed at a time (1960–1961) when antibiotic "prophylaxis," if administered, was usually initiated postoperatively.[13] Classification criteria in 1960–1961 were less restrictive in that cholecystectomies, appendectomies, hysterectomies, and urinary tract operations were included as "clean" if no inflammation was present at the time of operation. Contaminated wounds were also subdivided into "contaminated" and "dirty"; the latter included old traumatic wound and those wounds involving abscesses or perforated viscus.

[b] Data obtained from a prospective single-center study of 20,000 wounds[66] in which a fall in infection rates over a 5-year period was attributable to an increasing use of preoperative antibiotics.

Microbial Concentration and Virulence • Injury to Wound Tissues • Foreign Material
_________________________________ ≈ **Surgical Wound Infection**
General and Local Host Immunity • Peri-Operative Antibiotics

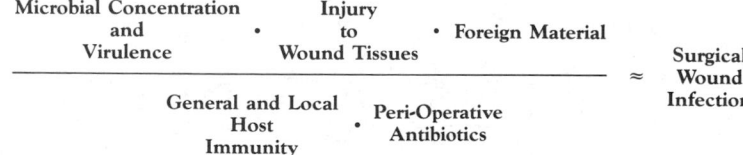

FIG. 2. Determinants of surgical wound infection. The risk for postoperative infection increases as the degree of bacterial contamination and the virulence of the contaminating bacteria increase. The presence of foreign material and highly traumatized tissue also potentiates the risk of infection. In contrast, a healthy local systemic immune system and appropriately administered prophylactic antibiotics are important factors in maintaining an infection-free incision.

suture material with the intradermal staphylococcal inoculum, the number of organisms required to establish a skin pustule could be reduced 10,000-fold relative to lesions without sutures (i.e., a fall from 5×10^6 organisms to 3×10^2 organisms in the inoculum). These investigators further suggested that "other circumstances may lead to the unhindered growth of small inocula, including heavily traumatized tissues, burns, or devitalized tissues distal to the ligated vessels. This may be the explanation of the traditional surgical view that untidy operative techniques predispose to infection."[12] Nevertheless, a healthy and active immune system has an incredible capacity to contain widespread bacterial contamination of deep tissue planes, rendering a surgical wound infection free.

Host Risk Factors

A variety of host factors historically have been associated with an increased risk of infection: extremes of age, diabetes mellitus, concomitant steroid therapy, severe obesity or malnutrition, and the presence of remote infection at the time of surgery.[13] Cigarette smoking has recently been added to the list of risk factors in patients undergoing cardiac surgery.[14] Inadequate immune function is the most likely explanation for the observed increase in infection rates in the elderly and malnourished. The delayed or absent reactivity to skin tests (anergy) that is frequently recorded in such patients is a marker for altered host resistance, sepsis, and increased mortality.[15]

Routes of Bacterial Contamination

Although numerous sources of bacterial contamination of surgical wounds have been described (Table 2), it is virtually impossible to identify, with certainty, the source(s) and route(s) of contamination of postoperative infection. Ketcham et al.[16] noted a highly significant correlation between the presence of nasal carriage of *S. aureus* and the incidence of postoperative *S. aureus* surgical wound infection (29 *S. aureus* wound infections among 108 nasal carriers versus 15 infections among 249 noncarriers, $p < 0.001$). Bacteriophage typing of *S. aureus* isolates revealed a high correlation between the organisms isolated from the nasal cultures and the subsequent infecting pathogens. These and other data that indicate a reduction in wound infections associated with the elimination of staphylococcal nasal colonization[17,18] strongly suggest that the *S. aureus* that colonized the anterior nares of patients are a major reservoir for the infecting organisms. However, the route of wound contamination remains undetermined. Among other sources and routes of spread, the patient's skin, closely juxtaposed to the operative field, may serve as a likely reservoir for the contaminating bacteria. A variety of antiseptics have proved effective in decontaminating the so-called transient flora of the skin's surface, but strategies are not available to eliminate the deeply placed resident flora (Fig. 3). The resident flora, located within sebaceous glands and hair follicles, represent at least 20 percent of the total microbial flora of the skin. After effective decontamination of the surface of the skin, the resident bacteria not only repopulate the superficial skin surface but also may be carried on surgical instruments directly into the wound during the operative procedure.

The relative importance of airborne contamination of the surgical wound versus direct contamination via hands, skin, and surgical instruments has been widely debated for a number of years. Several outbreaks of group A streptococcal wound infection have been traced to the anal or vaginal carriage of this organism by operating room personnel.[19,20,20a] Epidemiologic investigation of these outbreaks indicated that airborne contamination of the operative field had occurred. More importantly, the prospective controlled study by Lidwell et al.[21] demonstrated a remarkable decrease in infection rates in total hip and knee procedures associated with operating in an ultraclean operating room environment. However, the value of ultraclean or laminar flow environments in decreasing wound infections may be lessened when surgery occurs in modern operating room environments where high rates of air exchange and perioperative antibiotic use are routine.[22]

TABLE 2. Sources of Microbial Contamination of Surgical Wounds

Source	*Estimated Frequency of Occurrence*
Direct inoculation	
At time of surgery	
Residual flora of patient's skin	Common
Hands of surgical team members (via torn gloves)	Occasional
Contaminated surgical material	Rare
Contaminated or infected host tissues (during contaminated procedures)	Common
During the postoperative period[a]	
Drains and irrigating catheters	Occasional
Transient and residual skin flora of patient (via unstable incision sites, e.g., unstable sternum)	Rare
Contaminated or infected tissues (after contaminated procedures)	Occasional
Airborne contamination	
At time of surgery	
Skin, mucous membranes, and clothing of patient	Occasional
Skin, mucous membranes, and clothing of operating room staff	Occasional
Inanimate operating room environmennt	Rare
Air filtration equipment (malfunctioning)	Rare
During postoperative period	
Theoretically unimportant except for open wounds and burns	
Hematogenous-lymphatic seeding	
At time of surgery	
Pre-existing infection of nonwound sites (e.g., pneumonia, urinary tract infection)	Rare
Intravenous lines or equipment with intravascular access (e.g., bypass perfusion apparatus, cell-saver devices)	Rare
During the postoperative period[b]	
Intravenous lines or equipment with intravascular access (e.g., Swan-Ganz catheter)	Rare
Postoperative infection involving nonwound sites	Rare

[a] Sources of contamination are only evaluated for primarily closed wounds. Wounds left open (secondary closure) and burn wounds are also vulnerable to contamination from a variety of personnel and environmental sources.
[b] Incidental or transient bacteremia from a variety of sources (e.g., mucous membranes, superficial skin infections) has been implicated in the late hematogenous seeding of implanted prosthetic material.

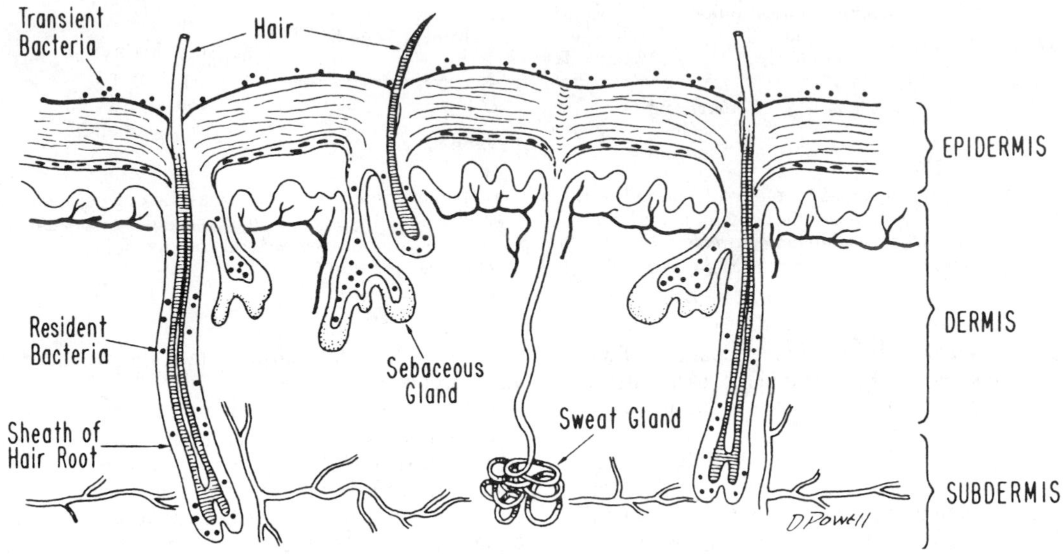

FIG. 3. Schematic diagram of the skin demonstrating the location of the transient bacteria on the skin surface, which are easily removed, and the deep resident bacteria, which cannot be destroyed by skin antiseptics. (From Postlethwaite,[140] with permission.)

More controversial still is the relative importance of hematogenous seeding of the surgical wound. It is generally accepted that after surgery, prosthetic valves and hips are at risk for an indefinite period of time for hematogenous seeding and infection. It is difficult, however, to be certain if a late postoperative infection results from intraoperative bacterial seeding of the prosthetic device with prolonged dormancy or from a true postoperative hematogenous event. For prosthetic valve endocarditis, the shift in bacterial etiology from primarily staphylococcal to a streptococcal spectrum supports the concept that late hematogenous seeding of the prosthetic valves occurs.[23,24] On the other hand, in a random prospective controlled study of antibiotic prophylaxis in total hip replacement, Carlsson et al.[25] demonstrated that deep wound infections that developed over 2.5 years after surgery were more likely to have occurred among placebo versus cloxacillin recipients (13.7 percent versus 3.3 percent, respectively, $p < 0.05$, one-tailed Fisher's exact test). These data strongly suggest that bacteria inoculated into wounds at the time of surgery lie dormant for years, rendering differentiation of the precise source of late wound infection virtually impossible. This is even less information regarding the possibility of hematogenous seeding of nonprosthetic surgical wounds during the postoperative period. Postoperative urinary tract infections were implicated as a source of postoperative surgical wound infection in one study, although the route of contamination was not discussed.[26] A report of acute pneumococcal osteomyelitis of the sternum occurring 3 months after coronary artery bypass surgery supports the concept that a surgical incision that does not contain a prosthetic device can also be seeded hematogenously during the postoperative period.[27] If late hematogenous seeding of a surgical wound with or without prosthetic material can occur, it is reasonable to assume that wounds are even more vulnerable to seeding and secondary infection during the immediate postoperative periods. During this time, surgical incisions are hyperemic from the trauma of the surgery and endothelialization of intravascular prosthetic materials has not yet had time to occur. Moreover, the regular use of indwelling intravascular access devices and lines makes the risk of bacteremia likely. However, information with which to judge the relative contribution of intraoperative versus postoperative hematogenous seeding of the surgical incision is unavailable.

Infection Caused by Multiply Resistant Pathogens

Among the more important challenges in the prevention of surgical wound infection is the problem of increasing antimicrobial resistance among infecting pathogens. As cephalosporins have been the mainstay of prophylaxis for over a decade, the concern has focused primarily on cephalosporin-resistant organisms. Surgical wound infection resulting from methicillin-resistant *S. aureus* (MRSA), methicillin- and cephalosporin-resistant coagulase-negative *S. aureus* (MR-CNS), cephalosporin- and gentamicin-resistant gram-negative rods, and fungi are being reported with increasing frequency, particularly in those procedures traditionally regarded as clean.[28–32] It is not clear, however, whether there has been a change in surgical wound infection rates or only a shift in the spectrum of infecting organisms. Data from the Centers for Disease Control National Nosocomial Infection Survey indicate that while nosocomial infections due to MRSA are increasing, the overall surgical wound infection rates have remained virtually unchanged over the past decade.[33–35] Nevertheless, numerous recent reports of nosocomial infections due to multiply resistant organisms, primarily MRSA and MR-CNS, suggest that whether or not the incidence of surgical wound infection has changed, strategies must be devised to contain these pathogens.

Recently reported cefazolin failures in cardiac surgery also deserve mention. A significantly higher incidence of deep would infection due to methicillin-sensitive staphylococci was observed in cefazolin recipients compared with cefamandole and cefuroxime recipients in one study[36] or with cefamandole recipients in another.[37] Preliminary data suggest that the *S. aureus* causing wound infection despite cefazolin prophylaxis are from a subset of methicillin-sensitive *S. aureus* that produce β-lactamase(s) that is more effective in hydrolyzing cefazolin than either cefamandole or cefuroxime.[38] One of the reports of cefazolin failure is from a hospital where an earlier prospective study of cefazolin prophylaxis in vascular surgery had encountered no *S. aureus* infection among 225 cefazolin recipients versus 11 such infections among 237 placebo recipients.[39] Whether the phenomenon of methicillin-sensitive *S. aureus* infection resisting cefazolin prophylaxis is new or only newly recognized, the role of cefazolin in prophylaxis of clean surgery has come under scrutiny.

Colonization and secondary infection with cephalosporin- and gentamicin-resistant bacteria are thought to follow exposure of the patient to the highly resistant hospital flora. Epidemiologic investigations indicate that multiply resistant bacteria are scattered throughout the hospital environment and transmitted via the hands of hospital personnel. Concomitant use of antibiotics has been thought to enhance the colonization process once exposure has occurred.[40] Recent studies also indicate that many patients are actually colonized with small numbers of resistant bacteria (e.g., MR-CNS, gentamicin-resistant *Pseudomonas*) on admission to the hospital.[41,42] After exposure to prophylactic or therapeutic antibiotics, these organisms proliferate on the skin and within the colon, eventually dominating the colonizing flora of a given patient (Fig. 4). Once patients are colonized, resistant pathogens apparently find their way into the surgical incision by a variety of routes (Table 2).

Whether colonization with resistant pathogens occurs by acquisition or by emergence (or, with rifampin, by mutational resistance),[40] antibiotic use, and specifically prophylactic antibiotic use, has been shown to have a critical role in the process. This, of course, has profound implications for a continued or expanded role of prophylactic antibiotics in surgery. In view of the improvement in overall surgical would infection rates over the past 2 decades (Table 1), the consensus is that prophylactic antibiotics are clearly worth this potential side effect. Moreover, although methicillin- and gentamicin-resistant coagulase-negative staphylococci can be detected in high numbers on the skin of surgical patients within 5 days of exposure to perioperatively administered cephalosporins, it is not yet clear whether such bacteria are able to dominate the colonizing flora in time to contaminate the surgical incision at the time of surgery.[43] In one recent study, however, patients who were randomized to receive a single dose of gentamicin in addition to perioperative cephalosporins at the time of coronary artery bypass surgery were more likely to acquire a wound infection with gentamicin-resistant pathogens than patients receiving only cephalosporin prophylaxis.[37] Antibiotic use in any circumstance has been associated with a rising prevalence of antibiotic-resistant bacteria, and authorities have stressed the importance of limiting prophylactic antibiotic use to proven agents and durations of administration.

In institutions where cephalosporin-resistant pathogens are being encountered with increasing frequency, a concomitant rise in the use of vancomycin and aminoglycosides is often observed. One would predict, however, that increasing reliance on our most potent antibiotics in prophylaxis will be associated in time with further increases in the incidence of difficult or impossible to treat surgical wound infection. For example, Roberts and Douglas[44] noted a marked increase in gentamicin resistance among nosocomial pathogens during a time when gentamicin was routinely used in prophylaxis in cardiac surgery. More recently, the emergence of vancomycin-resistant enter-

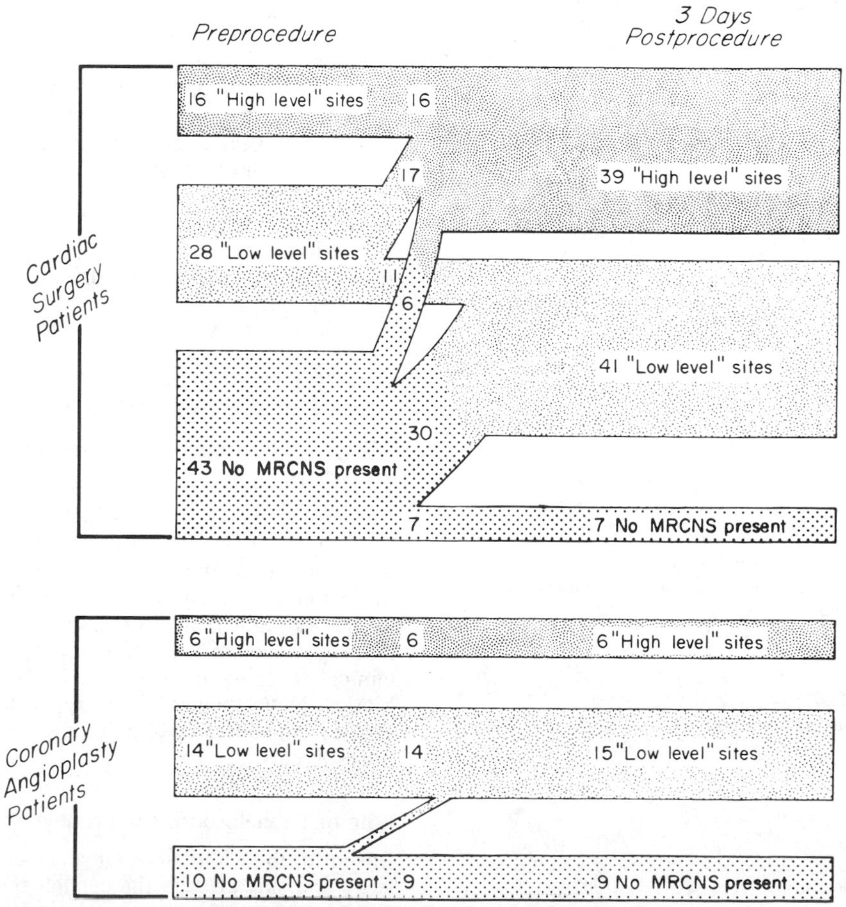

FIG. 4. Relationship of preprocedure to postprocedure recovery of methicillin-resistant coagulase-negative staphylococci (MR-CNS) in 29 cardiac surgery and 10 coronary angioplasty patients. After cardiac surgery and perioperative antibiotic prophylaxis, most sites either became colonized or demonstrated increasing levels of colonization with MR-CNS. Plasmid analysis indicated that the increased colonization with MR-CNS in the postoperative period was often due to strains that were present in low numbers in the preoperative period and that "emerged" to dominate the skin flora in the postoperative period. As indicated, little change in the skin flora was noted for the angioplasty patient who did not receive prophylactic antibiotic. (Data from Kernodle et al.[41])

ococci in association with the routine use of vancomycin prophylaxis has been reported.[45] It may be that by increasing the emphasis on antisepsis and decreasing our reliance on perioperative antibiotics, the problem of emerging resistance can be minimized. For the present, however, an all-inclusive solution to the problem of emerging resistance among pathogens causing surgical wound infection does not exist.

Pathophysiology of Surgical Wound Infection

A limiting factor in reducing further the incidence of surgical wound infection caused by sensitive as well as multiply resistant pathogens has been the paucity of new information regarding the pathophysiology of the infecting process. This is particularly true for clean infections in that a model of wound infection with low inoculi of bacteria has never been developed. During the 1950s great strides in understanding wound infection were made as Miles and Niven[46] and Burke and Miles[47] explored a multitude of variables important to the infecting process in experimental surgical incisions (Table 3). Elek and Coneh[12] added important new information regarding *S. aureus* infections in human volunteers. The importance of the timing of antibiotic administration in prophylaxis of surgical wound infection was focused by the work of Burke[8] in the early 1960s. First described by Howes[7] in 1946, the "effective period" of prophylactic antibiotic activity was quantified by Burke[8] to be a narrow period of 1–3 hours. Once bacterial contamination of tissues had occurred, antibiotics administered after this effective period exhibited little to no prophylactic efficacy. From another viewpoint, bacterial infection of surgical tissues demonstrated an "incubation period" during which the bacteria are highly vulnerable to prophylactic antibiotics and after which the bacteria appear to be well established within the wound tissues and resistant to the effect of antimicrobial prophylaxis. As important as these observations were, only a modicum of research explored the pathophysiology of these phenomena in the 1960s and 1970s. In contrast, over this same period, important contributions were made in understanding the pathophysiology of a variety of other infectious processes. Bacterial attachment and invasion of host tissues, evasion of local and systemic immune processes, and production of toxins and exoproteins have been explored in animal and tissue models of peritonitis, endocarditis, gastroenteritis, meningitis, and urethritis. A return of interest in the pathophysiology of surgical wound infection is evidenced by recent publications (Table 3). Investigations into the importance of tissue oxygenation, an increased understanding of the bacteria–leukocyte interaction in wound infection, and investigations into the role of bacterial exopolymers and capsular antigen are tantalizing. It is likely that further gains in limiting postoperative wound infection will await continued systematic investigations into the pathophysiology of the infecting process.

TABLE 3. Contributions of Investigational Models to an Understanding of the Pathophysiology of Surgical Wound Infection

Investigative Findings	*Model*	*Author(s) (Date)*
Adverse effect of dehydration, adrenalin, and heparin on infection resistance of contaminated wounds.	Subcutaneous infection in guinea pigs using a variety of aerobic and anaerobic bacteria.	Miles and Niven[46] (1950) Burke and Miles[47] (1958)
Importance of early administration of antibiotics in preventing wound infection.	Subcutaneous and intradermal infection in guinea pigs with *S. aureus*.	Howes[7] (1946) Burke[8] (1961)
Importance of foreign material in enhancing *S. aureus* infections.	Intradermal and subcutaneous infection in human volunteers.	Elek and Coneh[12] (1958)
Development of muscle infection model and exploring the role of iron in enhancing the infecting process.	Muscle infection in mice using *E. coli* with nonreplicating phage.	Polk and Miles[67] (1971)
Role of lymphatic clearance of bacteria in host defenses.	Subcutaneous infection in rabbits with *S. aureus* and anaerobic gram-negative rods.	Delong and Simmons[68] (1982)
Development of a model of subcutaneous tissue cage infection.	Subcutaneous infection in guinea pigs with *S. aureus*	Zimmerli et al.[69] (1982)
Development of a model for infected subcutaneous foreign body granuloma.	Subcutaneous infection in guinea pigs with *S. aureus* and aerobic gram-negative rods.	Grappel et al.[70] (1983)
Development of intra-abdominal abscess model.	Intraperitoneal infection in rats with *Escherichia coli* and *Bacteroides fragilis*.	Bartlett[71] (1984)
Importance of early administration of topical antiseptics and antibiotics in preventing wound infection.	Subcutaneous infection in guinea pigs with *S. aureus, E. coli,* and *B. fragilis*	Platt and Bucknall[72] (1984)
Importance of oxygen in preventing wound infection.	Intradermal infection in guinea pigs with *E. coli*.	Knighton et al.[62] (1984)
Role of fibrin in enhancing abscess formation.	Intraperitoneal infection in rats with *E. coli* and *B. fragilis*.	Hau et al.[73] (1986)
Importance of granulocytes in antibiotic prophylaxis.	Muscle infection of mice with *S. aureus*.	Hoogeterp et al.[74] (1987)
Quantitation of *S. aureus* capsular polysaccharide.	Subcutaneous graft infection in guinea pigs with *S. aureus*.	Arbeit and Dunn[75] (1987)
Quantitation of *S. aureus* exopolymers.	Subcutaneous tissue cage infection in guinea pigs with *S. aureus*.	Falcieri et al.[76] (1987)

PRACTICE OF SURGICAL WOUND INFECTION PREVENTION AND ANTIBIOTIC PROPHYLAXIS

Perioperative Antibiotics in Prevention of Surgical Wound Infection

Although mechanisms by which antibiotics provide prophylactic efficacy when administered early in the infecting process are not understood, their efficacy is unquestioned. Not only have the benefits of early antibiotic administration been duplicated by numerous investigators using different animal models, different pathogens, and different antibiotics, literally hundreds of clinical trials have verified the efficacy of perioperative antibiotics. Nevertheless, issues regarding the optimal choice, frequency, and duration of perioperative antibiotic prophylaxis are unresolved.

Role of Cephalosporins in Prophylaxis

Based on their antibacterial spectrum and low incidence of allergy and side effects, the cephalosporins have emerged as the drugs of choice for the vast majority of operative procedures. With a reasonably long half-life, cefazolin has been the dominant choice for clean procedures.[48] Even in clean-contaminated procedures such as hysterectomy and cholecystectomy in which cephalosporins with improved in vitro activity against anaerobic bacteria are often advocated, clinical studies indicate that cefazolin is equivalent in its prophylactic efficacy.[27] However, recently noted failures of this antibiotic in preventing infection by methicillin-sensitive *S. aureus* in cardiac surgery have forced investigators to consider alternatives, especially in clean surgical procedures in which *S. aureus* is the principal pathogen. Perhaps of more importance, increasingly frequent reports of MRSA, MR-CNS, and cephalosporin-resistant gram-negative rods have prompted an increasing use of vancomycin and aminoglycosides in routine prophylaxis. Clinical studies are, for the most part, too cumbersome to detect differences in efficacy between prophylactic regimens.[49] For example, in clean elective surgical procedures, infection rates with routine cephalosporin prophylaxis are already low, 5 percent or lower. In attempting to evaluate clinically the superiority of a different antibiotic regimen, randomization of approximately 900 patients would be necessary before a 50 percent reduction in infection rate could be demonstrated at the $p = 0.05$ level. Many more patients would require study to demonstrate reliably that differences did not exist.

Timing of Administration of Prophylactic Antibiotics

The timing of administering the prophylactic antibiotic is a matter of active clinical investigation. Except in elective colonic surgical procedures in which oral antibiotics must be administered several hours before the procedure, there is general agreement that the initial dose of systemically administered antibiotics need not be given until the onset of the procedure. The induction of anesthesia represents a convenient point for initiating antibiotic prophylaxis in major surgical procedures. However, the value of subsequent intraoperative or postoperative doses of antibiotic is a subject of considerable disagreement. There are theoretical reasons to ensure that adequate serum and tissue levels of antibiotics are maintained throughout the surgical procedure. The Burke guinea pig model demonstrated remarkable efficacy of antibiotics when they were administered as a single dose at or shortly before bacterial contamination.[8] In this model, the bacterial contamination of the intradermal tissues occurred at a single moment via an injection of viable microorganisms (Fig. 1). In the clinical arena, however, one cannot predict with certainty when bacterial contamination of the operative site will occur. It is quite possible that low-level contamination occurs continuously throughout the surgical procedure. The period of highest risk for bacterial contamination is most likely the close, not the beginning, of surgery. In prolonged procedures or with antibiotics with short half-lives, patients may be inadequately protected if redosing is not routinely provided.[49a] Goldmann et al.[50] noted a significantly higher infection rate among cardiac surgical patients whose antibiotic serum levels were undetectable by the close of surgery.

When designing a prophylactic regimen for a given antibiotic, the effect of disease or therapeutic interventions (e.g., cardiopulmonary bypass) on the metabolism and excretion of the antibiotic(s) must be considered. In addition, it may be important to consider the ranges, not just the means, of serum levels that have been observed at various times after the administration of prophylactic antibiotics. Pharmacokinetic studies of a given first- or second-generation cephalosporin, for example, invariably identify wide variations in the serum levels obtained 3 to 6 hours after the initial dose. Even greater variations in tissue levels may be seen. In one study, frequent intraoperative redosing of cefamandole, 1 g every 2 hours, was required to predictably maintain serum levels above 10 μg/ml.[37] This issue is complicated by the recent emphasis on cost reduction in hospitals. Redosing antibiotics every 8 to 24 hours is often recommended in an effort to reduce the cost of prophylaxis. Unfortunately, such regimens may be associated with inadequate intraoperative serum and tissue levels. Studies evaluating infrequent dosing of perioperative antibiotics have invariably contained small numbers of patients, precluding any meaningful evaluation of relative prophylactic efficacy. Third-generation cephalosporins with prolonged half-lives have been advocated for prophylaxis to ensure that adequate serum levels will be maintained throughout the surgical procedure and to decrease the cost and inconvenience associated with frequent redosing of antibiotics. However, these antibiotics, in general, exhibit inferior in vitro activity against *S. aureus*, clouding their potential for routine prophylactic use in clean and clean-contaminated surgery.

Antibiotics given preoperatively and intraoperatively for prophylaxis are often continued for one to several days into the postoperative period. This practice currently represents the most controversial area of antimicrobial prophylaxis. Studies comparing short-course versus long-course prophylaxis have reflected no increase in infection rates among the short-course recipients (Table 4). One comparative study of cesarean sections did detect a significantly higher incidence of endometritis in patients randomized to receive the short (18 hour) versus the long (3 day) course of perioperative ampicillin prophylaxis,[51] and Gatell et al.[52] noted a significantly higher infection rate in major joint repairs among patients receiving one versus five doses of perioperative cefamandole. Prolonged antimicrobial prophylaxis did not improve infection rates in separate studies in cardiac surgery, but all three studies involved small numbers of patients or low infection rates. The ultimate implications of the duration of postoperative antibiotics remain to be determined. Surgeons have justified continuing postoperative antibiotics for 2 or 3 days in patients who have undergone major surgical procedures and are being monitored with invasive devices on the basis that hematogenous seeding of the operative wound may occur. Data are simply not available to quantitate the relative risk and benefits of prolonged postoperative antibiotic prophylaxis in this setting. Large-scale studies with careful attention to infection rates and antimicrobial resistance patterns of infecting pathogens are clearly needed to resolve this issue.

Side Effects of Prophylaxis

Although the emergence of resistant bacteria has been a main concern in evaluating the deleterious effects of prophylactic antibiotics, a number of other side effects have been reported. Pseudomembranous colitis has been noted with a wide variety of prophylactic agents including oral erythromycin and neomycin, parenteral aminoglycosides, metronidazole, cephradine, cephaloridine, and cefoxitin.[53] However, in view of the extensive use of prophylaxis in this country and judging from the infrequency of published reports, pseudomembranous colitis remains an unusual complication of prophylactic therapy.

A bleeding disorder occasionally associated with the therapeutic use of certain β-lactam antibiotics represents a potential side effect in prophylaxis.[54] Hypoprothrombinemia is related to a methylthiotetrazole substitution in the β-lactam molecule, and impaired platelet function has been associated with the α-carboxyl substitution. The use of cefamandole possessing the methylthiotetrazole substitution was associated with an increased sensitivity to warfarin therapy in one retrospective study.[55] However, possibly associated with the relatively short duration of exposure associated with prophylactic antibiotic use, bleeding disorders have not been recognized as a complication of perioperative cephalosporin prophylaxis and concerns remain primarily theoretical.

The other side effect of note is profound hypotension associated with vancomycin prophylaxis.[56] Although the risk of this potentially reversible complication has been associated with rapid infusions of the antibiotic, others have encountered clinically significant hypotension despite exercising care to maintain slow vancomycin infusion rates.[57]

Prophylactic antibiotics add considerable cost to the routine care of surgical patients. In major surgical centers, the perioperative use of antibiotics may represent almost half of the phar-

TABLE 4. Prospective Randomized Comparisons of Long Versus Short Courses of Perioperative Prophylaxis

Surgical Procedure and Antibiotic Regimen	Duration: Short Course	Duration: Long Course	Total No. of Patients Studied	% Wound Infections: Short Course	% Wound Infections: Long Course	p Value
Major joint repair						
Nafcillin, 1 g q6h[77]	24 hr	72 hr	358	1.6	2.3	NS
Cefamandole, 2 g initially, then 1 g q6–10h[52]	Initial dose only	24 hr	717	5.2	0.9	<0.001
Cesarean section						
Cefuroxime, 0.75 g q8h[78]	24 hr	5 days	39	0[a]	10	NS
Ampicillin, 2 g initially, then 1 g q6h[51]	18 hr	72 hr	83	28[a]	8	<0.05
Vaginal hysterectomy						
Cefazolin, 1 g q6h[79]	Initial dose only	18 hr	90	8.9[b]	4.4	NS
Median sternotomy						
Cephalothin, 1 g q6h[80]	Initial dose only	4 days	64	6.6[c]	2.9	NS
Cephalothin, 2 g q6h[50]	48 hr	6 days	200	2.1[d]	2.8	NS
Median sternotomy						
Cephalothin, 12 mg/kg, plus kanamycin, 7 mg/kg, with or without oral cephalexin, 1 g q6h × 3 days[81]	48 hr	48 hr + oral cephalexin	160	2.5	1.2	NS

Abbreviation: NS: not significant.
[a] Endometritis.
[b] Cuff cellulitis.
[c] Includes one case of endocarditis.
[d] More urinary tract infections developed in 2-day (17.0%) versus 6-day (8.5%) patients ($p = 0.07$).

macy's expenditures for antibiotics, and surgeons are often encouraged to reduce or eliminate antibiotics given for prophylaxis in certain settings. For example, in carotid endarterectomy and cholecystectomy, infections develop only infrequently, are seldom life-threatening, and may cost more to prevent than to treat. However, it seems inappropriate to evaluate antibiotic use on the basis of cost alone. When prophylaxis or a particular form of prophylaxis offers a clear advantage to the patient, the health care system should advocate the better treatment without consideration of its cost. Moreover, an analysis of the cost of prophylactic antibiotics can be complicated. Not only the cost of the antibiotic per se but the cost of preparing, transporting, and administering multiple doses of antibiotic must be included. Perhaps of more importance, the cost of managing wound infections that develop when using inadequate prophylaxis must be considered. For example, in a recent comparative study of cefazolin versus cefamandole in cardiac surgery, the higher cost and more frequent dosing requirements of cefamandole resulted in a twofold increase in the cost of perioperative prophylaxis among patients randomized to receive cefamandole. However, because of a significantly higher infection rate among cefazolin recipients and the associated hospital cost for managing these excess infections, the total cost of prophylaxis and wound management was projected to be twice as high or $150,000 more in 500 patients randomized to receive cefazolin.[58]

Perioperative Management

Appropriate perioperative management of the surgical patient requires diligent attention to aseptic technique and a rational approach to the choice and use of prophylactic antibiotics (Table 5). Preoperative showering with a detergent containing the antiseptic chlorhexidine has been shown to suppress skin colonization for several hours, and the suppressive activity is enhanced by immediately reshowering or by repeated showers over several days.[59] It is not clear, however, whether this practice is associated with a corresponding decrease in infection rates. The preoperative hospital stay should be as short as possible, and the use of any antibiotic in the preoperative period should be avoided whenever possible. Recent information suggests that infection rates are lower in patients in whom hair is removed primarily by clipping rather than by shaving.[60] Other studies have suggested that if shaving for hair removal at the operative site is required, it should be performed as close to the time of surgery as possible. Infection at sites remote from the operative field, malnutrition, and cigarette use represent three identified host risk factors for postoperative infection that are potentially correctable.[14,15,61] However, except in unusual circumstances, it would be difficult to delay surgery awaiting the resolution of these factors.

Every effort should be made to ensure that adequate antibiotic levels are maintained throughout the surgical procedure. Most authorities have emphasized, however, that the single most important factor in ensuring a noninfected wound is surgical technique. Gentle handling of wound tissues, avoidance of dead space, devitalized tissues, and hematomas, and careful

TABLE 5. "Interventional" Manuevers of Proved or Theoretical Benefit in Diminishing the Risk of Surgical Wound Infection

Maneuvers to diminish inoculation of virulent or antimicrobial-resistant bacteria into wound

Preoperative factors
- Avoid preoperative antibiotic use
- Minimize preoperative hospitalization
- Eliminate nasal colonization with *S. aureus*
- Treat remote sites of infection
- Avoid shaving or delay shaving at operative site until time of surgery
- Routinely have patient shower or bathe preoperatively with chlorhexidine-containing soap

Intraoperative and postoperative factors
- Carefully prepare patient's skin with povidone-iodine or chlorhexidine-containing solution
- Rigorously adhere to routine aseptic techniques
- Maintain high flow of filtered air
- Consider laminar flow environment
- Consider irrigation of wound with antibiotic-containing solution
- Isolate clean from contaminated surgical fields (e.g., reglove and change instruments used to harvest saphenous vein before participating in intrathoracic field)
- Minimize use of drains
- Drains, if used, should be brought through a separate stab wound
- Minimize use of catheters and intravascular lines postoperatively

Maneuvers to improve host containment of contaminating bacteria

Preoperative factors
- Resolve malnutrition or obesity
- Discontinue cigarette smoking
- Maximize diabetes control

Intraoperative and postoperative factors
- Minimize dead space, devitalized tissue, and hematomas
- Maintain adequate hydration, oxygenation, and nutrition

approximation of tissue planes are all thought to be critical in maintaining an infection-free incision. Although a number of studies in the past have indicated that prolonged surgical procedures are associated with a higher infection rate, this association has not been noted in recent studies in cardiac surgery.[14,37] It may be that inadequate intraoperative redosing of prophylactic antimicrobials contributed to the previously noted deleterious effect of prolonged procedures.

Postoperatively, there is experimental evidence supporting the value of maintaining adequate perfusion and oxygenation of tissues.[62] Maintaining adequate nutrition in the postoperative period is also an important aspect of infection prevention. Drains and intravascular devices should be removed as quickly as possible to avoid the risk of, respectively, direct and hematogenous seeding of the operative site.

Surgical Wound Infection Surveillance

An effective infection control program is an essential part of surgical wound prevention. Such a program should provide accurate analysis of pathogens and their antibiograms. A surveillance system must be in place to readily identify epidemiologic foci of surgical wound infection. Representatives from the surgical attending staff should ideally be involved in the analysis of surveillance data for appropriate input and response. Data from surveillance activities must be critically evaluated, often with the aid of computerization, so that variations and trends in the antimicrobial susceptibility pattern of surgical wound pathogens can be detected.[63]

In collecting information on surgical wound infections, criteria for the definition of a wound infection must be established and endorsed by both infection control and surgical advisory committees. The presence of purulence within a surgical incision generally serves as evidence of a surgical wound infection. On the other hand, culture results of surgical wounds or exudates should not be used as a guide to the presence or absence of infection. Surgeons and hospital epidemiologists have recently emphasized the importance of stratifying surgical wound infections according to the depth of the infection. For example, delineation of surgical wound infection into four classes or degrees of infection have been recommended[63a] (Fig. 5). The differentiation between class I and class II wound infections is often made on an operational basis: purulence involving the subcutaneous tissues is classified as class II if surgical debridement or altered postoperative management (prolonged hospital stay or frequent outpatient visits) is required to manage the infection. The class I infections require little to no change in postoperative management of the patient. Class I infections, by definition, produce little morbidity. The pathophysiology of superficial and deep infections may be quite different, and it is reasonable to maintain a detailed analysis of infection rates by class of infection. For example, the less virulent coagulase-negative staphylococci tend to be isolated with more frequency from the more superficial infections.

In health care settings associated with a high volume of surgical procedures, surgical wound isolates should be maintained, if possible, for 2 to 3 weeks after isolation. Clusters or outbreaks of surgical wound infections due to a common pathogen are usually identified retrospectively, and the availability of infecting pathogens such as *S. aureus* (for phage typing) or coagulase-negative staphylococci (plasmid analysis) may be instrumental in identifying and eliminating the cause of the outbreak.

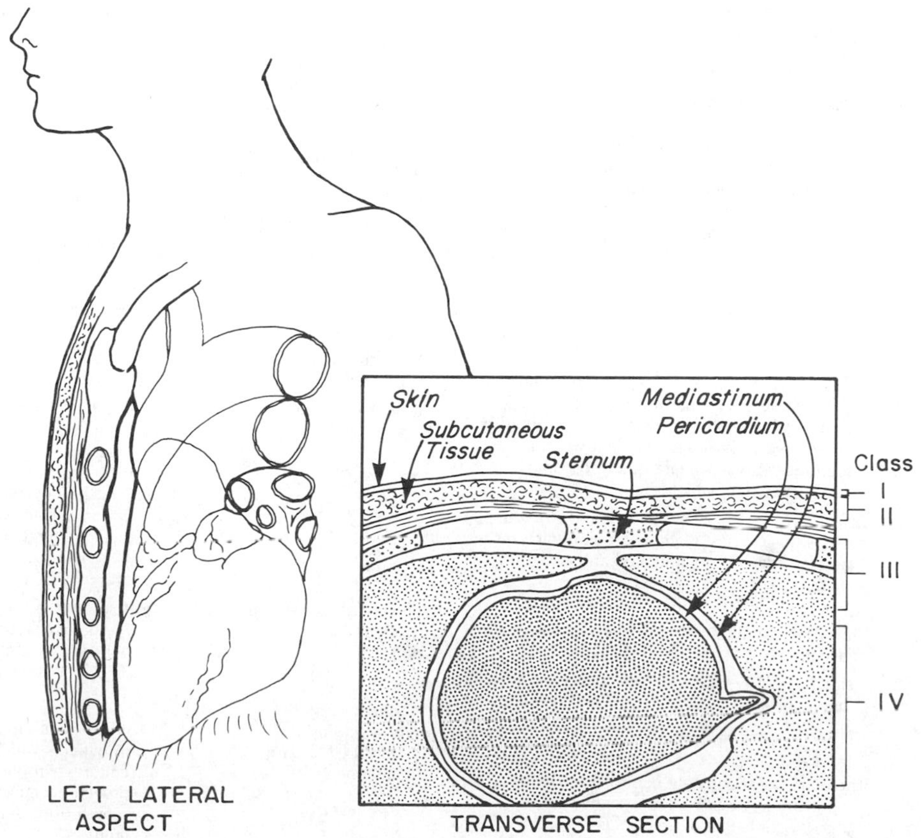

FIG. 5. Schematic of the mediastinum and a proposed classification of the severity of infection after surgery involving a median sternotomy incision. The morbidity, mortality, and cost related to infection increase substantially as the depth (or class) of infection increases.

There have been recent recommendations to maintain and even publicize surgeon-specific infection rates in an effort to indirectly cause a decrease in surgical wound infections.[64] Such data may identify unsuspected problems among the surgical staff or may encourage individual surgeons to rigorously adhere to standards of perioperative aseptic techniques. If such a program is used, it is vital that any analysis include an assessment of procedure-specific infection rates. Wide differences in infection rates exist among surgical procedures, even among those procedures within the same surgical subspecialty and category of bacterial contamination. For example, infection rates in vascular surgery after carotid endarterectomy are exceedingly low, less than one-tenth of 1 percent. On the other hand, bypass grafting in the femoral popliteal area may be associated with an infection rate of 2–3 percent despite the fact that both procedures are clean and may be performed by the same vascular surgeons. Other important variables such as the age and condition of the patients must also be considered before comparing infection rates among surgeons.

Selection of Prophylactic Regimens

Based on prospective studies of antibiotic prophylaxis, prophylactic regimens can be recommended for a wide variety of surgical procedures (Table 6). However, marked variations in the spectrum of infecting pathogens and in the degree of antimicrobial resistance exist among various hospitals. Moreover, variations in infecting pathogens and resistance patterns can and do occur over time within a given institution. Physicians and individual health care institutions must tailor routine prophylactic regimens based on carefully collected epidemiologic data regarding surgical wound infection. Equally important, many surgical procedures are far from routine, and numerous variations in perioperative circumstances will dictate deviations

TABLE 6. Recommended Antibiotic Prophylaxis for the Most Commonly Performed Surgical Procedures

Surgical Procedure[a]	*Recommended Prophylactic Regimen*[b]
Gynecologic surgery	
Cesarean section[82–87]	Cefazolin,[c] 1 g iv after clamping the cord and 6 and 12 hours later. Prophylaxis is not required in elective, uncomplicated cases. Uterine irrigation with antibiotics may be comparable to systemic therapy. If irrigating antibiotics are used, 2 g of cefoxitin in 1 liter of normal saline is effective. With β-lactam allergy, metronidazole, 500 mg iv after clamping cord, is effective.
Dilatation and curettage and abortion[88–90]	Prophylactic antimicrobials are not recommended for uncomplicated dilatation and curettage. In second-trimester instillation abortion, 1 g of cefazolin[c] preprocedure and 1 g q6h for 2 doses is effective. With β-lactam allergy, metronidazole, 400 mg po preprocedure and q4h for 2 doses, is effective. For induced abortion in the first trimester in patients with a history of pelvic inflammatory disease, 2 million IU of penicillin G im before and 3 hours after the procedure is effective.[d]
Hysterectomy, abdominal or vaginal[91–94]	Cefazolin,[c] 1 g iv preoperatively and 6 and 12 hours later. Second- or third-generation cephalosporins have not proved more effective. With β-lactam allergy, doxycycline, 200 mg iv, preoperatively as a single dose is effective in vaginal hysterectomy.
Bilateral occlusion of fallopian tubes	Data to recommend prophylaxis are not available.
Repair of cystocele and rectocele[95]	Prophylactic antibiotics have not proved effective.
Orthopedic surgery	
Arthroplasty of joints, including replacement[77,96,97]	For major joint (hip, knee) repair, cefazolin,[c] 1 g iv preoperatively and every 6 hours for 3 doses. A higher cefazolin dose (2 g) should be considered in knee replacement when a tourniquet is used. Data in arthroscopic surgery are not available.
Open reduction of fracture[98,99]	Cefazolin,[c] 1 g iv preoperatively and every 6 hours for 3 doses. Complex (open) fractures are considered contaminated and cefazolin therapy, 1 g every 8 hours for 10 days, beginning on admission, is indicated.
Laminectomy and spinal fusion[100,101]	Prophylactic antimicrobials have not proved beneficial.
Lower limb amputation[102]	Cefoxitin, 2 g iv preoperatively and every 6 hours for 4 doses.
Ophthalmic surgery	
Extraction of lens, including insertion of prosthesis[103]	There are no adequately controlled trials in ophthalmic surgery. Retrospective review of data suggests that antibiotics or topical antiseptics may be efficacious, but there is no consensus regarding efficacy or choice of therapy.
General surgery	
Cholecystectomy[104–106]	Cefazolin,[c] 2 g iv preoperatively in high-risk patients: age >60, previous biliary surgery, h/o acute symptoms, or presence of jaundice. With β-lactam allergy, gentamicin, 80 mg iv preoperatively and every 8 hours iv for 3 doses, is effective.
Inguinal hernia repair	Data to recommend prophylaxis are not available.
Colon surgery[107–109]	Neomycin and erythromycin base, 1 g of each po at 1, 2, and 11 PM on the day before surgery. For emergency colon surgery or situations precluding preoperative oral prophylaxis, cefoxitin, 2 g iv preoperatively and every 4 hours for 3 doses, is effective. With β-lactam allergy, metronidazole, 500 mg iv, and gentamicin, 1.7 mg/kg iv, preoperatively and every 8 hours postoperatively for 3 doses are effective.
Division of adhesions, laparotomy, and abdominal surgery not involving a viscus	Data to recommend prophylaxis are not available.
Primary appendectomy[95,110–113]	Cefoxitin, 2 g iv preoperatively and every 6 hours for 3 doses in nonperforated appendices; in perforated appendices, continue therapy for 3–5 days. Although combined aerobic and anaerobic coverage appears preferable, with β-lactam allergy, metronidazole, 500 mg iv preoperatively, is effective. With perforated appendices, continue metronidazole every 8 hours iv or po for 3–5 days.
Mastectomy, total or partial	Data to recommend prophylaxis are not available.
Gastric resection[114–116]	Cefazolin,[c] 1 g preoperatively in high-risk patients only: bleeding gastric or duodenal ulcer, obstructive duodenal ulcer, gastric ulcer, gastric malignancy, or morbid obesity (i.e., prophylaxis is not indicated in chronic uncomplicated duodenal ulcer). With β-lactam allergy, a single preoperative iv dose of gentamicin, 120 mg, and clindamycin, 600 mg, may be effective, but data are limited.
Surgery for penetrating abdominal trauma[117,118]	Cefoxitin, 2 g iv upon admission to the hospital. For patients found to have intestinal perforation, 2 g of cefoxitin iv q6h for 2–5 days is effective.
Urologic surgery	
Prostatectomy, transurethral and peritoneal[119–121]	Antimicrobial prophylaxis is not recommended in patients with sterile preoperative urine cultures. Prophylactic antibiotics have not proven effective in transperitoneal needle biopsy of prostate with sterile preprocedure cultures.
Dilatation of urethra	Data to recommend prophylaxis are not available.

(Continued)

TABLE 6. *(Continued)*

Surgical Procedure[a]	*Recommended Prophylactic Regimen*[b]
Surgery on nose, mouth, and pharynx	
Tonsillectomy with or without adenoidectomy	Data to recommend prophylaxis are not available.
Major head, neck, and oral surgery[122–124]	In major surgical procedures involving an incision through oral or pharyngeal mucosa, a combination of gentamicin, 1.7 mg/kg, and clindamycin, 300 mg iv, preoperatively and every 8 hours for 2 doses. Cefazolin and third-generation cephalosporins have also demonstrated effectiveness when given over a 24-hour period perioperatively.
Rhinoplasty and repair of nose[125]	Prophylactic antimicrobials have not proved effective.
Cardiothoracic and vascular surgery	
Median sternotomy, coronary artery bypass grafting, and valve surgery[36,37]	Although cefazolin,[c] 1 g iv preoperatively, followed by 1 g iv every 4 to 6 hours intraoperatively is commonly used, persistent *S. aureus* wound infections have been reported to be a problem in some institutions despite use of cefazolin prophylaxis. Cefuroxime, cefamandole, and vancomycin alternatives as outlined in the footnote should be considered in institutions where *S. aureus* wound infections continue to occur despite cefazolin prophylaxis. Antibiotic administration is generally continued into the postoperative period for 48 or 72 hours although the optimal duration of postoperative prophylaxis has not been extablished.
Pacemaker insertion[126]	Cefazolin,[c] 1 g preoperatively and every 6 hours postoperatively for 24 hours. With β-lactam allergy, no prophylaxis may be a reasonable alternative given the low incidence of infection.
Thoracic surgery procedure including lobectomy and pneumonectomy[127–130]	Cefazolin,[c] 1 g preoperatively and every 6 hours postoperatively for 24 hours. The optimal duration of postoperative prophylaxis had not been established. In penetrating thoracic trauma and in the placement of chest tubes in trauma management, prophylactic antibiotics have not been effective.
Peripheral vascular surgery[39]	Cefazolin,[c] 1 g preoperatively and every 6 hours postoperatively for 24 hours. The utility of antibiotic prophylaxis in carotid artery surgery has not been established, but when infection rates are high, cefazolin[c] as above should be used.
Neurosurgical procedures	
(See section on orthopedic surgery for recommendations regarding laminectomy and spinal fusion)	
CSF shunting procedures[131–133]	Antibiotic prophylaxis is not indicated in institutions with low infection rates (<10%). Trimethoprim (160 mg)-sulfamethoxazole (800 mg) iv preoperatively and every 12 hours for 3 doses has proved beneficial in institutions with high infection rates (>20%).
Craniotomy[134,135]	For high risk procedures (e.g., reexploration, microsurgery), clindamycin, 300 mg iv preoperatively and at 4 hours, has proved effective. Vancomycin 10 mg/kg (maximum of 500 mg) iv, and gentamicin 2 mg/kg (maximum of 120 mg) iv, plus an aminoglycoside irrigating solution, has also proved effective.
Miscellaneous	
Simple hand laceration[136–138]	Prophylactic antibiotics have not proved effective. However, in animal (cat) bites, amoxicillin/clavulanate[e] (50 mg/125 mg) po every 6 hours for 5 days may be effective.

[a] Procedures are ranked in approximately descending order at the frequency with which they were performed in patients discharged from federal short-stay hospitals, 1984. (National Center for Health Statistics, 1984 summary. National Hospital Discharge survey: Advance data from vital and health statistics. No. 112. Hyattsville, MD: Public Health Service; 1985 [DHHS publication no. (PHS) 85-1250].)
[b] Unless otherwise noted, the preoperative dose of intravenous (iv) antibiotic should be administered at the appoximate time of the operative incision. Preoperative intramuscular (im) antibiotic should be administered ½ to 1 hour before the time of the operative incision.
[c] Because of its superior half-life, cefazolin is recommended at the indicated dosing schedule although another dose of cefazolin, another cephalosporin, or a semisynthetic penicillin was evaluated in the referenced article. However, if methicillin-sensitive *S. aureus* infections continue to occur despite cefazolin prophylaxis, consider substituting cefuroxime, 1500 mg iv at the induction of anesthesia and 750 mg q 4–6 hr throughout the procedure, or, cefamandole, 2 g at induction of anesthesia and 1 g q 2 hr throughout the operative procedure. If coagulase-negative staphyloccocal infections are occurring, consider substituting cefamandole, 2 g at induction of anesthesia and 1 g q 2 hr throughout the operative procedure. If methicillin-resistant staphylococcal infections become frequent, vancomycin 15 mg/kg preoperatively, 10 mg/kg during surgery, and q 8 hr thereafter should be considered.[139]
[d] In the referenced article, pivampicillin, 350 mg po tid for 4 days, was also given postprocedure to patients in the prophylaxis group. Whether ampicillin, 500 mg po tid, can be substituted or whether a postprocedure oral antibiotic is necessary at all is not known.
[e] Ampicillin-clavulanate is recommended, although oxacillin was evaluated in the referenced article.
(Adapted from Kaiser,[48] with permission.)

from established prophylactic regimens. Early reexplorations for postoperative bleeding, a history of penicillin or cephalosporin allergy, trauma and other emergency surgery, and existing preoperative infections of nonwound sites (e.g., urinary tract infections, decubitus ulcers) are important variables that may influence the choice and duration of perioperative prophylaxis. Studies are not available that can provide guidelines for such situations. A continuous assessment of failures of prophylaxis and a willingness to alter antiseptic and perioperative antibiotic protocols based on local observations or published data are essential aspects of surgical wound prevention and antimicrobial prophylaxis.

REFERENCES

1. McDermott W, Rogers DE. Social ramifications of control of microbial disease. Johns Hopkins Med J. 1982;151:301–12.
2. Rice LB, Karchmer AW. Artificial heart implantation: What limitations are imposed by infectious complications? JAMA. 1988;259:894–5.
3. Finland M. Antibacterial agents: Uses and abuses in treatment and prophylaxis. Rhode Island Med J. 1960;43:499–520.
4. Culbertson WR, Altemeier WA, Gonzalez LL, et al. Studies on the epidemiology of postoperative infection of clean operative wounds. Ann Surg. 1961;154:599–610.
5. Howe CW, Marston AT. A study on sources of postoperative staphylococcal infection. Surg Gynecol Obstet. 1962;115:266–75.
6. Burke JF. Identification of the sources of staphylococci contaminating the surgical wound during operation. Ann Surg. 1963;158:898–904.
7. Howes EL. Prevention of wound infection by the injection of nontoxic antibacterial substances. Ann Surg. 1946;124:268–76.
8. Burke JF. The effective period of preventive antibiotic action in experimental incisions and dermal lesions. Surgery. 1961;50:161–8.
9. Sanchez-Ubeda R, Fernand E, Rousselot LM. Complication rate in general surgical cases: The value of penicillin and streptomycin as postoperative prophylaxis—a study of 511 cases. N Engl J Med. 1958;259:1045–50.
10. Johnstone FRC. An assessment of prophylactic antibiotics in general surgery. Surg Gynecol Obstet. 1963;116:1–10.
11. Aglietti P, Salvati EA, Wilson PD Jr, et al. Effect of a surgical horizontal unidirectional filtered air flow unit on wound bacterial contamination and wound healing. Clin Orthop 1974;101:99–104.
12. Elek SD, Coneh PE. The virulence of *Staphylococcus pyogenes* for man. A study of the problems of wound infection. Br J Exp Pathol. 1958;38:573–86.
13. Ad Hoc Committee of the Committee on Trauma, National Research Council Division of Medical Sciences. Postoperative wound infections: The influence of ultraviolet irradiation of the operating room and of various other factors. Ann Surg. 1964;160(2).
14. Nagachinta T, Stephens M, Reitz B. Risk factors for surgical-wound infection following cardiac surgery. J Infect Dis. 1987;156:967–73.
15. Meakins JL, Pietsch JB, Bubenick O, et al. Delayed hypersensitivity: Indicator of acquired failure of host defenses in sepsis and trauma. Ann Surg. 1977;186:241–50.
16. Ketcham AS, Lieberman JE, West JT. Antibiotic prophylaxis in cancer surgery and its value in staphylococcal carrier patients. Surg Gynecol Obstet. 1963;117:1–6.
17. Brunn JN. Post-operative wound infection: Predisposing factors and the effect of a reduction in the dissemination of staphylococci. Acta Med Scand. 1970; 188(Suppl 514):9.
18. Yu VL, Goetz A, Wagener M, et al. *Staphylococcus aureus* nasal carriage

and infection in patients on hemodialysis: Efficacy of antibiotic prophylaxis. N Engl J Med. 1986;315:91–6.
19. Schaffner W, Lefkowitz LB, Goodman JS. Hospital outbreak of infections with group A streptococci traced to an asymptomatic anal carrier. N Engl J Med. 1969;280:1224–5.
20. Stamm WE, Feeley JC, Facklam RR. Wound infections due to group A *Streptococcus* traced to a vaginal carrier. J Infect Dis. 1978;138:287–92.
20a. Berkelman RL, Martin D, Graham DR, et al. Streptococcal wound infections caused by vaginal carrier. JAMA 1982;247:2680–2.
21. Lidwell OM, Lowbury EJL, Whyte W, et al. Effect of ultraclean air in operating rooms on deep sepsis in the joint after total hip or knee replacement: A randomized study. Br Med J. 1982;185:10–4.
22. Marotte JH, Lord GA, Blanchard JP, et al. Infection rate in total hip arthroplasty as a function of air cleanliness and antibiotic prophylaxis: 10-year experience with 2,384 cementless Lord Madreporic prostheses. J Arthroplasty. 1987;2:77–82.
23. Dismukes WE, Karchmer AW, Buckley MJ, et al. Prosthetic valve endocarditis: Analysis of 38 cases. Circulation. 1973;48:365–77.
24. Slaughter L, Morris JE, Starr A. Prosthetic valvular endocarditis: A 12-year review. Circulation. 1973;48:1319–26.
25. Carlsson AS, Lidgren L, Lindberg L. Prophylactic antibiotics against early and late deep infections after total hip replacements. Acta Orthop Scand. 1977;48:405–10.
26. Krieger JN, Kaiser DL, Wenzel RP. Nosocomial urinary tract infections cause wound infections postoperatively in surgical patients. Surg Gynecol Obstet. 1983;156:313–8.
27. Kaiser AB. Overview of cephalosporin prophylaxis. Am J Surg. 1988;155 (Suppl 5A):52–5.
28. Karchmer AW, Archer GL, Dismukes WE. *Staphylococcus epidermidis* causing prosthetic valve endocarditis: Microbiologic and clinical observations as guides to therapy. Ann Intern Med. 1983;98:447–55.
29. Ward TT, Winn RE, Hartstein AI, et al. Observations relating to an interhospital outbreak of methicillin-resistant *Staphylococcus aureus*: Role of antimicrobial therapy in infection control. Infect Control. 1981;2:453–9.
30. Palmer DL, Kuritsky JN, Lapham SC, et al. *Enterobacter* mediastinitis following cardiac surgery. Infect Control. 1985;6:115–9.
31. Bartzokas CA, Paton JH, Gibson MF, et al. Control and eradication of methicillin-resistant *Staphylococcus aureus* on a surgical unit. N Engl J Med. 1984;311:1425–7.
32. Houang ET, Marples RR, Weir I, et al. Problems in the investigation of an apparent outbreak of coagulase-negative staphylococcal septicaemia following cardiac surgery. J Hosp Infect. 1986;8:224–32.
33. Centers for Disease Control. Nosocomial infection surveillance. 1980–1982. In: Surveillance Summaries (published four times a year). 1983;32(No. 4SS):1SS–16SS.
34. Centers for Disease Control. Nosocomial infection surveillance, 1983. In: Surveillance Summaries (published four times a year). 1984;33(No. 2SS): 9SS–21SS.
35. Centers for Disease Control. Nosocomial infection surveillance, 1984. In: Surveillance Summaries (published four times a year). 1986;35(No. 1SS):17SS–29SS.
36. Slama TG, Sklar SJ, Misinski J, et al. Randomized comparison of cefamandole, cefazolin, and cefuroxime prophylaxis in open-heart surgery. Antimicrob Agents Chemother. 1986;29:744–7.
37. Kaiser AB, Petracek MR, Lea JW IV, et al. Efficacy of cefazolin, cefamandole, and gentamicin as prophylactic agents in cardiac surgery. Ann Surg. 1987;206:791–7.
38. Kernodle DS, Kaiser AB. *Staphylococcus aureus* infections failing cefazolin or cefamandole prophylaxis in cardiac surgery: Clinical relevance of β-lactamase production (Abstract no. 87). In: Program and Abstracts of the 27th Interscience Conference on Antimicrobial Agents and Chemotherapy. New York: American Society for Microbiology; 1987.
39. Kaiser AB, Clayson KR, Mulherin JL Jr, et al. Antibiotic prophylaxis in vascular surgery. Ann Surg. 1978;188:283–9.
40. Archer GL, Armstrong BC. Alteration of staphylococcal flora in cardiac patients receiving antibiotic prophylaxis. J Infect Dis. 1983;147:642–9.
41. Kernodle DS, Barg NL, Kaiser AB. Low-level colonization of hospitalized patients with methicillin-resistant coagulase-negative staphylococci and their emergence during surgical antimicrobial prophylaxis. Antimicrob Agents Chemother. 1988;32:202–8.
42. Olson B, Weinstein RA, Nathan C, et al. Occult aminoglycoside resistance in *Pseudomonas aeruginosa*: Epidemiology and implications for therapy and control. J Infect Dis. 1985;152:769–74.
43. Archer GL, Tenenbaum MJ. Antibiotic-resistant *Staphylococcus epidermidis* in patients undergoing cardiac surgery. Antimicrob Agents Chemother. 1980;17:269.
44. Roberts NJ Jr, Douglas RG Jr. Gentamicin use and *Pseudomonas* and *Serratia* resistance: Effect of a surgical prophylaxis regimen. Antimicrob Agents Chemother. 1978;13:214–20.
45. Uttley AHC, Collins CH, Naidoo J, et al. Vancomycin-resistant enterococci. Lancet. 1988;1:57–8.
46. Miles AA, Niven JSF. The enhancement of infection during shock produced by bacterial toxins and other agents. Br J Exp Pathol. 1950;31:73.
47. Burke JF, Miles AA. The significance of vascular events in early infective inflammation. J Pathol Bacteriol. 1958;76:1–19.
48. Kaiser AB. Drug therapy: Antimicrobial prophylaxis in surgery. N Engl J Med. 1986;315:1129–38.
49. Evans M, Pollock AV. Trials on trials: A review of trials of antibiotic prophylaxis. Arch Surg. 1984;119:109–13.
49a. Platt R, Munoz A, Stella J, et al. Antibiotic prophylaxis for cardiovascular surgery: Efficacy with coronary artery bypass. Ann Intern Med. 1984;101:770–4.
50. Goldmann DA, Hopkins CC, Karchmer AW. Cephalothin prophylaxis in cardiac valve surgery: A prospective, double-blind comparison of two-day and six-day regimen. J Thorac Cardiovasc Surg. 1977;73:470–9.
51. Elliott JP, Freeman RK, Dorchester W. Short versus long course of prophylactic antibiotics in cesarean section. Am J Obstet Gynecol. 1982; 143:740–4.
52. Gatell JM, Garcia S, Lozano L, et al. Perioperative cefamandole prophylaxis against infections. J Bone Joint Surg. 1987;8:1189–93.
53. Block BS, Mercer LJ, Ismail MA, et al. *Clostridium difficile*-associated diarrhea follows perioperative prophylaxis with cefoxitin. Am J Obstet Gynecol. 1986;153:835–8.
54. Sattler FR. Weitekamp MR, Ballard JO. Potential for bleeding with the new beta-lactam antibiotics. Ann Intern Med. 1986;105:924–31.
55. Angaran DM, Dias VC, Arom KV, et al. The influence of prophylactic antibiotics on the warfarin anticoagulation response in the postoperative prosthetic cardiac valve patient. Ann Surg. 1983;199.107–11.
56. Dajee H, Laks H, Miller J, et al. Profound hypotension from rapid vancomycin administration during cardiac operation. J Thorac Cardiovasc Surg. 1984;87:145–6.
57. Odio C, Mohs E, Sklar FH, et al. Adverse reactions to vancomycin used as prophylaxis for CSF shunt procedures. Am J Dis Child. 1984;138:17–9.
58. Kaiser AB. Clinical implications of β-lactamases in surgical prophylaxis. Contemp Surg. 1988;32(Suppl 3A):30–8.
59. Kaul AF, Jewett JF. Agents and techniques for disinfection of the skin. Surg Gynecol Obstet. 1981;152:677–85.
60. Alexander JW, Fischer JE, Boyajian M, et al. The influence of hair-removal methods on wound infections. Arch Surg. 1983;118:347–52.
61. Valentine RJ, Weigelt JA, Dryer D, et al. Effect of remote infections on clean wound infection rates. Am J Infect Control. 1986;14:64–8.
62. Knighton DR, Halliday B, Hunt TK. Oxygen as an antibiotic. Arch Surg. 1984;119:199–204.
63. Moellering RC Jr, Kunz LJ, Poitras JW, et al. Microbiologic basis of the rational use of prophylactic antibiotics. South Med J. 1977;70:8–14.
63a. Kaiser AB. The use of antibiotics in cardiac and thoracic surgery in Sabistan/Spencer (eds): *Gibbon's Surgery of the Chest*, 5th edition. Philadelphia, WB Saunders, 1989.
64. Condon RE, Haley Rw, Lee JT Jr, et al. Does infection control control infections? Arch Surg. 1988;123:250–6.
65. Altemeier WA, Burke JF, Pluitt BA Jr, et al. Manual on control of infection in surgical patients. Philadelphia: JB Lippincott; 1976:29–30.
66. Olson M, O'Connor M, Schwartz ML. Surgical wound infections: A 5-year prospective study of 20,193 wounds at the Minneapolis VA Medical Center. Ann Surg. 1984;199:253–9.
67. Polk HC Jr, Miles AA. Enhancement of bacterial infection by ferric iron: kinetics, mechanisms, and surgical significance. Surgery. 1971;70:71–7.
68. DeLong TG, Simmons RL. Role of lymphatic vessels in bacterial clearance from early soft tissue infection. Arch Surg. 1982;117:123–8.
69. Zimmerli W, Waldvogel FA, Vaudaux P, et al. Pathogenesis of foreign body infection: Description and characteristics of an animal model. J Infect Dis. 1982;146:487–97.
70. Grappel SF, Phillips L, Lewis HB, et al. Prophylactic activity of cephalosporins in a mouse model of surgical wound infections. J Antibiot. 1983; 36:161–6.
71. Bartlett JG. Experimental aspects of intraabdominal abscess. Am J Med. 1984;75:91–8.
72. Platt J, Bucknall RA. An experimental evaluation of antiseptic wound irrigation. J Hosp Infect. 1984;5:181–8.
73. Hau T, Jacobs DE, Hawkins NL. Antibiotics fail to prevent abscess formation secondary to bacteria trapped in fibrin clots. Arch Surg. 1986; 121:163–7.
74. Hoogeterp JJ, Mattie H, Krul AM, et al. Quantitative effect of granulocytes on antibiotic treatment of experimental staphylococcal infection. Antimicrob Agents Chemother. 1987;31:930–4.
75. Arbeit RD, Dunn RM. Expression of capsular polysaccharide during experimental focal infection with *Staphylococcus aureus*. J Infect Dis. 1987;156:947–52.
76. Falcieri E, Vandaux P, Huggler E, et al. Role of bacterial exopolymers and host factors on adherence and phagocytosis of *Staphylococcus aureus* in foreign body infections. J Infect Dis. 1987;155:524–31.
77. Nelson CL, Green TG, Porter RA, et al. One day *versus* seven days of preventive antibiotic therapy in orthopedic surgery. Clin Orthop. 1983;176:258–63.
78. Scarpignato C, Caltabiano M, Condemi V, et al. Short-term versus long-term cefuroxime prophylaxis in patients undergoing emergency cesarean section. Clin Ther. 1982;5:186–92.
79. Soper DE, Yarwood RL. Single-dose antibiotic prophylaxis in women undergoing vaginal hysterectomy. Obstet Gynecol. 1987;69:879–82.
80. Conte JE Jr, Cohen SN, Roe BB, et al. Antibiotic prophylaxis and cardiac surgery: A prospective double-blind comparison of single-dose versus multiple-dose regimens. Ann Intern Med. 1972;76:943–9.
81. Hillis DJ, Rosenfeldt FL, Spicer WJ, et al. Antibiotic prophylaxis for cor-

onary bypass grafting: Comparison of a five-day and a two-day course. J Thorac Cardiovasc Surg. 1983;86:217.
82. Elyan A, Mahran M, el-Maraghy M, et al. Prophylactic intravenous metronidazole in cesarean section. Chemioterapia. 1984;3:67–70.
83. Stiver HG, Forward KR, Livingstone RA, et al. Multicenter comparison of cefoxitin versus cefazolin for prevention of infectious morbidity after nonelective cesarean section. Am J Obstet Gynecol. 1983;145:158–63.
84. Harger JH, English DH. Selection of patients for antibiotic prophylaxis in cesarean section. Am J Obstet Gynecol. 1981;141:752–8.
85. Hawrylyshyn PA, Bernstein P, Papsin FR. Short-term antibiotic prophylaxis in high-risk patients following cesarean section. Am J Obstet Gynecol. 1983;145:285–9.
86. Elliott JP, Flaherty JF. Comparison of lavage or intravenous antibiotics at cesarean section. Obstet Gynecol. 1986;67:29–32.
87. Conover WB, Moore TR. Comparison of irrigation and intravenous antibiotic prophylaxis at cesarean section. Obstet Gynecol. 1984;63:787–91.
88. Heisterbert L, Petersen K. Metronidazole prophylaxis in elective first trimester abortion. Obstet Gynecol. 1985;65:371–4.
89. Sonne-Holm S, Heisterberg L, Hebjorn S, et al. Prophylactic antibiotics in first-trimester abortions: A clinical, controlled trial. Am J Obstet Gynecol. 1981;139:693–6.
90. Spence MR, King TM, Burkman RT, et al. Cephalothin prophylaxis for midtrimester abortion. Obstet Gynecol. 1982;60:502–5.
91. Polk BF, Tager IB, Shapiro M, et al. Randomised clinical trial of perioperative cefazolin in preventing infection after hysterectomy. Lancet. 1980;1:437–41.
92. Hemsell DL, Hemsell PG, Nobles BJ. Doxycycline and cefamandole prophylaxis for premenopausal women underoing vaginal hysterectomy. Surg Gynecol Obstet. 1985;161:462–4.
93. Hemsell DL, Johnson ER, Bawdon RE, et al. Ceftriaxone and cefazoline prophylaxis for hysterectomy. Surg Gynecol Obstet. 1985;161:197–203.
94. Tuomala RE, Fischer SG, Munoz A, et al. A comparative trial of cefazolin and moxalactam as prophylaxis for preventing infection after abdominal hysterectomy. Obstet Gynecol. 1985;66:372–6.
95. Lau WY, Fan ST, Yui TF, et al. Prophylaxis of postappendicectomy sepsis by metronidazole and cefotaxime; a randomized, prospective and double blind trial. Br J Surg. 1983;70:670–2.
96. Cunha BA, Gossling HR, Pasternak HS, et al. Penetration of cephalosporins into bone. Infection. 1984;12:80–4.
97. Hill C, Flamant R, Mazas F, et al. Prophylactic cefazolin versus placebo in total hip replacement. Lancet. 1981;1:795–7.
98. Gatell JM, Riba J, Lozano ML, et al. Prophylactic cefamandole in orthopaedic surgery. J Bone Joint Surg. 1984;66:1219–22.
99. Patzakis MJ, Harvey P, Ivler D. The role of antibiotics in the management of open fractures. J Bone Joint Surg. 1974;56:532–41.
100. Geraghty J, Feely M. Antibiotic prophylaxis in neurosurgery: A randomized controlled trial. J Neurosurg. 1984;60:724–6.
101. Strohecker J, Piotrowski WP, Lametschwandtner A. The intra-operative application of povidone-iodine in neurosurgery. J Hosp Infect. 1985;6:532–41.
102. Sonne-Holm S, Boeckstyns M, Mench H, et al. Prophylactic antibiotics in amputation of the lower extremity for ischemia. J Bone Joint Surg. 1985;67:800–3.
103. Starr MB. Prophylactic antibiotics for ophthalmic surgery. Surv Ophthalmol. 1983;27:353–73.
104. Kaufman Z, Engelberg M, Eliashiv A, et al. Systemic prophylactic antibiotics in elective biliary surgery. Arch Surg. 1984;119:1002–4.
105. Lewis RT, Allan CM, Goodall RG, et al. A single preoperative dose of cefazolin prevents postoperative sepsis in high-risk biliary surgery. Can J Surg. 1984;27:44–7.
106. Lykkegaard Nielsen M, Moesgaard F, Justesen T, et al. Wound sepsis after elective cholecystectomy: Restriction of prophylactic antibiotics to risk groups. Scand J Gastroenterol. 1981;16:937–40.
107. Kaiser AB, Herrington JL Jr, Jacobs JK, et al. Cefoxitin versus erythromycin, neomycin, and cefazolin in colorectal operations: Importance of the duration of the surgical procedure. Ann Surg. 1983;198:525–30.
108. McDonald PJ, Karran SJ. A comparison of intravenous cefoxitin and a combination of gentamicin and metronidazole as prophylaxis in colorectal surgery. Dis Colon Rectum. 1983;26:661–4.
109. Clarke JS, Condon RE, Bartlett JG, et al. Preoperative oral antibiotics reduce septic complications of colon operations: Results of prospective randomized, double-blind clinical study. Ann Surg. 1977;186:251–9.
110. Chant AD, Turner DTL, Machin D. Metronidazole v ampicillin: Differing effects on the postoperative recovery. Ann R Coll Surg Engl. 1984;66:96–7.
111. Greenall MJ, Bakran A, Pickford IR, et al. A double-blind trial of a single intravenous dose of metronidazole as prophylaxis against wound infection following appendicectomy. Br J Surg. 1979;66:428–9.
112. Morris WT, Innes DB, Richardson RA, et al. Prevention of post-appendicectomy sepsis by metronidazole and cefazolin: A controlled double blind trial. Aust NZ J Surg. 1980;50:429–33.
113. Winslow RE, Dean RE, Harley JW. Acute nonperforating appendicitis. Arch Surg. 1983;118:651–5.
114. LoCicero J III, Nichols RL. Sepsis after gastroduodenal operations: Relationship to gastric acid, motility, and endogenous microflora. South Med J. 1980;73:878–90.
115. Richards DG, Clark RG, Rowland BJ, et al. Antibiotic prophylaxis against wound infection in emergency abdominal surgery. J R Coll Surg Edinb. 1981;26:232–7.
116. Stone HH, Hooper CA, Kolb LD, et al. Antibiotic prophylaxis in gastric, biliary and colonic surgery. Ann Surg. 1976;184:443–52.
117. Gentry LO, Feliciano DV, Lea AS, et al. Perioperative antibiotic therapy for penetrating injuries of the abdomen. Ann Surg. 1984;200:561–6.
118. Nichols RL, Smith JW, Klein DB, et al. Risk of infection after penetrating abdominal trauma. N Engl J Med. 1984;311:1065–70.
119. Ferrie BG, Scott R. Prophylactic cefuroxime in transurethral resection. Urol Res. 1984;12:279–81.
120. Quist N, Christiansen HM, Ehlers D. Severe Vibrio cholerae sepsis and meningitis in a young infant. Urol Res. 1984;12:275–7.
121. Packer MG, Russo P, Fair WR. Prophylactic antibiotics and Foley catheter use in transperineal needle biopsy of the prostate. J Urol. 1984;131:687–9.
122. Johnson JR, Yu VL, Myers EN, et al. Efficacy of two third-generation cephalosporins in prophylaxis for head and neck surgery. Arch Otolaryngol. 1984;110:224–7.
123. Seagle MB, Duberstein LE, Gross CW, et al. Efficacy of cefazolin as prophylactic antibiotic in head and neck surgery. Otolaryngology. 1979;85:568–72.
124. Slight PH, Gundling K, Plotkin SA, et al. A trial of vancomycin for prophylaxis of infections after neurosurgical shunts. N Engl J Med. 1985; 312:921.
125. Weimert TA, Yoder MG. Antibiotics and nasal surgery. Laryngoscope. 1980;90:667–72.
126. Muers MF, Arnold AG, Sleight P. Prophylactic antibiotics for cardiac pacemaker implantation: A prospective trial. Br Heart J. 1981;46:539–44.
127. Frimodt-Moller N, Ostri P, Pendersen IBK, et al. Antibiotic prophylaxis in pulmonary surgery: A double-blind study of penicillin versus placebo. Ann Surg. 1982;195:444–50.
128. Kvale PA, Ranga V, Kopacz M, et al. Pulmonary resection. South Med J. 1977;70:64–8.
129. LeBlanc KA, Tucker WY. Prophylactic antibiotics and closed tube thoracostomy. Surg Gynecol Obstet. 1985;160:259–63.
130. Mandal AK, Montano J, Thadepalli H. Prophylactic antibiotics and no antibiotics compared in penetrating chest trauma. J Trauma. 1985;25:639–43.
131. Blomstedt GC. Results of trimethoprim-sulfamethoxazole prophylaxis in ventriculotomy and shunting procedures: A double-blind randomized trail. J Neurosurg. 1985;62:694–97.
132. Wang EEL, Prober CG, Hendrick BE, et al. Prophylactic sulfamethoxazole and trimethoprim in ventriculoperitoneal shunt surgery: A double-blind, randomized, placebo-controlled trial. JAMA. 1984;251:1174–77.
133. Schmidt K, Gjerris F, Osgaard O, et al. Antibiotic prophylaxis in cerebrospinal fluid shunting: A prospective randomized trial in 152 hydrocephalic patients. Neurosurg. 1985;17:1–5.
134. Savitz MH, Malis LI. Prophylactic clindamycin for neurosurgical patients. NY State J Med. 1976;76:64–7.
135. Shapiro M, Wald U, Simchen E, et al. Randomized clinical trial of intraoperative antimicrobial prophylaxis of infection after neurosurgical procedures. J Hosp Infect. 1986;8:283–95.
136. Elenbaas RM, McNabney WK, Robinson WA. Evaluation of prophylactic oxacillin in cat bite wounds. Ann Emerg Med. 1984;13:155–7.
137. Grossman JAI, Adams JP, Kunec J. Prophylactic antibiotics in simple hand lacerations. JAMA. 1981;245:1055–6.
138. Haughey RE, Lammers RL, Wagner DK: Use of antibiotics in the initial management of soft tissue hand wounds. Ann Emerg Med. 1981;10:187–92.
139. Farber BF, Karchmer AW, Buckley MJ, et al. Vancomycin prophylaxis in cardiac operations: Determination of an optimal dosage regimen. J Thorac Cardiovasc Surg. 1983;85:933–40.
140. Postlethwaite RW. Principles of operative surgery: Antisepsis, technique, sutures, and drains. In: Sabistan DC, ed. Davis-Christopher Textbook of Surgery. 11th ed. Philadelphia: WB Saunders; 1977.

SECTION B. INFECTIONS IN SPECIAL HOSTS

286. INFECTIONS IN THE COMPROMISED HOST—AN OVERVIEW

STEPHEN C. SCHIMPFF

The term "compromised host" has come to mean an individual who has one or more defects in the body's natural defense mechanisms, defects sufficiently significant that the individual is rendered predisposed to severe, often life-threatening infection. Principal examples of compromised patients are those with acute leukemia (granulocytopenia, altered microbial flora, and damage to anatomic barriers to microbial invasion), lymphoma, transplant, or acquired immunodeficiency (AIDS) (T-cell dysfunction), carcinomas or sarcomas (obstruction to natural passages), intravenous drug abuse (direct venous access by microbes in addition to altered defense mechanisms), myeloma or chronic lymphocytic leukemia (loss of normal antibody function), brain tumors (loss of gag reflex and impaired micturition), and the seriously traumatized vehicular accident victim (anatomic barriers). The subjects of acute leukemia, AIDS, and organ transplantation are discussed in other chapters and will not be included here.

FACTORS PREDISPOSING TO INFECTION

The following are some of the most important factors that predispose to infection: (*1*) granulocytopenia, (*2*) cellular immune dysfunction, (*3*) humoral immune dysfunction, (*4*) anatomic-barrier damage, that is, mucosal or integumentary damage, (*5*) obstructive phenomena, (*6*) central nervous system dysfunction, and (*7*) various medical procedures. Table 1 lists these factors with examples of their most common associated infections.

TABLE 1. Factors Predisposing to Infection and the Most Common Pathogens

Granulocytopenia
Bacteria
Gram-negative bacilli
Escherichia coli
Pseudomonas aeruginosa
Klebsiella pneumoniae
Gram-positive cocci
Staphylococcus epidermidis
Staphylococcus aureus
Yeasts
Candida
Filamentous fungi
Aspergillus
Agents of mucormycosis
Cellular immune dysfunction
Bacteria
Listeria monocytogenes
Salmonella
Mycobacterium
Nocardia asteroides
Legionella
Fungi
Cryptococcus neoformans
Histoplasma capsulatum
Coccidioides immitis
Viruses
Varicella zoster
Cytomegalovirus
Herpes simplex
Protozoa
Pneumocystis carinii
Toxoplasma gondii
Cryptosporidium
Helminth
Strongyloides stercoralis
Humoral immune dysfunction
Bacteria
Streptococcus pneumoniae
Haemophilus influenzae

GRANULOCYTOPENIA AND DEFECTS IN PHAGOCYTIC DEFENSES

Granulocytopenia is particularly common in patients with acute leukemia (Chapter 287), following intensive myelosuppressive drug or radiation therapy for other malignancies or bone marrow transplantation (Chapter 291), or as a result of aplastic anemia. The incidence and severity of infection are inversely proportional to the absolute granulocyte count.[1] Figure 1 graphically displays the incidence of all infections among 64 consecutive patients with acute nonlymphocytic leukemia admitted to the University of Maryland Cancer Center for their initial remission induction therapy. The incidence of infection began to rise as the granulocyte count fell below 500/μl, with a very substantial rise when the granulocyte count approached zero. Most severe infections and nearly all bacteremias occurred when the granulocyte count was less than 100/μl.

The recognition that most infections and nearly all severe infections occur at polymorphonuclear (PMN) levels of less than 100/μl is critical to both therapy and prevention strategies. Decisions on selection of antibiotics (monotherapy vs. combination therapy, spectrum against bacteria, fungi, etc.) may vary, depending upon the granulocyte count, trend, and duration. Similarly, one would probably not consider oral prophylactic antimicrobial agents for a patient not expected to have a prolonged (10 days or greater) period of profound (less than 100 PMN/μl) granulocytopenia. An additional factor, not indicated by Figure 1, is the effect of the rate of fall of the granulocyte count; rapid declines were more often associated with infection.

Not only does the level and rapidity in decline of the granulocyte count correlate with infection, but also the duration of the aplastic phase. The current approach to initial remission induction therapy of acute nonlymphocytic leukemia is such that patients will become and remain granulocytopenic for about 20–25 days, with about one-half of that time spent with an absolute level of circulating neutrophils of less than 100/μl. Likewise, patients who receive bone marrow transplants will have a period of approximately 3 weeks with essentially no circulating granulocytes and, as a result, are at an exceedingly high risk of infection during that time. For the majority of carcinomas, most current standard approaches to cytotoxic therapy do not result in either long-term or very profound levels of granulocytopenia. However, the treatment of small-cell carcinoma of the lung, testicular carcinoma, and some sarcomas and lymphomas is highly myelosuppressive, although granulocytopenia is usually limited to intermittent periods of 7–10 days.

It is important to point out that although granulocytopenia clearly predisposes to infection, the occurrence of infection in

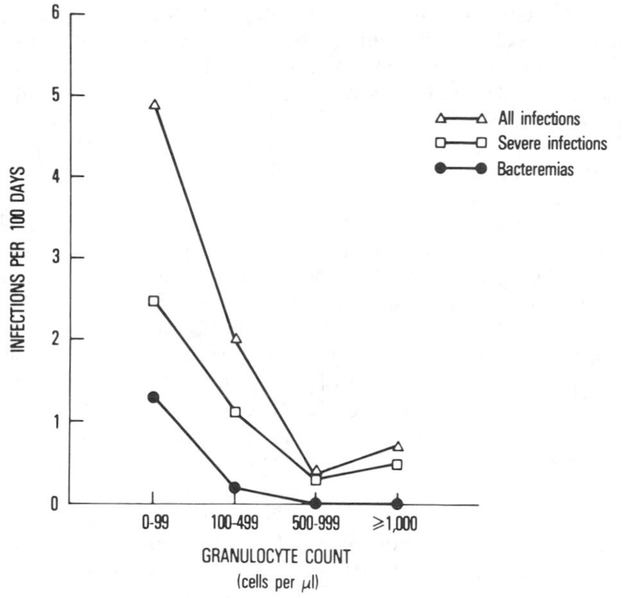

FIG 1. Incidence of infection in acute nonlymphocytic leukemia during induction therapy. The incidence of infection rises as the absolute granulocyte count is reduced. The graph is based on 64 newly diagnosed patients with acute nonlymphocytic leukemia treated with intensive chemotherapy at the University of Maryland Cancer Center between 1974 and 1977.

the setting of granulocytopenia is dependent upon the presence or absence of other associated predisposing factors, which act in concert with the absence of granulocytes. When cancer chemotherapy damages mucosal membranes, the opportunity for development of pharyngitis or perianal lesions is accentuated. Damage to the integument by venipuncture, indwelling vascular access catheter, hemorrhage, or axillary shaving may lead to infection. Damage to the mucosa of the trachea and bronchi, along with damage to ciliary function due to cancer chemotherapy, may offer the opportunity for pneumonia to develop. Any form of obstructive phenomenon can interact with granulocytopenia to encourage infection, such as the development of a urinary tract infection in a patient with tumor infiltration of the prostate, otitis media following an enlargement of adenoid tissue in patients with lymphocytic leukemia, or the development of axillary lesions in patients who use occlusive antiperspirants.

The most common sites of infection in granulocytopenic patients are the periodontium, oropharynx, lung, distal esophagus, colon, perianal area, and skin. As a general rule, the organism that causes infection has colonized (not just transiently present) the area that becomes infected.[2] In the presence of a damaged mucosal barrier, ciliary dysfunction, obstruction, etc., and in the absence of normal numbers of granulocytes, it then becomes possible for that organism of otherwise low pathogenicity to invade. Thus pneumonias are usually caused by organisms that have been colonizing the patient's oronasopharynx, and perianal lesions are caused by one or more of the organisms colonizing the lower intestinal tract.[2] The combination of anatomic barrier damage and absence of granulocytes allows for rapid progression to blood stream invasion, sepsis, and death. It is important to recognize that, although most infections are caused by organisms already colonizing the patient, they may well be organisms that have been acquired by the patient subsequent to admission to the hospital, that is, they are not truly part of the patient's normal endogenous flora. These pathogens may prove to be more virulent or more resistant to commonly utilized antibiotics, or both.

Qualitative abnormalities in phagocyte function occurring as a consequence of corticosteroid therapy, cancer chemotherapy, or irradiation may also be important in predisposing to infection. Furthermore, although certain antineoplastic agents, like daunorubicin, methotrexate, and vincristine, can inhibit phagocytosis, some of these agents in combination can inhibit granulocyte bactericidal activity. Children with acute lymphocytic leukemia who receive craniospinal irradiation have a higher incidence of infections in the period following irradiation than do nonirradiated children. This seems to be due to a transient impairment of bactericidal activity, although phagocytosis remains intact.

An appreciation of the types of organisms that cause infection in the setting of profound granulocytopenia and a recognition that many, if not most, are hospital-acquired is fundamental to the clinician's decision-making process for diagnosis, treatment, and prevention in this highly infection-prone patient population.

Equally important is the recognition that due to the impaired inflammatory response, the usual signs and symptoms of infection are muted, although fever is nearly universal as early evidence of infection.[3]

CELLULAR IMMUNE DYSFUNCTION

The term "cellular immune dysfunction" is a very broad generalization but is useful as an initial means of subclassifying the compromised host with regard to factors that predispose to infection. Certain diseases such as Hodgkin's disease or AIDS have an associated dysfunction of cellular immunity as an integral aspect of their disease, whereas patients with renal transplants[4,5] or acute lymphocytic leukemia in long-term maintained remission,[6] or patients who have a successful engraftment following bone marrow transplantation[7] all have substantial dysfunction of cellular immunity as a result of specific immunosuppressive therapy. Irradiation and drugs such as azathioprine, cyclosporine, corticosteroids, and cytotoxic agents have varying types and degrees of effects on cellular frame function and, in conjunction with the status of the underlying disease, interact to predispose to specific infections.

The end product of cellular immune defense is the activated macrophage or monocyte, which is key to the ingestion and killing of intracellular pathogens.[8] The precursors of these cells, the promonocytes, originate in the marrow, are stimulated to differentiate into monocytes by granulocyte–macrophage colony stimulating factor (GM-CSF) and M-CSF. These monocytes rapidly leave the marrow and circulate in the blood stream for about 3–5 days before migrating to tissues. Tissue-specific factors induce transformation to macrophages, which then persist in that site (liver, lung, spleen, intestinal wall, connective tissue, etc.) for about 3 months. Activation (i.e., an augmented capacity to destroy facultative intracellular microbes) of macrophages depends upon T_4-helper cell-derived lymphokines such as γ-interferon, tumor necrosis factor, or GM-CSF. T-cell release of lymphokines follows antigen stimulation of the committed sensitized lymphocyte.[9]

A defect anywhere in the T-lymphocyte or mononuclear–phagocytic system can lead to susceptibility to infection. A variety of diseases has been shown to result in impaired T-lymphocyte response (chronic and acute lymphocytic leukemia, renal, cardiac, and bone marrow transplantation, Hodgkin's disease, trauma, and HIV infection). Well-recognized defects in the mononuclear–phagocytic system can be found in patients with monocytic leukemia (impaired phagocytosis along with excess production of interleukin 1 with high fevers), chronic granulomatous disease (defect in oxidative killing), corticosteroid therapy, and some viral infections (e.g., cytomegalovirus [CMV]).

An array of opportunistic pathogens can produce infection in the setting of defective cellular immunity. (Table 1) In the general population, clinical infections caused by most of these organisms are infrequent, except for tuberculosis, childhood varicella, and recurrent herpes labialis. Many of the infecting organisms are common pathogens that can cause significant, but seldom disseminated or life-threatening infections in patients who are immunocompetent (for example, varicella-zoster virus, herpes simplex, or *Toxoplasma gondii*). Other organisms essentially never cause clinically recognized infection in immunocompetent individuals (for example, *Pneumocystis carinii*) or infection among specific groups (such as herpes simplex and CMV in the homosexual population), which may help to explain their transmission but not their virulence. It is worth noting that the organisms given in Table 1 as occurring in the patient with cellular immune deficiency do not occur in all patient groups with the same frequency. For example, the patient with Hodgkin's disease and recent radiation therapy has a nearly 25 percent likelihood of developing herpes zoster, yet the frequency of this infection is well under 10 percent in the patient with renal transplantation. The Hodgkin's disease patient rarely develops *P. carinii* infection, whereas the young child with acute lymphocytic leukemia receiving very intensive maintenance chemotherapy may have a 20 percent chance or greater of developing *Pneumocystis*, and the patient with AIDS (in part by definition) has an extremely high likelihood of developing *P. carinii* pneumonia. *Mycobacterium avium/M. intracellulare* is a fairly frequent cause of infection in AIDS patients and has been seen more frequently in the last decade in patients with non-Hodgkin's lymphoma receiving intensive cytotoxic therapy, whereas *Mycobacterium kansasii* has been found to be more common in hairy cell leukemia.

In general, most patients with cellular immune deficiency (with the notable exception of AIDS patients) have few infections caused by organisms commonly recognized as associated with cellular immune deficiency. Thus, if one looks at a large population of, say, Hodgkin's disease patients, and follows them over time, very few such infections, other than herpes zoster, will be documented. However, if one evaluates from the "organism point of view," then one will find that these organisms tend to cause infection or at least severe or life-threatening infection only in the setting of the cellular immune-deficient individual. For example, lymphoma and transplant patients uncommonly are infected with *Salmonella*, but a review of all *Salmonella* infections at Roswell Park Memorial Institute demonstrated that about one-half of those bacteremias occurred in patients who presumably had some form of cellular immune deficiency (e.g., lymphoma); the others had tumors with an anatomic effect on the colon.[10]

The intensity of immunosuppressive therapy that is continued for a prolonged period has a direct bearing on the frequency of infection. An excellent example was the demonstration of varying frequencies of *P. carinii* infection in children with acute lymphocytic leukemia randomly allocated to one of four remission maintenance regimens.[11] Group A received methotrexate alone; group B, methotrexate plus 6-mercaptopurine; group C, methotrexate, 6-mercaptopurine plus cyclophosphamide; and group D, the three drugs plus cytosine arabinoside. A final group (M), those who had presented with large mediastinal masses, received the three drug regimens plus mediastinal radiation. The incidence of infection was as follows:

Maintenance therapy group	A	B	C	D	M
P. carinii infection (%)	5	2	2	22	43
Varicella-zoster infection (%)	10	12	18	19	29

HUMORAL IMMUNE DYSFUNCTION

Patients with agammaglobulinemia have a fairly predictable spectrum of infections related to the fact that they do not have opsonizing antibodies in their serum to the common encapsulated pyogenic bacteria. This impairs the activity of all phagocytic cells including granulocytes, monocytes, and macrophages. Multiple myeloma is the prototype malignancy for demonstrating the infections associated with humoral immune deficiency.[12] The patient with multiple myeloma may or may not fit into such a category, depending on whether the disease had led to reduction of the specific opsonizing antibodies needed to defend against infection caused by the encapsulated pathogens, such as *Streptococcus pneumoniae* and *Haemophilus influenzae*. As a result, some patients with multiple myeloma will have no infections with *S. pneumoniae*, whereas others will have multiple recurrent episodes of pneumococcal infections caused by the same or different serotypes. It is apparent, however, from a number of studies attempting to discern the pattern of immunodeficiency in patients with myeloma that, rather than a generalized suppression of host immunity, only the humoral response is consistently and markedly suppressed. Polyclonal immunoglobulins (IgM, IgG, and IgA) are suppressed in most myeloma patients, and the level of immunosuppression appears to progress with the severity of the disease. Patients with chronic lymphocytic leukemia are often hypogammaglobulinemic and, as a result, also suffer from infections by encapsulated bacteria.

SPLENECTOMY

Infections following splenectomy are usually due to *S. pneumoniae* and, occasionally, to *H. influenzae* or *Neisseria meningitidis*; the aptly named "overwhelming pneumococcal sepsis syndrome" is much more common in splenectomized children and is relatively rare in adults, including those with lymphomas who have had staging laparotomies with splenectomy.[13] Nevertheless, it is a real phenomenon in adults and can be a devastating, often rapidly fatal infection when it does occur.

The spleen has at least two major anti-infective roles: clearing the blood stream of bacteria through its mononuclear–phagocyte function and the production of antibody. Although the liver is very efficient at removing opsonized bacteria, the spleen, through its ability to sequester particles, is more efficient in removing nonopsonized bacteria. Thus the spleen is of critical importance in the individual confronted with infection by a serotype of pneumococci to which he/she has had no prior contact and is nonimmune.

Splenectomized children have a high frequency of bacteremia due to *S. pneumoniae, H. influenzae*, and, occasionally, *N. meningitidis*. An adult, splenectomized following blunt trauma, but otherwise healthy, also is at risk for the overwhelming pneumococcal sepsis syndrome, albeit at a much lower incidence. Presumably, this lower incidence relates to the adult's prior contact with most strains of the encapsulated bacteria and hence his immune status, which allows the rest of the mononuclear–phagocytic system to be effective.

Recognition that adults as well as children are at increased risk of infection years after splenectomy has led to consideration of spleen-sparing surgical approaches after trauma. An animal model using an intravenous *S. pneumoniae* challenge has demonstrated the value of partial splenic preservation. Controls had a 4 percent mortality, splenectomized rats 63 percent, and a partial splenectomy resulted in 4 percent mortality.[14]

OBSTRUCTIVE PHENOMENA

The adage in pathology "obstruction leads to infection" pertains also the compromised host. For example, bronchogenic carcinoma with partial obstruction of a bronchus may lead to postobstructive pneumonia; partial urethral obstruction secondary to prostatic carcinoma may lead to urinary tract infection; and partial obstruction of the biliary tract secondary to lymphoma may lead to ascending cholangitis. In all these situations, the etiologic agent is usually one or more of the organisms that are colonizing at or near the area of obstruction.

Thus the pneumonia may be caused by pharyngeal flora, the urinary infection may be caused by colonic flora, and the cholangitis will be caused by intestinal flora. Recall, however, that the normal resident flora in seriously ill individuals will have changed (see below).

CENTRAL NERVOUS SYSTEM DYSFUNCTION

There will be some degree of aspiration with resultant potential for pneumonia in any situation in which there is complete or partial loss of the gag reflex. Similarly, neurologic dysfunction can lead to impaired micturition, with residual retained urine and resultant urinary tract infection. These situations can be caused by a primary central nervous system (CNS) tumor, metastatic tumor, or meningeal involvement by tumor in addition to metabolic, embolic, or hemorrhagic causes. Patients with brain tumors frequently receive very high doses of corticosteroids for prolonged periods, yet they have remarkably few infections of the type associated with cellular immune dysfunction. Meningitis, encephalitis, and brain abscess are uncommon unless related to problems of surgery.

MEDICAL PROCEDURES

Some of the most important factors that predispose to infection in the compromised host are those initiated by the health care team themselves. Integumentary and mucosal barriers to infection, provided by the intact skin, alimentary tract mucosa, and respiratory mucosa make up the host's primary defenses against organism invasion. The patient with multiple trauma or the patient with acute leukemia undergoing induction chemotherapy are examples that epitomize the surgical and medical patient in whom damage to anatomic barriers is an important predisposing factor to infection. Physical barriers in these and other compromised patients can be disrupted or bypassed completely in a variety of ways. These include indwelling urinary and venous catheters, contaminated intravenous infusion equipment, and trauma to the patient's integument by venipuncture, bone marrow aspiration, or damage to mucosa by endoscopy. The mucosal damage and ciliary dysfunction, as well as the induction of granulocytopenia or cellular immune deficiency by drug therapy, must be considered iatrogenic.

Surgery, especially when extensive, can result in anatomic barrier breaks and extravasation of material either already containing bacterial flora or supportive of organism growth. Surgical removal of the spleen can result in further immunologic defects (see above). Therapeutic irradiation, especially of lymph node areas, can depress cell-mediated immunity and antibody production. Postirradiation tissue damage of the respiratory, gastrointestinal, or urinary tracts can predispose to secondary infections. Total body irradiation predictably results in substantial depression of cellular immune function for months to years.

Implanted Vascular Catheters

The past decade has witnessed the introduction and widespread use of implanted vascular catheters. Although many types are marketed, the most commonly utilized is the Hickman or similar catheter. This catheter, which may be single-, double-, or triple-lumened, has many advantages for patient, doctor, and nurse (Fig. 2). It avoids the need for venipunctures for blood sampling, it allows for continuous infusion of chemotherapeutic agents or antibiotics when pharmacokinetic principles so dictate, it allows sclerosing agents to be deposited into large vessels with high flow, thus protecting peripheral veins, and it permits easy access for blood products, antibiotics, and other supportive medications. These catheters are not without risk, however, and the major risk is infection[15] (see Chapter 291).

Three separate infection types occur: exit site infection, tunnel infection, and catheter-related bacteremia/fungemia. Over the past 10 years at the University of Maryland Cancer Center (UMCC), 690 Hickman catheters were placed in 593 patients. This experience includes 160 separate exit site infections mostly occurring during episodes of neutropenia and usually caused by *Staphylococcus epidermidis* or *S. aureus*. Treatment for all exit site infections included antibiotics, usually vancomycin, with only 10 of 160 infections requiring catheter removal for management. Forty-six tunnel infections occurred, and, despite appropriate antibiotic therapy, 24 required catheter removal for infection control. Finally, these patients had numerous bacteremias from multiple sources, only a minority apparently arising from the catheter. The majority of presumed catheter-associated bacteremias, usually *S. epidermidis*, were treated effectively with vancomycin or other antimicrobials without catheter removal. Exceptions were *Bacillus* bacteremias and *Candida* fungemias. Examination of catheters by scanning electron microscopy demonstrates that most will develop a biofilm along the inner lumenal wall within about 1 month of placement. Gram-positive cocci will be found embedded in this glycocalyx (Fig. 3).[16]

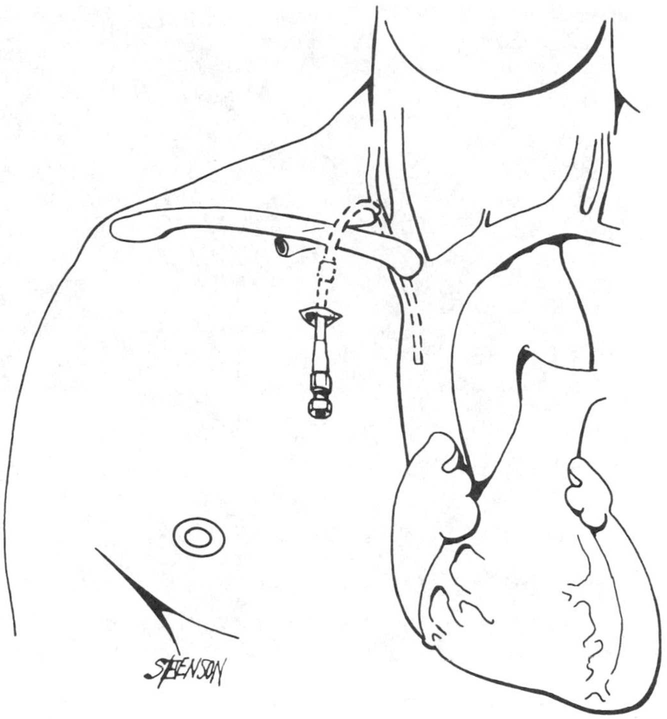

FIG 2. Hickman catheter showing placement through the jugular vein. (From Schimpff,[30] with permission.)

ALTERATIONS IN MICROBIAL FLORA/ ACQUISITION OF NEW ORGANISMS

Disease and the general debilitation that occurs as a consequence of any severe or chronic illness is likely to perturb indigenous flora. Shifts in normal oropharyngeal flora toward gram-negative aerobes have been documented with increasing severity of illness.[17] Similar changes in microbial flora have also been observed with chronic alcoholism and diabetes mellitus. The pathophysiology of this change in binding by the epithelial cell surface is not entirely clear but may be related to alterations in fibronectin content at the cell surface and its propensity to assist binding by gram-positives as opposed to aerobic gram-negative rods.[18]

Stasis, another important factor in the regulation of microbial populations, and medical procedures (in predisposing to infection by alteration in microbial flora) have been referred to

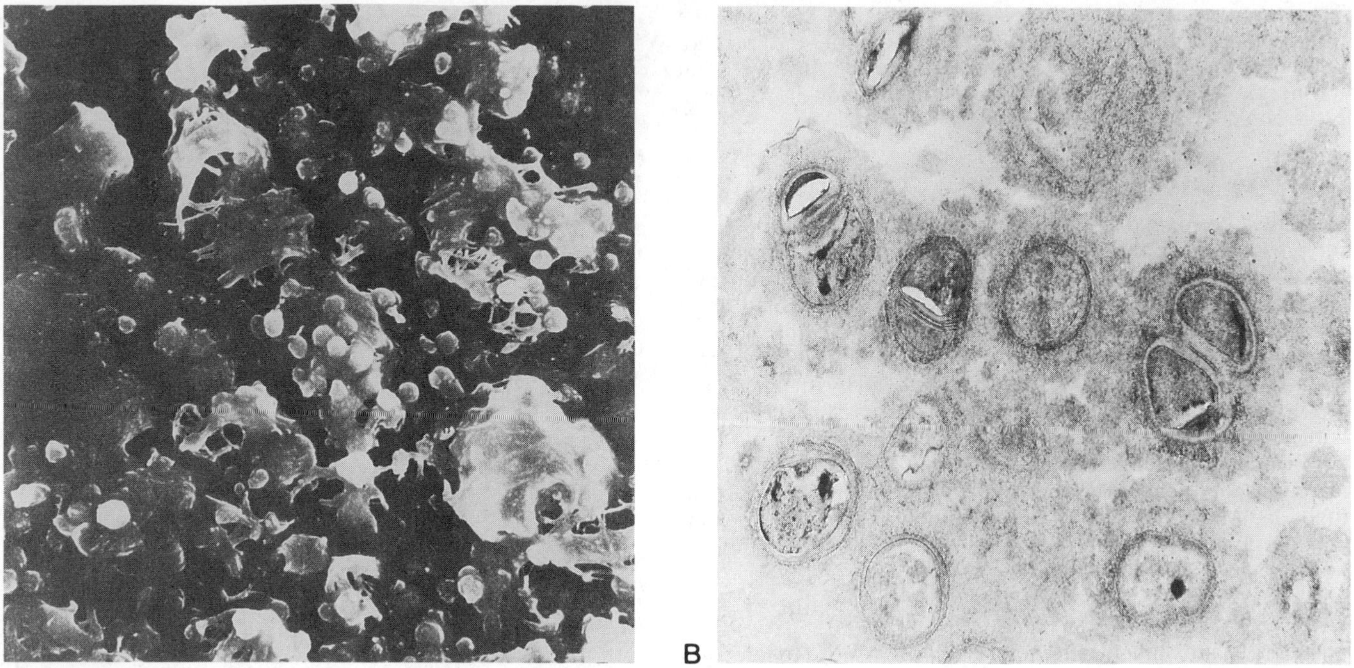

A B

FIG. 3. **(A),** Scanning electron microscope image of biofilm (bacteria and glycocalyx) on lumenal surface of segment of Hickman catheter. **(B)** Transmission electron micrograph of section of preparation of material scraped from surface of Hickman catheter demonstrating gram-positive cocci and glycocalyx. (Fig. A from Tenney et al.,[16] with permission.)

above. Of all exogenous influences, however, antimicrobial agents have the most dramatic effect on indigenous flora and cause both rapid and radical changes. Broad-spectrum antibiotics can suppress the noninvasive and potentially beneficial normal flora that provide a degree of protection against colonization and hence infection by more pathogenic microorganisms. Suppression of alimentary canal anaerobes reduces this means of endogenous microbial protection, termed colonization resistance.

The compromised host may spend substantial time in the hospital or clinic and, as a result, has an opportunity to acquire potential pathogens from this environment.[19] The organisms colonizing a patient at the time of infection may, however, have been acquired only subsequent to patient admission. This is of considerable importance because the organisms that a patient is likely to acquire in the hospital are more likely to be resistant to various therapeutically useful antibiotics and may be acquired in a manner that is particularly conducive to infection (bacteremia from intravenous catheters, hepatitis associated with blood products, pneumonia due to organisms transported to the lung via respirators). Potentially invasive diagnostic procedures, such as endoscopy, barium enema, sigmoidoscopy, and genitourinary tract manipulation, can either introduce potential pathogens from the hospital environment, which can then colonize and result in local infection, or can induce or encourage transient bacteremia by pathogens already colonizing patients.

Table 2 reviews the infections in a group of 48 patients with acute nonlymphocytic leukemia.[2] Seventy-five of 87 microbiologically documented infections were shown by surveillance cultures to have been caused by organisms that were colonizing the patients before the onset of infection. The nose, gingiva, axilla, and rectum were cultured upon admission and twice weekly thereafter throughout hospitalization. Infection nearly always occurred at the time of granulocytopenia, the infecting organism being the one colonizing the patient at or near the site where infection ultimately developed. Nearly one-half of these 75 pathogens had been acquired by the patient subsequent to admission to the hospital. Some of these organisms, such as *P. aeruginosa*, had a very high propensity to cause a subsequent infection in the presence of granulocytopenia, whereas others, such as the other species of *Pseudomonas, Proteus* sp., and

TABLE 2. Potential Pathogens: Acquisition and Subsequent Infections

	Baseline[a]		*Acquired*[a]	
	Patients Colonized	*Subsequent Bacteremia*[b]	*Patients Colonized*	*Subsequent Bacteremia*[b]
Pseudomonas aeruginosa	9	3	22	13
Pseudomonas sp. (non-*aeruginosa*)	4	0	25	0
Enterobacter cloacae	11	0	22	0
Klebsiella sp.	25	4	17	2
Serratia sp.	5	2	4	1
Proteus sp.	29	0	12	0
Citrobacter sp.	7	0	16	0
Haemophilus sp.	20	0	22	0
Candida albicans	21	1	18	1
Total all potential pathogens[c]	265	17	285	22

[a] Baseline organisms were those colonizing the patient at the time of admission as detected by two sets of surveillance cultures from nose, gingiva, axilla, and rectum. Acquired organisms were those first detected by subsequent surveillance cultures taken twice weekly during hospitalization.
[b] Bacteremia is defined as one or more positive blood cultures in association with definitive signs and symptoms of infection.
[c] Total potential pathogens greater than sum of data presented due to occurrence of less common organisms, which were not listed.
(Modified from Schimpff et al.,[2] with permission.)

Citrobacter sp., had relatively little virulence for this patient population despite their acquisition and colonization by these granulocytopenic, mucosally damaged patients. These observations demonstrate that even in this high-risk group, some colonizing organisms are more likely to proceed to infection than others. The biologic nature of this variation in virulence is not known.

There is considerable controversy as to whether "routine" surveillance cultures are helpful to the clinician in day-to-day care of neutropenic patients. The author's view is that they can be helpful to alert one to the presence or absence of *S. aureus* in the nares, *Aspergillus* in the nares, resistant gram-negative rods in the throat or anorectum, heavy colonization by *Candida* in the throat or anorectum, or heavy colonization of *S. epidermidis* or resistant *Corynebacterium* in nares, throat, or rectum.[20–22]

Animal models have demonstrated that bacteria can cross the intact intestinal mucosa, proceed to regional lymph nodes, and reach the blood stream if the normal balance of the microbial flora is severely altered.[23] For example, suppression of the anaerobic flora will allow *P. aeruginosa* to translocate in a rat or mouse model. Translocation can also occur in an immunosuppressed animal. This process suggests that microbial alterations in the intestinal tract in the presence of granulocytopenia could readily lead to *P. aeruginosa* (or other) translocation with progression to overwhelming bacteremia in the absence of detectable mucosal alterations. This may explain some cases of bacteremia of unknown origin in these patients.

SPECIFIC COMPROMISED HOSTS

Cancer

Acute Leukemia. Acute leukemia is dealt with in detail in Chapter 287. For purposes of this introductory chapter, the following concepts are offered. Infection relates to the predisposing factors and hence the astute clinician will pay close attention to the time course of the disease and its therapy, recognizing the implications of the length and depth of granulocytopenia, the shifts of microbial flora due to the disease and antimicrobial therapy (or prophylaxis), the presence and time in use of vascular catheters (e.g., Hickman), and the environmental situation (known reservoirs of *P. aeruginosa, Aspergillus flavus, Legionella pneumophilia*).

One must be very cautious in interpreting the literature to be certain that a specific recommendation fits the patient population and time course with which one is dealing. All episodes of neutropenia are not the same. The initial remission induction period is a time of intense granulocytopenia lasting about 2–3 weeks. Infections in this period are usually caused by gram-negative (especially *Escherichia coli, P. aeruginosa*, and *Klebsiella pneumoniae*) and gram-positive (especially *S. epidermidis* and *S. aureus*) aerobes that have colonized (over 50 percent acquired in the hospital) and invaded along the alimentary canal at points of mucosal disruption or at sites of skin damage (bone marrow aspiration) or in association with vascular access catheters. The patient who requires a second course of chemotherapy is at risk for the same infections but has now been exposed to the hospital environment for a longer period, has probably received many days of broad-spectrum antibiotics, has a resident flora that has probably shifted substantially toward more resistant gram-negative rods, heavy colonization with *Candida*, possible colonization with environmental contaminants such as *Aspergillus*, and may have reactivation of latent viruses such as herpes simplex and CMV.

The clinician needs to take these and other factors into consideration in planning diagnostic and treatment modalities.

Myeloma. This disease leads to both a decrease in synthesis and an increase in catabolism of normal immunoglobulins, leading to an absolute decrease in antibodies against the encapsulated pyogenic bacteria. The degree of immune suppression increases as the tumor burden increases, apparently as an exaggerated expression of natural control mechanism due to suppression of the remaining normal B-lymphocyte and plasma cells by suppressor macrophages. In addition, myeloma patients generally are deficient in functional complement activity. These patients may also demonstrate some cellular immune impairment, e.g., limited response to dinitrofluorobenzene, and granulocyte function (in vitro adherence, in vivo migration) may be impaired, especially in advanced disease.

Infections in myeloma patients, in the absence of chemotherapy, are caused largely by *S. pneumoniae*, consistent with the reduction of both normal opsonizing circulating antibody and the complement deficiency. Other causes of infection include *H. influenzae, N. meningitidis*, and *E. coli*, organisms for which host resistance depends upon complement and, for the first two, circulating antibody.

With disease progression, the bone marrow is unable to produce adequate numbers of granulocytes, with consequent increased prevalence of gram-negative infection. Similarly, as the chemotherapy of myeloma has become more aggressive, granulocytopenia-associated infections (i.e., gram-negative bacteremia, candidiasis, aspergillosis) have become more common. Infections characteristically associated with cellular immune dysfunction are not common.[12]

Chronic Lymphocytic Leukemia. The principle predisposing factor to infection is hypogammaglobulinemia. Many patients have normal serum levels of immunoglobulin at presentation but over time or with advanced stages, the serum IgG level usually is below the normal range and, unlike multiple myeloma, does not tend to revert following chemotherapy.

The vast majority of infections in chronic lymphocytic leukemia are caused by bacterial invasion of the upper and lower respiratory tract (sinusitis, otitis, pneumonia), skin, and urinary tract. As in other hypogammaglobulinemia states, *S. pneumoniae*, the other encapsulated pyogenic bacteria, and *E. coli* predominate. Intravenous immunoglobulin should theoretically reduce the incidence of these infections; reports of ongoing prospective studies are not yet available.[24]

Patients with advanced disease may require splenectomy, which further exacerbates the potential for severe pneumococcal infection.

Hairy Cell Leukemia. This rare lymphoproliferative malignancy of B-cell origin leads to infection due to monocytopenia, granulocytopenia, impaired monocyte function, and defective T-cell function.

Gram-negative infections, especially *P. aeruginosa* bacteremia, are common in association with granulocytopenia. Splenectomy, the therapy of choice until recently, often improves granulocyte levels sufficiently to negate this risk, although splenectomy creates its own infection predisposition. The cellular immune and monocyte defects predispose to opportunists, including occasional herpes simplex, cytomegalovirus, *Candida, Pneumocystis, Salmonella, Listeria*, and *Cryptococcus* infections. More common is infection with *M. kansasii* or *M. avium/M. intracellulare*, occasionally localized to lymph nodes or lungs but usually widely disseminated.[25]

α-Interferon has been found to produce dramatic and long-lasting remissions of hairy cell leukemia and is now the treatment of choice. Granulocytopenia and monocytopenia resolve, with consequent reduction of infectious risk.[26]

Brain Tumors. Whether primary or metastatic, the patient with a brain tumor develops infections that result from the neurologic impairments that alter host defenses. Aspiration pneumonia (loss of gag reflex), urinary tract infections (impaired micturition), and decubitus infections (impaired mobility) are particularly common. Infections of the CNS (meningitis, encephalitis, brain abscess) are uncommon.

SEVERE TRAUMA

Outside of wartime combat, the most common cause of severe trauma is vehicular accidents, often involving young adults. These represent individuals who were, in general, healthy hosts (apart from the effects of substance abuse, especially alcohol) who suddenly became compromised. The experience of the Shock Trauma Center at the University of Maryland is a cross-sectional example of the infections that occur in these patients and the factors that predispose to these infections.[27,28]

The paramedic on the scene determines the level of trauma and, if sufficiently severe, orders helicopter transportation to the Shock Trauma Center. The key to survival is arrival within less than 1 hour of injury. Patients tend to have multiple sites of trauma, including head, chest, abdomen, and extremities. Initial steps are to assure respiratory support with intubation and use of a volume-controlled respirator, placement of two long venous access lines, an arterial line for monitoring purposes, and a urinary catheter. The second step is to deal with emergent CNS trauma such as skull fracture, often with placement of a CNS ventricular pressure monitor. Third is further correction of cardiopulmonary status such as evacuation of hemo- or pneumothorax or flail chest. Fourth is attention to abdominal trauma, especially splenic rupture, and, fifth, initial attention to extremity trauma. This involves multiple surgical teams working at once under less than ideal aseptic conditions. The obvious result is an individual at high risk for infection due to the trauma itself (e.g., damage to anatomic barriers, forced entry of dirt and debris at the sites of trauma, hematomas), and to the myriad of foreign bodies inserted. Not surprisingly, infection occurs at a limited number of sites, all related to the trauma and its therapy.

Recognition of the site of infection is difficult for the inexperienced clinician. It is difficult to examine these patients in the usual thorough manner because of all of the equipment and devices in and about the patient, the inability to turn the patient for better examination, and, frequently, the inability to move the patient for certain types of diagnostic evaluation such as imaging. Fever and leukocytosis are almost universal in these patients because of blood in the retroperitoneal space, transient atelectasis, acute inflammation, or a reaction to medications or blood products. High doses of corticosteroids are often used for brain-injured patients, and this may have an effect on the febrile response. This combination of difficulty in examining the patient in association with the frequent presence of both fever and leukocytosis makes for difficult clinical decision-making and tends to prompt overuse of broad-spectrum antibiotics. However, injudicious use of antibiotics can be very much to the patient's disadvantage because of the further shifting of the microbial flora in an individual with major damage to body barriers to microbes in a setting where hospital acquisition of further potential pathogens is enormous.

Table 3 indicates the distribution of infections occurring in 10,308 multiply traumatized patients at the Shock Trauma Center. Respiratory tract infections, including pneumonia and empyema, made up 22 percent of the infections, followed by urinary tract (17 percent), vascular (14 percent), surgical wound (12 percent), and primary bacteremia (8 percent). Specific comments follow:

TABLE 3. Distribution of Infections Occurring in 10,308 Multiply Traumatized Patients

Site or Type of Infection	*Number*	*Percent*
Primary bacteremia	196	8
Vascular		
Phlebitis	262	11
Arterial line	59	3
Sinusitis	168	7
Lower respiratory		
Pneumonia	336	15
Empyema	172	7
Urinary tract	387	17
Central nervous system	95	4
Intra-abdominal	205	9
Surgical wound	267	12
Other	163	7
Total	2310	100

Pneumonia

Pneumonia is the most serious infection in these patients. Physical examination of the chest is frequently deceptive, so that a portable upright chest x-ray film should be done daily. Pneumonia can then be diagnosed by a combination of the usual signs and symptoms of infection and the presence of a new pulmonary infiltrate in association with a Gram stain of tracheal secretions that demonstrates both many polymorphonuclear leukocytes and many microbes of an apparent single morphologic type. It is important to note that atelectasis is common in these patients, and so before a diagnosis of pneumonia is made, even with all of the criteria noted above, one should first pursue aggressive physical therapy with repeat x-ray films in 3–6 hours. Infiltrates, if approached aggressively, will often resolve rapidly, with reduction in fever and change in tracheal secretions in the absence of antibiotics. This suggests that these cases represent atelectasis and not pneumonia.

In this group, most patients with pneumonia had an associated chest trauma and most had been on respirators at the time pneumonia developed. Nearly all deaths secondary to pneumonia were pneumonias caused by gram-negative rods, especially *P. aeruginosa*. Very few of the patients with a gram-positive coccal pneumonia had received prior antibiotics, whereas the majority of the gram-negative rod pneumonias occurred following use of broad-spectrum antibiotics.

Thoracic empyema is nearly as common as pneumonia, probably due to barotrauma with contamination of the pleural space with upper respiratory organisms that proceed to cause infection. The typical patient is one who has had a pneumothorax resolve with the use of a chest tube with development of otherwise unexplained pleural effusion a few days after chest tube removal. Examination of pleural fluid will show frank empyema with growth of upper airway microbes. Treatment includes both drainage and antibiotics.

Urinary Tract Infections

Urinary infections are very common because of the nearly universal use of urinary catheters. The approaches described elsewhere in this text should be utilized similarly for these patients. Interestingly, despite the frequency of urinary tract infection, the urinary tract is an uncommon source of bacteremia in the multitraumatized patient. That is, the urinary tract itself is usually not traumatized, and hence the risk of bacteremia from bladder catheterization is only modestly greater in these patients than in any patient who is catheterized.

Vascular Catheter-Associated Infection

It is frequently impossible to change indwelling vascular catheters, so that one must be highly attentive to careful monitoring for this complication (see Chapter 279).

Primary Bacteremia

Primary bacteremia (two positive blood cultures with systemic signs of infection from which the same organism is not isolated from any apparent site) in this patient population accounted for about 8 percent of infections. Nearly all were caused by *S. aureus* or a gram-negative rod, particularly *Klebsiella*. *Candida* has been an exceptionally infrequent isolate despite frequent use of parenteral hyperalimentation. It is believed that most of these primary bacteremias are related to intravascular lines, which, in turn, is consistent with the frequency of *S. aureus* and *Klebsiella* as agents. The best preventive measure is frequent changing of lines, limitation of unnecessary use of broad-spectrum antibiotics, and meticulous attention to protocols for hyperalimentation.

CNS Infection

CNS infection represented 4 percent of the infections. Brain abscesses, meningitis, and intraventricular catheter-related infection were most common. One should consider CNS infection following penetrating injury of the CNS (brain abscess), as a complication of lung abscess (brain abscess), meningitis (secondary to staphylococcal bacteremia), or intraventricular pressure monitoring device. The risk of infection due to the latter cause increases substantially if the monitoring devise is in place for more than 4 days. It is of note that the risk of infection should be low in open CNS injury. Prophylactic antibiotics have not been demonstrated to be efficacious in this setting; rather, meticulous surgical technique to removal all foreign and devitalized tissue is critical.

Sinusitis

Although sinusitis accounted for only 7 percent of all infections, its cryptic nature of presenting with fever and leukocytosis but with few other signs or symptoms makes it worth notation. Patients with nosocomial sinusitis are frequently unconscious, paralyzed, have a nasal tube in place (nasogastric or nasotracheal), and may be receiving corticosteroids. Purulent nasal discharge occurs in less than one-half of these patients. Diagnosis requires a portable x-ray film of the paranasal sinuses. The nasal tube must be removed and antibiotics are instituted based upon examination of a gram-stained sinus aspirate.[29]

Surgical Wound Infections

Infections that manifest within the first 24 hours may be due to β-hemolytic streptococci or *Clostridium* species, are unusually fulminant, and must be identified and treated aggressively. The more common infections, usually *S. aureus*, are those that occur more than 48 hours after surgery. Although gram-negative rods are not frequent, a Gram stain of the purulent material should be examined as a guide to instituting appropriate antibiotics in addition to the necessary surgical management.

REFERENCES

1. Bodey GP, Buckley M, Sathe YS, et al. Quantitive relationships between circulating leukocytes and infection in patients with acute leukemia. Ann Intern Med. 1966;64:328–40.
2. Schimpff SC, Young VM, Greene WH, et al. Origin of infection in acute nonlymphocytic leukemia; significance of hospital acquisition of potential pathogens. Ann Intern Med. 1972;77:707–14.
3. Sickles EA, Greene WH, Wiernik PH. Clinical presentation of infection in granulocytopenic patients. Arch Intern Med. 1975;135:715–9.
4. Ramsey PG, Rubin RM, Tolkoff-Rubin NE, et al. The renal transplant patient with fever and pulmonary infiltrates; etiology, clinical manifestations and management. Medicine (Baltimore). 1980;59:206–22.
5. Rubin RH, Wolfson JS, Cosimi AB, et al. Infection in the renal transplant recipient. Am J Med. 1981;70:405–11.
6. Hughes WT, Townsend TR. Nosocomial infections in immunocompromised children. Am J Med. 1981;70:412.
7. Winston DJ, Gale RP, Meyer DV, et al. Infectious complications of human bone marrow transplantation. Medicine (Baltimore). 1979;58:1–31.
8. Johnston RB. Monocytes and macrophages. N Engl J Med. 1988; 318:747–52.
9. Murray HW. Interferon-gamma, the activated macrophage, and host defense against microbial challenge. Ann Intern Med. 1988;108:595–608.
10. Han T, Sokal JE, Neter E. Salmonellosis in disseminated malignant diseases—a seven year review (1959–1965). N Engl J Med. 1967;276:1045–52.
11. Hughes WT, Feldman S, Aur RJA, et al. Intensity of immunosuppressive therapy and the incidence of *Pneumocystis carinii* pneumonitis. Cancer. 1975;36;2004–9.
12. Jacobson DR, Zolla-Prazner S. Immunosuppression and infection in multiple myeloma. Semin Oncol 1986;13:282–90.
13. Gopal V, Bisno AL. Fulminant pneumococcal infections in "normal" asplenic hosts. Arch Intern Med. 1977;137:1526–30.
14. Steely WM, Satava RM, Harris RW, et al. Comparison of omental splenic autotransplant to partial splenectomy. Am J Med. 1987;12:702–5.
15. Reed WP, Newman KA, de Jongh CA, et al. Prolonged venous access for chemotherapy by means of the Hickman catheter. Cancer. 1983;52:185–92.
16. Tenney JH, Moody MR, Newman KA, et al. Adherent microorganisms on lumenal surfaces of long-term intravenous catheters. Importance of *Staphylococcus epidermidis* in patients with cancer. Arch Intern Med. 1986;146:1949–54.
17. Johanson WG, Pierce AK, Sanford JP. Changing pharyngeal bacterial flora of hospitalized patients. Emergence of gram-negative bacilli. N Engl J Med. 1969;281:1137–40.
18. Proctor RA. Fibronectin: a brief overview of its structure, functiona, and physiology. Rev Infect Dis. 1987;9:S317–21.
19. Young LS. Nosocomial infections in the immunocompromised adult. Am J Med. 1981;70:394.
20. Schimpff SC. Surveillance cultures. J Infect Dis. 1981;144:81–4.
21. Newman KA, Schimpff SC, Young VM, et al. Lessons learned from surveillance cultures from patients with acute nonlymphocytic leukemia: usefulness for epidemiologic, preventive and therapeutic research. Am J Med. 1981;70:423–31.
22. Wells CL, Ferrieri P, Weisdorf DJ, et al. The importance of surveillance stool cultures during periods of severe neutropenia. Infect Control. 1987;8:317–9.
23. Deitch EA, Winterton J, Berg R. Effect of starvation, malnutrition, and trauma on the gastrointestinal tract flora and bacterial translocation. Arch Surg. 1987;122:1019–24.
24. Chapel HM, Bunch C. Mechanisms of infection in chronic lymphocytic leukemia. Semin Hematol. 1987;24:291–6.
25. Bennett C, Vardiman J, Golomb H. Disseminated atypical mycobacterial infection in patients with hairy cell leukemia. Am J Med. 1986;80:891–6.
26. Ratain MJ, Golomb HM, Vardiman JW, et al. Treatment of hairy cell leukemia with recombinant $alpha_2$ interferon. Blood. 1985;65:644–8.
27. Schimpff SC, Miller RM, Polakavetz S, et al. Infection in the severely traumatized patient. Ann Surg. 1974;179:352–7.
28. Stillwell M, Caplan ES. The septic multiple-trauma patient. Crit Care Clin. 1988;4:345–73.
29. Grindlinger GA, Niehoff J, Hughes SL, et al. Acute paranasal sinusitis related to nasotracheal intubation of head-injured patients. Crit Care Med. 1987;15:217.
30. Schimpff SC. Infection in the leukemia patient: diagnosis, therapy, and prevention. In: Henderson ES, ed. Leukemia, 5th ed. New York: Grune & Stratton; in press.

287. INFECTIONS IN PATIENTS WITH ACUTE LEUKEMIA AND LYMPHOMA

FRANÇOISE MEUNIER

Infections remain of major concern in the management of patients with hematologic malignancies. These complications are frequent, potentially life-threatening, and particularly worrisome, since the prognosis for patients with acute leukemia and lymphoma has improved significantly over the last decade. The better outcome of these patients is mainly due to more aggressive antineoplastic chemotherapy including procedures such as bone marrow transplantation. These intensive treatments induce severe alterations in various host defense mechanisms and therefore lead to an increased risk of infection. Tremendous progress has been achieved in the control of other major complications (such as hemorrhage), as well as in supportive care, resulting in an improved quality of life and even reproductive capacity for these immunocompromised hosts.[1,2]

Overall, the prognosis for patients with acute leukemia varies according to the age of the patient and the type of leukemia. Acute lymphoblastic leukemia (ALL) accounts for approximately 15 percent of acute leukemia in adults, and using currently available antineoplastic therapeutic approaches, a cure rate of 50 percent is expected.[3] In contrast to adults, ALL is the most common leukemia in children and has a cure rate as high as 60 percent.[1] Acute nonlymphocytic leukemia (ANLL) is more difficult to treat. The median duration of remission generally ranges from 1 to 2 years, with 5-years disease-free survival rates of 10–25 percent in adults and up to 45 percent in children.[4] The outcome of patients with other hematologic malignancies has also changed dramatically over the last decade. In Hodgkin's disease, over 70 percent of patients are cured, as well as 50–60 percent of those with lymphomas.[5] However, one of the major drawbacks of intensive and aggressive antineoplastic regimens is the increased risk of infections. The types of infections and the offending pathogens have been well characterized and are often predictable because they are related to various predisposing factors, such as granulocytopenia, defects in cell-mediated immunity, splenectomy, breaks in the mucocutaneous membranes (body barriers), or other deficits in host defense mechanisms. During the last decade, intensive antineoplastic chemotherapy has been administered not only to patients with acute leukemia but also to those with lymphoma or Hodgkin's disease. The various sites of infection, the organisms encountered, and current clinical approaches to diagnosis and therapy will be reviewed separately for patients with granulocytopenia and those with defects in cell-mediated immunity. Prevention and empiric therapy are discussed in Chapter 293.

INFECTIONS IN GRANULOCYTOPENIC PATIENTS

The incidence of infections is directly related to the granulocyte count.[6,7] Patients with fewer than 1000 polymorphonuclear cells/mm^3 are considered at risk. However, several studies have shown that there is a particular subgroup of patients with an increased risk of life-threatening complications (i.e., those with fewer than 500 polymorphonuclear neutrophils/mm^3). For those patients who have extremely low granulocyte counts (<100/mm^3) for prolonged periods of time, rapidly fatal infectious complications (mainly septicemia caused by gram-negative bacilli) have been well documented and account for 10–20 percent of febrile episodes.[8,9] Therefore, close medical surveillance is essential. Rapid initiation of empiric antimicrobial therapy at the onset of fever is mandatory and should occur within 60 minutes of the first signs or symptoms of infection.[10] This systematic approach has been shown to decrease the mortality due to septicemia caused by gram-negative bacilli.[11,12] The common microorganisms encountered in granulocytopenic patients are bacteria and fungi, but viruses and protozoa may also be implicated. The pattern of documented infections has been well described in granulocytopenic patients, the first febrile episode often being due to a bacterial infection, particularly that caused by endogenous pathogens. During prolonged and profound granulocytopenia, fungal infection or superinfection caused by resistant bacteria also occurs. Occasionally, dramatic fungal complications (such as invasive aspergillosis) have been described during the first induction therapy course.

For most febrile episodes observed in granulocytopenic patients, the specific microorganism is difficult to predict at the onset of fever. Despite extensive cultures, only 20 percent of febrile patients have a microbiologically documented infection with septicemia. The other febrile episodes are classified as microbiologically documented infection without septicemia, as clinically documented infection (if a site of infection is present and no pathogen has been isolated), or as possible infection (if no site or microorganism is identified). In addition, febrile episodes related to drugs, to the underlying disease, or to transfusion of blood products are usually classified as doubtful infection.[9,13] These criteria are of major importance in evaluating data from the literature, particularly to compare various therapeutic approaches, considering that the prognosis as well as the final outcome of these patients is dependent upon the severity of infection.[9,13–16]

Infections among 3295 febrile, granulocytopenic patients observed during five consecutive trials of the European Organization for the Research and Treatment of Cancer (EORTC) international antimicrobial therapy cooperative group are listed in Table 1. The common sites of infection identified in these patients are given in Table 2. Tremendous progress has been achieved in the management of infections in granulocytopenic patients. However, the overall survival is dependent mainly upon the recovery of an adequate granulocyte count, as well as remission of the underlying disease.

The Pathogens

Bacteria. The incidence of documented bacterial infections is increased in patients with severe, persistent granulocytopenia. The classic pathogens isolated in these circumstances are gram-negative bacilli. Most observations from large studies evaluating febrile episodes in granulocytopenic patients have stressed the high incidence of life-threatening complications caused by gram-negative bacillary septicemia.[6,8,9,12,16–20] The common pathogens associated with a high mortality rate are Enterobacteriaceae (*Escherichia coli, Klebsiella* species, *Proteus* species) and *Pseudomonas aeruginosa*. The infections usually occurred within the first 2 weeks after the initiation of antineoplastic chemotherapy and are considered a consequence of the rapid decrease in the granulocyte count. However, recently, most investigators have pointed out the decreased incidence of septicemia caused by gram-negative pathogens and a significant increase in documented infections caused by gram-positive cocci, mainly *Staphylococcus epidermidis* and streptococci.[20–25] The percentages of single gram-negative bacteremia and single gram-positive bacteremia documented among

TABLE 1. Documentation of infections in 3295 Febrile Granulocytopenic Patients[a]

Infection	*Percent*
Single-organism, gram-negative bacteremia	13.6
Single-organism, gram-positive bacteremia	10.6
Polymicrobial bacteremia	3
Microbiologically documented infections	11
Clinically documented infections	24.4
Possible infections	32.5
Viral or fungal infections	4.6

[a] Doubtful infection, protocol-inadherent, and nonevaluable patients are excluded.

TABLE 2. Common Sites of Infections Identified in Febrile, Granulocytopenic Patients

Site	*Percent*
Mouth and pharynx	25
Respiratory tract	25
Skin, soft tissue, and intravascular catheters	15
Perineal region	10
Urinary tract	5–10
Nose and sinuses	5
Gastrointestinal tract	5
Others	5–10

3295 febrile granulocytopenic patients during five consecutive trials of the EORTC international antimicrobial therapy cooperative group are reported on Table 3.

The exact reason for this epidemiologic change remains unclear. Several hypotheses have been elaborated. Prompt empiric antimicrobial therapy against gram-negative pathogens may be effective in decreasing the recovery rate of those pathogens from blood cultures; improved prophylaxis using oral absorbable antibiotics that are better tolerated (such as trimethoprim-sulfamethoxazole or the fluoroquinolones) has also been shown effective in reducing the incidence of gram-negative bacillary septicemia in high-risk patients.[26–33] However, the selection of streptococci has been well documented, particularly with the use of the fluoroquinolones. These agents are poorly effective against species such as *Streptococcus pneumoniae* or the viridans group of *Streptococcus*. In addition, most patients treated with an intensive antineoplastic regimen for hematologic malignancy have at least one central venous catheter or another intravascular device (including those for total parenteral nutrition), which may also constitute a source of infection caused mainly by staphylococci. In addition, other potential sources of gram-positive cocci in granulocytopenic patients have also been suggested, including the gastrointestinal tract[34] and the oropharynx. Severe mucositis is more common in patients treated with current antineoplastic regimens. The mouth may also represent an important source of infection caused by gram-positive cocci, particularly streptococci. However, despite the recently documented increased incidence of septicemia caused by gram-positive cocci, the overall mortality related to these complications is much lower than that associated with gram-negative bacillary septicemia.[20] Nevertheless, the optimal management of infections caused by gram-positive cocci remains controversial. In cases of catheter-related septicemia, the removal of the catheter (such as the Hickman, Broviac, or Port-a-Cath catheter) may constitute a problem, particularly for those patients with low platelet counts. In addition, severe complications associated with pulmonary infiltrates have been recently reported in patients with catheter-acquired septicemia caused by gram-positive cocci.

Beside the classic pathogens encountered, other recently identified factors have also been advocated as potential sources for various types of infection caused by less common pathogens in granulocytopenic patients. The selective pressure of systemic antimicrobial agents frequently administered to these patients (mainly third-generation cephalosporins) may be responsible for the frequent recovery of pathogens such as *Corynebacterium* J.K., *Serratia* species, *Enterobacter cloacae, Acinetobacter anitratus, Pseudomonas cepacia,* and *Pseudomonas* (*Xanthomonas*) *maltophilia*. In addition, transfusions of blood products have been reported as the source of septicemia caused by *Pseudomonas fluorescens,*[35] and extended storage of platelets has been associated with gram-positive bacteremia.[36]

Empiric therapy for a febrile episode should always take into account these epidemiologic factors, as well as previous exposure to antimicrobial agents. While the mortality caused by gram-negative bacillary septicemia has been reduced with improved empiric antimicrobial therapy, as well as optimal management of febrile episodes, the morbidity from infections caused by gram-positive cocci should not be underestimated, because these infections are associated with delay in the administration of maintenance or consolidation antineoplastic therapy, as well as prolonged hospitalization. Interestingly enough, infections caused by anaerobes (such as *Clostridium* species) are infrequent in granulocytopenic patients and represent less than 1 percent of the bacteremic isolates.

TABLE 3. Single Gram-Negative Bacteremia (SGNB) and Single Gram-Positive Bacteremia (SGPB) in 3295 Febrile, Granulocytopenic Patients

	Percent with SGNB	*Percent with SGPB*
EORTC Trial I	15.7	5.8
EORTC Trial II	15.7	7.8
EORTC Trial III	12.9	9
EORTC Trial IV	14.5	10.1
EORTC Trial V	10.5	17.7

Fungi. Invasive fungal infections are presently a major cause of morbidity and mortality in granulocytopenic patients, and the incidence of these life-threatening complications is increasing. Numerous reports from cancer centers provide evidence of invasive fungal infections documented by histopathology in 10–40 percent of autopsies of patients with hematologic malignancy.[37–40] Many predisposing factors have been identified, including prolonged hospitalization, previous exposure to antimicrobial agents (which are known to induce changes in the normal flora and favor fungal overgrowth), corticosteroids, invasive procedures requiring central venous catheters and total parenteral nutrition for supportive care, as well as lack of control of the underlying disease. All these conditions enhance fungal colonization, alter host defense mechanisms, and should be recognized as potential sources of fungal complications. Nevertheless, invasive mycoses are usually considered the result of severe, prolonged granulocytopenia. It should be emphasized that polymorphonuclear leukocytes play a major role in controlling infection due to *Candida* and *Aspergillus* species.

The common offending fungal pathogens in granulocytopenic patients are species of *Candida*[41–43] and *Aspergillus*.[44–46] Less frequently, *Torulopsis glabrata,*[47] *agents of mucormycosis,*[48] *Trichosporon,*[49–50] *Fusarium* species,[51] and *Pseudallescheria boydii*[52] have been isolated from granulocytopenic patients. Species of fungi previously considered contaminants have been described in such circumstances and should not be ignored by physicians, particularly for those patients receiving prophylaxis or treatment with various antifungal agents known to favor colonization with unusual fungal organisms. In addition, invasive infections caused by dimorphic fungi (such as disseminated histoplasmosis) have also been described occasionally in granulocytopenic patients. Previous exposure to such pathogens in an endemic area should be taken into consideration.

Candidiasis and aspergillosis usually have a characteristic clinical setting in granulocytopenic patients; however, accurate diagnosis remains extremely difficult to ascertain at the bedside, and invasive fungal infection is still too often an autopsy discovery. Thrombocytopenia may make biopsy a high-risk procedure. Nevertheless, definite histologic proof is mandatory to establish the exact role of yeasts isolated from such sites as sputum, throat, and urine due to the frequent colonization of these patients by yeasts. False-positive and false-negative results are routinely observed in surveillance cultures. The clinical relevance of such cultures remains a matter of controversy, particularly with *Candida albicans*.[47,53–55] Except for positive blood cultures for yeasts, all other positive cultures obtained from sputum, urine, the mouth, and stool should not be considered definite proof of invasive candidiasis. However, approximately 50 percent of patients with autopsy-proven fungal invasion do not have a single positive blood culture premortem.[37,38] Catheter-related fungemia may constitute a separate clinical entity that does not necessarily require prolonged antifungal therapy. Nevertheless, a single positive blood culture for yeasts should not be overlooked, and invasive candidiasis should be suspected in all fungemic, granulocytopenic patients. Specific therapy should always be considered. In contrast to *Candida*, the role of surveillance cultures performed in high-risk patients in order to detect nasal colonization by *Aspergillus* species has been advocated.[56] Moreover, isolation of *Aspergillus* from respiratory secretions or bronchoalveolar lavage in febrile, granulocytopenic patients should suffice to initiate antifungal therapy pending further documentation.[57,58] This approach has improved the prognosis of patients with invasive aspergillosis.[45,59] In addition, thoracic computed tomography (CT) scans have been found to be useful for early recognition of cavitation in lesions of invasive aspergillosis.[60,61]

Complete identification of fungal species isolated in immunocompromised patients should always be obtained. Recent observations have shown that infection caused by the ubiquitous soil saprophyte, *Scopulariopsis*, in patients with leukemia present a clinical picture identical to that of invasive aspergillosis.[62] For some fungal pathogens, including *P. boydii* and *Scopulariopsis,* the optimal antifungal agent may not be amphotericin B.[49,51,62–64]

Today there is no commercially available, reliable test to allow accurate serodiagnosis early in the evolution of the disease by detecting either specific antibodies or circulating fungal antigens or metabolites.[65] Invasive fungal infection should be suspected and empiric antifungal therapy considered for any febrile, granulocytopenic patient remaining microbiologically undocumented and not responding to empiric broad-spectrum antimicrobial therapy.[66–71] This clinical approach has been shown to be beneficial in some patients. It is obvious that not all unresponsive febrile episodes observed in granulocytopenic patients are clearly related to occult fungal infections. However, the patients who seem to be at higher risk are those with prolonged, profound granulocytopenia or with a clinically documented site of infection (esophagitis or pulmonary infiltrate), or those who did not receive previous antifungal prophylaxis.[69]

Viruses. Viral infections are also common in granulocytopenic patients with acute leukemia or lymphoma. Herpesviruses are frequently identified, particularly herpes simplex,[72] varicella-zoster virus,[73] and cytomegalovirus, the last isolated mainly in patients undergoing bone marrow transplantation.[74] Infections caused by adenoviruses have also been reported.[75]

Infections caused by herpes simplex virus are the most frequent viral infections in patients with acute leukemia and lymphoma. Numerous studies have documented the high incidence of isolation of herpes simplex virus in patients receiving antineoplastic chemotherapy, mainly from mouth rinses[76] or in urine. Reactivation of herpes simplex virus infection is often observed in these patients. In particular, severe mucositis is common, resulting in extensive ulcerations of the oral mucosa, which predispose to bacterial and/or fungal colonization as well as invasion. In addition, these lesions are particularly painful and significantly alter the quality of life of these patients. A major complication of herpes simplex infection in granulocytopenic patients is the extension of lesions to the esophagus, with signs and symptoms suggesting *Candida* esophagitis.[77] Accurate diagnosis is often very difficult and requires invasive procedures such as endoscopy to obtain a biopsy specimen for histologic examination and culture. Occasionally, esophagitis may occur without oropharyngeal involvement and without symptoms. Infections caused by herpes simplex virus localized to other sites (genital or perineal areas) have also been described but are less common. Dissemination of herpes simplex virus to visceral organs (liver, spleen, lungs, kidneys) also occurs in granulocytopenic patients[72,78] but is rare. Varicella is a classic opportunistic infection in children with ALL or lymphoma, particularly during antineoplastic chemotherapy.[79–81] Viral hepatitis (including infection caused by hepatitis B virus and non-A, non-B hepatitis) is also a frequent complication in patients with leukemia undergoing remission induction therapy.[82–84]

Parasites and Protozoa. Malaria has been described occasionally in granulocytopenic patients either as reactivated disease or acquired by fresh blood products. Epidemiologic factors including a history of travel or previous symptomatic disease should also be taken into consideration when caring for patients with hematologic malignancies. However, most parasitic and protozoan infections occur in patients with compromised cell-mediated immunity and will be discussed in the next section.

Characteristics of Common Clinical Infections in Granulocytopenic Patients

Septicemia. Blood stream infections are often life-threatening in these patients. In 30 percent of patients, a source of infection is not identified despite positive blood cultures for gram-negative bacilli, gram-positive cocci, or fungi. Occasionally, viremia is documented in febrile, granulocytopenic patients.

It is of major importance to document septicemia because the agent chosen for empiric therapy may be inappropriate. In addition, several studies have demonstrated a lower response rate to empiric antimicrobial therapy for patients with proven septicemia compared to those with clinically documented infection or possible infection. Persistent, profound granulocytopenia is a major prognostic factor.[8,9,16,41,42,85] In particular, the outcome of granulocytopenic patients with gram-negative septicemia or fungemia is uniformly poor unless the granulocyte count is rising and the underlying disease is controlled.

Clinical manifestations of sepsis have been well described,[86] but there are no pathognomonic signs. In a large study evaluating 410 episodes of *Pseudomonas* bacteremia,[87] shock occurred in 33 percent. For most cases of septicemia without an obvious focus of infection, it has been postulated that microorganisms invade and disseminate from the gastrointestinal tract through mucosal ulcerations caused by antineoplastic chemotherapy.

Blood cultures should be obtained for each episode with fever greater than 38.5°C or when infection is suspected on the basis of other clinical findings. Particularly for patients already receiving antimicrobial therapy who have failed to respond due to persisting fever, fungemia should be ruled out using the lysis-centrifugation or comparable blood culture systems[88–90] (see Ch. 13).

While the clinical relevance of a positive blood culture for gram-negative bacilli is not a matter of controversy, the significance of recovery of some gram-positive cocci, particularly by *S. epidermidis,* or *Corynebacterium* JK in blood samples is more difficult to ascertain. Single blood culture isolates of *Staphylococcus aureus, Streptococcus pneumoniae,* and *Enterococcus faecalis* identified in granulocytopenic patients should be considered significant. While viridans streptococci are common contaminants in the general population, a single positive blood culture obtained in patients with severe oral mucositis should probably not be disregarded. For other gram-positive organisms (coagulase negative *Staphylococcus* and *Corynebacterium* JK), the isolation from at least two blood cultures (two sets) drawn on 2 separate days or from two or more cultures drawn on the same day from separate venipunctures appears to be a useful criterion for clinical significance. In addition, a positive blood culture associated with a positive culture from a source other than blood (such as exudate) should also be considered significant.

Pending the results of blood cultures, empiric antibiotics should be administered to all febrile, granulocytopenic patients, using agents with adequate coverage against most gram-negative bacilli (due to the high mortality rate from this complication) as well as against gram-positive cocci. The optimal empiric regimen for this purpose is still controversial[16,24,91–93] and will be discussed in Chapter 293.

Oropharyngeal Infections. Numerous infectious complications of the upper gastrointestinal tract occur during the course of antineoplastic chemotherapy for hematologic malignancy.[94] Severe stomatitis is a common finding in patients receiving intensive therapy; these lesions are painful and impair food intake. In addition, mucosal ulcerations are frequently colonized by the oropharyngeal flora, leading to local invasion as well as dissemination. Gingivostomatitis and periodontal lesions are extremely frequent in patients with acute leukemia,[95] and optimal dental care as well as appropriate hygienic measures should be provided before the initiation of antineoplastic chemotherapy.

The pathogens encountered in granulocytopenic patients with mucositis are numerous and include herpes simplex virus, usually as a result of reactivation; bacteria (gram-negative bacilli, streptococci, and anaerobes); and *Candida* species. Mixed infections also occur. Asymptomatic excretion of herpes simplex virus is frequent and seems to be predictive of clinical signs and symptoms of oropharyngeal infection. Herpes simplex stomatitis is usually more extensive and protracted in granulocytopenic patients than in nonimmunocompromised hosts. Relapses are common.[76,96] Herpetic lesions predispose to fungal or bacterial invasion of the mucosa and are potential sources of bacteremia. Occasionally, unusual pathogens such as *Aerococcus* have been encountered in patients with mucositis.[97]

Oropharyngeal candidiasis is frequent and presents with characteristic clinical and pathologic features in granulocytopenic patients.[98] Various attempts to prevent yeast colonization in the mouth have been less successful than in stool. Extension of oral thrush to the esophagus is common.[99] Autopsy studies have revealed widespread *Candida* esophagitis in asymptomatic patients. At endoscopy, *Candida* esophagitis can be difficult to distinguish from lesions of herpes simplex virus, cytomegalovirus, peptic esophagitis, or bacterial esophagitis.[100–104] Brushings from the lesion should be smeared to look for pseudohyphae. Cultures for fungus are not helpful. At autopsy, disseminated candidiasis may be found with no other obvious portal than esophageal lesions. Considering the insensitivity of blood cultures in detecting disseminated candidiasis in neutropenic patients, the diagnosis of *Candida* esophagitis should raise the question of disseminated candidiasis in febrile, neutropenic patients. Unusual manifestations of candidiasis in the oropharynx include epiglottitis,[105] laryngitis, and cervical lymphadenitis following oral mucositis.[106]

Pulmonary Infections. Clinical signs and symptoms of pulmonary infections are frequently found in granulocytopenic patients, either as a primary focus of infection or as a complication of septicemia. Chest x-ray studies performed early in the evolution of infection usually fail to show significant lung infiltrates. Granulocytopenic patients who present with pulmonary infections caused by such pathogens as gram-negative bacilli (such as *Pseudomonas aeruginosa*), gram-positive cocci (such as *S. aureus* and streptococci), or fungi have a poor prognosis. Adult respiratory distress syndrome can occur in bacteremic patients with granulocytopenia.[107,108]

The outcome of invasive pulmonary aspergillosis appears to be dependent upon prompt diagnosis, an aggressive therapeutic approach, adequate control of the underlying disease, and/or recovery of the granulocyte count.[45,59,61] Pulmonary consolidation with progressive cavitation is highly suggestive of pulmonary aspergillosis, but mucormycosis may cause identical signs.[109] A CT scan has the potential of demonstrating cavitation earlier than conventional x-ray films and is useful in suggesting the diagnosis of aspergillosis or mucormycosis.[60] Although *Aspergillus* is ubiquitous, its isolation from pulmonary secretions or even from surveillance cultures in granulocytopenic patients should not be ignored.[56–58]

Eradication of pulmonary aspergillosis is particularly difficult to achieve, and relapses are frequent in patients with acute leukemia undergoing multiple courses of intensive chemotherapy.[110] The major complication of pulmonary aspergillosis is cerebral abscess.[44,70]

Viral pathogens (mainly cytomegalovirus) have also been identified as causative agents of widespread pulmonary infections, particularly in patients undergoing bone marrow transplantation.

The critical decision faced by the clinician at the bedside of patients with pulmonary infections is whether or not to perform invasive procedures such as fiberoptic bronchoscopy (with or without bronchoalveolar lavage), transbronchial biopsy, transthoracic aspiration, or open lung biopsy. The exact role of such diagnostic approaches for the management of the patient is still controversial[111,112] and depends upon the collaboration and skill of various specialists. In addition, these patients usually have severe thrombocytopenia, which precludes invasive diagnostic procedures. The alternative approach consists of treating these patients empirically. In a study evaluating the causes of initial remission-induction failure in patients with ANLL, 70 percent of all fatal infections were pneumonia, with or without septicemia.[113] However, it should be recognized that pulmonary infiltrates occurring in granulocytopenic patients may have noninfectious causes such as hemorrhage, leukemic infiltrates, emboli, edema, or leukoagglutinin reactions.

Skin, Soft Tissue, and Catheter-Related Infections. Cutaneous signs of infection in granulocytopenic patients are numerous and may be localized or widespread.[114] These manifestations may also represent the primary focus of infection (cellulitis) or may occur as the result of dissemination (septic emboli).

A common localized cutaneous infection in granulocytopenic patients with acute monocytic or myelomonocytic leukemia is perianal cellulitis presenting with painful lesions without abscess formation. A careful examination and history should be obtained in these patients, and antimicrobial therapy should be promptly initiated, since this clinical entity is a potential source of gram-negative bacillary bacteremia. Localized dermatologic manifestations on the face are usually caused by *S. aureus* or by mucormycosis. Facial mucormycosis usually represents an extension from the paranasal sinuses.[115]

In patients with severe herpetic stomatitis, lesions also involve the lips and may spread around the mouth. Extension of genital herpetic lesions to the thighs and perineal area has also been observed in these patients.

In granulocytopenic patients, cutaneous punctures (needle sticks, venipunctures, bone marrow aspiration punctures) and minor abrasions (in the axillae) may result in severe infection caused by staphylococci or *Corynebacterium* JK, as well as by colonizing Enterobacteriaceae or *Ps. aeruginosa*. Minor trauma should be recognized as a potential source of bacteremia.

Ecthyma gangrenosum represents a characteristic entity in patients with *Ps. aeruginosa* septicemia, resulting from hematogenous spread and causing extensive cutaneous necrosis. In a recent review of 410 episodes of *Ps. aeruginosa* bacteremia,[87] these cutaneous manifestations were reported in only 2 percent. Various other pathogens have also been reported as causative agents of similar lesions; aspiration or biopsy should be performed early. Lesions similar to ecthyma gangrenosum have been observed in patients with disseminated candidiasis and mucormycosis.[116,117] Other unusual manifestations (intradermal bullous dermatitis) of invasive candidiasis have been reported in patients with lymphoma.[118] Ecthyma gangrenosum should be distinguished from pyoderma gangrenosum, which is a noninfectious process also occurring in patients with myeloid malignancy.[119] The presence of widespread papules or nodules may be helpful in diagnosing fungemia; myalgias and muscle tenderness have also been reported in patients with disseminated candidiasis.

Life-threatening varicella virus leading to visceral dissemination is a frequent and well-characterized complication, particularly among leukemic children.[73,80,81]

Thrombosis of major blood vessels is a complication of widespread infection caused by *Aspergillus* species, leading occasionally to severe ischemia and necrosis of toe(s) or finger(s).

Intravenous indwelling catheters are another major source of infections in granulocytopenic patients caused mainly by organisms colonizing the skin. Long-term intravascular devices such as Hickman or Broviac catheters are more frequently used in leukemic patients, resulting in a significant number of catheter-related infections, either localized to the site of insertion or disseminated with septicemia. Recognition of these complications is important. Fortunately, such infections do not necessarily require the removal of the catheters.[120,121] This constitutes a major advance because with most infectious diseases occurring in the presence of a foreign material, catheter removal was once considered mandatory. Coagulase-negative staphylococci, as well as *S. aureus,* are the leading cause of catheter-related infection. Other reported pathogens include *Ps. maltophilia, Ps. cepacia, Ps. putida,*[122] *Corynebacterium* JK, *Candida* species and even *Aspergillus* species.[123,124]

Strict criteria should be used to define a catheter-related infection.[125] Recently, the magnitude of bacteremia caused by *S. aureus* evaluated by colony count determination has been reported to be useful for the management of catheter-related infection.[126]

Despite the increased incidence of septicemia caused by *S. epidermidis,* all these cases do not seem to be the result of catheter-related infection.[34,127]

Finally, although the incidence of endocarditis appears to be extremely low in granulocytopenic patients, particularly those with *S. aureus* bacteremia,[128] chronic right atrial catheters have been reported to be the source of endocarditis in patients with *S. epidermidis* septicemia.[129]

Other Sites of Infection. Infectious hepatitis is a common complication in patients with acute leukemia and has been related to several agents, including hepatitis A virus, hepatitis B virus, and non-A, non-B hepatitis, as well as δ hepatitis.[82,84,130] The exact influence of hepatitis B virus infection on the duration of remission and the survival of patients with leukemia remains controversial.[82,83,131]

Focal hepatic candidiasis has mainly been reported in patients with leukemia and resolving granulocytopenia. These patients present with fever refractory to broad-spectrum antibiotics, hepatomegaly, nonspecific gastrointestinal symptoms such as diarrhea (in 80 percent), and laboratory signs of liver involvement with elevation of alkaline phosphatase activity.[132–135] This clinical entity is particularly difficult to treat, and eradication of microabscesses is difficult to achieve. However, prolonged therapy with amphotericin B or amphotericin B incorporated in liposomes,[136] has shown promise.

A gastrointestinal focus of infection can also occur in granulocytopenic patients and may be responsible for septicemia caused by unusual pathogens, mainly *Clostridium* species.[137–139]

Diarrhea is common in leukemic patients and may result from many different causes. Fecal carriage of *Clostridium difficile* varies considerably among institutions, perhaps reflecting nosocomial acquisition.[140–145] Pseudomembranous colitis from *C. difficile* can be severe and even fatal.[143] Relapse is not rare and may follow cancer chemotherapy.[145] Stool should be tested for *C. difficile* toxin if the diagnosis is being considered. Occasionally, *Cryptosporidium* has also been identified as causal agent of diarrhea in patients under treatment for acute leukemia.[146]

Therapy of Documented Infection in Granulocytopenic Patients

Optimal management of established infection is mandatory to improve the outcome of granulocytopenic patients. When data obtained from blood cultures performed at initiation of empiric therapy are available, appropriate changes should be considered according to the identity and susceptibility pattern of the offending pathogen, as well as the clinical course of the patient. In particular for patients with documented gram-negative bacteremia who remain granulocytopenic for prolonged periods of time, the administration of a combined regimen (usually a β-lactam plus an aminoglycoside) seems to be optimal.[10,12,13,16,20,85,92,147] Improved survival of those patients treated with two agents active against the offending pathogen has also been observed.[85,148–150] The beneficial role of synergistic combinations has also been extensively demonstrated in these patients,[85,148–150] as well as the correlation between favorable outcome and high serum bactericidal activity in patients with gram-negative bacteremia.[151] Overall these parameters are useful tools to guide the clinician facing life-threatening infections in patients with profound granulocytopenia. The recovery of a normal granulocyte count is of major importance for a favorable prognosis in these patients.

Currently, indications for granulocyte transfusions are limited to infections not responding to conventional therapy (usually gram-negative bacilli or fungi).[147,152,153] In patients allergic to β-lactam antibiotics, the combination of trimethoprim-sulfamethoxazole plus an aminoglycoside may be useful, provided that the microorganism identified is not *Ps. aeruginosa.*[154] The exact role of monobactams, carbapenems, and fluoroquinolones is presently under investigation.[155–157] The control of polymicrobial septicemia is particularly difficult, especially if pneumonia is present.[158]

A remaining question for the management of infection in granulocytopenic patients is the optimal duration of antibiotic therapy in patients remaining markedly granulocytopenic.[66,159] It does not appear necessary to maintain broad-spectrum antibiotic therapy until recovery of the granulocyte count, provided that the patient is afebrile and has been treated adequately for 7–9 days. There is increased evidence that prolonged antimicrobial therapy leads to a high incidence of superinfection caused either by resistant microorganisms or opportunistic pathogens such as fungi.[9,66,159,160] For those patients with documented bacteremia, the spectrum of antimicrobial therapy should not be restricted to antibiotics active only against the isolated pathogen; particularly if gram-positive cocci have been isolated from blood cultures and if the patient remains granulocytopenic, appropriate coverage against gram-negative bacilli should also be administered. Rapidly fatal breakthough bacteremia caused by gram-negative bacilli has been observed in such circumstances. Treatment of infection in leukemic children is similar to that in adults.[161]

Unfortunately, there are few commercially available effective antifungal compounds.[70] The optimal therapy for most documented fungal infections remains amphotericin B, with the exception of *P. boydii, Fusarium* species, and occasional other unusual fungi that seem more susceptible to imidazoles.

Recently, the combination of amphotericin B and 5-flurocytosine has been suggested to be more effective to treat fungemia caused by *Candida tropicalis.*[43] Further studies should be initiated to evaluate the potential role of this regimen for this group of patients. Extensive studies are presently underway with various preparations of liposome-encapsulated amphotericin B.[136,162–164] These preparations are much better tolerated than conventional amphotericin B, and large, randomized, controlled studies should be performed to estimate the potential benefit of this approach.

Ketoconazole has been extensively studied, mainly for prophylaxis.[165] Its therapeutic use in granulocytopenic patients[166] is limited to oropharyngeal candidiasis or esophagitis. In addition, ketoconazole is available only for oral administration, its absorption varies from patient to patient, and high doses (i.e., 400–600 mg daily) are probably necessary. Moreover, besides having an unpredictable pharmacokinetic profile, various endocrine side effects and interactions with several drugs (e.g., cyclosporine A, rifampin, and anticoagulants) constitute potential problems in these patients. Other major drawbacks of ketoconazole are the selection of *T. glabrata* and the lack of activity against *Aspergillus* species.

There are also major developments of new triazoles such as itraconazole and fluconazole, but their specific indications in granulocytopenic patients with documented fungal infections are not yet clearly established.[167] Itraconazole is also poorly water soluble; it is available only for oral administration; and low serum concentrations have been measured after oral use. However, the activity of this new triazole against *Aspergillus* species is encouraging. Fluconazole, another new triazole, which is water soluble and has significant pharmacologic advantages, is also currently under investigation for several indications. So far, the clinical efficacy of fluconazole has been documented for cryptococcal meningitis in patients with the acquired immunodeficiency syndrome (AIDS) or other immunosuppressed hosts, as well as for oropharyngeal candidiasis in patients with malignancy. Further studies are needed, particularly in fungemic patients, since an intravenous formulation is available for fluconazole.

Antiviral drugs effective in granulocytopenic patients are also limited. Acyclovir constitutes a major advance in therapy of herpes simplex and herpes zoster infections.[73,81,168]

INFECTIONS IN PATIENTS WITH ALTERED CELL-MEDIATED IMMUNITY

The Pathogens

The spectrum of infectious complications occurring in patients with leukemia or lymphoma without granulocytopenia differs significantly from that described in the previous section.[38,70,79,169,170] These infections are usually related to defects in cell-mediated immunity, secondary either to the underlying disease or to medications such as antineoplastic chemotherapeutic agents or corticosteroids. In addition, patients who have undergone splenectomy are also predisposed to overwhelming infections, mainly caused by encapsulated pathogens such as *Strep. pneumoniae* and *Haemophilus influenzae*.[171] These patients should be informed of the risks of infection as well as of the need for prompt medical consultation and antimicrobial therapy if fever or symptoms suggesting infection do occur.[147]

Bacteria. The classic pathogens identified in patients with defects in cell-mediated immunity are *Listeria monocytogenes*, *Legionella pneumophila*, *Salmonella* species, *Mycobacterium tuberculosis*, and nontuberculous mycobacteria, as well as *Nocardia* species. Outbreaks of legionellosis have been well characterized in compromised patients hospitalized in heavily contaminated units.[172,173] *L. pneumophila* is a gram-negative bacillus requiring specific staining methods and culture media to be recognized.

So far, there has been no increased incidence of listeriosis in patients with Hodgkin's disease or lymphoma. However, recent epidemics of septicemia and meningitis caused by *L. monocytogenes*-contaminated milk and cheese indicate that patients who are at risk (i.e., those with altered cell-mediated immunity) should be informed about potential sources of infection. The incidence of salmonellosis varies greatly worldwide, as does that of tuberculosis.[147] Tuberculous lymphadenitis is rare in those patients who present more often either with reactivation of pulmonary tuberculosis or with a widespread infection (miliary tuberculosis). Skin testing with purified protein deviative (PPD) to evaluate previous contact with *M. tuberculosis* is difficult to interpet in patients with abnormal lymphocytic functions and/or anergy. Compared to the high incidence of recovery of nontuberculous mycobacteria in patients with AIDS, these pathogens are unusual in patients with lymphoma.

Nocardiosis is also a classic complication in these patients, who present with lesions localized to the lungs, the skin, and soft tissues or with brain abscesses.[174]

Fungi. The common fungal infection in these patients is cryptococcal meningitis. *Cryptococcus neoformans* is a yeast, the fungus being inhaled from sites in nature. The pulmonary focus usually remains asymptomatic. During severe immunosuppression, dissemination occurs, resulting in meningitis with or without a cerebral cryptococcoma. Occasionally, cutaneous lesions also occur.

Protozoa and Parasites. Patients with defects in cell-mediated immunity are highly predisposed to severe infections caused by *Pneumocystis carinii*. This pathogen is responsible for life-threatening pneumonia.[175] Most children have detectable serum antibodies, and it appears that these infections are the result of reactivation of latent pathogens. Intermittent chemoprophylaxis with trimethoprim-sulfamethoxazole has now been proven effective in reducing the incidence of pneumocystis, particularly in children with ALL.[176] *Toxoplasma gondii* can also reactivate, leading to chorioretinitis or cerebral abscesses.[177] *Strongyloides stercoralis* can cause diarrhea, as well as life-threatening hyperinfection.[178] In areas where this pathogen is endemic, stool examination to rule out asymptomatic carriage should be performed before the administration of immunosuppressive chemotherapy. Occasionally, *Cryptosporidium* has been identified as the cause of enteropathy in immunocompromised hosts without AIDS.

Viruses. Common viral infections in these patients are caused by herpes zoster virus, causing either varicella or herpes zoster infection. Varicella is a life-threatening infection in children with ALL.[179,180] Prophylactic vaccination has been recommended.[179,181,182] Reactivation leading to herpes zoster infection is common in patients with altered cell-mediated immunity. Cytomegalovirus is responsible for interstitial pneumonia, as well as viremia, viruria, hepatitis, and chorioretinitis in patients with defects in cell-mediated immunity. However, this agent is more commonly encountered in patients undergoing transplantation and will be discussed in Chapter 291.

Characteristics of Common Clinical Infections in Patients with Defects in Cell-Mediated Immunity

Septicemia. The clinical signs and symptoms of septicemia in patients with leukemia or lymphoma who have adequate granulocyte counts are similar to those observed in other patients. It should be mentioned, however, that corticosteroids may decrease or even abolish fever. In splenectomized patients, even in the absence of granulocytopenia, fulminant bacteremia has been observed and prompt initiation of antimicrobial therapy is mandatory. Septicemia caused by *S. pneumoniae* has a 30 percent mortality in immunosuppressed patients. Persistent fecal carriage of *Salmonella* species has also been observed in these patients with relapsing septicemia. Genitourinary tract infections resulting from obstruction caused by lymphomatous masses may also lead to bacteremia. Occasionally, blood cultures are positive for *L. monocytogenes* or *C. neoformans* before the development of neurologic symptoms. The recovery of one of these two pathogens from blood culture in an immunocompromised host should always lead to a lumbar puncture, provided that no intracranial hypertension is detected.

Pulmonary Infections. *Pneumocystis* pneumonia presents in these patients as fever, progressive pulmonary symptoms with dry cough, and dyspnea. Early in its evolution, the chest x-ray film usually shows discrete infiltrates progressing to interstitial pneumonia. The patient develops progressive hypoxemia. Clinical signs and symptoms often begin when corticosteroids have been discontinued within the last few weeks. While diffuse pneumonia caused by *P. carinii* is a well-known entity, occasionally this infection occurs with nonspecific symptoms and without typical chest x-ray bindings.[175] Other pulmonary infections may also be present, complicating diagnosis. A correct and specific etiology is difficult to establish without the use of invasive procedures. However, the diagnostic value of bronchoalveolar lavage in such circumstances has been well documented.[183] Pneumonia caused by *L. pneumophila* presents usually with a different clinical picture, as well as with chest x-ray signs of consolidation.[172] Other systemic manifestations such as headache, gastrointestinal symptoms, and renal insufficiency may also be present. The diagnosis can also be based on direct examination of bronchopulmonary secretions, using immunofluorescent staining. Confirmation by culture should be sought. Seroconversion is usually delayed and is of little help in management.[184]

Tuberculosis may be difficult to diagnose, particularly in patients who do not produce sputum. However, the overall incidence of tuberculosis in patients with leukemia is rather low. This infection is somewhat more frequent in patients with lymphoma or Hodgkin's disease.[147]

Meningitis and Other Neurologic Manifestations. Insidious onset of fever, headache, and confusion should alert the physician to rule out meningitis, particularly in patients with lymphoma or Hodgkin's disease. The cerebrospinal fluid (CSF) is usually clear, with a slight increase in white blood cells and a moderate elevation in protein concentration. In patients with a low glucose level, tuberculous meningitis should be considered; however, the most common pathogens in these circumstances are *L. monocytogenes* and *C. neoformans*.[185] *L. monocytogenes* is a gram-positive bacillus that may be erroneously considered as a *Corynebacterium* species. Such isolates should not be discarded as contaminants. The diagnosis of cryptococcal meningitis is more difficult to ascertain in patients with lymphoma or Hodgkin's disease than in those with AIDS due to a significantly lower inoculum of yeast in the CSF. In patients with malignant disease, the sensitivity of the India ink examination is poor (50 percent) but the sensitivity of antigen detection is much higher (95 percent). Efforts to grow *C. neoformans* should be pursued, but occasionally large amounts of CSF and repeated punctures may be required. Intracerebral cryptococcoma has also been described. Favorable prognostic factors have been identified and should serve as guidelines for optimal management.[186] Other neurologic problems in these patients consist of single or multiple cerebral abcesses.[185] Common pathogens in these circumstances are *T. gondii*,[177] *Nocardia* species,[174] or, less commonly, *M. tuberculosis*.

Skin and Soft Tissue Infections. Numerous opportunistic pathogens cause cutaneous manifestations in these patients. Lesions of cryptococcosis or nocardiosis have occasionally been described. However, the major dermatologic complication in patients with defects in cell-mediated immunity is herpes zoster.[72,73,179,180,187]

Another clinical entity causing abrupt onset of fever associated with cutaneous plaques and leukocytosis in patients with hematologic malignancy is called *acute febrile neutrophilic dermatosis* (or *Sweet syndrome*) and should also be recognized, since these manifestations respond to corticosteroids.[188] In addition to developing these rather specific clinical pictures, such patients are also predisposed to more classic infections during long-term ambulatory antineoplastic chemotherapy.

Therapy of Infections in Patients with Defects in Cell-Mediated Immunity

The optimal management of infections in this group of patients usually requires a different approach than for granulocytopenic patients. Despite the severity of the infections occurring in patients with Hodgkin's disease or lymphoma, the degree of emergency required to initiate empiric antimicrobial therapy is less than that in granulocytopenic or splenectomized patients. In all other circumstances, a specific etiology should be established, using various diagnostic procedures before the initiation of specific therapy. Prolonged therapy is required for some bacterial infections, particularly listeriosis[185] or nocardiosis.[189] The optimal antimicrobial regimen for *L. monocytogenes* includes 2–4 weeks of ampicillin plus a short course of aminoglycoside.[185] Trimethoprim-sulfamethoxazole is also a useful agent in treating *Listeria* meningitis and nocardiosis. For those immunocompromised patients with infection caused by *Nocardia*, therapy should be continued for 12 months.[189] Numerous studies have shown satisfactory results with trimethoprim-sulfamethoxazole in treating pneumonia caused by *P. carinii*,[190,191] without the numerous side effects encountered with this agent administered to patients with AIDS. The poor tolerance of pentamidine and the efficacy of trimethoprim-sulfamethoxazole in this population have almost eliminated the use of pentamidine in patients with neoplastic disease.

Optimal therapy of *S. pneumoniae* has remained unchanged over the years[192] and is still penicillin in most parts of the world. Erythromycin remains the drug of choice in treating legionellosis.[172]

In cryptococcal meningitis, amphotericin B plus 5-fluorocytosine remains the standard therapy. There are still major controversies regarding the duration of therapy, although a recent study[186] has defined a subgroup of patients who may benefit from a 4-week regimen. Other unanswered questions concern the exact role of and indications for intrathecal and intraventricular administration of amphotericin B.[185] This approach should be considered for those patients with severe infection at the onset (such as comatose patients) and for patients with relapse. Recently, fluconazole has been investigated for therapy of cryptococcal meningitis. Preliminary data are encouraging. Effective therapy for cryptosporidiosis is still lacking.[193] The management of disseminated strongyloidiasis is also extremely difficult and relies on thiabendazole.[178] The management of toxoplasmosis includes prolonged administration of sulfonamides with pyrimethamine. The value of trimethoprim-sulfamethoxazole for this disease remains controversial.[177]

Over the last decade, great progress has been achieved in the therapeutic approaches to viral infections. Although vidarabine has been shown effective in treating varicella infections in immunosuppressed children,[194] as well as herpes zoster infections in adults,[195] this agent is presently less commonly used than acyclovir. Acyclovir is highly effective and is considered to be the drug of choice for both herpes simplex and varicella-zoster.[168] It has been shown to be superior to vidarabine for herpes simplex encephalitis,[196] is significantly less toxic, and is easier to administer. However, relapse following acyclovir therapy has also been documented, and prolonged therapy may be necessary in immunocompromised patients.[197] A recent placebo-controlled study performed in immunocompromised children[198] has shown the benefit of acyclovir therapy in preventing dissemination of varicella and in reducing the duration of its rash. In addition, several new antiviral compounds are under development for herpes zoster, including bromovinyl deoxyuridine.[199] Gancyclovir and foscarnet are being evaluated in the treatment of cytomegalovirus infection.[200]

Finally, the exact value of immunoglobulin therapy in this group of patients remains controversial, except as prevention after exposure to varicella virus.[201]

REFERENCES

1. Chessels JM. Acute leukaemia in children. Clin Hematol. 1986;15:727–53.
2. Schleuning M, Clemm C. Chromosomal aberrations in a newborn whose mother received cytotoxic treatment during pregnancy. N Engl J Med. 1987;317:1666–7.
3. Prentice HG, Grob JP. Acute lymphoblastic leukaemia in adults. Clin Hematol. 1986;15:755–80.
4. Champlin R, Gale RP. Acute myelogenous leukemia: Recent advances in therapy. Blood. 1987;69:1551–61.

5. Freireich EJ, Keating M, Cabanillas F, et al. The hematologic malignancies: Leukemia, lymphoma and myeloma. Cancer. 1984;54:2741–50.
6. Bodey GP, Buckley M, Sathe YS, et al. Quantitative relationships between circulating leukocytes and infection in patients with acute leukemia. Ann Intern Med. 1966;64:328–40.
7. Schimpff SC, Hahn DM, Brouillet MD, et al. Infection prevention in acute leukemia. Comparison of basic infection prevention techniques, with standard room reverse isolation or with reverse isolation plus added air filtration. Leuk Res. 1978;2:231–40.
8. Schimpff SC. Therapy of infection in patients with granulocytopenia. Med Clin North Am. 1978;61:1101–18.
9. EORTC international antimicrobial therapy cooperative group. Three antibiotic regimens in the treatment of infection in febrile granulocytopenic patients with cancer. J Infect Dis. 1978;137:14–29.
10. Young LS. Fever and septicemia. In: Rubin RH, Young LS, eds. Clinical Approach to Infection in the Compromised Host. 2nd ed. New York: Plenum Medical; 1988:75–114.
11. Bodey GP, Rodriguez V. Advances in the management of *Pseudomonas aeruginosa* infections in cancer patients. Eur J Cancer. 1973;9:435–41.
12. Love LJ, Schimpff SC, Schiffer CA, et al. Improved prognosis for granulocytopenic patients with gram-negative bacteremia. Am J Med. 1980; 68:643–8.
13. Schimpff S, Satterlee WM, Young VM, et al. Empiric therapy with carbenicillin and gentamicin for febrile patients with cancer and granulocytopenia. N Engl J Med. 1971;284:1061–5.
14. EORTC international antimicrobial therapy project group. Combination of amikacin and carbenicillin with or without cefazolin as empirical treatment of febrile neutropenic patients. J Clin Oncol. 1983;1:597–603.
15. EORTC international antimicrobial therapy cooperative group. Prospective randomized comparison of three antibiotic regimens for empirical therapy of suspected bacteremic infection in febrile granulocytopenic patients. Antimicrob Agents Chemother. 1986;29:263–70.
16. EORTC international antimicrobial therapy cooperative group. Ceftazidime combined with a short or long course of amikacin for empirical therapy of gram-negative bacteremia in cancer patients with granulocytopenia. N Engl J Med. 1987;317:1692–8.
17. Singer C, Kaplan MH, Armstrong D. Bacteremia and fungemia complicating neoplastic disease. A study of 364 cases. Am J Med. 1977;62:731–42.
18. Bodey GP, Rodriguez V, Chang HY, et al. Fever and infection in leukemic patients. Cancer. 1978;41:1610–22.
19. Schimpff SC, Greene WH, Young VM, et al. Pseudomonas septicemia: Incidence, epidemiology, prevention and therapy in patients with advanced cancer. Eur J Cancer. 1973;9:449–55.
20. Klastersky J, Zinner SH, Calandra T, et al. Empiric antimicrobial therapy for febrile granulocytopenic cancer patients: Lessons from four EORTC trials. Eur J Cancer Clin Oncol. 1988;24:S35–S45.
21. Pizzo PA, Ladisch S, Simon RM, et al. Increasing incidence of gram-positive sepsis in cancer patients. Med Pediatr Oncol. 1978;5:241–4.
22. Wade JC, Schimpff SC, Newman KA, et al. *Staphylococcus epidermidis*: An increasing cause of infection in patients with granulocytopenia. Ann Intern Med. 1987;97:503–8.
23. Winston DJ, Dudnick DV, Chapin M, et al. Coagulase negative staphylococcal bacteremia in patients receiving immunosuppressive therapy. Arch Intern Med. 1983;143:32–6.
24. Karp JE, Dick JD, Angelopulos C, et al. Empiric use of vancomycin during prolonged treatment-induced granulocytopenia. Am J Med. 1986;81:237–42.
25. Whimbey E, Kiehn TE, Brannon P, et al. Bacteremia and fungemia in patients with neoplastic disease. Am J Med. 1987;82:723–9.
26. Wade JC, Schimpff SC, Hargadon MT, et al. A comparison of trimethoprim-sulfamethoxazole plus nystatin with gentamicin plus nystatin in the prevention of infections in acute leukemia. N Engl J Med. 1981;304:1057–66.
27. Wade JC, De Jongh CA, Newman KA, et al. Selective antimicrobial modulation on prophylaxis against infection during granulocytopenia with trimethoprim-sulfamethoxazole versus nalidixic acid. J Infect Dis. 1983; 147:624–34.
28. EORTC international antimicrobial therapy project group. Trimethoprim-sulfamethoxazole in the prevention of infection in neutropenic patients. J Infect Dis. 1984;150:372–9.
29. Henry SA. Chemoprophylaxis of bacterial infections in granulocytopenic patients. Am J Med. 1984;76:645–51.
30. Rozenberg-Arska M, Dekker AW, Verhoef J. Ciprofloxacin for selective decontamination of the alimentary tract in patients with acute leukemia during remission induction treatment. J Infect Dis. 1985;152:104–7.
31. Winston DJ, Winston GH, Nakao SL, et al. Norfloxacin versus vancomycin polymyxin for prevention of infections in granulocytopenic patients. Am J Med. 1986;80:884–90.
32. Dekker AW, Rozenberg-Arska M, Verhoef J. Infection prophylaxis in acute leukemia: A comparison of ciprofloxacin with trimethoprim-sulfamethoxazole and colistin. Ann Intern Med. 1987;106:7–12.
33. Karp JE, Merz WG, Hendricksen C, et al. Oral norfloxacin for prevention of gram-negative bacterial infections in patients with acute leukemia and granulocytopenia. Ann Intern Med. 1987;106:1–7.
34. Khabbaz RF, Cooksey RC, Saba G, et al. The alimentary tract as a source of *S. epidermidis* bacteremia in patients with cancer: Clues from molecular epidemiology. (Abstract 1036). In: Abstracts of the Twenty-Seventh Interscience Conference on Antimicrobial Agents and Chemotherapy. New York: American Society for Microbiology; 1987:271.
35. Khabbaz RF, Arnow PM, Highsmith AK, et al. *Pseudomonas fluorescens* bacteremia from blood transfusion. Am J Med. 1984;76:62–7.
36. Anderson KC, Lew MA, Gorgone BC, et al. Transfusion-related sepsis after prolonged platelet storage. Am J Med. 1986;81:405–11.
37. Bodey G. Fungal infections complicating acute leukemia. J Chronic Dis. 1966;19:667–87.
38. Krick J, Remington J. Opportunistic fungal infection in patients with leukemia and lymphoma. Clin Hematol. 1976;5:249–310.
39. De Gregorio M, Lee W, Linker C, et al. Fungal infections in patients with acute leukemia. Am J Med. 1982;73:543–8.
40. Hawkins C, Armstrong D. Fungal infections in the immunocompromised host. Clin Haematol. 1984;13:599–630.
41. Wingard J, Merz W, Saral R. *Candida tropicalis*: A major pathogen in immunocompromised patients. Ann Intern Med. 1979;91:539–43.
42. Meunier-Carpentier F, Kiehn T, Armstrong D. Fungemia in the immunocompromised host: Changing patterns, antigenemia, high mortality. Am J Med. 1981;1:363–70.
43. Horn R, Wong B, Kiehn TE, et al. Fungemia in a cancer hospital: Changing frequency, earlier onset, and results of therapy. Rev Infect Dis. 1985;7:646–55.
44. Young RC, Bennett JE, Vogel CL, et al. Aspergillosis: The spectrum of the disease in 98 patients. Medicine. 1970;49:143–7.
45. Fischer BS, Armstrong D, Yu B, et al. Invasive aspergillosis: Progress in early diagnosis and treatment. Am J Med. 1981;71:571–7.
46. Gerson SL, Talbot GH, Hurwitz S, et al. Prolonged granulocytopenia: The major risk factor for invasive pulmonary aspergillosis in patients with acute leukemia. Ann Intern Med. 1984;100:345–51.
47. Aisner J, Schimpff S, Sutherland J, et al. *Torulopsis glabrata* infections in patients with cancer; increasing incidence and relationship to colonization. Am J Med. 1976;61:23.
48. Meyer RD, Rosen P, Armstrong D. Phycomycosis complicating leukemia and lymphoma. Ann Intern Med. 1972;77:871–9.
49. Gold J, Poston W, Mertelsmann R, et al. Systemic infection with *Trichosporon cutaneum* in a patient with acute leukemia. Cancer. 1981;48:2163–7.
50. Walling DM, McGraw DJ, Merz WG, et al. Disseminated infection with *Trichosporon beigelii*. Rev Infect Dis. 1987;9:1013–9.
51. Blazar BR, Hurd DD, Snover DC, et al. Invasive *Fusarium* infections in bone marrow transplant recipients. Am J Med. 1984;77:645–51.
52. Yoo D, Lee HS, Kwong-Chung KJ. Brain abscesses due to *Pseudallescheria boydii* associated with primary non-Hodgkin's lymphoma of the central nervous system: A case report and literature review. Rev Infect Dis. 1985; 7:272–7.
53. Sanford GR, Merz WG, Wingard JR, et al. The value of fungal surveillance cultures as predictors of systemic fungal infections. J Infect Dis. 1980;142:503–9.
54. Kramer BS, Pizzo PA, Robichaud KJ, et al. Role of serial microbiologic surveillance and clinical evaluation in the management of cancer patients with fever and granulocytopenia. Am J Med. 1982;72:561–8.
55. Haupt HM, Merz WG, Beschorner WE, et al. Colonization and infection with *Trichosporon* species in the immunosuppressed host. J Infect Dis. 1983;147:199–203.
56. Aisner J, Murillo J, Schimpff SC, et al. Invasive aspergillosis in acute leukemia: Correlation with nose cultures and antibiotic use. Ann Intern Med. 1979;90:4–9.
57. Nalesnik MA, Myerowitz RL, Jenkins R, et al. Significance of *Aspergillus* species isolated from respiratory secretions in the diagnosis of invasive pulmonary aspergillosis. J Clin Microbiol. 1980;11:370–6.
58. Yu VL, Muder RR, Poorsattar A. Significance of isolation of *Aspergillus* from the respiratory tract in diagnosis of invasive pulmonary aspergillosis. Am J Med. 1986;81:249–54.
59. Aisner J, Schimpff SC, Wiernik PH. Treatment of invasive aspergillosis: Relation of early diagnosis and treatment to response. Ann Intern Med. 1977;86:539–43.
60. Kuhlman JE, Fishman EK, Siegelman SS. Invasive pulmonary aspergillosis in acute leukemia: Characteristic findings on CT, the CT halo sign, and the role of CT in early diagnosis. Radiology. 1985;157:611–4.
61. Burch PA, Karp JE, Merz WG, et al. Favorable outcome of aspergillosis in patients with acute leukemia. J Clin Oncol. 1987;5:1985–93.
62. Neglia JP, Hurd DD, Ferrieri P, et al. Invasive scopulariopsosis in the immunocompromised host. Am J Med. 1987;83:1163–6.
63. Lutwick LI, Galgiani JN, Johnson RH, et al. Visceral fungal infections due to *Petriellidium boydii* (*Allescheria boydii*). In vitro sensitivity studies. Am J Med. 1976;61:632–40.
64. June CH, Beatty PG, Shulman HM, et al. Disseminated *Fusarium moniliforme* infection after allogeneic marrow transplantation. South Med J. 1986;79:513–5.
65. Bennett JE. Rapid diagnosis of candidiasis and aspergillosis. Rev Infect Dis. 1987;9:398–402.
66. Pizzo PA, Robichaud KJ, Gill FA, et al. Empiric antibiotic and antifungal therapy for cancer patients with prolonged fever and granulocytopenia. Am J Med. 1982;72:101–11.
67. Cohen J. Empiric antifungal therapy in neutropenic patients. J Antimicrob Chemother. 1984;13:409–11.
68. Schwartz RS, Mackintosch FR, Schrier SL, et al. Multivariate analysis of factors associated with invasive fungal disease during remission induction therapy for acute myelogenous leukemia. Cancer. 1984;53:411–9.
69. EORTC antimicrobial therapy cooperative group. Empiric therapy with fun-

gizone in febrile neutropenic patients. (Abstract 681). In: Abstracts of the Twenty-Sixth Interscience Conference on Antimicrobial Agents and Chemotherapy. New Orleans: American Society for Microbiology; 1986:222.
70. Meunier F. Fungal infections in the compromised host. In: Rubin RH, Young LS, eds. Clinical Approach to Infection in the Compromised Host. 2nd ed. New York: Plenum Medical; 1988;193–220.
71. Talbot GH, Provencher M, Cassileth PA. Persistent fever after recovery from granulocytopenia in acute leukemia. Arch Intern Med. 1988;148:129–35.
72. Corey L, Spear PG. Infections with herpes simplex viruses. N Engl J Med. 1986;314:686–91 (Part I); 1986;749–57 (Part II).
73. Strauss SE, moderator. Varicella zoster virus infections: Biology, natural history, treatment and prevention. Ann Intern Med. 1988;108:221–37.
74. Meyers JD, Flournoy N. Risk factors for cytomegalovirus infection after human marrow transplantation. J Infect Dis. 1986;153:478–88.
75. Zahradnik JM, Spencer MJ, Porter DD. Adenovirus infection in the immunocompromised patient. Am J Med. 1980;68:725–32.
76. Rand KH, Kramer B, Johnson AC. Cancer chemotherapy associated symptomatic stomatitis: Role of herpes simplex virus. Cancer. 1982;50:1262–5.
77. Buss DH, Scharyj M. Herpes virus infection of the esophagus and other visceral organs in adults: Incidence and clinical significance. Am J Med. 1979;66:457–62.
78. Ramsey PG, Fife KH, Hackman RC, et al. Herpes simplex virus pneumonia: Clinical, virologic and pathologic features in 20 patients. Ann Intern Med. 1982;97:813–9.
79. Feld R, Bodey GP. Infections in patients with malignant lymphoma treated with combination chemotherapy. Cancer. 1977;39:1018–25.
80. Miliauskas JR, Webber B. Disseminated varicella at autopsy in children with cancer. Cancer. 1984;53:1518–25.
81. Weller TH. Varicella and herpes zoster: Changing concepts of the natural history, control and importance of a not-so-benign virus. N Engl J Med. 1983;1:1362–8 (Part I); 1983;1434–40 (Part II).
82. Wade JC, Gaffey M, Wiernik PH, et al. Hepatitis in patients with acute nonlymphocytic leukemia. Am J Med. 1983;75:413–21.
83. Ratner L, Peylan-Ramu N, Wesley R, et al. Adverse prognostic influence of hepatitis B virus infection in acute lymphoblastic leukemia. Cancer. 1986;58:1096–1100.
84. Dienstag JL. Viral hepatitis in the compromised host. In: Rubin RH, Young LS, eds. Clinical Approach to Infection in the Compromised Host. 2nd ed. New York: Plenum Medical; 1988:325–45.
85. De Jongh CA, Joshi JH, Newman KA, et al. Antibiotic synergism and response in gram-negative bacteremia in granulocytopenic cancer patients. Am J Med. 1986;80:96–100.
86. Harris RL, Muscher DM, Bloom K, et al. Manifestations of sepsis. Arch Intern Med. 1987;147:1895–1906.
87. Bodey GP, Jadeja L, Elting L. Pseudomonas bacteremia: Retrospective analysis of 410 episodes. Arch Intern Med. 1985;145:1621–9.
88. Bille J, Stockman L, Roberts GD, et al. Evaluation of a lysis–centrifugation system for recovery of yeasts and filamentous fungi from blood. J Clin Microbiol. 1983;18:469–71.
89. Guerra-Romero L, Edson RS, Cockerill FR III, et al. Comparison of DuPont isolator and Roche Septi-Check for detection of fungemia. J Clin Microbiol. 1987;25:1623–5.
90. Whimbey E, Wong B, Kiehn TE, et al. Clinical correlations of serial quantitative blood cultures determined by lysis–centrifugation in patients with persistent septicemia. J Clin Microbiol. 1984;19:766–71.
91. Pizzo PA, Hathorn JW, Hiemenz J, et al. A randomized trial comparing ceftazidime alone with combination therapy in cancer patients with fever and neutropenia. N Engl J Med. 1986;315:552–8.
92. Young LS. Empirical antimicrobial therapy in the neutropenic host. N Engl J Med. 1986;315:580–1.
93. Rubin M, Hathorn JW, Marshall D, et al. Gram positive infections and the use of vancomycin in 350 episodes of fever and neutropenia. Ann Intern Med. 1988;108:30–5.
94. Sonis ST. Oral complications of cancer therapy. In: Devita VT, Hellman S, Rosenberg SA, eds. Cancer, Principles and Practice of Oncology. 2nd ed. Philadelphia: JB Lippincott; 1985:2014–21.
95. Overholser CD, Peterson DE, William LT, et al. Periodontal infections in patients with acute nonlymphocytic leukemia: Prevalence of acute exacerbations. Arch Intern Med. 1982;142:551–4.
96. Hirsch MS. Herpes group virus infections in the compromised host. In: Rubin RH, Young LS, eds. Clinical Approach to Infection in the Compromised Host. 2nd ed. New York: Plenum Medical; 1988;347–66.
97. Kern W, Vanek E. Aerococcus bacteremia associated with granulocytopenia. Eur J Clin Microbiol. 1987;6:670–3.
98. Epstein J, Truelove E, Izutzu K. Oral candidiasis: Pathogenesis and host defense. Rev Infect Dis. 1984;6:96–106.
99. Trier JS, Bjorkman DJ. Esophageal, gastric and intestinal candidiasis. Am J Med. 1984;77:39–43.
100. Eras P, Goldstein M, Sherlock P. Candida infection of the gastrointestinal tract. Medicine. 1972;51:367–79.
101. Jones J. Necrotizing candida oesophagitis. Failure of symptoms and roentgenographic findings to reflect severity. JAMA. 1980;244:2190–1.
102. Buss DH, Schary JM. Herpesvirus infection of the esophagus and other visceral organs in adults. Incidence and clinical significance. Am J Med. 1979;66:457–62.
103. Onge GS, Bezahler GH. Giant esophageal ulcer associated with cytomegalovirus. Gastroenterology. 1982;83:127–30.
104. Walsh TJ, Belitsos NJ, Hamilton SR, et al. Bacterial esophagitis in immunocompromised patients. Arch Intern Med. 1986;146:1345–8.
105. Cole S, Zawin M, Lundberg B, et al. Candida epiglottitis in an adult with acute nonlymphocytic leukemia. Am J Med. 1987;82:662–4.
106. Shenep JL, Kalwinski DK, Feldman S, et al. Mycotic cervical lymphadenitis following oral mucositis in children with leukemia. J Pediatr. 1985;106:243–6.
107. Ognibene FP, Martin SE, Parker MM, et al. Adult respiratory distress syndrome in patients with severe neutropenia. N Engl J Med. 1986;315:547–51.
108. Laufe MD, Simon RH, Flint A, et al. Adult respiratory distress syndrome in neutropenic patients. Am J Med. 1986; 80:1022–6.
109. Funada H, Misawa T, Nakao S. The air crescent sign of invasive pulmonary mucormycosis in acute leukemia. Cancer. 1984;53:2271–3.
110. Robertson MJ, Larson RA. Recurrent fungal pneumonias in patients with acute nonlymphocytic leukemia undergoing multiple courses of intensive chemotherapy. Am J Med. 1988;84:233–9.
111. Rubin RH, Greene R. Etiology and management of the compromised patient with fever and pulmonary infiltrates. In: Rubin RH, Young LS, eds. Clinical Approach to Infection in the Compromised Host. New York: Plenum Medical; 1988:131–57.
112. McCabe RE, Brooks RG, Mark JB, et al. Open lung biopsy in patients with acute leukemia. Am J Med. 1985;78:609–16.
113. Estey EH, Keating MJ, McCredie KB, et al. Causes of remission induction failure in acute myelogenous leukemia. Blood. 1982;60:309–15.
114. Wolfson JS, Sober AJ. Dermatologic manifestations of infection in the compromised host. In: Rubin RH, Young LS, eds. Clinical Approach to Infection in the Compromised Host. 2nd ed. New York: Plenum Medical; 1986:115–30.
115. Berkow RL, Weisman SJ, Provisor AJ, et al. Invasive aspergillosis of paranasal tissues in children with malignancies. J Pediatr. 1983;103:49–53.
116. Bodey GP, Luna M. Skin lesions associated with disseminated candidiasis. JAMA. 1974;229:1466–8.
117. Fine JD, Miller JA, Harrist TJ, et al. Cutaneous lesions in disseminated candidiasis mimicking ecthyma gangrenosum. Am J Med. 1981;70:1133–5.
118. Suster S, Rose LB. Intradermal bullous dermatitis due to candidiasis in an immunocompromised patient. JAMA. 1987;258:2106–7.
119. Hay CRM, Messenger AG, Cotton DWK, et al. Atypical bullous pyoderma gangrenosum associated with myeloid malignancies. J Clin Pathol. 1987; 40:387–92.
120. Hiemenz J, Skelton J, Pizzo PA. Perspective on the management of catheter-related infections in cancer patients. Pediatr Infect Dis. 1986;5:6–11.
121. Johnson PR, Decker MD, Edwards KM, et al. Frequency of Broviac catheter infections in pediatric oncology patients. J Infect Dis. 1986;154:570–8.
122. Anaissie E, Fainstein V, Miller P, et al. *Pseudomonas putida*. Newly recognized pathogen in patients with cancer. Am J Med. 1987;82:1191–4.
123. Grossman ME, Fithian EC, Behrens C, et al. Primary cutaneous aspergillosis in six leukemic children. J Am Acad Dermatol. 1985;12:313–8.
124. Allo MD, Miller J, Townsend T, et al. Primary cutaneous aspergillosis associated with Hickman intravenous catheters. N Engl J Med. 1987;317: 1105–8.
125. Maki DG. Infections associated with intravascular lines. In: Remington JS, Swartz MN, eds. Current Clinical Topics in Infectious Diseases. v. 3. New York: McGraw-Hill; 1982:309–63.
126. Whimbey E, Kiehn TE, Brannon P, et al. Clinical significance of colony counts in immunocompromised patients with *Staphylococcus aureus* bacteremia. J Infect Dis. 1987;155:1328–30.
127. Friedman LE, Brown AE, Miller DR, et al. *Staphylococcus epidermidis* septicemia. Am J Dis Child. 1984;138:714–9.
128. Sotman SB, Schimpff SC, Young VM. *Staphylococcus aureus* bacteremia in patients with acute leukemia. Am J Med. 1980;69:814–8.
129. Liepman MK, Jones PG, Kauffman CA. Endocarditis as a complication of indwelling right atrial catheters in leukemic patients. Cancer. 1984;54: 804–7.
130. Ratner L. Delta hepatitis outbreak in a group of patients with leukemia. Ann Intern Med. 1986;105:972.
131. Foon KA, Yale C, Clodfelter K, et al. Posttransfusion hepatitis in acute myelogenous leukemia: Effect on survival. JAMA. 1980;244:1806–7.
132. Moseley RH, Kris G, Einzig A, et al. Respiratory alkalosis and abdominal pain heralding *Candida* hepatitis: Occurrence in patients with acute leukemia in remission. Arch Intern Med. 1982;142:1495–7.
133. Tashjian LS, Abramson JS, Peacock JE. Focal hepatic candidiasis: A distinct clinical variant of candidiasis in immunocompromised patients. Rev Infect Dis. 1984;6:689–703.
134. Haron E, Feld R, Tuffnell P, et al. Hepatic candidiasis: An increasing problem in immunocompromised patients. Am J Med. 1987;83:17–26.
135. Thaler M, Pastakia B, Shawker TH, et al. Hepatic candidiasis in cancer patients: The evolving picture of the syndrome. Ann Intern Med. 1988; 108:88–100.
136. Lopez-Berestein G, Bodey GP, Frankel LS, et al. Treatment of hepatosplenic fungal infections with liposomal amphotericin B. J Clin Oncol. 1987;5:310–7.
137. Grützmeier S. *Clostridium perfringens* septicemia and acute leukemia. Acta Med Scand. 1985;218:341–3.

138. Thaler M, Gill V, Pizzo PA. Emergence of *Clostridium tertium* as a pathogen in neutropenic patients. Am J Med. 1986;81:596–600.
139. Tikko SK, Distenfield A, Davison M. *Clostridium septicum* septicemia with identical metastatic myonecroses in a granulocytopenic patient. Am J Med. 1985;79:256–8.
140. Rampling A, Warren RE, Bevan PC, et al. *Clostridium difficile* in haematological malignancy. J Clin Pathol. 1985;38:445–51.
141. Delmée M, Vandercam B, Avesani V, et al. Epidemiology and prevention of *Clostridium difficile* infection in a leukemia unit. Eur J Clin Microbiol. 1987;6:623–7.
142. Gerard M, Defresne N, Daneau D, et al. Incidence and significance of *Clostridium difficile* in hospitalized cancer patients. Eur J Clin Microbiol Infect Dis. 1988;7:274–8.
143. Milligan DW, Kelly JK. Pseudomembranous colitis in a leukaemia unit: A report of five fatal cases. J Clin Pathol. 1979;32:1237–43.
144. Fainstein V, Bodey GP, Fekety R. Relapsing pseudomembranous colitis associated with cancer chemotherapy. J Infect Dis. 1981;143:865.
145. Heard SR, O'Farrell S, Holland D, et al. The epidemiology of *Clostridium difficile* with use of a typing scheme: Nosocomial acquisition and cross-infection among immunocompromised patients. J Infect Dis. 1986;153:159–62.
146. Lewis JI, Hart CA, Baxby D. Diarrhoea due to *Cryptosporidium* in acute lymphoblastic leukaemia. Arch Dis Child. 1985;60:60–2.
147. Young LS. Management of infections in leukemia and lymphoma. In: Rubin RH, Young LS, eds. Clinical Approach to Infection in the Compromised Host. 2nd ed. New York: Plenum Medical; 1988:467–501.
148. Young LS. Combination or single drug therapy for gram-negative sepsis. In: Remington JS, Swartz MN, eds. Current Clinical Topics in Infectious Diseases. v. 3. New York: McGraw-Hill; 1982:177–205.
149. Klastersky J, Cappel R, Daneau D, et al. Clinical significance of in vitro synergism between antibiotics in gram-negative infections. Antimicrob Agents Chemother. 1972;2:470–5.
150. Klastersky J, Meunier-Carpentier F, Prevost J, et al. Significance of antimicrobial synergism for the outcome of gram negative sepsis. Am J Med Sci. 1977;273:157–67.
151. Sculier JP, Klastersky J. Significance of serum bactericidal activity in gram negative bacillary bacteremia in patients with and without granulocytopenia. Am J Med. 1984;76:429–36.
152. Wade JC, Schimpff SC. Approaches to therapy of bacterial infections in the granulocytopenic patient. In: Klastersky J, ed. Infections in Cancer Patients. New York: Raven Press; 1982:105–29.
153. Schiffer CA. Current status of granulocyte transfusion therapy. In: Remington JS, Swartz MN, eds. Current Clinical Topics in Infectious Diseases. v. 5. New York: McGraw-Hill; 1984:189–209.
154. Young LS, Hindler J. Use of trimethoprim-sulfamethoxazole singly and in combination with other antibiotics in immunocompromised patients. Rev Infect Dis. 1987;9(Suppl 2):S177–83.
155. Jones PG, Rolston KV, Fainstein V, et al. Aztreonam therapy in neutropenic patients with cancer. Am J Med. 1986;81:243–8.
156. Wade JC, Standiford HC, Drusano GL, et al. Potential of imipenem as single-agent empiric antibiotic therapy of febrile neutropenic patients with cancer. Am J Med. 1985;78(Suppl 5A):62–72.
157. Webster A, Gaya H. Quinolones in the treatment of serious infections. Rev Infect Dis. 1988;10:S225–33.
158. Elting LS, Bodey GP, Fainstein V, et al. Polymicrobial septicemia in the cancer patient. Medicine. 1986;65:218–25.
159. Joshi JH, Schimpff SC, Tenney JH, et al. Can antibacterial therapy be discontinued in persistently febrile granulocytopenic cancer patients? Am J Med. 1984;76:450–7.
160. Dinubile MJ. Stopping antibiotic therapy in neutropenic patients. Ann Intern Med. 1988;108:289–92.
161. Pizzo PA. Diagnosis and management of infectious disease problems in the child with malignant disease. In: Rubin RH, Young LS, eds. Clinical Approach to Infection in the Compromised Host. 2nd ed. New York: Plenum Medical; 1988:433–66.
162. Lopez-Berestein G. Liposomes as carriers of antimicrobial agents. Antimicrob Agents Chemother. 1987;31:675–8.
163. Sculier JP, Coune A, Meunier F, et al. Pilot study of amphotericin B entrapped into sonicated liposomes in cancer patients with fungal infections. Eur J Cancer Clin Oncol. 1988;24:527–38.
164. Meunier F, Klastersky J. Recent developments in prophylaxis and therapy of invasive fungal infections in granulocytopenic cancer patients. Eur J Cancer Clin Oncol. 1988;24:539–43.
165. Meunier F. Prevention of opportunistic mycoses in immunocompromised patients. Rev Infect Dis. 1987;9:408–16.
166. Fainstein V, Bodey GP, Elting L, et al. Amphotericin B or ketoconazole therapy of fungal infections in neutropenic patients. Antimicrob Agents Chemother. 1987;31:11–5.
167. Saag MS, Dismukes WE. Azole antifungal agents: Emphasis on new triazoles. Antimicrob Agents Chemother. 1988;32:1–8.
168. Dorski DI, Crumpacker CS. Drugs five years later: Acyclovir. Ann Intern Med. 1987;107:859–74.
169. Notter DT, Grossman PL, Rosenberg SA, et al. Infections in patients with Hodgkin's disease: A clinical study of 300 consecutive adult patients. Rev Infect Dis. 1980;2:761–801.
170. Bishop JF, Schimpff SC, Diggs CH, et al. Infections during intensive chemotherapy for non-Hodgkin's lymphoma. Ann Intern Med. 1981;95:549–55.
171. Schimpff SC, O'Connel MJ, Greene WH, et al. Infections in 92 splenectomized patients with Hodgkin's disease. Am J Med. 1975;59:695–701.
172. Ampel NM, Wing EJ. Legionellosis in the compromised host. In: Rubin RH, Young LS, eds. Clinical Approach to Infection in the Compromised Host. 2nd ed. New York: Plenum Medical; 1988:305–19.
173. Muder RR, Yu VL, Woo AH, et al. Mode of transmission of *Legionella pneumophila*. Arch Intern Med. 1986;146:1607–12.
174. Young LS, Armstrong D, Blevins A, et al. *Nocardia asteroides* infection complicating neoplastic disease. Am J Med. 1971;50:356–67.
175. Young LS. Clinical aspects of pneumocystosis in man: Epidemiology, clinical manifestations, diagnostic approaches, and sequelae. In: Young LS, ed. *Pneumocystis carinii* Pneumonia: Pathogenesis, Diagnosis, Treatment. v. 22. New York: Marcel Dekker; 1984:139–68.
176. Hugues WT, Rivera GK, Schell MJ, et al. Successful intermittent chemoprophylaxis for *Pneumocystis carinii* pneumonitis. N Engl J Med. 1987; 316:1627–32.
177. Luft BJ, Remington JS. Toxoplasmosis of the central nervous system. In: Remington JS, Swartz MN, eds. Current Clinical Topics in Infectious Diseases. v. 6. New York: McGraw-Hill; 1985:315–58.
178. Longworth DL, Weller PF. Hyperinfection syndrome with strongyloidiasis. In: Remington JS, Swartz MN, eds. Current Clinical Topics in Infectious Diseases. v. 7. New York: McGraw-Hill; 1986:1–26.
179. Brunell PA, Taylor-Wideman J, Geiser FS, et al. Risk of herpes zoster in children with acute leukemia: Varicella vaccine compared with history of chickenpox. Pediatrics. 1986;77:53–6.
180. Bookman MA, Longo DL. Concomitant illness in patients treated for Hodgkin's disease. Cancer Treat Rev. 1986;13:77–111.
181. Gerson AA, Steinberg SP, Gelb L, et al. Live attenuated varicella vaccine use in immunocompromised children and adults. Pediatrics. 1986;73:757–62.
182. Lawrence R, Gershon AA, Holzman R, et al. The risk of zoster after varicella vaccination in children with leukemia. N Engl J Med. 1988;318:543–8.
183. Stover DE, Zaman MB, Hadju SI, et al. Bronchoalveolar lavage in the diagnosis of diffuse pulmonary infiltrates in the immunocompromised host. Ann Intern Med. 1984;101:1–7.
184. Kovatch AL, Jardine DS, Dowling JN, et al. Legionellosis in children with leukemia in relapse. Pediatrics. 1984;73:811–5.
185. Armstrong D, Polsky B. Central nervous system infections in the compromised host. In: Rubin RH, Young LS, eds. Clinical Approach to Infection in the Compromised Host. 2nd ed. New York: Plenum Medical; 1988:165–91.
186. Dismukes WE, Cloud G, Gallis HA, et al. Treatment of cryptococcal meningitis with combination amphotericin B and flucytosine for four as compared with six weeks. N Engl J Med. 1987;317:334–41.
187. Miliauskas JR, Webber BL. Disseminated varicella at autopsy in children with cancer. Cancer. 1984;53:1518–25.
188. Cohen PR, Kurzrock R. Sweet's syndrome and malignancy. Am J Med. 1987;82:1120–6.
189. Filice GA, Simpson GL. Management of nocardia infections. In: Remington JS, Swartz MN, eds. Current Clinical Topics in Infectious Diseases. v. 5. New York: McGraw-Hill; 1984:49–64.
190. Young LS. Treatment and prevention of *Pneumocystis carinii* infection. In: Young LS, eds. *Pneumocystis carinii* Pneumonia: Pathogenesis, Diagnosis, Treatment. v. 22. New York: Marcel Dekker; 1984:175–91.
191. Ruskin J. Newer developments in diagnosis and treatment of pneumocystis infections. In: Remington JS, Swartz MN, eds. Current Clinical Topics in Infectious Diseases. v. 7. New York: McGraw-Hill; 1986:194–215.
192. Meunier F, Van der Auwera P. Pneumococcal diseases. In: Balows A, Hausler WJ, Lennette EH, eds. Laboratory Diagnosis of Infectious Diseases. New York: Springer-Verlag; 1988:420–34.
193. Ma P. Cryptosporidiosis and immune enteropathy: A review. In: Remington JS, Swartz MN, eds. Current Clinical Topics in Infectious Diseases. v. 8. New York: McGraw-Hill; 1987:99–153.
194. Whitley RJ, Haynes R, Bryson Y, et al. Vidarabine therapy of varicella in immunosuppressed patients. Pediatrics. 1982;101:125–31.
195. Whitley R, Soong SJ, Dolin R, et al. Early vidarabine therapy to control the complications of herpes zoster in immunosuppressed patients. N Engl J Med. 1982;307:971–5.
196. Whitley RJ, Alford CA, Hirsch MS, et al. Vidarabine versus acyclovir therapy in herpes simplex encephalitis. N Engl J Med. 1986;314:144–9.
197. Rothman AL, Cheeseman SH, Nusinoff Lehrman S, et al. Herpes simplex encephalitis in a patient with lymphoma: Relapse following acyclovir therapy. JAMA. 1988;259:1056–7.
198. Nyerges G, Meszner Z, Gyarmati E, et al. Acyclovir prevents dissemination of varicella in immunocompromised children. J Infect Dis. 1988;157:309–13.
199. Wildiers J, de Clercq E. Oral (E)-5(2-bromovinyl)-2′-deoxyuridine treatment of severe herpes zoster in cancer patients. Eur J Cancer Clin Oncol. 1984;29:471–6.
200. De Clercq E. Antiviral chemotherapy: Potential drugs for the treatment of severe virus infection. In: Vincent JL, ed. Update in Intensive Care and Emergency Medicine. v. 3. New York: Springer-Verlag; 1987:77–85.
201. Winston DJ, Haas A, Gale RP, et al. Intravenous immunoglobulins as therapeutic agents. Ann Intern Med. 1987;107:367–82.

288. INFECTIONS IN PARENTERAL DRUG ABUSERS

JAY F. DOBKIN

Recognition and management of the numerous infectious complications traditionally associated with parenteral drug abuse have been overshadowed and complicated by the advent of the acquired immunodeficiency syndrome (AIDS) and the range of opportunistic infections it brings. Since 50 percent or more of parenteral drug abusers in several cities in the northeast United States have been infected by the human immunodeficiency virus (HIV),[1] and since addicts almost anywhere are at substantial risk of such infection, virtually any illness in a parenteral drug abuser raises the possibility of an HIV-related process.

Infectious complications of parenteral drug abuse are linked by the use of injection equipment contaminated by environmental organisms or blood-borne pathogens from previous users of the "works." An estimated one-fourth of hospital admissions of drug abusers are for infections.[2] Traditionally encountered are bacterial and fungal sepsis, endocarditis with its embolic complications, hematogenous infection of bones and joints, and an array of local soft tissue and vascular infections. The unusual organisms associated in the past with endocarditis and osteomyelitis in drug abusers were attributable to environmental contamination[3] rather than to altered immunity, even though prior to AIDS several reports of immune dysfunction in addicts had appeared.[4–6]

In the AIDS era the differential diagnosis for many clinical presentations in parenteral drug abusers is vastly broadened (Table 1). Correspondingly, the relatively straightforward approach to AIDS manifestations in nonaddicts is complicated in addicts by the numerous non-AIDS etiologies for such problems as diffuse lung disease, altered mental status, or central nervous system (CNS) masses. For a given illness in a potential AIDS victim who is a drug abuser, the difficulty of diagnosis, need for invasive procedures, requirement for multiple empiric treatments, and hence costs are likely to be greater than in nonaddicts.

TABLE 1. Clinical Syndromes in Drug Abusers: AIDS vs. Non-AIDS-Related Etiologies

Syndrome	*AIDS-Related*	*Non-AIDS-Related*
Diffuse pulmonary infiltrates, dyspnea, hypoxia	*P. carinii* pneumonia Kaposi sarcoma Lymphoid interstitial pneumonia Cytomegalovirus pneumonia	Septic pulmonary emboli Disseminated tuberculosis Opiate pulmonary edema Sepsis with shock lung Talc granulomatosis
Altered mental status	AIDS dementia Cryptococcal meningitis	Drug/alcohol intoxication or withdrawal Bacterial meningitis
Focal CNS lesion	Toxoplasmosis Cryptococcoma Lymphoma	Septic embolic infarct Brain abscess Tuberculoma Hemorrhage
Skin or mucous membrane petechiae/purpura	Idiopathic thrombocytopenic purpura	Sepsis and/or DIC Endocarditis
Lymphadenopathy	HIV adenopathy	Regional adenopathy from injecting (axillary, groin, neck)
Hepatitis	Cytomegalovirus Epstein-Barr syndrome	Viral hepatitis: A, B, delta, non-A/non-B

Abbreviation: DIC: disseminated intravascular coagulation.

Heroin has been the most widely abused agent during the post-World War II and especially post-Vietnam war surge of intravenous drug abuse. In recent years cocaine abuse has increased dramatically, often combined with heroin as a "speedball." A wide variety of other drugs are injected as well, with some clinically important geographic variation such as the use of tripelennamine with pentazocine ("Ts and blues") in the midwest.

In general the infectious complications of parenteral drug abuse derive from unsterile injection equipment and techniques. *Pseudomonas* infections may be more common in those injecting "Ts and blues" because this mixture, unlike heroin, does not require boiling to dissolve it before injection. Cocaine injection may predispose to necrotizing, mixed anaerobic soft tissue infection because of its capacity to constrict small vessels leading to local necrosis, especially after intradermal injection ("skin popping").

HOST DEFENSES

Despite numerous demonstrations of immunologic dysfunction induced by opiates in animal models or with human cells in vitro,[4,5,7,8] the clinical significance of these findings is unclear and appears to play at most a secondary pathogenic role compared with repeated, unsterile injections. In addition to producing local infection, the effect of repeated needle puncture has been held to increase skin carriage of *Staphylococcus aureus*[9] although this finding was not reproduced by others.[10] Polyclonal hypergammaglobulinemia is a frequent finding, probably related to recurrent stimulation by injected foreign antigens or to chronic alcoholic or viral liver disease. Although decreased number and in vitro function of T cells has been associated with intravenous opiate abuse, the occurrence of opportunistic infections typical of T-cell deficiency was rare prior to the AIDS epidemic.

Many addicts abuse several types of drugs besides opiates with possible immunodepressant capacity such as marijuana,[11] phencyclidine,[12] and alcohol.[13] Alcohol has direct effects on granulocyte function acutely and bone marrow function with chronic abuse.[14] Use of antibiotics, either prescribed or self-administered, is common[15,16] and may alter the defense function of the normal bacterial flora as well as predisposing toward colonization and infection with more resistant organisms like methicillin-resistant *S. aureus* (MRSA).[17]

Associated diseases, especially hepatitis and cirrhosis from alcohol or viral hepatitis, may lead to immune dysfunction involving hyperglobulinemia, depressed delayed hypersensitivity, and phagocytic abnormalities. Finally, the living conditions and environment associated with drug abuse, including poor nutrition and hygiene, frequent homelessness, and imprisonment, are important factors in exposure to agents such as *Mycobacterium tuberculosis*.

SOFT TISSUE INFECTIONS

Local skin infections, including cellulitis, superficial abscesses, and areas of deep subcutaneous suppuration, often develop at sites of needle injection. These lesions may be the result of directly inoculating microorganisms, the carrying of skin flora into the tissue, or secondary infection of areas traumatized by sclerosing drugs or diluents. Gram-positive aerobes such as *Streptococcus pyogenes* and *S. aureus* are the commonest organisms implicated in these infections, although a wide range of gram-negative bacilli and anaerobes have also been encountered, and polymicrobial infection is common.[18,19] Staphylococci of the same phage type as the infecting strain have often been recovered from nasal or skin carriage sites, indicating that the drug abuser is usually infected with his own flora rather than by microbially contaminated drugs.[3,9,19,20]

The severest soft tissue infections associated with drug abuse include necrotizing processes such as necrotizing fasciitis, in which small entry wounds or local infections give rise to extensive, spreading necrosis of underlying fascia and sometimes muscle or other structures. Initial manifestations may be indistinguishable from simple cellulitis, but severe pain and systemic toxicity are important distinguishing features. Development of cutaneous necrosis, crepitus, or the observation of soft tissue gas by x-ray film are more dramatic but often late signs. Many infections are of mixed etiology, with *S. pyogenes, S. aureus,* enteric gram-negative rods, and anaerobes often involved. Drug abuse accounted for almost one-third of necrotizing fasciitis cases in a recent series[21] and a specific association with injection of cocaine has been suggested.[22] Early detection and aggressive surgical management of this entity are crucial in preventing amputation or death.

BACTEREMIC INFECTIONS

Bacteremia

Blood stream infections constitute a major cause of morbidity and mortality in drug abusers. Unsterile injection accounts for the introduction of a wide array of microorganisms into the circulation. Other factors such as damage of the tricuspid valve by injected particulates and direct needle trauma to blood vessels are probably involved in the pathogenesis of such characteristic entities as tricuspid endocarditis and mycotic aneurysms.[2] Various associations of particular drugs with an increased frequency of endocarditis have been suggested: cocaine use in one report was strongly predictive of this diagnosis while amphetamine use was not.[23] Others, however, have associated amphetamines with increased risk of endocarditis.[2]

Although geographic variation in the microbial species involved in blood stream infections of addicts has been frequently documented, staphylococci continue to be the predominant pathogens. Streptococci, enteric gram-negative rods, *Pseudomonas* species, *Candida*, and an assortment of bizarre organisms account for the remaining cases. Contamination of the drugs or injection equipment has been reported as the likely source for some organisms like *Pseudomonas*, while skin carriage appears to be the source for others like *S. aureus*. The rising frequency of methicillin-resistant *S. aureus* infections in drug abusers markedly complicates their therapy and presents hospitals with substantial infection control problems.

Bacteremia has been found in 15 percent of hospital admissions of narcotic addicts. Soft tissue infection and endocarditis were the most frequent sources.[16] *Staphylococcus aureus* was recovered in 57 percent of patients, all gram-positive cocci together representing 80 percent of cases in this series.[16] Polymicrobial bacteremia is common in drug abusers and may imply a poorer prognosis.[24] In hospitalized drug abusers, nosocomial bacteremia may indicate that the patient is manipulating the intravenous line to inject drugs brought in by visitors. Restriction of visitors or removal of the iv line if possible may be beneficial.

Endocarditis

Diagnosis. Endocarditis occurs in a variety of forms in drug abusers, but two presentations predominate: *S. aureus* infection of the tricuspid valve, presenting with stigmata of septic pulmonary embolization; and left-sided endocarditis due to staphylococci, streptococci, or various other organisms, leading to systemic embolization and valve destruction.

Tricuspid valve infection accounts for 50 percent[27] to 78 percent[24] of endocarditis episodes in drug abusers. As originally described, this was a frequently lethal syndrome prominently complicated by systemic septic complications.[25,26] Recent reports, however, uniformly describe a relatively benign process with minimal sepsis beyond the pulmonary bed and a mortality rate of 10 percent.[27] Widespread appreciation of this entity and early hospitalization and treatment of febrile drug abusers probably accounts for the improvement.

The aortic and mitral valves are each infected in 15–20 percent of cases, and bivalvular disease or concomitant right- and left-sided endocarditis occurs in about 5 percent. Less than 1 percent of patients have isolated pulmonic valve infection.[27] *Staphylococcus aureus* is the most frequently isolated organism in addicts with endocarditis (about 60 percent of cases). Streptococci, including groups A, D, and G as well as viridans, are next most common. *Pseudomonas aeruginosa, Serratia marcescens*, and other aerobic gram-negative bacilli (10 percent), *Candida* sp. (5 percent), and miscellaneous bacteria (5 percent) comprise the remainder of identified pathogens.[24,27] In some reports, infecting species are strongly associated with tricuspid (89 percent *S. aureus*) or left-sided (60 percent streptococci) valves.[24] Unusual organisms include *Bacillus* sp., diphtheroids, *P. cepacia, P. maltophilia, Acinetobacter* sp., microaerophilic streptococci, various *Neisseria* species, and *Eikenella corrodens*. Polymicrobial endocarditis, especially common in addicts with *P. aeruginosa* infection, occurs in 5 percent of cases, and culture-negative endocarditis has been observed in 5–10 percent, often due to prior antibiotics. Bilateral endocarditis also may be associated with unusual pathogens like *P. aeruginosa*.[27]

Left-sided endocarditis is frequently associated with underlying valvular damage, as in nonaddicts. Clinical features of the disease are similar as well: systemic embolization, cutaneous stigmata, and valve destruction leading to heart failure in a large proportion of cases. Skin lesions, especially multiple petechiae and Janeway lesions may be early and virtually diagnostic findings of left-sided staphylococcal endocarditis in a febrile drug abuser with a heart murmur.

Tricuspid valve infection may be a distinctive process with a characteristic pattern of septic pulmonary embolization as the hallmark. Illness begins with fever for several days followed by symptoms of pulmonary embolization including dry cough, dyspnea, and pleuritic chest pain. Over a few days initially normal or nondiagnostic chest x-ray films reveal successive crops of bilateral infiltrates, which may evolve to cavitation. Coincident with the evolving chest x-ray pattern, the cough may become purulent or bloody, and the same bacterial strain may be recovered from sputum as from blood cultures. Patients can follow either a benign or complicated course. Peripheral emboli that cavitate near the pleura can lead to empyema or pyopneumothorax.[28] Recurrent bouts of embolization from the right heart may initiate the entire process all over again. The murmur of tricuspid insufficiency is often absent on presentation,[2,24] and its characteristic increased intensity with inspiration is infrequently detectable in otherwise well-documented cases.

Endocarditis involving any valve may present with only fever and chills.[2] The high frequency of abnormal chest x-ray films and arterial blood gas values in intravenous drug abusers further obscures the diagnosis.[29] Often the distinction between tricuspid endocarditis and *S. aureus* bacteremia in a drug abuser can be made only by documenting continuous bacteremia and an abnormal echocardiogram. Subtle features of left-sided endocarditis such as hematuria or initially small peripheral embolic skin lesions must be carefully sought in febrile drug abusers to avoid the pitfall of assuming the presence of tricuspid and therefore "benign" endocarditis.

Echocardiographic diagnosis of tricuspid endocarditis has a reported sensitivity as low as 40 or 50 percent[24] and as high as 90 percent.[30] Even a clearly positive study may be misleading, however, since residual vegetations from a prior endocarditis episode may be present in a febrile or bacteremic drug abuser.[31]

Since *S. aureus* and gram-negative bacilli may quickly seed to virtually any organ, patients with endocarditis may also present initially with complaints or areas of suppurative involvement that direct attention away from the heart. Examples include brain abscess or meningitis, septic arthritis or osteomyelitis, endophthalmitis, septic pulmonary infarcts, lung abscess, empyema, mycotic aneurysms, or a deep soft tissue or visceral abscess.

Medical Therapy. The urgency for initiating antibiotic therapy in a parenteral drug abuser with suspected endocarditis is determined by the clinical features of each case. In addicts, as with other patients, the greatest urgency is produced by left-sided endocarditis. Patients with syndromes suggesting systemic embolization should be presumed to have aortic or mitral involvement and should be treated aggressively, with cardiac monitoring strongly advised. Initial therapy for presumed left-sided endocarditis in drug abusers must include coverage for *S. aureus* with either a semisynthetic penicillinase-resistant penicillin (oxacillin or nafcillin) and/or vancomycin. Single agent therapy is effective for *S. aureus* endocarditis.[32,33] Addition of an aminoglycoside is reasonable, especially in a critically ill patient pending blood culture results. Gram-negative bacilli may be recovered from the blood. In addition, several days of aminoglycosides appears to produce more rapid blood stream clearance and defervescence in addicts with staphylococcal endocarditis.[33]

If left-sided disease seems unlikely, the urgency to treat depends on the evidence for right-sided involvement. Clearly established tricuspid endocarditis syndromes call for prompt antistaphylococcal therapy. In many cases of febrile drug abusers, there is little evidence on which to distinguish those with bacteremic disease from those without.[34] Some authors recommend routine antibiotic coverage at least for staphylococci in this setting, with treatment stopped if blood cultures are found negative.[2] Observation without antibiotics also appears reasonable in well-selected cases. Endocarditis therapy in drug abusers requires 4–6 weeks, as for other patients. In the tricuspid endocarditis–septic embolization syndrome, the resolution of intrathoracic complications is often the limiting factor. For the patient with *S. aureus* bacteremia but no evidence for endocarditis or other visceral seeding, the length of treatment is controversial. Some recommend 2 weeks of therapy, provided antibodies to teichoic acid are not elevated.[35] Prolongation of therapy may be warranted in some cases, especially if close observation following hospitalization is unlikely.

In hospitals where methicillin-resistant *S. aureus* is encountered, vancomycin 2 g/day may be appropriate initial therapy until blood culture susceptibility studies are completed, particularly for patients with left-sided endocarditis.[36,37] First-generation cephalosporins can be used in methicillin-sensitive but not methicillin-resistant *S. aureus* endocarditis. Intramuscular cephalosporins may be useful when vascular access is difficult.[38] When endocarditis is found to be due to methicillin-resistant *S. aureus*, there are no well-accepted alternatives to vancomycin. Regimens under evaluation include one of the fluoroquinolones such as ciprofloxacin, with or without rifampin, or teichoplanin.

Surgical Therapy. Indications for surgical intervention in drug abusers with endocarditis do not differ from those of other patients. Tricuspid endocarditis only occasionally necessitates valve surgery. Potential indications include resistant bacteria, fungal infection, or inability to clear the blood of an apparently sensitive organism after 10–14 days of appropriate antibiotics.[39,40]

Two aspects of valve surgery for endocarditis in drug abusers are controversial. First, there is a high frequency of prosthetic valve infection and death in those who continue to abuse drugs.[41] Therefore, when the patient has recently abused drugs and the indications for surgery are marginal, deferral of the procedure may be in the patient's interest. Second, the prospect of valve replacement in a potentially HIV-infected patient raises several issues: should the procedure be done at all, given the prognosis of AIDS; does HIV infection predispose the patient to serious surgical complications; and must the surgeon know the HIV status in order to take appropriate precautions? HIV seropositivity alone should not preclude potentially life-saving surgery. Patients at the asymptomatic stage of HIV infection can tolerate such surgery well, and their prognosis is at least equal to many patients with other severe chronic diseases who undergo open heart procedures. Patients with advanced manifestations of AIDS clearly must be evaluated individually. Preoperative testing for HIV should not, however, determine eligibility for surgery.

If valve surgery is to be done, careful attention should be paid to correcting potential sites of postoperative bacterial seeding of the prosthesis, especially infected skin lesions and carious teeth.

Peripheral Vascular Infections

Any vessel used for injection may become infected. As arm veins become scarred and unusable, addicts will utilize the femoral, axillary, and neck vessels, usually injecting into the large veins in these sites. Occasionally an artery is punctured deliberately or inadvertently. The range of vascular lesions is broad: hematoma, thrombosis, septic thrombophlebitis, mycotic aneurysm, and traumatic arteriovenous fistula.[42–44] Pain and fever are common findings, which, along with bacteremia, should suggest these diagnostic possibilities. As in other syndromes in drug abusers, gram-positive cocci are the predominant pathogens, with a range of gram-negatives and other organisms encountered as well.

If the involved vessels are deep, as in the groin or neck, little evidence of an otherwise severe infection may be visible. Persistent fever and tenderness in the groin may represent an aneurysm proceeding toward rupture. Similarly, differentiation of abscess in the neck from mycotic aneurysm must often be made radiologically.[45] Prompt diagnosis and surgical repair are vital. Septic pulmonary embolization appears to occur with high frequency in septic thrombophlebitis and may therefore closely mimic tricuspid endocarditis.[24] Drug abusers on hemodialysis may inject into the vascular access site, leading to recurrent sepsis or septic thrombophlebitis with pulmonary emboli.[46]

Peripheral veins in addicts are commonly scarred and thrombosed. In the setting of possible septic phlebitis, any fluctuant, inflamed, or tender peripheral venous site should be aspirated by needle. The recovery of frank pus is diagnostic and may indicate the need for open surgical drainage or resection of the vein. Treatment includes parenteral antibiotics as well as local drainage if a focus is identified. Anticoagulation is not routinely advised. In the case of lower extremity deep venous obstruction, which is encountered after groin injection, the risks of short-term anticoagulation may be outweighed by the embolic threat.

PULMONARY INFECTIONS

The lungs of drug abusers are assaulted by the foreign matter they inject, by septic emboli and by a higher frequency of tuberculosis, aspiration pneumonia, and lung abscess.[47] Pneumonia was the single commonest diagnosis (38 percent) in a series of febrile drug abusers.[34] Baseline abnormalities of chest x-ray films and arterial blood gases may cause diagnostic confusion in febrile addicts. Tuberculosis is a major problem in HIV-infected drug abusers, since the poor and minority communities from which they come typically have several times the tuberculosis incidence of more affluent areas. Homelessness and therapeutic noncompliance in this group further compounds the problem. The pulmonary complications of AIDS, especially *Pneumocystis carinii* pneumonia must also be considered in febrile addicts with pulmonary abnormalities. Initial management of such patients will often involve multiple drugs to cover several likely pathogens. Some agents such as trimethoprim–sulfamethoxazole provide activity against *P. carinii*, and many gram-negative rods. Pentamidine, however, offers only *Pneumocystis* activity. Empiric coverage for tuberculosis may be needed in critically ill patients or those unable to produce sputum for examination.

CENTRAL NERVOUS SYSTEM AND EYE INFECTIONS

Although bacterial meningitis due to the common pathogens may occur in drug abusers, *S. aureus* endocarditis leading to meningitis must be strongly suspected when an addict presents with clinical or cerebrospinal fluid features of meningitis. Antistaphylococcal therapy should be included in the initial regimen. Often patients with left-sided endocarditis have "sterile" meningitis, reflecting the finding on computed tomography (CT) scan of multiple enhancing, cerebral lesions. Although initially confused with frank abscesses, these CT lesions probably represent septic embolic infarction and usually resolve on antibiotic therapy alone without surgical drainage.[48] Other etiologies for meningitis include tuberculosis, cryptococcal infection, and leaking mycotic aneurysm. The differential diagnosis for encephalopathy includes drug intoxication or overdose and alcohol-induced hepatic coma.

Prominent headache or microscopic bleeding in the spinal fluid in an addict with suspected left-sided endocarditis should prompt consideration of mycotic aneurysm. CNS mass lesions detected on CT scan or presenting with focal signs may represent frank brain abscess associated with aspiration lung abscess or infrequently with endocarditis. Additional considerations are tuberculoma, intracerebral bleeding from a mycotic aneurysm, and the various mass lesions associated with AIDS: toxoplasmosis, cryptococcosis, lymphoma, and nocardiosis.

Fungal endophthalmitis has been recognized for many years as a complication of illicit drug injection.[49] A number of reports from France, Spain, and Australia have described disseminated *Candida* infection with eye, bone, and skin lesions in heroin users. These reports underscore the role of contamination rather than immunoincompetence in the pathogenesis of this process.[50]

BONE AND JOINT INFECTIONS

Hematogenous seeding of both bacteria and fungi to vascular areas, such as the axial skeleton and joints, is a common problem in drug abusers. The original source of these infections may be inapparent or represent a metastatic complication of endocarditis. Addicts are particularly prone to osteomyelitis of the cervical and lumbosacral spine and septic arthritis in unusual areas, such as the sternoclavicular and sternoarticular joints and pubic symphysis.[51–53] The wrist, knee, shoulder, hip, and sacroiliac joints can also be involved. Vertebral osteomyelitis may extend to the epidural space and cause abscess formation with cord compression. Bone and joint infections in addicts are caused by virtually any organism, including *S. aureus* and gram-negative bacilli (particularly *P. aeruginosa*). Some infections are polymicrobial. Tuberculous spondylitis must be considered in any drug abuser with spinal destruction seen on x-ray film.[54] Biopsy is mandatory, since pyogenic infection cannot be ruled out even with radiologic features of Pott's disease.

Contiguous osteomyelitis occurs frequently in "skin poppers" or others with chronic cutaneous ulcers on the extremities. Any organism in the environment may be involved in this syndrome. Either contiguous or hematogenous osteomyelitis in drug abusers often presents in an indolent fashion, with pain or impaired movement sometimes the only initial manifestation. Fever, signs of sepsis, leukocytosis, and radiologic changes may all be absent. Because of the wide spectrum of bacteria that may be involved (especially aerobic gram-negative bacilli), needle aspiration is warranted in all cases to obtain material for smear and culture. Drug abusers with documented bacteremia and probable hematogenous osteomyelitis should still undergo aspiration or biopsy, since the bone and blood stream infections may represent two separate processes. Infections caused by gram-negative bacilli or fungi often require 4–6 weeks of antibiotics, drainage of the joint, and débridement or resection of infected bone.

A musculoskeletal syndrome, thought to represent a noninfectious hypersensitivity reaction to heroin contaminants ("brown heroin"), can also present with fever, paraspinal myalgias, arthralgias, and periarticular tenderness and swelling.[55]

HEPATITIS

By virtue of exposure to any one of a number of viral pathogens or hepatotoxins, hepatitis is extremely common in drug addicts.[56] After only 2 or 3 years of parenteral drug abuse, approximately 90 percent of addicts demonstrate serum markers of hepatitis B infection.[57,58] Liver biopsy in asymptomatic addicts with chronic transaminase elevations showed evidence of chronic viral hepatitis in 75 percent and alcoholic hepatitis in 16 percent.[57] Delta hepatitis, was shown in a retrospective analysis to have been present in 10 percent of addicts with transaminase elevations in the mid-1970s (42 percent of those with hepatitis B surface antigen).[57] Non-A, non-B hepatitis[57,58] and hepatitis A[59] may play more significant roles in the etiology of hepatic disease in U.S. addicts than previously recognized. Epstein-Barr virus and cytomegalovirus are considerations in possibly HIV-infected addicts.

SUMMARY

AIDS has added substantially to the already complex pattern of infections of intravenous drug abusers. Soft tissue and endovascular infections with *S. aureus* remain common. Methicillin-resistant staphylococci are widespread and must be covered empirically in the severely ill. It is unclear whether HIV infection alters the course of common drug abuse-related infections, but it is apparent that the extent of diagnostic evaluation and the amount of initial empiric therapy for febrile drug abusers has been greatly increased. The importance of effective management of these problems will grow as the AIDS epidemic in the United States becomes increasingly centered on intravenous drug abusers.

REFERENCES

1. Curran JW, Jaffe HW, Hardy AM, et al. Epidemiology of HIV infection in the United States. Science. 1988;239:610–6.
2. Sheagren JN. Endocarditis complicating drug abuse. In: Remington J, Swartz M, eds. Current Clinical Topics in Infectious Diseases, v. 2. New York: McGraw-Hill; 1982:211.
3. Tuazon CU, Hill R, Sheagren JN. Microbiologic study of street heroin and injection paraphernalia. J Infect Dis. 1974;129:327–29.
4. Brown SM, Stimmel B, Taub RN, et al. Immunologic dysfunction in heroin addicts. Arch Intern Med. 1974;134:1001–6.
5. McDonough RJ, Madden JJ, Falek A, et al. Alteration of T and null lymphocyte frequencies in the peripheral blood of human opiate addicts: in vivo evidence for opiate receptor sites on T lymphocytes. J Immunol. 1980;125:2539–43.
6. Cherubin CE, Millian SJ. Serologic investigations in heroin addicts: I. Syphilis, lymphogranuloma venereum, herpex simplex, and Q fever. Ann Intern Med. 1968;69:739–42.
7. Tubaro E, Borelli G, Croce C, et al. Effect of morphine on resistance to infection. J Infect Dis. 1983;148:656–66.
8. Peterson PK, Sharp B, Gekker G, et al. Opioid-mediated suppression of interferon gamma production by cultured peripheral blood mononuclear cells. J Clin Invest. 1987;80:824–31.
9. Tuazon CU, Sheagren JN. Increased rate of carriage of *Staphylococcus aureus* among narcotic addicts. J Infect Dis. 1974;129:725–7.
10. Berman DS, Schaefler S, Simberkoff M, Rahal JJ. *Staphylococcus aureus* colonization in intravenous drug abusers, dialysis patients, and diabetics. J Infect Dis. 1987;155:829–31.

11. Cabral GA, Lockmuller JC, Mishkin EM. Delta 9 tetrahydrocannabinol decreases alpha/beta interferon response to herpes simplex virus type 2 in the B6C3F1 mouse. Proc Soc Exp Biol Med. 1986;181:305–11.
12. Khansari N, Whitten HD, Fudenberg HH. Phencyclidine-induced immunodepression. Science. 1984;225:76–8.
13. Brown B, Kozel NJ, Meyers MB, DuPont RL. Use of alcohol by addict and nonaddict populations. Am J Psychiatr. 1973;130:599–601.
14. MacGregor RR. Alcohol and immune defense. JAMA. 1986;256:1474–9.
15. Novick DM, Ness GL. Abuse of antibiotics by abusers of parenteral heroin or cocaine. South Med J. 1984;77:302–3.
16. Crane LR, Levine DP, Zervos MJ, Cummings G. Bacteremia in narcotic addicts at the Detroit Medical Center. I. Microbiology, epidemiology, risk factors, and empiric therapy. Rev Infect Dis. 1986;8:364–73.
17. Sarovalatz LD, Markowitz N, Arking L, et al. Methicillin resistant *Staphylococcus aureus*. Epidemiologic observations during a community-acquired outbreak. Ann Intern Med. 1982;96:11–16.
18. Webb D, Thadepalli H. Skin and soft tissue infections from intravenous abuse of drugs. West J Med. 1979;130:200–4.
19. Orangio GR, Pitlick SD, Della Latta P, et al. Soft tissue infections in parenteral drug abusers. Ann Surg. 1984;199:97–100.
20. Tuazon CU, Sheagren JN. Staphylococcal endocarditis in parenteral drug abusers: source of the organism. Ann Intern Med. 1975;82:788–90.
21. Sudarsky LA, Laschinger JC, Coppa GF, Spencer FC. Improved results from a standardized approach in treating patients with necrotizing fasciitis. Ann Surg. 1987;206:661–5.
22. Jacobson JM, Hirschman SZ. Necrotizing fasciitis complicating intravenous drug abuse. Arch Intern Med. 1982;142:634–5.
23. Chambers HF, Morris DL, Tauber MG, Modin G. Cocaine use and the risk for endocarditis in intravenous drug users. Ann Intern Med. 1987;106:833–6.
24. Levine DP, Crane LR, Zervos MJ. Bacteremia in narcotic addicts at the Detroit Medical Center: II. Infectious endocarditis: a prospective, comparative study. Rev Infect Dis. 1986;8:374–96.
25. Olsson RA, Romansky MJ. Staphylococcal triscupid endocarditis in heroin addicts. Ann Intern Med. 1962;57:755–62.
26. Hussey HH, Kelliher TF, Schaeffer BF, et al. Septicemia and bacterial endocarditis resulting from heroin addiction. JAMA. 1944;126:535–8.
27. Reisberg BE. Infective endocarditis in the narcotic addict. Prog Cardiovasc Dis. 1979;22:193–204.
28. Jaffe RB, Koschmann EB. Septic pulmonary emboli. Radiology. 1970;96:527–32.
29. Overland ES, Nolan AJ, Hopewell PC. Alterations of pulmonary function in intravenous drug abusers. Am J Med. 1980;68:231–7.
30. Ginzton LE, Siegel RJ, Criley JM. Natural history of tricuspid valve endocarditis: a two dimensional echocardiographic study. Am J Cardiol. 1982;49:1853–9.
31. Dubois RW, Ginzton LE. Role of echocardiography in suspected infective endocarditis in intravenous drug abusers. Am J Cardiol. 1986;58:649–50.
32. Abrams B, Sklaver A, Hoffman T, et al. Single or combination therapy of staphylococcal endocarditis in intravenous drug abusers. Ann Intern Med. 1979;90:789–91.
33. Korzeniowski D, Sande MA. Combination therapy for *Staphylococcus aureus* endocarditis in patients addicted to parenteral drugs and in non-addicts. A prospective study. Ann Intern Med. 1982;97:496–503.
34. Marantz PR, Linzer M, Feiner CJ, et al. Inability to predict diagnosis in febrile intravenous drug abusers. Ann Intern Med. 1987;106:823–8.
35. Bayer AS. Staphylococcal bacteremia and endocarditis. Arch Intern Med. 1982;142:1169–77.
36. Faville RJ Jr, Zaske DE, Kaplan EL, et al. *Staphylococcus aureus* endocarditis. Combined therapy with vancomycin and rifampin. JAMA. 1978;240:1963–5.
37. Gopal V, Bisno AL, Silverblatt FJ. Failure of vancomycin treatment on *Staphylococcus aureus* endocarditis. JAMA. 1976;236:1604–6.
38. Greenman RL, Arcey SM, Gutterman DA, et al. Twice-daily ceforanide therapy of *Staphylococcus aureus* endocarditis in parenteral drug abusers. Antimicrob Agents Chemother. 1984;25:16–9.
39. Barbour DJ, Roberts WC. Valve excision only versus valve excision plus replacement for active infective endocarditis involving the tricuspid valve. Am J Cardiol. 1986;57:475–8.
40. Stern HJ, Sisto DA, Strom JA, et al. Immediate tricuspid valve replacement for endocarditis. J Thorac Cardiovasc Surg. 1986;91:163–7.
41. Hubbell G, Cheitlin MD, Rapaport E: Presentation, management, and follow-up evaluation of infective endocarditis in drug addicts. Am Heart J. 1981;102:85.
42. Merhar GL, Colley DP, Clark RA, et al. Computed tomographic demonstration of cervical abscess and jugular vein thrombosis; a complication of intravenous drug abuse in the neck. Arch Otolaryngol. 1981;107:313–5.
43. Pace BW, Doscher W, Margolis I. The femoral triangle. A potential death trap for the drug abuser. NY State J Med. 1984;84:596–8.
44. Yeager RA, Hobson RW 2d, Padberg FT, et al. Vascular complications related to drug abuse. J Trauma. 1987;27:305–8.
45. Espiritu MB, Medina JE. Complications of heroin injections of the neck. Laryngoscope. 1980;1111–9.
46. Dobkin JF, Miller MH, Steigbigel NH. Septicemia in patients on chronic hemodialysis. Ann Intern Med. 1978;88:28–33.
47. Pare JP, Fraser RG, Hogg JC, et al. Pulmonary "mainline" granulomatosis: talcosis of intravenous methadone abuse. Medicine. 1979;58:229–39.
48. Dobkin JF, Healton EB, Dickinson PCT, et al. Nonspecificity of ring enhancement in "medically cured" brain abscess. Neurology. 1984;34:139–44.
49. Sugar HS, Mandell GH, Shalev J. Metastatic endophthalmitis associated with injection of addictive drugs. Am J Ophthalmol. 1971;71:1055–8.
50. Sorrell TC, Dunlop C, Collignon PJ, et al. Exogenous ocular candidiasis associated with intravenous heroin abuse. Br J Ophthalmol. 1984;68:841–5.
51. Holzman RS, Bishko F. Osteomyelitis in heroin addicts. Ann Intern Med. 1971;75:693–6.
52. Sapico FL, Montgomerie JZ. Vertebral osteomyelitis in intravenous drug abusers: report of three cases and review of the literature. Rev Infect Dis. 1980;2:196–206.
53. Sequeira W, Jones E, Siegel ME, et al. Pyogenic infection of the pubic symphysis. Ann Intern Med. 1982;96:604–6.
54. Forlenza SW, Axelrod JL, Grieco MH. Pott's disease in heroin addicts. JAMA. 1979;241:379–80.
55. Pastan RS, Silverman SL, Goldenberg DL: A musculoskeletal syndrome in intravenous heroin users: association with brown heroin. Ann Intern Med. 1977;87:22.
56. Gelb AM, Mildvan D, Stenger RJ: The spectrum and causes of liver disease in narcotic addicts. Am J Gastroenterol. 1977;67:314.
57. Ponzetto A, Seeff LB, Buskell-Bales Z, et al. Hepatitis B markers in United States drug addicts with special emphasis on the delta hepatitis virus. Hepatology. 1984;4:1111–5.
58. Weller IVD, Cohn D, Sierralta A, et al. Clinical, biochemical, serological, histological, and ultrastructural features of liver disease in drug abusers. Gut. 1984;25:417–23.
59. Hepatitis A among drug abusers. MMWR. 1988;37:297–305.

289. INFECTIONS IN HOMOSEXUAL MEN

HENRY MASUR

Homosexuality as a sexual orientation does not inherently predispose an individual to infection. A variety of mechanical and sociologic factors that are integral parts of the life-styles of many homosexuals do, however, predispose to the greatly augmented risks that certain homosexuals have for developing a broad range of disorders.[1] The spectrum of intestinal and rectal diseases that are uniquely or very frequently recognized in homosexual men has been termed the "gay bowel syndrome" and is described in this chapter.[1–3] Detailed descriptions of the infectious processes caused by individual microorganisms are discussed in other chapters. The acquired immunodeficiency syndrome (AIDS) is described in Chapters 105–111. The epidemic of AIDS has led to a greater emphasis on education about sexually transmitted diseases and "safer" sex practices. This emphasis appears to be modifying the frequency of many of these sexually transmitted diseases.

Specific sexual practices have a particularly important influence on the development of gastrointestinal infection and inflammation in homosexual men. Any practice that facilitates direct or indirect oral–rectal contact will enable rectal and fecal microorganisms to be ingested by the sexual partner. Anilingus, practiced by at least 75 percent of gay men, provides a direct route for rectal flora to be ingested.[4] Anilingus has been specifically identified as a risk factor for the acquisition of hepatitis, gonorrhea, and amebiasis.[5–7] Genital–rectal sex followed by genital–oral sex or genital–rectal intercourse with one partner followed by genital–rectal sex with another partner allows the penis to serve as a vector for indirect transmission of enteric organisms. Fomite transmission may also contribute to enteric infections when unsterile equipment is used for douching, colonic irrigation, or rectal manipulation.

Multiple sexual partners and anonymous sex also facilitate transmission of infection. Anonymity of sexual encounters makes it unlikely that an individual will have any knowledge of the health status of his partner or that his partner can be traced if the homosexual discovers that he has a sexually transmissible disease. Other major factors that complicate the identification of infected individuals are the high frequency of asymptomatic rectal or oropharyngeal processes, such as gonorrhea, syphilis, chlamydia, and herpes simplex, and the lack of sophistication of many physicians in screening, diagnosing, and treating sexually transmissible diseases in homosexual men.

The plethora of microbial processes that are especially associated with homosexuality has acquired new significance since the advent of the human immunodeficiency virus (HIV). These microbial processes may conceivably serve as cofactors for HIV infection by modulating immune function in a way that is permissive to the acquisition of HIV or the replication of this retrovirus after it is acquired.[8] Certain of these pathogens may break down mucosal or epithelial barriers to HIV, thereby enhancing the likelihood that exposure will result in infection.[9] Certain of these pathogens such as herpes simplex, *Salmonella*, and cryptosporidia also acquire enhanced importance when HIV-infected patients become significantly immunosuppressed since at that point they can cause particularly severe or persistent disease.

Rectal symptoms can be caused or exacerbated by trauma. Trauma to the rectum can be caused by multiple partners, by violent behavior, or by foreign objects. Fisting, the practice of inserting a fist into the rectum, sometimes up to the elbow, is a commonly performed sex act, as is the insertion of bottles, bats, and a wide variety of prosthetic devices. Such behavior inflames, erodes, and tears the rectal mucosa, thereby making these surfaces especially susceptible to microorganisms. This behavior can also cause ulcers and perforations that can hemorrhage, cause pain, or lead to a sterile or infected discharge.

Lesbians do not appear to have a substantial increase in the frequency of enteric sexually transmitted diseases.[10] Their relative monogamy and their different range of sexual practices as compared with homosexual men probably explain this decreased susceptibility, although it is important to recognize that female homosexuals have not been so thoroughly studied as have male homosexuals.

PROCTITIS AND PROCTOCOLITIS

Homosexual men with proctitis or proctocolitis usually complain of an acute episode of anorectal pain (about 80 percent) or a change in bowel habits (about 50 percent).[2,3,11] The anorectal pain can be associated with a mucoid or bloody discharge, tenesmus, or abdominal pain. The change in bowel habits can be manifested as either diarrhea or constipation. Sigmoidoscopy may be helpful in identifying chancres, ulcers, condyloma, or rectal tears. Some patients with symptomatic proctitis will have friable to ulcerated mucosa, whereas others will have only mucosal erythema, loss of the vascular pattern, or even normal-appearing mucosa. Almost all patients in the latter two groups will have inflammatory cells on biopsy or on rectal swabs. The distribution of the inflammatory response is diagnostically useful, as are the smears and cultures obtained at proctoscopy. Histologic evidence of proctitis can also be present in 27 percent of asymptomatic homosexual men, and 11–30 percent of asymptomatic men will have one or more enteric pathogens recovered by stool examination.[12,13] All homosexual men with anorectal or intestinal symptoms should undergo anoscopy or sigmoidoscopy with culture and Gram stain of rectal discharge and a serologic test for syphilis. If inflammation is limited to the distal 15 cm, the most likely pathogens are *Neisseria gonorrhoeae*, herpes simplex, and *Chlamydia trachomatis*. If ulcers are present in this area, herpes simplex or syphilis should be considered as well as lymphogranuloma venereum (LGV). Inflammation beyond 15 cm should encourage consideration of *C. trachomatis, Shigella* sp., *Campylobacter* sp., and *Entamoeba histolytica*.[3,12,13]

Early studies of proctitis in homosexual men emphasized traditional sexually transmissible diseases such as syphilis, gonorrhea, and condyloma, or they emphasized noninfectious causes such as trauma.[2] In recent studies of homosexual men with proctitis, the associated infectious agents were herpes simplex (29–30 percent), *N. gonorrhoeae* (13–17 percent), *Treponema pallidum* (11 percent), *Giardia lamblia* (6–7 percent), *E. histolytica* (7–9 percent), *C. trachomatis* (3–15 percent), and *Neisseria meningitidis* (0–2.9 percent).[3,11,13] Two or more pathogens were isolated from 11 percent of the patients. The identification of a pathogen obviously did not unequivocally establish that it was the cause of proctitis. In more than 34–42 percent of the episodes of proctitis, no infectious pathogen could be recognized.

Neisseria Gonorrhoeae

Rectal gonorrhea is usually asymptomatic. About 6–12 percent of homosexuals attending bath houses and 13–55 percent of homosexuals attending sexually transmitted disease clinics have positive rectal cultures, although the frequency of rectal gonorrhea among homosexual men appears to be declining.[14–16] The fraction of infected patients who ultimately develop symptoms is difficult to determine, particularly since other pathogens are often present concurrently. Symptomatic gonococcal proctitis can manifest itself as mild anorectal pain or occasionally as severe pain with mucoid discharge, fever, malaise, or a change in bowel habits, most often constipation.

Diagnostically, sigmoidoscopy can show either normal mucosa or edematous and friable mucosa. On occasion rectal ulcerations can be seen, and rarely, fistulas, strictures, and perirectal abscesses can form. Gram stain of the rectal discharge or mucus can diagnose only 50–85 percent of cases, so careful cultures of the rectum must be performed.[14] Treatment should consist of ceftriaxone, 125 mg or 250 mg im once, or alternatively, spectinomycin hydrochloride, 2.0 g im once. Treatment of concurrent *Chlamydia* is recommended as a routine without necessarily performing a diagnostic test for *Chlamydia*.[16,17] Regardless of the regimen employed, however, follow-up rectal cultures 10–14 days after therapy are indicated. If the proctitis does not respond to the antimicrobial therapy, diagnostic evaluation must be repeated to determine whether the antigonococcal treatment failed, whether another pathogen is present, or whether the patient has been reinfected.

Neisseria Meningitidis

Meningococci can be found in rectal cultures of homosexual men. Some studies have shown meningococci to be more commonly isolated than gonococci are.[18,19] Currently, it is unclear whether or not these meningococci can cause rectal disease or can cause disseminated infection and meningitis. Until these questions are answered, it seems appropriate to treat these isolates by using the same regimens suggested for rectal gonorrhea.

Treponema Pallidum

Although over half of all reported cases of syphilis involved homosexual or bisexual men in the United States in the 1970s, the rate of syphilis in this population appears to be declining in the 1980s.[20–22] Most rectal chancres are probably missed because physicians fail to examine the rectum or fail to recognize the chancre. Most rectal chancres are probably asymptomatic, but tenesmus, urgency, and mucoid or sanguineous discharge have been attributed to these lesions. Superinfection by fecal flora can probably cause cryptitis or small abscesses.

The diagnosis of rectal chancres is based on serology and direct visualization. Rectal chancres are indurated, circular lesions that can be 2–3 cm in diameter, and they may be tender. Darkfield microscopy is not useful for rectal lesions because *T. pallidum* cannot be distinguished morphologically from nonpathogenic spirochetes that are normally present in bowel flora; for anal and perianal lesions this technique is effective.

Treatment of anorectal chancres is benzathine penicillin G, 2.4 million units im once, or tetracycline hydrochloride, 500 mg orally four times daily for 15 days.[17] Serologic response and lesion resolution need to be followed regularly.

Chlamydia Trachomatis

Chlamydia trachomatis is more common in homosexual men than in heterosexuals. Both lymphogranuloma venereum (LGV) and non-LGV serotypes have been reported to occur in 5–16 percent of homosexual men with symptomatic anorectal disease. *Chlamydia* proctitis caused by non-LGV serotypes is usually asymptomatic or mild, similar to that caused by *N. gonorrhoeae*, and is more common than is the proctitis caused by LGV serotypes, which is more severe.[23–25] LGV causes destructive granulomas of the distal colon with boggy, friable mucosa being seen on sigmoidoscopic examination and crypt abscesses, granulomas, and inflammatory cells on biopsy. Fistulas, strictures, and rectal masses may result and produce a gross and microscopic picture similar to Crohn's disease.

Chlamydia proctitis is not reliably documented by skin testing. Some serologic tests are relatively sensitive for diagnostic purposes. The hallmark of diagnosis is culturing the organism in a tissue culture system.

The treatment of choice is tetracycline hydrochloride, 500 mg orally four times daily for at least 7–10 days for non-LGV strains and for 14–28 days for LGV strains.[21]

Shigella and Campylobacter Species

Shigella and *Campylobacter* sp. have been documented to cause proctitis as well as diarrhea.[26–29] *Shigella* sp. and *C. jejuni* in particular (and perhaps other *Campylobacter*-like organisms) can cause tenesmus, pain, and a purulent or bloody discharge, which may not be associated with diarrhea. In severe cases of *Shigella* proctitis the mucosa can be friable, hyperemic, and ulcerated. Diagnosis depends on culturing at least three separate specimens.

These bacterial processes may remit without therapy, but specific antimicrobial therapy will hasten resolution of the disease in severe episodes. Shigellosis can be treated with ampicillin (500 mg orally four times daily), chloramphenicol (500 mg orally four times daily), or trimethoprim-sulfamethoxazole (trimethoprim, 80 mg, and sulfamethoxazole, 400 mg orally twice daily) depending on the susceptibility of the organism.[28] *Campylobacter* proctitis will respond to erythromycin (500 mg orally four times daily) for 7 days.[17,29]

Herpes Simplex

Herpes simplex can be cultured from 20–32 percent of homosexual men with anorectal symptoms. Herpes simplex can cause a clinically severe proctitis characterized by fever, anorectal pain, rectal discharge, hematochezia, and inguinal adenopathy, especially at the time of the first episode.[30,31] The pain can be very severe and may be associated with reflex spasm of the anal and urethral sphincters and with sacral root signs manifested by posterior thigh pain or sacral and buttock paresthesias. The pathogenesis of the neurologic complications is not well understood.

Sigmoidoscopic examination can show mild mucosal erythema or severe mucosal friability and ulceration. These lesions are usually confined to the rectum, in contrast to other infectious causes of proctitis when the lesions extend to the sigmoid. Vesicular or pustular lesions may be seen. Histopathology shows multinucleated giant cells or herpetic inclusion bodies in a minority of cases. Viral isolation is a sensitive and definitive method of diagnosis. Tzanck preparations of the scrapings of an ulcer can also be useful. Most isolates have been herpes simplex virus 2 (HSV-2), but a few HSV-1 organisms have been reported. Recurrences of herpetic proctitis occur.

Oral acyclovir (400 mg four times daily for 10 days) will shorten the duration of viral shedding and rectal lesions.[31]

Entamoeba Histolytica

For reasons that are not certain, *Entamoeba histolytica* infections in homosexual men are often asymptomatic.[32–34]

Amebiasis can cause a mild change in bowel habits or a severe enterocolitis or proctitis. In severe cases, patients with amebic proctitis may have fever, tenesmus, severe rectal pain, cramps, a mucopurulent discharge, or rectal bleeding.[32]

Sigmoidoscopic examination can show mild mucosal erythema, but deep perforating ulcers are often seen. The highest yield for demonstrating amebic trophozoites is in fluid aspirated from the ulcers. Amebic proctitis can also be diagnosed by careful examination of at least three stool specimens. Amebic serology is not reliably positive in amebic bowel disease.

Therapy for amebic proctitis or colitis includes both metronidazole (750 mg orally three times daily for 5–10 days) and diiododohydroxyquin (650 mg orally three times daily for 20 days). For life-threatening cases (which rarely occur when amebiasis is acquired by a sexual route) it may be necessary to use dehydroemetine, 1.0–1.5 mg/kg body weight (maximum dose, 90 mg) im once daily for 3–5 days.

Condyloma Acuminata

Anal and rectal warts caused by papillomaviruses can occur in over 50 percent of males who practice anal intercourse. These lesions can cause pruritus or discomfort. Occasionally they become macerated and superinfected, especially when they are rectal in location. Squamous cell anal cancer is strongly associated with a history of genital warts, thus suggesting that papillomavirus infection is a cause of anal cancer.[35]

DIARRHEA

Homosexual men frequently complain of abdominal pain, cramps, bloating, flatulence, nausea, or vomiting.[2,3,21,36] They may notice a change in their bowel habits, with several soft stools per day for long periods of time. Episodic diarrhea also occurs. In some instances an infectious origin can be documented.

Many of the enteric organisms listed in Table 1 can cause diarrhea. In a recent series the frequency of identifiable pathogens in homosexual men with diarrhea were *Campylobacter* species, 23 percent; *Giardia*, 14 percent; herpes simplex virus, 14 percent; *Shigella* species, 11 percent; *Neisseria gonorrhoeae*, 9 percent; *Clostridium difficile* toxin, 6 percent; *Chlamydia* species, 3 percent; cryptosporidia, 3 percent; and *Vibrio parahaemolyticus*, 3 percent. No enteric pathogen could be isolated in 37 percent of patients.[12] There are no pathognomonic symptoms or signs predicting a specific organism as the obvious cause. Certain clinical features do characterize some microorganisms, however.

Giardia lamblia is a small bowel pathogen that is a common cause of diarrhea among homosexuals.[37] The diarrhea is usually copious (often with more than a dozen stools daily) and watery and may be associated with cramps or nausea. Systemic symptoms are unusual. Amebic bowel disease is typically colonic in nature. Mucoid discharge, bloody diarrhea, fever, and prostration characterize severe disease. For patients with mild abdominal complaints or moderate changes in bowel habits, the presence of ameba or *Giardia* in the stool is of uncertain clinical importance, although epidemiologically such reservoirs undoubtedly facilitate spread of these infections and thus merit therapy in the United States.

TABLE 1. Enteric Infections and Trauma in Homosexual Men: The Gay Bowel Syndrome

Etiology	*Common Enteric Manifestations*[a]
Infections	
Bacteria	
N. gonorrhoeae	Proctitis
N. meningitidis	?
T. pallidum	Chancres, proctitis
C. trachomatis	Proctocolitis, strictures, fistulase
Shigella sp.	Proctitis, diarrhea
Salmonella sp.	Diarrhea
Campylobacter sp.	Diarrhea, proctitis
Haemophilus ducreyi	Perianal pain, discharge
Donovanosis	Anal pain, hemorrhage, discharge
Fungi	
Candida sp.	Proctitis
Viruses	
Hepatitis viruses (A, B)	Hepatitis
Herpes simplex	Proctitis, sphincter spasm
Condyloma acuminata	Warts
Protozoa and helminths	
G. lamblia	Diarrhea
E. histolytica	Proctocolitis, diarrhea
Cryptosporidium	Diarrhea
Strongyloides	Abdominal pain, diarrhea
Enterobius vermicularis	Rectal pruritus
Trauma	
Anal fissure	Pain, hemorrhage
Anal fistula	Pain, discharge
Rectal ulcer	Pain, hemorrhage
Rectal tear	Pain, hemorrhage, peritonitis
Perirectal abscess	Pain, fever, sepsis
Colonic perforation	Hemorrhage, peritonitis
Nonspecific proctitis	Pain, discharge
Prolapsed hemorrhoids	Hemorrhage, incontinence, pain

[a] Manifestations of AIDS are excluded.

Entamoeba histolytica can be found in 25–40 percent of homosexual men: half the patients are asymptomatic, and half have enteric symptoms of mild to moderate severity. Extraintestinal manifestations are rare.

Shigella sp. can cause a nonspecific diarrhea that can be mild or fulminant. Often the patient initially has nausea and vomiting followed temporally by colitis symptoms. Fever and prostration can be part of the syndrome. Salmonellosis and *Campylobacter* disease can be associated with diarrhea and constitutional symptoms.

Blastocystis hominis and nonpallidum treponemes are among the microorganisms that can be isolated from the bowel contents of homosexual men: their importance in causing clinical disease is not clear.[38] Cryptosporidia are occasionally recognized as a cause of self-limiting diarrhea in immunocompetent homosexual men.[39] Diagnosis of the origin of the diarrhea depends on careful microbiologic examination of up to three fresh stool specimens. For diagnostically difficult cases, stools should be collected at 3- to 4-day intervals over a period of 10–14 days. Sigmoidoscopy is useful diagnostically, particularly for aspirating fluid from ulcers for parasitologic examination. If the diarrhea is small bowel in nature, aspiration of duodenal contents may be useful in searching for *Giardia* or *Strongyloides*. The string test is rarely helpful, but a small bowel biopsy specimen may show organisms that were not apparent on stool examination or on study of duodenal contents.

Therapy for most of these agents has been indicated in the section on proctitis. Therapy for *Giardia* should be metronidazole (250 mg orally three times daily for 7–10 days) or quinacrine hydrochloride (100 mg orally three times daily for 5–10 days). An empirical trial of metronidazole may be appropriate if microbiologic studies are unrevealing before proceeding to barium studies and endoscopy. Radiologic studies, endoscopy, and biopsies of the small bowel or rectum are usually indicated if a microbiologic cause is not documented so that inflammatory and neoplastic bowel disease can be excluded.

HEPATITIS

Homosexual men have an extraordinary frequency of clinical and subclinical hepatitis B. Serologic evidence suggests that 40–75 percent of homosexual men have hepatitis B antigen or antibody. Activities that abrade rectal mucosa (passive rectal intercourse, insertion of fingers into the rectum, and rectal douching) are more important risk factors than are the number of male partners or years of sexual activity.[30] The natural history and sequelae of hepatitis B are described in Chapter 125. An impression of many clinicians is that chronic hepatitis is relatively common among antigen-positive homosexuals, but that the clinical sequelae of such infection tends to be mild.[31,32]

Hepatitis A infection probably occurs with increased infection in homosexual men. Studies have yielded conflicting results, but when age and epidemiologic trends are considered, the yearly incidence of hepatitis A is probably greater in homosexual men. Cases of hepatitis due to cytomegalovirus or herpes simplex virus are rare in homosexuals and in heterosexuals.

REFERENCES

1. Owen WF. Sexually transmitted diseases and traumatic problems in homosexual men. Ann Intern Med. 1980;92:805–9.
2. Sohn N, Robilotti JG. The gay bowel syndrome. A review of colonic and rectal conditions in 200 male homosexuals. Am J Gastroenterol. 1977;67:478–84.
3. Quinn TC, Stamm WE, Goodell SE, et al. The polymicrobial origin of intestinal infections in homosexual men. N Engl J Med. 1983;309:576–82.
4. Phillips SC, Mildvan D, Williams DC. Sexual transmission on enteric protozoa and helminths in a venereal disease clinic population. N Engl J Med. 1981;305:603–6.
5. Corey L, Holmes KK. Sexual transmission of hepatitis A in homosexual men: Incidence and mechanisms. N Engl J Med. 1980;302:435–8.
6. Owen RL, Hill JL. Rectal and pharyngeal gonorrhea in homosexual man. JAMA. 1972;220:1315–8.
7. Pomerantz BM, Marr JS, Goldman WD. Amebiasis in New York City 1958–1978: Identification of the male homosexual high risk population. Bull NY Acad Med. 1980;56:232–44.
8. Quinn TC, Piot P, McCormick JB, et al. Serologic and immunologic studies in patients with AIDS in North America and Africa—the potential role of infectious agents as co-factors in human immunodeficiency virus infection. JAMA. 1987;257:2617–21.
9. Greenblatt RM, Lukehart SA, Plummer FA. Genital ulceration as a risk factor for human immunodeficiency virus infection. AIDS. 1988;2:47–50.
10. Robertson R, Schacter J. Failure to identify venereal disease in a lesbian population. Sex Transm Dis. 1981;8:75–9.
11. Quinn TC, Corey L, Chaffee RG. Campylobacter proctitis in a homosexual man. Ann Intern Med. 1980;93:458–9.
12. Laughon BE, Druckman DA, Vernon A, et al. Prevalence of enteric pathogens in homosexual men with and without acquired immunodeficiency syndrome. Gastroenterology. 1988;94:984–93.
13. Surawicz CM, Goodell SE, Quinn TC, et al. Spectrum of rectal biopsy abnormalities in homosexual men with intestinal symptoms. Gastroenterology. 1986;91:651–9.
14. Judson FN, Miller KG, Schaffnit TR. Screening for gonorrhea and syphilis in the gay baths—Denver, Colorado. Am J Public Health. 1977;67:740–2.
15. Merino HI, Richards JB. An innovative program of venereal disease casefinding treatment and education. Sex Transm Dis. 1977;4:50–2.
16. Antibiotic-resistant strains of *Neisseria gonorrhoeae*—policy guidelines for detection, management, and control. MMWR. 1987;36(Suppl 5):1S–18S.
17. Centers for Disease Control. Sexually transmitted diseases treatment guidelines. MMWR. 1985;34(Suppl 4):83–6.
18. Faur YC, Weisburd MH, Wilson ME. Isolation of *Neisseria meningitidis* from the genitourinary tract and anal canal. J Clin Microbiol. 1975;2:178–82.
19. Beck A, Flukes JL, Platt DJ. *Neisseria meningitidis* in urogenital infection. Br J Vener Dis. 1974;50:367–9.
20. Centers for Disease Control. Continuing increase in infectious syphilis—United States. MMWR. 1988;37:35–38.
21. Quinn TC. Clinical Approach to infections in homosexual men. Med Clin North Am. 1986;70:611–34.
22. Smith D. Infectious syphilis of the anal canal. Dis Colon Rectum. 1963;6:7–14.
23. Quinn TC, Goodell SE, Mkrtichian E. *Chlamydia trachomatis* proctitis. N Engl J Med. 1981;305:195–200.
24. Rompalo AM, Price CB, Roberts PL, et al. Potential value of rectal-screening cultures for *Chlamydia trachomatis* in homosexual men. J Infect Dis. 1986;153:888–92.
25. Barnes RC, Rompalo AM, Stamm WE. Comparison of *Chlamydia trachomatis* serovars causing rectal and cervical infections. J Infect Dis. 1987;156:953–8.

26. Dritz SK, Back AF. *Shigella* enteritis venerally transmitted. N Engl J Med. 1974;291:1194.
27. Drusin LM, Genvert G, Topf-Olstein B, et al. Shigellosis: Another sexually transmitted disease?. Br J Vener Dis. 1976;52:348–50.
28. Quinn TC, Corey L, Chaffee RG. *Campylobacter* proctitis in a homosexual man. Ann Intern Med. 1980;93:458–9.
29. Blaser MJ, Berkowitz ID, Laforce FM. *Campylobacter* enteritis: Clinical and epidemiologic features. Ann Intern Med. 1979;91:179–85.
30. Goodell SE, Quinn TC, Mkrtichian PA. Herpes simplex virus proctitis in homosexual men. Clinical, sigmoidoscopic, and histopathological features. N Engl J Med. 1983;308:868–71.
31. Rompalo AM, Mertz GJ, Davis LG, et al. Oral acyclovir for treatment of first-episode herpes simplex virus proctitis. JAMA. 1988;259:2879–81.
32. Schmerin MJ, Gelston A, Jones TC. Amebiasis—an increasing problem among homosexuals in New York City. JAMA. 1977;238:1386–7.
33. Goldmeter D, Sargeaunt PG, Price AB. Is *Entamoeba histolytica* in homosexual men a pathogen. Lancet. 1986;1:641–4.
34. Allason-Jones E, Mindel A, Sargeaunt P. *Entamoeba histolytica* as a commensal intestinal parasite in homosexual men. N Engl J Med. 1986;315:353–6.
35. Daling JR, Weiss NS, Hislop G. Sexual practices, sexually transmitted diseases, and the incidence of anal cancer. N Engl J Med. 1987;317:973–7.
36. Baker RW, Peppercorn MA. Gastrointestinal ailments of homosexual men. Medicine (Baltimore). 1982;61:390–405.
37. Schmerin MJ, Jones TC, Klein H. Giardiasis: Association with homosexuality. Ann Intern Med. 1978;88:801–3.
38. Jones MJ, Miller JN, George WL. Microbiological and biochemical characterization of spirochetes isolated from the feces of homosexual males. J Clin Microbiol. 1986;24:1071–4.
39. Soave R, Armstrong D. *Cryptosporidium* and Cryptosporidiosis. Rev Infect Dis. 1986;8:1012–23.
40. Schreeder MT, Thompson SE, Hadler SC, et al. Epidemiology of hepatitis B infection in gay men. J Homosex. 1980;5:307–310.
41. Shah N, Ostrow D, Baker H. Frequency and spectrum of chronic hepatitis B in homosexual males. (Abstract) Gastroenterology 1981;80:1348.
42. Szmuness W, Stevens CE, Harley EJ, et al. Hepatitis B vaccine. Demonstration of efficacy in a controlled clinical trial in a high-risk population in the United States. N Engl J Med. 1980;303:833–841.

290. RISK FACTORS AND APPROACHES TO INFECTIONS IN TRANSPLANT RECIPIENTS

MONTO HO
J. STEPHEN DUMMER

Since 1980 the field of organ transplantation has expanded dramatically, stimulated by the introduction of cyclosporine and marked by the growth and development of heart and liver transplantations, once the province of only a few academic centers.[1] It is now likely that an average physician may be called on to manage different types of transplant recipients in his or her practice.

Except for medical and surgical problems related to the function and rejection of the transplanted organ, infections are the most important problem after transplantation. The clinical manifestations of infection are quite variable and depend on the infecting pathogen, the prior immune status of the host, the time after transplantation, the level of pharmacologic immunosuppression, and many other factors. With this complexity in mind it is useful to address some general principles which may aid in the diagnosis, management, and understanding of infections after transplantation.

Infections require a susceptible host and an available pathogen. The susceptibility of transplant recipients is not the same for all pathogens. For instance, most respiratory viruses and enteroviruses do not appear to infect the transplant recipient with greater frequency or severity than a normal host. Or a transplant recipient may be quite susceptible to a given pathogen but have a low risk of infection because of lack of exposure to the pathogen. Thus despite the apparent vulnerability of transplant recipients to tuberculosis, the disease is a relatively minor problem at most transplant centers.[2] Likewise the kidney recipient with no past exposure to cytomegalovirus (CMV) who receives a kidney from a CMV-seronegative donor and has few blood transfusions is at very low risk for CMV infection (Chapter 120).[3] In practice the clinician can and should utilize such information and available clinical tools to assess each individual patient's susceptibility to important pathogens.

Most important and life-threatening infections tend to occur in the first 3 or 4 months after transplantation. This is the period when all the risk factors for infection (Table 1) may be fully operative. The patient may still be suffering from direct or indirect effects of his underlying disease. He will have undergone major surgery and possibly intensive care with the attendant risk of wound and other nosocomial infections (Chapter 285). Large amounts of immunosuppressive drugs will have been started and the allograft may be malfunctioning as a result of rejection or other factors. This early period also covers the usual incubation period of herpesviruses (CMV, herpes simplex virus [HSV], EBV), *Pneumocystis*, and *Toxoplasma*, which may be either transmitted by the donated organ or blood products at the time of transplantation or activated from endogenous sources with onset of immunosuppression. After the first 3 to 4 months, those infections that are related to surgery become less important. Meanwhile allograft reactions become less frequent and levels of immunosuppression can be kept at lower maintenance levels. Although the risk of serious infection never disappears, mortality declines to acceptable levels in the late post-transplant period 6 months after surgery.[1,4]

HOST FACTORS OF INFECTION

Underlying chronic diseases of the transplant recipient may contribute to infections after transplantation (Table 1). The

TABLE 1. Factors That Contribute to Infections after Transplantation

Pretransplant host factors	
Underlying medical condition	Conditions that persist or recur (hepatitis B, diabetes) Conditions that exacerbate (chronic bronchitis, gall bladder disease)
Lack of specific immunity	Leads to important primary infections (i.e., CMV, EBV, HSV, toxoplasmosis)
Prior colonization	Nosocomial gram-negative agents, *Candida*, staphylococci
Prior latent infection	Activation produces tuberculosis, ?pneumocystis, CMV, VZV, HSV
Prior medications	Immunosuppressive drugs and antibiotics affect post-transplant colonization susceptibility
Transplantation factors	
Type organ or tissue transplant	Site of transplantation and allograft are most common sites of infection Allograft may suffer from ischemia, injury, poor function, carried infection, or allograft reaction
Trauma of surgery	Surgical stress, duration of surgery
Immunosuppression	
Immunosuppressive agents	Corticosteroids, azathioprine, and other cytotoxic agents; cyclosporine; polyclonal and monoclonal antilymphocyte serums
Other measures	Pretransplant blood, total body irradiation
Infective immunosuppression	Primary CMV infections contribute to more bacterial and fungal infection
Allograft reactions	
Graft–vs.–host reaction	Cofactor in CMV interstitial pneumonia in bone marrow recipients
Host–vs.–graft reaction	?Cofactor in allograft infections

basic disease or organ dysfunction that led to transplantation may be corrected by the procedure, but occasionally it is not. Hepatitis B cannot be cured by removing the liver.[5] Diabetes mellitus continues to be a major problem in the diabetic renal transplant recipient, including the propensity of such patients to develop infections. Liver transplant recipients with hepatitis B or a cancer in the liver or biliary tract may not be cured. Underlying medical conditions such as gallbladder disease, diverticulosis, or chronic bronchitis may be clinically insignificant before transplantation and first become manifest in the post-transplant period, when their management is complicated by chronic immunosuppressive therapy.

Along with the patient's underlying condition, medications, particularly antibiotics and immunosuppressive agents such as corticosteroids, have an effect on the type and severity of subsequent infections in the early post-transplant period. For example, liver transplant recipients who received antibiotics or corticosteroids were more likely to develop systemic candida infections after transplantation.[6]

EFFECT OF TYPE OF TRANSPLANTATION

The type of transplantation is an important determinant of the type of infection occurring after transplantation, particularly during the first 3 months. There are a number of reasons why the transplanted organ and the surrounding structures are the most frequent and most important sites of infection. Sites of major surgery are particularly vulnerable to bacterial and fungal infection either during or shortly after surgery. The transplanted organ must establish a vascular supply and regain its functional integrity. Ischemia and improper function are potent factors contributing to infection. Allograft reactions of the host-vs.-graft or graft-vs.-host type may occur (Table 1, Allograft reactions). These reactions are known to reduce resistance to infection by viruses and contribute to the graft's being a locus minoris resistentiae.[7] Thus, the most common site of infection is the urinary tract in renal transplant patients. The abdomen, including the liver and biliary tree, is the most commonly infected site in liver recipients, as are the lung and chest cavity in heart and lung recipients.[8] (For details, see Chapter 291). Bone marrow transplant recipients do not have vulnerable surgical sites but are unique because leukopenia and depressed humoral immunity are superimposed on depressed T-cell immunity common to other transplantation during the first 30 to 40 days after transplantation. This leads to a very heightened vulnerability to additional varieties of infection (Chapter 291).

The contribution of surgical factors to infection is best illustrated by liver transplantation. With this type of surgery, the Achilles' heel is viable function of the biliary and vascular anastamoses. For example, the type of biliary drainage constructed at surgery was an important determinant of abdominal infection.[9] Choledochojejeunostomy was associated with three times as many infections as choledochocholedochostomy if the patient had more than one transplant. There was also a striking correlation between total hours spent in the operating room and mean episodes of infection per patient (Fig. 1). Patients who spent more than 25 hours in the operating room had 3 episodes, while those who spent 5–10 hours in the operating room had less than 1 episode of infection.[9] The duration of operation may

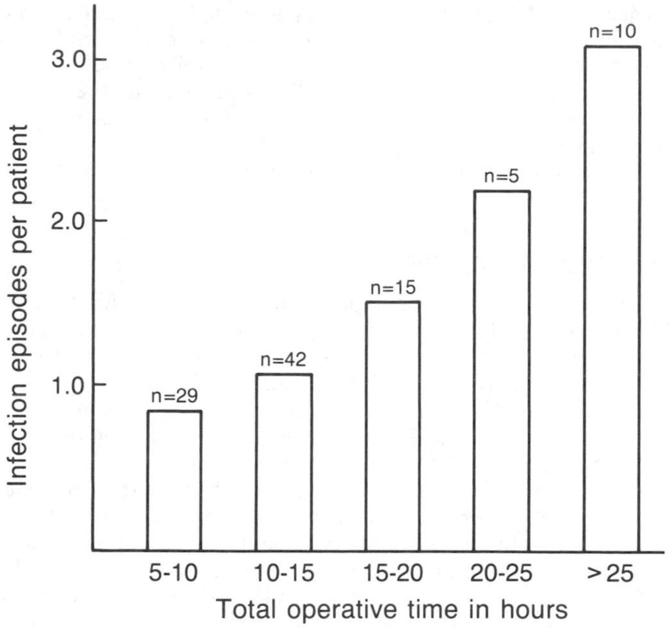

FIG. 1. Frequency of severe infections in relation to time spent in liver transplant surgery. (From Kusne et al.,[9] with permission.)

reflect the effects of surgical trauma and stress resulting from blood and body fluid loss, vascular bypass procedures, temporary loss of vital functions, metabolic derangements, and tissue damage. In kidney transplantation, complications of surgery may lead to perinephric infection. Lymphoceles with possible superinfection may result from interruption of lymphatic drainage. In transplantation of the lung, peritracheal infection may follow breakdown of end-to-end tracheal anastomoses. Lung infections are more frequent and more severe in heart and heart–lung transplant recipients.[10]

The susceptibility of the grafted organ to CMV infection is a striking example of the vulnerability of allografts to infection. Severe CMV hepatitis has been identified as a major problem in patients who undergo liver transplantation.[11] In other patients with CMV infection hepatitis is a common manifestation of infection, but it is almost always mild and usually only detected by laboratory measures.[3] CMV hepatitis in liver transplant recipients is frequently severe and may necessitate retransplantation. CMV pneumonia is a particularly important problem in heart–lung transplantation.[10] Table 2 summarizes data on four different types of transplant recipients in Pittsburgh, all of whom were on regimens of cyclosporine–prednisone immune suppression.[10,12] While the CMV infection rates were all high, the numbers of symptomatic patients and especially those who contracted CMV pneumonia were quite different: They were lowest in patients with kidney transplants and highest in those who received heart–lung transplants (32 percent). The cause of these differences is unknown. It is possible that the infection is carried by the graft and activated in the recipient. It has been demonstrated that the graft-vs.-host reaction, such as seen in bone marrow recipients,[13] is related to the frequency and se-

TABLE 2. Infection and Morbidity of CMV Infection in Different Transplant Groups in Pittsburgh after 1981

Type Transplant	Total No. Patients	No. Patients with Infections (% of Total)	No. Symptomatic Patients		No. Patients with CMV Pneumonia	
			Infected (%)	Total (%)	Infected (%)	Total (%)
Kidney	131	79/131(60)	13	8	4	2
Liver	93	55/93 (59)	49	29	5	3
Heart	48	44/48 (92)	27	25	9	8
Heart–Lung	31	22/31 (71)	55	39	45	32

(Data from Dummer et al.[10] and Ho.[12])

verity of CMV pneumonia (see Chapters 120 and 291). CMV pneumonia is one of the most important causes of death in this group (also see Chapter 291). Possibly a similar type or other types of allograft reaction may also contribute to the pathogenesis of CMV disease in liver and heart–lung recipients. Additional factors may include ischemic injury, loss of innervation, and lack of function unique to lung allografts.

IMMUNOSUPPRESSION

Of all the factors contributing to the occurrence of infections in transplant recipients, the most obvious and probably the most important is iatrogenic immunosuppression.[14] This becomes even more apparent as surgical techniques improve and infections due to surgical trauma, whether local or general in nature, are gradually reduced. Despite significant broadening of available immunosuppressive agents after the introduction of cyclosporine in 1981, the ideal suppressive regime that prevents rejection but preserves antimicrobial immunity remains elusive.

The major immunosuppressive agents may be divided into several categories. Corticosteroids have remained a part of the immunosuppressive regime although they alone are inadequate to sustain graft survival. Prednisone, especially in high doses, affects all aspects of immunity, including antibody formation, cellular immunity,[15,16] and impairment of inflammatory responses.[17] High doses of prednisone and hyperglycemia were found to be significant factors in causing infections in kidney transplant recipients and in infections causing death.[18] Doses of prednisone greater than 60 mg/day have been associated with the occurrence of clinical fungus infection in kidney recipients.[19] The general reduction of the dosage of prednisone in immunosuppressive regimens after 1966 was associated with reduction of significant infections in renal transplant recipients.[18,20]

Some infections do not usually occur with administration of corticosteroids alone. The prime example is CMV infection, which became a problem in transplantation only after cytotoxic drugs were added to the immunosuppressive regime.[21] Other evidence indicates that corticosteroids alone do not strongly predispose to CMV infection. In a study of 37 patients on chronic corticosteroids for various connective tissue diseases, such as rheumatoid arthritis, none had direct evidence of active CMV infection such as viruria or viremia.[22] On the other hand, the use of a cytotoxic drug such as cyclophosphamide alone was sufficient to reactivate CMV infections in seropositive subjects. A major advance in adequate immunosuppression drugs was the introduction of cytotoxic drugs, such as methotrexate, cyclophosphamide, actinomycin D, and azathioprine. All of these drugs are marrow suppressants and produce leukopenia when administered in large doses. Azathioprine became the mainstay and was effective in doses of 2 mg/kg or less per day without producing leukopenia. Higher doses were associated with leukopenia $<3000/mm^3$ and produced more bacterial and fungal infections.[18]

Cyclosporine introduced in 1980 a new era in transplant immunosuppression.[1] Without suppressing the bone marrow, it has a more focused effect on T-lymphocyte function than cytotoxic drugs. Its main activity appears to be inhibition of the antigen-directed elaboration of interleukin-2 by T-helper cells, with relative sparing of suppressor cell function.[23] Concentrations of the drug as low as 100 ng/ml effectively inhibit mixed lymphocyte reaction. It is striking that patients treated with cyclosporine alone for various autoimmune diseases have shown very low rates of clinical infection,[24] suggesting the possible importance of corticosteroids and other cofactors for infection (Table 1). Whether cyclosporine or azathioprine used together with corticosteroids in transplant recipients leads to less frequent and less severe infections is less clear. Most studies—whether randomized or historically controlled—appear to demonstrate lower rates of infection in cyclosporine-treated heart and kidney recipients. Thus, studies comparing azathioprine and cyclosporine showed reduction of bacterial infections in Pittsburgh[25] and reduction of CMV infection in Minnesota[26] and in Canada.[27] No differences were found in bacterial and viral infections in the European trial.[28] The two trials which showed more CMV infection in the azathioprine group included the use of antilymphocyte globulin, a key factor in enhancing of the morbidity of CMV (see below). The main advantage of cyclosporine was that there was a strong improvement in actuarial survival in kidney and liver recipients coincident with the introduction of cyclosporine.[1,29]

Antilymphocyte serums (ALSs) and antithymocyte globulins (ATGs) have been popular adjuncts for the prophylaxis or treatment of rejection. Excellent results on graft survival following its routine use as immunosuppressants have been reported.[26] Mason et al.[30] have shown a significant increase in infection rates in the 3 months following use of ATG for treatment of rejection of the heart. There are also many reports testifying to the enhancing role of ALS or ATG on CMV disease in renal transplant recipients,[3,31–33] and one report describes an increased rate of post-transplant lymphoproliferative disease in heart patients on high-dose cyclosporine and rabbit ATG.[34] Table 3 compares the frequency of CMV pneumonia as an indicator of significant CMV disease in various transplant groups on different immunosuppressive regimes. Kidney transplant recipients in Pittsburgh were routinely placed on azathioprine and prednisone before 1981 and on cyclosporine and prednisone after 1981–1983.[12] During these two periods, ATG was not used routinely and the frequency of CMV pneumonia (2–2.2 percent) did not change. This rate was also similar to the CMV pneumonia rate in kidney recipients who received cyclosporine and prednisone in Minnesota (2.6 percent).[35] However, the CMV pneumonia rate under their older regimen, which included routine use of ATG with azathioprine and prednisone, led to significantly more CMV pneumonia (8.3 percent).

The effect on infections of recently developed monoclonal anti-T-cell globulins is at this point less clear. Recent studies at our institution showed that liver transplant recipients who received OKT3 monoclonal antibodies for rejection had more instances of herpes superinfections and disseminated CMV disease and pneumocystis infection.[36] Much more needs to be done to define the capacity of these agents to enhance morbidity due to infections.

It appears unlikely that polyclonal or monoclonal antilymphocyte serums will be displaced, as they are the most useful agents for treating severe rejections and for reducing the dose of cyclosporine and its renal toxicity.[23] Part of the "cost" of their use may be a higher frequency of CMV disease and other infections. The history of using immunosuppressants has taught us that dosages are as important as the agent itself. It is possible that such agents may be used for relative impunity if restricted in dosage and frequency.[10] Only careful prospective clinical studies can provide the necessary data on which to make decisions.

TABLE 3. Effect of Types of Immunosuppression on Incidence of CMV Pneumonia in Kidney Recipients

Transplant Center	*Immunosuppression*	*No. Patients*	*No. CMV Pneumonia*	*%*
Pittsburgh	AZ–P	138	3	2.2
Pittsburgh	Cs–P	131	3	2.0
Minnesota	AZ–P–ATG	349	29	8.3[a]
Minnesota	Cs–P	76	2	2.6

Abbreviations: AZ: azathioprine; P: prednisone; Cs: cyclosporine; ATG: antithymocyte globulin.
[a] Significantly different.
(From Peterson et al.,[35] with permission.)

INFECTING MICROBIAL AGENTS

The sources of microbial agents and their methods of transmission in transplant recipients are listed in Table 4, and the major infecting organisms in Table 5.

There are two types of endogenous flora. One represents flora of extracorporeal lumina that colonize the mucous membranes of the gastrointestinal tract, including the oropharynx, the mouth, and the skin adjacent to the oral and anal orifices. This is the source of the most important potential pathogens represented by some of the more common gram-negative and gram-positive organisms listed in Table 5. These organisms may produce local infections by contaminating adjacent wound sites or may infect systemically by invading blood vessels or lymphatics. They may also be transmitted from one site or to another in the same patient by a surgical procedure or by contaminated instruments and hands.

TABLE 4. Sources of Microbial Agents and Methods of Transmission

Endogenous sources
Extracorporeal lumina (candida, enteric bacteria)
Latent tissue infection (herpesviruses, ?pneumocystis, toxoplasma, tubercle bacillus)
Exogenous sources
From physical environment (aspergillus, nocardia, legionella)
From human environment (all respiratory and enteric agents and viruses)
Transmission by donated organs
Transmission by blood and blood products

TABLE 5. Common Types of Infecting Microbial Agents after Transplantation

Bacteria	
Gram-negative bacteria Enteric bacteria (*E. coli, Enterobacteriaceae, Klebsiella*) *Pseudomonas* *Acinetobacter* *Serratia* Bacteroides and other anaerobes	This group of organisms can cause superficial wound infections or infections of the blood and deeper tissues of the urinary tract, lung, thorax, and abdomen. Despite a succession of highly effective antibiotics, these remain the most frequent causes of bacterial infection.
Legionella	Nosocomial from water supply.
Gram-positive aerobes *Staphylococcus aureus* *Staphylococcus epidermidis* *Streptococcus* *Enterococcus* *Pneumococcus* *Haemophilus influenzae* *Listeria monocytogenes* *Nocardia*	*S. epidermidis* has increased in frequency as other gram-positive organisms have been controlled by antibiotics. *Listeria* is an important cause of meningitis.
Fungi	
Candida spp. *Nocardia* *Aspergillus* *Cryptococcus* *Mucor*	*Candida* are the most common endogenous fungi. Systemic candida infection may be a particular problem after liver transplantation.
Histoplasmosis	Important in endemic areas.
Coccidioidomycosis	Important in Southwest United States.
Viruses	
Herpesvirus group Herpes simplex, I and II Cytomegalovirus Varicella-zoster virus Epstein-Barr virus	Herpesviruses are most common after transplantation because subjects are latently infected with one or more types, which reactivate after transplantation. They may also be transmitted by organs.
Human immunodeficiency virus	
Adenovirus	Pediatric.
Rotavirus	Pediatric.
BK virus (papovavirus) Papilloma virus Hepatitis B Non-A, non-B hepatitis	
Mycoplasma *M. hominis*	*M. hominis* may cause severe mediatinal wound infection after heart transplantation as well as other types of systemic infection, including arthritis, meningitis, and peritonitis.
Protozoa and Parasites	
Pneumocystis carinii	Probably latent in humans.
Toxoplasma gondii	
Strongyloides stercoralis	May reactivate as a visceral infection.

Candida, a frequent component of normal gastrointestinal tract flora, is the most important fungal pathogen. Superficial mucosal infection is common in the mouth and urinary tract. Candidemia and visceral infection may be associated with liver transplantation and occasionally in other transplant recipients in an intensive care setting.

The other type of endogenous flora comes from latent tissue infection. Such infections may reactivate, and the latent microbial agents may proliferate when the patient is immunosuppressed. The existence of this type of "flora" is best demonstrated in the case of herpesviruses, toxoplasmosis, and the tubercle bacilli. Their latent presence in tissues may be detected by serologic or immunologic tests. The presence of IgG antibodies against herpesvirus and toxoplasma also accurately indicates latent infection by these organisms. A positive purified protein derivative (PPD) skin test signals possible latent tissue infection by *Mycobacterium tuberculosis*. The situation is less clear in the case of *Pneumocystis carinii* since validated microbiologic or serologic tests for latent infection are still not available. In the absence of an environmental source for this protozoa, and in view of the remarkable frequency of *Pneumocystis* pneumonia in the acquired immunodeficiency syndrome (AIDS), one assumes that latent infection by this organism is common if not ubiquitous.

A number of organisms are transmitted airborne from the physical environment, particularly fungi such as *Aspergillus*, *Coccidioides*, *Histoplasma*, and *Cryptococcus*. Aspergillus, cryptococcal, and nocardial infections are seen in all geographic regions but post-transplant coccidioidomycosis is uniquely a problem of certain endemic regions such as the arid Southwest.

The most frequent source of infectious agents in the patient's environment is still other human beings. In the postoperative period, nosocomial transmission of common gram-positive and gram-negative organisms occurs by contaminated hands and via hospital vectors such as respiratory equipment, endoscopes, intravascular lines, and urinary catheters. Such equipment may at times amplify the agent if organisms are permitted to grow in reservoirs such as water baths and humidifiers. More virulent and fastidious microbial agents, such as encapsulated bacteria, viruses, and protozoa, are not likely to infect via the physical environment or be transmitted in the hospital setting but are transmitted directly from other human beings.

Some bacteria listed in Table 5 probably have exogenous sources but these are often undefined. *Pseudomonas* may come from the environmental water sources or raw vegetables.[37] *Listeria* may arise from contaminated food sources,[38] but a source is rarely identified in the sporadic cases of meningitis seen in the transplant population. The *Legionella*, including *Legionella pneumophila* and *Legionella micdadei* are important and well described causes of penumonia in transplant recipients. The predominant source of legionella is contaminated water supplies, particularly hot water supplies.[39,40] However, we have been unable to eliminate all nosocomial cases of legionella in our transplant population by hyperchlorination of the water supply despite our inability to detect the organism in either the hot water tanks or faucets and other plumbing fixtures in the patients' rooms.

An important source of infection unique to the transplant recipient is the donated organ (Table 6). With the development of more sophisticated methods to detect latent infection, it is possible that more agents will be found to be transmitted by the

TABLE 6. Transmission of Infective Agents by Donated Tissues, Blood, and Blood Products

Type Tissue	*Infective Agent*	*References*
Kidney, heart, liver, bone marrow	Cytomegalovirus	(3, 13, 36, 41)
Heart, kidney	Toxoplasmosis	(42)
Kidney	Herpes simplex virus	(43)
Kidney, heart, liver	HIV	(44)
Kidney	HBV	(45)
Blood[a]	CMV, EBV, HIV, HBV, HAV, HDV, NANB, HTLV-1	(46, 47, 48)
Leukocytes	CMV, HIV	

Abbreviations: HIV: human immunodeficiency virus; HBV: hepatitis B virus; CMV: cytomegalovirus; EBV: Epstein-Barr virus; HAV: hepatitis A virus; HDV: delta hepatitis virus; NANB: non-A, non-B hepatitis virus.

[a] On rare occasion, Chagas disease, malaria, babesiosis, and syphilis have been transmitted by blood transfusion.

allograft. At this time, the best evaluated agent is CMV. The allograft is the most important source of exogenous CMV and hence of primary CMV infection. (For details see Chapter 120 on CMV and Chapter 292 on solid organ transplants.) Both toxoplasmosis[42] and herpes simplex infections[43] have been transmitted from seropositive donor to seronegative recipients. It is not clear how important these methods of transmission are, but there is not enough evidence to exclude donors by testing for toxoplasma or herpes simplex antibody. This is different in the case of the AIDS virus (HIV), which though infrequently transmitted by organs[44] should be tested for in donors because of its unacceptable morbidity. There is some evidence that hepatitis B virus (HBV) may be transmitted by a donor kidney.[45] This would be an important consideration in countries where the HBsAg carrier rate is high.

The risk of transmission of microbial agents by blood and blood products to transplant recipients is the same as in other patient groups and is proportional to the number of transfusions and the efficacy of screening of blood donations. Screening is well in place for HBV and HIV, but it is still unsatisfactory for non-A, non-B hepatitis. (See Chapter 292.)

Since CMV is one of the most important of these pathogens in terms of frequency of transmission by organs and blood products it would be theoretically desirable to provide seronegative transplant recipients with organs and blood products only from seronegative donors. In view of the shortage of donors, varying morbidity of CMV, and logistic problems involved with maintaining organ survival, donor selection is difficult. This is particularly true for donors of marrow, liver, hearts, and hearts–lungs. These measures are practiced sporadically for some high-risk recipients, such as marrow recipients (Ch. 291) and pediatric seronegative renal recipients. Seronegative blood is used for heart–lung recipients in Pittsburgh (data unpublished).

DIAGNOSIS AND CONTROL OF INFECTIONS

Given a susceptible host and the types of microbial agents described, what can be done to facilitate diagnosis and control of infections? A proper approach to diagnosis and management of infections in transplant recipients requires a knowledge of the predominant nosocomial bacteria in each hospital and their antibiotic sensitivities. Some infections are theoretically preventable, but practically speaking, prevention may be difficult to carry out or not cost-effective. Legionella infection is preventable or at least reduced if one can eradicate the organism from the environment, particularly the water supply (see above). If one could prevent the transplantation of latently infected organs or the transfusion of contaminated blood, primary infection caused by CMV, EBV, HBV, HSV, HIV, and possibly toxoplasma might be prevented. Except for screening for HBV and HIV, which is now widespread for organ and blood donors, there is no accepted approach to this problem, particularly in the case of CMV.

The prompt and accurate diagnosis of some infections may be substantially aided if a serum is available to test the pretransplant serologic status. Table 7 lists in the first column those microbial agents that belong to this group. One sample of serum collected before transplantation is sufficient to determine the transplant recipient's acquired immunity to any one of the specific pathogens listed and to provide a baseline for testing after transplantation.

Practically speaking, we have most frequently made use of such serum collections in the diagnosis of infections with herpesviruses or *Toxoplasma gondii*. Herpesviruses include herpes simplex types I and II (HSV-1, HSV-2), cytomegalovirus (CMV), Epstein-Barr virus (EBV), and varicella-zoster virus (VZ). Patients who are seronegative or immunologically naive with respect to these agents prior to transplantation have not been previously exposed and are susceptible to primary or de novo infection around the time of transplantation. Under these conditions, a seropositive sample after transplantation is diagnostic of primary infection. Such infections are clinically more severe than secondary or reactivation infections. (For details see Chapter 292.) If the patient is seropositive before transplantation, he possesses specific immunity against that agent and will not develop a primary infection. However, seropositivity is also a sign of latent infection in the case of herpesviruses and toxoplasma. With immunosuppression seropositive subjects frequently have a reactivation of that infection, usually indicated by a serologic rise. Although reactivation infections are usually less severe than primary infections, in some cases they may cause serious clinical problems and are occasionally lethal (see Chapter 120).

It is also useful to save routinely a sample of serum from the donor, which can be used to determine agents to which the donor has been exposed and which may be carried by the donated organ (Table 6). The potential infectivity of the allograft may be indicated by the serologic state of the donor. We have used donor serum to trace an outbreak of severe herpes simplex infection in multiple recipients of donor organs.[43]

At times a negative test may not only mean a lack of acquired immunity but also predict a low risk of infection. For example, a negative tuberculin or PPD skin test indicates that the subject is susceptible to primary infection by the tubercle bacillus. But since infection by the organism is no longer common in the usual American community, the usual PPD-negative transplant candidate is unlikely to develop tuberculosis after transplantation. On the other hand, PPD-positive recipients may have a substantial risk of reactivation after transplantation if not previously treated (see Chapter 229). The management of a patient with a positive PPD test before transplantation is still controversial. While we advise testing, we feel the decision on prophylactic treatment should be individualized. Rubin[49] advises against prophylactic treatment because of the potential hepatotoxicity of isoniazid, particularly in the presence of other causes of liver failure after organ transplantation, such as drugs and infection.

TABLE 7. Routine Laboratory Studies before and after Transplantation

Before Transplantation[a]	*After Transplantation*
Cytomegalovirus IgG antibody	Viral surveillance cultures
Epstein-Barr virus IgG antibody	Antibody studies (as indicated)
Herpes simplex (types I and II) antibody	
Varicella-zoster IgG antibody	
Toxoplasma IgG antibody	
Legionella antibody	
Hepatitis B screen	
Human immunodeficiency virus antibody	
Tuberculin skin test	
Stool for ova and parasites[b]	

[a] For serologic studies, it is most important to collect serum before transplantation. Studies may then be done as clinically indicated. Not all tests need to be done on all patients.

[b] Particularly useful for residents of tropical and subtropical regions.

We now require in our institution that all transplant donors and recipients be tested for HIV antibodies. The presence of such antibodies indicates ongoing infection. We found in a survey of 583 donors and 1043 recipients that 2 donors (0.34 percent) and 18 (1.7 percent) recipients were positive by the enzyme-linked immunosorbent assay (ELISA) and Western blot test.[44] The donor organ should not be used until the result of the HIV test is known. The frequency of HIV seropositivity in recipients was significantly higher than that in the general population.[50] Two-thirds became positive after transplantation, and transmission by blood was suggested. The rationale for testing at our institution is that the results are needed to evaluate the patient fully. A positive test result also mandates the institution of proper precautions for the safety of the hospital personnel, although this may become a secondary indication with the gradual adoption of "universal precautions" by hospitals in this country. The HIV test may also be important for proper post-transplant evaluation and management of the patient who is susceptible to opportunistic infections and tumors from two potential sources: HIV infection and iatrogenic immunosuppression. Finally it is crucial to obtain accurate information on the outcomes of transplantation of HIV-infected individuals in order to formulate rational policies on the utilization of this limited resource.

CULTURE MONITORING

Routine surveillance cultures are probably of limited benefit, at least in most solid organ transplant recipients. One exception may be routine viral surveillance cultures for CMV and HSV. We order them every 2 to 4 weeks for the first 3 months after transplantation. Although many patients shed virus without any clinical manifestation, knowledge of whether a patient is shedding virus is helpful in formulating a differential diagnosis if the patient acquires a febrile illness. A diagnosis of symptomatic CMV infection is much less likely in a transplant patient who has repeatedly negative viral cultures for CMV. Prospective CMV cultures may also be useful if treatment with ganciclovir or other experimental antivirals is anticipated. Sometimes viral cultures also provide unsuspected new information. In a few instances a positive urine culture for herpes simplex virus led to the diagnosis of severe genital herpes. In these cases the patient was too embarrassed by genital lesions to report the symptoms. Another exception might be the routine surveillance of sputum of heart–lung recipients who are intubated in the intensive care unit. They are unusually susceptible to infection and breakdown at the site of tracheal anastomosis.

PROPHYLACTIC MEASURES

At present there is intense interest but no consensus on prophylactic regimens to prevent infection in transplant recipients. Many clinicans would advocate the routine use of pneumococcal and influenza vaccinations in transplant recipients; it has been demonstrated that most renal transplant recipients will mount an antibody response to these vaccinations but it is diminished.[51] Their clinical effectiveness has not been demonstrated in this population. We do recommend that transplant recipients keep up their immune status with killed vaccines, but not live vaccines (see Chapter 296). Most surgeons give a short course of parenteral antibiotics to prevent intraoperative sepsis and wound infections immediately before and shortly after surgery. The type of antibiotic used varies greatly (see Chapter 285). Preventive measures for CMV have been discussed. Prophylaxis with intravenous γ-globulin is covered in Chapters 120 and 291.

The use of oral antibiotics to prevent infection has been advocated by some groups. The most commonly used prophylactic antimicrobial is trimethoprim–sulfamethoxazole (TMP–SMX). This drug may decrease the rate of urinary tract infections and pneumonia[52] and perhaps decrease other gram-positive and gram-negative bacterial infections. Tolkoff-Rubin et al.[53] found in a controlled study of 52 patients that daily administration of 160 mg trimethoprim and 800 mg sulfamethoxazole for the first 4 months after renal transplantation reduced the incidence of urinary tract infection. More recently Fox, Maki et al. (personal communication) reported a double-blind placebo-controlled study of 132 renal recipients in which the treatment group received 320 mg trimethoprim and 1600 mg sulfamethoxazole while in the hospital and one-half of this dose after discharge. After at least 3 weeks of prophylaxis, the group who received TMP–SMX had significantly fewer urinary tract infections and blood stream infections and fewer infections caused by enteric gram-negative bacteria, enterococci, and *Staphylococcus aureus*. The reduction in urinary tract infection was most evidence after hospitalization. The drug was well tolerated, but in the presence of cyclosporine, drug recipients had 25 percent higher creatinine levels, which, however, were reversible.

Acyclovir is quite effective in preventing herpes simplex infection in the early post-transplant period and is probably indicated in bone marrow recipients, whose risk of severe herpes visceral disease is high.[54] Its role in solid organ recipients is less sure since most of the mucocutaneous infections that occur in those populations are easily diagnosed and managed when they occur. Acyclovir given intravenously at 500 mg/m^2 three times a day also reduced to some extent the frequency and severity of reactivated CMV infections in marrow transplant recipients.[55] It is probably not indicated for this purpose in other organ recipients. Recent evidence that acyclovir resistant strains of herpes simplex virus have appeared suggests that overuse should be discouraged.[56]

Since liver transplantation involves opening the potentially infected gastrointestinal tract, some groups advocate decontamination as a method to decrease bacterial and fungal sepsis.[57] Selective decontamination was achieved by oral administration of nonabsorbable polymyxin E, gentamicin, and nystatin and a diet free of raw foods and cheese 3 days prior to donor search and 21 days after transplantation. Surveillance cultures showed reduction of bacteria and fungi. Infection rates in an uncontrolled trial decreased. Apart from an unpleasant taste such regimens appeared to have little toxicity. Further studies are needed.

APPROACH TO FEVER IN THE TRANSPLANT PATIENT

Although immunosuppressive drugs can sometimes blunt the febrile response to infection, most transplant recipients with clinical infections have temperature elevations, often the first indication that something is awry.[58] When faced with a febrile patient the first task is to identify possible sites and sources of infection and assess the severity of illness. Patients with typical upper respiratory infection and low-grade fevers (<38.0°C) can generally be followed clinically. Cyclosporine seems to predispose patients to sinus infections. If suspected, it is often wise to order sinus radiographs. If the patient becomes febrile with a temperature elevated higher than 38.0°C, a medical evaluation should be made. If there are symptoms suggesting a serious localized infection even in the absence of demonstrable fever, the patient should also be evaluated.

The most important parts of this work-up are an examination of the chest and a chest radiograph to establish whether there is evidence for infection in the lungs. Patients with pulmonary infiltrates, or with persistent fevers greater than 38.5°C, should be hospitalized for further work-up. Most patients who cannot go about their normal daily activities should probably also be evaluated in the hospital unless the cause of their dysfunction is apparent and can be managed at home. Initial evaluation should include blood and urine cultures, examination of respiratory secretions (if pnemonia is suspected), white blood cell count and differential, liver function tests, and microscopic examination of the urine. Viral studies need only be ordered initially if there is strong reason to believe that the patient's disease is due to viral infection. Antibiotics may be withheld in patients who appear well and in whom no source of infection has emerged from the preliminary work-up. Although lumbar puncture need not be a routine part of the work-up of febrile transplant patients, one should have a low threshold for obtaining a sample of spinal fluid for culture and analysis in patients with headache and other neurologic complaints.

In a patient with a clear site of infection evaluation should focus on quickly obtaining adequate samples for culture and smears from that site. The patient who has persistent fever (≥7 days) without positive cultures or an apparent site of infection presents a diagnostic and therapeutic conundrum.

Relatively few clinical entities appear to account for the majority of these "fevers of unknown origin," the most important of which are viral syndromes caused by cytomegalovirus or occasionally Epstein-Barr virus. Other infections that present in this fashion are systemic toxoplasmosis and smoldering pneumocystis infection with a normal chest radiograph. Deep tissue abscesses almost always occur in or near the anatomic site of previous surgery or may be caused by systemic candidiasis. Disseminated candidiasis occurs largely in patients who are either neutropenic or long-term residents of the intensive care unit who have received broad-spectrum antibiotics and have multiple intravenous lines. Liver transplant recipients appear to be at higher risk for both *Candida* abscesses and disseminated candidiasis than heart, heart–lung, or kidney transplant recipients.

Not all fevers are caused by infections. The most common causes of noninfectious fevers in transplant recipients in our experience are drug reactions (especially reactions to anti-T-cell globulins) and rejection. The frequency with which rejection causes fever appears to vary widely among different transplant recipient groups. For instance, heart rejection rarely causes fever, but acute lung rejection is often associated with temperature elevations. Renal and hepatic transplant recipients appear to have an intermediate risk of fever with rejection.

Other noninfectious causes of fever are deep venous thrombosis (or pulmonary embolism), organ ischemia from infarction, or inadequate preservation and hemolytic reactions.

Finally it must be also be noted that infections may occur without any fever in transplant patients. At times this appears to be related to the use of high-dose corticosteroids; at other times severe organ failure (heart, liver, or kidney) appears to be implicated. There are some infections, such as progressive multifocal leukoencephalopathy, that almost never cause fever and others that frequently do not. Notable examples of the latter are pneumocystis pneumonia, which may present only with cough and dyspnea, or crytptoccocal meningitis, which may present with only headache and subtle neurologic symptoms. A good caveat for the physician approaching the transplant recipient is always to consider infection a possible cause of any new symptom or sign.

REFERENCES

1. Starzl TE, Klintmalm GBG, Porter KA, et al. Liver transplantation with use of cyclosporin A and prednisone. N Engl J Med. 1981;305:266–9.
2. Lichtenstein IH, Mac Gregor RR. Mycobacterial infections in renal transplant recipients: Report of 5 cases and review of literature. Res Infect Dis. 1983;5:216–26.
3. Ho M. Cytomegalovirus: Biology and Infection. New York: Plenum; 1982:309.
4. Shaw BW Jr, Martin DJ, Marquez JM, et al. Venous bypass in clinical liver transplantation. Ann Surg. 1984;200:524–34.
5. Van Thiel D, Schade RR, Gavaler JS, et al. Medical aspects of liver transplantation. Hepatology 1984;4:795–835.
6. Wajszczuk CP, Dummer JS, Ho M, et al. Fungal infections in liver transplant recipients. Transplantation. 1985;40:347–53.
7. Meyers JD, Spencer HC Jr, Watts JC, et al. Cytomegalovirus pneumonia after human marrow transplantation. Ann Intern Med. 1975;82:181–8.
8. Ho M, Wajszczuk CP, Hardy A, et al. Infections in kidney, heart and liver transplant recipients on cyclosporine. Transplant Proc. 1983;15:2768–72.
9. Kusne S, Dummer JS, Ho M, et al. Infections after liver transplantation: An analysis of 101 consecutive cases. Medicine. 1988;67:132–43.
10. Dummer JS, White LT, Ho M, et al. The morbidity of cytomegalovirus infection in heart and heart–lung transplant recipients on cyclosporine. J Infect Dis. 1985;152:1182–91.
11. Bronsther O, Makowka L, Jaffe R, et al. The occurrence of cytomegalovirus hepatitis in liver transplant patients. J Med Virol. 1988;24:423–34.
12. Ho M. Infection and organ transplantation. In: Gelman S, ed. Anesthesia and Organ Transplantation. Philadelphia: Saunders; 1987:49–60.
13. Meyers JD, Flournoy N, Thomas ED. Risk factors for cytomegalovirus infection after human marrow transplantation. J Infect Dis. 1986;153:478–88.
14. Ho M. Virus infections after transplantation in man. Arch Virol. 1977;55:1–24.
15. Saxon A, Stevens RH, Ramer SJ, et al. Glucocorticoids administered in vivo inhibit human suppressor T lymphocyte function and diminished B lymphocyte responsiveness in in vitro immunoglobulin synthesis. J Clin Invest. 1978;61:922–30.
16. Bovarnkitti S, Kangsadal P, Sathirapat P, et al. Reversion and reconversion rate of tuberculin skin reactions in correlation with the use of prednisone. Dis Chest. 1960;38:51–55.
17. Haynes BF, Fauci AS. The differential effect of in vivo hydrocortisone on the kinetics of subpopulations of human peripheral blood-derived lymphocytes. Blood. 1975;46:235–43.
18. Anderson RJ, Schafer LA, Olin DB, et al. Infectious risk factors in the immunosuppressed host. Am J Med. 1973;54:453–60.
19. Rifkind D, Marchioro T, Schneck S, et al. Systemic fungal infection complicating renal transplantation and immunosuppression therapy. Am J Med. 1967;43:28–38.
20. Rubin RH. Infection in the renal and liver transplant patient. In Rubin RH, and Young LS, eds. Clinical Approach to Infection in the Compromised Host. 2d ed. New York: Plenum; 1988:557–621.
21. Kanich RE, Craighead JE. Cytomegalovirus infection and cytomegalic inclusion disease in renal homotransplant recipients. Am J Med. 1966;40:874–82.
22. Dowling JN, Saslow AR, Ho M, et al. Cytomegaloviurs infection in patients receiving immunosuppressive therapy for rheumatologic disorders. J Infect Dis. 1976;133:399–408.
23. Kahan BD, Van Buren CT, Flechner SM, et al. Clinical and experimental studies with cyclosporine in renal transplantation. Surgery. 1985;97:125–40.
24. Palestine AG, Nussenblatt RB, Chan CC. Side effects of systemic cyclosporine in patients not undergoing transplantation. Am J Med. 1984;77:652–6.
25. Dummer JS, Hardy A, Ho M, et al. Early infections in kidney, heart and liver transplant recipients on cyclosporine. Transplantation. 1983;36:259–67.
26. Najarian JS, Fryd DS, Strand M, et al. A single institution, randomized, prospective trial of cyclosporine versus azathioprine–antilymphocyte globulin for immunosuppression in renal allograft recipients. Ann Surg. 1985;201:142–57.
27. Canadian Multicentre Transplant Study Group. A randomized clinical trial of cyclosporine in cadaveric renal transplantation. N Engl J Med. 1983;309:809–15.
28. European Multicentre Trial. Cyclosporin A as a sole immunosuppressive agent in recipients of kidney allografts from cadaver donors. Lancet 1982;2:57–60.
29. Starzl TE, Klintmalm GBG, Weil R III, et al. Cyclosporin A and steroid therapy in sixty-six cadaver kidney recipients. Surg Gynecol Obstet. 1981;153:486–94.
30. Mason JW, Stinson EB, Hunt SA, et al. Infections after cardiac transplantation: Relation to rejection therapy. Ann Intern Med. 1976;85:69–72.
31. Peterson PK, Balfour HH Jr, Marker SC, et al. Cytomegalovirus disease in renal allograft recipients: A prospective study of the clinical features, risk factors and impact on renal transplantation. Medicine. 1980;59:283–300.
32. Bia MJ, Andiman W, Gaudio K, et al. Effect of treatment with cyclosporine versus azathioprine on incidence and severity of cytomegalovirus infection posttransplantation. Transplantation. 1985;40:610–14.
33. Rubin RH, Tolkoff-Rubin NE, Oliver D, et al. Multicenter seroepidemiologic study of the impact of cytomegalovirus infection on renal transplantation. Transplantation. 1985;40:243–9.
34. Bieber CP, Herberling Rl, Jamieson SW, et al. Lymphoma in cardiac transplant recipients associated with cyclosporin A, prednisone and anti-thymocyte globulin (ATG). In Purtilo DT, ed. Immune Deficiency and Cancer. New York: Plenum; 1984:309–20.
35. Peterson PK, Balfour HH Jr, Fryd DS, et al. Risk factors in the development of cytomegalovirus-related pneumonia in renal transplant recipients. J Infect Dis. 1983;148:1121.
36. Singh N, Dummer JS, Ho M, et al. Infections with cytomegalovirus and other herpesviruses in 121 liver transplant recipients: Transmission by donated organ and the effect of OKT3 antibodies. J Infect Dis. 1988;158:124–31.
37. Kominos SD, Copeland CE, Brosiak B, et al. Introduction of *Pseudomonas aeruginosa* into a hosptial via vegetables. Appl Microbiol. 1972;24:567–70.
38. Schlech WF III, Lavigne PM, Bortolussi RA, et al. Epidemic listeriosis—evidence for transmission by food. Med Intel. 1983;308:203–6.
39. Shands K, Ho J, Meyer R, et al. Potable water as a source of Legionnaires' disease. JAMA. 1985;253:1412–16.

40. Muder RR, Yu VL, Woo AH. Mode of transmission of *Legionella pneumophila*. Arch Intern Med. 1986;146:1607–12.
41. Pollard R, Rand KH, Arvin AM, et al. Cell-mediated immunity to cytomegalo virus infection in normal subjects and cardiac transplant patients. J Infect Dis. 1978;137:541–49.
42. Luft BJ, Naot Y, Araujo FG, et al. Primary and reactivated toxoplasma infection in patients with cardiac transplants. Ann Intern Med. 1983;99:27–31.
43. Dummer JS, Armstrong J, Ho M, et al. Transmission of infection with herpes simplex virus by renal transplantation. J Infect Dis. 1987;155:202–6.
44. Dummer JS, Erb S, Breinig MK, et al. Infection with human immunodeficiency virus in the Pittsburgh transplant population: A study of 583 donors and 1043 recipients, 1981–86. Transplantation. 1989;47:134–9.
45. Wolf JL, Perkins HA, Schreeder MT, et al. The transplanted kidney as a source of hepatitis B infection. Ann Intern Med. 1979;91:412–3.
46. Gerber P, Wash JH, Rosenblum EN, et al. Association of EB-virus infection with the post-perfusion syndrome. Lancet 1969;1:593–6.
47. Greenwalt TJ, Jamieson GA. Transmissible Disease and Blood Transfusion. New York: Grune and Stratton; 1974:298.
48. Winston DJ, Ho WG, Howell CL, et al. Cytomegalovirus infections associated with leukocyte transfusions. Ann Intern Med. 1980;93:671–5.
49. Rubin RH. Tuberculosis and atypical mycobacterial infection in the renal transplant patient. In Rubin RH, Young LS, eds. Clinical Approach to Infection in the Compromised Patient. 2d Ed. New York: Plenum; 1988:599–600.
50. Centers for Disease Control. Human immunodeficiency virus infection in the United States: A review of current knowledge. MMWR. 1987;28–29.
51. Huang K, Armstrong JA, Ho M. Antibody response after influenza immunization in renal transplant patients receiving cyclosporine A or azathioprine. Infect Immun. 1983;40:421–4.
52. Hardy AM, Wajszczuk CP, Suffredini AF, et al. *Pneumocystic carinii*: Pneumonia in renal transplant recipients treated with cyclosporine and steroids. J Infect Dis. 1984;149:143–7.
53. Tolkoff-Rubin NE, Cosima AB, Russell PS, et al. A controlled study of TMP–SMZ prophylaxis of urinary tract infections in renal transplant recipients. Rev Infect Dis. 1982;4:614–8.
54. Saral R, Burns WH, Laskin OL, et al. Acyclovir prophylaxis of herpes-simplex-virus infections: A randomized, double-blind, controlled trial in bone-marrow transplant recipients. N Engl J Med. 1981;305:63–7.
55. Meyers JD, Reed EC, Shepp DH, et al. Acyclovir for prevention of cytomegalovirus infection and disease after allogeneic marrow transplantation. N Engl J Med. 1988;318:70–5.
56. Erlich KS, Mills J, Chatis P, et al. Acyclovir-resistant herpes simplex virus infections in patients with the acquired immunodeficiency syndrome. New Engl J Med. 1989;320:293–6.
57. Wiesner RH, Hermans PE, Rakela J, et al. Selective bowel decontamination to decrease gram-negative aerobic bacterial and candida colonization and prevent infection after orthotopic liver transplantation. Transplantation. 1988;45:570–4.
58. Peterson PK, Anderson RC. Infection in renal transplant recipients: Current approaches to diagnosis, therapy and prevention. Am J Med. 1986;81(Suppl 1A):2–10.

291. INFECTIONS IN MARROW TRANSPLANT RECIPIENTS

JOEL D. MEYERS

Marrow transplantation is increasingly used as therapy for aplastic anemia, hematologic malignancy, immunodeficiency syndromes, and thalassemia and is of theoretical use as the vector for gene replacement therapy (e.g., adenosine deaminase deficiency) and among patients with acquired immunodeficiency syndrome (AIDS). Transplant involves ablation of the patient's (host's) hematopoietic and immune systems and replacement with those of the marrow donor. The usual marrow donor is an human leukocyte antigen (HLA) and mixed leukocyte culture (MLC) matched sibling (allogeneic transplant). Related donors who are not fully matched with the patient and fully matched but unrelated donors have also been used.

Major complications after transplant include toxicity from conditioning, graft-vs.-host disease (GvHD), and infection. GvHD is the reaction of the transplanted immune system against host tissues. Immunosuppression is given for 100 days or more after allogeneic transplant to prevent GvHD, whereas it is not needed with identical twin (syngeneic) donors or among patients who receive their own, previously stored marrow (autologous transplant). Patients with GvHD are treated with additional immunosuppression. Both GvHD and its treatment increase the risk of infection. The advent of cyclosporine immunosuppression and, more recently, the use of cyclosporine with methotrexate have decreased the incidence of GvHD, although the benefits have not been as profound as after solid organ allografting (Chapter 292). An alternative approach for prevention of GvHD is depletion of T cells from the donor marrow before transplant; this procedure has a greater risk of graft failure or rejection and of prolonged neutropenia. Despite these complexities, extremely good results have been achieved with transplantation for severe aplastic anemia and acute nonlymphocytic leukemia in first remission, as well as for other diseases.

RISK FACTORS AND TEMPORAL PATTERN OF INFECTION

The marrow transplant recipient resembles both the patient receiving cytotoxic chemotherapy for acute leukemia and the patient whose cell-mediated immunity is suppressed for organ allografting. The initial ablation and sequential recovery of host defenses determine the characteristic pattern of infections (Fig. 1). Conditioning both damages anatomic barriers, producing sites of entry for resident flora, and causes severe neutropenia lasting from approximately 1 week before to 3 weeks after transplant. During this period the marrow transplant recipient is at risk of infection primarily with bacteria or fungi, similar to leukemic patients undergoing induction therapy. Viral infections other than herpes simplex virus (HSV) are less common. The previous experience of the patient may also influence the risk of infection. For example, patients with prolonged neutropenia before transplant (e.g., those with aplastic anemia) or previous infection with *Candida* or *Aspergillus* may be more likely to develop these infections after marrow transplant. The risk of bacterial infection decreases after quantitative recovery of neutrophils. However, neutrophil and macrophage function remains abnormal.[1,2]

Between the neutropenic period and approximately day 100 after transplant infection with opportunistic pathogens, such as cytomegalovirus (CMV) or *Aspergillus*, becomes more common. The syndrome of interstitial pneumonia occurs most commonly during this period. As with recipients of solid organ allografts, previous infection with agents which become latent such as CMV or *Toxoplasma gondii*, as documented by positive serologies before transplant, identifies the patient at higher risk

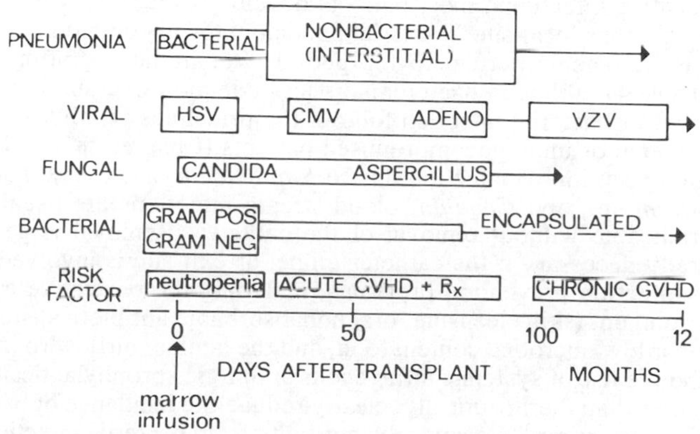

FIG. 1. Predisposing risk factors and common infections by time after marrow transplant.

of these infections after transplant. Infections are also more common among patients with acute GvHD. This period is marked by the slow return of antigen-specific immune responses. Nonspecific cytotoxic cells, such as natural killer cells, recover quantitatively and functionally soon after transplant[3]; the importance of these responses in defense against infection is uncertain. Specific immune responses remain suppressed for a longer period. Although T-cell numbers recover relatively soon, the number and function of helper–inducer cells remain low while suppressor–cytotoxic cells are relatively or absolutely increased, especially among patients with GvHD or viral infection.[4] Patients can develop T-cell activity against specific viruses after active infection, and cytotoxic T-cell activity has been associated with recovery from CMV infection.[5] Similarly, although total immunoglobulin levels may recover by 3 to 4 months after transplant, B-lymphocyte response to certain antigens remains depressed.[6] Whereas new antibody production to some viruses may occur very soon after transplant, antibody to other antigens such as pneumococcal polysaccharide remains low for as long as 2 years after transplant.[6,7] Both B- and T-helper cell failure as well as T-cell suppression of antibody production have been described.[8] Immunization of both marrow donor and recipient in order to "transfer" humoral responses is under study.[9] Many of these immunologic abnormalities are more severe or persist longer in patients with GvHD. The occurrence of infection after the initial neutropenic period is determined by the rapidity of maturation of the regenerating immune system.

After day 100, some patients remain at risk of infection with agents with a longer incubation period (e.g., varicella-zoster virus) or that occur predominantly among patients with chronic GvHD (e.g., *Streptococcus pneumoniae*). Infection due to sporadic or epidemic agents from either the community (e.g., *Influenza*) or the hospital (e.g., *Legionella*) may be superimposed on this pattern. A major difference between marrow and organ allograft patients from those with acquired immunodeficiency syndrome (AIDS) is that the marrow allograft patient will eventually develop normal immunity if GvHD can be prevented.

TABLE 1. Representative Organisms Recovered from Blood Cultures during and after the Neutropenic Period among Patients Transplanted for Hematologic Malignancy

	Before Engraftment[a]	*After Engraftment*[b]
Number of patients	342	278
Gram-postive organisms		
Staphylococcus		
Coagulase-positive	7	3
Coagulase-negative	41	28
Streptococcus sp.	16	3
Enterococcus	3	0
Corynebacteria	3	4
Clostridium sp.	0	1
Other	3	5
Total isolates	73	44
Total patients	63 (18%)	Not available
Gram-negative organisms		
Pseudomonas sp.	8	0
Escherichia coli	4	0
Klebsiella sp.	4	3
Enterobacter sp.	2	3
Bacteroides sp.	4	1
Other	6	4
Total isolates	28	11
Total patients	26 (8%)	Not available
Yeasts	19	5
All isolates	120	60
All patients	87 (25%)	39 (14%)

[a] Includes patients treated in 1984–1986 who received various modalities of infection prevention.
[b] Includes patients transplanted 1976–1984.

BACTERIAL INFECTIONS

The spectrum of bacterial infection during the initial neutropenic period is similar to that in other patients with acute neutropenia (Chapter 287). Representative organisms are shown in Table 1. The preponderance of gram-positive organisms may be related to the universal use of long-term central venous lines providing entry for skin organisms, oropharyngeal mucosal breakdown providing access for mouth organisms (e.g., *Streptococcus* sp.), frequent use of antibiotics effective against most gram-negative organisms, and possibly colonization of the gut with coagulase-negative *Staphylococcus*. Although the gut presumably serves as an initial site of infection for many gram-negative infections, most patients develop bacteremia without an obvious local site. Bacterial pneumonia is uncommon. Similar statements pertain to the period after initial engraftment (Table 1), although bacteremia is less common overall. Treatment of bacterial infection follows the principles in other neutropenic or immunocompromised patients (Chapter 287). With the exception of infection due to *Staphylococcus, Corynebacterium* sp., and *Candida*, blood stream infections are usually eradicable without removal of the catheter. Removal is generally necessary if the catheter tunnel or exit site is involved.

Infection prevention programs, including the protective environment (skin cleansing, oral nonabsorbable antibiotics, sterile or low microbial content food, and the laminar airflow room) and the use of systemic intravenous antibiotics prophylactically rather than therapeutically, clearly reduce the incidence of bacterial infection.[10] Because the mortality from bacterial infection is low, however, there has been less impact on survival. A delay in onset and a reduction in incidence and severity of GvHD were observed among aplastic anemia patients transplanted in the protective environment[11]; however, this benefit is less clear in more recent studies in both aplastic and leukemic individuals. Whether gut decontamination in patients with acute GvHD would reduce the incidence of bacterial infection is speculative. Other recent approaches to infection prevention include selective decontamination using the fluorinated quinolones and prophylactic intravenous immunoglobulins.[12,13] The latter may be applicable both to the early periods after transplant and especially to the period after day 100 when infection with encapsulated bacteria has been related to deficits in opsonizing antibody.[6,7]

FUNGAL INFECTION

Invasive fungal infection, primarily *Candida* and *Aspergillus*, is of increasing importance after marrow transplant.[14] Review of 1500 patients transplanted between 1980 and 1987 revealed an incidence of invasive *Candida* and *Aspergillus* infection of 11 and 4 percent, respectively. Incidence was higher in more recent years. The mortality rate of both *Aspergillus* and proven tissue candidal infection was 85 to 90 percent, whereas candidemia alone had a mortality of 50 percent. *Candida* infection occurred earlier than *Aspergillus*, with a median onset of 2 and 3 weeks after transplant, respectively, for candidemia and proven tissue infection compared with 6 weeks for aspergillosis. Putative risk factors for fungal infection include prolonged neutropenia and GvHD. Whether the use of corticosteroids adds to this risk is unknown. T-cell depletion of marrow has been identified as a risk factor independent of neutropenia.[15] Fungal surveillance cultures may be of help in predicting invasive candidiasis during the neutropenic period.

Treatment of proven infection is with amphotericin B. The use of 5-fluorocytosine is infrequent because of possible marrow toxicity, and insufficient data are available to evaluate miconazole, ketoconazole, or the addition of rifampin. Ketoconazole may increase blood levels of cyclosporine. Nystatin, oral amphotericin B, ketoconazole, and even miconazole have been used for prophylaxis in various centers, but there is no standard approach to prevention of fungal infection.

VIRAL INFECTION

Herpesvirus infections have been most prominent after marrow transplant. Herpes simplex virus (HSV) infection occurs within the first few weeks after transplant, cytomegalovirus (CMV) infection occurs 1 to 3 months after transplant, and varicella-zoster virus (VZV) infection occurs 3 months or more after transplant (Fig. 2). Infections with Epstein-Barr virus (EBV) or adenoviruses also appear to be common, and lymphoproliferative syndromes associated with EBV have been observed after marrow transplant.

Both HSV and VZV infections are due primarily to reactivation of latent virus, occurring in 75 percent of patients with previous HSV infection and 35 percent of patients with previous VZV infection. Infection with HSV occurs at the time of maximal mucosal damage from radiation and chemotherapy and may cause locally severe disease. In some patients contiguous spread of virus results in HSV pneumonia or esophagitis. Acyclovir is effective for the treatment and prophylaxis of HSV infection after marrow transplant and should be used in patients at risk for severe local disease. Most patients with VZV infection develop dermatomal herpes zoster, although one-third of these have subsequent cutaneous dissemination; 15 percent of patients have a generalized rash without initial localization. The mortality rate without antiviral treatment is approximately 10 percent. All patients with VZV infection within the first 12 months after transplant and any patient with cutaneous dissemination should be treated with acyclovir. Second cases of VZV infection have been uncommon, attributed to restoration of the immune response to this virus.[16]

Cytomegalovirus infection occurs in 30 to 40 percent of seronegative patients who receive unscreened blood products and up to 80 percent of seropositive patients who reactivate latent, endogeous virus. As in recipients of solid organs (Chapter 292), seronegative patients may also acquire primary CMV infection from the transplanted marrow. The incidence of CMV infection is increased among patients who develop GvHD.[17,18] The most important syndromes are pneumonia and infection of the gastrointestinal (GI) tract; retinitis is rare. One-third of patients with CMV infection develop CMV pneumonia. The risk of CMV pneumonia is increased among older patients and those with GvHD; this effect of GvHD is independent of the increased risk of infection.[17] It is hypothesized that the pathogenesis of CMV pneumonia is related to abnormal immune responses in patients with GvHD.[19] Treatment of CMV infection with the new agents ganciclovir and foscarnet is under study. Previously CMV pneumonia was fatal in 85 percent of patients with proven disease. Although treatment of CMV pneumonia with ganciclovir alone or combined with corticosteroids was not successful,[20] the combination of ganciclovir and intravenous immune globulin produced survival of 50 percent or greater.[21,22] Among seronegative patients, primary CMV infection can be prevented by screening of donors and blood products[23]; use of immunoglobulins for prevention of CMV infection after marrow transplant remains controversial.[23,24] Intravenous acyclovir given for the first month after transplant reduced CMV disease by 50 percent[25]; ganciclovir or foscarnet should provide better results.

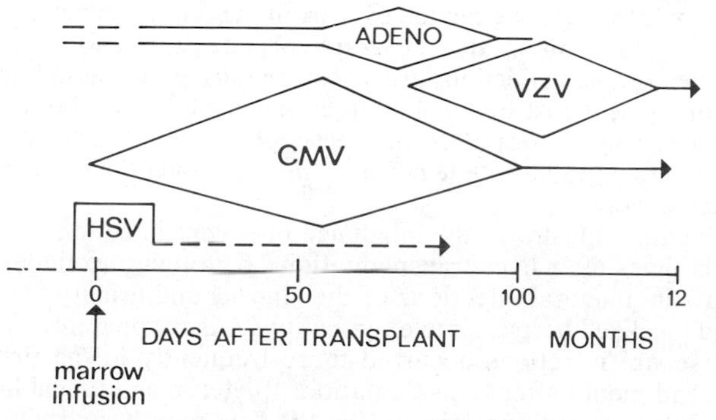

FIG. 2. Timing and relative significance of virus infections by time after marrow transplant.

Infections with papovaviruses, enteroviruses, and respiratory viruses have also been recognized after marrow transplant and have caused serious disease. Carriage of hepatitis B appears not to confer an increased risk of severe or fatal hepatic disease. Although live virus vaccines have not been used because of concern about disseminated infection, use of vaccines in donors before transplant or in patients after transplant to transfer or restore specific immunity is an area of future research.[9]

PROTOZOAN INFECTIONS

Pneumocystis carinii was previously a common cause of interstitial pneumonia, but is now rare because of trimethoprim–sulfamethoxazole (TMP–SMX) prophylaxis. A regimen of TMP–SMX given twice weekly at a dose of 1 double-strength tablet bid is quite effective. *Toxoplasma gondii* occurs rarely. Of 11 cases observed in our institution, only 1 had discrete brain abscesses on computed tomography (CT) scan. In contrast to the situation after heart transplant (Chapter 292), almost all cases after marrow transplant appear to be due to reactivation of latent organisms.

INTERSTITIAL PNEUMONIA

The one syndrome that is of special note after marrow transplant is pneumonia due to causes other than bacterial or fungal infection, commonly referred to as *interstitial pneumonia,* which occurs in up to 40 percent of patients with allografts for leukemia.[26,27] Most cases are due to CMV. The incidence of CMV pneumonia is markedly lower in patients receiving syngeneic or autologous transplants and in patients transplanted for aplastic anemia who do not receive total body irradiation. The usual onset is 60 (±30) days after transplant. Bronchoalveolar lavage combined with the technique of centrifugation culture for rapid detection of CMV has been shown to be both highly sensitive and specific for diagnosis of CMV pneumonia, obviating need for an open lung biopsy. One-third of cases are classified as "idiopathic interstitial pneumonia" and appear to be due to chemoradiation toxicity. Diffuse infiltrates occurring within the first 30 days after transplant are more commonly idiopathic pneumonia and uncommonly due to infection, although early respiratory syncytial virus infection has been observed. Idiopathic pneumonia has decreased as a result of fractionation of the dose of total body irradiation and of use of slower dose rates.[26,27]

LATE INFECTION

Infections beyond 100 days after transplant generally occur in patients being treated for chronic GvHD.[28] Infections commonly involve respiratory sites (sinusitis, bronchitis, pneumonia), oropharynx (pharyngitis, otitis media), skin (viral exanthems, cellulitis), the conjunctiva, or the urinary tract or present as bacterial sepsis without an apparent site. Late interstitial pneumonia may also occur. The preponderance of respiratory infections may be due to the bronchopulmonary sicca characteristic of chronic GvHD. Although incidence figures are not available, infection with *Streptococcus pneumoniae*, including sepsis and meningitis, occurs at an unusually high rate.[7] Anecdotal observations suggest that trimethoprim–sulfamethoxazole prophylaxis is effective for the prevention of pneumococcal infection, although infection with resistant pneumococci has been observed. Trimethoprim–sulfamethoxazole use also predisposes to oral candidiasis. The prophylactic use of penicillins is being investigated, as is the use of monthly immunoglobulin infusions. Decrease in the risk of late infections will depend both on improvement in the treatment or prevention of chronic GvHD and on measures to improve immune responsiveness.

REFERENCES

1. Clark RA, Johnson FL, Klebanoff SJ, et al. Defective neutrophil chemotaxis in bone marrow transplant patients. J Clin Invest. 1976;58:22–31.
2. Winston DJ, Territo MC, Ho WG, et al. Alveolar macrophage dysfunction in human bone marrow transplant recipients. Am J Med. 1982;73:859–66.
3. Livnat S, Seigneuret M, Storb R, et al. Analysis of cytotoxic effector cell function in patients with leukemia or aplastic anemia before and after marrow transplantation. J Immunol. 1980;124:481–90.
4. Atkinson K, Hansen JA, Storb R, et al. T-cell subpopulations identified by monoclonal antibodies after human marrow transplantation: I. Helper–inducer and cytotoxic–suppressor subsets. Blood. 1982;59:1292–8.
5. Quinnan GV, Kirmani N, Rook AH, et al. Cytotoxic T cells in cytomegalovirus infection. N Engl J Med. 1982;307:7–13.
6. Witherspoon RP, Storb R, Ochs HD, et al. Recovery of antibody production in human allogeneic marrow graft recipients: Influence of time posttransplantation, the presence or absence of chronic graft-versus-host disease, and antithymocyte globulin treatment. Blood. 1981;58:360–8.
7. Winston DJ, Schiffman G, Wang DC, et al. Pneumococcal infections after human bone-marrow transplantation. Ann Intern Med. 1979;91:835–41.
8. Lum LG. The kinetics of immune reconstitution after human marrow transplantation. Blood. 1987;60:369–80.
9. Wimperis JZ, Brenner MK, Prentice HG, et al. Transfer of a functioning humoral immune system in transplantation of T-lymphocyte-depleted bone marrow. Lancet. 1986;1:339–43.
10. Petersen FB, Buckner CD, Clift RA, et al. Laminar air flow isolation and decontamination: A prospective randomized study of the effects of prophylactic systemic antibiotics in bone marrow transplant patients. Infection. 1986;14:115–21.
11. Storb R, Prentice RL, Buckner CD, et al. Graft-versus-host disease and survival in patients with aplastic anemia treated by marrow grafts from HLA-identical siblings. Beneficial effect of a protective environment. N Engl J Med. 1983;308:302–7.
12. Winston DJ, Ho WG, Gale RP, et al. Prevention and treatment of infections after bone marrow transplantation. In: Baum SJ, Santos GW, Takaku F, eds. Experimental Hematology Today—1987: Recent Advances and Future Directions in Bone Marrow Transplantation. New York: Springer-Verlag; 1987:177–84.
13. Petersen FB, Bowden RA, Thornquist M, et al. The effect of prophylactic intravenous immune globulin on the incidence of septicemia in marrow transplant recipients. Bone Marrow Transplantation. 1987;2:141–8.
14. Peterson PK, Ramsay NKC, et al. A prospective study of infectious diseases following bone marrow transplantation. Infect Control. 1983;4:81–9.
15. Pirsch JD, Maki DG. Infectious complication in adults with bone marrow transplantation and T-cell depletion of donor marrow: increased susceptibility to fungal infections. Ann Intern Med. 1986;104:619–31.
16. Locksley RM, Flournoy N, Sullivan KM, et al: Varicella-zoster virus infection after marrow transplantation. J Infect Dis. 1985;152:1172–81.
17. Meyers JD, Flournoy N, Thomas ED. Risk factors for cytomegalovirus infection after human marrow transplantation. J Infect Dis. 1986;153:478–88.
18. Miller W, Flynn P, McCullough J, et al. Cytomegalovirus infection after bone marrow transplantion: An association with acute graft-v-host disease. Blood. 1986;4:1162–7.
19. Grundy JE, Shanley JD, Griffiths PD. Is cytomegalovirus interstitial pneumonitis in transplant recipients an immunopathological condition? Lancet. 1987;2:996–9.
20. Shepp DH, Dandliker PS, de Miranda P, et al. Activity of 9-[2-hydroxy-1-(hydroxymethyl)ethoxymethyl]guanine (BW B759U) in the treatment of cytomegalovirus pneumonia. Ann Intern Med. 1985;103:368–3.
21. Emanuel D, Cunningham I, Jules-Elysee K, et al. Cytomegalovirus pneumonia after bone marrow transplantation successfully treated with the combination of ganciclovir and high-dose intravenous immune globulin. Ann Intern Med. 1988;109:777–88.
22. Reed EC, Bowden RA, Dandliker PS, et al. Treatment of cytomegalovirus pneumonia with ganciclovir and intravenous cytomegalovirus immunoglobulin in patients with bone marrow transplantation. Ann Intern Med. 1988;109:783–8.
23. Bowden RA, Sayers M, Flournoy N, et al. Cytomegalovirus immune globulin and seronegative blood products to prevent primary cytomegalovirus infection after marrow transplantation. N Engl J Med. 1986;314:1006–10.
24. Winston DJ, Ho WG, Lin C-H, et al. Intravenous immune globulin for prevention of cytomegalovirus infection and interstitial pneumonia after bone marrow transplantation. Ann Intern Med. 1987;106:12–8.
25. Meyers JD, Reed EC, Shepp DH, et al. Acyclovir for prevention of cytomegalovirus infection and disease after allogeneic marrow transplantation. N Engl J Med. 1988;318:70–5.
26. Meyers JD, Flournoy N, Wade JC, et al. Biology of interstitial pneumonia after marrow transplantation. In: Gale RP, ed. Recent Advances in Bone Marrow Transplantation. New York: Alan R. Liss; 1983:405–23.
27. Weiner RS, Bortin MM, Gale RP, et al. Interstitial pneumonitis after bone marrow transplantation. Ann Intern Med. 1986;104:168–75.
28. Atkinson K, Farewell V, Storb R, et al. Analysis of late infection after human bone marrow transplantation: Role of genotypic nonidentity between marrow donor and recipient and of nonspecific suppressor cells in patients with chronic graft-versus-host disease. Blood. 1982;60:714–20.

292. INFECTIONS IN SOLID ORGAN TRANSPLANT RECIPIENTS

MONTO HO
J. STEPHEN DUMMER
PHILLIP K. PETERSON
RICHARD L. SIMMONS

Since the introduction of cyclosporine as a major immunosuppressant, there has been a marked increase in the numbers and types of organ transplantations. Liver, heart, and heart–lung transplantations have advanced from being experimental procedures to become established therapeutic modalities similar to transplantation of the kidney.[1,2] In three of the four types of transplantation, 1 year survival exceeds 70 percent; the exception is heart–lung transplantation, for which the rate it is still around 50 percent.[3] Other improvements have accompanied better immunosuppression. For example, 1 year survival after liver transplantation prior to the availability of cyclosporine was 32 percent.[4] When we first reviewed infections after liver transplantation after cyclosporine in 1981–83 the 6 month survival was 63 percent,[5] whereas more recently 5 year survival rates were 74 and 64 percent.[6,7] These improvements are probably related to better regulation of immunosuppression, better selection of candidates, technical advances such as introduction of venous–venous bypass during surgery, and clinical experience at all levels of the surgical and medical staff achieved with the performance of larger numbers of transplant procedures.[6]

Advances have also been made in pancreas transplantation although technical failure remains a major obstacle to graft survival. Of these failures infection and thrombosis are the most frequent.[8] One year actuarial graft and patient survivals are 30 and 86 percent.[8]

TIME OF OCCURRENCE OF INFECTIONS AFTER TRANSPLANTATION

Most infections occur within 4 months after transplantation. Petersen et al.[9] point out that 64 percent (125/194) of all febrile episodes occurring after renal transplantation were seen within 14 to 120 days after transplantation. The major infections in the first month are those carried over from the pretransplant period, such as hepatitis, and postsurgical infections. Reactivated herpes simplex infections are also seen during this period. Most of the typical post-transplant infections occur during the second period, which extends from the second to the fourth month. The third period, or "late period," includes infections occurring after 4 months.

Figure 1 illustrates the incidence of severe infections at various times after liver transplantation.[6] The figure excludes superficial mucosal infections of the sinuses and urinary bladder and localized herpes simplex infections. As is apparent, almost all severe infections occurred more frequently in the first or second month after transplantation. Bacterial and fungal infections were most common during the first month, and viral infections (mostly cytomegalovirus [CMV] infections) were most

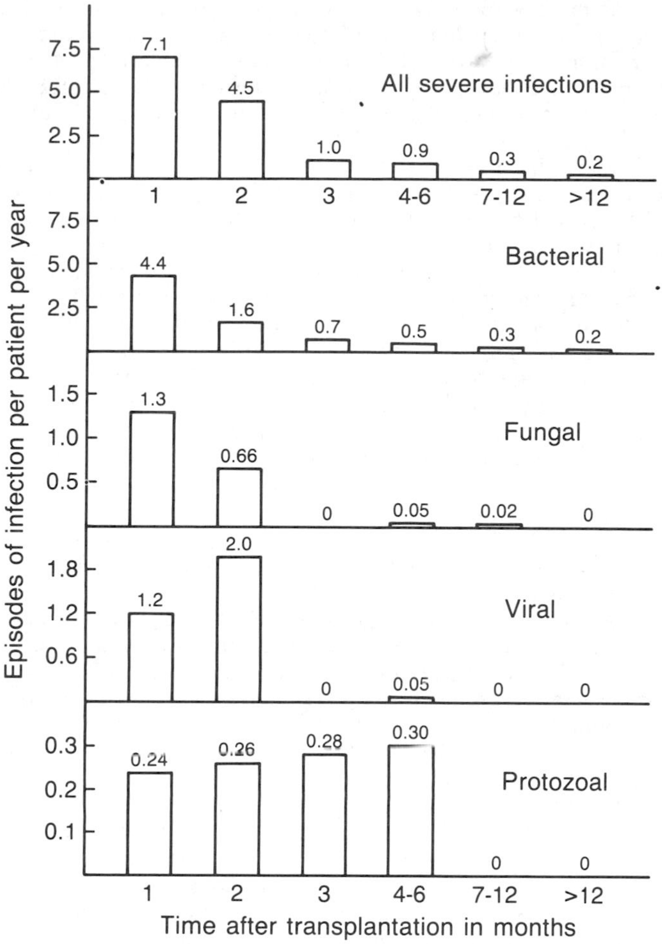

FIG. 1. Incidence and timing of severe infections expressed in episodes of infection per liver transplant patient per year at different times after transplantation. Data on all severe, bacterial, fungal, viral, and protozoal (mostly *Pneumocystis*) infections are included.

common during the second month. The exception was protozoal (mostly *Pneumocystis*) infections, which occurred at a steady frequency during the first 6 months. Scattered bacterial and fungal infections continued to occur after the first 6 months, but no viral or protozoal infections were observed. The timing of infections is quite similar after renal,[9] heart,[10] heart–lung,[11] and pancreas transplantation,[8] although the type, frequency, and severity of infections do vary considerably with the nature of transplantation, as will be discussed below.

What are some of the "late" infections that occur after the first 6 months of transplantation? These may be divided into three types. First, some infections persist after the early post-transplant period and are not resolved. For example, Dummer[11] found that heart–lung allograft recipients may suffer from chronic relaping bronchitis caused by *Pseudomonas*. Renal transplant recipients may suffer from chronic or recurring urinary tract infections.[12] Chronic or relapsing bacterial cholangitis may complicate liver transplantation.[6] Unlike other forms of CMV disease, which are mainly problems of the first 3 or 4 months, CMV retinitis may occur months or years after the initial infection.[13]

Second, other infections may represent de novo recurrences related to the altered immune state. Eruptions of herpes zoster may occur any time after transplantation.[14,15] Papovaviruses (BK and JC) may reactivate after the first 6 months of transplantation, at which time they may be associated with urethral stricture or hemorrhagic cystitis.[16] Subacute or chronic hepatitis, particularly of the non A, non B type, may also manifest itself after the first year.[17] A number of virus-related tumors may also occur late. The most frequent may be common warts (verruca vulgaris). Some Epstein-Barr virus- (EBV)-related lymphomas and lymphoproliferative syndromes may occur after 6 months or 1 year, particularly CNS lymphoma.[18,19] Cryptococcal meningitis typically occurs later.[20]

Third, some infections occurring in the late period are simply common infections found in any population. Diverticulitis, cholecystitis, cholangitis, and common respiratory infections are not transplant-specific but because of immune suppression may present in an altered fashion or have more severe sequelae.

TYPES OF TRANSPLANTS AND CHARACTERISTIC INFECTIONS

Table 1 presents the type, severity, and characteristic sites of infections in 315 kidney, heart, and heart–lung,[10,11,21] and liver transplant recipients[6,22] at the University of Pittsburgh observed during the first year after transplantation. The statistics will vary from center to center, and they have varied in Pittsburgh from time to time. They do, however, highlight salient features of post-transplantation infections in which cyclosporine and prednisone were the main immunosuppressive agents and antilymphocyte serum was not routinely used.

While the number of infections was high in all transplant recipients, the type of infection, its severity, and its mortality vary widely with the organ(s) transplanted. The mean number of episodes of infection per patient was lowest in the renal group (0.98), and none of these patients died of infection. The heart–lung recipients had the largest number of episodes (3.19) and the largest number of deaths associated with infection (45 percent). The frequency of bacteremia may be used as an indicator of serious bacterial infection. It was highest in the liver transplant group, and the most common origin of bacteremia in this group was the abdomen and biliary tract. As many as 75 percent of the heart–lung recipients had serious lung infections and 32 percent of these patients became ill with CMV pneumonia. In comparison, symptomatic CMV disease, including CMV pneumonia, was relatively uncommon in the renal recipients. It is striking how much better the outcome was for heart recipients

TABLE 1. Frequency, Severity, and Type of Infections Occurring in the First Year after Transplanation

Type of Transplant	*N*	*Infection per Patient*	*Infection-Associated Mortality (%)*	*Patients with Bacteremia (%)*	*Patients with Symptomatic CMV (%)*	*Patients with Invasive Fungal Infections (%)*	*Most Common Site*	
							Site	*All Infections (%)*
Renal	64	0.98	0	5	8 (5)[a]	0	Urinary tract	41
Heart	119	1.36	15	13	16 (5)	8	Lung	27
Heart–lung	31	3.19	45	19	39 (32)	23	Lung	57
Liver	101	1.86	23	23	22 (5)	16	Abdomen, GI	23

[a] Percentage of all patients with CMV pneumonia.
(Data on the four transplant groups are from the Pittsburgh experience, compiled from Ho,[21] Dummer,[10,11] Kusne et al.,[6] and Singh et al.[22])

than for heart–lung recipients even though they were similar in having many serious pulmonary infections after transplantation. Invasive fungal infections, most commonly due to *Candida* and *Aspergillus*, are no longer a serious problem in renal recipients now, as opposed to the 1960s, when half of one series of deaths in renal transplant recipients had serious fungal infection[23] (see Chapter 290). However, they are still a serious problem in heart–lung and liver recipients. Finally Table 1 shows that the sites of infections after transplantation were closely related to the site of surgery.

Infections after pancreas transplantation are especially closely related to the nature of the transplant and type of operation undertaken (see below).

Kidney Recipients

Urinary tract infections are clinically more important in renal recipients than in recipients of other types of organs.[24] They are discussed here even though most of what is said applies to other transplant groups as well.

Isolates are similar to those seen in urinary tract infections in other groups: *Escherichia coli*, *Klebsiella*, Enterobacteriaceae, *Pseudomonas aeruginosa*, *Enterococcus*, and *Candida*. Once a major source of fatal bacteremia,[25,26] infections of the urinary tract are now associated with considerably less morbidity and mortality. Elimination of structural problems before or after transplantation is an important factor, as is appropriate antibiotic treatment. Improvement may also be related to the availability of more effective antimicrobial agents and to the careful monitoring of aminoglycoside therapy.[27] Data from controlled studies have shown that trimethoprim–sulfamethoxazole can prevent urinary tract infection in recipients of renal allografts[28] (see Chapter 290). Chronic and recurrent urinary tract infections remain problematic. Abnormalities such as urethral strictures, ureteral reflux, strictures at the ureterovesicle junction, or neurogenic bladder, must be sought in patients with recurrent infections. However, many of the late, chronic, or recurrent urinary tract infections seen in renal transplant recipients may be benign. Griffin and Salaman[29] assessed the effect of urinary tract infections in 86 patients who had functional grafts for more than 1 year. One-fifth of the patients acquired infection in the first 6 months and a further fifth acquired it later. Recurrent or persistent infection was common but had no observable effect on graft function or survival of patients or grafts. On the other hand, acute pyelonephritis that is not related to rejection may occur in a stable transplanted patient and cause acute renal failure. It is reversible after treatment.[30]

Viral infections of the urinary tract are common but frequently asymptomatic. Infection of papovaviruses, of either the BK or JC type, may occur after renal transplantation as a result of primary or reactivation infection.[16,31] Papovaviruses may be detected by culture, viral cytology, or antibody rises. Unlike CMVs, these viruses may cause reactivation or primary infection after the third month after transplantation. In a prospective study of 48 patients, Gardner et al.[16] found that half of the 31 BK and JC virus infections occurred in the first 3 months after transplantation and the remainder as long as 1 or 2 years thereafter. Three patients had symptoms possibly associated with papovavirus infection. One BK infection was associated with ureteral stenosis, a complication that numerous other authors have described as connected with BK infection.[31] One patient with BK infection developed malaise and vomiting. One with JC infection developed pericarditis and pleural fusion. The specificity of these latter findings and their association with the viruses have not been firmly established. However, in view of the fact that JC virus is the cause of progressive multifocal leukoencephalopathy and can produce a systemic infection involving monocytes,[32] new types of pathology in immunosuppressed subjects may be expected.

One must be alert also to other unusual pathogens. We have seen, for example, in the first 2 weeks after transplantation urinary tract tuberculosis that arose from a focus in the native kidneys. We have also seen *Mycoplasma hominis* infection cause a breakdown of uretero-vesicle anastamosis and subsequent graft loss.

While Table 1 lists no deaths due to infections in renal transplant recipients, some deaths due to infections may be expected after renal transplantation. This mortality is often related to primary CMV infection and probably to the use of antilymphocyte serums.[33,34] The problem of such infections and methods of prevention is discussed in Chapters 290 and 120.

Rubin[35] points out that some renal transplant recipients continue to have infection problems even after the first 6 months. These are patients who have a serum creatinine greater than 2 mg/dl, a daily prednisone dose greater than 20 mg, a history of multiple antirejection therapy, and a high incidence of chronic viral infection, such as CMV and non-A, non-B hepatitis.

Heart Recipients

Heart recipients have more infections and are more affected by them than kidney recipients.[10,24] As shown in Table 1, pulmonary infections are the most important infections in heart recipients in terms of frequency and clinical significance.[10,36] Most of these infections are due to common pathogenic bacteria (see Table 3). Although the prepondernance occur in the first few months after transplantation, bacterial pneumonias continue to occur sporadically in the late post-transport period after the immediate trauma of surgery is past.

Mediastinitis is a unique postoperative complication of heart and heart–lung transplant recipients. The pathogens seen are similar to those observed in other patients undergoing cardiac surgery, with *Staphylococcus aureus* and *Staphylococcus epidermidis* predominating. The clinical presentation may be subtle with only unspecific clinical signs such as low-grade fever or an elevated white count presenting for a number of days before specific signs such as erythema, tenderness, or drainage along the sternal incision develop.[37] Mediastinitis due to *Mycoplasma hominis* should be considered when clinical mediastinitis and apparently negative bacterial cultures are observed.[38] Although these mycoplasma species may grow anaerobically on some laboratory media, they can be identified better on mycoplasma agar such as A7, and one should culture specifically for mycoplasma in "culture-negative" mediastinitis. Our cases are characterized by fairly mild systemic symptoms coupled with severe destruction of bone, which in two instances required muscle-flap grafting for repair. All cases responded microbiologically to treatment with doxycycline and clindamycin. Recently Griffith et al.[39] reported a high rate of mediastinitis in patients in whom an artificial heart device was used as a bridge to transplantation. Most cases did not occur while the device was in place but after it was removed and replaced with a transplant.

It should be mentioned that surgical drainage is crucial to the success of treatment of any type of mediastinitis in the transplant patient. There is considerable controversy over the best mode of drainage. Relatively good results have been obtained using irrigation of the chest with 5% povidone–iodine solution after closure of the chest over irrigating catheters.

A number of other infections appear to be more common in heart recipients than in other types of transplant recipients. These include systemic toxoplasmosis, nocardiosis, and lymphoproliferative disease related to Epstein-Barr virus infection.[40–44] The importance of toxoplasmosis in heart recipients is likely due to transmission of an infection by the organisms encysted in the allograft[45] (see also Chapter 290). The cause of the apparent increase in the other infections is not clear.

Despite frequent trauma to the tricuspid valve and right ventricular endocardium from repeated endomyocardial biopsies, a common post-transplant practice, heart transplant recipients do not appear to be at substantial risk of endocarditis.

Heart–Lung Recipients

As a result of a shortage of suitable donors, the field of heart–lung transplantation has progressed at a slower rate than others. In many respects, the heart–lung recipients have similar infection problems to those of heart recipients but infections that are more severe. Early reports stressed the high incidence of bacterial lung infections.[11,46] We have found that these patients also have higher rates of mediastinitis, *Pneumocystis* lung infection, and cytomegalovirus pneumonia than comparable heart recipients.[11,47] Besides pneumonias other serious infections are systemic viral or fungal infections that involve the lung.[11]

The unusual vulnerability of the lungs to infection in these patients is probably multifactorial. Besides the factors related to immunosuppression, allograft reactions, anastamomic breakdown, and allograft rejection (see Chapter 290), other local factors such as ablation of the cough reflex below the tracheal anastamosis are implicated. A substantial subset of patients in the late post-transplant period develop obliterative bronchiolitis.[48,49] This is thought to arise from chronic rejection and many of these have associated recurrent pulmonary infections.[48]

Liver Transplant Recipients

Mortality associated with infections in liver recipients has decreased significantly from 47 percent[5] in the early 1980s to 23 percent[6] in the late 1980s. Still, infections remain a major problem. In a study of 101 patients, most patients have at least one bacterial infection, and two-thirds have had at least one severe infection.[6] The great of majority of serious infections in liver transplant recipients are bacterial and fungal infections in the abdomen and gastrointestional tract (see below). There were 7 cases of peritonitis, 16 intra-abdominal abscesses, and 15 cases of bacterial pneumonias.

Liver transplant recipients illustrate particularly well the dynamics of deep candidal infections. Candidal infections frequently accompany or follow serious bacterial infections, excess use of antibiotics, and excess immunosuppression. This can be seen in other transplant groups. In addition, liver transplantation involves major surgery on the GI tract, which is well known as a major significant risk factor for candidal infections.[50] In an earlier series of 1983, 42 percent of liver recipients developed one or more episodes of deep fungal infection, mostly by candida.[5] The comparable rate in a more recent series was decreased to 16 percent.[6] Patients who were on antibiotics or steroids before surgery or on prolonged antibiotic therapy after surgery and those whose operations were prolonged were at greater risk. Those whose underlying disease was primarily biliary cirrhosis had less fungal disease than others. The reasons for the recent decrease are probably related to better monitoring of immunosuppressants, particularly cyclosporine; improvement of surgical techniques; and institution of venous–venous bypass.

Abdominal Infections in Liver Transplant Recipients. Transplantation of the liver differs from other transplant operations in the length and technical difficulty of the surgery, the necessity of making anastamosis to nonsterile sites (biliary tract, gut), and the frequency of serious bleeding problems. In addition many liver transplant recipients suffer from poor nutrition and severe metabolic difficulties. Abdominal infections after liver transplantation may be a result of technical aspects of the operation and their complications. For example, a choledochojejunostomy with anastomosis of the biliary duct to a Roux-en-Y jejunal bowel loop is associated with more fungal infections than a choledochocholedochostomy with primary anastomosis of the donor to the recipient's common bile duct.

Most *liver abscesses* in the liver transplant recipient are related to biliary or vascular obstruction caused by an anatomic problem such as biliary stricture, biliary sludge, hepatic artery thrombosis, or stenosis. The abscesses may be either solitary or multiple. They present as a febrile illness with bacteremia and leukocytosis with a shift to the left. The organisms responsible for enterococcus, gram-negative bowel organisms, and anaerobes. The diagnosis may usually be made by ultrasound or CT scan. Treatment with drainage and intravenous antibiotics is usually successful if biliary abnormalities are corrected. In the case of hepatic artery thrombosis, retransplantation is generally necessary.

Cholangitis may also result from technical problems. Two situations after liver transplantation predispose to cholangitis. The first is biliary stricture. Patients with strictures may have periodic bouts of cholangitis. Some improve after dilation procedures, but in others retransplantation is necessary. The second situation is that of cholangitis after radiologic study of the biliary tract such as T-tube cholangiogram or endoscopic retrograde cholangiopancreatography (ERCP).

Cholangitis may not be easy to diagnose because many cases do not present with the classic "Charcot triad" of fever, abdominal pain, and jaundice. The clinical presentation may be difficult to distinguish from that of rejection. The diagnosis is more reliable if there is bacteremia or if a liver biopsy indicates pericholangitis with classic aggregates of neutrophils around bile ducts. It is important to choose antibiotics to cover gram-negative enteric and anaerobic bacteria when cholangitis is suspected. Since procedures such as T-tube cholangiograms and ERCP may be followed by cholangitis and bacteremia, prophylactic antibiotics are recommended.

Peritonitis can accompany other abdominal infections such as abdominal abscesses and cholangitis and frequently complicates biliary leaks or disruption of an abdominal visucs. Bile peritonitis may occur after extraction of a T-tube. This is often well tolerated and may resolve by itself, but occasionally the leak persists and the chemical peritonitis becomes secondarily infected. The most common organisms involved in peritonitis are enterococcus and aerobic enteric gram-negative rods, but staphylococcal and candida infections are not infrequent. In established peritonitis prolonged antibiotic therapy is indicated together with drainage of associated abscesses and repair of technical problems such as biliary leaks.

Abdominal abscesses are more common in patients who have had frequent or lengthy abdominal operations. Only about one third of abdominal abscesses are associated with bacteremia. The location may be not only in the vicinity of the liver but splenic, pericolic, and pelvic abscesses are also seen. Most patients with abscesses have had an abdominal operation in the preceding 30 days. One-third of abscesses are polymicrobial, and although anaerobes and gram-negative enteric organisms cause most abscesses, they may be caused by coagulase-positive and coagulase-negative staphylococci. Usually radiologic studies (CT scan, ultrasound) define the location of the abscess, but occasionally the abscess is discovered only at laparotomy. As with any other abscesses, the appropriate treatment is a combination of drainage and antibiotics directed against the responsible pathogens.

CMV hepatitis occurs in about 4 percent of liver recipients.[51] Tissue obtained by liver biopsy is essential for diagnosis. Patients with isolated CMV hepatitis or enteritis often resolve their infections, but those who have disseminated disease often succumb. CMV hepatitis may be severe enough to necessitate retransplantation[51] (see Chapter 120). There is no approved therapy for CMV infection, but drugs, particularly ganciclovir, are being investigated.[52] Herpes simplex virus infection, particularly of the systemic type and of the liver, may also be more frequent after liver transplantation.[22] They also occur after renal transplantation.[53,54] There may not be any other obvious systemic or skin involvement. Biopsy diagnosis is helpful for hepatitis. If the infection is detected early in the hepatitis course, it responds well to acyclovir therapy.

Pancreas Transplant Recipients

Pancreas transplantation will almost certainly play an important role in organ transplantation in the next decade. It can potentially prevent the secondary and tertiary complications of type I diabetes mellitus by restoring physiologic titration of insulin in accordance with metabolic needs. In exchange for perfect diabetic management and prevention of complications, however, at present one assumes the risks of major operation, its complications, and the problems of long-term immunosuppression. The experience so far comes largely from patients with kidney transplants who desire to be freed of recurrent diabetes nephropathy in the transplanted kidney. It indicates that pancreas transplantation may be technically successful, but long-term graft survival is still not ideal. There is the usual incidence of opportunistic infectious complications associated with immunosuppression, but the most important infections are surgical abdominal infections peculiar to this type of transplantation.

Review of 116 pancreas transplants over a 7 year period in Minnesota indicates that intra-abdominal infections occurred in 22 percent of the transplant recipients 20 ± 12 days after transplantation.[8] They occurred equally in patients when exocrine secretion was managed by enteric drainage or by full drainage into the peritoneal cavity. While patient survival was generally high, 27 percent of those who contracted such infections died. This high incidence of parapancreatic deep wound infections with occasional mycotic aneurysm and hemorrhage is due to two factors: pancreatitis in the allograft and contamination of the wound with enteric organisms from the transplant duodenum or from the pancreatinojejunostomy utilized to drain off pancreatic exocrine secretions. Other methods of managing the pancreatic exocrine secretions carry a lower infection complication ratio. The pancreatic duct can be injected with a number of polymers, including Neoprene, which plug the duct. Alternatively, the duct can be left open to drain into the peritoneal cavity and cleared by the peritoneal lymphatics. These two techniques enjoy a low infection ratio. Unforunately, the former leads to pancreatic fibrosis and the later to a sterile peritonitis. The most successful solution to the problem has been to anastomose the ampulla of Vater to the urinary bladder. This technique has a much lower incidence of deep wound infection because intraoperative enteric contamination is reduced.

SITES AND TYPES OF INFECTION

Infections of the Skin and Wound Infection

Infections of the skin are extremely common after transplantation but rarely life-threatening. They constitute a significant nuisance to the transplant recipient, and they may indicate the presence of serious systemic infection. The most common pathogens are listed in Table 2.

All transplant recipients who undergo surgical procedures are at risk for wound infections. The reported incidence of wound infections after transplantation varies widely from center to center and appears to be highest in liver transplant recipients, lower in heart and heart–lung transplant recipients, and lowest in renal transplant recipients and bone marrow recipients. The most common isolate is *Staphylococcus aureus*, but infections with gram-negative enteric bacteria, *Staphylococcus epidermidis*, *Candida* species, and *Mycoplasma hominis* may also be seen.[38] Sternal wound infections following heart or heart–lung transplantation may be particularly devastating if they extend to the mediastinum (see above).

TABLE 2. Common Skin Pathogens in Transplant Recipients

Staphylococcus aureus
Herpes simplex virus
Varicella-zoster virus
Papillomavirus
Dermatophytes
Candida species

The most common viral infections of the skin are those caused by herpes simplex virus (HSV) and varicella-zoster virus. HSV-1 and HSV-2 may cause typical mucocutaneous lesions in the oral and perineal regions. These are usually benign but may at times be harbingers of a disseminated infection.[55] Herpes zoster occurs in 7–16 percent of renal and cardiac recipients[10,14,15,36] and may extend beyond the immediate post-transplant period. Warts are usually treated with surgery, including electro- or cryosurgery, or by the application of agents such as podophyllum. Dermatophyte infections usually respond to topical antifungals such as clotrimazole and miconazole.

The skin is often a target organ for many systemic infections. Systemic bacterial, candidal, cryptococcal, aspergillus, nocardial, atypical mycobacteria, and CMV infections may present with skin manifestations. As a rule one should be aggressive about investigating any new or unusual skin lesion by biopsies in transplant recipients.

Infections of the Urinary Tract

Urinary tract infections are discussed under "Kidney Recipients."

Infections of the Blood Stream

Bacteremia. The basic approach to the patient with bacteremia is the same whether or not one is dealing with transplant recipients. Usually one is dealing with a life-threatening infection. The first step is to ascertain the source of the bacteremia. Common sites producing bacterial blood stream infections are the lung, urinary tract, abdomen (including the biliary tract), skin, and soft tissues. The sinuses, upper airway structures, and bones are relatively uncommon sources of bacteremia, and the central nervous system is rarely a source, although it may be secondarily invaded. A thorough history, physical exam with basic laboratory studies, cultures, and radiographic studies can usually pinpoint likely primary sites producing bacteremia.

The sources of bacteremias reflect the common sites of infection, which vary with the type of transplantation (Table 1). For example, 62 percent of the bacteremias in kidney recipients came from the urinary tract or from perinephric abscesses.[21,25]

In 101 liver transplant recipients, 33 bacteremias occurred in 26 patients.[6] Twelve (36 percent) of the bacteremias had a fatal outcome. The most common source was the abdomen (33 percent), followed by the urinary tract (21 percent). The other bacteremias with a known source arose from wound infection (9 percent), intravenous catheters (6 percent), pneumonia (6 percent), and endocarditis (3 percent). Twenty-one percent of the bacteremias did not have a known source. It is likely that most of these also originated in the abdomen. Fifty-one percent of the blood cultures with single isolates were gram-negative aerobic bacteria, including *Pseudomonas*, 27 percent were gram-positive aerobic organisms, and 9 percent were anaerobes. Twelve percent of positive cultures had multiple isolates.

Hofflin et al.[56] compared the infectious complications of heart transplant recipients on either azathioprine or cyclosporine supplemented with corticosteroids and noted that bacteremias occurred in 29 and 15 percent of the respective groups. The source of 3 of the 11 cases of bacteremias in the cyclosporine group was unidentified; 2 were due to vascular catheters. The most frequent isolates were enterococci (3), *Pseudomonas aerugi-*

nosa (2), *Escherichia coli* (1), *Staphylococcus aureus* (1), *S. epidermidis* (1), *Klebsiella pneumoniae* (1), and anaerobes (1).

Blood-borne Infection with Nonbacterial Agents. The only *fungi* that are isolated from the blood stream of transplant patients with any frequency are candida and cryptococci. Self-limited catheter-related sepsis with candida is a well recognized entity in normal hosts that can often be treated by catheter removal and observation. However, detection of candida in the blood stream of transplant recipients often signifies invasive infection requiring amphotericin therapy. Metastatic lesions to the skin or retina may occur in patients with disseminated candidiasis. Cryptococcemia is frequently associated with cryptococcal infection elsewhere, most often the central nervous system, and carries a poor prognosis.[57] If routine viral cultures of buffy coat specimens are performed on transplant recipients, viremia with cytomegalovirus will be found in from 25 to 50 percent of all of the patients during the first 2 months after transplantation.[58] Less than half of these patients have a clinical illness due to cytomegalovirus so that the detection of CMV in the blood does not have a very high positive predictive value for disease.[24,58] However, significant CMV disease usually does not usually occur in the absence of CMV viremia. Both varicella-zoster virus and herpes simplex virus may be sometimes detected in buffy coat cultures during disseminated disease with these agents. Viremia with herpes simplex virus is usually associated with fulminant and often fatal disease.[53,54]

Infections in the Chest

Pulmonary Infections. The lung is the most common site of serious infection in heart and heart–lung transplant recipients, and pulmonary infections are also of great importance in other transplant recipient groups as well.

The usual microbial causes of pneumonia in the transplant recipient are listed in Table 3. They are subdivided according to whether the pneumonia occurs in the first month after transplantation or later and whether they are common or less common. The key to the management of pneumonia in transplant recipients is to identify rapidly the responsible pathogen and initiate specific therapy. Patients with a brief duration (≤3 days) of symptoms, who have a focal chest infiltrate, and who are producing sputum that shows neutrophils and a predominant bacterial population on Gram stain are more likely to have a routine bacterial pneumonia, and therapy to cover the bacteria found in the sputum can usually be begun. The presence of diffuse infiltrates (or nodular lesions), a nonproductive cough, or a long (≥7 days) duration of symptoms favors the presence of an unusual or "opportunistic" pathogen, and consideration should be given to the use of invasive techniques to make the diagnosis.

TABLE 3. Microbial Causes of Pneumonia in Transplant Recipients

Early Pneumonia (≤30 days)	*Late Pneumonia (>30 days)*
Common causes	
Gram-negative enteric bacilli	*Pneumococcus*
Staphylococcus	*Haemophilus influenzae*
Aspiration	*Pneumocystis*
	Cytomegalovirus
	No cause identified
Less common causes	
Aspergillus	*Nocardia*
Herpes simplex virus	*Legionella*
Legionella	*Aspergillus*
Toxoplasma	*Gram-negative enteric bacilli*
	Staphylococcus
	Aspiration
	Varicella
	Tuberculosis
	Coccidioidomycosis
	Histoplasmosis

Transtracheal aspiration was used for many years to obtain uncontaminated respiratory secretions for the diagnosis of pulmonary infection[56,59] but has largely been abandomed. More recently, bronchoscopy with bronchoalveolar lavage (BAL) has been promoted as a means of diagnosing infectious lung disease in the immunocompromised host. The major advantage of BAL appears to be its excellent sensitivity (90 percent) in diagnosing pneumocystis infection.[60]

Patients who present with the new appearance of peripheral lung nodules or cavities on chest radiograph may undergo percutaneous aspiration of these lesions with radiographic guidance (CT scan or fluoroscope) to obtain diagnostic material. Lung biopsy is usually reserved for those patients in whom the procedures listed above do not yield a strong presumptive diagnosis.

The frequency of *Legionella* infection may vary widely, depending on its endemicity in the hospital and sensitivity of diagnostic methods (see Chapter 290). It is possible, however, that sporadic cases will continue to occur in transplant patients despite hyperchlorination of the hot water system. *Legionella* pneumonia cannot be diagnosed unless specifically sought, since special laboratory procedures are necessary. The most specific method of diagnosis is isolation of the organism on special medium, but other methods, such as direct visualization by fluorescein labeled antiserum, serodiagnosis, and nucleic acid probing are also helpful. Even though specific treatment with erythromycin is available, a fatal outcome may result.[61] We have seen *Legionella* infection present as pneumonia, frequently with globular pleural based lesions, lung abscess, pleural effusion, and pericardial effusion. Any one of the serotypes of *Legionella pneumophila* or *Legionella micdadei* may be involved.[62] *Aspergillus* or *Nocardia* infection may also be relatively common in some localities. The factors required in the local environment for these occurrences are poorly understood.

Although a microbial cause is usually found for most pneumonias, particularly in the early post-transplant period, a definite etiologic agent is not always found later.

Abdominal and Gastrointestional Infections

Abdominal infections in liver transplant patients have already been discussed. They are less frequent after transplant operations that do not involve the abdomen. When they do occur they are often related to preexisting pathologic conditions such as biliary stones and diverticulosis. The presentation of these illnesses may be atypical in patients receiving corticosteroids, so one should have a low threshold for investigating abdominal symptoms in transplant recipients. CMV gastritis and enteritis do not appear to be related to type of surgery and may occur in all transplant groups. Their frequency is not well defined because endoscopic and tissue studies are needed for a definite diagnosis. One finds small ulcers or occasionally erythematous papules in the gastrointestinal mucosa anywhere from the distal esophagus to the rectum (see Chapter 120). There may be associated abdominal pain, diarrhea, or gastrointestinal bleeding, but the patients occasionally may be asymptomatic. Herpes simplex virus and *Candida* may also cause esophageal and occasionally gastric or duodenal ulcers. *Candida esophagitis* may respond to intensive oral therapy with nystatin, but patients sometimes need systemic therapy with amphotericin B. We have avoided ketoconazole therapy because of its reported interference with cyclosporine metabolism, although it may be useful in some circumstances. Herpetic esophagitis usually responds rapidly to intravenous acyclovir.

Hepatitis. La Quaglia et al.[17] report that 10 percent of 402 consecutive renal transplant recipients developed hepatitis; 12 percent were due to hepatitis B, 24 percent to CMV, 2 percent to azathioprine toxicity, and the remainder (52 percent) presumably to non-A, non-B hepatitis. The mortality in this group was significantly higher than in controls without hepatitis (45 versus 16 percent), but only 1 patient died of liver failure. The majority died of unrelated infections, perhaps as a result of the nonspecific immunosuppressive effect of a non-A, non-B virus. In accordance with this hypothesis, allograft survival in patients with hepatitis was actually better (73 versus 50 percent).

Herpes simplex virus,[22] adenovirus type 5,[63] and varicella-zoster all can cause hepatitis in the transplant setting. The most fulminant hepatitis is caused by herpes simplex virus, but it is also the most treatable if an early diagnosis is made. The liver can also be involved in systemic fungal infection such as disseminated candida infection. Rarely other fungi such as *Histoplasma* or *Aspergillus* can be seen. Liver "failure" is not usually observed with these infections, but hepatic enzyme elevations are frequent. Diagnosis of each of these liver infections requires a biopsy.

Infections of the Central Nervous System

CNS infections in transplant patients are an important cause of morbidity and mortality. They require prompt evaluation and diagnosis and early appropriate therapy. Any of the common pathogens that produce meningitis or cerebritis may afflict the transplant patient, but Table 4 presents in order of approximate frequency a list of the most commonly seen agents in our experience and that of others.[35,64] Notably absent on the list are the pyogenic bacteria and the herpesviruses, which are common pathogens at other sites in transplant recipients. As in the case of other infections, the highest risk for opportunistic CNS infection is present 1–6 months after transplantation; however, there are exceptions. For example, cryptococcal meningitis, for unknown reasons, is usually a "late" event.[20] The clinical presentation of CNS infection may be subtle even with life-threatening infection. During evaluation special attention should be directed to the fundoscopic exam, the paranasal exam, and the presence of pulmonary or skin lesions.

Listeria monocytogenes is a gram-positive rod that typically causes bacteremia, meningitis, and at times cerebritis in the immunosuppressed transplant patient. Fever and headache are frequent complaints; mild alterations in consciousness occur in 70 percent of the patients, but meningeal irritation may be absent. The Gram stain of the spinal fluid is negative in over half the cases. Usually the diagnosis is made by culturing the organism from cerebrospinal fluid or blood. All patients with *Listeria* bacteremia should have lumbar punctures even in the absence of CNS signs. Although most cases of listeriosis are sporadic, cluster outbreaks of *Listeria* infection among transplant patients have occurred; a common source is usually not found.[65]

Aspergillus fumigatus is a ubiquitous fungus that is an important cause of infection in immunocompromised patients. The most common portal of entry is the lung; invasive sinus infection also occurs but is less common. *Aspergillus* infections in solid organ transplant recipients usually occur 1–4 months after transplantation. Bone marrow transplant recipients usually have fungal infection during the periods of profound neutropenia in the first 30 days after transplantation. *Aspergillus* invades blood vessels, and metastatic spread may occur early in the infection. The onset of CNS infection by aspergillus is usually more acute than that of cryptococcosis, and it should be suspected in a patient who becomes disoriented, develops seizures, or exhibits focal neurologic findings such as hemiparesis. Examination of the CSF is not usually helpful in establishing the diagnosis; the fluid may be normal or have the characteristics of a parameningeal focus with elevated protein, with or without a pleocytosis.[66] The CT scan reveals single or multiple low-density, nonenhancing lesions. The prognosis of CNS aspergillus infections is dismal, and the only hope is to begin high-dose amphotericin B therapy as early as possible. If the lesions are in less critical areas of the brain, consideration should be given to drainage or resection.

TABLE 4. Pathogens of the Central Nervous System in Transplant Patients

Listeria monocytogenes
Aspergillus fumigatus
Cryptococcus neoformans
Toxoplasma gondii
Nocardia asteroides
Mucoraceae
Progressive multifocal leukoencephalopathy
Candida
Varicella-zoster

Cryptococcal meningitis usually presents subacutely, often with only headache or low-grade fever.[20,35] Meningeal signs and focal neurologic signs are infrequent until later in the course. Pulmonary disease due to *Cryptococcus* coexists in about 40 percent of the cases. A lumbar puncture should be performed in any cryptococcal infection even if no CNS signs are present. The spinal fluid usually contains a white blood cell count (WBC) less than 500 per cubic mm. predominantly lymphocytes, a moderate elevation in protein, low glucose concentration, and positive cryptococcal antigen. India ink preparations reveal positive findings in about 40 percent of patients. Cerebrospinal fluid (CSF) cultures are usually positive for *Cryptococcus* in 48–72 hours. CT scan of the head is usually normal, although occasionally a mass lesion, a cryptococcoma, is found. Blood and urine cultures should be submitted. Treatment is described elsewhere (see Chapter 241).

Toxoplasma gondii is a protozoan that can cause a nonspecific encephalopathy, diffuse meningoencephalitis, or progressive single or multiple brain lesions. It has been reported in renal, cardiac, liver, and bone marrow transplant recipients.[40,67–69] Toxoplasmosis may result from reactivation of latent infection or from new acquisition of the organism. The cardiac allograft has been shown to be a potential source of infection.[40] The patient may present with persistent fever without a defined source or with various foci of infection, including the central nervous system, myocardium, and lungs. The neurologic manifestations of a *Toxoplasma* infection are seizures, visual disturbances, headache, photophobia, and focal neurologic findings. Examination of the CSF classically reveals a slight mononuclear pleocytosis and an elevated protein with a normal glucose concentration. Serology should be performed on cardiac donors and recipients to identify patients at risk for allograft transmitted disease. Definitive diagnosis usually requires tissue biopsy, though occasionally the organism may be isolated from peripheral blood cells in tissue culture. The fatality rate is high and often the diagnosis is not established until autopsy.

Nocardia asteroides is a gram-positive, beaded, branching rod that may cause CNS lesions. The pulmonary disease may occur for unknown reasons more commonly in certain centers than others.[70] The primary route of infection is pulmonary with metastatic spread to bone, skin, and central nervous system. It is possible to have single or multiple brain abscesses, but meningitis is rare. Evaluation of the transplant patient in whom *Nocardia* is suspected should include a chest radiograph, CT scan of the head, bronchoscopy (if infiltrates are present), bone scan, and biopsy of any new cutaneous nodules. *Nocardia* brain abscesses may benefit from stereotactic aspiration biopsy, and surgical drainage in addition to long-term (9 months), high-dose (6–8 g qd) sulfonamide therapy.[71,72] We usually use sulfisoxazole. It is helpful to monitor sulfa levels periodically. The most common side effect of sulfa therapy is gastrointestinal distress. Possibilities for alternative therapy include minocycline and trimethoprim–sulfamethoxazole, amikacin, and a cephalosporin such as cefotaxime sodium.

SPECIFIC PROBLEMS OF HERPESVIRUS INFECTIONS

Herpes Simplex Virus Infections

Most herpes simplex infections occurring after transplantation represent reactivation infections in previously seropositive subjects.[73] As in immunologically healthy people, these infections usually involve the oral or genital mucocutaneous area. They are frequently more severe and protracted in transplant recipients than in healthy people, and in some groups prevention may be desirable. Many centers use oral or intravenous prophylactic acyclovir for the first 3 or 4 weeks after bone marrow transplantation. We do not use this measure in solid organ transplant recipients since such infections are generally easily identified and self-limited. In some cases the localized infections may spread to other parts of the body or there may be evidence of systemic spread. In either protracted local disease or the presence of systemic spread, intravenous acyclovir at intermediate doses, 5 mg/kg three times a day for 1 week to 10 days, is indicated. Oral therapy may be sufficient for milder forms of local disease including some cases of esophagitis.

Primary herpes accompanied by systemic spread occurred in two kidney recipients who were seronegative before transplantation in each case.[54,55] On two occasions, the common donor of the allograft kidneys was seropositive and the virus isolates from the two recipients were identical by restriction endonuclease analysis, implicating the donor as the source. How important the kidney is as a vehicle for herpes simplex infection is still unclear.

As in the neonate the most important indicator of systemic spread of herpesvirus may be sudden onset of severe hepatitis. There may be fever, dramatic rise of liver enzymes, and even disseminated intravascular coagulation. All of this occurs within 1 month after transplantation at a time when other types of viral hepatitis are unusual. CMV and hepatitis B infections generally require an incubation period of 1 month or more. Usually a biopsy is needed to diagnose any viral hepatitis, particularly in the case of liver transplantation or where rejection must be ruled out. Herpes simplex hepatitis shows severe necosis, and the virus is easily demonstrated by culture, immunofluorescence, or enzyme-linked antibody determinations. Herpes simplex hepatitis was previously uniformly fatal, but we have had cures after prompt institution of acyclovir therapy. The spread of the herpes simplex virus to the central nervous system is not common in transplant patients even in the presence of disseminated infection.

Cytomegalovirus Infections

Almost all seropositive graft recipients experience reactivation of latent CMV infections, and the majority of seropositive recipients develop primary infections (see also Chapter 120). Primary infections are more likely to be symptomatic.[74,75] The proportion of infected patients who become symptomatic is also a function of the intensity of immunosuppression.

The most common and least serious type of CMV disease is a mononucleosis syndrome characterized by fever, frequently of prolonged duration. There may be abnormalities of the liver function tests, though rarely jaundice, and often leukopenia and atypical lymphocytes may be present. Occasionally these may be absent or low (less than 10 percent) in number. Other manifestations, such as arthralgias, myalgias, and skin rash, are less frequent. Lymphadenopathy and organomegaly are uncommon.[75]

Interstitial pneumonia is the most common serious complication of CMV infection. There are no pathognomonic signs of this disease, and a tissue diagnosis by bronchoalveolar lavage or lung biopsy is required.[60] CMV pneumonia may coexist with other pathogens, particularly *Pneumocystis*.

One of the more troublesome manifestations of CMV disease is ulcerations in the gastrointestinal tract, although this is less apparent in transplant patients than in AIDS patients. These ulcerations are often multiple and may be found anywhere from the esophagus to the rectum. Bleeding, signs of peptic ulceration, or perforation may result. CMV disease should be considered in the event of an acute abdomen after transplantation, especially if no recent operation involving the abdomen has taken place. The diagnosis may not always be clear. Tissue evidence of local infection is essential but not always conclusive, as such infection may occur without being the cause of local symptoms.

Severe hepatitis due to CMV is unusual despite the ubiquity of chemical hepatitis in CMV disease. It may, however, occur in liver transplant recipients.[51] As in hepatitis due to herpes simplex virus, there may be difficulty distinguishing CMV hepatitis from rejection. Biopsy and tissue diagnosis are essential. (For further discussion of CMV, see Chapter 120.)

Varicella-Zoster Virus Infection

Children who are susceptible and are transplant recipients may suffer from severe varicella like other immunosuppressed children. Varicella-zoster immune globulin (VZIG) should be administered to such children within 72 hours after known contact with chickenpox. Once symptoms have developed, it is useless, and intravenous acyclovir, 500 mg/m^2 q8h or 10 mg/kg q8h iv should be instituted.

Herpes zoster may occur in 7–16 percent of transplant recipients, most often in the first 6 months after transplantation, but it may occur at any time.[10,14,15] Like herpes zoster in other immunosuppressed patients, these episodes are usually self-limited, but in the more severely immunosuppressed individuals severe morbidity due to local or systemic dissemination may occur.

Epstein-Barr Virus Infections and Associated Disorders

EBV infection, like CMV infection, occurs as a primary infection in a seronegative recipient or a secondary infection in a seropositive recipient. Among children 50 percent are seronegative and among adults, only 8.2 percent are seronegative.[21,76] Primary infection occurs in about two-thirds of susceptible children and adults. Thirty-three percent of seropositive patients develop secondary infections.[21] Most infections occur within the first 4 months after transplantation.[21,76] The most important disease associated with EBV infections is EBV-related lymphoproliferative syndrome observed in the patient population. We have found, in both pediatric and adult patients, that the highest risk for lymphoproliferative syndromes occurs in patients who develop primary EBV infection within the first 3 months after transplantation.[44,77] These individuals may be identified if a pretransplant serum for antibodies against EBV is available. Most, though not all, of the remaining patients with lymphoproliferative syndrome have evidence of reactivation EBV infection, usually significant rises in IgG antibody to virus capsid antigen. In some patients a mononucleosis syndrome similar to the CMV mononucleosis syndrome may occur, except that sore throat and lymphadenopathy may be seen in addition to fever, biochemical hepatitis, and mononucleosis.

The lymphoproliferative syndrome consists of three general

types.[44] First, it may be an isolated or recurrent severe mononucleosis-like syndrome without evidence of tissue involvement except in tonsils and peripheral lymph nodes. The second manifestation is a diffuse polymorphous B-cell infiltration in many visceral organs. This type is usually preceded by a "mono-like" episode, which may evolve directly into the tissue infiltrative process or be temporarily separated from it. It is similar to the lethal X-linked lymphoproliferative syndrome described in children with a congenital susceptibility to EBV.[78] Terminal hepatitis with disseminated intravascular coagulation, other clotting defects, and deficient immunoglobulin levels have been seen.[44] The third clinical presentation is the appearance of localized tumors in the gastrointestinal tract, neck, thorax, or other parts of the body. Tumors in the brain have also been described.[18] These tumors have the microscopic appearance of lymphomas and contain EBV genomes detectable by nucleic acid hybridization or EBV-specific antigens, such as nuclear antigen. These tumors are monoclonal or oligoclonal in type as determined by IgG light chain phenotype or immunoglobulin gene rearrangement.[79,80] Involved tissues of the other two clinical types of lymphoproliferative syndrome also contain evidence of EBV infection demonstrated by presence of EBV nuclear antigen or by EBV genomes.[44] Acyclovir has no proven efficacy either in the mononucleosis syndrome or in prevention or amelioration of these lymphoproliferative syndromes. It has, however, been used empirically.[81] Diagnosis of EBV-associated lymphoproliferative syndrome requires first either an active or a preceding EBV infection. Its presence may be determined by pretransplant and present serum for antibodies to EBV antigens, at least viral capsid antigen (VCA). Secondly, EBV nuclear antigen and/or EBV DNA should be demonstrated in tumor tissues by immunofluorescence or nucleic acid hybridization.

Although mononucleosis syndrome may resolve and tumors may regress after reduction or elimination of immunosuppression, there is currently no reliable prognostic indicator of when patients will respond to this mode of therapy. Lymphoproliferative lesions have also been reported to relapse after an interval of well-being.[44]

REFERENCES

1. Starzl TE, Klintmalm GBG, Porter KA, et al. Liver transplantation with use of cyclosporin A and prednisone. N Engl J Med. 1981;305:266–9.
2. Kahan BD, Van Buren CT, Flechner SM, et al. Clinical and experimental studies with cyclosporine in renal transplantation. Surgery. 1985;97:125–40.
3. Solis E, Kaye MP. The registry of the International Society for Heart Transplantation: Third official report—June 1986. J Heart Transplant. 1986;5:2–5.
4. Starzl TE, Koep LJ, Halgrimson CG, et al. Fifteen years of clinical liver transplantation. Gastroenterology. 1979;77:375–88.
5. Wajszczuk CP, Logan TF, Ho M, et al. Intra-abdominal actinomycosis presenting with sulfur granules in the urine. Am J Med. 1984;77:1126–8.
6. Kusne S, Dummer JS, Ho M, et al. Infections after liver transplantation: An analysis of 101 consecutive cases. Medicine. 1988;67:132–43.
7. Iwatsuki S, Starzl TE, Todo RD, et al. Experience in 1000 liver transplants under cyclosporine-steroid therapy: A survival report. Transplant Proc. 1988;20:498–504.
8. Hesse UJ, Sutherland DER, Najarian JS, et al. Intra-abdominal infections in pancreas transplant recipients. Ann Surg. 1985;203:153–62.
9. Peterson PK, Balfour HH, Fryd DS, et al. Fever in renal transplant recipients: Causes, prognostic significance and changing patterns at the University of Minnesota Hospital. Am J Med. 1981;345–51.
10. Dummer JS. Infectious complications of transplantation. In: Brest AN, ed. Cardiovascular Clinics. 1988. In press.
11. Dummer JS. Infectious complications of heart–lung transplantation. In: Cooper DKC, ed. Heart and Lung Replacement. Medical and Technical Press Ltd: 1988. In press.
12. Pearson JC, Amend WJ, Vincenti FG, et al. Post-transplantation pyelonephritis: Factors producing low patient and transplant morbidity. J Urol. 1980;123:153–6.
13. Egbert PR, Pillard RB, Gallagher JB, et al. Cytomegalovirus retinitis in immunosuppressed hosts. Ann Intern Med. 1980;93:664–70.
14. Rifkind D. The activation of varizella-zoster virus infections by immunosuppressive therapy. J Lab Clin Med. 1966;68:463.
15. Spenser ES, Anderson HK. Clinically evident, non-terminal infection with herpesvirus and wart virus in immunosuppressed renal transplant recipients. Br Med J. 1970;3:251–4.
16. Gardner SD, Mackenzie EFD, Smith C, et al. Prospective study of the human polyomaviruses BK and JC and cytomegalovirus in renal transplant recipients. J Clin Pathol. 1984;37:578–86.
17. La Quaglia MP, Tolkoff-Rubin NE, Dienstag JL, et al. Impact of hepatitis on renal transplantation. Transplantation. 1981;32:504–7.
18. Hanto D, Frizzera G, Gajl-Peczalska K, et al. Epstein-Barr virus, immunodeficiency, and B cell lymphoproliferation. Transplantation. 1985;39:461–72.
19. Ho M, Miller G, Atchison RW, et al. Epstein-Barr virus infections and DNA hybridization studies in post-transplantation lymphoma and lymphoproliferative lesions: Role of primary infection. J Infect Dis. 1985;152:876–86.
20. Hooper DC, Pruitt AA, Rubin RH. Central nervous system infection in the chronically immunosuppressed. Medicine. 1982;61:166–85.
21. Ho M. Infection and organ transplantation. In: Gelman S, ed. Anesthesia and Organ Transplantation. Philadelphia: Saunders; 1987:49–60.
22. Singh N, Dummer JS, Ho M, et al. Infections with cytomegalovirus and other herpesviruses in 121 liver transplant recipients: Transmission by donated organ and the effect of OKT3 antibodies. J Infect Dis. 1988;158:124–31.
23. Rifkind D, Marchioro TL, Schneck SA, et al. Systemic fungal infections complicating renal transplantation and immunosuppressive therapy. Am J Med. 1967;43:28–38.
24. Ho M, Wajszczuk CP, Hardy A, et al. Infections in kidney, heart and liver transplant recipients on cyclosporine. Transplant Proc. 1983;15:2768–72.
25. Myerowitz RL, Medeiros AA, O'Brien TF. Bacterial infection in renal homotransplant recipients: A study of fifty-three bacteremic episodes. Am J Med. 1972;53:308–14.
26. Anderson RJ, Schafer LA, Olin DB, et al. Septicemia in renal transplant patients. Arch Surg. 1973;106:692–4.
27. Tofte RW, Canafax DM, Simmons RL, et al. Aminoglycoside dosing in renal transplant patients: Comparison of nomogram and individualized pharmacokinetic methods in patients with shifting renal function. Ann Surg. 1982;195:287–93.
28. Tolkoff-Rubin NE, Cosima AB, Russell PS, et al. A controlled study of TMP–SMZ prophylaxis of urinary tract infections in renal transplant recipients. Rev Infect Dis. 1982;4:614–8.
29. Griffin PJA, Salaman JR. Urinary tract infections after renal transplantation: Do they matter: Br Med J. 1979;1:710–1.
30. Gillum DM, Kelleher SP. Acute pyelonephritis as a cause of late transplant dysfunction. Am J Med. 1985;78:156–8.
31. Hogan TF, Borden EC, McBain JA, et al. Human polyomavirus infections with JC virus and renal transplant patients. Ann Intern Med. 1980;92:373–8.
32. Houff SA, Major EO, Katz DA, et al. Involvement of JC virus-infected mononuclear cells from the bone marrow and spleen in the pathogenesis of progressive multifocal leukoencephalopathy. N Engl J Med. 1988;318:301–5.
33. Snydman DR, Werner BG, Heinze-Lacey B, et al. Use of cytomegalovirus immune globulin to prevent cytomegalovirus disease in renal-transplant recipients. N Engl J Med. 1987;317:1049–54.
34. Najarian JS, Fryd DS, Strand M, et al. A single institution, randomized, prospective trial of cyclosporine versus azathioprine–antilymphocyte globulin for immunosuppression in renal allograft recipients. Ann Surg. 1985;201:142–57.
35. Rubin RH. Infection in the renal and liver transplant patient. In: Rubin RH, Young LS, eds. Clinical Approach to Infection in the Compromised Host, 2d ed. New York: Plenum; 1988;557–621.
36. Copeland JG, Stinson EB. Human heart transplantation. In: Harvey WP, ed. Current Problems in Cardiology. Chicago: Year Book Medical; 1980:3–49.
37. Trento A, Bahnson HT, Dummer JS, et al. Mediastinitis following heart transplantation: Incidence, treatment, and results. Heart Transplant. 1984;3:336–40.
38. Steffenson DO, Dummer JS, Granick MS, et al. *Mycoplasma hominis* median sternotomy infections. Ann Intern Med. 1987;106:204–8.
39. Griffith BP, Kormos RL, Hardesty RL, et al. The artificial heart: Infection-related morbidity and its effect on transplantation. Ann Thoracic Surg. 1988;45:409–15.
40. Luft BJ, Naot Y, Araujo FG, et al. Primary and reactivated toxoplasma infection in patients with cardiac transplants. Ann Intern Med. 1983;99:27–31.
41. Wreghitt TG, Hakim M, Cory-Pearce R, et al. The impact of donor-transmitted CMV and *Toxoplasma gondii* disease in cardiac transplantation. Transplant Proc. 1986;18:1375–6.
42. Simpson GL, Stinson EB, Egger MJ, et al. Nocardial infections in the immunocompromised host: A detailed study in a defined population. Rev Infect Dis. 1981;3:492 507.
43. Beveridge T, Krupp P, McKibbin C. Lymphomas and lymphoproliferative lesions developing under cyclosporine therapy (Letter). Lancet. 1984;1:788.
44. Ho M, Jaffe R, Miller G, et al. The frequency of Epstein-Barr virus infection and associated lymphoproliferative syndrome after transplantation and its manifestations in children. Transplantation. 1988;45:719–27.
45. Ruskin J, Remington JS. Toxoplasmosis in the compromised host. Ann Intern Med. 1976;84:193–9.
46. Brooks RG, Hofflin JM, Jamieson SW, et al. Infectious complications in heart–lung transplant recipients. Am J Med. 1985;79:412–22.
47. Dummer JS, Montero CG, Griffith BP, et al. Infection in heart–lung transplant recipients. Transplantation. 1986;41:725–9.
48. Burke CM, Dawkins KD, Blank N, et al. Post-transplant obliterative bron-

chiolitis and other late lung sequelae in human heart–lung transplantation. Chest. 1984;86:824–9.
49. Yousem SA, Burke CM, Billingham ME. Pathologic pulmonary alterations in long-term human heart–lung transplantation. Hum Pathol. 1985;16:911–22.
50. Louria DB, Stiff DP, Bennet B. Disseminated moniliasis in the adult. Medicine. 1962;41:307–37.
51. Bronsther O, Makowka L, Jaffe R, et al. The occurrence of cytomegalovirus hepatitis in liver transplant patients. J Med Virol. 1988;24:423–34.
52. Shepp DH, Dandliker PS, De Miranda P, et al. Activity of 9-(2-hydroxy-1-(hydroxymethyl)ethoxymethyl) guanine in the treatment of cytomegalovirus pneumonia. Ann Intern Med. 1985;103:368–73.
53. Taylor RJ, Saul SH, Ho M, et al. Primary disseminated herpes simplex infection with fulminant hepatitis following renal transplantation. Arch Intern Med. 1981;141:1519–21.
54. Koneru B, Tzakis AG, Depuydt LE, et al. Transmission of fatal herpes simplex infection through renal transplantation. Transplantation. 1988;45:653–6.
55. Dummer JS, Armstrong J, Ho M, et al. Transmission of infection with herpes simplex virus by renal transplantation. J Infect Dis. 1987;155:202–6.
56. Hofflin JM, Potasman I, Baldwin JC, et al. Infectious complications in heart transplant recipients receiving cyclosporine and corticosteroids. Ann Intern Med. 1987;106;209–16.
57. Diamond RD, Bennett JE. Prognostic factors in cryptococcal meningitis: A study in 111 cases. Ann Intern Med. 1974;80:176–81.
58. Dummer JS, Hardy A, Ho M, et al. Early infections in kidney, heart and liver transplant recipients on cyclosporine. Transplantation. 1983; 15:2768–72.
59. Bartlett JG, Gorbach SL, Finegold SM. The bacteriology of aspiration pneumonia. Am J Med. 1974;56:202–7.
60. Stover DE, White DA, Romano PA, et al. Diagnosis of pulmonary disease in acquired immune deficiency syndrome (AIDS): Role of bronchoscopy and bronchoalveolar lavage. Am Rev Respir Dis. 1984;130:659–62.
61. Kugler JW, Armitage JO, Helms CM, et al. Nosocomial Legionnaires' disease: Occurrence in recipients of bone marrow transplants. Am J Med. 1983; 74:281–8.
62. Meyerowitz RL, Pasculle AW, Dowling JN, et al. Opportunistic lung infection due to "Pittsburgh Pneumonia Agent." N Engl J Med. 1979;301:953–8.
63. Koneru B, Jaffe R, Esquivel CO, et al. Adenoviral infections in pediatric liver transplant recipients. JAMA. 1987;258:489–92.
64. Britt RH, Enzmann Dr, Remington JS. Intracranial infection in cardiac transplant recipients. Ann Neurol. 1981;9:107–19.
65. Stamm AM, Dismukes WE, Simmons BP, et al. Listeriosis in renal transplant recipients: Report of an outbreak and review of 102 cases. Rev Infect Dis. 1982;4:665–82.
66. Weiland D, Ferguson RM, Peterson PK, et al. Aspergillosis in 25 renal transplant patients. Ann Surg. 1983;198:623–9.
67. Mason JC, Ordelheide KS, Grames GM, et al. Toxoplasmosis in two renal transplant recipients from a single donor. Transplantation. 1987;44:588–91.
68. Kusne S, Dummer JS, Ho M, et al. Self-limited toxoplasma parisitemia after liver transplantation. Transplantation. 1987;44:457–8.
69. Shepp DH, Hackman RC, Conley FK, et al. *Toxoplasma gondii* reactivation identified by detection of parasitemia in tissue culture. Ann Intern Med. 1985;103:218–21.
70. Krick JA, Stinson EB, Remington JS. *Nocardia* infection in heart transplant patients. Ann Intern Med. 1975;82:18–26.
71. Hall WA, Martinez AJ, Dummer JS, et al. Nocardial brain abscess: Diagnosis and therapeutic use of stereotactic aspiration. Surg Neurol. 1987;28;114–8.
72. Palmer DL, Harvery RL, Wheeler JK. Diagnostic and therapeutic considerations in *Nocardia asteroides* infection. Medicine. 1974;53:391–401.
73. Armstrong JA, Evans AS, Rao N, et al. Viral infections in renal transplant recipients. Infect Immun. 1976;14:970–5.
74. Ho M, Suwansirikul S, Dowling JN, et al. The transplanted kidney as a source of cytomegalovirus infection. N Engl J Med. 1975;293:1109–12.
75. Suwansirikul S, Rao N, Ho M, et al. Primary and secondary cytomegalorivus infection. Arch Intern Med. 1977;137:1026–9.
76. Breinig MK, Zitelli B, Ho M, et al. Epstein-Barr virus, cytomegalovirus, and other viral infections in children after liver transplantation. J Infect Dis. 1987;156:273–9.
77. Ho M, Miller G, Atchison RW, et al. Epstein-Barr virus infections and DNA hybridization studies in post-transplantation lymphoma and lymphoproliferative lesioins: Role of primary infection. J Infect Dis. 1985;876–86.
78. Purtilo D, Sakamoto K, Saemundsen A, et al. Documentation of Epstein-Barr virus infection in immunodeficient patients with life-threatening lymphoproliferative disease by clinical, virological, and immunopathological studies. Cancer Res. 1981;41:4226–35.
79. Starzl T, Nalesnik M, Porter K, et al. Reversibility of lymphomas and lymphoproliferative lesions developing under cyclosporine-steroid therapy. Lancet. 1984;1:583–7.
80. Cleary ML, Sklar J. Lymphoproliferative disorders in cardiac transplant recipients are multiclonal lymphomas. Lancet. 1984;2:489–93.
81. Hanto D, Frizzera G, Gajl-Peczalska K, et al. Epstein-Barr virus-induced B-cell lymphoma after renal transplantation. N Engl J Med. 1982;306:913–8.

293. EMPIRICAL THERAPY AND PREVENTION OF INFECTION IN THE IMMUNOCOMPROMISED HOST

PHILIP A. PIZZO

RATIONALE AND EVOLVING CONCEPTS FOR EMPIRICAL ANTIBIOTIC THERAPY

Empirical antibiotic therapy in febrile–granulocytopenic cancer patients became well established during the early 1970s because of the high mortality observed when antibiotics were withheld until an infectious cause could be proved.[1] Although this approach has reduced infectious morbidity and mortality, the changes in the organisms responsible for infection, the hosts susceptible to them, and the antimicrobial agents available to treat them have expanded the use of empirical therapy and have prompted the need for a continuing critical evaluation.[2]

The original targets of empirical antibiotics were gram-negative bacteria, particularly *Pseudomonas aeruginosa*. Although gram-negative bacillary infections (especially *Escherichia coli* and *Klebsiella* sp.) still predominate in some cancer centers, infections due to *P. aeruginosa* have inexplicably declined. In contrast, infections due to gram-positive cocci (*Staphylococcus aureus, Staphylococcus epidermidis*) have increased in recent years, particularly with the more widespread use of indwelling intravenous catheters,[3,4] and in many centers are the most common isolates. These organisms are less adequately covered by many empirical regimens. In some centers, methicillin-resistant *S. aureus* represents a considerable problem,[5] and in virtually all centers, the coagulase-negative staphylococci have become increasingly resistant to methicillin, making vancomycin a component of many therapeutic regimens. Of concern, isolates of coagulase-negative staphylococci that are resistant to vancomycin have also been described.[6] It should be noted, however, that the distribution of predominant pathogens often varies at different hospitals and may change at the same hospital over time, influencing both the selection and the success of empirical antibiotics.

Empirical antimicrobial management was originally formulated for patients with acute leukemia. Modern cancer therapy now renders patients with lymphomas and solid tumors as granulocytopenic as patients with leukemia, raising the question of whether these patients also require empirical antimicrobial therapy when they become febrile.

Until recently, the antibiotics used for empirical therapy consisted of first-generation cephalosporins, aminoglycosides, and/or antipseudomonal penicillins. The development of the third-generation cephalosporins, extended-spectrum penicillins, carbapenems, and quinolones offers new therapeutic options.

Although empirical therapy was initially focused on preventing death from an undiagnosed bacterial infection, patients who remain granulocytopenic for extended periods are also at risk for second infections and superinfections, particularly those due to fungi. Evidence of fungal invasion can be found at postmortem examination in 8–69 percent of patients who die with prolonged granulocytopenia, often without antemortem evidence of infection.[7–9] Whether these invasive fungal infections are a consequence of broad-spectrum antibiotics, prolonged granulocytopenia, or both remains unclear. Nonetheless, the excessive mortality related to these infections has prompted empirical antifungal therapy in some high-risk patients, although the risk–benefit ratio of current antifungal agents is suboptimal.[10,11]

Empirical antibiotics have also been used for patients who have clinically defined sites of infection when the risks of establishing a microbiologic diagnosis with an invasive diagnostic procedure appear prohibitive. The granulocytopenic patient with a new pulmonary infiltrate is such an example, since a trial of antibiotics may be preferable to immediate bronchoscopy or biopsy.

Thus, empirical antimicrobial therapy in the immunocompromised host is both multifaceted and evolving in its formulation and application. Currently relevant questions include the following: Who should receive empirical therapy and when should it be started? What constitutes appropriate initial empirical therapy? How should the initial therapy be modified for patients who remained granulocytopenic or who do not respond to the initial regimen? How long should empirical antibiotics be continued?

GUIDELINES FOR EMPIRICAL THERAPY

Candidates

As noted in Chapter 286, granulocytopenia is the single most important risk factor for infection in cancer patients. This risk, however, is also influenced by the depth and duration of the granulocytopenia as well as by qualitative abnormalities in phagocyte function, alterations in cellular or humoral immunity, and changes in physical defense barriers. Since more than 80 percent of the primary bacterial infections arise from the patient's endogenous microbial flora,[12] the spectrum and virulence of the host's colonizing flora can influence the risk for developing an infection as well as the need, selection, and success of empirically administered antibiotics.[13,14]

Whether or not all granulocytopenic patients deserve prompt empirical antibiotic management when they become febrile has been addressed in a number of recent studies. Adults with solid tumors (e.g., small cell lung cancer, testicular cancer) are at risk for fever when rendered neutropenic and appear to do well when treated empirically with antibiotics.[15] In a survey of 1001 consecutive episodes of fever in 324 pediatric and young adult cancer patients treated at the National Cancer Institute,[16] 39.5 percent had at least one febrile episode when they were granulocytopenic (defined as less than 500 polymorphonuclear leukocytes [PMNs] and band forms per cubic millimeter). Importantly, there was no apparent difference in the incidence, pattern, or severity of infectious complications that occurred, regardless of the patients' underlying malignancy, once they became granulocytopenic. Thus, as a matter of practice, all granulocytopenic patients should be considered to be at risk for infection and, once febrile, are candidates for early empirical therapy.

The level of granulocytopenia that should prompt empirical therapy is somewhat arbitrarily interpreted. Although some recommend starting antibiotics when the neutrophil count falls below 1000/mm^3, most would wait until the granulocyte count is less than 500/mm^3. Some studies have suggested that the incidence of bacteremia is significantly increased when the neutrophil count is less than 200/mm^3.[17] Perhaps more important than the absolute nadir is the rate at which the counts are falling. For example, only 17 percent of the fevers that occurred in cancer patients whose neutrophil counts are greater than 500/mm^3 could be attributed to infection. In contrast, the likelihood of an infectious cause of a fever was increased if the patient's neutrophil count was falling rapidly because of antecedent chemotherapy.[16]

The level of fever that should prompt therapy is also arbitrarily defined. In general, two or three low-grade elevations above 38°C (oral) or a single elevation above 38.5°C, in concert with a granulocyte count of less than 500/mm^3, is sufficient criterion to begin empirical therapy. Fever should not be attributable to blood products, cancer, or medications, and note should be taken to whether the patient is receiving drugs that might mask a febrile response (e.g., steroids, antipyretic containing analgesics). It is optimal to have institutional criteria for fever and granulocytopenia both predefined and rigidly adhered to. Such a policy plays an important role in reducing infection-related morbidity (e.g., shock, perianal cellulitis) and mortality.[18–20]

Preantibiotic Evaluation

The diminished inflammatory capability of the granulocytopenic patient can mask the usual signs and symptoms of infection.[21] In a prospective evaluation of 140 febrile–granulocytopenic patients,[16] it was not possible to differentiate patients with bacteremia from those with unexplained fever according to their age, sex, underlying malignancy, or types of therapeutic modalities or invasive diagnostic procedures they had received. Moreover, the absence of physical findings suggestive of infection did not exclude a potentially life-threatening bacteremia, since more than half of the bacteremic patients in this study exhibited no specific physical findings. Alternatively, even minimal signs suggesting infection must be carefully pursued.

Patients about to receive empirical therapy should have a baseline chest radiograph, a urinalysis, at least two sets of preantibiotic blood cultures, and aspirate (or biopsy) cultures from any accessible sites suggestive of infection. If blood cultures are obtained from an indwelling sialastic catheter, it is important to also obtain additional cultures(s) percutaneously from a peripheral vein. Furthermore, it is important to obtain blood cultures from each port in patients with multilumen catheters.[22]

Although the organisms ultimately responsible for infection are frequently part of the patient's colonizing flora, routine surveillance cultures from asymptomatic body sites do not appear helpful in guiding initial empirical therapy.[23] This is because no one body site is consistently positive and because multiple organisms are usually isolated from any one site, making prospective predictions of the true pathogen difficult. Moreover, the time lag for surveillance cultures to become positive does not make them prospectively useful or cost-effective. The role of surveillance cultures in guiding management decisions in patients already receiving antibiotics is also limited. Specific exceptions may be patients in protected isolation (where stool cultures may be of use) or centers with a high incidence of *Aspergillus flavus* infections (where nasal swabs may be helpful in identifying high-risk patients).[24,25]

Nuclear scanning with autologous or human leukocyte antigen (HLA)-matched allogeneic indium 111 labeled leukocytes has been used for the evaluation of the febrile–granulocytopenic cancer patient.[26] Even when positive, however, such scans are nonspecific; false-negatives make them of more limited use. Unfortunately, current attempts to develop rapid diagnostic assays to detect circulating bacterial or fungal antigens or enzymatic products have not had reliable predictability.[27]

Antibiotic Formulations for Initial Therapy

Since both gram-positive and gram-negative bacteria (as well as mixed infections) can be responsible for these initial infections, the empirical regimen must be broad in spectrum, ideally achieve high bactericidal levels, and be as nontoxic and as simple to administer as possible. This has usually necessitated the combination of two or more antibiotics. The availability of third-generation cephalosporins and carbapenems may offer an alternative to combination regimens, since a number of these antibiotics provide, as single agents, an exceedingly broad range of activity (including both gram-positive and gram-negative bacteria) as well as high bactericidal levels.[28–30] Moreover, unlike the aminoglycosides, these newer β-lactam antibiotics do not require the monitoring of serum levels and have minimal toxicity.

At present, an aminoglycoside plus a β-lactam containing regimen (e.g., ceftazidime plus amikacin) is considered by many the standard of care, particularly for patients with documented gram-negative infection.[31] However, no particular combination regimen has been shown to be clearly superior, and the one that is chosen at a given institution should reflect specific epidemiologic considerations (e.g., "local" resistance patterns) as well as cost.

Despite the proven efficacy of combination therapy, the potential of a single antibiotic ("monotherapy") for the empirical management of the febrile neutropenic patient is attractive for its ease of administration, cost, and lack of toxicity. To assess the efficacy of a monotherapeutic regimen, a prospective randomized trial was initiated at the National Cancer Institute that compared monotherapy with ceftazidime to combination therapy with cephalothin, carbenicillin, and gentamicin for the initial empirical management of 550 episodes of fever and neutropenia.[32] The antibiotic regimens were evaluated at both an "early" and an "overall" evaluation point. The early evaluation (at 72 hours) was specifically performed to assess the efficacy of the antibiotics during the period when they were truly utilized in an "empirical" manner (i.e., prior to the availability of definitive microbiologic data). The overall evaluation was performed at the resolution of the neutropenic episode. The responses were categorized as "successful" (with or without modification of the initial regimen) if the patient survived the episode of neutropenia and as "failures" if the patient died while neutropenic.

In this study, there was no significant difference in terms of success (with or without modifications) for patients randomized to ceftazidime or the combination regimen among patients classified as having either a fever of unknown origin (FUO) or a clinically or microbiologically documented infection. A significantly greater number of modifications were required, however, among the patients randomized to ceftazidime (58 of 282 [21 percent]) versus 29 of 268 (11.5 percent] $p = 0.002$ by chi-square test). This increased need for antibiotic modifications at the early evaluation reflected the necessity of anaerobic coverage among the patients randomized to ceftazidime who developed necrotizing gingivitis or perirectal cellulitis as well as the greater need for vancomycin for patients with documented gram-positive infections (especially those due to *Staphylococcus epidermidis*).

The results at the "overall evaluation" demonstrated equivalent success rates for the two regimens for patients classified as having either a fever of unknown origin (FUO) or a documented infection. The percentage of patients treated successfully without the need for modification of the initial antimicrobial therapy was predictably less than that at the early evaluation. Patients with documented infections required changes in antimicrobial therapy more often than those with FUO but the overall need for modification of the initial therapy for all patients randomized to monotherapy (59 percent) and those randomized to combination therapy (59 percent) was similar. Therefore, in terms of the overall outcome and the frequency with which modifications of the initial empirical regimen were necessary, monotherapy with ceftazidime was as effective as combination therapy with cephalothin, carbenicillin, and gentamicin for this population of patients.

Despite these results and the encouraging findings of other investigators, several concerns must be raised.[33–35] First the relative lack of activity of third-generation cephalosporins against gram-positive organisms (particularly the coagulase-negative staphylococci) has prompted a number of investigators to advocate that vancomycin be included in the primary empirical regimen.[36–38] Second, several investigators have argued for the inclusion of an aminoglycoside in the initial regimen, not only to maximize the activity against gram-negative pathogens but also to decrease the emergence of resistant organisms.[31] However, analysis of the National Cancer Institute (NCI) data does not substantiate these concerns. Without doubt, gram-positive bacteria have become increasingly problematic in recent years and were isolated in 75 of the 550 episodes (14 percent) in the recent NCI study. Fifty-three of these 75 isolates were from the "preantibiotic" evaluation (i.e., "primary" infections). The remaining 22 gram-positive isolates were responsible for "secondary" (or "breakthrough") infections. Vancomycin was ultimately required in 26 of the 53 (49 percent) primary infections, but was added after the identification of a resistant isolate in 14 of 17 cases. There was neither mortality nor significant morbidity associated with the addition of vancomycin *after* the identification of an organism resistant to the initial empirical regimen. Thus, the routine inclusion of vancomycin as a component of the initial empirical therapy would have overtreated the vast majority of patients, needlessly exposed them to a potentially toxic compound, and increased the cost of therapy without improving the overall clinical response. Thus, it seems more appropriate to withhold vancomycin until the pathogen is identified.[39] On the other hand, if there is a high incidence of *Staphytococcus aureus* that are methicillin-resistant at a given center, the initial inclusion of vancomycin in the antibiotic regimen would be appropriate.

In addition to gram-positive coverage, 36 of 282 patients (13 percent) randomized to ceftazidime in the NCI study required an aminoglycoside at some time during the episode of neutropenia.[32,40] The majority of these patients (24 of 36 [67 percent]) received the aminoglycoside because of prospectively designed protocol modifications for clinical deteriorations or "breakthrough" bacteremias. Patients with documented infections received aminoglycosides somewhat more frequently than did patients with unexplained fevers (16 of 92 [17 percent] compared to 20 of 190 [11 percent], respectively). Clearly, however, most patients (i.e., 87 percent) never required an aminoglycoside as a component of their antimicrobial regimen and the inclusion of an aminoglycoside as part of the initial empirical therapy would have unnecessarily exposed the patients to potentially ototoxic and nephrotoxic agents.

Ultimately, the decision regarding the appropriate regimen must be individualized at each institution. Oncology centers have different patterns of microbial isolates and antibiotic resistance patterns that must be taken into account. Nevertheless, there is mounting evidence that the initial empirical management of a febrile, neutropenic cancer patient may be accomplished with a single antibiotic. In addition to ceftazidime, imipenem-cilastatin is a potential candidate for monotherapy and is now under study. Regardless of the empirical regimen chosen, however, the clinician must recognize the indications for, and appropriately employ, the modifications of therapy essential to ensure a successful outcome for a neutropenic patient (Table 1).

Empirical Antibiotics for Clinically Defined Sites of Infection

Antibiotics are also administered empirically to granulocytopenic patients who have clinically defined sites of infection (e.g., a pulmonary infiltrate) but for whom a microbiologic diagnosis cannot be established without an invasive procedure. Two caveats should guide such therapy: First, a defined end point for empirical trial of antibiotics should be established. For example, if broad-spectrum antibiotics are begun in a granulocytopenic patient with a localized pulmonary infiltrate, a trial lasting 48–72 hours is generally appropriate. If the patient has not stabilized or improved by that time, an aggressive attempt to establish the diagnosis should be pursued, even if this requires an open lung biopsy.[41] Second, the choice of empirical antibiotics should closely approximate the probable causes of

TABLE 1. Modification of the Initial Antimicrobial Regimen for Febrile Neutropenic Cancer Patients

Clinical Event	*Possible Modifications of Therapy*
Breakthrough bacteremia	If gram-positive isolate (e.g., *Staphylococcus epidermidis*), add vancomycin.
	If gram-negative isolate (i.e., presumably resistant), switch to regimen containing non-cross-resistant antibiotics (e.g., aminoglycoside plus a carbapenem or extended-spectrum penicillin).
Catheter-associated infection	Add vancomycin (as well as gram-negative coverage) if not already being given.
Severe oral mucositis or necrotizing gingivitis	Add specific antianaerobic agent (e.g., clindamycin or metronidazole).
Esophagitis	Begin trial of oral clotrimazole, ketoconazole, or iv amphotericin B.
Pneumonitis	
Diffuse or interstitial	Begin trial of trimethoprim–sulfamethoxazole and erythromycin (plus broad-spectrum antibiotics if patient is granulocytopenic).
New infiltrate in a granulocytopenic patient also receiving antibiotics	If granulocyte count is rising, watch and wait.
	If granulocyte count is not recovering, biopsy to establish diagnosis; if biopsy cannot be done, add amphotericin B empirically.
Perianal tenderness	If patient is already receiving broad-spectrum antibiotics, add a specific antianaerobic agent.
	If patient is not on antibiotics, begin broad-spectrum therapy with anaerobic coverage.
Persistent fever and neutropenia	Continue antibiotics after 1 wk of persistent fever and neutropenia; add systemic antifungal therapy empirically.

the putative infectious process. For example, a diffuse interstitial pneumonitis in a nongranulocytopenic child with leukemia in remission is most likely due to *Pneumocystis carinii* and a trial of trimethoprim–sulfamethoxazole might be the appropriate empirical selection. If, however, the patient was neutropenic when the infiltrate appeared, the empirical regimen should include broad-spectrum antibiotics to cover possible bacterial causes of the diffuse pulmonary infiltrate in addition to trimethoprim–sulfamethoxazole and erythromycin.[42] Furthermore, if the patient was granulocytopenic and had already been on antibiotics when the infiltrate appeared, empirical therapy would have to include trimethoprim–sulfamethoxazole, erythromycin, broad-spectrum antibiotics, and antifungal therapy.[43] Moreover, if the patient is neutropenic, is febrile, and has a new pulmonary infiltrate, the presence of *Aspergillus* either in the sputum or in bronchoalveolar lavage (BAL) is highly associated with aspergillus pneumonia.[44] Furthermore, if the patient has had a prior fungal pneumonia and is again rendered neutropenic, the risk for recurrence of a fungal pneumonia may be high.[45] Clearly, the merits of such empiric management must be balanced against the risks of polypharmacy. The likely yield and liability of an invasive diagnostic procedure are additional considerations.

Empirical Antifungal Therapy

The situation is often complicated for patients who remain persistently febrile and granulocytopenic in spite of antibiotic therapy. In a randomized clinical trial, we observed that 56 percent of the FUO patients who had remained febrile even after receiving empirical antibiotics developed complications within 3 days of stopping therapy. Of these, 38 percent became hypotensive once antibiotic therapy was stopped. However, simply continuing antibiotics alone in FUO patients with persistent fever and granulocytopenia was not satisfactory, since 31 percent of these patients eventually developed invasive fungal infections. It is not possible to determine whether these fungal infections were the cause of the patient's persistent fever or a consequence of their continued antibiotic therapy and prolonged granulocytopenia. However, patients with persistent fever and granulocytopenia appeared to do best when their antibiotics were continued and amphotericin B was added empirically.

Thus, the rationale for the empirical utilization of an antifungal compound is based upon several lines of reasoning. First, the antemortem diagnosis of disseminated fungal disease is difficult in an immunocompromised host. Withholding antifungal therapy until the establishment of a definitive diagnosis frequently allows dissemination to occur prior to the institution of therapy.[46] It also appears that the outcome of a fungal infection in an immunocompromised patient is favorably improved with the early institution of effective therapy. Finally, it is possible to identify patients who are at greatest risk for the development of an invasive mycosis. Thus, neutropenic patients who remain febrile despite a 4–7 day trial of broad-spectrum antimicrobial therapy are particularly prone to fungal disease.[47,48] The utilization of empirical antifungal therapy would be expected to provide a dual benefit: the suppression of fungal overgrowth that inevitably accompanies broad-spectrum antimicrobial therapy and the early treatment of subclinical, localized mycotic disease.

Further support for the empirical institution of antifungal therapy comes from several retrospective studies. Bruke and coworkers utilized amphotericin B in patients with acute leukemia with recurrent or persistent fever despite antibiotic coverage with gentamicin and carbenicillin.[47] Stein and colleagues employed amphotericin B for patients with persistent or recrudescent fever following a week of antimicrobial therapy during induction therapy for acute myelogenous leukemia.[48] Both of these studies reported a decrease in deaths due to invasive mycoses relative to historic control groups.

Despite the theoretical and clinical evidence substantiating the efficacy of empirical antifungal therapy, the widespread acceptance and clinical use of this information have been hindered by the significant toxicity associated with amphotericin B. Fever, nephrotoxicity, hepatotoxicity, chills, and electrolyte imbalances (particularly hypokalemia) are frequently associated with the administration of amphotericin B. Less toxic alternatives to amphotericin B are desirable. The imidazoles are a new class of antifungal agents that are broad in spectrum, low in toxicity, and capable of being easily delivered.[49,50] A National Cancer Institute study randomized 72 patients who remained febrile and neutropenic after 7 days of antimicrobial therapy to receive either amphotericin (at 0.5 mg/kg/day) or ketoconazole (800 mg/day).[51] The results were similar in terms of the duration of fever after the antifungal randomization, the number of documented fungal infections, the number of patients requiring crossover because of intolerance, and to overall outcome scored as success (i.e., survival) or failure (i.e., death due to an invasive fungal infection). However, once the diagnosis of an invasive fungal infection was documented, disease progression was likely unless the patient received amphotericin B. Fainstein et al. corroborated these findings in a study of 172 neutropenic patients who remained febrile for 72–96 hours after the institution of empirical antibiotic therapy and who were randomized to receive either amphotericin B (at 0.6–1.0 mg/kg/day) or ketoconazole (200 mg orally every 6 hours).[52] In this study, there were no differences between the two regimens in the response of patients with documented "probable" or "possible" fungal infections. However, patients with documented infections due to *C. tropicalis* responded more often to amphotericin B (5 to 8 patients) than to ketoconazole (0 of 8 patients). Unfortunately, the unusual design and response criteria utilized for this study hinder its correlation with previously established data. It is important to emphasize that treatment failures as well as toxicity (e.g., adrenal and testosterone suppression) have been observed with prolonged ketoconazole use.[53,54] Recently, Wingard et al. evaluated parenteral miconazole as an empirical antifungal agent (versus a placebo) and demonstrated a significant reduction in the incidence of invasive mycoses.[55]

Questions still remain regarding the optimal point at which to initiate antifungal therapy. The arbitrary designation of day 7 avoids the overutilization of antifungal agents in patients who are slow to defervesce after empirical antibiotics or those who recover their granulocyte counts prior to day 7. The potential value of alternative antifungal compounds (e.g., liposome-encapsulated amphotericin B,[56,57] itraconazole,[58,59] fluconazole[60,61]) remains to be established by prospectively randomized clinical trials.

Thus, in summary, empirical antifungal therapy is indicated for those patients who remain neutropenic and febrile (or who recrudesce a fever) despite 1 week of broad-spectrum antibiotic therapy. The optimal duration of antibiotic antifungal therapy is based upon the dictum of clinical experience. For patients who remain neutropenic, antifungal therapy should be continued until the resolution of granulocytopenia. Persistence or recrudescence of fever should prompt a meticulous investigation for nonfungal infectious causes (e.g., bacterial or viral superinfections). Patients who develop a documented fungal infection should be treated according to established clinical guidelines for the offending pathogen (generally 2 g of amphotericin B). Neutropenic patients with aspergillus pneumonia may benefit from daily doses of amphotericin in the range of 1–1.5 mg/kg.[62]

Duration of Empirical Antibiotic Therapy

Having started antibiotics empirically, the question of how long to continue them when a site of infection has not been defined is often problematic. Stopping antibiotics too early can lead to clinical deterioration in patients who remain granulocytopenic, particularly when they are persistently febrile.

Patients with fever of unexplained origin (FUO) can be divided into low-risk and high-risk groups. Low risk FUO patients resolve their granulocytopenia within 1 week of starting antibiotics and do well when their antibiotics are continued simply until the time of recovery of their granulocyte count to about $500/mm^3$.[13]

The major dilemma pertains to the high-risk FUO patients, who remain neutropenic for more than 1 week. The management of these patients has been addressed in a series of prospective clinical studies, stratifying them according to whether they had defervesced after the initiation of broad-spectrum therapy or whether they remained persistently febrile in spite of empirical antibiotics.[63,64] Within 3 days of stopping antibiotics on day 7 in patients who had defervesced on therapy but who remained afebrile, 41 percent again became febrile; the isolate(s) obtained when these patients became febrile again were sensitive to the antibiotics that had been discontinued. By contrast, no subsequent infections are observed in the patients who simply continued on antibiotics. However, these data did not define whether antibiotics should be continued until the final resolution of neutropenia or whether a defined but limited course of antibiotic therapy, as if the patient had an occult site of infection, might suffice. Therefore, in an ongoing study, we have tried to evaluate further the appropriate duration of antibiotic therapy by continuing antibiotics for afebrile but persistently granulocytopenic FUO patients for a full 14-day treatment course (as if they had an occult infectious etiology for their fever) and then randomizing them either to stop antibiotics or to continue treatment until the resolution of the granulocytopenia. We have observed that after day 14, approximately one-third of the patients either stopping or continuing antibiotic therapy will become febrile again; since patients randomized to discontinue antibiotics responded to the reinstitution of therapy when the new fever developed, it seems reasonable simply to continue FUO patients on a standard 14-day treatment course if they remain granulocytopenic and then to stop and antibiotics, recognizing that approximately 30 percent of the patients will require further intervention.

SUMMARY

Empirical antibiotics appear to play a role throughout the episode of granulocytopenia since the patient remains at risk for multiple infectious events during this period. Although the need for the prompt initiation of empiric antibiotics when the granulocytopenic patient first becomes febrile is well established, current data suggest that continuing the empiric antibiotic regimen and modifying it (i.e., adding empirical antifungal therapy) if the patient remains febrile and granulocytopenic are also important. In the patient with prolonged granulocytopenia, empirical antibiotics may have a prophylactic as well as a therapeutic role.

PREVENTION OF INFECTION

Despite a multitude of clinical trials investigating the efficacy of various measures to prevent or reduce the occurrence of infection, the most important anti-infective measure identified has been the simplest: careful hand washing practices.[65] A number of approaches have been taken to decrease the acquisition of new organisms or suppress those already colonizing the cancer patient (Table 2). Unfortunately, no method has stood out as singularly effective, each having promise and problems (Tables 3 and 4). Unfortunately, as new preventive strategies are evaluated, they initially appear promising, but as additional studies are conducted, their beneficial results become less convincing.[66]

Preventing the Acquisition of New Organisms

Since it has been well documented that nearly 85 percent of the organisms responsible for infections among patients with cancer are derived from the endogenous flora, and that nearly half of these are acquired from the hospital environment, much attention has been directed toward mechanisms to prevent the acquisition of potential pathogens.

TABLE 2. Methods for Preventing Infection in Cancer Patients

Prevent Acquisition and/or Suppress or Eliminate the Microbial Flora	*Improve or Modify Host Defenses*
Isolation	Immunization
Simple or reverse isolation	Active
Isolation with HEPA air filtration	*Pseudomonas*
Prophylactic antibiotics	*Pneumococcus*
Nonabsorbable antibiotics	Passive
Trimethoprim–sulfamethoxazole	J5 core glycolipid
Selective decontamination	Pooled immunoglobulins
Quinolones	Specific
Prophylactic antivirals	Cell-component replacement
Acyclovir	Leukocyte transfusions
Amantadine	Acceleration of granulocyte recovery
Prophylactic antifungals	Lithium
Nystatin	GM-CSF
Imidazoles	
Prophylactic antiparasitics	
Thiabendazole	
Trimethoprim–sulfamethoxazole	
Combination-comprehensive	
Total protected isolation	

TABLE 3. Efficacy of Preventive Regimens in Reducing Acquisition of New Organisms or Suppressing Endogenous Microflora

	Total Protected Environment	*Nonabsorbable Antibiotics*	*Trimethoprim–Sulfamethoxazole*	*Selected Decontamination*	*Quinolones*
Exogenous Sources					
(Air, food, water, contacts)	Yes	No	No	No	No
Endogenous Sources					
Nares	Yes	No	No	No	Yes
Oropharynx	Yes	±	No	Yes	Yes
Lower respiratory tract	±	No	±	±	Yes
Gastrointestinal tract	Yes	Yes	Yes	Yes	Yes
Perianal area	Yes	±	±	±	±
Skin	Yes	No	No	No	No
Central venous catheter	No	No	No	No	No
Peripheral catheters	No	No	No	No	No
Systemic effect	±	No	Yes	Yes	Yes

Key: Yes: the regimen is effective; No: the regimen is not effective; ±: the regimen is partially effective or debatable.
(Modified from Pizzo,[66] with permission.)

TABLE 4. Effectiveness of Preventive Strategies Rated for Usefulness, Tolerance, Safety, and Cost-Effectiveness

	Total Protected Environment	*Nonabsorbable Antibiotics*	*Trimethoprim–Sulfamethoxazole*	*Selected Decontamination*	*Quinolones*
Efficacy					
Reduced infection	Yes	No	±	±	Yes
Decreased fever	Yes	No	No	No	No
Decreased or shortened need for antibiotics and antifungals	No	No	No	±	Yes
Contibuted to survival	No	No	No	No	No
Compliance					
Well tolerated?	No	No	±	±	Yes
Impact on efficacy	Yes	Yes	Yes	±	No
Liabilities					
Emergence of resistant organisms	Yes	Yes	Yes	Yes	Yes
Organ side effects					
Interference with other drugs	Yes	Yes	Yes	No	No
Bone marrow suppression	No	No	Yes	Yes	No
Specific organ toxicity	No	No	Yes	Yes	Yes
Cost					
For the drugs or regimens	Yes	Yes	No	Yes	Yes
For surveillance or monitoring	Yes	Yes	Yes	Yes	Yes
Reducing need for hopitalization or drugs	No	No	No	±	?

Key: Yes: the regimen is effective; No: the regimen is not effective; ±: the regimen is partially effective or debatable; ?: unknown.
(Modified from Pizzo,[66] with permission.)

Inanimate objects within the hospital environment (i.e., faucet aerators, shower heads, respirators, plants, floor) are reservoirs of pathogenic organisms. However, most epidemiologic studies (albeit most commonly investigating nonimmunocompromised patients) suggest that transmission from such inanimate sources usually requires a human vector. Therefore, the simplest yet most efficacious intervention that can be performed is adherence to strict handwashing precautions.[65] In reality, the easiest way to enforce such a policy is to educate the patient or family to disallow contact with individuals who have neglected to wash their hands.

A second maneuver to decrease the acquisition of new organisms is to maintain a cooked diet during periods of granulocytopenia, with avoidance of fresh fruits and vegetables and nonprocessed dairy products, since these foods are naturally contaminated with gram-negative bacteria (especially *Klebsiella pneumoniae, Escherichia coli,* and *Peudomonas aeruginosa*).[67,68]

Environmental sources can contribute to fungal (especially *Aspergillus* spp.) and bacterial (*Legionella*) colonization and infection. In centers where *Aspergillus* is a significant problem, special air filtration systems (e.g., high-efficiency particulate air filters [HEPAs] or water purification systems may prove helpful.

Although the technique of ''reverse isolation'' has often been used, it does not significantly reduce the acquisition of new organisms in an environment where hand washing techniques are strictly followed.[69] Therefore, there is no compelling reason to enforce this policy, particularly since the extra expense, time consumption, and inconvenience are not balanced by a beneficial effect.

The Total Protective Environment (TPE) is a comprehensive anti-infective regimen designed to reduce the patient's endogenous microbial burden while preventing the acquisition of new organisms (see Table 3). A sterile environment is created in a clean air room with constant positive airflow and is maintained by an aggressive program of surface decontamination, sterilization of all objects that enter the room, and an intensive regimen to disinfect the patient (including oral nonabsorbable antibiotics, skin antiseptics, antibiotic sprays and ointments, and a low microbial diet). Indeed, a number of studies have documented that the TPE can reduce the number of infections in profoundly granulocytopenic individuals.[70] However, the TPE is expensive, and because of improvements in treating established infections, it does not offer a clear survival advantage to patients. Thus, total protected isolation is not necessary for the routine care of cancer patients (Table 4).

An interesting application of the TPE is derived from the observation that patients with aplastic anemia undergoing allogeneic marrow transplant had a lower incidence of acute graft-vs.-host disease (GvHD). A similar effect has been more difficult to demonstrate among patients transplanted for hematologic malignancy, and additional studies are needed.

Prophylactic Antibiotics

A large number of clinical trials have been conducted to investigate the utility of prophylactic antibiotic regimens in immunocompromised patients. A number of strategies have been explored, including systemic prophylaxis, gastrointestinal decontamination, and selective gastrointestinal decontamination (i.e., maintenance of "colonization resistance"). Unfortunately, the interpretation of many of these trials is difficult as a result of poor study design (many are uncontrolled trials), nonuniform patient groupings, and failure to report or document compliance with the prophylactic regimens.[71]

Because the gastrointestinal tract is the source of many of the pathogens causing microbiologically defined infections, investigators have evaluated the efficacy of reducing the endogenous gastrointestinal flora by the administration of oral nonabsorbable antibiotics. This technique has been found not to be especially valuable and is fraught with a number of problems. The antimicrobial agents utilized (e.g., vancomycin, gentamicin, polymyxin B, nystatin, framycetin, and colistin) are unpalatable and are generally poorly tolerated, making compliance a significant liability (especially among patients receiving emetogenic chemotherapy) (see Table 3). Equally disturbing has been the emergence of resistant bacterial strains when aminoglycoside-containing regimens have been utilized. Therefore, prophylactic regimens aimed solely at reducing the endogenous gastrointestinal flora cannot be recommended (Table 4).

A modified technique is the "selective decontamination" of the gastrointestinal tract, employing antibiotics that preserve the anaerobic flora while reducing the aerobic bacteria. This is based upon experimental data showing that the preservation of the anaerobic flora of the GI tract provides a "colonization resistance" against aerobic and fungal organisms.[72,73] Although initial clinical trials provided evidence of a reduction of infections in patients undergoing induction therapy for acute leukemia,[74,75] clearly defined efficacy has not been definitely established. The most commonly investigated agent utilized for selective decontamination has been trimethoprim–sulfamethoxasole (TMP–SMX). Early trials investigating the utility of this antibiotic in children and adults demonstrated a reduction in all infections and in bacteremic episodes. However, a large number of follow-up clinical trials have yielded conflicting results.[71,76–82] The reasons for the contradictory results are unclear, although factors such as variability in study design, nonuniform patient populations, and failure to properly monitor compliance have played a part. The potential for reduction in infectious morbidity and mortality must be balanced against the prolongation of granulocytopenia and emergence of resistant organisms noted with the prophylactic utilization of TMP–SMX.[83] Successful utilization of this approach require close microbiologic monitoring in order to adjust the antimicrobial regimen properly for resistant or newly emerging species. Such surveillance is costly in terms of both time and money.

More recently, prophylactic antibiotic trials employing a derivative of nalidixic acid, the quinolone antibiotic norfloxacin, have shown promising results in a population of bone marrow transplant patients.[84] Additional clinical trials will be needed to assess the generalized applicability of these results to other immunocompromised patients. Similar studies with other fluorinated quinolones (e.g., ciprofloxacin) have also shown promising results, but confirmatory studies in larger numbers of patients are necessary.[85] At present, the quinolones cannot be used in children less than 18 years old because of putative joint toxicity.

Antifungal Prophylaxis

Because of the increasing incidence of invasive mycoses in immunocompromised hosts, antifungal prophylaxis has also been studied. The most frequently evaluated antifungal agents have included nystatin, amphotericin B, miconazole, clotrimazole, and ketoconazole. It is important to realize that the majority of prophylactic regimens have been aimed at a reduction of invasive infections due to *Candida* species and, by virtue of the antifungal activity of the agents employed, would not be expected to have a significant impact against aspergillus or mucormycosis.

Like antibiotic prophylaxis, interpretation of existing data is difficult, since studies suffer from variable patient inclusion criteria, disparate dosage regimens, nonuniform response criteria, and lack of appropriate controls. An added problem is the inherent difficulty in the definitive diagnosis of a fungal infection in an immunocompromised host.

Within the context of these limitations, however, several conclusions regarding antifungal prophylaxis can be put forth: First, when an adequate dose of antifungal agent has been administered (e.g., oral amphotericin B, ketoconazole, or clotrimazole), there has been a consistent decrease in fungal colonization (especially due to *Candida* spp.)[86] Decreased colonization has not clearly resulted, however, in a decreased incidence of invasive mycotic disease (although a decrease in superficial infection has been noted in some studies). Second, several studies employing prophylactic (and empirical) antifungal regimens have noted a shift in the colonization pattern of fungal organisms. In general, these shifts have been toward more resistant fungi. Thus, the prophylactic regimens may successfully eradicate the susceptible fungi (particularly *C. albicans*) but may permit the overgrowth and ultimate invasion by more resistant species, especially *Aspergillus*. This trend will have to be closely monitored in future studies.[87]

Overall, the potential benefits of prophylactic antifungal therapy must be balanced against the toxicities, epidemiologic considerations, and relative efficacy of the regimen employed. Until clear benefit can be proved, widespread chemoprophylaxis against fungi should not be attempted.

Antiviral Prophylaxis

Of considerable interest are the observations that both intravenous and oral formulations of acyclovir can prevent reactivation of HSV and resultant stomatitis among patients undergoing induction therapy for leukemia or lymphoma or marrow allografting.[88,89] Twice daily administration of intravenous acyclovir appears to be nearly as effective as three times daily use and is both more convenient and less expensive. Prophylactic acyclovir may also reduce the likelihood of development of acyclovir resistance.[90] Prevention of cytomegalovirus infection has been more problematic. Although primary CMV infection among seronegative patients can be prevented by use of screened seronegative blood products, use of CMV immune globulins or the licensed intravenous immune globulins remains controversial.[91,92] Leukocyte interferon has been shown to have a prophylactic benefit in renal allograft patients, although this effect was not reproduced in one study among marrow allograft recipients.[93,94] Recent studies suggest that intravenous acyclovir may have some effect against CMV when used prophylactically. Greater benefit might be anticipated with ganciclovir if marrow suppression can be circumvented or with forscarnet.

Antiparasitic Prophylaxis

In centers where *Pneumocystis carinii* occurs with some frequency, the administration of trimethoprim–sulfamethoxazole has been convincingly demonstrated to reduce the incidence of infection. However, not all children undergoing cancer treatment require prophylactic TMP–SMX. Rather, this should be influenced by the patients' underlying disease (e.g., leukemia versus solid tumors), the intensity of immunosuppression of the therapy being delivered, and the center where treatment is being administered.[95] Although the initial recommendations were for daily prophylactic therapy, recent studies have suggested that an intermittent (i.e., twice or thrice weekly) dosage schedule is effective and less toxic.[96]

Recently, aerosolized pentamidine has been evaluated in acquired immunodeficiency syndrome (AIDS) patients to prevent pneumocystis pneumonia. The results have been encouraging and may be applicable to patients with cancer.

Active and Passive Immunization

As a general rule, live attenuated viral vaccines should not be administered to immunosuppressed children. Although an initial antibody response may be elicited, the concurrent administration of cytotoxic chemotherapy is associated with a rapid decline of titers. Recently, a live varicella vaccine has been successfully administered to children with acute leukemia; only patients receiving maintenance chemotherapy have received the vaccine.[97]

Trials investigating the role of active immunization have evaluated the efficacy of immunization against commonly encountered pathogens such as the influenza virus, and *Haemophilus influenzae*, and *Streptococcus pneumoniae*. Such trials have been only partially successful because of the inability to maintain an adequate degree of protection in the fact of repeated immunosuppressive insults. However, these vaccines are safe and some investigators recommend their use between cycles of chemotherapy.

Passive immunization with varicella-zoster immunoglobulin (VZIG) reduces the incidence of pneumonitis and encephalitis and decreases the mortality (from 5–7 percent to 0.5 percent) in seronegative immunocompromised patients exposed to varicella infection. Immunosuppressed children who are seronegative or possess low-titer antivaricella antibody should receive VZIG (one vial/15 kg of body weight) within 72 hours of exposure to a potentially infectious source.[98–100]

A number of investigators have evaluated the efficacy of passive immunization with either high-titer antibody directed against the core glycolipid of Enterobacteriaceae (J-5 antisera) or pooled intravenous γ-globulin preparations. The rationale for this approach is drawn from several observations. First, patients with defective antibody production (e.g., chronic lymphocyte leukemia, multiple myeloma) are known to have an enhanced susceptibility to bacterial infection.[101] Second, antibody levels fall in patients receiving cytotoxic chemotherapy, and patients who develop gram-negative bacteremia have lower levels of antibody than those who do not develop infections.[102] The results of early clinical trials with the J-5 antisera have been encouraging. A double-blind, randomized, placebo-controlled trial involving patients with documented gram-negative bacteremia demonstrated enhanced survival among patients receiving the antisera.[103] A second placebo-controlled study using prophylactic J-5 antisera in surgical patients at high risk for gram-negative bacteremia demonstrated a reduction in infectious complications among the J-5 recipients, but not a survival advantage.[104] Unfortunately, preparation of such an antiserum is time- and labor-intensive and quite costly, and passive immunization with the J-5 antisera will remain an investigational approach until a clear advantage can be defined.

Pooled immunoglobulin preparations have antibody titers to a wide spectrum of potential pathogens. To test whether such preparations could reduce the incidence of fever and infection in neutropenic patients and alter the outcome of the infection that did occur, we conducted a double-blind, placebo-controlled trial in which adults and children who received chemotherapy regimens that would render them neutropenic for more than a week were randomized to receive either weekly intravenous immunoglobulin (500 mg/kg/wk) or an albumen placebo until their neutropenia resolved. With more than 70 entries in this study, no difference in the incidence of fever, type of infection, or outcome has been observed between the intravenous immunoglobulin arm and the placebo control.

Other investigators are evaluating hyperimmune antisera or monoclonal antibodies to prevent or treat bacterial infection.

Perhaps the most exciting development is the recent cloning and purification of molecules that can activate neutrophils or monocytes (e.g., interferons, tumor necrosis factor) or accelerate recovery from neutropenia (granulocyte macrophage-colony stimulating factor [GM-CSF]).[105–108] The utilization of these agents offers the prospect of abbreviating or attenuating the risk for serious infection in patients receiving cytotoxic chemotherapy. Moreover, if these agents are successful in reducing serious infectious complications, they may permit the delivery of chemotherapy in schedules that might maximize tumoricidal activity while minimizing toxicity.

REFERENCES

1. Schimpff SC, Saterlee W, Young VM, et al. Empiric therapy with carbenicillin and gentamicin for febrile patients with cancer and granulocytopenia. N Engl J Med. 1971;284:1061.
2. Pizzo PA. Infectious complications in children with cancer: I. Pathophysiology of the compromised host and initial evaluation and management of the febrile cancer patient. J Pediatr. 1981;98:341.
3. Pizzo PA, Ladisch S, Simon R, et al. Increasing incidence of gram positive sepsis in cancer patients. Med Pediatr Oncol. 1978;5:241.
4. Wade JL, Schimpff SC, Newman KA, et al. *Staphylococcus epidermidis:* An increasing cause of infection in patients with granulocytopenia. Ann Intern Med. 1982;97:503.
5. Walsh TJ, Vlahov D, Hansen SL, et al. Prospective surveillance in control of nosocomial methicillin-resistant staphyloccus aureus. Infect Control. 1987;8:7.
6. Schwabe RS, Stapleton JT. Emergence of vancomycin resistance in coagulase-negative staphylococci. N Engl J Med. 1987;316:927.
7. Cho SY, Choi HY. Opportunistic fungal infection among cancer patients. Am J Clin Pathol. 1979;72:617.
8. Krick JA, Remington JS. Opportunistic invasive fungal infections in patients with leukemia and lymphoma. Clin Haematol. 1976;5:249.
9. Meunier-Carpentier F, Kiehn T, Armstrong D. Fungemia in the immunocompromised host: Changing patterns, antigenemia, high mortality. Am J Med. 1981;71:363.
10. Walsh TJ, Pizzo PA. Nosocomial fungal infections and mycoses arising from endogenous flora or reactivation. Annu Rev Microbiol. 1988;42:517.
11. Commers JR, Pizzo PA. Empiric antifungal therapy in the management of the febrile–granulocytopenic cancer patient. Pediatr Infect Dis. 1983;2:56.
12. Schimpff SC, Young VM, Greene WH, et al. Origin of infection in acute nonlymphocytic leukemia: Significance of hospital acquisition of potential pathogens. Ann Intern Med. 1972;77:707.
13. Schimpff SC, Greene WH, Young VM, et al. Significance of *Pseudomonas aeruginosa* in the patient with leukemia or lymphoma. J Infect Dis. 1974;130:524.
14. Kurrle E, Bhaduri S, Krieger D, et al. Risk factors for infections of the oropharynx and the respiratory tract in patients with acute leukemia. J Infect Dis. 1981;144:128.
15. Markman M, Abeloff MD. Management of hematologic and infectious complications of intensive induction therapy for small cell carcinoma of the lung. Am J Med. 1983;74:741.
16. Pizzo PA, Robichaud KJ, Wesley R, et al. Fever in the pediatric and young adult patient with cancer: A prospective study of 1001 episodes. Medicine. 1982;61:153.
17. Love LJ, Schimpff SC, Schiffer CA, et al. Improved prognosis for granulocytopenic patients with gram-negative bacteremia. Am J Med. 1980;68:643.
18. EORTC International Antimicrobial Therapy Project Group. Three antibiotic regimens in the treatment of infection in febrile granulocytopenic patients with cancer. J Infect Dis. 1978;137:14.
19. Schimpff SC. Overview of empiric antibiotic therapy for the febrile neutropenic patient. Rev Infect Dis. 1985;7(Suppl 4):5734.
20. Pizzo PA. Infectious complications in children with cancer: II. Management of specific organisms. J Pediatr. 1981;98:513.
21. Sickles EA, Green WH, Wiernik PIT. Clinical presentation of infection in granulocytopenic patients. Arch Intern Med. 1975;135:715.
22. Hiemenz J, Skelton J, Pizzo, PA. Perspective on the management of catheter-related infections in cancer patients. Pediatr Infect Dis. 1986;5:6.
23. Kramer BS, Pizzo PA, Robichaud KJ, et al. Role of serial microbiologic surveillance and clinical evaluation in the management of cancer patients with fever and granulocytopenia. Am J Med. 1982;72:561.
24. Aisner J, Murillo J, Schimpff SC, et al. Invasive aspergillosis in acute leukemia: Correlation with nose cultures and antibiotic use. Ann Intern Med. 1979;90:4.
25. Schimpff SC. Surveillance cultures. J Infect Dis. 1981;144:81.
26. McDougall IR. The use of white blood cell scanning techniques in infectious disease. In: Remington JS, Swartz MN eds. Current Clinical Topics in Infectious Disease v. 4. New York: McGraw-Hill; 1983:130.
27. Hill HR, Matsen JN. Enzyme-linked immunosorbent assay and radioimmunoassay in the serologic diagnosis of infectious diseases. J Infect Dis. 1983;147:258.
28. Pizzo PA, Thaler M, Hathorn J, et al. New β-lactam antibiotics in the gran-

ulocytopenic patient: New options and new questions. Am J Med. 1985;79:75.
29. Birnbaum J, Kaham FM, Kropp H, et al. Carbapenems, a new class of β-lactam antibiotics: Discovery and development of Imipenem/Cilastatin. Am J Med. 1985;78(Suppl 16A):3021.
30. Neu HC. β-lactam antibiotics: Structural relationships affecting in vitro activity and pharmacologic properties. Rev Infect Dis. 1986;8(Suppl 3):S237.
31. The EORTC International Antimicrobial Therapy Cooperative Group. Ceftazidime combined with a short or long course of amikacin for empirical therapy of gram-negative bacteremia in cancer patients with granulocytopenia. N Engl J Med. 1987;317:1692.
32. Pizzo PA, Hathorn JW, Hiemenz JW, et al. A randomized trial comparing ceftazidime alone with combination antibiotic therapy in cancer patients with fever and neutropenia. N Engl J Med. 1986;315:552.
33. Pizzo PA. After empiric therapy: What to do until the granulocyte comes back. Rev Infect Dis. 1987;9:214.
34. de Pauw BE, Kauw F, Muytjens H, et al. Randomized study of ceftazidime versus gentamicin plus cefotaxime for infections in severely granulocytopenic patients. J Antimicrob Chemother. 1983;12(Suppl A):593.
35. Young L. Empirical antimicrobial therapy in the neutropenic host. (Editorial). N Engl J Med. 1986;315:580.
36. Karp JE, Dick JD, Angelopoulos C, et al. Empiric use of vancomycin during prolonged treatment-induced granulocytopenia: Randomized, double-blind, placebo-controlled clinical trial in patients with acute leukemia. Am J Med. 1986;81:237.
37. Kramer BJ, Ramphal R, Rand K. Randomized comparison between two ceftazidime containing regimens and cephalothin–gentamicin–carbenicillin in febrile granulocytopenic cancer patients. Antimicrob Agents Chemother. 1986;30:64.
38. Anaissie E, Fainstein V, Bodey G, et al. Randomized trial of β-lactam regimens in febrile neutropenic cancer patients. Am J Med. 1988;84:581.
39. Rubin M, Hathorn JW, Marshall D, et al. Gram-positive infections and the use of vancomycin in 550 episodes of fever and neutropenia. Ann Intern Med. 1988;108:30.
40. Hathorn JW, Rubin M, Pizzo PA. Empirical antibiotic therapy in the febrile neutropenic cancer patient: Clinical efficacy and impact of monotherapy. Antimicrob Agents Chemother. 1987;31:971.
41. Burt ME, Flye MN, Webber BL, et al. Prospective evaluation of aspiration needle, cutting needle, transbronchial and open lung biopsy in patients with pulmonary infiltrate. Ann Thorac Surg. 1981;32:146.
42. Browne MJ, Potter D, Gress J, et al. A randomized trial of open lung biopsy versus empiric antimicrobial therapy in cancer patients with pulmonary infiltrates. J Clin Oncol. In press.
43. Commers JR, Robichaud KJ, Pizzo PA. New pulmonary infiltrates in granulocytopenic cancer patients being treated with antibiotics. Pediatr Infect Dis. 1984;3:423.
44. Yu VL, Muder RR, Poorsattar A. Significance of isolation of *Aspergillus* from the respiratory tract in diagnosis of invasive pulmonary aspergillosis: Results from a three-year prospective study. Am J Med. 1986;81:249.
45. Robertson MJ, Larson RA. Recurrent fungal pneumonias in patients with acute nonlymphocytic leukemia undergoing multiple courses of intensive chemotherapy. Am J Med. 1988;84:233.
46. Pennington JE. Successful treatment of *Aspergillus* pneumonia in hematologic neoplasia. N Engl J Med. 1976;295:426.
47. Burke PJ, Braine HG, Rathbun HK, et al. The clinical significance and management of fever in acute myelocytic leukemia. Johns Hopkins Med J. 1976;139:1.
48. Stein RS, Kayser J, Flexner J. Clinical value of empirical amphotericin B in patients with acute myelogenous leukemia. Cancer. 1982;50:2247.
49. Drouhet E, Dupont B. Evolution of antifungal agents: Past, present and future. Rev Infect Dis. 1987;9:S4.
50. Walsh TJ, Pizzo PA. Treatment of systemic fungal infections: Recent advances and current problems. Eur J Clin Microbiol Infect Dis. 1988;7:460.
51. Hathorn JW, Gress J, Thaler M, et al. Empirical antifungal therapy among febrile neutropenic cancer patients: Amphotericin B versus ketoconazole. In press.
52. Fainstein V, Bodey GP, Elting L, et al. Amphotericin B or ketoconazole therapy of fungal infections in neutropenic cancer patients. Antimicrob Agents Chemother. 1987;31:11.
53. Brooks J, Williams WL, Sanders CV, et al. Apparent ketoconazole failure in candidal cholecystitis. Arch Intern Med. 1982;142:1934.
54. Best TR, Jenkins JK, Murphy FY, et al. Persistent adrenal insufficiency secondary to low-dose ketoconazole therapy. Am J Med. 1987;82:676.
55. Wingard JR, Vaughan WP, Braine HG, et al. Prevention of fungal sepsis in patients with prolonged neutropenia: A randomized double-blind, placebo-controlled trial for intravenous miconazole. Am J Med. 1987;83:1103.
56. Lopez-Berestein G, Hopfer RL, Mehta R, et al. Liposome-encapsulated amphotericin B for treatment of disseminated candidiasis in neutropenic mice. J Infect Dis. 1984;150:278.
57. Lopez-Berestein G, Bodey GP, Frenkel LS, et al. Treatment of hepatosplenic candidias with liposomal-amphotericin B. J Clin Oncol. 1987;5:310.
58. Ganer A, Arathoon E, Stevens DA. Initial experience in therapy for progressive mycoses with intraconazole, the first clinically studied triazole. Rev Infect Dis. 1987;9:S77.
59. Phillips P, Fetchick R, Weisman I, et al. Tolerance to and efficacy of intraconazole in treatment of systemic mycoses: Preliminary results. Rev Infect Dis. 1987;9:S87.
60. Perfect JR, Savani DV, Durack DT. Comparison of intraconazole of fluconazole in treatment of cryptococcal meningitis and candida pyelonephritis in rabbits. Antimicrob Agents Chemother. 1986;29:579.
61. Arndt C, Walsh TJ, McCally CL, et al. Cerebrospinal fluid penetration of fluconazole. J Infect Dis. 1988;157:178.
62. Burch PA, Karp JE, Merz WG, et al. Favorable outcome of invasive aspergillosis in patients with acute leukemia. J Clin Oncol. 1987;5:1985.
63. Pizzo PA, Robichaud KJ, Gill FA, et al. Duration of empiric antibiotic therapy in granulocytopenic cancer patients. Am J Med. 1979;67:194.
64. Pizzo PA, Robichaud KJ, Gill FA, et al. Empiric antibiotic and antifungal therapy for cancer patients with prolonged fever and granulocytopenia. Am J Med. 1982;72:101.
65. Albert RK, Condie F. Handwashing patterns in medical intensive care units. N Engl J Med. 1981;304:1465.
66. Pizzo PA. Considerations for preventing infectious complication in cancer patients. Rev Infect Dis. In press.
67. Remington JS, Schimpff SC. Please don't eat the salads. N Engl J Med. 1981;304:433.
68. Pizzo PA, Purvis D, Waters CW. Microbiological evaluation of food items for patients undergoing gastrointestinal decontamination and protected isolation. J Am Diet Assoc. 1982;81:272.
69. Nauseef WM, Maki DG. A study of the value of simple protective isolation in patients with granulocytopenia. N Engl J Med. 1981;304:448.
70. Pizzo PA. Do results justify the expense of protected environments? In Wiernik P, ed. Controversies in Oncology. New York: John Wiley & Sons; 1982;267.
71. Pizzo PA. Antimicrobial prophylaxis in the immunosuppressed cancer patient. In Remington JS, Swartz MN, eds. Current Clinical Topics in Infectious Diseases. v. 4. New York: McGraw-Hill; 1983:153.
72. van der Waaij D, Berghuis de Vries JN, Lekkerkerrk, et al. Colonization resistance of the digestive tract in conventional and antibiotic treated mice. J Hyg (Camb). 1971;69:405.
73. van der Waaij D, Berghuis de Vries J. Selective elimination of enterobacteriaceae species from the digestive tract in mice and monkeys. J Hyg (Camb). 72:205, 1974.
74. Guiot HFL, van der Brock PJ, van der Meer JWM, et al. Selective antimicrobial modulation of the intestinal flora of patients with acute nonlymphocytic leukemia: A double-blind placebo controlled study. J Infect Dis. 1983;147:615.
75. Sleijfer DT, Mulder NK, de Vries-Hospers HG, et al. Infection prevention in granulocytopenic patients by selective decontamination of the digestive tract. Eur J Cancer 1980;16:859.
76. Gurwith MJ, Brunton J, Lank B, et al. A prospective controlled investigation of prophylactic trimethoprim/sulfamethoxazole in hospitalized granulocytopenic patients. Am J Med. 1979;66:248.
77. Pizzo PA, Robichaud KJ, Edwards BK, et al. Oral antibiotic prophylaxis in patients with cancer: A double-blind randomized placebo-controlled trial. J Pediatr. 1983;102:125.
78. Weiser B, Lange M, Fialk M, et al. Prophylactic trimethoprim–sulfamethoxazole during consolidation chemotherapy for acute leukemia: A controlled trial. Ann Intern Med. 1981;95:436.
79. Dekker A, Rozenberg-Arska M, Sixma JJ, et al. Prevention of infection by trimethoprim–sulfamethoxazole plus amphotericin B in patients with acute nonlymphocytic leukemia. Ann Intern Med. 1981;95:555.
80. Kauffman CA, Liepman MJ, Bergman AG, et al. Trimethoprim–sulfamethoxazole prophylaxis in neutropenic patients: Reduction in infections and effect on bacterial and fungal flora. Am J Med. 1983;74:599.
81. Gaultieri RJ, Donowitz GR, Kaiser CE, et al. Double-blind randomized study of prophylactic trimethoprim–sulfamethoxazole in granulocytopenic patients with hematologic milignancies. Am J Med. 1983;74:934.
82. Wade J, deJongh CA, Newman KA, et al. Selective antimicrobial modulation as prophylaxis against infection during granulocytopenia: Trimethoprim–sulfamethoxazole versus nalidixic acid. J Infect Dis. 1983;147:624.
83. Wilson JM, Guinery DG. Failure of oral trimethoprim–sulfamethoxazole prophylaxis in acute leukemia: Isolation of resistant plasmids from strains of enterobacteriaceae causing bacteremia. N Engl J Med. 1982;306:16.
84. Karp JE, Merz WG, Hendricksen C, et al. Oral Norfloxacin for prevention of gram-negative bacterial infections in patients with acute leukemia and granulocytopenia. Ann Intern Med. 1987;106:1.
85. Dekker AW, Rozenberg-Arska M, Verhoef J. Infection prophylaxis in acute leukemia: A comparison of cifrofloxacin with trimethoprim–sulfamethaxozole and colistin. Ann Intern Med. 1987;106:7.
86. Meunier F. Prevention of mycoses in immunocompromised patients. Rev Infect Dis 1987;9:408.
87. Powderly WG, Kobayashi GS, Herzig GP, et al. Amphotericin B resistant yeast infection in severely immunocompromised patients. Am J Med. 1988;84:826.
88. Saral R, Ambinder RF, Burns WH, et al. Acyclovir prophylaxis against herpes simplex virus infection in patients with leukemia. Ann Intern Med. 1983;99:773.
89. Saral R, Burns WH, Laskin OL, et al. Acyclovir prophylaxis of herpes simplex virus infections: A randomized double-blind controlled trial in bone marrow–transplant recipients. N Engl J Med. 1981;305:63.
90. Ambinder RF, Burns WH, Lietman PS, et al. Prophylaxis: A strategy to minimize antiviral resistance. Lancet. 1984;1:1154.
91. Bowden RA, Sayers M, Flournoy N, et al. Cytomegalovirus immune glob-

ulin and seronegative blood products to prevent primary cytomegalovirus infection after marrow transplantation. N Engl J Med. 1986;314:1006.
92. Winston DJ, Ho WG, Lin CH, et al. Intravenous immune globulin for prevention of cytomegalovirus infection and interstitial pneumonia after bone marrow transplantation. Ann Intern Med. 1987;106:12.
93. Cheeseman SH, Rubin RH, Stewart JA, et al. Controlled clinical trial of prophylactic human-leukocyte interferon in renal transplantation: Effects on cytomegalovirus and herpes simplex virus infections. N Engl J Med. 1979;300:1345.
94. Hirsch MS, Schooley RT, Cosimi AB, et al. Effects of interferon-α on cytomegalovirus reactivation syndromes in renal-transplant recipients. N Engl J Med. 1983;308:1489.
95. Browne M, Hubbard S, Longo DL, et al. Excess prevalence of *Pneumocystis carinii* pneumonia in lymphoma patients treated with chemotherapy. Ann Intern Med. 1986;104:338.
96. Hughes WT, Rivera GK, Schell MJ, et al. Successful intermittent chemoprophylaxis for *Pneumocystis carinii* pneumonitis. N Engl J Med. 1987;316:1627.
97. Gershon A. Live attenuated varicella vaccine. J Pediatr 1987;110:154.
98. Paryani SG, Arvin AM, Koropchak CM, et al. Varicella zoster antibody titers after administration of intravenous serum globulin or varicella zoster immune globulin. Am J Med. 1984;76(Suppl 3A).124.
99. Gershon AA, Steinberg S, Brunnell PA. Zoster immune globulin: A further assessment. N Engl J Med. 1975;290:243.
100. Geiser CF, Bishop Y, Myers M, et al. Prophylaxis of varicella in children with neoplastic disease: Comparative results with zoster immune plasma and gamma globulin. Cancer. 1975;35:1027.
101. Jacobson DR, Zolla-Pazner S. Immunosuppression and infection in multiple myeloma. Semin Oncol. 1986;13:282.
102. Peter G, Pizzo PA, Robichaud KR, et al. Possible protective effect of circulating antibodies to the shared glycolipid of enterobacteriaceae in children with malignancy. Pediatr Res. 1979;13:466.
103. Ziegler EJ, McCutchan JA, Fierer S, et al. Treatment of gram-negative bacteremia and shock with human antiserum to a mutant UPD-GAL epimerase-deficient mutant *Escherichia coli*. New Engl J Med. 1982;307:1225.
104. Baumgartner JD, Gauser MP, McCutcheon JA, et al. Prevention of gram-negative shock and death in surgical patients by antibody to endotoxin core glycolipid. Lancet. 1985;2:59.
105. Sieff CA. Hematopoietic growth factors. J Clin Invest. 1987;79:1549.
106. Metcalf D. The molecular biology and function of the granulocyte-macrophage colony-stimulating factors. Blood. 1986;67:257.
107. Brandt SJ, Peters WP, Atwater SK, et al. Effect of recombinant human granulocyte-macrophage colony-stimulating factor on hematopoietic reconstruction after high-dose chemotherapy and autologous bone marrow transplantation. N Engl J Med. 1988;318:869.
108. Gabrilove JL, Jukubowski A, Scher H, et al. Effect of granulocyte-colony-stimulating factor on neutropenia and associated morbidity due to chemotherapy for transitional-cell carcinoma of the urothelium. N Engl J Med. 1988;318:1414.

294. INFECTIONS IN PATIENTS WITH SPINAL CORD INJURY

BARRETT SUGARMAN

Some 10,000 people survive spinal cord injuries each year in the United States, and their life expectancy continues to increase toward normal.[1] Initially, these individuals are prone to develop nosocomial infections because of their multiple injuries, prolonged hospital stay, frequent procedures, and other factors present in acutely ill, traumatized individuals.[2] Once stable, the presence of a neurogenic bladder, prosthetic devices, altered sensation, and other factors predispose these people to an increased incidence of infection throughout their lives.[3] Data are biased by the population seen at a particular center; however, infections occur in the majority of initially hospitalized spinal cord-injured people (SCIP), and they are a frequent cause of morbidity and mortality for many years after injury.[2–4]

INFECTIOUS CAUSES OF SPINAL CORD INJURY

Trauma is the cause of the overwhelming majority of cases of spinal cord damage.[1,2] Epidural abscesses remain a cause of spinal cord injury in a small percentage of SCIP and are usually caused by *Staphylococcus aureus*.[2,5–7] A variety of other common bacteria cause most other cases of epidural space infection, but brucellosis, tuberculosis, blastomycosis, coccidioidomycosis, cryptococcosis, schistosomiasis, gnathostomiasis, echinococcosis, and other infections may cause spinal cord injury.[5,6]

Spastic paraparesis of unknown cause remains a significant problem in parts of the world as diverse as the Caribbean, Africa, India, and South America but not North America. Preliminary, small studies suggest that 59–100 percent of these patients have antibodies to a retrovirus, human T-lymphotropic virus, type 1 (HTLV-I). The low prevalence of antibody in control patients (less than 5 percent) suggests that this retrovirus might be a factor in the development of certain types of spinal cord injury.[8,9] Furthermore, with newer techniques, viral antigens, viral DNA, and cultivable HTLV-I-like retrovirus have been found in spastic paraparesis patients (including a few from the United States) in small series published in 1988.[9a,9b] Viral causes of (transverse) myelitis are discussed in Chapter 68.

Unique Considerations in Evaluation of SCIP for Infection

Initial hospitalization with its frequent intensive care unit stays, associated surgery, insertion of various catheters, prolonged hospitalization, and other causes all make SCIP especially prone to develop nosocomial infections Table 1. Inadequate ventilation due to diaphragmatic paralysis in quadriplegics predisposes to pneumonia, the presence of a neurogenic bladder and bladder catheters predispose to urinary tract infections, and other prosthetic devices such as fracture fixation devices and vascular catheters allow the development of associated infections.[2,10,11] Often, more than one source of infection is identified: a referral infectious diseases service identified more than one likely source of infection in 70 percent of febrile SCIP for whom consultations were requested.[2]

Altered sensation in SCIP lessens the effectiveness of the history and physical examination in the evaluation for infection. This is dependent upon the type, completeness, and level of spinal cord injury. Pain in an area may lead one to focus on an evaluation of that area when in fact the cause of the pain is central (neurogenic pain is a frequent complication in SCIP[3]). More importantly, decreased or absent sensation may mask important symptoms that would otherwise be present. Patients may have no or nominal abdominal symptoms, but an acute abdomen may be present.[2,12] Soft tissue abscesses and other infections such as osteomyelitis might be present, but the absence of pain requires careful evaluation so as not to miss these potential foci of infection. Drug absorption and disposition are altered in SCIP.[13,14] It is not clear how much of this is uniquely due to spinal cord injury vs. what can occur in anyone under

TABLE 1. Special Infectious Considerations in the Spinal Cord-Injured Patient

High risk of nosocomial infection
Neurogenic bladder and frequent bladder catheterization
Frequency of insertion of other catheters and prosthetic devices
Prolonged hospital stay
Frequent stays in intensive care units
Frequent surgical procedures
Antimicrobial-resistant organisms
Multiple infections at the same time (e.g., urinary tract infection and an infected pressure sore)
Lack of sensation, which may mask symptoms of infection or allow an infection to progress to an advanced stage before diagnosis
Altered aminoglycoside and other drug disposition
Increased frequency of certain infections (e.g., infected urinary tract stones, osteomyelitis)
Noninfectious conditions that can mimic infection in SCIP

similar stresses with other injuries or illnesses. Months to years after spinal cord injury the decreased muscle mass and increased body fat-to-total body weight ratio may significantly alter dosing of drugs such as aminoglycosides and requires careful monitoring of toxic drugs.[3,14]

Certain conditions occur essentially only in SCIP, or they can occur in others but are so common in SCIP that they must be part of the initial differential diagnosis in the evaluation of SCIP for infection. Overall, the most common sites of infection in SCIP are the urinary tract, infected pressure sores and other soft tissue infections, and pneumonia (especially in quadriplegics). The progression from initially sensitive pathogens to multiple antimicrobial-resistant organisms over long hospitalizations remains a major problem.

Complications Most Common Soon After Spinal Cord Injury

Any traumatized individual may develop pulmonary complications; however, these represent a significant problem in the SCIP, especially the quadriplegic[10,15] (Table 2). Generalized lack of muscle movement predisposes to venous thrombi and pulmonary emboli; diaphragmatic/intercostals/abdominal muscle paralysis predisposes to the development of atelectasis and pneumonia in the patient with high-level spinal cord injury. Even when a tracheostomy is present and the SCIP is suctioned regularly, the propensity for catheters passed down the trachea to enter the right bronchus due to its anatomy makes it difficult to adequately suction the left bronchus, and atelectasis often develops on the left side in quadriplegics.[15] This atelectasis may be confused with pneumonia. Decreased pulmonary function in high-level SCIP may predispose to a lifetime of pulmonary complications and often necessitates interventions including tracheostomies, portable ventilators, and even diaphragmatic pacer insertion.

While abdominal pathology can occur at any time, it is most common within a few weeks after spinal cord injury. Abdominal distension is often present after spinal cord injury due to a loss of muscle tone alone, which makes evaluation of the abdomen challenging.[12,16] Abdominal organ injury associated with the spinal cord injury makes abdominal pathology a frequent concomitant. Any type of perforated viscus and secondary infection can develop. Pancreatitis has also been reported to occur, whether caused by trauma or some other mechanism such as alterations in innervation.[17] Unexplained fever and tachycardia are usually prominent in SCIP with an acute abdominal process, and localized abdominal spasticity may be present, depending upon the type and level of spinal cord injury. Further, many SCIP will have some type of sensation and may complain of abdominal pain or vague discomfort. Autonomic dysreflexia signs may also be present (see below).[12,16]

Thermoregulation problems in SCIP may readily be confused with infection.[18] Abnormalities including a diminished or lack of sweating and muscular activity below the level of spinal cord injury alter thermoregulation, especially in high-level SCIP.[18] Quadriplegics may sweat only in the uppermost body parts and upon evaluation appear infected because of a flushed face and profuse sweating, which is actually their physiologic method of thermoregulation. Rarely, prolonged exposure to low or high ambient temperatures is enough to make a high-level SCIP hypothermic or febrile.[18] A unique syndrome of unexplained fever also occurs in recently injured quadriplegics.[19,20] Within hours to the first few days after spinal cord injury these patients develop fever. Ambient temperature, altered sweating, and altered muscular activity do not explain this condition. It simply is not known what causes this.[20] Helpful diagnostic hints include the rapidity with which fever develops after injury, a usually normal peripheral white blood cell count, and a lack of identifiable infectious foci or lack of response to treatment for presumed infection.[20] Fever persists for weeks to months. This condition occurred in 2 of 19 recently injured quadriplegics and 0 of 22 recently injured paraplegics followed prospectively in one study and often required prolonged and repeated evaluation to make sure that infection was not present.[20]

Sequelae of central nervous system (CNS) trauma can be confused with infection. Spinal cord injury or associated surgery may cause cerebrospinal fluid (CSF) abnormalities such as pleocytosis and elevated protein levels for several weeks. If CSF is obtained as part of a procedure (e.g., myelogram) or diagnostic evaluation, these changes can be confused with meningitis; Gram stain, CSF glucose determination, and culture are used for differentiation. Concomitant head injury (e.g., hematoma) or a large hematoma involving the spinal cord may be difficult to distinguish from an abscess and require surgical exploration. CNS infections are not common complications in SCIP, especially soon after surgery.[2–4,20]

TABLE 2. Infections and Conditions that Mimic Infection and Are Most Common the First 2 Months after Spinal Cord Injury

Respiratory complications (especially in quadriplegics)
Pulmonary emboli
Pneumonia
Atelectasis (especially of the left lung)
Abdominal pathology
Ruptured viscus with or without an abscess
Pancreatitis
Unexplained fever in recently injured quadriplegics
CNS complications
Abnormal CSF due to spinal cord injury or surgery
Concomitant head injury
Nosocomial infections
Urinary tract infections
Catheter- and prosthetic device-associated infections

CHRONIC AND RECURRENT INFECTIONS IN SCIP

Urinary bladder emptying procedures vary greatly with different SCIP. Soon after the initial injury, most patients have bladder catheters and frequently develop nosocomial, antimicrobial-resistant urinary tract infections. A combination of trial-and-error and sophisticated urodynamic evaluation leads to bladder retraining varying from the catheter-free state (with or without sphincterotomy) to chronic indwelling catheterization. Intermittent bladder catheterization is also quite frequently used. This technique is generally considered to lessen the incidence of infectious complications as compared with an indwelling catheter; however, controlled prospective studies have not been published that substantiate this statement.[3,21] Because of the extra costs (skilled time and supplies), this technique cannot yet be unhesitatingly recommended for all people who require bladder catheterization.

Chronic bladder catheterization is associated with recurrent lower and upper tract infections, abscesses throughout the urinary tract, stones throughout the urinary tract, particularly in the kidney, and renal failure.[22] Relief of any obstruction present and the judicious use of antimicrobial therapy for symptomatic infections form the basis of treatment. Bacteriuria alone does not justify antimicrobial therapy. Because the SCIP may have altered sensation, the ability to thermoregulate, etc., bacteriuria with gross pyuria or white blood cell casts probably should also be treated. No regimen of prophylactic or suppressive antimicrobials is generally accepted to lessen the long-term recurrences of urinary tract infections in SCIP with neurogenic bladders. In fact, such use of antimicrobials more likely merely causes the selection of antimicrobial-resistant organisms.[3,22,23]

The presence of urinary tract stones, particularly calcium phosphate—magnesium ammonium phosphate (struvite), often requires more than antimicrobials for their eradication and can be a cause of chronic and recurrent urinary tract infections and renal failure; they can occur anywhere in the urinary tract.[3,22]

Regular evaluation for the presence of stones, especially if difficult-to-eradicate infection is present, should be part of the routine evaluation of SCIP. A prospective study of 500 SCIP noted the development of bladder stones in 36 percent within 8 years of injury.[24] Treatment consists of relief of obstruction (if present), removal of significant (because of their size or associated infection) stones via surgery or lithotripsy when possible, and the appropriate use of antimicrobials for an associated infection.

The majority of SCIP develop pressure sores at some time.[3,25] Lack of sensation, decreased movement, and alterations in skin innervation all predispose SCIP to develop pressure sores. With prompt removal of pressure from the area they rapidly heal; however, they often become infected.[25–27] In one prospective study of 209 hospitalized SCIP, 119 (57 percent) developed at least one pressure sore during hospitalization; 21 of these 119 patients (18 percent) developed drainage of grossly purulent material, extensive surrounding inflammation, or both and were defined as having clinically infected sores.[25] Optimal conditions in specialized centers can significantly lessen the frequency of this and other complications.[28] Soft tissue abscesses complicate up to 10 percent of infected pressure sores.[25] This may be difficult to diagnose because the patient complains of no pain and the superficial, visible areas do not appear to be infected. Such infection can burrow deep and cause osteomyelitis of the underlying bone[26,27] or, rarely, be associated with remote infection via a fistulous tract.[25] Bone infection beneath pressure sores is particularly difficult to diagnose because pressure can cause abnormalities of bone that are indistinguishable from bone infection by radiographic and nuclear imaging analysis.[26,27] Bone scans, when there are normal findings, are helpful in eliminating the diagnosis of osteomyelitis; however, these studies frequently show abnormalities, and biopsy may be necessary to determine whether bone infection is present. Fortunately, only about one-third of the deep pressure sores that seem likely to be associated with underlying bone infection have evidence of osteomyelitis on histologic examination of bone.[26,27] Sinograms are helpful if they establish a fistulous connection to an abscess or distant area but may be nondiagnostic if they are blocked by debris present in the tract. Deep débridement or aspiration is often necessary before a deep soft tissue abscess can be eliminated as a diagnostic possibility.

Combinations of gram-negative bacilli (often multiple antimicrobial-resistant), anaerobes, streptococci, and staphylococci cause most of these soft tissue and bone infections; in one study deep pressure sore cultures grew a mean of 4.1 organisms and infected bone, 2.3 organisms.[26] Treatment of infected pressure sores with removal of pressure from the area, débridement, and topical antimicrobial therapy (e.g., povidone-iodine) is often adequate, but systemic antimicrobial therapy is sometimes needed (e.g., for associated sepsis, deep tissue infection).[25] Underlying osteomyelitis, if present, should be treated for at least 4 weeks with appropriate systemic antimicrobial(s) and requires associated surgery (débridement, grafting, amputation, etc.) in the majority of patients to effect a cure.[26,27]

NONINFECTIOUS CONDITIONS IN SCIP

Thermoregulatory problems, pulmonary emboli and atelectasis, pancreatitis, and CNS abnormalities have already been mentioned. Two additional specific problems in SCIP that can mimic infection are autonomic dysreflexia and ectopic bone formation.

Autonomic dysreflexia (hyperreflexia) is limited almost exclusively to SCIP with midthoracic or higher lesions.[3,29] It usually first appears 2–8 months after injury, occurs in up to 50 percent of at-risk SCIP, and can range from a minor inconvenience to a life-threatening problem. Triggering stimuli that would normally only cause minor physiologic alterations cause generalized autonomic hyperactivity in this condition. Bladder distension or catheterization, bowel distention or stimulation, cutaneous stimuli, etc., may cause significant autonomic hyperactivity that produces symptoms and signs such as a rise in blood pressure, sweating, headache, changes in skin temperature, and rarely fever. The presence of other signs of autonomic dysfunction such as pupilary dilation, bradycardia, goose bumps, etc., are helpful in differentiation from infection. Further, removal of the triggering stimuli (completion of bladder emptying, bowel emptying, etc.) is usually associated with the prompt resolution of symptoms, but sometimes antihypertensive therapy is necessary. A prior history of similar episodes is also helpful in making the diagnosis; however, initial severe episodes may well be confused with infection if the triggering stimulus, such as a distended bowel or bladder, is overlooked.

Ectopic (heterotopic) ossification is present in up to one-half of SCIP. This complication occurs below the level of injury, usually around the shoulders, elbows, hips, or knees. It first appears weeks to months after injury and is usually asymptomatic or can cause decreased mobility of the involved joint. However, occasionally it presents as an acute process with swelling, erythema, and warmth around the area that suggests cellulitis or venous thrombosis.[3,30] This condition can often be diagnosed with a simple x-ray film; the alkaline phosphatase concentration is usually elevated, and bone scan findings are usually abnormal even before the x-ray film shows abnormalities. Treatment usually consists of a combination of motion exercises of the involved joints and the oral diphosphonate, etidronate disodium.[3,31] The erythematous extremity in the SCIP may represent cellulitus (especially if a nearby pressure sore or implanted prosthetic device is present) or venous thrombosis, but x-ray evaluation of the extremity is often helpful in the SCIP to also look for ectopic bone formation or a bone fracture. The osteoporotic bones of SCIP are more prone to fracture, and pain is often absent once fracture occurs.

EVALUATION OF FEBRILE SCIP

Careful evaluation of the patient usually reveals a likely source of infection. Evaluation should be completed even if one focus of infection is identified because so many of these individuals have more than one focus of infection. An altered sensation requires a complete physical examination so as not to miss an infected focus. Laboratory studies may show abnormalities that, while suggestive of infection, are actually due to noninfectious causes such as recent surgery, the presence of a prosthetic device, or trauma. Invasive procedures such as deep débridement, aspiration, and biopsy with aerobic and anaerobic cultures are often necessary to determine whether infection is present and accurately identify the causative organism(s). Survivors of severe head injuries often face the same complications as SCIP and can be evaluated similarly. Care of SCIP offered in specialized units familiar with these problems seems to lessen the frequency and severity of such complications.[2,28]

During the evaluation of SCIP, a key question to consider is whether further infectious complications can be prevented. SCIP should be evaluated to determine whether skin breakdown and subsequent infection might be prevented by the use of a different turning schedule, by the use of special beds or pads designed to relieve pressure, or by better control of the recurrent spasms that frequently complicate spinal cord injury and can damage skin.[3] The urinary tract should be evaluated to decide how to best minimize catheterization. Any struvite stones present in the urinary tract are easier to treat when small and may respond to acetohydroxamic acid, surgery, or numerous newer techniques of stone removal or dissolution.[3,32] SCIP with high thoracic or cervical lesions should be evaluated for significant atelectasis. Careful evaluation of SCIP coupled with appropriate therapy and preventive care usually yields gratifying results.

REFERENCES

1. Kraus JF. A comparison of recent studies on the extent of the head and spinal cord problem in the United States. J Neurosurg. 1980;53(Suppl):35–43.
2. Sugarman B, Brown D, Musher D. Fever and infection in spinal cord injury patients. JAMA. 1982;248:66–70.
3. Sugarman B. Medical complications of spinal cord injury. Q J Med. 1985:54:3–18.
4. Vaziri ND, Cesario T, Mootoo K, et al. Bacterial infection in patients with chronic renal failure. Occurrence with spinal cord injury. Arch Intern Med. 1982;142:1273–6.
5. Baker AS, Ojemann RG, Swartz MN, et al. Spinal epidural abscess. N Engl J Med. 1975;293:463–8.
6. Danner RL, Hartman BJ. Update of spinal epidural abscess: 35 cases and review of the literature. Rev Infect Dis. 1987;9:265–74.
7. Sugarman B. Osteomyelitis in spinal cord injury. Arch Phys Med Rehabil. 1984;65:132–4.
8. Gessain A, Vernant JC, Maurs L, et al. Antibodies to human T-lymphotropic virus type-I in patients with tropical spastic paraparesis. Lancet. 1985;2:407–10.
9. Newton M, Miller D, Rudge P, et al. Antibody to human T-lymphotropic virus type 1 in west-Indian-born UK residents with spastic paraparesis. Lancet. 1987;1:415–6.
9a. Bhagavati S, Ehrlich G, Kula RW, et al. Detection of human T-cell lymphoma/leukemia virus type I DNA and antigen in spinal fluid and blood of patients with chronic progressive myelopathy. New Engl J Med. 1988;318:1141–7.
9b. Jacobson S, Raine C, Mingioli ES, et al. Isolation of HTLV-I-like retrovirus from patients with tropical spastic paraparesis. Nature. 1988;331:540–3.
10. Bellamy R, Pitts FW, Stauffer ES. Respiratory complications in traumatic quadriplegia. J Neurosurg. 1973;39:596–600.
11. Sugarman B. Infections and prosthetic devices. Am J Med. 1986;81(Suppl 1A):78–84.
12. Charney KJ, Juler GL, Comarr AE. General surgery problems in patients with spinal cord injuries. Arch Surg. 1975;110:1083–8.
13. Halstead LS, Feldman S, Claus-Walker J, et al. Drug absorption in spinal cord injury. Arch Phys Med Rehabil. 1985;66:298–301.
14. Segal JL, Gray DR, Gordon SK, et al. Gentamicin disposition kinetics in humans with spinal cord injury: A preliminary report. J Am Paraplegia Soc 1983;6:41–2.
15. Sugarman B. Atelectasis in spinal cord injured people after initial medical stabilization. J Am Paraplegia Soc 1985;8:47–50.
16. Juler GL, Eltorai IM. The acute abdomen in spinal cord injury patients. Paraplegia. 1985;23:118–23.
17. Cary ME, Nance FC, Kirgis HD, et al. Pancreatitis following spinal cord injury. J Neurosurg. 1977;47:917–22.
18. Guttmann JS, Wyndham CH. Thermoregulation in spinal man. J Physiol. 1958;142:406–19.
19. Weber H. Two cases of lesion of the cervical portion of the spinal marrow, exhibiting the phenomena of heat-stroke. Trans Clin Soc Lond. 1868;1:163–7.
20. Sugarman B. Fever in recently injured quadriplegic persons. Arch Phys Med Rehabil. 1982;63:639–40.
21. Warren JW. Infections associated with urological devices. In: Sugarman B, Young EJ, eds. Infections Associated with Prosthetic Devices, Boca Raton, FL: CRC Press; 1984;219–41.
22. Warren JW, Muncie HL Jr, Bergquist EJ, et al. Sequelae and management of urinary infection in the patient requiring chronic catheterization. J Urol. 1981;125:1–8.
23. Warren JW, Anthony WC, Hoopes JM, et al. Cephalexin for susceptible bacteriuria in afrebile, long-term catheterized patients. JAMA. 1982;248:454–8.
24. DeVivo MJ, Fine PR, Cutter GR, et al. The risk of bladder calculi in patients with spinal cord injuries. Arch Intern Med. 1985;145:428–30.
25. Sugarman B. Infection and pressure sores. Arch Phys Med Rehabil. 1985;66:177–9.
26. Sugarman B, Hawes S, Musher DM, et al. Osteomyelitis beneath pressure sores. Arch Intern Med. 1983;143:683–8.
27. Sugarman B. Pressure sores and underlying bone infection. Arch Intern Med. 1987;147:553–5.
28. Donovan WH, Carter RE, Bedbrook GM, et al. Incidence of medical complications in spinal cord injury: Patients in specialised, compared with non-specialised centres. Paraplegia. 1984;22:282–90.
29. Johnson B, Thomason R, Pallares V, et al. Autonomic hyperreflexia: A review. Milit Med. 1975;140:345–9.
30. Nicholas JJ. Ectopic bone formation in patients with spinal cord injury. Arch Phys Med Rehabil. 1973;54:354–9.
31. Freed JH, Hahn H, Menter R, et al. The use of the three-phase bone scan in the early diagnosis of heterotopic ossification (HO) and in the evaluation of didronel therapy. Paraplegia. 1982;20:208–16.
32. Williams JJ, Rodman JS, Peterson CM. A randomized double-blind study of acetohydroxamic acid in struvite nephrolithiasis. N Engl J Med. 1984;311:760–4.

295. INFECTIONS IN THE ELDERLY

ROBERT B. BREITENBUCHER
PHILLIP K. PETERSON

Age has been recognized as an important factor in the pathogenesis of infectious diseases from the inception of this medical discipline. While numerous investigators have provided great insight at the pediatric end of the age spectrum, understanding is only beginning to emerge as to age-related mechanisms influencing the etiology, outcome, and response to preventive measures of infection. Special interest in infections in the elderly has been heightened by the "geriatric demographic imperative."[1] The world population is graying, and the elderly are receiving an increasing portion of health care expenditures.

The risk of developing or dying from most serious infectious diseases is increased in the elderly. The reasons for this are complex and only incompletely understood. While mounting evidence supports the involvement of age-related immunodeficiency,[2] cofactors such as underlying medical conditions, environmental exposures, nutritional deficiencies, and alteration of nospecific or mechanical defense factors are also contributory. Infections in the elderly are, by and large, inextricably related to other diseases of aging.

Most research in aging has emphasized age-related losses and neglected the heterogeneity of older persons. Clearly, physiologic age and chronologic age are not always concordant, and those who age successfully may not be at any greater risk of developing serious infection than young healthy individuals. Indeed, because of the physiologic heterogeneity of older persons, defining the "elderly" in terms of 70 years or older is somewhat arbitrary. It is our intent in this chapter to highlight aspects of various infections that are relatively unique to "the elderly." By doing so, we may not be portraying all older individuals, e.g., those who have aged successfully. Material elsewhere in this volume will probably be more pertinent to these individuals.

URINARY TRACT INFECTIONS

Urinary tract infection is predominantly a female disease starting from childhood.[3] Starting in the second decade of life, the incidence of bacteriuria in females increases by about 1% per decade, with little increase in males until the seventh decade of life when there is a sharp and rapidly progressing increase in both sexes but more notable in males.[4,5] Variances in the prevalance of bacteriuria in different reports probably relate more to differences in factors such as chronic disease, specific urologic disease, and factors bearing upon the reliability of voided urine cultures in many elderly women with decreased cognition and functional status rather than age per se. The prevalence of true bacteriuria in the United States is probably about 5–15 percent in males and 15–30 percent in females over the age of 65 years.[6]

Complicated urinary tract infections increase with aging, but the most common type of bacteriuria seen in the elderly is asymptomatic bacteriuria, which waxes and wanes in individuals with frequent species changes over time.[5]

Important differences in the etiology of urinary tract infections in the elderly are seen. In noninstitutionalized elderly over 65 years old, *Escherichia coli* is found in about 75 percent, with lower incidences of *Proteus, Klebsiella,* and staphylococci; *Pseudomonas aeruginosa* is an unusual pathogen. The same is true in noninstitutionalized persons less than 65 years old. For institutionalized elderly over 65 years old, however, there is a marked change in pathogens, with about a third of cases of bacteriuria caused by *E. coli* and about as many caused by *Proteus*. Also there is more than a sixfold increase in *Klebsiella* and *P. aeruginosa* when compared with noninstitutionalized persons. Urea-splitting *Proteus* infections are a special problem for the elderly. Thus, it appears that changes in urinary pathogens accompany debilitating diseases in patients with functional incapacities. In addition, the frequent use of antibiotics in long-term care institutions is undoubtedly a factor altering the bacterial flora. Antibiotic-resistant bacteria are frequently cultured from the urine of long-term care residents who have never themselves been exposed to the antibiotics.

Even if a bacteriuric person is asymptomatic, the question of whether the bacteriuria may be harmful has led to several studies.[7–9] Though some studies have shown a correlation between increased mortality with asymptomatic bacteriuria, the frequency of death caused by diseases that might in some way be attributed to bacteriuria (sepsis, pyelonephritis, renal failure, hypertension) was no different in those with or without bacteriuria. From present evidence, it is reasonable to assume that there are two coinciding factors: functionally disabled elderly are more prone to have bacteriuria, and they are also more apt to die from the cause of their primary disability.[9] Controlled studies of elderly bacteriuric men and women have not shown decreased survival in the untreated.[8]

There is a tendency to overuse long-term indwelling catheters in nursing homes for the treatment of urinary incontinence. Their use always results in a chronic urinary tract infection associated with constantly changing and predominantly polymicrobial flora with the danger of recurrent symptomatic urinary tract infections and the risk of death from sepsis. Urinary tract infections are the most common nosocomial infections seen in the elderly. They tend to occur in debilitated patients and are associated with a higher mortality than in younger patients.

Empirical treatment of symptomatic urinary tract infections depends upon the clinical assessment of several factors, e.g., upper tract involvement, community or institutionally acquired infection, or association with long-term catheterization. Single-dose treatment for acute symptomatic infections in the elderly is less likely to be effective than in younger persons but may be worth trying. Seven- to ten-day treatment courses may be necessary. Recurrences with the same organism can be treated with a 2 week course of antibiotics. See Chapter 58 for a more detailed discussion.

No clear evidence supports the treatment of asymptomatic bacteriuria.[10] Although treatment will usually result in a sterile urine, recurrence of bacteriuria with the same or different organism is expected. Prolonged or frequent treatment of asymptomatic bacteriuria often results in emergence of antibiotic-resistant bacteria. Although the majority of elderly institutionalized women with asymptomatic bacteriuria may have upper tract involvement, there are no clear guidelines for determining who should be treated and no good evidence that treatment will significantly alter their course.[11]

PNEUMONIA

Pneumonia is the fourth leading cause of death in the elderly[1] and causes substantial morbidity and health care expenditure.[12] Increased mortality has been ascribed to defects in host defense, coexistent medical disorders, atypical presentation resulting in delayed diagnosis, and increased oropharyngeal colonization with gram-negative bacilli and related increases in gram-negative pulmonary infections.[13] Pneumonia is especially prevalent in nursing homes with mortalities as high as 40 percent. However, a recent nursing home pneumonia study with overall mortality less than 10 percent[14] suggests that high mortality may not be inevitable and that prompt diagnosis and treatment is a major factor in a favorable outcome.

Clinical features of pneumonia in the elderly may be quite different from those observed in younger patients.[15] Fever, productive cough, or any cough at all may be absent. Chest examinations are frequently nondiagnostic, and leukocytosis may not be present.[15,16]

Since the pathogenesis of pneumonia is commonly related to subclinical aspiration, the composition of the oropharyngeal bacterial flora is important. Changes in health status may be more important factors than aging per se in relation to changes noted from a predominantly gram-positive to gram-negative oropharyngeal bacillary flora in many elderly people.[13,16,17] Thus, the incidence of pneumococcal pneumonia is markedly less, and there is a concomitant increase in the incidence of gram-negative pneumonias and those of mixed etiology. There is also an increase in pneumonias attributed to *Haemophilus influenzae*, staphylococci, and *Branhamella catarrhalis*.

The elderly have a distinct predilection for developing nosocomial infection. Pneumococci may cause pneumonia in 10–20 percent of nosocomial cases. Nearly one-half of nosocomial cases will be caused by gram-negative bacteria, with *Klebsiella* and *P. aeruginosa* causing one-half of these. Staphylococci are also prominent causes of nosocomial pneumonias. With notable exceptions, *Legionella* is not frequently involved in nosocomial pneumonia, although the disease has a predilection for the elderly. Aspiration pneumonia secondary to defects in swallowing is frequently seen in debilitated, poststroke, hospitalized, or nursing home patients and is usually caused by gram-negative bacteria or anaerobes.

The diagnosis of pneumonia in the elderly is frequently missed. It begins with a high index of suspicion and knowledge that characteristic signs and symptoms may be absent. The onset of dilirium, agitation, confusion, anorexia, lethargy, or falls may be the only signals of the onset of an infection. There may be considerable difficulty in getting the patient to expectorate a satisfactory specimen for Gram stain and culture. Although transtracheal aspiration may yield satisfactory specimens, the elderly patient frequently does not fit the criteria for safe performance of this procedure. Sputum induction by aerosolized hypertonic saline is simple, useful, and safe.

An attempt should always be made to make a definitive etiologic diagnosis by sputum examination and blood culture. Because of the lethal nature of pneumonia and increased mortality when treatment is delayed, empirical treatment should always be given with the intent of providing antibiotic coverage for the most likely pathogens while at the same time avoiding the adverse consequences of overzealous multiple antibiotic treatment. Because of the lower incidence of pneumococcal pneumonia in the elderly, penicillin is not recommended unless the clinical and laboratory data are highly supportive of a community-acquired pneumococcal infection. Expanded spectrum cephalosporins give broad coverage against the most likely gram-negative and gram-positive pathogens. In situations where *P. aeruginosa* is of major concern such as nosocomial pneumonia, an agent with activity against this organism should be administered. The radiographic resolution of pneumococcal pneumonia, and probably other types as well, is much slower in those older than 50 years than under 50 years of age (12 weeks vs. 4 weeks for 100 percent resolution). Though proof of efficacy for pneumococcal vaccine use in the elderly has been difficult to establish, it is recommended on the basis of evidence available.[18] The value of annual vaccination for influenza is established and should be encouraged for everyone over 65 years old.

TUBERCULOSIS

Though the incidence of tuberculosis has declined markedly in this century, the rate of new cases and deaths is highest in the elderly.[19] The role of declining immunity with aging is possibly of pathogenic importance; an association with concomitant disease also has been noted.[20] The potential risk for the development of active tuberculosis and spread of disease to susceptibles is great in nursing homes.[21]

Clinical syndromes in the elderly include all types of tuberculosis seen at younger ages. Primary infection with mid and lower lung infiltrates and large tuberculin skin test reactions may be seen in elderly persons with primary infection or, having outlived prior infecting organisms, reinfected with new organisms.[22] Tuberculous pleurisy with effusion is seen with increasing frequency in elderly people. Reactivation pulmonary tuberculosis is the most common form seen in elderly patients, but the diagnosis is often delayed or missed. Reasons for this include a failure to include tuberculosis in the differential diagnosis, infrequency of respiratory symptoms, the presence of underlying pulmonary or other disease, and atypical radiographic findings. Weight loss is evident in less than half of the patients. Hemoptysis is unusual. Nonspecific symptoms such as weakness, confusion, and anorexia predominate in about one-half. Fever is the most constant finding but may be misinterpreted as being caused by other types of pneumonia, particularly when there are lower or midlung infiltrates. With ill-defined symptoms and signs in setting of radiographic evidence of cavitation or infiltrates that are progressing despite an appropriate antibiotic regimen for other bacteria, there should be a high index of suspicion for tuberculosis.

Late generalized tuberculosis resulting from hematogenous dissemination occurs more frequently in elderly patients and is difficult to diagnose.[19,20] Most undiagnosed and fatal cases of miliary tuberculosis occur in persons over 60 years of age. Identifiable pulmonary disease and symptoms and signs usually associated with miliary tuberculosis are frequently absent, as may be the case in other forms of extrapulmonary tuberculosis. Bone and joint tuberculosis should be suspected in elderly patients with unexplained unifocal inflammation or destruction of bone and joint.

The numbers of people with waning skin test reactivity increases with age, starting about the fourth decade of life. Tuberculin skin testing can reestablish hypersensitivity in patients whose reactivity has decreased over many years. This booster effect, described in more detail in Chapter 228, causes repeated skin tests to give larger reactions, as if the patients had been recently exposed.

Therapy for active tuberculosis in the elderly follows established regimens for other age groups. A regimen of isoniazid (INH) and rifampin is usually well tolerated. Since elderly persons have most frequently acquired organisms causing their disease in the preantibiotic era, it is rare to find organisms that are insensitive to the standard regimen.

The decision to treat elderly patients with INH for a positive purified protein derivative (PPD) reaction but without identifiable active disease involves balancing the potential liver toxicity of INH against the probability of developing active tuberculosis. The incidence of liver toxicity increases with age up to 64 years but not beyond. For older persons with a recent PPD conversion, INH therapy is usually indicated. Monthly determinations of serum transaminase levels are recommended for all elderly patients receiving INH. For those with previously acquired positive PPD and no evidence of disease, no therapy for elderly persons is recommended. However, annual chest x-ray surveillance is recommended for all elderly PPD reactors, particularly for nursing home patients. For those with old scarring, there is no clear-cut decision. A decision analysis for nursing home patients suggests that the number of active cases of tuberculosis would diminish in patients given INH therapy; hence, a reduction in new cases. On the other hand, no increase was projected in the 5-year survival rate of the patients so treated.[23]

PRESSURE SORES/SKIN INFECTIONS

Pressure sores are the scourge of disabled elderly. Of a number of factors, the primary is prolonged pressure on tissues that results in ischemic necrosis. The resulting long-term sore brings about the potential for a number of infectious complications including local wound infection, cellulitis of the surrounding tissue, contiguous osteomyelitis, tetanus, and intermittent bacteremia with seeding of other organs.

Rational treatment should follow well-established medical and surgical principles in terms of pressure relief, nutritional repletion, medical or surgical débridement, etc. Though frequently used, povidone-iodine antiseptic solution offers no protection from infection of these wounds. Aqueous iodine, povidone-iodine surgical scrub solution, and hydrogen peroxide are actually damaging to newly formed granulation tissue and result in increased infection and prolonged healing.[24] Topical antimicrobial agents have not been shown to be effective.[25] Similarly, long-term systemic prophylactic antibiotic therapy is to be discouraged because of ineffectiveness in preventing infection and the likely possibility that the bacterial flora may be changed to a more undesirable one. Simply covering the wound with a hydroactive dressing is often the most effective therapy.

A variety of gram-positive and gram-negative organisms may be found when culturing these wounds. Most common aerobic organisms include *Proteus mirabilis*, group D streptococci, *E. coli*, staphylococci, and *Pseudomonas* species. Anaerobic organisms most frequently isolated include *Peptostreptococcus* and *Peptococcus* species, *Bacteroides fragilis*, and *Clostridium perfringens*. Because of an inability to permit differentiation of bacteria colonizing the ulcer base from pathogens invading deeper tissues, swab cultures of these wounds are often not helpful. Techniques using needle aspiration of the ulcer margin through intact skin may be more rewarding. Antibiotic therapy for pressure sores should be initiated only upon clinical signs of infection. Although anaerobes are frequently found in these ulcers, unless there are clinical signs suggesting an anaerobic infection, specific anaerobic antibiotic coverage is usually not necessary. Pressure sores are a fairly frequent source of sepsis in the elderly and occasionally may be a source of endocarditis or meningitis.[26] Contiguous osteomyelitis in the underlying bone should be considered in pressure sores that fail to heal properly.[27]

Common types of cellulitis (due to group A β-hemolytic *Streptococcus* and *Staphylococcus aureus*) and less common types (necrotizing or synergistic bacterial infections) are associated with greater morbidity and mortality in the elderly. Because of this, cellulitis should be treated as a potentially life-threatening infection. Antibiotic therapy should be initiated after appropriate cultures are taken, and if there is any clinical evidence to suggest necrotizing infection, prompt surgical intervention should be considered. One of the most common and often debilitating infections involving the skin is herpes zoster (shingles), the pathogenesis and therapy of which is dealt with elsewhere in this volume.

BACTEREMIA

More elderly patients are being seen with bacteremia associated with a fatality rate of 40–60 percent.[16] In contrast to younger ages where mortality in nosocomial bacteremia is greater than in community-acquired bacteremia, the mortality is the same in these two settings in the elderly.

Most frequent sources of community-acquired bacteremia in order of decreasing frequency are the urinary tract, biliary tract, and lungs. In long-term care facilities, the urinary tract is the most frequent source, followed by skin and subcutaneous tissue and the respiratory tract. Other sources to be considered include the abdomen, heart valves, meninges, colon, and female genital tract.[16] Organisms derived most frequently from skin sources are *Staphylococcus aureus, Staphylococcus epidermidis*, gram-negative enteric bacteria, and anaerobes. Bacteria from the urinary tract are usually gram-negative enterics or enterococci; from the biliary tract, gram-negative enterics or anaerobes; and from the respiratory tract, *H. influenzae, S. pneumoniae*, group B *Streptococcus*, or gram-negative enterics.

The clinical presentation of bacteremia in the elderly is often atypical, with a lack of fever reported in as many as 13 percent.[28] Changes in mental status, lethargy, or nonspecific gastrointestinal symptoms may predominate. Although most will have a left shift on a differential white blood cell count, the total white cell count will not be increased in as many as 30 percent. Unexplained acidosis or hypoglycemia may suggest the diagnosis.

INFECTIVE ENDOCARDITIS

Since the preantibiotic era, there has been a significant change in the age-related prevalence of bacterial endocarditis.[29] In the preantibiotic era, the average age of patients with infective endocarditis was 31.2 years, with less than 5 percent 60 years or older. In the period 1950–1977, the average age rose to 47.7 years, with 28 percent 60 years or older. In two series encompassing the 1970s and 1980s, 34 percent in one and 55 percent in the other have been 60 years or older.[30]

There are several reasons for the demographic shift in prevalence of endocarditis, one of which is the increasing numbers of elderly with various forms of degenerative cardiovascular disease. There has been a decline in the incidence of newly acquired rheumatic valvular heart disease in younger generations, and many older patients with this disease have had their lives prolonged by prosthetic heart valves. Also, hospitalization for serious diseases requiring the use of a variety of intravenous catheters and monitoring devices is more frequent in the elderly and results in an increased risk for nosocomial endocarditis. The use of a variety of surgically implanted devices in elderly people provides the opportunity for a nidus of infection that may lead to bacteremia and endocarditis. Urinary tract infection and urologic manipulations, more prevalent in older men, may lead to bacteremia and endocarditis. Enterococcal endocarditis is usually secondary to urinary tract sources in the elderly. Finally, gastrointestinal diseases that predispose to *Streptococcus bovis* endocarditis are common in the elderly. Nonenterococcal group D *Streptococcus bovis* is an increasingly important cause of endocarditis in patients over 55 years of age.

Elderly patients with endocarditis frequently present with vague symptoms such as weakness, malaise, weight loss, confusion, and musculoskeletal symptoms such as arthritis, arthralgia, myalgia, and low back pain. Neurologic manifestations of infective endocarditis are more common in elderly patients, with patients presenting with mental confusion, coma, aphasia, hemiplegia, personality change, and seizures from subarachnoid hemorrhage, embolism, mycotic aneurysm, or brain abscess. Peripheral vascular signs and splenomegaly are seen much less frequently in the elderly than in younger patients. Fever is usually present at some time during the illness but may be low grade or intermittent. Murmurs are usually present but may be misinterpreted as benign murmurs of calcific or sclerotic valves.

Autopsy series have shown that the antemortem diagnosis of infective endocarditis in the elderly is frequently missed. Nonspecific symptoms may be attributed to the vagaries of old age. Musculoskeletal complaints, changes in mental status, and neurologic manifestations, common in the elderly, may be attributed to causes other than endocarditis.

In the elderly, cardiac complications such as congestive heart failure are increased by nonvalvular causes of decompensation such as myocardial infarction, conduction abnormalities, arrhythmia, and myocarditis or an abscess. Elderly persons are prone to arterial embolization, the second most common complication of infective endocarditis. The mortality for infective endocarditis is substantially greater in elderly than in younger patients, and permanent disability and the need for long-term care are common outcomes.

INFECTIOUS DIARRHEA

There is increased mortality from infectious diarrhea in children under 1 year of age and adults older than 60 years.[16] Possible host factors increasing the incidence of *Salmonella* infections with age include achlorhydria, decreased intestinal motility associated with drugs and diseases prevalent in the elderly, and the more frequent use of antibiotics. Unlike their younger healthy counterparts with uncomplicated *Salmonella* gastroenteritis, those over 50 years old should be considered for antibiotic therapy because they may not tolerate enteric infection well and because of the risk of endarteritis and endocarditis.[16]

Since antibiotics shorten the duration of *Shigella* gastroenteritis, therapy is often indicated to abbreviate the risk of fluid and electrolyte imbalance so poorly tolerated by the elderly. Antibiotic therapy should also be considered for diarrhea caused by *Campylobacter jejuni*, invasive *E. coli, Vibrio parahaemolyticus*, and *Yersinia enterocolitica*. Because of the increased prevalence of antibiotic exposure for elderly nursing home patients, pseudomembranous colitis must be considered in this setting.

Both the Norwalk virus and rotavirus have produced well-described outbreaks of acute gastroenteritis in elderly patients, particularly in nursing homes. Differentiating these self-limited diseases from those requiring specific therapy is important. There has been an increasing number of outbreaks of *E. coli* 0157:H7-associated hemorrhagic colitis in nursing homes.[31] Infection with this verotoxin-producing *E. coli* is more prevalent in the very old and the very young. It is frequently associated with the hemolytic–uremia syndrome, with a very high mortality in the elderly.

MENINGITIS

Meningitis in neonates and the elderly is apt to be caused by unusual bacteria (*Listeria monocytogenes*, gram-negative bacilli, and *S. aureus*) with a high mortality.[32]

Atypical presentation of meningitis in the elderly or postneurosurgical status may cause delays in diagnosis, and age-related physiologic dysfunction may contribute to increased mortality. Pitfalls in the diagnosis primarily result from attributing mental status changes to dementia and neck stiffness to degenerative joint disease. Deaths from meningitis in the elderly do not seem to be particularly related to identifiable immune dysfunction or terminal debilitated status. With increasing rates of hospitalization and neurosurgical procedures, the elderly are more subject to nosocomial meningitis. Endocarditis and pneumonia are the common sources in the elderly.

Laboratory diagnostic features are not different in the elderly except for occasional cases where there is relatively little spinal fluid pleocytosis. Over one-half of the cases are caused by *S. pneumoniae*. Gram-negative bacillary meningitis may be "spontaneous," with no identifiable predisposing condition, or follow head trauma or neurosurgical procedures. *L. monocytogenes* infections are prone to occur in patients who are receiving immunosuppressive therapy for a lymphoproliferative disease or who are taking steroids but may occur in elderly who are otherwise healthy. *L. monocytogenes* meningitis carries a very high mortality in the elderly. *S. aureus* meningitis is commonly associated with neurosurgery and has a poor prognosis. Enterococcal and viridans streptococcal meningitis are uncommon but most frequently associated with endocarditis. Meningitis from anaerobes is usually secondary to otitis media or mastoiditis or is associated with head and neck malignancy.

SEPTIC ARTHRITIS

At present, 25–32 percent of persons with septic arthritis are over the age of 60.[33,34] Their mortality is higher and recovery of joint function is less satisfactory. Degenerative arthritis frequently antedates septic arthritis. Septic arthritis is also commonly associated with pre-existing rheumatoid arthritis. This association as well as that with diseases such as diabetes mellitus, malignancy, and cytotoxic or systemic corticosteroid therapy suggests that immunologic defects may play an important role in the pathogenesis of septic arthritis in the elderly. The frequency with which bacteremia occurs in elderly persons is undoubtedly a factor.

The knee is the joint most frequently involved, followed by the wrist and shoulder. Although most elderly patients complain of a painful, swollen joint, in contrast to younger patients they are seldom totally immobilized by pain, and muscle spasm is infrequent. As in younger patients, the most commonly isolated organism is *S. aureus*. Unlike younger patients, gram-negative rods are frequent causes in the elderly. In addition, septic arthritis is associated more frequently with osteomyelitis in the older patient.

OBSCURE FEVER

Many elderly persons have lower body temperatures than are traditionally accepted as normal for human beings and consequently have a diminished febrile response to infection.[35] However, 95 percent of elderly patients who have infection will show some febrile response by electronic thermometer measurement.[36] The criterion of fever in the elderly should be at least a degree below the usual criterion of 101°F (38.3°C). Using the usual criterion of fever, Esposito and Gleckman found that 36 percent of their elderly patients with fever of undetermined origin (FUO) had infection.[37] Abdominal infection was the most common infectious cause of FUO in their series.

Abdominal infections may be difficult to diagnose in some elderly patients because of a vague history and atypical physical findings. Infections of the biliary tract, liver abscess, appendicitis, diverticulitis of the colon, and an intra-abdominal abscess secondary to a perforated viscus are frequent causes of intra-abdominal infection.[16]

Fifty percent of the FUOs in the series of Esposito and Gleckman were caused by neoplasm and connective tissue disorders in about equal numbers.[37] Over half of the neoplasms were lymphomas, two-thirds of which were diagnosed on laparotomy. Most other neoplasms were renal or hepatobiliary in origin. Sixty-five percent of the connective tissue diseases were giant cell arteritis, predominantly in females. Polyarteritis nodosa was diagnosed in 20 percent.

PHARMACOLOGIC CONSIDERATIONS

Although the elderly are the age group most likely to receive antibiotic therapy when hospitalized and in nursing homes (where the number of beds now exceeds total hospital beds in the United States), there has been little accurate information about the effects of aging on the pharmacokinetics and toxicity of antimicrobial agents until recently.[38,39] Physiologic changes that accompany advanced age may significantly affect the absorption, distribution, plasma protein binding, metabolism, and elimination of many antibiotics. For example, a physiologic reduction in renal function requires a modified dosage of aminoglycosides to prevent ototoxicity or further renal impairment. The risk of toxicity of many other antibiotics is also increased in the elderly. The phenomenon of "polypharmacy," which is so common in this age group, greatly increases the chances for drug interactions. Although a detailed discussion of geriatric pharmacology is beyond the scope of this chapter, suffice it to say that special consideration of pharmacokinetics and toxicity is imperative when administering antibiotics to older individuals.

REFERENCES

1. Garibaldi RA, Nurse BA. Infection in the elderly. Am J Med. 1986;81(Suppl 1A):53–8.
2. Saltzman RL, Peterson PK. Immunodeficiency of the elderly. Rev Infect Dis. 1987;9:1127–39.
3. Kunin CM. Natural history of recurrent bacteriuria in school girls. N Engl J Med. 1970;282:1443–8.
4. Kasviki-Charvati P, Drolette-Kefakis B, Papanayiotou PC, et al. Turnover of bacteriuria in old age. Age Ageing. 1982;11:169–74.
5. Boscia JA, Kobasa WD, Knight RA, et al. Epidemiology of bacteriuria in an elderly ambulatory population. Am J Med. 1986; 80:208–14.
6. Lane T. Urinary tract infections in the elderly. In: McCue JD, ed. Medical Care of the Elderly. Lexington, MA: Collamore Press; 1983.
7. Nicolle LE, Mayhew WJ, Bryan L. Prospective randomized comparison of therapy and no therapy for asymptomatic bacteriuria in institutionalized elderly women. Am J Med. 1987;83:27–33.
8. Nicolle LE, Henderson E, Bjornson J, et al. The association of bacteriuria with resident characteristics and survival in elderly institutionalized men. Ann Intern Med. 1987;106:682–6.
9. Nordenstam GR, Brandberg CA, Oden AS, et al. Bacteriuria and mortality in an elderly population. N Engl J Med. 1986;314:1152–6.
10. Boscia JA, Abrutyn E, Kaye D. Asymptomatic bacteriuria in elderly persons: Treat or do not treat? Ann Intern Med. 1987;106:764 6.
11. Nicolle LE, Muir P, Harding GKM, et al. Localization of urinary tract infection in elderly, institutionalized women with asymptomatic bacteriuria. J Infect Dis. 1988;157:65–70.
12. Fedullo AJ, Swinburne AJ. Relationship of patient age to clinical features and outcome for in-hospital treatment of pneumonia. Gerontology. 1985;40:29–33.
13. Valenti WM, Trudell RG, Bentley DW. Factors predisposing to oropharyngeal colonization with gram(−) bacili in the aged. N Engl J Med. 1978;298:1108–11.
14. Peterson PK, Stein D, Guay DRP, et al. Prospective study of lower respiratory tract infections in an extended care nursing home program: Potential role of oral ciprofloxacin. Am J Med. 1988;85:164–71.
15. Austrian R. Pneumonia in the later years. J Am Geriatr Soc. 1981;29:481–9.
16. Gleckman RA, Gantz NM. Infections in the Elderly. Boston: Little, Brown; 1983.
17. Garb JL, Brown RB, Garb JR, et al. Differences in etiology of pneumonias in nursing home and community patients. JAMA. 1978;240:2169–72.
18. Sims RV, Steinmann WC, McConville JH, et al. The clinical effectiveness of pneumococcal vaccine in the elderly. Ann Intern Med. 1988;108:653–7.
19. Nogomi PH, Yoshikawa TT. Tuberculosis in the geriatric patient. J Am Geriatr Soc. 1983;31:356–63.
20. Slavin RE, Walsh TJ, Pollack AD. Late generalized tuberculosis. Medicine (Baltimore). 1980;59:352–66.
21. Stead WW, To T. The significance of tuberculin testing in elderly persons. Ann Intern Med. 1987;107:837–42.
22. Stead WW, Lofgren JP, Warren E, et al. Tuberculosis as an epidemic and nosocomial infection among the elderly in nursing homes. N Engl J Med. 1985;312:1483–7.
23. Cooper JK. Decision analysis for tuberculosis preventive treatment in nursing homes. J Am Geriatr Soc. 1986;34:814–7.
24. Rodeheaver G, Bellamy W, Kody M, et al. Bactericidal activity and toxicity of iodine-containing solutions in wounds. Arch Surg. 1982;117:181–6.
25. Geronemus RG, Mertz PM, Eaglstein WH. Wound healing: The effects of topical antimicrobial agents. Arch Dermatol. 1979;115:1311–4.
26. Bryan CS, Dew CE, Reynolds KL. Bacteremia associated with decubitus ulcers. Arch Intern Med. 1983;143:2093–5.
27. Sugarman B. Pressure sores and underlying bone infection. Arch Intern Med. 1987;147:553–5.
28. Gleckman R, Hibert D. Afebrile bacteremia: A phenomenon in geriatric patients. JAMA. 1982;248:1478–81.
29. Cantrell M, Yoshikawa TT. Aging and infective endocarditis. J Am Geriatr Soc. 1983;31:216–22.
30. Terpenning MS, Buggy BP, Kauffman CA. Infective endocarditis: Clinical features in young and elderly patients. Am J Med. 1987;83:626 34.
31. Ryan CA, Tauxe RV, Hosek GW, et al. *Escherichia coli* 0157:87 diarrhea in a nursing home: Clinical, epidemiological, and pathological findings. J Infect Dis. 1986;154:631–8.
32. Gorse GJ, Thrupp LD, Nudleman KL, et al. Bacterial meningitis in the elderly. Arch Intern Med. 1984;144:1603–7.
33. McGuire NM, Kauffman CA. Septic arthritis in the elderly. J Am Geriatr Soc. 1985;33:170–4.
34. Norman DC, Yoshikawa TT. Responding to septic arthritis. Geriatrics. 1983;38:83–91.

35. Fox RH, MacGibbon R, Davies L, et al. Problem of the old and the cold. Br Med. J. 1973;1:21–4.
36. McAlpine CH, Martin BJ, Lennox IM, et al. Pyrexia in infection in the elderly. Age Ageing. 1986;15:230–4.
37. Esposito AL, Gleckman RA. Fever of unknown origin in the elderly. J Am Geriatr Soc. 1978;26:498–505.
38. Norrby SR. Antibiotic therapy in aging patients. Bull NY Acad Med. 1987;63:519–32.
39. Guay DRP, Obaid S, Breitenbucher R. Antibiotic use in the elderly. In: Peterson PK, Verhoef J, eds. The Antimicrobial Agents Annual 2. Amsterdam: Elsevier; 1987:422–41.

SECTION C

296. IMMUNIZATION

ALAN R. HINMAN
WALTER A. ORENSTEIN
KENNETH J. BART
STEPHEN R. PREBLUD

The two most effective means of preventing disease, disability, and death from infectious diseases have been sanitation and immunization. Both of these approaches antedated understanding of the germ theory of disease. Artificial induction of immunity began centuries ago with variolation, the practice of inoculating fluid from smallpox lesions into the skin of susceptible persons. Although this technique usually produced mild illness without complications, spread of disease did occur, with occasional complications. In 1796, Jenner demonstrated that milk maids who had contracted cowpox (vaccinia) were immune to smallpox. He inoculated the vesicular fluid from cowpox lesions into the skin of susceptible individuals and induced protection against smallpox, thus beginning the era of immunization.

Immunization is the act of artificially inducing immunity or providing protection from disease; it can be active or passive. Active immunization consists of inducing the body to develop defenses against disease. This is usually accomplished by the administration of vaccines or toxoids that stimulate the body's immune system to produce antibodies that protect against the infectious agent. Passive immunization consists of providing temporary protection through the administration of exogenously produced antibody. Two situations in which passive immunization commonly occurs are through the transplacental transmission of antibodies to the fetus, which may provide protection against several diseases for the first 3–6 months of life, and the injection of immune globulin for specific preventive purposes. A more detailed description of the immune mechanisms involved follows.

Immunizing agents include vaccines, toxoids, and antibody containing preparations from human or animal donors. Some important definitions follow.[1]

1. Vaccine: A suspension of attenuated live or killed microorganisms (bacteria, viruses, or rickettsiae), or fractions thereof, administered to induce immunity and thereby prevent infectious disease.
2. Toxoid: A modified bacterial toxin that has been rendered nontoxic but retains the ability to stimulate the formation of antitoxin.
3. Immune globulin (IG): A sterile solution for intramuscular administration containing antibody from human blood. It contains 10–18 percent protein obtained by cold ethanol fractionation of large pools of blood plasma. It is primarily indicated for routine maintenance of certain immunodeficient persons and for passive immunization against measles and hepatitis A. Immune globulin intravenous (IGIV), a specialized preparation allowing intravenous administration, contains approximately 5% protein and is indicated primarily for replacement therapy in immunodeficient children.
4. Specific immune globulin: Special preparations obtained from donor pools preselected for a high antibody content against a specific disease, for example, hepatitis B immune globulin (HBIG), varicella-zoster immune globulin (VZIG), rabies immune globulin (RIG), and tetanus immune globulin solution (TIG).

The constituents of immunizing agents include:

1. Suspending fluid: This frequently is as simple as sterile water or saline, but it may be a complex fluid containing small amounts of proteins or other constituents derived from the medium or biologic system in which it is produced (serum proteins, egg antigens, cell culture derived antigens).
2. Preservatives, stabilizers, antibiotics: These components of vaccines are used (*a*) to inhibit or prevent bacterial growth in viral culture or the final product or (*b*) to stabilize the antigen. They include such materials as mercurials and specific antibiotics. Allergic reactions may occur if the recipient is sensitive to any of these additives.
3. Adjuvants: An aluminum salt is used in some vaccines to enhance the immune response to vaccines containing inactivated microorganisms or their products (e.g., toxoids and hepatitis B vaccine). Vaccine with such adjuvants must be injected deeply into muscle masses, since subcutaneous or intracutaneous administration can cause local irritation, inflammation, granuloma formation, or necrosis.

THE IMMUNE RESPONSE AND IMMUNIZATION

Two major approaches to active immunization have been employed: the use of live (generally attenuated) infectious agents or the use of inactivated, or detoxified, agents or their extracts. For many diseases (including influenza, poliomyelitis, measles) both approaches have been employed. Live attenuated vaccines are believed to induce an immunologic response more nearly like that resulting from natural infection than do killed vaccines. Inactivated or killed vaccines can consist of inactivated whole organisms (e.g., cholera, pertussis), detoxified exotoxins either alone or linked to carrier proteins (e.g., diphtheria and tetanus toxoids), soluble capsular material (e.g., pneumococcal polysaccharide), or extracts of some component (e.g., hepatitis B) or components of the organism (e.g., subunit influenza).

Since the organisms in live vaccines multiply in the recipient, antigen production generally increases logarithmically until checked by the onset of the immune response it is intended to induce. The live attenuated viruses (e.g., measles, mumps, rubella) generally are believed to confer lifelong protection with one dose. By contrast, nonpolysaccharide killed vaccines have generally not been shown to induce permanent immunity with one dose, making repeated vaccination and boosters necessary to develop and maintain high levels of antibody (e.g., diphtheria, tetanus, rabies, typhoid). Although the amount of antigen initially introduced is greater with inactivated vaccines, the multiplication of organisms in the host results in a cumulatively greater antigenic input with live vaccines.

The nature and extent of the response to vaccine or toxoid are determined by the chemical and physical states of the antigen, the mode of administration, the metabolic fate of the antigen, the genetic characteristics of the recipient, and various host factors. There is a dose–response curve relationship between antigen dose and peak response obtained beyond a threshold.[2]

The route of administration may determine the rapidity and nature of the immune response to a vaccine or toxoid. For example, parenterally administered Cendehill and HPV 77 strains of rubella vaccines do not produce detectable rubella-specific secretory IgA, whereas the RA 27/3 strain given intranasally stimulates the production of IgA in nasal secretions.

The age of an individual may determine to some extent the response to a vaccine. The recommended schedule by age for routine immunization is based on the age-dependent response. Differences in response capability exist during early infancy and senescence. The presence of high levels of passively acquired maternal antibody in the first few months of life impairs the initial immune response to some vaccines. In the elderly the response to antigenic stimulation may be diminished. Larger amounts of antigen may be required to produce the desired response (e.g., influenza).

The immune response to some vaccines or toxoids can be potentiated by the addition of adjuvants, such as aluminium salts. They are particularly useful with such inactivated products as diphtheria and tetanus toxoids and pertussis and hepatitis B vaccines. The mechanism of enhancement of antigenicity is not totally defined; however, adjuvants render a soluble antigen particulate (making it immunogenic), mobilize phagocytes to the site of antigen deposition, and delay the release of antigen.

Many of the structural constituents of microorganisms and exotoxins are antigenic. Antigens usually require the interaction of B and T cells to generate an immune response (e.g., measles, varicella) or may be able, on occasion, to initiate B-cell proliferation and antibody production without the help of T cells (e.g., pneumococcal type III polysaccharide, *Haemophilus influenzae* type b polysaccharide). After vaccination, antibodies formed to each of these constituents may be of any of the immunoglobulin classes. These antibodies may function alone or in conjunction with other components of the immune system (e.g., complement, opsonins): (*1*) by participating directly in the neutralization of toxin (e.g., diphtheria); (*2*) by opsonization of virus (e.g., poliovirus); (*3*) by initiating or combining with complement and promoting phagocytosis (e.g., pneumococcus, cholera); (*4*) by reacting with nonsensitized lymphocytes to stimulate phagocytosis (e.g., *Salmonella typhosa, Brucella*); (*5*) by sensitizing macrophages to stimulate phagocytosis (e.g., *Salmonella typhosa*). Cell-mediated and humoral immunity may act simultaneously. All five mechanisms may act separately or in combination.[3–6]

Independent of antibody production, the stimulation of the immune system by vaccination may, on occasion, elicit a hypersensitivity response. Killed measles vaccine, in use in the United States between 1963 and 1967, induced incomplete humoral immunity and cell-mediated hypersensitivity resulting in the development of a syndrome of atypical measles in some children upon subsequent challenge.

On first exposure to a vaccine antigen, the primary response requires a latent period of several days before humoral and cell-mediated immunity can be detected. When the antigen is thymus dependent, IgM and IgG classes of antibody are initially secreted by the B cells, with IgM appearing first. IgM antibodies may fix complement, making lysis and phagocytosis possible. As the titer of IgG rises during the second week after immunogenic stimulation, the IgM titer falls.[3] IgG antibodies are produced in large amounts and function in the neutralization, precipitation, and fixation of complement. The antibody titer reaches a peak in approximately 1–2 weeks and then falls gradually. The switch from IgM synthesis to predominantly IgG synthesis in B cells requires T-cell cooperation.

Many pathogens replicate at mucosal surfaces before host invasion and may induce secretory IgA along the respiratory and gastrointestinal mucous membranes and at other localized sites (e.g., polio, rubella, influenza, adenovirus). IgA antibodies are efficient at virus neutralization (e.g., polio), fix complement through the alternative pathway (e.g., cholera), prevent adsorption of organisms to the intestinal wall (e.g., *Escherichia coli*, cholera), and (with the aid of both complement and lysozyme) can lyse gram-negative bacteria.[7]

After a second exposure to the same antigen, heightened humoral or cell-mediated responses are observed. These secondary responses occur sooner than the primary response, usually within 4–5 days, and depend on a marked proliferation of antibody producing cells or effector T cells of cell-mediated immunity. The secondary response depends on immunologic memory mediated by both T and B cells. Polysaccharide vaccines such as *Haemophilus* b polysaccharide vaccine (HbPV) tend to evoke immune responses independent of T cells. Thus booster responses are not seen or repeat administration. Linking polysaccharides to proteins can convert them to T-cell dependent antigens that have the capacity to induce immunologic memory and secondary responses on repeat vaccination.[8] Infection with measles or varicella evokes a cell-mediated as well as a humoral response.

Response to vaccines is often gauged by measuring the concentration of the specific antibody in the serum. For some viral vaccines, such as measles and rubella, the presence of circulating antibodies correlates with clinical protection.[9] While this has served as a dependable indicator of immunity, seroconversion measures only one parameter of the immune response. Although a fall in titer takes place for some vaccines over time (e.g., measles and rubella), upon revaccination or challenge a secondary response is observed in IgG antibodies with little or no detectable IgM response, suggesting prior protection.[9] Thus, the absence of measurable antibody may not mean that the individual is unprotected. By contrast, with some vaccines and toxoids, the mere presence of antibodies is not sufficient to assure clinical protection, but rather a minimal circulating level of antibody is required (e.g., 0.01 International unit/ml of tetanus antitoxin).

General Principles of Immunization

Introduction and widespread use of vaccines have resulted in the global eradication of smallpox and dramatic reductions in the incidence rates of other diseases (see Table 1). Measles, poliomyelitis, diphtheria, and rubella have been eliminated or are in the process of being eliminated. Modern vaccines are very safe and very effective; however, they are not completely so. Each vaccine is associated with some adverse effects, which may range from very mild to life-threatening, and each vaccine falls short of 100 percent effectiveness. Consequently, some persons who have received a full course of vaccine or toxoid may develop disease on exposure.

In the development of vaccines, the initial experiments are typically carried out in animal models to demonstrate protection (or at least production of antibodies) and relative safety; then limited numbers of doses are administered to humans to demonstrate antibody production and safety. After this stage, clinical trials in humans are typically carried out in a limited number of individuals (several thousand) to demonstrate further safety and efficacy. Because of their limited size, these field trials can only be expected to detect adverse events that could occur relatively frequently. After clinical trials, licensure may be sought. Vaccine production is strictly regulated by the Center for Biologics Evaluation and Research, Food and Drug Administration. Only after a vaccine is found to be safe and effective is it licensed for use. Postmarketing surveillance is necessary to detect rare adverse events associated with vaccination.

TABLE 1. Comparison of Maximum and Current Morbidity Vaccine-Preventable Diseases

	Maximum Cases	(Year)	1988 Prov.	Percentage Change
Diphtheria	206,939	(1921)	1	−99.999
Measles	894,134	(1941)	2,933	−99.67
Mumps[a]	152,209	(1968)	4,730	−96.89
Pertussis	265,269	(1934)	3,000	−98.87
Polio (paralytic)	21,269	(1952)	2[b]	−99.99
Rubella[c]	57,686	(1969)	221	−99.62
CRS[d]	20,000[c]	(1964–1965)	4	−99.98
Tetanus[e]	601	(1948)	49	−91.85

[a] First reportable in 1968.
[b] Small number of cases under investigation.
[c] First reportable in 1966.
[d] Congenital rubella syndrome.
[e] First reportable in 1947.

The decision to use a vaccine involves assessment of the risks of disease, the benefits of vaccination, and the risks associated with vaccination. The relative balance of risks and benefits may change over time; consequently, continuing assessment of vaccines is essential. Recommendations for vaccine use are developed by several different bodies: The Public Health Service Immunization Practices Advisory Committee (ACIP) develops recommendations for vaccines with primary orientation toward the public health sector. The Committee on the Infectious Diseases of the American Academy of Pediatrics (the "Red Book" committee) develops recommendations for vaccine use in private pediatric practice.[10] The Committee on Immunization of the American College of Physicians has developed recommendations for vaccination of adults in the private sector, and the American Academy of Family Physicians is currently developing recommendations for immunizations.[11]

CURRENTLY AVAILABLE IMMUNIZING AGENTS

Tables 2 and 3 list currently licensed immunizing agents and immune globulins, along with the year in which they were first licensed. This section will present brief information about each, including the type of immunizing agent it represents, the primary indications for its use, its relative efficacy, the number and spacing of doses required, known adverse effects, and precautions and contraindications for use. Package inserts and specific references and recommendations should be consulted for more detailed information. In addition to these licensed products, several other vaccines are under development and may soon become available (e.g., varicella, improved pertussis).

Vaccines

Adenovirus Vaccine, Types 4 and 7. Types 4 and 7 adenovirus vaccines contain unattenuated living adenoviruses within a capsule, which is administered orally.[12,13] Release of the organisms in the gastrointestinal tract leads to local reproduction and induction of immunity without development of symptoms associated with infection via the nasopharyngeal route. Although licensed for general use, these vaccines are currently used exclusively in military recruits, in whom adenovirus infections have been an important cause of acute respiratory disease. Vaccine efficacy is in excess of 90 percent, and only a single dose is required. Adverse effects are essentially nonexistent, and the only known contraindications relate to use in immunocompromised individuals. On theoretical grounds these vaccines should not be given to pregnant women.[12,13]

Anthrax Vaccine. Anthrax vaccine is prepared from microaerophilic cultures of an avirulent nonencapsulated strain of *Baccilus anthracis*. The cultures are grown in a synthetic medium, and the organism elaborates the antigen that induces protective antibodies during the growth period. The vaccine is indicated only for those at high risk of exposure to anthrax, such as persons who may come in contact with imported animal

TABLE 2. Currently Available Vaccines and Toxoids and Year Licensed[a]

Product	Year Licensed
Adenovirus vaccine, live, oral, type 4	1980
Adenovirus vaccine, live, oral, type 7	1980
Anthrax vaccine absorbed	1970
BCG vaccine	1950
Cholera vaccine	1914
Diphtheria and tetanus toxoids and pertussis vaccine adsorbed	1949
Diphtheria and tetanus toxoids adsorbed (pediatric use, DT)	1949
Diphtheria toxoid	1927
Diphtheria toxoid adsorbed	1952
Haemophilus b polysaccharide vaccine	1985
Haemophilus b conjugate vaccine	1987
Hepatitis B vaccine	1981
Hepatitis B recombinant vaccine	1987
Influenza virus vaccine	1945
Measles and mumps virus vaccine, live	1973
Measles and rubella virus vaccine, live	1971
Measles virus vaccine, live, attenuated	1963
Measles, mumps, and rubella virus vaccine, live	1971
Meningococcal polysaccharide vaccine, group A	1975
Meningococcal polysaccharide vaccine, group C	1975
Meningococcal polysaccharide vaccine, groups A and C combined	1975
Meningococcal polysaccharide vaccine, groups A, C, Y, W135 combined	1981
Mumps virus vaccine, live	1967
Pertussis vaccine adsorbed	1948
Plague vaccine	1911
Pneumococcal vaccine, 23 valent	1983
Poliomyelitis vaccine (inactivated, enhanced potency)	1987
Poliovirus vaccine, live, oral, trivalent	1963[b]
Polyvalent bacterial vaccines with "No U.S. Standard of Potency"	1914
Rabies vaccine (human diploid)	1980
Rubella and mumps virus vaccine, live	1970
Rubella virus vaccine, live	1969
Smallpox vaccine	1903
Tetanus and diphtheria toxoids adsorbed (adult use Td)	1955
Tetanus toxoid	1933
Tetanus toxoid adsorbed	1949
Typhoid vaccine	1914
Yellow fever vaccine	1953

[a] As of June 1, 1988.
[b] Monovalent forms licensed 1961.

hides, furs, bone meal, wool, hair (especially goat hair), and bristles; for all personnel in factories handling these materials; and for laboratory workers contemplating investigational studies with the organism. Clinical efficacy is not known with certainty, but it induces antibodies in 90 percent or more of those who receive the primary course of six subcutaneous injections given at time zero, 2 weeks, 4 weeks, 6 months, 12 months, and 18 months. Annual boosters are necessary. Local reactions at the site of injection are infrequent. No serious untoward effects are known. This vaccine is currently available only through the Michigan Department of Public Health.[14]

BCG Vaccine. BCG vaccine contains living Calmette-Guérin bacillus, an attenuated strain of *Mycobacterium bovis*. In many countries it is widely used in infants and young children to prevent disseminated tuberculosis infection. In the United States,

TABLE 3. Current Available Immune Globulins and Year First Licensed[a]

Product	Year Licensed
Hepatitis B immune globulin (human)	1977
Immune globulin intravenous (human)	1981
Immune serum globulin (human)	1943[b]
Pertussis immune globulin (human)	1958
Rabies immunne globulin (human)	1974
$Rh_0(D)$ immune globulin (human)	1968
Tetanus immune globulin (human)	1957
Vaccinia immune globulin (human)	1968
Varicella zoster immune globulin (human)	1980

[a] As of June 1, 1988.
[b] Immune globulin (human) licensed 1934.

the risk of tuberculosis infection is so low that use of the vaccine is not recommended except in very special circumstances, particularly since BCG vaccination results in conversion of the tuberculin skin test, thereby removing one of the most important indicators of tuberculosis infection (tuberculin conversion). Although it is widely used throughout the world, there has been much controversy regarding efficacy. Recent studies suggest that the vaccine is effective particularly for preventing complications of disseminated tuberculosis in young children.[15] The only situations in which BCG use might be considered in the United States would be (*1*) for individuals, such as infants, who are skin test-negative who have prolonged close contact with patients with active tuberculosis who are untreated, are ineffectively treated, or have antibiotic-resistant infection; (*2*) for hospital staff where other tuberculosis control measures do not prevent an annual skin test conversion rate in excess of 1 percent; and (*3*) for groups in which an excessive rate of new infections can be demonstrated, and the usual surveillance and treatment programs have failed or are not feasible.

A single dose of vaccine is administered intradermally or subcutaneously. Known adverse effects include regional adenitis, disseminated BCG infection, and ostetitis due to the BCG organism. Adenitis occurs in approximately 1–10 percent of vaccinees, and disseminated infections and osteitis are apparently quite rare (approximately one case per million vaccines). Immunocompromised individuals should not receive the vaccine because of increased risk of disseminated BCG infection.[16]

Cholera Vaccine. Cholera vaccine is a killed suspension of *Vibrio cholerae* that can be administered intramuscularly, subcutaneously (for persons 6 months of age or older), or intradermally (for persons 5 years of age or older). The immunizing course consists of two doses given at least 1 week apart. Boosters are required every 6 months to maintain protection. Dosage varies, depending on route of administration and age of the recipient. The efficacy of this vaccine is on the order of 50 percent, and protection lasts only about 6 months. It is currently recommended for use only in order to satisfy the immunization requirements for entry to certain countries. For these purposes, a single dose is sufficient. The traveler's best protection against cholera, as well as against many other enteric diseases, is to avoid food and water that might be contaminated. Adverse effects from cholera vaccine include frequent local reactions and fever. Serious side effects are very rare.[17]

Diphtheria Toxoid. Diphtheria toxoid is a purified preparation of inactivated diphtheria toxin. It is highly effective in inducing antibodies that will prevent disease, although they may not prevent acquisition or carriage of the organism. The toxoid is available in fluid or adsorbed form; the adsorbed form is recommended because of its greater immunogenicity. Two dosage formulations are generally available, one for use up to the seventh birthday, and one for subsequent use. The adult formulation has a lower concentration of diphtheria toxoid than the pediatric formulation, since local reactions are thought to relate to both age and dosage. Diphtheria toxoid is usually administered in combination with tetanus toxoid (DT for children, Td for adults) and, in children younger than 7 years old, with pertusis vaccine also (DTP). The efficacy of both preparations is in excess of 95 percent.

Immunization against diphtheria is recommended for all residents in the United States. The primary immunizing series of DT (for children 1–6 years of age) or Td (for older children and adults) consists of at least two doses administered 4–8 weeks apart followed by a third dose 6–12 months later. For children younger than 7 years old with no contraindication to pertussis immunization, DTP is recommended, and the primary series is three doses administered 4–8 weeks apart followed by a fourth dose 6–12 months later. For infants with contraindications to pertussis vaccine, DT is administered in the same schedule as DTP. (See "Pertussis Vaccine" and Tables 4 and 5.) There is no need to restart a series if the schedule is interrupted; the next dose in the series should be given. Booster doses of Td should be given every 10 years. Known adverse effects include local reactions (frequent) and systemic reactions or fever, which occur rarely. The only known contraindication is in individuals who have previously had neurologic or severe hypersensitivity reactions after diphtheria toxoid.[18,19]

Haemophilus B Vaccine. There are two generic types of *Haemophilus* b vaccines available in the United States. *Haemophilus* b polysaccharide vaccine (HbPV) was licensed in the United States in 1985; a single dose of vaccine is recommended for routine use in infants 24 months of age. This recommendation is based on Finnish field trial data indicating that efficacy in children vaccinated once at 18–71 months of age was 90 percent. However, efficacy in children immunized at 18–23 months of age could not be assessed accurately. Little protection was afforded if vaccine was administered before 18 months of age.

Conjugate vaccines (HbCV) were first licensed at the end of 1987 and are now the preferred vaccines because they elicit substantially higher antibody titers than the HbPV. One product is conjugated to diphtheria toxoid while a second product is conjugated to a mutant nontoxic diphtheria toxin (CRM). On the basis of immunogenicity data, approximately 90 percent of children 18 months of age will be expected to be protected after a single dose of this vaccine. Accordingly, HbCV is intended for all children 18 months of age. All children 19–23 months should also be vaccinated. Children 18–23 months of age who have already received the polysaccharide vaccine should be revaccinated (with a minimum interval of 2 months) with a con-

TABLE 4. Recommended Schedule for Active Immunization of Normal Infants and Children[a]

Recommended Age[b]	*Vaccine(s)*[c]	*Comments*
2 months	DTP-1,[d] OPV-1[e]	Can be given earlier in areas of high endemicity.
4 months	DTP-2, OPV-2	6-week to 2-month interval desired between OPV doses to prevent interference.
6 months	DTP-3	Additional dose of OPV optional in areas with high risk of polio exposure.
15 months[f]	MMR,[g] DTP-4, OPV-3	Completion of primary series of DTP and OPV.
18 months	*Haemophilus* b conjugate[h,i]	
4–6 years	DTP-5[j] OPV-4	At or before school entry.
14–16 years	Td[k]	Repeat every 10 years throughout life.

[a] See Table 5 for the recommended immunization schedules for infants and children up to their seventh birthday not immunized at the recommended time in early infancy.

[b] These recommended ages should not be construed as absolute (i.e., 2 months can be 6–10 weeks, etc.) However, MMR should not be given to children less than 1 year of age. Single measles antigen vaccine can be administered as early as 6 months of age if exposure to measles disease is considered likely. *Haemophilus influenzae* b conjugate vaccine should not be given to children less than 18 months of age.

[c] For all products used, consult the manufacturer's package enclosure for instructions regarding storage, handling, dosage, and administration. Immunobiologics prepared by different manufacturers can vary, and those of the same manufacturer can change from time to time. The package insert is a useful reference for a specific product, but it may not always be consistent with ACIP and AAP concomitant immunization schedules.

[d] DTP: diphtheria and tetanus toxoids and pertussis vaccine adsorbed. DTP may be used up to the seventh birthday. The first dose can be given at 6 weeks of age and the second and third doses at 4–8 weeks after the preceding dose.

[e] OPV: Poliovirus vaccine live oral, trivalent; contains poliovirus types 1, 2, and 3.

[f] Provided at least 6 months has elapsed since DTP-3 or, if fewer than three DTPs have been received, at least 6 weeks since last previous dose of DTP or OPV. MMR vaccine should not be delayed to allow simultaneous administration with DTP and OPV. Administering MMR at 15 months and DTP-4 and OPV-3 at 18 months continues to be an acceptable alternative.

[g] MMR: measles, mumps, and rubella virus vaccine, live.

[h] *Haemophilus influenzae* b conjugate vaccine.

[i] If *Haemophilus* b conjugate vaccine is not available, an acceptable alternative is *Haemophilus* b polysaccharide vaccine given at 24 months of age. Children previously vaccinated with polysaccharide vaccine between 18 and 23 months should be revaccinated with a single dose of conjugate vaccine at least 2 months after the initial dose of polysaccharide vaccine.

[j] Up to the seventh birthday.

[k] Td: tetanus and diphtheria toxoids adsorbed (for adult use); contains the same dose of tetanus toxoid as DTP or DT and a reduced dose of diphtheria toxoid.

(From Centers for Disease Control.[1])

TABLE 5. Recommended Immunization Schedule for Infants and Children up to Seventh Birthday Not Immunized at the Recommended Time in Early Infancy[a]

Timing	*Vaccine(s)*	*Comments*
First visit	DTP-1[b] OPV-1[c] (if child is ≥15 mo., MMR[d]); if child is ≥18 mo, *Haemophilus* b conjugate[e,f])	DTP, OPV, and MMR should be administered simultaneously to children ≥15 mo if appropriate. *Haemophilus* b conjugate vaccine can be added for simultaneous administration for children 18 mo or older.
2 mo after DTP-1, OPV-1	DTP-2[g], OPV-2	
2 mo after DTP-2	DTP-3[g]	An additional dose of OPV at this time is optional in areas with a high risk of polio exposure.
6–12 mo after DTP-3	DTP-4, OPV-3	
Preschool[h] (4–6 yr)	DTP-5,[i] OPV-4	Preferably at or before school entry.
14–16 yr	Td[j]	Repeat every 10 years throughout life.

[a] If initiated in the first year of life, give DTP-1, 2, and 3; OPV-1 and -2 according to this schedule and give MMR when the child becomes 15 months old.
[b] DTP: diphtheria and tetanus toxoids with pertussis vaccine absorbed. DTP can be used up to the seventh birthday.
[c] OPV: poliovirus vaccine live oral, trivalent; contains poliovirus types 1, 2, and 3.
[d] MMR: measles, mumps, and rubella virus vaccine, live.
[e] *Haemophilus* b conjugate vaccine.
[f] If *Haemophilus* b conjugate vaccine is not available, an acceptable alternative is to give *Haemophilus* b polysaccharide vaccine at 24 months of age. Children previously vaccinated with polysaccharide vaccine should be revaccinated with a single dose of conjugate vaccine at least 2 months after the initial dose of polysaccaride vaccine. Either of the *Haemophilus* b vaccines can be administered up until the fifth birthday but is not generally recommended for persons 5 years and older.
[g] The second and third dosages of DTP can be given 4–8 weeks after the preceding dose.
[h] The preschool dosages are not necessary if the fourth dose of DTP and third dose of OPV are administered after the fourth birthday.
[i] Up to the seventh birthday.
[j] Td: tetanus and diphtheria toxoid absorbed (for adult use), contains the same dose of tetanus toxoid as DTP or DT and a reduced dose of diphtheria toxoid.
(From Centers for Disease Control.[1])

jugate vaccine. While the observed efficacy of the polysaccharide vaccine in the United States has not been consistently as high as that reported in the Finnish field trial, revaccination of children who received the polysaccharide vaccine at 24 months of age or older is optional. Although preliminary data indicate that three doses of conjugate vaccine administered in infancy is highly protective, further data are needed before conjugate vaccines are licensed for use in infants.

On the basis of the epidemiology of invasive *Haemophilus influenzae* type b infection in the United States, vaccination is not routinely recommended beyond the fifth year of life. Although vaccine is not indicated for children who had documented invasive *Haemophilus influenzae* type b infection at 2 years of age or older, it is indicated for younger children because of their inadequate antibody response after natural infection.

The vaccines appear to be quite safe. Local reactions at the injection site and moderate to high fever have been noted in approximately 10 percent and less than 1 percent of vaccinees, respectively. They can be administered simultaneously with MMR, DTP, and OPV with no increased risk of adverse reactions or compromise in efficacy of any of the vaccines. The vaccines should not be administered if there is a history of anaphylaxis to diphtheria toxoid (conjugate only) or other vaccine components such as thimerosal. Since vaccination does not prevent carriage and since it is not 100 percent effective, vaccination does not preclude use of rifampin when indicated. Although there has been conflicting information about the possibility of a slight increased risk of *Haemophilus influenzae* type b infection shortly after receipt of the polysaccharide vaccine, this problem has not been reported with conjugate vaccines.[18–21]

Hepatitis B Vaccine. Hepatitis B vaccine consists of purified inactivated hepatitis B surface antigen (HBsAg) particles obtained either from the plasma of chronic carriers or from yeast through recombinant DNA technology. The plasma derived vaccine undergoes three separate inactivation procedures that, in sum, are effective in inactivating all known viruses, including human immunodeficiency virus (HIV). The vaccine is indicated for individuals at high risk of exposure to hepatitis B, including certain categories of health care workers (those with risk of exposure to blood or blood products), hemodialysis patients, recipients of certain blood products, homosexual males, certain institutionalized individuals, and household or sexual contacts of chronic arriers of HBsAg. All pregnant women should be routinely screened for HBsAg, preferably during an early prenatal visit.[24] The vaccine should be administered to infants born of carrier mothers. The immunizing course consists of three doses given intramuscularly at time zero, 1 month, and 6 months. Infants born to carrier mothers should ideally receive the first dose within 12 hours of birth with HBIG at another site. Additional experience will be necessary to know whether there will be any need for boosters after several years. In carefully designed field trials, vaccine efficacy has been 80–95 percent in the 2 years following vaccination in immunocompetent persons. Follow-up for more than 5 years has shown the virtual absence of clinically significant infections in persons who initially achieved antibody titers ≥10 SRU by RIA. Efficacy may be lower in immunocompromised patients. The vaccine should be administered to adults intramuscularly in the deltoid region. Gluteal administration is associated with poorer antibody responses.

Adverse effects associated with hepatitis B vaccine have been very few; they consist primarily of local reactions or low-grade fever. Serious reactions have been very few and not convincingly established to have been associated with vaccination. Guillain-Barré syndrome following hepatitis B vaccination has been reported, although it is not clear that the incidence exceeds background or expected rates in the absence of vaccination.[25] Regardless, the benefits of hepatitis B vaccine in target populations clearly outweigh any risks. There is no evidence to indicate that hepatitis B vaccination is associated with subsequent development of acquired immune deficiency syndrome (AIDS). There are no known contraindications to the use of hepatitis B vaccine. It is not effective in eliminating the carrier state, but there is no known risk of vaccinating individuals who are carriers or who are already immune.[26,27]

Influenza Virus Vaccine. Influenza virus vaccine is composed of inactivated whole or disrupted ("split") influenza viruses. Because of the frequent antigenic changes in the influenza viruses, the antigenic content of influenza virus vaccine is changed annually to reflect the influenza A and B virus strains in circulation. Annual immunization is recommended for those who receive influenza vaccine. The efficacy of the vaccine in protecting against influenza is directly related to the degree of concordance between the virus strains included in the vaccine and the strains that are circulating in the community. When periodic major shifts in antigenic structure of influenza viruses occur, vaccine containing antigens representative of prior viruses has little or no effectiveness. In recent years, influenza vaccine has typically been 60–80 percent effective, except in nursing home settings, where efficacy has often been substantially lower, on the order of 20–30 percent. However, prevention of complications of influenza in such settings had been considerably higher, averaging about 60 percent in preventing pneumonia to 85 percent in preventing death.[28]

Influenza immunization strategy in the United States is directed at reducing the complications and mortality associated with influenza. Since this occurs primarily in the chronically ill and the elderly, these groups are most strongly advised to receive vaccine. Specifically, annual immunization is most strongly recommended for those with chronic cardiovascular or pulmonary disorders requiring regular medical follow-up or those hospitalized in the preceding year and residents of nursing homes and other facilities housing patients with chronic medical conditions. A second order of priority includes healthy persons 65 years of age and older; those with chronic metabolic disease (including diabetes mellitus), renal dysfunction, anemia, or immunosuppression; and children on long-term aspirin therapy. Finally, physicians and other personnel caring for high-risk persons should be vaccinated to reduce the chances that such patients will be exposed to influenza. Many of the persons in need of influenza vaccine are hospitalized frequently and should be vaccinated on discharge if hospitalized during the autumn.

If an individual is thought not to have had any prior exposure to influenza virus of the type circulating (as might occur with young children) two doses of vaccine are recommended with an interval of at least 4 weeks between them; otherwise, only a single dose is needed. Adverse events associated with current influenza vaccines are infrequent. Of recipients 3–5 percent report local tenderness or low-grade fever. Because reactions in children are more frequent when whole virus vaccines are used, only split virus vaccines are recommended for use in children. During the swine influenza immunization program of 1976, an elevated incidence rate of Guillian-Barré syndrome was noted in recipients of the swine flu vaccine. This has not been reported with other influenza vaccines. The only known contraindication of influenza vaccine is anaphylactic hypersensitivity to eggs.[29]

Measles Vaccine. Measles vaccine is a live attenuated virus vaccine recommended for use in all children who do not have contraindications. When it is administered to a child 15 months of age or older, efficacy is greater than 95 percent. Only a single dose is needed to provide long-lasting, probably lifelong, immunity. Immunization is recommended for all individuals not known to be immune. Since individuals born before 1957 are likely to have been infected naturally, they are commonly considered immune. Otherwise, individuals should be considered susceptible if they do not have documentary evidence of having received live virus measles vaccine on or after the first birthday or of having a physician diagnosed case of measles. Since measles is much more prevalent abroad, a one-time dose is recommended for all travelers born after 1956 regardless of prior vaccination history.

Recent evidence suggests that in rare instances, measles transmission can be sustained among vaccinated persons who failed to seroconvert following an initial dose of vaccine. Persons vaccinated between 12 and 14 months of age and persons vaccinated prior to 1980 may be at slightly increased risk of failure than other persons although the vast majority of such vaccinees are immune. Based on this evidence, no change in routine immunization is indicated. However, during outbreaks in school-age populations, persons at risk, particularly those in affected schools, who were vaccinated prior to 1980, should be revaccinated. Limiting revaccination to persons originally vaccinated at 12 to 14 months of age is acceptable. Recurrent measles transmission has also been reported among some preschool populations particularly in inner cities. In areas with recurrent preschool transmission, a two-dose schedule is recommended with the first dose at 9 months or soon thereafter. An acceptable alternative is a single dose at 12 months of age.

Untoward reactions associated with measles vaccine include fever of 39.4°C or greater in 5–15 percent of recipients and transient rashes in approximately 5 percent of vaccines. Encephalitis has been reported in vaccine recipients with a frequency of less than 1 in approximately 1 million vaccinations. Measles vaccine is contraindicated for pregnant women and persons in an immunocompromised state, with the exception of those infected with HIV. Such infected persons whether symptomatic or asymptomatic may be vaccinated. Persons with a history of anaphylactic reactions to eggs may be vaccinated with extreme caution using special protocols.[30–32a]

Meningococcal Polysaccharide Vaccine. A vaccine containing purified meningococcal polysaccharides of groups A, C, Y, and W135 is now available for use in the United States. These are highly purified antigen preparations that are primarily indicated for individuals at high risk of exposure such as might occur during epidemic disease or in military encampments. The vaccine is routinely indicated for high-risk groups such as persons with terminal complement component deficiencies and those with anatomic and functional asplenia. It may be of benefit to travelers to countries with endemic or hyperendemic disease who are expected to have prolonged contact with the local population. A single intramuscular injection induces protective levels of antibody in 90 percent or more of recipients 2 years of age and older. Booster doses after 2–3 years may be indicated for high-risk children, especially those vaccinated at <4 years of age. Booster doses are not currently recommended for older children and adults. Adverse effects associated with meningococcal polysaccharide vaccine are rare; local reactions are observed in less than 5 percent of recipients. There are no known contraindications to the use of this vaccine.[33]

Mumps Vaccine. Mumps vaccine is a live attenuated virus vaccine that is recommended for use in all children who do not have contraindications. When it is administered on or after the first birthday, 90 percent or more of recipients can be expected to develop protective antibodies. Protection is thought to be lifelong. Only a single dose of vaccine is necessary. As with measles, most persons born before 1957 are likely to have been infected naturally by mumps virus and can generally be considered to be immune; otherwise, individuals should be considered susceptible unless they have documentation of having received live mumps vaccine on or after the first birthday or a history of physician diagnosed mumps disease. Adverse events associated with mumps vaccine are very few. Parotitis and orchitis have been reported rarely. Contraindications to mumps vaccine are pregnancy and immunocompromised state. Persons with a history of anaphylactic reactions to eggs may be vaccinated with extreme caution using special protocols.[31,34]

Pertussis Vaccine. Pertussis vaccine is a suspension of killed whole *Bordetella pertussis*. It is usually given in combination with diphtheria and tetanus toxoids as DTP. The primary immunizing course consists of three doses administered intramuscularly at 4- to 8-week intervals with a fourth dose given approximately 1 year later. These doses are typically given at 2, 4, 6, and 18 months of age. A booster dose is given at 4–6 years of age. Pertussis vaccine is usually not recommended for administration to individuals after the seventh birthday because the risk of pertussis and pertussis complications appears to be substantially lower, and reactions may be more frequent in older individuals. Recent experience with pertussis vaccine in the United States indicates a vaccine efficacy of 80 percent or greater. Pertussis vaccine is associated with a higher rate of adverse events following vaccination than are most other vaccines in routine use.[18]

In a large prospective study, more than 60 percent of recipients had local reactions or fever.[35] Prolonged crying occurred in approximately 3 percent, and a high-pitched, unusual cry was noted at a frequency of 1 in 1000 doses given. The incidence rate of convulsions was 1 in 1750 vaccinations, as was that of hypotonic hyporesponsive collapse. These conditions were temporary and apparently unassociated with long-term ill effects.[36] However, pertussis vaccine has also been associated with acute encephalopathy with permanent brain damage. In a large case–control study in the United Kingdon,[37] the occurrence of serious neurologic illness associated with pertussis vaccination was estimated at 1 in 140,000 vaccinations; the risk of damage approximately 1 year after immunization was 1 in 330,000 injections. Recent reviews have disputed the relationship of pertussis vaccine and permanent brain damage.[38] Contraindications to pertussis vaccinations include history of a reaction to a previous dose, including a fever greater than 40.5°C; collapse; convulsions; prolonged or abnormal screaming; or encephalopathy. An evolving neurologic disorder is also a contraindication to vaccination. Children with a personal or family history of convulsions appear to be at higher risk of seizures after pertussis vaccination than the general population.[19] However, the benefits of vaccination outweigh the risks. Children with stable seizure disorders or with family histories of seizures may be vaccinated. Use of acetaminophen 15 mg/kg at the time of vaccination, 4 hours later, 8 hours later, then as needed reduces the risk of fever after pertussis and may decrease the likelihood of postvaccination seizures.

Because of the adverse reactions known or suspected to be associated with pertussis vaccine, there has been considerable controversy about the necessity of continuing its routine use. As a result, pertussis vaccine uptake in the United Kingdom declined markedly in the period 1974–1978. The result was a major epidemic of pertussis in the years 1977–1979, with a second epidemic in 1982. These episodes, and a similar one in Japan, illustrate the necessity for maintaining protection against pertussis, even while searching for improved vaccines.

Plague Vaccine. Plague vaccine is a suspension of killed *Yersinia pestis*. It is recommended for use only in individuals who are at substantial risk of plague infection, such as those who work in laboratories with plague organisms or who work with wild animals, in plague enzootic areas (e.g., New Mexico, Arizona). The efficacy of plague vaccine has never been measured precisely. After a primary immunizing course of three doses administered at time zero, 4 weeks, and 6 months, about 93 percent develop antibody to fraction 1 capsular antigen. A few fail to develop a reciprocal titer of 128, the level correlated with immunity in experimental animals. Boosters are given at 6-month to 1-year intervals thereafter. Adverse effects include local reactions and fever in approximately 10 percent of recipients. Sterile abscesses and sensitivity reactions have rarely been reported. Contraindications to its use include known hypersensitivity to any of the constituents and severe reactions to a previous dose.[39]

Pneumococcal Polysaccharide Vaccine. Pneumococcal polysaccharide vaccine was initially licensed as a purified preparation of 14 different serotypes of pneumococcal capsular polysaccharide in 1979. Since 1983 vaccine containing 23 types has replaced the earlier version. The types included in the current vaccine and immunologically related types account for approximately 85 percent of all bacteremic pneumococcal disease in the United States. Demonstrable antibody rises are noted in 80–95 percent or more of normal recipients to the serotypes contained in the vaccine. The vaccine has been highly effective in reducing pneumococcal disease among South African gold miners (a group at particularly high risk) and in military recruits. In randomized trials in some populations at high risk of pneumococcal infections, such as the elderly and those with high-risk medical conditions, efficacy has not been convincingly demonstrated in part because determining the etiology of pneumonia from sputum specimens may be difficult and because the studies were too small to evaluate infections associated with bacteremia.[40] However, studies of patients with isolates from normally sterile body fluids have generally reported efficacies of 60–80 percent overall with lower efficacy in persons who have compromised immune systems or cirrhosis or renal failure.[41] Vaccine is primarily recommended for adults at high risk of complications from respiratory infections, particularly those with cardiovascular and chronic pulmonary disease; adults and children ≥2 years of age at high risk of pneumococcal disease (e.g., splenic dysfunction or anatomic asplenia, Hodgkin's disease, multiple myeloma, cirrhosis, alcoholism, renal failure, cerebrospinal fluid leaks, and immunocompromised state); and the otherwise healthy elderly (≥65 years of age).

A single dose is administered by intramuscular injection; routine boosters are not recommended at this time. This recommendation currently includes most persons who received the 14-valent vaccine. However, revaccination should be strongly considered for persons who received the 14 valent vaccine if they are at the highest risk of fatal pneumococcal disease (e.g., asplenia). Revaccination should also be considered for adults at highest risk if 6 or more years have elapsed since receipt of the 23 valent vaccine and for adults known to rapidly lose pneumococcal antibody (e.g., patients with nephrotic syndrome, renal failure, or transplant recipients). Revaccination should also be considered for children with nephrotic syndrome, asplenia, or sickle cell anemia if 3 to 5 years have elapsed since their last dose and they are now 10 years of age or younger. Individuals revaccinated within 5 years may have had exaggerated local reactions. In some studies but not in others, mild reactions, such as erythema and mild pain at the site of injection, occur in approximately one-half of recipients. Anaphylactic reactions have rarely been reported. No contraindications are known, although its safety in pregnant women has not been evaluated.[41]

Polio Vaccine. Two types of polio vaccine are available in the United States: live attenuated oral polio vaccine (OPV) and inactivated polio vaccine (IPV). The primary course of OPV involves two doses administered at an interval of 6–8 weeks followed by a third dose at least 6 weeks later (typically 8–12 months later). A fourth dose is given to young children approximately 3 years later to ensure seroconversion to all three virus types. There is no evidence that booster doses of OPV are needed once seroconversion to a particular type has occurred. IPV is administered by subcutaneous injection. A new more potent IPV that has recently been licensed gives almost 100 percent seroconversion to all three types after two doses. The recommended schedule for this enhanced potency IPV is two doses at 4- to 8-weeks intervals followed by a third dose approximately 1 year later. The need for boosters has not been established.

Both IPV and OPV are highly effective and associated with protection of at least 95 percent. Because OPV induces local intestinal immunity and because OPV virus may spread from vaccinated individuals to contacts and thereby immunize the contacts, OPV is currently considered the preparation of choice for routine immunization in the United States. However, on rare occasions OPV is associated with paralysis either in the vaccine recipient or in contacts of vaccine recipients (overall risk 1 in every 2.6 million doses distributed). Almost the entire risk to both recipients and contacts is associated with administration of the first dose to the recipient (overall risk 1 in every 520,000 first doses[42]. In addition if OPV is given to an immunocompromised individual, it may result in paralysis. Because the risk of vaccine-associated polio is somewhat higher in adults, IPV is the vaccine of choice for individuals beyond secondary school age (generally 18 years of age and older). However, during control of an epidemic OPV should be used. With either vaccine, there is no need to restart a series if the primary immunization schedule is interrupted; the next dose in the series should be given. Contraindications to the use of OPV are an immunocompromised state, pregnancy (on theoretical grounds), or living in the same household with an immunocompromised individual. No significant adverse effects have been reported with current IPV and, except for pregnancy (when vaccine is contraindicated on theoretical grounds), there are no known contraindications to its use.[43,44] OPV is the vaccine of choice for pregnant women if immediate protection is needed. The availability of the more potent IPV has stimulated discussion about polio vaccine policy in the United States, including combined schedules using IPV first to induce systemic immunity and prevent paralysis in recipients, then OPV to obtain the benefits of gut immunity and perceived lifelong immunity, by many experts. These discussions may lead to a policy change in the near future.[45,46]

Polyvalent Bacterial Antigen with "No U.S. Standard of Potency." This vaccine contains a mixture of bacterial antigens, including streptococci and staphylococci. Its efficacy has not been established, and there are no recommendations for its use.[47]

Rabies Vaccine. Rabies vaccine is an inactivated virus vaccine prepared in human diploid cell culture. Rabies vaccination is recommended in two situations: as a routine in individuals likely to be exposed to rabies (e.g., veterinarians, forest rangers) and after exposure to animals known or suspected to be rabid. The primary pre-exposure immunizing course is three doses of rabies vaccine given intramuscularly or intradermally at time 0, 7 days, and 21–28 days. This course results in formation of protective levels of antibodies in virtually 100 percent of vaccinees. Boosters are recommended every 2 years for those in whom the possibility of exposure continues. In the postexposure setting, five doses of rabies vaccine are given intramuscularly in a relatively short period (on days 0, 3, 7, 14, and 28) to previously unimmunized persons. In such postexposure settings, rabies vaccine should always be used in conjunction with rabies immune globulin (see "Rabies Immune Globulin" below). Adverse events associated with current rabies vaccine include local reactions in approximately 25 percent of recipients. As many as 6 percent of persons may develop illnesses 2–21 days after boosters consisting of arthralgia, arthritis, angioedema, nausea, vomiting, fever, and malaise. There have been rare reports of transient neurologic reactions; in association with the current vaccine, however, a causal relationship has not been demonstrated. There are no known contraindications to rabies vaccination in persons at risk or exposed.[48,49] (See Chapter 140 for more details.)

Rubella Vaccine. Rubella vaccine contains live attenuated rubella virus vaccine grown in human diploid cells (RA 27/3). Other substrates, such as duck embryo cells or rabbit kidney cells, have also been used for rubella vaccines. When it is administered to an individual on or after the first birthday, 95 percent or more of recipients can be expected to become immune. Immunity following a single dose is long-lasting and appears likely to be lifelong. Boosters are not necessary. Rubella vaccine is recommended for all individuals on or after the first birthday except those who have documentation of having received live rubella vaccine and those who have laboratory documentation of immunity to rubella. It is particularly important to ensure that women of childbearing age are immune to rubella. Rubella vaccine virus is known to be able to cross the placenta and infect fetal tissue. There have been no instances of congenital rubella syndrome in the offspring of 210 susceptible women who received RA 27/3 rubella vaccine within 3 months of conception and who carried their pregnancies to term.[50] This indicates that the risk of congenital rubella syndrome from vaccine virus is so small as to be negligible. The Public Health Service Immunization Practices Advisory Committee recommends that "rubella vaccination during pregnancy should not be a reason to routinely recommend interruption of pregnancy."[51] Notwithstanding the fact that no observable risk has been associated with rubella vaccine administered during pregnancy, rubella vaccine should not knowingly be administered to a pregnant women. A reasonable approach is to ask women whether they are pregnant or may become pregnant within the next 3 months, exclude those who answer affirmatively, and vaccinate the others, after explaining the theoretical risk to them.

Known adverse events associated with rubella vaccine include low-grade fever and rash in 5–10 percent of recipients and joint pains with or without objective manifestations of arthritis. The latter occur with increasing frequency in older individuals; as many as 40 percent of susceptible adult females may have transient arthralgia after rubella vaccination. Frank arthritis is rarely seen, and only a single case of joint deformities has been reported.[52] The risk of arthritis after rubella vaccine is substantially lower than the risk after natural rubella.

Previous experience with programs involving serologic screening and subsequent vaccination of susceptible individuals has demonstrated a very disappointing rate of vaccination of identified susceptible persons (typically on the order of 30–50 percent). Because of the importance of ensuring that adult women are immune to rubella and because reactions appear to occur only in susceptible individuals, it is recommended that women be vaccinated without serologic testing unless it can be assured that they can be contacted and recalled for vaccination if serologic testing indicates they are susceptible. Contraindications to rubella vaccination are pregnancy and immunocompromised state.[51]

Smallpox Vaccine. Effective use of smallpox vaccine has eradicated smallpox from the earth. The vaccine is a live unattenuated preparation of vaccinia virus that induces protection against smallpox virus in 95 percent or more of recipients. It is also highly effective in providing protection against vaccinia and other orthopox viruses. The only indication for the use of smallpox vaccine in the United States is for individuals working with vaccinia or other orthopox viruses. Smallpox vaccine is not effective in the treatment of herpes. Vaccinia vector vaccines, in which DNA coding for antigens from various microorganisms is grafted onto vaccinia virus DNA, may lead to greater use of these types of vaccines in the future. Known adverse events associated with smallpox vaccine are rare and include disseminated vaccinia, vaccinia necrosum, encephalitis, and death. Although rare, the fact that smallpox no longer exists makes these reactions unacceptable and contravenes the use of smallpox vaccine in any but the limited circumstances described above.[53] In May 1983, Wyeth Laboratories Inc., the only active licensed producer in the United States, discontinued general distrubition of smallpox vaccine, making it no longer available for general civilian use.

Tetanus Toxoid. Tetanus toxoid, a purified preparation of inactivated tetanus toxin, is one of the most effective immunizing agents known. The preferred preparation is adsorbed (alum precipitated) because it is more immunogenic. A primary course of two doses administered 4–8 weeks apart with a third dose given 6–12 months later induces protective antibodies in more than 95 percent of recipients. When it is given to children under 7 years of age as DTP, the primary course includes four doses (see "Pertussis" section and Tables 4 and 5). It is recommended for use in all residents of the United States for whom contraindications do not exist. It should always be used in combination with diphtheria toxoid to ensure protection against both diseases. Common adverse effects include local reactions and fever. In some individuals who have received multiple doses of tetanus toxoid, Arthus-like reactions have been described. Consequently, it is recommended that individuals receive boosters only every 10 years, unless a particularly tetanus-prone wound has been incurred (see "Tetanus Immune Globulin" below). The only contraindication is in individuals who have previously had neurologic or severe hypersensitivity reactions following teatanus toxoid. Table 6 summarizes an approach to postexposure prophylaxis of tetanus.[18]

TABLE 6. Summary Guide to Tetanus Prophylaxis in Routine Wound Management: United States[a]

History of Absorbed Tetanus Toxoid (Doses)	*Clean, Minor Wounds* Td[c]	*Clean, Minor Wounds* TIG	*All Other Wounds*[b] Td[c]	*All Other Wounds*[b] TIG
Unknown or three	Yes	No	Yes	Yes
Three[d]	No[e]	No	No[f]	No

[a] Important details are in the text.
[b] Such as, but not limited to, wounds contaminated with dirt, feces, soil, saliva, etc; puncture wounds; avulsions; and wounds resulting from missiles, crushing, burns, and frostbite.
[c] For children under 7 years old DTP (DT if pertussis vaccine is contraindicated) is preferred to tetanus toxoid alone. For persons 7 years and older, Td is preferred to tetanus toxoid alone.
[d] If only three doses of *fluid* toxoid have been received, a fourth dose of toxoid, preferably an adsorbed toxoid, should be given.
[e] Yes, if more than 10 years since last dose.
[f] Yes, if more than 5 years since last dose. (More frequent boosters are not needed and can accentuate side effects.)

Typhoid Vaccine. Typhoid vaccine is a suspension of killed *Salmonella typhosa*. It is administered subcutaneously in a two dose series with the second dose administered 4 weeks or more after the first. The vaccine appears to be 70–90 percent effective in preventing typhoid. Because the risk of typhoid is so low in the United States, its only current recommended domestic use is for household contacts of chronic typhoid carriers. Individuals traveling in countries where typhoid is common may wish to consider use of the vaccine. Local and mild systemic reactions associated with typhoid vaccine are quite common. More severe systemic reactions are quite rare. There are no known contraindications to its use.[54]

Yellow Fever Vaccine. Yellow fever vaccine is a live attenuated virus preparation that is highly effective in inducing protection in recipients. It is indicated for use in travelers going to yellow fever endemic areas and may be required for entry into some countries. Only a single dose of vaccine is required; it is administered by subcutaneous inoculation. Boosters are recommended every 10 years, although their need has not been conclusively established. Local and mild systemic reactions occur in 2–5 percent of recipients 5–10 days after vaccination; more severe reactions, primarily encephalitis and encephalopathy, are rare. Contraindications include anaphylactic hypersensitivity to eggs, age less than 4 months, and immunocompromised states. Pregnancy is not considered an absolute contraindication; however, it is recommended that administration of the vaccine be postponed until after completion of pregnancy, if possible.[55]

Immune Globulins

Hepatitis B Immune Globulin (HBIG). HBIG is prepared from plasma preselected for high titer of antibody to hepatitis B surface antigen (HBsAg). In the United States, HBIG has an anti-HBs titer of greater than 1 : 100,000 by radioimmunoassay. It is recommended for use in postexposure settings for individuals who have been exposed by infected sexual partners or to blood containing HBsAG by percutaneous or mucous membrane route. The dosage is 0.06 ml/kg given immediately for sexual contacts. A second identical dose 1 month later is recommended for those with percutaneous exposure. HBIG is also recommended for infants born to HBsAg-positive women. A dose of 0.5 ml should be given within 12 hours of delivery in conjunction with a dose of hepatitis B vaccine. Additional doses of vaccine are indicated at 1 month and 6 months. The only known adverse effect is local discomfort at the site of injection. There are no known precautions or contraindications.[26]

Immune Globulin. Immune globulin is a preparation of pooled human immune globulins containing antibodies to several diseases, including hepatitis A, hepatitis B, and measles. Although not specifically checked for the presence of antibodies to other diseases, recent lots of immune globulin in the United States have also contained antibodies to yellow fever. Immune globulin is effective in preventing hepatitis A when administered within 14 days of exposure (dosage 0.02 ml/kg) or when given before exposure in somewhat larger quantities (dosage 0.02 ml/kg is acceptable for trips less than 2 months, 0.6 ml/kg every 5 months for longer trips). It may also prevent or modify measles if administered within 6 days of exposure (dosage 0.25 ml/kg for normal persons, 0.5 ml/kg for those who are immunocompromised, up to a maximum of 15 ml). Adverse effects include local tenderness and, rarely, arthus-type or anaphylactic reactions. Other than prior anaphylactic reactions, there are no known contraindications to use of the product. Ordinary immune globulin should not be administered intravenously.[26,30] Immune globulin intravenous (IGIV) is designed for intravenous use primarily as a maintenance preparation for individuals with hypogammaglobulinemia. In addition, it may also be useful to decrease infections in other immunodeficiency states such as HIV infection and may provide postexposure protection against measles and other infections.[32] The reader is referred to Chapter 137 for further discussion.

Pertussis Immune Globulin. Pertussis immune globulin has been administered to contacts of patients with pertussis. Its efficacy has not been established, and there are no recommendations for its use.[26]

Rabies Immune Globulin. Rabies immune globulin (RIG) is a hyperimmune serum prepared from humans who have been immunized against rabies and have very high titers of antibodies to rabies. It is designed for management of individuals who have been exposed to rabid animals. Rabies immune globulin should always be used in conjunction with rabies vaccine in vaccinated persons. However, if more than 8 days has elapsed since the first dose of rabies vaccine, RIG is unnecessary since an active antibody response to the vaccine has presumably begun. Experience to date indicates that administration of a full course of human diploid cell rabies vaccine with rabies immune globulin is 100 percent effective in preventing the development of rabies after exposure to known rabid animals. It is commonly administered with half of the dose given intramuscularly and the remainder infiltrated around the site of the wound. Adverse effects include minor local discomfort. There are no known contraindications.[48]

Rh Immune Globulin. Rh immune globulin is a hyperimmune globulin prepared for use in Rh-negative women who have just delivered Rh-positive babies or have undergone miscarriage or abortion of an Rh-positive fetus. When administered within 24 hours of the time of delivery or abortion it is highly effective in preventing sensitization of the mother to Rh-positive red blood cells that might be present in a future pregnancy. The appropriate administration of Rh immune globulin has reduced the occurrence of Rh hemolytic disease of the newborn in the United States to very low levels. Further reductions will require more careful attention to the administration of the product after abortion or delivery in all women for whom it is indicated. There are essentially no adverse effects associated with the product, and there are no known contraindications.[56]

Tetanus Immune Globulin. Tetanus immune globulin is a hyperimmune globulin indicated for management of tetanus-prone wounds in individuals who have no prior history of tetanus immunization. The standard dosage is 250 units intramuscularly. Local reactions are rare, and there are no known contraindications. If used, it should be administered simultaneously with, but at a different site from, combined tetanus–diphtheria toxoid. Primary immunization against tetanus and diphtheria should then be completed using the routine schedule. Table 6 summarizes an approach to postexposure prophylaxis of tetanus.[18]

Vaccinia Immune Globulin. Vaccinia immune globulin is a hyperimmune globulin prepared for use in individuals exposed to vaccinia virus who are at risk of complications associated with it by virtue of being immunocompromised. The need for this product should be very rare in this country because smallpox vaccine should only be used in very rare circumstances.[53]

Varicella-Zoster Immune Globulin. Varicella-zoster immune globulin is prepared by selection of serum containing high titers of varicella-zoster antibodies. It is indicated for administration to susceptible immunocompromised individuals and certain others who have recently been exposed to varicella, including newborns whose mothers develop varicella within 5 days before to 48 hours after delivery. It should be administered within 96 hours of exposure, but ideally as soon after exposure as possible. Some believe it may also be useful in ameliorating the expression of varicella in susceptible adults, particularly susceptible pregnant females who are at increased risk of complications from varicella infection after exposure to the virus. The product may not prevent infection; however, if infection occurs it is usually subclinical or mild. Local reactions are rare, and there are no known contraindications.[57]

USE OF VACCINES

Routine

Children. The recommended schedules for administration of vaccines to children are shown in Tables 4 and 5. It is currently recommended that children receive DTP, polio, measles, mumps, rubella, and HbCV or HbPV vaccines unless contraindications exist. Four doses of DTP and three doses of OPV constitute the primary series. A fifth dose of DTP should be given at 4–6 years of age with Td boosters administered every 10 years thereafter. A fourth dose of OPV is also recommended at 4–6 years of age. A single dose of combined measles, mumps, and rubella at 15 months of age or older provides long-lasting, probably lifelong, immunity in more than 95 percent of recipients.[1,10] DTP, MMR, and OPV may be given stimultaneously at 15 months without increasing reaction rates or impairing immune responses. HbCV is the preferred vaccine for prevention of disease due to *Haemophilus influenzae* type b and should be administered in a single dose at 18 months of age. If HbCV is unavailable, use of HbPV is acceptable, beginning at 2 years of age.[20,22] Either may be given simultaneously with DTP, MMR, and OPV.[58,59]

Adults. Routine immunizations for adults have received very little attention in recent years. All adults should be immune to diphtheria and tetanus and if not previously immunized should be given a primary immunizing course (three doses of Td administered at time zero, 4–8 weeks, and 12 months) with boosters administered every 10 years thereafter. Routine immunization against polio is not recommended for adults unless they are at particular risk of exposure. All individuals should be immune to measles, mumps, and rubella. For practical purposes, those born before 1957 can generally be considered to be immune to measles and mumps. All other individuals should be vaccinated unless it can be documented that they have either received vaccine on or after the first birthday or have had physician-diagnosed disease. Rubella vaccine should be administered to all individuals, particularly women of childbearing age, unless they have documentary proof of having received rubella vaccine on or after the first birthday or laboratory evidence of immunity. A history of prior rubella disease is unreliable and should not be accepted. Influenza vaccine is recommended for routine annual administration to adults 65 years of age and older and to individuals at any age who have chronic illness. Pneumococcal polysaccharide vaccine is recommended for administration to the elderly and the chronically ill. Hepatitis B virus vaccine is recommended for individuals at high risk of exposure to hepatitis B virus. These include primarily health care personnel at high risk of contact with blood that might be infected with hepatitis B virus, homosexuals, users of illicit injectable drugs, and individuals living and working in institutions for the mentally retarded and household contacts of carriers of HBsAg.[11,60] Table 7 summarizes adult immunizations.

Special Circumstances

Travel. The International Sanitary Regulations allow countries to impose requirements for yellow fever and cholera vaccines as a condition for admission. Consequently, travelers should be aware of whether these vaccines are required for entry into the country of their destination. This information is summarized in *Health Information for International Travel*[61]

TABLE 7. Recommended Immunizations for Adults

	Routine				Special Circumstances						
	Age Group[a]										
Vaccine	18–24	25–49	50–64	≥5[b]	Military Recruits	Travelers	Health Care Workers	Occupation	Immunocompromised	Pregnancy	Chronic Illness
Adenovirus 4 and 7					X						
Anthrax								S			
BCG							S±				
Cholera						S					
Diphtheria	X	X	X	X	X	X	X	X	X	X	X
Hepatitis B						S	X	S			
Influenza				X			X		X		X
Measles	X	X[c]			X	X	X		0	0	
Meningococcal					X	S					
Mumps	X	X[c]							0	0	
Pertussis											
Plague						S		S			
Pneumococcal				X					X		X
Polio-inactivated						S	S				
Polio-oral					X	S	S		0		
Polyvalent bacterial											
Rabies						S		S			
Rubella	X	X			X	X	X		0	0	
Smallpox	0	0	0	0		0	0	S	0	0	0
Tetanus	X	X	X	X	X	X	X	X	X	X	X
Typhoid						S		S			
Yellow fever						S		S	0		

Symbols: X: recommended; ±: divided opinion; 0: contraindicated; S: selected risk situations.
[a] Unless contraindications exist.
[b] Measles, mumps, and rubella vaccines should be considered for persons with symptomatic HIV infection. They are routinely indicated for persons with asymptomatic HIV infection.
[c] If susceptible and born after 1956.

(see Sources of Information below) and can also be obtained by calling local health departments. Other vaccines commonly considered for travelers include measles vaccine, polio vaccine, and boosters for tetanus and diphtheria. In addition, travelers to specified areas may wish to consider plague vaccine, typhoid vaccine, and immune globulin as protection against hepatitis A.

Occupational Exposure. A complete set of recommendations for vaccination for most occupation groups has not been developed. Specific recommendations are available for health care workers.[62] Those at particular risk of exposure to hepatitis B (e.g., laboratory technicians dealing with blood products, surgeons) should be protected against hepatitis B. It is clear that transmission of rubella in medical facilities can occur to or from health care workers. Consequently, it is important that all health care workers who might transmit rubella to pregnant patients be immune to rubella. Health care workers are at greater risk from measles than the general public. All workers likely to come in contact with measles patients should be immune. Since health care workers caring for patients with chronic diseases may transmit influenza to their patients, such workers should be vaccinated annually.

Pregnancy. Because of unknown but theoretical risks to the fetus, immunization of pregnant women is generally avoided. However, it is important to ensure that pregnant women are immune to tetanus, since transfer of maternal antibodies to tetanus toxin is an important means of prevention of neonatal tetanus. Pregnant women can receive combined tetanus–diphtheria toxoids. In general, live virus vaccines are contraindicated in pregnancy with the exceptions of polio and yellow fever virus vaccines, which may be administered if the risk of exposure to the diseases is great. If indicated, some inactivated vaccines, such as influenza, can be administered to pregnant women under the same circumstances as to nonpregnant individuals.[1]

Immunocompromised States. Immunocompromised individuals are particularly susceptible to many infections. It is feared that they may also be more susceptible to adverse effects from live virus vaccines. Consequently, in general live virus vaccines are not administered to immunocompromised individuals, although inactivated vaccines may be. It is particularly important to avoid administration of oral polio virus vaccine to immunocompromised individuals or their household contacts. The efficacy of inactivated vaccines in immunocompromised individuals may be less than that in healthy patients.

Immunization and Human Immunodeficiency Virus Infection. Human immunodeficiency virus (HIV) infection can cause a variety of clinical manifestations from completely asymptomatic infection to severe immunosuppression. However, limited studies in HIV infected persons have failed to show an increased risk of adverse events from live or inactivated vaccines.[63–65] Except for polio vaccination, known HIV infected persons who are asymptomatic should be vaccinated in the same manner as other persons, including administration of live, attenuated MMR vaccine (Table 8).[32,63] IPV should be used in place of OPV to prevent spread of polio vaccine virus to other potentially immunocompromised household contacts of HIV infected persons. For asymptomatic persons presenting for immunization, serologic testing to determine HIV infection is not necessary for making decisions about immunization.

Live, attenuated vaccines would normally be contraindicated in immunocompromised persons, such as those with symptomatic HIV infection. Thus, IPV should be used in these patients when vaccination against polio is indicated (Table 8). However, because of reports of severe measles disease, including death, in symptomatic HIV infected children, it is now recommended that measles vaccine, alone or preferably with mumps and rubella vaccines, be considered for all symptomatic HIV infected

TABLE 8. Recommendations for Routine Immunization of HIV Infected Persons—United States

	HIV Infection	
Vaccine	*Known Asymptomatic*	*Symptomatic*
DTP[a]	Yes	Yes
OPV[b]	No	No
IPV[c]	Yes	Yes
MMR[d]	Yes	Yes[e]
HbCV[f]	Yes	Yes
Pneumococcal	Yes	Yes
Influenza	Yes[e]	Yes

[a] DTP: diphtheria and tetanus toxoids and pertussis vaccine.
[b] OPV: oral, attenuated poliovirus vaccine; contains poliovirus types 1, 2, and 3.
[c] IPV: inactivated poliovirus vaccine; contains poliovirus types 1, 2, and 3.
[d] MMR: live, attenuated measles, mumps, and rubella vaccines in a combined vaccine.
[e] Vaccination should be considered.
[f] HbCV: *Haemophilus* b conjugate vaccine; preferred over polysaccharide vaccine.
(From Centers for Disease Control.[32,63])

persons.[32,66] The reader is referred to Chapter 137 for further information on the use of IG and IGIV in HIV infected persons exposed to measles. Recommendations for administration of other inactivated vaccines are listed in Table 8. While a protective immune response to receipt of vaccines and toxoids cannot be assured in these patients, some protection may be provided.

Postexposure Immunization. For certain diseases, administration of vaccine or immunoglobulin soon after exposure can prevent or attenuate the expression of the disease. For example, administration of immune globulin within 2 weeks of exposure to hepatitis A is likely to prevent clinical illness. Similarly, the administration of rabies immune globulin and rabies vaccine in the immediate postexposure period is highly effective in preventing the development of rabies. Individuals who have received a complete course of immunization against tetanus are in general well protected against the development of tetanus, particularly if a booster dose has been administered within 10 years. More problematic is the situation with individuals who cannot recall their immune status or who have not been immunized at all. Table 6 depicts an approach to postexposure prophylaxis of tetanus. Immune globulin administered within 6 days of exposure may be effective in preventing measles or modifying it so that the illness is very mild. Although overt manifestations of rubella can be minimized by postexposure administration of immune globulin, this may not prevent viremia and fetal infection with rubella. Therefore, the administration of immune globulin is recommended only for individuals who develop rubella during prenancy who will not consider induced abortion under any circumstances. There is also evidence that administration of measles vaccine within the first few days after exposure may prevent manifestation of the illness. In addition, if the exposure did not result in infection, the vaccination will provide protection against future exposure.

Other Considerations

Assessing the Need for Immunization. Immunization has traditionally been viewed as the task of the pediatrician, but all health care providers should assess the immunization status of their patients at first contact and, depending on immunization status and age, at selected contacts thereafter. In general, individuals should be viewed as susceptible unless they can prove immunity either through documentation of having received vaccine, laboratory evidence of immunity, or, for some diseases, documentation of physician diagnosed disease.

A high proportion of elderly individuals in the United States have never been immunized against tetanus or diphtheria. This is reflected in the fact that 59 percent of all cases of tetanus in the United States in the period 1982–1986 have occurred in individuals over the age of 60 years. Internists and other physicians caring for adults and elderly individuals should be particularly attuned to the need for administering tetanus toxoid to these individuals. Similarly, studies repeatedly demonstrate that only approximately 20 percent of targeted individuals receive influenza immunization in a given year. Only an estimated 10 percent have received pneumococcal vaccine and only about 20 percent of target populations have received hepatitis B vaccine. It is vital that internists and family practitioners remind themselves and their patients of the need for annual influenza immunization of the chronically ill and elderly.

Immunization Records. Every individual should have an immunization record that is up-to-date and that contains information about each dose of vaccine received, including the date. Patients should be asked to bring this record with them to all health care visits, and the record should be reviewed to ensure that it is up-to-date. Official immunization record cards should be used; they are available through local or state health departments. Effective March 22, 1988, the National Childhood Vaccine Injury Act requires that all providers of DTP or components, OPV, or IPV, and MMR or components record on the patient's permanent medical record the date, manufacturer, and lot number of each dose of vaccine administered and the name of the person giving the vaccine. This information should be recorded for other vaccines as well.

Parent and Patient Education. All patients (or their parents or guardians) should be informed of the benefits and the risks associated with vaccination. The discussion should be carried out in language that is comprehensible to the recipient, and ample opportunity for questions and discussion given. The Public Health Service has developed forms that explain the benefits as well as the risks of vaccination for use with the usual childhood vaccines. Interested health care providers can receive copies of these forms through local health departments. The National Childhood Vaccine Injury Act requires that specified information be provided by all providers of DTP or components, OPV, or IPV, and MMR or components. As of April 1989, vaccine information materials required by the law were being developed.

Simultaneous Administration and Intervals between Immunizations. Most of the widely used antigens can be given safely and effectively at the same time. In general, inactivated vaccines can be administered simultaneously at separate sites, and field observations indicate that simultaneous administration of the most widely used live virus vaccines has not resulted in impaired antibody response or increased rate of adverse reactions. However, simultaneous administration of immune globulins and measles, mumps, and rubella virus vaccines should be prevented since this may result in interference with antibody response. With those vaccines, immune globulin should not be given for at least 2 weeks after vaccination or vaccination should be delayed at least 3 months after immune globulin. Immune globulin does not appear to interfere with the response to OPV or yellow fever vaccines.[67] In general, the antigenic mass of inactivated vaccines is so great that immune globulins will not interfere with the antibody response. Because of the theoretical possibility of interference in the development of antibody response to live vaccines administered at intervals of 3–14 days, the advisable approach, if more than one vaccine is needed, is to administer needed vaccines simultaneously or to allow an interval of approximately 1 month between doses of different vaccines. In general, there are no restrictions on intervals between doses of inactivated vaccines or inactivated and live vaccines. The only exceptions are cholera and yellow fever vaccines, which should ideally be administered at least 3 weeks apart to achieve maximal immune responses to both antigens.

Reporting of Disease and Adverse Events. Each state has laws requiring the reporting of certain communicable diseases. The list of reportable diseases generally includes all or most of the diseases preventable by vaccination. Health care providers should ensure that each suspected case of vaccine preventable disease is reported promptly to the local health department. Similarly, serious adverse events following immunization should be reported to either the local health department, the vaccine manufacturer, or the Food and Drug Administration. The National Childhood Vaccine Injury Act requires providers to report specified adverse events. Tables 9 and 10 show which events must be reported to which Federal Agency.[68] Only through accurate reporting of both disease and adverse vaccine effects can we properly assess the changing balance of benefits and risks of vaccination.

Tickler–Recall Systems. Virtually all infants in the United States begin a course of immunization, but a substantial number

TABLE 9. Reportable Events Following Immunization

Vaccine	Event	Interval from Vaccination
DTP; P; DTP/polio combined	Anaphylaxis or anaphylactic shock	24 hours
	Encephalopathy (or encephalitis)[a]	7 days
	Shock collapse or hypotonic–hyporesponsive collapse[a]	7 days
	Residual seizure disorders[a]	
	Any acute complication or sequela (including death) of above events	[a]No limit
	Events in vaccinees described in manufacturer's package insert as contraindications to additional doses of vaccine[b] (such as convulsions)	(See package insert)
Measles, mumps, and rubella; DT, Td, tetanus toxoid	Anaphylaxis or anaphylactic shock	24 hours
	Encephalopathy (or encephalitis)[a]	15 days for measles, mumps, and rubella vaccines; 7 days for DT, Td, and T toxoids
	Residual seizure disorder[a]	
	Any acute complication or sequela (including death)	[a]No limit
	Events in vaccinees described in manufacturer's package insert as contraindications to additional doses of vaccine[b]	(See package insert)
Oral polio vaccine	Paralytic poliomyelitis	
	In a nonimmunodeficient recipient	30 days
	In an immunodeficient recipient	6 months
	In a vaccine associated community acquired infection	No limit
	Any acute complication or sequela (including death) of above events	No limit
	Events in vaccinees described in manufacturer's package insert as contraindications to additional doses of vaccine[b]	(See package insert)

(Continued)

TABLE 9. *(Continued)*

Inactivated polio vaccine	Anaphylaxis or anaphylactic shock	24 hours
	Any acute complication or sequela (including death) of above event	No limit
	Events in vaccinees described in manufacturer's package insert as contraindications to additional doses of vaccine[b]	(See package insert)

[a] Aids to interpretation:

Shock collapse or hypotonic–hyporesponsive collapse may be evidenced by signs or symptoms such as decrease in or loss of muscle tone, paralysis (partial or complete), hemiplegia, hemiparesis, loss of color or turning pale white or blue, unresponsiveness to environmental stimuli, depression of or loss of consciousness, prolonged sleeping with difficulty arousing, or cardiovascular or respiratory arrest.

Residual seizure disorder may be considered to have occurred if no other seizure or convulsion unaccompanied by a fever or accompanied by a fever of less than 102°F occurred before the first seizure or convulsion after the administration of the vaccine involved,

and, if in the case of measles, mumps, or rubella containing vaccines, the first seizures or convulsion occurred within 15 days after vaccination *or* in the case of any other vaccine, the first seizures or convusion occurred within 3 days of vaccination,

and, if two or more seizures or convusions unaccompanied by fever or accompanied by a fever of less than 102°F (38.9°C) occurred within 1 year after vaccination.

The terms *seizure* and *convusion* include grand mal, petit mal, absence, myoclonic, tonic–clonic, and focal motor seizures and signs. Encephalopathy means any significant acquired abnormality of, injury to, or impairment of function of the brain. Among the frequent manifestations of encephalopathy are focal and diffuse neurologic signs, increased intracranial pressure, or changes lasting at least 6 hours in level of consciousness, with or without convulsions. The neurologic signs and symptoms of encephalopathy may be temporary with complete recovery, or they may result in various degrees of permanent impairment. Signs and symptoms such as high-pitched and unusual screaming, persistent unconsolable crying, and bulging fontanelle are compatible with an encephalopathy but in and of themselves are not conclusive evidence of encephalopathy. Encephalopathy usually can be documented by slow wave activity on an electroencephalogram.

[b] The health care provider who administered the vaccine must refer to the contraindication section of the manufacturer's package insert for each vaccine.

fail to complete the series. There are many reasons for this, including forgetfulness and illness on the day vaccine is due to be received. To ensure that patients receive immunizations on schedule, practitioners should establish systems that will allow them to ascertain rapidly which patients should be vaccinated and whether the needed vaccine has been received. Such tickler or recall systems can be very simple or very complex and computer assisted. Many children and adults are not up-to-date for immunizations because providers do not use every opportunity to check immunizations and provide vaccine. At least two types of missed opportunities exist: (*1*) When the patient receives some vaccines because the provider is unaware that many vaccines can be administered simultaneously and (*2*) when the patient presents for another reason such as trauma and immunization status is not reviewed. Minimizing the missed opportunities will help assure that the patient does not return later with a vaccine preventable disease.

TABLE 10. Reporting of Events Occurring after Vaccination

Vaccine Sources	*Vaccine Purchased with Public Funds*	*Vaccine Purchased with Private Funds*
Who reports	Health care provider who administered the vaccine	Health care provider who administered the vaccine
What products to report	Products listed in Table 9 (DTP, P, measles, mumps, rubella, DT, Td, TT, OPV, IPV, and DTP/polio combined)	Products listed in Table 9
What reactions to report	Events listed in Table 9 including contraindicating reactions specified in manufacturers' package inserts	Events listed in Table 9 including contraindicating reactions specified in manufacturers package inserts
How to report	Initial report taken by local, county, or state health department. State health department completes CDC form 71.19.	Health care provider completes Adverse Reaction Report—FDA form 1639 (include interval from vaccination, manufacturer, and lot number on form)
Where to report	State health departments send CDC form 71.19 to: MSAEFI/IM (E05) Centers for Disease Control Atlanta, GA 30333	Send completed FDA form 1639 to: Food and Drug Administration (HFN-730) Rockville, MD 20857
Where to obtain forms	State health departments	FDA and publications

Sources of Information. Important sources for information about vaccines include the following:

OFFICIAL PACKAGE CIRCULAR. Manufacturers provide product-specific information along with each vaccine; some of these are reproduced in their entirety in the *Physicians' Desk Reference* (*PDR*) and are dated.

MORBIDITY AND MORTALITY WEEKLY REPORT (MMWR). This report is published weekly by the Centers for Disease Control (CDC) and contains vaccine recommendations, reports of specific disease activity, policy statements, and regular and special recommendations of the ACIP. The *MMWR* will contain any necessary updated information on the ACIP recommendations. Subscription information is available from MMWR, Superintendent of Documents, U.S. Government Printing Office, Washington, D.C. 20402.

HEALTH INFORMATION FOR INTERNATIONAL TRAVEL. CDC publishes an annual booklet as a guide to requirements and recommendations for specific immunizations and health practices for travel to various countries. It can be obtained from the Superintendent of Documents, U.S. Government Printing Office, Washington, D.C. 20402.

ADVISORY MEMORANDA. Memoranda are published when necessary by CDC to advise international travelers or those who provide information to travelers about specific outbreaks of communicable diseases abroad. These memoranda include health information for prevention and specific recommendations for immunization and may be obtained at present at no cost by writing to the Division of Quarantine, Centers for Disease Control, Atlanta, Georgia 30333, to request placement on the mailing list.

THE REPORT OF THE COMMITTEE ON INFECTIOUS DISEASES OF THE AMERICAN ACADEMY OF PEDIATRICS (*RED BOOK*). The full report containing recommendations on all licensed vaccines is usually updated every 4–5 years. The most recent Red Book was published in 1988. It can be ordered from American Academy of Pediatrics, 141 Northwest Point Blvd, P.O. Box 927, Elk Grove Village, IL 60009–0927.

CONTROL OF COMMUNICABLE DISEASES IN MAN. The American Public Health Association publishes a manual at approximately 5-year intervals. The 14th edition (1985) is currently available and a revision is in progress. The manual contains valuable information concerning infectious diseases; their occurrence worldwide; immunization, diagnostic, and therapeutic information; and up-to-date recommendations on isolation and other control measures for each disease presented. It can be ordered from the American Public Health Association, 1015 Fifteenth Street, N.W., Washington, D.C. 20005.

GUIDE FOR ADULT IMMUNIZATION. In 1985 the American College of Physicians produced a guide for physicians caring for adults (an update is in progress). It can be ordered from the American College of Physicians, Division of Scientific Activities, Health and Public Policy, 4200 Pine Street, Philadelphia, PA 19104.

TECHNICAL BULLETINS OF THE AMERICAN COLLEGE OF OBSTETRICIANS AND GYNECOLOGISTS (ACOG). ACOG bulletins, which are updated periodically, contain important information on immunization of pregnant women. A set can be ordered from American College of Obstetricians and Gynecologists, Attention: Resource Center, 409 12th Street S.W., Washington, D.C. 20024.

HEALTH DEPARTMENTS. Most state and many local health departments provide routine immunizations, immunization cards, and schedules to patients. They also send out routine reports of disease incidence.

ADDITIONAL INFORMATION. Additional information can be obtained from city, county, or state health departments; medical schools; and large hospitals. Specific questions can be addressed to the Division of Immunization, Centers for Disease Control, Atlanta, Georgia 30333.

REFERENCES

1. Centers for Disease Control. Recommendation of the Immunization Practices Advisory Committee (ACIP): General recommendation on immunization. MMWR. 1989;38:205–14, 219–27.
2. Edsall G. Immunoprophylaxis of bacterial diseases. In: Gell PGH, Coombs RRA, Lachmann PJ, eds. Clinical Aspects of Immunology. Oxford: Blackwell Scientifica; 1975:1601.
3. Benacerraf B, Unanaue ER. Textbook of Immunology. Baltimore: Williams and Wilkins; 1979.
4. Beal AJ. Immunoprophylaxis of Viral Disease. In: Gell PGH, Coombs RRA, Lachmann PJ, eds. Clinical Aspects of Immunology. Oxford: Blackwell Scientific; 1975:1631.
5. Bellanti JA, ed. Immunology II. Philadelphia: WB Saunders; 1978.
6. Rocklin RE. Mediators of cellular immunity. In: Fudenberg HH, Sites DP, Caldwell JL, et al. eds. Basic and Clinical Immunology. Los Altos, Calif.: Lange Medical; 1980.
7. Hanson LA, Ahlstedt S, Anderson B, et al. Mucosal immunity. In McGhee JR, Mestecky J, eds. The Secretory Immune System. Ann NY Acad Sci. 1983;409:1.
8. Schneerson R, Barrera O, Sutton A, et al. Preparation, characterization, and immunogenicity of *Haemophilus influenzae* type b polysaccharide–protein conjugates. J Exp Med. 1980;152:361–76.
9. Milgrom F, Abeyounis CJ, Kano K. Principles of Immunological Diagnosis in Medicine. Philadelphia; Lea & Febiger; 1981.
10. Committee on infectious Diseases, American Academy of Pediatrics. Report of the Committee on Infectious Diseases. 21st ed. Elk Grove Village, Ill: American Academy of Pediatrics; 1988.
11. Committee on Immunization, Council of Medical Societies, American College of Physicians. Guide for Adult Immunization. Philadelphia: American College of Physicians; 1985.
12. Wyeth Laboratories. Package insert, adenovirus vaccine, live, oral, type 4: Tablet for oral administration. Marietta, Penn.: Wyeth Laboratories; 1985.
13. Wyeth Laboratories. Package insert, adenovirus vaccine, live, oral, type 7: Tablet for oral administration. Marietta, Penn.: Wyeth Laboratories; 1985.
14. Michigan Department of Public Health. Package insert, anthrax, vaccine adsorbed. Lansing: Michigan Department of Public Health; 1979.
15. Snider DE, Rieder HL, Combs D, et al. Tuberculosis in children. Pediatr Infect Dis J. 1988;7:271–8.
16. Centers for Disease Control. Recommendation of the Immunization Practices Advisory Committee (ACIP): Use of BCG vaccines in the control of tuberculosis: A joint statement by the ACIP and the Advisory Committee for elimination of tuberculosis. MMWR. 1988;663–4, 669–75.
17. Centers for Disease Control. Recommendation of the Immunization Practices Advisory Committee (ACIP): Cholera vaccine. MMWR. 1988;617–24.
18. Centers for Disease Control. Recommendation of the Immunization Practices Advisory Committee (ACIP): Diphtheria, tetanus, and pertussis: Guidelines for vaccine prophylaxis and other preventive measures. MMWR. 1985;34:405–14, 419–26.
19. Centers for Disease Control. Recommendation of the Immunization Practices Advisory Committee (ACIP): Pertussis immunization, family history of convulsions and use of antipyretics—supplementary ACIP statement. MMWR. 1987;36:281–2.
20. Centers for Disease Control. Recommendations of the Immunization Practices Advisory Committee (ACIP): Polysaccharide vaccine for prevention of *Haemophilus influenzae* type b disease. MMWR. 1985;34:201–5.
21. Centers for Disease Control. Recommendations of the Immunization Practices Advisory Committee (ACIP): Update: Prevention of *Haemophilus influenzae* type b disease. MMWR. 1986;35:170–4, 179–80.
22. Centers for Disease Control. Recommendations of the Immunization Practices Advisory Committee (ACIP): Update: Prevention of *Haemophilus influenzae* type b disease. MMWR. 1988;37:13–6.
23. Centers for Disease Control. FDA workshop on *Haemophilus* b polysaccharide vaccine—a preliminary report. MMWR. 1987;36:529–31.
24. Centers for Disease Control. Recommendations of the Immunization Practices Advisory Committee: Prevention of perinatal transmission of hepatitis B virus: Prenatal screening of all pregnant women for hepatitis B surface antigen. MMWR. 1988;37:341–6, 351.
25. Shaw FE Jr, Graham DJ, Guess HA, et al. Postmarketing surveillance for neurologic adverse events reported after hepatitis B vaccination: Experience of the first three years. Am J Epidemiol. 1988;127:337–52.
26. Centers for Disease Control. Recommendation of the Immunization Practices Advisory Committee (ACIP): Recommendation for prevention against viral hepatitis. MMWR. 1985;34:313–24, 329–35.
27. Centers for Disease Control. Recommendation of the Immunization Practices Advisory Committee (ACIP): Update on hepatitis B prevention. MMWR. 1987;36:353–60, 366.
28. Patriarca PA, Arden NH, Koplan JP, et al. Prevention and control of type A influenza infections in nursing homes: Benefits and costs of four approaches using vaccination and amantadine. Ann Intern Med. 1987;107:732–40.
29. Centers for Disease Control. Recommendations of the Immunization Practices Advisory Committee (ACIP): Prevention and control of influenza. MMWR. 1988;37:361–4, 369–73, 390.
30. Centers for Disease Control. Recommendation of the Immunization Practices Advisory Committee (ACIP): Measles prevention. MMWR. 1987;36:409–18, 423–5.
31. Herman JJ, Radin R, Schneiderman R. Allergic reactions to measles (rubeola) vaccine in persons hypersensitive to egg protein. J Pediatr. 1983;102:196–9.
32. Centers for Disease Control. Recommendation of the Immunization Practices Advisory Committee (ACIP): Immunization of children infected with human immunodeficiency virus—supplementary ACIP statement. MMWR. 1988;37:181–3.

32a. Centers for Disease Control. Recommendations of the Immunization Practices Advisory Committee. Measles prevention: Supplementary statement. MMWR. 1989;38:11–14.

33. Centers for Disease Control. Recommendation of the Immunization Practices Advisory Committee (ACIP): Meningococcal polysaccharide vaccines. MMWR. 1985;34:255–9.
34. Centers for Disease Control. Recommendation of the Immunization Practices Advisory Committee (ACIP): Mumps vaccine. MMWR. 1982;31:617–25.
35. Cody CL, Baraff LJ, Cherry JD, et al. The nature and rate of adverse reactions associated with DTP and DT immunization in infants and children. Pediatrics. 1981;68:650–60.
36. Baraff LJ, Shields WD, Beckwith L, et al. Infants and children with convulsions and hypotonic–hyporesponsive episodes following diphtheria–tetanus–pertussis immunization: Follow-up evaluation. Pediatrics. 1988;81:789–94.
37. Miller D, Wadsworth J, Diamond J, et al. Pertussis vaccine and whooping cough as risk factors in acute neurological illness and death in young children. Dev Biol Stand. 1985;61:389–94.
38. Brahams D. Pertussis vaccine: Court finds no justification for association with permanent brain damage. Lancet. 1988;1:837.
39. Centers for Disease Control. Recommendation of the Immunization Practices Advisory Committee (ACIP): Plague vaccine. MMWR. 1982;31:301–4.
40. LaForce FM, Eickhoff TC. Pneumococcal vaccine: An emerging consensus. Ann Intern Med. 1988;108:757–9.
41. Centers for Disease Control. Recommendation of the Immunization Practices Advisory Committee (ACIP): Pneumococcal polysaccharide vaccine. MMWR. 1989;64–8, 73–6.
42. Nkowane BM, Wassilak SGF, Orenstein WA, et al. Vaccine-associated paralytic poliomyelitis. JAMA. 1987;257:1335–40.
43. Centers for Disease Control. Recommendation of the Immunization Practices Advisory Committee (ACIP): Poliomyelitis prevention. MMWR. 1982;31:22–6, 31–4.
44. Centers for Disease Control. Recommendation of the Immunization Practices Advisory Committee (ACIP): Poliomyelitis prevention: Enhanced potency inactivated poliomyelitis vaccine—supplementary statement. MMWR. 1987;36:795–8.
45. McBean AM, Modlin JF. Rationale for the sequential use of inactivated poliovirus vaccine and live attenuated poliovirus vaccine for routine poliomyelitis immunization in the United States. Pediatr Infect Dis J. 1987;6:881–7.
46. Institute of Medicine. Report of a study: An Evaluation of Poliomyelitis Vaccine Policy Options 1988. Washington D.C.: National Academy of Sciences; 1988.
47. Bacterial vaccines and bacterial antigens with no U.S. Standards of potency: Implementation of efficacy review proposal. Federal Register. 1977;42(Nov 8):58266.
48. Centers for Disease Control. Recommendation of the Immunization Practices Advisory Committee (ACIP): Rabies prevention in the United States. MMWR. 1984;33:393–402, 407–8.
49. Centers for Disease Control. Rabies post exposure prophylaxis with human diploid cell rabies vaccine: Lower neutralizing antibody titers with Wyeth vaccine. MMWR. 1985;34:90–2.
50. Centers for Disease Control. Rubella vaccination during pregnancy—United States, 1971–88. MMWR. 1989;38:289–93.
51. Centers for Disease Control. Recommendation of the Immunization Practices Advisory Committee (ACIP): Rubella prevention. MMWR. 1984;33:301–10.
52. Tingle AJ. Postpartum rubella immunization. J Infect Dis. 1986;154:368–9.
53. Centers for Disease Control. Recommendation of the Immunization Practices Advisory Committee (ACIP): Smallpox vaccine. MMWR. 1985;34:341–2.
54. Centers for Disease Control. Recommendation of the Immunization Practices Advisory Committee (ACIP): Typhoid vaccine. MMWR. 1978;27:231–3.
55. Centers for Disease Control. Recommendation of the Immunization Practices Advisory Committee (ACIP): Yellow fever vaccine. MMWR. In press.
56. American College of Obstetricians and Gynecologists (ACOG). Selective Rho (D) Immune Globulin (RHIG). Technical Bulletin no. 61. Chicago; American College of Obstetricians and Gynecologists; 1981.
57. Centers for Disease Control. Recommendation of the Immunization Practices Advisory Committee (ACIP): Varicella zoster immune globulin. MMWR. 1984;33:84–90, 95–100.
58. Deforest A, Long SS, Lischner HW, et al. Simultaneous administration of

58. Deforest A, Long SS, Lischner HW, et al. Simultaneous administration of measles–mumps–rubella vaccine with booster doses of diphtheria–tetanus–pertussis and poliovirus vaccines. Pediatrics. 1988;81:237–46.
59. Centers for Disease Control. Recommendation of the Immunization Practices Advisory Committee (ACIP): New recommended schedule for active immunization of normal infants and children. MMWR. 1986;35:577–9.
60. Centers for Disease Control. Recommendation of the Immunization Practices Advisory Committee (ACIP): Adult immunization. MMWR. 1984;33:1S–68S.
61. Centers for Disease Control. Health Information for International Travel, 1988. Washington, D.C.; U.S. Government Printing Office; 1988.
62. Williams WW. Centers for Disease Control guideline for infection control in hospital personnel. Infect Control. 1983;4(Suppl):326–48.
63. Centers for Disease Control. Recommendation of the Immunization Practices Advisory Committee (ACIP): Immunization of children infected with human T-lymphotrophic virus type III/lymphadenopathy associated virus. MMWR. 1986;35:595–8, 603–6.
64. von Reyn CF, Clements CJ, Mann JM. Human immunodeficiency virus infection and routine childhood immunization. Lancet. 1987;2:669–72.
65. Onorato IM, Markowitz LE, Oxtoby MJ. Childhood immunization, vaccine-preventable diseases and HIV infection. Pediatr Infect Dis J. 1988;7:588–95.
66. Centers for Disease Control. Measles in HIV-infected children, United States. MMWR. 1988;37:183–6.
67. Kaplan JE, Nelson DB, Schonberger LB, et al. The effect of immune globulin on trivalent oral polio and yellow fever vaccinations. Bull WHO. 1984;62:585–90.
68. Centers for Disease Control. National Childhood Vaccine Injury Act: Requirements for permanent vaccination records and for reporting of selected events after vaccination. MMWR. 1988;37:197–200.

SECTION D

297. PROTECTION OF TRAVELERS

MARTIN S. WOLFE

It is necessary for the physician dealing with traveling patients to be familiar with the potential diseases to which the traveler might be exposed. Advice on immunizations and general preventive measures must be given before travel, and on the traveler's return the physician must be aware of and recognize problems resulting from travel.

PRETRAVEL ADVICE

Preparations for Travel

Anyone with a pre-existing medical condition should be examined by, or at least have a consultation with, his or her physician approximately 1 month before beginning the trip. Special precautions are necessary for those with allergies, gastrointestinal conditions, diabetes, or cardiovascular or pulmonary disease. A brief medical summary and a recent copy of the patient's electrocardiogram or chest x-ray film, if pertinent, should be taken along. Engraved bracelets with a brief description of a potentially dangerous medical condition are available from a number of sources. For those requiring care by a particular specialist while abroad, a directory of that specialty should be consulted. A pocket directory is available from the nonprofit International Association for Medical Assistance to Travelers (IAMAT, 736 Center St., Lewiston, NY 14092), listing doctors worldwide who speak English, have attained respected qualifications, and understand U.S. medical techniques and practices. A regular visit to the dentist should be scheduled before traveling. If glasses or contact lenses are worn, an extra pair should be taken, as well as a prescription for replacement of eyeglasses. Travelers should be certain that their health insurance policy covers medical care, hospitalization, or medical evacuation in foreign countries. If not, special policies are available for such coverage.

Supply of Necessary Drugs

Patients with chronic illnesses who are taking medications such as digitalis, insulin, or anticoagulants should carry a sufficient supply. Since drugs sold abroad may have different names and may vary in potency, prescriptions should be clearly written, giving the trade, generic, and chemical names of the drug and the dosage.

Many drugs may be purchased over the counter in foreign countries, and these often lack label warnings. Travelers should be warned that potentially dangerous drugs such as chloramphenicol, sulfas, butazolidin, and aminopyrine may be included in cold or antidiarrheal preparations. In some countries injections are given in pharmacies, and it is important to avoid questionably sterile needles and syringes and where possible, to purchase or bring along disposable needles and syringes.

Components of a traveler's medical kit might include a thermometer, bandages and gauze, adhesive tape, an antiseptic or bactericidal soap solution, aspirin, antacids, an antimotion sickness drug such as dimenhydrinate, and a mild oral laxative or suppository for constipation. A decongestant should be carried while in the aircraft cabin for those prone to nasal congestion, and saline nose drops are useful to prevent nasal dryness from the low humidity of aircraft cabins. An antihistamine should be taken for allergies. Cough medication and other liquids should be carried in a tightly stoppered plastic bottle. A small amount of a nonnarcotic pain medication, or perhaps a codeine preparation, should be carried. Antibiotic and antifungal ointments and perhaps a foot powder should be included. In general, broad-spectrum antibiotics should not be given to travelers, since if they are sufficiently ill to require these medications, they would be better served by consulting a recommended physician. An exception to this may be made for those travelers who will be in remote areas in which immediate medical assistance may be unavailable; a tetracycline, a quinolone, or trimethoprim-sulfamethoxazole may then be given with clearly written instructions on indications, dosage, and possible side effects. Salt tablets may be useful in hot, humid climates.

Particularly useful drugs such as antimalarials and antidiarrheals, water purification tablets, insect repellants, and sunscreens will be discussed in detail in appropriate sections.

IMMUNIZATIONS

Required Immunizations

There are two immunizations that have been compulsory for entry into certain countries—yellow fever and cholera. Vaccination Certificate Requirements of various countries are listed in a U.S. Public Health Service booklet, *Health Information for International Travel* 1988, [HHS Publication No. (CDC) 88–8280].[1] This is revised yearly and is available from the Superintendent of Documents, U.S. Government Printing Office, Washington, DC 20402. The Foreign Quarantine Division of the Centers for Disease Control (CDC) in Atlanta also publishes a weekly "Blue Sheet" indicating changes in the requirements of countries for required vaccinations to supplement the yearly publication. The World Health Organization (WHO) in Geneva also publishes a booklet each January, *International Travel and Health: Vaccination Requirements and Health Advice*,[2] which gives a country-by-country listing of the required immunizations and the malaria situation. This information is supplemented on a weekly basis by the WHO *Weekly Epidemiological Record*. Subscriptions for these publications may be ordered in the United States from the WHO Publications Center USA, 49 Sheridan Avenue, Albany, NY 12210. Since vaccination certificate requirements can be very changeable, physicians frequently required to advise travelers should subscribe to these publications. Advice is also available from local health departments and specialized travel clinics.

Physicians and travelers must be advised that the requirements of countries of arrival are related not only to the infections present in the country of departure but also to conditions in countries in which the traveler may disembark during the journey. International Certificates of Vaccination are individual certificates and cannot be used collectively. Thus, separate certificates must be issued for children; the information cannot be incorporated in the mother's certificate. Travelers who do not have the required vaccinations upon entering a country may be subject to vaccination, medical follow-up, and/or isolation, and in some countries they may be denied entry. Vaccinations may be given under the supervision of any licensed physician. Certificates must be signed by a licensed physician or a designee under his or her supervision. Validation of the certificate can be from the "uniform stamp" of the vaccinating physician or from the local health department. Failure to have proper validation may cause the traveler to be revaccinated or quarantined. The date of vaccination should be recorded on the certificate in the following sequence: day, month, year—the month to be written out. Certificates of children who cannot write must be signed by a parent. The origin and batch number of the vaccine must be recorded on the certificate.

There are no vaccination requirements for travel directly between the United States and Europe, Canada, Mexico, and the Caribbean countries unless an outbreak of yellow fever or cholera occurs in any of these countries. If travelers visit a country reporting one of these diseases, countries remaining on their itinerary may require particular vaccination certificates. Even if travelers are coming from a country reporting yellow fever or cholera, no vaccination requirements are in effect for re-entry into the United States.

TABLE 1. Doses of Commonly Used Vaccines for International Travel

Vaccine	Age	Route	Dose	Booster
Cholera	6 mo–4 yr	Subq or	0.2 ml	0.2 ml
	5–10 yr	IM	0.3 ml	0.3 ml
	>10 yr		0.5 ml	0.5 ml
Yellow fever	>1 yr	Subq	0.5 ml	0.5 ml
Typhoid	<10 yr	Subq	1 and 2–0.25 ml	0.25 ml
	>10 yr		1 and 2–0.50 ml	0.50 ml
Polio (TOPV)	All ages	Oral	3 doses	1 dose[a]
(IPV)	All ages	IM	4 doses	1 dose[a]
Tetanus-diphtheria	>7 yr	IM	3 doses	1 dose[a]
		Long-term residence:		
Immune serum globulin	<23 kg	IM	1.0 ml	Every
(Hepatitis A	23–45 kg		2.5 ml	4–6 mo
prophylaxis)	>45 kg		5.0 ml	
		Short-term travel (<3 mo):		
	<23 kg		0.5 ml	
	23–45 kg		1.0 ml	
	>45 kg		2.0 ml	

[a] See manufacturer's recommended dose.

Yellow Fever

Yellow fever occurs in parts of tropical Africa and South America. Immunization can be required both for protection against infection and for entry when traveling to countries in these regions. A valid yellow fever vaccination certificate may also be required for entry into other countries from all travelers coming from a yellow-fever-infected area or, in some cases, from a country in which any part is infected (e.g., travelers transiting tropical Africa en route to India or Pakistan). Children below age 1 year are usually exempt from these requirements. Single primary or booster doses are valid for 10 years beginning 10 days after primary vaccination or revaccination. Unlike other immunizations, yellow fever vaccine must be administered at a designated yellow fever vaccination center, the locations of which can be obtained from local health departments.

From 2 to 10 percent of vaccinees have mild headache, myalgias, low-grade fever, or other minor symptoms 5–10 days after vaccination. Yellow fever vaccine should not be administered to anyone with a documented hypersensitivity to eggs or with an altered immune state. These people, as well as children below age 1 year and pregnant women who are not at risk of infection, should receive a letter of contraindication. Ideally, yellow fever vaccine should not be given to a known pregnant woman, but if she travels to an area in which there is any risk of infection, it should best be administered. If yellow fever and cholera vaccines are given within 3 weeks of each other, antibody response may not be optimal. See Table 1 for vaccine doses.

Cholera

The requirement of a cholera vaccination for entry into a country is considered excessive by WHO and by those countries bound by the International Health Regulations. As of January 1989, only five countries required a cholera certificate for travelers arriving from cholera-infected areas. Currently available cholera vaccines are considered of limited usefulness, providing about 50 percent effectiveness for about 3–6 months in reducing clinical illness. The risk of contracting cholera is considered to be so low for the usual traveler that many authorities question the benefit of vaccine and have recommended it only for travel to those countries requiring vaccination. Proper attention to food and water hygiene is considered much better protection against contracting cholera than is the vaccine. In 1988 WHO issued a modified International Certificate of Vaccination that no longer provides space for cholera vaccination with the official stamp of the vaccinating center. This is part of an effort to dissuade countries that still require a cholera vaccination from maintaining this requirement. Vaccination against cholera cannot protect any country from the introduction of this disease. It is likely that knowledge and acceptance of the new WHO regulations may take some time. Also, some countries may still require vaccination for travelers arriving from cholera endemic areas. A single cholera injection meets this requirement, as does a note of contraindication from a physician on letterhead stationery. If vaccination is given, it should be entered in the card under "Other vaccinations." Local reactions may occur, but serious reactions are very rare. Anyone experiencing a serious reaction should not receive this vaccine again. A cholera certificate is valid for 6 months, beginning 6 days after injection of one dose of vaccine or on the date of revaccination if within 6 months of the first injection. Booster doses can be required every 6 months.

Smallpox

The last reported case of endemic smallpox occurred in October 1977. WHO has amended the International Health Regulations to remove smallpox from the diseases subject to the regulations. As of January 1984, all countries had advised WHO that a smallpox vaccination certificate was not required from any traveler. As the risk of contracting smallpox is now virtually nil and since smallpox vaccine may rarely cause very serious or even fatal reactions, there is at this time no justification for administering smallpox vaccine to any traveler. The risk of vaccination clearly exceeds any benefit.

RECOMMENDED IMMUNIZATIONS

Although not required by international regulations, several other vaccines are recommended for protection against diseases more prevalent in certain areas of the world. For children, routine childhood vaccines should also be up-to-date before traveling.

Poliomyelitis

Polio remains a definite hazard to travelers to the developing world, and unprotected adults are particularly susceptible to paralytic complications. Many travelers have had the basic series of three doses of trivalent oral polio vaccine or four doses of inactivated polio vaccine. A single booster dose is recommended in this situation before traveling to areas of increased polio risk. The need for further supplementary booster doses has not been established. Those who have been unvaccinated or partially vaccinated should complete a polio vaccination series. Oral vaccine is preferred for most people, but previously unvaccinated adults and those who are immunocompromised should receive inactivated injectable vaccine, since the risk of vaccine-associated paralysis in adults is less with this vaccine. An enhanced potency, inactivated, injectable vaccine has recently been licensed in the United States. The older inactivated vaccine is manufactured in Canada and still licensed in the United States. This older vaccine may become obsolete. Oral polio vaccine is still recommended for routine use in infants and children. If less than 4 weeks are available before protection is needed for an unvaccinated person, a single dose of vaccine should be given; when time permits, the remaining doses can be administered. A pregnant woman intending to travel to a developing area should receive either oral or inactivated vaccine, as appropriate, since there is no convincing evidence documenting adverse effects on the developing fetus or pregnant woman.

Typhoid

Typhoid fever is endemic in much of the developing world, and vaccine is recommended for travelers to those areas in which it is difficult to use a reliable nonvaccine alternative method to prevent this infection. Certainly those travelers to typhoid epidemic areas and those traveling overland or off the beaten track should receive this vaccine. The basic adult series consists of two 0.5-ml doses given 4 or more weeks apart. When there is insufficient time for two doses at the recommended interval, three doses of the same volumes may be given at weekly intervals, although this schedule may be less effective. It is possible that even a single dose may provide some immunity for those leaving immediately. Booster doses need not be given more frequently than every 3 years, even in the presence of epidemic conditions or natural disasters. Generally, less reaction occurs when boosters are given as 0.1-ml intradermal doses, but only the heat-phenol killed vaccine (and *not* the acetone-killed and dried vaccine) may be given intradermally. Immunization frequently results in 1–2 days of local discomfort, which may be accompanied by fever, malaise, and headache. In children below age 10, febrile reactions are more common, and an antipyretic may be needed. Those with severe reactions to typhoid vaccine should subsequently best not receive it. Where practical, typhoid vaccination should ideally not be done in conjunction with any other vaccine apt to produce similar reactions. In the United States, paratyphoid A and B (TAB) vaccines are no longer combined with typhoid vaccine. Combined TAB vaccines are used abroad but are not recommended. Live oral typhoid vaccines used abroad are not recommended until they receive further controlled evaluations.[3] It is anticipated that oral vaccine will be licensed in the United States in the near future.

Tetanus–Diphtheria

Most travelers will have received the basic series with diphtheria, pertussis, tetanus (DPT) during childhood, and boosters are recommended every 10 years to offer continued protection against tetanus and diphtheria. Tetanus and diphtheria toxoid (Td) is the vaccine of choice for children over 7 years and adults, since it has only 10–20 percent of the amount of diphtheria toxoid present in standard DPT preparations and leads to fewer febrile reactions in those above age 7.

Measles

People born after 1956 who travel abroad should be protected against measles, which is endemic in many parts of the world. No immunization or record of immunization is required for entry into the United States. However, it is recommended that international travelers have immunity to measles, consisting of a physician's verification of prior measles disease, laboratory evidence of measles immunity, or verified measles vaccination on or after the first birthday. Since the risk of serious complications and death is greater for adults, it is especially important to protect young adults who have escaped measles disease and have not been vaccinated. Most people born before 1957 need not be considered susceptible.[4]

In the United States, measles vaccine is recommended for children at least 15 months of age. However, younger children traveling to measles endemic countries, where the risk of contracting measles is far greater than in the United States, should be protected, and such children should be given live measles vaccine after 6 months of age. These children should then receive another dose of measles-mumps-rubella (MMR) vaccine at approximately 15 months of age.

Rabies

Relatively few countries can be considered rabies free (these are listed in Ref. 1). Pre-exposure vaccination is recommended for high-risk groups for possible rabies exposure in rabies endemic areas, where rabies is a constant threat. These might include young children, veterinarians, animal handlers, field workers, and others with any significant risk of exposure to potentially rabid animals. Although adequate pre-exposure vaccination offers added protection when rabies exposure occurs, it does not eliminate the need for additional vaccine therapy. It does eliminate the need for the often difficult to obtain human rabies immune globulin. Present pre-exposure recommendations call for a series of three 1-ml intramuscular (administered over the deltoid) doses of human diploid cell vaccine (HDCV) on days 0, 7, 21, or 28. Administration of routine booster doses of vaccine depends on the exposure risk category given in Reference 1. Local reactions such as redness, pain, and itching are common. Systemic effects may also occur, and allergic reactions and neurologic complications have been very rarely reported. Since antibody titer determinations are no longer easily obtainable, those requiring protection who received rabies duck embryo vaccine or a vaccine other than HDCV in the past should best receive a full pre-exposure HDCV series. Duck embryo vaccine is no longer available in the United States. In Latin America, a suckling mouse brain vaccine, in a series of three doses given on alternative days, is favored, but this appears to be relatively less safe than HDCV.

RARELY INDICATED IMMUNIZATIONS

Certain vaccines are indicated only for very particular situations or for travel to specific remote locations.

Plague

Plague vaccination is not required for entry into any country and is recommended only for plague-infected areas. Plague is sporadically reported from the former Indochina area of Southeast Asia and Burma and in remote areas of enzootic plague in Asia, South America, and Africa. Vaccination is not indicated for most travelers to countries reporting cases, particularly if their travel is limited to urban areas with modern accommodations. Selected people engaged in field work in plague-enzootic or plague-epidemic rural areas might benefit from vaccination. The primary series consists of two immunizations 4 or more weeks apart and a third dose 4–12 weeks after dose two, with boosters required every 6–12 months where exposure risk persists. Mild reactions such as pain, erythema, and edema at the injection site are frequently recognized. Sterile abscesses rarely occur. The incidence and severity of reactions increase with the number of injections received, and the vaccine should not be given to people who previously experienced serious side effects from it.

Typhus

No epidemic typhus cases have been reported in U.S. travelers since 1950. Production of typhus vaccine has been discontinued in the United States, and the vaccine is no longer available or recommended.

Meningococcal Meningitis

Meningococcal disease is endemic throughout the world. In certain areas, particularly the Sahel region of West Africa, epidemics of meningococcal meningitis occur almost yearly in the winter and early spring months. Epidemics have recently occurred in Nepal and parts of India and in Saudi Arabia. Although meningitis is extremely uncommon in travelers or resident expatriates, even in epidemic situations, vaccination is often a more reasonable protective measure than drug prophylaxis. A quadrivalent A/C/Y/W-135 vaccine is available. A single dose in the volume indicated by the manufacturer is administered. The duration of immunity is unknown but appears to be at least 3 years in those 4 years of age or older. Serogroup A vaccine has not been shown to be effective in children less than 3 months of age and may be less than fully effective in children 3–11 months of age. Adverse reactions, consisting of localized erythema for 1–2 days, are uncommon. Although not proven dangerous in pregnant women, it is prudent not to use these vaccines unless there is a substantial risk of infection.

Influenza

Those considered at high risk of contracting influenza and traveling to parts of the world in which influenza is epidemic should receive influenza vaccine.

Pneumococcal Vaccine

The pneumococcal capsular polysaccharide vaccine is recommended for the prevention of pneumococcal infection only in high-risk patients who would receive it in the United States.

Calmette-Guérin Bacillus

Tuberculosis is a potential hazard to visitors to the developing world, and Calmette-Guérin bacillus (BCG) is sometimes recommended for travelers to highly endemic areas. However, its use in this situation remains controversial, and the weight of expert opinion presently seems to be against its use. The troublesome side effects of BCG, questionable efficacy of certain batches, and possible loss of skin test sensitivity lead the majority of workers to rely on skin test screening and the treatment of the relatively few people infected.

Japanese B Encephalitis

Rare cases of Japanese B encephalitis have occurred in resident expatriates in certain endemic areas of the Far East and Southeast Asia. The risk to travelers who confine their travel to urban centers is low, as is the risk in rural areas when the traveler stays for only a few weeks. The only recognized reliable, effective, and safe vaccine is manufactured in Japan. The vaccine has been available intermittently in the United States on an investigational basis. Currently, the vaccine is not available.

Tickborne Encephalitis

Tickborne encephalitis is a viral infection of the central nervous system occurring in forested areas of Central and East Europe. An effective vaccine may be obtained in Europe from Immuno, Vienna, Austria.[5] Present data do not support a recommendation for its use in travelers to endemic countries, but it can be considered in longer-term residents with exposure risk in forests.

HEPATITIS PREVENTION

Immune globulin (γ-globulin) is extremely valuable in protecting against type A hepatitis, which appears to be the most common form of hepatitis to which travelers will likely be exposed in the developing world through contaminated food or water. Some protection against the much less commonly acquired type B hepatitis and, possibly, against enterically transmitted non-A, non-B hepatitis may be provided by this product. Experience at the State Department and Peace Corps has shown that the administration of immune globulin every 4–6 months while residing or traveling in the developing world offers excellent protection against clinical illness from viral hepatitis. Some authorities do not recommend immune globulin for children below about age 12, since the disease is usually mild in children. Since it is usually difficult to completely avoid exposure to type A hepatitis and since immune globulin is effective, inexpensive, and safe, it should be recommended for both short-term travelers to and longer-term residents in hepatitis endemic areas. For travel of less than 2 months, a 2-ml dose is given. For longer-term travel or residence, adults should receive 5 ml every 4–6 months. If possible, immune globulin should not be given for 3 months before or at least 2 weeks after a live viral vaccine; data indicate, however, that immune globulin does not interfere with the immune response to yellow fever or oral polio virus vaccines. Local discomfort may occur at the injection site, and rare hypersensitivity reactions have been reported. Immune globulin is recommended and is considered safe for pregnant women requiring protection. Immune globulins prepared in the United States have never been shown to transmit infectous agents, including human immunodeficiency virus.

Hepatitis B immune globulin is not routinely recommended for travelers. It does not appear that the usual traveler to or expatriate resident in type B hepatitis endemic areas requires hepatitis B vaccine. Three doses over a 6-month period are necessary to give satisfactory protection, and the vaccine is quite expensive. At this time, the use of this vaccine should be particularly recommended for certain high-risk individuals, such as medical personnel in contact with blood and those who expect to have sexual contacts while abroad. Prevaccine antibody susceptibility testing may be cost effective in particular individuals.

VACCINATION DURING PREGNANCY

Pregnancy is a theoretical contraindication to all live virus vaccines. However, if there is a substantial risk of exposure to natural infection, including polio and yellow fever, vaccines should be administered. If there is no risk of infection, it is best to give a letter of contraindication. Pregnancy and breast-feeding are not contraindications to administration of immune serum globulin, toxoid vaccines, or killed or inactivated vaccines.[6]

GENERAL VACCINE RECOMMENDATIONS

People who have anaphylactic reactions to avian products should not receive vaccines containing egg products.

Some vaccines contain preservatives or trace amounts of antibiotics, such as neomycin or streptomycin, to which certain people may be hypersensitive. Vaccine label information should be reviewed with this in mind before deciding whether these vaccines should be administered to those with known hypersensitivity to these products.

An inactivated and a live attenuated virus vaccine can be administered simultaneously at separate sites.

Virus replication after administration of live attenuated virus vaccine can be potentiated by an immunosuppressed state, and immunosuppressed patients should not be given these vaccines.

Vaccination of people with a severe febrile illness should generally be deferred until recovery. Minor illnesses, such as upper respiratory infections, do not necessarily preclude vaccination.

Vaccines for routine preventable diseases in childhood (mumps, rubella, polio, diphtheria, tetanus, pertussis, and *Haemophilus influenzae* type B meningitis) should be administered to children going abroad according to recommended schedules for the United States (see Ref. 1).

ADVICE WHILE TRAVELING

General Advice

Flying. Since long-distance travel today is almost always by air, the traveler must be prepared for the effects of jet lag due to disturbance in circadian body rhythm. The average traveler requires about 1 day to readjust for every 1 or 2 hours of time change. Mild sedatives may be required to assist sleeping on the first night or two after arrival at the destination. Motion sickness may be prevented by agents such as dimenhydrinate (Dramamine) or meclizine (Bonine). A small plastic disk for continuous administration of scopolamine (Transderm-V [CIBA]) through the skin is available for treatment of motion sickness, but it takes several hours or longer to be effective and can cause dry mouth and drowsiness.[7] Moderation in the intake of alcoholic and carbonated beverages and the avoidance of excessive food intake lead to a more comfortable trip. Prolonged sitting should be avoided since this can lead to postural hypotension, abdominal distension, or venous stasis. The latter can predispose to pulmonary embolization. It is therefore essential for the traveler to walk about the plane periodically. If flying is necessary with a cold, nasal decongestants should be used.

Acclimatization. Going to high altitudes requires time for acclimatization, and it is best to avoid alcoholic beverages, tobacco, excessive food, and exercise and to take more frequent rests for the first few days at altitude. Similar adaptations and restrictions are necessary on arrival into a tropical area.

Water. A great hazard to the traveler to the developing world is contaminated water and ice. Unless it is absolutely certain that piped water is potable or that the water in a major chain hotel is assuredly safe, it is necessary to boil water for 5 minutes or to treat all water chemically for drinking or making ice. Iodine compounds such as Potable aqua tablets, 2% iodine tincture or Lugol's solution, or liquid chlorine bleach are satisfactory under most conditions but may be less effective in cloudy or very cold water, and an increased amount of disinfectant or contact time may be required.[8] The Water Tech Purifier Cup, containing a resin, is also useful. Hot water from the tap, although relatively safer than cold water, may still contain dangerous organisms and cannot be considered completely safe for drinking or for brushing teeth. No presently available simple water filter renders water sterile of all potential pathogenic organisms, and these should not be relied on by themselves. If they are used, the water should be first filtered and then boiled. It is possible for community-treated water to be coliform-free but yet capable of transmitting protozoa such as cysts of *Giardia lamblia*. Bottled commercial water is generally safer than untreated tap water, but this water may also occasionally be contaminated.

Food and Beverages. If well-cooked hot foods are eaten, most food-borne infections can be avoided. Cold foods and salads are much more easily contaminated by infected food handlers or may be prepared with contaminated water. Raw fruits should be eaten only when they have an unbroken skin and are peeled by the eater. Raw vegetables and green salads are often contaminated with bacteria, protozoan cysts, and helminth eggs from night soil used as fertilizer or from contaminated water used in growing or in preparation. Scrubbing of green leafy vegetables with a detergent solution and then soaking them in strong iodine or chlorine solutions can eliminate most but perhaps not all organisms. Dairy products should be eaten only if they are known to be prepared hygienically and properly refrigerated. Custards, cream pastries, salads made with mayonnaise, and raw or poorly cooked shellfish should be avoided, since these are excellent vehicles for propagation of pathogenic organisms. Eating raw or undercooked local beef, pork, sausage, or fish can lead to trichinosis, tapeworms, or fluke infections. Smoking, salting, pickling, or drying meat or fish alone is not effective, but heating these to at least 55°C for 1 hour or freezing at −10°C for 20 days will kill infective-stage parasites. Ciguatera and scombroid fish poisoning and shellfish poisoning may occur from eating apparently normal large marine fishes and shellfish in tropical areas and occasionally in temperate areas.[9] When fresh fruits and vegetables cannot be obtained or eaten, multivitamins should be taken.

Iced drinks, juices mixed with water, and noncarbonated bottled fluids should be avoided. Canned or bottled name-brand carbonated beverages are usually safe, as are coffee and tea made with boiled water and hot milk, beer, and wine.

Sunstroke and Heat Exhaustion. These can be avoided by abstaining from prolonged exposure to the sun or overly strenuous exercises. It is important to drink more fluids and to add salt to food or to use salt tablets. Formulations of 5% *p*-aminobenzoic acid (PABA) in ethanol, such as Pre-Sun or Pabanol, are the most effective nonopaque sunscreens. These should be applied in the morning after washing, particularly on exposed parts of the body, and again 30 minutes before exposure to combine with the skin keratin.

Insects. Since insects are important carriers of disease, as well as being a great nuisance, windows should be screened. In situations in which this is not possible, mosquito netting of 16 × 18 mesh should be used. Outdoors, mosquito exposure may be lessened by wearing clothing that covers the arms and legs and by applying an insect repellant to exposed areas of the skin and on clothing. The recommended repellant is one containing about 32 percent diethyl-meta-toluamide (Deet). A pyrethrum-containing flying-insect spray should be used in living and sleeping areas during evening and nighttime hours.

Snakes. Snakes are usually nocturnal in their habits and will generally bite during the day only if they are attacked or surprised. When walking in areas in which snakes are commonly found, boots with long trousers tucked into them should be worn. When going into remote areas, a snake-bite kit containing antivenom against local snakes or scorpions should be taken along.

Schistosomiasis and Other Water-Borne Organisms. Where schistosomiasis occurs, in parts of Africa, the Middle East, South America, and the Caribbean, all bodies of fresh water must be considered to be infected with these parasites, and contact with this water must be avoided. However, these parasites cannot be contracted in salt water or adequately chlorinated swimming pools. Some attractive bathing beaches, particularly in urban areas, may be highly polluted. Corals, jelly fish, and other biting and stinging aquatic creatures are a hazard to bathers.[10]

Sleeping Sickness. Only a handful of cases of sleeping sickness have occurred in U.S. travelers, and most of these have been contracted in game parks of East Africa and northern Botswana. Drug prophylaxis with pentamidine injections is not recommended,[11] but long sleeves and trousers may decrease the risk of bites from the tsetse fly vector.

Malaria Prophylaxis

One of the greatest risks to travelers in many parts of the developing world is malaria, and appropriate prophylactic drugs must always be taken when going to an area in which malaria transmission occurs. Country-by-country guides to the need for malaria prophylaxis and specific areas of chloroquine-resistant falciparum malaria are published by WHO[2] and the CDC.[1]

Chloroquine-resistant *Plasmodium falciparum* (CRPF) malaria presently occurs in most of tropical Africa, Southeast Asia, Oceania, the para-Amazon region of South America, and sporadically in South Asia. The continued extension of CRPF has reduced the number of effective drugs for malaria prophylaxis. Also, some alternative drugs to chloroquine have been associated with serious side effects, which limits their usefulness. Guidelines for prophylaxis must consider the exposure risk to malaria, the safety and effectiveness of available antimalarial drugs, and the use of personal protective measures (see above under "Insects"). Recommendations for the prevention of malaria must be periodically revised because of geographic spread of CRPF, new information on the efficacy and safety of prophylactic drugs, and the availability of new drugs. At this time, there is no available drug or combination of drugs with proven efficacy or safety to prevent all malaria infections. A variety of recommendations made in different countries has resulted, which has led to confusion. The following recommendations are considered most appropriate at the present time, as offering the best combination of safety and relative effectiveness. It must also be emphasized to travelers that regardless of the methods employed, malaria can still be contracted. Those who have symptoms of malaria must seek prompt medical attention. (See also Chapter 250 for a discussion of prophylaxis.)

For areas with chloroquine-sensitive malaria species or those where only low-level or focal CRPF has been reported, the drug of choice is chloroquine. This is taken in an adult dose of 300 mg base (equal to 500 mg salt) once weekly, beginning 2 weeks before departure to assure tolerance, regularly while in the malarious area, and for 4 weeks after leaving. For young children the dose is 5 mg/kg of base weekly. Liquid chloroquine preparations are available overseas but not in the United States. Although minor side effects are common, marked intolerance is unusual. Chloroquine is considered safe for infants and pregnant women.[12] Serious eye damage has very rarely been confirmed in those taking the recommended dose for malaria prophylaxis.[13] Only rarely should malaria develop in those taking regular suppressive chloroquine in areas where resistance to it does not occur; most malaria infections occur in those who have either not taken any suppression, have taken it irregularly, or have ceased taking it prematurely on leaving the malarious area.

For travelers to areas where CRPF is endemic, chloroquine taken weekly, as above, is recommended. Some experts recommend that proguanil (Paludrine), 200 mg daily, be taken in addition to chloroquine. Limited data suggest that proguanil is effective in tropical Africa, but not in Thailand or Papua New Guinea. No current data are available on its efficacy in other CRPF areas. Proguanil is presently not approved in the United States by the Food and Drug Administration, but is is available in England, Holland, Kenya, and many other places in Africa. Proguanil is one of the best tolerated of all antimalarial drugs and is safe in pregnancy. A third drug, pyrimethamine-sulfadoxine (Fansidar), in a three-tablet treatment dose, should also be carried during travel (unless one is allergic to sulfa) and should be promptly taken in the event of a febrile illness during travel when professional medical care is not readily available. It must be emphasized that such presumptive self-treatment of a possible malarial infection is only a temporary measure and that prompt medical evaluation is imperative. In some malarious areas with multidrug resistance by *P. falciparum,* doxycycline alone, 100 mg daily, can be considered for short-term travelers. A new antimalarial drug, mefloquine (Lariam), is currently undergoing review by the Food and Drug Administration. Mefloquine is available in Switzerland and France. It can be considered for use by travelers to areas with CRPF and particularly by those with multidrug resistance. Currently available information suggests that the adult prophylactic dose is 250 mg weekly.

Amodiaquine and pyrimethamine plus dapsone (Maloprim) are recommended by some experts abroad. Neither is available in the United States. Both have been associated with bone marrow problems and are not recommended.

To prevent potentially later relapsing malaria with persisting liver forms of *Plasmodium vivax* and *P. ovale,* which can occur for up to 3 years after leaving most malarious areas, primaquine can be considered. This is particularly important in those who have prolonged exposure in malarious areas. The drug is taken after the conclusion of terminal suppressive therapy with chloroquine and/or other drugs. There is no need to take combined choloroquine-primaquine prophylaxis while in malarious areas. The dose of primaquine is 15 mg base daily for 14 days (0.3 mg base/kg/day, not to exceed 15 mg, in young children). As primaquine may cause severe hemolysis in glucose-6-phosphate dehydrogenase deficiency, this deficiency must be ruled out before using primaquine. Primaquine is not recommended in pregnancy.

The above recommendations are detailed in a recent publication from the Malaria Branch of the CDC.[14]

Travelers' Diarrhea

Some of the diarrheas that affect travelers may be noninfectious and self-limited, related to eating strange foods, nervous tension, fatigue, altitude, or other factors. Acute viral infections, caused mainly by rotavirus and Norwalk agent, are other common causes of undiagnosed diarrhea. Enterotoxigenic *Escherichia coli* is the leading cause of travelers' diarrhea, causing more cases than all other causes combined. *Campylobacter* infections may cause more diarrhea in travelers than *Shigella* and *Salmonella* infections combined. Amebiasis, giardiasis, and tropical enteropathy are other relatively likely possible causes.

The avoidance of contaminated food and water will help prevent many diarrhea diseases.

The most important factor in treating any diarrhea is the replacement of lost fluids by drinking water, tea, broth, and carbonated beverages. Electrolyte replacement is also important, and commercial oral rehydration solutions can be mixed with a liter of potable water to prepare a more ideal replacement fluid.[15] Alternatively, a home preparation can be made from fruit juice, sodium chloride, sodium bicarbonate, and glucose. Bananas and oranges are a good source of potassium. The accompanying diet should be bland, with the particular avoidance of alcohol and fats.

Useful drugs to relieve excessive diarrhea or cramps include loperamide (Imodium) and diphenoxylate (Lomotil). These drugs are not recommended for young children and should be stopped if diarrhea becomes intractable after 3 days, if blood or mucus occurs in the stool, or if there is high fever and chills or severe cramps. A physician must then be contacted for appropriate diagnosis and treatment. Bismuth subsalicylate liquid (Pepto-Bismol) taken in a dose of 30 ml every half-hour until eight doses are taken has been shown to have a favorable effect on the course of diarrhea caused by toxigenic *E. coli*.[16] Antibiotics are usually not required with acute watery diarrheas, which are usually self-limited with supportive treatment. If it is important to shorten the course or decrease the severity of moderate to severe travelers' diarrhea, antimicrobial agents may be taken. After three or more loose stools with symptoms, consideration can be given to a short course of trimethoprim-sulfamethoxazole, doxycycline,[17] or ciprofloxacin.

Possible preventive measures for travelers' diarrhea include food and beverage hygiene, immunization, use of nonantimicrobial medications, and prophylactic antimicrobial drugs. Meticulous attention to food and beverage preparation can decrease the likelihood of developing travelers' diarrhea, but this is admittedly difficult to accomplish. No available vaccines and none that are expected to be available in the next few years are effective against travelers' diarrhea. The only nonantimicrobial agent found useful in preventing travelers' diarrhea is bismuth subsalicylate; the dosage of two tablets four times daily (2.1 g/day) appears to be a safe and effective means of reducing by about 65 percent the occurrence of travelers' diarrhea among persons at risk for periods of up to 3 weeks.[18] On the basis of apparent risk-benefit ratios, prophylactic antimicrobial agents are not recommended for travelers. Some travelers may wish to consult with their physician and may elect to use prophylactic antimicrobial agents for travel under special circumstances once the risks and benefits are clearly understood.[17] The use of halogenated hydroxyquinolone derivatives (e.g., Entero-Vioform, Mexaform, Clioquinol, and others) as a prophylactic is not recommended, since these drugs have never been proven to be effective for this purpose and their use has been associated with a syndrome of subacute myelo-optic neuropathy.[19] Entero-Vioform has been removed from the U.S. market, but it and related drugs are still available over the counter in many foreign countries.

ADVICE ON RETURN FROM TRAVEL

Even though apparently healthy, the traveler returning from exotic parts of the world should have certain routine screening procedures performed for exotic infections. These include a urinalysis, liver function tests, tuberculosis skin test or chest x-ray examination, and a complete blood cell count for evidence of anemia, leucocytosis, leukopenia, or eosinophilia. The last is an indicator of possible intestinal or systemic helminthic infection and is seldom caused by protozoal infections. A series of three stool tests should be carried out, including direct saline and iodine smears, concentration examination, and a stained slide when indicated by the finding of suspicious parasites. When stool specimens cannot be brought to the laboratory, preserved specimens can be sent using merthiolate-formalin, formalin, or polyvinyl alcohol. In interpreting a negative stool examination, it must be remembered that many preparations can cause a transient disappearance of parasites from the stool or can interfere with their recognition. These include antibiotics, sulfa drugs, antacids, kaolin products, barium, most enema products, and oily laxatives. It is necessary to wait for at least a week after a course of antibiotics and for at least 3–4 days after the use of other products, particularly when searching for protozoal parasites. A single negative stool is not sufficient to rule out parasitic infection, but three adequately performed negative examinations carried out on alternative days indicate approximately 70 percent certainty of the absence of infection.

In the febrile returnee, leading considerations are malaria, enteric fever, hepatitis, and amebic liver abscess. Returnees with significant eosinophilia and a possible exposure history for helminths should be evaluated for infections such as filariasis, schistosomiasis, strongyloidiasis, and other intestinal helminths. In situations in which there is a history of possible exposure, serologic screening tests are available for certain parasitic infections; those for schistosomiasis and amebiasis are particularly useful. Serologic testing may not be routinely available but can be obtained through some state health laboratories or at the CDC.

As certain exotic infections, including malaria, hepatitis, schistosomiasis, and intestinal parasites, may manifest themselves months or, rarely, years after the traveler's return, it is necessary for both the traveler and his or her physician to consider the possible relationship of the symptoms to earlier travel.

REFERENCES

1. Centers for Disease Control. Health Information for International Travel, 1988. Atlanta, GA.
2. World Health Organization. International Travel and Health: Vaccination Requirements and Health Advice, 1989. Geneva: 1989.
3. Hirschl B, Wüthrich R, Somaini B, et al. Inefficacy of the commercial live oral Ty21a vaccine in the prevention of typhoid fever. Eur J Clin Microbiol. 1985;4:295–8.
4. Centers for Disease Control. Measles prevention. MMWR. 1987;36:409–25.
5. Kunz C, Heinz FX, Hofmann H. Immunogenicity and reactogenicity of a highly purified vaccine against tick-borne encephalitis. J Med Virol. 1980; 6:103–9.
6. American College of Obstetricians and Gynecologists. Immunization during Pregnancy. Technical Bulletin No. 64. Washington, DC: May 1982.
7. Transdermal scopolamine for motion sickness. Med Lett Drugs Ther. 1981;23:89–90.
8. Jarroll EL, Bingham AK, Meyer EA. Giardia cyst destruction: Effectiveness of six small-quantity water disinfection methods. Am J Trop Med Hyg. 1980;29:8–11.
9. Dembert ML. Common diseases of fish and shellfish ingestion: Hazards of overseas travel and an underseas appetitie. Travel Med Int. 1988;6:1–9.
10. Jaws that bite, things that sting. Emergency Med. 1978;10:25–59.
11. Barrett-Connor E. Chemoprophylaxis of amebiasis and African trypanosomiasis. Ann Intern Med. 1972;77:797–805.
12. Wolfe MS, Cordero JF. Safety of chloroquine in chemosuppression of malaria during pregnancy. Br Med J. 1985;290:1466–7.
13. Appleton B, Wolfe MS, Mishtowt GI. Chloroquine as a malarial suppressive: Absence of visual effects. Milit Med. 1973;138:225–6.
14. Centers for Disease Control. Recommendations for the prevention of malaria in travelers. MMWR. 1988;37:277–84.
15. Oral fluids for dehydration. Med Lett Drugs Ther. 1987;29:63–4.
16. Johnson PC, Ericsson CD, Dupont HL, et al. Comparison of loperamide with bismuth subsalicylate for treatment of acute travelers' diarrhea. JAMA. 1986;255:757–60.
17. Gorbach SL, Edelman R, eds. Travelers' Diarrhea: National Institutes of Health Consensus Development Conference. J Infect Dis. 1986;8:S109–227.
18. Du Pont HL, Ericsson CD, Johnson PC, et al. Prevention of travelers' diarrhea by the tablet formulation of bismuth subsalicylate. JAMA. 1987; 257:1347–50.
19. Wolfe MS, Mishtowt GI. Enterovioform in travelers' diarrhea. JAMA. 1972;220:275–6.

INDEX

Page numbers in *italic* indicate tables and figures.